Bonica's
Management of
Pain

FIFTH EDITION

Bonica's
Management of
Pain

FIFTH EDITION

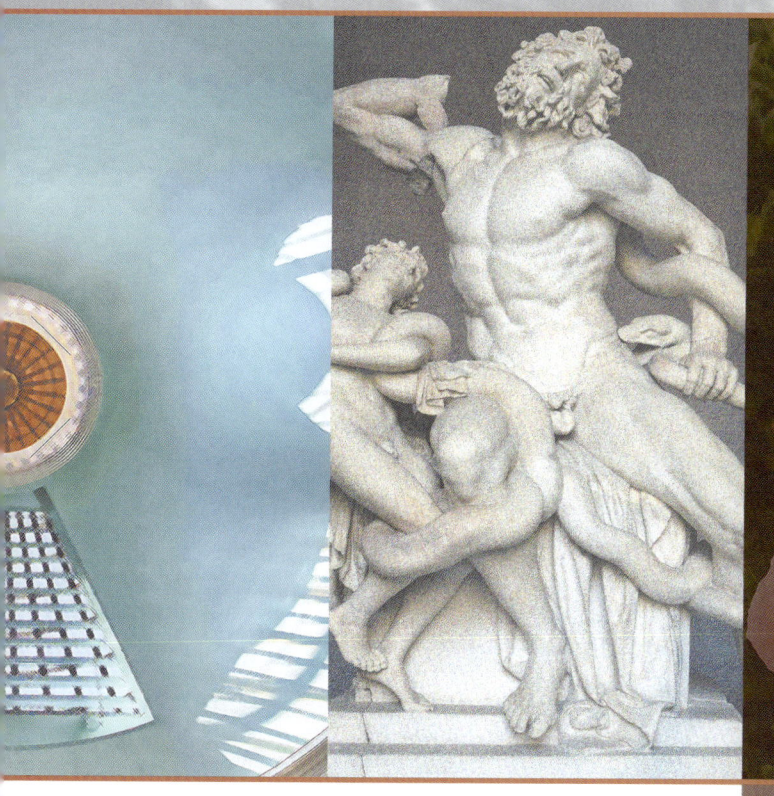

EDITORS

Jane C. Ballantyne, MD, FRCA
Professor of Anesthesiology and Pain Medicine
University of Washington
Seattle, Washington

Scott M. Fishman, MD
Fullerton Endowed Chair of Pain Medicine
Chief, Division of Pain Medicine and Professor of Anesthesiology
Director, Center for Advancing Pain Relief
Department of Anesthesiology and Pain Medicine
University of California, Davis School of Medicine
Sacramento, California

James P. Rathmell, MD
Chair, Department of Anesthesiology, Perioperative and Pain Medicine
Brigham and Women's Hospital
Leroy D. Vandam Professor of Anaesthesia, Harvard Medical School
Boston, Massachusetts

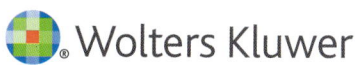
. Wolters Kluwer

Philadelphia · Baltimore · New York · London
Buenos Aires · Hong Kong · Sydney · Tokyo

Acquisitions Editor: Keith Donnellan
Product Development Editor: Rebeca Barroso/Elizabeth Schaeffer
Editorial Coordinator: Jeremiah Kiely
Editorial Assistant: Levi Bentley
Marketing Manager: Rachel Mante-Leung
Production Project Manager: Marian Bellus
Design Coordinator: Elaine Kasmer
Manufacturing Coordinator: Beth Welsh
Prepress Vendor: Absolute Service, Inc.

5th edition

Cover Figure Credits:
Top: fMRI of cognitive modulation of pain, Sean Mackey, MD, PhD, Stanford University
Left: Cupola of the Etherdome at Massachusetts General Hospital (inside), James P. Rathmell
Left Center: Laocoön and his sons in the Vatican. Marble, copy after an Hellenistic original from ca. 200 BC. Found in the Baths of Trajan, 1506, [Public domain], via Wikimedia Commons
Right Center: *Papaver orientale*, ornamental relative of *Papaver somniferum*, the opium poppy, James P. Rathmell
Right: *Capsicum chinese var. Habenero*, Les Ferme Lufa, Montréal, Québec

Cover Design: James P. Rathmell

9 8 7 6 5 4 3 2

Printed in China

Library of Congress Cataloging-in-Publication Data

Names: Ballantyne, Jane, 1948- editor. | Fishman, Scott, 1959- editor. |
   Rathmell, James P., editor.
Title: Bonica's management of pain / editors, Jane C. Ballantyne, Scott M.
   Fishman, James P. Rathmell.
Description: Fifth edition. | Philadelphia : Wolters Kluwer Health, [2019] |
   Includes bibliographical references and index.
Identifiers: LCCN 2018038021 | ISBN 9781496349033 (hardback)
Subjects: | MESH: Pain Management
Classification: LCC RB127 | NLM WL 704.6 | DDC 616/.0472—dc23 LC record
available at https://lccn.loc.gov/2018038021

shop.lww.com

TO THE LASTING MEMORY OF JOHN BONICA AND HIS ENDURING QUEST TO END NEEDLESS PAIN.

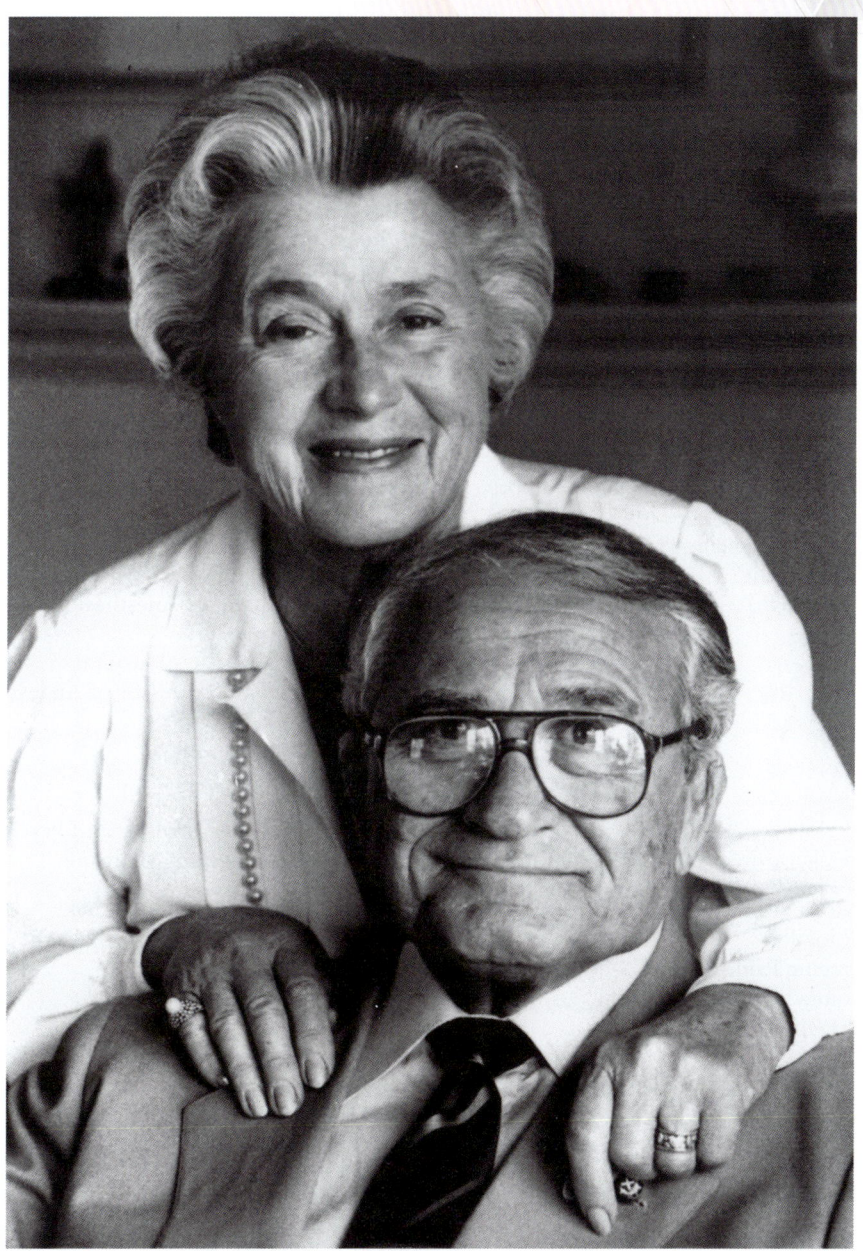

John and Emma L. Bonica

Section Editors

Jane C. Ballantyne, MD, FRCA
Professor of Anesthesiology and Pain Medicine
University of Washington
Seattle, Washington

Nikolai Bogduk, BSc(Med), MB, BS, MD, PhD, DSc, MMed, FAFRM, FFPM(ANZCA)
Emeritus Professor of Pain Medicine
The University of Newcastle
Newcastle, New South Wales, Australia

David J. Copenhaver, MD, MPH
Associate Professor
Department of Anesthesiology and Pain Medicine
Department of Neurological Surgery
Associate Director, Center for Advancing Pain Relief
Director, Cancer Pain Management
University of California at Davis
Sacramento, California

Emad N. Eskandar, MD
Professor
Department of Neurosurgery
Harvard Medical School
Boston, Massachusetts

Scott M. Fishman, MD
Fullerton Endowed Chair of Pain Medicine
Chief, Division of Pain Medicine and
    Professor of Anesthesiology
Director, Center for Advancing Pain Relief
Department of Anesthesiology and Pain Medicine
University of California, Davis School of Medicine
Sacramento, California

Rollin M. Gallagher, MD, MPH
Clinical Professor
Psychiatry and Anesthesiology
Perelman School of Medicine, University of Pennsylvania
Philadelphia, Pennsylvania

G.F. Gebhart, PhD (Retired)
Professor (emeritus)
Department of Pharmacology
Carver College of Medicine
University of Iowa
Iowa City, Iowa

Arthur G. Lipman†, PharmD
Professor Emeritus
Pharmacotherapy
University of Utah School of Medicine
Adjunct Professor of Anesthesiology and Director of Clinical
    Pharmacology
Pain Management
University of Utah
Salt Lake City, Utah

Timothy J. Ness, MD, PhD
Simon Gelman Endowed Professor of Anesthesiology
Department of Anesthesiology and Perioperative Medicine
University of Alabama at Birmingham
Birmingham, Alabama

James P. Rathmell, MD
Chair, Department of Anesthesiology, Perioperative and
    Pain Medicine
Brigham and Women's Hospital
Leroy D. Vandam Professor of Anaesthesia, Harvard
    Medical School
Boston, Massachusetts

Steven H. Richeimer, MD
Professor of Anesthesiology and Psychiatry
Chief, Division of Pain Medicine
Department of Anesthesiology
Keck School of Medicine
University of Southern California
Los Angeles, California

Virtaj Singh, MD
Clinical Assistant Professor
Department of Rehabilitation
University of Washington
Medical Director
Seattle Spine and Sports Medicine
Seattle, Washington

Mark S. Wallace, MD
Professor of Clinical Anesthesiology
Chair, Division of Pain Medicine
Department of Anesthesiology
University of California San Diego
La Jolla, California

Christopher L. Wu, MD
Clinical Professor of Anesthesiology
Department of Anesthesiology
The Hospital for Special Surgery, Weill Cornell Medical College
New York, New York

---

†Deceased.

Contributing Authors

Alaa Abd-ElSayed, MD
Assistant Professor/Medical Director
University of Wisconsin-Madison
Madison, Wisconsin

Roger J. Allen, PhD, PT
Distinguished Professor
School of Physical Therapy
Neuroscience Program
University of Puget Sound
Tacoma, Washington

Kevin N. Alschuler, PhD
Associate Professor
Department of Rehabilitation Medicine
University of Washington School of Medicine
Rehabilitation Psychologist
UW Medicine Multiple Sclerosis Center
University of Washington Medical Center
Seattle, Washington

David Arcella, MD
Private Practice
Trident Pain Center
Charleston, South Carolina

Charles E. Argoff, MD
Professor of Neurology
Albany Medical College
Director, Comprehensive Pain Center and
    Pain Management Fellowship
Albany Medical Center
Albany, New York

Paul M. Arnstein, PhD, RN, FAAN
Adjunct Associate Professor
Nursing
MGH Institute for Health Professions
Clinical Nurse Specialist for Pain Relief
Institute for Patient Care
Massachusetts General Hospital
Boston, Massachusetts

Desiree Azizoddin, PsyD
Pain Psychology Fellow
Department of Anesthesiology, Perioperative and
    Pain Medicine
Stanford University
Palo Alto, California

Miroslav Backonja, MD
Clinical Professor
Neurology
University of Washington
Seattle, Washington
Emeritus Professor
Department of Neurology
University of Wisconsin
Madison, Wisconsin

Matthew J. Bair, MD, MS
Associate Professor of Medicine
Medicine
Indiana University School of Medicine
Core Investigator
Center for Health Information and Communication
Rondebush VA Medical Center
Indianapolis, Indiana

Zahid H. Bajwa, MD, FAHS
Director, Boston Headache Institute
Director, Clinical Research, Boston PainCare Center
Waltham, Massachusetts
Tufts University School of Medicine
Boston, Massachusetts

Samir K. Ballas, MD, FACP, FASCP, DABPM, FAAPM
Emeritus Professor of Medicine and Pediatrics
Department of Medicine, Cardeza Foundation for
    Hematologic Research
Thomas Jefferson University
Honorary Staff Member
Medicine, Division of Hematology
Sidney Kimmel Medical College
Philadelphia, Pennsylvania

Andrew Baranowski, BScHons, MBBS, FRCA, MD, FFPMRCA
Honorary Senior Lecturer
Department of Pain Medicine
University College London
Consultant
Pain Medicine
University College London Hospitals
London, United Kingdom

Andrei Barasch, DMD, MDSc
Associate Professor
Medicine
Weill Cornell Medical College
Attending
Medicine
New York Presbyterian Hospital
New York, New York

David Barnard, PhD, JD
Retired Miles J. Edwards Chair in Professionalism and
 Comfort Care
Center for Ethics in Health Care
Oregon Health & Science University
Portland, Oregon

Kelly Barth, DO
Associate Professor
Department of Psychiatry and Behavioral Sciences
Medical University of South Carolina
Charleston, South Carolina

William C. Becker, MD
Associate Professor
Department of Internal Medicine
Yale School of Medicine
New Haven, Connecticut

Sharona Ben-Haim, MD
Assistant Professor
Department of Neurosurgery
University of California, San Diego
San Diego, California

Charles Berde, MD, PhD
Professor
Anesthesia
Harvard Medical School
Sara Page Mayo Chair and Chief, Division of Pain Medicine
Anesthesiology, Critical Care and Pain Medicine
Boston Children's Hospital
Boston, Massachusetts

Sarah K. Bick, MD
Resident
Department of Neurosurgery
Massachusetts General Hospital
Boston, Massachusetts

Klaus Bielefeldt, MD, PhD
Professor of Medicine
Medicine
University of Utah
Section Chief, Gastroenterology
Medicine
George E. Wahlen VAMC
Salt Lake City, Utah

**Nikolai Bogduk, BSc(Med), MB, BS, MD, PhD, DSc, MMed,
FAFRM, FFPM(ANZCA)**
Emeritus Professor of Pain Medicine
The University of Newcastle
Newcastle, New South Wales, Australia

Christina Elise Bokat, MD
Assistant Professor
Anesthesiology
University of Utah
Salt Lake City, Utah

Michael M. Bottros, MD
Associate Professor
Department of Anesthesiology, Division of Pain Medicine
Washington University School of Medicine
St. Louis, Missouri

Gary J. Brenner, MD, PhD
Associate Professor
Department of Anesthesia, Critical Care and Pain Medicine
Harvard Medical School
Director, Massachusetts General Hospital Pain Medicine
 Fellowship
Department of Anesthesia, Critical Care and Pain Medicine
Massachusetts General Hospital
Boston, Massachusetts

Shane E. Brogan, MB, BCH
Director of Pain Medicine
Anesthesiology
Huntsman Cancer Hospital
Salt Lake City, Utah

Chad Brummett, MD
Associate Professor of Anesthesiology
Director, Clinical Anesthesia Research
University of Michigan
Ann Arbor, Michigan

Kelly A. Bruno, MD
Pain Medicine Fellow
Department of Anesthesiology and Pain Medicine
University of California, San Diego
San Diego, California

Thomas N. Bryce, MD
Professor
Rehabilitation Medicine
Icahn School of Medicine
Attending Physician
Rehabilitation Medicine
Mount Sinai Hospital
New York, New York

Asokumar Buvanendran, MD
Professor, Department of Anesthesiology
William Gottschalk, Endowed Chair of Anesthesiology
Vice Chair Research and Director of Orthopedic Anesthesia
Rush University Medical Center
Chicago, Illinois

Jacqueline Casillas, MD, MSHS
Professor
Pediatrics Division of Hematology-Oncology
University of California, Los Angeles
Los Angeles, California
Medical Director
Pediatric Hematology-Oncology
Miller Children's Hospital
Long Beach, California

Ausim Chaghtai, MD
Neurology Resident
Albany Medical Center
Albany, New York

Wilson J. Chang, MD, MPH
Pain Specialist
Pain Services
Swedish Medical Center
Seattle, Washington

C. Richard Chapman, PhD
Professor Emeritus
Pain Research Center
Department of Anesthesiology
University of Utah
Salt Lake City, Utah

Martin D. Cheatle, PhD
Associate Professor
Department of Psychiatry
Perelman School of Medicine, University of Pennsylvania
Philadelphia, Pennsylvania

Srinivas Chiravuri, MD
Clinical Associate Professor
Department of Anesthesiology
University of Michigan Medical School
Ann Arbor, Michigan

Roger Chou, MD
Professor
Department of Medical Informatics and Clinical Epidemiology,
    Department of Medicine
Oregon Health & Science University
Portland, Oregon

Thomas Tai Chung, MD
Clinical Assistant Professor
Physical Medicine and Rehabilitation
University of Washington School of Medicine
Staff
Physical Medicine and Rehabilitation
Swedish Medical Center
Seattle, Washington

Michael R. Clark, MD, MPH, MBA
Chair, Department of Psychiatry and Behavioral Health
Inova Health System
Falls Church, Virginia

Daniel J. Clauw, MD
Professor
Department of Anesthesiology, Medicine (Rheumatology),
    and Psychiatry
University of Michigan
Director
Chronic Pain and Fatigue Research Center, Department of
    Anesthesiology
Michigan Medicine
Ann Arbor, Michigan

James F. Cleary, MD, FRACP, FAChPM
Professor
Medicine
University of Wisconsin School of Medicine and Public Health
Madison, Wisconsin

Richard F. Cody Jr., MD
Neuroradiology Fellow
Department of Radiology
University of Washington School of Medicine/Harborview
    Medical Center
Seattle, Washington

Peggy Compton, RN, PhD, FAAN
Associate Professor
School of Nursing
University of Pennsylvania
Philadelphia, Pennsylvania

David S. Craig, PharmD
Pharmacist Lead, Supportive Care Medicine and Acute Pain
Department of Pharmacy
Moffitt Cancer Center and Research Institute
Tampa, Florida

Lara Wiley Crock, MD, PhD
Research and Clinical Fellow
Department of Anesthesiology
Washington University School of Medicine
St. Louis, Missouri

Taylor Crouch, PhD
Instructor
Department of Psychiatry and Behavioral Sciences
Medical University of South Carolina
Charleston, South Carolina

Michele Curatolo, MD, PhD
Professor of Anesthesiology and Pain Medicine
Endowed Professor in Medical Education and Research
Department of Anesthesiology & Pain Medicine
University of Washington
Seattle, Washington

Melissa A. Day, PhD
NHMRC Early Career Fellow
School of Psychology
The University of Queensland
Brisbane, Australia

Jennifer J. DeBerry, PhD
Assistant Professor
Anesthesiology + Perioperative Medicine
University of Alabama at Birmingham
Birmingham, Alabama

Richard A. Deyo, MD, MPH
Professor
Family Medicine and Internal Medicine
Oregon Health & Science University
Portland, Oregon

Jan Dommerholt, PT, DPT, DAIPM
Associate Professor
Fisioterapia
Universidad CEU Cardenal Herrera
Valencia, Spain
President/Chief Executive Officer
Bethesda Physiocare Inc
Bethesda, Maryland

Robert H. Dworkin, PhD
Professor of Anesthesiology, Neurology, and Psychiatry
Department of Anesthesiology
University of Rochester School of Medicine and Dentistry
Rochester, New York

Robert Edwards, PhD, MSPH
Associate Professor
Anesthesiology
Harvard School of Medicine
Psychologist
Anesthesiology
Brigham and Women's Hospital
Boston, Massachusetts

Elon Eisenberg, MD
Professor of Neurology and Pain Medicine
Rappaport Faculty of Medicine
Technion—Israel Institute of Technology
Head, Pain Research Unit
Institute of Pain Medicine
Rambam Health Care Campus
Haifa, Israel

Andrew J. Engel, MD
Affordable Pain Management
Chicago, Illinois

Joyce M. Engel, PhD, OT
Professor
Occupational Science and Technology
College of Health Sciences
University of Wisconsin-Milwaukee
Milwaukee, Wisconsin

Joel Brian Epstein, DMD, MSD
Professor
Department of Surgery
Cedars-Sinai Health System
Los Angeles, California
Medical Director, Dentistry
Department of Surgery
City of Hope National Medical Center
Duarte, California

Emad N. Eskandar, MD
Professor
Department of Neurosurgery
Massachusetts General Hospital
Harvard Medical School
Boston, Massachusetts

Svetlana Faktorovich, MD
Clinical Neurophysiology Fellow
Department of Neurology
Icahn School of Medicine at Mount Sinai
New York, New York

Ronnie Fass, MD
Professor of Medicine
Medicine
Case Western Reserve University
Medical Director, Digestive Health Center
Medicine
MetroHealth Medical Center
Cleveland, Ohio

Roger B. Fillingim, PhD
Distinguished Professor
Pain Research and Intervention Center of Excellence
University of Florida
Gainesville, Florida

Ezekiel Fink, MD
Triple Board Certified in Neurology, Pain Management, and
    Brain Injury Medicine
Medical Director of Pain Management
Houston Methodist Hospital
Houston, Texas
Assistant Clinical Professor
David Geffen School of Medicine at UCLA
Los Angeles, California

Nanna Brix Finnerup, MD, Phd
Professor
Department of Clinical Medicine, Danish Pain
    Research Center
Aarhus University
Aarhus, Denmark

Scott M. Fishman, MD
Fullerton Endowed Chair of Pain Medicine
Chief, Division of Pain Medicine and
    Professor of Anesthesiology
Director, Center for Advancing Pain Relief
Department of Anesthesiology and Pain Medicine
University of California, Davis School of Medicine
Sacramento, California

Dermot Fitzgibbon, MB, BCh
Professor
Department of Anesthesiology and Pain Medicine
University of Washington School of Medicine
Medical Director, Pain and Anesthesia Services
Seattle Cancer Care Alliance
Seattle, Washington

Gregory C. Gardner, MD, FACP
Gilliland-Henderson Professor of Medicine
Division of Rheumatology
Adjunct Professor of Orthopedics and
    Rehabilitation Medicine
University of Washington
Seattle, Washington

Robert J. Gatchel, PhD, ABPP
Distinguished Professor and Director, Center of Excellence for
    the Study of Health and Chronic Illnesses, Nancy P. and John
    G. Penson Endowed Professor of Clinical Health Psychology
Department of Psychology, College of Science
University of Texas at Arlington
Arlington, Texas

G.F. Gebhart, PhD (Retired)
Professor (emeritus)
Department of Pharmacology
Carver College of Medicine
University of Iowa
Iowa City, Iowa

Youssef Ghabrial, MB, ChB, MOrth, DS, FRCS, FRACS
Professor of Orthopedic Surgery
School of Medicine and Public Health
Faculty of Health and Medicine
The University of Newcastle
Staff Specialist
Department of Orthopedic Surgery
John Hunter Hospital
Newcastle, New South Wales, Australia

Kimberly Varney Gill, PharmD, BCPS, BCCCP
Clinical Pharmacy Specialist, Critical Care, Medical
  Respiratory ICU, VCU Medical Center
Associate Clinical Professor of Pharmacy, VCU School of
  Pharmacy
Assistant Clinical Professor of Medicine, VCU Department of
  Internal Medicine
Richmond, Virginia

Christopher Gilligan, MD, MBA
Assistant Professor
Anesthesia
Harvard Medical School
Chief, Division of Pain Medicine
Department of Anesthesiology, Perioperative and
  Pain Medicine
Brigham and Women's Hospital
Boston, Massachusetts

Aaron M. Gilson, MS, MSSW, PhD
Research Program Manager/Senior Scientist
Carbone Cancer Center
University of Wisconsin School of Medicine and Public Health
Madison, Wisconsin

Lee Glass, MD, JD
Associate Medical Director
Department of Labor and Industries
Olympia, Washington

Peter J. Goadsby, MD, PhD, DSc, FRACP, FRCP, FMedSci
Professor of Neurology
Institute of Psychiatry, Psychology and Neuroscience
King's College London
London, United Kingdom

Layne A. Goble, PhD
Clinical Psychologist
Anesthesia
Charleston VA Medical Center
Associate Professor
Anesthesia and Perioperative Medicine
Medical University of South Carolina
Charleston, South Carolina

Michael S. Gold, PhD
Professor of Neurobiology
Department of Neurobiology
University of Pittsburgh School of Medicine
Pittsburgh, Pennsylvania

Douglas L. Gourlay, MD, MSc, FRCP(C), DFASAM
Educational Consultant
Ontario, Canada

Benjamin L. Grannan, MD
Resident Physician
Department of Neurosurgery
Massachusetts General Hospital
Boston, Massachusetts

Robert Griffin, MD, PhD
Clinical Assistant Professor
Anesthesiology
Weill Cornell Medical College
Assistant Attending Anesthesiologist
Anesthesiology, Critical Care, and Pain Management
Hospital for Special Surgery
New York, New York

Narasimha R. Gundamraj, MD
Assistant Professor
College of Human Medicine
Michigan State University
Physician
Pain Management Center
Sparrow Hospital
East Lansing, Michigan

Muhamed Hadzipasic, MD, PhD
Resident Physician
Department of Neurosurgery
Massachusetts General Hospital
Boston, Massachusetts

Neil A. Hagen, MD, FRCPC
Professor Emeritus
Departments of Oncology, Clinical Neurosciences and
  Medicine
Cumming School of Medicine, University of Calgary
Calgary, Canada

Emily Hagn, MD
Assistant Professor
Department of Anesthesiology
University of Utah
Salt Lake City, Utah

Marie N. Hanna, MD, MEHP
Associate Professor, Chief Division of Regional Anesthesia
  and Acute Pain Management
Deparment Anesthesia and Critical Care Medicine
Johns Hopkins University
Baltimore, Maryland

Robert Norman Harden, MD
Professor
Rehabilitation Institute of Chicago
Northwestern University
Chicago, Illinois

Simon Haroutounian, PhD, MSc Pharm
Assistant Professor
Department of Anesthesiology
Washington University School of Medicine
St. Louis, Missouri

Michael Hauck, MD, PhD
Research Fellow
Institute of Pathophysiology and Neurophysiology
University Medical Center Hamburg-Eppendorf
Attending Physician
Department of Neurology
University Medical Center Hamburg-Eppendorf
Hamburg, Germany

Howard A. Heit, MD, FACP, FASAM
Educational Consultant
Reston, Virginia

Jeanne Hernandez, PhD, MSPH
Director of Behavioral Medicine, Assistant Professor (Retired)
Department of Anesthesiology
School of Medicine, University of North Carolina Chapel Hill
Chapel Hill, North Carolina

Keela Herr, PhD, RN, AGSF, FGSA, FAAN
Professor and Associate Dean for Faculty
College of Nursing
University of Iowa
Iowa City, Iowa

Anita H. Hickey, MD
Pain Management Physician
Naval Medical Center San Diego
San Diego, California

Joseph Gregory Hobelmann, MD, MPH
Adjunct Faculty
Department of Psychiatry and Behavioral Sciences
Johns Hopkins University
Baltimore, Maryland
Chief Medical Officer
Ashley Addiction Treatment
Havre de Grace, Maryland

Pamela J. Hughes, DDS
Associate Professor and Department Chair
Oral and Maxillofacial Surgery
Oregon Health and Science University
Portland, Oregon

Robert W. Hurley, MD, PhD
Professor
Section Chief of Pain Medicine
Anesthesiology and Public Health Sciences
Wake Forest University
Executive Director
Pain Service Line
Wake Forest Baptist Health
Winston-Salem, North Carolina

S. Asra Husain, JD, MA
Legal and Policy Analyst
UW Carbone Cancer Center
Pain & Policy Studies Group
University of Wisconsin
Madison, Wisconsin

Charles E. Inturrisi, PhD
Professor
Department of Pharmacology
Weill Cornell Medicine
New York, New York

Gordon Irving, MB, BS, MSc (Med), MMED, FFA(SA)
Attending
Swedish Pain Services
Swedish Medical Center
Seattle, Washington

Robert N. Jamison, PhD
Professor
Departments of Anesthesia and Psychiatry
Harvard Medical School
Boston, Massachusetts
Pain Management Center
Brigham and Women's Hospital
Chestnut Hill, Massachusetts

Nora Janjan, MD, MPSA, MBA
Senior Fellow
National Center for Policy Analysis
Dallas, Texas

Mark P. Jensen, PhD
Professor and Vice Chair for Research
Rehabilitation Medicine
University of Washington
Seattle, Washington

Kaj Johansen, MD, PhD
Clinical Professor of Surgery
Department of Surgery
University of Washington School of Medicine
Staff Vascular Surgeon
Department of Surgery
Swedish Medical Center
Seattle, Washington

Anand B. Joshi, MD, MHA
Assistant Professor
Orthopedic Surgery
Duke University School of Medicine
Assistant Professor
Orthopedic Surgery
Duke Health
Durham, North Carolina

James D. Kang, MD
Chairman
Orthopedic Surgery
Harvard Medical School
Brigham and Women's Hospital
Boston, Massachusetts

Roy L. Kao, MD
Assistant Clinical Professor
Pediatrics
David Geffen School of Medicine at UCLA
Los Angeles, California
Pediatric Hematologist/Oncologist
Miller Children's and Women's Hospital
Long Beach, California

Michael L. Kent, MD
Assistant Professor
Department of Anesthesiology
Uniformed Services University
Staff Anesthesiologist
Department of Anesthesiology
Walter Reed National Military Medical Center
Bethesda, Maryland

Wade King, MB, BS, MMedSc, MMed (Pain Mgt.), GDMuscMed, FAFMM
Pain Physician
Mayo Multidisciplinary Pain Clinic
Mayo Private Hospital
Taree, New South Wales, Australia

Nancy D. Kishino, OTR/L, CVE
Director
West Coast Spine Restoration Center
Riverside, California

Claudia Kohner, PhD
Licensed Clinical Psychologist
Private Practice
Encino, California

Kristen Lynn Labovsky, MD
Assistant Professor
Department of Anesthesiology
Medical College of Wisconsin/Children's Hospital of Wisconsin
Milwaukee, Wisconsin

Irfan Lalani, MD
Assistant Professor
Department of Anesthesiology and Pain Medicine
University of Texas M.D. Anderson Cancer Center
Houston, Texas

Hai V. Le, MD
Resident Physician
Orthopedic Surgery
Harvard Medical School
Brigham and Women's Hospital
Boston, Massachusetts

David Justin Levinthal, MD, PhD
Assistant Professor
Department of Medicine, Division of Gastroenterology, Hepatology, and Nutrition
University of Pittsburgh School of Medicine
Director, Neurogastroenterology and Motility Center
Department of Medicine, Division of Gastroenterology, Hepatology, and Nutrition
University of Pittsburgh Medical Center
Pittsburgh, Pennsylvania

Bengt Linderoth, MD, PhD
Professor Emeritus
Department of Clinical Neuroscience
Karolinska Institutet
Retired Professor of Functional Neurosurgery
Department of Neurosurgery
Karolinska University Hospital
Stockholm, Sweden

Arthur G. Lipman[†], PharmD
Professor Emeritus
Pharmacotherapy
University of Utah School of Medicine
Adjunct Professor of Anesthesiology and Director of Clinical Pharmacology
Pain Management
University of Utah
Salt Lake City, Utah

Dave Loomba, MD
Assistant Professor
Director of Resident Education
Department of Anesthesiology and Pain Medicine
University of California
UC Davis Health System
Sacramento, California

Jürgen Lorenz, MD, PhD
Professor
Faculty of Life Sciences
Hamburg University of Applied Sciences
University Clinic Hamburg-Eppendorf
Institute of Neurophysiology and Pathophysiology
University of Hamburg
Hamburg, Germany

John MacVicar, MB, ChB, MPainMed
Medical Director
Southern Rehab
Christchurch, New Zealand

Gagan Mahajan, MD
Professor
Anesthesiology and Pain Medicine
University of California, Davis
Sacramento, California

Muhammad Hassan Majeed, MD
Research Scholar
Pain Management
Boston PainCare
Waltham, Massachusetts
Attending Psychiatrist
Psychiatry
Natchaug Hospital
Mansfield Center, Connecticut

Athar N. Malik, MD, PhD
Resident Physician
Department of Neurosurgery
Massachusetts General Hospital
Harvard Medical School
Boston, Massachusetts

Georgios Manousakis, MD
Assistant Professor
Department of Neurology
University of Minnesota
Minneapolis, Minnesota

Kenneth R. Maravilla, MD
Professor Radiology and Neurological Surgery
Radiology
University of Washington
Attending Neuroradiologist
Radiology
University of Washington Medical Center
Seattle, Washington

Michael T. Massey, DO
University of Washington
Seattle, Washington

[†]Deceased.

Martha A. Maurer, PhD, MPH, MSSW
Associate Scientist
UW Carbone Cancer Center
Pain & Policy Studies Group
University of Wisconsin—Madison
Madison, Wisconsin

Timothy Philip Maus, MD
Professor
Department of Radiology
Mayo Clinic College of Medicine
Rochester, Minnesota

Lance M. McCracken, PhD
Professor of Behavioral Medicine
King's College London
Health Psychology Section
Psychology Department
Institute of Psychiatry, Psychology and Neuroscience (IoPPN)
London, United Kingdom

Ellen McGough, PT, PhD
Associate Professor
Department of Rehabilitation Medicine
University of Washington
Seattle, Washington

Matthew K. Mian, MD
Chief Resident
Department of Neurosurgery
Massachusetts General Hospital
Harvard Medical School
Boston, Massachusetts

Kristin Miller, MD, MS
Assistant Professor
Division of Pulmonary Disease and Critical Care Medicine
Virginia Commonwealth University Health System, Medical
    College of Virginia
Associate Medical Director
Medical Respiratory Intensive Care Unit
Department of Internal Medicine
Virginia Commonwealth University Health System
Richmond, Virginia

James R. Miner, MD, FACEP
Professor
Department of Emergency Medicine
University of Minnesota
Chief
Department of Emergency Medicine
Hennepin County Medical Center
Minneapolis, Minnesota

Asako Miyakoshi, MD
Radiologist
Radiology
Southern California Permanente Medical Group/Kaiser
    Permanente
San Diego, California

Jane Moore, MBBS, MRCOG
Consultant Gynecologist
Nuffield Department of Women's and Reproductive Health
University of Oxford
Oxford, United Kingdom

David B. Morris, PhD
University Professor (Retired)
University of Virginia
Richmond, Virginia

James Michael Mossner, BS
Medical Student
University of Michigan Medical School
Ann Arbor, Michigan

Jennifer L. Murphy, PhD
Clinical Assistant Professor
Department of Neurology
University of South Florida College of Medicine
Supervisory Psychologist, Pain Section
Mental Health and Behavioral Sciences
James A. Haley Veterans' Hospital
Tampa, Florida

Timothy J. Ness, MD, PhD
Simon Gelman Endowed Professor of Anesthesiology
Department of Anesthesiology and Perioperative Medicine
University of Alabama at Birmingham
Birmingham, Alabama

Maureen Young Shin Noh, MD
Adjunct Professor
Orthopedics
Duke University
Staff Physician
Physical Medicine and Rehabilitation Services
VA Medical Center
Durham, North Carolina

Richard B. North, MD
Professor of Neurosurgery (Retired)
Anesthesiology and Critical Care Medicine
Johns Hopkins University School of Medicine
President
The Neuromodulation Foundation Inc
Baltimore, Maryland

Kenneth C. Nwosu, MD
Spine Fellow
Orthopedic Surgery
Harvard Medical School
Brigham and Women's Hospital
Boston, Massachusetts

Akiko Okifuji, PhD
Professor
Anesthesiology, Pain Research and Management Center
University of Utah
Salt Lake City, Utah

John E. Olerud, MD
Professor Emeritus
University of Washington Division of Dermatology
Seattle, Washington

Jean-Pierre P. Ouanes, DO
Assistant Professor
Anesthesiology and Critical Care Medicine
The Johns Hopkins University School of Medicine
Clinical Faculty
Anesthesiology and Critical Care Medicine
The Johns Hopkins Hospital
Baltimore, Maryland

Judith A. Paice, PhD, RN
Research Professor of Medicine
Feinberg School of Medicine
Northwestern University
Director, Cancer Pain Program
Division of Hematology-Oncology
Northwestern Medicine
Chicago, Illinois

Tonya M. Palermo, PhD
Professor
Anesthesiology and Pain Medicine
University of Washington School of Medicine
Associate Director
Center for Child Health, Behavior and Development
Seattle Children's Research Institute
Seattle, Washington

Parag G. Patil, MD, PhD
Associate Professor and Associate Chair
Departments of Neurosurgery, Neurology, Anesthesiology and
    Biomedical Engineering
University of Michigan Medical School
Ann Arbor, Michigan

David M. Peterson, PharmD
Adjunct Associate Professor
Department of Pharmacotherapy
University of Utah College of Pharmacy
Drug Information Specialist
Department of Pharmacy Services
University of Utah Hospital
Salt Lake City, Utah

Stacy J. Peterson, MD
Assistant Professor
Anesthesiology, MCW Pain Management Center
Medical College of Wisconsin
Milwaukee, Wisconsin

Ravi Prasad, PhD
Clinical Associate Professor
Department of Anesthesiology, Perioperative and
    Pain Medicine
Stanford University
Stanford, California

Amir Ramezani, PhD
Psychologist
Surgery
University of California, Davis
Sacramento, California

Alan Randich, PhD
Professor Emeritus
Anesthesiology
University of Alabama at Birmingham
Birmingham, Alabama

Ahmed M.T. Raslan, MD
Associate Professor of Neurological Surgery
School of Medicine
Neuroscience Quality Director
Oregon Health & Science University
Portland, Oregon

James P. Rathmell, MD
Chair, Department of Anesthesiology, Perioperative and
    Pain Medicine
Brigham and Women's Hospital
Leroy D. Vandam Professor of Anesthesia, Harvard
    Medical School
Boston, Massachusetts

Maria Regina Reyes, MD
Associate Professor
Department of Rehabilitation Medicine
University of Washington
Staff Physician
Spinal Cord Injury Service
Department of Veterans Affair VA Puget Sound Health
    Care System
Seattle, Washington

Ben A. Rich, JD, PhD
Emeritus Chair and Professor of Bioethics
Internal Medicine and Anesthesiology and Pain Medicine
UC Davis School of Medicine
Sacramento, California

Steven H. Richeimer, MD
Professor of Anesthesiology and Psychiatry
Chief, Division of Pain Medicine
Department of Anesthesiology
Keck School of Medicine
University of Southern California
Los Angeles, California

Bobbie L. Riley, MD, FAAP
Instructor
Anesthesia
Harvard Medical School
Staff
Anesthesiology, Critical Care and Pain Medicine
Boston Children's Hospital
Boston, Massachusetts

James P. Robinson, MD, PhD
Clinical Professor
Department of Rehabilitation Medicine
University of Washington
Seattle, Washington

Edgar Ross, MD
Associate Professor
Anesthesia
Harvard Medical School
Brigham and Women's Hospital
Boston, Massachusetts

Nathan J. Rudin, MD, MA
Professor
Department of Orthopedics and Rehabilitation
University of Wisconsin School of Medicine and Public Health
Madison, Wisconsin

Ramsey Saba, MD
Resident PGY4
Anesthesia
Harvard Medical School
Department of Anesthesiology, Perioperative and
    Pain Medicine
Brigham and Women's Hospital
Boston, Massachusetts

Friedhelm Sandbrink, MD
Clinical Associate Professor
Department of Neurology
Uniformed Services University
Bethesda, Maryland
Director Pain Management Program
Department of Neurology
Washington DC VA Medical Center
Washington, DC

Andrew J. Saxon, MD
Professor
Department of Psychiatry and Behavioral Sciences
University of Washington
Director, Center of Excellence in Substance Abuse Treatment
    and Education
Mental Health
VA Puget Sound Health Care System
Seattle, Washington

Michael E. Schatman, PhD
Adjunct Clinical Assistant Professor
Department of Public Health and Community Medicine
Tufts University School of Medicine
Boston, Massachusetts
Director
Research and Network Development
Boston Pain Care
Waltham, Massachusetts

Neil L. Schechter, MD
Associate Professor
Anesthesiology
Harvard Medical School
Director, Chronic Pain Clinic
Anesthesiology, Critical Care, Pain Medicine
Boston Children's Hospital
Boston, Massachusetts

Jerome Schofferman, MD
Founder and Current Member
Section on Rehabilitation, Interventions and Medical Spine
Immediate Past Chair, Committee on Ethics and Professionalism
North American Spine Society
Private Practice (Retired)
Sausalito, California

Curtis N. Sessler, MD, FCCP, FCCM
Orhan Muren Distinguished Professor of Medicine
Department of Internal Medicine
Virginia Commonwealth University
Director, Center for Adult Critical Care
Medical Director, Critical Care
Medical Director, Medical Respiratory ICU
Virginia Commonwealth University Health System
Richmond, Virginia

Jay P. Shah, MD
Affiliate Professor
Bioengineering Department
George Mason University
Fairfax, Virginia
Senior Staff Physiatrist and Clinical Investigator
Rehabilitation Medicine Department, Clinical Center
National Institutes of Health
Bethesda, Maryland

Sam R. Sharar, MD
Professor, Vice Chair for Faculty Affairs and Development
Anesthesiology and Pain Medicine
University of Washington School of Medicine
Attending Anesthesiologist
Anesthesiology
Harborview Medical Center
Seattle, Washington

Charles A. Simpson, DC, DABCO
Senior Clinical Advisor
Clinical Services
The CHP Group
Beaverton, Oregon

David M. Simpson, MD, FAAN
Professor of Neurology
Director, Clinical Neurophysiology Laboratories
Director, Neuromuscular Division
Director, Neuro-AIDS Program
Icahn School of Medicine at Mount Sinai
New York, New York

Jill Sindt, MD
Assistant Professor
Department of Anesthesiology
University of Utah
Associate Director Pain Medicine
Huntsman Cancer Hospital
Salt Lake City, Utah

Christopher D. Sletten, PhD, ABPP
Clinical Director, MCPRC
Assistant Professor of Psychology
Department of Pain Medicine
Mayo Medical School
Mayo Clinic Florida
Jacksonville, Florida

Howard S. Smith[†], MD
Associate Professor & Academic Director of
    Pain Management
Department of Anesthesiology
Albany Medical College
Albany, New York

Benjamin C. Soydan, PT, DPT, OCS, CSCS
Physical Therapist
Physical Medicine and Rehabilitation Services
VA Medical Center
Durham, North Carolina

Pamela Squire, MD
Associate Clinical Professor
Department of Medicine
University of British Columbia
Vancouver, Canada

Steven P. Stanos, DO
Physiatrist
Pain Medicine, Physical Medicine and Rehabilitation
Swedish Pain Services—First Hill
Seattle, Washington

[†]Deceased.

Milan P. Stojanovic, MD
Anesthesiology
Critical Care and Pain Medicine Service
VA Boston Healthcare System
Harvard Medical School
Boston, Massachusetts
Edith Nourse Rogers Memorial Veterans Hospital
Bedford, Massachusetts

Mark D. Sullivan, MD, PhD
Professor
Department of Psychiatry and Behavioral Sciences
University of Washington
Attending Physician
Psychiatry
University of Washington Medical Center
Seattle, Washington

Lalitha Sundararaman, MBBS, MD
Clinical Instructor
Department of Anesthesiology
Brigham and Women's Hospital
Clinical Instructor
Anesthesiology
Brigham and Women's Hospital, Harvard Medical School
Boston, Massachusetts

Kimberly Shawn Swanson, PhD
Psychologist
Behavioral Health
St. Charles Medical Center
Bend, Oregon

Pratik A. Talati, MD, PhD
Resident
Department of Neurosurgery
Harvard Medical School
Massachusetts General Hospital
Boston, Massachusetts

Rajbala Thakur, MBBS
Professor of Anesthesiology and Physical Medicine and
    Rehabilitation
Department of Anesthesiology
University of Rochester
Rochester, New York

Siddarth Thakur, MD
Instructor, Research Faculty
Pain Medicine
The University of Texas MD Anderson Cancer Center
Houston, Texas

Brian R. Theodore, PhD
Research Scientist II
Kaiser Permanente
Kaiser Foundation Rehabilitation Center
Vallejo, California

George I. Thomas, MD
Emeritus Clinical Professor
Surgery
University of Washington School of Medicine
Seattle, Washington

Beverly E. Thorn, PhD
Professor Emerita
Department of Psychology
The University of Alabama
Tuscaloosa, Alabama

Vicente Garcia Tomas, MD
Assistant Professor
Director, Acute Pain Service at Bayview Medical Center
Division of Regional Anesthesia and Acute Pain Medicine
Johns Hopkins University
Baltimore, Maryland

Dennis C. Turk, PhD
John and Emma Bonica Endowed Chair and Professor of
    Anesthesiology and Pain Research
Department of Anesthesiology and Pain Medicine
University of Washington
Seattle, Washington

Jan Van Zundert, MD, PhD, FIPP
Associate Professor Anesthesiology and Pain Management
Ziekenhuis Oost-Limburg
Genk, Belgium
Maastricht University Medical Center
Maastricht, The Netherlands

Mary Alice Vijjeswarapu, MD
Assistant Program Director, Pain Medicine Anesthesia
    Fellowship Program
Department of Anesthesiology
Cedars-Sinai Medical Center
Los Angeles, California

Katy Vincent, MRCOG, DPhil
Senior Pain Fellow
Nuffield Department of Women's and Reproductive Health
University of Oxford
Consultant Gynecologist
Department of Obstetrics and Gynecology
John Radcliffe Hospital, Oxford University Foundation Trust
Oxford, United Kingdom

Ashwin Viswanathan, MD
Associate Professor
Department of Neurosurgery
Baylor College of Medicine
Houston, Texas

Yakov Vorobeychik, MD, PhD
Professor
Department of Anesthesiology and Perioperative Medicine
Penn State Milton S. Hershey Medical Center
Hershey, Pennsylvania

Simon Vulfsons, MD
Director, Institute for Pain Medicine
Rambam Health Care Campus
Technion—Israel Institute of Technology
Haifa, Israel

Gary A. Walco, PhD
Professor
Anesthesiology and Pain Medicine
University of Washington
Director
Pain Medicine
Seattle Children's Hospital
Seattle, Washington

David Walk, MD
Associate Professor
Department of Neurology
University of Minnesota
Minneapolis, Minnesota

Ajay D. Wasan, MD, MSc
Vice Chair for Pain Medicine
Department of Anesthesiology
Professor of Anesthesiology and Psychiatry
University of Pittsburgh School of Medicine
Pittsburgh, Pennsylvania

Faye M. Weinstein, PhD
Associate Professor
Anesthesiology and Psychiatry
University of Southern California
Los Angeles, California

Steven J. Weisman, MD
Jane B. Pettit Chair in Pain Management
Children's Hospital of Wisconsin
Professor of Anesthesiology and Pediatrics
Medical College of Wisconsin
Milwaukee, Wisconsin

Shelley A. Wiechman, PhD, ABPP (Rp)
Associate Professor
Rehabilitation Medicine
University of Washington
Attending Psychologist
University of Washington Burn Center
Harborview Medical Center
Seattle, Washington

Matthew S. Willsey, MD
Resident in Neurosurgery
University of Michigan Medical School
Ann Arbor, Michigan

Hilary D. Wilson, PhD
Research Scientist
Outcomes Research
Evidera
Seattle, Washington

Cynthia A. Wong, MD
Professor, Chair and Department Executive Officer
Department of Anesthesia
University of Iowa Carver College of Medicine
Iowa City, Iowa

R. Joshua Wootton, MDiv, PhD
Assistant Professor
Anesthesia
Harvard Medical School
Boston, Massachusetts
Director of Pain Psychology
Department of Anesthesia, Critical Care and Pain Medicine
Beth Israel Deaconess Medical Center
Brookline, Massachusetts

Christopher L. Wu, MD
Clinical Professor of Anesthesiology
Department of Anesthesiology
The Hospital for Special Surgery, Weill Cornell
   Medical College
New York, New York

Takahisa Yamasaki, MD, PhD
Research Fellow
Division Gastroenterology and Hepatology
MetroHealth Medical Center
Visiting Scholar
Case Western Reserve University
Cleveland, Ohio

Jimmy Chen Yang, MD
Clinical Fellow
Department of Neurosurgery
Harvard University
Resident Physician
Department of Neurosurgery
Massachusetts General Hospital
Boston, Massachusetts

Lynda J. Yang, MD, PhD
Clinical Professor
Department of Neurosurgery
University of Michigan Medical School
Ann Arbor, Michigan

Shelley Yang, MD
Dermatology Chief Resident
University of Washington Division of Dermatology
Seattle, Washington

Adam C. Young, MD
Assistant Professor, Department of Anesthesiology
Director of Acute Pain Management
Rush University Medical Center
Chicago, Illinois

Lin Yu, PhD
Researcher
Pain Management Centre
Guy's and St. Thomas NHS Foundation Trust
London, United Kingdom

Fadel Zeidan, PhD
Assistant Professor
Department of Neurobiology and Anatomy
Associate Director of Neuroscience
Center for Integrative Medicine
Wake Forest School of Medicine
Winston Salem, North Carolina

Lonnie Zeltzer, MD
Distinguished Professor
Pediatrics, Anesthesiology, Psychiatry and Behavioral Sciences
David Geffen School of Medicine at UCLA
Director Pediatric Pain & Palliative Care Program
Pediatrics
UCLA Center for Health Sciences
UCLA Mattel Children's Hospital
Los Angeles, California

Foreword

This, the fifth edition of *Bonica's Management of Pain*, continues the tradition that John J. Bonica, MD, started with the publication of the first edition in 1953. That was a herculean endeavor and a monumental achievement, as no one had ever attempted to comprehensively describe all that was known about pain and how to diagnose and treat it. The first edition was almost exclusively the work of Dr. Bonica; only minor sections were contributed by his colleagues. It took him 30 years to bring out the second edition, which was the product of not only Bonica but also of a long list of contributors who in fact wrote more than half of the pages. This edition was characterized by extensive consideration of the anatomy and physiology underlying pain and by the discussion of multidisciplinary pain management and pain clinics.

The field of pain medicine, launched by Bonica's own practice and teaching and by his founding of the International Association for the Study of Pain, had flourished by the time of the second edition, as pain medicine and research were developing rapidly. Bonica knew that another edition of the *Bonica's Management of Pain* would have to be written to keep his textbook current. Unfortunately, his health limited his ability to undertake this task. Shortly before he died, I promised him that there would be a third edition that I would edit with the help of colleagues at the University of Washington. This was published in 2000, firmly based on the format of the prior editions but expanding the content to keep up with developments in both basic science and clinical pain management.

Another decade passed; the sciences basic to pain and clinical practice continued to rapidly expand. The fourth edition of this great book was produced by new editors who assembled an all-star group of contributors to continue what Bonica began over 60 years ago. Now, it is time for the fifth edition to be created to set the pace for the coming decade of pain research, teaching, and patient care.

Whereas everyone active in pain research or patient care knew John Bonica in the last 30 years of the 20th century, we now have spawned a generation or two of workers in this field who know him only through his publications or the occasional prophetic story. Although this is an understandable reality, it is unfortunate. John Bonica was a truly great man whose efforts almost single-handedly caused pain to be put on the road maps of both basic science and health care. As I wrote in his obituary published in *Pain*[1]:

"He cared about his patients for whom he tirelessly worked. He cared about the research that scientists undertook to understand the mechanisms of pain. He cared about those who suffered in far-away places; he wanted their doctors to learn about pain management. He cared about how governments impacted the delivery of pain management services. He cared about his students, trainees, and colleagues. He really cared about those who attempted to continue what he had started. He cared about his children and his wife, although his career took time away from them."[(p2)]

More than an inscription on his gravestone, the continued life of *Bonica's Management of Pain* tells us of his accomplishments. It was a privilege to have known him and his family. Working for and with him and carrying on the traditions that he launched has been an honor. JJB, as he was known to all who worked alongside him, would have been thrilled to see the advances that he inspired. His greatness will live on through the publication of this fifth edition.

JOHN D. LOESER, M.D.
June 2018

---

[1]Loeser JD. Obituary: John J Bonica, M.D. and Emma B. Bonica. *Pain* 1994;59:1–3.

Preface to the Fifth Edition (2019)

This book was first introduced 66 years ago, at a time that many believe marks the beginning of the multidisciplinary field of pain management. The idea for a clinical textbook devoted to the management of pain came from John Bonica, and in its first edition, he wrote that the book offers a synthesis of information from disparate disciplines to form a complete discussion on pain and its management. Such a book, he believed, would strengthen the field of medicine by assimilating new insights and growing knowledge from many interested disciplines. Since the first edition in 1953, the purpose of the book has remained the same despite extraordinary growth in the science and practice of pain management and the emergence of pain medicine as its own discipline. The book has remained a key reference for clinicians largely because of the high quality of the original book and its ability to attract world-class experts to engage in his project, even years after Dr. Bonica's death in 1994. It was with trepidation and pride that we, the three chief editors, first accepted the task of shepherding the fourth edition of this essential book to publication. We quickly realized that we were no match for Bonica, who formulated and wrote large parts of the original book himself, and from the start, we solicited help from expert subeditors. As an editorial group, we made several key decisions: that we would keep the book near its original manageable size, that understanding anew the key role played by central mechanisms in pain, that we would shift the book's emphasis from its focus on peripheral (anatomically based) mechanisms to one with a greater focus on neural (global) mechanisms, and that we would include new or updated chapters on issues that impact clinical pain management such as pain training, regulatory and political issues, and conducting clinical trials.

In his first edition, John Bonica tells us that he was called to write his book out of the ". . . deep feeling for those who are afflicted with intractable pain, and by an intense desire to contribute something toward the alleviation of their suffering." This commitment originated from his experiences in treating wounded soldiers with intractable pain during the Second World War. It is sad and ironic that this fourth edition was published in 2009 at a time when inadequate treatment of pain had come to be more widely recognized than ever and, in part, informed by wounded soldiers returning from the wars in Iraq and Afghanistan. In the year just prior to publishing the fourth edition, the US Congress passed, and the President of the United States signed into law, two bills that aimed to improve pain care for active military personnel and veterans, respectively. More than 50 years after Bonica began to raise awareness about the plight of those in pain, our society was coming to increasingly value safe and effective control of pain, and the trend echoed Bonica's vision of a world free of suffering from treatable pain. Over the past 9 years, since the publication of the fourth edition of the textbook, there has been widespread recognition of a devastating crisis in opioid abuse and deaths as well as excessive prescribing of opioids. Much controversy has arisen regarding the use of opioids, particularly opioids for chronic pain. This controversy plays out in the pages of this the

fifth edition, and you will find opposing and at times mutually exclusive opinions expressed. We, the editors, did not try to align the opinions of all of the experts expressed in the text. We allow readers to consider the disparate opinions on their own while we await the science we need to point us toward the best practices.

The fourth edition of the textbook remained faithful to Bonica's original intent that his book should provide a comprehensive reference for practicing clinicians across all disciplines. In 1953, Bonica was one of few experts in a nascent new field that would become pain medicine, and he almost single-handedly undertook the task of producing the first clinical textbook. Now, there are many experts with a remarkable depth of knowledge. It is a testament to Bonica that the many leading authorities contributing to the fourth and now this fifth edition as authors and section editors feel sincerely indebted to him, and they have willingly given of their time to maintain his legacy. Through its second and third editions, the book maintained a structure and organization similar to the first edition. In the fourth edition, every chapter was revised, substantially rewritten, or represented a completely new chapter and or topic. With a text of such broad scope, some degree of overlap was inevitable; indeed, we have often allowed significant overlap, so that each chapter would stand on its own during independent perusal or study.

Like the fourth edition, this fifth edition of the book is divided into six parts: (1) Basic Considerations; (2) Economic, Political, Legal, and Ethical Considerations; (3) Evaluation of the Pain Patient; (4) Pain Conditions; (5) Methods for Symptomatic Control; and (6) Provision of Pain Treatment. Basic Considerations offers an orientation to the history of pain management and the concepts and paradigms fundamental to this field, including taxonomy, basic science, anatomy, physiology, psychology, and social science. Economic, Political, Legal, and Ethical Considerations represents new content for this textbook, reflecting the emerging social impact of pain and pain management. Evaluation of the Pain Patient covers physical and psychological assessment and use of imaging and other technology-based testing as well as special assessment for function, disability, addiction, and multidisciplinary care. Pain Conditions is the largest single part of the text, comprising 9 sections and 53 chapters. These sections include neuropathic pain syndromes; psychological contributions to pain; vascular, cutaneous, and musculoskeletal pains; pain due to cancer; acute pain; pain in special populations; visceral pain; regional pain; and neck and low back pain. The section on pain in special populations addresses populations such as children, older persons, and those with pain and addiction. The regional pain section is a holdover from past editions and covers pain disorders that are associated with discrete parts of the body such as facial pain, cranial neuralgias, and pain syndromes associated with upper or lower extremities. Methods of Symptomatic Control is another large part of the text which is partitioned into the following six sections: pharmacologic therapies, psychological techniques, physical and other noninterventional therapeutic modalities, implanted electrical stimulators, interventional pain management, and surgical approaches. Provision of Pain Treatment is the final part of this text, addressing systems for delivery of care and means for training pain specialists. Special areas of medicine in which pain has a prominent role are addressed, including primary care, end-of-life care, intensive care, and emergency care. The text concludes with a brief view toward the future of pain management.

This book would not be possible without the extensive contributions of the section editors and particularly the efforts of the chapter authors; the success of this work is directly attributable to these individuals. The editors are indebted to Brian Brown and Keith Donnellan of Wolters Kluwer who served critical roles in shepherding this project into existence and managed its development with skill and diplomacy.

As the field of pain medicine has evolved, so has this text. Despite much that is new or revised, the text remains incomplete, a reflection of an emerging field that awaits profound discoveries and development. Through the many chapters and pages of this new fifth edition of his classic text, we hope that John Bonica's passion for an integrated, coherent, and compassionate field will live on. Like Bonica, our central purpose is to assist students and practitioners across all medical disciplines, advance their knowledge of pain medicine, and relieve suffering.

Preface to the First Edition (1953)

The purpose of this book is to present within one volume a concise but complete discussion of the fundamental aspects of pain, the various diseases and disorders in which pain constitutes a major problem, and the methods employed in its management, with special emphasis on the use of analgesic block as an aid in the diagnosis, prognosis, and therapy. Although several books dealing with certain phases of this problem are available, none is complete from the standpoint of the practitioner; for it is necessary for him to consult several texts in order to obtain information regarding the cause, characteristics, mechanisms, effects, diagnosis, and therapy of pain and management of its intractable variety with analgesic block and certain adjuvant methods. The present volume is the product of the author's desire to facilitate the task of the busy practitioner and to supply him easily accessible information with the conviction that this will induce more clinicians to employ these methods of diagnosis and therapy.

One need not elaborate on the reasons for writing on the management of pain, for reflection emphasized that this age-old problem is still one of the most difficult and often vexing phases of medical practice—a fact well appreciated by most physicians. This fact, as well as other reasons, are presented in the introduction and are emphasized throughout the book, particularly in Chapter 5.

I have been motivated to write this volume by a deep feeling for those who are afflicted with intractable pain, and by an intense desire to contribute something toward the alleviation of their suffering. The plan for its writing was germinated almost a decade ago during the Second World War, while I was Chief of the Anesthesia Section of a large Army hospital, where I was afforded the opportunity to observe and manage an unusually large number of patients with severe intractable pain. The gratifying results obtained with analgesic block in some instances impressed me with the efficacy of this method in selected cases. In addition, the fact that these procedures effected relief which frequently was not only dramatic, but outlasted by hours and days the transient physiochemical interruption of nerve impulses, fascinated me and aroused my interest. Perusal of the literature revealed a paucity of material on this subject—a situation which has not changed much since then and which clearly indicated an obvious need for a practical source of information about this perplexing phenomenon and the application of analgesic block to its management.

This book is composed of three parts. The first part includes a discussion of the fundamental aspects of pain. While some of the material, on superficial thought, might be considered too detailed or entirely unnecessary, it has been included because of my conviction that in order to manage pain properly its anatomical, physiological and psychological bases must be understood. As is true in all fields of endeavor, a thorough knowledge of fundamental principles is an essential prerequisite without which optimal results are precluded. In order to diagnose and treat it properly, the physician must know the course of pain from its place of origin to the apperception centers in the brain and must be well versed in all the essentials and components

of which pain consists; he must know its causes, mechanisms, characteristics, varieties, its localizations and significance, and the mental and physical effects it produces.

The second part deals with methods and techniques of managing pain. It was originally planned to include only the method which is the central theme of the book—analgesic block. However, it was soon realized that while this important phase is, to be sure, here treated in a comprehensive manner, it does not present the complete story of the management of pain; because frequently other adjuvant methods are employed in conjunction with nerve blocking. To illustrate the point, trigeminal neuralgia is frequently treated with neurolytic blocks, but sometimes this does not afford sufficiently long relief, and neurotomy is resorted to. The pain associated with malignancy is managed with alcohol nerve block, but roentgen therapy is frequently employed as an adjuvant. Moreover physical and/or psychiatric therapy constitute integral phases of the management of pain without which optimal results cannot be hoped for. After careful consideration, it was decided to include another section in Part II in which are presented methods that are frequently employed in conjunction with analgesic block. It is hoped that such inclusion will give the book a wider scope and greater usefulness.

In the third part are presented various diseases or disorders with painful syndromes which have been and can be managed with analgesic block with or without the aid of other methods. The arrangement of this part is explained in detail on page 671. It is suggested that the reader refer to that page before proceeding further to read any on the pain syndromes. Though the material in this part mainly represents my observations, clinical impressions, and opinions, obtained or developed from experience with, and statistical analysis of, many thousands of cases, it also includes unpublished data of several outstanding authorities who have kindly placed them at my disposal. Moreover, it includes the published views and clinical experiences of others, with credit given where it is due.

In writing this comprehensive treatise, which has involved no small amount of time and effort, the one principle which has always been kept in mind and adhered to has been to present the fundamental considerations and principles of the problem before the practical aspects are discussed.

I have endeavored to make this book as complete as possible, and to this end have thoroughly searched the literature, both English and foreign, and have taken from it all that I thought might be valuable to the reader. In order to comply with the aim of completeness and still keep the book concise and within reasonable size, the material has been selected with care and discretion. In a field so vast and complex as pain, it is unavoidable that what might be thought sufficiently important to deserve detailed discussion is presented in an abbreviated manner or entirely omitted. In other instances, mere mention or omission represents a reluctant compliance with the requirements dictated by the size of the volume. Nonetheless, I believe thoroughness and important detail have not been sacrificed. The bibliography represents the most important references, and many excellent articles on each subject were also reluctantly omitted for that reason.

The book is intended for practitioners of every field of medicine, because pain is universal and provides the main reason why patients seek the aid of the doctor. It is hoped that it will prove useful, not only to the anesthesiologist, neurologist, neurosurgeon, orthopedist, and physiatrist to whom especially is relegated the task of caring for patients with intractable pain, but also to the general practitioner, surgeon, internist, psychiatrist, and any other physician who may be confronted with this problem. It is especially intended for general practitioners, particularly those practicing in smaller communities where the services of a specialist in analgesic blocking are not available. With this aim in mind the techniques of analgesic block are presented in such a manner that most of them may be effectively accomplished by any physician, even though he may be a novice with regional analgesia. In order to facilitate the task of the busy reader, less relevant facts—material which has been included because of its academic importance, for the sake of completeness, or for consumption by students and those who wish to delve deeper into the problem—are presented in small type. These can be omitted without losing continuity of thought. In this manner, while completeness, detail, and thoroughness are not sacrificed, emphasis is laid on the practical aspects of the problem at hand.

The unusually large number of illustrations, many of which are original and composed from dissected material or clinical cases, have been included with the conviction that these frequently tell the story much better than words.

A book of this nature is made possible only by the contribution of many individuals. The information set forth in the first part of the volume represents the fruition of the joint effort of anatomists, physiologists, pharmacologists, neurologists, neurosurgeons, anesthesiologists, psychiatrists, and many other laboratory and clinical investigators who have spent untold time, labor, and effort to discover the mystery of pain. I am grateful for their elucidating knowledge. To clinicians who have reported their experiences, and to others who have placed at my disposal unpublished data, observations, and opinions, my

sincere thanks. I am particularly obliged to General Maxwell Keeler, and Col. Clinton S. Lyter, of Madigan Army Hospital for their continuous cooperation in obtaining much of the clinical data embraced in this volume. I want to express my gratitude to Mr. Harold Woodworth for his friendship, sympathetic understanding and devotion to the cause of medicine. I also want to thank the other members of the Board of Trustees of Tacoma General Hospital, but particularly Mr. Alex Babbit, and Mr. Walter Heath and John Dobyns, Directors of the hospital. Their continuous cooperation has facilitated the activities of the Department of Anesthesia, Nerve Block Clinic, and Pain Clinic.

I am very grateful to Dr. Robert Johnson, Associate Professor of Anatomy of the University of Washington School of Medicine, for his encouragement and criticism of some parts of the manuscript; to Doctor Frederick Haugen for his assistance, criticism and suggestion.

My collaborators, Professor Robert Ripley, Doctors Wendell Peterson, Frank Rigos, John T. Robson, Col. Clark Williams, M.C., and Lieut. Col. Walter Lumpkin, M.D., have my heartfelt thanks for their contributions and cooperation.

My appreciation is extended to Miss Joy Polis, Miss Virginia Coleman, and other artists for the illustrations and to Mr. Kenneth Ollar for the photography; to Mrs. Louise Cameron for her cooperation in obtaining the roentgenograms; to Mrs. Katherine Rogers Miller, Miss Eleanor Ekberg and the late Mrs. Blanch DeWitt of Tacoma, Miss Bertha Hallam, Portland, and Mr. Alderson Fry, Seattle—all librarians whose cooperation has facilitated a difficult task, and to Mr. John Morrison for editorial work.

This preface would be incomplete if I did not acknowledge my indebtedness to my secretaries, Miss Katherine Stryker and Mrs. Dorothy Richmond, for the inestimable aid they have given me in the preparation of the manuscript.

My appreciation is extended to my publishers for their courtesy, cooperation, and considerateness throughout the preparation of this volume.

JOHN J. BONICA
Tacoma, Washington

Acknowledgments

Jane C. Ballantyne and James P. Rathmell thank Dr. Warren Zapol, immediate past Chair of the Department of Anesthesiology and Critical Care at Massachusetts General Hospital, for his encouragement and support.

Scott M. Fishman thanks the exceptional faculty of the Division of Pain Medicine and Dr. Richard Applegate, Chair of the Department of Anesthesiology and Pain Medicine at the University of California, Davis, for encouragement and support.

Contents

CHAPTER **1**

Intellectual Milestones in Our Understanding and Treatment of Pain

G.F. GEBHART

> In order to treat something we first must learn to recognize it.
> —Sir William Osler[1]

Through the ages, pain and suffering have been the primary reasons why patients sought medical care. But what pain is (an independent sense, an emotion, an experience, . . .) has been considered and argued by philosophers and investigators alike to the present day. The International Association for the Study of Pain (www.iasp-pain.org) defines pain as "an unpleasant sensory and emotional experience associated with actual or potential tissue damage, or described in terms of such damage." Pain is always a subjective, personal, and unpleasant experience. This chapter reviews ideas and concepts about pain, including how our mental constructs shape our understanding, and then treatment of this complex experience we call pain. This chapter closes with a discussion of how the medical subspecialty is evolving within the broader context of medical specialization and thoughts for future development.[2]

Pain Understood as Part of a Larger Philosophy or Worldview

Since the beginning of time, humans have been born through a painful process, and the experience of suffering remains universal. The meaning of pain reflects the contemporary spirit of the age and, therefore, has changed over recorded history as worldviews changed. Among the earliest systems of pain management, dating back to the Stone Age, was Chinese acupuncture, theoretically based on the philosophy of imbalances of yin and yang affecting qi and blood flow. Thousands of years ago, Egyptians considered the experience of pain to be a god or disincarnate spirit afflicting the heart, which was conceptualized as the center of emotion. Galen, and later Aristotle, described pain as an emotional experience, or "a passion of the soul."[3]

An important concept dating from antiquity that persisted until the 19th century was the theory of importance of the four humors. This worldview was espoused by Greek philosophers in approximately 400 BC and later applied to medicine by Hippocrates, who described humors as related to one of the four constitutions, shown in Table 1.1. Seasonal changes evoked pain, and certain disorders, such as migraine, were associated with specific humors (e.g., excessive cold humors thought to result in a mucus discharge requiring application of "hot effusions" to the head).

Consistent with this ideology was the custom of treating pain by applying "opposites" such as hot applications to the head to counterbalance and evacuate "cold" humors of headaches.[5] Based on the humor theory and treatment by "opposites" was a technique called cupping. Warm suction cups were applied to the skin that on cooling resulted in raised reddened welts thought to "draw out" any unbalanced humors.[6]

Later, during the Middle Ages, coincident with the spread of Christianity, pain, not surprisingly, was explained in a spiritual, religious context. Medieval life has been described as short, cheap, and brutish, especially for the lower classes, with pain accepted as the universal lot of mankind. Little is known of how pain was actually treated during this period, but a suffering Christ, martyred saints, and the concept of physical pain in purgatory originated around the 12th century AD.[6,7] Commonly revered was the iconography of tortured saints with ecstatic faces depicting pain as a spiritual discipline bringing the saints closer to God, relieved primarily by prayer and meditation. A clear example of pain as ennobling was St. Ignatius Loyola's habit of wearing ropes and chains cutting into the skin and encouraging other humiliations of the flesh to enhance his spiritual development.[3]

An interesting example of pain as a function of the sociologic concepts of the day is the rise and fall of the diagnosis of hysteria, common in the 17th century and virtually nonexistent today. Thomas Sydenham (Fig. 1.1), in 1681, wrote, "Of all chronic diseases hysteria—unless I err—is the commonest."[8] The cardinal symptom of this condition was unexplained pain. In mid-19th century Europe and America, hysteria was virtually everywhere, found in every community. Invalids, mostly females, filled homes, spas, and convalescent facilities at the turn of the 19th century. This mysterious syndrome, afflicting

TABLE 1.1 Relationships in Antiquity between the Four Humors, Elements, Constitutions, and Seasons[4]

Black bile	Blood	Phlegm	Yellow bile
Earth	Air	Water	Fire
Dry, cold	Hot, wet	Cold, wet	Hot, dry
Autumn	Spring	Winter	Summer

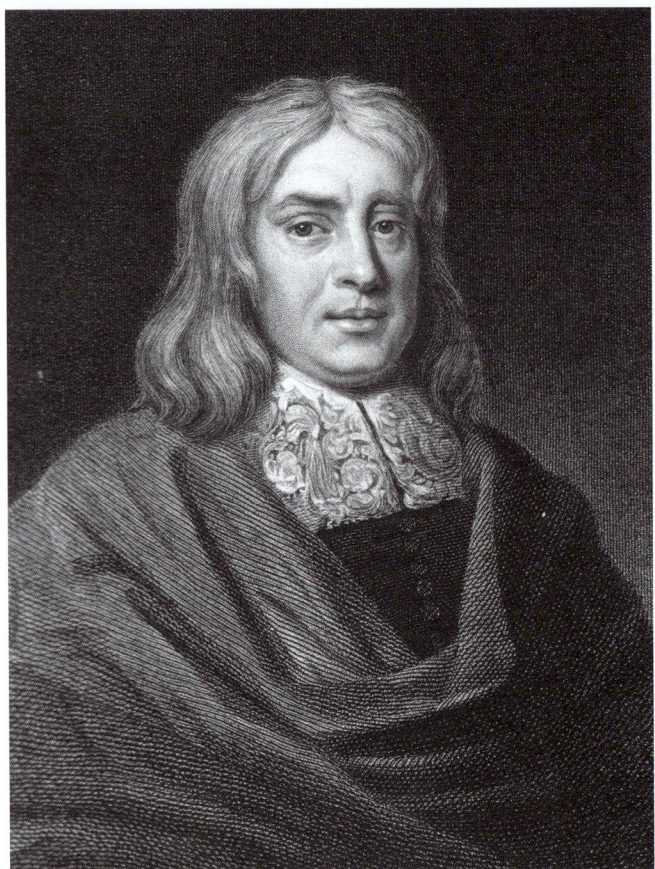

FIGURE 1.1   Thomas Sydenham. *(Courtesy of the National Library of Medicine.)*

only middle and upper class females, was treated by complete social isolation, confinement to bed, and a total prohibition on any form of intellectual activity, even sewing or reading (CP Gilman as quoted in Rey[9]). As the social situation and educational opportunities for women improved, this disorder almost totally disappeared, a public health success on the order of magnitude of the eradication of yellow fever. In the 21st century, fibromyalgia, although a commonly diagnosed condition in Western countries, interestingly enough, is either underreported or not significantly present in Asian and developing country populations.

Another very clear link between mental state and the perception and control of pain is apparent in the work of the German physician Franz Anton Mesmer. In 1766, he published his doctoral dissertation entitled "On the Influence of the Planets on the Human Body," describing animal (or life spirit) magnetism as a force to cure many ills.[10] He used iron magnets to treat various diseases, amplifying the magnetic fields with room-sized Leyden jars. His demonstrations of his technique, combining hypnotism with spectacle, included the wearing of brightly colored robes in dimly lit ritualistic séances, with soft music playing from a glass harmonium. He invoked magnetic power with poles either held or waved over the patient and his techniques were an early rival to ether anesthesia as a way to relieve pain during surgical procedures.[11] Mesmerism was such a common form of pain therapy during his day that Robert Liston reportedly exclaimed after the successful administration of ether anesthesia in an early above-knee operation, "This Yankee Dodge beats mesmerism hollow."[12] Mesmerism was based on the larger generally accepted theory of vitalism which posited that every part of a living thing was endowed with sensibility. The energy or force

which animated a living organism was capable of being stimulated or consumed. In disease, pain was necessary to produce a "crisis" which rid the patient of original pain by stimulating the diminishing energy.[6]

A further development of the link between mind and body and the understanding of pain was the landmark development of Freudian theory in understanding subconscious influences on pain perception and behavior. The link between the unconscious mind and physical sensation in hysterical conversion disorders was posited as an explanation for psychogenic pain and continues to be influential today. This conceptual paradigm was expanded in the 1970s by the psychiatrist George L. Engel who demonstrated the link between chronic pain and psychiatric illness.[13] Later, psychiatrists, psychologists, and social scientists, including Thomas Szasz,[14] Allan Walters,[15] and Harold Merskey,[16] explored social situations, psychological character traits, and the effects of past life experiences in understanding chronic pain in patients. Depression, stress, and personality, in addition to physiologic mechanisms, have proven to be critical grounds for investigation and therapy. From these early studies, investigating the mind–body interface of pain grew the cognitive-behavioral school of pain therapy in the 1980s that is widely employed today, emphasizing the development of coping mechanisms to deal with chronic pain as a basic component of interdisciplinary pain programs. The concept of pain, not only as a physiologic response to stimuli but as a more complicated construct, incorporating social, behavioral, and psychological responses as well, is an intellectual milestone that has inspired a wealth of investigations and patient treatment options. New areas of investigation now include pain in relationship to social setting, gender, national, ethnic, and racial background as well as differences in coping ability and psychiatric comorbidities. Considerations of vocational and legal environment as well as family and interpersonal dynamics are also relevant to the understanding and care of individual patients.

This global philosophy of pain as only part of an entire life experience can best be summed up in the words of Alexander Pope in his *Essay on Man* in 1733:

> Say what the use, were finer optics giv'n,
> T' inspect a mite, not comprehend the heav'n?
> Or touch, if tremblingly alive all o'er,
> To smart and agonize at ev'ry pore?
> Or, quick effluvia darting thro' the brain,
> Die of a rose in aromatic pain?[17]

Mechanistic Views of Pain

In counterpoint to the holistic philosophical consideration of pain was mechanism, the philosophical mind set suggesting that the human body functions as a simple machine with pain being the result of its malfunction.[18] This viewpoint is clearly seen in Descartes' *Passions of the Soul* in 1649 where he compares a human being to a watch:

> [T]he difference between the body of a living man and that of a dead man is just like the difference between, on the one hand, a watch or other automaton (that is, a self-moving machine) when it is wound up and contains in itself the corporeal principle of the movements for which it is designed . . . ; and, on the other hand, the same watch or machine when it is broken and the principle of its movement ceases to be active.[19]

How did the mechanistic view of the body develop and even supersede traditional theologic and philosophical explanations for pain? Early anatomical studies were conducted beginning with Galen of Pergamum (130–201 AD) and Avicenna (Fig. 1.2), the Persian Muslim polymath

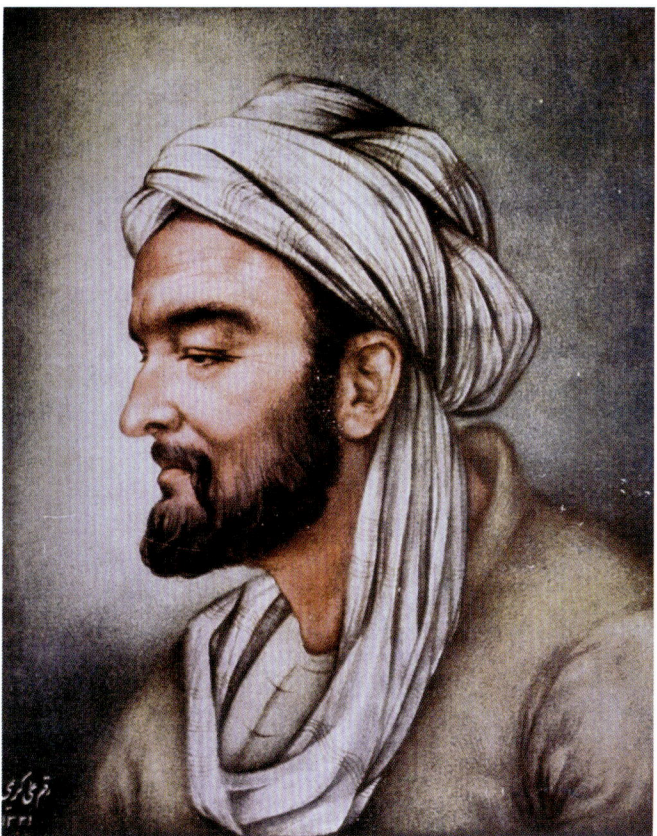

FIGURE 1.2   Avicenna. *(Courtesy of the National Library of Medicine.)*

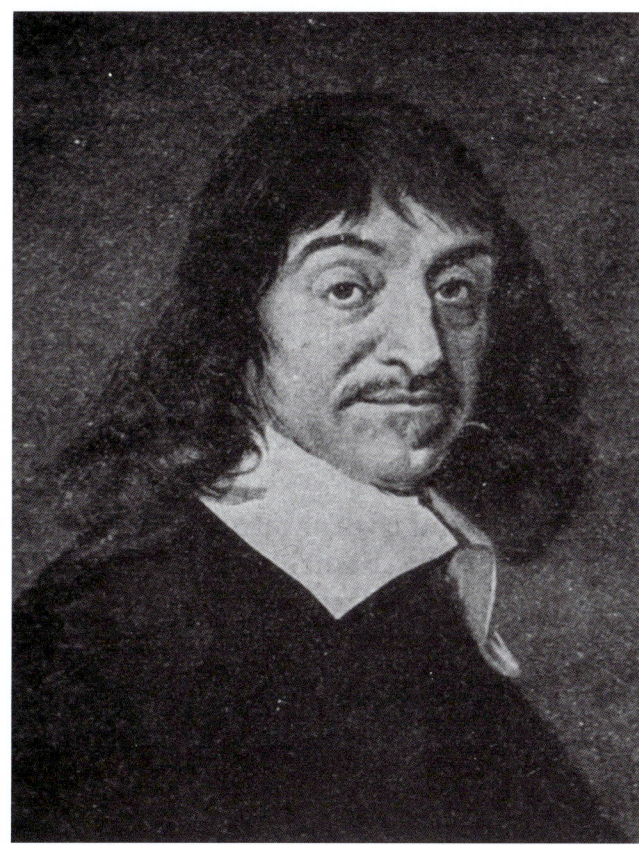

FIGURE 1.3   René Descartes. *(Courtesy of the National Library of Medicine.)*

(980–1037 AD), forming an intellectual basis for pain as an actual physical sensation rather than as a mental, spiritual dilemma. Later, in the 14th through 17th centuries, the Renaissance cultural movement questioned the basis of all knowledge, including ideas about the human body and the experience of pain. Empiricism and the development of scientific inquiry with direct observation into the mysteries of life became the basis for advances in both medical understanding and treatment, including the now commonly accepted neurologic basis of pain. Extended wars on the continent between France and Spain resulted in bullet and musket ball injuries that tore the skin, forcing surgical removal and amputation. Wounds were bound and foreign bodies extracted, originally posited to prevent leakage of the "vital force" or to inhibit the entrance of animal spirits into the injured body. Gradually, direct observation of the circulation of the blood by William Harvey[20] in 1628 and the direct anatomical studies of Descartes (Fig. 1.3)[19] in 1662, elucidating sensory physiology became the theoretical basis for further exploration in the 18th and 19th centuries.

19TH CENTURY—PAIN AS A SPECIFIC SENSE

In 1811, Charles Bell (Fig. 1.4), an anatomist in Edinburgh, Scotland, published a monograph in which he described new and important evidence for the specificity of function of peripheral nerves. Bell proposed differences in function between the dorsal and ventral roots of the spinal cord, writing that ". . . the nerves of sense and nerves of motion . . . are distinct . . ."[21] Bell's discovery that ventral root stimulation controlled muscle contraction was followed by François Magendie's (Fig. 1.5) report in 1822 that sectioning posterior (dorsal) nerve roots resulted in paralysis and insensibility of the corresponding

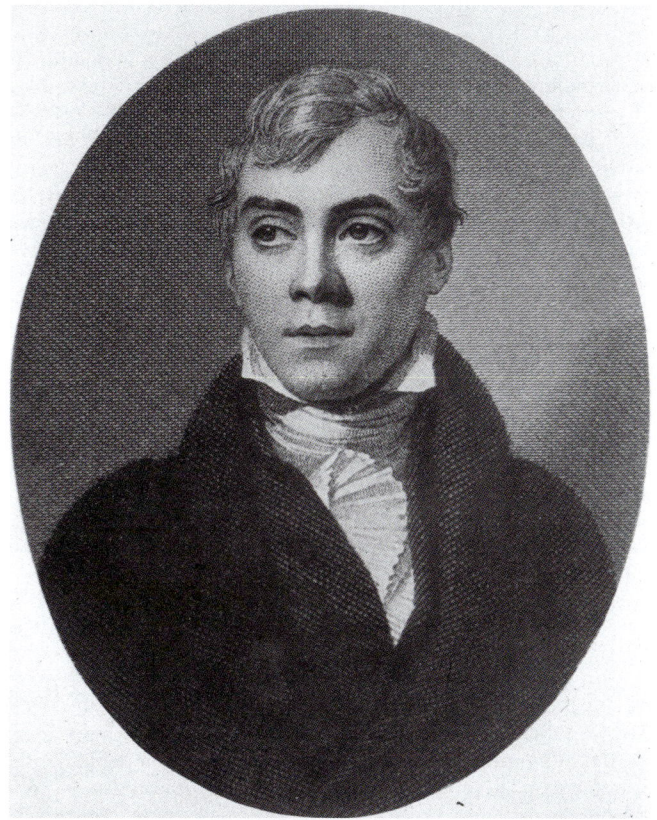

FIGURE 1.4   Sir Charles Bell. *(Courtesy of the National Library of Medicine.)*

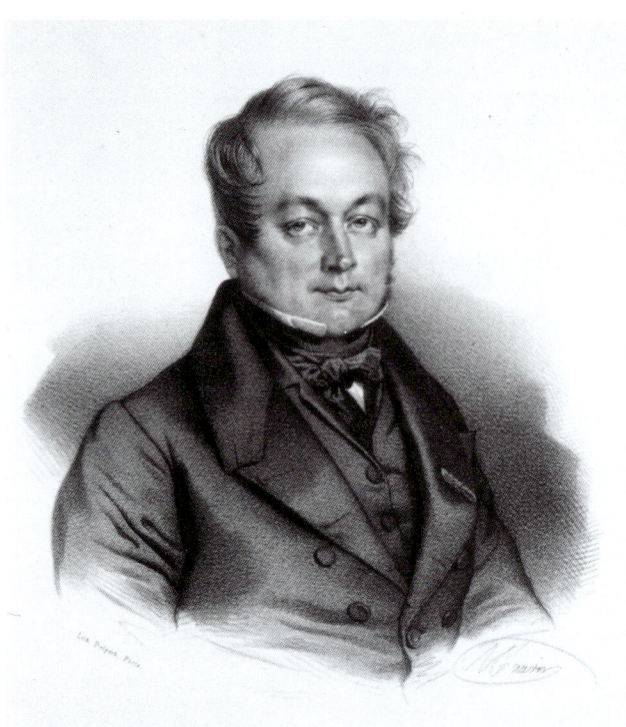

FIGURE 1.5 François Magendie. *(Courtesy of the National Library of Medicine.)*

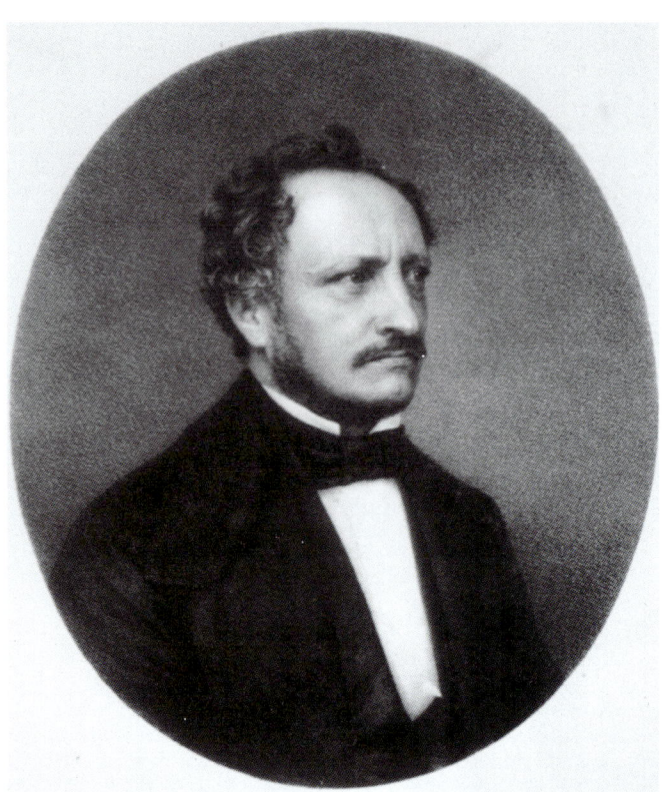

FIGURE 1.6 Johannes Müller. *(Courtesy of the National Library of Medicine.)*

limbs, confirming that the dorsal roots are afferent.[22] The result of these discoveries regarding the functions of the spinal roots is now known as the Bell-Magendie law (confirmed in 1831 by Johannes Müller).

Johannes Müller (Fig. 1.6)[23] was a precocious and influential German investigator who advanced in 1826 at the age of 25 years the Law of Specific Nerve Energies, which laid out the basic concept of modern sensory physiology (cf. Handwerker and Brune[24]). Müller's "law" emphasized that the quality of sensation depends not on the stimulus but on the sense organ and sensory pathway stimulated. Müller's law was not advanced in the context of pain as he was studying at that time vision. He considered the sensation of sound to be the "specific energy" of the acoustic nerve, and the sensation of light the particular "energy" of the visual nerve. In 1858, Moritz Schiff[25] established, based on studies of the effects of spinal cord lesions, that separate spinal pathways conveyed tactile, temperature, and pain sensations. On the basis of his studies, Schiff proposed that pain was an independent sensation (a specific sense). Schiff's findings were subsequently confirmed and extended by Charles-Édouard Brown-Séquard and Sir William Richard Gowers, establishing the importance of spinal pathways for conducting information about painful stimuli applied in the periphery.

Alfred Goldscheider (Fig. 1.7) and Max von Frey (Fig. 1.8) were contemporaries, adversaries, and also important to the history of pain research.[24] Their divergent interpretations and conclusions from their research fostered and supported debate about the "pain" sensitivity of pressure points in skin well into the 20th century. In 1881, Goldscheider, a German army physician, demonstrated in his dissertation (and independently of the Swedish physiologist Magnus Blix), spatially discontinuous warm and cold spots in the skin, thus confirming

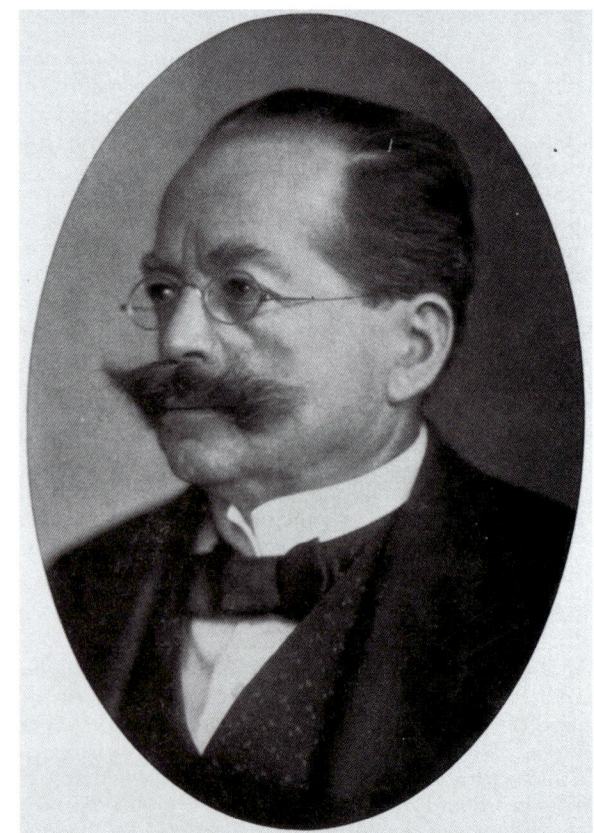

FIGURE 1.7 Alfred Goldscheider. *(Courtesy of the National Library of Medicine.)*

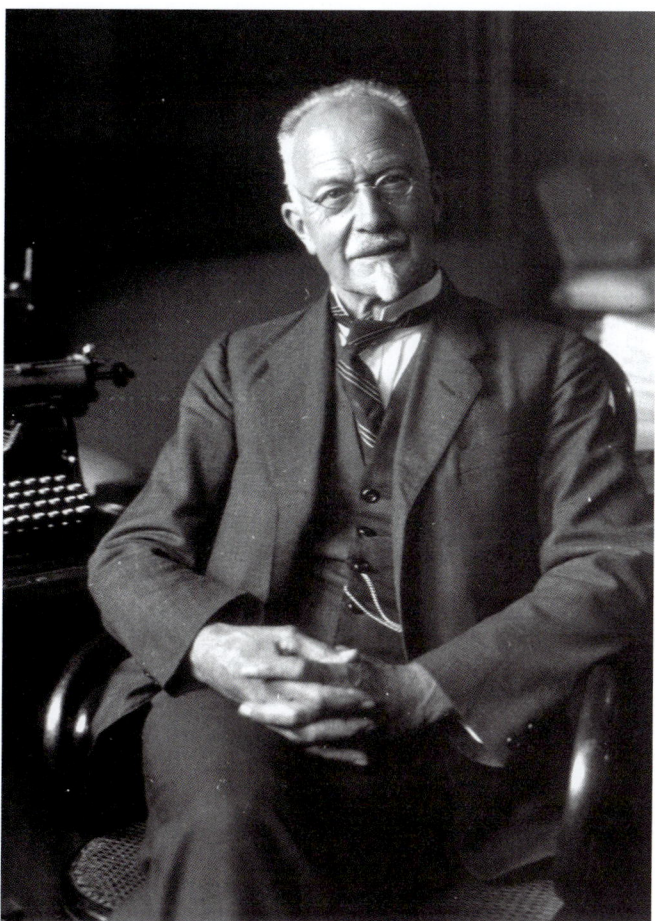

FIGURE 1.8   Max von Frey. *(Courtesy of the National Library of Medicine.)*

Müller's Law of Specific Nerve Energies. Goldscheider reported that stimulation of a cold point always produced the sensation of cold whether activated by a cold metal rod or by electrical stimulation. Goldscheider also reported that stimulation of temperature points did not produce a sensation of pain

and advanced therefore the existence of tactile and pain points in skin.[24,26]

Max von Frey was a systematic and methodical investigator interested in the skin as a sense organ and who today is largely (and incorrectly) credited with first documenting "pain points" in skin (Fig. 1.9). Using pig bristles and horsehairs of various diameters and stiffness, thus requiring different forces to bend when applied perpendicular to the skin, von Frey carefully mapped pressure points (Druckpunkte) and pain points (Schmerzpunkte) on the back of the hand.[24,27] Max von Frey believed that the critical event producing pain from the skin was excitation of pain-conducting nerve fibers in peripheral nerves and that different types of sensory spots (warm, cool, pressure, pain) were associated with distinct structural elements in the skin. In the aggregate, at the turn of the 20th century, it was generally agreed that skin contained a number of nonuniformly distributed, distinct receptive end organs, each representing a particular kind of sensibility—pressure, warmth, cold and pain—and each responding only to its appropriate stimulus (termed subsequently by Sherrington as its *adequate stimulus*).

AFFERENT SIGNALING

In the latter part of the 19th century and into the 20th century, however, arguments against pain as a specific skin sense were advanced. In particular, the advent of electrophysiology as a research approach contributed specific information about afferent fiber types (i.e., A and C fibers) and their responses to applied stimuli. The pioneering contributions of anatomists and physiologists in this period of time, several of whom were subsequently recognized with Nobel Prizes for revealing the structure and physiology of the nervous system (e.g., Adrian, Erlanger, Gasser, Golgi, Ramón y Cajal, Sherrington), were relevant to but did not specifically focus on pain (cf. Perl[28]). The contributions of the eminent British physiologist, Charles Scott Sherrington (Fig. 1.10), however, are remarkable for several reasons. Aware that pain commonly arises from injured tissue, Sherrington avoided labeling stimuli based on their physical character, instead naming stimuli that threatened or caused tissue damage "nocuous" (noxious). Importantly, he understood the distinction between pain and the neural encoding of noxious events, which he termed *nociception*, and

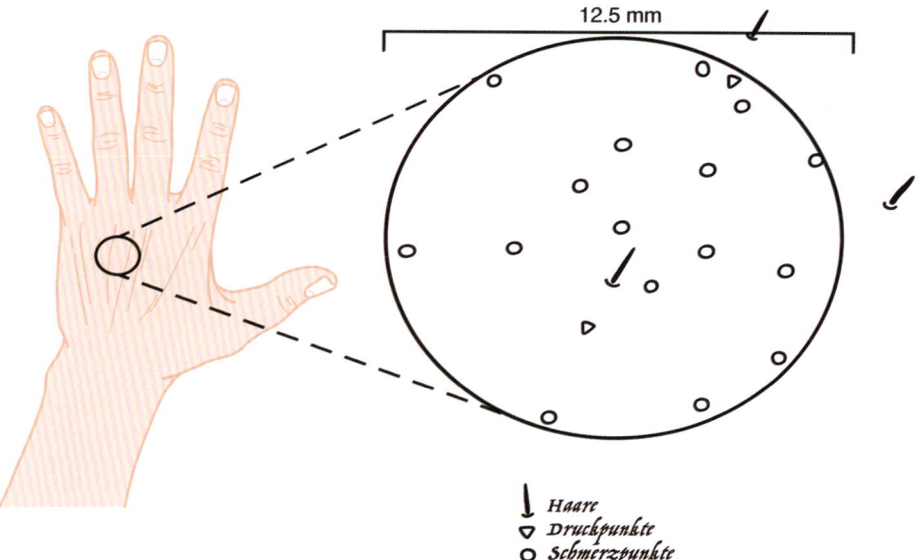

FIGURE 1.9   Pain points in the skin.

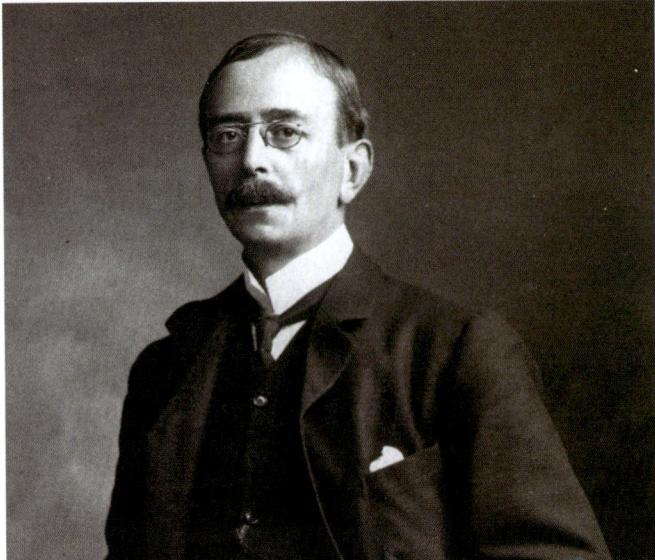

FIGURE 1.10   Charles Scott Sherrington. *(Courtesy of the National Library of Medicine.)*

named the sense organ in skin that responded to noxious stimuli a *nociceptor*.[29],*

Alfred Goldscheider, who initially supported the existence of pain sensory points, subsequently denied their existence and instead adopted the idea that pain arose from intense stimulation of pressure points. This "intensity theory" did not survive evidence that intense, even maximal stimulation of sense organs that respond to *in*nocuous stimuli does not generate pain-associated reactions. In light of these and other evidence, John Paul Nafe, an American psychologist, formalized what became referred to as pattern theory. He posited that all sensation arises from the spatial and temporal patterns of responses of afferent neurons rather than the result of activation of specific receptors or pathways.[30] In 1955, Sinclair[31] and Weddell[32] expanded the concept, emphasizing that all afferent endings, except those innervating hair follicles, are similar, and it is only the pattern that is important in sensory discrimination.

Based largely on clinical observations, other investigators focused on the role of the spinal dorsal horn, suggesting that pain resulted from the "summation" of afferent inputs rather than the "intensity" of the input or its spatiotemporal pattern. The American physician, William K. Livingston, suggested that pathologic input from the body activates reverberating circuits in spinal interneurons that subsequently can be triggered by normally innocuous afferent input (cf. Melzack and Wall[33]). The concept of central summation, coupled with growing appreciation of spinal modulation of afferent input, led to the introduction in 1965 by Ronald Melzack and Patrick Wall of a new theory of pain, the gate control theory.

GATE CONTROL THEORY

As reviewed earlier, specificity, intensity, and pattern theories about pain were not entirely exclusive in the writings of Goldscheider and von Frey. Even Müller, whose "laws" underlie the foundation of "specificity theory," understood that peripheral nerves did not feel pain and that it was their excitation

of the central nervous system that determined modality and quality of sensation. Although Goldscheider embraced concepts of "intensity theory," he also was aware of the notion of central inhibition, a component of pattern and summation theories of pain. The complexity of pain, today recognized as comprising sensory, emotional, and drive state components, however, could not be adequately explained as either a specific ("labeled line") pathway, spatiotemporal pattern of afferent input, or central summation of inputs. These often conflicting paradigms were reviewed and critically evaluated, and the prevailing basic and clinical evidence formulated as a new theory of pain by the Canadian psychologist Melzack and the British physiologist Wall (Figs. 1.11 and 1.12) while working together at the Massachusetts Institute of Technology.[33] The gate control theory most directly challenged specificity theory and generated both high praise and strong opposition to the underlying assumptions on with the theory was based (cf. Perl[28]). The gate control theory was (and remains) heuristically important, providing (1) a conceptual framework that challenged long-held views about pain mechanisms as well as (2) an experimentally testable model that continues to the present day to stimulate research into mechanisms of pain. The basic proposition of the theory is that information arriving in the spinal cord via C fibers is modulated through presynaptic inhibition exerted by Aβ fibers. The gate was placed by Melzack and Wall in the substantia gelatinosa and, importantly, its output modulated by supraspinal influences.[34] Many of the underlying assumptions of the gate control theory were immediately challenged and then or since shown to be incorrect (cf. Perl[28]). For example, specific end organs that encode intensities of noxious stimuli (nociceptors) have been widely documented in virtually all tissues, the roles of A and C fibers in pain are far more complex than envisioned in 1965, and the spinal dorsal horn substantia gelatinosa is not the location of a presynaptic "gate" for pain. Like Müller's Law of Specific Nerve Energies, introduction of the gate control theory was a seminal event in the pain field that has shaped thinking and research to the present day. It is now more than 50 years since its introduction, having been cited nearly 5,500 times through 2017, and remains a facile means of "explaining" pain to the layman.

Treatments for Pain

The rationale for choosing one form of pain treatment over another more often reflects the philosophical worldview of the physician more than the patient's presenting condition. Physicians who are focused on the patient's adaptation to life might focus on issues of lifestyle, stress, and emotional upheaval and assist the patient to work toward more adaptive behavioral responses to their pain. Physicians who see pain in mechanistic terms most likely will look for the anatomic foci of pain and be confounded if the source of the suffering is unclear. In the first, older, historical paradigm, pain is a part of an entire life and the enhancing adaptation to life is also needed to manage painful conditions. In the second, a specific anatomical or physiologic lesion is sought with therapy specifically directed toward the underlying pathology.

Cognitive Treatment for Pain

The fundamental significance of the word *pain* in English is derived from the Latin word *poena*, meaning punishment, and its relief was through prayer.[35] This reflects the supposed cause of the pain being harm inflicted by the powers above for putative wrongdoing. Prior to the 18th century, nonspecific therapies were employed for many types of pain, including acupuncture, the application of humoral opposites, bloodletting, purging, topical and oral herbal compounds, and distraction by creating a competing, more severe pain. To better define why patients

---

*It should be appreciated that theories about pain as a specific sense were advanced largely based on stimulation of the skin and assumed/implied to apply generally to other tissues. It is now known that stimuli adequate to produce pain differ in different tissues and that nociceptors are heterogeneous.

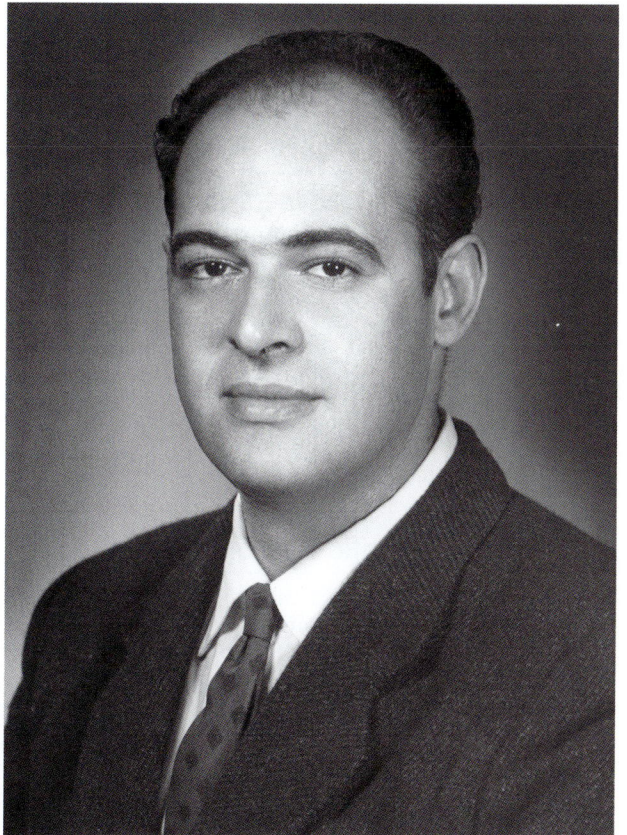

FIGURE 1.11 Ronald Melzack, PhD. *(Courtesy of MIT Museum.)*

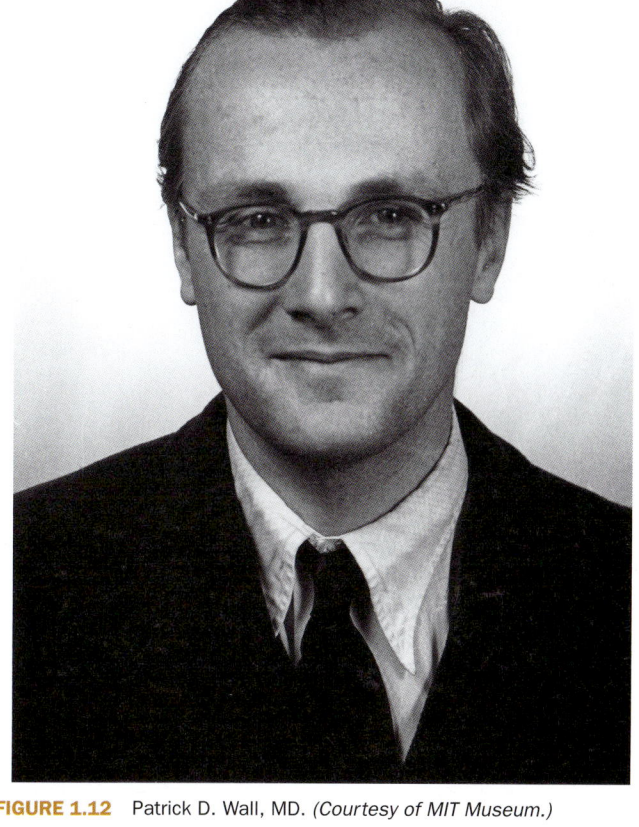

FIGURE 1.12 Patrick D. Wall, MD. *(Courtesy of MIT Museum.)*

experienced pain and, presumably, how to treat it, physicians attempted classification by causes. However, treatment options were still limited. During the Roman emperor Trajan's time, a noted physician recorded 13 causes of pain. Avicenna, a noted Muslim healer in the early 11th century, described 15 separate causes. And Hahnemann, the founder of homeopathy, listed 75.[36] However, nonspecific treatments such as mesmerism and hypnotism, and even general anesthetics, were based on a whole body cure rather than a mechanistic view of pain. Later, cognitive-behavioral therapy and palliative care focused on the care of the whole person as a human being in need of adaptive coping skills. Early work in the 1950s by Engel, based on Freud's theoretical ideals, explored the link between suffering from pain and psychiatric diagnosis. Merskey and Spear, in the mid-1960s, confirmed that chronic pain patients also often had coexisting psychiatric morbidity.[13] Henry Beecher, in the battlefields of World War II, observed that seriously wounded soldiers reported less pain than civilian patients in the Massachusetts General Hospital recovery room. Their injury may have been subjectively interpreted as a cause of removal from harm and their return home as a war survivor. Later, however, these same patients would complain loudly about a minor insult such as venous puncture, causing Beecher to conclude that the experience of pain was derived from a complex interaction between physical sensation, cognition, and an emotional reaction.[37]

Dame Cicely Saunders (Fig. 1.13), founder of the hospice movement in Great Britain and throughout the world, championed the idea of "total pain" emphasizing the holistic concept of patient-centered pain management.[38] Similarly, John Bonica (Fig. 1.14) instituted in 1947 a multidisciplinary approach to treat pain in World War II veterans with complex multifocal persistent pain. Cultivating the multidisciplinary approach to pain management, Bonica later organized a multidisciplinary conference held in Issaquah, Washington, in May

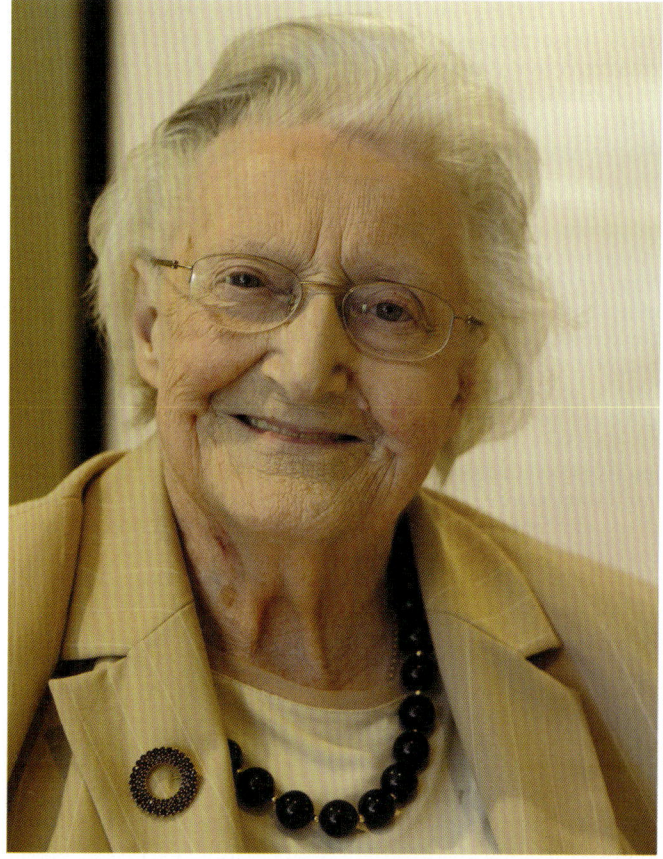

FIGURE 1.13 Dame Cicely Saunders. *(Courtesy of St Christopher's Hospice.)*

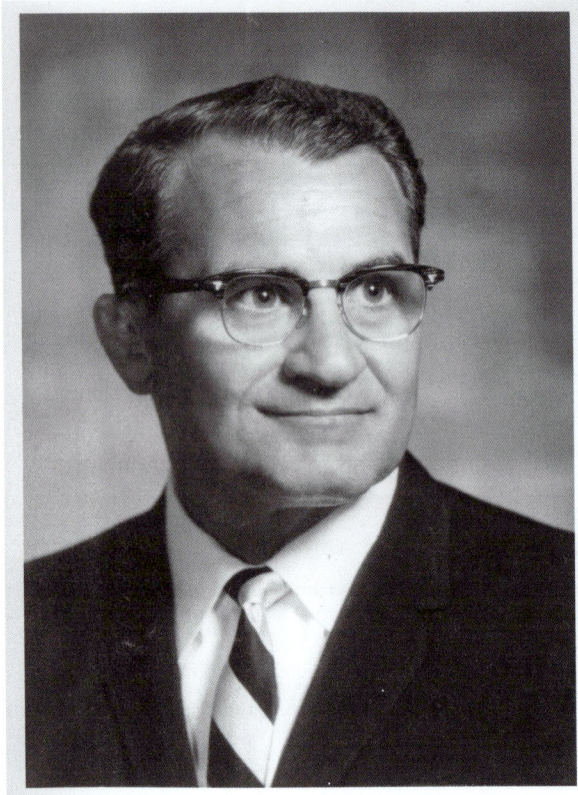

FIGURE 1.14   Dr. John J. Bonica. *(Courtesy of the Wood Library Museum of Anesthesiology.)*

1973 that was attended by more than 300 pain clinicians and researchers of various disciplines. Discussions among attendees at this meeting provided the impetus for the foundation on which the International Association for the Study of Pain was established.[39]

Pharmacologic Treatment of Pain

The development of pharmacology as a science parallels the treatment of painful conditions by medications. Alcohol and morphine were proven antidotes to pain. In the mid-17th century, Thomas Sydenham concocted laudanum, the ubiquitous mix combining sherry, wine, opium, saffron, cinnamon, and clove and used to treat everything from dysentery to hysteria and gout. In South America, coca leaves were in common use, both as an orally chewed remedy for altitude sickness and physical pain and as a topical treatment. The alkaloid cocaine was isolated by Albert Niemann[40] in his 1860s autoexperimentation and was originally touted as a cure for alcohol and morphine addiction. Carl Koller,[41] in 1884, demonstrated the local anesthetic effects of cocaine in reducing corneal movement during eye surgery.

As chemical analysis became more sophisticated, opium, a long known treatment for pain, was studied by the pharmacist Serturner who isolated "the soporific principle" from the compound in 1806. Despite being well-known to herbalists, the first scientific report of the power of willow derivatives was reported in a paper to the Royal Society of Medicine in London in 1763 by the Reverend Edmund Stone from Chipping Norton, Oxfordshire.[42] The overuse of quinine in the early 19th century led to a shortage of the Peruvian cinchona trees, and therefore, there were increased efforts to isolate, characterize, and then commercially synthesize pain-relieving compounds. In 1829, the French pharmacist Henri Leroux

extracted the active compound in willow leaves and bark that had been used in application to painful joints.

Later, in 1873, Charles von Gerhardt prepared salicylic acid by combining sodium salicylate with acetyl chloride to produce acetylsalicylic acid, or aspirin. The benefit of adding the acetyl group was decreased irritation to mucous membranes of the mouth, esophagus, and stomach and avoidance of the bitter alkaloid taste.[43] Clinically, the benefits of this newly synthesized product were reported in treating acute rheumatism by Thomas J. MacLagan in 1876, over a century after Reverend Stone's first report.[44]

Two other landmarks that marked clear leaps forward in the pharmacologic treatment of pain were the development of the hypodermic needle by Rynd[45] and the syringe by Wood (RD Mann as cited in Birk[46]), permitting injection of analgesics and anesthetics. Morton's 1846 landmark demonstration of ether anesthesia, following Crawford Long's earlier application of ether anesthesia in 1843, marked a new era of surgical anesthesia.

Anatomically Specific Treatments for Pain

In contrast, the majority of the treatment options for pain in the last two centuries have been inspired by specificity theory and its refined derivatives. Surgical cures have been employed for pain relief by interruption of specific sensory tracts in neurotomies, division of the anterolateral column of the spinal cord, dorsal roots excision, thalamectomy, mesencephalic lesioning, psychosurgical lobotomies, and other procedures that specifically alter the anatomy of the central nervous system. This paradigm shift developed over time, paralleling the scientific advances in understanding the mechanisms of pain transmission.

As knowledge of the importance of the central nervous system in the transmission of pain increased, cures based on this new science proliferated. An early treatment, neurocompression, was developed by James Moore, a Glasgow-born London surgeon. In 1784, he demonstrated that compression of specific nerves provided anesthesia in patients via clamps in both upper and lower limbs, inducing reversible neurapraxia to anesthetize a limb.[47]

Before his time, Ambroise Paré (1510–1590), the great French surgeon of the Renaissance and "physician to the kings of France," linked observable injury to the development of chronic pain. He not only sustained a prolific medical practice but wrote 10 books of surgery (*Dix Livres de la Chirurgie*). These books were based on his extensive experience in treating gun and sword wounds and the pain that attended them.[48] He was the first to describe pain after the amputation of limbs, 300 years before the conceptualization of "phantom limb pain" was ever expressed. Remarkably, contrary to the current philosophy of his time, he resisted the prevailing wisdom that pain was either inevitable and to be passively tolerated or in some way the will of God to be accepted by man as a path to holiness by actively treating pain in his suffering patients. Some of his innovations included the development of prosthetic devices for missing limbs, a steam bath chair for urethral stone pain, and combinations, called "allodynes," of opium and other drugs to treat the symptoms of pain.[11]

Other compassionate physicians observing their tormented pain patients, primarily as a result of catastrophic war injuries, continued to develop options to treat pain out of necessity. The US Civil War resulted in untold numbers of soldiers who suffered damaged nerves after amputation and injury, with resultant chronic "nerve" disease. The persistent burning pain long after the initial injury was first called *reflex paralysis* by Silas Weir Mitchell (Fig. 1.15) in 1864. Dr. Mitchell, born in Philadelphia as the seventh physician within three generations, was told at an early age by his physician father, "You are wanting in nearly all the qualities that go to make a success in

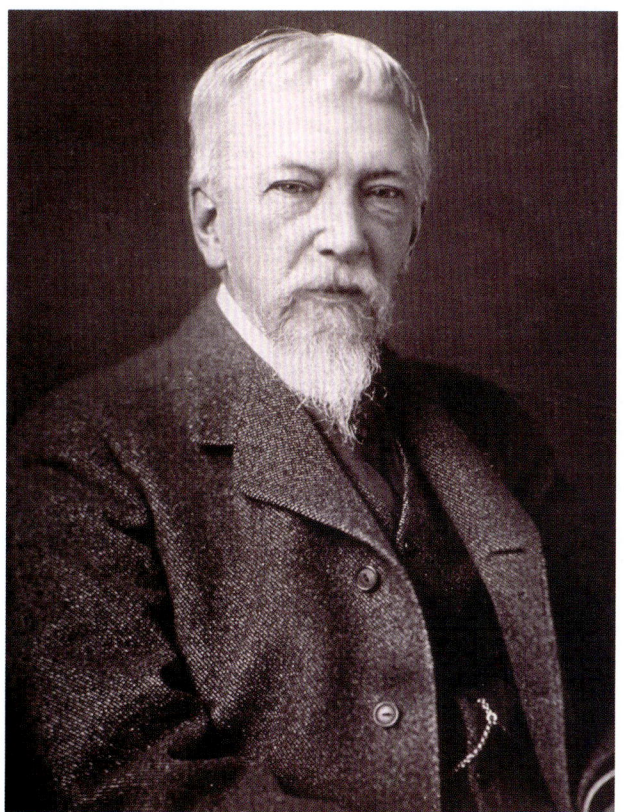

FIGURE 1.15 Silas Weir Mitchell, MD. *(Courtesy of the National Library of Medicine.)*

medicine." Despite this, he graduated from Jefferson Medical College in 1848 and, at the outbreak of hostilities in 1861, was placed in charge of Turner's Lane Hospital in Philadelphia, a 400-bed hospital for nervous diseases. With colleagues, William Williams Keen Jr. and George Read Morehouse, he personally transported railroad cars full of wounded soldiers from the Gettysburg battlefield and undertook their care. Based on daily patient observation and review of literally thousands of pages of careful clinical notes, he described causalgia for the first time in 1864 in the work *Gunshot Wounds and Other Injuries of Nerves*.[49–51]

An early example of injecting specific nerves to produce analgesia was the work of Schloesser in 1903. He injected alcohol to produce long-lasting interruption of neural conduction in patients with convulsive facial tics, obtaining paralysis that lasted from days to a month. He recommended lytic injections for the patients with clinical supraorbital neuralgia and tic douloureux.[52]

Later, war injuries in World War I soldiers inspired a practical French surgeon, René Leriche, to study pain and its treatment in various forms of pathology. He identified patients with sympathetic nerve injuries—his "pariahs of pain"—that he treated by injecting the local anesthetic procaine and surgical sympathectomy, which later became standard therapy in the 1930s. He was a clinician's clinician, describing pain from direct personal observation: "Physical pain is not a simple affair of an impulse, traveling at a fixed rate along a nerve. It is the resultant of a conflict between a stimulus and the whole individual."[53]

Following the theory of pain arising from specific nerve injuries, surgeons in the 1920s performed nerve ablation procedures for chronic unexplained pain syndromes. Following this model, anesthesiologists experimented with various local anesthetic nerve blocks to provide analgesia for surgery. The first nerve block clinic for pain relief was started by Emery Rovenstine at Bellevue Hospital in New York City, New York, in 1936.[54] Eleven years later, the first nerve block clinic in the United Kingdom was established at University College Hospital in London.[55]

Current therapies based on central nervous system plasticity modulating input from peripheral nerves include spinal cord stimulation, sympathetic nerve blocks, radiofrequency modulation (both pulsed and lesioning), and cognitive therapies and are now commonly available in modern pain practice.

The Specialty of Pain Medicine

How did pain as a medical specialty and physicians specializing in the diagnosis and treatment of pain conceive of chronic pain as an original and new field of clinical practice? A sociologist, Isabelle Baszanger, observed two clinics in Paris that had very different constructs of pain and pain treatment, which she described as the two poles of pain. The first—"curing through techniques"—considers pain as a function of physiologic abnormalities, with diagnosis aimed at confirming the pathology and using medication and technical therapies to treat it. As more technologic possibilities develop, the treatments become more focused and sophisticated. The second pole is "healing through adaptation," which considers pain a poorly adaptive behavior, and therefore, behavioral and cognitive therapies are necessary to alleviate pain and suffering.[56]

Whereas Emery A. Rovenstine established in 1936 one of the first outpatient clinics devoted to the treatment of chronic pain,[57] the founding father of interdisciplinary pain care was John J. Bonica, who established in 1947 in Seattle the first multidisciplinary clinic to treat the pain in wounded World War II veterans. He published the first edition of his comprehensive textbook, *Management of Pain*, in 1953.[7] His clinical practice increased and gained support after aligning with the University of Washington in Seattle in 1960. As his reputation grew, he encouraged other centers to recognize and treat pain as an integral part of health care.[58] He then proceeded to work internationally to foster the study and treatment of pain. He was the driving force behind the Issaquah, Washington, multidisciplinary pain conference in 1973 which, as noted earlier, led to the subsequent establishment of the International Association for the Study of Pain. This association currently represents over 60 scientific disciplines in active research and clinical practice in a wide variety of pain related fields. The journal, *Pain*, supported by this organization, foreshadowed the numerous peer reviewed scholarly publications now focused on all levels of pain research.[59] The American Board of Anesthesiology (ABA) approved a certificate of added qualification in pain management in 1991, followed by subspecialty certification from the American Board of Psychiatry and Neurology (ABPN) and the American Board of Physical Medicine and Rehabilitation (ABPMR) in 2000.[60]

It is an exciting time for the study and treatment of pain. New research approaches, including elegant molecular biologic and genetic approaches and imaging techniques that allow real-time investigation of information processing in the nervous system with improved resolution and power, are informing our improved understanding of pain mechanisms and central nervous system contributions to the experience of pain. The chapters that follow in this, the 5th edition of *Bonica's Management of Pain*, highlight the impressive developments in the understanding and managing of pain.

ACKNOWLEDGMENTS

This is an updated version of this chapter written originally by Dr. Doris Cope for the 4th edition of *Bonica's Management of Pain*.

References

1. Weiner RS. *Innovations in Pain Management: A Practical Guide for Clinicians*. Orlando, FL: Paul M. Deutsch Press, Inc; 1990.
2. Benedelow GA, Williams SJ. Transcending the dualisms toward a study of pain. *Soc Health Ill* 1995;17(2):139–165.
3. Birk RK. The history of pain management. *Hist Anesth Soc Proc* 2006;36: 37–46.
4. Keirsey D. *Please Understand Me II: Temperament, Character, Intelligence*. Del Mar, CA: Prometheus Nemesis Book Co, Inc; 1998.
5. King H. The early anodynes: pain in the ancient world. In: Mann RD, ed. *The History of the Management of Pain*. Lancaster, United Kingdom: Parthenon Publishing Group Ltd; 1988:51–60.
6. Rey R. Christianity and pain in the Middle Ages. In: *The History of Pain*. Cambridge, MA: Harvard University Press; 1955:48–49.
7. Bonica JJ. *The Management of Pain*. Philadelphia: Lea & Febiger; 1953:23.
8. Epistolary dissertation (1681). In: RG Latham, trans-ed. *The Works of Thomas Sydenham, M.D.* London: Sydenham Society; 1848–1850:85.
9. Rey R. The history of pain. Gilman CP, ed. *The Living of Charlotte Perkins Gilman: An Autobiography*. New York: D. Appleton-Century Co; 1935:96.
10. Colquhoun JC, ed. *Report of the Experiments on Animal Magnetism Made by a Committee of the Medical Section of the French Royal Academy of Sciences, Read at the Meetings of the 21st and 28th of June 1831*. Edinburgh: Whittaker; 1833.
11. Zimmermann M. The history of pain concepts and treatment before IASP. In: Merskey H, Loeser JD, Dubner R, eds. *The Paths of Pain, 1975–2005*. Seattle, WA: IASP Press; 2005:1–21.
12. Squire WW. On the introduction of ether inhalation as an anesthetic in London. *Lancet* 1888;22:1220–1221.
13. Engel GL. Psychogenic pain. *Med Clin North Am* 1958;42(6):1481–1496.
14. Szasz TS. *Pain and Pleasure: A Study of Bodily Feelings*. London: Taistock; 1957.
15. Walters A. Psychogenic regional pain alias hysterical pain. *Brain* 1961;84:1–18.
16. Merskey H. Psychiatric patients with persistent pain. *J Psychosom Res* 1965;9:299–309.
17. Pope A. *An Essay on Man. Epistle I. An Essay on Man in Four Epistles*. Whitefish, MT: Kessinger Publishing, LLC; 2004.
18. Sawday J. *Engines of the Imagination: Renaissance Culture and the Rise of the Machine*. London: Routledge; 2007.
19. Descartes R. *L'Homme*. Paris, France: C. Angot; 1664.
20. Harvey W. *Exercitatio Anatomica de Motu Cordis et Sanguinis in Animalibus*. Padua, Italy: University of Padua; 1628.
21. Bell C. *Idea of a New Anatomy of the Brain: Submitted for the Observations of His Friends*. London: Strahan & Preston; 1811.
22. Magendie F. Experiments on the spinal nerves. *J Exp Phys Pathol* 1822;2: 276–279.
23. Müller J. *Handbuch der Physiologie des Menschen*. Koblenz, Germany: J Hölscher; 1837.
24. Handwerker HO, Brune K. *Deutschsprachige Klassiker der Schmerzforschung* [Classical German contributions to pain research]. Haßfurt, Germany: Tagblatt-Druckerei KG; 1987.
25. Schiff M. *Lehrbuch der Physiologie des Menschen. I. Muskel und Nervenphysiologie*. Lahr, Germany: Verlag von M. Schauenburg & Co; 1859.
26. Goldscheider A. Die spezifische Energie der Gefühlsnerven der Haut. *Prakt Derm* 1884;3:283.
27. Rey R. Von Frey and the theory of specificity. In: Rey R, ed. *The History of Pain*. Cambridge, MA: Harvard University Press; 1955:215–218.
28. Perl E. Pain mechanisms: a commentary on concepts and issues. *Prog Neurobiol* 2011;94:20–38.
29. Sherrington CS. *The Integrative Action of the Nervous System*. Cambridge, United Kingdom: Cambridge University Press; 1906.
30. Nafe JP. A quantitative theory of feeling. *J Gen Psychol* 1929;2:199–211.
31. Sinclair DC. Cutaneous sensation and the doctrine of specific energy. *Brain* 1955;78:584–614.
32. Weddell G. Somesthesis and the chemical senses. *Ann Rev Psychol* 1955;6: 119–136.
33. Melzack R, Wall PD. Pain mechanisms: a new theory. *Science* 1965;150: 971–979.
34. Mendell L. Constructing and deconstructing the gate theory of pain. *Pain* 2014; 155:210–216.
35. Parris W. The history of pain medicine. In: Raj PP, ed. *Practical Management of Pain*. 3rd ed. St. Louis, MO: Mosby; 2000:4.
36. Fülöp-Miller R. *Triumph Over Pain*. Paul E, Paul C, trans-eds. New York: Literary Guild of America; 1938.
37. Beecher HK. Pain in men wounded in battle. *Ann Surg* 1946;123:96–105.
38. Clark D. Total pain: disciplinary power and the power in the work of Cicely Saunders, 1958–1967. *Soc Sci Med* 1999;49:727–736.
39. Liebeskind JC, Meldrum ML. John J. Bonica. World champion of pain. In: Jensen TS, Turner JA, Wiesenfeld-Hallin Z, eds. *Proceedings of the Eighth World Congress on Pain: Progress in Pain Research and Management*. Vol 8. Seattle, WA: IASP Press; 1997:19–32.
40. Niemann A. Über einer organische Base in der Coca. *Annalen Chemie* 1860;114:213.
41. Koller C. On the use of cocaine for producing anaesthesia on the eye. *Lancet* 1884;2:990.
42. Leake CD. *An Historical Account of Pharmacology to the Twentieth Century*. Springfield, IL: Charles C. Thomas; 1975.
43. Fairley P. *The Conquest of Pain*. London: Michael Joseph; 1978.
44. Andermann AAJ. Physicians, fads, and pharmaceuticals: a history of aspirin. *McGill J Med* 1996;2(2):1–19.
45. Rynd F. Neuralgia—introduction of fluid to the nerve. *Dublin Med Press* 1845;13:167.
46. Birk RK. The history of pain management. *Hist Anesth Soc Proc* 2006; 36:37–46.
47. Moore J. *A Method of Preventing or Diminishing Pain in Several Operations of Surgery*. London: T. Cadell; 1784.
48. Malgaigne JF. *Oeuvres completes d'Ambroise Paré*. Paris, France: Baillière; 1840–1841.
49. Mitchell SW, Morehouse GR, Keen WW. *Gunshot Wounds and Other Injuries of Nerves*. Philadelphia: J.B. Lippincott & Co; 1864.
50. Mitchell SW. Civilization and pain. *JAMA* 1892;18:108.
51. Mitchell SW. *Injuries to Nerves and Their Consequences*. Philadelphia: J.B. Lippincott & Co; 1872.
52. Schloesser. Heilung periphärer Reizzustände sensibler und motorischer Nerven. *Klin Monatsbl Augenheilkd* 1903;41:244.
53. Leriche R. *La Chirurgie de la Douleur*. Paris, France: Masson; 1937.
54. Rovenstine EA, Wertheim HM. Therapeutic nerve block. *JAMA* 1941;117: 1599–1603.
55. Swerdlow M. The early development of pain relief clinics in the UK. *Anaesthesia* 1992;47:977–980.
56. Baszanger I. Deciphering chronic pain. *Soc Health Ill* 1992;14(2):181–215.
57. Cousins M. History of neural blockade and pain management. In: Cousins MJ, Bridenbaugh PO, eds. *Neural Blockade in Clinical Anesthesia and Management of Pain*. 3rd ed. Philadelphia: Lippincott-Raven; 1998: 21–22.
58. Bonica JJ. Basic principles in managing chronic pain. *Arch Surg* 1977; 112(6):783.
59. Bond MR, Dubner R, Jones LE, et al. The history of the IASP: progress in pain since 1975. In: Merskey H, Loeser JD, Dubner R, eds. *The Paths of Pain, 1975–2005*. Seattle, WA: IASP Press; 2005:23–32.
60. Fishman S, Gallager RM, Carr DB, et al. The case for pain medicine. *Medicine* 2004;5(3):281–286.

CHAPTER 2

Pain Terms and Taxonomies of Pain

DENNIS C. TURK and **AKIKO OKIFUJI**

The inherent subjectivity of pain presents a fundamental impediment to increased understanding of its mechanisms and control. The language used by any two individuals attempting to describe a similar injury and their pain experience often varies markedly. Similarly, clinicians and clinical investigators commonly use multiple terms that at times have idiosyncratic meanings. Needless to say, appropriate communication requires a common language and a classification system that is used in a consistent fashion. Thus, we have two primary goals in this chapter: (1) to provide definitions for many commonly used terms in the pain literature, in an effort to bring about consistency and thereby improve communication, and (2) to describe and discuss different classification systems or taxonomies that have been used or proposed, in an attempt to improve communication and bring consistency to research and treatment of patients reporting pain.

Definition of Commonly Used Pain Terms

Discussions of pain involve many terms. The meaning and connotation of these different terms may vary widely. For example, some authors use the term *pain* to relate to a stimulus, others to a thing, and still others to a response. Such inconsistent usage creates difficulties in communication. As Merskey[1] noted, it would be most convenient and helpful if there were some consensus on technical meanings and usage. Based on this belief, the editors of the two editions of the International Association for the Study of Pain (IASP) *Classification of Chronic Pain* included a set of definitions of commonly used pain terms[2,3] (note that a third adaptation of chronic pain for the International Classification of Diseases 11th revision [ICD-11] does not include any listing of definitions).[4] In the second edition of this text, Bonica reproduced a list of the terms and in some cases provided annotations. We adopt a similar strategy. We follow the convention of IASP; we begin with the definition of pain and then proceed alphabetically. Terms preceded by an asterisk come directly from the IASP descriptions of pain terms.[3]

*Pain: An unpleasant sensory *and* emotional experience associated with *actual or potential* tissue damage, or described in terms of such damage (emphasis added). It should be noted that some have argued that inclusion of the phrase "described in terms of such damage" is problematic because it assumes an ability to verbally communicate that may not be present in very young children and individuals with limitations in their verbal abilities.[5] They also suggest that the use of the term *unpleasant* may trivialize the experience which may greatly exceed the unpleasant nature of the experience. Moreover, the original IASP definition fails to incorporate advanced knowledge as to the important role of cognitive, social, and contextual factors. Williams and Craig[5] suggest a revised definition, "Pain is a distressing experience associated with actual or potential tissue damage with sensory, emotional, cognitive, and social components,"[(p2420)] to take these factors into consideration.

Pain, acute/chronic[†]: Definitions of acute, chronic, recurrent, and cancer pain are not specifically included in the IASP list of pain terms. We believe, however, that it is important to clarify these because they are commonly used in the literature.

Traditionally, the distinction between acute and chronic pain has relied on a single continuum of time, with some interval since the onset of pain used to designate the onset of acute pain or the transition point when acute pain becomes chronic. The two most commonly used chronologic markers used to denote chronic pain have been 3 months and 6 months, most recently by IASP as lasting longer than 3 months[4] since the initiation of pain; however, these distinctions are arbitrary. Moreover, these criteria do not take into consideration intensity of pain, the severity and nature of its impact on functioning or treatment-seeking behaviors, or whether pain must be present every day or how frequent it occurs in this interval. These features are important because they may influence estimates of the prevalence of pain and effects on physical activity and treatment requirements and may explain some of the inconsistencies reported.

Another criterion for chronic pain is "pain that extends beyond the expected period of healing." This is relatively independent of time because it considers pain as chronic even when it has persisted for a relatively brief duration. Unfortunately, how long the expected process of healing will (or should) take is ambiguous. One suggestion has been to differentiate "chronic pain" from "impactful chronic pain."[6,7]

Some hold that pain that persists for long periods of time in the presence of ongoing pathology should be considered an extended "acute" pain state. In this case, treatment targets the underlying pathology. This is not to encourage a Cartesian dualistic perspective of pain that treats mind and body as independent entities with distinctive functions. Historically, such distinction led to a faulty assumption of acute pain as "real," whereas chronic pain without known pathology was suspect and viewed as being merely "functional." As the IASP definition clearly states, any pain, acute or chronic, regardless of the presence of identifiable tissue damage, is an unpleasant experience, inherently influenced by various cognitive, affective, and environmental factors. We hold that the weighing of psychological and environmental factors is often greater in chronic pain than acute pain, and the importance of these factors escalates over time, contributing to the experience of pain and associated disability.[8]

We propose conceptualizing acute and chronic pain on two dimensions: time and physical pathology. Figure 2.1 schematically depicts this two-dimensional conceptualization of acute and chronic pain. From this perspective, any case falling above the diagonal line (short duration or high physical pathology) is acute pain, whereas cases falling below the diagonal line (low physical pathology or long duration) suggest chronic pain. The perspective presented in Figure 2.1 leads to the following definitions of acute and chronic pain.

Acute pain: Acute pain is the physiologic response to and experience of noxious stimuli that can become pathologic, is normally sudden in onset, is time-limited, and motivates behaviors to avoid potential or actual tissue injury.[9] Pain is elicited by the injury of body tissues and activation of nociceptive transducers at the site of local tissue damage. The local injury alters the

---

[†]The discussion describing the distinction between acute and chronic pain reflects on deliberations among the editors of the third edition of this volume.

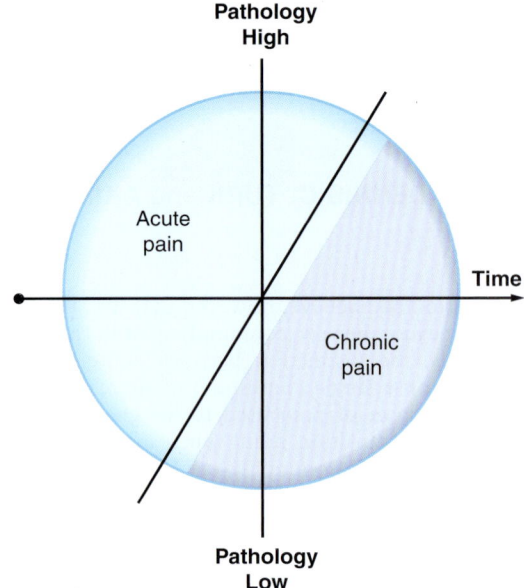

FIGURE 2.1 Pictorial representation of acute and chronic pain.

response characteristics of the nociceptors and perhaps their central connections and the autonomic nervous system in the region. In general, the state of acute pain lasts for a relatively limited time and remits when the underlying pathology resolves (however, see the following definition of *central sensitization*). This type of pain often serves as the impetus to seek health care, and it occurs following trauma, some disease processes, and invasive interventions.

Chronic pain: May be elicited by an injury or disease but is likely to be perpetuated by factors that are both pathogenetically and physically remote from the originating cause. Chronic pain extends for a long period of time and/or represents low levels of underlying pathology that does not explain the presence and extent of pain (e.g., mechanical back pain, fibromyalgia [FM] syndrome). There have been suggestions that chronic pain in the apparent absence of pathology may be attributable to modification of nerves and sensitization of the peripheral or central nervous system. There have also been suggestions that genetic factors and prior life experiences might predispose some to develop chronic pain problems following an initiating insult that resolves in others who do not have the predisposition. Just as the brain is modified by experience, especially in early life, the brain may alter the way noxious information is processed to reduce or augment its impact on subjective awareness.

Chronic pain frequently is the impetus for people to seek health care. Currently available treatments are rarely capable of totally eliminating the noxious sensations and thereby "curing" chronic pain. Because the pain persists, it is likely that environmental, emotional, and cognitive factors will interact with the already sensitized nervous system, contributing to the persistence of pain and associated illness behaviors (see following description of pain behaviors). It is also possible that, just as the brain is modified by experience, especially in early life, the brain may alter the way noxious information is processed to reduce or augment its impact on subjective awareness.

The acute–chronic pain continuum is based solely on duration. There is an implication that those with chronic pain will have progressed from an acute pain state to a chronic pain state and that once the threshold to chronic pain is crossed, it becomes fixed and relatively immutable with the implication that worsening, and deterioration over time is inevitable. The reality in contrast is there in the presence of considerable variability

within individuals who have transitioned into the classification based on arbitrary time points. A range of psychosocial, behavioral, and contextual factors as well as physical ones will influence the adaptation and responses to pain.[8]

Cancer pain: Pain associated with cancer includes pain associated with disease progression as well as treatments (e.g., chemotherapy, radiotherapy, surgery) that may damage the nervous system. Although some contend that pain associated with neoplastic disease is unique, in the majority of instances, we view it as fitting within our description of acute and chronic pain, as depicted in Figure 2.1. Moreover, pain associated with cancer can have multiple causes, namely, disease progression, treatment, and co-occurring diseases (e.g., arthritis). Regardless of whether the pain associated with cancer stems from disease progression, treatment, or a co-occurring disease, it may be either acute or chronic. Thus, we do not advocate a separate classification of cancer pain as distinct from acute and chronic pain.

Some concerns have also been raised regarding the common usage of chronic malignant and chronic benign pain[4]; often, pain unrelated to cancer is implicitly view as "benign" to distinguish it from cancer-related pain. Certainly, people who have pain associated with neoplastic disease experience a unique and disease-specific situation, but from a mechanistic perspective, there may be little to substantiate continued use of this dichotomy. Moreover, patients who have chronic noncancer pain who are told that their pain is "benign" may feel denigrated because, from their perspective, the inference is that their pain is not a serious concern.

Recurrent pain: Episodic or intermittent occurrences of pain, with each episode lasting for a relatively short period of time but recurring across an extended period of time (e.g., migraine headaches, tic douloureux, sickle cell crisis, dysmenorrhea). Our distinction between acute and chronic pain using the integration of the dimensions of time and pathology does not specifically include recurrent pain. In the case of recurrent pain, patients may experience episodes of pain interspersed with periods of being completely pain-free. Although recurrent pain may seem acute because each pain episode (e.g., headache) is of relatively short duration, the pathophysiology of many recurrent pain disorders (e.g., migraine) is not well understood. Syndromes characterized by recurrent acute pain share features in common with both acute and chronic pain. The fact that these syndromes extend over time, however, suggests that psychosocial and behavioral factors, not only physical pathology, may be major contributors to emotional and behavioral responses. IASP[4] now includes recurrent pain lasting longer than 3 months within its definition of chronic pain. However, it is not clear whether multiple episodes lasting several days within 3 months would meet the chronic pain criterion or whether the pain must last at least 3 months. That is, would multiple migraines in a 3-month period be chronic even if there were pain-free periods within the 3 month period?

Transient pain: Pain elicited by activation of nociceptors in the absence of any significant local tissue damage. This type of pain is ubiquitous in everyday life and is rarely a reason to seek health care. It is seen in the clinical setting and only in incidental or procedural pain, such as during a venipuncture or injection. This type of pain ceases as soon as the stimulus is removed. There are situations where sources of transient pain may be treated by providers with preventive analgesic or topical medication.

Acceptance: A choice to acknowledge pain experiences (intensity, thoughts, emotions) and to cease efforts to control them while simultaneously engaging in valued behaviors, particularly when control efforts have let to restrictions.

Addiction: A behavioral pattern of substance, including prescribed medication, abuse characterized by overwhelming involvement with the use of a drug (i.e., compulsive use), the securing of its supply, and a high tendency to relapse. The compulsive use of the drug results in physical, psychological, and/or social harm to the user, and use continues despite this harm. (See also *physical dependence*.)

*Allodynia: Pain due to a stimulus that does not normally provoke pain.

Analgesia: Absence of the spontaneous report of pain or pain behaviors in response to stimulation that would normally be expected to be painful. The term implies a defined stimulus and a defined response. Analgesic responses can be tested in nonhuman as well as humans.

*Anesthesia dolorosa: Spontaneous pain in an area or region that is anesthetic.

Breakthrough pain: A transient increase in pain to greater than moderate intensity superimposed on baseline pain that is fairly well managed. Breakthrough pain includes (1) incident pain that may arise from some activity or physical function (e.g., coughing, ambulating), (2) pain that routinely increases as the duration of analgesic medication is reaching its limit (end-of-dose failure), and (3) spontaneous exacerbation of a stable level of pain for nonspecific reasons.

Catastrophizing: A cognitive and emotional process that involves magnification of pain-related stimuli, feelings of helplessness, and a negative orientation to pain and life circumstances. Catastrophizing has been shown to be an important predictor of response to both acute and chronic pain.[10]

*Central pain: Pain initiated or caused by a primary lesion or dysfunction in the central nervous system.

Central sensitization: Increase in the excitability and responsiveness of neurons in the spinal cord. Central sensitization may explain the persistence of pain beyond the removal or resolution of the initiating stimulus.

Chronic widespread pain: A complex condition with a range of disabling physical and psychological symptoms that does not fit neatly into any medical specialty and has a myriad of possible causes and triggers, both physical and psychological. A set of disparate disorders is often lumped into chronic widespread pain including nonradicular back pain, FM, irritable bowel syndrome, pelvic pain, temporomandibular disorders (TMD), and tension-type headache. This diagnosis is based on the presence and distribution of symptoms in the absence of another defined pathologic process: The features in the history or clinical examination are generally more important than laboratory investigations.

*Complex regional pain syndrome type 1 (formerly reflex sympathetic dystrophy): A syndrome that usually develops after an initiating noxious event, is not limited to the distribution of a single peripheral nerve, and is apparently disproportionate to the inciting event. It is associated at some point with evidence of edema, changes in skin blood flow, abnormal pseudomotor activity in the region of the pain, or allodynia or hyperalgesia. Specific criteria for the diagnosis of complex regional pain syndrome (CRPS) have been proposed.[11]

*Complex regional pain syndrome type 2 (formerly causalgia): A syndrome of sustained burning pain, allodynia, and hyperpathia following a traumatic nerve lesion, often combined with vasomotor dysfunction and later trophic changes.

Conditioned pain modulation: Altered endogenous pain modulation is considered as a mechanism involved with diverse chronic pain syndromes (e.g., TMD, FM, chronic tension-type headache, and irritable bowel syndrome). It is assessed by measuring phasic pain response after a conditioned tonic pain stimulus. Conditioned pain modulation is at least partially mediated by the diffuse noxious inhibitory control (DNIC) system characterized by inhibition of wide dynamic range neurons in the dorsal horn of the spinal cord by heterosegmental noxious afferent input.[12]

Cost–benefit analysis: Evaluation of the costs and effects of an intervention in a common, usually monetary unit. The standardization of unit has an advantage because it permits comparisons across dissimilar intervention programs. On the other hand, the conversion of treatment effects to monetary units may not always be feasible. Estimation of the cost to outcome ratio is possible, as are comparisons between interventions using the rates of improvement (e.g., return to work) with common denominators.

Cost-effectiveness analysis: Estimation of treatment outcome entails criteria other than monetary terms, such as lives saved or return to work. An intervention is cost-effective when it satisfies one of the following conditions:

1. It is more effective than an alternative modality at the same cost;
2. It is less costly and at least as effective as an alternative modality;
3. It is more effective and more costly than an alternative treatment, but the benefit exceeds the added cost; or
4. It is less effective and less costly, but the added benefit of the alternative is not worth the additional cost.

Disability: Any restriction or loss of capacity to perform an activity in the manner or within the range considered normal for a human being, such as climbing stairs, lifting groceries, or talking on a telephone. It is a task-based concept that involves both the person and the environment. Disability is essentially a social and not a medical term or classification. Level of disability should be determined only after a patient has reached maximum medical improvement following appropriate treatment and rehabilitation.

*Dysesthesia: An unpleasant abnormal sensation, whether spontaneous or evoked.

*Hyperalgesia: An increased response to a stimulus that is normally painful.

*Hyperesthesia: Increased sensitivity to stimulation, excluding special senses.

*Hyperpathia: A painful syndrome characterized by an abnormally painful reaction to a stimulus, especially a repetitive stimulus, as well as an increased threshold.

*Hypoalgesia: Diminished pain in response to a normally painful stimulus.

Hypochondriasis: An excessive preoccupation with bodily sensations and fears that they represent serious disease despite reassurance to the contrary.

Impairment: Any loss of use of, or abnormality of, psychological, physiologic, or anatomical structure or function that is quantifiable. It is not equivalent to disability. Impairment is to disability as disease is to illness.

Malingering: A conscious and willful feigning or exaggeration of a disease or effect of an injury in order to obtain a specific external gain. It is usually motivated by external incentives such as financial compensation, avoiding work, or obtaining drugs.

Maximum medical improvement: The state beyond which additional medical treatment is unlikely to produce an improvement in function.

Minimum clinically important difference (MCID): The magnitude of reduction in pain or related problems that a patient would consider minimally important. In considering the determination of clinically important differences, two different aspects of the interpretation of clinical trial results must be distinguished. One is establishing the difference in the magnitude of response between the treatment and control groups that will be considered large enough to establish the scientific or therapeutic importance of the results. The other is establishing what change in the outcome measure represents a meaningful difference for patients. This later consideration has come to be referred to as the minimum clinically important difference. The development of criteria for determining what are important changes in an individuals' scores on the outcome measures used in chronic pain trials would provide clinicians and researchers with essential methods for evaluating treatment responses of individuals in clinical trials and clinical practice. Such individual-level criteria make it possible to conduct responder analyses that classify each trial participant as "improved," "stable," or "worse" on the basis of validated criteria of important change. (See description of *patient global impression of change*.)

Multidisciplinary (interdisciplinary) pain center: An organization of health care professionals and basic and applied scientists that includes research, teaching, and patient care related to acute and chronic pain. It includes a wide array of health care professionals including physicians, psychologists, nurses, physical therapists, occupational therapists, and other specialty health care providers. Multiple therapeutic modalities are available. These centers provide evaluation and treatment and are usually affiliated with major health science institutions.

*Neuralgia: Pain in the distribution of a nerve or nerves.

*Neuritis: Inflammation of a nerve or nerves.

*Neurogenic pain: Pain initiated or caused by a primary lesion, disease, dysfunction, or transitory perturbation in the somatosensory nervous system.[13] It may be spontaneous or evoked, as an increased response to a painful stimulus (hyperalgesia), a painful response to a painful stimulus (hyperalgesia), or a painful response to a normally nonpainful stimulus (allodynia).

Neuropathic pain: Pain arising as a direct consequence of a lesion or disease affecting the somatosensory system.[14]

*Neuropathy: A disturbance of function or pathologic change in a nerve: in one nerve, mononeuropathy; in several nerves, mononeuropathy multiplex; if diffuse and bilateral, polyneuropathy.

Nocebo: Negative treatment effects induced by a substance or procedure containing no toxic or detrimental substance.

Nociception: Activation of sensory transduction in nerves by thermal, mechanical, or chemical energy impinging on specialized nerve endings. The nerve(s) involved conveys information about tissue damage to the central nervous system.

*Nociceptor: A receptor preferentially sensitive to tissue trauma or to a stimulus that would damage tissue if prolonged.

*Noxious stimulus: A stimulus that is capable of activating receptors for tissue damage.

Pain behavior: Verbal or nonverbal actions understood by observers to indicate that a person may be experiencing pain and suffering. These actions may include audible emissions (e.g., signs, moans); facial expressions (e.g., grimacing); abnormal postures or gait (e.g., limping, bracing, moving in a guarded fashion); motor behavior (e.g., rubbing a body part); use of prosthetic devices; avoidance of activities; and verbal indications of pain, distress, and suffering. An important feature is the observable nature of these behaviors that can be subjected to the conditioning process. Once conditioned, the same behavior is exhibited as a learned response rather than expression of actual pain experience. Thus, pain behavior can either reflect internal experience of pain or is exhibited as a learned behavior in response to certain cues.

Pain clinic: Facilities focusing on diagnosis and management of patients with pain problems. It may specialize in specific diagnoses or pain related to a specific area of the body.

Pain relief: Report of reduced pain after a treatment. It does not require reduced response to a noxious stimulus and is not a synonym for analgesia. The term applies only to humans.

Pain threshold: The least level of stimulus intensity perceived as painful. In psychophysics, this is defined as a level of stimulus intensity that a person recognizes as painful 50% of time.

*Pain tolerance level: The greatest level of noxious stimulation that an individual is willing to tolerate.

Pain sensitivity range: The difference between the pain threshold and the pain tolerance level.

*Paresthesia: An abnormal sensation whether spontaneous or evoked.

Patient global impression of change (PGIC): Patients' overall evaluation of improvement or worsening of symptoms over the course of treatment. This measure is often a single-item rating by patients on a scale, often 5-point or 7-point scale that ranges from "very much improved" to "very much worse" with "no change" as the midpoint.

*Peripheral neurogenic pain: Pain initiated or caused by a primary lesion or dysfunction or transitory perturbation in the peripheral nervous system.

Physical dependence: A pharmacologic property of a drug (e.g., opioid) characterized by the occurrence of an abstinence syndrome following abrupt discontinuation of the substance or administration of an antagonist. It does not imply an aberrant psychological state or behavior or addiction.

Placebo: An inert substance or procedure without a specified therapeutic ingredient that is provided as a treatment. It is frequently used to control patients' expectations for the efficacy in testing a treatment.

Placebo effects: Refers to the positive benefit(s) from a placebo (i.e., inert) preparation or procedure when such benefit is generally achieved only with an active treatment intervention. Active treatments also are likely to have a placebo component that augments the active component associated with the treatment.

Plasticity, neural: Nociceptive input leading to structural and functional changes that may cause altered perceptual processing and contribute to pain chronicity.

Pseudoaddiction: Refers to drug-seeking behavior or misuse by patients who have severe pain and are undermedicated or who have not received other effective pain treatment interventions. Such patients may appear preoccupied with obtaining opioids, but the preoccupation reflects a need for pain relief and not drug addiction. Pseudoaddictive behavior differs from true addictive behavior because when higher doses of opioid are provided, the patient does not use these in a manner that persistently causes sedation or euphoria, the level of function is increased rather than decreased, and the medications are used as prescribed without loss of control over use.

Psychogenic pain: Report of pain attributable primarily to psychological factors usually in the absence of any objective physical pathology that could account for pain. This term is commonly used in a pejorative sense. It often suggests a Cartesian dualism and is not usually a helpful method of describing a patient.

Quality of life/health-related quality of life: Quality of life (QOL) refers to an individual's perception of his or her position in life in the context of the culture and value systems in which he or she lives and in relation to his or her goals, expectations, standards, and concerns. Concerns with this all-encompassing description have led a number of investigators to use a more circumscribed construct, *health-related quality of life* (HRQOL). Although *HRQOL* has been used interchangeably with terms such as *health status* and *functional status*, *HRQOL* is a narrower term than *QOL* because it does not include aspects of work, environmental conditions, housing, and other variables that are often considered relevant to QOL but that do not involve health directly.[7]

Rehabilitation: Restoration of an individual to maximal physical and mental functioning in light of his or her impairment.

Residual functional capacity: The capacity to perform specific social and work-related physical and mental activities following rehabilitation related to impairment or when a condition has reached a point of maximum medical improvement.

Resilience: Capacity and dynamic process of adaptively overcoming stress and adversity while maintaining normal psychological and physical functioning.[15]

Summed pain intensity difference (SPID): A strategy for combining relief magnitude and duration in a single score. It is calculated by the sum of the time-weighted pain intensity difference (difference between current pain and pain at baseline) multiplied by the interval between ratings.

Symptom magnification: Conscious or unconscious exaggeration of symptom severity in an attempt to convince an observer that one is truly experiencing some level of pain. It differs from malingering as it is an effort to be believed, not necessarily to achieve a positive outcome (i.e., secondary gain) such as financial compensation.

Suffering: Reaction to the physical or emotional components of pain with a feeling of uncontrollability, helplessness, hopelessness, intolerability, and interminability. Suffering implies a threat to the intactness of an individual's self-concept, self-identify, and integrity.

Tolerance, drug: A physiologic state in which a person requires an increased dosage of a psychoactive substance to sustain a desired effect.

Total pain relief (TOPAR): Is used in clinical trials to assess pain relief over time. It is a cumulative measure that is composed of the sum of time-weighted pain relief score multiplied by the interval between ratings. TOPAR is frequently used in clinical trials of medications designed to ameliorate pain.

Wind-up: Slow temporal summation of pain mediated by C fibers due to repetitive noxious stimulation at a rate faster than one stimulus every 3 seconds. It may cause the person to experience a gradual increase in the perceived magnitude of pain.

Taxonomies

The lack of a classification of chronic pain syndromes that is used on a consistent basis inhibits the advancement of knowledge and treatment of chronic pain and makes it hard for investigators as well as practitioners to compare observations and results of research. Bonica[16] referred to this language ambiguity as "a modern tower of Babel."

In order to identify target groups, conduct research, prescribe treatment, evaluate treatment efficacy, and for policy and decision making, it is essential that some consensually validated criteria are used to distinguish groups of individuals who share a common set of relevant attributes. The primary purpose of such a classification is to describe the relationships of constituent members based on their equivalence along a set of basic dimensions that represent the structure of a particular domain. Infinite classification systems are possible, depending on the rationale about common factors and the variables believed to discriminate among individuals. The majority of the current taxonomies of pain are "expert-based" classifications.

EXPERT-BASED CLASSIFICATIONS OF PAIN

Classifications of disease are usually based on a preconceived combination of characteristics (e.g., symptoms, signs, results of diagnostic tests), with no single characteristics being both necessary and sufficient for every member of the category, yet the group as a whole possesses a certain unity.[17] Most classification systems used in pain medicine (e.g., ICD,[18] classification and diagnostic criteria for headache disorders, cranial neuralgias, and facial pain,[19] IASP Classification of Chronic Pain,[2,4] CRPS,[11] whiplash-associated disorders,[20] and the Analgesic, Anesthetic, and Addiction Clinical Trial Translations, Innovations, Opportunities, and Networks [ACTTION]-American Pain Society Pain Taxonomy [AAPT][21] and ACTTION-American Pain Society-American Academy of Pain Medicine [AAPM] Pain Taxonomy [AAAPT][22]) and dentistry (i.e., Research Diagnostic Criteria [RDC] for Temporomandibular Disorders[23,24]) are based on the consensus arrived at by a group of "experts." In this sense, they reflect the inclusion or elimination of certain diagnostic features depending on agreement.

"Expert-based" classification tends to result in preconceived categories and "force" individuals into the most appropriate one even if not all characteristics defining the category are present. Expert-based classification systems do not explicitly state the mathematical rules that should exist among the variables used in order to assign a case to a specific category.

In an ideal classification, the categories comprising the taxonomy should be mutually exclusive and completely exhaustive for the data to be incorporated. Every element in a classification should fit into one, and only one, place, and no other element should fit into that place. An example of such an ideal, natural taxonomy is the periodic table in chemistry. We can also develop artificial classifications such as a telephone directory. The criterion for the classification, namely, the sequence of letters in the alphabet, bears no relation to the people, addresses, and telephone numbers being classified; but it is quite satisfactory for the intended purpose.[3] No classification in medicine or dentistry has achieved such aims. For example, the RDC (now Diagnostic Criteria as the RDC has been adopted for clinical diagnostic purposes based on the research evidence) for Temporomandibular Disorders[23,24] includes eight different diagnoses. In one study, over 50% of the sample received three or more RDC diagnoses.[25] Thus, the classifications or diagnoses are not mutually exclusive.

The most commonly used classification system of pain is the ICD published by the World Health Organization. In the most recent draft edition, the ICD-10,[22] conditions are classified along a number of different dimensions including causal agent; body system involved; pattern and type of symptoms; and whether or not they are related to the artificial intervention of an operation, time of occurrence or grouped as signs, symptoms, and abnormal clinical and laboratory findings. Within major groups, there are subdivisions by symptom pattern, the presence of hereditary or degenerative disease, extrapyramidal and movement disorders, location, and etiology. Overlapping occurs repeatedly in such approaches to categorization; thus, they are not ideal even if they serve a useful function. Recently, IASP has created its adaptation of the original IASP classification[2] (described in the following discussion) in an effort to have chronic pain included within the ICD-11[4] (described in the following discussion).

Further complications arise when clinicians require a separate coding system. In the United States, for example, in addition to the ICD codes, a clinician must select current procedural terminology (CPT) coding schemes for billing purposes. This has created a tendency where the fulfillment of the CPT coding may dictate the ICD selections to justify the procedures. Such practices often needlessly create diagnoses and additional treatments for billing purposes only.

It is clear that the classification of pain cannot approach the ideal found in chemistry or telephone books, but this is not unique to pain; it characterizes medical classification systems in general. Classification in medicine, dentistry, and psychology is pragmatic. It does not provide absolute truth but rather provides categories with which we can work to identify individuals with similar phenomena, prognoses, or causes.[3] Currently, the majority of pain classifications in pain medicine rely on various parameters of pain experience such as anatomy, system, severity, duration, and etiology.

CLASSIFICATION BASED ON ANATOMY

Several pain syndromes are classified by body location. For example, low back pain, pelvic pain, and headache, each refers to the specific location of symptoms. However, the extent to which the anatomy-based classification of pain is clinically meaningful is limited, at least partially, due to the lack of anatomically defined specificity in the neurophysiology of pain.

CLASSIFICATION BASED ON DURATION

As previously discussed, one common way to classify pain is to consider it along a continuum of duration. Thus, pain associated with tissue damage, inflammation, or a disease process that is of relatively brief duration (i.e., hours, days, or even weeks), regardless of how intense, is frequently referred to as acute pain (e.g., postsurgical pain). Many pain problems can be classified as chronic. For example, pain that persists for extended periods of time (i.e., months or years), accompanies a disease process (e.g., rheumatoid arthritis), or is associated with an injury that has not resolved within an expected period of time (e.g., low back pain, phantom limb pain) are all referred to as chronic. As noted, however, a single dimension of duration is inadequate because pathologic factors may be relatively independent of duration.

CLASSIFICATION BASED ON THE ETIOLOGY OF PAIN

Another way to classify pain is based on etiology, by lumping a range of potentially disparate diagnoses within general categories, for example, somatogenic-psychogenic, nociceptive-neuropathic, and nociceptive-neuropathic-widespread.

Historically, crude efforts were made to subdivide or classify patients reporting pain dichotomously based on the putative basis for their report. A classical approach to classify patients based the presence of physical pathology that to which the pain report was attributed—somatogenic versus pain with unknown physical pathology and with the implication on nonphysical causal mechanism such as psychopathology (psychogenic) or motivation to achieve some desired outcome such as disability attention or disability compensation (i.e., malingering), seeking of mood altering drugs, or avoidance of undesirable activities (e.g., work, homemaking responsibilities) (reinforcement). The processes by which clinicians determine whether pain is somatogenic or psychogenic are distinctive. The classification of somatogenic pain is established by identification of positive organic findings, whereas psychogenic pain is indicated only in the absence of positive signs.

More recently, a dichotomous classification has been advocated by the AAPM[26] with the somewhat analogous concepts of "eudynia" (good pain) and "maldynia" (bad pain). Eudynia (nociceptive pain) conceptualizes pain that serves as an alarm signal and that is mediated by specialized primary sensory neurons that respond to sufficiently intense thermal, mechanical, or chemical stimuli and transmit signals via well-defined pathways in the central nervous system. Eudynia is triggered and maintained by the presence of noxious stimuli. When local inflammation ensues, certain features of the nociceptive response are modified and magnified to aid healing and repair; hence, good pain. Little consideration is given to the involvement of psychosocial, behavioral, or contextual factors in the development, amplification, or maintenance of symptom or response to treatment. In contrast, maldynia is classified when pain is reported to be present when neural tissues in the peripheral or central nervous system are directly damaged or become dysfunctional. Here, in contrast to eudynia, different sequence of events unfolds. Under these conditions, pain can manifest and eventually persist in the absence of typical nociceptive generators. Such pain can be considered maladaptive because it occurs in the absence of ongoing noxious stimuli and does not promote healing and repair. In the instance of maldynia, there is an acknowledgment that psychosocial, behavioral, and contextual factors may become enmeshed. Accordingly, the AAPM and other proponents in the pain medicine community have advanced the notion that under such conditions, pain becomes the disease process itself.

Other variations on the dichotomous somatogenic versus psychogenic classification exist. For example, Portenoy[27] proposed that three primary categories of pain be used: nociceptive, neuropathic, and psychogenic. In this system, somatogenic pain is subdivided into two subtypes that contrast with psychogenic pain. More recently, a suggested broad classification into subgroups has proposed three categories, namely, nociceptive, neuropathic, and widespread (sometimes referred to as central sensitivity syndromes, with the causal mechanisms of central nervous system plasticity and the resulting central sensitization, combining such apparently disparate diagnoses as back pain, FM, irritable bowel syndrome, pelvic pain, TMD, tension-type headaches).[28,29]

CLASSIFICATION BASED ON BODY SYSTEM

Classification may focus on the body system involved. For example, Friction[30] proposed the use of five categories, namely, myofascial, rheumatic, causalgic, neurologic, or vascular. In this case, patients are assigned to one of five rather than two or three categories as proposed by Portenoy.[27] However, the decision regarding classification is still based on a single dimension system for the experience of pain.

CLASSIFICATION BASED ON SEVERITY

Frequently, pain is classified unidimensionally on the basis of severity (0- to 10-point scale with 0 = no pain and 10 = the worst pain that can be imagined). That is, regardless of the scale's level of measurement—nominal, ordinal, or interval—the construct involves a single dimension. When pain is classified on the basis of severity, it is dependent on the subjective report of patients. Assuming pain threshold is normally distributed, there will be significant variability among patients' rating severity of what might be objectively the same nociceptive stimulation.

Ratings of pain severity will be anchored to how questions are asked, and responses may vary widely depending on the question. For example, if the ratings associated with "pain right now," "over the past week?" "usual severity," "severity at its worst," "severity at its lowest," "during specific movements," or "at rest?" pain severity may be very useful in evaluating individual patients but less so for comparison among groups.

CLASSIFICATION BASED ON FUNCTIONING

The International Classification of Functioning, Disability and Health (ICF)[31] aims to provide a standard framework for the comparison and understanding of health outcomes. For any given health outcome, including chronic pain, the ICF identified three main outcomes: impairment, activity limitations, and participation restrictions. To date, the efforts of the ICF have been largely focused on identification of common domains across measures that can be used to evaluate patients and treatment outcomes. It has less emphasis on classification of patients, but it can be used for this purpose. The empirical approach described in the following discussion can be readily applied to the ICF conceptual model.

CLASSIFICATION BASED ON INTENSITY AND FUNCTIONING

The Emory Pain Estimate Model (EPEM) was the first attempt to integrate the biophysiologic and psychosocial domains in classifying pain patients.[32,33] Brena and colleagues[32,33] arbitrarily labeled the dimensions "pathology" and "behavior." The pathology dimension included the quantification of physical examination procedures (e.g., ratings of joint mobility, muscle strength) as well as assigning numerical indices to reflect the extent of abnormalities determined from diagnostic procedures such as radiographic studies. The behavioral dimension comprises a composite of activity levels, pain verbalizations, drug use, and measures of psychopathology based on the elevations of scales of the Minnesota Multiphasic Personality Inventory (MMPI).

Using median divisions on the pathology and behavior dimensions, the EPEM defines four classes of chronic pain patients. Class I patients are characterized by higher scores on the behavior dimension and lower scores on the pathology dimension. The EPEM describes these patients as displaying low activity levels, high verbalizations of pain, prominent social and psychological malfunctions, and frequent misuse of medications. Class II patients are those who display lower scores on both the pathology and behavioral dimensions. These patients are described as displaying dramatized pain complaints with ill-defined anatomical patterns. However, they do not display significant behavioral dysfunction. Class III represents patients with higher scores on both dimensions, characterized as showing clear evidence of physical pathology and high intensity illness behavior. Finally, Class IV patients are those who have higher scores on the pathology dimension and a lower score on the behavior dimension, thus demonstrating competent coping in the presence of a physical pathologic condition.

Although Brena and his colleagues[32,33] appropriately emphasized the importance of integrating physical and psychological data in order to develop a classification system for chronic pain patients, some of the basic theoretical and quantitative characteristics of the EPEM are problematic. We see this framework as a conceptual model rather than an adequately operationalized empirical one. For example, from a theoretical standpoint, the inclusion of activity levels, pain verbalizations, and measures of psychopathology under a single dimension labeled "behavioral" is troubling because research shows that there is little association between pain behaviors and psychopathology. Thus, the behavioral dimension is most likely not unidimensional and, therefore, cannot measure behavior directly.

Von Korff and colleagues[34] developed a similar model, the Chronic Pain Grade, which integrates the conceptual approach of the EPEM but adds greater emphasis of empirical determination of criteria for subgroup classification and empirical validation. The Chronic Pain Grade classifies patients into one of five categories: (1) pain-free, (2) low pain intensity and low disability, (3) high pain intensity and low disability, (4) low pain intensity and high disability, and (5) high pain severity and high disability. More recently, Deyo et al.[6] have based the core data set that they recommend for research on back pain on the Chronic Pain Grade.

CLASSIFICATION BASED ON PROGNOSIS

Chronic pain is typically viewed by definition as being fixed with progressive dysfunction over time; however, there is considerable variability in its course. An alternative view, based on prognosis such that chronic pain is defined by the *risk*, that clinically significant pain and associated dysfunction will be present at some future time point, where the likelihood of future pain and dysfunction is predicted by multiple biopsychosocial prognostic factors.[35,36] As a consequence, subgroups of pain patient should be based on prognosis. This approach is based on several propositions. The first proposition is that chronic pain is better characterized by a failure of the resolution of pain and associated dysfunction rather than progression based on time. The argument is that severe pain, pain-related activity limitations, and emotional distress often used to characterize chronic pain are observable soon after pain onset. What typically differentiates "chronic pain" from "acute pain" is the lack of meaningful improvement. The second proposition is that the seeds of chronic pain can be observed early in the pain course. The third proposition is that varied prognostic indicators can be combined into a prognostic risk score and this risk score will predict clinically significant pain and dysfunction in the future better than pain

duration in isolation. In this view, risk of future clinically significant pain is probabilistic and not immutable. In contrast, chronic pain status can change over time and that, rather than being hopeless, it can improve.

We must exercise caution, however, because duration does have some prognostic value.[37] Some classification system has included duration alongside prognostic indicators.[38] Other classifications are consistent with the prognostic approach.[34,39]

MECHANISM-BASED CLASSIFICATION OF PAIN

The conventional classifications of pain disorders based on anatomy, duration, and systems have drawn criticism for their deficiency in sensibility for guiding treatment or research.[40] Woolf et al.[40] support developing a mechanism-based classification of pain, proposing a potential list of pain mechanisms (Table 2.1). They argue that the list needs to include affective, behavioral, and cognitive factors relevant to pain, although they do not specify what these factors may be or how they would be incorporated within the proposed classification system.

The mechanism-based classifications of pain differ from the conventional classification in that the former frees pain from diseases that may accompany reports of pain. Mechanism-based classification groups patients who are homogeneous in pain mechanisms but heterogeneous in disease conditions or diagnoses. Woolf et al.[40] emphasize that their proposal is not to replace but rather to supplement the current system.

The basic premise underlying the mechanism-based classification of pain[40] is helpful, both in guiding treatment and in bridging research to clinical practice in pain medicine. However, such a system is still at the conceptual stage. Ongoing efforts to synthesize findings from various areas of pain research will help to formulate this new classification system.

This approach contrasts with our description of the use of two dimensions, time and severity, to distinguish acute and chronic pain (see Fig. 2.1). An explication of attempts to develop multidimensional classification systems incorporating features of several of the classifications is reviewed in the next section.

TABLE 2.1 Categories of Pain and Possible Mechanisms
Transient Pain
Nociceptor specialization
Tissue Injury Pain
Primary Afferent
Sensitization
Recruitment of silent nociceptors
Alteration in phenotype
Hyperinnervation
CNS Mediated
Central sensitization recruitment, summation, amplification
Nervous System Injury Pain
Primary Afferent
Acquisition of spontaneous and stimulus-evoked activity by nociceptor axons and somata at loci other than peripheral terminals
Alteration in phenotype
CNS Mediated
Central sensitization
Deafferentation of second-order neurons
Disinhibition
Structural reorganization

CNS, central nervous system.
Adapted with permission from Woolf CJ, Bennett GJ, Doherty M, et al. Towards a mechanism-based classification of pain? (editorial). *Pain* 1998;77(3):227–229.

Multiaxial Classifications

Ever since the gate control model underscored the importance of cognitive–evaluative and motivational–affective factors in the process of pain experience, the importance of integrating the psychosocial domains in the classification of pain has been proposed by a number of clinical investigators. However, as in other domains of pain medicine, the psychosocial classifications of pain have largely depended on psychiatric diagnoses to identify psychopathology. Although the psychiatrically defined classification of pain patients may help identify patients with specific psychiatric disorders, thereby directing treatments for those disorders, psychological classification systems aim to identify the specific psychosocial and behavioral contributions.

Empirically Based Classification of the Psychological Components of Pain

Many taxonomies of pain recognize that the conceptualization and operationalization of cognitive, affective, and behavioral factors associated with pain merit consideration (e.g., IASP,[4] AAPT[21]/AAAPT[22] described in the following discussion). Numerous instruments assess pain-related psychosocial constructs, but most are unidimensional, inadequate for pain populations, or lack predictive validity for treatment outcomes. We describe one specific multidimensional, psychosocial classification system used primarily with patients with chronic pain conditions.

The Multidimensional Pain Inventory (MPI)[41] consists of a set of empirically derived scales designed to assess chronic pain patients' (1) pain severity, (2) pain interferes, (3) their dissatisfaction with present levels of functioning in main life domains, (4) appraisals of support received from significant others, (5) perceived life control, (6) their affective distress, and (7) activity levels.

Turk and Rudy[39] performed cluster analyses on a heterogeneous sample of chronic pain patients' responses on the MPI scales. Three distinct profiles were identified: (1) dysfunctional (DYS): patients who perceived the severity of their pain to be high, reported that pain interfered with much of their lives, reported a higher degree of psychological distress due to pain, and reported low levels of activity; (2) interpersonally distressed (ID): patients with a common perception that significant others were not very supportive of their pain problems; and (3) adaptive copers (AC): patients who reported high levels of social support, relatively low levels of pain and perceived interference, and relatively high levels of activity. Reliable, external scales supported the uniqueness of each of the three subgroups of patients. Performing a 12-dimension Bayesian calculation to test goodness of fit can identify the profile that best fits a patient.

The empirical–statistical approach has a distinct advantage of permitting judgments about how well an individual patient matches the central features of that classification. This is especially useful in complex pain syndromes that involve various clinical characteristics with large individual variability even within a single diagnostic group. Based on a set of patient characteristics, signs, and symptoms, a prototype for a diagnosis can be established. It is possible to statistically determine how close an individual case matches that prototype. Assume that a perfect match to a prototype is 0.99. A particular case may fit within the diagnosis but not be a perfect fit; thus, the fit might be 0.80. Some statistical rule can decide the minimum fit to the characteristics of the diagnosis; for example, 0.67. Thus, any two individuals with the same diagnosis must share certain characteristics but not necessarily all; the similarity of two patients with the same diagnosis has a statistical definition.

Subsequent testing of the MPI profiles across various pain disorders suggests that the MPI psychosocial classification is independent of the conventionally defined pain syndromes, such as low back pain, TMD, migraine headaches, FM, and pain associated with cancer. In other words, two patients whose pain pathologies are likely to differ (e.g., cancer and migraine headaches) could have a homogeneous psychological classification of pain. On the other hand, two patients, both having same type of TMD based on the RDC[24] for comparable duration, may fare differently in the psychological classification of pain. Clinical trials using the MPI-based classification have yielded differential responses to a cognitive-behavioral approach.[42,43] Such results strongly suggest that the psychosocial treatment components need to conform to the psychological classification of pain.[44]

A number of other empirical classifications based on patterns of psychosocial and behavioral factors have been reported.[45,46] These approaches are similar but as with any empirically derived system that classification will depend on the variables assessed and entered into classification algorithms.

We suggest that disease classification should reflect physical assessment leading to medical/physical treatment plans (e.g., 2), whereas that a psychosocial–behavioral taxonomy should determine complementary psychological treatment strategies. Both physical and psychosocial diagnoses are important in the person with a chronic pain syndrome. Several groups[24,46,47] have proposed the use of a dual-diagnostic approach, whereby two diagnoses are assigned concurrently: physical and psychosocial–behavioral. Treatment could then target both simultaneously. A chronic pain patient might have diagnoses on two different but complementary taxonomies; for example, IASP and MPI-based classification. Thus, a patient might be classified as having CRPS type 1 of the upper extremity (203.X1, Axis I Region = upper shoulder and upper limbs, Axis II Systems = nervous, Axis III Temporal Characteristics of Pain: Pattern of Occurrence = none of the codes listed, Axis IV Intensity and Time of Onset = based on patient report, Axis V Etiology = trauma) on the IASP taxonomy and be classified DYS on the MPI-based taxonomy. Note that not all CRPS type 1 patients would be classified as DYS and not all DYS patients would have CRPS type 1. A second patient might have the same IASP diagnosis CRPS type 1 but be ID on the MPI-based classification. Conversely, patients might have quite different classifications on the IASP system but have an identical MPI-based classification. The most appropriate treatment for these different groups might vary, with different complementary components of treatments addressing the physical diagnosis (IASP) and the psychosocial diagnosis (MPI-based).

COMPREHENSIVE, MULTIDIMENSIONAL CLASSIFICATION OF PAIN: INTERNATIONAL ASSOCIATION FOR THE STUDY OF PAIN TAXONOMY

An alternative to the unidimensional approaches is a multidimensional approach that uses several relevant rather than a single dimension as the basis for developing the classification system and for assigning patients to a particular subgroup or diagnosis. The IASP has published an expert-based multiaxial classification of chronic pain[1,2] intended to standardize descriptions of relevant pain syndromes and to provide a point of reference. The published taxonomy classifies chronic pain patients according to five axes based on the best published information and consensus:

1. **Region** of the body (Axis I),
2. **System** whose abnormal functioning could conceivably produce the pain (Axis II),
3. **Temporal characteristics of pain and pattern of occurrence** (Axis III),
4. **Patient's statement of intensity and time since onset of pain** (Axis IV), and
5. Presumed **etiology** (Axis V) (Table 2.2).

TABLE 2.2	International Association for the Study of Pain (IASP): Scheme for Coding Chronic Pain Syndromes	

Axis I: Regions

Head, face, and mouth	000
Cervical region	100
Upper shoulder and upper limbs	200
Thoracic region	300
Abdominal region	400
Lower back, lumbar spine, sacrum, and coccyx	500
Lower limbs	600
Pelvic region	700
Anal, perineal, and genital region	800
More than three major sites	900

Axis II: Systems

Nervous system (central, peripheral, and autonomic) and special senses; physical disturbance or dysfunction	00
Nervous system (psychological and social)	10
Respiratory and cardiovascular systems	20
Musculoskeletal system and connective tissue	30
Cutaneous and subcutaneous and associated glands (breast, apocrine, etc.)	40
Gastrointestinal system	50
Genito-urinary system	60
Other organs or viscera (e.g., thyroid, lymphatic hemopoietic)	70
More than one system	80
Unknown	90

Axis III: Temporal Characteristics of Pain: Pattern of Occurrence

Not recorded, not applicable, or not known	0
Single episode, limited duration (e.g., ruptured aneurysm, sprained ankle)	1
Continuous or nearly continuous, nonfluctuating (e.g., low back pain)	2
Continuous or nearly continuous, fluctuating (e.g., ruptured intervertebral disc)	3
Recurring irregularly (e.g., headache, mixed type)	4
Recurring regularly (e.g., premenstrual pain)	5
Paroxysmal (e.g., tic douloureux)	6
Sustained with superimposed paroxysms	7
Other combinations	8
None of the above	9

Axis IV: Patient's Statement of Intensity: Time Since Onset of Pain

Not recorded, not applicable, or not known	.0
Mild—1 mo or less	.1
Mild—1 to 6 mo	.2
Mild—more than 6 mo	.3
Medium—1 mo or less	.4
Medium—1 to 6 mo	.5
Medium—more than 6 mo	.6
Severe—1 mo or less	.7
Severe—1 to 6 mo	.8
Severe—more than 6 mo	.9

Axis V: Etiology

Genetic or congenital disorders (e.g., congenital dislocations)	.00
Trauma, operation, burns	.01
Infective, parasitic	.02
Inflammatory (no known infective agent), immune reaction	.03
Neoplasm	.04
Toxic, metabolic (e.g., alcoholic neuropathy) anoxia, vascular, nutritional, endocrine, radiation	.05
Degenerative, mechanical	.06
Dysfunctional (including psychophysiologic)	.07
Unknown or other	.08
Psychological origin (e.g., conversion hysteria, depressive hallucination)	.09

IASP Chronic Pain Syndromes

A. Relatively generalized syndromes
B. Relatively localized syndromes of the head and neck
    I. Neuralgias of the head and face
    II. Craniofacial pain of musculoskeletal origin
    III. Lesions of the ear, nose, and oral cavity
    IV. Primary headache syndromes, vascular disorders, and cerebrospinal fluid syndromes
    V. Pain of psychological origin in the head, face, and neck
    VI. Suboccipital and cervical musculoskeletal disorders
    VII. Visceral pain in the neck
C. Spinal pain—spinal and radicular pain syndromes
D. Spinal pain—spinal and radicular pain syndromes of the cervical and thoracic regions
E. Local syndromes of the upper limbs and relatively generalized syndromes of the upper and lower limbs
    I. Pain in the shoulder, arm, and hand
    II. Vascular disease of the limbs
    III. Collagen disease of the limbs
    IV. Vasodilating functional disease of the limbs
    V. Arterial insufficiency in the limbs
    VI. Pain of psychological origin in the lower limbs
F. Visceral and other syndromes of the trunk apart from spinal and radicular pain
    I. Visceral and other chest pain
    II. Chest pain of psychological origin
    III. Chest pain referred from abdomen or gastrointestinal tract
    IV. Abdominal pain of neurologic origin
    V. Abdominal pain of visceral origin
    VI. Abdominal pain syndromes of generalized diseases
    VII. Abdominal pain of psychological origin
    VIII. Diseases of the bladder, uterus, ovaries, and adnexa
    IX. Pain in the rectum, perineum, and external genitalia
G. Spinal pain—spinal and radicular pain syndromes of the lumbar, sacral, and coccygeal regions
    I. Lumbar spinal or radicular pain syndromes
    II. Sacral spinal or radicular pain syndromes
    III. Coccygeal pain syndromes
    IV. Diffuse or generalized spinal pain
    V. Low back pain or psychological origin with referral
H. Local syndromes of the lower limbs
    I. Local syndromes in the leg or foot: pain of neurologic origin
    II. Pain syndromes of the hip and thigh of musculoskeletal origin
    III. Musculoskeletal syndromes of the leg

This system establishes a five-digit code that assigns to each chronic pain diagnosis, a unique number. For example, the code for carpal tunnel syndrome is 204.X6. Thus,

- 200 = REGION: upper shoulder and upper limbs
- 00 = SYSTEM: the abnormal functioning is attributed to the nervous system
- 4 = TEMPORAL CHARACTERISTICS: symptoms occur irregularly
- X = PATIENT'S STATEMENT OF INTENSITY AND TIME SINCE ONSET: this will vary by patient
- 06 = ETIOLOGY: degenerative, mechanical

Table 2.3 contains the IASP scheme developed for the coding of chronic pain diagnoses.

The IASP classification is the most comprehensive approach to classification of chronic pain syndromes. By design, the IASP classification is a heuristic, multiaxial guide that emphasizes the consideration of both signs and symptoms. Unfortunately, it excludes assessment of psychosocial or behavioral data. Moreover, to be useful, any classification system must be reliable and valid, but as yet little published research has evaluated the reliability, validity, or utility of the IASP classification. What little evidence is available[48] indicates that, although

TABLE 2.3   List of Descriptions in Each Syndrome in the IASP Classification

Definition

Site

System(s) involved

Main features of the pain including its prevalence, age of onset, sex ratio if known, duration, severity, and quality

Associated features; aggravating and relieving agents

Signs

Laboratory findings

Natural course

Complications

Social and physical disability

Pathology or other contributing factors

Essential features and diagnostic criteria

Differential diagnosis

Code based on the five axes

References (optional)

Axis I (body region) demonstrated reliable coding across examiners, Axis V (etiology) failed to achieve acceptable interrater reliability. The consistency (test–retest reliability) of the IASP taxonomy has yet to be established. Further research is needed in order to evaluate the psychometric properties of the classification system and to facilitate refinements of the system. The classifications we have described are only a few examples and are definitely not exhaustive. Specialists can arrive at classification categories based on clinical experience, published data, and consensus[6,43] There is no single system for classifying pain patients that is universally accepted by clinicians or researchers. Furthermore, several problems associated with the current classification systems have generated debate and research concerning an alternative classification of pain. We provide several examples to illustrate different attempts to devise alternative taxonomies of pain and chronic pain patients.

Recently, IASP proposed a classification of chronic pain for inclusion in the ICD-11.[4] The classification includes seven categories (i.e., "primary", cancer, postsurgical/posttraumatic, neuropathic, headache and orofacial, visceral, and musculoskeletal). The primary category is somewhat of a mixed back pain that cannot be explained by other chronic pain conditions and includes back pain that is neither identified as musculoskeletal or neuropathic, chronic widespread pain, FM, or irritable bowel syndrome. The primary category is consistent with the lumping of this set of disorders in the category of AAPM's diagnosis of maldynia and central sensitivity disorders advocated by Clauw[28] and Yunus[29] among others. There may be some concern that this poorly defined category may imply the discredited psychogenic classification; that is, an artificial dichotomy where either the condition has a physical basis (somatogenic) or in the absence is psychogenic.

COMPREHENSIVE, MULTIDIMENSIONAL CLASSIFICATION OF PAIN: ACTTION-AMERICAN PAIN SOCIETY AND ACTTION-AMERICAN PAIN SOCIETY-AMERICAN ACADEMY OF PAIN MEDICINE

Recently, a consortium composed of ACTTION partnering with the American Pain Society to create chronic pain taxonomy (AAPT)[21] and with the AAPM (AAAPT)[22] to create an acute pain taxonomy.

AAPT and AAAPT are evidence-based pain taxonomy in which a multidimensional diagnostic framework has been applied to the most prevalent and important chronic and acute pain conditions. A major impetus for the AAPT/AAAPT initiative derived from observing the transformative impact of evidence-based diagnostic classifications in related medical specialties.

An essential characteristic of the AAPT multidimensional framework, taxonomy, and diagnostic criteria is that they are based on the best available evidence regarding symptoms, signs, mechanisms, and consequences rather than on expert opinion alone. This coordinated effort can be applied across all chronic pain conditions, and as has been true of other diagnostic criteria, AAPT will be revised periodically on the basis of accumulating evidence. Another critical aspect of the AAPT is that it reflects the multidimensional, biopsychosocial nature of chronic pain, in which psychological and social risk factors and consequences are integrated with neurobiologic mechanisms and outcomes. In addition, an essential characteristic is that the taxonomy is intended to be applicable for both research and clinical settings; it is recognized, however, that widespread clinical use is likely to develop gradually as the clinical utility of the criteria become apparent and as the evidence base increases. Finally, the initial version of AAPT is based on currently available evidence, and the goal is to systematically update the criteria on the basis of new evidence, especially the results of studies of reliability, validity, and neurobiologic mechanisms.

AAPT therefore categorizes chronic pain conditions by organ system and anatomic structure, distinguishing peripheral and central neuropathic pain, musculoskeletal pain, spine pain, orofacial and head pain, and abdominal/pelvic/urogenital pain (Table 2.4). Because certain types of chronic pain cannot be included in one of these groups, an additional category for disease-related pain not classified elsewhere includes pain associated with cancer and pain associated with sickle cell disease (pain associated with Lyme disease and with leprosy, among other conditions, would also be included in this group). It is important to emphasize that all types of headache were intentionally excluded from AAPT because the International Classification of Headache Disorders (ICHD)[20] provides systematic, valid, and widely used diagnostic criteria for these conditions.

The AAPT multidimensional framework comprises five dimensions that can be applied to *all* chronic pain conditions. This can be contrasted with the new IASP taxonomy where psychosocial factors are "optional specifiers" for each diagnoses beyond the classification of "chronic primary pain" where it is given a prominent role along with interference with activities and participation in social roles (somewhat of a departure from the original IASP taxonomy). An overview of these dimensions is presented in Table 2.4, and each is briefly summarized in this section (see also Fillingim et al.[21]). Other than prioritizing core diagnostic criteria, which is the first AAPT dimension, the order of the dimensions does not reflect their importance. Indeed, as noted earlier, it is anticipated that AAPT diagnostic criteria will ultimately be based on the mechanisms of the specific chronic pain conditions, whereas in the current version of the taxonomy, these mechanisms constitute the final dimension.

Like the IASP classification, the AAPT also includes seven but somewhat different categories of chronic pain (i.e., peripheral nervous systems; central nervous system; spine; musculoskeletal; orofacial and head; visceral, pelvic, and urogenital; other [e.g., cancer, sickle cell]). Within the AAPT classification, psychological and behavioral factors are identified with all of the seven categories. Specifically, the AAPT classification incorporates five dimensions for each condition within the seven categories (Table 2.5). The AAAPT is being extended to acute pain, incorporating the same five dimensions, in this application for eight acute pain sets of conditions (i.e., acute surgical/procedural pain; acute trauma pain; acute musculoskeletal pain; acute visceral pain; cancer/immune-mediated acute pain; acute neuropathic pain; acute orofacial pain; acute pain in pediatric, geriatric, and special populations).[22]

TABLE 2.4 ACTTION-American Pain Society Pain Taxonomy (AAPT) for Chronic Pain

Peripheral Nervous System

Complex regional pain syndrome
Painful peripheral neuropathies associated with diabetes, impaired glucose tolerance, and human immunodeficiency virus
Postherpetic neuralgia
Posttraumatic neuropathic pain, including chronic pain after surgery
Trigeminal neuralgia

Central Nervous System

Pain associated with multiple sclerosis
Poststroke pain
Spinal cord injury pain

Spine Pain

Chronic axial musculoskeletal low back pain
Chronic lumbosacral radiculopathy

Musculoskeletal Pain

Fibromyalgia and chronic myofascial and widespread pain
Gout
Osteoarthritis
Rheumatoid arthritis
Spondyloarthropathies

Orofacial and Head Pain

Headache disorders (see International Classification of Headache Disorders)
Temporomandibular disorders

Abdominal, Pelvic, and Urogenital Pain

Interstitial cystitis
Irritable bowel syndrome
Vulvodynia

Disease-Associated Pain Conditions Not Classified Elsewhere

Pain associated with cancer: cancer-induced bone pain, chemotherapy-induced peripheral neuropathy, and pancreatic cancer pain
Pain associated with sickle cell disease

NOTE: The specific chronic pain conditions listed within each of the seven categories are those for which diagnostic criteria are included within AAPT and are not all of the chronic pain conditions that occur within these categories. This table is updated from (Fillingim et al.[21]).
Reprinted from Dworkin RH, Bruehl S, Fillingim RB, et al. Multidimensional diagnostic criteria for chronic pain: introduction to the ACTTION-American Pain Society Pain Taxonomy (AAPT). *J Pain* 2016;17(9 Suppl):T1–T9. Copyright © 2016 by the American Pain Society. With permission.

INDUCTIVE EMPIRICALLY BASED CLASSIFICATIONS OF PAIN

Those who advocate the use of empirically derived taxonomies maintain that quantitative analysis should define the relationships of contiguity and similarity among individuals. That is, the taxonomic system must reflect clinically relevant characteristics that exist in nature, defined by empirical methods rather than based on expert judgment and consensus.

The American College of Rheumatology (ACR) proposed the first standard criteria that were empirically derived for the classification of FM in 1990. In a multicenter study,[49] a group of FM experts from several medical centers collected FM-related variables and used those variables in an attempt to differentiate FM patients from patients with other types of chronic pain syndromes. The acceptable sensitivity and specificity were achieved by two criteria: presence of widespread pain (i.e., above and below the waist, right and left side of the body, and along the midline) and at least 11 of 18 positive tender points upon palpation. Other symptoms commonly reported by FM patients, such as fatigue and stiffness, did not differentiate between FM and other types of chronic pain. Since publication, most subsequent research seems to conform to this classification system, making it a bit easier to compare results across studies. Nonetheless, debate remains about the extent that this classification contributes to clinical practice and the meaning of tender points and the necessity of the tender point criterion.[50]

Although the criteria were well acknowledged as the important step to standardize the nature of FM population, they were criticized by many as not quite capturing the disease entity well. It is important to acknowledge that all relevant factors cannot be measured by a single classification system. The use of an inductive approach depends on what the investigator chooses to include within the statistical analysis. Thus, in practice, the inductive approach to classification is not a totally objective process that is completely atheoretical. Furthermore, there are significant difficulties in defining a "pure" syndrome that is distinct from all the relevant illnesses when the syndrome itself is a multisymptom disorder. In a case of FM, one of the major criticisms of the empirically driven 1990 ACR criteria is that they fail to incorporate main feature of FM, such as fatigue, cognitive problem, and sleep disturbance. These main features are common in other disorders and do not necessarily differentiate FM from others; nevertheless, not taking these features into account seemed to diminish the validity

TABLE 2.5 The ACTTION-American Pain Society Pain Taxonomy Multidimensional Framework for Chronic Pain

Dimension Description	
1. Core diagnostic criteria	Symptoms, signs, and diagnostic test findings required for the diagnosis of the chronic pain condition. Includes differential diagnosis considerations.
2. Common features	Additional information regarding the disorder, including common pain characteristics (e.g., location, temporal qualities, descriptors), nonpain features (numbness, fatigue), the epidemiology of the condition, and life span considerations, including those specific to pediatric and geriatric populations. These features are important in describing the disorder but are not components of the core diagnostic criteria.
3. Common medical and psychiatric comorbidities	Medical and psychiatric disorders that commonly occur with the chronic pain condition. For example, major depression is comorbid with many chronic pain conditions. Also includes chronic overlapping pain conditions, that is, those chronic pain conditions that are comorbid with each other.
4. Neurobiological, psychosocial, and functional consequences	Neurobiological, psychosocial, and functional consequences of chronic pain. Examples include sleep and mood disorders and pain-related interference with daily activities.
5. Putative neurobiological and psychosocial mechanisms, risk factors, and protective factors	Putative neurobiological and psychosocial mechanisms contributing to the development and maintenance of the chronic pain condition, including risk and protective factors. Examples include central sensitization, decreased descending inhibition, and somatosensory amplification.

Reprinted from Dworkin RH, Bruehl S, Fillingim RB, et al. Multidimensional diagnostic criteria for chronic pain: introduction to the ACTTION-American Pain Society Pain Taxonomy (AAPT). *J Pain*. 2016;17(9 Suppl):T1–T9. Copyright © 2016 by the American Pain Society. With permission.

of the classification. Purely inductive approach to empirically delineate a clinical syndrome may benefit therefore from incorporating clinically and theoretically meaningful approaches.

PSYCHOMETRIC CONSIDERATIONS

The general utility of any proposed empirical taxonomy links closely to the psychometric properties (i.e., reliability, validity, and utility) of the measures, scales, or instruments used to derive the classification system. Because these are the building blocks used to generate profiles or clusters, the reliability and validity of the classification system depends, in part, on the psychometric quality of the measures used. Because reliability and validity coefficients are generic terms, the specific psychometric techniques used to evaluate a measure's "psychometric properties" require consideration. There are multiple ways to demonstrate the reliability and validity of measures. Therefore, the more psychometric support there is for a measure, the more likely it will perform well when used in taxometric identification and classification procedures. Additionally, replication of classification accuracy on new samples and demonstrating substantial, statistically significant differences across patient profiles for conceptually related measures *external* to the measures used to develop the profiles are some of the best ways to demonstrate the reliability and validity of empirically derived profiles. Evaluation of any classification should demonstrate reliability, validity, and utility prior to widespread adoption.

Conclusion

Pain management specialists have witnessed rapid advances in the basic sciences and clinical arenas of pain medicine over the past three decades. Many pain-related terms, once a major source of confusion, have received clear definitions, aiding efficient and productive communication among researchers and clinicians. The classification systems that direct our research and clinical practice need to reflect the progress in our understanding of mechanisms, multifactorial integration, and outcome predictability of classification criteria. In this chapter, we have reviewed several conventional classifications as well as emerging classification systems that can supplement the conventional ones. The review of various classification systems suggests that the comprehensive taxonomy of pain require multifactorial assessments including physical, psychosocial, and behavioral components (see Table 2.5).

The utility of any classification system depends on application. The important question is whether assignment of an individual to a class truly facilitates treatment decisions or predictions of future behavior. Several of the taxometric systems have demonstrated their utility to predict treatment outcome.[45] The prognostic approach has some data supporting its use as an alternative to the traditional approach based on the acute–chronic duration continuum. In support of this, the multiaxial RDC for Temporomandibular Disorders has acquired sufficient data to warrant it being adopted as Diagnostic Criteria for Temporomandibular Disorders.[24] Research is needed to demonstrate the validity of the newer IASP[4] and AAPT[21]/AAAPT[22] taxonomies.

References

1. Merskey H. Classification of chronic pain. Descriptions of chronic pain syndromes and definitions. *Pain* 1986;(suppl 3):345–356.
2. Merskey H, Bogduk N. *Classification of Chronic Pain: Descriptions of Chronic Pain Syndromes and Definitions of Pain Terms.* 2nd ed. Seattle, WA: IASP Press; 1994.
3. Merskey H. Classification and diagnosis of fibromyalgia. *Pain Res Manag* 1996;1:42–44.
4. Treede RD, Rief W, Barke A, et al. A classification of chronic pain for the ICD-11. *Pain* 2015;156:1003–1007.
5. Williams AC, Craig KD. Updating the definition of pain. *Pain* 2016;157:2420–2423.
6. Deyo RA, Dworkin SF, Amtmann D, et al. Report of the NIH Task Force on research standards for chronic low back pain. *J Pain* 2014:15:569–585.
7. Von Korff M, Dunn KM. Chronic pain reconsidered. *Pain* 2008;138:267–276.
8. Turk DC, Murphy TB. Chronic pain. In: Carr A, McNulty M, eds. *The Handbook of Adult Clinical Psychology: An Evidence-Based Practice Approach.* 2nd ed. London: Routledge; 2016:635–685.
9. Turk DC. Remember the distinction between malignant and benign pain? Well, forget it. *Clin J Pain* 2002;18:75–76.
10. Sullivan MJ, Thorn B, Haythornthwaite JA, et al. Theoretical perspectives on the relation between catastrophizing and pain. *Clin J Pain* 2001;17:52–64.
11. Harden RN, Bruehl S, Stanton-Hicks M, et al. Proposed new diagnostic criteria for complex regional pain syndrome. *Pain Med* 2007;8:326–331.
12. Yarnitsky D, Arendt-Nielsen L, Bouhassira D, et al. Recommendations on terminology and practice of psychophysical DNIC testing. *Eur J Pain* 2010;14:339.
13. Jensen TS, Baron R, Haanpää M, et al. A new definition of neuropathic pain. *Pain* 2011;152:2204–2205.
14. Treede RD, Jensen TS, Campbell JN, et al. Neuropathic pain: redefinition and a grading system for clinical and research purposes. *Neurology* 2008;70:1630–1635.
15. Southwick SM, Bonanno GA, Masten AS, et al. Resilience definitions, theory, and challenges: interdisciplinary perspectives. *Eur J Psychotraumatol* 2014;5:25338.
16. Bonica JJ. The need of a taxonomy. *Pain* 1979;6:247–248.
17. Baron DN, Fraser PM. Medical applications of taxonomic methods. *Br Med Bull* 1968;24:236–240.
18. World Health Organization, ed. *ICD-10: International Statistical Classification of Diseases and Related Health Problems.* Vol 1. 10th rev ed. Geneva, Switzerland: World Health Organization; 1992. Available at: http://www.who.int/classifications/icd/revision/contentmodel/en/. Accessed October 1, 2014.
19. Classification and diagnostic criteria for headache disorders, cranial neuralgias and facial pain. Headache Classification Committee of the International Headache Society. *Cephalalgia* 1988;(8)(suppl 7):1–96.
20. Spitzer WO, Skovron ML, Salmi LR, et al. Scientific monograph of the Quebec Task Force on whiplash-associated disorders: redefining "whiplash" and its management. *Spine (Phila Pa 1976)* 1995;20(8)(suppl):1S–73S.
21. Fillingim RB, Bruehl S, Dworkin RH, et al. The ACTTION-American Pain Society Pain Taxonomy (AAPT): an evidence-based and multi-dimensional approach to classifying chronic pain conditions. *J Pain* 2014;15:241–249.
22. Kent ML, Tighe PJ, Belfer I, et al. The ACTTION-APS-AAM Pain Taxonomy (AAAPT) multidimensional approach to classifying acute pain conditions. *J Pain* 2017;18:479–489.
23. Dworkin SF, LeResche L. Research diagnostic criteria for temporomandibular disorders: review, criteria, examinations and specifications, critique. *J Craniomandib Disord* 1992;6:301–355.
24. Schiffman E, Ohrbach R, Truelove E, et al. Diagnostic criteria for temporomandibular disorders (DC/TMD) for clinical and dental research applications: recommendations of the International RDC/TMD Consortium Network and Orofacial Pain Special Interest Group. *J Oral Facial Pain Headache* 2014;28:6–27.
25. Zaki H, Rudy T, Turk D, et al. Reliability of Axis I research diagnostic criteria for TMD [abstract]. *J Dent Res* 1994;73:186.
26. Dickinson BD, Head CA, Gitlow S, et al. Maldynia: pathophysiology and management of neuropathic and maladaptive pain—a report of the AMA Council on Science and Public Health. *Pain Med* 2010;11:1635–1653.
27. Portenoy RK. Mechanisms of clinical pain. Observations and speculations. *Neurol Clin* 1989;7:205–230.
28. Clauw DJ. Fibromyalgia and related conditions. *Mayo Clinic Proc* 2015;90:680–692.
29. Yunus MB. Central sensitivity syndromes: a new paradigm and group nosology for fibromyalgia and overlapping conditions, and the related issue of disease versus illness. *Semin Arthritis Rheum* 2008;37:339–352.
30. Friction J. Medical evaluation of patients with chronic pain. In: Barber J, Adrian C, eds. *Psychological Approaches to the Management of Pain.* New York: Brunner/Mazel; 1982:37–61.
31. World Health Organization. *International Classification of Functioning, Disability and Health: ICF.* Geneva, Switzerland: World Health Organization; 2001.
32. Brena S, Koch D. A "pain estimate" model for quantification and classification of chronic pain states. *Anesth Rev* 1975;2:8–13.
33. Brena S, Koch D, Moss R. Reliability of the "pain estimate" model. *Anesth Rev* 1976;3:28–29.
34. Von Korff M, Ormel J, Keefe FJ, et al. Grading the severity of chronic pain. *Pain* 1992;50:133–149.
35. Dunn KM, Von Korff M, Croft PR. Defining chronic pain by prognosis. In: Hasenbring MI, Rusu AC, Turk DC, eds. *From Acute to Chronic Back Pain: Risk Factors, Mechanisms, and Clinical Implications.* Oxford, England: Oxford University Press; 2012:21–39.
36. Von Korff M, Miglioretti DL. A prognostic approach to defining chronic pain. *Pain* 2005;117:304–313.
37. Elliott AM, Smith BH, Hannaford PC, et al. Assessing change in chronic pain severity: the Chronic Pain Grade compared with retrospective perception. *Br J Gen Pract* 2002;52:269–274.

38. Spitzer WO, LeBlanc FE, Dupuis M, et al. Scientific approach to the assessment and management of activity-related spinal disorders: a monograph for clinicians. Report of the Quebec Task Force on Spinal Disorders. *Spine (Phila Pa 1976)* 1987;12(7)(suppl):S1–S59.

39. Turk DC, Rudy TE. Towards a comprehensive assessment of chronic pain patients. *Behav Res Ther* 1987;25:237–249.

40. Woolf C, Bennett G, Doherty M, et al. Towards a mechanism-based classification of pain? *Pain* 1998;77:227–229.

41. Kerns RD, Turk DC, Rudy TE. The West Haven-Yale Multidimensional Pain Inventory (WHYMPI). *Pain* 1985;23:345–356.

42. Turk DC, Okifuji A, Sinclair JD, et al. Differential responses by psychosocial subgroups of fibromyalgia syndrome patients to an interdisciplinary treatment. *Arthritis Care Res* 1998;11:397–404.

43. Turk DC, Rudy TE, Kubinski JA, et al. Dysfunctional patients with temporomandibular disorders: evaluating the efficacy of a tailored treatment protocol. *J Consult Clin Psychol* 1996;64:139–146.

44. Turk DC. Customizing treatment for chronic pain patients: who, what, and why? *Clin J Pain* 1990;6:255–270.

45. Rusu A, Boersma K, Turk DC. Reviewing the concept of subgroups in subacute and chronic pain and the potential of customizing treatments. In: Hasenbring MI, Rusu AC, Turk DC, eds. *From Acute to Chronic Back Pain: Risk Factors, Mechanisms, and Clinical Implications*. Oxford, United Kingdom: Oxford University Press; 2012:485–511.

46. Turk DC. The potential of matching treatments to characteristics of chronic pain patients: lumping versus splitting. *Clin J Pain* 2005;21:44–55.

47. Scharff L, Turk DC, Marcus DA. Psychosocial and behavioral characteristics in chronic headache patients: support for a continuum and dual-diagnostic approach. *Cephalalgia* 1995;15:216–223.

48. Turk DC, Rudy TE. Toward an empirically derived taxonomy of chronic pain patients: integration of psychological assessment data. *J Consult Clin Psychol* 1988;56:233–238.

49. Wolfe F, Smythe HA, Yunus MB, et al. The American College of Rheumatology 1990 Criteria for the Classification of Fibromyalgia. Report of the Multicenter Criteria Committee. *Arthritis Rheum* 1990;33:160–172.

50. Clauw DJ. Fibromyalgia: update on mechanisms and management. *J Clin Rheumatol* 2007;13:102–109.

CHAPTER 3

Peripheral Pain Mechanisms and Nociceptor Sensitization

MICHAEL S. GOLD

Pain has been categorized by duration (acute vs. chronic), location (superficial or deep; cutaneous, bone/joint, muscle, or viscera), and cause or type (inflammatory, neuropathic, cancer). Generally, activation of and/or ongoing activity in specific subpopulations of primary afferent neurons underlies the experience of pain regardless of how it is categorized. Accordingly, primary afferents are key players in understanding mechanisms of, and managing, pain.

Sir Charles Sherrington anticipated by many decades the existence sensory receptors that respond to noxious stimuli, that he called nociceptors and thereby provided for us the operational definition of stimuli that are noxious (i.e., stimuli that damage or threaten damage of tissue). Two considerations are important to this discussion. First, Sherrington functionally defines the nociceptor by its response to a noxious stimulus (e.g., a nociceptive withdrawal reflex, pain). Second, the definition of an applied stimulus as noxious is based on the response to the stimulus applied to skin and subcutaneous structures.

Sherrington's definition of a nociceptor continues to the present day. However, the term has undergone change and challenge over the past 100 years and may be nearing the end of its utility in the face of the growing understanding of the heterogeneity in the neurons that may not fit so comfortably under this umbrella term. It is therefore important to consider, within the context of our current knowledge, how a nociceptor is defined, identified, and studied, as the interpretation of this information will directly affect the management of pain.

All would agree that a nociceptor is a sensory receptor which, when activated or active, can contribute to the experience of pain. Nociceptors are present in skin, muscle, joints, and viscera, although the density of innervation (i.e., the number and distribution of sensory endings) varies between and within tissues. As originally described by Sherrington, a nociceptor is the peripheral sensory terminal (i.e., the site of energy transduction—see following section), although commonly the term is used to also include the cell body (in a dorsal root, trigeminal, or nodose ganglion) and its central termination in the spinal cord or brainstem. Beyond this, agreement about important features of nociceptors is less uniform. One of the best examples of why this definition is becoming problematic is the observation that injury-induced changes in the central nervous system underlie the emergence of allodynia, pain in response to normally innocuous stimuli. Allodynia is problematic for this definition of nociceptor because pain is mediated by activity in low-threshold afferents that in the absence of tissue injury would, if anything, contribute to the suppression of pain. That is, these afferents would not be considered nociceptors despite the fact that they contribute to the experience of pain.

Furthermore, because stimuli adequate for activation of nociceptors differ between tissues (e.g., tissue damage is not always required), defining a noxious stimulus has become a challenge. For example, some nociceptors in skin and joints and most nociceptors in the viscera have low thresholds for mechanical activation that do not conform to the condition that stimulus intensity must be either damaging or threaten damage. Further, so-called "silent" or "sleeping" nociceptors are unresponsive to intense mechanical stimulation (and are better denoted as mechanically insensitive nociceptors) but develop spontaneous activity and mechanosensitivity after exposure to inflammatory and other endogenous mediators. These types of nociceptors—low threshold and sleeping—as well as other subpopulations of sensory neurons that may contribute to the sensation of pain following tissue injury are considered further in the discussion of sensitization in the following section.

Functional Characterization of Nociceptors

As suggested earlier, there are many types of nociceptors, our knowledge of which has been advanced by human psychophysical studies while recording from afferent fibers (Box 3.1). In human skin, for example, there exist nociceptors that respond only to mechanical, only to cold thermal, or only to hot thermal stimuli as well as those that are insensitive to both mechanical and heat stimuli (mechanically insensitive or sleeping nociceptors).[1,2] The most abundant is the polymodal nociceptor, which responds to mechanical, thermal, and chemical stimuli. In general, nociceptors that innervate skin have the broadest range of modality selectivity, whereas nociceptors innervating deeper structures tend to be less modality-selective and more polymodal in character.[3] For example, mechanical sensitivity is a prominent feature of visceral and joint nociceptors because stimuli adequate for their activation include hollow organ distension and overrotation, respectively. Many of these nociceptors also respond to chemical and/or thermal stimuli as well, although the functional significance of thermal sensitivity in deep tissues is uncertain. An important characteristic of polymodal nociceptors, whether the modalities of stimulation to which they respond are two or all three, is that when sensitized (e.g., by an inflammatory insult), responses to the other modality or modalities of stimuli to which it responds are all increased.[4] That is, it is not only the mechanosensitive modality, for example, that becomes sensitized, but other modalities to which it responds are sensitized as well.

With respect to mechanosensitivity, nociceptors at the opposite extremes of sensitivity are most illustrative of the limitations of even a functional definition of a nociceptor. Nociceptors with low mechanical thresholds for response and those with very high mechanical thresholds for response (i.e., sleeping nociceptors) are both clinically important. Mechanosensitive sensory neurons with low thresholds for response have long been classified as non-nociceptors (because it was considered that nociceptors had to have response thresholds in the noxious range). Some mechanosensitive skin, joint, and many visceral sensory neurons have low thresholds for response (i.e., in the nonnoxious range) but possess characteristics that suggest an important role in pain. First, they encode stimulus intensity well into the noxious range and, moreover, typically give greater responses to all intensities of stimulation than do nociceptors with high mechanical thresholds for response. Second, they sensitize after tissue insult. Unlike nociceptors with low mechanical thresholds, mechanically insensitive or sleeping nociceptors normally provide no information to the central nervous system but after tissue insult become spontaneously active and mechanosensitive.[5]

BOX 3.1   Microneurography

The development of a method to record from human nerve fibers in situ,[191,192] termed *microneurography*, provided an unparalleled opportunity to expand our knowledge about peripheral sensory receptors, including nociceptors. The method involves percutaneous insertion of the tip of a sharp, insulated metal microelectrode into a nerve (e.g., peroneal or radial nerve) and the application of search stimuli to sites distal to the electrode. In earlier work, mechanical search stimuli (e.g., von Frey filaments) were used, and accordingly, only mechanosensitive afferents were studied. An electrical search stimulus (surface electrode), however, has become favored because the electrical stimulus identifies afferent fibers independent of sensitivity to natural stimulation. After an afferent fiber is isolated, the innervation territory can be drawn on the skin and the adequate, natural stimulus/stimuli determined.

Because microneurography can be easily coupled with a psychophysical approach, human subjects are able to describe stimulus-produced experiences (e.g., pain) while recording from single afferent fibers. Microneurography also has been expanded to include intraneural electrical stimulation of the fiber through the recording electrode, providing additional insight into the qualities of sensation produced, for example, by low- and high-frequency stimulation in addition to qualities associated with natural stimulation. Microneurography has confirmed in psychophysical experiments sensations associated with activation of rapidly adapting (flutter, vibration) and slowly adapting (pressure) cutaneous mechanoreceptors, Aδ-mechanonociceptors (AM$_{[mechano]}$; sharp pain), C-polymodal nociceptors (CM$_{[mechano]}$H$_{[heat]}$; dull, burning [heat] pain), and group IV muscle nociceptors (cramping pain).

Electrical search strategies have revealed a wider range of nociceptors, including[190] A-mechanoheat (AMH), which have similar heat thresholds as CMH (C-polymodal) fibers and also typically respond to chemical stimuli; C-mechanonociceptors (CM), C-heat (CH); C-mechano- and heat-insensitive (CM$_i$H$_i$, or sleeping nociceptors); and C-mechanoinsensitive-histamine responsive (CM$_i$His+, or itch fibers[193]). Microneurography has also been extended to psychophysical study of pathologic pain states in humans. In a study of patients suffering from erythromelalgia, a condition characterized by painful, red, and hot extremities, a proportion of CM$_i$H$_i$ fibers were found to be spontaneously active or sensitized to mechanical stimuli. Because CM$_i$H$_i$ fibers also mediate the axon flare reflex, their hyperexcitability was considered to contribute to the patients' ongoing pain and tenderness as well as the redness and warming in this pain syndrome. In patients with painful peripheral neuropathy, Ochoa et al.[194] reported hyperexcitability in CMH and CM$_i$H$_i$ fibers. Signs of hyperexcitability included reduced thresholds to mechanical and heat stimuli, spontaneous activity, and increased responses to stimulation. In diabetic neuropathic pain patients, Ørstavik et al.[195] found that the ratio of CMH to CM$_i$H$_i$ fibers was reduced by about 50%, apparently due to loss of mechanical and heat responsiveness in CMH fibers.

These and future studies will help to understand which nociceptors (and non-nociceptors) in which conditions contribute to spontaneous, ongoing pain as well as stimulus-evoked pain and what therapeutic strategies are most effective.

Identification of Putative Nociceptors

As indicated earlier, nociceptors are defined classically in a functional context. However, in experimental situations where function cannot be assessed, other criteria to classify a neuron as a nociceptor have been advanced. These include the presence or absence of axon myelination, cell size, and/or cell content (e.g., peptide or ion channel) as well as central termination pattern. Sensory neurons commonly identified as nociceptors are those with unmyelinated (C-fiber) axons, small cell body diameters (<20 or 25 μm), that terminate in the superficial layers of the spinal cord dorsal horn. The presence or absence of certain markers (e.g., the tetrodotoxin (TTX)-resistant sodium channel NaV1.8, the transient receptor potential vanilloid receptor TRPV1) have been used to identify subsets of nociceptors. More recently, with the ability to analyze many genes expressed in a single cell, patterns of gene expression have been used to further define subpopulations of nociceptors.[6,7] With respect to cell body size and myelination, it should be appreciated that there exist some large diameter cells with heavily myelinated and rapidly conducting axons that have been documented functionally to be nociceptors.[8] Conversely, many non-nociceptors have unmyelinated axons, and thus, axon myelination or cell diameter cannot be applied as reliable criteria to define a nociceptor. Similarly, identifying nociceptors by content or by what genes they express has limitations. Two examples of this are that (1) cells other than nociceptors express TRPV1 and (2) the features of the subset of nociceptors in the mouse skin that stain positive for the isolectin B4 do not apply to the visceral innervation.[9] And although patterns of gene expression may enable identification of additional subpopulations of nociceptive sensory neurons,[10] the extent to which any particular pattern reliably reveals a neuron's function remains to be established.

The fact that no single criterion can be used to identify all nociceptors combined with the growing number of examples to the ways in which these neurons are heterogeneous is at the core of a growing concern over the utility of the term. In addition to the anatomical, biochemical, and physiologic heterogeneity in the afferent population, generally referred to as nociceptors, there is functional heterogeneity. As will be discussed later, this

functional heterogeneity is manifest both within the context of nociceptive signaling (i.e., subpopulations of nociceptors may underlie distinct "types" of pain such as cold allodynia or thermal hyperalgesia) and in the context of nonnociceptive function (i.e., such as the maintenance of tissue integrity).

Even the two functional properties that have been viewed as common to all nociceptors, that they encode stimulus intensity into the noxious range and they sensitize, are, at best, generalities. As noted earlier, the so-called mechanically insensitive afferents shown to play such a prominent role in visceral pain[11] and the burning pain associated with capsaicin[12] do not appear to code stimulus intensity in the noxious range. Similarly, a variety of nociceptive afferents may be desensitized under the appropriate conditions.[13–16] The link between the stimulus–response properties of a given subpopulation of afferents and the functional role of these neurons in the context of nociceptive signaling has been further complicated by results of selective ablation/silencing studies in mice, where modality specific deficits in nociceptive processing are associated with the silencing of specific subpopulations of afferents despite electrophysiologic data suggesting that the majority of the afferents silenced/ablated are polymodal. For example, the majority of cutaneous neurons in the mouse that express the Mas1-related G protein-coupled receptor D (MrgprD) are polymodal nociceptors,[17] yet mice in which this subpopulation of neurons has been ablated respond normally to changes in temperature, demonstrating, instead, a relatively selective mechanosensitivity deficit.[18] Conversely, the voltage-gated sodium channel (VGSC) NaV1.8 is enriched in nociceptive afferents that are responsive to both noxious thermal (TRPV1-expressing) and mechanical (MrgprD-expressing) stimuli, yet mice in which NaV1.8-expressing neurons have been ablated respond to noxious heat but not noxious mechanical pressure or cold stimuli.[19] Minimally, these results suggest that the behavioral response to noxious stimulation involves a number of factors in addition to the types of afferents that are activated.

All of this heterogeneity does not bode well for the development of broadly acting novel analgesics. That is, given our current understanding of the complexity of peripheral pain mechanisms, it seems unlikely that the range of intensities within any one modality (thermal, mechanical) that is encoded by a nociceptor and initiates nociceptive transmission involves only a single voltage- or ligand-gated channel. Similarly, even if the ability to sensitize is one means of functionally defining a peripheral neuron as a nociceptor, the endogenous mediators and factors that contribute to an increase in the excitability of nociceptors (i.e., sensitization) are numerous and synergetic and differ in different pain conditions (e.g., inflammation, nerve injury). A sampling of the complexities and contributors to sensitization are discussed in the following section.

Why include in a clinical textbook of pain management a chapter on peripheral pain mechanisms and nociceptors? There are many reasons. First, in most cases, blockage of peripheral nociceptor activity removes the "drive" for the experience of pain. Further, if a primary goal is to develop mechanism-based strategies for pain management, it is critical that characteristics of a key player—the nociceptor—are fully understood. Finally, nociceptor characteristics change as the local environment in which they reside changes (inflammation, nerve injury, etc.). I discuss in the following section how nociceptors are activated, differ in different tissues, and contribute to the experience of pain and how their behavior changes when they become sensitized. Where possible, we have added relevant clinical examples and have inserted text boxes to elaborate on key issues.

Nociceptor Characteristics

ANATOMY OF THE NOCICEPTOR

As stated earlier, nociceptors are sensory neurons with a cell body located in dorsal root, trigeminal, or nodose ganglia. All sensory neurons arising from these ganglia are pseudo-unipolar neurons with a central process terminating in the central nervous system (e.g., spinal dorsal horn) and a peripheral process terminating in a peripheral target such as the skin, muscle, or viscera. Both central and peripheral processes terminate in a branching pattern referred to as a terminal arbor. The extent of the peripheral arbor depends on the afferent type and site of innervation with the general rule that the higher the spatial resolution for sensory discrimination, the smaller the terminal arbor. In contrast to low-threshold afferents that are responsive to nonnoxious stimuli such as brush or vibration and which terminate in specialized structures, such as Ruffini endings or Merkel disks,[20,21] nociceptors are said to have "free" (unencapsulated) nerve endings because peripheral terminals of these afferents do not appear to be associated with any specific cell type.[22]

Both light and electron micrographic analyses of peripheral nociceptor terminals reveal complex anatomical structures. As suggested earlier, the structure of the terminal arbor varies with target of innervation. There is also evidence that subpopulations of nociceptive afferents have distinct terminal arbor patterns within the same structure. For example, the terminal arbor morphology of cutaneous C fibers varies according to whether the C fiber is peptidergic (i.e., expresses substance P or calcitonin gene-relative peptide) or expresses the MrgprD.[23] On the other hand, the terminal morphology of a subpopulation of high-threshold Aδ fibers that appear to mediate the pain associated with hair pull[24] is similar to that of a subpopulation of low-threshold mechanosensitive Aβ fibers that appear to underlie the sensation of gentle stroking of the skin.[25] Evidence also suggests that distinct but overlapping subpopulations of nociceptors may signal distinct aspects of the painful experience (i.e., sensory/discriminative vs. emotional/motivational),[26] suggesting that it may someday be possible to selectively treat the suffering associated with chronic pain while still enabling patients to appropriately respond to noxious stimuli in their environment.

Four distinct events are necessary for a nociceptor to convey information to the central nervous system about noxious stimuli impinging on peripheral tissues (Fig. 3.1—the events are discussed fully in the following paragraphs). First, "energy" from the stimulus (mechanical, thermal, or chemical) must be converted into an electrical signal. This process, referred to as signal transduction, results in a generator potential or depolarization of the peripheral terminal. Second, the generator potential must initiate an action potential, the rapid "all or nothing" change in membrane potential that constitutes the basic unit of electrical activity in the nervous system. This process is sometimes referred to as transformation. Third, the action potential must be successfully propagated from the peripheral terminal to the central terminal. And fourth, the propagated action potential invading the central terminal must drive a sufficient increase in intracellular calcium ions to enable release of enough transmitter to initiate the whole process once again in the second-order neuron. Distinct sets of proteins underlie each of these processes and are, therefore, the targets of a wide variety of therapeutic interventions.

STIMULUS TRANSDUCTION

An important implication of the fact that nociceptive afferents terminate in "free nerve endings" is that they are not dependent on other cell types for the transduction of a noxious stimulus. That is, proteins responsible for transduction should be intrinsic to the nociceptor. Consistent with this suggestion, isolated sensory neurons are responsive to thermal (both heating[27,28] and cooling[29,30]), mechanical,[31,32] and a wide variety of chemical stimuli, including both endogenous[33,34] and exogenous[35,36] compounds that activate nociceptors in vivo. Proteins involved in the transduction of each stimulus modality have been identified (see Gold[37] for review).

With the exception of transient receptor potential (TRP) channels (see the following discussion), two-pore potassium channels (K2P), and possibly the acid-sensing ion channels (ASICs), chemotransducers are, in general, only activated by chemical stimuli (and not also mechanical or thermal stimuli) and encompass various families of proteins that respond to specific molecules such as adenosine triphosphate (ATP)[38] and protons.[39] There is also compelling evidence to support the suggestion that different members of the TRP superfamily underlie thermal transduction of temperatures ranging from the very cold (TRPA1[40]) to the very hot (TRPV2[41]), with receptors for cool,[42] warm,[43,44] and hot[45] in between. Subsequent research, however, suggests that in contrast to traditional chemoreceptors, TRP family members are not modality-specific as all are activated by specific chemicals[46] and several contribute to mechanical transduction.[32,47,48]

Because the only sensation associated with TRPV1 activation is pain, this receptor has received considerable attention from pain researchers. Data from an array of studies paint a picture of TRPV1 as an excellent example of a polymodal receptor; it is activated by exogenous compounds such as capsaicin and resiniferatoxin, endogenous compounds ranging from protons to lipids, as well as noxious heat.[49] TRPV1 is also present on the central terminals of nociceptive afferents where it also facilitates transmission of noxious mechanical stimuli.[50-52] Furthermore, excessive activation of the receptor with compounds such as capsaicin results in desensitization of the nociceptive terminal to all modes of stimuli, a process that underlies the therapeutic efficacy of topical capsaicin application.[53] More recently, intrathecal application of resiniferatoxin has been used to selectively ablate the central terminals of TRPV1 containing nerve terminals, resulting in a sustained block of nociceptive transmission.[54,55] There is also evidence that TRPV1 receptor antagonists may have some analgesic efficacy, although their therapeutic potential may be limited by a small but significant hyperthermia associated with systemic administration of blood–brain barrier permeable analogs.[53]

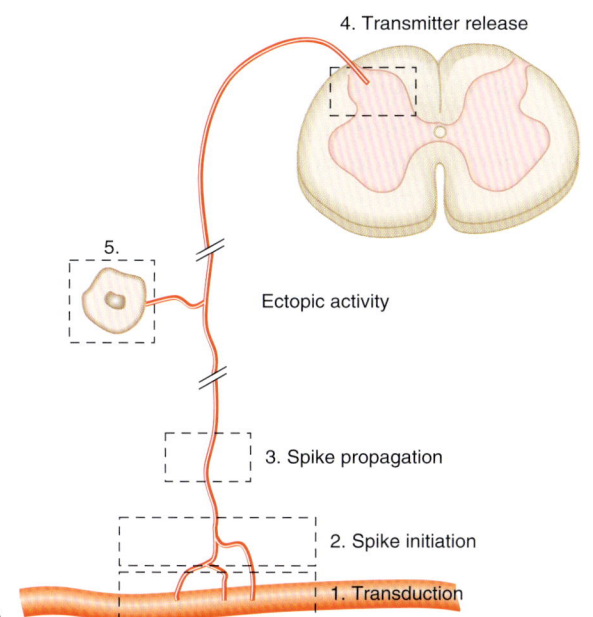

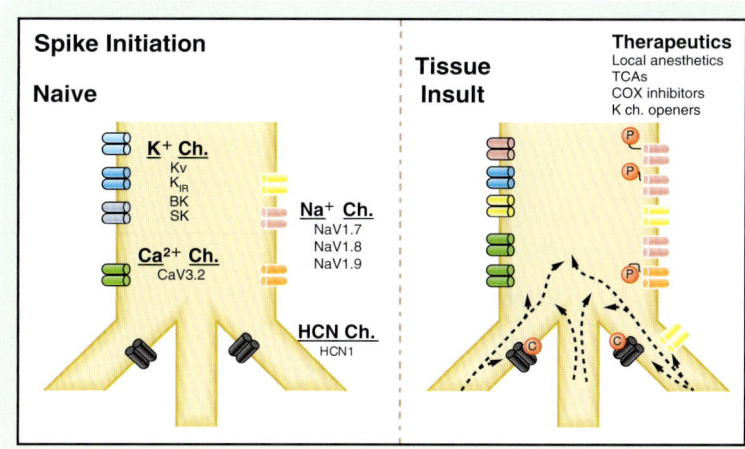

Transduction

FIGURE 3.1 Nociceptive afferents terminate as free nerve endings in skin and other tissues. **A:** Their principal sensory functions consist of (1) transduction of external or internal chemical or physical stimuli into generator potentials, (2) transformation of a generator potential into an action potential, (3) propagation of the action potential toward the central nervous system, and (4) release of neurotransmitters and neuromodulators into the superficial dorsal horn of the spinal cord or brainstem. Nociceptive afferents also release transmitters in the periphery, a process that contributes a neurogenic component to inflammation (not shown). The sensory neuron cell body (soma, 5) appears to be a site critical for the integration of neural activity. Proteins and signaling molecules are delivered to the soma via axonal transport mechanisms (not shown) under normal conditions, which may contribute to aberrant or ectopic activity under pathologic conditions. Many of the proteins responsible for each of these processes, both under normal and pathologic conditions, have been identified. Although not a complete list, several lines of data implicate each of the proteins and mediators illustrated in each subpanel. **B:** Transduction: In naive tissue, proteins thought to play a role in mechanotransduction include transient receptor potential vanilloid type 4 (TRPV4), acid-sensing ion channel type 3 (ASIC-3), and the low-threshold voltage-gated calcium channel (VGCC) CaV3.2. Several different classes of TRP channels are involved in transduction of changes in temperature from noxious cold (TRPA1, ankyrin type 1), cool (TRPM8, melastatin type 8), warm (TRPV4), and hot (TRPV1, vanilloid type 1). Many chemoreceptors are present in nociceptive afferents including those involved in the response to tissue acidosis (TRPV1 and ASIC-3), noxious organic compounds (e.g., aldehydes at TRPA1), and endogenous chemicals (e.g., ATP at P2X3, the ionotropic purine receptor type 3). A wide variety of other receptors for both pro- and anti-inflammatory (not shown) mediators are also present on the terminals of nociceptive afferents. These include G protein-coupled receptors (GPCRs) responsive to E-type prostaglandins (EP), bradykinin (B) types 1 and 2, and serotonin (5-HT) types 1A, 2, and 7. Tyrosine receptor kinases (TRK), responsive to trophic factors such as nerve growth factor (NGF) and artemin, are present as are receptors for cytokines such as TNF-α and interleukin 1-β. Also depicted are transmitters such as ATP stored in epithelial cells. Following tissue insult, there are changes in nociceptive terminals that result in both an increase in sensitivity to noxious stimuli as well as the emergence of membrane depolarization. There are increases in the density of several transducers as well as posttranslational modifications (depicted as phosphorylation, P) that increase channel activity or sensitivity such that the transducers are activated by lower intensity stimuli.

(continued)

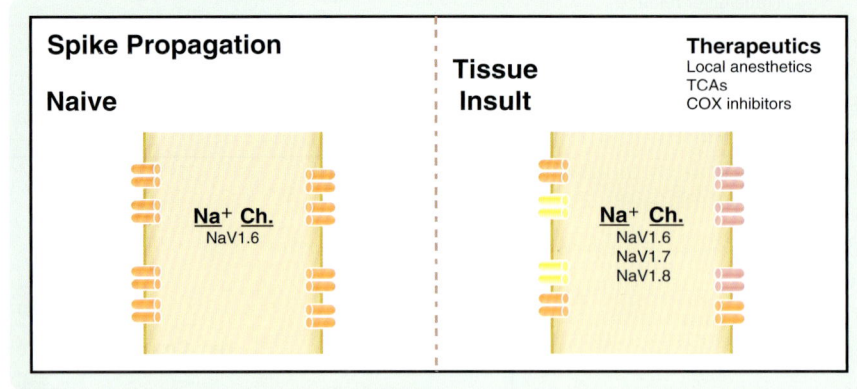

D

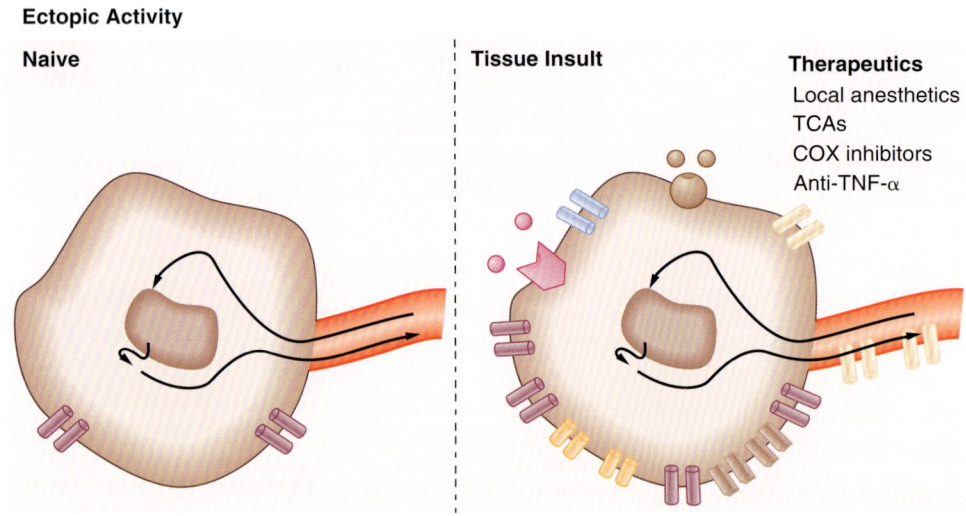

E

FIGURE 3.1 *(continued)* These changes are brought about by actions of inflammatory mediators such as ATP, prostaglandin E2, NGF, and TNF-α that can directly depolarize nociceptive terminals, drive posttranslational changes via the activation of second messenger cascades, and/or alter the expression of transducers via influencing transcription and/or translation. All of these processes may be facilitated as a result of an increase in the release of mediators from epithelial cells, resident (mast) cells, and recruited (macrophages) immune cells. Several therapeutics currently in use or in development act via suppressing the actions of proinflammatory mediators. The specific pattern of changes and mediators depends on many factors, including the type and site of injury, time after injury, and previous history of the injured tissue as well as age and sex, which also influence the relative efficacy of the therapeutic intervention. **C:** Spike initiation: The appropriate anatomical distribution of ion channels is critical for normal function. A number of ion channels play an important role in determining the threshold for spike initiation and upstroke of the spike. Action potential threshold appears to be critically regulated by potassium (K+) channels, which include voltage-gated K+ channels (KV), inward rectifying K+ channels (KIR), two-pore K+ channels (K2P), large-conductance calcium-modulated K+ channels (BK), and small conductance calcium-dependent K+ channels (SK). The nonselective inward rectifying cation channel (HCN) also contributes to action potential threshold. In some cases, the low-threshold calcium channel (CaV3.2) may contribute to action potential threshold, but when present, CaV3.2 appears to play a more prominent role in mediating burst activity. The voltage-gated sodium channel (VGSC) NaV1.9 may also contribute to establishing action potential threshold. Finally, the channels responsible for the upstroke of the action potential include the VGSCs NaV1.7 and NaV1.8. As with transduction, there are a number of changes in ion channels that affect action potential threshold and spike initiation to increase in the excitability of nociceptive afferents in the presence of insult. These changes include a decrease in K+ channel density and/or current and an increase in CaV3.2, HCN, and NaV channel density and/or activity. These changes are the result of both posttranslational modifications and/or changes in transcription driven by the same inflammatory mediators that influence transduction. Thus, several of the therapeutics listed under transduction may also act by inhibiting changes in channels underlying spike initiation. Other drugs may act via direct inhibition of the ion channels underlying spike initiation (which include local anesthetics, tricyclic antidepressants [TCAs], and several cyclooxygenase inhibitors). K+ channel openers such as retigabine may also have efficacy in increasing the threshold for spike initiation. **D:** Action potential propagation: The ion channels underlying action potential propagation are distinct from those underlying spike initiation. The channel most prominently implicated in action potential propagation is the VGSC NaV1.6. In myelinated axons, NaV1.6 is clustered at nodes of Ranvier, whereas in unmyelinated axons, the channel is distributed throughout the axon. Following insult, however, the pattern of channel expression can change, including redistribution of VGSCs NaV1.7 and/or NaV1.8 to the cell membrane. The dependence of action potential propagation on VGSCs confers the therapeutic efficacy of sodium channel blocking compounds such as local anesthetics, TCAs, and some cyclooxygenase (COX) inhibitors. **E:** Ectopic activity: As is true for all neurons in the absence of tissue insult, the soma serves as the supply depot for the rest of the neuron, synthesizing and packaging the proteins, transmitters, and lipids that will be used throughout the cell. Although the soma is capable of generating action potentials and is likely depolarized in response to neural activity in the axons, it is not necessary for action potentials to invade the soma for information to propagate from the periphery to the central nervous system. In nociceptive afferents, the VGSC NaV1.8 can be the primary, if not the only sodium channel in the cell underlying action potential generation. In the presence of nerve injury, however, changes in the soma and/or proximal axon can include an increase in transducer proteins that may make the soma responsive to mechanical, thermal, and chemical stimuli, an increase in sodium channels that may lead to membrane instability (manifesting as oscillatory behavior), and an increase in inflammatory mediators and their receptors. The result of such changes is that the soma and/or proximal axon may become a source of aberrant or ectopic activity. An important implication of this activity is that local administration of therapeutic agents to block activity arising from peripheral terminals may not provide pain relief. Given the source of much of this activity, therapeutic interventions designed to block sodium channels and/or inhibit the actions of inflammatory mediators are predicted to have the greatest efficacy.

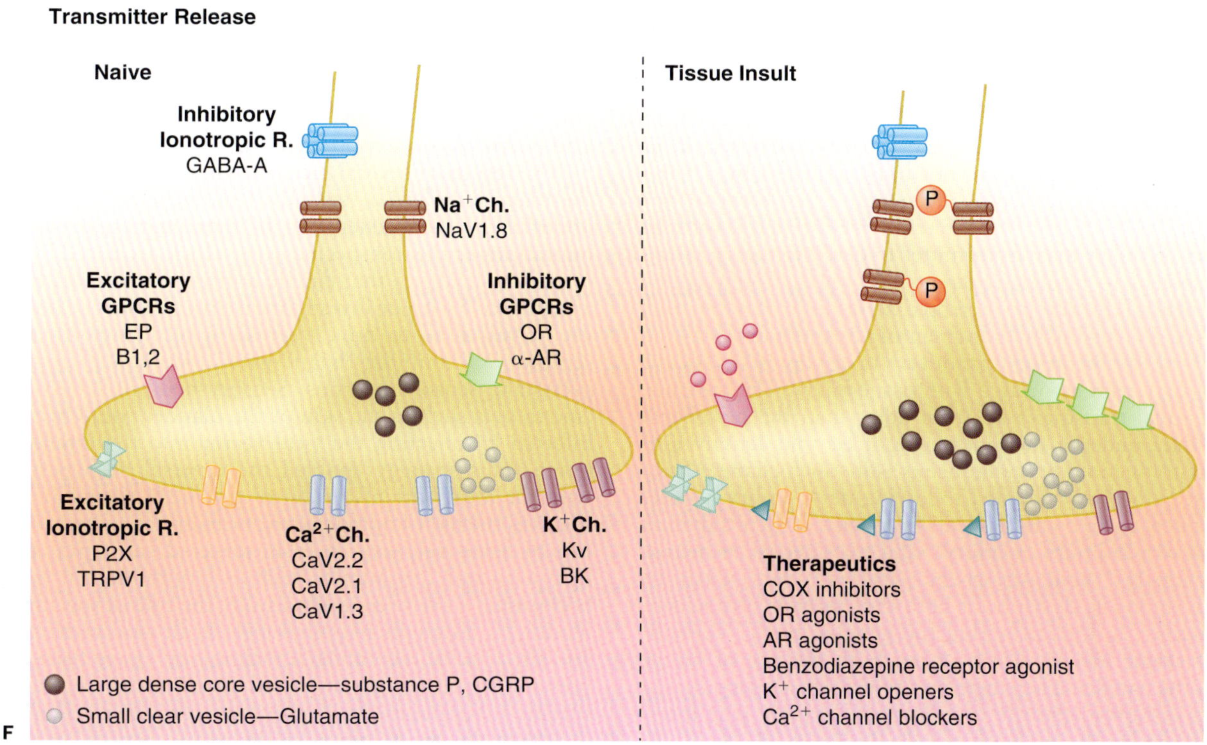

Transmitter Release

FIGURE 3.1 *(continued)* **F:** Transmitter release: The release of transmitter at the central terminals of nociceptive afferents is essential for transmission of nociceptive information to the central nervous system. This process is calcium-dependent—extracellular calcium enters the central terminal generally via high-threshold VGCCs that are activated following invasion of the action potential into the central terminals. N-type channels (CaV2.2) are the most abundant, but P/Q-type (CaV2.1) and L-type (CaV1.3) are also present. CaV2.2 is most readily modulated following activation of inhibitory GPCRs, serving as the primary mechanism for the therapeutic efficacy of intrathecal opioid receptor and alpha adrenergic receptor (α-AR) agonists. Transmitters present in nociceptive afferents are generally packaged in vesicles referred to as small clear vesicles, which generally contain the excitatory amino acid glutamate, and large dense-core vesicles, which contain, among other things, neuropeptides such as substance P and calcitonin gene-related peptide (CGRP). There are a number of excitatory ionotropic receptors, including P2X3 and TRPV1, that appear to facilitate transmitter release from the central terminals. Inhibition of the central terminal may involve activation of voltage-gated (KV) and calcium-modulated (BK) K+ channels. Under normal conditions, presynaptic ionotropic γ-aminobutyric acid (GABA) receptors (GABAA) play a major role in mediating presynaptic inhibition of the central terminals of nociceptive afferents. The VGSC that appears to play a major role in enabling spike invasion of the central terminals of nociceptive afferents is NaV1.8. Finally, excitatory GPCRs (e.g., EP and β1, β2 receptors) are also present. As with other steps in the process, a number of changes occur in the central terminals of nociceptive afferents after tissue insult that contribute to the transmission of nociceptive information. These include an increase in the $\alpha_2\delta_1$ subunit in VGSCs. This subunit is important for trafficking channels to the membrane and, importantly, is a binding site for gabapentin and pregabalin. There is also an increase in neuropeptide expression, the emergence of additional excitatory receptors, modulation of ion channels such as NaV1.8, and a decrease in K+ currents that facilitate nociceptive signaling. Interestingly, there is a growing body of evidence suggesting that there may be changes in GABAA receptor signaling as well such that activation of these receptors may become excitatory secondary to changes in the regulation of intracellular chloride. This issue is complicated by the fact that benzodiazepine receptor agonists may have therapeutic efficacy in the presence of tissue insult which appears to involve, at least in part, activation of presynaptic receptors. From the therapeutic perspective, it is important to note that following tissue insult, in particular that associated with inflammation, there may be an increase in the expression of inhibitory receptors, ultimately facilitating the therapeutic efficacy of opioid and adrenergic receptor agonists. Additional therapeutic interventions may also involve inhibitors of VGCCs, K+ channel openers, and inhibitors to inflammatory mediators.

Of the three modalities of noxious stimuli, molecular mechanisms of mechanotransduction remain the most elusive. Many mechanically sensitive proteins have been identified,[56] but none appears to be both necessary and sufficient for mechanotransduction in nociceptive afferents. Data from null mutant mice, where the deletion of a single putative mechanotransducer results in an increase in mechanosensitivity in one population of afferents and a decrease in others,[57–59] suggests that several different proteins are likely to work together in specific subpopulations of afferents to enable responses to specific forms of mechanical stimuli (e.g., stretch or compression). This picture is complicated further by the observation that some mechanotransducers such as piezo2 contribute to mechanotransduction in specific subsets of sensory neurons.[60] That even these more specialized forms of mechanosensitivity reflect intrinsic properties of afferents are suggested by the emergence of mechanosensitivity at the severed ends of a subpopulation of axons

within hours of transection.[61] Despite the slow progress in this area, identification of a nociceptor specific mechanotransducer blocker remains an active area of investigation because of its therapeutic potential in light of the fact that mechanical hypersensitivity is the primary complaint associated with the vast majority of chronic pain syndromes.[62–64]

Whereas mechanotransduction is an intrinsic property of many nociceptors, there is evidence that epithelial cells may also be mechanosensitive.[65–67] Because these cells may store and release transmitters such as ATP, it has been suggested that afferent activity evoked with mechanical stimulation of peripheral structures such as the bladder,[65] gastrointestinal tract,[68] and skin[66,67,69] may be secondary to the transduction event that has occurred in the epithelial cell that subsequently releases a chemical mediator capable of activating nearby nociceptor terminals. The implication of this mechanism from a therapeutic perspective is that it may be possible to attenuate mechanical hypersensitivity in several peripheral tissues with the appropriate antagonist of the responsible chemoreceptors on nociceptive afferents.[70] Consistent with this idea, there is evidence that mechanical hypersensitivity observed in several visceral structures can be attenuated with ATP receptor antagonists.[71] That a similar mechanism may contribute to chemotransduction, at least in the intestine, was recently suggested by the observation that enterochromaffin cells are not only activated by a variety of chemicals but are electrically excitable and form synaptic connections with primary afferents.[72] However, serotonin appears to be the primary transmitter underlying the signaling from these cells to primary afferents, possibly accounting for the therapeutic efficacy of inotropic serotonin receptor (i.e., 5-HT3) antagonists for the treatment of visceral pain[73]

Aberrant expression of transducers may play a significant role in chronic pain associated with tissue injury. The presence of a functional transducer at a site other than the peripheral terminal may underlie the emergence of ectopic activity and contribute to ongoing or spontaneous pain. Such changes have been most extensively detailed following nerve injury, where, as mentioned earlier, mechanical sensitivity is detectable in cut axons within hours of injury[61] and may persist in neuromas indefinitely.[74] Similarly, chemosensitivity, particularly to adrenergic agonists, develops at both the cut ends of nociceptive afferents[75] as well as within the ganglia itself,[76] contributing to ectopic activity arising from both the site of injury and from the ganglia. The emergence of ectopic activity arising from sites distant to the site of injury may explain why interventions targeting the site of injury are unsuccessful.

PASSIVE ELECTROPHYSIOLOGIC PROPERTIES AND THE SPREAD OF THE GENERATOR POTENTIAL

A generator potential at a primary afferent terminal ending is not equivalent to an action potential propagated along that afferent's axon. The generator potential decays over distance from the point of origin as a function of membrane resistance, membrane capacitance, and internal resistance of the nerve terminal and may or may not be propagated beyond the terminal ending. Generally considered stable properties, there is evidence for dynamic remodeling of the terminal arbor of central nervous system neurons[77] which may influence both membrane capacitance and internal resistance; it remains to be determined whether such changes may also impact passive conduction of generator potentials in peripheral terminals. In contrast, a number of ion channels have been identified that may establish resting membrane resistance and therefore the spread of the generator potential within the terminal arbor.[78] This issue is important to nociceptive signaling because action potential initiation does not always occur at the site of stimulus transduction.[79] Consequently, the magnitude of the generator potential at the site of action potential initiation must be greater than or equal to action potential threshold. Thus, at least in some fiber types, it may be possible to block nociceptor signaling and therefore pain, with manipulations such as the local administration of potassium (K^+) channels openers[80,81] that decrease membrane resistance and therefore spread the generator potential.

Although ion channels have been the focus of research into mechanisms controlling neuronal excitability of peripheral neurons, recent evidence suggests that ion pumps and exchangers may contribute as well. Some pumps and exchangers, such as the sodium/potassium ATPase and the sodium/calcium exchanger, are electrogenic; that is, they generate net flux of ions when active and therefore may contribute directly to resting membrane potential and consequently neuronal excitability. They may also contribute indirectly, via an influence on intracellular ion concentrations and consequently the activity and/or actions of other ion channels. For example, the sodium/calcium exchanger, and the calcium ATPase control intracellular calcium

levels in sensory neurons,[82,83] and intracellular calcium influences activity of calcium,[84] potassium,[85] and chloride[86] channels in sensory neurons. Conversely, the sodium/potassium/chloride cotransporter and the bicarbonate/chloride exchangers in sensory neurons influence intracellular chloride concentrations, which, in turn, influence the impact of type A γ-aminobutyric acid (GABAA) on sensory neurons.[87]

The results of several recent studies suggest that influencing the magnitude and/or spread of the generator potential may underlie the next generation of therapeutics. Because of the limitations of the nonspecific nerve block produced by local anesthetics, strategies that enable a more selective afferent block are an active area of investigation. In one such strategy, a viral vector was used to drive expression of an ionotropic glycine receptor, an inhibitory ligand-gated ion channel not normally present in sensory neurons. Sensory neurons innervating specific targets such as the skin or the bladder could be selectively infected by injecting the viral vector into the intended target tissue. This strategy enabled the reversal of hypersensitivity with the local administration of glycine.[88] A similar approach involves the use of optogenetics, or light-activated proteins that can be selectively expressed in targeted cell types. Inhibitory light-activated ion pumps, such as halorhodopsin or archaerhodopsin,[89] have been used to study the role of specific subpopulations of afferents in pain, where both viral vector-based[90–92] and site-specific recombinase technology[93] have been used. Expression of these light-activated proteins can be restricted to specific subpopulations of afferents via a variety of approaches including the site of infection, the virus serotype used,[90] as well as cell-specific promoters.[92] Given the spatial and temporal control of the afferent inhibition afforded by these strategies, combined with the ability to selectively target subpopulations of afferents, the therapeutic potential is tremendous.

ACTION POTENTIAL GENERATION

VGSCs are responsible for the upstroke of the action potential in virtually all excitable tissue. As their name implies, these channels are gated (opened and closed) by changes in membrane potential. VGSCs are generally composed of an α subunit and up to two β subunits. The α subunit is a large molecule (~200 kD) that contains all features necessary for a functional channel including voltage sensor, ion selectivity filter, channel pore, and inactivation gate.[94] Ten α subunits have been identified, nine of which form functional channels in heterologous expression systems. The channels encoded by each of these subunits can be distinguished by a combination of pharmacologic and biophysical properties. Eight of these nine α subunits are present in the nervous system, all eight of which are present in nociceptive afferents[95] at one point during development, with six of these detectable in the adult.[96] β Subunits influence channel gating properties as well as trafficking and localization in the plasma membrane.[97] Four β subunits have been identified, at least three of which are present in nociceptive afferents.[95]

The VGSC α subunit primarily responsible for action potential initiation in the majority of nociceptors is NaV1.8. This subunit is unique in several ways. First, it is normally only expressed in primary afferents[98,99] where it is primarily expressed in nociceptors.[100] This unique pattern of distribution, in combination with its primary function in spike initiation, makes it an ideal target for novel therapeutics.[101] Although in no way mitigating the therapeutic potential of this channel, recent evidence suggests that it may contribute to action potential propagation in the distal peripheral axon in addition to its role in action potential initiation.[102] Second, NaV1.8 has a relatively high threshold for activation. Whereas many other VGSCs begin to activate at membrane potentials between −50 and −40 mV, a depolarization to −30 mV or greater is necessary to activate NaV1.8.[103] This feature may explain, at least in part, why greater intensity stimuli are generally needed for nociceptor activation. Third, NaV1.8 is relatively resistant to steady-state inactivation, a voltage-dependent process whereby channels residing in a closed or resting state transition to an inactive state before they ever get a chance to open. Recovery from the inactivated state requires membrane hyperpolarization; thus, inactivated channels cannot contribute to the upstroke of the action potential. Even a small sustained depolarization to −50 mV can inactivate virtually all other VGSCs. However, NaV1.8 is still fully available for activation at this membrane potential.[103] Fourth, NaV1.8 recovers from inactivation rapidly.[104] These last two features enable the channel to underlie sustained activity in the face of a persistent depolarization that might be observed in the presence of inflammatory mediators. Fifth, NaV1.8 is resistant to cooling-induced inactivation.[105] Other VGSCs are completely inactivated at temperatures at or below 18° C. However, NaV1.8 is still functional at temperatures down to 4° C, enabling the burning pain associated with noxious cold stimuli. Sixth, in contrast to all but one other VGSC α subunit (NaV1.9), NaV1.8 is resistant to TTX and is therefore referred to as a TTX-resistant channel.

Whereas NaV1.8 is critical for action potential initiation in nociceptors, data from the study of rodent sensory neurons suggests that in many of these afferents, NaV1.8 works in concert with another VGSC α subunit, NaV1.7.[106] The NaV1.7 subunit has unique features enabling it to play a significant role in spike initiation.[107] That this channel may play a critical role in nociceptor activity is suggested by the recent discovery of individuals possessing both gain-of-function and loss-of-function point mutations in this subunit. Strikingly, two distinct pain syndromes—primary erythermalgia (PE) and paroxysmal extreme pain disorder (PEPD)—reveal the specific impact of gain-of-function mutations.[108] PE is associated with burning pain in the hands and feet, and PEPD is initially associated with pain in the rectum that ultimately progresses to include trigeminal structures including the eye and jaw. The unique distribution of these pain syndromes, in light of the widespread distribution of NaV1.7 in the peripheral nervous system as well as neuroendocrine tissues, highlights the importance of other channels in sculpting the response properties of sensory neurons. Furthermore, in contrast to the impact of the gain-of-function mutations, loss-of-function mutations that result in nonfunctional channels are associated with a complete insensitivity to pain.[109] Although the data from patients with these rare genetic mutations is intriguing, recent evidence suggests the role of NaV1.7 in nociceptive processing may be more complicated than originally anticipated. That is, evidence from null mutant mice suggests that the loss of function phenotype may not only involve sympathetic postganglionic neurons[110] but a compensatory upregulation of the endogenous opioid enkephalin in primary afferents.[111] Furthermore, electrophysiologic analysis of nociceptive afferents in patients with gain-of-function mutations in these channels suggests that at least at rest, the afferents are hypoexcitable.[112] These observations raise the possibility that the pain phenotypes associated with mutations in NaV1.7 reflect developmental processes independent of any ongoing influence of the channel in controlling afferent excitability. Furthermore, in contrast to isolated sensory neurons from the rat, where NaV1.7 appears to contribute to action potential initiation, recent evidence suggests that this may not be the case in human sensory neurons.[113]

Low voltage–activated, or T-type, calcium channels may also contribute to spike initiation in the periphery.[114] Whereas there is compelling evidence that these channels are present in high density in low-threshold D-hair afferents,[115] there is also evidence that they may be present in a subpopulation of nociceptors as well.[116] The biophysical properties of these channels enable them to play a particularly important role in mediating bursting activity, as the channels underlie a sustained membrane depolarization after a single action potential that provides the driving force for the initiation of subsequent action potentials.[117] This feature has led some to speculate that selective T-type channel blockers may be particularly effective for treating paroxysmal pain[116] such as that associated with trigeminal neuralgia.

The focus on NaV1.8 has been on its role in action potential initiation in the periphery. Nevertheless, there is also evidence that the channels are present and functional at central nociceptor terminals.[118,119] At the central terminal, the channel appears to facilitate the spread of the invading action potential throughout the terminal arbor and consequently the release of transmitter from the primary afferent. There is also a growing body of evidence suggesting that action potentials may also be initiated at the central terminals of nociceptors, where they are conducted antidromically to the periphery.[120] This activity, referred to as the dorsal root reflex, appears to play a significant role in the neurogenic inflammation that develops following tissue injury.

ACTION POTENTIAL PROPAGATION

NaV1.8 and NaV1.7 underlie action potential generation and even propagation over the first 5 to 10 mm of peripheral axon. However, a different set of VGSCs underlies action potential propagation into the central nervous system in the absence of tissue injury. NaV1.6 appears to be the subunit primarily responsible for propagation in both myelinated and unmyelinated axons of both nociceptive and nonnociceptive afferents,[121] although data from a small molecule inhibitor of NaV1.7 suggests this channel may contribute to action potential conduction as well[122] (but see Zhang et al.[113] for data suggesting this channel may not be as selective as originally thought). Unfortunately, the distribution of NaV1.6 in the peripheral nervous system in combination with its widespread expression in the central nervous system precludes selective block of propagation in nociceptors via a NaV1.6 specific mechanism. Nevertheless, block of these channels with local anesthetics and/or TTX, or more recently small interfering RNA knockdown,[123] remains an effective means of blocking input into the central nervous system.

TRANSMITTER RELEASE

Voltage-gated calcium channels (VGCC) are primarily responsible for the initial influx of calcium necessary for initiation of machinery underlying the release of neurotransmitters. Like VGSCs, these multisubunit channels consist of a large α subunit that contains all of the features necessary for a functional channel as well as a β subunit. Ten α subunits have been identified, encoding channels that are commonly defined by their threshold for activation or pharmacologic properties.[124] T-type channels (CaV3.1 to CaV3.3), as mentioned earlier, have a low threshold for activation, whereas all others have a high threshold for activation. The high-threshold channels are further subdivided based on their sensitivity to specific channel blockers: L-type channels (CaV1.1 to CaV1.4) are blocked by dihydropyridines such as nimodipine, N-type channels (CaV2.2) are blocked by the snail toxin ω-conotoxin GVIA, P/Q-type channels (CaV2.1) are blocked by the spider toxin ω-agatoxin IVA, and R-type channels (CaV2.3) are blocked by the spider toxin SNX-482.[125] In contrast to VGSCs, VGCCs are not effectively targeted to the plasma membrane in the absence of the $\alpha_2\delta$ subunit complex.[126] A single β subunit also appears to be important for efficient gating.[127] All VGCC subtypes are present in nociceptors. And whereas there is evidence that all high-threshold calcium channels may contribute to transmitter release, N-type channels appear to play a dominant role in the release of transmitter from nociceptors.[128]

The dominant role N-type channels play in mediating transmitter release from nociceptive afferent terminals makes them an ideal target for both endogenous and exogenous analgesics. Opioid and adrenergic receptor agonists act through inhibitory G protein-coupled receptors which enable inhibition of VGCCs via two major intracellular pathways. The first is a rapid, membrane delimited pathway involving G protein βγ-subunit displacement of the VGCC β subunit, resulting in a "sleepy" or "unwilling" channel that requires a larger membrane depolarization for channel opening.[127] The second pathway involves more traditional second messenger kinase dependent signaling with a slower onset and offset.[129] Interestingly, neither pathway results in complete VGCC block, yet both result in a dramatic inhibition of transmitter release. This amplification effect reflects the fact that there is considerable cooperativity of calcium in mediating vesicle fusion to the cell membrane that is necessary for transmitter release; four to five calcium ions are needed to trigger vesicle fusion.[130] This amplification effect is also likely to facilitate the use of relatively low concentrations of the N-type channel blocker SNX-111 (Prialt), enabling the block of transmitter release from nociceptive afferent terminals in the superficial dorsal horn while minimizing side effects associated with block of channels at more distant sites. Finally, although additional mechanisms likely contribute to the therapeutic efficacy of drugs like gabapentin and pregabalin, that have been shown to bind to the $\alpha_2\delta$ subunit, the most compelling model involves the inhibition of membrane trafficking of the α subunit. That is, following nerve injury, there is a dramatic increase in $\alpha_2\delta_1$ subunit expression in nociceptive afferents.[131] This increase in expression appears to facilitate the trafficking of VGCC α subunits to nociceptive afferent central terminals, which in turn, appears to facilitate transmitter release and consequently the increase in pain associated with nerve injury. These compounds block the increase in α subunit trafficking via an $\alpha_2\delta_1$-dependent mechanism.[132]

Although VGCCs play a dominant, if not essential, role in the increase in intracellular calcium needed for transmitter release, recent evidence suggests other calcium regulatory proteins contribute to the regulation of the amplitude and duration of the increase in intracellular calcium and, consequently, transmitter release. These include the sarco-endoplasmic reticulum ATPase/ryanodine receptor system,[133,134] the plasma membrane calcium ATPase,[135] mitochondria,[135] and the sodium/calcium exchanger.[83] Consistent with the suggestion, these calcium regulatory proteins influence nociception, selective genetic knockdown of the sodium/calcium exchanger, a regulatory protein that attenuates the calcium transient, in a subpopulation of nociceptive afferents decreases nociceptive threshold.[83]

Nociceptor Sensitization

Sensitization is a characterizing feature of nociceptors; nonnociceptors do not sensitize following tissue insult. Sensitization represents an increase in nociceptor excitability, which is expressed and defined as an increase in response to a noxious stimulus. Sensitization is also typically accompanied by a reduction in the threshold for activation and occasionally by the development of ongoing, spontaneous activity. Nociceptor sensitization is the cause of primary hyperalgesia (i.e., increased pain produced by stimulation at the site of tissue insult) and is important because nociceptor sensitization is the trigger for initiation of an increase in excitability of central neurons in the nociceptive pathway, an event termed *central sensitization*.

An increase in nociceptor excitability is a reflection of changes in the behavior of nociceptor voltage- and/or ligand-gated ion channels produced by actions of endogenous substances either released or synthesized at the site of tissue insult or attracted there. Endogenous substances considered classically to contribute

to sensitization include products of arachidonic acid metabolism (e.g., prostaglandin E2 [PGE$_2$]), histamine, serotonin, protons and ATP, but the list has grown quite extensively and now also includes cytokines, chemokines, growth factors, peptides, etc., some of which are released from immune competent cells attracted to the site of insult (e.g., macrophages), from nearby cells (e.g., mast cells), or from nociceptor (and other) nerve terminals (e.g., peptides). Interestingly, despite the variety of mediators capable of producing nociceptor sensitization, several appear to play particularly important roles. This list includes prostanoids, as evidenced by the antihyperalgesic efficacy of nonsteroidal anti-inflammatory drugs (NSAIDs) that act via inhibition of cyclooxygenase and thus prostanoid synthesis.[136,137] More recently, the importance of tumor necrosis factor alpha (TNF-α) in chronic inflammatory conditions has been highlighted by the antinociceptive efficacy of compounds such as etanercept which are designed to bind and inactivate TNF-α released at sites of inflammation.[138,139] Finally, nerve growth factor (NGF) appears to play a major role in orchestrating a variety of signaling cascades necessary for an inflammatory response and therefore has also been targeted with antibody-based strategies.[140–144]

The mechanisms that trigger changes in nociceptor excitability are not fully known. A growing body of evidence suggests that despite what appears to be a bewildering assortment of mediators and membrane receptors, there are a relatively small number of intracellular pathways that underlie their actions. For example, both prostaglandins and bradykinin, which are among the most extensively studied inflammatory mediators, act at G protein-coupled receptors. Two major G protein-dependent pathways have been implicated. One involves a stimulatory G protein, Gs, which drives activation of adenylate cyclase, resulting in an increase in cyclic adenosine monophosphate (cAMP) and the activation of protein kinase A (PKA).[145,146] The other involves a Gq-dependent pathway, resulting in the activation of phospholipase C, the liberation of diacylglycerol (DAG) and IP3, and the subsequent activation of protein kinase C (PKC).[147,148] The PKC-ε isoform appears to play a particularly important role in nociceptor sensitization. Other mediators that appear to play important roles in nociceptor sensitization, such as TNF-α and interleukin (IL) 1β, utilize a mitogen-activated protein kinase (MAPK)-dependent pathway ultimately resulting in the activation of p38.[149] Still other mediators directly activate ion channels. For example, protons (which increase in concentration during inflammation) act at TRPV1 and ASICs. ASIC-3 is important to pain associated with ischemia, such as that which occurs during angina, and deep muscle pain where protons and lactic acid accumulate. In contrast, ATP and its metabolites act at ionotropic P2X and metabotropic P2Y receptors to modulate nociceptor excitability.

The relatively novel, if not paradoxical, mechanism of sensitization involving ionotropic GABAA receptors that we described in the action potential generation section serves as an example of the dynamic interplay between second messenger signaling cascades and the regulation of ion channels. Activation of these receptors are normally inhibitory, even in nociceptive afferents where they drive membrane depolarization, because of the relatively high intracellular chloride concentration maintained in these neurons.[150] The GABAA-mediated depolarization in these neurons is inhibitory, as suggested earlier, because of the decrease in membrane resistance, referred to as shunting, as well as the depolarization-induced activation of low-threshold voltage-gated potassium channels.[151] In the presence of persistent inflammation, there is a constitutive shift in the balance of tyrosine kinase to tyrosine phosphatase activity, such that there is a net increase in protein phosphorylation. This increase results in a net increase in functional GABAA receptors in the plasma membrane because of a decrease in receptor internalization.[152]

The result is an increase in GABA-evoked current and an increase in the magnitude of the GABA-evoked depolarization. These changes are further augmented by a decrease in the density of low-threshold potassium current.[151] The result is a shift in GABA signaling, from inhibition to excitation.

This picture gets a little more complicated when one considers the ceramide/sphingosine 1-phosphate (S1P) system because ceramide, a potent proinflammatory sphingolipid-generated de novo from hydrolysis of sphingomyelin or synthesis from serine and palmityl CoA, can directly activate protein kinases and phosphatases as well as serve as a precursor to S1P, which acts via G protein-coupled receptors to sensitize nociceptive neurons.[153] And although a common set of second messengers, including phosphatidylinositol 3-kinase, phospholipase Cγ, and extracellular signal-regulated kinase (ERK), underlie the acute sensitizing actions of trophic factors such as NGF, these mediators signal via a distinct class of receptors that contain intrinsic tyrosine kinase activity, referred to as tropomyosin receptor kinase, or Trk receptors.[154] Channels underlying transduction and spike initiation, in particular TRPV1 and NaV1.8, respectively, appear to be final common targets for this diverse array of mediators and second messenger pathways.[155] Phosphorylation of specific residues on the channel or associated proteins results in increases in channel density and/or increases in channel function. Importantly, many inflammatory mediators including ceramide/SP1 and NGF drive long-term increases in nociceptor excitability via changes in gene expression, and mechanisms contributing to long-term changes in gene expression, such as alterations in DNA acetylation and methylation, have emerged as potential therapeutic targets.[156,157]

Although mechanisms underlying changes in gene expression associated with the emergence of persistent pain have received considerable attention, there is a growing body of evidence suggesting that changes in protein translation are also important. One of the first studies to implicate a change in the regulation of protein translation per se in manifestation of persistent pain was focused on the role of TRPV1 in persistent inflammatory pain. The authors observed that inflammation is associated with an increase in TRPV1 protein in the absence of a detectable increase in messenger RNA.[158] It was subsequently demonstrated that inflammatory mediators such as NGF and IL-6 could rapidly increase protein translation via the phosphorylation of proteins responsible for control over the rate-limiting step of protein translation, that of the initiation of protein synthesis.[159] The protein initiation step involves the assembly of a complex of eukaryotic initiation factors (eIF) eIF4E and G among others, as well as the dissociation of the eIF4E binding protein (4BP), from eIF4E. At least two distinct signaling pathways have been identified underlying the actions of NGF and IL-6. In addition to the activation of PI3K, NGF activation of TrkA drives the activation of PI3K which subsequently activates Akt (also known as protein kinase B). Akt then activates the mammalian target of rapamycin (mTOR), which facilitates the initiation of translation via facilitating the dissociation of 4BP from eIEF4E, as well as the activation of eIF4G, via the phosphorylation of both proteins. In contrast, IL-6 drives the activation of ERK, which subsequently activates MAP-kinase interacting kinase (MNK), which facilitates the initiation of translation via the phosphorylation of eIF4E (which facilitates the eIF4E/G complex formation).[159] Interestingly, this rapid regulation of translation contributes not only to the magnitude and duration of both the mechanical and thermal hypersensitivity associated with acute inflammation and the actions of inflammatory mediators like NGF and IL-6 but also the manifestation of more persistent changes in nociceptive processing, referred to as hyperalgesic priming.[160]

Hyperalgesic priming is the term used to describe the changes in nociceptive processing associated with an initial inflammatory insult, such as that associated with the subcutaneous injection of carrageenan, or inflammatory mediators such as IL-6.[148] These changes were manifest up to weeks after the complete resolution of hypersensitivity associated with the initiating stimulus and were most prominently manifest as a dramatic increase in the duration of the hypersensitivity associated with a subsequent challenge, although an increase in the magnitude of the hypersensitivity has also been described. That is, although the intradermal injection of PGE$_2$ into naive skin results in a relatively transient hypersensitivity lasting ~1 hour, the same injection into primed skin results in hypersensitivity detectable for more than 24 hours. This phenomenon has been proposed to contribute to the transition from acute to chronic pain.[161]

In the context of a discussion of mechanisms underlying nociceptor sensitization, the mechanisms implicated in the manifestation of hyperalgesic priming are notable for several reasons. First, although there are data suggesting changes within the central nervous system, notably involving a descending dopaminergic input to the superficial dorsal horn, contribute to the manifestation of hyperalgesic priming,[162] the bulk of data generated so far suggest that changes in nociceptive afferents may play a critical role in the emergence of chronic pain. Second, as further evidence of the differential role of distinct subpopulations of nociceptive afferents in nociceptive signaling, two distinct forms of hyperalgesic priming have been described, where type I depends on a subpopulation of neurons that do not express the neuropeptides calcitonin gene-related peptide (CGRP) or substance P and bind the plant lectin IB4,[163] whereas type II depends on a subpopulation of neurons that do express these neuropeptides and do not bind IB4.[164] Third, there appear to be sex differences in the mechanisms underlying both the initiation (type I)[165] and maintenance (type II)[164] of the primed state. And fourth, although a cAMP response element binding protein (CREB)-dependent change in gene expression appears to be necessary for the *establishment* of the primed state, local translation appears to be critical for the *manifestation* of the more robust response observed in primed state, at least for type I priming.[166] Given the length of some nociceptive afferents, in particular those innervating the distal appendages, local control of translation may prove to be an important therapeutic target for the treatment of pain.

Clinical Implications of Nociceptor Function

As researchers have begun to explore the basis for chronic pain syndromes generally associated with specific body regions and/or organs (e.g., temporomandibular joint disorder [TMJD], inflammatory bowel disease [IBD], irritable bowel syndrome [IBS], or painful bladder syndrome [formerly interstitial cystitis or IC]), a number of common themes have emerged that are likely to impact future treatment approaches. First, specific mechanisms underlying injury-induced sensitization of nociceptors vary as a function of target of innervation. For example, inflammation-induced sensitization of masseter muscle afferents appears to reflect a decrease in a specific subpopulation of voltage-gated potassium channels.[167] The same channels do not appear to contribute to the sensitization of TMJ afferents.[168] Similarly, inflammation-induced increases in the excitability of bladder sensory neurons appear to reflect one pattern of changes in voltage-gated[169] ion channels, whereas the inflammation-induced increase in the excitability of sensory neurons innervating the stomach,[170–172] ileum,[173,174] or colon[175] reflect other patterns. Although tissue-specific patterns of inflammation may contribute to these differences between subpopulations of afferents, differences persist when the response to inflammatory mediators is studied in vitro.[176,177] These observations imply that it may be possible, if not necessary, to treat pain arising from a specific structure with a specific intervention. Second, specific mechanisms underlying insult-induced sensitization of nociceptors also vary as a function of the type of insult. For example, acute phosphorylation-dependent modulation of the voltage-gated sodium channel NaV1.8 results in an increase in current which contributes to an inflammation-induced increase in nociceptor excitability.[178,179] In contrast, following traumatic nerve injury, redistribution of NaV1.8 to the axons of uninjured afferents appears to be necessary for the expression of mechanical hypersensitivity associated with nerve injury.[180] The dynamic allodynia that often develops after nerve injury, however, likely represents more than only a redistribution of NaV1.8 (Box 3.2).

With respect to the viscera, because each organ receives innervation from two nerves, the effect of organ insult can be different in the two groups of sensory neurons that innervate the organ (e.g., Wang et al.,[181] Traub[182]). These observations underscore the importance of developing diagnostic criteria that enable identification of the factors primarily responsible for ongoing pain. Third, as clearly indicated by the discussion of hyperalgesic priming, the history of the nociceptor influences the response to subsequent challenge. Furthermore, there is evidence of a developmental window within which injury may produce permanent changes in nociceptors.[183,184] With the development of more specific therapeutic tools, patient history may become a critical factor in the identification of the most appropriate intervention. Fourth, there is evidence for sex differences in both the excitability of different groups of nociceptors[185] as well as the response to tissue injury.[186,187] These differences appear to be mediated, at least in part, through the actions of gonadal hormones and may contribute to sex differences in the manifestation of a number of chronic pain syndromes. There is also evidence for age-dependent changes in nociceptor function.[188] Given the ever-growing proportion of aging adults, this particular issue in is need of further investigation. Finally, all of these factors interact with what are clearly genetic differences in pain and analgesic mechanisms.[189]

As indicated earlier, the consequences of tissue insult are not limited only to changes in the excitability of nociceptors and the awakening of sleeping nociceptors. Because sensitization leads to an increased response to noxious stimuli and a decrease in response threshold, previously nonnoxious intensities of stimulation also are now able to activate nociceptors. In addition, spontaneous activity may develop. In the aggregate, central nervous system input from sensitized nociceptors, awakened sleeping nociceptors, and spontaneously active nociceptors is significantly increased. For example, approximately 24% of human cutaneous C fibers are sleeping nociceptors,[190] comprising significant new input to the central nervous system if awakened. Consequently, the amount of neurotransmitters (as well as perhaps their relative proportions) released onto central neurons is increased, which in turn alters the excitability of central neurons. The increase in excitability of central neurons is manifest as an increase in the size of the cutaneous receptive field (i.e., secondary hyperalgesia) or area of tenderness referred from deep structures, particularly the viscera. Although the principal focus of study of mechanisms of central sensitization has been the spinal cord, it should be appreciated that nociceptor-driven changes in central excitability extend throughout the central nervous system.

References

1. Torebjork E. Nociceptor activation and pain. *Philos Trans R Soc Lond B Biol Sci* 1985;308(1136):227–234.
2. Torebjork E. Human microneurography and intraneural microstimulation in the study of neuropathic pain. *Muscle Nerve* 1993;16(10):1063–1065.
3. McGuire C, Boundouki G, Hockley JRF, et al. Ex vivo study of human visceral nociceptors. *Gut* 2018;67:86–96.
4. Hockley JR, Tranter MM, McGuire C, et al. P2Y receptors sensitize mouse and human colonic nociceptors. *J Neurosci* 2016;36(8):2364–2376.
5. Weidner C, Schmelz M, Schmidt R, et al. Functional attributes discriminating mechano-insensitive and mechano-responsive C nociceptors in human skin. *J Neurosci* 1999;19(22):10184–10190.
6. Goswami SC, Thierry-Mieg D, Thierry-Mieg J, et al. Itch-associated peptides: RNA-Seq and bioinformatic analysis of natriuretic precursor peptide B and gastrin releasing peptide in dorsal root and trigeminal ganglia, and the spinal cord. *Mol Pain* 2014;10:44.
7. Hu G, Huang K, Hu Y, et al. Single-cell RNA-seq reveals distinct injury responses in different types of DRG sensory neurons. *Sci Rep* 2016;6:31851.
8. Djouhri L, Lawson SN. Abeta-fiber nociceptive primary afferent neurons: a review of incidence and properties in relation to other afferent A-fiber neurons in mammals. *Brain Res Brain Res Rev* 2004;46(2):131–145.
9. La JH, Feng B, Kaji K, et al. Roles of isolectin B4-binding afferents in colorectal mechanical nociception. *Pain* 2016;157(2):348–354.
10. Usoskin D, Furlan A, Islam S, et al. Unbiased classification of sensory neuron types by large-scale single-cell RNA sequencing. *Nat Neurosci* 2015;18(1):145–153.
11. Feng B, La JH, Schwartz ES, et al. Long-term sensitization of mechanosensitive and -insensitive afferents in mice with persistent colorectal hypersensitivity. *Am J Physiol Gastrointest Liver Physiol* 2012;302(7):G676–G683.
12. Wooten M, Weng HJ, Hartke TV, et al. Three functionally distinct classes of C-fibre nociceptors in primates. *Nat Commun* 2014;5:4122.
13. Weng Y, Batista-Schepman PA, Barabas ME, et al. Prostaglandin metabolite induces inhibition of TRPA1 and channel-dependent nociception. *Mol Pain* 2012;8:75.
14. Giniatullin R, Nistri A. Desensitization properties of P2X3 receptors shaping pain signaling. *Front Cell Neurosci* 2013;7:245.
15. Lukacs V, Yudin Y, Hammond GR, et al. Distinctive changes in plasma membrane phosphoinositides underlie differential regulation of TRPV1 in nociceptive neurons. *J Neurosci* 2013;33(28):11451–11463.
16. Smith TP, Smith SN, Sweitzer SM. Endothelin-1 induced desensitization in primary afferent neurons. *Neurosci Lett* 2014;582:59–64.
17. Rau KK, McIlwrath SL, Wang H, et al. Mrgprd enhances excitability in specific populations of cutaneous murine polymodal nociceptors. *J Neurosci* 2009;29(26):8612–8619.
18. Cavanaugh DJ, Lee H, Lo L, et al. Distinct subsets of unmyelinated primary sensory fibers mediate behavioral responses to noxious thermal and mechanical stimuli. *Proc Natl Acad Sci USA* 2009;106(22):9075–9080.
19. Abrahamsen B, Zhao J, Asante CO, et al. The cell and molecular basis of mechanical, cold, and inflammatory pain. *Science* 2008;321(5889):702–705.
20. Johnson KO. The roles and functions of cutaneous mechanoreceptors. *Curr Opin Neurobiol* 2001;11(4):455–461.
21. Mearow KM, Diamond J. Merkel cells and the mechanosensitivity of normal and regenerating nerves in Xenopus skin. *Neuroscience* 1988;26(2):695–708.
22. KruMger L, Kavookjian A, Kumazawa T, et al. Nociceptor structural specialization in canine and rodent testicular "free" nerve endings. *J Comp Neurol* 2003;463(2):197–211.
23. Zylka MJ, Rice FL, Anderson DJ. Topographically distinct epidermal nociceptive circuits revealed by axonal tracers targeted to Mrgprd. *Neuron* 2005;45(1):17–25.

BOX 3.2 Afferent Contributions to Neuropathic Pain and Allodynia

One of the most striking positive symptoms of neuropathic pain is *dynamic mechanical allodynia*, a term used to describe pain resulting from light tactile stimuli that would never be considered noxious in the absence of nervous system injury. This phenomena can be recapitulated with a subcutaneous injection of capsaicin.[196] Data from detailed psychophysical analysis in combination with microneurography[197] and dorsal horn recording in animal models[198] all suggest that dynamic mechanical allodynia reflects activity in low-threshold afferents that signal pain as a result of changes in the central nervous system. The exact nature of these changes, generally referred to as central sensitization, is still debated (e.g., see Polgar and Todd[199] and Schoffnegger et al.[200]), but it is clear that they depend on activity in nociceptive afferents. Another possibility, however, is that low-threshold afferents undergo a phenotypic switch such that they begin to transmit information to the central nervous system as if they were nociceptive afferents. Consistent with this possibility, there is evidence following peripheral nerve injury that a subpopulation of putative nonnociceptive afferents begins to express the neuropeptide, substance P[201] although this change does not appear to be necessary for the expression of allodynia.[202] Evidence of a third possibility, which would involve sprouting of nonnociceptive afferents into more superficial layers of the dorsal horn to enable low threshold drive of nociceptive dorsal horn neurons,[203] remains largely unsubstantiated.[204–206]

24. Ghitani N, Barik A, Szczot M, et al. Specialized mechanosensory nociceptors mediating rapid responses to hair pull. *Neuron* 2017;95(4): 944.e4–954.e4.

25. Bai L, Lehnert BP, Liu J, et al. Genetic identification of an expansive mechanoreceptor sensitive to skin stroking. *Cell* 2015;163(7):1783–1795.

26. Braz JM, Nassar MA, Wood JN, et al. Parallel "pain" pathways arise from subpopulations of primary afferent nociceptor. *Neuron* 2005;47(6):787–793.

27. Cesare P, McNaughton P. A novel heat-activated current in nociceptive neurons and its sensitization by bradykinin. *Proc Natl Acad Sci U S A* 1996;93:15435–15439.

28. Reichling DB, Levine JD. Heat transduction in rat sensory neurons by calcium-dependent activation of a cation channel. *Proc Natl Acad Sci U S A* 1997;94(13):7006–7011.

29. Reid G, Flonta ML. Physiology. Cold current in thermoreceptive neurons. *Nature* 2001;413(6855):480.

30. Thut PD, Wrigley D, Gold MS. Cold transduction in rat trigeminal ganglia neurons in vitro. *Neuroscience* 2003;119(4):1071–1083.

31. McCarter GC, Reichling DB, Levine JD. Mechanical transduction by rat dorsal root ganglion neurons in vitro. *Neurosci Lett* 1999;273(3):179–182.

32. Vilceanu D, Stucky CL. TRPA1 mediates mechanical currents in the plasma membrane of mouse sensory neurons. *PLoS One* 2010;5(8):e12177.

33. Bevan S, Yeats J. Protons activate a cation conductance in a sub-population of rat dorsal root ganglion neurones. *J Physiol* 1991;433:145–161.

34. Krishtal OA, Marchenko SM, Obukhov AG. Cationic channels activated by extracellular ATP in rat sensory neurons. *Neuroscience* 1988;27(3):995–1000.

35. Heyman I, Rang HP. Depolarizing responses to capsaicin in a subpopulation of rat dorsal root ganglion cells. *Neurosci Lett* 1985;56:69–75.

36. Bautista DM, Jordt SE, Nikai T, et al. TRPA1 mediates the inflammatory actions of environmental irritants and proalgesic agents. *Cell* 2006;124(6):1269–1282.

37. Gold MS. Molecular biology of sensory transduction. In: McMahon SB, Koltzenburg M, Tracey I, et al, eds. *Wall and Melzack's Textbook of Pain*. 6th ed. London: Elsevier; 2013:31–47.

38. Burnstock G. Physiology and pathophysiology of purinergic neurotransmission. *Physiol Rev* 2007;87(2):659–797.

39. Wemmie JA, Price MP, Welsh MJ. Acid-sensing ion channels: advances, questions and therapeutic opportunities. *Trends Neurosci* 2006;29(10):578–586.

40. Story GM, Peier AM, Reeve AJ, et al. ANKTM1, a TRP-like channel expressed in nociceptive neurons, is activated by cold temperatures. *Cell* 2003;112(6):819–829.

41. Caterina MJ, Rosen TA, Tominaga M, et al. A capsaicin-receptor homologue with a high threshold for noxious heat. *Nature* 1999;398(6726):436–441.

42. McKemy DD, Neuhausser WM, Julius D. Identification of a cold receptor reveals a general role for TRP channels in thermosensation. *Nature* 2002;416(6876):52–58.

43. Xu H, Ramsey IS, Kotecha SA, et al. TRPV3 is a calcium-permeable temperature-sensitive cation channel. *Nature* 2002;418(6894):181–186.

44. Güler AD, Lee H, Iida T, et al. Heat-evoked activation of the ion channel, TRPV4. *J Neurosci* 2002;22(15):6408–6414.

45. Caterina MJ, Schumacher MA, Tominaga M, et al. The capsaicin receptor: a heat-activated ion channel in the pain pathway. *Nature* 1997;389(6653): 816–824.

46. Venkatachalam K, Montell C. TRP channels. *Annu Rev Biochem* 2007;76: 387–417.

47. Kwan KY, Allchorne AJ, Vollrath MA, et al. TRPA1 contributes to cold, mechanical, and chemical nociception but is not essential for hair-cell transduction. *Neuron* 2006;50(2):277–289.

48. Alessandri-Haber N, Joseph E, Olayinka D, et al. TRPV4 mediates pain-related behavior induced by mild hypertonic stimuli in the presence of inflammatory mediator. *Pain* 2005;118(1–2):70–79.

49. Mickle AD, Shepherd AJ, Mohapatra DP. Sensory TRP channels: the key transducers of nociception and pain. *Prog Mol Biol Transl Sci* 2015;131:73–118.

50. Honore P, Wismer CT, Mikusa J, et al. A-425619 [1-isoquinolin-5-yl-3-(4-trifluoromethyl-benzyl)-urea], a novel transient receptor potential type V1 receptor antagonist, relieves pathophysiological pain associated with inflammation and tissue injury in rats. *J Pharmacol Exp Ther* 2005;314(1): 410–421.

51. Mrozkova P, Spicarova D, Palecek J. Hypersensitivity induced by activation of spinal cord par2 receptors is partially mediated by trpv1 receptors. *PLoS One* 2016;11(10):e0163991.

52. Nishio N, Taniguchi W, Sugimura YK, et al. Reactive oxygen species enhance excitatory synaptic transmission in rat spinal dorsal horn neurons by activating TRPA1 and TRPV1 channels. *Neuroscience* 2013;247:201–212.

53. Moran MM, Szallasi A. Targeting nociceptive transient receptor potential channels to treat chronic pain: current state of the field [published online ahead of print September 19, 2017]. *Br J Pharmacol*. doi:10.1111/bph.14044.

54. Karai L, Brown DC, Mannes AJ, et al. Deletion of vanilloid receptor 1-expressing primary afferent neurons for pain control. *J Clin Invest* 2004; 113(9):1344–1352.

55. Brown DC, Agnello K, Iadarola MJ. Intrathecal resiniferatoxin in a dog model: efficacy in bone cancer pain. *Pain* 2015;156(6):1018–1024.

56. Delmas P, Hao J, Rodat-Despoix L. Molecular mechanisms of mechanotransduction in mammalian sensory neurons. *Nat Rev Neurosci* 2011;12(3): 139–153.

57. Price MP, Lewin GR, McIlwrath SL, et al. The mammalian sodium channel BNC1 is required for normal touch sensation. *Nature* 2000;407(6807): 1007–1011.

58. Shin JB, Martinez-Salgado C, Heppenstall PA, et al. A T-type calcium channel required for normal function of a mammalian mechanoreceptor. *Nat Neurosci* 2003;6(7):724–730.

59. Kwan KY, Glazer JM, Corey DP, et al. TRPA1 modulates mechanotransduction in cutaneous sensory neurons. *J Neurosci* 2009;29(15):4808–4819.

60. Ranade SS, Woo SH, Dubin AE, et al. Piezo2 is the major transducer of mechanical forces for touch sensation in mice. *Nature* 2014;516(7529): 121–125.

61. Michaelis M, Blenk KH, Vogel C, et al. Distribution of sensory properties among axotomized cutaneous C-fibres in adult rats. *Neuroscience* 1999;94(1):7–10.

62. Drew LJ, Rugiero F, Cesare P, et al. High-threshold mechanosensitive ion channels blocked by a novel conopeptide mediate pressure-evoked pain. *PLoS One* 2007;2:e515.

63. Park SP, Kim BM, Koo JY, et al. A tarantula spider toxin, GsMTx4, reduces mechanical and neuropathic pain. *Pain* 2008;137(1):208–217.

64. St. Sauver JL, Warner DO, Yawn BP, et al. Why patients visit their doctors: assessing the most prevalent conditions in a defined American population. *Mayo Clin Proc* 2013;88(1):56–67.

65. Birder LA. More than just a barrier: urothelium as a drug target for urinary bladder pain. *Am J Physiol Renal Physiol* 2005;289(3):F489–F495.

66. Baumbauer KM, DeBerry JJ, Adelman PC, et al. Keratinocytes can modulate and directly initiate nociceptive responses. *Elife* 2015;4. doi:10.7554 /eLife.09674

67. Zappia KJ, Garrison SR, Palygin O, et al. Mechanosensory and ATP release deficits following keratin14-Cre-Mediated TRPA1 deletion despite absence of TRPA1 in murine keratinocytes. *PLoS One* 2016;11(3):e0151602.

68. Wynn G, Rong W, Xiang Z, et al. Purinergic mechanisms contribute to mechanosensory transduction in the rat colorectum. *Gastroenterology* 2003;125(5):1398–1409.

69. Mizumoto N, Mummert ME, Shalhevet D, et al. Keratinocyte ATP release assay for testing skin-irritating potentials of structurally diverse chemicals. *J Invest Dermatol* 2003;121(5):1066–1072.

70. Burnstock G. Purinergic P2 receptors as targets for novel analgesics. *Pharmacol Ther* 2006;110(3):433–454.

71. Xu GY, Shenoy M, Winston JH, et al. P2X receptor-mediated visceral hyperalgesia in a rat model of chronic visceral hypersensitivity. *Gut* 2008;57(9):1230–1237.

72. Bellono NW, Bayrer JR, Leitch DB, et al. Enterochromaffin cells are gut chemosensors that couple to sensory neural pathways. *Cell* 2017;170(1):185. e16–198.e16.

73. Mawe GM, Hoffman JM. Serotonin signalling in the gut—functions, dysfunctions and therapeutic targets. *Nat Rev Gastroenterol Hepatol* 2013;10(8): 473–486.

74. Janig W, Grossmann L, Gorodetskaya N. Mechano- and thermosensitivity of regenerating cutaneous afferent nerve fibers. *Exp Brain Res* 2009;196:101–114.

75. Korenman EM, Devor M. Ectopic adrenergic sensitivity in damaged peripheral nerve axons in the rat. *Exp Neurol* 1981;72:63–81.

76. Devor M, Janig W, Michaelis M. Modulation of activity in dorsal root ganglion neurons by sympathetic activation in nerve-injured rats. *J Neurophysiol* 1994;71(1):38–47.

77. Mantyh PW, DeMaster E, Malhorta A, et al. Receptor endocytosis and dendrite reshaping in spinal neurons after somatosensory stimulation. *Science* 1995;268(5217):1629–1632.

78. Gold MS, Gebhart GF. Nociceptor sensitization in pain pathogenesis. *Nat Med* 2010;16(11):1248–1257.

79. Carr RW, Pianova S, Brock JA. The effects of polarizing current on nerve terminal impulses recorded from polymodal and cold receptors in the guinea-pig cornea. *J Gen Physiol* 2002;120(3):395–405.

80. Zhang XF, Gopalakrishnan M, Shieh CC. Modulation of action potential firing by iberiotoxin and NS1619 in rat dorsal root ganglion neurons. *Neuroscience* 2003;122(4):1003–1011.

81. Passmore GM, Selyanko AA, Mistry M, et al. KCNQ/M currents in sensory neurons: significance for pain therapy. *J Neurosci* 2003;23(18):7227–7236.

82. Gemes G, Oyster K, Pan B, et al. Painful nerve injury increases plasma membrane Ca^{2+}-ATPase activity in axotomized sensory neurons. *Mol Pain* 2012;8:46.

83. Scheff NN, Yilmaz E, Gold MS. The properties, distribution and function of Na(+)-Ca(2+) exchanger isoforms in rat cutaneous sensory neurons. *J Physiol* 2014;592(pt 22):4969–4993.

84. Tang Q, Bangaru ML, Kostic S, et al. Ca^{2+}-dependent regulation of Ca^{2+} currents in rat primary afferent neurons: role of CaMKII and the effect of injury. *J Neurosci* 2012;32(34):11737–11749.

85. Zhang X-L, Mok L-P, Katz EJ, et al. BK$_{Ca}$ currents are enriched in a subpopulation of adult rat cutaneous nociceptive dorsal root ganglion neurons. *Eur J Neurosci* 2010;31:450–462.

86. Vaughn AH, Gold MS. Ionic mechanisms underlying inflammatory mediator-induced sensitization of dural afferents. *J Neurosci* 2010;30(23):7878–7888.

87. Zhu Y, Zhang XL, Gold MS. Activity-dependent hyperpolarization of EGABA is absent in cutaneous DRG neurons from inflamed rats. *Neuroscience* 2014;256:1–9.

88. Goss JR, Cascio M, Goins W, et al. HSV delivery of a ligand-regulated endogenous ion channel gene to sensory neurons results in pain control following channel activation. *Mol Ther* 2011;19(3):500–506.

89. Rivnay J, Wang H, Fenno L, et al. Next-generation probes, particles, and proteins for neural interfacing. *Sci Adv* 2017;3(6):e1601649.

90. Boada MD, Martin TJ, Peters CM, et al. Fast-conducting mechanoreceptors contribute to withdrawal behavior in normal and nerve injured rats. *Pain* 2014;155(12):2646–2655.

91. Iyer SM, Montgomery KL, Towne C, et al. Virally mediated optogenetic excitation and inhibition of pain in freely moving nontransgenic mice. *Nat Biotechnol* 2014;32(3):274–278.

92. Li B, Yang XY, Qian FP, et al. A novel analgesic approach to optogenetically and specifically inhibit pain transmission using TRPV1 promoter. *Brain Res* 2015;1609:12–20.

93. Daou I, Beaudry H, Ase AR, et al. Optogenetic silencing of Nav1.8-positive afferents alleviates inflammatory and neuropathic pain. *eNeuro* 2016;3(1). doi:10.1523/ENEURO.0140-15.2016.

94. Catterall WA, Hulme JT, Jiang X, et al. Regulation of sodium and calcium channels by signaling complexes. *J Recept Signal Transduct Res* 2006;26(5–6):577–598.

95. Gold MS. Ion channels: recent advances and clinical applications. In: Flor H, Kaslo E, Dostrovsky JO, eds. *Proceedings of the 11th World Congress on Pain*. Seattle, WA: IASP Press; 2006:73–92.

96. Ho C, O'Leary ME. Single-cell analysis of sodium channel expression in dorsal root ganglion neurons. *Mol Cell Neurosci* 2011;46(1):159–166.

97. Isom LL. Sodium channel beta subunits: anything but auxiliary. *Neuroscientist* 2001;7(1):42–54.

98. Sangameswaran L, Delgado SG, Fish LM, et al. Structure and function of a novel voltage-gated, tetrodotoxin-resistant sodium channel specific to sensory neurons. *J Biol Chem* 1996;271(11):5953–5956.

99. Akopian AN, Sivilotti L, Wood JN. A tetrodotoxin-resistant voltage-gated sodium channel expressed by sensory neurons. *Nature* 1996;379(6562):257–262.

100. Djouhri L, Fang X, Okuse K, et al. The TTX-resistant sodium channel Nav1.8 (SNS/PN3): expression and correlation with membrane properties in rat nociceptive primary afferent neurons. *J Physiol* 2003;550(pt 3):739–752.

101. Jarvis MF, Honore P, Shieh CC, et al. A-803467, a potent and selective Nav1.8 sodium channel blocker, attenuates neuropathic and inflammatory pain in the rat. *Proc Natl Acad Sci USA* 2007;104(20):8520–8525.

102. Klein AH, Vyshnevska A, Hartke TV, et al. Sodium channel Nav1.8 underlies TTX-resistant axonal action potential conduction in somatosensory C-fibers of distal cutaneous nerves. *J Neurosci* 2017;37(20):5204–5214.

103. Elliott AA, Elliott JR. Characterization of TTX-sensitive and TTX-resistant sodium currents in small cells from adult rat dorsal root ganglia. *J Physiol (Lond)* 1993;463(39):39–56.

104. Gold MS, Zhang L, Wrigley DL, et al. Prostaglandin E(2) Modulates TTX-R I(Na) in Rat Colonic Sensory Neurons. *J Neurophysiol* 2002;88(3):1512–1522.

105. Zimmermann K, Leffler A, Babes A, et al. Sensory neuron sodium channel Nav1.8 is essential for pain at low temperatures. *Nature* 2007;447(7146):855–858.

106. Rush AM, Dib-Hajj SD, Liu S, et al. A single sodium channel mutation produces hyper- or hypoexcitability in different types of neurons. *Proc Natl Acad Sci U S A* 2006;103(21):8245–8250.

107. Cummins TR, Dib-Hajj SD, Waxman SG. Electrophysiological properties of mutant Nav1.7 sodium channels in a painful inherited neuropathy. *J Neurosci* 2004;24(38):8232–8236.

108. Dib-Hajj SD, Geha P, Waxman SG. Sodium channels in pain disorders: pathophysiology and prospects for treatment. *Pain* 2017;158(suppl 1):S97–S107.

109. Cox JJ, Reimann F, Nicholas AK, et al. An SCN9A channelopathy causes congenital inability to experience pain. *Nature* 2006;444(7121):894–898.

110. Minett MS, Nassar MA, Clark AK, et al. Distinct Nav1.7-dependent pain sensations require different sets of sensory and sympathetic neurons. *Nat Commun* 2012;3:791.

111. Minett MS, Pereira V, Sikandar S, et al. Endogenous opioids contribute to insensitivity to pain in humans and mice lacking sodium channel Nav1.7. *Nat Commun* 2015;6:8967.

112. Kist AM, Sagafos D, Rush AM, et al. SCN10A mutation in a patient with erythromelalgia enhances C-fiber activity dependent slowing. *PLoS One* 2016;11(9):e0161789.

113. Zhang X, Priest BT, Belfer I, et al. Voltage-gated Na+ currents in human dorsal root ganglion neurons. *Elife* 2017;6. doi:10.7554/eLife.23235.

114. Snutch TP, Zamponi GW. Recent advances in the development of T-type calcium channel blockers for pain intervention [published online ahead of print July 12, 2017]. *Br J Pharmacol*. doi:10.1111/bph.13906.

115. Bernal Sierra YA, Haseleu J, Kozlenkov A, et al. Genetic tracing of Cav3.2 T-type calcium channel expression in the peripheral nervous system. *Front Mol Neurosci* 2017;10:70.

116. Todorovic SM, Jevtovic-Todorovic V. The role of T-type calcium channels in peripheral and central pain processing. *CNS Neurol Disord Drug Targets* 2006;5(6):639–653.

117. White G, Lovinger DM, Weight FF. Transient low-threshold Ca²⁺ current triggers burst firing through an after depolarizing potential in an adult mammalian neuron. *Proc Natl Acad Sci USA* 1989;86:6802–6806.

118. Gu JG, MacDermott AB. Activation of ATP P2X receptors elicits glutamate release from sensory neuron synapses. *Nature* 1997;389(6652):749–753.

119. Jeftinija S. The role of tetrodotoxin-resistant sodium channels of small primary afferent fibers. *Brain Res* 1994;639(1):125–134.

120. Willis WD Jr. Dorsal root potentials and dorsal root reflexes: a double-edged sword. *Exp Brain Res* 1999;124(4):395–421.

121. Wittmack EK, Rush AM, Craner MJ, et al. Fibroblast growth factor homologous factor 2B: association with Nav1.6 and selective colocalization at nodes of Ranvier of dorsal root axons. *J Neurosci* 2004;24(30):6765–6775.

122. Alexandrou AJ, Brown AR, Chapman ML, et al. Subtype-selective small molecule inhibitors reveal a fundamental role for Nav1.7 in nociceptor electrogenesis, axonal conduction and presynaptic release. *PLoS One* 2016;11(4):e0152405.

123. Xie W, Strong JA, Zhang JM. Local knockdown of the NaV1.6 sodium channel reduces pain behaviors, sensory neuron excitability, and sympathetic sprouting in rat models of neuropathic pain. *Neuroscience* 2015;291:317–330.

124. Catterall WA, Perez-Reyes E, Snutch TP, et al. International Union of Pharmacology. XLVIII. Nomenclature and structure-function relationships of voltage-gated calcium channels. *Pharmacol Rev* 2005;57(4):411–425.

125. Dolphin AC. Voltage-gated calcium channels and their auxiliary subunits: physiology and pathophysiology and pharmacology. *J Physiol* 2016;594(19):5369–5390.

126. Davies A, Hendrich J, Van Minh AT, et al. Functional biology of the alpha(2)delta subunits of voltage-gated calcium channels. *Trends Pharmacol Sci* 2007;28(5):220–228.

127. Ikeda SR. Voltage-dependent modulation of N-type calcium channels by G-protein beta gamma subunits. *Nature* 1996;380(6571):255–258.

128. Rycroft BK, Vikman KS, Christie MJ. Inflammation reduces the contribution of N-type calcium channels to primary afferent synaptic transmission onto NK1 receptor-positive lamina I neurons in the rat dorsal horn. *J Physiol* 2007;580(pt 3):883–894.

129. Ewald DA, Matthies HJ, Perney TM, et al. The effect of down regulation of protein kinase C on the inhibitory modulation of dorsal root ganglion neuron Ca2+ currents by neuropeptide Y. *J Neurosci* 1988;8(7):2447–2451.

130. Schneggenburger R, Neher E. Presynaptic calcium and control of vesicle fusion. *Curr Opin Neurobiol* 2005;15(3):266–274.

131. Luo ZD, Chaplan SR, Higuera ES, et al. Upregulation of dorsal root ganglion $\alpha_2\delta$ calcium channel subunit and its correlation with allodynia in spinal nerve-injured rats. *J Neurosci* 2001;21(6):1868–1875.

132. Bauer CS, Nieto-Rostro M, Rahman W, et al. The increased trafficking of the calcium channel subunit alpha2delta-1 to presynaptic terminals in neuropathic pain is inhibited by the alpha2delta ligand pregabalin. *J Neurosci* 2009;29(13):4076–4088.

133. Cheng LZ, Lü N, Zhang YQ, et al. Ryanodine receptors contribute to the induction of nociceptive input-evoked long-term potentiation in the rat spinal cord slice. *Mol Pain* 2010;6:1. doi:10.1186/1744-8069-6-1.

134. Duncan C, Mueller S, Simon E, et al. Painful nerve injury decreases sarco-endoplasmic reticulum Ca²⁺-ATPase activity in axotomized sensory neurons. *Neuroscience* 2013;231:247–257.

135. Shutov LP, Kim MS, Houlihan PR, et al. Mitochondria and plasma membrane Ca2+-ATPase control presynaptic Ca2+ clearance in capsaicin-sensitive rat sensory neurons. *J Physiol* 2013;591(pt 10):2443–2462.

136. Gupta A, Bah M. NSAIDs in the treatment of postoperative pain. *Curr Pain Headache Rep* 2016;20(11):62.

137. Eccleston C, Cooper TE, Fisher E, et al. Non-steroidal anti-inflammatory drugs (NSAIDs) for chronic non-cancer pain in children and adolescents. *Cochrane Database Syst Rev* 2017;(8):CD012537.

138. Willrich MA, Murray DL, Snyder MR. Tumor necrosis factor inhibitors: clinical utility in autoimmune diseases. *Transl Res* 2015;165(2):270–282.

139. Jing S, Yang C, Zhang X, et al. Efficacy and safety of etanercept in the treatment of sciatica: a systematic review and meta-analysis. *J Clin Neurosci* 2017;44:69–74.

140. Jimenez-Andrade JM, Martin CD, Koewler NJ, et al. Nerve growth factor sequestering therapy attenuates non-malignant skeletal pain following fracture. *Pain* 2007;133(1–3):183–196.

141. Koewler NJ, Freeman KT, Buus RJ, et al. Effects of a monoclonal antibody raised against nerve growth factor on skeletal pain and bone healing after fracture of the C57BL/6J mouse femur. *J Bone Miner Res* 2007;22(11):1732–1742.

142. Sabsovich I, Wei T, Guo TZ, et al. Effect of anti-NGF antibodies in a rat tibia fracture model of complex regional pain syndrome type I. *Pain* 2008;138(1):47–60.

143. Wild KD, Bian D, Zhu D, et al. Antibodies to nerve growth factor reverse established tactile allodynia in rodent models of neuropathic pain without tolerance. *J Pharmacol Exp Ther* 2007;322(1):282–287.

144. Denk F, Bennett DL, McMahon SB. Nerve growth factor and pain mechanisms. *Annu Rev Neurosci* 2017;40:307–325.

145. Gold MS, Levine JD, Correa AM. Modulation of TTX-R INa by PKC and PKA and their role in PGE2-induced sensitization of rat sensory neurons in vitro. *J Neurosci* 1998;18(24):10345–10355.

146. Taiwo YO, Bjerknes LK, Goetzl EJ, et al. Mediation of primary afferent peripheral hyperalgesia by the cAMP second messenger system. *Neuroscience* 1989;32(3):577–580.

147. Ahlgren SC, Levine JD. Protein kinase C inhibitors decrease hyperalgesia and C-fiber hyperexcitability in the streptozotocin-diabetic rat. *J Neurophysiol* 1994;72(2):684–692.

148. Aley KO, Messing RO, Mochly-Rosen D, et al. Chronic hypersensitivity for inflammatory nociceptor sensitization mediated by the epsilon isozyme of protein kinase C. *J Neurosci* 2000;20(12):4680–4685.

149. Jin X, Gereau RW. Acute p38-mediated modulation of tetrodotoxin-resistant sodium channels in mouse sensory neurons by tumor necrosis factor-alpha. *J Neurosci* 2006;26(1):246–255.

150. Price TJ, Cervero F, Gold MS, et al. Chloride regulation in the pain pathway. *Brain Res Rev* 2009;60(1):149–170.

151. Zhu Y, Lu SG, Gold MS. Persistent inflammation increases GABA-induced depolarization of rat cutaneous dorsal root ganglion neurons in vitro. *Neuroscience* 2012;220:330–340.

152. Zhu Y, Dua S, Gold MS. Inflammation-induced shift in spinal GABA(A) signaling is associated with a tyrosine kinase-dependent increase in GABA(A) current density in nociceptive afferents. *J Neurophysiol* 2012;108(9):2581–2593.

153. Salvemini D, Doyle T, Kress M, et al. Therapeutic targeting of the ceramide-to-sphingosine 1-phosphate pathway in pain. *Trends Pharmacol Sci* 2013;34(2):110–118.

154. Kelleher JH, Tewari D, McMahon SB. Neurotrophic factors and their inhibitors in chronic pain treatment. *Neurobiol Dis* 2017;97(pt B):127–138.

155. Gold MS, Caterina MJ. Molecular biology of nociceptor transduction. In: Basbaum AI, Bushnell MC, eds. *The Senses: A Comprehensive Reference.* San Diego, CA: Academic Press; 2008:43–74.

156. Denk F, McMahon SB. Chronic pain: emerging evidence for the involvement of epigenetics. *Neuron* 2012;73(3):435–444.

157. Niederberger E, Resch E, Parnham MJ, et al. Drugging the pain epigenome. *Nat Rev Neurol* 2017;13(7):434–447.

158. Ji RR, Samad TA, Jin SX, et al. p38 MAPK activation by NGF in primary sensory neurons after inflammation increases TRPV1 levels and maintains heat hyperalgesia. *Neuron* 2002;36(1):57–68.

159. Melemedjian OK, Asiedu MN, Tillu DV, et al. IL-6- and NGF-induced rapid control of protein synthesis and nociceptive plasticity via convergent signaling to the eIF4F complex. *J Neurosci* 2010;30(45):15113–15123.

160. Moy JK, Khoutorsky A, Asiedu MN, et al. The MNK-eIF4E signaling axis contributes to injury-induced nociceptive plasticity and the development of chronic pain. *J Neurosci* 2017;37(31):7481–7499.

161. Reichling DB, Levine JD. Critical role of nociceptor plasticity in chronic pain. *Trends Neurosci* 2009;32(12):611–618.

162. Kim JY, Tillu DV, Quinn TL, et al. Spinal dopaminergic projections control the transition to pathological pain plasticity via a D1/D5-mediated mechanism. *J Neurosci* 2015;35(16):6307–6317.

163. Joseph EK, Levine JD. Hyperalgesic priming is restricted to isolectin B4-positive nociceptors. *Neuroscience* 2010;169(1):431–435.

164. Araldi D, Ferrari LF, Levine JD. Hyperalgesic priming (type II) induced by repeated opioid exposure: maintenance mechanisms. *Pain* 2017;158(7):1204–1216.

165. Joseph EK, Parada CA, Levine JD. Hyperalgesic priming in the rat demonstrates marked sexual dimorphism. *Pain* 2003;105(1–2):143–150.

166. Ferrari LF, Bogen O, Reichling DB, et al. Accounting for the delay in the transition from acute to chronic pain: axonal and nuclear mechanisms. *J Neurosci* 2015;35(2):495–507.

167. Harriott AM, Dessem D, Gold MS. Inflammation increases the excitability of masseter muscle afferents. *Neuroscience* 2006;141(1):433–442.

168. Flake NM, Gold MS. Inflammation alters sodium currents and excitability of temporomandibular joint afferents. *Neurosci Lett* 2005;384(3):294–299.

169. Yoshimura N, de Groat WC. Increased excitability of afferent neurons innervating rat urinary bladder after chronic bladder inflammation. *J Neurosci* 1999;19(11):4644–4653.

170. Bielefeldt K, Ozaki N, Gebhart GF. Mild gastritis alters voltage-sensitive sodium currents in gastric sensory neurons in rats. *Gastroenterology* 2002;122(3):752–761.

171. Dang K, Bielefeldt K, Gebhart GF. Gastric ulcers reduce A-type potassium currents in rat gastric sensory ganglion neurons. *Am J Physiol Gastrointest Liver Physiol* 2004;286(4):G573–G579.

172. Sugiura T, Dang K, Lamb K, et al. Acid-sensing properties in rat gastric sensory neurons from normal and ulcerated stomach. *J Neurosci* 2005;25(10):2617–2627.

173. Moore BA, Stewart TM, Hill C, et al. TNBS ileitis evokes hyperexcitability and changes in ionic membrane properties of nociceptive DRG neurons. *Am J Physiol Gastrointest Liver Physiol* 2002;282(6):G1045–G1051.

174. Stewart T, Beyak MJ, Vanner S. Ileitis modulates potassium and sodium currents in guinea pig dorsal root ganglia sensory neurons. *J Physiol* 2003;552(pt 3):797–807.

175. Beyak MJ, Ramji N, Krol KM, et al. Two TTX-resistant Na+ currents in mouse colonic dorsal root ganglia neurons and their role in colitis-induced hyperexcitability. *Am J Physiol Gastrointest Liver Physiol* 2004;287(4):G845–G855.

176. Gold MS, Traub RJ. Cutaneous and colonic rat DRG neurons differ with respect to both baseline and PGE2-induced changes in passive and active electrophysiological properties. *J Neurophysiol* 2004;91(6):2524–2531.

177. Harriott AM, Gold MS. Electrophysiological properties of dural afferents in the absence and presence of inflammatory mediators. *J Neurophysiol* 2009;101(6):3126–3134.

178. Fitzgerald EM, Okuse K, Wood JN, et al. cAmp-dependent phosphorylation of the tetrodotoxin-resistant voltage- dependent sodium channel Sns. *J Physiol (Lond)* 1999;516(pt 2):433–446.

179. Gold MS, Reichling DB, Shuster MJ, et al. Hyperalgesic agents increase a tetrodotoxin-resistant Na+ current in nociceptors. *Proc Natl Acad Sci USA* 1996;93(3):1108–1112.

180. Gold MS, Weinreich D, Kim CS, et al. Redistribution of Na(V)1.8 in uninjured axons enables neuropathic pain. *J Neurosci* 2003;23(1):158–166.

181. Wang G, Tang B, Traub RJ. Differential processing of noxious colonic input by thoracolumbar and lumbosacral dorsal horn neurons in the rat. *J Neurophysiol* 2005;94(6):3788–3794.

182. Traub RJ. Evidence for thoracolumbar spinal cord processing of inflammatory, but not acute colonic pain. *Neuroreport* 2000;11(10):2113–2116.

183. Ruda MA, Ling QD, Hohmann AG, et al. Altered nociceptive neuronal circuits after neonatal peripheral inflammation. *Science* 2000;289(5479):628–631.

184. Ren K, Anseloni V, Zou SP, et al. Characterization of basal and re-inflammation-associated long-term alteration in pain responsivity following short-lasting neonatal local inflammatory insult. *Pain* 2004;110(3):588–596.

185. Cairns BE, Hu JW, Arendt-Nielsen L, et al. Sex-related differences in human pain and rat afferent discharge evoked by injection of glutamate into the masseter muscle. *J Neurophysiol* 2001;86(2):782–791.

186. Bartley EJ, Fillingim RB. Sex differences in pain: a brief review of clinical and experimental findings. *Br J Anaesth* 2013;111(1):52–58.

187. Mogil JS, Bailey AL. Sex and gender differences in pain and analgesia. *Prog Brain Res* 2010;186:141–157.

188. Wang S, Davis BM, Zwick M, et al. Reduced thermal sensitivity and Nav1.8 and TRPV1 channel expression in sensory neurons of aged mice. *Neurobiol Aging* 2006;27(6):895–903.

189. Foulkes T, Wood JN. Pain genes. *PLoS Genet* 2008;4(7):e1000086.

190. Schmidt R, Schmelz M, Forster C, et al. Novel classes of responsive and unresponsive C nociceptors in human skin. *J Neurosci* 1995;15(1, pt 1):333–341.

191. Hagbarth KE, Vallbo AB. Mechanoreceptor activity recorded percutaneously with semi-microelectrodes in human peripheral nerves. *Acta Physiol Scand* 1967;69(1):121–122.

192. Hagbarth KE, Vallbo AB. Afferent response to mechanical stimulation of muscle receptors in man. *Acta Soc Med Ups* 1967;72(1):102–104.

193. Schmelz M, Schmidt R, Weidner C, et al. Chemical response pattern of different classes of C-nociceptors to pruritogens and algogens. *J Neurophysiol* 2003;89(5):2441–2448.

194. Ochoa JL, Campero M, Serra J, et al. Hyperexcitable polymodal and insensitive nociceptors in painful human neuropathy. *Muscle Nerve* 2005;32(4):459–72.

195. Ørstavik K, Namer B, Schmidt R, et al. Abnormal function of C-fibers in patients with diabetic neuropathy. *J Neurosci* 2006;26(44):11287–11294.

196. Baumann TK, Simone DA, Shain CN, et al. Neurogenic hyperalgesia: the search for primary cutaneous afferent fibers that contribute to capsaicin-induced pain and hyperalgesia. *J Neurophysiol* 1991;66(1):212–227.

197. Torebjörk HE, Lundberg LE, LaMotte RH. Central changes in processing of mechanoreceptive input in capsaicin-induced secondary hyperalgesia in humans. *J Physiol (Lond)* 1992;448:765–780.

198. Weng HR, Dougherty PM. Response properties of dorsal root reflexes in cutaneous C fibers before and after intradermal capsaicin injection in rats. *Neuroscience* 2005;132(3):823–831.

199. Polgar E, Todd AJ. Tactile allodynia can occur in the spared nerve injury model in the rat without selective loss of GABA or GABA(A) receptors from synapses in laminae I-II of the ipsilateral spinal dorsal horn. *Neuroscience* 2008;156(1):193–202.

200. Schoffnegger D, Ruscheweyh R, Sandkuhler J. Spread of excitation across modality borders in spinal dorsal horn of neuropathic rats. *Pain* 2008;135(3):300–310.

201. Noguchi K, Dubner R, De Leon M, et al. Axotomy induces preprotachykinin gene expression in a subpopulation of dorsal root ganglion neurons. *J Neurosci Res* 1994;37(5):596–603.

202. Hughes DI, Scott DT, Riddell JS, et al. Upregulation of substance P in low-threshold myelinated afferents is not required for tactile allodynia in the chronic constriction injury and spinal nerve ligation models. *J Neurosci* 2007;27(8):2035–2044.

203. Woolf CJ, Shortland P, Coggeshall RE. Peripheral nerve injury triggers central sprouting of myelinated afferents. *Nature* 1992;355(6355):75–78.

204. Hughes DI, Scott DT, Todd AJ, et al. Lack of evidence for sprouting of Abeta afferents into the superficial laminas of the spinal cord dorsal horn after nerve section. *J Neurosci* 2003;23(29):9491–9499.

205. Shehab SA, Spike RC, Todd AJ. Do central terminals of intact myelinated primary afferents sprout into the superficial dorsal horn of rat spinal cord after injury to a neighboring peripheral nerve? *J Comp Neurol* 2004;474(1):427–437.

206. Woodbury CJ, Kullmann FA, McIlwrath SL, et al. Identity of myelinated cutaneous sensory neurons projecting to nocireceptive laminae following nerve injury in adult mice. *J Comp Neurol* 2008;508(3):500–509.

CHAPTER 4

Substrates of Spinal Cord Nociceptive Processing

JENNIFER J. DEBERRY, ALAN RANDICH, and TIMOTHY J. NESS

The spinal cord and brainstem nuclei are home to second-order neurons, the first step of central nervous system (CNS) processing. As the first site of sensory integration and modulation, second-order neurons are more than a simple relay, and any plan for the treatment of nociception must understand the critical role these neurons play in the formation of painful sensation. The second-order neuron encodes afferent input from multiple sites and often multiple modalities into a message that is sent to other parts of the CNS. Those other parts of the CNS, in turn, modify the second-order neuron through both excitatory and inhibitory mechanisms. These modifying influences are the subject of the next chapter, whereas the present chapter focuses on the neuroanatomical and neurochemical characteristics of these spinal substrates.

Although it seems like a simple statement that pain-related second-order neurons are the neurons which receive primary afferent input related to tissue damage (i.e., from nociceptors), it must be accepted that this statement may or may not be wholly true because in certain pathologic states, pain can be evoked by non–tissue-damaging stimuli (allodynia). It is unfortunate that there has been a tendency in pain-related research to turn common observations into overgeneralizations, and so an attempt will be made in this chapter to be precise when possible. Sometimes, "assumptions" related to neuronal substrates of sensation have been necessarily used as "premises" on which to build scientific logic. The primary premise on which this chapter is based is that all nociceptive second-order neurons receive nociceptive primary afferent input as *one* of their excitatory modalities. If one can accept that premise, then one can identify where the neurons receiving such input are located and can further identify where these neurons send the information.

Defining Nociceptive Systems

MODELS OF PAIN PROCESSING

Pain is both a sensation and responses to that sensation. The sensory component of pain is described in terms of tissue damage (e.g., cutting, burning, rending) even when tissue damage is not occurring, and so the sensation of pain is defined as nociception. The sensory systems of our body which encode for nociception can be modeled in two main ways: (1) as a system which is specific for pain (specificity theory) or (2) as a system that requires a pattern of neuronal activation to occur for the experience of pain to be generated (pattern theory). The simplest and oldest of the pattern theories is that which suggests pain is due to high intensities of input that are independent of modality (intensity theory). Each of these theories (or the multiple variants thereof) has prominent proponents who can make persuasive arguments that focus on subsets of data that support their particular view. Each knowledgeable person must derive their own model system which is ideally based on characterized human phenomena and which must clearly go beyond simple models.

As is apparent from the preceding chapter, primary afferent neurons with sensory endings have been characterized using functional and neurochemical methods. A subset of these primary afferents with sensory endings in cutaneous tissues is only activated by (and so *specific* for) pain-producing stimuli. Although these afferents may be polymodal, that is, encode for multiple different stimuli, the stimuli that excite these primary afferents have in common the potential for producing tissue damage. They have therefore been defined as *nociceptors*. Primary afferent nociceptors are thinly myelinated or nonmyelinated and so fall into the Aδ- and C-fiber classes. Human psychophysical data support that when Aδ- and/or C-fiber function is disrupted by ischemia or pharmacologic agents, then cutaneous sensations associated with immediate (first) or briefly delayed (second) pains are similarly disrupted. Unfortunately (for the sake of easy logic), there are also many primary afferents that do not encode for tissue-damaging stimuli (e.g., "warm" receptors) but which are also of the Aδ- and C-fiber classes. Hence, it is a flawed logic that interprets all Aδ- and C-fiber–related input to second-order neurons as nociceptive. Existent literature constrains further definition of specific nociceptor neurochemical and localization characteristics except on an anecdotal (single unit) basis. With that caveat, there are basic patterns that appear common to most Aδ and C fibers, and generalizations related to these fiber groups have some validity as being representative of nociceptor localization and neurochemical content.

METHODS OF NEURONAL CHARACTERIZATION

To definitively describe the structure and function of CNS structures is a daunting task. As with nociceptors, standard histologic, ultrastructural, and neurochemical methods used to examine CNS structure have allowed for precise definition of axons, dendrites, and neurotransmitter content, but, unfortunately, they do not allow for the precise definition of function. Studies of neuronal function typically utilize electrophysiologic techniques to measure the real-time electrochemical activity of single neuronal units (e.g., action potentials) which may be evoked by multiple manipulations. These neurophysiologic measures utilize electrodes placed either extracellularly or intracellularly. When the former technique is utilized, correlative anatomic localization is possible but little more. Electrophysiologic techniques such as retrograde activation of axonal extensions can define some of the neuronal anatomy, but true morphology is only certain with the intracellular injection of a dye. Immunohistochemical characterization of intracellularly labeled neurons is methodologically feasible, and so it is possible to quantitatively define sensory elements. However, such studies are sufficiently tedious and subject to interpretive concerns related to sampling error and preparation effects (i.e., anesthesia) that, to date, these types of experiments have only been performed at a rudimentary level. A compromise microscopic analysis technique is that which uses induction of the c-*fos* gene or phosphorylation of extra cellular signal-related kinase (pERK) in response to neuronal activation to functionally identify neurons excited by a noxious stimulus. A proto-oncogene, c-*fos*, is activated after potentially tissue-damaging stimuli are applied to most tissues. The expressed product, Fos protein, is immunohistochemically identifiable within hours of stimulation. As a consequence, mapping of gene induction or Fos protein in the nucleus of activated neurons can be used to indirectly functionally define these neurons as "nociceptive."[1] However, a systematic comparison study of Fos and pERK as markers of spinal nociceptive activation revealed greater specificity for activity in nociceptive pathways (vs. nonnociceptive activation) using pERK.[2] Labeled neurons can then be colabeled with antibodies against neurotransmitters or important cell proteins or specific histologic stains to further characterize the neurons. Analgesic pharmacologic manipulations such as systemic morphine reduce both the total number of labeled neurons and the total Fos or pERK content of the spinal cord following a noxious stimulus. Even newer technologies have been able to identify a changed form of receptors following neuronal activation by noxious stimuli. For example, the internalization of neurokinin 1 (NK1) receptors following activation by substance P[3] or the phosphorylation of glutamate receptor subtypes[4] has been used as surrogates for neuronal excitation. Macroscopic examination of CNS activation sites using magnetic resonance imaging technologies have allowed confirmation of microscopic techniques and further demonstrated the functional complexity of spinal and supraspinal connections. At a microscopic level, "tracer" dyes which are taken up by the terminal endings of axons of neurons and transported back to the neuron somata allow for a histologic identification of axonal projections of spinal neurons that is dependent on the site of dye injections (e.g., spinothalamic neurons are retrogradely labeled to the spinal cord by injections in the thalamus). Such labeling techniques, when coupled together with functional techniques, have made it possible to construct a quantitative but nonspecific "global" neuroanatomic view of spinal cord nociceptive processing that appears to agree with anecdotal, definitive evidence generated by single-unit studies.

DEFINING NOCICEPTIVE SECOND-ORDER NEURONS

Strict proponents of specificity theory state that all discussion related to pain should only involve CNS neurons excited *exclusively* by primary afferent nociceptors. Such specific second-order neurons are a small but an obviously important minority of the total sample of spinal neurons receiving input from primary afferent nociceptors. One can also argue that the presence of primary afferent neurons with specificity for pain-producing stimuli does not necessitate that the second-order neurons responsible for pain sensation have a similar specificity. For purposes of the present discussion, the primary premise of the rest of this chapter is that such excitatory input is a *necessary* requirement of pain-related second-order neurons, but it is notable that most second-order neurons receiving such input receive other types of sensory input. Excitation of second-order neurons may come from primary afferent pathways or from segmental (interneurons), propriospinal (nonsegmental intraspinal), and supraspinal sources. Inhibition arises from the same CNS sources and can promote neuronal specificity by selectively reducing responsiveness to nonnociceptive inputs. It is for this reason that proponents of pattern theory argue that all second-order neurons receiving nociceptive inputs should be considered as candidates for inclusion in pain-processing pathways.

DEVELOPMENT OF SENSORY SYSTEMS

The embryologic development of the nervous system suggests reasons that differences can exist between peripheral and central phenomena because excitatory systems develop before inhibitory systems. The edges of the neural plate that come together to form the neural tube split off to become the migratory cells of the neural crest. These cells spread to form the sensory components of the peripheral nervous system. At a spinal cord level, substances from the ventrally located notochord induce the formation of motoneurons with axonal extensions extending to the periphery. The dorsal aspect of the spinal cord, lacking effects of the notochord, forms short connections (local connectivity) or develops axonal projections attracted to distant spinal cord and/or brainstem sites. Sensory structures that develop from the neural crest send axonal projections both to the periphery as well as into the dorsal aspect of the spinal cord and contain neurotransmitters that are predominantly excitatory. At birth, sensory systems have very little inhibitory connectivity. This changes during development until inhibitory connections become the predominant form of CNS communication.

In humans, the precise timing of both excitatory and inhibitory system maturation is not fully known, but based on experiments in nonhuman animals, these systems appear highly plastic with cell death processes as important as cell growth processes in relation to the final product.[5] Specific transcriptional factor expression has been used to track neuronal subgroup development and has demonstrated a profound role for pathologic modification of nociceptive circuitry.[6] The general phenomenon of use-dependent growth (or preservation) appears to hold in multiple sensory systems ranging from taste to vision with the nociceptive systems notwithstanding. Ruda and colleagues[7] have demonstrated that injury during critical periods of development, such as the neonatal period, can have profound effects on the subsequent development of nociceptive systems. In humans, critical periods of neuronal outgrowth and myelination occur in childhood, during puberty, and following events that injure nervous system structures.

Targets of Primary Afferent Input

GROSS ANATOMY OF THE SPINAL CORD

The spinal cord is segregated into areas that, on gross examination, appear as white and grey matter and consist of predominantly myelinated nerve fiber tracts and cell bodies, respectively. Wrapped in protective pial, arachnoid, and dural meninges, the spinal cord is continually being penetrated by centrally directed axons of primary afferent neurons whose cell bodies reside within the neighboring dorsal root ganglia. These axons enter as the dorsal roots and may traverse several spinal segments rostrally or caudally in the dorsolaterally located Lissauer's tract before entering the grey matter for synaptic contact. The spinal cord white matter is divided into multiple subdivisions with component "tracts" consisting of ascending or descending axonal fibers of various origins and destinations. There is significant overlap of these tracts, such that any lesion of white matter is likely to interrupt fibers of passage with multiple origins and multiple sites of termination. The white matter gets larger as one ascends the spinal cord from sacral to cervical levels as additional ascending fibers to the brain add to the white matter and progressive numbers of descending fibers to spinal targets drop out to form synaptic connection. Grey matter is largest at the cervical and lumbar enlargements due to association with sensation and motor control of the limbs. The most notable divisions of the white matter that are important to pain sensation are the dorsal columns, the dorsolateral fasciculus, and the ventrolateral (anterolateral) fasciculus and their associated subdivision into tracts (Fig. 4.1).

SPINAL LAMINAE

The morphology of neurons in the grey matter of the spinal cord differs depending on location. Using Rexed's cytoarchitecture-based classification system, there are at least 10 different layers or laminae of neurons—of which the first six (I to VI) are termed the *dorsal horn of the spinal cord* (Fig. 4.2). These laminae, plus the area around the central canal (lamina X), receive a bulk of primary afferent inputs. Spinal dorsal horn neurons receiving excitatory inputs from nociceptive afferents have been demonstrated to be present throughout the dorsal horn but with particular localization to laminae I, II,

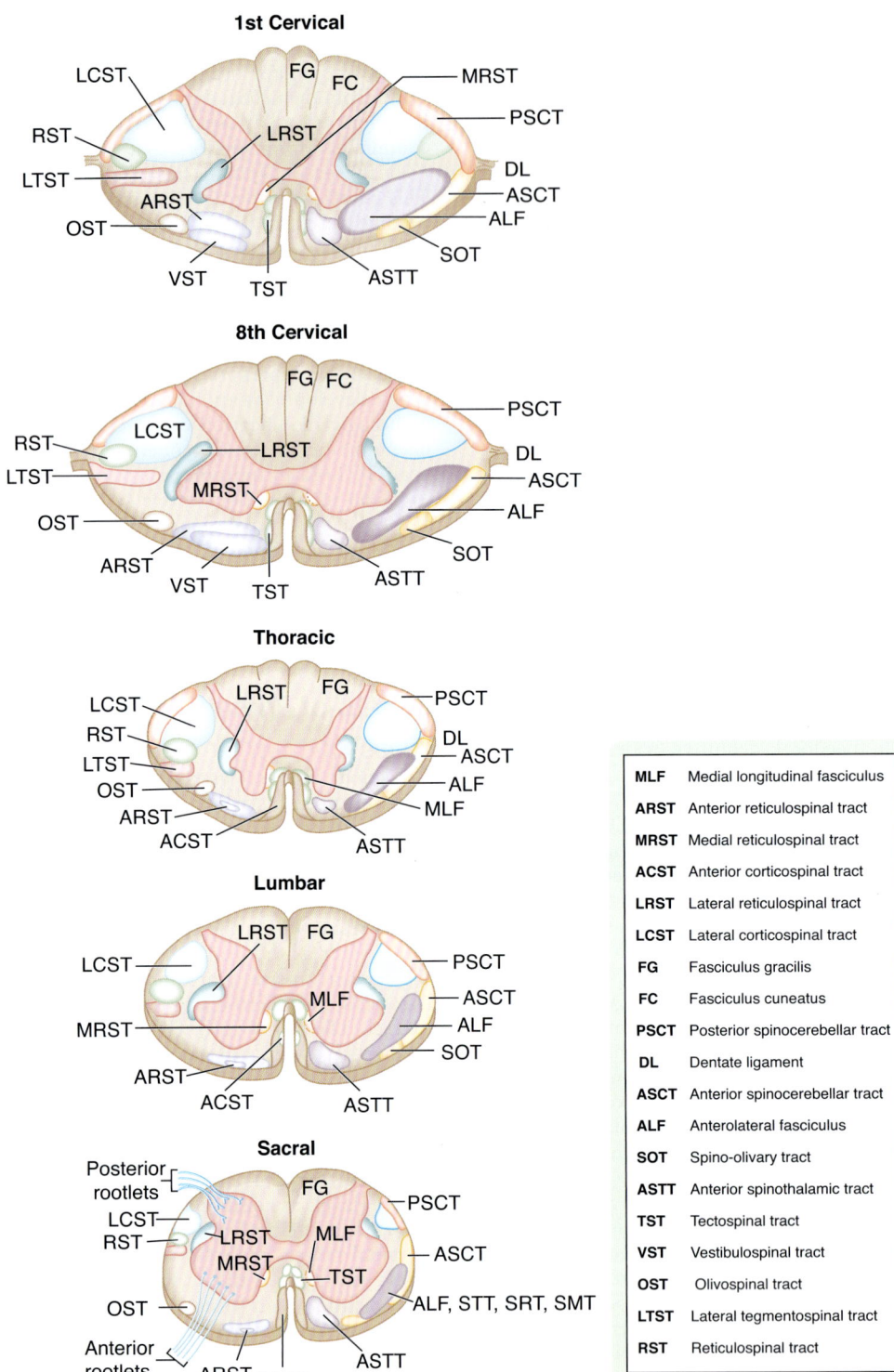

MLF	Medial longitudinal fasciculus
ARST	Anterior reticulospinal tract
MRST	Medial reticulospinal tract
ACST	Anterior corticospinal tract
LRST	Lateral reticulospinal tract
LCST	Lateral corticospinal tract
FG	Fasciculus gracilis
FC	Fasciculus cuneatus
PSCT	Posterior spinocerebellar tract
DL	Dentate ligament
ASCT	Anterior spinocerebellar tract
ALF	Anterolateral fasciculus
SOT	Spino-olivary tract
ASTT	Anterior spinothalamic tract
TST	Tectospinal tract
VST	Vestibulospinal tract
OST	Olivospinal tract
LTST	Lateral tegmentospinal tract
RST	Reticulospinal tract

FIGURE 4.1   Diagram of the white matter of the spinal cord. The ascending tracts are emphasized on the right side and the descending tracts on the left side. The anterolateral (ventrolateral) funiculus, which is composed of the anterolateral fasciculus (ALF), composed of the spinothalamic (STT), spinore-ticular (SRT), and spinomesencephalic (SMT) tracts in the spinal cord. As it ascends, the ALF becomes progressively larger, the largest part being in the upper cervical region. This is not only because the STT continues to add axons but also because there are more SRT cell bodies (and hence axons) in the cervical enlargement than in the lumbosacral enlargement. Throughout the course of the ALF in the spinal cord, the three nociceptive pathways are situated medial to the anterior (ventral) spinocerebellar tract, lateral to the ventrolateral and ventral horns, and posterolateral to the spino-olivary tract. The anterior spinothalamic tract (ASTT), which may be an alternate nociceptive pathway, is separate from the three tracts of the ALF. Because a cordotomy lesion in the upper thoracic or cervical segments usually extends from the dentate ligament medially, the ASTT and some of the descending tracts are likely to be inter-rupted with the operation. In the cervical region, the ALF is shaped as a somewhat flat triangle with the apex medial and the base lateral. At successively higher cervical levels, there is a gradual dorsolateral shift of the ALF.

V, VI, and X. One must remember that laminar assignment is based on the central location of the neuronal soma. However, dendritic extensions of these neurons may extend throughout numerous laminae such that the immunohistochemical demonstration of primary afferent neuron terminations in specific laminae does not limit connectivity to just neurons of those laminae. Furthermore, although both myelinated and unmyelinated nociceptive afferent fibers project predominately to the laminae described earlier, there exist projections in those laminae from afferent fibers that transmit innocuous sensory information. Mapping of individual C-fiber primary afferents encoding for cutaneous nociception has demonstrated sites of connectivity that are highly localized into tight "baskets" typically located in superficial laminae of a single spinal segment. In contrast, single primary C-fiber afferents from deep, visceral structures have been demonstrated to travel via Lissauer's tract to multiple spinal segments and multiple laminae (I, V, X, and even contralateral sites) (Fig. 4.3).[8] Fine muscle afferents and articular afferents have sites of termination similar to those of visceral afferents. By using intracellular recording and labeling techniques, it has been possible to determine that nociceptive afferents connect with second-order neurons that have many different morphologies—some of which correlate with electrophysiologic characteristics (see Morris et al.[9] and Grudt and Perl[10]). The morphology and neurotransmitter content of each lamina will be briefly discussed.

Lamina I: Termed the *marginal zone* as it forms the outermost layer of the dorsal horn. This single lamina contains a heterogeneous population of neurons with morphologic studies identifying neurons with pyramidal, fusiform, and multipolar shapes, some with smooth and some with spiny dendrites. Morphology and function are correlated in at least a subset of these neurons. Lamina I and the adjoining lamina II are the predominant location of excitatory neuropeptide input from primary afferent neurons with heavy immunohistochemical labeling for substance P and calcitonin gene-related peptide (CGRP). Axonal projections of a subset of lamina I neurons extend to supraspinal structures such as the medulla, midbrain, and/or thalamus. Fos and pERK induction in response to noxious stimuli have consistently been reported to occur in lamina I with double-labeling noted in association with antibodies to preproenkephalin, dynorphin, glutamate, N-methyl-D-aspartate (NMDA) receptors, γ-aminobutyric acid (GABA), glycine, GABA-B receptors, NK1 receptors, calbindin, glucocorticoid receptors, and estrogen receptor α.[1]

Lamina II: Called the substantia gelatinosa due to its gross jellylike appearance in fresh cut tissue. The neurons of this lamina are generally small with five distinct morphologies, two of which are viewed as important to the local processing of nociceptive information: stalked and islet cells (using the terminology of Gobel[11]). Stalked cells have soma at the outer edge of lamina II with centrally arborizing dendrites and axons that synapse with lamina I projection neurons. Islet cells have fusiform cell bodies with extensive dendritic and axonal arborizations containing inhibitory neurotransmitters such as GABA or enkephalin.[12,13] Axodendritic, dendrodendritic, and axoaxonic synapses are manifest throughout lamina II on ultrastructural analysis demonstrating a profound potential for neuronal interaction and signal processing. Primary afferent input from both nociceptive and nonnociceptive neurons has been noted; particularly, input from a population of nonpeptidergic, nociceptive primary afferents, is received in a narrow band within lamina II. Descending axonal connections are also present with evidence of serotonergic and noradrenergic inputs to lamina II neurons. A distinction is frequently made between lamina II-outer (II$_o$) and lamina II-inner (II$_i$) with II$_o$ commonly combined with lamina I in discussions of the superficial dorsal horn.

Lamina III and lamina IV: Known as the nucleus proprius as both receive highly myelinated low-threshold primary afferent neuronal inputs that include proprioceptors. Whereas lamina III consists mainly of small neurons with morphologies similar to lamina II, lamina IV has a subpopulation of large cells with extensive dendritic extensions that reach superficially. Laminae III and IV also have neurons with axonal projections extending up ascending pathways including the spinothalamic tract and the dorsal columns.

Lamina V: Neurons receive input from Aδ- and C-fiber nociceptors as well as myelinated afferents carrying low-threshold information. Cell bodies are frequently moderately sized pyramidal cells and may have dendritic extensions through the entire dorsal horn reaching to lamina I and II sites of synaptic contact as well as laterally. Neurons of this lamina have been demonstrated to receive input from all somatic, muscle, and visceral afferent types. Axonal projections of lamina V neurons to supraspinal sites are common.

Lamina VI: Neurons are small neurons present in the cervical and lumbar enlargements but largely missing in the rest of the spinal cord. Low-threshold muscle afferents and both low- and high-threshold cutaneous afferents reach to this lamina.

Laminae VII to IX: Represent neurons of the ventral horn.

Lamina X: Neurons are arranged around the central canal of the spinal cord. They receive bilateral inputs of unmyelinated, poorly myelinated, and highly myelinated afferents. Cell bodies are of moderate size with local dendritic arborizations. Some neurons in the dorsal aspects of lamina X have axonal projections extending up the dorsal columns to reach medullary targets. Peptidergic inputs are extensive and immunohistochemical localization of noradrenergic and serotonergic inputs

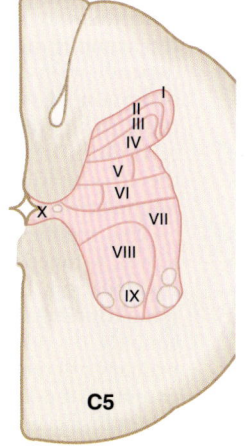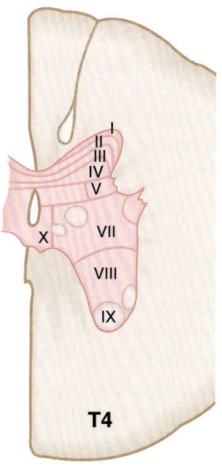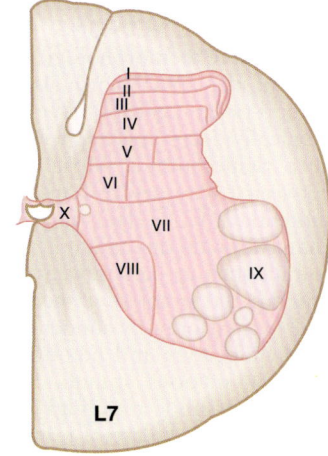

FIGURE 4.2 Diagrams showing Rexed's laminar histologic organization of the cat spinal cord grey matter at three levels. The dorsal horn corresponds to laminae I through VI inclusive. *(Redrawn after Rexed B. The cytoarchitectonic organization of the spinal cord in the cat. J Comp Neurol 1952;96(3): 415–495. Copyright © 1952 The Wistar Institute of Anatomy and Biology. Reprinted by permission of John Wiley & Sons, Inc.)*

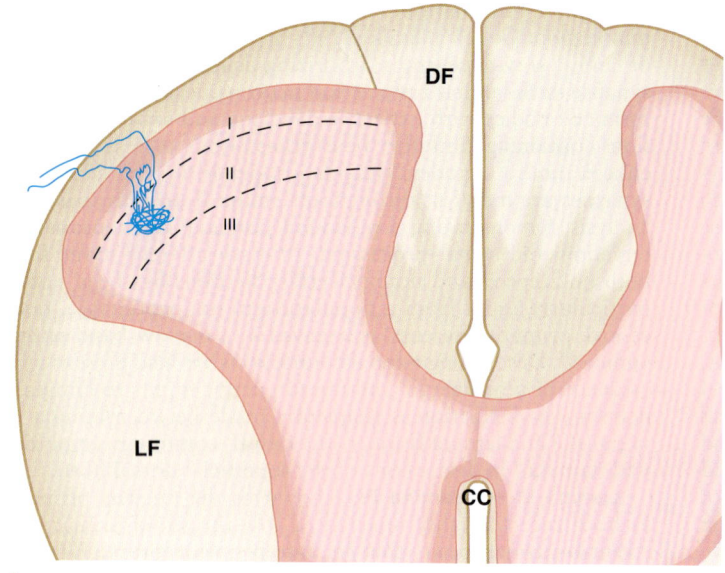

A

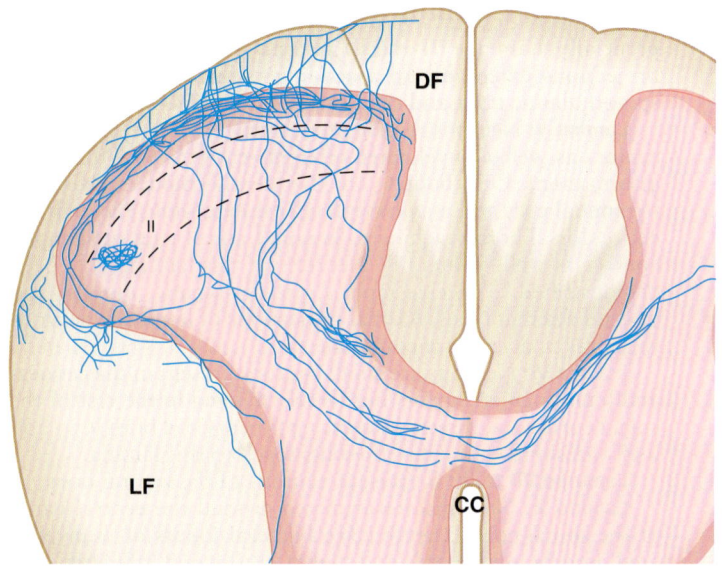

B

have been identified. Inhibitory neurons with immunohistochemical identification of glycinergic and GABAergic enzymes are locally present.

FUNCTIONAL CHARACTERIZATION OF NOCICEPTIVE NEURONS

In addition to morphologic heterogeneity, the multiple laminae of the spinal cord also have functional heterogeneity. Second-order neurons have been characterized electrophysiologically according to their responsiveness to cutaneous and deep tissue stimuli. Most commonly, a distinction is made between excitatory responses that are produced by noxious (potentially tissue-damaging) stimuli such as high-intensity mechanical or thermal stimuli and those produced by innocuous stimuli such as hair movement or vibration. Using these two criteria, the simplest nomenclature defines neurons as Class 1 if excited only by innocuous stimuli, Class 2 if excited by both innocuous and noxious stimuli, and Class 3 if excited only by noxious stimuli. Similar nomenclatures, but with additional subtle meanings implied by their original descriptions, include the use of terms such as *low threshold* for Class

1 neurons, *wide-dynamic-range*[14] or *convergent*[15] for Class 2 neurons, and *high threshold* or *nociceptive-specific* for Class 3 neurons. A fourth *nonresponder* group also must be factored in for neurons that fail to be excited by any of the employed stimuli. Despite the "clean" nature of this categorization, there unfortunately appears to be a spectrum of responses to all afferent input modalities with varying overlap that is somewhat dependent on the precise stimuli and definitions employed. The definition of neurons according to excitatory stimuli also appears to be preparation-dependent, as extracellular dorsal horn recordings of spinal neurons in cats have demonstrated that the classification of an individual neuron may change with the administration of anesthesia.[16]

The number of neuronal subgroups in any classification system is a function of the number of criteria employed for that classification. Despite this, it has been suggested that the use of inhibitory inputs as part of a classification criterion might actually simplify overall schema. Some neurons are inhibited following primary afferent activation. Inhibitory neurotransmitters are uncommon, if not absent, in primary afferents and so inhibition has generally been interpreted as due to a "modulatory" influence.

One such modulatory inhibitory influence used in classification is known as *diffuse noxious inhibitory controls* (DNIC) which is proposed to be an endogenous inhibitory system activated by a nonsegmental noxious stimulus. DNIC produces inhibition of ongoing or evoked dorsal horn neuronal activity, and according to its original description,[17,18] DNIC is specific for Class 2 (wide dynamic range [WDR], convergent) neurons and has no effect on Class 3 (nociceptive-specific [NS]) neurons. Subsequent studies of DNIC would support the general statement that DNIC effects are highly *selective* for Class 2 neurons with lesser effect on Class 3 neurons. Nomenclatures using a combination of responses to excitatory and inhibitory inputs have not been universally accepted.

CLASSIFICATION ACCORDING TO SITE OF PROJECTION

Second-order nociceptive spinal dorsal horn neurons frequently have axonal extensions projecting to rostral (and caudal) sites of termination. These sites include other segments of the spinal cord and supraspinal structures such as the thalamus, the hypothalamus, the midbrain, the pons, and the medulla. These axons travel predominantly within the white matter of the spinal cord in two main sites: the ventrolateral quadrants and the dorsal midline. Ascending fiber tracts in the dorsolateral funiculus have also been described. Decussation of fibers to the contralateral ventrolateral white matter occurs for axons projecting to the thalamus and most other brainstem sites, although many axons with sites of termination in "reticular" structures remain in the ipsilateral ventrolateral white matter. Dorsal column pathways have sites of termination in the gracile or cuneatus nucleus of the medulla. Intraspinal pathways that may stay within the grey matter have also been demonstrated as well as extensive collateralization of axons with multiple sites of termination at supraspinal and intraspinal sites.

Targets of Axonal Projections

INTRASPINAL PATHWAYS

Multiple interconnections occur between spinal neurons. On a segmental level, this is referred to as *interneuron connectivity*. When connections are more distant, the pathways of connection are termed *propriospinal* based on the initial demonstration of a coordinating connectivity between the cervical and lumbar enlargements of quadrupeds that allowed for coordinated motion. Intraspinal connectivity has also been demonstrated in the case of neurons receiving afferent input from pelvic structures with a dual innervation through thoracolumbar sympathetic and sacral pelvic nerves. These intraspinal connections appear to coordinate autonomic functions related to the pelvic organs.[19,20] A precise white matter localization of the axonal extensions of propriospinal nociceptive neurons has not been performed, but they are presumed to follow the paths of other propriospinal neurons which include dorsally located white matter paths and some within grey matter extensions. Collateral intraspinal extensions of ascending axons located within the ventrolateral white matter have also been demonstrated.

A separate system of intraspinal connections, the multisynaptic ascending system, may have particular relevance to chronic pain. In concepts championed by Noordenbos[21] but first proposed by Goldschneider, long chains or "webs" of neuronal connections extend through the length of the spinal cord and carry nociceptive information in a slow but progressive fashion to the brain by short "hops." Support for this concept is given by animal experiments, in which opposing hemisections performed at differing spinal levels fail to block nociceptive behaviors, but total transections at a single level are effective.[22] Traditionally described as an ascending pathway, bidirectionality of signaling is possible with a potential for the generation of "reverberatory" circuits.

SPINOTHALAMIC TRACT
Ventrolateral (Anterolateral) Axonal Pathways

The most studied spinal projection pathway is the spinothalamic tract which is located within the ventrolateral white matter of the spinal cord. Both ipsilateral and contralateral localization of axon pathways have been demonstrated en route to supraspinal sites, but the predominant path for axonal projections traveling to the ventrobasal thalamus resides on the contralateral side. Experiments utilizing lesions of the ventrolateral spinal white matter have demonstrated reduction or abolition of ventrobasal thalamic neuronal responses to most somatic noxious stimuli. Consistent with this observation, surgical or traumatic interruption of ventrolateral fiber pathways results in the lack of sensation to noxious cutaneous stimuli (i.e., pinprick) applied to the contralateral side of the body at spinal segments below the level of the lesion. The second-order neurons which project to the thalamus have been identified in rodent, feline, and primate models using neuroanatomical (retrograde dye labeling or chromatolytic responses to axonal section) and electrophysiologic (antidromic activation) methods. Neurophysiologic experiments have not always proven that the neurons of study had axonal projections that actually reach the thalamus but have always demonstrated that neurons of interest have axons present within the ventrolateral spinal white matter and so the term *spinothalamic tract* (STT) neurons is generally employed to describe the neurons rather than the more specific term *spinothalamic*.

Neospinothalamic versus Paleospinothalamic

There exist two different components of the spinothalamic tract—the neospinothalamic tract (nSTT) and the paleospinothalamic tract (pSTT), the former of which forms a direct, dedicated relay to the ventrobasal group of the thalamus and the latter of which has many neurons with one or more axonal bifurcations that form dichotomizing fibers ending in synaptic contact with medullary, pontine, midbrain, and medial thalamic structures. Ascending information transmitted through the pSTT produces activation of numerous limbic structures and has therefore been viewed as important to affective and motivational aspects of pain, whereas the nSTT, through relays in the ventrobasal and posterior thalamus, activates the somatosensory cortex and so has been viewed as important to localization and intensity coding of pain-related sensations. Axonal collateral branchings of pSTT neurons have been identified that correspond to multiple areas of limbic and autonomic activation which include medullary, pontine, mesencephalic, hypothalamic, and medial thalamic targets.

Laminar Distribution of Spinothalamic Tract Neurons

The cells of origin of the STT reside within all laminae of the spinal cord except motoneuronal layers and therefore can have multiple different morphologies. At lumbar levels in primates, the greatest number of nSTT neurons not only reside in laminae I and V but also are highly represented in laminae IV, VI, IX, and X with additional representation in III, VII, and VIII. In contrast, the neurons of the pSTT have soma in deeper laminae (VI to VIII) with a lesser representation in I, IV, and V. The axons of STT neurons typically decussate to the contralateral side via the dorsal commissure within one to two spinal segments of the neuronal soma, but at sacral and upper cervical levels, a significant number (up to 26%) of axons of STT neurons may remain ipsilateral.[23] A general somatotopic organization of the ascending fibers within the STT has been noted with an inner-to-outer progression of layers of fibers to the white matter from cervical to sacral levels (Fig. 4.4). A similar somatotopy is noted at medullary levels. The STT splits into two parts through the rostral medulla and pons to merge again at mesencephalic regions where an anterior-to-posterior somatotopic distribution

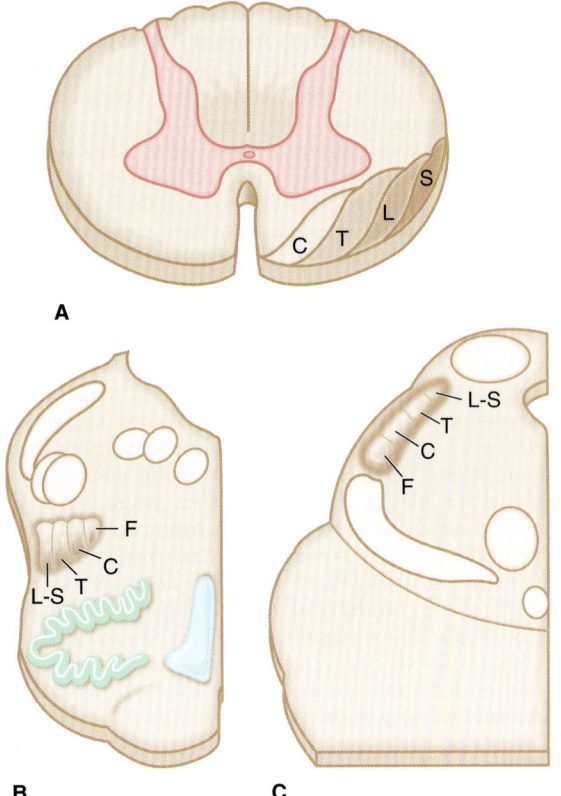

FIGURE 4.4 Schematic diagrams showing cross-section of the spinal cord, medulla, and midbrain, depicting the laminar arrangement of the ascending tracts in the ventrolateral funiculus in the upper part of the cervical spinal cord **(A)** and with the addition of the trigeminothalamic tract in the medulla **(B)** and midbrain **(C)**. *C*, cervical; *F*, face; *L*, lumbar; *S*, sacral; *T*, thoracic.

is noted. Differences in conduction velocity of subsets of STT neurons has been identified (lamina I STT neurons have slower conduction velocities than lamina V STT neurons) suggesting differences in axonal diameter and myelination processes. That, in turn, suggests a potential for temporally different delivery of sensory information to brain structures and differential susceptibility to pathologic processes.

Functional Characterization of Spinothalamic Tract Neurons

Quantitative electrophysiologic characterization of STT neurons has demonstrated a predominance for neurons processing nociceptive information. However, approximately 20% of STT neurons encode exclusively for nonnoxious light touch sensations,[13] and a small subset encodes for proprioceptive information. Multiple subsets of nociceptive neurons have been identified that have selective laminar localization. NS STT neurons, with slow adapting responses to noxious pinch, heat, or chemical stimulation, are commonly located in lamina I but are also present in deeper laminae. Noxious cold has been used as an additional characterizing stimulus[24] and allowed for the identification of additional subsets of lamina I NS STT neurons. WDR STT neurons, which demonstrate excitatory responses to multimodal sensory inputs (including both noxious and nonnoxious stimuli), are found extensively in lamina V but can also be found in all other laminae. Convergence of visceral, myofascial, articular, and cutaneous inputs is the rule rather than the exception when examining WDR STT neurons,[25] but similar convergence has been noted in NS STT neurons. Overall, with the possible exception of noxious cold inputs, the presence or absence of a particular group of sensory inputs has been of limited value in

identifying lamina-specific, morphologic, functional, or projection-related neuronal subsets. However, there are important generalities that are apparent in quantitative analyses of neuronal subsets[26]: Lamina I STT neurons tend to be NS neurons, lamina V (and other deep laminae) STT neurons tend to be WDR neurons, STT neurons with projections to the medial thalamus (pSTT) are more likely to be NS rather than WDR neurons and frequently have large receptive fields, STT neurons with projections to the lateral thalamus (nSTT) are more likely to be WDR rather than NS neurons and often have smaller receptive fields, and STT neurons with projections to both medial and lateral thalamus appear similar to neurons with projections only to the lateral thalamus.

Dorsolateral and Ventromedial Axonal Pathways

Spinothalamic neurons with soma primarily located within lamina I have been demonstrated to send axonal projections to the contralateral posterior nuclei of the thalamus via a contralateral dorsolateral pathway.[27,28] Estimated to form up to a quarter of all spinothalamic neurons,[29] these neurons have been identified electrophysiologically to be primarily NS neurons with small cutaneous receptive fields. Deeper laminae neurons and WDR neurons are also represented in this pathway. Many axons of spinothalamic neurons also travel within the ventromedial white matter of the spinal cord with soma located within laminae I, IV, V, VI, and VII.[30] Functional characterization of spinothalamic neurons with axons in the ventromedial white matter suggest a mixture of nonnociceptive and nociceptive neurons with supraspinal targets in the mesencephalon and intralaminar nuclei of the thalamus.

SPINORETICULAR AND SPINOMESENCEPHALIC TRACTS

Ventrolateral (Anterolateral) Axonal Pathways

As noted previously, ascending axonal fibers of nociceptive second-order neurons traveling to the thalamus may frequently branch and send collaterals into brainstem structures including the medulla, pons, and mesencephalon. However, numerous ascending fibers travel to these brainstem structures without having collaterals to the thalamus and collectively are described as spinoreticular if they reach medullary and pontine sites or spinomesencephalic if they reach midbrain targets. Subsets of spinoreticular neurons, defined by known targets for the axons, include spinomedullary, spinopontine, spinoolivary, spinosolitary, spinoraphe, and spinoparabrachial neuronal groups. Identification of these subgroups has been possible using focal injections of retrogradely transported neuronal dyes at supraspinal sites or antidromic electrical activation of axonal extensions. Although the former technique has reasonable localization potential, the latter does not always discriminate axons of passage from final sites of termination. The presence of collateralization of axons to multiple targets has been identified but not quantitatively defined, and so the overlap between the sampling of groups is not known. The spinal localization of spinoreticular and spinomesencephalic ascending axons overlap with those of the ventrolateral STT except for a greater propensity for remaining ipsilateral within the spinal cord and a slightly more medial line of passage upon entering the medulla. Spinomesencephalic neurons also utilize the dorsolateral funiculus for a subset of lamina I neurons in a fashion similar to that of similar spinothalamic neurons.

Features of Spinoreticular Neurons

The locations and functional characteristics of spinoreticular neurons in primates are virtually identical with the same features of STT neurons with projections to the medial thalamus. They demonstrate a predominant localization to deeper laminae of the spinal cord and tend to have large, sometimes whole-body, receptive fields of the NS and WDR types. Synaptic targets include many areas of the medulla and brainstem highly involved in autonomic regulation as well as the regulation of nociceptive systems. The potential for feedback control of nociceptive processing is therefore anatomically present. An important relay site is the parabrachial nucleus in the pons[31] which has extensive projections to limbic subcortical structures such as the amygdala.

Features of Spinomesencephalic Neurons

In contrast to spinoreticular neurons, the locations and functional characteristics of spinomesencephalic neurons in primates are similar to STT neurons with projections to the lateral thalamus, although significant differences are present. They demonstrate a predominant localization of soma to laminae I and V of the spinal cord with a small scattering to other deep laminae. Electrophysiologic characterization of spinomesencephalic neurons suggests a predominance of NS neurons. Synaptic targets include the periaqueductal gray, a site with known importance to the regulation of nociception as well as the collicular and cuneiformis nuclei.

POSTSYNAPTIC DORSAL COLUMN NEURONS

Recently, there has been increasing evidence for the existence of a spinal pathway in the midline of the dorsal spinal cord that carries the rostral transmission of deep tissue nociception. Traditionally, the dorsal columns have been viewed as transmitting information related to nonnociceptive information such as vibration or other light touch sensations. However, discrete neurosurgical lesions of this portion of the spinal cord have been demonstrated to relieve cancer-related pain in patients with pelvic visceral and deep muscle pathology.[32,33] Parallel studies in nonhuman animals have demonstrated that in this area of spinal white matter, there exist axons of postsynaptic dorsal column (PSDC) neurons receiving noxious excitatory input from the colon, bladder, and/or uterus. Excitatory responses of neurons located in the ventrobasal thalamus to noxious deep tissue stimuli are attenuated/abolished with lesions of the dorsal midline region of the spinal cord[32] but are only minimally affected by lesions of the traditional spinothalamic pathways (ventrolateral quadrant).

The soma of PSDC neurons are located predominantly in lamina III, IV, and X, and in a limited number of studies, the neurons have been demonstrated to be responsive to both somatic and visceral nociceptive inputs. Both NS and WDR neuronal types have been reported and their role in nociception is linked more to the secondary effects of dorsal column lesions than inherent neuronal characteristics. Targets for synaptic contact include the gracile and cuneatus nuclei of the medulla (dorsal column nuclei), but it is notable that the presence or absence of collaterals to other ascending tracts or other supraspinal targets has not been performed.

OTHER ASCENDING PATHWAYS

There exist other pathways to the brain apart from those noted. The spinocervicothalamic tract is important in other species but appears minimal or absent in humans. Direct projection pathways to the hypothalamus, amygdala,[31] and cerebellum have also been identified with presumed roles in autonomic function, affective-emotional modulation, and motor coordination, respectively. Extraspinal pathways for peripheral primary afferents exist and can sometime lend confusion to studies of central pathways. Vagal afferents can reach the brainstem carrying extensive information from visceral and other deep tissue structures leaving brainstem-mediated responses intact despite the interruption of spinal pathways. Similarly, primary afferents from deep structures including the viscera and peripheral vasculature can travel via the sympathetic chain to enter the spinal cord at levels much higher than expected and so can "bypass" selective spinal lesions of ascending pathways forming synaptic contact at levels above the lesions. Clinically, these other pathways sometimes prove important to consider, particularly in conditions of spinal cord injury.

Neurochemistry of Second-order Neurons

NEUROTRANSMITTERS FROM PRIMARY AFFERENTS

Excitatory neurotransmission of second-order spinal neurons is produced predominantly by the release of excitatory amino acids (EAAs), such as glutamate and aspartate, from primary afferent neurons. Various other neurotransmitters lead to neuroexcitatory effects by channel activation or sometimes via second messenger systems, but in most cases, these other neurotransmitters appear to have the augmentation of EAA-induced excitatory responses as their primary function. Most notable of these neurotransmitters are CGRP, substance P, and NK-A, but roles for serotonin, adenosine triphosphate (ATP), and cholecystokinin (CCK) have been identified. The inhibitory neuropeptides galanin and somatostatin are also released from primary afferents, but they are small in number and with limited effects on second-order neurons. A summary of spinal cord dorsal horn neurotransmitter location and associated receptors is given in Table 4.1.

Excitatory Amino Acids: Ionotropic Receptor/Channels

EAAs not only act on ligand-activated ion channels to produce immediate excitatory postsynaptic potentials (EPSPs) but also act at metabotropic receptors to alter intracellular second messenger systems (discussed in the following text). Three different EAA-activated ion channels have been characterized: α-amino-3-hydroxy-5-methyl-4-isoxazolepropionic acid (AMPA) receptors, NMDA receptors, and kainate (KA) receptors. These receptors have differential functions despite frequent colocalization on the same neurons due to differences in their regulation by baseline membrane potentials. As different receptors/channels, they are also differentially affected by the presence of other agonists and ions such as magnesium.

Activation of AMPA receptors immediately allows selective sodium ion flow through the extracellular membrane and is responsible for a majority of the "fast" transmission in nociceptive systems. AMPA receptors are unaffected by the baseline depolarization state of the second-order neuron. In contrast, NMDA receptors are both voltage- and ligand-gated and allow permeability to both sodium and calcium ions. Magnesium ions act to block the channels of NMDA receptors, which are unblocked following a sustained depolarization of the extracellular membrane. Such a sustained alteration in membrane potential enables the magnesium ion to disengage intracellularly which then allows the opening and activation of the NMDA receptor/channel complex, which, in turn, results in a *very* sustained depolarization. Because the NMDA receptor/channel is permeable to calcium, its sustained activation can produce alterations in intracellular second messenger functions of calcium.

Two phenomena have been clearly linked to NMDA receptor activation: "wind-up" (increasing responses to repeated stimuli of equal intensity) and "central sensitization" (decreased thresholds for response and/or increased vigor of responses due to a sensitizing event). NMDA antagonists will block/blunt both phenomena, but these phenomena can also be stopped prior to their development by pharmacologic antagonists that block the initial event that led to the sustained depolarization that allowed the NMDA receptor activation. As a consequence, the antagonism of other excitatory systems (i.e., AMPA receptors) or the activation of endogenous inhibitory systems may also blunt or block these "hyperalgesic" phenomena. Clinical use of NMDA receptor antagonists such as ketamine or dextromethorphan has been

TABLE 4.1   Location of Substrates of Nociception

Neurotransmitter (Receptor)	Primary Afferent Neuron (Presynaptic)	Dorsal Horn Neuron (Second-order, Interneuron)	Descending Fibers
Glutamate/aspartate	x	x	x
AMPA	+	+	
NMDA	+	+	
KA	+	+	
mGluR1–8	+	+/−	
iGluR	−		
GABA		x	x
GABA$_A$	−	−	
GABA$_B$	−	−	
Glycine		x	x
Strych-sensitive	−	−	
Strych-insensitive	−	−	
NMDA bind site	+	+	
Substance P	x	x	x
NK1		+	
Neurokinin A, B	x(A)	x(A), x(B)	x(A)
NK2		+	
CGRP	x		
CGRP-R		+	
ATP	x	x	x
P2X	+	+	
P2Y	+		
Adenosine		x	
A1		−	
Serotonin		x	x
5-HT$_2$		−	
5-HT$_3$	+/−	+	
Norepinephrine			x
α_1		+	
α_2	−	−	
Acetylcholine		x	
nACh	−	+	
mACh	−		
Cholecystokinin	x	x	x
CCK-A		+	
CCK-B	+	+	
Galanin	x	x	
Gal1	−		
Gal2		−	
Somatostatin	**x**	x	
SSN-R2		−	
SSN-R4	−		
VIP	x		
VIP-R		+	
Enkephalin		x	x
Dynorphin	x	x	
MOR	−	−	
DOR	−	−	
KOR	−	+/−	
Nociceptin		x	
ORL1	+/−	−	
NPY	x	x	
NPY-1	−	−	
Bombesin		x	
NM	+		
Other neurotransmitters implicated in central modulation of nociception			
Dopamine			x (−)
Oxytocin			x (−)
CRF and urocortins		x (+/−)	x (+/−)
Growth factors			
BDNF	x (+/−)	x (+)	
NGF	x (+)		
GDNF	x (+/−)		
ARTN	x (+/−)		

TABLE 4.1   (Continued)

Neurotransmitter (Receptor)	Primary Afferent Neuron (Presynaptic)	Dorsal Horn Neuron (Second-order, Interneuron)	Descending Fibers
Nitric oxide		x (+)	
Neurotensin		x (−)	
NFF		x (+/−)	
TRH		x (+)	x (+)
Other receptors implicated in central modulation of nociception			
(TRPV1)	+		
(TRPA1)	+		
(TRPM8)	+/−		
(B2)	+		
(CB1)	−		
(TrkA-C)	+(A), +(B)	+(A), +(B), +(C)	
(GFR1–3)	+/− (1, 2, 3)	+ (1, 3)	

NOTE: Pharmacologic systems thought to contribute to the transmission and modulation of second-order nociceptive neurons in the dorsal horn of the spinal cord. The various neurochemicals and receptors depicted each has its own pharmacologic profile and may represent independent populations of neurons and fibers but more commonly coexist and interact with each other at individual synapses. Interactions may take place at presynaptic terminals, dendrites, and somata.

x, origin of neurotransmitter; +, pronociceptive effect; −, antinociceptive effect; α_1, α_2, alpha adrenoceptors; A1, adenosine receptor 1; AMPA, α-amino-3-hydroxy-5-methyl-4-isoxazolepropionate; ARTN, artemin; ATP, adenosine triphosphate; B2, beta 2; BDNF, brain-derived neurotrophic factor; CB1, cannabinoid receptor 1; CCK, cholecystokinin; CGRP, calcitonin gene-related peptide; CRF, corticotropin-releasing factor; DOR, δ-opioid receptor; 5-HT, 5-hydroxytryptamine; GABA, γ-aminobutyric acid; Gal1, galanin receptors type 1; Gal2, galanin receptors type 2; GDNF, glial cell line-derived neurotrophic factor; GFR, GDNF family receptors; iGluR, ionotropic glutamate receptor; KA, kainate receptors; KOR, κ-opioid receptor; mACh, muscarinic acetylcholine; mGluR, metabotropic glutamate receptor; MOR, μ-opioid receptors; nACh, nicotinic acetylcholine; NFF, neuropeptide FF; NGF, nerve growth factor; NK1, neurokinin 1 receptor; NK2, neurokinin 2 receptor; NM, neuromedin receptor; NMDA, N-methyl-D-aspartate. NPY, neuropeptide Y; ORL1, nociceptin/orphanin FQ peptide receptor; SSN-R2, somatostatin receptor 2; SSN-R4, somatostatin receptor 4; TRH, thyrotropin-releasing hormone; TrkA-C, receptor tyrosine kinase C; TRPA1, transient receptor potential cation channel subfamily A member 1; TRPM8, transient receptor potential cation channel subfamily M member 8; TRPV1, transient receptor potential cation channel subfamily V member 1; VIP, vasoactive intestinal polypeptide.

From Gao and Ji[2]; Nauta et al.[33]; Gerber et al.[34]; Wiesenfeld-Hallin and Xu[35]; Pan et al.[36]; Gu and MacDermott[37]; Gu et al.[38]; Chiou et al.[39]; Mollereau et al.[40]; Pertovaara[41]; Obata and Noguchi[42]; Yaksh[43]; Dickenson[44]; Terman et al.[45]; Ness and Brennan[46]; Millan[63]; Korosi et al.[64]; Vasconcelos et al.[65]

demonstrated to produce prolonged analgesic effects when co-administered with opioids or as part of a perioperative regimen.

The third ligand-activated ion channel, the KA channel, is not well-understood but is likely to affect nociceptive systems in a yet-to-be-defined fashion. Metabotropic effects (second messenger–mediated) of the KA receptor that are in addition to its primary ionotropic effects have been observed in CNS sites such as the hippocampus. Evidence of participation in intracellular signaling cascades and G protein activation that lead to the modulation of GABA release suggest that KA receptors could have a role in nociceptive processing.[47]

Metabotropic Glutamate Receptors
Acting via second messenger systems rather than channel activation, the eight different metabotropic glutamate receptors (mGluRs) can be classified into three groups on the basis of sequence similarity and whether they positively couple to the phospholipase C cascade or negatively couple to the adenyl cyclases.[34] Group I (mGluR1 and mGluR5) has been linked to nociceptive processing as these receptors produce alterations in NMDA receptor/channel opening. As such, they have been implicated in processes of central sensitization and persistent pain. Group II (mGluR2 and mGluR3) has also been used to modify nociceptive behavioral responses in models of neuropathic and inflammatory pain. Group III (mGluR6, mGluR7, and mGluR8) has not yet had a clearly defined role in nociception.

Substance P
This neuropeptide has long been attributed a special role in pain processing as it is located in small diameter primary afferents and is released following cutaneous noxious stimuli.[48,49] Substance P acts by binding to NK1 receptors on second-order neurons, thereby affecting intracellular G protein-related phosphorylation processes. It is often colocalized with, and so coreleased with, glutamate from primary afferents and promotes membrane depolarization produced by glutamate. In this way, it modifies the gain of nociceptive transmission. It is important in conditions of inflammation, particularly neurogenic inflammation, where it is released from peripheral axons and produces

a local tissue effect. However, substance P may not be necessary for acute nociceptive transmission because the pharmacologic or genetic "knock-out" of the NK1 receptor has minimal effect on acute responses to most nociceptive stimuli. Substance P is present in highest concentration in laminae I and II$_\text{o}$ as well as in laminae V and VI. Other neurokinin receptors also exist which bind other neuropeptides such as NK-A, which has physiologic effects similar to substance P. Neuropeptide antagonists such as the NK1 antagonists have proved to have disappointing results in clinical trials when pain was the clinical endpoint,[50] although efficacy has been noted in association with nausea therapy.

Calcitonin Gene-Related Peptide
The most commonly located neuropeptide in afferent systems (CGRP) has a poorly defined role in nociceptive processing with mixed results from depletion, augmentation, and antagonism studies.[51] At present, its most important effects appear to be related to peripheral vasodilation that is associated with the generation of headaches.[52] Electrophysiologic studies of spinal WDR second-order neurons have demonstrated an augmentation of nociceptive responses due to direct application of CGRP in a neuromodulatory fashion similar to substance P and NK1 receptor activation.[53] Like substance P, the knockout of CGRP synthesis has little effect on acute experimental models. CGRP localizes in primary afferent terminals in laminae I, II, and V. Human and nonhuman animal studies suggest that CGRP may be most important in relation to neurogenic inflammatory processes—particularly those associated with migraine headache. There is a clear association between headache symptomatology and the peripheral release of CGRP and antagonists to the CGRP receptor have been reported as efficacious for the relief of acute migraine attacks.[54] For these reasons, CGRP may not be as important as a substrate for spinal cord processing as it is for the peripheral effects of nociceptor activation.

Cholecystokinin
A peptide present in primary afferent neurons, CCK has little effect in animals without pathology, but the neuropeptide increases in content and its receptors in number following

nerve injury.[35,55] Opioid receptor function and CCK receptor activation are also related in a complex fashion as CCK receptor antagonists may promote opioid analgesia and slow morphine tolerance development at spinal levels. Consistent with this, CCK receptor antagonists may be analgesic in neuropathic pain models, and this analgesia is antagonized by naloxone. CCK is localized predominantly to laminae I, II, IV, and X and is a neurotransmitter present in both primary afferents and interneurons.

Other Neuropeptides

Multiple other neuropeptides that are in primary afferent neurons or which have receptors on the central terminals of primary afferent receptors have been implicated in nociceptive spinal processing. These include vasoactive intestinal polypeptide (VIP), bombesin, gastrin-releasing peptide, neuromedin B, neuromedin C, neuropeptide YY, and thyrotropin-releasing hormone (TRH). Action of most of these neurotransmitters on nociceptive systems appears to be predominantly a facilitatory presynaptic action on primary afferent neurotransmitter release. VIP has a presence in the ventral horn of the spinal cord, but the predominant source of VIP to the dorsal horn is primary afferents with strong localization in lamina I and a sparse representation in lamina V. Two neuropeptides located in primary afferent terminals, galanin and somatostatin, have inhibitory influences on second-order neurons.[35,36] Trophic factors such as nerve growth factor and brain-derived neurotrophic factor (BDNF) also act as influences to the second-order neurons, particularly in conditions of nerve injury or death.

Adenosine Triphosphate

Present in many primary afferents, ATP, as a neurotransmitter, is known to activate the ligand-gated ion channels of the P2X family as well as the metabotropic P2Y family of receptors. P2X receptor activation both potentiates glutamatergic transmission and produces fast transmission related to nociceptor activation.[37,38] Ubiquitous as the compound used to drive most energy-requiring processes of metabolism, ATP also has breakdown products that may serve as agonists to other purinergic receptors (A1, A2) located both extracellularly and intracellularly on second-order neurons.

Colocalization of Neurotransmitters

Corelease of neurotransmitters from primary afferent neurons is the typical rule rather than exception in relation to small diameter fibers. EAAs coexist with ATP, substance P, NK-A, CGRP, and other neuropeptides. These neuropeptides coexist in nerve terminals in varying combinations with each other with all possible mixtures described in overlap. CGRP is the most ubiquitous of the neuropeptides located within C fibers and so commonly colocalized with other neurotransmitters. The mechanisms of corelease are poorly understood and could involve selective release of one of the neurotransmitters.

NEUROTRANSMITTERS FROM INTERNEURONS

Whereas the predominant effect of primary afferent neurotransmitter release on second-order spinal neurons is excitation, the predominant effect of interneuron neurotransmitter release is inhibition. Second-order neurons may act as interneurons and at the same time may also be third, fourth, or higher order neurons responsible for excitatory and/or inhibitory effects on other second-order neurons. This is apparent in intermediate laminae neurons which have complex cutaneous receptive fields that represent the total body when both excitatory and inhibitory influences are considered.[15] Interneurons utilize many of the same excitatory neurotransmitters as primary afferents but, in addition, utilize many other neurotransmitters to produce inhibitory influences.

These fall mainly into the amino acid, neuropeptide, and small molecule groups. A listing of these neurotransmitters is also given in Table 4.1.

Inhibitory Amino Acids

GABA and glycine are the two main inhibitory amino acids of the CNS. GABAergic systems appear to be more predominant at supraspinal sites and glycine at spinal sites, but both are present throughout the CNS. GABA acts through a "fast" ligand-activated ion channel that allows chloride ion flow, which in turn produces hyperpolarization of the neuronal membrane. Termed the *GABA_A receptor*, it has associated structures that allow benzodiazepine or barbiturate binding to alter the GABA affinity and channel activation characteristics of the receptor/channel complex. The "slow" metabotropic receptor for GABA, the $GABA_B$ receptor is the binding site for baclofen and works via G protein-linked systems to alter potassium (promotes) and calcium (inhibits) ion channel flow. Via actions on motoneurons, $GABA_B$ receptor activation leads to decreased spasticity and muscle tone. At brainstem levels, in association with cranial nerve function, $GABA_B$ activation may be analgesic and so is indicated in the treatment of various cranial neuralgias. A putative $GABA_C$ receptor which is ionotropic has been described but with an uncertain role in sensory systems.

Glycine acts through both strychnine-sensitive and strychnine-insensitive receptors. The former, a ligand-gated anion channel very similar to the $GABA_A$ complex, is diffusely located but with particular effect in the ventral horn of the spinal cord such that the administration of strychnine can lead to spontaneous muscle contractions. Also present in spinal sensory systems, the antagonism of glycine effects with strychnine in animal models leads to motor and autonomic hyperreflexia. Paradoxically, glycine can also have excitatory effects via binding as a coagonist to a separate site of the NMDA receptor. Because of their multiple nonspecific effects, anti- or pro-glycinergic drugs have not been employed clinically, although theoretical uses are present. Selective delivery of agents to focused CNS sites might be able to overcome some of these nonspecific effects.

Opioids

Endogenous opioids form the most prominent family of inhibitory neuropeptides in the dorsal horn. Arising from intrinsic spinal interneurons, enkephalins, dynorphin, and β-endorphin bind to G protein-related receptor complexes that fall into three major classes: the μ-opioid receptors (MOR), the κ-opioid receptors (KOR), and the δ-opioid receptors (DOR). Exogenously administered MOR agonists are the mainstay of analgesic therapy for severe pain today with actions at both spinal and supraspinal sites. Spinal effects arising from supraspinal actions of MOR agonists are via descending serotonergic and noradrenergic mechanisms. MOR agonists administered to spinal sites act both presynaptically on primary afferents to inhibit release of excitatory neurotransmitters and postsynaptically to directly inhibit second-order neurons. KOR agonists, such as the endogenous dynorphins, have been demonstrated to be neurotoxic when administered in high concentrations. Peripherally, these same agents appear to produce analgesia particularly in the realm of deep tissue afferents. DOR agonists hold great promise with many of the favorable characteristics of MOR agonists. However, to date, study of selective DOR agonists have been hampered by the lack of highly selective, nontoxic drugs for use.

An opioid receptor–related neurotransmitter is the substance nociceptin and its receptor, the nociceptin/orphanin FQ (N/OFQ) peptide receptor. Due to the technology of functional genomics, this receptor, formerly known as the opioid receptor like orphan receptor-1, was the first of hundreds of G protein-coupled receptors identified which had no known endogenous ligand or function. Subsequently, nociceptin (orphanin FQ) was identified and functional pharmacology performed with agonists to the N/OFQ peptide receptor showing some promise in relation to the treatment of anxiety, stress-induced anorexia, cough, neurogenic bladder, edema, drug dependence, cerebral ischemia, and epilepsy.[39] The precise role of nociceptin in pain processing is still being determined with both antiopioid and opioid-potentiating modulatory properties demonstrated.[40]

Acetylcholine

A rediscovered and so developing, novel pharmacology important to nociceptive processing is that involving the cholinergic systems. Numerous dorsal horn interneurons label positive for enzymes associated with acetylcholine synthesis and/or degradation and pharmacologic effects have been noted in relation to both nicotinic and muscarinic subtypes. Use of neuraxially delivered cholinesterase inhibitors, which leads to the increased activation of both nicotinic and muscarinic receptors, not only clearly produces analgesia in nonhuman animal models but also produces intractable nausea in clinical studies (which reduces enthusiasm for their use). Cholinergic interneurons may act as intermediary steps for other analgesic treatments such as descending norepinephrine-related inhibitory systems.

Other Neurotransmitters within Interneurons

Numerous other neuropeptides and small molecules have been localized to interneurons which include thyroid-stimulating hormone (TSH), neurotensin, neuropeptide FF, neuropeptide Y, somatostatin, galanin, and CCK. All of these have been demonstrated to have dorsal horn localization, and all produce neuromodulatory effects, many with mixed excitatory/inhibitory interactions with opioid systems.

NEUROTRANSMITTERS FROM SUPRASPINAL SOURCES

Spinal transection leads to a depletion of the content of several neurotransmitters within the dorsal horn of the spinal cord. Most notable of these are the monoamines serotonin and norepinephrine. Spinal transection still leaves residual serotonin content within the ventral horn indicating some local production of neurotransmitter that may be in addition to that circulating in blood components. Any residual noradrenergic content appears to be of sympathetic origin. As will be discussed in the next chapter, descending noradrenergic and serotonergic fibers originating in the brainstem produce robust inhibitory effects on second-order spinal neurons. It has also been recently appreciated that these same neurotransmitters may also produce excitatory effects and may therefore serve as the mechanisms of descending facilitation, another topic of the next chapter.

Serotonin (5-Hydroxytryptamine)

The pharmacologic characterization of responses to the endogenous substance, serotonin, has identified a highly complex interaction of this substance with multiple receptors, some with multiple subtypes. At last count, seven main families of 5-hydroxytryptamine (5-HT) receptors (most families further subdivided) have been identified, some with inhibitory and some with excitatory effects. The receptor of greatest relevance to pain production or excitatory phenomena is the 5-HT$_3$ receptor, the only one of the receptors which is a ligand-gated ion channel.[56] Excitatory responses to serotonin administered peripherally suggest that it can directly activate nociceptive primary afferent neurons. Actions on the dorsal roots have been postulated to be pronociceptive, antinociceptive, and pruritic. An increasing role for 5-HT$_{1A}$ has also been demonstrated as well as other serotonergic subsets. Boutons with serotonin content have been noted throughout the dorsal horn, and cell

bodies with serotonin have been identified in the ventral horn. A colocalization within synaptic boutons with the neuropeptide substance P has been commonly noted.

Noradrenaline

Adrenoceptors important to the spinal processing of pain appear to be of the α_1 or α_2 subtypes based on the use of agonists (i.e., clonidine) and antagonists administered spinally. Descending from brainstem noradrenergic neuronal nuclei (primarily A5, A6, and A7), known pharmacologic sites of action for norepinephrine include presynaptic terminals of nociceptive primary afferent neurons (α_2 inhibitory), second-order neurons (α_2 inhibitory), and interneurons (α_1 excitatory) and, as such, has been implicated in both descending inhibition and descending facilitation of nociceptive transmission.[41] Immunohistochemical localization of noradrenergic nerve fibers have found them widely dispersed throughout the dorsal horn and much of the release of neurotransmitter appears nonsynaptic in nature,[57] such that the neurotransmitter has to diffuse from its site of release to its site of action which may be neuronal or glial.[58] Extensive synaptic contact of noradrenergic nerve endings does occur within the ventral horn and intermediolateral grey.

Other Neurotransmitters in Descending Systems

Often colocalized with other neurotransmitters, certain neuropeptides and other monoamines are also in descending fibers that make contact with the spinal dorsal horn. These include substance P, CCK, corticotropin-releasing factor, urocortin 1, and TRH, which have excitatory neuromodulatory effects and dopamine, oxytocin, GABA, glycine, and endogenous opioids, which have inhibitory neuromodulatory effects. These descending fibers modulate more than just nociceptive sensory information but when exogenously administered to the spinal cord can produce profound autonomic and motor effects. TSH has been noted to have effects that are like CCK in that it appears to inhibit opioid analgesia.

NEUROTRANSMITTERS FROM GLIA OR UNKNOWN SOURCES

Numerous substances alter the excitability of second-order neurons to nociceptive input that are not from neural structures. For example, bradykinin, which is normally known for its peripheral nervous system effects, activates B2 receptors in the dorsal horn with the subsequent induction of hyperalgesia phenomena. Destruction of primary afferents results in the loss of two-thirds of these receptors, but the source of the activating bradykinin is unknown. Likewise, other substances associated with inflammation, such as prostanoids and cytokines, have similar neuromodulatory effects and the spinal administration of prostaglandin receptor agonists such those associated with prostaglandin E2 (PGE$_2$), prostaglandin D2 (PGD$_2$), or prostaglandin I2 (PGI$_2$) leads to hypersensitivity. Prostaglandin receptor activation may require other receptors for full expression of sensory phenomena as appears to be the case for PGE$_2$ which needs an intact NMDA receptor and a PGD$_2$ which requires intact NK1 receptors. Cytokines such as interleukin 1 beta (IL-1β), interleukin 6 (IL-6), and tumor necrosis factor-α, which are released by activated microglia and other neuroimmunologic cellular components of the CNS following nerve injury, have been appreciated as having neurotoxicity effects on nociceptive neurons that involve purinergic mechanisms.[59,60] Second-order neurons are sensitive to neurotrophin and glial cell line-derived neurotrophic factor (GDNF) families of ligands, released locally from multiple sources, including neural structures. Neuron responsiveness to these ligands is dependent on expression of high-affinity receptor tyrosine kinases (TrkA-C), the low-affinity receptor p75, GDNF family coreceptors (GDNF family receptor α [GFRα] 1 to 4), and the tyrosine kinase RET. The angiogenic growth factor, vascular endothelial growth factor (VEGF), and its receptors also modulate dorsal horn pain transmission. Receptor expression patterns, and thus growth factor sensitivity, are cell type–specific and produce trophic and phenotypic changes, but the specifics are beyond the scope of this chapter due to complexities related to developmental regulation and altered expression following tissue injury. Of note, however, is evidence that BDNF plays a substantial role in pain transduction by decreasing inhibition in dorsal horn neurons and descending inputs and increasing dorsal horn neuronal excitation. In addition to its pronociceptive actions mediated by TrkB, BDNF modulates a subset of NMDA receptors involved in the development and maintenance of central sensitization (discussed in the following chapter).[42,61,62]

OTHER IMPORTANT RECEPTORS/CHANNELS

Consideration needs to be given to the presence of receptors or channels that are either "universal" in that their pharmacologic modulation seemingly affects all spinal cord neurons in a relatively nondiscriminative fashion, or "selective" in that they are present in a subset and/or subsite of neurons such as the end terminals of primary afferent neurons. A particular group of ion channels that are in the *selective* group are the N-type calcium channels found on primary afferent neurons.[43] Calcium influx into the intercellular space due to receptor activation (ligand-gated) or due to membrane depolarization (voltage-gated) results in both membrane depolarization effects and second messenger cascade activation. In primary afferents, this calcium influx is associated with the release of neurotransmitter at synapses. There exist at least five families of voltage-gated channels (L, N, P/Q, R, and T) with differing pharmacologies and localization within the spinal cord. Some of the families share auxiliary subunits such as the L- and N-type channels which both have an $\alpha_2\delta$ subunit. This subunit is the site to which the drugs gabapentin and pregabalin bind with a subsequent reduction but not abolition of membrane excitability. The N-type calcium channels are located throughout the CNS but, at a spinal cord level, have particular localization to the nerve terminals of small diameter primary afferents. The ω-conotoxin ziconotide binds to and blocks ion flow through this channel and has found clinical utility in the control of pain when administered intrathecally.

Primary afferent sensory neurons also express voltage-gated sodium channels (VGSCs) that are fundamental to the generation and propagation of action potentials. Those VGSCs with subunits encoded by the genes for Nav1.8 and Nav1.9 are specific to sensory neurons, and Nav1.7 is expressed in nociceptive sensory neurons as well as other cell types. Changes in the expression of these channels or posttranslational modifications that alter their gating or trafficking impact nociceptive transmission, and thus, VGSCs expressed on sensory neurons have become targets for therapeutic strategies. Gain- and loss-of-function mutations that increase or decrease nociceptive transmission in animal models have been corroborated in humans; for example, gain-of-function mutations have been found in patients with painful neuropathy, erythermalgia, and paroxysmal extreme pain disorder, and loss-of-function mutations have been reported in families with congenital insensitivity to pain.

What Is Important to the Clinician

The substrates of nociception that exist at a spinal level are as complex as the phenomenon of pain itself. More than 30 different neurotransmitters acting at more than 50 different receptors have been identified as present in the spinal cord and associated with some pain-related phenomenon. Sensory pathways connecting the spinal cord to the brain have been identified that result in rapid transmission of information that is highly organized and site-specific, but similar pathways have also been identified which have slow transmission that is poorly organized and therefore resistant to attempts at ablation. The clinician must synthesize these diverse pieces of information into a general model of nociceptive processing and must accept that at this point in time, the model is incomplete. The effectiveness of therapeutic interventions intended to treat pain is dependent on the modulation of these substrates of nociception which forms the topic of the next chapter.

ACKNOWLEDGMENTS

The authors of this chapter are supported by DK51419, DK73218, and DK78655.

Note: The present chapter is intended as a summary of information important to pain clinicians and as a presentation of new information coupled with a simplification of previous presentations of similar information in this text and other sources.[44–46] As such, referencing has been lessened, although many of the primary sources of information may be found in the previous reviews.

References

1. Coggeshall RE. Fos, nociception and the dorsal horn. *Prog Neurobiol* 2005; 77:299–352.
2. Gao YJ, Ji RR. C-Fos and pERK, which is a better marker for neuronal activation and central sensitization after noxious stimulation and tissue injury? *Open Pain J* 2009;2:11–17.
3. Mantyh PW. Neurobiology of substance P and NK1 receptor. *J Clin Psychiatry* 2002;63(suppl 11):6–10.
4. Guo W, Wei F, Zou S, et al. Group 1 metabotropic glutamate receptor NMDA receptor coupling and signaling cascade mediate spinal dorsal horn NMDA receptor 2B tyrosine phosphorylation associated with inflammatory hyperalgesia. *J Neurosci* 2004;24:9161–9173.
5. Pattinson D, Fitzgerald M. The neurobiology of infant pain: development of excitatory and inhibitory neurotransmission in the spinal dorsal horn. *Reg Anesth Pain Med* 2004;29:36–44.
6. Zhang X, Bao L. The development and modulation of nociceptive circuitry. *Curr Opin Neurobiol* 2006;16:460–466.
7. Ruda MA, Ling QD, Hohmann AG, et al. Altered nociceptive neuronal circuits after neonatal peripheral inflammation. *Science* 2000;289:628–631.
8. Sugiura Y, Terui N, Hosoya Y. Difference in distribution of central terminals between visceral and somatic unmyelinated C-primary afferent fibers. *J Neurophysiol* 1989;62:834–840.
9. Morris R, Cheunsuang O, Stewart A, et al. Spinal dorsal horn neurone targets for nociceptive primary afferents: do single neurone morphological characteristics suggest how nociceptive information is processed at the spinal level. *Brain Res Rev* 2004;46:173–190.
10. Grudt TJ, Perl ER. Correlations between neuronal morphology and electrophysiological features in the rodent superficial dorsal horn. *J Physiol* 2002;540(pt 1):189–207.
11. Gobel S. Golgi studies of the neurons in layer II of the dorsal horn of the medulla (trigeminal nucleus caudalis). *J Comp Neurol* 1978;180:395–413.
12. Gobel S. Neural circuitry in the substantia gelatinosa of Rolando: anatomical insights In: Bonica JJ, Liebeskind J, Albe-Fessard D, eds. *Advances in Pain Research and Therapy.* Vol 3. New York: Raven Press; 1979:175–195.
13. Dubner R, Bennett GJ. Spinal and trigeminal mechanisms of nociception. *Ann Rev Neurosci* 1983;6:381–418.
14. Mendell LM, Wall PD. Responses of single dorsal cord cells to peripheral cutaneous unmyelinated fibres. *Nature* 1965;206:97–99.
15. Le Bars D. The whole body receptive field of dorsal horn multireceptive neurons. *Brain Res Revs* 2002;40:29–44.
16. Collins JG, Ren K. WDR response profiles of spinal dorsal horn neurons may be unmasked by barbiturate anesthesia. *Pain* 1987;28:369–378.
17. Le Bars D, Dickenson AH, Besson JM. Diffuse noxious inhibitory controls (DNIC): I. Effects on dorsal horn convergent neurones in the rat. *Pain* 1979;6:283–304.
18. Le Bars D, Dickenson AH, Besson JM. Diffuse noxious inhibitory controls (DNIC): II. Lack of effect on non-convergent neurones, supraspinal involvement and theoretical implications. *Pain* 1979;6:305–321.
19. McMahon SB, Morrison JF. Two group of spinal interneurones that respond to stimulation of the abdominal viscera of the cat. *J Physiol* 1982;322:21–34.
20. McMahon SB, Morrison JF. Spinal neurones with long projections activated from the abdominal viscera of the cat. *J Physiol* 1982;322:1–20.
21. Noordenbos W. *Pain.* Amsterdam, The Netherlands: Elsevier; 1959.
22. Basbaum AI. Conduction of the effects of noxious stimulation by short-fiber multisynaptic systems of the spinal cord in the rat. *Exp Neurol* 1973;40:699–716.

23. Willis WD, Kenshalo DR Jr, Leonard RB. The cells of origin of the primate spino-thalamic tract. *J Comp Neurol* 1979;188:543–573.
24. Han ZS, Zhang ET, Craig AD. Nociceptive and thermoreceptive lamina I neurons are anatomically distinct. *Nat Neurosci* 1998;1:218–225.
25. Willis WD, Westlund KN. Neuroanatomy of the pain system and the pathways that modulate pain. *J Clin Neurophysiol* 1997;14:2–31.
26. Giesler GJ Jr, Yezierski RP, Gerhart KD, et al. Spinothalamic tract neurons that project to medial and/or lateral thalamic nuclei: evidence for a physiologically novel population of spinal cord neurons. *J Neurophysiol* 1981;46:1285–1308.
27. Ralston HJ III, Ralston DD. The primate dorsal spinothalamic tract: evidence for a specific termination in the posterior nuclei (Po/SG) of the thalamus. *Pain* 1992;48:107–118.
28. Martin RJ, Apkarian AV, Hodge CJ Jr. Ventrolateral and dorsolateral ascending spinal cord pathway influence on thalamic nociception in cat. *J Neurophysiol* 1990;64:1400–1412.
29. Apkarian AV, Hodge CJ. Primate spinothalamic pathways: II. The cells of origin of the dorsolateral and ventral spinothalamic pathways. *J Comp Neurol* 1989;288:474–492.
30. Kerr F. Segmental circuitry and ascending pathways of the nociceptive systems In: Beers RF, Bassett EJ, eds. *Mechanisms of Pain and Analgesic Compounds.* New York: Raven Press; 1979:113–141.
31. Bernard JF, Bester H, Besson JM. Involvement of the spino-parabrachio, -amygdaloid and -hypothalamic pathways in the autonomic and affective emotional aspects of pain. *Prog Brain Res* 1996;107:243–255.
32. Hirschberg RM, Al-Chaer ED, Lawand NB, et al. Is there a pathway in the posterior funiculus that signals visceral pain? *Pain* 1996;67:291–305.
33. Nauta HJ, Soukup VM, Fabian RH, et al. Punctate midline myelotomy for the relief of visceral cancer pain. *J Neurosurg* 2000;92(suppl 2):125–130.
34. Gerber U, Gee CE, Benquet P. Metabotropic glutamate receptors: intracellular signaling pathways. *Curr Opin Pharmacol* 2007;7:56–61.
35. Wiesenfeld-Hallin Z, Xu XJ. Neuropeptides in neuropathic and inflammatory pain with special emphasis on cholecystokinin and galanin. *Eur J Pharmacol* 2001;429:49–59.
36. Pan HL, Wu ZZ, Zhou HY, et al. Modulation of pain transmission by G-protein-coupled receptors. *Pharmacol Ther* 2008;117:141–161.
37. Gu JG, MacDermott AB. Activation of ATP P2X receptors elicits glutamate release from sensory neuron synapses. *Nature* 1997;389:749–753.
38. Gu JG, Bardoni R, Magherini PC, et al. Effects of the P2-purinoceptor antagonists suramin and pyridoxal-phosphate-6-azophenyl-2′,4′-disulfonic acid on glutamatergic synaptic transmission in rat dorsal horn neurons of the spinal cord. *Neurosci Lett* 1998;253:167–170.
39. Chiou LC, Liao YY, Fan PC, et al. Nociceptin/orphanin FQ peptide receptors: pharmacology and clinical implications. *Curr Drug Targets* 2007;8:117–135.
40. Mollereau C, Roumy M, Zajac JM. Opioid-modulating peptides: mechanisms of action. *Curr Top Med Chem* 2005;5:341–355.
41. Pertovaara A. Noradrenergic pain modulation. *Prog Neurobiol* 2006;80:53–83.
42. Obata K, Noguchi K. BDNF in sensory neurons and chronic pain. *Neurosci Res* 2006;55:1–10.
43. Yaksh TL. Calcium channels as therapeutic targets in neuropathic pain. *J Pain* 2006;7:S13–S30.
44. Dickenson A, Besson JM, eds. *Pharmacology of pain.* New York: Springer; 1997.
45. Terman GW, Bonica JJ, Liebeskind JC. Spinal mechanisms and their modulation. In: Loeser JD, Butler SH, Chapman CR, et al, eds. *Bonica's Management of Pain.* 3rd ed. New York: Lippincott Williams & Wilkins; 2001:73–153.
46. Ness TJ, Brennan TJ. Sensory systems. In: Hemmings HC, Hopkins PM, eds. *Foundations of Anesthesia.* 2nd ed. London: Mosby Press; 2006.
47. Rodriguez-Moreno A, Sihra TS. Metabotropic actions of kainate receptors in the CNS. *J Neurochem* 2007;103:2121–2135.
48. Hill RG, Oliver KR. Neuropeptide and kinin antagonists. *Handb Exp Pharmacol* 2007;177:181–216.
49. Harrison S, Geppetti P. Substance P. *Int J Biochem Cell Biol* 2001;33:555–576.
50. Hill R. NK1 (substance P) receptor antagonists—why are they not analgesic in humans? *Trends Pharmacol Sci* 2000;21:244–246.
51. Van Rossum D, Hanisch UK, Quirion R. Neuroanatomical localization, pharmacological characterization and functions of CGRP, related peptides and their receptors. *Neurosci Biobehav Rev* 1997;21:649–678.
52. Brain SD, Cox HM. Neuropeptides and their receptors: innovative science providing novel therapeutic targets. *Br J Pharmacol* 2006;147:S202–S211.
53. Yu Y, Lundeberg T, Yu LC. Role of calcitonin gene-related peptide and its antagonist on the evoked discharge frequency of wide dynamic range neurons in the dorsal horn of the spinal cord in rats. *Regul Pept* 2002;103:23–27.
54. Edvinsson L, Petersen KA. CGRP-receptor antagonism in migraine treatment. *CNS Neurol Disord Drug Targets* 2007;6:240–246.
55. Wiesenfeld-Hallin Z, Xu XJ, Hökfelt T. The role of spinal cholecystokinin in chronic pain states. *Pharmacol Toxicol* 2002;91:398–403.
56. Färber L, Haus U, Späth M, et al. Physiology and pathophysiology of the 5-HT3 receptor. *Scand J Rheumatol Suppl* 2004;119:2–8.
57. Rajaofetra N, Ridet JL, Poulat P, et al. Immunocytochemical mapping of noradrenergic projections to the rat spinal cord with an antiserum against noradrenaline. *J Neurocytol* 1992;21:481–494.
58. Ridet JL, Rajaofetra N, Teilhac JR, et al. Evidence for nonsynaptic serotonergic and noradrenergic innervation of the rat dorsal horn and possible involvement of neuron-glia interactions. *Neuroscience* 1993;52:143–157.
59. Tsuda M, Inoue K, Salter MW. Neuropathic pain and spinal microglia: a big problem from molecules in "small" glia. *Trends Neurosci* 2005;28:101–107.
60. Inoue K. The function of microglia through purinergic receptors: neuropathic pain and cytokine release. *Pharmacol Ther* 2006;109:210–226.
61. Sah DW, Ossipov MH, Rossomando A, et al. New approaches for the treatment of pain: the GDNF family of neurotropic growth factors. *Curr Top Med Chem* 2005;5:577–583.
62. Bennett DL. Neurotrophic factors: important regulators of nociceptive function. *Neuroscientist* 2001;7:13–17.
63. Millan MJ. The induction of pain: an integrative review. *Prog Neurobio* 1999;57:1–164.
64. Korosi A, Kozicz T, Richter J, et al. Corticotropin-releasing factor, urocortin 1, and their receptors in the mouse spinal cord. *J Comp Neurol* 2007;502:973–989.
65. Vasconcelos LA, Donaldson C, Sita LV, et al. Urocortin in the central nervous system of a primate (*Cebus apella*): sequencing, immunohistochemical, and hybridization histochemical characterization. *J Comp Neurol* 2003;463:157–175.

CHAPTER 5

Modulation of Spinal Nociceptive Processing

TIMOTHY J. NESS, ALAN RANDICH, and **JENNIFER J. DEBERRY**

The preceding chapter addressed the neuroanatomy and neurochemistry of neurons located within the spinal cord that process information related to pain-related sensation. These neurons are highly regulated components of the central nervous system (CNS) with inhibitory and excitatory feedback mechanisms. Pain may be due to increased primary afferent input or may be the result of a failure of feedback regulation or a combination of the two. Too much "gain" or inadequate "braking" can both result in an excess of sensory transmission. In the normally functioning state, there are tonic influences present as well as evocable mechanisms whereby the responses of second-order neurons can be suppressed or facilitated dependent on other events important to the organism. Some modulatory effects are relatively "hardwired" occurring in a reliable and predictable fashion. Other modulators are less predictable and may be dependent on psychic/cognitive processes that vary from organism to organism and may involve learning, motivation, or emotional factors. In most cases, modulatory systems are adaptive in that they help an organism to function optimally. Unfortunately, with disease, some of these same modulatory systems have become maladaptive and serve to impede both physiologic and social processes of healing. The complex nature of these modulatory influences and the neurotransmitters involved are discussed in three parts beginning with a discussion of mechanisms based at spinal levels, followed by a discussion of mechanisms related to descending influences, and finally by a brief discussion of some "triggers" of spinal neuron hyperexcitability that may occur pathologically and/or iatrogenically which lead to hypersensitivity. These triggers are used as examples of the interactive nature of these modulatory forces. There is value in understanding endogenous modulatory systems because they are the systems which the clinician activates or suppresses by using exogenous modulators, such as electrical stimulation or pharmacologic agents. Modulation occurs at each step of processing within the CNS, but the focus of the present discussion is the modulation of the spinal second-order nociceptive neuron.

Spinal Cord–Based Modulatory Mechanisms

ACUTE SEGMENTAL MODULATORY EFFECTS

Sensory inputs to the spinal cord and trigeminal nucleus begin to interact at the very first steps of transmission. Activation of large diameter afferents (Aβ) produces an inhibitory effect on the processing of signals from small diameter (Aδ and C-fiber) afferents. This effect has been documented since ancient times and is relearned by every child who rubs or massages injured parts of their bodies in order to achieve pain relief. The mechanism of this manipulation has been more difficult to explain than the time-honored efficacy of the effect.[1] What is clear is that second-order neurons of the spinal cord have both excitatory and inhibitory "receptive fields." Namely, stimulation of different parts of the body using one or more types of stimuli (e.g., noxious heat, low threshold mechanical, high threshold mechanical) results in the depolarization or hyperpolarization of individual second-order neurons. Inhibition of second-order

neurons which is produced by noxious stimuli can be evoked from heterosegmental sites and so is discussed separately later. Inhibition of second-order neurons which is produced by nonnoxious stimulation appears to be predominantly segmentally organized. Theoretically formulated as the initial gate control theory of Melzack and Wall,[2] this effect was hypothesized to occur because of a combination of presynaptic inhibition and the actions of inhibitory interneurons located in lamina II (substantia gelatinosa) of the spinal cord which are activated by large diameter afferents (Fig. 5.1). Although the specifics of this theory have evolved further to include nonsegmental effects, its general description has served as the theoretical underpinnings for the clinical effects of neuromodulatory (electrostimulatory analgesic) techniques ranging from transcutaneous electrical nerve stimulation to spinal cord stimulation and aspects of acupuncture.[3]

Numerous electrophysiologic studies of second-order neurons have observed that low-intensity, high-frequency electrical stimulation of nerves or somatic tissues located at the same segmental level as the neuron produces an inhibitory effect which is not reduced by naloxone (nonopioidergic) but which may involve GABAergic or glycinergic mechanisms. This phenomenon is present in both spinally transected and intact animals and so does not necessarily involve a brainstem mechanism. Dorsal column stimulation, which produces retrograde activation of Aβ fiber inputs to the spinal cord (but may also activate descending modulatory pathways), produces similar nonopioid, GABAergic, and/or glycinergic inhibition of spinal nociceptive processing.

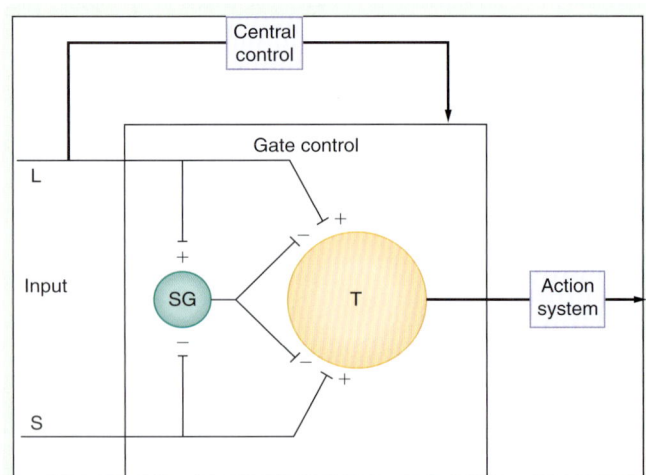

FIGURE 5.1 Gate control theory as originally schematically described by Melzack and Wall[2] where large-diameter (L) and small-diameter (S) primary afferent fibers project to substantia gelatinosa (SG) and second-order transmission (T) neurons in the spinal dorsal horn. The inhibitory effect of SG neuronal activity is increased by L and decreased by S fiber activity. T neurons transmit information to the brain and other action sites. Activation of peripheral or central projections of L fibers using transcutaneous nerve stimulation, peripheral nerve stimulators, or dorsal column stimulators would all be expected to produce inhibition of S fiber input to the T cells.

HETEROSEGMENTAL MODULATORY SYSTEMS

Both excitatory and inhibitory effects can occur at one spinal level when stimuli are presented to distant portions of the body. Excitatory effects have generally been described in imprecise terms as *extended connectivity* or as *propriospinal* pathways that are just one component of the systems that alter the "gain control" mechanisms of nociceptive systems.[4] Some of these intraspinal networks serve to integrate both sensory and motor functions involving the upper and lower extremities with an example being crossed flexion–extension reflex responses to noxious stimuli. A coordination of pelvic organ function also relies on intraspinal excitatory and inhibitory connections that link processing of sensory information from afferents traveling in the pelvic nerve to the lumbosacral cord with that of afferents traveling in sympathetic nerves to the thoracolumbar spinal cord. Intraspinal networks of neurons, which form a reticular network in the deeper parts of the spinal dorsal horn, have been described in the context of the multisynaptic ascending system of Noordenbos.[5] This same network could just as easily serve as the substrates for multisynaptic descending modulatory influences.

The most formally studied heterosegmental interaction related to nociception is the phenomenon known as *diffuse noxious inhibitory controls* (DNIC). This endogenous inhibitory system is activated by noxious stimuli presented to a distant nonsegmental site and results in the inhibition of ongoing or evoked dorsal horn neuronal activity. The mechanisms of DNIC are postulated to involve the activation of brainstem nuclei that subsequently produce inhibition of spinal dorsal horn neurons through a descending modulatory mechanism, but it is notable that the neurophysiologic phenomena associated with DNIC have been demonstrated in spinally transected preparations. These "propriospinal" phenomena represent a general inhibitory system activated by heterosegmental noxious conditioning stimuli which is either synonymous with or highly augmented by the presence of a brainstem and mechanisms of DNIC. According to its original description by Le Bars et al.,[6,7] DNIC results in the inhibition of class II (wide dynamic range [WDR]; convergent) neurons and has no effect on class III (nociceptive specific) neurons. A consistency of many studies related to DNIC (and propriospinal heterosegmental inhibition) is that they have identified that most spinal neurons responsive to noxious stimuli effectively have "total body" receptive fields in that noxious stimuli will produce excitation or inhibition that is dependent on precise body site. DNIC-sensitive neurons have a resultant "inhibitory surround" effect where all noxious inputs outside of a defined area are inhibitory to the individual neurons. Human studies of the similar, but more general, phenomenon of conditioned pain modulation have described the potential for complex interactions of heterosegmental stimuli in which one pain typically inhibits other pains (as in DNIC) except in case of pathologic pain disorders where the expected inhibition may be absent or facilitation may be noted instead.[8]

C-FIBER WIND-UP AND CENTRAL SENSITIZATION

Changes in excitability occur in second-order neurons when repetitive or prolonged high-intensity input is received from primary afferent C-fibers. One of these changes in excitability is termed C-fiber *wind-up*. Noted by Mendell[9] when recording from ascending axons of spinal dorsal horn neurons, wind-up is the phenomenon whereby repeated electrical C-fiber activation at certain rates (i.e., ≥1 Hz) leads to a sequential increase in the number of action potentials evoked by each stimulus (Fig. 5.2). Slower stimulus rates do not produce progressive increases in activation. Mechanical and thermal stimuli at intensities sufficient to activate C-fibers also produce similar wind-up. This sequential increase in response can be blunted through use of N-methyl-D-aspartate (NMDA) receptor antagonists and the effect disappears after a few seconds of nonstimulation.

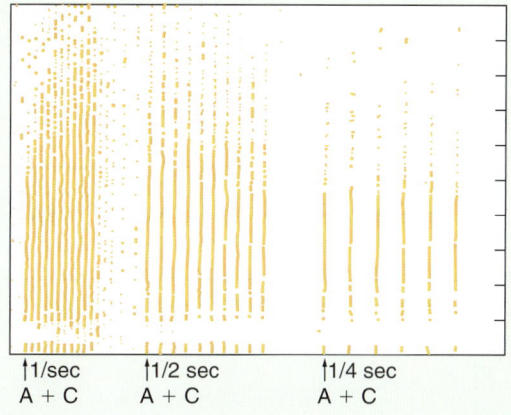

FIGURE 5.2 Wind-up responses of single dorsolateral column axon to repeated stimulation of the sural nerve at sufficient intensity to activate A and C fibers (no wind-up seen with A-fiber stimulation by itself). The *vertical time markers* on the far right represent 100 milliseconds. Each *mark* at the bottom of the *time line* represents the stimulation artifact and the burst of activity immediately above each of these stimulations is the response to A-fiber stimulation (each *dot* represents an action potential). The more delayed responses are to the more slowly conducting C-fiber inputs. Response to stimulation shows increasing C-fiber wind-up responses on to 1 per second stimulation (not to 1 every 2 or 1 every 4 second stimulation rates at right). Wind-up lasts for only several seconds following the stimulation as seen by transient increase in spontaneous activity. *(Redrawn from Mendell LM. Physiological properties of unmyelinated fiber projections to the spinal cord.* Exp Neurol *1966;16:316–332.)*

Another general category of increased neuronal excitability is termed *central sensitization*. This term has been used in a focused manner to describe acute changes in the responsiveness of second-order neurons following high-intensity or prolonged stimuli such as those that occur with nonneuronal tissue injury and subsequent inflammation. The term has also been used to describe phenomena such as delayed-onset nerve injury–related hypersensitivity and, in that case, is more subacute or chronic in nature with a potential for morphologic as well as biochemical alteration of second-order neurons. For purposes of the present discussion, injury-induced central sensitization as described by Woolf[10] is used as the archetype model of central sensitization (Fig. 5.3). Multiple studies have demonstrated that tissue injury produces an augmentation of nociceptive reflexes that is NMDA receptor–dependent. In preclinical models, pharmacologic treatment has the greatest effect if given prior to injury and a blocking of afferent input serves to delay the onset of development of hypersensitivity. Extrapolating from this data and coupling it with evidence of long-term potentiation (LTP) of synaptic efficacy in the spinal cord after even brief bouts of NMDA receptor activation and interaction with glia,[11] some have further extrapolated these laboratory data to the clinical concept of "preemptive analgesia." Treating pain before (and after) it begins has a clear potential for clinical benefit, although the true clinical significance of early intervention has proven difficult to define. On a neurophysiologic basis, an expansion of cutaneous excitatory receptive fields has been noted following tissue injury which follows a similar pharmacology, but specific results have been model- and species-dependent.

Supraspinal Modulatory Systems

TONIC DESCENDING INFLUENCES

A characteristic of spinal nociceptive systems is that they are under tonic descending inhibition such that a common effect of injury to spinal pathways is a release from this inhibition. Hyperreflexive states with secondary spasticity and autonomic

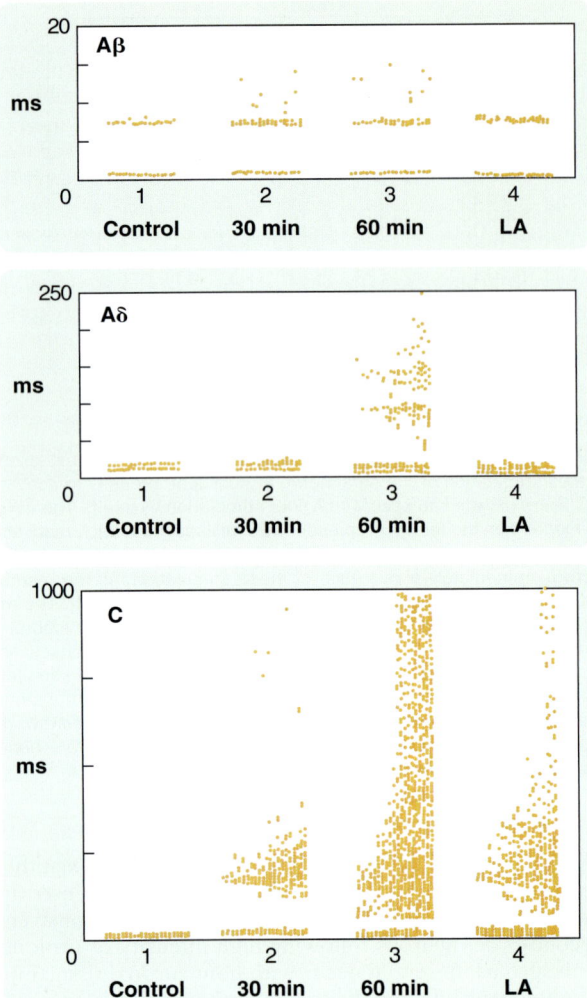

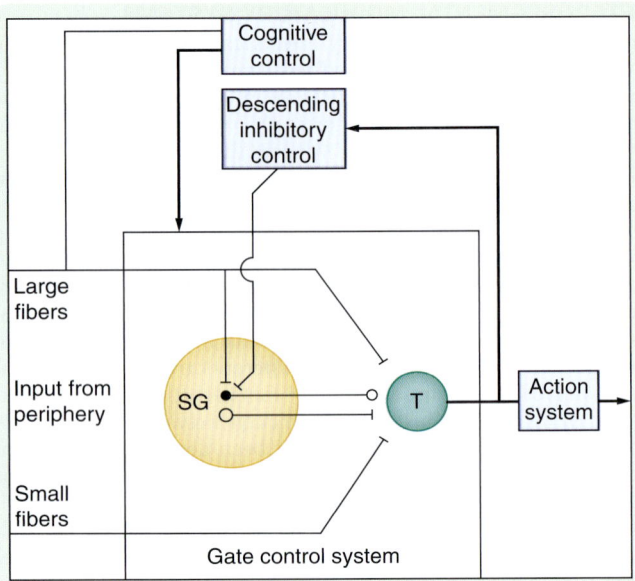

FIGURE 5.4 A modification of the gate control theory schematic models includes excitatory (*white circle*) and inhibitory (*black circle*) links from the substantia gelatinosa (SG) to the transmission (T) cells as well as descending inhibitory control from brainstem systems. The round knob at the end of the inhibitory link indicates that its actions may be presynaptic, postsynaptic, or both. All connections are excitatory except the inhibitory link from SG to T cells. (*Redrawn after Melzack R, Wall PD. The Challenge of Pain.* New York: Basic Books; 1983.)

FIGURE 5.3 *Raster dot* displays of a single biceps femoris unit activated by stimulation of the sural nerve once every 2 seconds before an ipsilateral thermal injury (Control), 30 and 60 minutes postinjury, and 10 minutes after the injured foot has been completely anesthetized with local anesthetic (LA). Each *dot* represents a unit discharge. The vertical scale is the latency of the responses after sural nerve stimulation, and the stimulus artifact can be seen at time 0. Stimulation strengths were sufficient to activate Aβ, Aδ, and C fibers. Note the different time scales used in the three panels to record the activity evoked by the three different fiber populations. In the preinjury state, only Aβ input was evoked. Thirty minutes after injury, a C-fiber response begins to occur, whereas at 60 minutes, both Aδ and C-fiber evoked responses are present (the C-fiber responses with wind-up). Ten minutes after LA, the C-fiber evoked responses remain higher than before the injury suggesting a central component of the sensitization. (*Redrawn from Woolf CJ. Evidence for a central component of post-injury pain hypersensitivity.* Nature *1983;306:686–688.*)

lability can occur. The precise neurophysiologic circuits associated with this descending inhibition is of significant debate, but known inhibitory neurotransmitters such as norepinephrine (NE) and serotonin (5-hydroxy-tryptophan; 5-HT) are synthesized in the brainstem and transported to the spinal cord from multiple supraspinal sites. This role for supraspinal structures in providing descending influences on spinal reflexes has long been recognized. In 1915, Sherrington and Sowton[12] demonstrated enhanced flexion reflexes following spinal transection. Later in 1926, Fulton[13] suggested that this effect reflected removal of tonic descending inhibitory modulation of spinal interneurons mediating those reflexes. Descending control of flexion reflexes was extensively studied in ensuing years,[14] but these studies did not target the issue of how the brain might

specifically modulate incoming nociceptive signals from peripheral tissue.

A series of seminal events in the late 1960s and early 1970s led to a full-fledged appreciation and analysis of descending modulation of spinal nociceptive processing. These included a modification of the original gate control theory to include supraspinal systems (Fig. 5.4). This change was prompted by studies which showed that spinal dorsal horn neurons were subject to tonic descending inhibitory influences[15] and Reynolds's[16] demonstration that electrical stimulation of the midbrain periaqueductal grey (PAG) produced analgesia sufficient to perform abdominal surgery in a rat. This last phenomenon was referred to as "stimulation-produced analgesia" (SPA).[17,18] SPA can also be produced in humans[19] in the form of deep brain stimulation, and it suggests the existence of endogenous systems that can selectively modulate pain. This served as the impetus for the extensive, formal analyses of supraspinal structures involved in descending modulation of spinal nociceptive processing that continues today. Later, a number of investigators found that electrical or chemical stimulation of other brain regions could also promote *facilitation* of nociceptive processing,[20,21] suggesting the existence of similar descending facilitatory systems.

SUPRASPINAL SUBSTRATES MEDIATING THE DESCENDING MODULATION OF PAIN
Periaqueductal Grey of the Mesencephalon and the Rostral Ventral Medulla
The midbrain PAG and the rostral ventral medulla (RVM), in particular the medullary nucleus raphe magnus (NRM) figured prominently in the original analyses of descending modulation of pain. Indeed, they are often viewed as the "backbone" of the pain modulatory system[22] and have been more extensively studied than any other brain regions. Yet, other brainstem nuclei/cell groups also serve in this role and include the nucleus gigantocellularis (NGC), nucleus reticularis gigantocellularis pars alpha (NGCα), nucleus paragigantocellularis (NpGC),

midbrain reticular formation, locus coeruleus/A6 cell group (LC/A6), the A5 cell group, the lateral reticular nucleus (LRN) and nearby A1 and C1 cell groups, the parabrachial nucleus/A7 cell group (PBN/A7) and the nucleus tractus solitarius (NTS). A limited amount of information is also available on cortical and limbic systems such as the anterior cingulate cortex (ACC), the amygdala, and hypothalamus that contribute to descending modulation. It is the investigation of these structures that has led to our current understanding of how descending pain modulatory systems affect pain perception. This topic has been well reviewed.[1,23–29] Table 5.1 summarizes results related to many of these areas separately along with the neurotransmitters associated with their putative inhibitory versus facilitatory effects on nociceptive transmission. A summary of the most important components is described in Figure 5.5.

The PAG was the initial site of investigation for endogenous pain control systems and is still viewed as an integral component of these systems. Antinociception produced by electrical stimulation of the PAG (SPA) is profound and comparable to that produced by a high dose of morphine. It eliminates behavioral and spinal dorsal horn neuronal responses to noxious stimuli including electric shock applied to the tooth pulp or limbs, noxious heating of the tail and hind paws, noxious pinching of the limbs, and injection of irritants into the viscera. The effects of SPA are produced almost immediately after the onset of stimulation and may last from a few seconds to hours after termination of stimulation. Microinjection of opiates into the PAG also produces behavioral antinociception and inhibition of spinal nociceptive transmission via disinhibition of inhibitory interneurons in the PAG. The subsequent discovery of endogenous opioid receptors and peptides[56–59] and demonstration of the presence of opioid receptors throughout the brainstem[60] further established a role for the PAG in pain modulation. Similarities were also observed between phenomena associated with PAG-derived inhibitory effects and opiate-induced analgesia, including tolerance and cross tolerance.[61] SPA- and morphine-induced antinociception from the PAG also involve a spinal release of 5-HT and NE and mediation by both spinal 5-HT receptors and α_2 adrenoreceptors suggesting the need for a relay through serotonergic and noradrenergic brainstem sites. Anatomical studies reveal relatively few fibers that descend from the PAG directly to the spinal cord.[28] However, the PAG does have strong projections to the NRM and adjacent areas of the RVM. Attention has therefore been focused on the NRM as the primary relay in mediating the antinociceptive effects of activation of PAG neurons. Studies of the NRM were performed in a manner analogous to those performed in the PAG and often with comparable results.[28,29] Electrical stimulation of sites within the PAG or NRM produces inhibitory postsynaptic potentials (IPSPs) in dorsal horn neurons including those with ascending projections.[62] Lesions of the dorsolateral funiculi (DLFs) of the spinal cord eliminate this inhibition and so this white matter pathway has been viewed as the primary spinal locus for descending fibers from the RVM.[63] Ventrolateral funiculi (VLFs) have also been implicated as the spinal pathways by which descending systems access the spinal dorsal horn (e.g., from the LRN), but there is greater evidence for these descending paths to promote facilitatory influences as opposed to inhibitory influences.

TABLE 5.1 Central Nervous System (CNS) Sites Modulating Nociceptive Transmission (NT)

CNS Site	Direct Projection to Spinal Segments	Possible Relay Sites	Facilitation NTs	Inhibition NTs
Spinal Cord				
Segmental	NA	Multisegmental	GLUT	GABA, glycine
Propriospinal	Many	Multisegmental	GLUT	GABA, glycine, opioid, ACh
Heterosegmental	Many	Multisegmental-RVM-DRt	GLUT	Opioid, 5-HT, NE, GABA
Medulla				
NTS	Few	RVM, LC, PAG, A5, cortex	GLUT	NE and 5-HT together
RVM (region)	Many		5-HT2, 5-HT3, NE (α1), GLUT, ACh	5-HT1A, 5-HT1B, 5-HT1D, 5-HT7, opioid, NE (α2), ACh, GABA, glycine
NRM	Many		5-HT2, 5-HT3	5-HT, opioid, ACh, GABA
NGC, NGCα, NpGC	Many	LC	GLUT, 5-HT, CCK-B, NE (α1)	5-HT, NE(α2)
LRN	Some	LC, RVM, A5		NE (α2)
A1	Few		NE (α1)	NE (α2)
DRt	Many		GLUT	
Pons				
LC/A6/A5	Many		NE (α1)	NE (α2)
PBN/A7	Many/few	PAG, RVM	NE (α1)	NE (α2), oxytocin?
Mesencephalon				
PAG	Few	RVM, LC	NE (α1), 5-HT	5-HT, NE (α2), opioid, ACh
Diencephalon Cortex				
Hypothalamus	Some	RVM, PAG	GLUT	5-HT, NE(α2), DA
Amygdala	Some	PAG, PBN	GLUT, oxytocin? CRF-related?	NE(α2), oxytocin? CRF-related?
ACC	Few	RVM, PAG	GLUT, 5-HT	
Sensory cortex	Few	RVM	GLUT	5-HT, NE(α2), opioid
Sensory cortex	Few	?	GLUT	5-HT, NE(α2), opioid
VLO	Few	RVM, PAG	GLUT	5-HT, NE(α2), opioid

NOTE: A1 to A7 designation are noradrenergic nuclei as defined by Dahlström and Fuxe.[64]

5-HT, serotonin; ACC, anterior cingulate cortex; ACh, acetylcholine; CCK, cholecystokinin; CRF, corticotropin-releasing factor; DA, dopamine; DRt, dorsal reticular nucleus; GABA, γ-aminobutyric acid; GLUT, glutamate; LC, locus coeruleus; LRN, lateral reticular nucleus; NA, not applicable; NE, norepinephrine; NGC, nucleus gigantocellularis; NGCα, nucleus reticularis gigantocellularis pars alpha; NpGC, nucleus paragigantocellularis; NRM, nucleus raphe magnus; NTS, nucleus tractus solitarius; PAG, periaqueductal gray; PBN, parabrachial nucleus; RVM, rostral ventrolateral medulla; VLO, ventrolateral orbital cortex.

From Randich and Ness[1]; Mendell[3]; Le Bars et al.[7]; Zhuo[21]; Mason[22]; Boadas-Vaelllo et al.[23]; Lau and Vaughan[24]; Ossipov et al.[25]; Kwon et al.[26]; Peirs and Seal[27]; Basbaum and Fields[28,29]; Taylor and Westlund[30]; Tsuruoka et al.[31]; Stevens et al.[32]; Janss and Gebhart[33,34]; Randich and Aicher[35]; Ren et al.[36]; Aimone and Gebhart[37]; Neugebauer[38]; Senapti et al.[39]; Kuroda et al.[40]; Zhang et al.[41]; Zhang et al.[42]; Hutchinson et al.[43]; Millan[44]; Gebhart and Randich[45]; Thurston and Randich[46]; Urban et al.[47]; Schaible et al.[48]; Ren and Dubner[49]; Butler and Finn[50]; Jennings et al.[51]; Robbins and Ness[52]; Suzuki et al.[53]; Gao and Mason[54]; Kaplan and Fields[55]

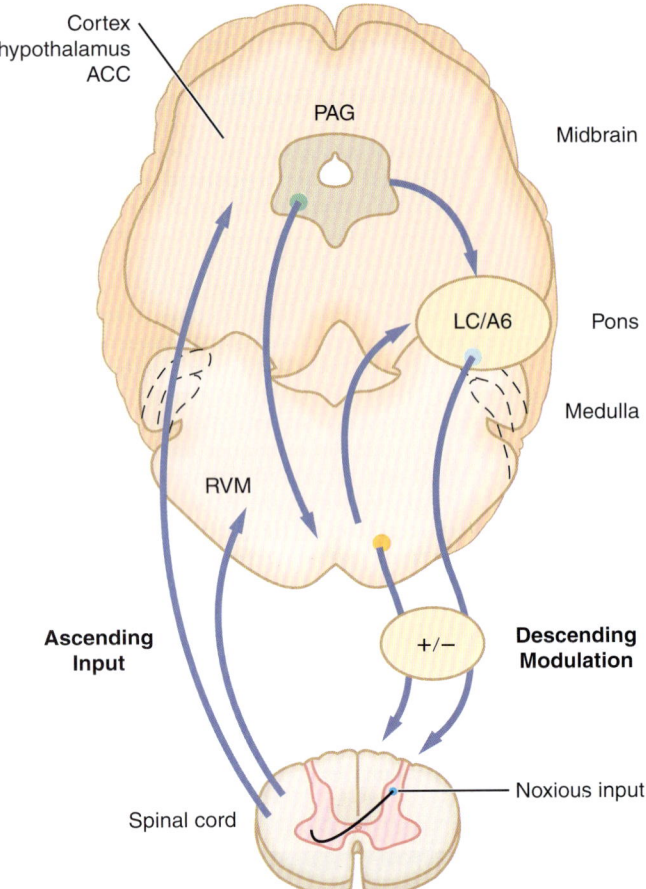

FIGURE 5.5 Schematic diagram of descending modulatory influences of spinal nociceptive processing. Multiple sites within the brain have been demonstrated to be of importance including the midbrain periaqueductal grey (PAG), locus coeruleus/A6 cell group (LC/A6), and the rostral ventromedial medulla (RVM). These sites are reciprocally interconnected, are activated by ascending nociceptive information, and serve as relays for other brain sites known to modulate spinal processing including the anterior cingulate cortex (ACC), other cortical sites (somatosensory, motor, insular, ventrolateral orbital), and the hypothalamus. Resultant modulatory effects on spinal dorsal horn processing can be inhibitory (−) or facilitatory (+) to nociceptive primary afferent input.

Detailed electrical stimulation mapping and intensity studies of the RVM, and the NGC and NGCα in particular, reveal that these regions not only support inhibition of nociceptive reflexes but also facilitation or enhancement of those reflexes under certain conditions.[21] In most cases, facilitatory effects were supplanted by inhibitory effects at a given site of stimulation when greater intensities of electrical stimulation were examined. The results of behavioral studies were paralleled by in-depth analyses of the effects of either electrical stimulation or glutamate microinjection into the NGC and NGCα on spontaneous activity and noxious heat-evoked activity of spinal dorsal horn neurons. The results are generally comparable in nature. Facilitatory effects are observed as a leftward shift in the stimulus–response functions (SRFs) to graded heat, whereas inhibition is manifested as a rightward shift or a decrease in the slope of the SRF to noxious stimuli. Multiple electrophysiologic studies, in conjunction with the behavioral studies, reinforced the notion that that activation of cell bodies in the NGC/NGCα can produce direct descending inhibitory effects via pathways traveling in the DLFs but that the facilitatory effects required at least another relay prior to passage in the VLFs of the spinal cord.[21]

Other Deep Brain Sites

Using the nomenclature of Dahlström and Fuxe,[64] the noradrenergic nuclei of the CNS are designated as "A" nuclei numbered in ascending order from the caudal medulla near the A1 to the lateral pons near the PBN (A7). One of the most important of these nuclei is the A6 nucleus which colocalizes with and is also ventral to the morphologic structure, the LC. This area has extensive direct axonal projections to the spinal cord. The effects of LC/A6 descending inhibition are independent of midbrain or medullary mediation, although the reverse is not necessarily true. The role of the LC/A6 in nociceptive modulation is complex, reminiscent of the role of the RVM with evidence of both inhibitory and facilitatory influences originating from the same site.[30,31,65] The PBN and adjacent Kölliker-Fuse/A7 area has also been examined in relation to descending pain modulation. The Kölliker-Fuse nucleus, which is lateral and ventral to the LC, is the principal source of descending NE-containing fibers in the cat and may play a comparable role to that of the LC/A6 noted earlier for rat and primate.[32] The PBN has long been known for its role in respiratory and cardiovascular function, taste and aversions, locomotion, and sleep. However, the PBN/A7 complex may have particular relevance to descending modulation of nociception as this site also receives extensive ascending nociceptive input directly from the spinal cord.

Occasional facilitation of nonnociceptive and nociceptive responses of trigeminal nociceptive neurons when stimulating in the PBN/A7 has also been observed. These facilitatory effects may bear on those described previously in the RVM but have not been systematically studied. The PBN/A7 has few direct projections to spinal cord but has multiple interconnections with PAG, NRM, NpGC, and the ventrolateral medulla. Electrical stimulation of the region of the A5 cell group in the ventrolateral pons produces antinociception that can be antagonized by intrathecal administration of NE receptor antagonists.[66] The A5 cells project to the spinal cord, although their overall contribution to the total NE innervation of the spinal cord is relatively small, and A5 neurons may exert their effects primarily on lamina X neurons.

The LRN is a bilateral structure located in the ventrolateral medulla and lies in close proximity to the A1 (norepinephrine-containing) and C1 (epinephrine-containing) cell groups, although most of the effects of C1 activation appear to be associated with hemodynamic changes and not with nociception. Like the PBN/A7, the LRN is of particular interest because is also a major relay center for ascending nociceptive information. Electrical and glutamate stimulation of the LRN inhibits spinal nociceptive reflexes and responses of spinal dorsal horn neurons to noxious stimuli.[33,34] These effects can be antagonized by spinal administration of α₂ receptor antagonists. The involvement of spinal adrenoreceptors in these antinociceptive effects suggests that the LRN relays to an NE-containing cell group to produce these outcomes because little or no NE-containing fibers descend from the LRN. The LRN is also innervated by the PAG, PBN, LC, and RVM regions, suggesting complex reciprocal interactions exist between all these regions.

Several studies have demonstrated that the NTS is a region that is both capable of modulating pain and may serve as a relay site for peripheral cardiopulmonary afferent influences on nociception. Input from vagal nerve stimulation relays through the NTS and has been demonstrate to produce both inhibition and excitation dependent on stimulation parameters.[35,36] The NTS has few direct spinal projections suggesting that changes in nociception derived from the NTS involved secondary relays including the RVM, LC/A6, PAG, A5 cell groups, and other forebrain loops.

Subcortical limbic structures have also been implicated in supraspinal modulation of nociception. Electrical stimulation of a variety of hypothalamic periventricular structures results in antinociception, although not necessarily with similar characteristics. The hypothalamus has connections with a variety of structures implicated in descending inhibitory influences including the PAG, NTS, and RVM, and these sites may be necessary for the effects of the hypothalamus on nociception.[37,67,68]

The amygdala is another limbic structure highly implicated in both the receipt of nociceptive input and the activation of sensation modulating phenomena. Evidence has been found that the amygdala mediates both stress responsiveness and nociceptive processing.[38,69] Pain-related plasticity within the amygdala has been demonstrated in rats in multiple systems including visceral, somatic, and neuropathic models of pain. Chemical stimulation of the central nucleus of the amygdala results in facilitation of nociceptive reflexes and dorsal horn neurons.[70,71] At the present time, the complex pharmacology and intricate connections that project to other brain sites such as the PBN/A7 and the PAG as well as the spinal cord itself preclude any definitive statements about pharmacologic mediators, except to say they include stress-related compounds such as oxytocin, corticotropin-releasing factor, urocortins, and adrenocorticoid receptors.[38] Recent optogenetic studies by Sadler et al.[72] suggest even greater complexity in terms of right versus left central amygdala influences on nociceptive responses with both facilitatory and inhibitory effects originating from amygdalar site.

Cortical Structures

The previously discussed literature related to the effect of supraspinal modulation of nociception has as its translational therapeutic correlate, the technique of deep brain stimulation—where an electrode is surgically, stereotaxically placed via a craniotomy into a CNS location for purposes of electrically evoking an analgesic effect. More superficial structures such as the cortex have allowed the application of noninvasive brain stimulation techniques such as transcranial direct current stimulation (tDC) and transcranial magnetic stimulation (TMS). Some of these techniques have clear and obvious benefit in association with effects on phenomena such as depression. Because they are also relatively noninvasive with limited adverse events,[73,74] they have found increasing use in the treatment of pain.[75]

Stimulation of both somatosensory cortex (SSC) and motor cortex (MC) have been used in the clinical treatment of neuropathic pain, central poststroke pain, and phantom limb pain. These have been achieved using either surgically implanted electrical stimulation methods or TMS. Although spinal influences of such treatments have been reported, there is reason to believe most of their effects are mediated at the supraspinal level.[76] These factors notwithstanding, there is evidence for SSC and other cortical influences in producing descending inhibition of spinal nociceptive transmission via various brainstem sites. Senapati et al.[39] provided one of the stronger demonstrations of cortical influences on spinal nociceptive transmission. They showed that electrical stimulation of either the ipsilateral or contralateral primary SSC of rats inhibited responses of L5–L6 WDR neurons to noxious pressure and pinch but not brush. In contrast, electrical stimulation of the secondary SSC has been reported to produce only a weak behavioral antinociception in the second phase of the formalin test and was without effect on responses to noxious thermal or mechanical stimuli.[40] There are reports that electrical stimulation of or glutamate microinjections into the ventrolateral orbital cortex (VLO) can inhibit nociceptive reflexes via the PAG,[41,42] but others have found pronociceptive effects of similar treatments.[43] Morphine administration in the VLO also has been reported to inhibit both the hot plate and paw withdrawal responses to noxious heat in intact rats, and the tactile allodynia, hot plate, and paw withdrawal responses in rats with peripheral mononeuropathy. The antinociceptive effects produced by VLO stimulation observed

in neuropathic rats were reversed by naloxone, whereas those observed in intact rats were not affected by naloxone. However, it cannot be ascertained from these studies whether descending inhibitory systems were activated by morphine because all of the response measures were organized at the supraspinal level.[77] Morphine microinjection in the rostral agranular insular cortex (RAIC), a structure immediately caudal to the VLO, also has been reported to inhibit nociceptive responses in the formalin test, reduce c-Fos expression in the spinal cord ipsilateral to a formalin stimulus, and produce a naloxone-reversible inhibition of spinal dorsal horn neuronal responses to a noxious thermal stimulus.[78] The influence on the RAIC on descending inhibitory influences may critically depend on dopamine acting on neurons in this region.[79]

There is also strong evidence that some cortical regions can provide descending facilitatory influences. Electrical, chemical, or optogenetic activation of the ACC produced significant facilitation of nociceptive reflexes with components both dependent and independent of a relay in the RVM.[21] It is notable that the ACC is one of the cortical sites reliably activated by ascending nociceptive inputs.

SUMMARY OF SUPRASPINAL INFLUENCES

There is overwhelming support for the structures discussed in the previous sections in mediating descending inhibitory and facilitatory influences on spinal nociceptive transmission. A striking feature of these systems is the Janus-like dual nature of almost all of the identified CNS sites. Those which receive ascending nociceptive information almost invariably are associated with a dual function of both inhibition and facilitation. There is also overwhelming support that activation of most of these structures involves spinal release of *both* 5-HT and NE in producing inhibitory phenomena but many other neurotransmitters including acetylcholine, γ-aminobutyric acid (GABA), glycine, substance P, corticotropin-releasing factor, urocortins, thyroid-stimulating hormone, and oxytocin, which have been described as part of both excitatory and inhibitory mechanisms.[44] Thus, "coactivation" or "recruitment" of more than a single system appears to be the rule rather than the exception.[45] It is quite surprising, therefore, that although the discovery of endogenous opioids prompted the intense study of descending modulatory systems, endogenous opioids per se have not figured prominently in the "system" side of the analyses. Rather, they appear far more critical in the local circuitries of specific brainstem or spinal regions that allow these systems to function. Furthermore, although the structures supplying these transmitters affecting spinal nociceptive transmission have been identified, for the most part, our general knowledge about how those structures interact in producing inhibitory and facilitatory effects is still not well understood.

ON, OFF, AND NEUTRAL CELLS

With the identification of CNS sites that could be stimulated to produce inhibitory and/or facilitatory effects at the spinal cord level came theories related to the neuronal constituents of those sites. Seminal studies performed by Fields and colleagues[80,81] demonstrated the existence of three types of neurons in the RVM that can be classified based on the neuron's response to noxious heat applied to the tail of a lightly anesthetized rat that elicited the tail flick reflex. ON cells were shown to increase their firing rate just before the occurrence of the tail flick, OFF cells decreased their firing rate just before the occurrence of the tail flick, and NEUTRAL cells showed no change in activity throughout the application of noxious heat. Importantly, the activity of ON and OFF cells, but not NEUTRAL cells, was shown to be affected by systemic administration of morphine. At doses of systemic morphine that inhibit the tail flick reflex, OFF cells became continuously active and failed to pause before reflex movements, whereas ON cell activity decreased.[81] These and other findings led to the proposition that OFF cells exert descending inhibitory effects on spinal nociceptive transmission. ON cells were hypothesized to exert a pronociceptive or facilitatory influence. NEUTRAL cells were purported to have no role in nociception.

Extensive studies have examined the role of ON and OFF cells in relation to other descending modulation-related phenomena such as spinal cord stimulation,[82] diffuse noxious inhibitory controls,[83] or the pain associated with diabetic neuropathy[84] with a mixture of results, but the role of a subpopulation of these neurons in pain modulation is firmly established. Neurons with the same characteristics as RVM ON and OFF cells have been identified in other CNS sites such as the PAG such that an exclusive role of the ON and OFF cells located in the RVM is unlikely. An exclusive association of ON and OFF cells with nociception is similarly unlikely. Mason[22] has argued using data that there is substantial evidence that these cells are involved in a variety of homeostatic control functions including micturition and arterial blood pressure control, and that they should be viewed as modulating a much broader spectrum of somatosensory inputs than nociception. Indeed, correlative data supporting a role of ON and OFF cells in control of arterial blood pressure is equally as compelling as for pain modulation.[46] Whether different subsets of ON and OFF cells serve different functions, or whether individual ON and OFF cells can subserve or coordinate many different functions, remains to be determined.

Triggers of Clinical Hypersensitivity

ALLODYNIA AND HYPERALGESIA

Clinically, there are at least four general etiologies producing hypersensitivity or sudden "flares" in pain experience. These include inflammation, stress, altered neurologic function (typically secondary to previous injury), and drug-related effects. Each of these etiologies is associated with mechanisms that include altered modulation of spinal dorsal horn processing. The terms *allodynia* and *hyperalgesia* are clinical terms that represent different forms of hypersensitivity. Defined using clinical terms, *allodynia* has been defined as "pain produced by a stimulus that does not normally cause pain." Similarly defined, *hyperalgesia* is "an increased response to a stimulus that is normally painful," which may mean either a lower threshold for evoking pain or a higher intensity of pain perception produced by a given intensity of a suprathreshold painful stimulus. Based on psychophysical experiments, hyperalgesia may be either "primary" when it is located at a site of injury such as a burn or "secondary" when altered sensations are evoked from uninjured tissue that typically surrounds the site of injury but, in some cases, could be physically distant. Primary hyperalgesia has generally been relegated to mechanisms involving the primary afferents and secondary hyperalgesia to spinal second-order neuron effects.

Notably, when studying hypersensitivity in nonhuman animal models, interpretive issues can be problematic, particularly when studying phenomena that have clinical definitions. For purposes of the present discussion, hyperalgesia is defined as augmented responses and/or lowered stimulus thresholds for response to a nociceptive stimulus. Allodynia is defined as the evocation of responses that would have been called nociceptive (e.g., flexion-withdrawal responses) to clearly nonnociceptive stimuli (e.g., light brushing).

INFLAMMATION-INDUCED HYPERSENSITIVITY AND INHIBITORY SYSTEMS

Tissue-damaging events can result in both the peripheral sensitization of primary afferent nociceptors and the central sensitization of spinal dorsal horn neurons. Historically, these two phenomena have played a fundamental role in accounting for primary and secondary hyperalgesia, respectively. These phenomena were viewed as either increased input to or increased responsiveness of second-order neurons with an emphasis on local spinal mechanisms. However, a role for brainstem descending control systems in both primary and secondary hyperalgesia phenomena are now receiving increasing attention and have led to a much better understanding of persistent pain states. There is now evidence that the RVM and the LC/A6 sites are responsible for exerting primarily descending inhibitory influences under conditions of primary hyperalgesia associated with either somatic or visceral tissue damage and primarily descending facilitatory influences under conditions of secondary hyperalgesia. These processes are not well understood, but spinobulbospinal loops are now being proposed to recognize that enhanced afferent input from the spinal dorsal horn ascends either directly or indirectly to the brainstem, which in turn, changes this balance and, ultimately, the perception of pain.

There is substantial evidence that RVM ON cells, originally hypothesized to exert a pronociceptive effect, may be responsible for contributing to the descending facilitatory influences that result in secondary hyperalgesia in persistent pain states. Acute inflammation produced by ipsilateral topical application of mustard oil above the knee of a rat increases ongoing ON cell discharge and decreases ongoing discharge of OFF cells. These changes correlate with a decrease in the withdrawal latency of the ipsilateral but not contralateral paw. This hyperalgesic effect could be blocked by either lidocaine infusion[85] or a local infusion of an NMDA-receptor antagonist[86] into the RVM suggesting the NMDA-receptor activation induced by inflammation contributes to the secondary hyperalgesia. The spinobulbospinal loop engaged by peripheral cutaneous inflammation and mediating secondary hyperalgesia may involve spinal release of cholecystokinin (CCK) because spinal intrathecal administration of CCK antagonists block these effects.[47]

Whereas secondary hyperalgesia may be augmented by descending facilitatory systems, primary hyperalgesia (increased primary afferent activity) associated with either acute or persistent inflammation may actively engage descending *inhibitory* influences. Schaible et al.[48] showed that a mixture of kaolin and carrageenan injected into the knee joint of the cat resulted in a progressive increase in both spontaneous activity and evoked activity of spinal dorsal horn neurons to innocuous and noxious stimuli. Reversible interruption of descending modulatory influences using spinal "cold block" further increased activity in a progressive fashion demonstrating that spinal descending inhibitory influences were being progressively engaged by inflammation. Ren and Dubner[49] showed that primary thermal hyperalgesia produced by carrageenan administration into the hind paw of the rat was increased by prior transections of the DLFs and that lidocaine microinjection in the RVM increased the spontaneous activity of nociceptive dorsal horn neurons and their responses to mechanical and thermal stimulation of the inflamed hind paw.

In the RVM, this enhancement of descending inhibitory influences may reflect inflammation-induced increases in the synthesis of enkephalins and/or enhanced efficacy of endogenous opioids acting at μ- and δ-opioid receptors such that the effectiveness of opioids is increased.[87,88] Mechanistically, these changes would be consistent with opioid inhibition of pronociceptive ON cells and disinhibition of pro-inhibitory OFF cells; the net outcome of which should be enhanced descending inhibition. They also depend on RVM glutaminergic influences and increased sensitivity to both NE and opioidergic spinal inhibitory mechanisms.

The LC/A6 region may play a comparable role to the RVM in attenuating the development of primary hyperalgesia induced by acute inflammatory pain but not necessarily persistent inflammatory pain. Upregulation of spinal α_2 adrenoreceptors under conditions of inflammation may also enhances the potency of this descending inhibitory influence.

That descending inhibitory influences are recruited from both the RVM and LC/A6 under conditions of inflammation are supported by studies of spinal cord lesions. Wei et al.[89] observed that the c-Fos expression observed in the L4–L5 spinal segments 24 hours after hind paw injection of complete Freund's adjuvant (CFA) was significantly increased on the side ipsilateral, but not contralateral, to the injection by either bilateral DLF or VLF lesions. The increases occurred in both superficial and deep laminae, as well as lamina III to IV, region of termination of mechanoreceptor afferents. Presumably, descending facilitatory influences accompanying the CFA-induced inflammatory state, and which should have been eliminated by these lesions, were masked by the descending inhibitory influences.

Following a common theme, these multiple examples illustrate that inflammation activates both inhibitory and facilitatory influences on spinal cord sensory processing with identical sites in the CNS responsible for the differing phenomena.

STRESS-INDUCED ANALGESIA AND HYPERALGESIA
Exposure to psychological stressors can produce *bidirectional* modulation of nociceptive responses, secondary to presumed mechanisms of descending inhibition and descending facilitation. These modulatory phenomena are termed *stress-induced analgesia* (SIA) and *stress-induced hyperalgesia* (SIH), respectively,[50,51] and are viewed as classic examples of descending modulation because they are thought to originate from supraspinal psychological processes. From a translational standpoint, SIA is relatively uncommon except when associated with acute injuries and the need for uninhibited motor activity (i.e. escape). It has been identified as having both opioid-related and opioid-independent components. SIH, on the other hand, is the more typical phenomenon when discussing clinical pain, as psychologically stressful events are commonly associated with increases in pain. Animal models of both stress and nociception have allowed a better understanding of the mechanisms underlying the pathophysiologic processes that produce and exacerbate chronic pain. SIH appears to be the result of a combination of intrinsic and extrinsic factors, including dysfunction in the hypothalamic-pituitary-adrenocortical (HPA) axis and activation of various neurotransmitter systems and anatomical sites, genes, and environment. Hyperalgesia following the experience of stress appears to occur particularly (but not exclusively) when exposure to a stressor is prolonged or exaggerated. Chronic stress can result in long-term and maladaptive physiologic changes. Interestingly, the two seemingly mutually exclusive phenomena of SIA and SIH can occur concomitantly (e.g., Robbins and Ness[52]). Particular vulnerability factors, such as genetics and perinatal environment, may play a predominant role in SIH. Known CNS sites of importance to HPA axis activation, SIA, and SIH are the amygdala, the hypothalamus, the PAG, and the RVM. Neurotransmitters of interest at a spinal level include oxytocin, endocannabinoids, corticotropin receptor agonists, 5-HT, and NE as well as the more typical opioids.

NEUROPATHIC PAIN
The injury of peripheral nerves has many consequences, one of which is an alteration in spinal dorsal horn neuron excitability. One of the recently identified mechanisms important to this is the activation of spinal microglia in male rats by substances such as fractalkine released by the central processes of the injured nerves. In female rats, similar astrocytic mechanisms appear to be ongoing. Subsequent release of cytokines, purines, and growth factors results in the sensitization of second-order nociceptive neurons[90] and subsequent increased excitability reflected as hyperalgesia and allodynia. These spinal mechanisms

are not the whole phenomenon as there is clear evidence that supraspinal modulatory systems are also important to the development of hypersensitivity following nerve injury. The RVM is now believed to significantly contribute to neuropathic pain produced by such experimental treatments such as loose ligation of L5–L6 spinal and chronic sciatic nerve transection. For example, inactivation of the RVM with lidocaine injections enhanced both the withdrawal response and the thermal and tactile hypersensitivity produced by peripheral nerve injury.[91,92] Various lines of evidence suggest that RVM ON cells may be critical for sustaining neuropathic pain. Selective lesions of ON cells block the thermal hyperalgesia and tactile allodynia produced by peripheral nerve injury.[92] Other evidence suggests that the effect of ON cells in contributing to neuropathic pain may reside in spinal release of 5-HT and a presynaptic action on 5-HT$_3$ receptors located on substance P–containing terminals.[53] The precise details relating ON cell activation to spinal 5-HT release remain to be worked out because some studies have reported that neither ON nor OFF cells contain 5-HT.[54] In neuropathic pain, the influence of the LC/A6 may be reduced leading to increased pain. For example, following rhizotomy, the antinociceptive effect produced by LC/A6 stimulation is reduced.[93]

OPIOID-INDUCED HYPERALGESIA
Opiates remain the primary treatment for a wide variety of pain disorders in both acute and chronic clinical pain disorders. Prolonged administration of opiates can be associated with significant reactive processes including the development of tolerance to the analgesic effects of the drugs such that greater doses of drug are required to achieve adequate pain relief. Recently, it has been recognized that exposure to opioids can also result in paradoxical pain including regions not described in the initial pain complaint,[94] a phenomenon commonly referred to as "opioid-induced hyperalgesia."[94,95] Many substances delivered spinally can reverse or block antinociceptive tolerance as well as opioid-induced hyperalgesia, which include NMDA receptor antagonists, phosphokinase C inhibitors, cyclo-oxygenase inhibitors, and use of differing opioid receptor subtype agonists/antagonists.[94,95] It is also clear that there is an effect of chronic opioids on descending pain modulatory systems that is critical to the development of the spinal cord changes mediating paradoxical pain and antinociceptive tolerance. These drugs have known neuroexcitatory effects arising within the RVM and PAG when the effects of opioids are rapidly reversed by naloxone or other substances interacting with opioid systems. Additional evidence that supraspinal modulatory systems are involved in the mechanisms of opioid-induced hyperalgesia includes the demonstration that animals with lesions of the DLF of the spinal cord do not appear to develop abnormal pain or antinociceptive tolerance that are normally a consequence of prolonged opiate administration.[96,97] Furthermore, the effects of both acute and prolonged exposure to morphine (tactile hyperesthesia, thermal hyperalgesia, and antinociceptive tolerance) are abolished by local anesthesia blockade of the RVM.[55,96,97] Thus, opioid-induced pain and tolerance in these circumstances may be mediated in part by activation of descending facilitatory mechanisms arising in the RVM. This, in turn, has been suggested to act as a trigger for the upregulation of spinal dynorphin that serves to promote enhanced input from nociceptors.[98] An underlying assumption related to these studies has been that opioid-induced hyperalgesia requires the activation of opioid receptors. However, it is possible that opioid drugs may also be acting by nonopioid mechanisms to produce their physiologic effects. The demonstration that opioid-induced hyperalgesia can be elicited in mice without functional μ-, κ-, or δ-opioid receptors supports this possibility.[99] At this point in time, it is clear that the use of opioids for the treatment of pain leads to a series of complicated interactions in spinal pain

processing systems such that the resultant physiologic effects may be at times beneficial (analgesic) and at other times detrimental to the function of the organism.

Conclusion

The original proposition of gate control theory of Melzack and Wall[2] that nociceptive input to spinal dorsal horn neurons could be modulated by a number of systems prompted investigations of the systems that modulate our perception of pain. One could hardly have envisioned both the diversity and complexity of the systems that have been identified with evidence of positive feedback loops, negative feedback loops, and tonic effects that may be either inhibitory or facilitatory. As a consequence, the original notions of systems descending from supraspinal sites to the spinal cord to inhibit pain have been expanded to include descending systems that also enhance our perception of pain. At the present time, our analyses indicate these two systems are functionally and anatomically intertwined and appear to operate as a unit rather than as separate entities. The ultimate perception we develop following exposure to noxious events represents some balance between these two systems. It is possible that these systems attenuate or amplify responses to noxious stimuli in order to enhance our ability to localize and attend to peripheral stimuli that threaten us. Studies of stress, inflammation, neuropathic pain, drug-induced hypersensitivity, or other mechanisms leading to chronic pain states have begun to demonstrate that deficits in descending inhibition and/or activation of descending facilitation-related systems may also serve as mechanisms of pain generation or amplification.

Studies related to the neurotransmitters of modulation have consistently identified NE, 5-HT, GABA, and endogenous opioids to be key substances involved in the balance of inhibitory and excitatory influences. It should come as no small wonder then, that the drugs clinicians find useful in the treatment of hypersensitivity and pain are associated with noradrenergic, serotonergic, GABAergic, and opioidergic function within the CNS. It is the subtleties of the pharmacology that will define future refinements in therapeutics and many of these subtleties are only now being defined.

References

1. Randich A, Ness TJ. Modulation of spinal nociceptive processing. In: Fishman SM, Ballantyne JC, Rathmell JP, eds. *Bonica's Management of Pain*. Philadelphia: Lippincott William & Wilkins; 2009:48–60.
2. Melzack R, Wall PD. Pain mechanisms: a new theory. *Science* 1965;150: 971–979.
3. Mendell LM. Constructing and deconstructing the gate theory of pain. *Pain* 2014;155:210–216.
4. Treede RD. Gain Control mechanisms in the nociceptive system. *Pain* 2016;157(6):1199–1204.
5. Noordenbos W. *Pain*. Amsterdam, The Netherlands: Elsevier; 1959.
6. Le Bars D, Dickenson AH, Besson JM. Diffuse noxious inhibitory controls (DNIC). I. Effects on dorsal horn convergent neurones in the rat. *Pain* 1979;6:283–304.
7. Le Bars D, Dickenson AH, Besson JM. Diffuse noxious inhibitory controls (DNIC). II. Lack of effect on non-convergent neurons, supraspinal involvement and theoretical implications. *Pain* 1979;6:305–327.
8. Yarnitsky D. Role of endogenous pain modulation in chronic pain mechanisms and treatment. *Pain* 2015;156(suppl):S24–S31.
9. Mendell LM. Physiological properties of unmyelinated fiber projections to the spinal cord. *Exp Neurol* 1966;16:316–332.
10. Woolf CJ. Evidence for a central component of post-injury pain hypersensitivity. *Nature* 1983;306:686–688.
11. Sandkühler J, Gruber-Schoffnegger D. Hyperalgesia by synaptic long-term potentiation (LTP): an update. *Curr Opin Pharmacol* 2012;12:18–27.
12. Sherrington CS, Sowton SC. Observations on reflex responses to single break-shocks. *J Physiol* 1915;49:331–348.
13. Fulton JF. *Muscular Contraction and the Reflex Control of Movement*. Baltimore, MD: Williams & Wilkins; 1926.
14. Lundberg A. Supraspinal control of transmission in reflex paths to motoneurons and primary afferents. *Prog Brain Res* 1964;12:197–221.
15. Wall PD. The laminar organization of the dorsal horn and effects of descending impulses. *J Physiol* 1967;188:403–423.
16. Reynolds DV. Surgery in the rat during electrical analgesia induced by focal brain stimulation. *Science* 1969;164:444–445.
17. Mayer DJ, Liebeskind JC. Pain reduction by focal electrical stimulation of the brain: an anatomical and behavioral analysis. *Brain Res* 1974;68:73–93.
18. Mayer DJ, Wolfle TL, Akil H, et al. Analgesia from electrical stimulation in the brainstem of the rat. *Science* 1971;174:1351–1354.
19. Adams JE. Naloxone reversal of analgesia produced by brain stimulation in the human. *Pain* 1976;2:161–166.
20. Haber LH, Martin RF, Chung JM, et al. Inhibition and excitation of primate spinothalamic tract neurons by stimulation in the region of nucleus reticularis gigantocellularis. *J Neurophysiol* 1980;43:1578–1593.
21. Zhuo M. Descending facilitation: from basic science to the treatment of chronic pain. *Molecular Pain* 2017;13:1–12.
22. Mason P. Ventromedial medulla: pain modulation and beyond. *J Comp Neurol* 2005;493:2–8.
23. Boadas-Vaelllo P, Castany S, Homs J, et al. Neuroplasticity of ascending and descending pathways after somatosensory system injury: reviewing knowledge to identify neuropathic pain therapeutic targets. *Spinal Cord* 2016;54: 330–340.
24. Lau BK, Vaughan CW. Descending modulation of pain: the GABA disinhibition hypothesis of analgesia. *Curr Opin Neurobiol* 2014;29:159–164.
25. Ossipov MH, Morimura K, Porreca F. Descending pain modulation and chronification of pain. *Curr Opin Support Palliat Care* 2014;8:143–153.
26. Kwon M, Altin M, Duenas H, et al. The role of descending inhibitory pathways on chronic pain modulation and clinical implications. *Pain Practice* 2014;14:656–667.
27. Peirs C, Seal RP. Neural circuits for pain: recent advances and current views. *Science* 2016;354:578–584.
28. Basbaum AI, Fields HL. Endogenous pain control systems: review and hypothesis. *Ann Neurol* 1978;4:451–462.
29. Basbaum AI, Fields HL. Endogenous pain control systems: brainstem spinal pathways and endorphin circuitry. *Annu Rev Neurosci* 1984;7:309–338.
30. Taylor BK, Westlund KN. The noradrenergic locus coeruleus as a chronic pain generator. *J Neurosci Res* 2017;95:1336–1346.
31. Tsuruoka M, Tamaki J, Maeda M, et al. Biological implications of coeruleospinal inhibition of nociceptive processing in the spinal cord. *Front Int Neurosci* 2012;6:1–10.
32. Stevens RT, Hodge CJ Jr, Apkarian AV. Kölliker-Fuse nucleus: the principal source of pontine catecholaminergic cells projecting to the lumbar spinal cord of the cat. *Brain Res* 1982;239:589–594.
33. Janss AJ, Gebhart GF. Quantitative characterization and spinal pathway mediating inhibition of spinal nociceptive transmission from the lateral reticular nucleus in the rat. *J Neurophysiol* 1988;59:226–247.
34. Janss AJ, Gebhart GF. Brainstem and spinal pathways mediating descending inhibition from the medullary lateral reticular nucleus in the rat. *Brain Res* 1988;440:109–122.
35. Randich A, Aicher SA. Medullary substrates mediating antinociception produced by electrical stimulation of the vagus. *Brain Res* 1988;335:68–76.
36. Ren K, Randich A, Gebhart GF. Modulation of spinal nociceptive transmission from nuclei tractus solitarii: A relay for effects of vagal afferent stimulation. *J Neurophysiol* 1990;63:971–986.
37. Aimone LD, Gebhart GF. Serotonin and/or an excitatory amino acid in the medial medulla mediates stimulation-produced antinociception from the lateral hypothalamus in the rat. *Brain Res* 1988;450:170–180.
38. Neugebauer V. Amygdala pain mechanisms. *Hanb Exp Pharmacol* 2015;227:261–284
39. Senapti AK, Huntington PJ, LaGraize SC, et al. Electrical stimulation of the primary somatosensory cortex inhibits spinal dorsal horn neuron activity. *Brain Res* 2005;1057:134–140.
40. Kuroda R, Kawabata A, Kawao N, et al. Somatosensory cortex stimulation-evoked analgesia in rats: potentiation by NO synthase inhibition. *Life Sci* 2000;66:PL271–PL276.
41. Zhang YQ, Tang JS, Yuan G, et al. Inhibitory effects of electrically evoked activation of ventrolateral orbital cortex on the tail-flick reflex are mediated by the periaqueductal gray in rats. *Pain* 1997;72:127–135.
42. Zhang S, Tang JS, Yuan G, et al. Involvement of the frontal ventrolateral orbital cortex in descending inhibition of nociception mediated by the periaqueductal gray in rats. *Neurosci Lett* 1997;224:142–146.
43. Hutchinson WD, Harfa L, Dostrovsky JO. Ventrolateral orbital cortex and periaqueductal gray stimulation-induced effects on- and off-cells in the rostral medial medulla in the rat. *Neuroscience* 1996;70:391–407.
44. Millan MJ. Descending control of pain. *Prog Neurobiol* 2002;66:355–474.
45. Gebhart GF, Randich A. Brainstem modulation of nociception. In: Klemm WR, Vertes RP, eds. *Brainstem Mechanisms of Behavior*. New York: John Wiley and Sons, Inc; 1990:315–352.
46. Thurston CL, Randich A. Effects of vagal afferent stimulation on ON and OFF cells in the rostroventral medulla: relationships to nociception and arterial blood pressure. *J Neurophysiol* 1992;67:180–196.
47. Urban MO, Zahn PK, Gebhart GF. Descending facilitatory influences from the rostral medial medulla mediate secondary, but not primary hyperalgesia in the rat. *Neuroscience* 1999;90:349–352.
48. Schaible HG, Neugebauer V, Cervero F, et al. Changes in tonic descending inhibition of spinal neurons with articular input during the development of acute arthritis in the cat. *J Neurophysiol* 1991;66:1021–1032.

49. Ren K, Dubner R. Enhanced descending modulation of nociception in rats with persistent hindpaw inflammation. *J Neurophysiol* 1996;76:3025–3037.
50. Butler RK, Finn DP. Stress-induced analgesia. *Prog Neurobiol* 2009;88: 184–202.
51. Jennings EM, Okine BN, Roche M, et al. Stress-induced hyperalgesia. *Prog Neurobiol* 2014;121:1–18.
52. Robbins MT, Ness TJ. Footshock-induced urinary bladder hypersensitivity: role of spinal corticotropin-releasing factor receptors. *J Pain* 2008;9:991–998.
53. Suzuki R, Rygh LJ, Dickenson AH. Bad news from the brain: descending 5-HT pathway that control spinal pain processing. *Trends Pharm Sci* 2004;25(12):613–617.
54. Gao K, Mason P. Serotonergic raphe magnus cells that respond to noxious tail heat are not ON or OFF cells. *J Neurophysiol* 2000;84:1719–1725.
55. Kaplan H, Fields HL. Hyperalgesia during acute opioid abstinence: evidence for a nociceptive facilitating function of the rostral ventromedial medulla. *J Neurosci* 1991;11:1433–1439.
56. Pert CB, Snyder SH. Opiate receptor: demonstration in nervous tissue. *Science* 1973;179:1011–1014.
57. Cox BM, Opheim KE, Teschemacher H, et al. A peptide-like substance from pituitary that acts like morphine. 2. Purification and properties. *Life Sci* 1975;16:1777–1782.
58. Hughes J, Smith TW, Kosterlitz HW, et al. Identification of two related pentapeptides from the brain with potent opiate agonist activity. *Nature* 1975;258:577–580.
59. Simantov R, Snyder SH. Morphine-like peptides in mammalian brain: isolation, structure elucidation, and interactions with the opiate receptor. *Proc Natl Acad Sci U S A;* 1976;73:2515–2519.
60. Atweh S, Kuhar MJ. Autoradiographic localization of opiate receptors in rat brain. II. The brain stem. *Brain Res* 1977;129:1–12.
61. Mayer DJ, Hayes RL. Stimulation-produced analgesia: development of tolerance and cross-tolerance to morphine. *Science* 1975;188(4191):961–962.
62. Gerhart KD, Wilcox TK, Chung JM, et al. Inhibition of nociceptive and nonnociceptive responses of primate spinothalamic cells by stimulation in medial brain stem. *J Neurophysiol* 1981;45:121–136.
63. Basbaum AI, Clanton CH, Fields HL. Three bulbospinal pathways from the rostral medulla of the cat: an autoradiographic study of pain modulating systems. *J Comp Neurol* 1978;178:209–224.
64. Dahlström A, Fuxe K. Evidence for the existence of monoamine-containing neurons in the central nervous system. I. Demonstration of monoamines in the cell bodies of brainstem neurons. *Acta Physiol Scand Suppl* 1964;(suppl 62):1–55.
65. Llorca-Torralba, Borges G, Neto F, et al. Noradrenergic locus coeruleus pathways in pain modulation. *Neuroscience* 2016;338:93–113.
66. Burnett A, Gebhart GF. Characterization of descending modulation of nociception from the A5 cell group. *Brain Res* 1991;546:271–281.
67. Behbehani MM, Park MR, Clement ME. Interactions between the lateral hypothalamus and the periaqueductal gray. *J Neurosci* 1988;8:2780–2787.
68. Carstens E. Hypothalamic inhibition of rat dorsal horn neuronal responses to noxious skin heat. *Pain* 1986;25:97–107.
69. LeDoux J. The amygdala. *Current Biol* 2007;17:R868–R874.
70. Nishii H, Nomura M, Aono H, et al. Up-regulation of galanin and corticotropin-releasing hormone mRNAs in the key hypothalamic and amygdaloid nuclei in a mouse model of visceral pain. *Regul Pept* 2007;141:105–112.
71. Qin C, Greenwood-Van Meerveld B, Foreman RD. Visceromotor and spinal neuronal responses to colorectal distension in rats with aldosterone onto the amygdala. *J Neurophysiol* 2003;90:3–11.
72. Sadler KE, McQuaid NA, Cox AC, et al. Divergent functions of the left and right central amygdala in visceral nociception. *Pain* 2017;158:747–759.
73. Yavari F, Jamil A, Samani MM, et al. Basic and functional effects of transcranial electrical stimulation (tES)—an introduction. *Neurosci Behav Revs* 2017;85:81–92.
74. Antal A, Aleckseichuk I, Bikson M, et al. Low intensity transcranial electric stimulation: safety, ethical, legal regulatory and application guidelines. *Clin Neurophysiol* 2017;128:1774–1809.
75. Klein MM, Treister R, Raij T, et al. Transcranial magnetic stimulation of the brain: guidelines for pain treatment research. *Pain* 2015;156:1601–1614.
76. Ohara PT, Vit JP, Jasmin L. Cortical modulation of pain. *Cell Mol Life Sci* 2005;62:44–52.
77. Al Amin HA, Atweh SF, Baki SA, et al. Continuous perfusion with morphine of the orbitofrontal cortex reduces allodynia and hyperalgesia in a rat model for mononeuropathy. *Neurosci Lett* 2004;364:27–31.
78. Burkey AR, Carstens E, Wenniger JJ, et al. An opioidergic cortical antinociception triggering site in the agranular insular cortex of the rat that contributes to morphine antinociception. *J Neurosci* 1996;16:6612–6623.
79. Burkey AR, Carstens EJ. Dopamine reuptake inhibitor in the rostral agranular insular cortex produces antinociception. *J Neurosci* 1999;19:4169–4179.
80. Fields HL, Bry J, Hentall I, et al. The activity of neurons in the rostral medulla of the rat during withdrawal from noxious heat. *J Neurosci* 1983;3:2545–2552.
81. Fields HL, Vanegas H, Hentall I, et al. Evidence that disinhibition of brain stem neurons contributes to morphine analgesia. *Nature* 1983;306:684–686.
82. Song Z, Ansah OB, Meyerson BA, et al. The rostroventromedial medulla is engaged in the effects of spinal cord stimulation in a rodent model of neuropathic pain. *Neuroscience* 2013;247:134–144.
83. Chebbi R, Boyer N, Monconduit L, et al. The nucleus raphe magnus OFF-cells are involved in diffuse noxious inhibitory controls. *Exp Neurol* 2014;256:39–45.
84. Silva M, Costa-Pereira JT, Martins D, et al. Pain modulation from the brain during diabetic neuropathy: uncovering the role of the rostroventromedial medulla. *Neurobio Dis* 2016;96:346–356.
85. Kincaid W, Neubert MJ, Xu M, et al. Role for medullary pain facilitating neurons in secondary thermal hyperalgesia. *J Neurophysiol* 2006;95:33–41.
86. Urban MO, Coutinho SV, Gebhart GF. Involvement of excitatory amino acid receptors and nitric oxide in the rostral ventromedial medulla in modulating secondary hyperalgesia produced by mustard oil. *Pain* 1999;81:45–55.
87. Hurley RW, Hammond DL. The analgesic effects of supraspinal mu and delta opioid receptor agonists are potentiated during persistent inflammation. *J Neurosci* 2000;20:1249–1259.
88. Hurley RW, Hammond DL. Contribution of endogenous enkephalins to the enhanced analgesic effects of supraspinal mu opioid receptor agonists after inflammatory injury. *J Neurosci* 2001;21:2536–2545.
89. Wei F, Ren K, Dubner R. Inflammation-induced Fos protein expression in the rat spinal cord is enhanced following dorsolateral or ventrolateral funiculus lesions. *Brain Res* 1998;782:136–141.
90. Scholz J, Woolf CJ. The neuropathic pain triad: neurons, immune cells and glia. *Nat Neurosci* 2007;10:1361–1368.
91. Kovelowski CJ, Ossipov MH, Sun H, et al. Supraspinal cholecystokinin may drive tonic descending facilitation mechanisms to maintain neuropathic pain in the rat. *Pain* 2000;87:265–273.
92. Burgess SE, Gardell LR, Ossipov MH, et al. Time-dependent descending facilitation fm the rostral ventromedial medulla maintains, but does not initiate, neuropathic pain. *J Neurosci* 2002;22:5129–5136.
93. Hodge CJ Jr, Apkarian AV, Owen MP, et al. Changes in the effects of stimulation of locus coeruleus and nucleus raphe magnus following dorsal rhizotomy. *Brain Res* 1983;288:325–329.
94. Roeckel LA, LeCoz GM, Gaveriaux-Ruff C, et al. Opioid-induced hyperalgesia: cellular and molecular mechanisms. *Neuroscience* 2016;338: 160–182.
95. Angst MS, Clark JD. Opioid-induced hyperalgesia: a qualitative systematic review. *Anesthesiology* 2006;104:570–587.
96. Vanderah TW, Suenaga NM, Ossipov MH, et al. Tonic descending facilitation from the rostral ventromedial medulla mediates opioid-induced abnormal pain and antinociceptive tolerance. *J Neurosci* 2001;21:279–286.
97. Vanderah TW, Ossipov MH, Lai J, et al. Mechanisms of opioid-induced pain and antinociceptive tolerance: descending facilitation and spinal dynorphin. *Pain* 2001;92:5–9.
98. Ossipov MH, Lai J, King T, et al. Underlying mechanisms of pronociceptive consequences of prolonged morphine exposure. *Biopolymers* 2005;80: 319–324.
99. Juni A, Klein G, Pintar JE, et al. Nociception increases during opioid infusion in opioid receptor triple knock-out mice. *Neuroscience* 2007;147:439–444.

CHAPTER 6

Supraspinal Mechanisms of Pain and Nociception

MICHAEL HAUCK and **JÜRGEN LORENZ**

The preceding chapters addressed the peripheral and spinal mechanisms of nociceptive processing. Neither normal nor pathologic pain can be understood without knowledge about supraspinal mechanisms. The multidimensionality of pain with mainly sensory-discriminative and emotional-affective components has its anatomic counterparts in a variety of supraspinal areas, which are involved in pain processing. Hence, the experience of pain is formed in a distributed network which gates the transformation of peripheral nociceptive input to conscious pain.[1] Supraspinal structures include the hindbrain (lower and upper brainstem and cerebellum) and the forebrain. The forebrain has two major divisions, the lower diencephalon involving hypothalamus and thalamus and the cerebrum involving the cortex, basal ganglia, and the limbic system (cingulate cortex, amygdala, hippocampus, Fig. 6.1). In humans, the forebrain anatomically dominates and physiologically controls much more than in other species nociceptive processing. Because of the large proportion of the human forebrain of the entire central nervous system (CNS) volume (85%) when compared to that of the spinal cord (2%), descending modulatory influences assume much greater importance than for example in the rat in which the forebrain comprises 44% and the spinal cord 35% of CNS volume.[2,3] Thus, the great variety of psychological phenomena characterizing normal and abnormal pain in humans can only be studied in humans, although anatomic tracing and electrophysiologic techniques and behavioral studies in rodents and primates contributed significantly to our current knowledge about the pathways connecting the dorsal horn with supraspinal structures.

Functional Imaging of Pain in Humans

Since release of the early editions of this handbook, functional brain imaging in human volunteers and patients addressed many questions pertaining to brain structures involved in pain processing. Before going into the details of supraspinal regions engaged in pain processing and perception, we will therefore briefly describe the methodologic basis of these technologies.

METHODOLOGIES OF NONINVASIVE AND INVASIVE FUNCTIONAL BRAIN IMAGING IN PAIN

Functional imaging techniques applied for the study of pain are positron emission tomography (PET), functional magnetic resonance imaging (fMRI), near-infrared spectroscopy (NIRS), multi-channel electroencephalography (EEG) and magneto-encephalography (MEG), and intracranial recordings. PET measures cerebral blood flow, glucose metabolism, or neurotransmitter kinetics. A very small amount of a labeled compound (called the *radiotracer*) is intravenously injected into the patient or volunteer. During its uptake and decay in the brain, the radionuclide emits a positron, which, after traveling a short distance, "annihilates" with an electron from the surrounding environment. In case of the most common use of O^{15}-water injection, counting and spatial reconstruction of these occurrences within the brain anatomy allow visualization of the regional cerebral blood flow response (rCBF) as an indicator of neuronal activity. Radio-labeled fluorodeoxyglucose (FDG) is applied to measure regional energy consumption as a function of metabolic rate. An interesting refinement of PET technology represents the use of neurotransmitters as tracers to investigate binding mechanisms and kinetics, for example, in the opioidergic system.

One method of fMRI images blood oxygenation, a technique called blood oxygen level-dependent (BOLD), which exploits the phenomenon that oxygenated and deoxygenated hemoglobin possess different magnetic properties resulting in different relaxation behavior following radiofrequency pulses inside the magnet. An additional fMRI technique called arterial spin labeling (ASL) uses a radio pulse to magnetically "label"

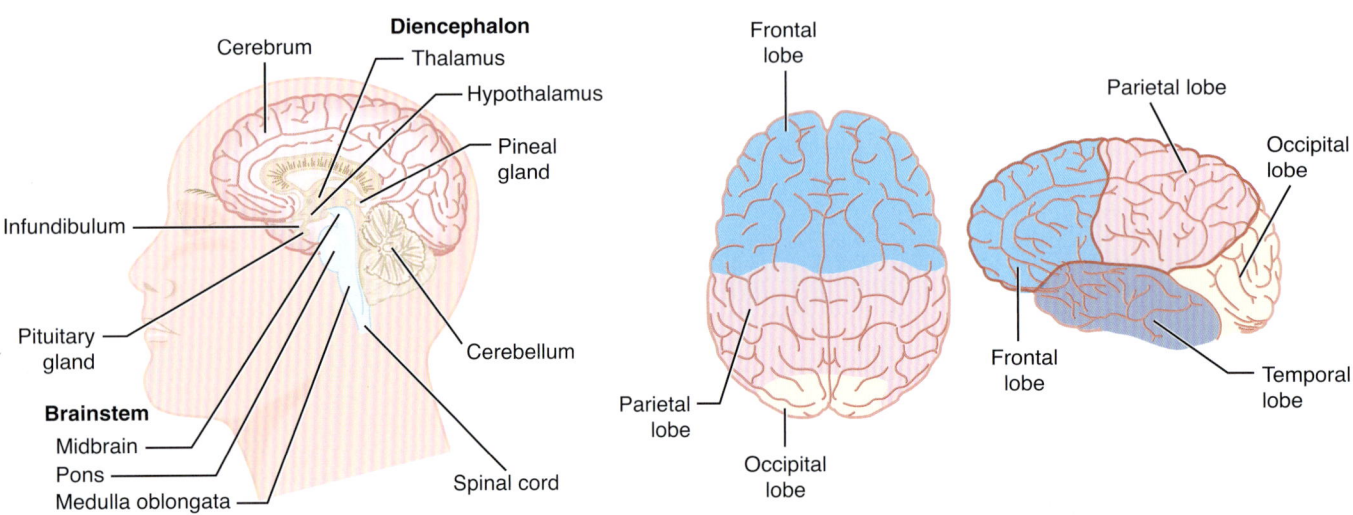

FIGURE 6.1 Structure of the brain.

hydrogen atoms ascending through the vasculature and then determines alterations in paramagnetic characteristics as the labeled blood perfuses the brain. The rCBF measures using O^{15}-water PET, the BOLD technique, and the ASL technique rely on neurovascular coupling mechanisms that are not yet fully understood, but which overcompensate local oxygen consumption, thus causing a flow of oxygenated blood into neuronally active brain areas in excess of that used.[4]

NIRS is an optical approach that also analyses changes in hemoglobin oxygenation levels by using light in the near infrared range (650 to 950 nm). Shortly, NIRS measures the attenuation of light over the cortex and can be applied noninvasively through the skull. Another advantage is the portability of NIRS systems and the possibility to measure in different environments. However, the spatial and temporal resolution in noninvasive measurements is low for NIRS.[5]

EEG and MEG are noninvasive neurophysiologic techniques that measure the respective electrical potentials and magnetic fields generated by neuronal activity of the brain and propagated to the surface of the skull where they are picked up with EEG electrodes or, in the case of its magnetic counterpart, received by supra conducting quantum interference device (SQUID) sensors located outside the skull. Compared with PET and fMRI, EEG and MEG are direct indicators of neuronal activity and yield a higher temporal resolution of investigated brain function. The spatial distributions of EEG potentials and MEG fields at characteristic time points following noxious stimulation are analyzed using an inverse mathematical modeling and spatial filtering to estimate the anatomic origin of the recorded pain-related activity. The spatial acuity of MEG is higher than that of EEG because the latter measures the extracellular volume currents that are distorted by the differentially conducting tissues such as gray and white matter, cerebrospinal fluid, durae, and bone. In contrast, MEG measures the magnetic field perpendicular to the intracellular currents undistorted by the surrounding tissue.

Invasive recordings, which are assessed during neurosurgical interventions in patients ongoing epileptic surgery, or deep brain stimulation (DBS) procedures (most common in Parkinson disease), are extremely helpful to directly measure supraspinal pain signals. Different invasive recording techniques, namely, depth electrodes, subdural grids, subdural strips, and stereoencephalography, are used today.[6] Advantage of all these invasive recordings is that the neuronal activity is picked up directly from the neurons and not being distorted by the cerebrospinal fluid, durae, and bone as in EEG or MEG. Disadvantage lies in the invasive nature of the procedure and the only limited area that can be investigated using invasive recordings.

Brainstem

The brainstem represents the connection of the spinal cord with the diencephalon (hypothalamus and thalamus). It comprises the rhombencephalon (pons and medulla) and the mesencephalon (midbrain, see Fig. 6.1). A major rhombencephalic structure is the reticular formation (RF) which encompasses a distributed network of small and large nerve fibers and extends from the medulla up to the level of the thalamus. It has manifold local interneuronal connections within the brainstem and contains both ascending and descending projecting systems. It is divided into three vertical zones. The medial magnocellular zone contains the ascending reticular activating system (ARAS), a major pathway to the thalamus, hypothalamus, and basal forebrain (a group of structures at the base of the frontal lobe, including the nucleus basalis, diagonal band, medial septum, and substantia innominata). The median and paramedian zones contain the raphe nuclei of serotonergic projection neurons. The lateral parvocellular zone receives afferents from

amygdala and hypothalamus. RF and basal forebrain have reciprocal connection with virtually all cortical and subcortical structures through cholinergic (from the basal forebrain), noradrenergic (from the locus coeruleus), dopaminergic (from the substantia nigra [SN] and ventral tegmentum [VTA]), and serotoninergic (from the raphe) pathways. Reciprocal connections with the spinal cord mediate motor, respiratory, and cardiovascular functions and pain modulation.

The RF is an important mediator of consciousness and arousal. The stream of information about the outer world that reaches specific nuclei of the thalamus and cortex through the sensory pathways of vision, audition, gustation, and somatosensation is blocked when the activity of the mesencephalic RF, which drives nonspecific thalamic sites, drops below a critical level, such as, for example, during slow wave sleep or certain types of absence epilepsies.[7] Wakefulness and arousal are thus closely coupled to the RF, which act as the "energetic supplier" of conscious perception and behavior. Widespread areas of the RF are responsive to noxious stimuli.[8] The gigantocellular and magnocellular fields of the medullar RF, that is, the bulboreticular region, mediate escape behavior following acute painful stimuli[9,10] and respond neurochemically during persistent pain.[11] The close relationship of nociception and pain with arousal and consciousness guarantees optimal alertness and readiness to avoid bodily harm. Sleep is therefore disrupted by the awakening nature of pain through its influence on the RF. Similarly, opioid-induced sedation is antagonized by residual pain. These aspects will be discussed in more detail later.

A view of the RF as a "diffuse arousal network"[12] has been replaced by the acknowledgement of localized reticular cell groups with highly specific functions and connections in the coordination of head and eye movements, postural orientation, and autonomic visceral control.[13] Also, the understanding of RF in pain has become more differentiated. The subnucleus reticularis dorsalis (SRD) represents a homogenous population of neurons in the caudal-dorsal medulla whose axons form both ascending and descending collaterals to the thalamus and spinal cord, respectively. SRD neurons are strongly activated by noxious cutaneous and visceral stimuli from any part of the body.[14] It is regarded a medullary substrate of the link between nociceptive and motor activities. SRD has also been suggested as major supraspinal site mediating the "pain-inhibits-pain," or counterirritation, phenomenon as formulated in the concept of diffuse noxious inhibitory controls (DNIC).[15] As part of a spinal-bulbospinal feedback loop, SRD is proposed to facilitate the extraction of nociceptive information by increasing the signal-to-noise ratio between a pool of deep dorsal horn neurons activated by a tonic painful focus and the remaining population of such neurons, which are inhibited for simultaneous phasic noxious input. Youssef et al.[16] used fMRI in healthy test participants and observed that the magnitude of signal reduction in SRD following repetitive phasic heat stimuli applied to the right lip correlated with magnitude of analgesia produced by a conditioning pain exerted by injection of hypertonic saline into the tibialis anterior muscle.

PERIAQUEDUCTAL GRAY MATTER—A KEY STRUCTURE OF ENDOGENOUS ANALGESIA

The periaqueductal gray (PAG) is a midbrain territory located medially adjacent to the RF surrounding the cerebral aqueduct in a horse shoe–shaped manner by sparing ventral regions subserving distinct ocular-motor functions unrelated to pain.[17] The PAG plays a critical role in the expression of a variety of emotion-related behaviors including pain.[18] It represents a key structure in relaying descending pathways from the limbic system (prefrontal cortex, amygdala, and hypothalamus) to midbrain (e.g., inferior and superior colliculi), pons (e.g., locus coeruleus, lateral parabrachial nucleus, dorsolateral pontine tegmentum), the raphe nuclei of the rostroventral medulla (RVM) and the deeper layers of the spinal cord (Rexed layers V, VII, VIII). Midbrain, pontine, medullar, and spinal connections are all reciprocal, such that the PAG is connecting afferents from these origins to medial thalamic nuclei and hypothalamus.[19] Early systematic studies identified PAG and RVM as brainstem sites that elicit powerful surgical levels of analgesia through focal brain stimulation,[20] subsequently more elaborated and referred to as *stimulus-induced analgesia*.[21-23] A milestone contribution to the understanding of the interaction between PAG and RVM and its role in opioid analgesia was delivered by Fields and colleagues'[24] working group who identified two classes of pain modulatory cells in the RVM exerting inhibitory and facilitatory actions through respective off- and on-cells. Off-cells are activated by local infusion of μ-opioid agonists, and their activity inhibits nociceptive transmission. In contrast, on-cells facilitate nociceptive transmission, are inhibited by local μ-opioids, and are activated by naloxone and morphine abstinence. Approximately 15% of RVM neurons are serotonergic and are neither on- nor off-cells and do not respond to opioids.[25] Some respond to baroreceptor input integrating cardiovascular and nociceptive function.[26] Descending serotonergic fibers from the RVM project to dorsal horn neurons via the dorsolateral funiculus and mediate the analgesic effect of opioid receptor activation. Also noradrenergic structures in the brainstem, namely, the locus coeruleus, are regarded to be pain inhibitory through activation of α_2-adrenoceptors on central terminals of primary afferent nociceptors (presynaptic inhibition), by direct α_2-adrenergic action on spinal pain-relay neurons (postsynaptic inhibition), and by α_2-adrenergic activation of inhibitory interneurons.[27] However, the central as well as the peripheral efficacy of pain inhibition can vary depending on neuroplastic changes following inflammation and injury.[27] Taylor and Westlund[28] recently reviewed evidences that argue for a pain facilitatory action of locus coeruleus neurons under conditions of neuropathic pain, especially at later stages after the traumatic lesion.

The biologic significance of endogenous pain control is generally seen in the context of behavioral conflicts in which the subject needs to disengage from pain in order to fight or escape at the presence of body injury. Analogous human life situations are sporting competition or combat, during which a subject may fail to be aware of even severe tissue damage, which becomes painful when the victim releases engagement in these activities. Thus, forebrain input to the PAG mediates contextual information, from the prefrontal cortex, the amygdala, the anterior cingulate cortex (ACC), and the hypothalamus about momentary behavioral goals, past experience, and bodily needs. Evidence furthermore indicates that injury and inflammation causing increased sensitivity toward painful stimuli (primary hyperalgesia) triggers the RVM as key structure of a feedback pain inhibiting circuitry.[29] There is solid evidence by fMRI that PAG and RVM are also mediating the placebo response in humans.[30,31]

Using the expression of the immediate early gene, c-*fos*, as a marker of neuronal activation, an interesting regional distinction for deep versus cutaneous pain had been demonstrated within the midbrain PAG. Noxious stimulation of a range of deep somatic and visceral structures evoked a selective increase in Fos expression in the ventrolateral PAG column (vlPAG), whereas, noxious cutaneous stimulation evoked Fos expression predominantly in the lateral PAG column (lPAG).[32] vlPAG and lPAG areas are suggested to represent different modes of behavioral adaptation characterizing inescapable and escapable types of pain, respectively. Earlier studies showed that both deep pain as well as microinjection of excitatory amino acids (EAA) into the vlPAG of freely moving animals evoked a response of quiescence, decreased vigilance, decreased reactivity, hypotension, and bradycardia. In contrast, cutaneous pain as well as activation of the lPAG-evoked fight-and-flight behavior, increased vigilance, hyperreactivity, hypertension, and tachycardia. Lumb et al.[33,34] presented evidence that differential representation of escapable and inescapable pain in the PAG extends to distinct representations of "first" and "second" pain, as indicated by the columnar distribution of neurones activated by inputs from respective Aδ and C nociceptors. Furthermore, the functional organization of projections from circumscribed regions of the hypothalamus to the different columns of the PAG indicates that the behavioral significance of the pain signal is also represented in brain regions other than the PAG. Such specificity may coordinate antinociception with adequate behavioral and autonomic responses to prevent damage, in case of an imminent threat, or promote healing when an injury is already manifest.

Finally, the PAG is a promising target in invasive DBS to treat chronic pain, first applied by Hosobuchi et al.[35] and Richardson and Akil[36] in humans. However, its use is limited due to loss of efficacy over time and intolerable side effects. It remains to be cleared whether more precise electrode positioning and simultaneous stimulation of distinct locations[37] or a better understanding of pain mechanisms that are sensitive or insensitive to DBS will help to achieve better outcome. In chronic neuropathic and central pain syndromes, DBS of the PAG appears less effective than nociceptive pain.[38]

MESOLIMBIC DOPAMINE SYSTEM

The mesolimbic system comprises dopaminergic brainstem sites, that is, the VTA and the SN projecting to the striatum. Neurons originating in the SN pars compacta innervate D1- and D2-receptors of the dorsal striatum (putamen and caudate nucleus) that are functionally integrated into the motor loop of the basal ganglia (see the following text). The nucleus accumbens of the ventral striatum is regarded the key structure of a mesolimbic circuitry receiving input from SN and VTA mediating motivational salience and valence of painful stimuli to drive pain avoidance and pain endurance depending on the situational context.[39] The mesolimbic circuitry is furthermore regarded important for the encoding of the rewarding effect of pain relief.[40] Chronic fibromyalgia and low back pain have been observed to be associated with reduced responses of the mesolimbic circuitry to salient stimuli[41,42] that could account for the depressive comorbidity in these patients.[39]

Hypothalamus

The hypothalamus occupies the ventral half of the diencephalon below the thalamus on either side of the third ventricle. It lies just above the pituitary gland with which it is intimately coupled for various neuroendocrine secretions subserving autonomic functions. Neurosecretory neurons are mainly located in periventricular and supraoptic nuclei. Fiber tracts to the pituitary gland are subdivided into two parts: (1) magnocellular secretory cells expressing vasopressin and oxytocin innervate the posterior pituitary gland and (2) parvocellular secretory cells expressing gonadotropins, releasing and inhibiting hormones that innervate the anterior pituitary gland. The hypothalamus receives nociceptive inputs from the midbrain parabrachial nucleus, the ventrolateral medulla, and the spinal and trigeminal dorsal horn.[43,44] The nucleus of the solitary tract (NTS), a major relay of cardiorespiratory, visceral, and gustatory information, is also connected with the hypothalamus. Its role in nociception is not quite clear, but the convergence of autonomic, visceral, and nociceptive information in the hypothalamus underpins the importance of it for the control of homeostasis as part of the brain's defense system. More recent research points to a pain inhibitory role of hypothalamic orexin neurons (orexin-A and orexin-B), similar to opioidergic neurons, acting on the

PAG as the most important supraspinal site.[45,46] Interestingly, hypothalamic orexin neurons mediate analgesia induced by odorants in mice.[47]

Thalamus

The thalamus is the major structure of the diencephalon, which additionally contains, in relation to thalamus, basally the hypothalamus, laterally the globus pallidus and nucleus subthalamicus, and medially the third ventricle. With the exception of the olfactory system, all sensory systems send afferent input to the thalamus from where it is projected into the specific cortical representation areas. This is why the thalamus is often referred to as *the gate to consciousness*. The intralaminar and ventral motor nuclei are the main targets of thalamic inputs from the striatum (putamen and caudate nucleus). Corticostriatal and striatothalamocortical connections form the sensory-motor loop of the basal ganglia which is under control of dopaminergic input from the midbrain SN pars compacta (see earlier discussion). The thalamic extension of the ARAS contributes to arousal and wakefulness driven by the midbrain RF (see earlier discussion). The multidimensional nature of pain as composed of sensory-discriminative and affective-motivational determinants first introduced by Melzack and Casey[48] four decades ago formed a conceptual framework that guided many research groups studying supraspinal pain mechanisms. One of their postulates was that sensory and affective pain dimensions are anatomically represented by spinal pathways that differentially target respective lateral and medial nuclei of the dorsal thalamus.

THE LATERAL PAIN SYSTEM—THE SENSORY-DISCRIMINATIVE PATHWAY

The cell bodies of spinothalamic tract (STT) fibers are located in the most superficial layers, lamina I, the outer region of lamina II, and deeper laminae V to VI[49] according to the Rexed scheme. STT axons cross via the anterior commissure to the anterolateral portion of the contralateral hemisphere and have their main thalamic targets in lateral nuclei, namely, ventral posterolateral (VPL; from the body) and posteromedial (VPM; from the face) nuclei and the ventral posterior inferior (VPI) nucleus. These fibers contribute to thermal and pain sensation. The lateral thalamic nuclei have small receptive fields and mostly gradual stimulus response functions over nonnoxious and noxious intensities, representing the "wide-dynamic-range," or to a lesser extent, over noxious range only, representing the "nociceptive-specific" type of cells. These features render lateral thalamic targets of spinal nociceptive afferents ideally suited for the encoding of spatial localization and intensity of painful stimuli, similar to the properties of touch. The sensory-discriminative determinant of pain is thus governed by a spinal afferent pathway that mainly reaches lateral thalamic nuclei, from where neuronal activity is projected into the contralateral primary (SI) and bilateral secondary (SII) somatosensory cortices and mid and posterior sections of the insula (see the following text). Invasive DBS of the VPL demonstrated improvement of chronic neuropathic and central pain.[50]

SPINAL CONNECTIONS TO BRAINSTEM AND MEDIAL THALAMUS—THE AFFECTIVE PATHWAY

Although direct connections of lamina I STT cells exist with medial thalamic nuclei, namely, the central lateral nucleus and intralaminar complex,[51–53] the major source of nociceptive input to the medial thalamus is likely indirect through the brainstem that relays spinoreticular, spinomesencephalic, and spinoparabrachial input from both superficial and deeper dorsal horn. Medial thalamic nuclei project densely into key structures of the limbic system, such as the ACC, the amygdala, the hippocampus, the anterior insula, and prefrontal cortex, which represent the perceived intrusion and threat by pain, referred to as *affective-motivational* and *cognitive-evaluative* determinants of pain.[48]

The contention that slowly and rapidly conducting nociceptors project differentially to respective medial and lateral thalamic nuclei had been recently challenged. Using intracerebral recordings of laser-evoked potentials in patients receiving neurosurgery due to refractory partial epilepsy, Bastuji et al.[54] identified three major thalamic regions, namely, the centrolateral (CL), VPL, and anterior pulvinar responding equally and simultaneously to phasic nociceptive laser input. The authors conclude that at least part of the nociceptive input driven by rapidly conducting Aδ fibers reaches both lateral and medial thalamic regions arguing for rapid medial thalamic projection to cingulate structures to subserve rapid orienting reactions to, and withdrawal from, the noxious stimulus. This suggests that both medial and lateral thalamic sites contribute to the exteroceptive function of escapable pain.

In contrast, Craig[55] hypothesized that pain is a purely interoceptive perception such as hunger, thirst, or itch. It originates in specific lamina I neurons which impinge on specific thalamic nuclei, such as the posterior part of the ventral medial nucleus (VMpo) and the ventral caudal part of the mediodorsal nucleus (MDvc). These distinct thalamic nuclei relay afferent input to the dorsal posterior insula and caudal ACC, respectively, and form separate pathways regarded as important elements of a hierarchical system subserving homeostasis, linking thermal sensation and pain contributing to the sense of the physiologic condition of the body (interoception) with subjective feelings and emotion.

Cortex

The human cortex is divided according to functional and anatomic criteria. The German neuroanatomist and psychiatrist Brodmann[56] introduced a systematic classification of the human cortex based on cytoarchitectonic properties, which, in refined modification, is still often referred to in the neuroimaging literature. Functional classifications consider the specific relevance of different cortical structures for motor, sensory, cognitive, emotional, or autonomic information processing. These functional areas can be divided into hierarchically organized subregions, for example, primary and secondary projection areas or network systems consisting of distributed areas. The current view is that higher order projection areas and distributed networks rather than a unique "pain center" represent the cortical substrate of pain perception. This view is consistent with the multidimensional definition of pain[48,57] which postulates differential projection of lateral and medial thalamic pathways to respective sensory and limbic cortical structures in addition to cortico-cortical as well as cortico-subcortical interactions for the composition of sensory-discriminative, affective-motivational, and cognitive-evaluative determinants (see earlier discussion). According to this concept, the primary (SI) and secondary somatosensory (SII) cortices receiving input from lateral thalamic nuclei are responsible for sensory-discriminative processing. Emotional content and aversive quality to noxious stimuli motivating escape and avoidance behavior are linked to limbic areas. The limbic system involves cortical and subcortical areas from the frontal, parietal, and temporal lobe that from a ring (limbus) around the upper brainstem and diencephalon, first regarded by Papez[58] as important for emotion. It includes the cingulate cortex, the insula, the prefrontal cortex, and, as subcortical structures, amygdala, hippocampus, medial thalamus, and hypothalamus. Taken together, it is important to highlight that the multidimensionality of pain is neuroanatomically reflected in multiple cortical sites being involved in pain processing.

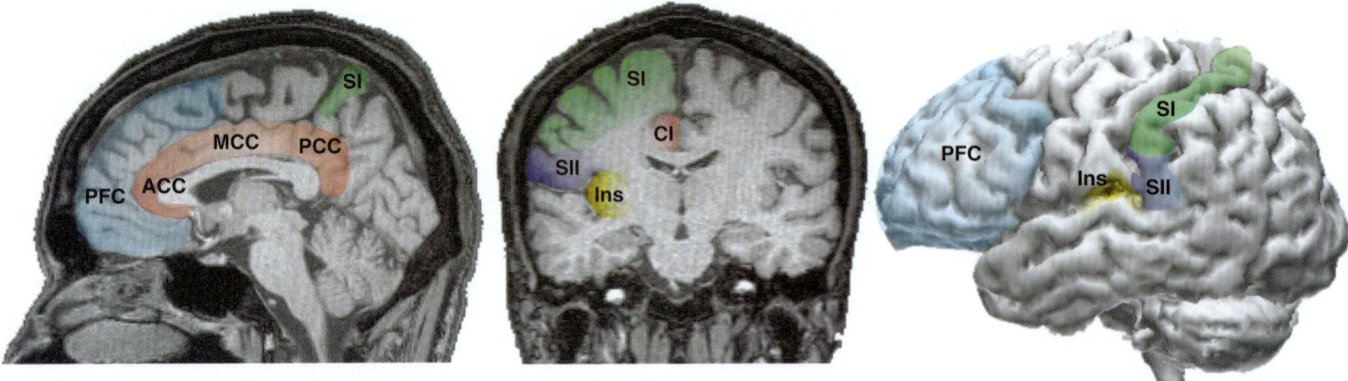

FIGURE 6.2   Schematic anatomic localization of cortical areas, which are regarded as important for pain processing. Somatosensory areas, which are responsible for sensory-discriminative pain processing such as intensity and stimulus decoding, are the primary (SI) and secondary somatosensory cortex (SII). Adjacent to SII is the insula (Ins), which belongs to the limbic system and is involved in emotional-affective pain processing. Other limbic structures include the cingulate gyrus (CI) with its subdivisions anterior cingulate cortex (ACC), midcingulate cortex (MCC), and posterior cingulate gyrus (PCC). Finally, the prefrontal cortex (PFC) plays an important role in cognitive-evaluative pain processing especially for the organization of context-dependent pain behavior.

SENSORY AREAS
Primary Somatosensory Cortex

The primary somatosensory cortex (SI) is located in the parietal lobe within the postcentral gyrus (Fig. 6.2). It includes the Brodmann areas 1, 2, 3a, and 3b, the latter two occupying the depth and the posterior wall of the central sulcus and generally considered to be the major recipient of cutaneous somatosensory input. Early studies of patients with cortical lesions reported controversial results. Whereas Head and Holmes[59] did not find deficits in pain sensitivity following cortical lesions, studies on World War I and II injury victims with lesion of SI (area 3a) reported loss of cutaneous pain sensibility.[60–62] Experimental data using single-cell recordings in awake monkeys revealed a strong correlation between SI firing rate and stimulus intensity and duration of painful stimuli.[63] Patients with subdural electrodes implanted for surgical treatment of intractable epilepsy showed encoding of intensity of painful stimuli within SI.[64] Direct intracerebral electrical stimulation of SI in awake patients, however, failed to elicit painful sensations.[65,66] Thus, it appears that SI processes nociceptive input, but it is not sufficient to cause a pain sensation. Due to its spatial and intensity-encoding properties, SI is regarded to contribute to discriminative analysis of painful stimuli but does obviously not cause the aversive nature of pain perception.

Consistent evidence for SI involvement in pain processing is derived from other functional neuroimaging studies in humans.

SI is organized somatotopically; that is, neighboring peripheral skin areas are also represented by neighboring cortical sites. Human imaging studies established a somatotopic organization of SI for painful laser stimuli (Fig. 6.3).[67] Accordingly, laser stimuli at the foot and hand activated SI regions medially, near the interhemispheric gap, or more laterally, respectively. Ploner et al.[68] and Tran et al.[69] showed that laser-evoked MEG responses to Aδ- and C-fiber activation, respectively, appeared simultaneously in SI and SII, a finding which contrasts with the sequential activation of SI and SII following tactile stimuli. Kanda et al.[70] confirmed these results by using implanted subdural electrodes. Yet, not all functional imaging studies revealed SI activation related to pain. PET and fMRI studies exhibited robust SI activity following painful stimuli when using contact heat,[71–73] laser radiant heat,[67,74] or electrical pain[75,76] but less consistently during spontaneous or provoked clinical pain states.[77,78] Casey et al.[79] noted a clear temporal dynamic of SI activity following painful contact heat using PET. Notably, hypnotic suggestion of sensory pain quality enhanced SI activity following thermal stimulation,[80] whereas that of the affective pain quality did not.[81] This latter result with experimental pain stimuli fits with clinical observation that SI lesions alter sensory qualities but leave affective or cognitive aspects of pain, especially chronic pain largely unchanged.[82] Furthermore, pain-induced BOLD activations in SI are more likely correlated with stimulus intensity than perceived pain,[83] although other authors

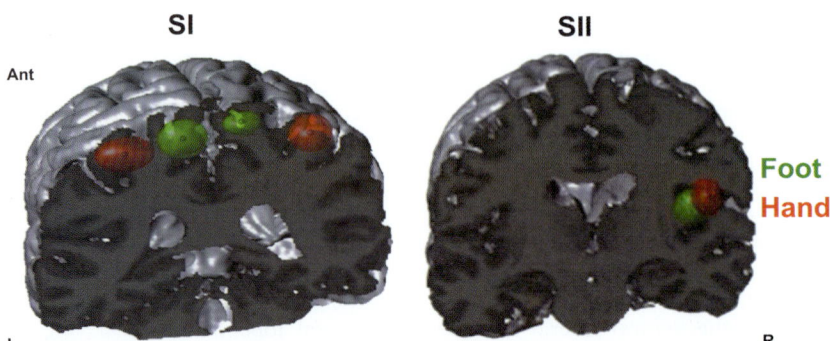

FIGURE 6.3   Somatotopic organization of somatosensory areas. Experimental pain was induced using an infrared laser, which elicits a short burning and pinprick-like pain sensation. Laser stimuli were given at both hands and feet, before pain-induced activation of the primary (SI) and secondary somatosensory (SII) areas were localized using functional magnetic resonance imaging (fMRI) technique. Pain-induced activation after hand stimulation (*red*) was found in SI near the interhemispheric gap, whereas foot stimulation (*green*) elicits more lateral activation of SI. Pain-induced localization in SII is less spatially separated between hand and foot stimulation. The *center of the colored circles* is the mean coordinate of the subjects, whereas the *radius of the circle* is the standard deviation. L, left; R, right. (*Reprinted from Bingel U, Lorenz J, Glauche V, et al. Somatotopic organization of human somatosensory cortices for pain: a single trial fMRI study. Neuroimage 2004;23[1]:224–232. Copyright © 2004 Elsevier. With permission.*)

showed that gamma oscillations in SI reflect pain perception and not the stimulus intensity.[84] Collective evidence thus indicates that noninvasive imaging methods strongly support the participation of SI in sensory-discriminative aspects of pain perception, although temporal aspects of the applied stimulus method and imaging technique and attentional and cognitive factors can significantly modify SI activity.[79,85,86]

Secondary Somatosensory Cortex

The existence of a secondary somatosensory cortex (SII) was introduced for the first time by Adrian[87] in the cat. SII is situated lateral and posterior to SI and occupies the posterior parietal operculum at the upper bank of the Sylvian fissure (see Fig. 6.1), encompassing Brodmann areas 40 and 43.[88] Because SII receives input from the thalamus via the spinothalamic projection into lateral nuclei (VPI, VPL, VPM) and sends output to the adjacent insula, SII is in a position to link nociceptive information to limbic cortical regions, such as the ACC and medial prefrontal cortex. Because of the robust generation of dipolar electric activity following noxious laser stimuli in SII that is oriented tangentially to the skull convexity, multichannel MEG recordings became an important functional brain imaging method to study pain-related SII activity in humans at high temporal resolution. The activity starts between 90 and 150 ms after the painful laser stimulus, depending on the body site and activated nerve fiber spectrum[89–91] and coincides with parallel SI activation.[68] Selective C-fiber activation also activates SII.[92] PET and fMRI revealed SII as one of the most consistent structure activated by pain.[82,93,94] Notably, the origin of painful somatosensory seizures could be assigned to the operculo-insular cortex including SII by intracerebral recordings.[95] Although less precise than SI, SII is also organized somatotopically (see also Fig. 6.3).[66,67,96] Patients with lesions within the SII cortex have been reported to exhibit elevated pain thresholds contralaterally,[97] sometimes associated with a central (neuropathic) pain syndrome.[98,99] Several authors point to the problem of differentiating SII from the adjacent posterior insula.[93] Recent evidence from intracerebral recording and stimulations in patients, however, indicates separate representations of nociceptive processing in SII and insula.[66,100] The functional role of SII is not clear. Given its coarse somatotopy, it unlikely represents a critical site for spatial discrimination but rather supplements SI in the organization of spatially guided defensive and protective behavior against bodily threat. Accordingly, SII seems to be involved in recognition, memory, and learning of painful events[101] in that it links a primordial sensory representation of pain with further cognitive evaluation and affective appraisal.

LIMBIC AREAS
Insular Cortex

As stated, the insula belongs to the limbic system and is located adjacent to SII and can be divided cytoarchitectonically into Brodmann areas 13 (anterior insula) and 41 (posterior insula). Functionally, the anterior insula, which lies rostral to the most lateral point of the central sulcus, mainly processes viscero-autonomic (intrapersonal) functions and is closely linked to gustation and olfaction, thus proximal senses. In contrast, the posterior part is related to distal senses such as audition, vision, and somatosensation and extrapersonal functions. Craig[55] attributes a key role to the insular cortex in the integration of thermosensation and pain for homeostatic feelings and behavior. Despite the already cited evidence of distinct representations of pain in SII and posterior insula (see the following text), there is not enough data to clearly delineate SII and posterior insula functionally. However, the anterior part appears to represent separate functions from posterior insula and SII, from where it receives input. Further input comes from the amygdala and brainstem nuclei. Projections from the anterior insula go to various limbic structures

such as the ACC and the entorhinal cortex of the temporal lobe (amygdala and hippocampus).

Lesion studies from patients are rare. Isolated anterior insula lesions without damage of the posterior insula and SII yield normal heat pain thresholds.[97] Others reported that damage of the anterior insula reduces pain affect and appropriate behavioral reactions to pain.[102] Functional imaging studies strongly confirmed the engagement of the anterior insula in pain and the ability to manipulate anterior and posterior insula differentially.[103] Using PET, Casey et al.[79] demonstrated that anterior insula responds early, whereas posterior insula is activated late following painful contact heat stimuli. This result is consistent with the dissociation of anterior and posterior insula according to respective anticipatory and real pain sensations.[104] Lorenz et al.[105] found stronger anterior insula activation with PET following heat stimuli applied on sensitized skin (heat allodynia) in comparison with equally intense heat stimuli applied on normal skin, whereas posterior insula and SII exhibited same activation across skin conditions. Thus, although both portions of the insula vary with pain intensity, anterior insula additionally represents subjective relevance and meaning of the pain in terms of its relation to an exteroceptive or interoceptive threat. This is also consistent with the role of the anterior insula in processing stimulus novelty.[106] On the other hand, besides multifactorial influences of pain such as pain-related anxiety, altered attention, and other nonspecific features, the posterior insula plays a major role in pain processing and can be regarded as pure nociceptive region in human pain processing (Fig. 6.4).[107] The insula also plays an important role in chronic pain processing because evidence exists that chronic pain disrupts functional connectivity of the insula cortex characteristic for resting state brain activity.[1]

Cingulate Cortex

The cingulate cortex represents a key structure of the limbic system. Anatomically, it is located in the medial portion of both hemispheres above the corpus callosum. Cytoarchitectonically, it is divided into distinct areas, the ACC (areas 24 and 25) and the posterior cingulate cortex (PCC, area 23). A more recent view additionally separates the midcingulate cortex (MCC, area 24) and the retrosplenial cortex (RSC). A major input to ACC comes from medial and intralaminar thalamic nuclei,[108] which places the ACC into the center of the medial pain system subserving affective-motivational and cognitive-evaluative pain determinants.[47] Anatomically distinct regions are thought to relate to different functions, some more specifically related to pain, and others to motor, autonomic, and cognitive functions (Fig. 6.5).[108] Whereas cingulotomy for intractable pain yielded only a modest relief from pain, it appeared that the degree to which pain interfered with other cognitive activities, behaviors, and social functions was significantly reduced.[109] Also cingulate lesions in animals revealed minimal deficits in discriminative pain function but robust changes in pain-related behavior and learning.[110,111] A multimodal integrative rather than a specific nociceptive role of the ACC is also underlined by its large receptive fields and the absence of somatotopy.[108] MEG activity following laser radiant heat pain demonstrates a preferential response of the ACC to C-fiber input, regarded as important for the sustained "suffering" component of pain associated with C- rather than Aδ-fiber activity.[112] Together with SII and insula, ACC is the most consistent region activated by pain.[90,94,103] However, imaging of subjects engaged in a variety of cognitive, affective, and motor tasks also revealed ACC as the most consistent brain area.[113] The MCC is involved in response selection, fear avoidance, and motor function. Despite the diversity of perceptual, emotional, cognitive, motor, and autonomic processes harbored within distinct or overlapping cingulate cortex structures as revealed from numerous functional imaging studies, a common

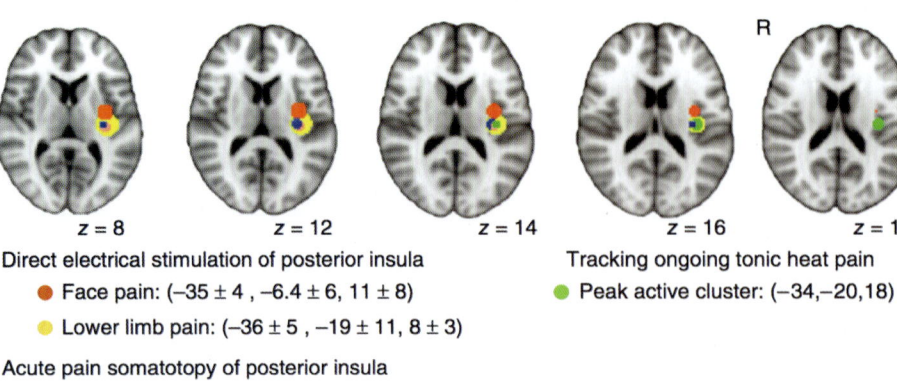

z = 8   z = 12   z = 14   z = 16   z = 18

Direct electrical stimulation of posterior insula

● Face pain: (-35 ± 4 , -6.4 ± 6, 11 ± 8)

● Lower limb pain: (-36 ± 5 , -19 ± 11, 8 ± 3)

Tracking ongoing tonic heat pain

● Peak active cluster: ($-34, -20, 18$)

Acute pain somatotopy of posterior insula

● Thermal stimulus applied to foot: (-35 ± 4 , -20.8 ± 6, 11 ± 5)

● Laser stimulus applied to foot: (-32 ± 2 , -20 ± 1.8, 12 ± 2.4)

FIGURE 6.4   Involvement of the insula in human pain studies. Activation clusters in *purple* and *blue* represent activation clusters triggered by acute painful stimulation of subjects' feet using heat or a laser. The activation clusters in *red* and *yellow* represent surgical coordinates at which direct electrical stimulation resulted in the perception of pain at a particular body site (red = face pain, yellow = lower limb pain). The activation clusters in *green* were derived by a newly developed stimulation procedure to identify true nociceptive input using contact heat stimulation with topical capsaicin treatment. Radiologic convention is used. L, left; R, right. *(Reprinted by permission from Nature: Segerdahl AR, Mezue M, Okell TW, et al. The dorsal posterior insula subserves a fundamental role in human pain. Nat Neurosci 2015;18[4]:499–500. Copyright © 2015 Springer Nature.)*

function to which all these processes converge may be seen in the awareness and monitoring of bodily threat or behavioral conflict demanding for executive control. Such view would explain why both the detrimental effects of pain on cognition as well as the beneficial effects of cognitive distraction on pain are represented in the ACC.[114,115] Thus, the reciprocity of pain and cognitive processes at the level of the ACC might significantly determine the degree by which pain interrupts cognitive performance and is intrinsically difficult to ignore.[116]

Prefrontal Cortex

The prefrontal cortex (PFC) is the anterior part of the frontal lobe and contains numerous neurons and a large volume (30%

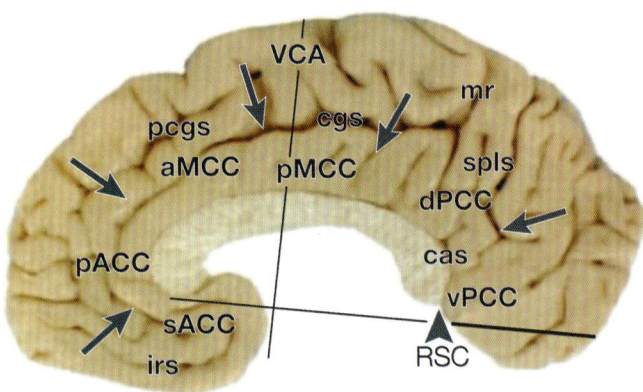

FIGURE 6.5   Region borders of the cingulate cortex according to Vogt. Subregions are marked with *arrows* and were determined based on postmortem cases that were coregistered to a stereotaxic atlas with the vertical plane at the anterior commissure (VCA) and the anteroposterior commissural line. A functional overview, derived from the analysis of a large volume of literature, is provided. This illustrates general regional function and, where known, subregional specializations. aMCC, anterior midcingulate cortex; cas, callosal sulcus; cgs, cingulate sulcus; dPCC, dorsal posterior cingulate cortex; irs, inferior rostral sulcus; mr, marginal ramus of cingulate sulcus; pACC, pregenual anterior cingulate cortex; pcgs, paracingulate sulcus; pMCC, posterior midcingulate cortex; RSC, retrosplenial cortex; sACC, subgenual anterior cingulate cortex; spls, splenial sulci; vPCC, ventral posterior cingulate cortex. *(Modified by permission from Nature: Vogt BA. Pain and emotion interactions in subregions of the cingulate gyrus. Nat Rev Neurosci 2005;6[7]:533–544. Copyright © 2005 Springer Nature.)*

of brain mass) and is farthest developed in humans compared to nonhuman species.[117] It can be divided into different subdivisions[113]: the mid-dorsal (area 9), dorsolateral (BA 46), ventrolateral, orbitofrontal, and medial frontal parts (BA 10, 11, 13, 14). All these frontal areas receive convergent input from different sensory modalities and again project to different associative sensory areas, motor areas, and limbic structures. The PFC is considered to be important for higher cortical functions that characterize the flexibility of human behavior, the ability to control attention, and the richness of intellectual and emotional competence. With respect to pain, PFC plays a major role in cognitive, attentional, and emotional processing of painful stimuli and recruitment of endogenous pain control. A particular part of the PFC, the dorsolateral prefrontal cortex (DLPFC), is important for continuous monitoring of the external world, maintenance of information in short-term memory, and governing efficient performance control in the presence of distracting or conflicting stimuli.[118,119] In turn, orbital and medial portions of the PFC are known to be important for mood and emotional behavior, for example, when guided by cues of reward or punishment as well as for visceral and autonomic homeostasis related to eating and drinking behavior.[120] The famous case of Phineas Gage demonstrated that lesions of the PFC can strongly interfere with the maintenance of an individual's personality, socially appropriate behavior, and learning capabilities.[121,122] There is evidence of elevated pain thresholds in patients with frontal lobe lesions.[123]

The PFC is activated in several, yet not all, functional imaging studies using experimental painful stimuli or clinical pain states. Older studies using blood flow–related analysis failed to show a clear pain-related stimulus–response function,[74,124] which led to the assumption that PFC activity mainly relates to the engagement of attention during pain processing.[93] On the other side, prefrontal gamma oscillations have shown to encode ongoing tonic pain,[125] which differed from the encoding of brief experimental pain. Further evidence indicates that the PFC, irrespective of pain intensity, integrates information about the psychological and bodily context of pain in order to allow disengagement from pain through activating endogenous pain control. Lorenz et al.[105,126] confirmed strong responses of dorsolateral PFC and orbitofrontal and medial PFC (OMPFC) during inflammatory pain (Fig. 6.6). They used O[15]-water injections in healthy volunteers to compare cerebral blood flow responses by PET following contact heat stimuli applied on

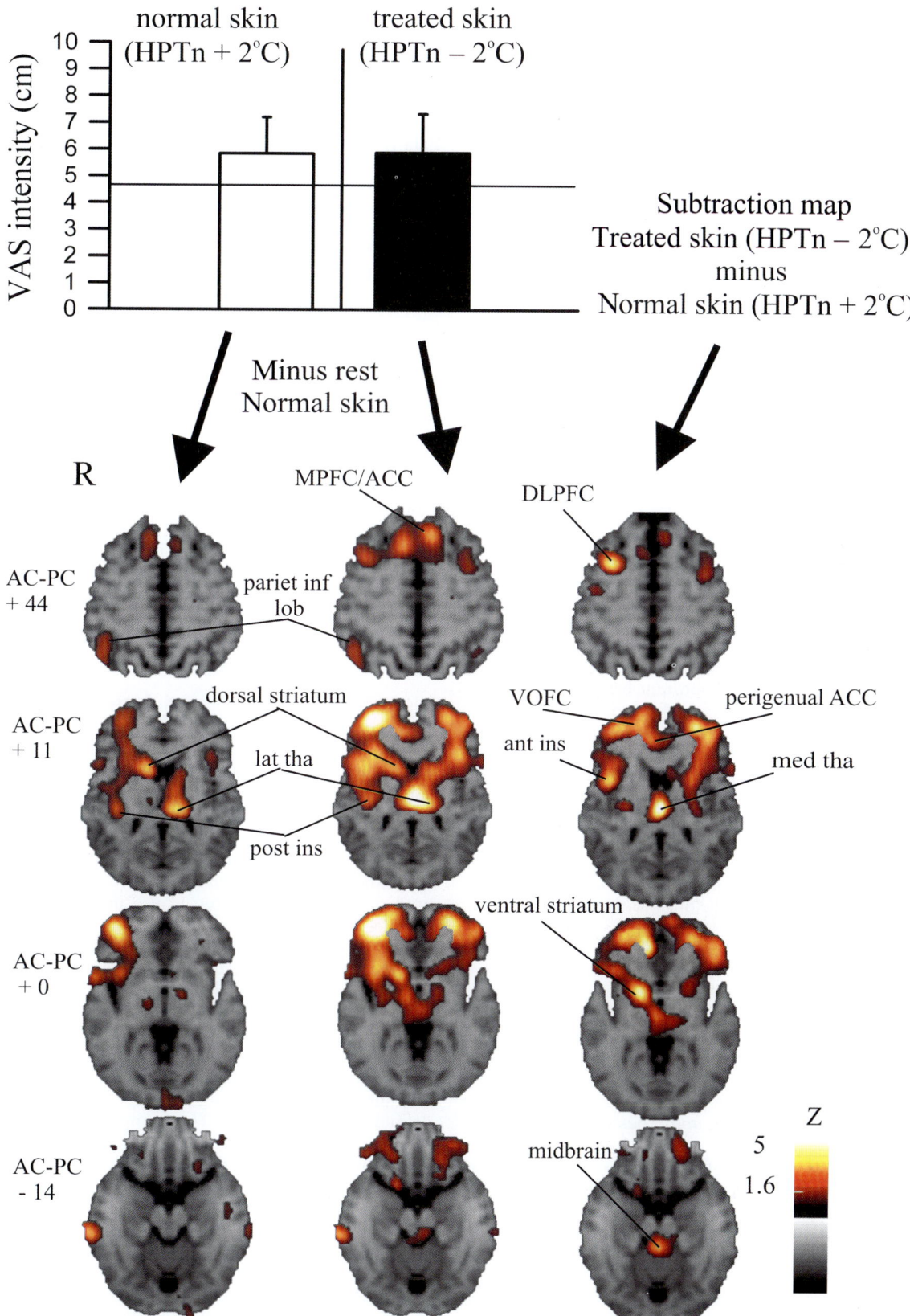

FIGURE 6.6 Regional brain activity during equally intense pains across normal and capsaicin-treated skin conditions. **Top:** Stimulation of the normal skin with the high-intensity stimulus yields the same pain intensity as stimulation with the low-intensity stimulus on capsaicin-treated skin. However, the O[15]-water positron emission tomography (PET) images during heat pain **(left)** and equally intense heat allodynia **(middle)** are different when compared against normal rest condition. Similar magnitudes of activity in the dorsal striatum, lateral thalamus (lat tha), and posterior insula (post ins) are removed in the image subtraction of heat allodynia minus heat pain **(right)** contrasting activity in the ventral striatum, medial thalamus (med tha), anterior insula (ant ins), midbrain, dorsolateral prefrontal cortex (DLPFC), medial prefrontal cortex (MPFC) and ventral/orbitofrontal cortex (VOFC), and perigenual anterior cingulate cortex (ACC) during heat allodynia. *(Reproduced from Lorenz J, Minoshima S, Casey KL. Keeping pain out of mind: the role of the dorsolateral prefrontal cortex in pain modulation. Brain 2003;126:1079–1091. Reproduced by permission of Guarantors of Brain.)*

normal skin with those following warm stimuli but equally painful on capsaicin-treated skins of the volar forearm. They found strong activation of the bilateral DLPFC and OMPFC during capsaicin-induced heat allodynia. Whereas DLPFC exhibited a negative, OMPFC yielded a positive relationship to the unpleasantness of perceived pain. Furthermore, the interregional correlation of activity between midbrain and medial thalamus was significantly reduced during high, compared to low, left DLPFC activity which could indicate a top–down mode of inhibition of effective synaptic connectivity between brainstem and medial thalamus as cause for the inverse relationship of DLPFC activity to pain unpleasantness. A role of the DLPFC in the initiation of endogenous pain control is further supported by its participation in placebo analgesia. Wager et al.[127] demonstrated that DLPFC responds to cues that inform test participants about an expected analgesic effect in a placebo experiment. The analgesic effect itself, however, goes along with stronger rostral ACC activation[127,128] being stronger coupled with the brainstem PAG.[30]

Other clinical studies lend further support for the association of the DLPFC with pain suppression. Apkarian et al.[129] observed a reduction of the gray matter density determined by morphometry of magnetic resonance scans in bilateral DLPFC and right thalamus in chronic back pain patients that was strongly related to pain characteristics. In agreement with the suggested role of DLPFC in pain control high-frequency transcranial magnetic stimulation (rTMS) over left DLPFC was able to ameliorate chronic migraine.[130] This is consistent with earlier studies in animals where electrical stimulation of fiber connections of the PFC to the midbrain mediates antinociceptive effects in rodents.[131] In summary, collective evidence suggests that the PFC represents an important brain substrate for the human ability to actively disengage from pain. Seminowicz and Moayedi[132] recently reviewed the neuroimaging literature regarding the role of the DLPFC as a therapeutic target for chronic pain conditions. Evidence indicates functional and structural abnormalities of the DLPFC and their reversal after successful interventions for chronic pain.

Amygdala

The amygdala is an almond-shaped structure deep in the midtemporal lobe (see Fig. 6.1) and belongs to the limbic system. The amygdala complex comprises about 13 nuclei, which are further divided into subregions.[133] These nuclei can also be grouped by functional properties in frontotemporal, autonomic, main, and accessory olfactory systems.[134] Tracer studies revealed that the amygdala gets multiple inputs from different cortical and subcortical structures and all sensory modalities. Cortical somatosensory and pain input arises directly from SI, SII, and the insula,[135] whereas subcortical pain signals arise among others from the thalamus and the brainstem parabrachial nucleus. In addition, numerous projections from the amygdala go back to the brainstem, the hippocampus, and cortical areas such as the PFC, whereas output connections to sensory areas are rare.[133] Numerous, but not all, imaging studies have revealed amygdala activation during pain perception. Furthermore, the amygdala is involved in the pathophysiology of migraine-related pain.[136] There is no steady increase of activity in the amygdala with stimulus intensity but rather a stepwise increase once stimulus intensity transits into pain.[74] This finding may point to learning following painful stimuli or to processing the emotional valence of pain stimuli. Amygdala activation during pain might also reflect activation of a "defensive behavioral system," which controls transmission of nociceptive experience to the brain through descending modulatory circuits.[137] Furthermore, the central nucleus of the amygdala is involved in emotional-affective behaviors and the modulation of defense behavior.[138] There are projections of the amygdala

to the PAG that might initiate antinociceptive function during emotional stress or pain expectation.[139–141] Lesions in the amygdala, also known as Klüver-Bucy syndrome, lead to flattened emotional reactivity and loss of fear conditioning but, similar to ACC lesions, do not impair pain discrimination but change the behavioral response to pain. It is conceivable that the amygdala is important for the memory storage of past pain experiences and their context in terms of the processes underlying fear conditioning to facilitate defensive autonomic reactions and behavior.

Hippocampus

The hippocampus forms, relative to the amygdala, the caudal extension of the deep medial temporal lobe. It can be subdivided into the dentate gyrus and the cornu ammonis (CA1 and CA2). Its major input comes from the entorhinal cortex, a network including the DLPFC and parietal association cortex. Reports of Patient H.M.[142,143] highlight the role of the hippocampus in learning and explicit memory. Moreover, the importance for the involvement in pain processing and learning pain related behavior is evident because associations between pain and predictive cues have fundamental adaptive value.[144] Furthermore, learning adverse effects can play an important role in chronic pain and chronic pain–related avoidance behavior. Functional imaging revealed hippocampus activity during mild and moderate heat pain,[137,145] in a pain-learning paradigm when pain was not expected and when pain stimuli were manipulated as to induce anxiety.[144] Together with the assumed role of the amygdala in pain, these findings show that medial temporal lobe structures participate in elaborating the experience of pain based on emotional state, expectation, and past experience.[82]

Vigilance, Arousal, and Attention in Pain Processing

Attention is not a single neurophysiologic entity. Among many authors, Parasuraman et al.[146] describe different major components of attention that rely on a finite set of brain processes being hierarchically organized and interacting with each other. A basic component serves the maintenance of behavioral goals over time and is largely synonymous to *arousal, vigilance, alertness,* or *sustained attention.* It also involves the regulation of the sleep–wakefulness cycle. Cholinergic and noradrenergic ascending systems originating in the RF (see the earlier text) and the locus coeruleus and dopaminergic projections into the striatum are regarded as important for this function referred to as "the vigilance network" by Posner and Petersen.[147] Another component concerns the bias or filtering of task-relevant against irrelevant information. It serves to cope with capacity limits of central information processing which cannot deal with the huge amount of input from a large variety of sensors in different modalities at the same time. This component is often referred to as *selective or focused attention* and, according to Posner and Pertersen,[147] depends on the posterior attention network that includes brain structures such as the superior colliculus, thalamic pulvinar, and the posterior parietal cortex. Selective attention is often metaphorically described by a "spotlight" or "cocktail party" effect, which emphasizes the phenomenon that the focus of awareness can momentarily fluctuate between sensory objects, features, or locations sometimes without overt orientation in the form of eye or head movements. It is believed that the gating of the afferent flow of information within attentional channels (i.e., the set of stimuli benefiting from selective attention) optimizes functional efficiency even at very early stages of modality-specific cortical processes. Closely linked to this function is a supervisory component of attention that temporarily intervenes into ongoing performance when called for by new relevant, unfamiliar, or potentially dangerous information, the detection of performance errors, or when internal representations need to be continuously updated, that is, during working memory operations. This component is often referred to as *executive attention*, largely governed by the anterior attention network *sensu*[147] that comprises the anterior cingulate, medial, and lateral PFC areas and the supplementary motor area.

Long-duration mental tasks yield a characteristic vigilance decrement that can be measured subjectively or by behavioral indicators such as reaction time.[146] Similarly, amplitudes of pain-related, evoked potentials after electrical stimuli, painful chemical stimulation of the nasal mucosa, and laser stimulation are strongly attenuated by habituation and decreases of vigilance over time.[148] Although pain generally enhances arousal, the laser-evoked potential (LEP) test situation is characterized by short durations of single laser stimuli, presented at long interstimulus intervals in quite monotonous long stimulus blocks, which contribute to the vigilance decrement in LEP amplitudes. Experimental pain studies therefore use study designs to avoid or control for habituation. Pain habituation can be observed not only during short-term pain experience but also during longer lasting pain after several days. fMRI experiments on the mechanisms of habituation revealed decreases of activation in major pain areas including the thalamus, insula, SII, and the putamen. Notably, an increase of activation was observed in the ACC.[149] One possible mechanism could be the involvement of the endogenous opioidergic pain control system (see earlier text). In an animal model of habituation, naloxone sufficiently prevents habituation to repeated electrical pain stimuli.[150] There are important interindividual differences regarding the strength of habituation that are not well understood. However, it is described that especially chronic pain patients show an impairment of habituation.[151–154]

Beydoun et al.[155] examined subjects who they allowed to fall asleep after 1 day of sleep deprivation to look for LEP during different sleep stages compared to normal wakefulness. They demonstrated the abolition of the N2 to P2 component at the vertex position during sleep stage II, defined by the appearance of sleep spindles, and its strong amplitude attenuation during sleep stage I, defined by dropout of α activity and appearance of lateral eye movements. It appears evident that there is a reciprocal relationship between sleep and pain allowing not only sleep to reduce pain but also pain to reduce or disturb sleep.[156] Furthermore, decreases of pain sensitivity also accompany sedation and drowsiness when induced pharmacologically using benzodiazepines,[157] clonidine,[158] or subanesthetic isoflurane.[159] It is therefore often difficult to differentiate drowsiness or sedation from analgesia.

Given the profound role of attention in conscious perception, it is clear that attention significantly impacts on behavior and pain experience.[116] Pain is a salient stimulus and draws attention for extended periods.[105] The manipulation of attention by distraction or focused attention has been used as a therapeutic intervention for several years[160,161] and reflects everyday life experience such as when a mother tries to distract her child when it is injured. Clinical evidence suggests that attentional mechanisms may be also involved in the amplification of some chronic clinical pain stages.[162] Patients with chronic pain problems seem to selectively attend to pain and the degree by which pain distracts attention from concurrent tasks appears to depend on the evaluation of pain stimuli as threatening or worrying.[116] In tasks where attentional shifts are required, anxious patients exhibit difficulties disengaging from painful stimuli.[163]

The neural mechanisms underlying attentional modulation of pain are not fully understood, but various areas of the pain matrix appear to be involved.[164] More recent studies using EEG and MEG have focused on cortical synchronization processes as indicators of attentional modulation of sensory input. Mainly derived from experiments with nonpainful stimuli, it is

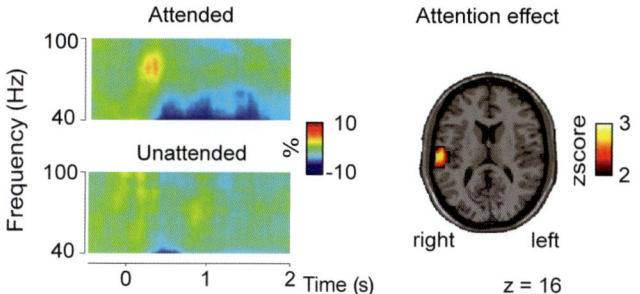

FIGURE 6.7 Pain modulation by attention. Attention to pain (Attended) was induced by evaluating the pain intensity at the attended finger while ignoring laser stimuli delivered to the other finger (Unattended). Electrophysiologic signals were recorded using electroencephalography (EEG). After time–frequency transformation, neuronal oscillations around 80 Hz (γ band) and with latencies around 270 ms indicated a difference for attention. This attention effect was localized in the contralateral SII/insula areas. *(From Hauck M, Domnick C, Lorenz J, et al. Top-down and bottom-up modulation of pain-induced oscillations.* Front Hum Neurosci *2015;9:375. doi: 10.3389/fnhum.2015.00375. Copyright © 2015 Hauck, Domnick, Lorenz, Gerloff, and Engel.)*

proposed that selective attention may act by modulating subthreshold oscillations in sensory assemblies and by enhancing the gain of oscillatory responses to stimuli that match stored contextual information.[165,166] A recent study indicates that during selective attention, enhanced oscillatory activity in the γ bandwidth of EEG (60 Hz rhythms), which was localized in the insula, which suggests a key role of γ-band oscillations in the integration of nociceptive input into the multidimensional experience of pain (Fig. 6.7)[167] One possible neuronal correlate of abnormal attentional amplification may therefore be suspected in an "oversynchronization" among pain-related cortical areas, leading to an uncontrolled spread of signals even in the case of weak or absent nociceptive inputs. Thus, the dynamic control of neuronal signal flow might be disturbed, preventing an appropriate context-dependent modulation of the gain of neural signals and reducing the capacity for descending control of nociceptive afferent inputs. As assumed for states of chronic pain, such an oversynchronization might be viewed as the result of central neuroplastic changes underlying a learning process.[168]

Pain Plasticity

The brain is an adaptive system, which has a high plasticity such that it can change excitability of its networks according to a variety of external and internal processes. The uniqueness of pain compared with other human senses is characterized by its enormous plasticity to adapt according to both the bodily and the psychological context in which pain occurs. Studies on acute pain models in animals and humans had long made clear that clinically important pains exhibit distinct neurophysiologic and pharmacologic properties due to alteration of impulse generation at the site of an injury and propagation into and through the CNS. Once tissue damage and inflammation occur, the production and release of chemical mediators excite and sensitize nociceptors rendering their axons much more responsive and giving rise to tenderness and hyperalgesia as well as spontaneous pain. Hyperexcitability also occurs at the level of the dorsal horn in the spinal cord following tissue damage and inflammation, further aggravating sensitization and even rendering innocuous tactile stimuli outside the lesion capable of producing pain through an increase of synaptic efficacy of local interneurons, a phenomenon called *allodynia*. Thus, the bodily context of normal versus damaged tissue dramatically determines the perception of pain.

Several pain states such as chronic pain or phantom pain can induce central cortical changes in the pain matrix. Patients suffering from cancer with intractable unilateral pain developed a decrease in metabolism within the contralateral thalamus, which was abolished after blocking nociceptive input by surgical hemicordotomy.[169] A smaller representation of the affected hand was found in somatosensory areas (SI and SII) for nonpainful stimulation that correlated with symptom severity in patients suffering from complex regional pain syndrome (CRPS),[170] whereas representation for nociceptive input is extended in somatosensory areas in these patients.[171] Similarly, other chronic pain states yielded exaggerated activation and occupied larger areas in somatosensory cortex as demonstrated for low back pain,[172] fibromyalgia,[173] and neuropathic pain.[174] Anatomic changes in gray matter density can be observed for chronic pain patients as well. Using MRI scans with voxel-based morphometry analysis, changes in white and gray matter can be compared between groups and within subject during different time points. Changes in different cortical areas were found for different pain syndromes. In chronic back pain patients,[129] atrophy in the thalamus and the PFC were observed (Fig. 6.8). Others describe atrophy in the hippocampus, the MCC, the frontal cortex, and the insula in fibromyalgia.[175] Similar findings have been observed in chronic headache.[176] Interestingly, these gray matter density changes occur in pain-related regions such as the PFC, thalamus (Fig. 6.8), the insula, and the cingulate cortex. However, it is still under debate if the brain atrophy is the reason or a consequence of ongoing pain. Another possible explanation for the decreased gray matter density in these disorders might be atrophy secondary to excitotoxicity and/or exposure to inflammation-related agents, such as cytokines.[129]

Summary and Conclusion

Noninvasive functional neuroimaging and invasive recordings of pain in human volunteers and patients has attracted an enormous interest and activity in pain research and significantly enriched our knowledge about the contribution of the brain in processing and modifying peripheral and spinal nociceptive signals. Supraspinal mechanisms of nociception and pain rely on a multilevel organization of brain structures involving the brainstem (medulla, pons, midbrain), diencephalon (thalamus, hypothalamus), primary (SI) and secondary (SII) somatosensory cortices, and frontolimbic circuits (PFC, ACC, insula, amygdala, hippocampus). Spinal nociceptive afferents that reach predominantly lateral thalamic nuclei convey nociceptive signals into the sensory cortex (SI, SII) and provide the individual with the capability to recognize intensity, location, and duration of noxious stimuli. This lateral pain system is therefore commonly referred to as the major brain anatomic substrate of the sensory-discriminative determinant of pain. Direct and multisynaptic projections from the dorsal horn and brainstem into medial thalamic nuclei transmit nociceptive signals into the limbic system (insula, ACC, PFC). This medial pain system predominantly comprises the affective-motivational determinant of pain. A pivotal role of the DLPFC in pain is its ability to coordinate nociceptive signals with momentary bodily needs and behavioral goals to account for the significance and threat value of pain. The multimodal connectivity of the DLPFC with sensory and motor systems allows the individual not only to maintain attention on pain but also to release it in favor of superior behavioral goals or in expectation of positive outcome through recruitment of endogenous pain control systems. A predominant feature of pain in comparison with other human senses is its enormous ability to adapt its response properties according to both the bodily and psychologic context. This plasticity implies fundamental changes in the course of pathologic processes underlying tissue damage and inflammation or in the course of memory processes and learning from past pain experiences. Supraspinal mechanisms thus contribute to such plasticity by integrating information about the nature and behavioral significance of pain by recruiting unique pathways during normal or sensitized conditions and by facilitating learned pain behaviors. Although in most instances such plasticity is adaptive to avoid actual bodily damage or promote the healing process, it also forms the basis for maladaptive consequences underlying chronic pain and neuropathic pain.

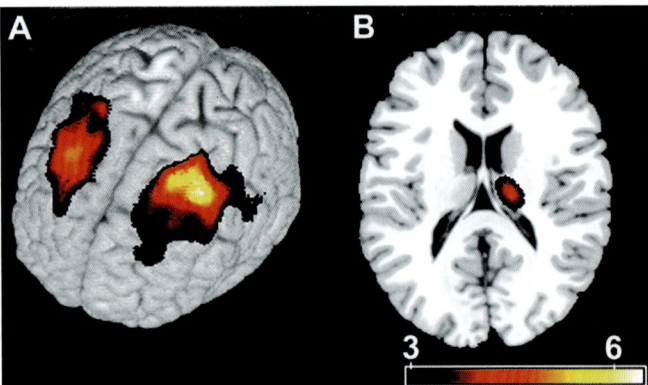

FIGURE 6.8 Regional gray matter density decreases in patients suffering from chronic back pain (CBP). A nonparametric comparison of voxel-based morphometry (VBM) between CBP and control subjects is shown. **A:** Gray matter density is bilaterally reduced in the dorsolateral prefrontal cortex (DLPFC). The result is from a VBM permutation-based pseudo–T-test and voxel-level contrasts when all brain gray matter voxels were compared between controls and CBP subjects. Pseudocolor highly positive values indicate regions where gray matter density was reduced in CBP subjects (controls, CBP). **B:** A nonparametric comparison spatially limited to the thalami revealed a significant decrease in gray matter density in the right anterior thalamus. A slice at the peak of decreased thalamic gray matter is shown. Pseudo–T-values are color-coded; range is 3 to 6. (Republished with permission of Society for Neuroscience from *Apkarian AV, Sosa Y, Sonty S, et al. Chronic back pain is associated with decreased prefrontal and thalamic gray matter density. J Neurosci 2004;24[46]:10410–10415;* permission conveyed through Copyright Clearance Center, Inc.)

References

1. Baliki MN, Apkarian AV. Nociception, pain, negative moods, and behavior selection. *Neuron* 2015;87(3):474–491. doi:10.1016/j.neuron.2015 .06.005.
2. Swanson LW. Mapping the human brain: past, present, and future. *Trends Neurosci* 1995;18(11):471–474.
3. Casey KL. Forebrain mechanisms of nociception and pain: analysis through imaging. *Proc Natl Acad Sci* 1999;96:7668–7674.
4. Gusnard DA, Raichle ME. Searching for a baseline: functional imaging and the resting human brain. *Nat Rev Neurosci* 2001;2(10):685–694.
5. Obrig H, Villringer A. Beyond the visible—imaging the human brain with light. *J Cereb Blood Flow Metab* 2003;23(1):1–18.
6. Kovac S, Vakharia VN, Scott C, et al. Invasive epilepsy surgery evaluation. *Seizure* 2017;44:125–136. doi:10.1016/j.seizure.2016.10.016.
7. Coenen AM. Neuronal phenomena associated with vigilance and consciousness: from cellular mechanisms to electroencephalographic patterns. *Conscious Cogn* 1998;7(1):42–53.
8. Bowsher D. Role of the reticular formation in responses to noxious stimulation. *Pain* 1976;2(4):361–378.
9. Casey KL, Morrow TJ. Effect of medial bulboreticular and raphe nuclear lesions on the excitation and modulation of supraspinal nocifensive behaviors in the cat. *Brain Res* 1989;501(1):150–161.
10. Casey KL. Somatosensory responses of bulboreticular units in awake cat: relation to escape-producing stimuli. *Science* 1971;173(991):77–80.
11. Wei F, Dubner R, Ren K. Nucleus reticularis gigantocellularis and nucleus raphe magnus in the brain stem exert opposite effects on behavioral hyperalgesia and spinal Fos protein expression after peripheral inflammation. *Pain* 1999;80:127–41.
12. Moruzzi G, Magoun HW. Brain stem reticular formation and activation of the EEG. *Electroencephalogr Clin Neurophysiol* 1949;1(4):455–473.
13. Horn AK, Adamczyk C. Reticular formation: eye movements, gaze and blinks. In: Mai JK, Paxinos G, eds. *The Human Nervous System*. 3rd ed. London: Academic Press; 2012:328–366.

14. Villanueva L, Bouhassira D, Le Bars D. The medullary subnucleus reticularis dorsalis (SRD) as a key link in both the transmission and modulation of pain signals. *Pain* 1996;67:231–240.

15. Villanueva L, Le Bars D. The activation of bulbo-spinal controls by peripheral nociceptive inputs: diffuse noxious inhibitory controls. *Biol Res* 1995;28(1):113–125.

16. Youssef AM, Macefield VG, Henderson LA. Pain inhibits pain; human brainstem mechanisms. *Neuroimage* 2016;124(pt A):54–62. doi:10.1016/j.neuroimage.2015.08.060.

17. Carrive P, Morgan MM. Periaqueductal gray. In: Mai JK, Paxinos G, eds. *The Human Nervous System*. 3rd ed. London: Academic Press; 2012:367–400.

18. Merker B. Consciousness without a cerebral cortex: a challenge for neuroscience and medicine. *Behav Brain Sci* 2007;30(1):63–81.

19. Morgan MM, Carrive P. Activation of the ventrolateral periaqueductal gray reduces locomotion but not mean arterial pressure in awake, freely moving rats. *Neuroscience* 2001;102(4):905–910.

20. Reynolds DV. Surgery in the rat during electrical analgesia induced by focal brain stimulation. *Science* 1969;164(878):444–445.

21. Mayer DJ, Wolfle TL, Akil H, et al. Analgesia from electrical stimulation in the brainstem of the rat. *Science* 1971;174(16):1351–1354.

22. Oliveras JL, Redjemi F, Guilbaud G, et al. Analgesia induced by electrical stimulation of the inferior centralis nucleus of the raphe in the cat. *Pain* 1975;1(2):139–145.

23. Basbaum AI, Fields HL. Endogenous pain control mechanisms: review and hypothesis. *Ann Neurol* 1978;4(5):451–462.

24. Fields HL, Vanegas H, Hentall ID, et al. Evidence that disinhibition of brain stem neurones contributes to morphine analgesia. *Nature* 1983;306(5944):684–686.

25. Potrebic SB, Fields HL, Mason P. Serotonin immunoreactivity is contained in one physiological cell class in the rat rostral ventromedial medulla. *J Neurosci* 1994;14:1655–1665.

26. Lima D, Albino-Teixeira A, Tavares I. The caudal medullary ventrolateral reticular formation in nociceptive-cardiovascular integration. An experimental study in the rat. *Exp Physiol* 2002;87(2):267–274.

27. Pertovaara A. The noradrenergic pain regulation system: a potential target for pain therapy. *Eur J Pharmacol* 2013;716(1–3):2–7. doi:10.1016/j.ejphar.2013.01.067.

28. Taylor BK, Westlund KN. The noradrenergic locus coeruleus as a chronic pain generator. *J Neurosci Res* 2017;95(6):1336–1346. doi:10.1002/jnr.23956.

29. Ren K, Ruda MA. Descending modulation of Fos expression after persistent peripheral inflammation. *Neuroreport* 1996;7(13):2186–2190.

30. Bingel U, Lorenz J, Schoell E, et al. Mechanisms of placebo analgesia: rACC recruitment of a subcortical antinociceptive network. *Pain* 2006;120(1–2):8–15.

31. Eippert F, Finsterbusch J, Bingel U, et al. Direct evidence for spinal cord involvement in placebo analgesia. *Science* 2009;326(5951):404. doi:10.1126/science.1180142.

32. Keay KA, Bandler R. Deep and superficial noxious stimulation increases Fos-like immunoreactivity in different regions of the midbrain periaqueductal grey of the rat. *Neurosci Lett* 1993;154(12):23–26.

33. Lumb BM. Inescapable and escapable pain is represented in distinct hypothalamic-midbrain circuits: specific roles for Adelta- and C-nociceptors. *Exp Physiol* 2002;87(2):281–286.

34. Lumb BM. Hypothalamic and midbrain circuitry that distinguishes between escapable and inescapable pain. *News Physiol Sci* 2004;19:22–26.

35. Hosobuchi Y, Adams JE, Linchitz R. Pain relief by electrical stimulation of the central gray matter in humans and its reversal by naloxone. *Science* 1977;197(4299):183–186.

36. Richardson DE, Akil H. Long term results of periventricular gray self-stimulation. *Neurosurgery* 1977;1(2):199–202.

37. Hollingworth M, Sims-Williams HP, Pickering AE, et al. Single electrode deep brain stimulation with dual targeting at dual frequency for the treatment of chronic pain: a case series and review of the literature. *Brain Sci* 2017;7(1):E9. doi:10.3390/brainsci7010009.

38. Bandler R, Shipley MT. Columnar organization in the midbrain periaqueductal gray: modules for emotional expression? *Trends Neurosci* 1994;17(9):379–389.

39. Taylor AM, Becker S, Schweinhardt P, et al. Mesolimbic dopamine signaling in acute and chronic pain: implications for motivation, analgesia, and addiction. *Pain* 2016;157(6):1194–1198. doi:10.1097/j.pain.0000000000000494.

40. Navratilova E, Porreca F. Reward and motivation in pain and pain relief. *Nat Neurosci* 2014;17(10):1304–1312. doi:10.1038/nn.3811.

41. Loggia ML, Berna C, Kim J, et al. Disrupted brain circuitry for pain-related reward/punishment in fibromyalgia. *Arthritis Rheumatol* 2014;66(1):203–212. doi:10.1002/art.38191.

42. Martikainen IK, Nuechterlein EB, Peciña M, et al. Chronic back pain is associated with alterations in dopamine neurotransmission in the ventral striatum. *J Neurosci* 2015;35(27):9957–9965. doi:10.1523/JNEUROSCI.4605-14.2015.

43. Bernard JF, Bester H, Besson JM. Involvement of the spino-parabrachio-amygdaloid and hypothalamic pathways in the autonomic and affective emotional aspects of pain. In: Holstege G, Bandler R, Saper CB, eds. *The Emotional Motor System*. Amsterdam, The Netherlands: Elsevier; 1996:243–255.

44. Burstein R, Falkowsky O, Borsook D, et al. Distinct lateral and medial projections of the spinohypothalamic tract of the rat. *J Comp Neurol* 1996;373(4):549–574.

45. Razavi BM, Hosseinzadeh H. A review of the role of orexin system in pain modulation. *Biomed Pharmacother* 2017;90:187–193. doi:10.1016/j.biopha.2017.03.053.

46. Roohbakhsh A, Alavi MS, Zarmehri HA. The orexinergic (hypocretin) system and nociception: an update to supraspinal mechanisms [published online ahead of print May 28, 2017]. *Curr Med Chem*. doi:10.2174/0929867324666170529072554.

47. Tashiro S, Yamaguchi R, Ishikawa S, et al. Odour-induced analgesia mediated by hypothalamic orexin neurons in mice. *Sci Rep* 2016;6:37129. doi:10.1038/srep37129.

48. Melzack R, Casey KL. Sensory, motivational, and central control determinants of pain. In: Kenshalo DR, ed. *The Skin Senses*. Springfield, IL: Charles C. Thomas; 1968:423–443.

49. Willis WD, Coggeshall RE. *Sensory Mechanisms of the Spinal Cord*. New York: Plenum Press; 1991.

50. Pereira EA, Green AL, Aziz TZ. Deep brain stimulation for pain. *Handb Clin Neurol* 2013;116:277–294. doi:10.1016/B978-0-444-53497-2.00023-1.

51. Mehler WR, Feferman ME, Nauta WJ. Ascending axon degeneration following anterolateral cordotomy. An experimental study in the monkey. *Brain* 1960;83:718–750.

52. Willis WD, Kenshalo DR Jr, Leonard RB. The cells of origin of the primate spinothalamic tract. *J Comp Neurol* 1979;188(4):543–573.

53. Apkarian AV, Shi T. Squirrel monkey lateral thalamus. I. Somatic nociresponsive neurons and their relation to spinothalamic terminals. *J Neurosci* 1994;14(11 pt 2):6779–6795.

54. Bastuji H, Frot M, Mazza S, et al. Thalamic responses to nociceptive-specific Input in humans: functional dichotomies and thalamo-cortical connectivity. *Cerebral Cortex* 2016;26:2663–2676.

55. Craig AD. How do you feel? Interoception: the sense of the physiological condition of the body. *Nat Rev Neurosci* 2002;3:655–666.

56. Brodmann K. Beiträge zur histologischen lokalisation der grosshirnrinde: dritte mitteilung: die rindenfelder der niederen affen. *J Psychologie Neurologie* 1905;4:177–226.

57. Price DD. Psychological and neural mechanisms of the affective dimension of pain. *Science* 2000;288:1769–1772.

58. Papez JW. A proposed mechanism of emotion. *Arch Neurol Psychiat* 1937;38:725–743.

59. Head H, Holmes G. Sensory disturbances from cerebral lesions. *Brain* 1911;34:102–254.

60. Kleist K. Kriegsverletzungen des gehirns in ihrer bedeutung für die hirnlokalisation und hirnpathologie. In: von Schjerning O, ed. *Handbuch der Ärztlichen Erfahrungen im Weltkriege 1914-1918. Geistes- und Nervenkrankheiten*. Vol 4. Leipzig, Germany: Barth; 1934:343–393.

61. Russel WR. Transient disturbances following gunshot wounds of the head. *Brain* 1945;68:79–97.

62. Marshall J. Sensory disturbances of cortical wounds with special reference to pain. *J Neurol Neurosurg Psychiat* 1951;14:187–204.

63. Kenshalo DR Jr, Chudler EH, Anton F, et al. SI nociceptive neurons participate in the encoding process by which monkeys perceive the intensity of noxious thermal stimulation. *Brain Res* 1988;454(1–2):378–382.

64. Ohara S, Crone NE, Weiss N, et al. Amplitudes of laser evoked potential recorded from primary somatosensory, parasylvian and medial frontal cortex are graded with stimulus intensity. *Pain* 2004;110(1–2):318–328.

65. Penfield W, Boldrey E. Somatic motor and sensory representation in the cerebral cortex of man as studied by electrical stimulation *Brain* 1937;60:389–443.

66. Mazzola L, Isnard J, Mauguière F. Somatosensory and pain responses to stimulation of the second somatosensory area (SII) in humans. A comparison with SI and insular responses. *Cereb Cortex* 2006;16(7):960–968.

67. Bingel U, Lorenz J, Glauche V, et al. Somatotopic organization of human somatosensory cortices for pain: a single trial fMRI study. *Neuroimage* 2004;23(1):224–232.

68. Ploner M, Schmitz F, Freund HJ, et al. Parallel activation of primary and secondary somatosensory cortices in human pain processing. *J Neurophysiol* 1999;81(6):3100–3104.

69. Tran TD, Inui K, Hoshiyama M, et al. Cerebral activation by the signals ascending through unmyelinated C-fibers in humans: a magnetoencephalographic study. *Neuroscience* 2002;113(2):375–386.

70. Kanda M, Nagamine T, Ikeda A, et al. Primary somatosensory cortex is actively involved in pain processing in human. *Brain Res* 2000;853(2):282–289.

71. Talbot JD, Marrett S, Evans AC, et al. Multiple representations of pain in human cerebral cortex. *Science* 1991;251(4999):1355–1358.

72. Coghill RC, Talbot JD, Evans AC, et al. Distributed processing of pain and vibration by the human brain. *J Neurosci* 1994;14(7):4095–4108.

73. Casey KL, Minoshima S, Morrow TJ, et al. Comparison of human cerebral activation pattern during cutaneous warmth, heat pain, and deep cold pain. *J Neurophysiol* 1996;76(1):571–581.

74. Bornhövd K, Quante M, Glauche V, et al. Painful stimuli evoke different stimulus-response functions in the amygdala, prefrontal, insula and somatosensory cortex: a single-trial fMRI study. *Brain* 2002;125:1326–1336.

75. Davis KD, Wood ML, Crawley AP, et al. fMRI of human somatosensory and cingulate cortex during painful electrical nerve stimulation. *Neuroreport* 1995;7(1):321–325.

76. Oshiro Y, Fujita N, Tanaka H, et al. Functional mapping of pain-related activation with echo-planar MRI: significance of the SII-insular region. *Neuroreport* 1998;9(10):2285–2289.

77. Rosen SD, Paulesu E, Frith CD, et al. Central nervous pathways mediating angina pectoris. *Lancet* 1994;344(8916):147–150.

78. Weiller C, May A, Limmroth V, et al. Brain stem activation in spontaneous human migraine attacks. *Nat Med* 1995;1(7):658–660.

79. Casey KL, Morrow TJ, Lorenz J, et al. Temporal and spatial dynamics of human forebrain activity during heat pain: analysis by positron emission tomography. *J Neurophysiol* 2001;85(2):951–959.

80. Rainville P, Duncan GH, Price DD, et al. Pain affect encoded in human anterior cingulate but not somatosensory cortex. *Science* 1997;277:968–971.

81. Hofbauer RK, Rainville P, Duncan GH, et al. Cortical representation of the sensory dimension of pain. *J Neurophysiol* 2001;86:402–411.

82. Casey KL. Cortical and limbic mechanisms mediating pain and pain-related behavior. In: Schmidt R, Willis WD, eds. *Encyclopedic Reference to Pain.* Heidelberg, Germany: Springer; 2007:465–477.

83. Moulton EA, Pendse G, Becerra LR, et al. BOLD responses in somatosensory cortices better reflect heat sensation than pain. *J Neurosci* 2012;32(17):6024–6031. doi:10.1523/JNEUROSCI.0006-12.2012.

84. Gross J, Schnitzler A, Timmermann L, et al. Gamma oscillations in human primary somatosensory cortex reflect pain perception. *PLoS Biol* 2007;5(5):e133.

85. Bushnell MC, Duncan GH, Hofbauer RK, et al. Pain perception: is there a role for primary somatosensory cortex? *Proc Natl Acad Sci U S A* 1999; 96(14):7705–7709.

86. Ploner M, Platzen J, Pollok B, et al. Evoked response amplitudes from somatosensory cortices do not determine reaction times to tactile stimuli. *Eur J Neurosci* 2007;25(12):3734–3741.

87. Adrian ED. Double representation of the feet in the sensory cortex of the cat. *J Physiol* 1940;98:16–18.

88. Eickhoff SB, Grefkes C, Zilles K, et al. The somatotopic organization of cytoarchitectonic areas on the human parietal operculum. *Cereb Cortex* 2007;17(8):1800–1811.

89. Hari R, Kaukoranta E. Neuromagnetic studies of somatosensory system: principles and examples. *Prog Neurobiol* 1985;24(3):233–256.

90. Treede RD, Kenshalo DR, Gracely RH, et al. The cortical representation of pain. *Pain* 1999;79(2–3):105–111.

91. Bromm B. Brain images of pain. *News Physiol Sci* 2001;16:244–249.

92. Opsommer E, Weiss T, Plaghki L, et al. Dipole analysis of ultralate (C-fibres) evoked potentials after laser stimulation of tiny cutaneous surface areas in humans. *Neurosci Lett* 2001;298(1):41–44.

93. Peyron R, Frot M, Schneider F, et al. Role of operculoinsular cortices in human pain processing: converging evidence from PET, fMRI, dipole modeling, and intracerebral recordings of evoked potentials. *Neuroimage* 2002;17(3):1336–1346.

94. Tracey I, Mantyh PW. The cerebral signature for pain perception and its modulation. *Neuron* 2007;55(3):377–391.

95. Montavont A, Mauguière F, Mazzola L, et al. On the origin of painful somatosensory seizures. *Neurology* 2015;10;84(6):594–601.

96. Burton H, Fabri M, Alloway K. Cortical areas within the lateral sulcus connected to cutaneous representations in areas 3b and 1: a revised interpretation of the second somatosensory area in macaque monkeys. *J Comp Neurol* 1995;355(4):539–562.

97. Greenspan JD, Lee RR, Lenz FA. Pain sensitivity alterations as a function of lesion location in the parasylvian cortex. *Pain* 1999;81(3):273–282.

98. Schmahmann JD, Leifer D. Parietal pseudothalamic pain syndrome. Clinical features and anatomic correlates. *Arch Neurol* 1992;49(10):1032–1037.

99. Horiuchi T, Unoki T, Yokoh A, et al. Pure sensory stroke caused by cortical infarction associated with the secondary somatosensory area. *J Neurol Neurosurg Psychiatry* 1996;60(5):588–589.

100. Frot M, Magnin M, Mauguière F, et al. Human SII and posterior insula differently encode thermal laser stimuli. *Cereb Cortex* 2007;17(3):610–620.

101. Schnitzler A, Ploner M. Neurophysiology and functional neuroanatomy of pain perception. *J Clin Neurophysiol* 2000;17(6):592–603.

102. Berthier M, Starkstein S, Leiguarda R. Asymbolia for pain: a sensory-limbic disconnection syndrome. *Ann Neurol* 1988;24(1):41–49.

103. Apkarian AV, Bushnell MC, Treede RD, et al. Human brain mechanisms of pain perception and regulation in health and disease. *Eur J Pain* 2005;9(4):463–484.

104. Ploghaus A, Tracey I, Gati JS, et al. Dissociating pain from its anticipation in the human brain. *Science* 1999;284:1979–1981.

105. Lorenz J, Cross DJ, Minoshima S, et al. A unique representation of heat allodynia in the human brain. *Neuron* 2002;35:383–393.

106. Downar J, Mikulis DJ, Davis KD. Neural correlates of the prolonged salience of painful stimulation. *Neuroimage* 2003;20(3):1540–1551.

107. Segerdahl AR, Mezue M, Okell TW, et al. The dorsal posterior insula subserves a fundamental role in human pain. *Nat Neurosci* 2015;18(4):499–500. doi:10.1038/nn.3969.

108. Vogt BA, Laureys S. Posterior cingulate, precuneus and retrosplenial cortices: cytology and components of the neural network correlates of consciousness. *Prog Brain Res* 2005;150:205–217.

109. Cohen RA, Kaplan RF, Moser DJ, et al. Impairments of attention after cingulotomy. *Neurology* 1999;53(4):819–824.

110. Vaccarino AL, Melzack R. Analgesia produced by injection of lidocaine into the anterior cingulum bundle of the rat. *Pain* 1989;39(2):213–219.

111. Gabriel M, Kubota Y, Sparenborg S, et al. Effects of cingulate cortical lesions on avoidance learning and training-induced unit activity in rabbits. *Exp Brain Res* 1991;86(3):585–600.

112. Ploner M, Gross J, Timmermann L, et al. Cortical representation of first and second pain sensation in humans. *Proc Natl Acad Sci U S A* 2002;99(19):12444–12448.

113. Miller EK, Cohen JD. An integrative theory of prefrontal cortex function. *Annu Rev Neurosci* 2001;24:167–202.

114. Bingel U, Rose M, Gläscher J, et al. fMRI reveals how pain modulates visual object processing in the ventral visual stream. *Neuron* 2007;55(1):157–167.

115. Valet M, Sprenger T, Boecker H, et al. Distraction modulates connectivity of the cingulo-frontal cortex and the midbrain during pain—an fMRI analysis. *Pain* 2004;109(3):399–408.

116. Eccleston C, Crombez G. Pain demands attention: a cognitive-affective model of the interruptive function of pain. *Psychol Bull* 1999;125:356–366.

117. Casey KL. The imaging of pain: background and rationale. In: Casey KL, Bushnell MC, eds. *Pain Imaging.* Seattle, WA: IASP Press; 2000:1–29.

118. Bunge SA, Ochsner KN, Desmond JE, et al. Prefrontal regions involved in keeping information in and out of mind. *Brain* 2001;124:2074–2086.

119. Sakai K, Rowe JB, Pasingham RE. Active maintenance in prefrontal area 46 creates distractor-resistant memory. *Nature Neurosci* 2002;5:479–484.

120. Price JL, Carmichael ST, Drevets WC. Networks related to the orbital and medial prefrontal cortex; a substrate for emotional behavior? *Prog Brain Res* 1996;107:523–536.

121. Damasio H, Grabowski T, Frank R, et al. The return of Phineas Gage: clues about the brain from the skull of a famous patient. *Science* 1994;264(5162):1102–1105.

122. Goodenough OR, Prehn K. A neuroscientific approach to normative judgment in law and justice. *Philos Trans R Soc Lond B Biol Sci* 2004;359(1451):1709–1726.

123. Daum I, Braun C, Riesch G, et al. Pain-related cerebral potentials in patients with frontal or parietal lobe lesions. *Neurosci Lett* 1995;197(2):137–140.

124. Coghill RC, Sang CN, Maisog JM, et al. Pain intensity processing within the human brain: a bilateral, distributed mechanism. *J Neurophysiol* 1999;82:1934–1943.

125. Schulz E, May ES, Postorino M, et al. Prefrontal gamma oscillations encode tonic pain in humans. *Cereb Cortex* 2015;25(11):4407–4414. doi:10.1093/cercor/bhv043.

126. Lorenz J, Minoshima S, Casey KL. Keeping pain out of mind: the role of the dorsolateral prefrontal cortex in pain modulation. *Brain* 2003;126(pt 5):1079–1091.

127. Wager TD, Rilling JK, Smith EE, et al. Placebo-induced changes in FMRI in the anticipation and experience of pain. *Science* 2004;303(5661):1162–1167.

128. Petrovic P, Kalso E, Petersson KM, et al. Placebo and opioid analgesia—imaging a shared neuronal network. *Science* 2002;295:1737–1740.

129. Apkarian AV, Sosa Y, Sonty S, et al. Chronic back pain is associated with decreased prefrontal and thalamic gray matter density. *J Neurosci* 2004;24(46):10410–10415.

130. Brighina F, Piazza A, Vitello G, et al. rTMS of the prefrontal cortex in the treatment of chronic migraine: a pilot study. *J Neurol Sci* 2004;227(1):67–71.

131. Hardy SG, Haigler HJ. Prefrontal influences upon the midbrain: a possible route for pain modulation. *Brain Res* 1985;339(2):285–293.

132. Seminowicz DA, Moayedi M. The dorsolateral prefrontal cortex in acute and chronic pain. *J Pain* 2017;18:1027–1035.

133. Sah P, Faber ES, Lopez De Armentia M, et al. The amygdaloid complex: anatomy and physiology. *Physiol Rev* 2003;83(3):803–834.

134. Swanson LW, Petrovich GD. What is the amygdala? *Trends Neurosci* 1998;21(8):323–331.

135. Shi CJ, Cassell MD. Cascade projections from somatosensory cortex to the rat basolateral amygdala via the parietal insular cortex. *J Comp Neurol* 1998;399(4):469–491.

136. Chen Z, Chen X, Liu M, et al. Altered functional connectivity of amygdala underlying the neuromechanism of migraine pathogenesis. *J Headache Pain* 2017;18(1):7. doi:10.1186/s10194-017-0722-5.

137. Bingel U, Quante M, Knab R, et al. Subcortical structures involved in pain processing: evidence from single-trial fMRI. *Pain* 2002;99(1–2):313–321.

138. Ji G, Zhang W, Mahimainathan L, et al. 5-HT2C receptor knockdown in the amygdala inhibits neuropathic-pain-related plasticity and behaviors. *J Neurosci* 2017;37(6):1378–1393. doi:10.1523/JNEUROSCI.2468-16.2016.

139. Borszcz GS, Streltsov NG. Amygdaloid-thalamic interactions mediate the antinociceptive action of morphine microinjected into the periaqueductal gray. *Behav Neurosci* 2000;114(3):574–584.

140. Fields HL. Pain modulation: expectation, opioid analgesia and virtual pain. *Prog Brain Res* 2000;122:245–253.

141. Mena NB, Mathur R, Nayar U. Amygdalar involvement in pain. *Indian J Physiol Pharmacol* 1995;39(4):339–346.

142. Scoville WB, Milner B. Loss of recent memory after bilateral hippocampal lesions. *J Neuropsychiatry Clin Neurosci* 2000;12(1):103–113.

143. Neylan TC. Neuropsychiatric consequences of traumatic brain injury: observations from Adolf Meyer. *J Neuropsychiatry Clin Neurosci* 2000;12(3):406.

144. Ploghaus A, Tracey I, Clare S, et al. Learning about pain: the neural substrate of the prediction error for aversive events. *Proc Natl Acad Sci U S A* 2000;97(16):9281–9286.

145. Derbyshire SW, Jones AK, Gyulai F, et al. Pain processing during three levels of noxious stimulation produces differential patterns of central activity. *Pain* 1997;73(3):431–445.

146. Parasuraman R, Warm JS, See JE. Brain systems of vigilance. In: Parasuramann R, eds. *The Attentive Brain.* Cambridge, MA: MIT Press; 1998: 221–256.

147. Posner MI, Petersen SE. The attention system in the human brain. *Ann Rev Neurosci* 1990;13:25–42.

148. Lorenz J, Garcia-Larrea L. Contribution of attentional and cognitive factors to laser evoked brain potentials. *Neurophysiol Clin* 2003;33:293–301.

149. Bingel U, Schoell E, Herken W, et al. Habituation to painful stimulation involves the antinociceptive system. *Pain* 2007;131(1–2):21–30.

150. Janicki P, Libich J, Gumulka W. Lack of habituation of pain evoked potentials after naloxone. *Pol J Pharmacol Pharm* 1979;31(3):201–205.

151. Peters ML, Schmidt AJ, Van den Hout MA. Chronic low back pain and the reaction to repeated acute pain stimulation. *Pain* 1989;39(1):69–76.

152. Demirci S, Savas S. The auditory event related potentials in episodic and chronic pain sufferers. *Eur J Pain* 2002;6(3):239–244.

153. Valeriani M, de Tommaso M, Restuccia D, et al. Reduced habituation to experimental pain in migraine patients: a CO_2 laser evoked potential study. *Pain* 2003;105(1–2):57–64.

154. Flor H, Diers M, Birbaumer N. Peripheral and electrocortical responses to painful and non-painful stimulation in chronic pain patients, tension headache patients and healthy controls. *Neurosci Lett* 2004;361(1–3):147–150.

155. Beydoun A, Morrow TJ, Shen JF, et al. Variability of laser-evoked potentials: attention, arousal and lateralized differences. *Electroencephalogr Clin Neurophysiol* 1993;88:173–181.

156. Moldofsky H. Sleep and pain. *Sleep Med Rev* 2001;5(5):385–396.

157. Zaslansky R, Sprecher E, Katz Y, et al. Pain-evoked potentials: what do they really measure? *Electroencephalogr Clin Neurophysiol* 1996;100(5):384–391.

158. Hauck M, Bischoff P, Schmidt G, et al. Clonidine effects on pain evoked SII activity in humans. *Eur J Pain* 2006;10(8):757–765.

159. Roth D, Petersen-Felix S, Bak P, et al. Analgesic effect in humans of subanaesthetic isoflurane concentrations evaluated by evoked potentials. *Br J Anaesth* 1996;76:38–42.

160. McCracken LM, Turk DC. Behavioral and cognitive-behavioral treatment for chronic pain: outcome, predictors of outcome, and treatment process. *Spine* 2002;27(22):2564–2573.

161. McCabe C, Lewis J, Shenker N, et al. Don't look now! Pain and attention. *Clin Med* 2005;5(5):482–486.

162. Vlaeyen JW, Linton SJ. Fear-avoidance and its consequences in chronic musculoskeletal pain: a state of the art. *Pain* 2000;85(3):317–332.

163. Van Damme S, Crombez G, Eccleston C, et al. Impaired disengagement from threatening cues of impending pain in a crossmodal cueing paradigm. *Eur J Pain* 2004;8:227–236.

164. Villemure C, Bushnell MC. Cognitive modulation of pain: how do attention and emotion influence pain processing? *Pain* 2002;95(3):195–199.

165. Engel AK, Fries P, Singer W. Dynamic predictions: oscillations and synchrony in top-down processing. *Nat Rev Neurosci* 2001;2(10):704–716.

166. Herrmann CS, Munk MH, Engel AK. Cognitive functions of gamma-band activity: memory match and utilization. *Trends Cogn Sci* 2004;8(8):347–355.

167. Hauck M, Domnick C, Lorenz J, et al. Top-down and bottom-up modulation of pain-induced oscillations. *Front Hum Neurosci* 2015; 9:375. doi:10.3389/fnhum.2015.00375.

168. Flor H, Diers M. Limitations of pharmacotherapy: behavioral approaches to chronic pain. *Handb Exp Pharmacol* 2007;177:415–427.

169. Di Piero V, Jones AK, Iannotti F, et al. Chronic pain: a PET study of the central effects of percutaneous high cervical cordotomy. *Pain* 1991;46(1):9–12.

170. Pleger B, Ragert P, Schwenkreis P, et al. Patterns of cortical reorganization parallel impaired tactile discrimination and pain intensity in complex regional pain syndrome. *Neuroimage* 2006;32(2):503–510.

171. Maihöfner C, Forster C, Birklein F, et al. Brain processing during mechanical hyperalgesia in complex regional pain syndrome: a functional MRI study. *Pain* 2005;114(1–2):93–103.

172. Flor H, Braun C, Elbert T, et al. Extensive reorganization of primary somatosensory cortex in chronic back pain patients. *Neurosci Lett* 1997; 224(1):5–8.

173. Montoya P, Pauli P, Batra A, et al. Altered processing of pain-related information in patients with fibromyalgia. *Eur J Pain* 2005;9(3):293–303.

174. Peyron R, Schneider F, Faillenot I, et al. An fMRI study of cortical representation of mechanical allodynia in patients with neuropathic pain. *Neurology* 2004;63(10):1838–1846.

175. Kuchinad A, Schweinhardt P, Seminowicz DA, et al. Accelerated brain gray matter loss in fibromyalgia patients: premature aging of the brain? *J Neurosci* 2007;27(15):4004–4007.

176. May A, Matharu M. New insights into migraine: application of functional and structural imaging. *Curr Opin Neurol* 2007;20(3):306–309.

CHAPTER 7

Psychological Aspects of Pain

DENNIS C. TURK, KIMBERLY SHAWN SWANSON, and **HILARY D. WILSON**

Advances in the knowledge of the neurophysiology of pain have resulted in the development of new pharmacologic agents, sophisticated surgical interventions, and the use of innovative technologies (e.g., spinal cord stimulation, implantable drug delivery systems) for the treatment of patients with chronic pain. Despite these advances, the cure of pain remains elusive. Regardless of the treatment, the amount of pain reduction averages only about 35%, and fewer than 50% of persons treated with these interventions obtain this result. The extent of improvement in emotional, physical, and social functioning is often below these dissatisfying levels.[1]

Notwithstanding the relatively modest track record for even "newer" chronic pain treatments, patients are often given an expectation, directly or indirectly, that they should expect significant improvements if not elimination of their pain. Although individuals with acute pain can often receive good relief from over-the-counter medications and treatments from their primary health care providers, people with persistent pain become enmeshed in the medical-legal system as they shuttle from doctor to doctor, diagnostic test to diagnostic test, in a frustrating quest to receive successful treatment. This experience of "medical limbo"—the presence of a painful condition that, in the absence of acceptable pathology, is either attributed to psychiatric causation or malingering on the one hand, or an undiagnosed but potentially progressive and untreatable disease on the other—is itself a source of significant and ongoing stress that can initiate high levels of emotional distress or aggravate a premorbid psychiatric condition.[2]

The person who has a chronic pain condition resides in a complex and costly world that is populated not only by themselves but also by their significant others, including health care providers, employers, and third-party payers. Family members feel increasingly hopeless and distressed as medical costs, disability, and emotional suffering mount while income and available treatment options decline. Health care providers grow increasingly frustrated and feel defeated and ineffective as available treatment options are exhausted while the pain condition remains a mystery and may worsen. They may come to question the veracity of their patients and their complaints. Employers, who are already resentful of growing worker's compensation benefits, pay higher costs while productivity suffers because the employee frequently calls out sick or is unable to perform at his or her usual level ("presenteeism"), often with coworkers having to pick up the slack. Third-party payers watch as health care expenditures soar with repeated diagnostic testing, often with inconclusive results. In time, the legitimacy of the individual's report of pain may be questioned because oftentimes, a medical etiology fails to substantiate the cause of the symptoms.

People with chronic pain may begin to feel that their health care providers, employers, and even family members are blaming them when their condition fails to respond to treatment as expected. Some may suggest that the individual is complaining excessively in an attempt to obtain prescriptions for centrally acting and reinforcing medications (e.g., opioids), to receive attention, to avoid undesirable activities, or to be relieved from onerous obligations (e.g., gainful employment, household chores). Others may suggest that the pain reported is not real, they are feigning or exaggerating their symptoms, and is "all in

their head"—"psychogenic." Third-party payers may even suggest that the claimant is intentionally exaggerating his or her pain in order to obtain financial gain, whereas others may attribute reported symptoms to the desire to obtain mood-altering drugs. In this way, people with chronic pain may come to be viewed as "wimps," "crocks," or "fakes." Those experiencing persistent pain may in turn come to view health care providers and claims adjustors as "quacks," "hacks," or "thieves." Often, the ensuing result is an unfortunate, inappropriate, and detrimental adversarial relationship.

As a result of the attitudes, and in the absence of cure or even substantial relief described, individuals experiencing chronic pain may withdraw from contacts; lose their sources of income; alienate family, friends, and coworkers; and become more and more isolated, despondent, depressed, and, in general, demoralized. They become angry, and frustration increases as their bodies, the health care system, legal system, and their significant other have all let them down. They may feel they have even let themselves down as they relinquish their usual activities and responsibilities due to symptoms that are intractable, yet often inscrutable, when not validated by objective pathologic findings. This emotional distress, however, can be exacerbated by a variety of other factors, including fear of disease progression and their vulnerability to escalating sets of symptoms and disability, inadequate or maladaptive support systems, inadequate personal and material coping resources, treatment-induced (iatrogenic) complications, overuse of potent drugs with significant adverse effects, inability to work, financial difficulties, prolonged litigation, disruption of usual activities, and sleep disturbance. In short, living with persistent pain conditions requires considerable emotional resilience and tends to deplete people's emotional reserves, taxing not only the individual sufferer but also the capacity of family, friends, coworkers, employers, and society to provide support.

Based on what we described earlier about the plight of the person with chronic pain, two conclusions are obvious: (1) Psychosocial and behavioral factors play a significant role in the experience, maintenance, and exacerbation of pain and potentially even the cause[3] and (2) because some level of pain persists in the majority of people with chronic pain regardless of treatment, self-management is an important complement to biomedical approaches.[4] In this chapter, we emphasize a set of important psychological constructs including dispositional, cognitive, affective, and behavioral factors. We discuss them individually for ease of explication. It is important to note, however, that although we describe these separately, there is considerable overlap and integration among them. We conclude with a discussion of integrative models and treatments of chronic pain.

Cognitive Factors: Predispositions, Appraisals, Beliefs, Perceived Control, and Self-efficacy

PREDISPOSITIONS

Temperament is, at least partly, putatively heritable and may show continuity throughout the entire life span. Personality in adulthood reflects the molding of underlying temperament by life experiences. Temperament and personality may predispose individuals toward misinterpretation of pain sensations and maladaptive pain beliefs, or they can have a protective role contributing to resilience in the face of adversity.

Among the potential vulnerability factors that have been proposed are negative affectivity, anxiety sensitivity (AS), and illness/injury sensitivity. Negative affectivity may be considered as heritable, stable, and promoting a tendency to experience a broad range of negative emotions and to view the world as threatening and distressing.[5] Negative affectivity has been associated with heightened vigilance to bodily sensations and interpretational biases toward ambiguous internal signals.[6,7] Studies in nonclinical populations have reported negative affectivity to predict lower pain tolerance.[8] However, studies in chronic pain populations have, to date, not provided consistent evidence for a role of trait negative affectivity. Thus, although negative affectivity has often been implicated as a vulnerability factor in chronic pain, convincing evidence is lacking.

More convincing has been the research on another potential vulnerability factor: AS. AS is defined as the fear of anxiety-related sensations and is conceived as a partly heritable personality trait.[9] Individuals with high AS interpret unpleasant physical sensations (such as rapid heart beating, feeling faint) more often as a sign of danger than individuals with low AS. There is growing evidence that AS may also be a risk factor for the maintenance and exacerbation of chronic pain and disability.[10] AS has been shown to correlate with measures of fear-avoidance (described in the following text) and is associated with distress, analgesic use, and impairment of physical and social functioning in patients across a wide range of different pain-related conditions.[11] Moreover, path analyses and mediation models suggest that AS exacerbates fear-avoidance beliefs and the negative interpretation of bodily sensations, which in turn leads to enhanced pain experience and pain avoidance.[12,13] Studies examining the predictive value of AS in relation to cognitive and behavioral reactions to experimentally induced pain support a causal, negative biasing role of AS in maladaptive cognitive and behavioral pain response.

In contrast to the extensive search after negative predisposing factors described, there has been relatively little research on protective factors for chronic pain and disability. Traditionally, research on resilience has focused on adaptive responses in the wake of significant adversity or challenge (e.g., developmental resilience, posttraumatic growth). In the context of pain, resilience might mean effective recovery from an injury, infection, or other painful experience, both from a physical and psychosocial standpoint (e.g., effective resilience in the wake of an injury might ideally mean total resolution of pain and resumption of normal functioning). However, in patients for whom resolution of pain is unlikely, behavioral, and cognitive responses to pain may have very different implications in terms of their adaptiveness. When a new and unfamiliar painful condition develops, a fearful and avoidant response may be protective; consistent with an evolutionary view of pain, new painful sensations may signal significant danger to the organism, such that mobilization of individual resources to escape pain and threat may prolong survival. However, prolongation of this fearful avoidant response tends to yield fewer benefits in cases of chronic pain and, instead, increase the risk of protracted physical disability, deconditioning, and psychosocial dysfunction.[14] Chronic pain resilience is a construct that has garnered a great deal of attention in recent years (e.g., Friborg et al.,[15] Hassett and Finan,[16] Ruiz-Parraga et al.,[17] Sturgeon and Zautra[18]).

Several investigators[18,19] have proposed a model of resilience in chronic pain that follows a "temporal" order of adaptation, manifesting in three interrelated factors: *sustainability*, or prolonged and positive functioning despite the immediate presence of pain; *recovery*, or expedient and effective recovery from the negative consequences of pain; and *growth*, or long-term learning or personal development that may result in new strengths, protective attitudes, or skills as a result of chronic pain.

Three potential resilience factors are particularly relevant in chronic pain: optimism, hope, and psychological flexibility. Review of the literature suggests that optimism may be one of the most important personality traits in relation to adjustment to chronic pain. Dispositional *optimism* is defined as "the tendency to believe that one will generally experience good outcomes in life" and is distinguishable from neuroticism and trait anxiety.[20] In cross-sectional and prospective studies, optimism was found to be associated with better general health, adaptation to chronic disease, and recovery after various surgical procedures.[21–23]

Only a few studies have explored the role of dispositional optimism or hope in adaptation to chronic pain. Novy[24] found that optimism was related to less catastrophizing and more use of active coping strategies in chronic pain patients. Affleck and Tennen[25] reported that dispositional optimism predicts pleasant daily mood in fibromyalgia but that it is not related to daily pain. Finally, in studying rheumatoid arthritis patients, Treharne and colleagues[26] found that optimism was associated with less depression and pain and higher life satisfaction for patients in the early and intermediate stages of disease.

The primary mechanism of the beneficial effect of optimism may be differences in coping behavior between optimistic and pessimistic people.[27] In general, pessimists turn to avoidant coping strategies and denial more often, where optimists employ more problem-focused coping strategies. When problem-focused coping is not possible, they turn to coping strategies such as acceptance, use of humor, and positive reframing of the situation.[20] Thus, it may not be the use of specific coping strategies but flexibility of coping that protects against disability and distress.[20] Snyder[28] has described a similar pathway for hope, with people with low hope showing a tendency to catastrophize, whereas people with high hope seek means to encounter future challenges and show flexibility in finding alternative life goals when their original goals are blocked.

Psychological flexibility manifests as an ability to effectively and flexibly adjust behavioral efforts at goal pursuit in a way that is consistent with one's own values[29] despite the presence of pain and associated problems. Psychological flexibility may act independently of reductions rumination about symptoms and impact on life and other negative patterns of thinking.[30]

Individuals with chronic pain who better sustain their optimism, hope, and flexibility appear to be more able to persist in painful behavioral tasks[31] and to be less susceptible to other pain-related difficulties, such as fatigue[32] and problematic opioid use.[33] Similarly, positive emotional states have been found to be predictors of better social[34] and physical functioning[35] in some individuals with chronic pain.

APPRAISAL AND BELIEFS

Specific appraisal and beliefs are largely shaped by an individual's learning history through direct experience, observational learning, or information acquired from others. These experiences may interact with an individual's enduring traits, sociocultural background, prior learning and experiences, and the current context in which they reside. That is, personality factors may predispose some people to make certain kinds of appraisals and to be more susceptible to some idiosyncratic beliefs than to others.

Pain appraisal refers specifically to the meaning ascribed to pain by each individual. In accordance with the transactional stress model,[36] a distinction can be made between primary appraisal (evaluation of the significance of pain as threatening, benign, or irrelevant) and secondary appraisal (evaluation of the controllability of pain and one's coping resources).

Beliefs refer to assumptions about reality that shape how one interprets events and can thus be considered as determinants of appraisal. Pain beliefs develop throughout the lifetime as a result of an individual's learning history and cover all aspects of the pain experience (e.g., the causes of pain, its prognosis, appropriate treatments).

Appraisal and beliefs about pain can have a strong impact on an individual's response to pain. If a pain signal is interpreted as harmful (threat), it may be perceived as more intense, more unpleasant and evoke more escape or avoidance behavior. For instance, Smith and colleagues[37] demonstrated that cancer patients who attributed pain sensations after physiotherapy directly to cancer reported more intense pain than patients who attributed this pain to other causes. Perception of danger of an experimental pain stimulus may also lead to avoidance of this stimulus. Arntz and Claassens[38] experimentally manipulated the appraisal of a mildly painful stimulus (a very cold metal bar placed against the neck) by suggesting that it was either very hot or very cold. As expected, participants rated the stimulus as more painful in the condition where they were informed that it was hot. The effect appeared to be mediated by the belief that the stimulus would be harmful. These studies demonstrate the important role of people's interpretations regarding the meaning of the pain.

Pain appraisal and pain beliefs are also prominent determinants of adjustment to chronic pain.[39] Pain that is viewed as a signal of damage, leads to disability, is uncontrollable, and is a permanent condition has been shown to affect individuals' responses,[40,41] and these beliefs are widespread.[42,43]

CATASTROPHIZING AND FEAR-AVOIDANCE BELIEFS

Pain catastrophizing can be defined as an exaggerated, negative cognitive and emotional orientation toward actual or anticipated pain experiences. Current conceptualizations most often describe it in terms of appraisal or as a set of maladaptive beliefs.[44] Pain-related catastrophizing thought patterns are fairly common in both acute and chronic pain and show significant relationship to pain intensity and functional disability.[45,46] For example, prospective studies indicated that catastrophizing might be predictive of the inception of chronic musculoskeletal pain in the general population.[47–49] For patients undergoing surgery, catastrophizing has been shown to predict postoperative pain severity, length of hospital stay, poor quality of life, greater postsurgical opioid use, opioid misuse,[50] as well as later development of chronic pain and disability (e.g., Khan et al.,[51] Theunissen et al.[52]). Catastrophizing has been associated with increased perceptions of pain severity in both acute[53] and chronic pain severity[54] and disability among groups with diverse pain diagnoses.[55,56] Catastrophizing also alters perception of noxious stimulation. In addition, catastrophizing is related to greater sensitivity to experimentally induced pain in pain-free volunteers and pain patients.[46,57,58] The relationship has been observed in healthy adults[54] as well as children.[59] In a systematic review, Wertli et al.[60] reported that catastrophizing was a prognostic factor predicting outcomes of patients with low back pain. Conversely, following treatment, reductions in catastrophizing were related to reduction in pain intensity and physical impairment and maintenance of treatment benefits.[61]

Imaging studies have shown how catastrophizing is associated with specific brain regions.[62–64] Several studies[65,66] used the diffuse noxious inhibitory control/conditioned pain modulation (DNIC/CPM) paradigm demonstrated that catastrophizing may influence the pain modulatory process in pain-free individuals and predict pain following surgery.[67] Catastrophizing has also been associated with immune function (i.e., interleukin-6) responses to acute pain[68] and stress hormones in response to laboratory-induced pain in individuals with chronic pain and pain-free individuals.[69]

People with chronic pain often anticipate that certain activities will increase their pain or induce further injury. These fears may contribute to avoidance of activity and subsequently greater physical deconditioning, emotional distress, and, ultimately, greater disability.[14] Their failure to engage in activities prevents them from obtaining any corrective feedback about the associations among activity, pain, and injury.

In addition to fear of movement, people with persistent pain may be anxious about the meaning of their symptoms for the future—will their pain increase, will their physical capacity diminish, will they have progressive disability where they ultimately end up in a wheelchair or bedridden? In addition to these sources of fear, people experiencing persistent pain may fear that on the one hand, people will not believe that they are suffering, and on the other, they may be told that they are beyond help and will "just have to learn to live with it." Such fears can contribute to additional emotional distress and to increased muscle tension and physiologic arousal that may directly exacerbate and maintain pain.

The role of catastrophizing and the belief that pain means harm and activity should be avoided has been most articulated in fear-avoidance models (FAMs) of chronic pain.[14,70] Although FAMs are multifaceted and include affective (fear) and behavioral (avoidance) components, cognitions are identified as the core determinants of entering into a negative pain cycle. The tenets of contemporary FAMs can be summarized as follows: When pain is perceived following injury, an individual's idiosyncratic beliefs will determine the extent to which pain is catastrophically interpreted. A catastrophic interpretation of pain gives rise to physiologic (arousal), behavioral (avoidance), and cognitive fear responses. The cognitive shift that takes place during fear enhances threat perception (e.g., by narrowing of attention) and further feeds the catastrophic appraisal of pain.[49,70]

There is substantial evidence that fear-avoidance beliefs are associated with disability and impaired physical performance in chronic pain.[14,37] A systematic review of the literature on psychological risk factors in back and neck pain indicated that the evidence for the association between fear-avoidance beliefs and increased pain and disability was of the highest level.[14,37] In addition, prospective studies have shown that fear-avoidance beliefs in patients seeking care for acute pain may be predictive of pain persistence, disability, and long-term sick leave.[71–73] A number of treatment approaches have been developed and implemented to address pain-related fear and anxiety in chronic pain patients (e.g., Bailey et al.[74]).

Fear-avoidance beliefs of health care providers have also been found to be related to their treatment behavior and their recommendation for engaging in physical activities.[75–77] The beliefs of patients and health care providers may further interact with each other in a mutually reinforcing way because a patient's beliefs may guide the choice of which health care provider is visited.[78]

PERCEIVED CONTROL AND SELF-EFFICACY

Perceived control over pain refers to the belief that one can exert influence on the duration, frequency, intensity, or unpleasantness of pain. Perceived controllability of a pain stimulus may modify the meaning of this stimulus and directly affect threat appraisal.[79] As a consequence, pain may be rated as less intense or less unpleasant, and pain tolerance may increase.

The belief that one has control over pain has a strong influence on disability in patients with chronic pain[40,80] and an increase in this belief after multidisciplinary pain treatment may predict pain reduction and decreases in disability[81–83] demonstrated that perceived control over the effects of pain was more strongly related to better adjustment and less disability than perceived control over pain itself.

Related to perceived control is the construct of self-efficacy. Self-efficacy is the conviction that one can successfully perform a certain task or produce a desirable outcome.[84] A major determinant of self-efficacy is prior mastery experience. In laboratory experiments, self-efficacy beliefs predict pain tolerance.[85,86] In chronic pain patients, self-efficacy positively affects physical and psychological functioning,[87,88] and improvements in self-efficacy after self-management and cognitive-behavioral interventions are associated with improvements in pain, functional status, and psychological adjustment. Recent reviews of psychological factors in chronic pain have concluded that the evidence for the role of self-efficacy across a broad range of pain populations is impressive (e.g., Jackson et al.,[39] Riddle et al.[89]). Moreover, self-efficacy also influences the prognosis after acute physical interventions like surgery.[89,90] Prospective studies in patients who underwent surgery demonstrated that high self-efficacy before the start of rehabilitation and larger increases over the course of rehabilitation speed recovery and predict better long-term outcome.[91,92] A preoperative intervention (an instruction video demonstrating movement and breathing skills) in hysterectomy patients was able to enhance preoperative self-efficacy and decrease pain associated with postoperative activities and promote earlier mobilization.[93] Perceived self-efficacy has been shown to have a direct effect on the body's opioid and immune systems[94] confirming the important association between psychological constructs and physiology.

COPING

Self-regulation of pain and its impact depend on people's specific ways of dealing with pain, adjusting to pain, and reducing or minimizing distress caused by pain; in other words, their coping strategies. Coping is assumed to involve spontaneously employed purposeful and intentional acts, and it can be assessed in terms of overt and covert behaviors. Overt behavioral coping strategies include rest, use of relaxation techniques, or medication. Covert coping strategies include various means of distracting oneself from pain, reassuring oneself that the pain will diminish, seeking information, and problem solving. Coping strategies are thought to act to alter both the perception of pain intensity and the ability to manage or tolerate pain, and to continue everyday activities (e.g., Skinner et al.,[4] Flor and Turk[95]). Some studies have found active coping strategies (efforts to function in spite of pain or to distract oneself from pain, such as engaging in activity or ignoring pain) to be associated with adaptive functioning, and passive coping strategies (such as depending on others for help in pain control and restricting one's activities) to be related to greater pain and depression (e.g., Benyon et al.,[87] Ip et al.,[96] Samwel et al.[97]). However, beyond this, there is no evidence supporting the greater effectiveness of any one active coping strategy compared to any other. It seems more likely that different strategies will be more effective than others for some people at some times but not necessarily for all people all the time.[98]

Stress and Autonomic Responses: Hypothalamic-Pituitary-Adrenal Axis Dysregulation

It is becoming clear that the pain experience is determined by a multitude of factors. Although the focus has historically been directed at sensory mechanisms, more attention is being placed on factors related to cognitive and homeostatic factors. The primary basis for including discussions of homeostatic factors is that chronic pain threatens the organism and produces a cascade of events that eventually contributes to the maintenance of such conditions. If one views pain as a primary threat to the organism, then mechanisms should be present to engage and motivate the organism to restore basic homeostatic function.[99] The major consequence of homeostatic imbalance is stress. Regardless of the source, stressors activate numerous systems such as the autonomic nervous system and the hypothalamic-pituitary-adrenal (HPA) axis. Prolonged activation of the stress system has disastrous effects on the body[100] and sets up a condition of a feedback loop between pain and stress reactivity.

During periods of short-term stress and homeostatic imbalance, the hypothalamus activates the pituitary gland to secrete adrenocorticotropic hormone, which acts on the adrenal cortex to secrete cortisol. Secretion of cortisol elevates blood sugar levels and enhances metabolism, an adaptive response that allows the organism to mobilize energy resources to deal with the threat and restore homeostatic balance (i.e., fight or flight response). The situation is much more serious during prolonged periods of stress and homeostatic imbalance that is associated with long-term psychological stress, chronic pain, and other pathologic conditions. Prolonged, elevated levels of cortisol are related to the exhaustion phase of Selye's[100] general adaptation syndrome. The negative effects of this stage of the adaptation syndrome include atrophy of muscle tissue, impairment of growth and tissue repair, and immune system suppression, which together might set up conditions for the development and maintenance of a variety of chronic pain conditions.[101,102] According to Melzack,[103] psychological stress, as well as sensory and cognitive events, modulates the neurosignature of the body–self neuromatrix which, as a consequence of altered neuromatrix output, is associated with chronic pain conditions. The concept of the neuromatrix has potentially important explanatory implications for brain function in general and also provides a theoretical framework for the biopsychosocial perspective of chronic pain. As will be discussed later, there is a growing literature demonstrating the importance of psychosocial factors (emotion and cognition) in this neuromatrix conceptualization.

Emotion

Pain is ultimately a subjective, private experience, but it is invariably described in terms of sensory and affective properties. As defined by the International Association for the Study of Pain, "[Pain] is unquestionably a sensation in a part or parts of the body but it is also always unpleasant and therefore also an *emotional experience* [emphasis added]."[104] The central and interactive roles of sensory information and affective state are supported by an overwhelming amount of evidence.[105] The affective component of pain incorporates many different emotions. Depression and anxiety have received the greatest amount of attention in chronic pain patients; however, anger and hostility have received considerable interest as a significant emotion in chronic pain patients (e.g., Burns et al.,[106] Burns et al.,[107] Burns et al.[108]). Additionally, the ability to maintain positive affect during times of stress has been investigated in relationship to pain.[109]

In addition to affect being one of the three interconnected components of pain, emotions and pain interact in a number of ways. Emotional distress may predispose people to experience pain, be a precipitant of symptoms, be a modulating factor amplifying or inhibiting the severity of pain, be a consequence of persistent pain, or a perpetuating factor. Moreover, these potential roles are not mutually exclusive, and any number of them may be involved in a particular circumstance interacting with cognitive appraisals. For example, the literature is replete with studies demonstrating that current mood state modulates reports of pain as well as tolerance for acute pain.[110] Levels of anxiety have been shown to influence not only pain severity but also complications following surgery and number of days of hospitalization.[111,112] Individual difference variables, such as AS, have also been shown to play an important predisposing and augmenting role in the experience of pain.[113] Level of depression has been observed to play a significant role in premature termination from pain rehabilitation programs.[114]

Emotional distress is commonly observed in people with chronic pain. As described previously, people with chronic pain often feel rejected by the medical system, believing that they are blamed or labeled as symptom magnifiers and complainers by their physicians, family members, friends, and employers when their pain condition does not respond to treatment. Although most of the literature has focused on the relationship between negative affect and pain, research has indicated the ability to maintain positive affect during stress is an important factor contributing to ongoing adaptation to chronic illness. Positive affect serves to decrease distress in chronic pain patients by broadening the individual's range of affective and cognitive responses permitting a wider range of experiences.[115] Positive affect can serve as psychological immunity in that chronic pain patients may experience more optimal functioning and improved quality of life while living with ongoing pain. Although we provide an overview of research on the predominant emotions—anxiety, depression, and anger—associated with pain individually, it is important to acknowledge that these emotions are not as distinct when it comes to the experience of pain. They interact and augment each other over time.

ANXIETY

It is common for patients with symptoms of pain to be anxious and worried. This is especially true when the symptoms are unexplained, as is often the case for chronic pain syndromes. For example, in a large-scale, multicenter study of fibromyalgia patients, between 44% and 51% of patients acknowledged that they were anxious.[116] In addition, up to 45% of patients with chronic pain will screen positive for an anxiety disorder.[117] Chronic pain patients with comorbid anxiety may have a lower pain tolerance, be more prone to medication side effects or fearful of having side effects, and be more fearful of pain itself.[118] One study indicated 40% of patients with panic disorder also had chronic pain, particularly head, shoulder, and lower back pain.[119] Panic disorder involves a hyperfocus on somatic sensations that might increase subjective pain sensations. Patients with both chronic pain and panic may engage in more "illness behaviors."[119]

Fear and anxiety will also relate to activities that people with pain anticipate will increase their pain or exacerbate whatever physical factors might be contributing to the pain. As noted in the discussion of the FAM previously, these fears may contribute to avoidance, motivate inactivity, and, ultimately, greater disability.[14] Continual vigilance and monitoring of noxious stimulation and the belief that it signifies disease progression may render even low-intensity aversive sensations less bearable. In addition, such fears will contribute to increased muscle tension and physiologic arousal that may exacerbate and maintain pain.

Threat of intense pain captures attention from which it is difficult to disengage. The experience of pain may initiate a set of extremely negative thoughts, as noted previously, and arouse fears—fears of inciting more pain and injury, fear of future impact.[14] Fear and anticipation of pain are cognitive-perceptual processes that are not driven exclusively by the actual sensory experience of pain and can exert a significant impact on the level of function and pain tolerance.[120,121] People are motivated to avoid and escape from unpleasant consequences; they learn that avoidance of situations and activities in which they have experienced acute episodes of pain will reduce the likelihood of reexperiencing pain or causing further physical damage. They may become hypervigilant to their environment as a way of preventing the occurrence of pain.

Investigators[122,123] have suggested that fear of pain, driven by the anticipation of pain and not by the sensory experience of pain itself, produces strong negative reinforcement for the persistence of avoidance behavior and the putative functional disability in pain patients. Avoidance behavior is reinforced in the short-term through the reduction of suffering associated with noxious stimulation.[124] Avoidance, however, can be a maladaptive response if it persists and leads to increased fear, limited activity, and other physical and psychological consequences that contribute to disability and persistence of pain.

Studies have demonstrated that fear of movement and fear of (re)injury are better predictors of functional limitations than biomedical parameters or even pain severity and duration.[125,126] For example, Crombez and colleagues[125] showed that pain-related fear was the best predictor of behavioral performance in trunk extension, flexion, and weight lifting tasks, even after partitioning out the effects of pain intensity. Moreover, Vlaeyen and colleagues[127] found that fear of movement/(re)injury was the best predictor of self-reported disability among chronic back pain patients and that physiologic sensory perception of pain and biomedical findings did not add any predictive value. The importance of fear of activity appears to generalize to daily activities as well as in the clinical experimental context. Approximately two-thirds of individuals with chronic nonspecific low back pain avoid back-straining activities because of fear of (re)injury.[125] For example, fear-avoidance beliefs about physical demands of a job are strongly related to disability and work lost during the previous year, even more so than pain severity or other pain variables.[128,129] Interestingly, reduction in pain-related anxiety predicts improvement in functioning, affective distress, pain, and pain-related interference with activity.[83] Clearly, fear, pain-related anxiety, and concerns about harm avoidance all play important roles in chronic pain and need to be assessed and addressed in treatment.

Pain-related fear and concerns about harm avoidance all appear to exacerbate symptoms.[123] Anxiety is an affective state that is greatly influenced by appraisal processes; to cite the stoic philosopher Epictetus, "there is nothing either bad or good but thinking makes it so." Thus, there is a reciprocal relationship between affective state and cognitive-interpretive processes. Thinking affects mood, and mood influences appraisals and, ultimately, the experience of pain.

DEPRESSION

Research suggests that 40% to 50% of chronic pain patients experience depressive symptoms.[130,131] Conversely, on average, 65% of depressed individuals also report pain symptoms.[132] Epidemiologic studies provide solid evidence for a strong association between chronic pain and depression but do not address whether chronic pain causes depression or depression causes chronic pain. Prospective studies of patients with chronic musculoskeletal pain have suggested that chronic pain can cause depression,[133] that depression can cause chronic pain,[134] and that they exist in a mutually reinforcing relationship.[135] A neuroanatomic link between depression and chronic pain via the hypothalamus, amygdala, and anterior cingulate gyrus pathway has been described. Reduced serotonin and norepinephrine are associated with both depression and increased pain sensation.[132]

One fact often raised to support the idea that pain causes depression is that the current depressive episode often began after the onset of the pain problem. The majority of studies appear to support this contention.[136] However, several studies have documented that many patients with chronic pain have often had prior episodes of depression that predated their pain problem by years.[137,138] One important prospective study[138] demonstrated that levels of depression predicted the development of low back pain 3 years following the initial assessment. Patients with depression were 2.3 times more likely to report back pain compared to those who did not report depression.

Depression was a much stronger predictor of incident back pain than any clinical or anatomic risk factors. This has led some investigators to propose that there may exist a common trait of susceptibility to dysphoric physical symptoms (including pain) and negative psychological symptoms (including anxiety as well as depression). They conclude that "pain and psychological illness should be viewed as having reciprocal psychological and behavioral effects involving both processes of illness expression and adaptation."[138,139] For example, those who experience both depression and chronic pain report more intense pain, less control of their lives, more unhealthy coping strategies, and reduced analgesic response to opiate medications.[132] In addition, negative thinking is a common feature of depression and chronic pain. Commonalities in thinking patterns between chronic pain and depression include catastrophic thinking, helplessness-hopelessness, and negative expectations regarding treatment outcome. These thinking patterns negatively impact how a person might respond to pain treatment interventions in that they lead to a reverse placebo/nocebo effect where the patient concludes "nothing works for me."[132]

Given the scenario of chronic pain just described, it is hardly surprising that chronic pain patients are depressed. It is interesting, however, to ponder the flip side of the coin—why are not *all* chronic pain patients depressed? Turk and colleagues[135,140] examined this question and determined that two factors appear to mediate the pain–depression relationship: patients' appraisals of the effects of the pain on their lives and appraisals of their ability to exert any control over their pain and lives. That is, those patients who believed that they could continue to function and that they could maintain some control despite their pain were less likely to become depressed. Here, we see the interdependence of cognition and affect.

As noted previously, in the majority of cases, depression appears to be reactive, although some have suggested that chronic pain is a form of "masked depression," whereby patients use pain to express their depressed mood because they feel it is more acceptable to complain of pain than to acknowledge that one is depressed. Once a person has a chronic pain diagnosis, it no longer matters which is the cause and which is the consequence—pain or depression. Both need to be treated.

ANGER AND HOSTILITY

Anger has been widely observed in people with chronic pain.[141] Even though chronic pain patients might present an image of themselves as even-tempered, Corbishley and colleagues[142] found that 88% acknowledged their feelings of anger when these were explicitly sought. Approximately 98% of the patients referred to a multidisciplinary pain rehabilitation center reported that they were feeling some degree of anger at the time of the assessment.[143] We must be cautious in interpreting data from patients recruited at pain centers, however, as there may be a referral bias such that the most distressed patients are sent to these facilities, and they do not represent the large number of people with persistent pain who are never evaluated in treatment facilities that specialize in pain management.

Because anger is frequently considered as socially undesirable, some patients in the studies cited previously may have found it difficult to admit that they were angry to the health care professionals. Thus, it is possible that the anger rates may actually be an underestimate. The high prevalence of anger observed is perhaps not surprising, given the frustrations related to persistence of symptoms, limited information on etiology, and repeated treatment failures along with anger toward others (employers, insurance companies, the health care system, family members) and anger toward themselves, perhaps, for their inability to alleviate their symptoms and to move on with their lives.[143] Several empirical studies provide preliminary support for the association between anger and pain intensity,[106,108]

unpleasantness of pain,[144] affective component of pain,[145] and emotional distress in chronic pain patients[146,147] as well as families of chronic pain patients.[141]

Anger in chronic pain has been considered by some to be attributable to enduring personality dispositions associated with unconscious conflicts,[148] whereas others have suggested that anger may be a reaction to the presence of recalcitrant symptoms that have been unsubstantiated by objective medical findings and unrelieved by medical treatments.[149] There is some evidence supporting the latter hypothesis. For example, a laboratory study[150] demonstrated that the mere anticipation of pain was sufficient to provoke angry behavioral responses in healthy individuals. Using the cross-lagged design with a clinical sample, Arena et al.[151] found that an increase in pain tends to precede anger, directly contradicting the anger–somatization association. Inhibition of anger seems to contribute to aversion of the chronic pain experience. Inhibition of anger has been found to be related to pain severity and overt pain behaviors[152] as well as to increased emotional distress.[146,153]

Denial of anger appears to be common among chronic pain patients. However, awareness of anger should not be confused with anger expression. For example, Corbishley et al.[142] observed that chronic pain patients tend to show strong reservations about expressing socially undesirable emotions that could create interpersonal conflict. For these individuals, it seems that expression of the emotion is under conscious control. They are aware of their anger but choose not to express it. On the other hand, some chronic pain patients may lack awareness of their angry feelings and have increased difficulties in recognizing and reporting these feelings.[154]

Fernandez and Turk[149] proposed that the specificity of targets toward which patients experience angry feelings may be important in understanding of the relationship between pain and anger. When a pain sufferer is angry, there are a range of possible targets (e.g., employer, insurance company, health care providers). The presence or intensity of anger toward different targets may be differentially related to chronic pain experience. That is, there may be some targets of anger that are more relevant to the chronic pain experience than others. As discussed later, Okifuji et al.[143] found that anger directed toward oneself was particularly common among chronic pain patients evaluated at a pain rehabilitation facility.

Although the effects of anger, hostility, and frustration on amplification of pain and treatment acceptance has not received as much attention as anxiety and depression, Kerns et al.[152] found that the suppressed feelings of anger accounted for a significant portion of the variance in pain intensity, perceived interference, and frequency of pain behaviors. Furthermore, Summers et al.[155] found that anger and hostility were powerful predictors of pain severity in people with spinal cord injuries.

It is thus reasonable to expect that the presence of anger may serve as a complicating factor, increasing autonomic arousal and blocking motivation and acceptance of treatments oriented toward rehabilitation and disability management rather than cure, which are often the only treatments available for chronic pain.[110] It would be reasonable to expect that the presence of anger may serve as a complicating factor, increasing autonomic arousal and blocking motivation and acceptance of treatments oriented toward rehabilitation and disability management rather than cure.

Frustrations related to persistence of symptoms, unknown etiology, and repeated treatment failures, along with anger toward employers, insurers, the health care system, family, and themselves, all contribute to the general dysphoric mood of patients.[143] Okifuji et al.[143] reported that 60% of patients expressed anger toward health care providers, 39% toward significant others, 30% toward insurance companies, 26% toward employers, and 20% toward attorneys. The target of anger most commonly acknowledged, however, was anger toward themselves (endorsed by approximately 70% of the sample). Internalization of angry feelings is strongly related to measures of pain intensity, perceived interference, and frequency of pain behaviors.[152] Overall, correlations between anger and pain severity have been shown to be statistically significant, ranging from 0.17 to 0.35.[152,156] Okifuji et al.[143] reported that anger was significantly correlated with pain intensity (correlations = .30 to .35). They also reported that anger was significantly correlated with disability (r = .26) and was highly associated with depression (r = .52).

The precise mechanisms by which anger and frustration exacerbate pain are not known. One reasonable possibility is that anger exacerbates pain by increasing autonomic arousal.[157,158] Anger and hostility may also interact with depression to modulate perceived severity of pain. In addition, anger may block motivation for, and acceptance of, treatments oriented toward rehabilitation and disability management rather than cure. Yet, rehabilitation and disability management are often the only treatments available for these patients.

In summary, it is important to be aware of the significant role of negative mood in chronic pain patients because it is likely to influence treatment motivation and compliance with treatment recommendations. For example, individuals experiencing pain who are anxious may fear engaging in what they perceive as demanding activities; patients who are depressed and who feel helpless may have little initiative or motivation to comply; and patients who are angry with the health care system are not likely to be motivated to respond to recommendations from yet another health care professional. Thus, clinicians who are treating people with persistent pain must focus on their mood states as well as physical pathology and somatic factors. Pain cannot be treated successfully without attending to the patient's emotional state. This is true for acute pain, such as pain associated with surgery, as well as persistent pain states.

Psychogenic Conceptualizations of Chronic Pain

As a result of the multiple psychosocial factors involved in the onset and maintenance of chronic pain, a number of different psychological perspectives on chronic pain have evolved. Many of the psychological treatments for chronic pain are based on different psychological principles that at times compete and differ from one another. Thus, it is important to consider the varying perspectives.

PSYCHOGENIC VIEW

Frequently in medicine, when physical explanations seem inadequate or when the results of treatment are inconsistent, reports of pain are attributed to a psychological etiology (and thus are "psychogenic"). Although psychogenic views of pain have been discussed since the formulation of psychodynamic theory, a psychodynamic perspective on chronic pain was first described systematically in the 1960s. During this time, people with pain were viewed as having compulsive and masochistic tendencies, inhibited aggressive needs, and feelings of guilt— "pain-prone personalities."[159] It was commonly held that people with pain had childhood histories fraught with emotional abuse, family dysfunction (e.g., parental quarrels, separation, divorce), illness or death of a parent, early responsibilities, and high orientation toward achievement.[160] Some current research has reported associations between chronic pain and childhood trauma, although the research is not consistent.[161] Based on the psychogenic perspective, assessment of persons with chronic pain is directed toward identifying the psychopathologic tendencies that instigate and maintain pain. It is assumed that

reports of pain will cease once the psychogenic mechanisms are resolved. Treatment is geared toward helping patients gain "insight" into the underlying maladaptive psychological contributors.[161,162]

Empirical evidence supporting the psychogenic view is scarce. A number of people with chronic pain do not exhibit significant psychopathology. Furthermore, insight-oriented psychotherapy has not been shown to be effective in reducing symptoms for the majority of patients with chronic pain.[163] Studies suggest that the emotional distress observed in patients with chronic pain more typically occurs in *response to* the persistence of pain and not as a causal agent[135,164] and may resolve once pain is adequately treated.[165] The psychogenic model has thus come under scrutiny and may be flawed in its view of chronic pain.[166]

Behavioral Formulations

CLASSICAL CONDITIONING

According to the classical or respondent conditioning model, if a painful stimulus is repeatedly paired with a neutral stimulus, the neutral stimulus will elicit a pain response. For example, a person who experienced pain after performing a treadmill exercise may become conditioned to experience a negative emotional response to the presence of the treadmill and to any stimulus associated with it (e.g., physical therapist, gym). The negative emotional reaction may instigate muscle tensing, thereby exacerbating pain, and further reinforcing the association between the stimulus and pain. Based on this, people with chronic pain may avoid activities previously associated with pain onset or exacerbation.

OPERANT CONDITIONING

In 1976, Fordyce[167] (for an update, see Main et al.[168]) introduced an extension of operant conditioning to chronic pain. This view proposes that acute pain behaviors (such as avoidance of activity to protect a painful area from additional pain) may come under the control of external contingencies of reinforcement (responses increase or decrease as a function of their reinforcing consequences) and thus develop into a chronic pain problem. Fordyce[167] underscored the fact that because there is no objective way to measure pain—no pain thermometer—the only way we can know of anyone's pain is by their behavior, whether verbal or nonverbal expressions. Overt pain behaviors include verbal reports, paralinguistic vocalizations (sighs, moans), motor activity, facial expressions, body postures and gesturing (limping, rubbing a painful body part, grimacing), functional limitations (reclining for extensive periods of time, inactivity), and behaviors designed to reduce pain (taking medication, use of the health care system).

The central features of pain behaviors are that they are (1) sources of communication and (2) observable. Observable behaviors are capable of eliciting a response and the consequences of behavior will influence subsequent behavior. Through a process of learning, responses that receive positive consequences, especially repeated desirable consequences, will more likely be maintained; behaviors that fail to activate positive consequences, or that receive negative consequences, will be less likely to occur (i.e., extinguished). Pain behaviors may be positively reinforced directly (e.g., attention from a spouse or health care provider, monetary compensation, avoidance of undesirable activity). Pain behaviors may also be maintained by the escape from noxious stimulation through the use of drugs or rest or the avoidance of undesirable activities such as work. In addition, "well behaviors" (e.g., activity, working) may not be positively reinforcing, and the more rewarding pain behaviors may, therefore, be maintained.

The operant conditioning model considers pain an internal subjective experience that can be directly assessed and may be maintained even after an initial physical basis of pain has resolved rather than the initial causes. The pain behavior originally elicited by organic factors caused by injury or disease may later occur, totally or in part, in response to reinforcing environmental events.

It is important, however, not to make the mistake of viewing pain behaviors as being synonymous with malingering. Malingering involves consciously and purposely faking a symptom such as pain for some gain, usually financial or to gain attention. Contrary to the beliefs of many third-party payers, there is little support for the contention that outright faking of pain for financial gain is prevalent.

There is some support for the operant model (e.g., Becker et al.,[169] Block et al.,[170] Doleys et al.,[171] Lousberg et al.[172]). For example, Romano et al.[173] videotaped patients and spouses in a series of cooperative household activities and recorded patients' pain behaviors. Sequential analyses showed that spouses' solicitous responses more frequently preceded and followed pain behaviors in patients than pain-free controls. At least a subset of patients do demonstrate high levels of pain behaviors and benefit from treatment targeting these behaviors (e.g., Thieme et al.,[174] Thieme et al.[175]).

SOCIAL (OBSERVATIONAL) LEARNING

The *social (observational) learning model* emphasizes the point that behavior can be learned not only by actual reinforcement of the individual's behavior but also by observation of how others respond and the consequences following responses. This is a powerful way of learning especially when the others being observed are judged to be similar to the observer. For example, a middle-aged man might learn what to expect by observing how other middle-aged men with similar medical problems are treated. People can acquire responses that were not previously in their behavioral repertoire by the observation of others performing these activities. Expectancies and actual behavioral responses to nociceptive stimulation are based, at least partially, on prior social learning history.

Another example of social learning occurs in children. Children develop attitudes about health and health care and the perception and interpretation of symptoms and physiologic processes from their parents and others they confront in their social environment. They learn how others respond to injury and disease and thus may be more or less likely to ignore or overrespond to symptoms they experience based on behaviors modeled in childhood. For example, children of chronic pain patients may make more pain-related responses during stressful times or exhibit greater illness behaviors (e.g., complaining, days absent, visit to school nurse) than children of healthy parents based on what they observed and learned at home.[176] Models can influence the expression, localization, and methods of coping with pain. Even physiologic responses may be conditioned during observation of others in pain.[177]

A central construct of the social learning perspective is that of self-efficacy.[84] Self-efficacy as described previously is a personal expectation that is important in patients with chronic pain. A self-efficacy belief is defined as a personal conviction that one can successfully execute a course of action (perform required behaviors) to produce a desired outcome in a given situation.[84] Given sufficient motivation to engage in a behavior, it is a person's self-efficacy beliefs that determine the choice of activities that he or she will initiate, the amount of effort that will be expended, and how long the individual will persist in the face of obstacles and aversive experiences. In this way, self-efficacy plays an important role in therapeutic change and compliance to psychological and medical regimes.[178]

Efficacy judgments are based on four sources of information regarding one's capabilities, listed in descending order of importance[84]: one's own past performance at the task or similar tasks; the performance accomplishments of others who are perceived to be similar to oneself; verbal persuasion by others that one is capable; and perception of one's own state of physiologic arousal, which is, in turn, partly determined by prior efficacy estimation. Performance mastery can then be created by encouraging people to undertake subtasks that are initially attainable but become increasingly difficult and subsequently approaching the desired level of performance. It is important to remember that coping behaviors are influenced by the person's beliefs that the demands of a situation do not exceed their coping resources.

How people interpret, respond to, and cope with illness is determined by cultural norms and perceptions of self-efficacy. These two sets of factors contribute to the marked variability in response to objectively similar degrees of physical pathology noted by health care providers.

GATE CONTROL THEORY

Although not a psychological formulation itself, the *gate control theory* (GCT)[179] was the first to popularize the importance of central, psychological factors in pain perception. Perhaps the most important contribution of the GCT is the way it changed thinking about pain perception. Melzack and Casey[180] differentiate three systems related to the processing of nociceptive stimulation—sensory-discriminative, motivational-affective, and cognitive-evaluative—all thought to contribute to the subjective experience of pain. Thus, the GCT specifically includes psychological factors as an integral aspect of the pain experience. It emphasizes the central nervous system (CNS) mechanisms and provides a physiologic basis for the role of psychological factors in chronic pain.

The GCT contradicts the notion that pain is *either* somatic *or* psychogenic. Instead, it postulates that both factors have potentiating and moderating effects. According to this theory, both the central and peripheral nervous systems interact to contribute to the experience of pain. It is not only these physical factors that guide the brain's interpretation of painful stimuli that is at the center of this model; psychological factors (e.g., thoughts, beliefs, emotions) are also painful stimuli.

Prior to the Melzack and Wall[179] formulation of the GCT, psychological processes were largely dismissed as reactions to pain. Although the physiologic details of the GCT have been challenged,[181] it has had a substantial impact on basic research and can be credited as a source of inspiration for diverse clinical applications to control or manage pain, including neurophysiologically based procedures (e.g., neural stimulation techniques from peripheral nerves and collateral processes in the dorsal columns of the spinal cord, pharmacologic advances, behavioral treatments, and those interventions that target modification of attentional and perceptual processes involved in the pain experience).

Cognitive-Behavioral Perspective

The *cognitive-behavioral perspective*, perhaps the most commonly accepted model for the psychological treatment of individuals with chronic pain,[182,183] incorporates many of the psychological variables previously described—namely, anticipation, avoidance, and contingencies of reinforcement—but suggests that cognitive factors rather than conditioning factors are of central importance. The model suggests that conditioned reactions are largely self-activated on the basis of learned expectations rather than automatically evoked. The model proposes that behaviors and emotions are influenced by interpretations of events, and emphasis is placed on how peoples' beliefs and attitudes interact with physical, affective, and behavioral factors. It proposes that conditioned reactions are largely activated by learned *expectations* rather than automatically evoked. In other words, it is the person's information processing that results in anticipatory anxiety and avoidance. The critical factor, therefore, is that people learn to anticipate and predict events and to express appropriate reactions.[184]

From the cognitive-behavioral perspective, people with pain are viewed as having negative expectations about their own ability to control certain motor skills without pain. Moreover, people with chronic pain tend to believe they have limited ability to exert any control over their pain. Such negative, maladaptive appraisals about the situation and personal efficacy may reinforce the experience of demoralization, inactivity, and overreaction to nociceptive stimulation. These cognitive appraisals and expectations are postulated as having an effect on behavior leading to reduced efforts and activity, which may contribute to increased psychological distress (helplessness) and subsequent physical limitations. If one accepts that pain is a complex, subjective phenomenon that is uniquely experienced by each person, then knowledge about idiosyncratic beliefs, appraisals, and coping repertoires becomes critical for optimal treatment planning and for accurately evaluating treatment outcome.

People with chronic pain's beliefs, appraisals, and expectations about pain; their ability to cope; social supports; their disorder; the medicolegal system; the health care system; and their employers are all important because they may facilitate or disrupt the individuals sense of control. These factors also influence patients' investment in treatment, acceptance of responsibility, perceptions of disability, adherence to treatment recommendations, support from significant others, expectancies for treatment, and acceptance of treatment rationale.

Cognitive interpretations also affect how individuals with pain present symptoms to others, including health care providers. Overt communication of pain, suffering, and distress will enlist responses that may reinforce pain behaviors and impressions about the seriousness, severity, and uncontrollability of pain. That is, complaining of pain may induce physicians to prescribe more potent medications, order additional diagnostic tests, and, in some cases, perform surgery. Significant others may express sympathy, excuse the person with chronic pain from responsibilities, and encourage passivity, thereby fostering further physical deconditioning. It should be obvious that the cognitive-behavioral perspective integrates the operant conditioning emphasis on external reinforcement and respondent view of conditioned avoidance within the framework of information processing.

People with persistent pain often have negative expectations about their own ability and responsibility to exert any control over their pain. Moreover, they often view themselves as helpless. Such negative, maladaptive appraisals about their condition, situation, and their personal efficacy in controlling their pain and problems associated with pain reinforce their experience of demoralization, inactivity, and overreaction to nociceptive stimulation. These cognitive appraisals are posited as having an effect on behavior, leading to reduced effort, reduced perseverance in the face of difficulty, reduced activity, and increased psychological distress.

The cognitive-behavioral perspective on pain management focuses on providing the patient with techniques to gain a sense of control over the effects of pain on his or her life as well as actually modifying the affective, behavioral, cognitive, and sensory facets of the experience. Behavioral experiences help to show individuals with pain that they are capable of more than they assumed, increasing their sense of personal competence. Cognitive techniques (e.g., self-monitoring to identify relationships among thoughts, mood, and behavior, distraction using imagery, and problem solving) help to place affective, behavioral, cognitive, and sensory responses under the person's control.

The assumption is that long-term maintenance of behavioral changes will occur only if the person with pain has learned to attribute success to his or her own efforts. There are suggestions that these treatments can result in changes of beliefs about pain, coping style, and reported pain severity as well as direct behavior changes. Treatment that results in increases in perceived control over pain and decreased catastrophizing also results in decreases in pain severity and functional disability. When successful rehabilitation occurs, there is a major shift from beliefs about helplessness and passivity to resourcefulness and ability to function regardless of pain and from an illness conviction to a rehabilitation conviction.

A number of studies have attempted to identify cognitive factors that contribute to pain and disability.[178,185] These studies have consistently demonstrated that a person's attitudes, beliefs, and expectancies about his or her plight, own self, coping resources, and the health care system affect reports of pain, activity, disability, and response to treatment. For example, people respond to medical conditions in part based on their subjective ideas about illness and their symptoms. When pain is interpreted as signifying ongoing tissue damage or a progressive disease, it is likely to produce considerably more suffering and behavioral dysfunction than if it is viewed as being the result of a stable problem that is expected to improve.

Once beliefs and expectancies are formed, they become stable and rigid and relatively impervious to modification. Pain sufferers tend to avoid experiences that could invalidate their beliefs (disconfirmations) and guide their behavior in accordance with these beliefs, even in situations where these beliefs are no longer valid. It is thus essential for people with chronic pain to develop adaptive beliefs about the relationships among impairment, pain, suffering, and disability and to deemphasize the role of experienced pain in their regulation of functioning.

Distorted thinking can also contribute to the maintenance and exacerbation of pain. A particularly potent and pernicious thinking style that has been observed among people with chronic pain is catastrophizing (holding negative thoughts about one's situation and interpreting even minor problems as major catastrophes).[186] Research has indicated that people who spontaneously use more catastrophizing thoughts report more pain than those who do not catastrophize.[186]

Coping strategies, or a person's specific ways of adjusting to or minimizing pain and distress, act to alter both the perception of pain intensity and one's ability to manage or tolerate pain and continue everyday activities. Overt behavioral coping strategies include rest, medication, and use of relaxation, among others. Covert coping strategies include various means of distracting oneself from pain, reassuring oneself that the pain will diminish, seeking information, and problem solving to list some of the most prominent.

Studies have found active coping strategies (efforts to function in spite of pain or to distract oneself from pain) to be associated with adaptive functioning and passive coping strategies (depending on others for help with pain control, avoiding activities because of fear of pain/injury, self-medication, alcohol) to be related to greater pain and depression.[187] Regardless of the type of coping strategy, if people with chronic pain are instructed in the use of adaptive coping strategies, their rating of intensity of pain decreases and tolerance of pain increases.[187] Thus, the perspective on how people function and the emphasis on facilitating self-management are more important than any specific cognitive or behavioral techniques that are used to bring about change in thinking and changes in behavior.

TREATMENTS BASED ON THE COGNITIVE-BEHAVIORAL PERSPECTIVE

A detailed description of treatments based on the cognitive-behavioral perspective is beyond the scope of this chapter and can be found in many recent publications (e.g., Turk[188]). There are a number of reports supporting the efficacy of cognitive-behavioral therapy (CBT) for treating various chronic pain conditions and with children[189] as well as adults (e.g., Ehde et al.[190]). A systematic review on CBT for chronic pain based on 35 randomized clinical trials (n = 4,788 patients) suggests that the treatment had modest benefits for pain and disability and a small to moderate range of benefit for mood and catastrophizing.[191]

Biopsychosocial, Contextual Model

Although Melzack and Wall's GCT described previously introduced the role of psychological factors in the maintenance of pain symptoms, it focused primarily on the basic anatomy and neurophysiology of pain. The biopsychosocial, contextual model, which expands the cognitive-behavioral perspective of pain, views illness as a dynamic and reciprocal interaction between biologic, psychological, sociocultural, and contextual variables that shape the person's response to pain.[95,192,193] What is unique about the perspective is that it takes into consideration the influence of higher order cognitions, including perception and appraisal and the environmental context in which these appraisals take place. It accepts that people are active processors of information and that behavior, emotions, and even physiology are influenced by interpretations of events rather than solely by physiologic factors.[95,192,193] People with chronic pain may therefore have negative expectations about their own ability and responsibility to exert any control over their pain. Moreover, behaviors of people with pain elicit responses from significant others that can reinforce both adaptive and maladaptive modes of thinking, feeling, and behaving.

Loeser[194] originally formulated a general model that delineated four dimensions associated with the concept of pain: nociception, the stimulation of nerves that convey information about possible tissue damage to the brain; pain, the subjective perception that is the result of transduction, transmission, and modulation of sensory information; suffering, the emotional responses that are triggered by nociception or some other aversive event associated with it, such as fear or depression; and pain behavior, those things that people do when they are suffering or in pain, such as avoiding activities or exercise for fear of (re) injury. Subsequently, Waddell[195] emphasized that pain cannot be comprehensively evaluated without an understanding of the individual who is exposed to the nociception. Waddell[195] also made a comparison between Loeser's[196] model of pain and the earlier discussed call by Engel[159] of the need for a new, more biopsychosocial model in medicine. Engel[159] proposed the important dimensions of the physical problem, distress, illness behavior, and the sick role, which correspond to Loeser's[196] dimensions of nociception, pain, suffering, and pain behavior, respectively. Thus, with this general perspective, a diversity of pain or illness can be expected (including its severity, duration, and psychosocial consequences). In order to fully understand a person's perception and response to pain and illness, the interrelationships among biologic changes, psychological status, and the sociocultural context all need to be considered. Any model that focuses on only one of these dimensions will be incomplete.

Families and Family Systems Perspective

In *family systems* (and this could be expanded to significant others and not only traditional conceptualizations of nuclear families), the family is viewed as an interactional unit, and family members profoundly impact each other's emotions, thoughts, and behaviors. Thus, the functioning of family members is interdependent, and family relationships are an important factor not only in psychological but also physical health.[197,198]

Increasingly, evidence supports family members contribute to behavioral risk factors to the development of numerous chronic illnesses such as smoking, lack of exercise, and poor diet.[198] Additionally, families influence the development and maintenance of chronic pain (e.g., Cano et al.[199]). One mechanisms that has been shown to be important is chronic pain is based on operant theory.[131,200] For example, expressions of acute pain (reporting pain, grimacing, avoidance of activity, and use of pain medication), because they are overt and observable, may be reinforced through expressions of concern from family members. Furthermore, in support of this idea, a number of investigators (e.g., Thieme et al.[174]) have found that spousal attentiveness to expressions of pain was positively correlated with higher levels of reported pain, pain behavior frequency, and disability. However, social interaction may not always be viewed negatively and may be important in building intimacy serving as a positive support for a person with pain who is distressed.[201] Marital satisfaction has also been identified as an important mediator of disability associated with chronic pain.[202]

The experience of chronic stress within the family has also been hypothesized to contribute to the development of chronic illness.[203] Specifically, chronic stress within the family may play an important role in sympathetic nervous system and endocrine dysregulation often found in chronic pain patients.

As noted previously, pain does not take place in isolation but in a social context. Pain does not occur solely in people's bodies, nor does it occur solely in their brains, but, rather, it occurs in their lives. The emphasis on the role of significant others is important, as it reminds us that to successfully treat chronic pain patients requires that we not only assess and treat the patient but must also target significant others that can either impede or facilitate rehabilitation.[204]

Conclusion

For the person experiencing chronic pain, there is a continuing quest for relief that often remains elusive, leading to feelings of helplessness, hopelessness, and outright depression. Emotional distress may be attributed to a variety of factors, including inadequate or maladaptive coping resources, iatrogenic complications, overuse of medication, disability, financial difficulties, litigation, disruption of usual activities, lack of social support, and sleep disturbance. Thus, chronic pain is a demoralizing situation that confronts the person not only with the stress created by pain but also with a cascade of ongoing stressors that compromise all aspects of the life of the sufferer. Living with chronic pain requires considerable emotional resilience and tends to deplete emotional reserve and taxes not only the individual experiencing chronic pain but also the capacity of significant others to provide support.

There is a large body of evidence to demonstrate that psychological factors can interfere with or hinder a person's ability to cope with the pain experience. As a result, psychological intervention in the assessment and treatment of chronic pain is becoming standard practice. Psychological treatments can focus on the emotional distress that accompanies chronic pain and provide education and training in the use of cognitive and behavioral techniques that may reduce perceptions of pain and related disability. Psychologists and psychological principles have played a major role in the understanding and treatment of people with pain, and psychologists have an important function in interdisciplinary pain rehabilitation programs (IPRPs) as clinicians and researchers.

None of the psychological treatments described are successful in eliminating pain completely; in fact, the same statement can be made in reference to the most commonly used pharmacologic, medical, and surgical interventions.[1] Consequently, the majority of people have to adapt to the presence of chronic pain and learn self-management in the face of persistent pain and accompanying symptoms. The various psychological interventions described in this chapter provide a general overview of different treatment strategies. By far, however, treatment with CBT alone or within the context of an IPRP holds the greatest empirical evidence for success. There is a substantial and overwhelming body of research supporting the effectiveness of various psychological approaches. At point, it seems prudent to consider the use of psychological treatments in combination with traditional medical interventions.

References

1. Turk DC, Wilson HD, Cahana A. Treatment of chronic noncancer pain. *Lancet* 2011;377:2226–2235.
2. Okifuji A, Turk DC. Assessment of patients with chronic pain with and without mental health problems. In: Machard S, Gaumond I, Saravane D, eds. *Mental Health and Pain.* New York: Springer; 2014:227–259.
3. Turk DC, Fillingim RB, Ohrbach R, et al. Assessment of psychosocial and functional impact of chronic pain. *J Pain* 2016;17(9)(suppl 2):T21–T49.
4. Skinner MS, Wilson HD, Turk DC. Cognitive-behavioral perspective and cognitive-behavioral therapy for people with chronic pain: distinctions, outcomes, and innovations. *J Cogn Psychother* 2012;26:93–113.
5. Watson D, Clark LA, Harkness AR. Structures of personality and their relevance to psychopathology. *J Abnorm Psychol* 1994;103:18–31.
6. Stegen K, Van Diest I, Van de Woestijne KP, et al. Negative affectivity and bodily sensations induced by 5.5% CO-sub-2 enriched air inhalation: is there a bias to interpret bodily sensations negatively in persons with negative affect? *Psychol Heath* 2000;15:513–525.
7. Stegen K, Van Diest I, Van de Woestijne KP, et al. Do persons with negative affect have an attentional bias to bodily sensations? *Cogn Emot* 2001;15:813–829.
8. Fillingim RB, Hastie BA, Ness TJ, et al. Sex-related psychological predictors of baseline pain perception and analgesic responses to pentazocine. *Biol Psychol* 2005;69:97–112.
9. Reiss S, Peterson RA, Gursky DM, et al. Anxiety sensitivity, anxiety frequency and the predictions of fearfulness. *Behav Res Ther* 1986;24:1–8.
10. Asmundson GJG, Wright KD, Hadjistavropoulos HD. Anxiety sensitivity and disabling chronic health conditions: state of the art and future directions. *Scand J Behav Ther* 2000;29:100–117.
11. Keogh E, Asmundson GJG. Negative affectivity, catastrophizing and anxiety sensitivity. In: Asmundson GJG, Vlaeyen JWS, Crombez G, eds. *Understanding and Treating Fear of Pain.* Oxford, NY: Oxford University Press; 2004:91–115.
12. Asmundson GJG, Taylor S. Role of anxiety sensitivity in pain-related fear and avoidance. *J Behav Med* 1996;19:577–586.
13. Keogh E, Hamid R, Hamid S, et al. Investigating the effect of anxiety sensitivity, gender and negative interpretative bias on the perception of chest pain. *Pain* 2004;111:209–217.
14. Vlaeyen JW, Linton SJ. Fear-avoidance and its consequences in chronic musculoskeletal pain: a state of the art. *Pain* 2000;85:317–332.
15. Friborg O, Hjemdal O, Rosenvinge JH, et al. Resilience as a moderator of pain and stress. *J Psychosom Res* 2006;61:213–219.
16. Hassett AL, Finan PH. The role of resilience in the clinical management of chronic pain. *Curr Pain Headache Rep* 2016;20:39.
17. Ruiz-Parraga GT, Lopez-Martinez AE, Esteve R, et al. A confirmatory factor analysis of the Resilience Scale adapted to chronic pain (RS-18): new empirical evidence of the protective role of resilience on pain adjustment. *Qual Life Res* 2015;24:1245–1253.
18. Sturgeon J, Zautra AJ. Resilience: a new paradigm for adaptation to chronic pain. *Curr Pain Headache Rep* 2010;14:105–112.
19. Yeung EW, Arewasikporn A, Zautra AJ. Resilience and chronic pain. *J Soc Clin Psychol* 2012;31:593–617.
20. Carver CS, Scheier MF, Segerstrom SC. Optimism. *Clin Psychol Rev* 2010;30:879–889.
21. Hansen MM, Peters ML, Vlaeyen JW, et al. Optimism lowers pain: evidence of the causal status and underlying mechanisms. *Pain* 2013;154:53–58.
22. Hetmann F, Kiongsgaard UE, Sandvik I, et al. Prevalence and predictors of persistent post-surgical pain 12 months after thoracotomy. *Acta Anaesth Scand* 2015;59:740–748.
23. Rasmussen HN, Scheier MF, Greenhouse JB. Optimism and physical health: a meta-analysis. *Ann Behav Med* 2009;37:239–256.
24. Novy DM. Psychological approaches for managing chronic pain. *J Psychopathol Behav Assess* 2004;26:279–288.
25. Affleck G, Tennen H. Construing benefits from adversity: adaptational significance and dispositional underpinnings. *J Pers* 1996;64:899–922.
26. Treharne GJ, Kitas GD, Lyons AC, et al. Well-being in rheumatoid arthritis: the effects of disease duration and psychosocial factors. *J Health Psychol* 2005;10:457–474.
27. Goodin BR, Bulls HW. Optimism and the experience of pain: benefits of seeing the glass as half full. *Curr Pain Headache Rep* 2013;17:1–9.
28. Snyder CR, Rand KL, Sigmond DR. Hope theory: a member of the positive psychology family. In: Snyder CR, Lopez SJ, eds. *Handbook of Positive Psychology.* Oxford, United Kingdom: Oxford University Press; 2005:257–276.
29. McCracken LM, Morley S. The psychological flexibility model: a basis for integration and progress in psychological approaches to chronic pain management. *J Pain* 2014;15:221–234.
30. Trompetter HR, Bohlmeijer ET, Fox JP, et al. Psychological flexibility and catastrophizing as associated change mechanisms during online Acceptance & Commitment Therapy for chronic pain. *Behav Res Ther* 2015;74:50–59.
31. Karsdorp PA, Ranson S, Nijst S, et al. Goals, mood and performance duration on cognitive tasks during experimentally induced mechanical pressure pain. *J Behav Ther Exper Psychiat* 2013;44:240–247.
32. Yeung EW, Davis MC, Aiken LS, et al. Daily social enjoyment interrupts the cycle of same-day and next-day fatigue in women with fibromyalgia. *Ann Behav Med* 2015;49:411–419.
33. Garland EL, Gaylord SA, Palsson O, et al. Therapeutic mechanisms of a mindfulness-based treatment for IBS: effects on visceral sensitivity, catastrophizing, and affective processing of pain sensations. *J Behav Med* 2012;35:591–602.
34. Park SH, Sonty N. Positive affect mediates the relationship between pain-related coping efficacy and interference in social functioning. *J Pain* 2010;11:1267–1273.
35. White DK, Keysor JJ, Neogi T, et al. When it hurts, a positive attitude may help: association of positive affect with daily walking in knee osteoarthritis. Results from a multicenter longitudinal cohort study. *Arthritis Care Res* 2012;64:1312–1319.
36. Lazarus RS, Folkman S. *Stress, appraisal, and coping.* New York: Springer; 1984.
37. Smith WB, Gracely RH, Safer MA. The meaning of pain: cancer patients' rating and recall of pain intensity and affect. *Pain* 1998;78:123–129.
38. Arntz A, Claassens L. The meaning of pain influences its experienced pain intensity. *Pain* 2004;109:20–25.
39. Jackson JT, Wang Y, Fan H. Associations between pain appraisals and outcomes: meta-analysis of laboratory and chronic pain literatures. *J Pain* 2014;15:586–601.
40. Turner JA, Jensen MP, Romano JM. Do beliefs, coping, and catastrophizing independently predict functioning in patients with chronic pain? *Pain* 2000;85:115–125.
41. Jensen MP, Turner JA, Romano JM, et al. Relationship of pain-specific beliefs to chronic pain adjustment. *Pain* 1994;57:301–309.
42. Balderson BH, Lin EH, Von Korff M. The management of pain-related fear in primary care. In: Asmundson GJG, Vlaeyen JWS, Crombez G, eds. *Understanding and Treating Fear of Pain.* Oxford, United Kingdom: Oxford University Press; 2004:267–292.
43. Ihlebaek C, Erikson HR. Are the "myths" of low back pain alive in the general Norwegian population? *Scand J Public Health* 2003;31:395–398.
44. Quartana PJ, Campbell CM, Edwards RR. Pain catastrophizing: a critical review. *Expert Rev Neurother* 2009;9:745–758.
45. Arnow BA, Blasey CM, Constantino MJ, et al. Catastrophizing, depression and pain-related disability. *Gen Hosp Psychiat* 2011;33:150–156.
46. Parr JJ, Borsa PA, Fillingim RB, et al. Pain-related fear and catastrophizing predict pain intensity and disability independently using an induced muscle injury model. *J Pain* 2012;13:370–376.
47. Picavet HS, Vlaeyen JWS, Schouten JS. Pain catastrophizing and kinesiophobia: predictors of chronic low back pain. *Am J Epidemiol* 2002;156:1028–1034.
48. Severeijns R, Vlaeyen JWS, van den Hout MA, et al. Pain catastrophizing and consequences of musculoskeletal pain: a prospective study in the Dutch community. *J Pain* 2005;6:125–132.
49. Linton SJ. A review of psychological risk factors in back and neck pain. *Spine* 2000;25:1148–1156.
50. Katz J, Buis T, Cohen L. Locked out and still knocking: predictors of excessive demands for postoperative intravenous patient-controlled analgesia. *Can J Anaesth* 2008;55:88–99.
51. Khan RS, Ahmed K, Blakeway E, et al. Catastrophizing: a predictive factor for postoperative pain. *Am J Surg* 2011;201:122–131.
52. Theunissen M, Peters ML, Bruce J, et al. Preoperative anxiety and catastrophizing. A systematic review and meta-analysis of the association with chronic postsurgical pain. *Clin J Pain* 2012;28:819–841.
53. Kapoor SH, White J, Thorn BE, et al. Patients presenting to the emergency department with acute pain: the significant role of pain catastrophizing and state anxiety. *Pain Med* 2016;17:1069–1078.
54. Edwards RR, Smith MT, Stonerock G, et al. Pain-related catastrophizing in healthy women is associated with greater temporal summation of and reduced habituation to thermal pain. *Clin J Pain* 2006;22:730–737.
55. Buitenhuis J, de Jong, PJ, Jaspers JP, et al. Catastrophizing and causal beliefs in whiplash. *Spine* 2008;33:2427–2433.
56. Menendez ME, Baker DK, Oladeji LO, et al. Psychological distress is associated with perceived disability and pain in patients presenting to a shoulder clinic. *J Bone Jt Surg Am* 2015;97:1999–2003.

57. Kjogx H, Kasch H, Zachariae R, et al. Experimental manipulations of pain catastrophizing influence pain levels in patients with chronic pain and healthy volunteers. *Pain* 2016;157:1287–1296.

58. Martel M, Trost Z, Sullivan MJ. The expression of pain behaviors in high catastrophizers: the influence of automatic and controlled processes. *J Pain* 2012;13:808–815.

59. Lu Q, Tsao JC, Myers CD, et al. Coping predictors of children's laboratory-induced pain tolerance, intensity, and unpleasantness. *J Pain* 2007;8:708–717.

60. Wertli MM, Eugster R, Heid U, et al. Catastrophizing—a prognostic factor for outcome in patients with low back pain: a systematic review. *Spine J* 2014;14:2639–2657.

61. Moore E, Thibault P, Adams H, et al. Catastrophizing and pain-related fear predict failure to maintain treatment gains following participation in a pain rehabilitation program. *Pain Rep* 2016;1:e567.

62. Gracely RH, Geisser ME, Giesecke T, et al. Pain catastrophizing and neural responses to pain among persons with fibromyalgia. *Brain* 2004;127:835–843.

63. Kucyi A, Moayedi M, Weisman-Fogel I, et al. Enhanced medial prefrontal-default mode network functional connectivity in chronic pain and its association with pain rumination. *J Neuroscience* 2014;34:3969–3975.

64. Seminowicz DA, Davis KD. Cortical responses to pain in healthy individuals depends on pain catastrophizing. *Pain* 2006;120:297–306.

65. Goodin BR, McGuire L, Allshouse M, et al. Associations between catastrophizing and endogenous pain-inhibitory processes: sex differences. *J Pain* 2009;10:180–190.

66. Weissman-Fogel I, Sprecher E, Pud D. Effects of catastrophizing on pain perception and pain modulation. *Exp Brain Res* 2008;186:79–85.

67. Grosen K, Vase L. Pilegaard JK, et al. Condition pain modulation and situation pain catastrophizing as preoperative predictors of pain following chest wall surgery: a prospective observation cohort study. *PLoS One* 2014;9:e90185.

68. Edwards RR, Kronfli T, Haythornthwaite JA, et al. Association of catastrophizing with interleukin-6 responses in acute pain. *Pain* 2008;140:135–144.

69. Quartana PJ, Buenaver LF, Edwards RR, et al. Pain catastrophizing and salivary cortisol responses to laboratory pain testing in temporomandibular disorder and healthy controls. *J Pain* 2013;11:186–194.

70. Asmundson GJ, Norton PJ, Vlaeyen JW. Fear-avoidance models of chronic pain: an overview. In: Asmundson GJ, Vlaeyen JW, Crombez G, eds. *Understanding and Treating Fear of Pain*. Oxford, United Kingdom: Oxford University Press; 2004:3–24.

71. Fritz JM, George SZ, Delitto A. The role of fear-avoidance beliefs in acute low back pain: relationships with current and future disability and work status. *Pain* 2001;94:7–15.

72. Boersma K, Linton SJ. Screening to identify patients at risk: profiles of psychological risk factors for early intervention. *Clin J Pain* 2005;21:38–43, 69–72.

73. Buer N, Linton SJ. Fear-avoidance beliefs and catastrophizing: occurrence and risk factor in back pain and ADL in the general population. *Pain* 2002;99:485–491.

74. Bailey KM, Carelton RN, Vlaeyen JW. Treatments addressing pain-related fear and anxiety in chronic musculoskeletal pain: a preliminary review. *Cogn Behav Ther* 2010;39:46–63.

75. Houben RM, Vlaeyen JWS, Peters ML, et al. Health care providers' attitudes and beliefs towards common low back pain: factor structure and psychometric properties of the HC-PAIRS. *Clin J Pain* 2004;20:37–44.

76. Houben RM, Ostelo RW, Vlaeyen JWS, et al. Health care providers' orientations towards common low back pain predict perceived harmfulness of physical activities and recommendations regarding return to normal activity. *Eur J Pain* 2005;9:173–183.

77. Linton SJ, Vlaeyen J, Ostelo R. The back pain beliefs of health care providers: are we fear-avoidant. *J Occup Rehabil* 2002;12:223–232.

78. Werner EL, Ihlebaek C, Skouen JS, et al. Beliefs about low back pain in the Norwegian general population: are they related to pain experiences and health professionals? *Spine* 2005;30:1770–1776.

79. Arntz A, Schmidt AJM. Perceived control and the experience of pain intensity. In: Steptoe A, Appels A, eds. *Stress, Personal Control and Health*. Oxford, United Kingdom: John Wiley & Sons; 1989:20–25.

80. Jensen MP, Karoly P. Control beliefs, coping efforts, and adjustment to chronic pain. *J Consult Clin Psychol* 1991;59:431–438.

81. Jensen MP, Turner JA, Romano JM. Changes in beliefs, catastrophizing, and coping are associated with improvement in multidisciplinary pain treatment. *J Consult Clin Psychol* 2001;69:655–662.

82. Spinhoven P, ter Kuile MM. Treatment outcome expectancies and hypnotic susceptibility as moderators of pain reduction in patients with chronic tension-type headache. *Int J Clin Exp Hypn* 2000;48:290–305.

83. Tan G, Jensen MP, Robinson-Whelen S, et al. Measuring control appraisals in chronic pain. *J Pain* 2002;3:385–393.

84. Bandura A. Self-efficacy: toward a unifying theory of behavioral change. *Psychol Rev* 1977;84:191–215.

85. Bandura A, O'Leary A, Taylor CB, et al. Perceived self-efficacy and pain control: opioid and nonopioid mechanisms. *J Pers Soc Psychol* 1987;53:563–571.

86. Keefe FJ, Lefebvre JC, Maixner W, et al. Self-efficacy for arthritis pain: relationship to perception of thermal laboratory pain stimuli. *Arthritis Care Res* 1997;10:177–184.

87. Benyon K, Hill S, Zadurian N, et al. Coping strategies and self-efficacy as predictors of outcome in osteoarthritis: a systematic review. *Musculoskel Care* 2010;8:224–236.

88. Sardá J Jr, Nicholas MK, Asghari A, et al. The contribution of self-efficacy and depression to disability and work status in chronic pain patients: a comparison between Australian and Brazilian samples. *Eur J Pain* 2009;13:189–195.

89. Riddle DL, Wade JB, Jiranek WA, et al. Preoperative pain catastrophizing predicts pain outcome after knee arthroplasty. *Clin Orthoped* 2010;468:798–806.

90. Abbott AD, Tyni-Lenne R, Hedlund R. The influence of psychological factors on pre-operative levels of pain intensity, disability and health related quality of life in lumbar spinal fusion patients. *Physiotherapy* 2010;98:213–221.

91. Dohnke B, Knäuper B, Muller-Fahrnow W. Perceived self-efficacy gained from, and health effects of, a rehabilitation program after hip joint replacement. *Arthritis Rheum* 2005;53:585–592.

92. Orbell S, Johnston M, Rowley D, et al. Self-efficacy and goal importance in the prediction of physical disability in people following hospitalization: a prospective study. *Br J Health Psychol* 2001;6:25–40.

93. Heye ML, Foster L, Bartlett MK, et al. A preoperative intervention for pain reduction, improved mobility, and self-efficacy. *Appl Nurs Res* 2002;15:174–183.

94. Weisenberg M. Cognitive aspects of pain and pain control. *Int J Clin Exp Hypn* 1998;46:44–61.

95. Flor H, Turk DC. *Chronic Pain: An Integrated Biobehavioral Perspective.* Seattle, WA: IASP Press; 2011.

96. Ip HY, Abrishami A, Peng PW, et al. Predictors of postoperative pain and analgesic consumption: a qualitative systematic review. *Anesthesiology* 2009;111:657–677.

97. Samwel HJ, Evers AW, Crul BJ, et al. The role of helplessness, fear of pain and passive pain-coping in chronic pain patients. *Clin J Pain* 2006;22:245–251.

98. Broderick JE, Keefe FJ, Schneider ST, et al. Cognitive behavioral therapy for chronic pain is effective, but for whom? *Pain* 2016;157:2115–2123.

99. LaGraize SC, Borzan J, Rinker MM, et al. Behavioral evidence for competing motivational drives of nociception and hunger. *Neurosci Lett* 2004;372:30–34.

100. Selye H. *Stress.* Montreal, Canada: Acta Medical Publisher; 1950.

101. McBeth J, Chiu YH, Silman AJ, et al. Hypothalamic-pituitary-adrenal stress axis function and the relationship with chronic widespread pain and its antecedents. *Arthritis Res Ther* 2005;7:R992–R1000.

102. McLean SA, Williams DA, Harris RE, et al. Momentary relationship between cortisol secretion and symptoms in patients with fibromyalgia. *Arthritis Rheum* 2005;52:3660–3669.

103. Melzack R. Evolution of the neuromatrix theory of pain. *Pain Pract* 2005;5:85–94.

104. Merskey H. Classification of chronic pain. Descriptions of chronic pain syndromes and definitions of pain terms. Prepared by the International Association for the Study of Pain, Subcommittee on Taxonomy. *Pain Suppl* 1986;3:S1–S226.

105. Gatchel RJ, Peng YB, Peters ML, et al. The biopsychosocial approach to chronic pain: scientific advances and future directions. *Psychol Bull* 2007;133:581–624.

106. Burns JW, Bruehl S, Quartana P. Anger management style and hostility among patients with chronic pain: effects on symptom-specific physiological reactivity during anger- and sadness-recall interviews. *Psychosom Med* 2006;68:786–793.

107. Burns JW, Quartana PJ, Bruehl S. Anger inhibition and pain: evidence and new directions. *J Behav Med* 2008;31:259–279.

108. Burns JW, Gerhart JI, Bruehl S, et al. Anger arousal and behavioral anger regulation in everyday life among people with chronic low back pain: relationships with spouses and negative affect. *Health Psychol* 2015;34:547–555.

109. Davis MC, Zautra AJ, Reich JW. Vulnerability to stress among women in chronic pain from fibromyalgia and osteoarthritis. *Ann Behav Med* 2001;23:215–226.

110. Fernandez E, Turk DC. Sensory and affective components of pain: separation and synthesis. *Psychol Bull* 1992;112:205–217.

111. DeGroot KI, Boeke S, van den Berg HJ, et al. Assessing short- and long-term recovery from lumbar surgery with pre-operative biographical, medical and psychological variables. *Br J Health Psychol* 1997;2:229–243.

112. Pavlin DJ, Rapp SE, Pollisar N. Factors affecting discharge time in adult outpatients. *Anesth Analg* 1998;87:816–826.

113. Asmundson GJG. Anxiety sensitivity and chronic pain: empirical findings, clinical implications, and future directions. In: Taylor S, ed. *Anxiety Sensitivity: Theory, Research, and Treatment of the Fear of Anxiety.* Mahwah, NJ: Lawrence Erlbaum Associates; 1999:269–285.

114. Kerns RD, Haythornthwaite JA. Depression among chronic pain patients: cognitive-behavioral analysis and effect on rehabilitation outcome. *J Consult Clin Psychol* 1988;56:870–876.

115. Finan P, Garland EL. The role of positive affect in chronic pain and its treatment. *Clin J Pain* 2015;31:177–187.

116. Wolfe F, Smythe HA, Yunnus MB, et al. The American College of Rheumatology 1990 criteria for the classification of fibromyalgia. Report of the Multicenter Criteria Committee. *Arthritis Rheum* 1990;33:160–172.

117. Pederson T. Anxiety symptoms often accompany chronic pain. Available at: https://psychcentral.com/news/2013/05/11/anxiety-symptoms-often-accompany-chronic-pain/54716.html. Accessed July 13, 2017.

118. Roy-Byrne PP, Davidson KW, Kessler RC, et al. Anxiety disorders and co-morbid medical illness. *Gen Hosp Psychiat* 2008;30:208–225.

119. Kuch KM, Evans RJ, Watson PC, et al. Road vehicle accidents and phobias in 60 patients with fibromyalgia. *J Anxiety Dis* 1991;5:273–280.

120. Feurstein M, Beattie P. Biobehavioral factors affecting pain and disability in low back pain: mechanisms and assessment. *Phys Ther* 1995;75:267–280.

121. Vlaeyen JW, Seelen HA, Peters M, et al. Fear of movement/(re)injury and muscular reactivity in chronic low back pain patients: an experimental investigation. *Pain* 1999;82:297–304.

122. Lenthem J, Slade PD, Troup JD, et al. Outline of a fear-avoidance model of exaggerated pain perception. *Behav Res Ther* 1983;21:401–408.

123. Vlaeyen JW, Kole-Snijders AM, Boeren RG, et al. Fear of movement/(re)injury in chronic low back pain and its relation to behavioral performance. *Pain* 1995;62:363–372.

124. McCracken LM, Gross RT, Sorg PJ, et al. Prediction of pain in patients with chronic low back pain: effects of inaccurate prediction and pain-related anxiety. *Behav Res Ther* 1993;31:647–652.

125. Crombez G, Vlaeyen JWS, Heuts PH. Pain-related fear is more disabling than pain itself: evidence of the role of pain-related fear in chronic back pain disability. *Pain* 1999;80:329–339.

126. Turk DC. Understanding pain sufferers: the role of cognitive processes. *Spine J* 2004;4:1–7.

127. Vlaeyen JWS, Kole-Snijders AM, Rooteveel A, et al. The role of fear/(re)injury in pain disability. *J Occupat Rehabil* 1995;5:235–252.

128. Asmundson GJG, Norton PJ, Norton GR. Beyond pain: the role of fear and avoidance in chronicity. *Clin Psychol Rev* 1999;19:97–119.

129. Vlaeyen JW, Crombez G. Fear of movement/(re)injury, avoidance, and pain disability in chronic low back pain patients. *Manl Ther* 1999;4:187–195.

130. Banks SM, Kerns RD. Explaining high rates of depression in chronic pain: a diathesis-stress framework. *Psychol Bull* 1996;119:95–110.

131. Romano JM, Turner JA, Jensen MP, et al. Chronic pain patient–spouse behavioral interactions predict patient disability. *Pain* 1995;63:353–360.

132. Surah A, Baranidharan G, Morley S. Chronic pain and depression. *Contin Educ Anaesth Crit Care Pain* 2014;14:85–89.

133. Atkinson JH, Slater MA, Patterson TL, et al. Prevalence, onset, and risk of psychiatric disorders in men with chronic low back pain: a controlled study. *Pain* 1991;45:111–121.

134. Magni G, Mreschi C, Rigatti Luchinie S, et al. Prospective study on the relationship between depressive symptoms and chronic musculoskeletal pain. *Pain* 1994;56:289–297.

135. Rudy TE, Kerns RD, Turk DC. Chronic pain and depression: toward a cognitive-behavioral mediational model. *Pain* 1988;35:129–140.

136. Brown GK. A causal analysis of chronic pain and depression. *J Abnorm Psychol* 1990;99:127–137.

137. Carragee EJ, Alamin TF, Miller JL, et al. Discographic, MRI and psychosocial determinants of low back pain disability and remission: a prospective study in subjects with benign persistent back pain. *Spine J* 2005;5:24–35.

138. Jarvik JG, Hollingworth W, Heagerty PJ, et al. Three-year incidence of low back pain in an initially asymptomatic cohort. Clinical and imaging risk factors. *Spine* 2005;30:1541–1548.

139. Van Korff MJ, Simon G. The relationship between pain and depression. *Br J Psychiat* 1996;168(suppl 30):101–108.

140. Turk DC, Okifuji A, Scharff L. Chronic pain and depression: role of perceived impact and perceived control in different age cohorts. *Pain* 1995;61:93–101.

141. Schwartz L, Slater MA, Birchler G, et al. Depression in spouses of chronic pain patients: the role of patient pain and anger, and marital satisfaction. *Pain* 1991;44:61–67.

142. Corbishley M, Hendrickson R, Beutler L, et al. Behavior, affect, and cognition among psychogenic pain patients in group expressive psychotherapy. *J Pain Symptom Manage* 1990;5:241–248.

143. Okifuji A, Turk DC, Curran SL. Evaluation of the relationship between depression and fibromyalgia syndrome: why aren't all patients depressed? *J Rheumatol* 1999;27:212–219.

144. Wade JB, Price DD, Hamer RM, et al. An emotional component analysis of chronic pain. *Pain* 1990;40:303–310.

145. Fernandez E, Milburn TW. Sensory and affective predictors of overall pain and emotions associated with affective pain. *Clin J Pain* 1994;10:3–9.

146. Duckro PN, Chibnall JT, Tomazic TJ. Anger, depression, and disability: a path analysis of relationships in a sample of chronic posttraumatic headache patients. *Headache* 1995;35:7–9.

147. Kinder BN, Curtiss G, Kalichman S. Affective differences among empirically derived subgroups of headache patients. *J Pers Assess* 1992;58:516–524.

148. Fromm-Reichman F. Contributions to the psychogenesis of migraine. *Psychoanalytic Rev* 1937;24:26–35.

149. Fernandez E, Turk DC. The scope and significance of anger in the experience of chronic pain. *Pain* 1995;61:165–175.

150. Berkowitz L, Thomas P. Pain expectation, negative affect, and angry aggression. *Motivation Emot* 1987;11:183–193.

151. Arena J, Blanchard E, Andrasik F. The role of affect in the etiology of chronic headache. *J Psychosom Res* 1984;28:79–86.

152. Kerns RD, Rosenberg R, Jacob MC. Anger expression and chronic pain. *J Behav Med* 1994;17:57–67.

153. Tschannen TA, Duckro PN, Margolis RB, et al. The relationship of anger, depression, and perceived disability among headache patients. *Headache* 1992;32:501–503.

154. Braha R, Catchlove R. Pain and anger: inadequate expression in chronic pain patients. *Pain Clinic* 1985;1:125–129.

155. Summers JD, Rapoff MA, Varghese G, et al. Psychosocial factors in chronic spinal cord injury pain. *Pain* 1991;47:183–189.

156. Burns JW, Johnson BJ, Devine J, et al. Anger management style and the prediction of treatment outcome among male and female chronic pain patients. *Behav Res Ther* 1998;36:1055–1062.

157. Burns JW. Anger management style and hostility: predicting symptom-specific physiological reactivity among chronic low back pain patients *J Behav Med* 1997;20:505–522.

158. Cacioppo JT, Berston GG, Klein DJ, et al. The psychophysiology of emotion across the lifespan. *Ann Rev Gerontol Geriatrics* 1997;17:27–74.

159. Engel GL. Psychogenic pain and the pain-prone patient. *Am J Med* 1959;26:899–918.

160. Frischenschlager O, Pucher I. Psychological management of pain. *Disabil Rehabil* 2002;24:416–422.

161. Davis DA, Luecken LJ, Zautra AJ. Are reports of childhood abuse related to the experience of chronic pain in adulthood? A meta-analytic review of the literature. *Clin J Pain* 2005;21:398–405.

162. Basler SC, Grzesiak RC, Dworkin RH. Integrating relational psychodynamic and action-oriented psychotherapies: treating pain and suffering. In: Turk DC, Gatchel RJ, eds. *Psychological Approaches to Pain Management: A Practitioner's Handbook.* 2nd ed. New York: Guilford; 2001:94–127.

163. Turk DC, Swanson K, Tunks E. Psychological approaches in the treatment of chronic pain patients—when pills, scalpels, and needles are not enough. *Can J Psychiatry* 2008;53:213–223.

164. Okifuji A, Turk DC, Sherman JJ. Evaluation of the relationship between depression and fibromyalgia syndrome: why aren't all patients depressed? *J Rheumatol* 2000;27:212–219.

165. Wallis BJ, Lord SM, Bogduk N. Resolution of psychological distress of whiplash patients following treatment by radiofrequency neurotomy: a randomised, double-blind, placebo-controlled trial. *Pain* 1997;73:15–22.

166. Sullivan M, Turk DC. Psychiatric disorders and psychogenic pain. In: Loeser JD, Butler SR, Chapman CR, et al., eds. *Bonica's Management of Pain.* 3rd ed. Baltimore, MD: Williams & Wilkins; 2001;483–500.

167. Fordyce WE. *Behavioral Methods for Chronic Pain and Illness.* St. Louis, MO: Mosby; 1976.

168. Main CJ, Keefe FJ, Jensen M, et al, eds. *Fordyce's Behavioral Methods for Chronic Pain and Illness.* Washington, DC: IASP Press; 2015.

169. Becker S, Kleinbohl D, Klossika I, et al. Operant conditioning of enhanced pain sensitivity by heat-pain titration. *Pain* 2008;140:104–114.

170. Block A, Kremer EF, Gaylor M. Behavioral treatment of chronic pain: the spouse as a discriminative cue for pain behavior. *Pain* 1980;9:243–252.

171. Doleys DM, Crocker M, Patton D. Response of patients with chronic pain to exercise quotas. *Phys Ther* 1982;62:1111–1114.

172. Lousberg R, Schmidt AJM, Groenman NH. The relationship between spouse solicitousness and pain behavior: searching for more experimental evidence. *Pain* 1992;51:75–79.

173. Romano JM, Turner JA, Friedman LS, et al. Sequential analysis of chronic pain behaviors and spouse responses. *J Consult Clin Psychol* 1992;50:777–782.

174. Thieme K, Gromnica-Ihle W, Flor H. Operant behavioral treatment of fibromyalgia: a controlled study. *Arthritis Reum* 2003;49:314–320.

175. Thieme K, Turk DC, Flor H. Responder criteria for operant and cognitive-behavioral treatment of fibromyalgia syndrome. *Arthritis Care Res* 2007;57:830–836.

176. Richard K. The occurrence of maladaptive health-related behaviors and teacher-related conduct problems in children of chronic low back pain patients. *J Behav Med* 1988;11:107–116.

177. Vaughan KB, Lanzetta JT. Vicarious instigation and conditioning of facial expressive and autonomic responses to a model's expressive display of pain. *J Pers Soc Psychol* 1980;38:909–923.

178. Turk DC. Cognitive-behavioral approach to the treatment of chronic pain patients. *Reg Anesth Pain Med* 2003;28:573–579.

179. Melzack R, Wall PD. Pain mechanisms: a new theory. *Science* 1965;150:971–979.

180. Melzack R, Casey KL. Sensory, motivational, and central control determinants of pain: a new conceptual model. In: Kenshalo D, ed. *The Skin Senses.* Springfield, IL: Charles C. Thomas Publishers; 1968:423–443.

181. Dickenson AH, Matthews EA, Suzuki R. Neurobiology of neuropathic pain: mode of action of anticonvulsants. *Eur J Pain* 2002;6(suppl A):51–60.

182. Morley S, Eccleston C, Williams A. Systematic review and meta-analysis of randomized controlled trials of cognitive behaviour therapy and behaviour therapy for chronic pain in adults, excluding headache. *Pain* 1999;80:1–13.

183. Turk DC, Meichenbaum D, Genest M. *Pain and Behavioral Medicine: A Cognitive-Behavioral Perspective.* New York: Guilford; 1983.

184. Turk DC, Robinson JP, Burwinkle TM. Prevalence of fear of pain and activity in fibromyalgia syndrome patients. *J Pain* 2004;5:483–490.

185. Okifuji A, Turk DC. Stress and psychophysiological dysregulation in patients with fibromyalgia syndrome. *Appl Psychophysiol Biofeedback* 2002;27:129–141.

186. Sullivan MJ, Rodgers WM, Kirsch I. Catastrophizing, depression, and expectancies for pain and emotional distress. *Pain* 2001;91:147–154.
187. Turk DC, Okifuji A. Psychological factors in chronic pain: evolution and revolution. *J Consult Clin Psychol* 2002;70:678–690.
188. Turk DC. A cognitive-behavioral perspective on the treatment of individuals experiencing chronic pain. In: Turk DC, Gatchel RJ, eds. *Psychological Approaches to Pain Management: A Practitioner's Handbook.* 3rd ed. New York: Guilford Press. In press.
189. Eccleston C, Palermo TM, Williams AC, et al. Psychological therapies for the management of chronic and recurrent pain in children and adolescents. *Cochrane Database Syst Rev* 2009;(2):CD003968.
190. Ehde DM, Dillworth TM, Turner JA. Cognitive-behavioral therapy for individuals with chronic pain: efficacy, innovations, and directions for research. *Am Psychol* 2014;69:153–166.
191. Williams AC, Eccleston C, Morley S. Psychological therapies for the management of chronic pain (excluding headache) in adults. *Cochrane Database Syst Rev* 2012;(11):CD007407.
192. Turk DC, Monarch ES. Biopsychosocial perspective on pain. In: Turk DC, Gatchel RJ, eds. *Psychological Approaches to Pain Management: A Practitioner's Handbook.* 3rd ed. New York: Guilford Press. In press.
193. Turk DC, Wilson HD, Swanson KS. The biopsychosocial model of pain and pain management. In: Ebert M, Kerns RD, eds. *Behavioral and Pharmacological Pain Management.* New York: Cambridge University Press; 2011:16–43.
194. Loeser JD. Low back pain. *Res Publ Assoc Res Nerv Ment Dis* 1980;58:363–377.
195. Waddell G. Clinical diagnosis of leg pain and nerve root involvement in low back disorders. *Acta Orthop Belg* 1987;53:152–155.
196. Loeser JD. The concepts of pain. In: Stanton-Hicks M, Boaz R, eds. *Chronic Low Back Pain.* New York: Raven Press; 1982:109–142.
197. Kerns RD. Family assessment and intervention. In: Nicassio PM, Smith TW, eds. *Managing Chronic Illness: A Biopsychosocial Perspective.* Washington, DC: American Psychological Association; 1995:207–244.
198. Schmaling K, Sher TG, eds. *The Psychology of Couples and Illness: Theory, Research, and Practice.* Washington, DC: American Psychological Association Press; 2000.
199. Cano A, Johansen AB, Franz A. Multilevel analysis of couple congruence on pain, interference, and disability. *Pain* 2005;118:369–379.
200. Thieme K, Spies C, Sinha P, et al. Predictors of pain behaviors in fibromyalgia syndrome patients. *Arthritis Care Res* 2005;53:343–350.
201. Cano A, Williams AC. Social interaction in pain: reinforcing pain behaviors or building intimacy? *Pain* 2010;149:9–11.
202. Cano A, Weisberg JN, Gallagher RM. Marital satisfaction and pain severity mediate the association between negative spouse responses to pain and depressive symptoms in a chronic pain sample. *Pain Med* 2000;1:35–43.
203. Groth T, Fehm-Wolfsdorf, Hahlweg K. Basic research on the psychology of intimate relationships. In: Schmaling K, Sher T, eds. *The Psychology of Couples and Illness: Theory, Research, and Practice.* Washington, DC: American Psychological Association Press; 2000:13–42.
204. Turk DC, Kerns RD, Rosenberg R. Effects of marital interaction on chronic pain and disability: examining the down-side of social support. *Rehab Psychol* 1992;37:357–372.

CHAPTER 8

Individual Differences in Pain: The Roles of Gender, Ethnicity, and Genetics

ROGER B. FILLINGIM

The experience of pain is characterized by tremendous interindividual variability.[1] Indeed, similar injuries, disease states, or noxious stimuli are often accompanied by pain responses that differ dramatically across people. Although it is inarguable that such individual differences in pain responses exist, their contributing factors and clinical importance remain important topics of study. This chapter aims to review the nature of individual differences in responses to pain and its treatment. After briefly highlighting several examples of individual differences, several individual difference factors are reviewed, emphasizing demographic variables (e.g., sex/gender and race/ethnicity) and genetic contributions to individual differences in pain. This chapter concludes by considering the interactions among different individual difference variables and discusses the clinical relevance of individual differences, including implications for treatment tailoring.

In the clinical setting, providers are well acquainted with individual differences in pain, as patients with the same pain condition often vary markedly in their self-reported pain and related symptoms. This variability is often attributed to differences in disease severity, based on the misguided assumption that the noxious stimulus itself is the primary determinant of the pain experience, despite considerable evidence suggesting otherwise. For example, the majority of individuals who show radiographic evidence of osteoarthritis (OA) are asymptomatic,[2] and even in symptomatic patients, radiographic measures of disease severity in OA account for a limited proportion of the interindividual variability in pain and disability.[3,4] Likewise, physical and diagnostic findings have limited value in predicting the occurrence or severity of low back pain.[5,6] Moreover, in the acute pain setting, patients undergoing similar surgical procedures report widely varying amounts of pain.[7–11] Thus, for many forms of clinical pain, the nature or magnitude of the noxious clinical stimulus appears to be a poor predictor of the degree of pain experienced.

Studying individual differences in the clinical setting is challenging because it is often difficult to quantify with any accuracy the noxious stimulus thought to be responsible for the patient's pain. Moreover, clinical pain reports are commonly influenced by previous or current therapies, creating additional sources of interindividual variability. In order to circumvent some of these issues, investigators have turned to the application of quantifiable and controllable painful stimuli in the laboratory setting. Interestingly, responses to experimentally induced pain are also marked by robust individual differences. For example, in a previous study of healthy adults undergoing an identical cold water stimulus, pain intensity ratings ranged from 0 to 100.[12] In subsequent analyses, the authors found that that the intensity of the noxious stimulus accounted for only 40% of the variance in pain ratings, with the remaining 60% accounted for by true individual differences. More recently, findings from 321 healthy young adults revealed that pain ratings in response to a 48° C heat stimulus ranged from 4 to 100.[1] Similarly, a prior study assessed 16 different experimental pain measures using identical methods in more than 200 healthy young females.[13]

They subsequently combined these measures into overall index scores by summing standardized (z scores) scores for each of the individual pain tests. This yielded a normal distribution of summary scores with a mean of 0, where positive and negative values indicated higher and lower pain sensitivity, respectively. They observed a range of summary scores from -20 to greater than 30 across the sample. These findings clearly demonstrate that even under experimental conditions in which stimulus intensity is carefully controlled, pain responses are marked by robust individual differences.

It is important to recognize that in addition to interindividual variability in pain responses, pain treatment outcomes are characterized by substantial individual differences. For example, a study of more than 3,000 patients undergoing different surgical procedures revealed that the number of morphine boluses required to produce adequate postoperative pain relief (Visual Analog Scale rating <30) ranged from 1 to 20.[7] A clinical trial of opioid therapy for chronic neuropathic pain showed that following treatment, patients reported changes in pain ranging from a 100% decrease to a nearly 70% increase in pain.[14] Likewise, even in laboratory pain studies, analgesic responses to opioids differ considerably across individuals.[15–17] In addition to variability in responses to medications, responses to nonpharmacologic pain treatments also vary widely from person to person. For example, a long-term (8 to 10 years) follow-up study of outcomes from surgical and nonsurgical management of spinal stenosis showed that approximately half of the patients in both treatment groups reported improvement in their symptoms over the follow-up period, whereas 20% to 25% reported no change and 20% to 25% reported that their symptoms had worsened.[18] Several other nonpharmacologic treatments have also been shown to confer widely varying amounts of pain relief across individuals, including acupuncture[19] and psychological interventions for pain.[20,21]

This brief overview of individual differences demonstrates that responses to pain and its treatment vary substantially from person to person. Although the study of this variability in pain responses has a long history,[22,23] recent years have witnessed substantially increased interest in individual differences, motivated in large part by the contemporaneous explosion of research on genetic determinants of health and disease. Although genetic factors contribute importantly to pain and analgesia, it is critical to remember that responses to pain and its treatment result from complex and dynamic interactions among numerous biologic, psychological, and social factors.[1] Thus, before discussing findings regarding the contribution of various demographic, genetic, and psychosocial factors to individual differences in pain, I provide a brief overview of the biopsychosocial model (Fig. 8.1), which represents the optimal model for conceptualizing individual differences in pain.

The biopsychosocial model emerged as an alternative to the unsatisfactory medical model, which reductionistically viewed health and symptoms as products of biologic disease.[24] In its application to pain, the model posits that the experience of and response to pain are determined by multiple biologic,

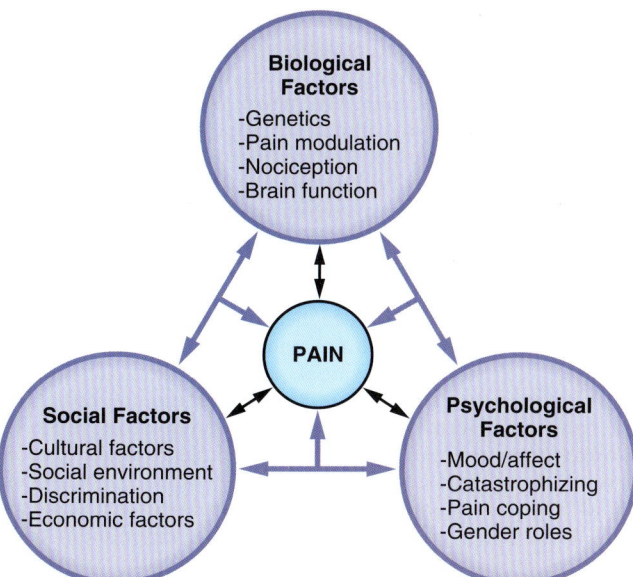

FIGURE 8.1 Biopsychosocial model of pain. The figure shows that pain experiences are influenced by the combined effects of biologic, psychological, and social factors. Although variables from each of the three domains can impact pain individually (as shown by small bidirectional arrows), biologic, psychological, and social factors also interact to produce complex and important influences on pain, as illustrated by the *large three-way arrows*. These interactions across numerous biopsychosocial factors produce myriad possible pain-modulating combinations of variables, resulting in tremendous interindividual variability of pain experiences. *(Modified with permission from Fillingim RB. Individual differences in pain: understanding the mosaic that makes pain personal.* Pain *2017;158[suppl 1]:S11–S18.)*

psychological, and social factors.[25] In addition to their individual contributions, an important tenet of the biopsychosocial model is that these factors interact dynamically to drive the pain experience. Of particular relevance to individual differences, this mosaic of pain-related biopsychosocial influences varies considerably from person to person. Hence, for each individual at a given point in time, a unique combination of biologic and psychosocial factors operates to sculpt the experience of pain.

Next, I discuss sex/gender and race/ethnicity as potentially important individual difference variables. I emphasize these demographic variables for several reasons. First, sex and ethnic differences in pain have tremendous public health implications, as they may contribute to differences in pain prevalence or severity that impact large population groups. Second, such demographic variables represent important proxies for a variety of other biopsychosocial factors that can influence pain, and the observation of group differences in pain is often the impetus for further exploration of these other pain-related factors. Finally, these demographic variables may be important moderators of the influence of other individual difference factors on pain, as discussed in the following text.

Sex and Gender Differences in Pain

CLINICAL PAIN

Although research addressing sex and gender differences in pain has a long history, interest in this topic has increased dramatically in the last two decades. Several recent reviews have addressed the topic from different perspectives and in varying levels of detail.[26–29] The importance of the topic is dictated by the abundance of epidemiologic and clinical research demonstrating that, compared to men, women are at greater risk for pain, tend to have higher levels of pain, and are more likely to seek

treatment for pain. Findings from myriad population-based studies demonstrate greater prevalence of chronic pain among females versus males. In a Canadian household survey, women reported higher rates of both temporary and persistent pain,[30] and a mail survey of more than 3600 adults in Scotland found that women were significantly more likely than men to report chronic pain.[31] Two Scandinavian studies found that multisite body pain was more common among women than men.[32,33] Similarly, in a survey of health maintenance organization enrollees in Seattle, Von Korff and colleagues[34] found that women were significantly more likely than men to report at least three of the following five pain conditions: headache, back pain, chest pain, abdominal pain, and facial pain. In our 2009 review article,[26] we summarized the findings of 10 population-based studies of general pain prevalence that were conducted in different geographical regions. These studies reported widely varying prevalences of pain for both women (11% to 59%) and men (10% to 49%). Every study reported higher pain prevalence among women, although the magnitude of the excess female prevalence varied considerably across studies, ranging from 1% to 14%. Subsequently, findings from the National Health Interview Survey (NHIS) revealed significantly higher frequency of persistent pain (i.e., pain on most days or every day for the past 3 months) among women (21.6%) than men (16.2%).[35,36] A recent meta-analytic review of epidemiologic studies reported an overall female-to-male prevalence ratio of 1.27, indicating that 27% more females than males reported chronic pain.[37] Overall, these findings from numerous population-based studies conducted in varied geographic regions across the world reveal a consistent pattern of higher prevalence of general chronic pain among women than men, although the magnitude of the sex difference varies across studies.

In addition to these data on general pain symptoms, considerable research suggests that specific pain conditions show sex differences in their prevalence. More than 30 years ago, the NUPRIN Pain Report, based on a telephone survey of 1,254 US adults, found that women were more likely to report headaches, stomach pain, joint pain, and back pain than men.[38] An abundance of epidemiologic evidence shows that several common chronic pain conditions are more common among women, including fibromyalgia (FM),[39] chronic widespread pain (CWP),[40] migraine headache,[41] temporomandibular disorder (TMD),[42,43] irritable bowel syndrome,[44] and low back pain.[45–47] Sex differences in the prevalence of specific pain conditions were recently summarized by examining findings from 47 studies that reported on sex differences in pain prevalence across the following pain conditions: back pain, migraine, musculoskeletal pain, neuropathic pain, oral pain, OA pain, and widespread pain.[27] For each comparison, the excess female prevalence was computed by subtracting the prevalence in men from that in women. Prevalence in females was greater than in males in 45 of 47 comparisons, and the average excess female prevalence across all of the pain conditions was 5.5%. Sex differences in back pain prevalence were examined in a more recent study of adults aged 50 years and older from six low- and middle-income countries conducted by the World Health Organization. These authors reported that back pain during the past month was significantly more frequent for women (34.9%) than men (24.2%), and women also had more severe pain.[48] Also, in a Canadian study, both knee and hip OA were more prevalent among women versus men.[49] A recent meta-analysis of 14 studies that reported sex-specific prevalence of CWP found that prevalence was approximately twice as great in women as men.[40] Also, Jones and colleagues[39] compared the prevalence of FM in females and males using three different diagnostic criteria. Prevalence was substantially higher in women, but the magnitude of the sex difference varied dramatically across diagnostic criteria. It is worth noting that these epidemiologic findings reflect the frequency of pain in the general population. The disproportionate impact of pain among women is even greater in the clinical setting due to their increased health care use for pain.[50–53] Taken together, these findings demonstrate that the frequency of pain is higher for women than men, particularly for pain conditions that are both common and associated with substantial societal costs.

These findings of greater pain prevalence among adults are somewhat mirrored by studies of children and adolescents. For example, a systematic review found that pain prevalence for most pain types was higher for girls than for boys, including headaches, abdominal pain, musculoskeletal pain, combined pain types, and general chronic pain.[54] Also, a recent study of children and adolescents (aged 10 to 17 years) found that females were more likely than males to transition from acute to persistent musculoskeletal pain.[55] However, several studies of acute pain report no sex differences in children, and age appears to be an important moderating factor, as sex differences generally become more pronounced as children age.[56–58] For example, LeResche and colleagues[59] reported increasing excess female prevalence of pain conditions as children progressed through pubertal development, implicating potential hormonal contributions.

The aforementioned findings speak to the frequency of pain but not to its impact or severity, which has been addressed in a number of clinical studies. Regarding acute pain, sex differences in postoperative pain have been inconsistent. In cohorts of patients undergoing mixed surgical procedures, results have shown greater pain among women[60–62] as well as greater pain among men.[63] Other studies have evaluated sex differences in pain after specific types of surgery. More severe pain has been observed for women after dental surgery in some[64,65] but not other studies.[66] Women have also been found to report higher pain levels following orthopedic[67–71] and cardiothoracic surgery[72] and after laparoscopic cholecystectomy.[73] A recent review of this literature concluded that women generally experience more severe postoperative pain, but the observed sex differences are often small and of limited clinical significance.[74] It should also be noted that persistent pain after surgery represents an important clinical concern, and several studies have shown that females are at greater risk for pain persistence than males.[72,75,76]

In addition to these findings addressing acute pain, sex differences in the severity of chronic pain have also been investigated. Women with arthritis have been found to report higher levels of pain and disability than their male counterparts.[77–79] In addition, in a cohort of people with mixed chronic pain conditions seeking treatment in a multidisciplinary pain clinic, women reported higher pain severity than men.[80] In a sample of patients with chronic musculoskeletal pain, pain ratings did not differ by sex; however, women's pain drawings showed a greater area of pain compared to men.[81] In contrast to these findings of sex differences in chronic pain severity and impact, many other studies have found little evidence for sex differences in the severity of chronic pain.[82–86] Moreover, in a treatment-seeking sample of patients composed largely of individuals with myofascial pain conditions, men reported more frequent and severe pain and greater disability compared to women.[87] Thus, the available evidence regarding sex differences in chronic pain severity is inconsistent and precludes firm conclusions. Perhaps this should not be surprising because most of the evidence regarding chronic pain derives from patients whose pain was severe enough to motivate treatment seeking, thereby increasing the likelihood of sampling bias. A handful of studies have examined sex differences in chronic pain severity in community-based samples, providing a less biased approach to the issue. A population-based study in Australia reported that among people reporting chronic pain, a greater proportion

of females than males characterized their pain as moderate to severe.[88] Among people reporting activity-limiting pain, pain frequency, pain-related negative affect, and disability were all greater for women compared to men.[89] In a community-based study of knee OA, Glass and colleagues[90] found that women reported higher pain levels that men across all grades of radiographic knee OA severity, but these differences were small in magnitude, and some became nonsignificant after controlling for confounders. Similarly, we recently reported no differences in clinical pain severity in women and men with knee OA; however, women reported pain in more body sites than did men.[91] A Scandinavian study revealed higher pain levels among women with musculoskeletal conditions compared to their male counterparts.[92] In a study of individuals with painful TMD, multiple comorbid pain conditions (e.g., headache/migraine, neck pain, low back pain, joint pain) were significantly more prevalent among women than men.[93] Recently, findings from a telephone survey showed that compared to men, women using chronic opioid therapy reported poorer pain-related adjustment.[94] Thus, when considering these findings from community-based studies of individuals with existing chronic pain, women appear to have higher impact pain than men.

EXPERIMENTAL PAIN

Although sex differences in clinical pain prevalence and severity are inevitably driven by multiple factors, one possible contributor could be sex differences in the functioning of pain processing systems. Indeed, altered nociceptive processing characterizes many of the female-predominant pain disorders, which adds further credibility to this argument.[1,26,95] Several reviews have examined the literature regarding sex differences in experimental pain sensitivity.[26–29] Overall, the findings reveal lower pain thresholds (i.e., the minimum stimulus intensity required to produce pain) and tolerances (i.e., the maximum stimulus intensity that the individual is willing to tolerate) among women relative to men, across multiple stimulus modalities. The direction of the findings has been highly consistent across studies; however, the magnitude of the sex difference has been quite variable. Some 20 years ago, our meta-analysis reported that the average effect size was moderate.[96]

Over the past two decades, multiple review articles have summarized existing findings related to sex differences in responses to laboratory pain stimuli. For example, in a 2009 review paper[97], we concluded that "current human findings regarding sex differences in experimental pain indicate greater pain sensitivity among females compared with males for most pain modalities, including more recently implemented clinically relevant pain models such as temporal summation of pain and intramuscular injection of algesic substances."[98] Shortly thereafter, based on examination of largely the same literature, Racine and colleagues[99] came to the contrasting conclusion that "10 years of laboratory research have not been successful in producing a clear and consistent pattern of sex differences in human pain sensitivity, even with the use of deep, tonic, long-lasting stimuli, which are known to better mimic clinical pain." In an effort to reconcile these discrepant conclusions, Mogil[27] conducted a careful analysis of the studies reviewed by Racine and colleagues, and his findings provided strong evidence of higher pain sensitivity among females. In another recent review article, the authors state that existing findings from laboratory pain studies of sex differences "represent trends, but, in most cases, the findings are more nuanced than the conclusions." So what is one to conclude from these widely varying views of the same literature?

The answer is both simple and complex. Regarding the former, the existing literature shows that sex differences in responses experimental pain stimuli are undeniably consistent in their direction in that females are consistently found to be more pain-sensitive than men. This pattern has been observed for multiple stimulus modalities, numerous body regions, and across all common pain sensitivity measures (i.e., pain threshold, pain tolerance, and suprathreshold pain ratings). In addition, more sophisticated measures of pain modulatory processes have demonstrated greater temporal summation of pain among women versus men, in response to different stimuli, including heat,[100] cutaneous mechanical,[101] and pressure stimuli.[102] Laboratory measures of pain inhibitory function seem to vary somewhat across assessment methods, with men showing greater conditioned pain modulation (CPM),[103] but sex differences have been less consistent using other assays of pain inhibition.[98] Findings from studies of children and adolescents reveal a pattern of results that is similar those observed in adults, but the differences in children are generally of lesser magnitude, and sex differences in pain responses are influenced by age, likely reflecting the influence of developmental stage.[104] Thus, the simple answer regarding sex differences in experimental pain sensitivity is that women are consistently more sensitive than men.[99] However, the complexity of the issue is reflected in the highly variable magnitude of the sex difference, which suggests important influences of methodologic and contextual factors. For example, brief, repeated thermal stimuli evoke greater temporal summation of pain among females than males, whereas, in response to sustained heat stimuli, females show greater attenuation of pain over time.[105] The study sample can also impact sex differences in pain sensitivity because in addition to sex, multiple individual difference factors are known to influence pain responses,[106] including other demographic factors. For example, race/ethnicity and age are known to affect experimental pain responses; therefore, the age and ethnic diversity of the study sample could influence the magnitude of the sex differences observed. Moreover, a variety of other biopsychosocial variables can impact pain responses, sometimes in a sex-dependent manner, which could modulate the magnitude of observed sex differences in pain sensitivity. Regarding contextual factors, some evidence suggests that experimenter sex/gender may affect pain responses in the laboratory setting,[107,108] and this could certainly contribute to the inconsistent magnitude of sex differences that have been reported.

Thus, studies of experimental pain reveal a consistent pattern of sex differences, with women showing more robust perceptual responses to painful stimuli than men. However, the magnitude of these differences varies considerably across studies, and the underlying mechanisms remain poorly understood.

RESPONSES TO PAIN TREATMENT

In addition to sex differences in clinical and experimental pain responses, whether women and men respond differently to pain treatment represents a topic of substantial interest. Before reviewing sex differences in treatment efficacy, it is important to consider whether there are differences in the provision of treatment to male and female patients. A gender bias in pain treatment has been previously described,[109] although the patterns of gender differences in pain treatment are complex. Indeed, a systematic review noted that although different pain treatments are often provided to women and men, the evidence does not demonstrate a consistent bias in pain treatment against women or men.[110] A study of veterans typifies this pattern, as the authors found that compared to males, females received pain care that was more consistent with clinical practice guidelines; however, sedatives were prescribed more often for females than males, which is not supported by guidelines.[111] When biases in pain treatment do occur, they emerge from a complex mosaic of factors, including characteristics of both the patient and the provider. In a recent study, after viewing a patient video, specialist physicians and medical students concluded that female patients had less pain and were more likely to exaggerate their

pain,[112] and providers were less likely to prescribe analgesics and more likely to recommend psychological treatment for female patients. Using computerized avatars to depict patients with chronic low back pain, Hirsh and colleagues[113] reported that female but not male health care providers and trainees were more likely to prescribe antidepressants and mental health treatments for female versus male patients. Thus, there appear to be some gender-related biases in pain treatment, but these biases are influenced by interactions among multiple contextual factors, including but not limited to the gender of both the patient and the provider.

Another important issue regarding pain treatment is whether the effectiveness of treatments differs for women versus men. The treatment that has been most extensively studied in this regard is opioid therapy. In their meta-analysis, Niesters and colleagues[114] examined whether responses to opioids differed across sex for both acute clinical pain and for experimental pain. Postoperatively, females consumed lower amounts of μ-opioid agonists than males, particularly for morphine administered via patient-controlled analgesia (PCA). The authors speculated that this pattern of results may have emerged because PCA studies often assess opioid use for a longer duration, which may increase detection of sex differences because morphine has a longer duration of action for women. Interestingly, a recent study reported sex differences in the daily rhythmicity of postoperative morphine consumption, with men using more morphine during the night.[115] It should be mentioned that because these findings are based on opioid consumption rather than analgesic efficacy, it is possible that other factors may have contributed to lower consumption in women. Indeed, increased side effects, including nausea and vomiting, and unpleasant cognitive-affective effects have been reported for females.[116] However, in experimental studies that directly measure analgesic responses, females showed greater analgesia in response to μ-opioids, with moderate effect sizes, which were larger than those observed for acute clinical pain. The authors also reviewed studies of mixed action opioids (e.g., pentazocine, nalbuphine, butorphanol), and in acute clinical pain, these agents produced considerably more robust analgesia in women. In contrast, studies of these medications tested against experimental pain models showed a striking absence of sex differences in analgesia. The most obvious explanation for these conflicting results lies in the characteristics of the pain models. Specifically, greater analgesic responses in women were observed for acute postoperative pain, which includes a strong inflammatory component, whereas the experimental pain models were decidedly noninflammatory. Taken together, the existing evidence suggests that women exhibit greater analgesic responses to μ-opioid agonists analgesia, whereas mixed-action opioid medications produce greater analgesia in females for postoperative but not experimental pain.

In the last 20 years, prescriptions of opioids for chronic pain have increased dramatically, resulting in a major public health crisis of opioid misuse and overdose in the United States.[117-119] Very little research has addressed whether males and females with chronic pain respond differently to opioid therapy; however, there is evidence that the opioid crisis is differentially impacting women versus men. Opioids are prescribed more often for women than men, in part due to the excess female prevalence of chronic pain.[120,121] Although even among individuals with chronic pain, women are more likely than men to use prescription opioids.[122-124] Also, among people with chronic pain using long-term opioids, women showed poorer overall chronic pain status.[94] However, nonmedical use of opioids is higher for males,[125] as are risks for dose escalation and opioid-related death.[126-128] Thus, despite more frequent opioid use in women with chronic pain, adverse outcomes are more common among males.

Scant research has addressed sex differences in responses to nonopioid therapies, and the inconsistent results of these studies defies general conclusions. For example, males exhibited greater analgesic responses to ibuprofen tested against experimental[129] but not postoperative pain.[64] Analgesic responses tested with electrical pain were more robust for males who expected to receive ibuprofen regardless of whether they received ibuprofen or placebo.[130] These findings suggesting that expectations induce greater analgesia in males are paralleled by other laboratory pain studies in which placebo analgesia has been found to be higher among males than females.[131,132] In contrast, women displayed greater placebo responses in another study,[133] and consistent findings were observed in a pediatric study that demonstrated increased placebo analgesia in girls compared to boys.[134] Additional research elucidating sex differences in placebo analgesia is warranted not only because such information influences clinical trial design and interpretation but also because sex differences in placebo analgesia could reflect sex differences in the engagement of endogenous analgesic mechanisms.

Research investigating sex differences in outcomes from nonpharmacologic pain treatments is even more limited, with variable results. As described in our previous review,[98] some evidence suggests more positive treatment effects in men, others show greater improvements among women; yet, others show similar outcomes across sex. A recent meta-analysis of sex differences in responses to psychological pain therapies in children and adolescents reported that boys and girls generally showed similar treatment responses.[135] Clearly, more research is needed to determine the extent to which nonpharmacologic pain treatments impact males and females differently and whether the mechanisms underlying treatment response differ by sex.

BIOPSYCHOSOCIAL MECHANISMS

The mechanisms responsible for sex differences in pain are complex and incompletely understood. Multiple biologic and psychosocial factors contribute to sex differences in pain, as previously reviewed by multiple authors.[26-29,136] Considerable evidence suggests that sex hormones may importantly influence pain responses and the effects of pain medications.[26,36,137,138] For example, both clinical pain severity and experimental pain sensitivity have been found to fluctuate across the female menstrual cycle.[139,140] Moreover, use of exogenous hormones, particularly estrogen replacement in postmenopausal women, is associated with greater risk for clinical pain in some studies[141-143] but not others.[144,145] However, the association of gonadal hormones with pain appears complex and bidirectional. In contrast to the earlier findings suggesting pain promoting effects of estrogen, other findings imply an antinociceptive role for estrogen. For example, pain-evoked brain responses were attenuated during menstrual phases characterized by high estrogen levels, particularly in brain regions subserving the affective dimension of pain.[146] Moreover, in healthy women, administration of exogenous estrogen reduced muscle pain sensitivity and increased pain-related brain μ-opioid receptor binding.[147] Thus, sex hormones clearly can influence pain responses; yet, the pattern and direction of hormonal effects on pain are complex and remain poorly understood.

Sex differences in pain responses are also influenced by psychosocial variables. Indeed, pain coping has been found to differ by sex, which may contribute to sex differences in both clinical and experimental pain responses.[148-150] Furthermore, females and males have been found to differ in emotional processes, and affective variables may relate to pain in a sex-dependent manner.[28] Also, traditional masculine versus feminine gender roles may influence pain responses, as the former may promote stoicism, whereas the latter may encourage increased reporting of pain.[136] Experimental studies suggest that both females and males report that willingness to report pain is higher for women than men, and adjustment for willingness to report pain has rendered sex differences in experimental pain responses nonsignificant in some studies.[151,152] Moreover, traditional gender role measures assessing masculinity and femininity predict lower and higher pain sensitivity, respectively,[153,154] and men who identified strongly with masculine gender norms had higher pain tolerance than men with low masculine identification.[155] The extent to which such gender roles contribute to sex differences in clinical pain has received little empirical attention.

Ethnic Group Differences in Pain

Racial and ethnic background is another important pain-relevant demographic factor, and there is an increasing need to understand its contribution to individual differences in pain given the growing ethnic diversity of the US population. Indeed, racial and ethnic disparities across multiple health conditions have been well documented, which represents an urgent public health concern.[156,157] That these ethnic/racial group differences extend to chronic pain conditions is increasingly appreciated.[158,159] Progress in research addressing racial and ethnic disparities in pain has been impeded by inconsistent definitional and conceptual approaches to studying health and disease across population groups.[160] Moreover, in contrast to sex differences, where individuals are relatively easily classified into one of two largely mutually exclusive groups, racial and ethnic categories are greater in number and overlap.

CLINICAL PAIN

The epidemiology of chronic pain across ethnic and racial groups has not been well characterized. Population-based studies in the United States generally show limited evidence suggesting consistent racial and ethnic differences in prevalence of general chronic pain.[161] Plesh and colleagues[162] reported lower incidence of common chronic pain conditions among African American young women compared to non-Hispanic white women. National Health and Nutrition Examination Survey (NHANES) data indicate lower prevalence of chronic pain among Mexican Americans compared to non-Hispanic black and white Americans.[163] Likewise, findings from the Health and Retirement Study revealed similar prevalence of high-impact chronic pain among Hispanic, non-Hispanic white, and non-Hispanic black adults older than age 50 years.[164] Using data from the NHIS, Nahin[165] found that non-Hispanic whites had somewhat higher prevalence of pain, particularly when compared to Asians and Hispanic whites, but group differences were also influenced by language preference. A recent review noted that chronic pain prevalence is generally lower among Hispanic Americans compared to non-Hispanic white and black individuals.[159] Thus, epidemiologic studies in the United States suggest that chronic pain prevalence may be slightly lower among individuals from minority ethnic and racial groups compared to non-Hispanic whites.

Other studies have moved beyond pain prevalence to examine whether racial and ethnic groups differ in the severity and impact of chronic pain. Studies in several clinical populations have reported greater pain among African Americans compared to non-Hispanic whites, including cancer[166] and back pain,[167,168] and in heterogeneous samples of people with chronic pain.[169-172] Similarly, higher pain levels have been observed among Hispanic patients with chronic pain.[159,173] Also, higher levels of pain-related disability have been observed among African Americans with back pain.[174] The most consistent evidence of racial and ethnic differences comes from studies of OA, where African American and Hispanic adults with OA consistently show greater pain and disability than their non-Hispanic white counterparts.[159,175-177] In addition to these findings derived from clinical samples, community-based research suggests that chronic pain may be more severe among African American and Hispanic individuals compared to non-Hispanic whites.[178] For example, the prevalence of severe joint pain is higher among these minority groups than in whites.[179] Not surprisingly, most of the available data have addressed the largest minority groups in the United States (African American and Hispanic); however, some investigators have also reported greater pain severity in other minority groups, including Asian Americans[180] and Native Americans.[181] In contrast to these findings, some population-based studies have observed minimal racial and ethnic group differences in chronic pain severity.[182,183] Most recently, Grol-Prokopczyk[184] examined data from the Health and Retirement Study and found that after adjusting for confounders, black older adults had lower pain severity than other racial or ethnic groups. Thus, the overall findings are variable, but the evidence suggests that among individuals with chronic pain, African American and Hispanic adults are at risk for more severe pain compared to non-Hispanic whites, with the strongest evidence emerging from studies of OA.

EXPERIMENTAL PAIN

Racial and ethnic group differences in clinical pain are influenced by multiple biologic and psychosocial factors. For example, socioeconomic variables (e.g., education and income) are associated with pain and its impact, and these factors may well contribute to the observed racial and ethnic disparities in pain.[184–186] Also, undertreatment of pain among African American and Hispanic patients represents another potential contributor to more severe pain in these individuals.[187] However, patient-level factors, such as group differences in pain perception, could potentially play a role in the observed differences in clinical pain severity. In this regard, numerous studies have investigated racial and ethnic differences in pain responses using quantitative sensory testing. These findings have been summarized in two relatively recent meta-analyses. Rahim-Williams and colleagues[188] reviewed findings from studies examining experimental pain responses in African Americans versus non-Hispanic whites. They concluded that African Americans displayed lower pain thresholds and tolerances, suggesting greater pain sensitivity. Effect sizes were generally small to moderate for group differences in pain threshold, but moderate to large for pain tolerance. A subsequent meta-analysis corroborated and extended these findings, concluding that African American, Hispanic, and Asian adults showed greater experimental pain sensitivity compared to non-Hispanic whites.[189] These findings demonstrate group differences in pain sensitivity; however, whether these experimental findings contribute to group differences in clinical pain remains unknown. Interestingly, we previously observed that African Americans reported higher levels of OA-related pain and disability as well as greater experimental pain sensitivity than non-Hispanic whites.[190] We also found that the relationship of pain sensitivity to clinical pain differed across race groups. Specifically, thermal pain sensitivity was related to clinical pain among non-Hispanic whites, whereas mechanical pain responses were associated with clinical pain among African Americans.

RESPONSES TO PAIN TREATMENT

Racial and ethnic group differences in clinical pain could in part be driven by differences in the provision or effectiveness of pain treatments. Several lines of evidence suggest that analgesic interventions are provided at lower doses and lower frequency for African American and Hispanic patients compared to non-Hispanic whites,[158,191–193] although some studies have shown no such disparity.[194–198] One recent emergency department study reported no race group differences in administration of any analgesic treatment; however, African Americans

were less likely than whites to receive an opioid for low back pain but not long bone fracture.[199] Regarding opioid prescriptions for chronic pain, North Carolina Medicare claims data revealed that black patients were significantly less likely to have filled an opioid prescription.[200] In contrast, data from the National Ambulatory Medical Care Survey showed that among patients with chronic pain, non-white individuals were more likely to have been prescribed an opioid.[201] Potential race differences in opioid treatment may be influenced by other factors. For example, Burgess and colleagues[202] found that among veterans with chronic pain, younger blacks were less likely to receive opioids, whereas older blacks were more likely to receive opioids, compared to whites. These clinical findings have been corroborated by experimental studies demonstrating that patient race influences decisions about analgesic treatments for chronic pain.[203–205]

Limited research has addressed whether effectiveness of analgesics differs across racial or ethnic groups. More than 30 years ago, Kaiko and colleagues[206] reported greater analgesic responses to morphine among African American patients with cancer-related chronic pain compared to white patients. Similarly, we found that African Americans exhibited more robust analgesia in response to both morphine and butorphanol using experimental pain stimuli to test analgesic efficacy.[17] Regarding opioid side effects, white patients showed greater opioid-induced nausea and vomiting than black patients.[207]

Given increasing concerns about opioid misuse and adverse outcomes, the possible importance of patient race and ethnicity in use of prescription opioids warrants some discussion. Among high school seniors, whites were significantly more likely to report both medical and nonmedical use of opioids compared to African Americans and Hispanics.[208] In the primary care setting, opioid risk reduction strategies were more often implemented for black than for white patients.[209] In contrast, white patients were more likely to be on a pain treatment agreement in one study[210] but not another.[211] Also, in this Veteran Affairs study, black veterans underwent significantly more urine drug tests than whites and were less likely to be referred to a pain specialist and more likely to be referred to a substance abuse specialist.[211] These findings suggest that race and ethnicity may impact the efficacy of opioids, as well as providers' behaviors related to opioid prescription, which could influence patterns of medical and nonmedical use in the general population. More research is needed to elucidate these issues.

BIOPSYCHOSOCIAL MECHANISMS

Consistent with sex differences, multiple biologic, psychological, and social factors contribute to racial and ethnic group differences in pain. The limited information related to biologic mediators of racial and ethnic differences in pain derives primarily from laboratory studies. For example, several biologic markers of stress reactivity appear to be more strongly associated with lower pain sensitivity among white versus African American individuals, implicating neuroendocrine responses in racial and ethnic differences in pain perception.[212–214] In a study of patients with knee OA, African Americans had lower vitamin D levels than non-Hispanic whites, and vitamin D mediated the greater mechanical and heat pain sensitivity observed in African Americans.[215] Genetic factors represent another potential biologic contributor to racial and ethnic group differences in pain, as discussed further in text. Thus, although limited, some evidence implicates biologic factors in racial and ethnic group differences in pain.

Several psychological and social factors also may contribute to race group differences in the experience of pain. For example, differences in pain coping have been observed across racial and ethnic groups. A recent meta-analysis found that black individuals used pain coping strategies more frequently overall compared to whites, particularly praying and catastrophizing, whereas white individuals engaged in higher levels of task persistence.[216] These authors subsequently conducted a study of experimental pain responses and found that the rumination component of pain catastrophizing mediated the lower pain tolerance of black participants.[217] Social factors also represent important drivers of variation in pain responses both within and between racial and ethnic groups. Lower socioeconomic status has been associated with increased risk for pain, and some findings suggest that race differences in pain are accounted for by the lower SES of certain minority groups.[164,184] Also, experiences of discrimination are a source of chronic stress that occurs more frequently among minority groups, and discrimination has been associated with increased pain severity.[218–221] In a sample of adults with knee OA, we found that African Americans reported more experiences of discrimination compared to whites, and discrimination mediated the lower heat pain tolerance observed among African American individuals.[222] Additional research is needed to further characterize the influence of social factors on pain responses and ethnic group differences therein.

Genetic Contributions to Pain

The genomic revolution spurred substantially increased interest in understanding how individual differences influence health, including pain, such that considerable research has addressed genetic contributions to individual differences in pain. The following discussion text highlights several examples of genetic associations with pain, including interactions between genetics and other individual differences factors, such as sex and racial or ethnic group. For more detailed reviews of this literature, the reader is referred elsewhere.[223–228]

CLINICAL PAIN

Increasing evidence from human research documents the importance of genetic influences in numerous clinical pain conditions. Twin studies, which estimate genetic contributions by comparing disease concordance rates for monozygotic versus dizygotic twins, demonstrate significant heritability for several common chronic pain conditions, including back pain, neck pain, headache, arthritis, CWP, and abdominal pain.[229–233] Numerous candidate gene studies and an increasing number of genome-wide association studies have identified specific genes that are associated with certain pain conditions[228]; however, these findings are often marked by small effect sizes and nonreplication.[234,235] Genetic associations could reflect the pathophysiologic processes of specific diseases that produce pain. For example, genes involved in cartilage biology could be associated with OA pain. Alternatively, genetic influences on pain perception or endogenous pain modulation could potentially underlie genetic associations with chronic pain conditions. This possibility is bolstered by findings that many of these heritable pain syndromes are characterized by enhanced pain sensitivity and/or altered endogenous pain modulation.[223,236] Indeed, a recent review identified several genes that have been associated with multiple chronic overlapping pain conditions across multiple studies. These genes primarily reflect biologic systems involved in pain processing, including catecholaminergic, serotonergic, and opioidergic function.[95]

EXPERIMENTAL PAIN

Abundant preclinical research implicates genetic factors in both nociceptive sensitivity and responses to analgesic drugs, and growing evidence from studies of experimental pain indicates important genetic contributions to human pain sensitivity.[27,227,237] The first twin study of experimental pain response estimated the heritability of pressure pain threshold to be 10%,

suggesting minimal genetic contribution.[238] However, statistical power in twin studies is often insufficient for multifactorial traits like pain sensitivity, and twin pairs were tested together in unblinded fashion in this study, likely increasing the effect of nongenetic factors. Subsequent twin studies of experimental pain responses reported heritability estimates ranging from 22% to 60% across different pain modalities, including heat pain, cold pain, and chemically induced pain.[12,15,239] Candidate gene approaches have identified several genes associated with experimental pain responses across multiple studies. The following discussion highlights three genes that have been associated with pain in numerous cohorts and across several pain phenotypes. It is important to note that although these genes have been associated with pain in multiple studies, numerous investigators have failed to find associations, as is common in genetic research, due to relatively small effect sizes and differences in methodology and study samples. Interested readers can find additional information in several recent reviews.[223–225,227]

The gene that encodes catechol-O-methyl-transferase (COMT), an enzyme that metabolizes catecholamines, has been the most frequently examined gene in pain studies. A commonly studied *COMT* single nucleotide polymorphism (SNP) involves the substitution of valine by methionine at codon 158 (*val158met*). This SNP produces a thermally unstable enzyme resulting in lower enzymatic activity. Zubieta and colleagues[240] investigated this SNP using a model of facial pain produced by injection of hypertonic saline into the masseter muscle. Individuals carrying the *val/val* genotype required a larger dose of hypertonic saline to produce moderate pain, suggesting that the *val/val* genotype confers lower pain sensitivity. Moreover, using positron emission tomography, the investigators found that the *val/val* genotype group showed significantly greater pain-related brain μ-opioid receptor activation, which indicates more robust endogenous opioid-mediated pain inhibition. Subsequently, Diatchenko and colleagues[13] identified three *COMT* haplotypes which were associated with experimental pain sensitivity in healthy young women. Interestingly, the haplotype that predicted lower pain sensitivity also was protective against future development of painful TMD. *COMT* has been associated with experimental pain sensitivity in several other studies[241–243] as well as with risk for or severity of clinical pain.[244,245]

Another frequently studied candidate gene is *OPRM1*, which encodes the μ-opioid receptor. The A118G SNP produces an amino acid substitution whose functional effects include altered binding affinity for β-endorphin[246] and changes in messenger RNA expression and protein yield.[247] The G allele has been associated with lower pressure pain sensitivity,[248] lower heat pain sensitivity,[249] and reduced pain-related evoked potential responses.[250] Regarding clinical pain, the G allele has shown lower frequency among patients with chronic pain compared to controls.[251,252] Also, patients homozygous for the A allele showed greater day-to-day pain variability compared to those with at least one G allele.[253] In addition to associations with experimental and clinical pain phenotypes, *OPRM1* may influence opioid analgesic responses. Recent meta-analytic reviews have found that carriers of the G allele of A118G require significantly higher postoperative opioid doses compared to patients homozygous for the A allele.[254,255] Also, the G allele was protective against morphine-induced respiratory depression following spine surgery.[256] G allele carriers also showed higher morphine requirements for management of cancer pain.[257] Thus, the A118G SNP of *OPRM1* has been consistently associated with basal pain sensitivity and opioid requirements.

The *GCH1* gene has also been associated with pain responses in multiple studies. *GCH1* encodes an enzyme (GTP cyclohydrolase or GCH) which is involved in production of tetrahydrobiopterin (BH4). BH4 is a cofactor involved in biosynthesis of several neurotransmitters, including serotonin, dopamine, and norepinephrine. Tegeder and colleagues[258] observed that upregulation of GCH and BH4 contributed to neuropathic and inflammatory pain in rodents. In a translational effort, these findings were extended to humans when a haplotype of the *GCH1* gene was found to be associated with lower levels of persistent pain following lumbar surgery for disk herniation and with reduced experimental pain sensitivity among healthy adults. Since this original paper, several studies have reported associations of *GCH1* with various pain phenotypes, including capsaicin-induced pain[259] and hyperalgesia,[260] HIV-associated neuropathic pain,[261] and outcomes following surgery for lumbar disk disease.[262]

Interactions among Individual Difference Factors

The earlier discussion addresses each individual difference factor independently; however, it is important to recognize that these and many other individual difference variables interact to influence pain responses. Unfortunately, such interactions are often not considered in research design and analysis. Indeed, although pain responses have been shown to differ markedly by sex and race, whether these two demographic factors interact to influence pain remains largely unexplored. On the other hand, interactions between genetic factors and sex have been examined in several studies. For example, a previous twin study reported that the heritability of neck pain was significantly higher among females (51%) compared to males (33%).[263] In a study of experimentally induced pain, the *OPRM1* gene interacted with sex to predict ratings of heat pain, such that the G allele was associated with lower pain ratings for men but higher ratings among women.[248] Interestingly, these findings were subsequently replicated in a clinical cohort in which the G allele predicted improved 12-month outcomes from lumbar disk herniation among men but worse outcomes among women.[264] Sex-dependent genetic associations have also been reported for both *COMT* and *GCH1*,[242,265] which further reinforces the importance of incorporating both males and females into study samples and considering potential interactions in the analytic approach.

Interactions between genes and racial or ethnic background have received far less attention, which is somewhat surprising given that allele frequencies for many SNPs are known to differ notably based on racial and ethnic background.[266–269] Regarding genes relevant to pain research, it has been reported that allele frequencies for the A118G SNP of *OPRM1* differ across ethnic groups, such that minor (G) allele frequency is substantially lower among African Americans compared to other racial and ethnic groups.[270,271] Because the G allele has been associated with lower pain sensitivity[248,249] and higher morphine requirements,[254,255] it is plausible that the previously reported increased pain sensitivity[188,189] and reduced morphine requirements[17,206] among African Americans could be due in part to the lower frequency of this minor allele of *OPRM1*. However, this speculation requires empirical confirmation. Beyond ethnic group differences in allele frequencies, an interaction could emerge if the strength or direction of a genetic association with a pain phenotypic differed across racial or ethnic groups. One such example emerged from a study examining associations of the A118G SNP of *OPRM1* with experimental pain responses.[271] The investigators report that Hispanic and non-Hispanic whites show similar minor allele frequencies; however, a gene by ethnic group interaction emerged. Specifically, the G allele was associated with lower pain sensitivity among non-Hispanic whites but with higher sensitivity among Hispanic participants. These findings highlight the importance of increasing the racial and ethnic diversity of samples used for genetic association studies and exploring potential race/ethnicity by genetic interactions in these designs.

Although psychological contributions to pain are beyond the scope of this chapter, it is important to consider interactions between psychological factors and other individual difference variables. For example, the *COMT* gene has been found to interact with pain catastrophizing to explain variability in both clinical and experimental models of shoulder pain. Specifically, among individuals with a high pain sensitivity *COMT* haplotype, catastrophizing is associated with greater pain severity or duration.[272–276] Another *COMT* by psychology interaction emerged from the Orofacial Pain Prospective Evaluation and Risk Assessment (OPPERA) study. Using a prospective design that included repeated measurements of perceived stress, these investigators found that increasing stress over time predicted development of TMD but only among people with a *COMT* haplotype that conferred low COMT activity.[277] Thus, stress-related increases in risk for TMD were observed only among those individuals whose *COMT* genotype would result in greater catecholaminergic drive.

Conclusion

Pain and analgesic responses are characterized by tremendous individual differences, which are driven by a complex mosaic of biologic and psychosocial factors. This chapter highlights the contributions of sex, racial and ethnic group, and genetic factors and their interactions. Females are at greater risk for clinical pain and show higher sensitivity to experimental pain compared to males. Some evidence also suggest that women show greater analgesic responses to μ-opioids. Racial and ethnic group differences in pain are more nuanced. Pain prevalence does not appear to differ greatly by racial or ethnic group, although some evidence suggests lower prevalence in minority groups compared to whites. However, among individuals experiencing chronic pain, African Americans and Hispanics generally reported greater pain and disability compared to their non-Hispanic white counterparts. African American and Hispanic individuals also display greater experimental pain sensitivity. These sex and racial/ethnic group differences are driven by multiple biologic and psychosocial mechanisms, and it is important to recognize that within-group differences are always greater than differences between groups. Additional research is needed to explain within-group variability in pain responses, especially considering that the mechanisms contributing to pain responses may differ substantially from one group to another. Thus, in addition to their role as individual differences factors, demographic group variables (e.g., sex, race group) may also moderate the effects of other pain-related individual difference factors. An important goal of research on individual differences in responses to pain and its treatment is to enable a priori predictions of an individual's projected pain experience or treatment response, which would inform personalized pain management. Ultimately, greater appreciation of the importance of individual differences in pain and continued research to elucidate the underlying biopsychosocial mechanisms will propel advancement toward improved diagnosis and treatment of pain.

ACKNOWLEDGMENTS
Preparation of this chapter was supported by National Institutes of Health grants R37AG033906, K07AG046371, and U01DE017018.

References

1. Fillingim RB. Individual differences in pain: understanding the mosaic that makes pain personal. *Pain* 2017;158(suppl 1):S11–S18.
2. Lawrence RC, Felson DT, Helmick CG, et al. Estimates of the prevalence of arthritis and other rheumatic conditions in the United States. Part II. *Arthritis Rheum* 2008;58(1):26–35.
3. Szebenyi B, Hollander AP, Dieppe P, et al. Associations between pain, function, and radiographic features in osteoarthritis of the knee. *Arthritis Rheum* 2006;54(1):230–235.
4. Carotti M, Salaffi F, Di Carlo M, et al. Relationship between magnetic resonance imaging findings, radiological grading, psychological distress and pain in patients with symptomatic knee osteoarthritis. *Radiol Med* 2017;122:934–943.

5. Carragee EJ, Alamin TF, Miller JL, et al. Discographic, MRI and psychosocial determinants of low back pain disability and remission: a prospective study in subjects with benign persistent back pain. *Spine J* 2005;5(1):24–35.

6. Chou R, Qaseem A, Owens DK, et al.; for Clinical Guidelines Committee of the American College of Physicians. Diagnostic imaging for low back pain: advice for high-value health care from the American College of Physicians. *Ann Intern Med* 2011;154(3):181–189.

7. Aubrun F, Langeron O, Quesnel C, et al. Relationships between measurement of pain using visual analog score and morphine requirements during postoperative intravenous morphine titration. *Anesthesiology* 2003;98(6):1415–1421.

8. Bisgaard T, Klarskov B, Rosenberg J, et al. Characteristics and prediction of early pain after laparoscopic cholecystectomy. *Pain* 2001;90(3):261–269.

9. Tighe PJ, Le-Wendling LT, Patel A, et al. Clinically derived early postoperative pain trajectories differ by age, sex, and type of surgery. *Pain* 2015;156(4):609–617.

10. Werner MU, Duun P, Kehlet H. Prediction of postoperative pain by preoperative nociceptive responses to heat stimulation. *Anesthesiology* 2004;100(1):115–119.

11. Gerbershagen HJ, Aduckathil S, van Wijck AJ, et al. Pain intensity on the first day after surgery: a prospective cohort study comparing 179 surgical procedures. *Anesthesiology* 2013;118(4):934–944.

12. Nielsen CS, Stubhaug A, Price DD, et al. Individual differences in pain sensitivity: genetic and environmental contributions. *Pain* 2008;136:21–29.

13. Diatchenko L, Slade GD, Nackley AG, et al. Genetic basis for individual variations in pain perception and the development of a chronic pain condition. *Hum Mol Genet* 2005;14(1):135–143.

14. Edwards RR, Haythornthwaite JA, Tella P, et al. Basal heat pain thresholds predict opioid analgesia in patients with postherpetic neuralgia. *Anesthesiology* 2006;104(6):1243–1248.

15. Angst MS, Phillips NG, Drover DR, et al. Pain sensitivity and opioid analgesia: a pharmacogenomic twin study. *Pain* 2012;153:1397–1409.

16. Sarton E, Olofsen E, Romberg R, et al. Sex differences in morphine analgesia: an experimental study in healthy volunteers. *Anesthesiology* 2000;93(5):1245–1254.

17. Sibille KT, Kindler LL, Glover TL, et al. Individual differences in morphine and butorphanol analgesia: a laboratory pain study. *Pain Med* 2011;12(7):1076–1085.

18. Atlas SJ, Keller RB, Wu YA, et al. Long-term outcomes of surgical and nonsurgical management of lumbar spinal stenosis: 8 to 10 year results from the Maine lumbar spine study. *Spine* 2005;30(8):936–943.

19. Chae Y, Park HJ, Hahm DH, et al. Individual differences of acupuncture analgesia in humans using cDNA microarray. *J Physiol Sci* 2006;56(6):425–431.

20. Broderick JE, Keefe FJ, Schneider S, et al. Cognitive behavioral therapy for chronic pain is effective, but for whom? *Pain* 2016;157(9):2115–2123.

21. Hoffman BM, Papas RK, Chatkoff DK, et al. Meta-analysis of psychological interventions for chronic low back pain. *Health Psychol* 2007;26(1):1–9.

22. Chapman WP, Jones CM. Variations in cutaneous and visceral pain sensitivity in normal subjects. *J Clin Invest* 1944;23:81–91.

23. Hardy JD, Wolff HG, Goodell H. *Pain Sensation and Reactions.* Baltimore, MD: Williams & Wilkins; 1952.

24. Engel GL. The need for a new medical model: a challenge for biomedicine. *Science* 1977;196(4286):129–136.

25. Gatchel RJ, Peng YB, Peters ML, et al. The biopsychosocial approach to chronic pain: scientific advances and future directions. *Psychol Bull* 2007;133(4):581–624.

26. Fillingim RB, King CD, Ribeiro-Dasilva MC, et al. Sex, gender, and pain: a review of recent clinical and experimental findings. *J Pain* 2009;10(5):447–485.

27. Mogil JS. Sex differences in pain and pain inhibition: multiple explanations of a controversial phenomenon. *Nat Rev Neurosci* 2012;13(12):859–866.

28. Racine M, Tousignant-Laflamme Y, Kloda LA, et al. A systematic literature review of 10 years of research on sex/gender and pain perception—part 2: do biopsychosocial factors alter pain sensitivity differently in women and men? *Pain* 2012;153(3):619–635.

29. Hashmi JA, Davis KD. Deconstructing sex differences in pain sensitivity. *Pain* 2014;155(1):10–13.

30. Crook J, Rideout E, Browne G. The prevalence of pain complaints in a general population. *Pain* 1984;18:299–314.

31. Elliott AM, Smith BH, Penny KI, et al. The epidemiology of chronic pain in the community. *Lancet* 1999;354(9186):1248–1252.

32. Andersson HI, Ejlertsson G, Leden I, et al. Chronic pain in a geographically defined general population: studies of differences in age, gender, social class, and pain localization. *Clin J Pain* 1993;9:174–182.

33. Kamaleri Y, Natvig B, Ihlebaek CM, et al. Number of pain sites is associated with demographic, lifestyle, and health-related factors in the general population. *Eur J Pain* 2008;12:742–748.

34. Von Korff M, Dworkin SF, LeResche L, et al. An epidemiologic comparison of pain complaints. *Pain* 1988;32:173–183.

35. Kennedy J, Roll JM, Schraudner T, et al. Prevalence of persistent pain in the U.S. adult population: new data from the 2010 National Health Interview Survey. *J Pain* 2014;15(10):979–984.

36. Craft RM. Modulation of pain by estrogens. *Pain* 2007;132:S3–S12.

37. Steingrimsdottir OA, Landmark T, Macfarlane GJ, et al. Defining chronic pain in epidemiological studies: a systematic review and meta-analysis. *Pain* 2017;158(11):2092–2107.

38. Sternbach RA. Survey of pain in the United States: the NUPRIN Pain Report. *Clin J Pain* 1986;2:49–53.

39. Jones GT, Atzeni F, Beasley M, et al. The prevalence of fibromyalgia in the general population—a comparison of the American College of Rheumatology 1990, 2010 and modified 2010 classification criteria. *Arthritis Rheumatol* 2015;67:568–575.

40. Mansfield KE, Sim J, Jordan JL, et al. A systematic review and meta-analysis of the prevalence of chronic widespread pain in the general population. *Pain* 2016;157(1):55–64.

41. Lipton RB, Stewart WF, Diamond S, et al. Prevalence and burden of migraine in the United States: data from the American Migraine Study II. *Headache* 2001;41(7):646–657.

42. Dworkin SF, Huggins KH, LeResche L, et al. Epidemiology of signs and symptoms in temporomandibular disorders: clinical signs in cases and controls. *J Am Dent Assoc* 1990;120:273–281.

43. LeResche L, Mancl LA, Drangsholt MT, et al. Predictors of onset of facial pain and temporomandibular disorders in early adolescence. *Pain* 2007;129(3):269–278.

44. Chang L, Heitkemper MM. Gender differences in irritable bowel syndrome. *Gastroenterology* 2002;123(5):1686–1701.

45. Chenot JF, Becker A, Leonhardt C, et al. Sex differences in presentation, course, and management of low back pain in primary care. *Clin J Pain* 2008;24(7):578–584.

46. Freburger JK, Holmes GM, Agans RP, et al. The rising prevalence of chronic low back pain. *Arch Intern Med* 2009;169(3):251–258.

47. Oksuz E. Prevalence, risk factors, and preference-based health states of low back pain in a Turkish population. *Spine* 2006;31(25):E968–E972.

48. Stewart Williams J, Ng N, Peltzer K, et al. Risk factors and disability associated with low back pain in older adults in low- and middle-income countries. Results from the WHO Study on Global AGEing and Adult Health (SAGE). *PLoS One* 2015;10(6):e0127880.

49. Plotnikoff R, Karunamuni N, Lytvyak E, et al. Osteoarthritis prevalence and modifiable factors: a population study. *BMC Public Health* 2015;15:1195.

50. Barsky AJ, Peekna HM, Borus JF. Somatic symptom reporting in women and men. *J Gen Intern Med* 2001;16(4):266–275.

51. Kaur S, Stechuchak KM, Coffman CJ, et al. Gender differences in health care utilization among veterans with chronic pain. *J Gen Intern Med* 2007;22(2):228–233.

52. Verbrugge LM. Sex differentials in health. *Public Health Rep* 1982;97(5):417–437.

53. Bertakis KD, Azari R, Helms LJ, et al. Gender differences in the utilization of health care services. *J Fam Pract* 2000;49(2):147–152.

54. King S, Chambers CT, Huguet A, et al. The epidemiology of chronic pain in children and adolescents revisited: a systematic review. *Pain* 2011;152(12):2729–2738.

55. Holley AL, Wilson AC, Palermo TM. Predictors of the transition from acute to persistent musculoskeletal pain in children and adolescents: a prospective study. *Pain* 2017;158(5):794–801.

56. Tsze DS, Hirschfeld G, Dayan PS, et al. Defining no pain, mild, moderate, and severe pain based on the Faces Pain Scale-Revised and color analog scale in children with acute pain [published online ahead of print May 25, 106]. *Pediatric Emerg Care.* doi:10.1097/PEC.0000000000000791.

57. Almeida GF, Longo DL, Trevizan M, et al. Sex differences in pediatric dental pain perception. *J Dent Child* 2016;83(3):120–124.

58. von Baeyer CL, Chambers CT, Eakins DM. Development of a 10-item short form of the parents' postoperative pain measure: the PPPM-SF. *J Pain* 2011;12(3):401–406.

59. LeResche L, Mancl LA, Drangsholt MT, et al. Relationship of pain and symptoms to pubertal development in adolescents. *Pain* 2005;118(1–2):20–29.

60. Periasamy S, Poovathai R, Pondiyadanar S. Influences of gender on postoperative morphine consumption. *J Clin Diagn Res* 2014;8(12):GC04–GC07.

61. Cepeda MS, Carr DB. Women experience more pain and require more morphine than men to achieve a similar degree of analgesia. *Anesth Analg* 2003;97(5):1464–1468.

62. Tighe PJ, Riley JL III, Fillingim RB. Sex differences in the incidence of severe pain events following surgery: a review of 333,000 pain scores. *Pain Med* 2014;15(8):1390–1404.

63. Chia YY, Chow LH, Hung CC, et al. Gender and pain upon movement are associated with the requirements for postoperative patient-controlled IV analgesia: a prospective survey of 2,298 Chinese patients. *Can J Anaesth* 2002;49(3):249–255.

64. Averbuch M, Katzper M. A search for sex differences in response to analgesia. *Arch Intern Med* 2000;160(22):3424–3428.

65. Grossi GB, Maiorana C, Garramone RA, et al. Assessing postoperative discomfort after third molar surgery: a prospective study. *J Oral Maxillofac Surg* 2007;65(5):901–917.

66. Gear RW, Gordon NC, Heller PH, et al. Gender difference in analgesic response to the kappa-opioid pentazocine. *Neurosci Lett* 1996;205(3):207–209.

67. Heyer EJ, Sharma R, Winfree CJ, et al. Severe pain confounds neuropsychological test performance. *J Clin Exp Neuropsychol* 2000;22(5):633–639.

68. Logan DE, Rose JB. Gender differences in post-operative pain and patient controlled analgesia use among adolescent surgical patients. *Pain* 2004;109(3):481–487.

69. Shabat S, Folman Y, Arinzon Z, et al. Gender differences as an influence on patients' satisfaction rates in spinal surgery of elderly patients. *Eur Spine J* 2005;14(10):1027–1032.

70. Storesund A, Krukhaug Y, Olsen MV, et al. Females report higher postoperative pain scores than males after ankle surgery. *Scand J Pain* 2016;12:85–93.

71. Zheng H, Schnabel A, Yahiaoui-Doktor M, et al. Age and preoperative pain are major confounders for sex differences in postoperative pain outcome: a prospective database analysis. *PloS One* 2017;12(6):e0178659.

72. Ochroch EA, Gottschalk A, Troxel AB, et al. Women suffer more short and long-term pain than men after major thoracotomy. *Clin J Pain* 2006;22(5):491–498.

73. Uchiyama K, Kawai M, Tani M, et al. Gender differences in postoperative pain after laparoscopic cholecystectomy. *Surg Endosc* 2006;20(3):448–451.

74. Pereira MP, Pogatzki-Zahn E. Gender aspects in postoperative pain. *Curr Opin Anaesthesiol* 2015;28(5):546–558.

75. Bjornnes AK, Parry M, Lie I, et al. Pain experiences of men and women after cardiac surgery. *J Clin Nurs* 2016;25(19–20):3058–3068.

76. Kehlet H, Jensen TS, Woolf CJ. Persistent postsurgical pain: risk factors and prevention. *Lancet* 2006;367(9522):1618–1625.

77. Affleck G, Tennen H, Keefe FJ, et al. Everyday life with osteoarthritis or rheumatoid arthritis: independent effects of disease and gender on daily pain, mood, and coping. *Pain* 1999;83(3):601–609.

78. Holtzman J, Saleh K, Kane R. Gender differences in functional status and pain in a Medicare population undergoing elective total hip arthroplasty. *Med Care* 2002;40(6):461–470.

79. Keefe FJ, Affleck G, France CR, et al. Gender differences in pain, coping, and mood in individuals having osteoarthritic knee pain: a within-day analysis. *Pain* 2004;110(3):571–577.

80. Fillingim RB, Doleys DM, Edwards RR, et al. Clinical characteristics of chronic back pain as a function of gender and oral opioid use. *Spine* 2003;28(2):143–150.

81. George SZ, Bialosky JE, Wittmer VT, et al. Sex differences in pain drawing area for individuals with chronic musculoskeletal pain. *J Orthop Sports Phys Ther* 2007;37(3):115–121.

82. Bush FM, Harkins SW, Harrington WG, et al. Analysis of gender effects on pain perception and symptom presentation in temporomandibular joint pain. *Pain* 1993;53:73–80.

83. Edwards R, Augustson E, Fillingim R. Differential relationships between anxiety and treatment-associated pain reduction among male and female chronic pain patients. *Clin J Pain* 2003;19(4):208–216.

84. Robinson ME, Wise EA, Riley JL III. Sex differences in clinical pain: a multi-sample study. *J Clin Psychol Med Settings* 1998;5:413–423.

85. Turk DC, Okifuji A. Does sex make a difference in the prescription of treatments and the adaptation to chronic pain by cancer and non-cancer patients? *Pain* 1999;82(2):139–148.

86. Rovner GS, Sunnerhagen KS, Bjorkdahl A, et al. Chronic pain and sex-differences; women accept and move, while men feel blue. *PloS One* 2017;12(4):e0175737.

87. Marcus DA. Gender differences in chronic pain in a treatment-seeking population. *J Gend Specif Med* 2003;6(4):19–24.

88. Miller A, Sanderson K, Bruno R, et al. The prevalence of pain and analgesia use in the Australian population: findings from the 2011 to 2012 Australian National Health Survey. *Pharmacoepidemiol Drug Saf* 2017;26(11):1403–1410.

89. Mullersdorf M, Soderback I. The actual state of the effects, treatment and incidence of disabling pain in a gender perspective—a Swedish study. *Disabil Rehabil* 2000;22(18):840–854.

90. Glass N, Segal NA, Sluka KA, et al. Examining sex differences in knee pain: the multicenter osteoarthritis study. *Osteoarthritis Cartilage* 2014;22(8):1100–1106.

91. Bartley EJ, King CD, Sibille KT, et al. Enhanced pain sensitivity among individuals with symptomatic knee osteoarthritis: potential sex differences in central sensitization. *Arthritis Care Res (Hoboken)* 2016;68(4):472–480.

92. Wranker LS, Rennemark M, Berglund J. Pain among older adults from a gender perspective: findings from the Swedish National Study on Aging and Care (SNAC-Blekinge). *Scand J Public Health* 2016;44(3):258–263.

93. Plesh O, Adams SH, Gansky SA. Temporomandibular joint and muscle disorder-type pain and comorbid pains in a national US sample. *J Orofac Pain* 2011;25(3):190–198.

94. LeResche L, Saunders K, Dublin S, et al. Sex and age differences in global pain status among patients using opioids long term for chronic noncancer pain. *J Womens Health (Larchmt)* 2015;24(8):629–635.

95. Maixner W, Fillingim RB, Williams DA, et al. Overlapping chronic pain conditions: implications for diagnosis and classification. *J Pain* 2016;17(9 suppl):T93–T107.

96. Riley JL, Robinson ME, Wise EA, et al. Sex differences in the perception of noxious experimental stimuli: a meta-analysis. *Pain* 1998;74:181–187.

97. Fillingim RB, Maixner W. Gender differences in the responses to noxious stimuli. *Pain Forum* 1995;4(4):209–221.

98. Fillingim RB, King CD, Ribeiro-Dasilva MC, et al. Sex, gender, and pain: a review of recent clinical and experimental findings. *J Pain* 2009;10(5):447–485.

99. Racine M, Tousignant-Laflamme Y, Kloda LA, et al. A systematic literature review of 10 years of research on sex/gender and experimental pain perception—part 1: are there really differences between women and men? *Pain* 2012;153(3):602–618.

100. Fillingim RB, Maixner W, Kincaid S, et al. Sex differences in temporal summation but not sensory-discriminative processing of thermal pain. *Pain* 1998;75(1):121–127.

101. Sarlani E, Grace EG, Reynolds MA, et al. Sex differences in temporal summation of pain and aftersensations following repetitive noxious mechanical stimulation. *Pain* 2004;109(1–2):115–123.

102. Graven-Nielsen T, Vaegter HB, Finocchietti S, et al. Assessment of musculoskeletal pain sensitivity and temporal summation by cuff pressure algometry: a reliability study. *Pain* 2015;156(11):2193–2202.

103. Popescu A, LeResche L, Truelove EL, et al. Gender differences in pain modulation by diffuse noxious inhibitory controls: a systematic review. *Pain* 2010;150(2):309–318.

104. Boerner KE, Birnie KA, Caes L, et al. Sex differences in experimental pain among healthy children: a systematic review and meta-analysis. *Pain* 2014;155(5):983–993.

105. Hashmi JA, Davis KD. Women experience greater heat pain adaptation and habituation than men. *Pain* 2009;145(3):350–357.

106. Fillingim RB. Individual differences in pain responses. *Curr Rheumatol Rep* 2005;7(5):342–347.

107. Kallai I, Barke A, Voss U. The effects of experimenter characteristics on pain reports in women and men. *Pain* 2004;112(1–2):142–147.

108. Levine FM, De Simone LL. The effects of experimenter gender on pain report in male and female subjects. *Pain* 1991;44:69–72.

109. Hoffmann DE, Tarzian AJ. The girl who cried pain: a bias against women in the treatment of pain. *J Law Med Ethics* 2001;29(1):13–27.

110. LeResche L. Defining gender disparities in pain management. *Clin Orthop Relat Res* 2011;469:1871–1877.

111. Oliva EM, Midboe AM, Lewis ET, et al. Sex differences in chronic pain management practices for patients receiving opioids from the Veterans Health Administration. *Pain Med* 2015;16(1):112–118.

112. Schäfer G, Prkachin KM, Kaseweter KA, et al. Health care providers' judgments in chronic pain: the influence of gender and trustworthiness. *Pain* 2016;157:1618–1625.

113. Hirsh AT, Hollingshead NA, Matthias MS, et al. The influence of patient sex, provider race, and sexist attitudes on pain treatment decisions. *J Pain* 2014;15(5):551–559.

114. Niesters M, Dahan A, Kest B, et al. Do sex differences exist in opioid analgesia? A systematic review and meta-analysis of human experimental and clinical studies. *Pain* 2010;151(1):61–68.

115. Cattaneo S, Ingelmo P, Scudeller L, et al. Sex differences in the daily rhythmicity of morphine consumption after major abdominal surgery. *J Opioid Manag* 2017;13(2):85–94.

116. Riley JL III, Hastie BA, Glover TL, et al. Cognitive-affective and somatic side effects of morphine and pentazocine: side-effect profiles in healthy adults. *Pain Med* 2010;11(2):195–206.

117. Ballantyne JC. Opioids for the treatment of chronic pain: mistakes made, lessons learned, and future directions. *Anesth Analg* 2017;125(5):1769–1778.

118. Stagnitti MN. *Trends in Prescribed Outpatient Opioid Use and Expenses in the U.S. Civilian Noninstitutionalized Population, 2002-2012.* Rockville, MD: Agency for Healthcare Research and Quality; 2015.

119. Sullivan MD, Howe CQ. Opioid therapy for chronic pain in the United States: promises and perils. *Pain* 2013;154(suppl 1):S94–S100.

120. Sites BD, Beach ML, Davis MA. Increases in the use of prescription opioid analgesics and the lack of improvement in disability metrics among users. *Reg Anesth Pain Med* 2014;39(1):6–12.

121. Darnall BD, Stacey BR. Sex differences in long-term opioid use: cautionary notes for prescribing in women. *Arch Intern Med* 2012;172(5):431–432.

122. Samuelsen PJ, Svendsen K, Wilsgaard T, et al. Persistent analgesic use and the association with chronic pain and other risk factors in the population-a longitudinal study from the Tromso Study and the Norwegian Prescription Database. *Eur J Clin Pharmacol* 2016;72:977–985.

123. Wright EA, Katz JN, Abrams S, et al. Trends in prescription of opioids from 2003-2009 in persons with knee osteoarthritis. *Arthritis Care Res* 2014;66(10):1489–1495.

124. Serdarevic M, Striley CW, Cottler LB. Sex differences in prescription opioid use. *Curr Opin Psychiatry* 2017;30(4):238–246.

125. Back SE, Payne RL, Simpson AN, et al. Gender and prescription opioids: findings from the National Survey on Drug Use and Health. *Addict Behav* 2010;35(11):1001–1007.

126. Kaplovitch E, Gomes T, Camacho X, et al. Sex differences in dose escalation and overdose death during chronic opioid therapy: a population-based cohort study. *PloS One* 2015;10(8):e0134550.

127. Brady JE, Giglio R, Keyes KM, et al. Risk markers for fatal and nonfatal prescription drug overdose: a meta-analysis. *Inj Epidemiol* 2017;4(1):24.

128. Gladstone EJ, Smolina K, Weymann D, et al. Geographic variations in prescription opioid dispensations and deaths among women and men in British Columbia, Canada. *Med Care* 2015;53(11):954–959.

129. Walker JS, Carmody JJ. Experimental pain in healthy human subjects: gender differences in nociception and in response to ibuprofen. *Anesth Analg* 1998;86(6):1257–1262.

130. Butcher BE, Carmody JJ. Sex differences in analgesic response to ibuprofen are influenced by expectancy: a randomized, crossover, balanced placebo-designed study. *Eur J Pain* 2012;16(7):1005–1013.

131. Aslaksen PM, Bystad M, Vambheim SM, et al. Gender differences in placebo analgesia: event-related potentials and emotional modulation. *Psychosom Med* 2011;73(2):193–199.

132. Compton P, Charuvastra V, Ling W. Effect of oral ketorolac and gender on human cold pressor pain tolerance. *Clin Exp Pharmacol Physiol* 2003;30(10):759–63.

133. Pud D, Yarnitsky D, Sprecher E, et al. Can personality traits and gender predict the response to morphine? An experimental cold pain study. *Eur J Pain* 2006;10(2):103–112.

134. Krummenacher P, Kossowsky J, Schwarz C, et al. Expectancy-induced placebo analgesia in children and the role of magical thinking. *J Pain* 2014;15(12):1282–1293.

135. Boerner KE, Eccleston C, Chambers CT, et al. Sex differences in the efficacy of psychological therapies for the management of chronic and recurrent pain in children and adolescents: a systematic review and meta-analysis [published online ahead of print December 15, 2016]. *Pain*. doi:10.1097/j .pain.0000000000000803.

136. Bernardes SF, Keogh E, Lima ML. Bridging the gap between pain and gender research: a selective literature review. *Eur J Pain* 2008;12(4):427–440.

137. Ribeiro-Dasilva MC, Shinal RM, Glover T, et al. Evaluation of menstrual cycle effects on morphine and pentazocine analgesia. *Pain* 2011;152(3):614–622.

138. Fillingim RB, Ness TJ. Sex-related hormonal influences on pain and analgesic responses. *Neurosci Biobehav Rev* 2000;24:485–501.

139. LeResche L, Mancl L, Sherman JJ, et al. Changes in temporomandibular pain and other symptoms across the menstrual cycle. *Pain* 2003;106(3):253–261.

140. Riley JL III, Robinson ME, Wise EA, et al. A meta-analytic review of pain perception across the menstrual cycle. *Pain* 1999;81:225–235.

141. Brynhildsen JO, Bjors E, Skarsgard C, et al. Is hormone replacement therapy a risk factor for low back pain among postmenopausal women? *Spine* 1998;23(7):809–813.

142. LeResche L, Saunders K, Von Korff MR, et al. Use of exogenous hormones and risk of temporomandibular disorder pain. *Pain* 1997;69(1–2):153–160.

143. Musgrave DS, Vogt MT, Nevitt MC, et al. Back problems among postmenopausal women taking estrogen replacement therapy. *Spine* 2001;26:1606–1612.

144. Macfarlane TV, Blinkhorn A, Worthington HV, et al. Sex hormonal factors and chronic widespread pain: a population study among women. *Rheumatology (Oxford)* 2002;41(4):454–457.

145. Macfarlane TV, Blinkhorn AS, Davies RM, et al. Association between female hormonal factors and oro-facial pain: study in the community. *Pain* 2002;97(1–2):5–10.

146. de Leeuw R, Albuquerque RJ, Andersen AH, et al. Influence of estrogen on brain activation during stimulation with painful heat. *J Oral Maxillofac Surg* 2006;64(2):158–166.

147. Smith YR, Stohler CS, Nichols TE, et al. Pronociceptive and antinociceptive effects of estradiol through endogenous opioid neurotransmission in women. *J Neurosci* 2006;26(21):5777–5785.

148. El-Shormilisy N, Strong J, Meredith PJ. Associations between gender, coping patterns and functioning for individuals with chronic pain: a systematic review. *Pain Res Management* 2015;20(1):48–55.

149. Edwards RR, Haythornthwaite JA, Sullivan MJ, et al. Catastrophizing as a mediator of sex differences in pain: differential effects for daily pain versus laboratory-induced pain. *Pain* 2004;111(3):335–341.

150. Unruh AM, Ritchie J, Merskey H. Does gender affect appraisal of pain and pain coping strategies? *Clin J Pain* 1999;15(1):31–40.

151. Robinson ME, Riley JL III, Myers CD, et al. Gender role expectations of pain: relationship to sex differences in pain. *J Pain* 2001;2:251–257.

152. Robinson ME, Wise EA, Gagnon C, et al. Influences of gender role and anxiety on sex differences in temporal summation of pain. *J Pain* 2004;5(2):77–82.

153. Myers CD, Riley JL III, Robinson ME. Psychosocial contributions to sex-correlated differences in pain. *Clin J Pain* 2003;19(4):225–232.

154. Myers CD, Robinson ME, Riley JL III, et al. Sex, gender, and blood pressure: contributions to experimental pain report. *Psychosom Med* 2001;63(4):545–550.

155. Pool GJ, Schwegler AF, Theodore BR, et al. Role of gender norms and group identification on hypothetical and experimental pain tolerance. *Pain* 2007;129(1–2):122–129.

156. Smedley BD, Stith AY, Nelson AR, eds. *Unequal Treatment*. Washington, DC: National Academies Press; 2003.

157. Meyer PA, Penman-Aguilar A, Campbell VA, et al. Conclusion and future directions: CDC Health Disparities and Inequalities Report—United States, 2013. *MMWR Suppl* 2013;62(3):184–186.

158. Anderson KO, Green CR, Payne R. Racial and ethnic disparities in pain: causes and consequences of unequal care. *J Pain* 2009;10(12):1187–1204.

159. Hollingshead NA, Ashburn-Nardo L, Stewart JC, et al. The pain experience of Hispanic Americans: a critical literature review and conceptual model. *J Pain* 2016;17(5):513–528.

160. Bhopal R. Race and ethnicity: responsible use from epidemiological and public health perspectives. *J Law Med Ethics* 2006;34(3):500–507.

161. Lavin R, Park J. A characterization of pain in racially and ethnically diverse older adults: a review of the literature. *J Appl Gerontol* 2014;33(3):258–290.

162. Plesh O, Gansky SA, Curtis DA. Chronic pain in a biracial cohort of young women. *Open Pain J* 2012;5:24–31.

163. Hollingshead NA, Vrany EA, Stewart JC, et al. Differences in Mexican Americans' prevalence of chronic pain and co-occurring analgesic medica-

164. Janevic MR, McLaughlin SJ, Heapy AA, et al. Racial and socioeconomic disparities in disabling chronic pain: findings from the Health and Retirement Study. *J Pain* 2017;18:1459–1467.

165. Nahin RL. Estimates of pain prevalence and severity in adults: United States, 2012. *J Pain* 2015;16(8):769–780.

166. Castel LD, Saville BR, Depuy V, et al. Racial differences in pain during 1 year among women with metastatic breast cancer: a hazards analysis of interval-censored data. *Cancer* 2008;112(1):162–170.

167. Carey TS, Freburger JK, Holmes GM, et al. Race, care seeking, and utilization for chronic back and neck pain: population perspectives. *J Pain* 2010;11(4):343–350.

168. Carey TS, Garrett JM. The relation of race to outcomes and the use of health care services for acute low back pain. *Spine* 2003;28(4):390–394.

169. Edwards RR, Doleys DM, Fillingim RB, et al. Ethnic differences in pain tolerance: clinical implications in a chronic pain population. *Psychosom Med* 2001;63(2):316–323.

170. Green CR, Baker TA, Sato Y, et al. Race and chronic pain: a comparative study of young black and white Americans presenting for management. *J Pain* 2003;4(4):176–183.

171. Green CR, Baker TA, Smith EM, et al. The effect of race in older adults presenting for chronic pain management: a comparative study of black and white Americans. *J Pain* 2003;4(2):82–90.

172. McCracken LM, Matthews AK, Tang TS, et al. A comparison of blacks and whites seeking treatment for chronic pain. *Clin J Pain* 2001;17(3):249–255.

173. Bates MS, Edwards WT, Anderson KO. Ethnocultural influences on variation in chronic pain perception. *Pain* 1993;52(1):101–112.

174. Jarvik JG, Comstock BA, Heagerty PJ, et al. Back pain in seniors: the Back pain Outcomes using Longitudinal Data (BOLD) cohort baseline data. *BMC Musculoskelet Disord* 2014;15:134.

175. Allen KD. Racial and ethnic disparities in osteoarthritis phenotypes. *Curr Opin Rheumatol* 2010;22(5):528–532.

176. Allen KD, Chen JC, Callahan LF, et al. Racial differences in knee osteoarthritis pain: potential contribution of occupational and household tasks. *J Rheumatol* 2012;39(2):337–344.

177. Dominick KL, Baker TA. Racial and ethnic differences in osteoarthritis: prevalence, outcomes, and medical care. *Ethn Dis* 2004;14(4):558–566.

178. Reyes-Gibby CC, Aday LA, Todd KH, et al. Pain in aging community-dwelling adults in the United States: non-Hispanic whites, non-Hispanic blacks, and Hispanics. *J Pain* 2007;8(1):75–84.

179. Barbour KE, Boring M, Helmick CG, et al. Prevalence of severe joint pain among adults with doctor-diagnosed arthritis—United States, 2002-2014. *MMWR Morb Mortal Wkly Rep* 2016;65(39):1052–1056.

180. Ahn H, Weaver M, Lyon DE, et al. Differences in clinical pain and experimental pain sensitivity between Asian Americans and whites with knee osteoarthritis. *Clin J Pain* 2017;33(2):174–180.

181. Barnes PM, Adams PF, Powell-Griner E. Health characteristics of the American Indian or Alaska Native adult population: United States, 2004-2008. *Natl Health Stat Report* 2010;(20):1–22.

182. Calvillo ER, Flaskerud JH. Evaluation of the pain response by Mexican American and Anglo American women and their nurses. *J Adv Nurs* 1993; 18(3):451–459.

183. Edwards RR, Moric M, Husfeldt B, et al. Ethnic similarities and differences in the chronic pain experience: a comparison of African American, Hispanic, and white patients. *Pain Med* 2005;6(1):88–98.

184. Grol-Prokopczyk H. Sociodemographic disparities in chronic pain, based on 12-year longitudinal data. *Pain* 2017;158(2):313–322.

185. Poleshuck EL, Green CR. Socioeconomic disadvantage and pain. *Pain* 2008;136:235–238.

186. Portenoy RK, Ugarte C, Fuller I, et al. Population-based survey of pain in the United States: differences among white, African American, and Hispanic subjects. *J Pain* 2004;5(6):317–328.

187. Tait RC, Chibnall JT. Racial/ethnic disparities in the assessment and treatment of pain: psychosocial perspectives. *Am Psychol* 2014;69(2):131–141.

188. Rahim-Williams B, Riley JL III, Williams AK, et al. A quantitative review of ethnic group differences in experimental pain response: do biology, psychology, and culture matter? *Pain Med* 2012;13(4):522–540.

189. Kim HJ, Yang GS, Greenspan JD, et al. Racial and ethnic differences in experimental pain sensitivity: systematic review and meta-analysis. *Pain* 2017;158(2):194–211.

190. Cruz-Almeida Y, Sibille KT, Goodin BR, et al. Racial and ethnic differences in older adults with knee osteoarthritis. *Arthritis Rheumatol* 2014;66(7):1800–1810.

191. Chen I, Kurz J, Pasanen M, et al. Racial differences in opioid use for chronic nonmalignant pain. *J Gen Intern Med* 2005;20(7):593–598.

192. Pletcher MJ, Kertesz SG, Kohn MA, et al. Trends in opioid prescribing by race/ethnicity for patients seeking care in US emergency departments. *JAMA* 2008;299(1):70–78.

193. Todd KH, Deaton C, D'Adamo AP, et al. Ethnicity and analgesic practice. *Ann Emerg Med* 2000;35(1):11–16.

194. Adams RJ, Armstrong EP, Erstad BL. Prescribing and self-administration of morphine in Hispanic and non Hispanic Caucasian patients treated with patient-controlled analgesia. *J Pain Palliat Care Pharmacother* 2004; 18(2):29–38.

tion and substance use relative to non-Hispanic white and black Americans: results from NHANES 1999-2004. *Pain Med* 2016;17(6):1001–1009.

195. Fuentes EF, Kohn MA, Neighbor ML. Lack of association between patient ethnicity or race and fracture analgesia. *Acad Emerg Med* 2002;9(9):910–915.

196. Yen K, Kim M, Stremski ES, et al. Effect of ethnicity and race on the use of pain medications in children with long bone fractures in the emergency department. *Ann Emerg Med* 2003;42(1):41–47.

197. Nafiu OO, Chimbira WT, Stewart M, et al. Racial differences in the pain management of children recovering from anesthesia. *Paediatr Anaesth* 2017;27(7):760–767.

198. Craven P, Cinar O, Fosnocht D, et al. Prospective, 10-year evaluation of the impact of Hispanic ethnicity on pain management practices in the ED. *Am J Emerg Med* 2014;32(9):1055–1059.

199. Dickason RM, Chauhan V, Mor A, et al. Racial differences in opiate administration for pain relief at an academic emergency department. *West J Emerg Med* 2015;16(3):372–380.

200. Ringwalt C, Roberts AW, Gugelmann H, et al. Racial disparities across provider specialties in opioid prescriptions dispensed to medicaid beneficiaries with chronic noncancer pain. *Pain Med* 2015;16(4):633–640.

201. Prunuske JP, St. Hill CA, Hager KD, et al. Opioid prescribing patterns for non-malignant chronic pain for rural versus non-rural US adults: a population-based study using 2010 NAMCS data. *BMC Health Serv Res* 2014;14:563.

202. Burgess DJ, Nelson DB, Gravely AA, et al. Racial differences in prescription of opioid analgesics for chronic noncancer pain in a national sample of veterans. *J Pain* 2014;15(4):447–455.

203. Hollingshead NA, Meints S, Middleton SK, et al. Examining influential factors in providers' chronic pain treatment decisions: a comparison of physicians and medical students. *BMC Med Educ* 2015;15:164.

204. Hirsh AT, Hollingshead NA, Ashburn-Nardo L, et al. The interaction of patient race, provider bias, and clinical ambiguity on pain management decisions. *J Pain* 2015;16(6):558–568.

205. Hoffman KM, Trawalter S, Axt JR, et al. Racial bias in pain assessment and treatment recommendations, and false beliefs about biological differences between blacks and whites. *Proc Natl Acad Sci USA* 2016;113(16):4296–4301.

206. Kaiko RF, Wallenstein SL, Rogers AG, et al. Sources of variation in analgesic responses in cancer patients with chronic pain receiving morphine. *Pain* 1983;15(2):191–200.

207. Cepeda MS, Farrar JT, Baumgarten M, et al. Side effects of opioids during short-term administration: effect of age, gender, and race. *Clin Pharmacol Ther* 2003;74(2):102–112.

208. McCabe SE, West BT, Teter CJ, et al. Medical and nonmedical use of prescription opioids among high school seniors in the United States. *Arch Pediatr Adolesc Med* 2012;166(9):797–802.

209. Becker WC, Starrels JL, Heo M, et al. Racial differences in primary care opioid risk reduction strategies. *Ann Fam Med* 2011;9(3):219–225.

210. Kay C, Wozniak E, Koller S, et al. Adherence to chronic opioid therapy prescribing guidelines in a primary care clinic. *J Opioid Manag* 2016;12(5):333–345.

211. Hausmann LR, Gao S, Lee ES, et al. Racial disparities in the monitoring of patients on chronic opioid therapy. *Pain* 2013;154(1):46–52.

212. Mechlin B, Heymen S, Edwards CL, et al. Ethnic differences in cardiovascular-somatosensory interactions and in the central processing of noxious stimuli. *Psychophysiology* 2011;48:762–773.

213. Mechlin B, Morrow AL, Maixner W, et al. The relationship of allopregnanolone immunoreactivity and HPA-axis measures to experimental pain sensitivity: evidence for ethnic differences. *Pain* 2007;131:142–152.

214. Mechlin MB, Maixner W, Light KC, et al. African Americans show alterations in endogenous pain regulatory mechanisms and reduced pain tolerance to experimental pain procedures. *Psychosom Med* 2005;67(6):948–956.

215. Glover TL, Goodin BR, Horgas AL, et al. Vitamin D, race, and experimental pain sensitivity in older adults with knee osteoarthritis. *Arthritis Rheum* 2012;64(12):3926–3935.

216. Meints SM, Miller MM, Hirsh AT. Differences in pain coping between black and white Americans: a meta-analysis. *J Pain* 2016;17(6):642–653.

217. Meints SM, Stout M, Abplanalp S, et al. Pain-related rumination, but not magnification or helplessness, mediates race and sex differences in experimental pain. *J Pain* 2017;18(3):332–339.

218. Dugan SA, Lewis TT, Everson-Rose SA, et al. Chronic discrimination and bodily pain in a multiethnic cohort of midlife women in the Study of Women's Health Across the Nation. *Pain* 2017;158(9):1656–1665.

219. Carlisle SK. Perceived discrimination and chronic health in adults from nine ethnic subgroups in the USA. *Ethn Health* 2015;20(3):309–326.

220. Burgess DJ, Grill J, Noorbaloochi S, et al. The effect of perceived racial discrimination on bodily pain among older African American men. *Pain Med* 2009;10(8):1341–1352.

221. Edwards RR. The association of perceived discrimination with low back pain. *J Behav Med* 2008;31(5):379–389.

222. Goodin BR, Pham QT, Glover TL, et al. Perceived racial discrimination, but not mistrust of medical researchers, predicts the heat pain tolerance of African Americans with symptomatic knee osteoarthritis. *Health Psychol* 2013;32(11):1117–1126.

223. Diatchenko L, Fillingim RB, Smith SB, et al. The phenotypic and genetic signatures of common musculoskeletal pain conditions. *Nat Rev Rheumatol* 2013;9:340–350.

224. Diatchenko L, Nackley AG, Tchivileva IE, et al. Genetic architecture of human pain perception. *Trends Genet* 2007;23(12):605–613.

225. Fillingim RB, Wallace MR, Herbstman DM, et al. Genetic contributions to pain: a review of findings in humans. *Oral Dis* 2008;14:673–682.

226. Young EE, Lariviere WR, Belfer I. Genetic basis of pain variability: recent advances. *J Med Genet* 2012;49(1):1–9.

227. Mogil JS. Pain genetics: past, present and future. *Trends Genet* 2012;28(6):258–266.

228. Zorina-Lichtenwalter K, Meloto CB, Khoury S, et al. Genetic predictors of human chronic pain conditions. *Neuroscience* 2016;338:36–62.

229. Kato K, Sullivan PF, Evengard B, et al. Importance of genetic influences on chronic widespread pain. *Arthritis Rheum* 2006;54(5):1682–1686.

230. Leboeuf-Yde C. Back pain—individual and genetic factors. *J Electromyogr Kinesiol* 2004;14(1):129–133.

231. Morris-Yates A, Talley NJ, Boyce PM, et al. Evidence of a genetic contribution to functional bowel disorder. *Am J Gastroenterol* 1998;93(8):1311–1317.

232. Spector TD, Macgregor AJ. Risk factors for osteoarthritis: genetics. *Osteoarthritis Cartilage* 2004;12(suppl A):S39–S44.

233. Nielsen CS, Knudsen GP, Steingrimsdottir OA. Twin studies of pain. *Clin Genet* 2012;82(4):331–340.

234. McCarthy MI, Hirschhorn JN. Genome-wide association studies: potential next steps on a genetic journey. *Human Mol Genet* 2008;17(R2):R156–R165.

235. McCarthy MI, Hirschhorn JN. Genome-wide association studies: past, present and future. *Human Mol Gent* 2008;17(R2):R100–R101.

236. Diatchenko L, Nackley AG, Slade GD, et al. Idiopathic pain disorders—pathways of vulnerability. *Pain* 2006;123(3):226–230.

237. Mogil JS. *The Genetics of Pain*. Seattle, WA: IASP Press; 2004.

238. Macgregor AJ, Griffiths GO, Baker J, et al. Determinants of pressure pain threshold in adult twins: evidence that shared environmental influences predominate. *Pain* 1997;73(2):253–257.

239. Trost Z, Strachan E, Sullivan M, et al. Heritability of pain catastrophizing and associations with experimental pain outcomes: a twin study. *Pain* 2015;156(3):514–520.

240. Zubieta JK, Heitzeg MM, Smith YR, et al. COMT val158met genotype affects mu-opioid neurotransmitter responses to a pain stressor. *Science* 2003;299(5610):1240–1243.

241. Nielsen LM, Olesen AE, Sato H, et al. Association between gene polymorphisms and pain sensitivity assessed in a multi-modal multi-tissue human experimental model—an Explorative Study. *Basic Clin Pharmacol Toxicol* 2016;119(4):360–366.

242. Belfer I, Segall SK, Lariviere WR, et al. Pain modality- and sex-specific effects of COMT genetic functional variants. *Pain* 2013;154(8):1368–1376.

243. Martinez-Jauand M, Sitges C, Rodriguez V, et al. Pain sensitivity in fibromyalgia is associated with catechol-O-methyltransferase (COMT) gene. *Eur J Pain* 2013;17(1):16–27.

244. Desmeules J, Chabert J, Rebsamen M, et al. Central pain sensitization, COMT Val158Met polymorphism, and emotional factors in fibromyalgia. *J Pain* 2014;15(2):129–135.

245. Orrey DC, Bortsov AV, Hoskins JM, et al. Catechol-O-methyltransferase genotype predicts pain severity in hospitalized burn patients. *J Burn Care Res* 2012;33(4):518–523.

246. Bond C, LaForge KS, Tian M, et al. Single-nucleotide polymorphism in the human mu opioid receptor gene alters beta-endorphin binding and activity: possible implications for opiate addiction. *Proc Natl Acad Sci U S A* 1998;95(16):9608–9613.

247. Zhang Y, Wang D, Johnson AD, et al. Allelic expression imbalance of human mu opioid receptor (OPRM1) caused by variant A118G. *J Biol Chem* 2005;280(38):32618–32624.

248. Fillingim RB, Kaplan L, Staud R, et al. The A118G single nucleotide polymorphism of the mu-opioid receptor gene (OPRM1) is associated with pressure pain sensitivity in humans. *J Pain* 2005;6(3):159–167.

249. Matic M, van den Bosch GE, de Wildt SN, et al. Genetic variants associated with thermal pain sensitivity in a paediatric population. *Pain* 2016;157(11):2476–2482.

250. Lotsch J, Stuck B, Hummel T. The human mu-opioid receptor gene polymorphism 118A > G decreases cortical activation in response to specific nociceptive stimulation. *Behav Neurosci* 2006;120(6):1218–1224.

251. Janicki PK, Schuler G, Francis D, et al. A genetic association study of the functional A118G polymorphism of the human mu-opioid receptor gene in patients with acute and chronic pain. *Anesth Analg* 2006;103(4):1011–1017.

252. Solak O, Erdogan MO, Yildiz H, et al. Assessment of opioid receptor mu1 gene A118G polymorphism and its association with pain intensity in patients with fibromyalgia. *Rheumatol Int* 2014;34(9):1257–1261.

253. Martire LM, Wilson SJ, Small BJ, et al. COMT and OPRM1 genotype associations with daily knee pain variability and activity induced pain. *Scand J Pain* 2016;10:6–12.

254. Hwang IC, Park JY, Myung SK, et al. OPRM1 A118G gene variant and postoperative opioid requirement: a systematic review and meta-analysis. *Anesthesiology* 2014;121(4):825–834.

255. Choi SW, Lam DMH, Wong SSC, et al. Effects of single nucleotide polymorphisms on surgical and postsurgical opioid requirements: a systematic review and meta-analysis. *Clin J Pain* 2017;33(12):1117–1130.

256. Chidambaran V, Mavi J, Esslinger H, et al. Association of OPRM1 A118G variant with risk of morphine-induced respiratory depression following spine fusion in adolescents. *Pharmacogenomics J* 2015;15(3):255–262.

257. Hajj A, Halepian L, Osta NE, et al. OPRM1 c.118A>G polymorphism and duration of morphine treatment associated with morphine doses and quality-of-life in palliative cancer pain settings. *Int J Mol Sci* 2017;18(4):E669.

258. Tegeder I, Costigan M, Griffin RS, et al. GTP cyclohydrolase and tetrahydrobiopterin regulate pain sensitivity and persistence. *Nat Med* 2006;12(11):1269–1277.

259. Campbell CM, Edwards RR, Carmona C, et al. Polymorphisms in the GTP cyclohydrolase gene (GCH1) are associated with ratings of capsaicin pain. *Pain* 2009;141(1–2):114–118.

260. Tegeder I, Adolph J, Schmidt H, et al. Reduced hyperalgesia in homozygous carriers of a GTP cyclohydrolase 1 haplotype. *Eur J Pain* 2008;12:1069–1077.

261. Wadley AL, Lombard Z, Cherry CL, et al. Analysis of a previously identified "pain-protective" haplotype and individual polymorphisms in the GCH1 gene in Africans with HIV-associated sensory neuropathy: a genetic association study. *J Acquir Immune Defic Syndr* 2012;60(1):20–23.

262. Kim DH, Dai F, Belfer I, et al. Polymorphic variation of the guanosine triphosphate cyclohydrolase 1 gene predicts outcome in patients undergoing surgical treatment for lumbar degenerative disc disease. *Spine* 2010;35(21):1909–1914.

263. Fejer R, Hartvigsen J, Kyvik KO. Sex differences in heritability of neck pain. *Twin Res Hum Genet* 2006;9(2):198–204.

264. Olsen MB, Jacobsen LM, Schistad EI, et al. Pain intensity the first year after lumbar disc herniation is associated with the A118G polymorphism in the opioid receptor mu 1 gene: evidence of a sex and genotype interaction. *J Neurosci* 2012;32(29):9831–9834.

265. Belfer I, Youngblood V, Darbari DS, et al. A GCH1 haplotype confers sex-specific susceptibility to pain crises and altered endothelial function in adults with sickle cell anemia. *Am J Hematol* 2014;89(2):187–193.

266. Mountain JL, Risch N. Assessing genetic contributions to phenotypic differences among 'racial' and 'ethnic' groups. *Nat Genet* 2004;36(11 suppl):S48–S53.

267. Gower BA, Fernandez JR, Beasley TM, et al. Using genetic admixture to explain racial differences in insulin-related phenotypes. *Diabetes* 2003;52(4):1047–1051.

268. Shriver MD. Ethnic variation as a key to the biology of human disease. *Ann Intern Med* 1997;127(5):401–403.

269. Shriver MD, Kennedy GC, Parra EJ, et al. The genomic distribution of population substructure in four populations using 8,525 autosomal SNPs. *Hum Genomics* 2004;1(4):274–286.

270. Gelernter J, Kranzler H, Cubells J. Genetics of two mu opioid receptor gene (OPRM1) exon I polymorphisms: population studies, and allele frequencies in alcohol- and drug-dependent subjects. *Mol Psychiatry* 1999;4(5):476–483.

271. Hastie BA, Riley JL III, Kaplan L, et al. Ethnicity interacts with the OPRM1 gene in experimental pain sensitivity. *Pain* 2012;153:1610–1619.

272. George SZ, Dover GC, Wallace MR, et al. Biopsychosocial influence on exercise-induced delayed onset muscle soreness at the shoulder: pain catastrophizing and catechol-o-methyltransferase (COMT) diplotype predict pain ratings. *Clin J Pain* 2008;24(9):793–801.

273. George SZ, Parr J, Wallace M, et al. Genetic and psychological risk factors are associated with pain and disability in an experimentally induced acute shoulder pain model. *J Pain* 2012;13(4)(suppl 1):s29.

274. George SZ, Parr JJ, Wallace MR, et al. Inflammatory genes and psychological factors predict induced shoulder pain phenotype. *Med Sci Sports Exerc* 2014;46:1871–1881.

275. George SZ, Wallace MR, Wu SS, et al. Biopsychosocial influence on shoulder pain: risk subgroups translated across preclinical and clinical prospective cohorts. *Pain* 2015;156(1):148–156.

276. George SZ, Wallace MR, Wright TW, et al. Evidence for a biopsychosocial influence on shoulder pain: pain catastrophizing and catechol-O-methyltransferase (COMT) diplotype predict clinical pain ratings. *Pain* 2008;136(1–2):53–61.

277. Slade GD, Sanders AE, Ohrbach R, et al. COMT diplotype amplifies effect of stress on risk of temporomandibular pain. *J Dent Res* 2015;94(9):1187–1195.

CHAPTER 9

Functional Neuroanatomy of the Nociceptive System

ROBERT GRIFFIN, EZEKIEL FINK, and **GARY J. BRENNER**

From the standpoint of the physician, there are two perspectives from which to view pain. One is as a symptom of a disease process that will inform about the underlying pathophysiology. The other is as the primary cause for suffering that requires treatment in its own right. These two views of pain often coexist when the pain reveals pathology whose treatment will not resolve the pain rapidly enough for the patient to tolerate. For example, in acute myocardial ischemia, the pain is the cardinal symptom of the underlying illness but in itself can provide an ongoing stimulus for a catecholaminergic state that will increase myocardial demand and potentially worsen the ischemic state. Both of these perspectives, either using the pain as a clue or addressing it as the primary aim of treatment,[1] are enhanced by considering the patient's report of their pain in light of the specific anatomic structures that collect information about noxious stimuli and communicate this information to the central nervous system (CNS) where pain is perceived and behavioral responses are generated.

Pain may be grouped according to several different parameters including acute versus chronic, physiologic versus pathologic, and somatic versus visceral. Full understanding of the nature of any pain complaint requires knowledge of the anatomic structures involved and the functional status of these structures. Chronicity of pain is determined by the duration of the irritating stimulus and by the plastic response of the peripheral and CNS to injury or ongoing stimulus. Pain may be either nociceptive, induced by high-threshold sensory stimuli required for activation of peripheral nociceptors, or pathologic, induced by low-threshold stimuli due to a heightened state of nervous system excitability brought on by either inflammatory cell–cell signaling (i.e., inflammatory pain) and signal transduction or by the extensive anatomic and physiologic alterations brought on by nerve injury (i.e., neuropathic pain).[2] Finally, pain may be somatic, transmitted by the somatosensory nervous system, or visceral, transmitted by splanchnic sympathetic and pelvic nerve afferent fibers (or by specific cranial nerves in the case of the head and neck).[3,4] This chapter touches on the specific anatomic structures that are involved in the transduction of physical stimuli into sensory responses, the conduction of sensory information to the CNS, and the processing and relay of this sensory information within the spinal cord and brain and discusses some of the major perturbations in these structures as related to clinical pain phenomena.

Organization of the Peripheral Nociceptive System

There are several major anatomic units involved in pain sensation. First, primary sensory neurons whose peripheral terminals respond to physical energy conduct action potentials along long axons bundled into peripheral nerves from the site of sensory stimulus to the CNS.[5] Next, nociceptive synaptic relay occurs at the dorsal horn of the spinal cord, where substantial sensory processing occurs.[6–8] Ascending fiber tracts carry this information to the brainstem and, from there, diverse brain regions. Descending fiber tracts project from the brainstem and

brain to the dorsal horn of the spinal cord and regulate the processing of incoming sensory information.[9]

The peripheral nerves that carry sensory information from visceral organs, bone, muscle, joint, or skin to the CNS may be either cranial nerves or spinal nerves. Cranial nerves carry sensory information to the brainstem,[10] whereas spinal nerves carry sensory information to the spinal cord and may bear axons for neurons that synapse within the spinal cord or brainstem.[11,12] Spinal nerves are mixed nerves that carry general somatic afferent fibers, general visceral afferent fibers, general somatic efferent fibers, and general visceral efferent fibers. Somatic afferents primarily carry information from skin, muscle, tendon, and joint, whereas visceral afferents carry information from the other tissues. The cell bodies of both the somatic and the visceral afferent fibers carried by spinal nerves reside in the dorsal root ganglia (DRG) of the spinal cord, whereas those carried by cranial nerves reside in the brainstem cranial nerve nuclei.[12]

The ability to localize painful stimuli depends on the topographic organization of the nervous system. The somatic afferent system and the visceral afferent system are strikingly different in this regard, with precise stimulus position detected and encoded by the somatic nervous system but only relatively diffuse information coming to conscious awareness from the visceral afferent system.[4] In the clinical setting, precise localization of pain is often considered as evidence that the pain is detected by somatic afferents rather than visceral afferents. For example, knifelike well-localized pain associated with inspiration is likely detected by somatic fibers innervating the parietal pleura.[13] In the abdomen, well-localized lower right quadrant pain occurring late in the course of acute appendicitis is likely due to spread of the periappendiceal inflammation that irritates the somatic nerves innervating the abdominal wall overlying the appendix.[14]

In the somatic system, the spinal cord is segmentally organized, such that each spinal segment receives afferent information about a specific cutaneous band or dermatome (Fig. 9.1).[15] This organization arises during embryonic development when the embryonic neural tube and adjacent mesodermal tissues segment into a series of rostrocaudally adjacent somites.[16] Each spinal nerve innervates tissue developing from a single somite.[17] Spinal nerves from several different spinal segments, such as axons from neurons with cell bodies located in several different DRG, join to give rise to peripheral nerves with cutaneous fields of innervation that span multiple dermatomes (Fig. 9.2).[18] The innervation of specific peripheral cutaneous nerves, as compared to the organization of the cutaneous dermatomes, is illustrated (Fig. 9.3).

Although there are many anatomic similarities between the somatic and autonomic afferent fibers, there are significant differences in the clinical presentation of visceral pain and somatic pain. Visceral pain is perceived as deep and is typically not well spatially localized. The clinical features of visceral as compared to somatic pain are summarized in Table 9.1. Pain symptoms resulting from visceral afferents are felt in a location different than the organ itself, such as the experience of arm pain with myocardial infarction.[19] A possible explanation for the clinical

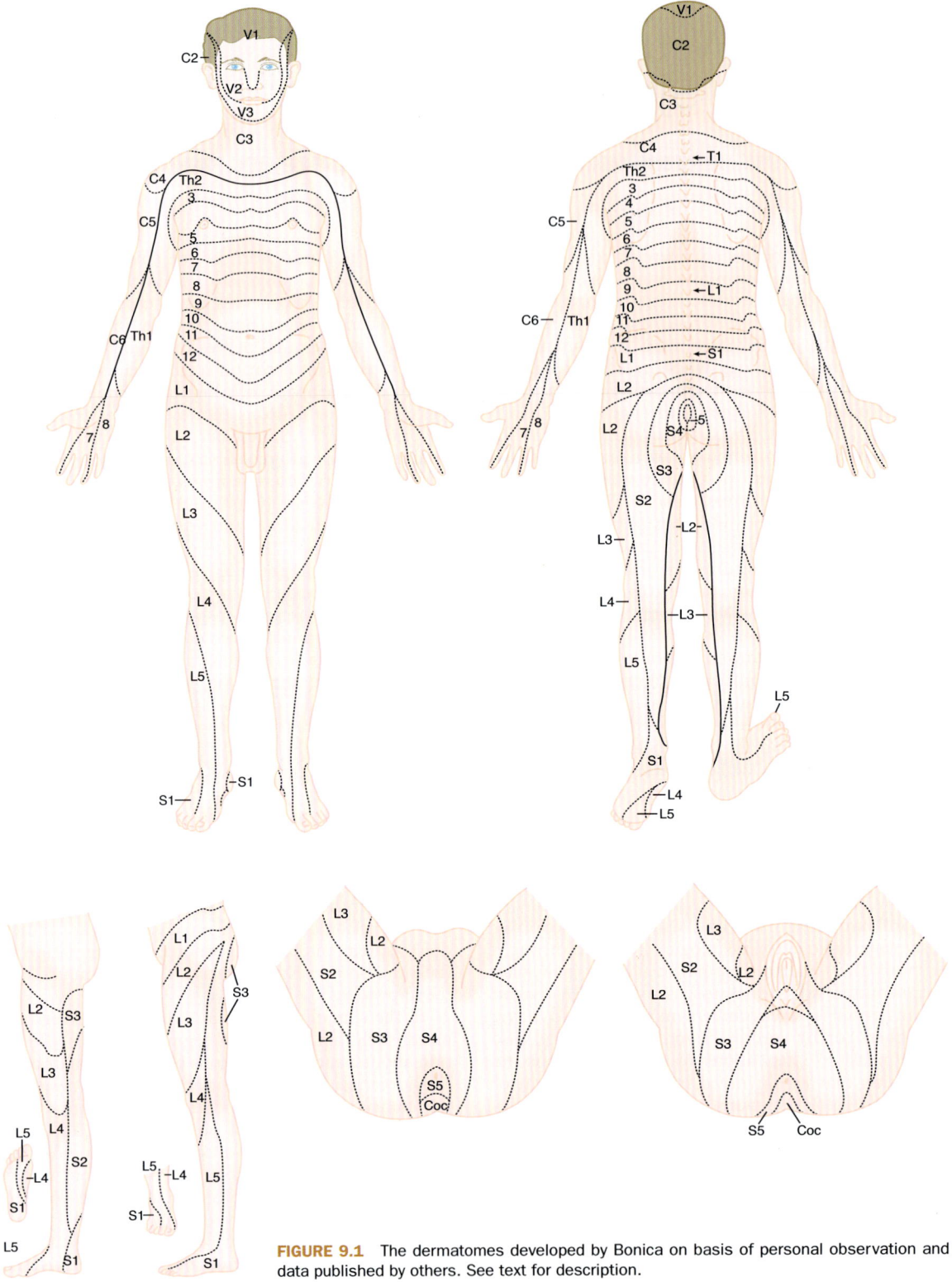

FIGURE 9.1   The dermatomes developed by Bonica on basis of personal observation and data published by others. See text for description.

symptoms of referred pain is that peripheral nociceptors from somatic and visceral origin converge on a single projection neuron in the dorsal horn. As a result, higher levels of the CNS cannot distinguish the source of the signal input and attribute the sensation to somatic structures by default because somatic sensory representation predominates in the CNS. Convergence occurs in the dorsal horn neurons in laminae I, IV, and V as well as in the intermediate gray matter in lamina X (Fig. 9.4)[20–22] as

well as other areas of the CNS including the brainstem, basal forebrain, thalamus, and cerebral cortex.[23] Functional neuroimaging studies have shown that regions of the cortex that are activated by noxious stimuli can also be activated by visceral stimuli.[24] In the thorax, substernal chest pain may be due to any of the visceral sensory afferents from the T1 to T6 spinal segments and may arise from the heart and great vessels, esophagus, lungs, or chest wall. Visceral pain in the abdomen

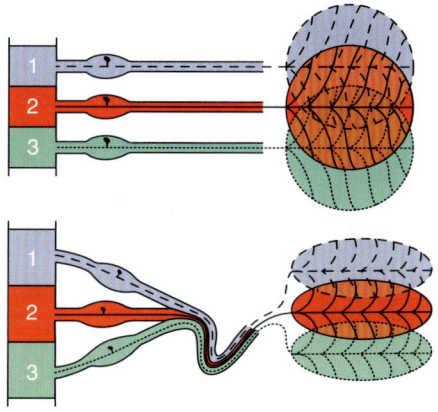

FIGURE 9.2 Simple diagrams to illustrate the overlap of cutaneous fields of segmental and peripheral nerves. In the **upper figure**, three intercostal (segmental) nerves extending from the periphery to the spinal cord are represented. The **lower figure** illustrates a somewhat analogous but less extensive overlap in the peripheral nerves.

tends to follow the structure of endodermal embryonic development with pain due to foregut structures (stomach, proximal duodenum, liver, biliary system, and pancreas) perceived in the epigastrium or upper abdomen, pain due to midgut structures (distal duodenum, small bowel, cecum, appendix, ascending colon, and proximal transverse colon) perceived in the periumbilical region, and pain due to hindgut structures (distal transverse colon, descending colon, sigmoid, rectum, and urinary bladder) perceived in the lower abdomen.[14]

The central processes of the visceral fibers synapse extensively above and below the segment where they entered, thus activating spinothalamic cells at multiple levels. Clinically, noxious stimulation of the viscera elicits an autonomic spinal reflex reaction, with sympathetic activation that causes symptoms such as excessive sweating and pronounced changes in circulatory system resulting in increased blood pressure. This reflex reaction tends to be more pronounced than what is seen with noxious stimulation of the skin. Noxious visceral stimulation can also result in hypotension and bradycardia by either reflex inhibition of sympathetic outflow or activation of the

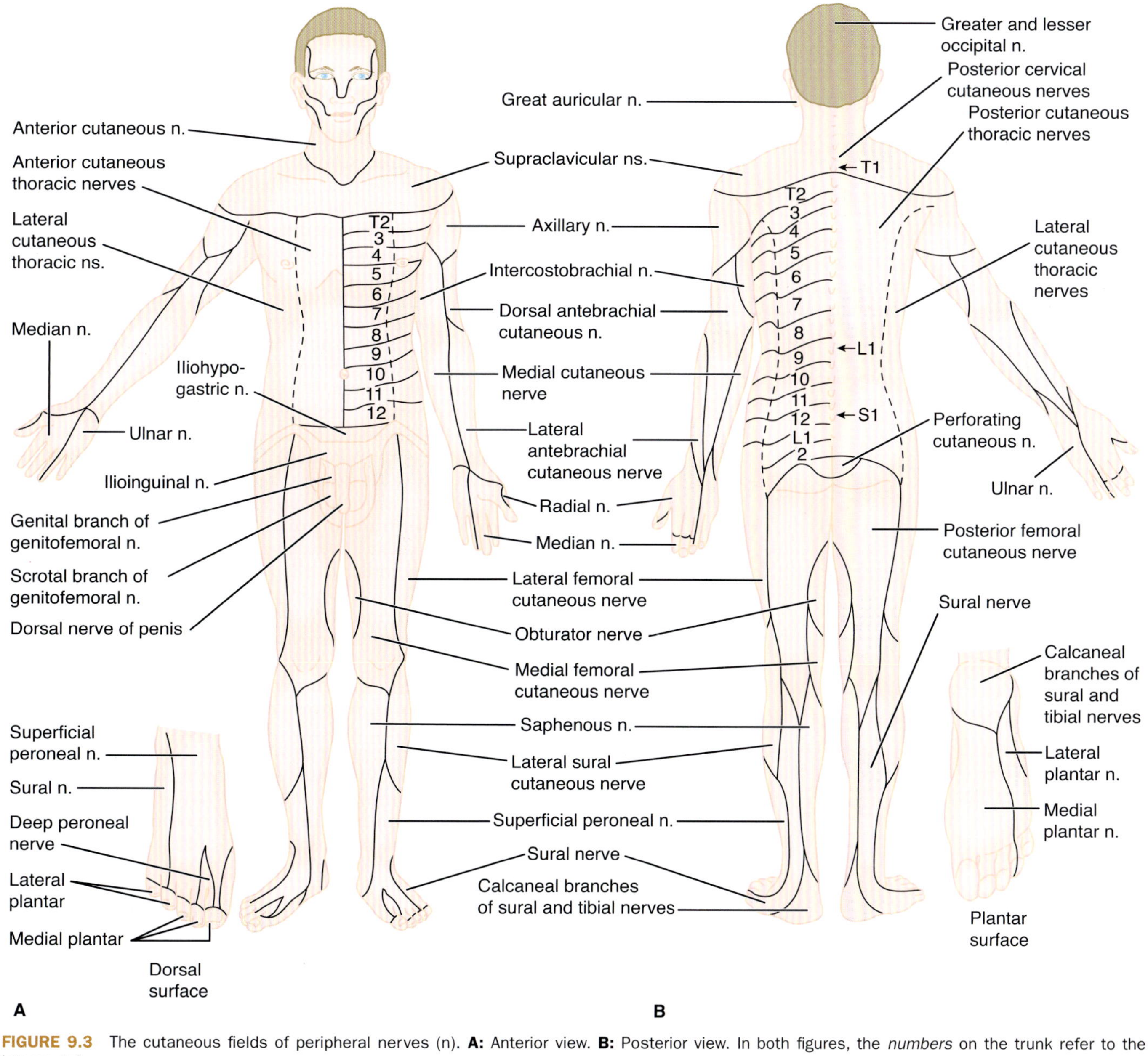

FIGURE 9.3 The cutaneous fields of peripheral nerves (n). **A:** Anterior view. **B:** Posterior view. In both figures, the *numbers* on the trunk refer to the intercostal nerves.

TABLE 9.1	Comparison of Somatic and Visceral Nociceptive Pain	
	Somatic Nociceptive Pain	**Visceral Nociceptive Pain**
Localization	More focused	More diffuse and poorly localized; pain felt in distribution innervated by the same spinal segment as organ; referred to other locations
Quality	Sharp, aching, burning, stabbing	Vague discomfort Hyperesthesia, hyperalgesia, allodynia
Associated symptoms	Accompanied by motor reflexes	Accompanied by motor and autonomic reflexes: associated muscle contraction/spasm, nausea/vomiting, faint sensation, circulatory changes in the region, decreased pulse/blood pressure, cold sweat
Triggers	Tissue injury	Distention, contraction, ischemia, inflammation; pain not evoked from all viscera (organs such as liver and kidneys are not sensitive to pain)

parasympathetic nervous system.[25] These reactions may be mediated by the periaqueductal gray matter (PAG) and the nucleus of the solitary tract. There are also protective reflexes that are directed toward reducing pain, such as the inhibition of visceral motility. Deregulation of this reflex as well as aberrant response by vagal afferents in the enteric system is thought to contribute to the pathophysiology of irritable bowel syndrome.[26] Coordination centers at higher levels of the CNS, such as the PAG, also mediate nausea and vomiting as well as complex somatic responses in the context of visceral pain.

Peripheral Nervous System Structures of Pain Sensation

Among the primary afferent neurons of the peripheral nervous system, there are several neuronal populations classified primarily according to caliber and myelination and secondarily according to the expression of chemical markers.[27] Large myelinated fibers comprise the A-beta (Aβ) population, which respond predominantly to low-energy, nonpainful mechanical stimuli and conduct action potentials rapidly. Small, thinly myelinated fibers make up the A-delta (Aδ) population, which respond to high-energy mechanical stimuli and have intermediate conduction velocity. Small, unmyelinated fibers are classified as the C-fiber population and have slow conduction velocity.[28]

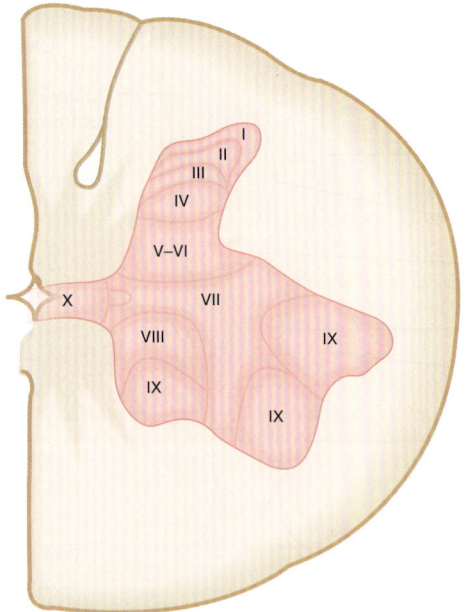

FIGURE 9.4 Schematic drawing of a cross-section of the cervical spinal cord highlighting the lamina. (*Modified from Kiernan JA. Barr's: The Human Nervous System: an Anatomical Viewpoint. 7th ed. Philadelphia: Lippincott Williams & Wilkins; 1998.*)

In general, C fibers can respond to chemical, thermal, and high-threshold mechanical stimuli, with several subclasses of C fibers exhibiting responses to various combinations of these stimulus categories.[29] Typical of electrically excitable cells, the conduction of action potentials along the axons of primary afferent sensory neurons depends on voltage-gated ion channels. The inward current of the action potential is carried by voltage-gated sodium ion channels. There are six types of these in the DRG neurons of which two, Nav1.8 and Nav1.9, have expression pattern limited to sensory neurons, with Nav1.8 limited to nociceptors.[30–32]

C-fiber neurons are further subdivided into two groups. One group expresses the nerve growth factor (NGF) receptor TrkA, as well as the neuropeptides substance P and calcitonin gene-related peptide (CGRP), whereas the other group of C fibers expresses the glial derived neurotrophic factor receptor c-ret and binds to the isolectin B4 (IB4).[33,34] Interestingly, recent data has demonstrated that the free nerve endings in the epidermis are anatomically structured such that the peptidergic fibers terminate in the stratum spinosum, whereas the nonpeptidergic fibers terminate in the more superficial stratum granulosum.[35] This topographic separation is maintained at the level of the dorsal horn of the spinal cord, where the peptidergic and nonpeptidergic afferents terminate in distinct Rexed laminae.

The peripheral terminals of DRG neurons are specialized to respond to thermal, mechanical, or chemical energy. Briefly, thermosensation depends on thermosensitive ion channels in the transient receptor potential (TRP) family, with TRPV1 and TRPV2 responsive to heat that is usually perceived as painful.[36,37] Recently, a specific inhibitor of TRPV1 has been identified that may eventually prove to have a role as a pain-specific local anesthetic agent.[38] Mechanosensation likely also depends on a set of mechanosensitive ion channels; however, the receptors responsible for transducing this information have yet to be unequivocally identified.[39–41] A wide range of chemical mediators can also act on the peripheral terminals of DRG neurons, acting either directly to activate nociceptors or indirectly by sensitizing the peripheral terminals to be activated at a lower stimulus threshold. Chemical mediators may be either exogenous (e.g., capsaicin, mustard oil, chemical acids, bee venom) or endogenous (e.g., many of the myriad inflammatory mediators). Endogenously released chemical mediators that cause pain directly are typically associated with tissue destruction that alters the chemical microenvironment, for example, H+ ions and adenosine triphosphate, or causes an inflammatory response, such as bradykinin.[42,43]

Functional Anatomy of the Central Nervous System

Pain is defined by not only the physiologic perception of nociception but also the affective and emotional response to that perception. Pain is a highly individual and subjective experience to the extent that the same stimulus can produce different responses in different individuals under the same conditions. The CNS is both the processing center for the perception of noxious stimulation and the primary regulator of adaptive and modulatory mechanisms to produce a pain behavior. Pain is primarily categorized by duration of symptoms (acute vs. chronic) and the origin of the pain signal (visceral vs. somatic and nociceptive vs. neuropathic). Understanding the anatomy and function of the pain structures and pathways in the CNS is essential to understanding and managing the different categories of pain.

DORSAL HORN

The dorsal horn represents the termination point of the dorsal root in the CNS. There is a correspondence between the functional and anatomic organization of the dorsal horn. It is arranged into 10 laminae, and distinct sensory modalities from the periphery terminate in distinct laminae (see Fig. 9.4).[44] Signals conducting nociceptive signals (Aδ and C fibers) terminate in the superficially located laminae I (also called the marginal layer) and II (also called the substantia gelatinosa). Many neurons from lamina I respond exclusively to noxious stimulation and project to higher levels of the CNS. Some neurons called wide dynamic range neurons respond in a stepwise fashion to peripheral stimulation. The neurons of lamina II are mostly interneurons and modulate nociceptive responses at the level of the dorsal horn. The Aδ fibers also terminate in lamina V which contains wide dynamic range neurons that project to higher levels of the CNS including the thalamus.[45] There is some convergence of somatic and visceral nociceptive input into lamina V, which may explain referred pain from visceral structures.[46] Single axons of all receptors give off ascending and descending branches after entering the spinal cord. In addition to synapsing at the level they enter, these branches give off multiple collaterals that end in the gray matter of the dorsal horns at one to two levels above and below where the axon entered the spinal cord.[47] Integration of signals from the periphery and higher levels of the CNS occur at the level of the dorsal horn through the dense network of dendrites and interneurons.

Synaptic transmission by nociceptive afferent neurons at the level of the dorsal horn is mediated primarily by the excitatory neurotransmitter glutamate. Both ionotropic and metabotropic glutamate receptors are located in high concentration in the substantia gelatinosa.[48] Many neuropeptides (e.g., substance P, vasoactive intestinal polypeptide, cholecystokinin, and CGRP), which are theorized to modulate synaptic action, are present in the neurons in the dorsal horn. The receptors for most of these neuropeptides are concentrated in the substantia gelatinosa, which suggests that they are involved in the transmission of pain. Among the neuropeptides, substance P and its receptor, neurokinin 1, are likely to be involved in the processing and modulating of pain signals in the dorsal horn. Substance P may increase the excitation from incoming sensory fibers by enhancing and prolonging the actions of glutamate. This has been demonstrated experimentally: Substance P and CGRP have been found to increase the release of glutamate; substance P induces the N-methyl-D-aspartate (NMDA) receptors to become more sensitive to glutamate. This unmasks normally silent interneurons and sensitizes second-order spinal neurons.[49] Blocking the neurokinin 1 receptors can prevent many of these effects. Substance P can also extend long distances within the spinal cord and sensitize dorsal horn neurons several segments away from the initial nociceptive signal. This results in an expansion of receptive fields and the activation of wide dynamic neurons by nonnociceptive afferent impulses.[50]

Sustained noxious stimulation or high-intensity nociceptive signals to the dorsal horn neurons may lead to increased neuronal responsiveness or central sensitization.[51] Hyperalgesia, which is an exaggerated perception of painful stimuli, is at least partially mediated through low-threshold mechanoreceptors (Aβ afferents) in the dorsal horn. Allodynia, which is a perception of innocuous stimuli as painful, is mediated through high-threshold nociceptors (Aδ or C fibers) in the dorsal horn. The factors that contribute to these hyperexcitable states include altered function of neurochemical and electrophysiologic systems as well as changes in the anatomy in the dorsal horn.[52]

"Wind-up" refers to a central spinal mechanism in which repetitive noxious stimulation results in a slow summation of these signals that is experienced as increased pain.[53] The amplification of the pain signal occurs in the spinal cord when nociceptive C fibers synapse on the dorsal horn nociceptive neurons activating the NMDA receptors.[54] A cascade of events ensues with the activation of nitric oxide synthase.[55] This ultimately leads to enhance the release of sensory neuropeptides, including substance P, from presynaptic neurons, contributing to the development of hyperalgesia and maintenance of central sensitization.[56] Wind-up can be elicited if identical nociceptive stimuli are applied at a frequency of 3 seconds or less.[57]

SPINOTHALAMIC TRACT

Prior to synapsing in the dorsal horn of the spinal cord, C and Aδ fibers may ascend or descend one to two spinal levels, forming a tract dorsal to the dorsal horn called the tract of Lissauer (Fig. 9.5); Lissauer's tract also contains axons of interneurons that may travel for several spinal segments. Following synapsing of the central projections of C and Aδ afferents, the axons of many of the second-order neurons cross the midline, forming the lateral spinothalamic tract which ascends without interruption from the dorsal horn through the brainstem to the thalamus. This somatotopically organized tract carries information from neurons about the location, intensity, and duration of nociceptive stimuli. This tract is also responsible for relaying the sensation of temperature and, to a lesser extent, it transmits touch and pressure sensation. A large proportion of the neurons that contribute fibers to the lateral spinothalamic tract originate in lamina I. There is also a dorsally located spinothalamic tract arising ipsilaterally from lamina I neurons, although this projection of second-order nociceptive neurons is less well described.

Lamina V also contributes a large group of neurons to the spinothalamic tract mostly composed of Aδ fibers. The anterior spinothalamic tract, which conveys information about the location of nociception, is largely composed of fibers from laminae VII and VIII. Conversely, lamina II sends very few fibers to the spinothalamic tracts despite being the destination for many C fibers. The fibers from lamina II modulate the spinothalamic cells in laminae I, V, VII, and VIII at the level of the nociceptive input as well as at spinal segments above and below via spinal interneurons that travel in the tract of Lissauer. This complex mesh of interneurons plays a significant role in determining whether signals from nociceptors will be propagated to higher levels of the nervous system or be inhibited. Spinal interneurons modulate the intensity of a stimulus and also establish connections with other spinal neurons to form somatic and autonomic reflex arcs at the level of the spinal cord. Whereas interruption of the spinothalamic tract results in immediate loss of pain and temperature perception in the contralateral side of the body, injuries of the spinothalamic tract can develop into central pain (CP) syndromes.

Nociceptive afferents from visceral organs and somatic structures terminate in the same population of spinothalamic cells in the spinal cord, which in turn synapse in the thalamus. The convergence of nociceptive signals in the spinal cord is segmentally arranged and may account for pain from visceral organs being referred to somatic structures; this topic is discussed in more detail later in the chapter. There are several

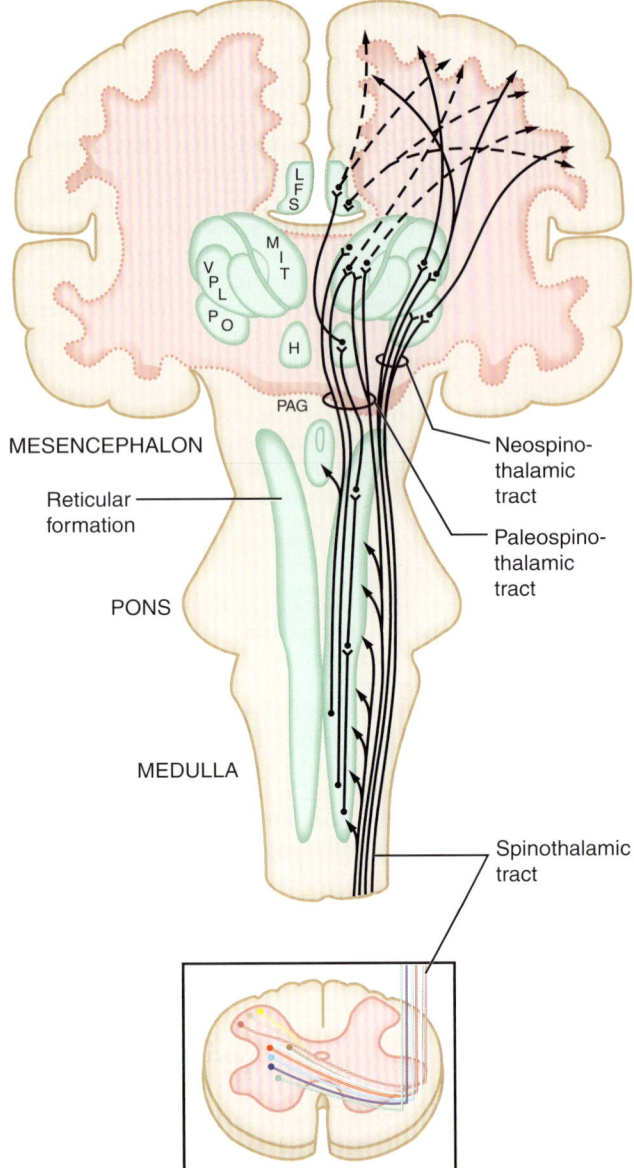

FIGURE 9.5 Simple diagram of the course and termination of the spinothalamic tract. Most of the fibers cross to the opposite side and ascend to the brainstem and brain, although some ascend ipsilaterally. The neospinothalamic part of the tract has cell bodies located primarily in laminae I and V of the dorsal horn, whereas the paleospinothalamic tract has its cell bodies in deeper laminae. The neospinothalamic fibers ascend in a more superficial part of the tract and project without interruption to the caudal part of the ventroposterolateral thalamic nucleus (VPL), the oral part of this nucleus, and the medial part of the posterior thalamus (PO). In these structures, they synapse with a third relay of neurons, which project to the somatosensory cortex (SI, SII, and retroinsular cortex) (*solid lines*). Some of the fibers of the paleospinothalamic tract pass directly to the medial/intralaminar thalamic nuclei, and others project to the nuclei and the reticular formation of the brainstem and thence to the periaqueductal gray matter (PAG), hypothalamus (H), nucleus submedius, and medial/intralaminar thalamic (MIT) nuclei. Once there, these axons synapse with neurons that connect with the limbic forebrain structure (LFS) via complex circuits and also send diffuse projections to various parts of the brain (*dashed lines*).

Labels in figure: LFS, MIT, VPL, PO, H, PAG, MESENCEPHALON, Reticular formation, PONS, MEDULLA, Neospinothalamic tract, Paleospinothalamic tract, Spinothalamic tract

other ascending tracts that supply nociceptive signals to higher levels of the CNS. The spinoreticular tract transmits nociceptive signals on the ipsilateral side of the spinal cord. This tract is clinically important as it may explain the persistence of pain after an anterior cordotomy.

THALAMUS

The majority of the second-order lateral spinothalamic tract fibers terminate in the lateral nuclear group of the thalamus which contains both the ventroposterior lateral (VPL) nucleus and the ventroposterior medial (VPM) nucleus. The VPL nucleus of the thalamus receives information from the lateral spinothalamic tract, whereas the VPM nucleus receives sensory information from the spinal trigeminal nucleus, which transmits sensory information from the face (Fig. 9.6). Spinothalamic fibers also terminate in areas of the intralaminar nuclei and in the mediodorsal nucleus. These fibers transmit signals to the limbic system which integrates autonomic and arousal responses and attention to the perception of pain. Many of the fibers originating in lamina I terminate in the ventromedial (VM) nucleus. Most of the neurons in VM are activated by nociceptors. Lesions of the thalamus, such as stroke, can result in severe CP syndromes on the contralateral side of the body.

With the exception of olfaction, all sensory pathways traveling from the periphery to the cerebral cortex synapse in the thalamus. The spinothalamic fibers terminate in multiple areas of the thalamus and subsequently are relayed to different areas of the cortex. VPL/VPM supplies the primary and secondary somatosensory cortex (S1, S2) with nociceptive signals. Spinothalamic fibers terminating in other areas of the thalamus influence other cortical areas, such as the insular cortex.

SENSORY CORTEX

Nociceptive signals from the thalamus terminate in multiple areas of the cerebral cortex and subcortical regions. The thalamic fibers project primarily to layer IV of the primary somatosensory cortex (S1) to transmit information about limb position, sense of touch, and discriminative aspects of sensation. This area of the cortex makes a limited contribution to the perception of nociception. The cortical association areas and secondary somatic sensory cortex are connected with S1 and help further process tactile information necessary for object recognition and spatial relationships.

Functional imaging has demonstrated that the insula and anterior cingulate gyrus are the areas most consistently linked with nociceptive stimulation.[58] The insular cortex receives direct projections from the medial thalamic nuclei as well as from the lateral nuclear group. This area of the cortex processes nociceptive information on the internal state of the body and regulates the autonomic component of the pain response. Patients with lesions of the insular cortex do not display appropriate emotional responses to pain as part of a syndrome termed *pain asymbolia*.[59] The anterior cingulate gyrus integrates the affective component of pain. To a lesser extent, S1, the premotor cortex, the prefrontal cortex, and posterior parietal cortex are activated with nociception. In the subcortical region, the amygdala, hypothalamus, PAG, basal ganglia, and cerebellum are all activated with nociception. Although there are multiple cortical regions that play significant roles in the perception of nociception, there is enough variability in the patterns of activation that, as of yet, there is not a defined area considered to be specific for nociceptive perception.

DESCENDING PATHWAYS OF THE CENTRAL NERVOUS SYSTEM

There are descending pathways from the cortex that modulate sensory impulses. For example, somatotopically organized fibers from the primary somatosensory cortex terminate in the

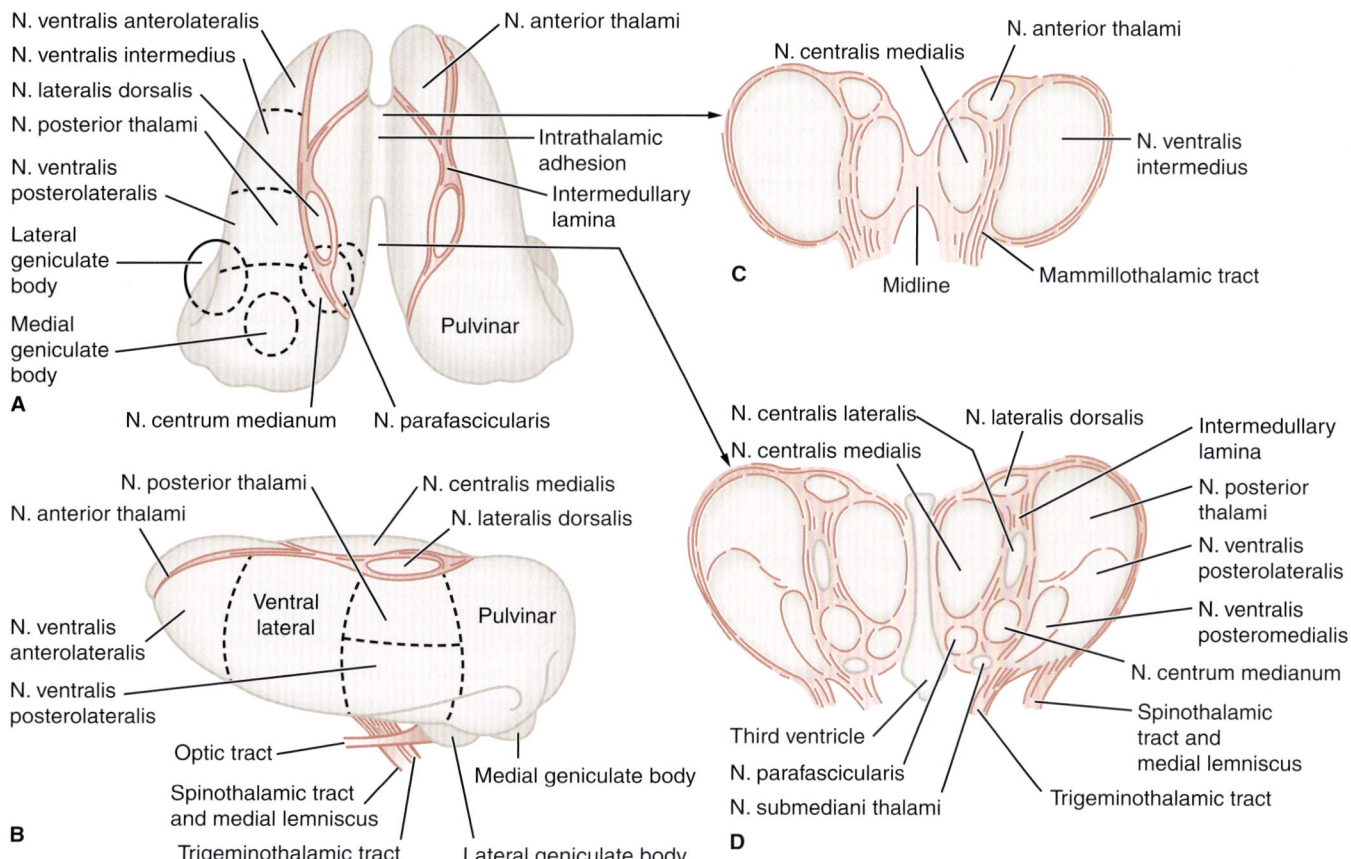

FIGURE 9.6 Schematic diagram of the human thalamus. **A:** Superior view. **B:** Lateral view shows the locations of the most important nuclei. **C:** Frontal section of the anterior part of the thalamus depicts the relationships of various nuclei. **D:** Frontal section of the middle part of the thalamus. Note that the spinothalamic tract and medial lemniscus terminate in nucleus (N.) ventralis posterolateralis, whereas the trigeminothalamic tract terminates in N. ventralis posteromedialis.

thalamus, brainstem, and spinal cord. Descending pathways may modulate sensory signals from specific receptors and/or areas of the body. The inhibitory effects are most common and are usually transmitted through inhibitory interneurons. The sensory system is designed to react to the dynamic nature of the environment. As a result, sensory signals are regulated at multiple levels of the nervous system.[60]

Collateral fibers from the periaqueductal gray, matter modulate both descending and ascending pain pathways. The PAG has been experimentally demonstrated to produce analgesia when stimulated and is felt to play a major role in modulating nociception at the level of the dorsal horn as well as at higher levels of the CNS.[61] The PAG receives signals from limbic and cortical centers involved in the affective component of pain. The descending signal from the PAG travels through the nucleus raphe magnus (NRM) in the medulla as well as the medullary reticular formation. The serotonergic NRM fibers descend to inhibit peripheral nociceptors in the dorsal horn in laminae I and II. Clinically, this descending system blocks the spinal withdrawal reflex at the level of the dorsal horn. The PAG has ascending connections which may modulate sensory signals at the level of the thalamus. The PAG also supplies the reticular activating system responsible for arousal to painful stimuli.

CENTRAL PAIN
CP is a term that includes dysesthesias, paresthesias, and even pruritus[62] initiated by a lesion that interferes with the pathway of nociceptive signals within the CNS from the spinothalamic tract to the parietal somatosensory areas. CP remains an underdiagnosed condition that occurs with damage to the CNS.

Studies suggest that up to 10% of all individuals who experience strokes (more correctly, cerebrovascular accidents),[63] up to two-thirds of spinal cord injury (SCI) patients,[64] 18% of patients with multiple sclerosis, and an undefined number of patients with other neurologic conditions suffer CP.[65]

CP is a complex complaint with several subtypes of pain that can be moderate to severe in intensity. Patients may complain of a constant pain often described as aching, burning, pricking, dysesthesias, paresthesias, or pruritus in isolation or in combination. Most of these patients also complain of stimulus-evoked pain. Patients may complain of spontaneous episodic pain superimposed on their chronic symptoms that is most commonly characterized as lancinating.[61] These uncomfortable sensations are difficult to treat and are often poorly tolerated, which leads to a decrease in quality of life.

Central poststroke pain was first described by Dejerine and Roussy[66] in 1906 who found that thalamic stroke on one side of the brain can cause a pain syndrome affecting the contralateral half of the body. This syndrome may occur after a stroke in any location in the CNS. There are several theories as to the mechanism of central poststroke pain. Interruption of the descending inhibitory pathway, hyperexcitability of the affected afferent sensory pathways, denervation hypersensitivity, as well as loss of balance between excitatory (glutamatergic) and inhibitory (GABAergic) neurotransmitters are all possible contributors.

CENTRAL PAIN AFTER SPINAL CORD INJURY
Chronic pain is a major complication of SCI, with approximately two-thirds of all SCI patients experiencing some type of chronic pain and up to one-third complaining of that their pain

is severe.[67] The prevalence of pain after SCI often increases with time after injury.[67] There are an estimated 40 cases per million population in the United States, or approximately 11,000 new individuals with SCI pain each year.[68] Research suggests that chronic pain in SCI patients significantly interferes with their rehabilitation and activities of daily living and therefore reduces quality of life. Attempts to manage these pain symptoms are costly, and success is often limited.[69]

In addition to CP, there are multiple types of pain that develop after SCI including musculoskeletal, visceral, and peripheral neuropathic pain. The etiology of pain in SCI is multifaceted and the various types of SCI pain differ with regard to clinical findings, pathophysiology, and therapy. The mechanisms involved in the development of CP after SCI are not fully elucidated, but continuing research has identified possible mechanisms for pain generation. CP has been reported with injury to all levels of the spinal cord.[70]

CP is a common sequelae of SCI. It has many descriptors; it is often characterized by patients as a continuous burning, shooting, aching, and tingling. The distribution of pain is usually bilateral and can involve multiple adjacent dermatomes or be regional in nature. In addition, many patients with SCI report feeling the phantom phenomenon of their body below the lesion, and it is described in a distorted fashion. This occurs despite most patients having no conscious appreciation of sensory input below the spinal cord lesion.[71] Central neuropathic pain after SCI has been categorized based on the location of the complaint as either at the level of the injury or below the level of the injury. Although it may be difficult to distinguish the two clinically (and both may be present in the same patient), CP that occurs at the level of injury is due to segmental spinal cord damage, not nerve root damage. CP that occurs at the level of injury can be within two dermatomal levels either above or below the level of injury.[72] CP associated with SCI may also be caused by syringomyelia.[71]

Physiologic changes occur to the nociceptive neurons in the dorsal horn following SCI, including an increase in abnormal spontaneous and evoked discharges from dorsal horn cells.[73,74] Noxious stimulation causes primary afferent C fibers to release excitatory amino acid neurotransmitters in the dorsal horn. Prolonged high-intensity noxious stimulation activates the NMDA receptors, which induces a cascade that may result in central sensitization.[75] The cascade includes upregulation of neurokinin receptors and activation of the intracellular cyclooxygenase-2, nitric oxide synthase, and protein kinase C enzymes.[76] Other neuroanatomic and neurochemical changes thought to impact CP in SCI include alteration in the activity of the neurotransmitter glutamate,[77] interruption of descending inhibitory pathways,[78] and dysfunction of the inhibitory GABAergic interneurons,[79] all at the level of the dorsal horn. On a molecular level, abnormal sodium channel expression within the dorsal horn (laminae I to VI) bilaterally has been implicated as a major contributor to hyperexcitability.

Thalamic neurons appear to undergo changes after SCI in both human and animal models. In the animal model, enhanced neuronal excitability in the VPL has been demonstrated

directly[80] as well as indirectly; enhanced regional blood flow has been found in the rat VPL after SCI, suggesting increased neuronal activity.[81] Magnetic resonance spectroscopy studies have demonstrated changes in metabolism of the neurons in human thalamus associated with pain in SCI.[82] Much like the neurons in the dorsal horn, the thalamic neurons after SCI show increased activity with noxious and nonnoxious stimuli. VPL neurons are spontaneously hyperexcitable following SCI without receiving input from the spinal cord neurons suggesting that the thalamus may act as a pain signal generator in CP accompanying SCI.[71]

There is emerging evidence that cortical reorganization may play a role in the development of phantom symptoms after loss of limbs, but little evidence of the cortical mechanisms at work with the development of phantom phenomena after SCI.[83] The full spectrum of anatomic, chemical, and physiologic changes contributing to central neuropathic pain after SCI is still being elucidated.

Autonomic Nervous System

At the turn of the 20th century, the Cambridge physiologist John Newport Langley[84] coined the term "autonomic nervous system" (ANS) to describe the portion of the nervous system that mediated the unconscious function of the internal organs. Soon afterward, the concept of two distinct components of the ANS, the sympathetic and parasympathetic systems, which antagonize each other to maintain homeostasis, was developed. The enteric system is also recognized as being a distinct part of the ANS. In addition to regulating the activity of visceral organs, vessels, and glands, the ANS has been found to play an active role in many pain states. Understanding the complexity of the pain–ANS interaction is essential to physicians managing all types of pain. The anatomy of the ANS with the current understanding of the interrelationship between these structures is shown in Figure 9.7. The ANS is composed of peripheral and central portions.

PERIPHERAL AUTONOMIC NERVOUS SYSTEM

The peripheral efferent pathways of both the sympathetic and parasympathetic nervous system have two components: a primary presynaptic or preganglionic neuron and a secondary postsynaptic or postganglionic neuron. Unlike the somatic motor system which has its motor neurons in the CNS, the motor neurons of the ANS are located in the periphery. As such, the transmission of autonomic signals from the CNS synapses at ganglia in the periphery prior to reaching the target organ (Fig. 9.8). The different locations of the cell bodies of the primary preganglionic neurons of the different divisions of the ANS are discussed later.

The cell bodies of the postganglionic neurons are arranged in aggregates known as ganglia, wherein the synapses between pre- and postganglionic neurons are located. As shown in Figure 9.7, there are four general groups of these ganglia, two within the sympathetic division and two within the parasympathetic division.

A typical feature of the ANS is that postganglionic fibers form nerve plexuses around their target organs composed of

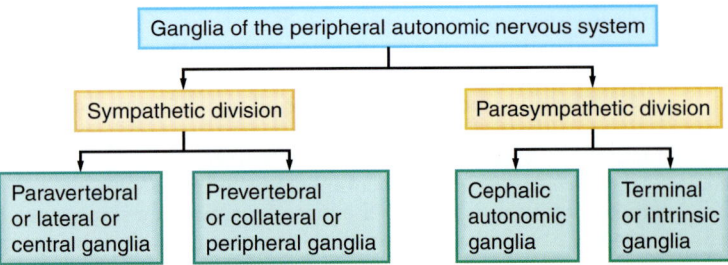

FIGURE 9.7 Ganglia of the peripheral autonomic nervous system.

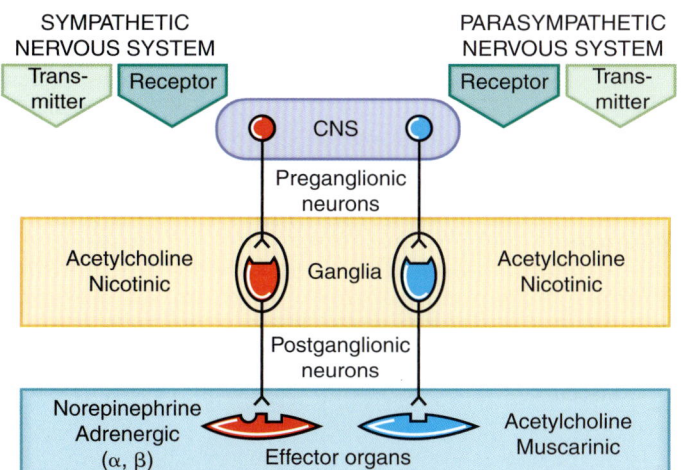

FIGURE 9.8 Transmitter substances in the peripheral autonomic nervous system. *(Modified by permission from Springer: Jänig W. The autonomic nervous system. In: Schmidt RF, Thews G, eds.* Human Physiology *1st ed. Berlin: Springer-Verlag; 1983:111–144. Copyright © 1983 Springer-Verlag Berlin · Heidelberg.)*

both sympathetic and parasympathetic fibers. Unlike their somatic efferent counterparts, the postganglionic fibers branch extensively, forming a network in the vicinity of their effector cells allowing one fiber to act on several effector cells.

PARASYMPATHETIC DIVISION

The parasympathetic preganglionic fibers travel from the CNS to synapse in ganglia located close to their target organs. In most areas, parasympathetic innervation tends to be more precise than sympathetic innervation. Parasympathetic fibers generally innervate visceral organs. Table 9.2 summarizes parasympathetic nerve supply to essential body structures.

CRANIAL PARASYMPATHETICS

The preganglionic parasympathetic neurons have their cell bodies in the gray matter of the brainstem, and their fibers travel with the oculomotor, facial, glossopharyngeal, and vagus nerves (Fig. 9.9).

The preganglionic fibers from the oculomotor, facial, and glossopharyngeal nerves synapse in the ciliary, sphenopalatine, otic, and submaxillary ganglia, all of which are located in the head. From these ganglia, the postganglionic fibers travel to the target organs (e.g., the lacrimal and salivary glands).

The preganglionic parasympathetic fibers in the vagus nerve descend from the brainstem to terminate in visceral organs. In the abdomen, many of these fibers synapse in a diffuse network of postganglionic neurons to form a plexus within the wall of the gastrointestinal tract. The postganglionic neurons within this plexus send short processes to innervate the smooth muscles and glands in the gastrointestinal tract. In the thorax, the vagus nerve supplies parasympathetic innervation to the heart (via the cardiac plexus) and airways. In the heart, the sinus node and atrioventricular node have significant parasympathetic innervation. This is in contrast to the ventricles, which are supplied with dense sympathetic innervation.[85]

SACRAL PARASYMPATHETICS

The sacral portion of the parasympathetic system consists of preganglionic neurons which have their cell bodies in the intermediolateral column of the gray matter of the S2–S4 spinal segments (see Figs. 9.9 and 9.10). The preganglionic fibers travel via the ventral roots to the corresponding spinal nerves for a short distance and then form the pelvic splanchnic nerves. These nerves form the pelvic plexuses which are in close proximity to the target organs (rectum, bladder, prostate gland in the male, cervix in the female). Many of these preganglionic fibers synapse in the plexus, whereas other fibers pass through the plexus without interruption and terminate in intramural ganglia of their target organs (e.g., urinary bladder, descending colon, sigmoid colon and rectum, and genital organs). All of the pelvic organs are innervated by postganglionic parasympathetic fibers. These fibers play an essential role in eliminating waste products from the bladder and rectum.[86]

SYMPATHETIC (THORACOLUMBAR) DIVISION

The peripheral sympathetic nervous system is composed of efferent and afferent fibers. The efferent portion of the sympathetic division of the ANS consists of preganglionic neurons, the two paravertebral (lateral) sympathetic chains, prevertebral and terminal ganglia, and postganglionic neurons (see Figs. 9.9 and 9.10).[87,88]

TABLE 9.2 Summary of Parasympathetic Nerve Supply to Essential Body Structures

	Parasympathetic Nerve Supply		
Region/Structure/Organ	Location of Cell Body/ Preganglionic Neurons in the Central Nervous System	Site of Synapse of the Preganglionic with Postganglionic Neurons	Action
Head and Neck			
Eye	Parasympathetic oculomotor nucleus/ Edinger-Westphal nucleus	Ciliary ganglion	Pupillary constriction, accommodation for near vision
Lacrimal gland	Superior salvatory nucleus	Pterygopalatine nucleus	Secretion
Parotid gland	Inferior salvatory nucleus	Otic ganglion	Secretion
Submandibular and sublingual glands	Superior salvatory nucleus	Submandibular ganglion	Secretion
Thoracic Viscera			
Heart	Dorsal motor vagus nucleus	Cardiac plexus	Decreased heart rate and cardiac output
Trachea, bronchi, and lungs	Dorsal motor vagus nucleus	Pulmonary plexus	Constriction of bronchial muscles and increased glandular secretion
Abdominal Viscera			
Stomach	Dorsal motor vagus nucleus	Gastric plexus	Increased motility and secretion, relaxed sphincter
Pancreas	Dorsal motor vagus nucleus	Periarterial plexus	Dilation of blood vessels and increased secretion
Pelvic Viscera			
Ureter	Sacral cord S3–S4	Pelvic plexus	Increased tone and motility
Bladder	Sacral cord S3–S4	Pelvic plexus	Contracted detrusor muscle

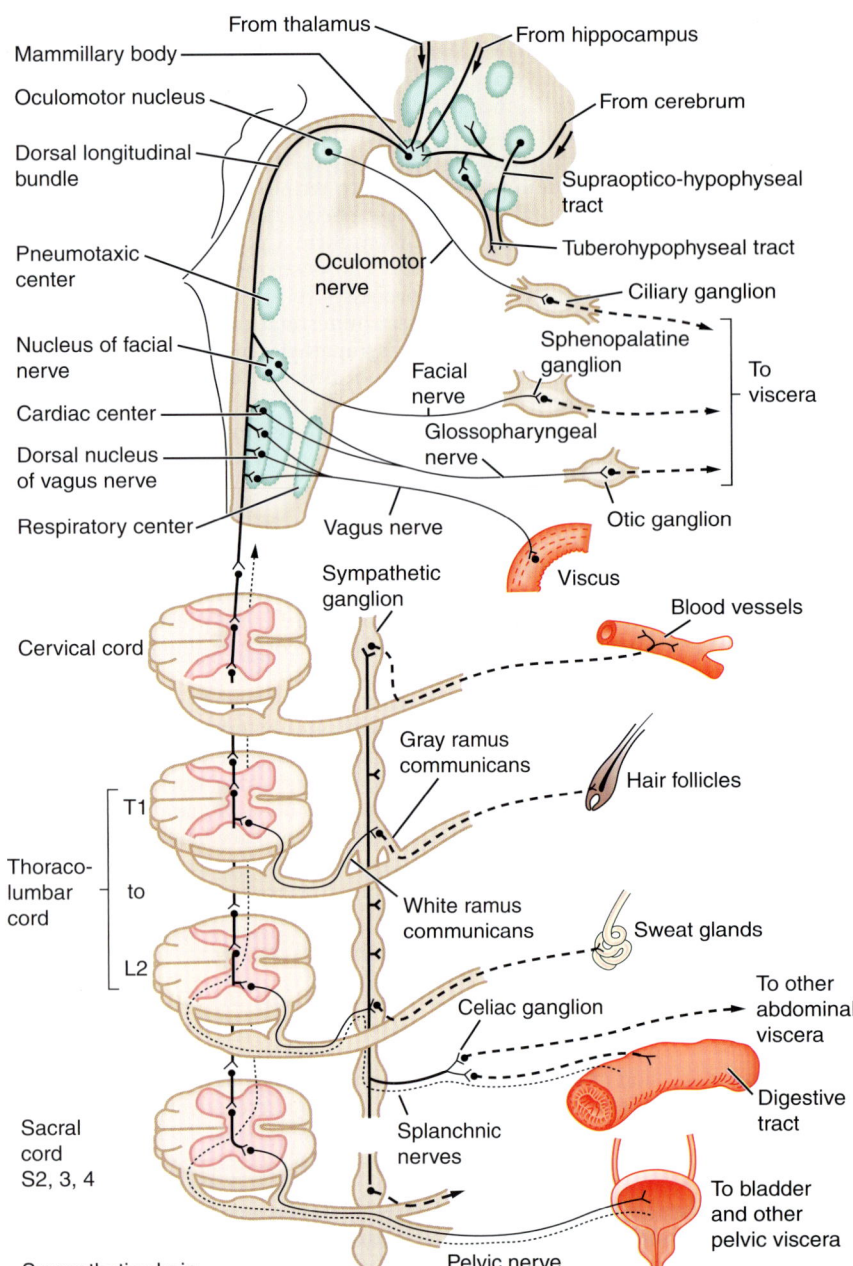

FIGURE 9.9 Schematic representation of autonomic pathways in the neuraxis and the efferent peripheral pathways. Note the connection among the various hypothalamic nuclei and between these structures and the nuclei and important autonomic centers in the brainstem and spinal cord. The dorsal longitudinal fasciculus (DLF) passes from the hypothalamus caudad through the central and tegmental portion of the mesencephalon and the tegmental portion of the pons to terminate in the reticular formation, the autonomic centers and cranial nerve nuclei in the brainstem, and in the intermediolateral cell column of the spinal cord. The DLF is composed of both crossed and uncrossed fibers, including some long ones and an extensive system of short fibers, which are arranged in the gray matter in frequent relays. Note also that the cell bodies of preganglionic sympathetic neurons are located only in spinal cord segments T1–L2, whereas the parasympathetic neurons are located in cranial nerves and in S2, S3, and S4. The *solid lines* represent preganglionic fibers, the *dashed lines* represent postganglionic fibers, and the *dotted lines* are afferent (sensory) fibers. Not shown are the sensory fibers contained in the facial, glossopharyngeal, and vagus nerves, which transmit nociceptive and other somatosensory information from the head.

Sympathetic Preganglionic Neurons

The cell bodies of the efferent preganglionic neurons are located in the intermediolateral column in the spinal cord from T1 to L2. The efferent fibers of these preganglionic neurons travel from the spinal cord into the periphery through the ventral roots accompanying the somatic fibers at these levels at the thoracolumbar spine. From this point, the preganglionic neurons diverge to provide inputs to ganglia in multiple locations. Each preganglionic fiber synapses on multiple postganglionic cells, thus serving to amplify the sympathetic outflow from the CNS.[89] Some of the sympathetic fibers leave the spinal nerve immediately after the ventral and dorsal roots fuse to form the white communicating ramus which synapses with postganglionic neurons in the sympathetic ganglia outside the neuraxis (see Fig. 9.10). The white rami are usually present only in the thoracic and upper two or three lumbar segments corresponding to the location of the intermediolateral column in the spinal cord (see Fig. 9.10). The white color of the rami is a result of the sympathetic fibers being myelinated.

The peripheral ganglia of the sympathetic nervous system are located close to the CNS. These paravertebral ganglia are segmentally arranged in two sympathetic trunks, each of which is a vertical row along the anterior margin of the vertebral column. Each trunk is composed of a longitudinal network of ganglia connected to each other by ascending and descending nerve fibers that extend the entire length of the spinal column. As each spinal segment develops in the embryo, one sympathetic ganglion is formed for every level on each side. Some of these ganglia fuse, so the final number of ganglia is usually less than the number of spinal segments.[90] This is most prominent in the cervical region where only the superior, middle, intermediate, and inferior cervical ganglia are present for seven cervical vertebrae. The middle cervical ganglion is often not present, and the inferior cervical ganglion commonly fuses with the upper thoracic ganglion forming the stellate ganglion. The cephalic end of the paravertebral ganglia continues beyond the cervical spine, traveling along the carotid nerve to eventually distribute sympathetic fibers within the head. The caudal end of the two

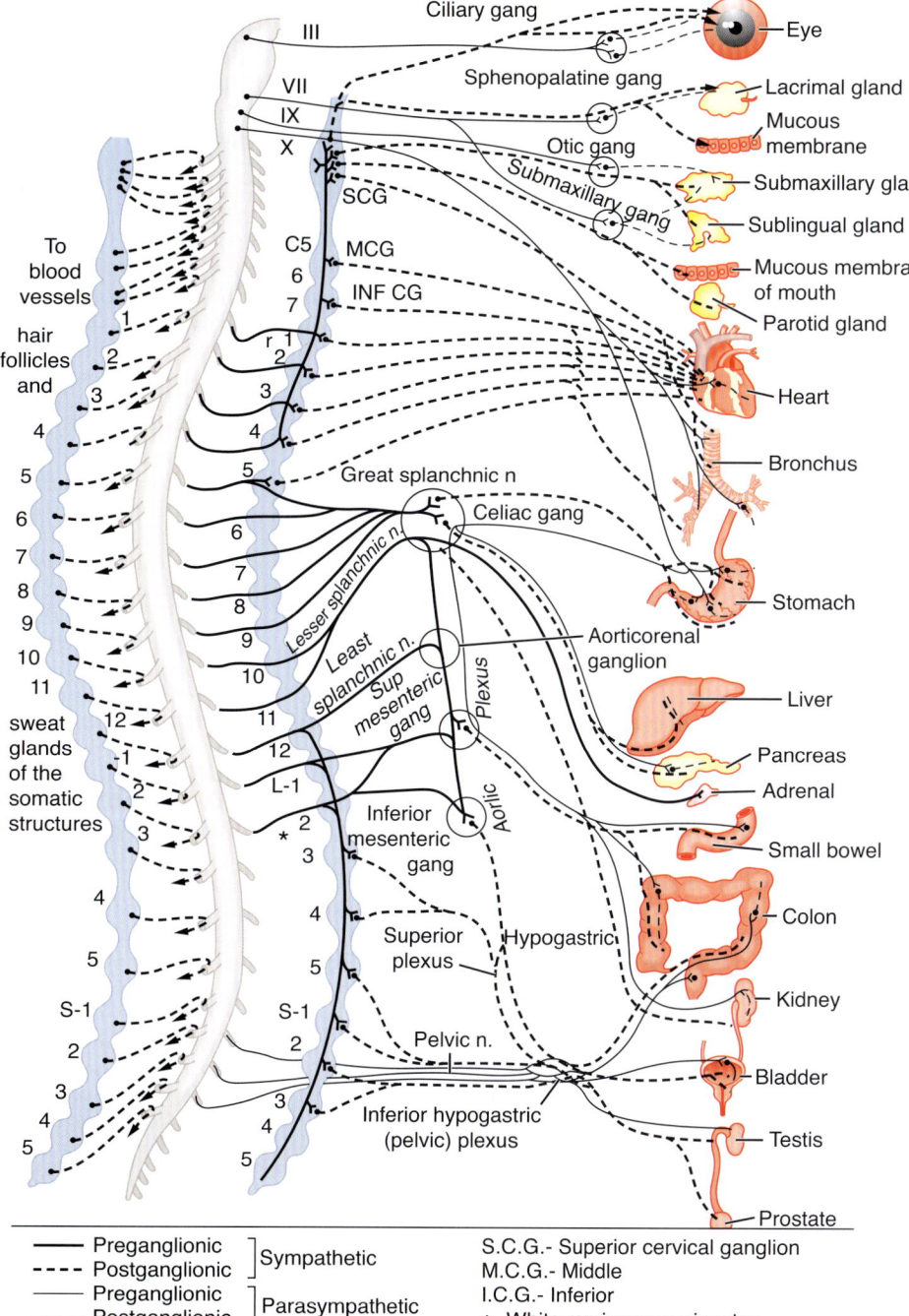

FIGURE 9.10 Distribution of peripheral autonomic nervous system to various structures of the body. On the reader's right are shown (from above downward) the four cranial nerves which contain preganglionic parasympathetic fibers, the axons of preganglionic sympathetic fibers (which pass from the anterior root to the paravertebral sympathetic chain), and the parasympathetic preganglionic axons in S2, S3, and S4. Note that the axons of all of the preganglionic sympathetic neurons pass via the white rami communicantes into the paravertebral chain, in which some synapse with postganglionic neurons, whereas others pass to the prevertebral sympathetic ganglia, in which they synapse with postganglionic fibers. On the reader's left are depicted the gray rami communicantes, containing postganglionic sympathetic fibers, which originate in the paravertebral chain and then pass to each of the spinal nerves to innervate blood vessels, hair follicles, and sweat glands in various parts of the body.

trunks converges and terminates in front of the coccyx as the ganglion impar.[87]

The paravertebral sympathetic ganglia are connected by interganglionic fibers forming the lateral sympathetic chain, which extends from the skull to the coccyx. On entering the sympathetic chain, some preganglionic axons synapse in the ganglia at the spinal level they exited the neuraxis. Other preganglionic fibers pass uninterrupted cephalad or caudad within the sympathetic trunk before they synapse to ensure that preganglionic fibers synapse at all levels of the sympathetic trunk.

Some preganglionic sympathetic fibers pass uninterrupted through the sympathetic chain to form splanchnic nerves that synapse within one of the prevertebral ganglia that are found at the junction of the celiac and mesenteric arteries and the abdominal aorta. The postganglionic fibers that travel from the prevertebral ganglion tend to follow arteries within the abdomen to

their target organs. The greater and lesser splanchnic nerves are formed from preganglionic fibers from the T6 to T10 levels, pass through the sympathetic chain without synapsing, and terminate in ganglia that innervate the abdominal viscera in the upper and middle part of the abdomen. Splanchnic nerves also contribute preganglionic fibers to the adrenal medulla. These fibers synapse within chromaffin cells, which are homologous to postganglionic neurons but release epinephrine into the bloodstream with sympathetic stimulation.[91]

Sympathetic Postganglionic Neurons

The axons of the postganglionic neurons travel via multiple pathways into the periphery. Some of the postganglionic neurons which have their cell bodies in the paravertebral chain reenter the spinal nerves via the gray communicating ramus, which, in distinction to the white rami, has a gray color because most of these postganglionic fibers are unmyelinated. Postganglionic sympathetic neurons from gray rami communicans travel in all spinal nerves. These postganglionic sympathetic fibers follow the spinal nerves into somatic areas innervating various somatic, sudomotor, and pilomotor structures, such as the sweat glands and smooth muscle fibers in hair follicles in the skin. The axons of other postganglionic neurons, which have their cell bodies in the paravertebral chain, travel largely along arteries to pass to the thoracic and pelvic viscera. This is in contrast to the preganglionic neurons that pass uninterrupted to the prevertebral ganglia via the greater and lesser splanchnic nerves and are distributed to the viscera in the upper and middle part of the abdomen. The visceral organs in the lower abdomen receive their sympathetic innervation from the lumbar splanchnic nerve which also synapses in prevertebral ganglia. The celiac ganglia is usually the largest of the prevertebral ganglia, and it surrounds the celiac artery at its juncture with the aorta. The sympathetic innervation of the heart originates in the cervical and thoracic ganglia and travels via the cardiac nerves to the heart. Table 9.3 summarizes the autonomic and nociceptive pathways to various body structures.

In addition to the gray rami, the sympathetic trunks give off postganglionic rami that supply the viscera of the head, chest, and abdomen. These rami include the carotid nerve; the superior, middle, and inferior cardiac nerves; the superior, middle, and inferior thoracic splanchnic nerves; and the lumbar and sacral splanchnic nerves.

Some preganglionic fibers synapse in the intermediary ganglia in the white communicating rami, ventral nerve roots, or the spinal nerves outside of the sympathetic chain.[87,88] These anomalous sympathetic pathways are most commonly found in the sympathetic trunk at the cervicothoracic juncture and the thoracolumbar juncture.[92–94] These pathways explain why surgical interruption of the sympathetic chain may not completely block sympathetic outflow. Conversely, these anatomic variations often respond to sympathetic blockade with a local anesthetic solution because it diffuses locally to affect these pathways.[92] A sympathetic block can therefore be a poor predictor of the efficacy of surgical sympathectomy. In cases of incomplete sympathectomy, a postsurgical sympathetic block that produces complete interruption of sympathetic outflow and pain relief in sympathetically dependent pain syndromes may suggest the presence of anomalous sympathetic ganglia.[92,93]

Sympathetic postganglionic neurons may be involved in the generation of pain, hyperalgesia, and inflammation in disease. Depending on the extent of the peripheral nerve lesion, plastic changes can occur at multiple levels of the ANS. Release of mediators (e.g., epinephrine, norepinephrine) from efferent sympathetic nerves both locally and systemically and upregulation of adrenoreceptors in nociceptive afferents contribute to the increased excitability of nociceptors and changes in local vasomotor and sudomotor activity.[95] This reorganization of the peripheral neurons may lead to chemical coupling between sympathetic and afferent neurons. This may be responsible for sensitization and/or activation of primary afferent neurons by the sympathetic neurons.[96]

SENSATION IN VISCERAL ORGANS

Visceral afferent fibers convey sensory information from the internal organs to the CNS. Sensory fibers from viscera follow autonomic nerves as they travel centrally; the majority of the fibers conducting nociceptive information travel along sympathetic nerves. The neurons of visceral afferent fibers are structurally similar to somatic afferent fibers and, like their somatic counterparts, have cell bodies in the DRG of spinal nerves. Their central processes pass to the spinal dorsal horn, primarily in laminae I and V, and from there, visceral information travel centrally via dorsal column pathways as well as by the spinothalamic and spinoreticular tracts. At the level of the

dorsal horn, some primary afferents make synaptic connections with somatic motor neurons, whereas others synapse with preganglionic neurons in the intermediolateral cell column, thus mediating complex visceral reflexes. These reflexes usually involve alteration of the function of the viscera, increase in skeletal muscle tension, and increase in sympathetic activity.

Visceral afferent fibers mediate reflexes such as coughing, cardiopulmonary reflexes, and emptying of the bladder. Most of the visceral receptors are free nerve endings with large receptive fields that are able to respond to varied stimuli. The receptors responsible for transmitting nociceptive signals are largely chemoreceptors that are sensitive to changes that disrupt the internal milieu such as ischemia, inflammation, or the presence of an irritant (e.g., bile, blood). Indeed, in inflammatory diseases of the viscera, such as Crohn's disease or ulcerative colitis, the peripheral nerve endings may become essentially engulfed in the inflammatory infiltrate that invades the mucosa. The visceral afferent fibers are sensitive to distension and contraction, not cutting or tearing of tissue like the somatic afferents. Although visceral sensations are for the most part not consciously perceived, nociceptive information is transmitted. These fibers also transmit information about the immune system and contribute to the development of fever in the presence of infection.[89,97]

Cervical spinothalamic cells receive input from cardiothoracic afferent fibers and transmit the information to autonomic and nociceptive centers higher in the CNS; these afferent fibers also activate propriospinal pathways in the cervical spine that modulate visceral input from lower levels of the spine.[98]

AUTONOMIC CENTERS IN THE CENTRAL NERVOUS SYSTEM

Unlike the peripheral ANS, distinctions between the somatic and autonomic structures and pathways are often difficult in the CNS. The cortex is the central integration center for both somatic and vegetative functions. Multiple cortical structures have been identified as playing a role in the pain–ANS interaction. The insula, in addition to being associated with the limbic system, is the primary cortex for the viscerosensory system and is involved in the discriminative aspect of pain sensation. It plays a role in the subjective experience of pain and has connections with multiple centers (amygdala, lateral hypothalamus, etc.) involved with autonomic outflow.[99,100] The anterior cingulate cortex receives nociceptive inputs and maintains broad connections with multiple areas of the central autonomic network. In addition to being included as part of the limbic system and being involved in goal related behavior, it plays an essential role in affective and motivational components of pain.[101] Surgical stimulation of this region elicits a range of autonomic responses.[102] The amygdala is composed of several nuclei with distinct functional properties. It plays an essential role in modulating the ANS and is closely linked to the hypothalamus. The amygdala plays a role in the subjective perception of pain as well as expression of emotional response to pain.[103] The PAG is a complex region of the CNS that has distinct anatomic and functional regions. Different areas of the PAG receive sensory information and help integrate and regulate autonomic responses to these signals and modulate the sympathetic nervous system in analgesia.[104] The PAG receives sensory signals from laminae I and V of the dorsal horn and helps regulate responses to cardiovascular and nociceptive input.

There are several autonomic centers in the brainstem that have been physiologically delineated. In addition to regulating vital functions such as breathing and circulation, aggregates of neurons in the medullary and pontine reticular formation regulate the ANS through ascending and descending tracts. In the medulla, the nucleus of the solitary tract is a control center of vegetative functions and also appears to contribute antinociceptive input to the dorsal horn.[24] The parabrachial nucleus integrates nociceptive and visceral information through

TABLE 9.3 Summary of Sympathetic and Nociceptive Nerve Supply to More Important Body Structures

Region, Structure	Sympathetic Nerve Supply			Nociceptive Pathways	
	Location of Cell Body in Spinal Cord and Course of Preganglionic Neurons	Site of Synapse of Preganglionic with Postganglionic Neurons	Course of Postganglionic Axons	Location of Primary Afferent Pathway	Entrance into Central Nervous System
Head and Neck					
Meninges and arteries of brain	T1, T2, (T3)[a] To and through cervical sympathetic chain	All cervical sympathetic ganglia	Plexuses around internal carotid and vertebral arteries	Cranial nerves (CN) V, IX, X C1–C3	Trigeminal subnucleus caudalis C1–C3 spinal segments
Eye[b]	T1, T2, T3, (T4) To and through cervical sympathetic chain	Superior cervical ganglion and ganglia in internal carotid plexus	Internal carotid and cavernosus plexuses → ciliary ganglion or nasociliary nerve → ciliary nerves or along ophthalmic artery	Ophthalmic branch of CN V	Trigeminal subnucleus caudalis
Lacrimal gland[b]	T1, T2 To and through cervical sympathetic ganglia	Superior cervical sympathetic ganglion	Internal carotid plexus → vidian nerve → sphenopalatine ganglion → maxillary nerve → zygomatic/lacrimal nerves	Lacrimal nerve → ophthalmic branch of CN V	As above
Parotid gland[b]	As above	All cervical sympathetic ganglia	External carotid plexus → internal maxillary and middle meningeal plexus → to auriculotemporal nerve and plexus and to the parotid arterial plexuses	Parotid nerve → auriculotemporal nerve of mandibular division of CN V	As above
Submandibular and sublingual glands[b]	As above	As above	External carotid plexus → facial plexus → submandibular ganglion → direct glandular filaments or via lingual nerves or directly to glands along vessels	Submandibular branch of lingual nerve → mandibular division of CN V	As above
Thyroid gland	T1–T4 To and through cervical sympathetic chain	Middle and inferior cervical sympathetic ganglia	Perivascular sympathetic plexuses accompanying superior and inferior thyroid arteries	Afferents accompanying sympathetic pathways	T1 and T2 spinal cord segments
Blood vessels of skin and somatic structures Sweat glands Hair follicles	T1–T4 To and through cervical sympathetic chain	All cervical sympathetic ganglia	In perivascular plexuses accompanying various branches of external and internal carotid arteries	Afferents accompanying sympathetic nerves CN V, IX, X C2–C4	T1–T4 spinal cord Subnucleus caudalis C2–C4 spinal cord segments
Thoracic Viscera					
Heart	T1–T4, (T5) To upper thoracic and cervical sympathetic chain	All cervical and upper four (five) thoracic ganglia	Superior, middle, and inferior cervical cardiac nerves and the four (five) thoracic cardiac nerves → cardiac plexuses	Afferents in middle and inferior cervical cardiac and the thoracic cardiac nerves	T1–T4 (T5)
Larynx	T1, T2 To and through cervical sympathetic chain	Superior cervical ganglion	Laryngeal branch of superior cervical ganglion → superior laryngeal nerve	Superior laryngeal nerve	Trigeminal subnucleus caudalis
Trachea, bronchi, and lungs	T2–T6, (T7) To upper thoracic sympathetic chain	T2–T6, (T7) Sympathetic ganglia	Pulmonary branches from sympathetic trunk → pulmonary plexuses	Afferents with sympathetics Afferents with vagus	T2–T6, (T7) Nucleus tractus solitarius (medulla)
Esophagus Cervical	T2–T4 To and through upper thoracic sympathetic chain	All cervical sympathetic ganglia and pharyngeal plexus	From cervical ganglia to recurrent laryngeal nerve	Afferents in vagus Afferents with sympathetics	Nucleus tractus solitarius T2–T4 (?)
Thoracic	T3–T6 To and through upper thoracic sympathetic chain	Stellate and upper thoracic ganglia	Direct esophageal branches and through cardiac sympathetic nerves	Afferents with vagus Afferents with sympathetics	Nucleus tractus solitarius T3–T6 (?)
Abdominal	T5–T8 To thoracic sympathetic chain—superior thoracic splanchnic nerve	Celiac ganglia	Via plexuses around left gastric and inferior phrenic arteries	Afferents with sympathetics Afferents with vagus	T5–T8 Nucleus tractus solitarius
Thoracic aorta	T1–T5, (T6) To thoracic sympathetic chain	Synapse upper five (six) thoracic sympathetic ganglia	Branches from cardiac sympathetic nerves and direct fibers from thoracic sympathetic chain	Afferents with sympathetic pathways	T1–T5, (T6)

(continued)

TABLE 9.3   (Continued)

Region, Structure	Sympathetic Nerve Supply			Nociceptive Pathways	
	Location of Cell Body in Spinal Cord and Course of Preganglionic Neurons	Site of Synapse of Preganglionic with Postganglionic Neurons	Course of Postganglionic Axons	Location of Primary Afferent Pathway	Entrance into Central Nervous System
Abdominal Viscera					
Abdominal aorta	T5–L2 Some through splanchnic nerves and direct branches	Celiac ganglia and paravertebral sympathetic chain	Fibers that contribute to the aortic plexus	Afferents associated with sympathetics	T5–L2
Stomach and duodenum	(T5), T6–T9, (T10), (T11) Superior (greater) and middle (lesser) thoracic splanchnic nerves and celiac plexus	Celiac ganglia	Right and left gastric and gastroepiploic plexuses	Afferents with sympathetics	(T5), T6–T9, (T10), (T11)
Gallbladder and bile ducts	(T5), T6–T9, (T10) Superior thoracic (greater) splanchnic nerves and celiac plexus	Celiac ganglia	Hepatic and gastroduodenal plexuses	Afferents associated with sympathetics	(T5), T6–T9, (T10)
Liver	(T5), T6–T9, (T10) Superior thoracic (greater) splanchnic nerves and celiac plexus	Celiac ganglia	Hepatic plexus	Afferents associated with sympathetics	(T5), T6–T9, (T10)
Pancreas	(T5), T6–T10, (T11) Superior thoracic (greater) splanchnic nerves and celiac plexus	Celiac ganglia	Direct branches from celiac plexus and offshoots from splenic, gastroduodenal, and pancreaticoduodenal plexuses	Afferents associated with sympathetics	T5–T10, (T11)
Small intestines	T8–T12 (right side) T8–T11 (left side) To superior (greater) and middle (lesser) thoracic splanchnic nerves to celiac plexus	Celiac and superior mesenteric ganglia	Superior mesenteric plexus → nerves alongside jejunal and ileal arteries	Follow sympathetic pathways through celiac and inferior mesenteric plexuses	(T8), T9, T10 T10, T11
Cecum and appendix[b]	T10–T12 Superior (greater) and middle (lesser) thoracic splanchnic nerves → celiac and superior mesenteric plexuses	Celiac and superior mesenteric ganglia	Nerves alongside ileocolic artery	Accompanying sympathetic pathways	T10–T12
Colon to splenic flexure[b]	T10–L1 Middle (lesser) and inferior (least) thoracic and first lumbar splanchnic nerves	Superior and inferior mesenteric ganglia	Mesenteric plexus → nerves alongside right, middle, and superior left colic arteries	Associated with sympathetics, pass through superior and inferior mesenteric plexuses and splanchnic nerves and to spinal cord	T10–L1
Splenic flexure to rectum[b]	L1, L2 (left side) S2–S4 Lumbar and sacral splanchnic nerves → inferior mesenteric and inferior hypogastric pelvic plexuses	Inferior mesenteric ganglion and ganglia in superior and inferior hypogastric plexuses	Nerves alongside inferior left colic and rectal arteries	Afferents with parasympathetic nerves and pudendal nerves	S2–S4

Structure	Spinal/splanchnic nerves	Ganglia	Plexus pathway	Afferent course	Spinal cord segments
Suprarenal (adrenal) glands[b]	(T7), T8–L1, (L2) Superior (greater), middle (lesser), and inferior (least) thoracic splanchnic nerves and first (second) lumbar splanchnic nerves	Chromaffin cells of adrenal medulla	Within the gland		
Kidneys[b]	T10–T12, L1, (L2) Middle (lesser) and inferior (least) thoracic splanchnic nerves and first (second) lumbar splanchnic nerves → celiac and renal plexuses	Celiac and aorticorenal ganglia	Along renal plexus	Accompanies sympathetic pathways	T10–L12, (L1, L2)
Ureters Upper two-thirds[b]	T(10), T11, T12, L1, L2 Middle and inferior thoracic splanchnic and upper two lumbar splanchnic nerves	Celiac and aorticorenal ganglia	Superior mesenteric and renal plexuses → superior and middle ureteric nerves	Associated with sympathetics	T10–T12, (L1, L12)
Ureters Lower one-third	T11–L1, S2–S4	Aorticorenal ganglion and sacral sympathetic ganglia	Aortic, superior hypogastric, and inferior hypogastric (pelvic) plexuses and sacral splanchnic nerves	Accompany sympathetic and parasympathetic nerves	T10–T12
Pelvic Viscera					
Bladder	(T11), T12, L1, L2 Middle and inferior thoracic splanchnic nerves	Inferior mesenteric ganglion and sacral paravertebral ganglia	Superior and inferior hypogastric plexuses and sacral splanchnic nerves to vesical plexus	Predominantly afferents of parasympathetic nerves; also some sympathetic afferents	S2–S4
Uterus	(T6–T9), T10–T12, L1, (L2) Splanchnic nerves to aortic and ovarian plexuses and superior and inferior hypogastric plexuses	Celiac ganglion and various paravertebral ganglia	Lumbar and sacral splanchnic nerves; superior, middle, and inferior hypogastric plexuses → uterine plexus	Accompanying sympathetic pathways	T11–L2
Testes, ductus deferens, epididymis, seminal vesicles, prostate	T10–L1 inclusive Splanchnic nerves → aortic and superior hypogastric plexus	Prevertebral ganglia and inferior mesenteric ganglion	Follow various vascular plexuses in sacral splanchnic nerves	Testes (ovaries) Prostate Parasympathetic afferents	T10 S2–S4
Trunks and Limbs (Innervation of Vessels, Sweat Glands, and Hair Follicles)					
Trunk	T1–T12	T1–T12 paravertebral sympathetic ganglia	Gray rami communicantes → thoracic spinal nerves	Primary afferents in spinal nerves	T2–L1
Upper extremities	T2–T8, (T9) To and through upper thoracic and lower cervical sympathetic chain	Middle and stellate ganglia; T2 and T3 ganglia	Gray rami communicantes to roots of brachial plexus → brachial plexus and its major nerves; some directly to plexuses around subclavian, axillary, and upper brachial arteries	Brachial plexus and its branches	C5–T1
Lower extremities	T10–T12, L1, L2 To and through lumbar and upper sacral sympathetic chain	L1–L5, S1–S3 paravertebral ganglia	Gray rami communicantes → lumbosacral plexus and its major nerves; direct branches to perivascular plexuses as far as upper femoral artery	Lumbosacral plexus	L1–S3

[a]Segments in parentheses are inconstant.
[b]Unilateral innervation.

TABLE 9.4	Autonomic Centers (AC) in Spinal Cord
Structure	**Location of AC in Spinal Cord**
Head and neck	T1–T4
Upper limb	T2–T8/T9
Upper trunk	T2–T8
Lower trunk	T9–L2
Lower limb	T10–L2
Viscera	
Thoracic (sympathetic)	T1–T5
Abdominal (sympathetic)	T5–L2
Pelvic (parasympathetic)	S2–T4

its extensive connections with the medulla, hypothalamus, and amygdala to maintain homeostasis. The autonomic centers in the brainstem give rise to the parasympathetic visceral efferent fibers of the cranial nerves.[105]

The spinal cord is a central area of integrating the somatic and autonomic functions. Through spinal reflexes, somatic nociception can exert a major impact on the autonomic system. Noxious stimulation to the skin induces a cascade of sympathetic responses, including increased sweat production and skin vasomotor responses.[106]

The location of the preganglionic neurons for the sympathetic and parasympathetic nervous systems in the CNS differ. The sympathetic preganglionic neurons are located in the T1–L2 spinal segments of the spinal cord. The parasympathetic preganglionic neurons are located in the brainstem and the S2–S4 spinal segments (see Figs. 9.9 and 9.10). The locations of the cell bodies of preganglionic sympathetic and parasympathetic neurons, which mediate their function in various parts of the body, are listed in Table 9.4. There are essential differences between the ganglia these neurons form. The sympathetic ganglia are distributed widely throughout the body, are located close to the CNS, and use epinephrine as the primary neurotransmitter. In contrast, the parasympathetic ganglia largely innervate visceral organs, which they are in close proximity to, and use acetylcholine as a neurotransmitter. Figure 9.9 depicts the autonomic pathways that connect the preganglionic neurons in the intermediolateral horn of the spinal cord with the hypothalamus and other brainstem structures.

TRANSMISSION IN THE PERIPHERAL AUTONOMIC NERVOUS SYSTEM

The majority of preganglionic neurons in the ANS are cholinergic, as are some sympathetic postganglionic neurons, such as sweat glands. Acetylcholine binds nicotinic receptors in the membrane of postganglionic neurons. Postganglionic parasympathetic neurons also release acetylcholine, which binds to muscarinic receptors in effector organs (e.g., cardiac and smooth muscle, glandular cells). There are drugs that selectively block each of these receptors (see Fig. 9.8).

Norepinephrine is the transmitter substance in the majority of sympathetic postganglionic nerve endings. The response of the effector cells is mediated by two types of receptors: the α- and β-adrenergic receptors. These receptors have different effects at different organs. For example, in the heart, norepinephrine binding to a β receptor causes an increase in heart rate, whereas in the bladder and airways, this same process causes a relaxation of smooth muscle cells. A variety of pharmacologic agents can either enhance or block the action of these receptor subtypes.

The cells in the adrenal medulla, which are homologues of the postganglionic neurons, mainly release epinephrine into the bloodstream with sympathetic stimulation. Although it has many of the same effects as norepinephrine, epinephrine stimulates the β receptors in the fat and liver cells accelerating metabolism of fat and glucose.

There are other neurotransmitters in the ANS. Most preganglionic neurons contain neuropeptides (enkephalin, somatostatin) of unclear functional purpose in addition to acetylcholine. Some autonomic neurons do not contain either acetylcholine or norepinephrine. These are primarily located in the gastrointestinal tract.

PHYSIOLOGY OF THE AUTONOMIC NERVOUS SYSTEM

The ANS regulates activities that are required for maintenance of the internal environment of an organism but which are not normally under voluntary or conscious control. This includes modulating functions such as metabolism, circulation, respiration, body temperature, digestion, sweating, circadian rhythm, and endocrine secretion. The ANS coordinates these physiologic processes to maintain homeostasis,[107] such as the constancy of the internal environment.

The effects of stimulating either portion of the ANS and its impact on various organs, visceral structures, and effector cells are summarized in Table 9.5. The sympathetic nervous system is focused on catabolic function and mobilizing the body's resources. In contrast to the sympathetic nervous system, the parasympathetic function is anabolic and dedicated to regulating functions that maintain an organism over the long term. Through regulation of the enteric system, it conserves and stores energy, it plays a central role in coordinating the muscular contraction of the bladder and rectum to eliminate waste products, and it maintains the basal heart rate and respiration under normal conditions.[90]

The functional balance that is normally maintained by the two divisions of the ANS can be disturbed in disease. Linkages exist between the autonomic and immune systems that may be important in the production of disease states and the response to neoplasia and other chronic disease that may lead to pain.[108] Pain itself may alter the immune response and thereby alter the progression of a disease.[109] Animal and human physiologic and pharmacologic studies of visceral as well as somatic pain have demonstrated both plasticity and functional characteristics that are far more complex than the basic anatomy described in this chapter; entire books have been written, for example, on visceral pain.[110]

ENTERIC NERVOUS SYSTEM

The enteric nervous system (ENS) is a highly dynamic division of the ANS often referred to as the "little brain" of the gut and contains as many neurons as the spinal cord. It controls gastrointestinal motility and secretion and is involved in visceral sensation. The digestive tract consists of two plexuses, the myenteric and submucous plexuses, formed from sympathetic and parasympathetic postganglionic neurons and a significant number of enteric neurons (Fig. 9.11).[111] Although these plexuses interact with the ANS ganglia in the periphery as well as the spinal cord, brainstem, and cortex, the ENS can function autonomously without input from the sympathetic and parasympathetic systems or the CNS.[112] Enteric neurons were once felt to be postganglionic parasympathetic fibers but are now felt to comprise an independent system in the ANS. The ENS regulates the gastrointestinal system to maintain homeostasis through control of peristalsis, blood vessels, and glandular activity. The ENS also has extensive interaction with the immune system. Disruption of this delicate relationship may be the cause of functional bowel disorders such as irritable bowel syndrome.[26] Enteric neurons appear able to change their function and phenotype, a phenomenon called neuronal plasticity, which contributes to the pathogenesis of visceral hypersensitivity.[111]

TABLE 9.5 Physiologic Responses to Autonomic Stimulation

Structures/Organs	Sympathetic Stimulation	Adrenergic Receptors	Parasympathetic Stimulation
Eye			
Ciliary muscle	Relaxed for far vision	β	Contraction (accommodation for near vision)
Pupillary muscles			
Dilator	Dilated (mydriasis)	α	—
Sphincter	—		Contraction (miosis)
Lacrimal gland	—		Secretion
Salivary glands			
Parotid	Sparse, thick secretion	α	Profuse serous secretion
Sublingual			
Submaxillary			
Thyroid gland	Stimulated		—
Tracheobronchial tree			
Bronchial muscles	Relaxed	β	Contracted
Bronchial glands	—(?)		Secretion
Heart			
Rate	Increased	β	Decreased
Output	Increased	β	Decreased
Esophagus			
Motility	Decreased	α and β	Increased
Sphincters	Contracted	α	Relaxed
Stomach			
Motility	Decreased	α and β	Increased
Sphincters	Contracted	α	Relaxed
Secretion	Inhibited	α	Increased
Liver	Glycogenolysis, gluconeogenesis	β	—
Gallbladder and biliary ducts	Relaxed	β	Contracted
Pancreas			
Blood vessels	Constriction		Dilation
Insulin secretion	Reduced	α	Increased
Spleen	Contraction of capsule	α	—
Intestines			
Motility	Decreased	α and β	Increased
Sphincters	Relaxed	β	Contracted
Secretion	Decreased	α	Increased
Adrenal gland	Secretion of 80% epinephrine /20% norepinephrine	α	—
Kidneys			
Arterioles	Constriction	α	Dilation
Ureter			
Tone and motility	Decreased	α	Increased
Urinary bladder			
Detrusor muscles	Relaxed	β	Contracted
Trigone and sphincter	Contracted	α	Relaxed
Genital organs			
Seminal vesicles	Contraction	α	—(?)
Vas deferens	Contraction	α	—(?)
Uterus	Contraction	α	Depends on species and hormonal status
	Relaxation	β	
Blood vessels			
Coronary arteries	Constriction	α	—
	Dilation(?)	β	—
Arteries in skeletal muscles	Constriction	α[a]	—
	Dilation	β	
Arteries in penis or clitoris	—(?)		Dilation
All other arteries	Constriction	α	Dilation
Veins	Constriction	α	—

[a]By circulating epinephrine only.

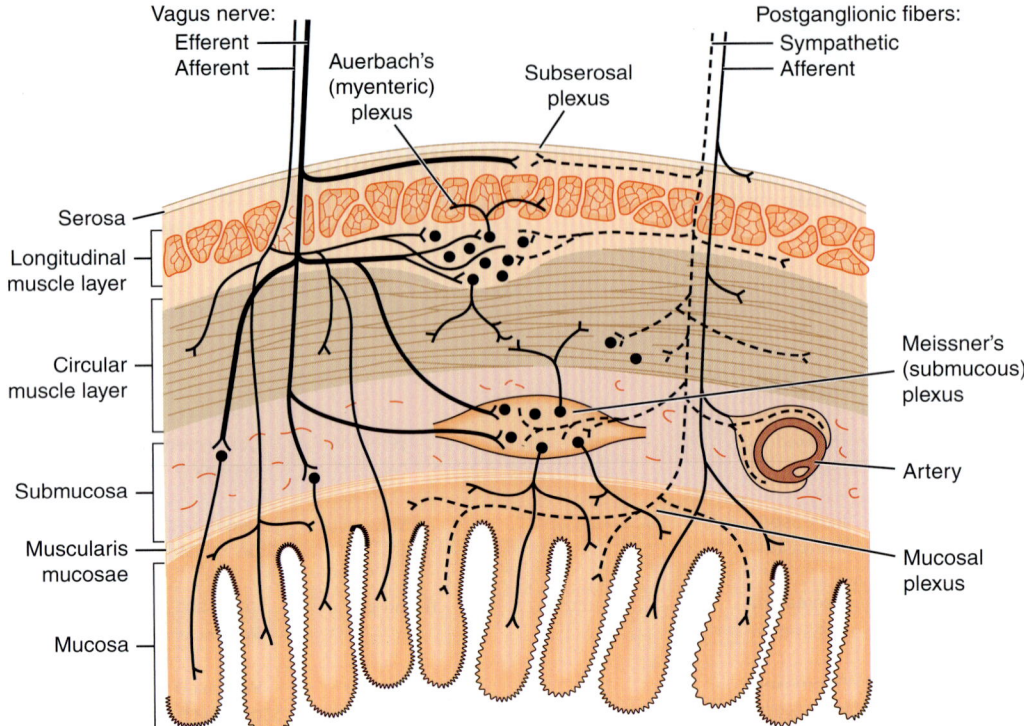

FIGURE 9.11 Arrangement of nerve cells and nerve fibers in the intramural plexuses in the intestine. The axonal endings of the parasympathetic preganglionic neurons synapse in the wall of the intestine, whereas the axonal endings of postganglionic sympathetic neurons are largely distributed to the intramural ganglia and the blood vessels. (*Modified from Kuntz A. Autonomic Nervous System. 4th ed. Philadelphia: Lea & Febiger; 1953:215.*)

Conclusion

Complete evaluation of individuals with persistent pain includes anatomic localization of the lesion or lesions responsible for both the initiation and maintenance of pain. It is necessary to distinguish between pain that is of peripheral, central, and mixed origin; it is necessary to determine whether pain is somatic or visceral. Thus, optimal evaluation and care of patients with persistent pain is dependent on a thorough knowledge of the anatomy of nociceptive systems. Future advances in our understanding of the anatomy and physiology of pain in conjunction with improvements in evaluative and diagnostic technologies (e.g., imaging, genetic) will no doubt enhance the care of individual patients.

References

1. Woolf CJ, Mannion RJ. Neuropathic pain: aetiology, symptoms, mechanisms, and management. *Lancet* 1999;353(9168):1959–1964.
2. Woolf CJ, Costigan M. Transcriptional and posttranslational plasticity and the generation of inflammatory pain. *Proc Natl Acad Sci USA* 1999;96(14):7723–7730.
3. Al-Chaer ED, Traub RJ. Biological basis of visceral pain: recent developments. *Pain* 2002;96(3):221–225.
4. Cervero F, Laird JM. Visceral pain. *Lancet* 1999;353(9170):2145–2148.
5. Almeida TF, Roizenblatt S, Tufik S. Afferent pain pathways: a neuroanatomical review. *Brain Res* 2004;1000(1–2):40–56.
6. Craig AD. Pain mechanisms: labeled lines versus convergence in central processing. *Annu Rev Neurosci* 2003;26:1–30.
7. Woolf CJ. Evidence for a central component of post-injury pain hypersensitivity. *Nature* 1983;306(5944):686–688.
8. Woolf CJ, Fitzgerald M. The properties of neurones recorded in the superficial dorsal horn of the rat spinal cord. *J Comp Neurol* 1983;221(3):313–328.
9. Saadé NE, Jabbur SJ. Nociceptive behavior in animal models for peripheral neuropathy: spinal and supraspinal mechanisms. *Prog Neurobiol* 2008;86:22–47.
10. Laine FJ, Smoker WR. Anatomy of the cranial nerves. *Neuroimaging Clin N Am* 1998;8(1):69–100.
11. White JC. Sensory innervation of the viscera. *Res Publ Assoc Nerv Ment Dis* 1943;23:373–390.
12. Nolte J, Sundsten JW. *The Human Brain: An Introduction to its Functional Anatomy.* 5th ed. St. Louis, MO: Mosby; 2002.
13. DeGowin RL, DeGowin EL, Brown DD, et al. *DeGowin & DeGowin's Diagnostic Examination.* 6th ed. New York: McGraw-Hill; 1994.
14. Silen W, Cope Z. *Cope's Early Diagnosis of the Acute Abdomen.* 21st ed. New York: Oxford University Press; 2005.
15. Lee MW, McPhee RW, Stringer MD. An evidence-based approach to human dermatomes. *Clin Anat* 2008;21(5):363–373.
16. Dequéant ML, Pourquié O. Segmental patterning of the vertebrate embryonic axis. *Nat Rev Genet* 2008;9(5):370–382.
17. Tannahill D, Britto JM, Vermeren MM, et al. Orienting axon growth: spinal nerve segmentation and surround-repulsion. *Int J Dev Biol* 2000;44(1):119–127.
18. Netter FH. *Atlas of Human Anatomy.* 4th ed. Philadelphia: Saunders/Elsevier; 2006.
19. Swap CJ, Nagurney JT. Value and limitations of chest pain history in the evaluation of patients with suspected acute coronary syndromes. *JAMA* 2005;294(20):2623–2629.
20. Cervero F, Laird JM, Pozo MA. Selective changes of receptive field properties of spinal nociceptive neurones induced by noxious visceral stimulation in the cat. *Pain* 1992;51(3):335–342.
21. Cervero F, Tattersall JE. Somatic and visceral inputs to the thoracic spinal cord of the cat: marginal zone (lamina I) of the dorsal horn. *J Physiol* 1987;388:383–395.
22. Foreman RD. Integration of viscerosomatic sensory input at the spinal level. *Prog Brain Res* 2000;122:209–221.
23. Saper CB. Pain as a visceral sensation. *Prog Brain Res* 2000;122:237–243.
24. Pappagallo M. *The Neurological Basis of Pain.* New York: McGraw-Hill; 2005.
25. Westlund KN. Visceral nociception. *Curr Rev Pain* 2000;4(6):478–487.
26. Bueno L. Neuroimmune alterations of ENS functioning. *Gut* 2000;47(suppl 4):iv63–iv65, discussion iv76.
27. Julius D, Basbaum AI. Molecular mechanisms of nociception. *Nature* 2001;413(6852):203–210.
28. Cain DM, Khasabov SG, Simone DA. Response properties of mechanoreceptors and nociceptors in mouse glabrous skin: an in vivo study. *J Neurophysiol* 2001;85(4):1561–1574.
29. Perl ER. Cutaneous polymodal receptors: characteristics and plasticity. *Prog Brain Res* 1996;113:21–37.
30. Wood JN, Akopian AN, Baker M, et al. Sodium channels in primary sensory neurons: relationship to pain states. *Novartis Found Symp* 2002;241:159–168, discussion 68–72, 226–232.
31. Rush AM, Cummins TR, Waxman SG. Multiple sodium channels and their roles in electrogenesis within dorsal root ganglion neurons. *J Physiol* 2007;579(pt 1):1–14.
32. Amaya F, Decosterd I, Samad TA, et al. Diversity of expression of the sensory neuron-specific TTX-resistant voltage-gated sodium ion channels SNS and SNS2. *Mol Cell Neurosci* 2000;15(4):331–342.

33. Fang X, Djouhri L, McMullan S, et al. Intense isolectin-B4 binding in rat dorsal root ganglion neurons distinguishes C-fiber nociceptors with broad action potentials and high Nav1.9 expression. *J Neurosci* 2006;26(27):7281–7292.

34. Luo W, Wickramasinghe SR, Savitt JM, et al. A hierarchical NGF signaling cascade controls Ret-dependent and Ret-independent events during development of nonpeptidergic DRG neurons. *Neuron* 2007;54(5):739–754.

35. Zylka MJ, Rice FL, Anderson DJ. Topographically distinct epidermal nociceptive circuits revealed by axonal tracers targeted to Mrgprd. *Neuron* 2005;45(1):17–25.

36. Jordt SE, McKemy DD, Julius D. Lessons from peppers and peppermint: the molecular logic of thermosensation. *Curr Opin Neurobiol* 2003;13(4): 487–492.

37. Levine JD, Alessandri-Haber N. TRP channels: targets for the relief of pain. *Biochim Biophys Acta* 2007;1772(8):989–1003.

38. Binshtok AM, Bean BP, Woolf CJ. Inhibition of nociceptors by TRPV1-mediated entry of impermeant sodium channel blockers. *Nature* 2007; 449(7162):607–610.

39. Lumpkin EA, Bautista DM. Feeling the pressure in mammalian somatosensation. *Curr Opin Neurobiol* 2005;15(4):382–388.

40. Wemmie JA, Price MP, Welsh MJ. Acid-sensing ion channels: advances, questions and therapeutic opportunities. *Trends Neurosci* 2006;29(10):578–586.

41. Christensen AP, Corey DP. TRP channels in mechanosensation: direct or indirect activation? *Nat Rev Neurosci* 2007;8(7):510–521.

42. Kohno T, Wang H, Amaya F, et al. Bradykinin enhances AMPA and NMDA receptor activity in spinal cord dorsal horn neurons by activating multiple kinases to produce pain hypersensitivity. *J Neurosci* 2008;28(17):4533–4540.

43. Wang H, Kohno T, Amaya F, et al. Bradykinin produces pain hypersensitivity by potentiating spinal cord glutamatergic synaptic transmission. *J Neurosci* 2005;25(35):7986–7992.

44. Cervero F. Dorsal horn neurons and their sensory inputs. In: Yaksh TL, ed. *Spinal Afferent Processing*. New York: Plenum Press; 1986:197–216.

45. Willis WD, Westlund KN. Neuroanatomy of the pain system and of the pathways that modulate pain. *J Clin Neurophysiol* 1997;14(1):2–31.

46. Jänig W. Neuronal mechanisms of pain with special emphasis on visceral and deep somatic pain. *Acta Neurochir Suppl (Wien)* 1987;38:16–32.

47. Brown AG, Fyffe RE. Form and function of dorsal horn neurones with axons ascending the dorsal columns in cat. *J Physiol* 1981;321:31–47.

48. Rustioni A. Modulation of sensory input to the spinal cord by presynaptic ionotropic glutamate receptors. *Arch Ital Biol* 2005;143(2):103–112.

49. Liu H, Brown JL, Jasmin L, et al. Synaptic relationship between substance P and the substance P receptor: light and electron microscopic characterization of the mismatch between neuropeptides and their receptors. *Proc Natl Acad Sci U S A* 1994;91(3):1009–1013.

50. Staud R. Evidence of involvement of central neural mechanisms in generating fibromyalgia pain. *Curr Rheumatol Rep* 2002;4(4):299–305.

51. Baranauskas G, Nistri A. Sensitization of pain pathways in the spinal cord: cellular mechanisms. *Prog Neurobiol* 1998;54(3):349–365.

52. DeLeo JA, Winkelstein BA. Physiology of chronic spinal pain syndromes: from animal models to biomechanics. *Spine* 2002;27(22):2526–2537.

53. Gracely RH, Grant MA, Giesecke T. Evoked pain measures in fibromyalgia. *Best Pract Res Clin Rheumatol* 2003;17(4):593–609.

54. Bennett GJ. Update on the neurophysiology of pain transmission and modulation: focus on the NMDA-receptor. *J Pain Symptom Manage* 2000;19(1 suppl):S2–S6.

55. Meller ST, Gebhart GF. Nitric oxide (NO) and nociceptive processing in the spinal cord. *Pain* 1993;52(2):127–136.

56. Luo ZD, Cizkova D. The role of nitric oxide in nociception. *Curr Rev Pain* 2000;4(6):459–466.

57. Price DD, Hu JW, Dubner R, et al. Peripheral suppression of first pain and central summation of second pain evoked by noxious heat pulses. *Pain* 1977;3(1):57–68.

58. Schnitzler A, Ploner M. Neurophysiology and functional neuroanatomy of pain perception. *J Clin Neurophysiol* 2000;17(6):592–603.

59. Masson C, Koskas P, Cambier J, et al. Left pseudothalamic cortical syndrome and pain asymbolia. *Rev Neurol (Paris)* 1991;147(10):668–670.

60. Vanegas H, Schaible HG. Descending control of persistent pain: inhibitory or facilitatory? *Brain Res Brain Res Rev* 2004;46(3):295–309.

61. Tasker R. Central pain states. In: Loeser JD, ed. *Bonica's Management of Pain*. 3rd ed. Philadelphia: Lippincott Williams & Wilkins; 2001:433–457.

62. Canavero S, Bonicalzi V, Massa-Micon B. Central neurogenic pruritus: a literature review. *Acta Neurol Belg* 1997;97(4):244–247.

63. Andersen G, Vestergaard K, Ingeman-Nielsen M, et al. Incidence of central post-stroke pain. *Pain* 1995;61(2):187–193.

64. Finnerup NB, Johannesen IL, Sindrup SH, et al. Pain and dysesthesia in patients with spinal cord injury: a postal survey. *Spinal Cord* 2001;39(5): 256–262.

65. Canavero S, Bonicalzi V. *Central Pain Syndrome: Pathophysiology, Diagnosis and Management*. Cambridge, United Kingdom: Cambridge University Press; 2007.

66. Dejerine J, Roussy G. Le syndrome thalamique. *Rev Neurol (Paris)* 1906;14: 521–532.

67. Waxman SG, Hains BC. Fire and phantoms after spinal cord injury: Na+ channels and central pain. *Trends Neurosci* 2006;29(4):207–215.

68. National Spinal Cord Injury Statistical Center. Spinal cord injury facts and figures at a glance. *J Spinal Cord Med* 2005;28(4):379–380.

69. Finnerup NB, Jensen TS. Spinal cord injury pain—mechanisms and treatment. *Eur J Neurol* 2004;11(2):73–82.

70. Siddall PJ, Loeser JD. Pain following spinal cord injury. *Spinal Cord* 2001;39(2):63–73.

71. Todor DR, Mu HT, Milhorat TH. Pain and syringomyelia: a review. *Neurosurg Focus* 2000;8(3):E11.

72. Ragnarsson KT. Management of pain in persons with spinal cord injury. *J Spinal Cord Med* 1997;20(2):186–199.

73. Loeser JD, Ward AA Jr, White LE Jr. Chronic deafferentation of human spinal cord neurons. *J Neurosurg* 1968;29(1):48–50.

74. Hains BC, Johnson KM, Eaton MJ, et al. Serotonergic neural precursor cell grafts attenuate bilateral hyperexcitability of dorsal horn neurons after spinal hemisection in rat. *Neuroscience* 2003;116(4):1097–1110.

75. Davies SN, Lodge D. Evidence for involvement of N-methylaspartate receptors in 'wind-up' of class 2 neurones in the dorsal horn of the rat. *Brain Res* 1987;424(2):402–406.

76. Yaksh TL, Hua XY, Kalcheva I, et al. The spinal biology in humans and animals of pain states generated by persistent small afferent input. *Proc Natl Acad Sci U S A* 1999;96(14):7680–7686.

77. Mills CD, Johnson KM, Hulsebosch CE. Group I metabotropic glutamate receptors in spinal cord injury: roles in neuroprotection and the development of chronic central pain. *J Neurotrauma* 2002;19(1):23–42.

78. Hains BC, Willis WD, Hulsebosch CE. Serotonin receptors 5-HT1A and 5-HT3 reduce hyperexcitability of dorsal horn neurons after chronic spinal cord hemisection injury in rat. *Exp Brain Res* 2003;149(2):174–186.

79. Drew GM, Siddall PJ, Duggan AW. Mechanical allodynia following contusion injury of the rat spinal cord is associated with loss of GABAergic inhibition in the dorsal horn. *Pain* 2004;109(3):379–388.

80. Hains BC, Saab CY, Waxman SG. Changes in electrophysiological properties and sodium channel Nav1.3 expression in thalamic neurons after spinal cord injury. *Brain* 2005;128(pt 10):2359–2371.

81. Morrow TJ, Paulson PE, Brewer KL, et al. Chronic, selective forebrain responses to excitotoxic dorsal horn injury. *Exp Neurol* 2000;161(1): 220–226.

82. Pattany PM, Yezierski RP, Widerström-Noga EG, et al. Proton magnetic resonance spectroscopy of the thalamus in patients with chronic neuropathic pain after spinal cord injury. *AJNR Am J Neuroradiol* 2002;23(6): 901–905.

83. Birbaumer N, Lutzenberger W, Montoya P, et al. Effects of regional anesthesia on phantom limb pain are mirrored in changes in cortical reorganization. *J Neurosci* 1997;17(14):5503–5508.

84. Langley JN. The autonomic nervous system. *Brain* 1903;26:1–26.

85. Longhurst JC. Cardiac receptors: their function in health and disease. *Prog Cardiovasc Dis* 1984;27(3):201–222.

86. Shefchyk SJ. Spinal cord neural organization controlling the urinary bladder and striated sphincter. *Prog Brain Res* 2002;137:71–82.

87. Mitchell GAG. *Anatomy of the Autonomic Nervous System*. Edinburgh: Livingstone; 1953.

88. Pick J. *The Autonomic Nervous System; Morphological, Comparative, Clinical, and Surgical Aspects*. Philadelphia: Lippincott; 1970.

89. Jänig W. Neurobiology of visceral afferent neurons: neuroanatomy, functions, organ regulations and sensations. *Biol Psychol* 1996;42(1–2):29–51.

90. Brodal P. *The Central Nervous System: Structure and Function*. 3rd ed. Oxford, United Kingdom: Oxford University Press; 2004.

91. Aunis D, Langley K. Physiological aspects of exocytosis in chromaffin cells of the adrenal medulla. *Acta Physiol Scand* 1999;167(2):89–97.

92. Cho HM, Lee DY, Sung SW. Anatomical variations of rami communicantes in the upper thoracic sympathetic trunk. *Eur J Cardiothorac Surg* 2005;27(2):320–324.

93. Murata Y, Takahashi K, Yamagata M, et al. Variations in the number and position of human lumbar sympathetic ganglia and rami communicantes. *Clin Anat* 2003;16(2):108–113.

94. Ramsaroop L, Partab P, Singh B, et al. Thoracic origin of a sympathetic supply to the upper limb: the 'nerve of Kuntz' revisited. *J Anat* 2001;199(pt 6): 675–682.

95. Sato J, Perl ER. Adrenergic excitation of cutaneous pain receptors induced by peripheral nerve injury. *Science* 1991;251(5001):1608–1610.

96. Jänig W, Levine JD, Michaelis M. Interactions of sympathetic and primary afferent neurons following nerve injury and tissue trauma. *Prog Brain Res* 1996;113:161–184.

97. Joshi SK, Gebhart GF. Visceral pain. *Curr Rev Pain* 2000;4(6):499–506.

98. Hobbs SF, Oh UT, Chandler MJ, et al. Evidence that C1 and C2 propriospinal neurons mediate the inhibitory effects of viscerosomatic spinal afferent input on primate spinothalamic tract neurons. *J Neurophysiol* 1992;67(4): 852–860.

99. Craig AD. Distribution of trigeminothalamic and spinothalamic lamina I terminations in the macaque monkey. *J Comp Neurol* 2004;477(2):119–148.

100. Craig AD. A new view of pain as a homeostatic emotion. *Trends Neurosci* 2003;26(6):303–307.

101. Vogt BA, Berger GR, Derbyshire SW. Structural and functional dichotomy of human midcingulate cortex. *Eur J Neurosci* 2003;18(11):3134–3144.

102. Oppenheimer SM, Gelb A, Girvin JP, et al. Cardiovascular effects of human insular cortex stimulation. *Neurology* 1992;42(9):1727–1732.

103. Davis M, Whalen PJ. The amygdala: vigilance and emotion. *Mol Psychiatry* 2001;6(1):13–34.

104. Benarroch EE. Pain-autonomic interactions. *Neurol Sci* 2006;27(suppl 2): S130–S133.
105. Bernard JF, Bester H, Besson JM. Involvement of the spino-parabrachio-amygdaloid and -hypothalamic pathways in the autonomic and affective emotional aspects of pain. *Prog Brain Res* 1996;107:243–255.
106. Janig W. The sympathetic nervous system in pain. *Eur J Anaesthesiol Suppl* 1995;10:53–60.
107. Cannon WB. *The Wisdom of the Body*. Rev and enl ed. New York: Norton; 1939.
108. Ader R, Cohen N, Felten D. Psychoneuroimmunology: interactions between the nervous system and the immune system. *Lancet* 1995;345(8942):99–103.
109. Page GG, Ben-Eliyahu S. The immune-suppressive nature of pain. *Semin Oncol Nurs* 1997;13(1):10–15.
110. Gebhart GF. *Visceral Pain*. Seattle, WA: IASP Press; 1995.
111. Boeckxstaens GE. Understanding and controlling the enteric nervous system. *Best Pract Res Clin Gastroenterol* 2002;16(6):1013–1023.
112. Hodgkiss JP. Intrinsic reflexes underlying peristalsis in the small intestine of the domestic fowl. *J Physiol* 1986;380:311–328.

CHAPTER 10

Clinical Trials

ROGER CHOU and **RICHARD A. DEYO**

Controversies abound in the clinical management of pain, and there are enormous geographic variations in care. Lumbar spine surgery rates historically vary fivefold among developed countries, with rates in the United States being highest and rates in the United Kingdom being among the lowest[1]—yet, patient outcomes appear to be broadly similar across countries. In smaller geographic areas, variations are also striking. Within the United States, rates of lumbar fusion surgery among Medicare enrollees vary more than 20-fold between regions, from 4.6 per 1,000 enrollees in Idaho Falls, Idaho, to 0.2 per 1,000 in Bangor, Maine.[2] Within Washington State, county back surgery rates vary more than sevenfold, even after excluding the smallest counties.[3]

Another problem in pain management is the successive uptake of a series of fads in treatment. Research has eventually discredited many of these, but they enjoyed widespread use, with substantial costs and side effects, before they were found to be ineffective. Examples include sacroiliac joint fusion for the treatment of low back pain, coccygectomy for coccydynia, bed rest and traction for back pain, and many others.[4] This phenomenon is prominent in the field of pain medicine but not unique to it. Examples of abandoned therapies from other areas of medicine include internal mammary artery ligation for treating angina pectoris, gastric freezing for duodenal ulcers, and vitamin E and hormone therapy for prevention of cardiovascular events.[5-7] Promoting such ineffective treatments drains resources from more useful interventions, produces side effects, and eventually damages professional credibility.

Despite welcome breakthroughs in basic science research on pain, increases in knowledge regarding optimal ergonomics of work tasks, and the development and use of more technologically advanced medical therapies, evidence indicates an increasing prevalence of chronic back pain and disability. In the state of North Carolina, the prevalence of chronic, impairing back pain more than doubled from 3.9% in 1992 to 10.2% in 2006.[8] A large and steady rise in use of opioids, surgery, and interventional therapies for low back pain has not been associated with improved health status but appears to be an important factor contributing to increases in health care expenditures associated with back pain.[9-11] Thus, despite impressive gains in our understanding of the molecular and cellular origins of pain, there is an important gap in translating this knowledge into effective clinical management. One reason may be the widespread reliance on inadequate research designs that lead to conflicting, confusing, or misinterpreted results. Biostatistical and epidemiologic methods make it possible to substantially improve this situation, but many key principles are not widely appreciated.

Uncontrolled Studies Paradigm

Historically, much of pain treatment research consisted simply of uncontrolled studies in which clinicians treated a group of patients and then reported mean pain scores or the proportion who improved. Such studies are often referred to as *case series*, although the alternative term *before-after study* or *treatment series* may help distinguish them from studies that identify "cases" based on an outcome (such as an adverse event) rather than an exposure (such as a medical intervention) and only assesses patients at one point in time.[12] The before-after study

design remains popular in part because it usually does not require extensive resources but is vulnerable to many pitfalls.[13]

First, many uncontrolled studies are retrospectively reported. After treating a certain number of patients, the clinician looks back at his or her experience and tries to summarize the characteristics, treatments, and outcomes of the patients studied. Unfortunately, in this retrospective approach, there is often incomplete baseline information on patient characteristics. For example, factors such as age, sex, previous surgery, disability compensation, neurologic deficits, psychological comorbidities, and pain duration often have a major influence on the outcomes of back surgery. Yet, in a systematic review of outcome studies on surgery for spinal stenosis, 74 relevant articles were found, but less than 10% mentioned all these patient characteristics.[7]

Another problem with the retrospective approach is that it can be difficult to identify an "inception cohort" of all patients (or a random sample) who met specified criteria and received the intervention. A systematic review of 72 uncontrolled studies of spinal cord stimulation for chronic low back pain or failed back surgery syndrome found that less than one-quarter clearly described evaluation of a consecutive or representative sample of patients.[14] In such studies, it is impossible to know if patients with poorer results were excluded for arbitrary reasons, or how many patients received the treatment but were lost to follow-up. If patients excluded from analysis or lost to follow-up were more likely to experience poor outcomes than those who were followed, this could result in serious overestimates of benefits.

A third problem with uncontrolled studies is that even if the researcher collects data prospectively, there is typically no blinding of patient, therapist, or outcome assessor to the nature of the treatment provided. This allows important unconscious—or conscious—biases to affect assessments. This is particularly important for outcomes related to pain, which by nature are subjective. Most of us would question the reliability of outcomes rated by a surgeon evaluating his or her own patients, and yet, this is the norm in much of the literature.

By definition, uncontrolled studies do not include control groups for comparison. The assumption seems to be that patients with painful conditions, especially chronic pain, will not improve unless effective treatment is given. However, there are many reasons why patients improve in the face of ineffective therapy, some of which are listed in Table 10.1. First, the natural history of many painful conditions is to improve spontaneously. This may be true even for patients with long-standing pain, who sometimes improve for unclear reasons. For acute conditions such as acute low back pain, rapid early improvement is the norm.[15] Second are placebo effects, which are not well understood but are consistently underestimated and may be particularly important when assessing pain.[7] Several factors may mediate placebo effects, including patient expectations,[16] learning and conditioning from previous treatments, reduction of anxiety, and endorphin effects. Placebo effects for pain treatments may be getting larger. In 1996, patients in US clinical trials reported that drugs relieved neuropathic pain 27% more than placebo, but by 2013, the difference had decreased to 9%,[17] a trend that appeared due to a stronger placebo response in the setting of stable drug effects.

TABLE 10.1 Why Patients May Improve with Ineffective Therapy

Natural history of a condition to improve
Placebo effects
Regression to the mean
Nonspecific effects: concern, conviction, enthusiasm, attention

Another poorly appreciated factor is *regression to the mean*.[18] This term was coined by statisticians who observed that in a group of patients who are assembled because of the extreme nature of some clinical condition, there is a tendency for the condition to return to some average level that is less severe over time. Figure 10.1 shows what we often assume to be the course of chronic pain problems, with a steady level of severity that falls after successful intervention. However, the second panel is more likely to represent the true natural history, with good days and bad days, and fluctuations being the norm.[19] Patients seek health care when their symptoms are most extreme. We might easily be misled into believing that improved outcomes are due to the intervention, when in fact, random fluctuations are why their symptoms have returned toward a more average level. As Sartwell and Merrell[20] pointed out, "the term chronic has a tendency to conjure up ideas of stability and unchangeability . . . it is changeability and variation, not stability, that is in fact the dominant characteristic of most long-lived conditions."

Imagined Course of LBP

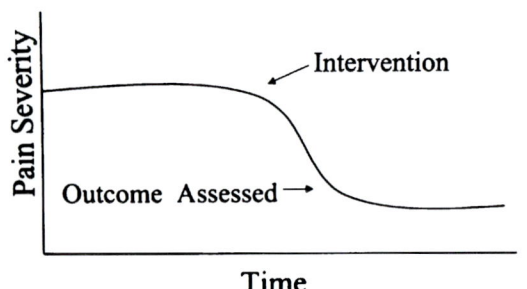

More Likely Course of LBP

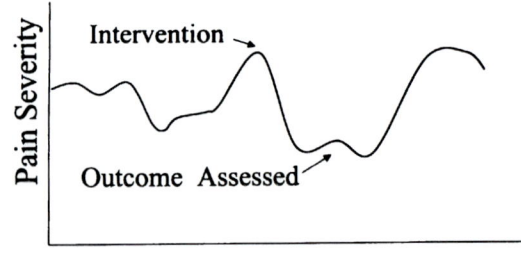

FIGURE 10.1 Hypothetical course of chronic low back pain (LBP). (Reprinted with permission from *Deyo RA. Practice variations, treatment fads, rising disability. Do we need a new clinical research paradigm? Spine 1993;18[15]: 2153–2162)*

TABLE 10.2 Therapeutic Trial for Patients with Chronic Low Back Pain: Mean Duration of 4 Years, n = 31

Outcome Measure	Score Improvement Baseline to 1-Month Follow-Up	*p* Value
Overall function (SIP)	32%	.002
Physical function	44%	.001
Pain severity (VAS)	33%	.006
Pain frequency (5-point scale)	20%	.000

SIP, Sickness Impact Profile; VAS, visual analog scale.
Reprinted with permission from Deyo RA. Practice variations, treatment fads, rising disability. Do we need a new clinical research paradigm? *Spine* 1993;18(15):2153–2162.

A host of other nonspecific effects also can affect assessments of patient improvement. Increased concern, conviction, enthusiasm, and attention of a therapist, a researcher, and a clinical staff may all have positive but nonspecific effects on patient outcomes. Table 10.2 shows a potential consequence of all these factors, using data from a clinical trial of patients with chronic low back pain.[19] The 31 patients in Table 10.2 have had back pain an average of 4 years. They received a clinical intervention that resulted in 20% to 44% improvements in pain frequency, severity, and function, all of which were highly statistically significant. However, this seemingly effective treatment for chronic pain was a sham transcutaneous electrical nerve stimulation (TENS) unit, along with hot packs twice a week. This was the control arm of a randomized trial and illustrates the substantial improvements that may occur among those with long-standing pain who receive ineffective treatments.

Finally, an issue that has begun to receive more attention is that uncontrolled studies are highly susceptible to publication bias.[21] There is little incentive for clinicians to publicize poor or even average results. Estimates of efficacy from uncontrolled studies that get published will therefore often overrepresent the most positive results.

There is considerable room for improvement in the design and conduct of uncontrolled studies of pain interventions.[14,22] However, even when conducted well, the ability of uncontrolled studies to provide reliable information about treatment efficacy will always be limited. Exceptions can occur when the relationship between an intervention and outcomes is obvious, the effects are immediate, and the effects are so dramatic that they cannot be explained by other factors.[23] Examples include surgery for appendicitis, eyeglasses for correction of refractive error, and cataract surgery. For nearly all pain conditions, however, there are many plausible alternative explanations for the observed changes in outcomes, and reliable conclusions about treatment efficacy require the use of more rigorous study designs. There is simply too much "noise" to sort out whether outcomes are due to the treatment or to other factors.[24]

CONTROL GROUPS: AN IMPROVEMENT OVER THE CASE SERIES

Given the variety of factors that may produce improvement with ineffective therapy, it is incumbent on investigators to have a comparison group of subjects with the same likelihood for improvement as a treatment group but who do not receive the active therapy. The goal should be to minimize the potential differences across groups in the effects of the various nonspecific causes for improvement that are listed in Table 10.1. With this goal in mind, the appropriate comparison group is unlikely to be one that receives no care at all. Patients in such a group would not experience placebo effects or the nonspecific effects of clinical concern and enthusiasm. The importance of having an adequate placebo is illustrated by a trial that found acupuncture more effective than no treatment for chronic low back pain but no more effective than sham acupuncture.[25] Similarly, using a "waiting list" control group is often suboptimal because these patients experience none of the placebo or nonspecific effects of the intervention group. A preferable control group would be one that receives other credible, appropriate care that does not include the specific treatment under study. This might consist of "usual care" supplemented by a placebo of some sort. The placebo should be difficult to distinguish from the intervention under study so that it is perceived as being as likely to help as the active therapy. This is the reason for providing inactive pills in the control groups of drug trials, but even for nondrug treatments, credible placebos should be provided when possible. Examples include the use of sham TENS units in trials of TENS, the use of sham injections in trials of interventional therapies, the use of subtherapeutic weight in trials of traction, or "misplaced needling" as a control for acupuncture.

In some cases, it may be unethical or impossible to provide a true placebo. Examples include many surgical interventions, psychological therapies, and rehabilitation interventions. In such situations, a reasonable alternative is to provide a control treatment that creates some sense that patients are receiving an additional intervention and attention but is not likely to have a strong effect on outcomes. One example might be a brief educational brochure.[26]

In addition to choosing an appropriate control intervention, it is also important to make the treatment and control groups as similar to each other as possible in other ways. Confounding is a critical concept that refers to variables associated with both the intervention being evaluated and observed outcomes. A classic example of confounding is the association between alcohol consumption and lung cancer. This association is confounded by smoking, which is associated with alcohol consumption and is also an independent risk factor for lung cancer. Examples of common confounders in pain research include severity of baseline pain or functional deficits, psychological and medical comorbidities, age, and use of other therapies. The consequence of confounding is that the observed treatment effect is a poor estimate of the true effect. The modifying effect of the confounding variables result in either an overestimate or underestimate of treatment benefits and can sometimes even result in a positive effect when the true effect is negative (or vice versa).

Selection of controls to minimize the potential for confounding is often a challenge. Control groups that are convenient to assemble are also unfortunately frequently associated with important pitfalls. For example, it would be unwise to choose patients who did not have adequate insurance coverage for the treatment being provided as a control group because insurance coverage is related to important sociodemographic characteristics. Patients with the best insurance are typically those with the highest salaries and the most satisfying jobs, are happier with their insurance, and are more likely to practice healthy behaviors. Failure to adjust for socioeconomic status in observational studies could have resulted in the subsequently disproven belief in the positive cardiovascular benefits of hormone replacement therapy.[27] Similarly, selecting patients nonadherent with intended therapy as a control group is a flawed strategy. In a large-scale study of cholesterol-lowering therapy, control patients were divided among those who took more than 80% of their placebo tablets and those who took less than 80%.[28] Even after adjusting for 40 coronary risk factors, there were enormous differences in mortality between the adherent and nonadherent groups. Patients who were adherent with their placebos had a 5-year mortality of only 16%, whereas those who were not adherent had a 5-year mortality rate of 26% ($P < .0001$).

These findings were probably related to important differences between the groups that were not reflected in their coronary risk factors. These may have included other health habits, behaviors, attitudes toward risk, and occupations. Thus, nonadherent patients are often strikingly different from adherent patients, and we cannot assume that any differences in outcome are related only to treatment effects.

Sometimes, the issues of proper selection of control patients and treatments are intertwined. A study that assigned patients with presumed discogenic low back pain to intradiscal electrothermal therapy (IDET) or rehabilitation therapy based on their insurance coverage for IDET reported an average 4.5-point improvement in pain scores.[29] Subsequent randomized trials found either no advantage of IDET or only a 1-point difference between IDET and sham treatment.[30,31] In addition to potential socioeconomic differences related to differential insurance coverage, patients who were denied IDET probably had lower expectations about the likely benefits of rehabilitation therapy, particularly because some had previously received this treatment but had not responded.

Confounding by indication is particularly important in studies that assess treatment efficacy. It refers to the strong, natural (and appropriate) tendency for clinicians to selectively use therapies in patients most likely to benefit. A striking example of confounding by indication is a study of new users of nonsteroidal anti-inflammatory drugs that found use of ulcer-healing drugs associated with a 10-fold *increase* in risk of gastrointestinal bleeding or perforations.[32] Obviously, ulcer-healing drugs do not cause ulcers. Rather, the increased risk of gastrointestinal complications in patients deemed appropriate for ulcer-healing drugs dwarfed any protective effect of the drugs.

There are ways to minimize or adjust for the effects of confounding. These include matching patient selection on the variables thought to be most important potential confounders, restricting enrollment to patients defined by a narrow set of inclusion criteria, and statistically adjusting and analyzing known confounders.[33] Nonetheless, the effects of confounding can be dramatic even when one or more of these strategies are employed. For example, confounding by indication was strong in the study on ulcer-healing drugs, even though it attempted to restrict enrollment to lower risk patients without a previous ulcer or who had even been previously prescribed an ulcer-healing drug.[32]

Matching also may not be enough to overcome effects of confounding. Table 10.3 shows how one might assemble two groups of objects that are well matched on five different characteristics and yet literally be comparing apples and oranges.[19] Table 10.4 shows real data from a comparison of outcomes of two groups of Medicare patients who underwent low back surgery. They were matched on diagnosis (all had spinal stenosis), gender, age, insurance (all Medicare), and surgical procedure (all had a laminectomy without fusion). Despite being well matched on these five characteristics, the likelihood of reoperations differed almost fourfold between the two groups.

TABLE 10.3	Why Not Find "Matching" Controls?	
	Apples	**Oranges**
Shape	Round	Round
Source	Tree	Tree
Edible?	Yes	Yes
Size	Handheld	Handheld
Weight	½ lb.	½ lb.

Reprinted with permission from Deyo RA. Practice variations, treatment fads, rising disability. Do we need a new clinical research paradigm? *Spine* 1993;18(15):2153–2162.

TABLE 10.4 Two Cohorts of Medicare Patients with Laminectomy for Stenosis (1985)

	Group A (n = 252)	Group B (n = 141)	Significance
% Women	57%	55%	NS
Mean age	71	72	NS
% Fusion	0	0	NS
4-Year reoperations	4%	15%	<.0005

NS, not significant.
Reprinted with permission from Deyo RA. Practice variations, treatment fads, rising disability. Do we need a new clinical research paradigm? *Spine* 1993;18(15):2153–2162.

TABLE 10.5 Bias in Studies of Myocardial Infarction

Allocation Method	Prognostic Maldistribution (%)	Difference Found in Case-Fatality (%)
Blinded randomization	14	9
Unblinded randomization	27	24
Nonrandomized	58	58

Data from Chalmers T, Celano P, Sacks HS, et al. Bias in treatment assignment in controlled clinical trials. *N Engl J Med* 1983;309:1358–1361 and Deyo RA. Practice variations, treatment fads, rising disability. Do we need a new clinical research paradigm? *Spine* 1993;18:2153–2162.

Differences of this magnitude might easily be attributed to some dramatic advantage of the treatment used in group A. However, these groups were intentionally assembled in such a way that group A was composed of African American patients who had not had prior surgery and group B was composed of white patients with prior surgery.[19] These two characteristics, which might have easily been overlooked, accounted entirely for the difference in reoperation rates. Unfortunately, it usually is not as simple as matching on a few critical and easily measured variables. The cholesterol-lowering placebo study described earlier shows how even matching (or adjusting) for 40 different risk factors may not capture important differences between two groups of patients.[28]

If waiting lists, patients with insufficient insurance coverage, nonadherent patients, or even carefully matched patients receiving appropriate placebo treatments make poor control groups, is there a better solution? Fortunately, the concept of random allocation provides an ideal method of establishing a comparison group that is likely to be similar in nearly all respects to an intervention group.

Randomized Allocation of Treatment and Control Groups

The term *randomized trial* has become familiar among clinicians and yet is often misunderstood. Some assume that a randomized trial is one in which patients are randomly selected from a population of interest. However, just the opposite may be true. Patients may be highly selected from a group of potential candidates based on specific characteristics that make the study treatment safe and likely to succeed. Randomization does not refer to the selection of patients to be studied but rather to the patients' allocation to the treatment or the control group.

Why is randomization such a desirable way of creating a control group? It is attractive because the problem of confounding is largely eliminated.[34] Because it is never possible to completely understand or measure all confounders, residual confounding is always a potential issue in studies that are not randomized.[35] With random allocation, we may not even know the important prognostic factors, but they will be equally distributed (given a fair randomization and enough patients) between the treatment and control groups. Effective randomization requires the generation of a truly unpredictable (random) allocation sequence as well as its successful implementation via allocation concealment.[36]

There is sometimes confusion about what constitutes randomization. Randomization requires using a list of random numbers that may be published or determined by a computer program. Each successive subject has an equal likelihood of being assigned to each treatment arm, although the order in which they are assigned is unpredictable.

Alternating assignment—that is, the first patient is assigned to treatment, the next to placebo, the next to treatment, and so on—is not random because it is predictable. Similarly, assigning patients without conscious bias, or haphazardly, is not the same as random allocation. Using hospital numbers, date of birth, or day of the week is also not randomization. If day of the week is used, a patient could simply come in (or be told to come in) on the day that the desired intervention will be offered. Allocation concealment means that the allocation sequence remains unknown until at least after patients have been assigned to therapy, thus preserving the actual randomization. A traditional method to help preserve allocation concealment is use of opaque sealed envelopes containing the treatment assignment. An increasingly common alternative is to have an offsite facility that keeps the random sequence, so research personnel cannot know the next assignment as a subject is enrolled.[37]

A dramatic example of the effects of randomization in pain research is a systematic review of TENS therapy for postoperative pain that found 15 of 17 randomized trials of efficacy showed no benefit.[38] By contrast, 17 of 19 nonrandomized studies showed a substantial positive treatment effect. Some investigators have also quantified the magnitude of bias that occurs when allocation concealment is inadequate. One such study, shown in Table 10.5, compared randomization with adequate allocation concealment with randomization with inadequate allocation concealment and with nonrandom allocation of controls.[39] The investigators examined a series of treatments for acute myocardial infarction and, as the table shows, demonstrated that maldistribution of prognostic factors was least with randomization with adequate allocation concealment and greatest with nonrandom allocation. Similarly, the likelihood of finding a substantial improvement in case fatality rate rose dramatically, from just 9% of trials with randomization and adequate allocation concealment to up to almost 60% of trials with nonrandom allocation. Other studies suggest that on average, inadequate allocation concealment inflates results by about 40% compared to studies with adequate allocation concealment.[37,40]

Why is allocation concealment so important? There are probably several reasons. Failure to conceal allocation makes it easy to subvert the randomization process. If this occurs, confounding by indication can be as much of a problem as in nonrandomized studies.[37] Some overt methods that have been used to bypass randomization include adjusting treatment assignments based on posted allocation sequences or ignoring allocation to treatments perceived as less desirable.[41] Inadequate allocation concealment can also have more subtle effects. If the investigator has a bias as to which treatment group is more effective—even a subconscious bias—he or she may approach the next subject differently based on knowledge of what the next treatment assignment will be. This may affect the way in which a clinical trial is presented to a patient, the enthusiasm with which consent is sought, or the rigor with which eligibility criteria are applied.

TABLE 10.6 Evaluating Articles about Therapy[42]
These criteria can be used as a guide for evaluating the validity of study results and treatment efficacy.
• Were patient assignments randomized and were those groups analyzed?
• Were patients properly accounted for and attributed?
• Was follow-up complete?
• Were all study participants (including study staff and health workers) "blind" to treatment?
• Were groups similar throughout the trial?
• Were groups treated equally (other than the intervention being studied)?
• What was the extent of the treatment's effect?
• Are the results applicable to my patient care?
• Do benefits of the treatment outweigh the risks and costs?

Other Methods for Reducing Bias in Clinical Trials

Randomization is a powerful method for minimizing the possibility of confounding, but does not protect against other types of bias, or systematic errors in measurement. The quality of a trial refers to how rigorously it employs measures to protect against bias. Table 10.6 lists criteria that have been proposed for critical readers to evaluate the quality of studies on treatment efficacy.[42,43] Lengthier and more detailed sets of criteria for evaluating clinical trials has been developed by the Cochrane Collaboration[44] and by the Cochrane Collaboration Back and Neck Group.[45] Additional guidance for clinical investigators includes recommendations on how to report the methods and results of randomized trials.[46] The list of criteria in Table 10.6 begins with random allocation, which was discussed in detail previously.

BASELINE SIMILARITY OF STUDY GROUPS

Randomization usually provides the best way to produce groups with equivalent prognoses. However, randomization may not always work, and investigators should present a comparison of baseline characteristics of patients in the treatment and control groups. In a properly randomized trial, any observed differences are chance occurrences but may still be sufficiently large to compromise the validity of the study. When this occurs, investigators sometimes adjust for baseline differences using statistical techniques. Such statistical adjustments should be based on how strongly the prognostic factor is thought to be associated with the outcomes and the clinical importance of baseline imbalances, not on the results of statistical tests for significant differences.[47] Statistical tests can be misleading, as small differences may be clinically trivial but statistically significant in large trials, and large differences may be clinically important but statistically nonsignificant in small trials.

Even if adjustment is appropriate, it cannot control for differences in unmeasured confounders. It is also important to consider whether baseline imbalances could be due to intentional subversion of randomization.[48] Minimization is a method for achieving balanced groups based on key predefined patient factors and the number of patients in each groups.[49] Although it is not truly random, because patient factors influence treatment assignments, minimization may provide better balance between treatment groups than standard randomization.

BLINDING

The importance of blinding is that it helps to create similar expectations on the part of patients and similar enthusiasm by the therapists. Furthermore, it ensures that the same level of attention and concern is provided to both a treatment and a control group. Blinding is particularly important in studies that assess subjective outcomes such as pain. In one study, lack of blinding inflated estimates of treatment effects by 30% in trials with subjective outcomes such as pain but had no effect on estimates in trials with objective outcomes.[50]

It is common to talk about *double-blind* trials, but the term is often used ambiguously.[51] Typically, it is meant to imply that the patient is unaware whether he or she is receiving active treatment or a placebo, and the person administering or prescribing the treatment is also unaware. In some cases, it may be impossible to "blind" patients or therapists, as in trials of surgical treatments or some rehabilitation and psychological interventions. There is also a third party that may be blinded—an independent assessor of outcomes. Maintaining such a blinded assessor should generally be feasible, even when it is impossible to blind patients and therapists. Trials should explicitly describe who was blinded rather than use nonspecific jargon such as "single-," "double-," or even "triple-blinded."[51]

As noted in the discussion of control groups, creativity can sometimes produce credible placebo or alternative treatments that at least help to maintain blinding. In many situations, it would be informative to test the success of blinding at the end of a study. This is not done frequently but is important for certain drugs and other interventions that have side effects or other characteristics that can give the treatment away.[52] In a trial of TENS therapy for low back pain, for example, sham treatment does not produce the same sensation as active therapy, so patients could know they are receiving sham rather than active therapy. This would essentially result in an unblinded trial. In fact, one trial of TENS found that patients and physicians were able to guess better than random chance whether individual patients were in the treatment or control group, but the magnitude of blinding failure was sufficiently modest that the results could be interpreted with some confidence.[53]

In trials of drug therapy, crossover designs have commonly been used because they help to reduce the effects of interpatient variability in baseline and outcome measures. For many pain treatments, however, such designs may be undesirable because patients would experience both treatments and could determine with a high level of certainty whether they were receiving active treatment or placebo. For example, maintenance of blinding would be very difficult in a crossover study from sham TENS to true TENS, or from subtherapeutic weight to therapeutic weight with traction, or from mild exercise to strenuous exercise. Because of the potential for loss of blinding and other issues such as carryover effects and loss to follow-up from one intervention period to another,[54] crossover trials may be undesirable for many types of pain therapy.

WERE GROUPS TREATED EQUALLY EXCEPT FOR THE EXPERIMENTAL TREATMENT?

Sometimes, patients in a treatment group are given multiple interventions, and yet, the authors or readers are tempted to ascribe the results to a single feature of the treatment. For example, a patient who receives a sclerosant injection into the spinal ligaments along with corticosteroids and spinal manipulation might be said to have improved because of the sclerosant therapy, and yet, much of the observed improvement might be due to the cotreatments.[55] Thus, it is important that any cotreatments also be given to the control group and that the intensity of the treatments is equal.[56]

Furthermore, use of multiple treatments for chronic painful conditions is common. Many patients obtain over-the-counter pain medications; visit multiple physicians; or seek alternative forms of therapy such as chiropractic care, acupuncture, or massage. In outpatient trials, it may be difficult to prevent patients from obtaining such cotreatments, and it may simply be necessary to inquire about these "cointerventions" and determine if they are roughly equivalent between two groups. Alternatively, investigators may make strenuous efforts to ensure that patients do not receive certain types of cointerventions, such as opioids or surgery. Even the nature of follow-up should be consistent between study groups. If one group has closer or more frequent follow-up, for example, more adverse events might be reported, or treatment might be given more intensively. Increased contact with a caring clinician can also have important nonspecific effects, as noted previously.

LOW LOSS TO FOLLOW-UP AND INTENTION-TO-TREAT ANALYSIS

The second item in the list in Table 10.6 concerns completeness of follow-up for patients who entered the trial. As discussed in the section on uncontrolled studies, investigators should attempt to follow up every patient who enters the study because those who drop out may be systematically different from patients who remain in the study, resulting in attrition bias. For example, disgruntled patients who have failed to improve may drop out of a trial, leaving an obvious bias in favor of the new treatment. On the other hand, patients with dramatic improvements may drop out because they are so much better they see no need for continued medical contact. Dropouts from clinical studies often differ systematically from those who remain in the study with regard to their baseline characteristics.

In highly mobile societies, such as the United States, obtaining complete follow-up can be difficult. Strategies for maximizing follow-up include gathering multiple telephone numbers at the time of enrollment for the patient, relatives, and friends; excluding patients who are planning to move in the near future; excluding patients who have no telephone; sending multiple mails of questionnaires; giving financial incentives to return data; maintaining contact with greeting cards or newsletters; using the briefest possible follow-up questionnaires; and using the Internet to track patients through public records.

A useful rule of thumb is that at least 80% to 85% of patients who enter a trial should be included at the end of the study to avoid attrition as a worrisome potential source of bias. Rates of attrition can be substantial in pain trials. For example, a systematic review of opioids for chronic low back pain found that attrition was >20% in all included trials, even though duration of follow-up was relatively brief.[57] Attrition tends to increase as the duration of follow-up increases. One way to ensure that the results are robust in the face of dropouts is to do a "worst-case analysis," in which one assumes that all dropouts from the treatment group failed to improve, whereas all dropouts from the comparison group improved substantially. If this worst-case analysis does not change the conclusion, one can be confident in the findings.[42] In one analysis, over half of trials that reported statistically significant results no longer reported statistically significant effects under a worst-case scenario.[58] However, it is implausible that all persons lost to follow-up will experience the worse outcome. Under more plausible assumptions regarding outcomes of persons lost to follow-up, results of 0% to 33% of trials were no longer significant.

An alternative approach for handling missing data is "baseline observation carried forward." This technique utilizes the baseline value for the outcome of interest for patients who are lost to follow-up.[59] Although it has the advantage over "worst-case analysis" of being based on "real" data, it is based on the flawed assumption that the baseline values will not change during the course of follow-up or as a result of treatment. "Last observation carried forward" has an advantage over

using baseline values in that it takes into account any recorded changes in outcomes. More sophisticated methods such as multiple imputation create several different plausible data sets for missing data based on the observed data and appropriately combine the results obtained from each of them.[60]

It is also important that patients be analyzed in the groups to which they were randomized ("intention-to-treat analysis") regardless of whether they received the intended treatment, how well they adhered to the assigned therapy, and whether they completed the trial.[61] We have seen the hazards of assuming that patients who are noncompliant are otherwise the same as compliant patients. Indeed, patients who do not receive the intended therapy may be systematically different from those who do. The only way to maintain the benefits of randomization and to avoid a biased comparison is to keep patients for analytic purposes in the group to which they were assigned. Intention-to-treat analyses take into account the fact that patients in clinical practice are autonomous and do not always follow the trial protocol to the letter—or at all. In some cases, intention-to-treat analyses can be difficult to interpret. In the Spine Patient Outcomes Research Trial of surgery, nearly 40% of patients crossed over from surgery to nonsurgical therapy and vice versa.[62] The intention-to-treat analysis still provides information about patient outcomes when they are advised to undergo surgery or nonsurgical therapy, even though many patients decided not to proceed with the recommended therapy. An as-treated analysis provides additional information based on which therapy the patients actually received. This can also be informative, so long as potential confounders are adjusted for and the high probability of some residual confounding is recognized.[63]

Other Issues in Clinical Trials

MEASUREMENT OF OUTCOMES

What outcomes should be measured in a clinical trial? In traditional clinical trials, investigators often seek the most objective possible outcomes for evaluation, such as joint range of motion, spinal fluid endorphins, or dynamometer measures of muscle strength. Although the search for objective outcome measures is appropriate for many medical conditions, pain is inherently a subjective phenomenon and one that often correlates only modestly with these physiologic measures. Table 10.7 illustrates several examples of dissociations between physiologic measures and pain or functioning.[64] Some researchers have argued that the essence of "hard" data is their reproducibility under the

---

TABLE 10.7 Examples of Dissociations between Various Outcome Measures

- Biofeedback reduces paraspinal electromyography activity but not pain.
- Tricyclic antidepressants relieve pain and depression but do not alter cerebrospinal fluid beta-endorphin levels or paraspinous electromyography activity.
- Statements of pain severity correlate poorly with medication use, health care use, and activity level.
- Reduced spinal mobility may be associated with improvement in pain and disability or lower risk of pain.
- Muscle function does not predict 10-year incidence of back symptoms.
- Correlations between lumbar spine mobility and modified Oswestry questionnaire are only .04–.17 (absolute value).
- In a clinical trial of rigid corset, improvements in symptoms with activity were observed but not in spine mobility or straight-leg raising.

Reprinted from Deyo RA. Measuring the functional status of patients with low back pain. *Arch Phys Med Rehabil* 1988;69(12):1044–1053Copyright © 1988 Elsevier. With permission.

same circumstances.[65] Happily, many subjective phenomena can be measured in reproducible fashion. A good example is the use of visual analog pain scales and other ordinal rating scales for quantifying pain.

For evaluation of therapies for chronic pain, trials should go beyond the self-report of pain to routinely examine patients' behavior and function in their daily lives.[66] Function should be considered a separate domain from pain and measured separately because improvements in pain and function often correlate only loosely with one another.[67] For example, trials of opioids for chronic noncancer pain and exercise therapy for low back pain both found considerably smaller benefits according to measures of function compared to measures of pain.[68,69] So how should function be assessed? Performance measures such as a series of timed tasks or an "obstacle course" may have the attraction of seeming objectivity, but performance can be highly influenced by motivation, mood, setting, financial incentives, and other nonphysical attributes of the patient and his or her environment. Such measures often do not correlate well with how a patient actually functions on a day-to-day basis. By contrast, a number of self-report measures of health status or functional status have been validated and are quite reproducible. Examples include the Sickness Impact Profile[70,71] the Brief Pain Inventory,[72] and the Medical Outcomes Study Short-Form-36[73] as well as condition-specific scales such as the Roland-Morris Disability Questionnaire and Oswestry Disability Index for patients with back pain,[74] the Arthritis Impact Measurement Scale,[75] the Western Ontario and McMaster Universities Osteoarthritis Index physical function subscale,[76] and many others. A simple three-item measure of pain and function adapted from the Brief Pain Inventory is the Pain, Enjoyment of Life, and General Activity (PEG) scale.[77]

To provide a full picture of the effects of pain interventions, the Initiative on Methods, Measurement, and Pain Assessment in Clinical Trials (IMMPACT) recommends that clinical trials routinely measure outcomes in multiple "core" domains. In addition to pain, physical functioning, and emotional functioning, IMMPACT recommends assessment of participant ratings of global improvement and satisfaction with treatment, symptoms and adverse events, and participant disposition.[66] A task force convened by the National Institutes of Health (NIH) Pain Consortium developed research standards for studies of chronic low back pain including reporting of outcomes addressing pain intensity, pain interference, physical function, depression, sleep disturbance, and catastrophizing.[78]

Work status is often used as an outcome measure for chronic pain treatment because of its clear relevance to both patients and to society. However, it has a number of drawbacks as an outcome measure, most important of which is that it is influenced by many nonmedical factors. For example, studies have demonstrated that the likelihood of return to work in the face of a painful medical condition varies depending on job satisfaction, relationships with fellow employees and supervisors, regional unemployment rates, the presence of another breadwinner in the family, proximity to retirement age, and physical job demands. Similarly, the duration of pain-related disability is strongly associated with the patient's educational status, income,[79] and the generosity of disability benefits. For many members of our society, including students, homemakers, and retired persons, return to employment is simply not available as an indicator of outcome. Thus, although this measure of outcome is important in many settings and is recommended by the NIH Task Force on Research Standards for Chronic Low Back Pain as part of the minimum data set,[78] it should be interpreted in light of these potentially confounding factors.

REPORTING THE RESULTS

Many clinical trials report mean outcome scores or mean differences in scores compared to baseline values. This can be difficult to interpret clinically, as a 10-point mean improvement on a 100-point scale could indicate that nearly all patients experienced only very mild improvement or that some proportion of patients experienced a clinically significant improvement, whereas others did not. The minimal important change, or the smallest change in outcome scores perceived by patients to be meaningful, is a key concept.[80] It refers to the smallest amount of improvement perceived by patients as being important. For low back pain, a consensus group recently proposed a 30% improvement from baseline in pain or function as the minimum important change.[81] A randomized trial found that the average difference between mindfulness-based stress reduction versus usual care was less than 1 point on a 0-to-10 pain bothersomeness scale at 1 year, indicating a relatively small average effect well below the threshold for clinical significance.[82] However, the proportion of patients who experienced $\geq$30% improvement was greater in the mindfulness group (48% vs. 31%; relative risk [RR], 1.56; 95% confidence interval [CI], 1.1 to 2.1), indicating that persons who respond to mindfulness therapy often experience clinically meaningful improvements. Therefore, reporting the proportion of patients that meet a certain threshold for improvement can be very helpful for interpreting the clinical significance of results. This is sometimes referred to as a *responder* analysis and is recommended by the NIH Task Force on Research Standards for Chronic Low Back Pain in addition to reporting mean outcome scores.[78]

In some studies, actual outcome measurements are not reported. Rather, only the *P* values for the significance of results are provided. A *P* value tells us the probability of obtaining a result that is at least as extreme as the one actually observed, assuming that the null hypothesis of no difference between treatments is true. However, this gives a reader no idea what the magnitude of treatment effects may have been.[83] In a very large trial, a difference between groups may achieve statistical significance even though the difference is too trivial to be clinically relevant. On the other hand, in a very small trial, a large treatment effect might fail to achieve statistical significance. Thus, the magnitude of treatment effect is somewhat independent of statistical significance and should be reported. An ideal way to present the results is to give the actual estimate of success rates or mean scores along with 95% confidence limits, which allows the reader to see the range of results that would be consistent with the study findings. The 95% confidence limits are closely related to *P* values but give readers a better understanding of the potential range of effects compatible with the data.

STATISTICAL POWER

When a trial shows "no statistically significant difference," it is often interpreted as meaning that it has proven that there is no difference between the intervention and control groups. However, this interpretation is often incorrect. In fact, most trials are too small to prove that there is no difference between groups—rather, they only show an absence of evidence of a difference.[84] This is a critical distinction. The likelihood that a true difference may not have been detected is referred to as type II (or β) error, in contrast to type I (or α) error (which is reflected in the *P* value).[85] Statistical power (calculated as $1 - \beta$) refers to the likelihood that a clinically relevant difference between groups will be identified. Larger sample sizes increase statistical power. On the other hand, statistical power decreases as the size of the clinical effect to be detected (typically the minimal important change) goes down. Nonstatistically significant results should always be interpreted in the context of the statistical power of the study.

GENERALIZABILITY OF RESULTS AND EFFICACY VERSUS EFFECTIVENESS

Even if a clinical trial is internally valid, its results may not be applicable (generalizable) to other patients and settings. Patients who enroll in low back pain clinical trials, for example, tend to be better educated, more frequently employed, and different in other prognostically important ways from patients in everyday practice.[86] Clinical trials often exclude patients with medical or psychological comorbidities or use run-in periods to identify and exclude patients who experience adverse events before randomizing them. For example, older patients have often been excluded from trials of arthritis drugs, even though they are the most likely to receive such drugs in actual practice. Patients enrolled in clinical trials are usually recruited from tertiary care settings, and the resources available in clinical trials to help maximize patient compliance and follow-up are rarely available to most clinicians. A number of other threats to generalizability have been described.[87] It is important for patients, treatments, and study conditions to be adequately reported so readers can determine whether they would be likely to apply to their own situations.

Related to generalizability is the concept of efficacy versus effectiveness. Most clinical trials are designed to evaluate efficacy: the benefits of an intervention in optimal populations and under ideal conditions. Such studies generally focus on narrow, short-term outcomes. Effectiveness studies, on the other hand, are designed to evaluate whether an intervention will actually work under conditions encountered in usual practice.[88] Of course, there is a continuum between efficacy and effectiveness, although most randomized trials fall squarely on the efficacy side of the spectrum. Factors that can enhance the ability of clinical trials to evaluate effectiveness are use of less stringent eligibility criteria, enrollment of patients from primary care populations, evaluation of multiple clinically relevant outcomes, and longer duration of follow-up.[89] Observational studies can also be helpful for evaluating effectiveness once efficacy has been established in randomized trials.

SUBGROUP ANALYSES

Sometimes, analyses are performed to examine whether the effects of an intervention differ in clinically relevant groups of patients defined by some factor (such as baseline pain score, sex, or age).[90] For example, a trial of glucosamine for osteoarthritis found no overall treatment benefit, but a subgroup analysis found that it was effective in patients with high baseline pain scores.[91] There is a great risk that subgroup analyses may be overinterpreted, as results could simply represent chance effects, particularly when data are "mined" to look for significant results. Confidence in subgroup analyses is enhanced if the treatment effects are large, are unlikely to have occurred by chance (low P value), occur in an analysis based on a prespecified and plausible hypothesis, come from a small number of subgroup analyses, and are replicated in other studies.

EFFECTS OF FUNDING SOURCE

Commercially funded clinical trials are consistently more likely to report results that favor the funder than trials that are not commercially funded.[92,93] This appears to be true for devices, such as surgical implants, as well as drugs.[94,95] Why might this be? One reason is publication bias. This refers to the differential tendency for studies to be published depending on the strength and direction of results.[96] Generally, studies that report statistically significant and more strongly positive results are more likely to be published compared to those that report statistically insignificant or less striking results. The result is inflated estimates of treatment effects. Publication bias can occur no matter what the source of funding is, but commercially funded clinical trials appear to be particularly susceptible due to either overt or more subtle pressures.[93,97,98] A related situation is the selective reporting of outcomes.[99–101] This leads to bias because more favorable results tend to be reported and publicized, and there is often no indication to readers that other (less favorable) outcomes were even assessed. Results can also be "spun" to appear more favorable than they really are. One study found that of 36 industry-sponsored new drug approval trials of antidepressants viewed by the U.S. Food and Drug Administration (FDA) as having negative or questionable results, 22 had not been published, and another 11 were reported in a way that conveyed positive outcomes.[102] Another questionable strategy that has begun to receive increased scrutiny is the practice of "seeding" trials following new drug approvals.[103] Such trials are framed as scientific research but in reality are marketing tools designed to increase familiarity and use of the medication by experienced clinicians and often utilize scientifically suspect study designs driven by marketing staff, recruit underqualified investigators who prescribe competing products, overcompensate investigators, and utilize poor data collection methods.[104]

This is not to say that commercially funded trials can not be conducted and reported rigorously. However, replication of results in non–commercially funded trials may be required to increase confidence in the findings of commercially funded trials, even when methodologic shortcomings are not readily apparent. Statistical and graphical methods are available to formally assess for the likelihood of publication bias, although all have some limitations.[105] The FDA Web site can be a useful resource for identifying unpublished trials and unreported outcomes, but data are often incomplete or redacted. Ideally, publication and selective outcomes reporting bias would not only be detected but would also not occur in the first place. The development of clinical trials registries and mandatory requirements for researchers to submit trial protocols and full results in order to be considered for journal publication or for new drug approvals may help reduce the effects of these biases.[106,107] The usefulness of clinical trials registries will depend on how assiduously and quickly researchers comply with reporting requirements.

ASSESSMENT OF HARMS

In order to generate balanced conclusions about an intervention, it is important to understand both its benefits and harms.[108] However, benefits have been accorded far greater prominence than harms when conducting and reporting clinical trials. In fact, most randomized trials lack prespecified hypotheses for harms. Rather, hypotheses are usually designed to evaluate beneficial effects, with assessment of harms a secondary consideration. As a result, the quality and quantity of harms reporting in clinical trials is often inadequate.[109]

There are other problems with relying solely on clinical trials to assess harms.[110] Few clinical trials have large enough sample sizes or are long enough in duration to adequately assess uncommon or long-term harms. For example, one systematic review found that trials of opioids for chronic noncancer pain averaged only 5 weeks in duration, even though patients frequently remain on these medications for years or indefinitely.[68] In addition, patients who are more susceptible to adverse events are often excluded from clinical trials, although they may commonly receive the therapy in clinical practice. For example, all trials of opioids for chronic noncancer pain that reported information on history of drug addiction excluded such patients.[68] Harms may also be downplayed or misrepresented if there is a vested interest in doing so.[111] Aggressive promotion of unsubstantiated claims of lower abuse, diversion, and withdrawal risks of OxyContin (Purdue Pharma, Stamford, CT), a sustained-release formulation of oxycodone, eventually resulted in a criminal conviction and $634 million fine against the Purdue Frederick Company, along with three company executives.[112]

Assessment and reporting of harms in clinical trials can certainly be improved. This is also an area where observational studies can be a very useful source of information. Unlike assessments of treatment benefits, confounding by indication is usually not an issue with unexpected or unpredictable adverse events because such outcomes are not related to the decision to use the therapy.[34,113] An example is observational studies on risk of myocardial infarction associated with cyclo-oxygenase-2 selective nonsteroidal anti-inflammatory drugs. Those conducted prior to knowledge regarding the cardiovascular risks of rofecoxib were unlikely to be affected by confounding by indication related to the baseline risk of heart disease. Observational studies can also provide important information on rare or long-term adverse events and in populations underrepresented in clinical trials (such as pregnant women, children, older adults, or those with important comorbidities). Even uncontrolled studies such as case reports have been invaluable for evaluating harms and may be the first or primary signal of a rare adverse event.

TRIAL-BASED COST-EFFECTIVENESS ANALYSIS

Even if the balance of benefits to harms of a treatment is acceptable, widespread implementation may not make sense if costs are very high. Clinical trials can also be designed to assess the question "Is it worth it?" by collecting cost data alongside clinical outcomes.[88] Unlike decision analytic studies that model costs and clinical outcomes, such trial-based cost-effectiveness analyses directly measure the cost per some increment of clinical utility (often a quality-adjusted life-year). A challenge with cost-effectiveness analyses of clinical trials is that cost data are often associated with large variability, so estimates can be imprecise unless sample sizes are large.[114] In addition, distributions of cost estimates are often quite skewed, which can pose a statistical challenge, and costs are frequently highly variable depending on locale and reimbursement factors and can rapidly change over time.

Alternative Study Designs

CLUSTER TRIALS

For certain interventions, it may be undesirable or unfeasible to randomly allocate individual patients to a treatment or a control group. For example, if one were testing a guideline that involved changes in clinic organization and changes in management by nurses or other ancillary staff, it might be extremely difficult to ensure that all involved gave one particular approach to some patients and not to others. Furthermore, individual physicians would have difficulty treating certain patients according to a guideline and others not according to the guideline, which could increase treatment group contamination. In such a circumstance, one might wish to allocate clusters of patients, such as entire clinics, to intervention or control arms. Such studies are referred to as *cluster randomized trials*.[115] When these designs are used, specific statistical methods are needed to account for the similarities among patients of a single physician or facility, which can inflate estimates of treatment effects. Analytic techniques such as the "cluster correlation correction" for such studies have been well described,[116] and computer software is available to perform these analyses.

CROSSOVER TRIALS

In a standard parallel group randomized clinical trial, patients are randomized to a single treatment out of two or more possibilities. In a crossover trial, patients each receive two or more treatments in a random order, typically separated by a washout period.[117] This allows a patient's response to one treatment to be compared with the same patient's response to another treatment. The crossover design confers a statistical efficiency advantage over parallel group trials because with the same number of subjects, the use of paired data enables more precise estimation of treatment effects. A key drawback of crossover trials is the potential for carryover effects, with effects of one treatment "carrying over" to the next. Thus, the washout period must take into account the likely duration of action for each treatment involved and may require testing for crossover effects. Attrition can also occur during the initial treatment period, making within-subject comparisons impossible for those persons lost to follow-up.[118] Other factors that may impact the interpretability of crossover trials are period effects (due to changes in the underlying condition over time) or sequence effects (due to changes in effectiveness of treatments based on the order in which they are given).[119] Crossover trials are most appropriate for chronic pain conditions in which the symptoms are relatively stable, generally inappropriate for acute pain, for which symptoms change rapidly, and should be reserved for treatments that do not have permanent effects on the underlying condition. Results of crossover trials tend to agree with those of parallel group trials, although some research indicates a trend toward larger effect estimates in crossover trials.[120]

FACTORIAL DESIGN

In a factorial design, patients are simultaneously randomized to receive or not receive two different treatments.[121] In the United Kingdom Back Pain Exercise and Manipulation (BEAM) trial, for example, patients were allocated to receive exercise therapy versus no exercise therapy and to receive spinal manipulation or no spinal manipulation.[122] Such factorial designs have important efficiencies if the dropout rate is low. If there is no statistical interaction between the two treatments (in this example, exercise therapy and spinal manipulation), then a factorial design provides an unbiased assessment of the effect of each treatment. Such designs might be useful in studying combinations of therapy such as an analgesic plus a muscle relaxant, drug therapy plus physical therapy, and other clinically relevant combinations. Indeed, factorial designs may be the best way to evaluate the multicomponent approach that is widely advocated for the treatment of chronic pain. If there is no synergy between treatments, the investigator essentially has two trials for the price of one. If there is synergy or additive effects between treatments, the factorial design can identify this effect. Factorial designs introduce analytical complexities that are avoided in simple parallel designs, but in some circumstances, the benefits may outweigh the disadvantages.[123]

New Directions in Clinical Trials

PRAGMATIC TRIALS

With increased attention to effectiveness has come an increased demand for "pragmatic" trials that attempt to inform routine clinical practice better than traditional efficacy trials. Key features of pragmatic trials are that they are set in normal practice settings rather than highly specialized or controlled settings, apply few exclusion criteria, allow flexibility in use of treatment interventions, and assess key, patient-centered outcomes.[124] For example, a pragmatic trial of acupuncture for chronic low back pain was conducted in general practice and private acupuncture clinics in the United Kingdom, enrolled anyone aged 18 to 65 years with nonspecific low back pain of 4 to 52 weeks duration (with few exclusion criteria), allowed acupuncturists to determine the content and number of treatments, and evaluated bodily pain as well as outcomes related to use of analgesics and patient satisfaction.[125]

ENRICHED ENROLLMENT RANDOMIZED WITHDRAWAL TRIALS

A design that has become increasingly common, particularly for evaluation of pharmaceuticals, is the enriched enrollment randomized withdrawal design. In this design, potential study participants all receive the study drug for a specified period of time during an open-label prerandomization phase.[126] Only persons who report benefits and can tolerate the drug proceed to the randomization phase, in which patients either continue to receive the medication or are randomized to a control (usually placebo). The enriched enrollment randomized withdrawal design has been proposed as a useful method for studying drugs for whom only a small proportion of patients benefit by focusing on those in whom the drug works and do not experience bothersome side effects.[127] However, this design could exaggerate treatment benefits and underestimate harms because the population enrolled is purposefully skewed toward those who have already demonstrated good outcomes and few side effects on the treatment; blinding may be ineffective because all patients are familiar with the treatment due to exposure during the prerandomization phase; and for certain medications (e.g., opioids), development of tolerance from prerandomization exposure could lead to withdrawal symptoms in persons randomized to placebo, confounding interpretation of results. One analysis of clinical trials of opioids for chronic pain found that compared to standard trials, the enriched enrollment randomized withdrawal design did not appear to bias results for efficacy but underestimated adverse effects.[126]

EXPERTISE-BASED TRIALS

For nonpharmacologic interventions such as surgery that are highly dependent on the skill and training of the clinician, "expertise-based" randomized controlled trials have been proposed.[128] In the traditional randomized controlled trial, participants are randomized to one of two interventions and individual clinicians provide intervention A to some patients and intervention B to others. In the expertise-based randomized trial, participants are randomized to individual clinicians with expertise in intervention A or to clinicians with expertise in intervention B. Proposed advantages of expertise-based randomized trials are that they can reduce the effects of differential expertise bias. In the case of surgery, this can be important, as many procedures require considerable experience to gain proficiency. In addition, the expertise-based design reduces potential effects of differential enthusiasm or skepticism for the different procedures, as each surgeon provides only the procedure that he or she believes is the best. As yet, however, there is relatively little evidence on the validity of expertise-based randomized trials.

COMPARATIVE EFFECTIVENESS

Another direction in clinical trials is toward increased evaluations of not just effectiveness of interventions versus placebo but comparative effectiveness of two or more interventions.[129] Head-to-head trials that compare two interventions are the most direct method for evaluating comparative effectiveness. However, head-to-head trials are not always available. An alternative method for evaluating comparative effectiveness is through indirect comparisons. This refers to assessments of the relative benefits and harms of competing interventions based on how well each performs against a common comparator (usually placebo). Methods are available for conducting indirect comparisons that preserve some of the benefits of randomization as well as for more complex network analyses and mixed treatment comparisons that incorporate both indirect and direct evidence.[130] In all cases, the validity of indirect comparisons is based on the critical assumption that treatment effects are consistent across all trials. This assumption can be violated due to a number of factors, including differences in study quality, patient populations, settings, outcomes, and other factors. In fact, large discrepancies between indirect and direct studies have been reported. For example, in patients with neuropathic pain, an indirect comparison found tricyclic antidepressants associated with a much higher likelihood of achieving pain relief compared to gabapentin, but head-to-head trials found no significant difference.[131] Indirect comparisons should only be used when the critical assumption of similarity of treatment effects is met and verified against results from head-to-head trials as they become available.

EQUIVALENCE AND NONINFERIORITY TRIALS

Traditional clinical trials are designed to determine whether an active treatment is superior to another treatment (often placebo). The null hypothesis is that there is no difference between the treatments being compared. In equivalence trials, on the other hand, the purpose is to determine whether one (typically new) intervention is therapeutically similar (equivalent) to another, usually established, treatment.[132] This requires testing of a different null hypothesis—specifically, the null hypothesis that there *is* a difference being treatments. Noninferiority trials are similar to equivalence trials but are designed to focus on whether a new treatment is no worse than (rather than therapeutically similar to) an established treatment. For either type of trial, boundaries for what will be considered "equivalent" or "noninferior" must be defined in order to perform appropriate hypothesis testing. Unfortunately, many trials that report equivalence do not define these boundaries, or are based on misapplied or misinterpreted statistical analyses, often based on standard superiority hypotheses or inadequate sample sizes.[133] Guidance is available to help improve the conduct, reporting, and interpretation of equivalence and noninferiority trials.[132]

STEPPED WEDGE DESIGN

The standard cluster randomized trial utilizes a parallel design, in which patients receive different interventions according to their cluster at roughly the same time. The stepped wedge design is a variant on the cluster framework in which each cluster begins in the control condition and receives the intervention by the end of the study.[134,135] The time to receive the intervention condition varies from cluster to cluster. The stepped wedge design may be more feasible to implement than a standard parallel group cluster design when the cost of implementing an intervention simultaneously in many clusters is high because the intervention is implemented across the clusters in a stepped fashion, or when withholding an intervention is considered unethical or may pose a barrier to recruitment because all clusters will receive the intervention by the end of the study. As in crossover trials, the crossover from the control condition to the intervention within each cluster allows for within-cluster comparisons that may increase statistical efficiency; similarly, stepped wedge studies must guard against carryover effects.

BAYESIAN STATISTICAL INFERENCE AND ADAPTIVE DESIGNS

Another direction in clinical trials is the use of Bayesian frameworks of statistical inference instead of the standard classical (frequentist) framework.[136] Although a full discussion of Bayesian statistical inference is beyond the scope of this chapter, in essence, the Bayesian framework incorporates new evidence or observations to update probabilities that a hypothesis might be true. Bayesian adaptive trials use Bayesian methods to incorporate data collected during the course of a trial in order to inform decisions regarding the need to update, modify, or stop the trial.[137]

Systematic Reviews

The relatively rapid advances in other fields of medicine, such as oncology and cardiology, occur because a succession of large randomized trials, typically implemented in multiple centers, results in cumulative knowledge. Such large, multicenter trials are still the exception rather than the rule in pain treatment, perhaps in part because of lower research funding for nonfatal conditions. Nonetheless, more pain research trials are being conducted, resulting in an ever-growing body of literature. This growth has been exponential. Between 1950 and 1990, more than 8,000 randomized controlled trials of pain research were published, with over 85% appearing during the last 15 years of that period.[138]

Given the amount of evidence, it is difficult for clinicians to keep up with the literature on even a circumscribed area of medicine. Review articles can be a useful way to summarize the evidence on a given topic. A systematic review is a particular type of review article that applies explicit methods to reduce bias and error when summarizing evidence.[139] This is in contrast with traditional or "narrative" reviews, which do not use explicit methods to identify, select, and assess evidence. Such review articles are relatively subjective and are apt to be based on incomplete, outdated, or flawed evidence. This increases the likelihood of incorrect or unsubstantiated conclusions.

A "systematic" review attempts to bring the same level of scientific rigor to the review article as should be used when conducting original research. Systematic reviews can be qualitative or quantitative. The latter are also referred to as meta-analyses, although strictly speaking, a meta-analysis is not necessarily based on systematic methods. Potential advantages of systematic review over traditional review articles are shown in Table 10.8. A high-quality systematic review minimizes bias and random error by using transparent, reproducible, and objective methods. In addition to summarizing existing data, systematic reviews can also increase statistical power for evaluating low-frequency events, provide more precise estimates of treatment effects, permit formal comparisons between studies, permit formal assessments of publication bias, and help delineate areas of uncertainty.

Before trusting the results of systematic reviews, it is important to critically evaluate whether rigorous methods were used. In fact, results of lower quality reviews can be misleading, as they are more likely than higher quality reviews to produce positive conclusions about the effectiveness of interventions.[138,140] Table 10.9 lists some factors that can influence whether a systematic review is likely to be reliable. A number of other methods for assessing the quality of systematic reviews are available, including the more detailed list of criteria in the Assessment of Multiple Systematic Reviews (AMSTAR)[141] and AMSTAR 2 tools.[142]

TABLE 10.8 Potential Advantages of Systematic Reviews over Narrative Reviews

Designed to address a focused clinical question

Describes explicit methods used to identify as many of the relevant trials as possible

Reports literature search dates

Describes and applies predefined study inclusion criteria

Formally assesses characteristics of studies associated with biases

Follows explicit methods for weighing and synthesizing studies

Can pool studies quantitatively, leading to more precise estimates and increased statistical power

Can test for statistical heterogeneity and explore reasons for heterogeneity through subgroup, sensitivity, and other analyses

Research gaps and areas of uncertainty more clearly delineated

Can test for and estimate effects of publication bias on results

Conclusions more directly linked to data and analyses

TABLE 10.9 Factors to Consider when Assessing Quality of Systematic Reviews

Was the search comprehensive?

Was selection of studies unbiased?

Is the systematic review current?

Was quality of included studies appropriately assessed?

Was evidence combined and summarized appropriately?

Was publication bias assessed?

Are the conclusions justified?

All quality rating methods are based on the idea that systematic reviews that are comprehensive, up-to-date, and use appropriate methods to identify, select, assess, and synthesize the literature are more likely to provide a complete and unbiased picture than those that use suboptimal methods.

The Cochrane Collaboration is an international effort to systematically review the results of multiple randomized clinical trials and make the results widely available via the Internet. The number of Cochrane reviews on pain topics is rapidly expanding, and many have been published in conventional journals as well as in the Cochrane Library.

Conclusion

Despite the rapid growth of research literature on the treatment of pain, there remain wide variations in care and the successive use of fads that are later demonstrated to be ineffective when well-designed studies are performed. Both the prevalence of painful conditions and their associated disability are increasing, and there is only a limited professional consensus on optimal approaches to many painful conditions. The disappointing pace of progress may be partly the result of few comprehensive theories that would guide treatment innovations. However, an equally important factor may be the methodologic inadequacy of the research used to justify the introduction of new or innovative therapies to clinical care. Flaws in research design jeopardize not only the internal validity of research results but also their generalizability to routine clinical practice. Greater attention to scientific principles in the design of clinical research should accelerate progress in this area, lead to more consistent clinical practices, and improve patient care.

References

1. Cherkin DC, Deyo RA, Loeser JD, et al. An international comparison of back surgery rates. *Spine* 1994;19:1201–1206.
2. Weinstein JN, Lurie JD, Olson PR, et al. United States' trends and regional variations in lumbar spine surgery: 1992-2003. *Spine* 2006;31:2707–2714.
3. Volinn E, Mayer J, Diehr P, et al. Small area analysis of surgery for low-back pain. *Spine* 1992;17:575–579.
4. Deyo RA. Fads in the treatment of low back pain. *N Engl J Med* 1991;325(14): 1039–1040.
5. Eidelman RS, Hollar D, Hebert PR, et al. Randomized trials of vitamin E in the treatment and prevention of cardiovascular disease. *Arch Intern Med* 2004;164:1552–1556.
6. Herrington DM, Howard TD. From presumed benefit to potential harm—hormone therapy and heart disease. *New Engl J Med* 2003;349:519–521.
7. Turner JA, Deyo RA, Loeser JD, et al. The importance of placebo effects in pain treatment and research. *JAMA* 1994;271:1609–1614.
8. Freburger JK, Holmes GM, Agans RP, et al. The rising prevalence of chronic low back pain. *Arch Intern Med* 2009;169:251–258.
9. Friedly J, Chan L, Deyo R. Increases in lumbosacral injections in the Medicare population. *Spine* 2007;32:1754–1760.
10. Martin BI, Deyo RA, Mirza SK, et al. Expenditures and health status among adults with back and neck problems. *JAMA* 2008;299:656–664.
11. Martin BI, Turner JA, Mirza SK, et al. Trends in health care expenditures, utilization, and health status among US adults with spine problems, 1997-2006. *Spine* 2009;34(19):2077–2084.
12. Briss PA, Zaza S, Pappaioanou M, et al. Developing an evidence-based guide to community preventive services—methods. The Task Force on Community Preventive Services. *Am J Prev Med* 2000;18(suppl 1):35–43.

13. Carey TS, Boden SD. A critical guide to case series reports. *Spine* 2003;28:1631–1634.
14. Taylor RS, Van Buyten J, Buscher E. Spinal cord stimulation for chronic back pain and leg pain and failed back surgery syndrome: a systematic review and analysis of progressive factors. *Spine* 2005;30(1):152–160.
15. Pengel LHM, Herbert RD, Maher CG, et al. Acute low back pain: systematic review of its prognosis. *BMJ* 2003;327:323–327.
16. Bingel U, Wanigasekera V, Wiech K, et al. The effect of treatment expectation on drug efficacy: imaging the analgesic benefit of the opioid remifentanil. *Sci Transl Med* 2011;3(70):70ra14.
17. Tuttle AH, Tohyama S, Ramsay T, et al. Increasing placebo responses over time in U.S. clinical trials of neuropathic pain. *Pain* 2015;156(12):2616–2626.
18. Whitney CW, Von Korff M. Regression to the mean in treated versus untreated chronic pain. *Pain* 1992;50:281–285.
19. Deyo RA. Practice variations, treatment fads, rising disability. Do we need a new clinical research paradigm? *Spine* 1993;18(15):2153–2162.
20. Sartwell P, Merrell M. Influence of the dynamic character of chronic disease on the interpretation of morbidity rates. *Am J Public Health* 1952;42:579–584.
21. Albrecht J, Meves A, Bigby M. Case reports and case series from Lancet had significant impact on medical literature. *J Clin Epidemiol* 2005;58:1227–1232.
22. Hartz A, Benson K, Glaser J, et al. Assessing observational studies of spinal fusion and chemonucleolysis. *Spine* 2003;28:2268–2275.
23. Eddy DM. Medicine, money, and mathematics. *Bull Am Coll Surg* 1992;77:36–49.
24. Glasziou P, Chalmers I, Rawlins M, et al. When are randomised trials unnecessary? Picking signal from noise. *BMJ* 2007;334:349–351.
25. Brinkhaus B, Witt CM, Jena S, et al. Acupuncture in patients with chronic low back pain. *Arch Intern Med* 2006;166:450–457.
26. Cherkin DC, Deyo RA, Street JH, et al. Pitfalls of patient education. Limited success of a program for back pain in primary care. *Spine* 1996;21(3):345–355.
27. Humphrey LL, Chan BK, Sox HC. Postmenopausal hormone replacement therapy and the primary prevention of cardiovascular disease. *Ann Intern Med* 2002;137:273–284.
28. Coronary Drug Project Research Group. Influence of adherence to treatment and response of cholesterol on mortality in the Coronary Drug Project. *N Engl J Med* 1980;303:1038–1041.
29. Bogduk N, Karasek M. Two-year follow-up of a controlled trial of intradiscal electrothermal anuloplasty for chronic low back pain resulting from internal disc disruption. *Spine J* 2002;2(5):343–350.
30. Freeman BJ, Fraser RD, Cain CM, et al. A randomized, double-blind, controlled trial: intradiscal electrothermal therapy versus placebo for the treatment of chronic discogenic low back pain. *Spine* 2005;30(21):2369–2377.
31. Pauza KJ, Howell S, Dreyfuss P, et al. A randomized, placebo-controlled trial of intradiscal electrothermal therapy for the treatment of discogenic low back pain. *Spine J* 2004;4(1):27–35.
32. McMahon AD. Observation and experiment with the efficacy of drugs: a warning example from a cohort of nonsteroidal anti-inflammatory and ulcer-healing drug users. *Am J Epidemiol* 2001;154:557–562.
33. Normand ST, Sykora K, Li P, et al. Readers guide to critical appraisal of cohort studies: 3. Analytical strategies to reduce confounding. *BMJ* 2005;330:1021–1023.
34. Miettinen OS. The need for randomization in the study of intended effects. *Stat Med* 1983;2:267–271.
35. Psaty BM, Koepsell TD, Lin D, et al. Assessment and control for confounding by indication in observational studies. *J Am Geriatr Soc* 1999;47:749–754.
36. Schulz KF, Grimes DA. Allocation concealment in randomised trials: defending against deciphering. *Lancet* 2002;359:614–618.
37. Schulz KF, Chalmers I, Hayes RJ, et al. Empirical evidence of bias. Dimensions of methodological quality associated with estimates of treatment effects in controlled trials. *JAMA* 1995;273(5):408–412.
38. Carroll D, Trawer M, McQuay H, et al. Randomization is important in studies with pain outcomes: systematic review of transcutaneous electrical nerve stimulation in acute postoperative pain. *Br J Anaesth* 1996;77:798–803.
39. Chalmers TC, Celano P, Sacks HS, et al. Bias in treatment assignment in controlled clinical trials. *New Engl J Med* 1983;309:1358–1361.
40. Moher D, Pham B, Jones A, et al. Does quality of reports of randomised trials affect estimates of intervention efficacy reported in meta-analyses? *Lancet* 1998;352(9128):609–613.
41. Schulz K. Subverting randomization in clinical trials. *JAMA* 1995;274:1456–1458.
42. Guyatt G. Users' guides to the medical literature: II. How to use an article about therapy or prevention. A. Are the results of the study valid? *JAMA* 1993;270(21):2598–2601.
43. Guyatt G. Users' guides to the medical literature: II. How to use an article about therapy or prevention. B. What were the results and will they help me in caring for my patients? *JAMA* 1994;271(1):59–63.
44. Higgins JP, Altman DG, Gotzsche PC, et al. The Cochrane Collaboration's tool for assessing risk of bias in randomised trials. *BMJ* 2011;343:d5928.
45. Furlan AD, Malmivaara A, Chou R, et al. 2015 Updated method guideline for systematic reviews in the Cochrane Back and Neck Group. *Spine* 2015;40(21):1660–1673.
46. Schulz KF, Altman DG, Moher D. CONSORT 2010 statement: updated guidelines for reporting parallel group randomised trials. *BMJ* 2010;340:c332.
47. Assmann SF, Pocock SJ, Enos LE, et al. Subgroup analysis and other (mis)uses of baseline data in clinical trials. *Lancet* 2000;355(9209):1064–1069.
48. Roberts C, Torgerson DJ. Baseline imbalance in randomised controlled trials. *BMJ* 1999;319:185.
49. Scott NW, McPherson GC, Ramsay CR, et al. The method of minimization for allocation to clinical trials. A review. *Control Clin Trials* 2002;23(6):662–674.
50. Wood L, Egger M, Gluud LL, et al. Empirical evidence of bias in treatment effect estimates in controlled trials with different interventions and outcomes: meta-epidemiological study. *BMJ* 2008;336:601–606.
51. Schulz KF, Chalmers I, Altman DG. The landscape and lexicon of blinding in randomized trials. *Ann Intern Med* 2002;136(3):254–259.
52. Machado LA, Kamper SJ, Herbert RD, et al. Imperfect placebos are common in low back pain trials: a systematic review of the literature. *Eur Spine J* 2008;17:889–904.
53. Deyo RA, Walsh NE, Schoenfeld LS, et al. Can trials of physical treatments be blinded? The example of transcutaneous electrical nerve stimulation for chronic pain. *Am J Phys Med Rehabil* 1990;69(1):6–10, comment 219–220.
54. Elbourne DR, Altman DG, Higgins JP, et al. Meta-analyses involving crossover trials: methodological issues. *Int J Epidemiol* 2002;31(1):140–149.
55. Ongley M, Klein R, Dorman T, et al. A new approach to the treatment of chronic low back pain. *Lancet* 1987;2(8551):143–146.
56. Klein R, Eek B, DeLong W, et al. A randomized double-blind trial of dextrose-glycerine-phenol injections for chronic, low back pain. *J Spine Disord* 1993;6(1):23–33.
57. Chaparro LE, Furlan AD, Deshpande A, et al. Opioids compared with placebo or other treatments for chronic low back pain: an update of the Cochrane Review. *Spine* 2014;39(7):556–563.
58. Akl EA, Briel M, You JJ, et al. Potential impact on estimated treatment effects of information lost to follow-up in randomised controlled trials (LOST-IT): systematic review. *BMJ* 2012;344:e2809.
59. Marston L, Sedgwick P. Randomised controlled trials: missing data. *BMJ* 2014;349:g4656.
60. Sterne JA, White IR, Carlin JB, et al. Multiple imputation for missing data in epidemiological and clinical research: potential and pitfalls. *BMJ* 2009;338:b2393.
61. Fisher LD, Dixon DO, Herson J, et al, eds. *Intention to Treat in Clinical Trials*. New York: Marcel Dekker; 1990.
62. Weinstein JN, Tosteson TD, Lurie JD, et al. Surgical vs nonoperative treatment for lumbar disk herniation: the Spine Patient Outcomes Research Trial (SPORT): a randomized trial. *JAMA* 2006;296(20):2441–2450.
63. Deyo RA. Back surgery—who needs it? *N Engl J Med* 2007;356:2239–2243.
64. Deyo RA. Measuring the functional status of patients with low back pain. *Arch Phys Med Rehabil* 1988;69:1044–1053.
65. Feinstein AR. Clinical biostatistics XLI. Hard science, soft data, and challenges of choosing clinical variables in research. *Clin Pharmacol Ther* 1977;22:485–498.
66. Dworkin RH, Turk DC, Farrar JT, et al. Core outcome measures for chronic pain clinical trials: IMMPACT recommendations. *Pain* 2005;113:9–19.
67. Carey TS, Mielenz TJ. Measuring outcomes in back care. *Spine* 2007;32(suppl 11):S9–S14.
68. Furlan AD, Sandoval JA, Mailis-Gagnon A, et al. Opioids for chronic noncancer pain: a meta-analysis of effectiveness and side effects. *CMAJ* 2006;174(11):1589–1594.
69. Hayden J, van Tulder M, Malmivaara A, et al. Exercise therapy for low-back pain. *Cochrane Database Syst Rev* 2005;(3):CD000335.
70. Bergner M, Bobbitt RA, Carter WB, et al. The Sickness Impact Profile: development and final revision of a health status measure. *Med Care* 1981;19:787–805.
71. Follick MJ, Smith TW, Ahern DK. Sickness Impact Profile: a global measure of disability in chronic low back pain. *Pain* 1985;21:67–76.
72. Cleeland CS, Ryan KM. Pain assessment: global use of the Brief Pain Inventory. *Ann Acad Med Singapore* 1994;23(2):129–138.
73. Ware JE, Sherbourne C. The MOS 36-item Short-Form Survey (SF-36). I. Conceptual framework and item selection. *Med Care* 1992;30:473–483.
74. Roland M, Fairbank J. The Roland-Morris Disability Questionnaire and the Oswestry Disability Questionnaire. *Spine* 2000;25:3115–3124.
75. Meenan RF, German PM, Mason JH. Measuring health status in arthritis: the Arthritis Impact Measurement Scales. *Arthritis Rheum* 1980;23:146–152.
76. Bellamy N, Buchanan WW, Goldsmith CH, et al. Validation study of WOMAC: a health status instrument for measuring clinically important patient relevant outcomes to antirheumatic drug therapy in patients with osteoarthritis of the hip or knee. *J Rheumatol* 1988;15:1833–1840.
77. Krebs EE, Lorenz KA, Bair MJ, et al. Development and initial validation of the PEG, a three-item scale assessing pain intensity and interference. *J Gen Intern Med* 2009;24(6):733–738.
78. Deyo RA, Dworkin SF, Amtmann D, et al. Report of the NIH Task Force on Research Standards for Chronic Low Back Pain. *Pain Med* 2014;15(8):1249–1267.
79. Deyo RA, Tsui-Wu WJ. Functional disability due to back pain: a population-based study indicating the importance of socioeconomic factors. *Arthritis Rheum* 1987;30:1247–1253.
80. Dworkin RH, Turk DC, Wyrwich KW, et al. Interpreting the clinical importance of treatment outcomes in chronic pain clinical trials: IMMPACT recommendations. *J Pain* 2008;9:105–121.

81. Ostelo RW, Deyo RA, Stratford P, et al. Interpreting change scores for pain and functional status in low back pain. *Spine* 2008;33:90–94.

82. Cherkin DC, Sherman KJ, Balderson BH, et al. Effect of mindfulness-based stress reduction vs cognitive behavioral therapy or usual care on back pain and functional limitations in adults with chronic low back pain: a randomized clinical trial. *JAMA* 2016;315(12):1240–1249.

83. Goodman S. Toward evidence-based medical statistics. 1: the P value fallacy. *Ann Intern Med* 1999;130(12):995–1004.

84. Altman DG, Bland JM. Absence of evidence is not evidence of absence. *BMJ* 1995;311:485.

85. Freiman JA, Chalmers TC, Smith HJ, et al. The importance of beta, the type II error and sample size in the design and interpretation of the randomized control trial. *N Engl J Med* 1978;299:690–694.

86. Deyo RA, Bass JE, Walsh NE, et al. Prognostic variability among chronic pain patients: implications for study design, interpretation, and reporting. *Arch Phys Med Rehabil* 1988;69:174–178.

87. Rothwell P. External validity of randomised controlled trials: "to whom do the results of this trial apply?" *Lancet* 2005;365(9453):13–14.

88. Haynes B. Can it work? Does it work? Is it worth it? *BMJ* 1999;319:652–653.

89. Gartlehner G, Hansen RA, Nissman D, et al. A simple and valid tool distinguished efficacy from effectiveness studies. *J Clin Epidemiol* 2006;59(10):1040–1048.

90. Rothwell P. Treating individuals 2. Subgroup analysis in randomised controlled trials: importance, indications, and interpretation. *Lancet* 2005;365(9454):176–186.

91. Clegg DO, Reda DJ, Harris CL, et al. Glucosamine, chondroitin sulfate, and the two in combination for painful knee osteoarthritis. *N Engl J Med* 2006;354:795–808.

92. Als-Nielsen B, Chen W, Gluud C, et al. Association of funding and conclusions in randomized drug trials. *JAMA* 2003;290(7):921–928.

93. Lexchin J, Bero LA, Djulbegovic B, et al. Pharmaceutical industry sponsorship and research outcome and quality: systematic review. *BMJ* 2003;326(7400):1167–1170.

94. Ezzet KA. The prevalence of corporate funding in adult lower extremity research and its correlation with reported results. *J Arthroplasty* 2003;18(7)(suppl 1):138–145.

95. Shah RV, Albert TJ, Bruegel-Sanchez V, et al. Industry support and correlation to study outcome for papers published in Spine. *Spine* 2005;30:1099–1104.

96. Easterbrook PJ, Berlin JA, Gopalan R, et al. Publication bias in clinical research. *Lancet* 1991;337:867–872.

97. Bekelman JE, Li Y, Gross CP. Scope and impact of financial conflicts of interest in biomedical research: a systematic review. *JAMA* 2003;289:454–465.

98. Lee K, Bacchetti P, Sim I. Publication of clinical trials supporting successful new drug applications: a literature analysis. *PLoS Med* 2008;5:1348–1356.

99. Chan A-W, Hróbjartsson A, Haahr MT, et al. Empirical evidence for selective reporting of outcomes in randomized trials: comparison of protocols to published articles. *JAMA* 2004;291(20):2457–2465.

100. Melander H, Ahlqvist-Rastad J, Meijer G, et al. Evidence b(i)ased medicine—selective reporting from studies sponsored by pharmaceutical industry: review of studies in new drug applications. *BMJ* 2003;326(7400):1171–1173.

101. Rising K, Bacchetti P, Bero L. Reporting bias in drug trials submitted to the Food and Drug Administration: review of publication and presentation. *PLoS Med* 2008;5:1561–1569.

102. Turner EH, Matthews AM, Linardatos E, et al. Selective publication of antidepressant trials and its influence on apparent efficacy. *N Engl J Med* 2008;358:252–260.

103. Hill KP, Ross JS, Egilman DS, et al. The ADVANTAGE seeding trial: a review of internal documents. *Ann Intern Med* 2008;149:251–258.

104. Kessler DA, Rose JL, Temple RJ, et al. Therapeutic-class wars—drug promotion in a competitive marketplace. *N Engl J Med* 1994;331(20):1350–1353.

105. Sterne JA, Egger M, Smith GD. Systematic reviews in health care: investigating and dealing with publication and other biases in meta-analysis. *BMJ* 2001;323:101–105.

106. Drazen JM, Morrissey S, Curfman GD. Open clinical trials. *N Engl J Med* 2007;357:1756–1757.

107. Laine C, Horton R, DeAngelis CD, et al. Clinical trial registration—looking back and moving ahead. *N Engl J Med* 2007;356:2734–2736.

108. Loke YK, Price D, Herxheimer A. Systematic reviews of adverse effects: framework for a structured approach. *BMC Med Res Methodol* 2007;7:32.

109. Ioannidis JP, Lau J. Completeness of safety reporting in randomized trials. *JAMA* 2001;285(4):437–443.

110. Chou R, Helfand M. Challenges in systematic reviews that assess treatment harms. *Ann Intern Med* 2005;142(12 pt 2):1090–1099.

111. Golder S, Loke YK. Is there evidence for biased reporting of published adverse effects data in pharmaceutical industry-funded studies? *Brit J Clin Pharmacol* 2008;66:767–773.

112. Van Zee A. The promotion and marketing of OxyContin: commercial triumph, public health tragedy. *Am J Public Health* 2009;99:221–227.

113. Psaty BM, Koepsell T, Lin D, et al. Assessment and control for confounding by indication in observational studies. *J Am Geriatr Soc* 1999;47:749–754.

114. Barber JA, Thompson SG. Analysis and interpretation of cost data in randomised controlled trials: review of published studies. *BMJ* 1998;317:1195–2000.

115. Campbell MK, Elbourne DR, Altman DG; for the CONSORT Group. CONSORT statement: extension to cluster randomised trials. *BMJ* 2004;328:702–708.

116. Donner A, Birkett N, Buck C. Randomization by cluster: sample size requirement and analysis. *Am J Epidemiol* 1981;114:906–914.

117. Sibbald B, Roberts C. Understanding controlled trials. Crossover trials. *BMJ* 1998;316(7146):1719.

118. Mills EJ, Chan AW, Wu P, et al. Design, analysis, and presentation of crossover trials. *Trials* 2009;10:27.

119. Reed JF III. Analysis of two-treatment, two-period crossover trials in emergency medicine. *Ann Emerg Med* 2004;43(1):54–58.

120. Lathyris DN, Trikalinos TA, Ioannidis JP. Evidence from crossover trials: empirical evaluation and comparison against parallel arm trials. *Int J Epidemiol* 2007;36(2):422–430.

121. Chalmers TC. A potpourri of RCT topics. *Control Clin Trials* 1982;3:285–298.

122. UK BEAM Trial Team. United Kingdom back pain exercise and manipulation (UK BEAM) randomised trial: effectiveness of physical treatments for back pain in primary care. *BMJ* 2004;329(7479):1377.

123. Brittain E, Wittes J. Factorial designs in clinical trials: the effects of non-compliance and subadditivity. *Stat Med* 1989;8:161–171.

124. Zwarenstein M, Treweek S, Gagnier JJ, et al. Improving the reporting of pragmatic trials: an extension of the CONSORT statement. *BMJ* 2008;337:a2390.

125. Thomas KJ, MacPherson H, Thorpe L, et al. Randomised controlled trial of a short course of traditional acupuncture compared with usual care for persistent non-specific low back pain. *BMJ* 2006;333(7569):623.

126. Furlan A, Chaparro LE, Irvin E, et al. A comparison between enriched and nonenriched enrollment randomized withdrawal trials of opioids for chronic noncancer pain. *Pain Res Manag* 2011;16(5):337–351.

127. Moore RA, Wiffen PJ, Eccleston C, et al. Systematic review of enriched enrolment, randomised withdrawal trial designs in chronic pain: a new framework for design and reporting. *Pain* 2015;156(8):1382–1395.

128. Devereaux PJ, Bhandari M, Clarke M, et al. Need for expertise based randomised controlled trials. *BMJ* 2005;330:88.

129. Lohr KN. Emerging methods in comparative effectiveness and safety: symposium overview and summary. *Med Care* 2007;45:S5–S8.

130. Glenny AM, Altman DG, Song F, et al. Indirect comparisons of competing interventions. *Health Technol Assess* 2005;9(26):1–134.

131. Chou R, Carson S, Chan BK. Gabapentin versus tricyclic antidepressants for diabetic neuropathy and post-herpetic neuralgia: discrepancies between direct and indirect meta-analyses of randomized controlled trials. *J Gen Intern Med* 2009;24:178–188.

132. Piaggio G, Elbourne DR, Altman DG, et al; for CONSORT Group. Reporting of noninferiority and equivalence randomized trials: an extension of the CONSORT statement. *JAMA* 2006;295(10):1152–1160.

133. Greene WL, Concato J, Feinstein AR. Claims of equivalence in medical research: are they supported by the evidence? *Ann Intern Med* 2000;132(9):715–722.

134. Barker D, McElduff P, D'Este C, et al. Stepped wedge cluster randomised trials: a review of the statistical methodology used and available. *BMC Med Res Methodol* 2016;16:69.

135. Hemming K, Haines TP, Chilton PJ, et al. The stepped wedge cluster randomised trial: rationale, design, analysis, and reporting. *BMJ* 2015;350:h391.

136. Goodman S. Toward evidence-based medical statistics. 2: the Bayes factor. *Ann Intern MEd* 1999;130(12):1005–1013.

137. Xiaoyu L, Sunil D. The application of Bayesian adaptive design in clinical trials. *Am J Math Stat* 2012;3(2):s67–s72.

138. Jadad AR, Carroll D, Moore A, et al. Developing a database of published reports of randomised clinical trials in pain research. *Pain* 1996;66:239–246.

139. Cook DJ, Mulrow CD, Haynes RB. Systematic reviews: synthesis of best evidence for clinical decisions. *Ann Intern Med* 1997;126:376–380.

140. Furlan AD, Clarke J, Esmail R, et al. A critical review of reviews on the treatment of chronic low back pain. *Spine* 2001;26(7):E155–E162.

141. Shea BJ, Grimshaw JM, Wells GA, et al. Development of AMSTAR: a measurement tool to assess the methodological quality of systematic reviews. *BMC Med Res Methodol* 2007;7:10.

142. Shea BJ, Reeves BC, Wells G, et al. AMSTAR 2: a critical appraisal tool for systematic reviews that include randomised or non-randomised studies of healthcare interventions, or both. *BMJ* 2017;358:j4008.

PART TWO

Economic, Political, Legal, and Ethical Considerations

CHAPTER **11**

Transdermal Pain: A Sociocultural Perspective

DAVID B. MORRIS

> "Chronic pain is a transdermal phenomenon and the environment is always a player in the chronic pain patient's predicament."
> —J. D. Loeser[1]

"A threshold has been crossed," writes sociologist Nikolas Rose.[2] Rose is director of the BIOS Centre for the Study of Bioscience, Biomedicine, Biotechnology and Society at the London School of Economics and Political Science. He wants to avoid what he calls "breathless epochalization"—hyperbolic claims that human history is undergoing a single, abrupt, massive upheaval—and he understands the present instead as the unfolding of "multiple histories" that emerge from the intersection of numerous "contingent pathways." Nonetheless, he also provides in *The Politics of Life Itself* (2007) an indispensable framework for considering how much has changed since the first edition of John Bonica's ground-breaking text *The Management of Pain* (1953). Pain too has changed, especially chronic pain, as pain has moved from the status of symptom to diagnosis, from the category of what humans passively endure (a mark of our changeless humanity) to what patients and health professionals together, as partnered agents of somatic change, now actively manage. These recent transformations in understanding pain hold important implications for pain management.

The dimension of change might be traced in the invention of the new discipline of pain medicine. "Prior to 1960," writes distinguished pain specialist John D. Loeser, "there were no pain specialists." He adds, "There were no journals devoted to pain, no dedicated research laboratories, and no funding programs aimed at pain research or training for clinicians. . . . Pain was always described as a byproduct of a disease state; the implication was that proper treatment of disease would relieve pain. The sensory nervous system was envisioned as a passive set of wires that conducted incoming impulses to the brain."[3] *The Management of Pain* in its first edition, reflecting this earlier and clearly imperfect state of knowledge, contained no discussion of relations between human pain and the sociocultural environment.

The rich biomedical literature currently exploring relations between human pain and the sociocultural environment is sometimes difficult to appreciate because we are in the midst of another momentous change. Nikolas Rose describes this change as what he calls "a molecular vision of life." Contemporary medicine and the biotechnologies on which it relies increasingly understand life at a subcellular level—with consequences that extend far beyond such familiar categories as illness and health, pathology and normality, and treatment and enhancement. The new techno-medicine, Rose argues, does not just cure disease or correct organic damage but, in its promise to refigure human vital processes at the molecular level, even changes "what it is to be a biological organism."

What it is to be a biological organism has always included vulnerability to pain, but it is not only our understanding of pain that has changed dramatically since 1953. Pain patients too have changed. A large subset of patients now regard themselves as well-informed, self-educated medical consumers, alert to the documented dilemma of medical error and actively embracing the apparent promise of what has been called our "genetic citizenship."[4] Women who carry the BRCA1 gene, for example, now understand that they face both an 87% risk of developing breast cancer and difficult medical options. Pain patients may expect that researchers simply need to find the gene for pain and knock it out—without understanding that most researchers do not seek a single specific "gene for" but rather variations in multiple loci within multiple gene systems. Although older infectious diseases have almost disappeared, chronic pain seems almost ineradicable, even on the rise, less a predictable companion of old age or an image of the human condition than an unaccountable failure of the molecular gaze to identify a local culprit neuron. It leaves the modern patient locked out from the molecular promise of somatic optimization. The "incrementalism" required for slow, steady improvement (that likely falls far short of cure) is also frequently difficult for doctors to grasp.[5] Thus, damage that chronic pain inflicts on body, mind, and spirit leaves many patients not at the threshold of a shining future but in a dark limbo or dystopia that negative psychosocial and sociocultural influences can turn into a prison or hell.

What follows, then, is an effort to place the new understandings of pain within a conflict-laced field where sociocultural and psychosocial forces may actively impede or assist treatment. In the new era of the molecular gaze, it is increasingly clear to health care professionals (if not to patients) that chronic pain in its numerous types, from migraine to cancer to garden-variety low back distress, is often more amenable to sociocultural analysis and to psychosocial therapies than to biomedical cure. Drugs and surgeries—perhaps the first choice of patients

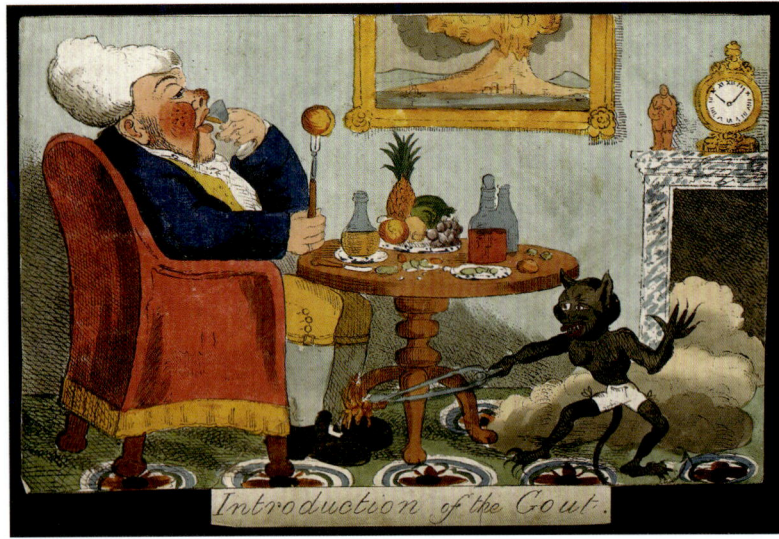

FIGURE 11.1 *Introduction of the Gout* by George Cruikshank, 1819 (this impression 1835). Colored etching. *(Courtesy of Wellcome Library, London.)*

or insurance providers—may be exactly the wrong approach. Pain specialist Scott Fishman puts it this way: "When somebody comes in with 25 years of chronic pain, I might sit with them for 90 minutes to get the beginning of the story, to really understand what is happening. The insurers would rather pay me $1,000 to do a 20-minute injection than pay me a fraction of that to spend an hour or two talking with a patient."[6] The pain that patients experience in certain medical settings, as new research unmistakably demonstrates, also reflects racial, ethnic, and provider biases in health care professionals that directly or indirectly affect real-world assessment and treatment.[7–11]

One quick caution. An attention to sociocultural and psychosocial influences on chronic pain does not imply rolling back decades of biomedical progress in which we now understand gout, for example, as a type of congenital arthritis and not—as in this 19th-century etching by satirist George Cruikshank (Fig. 11.1)—a justified moral punishment for luxurious aristocratic lifestyles.

Cruikshank, however, is not wholly wrong. The pain of gout correlates not only with molecular processes affecting serum uric acid levels but also with cultural and psychic forces underlying diet and socioeconomic position.[12] Even today, gout has a sociocultural impact on patients' lives that differs between African-American and Caucasian men and women.[13] Bottom line: What most patients do not know about chronic pain—especially its concealed link with social institutions, cultural practices, and individual personal belief—is exactly what evidence-based pain treatment in the era of the molecular gaze cannot ignore.

What Is Transdermal Pain?

Pain, especially chronic pain, is a transdermal phenomenon in that it occurs not only within an individual nervous system, including the brain, but also within a social and cultural environment. "Our concepts of pain, impairment, and disability," writes Wilbert E. Fordyce, "must consider environmental factors as well as the person."[14] Clinical practice frequently reduces environmental factors to three main stressors—employment, family, and alcohol or drugs—but this trio can serve as placeholder for a more extensive mix of sociocultural variables. The fundamental question is whether the sociocultural environment merely *influences* pain that already exists as a purely biologic phenomenon, simply modulating it, or, alternatively, if the sociocultural environment (beyond mere influence and modulation) helps to *construct* and to *constitute* pain.

The difference between influence and construction is important, but its significance for assessment and treatment is unclear because chronic pain often reflects multivariate influences. Some pain—often called psychogenic—seems produced almost wholly by the brain or with little more than an innocuous trigger from the environment. In one study, researchers attached volunteers to an electrical stimulator and told them that its current might possibly produce a headache. Volunteers were not told that the stimulator was set to produce nothing beyond a low humming sound. The result? Half the volunteers reported pain.[15] The environment need not cause or trigger pain in the way a hammer blow impacts a thumb. Positive or negative influences from the sociocultural environment may be as indirect as a whisper. Researchers, utilizing the molecular gaze, recently found that simply looking at the picture of a romantic partner reduced moderate pain by 40%.[16] The sociocultural environment, in contact with human consciousness, may not create or construct pain, but it clearly possesses a resource for pain management too important to neglect or dismiss, and its importance increases in proportion to acceptance of the now widespread recognition that distinguishes between nociception and pain.

The transmission of nociceptive impulses may at times generate autonomic responses, the human equivalent of a rodent's tail flick, but nociception alone does not constitute human pain. Pain, according to the prestigious International Association for the Study of Pain (IASP), is "always subjective" and "always a psychological state."[17] The subjective, psychological quality of pain, as human consciousness interacts with the sociocultural environment, is true in spades of chronic pain.

The crucial point here is that most pain specialists today attribute a significant role to the sociocultural environment—a truly historic change in thinking about pain and pain management.

Moreover, the new managers of pain, from a sociocultural perspective, are now doctors and health care professionals, working within complex interrelated systems in which health care costs in 2014 rose to 17.5% of the U.S. Gross Domestic Product.[18] Pain management now cannot be cordoned off from the surrounding medicalized culture and subcultures, where the molecular vision of life has (selectively but broadly) replaced a reliance on shaman, priest, or astrologer. This pervasive medicalization of pain, however, is not without consequences, especially when medical care seems to fail patients. Pain medicine thus is not a neutral or inevitable byproduct of scientific knowledge but rather a presence within the new sociocultural environment that influences pain. Many patients today, that is, experience pain only within a context that includes various specialists who deal with pain, from orthopedists, oncologists, and neurologists to acupuncturists, homeopaths, and practitioners of alternative and complementary medicine. Pain specialists cannot excuse themselves from discussion as if they were mere impartial technicians, objective researchers, or altruistic caregivers—who assess and treat pain but do not affect how patients understand or experience it. Lous Heshusius, a Canadian academic born in The Netherlands, suffered excruciating chronic pain in the aftermath of an automobile accident. Over an 11-year period, she lists some 240 appointments with doctors and specialists; nearly 500 appointments with alternative professionals; a dozen appointments for tests and assessments; and countless hours keeping track of prescriptions, bills, and insurance.[19] Pain specialists are among the key players in the new sociocultural environment that not only indirectly influences pain but also helps constitute the chronic pain patient's predicament.

The new active role for pain specialists is certainly driven by patient demand but not *solely* by patient demand, nor are its effects inconsequential. When clinicians employ evidence-based practices, chart pain as the fifth vital sign, or "game" insurance systems on behalf of their patients, such actions contribute to the maintenance of a significant sociocultural environment within which patients now experience pain. Although pain medicine did not invent insurance providers or disability systems, it operates today within a field of economic compensation that sets patients in a new relation to their pain. In a controversial recommendation, an IASP task force argues that chronic nonspecific low back pain in the workplace, in the absence of an organic lesion and under specified circumstances, should be reclassified not as a medical problem but as "activity intolerance."[20] *Activity intolerance* is less a diagnosis than a tone-deaf counter-narrative meant to contest the implicit sociocultural narrative that regards chronic low back pain as redeemable for disability payments or for time off. The almost seamless but culturally mandated transition from person-in-pain to pain patient—whose inner life is now under the implicit surveillance of the molecular gaze—also involves an invisible agenda of forms to fill out, waiting rooms, secretaries, insurance companies, drugs, side effects, referrals, more waiting rooms, indignities, task forces, protocols, and still more waiting rooms.[21] It situates pain and the pain patient within a web of sociocultural relations that reframe pain as transdermal.

Ethnicity, Race, Sex, Gender, Age: Whose Pain?

A molecular vision of life enfolds the modern pain patient within layers of unappreciated irony. That is, while patients increasingly adopt the expectations of a molecular gaze, pain medicine finds increasing evidence to support nonmolecular and sociocultural understandings of pain. Culture and biology both contribute to pain, of course, as the standard biopsychosocial model implies, but patients committed to the molecular gaze fail to grasp the extent to which human pain is not only always subjective but also always intersubjective. It intersects with shaping social systems from family, church, and nation to jobs and prisons, just as it meshes with variable cultural practices and beliefs from stoic dispassion to pharmaceutical trials. Such sociocultural environments are not necessarily material locales, like a doctor's office, but bear more resemblance to internalized, individual subsets of what anthropologists would call a *lifeworld*—a lifeworld that we experience as a state of body, mind, and emotion. Consciousness is the hard-to-define locus of such complex states, and chronic pain (as a classic mind/body state) is thus inextricable from the individual, intersubjective lifeworlds that shape as well as frame it.

The clearest instance of how sociocultural environments shape as well as frame pain comes in long-standing medical undertreatment for pain.[22,23] The hospital, that is, constitutes a distinctive microenvironment that demonstrates how sociocultural forces help alter the experience of pain. The prestigious 1996 SUPPORT study found that 50% of hospitalized seriously ill or dying patients failed (according to family members) to receive adequate pain medication.[24] Hospitals, like doctors, belong to the larger sociocultural environment where both drug abuse and fear of opioids have a strong presence, and the hospital as a distinctive microenvironment in some sense reproduces the mixed or self-contradictory beliefs and practices that surround it. Anesthesia belongs to the sociocultural environment of the hospital, where it is accepted as necessary, just as illegal street drugs belong to the environment of the street, where other necessities prevail. Pure pain—pain free from all direct or indirect sociocultural influences, including the artificial, scientific subculture of the laboratory—is a pain that exists nowhere except in theory. Pain as it inhabits the social world outside the laboratory proves always open to the modifying environmental influences of (among other often imprecise categories) race, ethnicity, sex, gender, and age.

Racial disparities in the assessment and treatment of pain are the focus of numerous medical studies.[25] Differences in pain tolerance provide conflicting data, as in laboratory studies about racial tolerance for thermal pain.[26] Some facts, however, are incontrovertible. In New York City, nonwhite patients who lived in disadvantaged neighborhoods (often black and Hispanic) had substantially less access to pharmacies than did white patients in more affluent neighborhoods. The pharmacies in disadvantaged areas moreover did not maintain adequate stocks of pain medication.[27] A sociocultural environment that reduces access to analgesia has an indirect but powerful impact on pain. Although reduced access does not *directly* cause pain, sociocultural practices that unfairly burden racial and ethnic minority populations *indirectly* both maintain currently unrelieved pain and, in effect, permit the emergence of new pain that does not exist in primarily white, affluent, more pharmacofriendly communities. There is even neurologic evidence indicating brain and autonomic correlates with empathetic responses to pain in persons of other races.[28] Fortunately, studies are now underway to improve clinician awareness concerning pain management disparities.[29,30]

Race and ethnicity, then, are frequently discussed in recent studies on pain—but discussion is often impeded by failures to clarify underlying concepts. Classic articles describe ethnocultural differences in the perception of pain and of chronic pain.[31,32] Numerous researchers report ethnic differences in the prevalence and severity of pain, and they find interethnic differences in tolerance levels for clinical and experimentally induced pains. For example, attitudes toward pain show sharp differences along ethnic lines among surgical patients in Australia.[33] Cancer pain among southwest Native Americans has its own specific ethnic signature.[34] Race affects how we view others' pain.[35] It influences analgesia use in pediatric emergency departments.[36] It affects analgesic access for acute abdominal pain in the emergency department.[37] Among patients with arthritis and rheumatic conditions, race and ethnicity even impact treatment outcomes.[38] Yet, exactly what *are* ethnicity and race?

Pain specialists need to engage with recent thinking about how to understand race and ethnicity. Bio-anthropologists contend that there is no genetic signature for race. In general, there is more genetic variation within (so-called) races than across races, which means that race and ethnicity are primarily sociocultural rather than genetic categories.[39] Skin color alone links population groups as diverse as their languages: say, Italians and Swedes, Scots and Russians, and Belgians and Croats. Blackness, as a supposed racial marker, links West Africans with the historically very different East Africans, as well as with Haitians, African Americans, some Hispanics, and various hyphenated groups identified, roughly, by the mere color of their skin. Migration, intermarriage, and global travel have produced a wave of mixed-race offspring. The census term "Asian" has a different meaning in Europe than in America, and census data in Western democracies now define race and ethnicity not through genes, skin color, or geography but rather as a matter of *self-identification*. In a movement away from reductive ideas of racial science, the most helpful recent turn in health care discussion emphasizes *population groups*, where biology and genetics are relevant but far from determinative. "Key, here," as Nikolas Rose explains, "is not so much race, but the belief that a particular community has specific health needs that may have a genomic basis, and that research on the genomic basis is essential if these needs are to be met."[40]

Pain assessment and pain management are caught up in the shifting sociocultural and historical web of attitudes and practices that envelop race and ethnicity. Over half of Hispanics who presented at emergency rooms with long bone fractures, for example, were twice as likely as similar white patients to go without pain medicine.[41,42] Hispanic ethnicity, according to a recent prospective 10-year evaluation, continues to impact pain management decisions in the emergency department.[8] We need not posit conscious racism on the part of health care providers, although its presence in medicine (whether conscious or nonconscious) is well documented.[43,44] It is enough to observe that medical degrees do not confer immunity from nonconscious acts of discrimination that reflect the racism of a surrounding culture. This fact should be cause for vigilance in health care settings. Although many blacks carry a gene that puts them at risk for sickle cell disease, their need for pain relief too often runs up against tacit medical stereotypes of drug-seeking behavior.[45,46] Like the infamous Tuskegee syphilis experiments on black airmen, the history of sickle cell pain warns that sociocultural *biases* concerning race and ethnicity—not race or ethnicity themselves—pose a significant continuing danger to the achievement of color-blind, discrimination-free, equitable pain management. A means to identify and combat racial bias in pain treatment is now an urgent ethical issue in medicine.[10]

Telltale absences of equitable pain management unfortunately continue to appear in multiple medical sites not limited to the pain clinic. African American cancer patients in nursing homes were 63% more likely than whites to receive no pain treatment.[47] Other minorities with cancer pain also experience inadequate pain relief.[48] The unequal worldwide distribution and consumption of morphine means that medication for pain is far more available to first-world and mostly white patients than to nonwhites in the developing world.[49,50] This difference is not mainly a function of income, although in the United States, there is a strong association between pain prevalence and socioeconomic position.[51] The US campaign against illegal drug trafficking makes inadequate pain relief for Mexican patients also political in origin.[52] Pain management teams, as they confront questions about clinical policy and research design, need to recognize that race and ethnicity are ill-defined, socially explosive classifications with little basis in genetic science. The laudable recent interest in developing "cultural competence" among health care professionals who treat patients in pain cannot allow generic descriptions of group traits to replace a focus on the individual patient.[53] Geronimo was not a typical Chiricahua Apache, and modern Apaches may share few cultural connections with modern southwestern pueblo peoples. Stereotypes based on race or ethnicity—often flawed or at least slippery concepts—are the enemy of good pain medicine.

Sex and gender raise additional complications in assessing sociocultural influences on pain. Sex differences appear real, if limited. Animal studies indicate differences between male and female rodents in pain processing, including a greater efficacy of μ-opioids in males. In humans, κ-opioids produce significantly greater analgesia in women than in men.[54] Even among women only, red-haired women (in a study that did not test men) show increased sensitivity to thermal pain and reduced responsiveness to subcutaneous lidocaine because of specific mutations of the melanocortin-1 receptor.[55,56] Biologically based sexual differences clearly play a role in women's pain across a range of chronic pain conditions from migraine to irritable bowel syndrome, although the precise mechanisms are often unclear.[57] Sex steroid hormones in men and women appear to modulate different nociceptive behaviors. Pregnancy, for example, whatever the television-dramatics associated with morning sickness and labor pain, creates an antinociception that involves δ-opioid and κ-opioid but not μ-opioid systems.[58] Such biologic differences, however, are likely modest when compared with the exaggerated and shifting sociocultural representations of female and male pain—from Freudian hysteria to John Wayne machismo—that undoubtedly have a shaping influence on the experience of pain.

Pain researchers have been slow to investigate potential differences due less to sex than to gender. Sex, that is, depends on the biology of male/female difference, whereas gender splinters the standard male/female binary into a rainbow of orientations from gay and lesbian to bisexual and transgender. One prominent argument in the field of gender studies holds that gender is largely performative, meaning, gender—no matter how individual, eccentric, or dependent on hormone therapies—constitutes a quasi-public social role.[59] The women whom Charcot in the 19th century photographed in his famous hysteria wards clearly "performed" their illness for the camera, even if unknowingly, and today women tend to perform specific gender roles (e.g., as overextended caregivers) that are sociocultural and not entirely unrelated to pain. Caregivers, for example, are at increased risk for multiple maladies, from depression to heart disease. Men, too, perform certain gender roles directly or indirectly related to the capacity to endure pain, where the power to endure pain is a sociocultural rather than biologic trait. A pain treatment program that recognizes the complicating sociocultural role of gender—in addition to well-known differences in sex, race, and ethnicity—will be best equipped to grasp the multiple lines of influence, both biologic and psychosocial, that so often converge in chronic pain.

Age might stand as an icon for the multiple biologic and sociocultural convergences that influence chronic pain. Pediatrics and geriatrics both depend on biologic changes that accompany human growth, but childhood and old age are both also the site of numerous, tacit, culturally specific expectations. Pain research has devoted considerable resources to children, whose limitations in language and in perception require ingenious techniques for assessment. Techniques such as drawings that indicate the location and intensity of pain depend equally on the biologic facts of human linguistic development and on the sociocultural skills and learning associated with graphic design. Pain treatment geared to children also requires, in addition to carefully age-adjusted medications, an attention to childhood fears and feelings that belong to particular cultures. Much like ethnicity and race, age (especially cultural stereotypes of the elderly) has an impact on pain management decisions.[60] Even in the emergency department, there appear to be disparities in pain treatment afforded to younger and older adults.[61] Old age, however, whether defined by chronology alone or by organic and developmental changes, has received less attention than childhood in pain research, although the new field of palliative medicine is bringing rapid change.[62] Indeed, one area in particular need of increased study is pain at the end of life.[63] Dying is clearly a biologic process, but the funeral industry alone indicates how far death and dying are endowed with significance that is both economic and sociocultural. American and European medical attitudes clearly differ about continuous deep sedation until death.[64] Clear ethical guidelines on pain treatment at the end of life are greatly needed. Edmund Pellegrino,[65] a giant of modern bioethics, defines the challenge to modern end-of-life pain medicine in what resembles a blunt, if indirect, ultimatum: "Not to relieve pain optimally is tantamount to moral and legal malpractice."

Why is it important for medicine to recognize the sociocultural influences on human pain as reflected in race, ethnicity, sex, gender, and age? First, although drugs and surgery sometimes erase or control pain associated with clear organic sources, many conditions such as chronic nonspecific low back pain expose the limits of drugs and surgery, especially where sociocultural influences—such as family, job, and disability—are involved. Furthermore, organic lesions do not map exactly onto pain. Most adults who complain of back pain have lumbar disk disease, but so do many adults without pain complaints.[66] In America, long-term functioning of patients treated for back pain is similar whether doctors prescribe medication and bed rest or self-care and education.[67] Pain simply does not provide an accurate report of tissue damage. "The truth is that pain is a very poor reporting system," writes Patrick Wall. He adds, "The doctrine that pain is a useful signal needs heavy qualification."[68] The erroneous belief that pain is a reliable alarm system not only justifies countless unnecessary surgeries but also cannot begin to explain why the two strongest signs predicting that an American worker will develop chronic back pain are job dissatisfaction and unsatisfactory social relations in the workplace.[69,70] It is as if the American low back is wired directly into the sociocultural work environment. A study covering 18 countries found large international variation in the prevalence of disabling forearm and back pain among occupational groups carrying out similar tasks.[71]

Second, the recognition of sociocultural influences on pain opens up possibilities for system-wide changes in pain management. In 1999, a memorandum directed to over 1,200 sites required the entire U.S. Veterans Health Administration to make policy and procedural changes implicit in the new principle that pain is the *fifth vital sign*.[72] In one VA outpatient clinic, this change produced no measurable improvement in pain management quality.[73] The possibilities for system-wide change are impressive, however, especially when hospital accreditation now depends on requirements to chart pain levels. A similar requirement altered policies in pain management and in palliative medicine throughout all the hospitals in the vast southwest region of the U.S. Indian Health Service.[74] Such changes acknowledge that pain management belongs to a surrounding sociocultural environment that includes the changing subculture of medicine. Systemic changes in pain management thus affect not only individual patients but also the wider sociocultural environments (from clinics and hospitals to digital media reports) within which both patients and nonpatients understand and experience pain.

The IASP in its glossary of terms describes pain as "always subjective" and "always a psychological state."[17] Pain, by implication, may change when a person's subjective, psychological state changes sufficiently. Systemic changes in the sociocultural environment of medicine—including efforts to reduce provider bias based on age, gender, sex, ethnicity, and race—can materially alter individual experience and help relieve pain. Such changes also recognize that a patient's race, ethnicity, sex, gender, and age have demonstrable effects on the experience of pain. Suppose that a woman from a minority group in a low-income neighborhood repeatedly fails to receive adequate pain medication from her local pharmacy. Frustration, humiliation, and rage, compounding the fear that she may already feel about her health, constitute a significant change in her

subjective state not unrelated to pain. Fear, as researchers show, elevates pain intensity.[75] Pain specialist Mark Sullivan[76] argues that pain itself is best understood *as* an emotion. Patient education and improved access to care offer two additional and specific areas for systemic change, with consequences that promise a difference in both the psychology of individual pain patients and in the surrounding, interpenetrating sociocultural environments within which people of any sex and gender—patients, doctors, nurses, adults, children, workers—understand and experience pain.

Across Cultures: Beliefs, Attitudes, Perceptions, Behaviors

Pain varies across individuals, cultures, and times. This strong claim contradicts the universalist view that pain is a changeless sensory signal, identical in everyone, everywhere. Dental research has identified an effect of culture on pain sensitivity.[77] Culture, of course, is a broad general concept and not a sufficient explanation for pain or for pain sensitivity. In women, sensitivity to a variety of experimental thermal, mechanical, and chemical pain-producing stimuli has a proven genetic contribution.[78] Individual variations in reported pain intensity produced by exposure to an identical noxious stimulus correlate directly with altered brain patterns, which can hardly be explained solely as an effect of culture.[79] Most researchers agree, however, that pain includes *both* sensory and affective components, and affective components of pain show wide variation across individuals and cultures. The 1950s era surgically lobotomized patients could still feel pain, reportedly, but said that the pain no longer *bothered* them. It may require a philosopher to decide if pain that fails to bother us still counts as pain. (It will not show up at pain clinics.) It did require philosophers to compile a volume of essays entitled *Cultural Ontology of the Self in Pain*[80] (a rough translation: *The Self in Pain as a Cultural Being*). Pain that is both affect-free and culture-free constitutes almost a self-contradiction because researchers agree that personal emotions—far from being bio-hardwired at birth—are fundamentally cultural.[81]

Real-world pain, then, is characterized by an affective quality of aversiveness open to wide modulation. This aversiveness depends on corticolimbic networks, much as anxiety correlates with activity in the septohippocampal system.[82] Emotions associated with aversiveness, however, also in part socially constructed and socially modified, need not prove static or unresponsive to additional sociocultural input. Stoic philosophers in the age of Nero exalted the use of reason to overcome pain, and many Greek texts retell the story of the Spartan boy (trained in courage and in military discipline) who remains silent as a fox hidden in his cloak gnaws him to death. Athletes, dancers, yogis, and religious celebrants continue to demonstrate how minds and emotions, as shaped by differing sociocultural environments, help to modify pain and pain behavior. Such sociocultural environments are not neutral containers for bodies in pain—like stage sets—but rather, the setting and its sociocultural forces shape the pain. Even pain clinics and research labs are, in a specialized sense, sociocultural spaces. They help to shape expectations and to reinvent pain as surely as ancient religions shaped and reinvented pain through authoritative teachings about demonic possession and original sin. Whatever the surrounding culture teaches us or shows us about pain (including false information, erroneous recommendations, and harmful tales) holds the power to modulate what we feel—for better or worse—with direct and indirect implications for the medical discipline of pain management.

Culture as a crucial force in shaping human pain across various eras, disciplines, and practices, from legal punishment to religion, is a subject of wide-ranging books and articles.[83–85] An evidence-based pain medicine can draw particularly persuasive data from cross-cultural studies. For example, researchers compared chronic low back pain patients in Japan with a similar group in the United States and found the Japanese patients to be significantly less impaired in social, psychological, vocational, and avocational function.[86] A cross-cultural comparison matching Portuguese chronic pain patients with English-speaking chronic pain patients showed strong similarities in associations between psychosocial factors and measures of pain experience: intensity, physical function, and psychological function.[87] Just as various psychosocial factors may differ across cultures, psychosocial factors themselves (likely rooted in particular cultures) regularly affect the experience of pain. Of course, pain evoked in a lab or studied in reviews of medical literature may not replicate everyday pain experienced outside various controlled environments, and real-world sociocultural environments include not only visible institutions such as families, schools, and workplaces but also less visible currents of thought and feeling conveyed in advertisements, songs, sports, and personal interactions. Even parental models have an influence on how individuals understand specific pain events.[88] Aboriginal people in Australia deal with pain in culturally specific ways.[89,90] Hispanics and non-Hispanics show significant differences in their knowledge about hospice care, with a resulting impact on pain management at the end of life.[91] Although similar illustrations might be greatly multiplied, they all tend to demonstrate how cultural attitudes and understandings permeate the experience of pain, especially chronic pain. Nowhere is the interpenetration of culture and chronic pain so clear as in the growing medical literature on so-called pain beliefs.

Pain beliefs exist in an individual mind, but they also reside within cultures so that cultures are the effective origin of most individual pain beliefs. We cannot name or discuss pain except in a natural language—English, Spanish, Farsi—that inevitably colors our understanding and subtly shapes our experience.[92] Pain thus comes always already interpreted, and pain beliefs silently infiltrate behavior through implicit cultural scripts or narratives, much as athletes often play out a prescribed role in which tolerance for pain affirms male courage, team loyalty, and physical strength. Such normative social practices and behaviors, like the beliefs that support them, often prove amenable to observation. In fact, observation of pain beliefs (mostly via questionnaire) is a robust subdiscipline within pain medicine. Research shows that specific beliefs affect the pain we experience, especially beliefs about cause, control, duration, outcome, and blame. These beliefs affect not only chronic pain but also acute pain and postoperative pain. Pain beliefs, moreover, are often linked with emotions: anger toward a negligent employer, fear of financial disaster, hope for monetary compensation, or the desire for caring attention from a spouse. Some pain beliefs strongly correlate with pain intensity. Patients function better, this research shows, who believe they have some control over their pain, who believe in the value of medical services, who believe that family members care for them, and who believe that they are not severely disabled. In one study, specific pain beliefs correlated directly with treatment outcomes.[93–97] If you believe that your pain is disabling, this internal pain belief (played out as human consciousness alters feeling and behavior) already predicts that you will be disabled by pain.

The pain belief research that got underway in the 1990s shows no sign of slowing down. The vocabulary sometimes shifts from beliefs to perceptions to attitudes—and the patients under study now reflect an extended ethnic and global reach—but the findings consistently recognize the effect of culture on the understanding and experience of pain. It is important for pain management professionals in the United States to understand African Americans' distinctive perceptions of pain

and pain management.[98] New Zealand practitioners need to understand the attitudes and beliefs about back pain shared by New Zealanders.[99] Studies of pain beliefs now extend to Somali women, inner city veterans, French Canadians, the general populace of India, as well as such distinctive groups as children and the obese.[100–104] Research still tends to focus on what we might call the big three pain beliefs—catastrophizing, control, and disability—but researchers are beginning to study more diverse cognitive/emotional states associated with religious faith and spiritual practices.[105] Especially important is pain-related research into attitudes about personal identity and self-efficacy.[106] One review article posed the crucial question whether pain-related beliefs influence adherence to multidisciplinary rehabilitation. Conclusion: Treatment adherence is determined by a combination of pain-related beliefs either supporting or inhibiting chronic pain patients' ability to adhere to treatment recommendations over time, and self-efficacy appears to be the most commonly researched predictor of treatment adherence, with its effects also influencing other pain-related beliefs.[107]

Future studies might well expand their methods and focus to include a larger sense of meaning—its presence, absence, or indeterminacy—as intrinsic to human pain. *Meanings of Pain* (2017), a collection of multiauthored essays with a philosophical turn, offers a rich lode of thought.[108] In adults, chronic pain often implies a continuous process of interpretation—conscious, nonconscious, personal, cultural—that both builds up and deconstructs meaning. Why me? Is it serious? Will I get better? Such questions about meaning as well as the responses that they elicit, even nonconscious responses, illustrate how meaning is not merely an add-on to pain. Meaning is intrinsic to pain even at the zero degree where patients (hooked on biomedical myths) assert the belief that pain is meaningless. Pain in its social functions often reverts to its etymologic (Latin) meaning of punishment. Childhood discipline, spouse abuse, and even self-punishing guilt belong to a punitive semantics of pain. Although drugs temporarily stop pain and bypass meaning, meaning does not therefore die out. The brief pharmaceutical erasure can simply perpetuate the belief that consumer purchases and drug therapies buy relief. Meaning here passes imperceptibly into cultural myth, and myths matter for pain management when the meanings that they encode prove harmful. A growing medical literature now explores false, erroneous, or harmful pain beliefs.[109,110] Such harmful pain beliefs are as damaging to patients as unsupervised multiple drug cocktails. Detoxification is often a necessary step in pain treatment programs, and it makes sense to consider various clinical techniques of semantic detox. Catastrophizing—a toxic compound of fears and of beliefs anticipating disastrous outcomes—proves the single most important predictor for lower quality of life in chronic pain patients.[111]

Transdermal pain, then, is not a subclass of pain, but rather an encompassing tautology: All pain, especially chronic pain, is transdermal. It is shaped, invisibly, by sociocultural and intersubjective forces. This counterintuitive claim seems berserk to a weekend handyman who has just hammered his thumb, but pain (in addition to various neural networks and organic systems) depends on developmental learning and cultural editing. Ice packs on a throbbing thumb invoke an elementary cultural education, as does the commonsense but erroneous belief that pain correlates directly with tissue damage. Chronic pain requires a personal and cultural reeducation in which talk of genetic susceptibilities and neurotransmitters is compatible with research into modulating sociocultural variables.[112] Even neuropathic pain in laboratory rats appears to show the impact of rodent-specific social variables.[113] The medical literature on sociocultural variables in pain is too vast to review here, but future researchers might wish to explore what it might mean for pain management when sociocultural perspectives expand far enough to put assessment and treatment in contact with quasi-philosophical issues as large as narrative, ethics, and globalization.

Pain and Narrative: Culture, Meaning, Ethics

Philosopher Alasdair MacIntyre[114] identifies the widest importance of narrative knowledge when he writes that "we all live out narratives in our lives" and "we understand our own lives in terms of the narratives that we live out." Life, as the discipline of narrative psychology puts it, is inherently "storied."[115,116] In acknowledgment of this so-called narrative turn, Rita Charon writing in *JAMA* describes a new clinical approach she calls "narrative medicine."[117] Narrative (from Latin *narrare = to tell*) can be defined as simply as "someone telling something to someone about something."[118] Narrative medicine sets out to reframe the everyday act of talking with patients. Charon also reframes narrative as a specific form of knowledge—*narrative* knowledge—as distinct from what she calls the *logicoscientific* knowledge so valued in medicine. Narrative knowledge, as Charon describes it, is not in conflict with logicoscientific knowledge but rather, especially as an instrument for understanding pain, offers a valuable supplement or complement to the molecular gaze. The IASP multi-authored collection *Narrative, Pain, and Suffering* (2005) explores a series of relevant and illustrative cases.[119]

Narrative can offer insights into human pain sometimes otherwise unavailable. As a vehicle for the communication of cultural beliefs and social practices, narrative clearly plays a role in transmitting attitudes and perceptions that pain patients may imagine to be strictly their own unique personal beliefs. A personal narrative may also convey fine nuances of meaning and troubling webs of self-contradiction that offer a significant tool for understanding treatment-related attitudes that elude the coarse grid of generic questionnaires. There is also a downside to narrative that affects pain management. Pain narratives, that is, sometimes encode mistaken beliefs, such as the dominant biomedical myth that regards pain as the invariable consequence and symptom of organic tissue damage. In truth, as the IASP explains, many people report pain "in the absence of tissue damage or any likely pathophysiological cause."[17] A narrative medicine for pain, as Rita Charon puts it, promises significant therapeutic benefits where other approaches fail or fall short.[120]

A narrative medicine for pain might find one specific use in explicating the dilemma that occurs when chronic pain engages patients in the dynamics of what anthropologists call *damaged* or *spoiled* identity. Narrative, in this instance, offers insight into a patient's experience of self and, in some cases, can provide a means for patients to construct a new or revised selfhood: an important step toward exiting the role of chronic pain sufferer.[121] The findings in a study of fibromyalgia patients, for example, suggest that narrative approaches helped participants both invent their own coping strategies and discover identities other than as pain patients.[122] Participants in experiments asked to write about trauma demonstrate the astonishing power of narrative to moderate pain. Rheumatoid arthritis patients who wrote in narrative form about stressful experiences, for example, showed significant symptom reduction.[123] Indeed, writing about trauma is associated with various measurable health benefits.[124,125] The beneficial writing very often takes the specific form of narration. "Using our computer analyses as a guide," explains psychologist James Pennebaker,[126] "we realized that the people who benefited from writing were constructing stories."

Narrative, like a scalpel or questionnaire, has limits to its uses as a therapeutic instrument.[127] Pain can push both narrative and meaning to an extreme point of collapse, where nothing can be written or spoken: a black hole from which meaning cannot emerge. Victims of torture may undergo experience so horrific and chaotic that it blocks any possible narration.[128] In less traumatic situations, however, stories offer helpful public and private uses through their explicit or inexplicit commerce with ethics. Narrative had no relevance to bioethics at its modern beginnings in the 1970s as a branch of analytic philosophy, wedded to a rationalist, universalist discourse of principles, often referred to as principlism. From a sociocultural perspective, ethics is not strictly a discourse about universal truths and timeless principles but, like medicine, an intersubjective project shot through with narrative meaning.[129] Although pain medicine has developed ethical guidelines concerning research on animals and on humans, there is room and need for an ethics of pain that moves beyond professional guidelines and beyond principlism.[130] Pain, like love, can call into question our relations with others, not only spouses or friends but also people who are *radically* other, nothing like us, enemies perhaps. Narrative ethics challenges us to understand pain as always embedded in the distinctive life-stories of individuals, where ethical choices may fail to map precisely onto a rationalist logic of universal principles. A narrative ethics can illuminate contingent choices and variable contexts in which universalized moral rules are less important for health than the clarification of contingent values.

Values, intricately layered with beliefs, have proven correlations with pain. Among adult patients in a pain management unit, success at living in accordance with one's values correlated with measures of disability, depression, and pain-related anxiety.[131] Religion and spirituality also engage value-based beliefs—relevant to pain—that narrative helps illuminate. Among predominantly white, Christian, mid-Western patients with chronic musculoskeletal pain, the religious and spiritual beliefs of patients differ from the beliefs of a healthy population, and long-time pain patients received less support than other patients from their church community, tending to lose hope and to grow bitter: angry at themselves, at society, and at God.[132] The *Journal of Pain and Symptom Management* in 2010 published an article evaluating the FICA tool for spiritual assessment.[133] In Europe, a spiritual-needs questionnaire has proved useful for treating patients with chronic pain and cancer pain.[134] Such instruments are not attuned to narrative meaning, but spiritual needs regularly imply an underlying narrative structure of belief. Pain narratives turn especially complex, however, when personal, spiritual, and social values clash. Should pain management—in such instances, or perhaps generally—be understood as a basic human right?[135] A response based on timeless principles or universal truths may prove less persuasive than extended discourse that identifies underlying narrative beliefs and ultimately hammers out a shared agreement on values. Pain management implicitly affirms a set of values perhaps less applicable to illness in general than specific to pain: values that attribute to pain the status of an imperative call. Pain in this sense—as in the familiar biblical narrative of the good Samaritan—calls out for (or requires) active assistance. Reason, like justice, is not timeless and universal but temporal and context-bound.[136] Pain management in an era of increased global diversity may find more common ground in shared professional narratives—narratives of human rights or of service to others—than in principles at odds with the values of a surrounding culture.

Beyond the Gate: Consciousness and the Limits of a Molecular Gaze

The molecular vision of life—or its precursor in Foucault's well-known *clinical gaze*—made its dramatic entry into pain studies in 1965 when anatomist Patrick Wall and psychologist

Ronald Melzack published their influential gate-control theory.[137] The gate-control theory focuses on the process of nociception and on neural impulses blocked or transmitted at specific organic locales, and it pays particular attention to the "gating mechanism" located in the dorsal horn of the spinal cord. This innovative gaze inside the anatomy of human pain certainly changed medical thinking in the latter half of the 20th century, when the gate-control theory achieved iconic explanatory status, and some 21st century pain specialists find the gate-control theory entirely adequate: It has stood the test of time.[138] The legacy of the gate-control theory can be traced, for example, in research into molecular approaches to treat neuropathic pain.[139] Others, however, remain quiet or uneasy. The uneasiness occurs in part because the gate-control theory applies far better to acute pain than to chronic pain. Ronald Melzack has radically revised or quietly abandoned talk of a dorsal-horn gate and now emphasizes what he calls a cortical "neuromatrix."[140] Distinguished pain specialist and neurosurgeon John D. Loeser—in a 1991 article entitled "What Is Chronic Pain?"—reflects a similar change in perspective when he asserts, "The brain is the organ responsible for all pain." "All sensory phenomena," he adds, "including nociception, can be altered by conscious and unconscious mental activity."[141]

Neuromatrix theory proposes numerous networked brain connections that, beyond nociception, call into play a range of conscious and nonconscious human mental–emotional activity often rooted in the sociocultural environment. A molecular gaze that focuses on a few anatomical "gates" may prove adequate for specific chronic conditions such as neuropathic pain, although treatment for neuropathic pain remains extremely difficult, but an explanatory theory that reduces all chronic pain to neural impulses blocked or passing through a spinal gate risks ignoring the complex mind/body interrelations characteristic of a transdermal perspective. The dilemma is clear: Insurers and peer reviewers want hard evidence, although chronic pain is often characterized by multiple influences not easily amenable to cellular repair or reducible to sound quantitative data. Research on chronic low back pain, for example, is mostly restricted to high-income countries, where rates of low back pain run 2 to 4 times higher than in low-income countries. Within low-income countries, rates of low back pain are higher in urban populations than in rural populations.[142] These socioeconomic variations suggest that low back pain—a signature instance of chronic pain—is not a likely candidate for molecular cure. Many multidisciplinary treatment programs now recognize the impact of psychosocial factors and emphasize cognitive-behavioral therapies, but "psychosocial factors"—reducible to the influence of families, jobs, and alcohol or drugs—often merely nestle uncertainly within a dominant, evidence-driven, biomedical model.

The challenge for pain management in the decades ahead is perfectly captured in the title of a recent research paper: "Cognitive Behavioral Therapy for Chronic Pain Is Effective, But for Whom?"[143] The authors point out that the oldest and most educated patients showed strong treatment effects, whereas younger and less educated patients did not. It will require extensive additional research to confirm and to explain these findings. Unless the impact of age and of education are due entirely to anatomical or neural development, however, it appears that even the success of cognitive-behavioral therapies depends in part on changes ascribable to a sociocultural environment. Success, most patients would agree, is the goal of any pain management program, and a totally pain-free state is no doubt an unrealistic definition of a successful outcome. Pain management programs may at times unknowingly prove countertherapeutic if they provide an official confirmation of disability status or rigorously transform people in pain into long-term pain patients. Patienthood as an official or unofficial status brings its own sociocultural baggage. In pursuit of success, there is value in studying communities in which people who do not seek medical care for chronic pain—by choice or because modern medical care is unavailable—nonetheless lead, by their own accounts, happy, productive, successful lives. How do they do it?

Success for a person living with pain ultimately is a matter of consciousness. Of course, consciousness is a concept difficult enough to occupy teams of philosophers, neurologists, and students of artificial intelligence, but success for people in pain ultimately plays out in their conscious and nonconscious mental lives. Even chronic pain patients who master coping skills have somehow changed their mental and emotional architecture. The new field of positive psychology argues persuasively for shifting focus away from dysfunction and instead seeking to understand what specific beliefs, attitude, and practices appear to promote effective function and personal happiness.[144] Positive psychology suggests that there is value in identifying "success stories": another narrative genre relevant to medicine.[145] Such success stories might be drawn not only from people in pain who benefit from cognitive-behavioral therapies but also, perhaps especially, from people in pain who lead successful lives and do not enter pain treatment programs or research protocols. Hope and fear take on unusual, even primal power when pain strikes, as reflected in both the placebo effect and the nocebo effect. ("Voodoo death" is a documented fact.) Prayer and the belief structure reinforced in a church-centered community suggest resources that a biomedical or gate-control model of pain too often ignores in its quest to identify organic processes. An additional danger or limitation in an unrevised gate-control theory is that it may excuse specialists from an opportunity—ethical or medical—to address social and political pain-related conditions *outside* the nervous system.

Pain and Globalization: Power, Money, Systems

Sociologist Elliott A. Krause[146] in *Power & Illness* (1977) shows how health and health care are "intimately involved with the political, economic, and social struggles of the present day." Krause[146] studied power as oppressive and coercive—a perspective that is relevant to current legal, military, and medical discussions of pain in torture, say, or in capital punishment. Michel Foucault,[147] however, moves beyond his early focus on power as oppressive, top–down, and hegemonic, expressed in prohibitions and restraints. In his later work, Foucault[147] views power as horizontal, distributed, even demotic, expressed as usable energies always circulating within a social system, like electricity coursing unseen and productively through the walls of medical facilities. This later perspective illuminates the recent, ongoing transformation of patients from passive (powerless) subjects of a colonizing biomedical gaze to active agents, whose limited but real powers range from noncompliance and litigation to undisclosed alternative and holistic modes of self-care.[148] Such changes, reflected in hospitals that openly post a patient's bill of rights to adequate pain relief, suggest that pain management inescapably takes place now within the vast, disruptive, social, and economic power shift called globalization.

Globalization holds potent implications for the sociocultural dimensions of pain and of pain management. It brings patients from far-flung nations whose indigenous belief systems and whose inabilities to handle spoken English create new challenges across medicine. It also alters the commercial landscape within which medical care and pain management occur. For example, the publicly owned, family-run, mid-Western US pharmaceutical company Upjohn, which marketed ibuprofen and its over-the-counter (OTC) spin-off, Motrin, merged in

1995 with European conglomerate Pharmacia, headquartered in Sweden; the merged company Pharmacia & Upjohn in 2000 merged with Monsanto and took the name Pharmacia Corporation; and in 2002, Pharmacia Corporation was bought by the international colossus Pfizer in pursuit of full rights to the (now disgraced) blockbuster pain drug Celebrex. Marketplace dominance consolidated in a few transnational monoliths that underwrite activities, journals, and organizations in support of pain specialists justifies Foucault's[149] concept of *biopower*. Biopower refers to a modern, medical, state-sponsored, and corporate-inflected authority over health-related activities from sexuality to population control. Nikolas Rose[150] proposes the related term *biopolitics* to describe a postmodern extension of biopower to far broader supra-state manipulations of human vitality, morbidity, and mortality. Pain management, not fully separable from the influence of a transnational pharmaceutical industry, cannot today be fairly represented as individual encounters between a patient and a caring doctor or health care provider. A full sociocultural analysis of modern pain management would need to situate the traditional doctor/patient dyad within a new supradyadic, globalized biopolitics as dominant (if unnoticed in most everyday affairs) as the force of gravity.

Money and pain? Pain patients are, of course, cared for largely within complex, high-tech, financially stable systems assuring—to put it crassly—that health care professionals are paid. Local compensation issues are often influenced by national or international forces, such as the traffic in illegal drugs and its effect on domestic licensing and disciplinary boards charged with regulating opioids.[151] Financial and political questions cannot be dismissed as merely crass in any full sociocultural perspective on pain. Who is eligible for treatment in a pain center or pain clinic? Political issues concerning citizenship and insurance coverage may be highly relevant. Is "likelihood of improvement" a formal criterion for enrolling patients? If insurance coverage is held to enhance the likelihood of improvement, then uninsured patients are de facto excluded. Some 10.4% of the US population still has no health insurance, despite recent changes, with percentages far higher among black and Latino minorities.[152] These bland statistics reveal pain silently enfolded within larger, invisible systems of biopower and of biopolitics.

Biopower and *biopolitics* are not soft concepts but hard realities that influence the profound inequalities (in access to care and in treatment of pain) that face individual patients as the consequences of race, socioeconomic status, and the fast-changing configuration of national and international health care systems. In Haiti, for example, anthropologist-physician Paul Farmer struggles against global pharmaceutical companies and cost-driven policies of the World Health Organization to provide medication for HIV/AIDS patients with multiple drug-resistant tuberculosis (TB).[153] Even national systems of universal health care cannot ignore cost in decisions about whom to treat and how. Among postoperative patients, patient-controlled analgesia (PCA) lessens pain, shortens hospital stays, and reduces pain medication, but it is also expensive, raising unresolved questions about cost-effectiveness, social justice, and access to care.[154] Who gets it? In a balancing act that weighs cost against temporary discomfort, many patients and systems cannot afford adequate pain control.[155] There is no mechanism for creating balance—indeed, no agreement about what constitutes balance. For HIV/AIDS patients in sub-Saharan Africa who may barely find enough to eat, pain medications and nondrug therapies alike are an unaffordable luxury.[156] Here, too, the operations of biopower and biopolitics in a non-Western sociocultural environment help bring to light the less obvious (more accepted) ways in which liberal democracies do or do not deal adequately in the management of pain.

The impact of changing worldwide health systems shows up in pain management as patient concern for alternative and complementary medicine. Patients today pick the latest secularized healing art from a menu of eclectic, health-related therapies marketed like vitamin pills to late-capitalist consumers in a new global "ethnomedicine."[157] In 1990, Americans made 425 million visits to providers of complementary and alternative medicine (CAM) or, as it was first called, "unconventional therapy."[158] This figure startled many analysts because it exceeded the population of the United States. It did not express an outright rejection of biomedicine, as 83% of these patients also sought treatment for the same condition from a medical doctor: Significantly, they also paid 75% of all costs out-of-pocket. A sense of the illicit nonetheless surrounded these excursions outside the biomedical model. The vast majority (72%) of patients who used unconventional therapies did not tell their physicians.

Official discourse and unofficial practice—including the practice and discourse of pain medicine—has begun to change in response to this new populist, eclectic self-care that draws its principles and therapies from around the globe. From 1990 to 1997, there was an almost 50% increase in visits to so-called "alternative medicine practitioners."[159] The number of visits soon exceeded the total visits to primary care physicians, and in 1998 the usually slow-footed US Congress established the National Center for Complementary and Alternative Medicine (NCCAM)—with a mandate to explore approaches to health and wellness "that the public is using, often without the benefit of rigorous scientific study."[160] CAM research increasingly supports the use of nontraditional treatments for symptom control among seriously ill and elderly patients.[161] No mere lifestyle fad, this change extends even to cancer patients, who show a high prevalence of CAM use, especially among patients who are well-educated, well-off, young, and female.[162] Three quarters of US medical schools now require coursework in CAM, and CAM therapies crossover to pain medicine with surprising ease. Among people reporting back or neck pain within the last 12 months, a national telephone survey in the United States found that 54% used complementary therapies (especially chiropractic, massage, and relaxation techniques), compared with 37% who saw a conventional provider.[163] Indeed, mind–body therapies have been shown both to cut the number of physician visits and to reduce arthritis pain.[164] As attitudes change and as science catches up, American physicians and patients can now consult research-based data on topics from acupuncture to zinc enfolded within the Internet site of a new National Center for Complementary and Integrative Health.

Pain is now the focus of significant research into CAM therapies, and today the NCCAM has an annual budget over $100 million, representing not only a major institutional shift but also changes in the application of biopower. Review articles give mixed reports concerning the cost-effectiveness and clinical benefit of CAM therapies for various pain syndromes, especially chronic low back pain.[165-167] Back pain is certainly the most common reason for visits to acupuncturists, chiropractors, and massage therapists.[168] Although CAM *mind–body* therapies are not a popular treatment for pain as yet, most patients with chronic back pain expressed at least an interest in CAM therapies.[169,170] The inconclusive and scattered data boil down to a strong initial preference among back pain patients for acupuncture, chiropractic, and massage: a view that pain management programs need to take into account not least because patient preferences encode pain beliefs and because beliefs as well as preferences change. Beyond an individual choice of therapies, however, a sociocultural perspective would emphasize how complementary and alternative therapies reflect changes in a globalized medical marketplace where drugs and surgeries for pain face increased competition from homeopaths, multicultural Internet remedies, mind–body meditation techniques, and assorted unconventional therapies. Consumer activism, global options, and perhaps even a discontent with traditional biomedicine are changing the culture of pain patients, and additional related changes are predictable for pain management.

The cultural system that has received most attention in its impact on chronic pain is disability insurance. Like most developed nations, for example, Scandinavian countries face rapidly mounting claims for pain associated with automobile accidents. Lithuania, however, which has no auto insurance, also shows no significant difference between accident victims and a control group in reports of headache and neck pain.[171] Chronic whiplash syndrome appears to be partly an artifact of social systems of accident and disability insurance. It is the systems, as much as persons in pain, that produce a call for pain treatment. This new post-1950s postmodern cash-driven disability narrative, however well intended, entails emotional costs for patients and financial costs for health care systems; it sometimes puts pain management programs in adversarial roles in relations to patients or to stage agencies; and it often makes successful treatment more difficult.[172–175]

Pain today, in short, exists inside cultures where national health care systems and third-party insurers may inadvertently establish potential careers for patients as damaging as hysteria in the 19th century. Even the decision to become a patient is a cultural artifact: In a small Aboriginal community in Australia, back pain is not regarded as a health issue, people do not show public pain behaviors, and sorcery is a standard resource.[176] Law as well as sorcery has an impact on pain. Some organizations require pain patients to sign contracts that transform prescription drug abuse into legal grounds for denial of treatment. Employers too play a role in reframing pain, as monotonous jobs and lack of workplace autonomy are predictors of chronic pain disability.[177] The category of repetitive stress injury shows how sociocultural changes create new patterns of pain. Older employees with lower education and lower occupational status appear at increased risk for disabling chronic pain.[178] Women of so-called "deprived" socioeconomic status run higher risk of pain and experience pain as more severe and disabling.[179]

Families as a sociocultural system, like jobs, add significant complications to pain.[180] Large-scale changes in family structure create new challenges for clinicians, as postmodern families emerge reconfigured as unstable, nuclear units fractured by divorce, blended across multiple marriages, mixed in race and gender, and marked by significant demographic shifts. The family dynamics of chronic pain has so far yielded inconclusive data.[181] Researchers agree, however, that pain and families exist in an intricate loop of reciprocal relations, such that the patient's pain affects the family and the family affects the patient's pain.[182,183] Among people with rheumatoid arthritis, spousal interaction has a complex influence on pain-related catastrophizing.[183] The precise family dynamics across specific disease conditions is less important here than identifiable links between family life and chronic pain patterns. As various emerging social roles and responses within the family structure grow clearer, pain specialists have particular reason to examine the related narratives and cultural forces that inescapably impinge on the individual experience of pain.

Conclusion: Summary and Synthesis

A sociocultural perspective is imperative for a full and adequate understanding of pain, especially chronic pain. The limitations of a molecular gaze for understanding chronic pain would seem clear in proposals that seek to reduce all pain to a single organic cause: for example, inflammation.[184] Inflammation is a biologic process common in chronic pain, but chronic pain is always both biologic and cultural. Neither inflammation nor any other single molecular process can wholly explain the peculiar difficulties of treating chronic pain in children, for example, where cognitive development, linguistic abilities, and family relations are central.[185] It cannot illuminate the challenges that face elderly chronic pain patients,[186] people with HIV/AIDS,[187,188] or dying patients.[189] Pain, from a transdermal perspective, is never simply a matter of molecules, nerves, or neurotransmitters, just as the practice of pain management is never just or entirely a matter of unambiguous evidence or of applied science.

Overdetermination, in psychoanalytic theory, refers to the concept that multiple causes combine to produce a single behavior, emotion, symptom, or dream. Chronic pain, usually overdetermined in spades, is often described today not as a symptom but as a disease, although it is less a classic disease state than a complex, changing, multivariate event staged within human consciousness as always open to and modified by the surrounding sociocultural environment. Contemporary Barcelona sculptor Jaume Plensa, in his gigantic figure entitled *Wonderland*, offers a powerful image of how we might reimagine the human figure in pain—not so much contorted in agony but rather (no matter what the outward expression) as semitransparent: embedded within a surrounding, interpenetrating, and changing sociocultural environment (Fig. 11.2).

The sociocultural environment today as it impinges on human pain includes skyscrapers, banking centers, multinational pharmaceutical corporations, civic plazas, monumental

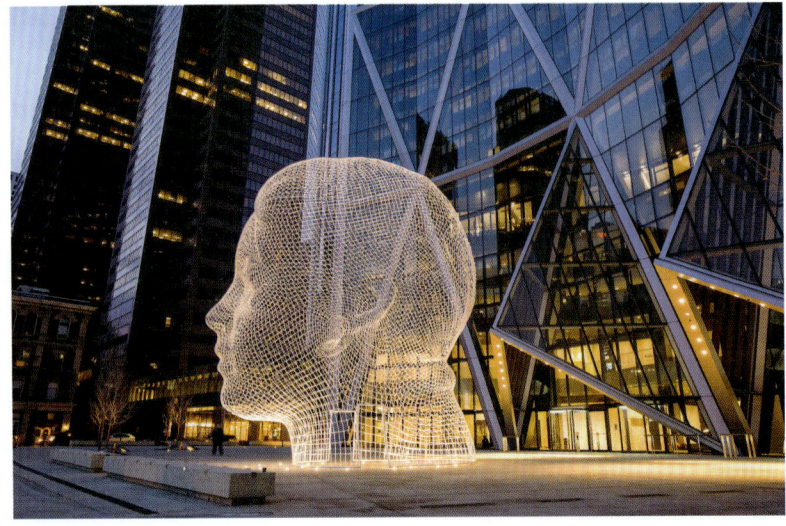

FIGURE 11.2 *Wonderland*, by Jaume Plensa, 2012. Calgary, Alberta. Painted stainless steel, 12 m high. *(Courtesy of the artist and Richard Gray Gallery, Chicago. Photographer: Thomas Porostocky.)*

artworks, and pain management programs even as it includes less tangible beliefs, attitudes, behaviors, and perceptions—all flowing through whatever individual organic neuromatrix or brain state gives rise to the phenomenon (as yet invisible to the molecular gaze) that we call consciousness. Human consciousness is ultimately where the organic processes of nociception culminate in pain.

Consciousness—arguably, an emergent property of human brains, but no matter how we define or imagine it—modifies and interprets nociceptive sensory input in ways consistently responsive to the changing sociocultural forces within an individual's immediate environment. It is an environment that for pain patients necessarily includes the clinician. Researchers recently confirmed, at least in electronic simulation, the hypothesis that patients who believe they share core beliefs and values with their clinician will report less pain than patients who do not.[189] Such findings extend our general understanding that chronic pain is open to significant modification—for better or worse—from workplace, gender, ethnicity, belief, emotion, money, age, racial stereotypes, and narrative, to name a few. Children, in part because of a distinctive cultural, social, and linguistic background, may experience pain very differently than adults do. First-generation immigrants may experience pain differently than their assimilated second-generation children do. Persons with HIV/AIDS may face a pain that is distinctive depending on how, in individual cases, a specific infectious disease engages the highly variable forces of geography, nation, social class, race, religion, stigma, and access to care. New media (such as Flickr and Tumblr) that combine visual images and multimodal elements are already extending and transforming traditional chronic pain narratives.[190] Future media and new social forces, as their energies flow through the open mesh of human consciousness, will doubtless bring new changes to the experience of intractable pain. Chronic pain, in short, cannot be reduced to a static diagram of cellular processes. It is the always extracellular, nonmolecular, sociocultural dimensions of chronic pain that promise to offer difficult and continually changing challenges that pain management programs in the 21st century will need to confront and to address effectively.

ACKNOWLEDGMENT

For his assistance, I am grateful to John Loeser, who attributes the phrase "transdermal pain" to his colleague Wilbert Fordyce. Many thanks as well to Daniel B. Carr.

References

1. Loeser JD. Economic implications of pain management. *Acta Anaesthesiol Scand* 1999;43(9):957–959.
2. Rose N. Introduction. In: *The Politics of Life Itself: Biomedicine, Power, and Subjectivity in the Twenty-First Century*. Princeton, NJ: Princeton University Press; 2007:1–8.
3. Loeser JD. The future: will pain be abolished or just pain specialists? *Pain Clin Updates* 2000;8(6):1–7.
4. Heath D, Rapp R, Taussig KS. Genetic citizenship. In: Nugent D, Vincent J, eds. *A Companion to the Anthropology of Politics*. Oxford, United Kingdom: Blackwell; 2004:152–167.
5. Gawande A. The heroism of incremental care. *The New Yorker*. January 2017. Available at: http://www.newyorker.com/magazine/2017/01/23/the-heroism-of-incremental-care.
6. Wallis C. The right (and wrong) way to treat pain. *Time Magazine*. February 2005. Available at: http://content.time.com/time/magazine/article/0,9171,1029836,00.html?iid=sr-link2.
7. Bartley EJ, Boissoneault J, Vargovich AM, et al. The influence of health care professional characteristics on pain management decisions. *Pain Med* 2015;16(1):99–111.
8. Craven P, Cinar O, Fosnocht D, et al. Prospective, 10-year evaluation of the impact of Hispanic ethnicity on pain manage practices in the ED. *Am J Emerg Med* 2014;32(9):1055–1059.
9. Dickason RM, Chauhan V, Mor A, et al. Racial differences in opiate administration for pain relief at an academic emergency department. *West J Emerg Med* 2015;16(3):372–380.
10. Drwecki BB. Education to identify and combat racial bias in pain treatment. *AMA J Ethics* 2015;17(3):221–228.
11. Goyal MK, Kuppermann N, Cleary SD, et al. Racial disparities in pain management of children with appendicitis in emergency departments. *JAMA Pediatr* 2015;169(11):996–1002.
12. Choi HK, Curhan G. Gout: epidemiology and lifestyle choices. *Curr Opin Rheumatol* 2005;17(3):341–345.
13. Singh JA. The impact of gout on patients' lives: a study of African-American and Caucasian men and women with gout. *Arthritis Res Ther* 2014;16(3):R132.
14. Fordyce WE, ed. *Back Pain in the Workplace: Management of Disability in Nonspecific Conditions*. Seattle, WA: IASP Press; 1995:4.
15. Bayer TE, Baer PE, Early C. Situational and psychophysiological factors in psychologically induced pain. *Pain* 1991;44:45–50.
16. Younger J, Aron A, Parke S, et al. Viewing pictures of a romantic partner reduces experimental pain: involvement of neural reward systems. *PLoS One* 2010;5(10):e13309. Available at: http://journals.plos.org/plosone/article?id=10.1371/journal.pone.0013309.
17. Merskey H, Bogduk N, eds. Pain terms: a current list with definitions and notes on usage. In: *Classification of Chronic Pain: Descriptions of Chronic Pain Syndromes and Definitions of Pain Terms*. 2nd ed. Seattle, WA: IASP Press; 1994:207–214.
18. Pianin E. US health care costs surge to 17 percent of GDP. *The Fiscal Times*. December 3, 2015. Available at: http://www.thefiscaltimes.com/2015/12/03/Federal-Health-Care-Costs-Surge-17-Percent-GDP.
19. Heshusius L. A life altered. In: *Inside Chronic Pain: An Intimate and Critical Account*. Ithaca, NY: Cornell University Press; 2009:1–13.
20. Fordyce WE, ed. *Back Pain in the Workplace: Management of Disability in Nonspecific Conditions*. Seattle, WA: IASP Press; 1995:xiii.
21. Becker DM. Through the looking glass: the patient's point of view. In: Mills AE, Chen DT, Werhane PH, et al, eds. *Professionalism in Tomorrow's Healthcare System: Towards Fulfilling the ACGME Requirements for Systems-Based Practice and Professionalism*. Hagerstown, MD: University Publishing Group; 2005:169–177.
22. American Pain Society Quality of Care Committee. Quality improvement guidelines for the treatment of acute pain and cancer pain. *JAMA* 1995;274:1874–1880.
23. Wee B, Hiller R. Pain control. *Medicine* 2011;39:639–644.
24. SUPPORT Principal Investigators. A controlled trial to improve care for seriously ill hospitalized patients. *JAMA* 1995;274(20):1591–1598.
25. Green CR, Anderson KO, Baker TA, et al. The unequal burden of pain: confronting racial and ethnic disparities in pain. *Pain Med* 2003;4(3):277–294.
26. Foster JB. Racial, ethnic variables shape the experience of chronic pain. *Appl Neurol* 2006;2(11):19–22.
27. Morris RS, Wallenstein S, Natale DK, et al. "We don't carry that"—failure of pharmacies in predominantly nonwhite neighborhoods to stock opioid analgesics. *N Engl J Med* 2000;342(14):1023–1026.
28. Azevedo RT, Macaluso E, Avenanti A, et al. Their pain is not our pain: brain and autonomic correlates of empathic resonance with the pain of same and different race individuals. *Hum Brain Mapp* 2013;34(12):3168–3181.
29. Bekanich SJ, Wanner N, Junkins S, et al. A multifaceted initiative to improve clinician awareness of pain management disparities. *Am J Med Qual* 2014;29(5):388–396.
30. Drwecki BB, Moore CE, Ward SE, et al. Reducing racial disparities in pain treatment: the role of empathy and perspective-taking. *Pain* 2011;152(5):1001–1006.
31. Wolff BB. Ethnocultural factors influencing pain and illness behavior. *Clin J Pain* 1985;1(1):23–30.
32. Bates MS, Edwards WT, Anderson KO. Ethnocultural influences on variation in chronic pain perception. *Pain* 1993;52(1):101–112.
33. Madjar I. Pain and the surgical patient: a cross-cultural perspective. *Aust J Adv Nurs* 1985;2(2):29–33.
34. Haozous EA, Knobf MT. "All my tears were gone": suffering and cancer pain in Southwest American Indians. *J Pain Symptom Manage* 2013;45(6):1050–1060.
35. Trawalter S, Hoffma KM, Waytz A. Racial bias in perceptions of others' pain. *PLoS One* 2012;7(11):e0048546. Available at: http://journals.plos.org/plosone/article?id=10.1371/journal.pone.0048546.
36. Rasooly IR, Mullins PM, Mazer-Amirshahi M, et al. The impact of race on analgesia use among pediatric emergency department patients. *J Pediatr* 2014;165(3):618–621.
37. Shah AA, Zogg CK, Zafar SN, et al. Analgesic access for acute abdominal pain in the emergency department among racial/ethnic minority patients: a nationwide examination. *Med Care* 2015;53(12):1000–1009.
38. Jordan JM. Effect of race and ethnicity on outcomes in arthritis and rheumatic conditions. *Curr Opin Rheumatol* 1999;11(2):98–103.
39. Morris DB. Ethnicity and pain. *Pain Clin Updates* 2001;9(4):1–8.
40. Rose N. Race in the age of genomic medicine. In: *The Politics of Life Itself: Biomedicine, Power, and Subjectivity in the Twenty-First Century*. Princeton, NJ: Princeton University Press; 2007:155–186.
41. Todd K, Samaroo N, Hoffman J. Ethnicity as a risk factor for inadequate emergency department analgesia. *JAMA* 1993;269(12):1537–1539.
42. Todd KH. Pain assessment and ethnicity. *Ann Emerg Med* 1996;27(4):421–423.
43. Hoberman J. *Black and Blue: The Origin and Consequences of Medical Racism*. Berkeley: University of California Press; 2012.

44. Chapman EN, Kaatz A, Carnes M. How doctors may unwittingly perpetuate health care disparities. *J Gen Int Med* 2013;28(11):1504–1510.
45. Ballas SK. *Sickle Cell Pain*. Seattle, WA: IASP Press, 1998.
46. Wailoo K. *Dying in the City of the Blues: Sickle Cell Anemia and the Politics of Race and Health*. Chapel Hill, NC: University of North Carolina Press; 2001.
47. Bernabei R, Gambassi G, Lapane K, et al. Management of pain in elderly patients with cancer. *JAMA* 1998;279(23):1877–1882.
48. Cleeland C, Gonin R, Baez L, et al. Pain and treatment of pain in minority patients with cancer: the Eastern Cooperative Oncology group minority outpatient pain study. *Ann Inter Med* 1997;127(9):813–816.
49. Joranson DE. Global opioid consumption: trends, barriers, and diversion. *IASP Newsletter*. September/October 1994: 4–5.
50. Pain and Policy Studies Group, University of Wisconsin-Madison Paul P. Carbone Comprehensive Cancer Center. Availability of morphine and pethidine in the world and Africa, with a special focus on Botswana, Ethiopia, Kenya, Malawi, Nigeria, Rwanda, Tanzania, Zambia. Available at: http://www.painpolicy.wisc.edu/publicat/monograp/africa06.pdf.
51. Riskowski JL. Associations of socioeconomic position and pain prevalence in the United States: findings from the National Health and Nutrition Examination Survey. *Pain Med* 2014;15(9):1508–1521.
52. DePalma A. For Mexicans, pain relief is both a medical and a political problem. *New York Times*. June 19, 1966:A4.
53. Martin EM, Barkley TW Jr. Improving cultural competence in end-of-life pain management. *Nursing* 2016;46(1):32–41.
54. Gear RW, Miaskowski C, Gordon NC, et al. Kappa-opioids produce significantly greater analgesia in women than in men. *Nat Med* 1996;2(11):1248–1250.
55. Liem EB, Lin CM, Suleman MI, et al. Anesthetic requirement is increased in redheads. *Anesthesiology* 2004;101(2):279–283.
56. Liem EB, Joiner TV, Tsueda K, et al. Increased sensitivity to thermal pain and reduced subcutaneous lidocaine efficacy in redheads. *Anesthesiology* 2005;102(3):509–514.
57. Buse DC, Loder EW, Gorman JA, et al. Sex differences in the prevalence, symptoms, and associated features of migraine, probable migraine and other severe headache: results of the American Migraine Prevalence and Prevention (AMPP) Study. *Headache* 2013;53(8):1278–1299.
58. Berkley KJ. Female pain versus male pain? In: Fillingim RB, ed. *Sex, Gender, and Pain*. Seattle, WA: IASP Press; 2000:373–381.
59. Butler J. Language, power, and the strategies of displacement. In: *Gender Trouble: Feminism and the Subversion of Identity*. New York: Routledge; 1990:25–33.
60. Phelan SM, Hardeman RR. Health professionals' pain management decisions are influenced by their role (nurse or physician) and by patient gender, age and ethnicity. *Evid Based Nurs* 2015;18(2):58.
61. Hwang U, Richardson LD, Harris B, et al. The quality of emergency department pain care for older adult patients. *J Am Geriatr Soc* 2010;58(11):2122–2128.
62. Giordana J, Gomez CF, Harrison C. On the potential role for interventional pain management in palliative care. *Pain Physician* 2007;10(3):395–398.
63. Morris DB. Pain at the end of life: optimal care. In: Moore R, ed. *Handbook of Pain and Palliative Care*. 2nd ed. New York: Springer. In press.
64. Anquinet L, Rietjens JAC, Seale C, et al. The practice of continuous deep sedation until death in Flanders (Belgium), The Netherlands, and the UK: a comparative study. *J Pain Symptom Manage* 2012;44(1):33–43.
65. Pellegrino ED. Emerging ethical issues in palliative care. *JAMA* 1998;279:1521–1522.
66. Jensen MC, Brant-Zawadzki MN, Obuchowski N, et al. Magnetic resonance imaging of the lumbar spine in people without back pain. *N Engl J Med* 1994;331(2):69–73.
67. Von Korff M, Barlow W, Cherkin D, et al. Effects of practice style in managing back pain. *Ann Inter Med* 1994;121(3):187–195.
68. Wall PD, Jones M. The causes of pain. In: *Defeating Pain: The War Against a Silent Epidemic*. New York: Plenum Press; 1991:31–68.
69. Bigos SJ, Battié MC, Spengler DM, et al. A prospective study of work perceptions and psychosocial factors affecting the report of back injury. *Spine* 1991;16(1):1–6.
70. Dwyer T, Raftery AE. Industrial accidents are produced by social relations of work: a sociological theory of industrial accidents. *Appl Ergon* 1991;22(3):167–178.
71. Coggon D, Ntani G, Palmer KT, et al. Disabling musculoskeletal pain in working populations: is it the job, the person, or the culture? *Pain* 2013;154(6):856–863.
72. Geriatrics and Extended Care Strategic Healthcare Group. *Pain as the 5th Vital Sign Toolkit*. Washington, DC: Veterans Health Administration; 2000.
73. Mularski RA, White-Chu F, Overbay D, et al. Measuring Pain as the 5th Vital Sign does not improve quality of pain management. *J Gen Intern Med* 2006;21(6):607–612.
74. Kitzes JA. Palliative medicine: facing the challenge of care beyond cure. *IHS Prim Care Provid* 1999;24(2):23–25.
75. Vlaeyen JWS, Crombez G. Fear and pain. *Pain Clin Updates* 2007;15(6):1–4.
76. Sullivan MD. Pain as emotion. *Pain Forum* 1996;5(3):208–209.
77. Norbury TA, MacGregor AJ, Urwin J, et al. Heritability of responses to painful stimuli in women: a classical twin study. *Brain* 2007;130(11):3041–3049.
78. Coghill RC, McHaffie JG, Yen YF. Neural correlates of interindividual differences in the subjective experience of pain. *Proc Natl Acad Sci USA* 2003;100(14):8538–8542.
79. Barrett LF. Why our emotions are cultural—not built in at birth. *The Guardian*. March 26, 2017. Available at: https://www.theguardian.com/lifeandstyle/2017/mar/26/why-our-emotions-are-cultural-not-hardwired-at-birth?CMP=Share_iOSApp_Other.
80. George SK, Jung PG, eds. *Cultural Ontology of the Self in Pain*. New York: Springer; 2016.
81. Gray JA. *The Neuropsychology of Anxiety: An Enquiry into the Functions of the Septo-Hippocampal System*. Oxford, United Kingdom: Clarendon Press; 1982.
82. Morris DB. *The Culture of Pain*. Berkeley: University of California Press; 1991.
83. King DW. African Americans and the culture of pain. Charlottesville, VA: University of Virginia Press; 2008.
84. Coakley S, Shekemay KK, eds. *Pain and Its Transformations: The Interface of Culture and Biology*. Cambridge, MA: Harvard University Press; 2008.
85. Brena SF, Sanders SH, Motoyama, H. American and Japanese chronic low back pain patients: cross-cultural similarities and differences. *Clin J Pain* 1990;6(2):118–124.
86. Ferreira-Valente MA, Pais-Ribeiro JL, Jensen, MP. Associations between psychosocial factors and pain intensity, physical functioning, and psychological functioning in patients with chronic pain: a cross-cultural comparison. *Clin J Pain* 2014;30(8):713–723.
87. Boissoneault J, Bunch JR, Robinson R. The roles of ethnicity, sex, and parental pain modeling in rating of experienced and imagined pain events. *J Behav Med* 2015;38(5):809–816.
88. Bernardes SF, Marques S, Matos M. Old and in pain: enduring and situational effects of cultural aging stereotypes on older people's pain experiences. *Eur J Pain* 2015;19(7):994–1001.
89. Lin I, O'Sullivan P, Coffin J, et al. "I can sit and talk to her:" Aboriginal people, chronic low back pain and healthcare practitioner communication. *Aust Fam Physician* 2014;43(5):320–324.
90. Strong J, Nielsen M, Williams M, et al. Quiet about pain: experiences of Aboriginal people in two rural communities. *Aust J Rural Health* 2015;23(3):181–184.
91. Carrion IV, Cagle JG, Van Dussen DJ, et al. Knowledge about hospice care and beliefs about pain management: exploring differences between Hispanics and Non-Hispanics. *Am J Hosp Palliat Care* 2015;32(6):647–653.
92. Sullivan MD. Pain in language: from sentience to sapience. *Pain Forum* 1995;4(1):3–14.
93. Williams DA, Thorn BE. An empirical assessment of pain beliefs. *Pain* 1989;36:351–358.
94. Williams DA. Acute pain management. In: Gatchel RJ, Turk DC, eds. *Psychological Approaches to Pain Management: A Practitioner's Handbook*. New York: Guilford Press; 1996:55–77.
95. Williams DA, Keefe FJ. Pain beliefs and the use of cognitive-behavioral coping strategies. *Pain* 1991;46:185–190.
96. Jensen MP, Karoly P. Pain-specific beliefs, perceived symptom severity, and adjustment to chronic pain. *Clin J Pain* 1992;8:123–130.
97. Shutty MS Jr, DeGood DE, Tuttle DH. Chronic pain patients' beliefs about their pain and treatment outcomes. *Arch Phys Med Rehabil* 1990;71:128–132.
98. Booker SQ. African Americans' perceptions of pain and pain management: a systematic review. *J Transcult Nurs* 2016;27(1):73–80.
99. Darlow B, Perry M, Stanley J, et al. Cross-sectional survey of attitudes and beliefs about back pain in New Zealand. *BMJ Open* 2014;4(5):e004725.
100. Finnström B, Söderhamn O. Conceptions of pain among Somali women. *J Adv Nurs* 2006;54(4):418–425.
101. Goldstein JN, Ibrahim SA, Frankel ES, et al. Race, pain, and beliefs associated with interest in complementary and alternative medicine among inner city veterans. *Pain Med* 2015;16(8):1467–1474.
102. Lacasse A, Connelly JA, Choinière M. The chronic pain myth scale: development and validation of a French-Canadian instrument measuring knowledge, beliefs, and attitudes of people in the community towards chronic pain. *Pain Res Manag* 2016;2016:5940206.
103. Pagare VK, Dhanraj T, Thakkar D, et al. Beliefs about low back pain: status quo in Indian general population. *J Back Musculoskelet Rehabil* 2015;28(4):731–737.
104. Miro J, Huguet A, Jensen MP. Pain beliefs predict pain intensity and pain status in children: usefulness of the pediatric version of the survey of pain attitudes. *Pain Med* 2014;15(6):887–897.
105. Torensma B, Thomassen I, van Velzen M, et al. Pain experience and perception in the obese subject systemic review (revised version). *Obes Surg* 2016;26(3):631–639.
106. Eccleston C, Williams AC, Rogers WS. Patients' and professionals' understandings of the causes of chronic pain: blame, responsibility and identity protection. *Soc Sci Med* 1997;43(5):699–709.
107. Thompson EL, Broadbent J, Bertino MD, Staiger PK. Do pain-related beliefs influence adherence to multidisciplinary rehabilitation? A systematic review. *Clin J Pain* 2016;32(2):164–178.
108. van Rysewyk S, ed. *Meanings of Pain*. New York: Springer; 2017.
109. Fishbain DA, Bruns D, Bruns A, et al. The perception of being a burden in acute and chronic pain. *Pain Med* 2016;17(3):530–538.
110. Hoffman KM, Trawalter S, Axt JR, et al. Racial bias in pain assessment and treatment recommendations, and false beliefs about biological differences between blacks and whites. *Proc Natl Acad Sci U S A* 2016;113(16):4296–4301.

111. Lame IE, Peters ML, Vlaeyen JW, et al. Quality of life in chronic pain is more associated with beliefs about pain, than with pain intensity. *Eur J Pain* 2005;9(1):15–24.

112. Loeser J. Socioeconomic factors in chronic pain and its management. In: Cousins M, Bridenbaugh P, Carr D, et al, eds. *Cousins and Bridenbaugh's Neural Blockade in Clinical Anesthesia and Management of Pain.* 4th ed. Philadelphia: Lippincott Williams & Wilkins; 2008: 644–650.

113. Raber P, Devor M. Social variables affect phenotype in the neuroma model of neuropathic pain. *Pain* 2002;97(1–2):139–150.

114. MacIntyre A. *After Virtue: A Study in Moral Theory.* Notre Dame, IN: Notre Dame University Press; 1981:197.

115. Sarbin TR, ed. *Narrative Psychology: The Storied Nature of Human Conduct.* New York: Praeger; 1986.

116. Crossley ML. *Introducing Narrative Psychology: Self, Trauma and the Construction of Meaning.* New York: McGraw-Hill; 2000.

117. Charon R. Narrative medicine: a model for empathy, reflection, profession, trust. *JAMA* 2001;286(15):1897–1902.

118. Kearney R. Where do stories come from? In: *On Stories.* New York: Routledge; 2002:3–14.

119. Carr DR, Loeser JD, Morris DB, eds. *Narrative, Pain, and Suffering.* Seattle, WA: IASP Press; 2005.

120. Charon R. Suffering, storytelling, and community: an approach to pain treatment from Columbia's Program in Narrative Medicine. In: Flor H, Kalso E, Dostrovsky JO, eds. *Proceedings of the 11th World Congress on Pain.* Seattle, WA: IASP Press; 2006:19–27.

121. Kelley P, Clifford P. Coping with chronic pain: assessing narrative approaches. *Soc Work* 1997;42(3):266–277.

122. Jackson JE. *Camp Pain: Talking with Chronic Pain Patients.* Philadelphia: University of Pennsylvania Press; 1999.

123. Smyth JM, Stone AA, Hurewitz A, et al. Effects of writing about stressful experiences on symptom reduction in patients with asthma or rheumatoid arthritis: a randomized trial. *JAMA* 1999;281(14):1304–1309.

124. Pennebaker JW, Beall SK. Confronting a traumatic event: toward an understanding of inhibition and disease. *J Abnor Psychol* 1986;95(3): 274–281.

125. Pennebaker JW, Seagal JD. Forming a story: the health benefits of narrative. *J Clin Psychol* 1999;55(10):1243–1254.

126. Pennebaker JW. *Opening Up: The Healing Power of Expressing Emotions.* New York: Guilford Press; 1997:103.

127. Nelson HL, ed. *Stories and Their Limits: Narrative Approaches to Bioethics.* New York: Routledge; 1997.

128. Waitzkin H, Magaña H. The black box in somatization: unexplained physical symptoms, culture, and narratives of trauma. *Soc Sci Med* 1997: 45(6):811–825.

129. Charon R, Montello M, eds. *Stories Matter: The Role of Narrative in Medical Ethics.* New York: Routledge; 2002.

130. Morris DB. Ethics beyond guidelines: culture, pain, and conflict. In: Dostrovsky JO, Carr DB, Koltzenburg M, eds. *Proceedings of the 10th World Congress on Pain.* Seattle, WA: IASP Press; 2003:37–48.

131. McCracken LM, Yang SY. The role of values in a contextual cognitive-behavioral approach to chronic pain. *Pain* 2006;123(1–2):137–145.

132. Rippentrop AE, Altmaier EM, Chen JJ, et al. The relationship between religion/spirituality and physical health, mental health, and pain in a chronic pain population. *Pain* 2005;116(3):311–321.

133. Borneman T, Ferrell B, Puchalski CM. Evaluation of the FICA tool for spiritual assessment. *J Pain Symptom Manage* 2010;40(2):163–173.

134. Buessing A, Balzat HJ, Heusser P. Spiritual needs of patients with chronic pain diseases and cancer—validation of the Spiritual Needs Questionnaire. *Eur J Med Res* 2010;15(6):266–273.

135. Brennan F, Carr DB, Cousins M. Pain management: a fundamental human right. *Anesth Analg* 2007;105(1):205–221.

136. MacIntyre A. *Whose Justice? Which Rationality?* South Bend, IN: University of Notre Dame Press; 1988.

137. Melzack R, Wall PD. Pain mechanisms: a new theory. *Science* 1965; 150(699):971–979.

138. Dickenson AH. Gate control theory of pain stands the test of time. *Br J Anaesth* 2002;88(6):755–757.

139. Siniscalco D, Rossi F, Maione S. Molecular approaches for neuropathic pain treatment. *Curr Med Chem* 2007;14(16):1783–1787.

140. Melzack R. From the gate to the neuromatrix. *Pain* 1999;82(suppl 1): S121–S126.

141. Loeser JD. What is chronic pain? *Theor Med* 1991;12:215–216.

142. Volinn E. The epidemiology of low back pain in the rest of the world: a review of surveys in low- and middle-income countries. *Spine* 1997;22(15): 1747–1754.

143. Broderick JE, Keefe FJ, Schneider S, et al. Cognitive behavioral therapy for chronic pain is effective, but for whom? *Pain* 2016;157(9):2115–2123.

144. Snyder CR, Lopez SJ, eds. *Handbook of Positive Psychology.* New York: Oxford University Press; 2002.

145. Morris DB. Success stories: narrative, pain, and the limits of storylessness. In: Carr DB, Loeser JD, Morris DB, eds. *Narrative, Pain, and Suffering.* Seattle, WA: IASP Press; 2005:269–285.

146. Krause E. *Power & Illness: The Political Sociology of Health and Medical Care.* New York: Elsevier; 1977:xi.

147. Foucault M. *Power/Knowledge: Selected Interviews and Other Writings 1972–1977.* Gordon C, Marshall L, Mepham J, et al, trans. New York: Pantheon Books; 1980:183–193.

148. Sullivan MD. *The Patient as Agent of Health and Health Care.* New York: Oxford University Press; 2017.

149. Foucault M. *The History of Sexuality: Volume I: An Introduction.* Hurley R, trans. New York: Random House; 1978:140–144.

150. Rose N. Politics. In: *The Politics of Life Itself: Biomedicine, Power, and Subjectivity in the Twenty-First Century.* Princeton, NJ: Princeton University Press; 2007:41–76.

151. Hill CS Jr. The negative influence of licensing and disciplinary boards and drug enforcement agencies on pain treatment with opioid analgesics. *J Pharm Care Pain Symp Control* 1993;1(1):43–62.

152. Barry-Jester AM, Casselman B. 33 million Americans still don't have health insurance. Available at: https://fivethirtyeight.com/features/33-million-americans -still-dont-have-health-insurance.

153. Farmer P. *Pathologies of Power: Health, Human Rights, and the New War on the Poor.* Berkeley: University of California Press; 2003.

154. Jacox A, Carr DB, Mahrenholz DM, et al. Cost considerations in patient-controlled analgesia. *Pharmacoeconomics* 1997;12(2 pt 1):109–120.

155. Viscusi ER, Schechter LN. Patient-controlled analgesia: finding a balance between cost and comfort. *Am J Health Syst Pharm* 2006;63(8 suppl 1):S3–S13.

156. Laurent S. No time to die. In: Carr DB, Loeser JD, Morris DB, eds. *Narrative, Pain, and Suffering.* Seattle, WA: IASP Press; 2005:243–248.

157. Herskovits EJ. *Sick at Heart: Modern Disease & Modern Therapeutics in Malaysia.* San Francisco, CA: University of California San Francisco; 1999:14–19.

158. Eisenberg DM, Kessler RC, Foster C, et al. Unconventional medicine in the United States: prevalence, costs, and patterns of use. *N Engl J Med* 1993;328(4):246–252.

159. Eisenberg DM, Davis RB, Ettner SL, et al. Trends in alternative medicine use in the United States, 1990-1997: results of a follow-up national survey. *JAMA* 1998;280(18):1569–1575.

160. Francis S, Collins FS. NIH Complementary and Integrative Health agency gets new name. Available at: https://www.nih.gov/news-events/news-releases /nih-complementary-integrative-health-agency-gets-new-name.

161. Luskin FM, Newell KA, Griffith M, et al. A review of mind/body therapies in the treatment of musculoskeletal disorders with implications for the elderly. *Altern Ther Health Med* 2000;6(2):46–56.

162. Cassileth BR, Vickers AJ. High prevalence of complementary and alternative medicine use among cancer patients: implications for research and clinical care. *J Clin Oncol* 2005;23(12):2590–2592.

163. Wolsko PM, Eisenberg DM, Davis RB, et al. Patterns and perceptions of care for treatment of back and neck pain: results of a national survey. *Spine* 2003;28(3):292–297.

164. Eisenberg DM, Post DE, Davis RB, et al. Addition of choice of complementary therapies to usual care for acute low pack pain: a randomized controlled trial. *Spine* 2007;32(2):151–158.

165. Sherman KJ, Cherkin DC, Connelly MT, et al. Complementary and alternative medical therapies for chronic low back pain: what treatments are patients willing to try? *BMC Complement Altern Med* 2004;4:9.

166. Kizhakkeveettil A, Rose K, Kadar GE. Integrative therapies for low back pain that include complementary and alternative medicine care: a systematic review. *Glob Adv Health Med* 2014;3(5):49–64.

167. Furlan AD, Yazdi F, Gross A, et al. A systematic review and meta-analysis of efficacy, cost-effectiveness, and safety of selected complementary and alternative medicine for neck and low-back pain. *Evid Based Complement Alternat Med* 2012;2012:953139.

168. Sherman KJ, Cherkin DC, Deyo RA, et al. The diagnosis and treatment of chronic back pain by acupuncturists, chiropractors, and massage therapists. *Clin J Pain* 2006;22(3):227–234.

169. Wolsko PM, Eisenberg DM, Davis RB, et al. Use of mind-body medical therapies. *J Gen Intern Med* 2004;19(1):43–50.

170. Tindle HA, Wolsko P, Davis RB, et al. Factors associated with the use of mind body therapies among United States adults with musculoskeletal pain. *Complement Ther Med* 2005;13(3):155–164.

171. Schrader H, Obelieniene D, Bovim G, et al. Natural evolution of late whiplash syndrome outside the medicolegal context. *Lancet* 1996;347(9010): 1207–1211.

172. Teasell RW. Compensation and chronic pain. *Clin J Pain* 2001;17(4 suppl): S46–S54.

173. Mendelson G. Compensation and chronic pain. *Pain* 1992;48(2):121–123.

174. Guest GH, Drummond PD. Effect of compensation on emotional state and disability in chronic back pain. *Pain* 1992;48(2):125–130.

175. Rohling ML, Binder LM, Langhinrichsen-Rohling J. Money matters: a meta-analytic review of the association between financial compensation and the experience and treatment of chronic pain. *Health Psychol* 1995;14(6): 537–547.

176. Honeyman PT, Jacobs EA. Effects of culture on back pain in Australian Aboriginals. *Spine* 1996;21(7):841–843.

177. Teasell RW, Bombardier C. Employment-related factors in chronic pain and chronic pain disability. *Clin J Pain* 2001;17(4 suppl):S39–S45.

178. Saastamoinen P, Leino-Arjas P, Laaksonen M, et al. Socio-economic differences in the prevalence of acute, chronic and disabling chronic pain among ageing employees. *Pain* 2005;114(3):364–371.

179. Jablonska B, Soares JJ, Sundin O. Pain among women: associations with socio-economic and work conditions. *Eur J Pain* 2006;10(5):435–447.

180. Payne B, Norfleet MA. Chronic pain and the family: a review. *Pain* 1986; 26(1):1–22.

181. Flor H, Turk DC, Rudy TE. Pain and families. II. assessment and treatment. *Pain* 1987;30(1):29–45.

182. Roy R. *The Family and Chronic Pain: A Special Issue of the International Journal of Family Therapy.* New York: Human Sciences Press; 1985.

183. Holtzman S, DeLongis A. One day at a time: the impact of daily satisfaction with spouse responses on pain, negative affect and catastrophizing among individuals with rheumatoid arthritis. *Pain* 2007;131(1–2):202–213.

184. Omoigui S. The biochemical origin of pain—proposing a new law of pain: the origin of all pain is inflammation and the inflammatory response. *Med Hypotheses* 2007;69(1):70–82.

185. McGrath PJ, Finley GA, eds. *Pediatric Pain: Biological and Social Context.* Seattle, WA: IASP Press; 2003.

186. Gibson SJ, Weiner DK, eds. *Pain in Older Persons.* Seattle, WA: IASP Press; 2005.

187. Breitbart W, Dibiase L. Current perspectives on pain in AIDS. *Oncology* 2002;16(6):818–829, 834–835.

188. Breitbart W, Dibiase L. Current perspectives on pain in AIDS. *Oncology* 2002;16(7):964–968, 972.

189. Losin EAR, Anderson SR, Wager TD. Feelings of clinician-patient similarity and trust: evidence from simulated clinical interactions. *J Pain.* In press.

190. Gonzalez-Polledo E, Tarr J. The thing about pain: the remaking of illness narratives in chronic pain expressions on social media. *New Media Soc* 2016;18(8):1455–1472.

CHAPTER 12

Ethical Issues in Pain Management

The fourth edition of this book was the first to include chapters specifically addressing the ethical dimensions of pain management. This is curious because the duty of physicians to relieve pain and suffering has been acknowledged for centuries. Indeed, this duty has been deemed an essential component of the ethos of medicine, as fundamental as the diagnosis and treatment of maladies. The rise of ethical discourse on the relief of pain and suffering in the late 20th century was prompted by a growing recognition that all too often pain was not adequately treated, and far too many patients unnecessarily endured the pain and suffering engendered by their illness. The fact that failure to adequately treat pain was not viewed until relatively recently as an ethical problem may have been due in large measure to the prevailing perception in medicine that pain was a necessary concomitant of illness which the "good" patient must bear with equanimity. Indeed, that is a common dictionary definition of the adjectival form of the word patient.

In light of the preceding text, one can argue that the traditional view of the ethics of pain management, to the extent that it was articulated at all in the professional literature, provided a basis for undertreating pain, particularly if what was required to adequately relieve pain involved the administration of opioid analgesics. From the time of its development and inclusion in the medical pharmacopeia, morphine, and subsequent synthetic derivatives, has been recognized as a two-edged sword, carrying both the benefit of pain relief and the burden of potential addiction. The widespread phenomenon of undertreated pain seemed to be a product of a risk/benefit calculation by physicians that the risks of addition to opioids were unacceptably high, whereas the benefits of pain relief were relatively inconsequential. Particularly, in the second half of the 20th century, the clinical focus was on formulating a diagnosis and implementing disease-directed therapies, not palliating symptoms.

During the last several decades, however, there has been a gradual but highly significant paradigm shift in the ethics of pain management. Until quite recently, as David Morris insightfully notes in his book, *The Culture of Pain*, "The everyday medical dealings with pain conceal unacknowledged ethical questions." Even in the care of cancer patients, Morris continues, the clinical ethos has been tainted by "an unacknowledged moral code expressing half-baked notions about the evil of drugs and the duty to bear affliction." He concludes with the grim observation that "the ethics of pain management, unfortunately, may not receive proper attention until the first doctor is successfully sued for failing to provide adequate relief."[1] There was a remarkable prescience to Morris's suggestion, for in the very year in which his book was published, a jury awarded millions of dollars in both compensatory and punitive damages to the family of a patient whose terminal cancer pain was undertreated. That case is discussed in detail in Chapter 15 of this book. Similarly, the ethical issues pertaining to the care of the dying patient are discussed in depth in Chapter 13, and the laws and policies relating to opioid analgesia are surveyed in Chapter 14.

In the decade and a half since the publication of *The Culture of Pain*, the ethics of pain management has finally begun to receive the attention, discussion, and debate that had been so starkly absent before. This was the result not only of a heightened sensitivity to the phenomenology of pain and the suffering which it can engender or exacerbate but also of recognition of its multiplicity of sequelae. Also during this period, there was a remarkable shift in the prevailing view about the risk of addiction associated with medically directed opioid use. It is this last item that has undergone yet another significant transformation in the years since the fourth edition of this book was published. In the sections that follow, I consider the evolutionary process of the ethics of pain management and the current state of affairs.

Pain, Suffering, and the Core Values of Health Care

For centuries, the core values of medicine and the other health professions never seemed to be in doubt. They were often, however, encapsulated in vague maxims of uncertain origin and authenticity such as *primum non nocere* (first do no harm) or "to cure when possible, to relieve often, and to comfort always." The core ethical principles on which these maxims were grounded—beneficence and nonmaleficence—were unquestionably formulated by physicians during the long reign of paternalism as the overarching paradigm for the professional–patient relationship. What constituted benefit and harm, and when the zealous pursuit of cure should yield to the provision of comfort, or more radically still, occur simultaneously, was for the physician, not the patient, to determine. In the latter half of the 20th century, particularly but certainly not exclusively in the United States, the evolution of medical jurisprudence and the revolution in bioethics challenged the legitimacy of the paternalistic paradigm. This challenge was grounded on an emerging principle of bioethics—respect for individual patient autonomy. Indeed, by the end of that century, paternalism had been almost completely discredited, replaced by a new paradigm grounded on the legal duty to obtain informed consent (and to accept an informed refusal) supported by and in turn operating in affirmation of the most recent bioethical principle.[2] The new paradigm for the professional–patient relationship became that of shared decision making.[3]

Although beneficence and nonmaleficence were retained among the core principles of modern bioethics along with a fourth justice, the clinician was no longer considered the ultimate authority on what constituted benefit and harm in the care of any particular patient. It is, after all, the patient who must endure the rigors of medical interventions and/or the burdens of disease. Thus, in the case of intractable disputes between clinician and patient, the patient has come to be recognized as the final arbiter. The dissenting clinician's option is to disengage from the relationship (but not precipitously to constitute abandonment) when and if respecting the patient's wishes compromises professional ethics or personal conscience.[4] The relief of pain and suffering, however, was not an integral part of this transformative process. Only quite recently have the legal, ethical, and public policy dimensions of pain management and palliative care begun to receive due consideration, thereby properly placing them within the emerging bioethical, jurisprudential, and sociocultural framework. Providing the details of this process is the task of this chapter, and the others in this section of this book.

THE DUTY TO RELIEVE PAIN AND SUFFERING

When, over three decades ago, Eric Cassell began his seminal article on suffering and medicine in *The New England Journal of Medicine*, he did not think it necessary to build an extensive case for the proposition that physicians have a duty to relieve pain and suffering. Nevertheless, his initial inquiries into the attitudes of physicians and patients about pain and suffering revealed a curious phenomenon: Contemporary patients and laypersons attached appreciably more significance to that duty than did his physician colleagues.[5] It is this disparity between laypersons and health care professionals in the prioritization of the need for and duty to provide not only treatment of disease but also relief of distress associated with it that caused, or at least significantly contributed to, the jury verdicts in legal cases alleging undertreatment of pain, which we consider in Chapter 15. If, in the ethos of ancient medicine, the relief of pain and suffering was the essence of beneficence (doing good) and nonmaleficence (avoiding harm), then something transformative took place in the transition to modern medicine. Otherwise, the opening passage of the preface to this book, which substantially expanded on Cassell's original article, would be incomprehensible. That passage, a remarkably stinging indictment of his own profession, reads, "The test of a system of medicine should be its adequacy in the face of suffering . . . modern medicine fails that test."[6] In it, he analyzes in great depth important distinctions between pain and suffering, including notable instances in which a person can experience pain but not suffer as well as suffer in the absence of pain. However, most pertinently to this chapter and book is his observation that pain is the most common cause of suffering, and people in pain experience suffering when it is severe, uncontrolled, and seemingly without end.

CURATIVE VERSUS PALLIATIVE PARADIGMS OF PATIENT CARE

Continuing with Cassell's analysis, the willful blindness that afflicts modern medicine with regard to pain and suffering (with the exception of those who specialize in pain management and palliative care) relates to the complex nature of persons and the reductionistic tendencies of modern medical science. He cogently expresses the nub of the problem when he declares, "Bodies do not suffer; persons suffer." The implications of this proposition are clear but nonetheless potentially controversial: If a clinician cannot relate to the patient as a person, rather than as a body that is merely the locus of some disease process, then he or she cannot even recognize suffering and certainly cannot begin to competently and compassionately respond to it. Unsurprisingly, many clinicians view this as a gross exaggeration, verging on caricature. However, other credible sources bolster Cassell's point. Consider, for example, the following panegyric of the late Yale surgeon and writer Sherwin Nuland[7] in his book *How We Die* the curative paradigm of medicine:

> . . . the challenge that motivates most persuasively; the challenge that makes each of us physicians continue ever trying to improve our skills; the challenge that results in the dogged pursuit of a diagnosis and a cure; the challenge that has resulted in the astounding progress of late-twentieth century clinical medicine—that foremost of challenges is not primarily the welfare of the individual human being, but rather, the solution of The Riddle of his disease.

Nuland[7] is describing, with only a bit of grandiosity, one of the essential elements of the curative model cogently presented several years later by Ellen Fox.[8] For ease of analysis, her

TABLE 12.1 Models of Patient Care	
Curative Model	**Palliative Model**
• Analytic and rational	• Humanistic and personal
• Clinical puzzle solving	• Patient as person
• Mind–body dualism	• Mind–body unity
• Disvalues subjectivity	• Privileges subjectivity
• Biomedical model	• Biocultural model
• Discounts idiosyncrasy	• Respects idiosyncrasy
• Death = failure	• Unnecessary suffering = failure

delineation of the essential features of the curative and palliative models of patient care is illustrated in Table 12.1.

As illustrated in the table, point by point, the core elements of the reigning curative model are the diametric opposite of those in the palliative model, the latter being the one that presumably must be followed in order to respond appropriately to the pain and suffering associated with both acute and chronic illness. The clinical puzzle-solving element is precisely what Nuland[7] waxes so euphorically about in his discussion of the zealous pursuit of "The Riddle," which he maintains is the primary motivator and the ultimate goal of the best clinicians.

As previously indicated, ethical issues in end-of-life care will be the special focus of Chapter 13 of this book. Nevertheless, it is worth noting the stark contrast in the perspective on death and dying between the two models. The view of many clinicians in the full grip of the curative model that a patient's death is the ultimate medical failure has led, as Nuland[7] himself admits, to situations in which medical specialists have "convinced patients to undergo diagnostic or therapeutic measures at a point in illness so far beyond reason that 'The Riddle' might better have remained unsolved." The type of clinical situations to which Nuland[7] refers, particularly when patients are intentionally deceived or kept in the dark about the grimness of their prognosis or the dismal prospect that additional disease-directed interventions will produce any benefit, constitute a form of what might reasonably be characterized not only as "medical futility" but also as "therapeutic belligerence."[9]

The Phenomenon of Undertreated Pain

The zealous, single-minded pursuit of a diagnosis and the relentless delivery of disease-directed interventions means, as a practical matter, that precious little professional time, energy, or attention is available for assessing and managing pain or suffering, even for those patients in the intensive care unit (ICU) who may be unlikely to leave the hospital alive. That is the bleak conclusion reached by the investigators in the formidable Study to Understand Prognoses, Preferences for Outcomes, and Risks of Treatments (SUPPORT) project in the mid-1990s.[10] The SUPPORT principal investigators sought to evaluate the quality of care in the ICUs of certain premier academic medical centers across the country. The ICU, of course, is the locus of patient care in which the curative (disease-directed) paradigm of high-technology patient care reigns supreme. The findings of the SUPPORT investigators are quite concerning with regard to such considerations as the relief of pain and suffering, the extent to which a patient's plan of care had been discussed with the patient or her proxy, or the likelihood that code status was consistent with what was known about the patient's wishes or values. For purposes of this discussion, at least three fundamental principles of bioethics were frequently violated in ICU care: respect for patient autonomy, beneficence, and nonmaleficence. More particularly, SUPPORT revealed that there was at best a 50–50 chance that the care provided to patients was consistent with their wishes, values, or written directives, and half of the patients studied were believed to be experiencing significant pain or distress in the last days of their lives.

Similar disappointing findings about pain and symptom management have been reported in the care of pediatric ICU patients,[11] nursing home patients,[12] and in outpatient care of cancer patients.[13] The pervasiveness of deficiencies in pain and symptom management encompasses virtually all patients regardless of age, type of disease, or locus of care and thus strongly suggests a problem that emanates from certain core issues in medicine and society to which we now must turn. Otherwise, we would be compelled to consider a highly implausible proposition; that is, that health care professionals are truly indifferent to the pain and suffering of their patients.

IDENTIFYING THE BARRIERS TO PAIN RELIEF

Beginning in the 1990s, an unprecedented amount of attention has been paid to the root causes of undertreated pain. A consistently cited set of barriers has been identified. At a basic level, these barriers exist with regard to all types of pain: acute, chronic noncancer, and pain associated with terminal illness. However, certain barriers are exacerbated in patients with chronic pain. The general categories into which these barriers are divided are professional, patient, and societal in nature and origin.

Professional Barriers

In one sense, as I will endeavor to make clear, the professional barriers to pain relief are the most ethically significant, given the fiduciary nature of the clinician–patient relationship. The key elements utilized in assessing professional competence are knowledge, skills, and attitudes. Deficiencies in any one of these elements can result in inadequate and hence substandard patient care. Deficiencies in more than one for any type of patient care will markedly increase the likelihood that substandard care will result. Marked deficiencies in each of these dimensions have been documented in physicians (of all specialties), nurses, and pharmacists.[14–16] What is most important from an ethical perspective is how deficiencies in one or more of these categories translate into behavior, that is, professional conduct. Given the pervasiveness of pain across the clinical spectrum, and the by now well-recognized sequelae of pain, only rarely may any clinician legitimately claim that such deficiencies pose no threat of harm to patients. As we shall further consider shortly, however, even clinicians who possess the requisite knowledge, skills, and attitudes may be reluctant to translate them consistently into effective pain management, particularly when what is clinically indicated may be opioid analgesia because of fears of regulatory scrutiny or other forms of potential legal liability. More recently, with the exponential increase in prescription drug abuse, addiction, and associated overdose deaths, deficiencies or other problems associated with a prescribing physician's knowledge, skills, or attitudes may also imperil the lives or well-being of patients by inappropriately prescribing or failing to properly monitor a patient's use of these medications.

None other than John Bonica himself pointed out many years ago that no medical school has been so bold and innovative as to establish and maintain a formal, required curriculum in assessing and treating the most common problem of patients who seek medical care—pain.[17] This glaring deficiency that he described nearly 20 years ago persists. In data ascribed to the Association of American Medical Colleges in 2003, only 3% of medical schools have a separate required course in pain management, and only 4% require students to take a course in end-of-life care.[18]

The absence of any solid evidence of a formal curriculum in the assessment and management of pain in most medical schools warrants the conclusion that none actually exists. Some defenders of the status quo have argued that the requisite knowledge, skills, and attitudes are imparted in other less formal but perfectly acceptable ways, such as in the care of actual patients in the clinical years of medical education. What undermines these assertions is the strong evidence that health care professionals continue to graduate and obtain licensure with major deficits in knowledge, skills, and attitudes concerning pain management and its relevance to quality in patient care.

The ethical significance of this phenomenon is the aforementioned "culpability of cultivated ignorance." The absence of a pain curriculum in medical and other educational programs in the health professions may be an important reason why pain is often undertreated but is not an excuse for it. Medical schools have been, and continue to be, major culprits in the epidemic of pain. Evidence of the persistence of this epidemic continues to accumulate. The 2011 Institute of Medicine report *Relieving Pain in America* conservatively estimated that one-third of the adult population of the United States experience chronic pain.[19] It is not merely an absence of required course work on up-to-date pain assessment and management techniques but also myths and misconceptions about the risks and purportedly unmanageable side effects of opioids that are deeply entrenched in the minds of clinical faculty and which are passed on from one generation of physicians to the next.[20] However, it is axiomatic that good ethics begins with good facts. In the past decade, further research and examination has suggested that with regard to the long-term use of opioids for the management of chronic pain, the purported benefits may have been exaggerated, whereas the real risks of abuse and addiction underestimated.[21]

Recognizing the curricular deficiencies in pain assessment and management that have plagued physician training for decades, when the American Medical Association developed the Education for Physicians on End-of-Life Care Project (EPEC), it adopted a train-the-trainer approach in the hope of maximizing the dissemination of current thinking on palliative care to experienced practitioners rather than medical students or residents.[22] Entering a profession entails a moral responsibility to ensure that one possesses and consistently applies the knowledge and skills essential to minimal competence. That one may in some instances enter the profession with certain deficiencies does not provide a legitimate basis for cultivating ignorance that may be originally attributable to curricular deficiencies. The medical school curriculum should reflect the current standard of care and anticipate future improvements to it, but it does not set that standard in any definitive sense.

In California, the continuing absence of a pain curriculum in medical schools, combined with increasing public awareness of and outrage over a national, indeed international, epidemic of undertreated pain, moved one crusading member of the California Assembly to introduce and successfully pursue a statute mandating two things: (1) that pain management and end-of-life care be part of the medical school curriculum for applicants seeking a license as a California physician after June 1, 2000, and (2) that inpatient health facilities include pain as a fifth vital sign assessed along with other vital signs and noted in the patient's medical record.[23] In yet another example of lawmakers interceding to address professional deficiencies, the California Assembly in 2001 enacted a statute requiring that all licensed physicians in the state (with the exception of radiologists and pathologists) receive a minimum of 12 hours of continuing medical education prior to January 1, 2007.[24] The statute, however, had a sunset provision. Because the California Assembly did not vote to extend it, this continuing medical education mandate is no longer in force.

These and the other legislative measures described hereinafter actually run counter to a well-established tradition in American government to leave the professions, particularly the health professions, virtually unfettered latitude and discretion to manage their affairs. Only when substantial evidence accumulates—and results in a high level of public concern—are lawmakers prompted to intercede. When morally troubling circumstances are allowed to persist by those who ostensibly have the power and authority to address them through nonlegal measures, the law has been invoked to address the problem. A graphic example was the Nuremberg Code that emerged from the Nuremberg tribunal's prosecution of the Nazi doctors. The first principle of the Nuremberg Code was the right of human research subjects to informed consent. Twenty-five years later, when the public became aware that a number of clinical trials conducted by prominent medical researchers in the United States were openly and notoriously violating the Code, which was an ethical–professional, not necessarily a legal mandate, the federal government stepped in with the first of what became many regulations of federally funded research involving human subjects.[25]

Similarly, in the early 1980s, a phenomenon known as "patient dumping" became the subject of significant public awareness and concern. When indigent or uninsured patients presented to emergency rooms, they were with increasing frequency shunted off to other (usually government-operated) hospitals for care, often with deleterious consequences from the delay in properly addressing an unstable medical condition. When neither the health professions nor national hospital organizations demonstrated any inclination to address the problem, the Congress of the United States passed the Emergency Medical Treatment and Active Labor Act (EMTALA), which imposed a mandate on all emergency departments to provide a medical screening examination to patients upon arrival, and to prohibit transfer of any patient found to be in an unstable medical condition prior to stabilization except under certain carefully described situations.[26] Notably, EMTALA recognized pain as an indication of an unstable medical condition requiring prompt attention and effective remediation. These instances indicate that it is often the failure or refusal of health care institutions and/or professionals to put their own houses in order that prompts major governmental intervention in order to address an otherwise seemingly intractable problem.

One must ask whether there is a causal connection between the failure of health professional schools to recognize the need for a pain curriculum and the failure of the health professions and the institutions in which health care is delivered to make the prompt, effective, and consistent assessment and management of pain a priority in patient care. We noted early in this chapter how Eric Cassell was perplexed by the seeming indifference to the phenomenon of suffering on the part of physicians given the traditional core values of medicine. The same is true for pain because another professional barrier has been characterized as the failure of health care institutions and professionals to make pain relief a priority in patient care. One of the primary objectives of many of the policies discussed in Chapter 14 of this book, particularly the Federation of State Medical Boards (FSMB) Model Policy and The Joint Commission Accreditation Manual standards on pain management, was to disabuse their target audience of the perception that effective pain management was not an essential element of sound patient care.

The final professional barrier to effective pain management is fear of regulatory scrutiny and potential legal liability (civil or criminal). There is little question that the nidus of this concern relates to opioid analgesia. There is quite simply no discussion about such concerns arising out of nonpharmacologic pain management strategies. When one looks at the record of disciplinary actions by state medical boards, those relating in any manner to pain management practices were invariably characterized as excessive prescribing of opioids. Such cases are addressed in detail in Chapter 15 of this book. It is for this reason that the previously mentioned FSMB policy is of such potential significance, for it seeks to shift the focus of medical boards from "overprescribing" or "underprescribing"

of opioids to inappropriate prescribing because both extremes pose risks to patients.

From an ethical perspective, it is a troubling state of affairs when clinicians fear that they are at risk of disciplinary action by their professional licensing board if they follow current national clinical practice guidelines on the use of opioid analgesics. Their concerns have not been without foundation, for an initial survey of the knowledge and attitudes of state medical licensing board members regarding opioids and pain management revealed significant knowledge deficits and attitudes that were at best unsupportive and at worst hostile toward the use of opioids, especially for patients with chronic noncancer pain.[27] One analysis of the prevailing attitude among medical board members concerning opioid analgesia characterized it as an "ethic of underprescribing."[28] A follow-up study conducted after the promulgation of FSMB guidelines on prescribing opioids and a series of workshops across the country on pain management for medical board members not only revealed some improvement in areas that might be reassuring to those whom boards are charged with regulating but also noted the need for further education and wider acceptance of the FSMB model guidelines/policy.[29]

When medical and other health professions' boards issue new and presumably more enlightened policies on pain management, one cannot presume that most affected clinicians will become aware of them. There is still less of a basis to expect that these policies will, in the short term, have a direct and immediate impact on clinical practice even among clinicians who become aware of them. In the event that these new or updated policies were to become part of a mandatory continuing professional education program, there is nevertheless reason for concern that they would in fact be likely to significantly improve the usual custom and practice of minimizing the clinical significance of pain that has been mentored, modeled, and followed by generations of professionals.[30] Concerted efforts must be made to reform practice patterns and the underlying clinical culture that sustains them by infusing more enlightened attitudes about the importance of pain relief to patient health and well-being.

The regulatory barriers also include the federal Controlled Substances Act, the policies and procedures of the U.S. Drug Enforcement Administration, and criminal prosecutions of physicians for drug diversion or trafficking when their prescribing practices are deemed far outside the ambit of mainstream medicine. These issues are dealt in depth in Chapters 14 and 15 of this book. The ethics of public policy formulation and law enforcement strategies and tactics are somewhat beyond the scope of this chapter. Nevertheless, such practices are fraught with moral implications because they affect the lives of many people. Much of the impetus for the new emphasis on balance intended to moderate between seemingly competing considerations of preventing drug abuse and diversion, on the one hand, and ensuring that patients in pain receive the analgesics they require for effective relief has been based on legitimate concerns that state and federal regulatory and law enforcement measures have been obsessively focused on the former and virtually indifferent to the latter. We consider the moral dimensions of pain policy and law further from the perspective of the health care professional in a subsequent section of this chapter as well, when we take up the demands of professionalism to make the patient's needs and interests primary in a fiduciary relationship.

As the full scope of the national opioid overdose epidemic became apparent, the political and societal pressure to discourage physicians from routinely and indiscriminately prescribing opioids has understandably increased. The statistics are striking. In 2014, roughly one in three accidental drug overdose deaths were related to prescription pain relievers.[31] This data calls into question one of the lynchpins of the original challenge to the ethic of underprescribing of opioids for chronic pain, which was that the risks of addiction or abuse of such medications was relatively low.

Patient Barriers

Patient barriers to effective pain relief are in important ways related to physician barriers. Traditionally, clinicians were the primary source of patient information on medicine and health. If they did not themselves possess accurate and up-to-date information about the risks and benefits of pharmacologic and nonpharmacologic modalities of pain relief, they would not be able to fulfill their professional responsibility to educate their patients. Indeed, that is why pain management has historically been an area of clinical practice in which truly informed patient consent was virtually nonexistent. Now, however, in the Internet age, patients and family members may actually access up-to-date information on pain and its management as or more often than their physicians.

Without adequate information concerning the available range of pain management interventions and their relative risks and benefits, patients had no basis on which to formulate reasonable expectations with regard to pain relief. A major public survey on pain in the United States conducted in 1997 revealed that not only is pain pervasive, but the most common reason why people avoid seeking medication to relieve their pain is fear of addiction or physical dependence.[32] Once again, recent data on prescription drug abuse and overdose deaths indicate that patient concerns about this risk are neither groundless nor frivolous. The clinical and ethical challenge for physicians is to accurately assess the risks and benefits of each pain relief option based on the patient's particular circumstances.

Patients may also avoid seeking medical care when they experience pain because they fear it may be caused by some serious, perhaps even life-threatening, condition. Finally, patients experiencing pain that is associated with conditions for which they are currently receiving treatment may not complain about their pain and seek more effective pain relief because of a mistaken assumption that pain is an unavoidable concomitant of therapy or that their physician would certainly be providing as much pain relief as possible. It is these latter perspectives that help explain how, until the legal cases discussed in Chapter 15 arose, no malpractice claims based on negligent pain management had been brought despite an epidemic of undertreated pain.[33]

Societal Barriers

Pain and suffering are not just immensely complex and highly individualized human experiences. They occur within familial and other interpersonal contexts as well as social, organizational, and governmental configurations. Pain in particular may not only be a symptom of an underlying condition, but it may also, in the case of chronic noncancer pain, become a condition itself, hence the appropriateness of the term *chronic pain syndrome*. These are often, as Arthur Kleinman[34] has observed, "Conditions in which the degree of pathology does not seem to explain the severity of perceived pain or the limitations in bodily functioning the pain produces." This marked disparity between the patient's pathophysiology and reports (often interpreted as complaints) of pain and disability produces a strong element of skepticism not only on the part of clinicians from whom the patient seeks care but also from family and friends. These doubts about the veracity of the patient's experience of chronic pain can exacerbate the feelings of isolation and abandonment that characterize the chronic pain patient. At the end of this chapter, we further consider the special challenges for the clinician posed by the chronic pain patient.

American culture in particular has precious little patience with or sympathy for the chronically ill. Indeed, much of the recent momentum within the disability rights movement has been an understandably strong reaction to the widespread perception among the healthy and able-bodied that certain profoundly disabling conditions are categorically incompatible with any quality of life whatsoever. In response to such pervasive attitudes, perhaps the most high-profile disability rights organization took the name "Not Dead Yet." Their message is clear to society in general and health professionals in particular: We do not seek your assistance in ending what *you* consider our miserable existence but rather in enhancing what *we* consider to be our quality of life and our ability to be active and engaged members of our community.

Ethical Implications of the Barriers

There is a new emphasis in both undergraduate and graduate medical education on professionalism and communication.[35] In some small measure, such curricular reforms may begin to address the larger and more fundamental problem identified by previously cited commentators such as Cassell, Fox, Kleinman, and Morris that is posed by medicine's predilection for biologic reductionism and obsession with diagnostic and disease-directed interventions. The none-too-subtle point is that one does not enter into a professional relationship with or provide care to a disease process. Although a certain cadre of clinicians may romanticize the pursuit of "The Riddle" of disease, the professional relationship (fiduciary in nature) and communication are necessarily with the personhood, not the disease of the patient. The assessment of pain, for example, is all about effective communication between patient and physician concerning the subjective experience of pain. If effective pain assessment is absolutely essential to providing effective pain relief, then the clinician must be able to understand and appreciate the patient's experience of illness in a manner and to an extent that may not be true for other aspects of patient care.

As previously noted, the concept of holding oneself out as a professional and the ethical demands of entering into a fiduciary relationship with another person entail the acquisition, utilization, and maintenance of the knowledge, skills, and attitudes necessary to ensure minimally sufficient competence. When a significant percentage of the practitioners of a profession such as medicine or nursing have been found to have major deficiencies in something as pervasive as pain and as integral to good patient care as are its assessment and management, invariably major ethical issues arise. It is in the recognition of these ethical issues that one demonstrates a grasp of the close relationship between ethics and professionalism. Yet, there was a period in the early years of the movement to address the widespread phenomenon of undertreated pain when there was little acknowledgment of, and hence attention to, the ethical dimensions of these professional deficiencies.

Turning from barriers associated with knowledge deficits and problematic attitudes toward the significance of pain and its relief to those associated with legal and regulatory concerns, we encounter a challenging ethical quandary. As described in detail in Chapter 14, the regulation of opioid analgesics created a hostile environment toward their widespread use in pain management. Regulatory barriers, including a pattern of medical board disciplinary actions against physicians for so-called "overprescribing" of opioids, have, as previously noted, caused physicians to feel at risk even if they are scrupulously following state-of-the-art clinical practice guidelines.

A fundamental ethical question posed by this situation is as follows: To what extent is it reasonable to expect, indeed to demand, that physicians routinely engage in acts of moral courage in order to ensure that their patients with pain receive the medications and/or other therapies that they require for relief? The essence of the duty imposed on a professional when entering into a fiduciary relationship is that the other person's interests become primary and any potential conflict of interest shall be resolved in favor of the person to whom the professional duty is owed. Therefore, prescribing inadequate doses of analgesics or opioids from a lower schedule of the Controlled Substances

Act (e.g., Schedules III to V) when those from a higher schedule (e.g., Schedule II) are medically indicated in order to avoid regulatory scrutiny would constitute a breach of fiduciary duty. It is also the case, however, that a public policy posture and regulatory regime that routinely demands acts of moral courage on the part of professionals is a fundamentally flawed system that is vulnerable to strong moral critique. Such a critique is at least implied in the Report Card on state and federal pain policies that has been issued by the Pain & Policy Studies Group and which is discussed in some detail in Chapter 14.

Embracing a New Ethic of Pain Relief

Although it is important to understand the historical context in which formerly prevailing attitudes toward pain and its relief with opioids developed and ultimately became so pervasive and persistent, continuing the momentum that has followed from more enlightened attitudes is necessary to address emerging ethical concerns. The clinical specialty of pain medicine has played a major role in the progress that has been achieved in the last two decades. Ultimately, however, each of the health professions has a responsibility to cultivate within its practitioners the knowledge, skills, and attitudes that are essential to the provision of effective pain management. The need for highly trained physicians and nurses in pain and palliative care will continue to grow but so too will the need for all physicians and nurses to possess certain minimal core competencies in the assessment and management of pain.

The clinical and ethical challenge of providing appropriate pain and symptom management has, if anything, increased in the last decade with the mounting evidence of two previously noted phenomenon: (1) the epidemic of prescription drug abuse and resulting deaths from overdose and (2) studies indicating that long-term high-dose opioid therapy in many instances is at best nonbeneficial and at worst harmful. Primary care physicians, on whom most patients must rely for management of their pain, find it increasingly difficult allocate the time and energy necessary to deliver state-of-the-art pain assessment and management. This potential conflict of commitment between fiduciary duties to individual patients and contractual duties to employer or health care institutional policy and procedural mandates or limitations is yet another source of ethical dilemmas.

One of the new shibboleths in pain management is "pharmacovigilance."[36] Of course, the judicious prescribing of medications is an essential element of sound clinical practice in all domains of medicine. However, with the prescription drug abuse epidemic primarily associated with opioid analgesics, the insistence on pharmacovigilance appears disproportionately in the pain management literature. The implicit premise of this concept is that clinicians are not truly confronted with a genuine moral dilemma of providing effective pain relief for patients or preventing drug abuse and diversion. The basic presupposition appears to be that the parameters delineated by pharmacovigilance, as conceived by some of the thought leaders in pain medicine, enable a responsible prescribing professional to provide appropriate and effective pain relief to patients while at the same time significantly minimizing the known risk of addiction posed by opioids or their diversion to persons who have no legitimate need for them. In other words, pharmacovigilant pain management recognizes the need in clinical practice for a kind of balance that is similar to the balance sought in laws, regulations, and public policies affecting opioid analgesics as discussed in Chapter 14 of this book.

Even within the domain of pain management, the term has most often been invoked in the context of chronic pain management. Patients who have just undergone major surgical procedures, who have been the victims of traumatic injury, or those who are facing terminal conditions do not encounter the same credibility problems when they report high levels of pain and seek relief. The phenomenon of pseudoaddiction, in which patients with genuine pain that has been undertreated engage in behaviors that cause them to appear to be drug seeking (in some illegitimate sense), is most prevalent in the population of chronic noncancer pain patients.[37] With regard to end-of-life care, it was once thought that undertreatment was the driving force behind the movement to legalize the prescribing of lethal doses of medication at the request of patients with terminal illnesses. However, the data accumulated as a result of the Oregon Death with Dignity Act reveal that undertreated pain is actually not even among the five most frequently cited reasons why dying patients seek a lethal prescription.[38]

Some of the practices that have come to be advocated with increasing frequency under the rubric of "pharmacovigilance" or "responsible opioid prescribing" are opioid contracts and random urine drug screens. Both approaches raise critical questions of an ethical nature about the role of trust in the clinician– patient relationship as well as questions about why patients with chronic pain are special cases that require such measures when other patients whose conditions necessitate treatment with potentially dangerous medications and strict adherence to clinician recommendations do not. We focus here particularly on the contracts/agreements that are being so widely promoted, the form that they take, the benefits that are claimed by their proponents, and the risks they pose to the establishment and maintenance of trust in the clinician–patient relationship.

There is an ethically more and less benign way in which to view and characterize the nature and role of these documents. The more benign approach is to simply consider the contract or agreement under the traditional rubric of a written informed consent document. Informed consent is a foundational concept in both medical ethics and medical jurisprudence and the primary mechanism by which respect for individual patient autonomy is demonstrated.[39] The execution by patients of consent forms is a routine practice for any invasive medical procedure or other therapeutic measure. Thus, to the extent that an opioid contract were nothing more than a patient's written informed consent to undergo opioid therapy, acknowledging thereby both the risks and benefits associated with it, there would be nothing remarkable about it and certainly nothing that would raise serious ethical concerns.

The authors of one important article on the subject state, "The contract is ideally intended to enhance the therapeutic relationship by initiating and supporting an alliance between the patient and the physician. It may enable a patient to have an active role in treatment. . . . "[40] The keyword in this passage may be "ideal," for there is growing concern among some that the primary reasons why opioid contracts are becoming routine among those physicians who are willing to consider opioid therapy for chronic noncancer pain patients relate to risk management and regulatory/law enforcement considerations rather than patient empowerment or well-being. For example, one review of opioid contracts that are currently in use revealed that over 90% had specific conditions warranting disciplinary termination of the agreement by the physician (e.g., if the patient were to violate a provision of the contract or miss appointments without adequate justification) and nearly 70% required submission to random drug screens, whereas only 5% stated the potential benefits of opioid therapy and just 3% provided general information regarding treatment.[40] Because the latter two elements are most typically found on consent forms, their absence seriously undermines the argument that these contracts are merely more elaborate or formal consent documents.

Such contract provisions emphasize the physician's power to impose conditions of treatment on patients rather than the autonomy of the patient to participate meaningfully in the consideration of therapeutic options according to the paradigm of shared decision making.[41] The American Academy of Pain Medicine (AAPM) features a sample "Consent for Chronic Opioid Therapy" on its Web site. This agreement/consent form includes the more common provisions such as obtaining all opioid prescriptions from a single physician and filling them at a single pharmacy. The form states that the patient agrees to such random urine or blood tests as well as pill counts as may be "requested."[41]

The absence of such detailed therapeutic agreements in most other clinical settings in which the modalities of treatment and the need for patient adherence to the therapeutic regimen are of equal importance to patient well-being (e.g., cancer chemotherapy) suggests that chronic noncancer pain patients who require opioid analgesia for effective relief warrant a heightened level of suspicion. Furthermore, the widespread and routine use of opioid contracts by many physicians for all of their chronic noncancer pain patients receiving opioid therapy, but not for acute pain or pain associated with terminal illness, implies that there is something intrinsically untrustworthy or suspicious about this category of patient.[42] Clearly, however, merely being a victim of chronic noncancer pain that happens to be refractory to nonopioid analgesics is not inherently suspicious. Such patients and syndromes exist, and a consensus of thought leaders in pain medicine has emerged in support of the position that opioid analgesia should generally be offered to these patients unless there are specific and significant contraindications.[43]

Recent acknowledgment that earlier estimations of the risk of addiction associated with opioid analgesia were much too low does not undercut this consensus view. The best current evidence is that the incidence of addictive disorders (of all types) in the general population ranges from 3% to 26%, whereas the rate for hospitalized patients is 19% to 25%, and for major trauma patients as high as 40% to 60%.[44] It is important to note that recently formulated model pain policies do not recommend the routine use of either opioid agreements or urine drug screens in all patients—even all chronic noncancer pain patients—but rather those patients who in the exercise of sound clinical judgment are deemed to pose a "high risk for medication abuse or have a history of substance abuse."[45] Approaches to screening for addiction prior to the initiation of chronic opioid therapy as well as assessing for addiction during therapy (exclusive of urine toxicology screening) have been identified and utilized.[46]

The imposition of random urine drug screening as one condition precedent to offering opioid therapy to a patient appears to have become a common practice among clinicians whose practice includes patients with persistent pain problems. As with opioid agreements themselves, random drug screens may be required of all patients who receive opioid analgesia for an extended period, not simply those whose histories raise questions or concerns about the likelihood that they will take the medications as directed. In this way, it might be argued that all patients for whom opioid analgesia is indicated are treated the same rather than certain patients being stigmatized by differential treatment that calls their capacity to adhere to the treatment protocol in question. Nonadherence to chronic opioid therapy may take a variety of forms, including consuming more (or less) than the amount of the prescribed drug directed by the prescribing clinician, using opioids obtained from other sources, and failing to take the drug prescribed, whether or not the drug is then sold or otherwise diverted from legitimate medical use.

Failure to comply with instructions concerning the taking of medication is not unique to chronic pain patients, and the risks of such behaviors by patients can have serious consequences in many different clinical settings, including diabetes, hypertension, epilepsy, and cancer therapy, to name only a few.[47] Nevertheless, it has not yet become routine to insist on prescription medication agreements and laboratory screening for those patients, even when studies suggest that in some patient populations nonadherence to therapeutic regimens may exceed 50%.[48,49]

One important distinction between nonadherence to opioid therapy and nonadherence to other pharmacologic regimens that do not involved prescription medications that are subject to diversion and abuse is the risk posed to society. A patient who must take a prescription medication for a serious medical condition but who fails to do so as directed in most instances places only himself or herself at risk of adverse consequences. However, when nonadherence to opioid therapy takes the form of selling or otherwise diverting these medications, there are significant adverse societal implications. There is no question that clinicians have responsibilities to their communities and the society at large and not only to their individual patients. Sometimes, as in the case of public health emergencies, there may be genuine conflicts between these two responsibilities. However, minimizing the risk of opioid addiction and diversion through the responsible use of treatment agreements and adherence monitoring enables the clinician to meet his or her obligations to both individual patient and society. As with the informed consent and information disclosure process itself, the manner in which such approaches are taken is as important as the details of the approach itself. Moreover, it may well be the case that the wider use of measures to warn patients about the risks of nonadherence to prescription medication regimens and to monitor such adherence may be a necessary and appropriate response by the health professions to the data documenting the extent to which patients fail to take their medications as prescribed. What is needed but presently does not exist are rigorous empirical studies evaluating the effects of patient agreements and drug screening on adherence to or the outcomes of treatment regimens.[40] This is a problem with regard to many other aspects of pain medicine as well in that in the absence of sufficient evidence, clinical practice guidelines are often consensus-based.

It would not be surprising to find that some of the high-profile federal prosecutions of physicians with very liberal prescribing practices described in detail in Chapter 15 of this book have fueled the widespread adoption of rigorous opioid contract provisions. Those physicians were alleged to have, among other things, engaged in a form of willful blindness to a host of red flags that some of their patients either had no legitimate medical need for opioids or were flagrantly abusing or selling their medications. The recordkeeping and monitoring by the physicians was poor to nonexistent.

Conclusion

The ethics of pain management are in a profound state of flux. Neither the term *evolution* nor *revolution* seems to be an apt characterization, for such terms suggest a gradual and organic development process on the one hand or a transformational paradigm shift on the other, neither of which can be supported by the existing evidence. Rather, the current state of affairs might well be characterized, without risk of serious exaggeration, as a battle for the soul of medicine. For as we noted at the very beginning of this chapter, seminal works on the place of pain and suffering in the context of the patient's experience of illness consistently remind us that their relief is a core value of medicine with roots running back to the very origins of the profession.[50] In the modern era, when organized medicine has confronted phenomena such as physician-assisted suicide (aid in dying) or physician participation in lethal injection, prominent voices in opposition to the legitimacy of the physician's role in such practices have consistently invoked statements of principle such as the following: "Healing the sick and alleviating suffering is the primary role of physicians in U.S. society."[51]

Yet, those same voices have, for the most part, been silent in the midst of an epidemic of undertreated pain that afflicts chronic noncancer pain patients disproportionately. It has fallen to organizations such as the World Health Organization (WHO) and the International Association for the Study of Pain (IASP) to call for the recognition of pain relief as a human right.[52]

In no other aspect of patient care has the fundamental role of trust in the clinician–patient relationship become more of a pivotal issue than in the care of patients with chronic noncancer pain. With the proliferation of detailed opioid contracts including provisions for routine urine drug screens and rigidly specified grounds for terminating the relationship for nonadherence, we may be at risk of distrust becoming the reigning paradigm.[53] A byword of the cold war era notably used by President Reagan but originally traced to Vladimir Lenin was "trust but verify." This approach may well have a place in patient care and the standard of care with which clinicians must comply. The challenge to the health professions posed by the current ambivalence toward patients requiring opioid analgesia for moderate to severe noncancer pain is formidable. On one hand are prominent voices such as the WHO and the IASP calling for recognition of a human right to pain relief for all patients. On the other hand are dire warnings to clinicians about deceptive, drug-seeking patients who must be engaged with extreme caution, a robust skepticism, and rigorous scrutiny as well as all of the other essential elements of pharmacovigilance. The establishment of a solid consensus among clinical and regulatory stakeholders as to where we ought to situate a healthy and reasonable balance between extreme, unrealistic naivete and a rigid, pervasive cynicism about the role of trust in the care of patients with persistent pain should become a high priority for all conscientious and caring professionals.

References

1. Morris DM. The uses of pain. In: *The Culture of Pain*. Berkeley: University of California Press; 1991:174–197.
2. Faden RR, Beauchamp TL, King NMP. *A History and Theory of Informed Consent*. New York: Oxford University Press; 1986.
3. Rothman DJ. *Strangers at the Bedside: A History of How Law and Bioethics Transformed Medical Decision Making*. New York: Basic Books; 1991.
4. Veatch RM. *The Patient-Physician Relationship: The Patient as Partner*. Bloomington, IN: Indiana University Press; 1991.
5. Cassell EJ. The nature of suffering and the goals of medicine. *N Engl J Med* 1982;306:639–645.
6. Cassell EJ. Preface. In: *The Nature of Suffering and the Goals of Medicine*. New York: Oxford University Press; 1991:vii–xiii.
7. Nuland SB. *How We Die: Reflections on Life's Final Chapter. The Lessons Learned*. New York: Knopf; 1994:248–249.
8. Fox E. Predominance of the curative model of medical care. A residual problem. *JAMA* 1997;278:761–763.
9. Pellegrino ED, Thomasma DM. *For the Patient's Good: The Restoration of Beneficence in Health Care*. New York: Oxford University Press; 1988.
10. The SUPPORT Principle Investigators. A controlled trial to improve care of seriously ill hospitalized patients. The study to understand prognoses and preferences for outcomes and risks of treatments (SUPPORT). *JAMA* 1995;274:1591–1598.
11. Wolfe J, Grier HE, Klar N, et al. Symptoms and suffering at the end of life in children with cancer. *N Engl J Med* 2000;342:326–333.
12. American Geriatrics Society. The management of persistent pain in older persons: AGS panel on persistent pain in older persons. *J Am Geriatr Soc* 1998;46:635–651.
13. Cleeland CS, Gonin R, Hatfield AK, et al. Pain and its treatment in outpatients with metastatic cancer. *N Engl J Med* 1994;330:592–596.
14. Von Roenn JH, Cleeland CS, Gonin R, et al. Physician attitudes and practices in cancer pain management. A survey from the Eastern Oncology Group. *Ann Intern Med* 1993;119:121–126.
15. Sanderson L. Review. Attitudes to and knowledge about pain and pain management of nurses working with children with cancer: a comparative study between UK, South Africa, and Sweden. *J Res Nurs* 2007;12:517–519.
16. Joranson DE, Gilson AM. Pharmacists' knowledge and attitudes about pain medication in relation to federal and state policies. *J Am Pharm Assoc (Wash)* 2001;41:213–220.
17. Weiner RS. An interview with John J. Bonica, MD. *Pain Pract* 1989;1:2.
18. Silverman J. Students need more pain management training: education effort underway. Available at: http://www.obgynnews.com/article/S0029-7434(03)70079-2/fulltext. Accessed October 15, 2003.
19. Institute of Medicine. *Relieving Pain in America: A Blueprint for Transforming Prevention, Care, Education, and Research*. Washington, DC: National Academies Press; 2011.
20. Hill CS Jr. When will adequate pain management be the norm? *JAMA* 1995;274:1881–1882.
21. Ballantyne JC, Shinn NS. Efficacy of opioids for chronic pain: a review of the evidence. *Clin J Pain* 2008;24:469–478.
22. Education in Palliative and End-of-life Care. Available at: http://www.epec.net/EPEC/Webpages/index.cfm. Accessed May 5, 2009.
23. Thomson H. A new law to improve pain management and end-of-life care. *West J Med* 2001;174:161–162.
24. California Business and Professions Code, § 2190.5.
25. Frankel MS. The policy-making environment. In: *The Public Health Service Guidelines Governing Research Involving Human Subjects: An Analysis of the Policy-Making Process*. Washington, DC: George Washington University Program of Policy Studies in Science and Technology; 1972:19–29.
26. Emergency Medical Treatment and Active Labor Act, 42 USC §1395dd (1986).
27. Joranson DE, Cleeland CS, Weissman DE, et al. Opioids for chronic cancer and non-cancer pain: a survey of state medical boards. *Fed Bull* 1992;79:15–49.
28. Martino AM. In search of a new ethic for treating patients with chronic pain: what can medical boards do? *J Law Med Ethics* 1998;26:332–349, 263.
29. Gilson AM, Joranson DE. Controlled substances and pain management: changes in knowledge and attitudes of state regulators. *J Pain Symptom Manage* 2001;21:227–237.
30. Max MB. Improving outcomes of analgesic treatment: is education enough? *Ann Intern Med* 1990;113:885–889.
31. American Society of Addiction Medicine. Opioid addiction: 2016 facts and figures. Available at: http://www.asam.org/docs/default-source/advocacy/opioid-addiction-disease-facts-figures.pdf. Accessed July 11, 2016.
32. Bostrom M. Summary of the Mayday Fund Survey: public attitudes about pain and analgesics. *J Pain Symptom Manage* 1997;13:166–168.
33. Dawson R, Spross JA, Jablonski ES, et al. Probing the paradox of patient's satisfaction with inadequate pain management. *J Pain Symptom Manage* 2002;23:211–220.
34. Kleinman A. Vulnerability of pain and the pain of vulnerability. In: *The Illness Narratives: Suffering, Healing & the Human Condition*. New York: Basic Books; 1988:56–74.
35. Whitcomb ME. Professionalism in medicine. *Acad Med* 2007;82:1009.
36. Fishman SM. *Responsible Opioid Prescribing: A Physician's Guide*. 2nd ed, Rev ed. Washington, DC: Waterford Life Sciences; 2014.
37. Weissman DE, Haddox JD. Opioid pseudoaddiction. *Pain* 1989;36:363–366.
38. Oregon Health Authority. Oregon Death with Dignity Act: 2015 data summary. Available at: https://public.health.oregon.gov/ProviderPartnerResources/EvaluationResearch/DeathwithDignityAct/Documents/year18.pdf. Accessed July 31, 2016.
39. Meisel A, Kuczewski M. Legal and ethical myths about informed consent. *Arch Intern Med* 1996;156:2521–2526.
40. Fishman SM, Bandman TB, Edwards A, et al. The opioid contract in the management of chronic pain. *J Pain Symptom Manage* 1999;18:27–37.
41. Arnold RM, Han PK, Seltzer D. Opioid contracts in chronic nonmalignant pain management: objectives and uncertainties. *Am J Med* 2006;119:292–296.
42. American Academy of Pain Medicine. Consent for chronic opioid therapy. Available at: http://www.painmed.org/files/consent-for-chronic-opioid-therapy.pdf. Accessed July 31, 2016.
43. Miller J. The other side of trust in health care: prescribing drugs with the potential for abuse. *Bioethics* 2007;21:51–60.
44. Savage SR. Assessment for addiction in pain-treatment settings. *Clin J Pain* 2002;18:S28–S38.
45. American Academy of Pain Medicine. Use of opioids for the treatment of chronic pain: a statement from the American Academy of Pain Medicine. Available at: http://www.painmed.org/files/use-of-opioids-for-the-treatment-of-chronic-pain.pdf. Accessed July 31, 2016.
46. Federation of State Medical Boards of the United States. Model policy for the use of controlled substances for the treatment of pain. Available at: http://www.fsmb.org/pdf/2004;usgrpol;usControlled;usSubstances.pdf. Accessed May 6, 2009.
47. Fishman SM, Wilsey B, Yang J, et al. Adherence monitoring and drug surveillance in chronic opioid therapy. *J Pain Symptom Manage* 2000;20:293–307.
48. Cramer JA, Mattson RH, Prevey ML, et al. How often is medication taken as prescribed? A novel technique. *JAMA* 1989;261:3273–3277.
49. Levine AM, Richardson JL, Marks G, et al. Compliance with oral drug therapy in patients with hematologic malignancy. *J Clin Oncol* 1987;5:1469–1476.
50. Beauchamp TL, Childress JF. *Principles of Biomedical Ethics*. 4th ed. New York, Oxford University Press; 1994:163–170.
51. Black L, Sade RM. Lethal injection and physicians: state law vs medical ethics. *JAMA* 2007;298:2779–2781.
52. World Health Organization. Pain relief a human right. Available at: http://www.who.int/mediacentre/news/releases/2004/pr70/en/. Accessed May 6, 2009.
53. Victor L, Richeimer SH. Trustworthiness as a clinical variable: the problem of trust in the management of chronic, nonmalignant pain. *Pain Med* 2005;6:385–391.

CHAPTER 13

Ethical Issues in the Care of Dying Patients

DAVID BARNARD

Introduction

THE QUEST FOR MORAL ORDER AMID EXISTENTIAL DISORDER

To the dying person, his doctor, however much he is trusted and regarded as a source of treatment, is no longer one with the power to cure; to the doctor, the patient has become one whose death, despite every possible effort, he is impotent to prevent. This gives rise to problems in the special professional relationship which often develops between a patient and his doctor, and besides that, they have the difficulties that face any two people trying to adjust to the fact that one of them is shortly going to die.[1]

This comment by John Hinton is a pointed reminder that the patient's nearness to death places the patient and the doctor in a challenging and disturbing place, both in their relationship with each other and in their sense of personal identity. The direct encounter with death—in the guise of the death of the patient—has the power to disrupt the doctor's relationship and communication with the dying person, throw rational decision making into confusion, and capsize carefully wrought treatment plans.

Robert Burt has commented on the "inherent unruliness of death and the persistence of individual and social ambivalence about death" as features that limit our ability to fashion social policies and practice guidelines that are free of moral ambiguity or the possibility for evil and abuse. At the conclusion of his study of the conflict-ridden policies governing abortion, the death penalty, and physician-assisted death in the United States during the last half-century, Burt writes,

> Here is the paradox that we must learn to live with in regulating death: that we must teach ourselves, through our rational intellectual capacities, that our rational intellect cannot adequately comprehend, much less adequately control, death. We are no more compassionate, honorable, or intelligent than our predecessors who embraced the pursuit of rational mastery over death and were led, without acknowledgment, into unreasoned evil. We would do better to admit, as W.H. Auden acknowledged, that "Death is not understood by Death; nor You, nor I."[2]

THE CONTRIBUTIONS AND LIMITATIONS OF ETHICAL ANALYSIS IN END-OF-LIFE CARE

Hinton and Burt suggest that the psychological and existential dimensions of the encounter with death destabilize the doctor–patient relationship and rational decision making. These dimensions also require that we acknowledge the limitations as well as the contributions of ethical analysis in end-of-life care. At the most general level, the discipline of ethics itself embodies the cacophony of voices, worldviews, cultural frameworks, and value systems characteristic of postmodernity. As philosophers such as McIntyre[3] and Englehardt[4] argue, no single, overarching standpoint or scale of values commands universal allegiance in a secular, pluralist society that is committed to the peaceable resolution of differences. Yet, without such a universally compelling standpoint, there is no means short of force to eliminate the contradictions between philosophical systems or the competing claims of multiple moral communities.

Two aspects of uncertainty more specifically related to clinical ethics near the end of life are worth particular note at the outset. Consider the commonly accepted public consensus on the ethics of end-of-life care. Its main points include the following:

1. Competent adults may refuse medical treatment.
2. Treatment refusals may include all forms of life-sustaining medical treatment, including artificially provided nutrition and hydration.
3. Complying with a competent adult's informed wishes to refuse or discontinue life-sustaining treatment should be considered neither homicide nor assisted suicide.
4. From a moral and legal point of view, there is no difference between withholding a treatment (not starting it) and withdrawing a treatment (stopping it after it has been started), if the treatment in question is inconsistent with a competent patient's informed preferences.
5. For a patient who is terminally ill and who values comfort over prolongation of life, symptom control that has as a side effect the shortening of life is morally permissible and is not the moral equivalent of active euthanasia.
6. Incompetent or otherwise nonautonomous people have the same rights as competent people in these matters, with their wishes expressed either in the form of an advance directive or by a person authorized to make health care decisions for them.

To call these points the "public consensus" means that they capture a broad agreement in the bioethics literature, policy statements of professional organizations, judicial decisions, and the actions of state legislatures on the matters in question.[5] It is probably safe to say that these points organize the notes of nearly every medical school and nursing school lecturer on the topic of "the ethics of end-of-life care" and that they are the guiding principles brought to bear on individual cases by the vast majority of clinical ethics consultants at large in the corridors of US hospitals. And yet, it must be admitted that the consensus, although undoubtedly broad-based intellectually and influential clinically, masks substantial differences and disagreements within the health professions and the larger society. These differences encompass matters such as the relative weight to be accorded to individual autonomy and the general welfare; the validity of the distinction between, say, "killing" and "allowing to die"; or the proper characterization of artificially provided nutrition and hydration as either "medical treatment" or "basic, humane care."

A second aspect of uncertainty stems from the potential disconnect between an individual health professional's espoused values and ethical commitments and his or her ability to act according to those commitments in specific clinical situations. To take one of many examples, since the 1960s, there has been an enormous shift in physicians' stated attitudes toward disclosing bad news to their patients. Whereas physicians have historically been reluctant to discuss bad diagnoses such as cancer directly with patients for fear of depressing them or eliminating hope,[6] by the late 1970s, physicians who responded to surveys overwhelmingly favored full disclosure of a cancer diagnosis to the patient.[7] Patients themselves, especially in Western societies, usually want to know the truth of their cancer diagnosis, and most also want a realistic estimate of how long they are likely to live. Yet, when Baile and his colleagues[8] surveyed more than 500 oncologists attending a meeting of the American Society of Clinical Oncology (ASCO), nearly one-half rated their ability to break bad news as only fair or poor, and two-thirds rated themselves as not very comfortable or uncomfortable dealing with their patients' resulting emotions. Only half had received any training in the subject.[8] These findings are consistent with the fact that although many studies report general satisfaction on the part of patients and families with the information disclosure process,[9] other studies report significant dissatisfaction with the level of information or emotional support that patients receive from their doctors.[10,11]

With these considerations and qualifications in mind, this discussion of ethical issues in end-of-life care attempts to bring to bear the public consensus mentioned earlier on four major themes:

1. The transition from curative to palliative and end-of-life care
2. Surrogate decision making
3. Responding to demands for nonbeneficial treatment
4. Physician-assisted death

Although ethical analysis cannot pretend to eliminate moral doubt and disagreement—particularly on some of the most contested issues in these domains—some goals are quite realistic. These include (1) providing a blueprint or template for careful and systematic ethical scrutiny of a clinical situation; (2) organizing the dialogue among the various parties to an ethical dispute, thereby assuring that the concerns and perceptions of everyone with a stake in the outcome of a clinical decision are taken seriously; (3) providing a method for isolating particular sources of ethical disagreement, thereby making possible either the marshalling of additional facts or arguments to produce agreement or allowing people unable to agree to recognize their mutual good faith; (4) pointing to areas of agreement as the basis for creative problem solving that leads to decisions and actions consistent with people's most important values; and (5) encouraging educational efforts for health professionals—especially in the realm of patient–provider communication—to bring professionals' behavior more fully in line with their avowed values and beliefs.

The Transition from Curative to Palliative and End-of-Life Care

Patients with serious disease and their physicians usually share three goals for the patient's care: cure or long-lasting remission, prolongation of survival, and comfort and quality of life. As prospects for the first and second goals dim with the progression of disease and the exhaustion of curative therapies, physicians have the opportunity, and the challenge, of recommending that the third goal become the main focus of the patient's continuing care. The World Health Organization[12] defines palliative care as "the active total care of patients whose disease is not amenable to curative treatment. Control of pain, of other symptoms, and of psychological, social, and spiritual problems is paramount. The goal of palliative care is the achievement of the best possible quality of life for patients and their families." J. Andrew Billings has suggested a more patient- and family-friendly definition:

> Palliative care is a special service, a team approach to providing comfort and support for persons living with a life-threatening illness and for their families. We are nurses, social workers, chaplains, and physicians who work with your current health-care team to assure that you and your

family receive excellent pain control and other comfort measures, get the information you want to participate in decisions about your care, receive emotional and spiritual support and practical assistance, obtain expert help in planning for care outside the hospital, continue getting good services in the community, and overall enjoy life as best you can, given your condition. We try to coordinate and tailor a package of services that best suits your values, beliefs, wishes, and needs in whatever setting you are receiving care.[13]

For the doctor, arriving at the decision to focus primarily on palliative care rather than active, disease-modifying therapy can be complicated. It usually combines scientific and technical skills related to prognosis and clinical judgment; communication skills, often involving bad news and the need to respond sensitively to the patient's emotions; and negotiation of treatment preferences. Billings' description of the doctor's role at this juncture is:

> The patient and the family need a doctor who respects their expertise and can help them clarify and choose what they want, yet who is authoritative, helping to bring clarity and control by saying, "Let's keep trying" or "Let's face the music, it's time to stop."[14]

Billings' formulation strikes a balance between the two poles that have characterized ethical debates about the doctor–patient relationship for the past several decades: the doctor as neutral respecter of patient autonomy and the doctor as authority figure under whose guidance patients suspend their own preferences in favor of the doctor's superior insight into their best interests. Despite the strong emphasis on patient autonomy and self-determination in the bioethics literature, when patients are faced with very serious disease and complicated choices, few want to be left completely on their own to make treatment decisions. Billings' formulation captures this reality by emphasizing both respect for the patient's ultimate decision-making authority and the commitment not to abandon the patient by withholding the physician's best professional judgment.

NEGOTIATING TREATMENT PREFERENCES: THE IDEAL DECISION-MAKING PROCESS

From the standpoint of ethics, treatment decisions near the end of life, as at any other juncture in health care, ought to be structured by the notion of informed consent.[15] To be valid, the patient's consent should be informed and free of duress or coercion and should reflect the patient's genuine values and preferences. An ideal decision-making process for medical care would include the following elements:

- *Joint participation* of doctor and patient, with additional participation of significant others of the patient's choice
- *Clear and truthful communication* by the physician
- *Clear and thoughtful deliberation* by the patient
- *Consideration*, by both doctor and patient, of medical and nonmedical factors, including
  - The patient's medical condition and options for treatment (including no treatment)
  - The reasonable probabilities that particular goals can be achieved
  - The reasonably expected proportion of benefits of treatment to harmful or painful side effects
  - The patient's values and life goals
  - The patient's assessment of his or her quality of life and the essential elements for a positive quality of life
  - The patient's tolerance for risks and uncertainty
- *So that*, the resulting decision
  - Reflects a reasonable accommodation to the medical facts
  - Is consistent with the patient's values and the physician's conscience

DEPARTURES FROM THE IDEAL

In the end-of-life context, several factors are likely to complicate the ideal. They can be divided into two large groups: factors related to the uncertainty of prognosis and clinical judgment and factors related to attitudes and values of both patients and physicians. After some discussion of each of these, this section concludes with some suggestions for approaching conversations with patients that attempt to accommodate both prognostic uncertainties and emotional reactions.

Prognosis and Clinical Judgment

There are now a number of resources available that provide prognostic information across a wide range of diseases and conditions, for example, in advanced cancer,[16] heart failure,[17] end-stage chronic obstructive pulmonary disease,[18] dementia,[19] cirrhosis,[20] and coma following cardiopulmonary resuscitation.[21] Although the general outcomes and trajectories of diseases that are the major causes of death in the United States are known, and a typical patient's survival (assuming accurate diagnosis) can usually be estimated within a known range of probabilities, when any particular individual will die remains an inexact prediction. *Most people appreciate this, however, and the inability to give very precise predictions of a patient's remaining life expectancy should not be a barrier to physicians' participating in discussions with patients who want to have some realistic idea of their situation.* As described further in the following text, the most important question for the physician is the level of information a patient desires to receive. The question "Doctor, how long am I going to live?" cannot be answered helpfully without some initial exploration of the meaning the question has to the patient, what has motivated the question, and the patient's preferred level of detail.

A physician's prognostic accuracy seems to vary inversely with the length of time the physician has known the patient. The longer the relationship, the more likely it is that the physician will overestimate the patient's remaining time.[22] Lamont and Christakis[23] comment in relation to this data that a palliative medicine specialist, or some other physician with relevant expertise but with no prior relationship to the patient, is likely to be a helpful resource to the treating physician in formulating prognostic information for individual patients.

Another tendency of physicians that can diminish the usefulness of prognostic information is to provide it solely in terms of the quantity of remaining life (weeks, months, or years), without attempting to describe the quality of life the patient is likely to enjoy. Especially for people with chronic, degenerative conditions or conditions for which available disease-modifying therapies have significant side effects, their remaining quality of life is likely to be as important as a bare estimate of survival. Some issues that are likely to be of particular interest to the patient include the pace and timing of decreases in functional and/or cognitive status, pain and discomfort and the availability of the means to relieve them, loss of independence, and the expected burden on caregivers. It bears repeating that the physician's offer to go into detail on any of these matters should be contingent on a signal from the patient that he or she does in fact want to discuss them. Some people would prefer *not* to have such a clear image of impending decline to look forward to, although they may wish someone in the family to have this information to be better prepared.

Patients' Attitudes and Values

The physician's first responsibility in preparing for a conversation about treatment preferences in the setting of end-of-life care is to assess the patient's emotional and cognitive capacity to participate in the conversation. Among the emotional and attitudinal factors that may cause patients to depart from the ideal decision-making process are the patient's denial of the seriousness of the disease, or the presence of depression or other psychiatric disorders, as well as other forms of cognitive impairment that may be related either to the disease or its treatment. Appropriate treatment of the underlying causes of the cognitive impairment should be the first order of business. If this is not possible, the physician should consider the availability of a surrogate decision maker, as discussed in the next section.

Other emotional factors short of psychiatric impairment can diminish the patient's capacity to participate meaningfully in these discussions. For example, some patients may appear determined to *continue* pursuing active treatment for their disease because they believe other people want them to do this, not because it is their own preference. Some patients may worry about family members' ability to cope with the patient's worsening illness or about their future security and well-being once the patient has died. Some patients may find it hard to reject treatments because they do not want to disappoint the doctor.

On the other hand, patients may *reject* further treatments not because they genuinely believe this is in their best interest but because treatment refusal is a language for expressing other concerns, such as fear (of being a burden to others, of the treatment, of the process of dying), anger, exhaustion, helplessness, mistrust, or unrelieved physical symptoms. A similar phenomenon can underlie patients' requests for physician-assisted death. Sensitive exploration of the background and motivations underlying the patient's stated preferences is essential before the physician concludes that he or she has a clear understanding of the patient's perspective.

Physicians' Attitudes and Values

Several factors on the physician's side can also cause a dialogue about treatment preferences to deviate from the ideal. The physician's counterpart to the patient's denial is the tendency for physicians to overestimate expected survival, especially for patients with whom they have had long-term relationships. It is often easier to perceive the deterioration in the patients of one's colleagues than in one's own patients.

A number of conceptual and philosophical commitments may also lead physicians to minimize or avoid open discussion with the patient about the transition from curative to palliative care. For example, medical training is primarily focused on providing the tools and skills necessary for the active investigation, diagnosis, and treatment of pathology. This instills an ideology of intervention, according to which any pathologic state or process that is potentially reversible *should* be reversed. To stand back and look at the "big picture"—to accompany a patient into death without investigating or treating conditions for which (at least short term) remedies are available—requires a shift in perspective that many physicians find very difficult and contrary to their professional identity.

A closely related issue, especially in academic medical centers, is the imperative of research and therapeutic innovation. From this perspective, it is precisely the point in the patient's illness when all known effective remedies have been exhausted that presents the greatest opportunity for scientific progress. The research imperative demands that these opportunities be seized for trials of new and unproven treatments to push back the boundaries of medical power. Many patients (especially if they are of a socioeconomic status that has entitled them to regular access to health care) are themselves caught up in the ideology of medical progress, having absorbed a lifetime of exhortations from doctors and hospitals to avail themselves of regular checkups and the very latest in medical technology to ensure a longer, happier life.

The power of medical technology to forestall the time of death, especially in the intensive care unit (ICU), gives rise, in Daniel Callahan's phrase, to "technological brinkmanship."[24]

This is the idea that we can and should employ our technology for its maximum life-extending benefit and then back off just at the point—but no later—when its marginal benefits begin to be outweighed by its burdens and costs. The reality is that the point of diminishing return is almost always only discernible in retrospect, after the patient has been subjected to a period of intensive and invasive treatments to no positive end and the family is left to wonder why the patient could not have enjoyed a more peaceful death.

The availability of technology to forestall death creates an additional psychological pressure that derives from the apparently observable fact that the death of any individual patient (especially in the ICU) almost always results from a decision to withhold or withdraw medical treatment. In other words, although in principle, we ought to be able to take comfort from the fact that death is natural and universal—as in the ancient syllogism, "Socrates is a man; all men are mortal, therefore Socrates is mortal"—death for *this* patient *now* seems always to be optional. Its psychological reality for the doctor is that the death occurred only because he or she brought it about when he or she recommended, or acquiesced when the patient or family requested, termination of treatment.

Finally, a very common concern for physicians faced with recommending the transition from curative to palliative care (identified by nearly 60% of the respondents to Baile and colleagues'[8] ASCO survey as the most difficult part of breaking bad news) is "being honest without taking away hope." This is particularly the case when "hope" is identified with cure or significantly extended life. In fact, there are many other objects of patients' and families' hope that physicians almost always can help them realize; for example, comfort and freedom from pain, companionship, completion of important tasks, and security for those who will be left behind.[25] Indeed, as suggested by Billings' previously quoted definition, these concerns are precisely the focus of palliative care. Nevertheless, the strong association of "giving up all hope" with the shift to palliation from active treatment can lead physicians to dread and put off serious discussion of a patient's end-of-life treatment preferences.

COMMUNICATION WITH PATIENTS ABOUT TREATMENT PREFERENCES NEAR THE END OF LIFE

The physician has four primary goals in the dialogue with a patient in the context of end-of-life decision making:

1. To learn about the patient's preferences for receiving information and to assess the patient's coping style when confronting threatening situations
2. To provide the patient with sufficient information about his or her current and projected medical situation and options for treatment and support to enable the patient to make choices that reflect his or her values and preferences
3. To establish rapport and trust in order to enhance the physician's credibility as a source of reliable information and interpersonal support
4. To balance genuine appreciation of the clinical situation with realistic optimism to empower the patient—by mobilizing his or her adaptive capacities and social supports—to maximize his or her quality of life for as long as possible

The goal of effective information transfer, although obviously of cardinal importance, is only one of these several goals. If the others are not also satisfied, information transfer itself may not successfully occur. For this reason, most expert opinion on communication with patients about bad news recommends that the physician address the interpersonal and emotional dimensions of communication as well as the clear presentation of scientific facts.

In an extensive literature review, Penelope Schofield and her colleagues[26] identified 10 major considerations for communication about the transition from curative cancer treatment to palliative care:

1. Preparation prior to the discussion
2. Eliciting the person's understanding of the illness and preferences for information transfer
3. Providing information
4. Responding to emotional reactions
5. Negotiating new goals of care
6. Arranging for continuity of care
7. Addressing family concerns
8. Acknowledging cultural and linguistic diversity
9. Concluding the discussion
10. Documenting the discussion and appropriately informing other members of the treatment team

Baile and colleagues[8] consolidate these dimensions in a six-step protocol with the mnemonic **SPIKES**. In their formulation, the physician's communication with the patient proceeds as follows:

- Step 1: SETTING UP the interview
  Mental rehearsal, arranging for a private setting, involvement of significant others, sitting down, making eye contact, and taking steps to avoid interruption
- Step 2: Assessing the patient's PERCEPTION
  Ask before telling: Ascertain what the patient knows, how they want to receive information; for example, "What have you been told about your medical condition so far?" or "What is your understanding of the reasons we did the MRI?"
- Step 3: Obtaining the patient's INVITATION
  Ask before telling: Ascertain the patient's preference for receiving information, recognizing that shunning information is a valid psychological response for some people. Asking this at the time of test ordering can help set the stage; for example, "How would you like me to give you the test results? Would you like all of the information, or just the big picture, with more time for us to talk about a treatment plan? Is there anyone else with whom you would prefer us to discuss this information?" Lamont and Christakis[23] suggest, "Some people want to know everything possible about their illness and others prefer to know very little. How much about your illness do you want to know from me today?"
- Step 4: Giving KNOWLEDGE and information to the patient
  Give a "warning shot." For example, "Unfortunately I've got some bad news to tell you. . . " Start at the patient's comprehension level, avoiding technical words (say "spread" rather than "metastasize"); give information in small chunks with pauses to check understanding; avoid phrases such as "there is nothing more we can do."
- Step 5: Addressing the patient's EMOTIONS with empathic responses
  Another mnemonic, **NURSE**, is helpful here.
  Name the emotion: You look (sound) as if this is a real shock to you.
  Understand: I cannot imagine what it is like to be so sick.
  Respect: I really appreciate how you have been coping with this.
  Support: I want you to know that regardless of what happens I will be there for you.
  Explore: Tell me more.
- Step 6: STRATEGY and SUMMARY
  Ask before telling: Determine whether the patient wants to discuss future treatment plans at the present time; check the patient's overall understanding of what has been said; present treatment options if appropriate in the moment; offer time for the patient to reflect; offer to be available for questions that may arise after the interview; schedule a follow-up appointment.

In summary, the physician–patient dialogue about the transition from active treatment to palliative care can help the physician fulfill several aspects of the ideal decision-making process. By acknowledging emotional aspects of the situation that are likely to be present on both sides, by offering patients the opportunity to receive information—or not—at their own pace, by examining one's professional biases and assumptions that may hinder an open discussion of the patient's circumstances, and by attention to the interpersonal as well as factual aspects of information transfer, the physician is most likely to support treatment decisions by patients that reflect their genuine values and also to strengthen the foundations for the physician's role as a supportive companion to the patient throughout the course of the illness.

Surrogate Decision Making

At the time end-of-life treatment decisions have to be made, patients may not be able to speak clearly for themselves. They may be too sick to speak, too confused to listen to medical information or to deliberate about preferences, or completely unconscious. Typical contexts when patients lack decisional capacity near the end of life include patients suffering from dementia or other long-term cognitive impairment; patients suffering from delirium as a consequence of their disease or side effects of its treatment (e.g., metabolic derangements, drug-induced delirium, "ICU psychosis"), severely depressed patients, patients with waxing and waning mental capacity, or who give inconsistent, contradictory answers to treatment-related questions within a short period of time; postoperative patients under the influence of anesthetics or medications to promote ventilator compliance; patients suffering loss of consciousness due to stroke, cardiac arrest, or other traumatic event; and patients in coma or persistent vegetative state.

Surrogate decision making is the process by which these patients may be brought as close as possible to the ideal decision-making process described earlier. It involves the following basic elements: (1) assessment of the patient's decisional capacity; (2) for patients deemed lacking in capacity, attempts to rule out or eliminate reversible causes; (3) identification of an appropriate surrogate; (4) clarifying the surrogate's roles and responsibilities; and (5) anticipating, where possible, future needs for surrogate decision making through a process of advance care planning.

ASSESSING DECISIONAL CAPACITY

Decisional capacity is task-specific. Someone may be properly judged capable of making some decisions—Jell-O or custard for dessert, baseball or NASCAR on TV—and incapable of making other decisions—financial investments, whether or not to enter a nursing home, or, most relevant here, the choice of medical treatments in the setting of advanced disease. For the latter, the patient's capacity should be assessed in terms of the following:

- **Understanding:** Does the patient understand the meaning of the diagnostic or prognostic information provided to him or her? Can the patient restate the information in his or her own words in a way that demonstrates this understanding?
- **Appreciation:** Does the patient appreciate the implications of the information for himself or herself? Does he or she appreciate that decisions have to be made from among alternative treatment plans and that his or her input is necessary for these decisions?
- **Deliberation:** Can the patient weigh the alternative treatments according to his or her personal goals and values?
- **Communication:** Can the patient communicate his or her treatment preferences in an understandable manner? Do the patient's stated preferences appear logically related to the patient's goals?

There is no rigid, quantifiable measure of the patient's abilities in these domains. In general, the more significant the decision that needs to be made—in terms of risks, benefits, and side effects—the more stringent our standards should be in satisfying ourselves that the patient has the requisite capacity.[27]

Contrary to common practice, especially in hospitals where psychiatric consultation is readily available, a formal psychiatric consultation is not required to assess a patient's decisional capacity. Nonpsychiatrist physicians ordinarily are capable of forming a reasonable judgment of the patient's abilities in these four domains. Moreover, even if a psychiatric consultant judges the patient to have capacity, it remains the attending physician's responsibility to satisfy himself or herself that the patient is in fact capable of giving informed consent before proceeding with treatment. Where psychiatric opinion is most relevant is when the physician suspects mental illness or delirium as the (possibly reversible) cause of the patient's lack of capacity or where appointment of a legal guardian is anticipated, in which case the court will be interested in authoritative medical opinion.

RULING OUT OR ELIMINATING REVERSIBLE CAUSES OF INCAPACITY

Reversible causes of incapacity can be biologic or situational. Biologic causes include transient delirium, treatable depression, or the side effects of anesthetic or analgesic medications. Situational causes include anxiety or fear as an immediate consequence of receiving bad news, confusion or anxiety due to the effects of hospitalization, the sensory overload of the ICU, and/or separation from familiar people. Before deciding that a patient's lack of capacity warrants turning to a surrogate, realistically assess the importance of making particular decisions right away. If urgent decisions are not required, attempt to diagnose and eliminate the patient's incapacity. This could entail adjustments of medication, psychosocial intervention, or simply the passage of time.

IDENTIFYING A SURROGATE

If the gold standard for ethical health care decision making is the thoughtful participation of an informed patient, the gold standard for surrogate decision making involves a surrogate who is:

- *Authorized* by the patient because the patient considers the surrogate to be trustworthy and in the best position to advocate for the patient's best interests
- *Willing* to accept the patient's trust and to fulfill the role of surrogate in good faith
- *Informed*, through prior acquaintance or explicit conversation with the patient, about the patient's values and preferences regarding medical care near the end of life
- *Capable* of understanding the physician's explanations of the patient's condition and weighing treatment options in light of the patient's preferences
- *Available* to represent the patient's interests at the time decisions have to be made

Since Congress passed the Patient Self-Determination Act in 1990 in the wake of the *Nancy Cruzan* decision of the US Supreme Court, there have been many local and national efforts to encourage people to identify a surrogate in case of their own future incapacity. All 50 states have adopted legislation authorizing health care decision making by surrogates. Despite these efforts, most people for whom end-of-life medical decisions must be made have not designated a surrogate in advance.[28]

A number of states have addressed this gap legislatively by prescribing, in lexical order, the persons who are empowered to act as the patient's surrogate in the absence of the patient's prior designation. A typical ordering begins with the patient's spouse and then moves in descending order through adult children, parents, adult siblings, adult grandchildren, and (only then) other adults who may be in a position to know the patient's beliefs about medical treatment. In states where this regime applies, physicians as well as patients may be faced with the situation where the prescribed surrogate does not fulfill the criteria noted earlier as well as someone lower on the list—or not on the list at all. Gay partners, for example, have legitimate reason to fear exclusion and disenfranchisement in decision making for each other under strict interpretations of these surrogacy laws.

From the point of view of ethics, the physician's primary responsibility as the patient's advocate is to identify the surrogate who meets those criteria to the greatest extent. In cases where that person is available and willing to serve in the role, but another, less qualified, person with lexical priority is expressing conflicting preferences for care, it is advisable for the physician to seek consultation from an ethics committee or from a hospital's legal counsel.

THE SURROGATE'S ROLES AND RESPONSIBILITIES

The surrogate's primary responsibility is to interpret the physician's recitation of the patient's medical condition and recommended treatment in light of what the surrogate has reason to believe are *the patient's* relevant values, preferences, and life goals. This is the "substituted judgment" standard for surrogate decision making. Unless the surrogate has been instructed differently by the patient, he or she ought to try to the best of his or her ability to express treatment preferences that reflect the patient's goals and values, and not the surrogate's, if there is a conflict between them. If the surrogate is not certain what the patient would prefer in a given situation, or if, despite a good faith effort on the part of all who are in a position to know, there is simply no evidence whatsoever of the patient's likely preference, the surrogate ought to make the decision that appears to be, from an objective point of view, in the patient's best interests. Ordinarily, this is determined by weighing, in the most informed manner possible, the likely benefits (to the patient) of various proposed treatments—or no treatment—against their likely burdens (again to the patient). This is (not surprisingly) the "best interests" standard for surrogate decision making.

Physicians and other members of the health care team have potential roles to play in helping surrogates do their job. Their most obvious role is to provide clear and helpful prognostic information and descriptions of proposed treatments according to the protocols outlined in the previous section. But they may also be able to enhance the surrogate's ability to represent the patient's interests and preferences by engaging in dialogue with the surrogate about the patient. The content of that dialogue is suggested by the discussion in the next section of the most useful elements of an advance directive for health care.

A REALISTIC PROCESS OF ADVANCE CARE PLANNING

Most commentators agree that policies to encourage people to use advance directives to prepare for future end-of-life decision making have been largely unsuccessful.[28,29] As noted earlier, only a minority (between 20% and 30%) of American adults have filled out an advance directive. Evidence suggests that even for those who have them, advance directives do not influence decision making. Most particularly, if people expect that filling out an advance directive will ensure that the medical decisions made during their future incapacity will match the choices they themselves would have made had they been able to participate in those decisions themselves, they will almost certainly be disappointed.

Common difficulties are that the documents cannot be located when they are needed, they are too vague to give useful guidance in the patient's actual circumstances, or the patient's stated preferences are ignored in favor of a course of action that physicians and/or family members believe is more in accord with the patient's present best interests. Hickman et al.[29] have listed some of the main factors that may explain these difficulties. These include:

1. An overemphasis on the patient's legal rights to refuse medical care, as opposed to the more general objective of enhancing people's ability to influence their care according to their goals and values
2. Insufficient efforts by health professionals to educate patients as to realistic outcomes of various medical interventions
3. Overemphasis on patients' preferences for specific medical interventions rather than the effort to ascertain the patient's views about goals and values and about what constitutes an acceptable quality of life
4. The assumption that the planning process is complete as soon as an advance directive has been filled out rather than viewing the process as ongoing and subject to periodic reassessment and revision in light of changing medical circumstances
5. Failure to involve family members or other important people in the patient's life in discussions about preferences for medical care
6. Absence of system-wide policies and procedures to ensure that patients' preferences for care are known and respected wherever the patient may be receiving care
7. Low community awareness of issues related to end-of-life planning
8. State advance directive laws that introduce barriers into the advance planning process

Three Basic Problems

As significant as Hickman and colleagues'[29] barriers are, there are three more basic problems with advance directives that frequently lead to frustration and disappointment even when patients have gone to the trouble of creating one. All three are related to the nature of medical care for the critically ill and the existential predicament of the person facing death. Stated briefly, and somewhat too simply, they are as follows.

Unpredictability

Because of the probabilistic and uncertain nature of prognosis, it is extremely unlikely that the scenarios a healthy person imagines when filling out his or her advance directive—either sitting at the kitchen table or in the doctor's office—will match the actual circumstances the patient or surrogate will face in the future. The more general the terms of the advance directive, in order to capture a range of possibilities broad enough to fit an unknown and unknowable future, the less use they will be in providing specific guidance about treatment preferences. This is a structural problem that no preprinted advance directive form—no matter how elaborately or imaginatively it has been constructed—can solve.

Uncertainty

Related to the unpredictability of the time and manner of death in general is a more specific uncertainty as to the potential benefit of any particular medical intervention or treatment that might be used near the end of the incapacitated person's life. Consider, for example, treatments such as antibiotics, oxygen therapy, blood transfusions, or even more invasive procedures such as kidney dialysis. All of these are typically among the items that, in advance directives, people indicate the desire *to refuse* in the case of terminal illness. Yet, each of these, although not capable of reversing the dying process, may be very useful for more particular goals such as alleviating pain, clearing mental confusion, or simply keeping a person alive long enough for family or friends to gather at the bedside for a final farewell. The question "If you were mentally incapacitated and terminally ill, would you want blood products or antibiotics?" for example, is practically meaningless when asked far in advance.[30]

Ambivalence

The desire for a gentle death, free of tubes and machines, co-exists in most of us with the powerful desire to stay alive. It is very difficult to predict how, in the moment of truth, a particular patient will respond to even a tiny chance of success for a life-prolonging treatment when the alternative to trying the treatment is likely to be imminent death. The difficulty of extrapolating a patient's real-time choices from previous discussions is compounded by the "framing effect," in which those choices will be strongly influenced by the way the alternatives are actually described.[31]

A Realistic Approach

Despite these difficulties, there are some very realistic and meaningful goals that advance care planning *can* help people achieve. One goal is to promote honest and open communication about important values and life goals within families and between patients, families, and health professionals in the face of serious illness. This type of communication is often of great intrinsic value whether or not it bears any relation to specific treatment choices. Another goal is to arrange for future medical decisions to be made, in case of future incapacity, by someone whose love and care the principal trusts—not on the assumption that this individual will infallibly make the "right" decision (if "right" means matching exactly the decision the principal would have made)—but, because *any* surrogate is apt to be "wrong," it is often of great comfort to know that the decision maker is someone who loves and cares about you and is doing his or her best to serve your best interests. Finally, advance planning is an opportunity to reflect on those qualities of life that make life worth holding onto and, conversely, those qualities that might be worse than death and to communicate those values to a surrogate, who can then compare the likely outcomes of real-time medical alternatives to those benchmarks and make choices in their light.[32]

A reasonable and useful advance care planning document should probably contain information along the following lines:

1. Identification of a preferred surrogate decision maker and at least one backup
2. Statement of the extent of the surrogate's authority and how much flexibility the surrogate has in responding to real-time circumstances in ways that might depart from any specific instructions
3. Evidence that the surrogate is aware of his or her appointment and understands the scope of his or her authority
4. A statement from the principal describing the qualities and aspects of life that the principal considers necessary for a minimally acceptable quality of life, accompanied by instructions to the surrogate to request the application or continuation of *any and all* medical treatments that have a reasonable likelihood—according to accepted medical judgment—of restoring to the principal that quality of life for a reasonable period of time. Similarly, the surrogate is instructed to decline or insist on the withdrawal of *any and all* medical treatments if those treatments do not have a reasonable chance—according to accepted medical judgment—of achieving or maintaining that quality of life for a reasonable period of time.
5. In general, the document should *not* specify particular treatments that the principal does or does not want. The statement in item 4 should provide sufficient guidance for the physician to make these specific treatment decisions

in light of the principal's overall criteria for an acceptable quality of life, combined with the principal's preference for resolving medical uncertainties—see item 7. However, there may be some special circumstances in which particular treatments should be mentioned; for example, a Jehovah's Witness may wish to decline blood or blood products, or a person who has previously been resuscitated and placed on a mechanical respirator may have become convinced by the experience that he or she would never want it to be repeated, or in states that require the administration of artificial nutrition and hydration unless they are explicitly included among treatments to be withheld. Otherwise, the broad statement of values (item 4) and preference for resolution of uncertainties (item 7) should suffice for most people.

6. A statement of the principal's willingness to undergo trial periods of medical treatments when physicians are uncertain of their likely benefit, as defined in item 4, accompanied by a clear statement of the surrogate's authority to stop those treatments after the agreed-on trial period has ended
7. A statement of the principal's preference either that genuine medical uncertainties be resolved in favor of *more* aggressive treatment or *less* aggressive treatment, with a clear additional statement that the surrogate has the ultimate authority to resolve disagreements between conflicting medical opinions
8. A statement by the principal that he or she wants all necessary measures to maintain comfort and to treat pain and that when medical treatments are deemed incapable of achieving the goals defined in item 4, pain and other symptoms should be treated aggressively even if adequate treatment carries the risk of hastening death. The statement should include the desire for treating physicians to consult with qualified specialists in pain management and palliative care whenever they or the surrogate deems it appropriate.

Beyond their value in suggesting what an advance directive should contain, these items are also intended to suggest some of the questions that physicians can ask—directly of patients in advance—or to help surrogates fulfill their roles in order to fashion a treatment plan more likely than not to respect patient values.

A further step beyond the preparation of an advance care planning document is the execution of a different sort of document, designed to turn a patient's statement of treatment preferences into *actionable medical orders* to be followed by clinicians and emergency medical technicians wherever the patient happens to be. The Physician Orders for Life-Sustaining Treatment (POLST), originated in Oregon, was the first such document—whose successful implementation requires intensive efforts to educate clinicians as well as patients about the indications for and scope of the document—although at the present time, well over 30 states have adopted similar programs.[33]

It should be said in conclusion that many people experience end-of-life decision making that is smooth and uncomplicated, and for many survivors, the death of a loved one, although sad, is neither chaotic nor traumatic. When things do go awry, leaving people anguished and bewildered by events that seem to be tumbling out of control, it is usually not the fault of a missing or poorly worded living will or durable power of attorney for health care. Recall the perspectives of Hinton and Burt in the introduction. Death carries enormous power to frighten us and to discombobulate the best laid plans. Despite our rhetoric of *management* of symptoms, or of *directing* our health care providers to do (or not to do) this or that, we do not control death. In its presence, we bear witness and do the best we can.

Responding to Demands for Nonbeneficial Treatment

The ethical consensus respecting a competent adult's right to *refuse* medical treatment—even life-sustaining treatment when the refusal is contrary to the physician's professional judgment—does not extend to the patient's or family's right to *demand* medical treatments that, in the physician's professional judgment, offer no prospect of patient benefit. This difference in the moral and legal status of refusals and demands occasionally gives rise to conflicts that are among the most vexing and emotionally draining that can occur in end-of-life care. Taken to their limit, these conflicts can be so destructive not only of the physician–patient–family relationship but also of the atmosphere and milieu of the patient's dying that loved ones will take with them in memory, that preventing them is the physician's foremost ethical responsibility. Preventive measures are not always successful, but their chances can be improved through systematic analysis of the nature of a conflict in its early manifestations ("differential diagnosis") and a range of communication and conflict resolution strategies.

THE ETHICAL BASIS OF THE CONFLICT

Ethically, the difference in physicians' obligations toward refusals of treatment and demands for treatment stems from the way ethics and law customarily interpret the concepts of autonomy and self-determination. In bioethics, respect for personal autonomy and self-determination is rooted in the ideas of privacy and bodily integrity. The idea is that—with very few exceptions, such as a potential public health emergency—a person ought to be able to control what is done to, with, or for his or her own body. This is the foundation for the requirement of informed consent and for the patient's right to say "No" to the physician's recommendations for (even life-saving) treatment. Courts have tested the claim of patient self-determination, or the patient's right to say "No," against potentially competing claims such as the state's interest in preserving life, the interests of third parties (e.g., spouses or minor children), the integrity of the medical profession, and the prevention of suicide. In every case, almost all courts have come down in favor of self-determination. The competing interests have been seen as too abstract, too remote, or too weak to override the individual's interests in preventing the violation of his or her bodily integrity and limiting the power of others to enforce values or life goals that he or she does not share.[34]

The matter is quite different for the person who demands a particular treatment. (This distinction applies equally to requests for physician-assisted death, which are discussed in the next section.) Here, it is no longer a question of an individual protecting his or her bodily integrity by drawing a boundary and saying, "Do not cross." Respecting this essentially negative right (the right to be let alone) requires physicians and everyone else simply to do nothing. The person who demands a treatment, however, would compel the physician, and potentially many other people, to act affirmatively to supply the treatment. Many more public and professional interests and resources are implicated in the positive satisfaction of a demand than in the negative respect for a refusal. And, especially when the demand is for a treatment that, according to accepted medical opinion, will not benefit the patient, ethical opinion is far more deferential to competing societal and professional interests than in the case of patients who are asserting their negative right to be let alone.

It is worth noting that only a very few courts have explicitly addressed the question of patients' demands for lifesaving treatments that are contrary to widely accepted medical opinion, and up to now, no clear judicial trend has emerged.[35] Among the most likely reasons for the relative lack of such cases is hospitals' reluctance—despite their desire to support their physicians' professional judgment—to face the costs and potential damage to their public image of going to court to force the removal of life-sustaining treatment over a family's vehement protests. However, as noted earlier, there are other, better reasons to avoid recourse to the very public, adversarial forum of a court of law to resolve these conflicts. Preserving a therapeutic relationship and protecting the special environment of the deathbed are very worthy motivations for the physician's efforts to find a more constructive resolution.

THE CLINICAL CONTEXT OF THE CONFLICT

Many clinical scenarios have the potential to bring doctors into conflict with patients or their families over the continuation of medical treatments of little or no likely patient benefit; for example, continuous blood transfusion for the patient with inoperable bleeding, full resuscitation efforts for the elderly patient with sepsis and multiorgan failure, and additional courses of high-toxicity anticancer treatment for the patient for whom both standard and experimental therapies have failed to slow the spread of the disease. The paradigm case, however, continues to be the noncommunicative, ventilator-dependent patient, kept alive by mechanical means while suffering inexorable bodily deterioration and discomfort with little prospect of improvement. This is the patient who, in K. Danner Clouser's words—as vividly applicable today as when he wrote them 40 years ago—"is on the borderline between treatment and torture, where therapeutic hope has vanished, and pain without point has taken over. The doctor's time-honored admonition to preserve life and lessen pain is at a stupefying impasse."[36]

Faced with a family's continuing insistence that "everything be done," including, if necessary, chest compressions and electric shocks to the heart in order to keep the patient alive, the medical team chafes in resentment at another "family that does not get it." Every evening, when the family arrives at the ICU, the same routine plays out: A physician from the team recites the grim medical facts, points to the patient's deteriorating body, and urges the family to allow them to withdraw the ventilator so the patient can die peacefully. The family listens to the explanations—the descriptions of failing organs, alarming laboratory values, hopelessly long odds—and insists that everything be done. The team wonders why a supposedly loving family is being so selfish and cruel and how it is possible for the obstinacy of one family to commandeer enormous medical resources that could and should be put to much better use. The family wonders why the doctors keep badgering them with their litany of doom and gloom when they should simply be about their business of keeping their loved one alive and how it is possible that the hospital can be so indifferent to the value of the life which the family has entrusted to it.

DIFFERENTIAL DIAGNOSIS OF THE CONFLICT

The frustrated medical team's epithet, "The family does not get it," is often shorthand for a common diagnosis of the cause of the impasse; namely, that for all of the medical team's efforts to be clear about the patient's serious medical condition and grim prognosis, the family has yet to fully comprehend. With every passing day, with its presentation of facts, laboratory values, and statistics, the team's hypothesis appears to be confirmed by the family's implacable opposition to changing the patient's level of care. Perhaps, the team reflects, we are using too many big words. Perhaps, this is not a very well educated family. Maybe English is not their native language. The team redoubles its efforts to educate the family about the seriousness of the situation, only to remain stuck with the same result.

In fact, there are several possible explanations for the conflict between the doctor and the family, of which a lack of intellectual understanding is only one and not the most common

TABLE 13.1 Conflicts Often Resolvable
• Lack of comprehension
• Emotional barriers to processing information
• Disagreement about the patient's preferences
• Narrow understanding of "hope" and "caring"
• Mistrust of health care team
• Team conflict and mixed messages

TABLE 13.2 Conflicts Often Intractable
• Disagreement on legitimate goals of medical care
• Disagreement on acceptable probabilities of success or trade-offs between potential benefits and burdens
• Disagreement on an acceptable quality of life
• Waiting for a miracle

in any event. But if lack of understanding is *not* the principal source of the conflict, repeated efforts to lecture the family about the medical facts are no more likely to resolve the impasse than a course of antibiotics is likely to succeed in treating a viral infection. From the outset, therefore, the ethics of prevention requires careful discrimination among the possibilities. Tables 13.1 and 13.2 suggest a differential diagnosis of physician–family conflicts surrounding medically nonbeneficial treatments.

The principal difference between the two tables is that, in principle at least, all of the issues in Table 13.1 are amenable to resolution through sensitive, therapeutic dialogue, whereas the issues in Table 13.2 represent potentially intractable clashes of values or worldviews. Therefore, a good first step for the team is to try to elicit as specifically and clearly as possible all apparent sources of disagreement, sorting them if possible into the two categories and choosing strategies of mediation or conflict resolution accordingly.[37]

In Table 13.1, for example, even though problems of intellectual comprehension are infrequently the cause of profound disagreements about life-sustaining treatment, the team has the responsibility (always implicit in our ideal decision-making process) of communicating information about the patient's illness in a language and in a setting that are conducive to patient/family comprehension. It is worthwhile cultivating the skill of inquiring, in a noncondescending way, whether a family can repeat back to the team the essence of the information the team has tried to convey. (A likely apocryphal story recounts the experience of a surgeon who hastily sketched the chambers of a baby's heart for a new mother, drawing a schematic diagram similar to that shown in Figure 13.1, in an effort to explain the need for a valve repair, only to overhear the mother report to the father that their baby's problem was that it had been born with a square heart.) Genuine misconceptions and misunderstanding usually can be corrected with appropriate educational strategies.

Other issues in Table 13.1 may deserve more consideration. For example:

- What may appear as a lack of intellectual comprehension may be a manifestation of emotional barriers to taking in information. The information may be too threatening, too unexpected, or too evocative of a deepest dread to be absorbed without the protective shields of numbing or denial. Most situations permit periods of supportive accompaniment of the shell-shocked, grief-stricken family before pressing forward with the team's recommendations to change the focus of care. Communication strategies discussed earlier, particularly under the SPIKES and NURSE mnemonics, can be of great value in this setting.
- The team and family may have different understandings, or evidence, of the patient's likely preferences. The patient may have expressed one view to the doctor and another to the family. Language in an advance directive may suggest one thing to the team but something quite different to family members who were present when the document was filled out. A tension-lowering approach in this setting is for someone (perhaps an ethics consultant) to open a physician–family conference with the statement,

"Everyone in this room is trying to do exactly the same thing, which is to give [your husband, father, brother] the care that he would want if he could speak with us now. Our challenge is to figure out what that is. Let's go over what each of us knows about his likely preferences at this point, and how we learned this information."

- Patients as well as physicians may equate "hope" exclusively with cure or prolongation of life and "care" with the provision of maximal medical treatment. Efforts to expand hope to include achievable goals more consistent with the patient's condition and suggestions to the family of ways to express love and care through their presence, voice, and touch may offer the family emotional space to adjust their expectations of the medical team.
- Especially for families from marginalized, economically disadvantaged communities, the recommendation to limit intensive medical care can appear to repeat long-standing patterns of social injustice and deprivation. The medical team may represent one more agent of an oppressive power structure. In this setting, the family is unlikely to trust the team's recommendations, even when they are made in good faith on the basis of solid scientific evidence. If the team suspects this dynamic may be at work, explicitly naming the lack of trust and offering to call in more trusted individuals from the family's community may diffuse the conflict and promote eventual agreement on a treatment plan.
- Perhaps most common of all preventable or remediable sources of conflict, especially in the ICU, are mixed messages to the family about the patient's condition. The attending physician may prepare the family for the patient's inevitable death based on the overall combination of downward-trending prognostic indicators only to have a specialist consultant come by later to tell the family that "the [lungs, kidneys, blood counts] look a bit better today." A team that repeatedly sends mixed signals to the family should not be surprised when the family holds fast to the most optimistic statements and insists on staying the course. The most urgent task is for the team to arrive at its own internal consensus.

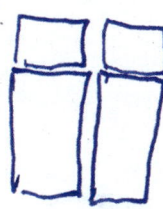

FIGURE 13.1 Physician's sketch of infant heart in apocryphal story of miscommunication.

TABLE 13.3 Checklist for the Team
• Do team members agree on diagnosis and prognosis?
• Have team members and family compared sources of information about the patient's preferences?
• Is the team speaking to the family with one voice?
• Has the team identified a spokesperson with the greatest rapport and credibility in the eyes of the family?

A brief checklist (Table 13.3) can be part of a preventive ethics strategy to help the team first ascertain whether it is in fact dealing with a Table 13.1 type of conflict and, second, maximize its chances of resolving it.

Table 13.2 conflicts are more difficult to resolve solely within the context of therapeutic dialogue. This is because the terms of the disagreement reflect value differences or worldviews that are not necessarily amenable to rational persuasion or supply disputants with individually convincing yet mutually incompatible interpretations of agreed on facts. Institutional policies for mediation, which may include mandatory consultations with an ethics committee and—if these efforts fail to break the impasse—offers to transfer the care of the patient either to another physician or to another institution, are options of almost last resort.[37] In the extreme case, where none of these options is feasible, the institution may be faced with the choice of going to court to obtain judicial authorization to stop the treatment—with no certainty of success but the virtual certainty of cementing the family's enduring resentment. Alternatively, it may recognize that there are (fortunately rare) instances where, for reasons of compassion, "professional medical judgment" and "the rational use of medical resources" may yield to a family's indomitable will. Although the team may view the patient's dying as needlessly prolonged and even horrible, in the circumstances of a family's passionate intransigence, it may be the least poor outcome. Support for the likely moral distress of the staff becomes another institutional responsibility in this situation.

Physician-Assisted Death

The vast attention paid to physician-assisted death in discussions of ethics at the end of life is far out of proportion to its actual significance in the experiences of most dying patients and their families. For most people, far more important issues are related to maintaining the energy and stamina to pursue valued activities and relationships amid the burdens of illness and obtaining timely, skilled help with pain, anxiety, and other symptoms. Even in Oregon, whose first-in-the-nation Death with Dignity Act legalizing physicians' prescriptions of lethal doses of medication for terminally ill patients spawned fears of a "suicide mecca" in the Pacific Northwest, the 133 deaths in 2016 that occurred under the law amounted to barely more than one-third of 1% of all deaths in the state that year.[38,39] Nevertheless, the issue commands attention in part because of legitimate public concerns about the quality of care that our society makes available to the dying and because active campaigns to expand legalization of the practice beyond Oregon are ongoing in many states across the United States. As of 2017, four states (Washington, Montana, Vermont, and California) have chosen to do so.[40]

TERMINOLOGY

As with many contested social practices, the language used to describe the various ways physicians can be involved in hastening the time of a patient's death has evolved through many phases and fashions, with people's preferred language often reflecting their prior moral evaluation of the practices in question. Thus, the literature abounds in discussions of the differences between "killing patients" and "allowing patients to die" or the differences between "passive euthanasia" and "active euthanasia,"[41] and—more recently—the preference of organizations such as the American Public Health Association[42] and the American Academy of Hospice and Palliative Medicine[43] for the term *physician-assisted dying* rather than *physician-assisted suicide*. What seems to be at issue in the debates about terminology is the recognition that *how we characterize* an action (or an omission) often predetermines judgments of its moral status.

Because "killing" is nearly universally condemned in all but very carefully circumscribed situations, proponents of physician actions (or omissions) that hasten a patient's death take pains to argue that those actions or omissions are not instances of "killing." Similarly, because "suicide" carries wide social stigma and is often associated with mental illness, patients who make use of physician-provided lethal prescriptions and the physicians who provide them prefer to characterize what they are doing in terms other than committing or aiding in "suicide." In fact, there is usually room for reasonable people to disagree about the most accurate characterization of many actions. This is one reason why, as mentioned at the beginning of this chapter, the public consensus on many aspects of end-of-life care masks considerable uncertainty and debate within society.

For convenience, the rest of this section will employ the term *physician-assisted death* to refer to a spectrum of actions and omissions by which physicians may influence the timing of an incurably ill patient's death so that it occurs sooner than it probably would have without the physician's involvement. There is a fairly strong public and professional consensus (with the qualifications previously mentioned) about the moral status of many points along the spectrum.

ETHICAL CONSIDERATIONS ALONG THE CLINICAL SPECTRUM

Requests for physician-assisted death confront physicians with troubling questions about the proper boundaries of medical practice and the nature of their duty to relieve suffering. There are at least six reasonably distinct actions or roles that a physician might take in the care of an incurably ill patient that could advance the timing of the patient's death. Two lie at opposite ends of the ethical and legal spectrum. Respecting a competent patient's wishes to forego or remove life-sustaining treatment is universally accepted ethically and legally in the United States. Administering a lethal injection with the intent of immediately ending the patient's life ("active euthanasia") is universally rejected legally in the United States and—although not universally condemned ethically—commands the least widespread support in the ethical literature. In between are four actions that remain somewhat controversial although in varying degrees, always allowing for the fact that characterizing an action as one of these four is itself often a morally significant choice.[44,45]

The four intermediate actions are:
- Aggressive symptom management, usually with opiates and sedatives, despite the risk of hastening the patient's death. The paradigm case is the use of large doses of morphine for pain relief that have the effect of causing fatal respiratory depression. In fact, this is an extremely *unlikely* side effect of skillful opioid administration to a patient who has been receiving chronic opioid therapy for pain relief for a period of time. Nevertheless, the scenario is frequently brought up in discussion of the "rule of double effect." This is the notion, originating in Catholic moral theology, that an action with foreseeable but unintended bad effects (here, the death of the patient) may under certain conditions be undertaken with the primary intent of bringing about its good effect (here, the relief of pain). The extensive debate over the philosophical coherence and clinical applicability of the rule of double

effect is beyond the scope of this chapter.[46–48] For present purposes, it is sufficient to note that the basic concept of treating patient suffering aggressively with appropriate medical therapies, even at the risk of the patient's earlier death as a side effect of the therapy, is well accepted clinical practice and appears also to have received the sanction of at least some justices of the U.S. Supreme Court.

- Sedating the consenting, terminally ill patient to the point of unconsciousness to protect the patient from otherwise intractable physical or emotional suffering while also withholding artificially provided nutrition and hydration. This sits on the borderline between the previous action (in combination with the universally accepted practice of respecting patient refusals of medical treatment), on the one hand, and the far more controversial action of injecting patients with a lethal dose of medication. The argument against the practice is that although the sedatives themselves are not administered in an intentionally lethal dose as in the case of "active euthanasia," when combined with the withholding of nutrition and hydration, the patient's death is as inevitable as it would be at the lethal dose. That it takes place more slowly, in this view, does not avoid the appropriate characterization of the action as ("slow") active euthanasia.[49] The rejoinder to this is that, unlike active euthanasia, with its clear intent for immediate death, "palliative sedation"—as the practice has come to be known—is in principle always reversible (sedatives can be lightened to give the patient the opportunity to interact and change course if desired) and remains focused on alleviation of discomfort rather than bringing about the patient's death.

- Counseling the patient about voluntarily stopping eating and drinking and, if the patient decides to do this, providing medication as needed to alleviate possible discomforts or anxiety over the ensuing period of the patient's death from dehydration. This is another borderline action. On the one hand, it seems to avoid the moral conundrum posed by physician-provided prescriptions for lethal injection because the patient is solely responsible for his or her lack of nutrition and hydration. Moreover, the determination required on the patient's part to persist in refusing to eat or drink until death is a safeguard against subtle manipulation or coercion of the patient. On the other hand, the physician clearly has played some significant role. Without the physician's education of the patient about the option, his or her assurances of providing comfort measures, and actually providing them, many people would probably never consider this option at all, much less pursue it to its conclusion.

- Providing a prescription for a lethal dose of medication at the patient's request and counseling the patient about how to take the medication to ensure a painless death, after ensuring the patient's mental competence, providing information about palliative care as an alternative, and requiring both oral and written requests separated by a waiting period. This is the Oregon Death with Dignity Act. As with the previous action, the patient takes all of the decisive steps to bring about his or her death and may decide at many points to change his or her mind—indeed, since Oregon's law was passed in 1997, a total of 1,749 people have had prescriptions written under the law, whereas only 1,127 have died from ingesting the medications.[38] Nevertheless, by calculating the effective dose, writing the prescription, and counseling the patient on how to ingest the medication, the physician is complicit in the patient's death in a way that he or she would not be were the patient to end his or her life in a completely private act.

TWO LEVELS OF RESPONSE: SOCIAL POLICY AND CLINICAL CARE

There are two important levels of response to the issue of physician-assisted death: the level of social policy (i.e., which actions along the clinical spectrum should be legally permitted or prohibited) and the level of clinical care (i.e., how individual physicians should respond to their patients who request help in advancing the time of their death).

Social Policy

At the level of social policy, there are once again two positions at the ends of a spectrum, with ongoing active debates about positions in between. One end is occupied by advocates of a thoroughgoing libertarianism: The choice to end one's life at the time and in the manner of one's own choosing is so bound up with personal privacy and self-determination that no limits should be set on the actions of fully informed, mentally competent adults, or on those of a physician willing to help a terminally ill, suffering patient achieve a swift and painless death. The other end views physicians' direct involvement in assisted death in the forms of providing prescriptions or injecting lethal medication as so contrary to the role and professional identity of the physician, and so destructive of important societal values, as to require universal and permanent legal prohibition. Physicians, on this view, should abstain from the practice even where it is legally permitted.[50]

The most active debate takes place between these extremes. The essential dispute is this: Given the improvement in the science and technique of palliative care and pain management over the last 20 years or so (much of which is documented elsewhere in this volume), is the number of people whose physical or existential anguish near the end of life is beyond the reach of effective palliation large enough to justify the societal risks that could accompany widespread legalization of physician-assisted death in its most direct and active forms? Those who say *no*—and at the state level that would include, as of now, all states in the United States *except* Oregon, Washington, Montana, Vermont, and California—worry that the possibilities for various types of abuse in a permissive legal system outweigh the benefits to the very small number of people who truly have no other acceptable options. These abuses might include acts of desperation by people without reliable access to medical care of any sort, much less state-of-the-art palliative care; subtle coercion of people to take advantage of legal means to end their lives, playing on their common desire not to be a burden on others; or misguided compassion of caregivers who are ignorant of comfort measures and social supports that could have provided the patient with more options for maintaining dignity and comfort.[2]

Those who say *yes* argue that these hypothetical, even if theoretically plausible, worries should not outweigh the actual suffering of identifiable people who are ravaged by disease and dying in uncontrolled misery or humiliation. Given what even most opponents concede that there are indeed some patients (small though their number might be) whose suffering is not remediable with standard measures of palliative care, proponents of legalization believe the more active forms of physician assistance should be available—and socially permissible—as a last resort.[45,51] They contend that the Oregon experience itself should reassure skeptics that safeguards against abuse can work[38]; and that, even if legally prohibited, physician-assisted death in its active forms is and will be carried out, whereas legalization will allow a more public, well-regulated practice to take the place of the "euthanasia underground."[52]

Clinical Care

Regardless of the resolution of these issues at the social and political level, individual physicians should be prepared to deal compassionately and therapeutically with patients who raise the possibility of physician-assisted death. Opponents and proponents of legalization of the more active forms of physician involvement usually agree that excellent palliative care—the active management and support for physical, psychosocial, and spiritual distress—is the standard of care for the seriously ill patient near the end of life. Quill and Arnold[53] outline a set of responses within the physician–patient relationship and the therapeutic dialogue that can help assess and respond to patients, independent of the physician's personal moral beliefs or the legal environment of his or her practice. They recommend that the physician who receives a request from a patient to help hasten death:

- **CLARIFY** what the patient is communicating: General thoughts about the desirability of ending his or her life? Wondering about the future if his or her condition deteriorates? Asking for help right now?
- **SUPPORT** the patient by giving reassurance that whatever the patient feels or desires, the physician is prepared to work together to find a mutually acceptable solution.
- **EVALUATE** the patient's mental state and decision-making capacity; whether the request seems commensurate with the level of unrelieved suffering; whether there is evidence of treatable depression.
- **EXPLORE** the many possible sources of intolerable suffering, for example, poorly controlled physical symptoms, loneliness, sleep disturbances and exhaustion, psychological or spiritual anguish.
- **RESPOND** to the emotions associated with the patient's request. Take them seriously while also trying to separate your own emotions from those of the patient.
- **INTENSIFY TREATMENT**, with the help of a multidisciplinary team, of any potentially reversible elements of the patient's suffering.

Only when all of these steps have been completed, Quill and Arnold[53] recommend, should the physician respond directly to a patient's persistent request for hastened death. Physicians who believe that affirmative assistance is justified beyond steps that fall within ethically or legally accepted practice have a genuine moral dilemma. Some may feel compelled to inform the patient that, despite their sympathy and solidarity, they cannot cross a particular legal or ethical boundary but may be willing to refer the patient to another physician. Others may be willing to, in Quill's words—cited in a very valuable essay by John Arras[54]—"take small risks for people [they] really know and care about."

Conclusion: Beyond the Patient–Physician Dyad

Good care for a dying patient depends on more than the skillful efforts of the most conscientious physician. Dying is both an intensely private and an inherently social process. The ramifications of the patient's illness spread throughout his or her social network, both in space—to family, intimate friends, workmates, and so on—and in time—lasting throughout the grief and bereavement of the survivors. Palliative care, which sets itself the task of ministering not only to the patient but also to the "family as the unit of care," necessarily raises ethical and policy questions beyond the patient–physician dyad.

Some of these issues are closely connected to some of the familiar topics of clinical ethics, such as protecting the confidentiality of medical information or weighing the preferences or needs of family members against potentially incompatible wishes of the patient (e.g., the patient who insists on remaining at home to die even as family members are pushed beyond their physical or emotional limits by the demands of home-based care). Issues such as these push against an individualistic ethic that places the physician's obligations to the best interests of his or her patient above all other moral considerations,[55] and they

often call for skills of negotiation and mediation that are not typically included in the interviewing and communication skills training in medical schools.

Other issues touch on broader questions of public policy and the allocation of society's resources. Excellent palliative care requires *systems* of care that can match the particular needs of patients and their families across all the sites of care typical of the prolonged, chronic illnesses that precede most deaths in our society.[28] These include, at a minimum:

- Systems to elicit and document meaningful information from patients about their values, preferences, and goals for medical care and to make sure the documentation accompanies the patient wherever they are in the health care system
- Systems to assure quality standards for the provision of palliative care in health care institutions, including hospitals, nursing homes, and personal care facilities
- Systems to train health professionals in the principles and practices of palliative care
- Systems for family and caregiver support that help families participate meaningfully in the lives and care of their dying loved ones without sacrificing their own physical, mental, and financial well-being
- Systems for financing care that reward professionals for the time-intensive nature of patient and family support and communication in palliative care

As has been mentioned more than once in this chapter, the disruptive power of death makes it impossible for even the best systems and most dedicated individuals to ensure that every person dies according to his or her ideals and hopes for meaning, dignity, and comfort. And the physician is only one actor—albeit a very significant one—in the universal human process of coming to terms with life's ending. Families, faith communities, neighborhoods, civic groups, employers, professional caregivers, and many others have the opportunity and responsibility to help a person die in ways that affirm the values and qualities that made his or her life itself worthwhile. The best social policies, laws, and regulations for the care of the dying will be those that make the efforts of all of these people easier rather than harder.

References

1. Hinton J. The dying and the doctor. In: Toynbee A, ed. *Man's Concern with Death*. St. Louis, MO: McGraw-Hill; 1969:36–45.
2. Burt RA. *Death Is That Man Taking Names: Intersections of American Medicine, Law, and Culture*. Berkeley: University of California Press; 2002.
3. McIntyre A. *After Virtue*. Notre Dame, IN: Notre Dame University Press; 1981.
4. Engelhardt HT Jr. *The Foundations of Bioethics*. 2nd ed. New York: Oxford University Press; 1996.
5. Meisel A. The legal consensus about forgoing life-sustaining treatment: its status and its prospects. *Kennedy Inst Ethics J* 1993:2(4):309–345.
6. Oken D. What to tell cancer patients. A study of medical attitudes. *JAMA* 1961;175:1120–1128.
7. Novack DH, Plumer R, Smith RL, et al. Changes in physicians' attitudes toward telling the cancer patient. *JAMA* 1979;241:897–900.
8. Baile WF, Buckman R, Lenzi R, et al. SPIKES—a six-step protocol for delivering bad news: application to the patient with cancer. *Oncologist* 2000;5:302–311.
9. Benbassat J, Pilpel D, Tidhar M. Patients' preferences for participation in clinical decision-making: a review of published surveys. *Behav Med* 1998;24:81–88.
10. Ford S, Fallowfield L, Lewis S. Can oncologists detect distress in their out-patients and how satisfied are they with their performance during bad news consultations? *Br J of Cancer* 1994;70:767–770.
11. Ford S, Fallowfield L, Lewis S. Doctor-patient interactions in oncology. *Soc Sci Med* 1996;42:1511–1519.
12. World Health Organization. *Cancer Pain Relief and Palliative Care*. Geneva, Switzerland: World Health Organization; 1990. Technical report series 804.
13. Billings JA. What is palliative care? *J Palliat Med* 1998;1(1):73–81.
14. Billings JA. On being a reluctant physician—strains and rewards in caring for the dying at home. In: Billings JA, ed. *Outpatient Management of Advanced Cancer*. Philadelphia: Lippincott; 1985:309–318.
15. Berg JW, Appelbaum PS, Lidz CW, et al. *Informed Consent: Legal Theory and Clinical Practice*. 2nd ed. New York: Oxford University Press; 2001.

16. Hauser CA, Stockler MR, Tattersall MH. Prognostic factors in patients with recently diagnosed incurable cancer: a systematic review. *Support Care Cancer* 2006;14:999–1011.

17. Levy WC, Mozaffarian D, Linker DT, et al. The Seattle Heart Failure Model: prediction of survival in heart failure. *Circulation* 2006;113:1424–1433.

18. Childers JW, Arnold RM, Curtis JR. Prognosis in end-stage chronic obstructive pulmonary disease #141. *J Palliat Med* 2007;10(3):806–807.

19. Mitchell SL, Kiely DK, Hamel MB, et al. Estimating prognosis for nursing home residents with advanced dementia. *JAMA* 2004;291:2734–2740.

20. D'Amico G, Garcia-Tsao G, Pagliaro L, et al. Natural history and prognostic indicators of survival in cirrhosis: a systematic review of 188 studies. *J Hepatol* 2006;44:217–231.

21. Wijdicks EF, Hijdra A, Young GB, et al. Practice parameters: prediction of outcome in comatose survivors after cardiopulmonary resuscitation (an evidence-based review): report of the Quality Standards Subcommittee of the American Academy of Neurology. *Neurology* 2006; 67:203–210.

22. Christakis NA, Lamont EB. Extent and determinants of error in doctors' prognoses in terminally ill patients: prospective cohort study. *BMJ* 2000; 320:469–474.

23. Lamont EB, Christakis NA. Complexities in prognostication in advanced cancer: "to help them live their lives the way they want to." *JAMA* 2003; 290(1):98–104.

24. Callahan D. *The Troubled Dream of Life: Living with Mortality*. New York: Simon & Schuster; 1993.

25. Herth K. Fostering hope in terminally-ill people. *J Adv Nurs* 1990;15: 1250–1259.

26. Schofield P, Carey M, Love A, et al. 'Would you like to talk about your future treatment options'? Discussing the transition from curative cancer treatment to palliative care. *Palliat Med* 2006;20:397–406.

27. Appelbaum PS, Grisso T. Assessing patients' capacities to consent to treatment. *N Engl J Med* 1988;319(25):1635–1638.

28. Institute of Medicine. *Dying in America: Improving Quality and Honoring Individual Preferences Near the End of Life*. Washington, DC: National Academies Press; 2014.

29. Hickman SE, Hammes BJ, Moss AH, et al. Hope for the future: achieving the original intent of advanced directives. *Hastings Cent Rep* 2005;35: S26–S30.

30. Brett AS. Limitations of listing specific medical interventions in advanced directives. *JAMA* 1991;266(6):825–828.

31. Tversky A, Kahneman D. The framing of decisions and the psychology of choice. *Science* 1981;211:453–458.

32. Barnard D. Advance care planning is not about "getting it right." *J Palliat Med* 2002;5:475–481.

33. National POLST Paradigm. Available at: http://polst.org. Accessed April 10, 2017.

34. Meisel A. *The Right to Die*. 2nd ed. New York: Aspen; 1985.

35. Helft PR, Siegler M, Lantos J. The rise and fall of the futility movement. *N Engl J Med* 2000;343:293–296.

36. Clouser KD. Allowing or causing: another look. *Ann Intern Med* 1977; 87:622–624.

37. Back AL, Arnold RM. Dealing with conflict in caring for the seriously ill: "it was just out of the question." *JAMA* 2005;293(11):1374–1381.

38. Oregon Public Health Division. Death with Dignity Act annual reports. Available at: https://public.health.oregon.gov/ProviderPartnerResources/Evaluation Research/DeathwithDignityAct/Pages/ar-index.aspx. Accessed April 17, 2017.

39. Oregon Public Health Division. Oregon death data. Available at: https://public.health.oregon.gov/BirthDeathCertificates/VitalStatistics/death/Pages/index.aspx. Accessed April 12, 2017.

40. Emanuel EJ, Onwuteaka-Philipsen BD, Urwin JW, et al. Attitudes and practices of euthanasia and physician-assisted suicide in the United States, Canada, and Europe. *JAMA* 2016;316:79–90.

41. Battin MP, Rhodes R, Silvers A, eds. *Physician-assisted Suicide: Expanding the Debate*. New York: Routledge; 1998.

42. American Public Health Association. Patients' rights to self-determination at the end of life. Available at: https://www.apha.org/policies-and-advocacy/public-health-policy-statements/policy-database/2014/07/29/13/28/patients-rights-to-self-determination-at-the-end-of-life. Accessed April 10, 2017.

43. American Academy of Hospice and Palliative Medicine. Statement on physician-assisted dying. Available at: http://aahpm.org/positions/pad. Accessed April 10, 2017.

44. Quill TE, Lee BC, Nunn S. Palliative treatments of last resort: choosing the least harmful alternative. University of Pennsylvania Center for Bioethics Assisted Suicide Consensus Panel. *Ann Intern Med* 2000;132:488–493.

45. Quill TE, Lo B, Brock DW. Palliative options of last resort: a comparison of voluntarily stopping eating and drinking, terminal sedation, physician-assisted suicide, and voluntary active euthanasia. *JAMA* 1997;278(23): 2099–2104.

46. Quill TE, Dresser R, Brock DW. The rule of double effect—a critique of its role in end-of-life decision making. *N Engl J Med* 1997;337:1768–1771.

47. Sulmasy DP, Pellegrino ED. The rule of double effect: clearing up the double talk. *Arch Intern Med* 1999;159:545–550.

48. Fohr SA. The double effect of pain medication: separating myth from reality. *J Palliat Med* 1998;1:315–328.

49. Billings JA, Block SD. Slow euthanasia. *J Palliat Care* 1996;12(4):21–30.

50. Pellegrino ED. Doctors must not kill. *J Clin Ethics* 1992;3:95–102.

51. Quill TE. Doctor, I want to die, will you help me? *JAMA* 1993;270: 870–873.

52. Magnusson RS. *Angels of Death: Exploring the Euthanasia Underground*. New Haven, CT: Yale University Press; 2002.

53. Quill TE, Arnold R. Fast fact and concept #156: evaluating requests for hastened death. Available at: https://www.mypcnow.org/fast-facts. Accessed April 10, 2017.

54. Arras JD. Physician-assisted suicide: a tragic view. In: Battin MP, Rhodes R, Silvers A, eds. *Physician-Assisted Suicide: Expanding the Debate*. New York: Routledge; 1998:63–72.

55. Randall F, Downie RS. *Palliative Care Ethics: A Companion for All Specialties*. 2nd ed. Oxford: Oxford University Press; 1999.

CHAPTER 14

Laws and Policies Affecting Pain Management in the United States

AARON M. GILSON and **JAMES F. CLEARY**

Introduction

PREVALENCE OF UNRELIEVED PAIN IS A PUBLIC HEALTH PROBLEM

In *The Mystery of Pain*, poet Emily Dickinson wrote,

Pain has an element of blank;

It cannot recollect
When it began, or if there were
A day when it was not.

It has no future but itself,
Its infinite realms contain
Its past, enlightened to perceive
New periods of pain.[1(p650)]

Dickinson's description personifies pain and reveals that the pain experience, conversely, depersonalizes the sufferer. As intense and prolonged pain becomes a defining trait of someone's life, pain and that person's existence become intertwined—defining not only the present and future but also the past. This loss of self, coupled with constant suffering, sheds light onto why some people feel hopelessness because of unremitting pain.[2,3] Pain is, in fact, one of the most common physical complaints on a person's admission into the health care system, and moderate to severe pain is frequently reported to be experienced throughout hospitalization, during treatment, and even after discharge. The Institute of Medicine (IOM) estimates that "at least 100 million Americans" live with chronic pain, including pain associated with the disease of cancer,[4] and recent research suggests that the prevalence of pain in people with cancer can vary considerably, depending on chronicity, severity, and site of the disease.[5] In addition, the national prevalence of chronic pain (defined as pain every day for the past 3 months) is estimated at approximately 11%, whereas around 16% reported a lot of pain or the most severe level of pain.[6] The costs of pain, both emotional and financial, can be enormous.[4] Untreated or undertreated severe pain from any condition or any stage of disease can limit a person's functioning, productivity, and ability to interact socially; sometimes, pain destroys the will to live.[2] A recent study from the Johns Hopkins Center for Health Disparities Solutions and Department of Health Policy and Management indicated that cumulative US health care costs associated with pain exceeded $560 billion in 2010 and calculated an estimate ranging between $299 and $335 billion per year in lost productivity and wages.[7] These estimates suggest that the financial cost of chronic pain has surpassed that of cancer, cardiovascular disease, or diabetes.[7] Increasingly, unrelieved pain has been recognized as a significant public health problem in the United States.[4,8,9]

Issues of public health demand a public health approach to develop informed and organized responses to these health problems.[10] A public health approach is intended to protect the community and enhance the health and quality of life of this population by making available effective and economical interventions.[11] Utilizing a social systems perspective, which incorporates input from various levels of the government (including administrative agencies), health care, education, and welfare systems, often is necessary to guide effective interventions.[12] As inadequate pain management becomes accepted as an important public health issue, efforts to rectify this situation will necessarily involve the systematic utilization of methods to measure outcomes of improved treatment. Some of the most frequent outcome measures, including reduction in pain scores and indicators of quality of life enhancement, must be considered alongside more long-term objectives that denote optimal levels of health status.[13] Before such approaches and outcomes can be conceptualized and achieved, however, the numerous factors that can combine to result in unrelieved pain for patients with chronic diseases or conditions must be understood.

BARRIERS TO THE SAFE AND EFFECTIVE USE OF OPIOID ANALGESICS FOR PAIN MANAGEMENT

Unlike most countries in the world, the problem of unrelieved pain in the United States is not a function of needed medications being unavailable (see Chapter 16 for more detail about global medication unavailability). Patients who experience chronic severe pain still often do not have access to prescription opioid analgesics, which are considered essential medications for treating this level of pain.[14] Of course, this does not mean that prescription opioid medications are to be considered the first-choice treatment option for every patient, a position that is apparent throughout this text, but rather one to be initiated and monitored when the clinical circumstances warrant.[13,15,16] Access to effective pain management requiring prescription opioids is a direct function of the equity of health care services, and the reasons for inequity relate to a variety of issues.

Health care organizations and national experts suggest that a number of diverse factors can interfere with the legitimate medical use of opioid analgesics for the treatment of pain and can negatively affect patients' access to safe and effective pain relief. Most studies have focused on issues in the patient or clinical domains, such as (1) patients' and family perceptions about the use of opioids for pain relief[17–26]; (2) patients' characteristics such as race or ethnicity, substance use history, or the community in which they live[27–34]; and (3) knowledge and attitudes of health care professionals about the legitimate use of opioids.[35–43]

When considering whether to treat pain with opioid analgesics, health care practitioners must determine how to maximize benefit and minimize harm,[15] which they have generally not been trained to do.[44–47] Such inadequate preparation contributes to an unfamiliarity with pain management in general and with relevant treatment modalities in particular, as well as inconsistent use of risk mitigation strategies for patients[48] and perceptions about regulatory or criminal sanctions resulting from prescribing the medications.[49] As a result, there remains an urgent need to enhance clinicians' skills and confidence and to explore the motivations and challenges to get both practitioners and patients involved in activities promoting pain management services.

Many of the clinical and patient factors previously mentioned can contribute to the high prevalence of unrelieved pain in the United States, including characteristics of the health care system and health care professionals.[50] Restrictive federal and state policies relating to drug control and health care practice (often referred to as *regulatory barriers*) also are recognized as potential impediments to pain management, especially considering the extent that practitioners know of and adhere to such policies. Since the early 1990s, national health care organizations have frequently voiced concern about the possible detrimental effects of regulatory barriers. In 1994, the Agency for Health Care Policy and Research (AHCPR) (now the Agency for Healthcare Research and Quality) published a clinical practice guideline on cancer pain relief, which recognized the existence of regulatory barriers, and recommended that laws and regulations aimed at preventing the abuse and diversion of opioids should not hamper their appropriate use in the treatment of cancer pain[51]; these messages were retained a decade later when the American Pain Society updated the guideline.[52] Around the time of the AHCPR guideline dissemination, the National Cancer Institute sponsored a workshop to define priorities in cancer pain–related research that included policy and regulatory issues.[53] The American Cancer Society (ACS) later convened a Cancer Pain Management Policy Review Group to discuss regulatory challenges facing cancer pain management, with an emphasis on ensuring access to appropriate treatment given the national attention on the nonmedical use of pain medications. The Review Group developed several policy statements about various aspects of cancer pain management,[54–56] including a description of regulatory barriers affecting quality pain treatment.[55] Calls for studies to improve pain management and identify the legal and regulatory impediments to appropriately using opioids for pain relief have come from the ACS[54] as well as the IOM[57] and the National Institutes of Health (NIH).[58] For the United States, this involves an understanding and examination of both federal and state laws.

POLICIES GOVERNING THE USE OF OPIOID ANALGESICS FOR PAIN MANAGEMENT

Governments, at both the federal and state levels, can create and change public policies that influence the health of the population. Laws reflect governmental decisions that are largely influenced by social values but provide the legal basis for actions that affect public health, including pain management. For example, given the increasing recognition of pain relief as a basic human right,[9,59] health care facility licensing regulatory standards (e.g., for hospitals, nursing homes, residential care units, and hospices) have even emphasized the pain care of their patients.[60] The World Health Organization (WHO) embraces the incorporation of human rights principles, acknowledging the need to "balance effective responses to disease risks" with respect for fundamental individual freedoms.[61] However, a patient receiving effective pain relief currently is viewed more as a right in the moral sense but generally not in the sense of law or regulatory content.[62]

Legislative bodies typically create laws (i.e., statutes) that are broad and general and depend on the relevant regulatory agency to interpret and implement the laws through regulations. In fact, legislatures that avoid making considerably detailed law would likely require less frequent amendments to such laws because the accompanying regulations contain the professional or technical details that would need to be revised periodically to keep pace with changing practice standards. For medicine, for example, the legislature grants authority to the state medical board to define and implement its laws through regulation (or administrative rules); regulations must be consistent with legislative provisions. Even given this structured process, pain-related law has not kept pace with advances in medical and scientific understanding. Although professional boards may revise their pain management policies in reaction to updated professional standards, legislation has been slow to change. This has particular implication for pain management, including opioid prescribing, where such legislation

tends to have extensive detail and may not reflect current medical standards (see "State Pain Policy Development: An Emerging Trend" section for examples).

In late 2016, *Pain Medicine* published Daniel Carr's President's Message to the American Academy of Pain Medicine readership, entitled "Patients with Pain Need Less Stigma, Not More."[63] According to Dr. Carr, who is the founding director of the Tufts Program on Pain Research, Education and Policy, the ubiquitous clinical scenario surrounding the treatment of patients with chronic pain (especially noncancer pain) is characterized by, among other things:

- "Stigma—shaming and shunning—continues to befall patients with chronic pain, as do inequities in access to care."[63(p1391)]
- "[The] most damaging barrier now facing patients with chronic pain [is] the unprecedented rise in illegal diversion and abuse of opioids, often involving prescription painkillers, with pervasive societal consequences from addiction, crime, overdose, and death . . . [despite the] general agreement that most patients prescribed opioids for chronic noncancer pain are not these problematic outliers."[63(p1392)]
- "Practice guidelines put forth or proposed by different governmental agencies are not uniform, leaving prescribers uneasy that by prescribing opioids at any dose, to any patient, they place themselves in harm's way . . . unleashing a torrent of blame and stigma directed towards all opioid prescriptions, prescribers, and patients."[63(p1392)]
- "Increasing numbers of legitimate patients are voicing personal narratives of long-term benefit from a chronic modest dose of an opioid, now finding such care terminated by policies based upon administrators' interpretations of group statistics never meant to guide individual care."[63(pp1392–1393)]

Within these statements, Dr. Carr recognizes that health care professionals must practice in an environment of legal and regulatory influences, one that can seem particularly ambiguous when it comes to chronic pain, opioid therapy, and risk of addiction or other serious harms. In such an environment, understanding current practice policy requirements is critical.

Although practitioners generally do not receive training in legal and regulatory issues related to prescribing of opioid analgesics and can be unfamiliar with the federal and state laws that govern their practice, there has been an increasing call for clinicians to acquire knowledge about the policies under which they practice.[13,16,64,65] This chapter attempts to create a resource to address this need by describing the three layers of laws in the United States that create the policy framework for both the diversion and legitimate medical use of opioid analgesics: (1) international treaties governing drug control; (2) federal laws and regulations governing drug control, which includes the legal parameters for prescribing controlled substances; and (3) state laws and regulations governing drug control and health care practice, including prescribing controlled substances. The chapter also discusses other policy considerations related to prescribing practices, highlights the need for communication and implementation as a means to improve practitioners' understanding of policy requirements, and suggests the influence that diversion of medications can have on opioid-related harms.

International Treaties: Establishing Balance between Drug Control and Medical Use

Treaties form the basic legal framework to control international and domestic production and distribution of drugs—including medications—that have a recognized abuse liability. The drugs subject to these more rigorous controls are therefore referred to as *controlled substances* and include, but are not limited to, opioid analgesics. The principal treaty establishing controls for prescription opioids used to treat pain is the Single Convention on Narcotic Drugs of 1961 (Single Convention).[66,67] It should be understood that the term *narcotic*, which includes opioid analgesics, is now primarily used in legal contexts, such as in reference to the international drug control treaty or relevant laws; *narcotic*, which generally is defined as an agent that produces stupor or insensibility, is not considered "useful in a pharmacological context" when describing opioid medications.[68(p486)] The Single Convention establishes a number of basic requirements for a country's laws and regulations to create effective measures against drug abuse and diversion. Many of these measures relate directly to the health care setting, including:

- A country's government must duly authorize everyone involved in the medical distribution of narcotic drugs (Article 30).
- Opioid medicines are to be possessed with only legal authority—that is, a valid prescription issued to a patient by a properly licensed practitioner for a legitimate medical purpose in the usual course of professional practice (Articles 30 and 33).
- All licensees are qualified and adhere to their obligation to prescribe and dispense controlled medicines in full and faithful execution of the law, as well as maintain records for medication manufacture, acquisition, and disposal (Article 34).[67]

Although established as international law aimed at preventing drug abuse, this treaty also recognizes that many controlled substances are indispensable to public health and that there is a need to ensure their availability for legitimate medical and scientific purposes (United Nations,[67] Preamble). Becoming a party to this treaty obligates a government to take steps to make controlled substances available in adequate amounts to effectively treat medical conditions. Most, but not all, of the world governments are parties to the Single Convention, including the United States, which means that they formally accept the obligation to develop a legislative and administrative framework to implement the treaty's objectives.[69]

The long-standing dual obligation of country governments to (1) establish a system of controls to prevent abuse, trafficking, and diversion of controlled substances and (2) simultaneously assure their medical availability, is referred to as *Balance*.[70] Balance maintains that opioid analgesics, although designated as controlled drugs, also are essential medicines, are absolutely necessary for adequate pain relief, and must be accessible to patients who need them for medical purposes. Within this framework, the status of these medications as "controlled substances" is not meant to diminish their medical usefulness or create the perception that practitioners should avoid their use when there is a clear clinical indication. Moreover, the principle of Balance does not sanction medication use outside an established system of control, recognizing that only properly licensed health care practitioners can use opioid analgesics for legitimate medical purposes in the course of professional practice.[67] Governments that achieve and implement balanced policy continue to maintain an opioids supply sufficient to meet medical demand and empower practitioners to rationally prescribe, dispense, and administer opioids in the course of professional practice and in response to individual patient needs. With these efforts, it is clear that medication availability is supposed to be limited exclusively to medical and scientific purposes.[67]

The International Narcotics Control Board (INCB), a United Nations–affiliated agency responsible for monitoring governments' implementation of the Single Convention, has historically observed, and continues to note that the global medical need for opioid analgesics is not being fully met.[71–73] Opioids remain insufficiently available to meet medical needs throughout the world for many reasons, including severely restrictive drug control policies[74–79]; the real and overriding concern about drug abuse and addiction also has motivated the creation of laws that when put into practice hamper the appropriate medical use of opioids, including for the treatment of cancer pain[74,77,80,81]:

> . . . the reaction of some legislators and administrators to the fear of drug abuse developing or spreading has led to the enactment of laws and regulations that may, in some cases, unduly impede the availability of opiates. The problem may also arise as a result of the manner in which drug control laws and regulations are interpreted or implemented.[71(p1)]

More recently, such international organizations as the Council of Europe,[82] the World Medical Association,[83] the WHO,[79] WHO HIV/AIDS,[84] the INCB,[75,85] the United Nations Commission on Narcotic Drugs,[86] and the United Nations Economic and Social Council[87,88] have called for governments to identify and address regulatory barriers in their narcotics control policies.

For example, a common requirement found in international drug control policies has been and continues to be the use of multiple-copy prescription forms (also commonly called "serialized forms"), which the Single Convention encourages when a country's government considers such a control measure necessary or desirable (United Nations,[67] Article 30(2)(b)(ii)). This requirement typically involves the need for physicians to issue prescriptions using a special form so that a designated regulatory or enforcement agency can monitor the prescribing and dispensing of certain drugs. These forms are designed and enacted primarily to prevent forgery of narcotic prescriptions and can vary in type, from the use of prescription pads with counterfoil or carbon pages to an extreme where the physician must complete the same required prescription information repeatedly on a number of separate forms. Serialized prescription forms are government-issued, but they may be difficult to obtain and can increase the health care and social stigma associated with prescribing opioid medications.[89–93] As early as 1990, the WHO Expert Committee on Cancer Pain Relief and Active Supportive Care addressed how special government-issued prescription forms can influence prescribing:

> Record-keeping and authorization requirements should not be such that, for all practical purposes, they eliminate the availability of opioids for medical purposes. Multiple-copy prescription programmes are cited as means of reducing careless prescribing and "multiple doctoring" (patients registering with several medical practitioners in order to obtain several prescriptions for the same, or similar drugs). There is some justification for [this], but the extent to which these programmes restrict or inhibit the prescribing of opioids to patients who need them should also be questioned.[94(p39)]

Some governments have concluded that multiple-copy prescription forms create burdens to physicians' practice that can unduly limit access to covered medications, and have changed the requirements of these forms to respond to these problems—this has occurred in such countries as Austria,[95] Italy,[96] and Mexico[97] and in numerous states in the United States.[98,99] These positive programmatic changes are not meant to undermine the drug control capacities inherent in the serialized forms but rather to make it less likely that they hinder patient care. Other ways that countries have established overly restrictive drug monitoring and control systems include establishing extremely short medication supply limits (e.g., 3 days)[90,100–104] and only allowing physicians with certain specialties to prescribe.[100–103,105,106] Again, countries' governments are addressing these potential barriers in law, which is described in detail in Chapter 16.

It is apparent that the international narcotics treaty is intended for drug control and to maintain drug availability for medical purposes, which the World Health Assembly[59,107–109] has historically reaffirmed. However, some countries have implemented the treaty too strictly, resulting in abuse/diversion mitigation while making the use of opioid medications for pain management difficult if not impossible.[110] Given this reality, it may help to understand the current status of national laws and regulations. The next section describes the extent that the United States is meeting its obligation to prevent medication diversion and abuse while continuing its responsibility to ensure the appropriate medical use of opioid analgesics.

US Federal Law: Preserving Balance between Drug Control and Medical Use

THE FEDERAL FOOD, DRUG, AND COSMETIC ACT

Under the authority of the Federal Food, Drug, and Cosmetic Act of 1962 (FFDCA), the U.S. Food and Drug Administration (FDA), which is part of the U.S. Department of Health and Human Services, is responsible for promoting public health by ensuring that all medications, including opioids and other controlled substances, are safe and effective for human use.[111] The FDA's approval decisions for marketing a particular drug always involve an assessment of the benefits and risks,[112] including its abuse liability. The drug manufacturer must provide to the FDA all relevant data related to safety by the time a new drug application is submitted.[113] When the benefits of a drug are considered to outweigh its risks, and when the labeling instructions allow for safe and effective use, only then does the FDA consider the drug safe for approval and marketing.[114] To further reduce opportunities for adverse events, patients also are expected to use the medications according to the prescriber's instructions.[115] Of course, use of any medication outside of the prescriber's instructions, for nonmedical purposes, or absent medical supervision, undermines the safety profile of that medication and increases the likelihood of harms.

When reviewing a new drug application, or after the FDA approves a medication, a determination can be made that the manufacturer also must submit plans for a risk evaluation and mitigation strategy (REMS) to ensure that the benefits of the medication outweigh its risks.[116] In the context of pain management, the FDA approved a shared class-wide REMS for long-acting (LA) and extended-release (ER) opioid analgesics in mid-2012, which has been updated with new products every year since[117]; as of this writing, this REMS program encompasses 65 separate generic or branded LA/ER products.[117] In addition, a REMS for transmucosal immediate-release fentanyl (TIRF) products was begun in 2011 and subsequently has been applied to additional products, at this time covering a total of ten TIRF medications.[118] Within the primary objective of REMS programs to enhance medication safety, there remains an explicit commitment to "enable patients to have continued access to such medicines by managing their safe use" (webinar statement).[116]

A REMS program contains steps to address morbidity and mortality and, according to law, requires a timetable to assess the strategy at 18 months, 3 years, and 7 years after the strategy is approved,[119] whereas the LA/ER REMS specifically mandates that assessments be submitted to the FDA at 6 months and 12 months and then every year thereafter.[120] Again, the goal of the REMS relates to reducing serious adverse outcomes from the misuse and abuse of, as well as to ensure appropriate access to, the covered medications.[120] Two components comprise the adopted REMS: (1) a medication guide and (2) elements to assure safe use. A one-page medication guide is designed for each covered opioid product, either generic or branded,[121] and are to be provided through the pharmacy when an LA/ER opioid is dispensed outside of a hospital setting. Elements to assure safe use are satisfied through voluntary REMS-compliant training

for prescribers, with the training content conforming to learning objectives outlined in the FDA Blueprint.[122] The learning objectives relate broadly to the consideration of medication-related risks and benefits throughout treatment, including during initial patient assessment; initiating, maintaining, or discontinuing opioid therapy; and counseling patients and their caregivers.[122] In addition, the training is designed to improve practitioners' general and specific understanding of LA/ER opioid medications.[122]

Various methods are being used to enhance prescribers' awareness of available REMS training opportunities, as a means to achieve explicitly defined performance goals.[120] Such methods include developing and maintaining a REMS-related Web site, sending letters to all practitioners registered to prescribe relevant medications, and requesting that informational letters be disseminated through state health care licensing and disciplinary boards (i.e., boards of medicine, nursing, and dentistry) as well as their national associations (i.e., the Federation of State Medical Boards of the United States [the Federation], the National Council of State Boards of Nursing, and the American Association of Dental Boards) and professional societies and associations.[120] Another important resource included in these methods is the availability of a one-page counseling document, which health care practitioners are expected to give to patients when treatment involves LA/ER opioids. It is clear that these LA/ER REMS characteristics conform to general programmatic elements defined in law to include a communications plan to health care practitioners about the medications, such as (1) sending letters, (2) disseminating information about the REMS to explain certain safety protocols or to encourage implementation by health care practitioners of applicable components of the REMS, and (3) using professional societies to disseminate information about serious drug risks and protocols to enhance safety.[123]

Available research suggests, cumulatively, that implementation of REMS-compliant prescriber training contributes to increases in practitioner knowledge; better patient awareness of mediation risks; and lower occurrence of abuse, overdose, and death while not creating a barrier to appropriate medication access.[36,124,125] When searched on March 22, 2017, almost 80 REMS-compliant continuing education (CE) training courses were available either at no cost or for a nominal fee, some extending into 2018 (https://search.er-la-opioidrems.com/Guest/GuestPageExternal.aspx), whereas Cepeda et al.[125] indicated that more than 500 such courses were offered in 2013 and 2014. Despite these opportunities, proportionally few prescribers have completed REMS-compliant training.[125] Many reasons account for this low completion rate, including the voluntary nature of the training, participation in non–REMS-compliant CE training (which does not cover all of the content outlined in the FDA Blueprint), and incomplete documentation such as failure to submit a posttest evaluation and the prescribing of an LA/ER opioid in the last year.[125]

The FDA is responsible for reviewing and sanctioning product labeling,[126] with the purpose of providing information for the patients' safe and effective use of the medication.[114] The FDA also has an obligation to ensure that postmarketing promotional materials are consistent with the approved labeling information.[127] Historically, the FDA's statutory authority applied primarily to the evaluation of premarketing testing and, after drug approval, the agency's role was limited. However, in September 2007, the FFDCA was expanded to comprise active postmarket risk identification for approved drugs.[128] Activities under this mandate include ongoing analysis of drug safety data from disparate data sources as well as adverse event surveillance using electronic data from the federal government (e.g., the FDA Adverse Event Reporting System) and the private sector (e.g., the Researched Abuse, Diversion and Addiction-Related

Surveillance [RADARS] system).[114] Information from these sources can lead to safety-related label changes to address new safety data. For example, in 2013, LA/ER opioid medications underwent an indication revision. As a result, LA/ER opioids are no longer indicated for the treatment of moderate to severe pain but rather "for the management of pain severe enough to require daily, around-the-clock, long-term opioid treatment and for which alternative treatment options are inadequate."[129] This change has the benefit of characterizing a more explicit clinical circumstance warranting opioid therapy and implicitly reinforces the standard that these medications are to be initiated only after other modalities have been at least considered and ruled out as unsatisfactory. Overall, the collaborative process engendered through the 2007 legislative change is designed to improve the quality and efficiency of postmarketing drug safety risk–benefit analysis and to allow for the public disclosure of safety and effectiveness data in a timely, systematic, and transparent manner.[114]

A potentially important contribution to the FDA regulatory process comes from a 2017 report from the National Academies of Sciences, Engineering, and Medicine on opioid medications and pain management.[130] The report contains a series of recommendations that, among other things, advises the FDA to conduct a full review of currently marketed and approved opioid products to further ensure the benefit and safety of those modifications both on patients and to public health.[130] Accomplishing this objective is further enhanced when the review is conducted within a framework of what is called a "comprehensive systems approach," in which the following factors are urged to be considered:

- "Benefits and risks to individual patients, including pain relief, functional improvement, the impact of off-label use, incident opioid use disorder (OUD), respiratory depression, and death;
- Benefits and risks to members of a patient's household, as well as community health and welfare, such as effects on family well-being, crime, and unemployment;
- Effects on the overall market for legal opioids and, to the extent possible, impacts on illicit opioid markets;
- Risks associated with existing and potential levels of diversion of all prescription opioids;
- Risks associated with the transition to illicit opioids (e.g., heroin), including unsafe routes of administration, injection-related harms (e.g., HIV and hepatitis C virus), and OUD; and
- Specific subpopulations or geographic areas that may present distinct benefit-risk profiles."[130(pp6–26)]

To the extent that this recommended approach is informed by available evidence that considers the benefit/risk profiles with those for whom the medications are indicated and prescribed, as well as those for whom the medications are not prescribed (e.g., use for nonmedical purposes), this would be a highly valuable and illustrative decision-making process. Another important consideration for an FDA review will be to ascertain whether the prescribing conforms to current practice standards, including patient risk stratification and ongoing treatment monitoring as well as whether patients were compliant with practitioner instructions or product labeling directions. Along with additional attention to illegal drug markets and diversion activity (see the "Taking Diversion into Account" section), there can be a more complete understanding of the degree to which demonstrated harms result from legitimate medical, compared to nonmedical, use.

Of course, prescribing decisions are part of medical practice. The FFDCA is intended neither to regulate medical practice[131] nor to interfere with the authority of a licensed health care practitioner to use controlled substances for a legitimate medical purpose.[132] It is the responsibility of the states, and not the US federal government to regulate professional health care practice. However, both the state and the federal government share drug control responsibilities.

US FEDERAL CONTROLLED SUBSTANCES LAW

Controlled substances laws provide an additional layer of control over the distribution of prescription drugs that have an abuse liability (i.e., using criteria related to the potential to produce psychological or physical dependence), establishing a closed distribution system to minimize their abuse, trafficking, and diversion. The federal Controlled Substances Act (CSA)[133] is part of the Comprehensive Drug Abuse Prevention and Control Act of 1970,[134] and is the principal drug control law in the United States and conforms to the international treaties—it establishes criminal penalties for the illicit possession, manufacture, and trafficking of controlled substances and prohibits their nonmedical use while, at the same time, recognizing that they are necessary for public health and that their medical availability must be ensured. The CSA creates a comprehensive regulatory framework designed to ensure that controlled substances are only produced and distributed through proper channels and for proper medical purposes. In fact, the CSA is a culmination of more than 50 pieces of federal legislation adopted since 1914 relating to drug control and diversion.[134]

The CSA specifies five classification schedules for controlled substances, each carrying different penalties for unlawful uses. A drug's medical usefulness and abuse liability form the basis for the decision to assign it to a particular schedule.[135] Schedule I drugs have no currently accepted medical use, no accepted safety for use under medical supervision, and a high potential for abuse (e.g., ecstasy; heroin, LSD, marijuana, methaqualone, and peyote) and are available only for scientific research. Drugs that have an FDA-approved medical use are placed in Schedules II through V according to potential for abuse in the following manner:

- Schedule II medications have the highest potential for abuse and include such opioids as codeine, fentanyl, hydrocodone (including combination products since 2014),[136] hydromorphone, meperidine, methadone, morphine, and oxycodone (including combination products) as well as nonopioids such as short-acting barbiturates (e.g., pentobarbital), amphetamine, methamphetamine, methylphenidate, and cocaine.
- Schedule III medications have a lower abuse potential than Schedule II drugs and include opioids such as dihydrocodeine and codeine combinations with aspirin or acetaminophen as well as nonopioids such as buprenorphine, intermediate-acting barbiturates (e.g., butalbital), and the synthetic cannabinoid dronabinol.
- Schedule IV medications have a lower abuse potential relative to drugs in Schedule III and include opioids such as dextropropoxyphene, pentazocine, and tramadol as well as nonopioids such as benzodiazepines (e.g., alprazolam and diazepam), LA barbiturates (e.g., phenobarbital), and certain nonamphetamine stimulants (e.g., pemoline).
- Schedule V medications have a lower abuse potential compared to drugs in Schedule IV and include compounds or preparations containing limited quantities of opioids such as codeine or opium, which may be used for over-the-counter preparations to treat cough or diarrhea, respectively, as well as antidiarrheals containing diphenoxylate and difenoxin, and pregabalin.

Under federal law, the Drug Enforcement Administration (DEA) is the primary federal agency responsible for enforcing the CSA and, thus, has regulatory authority over controlled substances. The DEA is an agency of the federal Department of Justice, headed by the attorney general of the United States.

To conduct research with, or manufacture, distribute, handle, dispense, administer, or prescribe, controlled substances, a person or business must be registered with the DEA (and, in some cases, also with the relevant state agencies).[137,138] Licensed and registered practitioners can prescribe, dispense, or administer controlled substances only for legitimate medical purposes and in the usual course of professional practice[139,140]; the DEA and federal courts have interpreted this to mean that prescriptions must be issued "in accordance with a standard of medical practice generally recognized and accepted in the United States."[141(p139)] Registrants' distribution of Schedule I and II controlled substances are made using a special order form (DEA Form 222) to monitor all transfers of these controlled substances within the "closed" system.[142,143]

A number of federal standards are relevant to pain treatment involving controlled medications. For example, prescriptions for Schedule II medications must be written and may not be refilled,[144,145] whereas five refills are permitted for drugs in Schedules III and IV.[146,147]

The requirement for a written prescription is additionally fulfilled through federal law's allowance of prescribers to issue electronic prescriptions for Schedule II controlled substances[148]; electronic prescriptions remain an option that is not designed to completely supplant written paper prescriptions. For this reason, pharmacists and health care facilities are required to have the technologic infrastructure to process e-prescriptions as a means to create a transparent environment that is auditable and DEA-compliant.[149] Regulatory requirements governing this process are quite elaborate. Every aspect of the technology requires certification by the DEA, such as supervised pre-enrollment, maintaining records, the cryptographic signing module, the authentication software and hardware, and the routing of the prescription to the pharmacies (with those pharmacies needing a certified technology platform).[148] Generally, many practitioner obligations involve maintaining information and transmission security, including the need to promptly report security breaches.[150] The same legal responsibilities exist when issuing electronic prescriptions as with hard-copy prescription forms for controlled substances, especially the need to issue for a legitimate medical purpose and in the course of professional practice. Clearly, electronic prescriptions must be issued in conformity to applicable laws, as with any other prescription. All states have modified their laws to accommodate this federal authorization,[151] and as of January 1, 2015, about 70% of pharmacies and 4% of practitioners have the ability to issue electronic prescriptions for controlled substances (Rick Camp, marketing director of Surescripts, as a comment to HealthIT Buzz's "The Electronic Prescribing of Controlled Substances Is on the Rise," https://www.healthit.gov/buzz-blog/health-information-exchange-2/electronic-prescribing-controlled-substances-rise/).

Federal law also allows oral or faxed (but not electronic) transmission of prescriptions for Schedule II controlled substances in medical emergencies under specific circumstances,[152] as well as for the partial dispensing and faxing (but not oral or electronic data transmission) of prescriptions under certain specific clinical circumstances.[153] There are penalties, both criminal and civil, for violating federal requirements.

Although prescriptions for certain controlled substances must be in writing, and refills are limited, the fact that a drug has been approved for medical use does not change when it becomes a controlled substance. This principle is conveyed by the CSA statement that

> many of the drugs included within this title have a useful and legitimate medical purpose and are necessary to maintain the health and general welfare of the American people.[154]

Overall, the legislative history, as well as language contained in the CSA itself (and its related regulations), makes it clear that efforts to prevent drug abuse and diversion are not to interfere with legitimate medical practice and appropriate patient care.[155]

The Controlled Substances Act Ensures Availability of Controlled Substances for Medical Purposes

The CSA authorizes the DEA to establish production quotas for a number of opioids and other controlled substances as a means to stem diversion resulting from excessive unused supplies.[156] Such quotas also must maintain sufficient supplies to accommodate all medical and scientific needs as well as to establish and maintain reserve stock.[140] Despite this apparent standard, however, insufficiently low quotas have occurred for various controlled substances. For example, 30 years ago, the DEA set a very low quota for methylphenidate to restrict its production in an effort to control diversion.[157] As a result, the methylphenidate supply was inadequate to treat patients with attention-deficit/hyperactivity disorder and narcolepsy, which are legitimate medical uses. An official statement was promulgated in response to this action, establishing the principle of an "undisputed proposition" of drug availability:

> The CSA requirement for a determination of legitimate medical need is based on the undisputed proposition that patients and pharmacies should be able to obtain sufficient quantities of methylphenidate, or of any Schedule II drug, to fill prescriptions. A therapeutic drug should be available to patients when they need it. To accomplish this, a smooth flow of distribution is required . . . the harshest impact of actual or threatened shortages falls on the patients who must take methylphenidate, not on the manufacturers to whom the quotas directly apply. Actual drug shortages, or even threatened ones, can seriously interfere with patients' lives and those of their families.[157(pp50593–50594)]

Following this statement, the DEA recalculated the methylphenidate quotas to accommodate its demand for medical purposes. The same situation later occurred for amphetamines as a treatment for attention-deficit/hyperactivity disorder.[158]

The DEA has, over time, expressed a willingness to grant additional quotas for controlled substances necessary to treat medical conditions, including prescription opioids for pain.[159-161] In fact, in response to concerns about natural disasters or other unanticipated situations resulting in prolonged interruption of medication availability:

> DEA included in all schedule II aggregate production quotas, and certain schedule I aggregate production quotas, an additional 25% of the estimated medical, scientific, and research needs as part of the amount necessary to ensure the establishment and maintenance of reserve stocks. The established aggregate production quotas reflect these included amounts.[1(p59980)]

However, the most recent proposed quotas have removed the 25% buffer that were in effect over the last few years, an action that some have interpreted to exemplify a potentially problematic supply reduction (see Anson[162] for example). It is possible, though, that activities such as increased sales to meet prescription demand or product development will prompt the DEA to revise the quotas. Such quota revisions are indeed permissible under federal law.[163]

The Controlled Substances Act Does Not Regulate Medical Practice

The CSA's legislative history demonstrates health care professionals' overriding concern that the drug control law ultimately would give law enforcement inappropriate authority over medical and scientific decisions[155]; abundant professional testimony resulted in Congress establishing a procedure in which the federal health agency (now the U.S. Department of Health and Human Services) makes medical determinations under the CSA. This history makes it apparent that the federal government is obligated to create criteria for drug control, including the legal parameters for prescribing controlled substances and to investigate intentional criminal conduct (e.g., issuing prescriptions *not* for a legitimate medical purpose and in the usual course of professional practice). That is, cases involving questionable prescribing are to be evaluated to determine whether the relevant practice is intentional criminal conduct or substandard professional practice.[64,164-166] Such a distinction historically has helped assure proper jurisdiction: Good faith professional practice, even if poor, can insulate a practitioner from criminal prosecution[167]; both state and federal case law supports this differentiation.[168] If a practitioner's conduct is intentionally outside legitimate professional practice, law enforcement interventions from federal, state, or local agencies seem warranted.[165] That is, a prescription issued or dispensed other than in good faith (i.e., the practitioner knew, or intended, that the prescription would not be used for a legitimate medical purpose) could form the basis for criminal sanctions.[165,169] By extension, unwarranted criminal charges against practitioners may become less frequent, at least in part, to the extent that investigations clearly and consistently consider criminal behavior as distinct from unprofessional conduct. Chapter 16 of this text provides much more descriptive detail about this legal foundation through a discussion of legal cases involving pain management within four primary domains of law: administrative proceedings, civil litigation, criminal litigation, and constitutional cases.

Given this context, the federal government clearly does not have the statutory authority to regulate medical practice. This authority belongs to the states and is based on the police power in state constitutions and underlies the medical practice acts that are designed to protect the public health and safety.[170] The CSA is not intended to supersede the authority of the FFDCA and provides no authority for the DEA to define or regulate medical practice,[133] including the treatment of pain or the indications for which a drug may be prescribed.

The DEA's enforcement authority is intended to relate to clinicians involved in unlawful distribution of controlled substances that is outside legitimate health care practice (i.e., behaviors that are clearly criminal in nature). To this end, a prescription for a controlled substance is only lawful when issued for a legitimate medical purpose and in the usual course of professional practice.[139] David Brushwood, a pharmacist and attorney and now professor emeritus from the College of Pharmacy at the University of Florida, Gainesville, has interpreted a useful distinction between the phrases "legitimate medical purpose" and "course of professional practice," which define the boundaries of practitioner investigations and prosecutions for the DEA:

"Legitimate medical purpose" has no meaning unless "illegitimate medical purpose" has meaning. Yet medicine is inherently legitimate; there is no such thing as "illegitimate medicine." A practice that is not medical is neither legitimate nor legal under the DEA regulation. A practice that is medical is legitimate and is legal under the DEA regulation. DEA does not regulate within medical practice but simply discerns whether a practice is medical or nonmedical. . . . The DEA regulation has nothing to do with the credentials or qualifications of a health care provider. It has everything to do with the *activities* of the health care provider. If those activities are not professional health care activities, then they are illegal under the DEA regulations; if they are professional health care activities, they are legal. DEA has no authority to pass judgment on the merits of a professional practice. Its role is limited to determining whether a practice is a professional practice.[171(p307)]

This critical distinction remains relevant today.

Further evidence that the CSA was not intended to interfere with legitimate medical practice is found when Congress enacted a law in 1978 to implement another international treaty (i.e., the Convention on Psychotropic Substances of 1971).[172] Consequently, the control of psychotropic substances such as benzodiazepines became a responsibility within the CSA to:

insure that the availability of psychotropic substances to manufacturers, distributors, dispensers, and researchers for useful and legitimate medical and scientific purposes will not be unduly restricted . . . and nothing in the Convention [on psychotropic substances] will interfere with ethical medical practice in this country as determined by the secretary of Health and Human Services on the basis of a consensus of the American medical and scientific community.[173]

The Controlled Substances Act Distinguishes Treatment of Addiction from Treatment of Pain, but Legal Definitions Create Confusion

Under the CSA, a separate registration by the federal government as an opioid treatment program (OTP) is required for the purpose of maintenance or detoxification of opioid addiction with certain opioid medications.[174] The use of medications approved for the purpose of addiction treatment, such as methadone and buprenorphine, must comply with federal and state regulations. Methadone and some buprenorphine products, however, are indicated for analgesic purposes according to the same laws for prescribing any other Schedule II or Schedule III opioids.

The accurate application of terminology is central to shaping a balanced policy on drug control and professional practice, especially in the United States where extended opioid therapy to maintain addiction (without a separate registration) is illegal. Addiction often is perceived as being based solely on the development of physical dependence or tolerance, both of which are expected physiologic consequences of using opioids for a prolonged period, which runs counter to current diagnostic nomenclature.[175] Practitioners who consider these related, but separate, phenomena as synonymous can inappropriately label a patient with pain who is receiving opioid therapy as an "addict," which can influence care decisions and inflate determinations about iatrogenic addiction. Given this situation, one must carefully differentiate between treating a patient's pain and maintaining or detoxifying a person with an addictive disease and to understand and use terms correctly.

The CSA defines *addict* as

an individual who habitually uses any narcotic drug so as to endanger the public morals, health, safety, or who is so far addicted to the use of narcotic drugs as to have lost power of self-control with reference to his addiction.[176]

This definition is characterized by the use of circular, imprecise, and outdated language and is not comparable to the WHO's current International Classification of Diseases [ICD10] concept of *dependence syndrome*,[177] the American Psychiatric Association's *Diagnostic and Statistical Manual of Mental Disorders (DSM)* classification of *substance use disorder*,[175] or the American Society of Addiction Medicine's definition of *addiction*.[178] Given its inconsistency with more recent nomenclature, the CSA could indeed be updated to conform more completely to current terminology and standards.

Although not contained in the CSA, in 1970, a definition of *drug-dependent person* was added to the federal Public Health Service Act (now the Public Health and Welfare Act).[179] The Interstate and Foreign Commerce Committee of the House of Representatives[180] considered the adopted definition as similar to the WHO's terminology of the time. *Drug-dependent person* was defined as

> a person who is using a controlled substance . . . and who is in a state of psychic *or physical dependence*, or both, arising from the use of that substance on a continuous basis. Drug dependence is characterized by behavioral and other responses which include a strong compulsion to take the substance on a continuous basis in order to experience its psychic effects or to avoid the discomfort caused by its absence [italics added].[179]

Although indeed similar, there is a critical interpretive distinction between the resulting US legal term and the WHO term from which it was adopted. Unlike the US definition, the WHO conceptualization did not provide the opportunity for physical dependence alone to characterize drug dependence. In 1998, the WHO reaffirmed this conceptualization when it replaced the term *drug dependence* with *dependence syndrome* and further emphasized the biopsychosocial nature of compulsive drug seeking.[181] Even given the medical and scientific evolution of addiction-related terminology that has occurred in the last 50 years, the 1970 Public Health and Welfare definition continues to have the potential to legally codify as "drug dependent" a patient with pain who has been taking opioids for a prolonged period.

Despite the inconsistent and incorrect use of addiction-related terminology in federal law, it remains lawful under federal law to use opioids to treat pain in patients, even when they have a history of substance use or current addictive disease. For example, in 1993, the DEA initiated action to revoke an Ohio physician's prescribing authority because prescriptions were issued to patients who were "known" drug abusers and drug traffickers. A DEA administrative law judge ruled, however, that the physician's controlled substances prescriptions were lawful because they were issued for legitimate medical purposes (e.g., pain relief, muscle spasm, and anxiety).[182] This ruling represented the critical distinction between a practitioner's ability to prescribe controlled substances to treat pain, even though the patient has an addictive disease, and clearly criminal behavior in which controlled substances are distributed without regard to their purposes or ultimate use. Such a judgment upholds the fundamental principle that, when considering the legality of a particular prescribing practice, the determination must be based, at least in part, on the purpose of the prescribing and not the type of patient being treated.

The Controlled Substances Act and Regulations Do Not Limit Prescription Amount or Duration

As stated previously, federal law establishes requirements for what constitutes a lawful controlled substances prescription.[139] At this time, neither the CSA nor the Code of Federal Regulations (CFR) sets limits on the amount or duration of medication for which a practitioner can prescribe, administer, or dispense at one time. This still holds true after the DEA amended the CFR in late 2007 to allow practitioners to issue multiple prescriptions of a Schedule II controlled substance, each issued on the same date and filled sequentially (called a "prescription series").[183]

A prescription series is a method for a practitioner to provide a patient with a large enough amount of a Schedule II medication, for example, for a 3-month supply, without using a single prescription. Rather, the practitioner can now issue several prescriptions, each for one-third of the total amount needed. These prescriptions, each issued on the same day and containing written instructions for the date on which they are to be dispensed, would be delivered to the pharmacist and then dispensed sequentially on the dates indicated on the prescriptions. This procedure allows patients access to the medications they need and results in fewer doses dispensed at a time, thereby

reducing the potential for diversion. A practitioner's ability to specifically issue a prescription series for Schedule II controlled substances was not previously authorized within the CSA; the CSA, when adopted in 1970, did not address this practice because continual pain treatment was uncommon at that time.[184]

The DEA said it wanted to reassure health care professionals and patients that it is legal for practitioners to provide a prescription series to individual patients during a single office visit,[184,185] and authorized multiple prescriptions for "a total of up to a 90-day supply of a Schedule II controlled substance."[183] The DEA clarified that allowing a 90-day prescription series did not alter the fact that the CSA and the CFR do not limit the quantity or number of days for which a single prescription for a Schedule II controlled substance can be written:

> The [Final] rule in no way changes longstanding federal law governing the issuance of prescription for controlled substances . . . the CSA and DEA regulations contain no specific limit on the number of days worth of a schedule II controlled substance that a physician may authorize per prescription.[183(pp64923–64924)]

In addition, the DEA verified that the new prescription series rule did not preclude additional practice standards to which health care professionals must conform, especially in relation to a practitioner's responsibility to minimize the potential for medication abuse and diversion[186]:

> Under this Final Rule, practitioners who prescribe controlled substances are subject to the same standard in preventing diversion as they always have been under the CSA and DEA regulations. Section 1306.12(b)(iii) of this Final Rule is intended to make clear that a practitioner may not simply comply with the other requirements of this Final Rule while turning a blind eye to circumstances that might be indicative of diversion. Thus, section 1306.12(b)(iii) merely underscores that the longstanding requirement of providing effective controls against diversion remains in effective when issuing multiple schedule II prescriptions in accordance with this Final Rule.[183(p64926)]

The intent of the CFR amendment is commendable, with the DEA wanting to reaffirm a practitioner's legal authority to issue a prescription series for Schedule II medications.[183,184,187] Multiple prescriptions for sequential dispensing permit health care professionals to better manage chronic pain in stable patients while exercising improved control over potential medication abuse and diversion, which is consistent with the principle of Balance.[188] The DEA also recognizes the need to maintain balanced policy:

> . . . DEA, through its enforcement of the CSA and its implementing regulations, must prevent the diversion and abuse of controlled substances while ensuring that there is an adequate supply for legitimate medical purposes. DEA supports the intent of this Final Rule to address patients' needs for schedule II controlled substances while preventing the diversion of those substances.[183(p64929)]

Indeed, the federal prescription series regulation was an important step to improve the regulatory environment for both diversion control and providing pain management and palliative care.

Regulations Implementing the Controlled Substances Act Now Authorize a Greater Variety of Secure Disposal Opportunities for Controlled Substances

An even more recent change to the CFR, effective on October 9, 2014, relates specifically to reducing the public health threats inherent in large volumes of unused medications.[189] Under federal law, certain entities who have a DEA registration to handle controlled substances now can volunteer to become a collector of controlled medications for the purpose of destruction using a variety of prescribed methods.[190,191] The DEA registrants permitted to become collectors are manufacturers, distributors, reverse distributors, OTPs, hospitals or clinics with an on-site pharmacy, and retail pharmacies.[190] These registrants can accept back the controlled substances using either mail-back programs or collection receptacles (also called "drop boxes"), or both.[192] In addition, authorized hospitals and clinics and retail pharmacies now have broader authority for maintaining drop boxes at long-term care facilities, when so authorized.[193,194] Finally, a reverse distributor can also acquire these drugs from law enforcement and from other collectors.[195] Of course, the new rule requires additional registration, security, methods of controlled substances destruction, and record-keeping procedures.[191]

Given the introduction into federal law of these disposal standards, now more than ever before there is an acknowledged need for ultimate users (i.e., patients or their caregivers) to have additional ways in which their controlled medications can be collected and destroyed. Although this new law does not give prescribers (e.g., physicians, osteopathic physicians, nurses, and physician assistances) the option to become a collector, there could be a way that these practitioners could help achieve the purpose for which these regulations were developed. If up-to-date resources were easily available that identified local collection opportunities, practitioners could at least advise their patients about the variety of disposal options within the vicinity. Such information could motivate patients to take advantage of the more widespread secure disposal system that may be present in their community. However, the authors are unaware of whether such data are available or even if data exist about the overall proportion of relevant registrants who have chosen to become authorized as collectors.

US State Laws: Striving for Balance between Drug Control and Medical Use

Both federal and state laws regulate the prescribing, dispensing, and administering of controlled medications as well as establish controls to mitigate the unlawful distribution and use of all controlled substances. Federal and state laws prohibit the nonmedical use of controlled substances; set potential penalties and sanctions for violations; and are enforced by local, state, or federal law enforcement. In addition, states are solely responsible for regulating health care practice, including medical, pharmacy, and nursing practice. State licensing boards establish minimum expectations (or standards) for health care practice and the use of controlled substances to treat pain and can discipline practitioners for unprofessional conduct. Given this reality, it is important for practitioners to understand the legal and regulatory framework for the treatment of pain, including when it involves the use of opioid analgesics or other controlled substances. State policies, historically, have not consistently supported the availability of needed medications to the extent of international treaties and federal law.[196] For example, most state laws do not specifically recognize the appropriate medical use of controlled medications as important to public health, which is a concept inherent in federal law.[154] Some state policies also establish more requirements on the prescribing and dispensing of opioids, compared to federal law, which can ultimately interfere with medical decision making, decision making that should be based both on the expertise of the practitioner and the individual patient needs.[197] Policy impediments at the state level have been known to contribute to inadequate pain management.[52,198–206] In response to this knowledge, both international organizations[74,94,207,208] and national organizations[55,57,58] have called for studies to improve pain management by identifying and addressing the legal and regulatory impediments to using opioids for pain relief. A number of governmental and national

authorities, such as Congress,[133] the National Conference of Commissioners on Uniform State Laws,[201,202,209] and the Federation,[210,211] have recommended controlled substances or medical practice policy that permits medication access to patients when needed while restricting nonmedical use by either patients or people to whom the medications are not prescribed.

STATE PAIN POLICY DEVELOPMENT: AN EMERGING TREND

Since the late 1980s, there have been an increasing number of state pain-specific policies, including legislatively issued statutes and health care regulatory board regulations and guidelines or policy statements. Such policy adoption typically promoted the safe and appropriate use of controlled substances when clinically warranted and recommended ways to reduce abuse or diversion of those medications. In some cases, however, these policies led to additional restrictions and requirements with the potential to create barriers to the effective treatment of pain.

As an early example of this occurrence, intractable pain treatment acts (IPTAs) were statutes that created immunity from regulatory sanctions for physicians who prescribe opioids to patients with intractable pain, and thus were intended to improve access to pain management; however, many IPTAs imposed additional requirements and restrictions on prescribing opioids to such patients.[196,212–215] IPTAs often implied that opioid use for "intractable pain" was outside of ordinary medical practice, which produced greater rather than less government regulation when treating pain with controlled substances. For physicians who prescribe to patients whose pain did not satisfy the definition of "intractable pain," there was question about whether an IPTA provides immunity and created ambiguity for the clinician. Many IPTAs did not contain clear statements supporting enhanced pain management or instructing practitioners about how to provide safe and appropriate access and maintenance to such care.

Some advocates have recently recognized the potential negative impact of these characteristics on patient care and have worked with the legislature to remove ambiguities and restrictions from their state's IPTA. Iowa and Michigan became the first states, in 2002, to delete the term *intractable pain* from law. More recently, Arizona, California, North Dakota, Oregon, Rhode Island, Tennessee, and Texas repealed a number of restrictive provisions from their IPTAs, including removing the term and definition of *intractable pain*; the resulting laws now govern treatment for all types of pain. Indeed, IPTAs were the first instance of legislation created specifically for the treatment of chronic pain (i.e., "intractable pain"), which differed from the approach commonly taken by regulatory boards at the time to address the issues related to pain management in general.

As an alternative approach to creating legislation, which often is difficult to modify to keep pace with evolutions in medical and scientific understanding, many states chose to develop health care regulatory board guidelines or regulations to encourage better pain management and to address physicians' expressed anxiety surrounding investigation and sanction.[196,216] Early reports suggested that concerns about regulatory scrutiny were prevalent and could hinder the availability of opioids for patients who may clinically benefit from these medications.[203,217–220] Apprehension about disciplinary action for opioid prescribing[221–224] has been documented for a variety of health care practitioners, including primary care physicians,[225–228] oncologists,[229] pain specialists,[230,231] medical residents,[232] pharmacists,[225,233] and nurses.[225,234–236] To address these concerns directly, for more than 30 years, health care regulatory boards have promulgated regulations, guidelines, and policy statements perpetuating the message that pain management, including the appropriate use of controlled substances, is an accepted part of professional practice; a typical goal of such policies was to reassure clinicians that they had nothing to fear from their licensing agency if reasonable professional practices are followed when using controlled substances for appropriate patient care.

State medical boards' issuance of recommendations for pain management was aided considerably when, in 1998, the Federation adopted a policy template to promote consistency in state medical board policy, entitled *Model Guidelines for the Use of Controlled Substances for the Treatment of Pain* (Model Guideline).[210] In May 2004, the Federation revised the Model Guideline as the *Model Policy for the Use of Controlled Substances for the Treatment of Pain* (Model Policy).[211] The 2004 Model Policy is substantially the same as the 1998 guideline but encouraged state boards to consider the failure to treat pain as worthy of disciplinary sanction; undertreated pain previously had been identified as an important clinical topic to address in state policy.[237] These models were later supplanted by the *Model Policy on the Use of Opioid Analgesics for the Treatment of Chronic Pain*[16] in 2013 and then, most recently, the 2017 *Guidelines for the Chronic Use of Opioid Analgesics*.[13] Interestingly, these newer templates relate specifically to the treatment of chronic pain related to noncancer conditions (i.e., excluding "acute pain, acute pain management in the perioperative setting, emergency care, cancer-related pain, palliative care, or end-of-life care"[13[p2]]) rather than offering guidance for pain management in general as was done in the previous versions. They do, however, offer a benefit by providing more descriptive recommendations than older templates about altering or discontinuing opioid treatment when clinical evidence supports such an approach. According to the Federation, most state medical and osteopathic boards have adopted policies based, at least in part, on these model templates (see https://www.fsmb.org/Media/Default/PDF/FSMB/Advocacy/GRPOL_Pain_Management.pdf).

EVALUATING THE QUALITY OF STATE PAIN POLICY

Since the early 2000s, a criteria-based policy research methodology has existed to evaluate federal and state drug control and health care regulatory policies related to pain management, palliative care, and end-of-life care (issued in a report called an Evaluation Guide).[98,188,238–242] The basis for this policy evaluation was the aforementioned principle called Balance, which is a fundamental and long-standing national and international principle of drug regulation and medical ethics. Balanced state policies maintain drug controls and avoid undue restrictions to appropriate health care practice and patient care and support pain treatment, including the use of controlled substances when warranted, as a component of quality medical practice.[98] Although additional efforts are necessary to assess the presence and effectiveness of current state-level drug control frameworks to minimize abuse and diversion, the purpose of this evaluation has been to characterize pain-related issues covered in state policies.

The principle of Balance was used to derive 16 evaluation criteria. Each criterion relates to one of two categories: (1) positive provisions—policy language that can *enhance* pain relief and (2) negative provisions—language that can *impede* pain relief. A complete description of the criteria, the evaluation methodology, and the policy language from all states (including the District of Columbia) that satisfies each criterion, can be found at http://www.painpolicy.wisc.edu.

Policy Evaluation Findings

Policy language was identified that promotes appropriate pain management; such language is common in the policies from state regulatory agencies rather than from legislative statutes. The frequency with which states' policies contained such language in 2015[60] is as follows:

- A statement that recognizes medical use of opioid as legitimate professional practice (in all states)
- A statement that recognizes pain management as part of general medical practice (in 45 states)

- A statement that encourages pain management (in 40 states)
- A statement that addresses practitioners' concerns about regulatory scrutiny (in 39 states)
- A definition or statement in which addiction is different from physical dependence or analgesic tolerance (in 38 states)
- A statement that recognizes medication amount or duration as insufficient to determine legitimacy of a prescription (in 32 states)

Policy language that appears less frequently than the earlier concepts, but that also promotes effective pain control and patient care, was identified and relates to three broad domains: (1) health care professional issues (e.g., encourages patient evaluation and discussion relating to potential benefits and risks of opioid treatment, recognizes that the goals of pain treatment should include improvements in patient functioning and quality of life, and recognizes the need for a multidisciplinary approach to pain management [integrative pain care]), (2) patient characteristics (e.g., assures that no person will be considered an "addict" based solely on taking a medication pursuant to a lawful prescription issued by a physician in the course of professional treatment for legitimate medical purposes and exempts certain patient populations from undue prescription requirements), and (3) regulatory or policy issues (e.g., encourages health care professionals to understand and follow federal and state laws governing their practice and specifically acknowledges that drug control policies should not interfere with legitimate medical use of controlled substances). A state's drug control laws, appropriately, focus on the abuse potential of controlled medications but often to the exclusion of recognizing their public health and medical benefit when used as directed for legitimate purposes unlike more positive provisions contained in federal law (see, for example, CSA[154]; Federal Food Drug and Cosmetic Act[243]).

It has been, and continues to be, possible to adopt state policies designed to prevent drug abuse and the transfer of medications to an illicit distribution system without creating ambiguity for health care decision making that conform to and do not conflict with current standards of professional practice, and that eschew imposing excessive burdens on patients. In 2015, however, the frequency with which states' policies contained such language is as follows:

- A definition or statement in which addiction is synonymous with physical dependence or analgesic tolerance (in 13 states)
- A statement that seems to require a specialist consultation for every patient who is prescribed Schedule II controlled substances (in 7 states)
- A statement that seems to completely prohibit prescribing of controlled substances to certain patients (in 5 states)
- A requirement that limits the amount of time that a Schedule II prescription is valid to less than 2 weeks (in 2 states) (see Table 14.1 for specific restrictions for each state)
- A requirement that limits the number of dosage units of pain medications that can be prescribed and dispensed at one time (in 1 state) (see Table 14.2 for the specific restriction)

These evaluations also consider, at least to a limited extent, laws that create and implement prescription monitoring program (PMP), which are primary diversion control mechanisms

TABLE 14.1 States with Laws Restricting Schedule II Prescription Validity Period (in days)	
Delaware	7
Hawaii	7

TABLE 14.2   State with a Law Restricting Schedule II Prescription Quantity or Duration

Utah	A Schedule II controlled substance may not be filled in a quantity to exceed a one-month's supply, as directed on the daily dosage rate of the prescriptions . . . (i) A practitioner licensed under this chapter may not prescribe or administer dosages of a controlled substance in excess of medically recognized quantities necessary to treat the ailment, malady, or condition of the ultimate user. (Utah Code Ann. § 58-37-6(B))

in the United States, specifically at the state level. PMPs historically were characterized as multiple-copy prescription programs (MCPPs), which use multiple-copy government-issued serialized prescription forms (usually required in triplicate or duplicate). The prescription forms were required for Schedule II medications only (i.e., the only medications indicated for severe pain) and the programs were administered by state law enforcement, such as the state Department of Justice. The purpose of early PMPs was to provide law enforcement and prescribers and dispensers with information on "doctor shoppers," "scammers," and dishonest physicians. Unfortunately, prescription information collected through MCPPs was not real-time and often took a considerable time to compile, which severely undermined their ability to actively monitor diversion or abuse activity. MCPPs also focused exclusively on Schedule II medications and used unique forms that practitioners had to order from the government to prescribe only those medications. Research suggested that linking the government-issued prescription form only to those medications in Schedule II often motivated practitioners to prescribe lower scheduled medications to avoid being monitored[244–248]; this phenomenon has come to be known as the *substitution effect*.[248] Of course, practices influenced by concerns about governmental oversight, rather than solely by patient needs and clinical circumstances, usually characterized the substitution effect as the potential for inappropriately treated pain. It is also true that decreased prescribing of Schedule II medications often has been interpreted, by itself, as evidence that the program was effective in reducing diversion,[249,250] rather than considering outcomes more descriptive of diversion.

MCPPs have been replaced by electronic data transfer (EDT) programs that collect prescription information about more than Schedule II controlled substances (usually Schedules II, III, and IV).[251–253] Monitoring multiple schedules minimizes a potential substitution effect because there are few other medications with which they could be replaced. EDT programs tend to be administered by state health agencies, such as the pharmacy board, and the policies that implement the programs generally emphasize that this effort to reduce abuse and diversion is not meant to interfere with appropriate patient care. The information from these programs is collected in a more timely fashion, although it is usually not real-time. However, there is still limited evidence to demonstrate the programs' effects either on practitioner prescribing or on incidents of medication abuse and diversion.

As of this writing, all but one state and the District of Columbia have a functional PMP that is an EDT system for a variety of medication schedules. Over half of these programs were created since the early 2000s, primarily as a result of the Harold Rogers Prescription Drug Monitoring Program grant program through the U.S. Department of Justice.[254] Requirements for states to apply for such grants has been described as "relatively simple."[255(p509)] At around the same time, an additional funding mechanism was introduced through the National All Schedules Prescription Electronic Reporting Act of 2005

(NASPER)[256] and administered through the U.S. Department of Health and Human Services. NASPER also provides grants to states to develop PMPs only if the programs are EDTs that apply to medications in at least Schedules II to IV; states can create programs with different characteristics, but they are not fundable under NASPER. Federal law mandates that the Secretary of Health and Human Services evaluates the safety and efficacy of the programs established through NASPER. In this context, "safety" refers to the extent that the programs avoid creating barriers to prescribing to patients for legitimate medical purposes, such as for pain management. "Efficacy" means the ability of the program to validly identify instances of abuse and diversion. Although there seems to be less chance for EDTs to restrict patient care, especially when compared to MCPPs, empirical documentation remains mixed about either the safety or efficacy of these programs.[257]

In addition to the discrete occurrences of policy language that can either enhance or impede the appropriate treatment of pain, including with opioid analgesics, some state policies contain requirements or concepts that are contradictory and can create ambiguous practice expectations. For example, as identified previously, policies in 38 states define addiction as a psychological/behavioral disorder that is not synonymous with either physical dependence or tolerance. Laws in 13 states also have a definition that could legally classify patients being treated chronically with opioids as "addicts" only because they are physically dependent. As a result, 8 states have at least one policy that defines addiction according to current official standards and another that defines the concept differently (see Table 14.3 for a listing of the discrepant definitions). There is no clear guidance for practitioners in these states about how patients with pain who are being treated with opioids are to be viewed, given the inconsistencies among the legal, regulatory, and health care classification. Achieving positive uniform policy often depends on potentially discrepant practice standards being identified and corrected.

A PROGRESS REPORT CARD TO MEASURE CHANGES IN THE QUALITY OF STATE PAIN POLICIES

The criteria-based evaluation of state pain policy also serves as the basis for a methodology to quantify a state's policy based on its quality, creating a single metric that can then be used to compare all states and track policy changes over time.[60,188,258–262] This metric, along with the content of the Evaluation Guide, has helped states identify policy provisions that could be considered for modification.[263]

In the latest report using cumulative policy data from the state profiles, grades were calculated for the state policies in effect in 2015.[60] The grades, and the methodology used to calculate the grades, are contained in the most recent report, entitled "Achieving Balance in State Pain Policy: A Progress Report Card" (Progress Report Card), and is available at https://www.acscan.org/sites/default/files/National%20Documents/Achieving%20Balance%20in%20State%20Pain%20Policy.pdf.

Grades can range from A to F, using midpoint grades (e.g., B+, C+, D+) to characterize more precisely each state's overall combination of positive and negative provisions. A higher grade means a state's policies have many positives and few negatives and are, therefore, more balanced in relation to appropriate pain management. An A is achieved only if a state has a high number of positive provisions and no instances of unduly restrictive or ambiguous language. A lower grade is associated with the presence of provisions that contradict current medical knowledge; are inconsistent with policy guidance recommendations from authoritative sources; or fail to communicate the appropriate messages about pain management to professionals, patients, and the public. An F results when a state has abundant negative provisions and no positive language.

TABLE 14.3	States with Laws Containing Conflicting Definitions of Addiction-Related Terminology	
State	**Definitions in Which Physical Dependence or Analgesic Tolerance Are _Not Confused_ with "Addiction"**	**Definitions in Which Physical Dependence or Analgesic Tolerance Are _Confused_ with "Addiction"**
Arizona	As discussed, physical dependence and tolerance are expected physiological consequences of extended opioid therapy for pain and in this context do not indicate the presence of addiction. (Medical Board: Reference for Physicians on the Use of Opioid Analgesics in the Treatment of Chronic Pain, in the Office Setting)	"Drug-dependent person" means a person who is using a controlled substance and who is in a state of psychic or physical dependence, or both, arising from the use of that substance on a continuous basis. Drug dependence is characterized by behavioral and other responses which include a strong compulsion to take the substance on a continuing basis in order to experience its psychic effects or to avoid the discomfort caused by its absence. (A.R.S. § 36-2501(A)(5))
Hawaii	Addiction—Addiction is a primary, chronic, neurobiologic disease, with genetic, psychosocial, and environmental factors influencing its development and manifestations. It is characterized by behaviors that include the following: impaired control over drug use, craving, compulsive use, and continued use despite harm. Physical dependence and tolerance are normal physiologic consequences of extended opioid therapy for pain and are not the same as addiction. (Medical Board: Pain Management Guidelines)	The term _narcotic-dependent person_ as used in this section means an individual who physiologically needs heroin or a morphine-like drug to prevent the onset of signs of withdrawal. (HRS § 329-40)
Louisiana	"Substance abuse" or "addiction" means a compulsive disorder in which an individual becomes preoccupied with obtaining and using a substance, despite adverse social, psychological, or physical consequences, the continued use of which results in a decreased quality of life. The development of controlled dangerous substance tolerance or physical dependence does not equate with substance abuse or addiction. (La. R.S. 40:961(38))	"Drug-dependent person" means a person who is using a controlled dangerous substance and who is in a state of psychic or physical dependence, or both, arising from administration of that controlled dangerous substance on a continuous basis. Drug dependence is characterized by behavioral and other responses which include a strong compulsion to take the substance on a continuous basis in order to experience its psychic effects or to avoid the discomfort of its absence. (La. R.S. 40:961(18))
Maryland	It is important to realize that habituation and tolerance to drugs are not the same as addiction. These are expected consequences of long-term analgesic therapy and do not have the characteristics of sociopathy and psychological dependence associated with addiction. (Medical Board: Prescribing Controlled Substances)	Drug-dependent person—"Drug-dependent person" means a person who (1) is using a controlled dangerous substance and (2) is in a state of psychological or physical dependence, or both, that (i) arises from administration of that controlled dangerous substance on a continuous basis and (ii) is characterized by behavioral and other responses that include a strong compulsion to take the substance on a continuous basis in order to experience its psychological effects or to avoid the discomfort of its absence. (Md. CRIMINAL LAW Code Ann. § 5-101(o))
Nebraska	Physicians should recognize that tolerance and physical dependence are normal consequences of sustained use of opioid analgesics and are not the same as addiction. (Medical Board: Guidelines for the Use of Controlled Substances for the Treatment of Pain)	Active addiction means current physical or psychological dependence on alcohol or a substance, which develops following the use of alcohol or a substance on a periodic or continuing basis. (Nebraska Admin. Code Title 172, Ch. 88, 88-002)
Nevada	Physicians should recognize that tolerance and physical dependence are normal consequences of sustained use of opioid analgesics and are not synonymous with addiction. (NAC 630.187)	"Narcotic addiction" means compulsion to continue taking or psychic or physical dependence on the effects of a narcotic drug. (Nev. Rev. Stat. Ann. § 453.099)
North Carolina	Addiction: A primary, chronic, neurobiologic disease with genetic, psychosocial, and environmental factors influencing its development and manifestations. Addiction is characterized by behaviors that include the following: impaired control over drug use, craving, compulsive use, and continued use despite harm. Physical dependence and tolerance are normal physiologic consequences of extended opioid therapy for pain and are not the same as addiction. (Medical Board: Policy for the Use of Opiates for the Treatment of Pain)	"Drug-dependent person" means a person who is using a controlled substance and who is in a state of psychic or physical dependence, or both, arising from use of that controlled substance on a continuous basis. Drug dependence is characterized by behavioral and other responses which include a strong compulsion to take the substance on a continuous basis in order to experience its psychic effects or to avoid the discomfort of its absence. (N.C. Gen. Stat. § 90-87(13))
Oklahoma	Physicians should recognize that tolerance and physical dependence are normal consequences of sustained use of opioid analgesics and are not the same as addiction. (Medical Board: Use of Controlled Substances for the Treatment of Pain)	"Drug-dependent person" means a person who is using a controlled dangerous substance and who is in a state of psychic or physical dependence, or both, arising from administration of that controlled dangerous substance on a continuous basis. Drug dependence is characterized by behavioral and other responses which include a strong compulsion to take the substance on a continuous basis in order to experience its psychic effects or to avoid the discomfort of its absence. (63 Okl. St. § 2-101(15)

Progress Report Card Findings

Results show that the quality of pain policies continues to vary across states as of December 31, 2015, which were reported in the most recent Progress Report Card[60] (see Table 14.4 for a list of each state's grade). In the aggregate, 13 states achieved an A. An A means that there is prevalent language in laws or regulatory policies, or both, that promote safe and effective pain management as well as there being no language that can create inflexible barriers or ambiguities for clinical decision making. Eighteen states had a B+, 13 states had a B, 6 states had a C+, and only 1 state had a grade of C. In terms of population coverage, the 13 states achieving an A comprise 19% of the total US population, and states with a B or B+ make up almost 65% of the US population. Another 16% of the US population live in the 7 states that have grade of C or C+.

A variety of policy changes contributed to these current grades. Within the past few years, a total of 11 states had adopted legislation or regulations mandating CE about prescribing controlled substances or opioid medications, pain management, or palliative care for licensees or for those who prescribe as staff of pain clinics. Eight states either adopted, adopted by reference or adopted based on, or updated to the Federation's 2013 *Model Policy on the Use of Opioid Analgesics in the Treatment of Chronic Pain*[16] (the most recent version of the Federation's models that was current at the time of the evaluation), whereas another 10 states added or updated other statutes or regulatory policies governing pain management, and an additional 2 states now require the development of rules governing prescribing for pain. Four states adopted legislative or regulatory language initiating or expanding their pain management, hospice, or palliative care standards in various health care facilities. Importantly, two states also added a law containing a statement that directly supports the principle of Balance. Further improvements were made through the following policy adoptions:

- A regulation for offering addiction treatment services in the office that provides a definition of "addiction" that not only distinguishes it from physical dependence or tolerance but also explicitly acknowledges that physical dependence occurring with a "patient on long-term opioid analgesics for pain" is distinct from ICD10 or *DSM* diagnostic classification systems.

- A statute governing a state PMP will now offer educational information to the program Web site and will regularly send updates of such information to registered program users, whereas another state's PMP regulations now offer training to practitioners and pharmacists and their delegates, as well as to other users, about how to use program information.

- A statute that appears to allow pharmacists to dispense up to a 10-day supply of a Schedule II or Schedule III opioid medication from a prescription issued by an out-of-state practitioner (while needing to notify the practitioner of the partial dispensing), rather than prohibiting any such prescriptions.

- A statute that initiated an interdisciplinary advisory council within the Department of Health as a mechanism to create, maintain, and evaluate state palliative care initiatives.

In addition to adopting policy language that promotes safe and effective pain management, a number of states further improved policy quality by repealing restrictive or ambiguous provisions from statutes or regulatory policy. Such recent abrogations involved a 1-week prescription validity period; the requirement that the standard for "unprofessional conduct" be met by a failure to strictly adhere to a clinical practice guideline, which does not allow for treatment flexibility based on reasonable cause; a prescription filling standard with broad interpretive latitude for pharmacists; an entire IPTA, along with the various requirements and ambiguities typically contained in such policies (see "State Pain Policy Development: An Emerging Trend" section); an immutable requirement for patients to undergo other treatment modalities before being prescribed opioids and other controlled substances, regardless of the clinical circumstances; and definitions of *drug-dependent person*, *chemical dependency*, and *dependence* that could be established by the presence of physical dependence only and, thus, could legally apply to a person who is being treated with opioid pain medications.

As with previous evaluations, only a very few states adopted any type of policy containing restrictive or ambiguous policy language. As such, states have generally avoided adopting new policies that could impede pain management and the medical use of controlled substances. Considering current policy content, states wanting to achieve an A can be classified into four domains. First, three states currently have no restrictive or ambiguous language in their state's pain policies and can change to an A simply by adopting additional positive language. Second, 32 states (84%) of the remaining 38 states that do not have an A can improve their grade only by repealing restrictive or ambiguous policy language. Of these states, six continue to not only have a considerable number of beneficial provisions but also have many potentially problematic provisions, which represent a noteworthy challenge. These particular states must

TABLE 14.4	States' Pain Policy Grades for 2015				
Alabama	A	Kentucky	B+	North Dakota	B
Alaska	B+	Louisiana	C+	Ohio	B+
Arizona	B+	Maine	A	Oklahoma	C+
Arkansas	B	Maryland	B+	Oregon	A
California	B+	Massachusetts	B	Pennsylvania	B+
Colorado	B	Michigan	A	Rhode Island	A
Connecticut	B+	Minnesota	B+	South Carolina	B+
Delaware	B+	Mississippi	B+	South Dakota	B
District of Columbia	B	Missouri	C	Tennessee	C+
Florida	B	Montana	C+	Texas	C+
Georgia	A	Nebraska	B	Utah	B+
Hawaii	B	Nevada	C+	Vermont	A
Idaho	A	New Hampshire	B+	Virginia	A
Illinois	B	New Jersey	B	Washington	A
Indiana	B+	New Mexico	B	West Virginia	B+
Iowa	A	New York	B	Wisconsin	A
Kansas	A	North Carolina	B+	Wyoming	B+

undertake a continued focus on reducing the number of restrictive or ambiguous provisions for any grade improvement to occur. Third, as of December 31, 2015, four states have neither medical nor pharmacy board policies addressing the treatment of pain (including the use of controlled substances), palliative care, or end-of-life care. In these states, clinicians are not provided guidance from their licensing agency about what is considered acceptable approaches related to patient pain care. Finally, when striving for an A, two states now face the challenge not only of adopting positive policies but also of removing restrictive or ambiguous language from legislation or regulations. Even for those 13 states that currently have an A, a potential remains for additional policy activity (however well-intentioned) to introduce policy provisions that ultimately can lower the state's grade. Continued state policy efforts to improve patient pain care, including through activities to address clinical and societal harms related to prescription opioids, can seek to maintain grade improvements.

THE IMPORTANCE OF IMPROVING STATE PAIN POLICY

In the aggregate, the last decade witnessed notable improvement in the quality of many states' drug control and professional practice laws and regulatory policies. This policy advancement was in response to continuing national and state acknowledgment that adopting positive policies governing health care practice and patient care is part of improving safe and effective pain treatments for patients with cancer, HIV/AIDS, and other chronic diseases or conditions. States typically have avoided adopting new policies that could inadvertently impede pain management, including treatment involving the medical use of controlled substances when clinically justified. Members of government and regulatory agencies, as well as health care professionals, are in a position to continue seeking policy approaches that eschew requirements that could confound medical decision making or lead to unintentional consequences on pain treatment. Such improvements, as evidenced by higher state policy grades, are a necessary part of an overall multifaceted plan to enhance pain and symptom management while stemming prescription medication abuse and diversion.[60,98]

Much of the positive content inherent in state pain policies has resulted historically from individual health care regulatory boards taking advantage of the Federation's policy templates to promote consistency in state medical board policy.[16,210,211] Throughout the templates, the importance of documenting various aspects of treatment is mentioned. These templates also have, at various points in time, encouraged safe and effective pain relief, perpetuated the message that pain management and the appropriate use of controlled substances was an accepted part of professional practice, and reassured clinicians that they should not be concerned about disciplinary action from their licensing agency if reasonable professional practices are followed when using controlled substances for patient care. In addition, the policies promote assessment of both potential benefits and risks when considering opioid treatment, especially for patients with more chronic conditions. Patient risk assessment, as well as the periodic monitoring for adverse events and the manifestation of abuse-, addiction-, and diversion-related behaviors, have been an explicit component of the Federation's templates since their first inception[264,265]; in fact, the clinical need for risk stratification strategies was emphasized even more in the most recent policies issued in 2013[16] and 2017.[13] Importantly, health care regulatory boards (e.g., medical, osteopathic, pharmacy, and nursing) in many states have worked together to adopt joint guidelines for pain management, palliative care, or end-of-life care.[60] Such policies tend to emphasize the value of an integrative multidisciplinary approach to treating pain; recognize that the goal of pain treatment should include improvements

in patient functioning and quality of life; and assure that a broader variety of health care practitioners can engage in practice that generally conforms to adopted treatment standards without being apprehensive about regulatory sanctions from their licensing board.

Given this notable regulatory progress, most states now can focus on maintaining policy improvement and consider efforts to remove long-outdated restrictive or ambiguous language from law, some of which has been present for over 30 years. This is especially the case with drug control laws that contain outdated definitions of "drug-dependent person" (or "addict") that are based on the concept of physical dependence and developing a withdrawal syndrome. Such definitions can, when interpreted strictly, legally classify as an addict any patient who is taking an opioid for analgesia (see Table 14.3 for examples of these types of definitions).[98] Repeal from law of decades-old restrictive language has received less attention compared to the work of professional licensing boards to adopt positive policy.[60] Avoiding such language ensures that patient care decisions requiring medical judgment are not overly limited by governmental laws.

The Need to Implement and Communicate Policy

Inadequately treated pain is a multifactorial phenomenon. As such, focusing solely on changing state policy is likely insufficient to guarantee better patient access to appropriate pain relief and symptom control.[266] Addressing this single factor, however, often remains a necessary activity to attain a supportive professional practice and regulatory environment for the appropriate treatment of pain. Adoption of such policies also requires broad dissemination and communication to relevant practitioners to help enhance compliance to the policy recommendations or requirements,[266] because an evaluation of practice should always involve a determination regarding adherence to applicable policy.[267]

Improving state policies covering pain-related issues requires a strategic approach, often beginning simply by determining the types of policies in need of improvement. For example, the revision of statutory law requires legislative activity, whereas a change in regulatory policy involves engaging with the relevant health care administrative agency such as the medical, pharmacy, or nursing board. Health care practitioners increasingly have assumed a leadership role in collaborating with legislators or members of administrative agencies to help construct state policy that avoids interfering with appropriate decision making or creating ambiguities, recognizes the professional obligation to treat pain, and promotes effective patient pain care.[266] This activity has been accomplished when practitioners have acted alone, in conjunction with a state pain initiative or other organization, or as a member of a legislatively created advisory committee.[263,268]

Considering Additional US Policies

The aforementioned policy evaluation reports synthesize the content of numerous state-level statutes and regulatory policies governing drug control and medical, pharmacy, and nursing practice. Because this evaluation was policy-specific, it did not consider reports or projects from federal or state agencies that related directly to pain, such as the IOM's *Relieving Pain in America*,[4] the U.S. Department of Health and Human Service's *National Pain Strategy*,[50] and the NIH's *Federal Pain Research Strategy* (https://iprcc.nih.gov/FPRS/FPRS.htm). The finalized methodology also was never meant to imply that the reviewed policies are the only policies relevant to pain management. In fact, various other policy types may affect patient pain care but ultimately fall outside the scope of the evaluation process. Examples of unevaluated policies include, but are not necessarily limited to, physician assistant's practice, controlled substances scheduling, advance directives or living wills, workers' compensation, institutional (including chain pharmacies) policies, and program grants to state agencies. Another unconsidered, but especially important, influence on treatment considerations is the multitude of federal and state laws establishing standards for reimbursement of therapeutic interventions, covering such areas as prior authorization, drug formularies, medication synchronization, and abuse-deterrent formulations for opioid medications. Efforts to understand the beneficial or potentially problematic ramifications of these policies, as well as the impact of such policy requirements on professional practice and patient care, are warranted.

It also is important to keep informed about the content of proposed statutes being introduced in the state legislature but which have not yet been signed into law (i.e., bills). Some recent bills, including some that have been drafted with the objective of improving public health and safety by reducing prescription medication abuse and diversion, may inadvertently create barriers to the availability of medications to people who use them therapeutically for pain relief and to maintain quality of life (see http://sppan.aapainmanage.org/legislation). Coordinated reactions to both draft and introduced legislative bills, and also to proposed regulatory policies whenever possible, can create opportunities to make policymakers aware of potential unintended consequences and recommendations for language modifications. Engagement with legislators and regulators during policy development can effectively reduce the prospect of future policy impediments and can even strengthen the policy's ability to achieve its stated objectives.

One of the most prevalently considered policies, which has been recently promoted to improve patients' pain care and reduce opioid-related overdoses and other harmful consequences, is dosing thresholds based on cumulative morphine equivalent daily dose (MEDD) milligram amounts. At this time, these thresholds typically are limited only to the treatment of patients with chronic noncancer pain and exempts patients with the disease of cancer and those undergoing palliative care or end-of-life care. These MEDD thresholds have been described as "a precautionary signal to get the prescriber to press pause before moving forward with dose escalation."[269(p1851)] Meeting or exceeding the dosage threshold is often coupled with a recommendation for the prescriber to obtain an expert consultation (see Paice and Von Roenn[270] for example). Washington was the first state (in 2007) to establish a recommended MEDD threshold, at 120 mg, in a clinical practice guideline.[271] Since that time, some states (including Washington) eventually established such amounts in law (see, for example, Washington Administrative Code[272]). Measures even were put into place to evaluate outcomes from codifying the Washington MEDD, with the goal of:

> [making] sure any interventions to prevent problematic use don't adversely affect the vast majority who are appropriately using their medications.[273(p2)]

An inherent by-product of codifying these dosage amounts into law is that this now establishes a legal liability for practitioners who fail to comply with the requirements. This concern was especially important for a state like Maine, which in 2016 adopted a 100-mg MEDD amount for treating chronic pain that generally could not be exceeded[274] but has since been modified to allow for therapeutic exceptions through a documentation of medical necessity.[275]

In addition to the MEDD threshold itself, the American Academy of Pain Management[276] (now the Academy of Integrative Pain Management) issued a statement reviewing requirements contained in the Washington law, and consequently also contained in similar policies adopted subsequently by other states, which could create uncertainty for practitioners attempting to comply to this distinctive regulation. Such provisions included (1) use of a written prescriber–patient agreement for those judged to be at a high risk of substance abuse, have a history of substance abuse, or have psychiatric comorbidities; (2) requiring certain prescribers to obtain a consultation with a "pain management specialist" under certain circumstances, including exceeding the dosing threshold; and (3) establishing qualifications for prescribers who can serve as adequately prepared specialist consultants.[276] Within this statement, though, the possibility was raised that any practitioner reluctance surrounding this law may relate more to perceptions based on an inaccurate understanding of the legal requirements, rather than being founded on a direct reaction to the mandatory conditions themselves.[276] That is, it is acknowledged that policy barriers to practice can occur as much from misinterpretations about policy requirements than from perceptions about legal liability based on actual policy content.

A more recent commentary by Ziegler[269] has identified additional substantive concerns related to policies establishing MEDD dosage thresholds. These potentially problematic issues include the implied emphasis on potential harms only at higher dosage levels (although risks are heightened at any dosage level,[277] especially without proper treatment monitoring); neglect of other, separate, factors that could contribute to clinical harms; nonstandard and erroneous conversion formulas for morphine equivalence; and an insufficient number of pain management specialists available for required consultations.[269] These considerations, as well as those mentioned earlier, support the need to thoroughly assess the various reasons for practitioners' reactions to such laws to help formulate ideas about addressing health care professionals' perceptions. This is especially feasible now because some of these policies have been in effect for a few years, so practitioner awareness should be higher than it would have been closer to the policy adoption. Ultimately, it can be determined whether any identified practitioner concerns are more likely remedied through modifying (to any degree) the requirements or recommendations contained in the laws or other regulatory policies, increasing resources to aid more broad and consistent implementation, or improving practitioners' understanding about the policy standards and promoting their clinical utility, or through a combination of approaches.

Taking Diversion into Account

In addition to efforts to promulgate pain policies that enhance benefits and minimize harms from treatments for patients with pain, drug control measures must be established, through both the same and separate policies, to reduce the potential for transferring prescription medications into illicit channels. Even given the numerous and varied legislative and regulatory requirements that have been implemented over time in the United States to govern the closed distribution of controlled medications, opioid analgesics can still be diverted from all levels of the distribution system.[278] Diverted opioid medications often become illegally available for illicit distribution and nonmedical use, which can contribute to harmful outcomes such as overdose and death. It should come as no surprise that using controlled medications obtained through means other than a valid prescription issued by a properly licensed practitioner for a legitimate medical purpose, or in ways that do not conform to practitioner instructions, compounds the risk of harmful consequences.

Given the risks inherent in all controlled substances, health care professionals who provide treatment with opioid medications have a responsibility to protect patient and public safety by taking actions to avoid contributing to abuse and diversion.

Prescribing or dispensing more dosage units than medically necessary is potentially problematic because these medications may go unused, accumulate in volume, and become susceptible to theft or perhaps accidental use by others.[279,280] When a practitioner's issuance of prescriptions reaches a level or pattern considered "excessive," in some states, it can fulfill the criteria for "unprofessional conduct" in which the practitioner is subject to license revocation or other civil penalties under law (see New Mexico Medical Board[281] as an example).

Patients receiving prescription-only controlled medications for pain treatment also share responsibilities under law, which has only recently begun receiving attention in earnest. Warnings on prescription labeling denote that it is a violation of law for patients to transfer the medications prescribed for them to any other person.[282] More generally, any person who possess controlled substances, including opioid analgesics, without a valid prescription, as well as someone who acquires these medications by theft, fraud, or misrepresentation, is in violation of federal and state laws. Opioids may even be prescribed legitimately but, when they are not stored securely in the patient's home, they are vulnerable to diversion through loss or theft. These scenarios reinforce the reality that learning whether a person acquired an opioid from peers or family, or even through a dispensed prescription, is often not enough information to inform a sufficient response—it is necessary to additionally consider the *circumstances* leading up to how the opioid was obtained initially.

There is a potential for opioid medications to be diverted from throughout the entire medication distribution system, including before they are prescribed. Consequently, there are many potential sources that feed the use of prescription opioids for illicit purposes. Examples of such activities, from each level of the distribution chain, include the following:

- *From the wholesale level*: Criminal diversions of large quantities are reported by manufacturers and distributors.
- *From the retail level*: Criminal activities by organizations and individuals, including some patients, to obtain opioid analgesics unlawfully
  - Armed robberies and night break-ins from pharmacies
  - Thefts, including employee pilferage, occurring from pharmacy supplies in nursing homes and hospitals
  - Fraud and misrepresentation, such as "doctor shopping" or prescription form theft, forgery, or alteration
  - "Script doctors" and "pill mills," which are illegal activities by rogue physicians who still have the necessary authority to prescribe, or to purchase and dispense, controlled substances
  - Misuse of Medicare and Medicaid drug coverage
- *From the ultimate user level*: Intentional or unintentional behaviors
  - Patient sharing with friends or family members
  - Patient selling to strangers
  - Caregiver stealing directly from patient
  - Stealing from unsecured amounts

Such a variety of diversion opportunities makes it clear that efforts to reduce nonmedical drug use should include, but must be more comprehensive than, focusing on prescribing and dispensing practices and patient access.

Although potential diversion sources can be identified through knowledge of the medication distribution system, little empirical evidence exists about the degree to which these numerous conceivable diversion activities are involved in prescription medication–related abuse, addiction, overdose, and death. However, understanding the multiple ways that diversion can occur substantiates use of a broad multifaceted approach for effectively addressing nonmedical use of prescription opioids. Such an approach is exemplified at a federal level by the Office of National Drug Control Policy's (ONDCP's)

Prescription Drug Abuse Prevention Plan,[283] which was unveiled in April 2011 and then updated each year as part of the US national drug control strategy (see ONDCP[284] for example). Under the ONDCP's Plan, multiple federal, state, and local regulatory and enforcement agencies are collaborating to address four distinct domains: (1) *Education*—to enhance practitioner and public awareness about the risks and benefits of prescription medications, to investigate the production of analgesics with less or no abuse liability, and to promote research to demonstrate changes in abuse trends; (2) *Tracking and monitoring*—to support the funding, breadth, and use of PMPs, to promote electronic prescribing of controlled substances and other treatment technologies, and to evaluate the utility of federal database for epidemiologic purposes; (3) *Proper medication disposal*—to reduce the volume of unused medications through enhanced disposal opportunities; (4) *Enforcement*—to train laws enforcement members and others to address pill mills and other drug-trafficking activities and to focus on doctor shopping or pharmacy hopping.[283] This collaborative and systematic strategy has the benefit of seeking to more comprehensively address the multiple means by which prescription medications can become available for illicit use, including through the practitioner–patient relationship. Such an approach, as well as detailed multiagency policy initiatives now underway in some states, symbolizes an apt appreciation for the intricate nature of the national public health problem of nonmedical drug use.[285-287]

Conclusions

In the United States, destructive consequences related to the use, misuse, and abuse of, as well as addiction to, prescription opioid analgesics have been increasing for more than a decade. These occurrences can create a potential to put at odds, and even conflate, the needs of those who are being harmed through the often-illicit use of prescription medications with patients who may benefit from their therapeutic use.[288] It is beneficial to contemplate, however, how current US legislative and regulatory policies can provide a critical reference point for considering the needs of these two separate, but sometimes overlapping, populations.

As has been described throughout this chapter, both US federal and state governmental and regulatory policies can contain language that establishes an effective drug control system that reduces the likelihood that these medications become available for inappropriate or unlawful use while also promoting medication access to patients when clinically warranted (i.e., Balance).[110] These dual objectives are promoted by many national and international entities and sanctioned by international treaty and federal law. Even given the substantial progress in reducing legal and regulatory barriers, there is a need to maintain ongoing vigilance to new or changing policy content. For this, the principle of Balance remains an unassailable conceptual framework to guide the continuing development of state policies governing health care practice and controlled substances prescribing.

Importantly, improved policy does not guarantee that the ideal outcomes of safe and effective pain management and reducing deaths and harm associated with the nonmedical use of controlled medications will be achieved. For example, it certainly is feasible that nonconformity to the recommendations inherent in a state-issued regulatory guideline could adversely affect the benefit/risk determinations necessary to best reach treatment decisions, as well as undermine the strategies offered in the policy to identify and address potential abuse or diversion behaviors. This scenario does not even account for the numerous factors within the health care system that can work against policies with balanced content, including a lack of understanding or misperceptions about a policy or poor or nonexistent implementation of a policy. Because of such influences, any policy improvement that is accomplished may not produce results that reflect its inherent Balance. Realizing *true* Balance requires an understanding of not only the actual policy content but also the extent of practice adherence to that policy content and then effectuating interventions based on this knowledge.

Although Balance is a principle conceived in, and intended for, policy development in an effort to maintain patient care with controlled medications during implementation of a broader abuse/diversion mitigation regulatory infrastructure, it has even been applied to activities outside of policy. This principle is useful for delineating the appropriate roles and responsibilities of health care professionals, members of regulatory agencies, and law enforcement officials regarding the issues of pain treatment and stemming the nonmedical use and prescription opioid–related harms. A practitioner's responsibility, of course, is patient health care—when providing pain treatment using opioid therapy, that practitioner is also expected to monitor for the abuse and diversion of the prescribed medications and to identify possible comorbidities and other patient factors that may have treatment implications; such an outcome represents Balance. Conversely, drug control is chiefly a responsibility of certain regulatory agencies and law enforcement—when planning efforts to curb abuse and diversion, these efforts can avoid interfering in legitimate medication availability, health care practice, or patient care; this, too, represents Balance. From this national and international medicolegal concept, it is clear that the actions of members of health care, regulation, and law enforcement often overlap in the obligations related to medication availability and efforts to minimize abuse and diversion.

In addition, recent national efforts to curb harms involving prescription medications, such as practitioner educational initiatives,[122] clinical practice guidelines,[15,289] and a Surgeon General's report,[290] have acknowledged the value of maintaining appropriate pain treatment. Clearly, these examples demonstrate a widespread belief in, as well as a commitment to, the ability to contemporaneously address the dual public health problems of undertreated pain and prescription medication abuse/diversion without sacrificing either. Attaining either objective at the expense of the other represents a failure of the drug control or health care regulatory systems, or both, that demands immediate corrective action. The laudable goals expressed through these activities will, hopefully, be demonstrated through the routine collection, assessment, and consideration of relevant outcomes to document whether implementation of any adopted approach effectively reduces harms and eschews deleterious unintended consequences for health care practitioners who provide pain management services using opioids.

Given these considerations, it is time to move beyond the call to evaluate policies. The increased research focus on degree of opioid prescribing concordance with clinical practice guidelines[291–296] establishes the precedent that attention must now turn toward determining the effect of pain policy content on clinical practice, including the assessment of factors influencing compliance with policy requirements or recommendations. Translating policy content into clinical practice and patient care outcomes representing both facets of Balance is necessary to optimize public safety as well as treatment safety and benefit for all patients requiring opioid therapy. This goal remains necessary until effective and readily available nondrug alternatives and nonopioid analgesics, as well as opioid analgesic products without an abuse potential, make such an approach obsolete. Certainly, achieving such an ideal treatment scenario is something that we can all support.

References

1. Dickinson E. *The Complete Poems of Emily Dickinson*. Boston, MA: Back Bay Books; 1976.
2. Fishbain DA, Lewis JE, Gao J. The pain-suffering association: a review. *Pain Med* 2015;16:1057–1072.
3. Rizvi SJ, Iskric A, Calati R, et al. Psychological and physical pain as predictors of suicide risk: evidence from clinical and neuroimaging findings. *Curr Opin Psychiatry* 2017;30:159–167.
4. Institute of Medicine Committee on Advancing Pain Research, Care, and Education. *Relieving Pain in America: A Blueprint for Transforming Prevention, Care, Education and Research*. Washington, DC: National Academies Press; 2011.
5. Neufeld NJ, Elnahal SM, Alvarez RH. Cancer pain: a review of epidemiology, clinical quality and value impact. *Future Oncol* 2017;13:833–841.
6. Nahin RL. Estimates of pain prevalence and severity in adults: United States, 2012. *J Pain* 2015;16:769–777.
7. Gaskin DJ, Richard P. The economic costs of pain in the United States. *J Pain* 2012;13:715–724.
8. Brennan F, Carr DB, Cousins M. Pain management: a fundamental human right. *Anesth Analg* 2007;105:205–221.
9. Brennan F, Carr D, Cousins M. Assess to pain management: still very much a human right. *Pain Med* 2017;17:1785–1789.
10. Brownson RC, Baker EA, Leet TL, et al. *Evidence-based Public Health*. New York: Oxford University Press; 2003.
11. Stjernswärd J, Foley K, Ferris FD. Integrating palliative care into national policies. *J Pain Symptom Manage* 2007;33:514–520.
12. Turnock BJ. *Public Health: What It Is and How It Works*. Boston, MA: Jones & Bartlett; 2004.
13. Federation of State Medical Boards of the United States. *Guidelines for the Chronic Use of Opioid Analgesics*. Euless, TX: Federation of State Medical Boards of the United States; 2017.
14. Inturrisi CE, Lipman AG. Opioid analgesics. In: Ballantyne JC, Rathmell JP, Fishman SM, eds. *Bonica's Management of Pain*. 4th ed. Philadelphia: Lippincott Williams & Wilkins; 2010:1172–1187.
15. Dowell D, Haegerich TM, Chou R. CDC guidelines for prescribing opioids for chronic pain: United States, 2016. *JAMA* 2016;315:1624–1645.
16. Federation of State Medical Boards of the United States. *Model Policy on the Use of Opioid Analgesics in the Treatment of Chronic Pain*. Euless, TX: Federation of State Medical Boards of the United States; 2013.
17. Chi NC, Demiris G. Family caregivers' pain management in end-of-life care: a systematic review. *Am J Hosp Palliat Care* 2017;34:470–485.
18. Dawson R, Sellers DE, Spross JA, et al. Do patients' beliefs act as barriers to effective pain management behaviors and outcomes in patients with cancer-related or noncancer-related pain? *Oncol Nurs Forum* 2005;32:363–374.
19. Duensing L, Eksterowicz N, Macario A, et al. Patient and physician perceptions of treatment of moderate-to-severe chronic pain with oral opioids. *Curr Med Res Opin* 2010;26:1579–1585.
20. McCracken LM, Hoskins J, Eccleston C. Concerns about medication and medication use in chronic pain. *J Pain* 2006;7:726–734.
21. Oliver DP, Washington K, Kruse RL, et al. Hospice family members' perceptions of and experiences with end-of-life care in the nursing home. *J Am Med Dir Assoc* 2014;15:744–750.
22. Reddy A, Yennurajalingam S, Bruera E. "Whatever my mother wants": barriers to adequate pain management. *J Palliat Med* 2013;16:709–712.
23. Schieffer BM, Pham Q, Labus J, et al. Pain medication beliefs and medication misuse in chronic pain. *J Pain* 2005;6:620–629.
24. Vallerand A, Nowak L. Chronic opioid therapy for nonmalignant pain: the patient's perspective. Part 1: life before and after opioid therapy. *Pain Manage Nurs* 2009;10:165–172.
25. Vallerand A, Nowak L. Chronic opioid therapy for nonmalignant pain: the patient's perspective. Part 2: barriers to chronic opioid therapy. *Pain Manage Nurs* 2010;11:126–131.
26. Wilkie DJ, Molokie R, Boyd-Seal D, et al. Patient-reported outcomes: descriptors of nociceptive and neuropathic pain and barriers to effective pain management in adult outpatients with sickle cell disease. *J Natl Med Assoc* 2010;102:18–22.
27. Barry DT, Irwin KS, Jones ES, et al. Opioids, chronic pain, and addiction in primary care. *J Pain* 2010;11:1442–1450.
28. Green CR, Hart-Johnson T. The adequacy of chronic pain management prior to presenting at a tertiary care pain center: the role of patient socio-demographic characteristics. *J Pain* 2010;11:746–754.
29. Green CR, Hart-Johnson T, Loeffler DR. Cancer-related chronic pain: examining quality of life in diverse cancer survivors. *Cancer* 2011;117:1994–2003.
30. Haozous EA, Knobf MT. "All my tears were gone": suffering and cancer pain in Southwest American Indians. *J Pain Symptom Manage* 2013;45:1050–1060.
31. Kapoor S, Thorn BE. Healthcare use and prescription of opioids in rural residents with pain. *Rural Remote Health* 2014;14:2879.
32. Monsivais DB, Engebretson JC. "I'm just not that sick": pain medication and identity in Mexican American women with chronic pain. *J Holist Nurs* 2012;30:188–194.
33. Passik SD, Kirsh KL, Donaghy KB, et al. Pain and aberrant drug-related behaviors in medically ill patients with and without histories of substance abuse. *Clin J Pain* 2006;22:173–181.

34. Stein KD, Alcaraz KI, Kamson C, et al. Sociodemographic inequalities in barriers to cancer pain management: a report from the American Cancer Society's Study of Cancer Survivors-II (SCS-II). *Psychooncology* 2016;25: 1212–1221.

35. Dobscha SK, Corson K, Flores JA, et al. Veterans Affairs primary care clinicians' attitudes toward chronic pain and correlates of opioid prescribing rates. *Pain Med* 2008;9:564–571.

36. Donovan AK, Wood GJ, Rubio DM, et al. Faculty communication knowledge, attitudes, and skills around chronic non-malignant pain improve with online training. *Pain Med* 2016;17:1985–1992.

37. Harle CA, Bauer SE, Hoang HQ, et al. Decision support for chronic pain care: how do primary care physicians decide when to prescribe opioids? A qualitative study. *BMC Fam Pract* 2015;16:48. doi:10.1186/s12875-015-0264-3.

38. Hollingshead NA, Meints S, Middleton SK, et al. Examining influential factors in providers' chronic pain treatment decisions: a comparison of physicians and medical students. *BMC Med Educ* 2015;15:164. doi:10.1186 /s12909-015-0441-z.

39. Leverence RR, Williams RL, Potter M, et al. Chronic non-cancer pain: a siren for primary care—a report from the PRImary Care MultiEthnic Network (PRIME Net). *J Am Board Fam Med* 2011;24:551–561.

40. Pearson AC, Eldrige JS, Moeschler SM, et al. Opioids for chronic pain: a knowledge assessment of nonpain specialty providers. *J Pain Res* 2016;9:129–135.

41. Riemondy S, Gonzalez L, Gosik K, et al. Nurses' perceptions and attitudes toward use of oral patient-controlled analgesia. *Pain Manage Nurs* 2016;17:132–139.

42. Salinas GD, Susalka D, Burton BS, et al. Risk assessment and counseling behaviors of healthcare professionals managing patients with chronic pain: a national multifaceted assessment of physicians, pharmacists, and their patients. *J Opioid Manag* 2012;8:273–284.

43. Trudeau KJ, Hildebrand C, Garg P, et al. A randomized controlled trial of the effects of online pain management education on primary care providers. *Pain Med* 2017;18:680–692.

44. Bradshaw YS, Patel Wacks N, Perez-Tamayo A, et al. Deconstructing one medical school's pain curriculum: I. Content analysis. *Pain Med* 2017;18:655–663.

45. Fishman SM, Young HM, Lucas AE, et al. Core competencies for pain management: results of an interprofessional consensus summit. *Pain Med* 2013;14:971–981.

46. Herr K, Marie BS, Gordon DB, et al. An interprofessional consensus of core competencies for prelicensure education in pain management: curriculum application for nursing. *J Nurs Educ* 2015;54:317–327.

47. Yanni LM, McKinney-Ketchum JL, Harrington SB, et al. Preparation, confidence, and attitudes about chronic noncancer pain in graduate medical education. *J Grad Med Educ* 2010;2:260–268.

48. Casty FE, Wieman MS, Shusterman N. Current topics in opioid therapy for pain management: addressing the problem of abuse. *Clin Drug Investig* 2013;33:459–468.

49. Webster LR, Grabois M. Current regulations related to opioid prescribing. *PMR* 2015;7:S236–S247.

50. Office of the Assistant Secretary for Health, U.S. Department of Health and Human Services. *National Pain Strategy: A Comprehensive Population Health-Level Strategy for Pain.* Washington, DC: U.S. Department of Health and Human Services; 2016.

51. Jacox A, Carr DB, Payne R, et al. *Management of Cancer Pain: Clinical Practice Guideline Number 9.* Rockville, MD: Agency for Health Care Policy and Research; 1994. AHCPR No. 94-0592.

52. Miaskowski C, Cleary J, Burney R, et al. *Guideline for the Management of Cancer Pain in Adults and Children: APS Clinical Practice Guidelines Series, No. 3.* Glenview, IL: American Pain Society; 2005.

53. Advisory Group on Cancer Pain Relief. *American Cancer Society Advisory Group on Cancer Pain Relief: Agenda, Patient Services.* Atlanta, GA: American Cancer Society; 1994.

54. Cancer Pain Management Policy Review Group. *American Cancer Society Policy Statement on Cancer Pain Management.* Atlanta, GA: National Government Relations Department, American Cancer Society; 2001.

55. Cancer Pain Management Policy Review Group. *American Cancer Society Position Statement on Regulatory Barriers to Quality Cancer Pain Management.* Atlanta, GA: National Government Relations Department, American Cancer Society; 2001.

56. Cancer Pain Management Policy Review Group. *American Cancer Society Position Statement on Medicaid Prior Authorization for Pain Medications.* Atlanta, GA: National Government Relations Department, American Cancer Society; 2001.

57. Institute of Medicine Committee on Care at the End of Life. *Approaching Death: Improving Care at the End of Life.* Washington, DC: National Academies Press; 1997.

58. National Institutes of Health Consensus Development Program. *Symptom Management in Cancer: Pain, Depression and Fatigue.* Bethesda, MD; National Institutes of Health; 2002.

59. World Health Assembly. *Cancer Prevention and Control. WHA 58.22.* Geneva, Switzerland: World Health Organization; 2005.

60. Pain & Policy Studies Group. *Achieving Balance in State Pain Policy: A Progress Report Card (CY 2015).* Madison, WI: University of Wisconsin Carbone Cancer Center; 2016.

61. World Health Organization. *Equitable Access to Essential Medicines: A Framework for Collective Action.* Geneva, Switzerland: World Health Organization; 2004.

62. Cousins MJ, Brennan F, Carr DB. Pain relief: a universal human right. *Pain* 2004;112:1–4.

63. Carr DB. Patients with pain need less stigma, not more. *Pain Med* 2016;17:1391–1393.

64. Bolen J. Enough about barriers and fear already: the pain community needs to be proactive and take steps to stop the "Roulette Wheel." *Pain Med* 2007;8:438–440.

65. Chou R, Fanciullo GJ, Fine PG, et al. Clinical guidelines for the use of chronic opioid therapy for chronic noncancer pain. *J Pain* 2009;10:113–130.

66. United Nations. *Single Convention on Narcotic Drugs, 1961.* Geneva, Switzerland: United Nations; 1961.

67. United Nations. *Single Convention on Narcotic Drugs, 1961, as Amended by the 1972 Protocol Amending the Single Convention on Narcotic Drugs, 1961.* New York: United Nations; 1972.

68. Jaffe JH, Martin WR. Opioid analgesics and antagonists. In: Gilman AG, Rall TW, Nies AS, et al, eds. *Goodman and Gilman's The Pharmacological Basis of Therapeutics.* 8th ed. New York: Pergamon Press; 1990:485–521.

69. International Narcotics Control Board. *Report of the International Narcotics Control Board for 2016.* New York: United Nations; 2017.

70. Cleary JF, Husain A, Maurer M. Increasing worldwide access to medical opioids. *Lancet* 2016;387:1597–1599.

71. International Narcotics Control Board. *Report of the International Narcotics Control Board for 1989: Demand for and Supply of Opiates for Medical and Scientific Needs.* Vienna, Austria: United Nations; 1989.

72. International Narcotics Control Board. *Report of the International Narcotics Control Board for 2006.* New York: United Nations; 2007.

73. International Narcotics Control Board. *Availability of Internationally Controlled Drugs: Ensuring Adequate Access for Medical and Scientific Purposes: Indispensable, Adequately Available and Not Unduly Restricted.* New York: United Nations; 2016.

74. International Narcotics Control Board. *Report of the International Narcotics Control Board for 1995: Availability of Opiates for Medical Needs.* New York: United Nations; 1996.

75. International Narcotics Control Board. *Report of the International Narcotics Control Board on the Availability of Internationally Controlled Drugs: Ensuring Adequate Access for Medical and Scientific Purposes.* New York: United Nations; 2011.

76. International Narcotics Control Board, World Health Organization. *Guide on Estimating Requirements for Substances Under International Control.* Vienna, Austria: United Nations; 2012.

77. World Health Organization. Guiding principles for small national drug regulatory authorities. *World Health Organ Drug Info* 1989;3:43–50.

78. World Health Organization. *Cancer Pain Relief: With a Guide to Opioid Availability.* 2nd ed. Geneva, Switzerland: World Health Organization; 1996.

79. World Health Organization. *Ensuring Balance in National Policies on Controlled Substances: Guidance for Availability and Accessibility of Controlled Medicines.* 2nd ed, Rev ed. Geneva, Switzerland: World Health Organization; 2011.

80. United Nations Office on Drugs and Crime. *The Non-medical Use of Prescription Drugs: Policy Direction Issues.* Vienna, Austria: United Nations; 2011.

81. Rwanda Ministry of Health. *Five Years (2010-2014) Strategic Plan for Palliative Care for Incurable Disease.* Kigali, Rwanda: Rwanda Ministry of Health; 2010.

82. Council of Europe. *Recommendation 24 of the Committee of Ministers to Member States on the Organisation of Palliative Care. Adopted by the Committee of Ministers on 12 November 2003 at the 860th Meeting of the Ministers' Deputies.* Strasbourg, France: Council of Europe; 2003.

83. World Medical Association. *WMA resolution on the access to adequate pain treatment.* Paper presented at: 62nd WMA General Assembly; October 2011; Montevideo, Uruguay.

84. World Health Organization. *A Community Health Approach to Palliative Care for HIV/AIDS and Cancer Patients in Sub-Saharan Africa.* Geneva, Switzerland: World Health Organization; 2004.

85. International Narcotics Control Board. *Report of the International Narcotics Control Board for 2004.* New York: United Nations; 2005.

86. United Nations Commission on Narcotic Drugs. *Resolution 54/6: Promoting Adequate Availability of Internationally Controlled Narcotic Drugs and Psychotropic Substances for Medical and Scientific Purposes While Preventing Their Diversion and Abuse.* Vienna, Austria: United Nations; 2011.

87. United Nations Economic and Social Council. Demand for and supply of opiates used to meet medical and scientific needs: resolution 2005-26. In: *Commission on Narcotic Drugs. Report on the Forty-eighth Session.* Geneva, Switzerland: United Nations; 2005:5–6.

88. United Nations Economic and Social Council. Promoting adequate availability of internationally controlled licit drugs for medical and scientific purposes while preventing their diversion and abuse: resolution 53/4. In: *Commission on Narcotic Drugs: Report of the Fifty-third Session.* Geneva, Switzerland: United Nations; 2010:12–15.

89. Cherny NI, Baselga J, De Conno F, et al. Formulary availability and regulatory barriers to accessibility of opioids for cancer pain in Europe: a report from the ESMO/EAPC Opioid Policy Initiative. *Ann Oncol* 2010;21:615–626.

90. Cleary J, Powell RA, Munene G, et al. Formulary availability and regulatory barriers to accessibility of opioids for cancer pain in Africa: a report from the Global Opioid Policy Initiative (GOPI). *Ann Oncol* 2013;24:14–23.

91. Dzierzanowski T, Cialkowska-Rysz A. Accessibility of opioid analgesics and barriers to optimal chronic pain treatment in Poland in 2000-2015. *Support Care Cancer* 2017;25:775–781.

92. Križanová K. Slovakia: cancer pain management and palliative care. *J Pain Symptom Manage* 2002;24:231–232.

93. United Nations Commission on Narcotic Drugs. *Ensuring Availability of Controlled Medications for the Relief of Pain and Preventing Diversion and Abuse.* Vienna, Austria: Commission on Narcotic Drugs; 2011.

94. World Health Organization. *Cancer Pain Relief and Palliative Care: Report of the WHO Expert Committee on Cancer Pain Relief and Active Supportive Care.* Geneva, Switzerland: World Health Organization; 1990. Technical report series 804.

95. Beubler E, Eisenberg E, Castro-Lopes J, et al. Prescribing policies of opioids for chronic pain. *J Pain Palliat Care Pharmacother* 2007;21:53–55.

96. Blengini C, Joranson DE, Ryan KM. Italy reforms national policy for cancer pain relief and opioids. *Eur J Cancer Care* 2003;12:28–34.

97. Human Rights Watch. Mexico: breakthrough for pain treatment: modernized system for prescribing strong medicines. Available at: https://www.hrw.org/news/2015/06/15/mexico-breakthrough-pain-treatment. Accessed April 12, 2018.

98. Pain & Policy Studies Group. *Achieving Balance in Federal and State Pain Policy: A Guide to Evaluation (CY 2013).* Madison, WI: University of Wisconsin Paul P. Carbone Cancer Center; 2014.

99. Center for Substance Abuse Treatment. *National All Schedules Prescription Electronic Reporting Act of 2005: A Review of Implementation of Existing State Controlled Substance Monitoring Programs.* Substance Abuse and Mental Health Services Administration, U.S. Department of Health and Human Services; 2005.

100. Cleary J, Radbruch L, Torode J, et al. Formulary availability and regulatory barriers to accessibility of opioids for cancer pain in Asia: a report from the Global Opioid Policy Initiative (GOPI). *Ann Oncol* 2013;24:24–32.

101. Cleary J, Simha N, Panieri A, et al. Formulary availability and regulatory barriers to accessibility of opioids for cancer pain in India: a report from the Global Opioid Policy Initiative (GOPI). *Ann Oncol* 2013;24:22–40.

102. Cleary J, De Lima L, Eisenchlas J, et al. Formulary availability and regulatory barriers to accessibility of opioids for cancer pain in Latin America and the Caribbean: a report from the Global Opioid Policy Initiative (GOPI). *Ann Oncol* 2013;24:41–50.

103. Cleary J, Silbermann M, Scholten W, et al. Formulary availability and regulatory barriers to accessibility of opioids for cancer pain in the Middle East: a report from the Global Opioid Policy Initiative (GOPI). *Ann Oncol* 2013;24:51–59.

104. Mosoiu D, Ryan KM, Joranson DE, et al. Reforming drug control policy for palliative care in Romania. *Lancet* 2006;367:2110–2117.

105. Government of Bangladesh, Department of Cancer Control. *Circular No. 1(20)/89-90/292(42).* Dhaka, Bangladesh: Government of Bangladesh; 1990.

106. Green K, Kinh LN, Khue LN. *Palliative Care in Viet Nam: Findings from a Rapid Situation Analysis in Five Provinces.* Hanoi, Vietnam: Ministry of Health; 2006.

107. World Health Assembly. *Ensuring Accessibility to Essential Medicines.* WHA 55.14. Geneva, Switzerland: World Health Organization; 2002.

108. World Health Assembly. *Cancer Prevention and Control. Resolution EB114.R2.* Geneva, Switzerland: World Health Organization; 2004.

109. World Health Assembly. *Access to Essential Medicines. WHA 67.22.* Geneva, Switzerland: World Health Organization; 2014.

110. Berterame S, Erthal J, Thomas J, et al. Use of and barriers to access to opioid analgesics: a worldwide, regional and national study. *Lancet* 2016;387:1644–1656.

111. Federal Food Drug and Cosmetic Act. Title 21 USCS §393.

112. Fain KM, Yu T, Boyd CM, et al. Evidence selection for a prescription drug's benefit-harm assessment: challenges and recommendations. *J Clin Epidemiol* 2016;74:151–157.

113. Federal Food Drug and Cosmetic Act. Title 21 USCS §355.

114. Gassman AL, Nguyen CP, Joffe HV. FDA regulations of prescription drugs. *N Engl J Med* 2017;376:674–682.

115. U.S. Food and Drug Administration. *Guidance for Industry: Premarketing Risk Assessment.* Rockville, MD: U.S. Department of Health and Human Services; 2005.

116. U.S. Food and Drug Administration. FDA Basics Webinar: a brief overview of risk evaluation and mitigation strategies (REMS). Available at: https://www.fda.gov/aboutfda/transparency/basics/ucm325201.htm. Accessed April 12, 2018.

117. U.S. Food and Drug Administration. Approved risk evaluation and mitigation strategies (REMS): extended-release and long-acting (ER/LA) opioid analgesics. Available at: http://www.accessdata.fda.gov/scripts/cder/rems/index.cfm?event=RemsDetails.page&REMS=17. Accessed April 12, 2018.

118. U.S. Food and Drug Administration. Approved risk evaluation and mitigation strategies (REMS): transmucosal immediate-release fentanyl (TIRF) products. Available at: http://www.accessdata.fda.gov/scripts/cder/rems/index.cfm?event=RemsDetails.page&REMS=60. Accessed April 12, 2018.

119. Federal Food Drug and Cosmetic Act. Title 21 USCS §355-1(d).

120. U.S. Food and Drug Administration. *Extended-Release (ER) and Long-Acting (LA) Opioid Analgesics Risk Evaluation and Mitigation Strategy (REMS).* Rockville, MD: U.S. Food and Drug Administration; 2012.

121. ER/LA Opioid Analgesics REMS. Products covered under the ER/LA Opioid Analgesics REMS Program. Available at: http://www.er-la-opioidrems.com/IwgUI/rems/products.action. Accessed April 12, 2018.

122. U.S. Food and Drug Administration. *FDA Blueprint for Prescriber Education for Extended-Release and Long-Acting Opioid Analgesics.* Silver Spring, MD: U.S. Food and Drug Administration; 2017.

123. Federal Food Drug and Cosmetic Act. Title 21 USCS §355-1(e)(3).

124. Alford DP, Zisblatt L, Ng P, et al. SCOPE of pain: an evaluation of an Opioid Risk Evaluation and Mitigation Strategy continuing education program. *Pain Med* 2016;17:56–63.

125. Cepeda MS, Coplan PM, Kopper NW, et al. ER/LA Opioid Analgesics REMS: overview of ongoing assessments of its progress and its impact on health outcomes. *Pain Med* 2017;18:78–85.

126. Code of Federal Regulations. Title 21 CFR Part 201 - Labeling.

127. Code of Federal Regulations. Title 21 CFR §202.1.

128. Federal Food Drug and Cosmetic Act. Title 21 USCS §355(k)(3).

129. U.S. Food and Drug Administration. *Classwide Labeling Changes for All Extended-release and Long-acting (ER/LA) Opioid Analgesics.* Silver Spring, MD: U.S. Food and Drug Administration; 2016.

130. Bonnie RJ, Ford MA, Phillips JK, eds. *Pain Management and the Opioid Epidemic: Balancing Societal and Individual Risks and Benefits of Prescription Opioid Use.* Washington, DC: The National Academies Press; 2017.

131. United States v Evers. 643 F2d 1043 5th Circuit, 1981.

132. Federal Food Drug and Cosmetic Act. Title 21 USCS §396.

133. Controlled Substances Act. Pub L No. 91-513, 84 Stat 1242.

134. United States House of Representatives. *Comprehensive Drug Abuse Prevention and Control Act of 1970.* Washington, DC: United States House of Representatives; 1970. House Report No 91-1444.

135. Controlled Substances Act. Title 21 USCS §812(c).

136. Drug Enforcement Administration. *Schedules of Controlled Substances: Rescheduling of Hydrocodone Combination Products from Schedule III to Schedule II.* Springfield, VA: Drug Enforcement Administration; 2014. Docket no. DEA-389.

137. Controlled Substances Act. Title 21 USCS §823(e).

138. Controlled Substances Act. Title 21 USCS §823(f).

139. Code of Federal Regulations. Title 21 CFR §1306.04(a).

140. Controlled Substances Act. Title 21 USCS §826(a).

141. United States v Moore. 96 S. Ct. 335, 423 U.S. 122, 1975.

142. Code of Federal Regulations. Title 21 CFR §1305.03.

143. Controlled Substances Act. Title 21 USCS §828(a).

144. Code of Federal Regulations. Title 21 CFR §1306.12.

145. Controlled Substances Act. Title 21 USCS §829(a).

146. Code of Federal Regulations. Title 21 CFR §1306.22.

147. Controlled Substances Act. Title 21 USCS §829(b).

148. Code of Federal Regulations. Title 21 CFR §1311.

149. Drug Enforcement Administration. *Electronic Prescriptions for Controlled Substances: Final Rule.* Springfield, VA: Drug Enforcement Administration; 2010. Docket No. DEA-218I.

150. Code of Federal Regulations. Title 21 CFR §1311.102.

151. Surescripts. E-prescribing of controlled substances now legal nationwide. Available at: http://surescripts.com/news-center/press-releases/!content/e-prescribing-of-controlled-substances-now-legal-nationwide. Accessed April 12, 2018.

152. Code of Federal Regulations. Title 21 CFR §1306.11(d).

153. Code of Federal Regulations. Title 21 CFR §1306.13.

154. Controlled Substances Act. Title 21 USCS §801(1).

155. United States of America Congressional Record. *Proceedings and Debates of the 91st Congress Second Session, Volume 116—Part 25.* Washington, DC: U.S. Government Printing Office; 1970.

156. Controlled Substances Act. Title 21 USCS §826(b).

157. Drug Enforcement Administration. *Ciba-Gelgy Corp. and MD Pharmaceutical Inc.; 1986 Aggregate Production Quota, 1986 Individual Manufacturing Quotas, and 1986 Disposal Allocations for Methylphenidate.* Springfield, VA: Drug Enforcement Administration; 1988.

158. Drug Enforcement Administration. *Controlled Substances: Proposed Adjustment to the Aggregate Production Quotas for 2012.* Springfield, VA: Drug Enforcement Administration; 2012.

159. Drug Enforcement Administration. *Controlled Substances: Established Initial 1995 Aggregate Production Quotas.* Springfield, VA: Drug Enforcement Administration; 1994.

160. Drug Enforcement Administration. *Controlled Substances: Proposed Revised Aggregate Production Quotas for 2007.* Springfield, VA: Drug Enforcement Administration; 2007.

161. Drug Enforcement Administration. *Established Aggregate Production Quotas for Schedule I and II Controlled Substances and Established Assessment of Annual Needs for the List I Chemicals Ephedrine, Pseudoephedrine, and Phenylpropanolamine for 2013.* Springfield, VA: Drug Enforcement Administration; 2012.

162. Anson P. DEA cutting opioid supply in 2017. Available at: https://www.painnewsnetwork.org/stories/2016/10/4/dea-cutting-opioid-supply-in-2017. Accessed April 12, 2018.

163. Controlled Substances Act. Title 21 USCS §826(e).
164. Brushwood DB. *Drug Control Policy Out of Balance*. Boston, MA: American Society of Law, Medicine and Ethics; 2003.
165. Jung B, Reidenberg MM. Physicians being deceived. *Pain Med* 2007;8:433–437.
166. Rich BA. Litigation involving pain management. In: Fishman SM, Ballantyne JC, Rathmell JP, eds. *Bonica's Management of Pain*. 4th ed. Lippincott Williams & Wilkins; 2010:183–193.
167. Ziegler SJ. Pain, patients, and prosecution: who is deceiving whom? *Pain Med* 2008;8:445–446.
168. Brushwood DB. The "general recognition and acceptance" standard of objectivity for good faith in prescribing: legal and medical implications. *J Pain Palliat Care Pharmacother* 2007;21:35–38.
169. Edmondson WAD, Rowe GS, Goddard T, et al. *Docket No. DEA-261: Comment on Dispensing of Controlled Substances for the Treatment of Pain*. Washington, DC: National Association of Attorneys General; 2005.
170. Annas GJ. Congress, controlled substances, and physician-assisted suicide: elephants in mouseholes. *N Engl J Med* 2006;354:1079–1084.
171. Brushwood DB. Defining "legitimate medical purpose." *Am J Health Syst Pharm* 2005;62:306–308.
172. United Nations. *Convention on Psychotropic Substances, 1971*. Geneva, Switzerland: United Nations; 1971.
173. Controlled Substances Act. Title 21 USCS §801a(3).
174. Controlled Substances Act. Title 21 USCS §823(g).
175. American Psychiatric Association. *Diagnostic and Statistical Manual of Mental Disorders (DSM-5)*. 5th ed. Arlington, VA: American Psychiatric Association; 2013.
176. Controlled Substances Act. Title 21 USCS §802(1).
177. World Health Organization. *The ICD-10 Classification of Mental and Behavioural Disorders: Clinical Descriptions and Diagnostic Guidelines. F1x.2 Dependence Syndrome*. Geneva, Switzerland; World Health Organization; 2006.
178. American Society of Addiction Medicine. *Public Policy Statement: Definition of Addiction*. Chevy Chase, MD: American Society of Addiction Medicine; 2011.
179. Public Health and Welfare Act. Title 42 USC §201.
180. United States House of Representatives. Public Law 91-513 Public Health Services Act. October 27, 1970.
181. World Health Organization. *WHO Expert Committee on Drug Dependence: Thirtieth Report*. Geneva, Switzerland: World Health Organization; 1998.
182. Drug Enforcement Administration. *David H. Gillis: Granting of Registration*. Springfield, VA: Drug Enforcement Administration; 1993.
183. Drug Enforcement Administration. *Issuance of Multiple Prescriptions for Schedule II Controlled Substances*. Springfield, VA: Drug Enforcement Administration; 2007. Docket no. DEA-287F.
184. Drug Enforcement Administration. *Issuance of Multiple Prescriptions for Schedule II Controlled Substances*. Springfield, VA: Drug Enforcement Administration; 2006. Docket no. DEA-287N.
185. Gilson AM, Joranson DE. The Federal Drug Enforcement Administration "prescription series" proposal: continuing concerns. *J Pain Palliat Care Pharmacother* 2007;21:21–24.
186. Gilson AM, Joranson DE. Is the DEA's new "Prescription Series" regulation balanced? *J Pain Palliat Care Pharmacother* 2008;22:218–220.
187. Heit H. Healthcare professionals and the DEA: restoring the balance. *J Opioid Manag* 2006;2:310–311.
188. Pain & Policy Studies Group. *Achieving Balance in Federal and State Pain Policy: A Guide to Evaluation*. 5th ed. Madison, WI: University of Wisconsin Paul P. Carbone Comprehensive Cancer Center; 2008.
189. Code of Federal Regulations. Title 21 CFR Part 1317 - Disposal.
190. Code of Federal Regulations. Title 21 CFR §1317.40(a).
191. Drug Enforcement Administration. *Final Rule on the Disposal of Controlled Substances*. Springfield, VA: Drug Enforcement Administration; 2014. Docket no. DEA-316.
192. Code of Federal Regulations. Title 21 CFR §1317.40(c).
193. Code of Federal Regulations. Title 21 CFR §1317.40(b)(2).
194. Code of Federal Regulations. Title 21 CFR §1317.80.
195. Code of Federal Regulations. Title 21 CFR §1304.11.
196. Gilson AM, Maurer MA, Joranson DE. State policy affecting pain management: recent improvements and the positive impact of regulatory health policies. *Health Policy* 2005;74:192–204.
197. De Lima L, Sakowski JA, Stratton HC, et al. Legislation analysis according to WHO and INCB criteria on opioid availability: a comparative study of 5 countries and the state of Texas. *Health Policy* 2001;56:99–110.
198. Fujimoto D. Regulatory issues in pain management. *Clin Geriatr Med* 2001;17:537–551.
199. Hill CS Jr. The negative effect of regulatory agencies on adequate pain control. *Prim Care Cancer* 1989;11:47–51.
200. Merritt D, Fox-Grage W, Rothouse M, et al. *State Initiatives in End-of-life Care: Policy Guide for State Legislators*. Washington, DC: National Conference of States Legislatures; 1998.
201. National Conference of Commissioners on Uniform State Laws. *Uniform Controlled Substances Act*. Washington, DC: National Conference of Commissioners on Uniform State Laws; 1990.
202. National Conference of Commissioners on Uniform State Laws. *Uniform Controlled Substances Act*. Washington, DC: National Conference of Commissioners on Uniform State Laws; 1994.
203. New York State Public Health Council. *Breaking Down the Barriers to Effective Pain Management: Recommendations to Improve the Assessment and Treatment of Pain in New York State*. Albany, NY: New York State Department of Health; 1998.
204. National Institutes of Health. *State-of-the-Science Conference Statement: Improving End-of-Life Care*. Bethesda, MD: National Institutes of Health; 2004.
205. Rich BA. An ethical analysis of the barriers to effective pain management. *Camb Q Healthc Ethics* 2000;9:54–70.
206. Tucker KL. A new risk emerges: provider accountability for inadequate treatment of pain. *Ann Long-Term Care* 2001;9:52–56.
207. World Health Organization. *Cancer Pain Relief and Palliative Care in Children*. Geneva, Switzerland: World Health Organization; 1998.
208. World Health Organization. *Achieving Balance in National Opioids Control Policy: Guidelines for Assessment*. Geneva, Switzerland: World Health Organization; 2000.
209. National Conference of Commissioners on Uniform State Laws. *Uniform Controlled Substances Act*. St. Louis, MO: National Conference of Commissioners on Uniform State Laws; 1970.
210. Federation of State Medical Boards of the United States. *Model Guidelines for the Use of Controlled Substances for the Treatment of Pain*. Euless, TX: Federation of State Medical Boards of the United States; 1998.
211. Federation of State Medical Boards of the United States. *Model Policy for the Use of Controlled Substances for the Treatment of Pain*. Euless, TX: Federation of State Medical Boards of the United States; 2004.
212. American Alliance of Cancer Pain Initiatives. *Statement on Intractable Pain Treatment Acts (IPTA)*. Madison, WI: American Alliance of Cancer Pain Initiatives; 2004.
213. Hill CS Jr. The intractable pain treatment act of Texas. *Tex Med* 1992;88:70–72.
214. Joranson DE. Intractable pain treatment laws and regulations. *Am Pain Soc Bull* 1995;5:1–3, 15–17.
215. Joranson DE, Gilson AM. State intractable pain policy: current status. *Am Pain Soc Bull* 1997;7:7–9.
216. Gilson AM, Joranson DE. U.S. policies relevant to the prescribing of opioid analgesics for the treatment of pain in patients with addictive disease. *Clin J Pain* 2002;18:S91–S98.
217. Clark HW. Policy and medical-legal issues in the prescribing of controlled substances. *J Psychoactive Drugs* 1991;23:321–328.
218. Dahl JL, Joranson DE, Weissman DE. The Wisconsin cancer pain initiative: a progress report. *Am J Hospice Care* 1989;6:39–43.
219. Hill CS Jr. The negative influence of licensing and disciplinary boards and drug enforcement agencies on pain treatment with opioid analgesics. *J Pharm Care Pain Symptom Control* 1993;1:43–62.
220. Weissman DE, Joranson DE, Hopwood MB. Wisconsin physicians' knowledge and attitudes about opioid analgesic regulations. *Wis Med J* 1991;671–675.
221. Hoffmann DE, Tarzian AJ. Achieving the right balance in oversight of physician opioid prescribing for pain: the role of state medical boards. *J Law Med Ethics* 2003;31:21–40.
222. Johnson SH. Disciplinary actions and pain relief: analysis of the Pain Relief Act. *J Law Med Ethics* 1996;24:319–327.
223. Martino AM. In search of a new ethic for treating patients with chronic pain: what can medical boards do? *J Law Med Ethics* 1998;26:332–349.
224. Richard J, Reidenberg M. The risk of disciplinary action by state medical boards against physicians prescribing opioids. *J Pain Symptom Manage* 2005;29:206–212.
225. Furstenberg CT, Ahles TA, Whedon MB, et al. Knowledge and attitudes of health-care providers toward cancer pain management: a comparison of physicians, nurses, and pharmacists in the State of New Hampshire. *J Pain Symptom Manage* 1998;15:335–349.
226. Nowels D, Lee JT. Cancer pain management in home hospice settings: a comparison of primary care and oncologic physicians. *J Palliat Care* 1999;15:5–9.
227. Weinstein SM, Laux LF, Thornby JI, et al. Physicians' attitudes toward pain and the use of opioid analgesics: results of a survey from the Texas Cancer Pain Initiative. *South Med J* 2000;93:479–487.
228. Zimbal M, Cleary J, Gilson AM, et al. Wisconsin physicians' beliefs and attitudes about the use of opioid analgesics. *J Pain* 2007;7 (suppl 2):597.
229. Von Roenn JH, Cleeland CS, Gonin R, et al. Physician attitudes and practice in cancer pain management: a survey from the Eastern Cooperative Oncology Group. *Ann Intern Med* 1993;119:121–126.
230. Grahmann PH, Jackson II KC, Lipman AG. Clinician beliefs about opioid use and barriers in chronic nonmalignant pain. *J Pain Palliat Care Pharmacother* 2004;18:7–28.
231. Turk DC. What position do APS's physician members take on chronic opioid therapy? *Am Pain Soc Bull* 1992;2:1–5.
232. Roth CS, Burgess DJ, Mahowald ML. Medical residents' beliefs and concerns about using opioids to treat chronic cancer and noncancer pain: a pilot study. *Journal of Rehabilitation Research & Development* 2007;44:263–270.
233. Joranson DE, Gilson AM. Pharmacists' knowledge of and attitudes toward opioid pain medications in relation to federal and state policies. *J Am Pharm Assoc* 2001;41:213–220.
234. Drayer RA, Henderson J, Reidenberg M. Barriers to better pain control in hospitalized patients. *J Pain Symptom Manage* 1999;17:434–440.
235. Hickman SE, Tolle SW, Tilden VP. Physicians' and nurses' perspectives on increased family reports of pain in dying hospitalized patients. *J Palliat Med* 2000;3:413–418.

236. Hollen CJ, Hollen CW, Stolte K. Hospice and hospital oncology unit nurses: a comparative survey of knowledge and attitudes about cancer pain. *Oncol Nurs Forum* 2000;27:1593–1599.

237. Tucker KL. Treatment of pain in dying patients (to the Editor). *N Engl J Med* 1998;338:1231.

238. Joranson DE, Gilson AM, Ryan KM, et al. *Achieving Balance in Federal and State Pain Policy: A Guide to Evaluation.* Madison, WI: University of Wisconsin Paul P. Carbone Comprehensive Cancer Center; 2000.

239. Pain & Policy Studies Group. *Achieving Balance in Federal and State Pain Policy: A Guide to Evaluation.* 2nd ed. Madison, WI: University of Wisconsin Paul P. Carbone Comprehensive Cancer Center; 2003.

240. Pain & Policy Studies Group. *Achieving Balance in Federal and State Pain Policy: A Guide to Evaluation.* 3rd ed. Madison, WI: University of Wisconsin Paul P. Carbone Comprehensive Cancer Center; 2006.

241. Pain & Policy Studies Group. *Achieving Balance in Federal and State Pain Policy: A Guide to Evaluation.* 4th ed. Madison, WI: University of Wisconsin Paul P. Carbone Comprehensive Cancer Center; 2007.

242. Pain & Policy Studies Group. *Achieving Balance in Federal and State Pain Policy: A Guide to Evaluation (CY 2012).* Madison, WI: University of Wisconsin Paul P. Carbone Comprehensive Cancer Center; 2013.

243. Federal Food Drug and Cosmetic Act. Title 21 USCS §355-1(f)(2).

244. Ross-Degnan D, Simoni-Wastila L, Brown JS, et al. A controlled study of the effects of state surveillance on indicators of problematic and non-problematic benzodiazepine use in a medicaid population. *Int J Psychiatr Med* 2004;34:103–123.

245. Simoni-Wastila L, Tompkins C. Balancing diversion control and medical necessity: the case of prescription drugs with abuse potential. *Subs Use Misuse* 2001;36:1275–1296.

246. Simoni-Wastila L, Ross-Degnan D, Mah C, et al. A retrospective data analysis of the impact of the New York triplicate prescription program on benzodiazepine use in Medicaid patients with chronic psychiatric and neurologic disorders. *Clin Ther* 2004;26:322–336.

247. Wagner AK, Soumerai SB, Zhang F, et al. Effects of state surveillance on new post-hospitalization benzodiazepine use. *Int J Qual Health Care* 2003;15:423–431.

248. Wastila LJ, Bishop C. The influence of multiple copy prescription programs on analgesic utilization. *J Pharm Care Pain Symptom Control* 1996;4:3–19.

249. United States General Accounting Office. *Prescription Drug Monitoring: States Can Readily Identify Illegal Sales and Use of Controlled Substances.* Washington, DC: United States General Accounting Office; 1992. GAO/HRD-92-115.

250. United States General Accounting Office. *Prescription Drugs: State Monitoring Programs Provide Useful Tool to Reduce Diversion.* Washington, DC: United States General Accounting Office; 2002. GAO-02-634.

251. American Alliance of Cancer Pain Initiatives. *Statement on State Prescription Monitoring Programs.* Madison, WI: American Alliance of Cancer Pain Initiatives; 2002.

252. Brushwood DB. Maximizing the value of electronic prescription monitoring programs. *J Law Med Ethics* 2003;31:41–54.

253. Joranson DE, Carrow GM, Ryan KM, et al. Pain management and prescription monitoring. *J Pain Symptom Manage* 2002;23:231–238.

254. Clark T, Eadie J, Kreiner P, et al. *Prescription Drug Monitoring Programs: An Assessment of the Evidence for Best Practices.* Waltham, MA: Prescription Drug Monitoring Program Center for Excellence, Heller School for Social Policy and Management, Brandeis University; 2012.

255. Wang J, Christo PJ. The influence of prescription monitoring programs on chronic pain management. *Pain Physician* 2009;12:507–515.

256. Alliance of States with Prescription Monitoring Programs. BJA announces 2009 PDMP grant solicitations. *Alliance Monit* 2009;1:1.

257. Finley EP, Garcia A, Rosen K, et al. Evaluating the impact of prescription drug monitoring program implementation: a scoping review. *BMC Health Serv Res* 2017;17:420. doi:10.1186/s12913-017-2354-5.

258. Pain & Policy Studies Group. *Achieving Balance in State Pain Policy: A Progress Report Card.* Madison, WI: University of Wisconsin Paul P. Carbone Comprehensive Cancer Center; 2003.

259. Pain & Policy Studies Group. *Achieving Balance in State Pain Policy: A Progress Report Card.* 2nd ed. Madison, WI: University of Wisconsin Paul P. Carbone Comprehensive Cancer Center; 2006.

260. Pain & Policy Studies Group. *Achieving Balance in State Pain Policy: A Progress Report Card.* 3rd ed. Madison, WI: University of Wisconsin Paul P. Carbone Comprehensive Cancer Center; 2007.

261. Pain & Policy Studies Group. *Achieving Balance in Federal and State Pain Policy: A Progress Report Card (CY 2012).* Madison, WI: University of Wisconsin Paul P. Carbone Comprehensive Cancer Center; 2013.

262. Pain & Policy Studies Group. *Achieving Balance in State Pain Policy: A Progress Report Card (CY 2013).* Madison, WI: University of Wisconsin Paul P. Carbone Comprehensive Cancer Center; 2014.

263. Twillman RK, Kirch R, Gilson A. Efforts to control prescription drug abuse: why clinicians should be concerned and take action as essential advocates for rational policy. *CA Cancer J Clin* 2014;64:369–376.

264. Fishman SM. *Responsible Opioid Prescribing: A Physician's Guide.* Washington, DC: Waterford Life Sciences; 2007.

265. Fishman SM. *Responsible Opioid Prescribing: A Clinician's Guide.* 2nd ed. Washington, DC: Waterford Life Sciences; 2012.

266. Gilson AM. Good state policy may not mean good pain care, but policy improvement offers hope for further progress: response to the Wahowiak article. *J Pain Palliat Care Pharmacother* 2015;29:169–172.

267. Brushwood DB, Rich BA, Coleman JJ, et al. Legal liability perspectives on abuse-deterrent opioids in the treatment of chronic pain. *J Pain Palliat Care Pharmacother* 2010;24:333–348.

268. Gilson AM, Joranson DE, Maurer MA. Improving state pain policies: recent progress and continuing opportunities. *CA Cancer J Clin* 2007;57:341–353.

269. Ziegler SJ. The proliferation of dosage thresholds in opioid prescribing policies and their potential to increase pain and opioid-related mortality. *Pain Med* 2015;16:1851–1856.

270. Paice JA, Von Roenn JH. Under- or overtreatment of pain in the patient with cancer: how to achieve the proper balance. *J Clin Oncol* 2014;32:1721–1726.

271. Agency Medical Director's Group. Washington State's draft guidelines for opioids for chronic non-cancer pain: frequently asked questions. Available at: http://www.agencymeddirectors.wa.gov/Files/2006FAQV8.pdf. Accessed April 12, 2018.

272. Washington State Legislature, *Pain Management—Intent.* Olympia, WA: WAC 246-919-850.

273. Magill-Lewis J. Washington State weighs limiting narcotic doses. *Drug Topics.* January 8, 2007.

274. Maine Revised Statutes. 32 M.R.S. §3300-F.

275. Maine Legislature. An Act to establish reasonable and clinically appropriate exceptions to opioid medication prescribing limits. SP0338 LD 1031, 128th Session, 2017.

276. American Academy of Pain Management. *State of Washington Pain Management Rules Opinions of the American Academy of Pain Management.* Chicago, IL: American Academy of Pain Management; 2011.

277. Bohnert AS, Logan JE, Ganoczy D, et al. A detail exploration into the association of prescribed opioid dosage and overdose deaths among patients with chronic pain. *Med Care* 2016;54:435–441.

278. Coleman JJ. The supply chain of medicinal controlled substances: addressing the Achilles heel of drug diversion. *J Pain Palliat Care Pharmacother* 2012;26:233–250.

279. Gray J, Hagemeir N, Brooks B, et al. Prescription disposal practices: a 2-year ecological study of drug drop box donations in Appalachia. *Am J Public Health* 2015;105:e89–e94.

280. Welham GC, Mount JK, Gilson AM. Type and frequency of opioid pain medications returned for disposal. *Drugs Real World Outcomes* 2015;2(2):129–135. doi:10.1007/s40801-015-0019-4.

281. New Mexico Medical Board. Title 16. Occupational and Professional Licensing. Chapter 10. Medicine and Surgery Practitioners. §16.10.8.8.

282. Kennedy-Hendricks A, Gielen A, McDonald E, et al. Medication sharing, storage, and disposal practices for opioid medications among U.S. adults. *JAMA Intern Med* 2016;176:1027–1029.

283. Office of National Drug Control Policy. *Epidemic: Responding to America's Prescription Drug Abuse Crisis.* Washington, DC: The White House; 2011.

284. Office of National Drug Control Policy. *National drug control strategy.* Washington, DC: The White House; 2013.

285. Becker WC, Tobin DG, Fiellin DA. Non-medical use of opioid analgesics obtained directly from physicians: prevalence and correlates. *Arch Intern Med* 2011;171:1034–1036.

286. Joranson DE, Gilson AM. Wanted: a public health approach to prescription opioid abuse and diversion [editorial]. *Pharmacoepidem Drug Safe* 2006;15:632–634.

287. Massachusetts Department of Public Health. *An Assessment of Opioid-related Deaths in Massachusetts (2013-2014).* Boston, MA: Massachusetts Department of Public Health; 2016.

288. PAINS Project. *Lost in Chaos: The State of Chronic Pain in 2016.* Kansas City, MO: PAINS Project; 2017.

289. Department of Veterans Affairs, Department of Defense. *VA/DoD Clinical Practice Guideline for Opioid Therapy for Chronic Pain.* Washington, DC: Department of Veterans Affairs, Department of Defense; 2017.

290. United States Department of Health and Human Services. *Facing Addiction in America: The Surgeon General's Report on Alcohol, Drugs, and Health.* Washington, DC: U.S. Department of Health and Human Services; 2016.

291. Corson K, Doak MN, Denneson L, et al. Primary care clinician adherence to guidelines for the management of chronic musculoskeletal pain: results from the study of the effectiveness of a collaborative approach to pain. *Pain Med* 2011;12:1490–1501.

292. Dorflinger L, Moore B, Goulet J, et al. A partnered approach to opioid management, guideline concordant care and the stepped care model of pain management. *J Gen Intern Med* 2014;29:S870–S876.

293. Gaither JR, Goulet JL, Becker WC, et al. The association between the receipt of guideline-concordant long-term opioid therapy and all-cause mortality. *J Gen Intern Med* 2016;31:492–501.

294. Gaither JR, Goulet JL, Becker WC, et al. The effect of substance use disorders on the association between guideline-concordant long-term opioid therapy and all-cause mortality. *J Addict Dis* 2016;10:418–428.

295. Gaither JR, Goulet JL, Becker WC, et al. Guideline-concordant management of opioid therapy among human immunodeficiency virus (HIV)-infected and uninfected veterans. *J Pain* 2014;15:1130–1140.

296. Krebs EE, Bergman AA, Coffing JM, et al. Barriers to guideline-concordant opioid management in primary care: a qualitative study. *J Pain* 2017;15:1148–1155.

CHAPTER 15

Litigation Involving Pain Management

BEN A. RICH

In recent decades, issues arising in the context of pain management have increasingly been raised in the context of law and public policy. Indeed, one of the major professional journals, *Pain Medicine*, now has an entire section devoted to this area of activity (i.e., forensic pain medicine). Although technically, forensic pain medicine encompasses all instances in which pain medicine and the law converge, this chapter focuses on the area of convergence that is most often associated with the term *forensic*—litigation. Other aspects of law and public policy affecting pain management are covered in the pain policy chapter of this book (Chapter 14).

American jurisprudence is divided into two broad categories of jurisdiction—state and federal—and four distinct domains within both categories: administrative, civil, criminal, and constitutional. Cases involving pain management have arisen in all four domains, and in this chapter, we will consider representative cases in each and identify the important lessons for practitioners. We will begin with administrative proceedings, all of which involve disciplinary actions by state medical licensing boards against physicians. In reviewing these cases, it will become clear how the pendulum has been swinging over the last 20 to 25 years. Beginning in the early 1990s, the long-standing concern about "overprescribing" of opioid analgesics was disrupted by several cases in which health care institutions and professionals were charged with substandard practice for their failure to provide seriously ill or dying patients with adequate management of pain and/or symptom distress. These proceedings reflect an emerging policy trend among licensing boards to emphasize the important role of pain management in patient care. With the ever-increasing evidence in the last 10 years that opioid overdose deaths have reached epidemic levels in some parts of the country, state boards and federal regulators have begun to revise policies and guidelines to reflect the current level of risk posed by the indiscriminate prescribing of opioids. These policy permutations are more fully discussed in the pain policy chapter (Chapter 14).

The aspect of civil litigation that most often involves health care professionals is medical malpractice. Such claims are a species of tort claim in which an injured party, the plaintiff, asserts that they have sustained compensable injury as a result of the negligence of the other party, the defendant. In order to be successful, medical malpractice claimants must establish four essential elements. The first element is the existence of a duty owed by the defendant to the plaintiff. The generic characterization of such a duty is "due care."[1] In professional liability cases, this translates to compliance with the prevailing standard of care. However, a health care professional–patient relationship must exist before such a duty may be deemed to have arisen.

The second element is breach of the duty owed, hence in medical malpractice litigation, a material departure from the standard of care. A dispute as to what constitutes the relevant standard of care by which the defendant professional's conduct is to be evaluated is usually the critical issue in a medical malpractice case, and the outcome often depends on whose expert witness or witnesses are deemed by the jury to be most convincing. Consequently, medical malpractice cases have come to be characterized as little more than a "battle of the experts." Traditionally, the usual custom and practice of physicians in the same or similar situations to the defendant has set the standard of care. Evidence of compliance by the defendant physician with the custom tended to create an irrefutable presumption that the applicable standard of care had been met. Over the last several decades, there has been a gradual trend by the courts toward a recognition of instances in which the custom and practice of clinicians has lagged noticeably far behind advances in medical science and technology, or physicians have failed to adopt safer or more effective clinical practices such as those advocated by national clinical guidelines. In such situations, the courts have acknowledged that rigid and unreflective adherence to the customary practice might demonstrate a failure to exercise appropriate clinical judgment. We will consider that issue further in the section of the chapter pertaining to civil litigation.

The third element of a tort claim is damage or injury. The breach of a duty of due care that fails to produce an injury or other harm is, from a strictly legal perspective, of no consequence. It is characterized in the law as *damnum absque injuria* (a wrong without injury). Such circumstances may be of interest to risk managers and quality improvement personnel, but they do not give rise to tort liability. The intriguing aspect of harm in the context of pain management is whether subjecting patients to unnecessary pain through substandard care would be deemed by juries as on the same level as medical errors that produce demonstrable physical injury or even death. The cases we will examine confirm that this is indeed the case, at least for patients who were at the end of life.

Finally, the plaintiff must establish that the breach of the duty of care by the defendant was the proximate (direct and immediate) cause of the damage or injury he or she sustained. In the cases we will be considering, the plaintiff must persuade the jury that pain management consistent with the standard of care would have, to a reasonable degree of medical probability, ensured that the patient did not suffer to the same extent as she did.

In the fourth section of the chapter, we will review criminal prosecutions by both the state and federal governments that concern the prescribing of opioid analgesics for terminal or chronic noncancer pain patients. Finally, in "Constitutional Cases" section, we will consider three US Supreme Court cases in which constitutional issues are raised in the context of cases related to pain management and/or end-of-life care.

Administrative Proceedings

Until recently, disciplinary actions by state medical licensing boards involving the prescribing of opioid analgesics targeted the phenomenon of "overprescribing," and it was the leading cause of both investigations and disciplinary actions.[2] Some of these actions were well-founded efforts to punish physicians who prescribed controlled substances inappropriately or without a legitimate medical purpose, thereby endangering their patients and/or society. Others, however, sought to punish physicians who were engaged in a good faith effort to manage chronic noncancer pain and demonstrated either a dismissal by the boards of the plight of chronic pain patients or an ignorance of the risks, side effects, and benefits of opioid analgesia.[3] We will consider two cases from the second group in which the practices of the accused physicians were ultimately vindicated by state appellate court decisions.

IN THE MATTER OF DILEO

Dr. Lucas DiLeo, a general practitioner, prescribed opioid analgesics for some of his patients with significant chronic nonmalignant pain. One of these patients, for example, was an ironworker who had fallen over 40 ft onto concrete and sustained 153 fractures, 93 in the face, as well as shattering his knees, ankles, and left femur. He underwent 10 operations, and continued thereafter to suffer with chronic pain. In 1992, the Louisiana Board of Medical Examiners filed an administrative complaint against Dr. DiLeo alleging that his prescribing of opioids to seven patients (an eighth patient was treated for obesity with a combination of benzphetamine [Didrex] and alprazolam [Xanax]) was not for a legitimate medical purpose, demonstrated incompetence, and fell outside acceptable standards of medical practice.

The board's expert witness, Dr. Linda Stuart, a board-certified family practitioner and addiction specialist, did not question that the seven patients receiving opioids had serious pain problems nor did she challenge the doses prescribed as excessive. However, she did testify that in her opinion, opioid analgesia was provided for too long a period of time, thereby posing an unacceptable risk of addiction and withdrawal symptoms. She acknowledged, however, that there were different schools of thought on this issue in the medical profession. As for the obesity patient, Dr. Stuart questioned the prescribing of Didrex and Xanax at the same time because she considered the former to be a stimulant, whereas the latter was a depressant.

Five of Dr. DiLeo's patients testified on his behalf, as did a physician whose specialty was internal medicine/endocrinology. The medical board ruled against Dr. DiLeo, and that ruling was affirmed by a trial court. The Louisiana Court of Appeals reversed and dismissed all charges against him after finding that no evidence had been presented by the board to support Dr. Stuart's assertion that the duration of Dr. DiLeo's prescriptions was excessive. Indeed, the Court of Appeals held that the board had failed to present any evidence as to what the relevant standard of medical practice was for prescribing opioids for chronic pain. In the absence of such evidence, the unsupported assertions of Dr. Stuart were insufficient to justify the disciplinary measures imposed on Dr. DiLeo, and the charges against him were deemed by the court to be arbitrary, capricious, and an abuse of the board's discretion.[4]

HOOVER V AGENCY FOR HEALTH CARE ADMINISTRATION

Katherine Hoover, MD, was a board-certified internist who had a number of chronic pain patients in her practice. For some of them, she elected to prescribe opioid analgesics for an extended period of time. The state medical board took a dim view of this and initiated disciplinary proceedings for "inappropriately and excessively" prescribing Schedule II drugs to seven patients. The board's case against Dr. Hoover consisted of two physicians who had reviewed pharmacy computer printouts documenting the prescriptions written for these patients by Dr. Hoover, and their opinions that the dosages she had prescribed were "excessive, perhaps lethal." None of these patients had, in fact, suffered any adverse effects from the prescriptions written by Dr. Hoover. Rather, they rallied to her support because she had diligently and successfully worked to manage their pain and restore their ability to function, whereas other physicians had either discounted their reports of pain or refused to prescribe opioids.

The board's experts did not review the medical records for any of these patients. Also, on cross-examination, these "experts" acknowledged that they did not treat chronic pain patients in their practice. Indeed, under the more stringent standards for expert testimony that have developed in the last 10 years, one could reasonably argue that the medical board's experts were not really experts in pain management. The hearing officer in the case may have taken the same view because she ultimately ruled that the evidence presented at the hearing supported a conclusion that Dr. Hoover's care of these patients was entirely appropriate. Nevertheless, the Board of Medicine took the remarkable step of disregarding the hearing officer's findings and conclusions and imposed sanctions that included an administrative fine of $4,000, continuing medical education (CME) on the prescribing of "abusable drugs," and 2 years of probation.

Dr. Hoover appealed, and in a scathing opinion by a three-judge panel of the Florida Court of Appeals, the ruling of the medical board was reversed. Noting a disturbing pattern and practice by the medical board, the opinion declared, "The board has once again engaged in the uniformly rejected practice of overzealously supplanting a hearing officer's valid findings of fact regarding a doctor's prescription practices with its own opinion in a case founded on a woefully inadequate quantum of evidence."[5] Elsewhere in the opinion, the court referred to the board's "draconian policy of policing pain prescription practice." Similar to the decision by the Louisiana Court of Appeals in DiLeo, the Florida Court of Appeals noted that the medical board had failed to introduce competent, credible evidence of the standard of care by which Dr. Hoover's prescribing practices could be evaluated.

One very important implication of the DiLeo and Hoover cases is that the courts will not simply sit back and allow medical boards to declare what the standard of care is in any particular clinical situation. Rather, the board must present persuasive evidence in support of the prevailing standard of care. Moreover, such cases as these appear to represent an "ethic of underprescribing" on the part of state medical boards that persisted for decades.[6] It was the deeply engrained and pervasive nature of this ethic that prompted some state legislatures to adopt the intractable pain treatment acts (IPTAs) that are discussed in Chapter 14. The thrust of such legislation was to send a message that the public policy of the state should not be to discourage physicians from providing effective pain management to patients with chronic nonmalignant pain, even if in some cases, that would involve the extended use of opioid analgesics. The Hoover case suggests how difficult it was to surmount the prevailing ethic in some boards because that case was brought shortly after the State of Florida had enacted an IPTA. The medical board rationalized its attempt to discipline Dr. Hoover by arguing that she had treated the patients in question prior to the effective date of the Florida law. The Florida Court of Appeals critiqued the cramped and legalistic way in which the board attempted to flaunt the statute, noting that what the board failed or refused to recognize was that the public policy of the state did not support its approach to punishing physicians who dared to prescribe opioids to patients with chronic noncancer pain.

As noted earlier, beginning in the mid-1990s, a few state medical boards adopted policies on pain management that were intended to reassure physicians that the board was not, in fact, hostile to good pain management practice and sought to outline how physicians could care for such patients in a manner that was consistent with good medical practice. Then, in 1998, the Federation of State Medical Boards (FSMB) promulgated model guidelines for the use of controlled substances for the treatment of pain.[7]

The gradual dissemination of medical board policies promoting effective pain relief as an essential component of quality patient care signaled the beginning of a paradigm shift.

Heretofore, the idea that if there could be such a thing as over-prescribing of opioids, then as a matter of logic and consistency, there must be an opposite side to the coin (i.e., underprescribing of opioids) seemed to be unintelligible to many medical boards. The inconsistency between perception and reality was truly remarkable. Whereas the medical literature in the 1980s and 1990s was replete with data indicating that pain was significantly undertreated in almost all patient care settings, no medical board had ever encountered a case in which underprescribing was deemed to constitute incompetent or unprofessional conduct.[8]

OREGON BOARD OF MEDICAL EXAMINERS V BILDER

Paul A. Bilder is a pulmonary specialist who in the late 1990s was practicing in a small Oregon community. In 1999, the Oregon Board of Medical Examiners (OBME) initiated disciplinary action against Bilder following an investigation of complaints concerning his alleged failure to properly manage the pain and other distressing symptoms of six patients over a period of 5 years. The disciplinary action ultimately led to a stipulated order in which Bilder agreed to certain remedial measures.[9] Two of the six were elderly patients with metastatic cancer who were enrolled in hospice. In each instance, the hospice nurse requested an increase in the dosage of pain medication in what turned out to be the last hours of the patient's life which Dr. Bilder refused to provide because he considered the amount requested excessive. In the other three cases, he refused to provide morphine or similar pain medication to a patient with congestive heart failure (CHF) who was do not resuscitate (DNR) and gasping for breath. The other three cases involved patients who were ventilator-dependent because of chronic obstructive pulmonary disease (COPD) or pneumonia. Dr. Bilder ordered paralytic agents but refused to order antianxiolytics or pain medication.

By the terms of the stipulated order, Dr. Bilder agreed to a 10-year probation, a formal reprimand, successful completion of the board's Physician's Evaluation Education Renewal Program, and an approved course in physician–patient communication as well as continuing psychiatric treatment with regular reports from the treating psychiatrist to the board. The Oregon Board once again found it necessary to take disciplinary action against Dr. Bilder 2 years later for similar instances of failure or refusal to appropriately respond to clear indications of patient suffering.[10]

ACCUSATION OF EUGENE WHITNEY, MD

In 2003, California became the second state to take disciplinary action against a physician for failure to provide appropriate pain relief. The patient in question was an 85-year-old man with advanced mesothelioma. The care of Lester Tomlinson in the last weeks of his life was the subject of both civil litigation and medical board disciplinary action. The civil litigation will be discussed in the next section of this chapter.

Mr. Tomlinson spent 5 days in a local hospital receiving treatment for pneumonia and pleural effusion. He was then transferred to a skilled nursing facility (SNF) and came under the care of Eugene B. Whitney, MD, for the duration of his stay, which ended with his death approximately 3 weeks later.[11] The care of Mr. Tomlinson at the SNF generated a great deal of contention between the members of his family (wife and daughter) and the caregivers. Each administration of pain medication, which began on the fourth day following his transfer from the hospital, was precipitated by a complaint from the family that he was in pain. Medication orders progressed from remazepam (Restoril) to hydrocodone/paracetamol (Vicodin) to various strengths of fentanyl transdermal (Duragesic) patch. Only after the family specifically requested morphine for Mr. Tomlinson's increasing pain did Dr. Whitney discontinue the hydrocodone/paracetamol (Vicodin) and ordered morphine (Roxanol) 20 mg, 10 mg orally every 6 hours.

Dr. Whitney saw Mr. Tomlinson only once during that period of time, 2 days after the first administration of Roxanol. He found the patient to be in pain and ordered morphine sulfate controlled-release (MS Contin) oral solution 10 mg every 4 hours as needed. As noted in the medical board charges against Dr. Whitney, MS Contin comes in tablet form only and should be provided on a regular schedule and not on an "as needed" basis. Dr. Whitney discontinued the prior order 2 days later and instead ordered MS Contin 5 mg every 2 hours for breakthrough pain. As further noted in the medical board accusation, halving the dose of an opioid analgesic and doubling the frequency of administration will not increase the analgesic potency. Nursing notes at the SNF in the subsequent 2 days until Mr. Tomlinson's death indicate uncontrolled pain and anxiety.

The Medical Board of California charged Dr. Whitney with unprofessional conduct and incompetence for his failure "to understand the unique properties of Roxanol solution and MS Contin tablets and to prescribe the medications properly."[11] The board and Dr. Whitney entered into a stipulation for public reprimand, the terms and conditions of which require that he obtain CME in pain management, the prescribing of opioid analgesics, and communication with patients and families.[12]

At this point, it is still too early to conclude that the medical board actions against Drs. Bilder and Whitney represent any sort of lasting paradigm shift in philosophy and practice of medical boards generally in regard to opioid prescribing by their licensees. Two cases do not constitute a trend. The FSMB Model Policy concerning controlled substances for pain relief has undergone a number of periodic updates, expansions, and revisions over the last two decades. In the most recent iteration (2013), it states that "evidence for the risk associated with opioids has surged, while the evidence for benefits has remained controversial and insufficient."[13] The current document admonishes prescribing professionals to recognize that appropriate pain management includes an ongoing risk–benefit assessment of opioid analgesia versus nonpharmacologic measures.

A majority of state medical boards had adopted the model policies or promulgated policies that emphasize the need to incorporate sound pain management practices into patient care.[14] To some extent, the shift in attitudes about the role of pain management in patient care, and the influence of those new attitudes in the formulation of medical practice guidelines and policies, can be traced to a few dramatic legal cases. We turn now to these cases and their role in informing public attitudes and policies about pain and its management.

Civil Litigation

Despite growing evidence in the clinical literature that pain is often undertreated, and a medical malpractice crisis purportedly arising out of a plethora of malpractice claims yielding significant monetary damage awards, prior to 1990, there had never been a malpractice suit seeking damages for failure to provide appropriate pain relief.

Although somewhat speculative, there are several possible explanations of this curious state of affairs. First, the phenomenon of widespread undertreated pain was not well known outside of the health professions. It had yet to become a featured topic in the print or electronic media. Moreover, laypersons held the erroneous belief that pain was the inevitable result of traumatic injury, serious illness, or a major surgical procedure. Finally, the generally high repute in which health care professionals were held presupposed that they would most certainly not allow a patient to experience unnecessary pain or suffering. The pervasiveness of pain in the clinical setting must, on this view, result from the sheer intractability of the pain associated with major illness and most certainly with the process of dying. From this perspective, the case we now consider is all that more remarkable in its outcome.

ESTATE OF HENRY JAMES V HILLHAVEN CORPORATION

Henry James was a 75-year-old man who carried the diagnosis of stage III adenocarcinoma of the prostate with metastasis to the lumbar sacral spine and left femur. In December of 1986 and January of 1987, he spent nearly 2 months in a local hospital receiving treatment for a pathologic hip fracture. During that hospitalization, in addition to bone debridement and radiation therapy, Mr. James was evaluated by hospice and received Roxanol 150 mg every 3 to 4 hours around the clock for his pain. Progress notes indicate that his pain was well controlled on this regimen.

After a very short stay at home, he was admitted to an SNF owned and operated by the Hillhaven Corporation. The continuing orders for pain medication included 150 mg per day of Roxanol, along with two tablets of acetaminophen (Tylenol) every 4 hours as needed and propoxyphene napsylate and acetaminophen (Darvocet-N) 100 mg. His family had ensured that he received the medication when he was at home and made certain that the nursing home staff was aware of it on his admission.[15]

In preparation of the SNF admission documents, a nurse offered the opinion that Mr. James was addicted to morphine and on that basis declared her intent to significantly reduce the amount of opioid analgesia and replace it with a tranquilizing agent. Remarkably, she was able to effectuate this change in the pain management regimen without the review and approval of the patient's physician. His family learned about the change only after he had been discharged from the facility and was interviewed by investigators for the North Carolina Department of Human Resources, the licensing agency for the facility. Their investigation revealed that at no time during his 23-day stay did he receive pain medication as ordered.[15]

Thereafter, the family consulted an attorney and suit was filed against the nurse and the facility for failure to properly treat Mr. James's pain.[16] In order to prevail in such a case, the plaintiff (Mr. James's estate) had to establish by a preponderance of the evidence that (1) a recognized standard of care for the management of his pain existed, (2) the standard was violated by the defendants, and (3) the departure from the standard of care caused him to experience pain to an extent that he would not had the standard been met. If the jury answered each of those questions in the affirmative, then it must proceed to determine what several weeks of unnecessary pain should be worth in monetary damages. During the course of the trial, expert witnesses called by the plaintiff challenged the position taken by the nurse at the Hillhaven facility that the dose of morphine prescribed for Mr. James was excessive and not necessary to control his pain.[17]

The jury answered each of the questions in the affirmative and awarded the plaintiff compensatory damages of $7.5 million. However, the jury did not stop with that award. In a civil action, when a defendant's conduct is sufficiently egregious to meet certain criteria, punitive damages may be awarded. The purpose of such damages, as the term suggests, is not to compensate the plaintiff, but rather to make a negative example of and punish the defendant. The jury in this case assessed another $7.5 million in punitive damages. Apparently, the jurors were convinced that there is or ought to be something like a right to effective pain relief, at least for patients in the circumstances of Mr. James, and that the defendant corporation and/or its agent consciously disregarded that right and in the process subjected an elderly, dying patient to unnecessary pain and suffering. In a subsequent section of this chapter, we will consider two cases in which the US Supreme Court appears to adopt a similar position as a matter of constitutional law.

Several years after the verdict and subsequent out-of-court (and confidential) settlement of the *Estate of Henry James v Hillhaven Corporation* case, North Carolina joined a number of other states in enacting tort reform legislation. Consequently, the same result could not be achieved today even in the same or a very similar case. Punitive damages are now capped at 3 times the amount of compensatory damages or $250,000, whichever is greater. Furthermore, punitive damages cannot even be sought unless the plaintiff can prove by clear and convincing evidence (a higher burden of proof than a preponderance of the evidence) one of the following aggravating factors: (1) the defendant acted out of malice, (2) fraudulently, or (3) in willful and wanton disregard of the rights or safety of the defendant. Punitive damages could not be recovered from a corporation (such as Hillhaven) unless the officers, managers, or directors participated in or condoned the conduct that constituted the aggravating factors.[18]

BERGMAN V CHIN, MD, AND EDEN MEDICAL CENTER

William Bergman was an 85-year-old man in severe pain when he arrived at the emergency department (ED) of Eden Medical Center. He had been taking the Vicodin prescribed by his physician but without receiving adequate relief. He was given morphine by the ED physician and experienced significant relief. In order to do a more extensive workup, he was admitted to the hospital and came under the care of a hospitalist, Wing Chin, MD. Out of concerns about the side effects of morphine, in particular respiratory depression, Dr. Chin discontinued it and wrote a standing order for meperidine (Demerol), 25 to 50 mg every 4 hours "as needed." This order remained in place throughout the 5-day hospital stay, during which the nurses charted pain levels in the range of 7 to 10 on the standard 10-point scale. On the date of Mr. Bergman's discharge, his numerical pain score was noted to be a 10; nevertheless, Dr. Chin planned to send him home with a prescription for Vicodin. When Mr. Bergman's daughter protested, Dr. Chin ordered another administration of Demerol and a fentanyl patch.

During the hospitalization, the medical workup was strongly suggestive of lung cancer, although Mr. Bergman refused to consent to a lung biopsy that Dr. Chin believed was indicated in order to make a definitive diagnosis. Despite a diagnosis Dr. Chin deemed less than definitive, shortly following his discharge, Mr. Bergman came under the care of a hospice nurse, who prevailed on another physician in the community to write a prescription for morphine after she found the fentanyl patch to be inadequate to manage Mr. Bergman's pain. He died 3 days following discharge. No autopsy was performed. The cause of death was considered to be complications from lung cancer.[19]

The children of William Bergman became convinced that the last days of their father's life were severely compromised by a clinical failure to provide effective pain relief. Their conviction resulted in part from a review of his medical record by an expert secured through the assistance of the organization Compassion in Dying (now Compassion and Choices). The family initially filed a complaint against Dr. Chin with the Medical Board of California. In an interesting approach to the case, the board's own investigation and independent expert review confirmed that the pain relief Dr. Chin provided to Mr. Bergman was inadequate. Nevertheless, the board notified the family that it would not take any adverse disciplinary action against Dr. Chin based on only one episode of inadequate patient care. Displeased by this response, and with continuing support from Compassion in Dying, the Bergman family secured legal counsel and filed a civil action against Dr. Chin and Eden Medical Center. The medical center settled with the plaintiffs prior to trial.

The complaint against Dr. Chin that was tried to a jury was unusual in that it was not a straightforward medical malpractice claim. Such a claim could not have any chance of success in California because, as a result of tort reform legislation, damages for pain and suffering resulting from medical malpractice can only be recovered by the patient; they are not deemed to "survive" such that they can be recovered following the patient's death by the personal representative. The only challenge to the medical care provided by Dr. Chin related to his alleged failure to properly manage Mr. Bergman's pain; hence, the only damages that could be awarded would be for unnecessary pain and suffering. However, if the pain and suffering can be proven to have resulted from acts or omissions that constitute "elder abuse," under California law, the personal representative of the "victim" of the abuse can recover damages. Consequently, the Bergman family's suit against Dr. Chin and the hospital alleged elder abuse.

Another complicating factor about an elder abuse claim in California is that it carries an elevated burden of proof. Rather than a mere preponderance of the evidence, the plaintiff must establish by "clear and convincing evidence" that the defendant was guilty of recklessness, fraud, or malice in perpetrating physical, financial, or fiduciary abuse or neglect.[20] Prior to this case, no physician had ever been accused of elder abuse, and the claim that failure of a health care professional to provide effective pain management might constitute a violation of the statute was an even further stretch. From all appearances, the trial of the case proceeded as would a typical medical malpractice claim. The plaintiffs offered the testimony of two physician expert witnesses, both of whom testified that there were serious problems with the type, dose, and schedule of administration of analgesia to Mr. Bergman while a patient at Eden Medical Center. In rebuttal, Dr. Chin called two physician expert witnesses who testified that in their opinion, the measures he employed in an effort to manage Mr. Bergman's pain did not constitute a material departure from the custom and practice of similar physicians caring for patients like Mr. Bergman.[21]

During the course of the trial, despite Dr. Chin's contention that there was no conclusive evidence that Mr. Bergman had lung cancer, the judge allowed the plaintiffs to introduce into evidence the Agency for Health Care Policy and Research Clinical Practice Guideline *Managing Cancer Pain*. That evidence tended to bolster the testimony of the plaintiff's experts that Dr. Chin's pain management strategy was deficient in significant ways. The guideline provides, for example:

- Treatment of persistent or moderate to severe pain should be based on increasing the opioid potency or dose.
- Medications for persistent cancer-related pain should be administered on an around-the-clock basis with additional "as needed" doses, because regularly scheduled dosing maintains a constant level of drug in the body and helps prevent recurrence of the pain.
- Meperidine (Demerol) should not be used if continued opioid use is anticipated.[22]

Dr. Chin testified that he had no familiarity with these or with the Medical Board of California's 1994 guidelines and policy on pain management. He also stated that he did not take the nurses' notes on Mr. Bergman's pain levels into account because he did not have any confidence in that form of pain assessment.

The nurses involved in the care of Mr. Bergman testified on behalf of Dr. Chin that whenever Mr. Bergman reported pain in the moderate to severe range, they administered another 25-mg dose of Demerol consistent with the standing order. Interestingly, however, they testified that the reason the medical record did not reflect what they insisted to have been consistent achievement of pain relief in response to these administrations was that at Eden Medical Center, pain was charted "by exception." In other words, pain was only noted when it was outside of normal limits. Such an approach begs the question of what constitutes an authoritative source for the "normal limits" of pain for any particular patient. This charting anomaly worked

against the defendant because the medical record was replete with pain levels in the moderate to severe range each day but not in the mild to nonexistent range that would have supported their claim that the opioids administered to Mr. Bergman during his hospitalization were sufficient to meet his needs.

Ultimately, the jury reached a verdict in favor of the plaintiffs and awarded $1.5 million in damages. They came within one vote of awarding an additional amount in punitive damages. The trial judge reduced the award to $250,000 on the theory that the statutory cap on monetary damage awards for medical malpractice claims applied even though this claim was filed pursuant to the elder abuse statute. The judge awarded nearly $1 million in attorney fees and litigation costs to the plaintiffs as well. Outstanding posttrial issues were resolved by confidential agreement between the parties; hence, no appeal was taken by either side.

News of the verdict in the *Bergman v Chin* case shook the medical community. The stark contrast between the reaction of the Medical Board of California to the allegations in the case and that of the lay jury seemed to support an observation by the physician Eric Cassell nearly 20 years earlier: "The relief of suffering, it would appear, is considered one of the primary ends of medicine by patients and lay persons, but not by the medical profession."[23] Because the verdict came in the context of an elder abuse claim against Dr. Chin, it seemed particularly punitive in nature and raised the issue of how to most appropriately and effectively "rehabilitate" physicians whose knowledge, skills, and/or attitudes were not conducive to the effective assessment and management of pain. We will revisit this issue after the discussion of the Tomlinson case that follows.

TOMLINSON V BAYBERRY CARE CENTER, ET AL.

We have previously discussed the Tomlinson case in the context of the elder abuse claims filed against both the acute and long-term care facilities in which the patient received care in the last month of his life as well as the physicians who were responsible for that care in both clinical settings. The claims in that case bore a striking resemblance to the claims in the *Bergman v Chin* case.[24] Perhaps, because of the jury verdict in the prior case, as noted, all of the defendants in Tomlinson settled prior to trial. Interestingly, as alluded to previously, the Medical Board of California took a much different position in dealing with the complaint by the Tomlinson family against Dr. Eugene Whitney, who was the responsible physician when Mr. Tomlinson was in the SNF (Bayberry Care Center) than it did with regard to the complaint filed by the Bergman family against Dr. Chin. The Medical Board of California sanctioned Dr. Whitney for his failure "to understand the unique properties of Roxanol solution and MS Contin tablets and to prescribe the medications properly" pursuant to a stipulated disciplinary order he entered into with the board. He was required to undergo an extensive evaluation of his professional knowledge and skills and work with the board in developing a detailed remediation plan.[25] Also, the California Department of Health Services issued a notice of deficiency against Bayberry Care Center based on the many problems with the care Mr. Tomlinson received at that facility.[26]

Just as one can speculate that the defendants in the elder abuse claims by the Tomlinson family were motivated to settle prior to trial because of the earlier jury verdict against Dr. Chin, it is also tempting to suggest that the decision of the Medical Board of California to take disciplinary action against Dr. Whitney in response to the complaint filed against him by the Tomlinson family was influenced by the highly negative public response to the board's refusal to take similar action against Dr. Chin, particularly when a lay jury deemed the same conduct not just malpractice but elder abuse and the California legislature was motivated to pass a law mandating CME in pain management for California physicians. It is certainly possible that one influenced the other, but there is no way to authoritatively establish that proposition.

More contemporaneously, some patients who have developed addiction to prescription opioids have initiated legal actions against their physicians. In a recent West Virginia Supreme Court ruling, a number of patients sued several physicians and a clinic alleging negligence in the prescribing of opioid analgesics. What is remarkable about the cases consolidated for review of questions submitted by the trial court was that the plaintiffs admitted not only that they had abused controlled substances before they sought treatment from the defendant physicians but also that they had engaged in criminal conduct involving opioids such as obtaining them through fraud. The West Virginia Supreme Court ruled that the plaintiffs criminal misconduct would not, under its interpretation of state law, act as a complete bar to their claims of negligence against the defendants.[27] Dissenting opinions in the case noted that in many other jurisdictions such wrongful conduct by a plaintiff would preclude the action from going forward.

One of the physician defendants in this case was Kathrine Hoover, whose ultimate legal victory over the Florida medical board was discussed earlier. She was alleged to be the number one prescriber of opioids in the state. The clinic where she practiced was raided by law enforcement, but she was never criminally charged.

Criminal Litigation

Criminal prosecutions of health care professionals for acts or omissions resulting in death or grave harm to patients are exceedingly rare.[28] By far, the most common means of imposing sanctions on health professionals for negligent or even reckless patient care are those we have already considered—disciplinary action by state licensing boards or professional liability (malpractice) claims. The exceptional case that prompts a criminal prosecution is almost invariably one involving the death of the patient and conduct by the professional that is considered egregious in nature or in the extent to which it departs from a consensus view of what constitutes the parameters of responsible professional conduct.

Because our focus is necessarily on pain management and palliative care, we will consider several instances in which physicians have been prosecuted in either state or federal court. Some of the more high-profile state prosecutions have involved the care of dying patients, whereas those in federal court have been pursuant to the Controlled Substances Act (CSA) and involved prescribing opioids for chronic noncancer pain patients. We begin with a highly instructive state prosecution.

STATE V NARAMORE

In 1994, the attorney general of Kansas filed a two-count criminal complaint against L. Stanley Naramore, D.O. Both counts related to his care of patients almost 2 years before who were facing terminal conditions. Early in 1996, a jury returned guilty verdicts related to each count and the court sentenced Dr. Naramore to concurrent terms of 5 to 20 years. We will focus on the case that gave rise to the first count and on the subsequent reversal of both convictions by the Kansas Court of Appeals.

The patient, Ruth Leach, was a 78-year-old woman suffering from advanced breast cancer that had metastasized to her bones, lungs, and brain. She had been hospitalized and her condition deteriorating. The fentanyl patches no longer controlled her pain, and she was restless and agitated. A nurse suggested to the family that Dr. Naramore be called and asked to prescribe stronger pain medication. Upon arriving at the hospital, he examined Ruth Leach and spoke with her two

adult children. Together, they reached a decision to increase her pain medication. Dr. Naramore explained that there was a risk of depressed respiration. He then administered 4 mg of midazolam (Versed) and 100 micromilligrams of fentanyl. Thereafter, the nursing notes indicate that the patient's respiration slowed and grew irregular.

From this point on, the accounts of what transpired take on a curious, disjointed quality. To the extent they are accurate, it is not difficult to understand why there was a failure to maintain a consensus among the family and caregivers concerning the goals of care and how each subsequent action would be consistent with the reasonable pursuit of those goals.

The patient's son, who had training as an emergency medical technician, is reported to have asked Dr. Naramore if his mother was dying, and Naramore was said to have observed that she was but that the effects of the fentanyl could be reversed by the administration of Narcan. This statement suggested to the patient's son and the nurse on duty that an overdose of pain medication must have been given. Thereafter, when Dr. Naramore began to prepare for continuing IV infusion of analgesics, the son insisted that he not administer any more and was quoted as saying, "I'd rather have my mother lay there and suffer for 10 more days than you do anything to speed up her death." In an effort to dissuade the son, Dr. Naramore told him that "it just gets terrible from here on out . . . the next few days are going to be absolutely terrible."[29] When the son remained intransigent and assured Dr. Naramore that he would hold the doctor accountable for anything that happened, Dr. Naramore withdrew from the case. The next day, Ruth Leach was transported to another hospital, where she was given morphine for her pain and died 3 days later of her underlying terminal illness.[29]

The patient's family became convinced, and they in turn persuaded the Kansas Attorney General that Dr. Naramore had intended to hasten her death through administration of excessive doses of analgesics. Dr. Naramore was charged with attempted first-degree murder. He was also charged with second-degree murder of another patient from about the same time period, Chris Willt.

In order to convict a defendant of attempted first-degree murder, the jury must find that the prosecution has proven beyond a reasonable doubt that the defendant (1) performed an overt act toward the commission of the crime, (2) did so with the intent to commit the crime of first-degree murder, and (3) failed to complete the commission of that crime. The elements of murder in the first degree include intent to kill a person, the intentional performance of an overt act toward that end that is both deliberate and premeditated.

The prosecution presented several medical experts. The director of Emergency Medicine at the University of Kansas Medical Center testified that in his opinion, Ruth Leach was near death after the administration of Versed and fentanyl and that she would have died if the morphine Dr. Naramore had ordered had in fact been administered. This view was similarly expressed by a specialist in anesthesiology and critical care medicine at the University of Vermont College of Medicine who had previously practiced in Kansas. He testified that a dose of Versed combined with that of the fentanyl were excessive and in short order would have caused the patient to stop breathing. An additional respiratory depressant such as morphine would simply have added to the certainty of her death.

In his defense, Dr. Naramore called several expert witnesses. One, a physician who had cared for Ruth Leach for 5 years prior to her death, noted that she had received a variety of medications for her pain, none of which had brought it under control. He found it to be "phenomenal" that anyone would accuse Dr. Naramore of trying to kill her under these circumstances. A family physician from another small Kansas community said that if Dr. Naramore had actually intended to kill

Ruth Leach, he would have used 10 times the dosage administered. He characterized the care provided as "concerned and compassionate."

Another witness for Dr. Naramore, the president of the Kansas Association of Osteopathic Medicine and a family medicine practitioner, characterized Dr. Naramore's efforts to control Ruth Leach's pain and distress as exemplary. Finally, another family physician who served on the peer-review committee for Blue Cross/Blue Shield of Kansas testified that given her significant history of opioid analgesia and the extent of her distress at the time, the dosages of Versed and fentanyl were reasonable and in no sense an overdose.

The convictions of Dr. Naramore for the attempted murder of Ruth Leach and for the second-degree murder of the other patient were reviewed and reversed by the Kansas Court of Appeals. In its opinion, the Court of Appeals made numerous references not only to the expert witness testimony on his behalf at trial but also to *amicus curiae* (friend of the court) briefs filed on behalf of Dr. Naramore by the Kansas Association of Osteopathic Medicine, the American Osteopathic Association, and the Kansas Medical Society. The court also noted that it had done its own substantial research on the subject of palliative care. Moreover, its review of the case law revealed "no criminal conviction of a physician for the attempted murder or murder of a patient which has ever been sustained on appeal based upon evidence of the kind presented here."[29]

In articulating the rationale for its decision that the criminal convictions must be reversed, the Court of Appeals declared,

> We have made a thorough review of the record [of the trial court proceedings], which contains a wealth of undisputed evidence and expert medical testimony. We find that no rational jury could find criminal intent and guilt beyond a reasonable doubt based on the record here. When the issue is whether there is reasonable doubt, a jury is not free to disbelieve undisputed facts. What occurred here is generally known. The jury was not free to disbelieve that there was substantial competent medical opinion in support of the proposition that Dr. Naramore's actions were not only noncriminal, but were medically appropriate.
>
> . . . When there is such strong evidence supporting a reasonable, noncriminal explanation for the doctor's actions, it cannot be said that there is no reasonable doubt of criminal guilt . . . All three *amicus* briefs . . . note that if criminal responsibility can be assessed based solely on opinions of a portion of the medical community which are strongly challenged by an opposing and authoritative medical consensus, we have criminalized malpractice, and even the possibility of malpractice. The instant case is a very good example of this.[29]

The quoted language of the court mentioned and subsequent statements in the court's decision regarding the absence of any jury instructions "relating to the medical and moral responsibilities of care givers for the critically or terminally ill patient" are of considerable consequence because of their implications for a wide range of criminal prosecutions of physicians for care provided in an effort to manage the pain and adverse symptoms associated with terminal or serious chronic conditions. Although physician fears persist concerning the risk of potential criminal prosecution for actions taken to relieve the distress of dying patients, such prosecutions are quite rare.[30]

Despite his ultimate vindication in these proceedings, Dr. Naramore's legal travails did not end. After relocating to Ohio, in late 2009, he plead guilty to conspiracy to distribute methadone to over 100 patients whom he acknowledged were likely distributing the pills, thereby promoting drug trafficking. He was sentenced to 48 months in prison.[31]

Several more recent cases reflect the mixed results of state criminal prosecutions of physicians for based on their prescribing of controlled substances. In October of 2015, southern California physician Hsiu-Ying "Lisa" Tseng was convicted of second-degree murder after three of her patients died as a result of drug overdoses. According to the prosecutor, this is the first time a physician has been convicted of murder for prescribing practices leading to overdose death. Dr. Tseng's defense was that at worst her conduct amounted to negligence, not criminal homicide. The prosecutor and the jury disagreed.[32] In February of 2016, Dr. Tseng was sentenced to 30 years to life in prison. In issuing the sentence, the trial judge criticized Dr. Tseng for blaming the patients, pharmacists, and even other physicians rather than accepting any responsibility. The prosecution had argued to the jury that despite having been notified by medical examiners or law enforcement of the death of a patient, Dr. Tseng did not change her prescribing practices.[33]

At about the same time, Florida physician Gerald Klein was acquitted of first-degree murder and other serious drug charges by a Palm Beach County jury. Although one of his patients died of a drug overdose, the jury did not find sufficient evidence to hold the prescribing physician responsible for it. Only one charge, "sale of alprazolam," resulted in a conviction. Interestingly, the patient in that transaction was at the time a chef for billionaire Donald Trump.[34]

Before concluding this discussion of civil and criminal cases against physicians at the local and state level, we should also note the multiplicity of ongoing litigation against major pharmaceutical companies concerning their marketing of prescription pain medications. The most frequent target of these cases is Purdue Pharma LP and its aggressive marketing of oxycodone HCl (OxyContin). In late December of 2015, the company settled a case filed by the State of Kentucky in 2007 charging it with misleading marketing of the drug to induce physicians and patients to discount its potential to lead to addiction. According to the terms of the settlement, Purdue Pharma will pay $24 million over a period of 8 years.[35]

In July of 2016, Pfizer entered into an agreement with the City of Chicago to adhere to a written code of conduct for marketing opioids. The code calls for disclosure that opioid analgesics may pose a serious risk of addiction in some patients even when used properly as well as an assurance that it will not promote opioids for "off-label" uses. The City of Chicago filed a lawsuit against Pfizer, Purdue Pharma, and several other pharmaceutical companies alleging misleading marketing of this type of medication.[36]

Federal Criminal Prosecutions

Recent federal criminal prosecutions of physicians pursuant to the federal CSA for prescribing practices in the care of chronic noncancer pain patients are not entirely aberrational. They follow in the history and tradition of earlier cases, and the appellate courts reviewing these cases cite the earlier decisions profusely as correctly interpreting and applying the intent of the Congress when enacting the CSA. It therefore behooves us to review key elements of one such precedent-setting case before taking up the contemporary examples.

UNITED STATES V ROSEN (1978)

Although Dr. Isadore Rosen was prosecuted under the CSA for prescribing controlled substances to patients for weight loss as part of an "obesity practice," and not for pain management, the language of the appellate court decision and its analysis of the CSA are often cited in later cases involving the prescribing of controlled substances for pain. Also, the prosecution of Dr. Rosen was based in large measure on the testimony of undercover law enforcement agents who came to him posing as patients seeking to lose weight. The use of such tactics generally gives rise to a claim of "entrapment" by the defendant; that is, that the government agents induced him to engage in one or more unlawful acts that he was not otherwise contemplating and in which he never would have engaged but for their inducement. As often happens, the court in *United States v Rosen* easily disposed of this defense by noting, "When a person is shown to be ready and willing to violate the law, the providing of an opportunity therefore by undercover agents or police officers is not entrapment."[37]

In order to convict Dr. Rosen of the 25 counts of distributing controlled substances in violation of the CSA with which he was charged, the government had to prove the following three elements of the offense beyond a reasonable doubt:

1. That he distributed or dispensed a controlled substance
2. That he acted knowingly and intentionally
3. That he did so other than for a legitimate medical purpose and in the usual course of his professional practice

Dr. Rosen conceded the first two elements but asserted as to the third that each of the agents who came to him posing as patients presented symptoms for which the drugs he prescribed or dispensed were medically appropriate. It is important to note that although the prescribing of certain types of medications for the purpose of weight reduction is subject to some controversy, for purposes of this decision, the court noted that all of the drugs prescribed by Dr. Rosen have legitimate therapeutic uses.

The crux of Dr. Rosen's argument on appeal of his criminal conviction was that the trial court relied on what it considered to be evidence of substandard medical practice as a basis for finding criminal intent. This point is critical as it will arise in the discussion of more recent prosecutions under the CSA. If the third element listed earlier is deemed to have been established beyond a reasonable doubt by the evidence, then the courts treat the physician not simply as a negligent, or even in some instances a reckless physician, but simply as a drug dealer. The court in *United States v Rosen* reviewed a number of earlier convictions under the CSA and identified the following list of "red flags" suggesting that a physician may be acting illegitimately or outside the course of professional practice.

1. An inordinately large quantity of controlled substances was prescribed.
2. Large numbers of prescriptions were issued.
3. No physical exam was given.
4. The physician warned the patient to fill the prescriptions at different pharmacies.
5. The physician issued prescriptions to a patient known to be delivering the drugs to others.
6. The physician prescribed controlled substances at intervals inconsistent with legitimate medical treatment.
7. The physician used street slang rather than medical terminology for the drugs prescribed.
8. There was no logical relationship between the drugs prescribed and treatment of the condition allegedly existing.
9. The physician wrote more than one prescription on occasions in order to spread them out.[37]

The routine followed by Dr. Rosen's weight loss "clinic" included many of these red flag elements according to the testimony of the government agents who posed as patients seeking to lose weight. In particular, Dr. Rosen did not take a medical history or perform a physical exam other than to have the patients weighed and their blood pressure taken on the first visit by a staff member who was not a nurse. He provided no instructions on how to take the medications or warnings of risks or side effects to be concerned about, nor did he schedule follow-up appointments. Based on this and other evidence at trial, the court of appeals ruled that the government had met its burden of proof that Dr. Rosen's prescribing or dispensing

of controlled substances to the undercover agents was not in good faith for legitimate medical purposes in the course of his professional practice.

UNITED STATES V HURWITZ

Dr. William Hurwitz was a medical doctor who operated a pain medicine practice in McLean, Virginia. So widespread was his reputation as a liberal prescriber of opioids that many of his patients came from great distances—39 states—seeking medications from him that other physicians would not prescribe. In 1992, he was reprimanded by the District of Columbia medical board because of his "liberal" prescribing practices, and in 1996, the Virginia board revoked his license and subsequently reinstated it with ongoing monitoring of his prescribing practices. Ostensibly, that monitoring was still taking place when, in 2004, a federal grand jury indicted him on 62 counts, including drug trafficking resulting in death and serious bodily injuries, health care fraud, and criminal forfeiture. He was subsequently convicted on 50 of those counts and sentenced to 25 years in prison.[38] Throughout the criminal process, Dr. Hurwitz was portrayed by the federal prosecutor and officials of the U.S. Drug Enforcement Administration (DEA) as "no different from a cocaine or heroin dealer peddling poison on the street corner."[39] At the trial, however, several nationally prominent experts in pain medicine testified on behalf of Dr. Hurwitz. During the trial, immediately following the testimony of the government's chief expert witness, six former presidents of the American Pain Society (APS) took the unprecedented step of sending a letter to the trial judge expressing their deep concerns about "serious misrepresentations" that had been made by the government's expert, who was also a past president of the APS.

When Dr. Hurwitz appealed his convictions to the Fourth Circuit Federal Court of Appeals, the American Academy of Pain Medicine, the American Pain Foundation, and a group of nationally prominent experts in pain management, among others, filed *amicus curiae* (friend of the court) briefs in support of his appeal. These briefs asserted, among other points, that "seriously erroneous rules of law and scientific theories [were] relied upon to convict [Dr. Hurwitz]."[40]

It is important to understand the significance one can reasonably attach to the willingness of these prominent organizations and individual members of the pain medicine community to go on record in this case. The government's position was that Dr. Hurwitz's prescribing of controlled substances had absolutely nothing to do with pain management. It was drug trafficking, pure and simple. The persons to whom he dispensed or prescribed these drugs were not patients but rather drug seekers who sought either to feed their addiction or further disseminate them in the illicit market for prescription drugs. The thrust of the argument on the other side was not that Dr. Hurwitz was practicing exemplary medicine, or in some instances, even prescribing within the minimal standard of acceptable care for chronic pain patients but rather that however far out of the mainstream his prescribing practices were, he was nevertheless a physician and not a drug dealer. The appropriate societal sanctions for physicians who practice negligently are medical malpractice liability claims or disciplinary action by licensing boards. In egregious circumstances, appropriate sanctions might include the permanent revocation of licensure. Nevertheless, physicians who practice substandard medicine are nonetheless physicians, and their patients remain patients in need of medical care, even if in some instances, the care they require is for addiction. The Fourth Circuit Court of Appeals reversed the Hurwitz conviction and remanded the case to the District Court for a new trial. In doing so, it sought to make clear where the trial judge had erred and how the retrial should be conducted to provide Dr. Hurwitz with a fair trial. At the end of the new trial, he was convicted of 16 counts of drug trafficking and sentenced to 57 months in prison.

UNITED STATES V MCIVER

Dr. Ronald McIver had approximately 1,000 patients in his South Carolina practice, most of whom saw him because of problems with chronic noncancer pain. In response to reports from the Columbia, South Carolina, police department about Dr. McIver's prescribing practices, the DEA initiated an investigation of his practice in 2002. Based on investigatory findings that among McIver's patients, there were those who regularly received prescriptions for what were characterized as "massive quantities" of oxycodone, hydromorphone hydrochloride (Dilaudid), OxyContin, methadone, and morphine; he was indicted on 15 counts of drug trafficking related to his treatment of 10 patients, 9 of whom testified for the government at his trial. The remaining patient was deceased, the cause of death having been characterized as an "oxycodone overdose."[41]

The major thrust of the prosecution's case at trial was based on the expert testimony of a Dr. Steven Storick, an anesthesiologist who the court deemed to be duly qualified as an expert in pain management. After reviewing the medical records of the patients in question, he concluded that Dr. McIver's treatment of several of them fell outside the parameters of legitimate medical practice. For example, in the case of a patient with a history of substance abuse, Dr. Storick asserted that prescribing opioids to such a patient was "like pouring gasoline on a fire." A Medicaid patient who sought treatment from Dr. McIver for fibromyalgia traveled almost 3 hours to see him, paid for his services in cash, and filled prescriptions for methadone, OxyContin, oxycodone, and morphine costing thousands of dollars. The patient testified that she sold the methadone and morphine and was addicted to oxycodone. With regard to her treatment, Dr. Storick testified that Dr. McIver's conduct was "way outside the course of legitimate medical treatment."[41]

The jury convicted Dr. McIver of multiple counts of unlawful distribution of a controlled substance and one that resulted in death. He was sentenced to 30 years in prison. On appeal to the Fourth Circuit Court of Appeals, the same court that granted Dr. Hurwitz a new trial, Dr. McIver's counsel attacked Dr. Storick's testimony as reflective of a hostile and suspicious approach to the care of chronic noncancer pain patients in that he insisted on objective signs of tissue damage before prescribing opioids, and he refused to acknowledge that physicians could be deceived by some patients' reports of pain and yet still be legitimately prescribing opioids for them based on a reasonable belief that they had significant pain.

The appeal also challenged the jury instructions, which Dr. McIver claimed suggested to the jury that he could be convicted if he "deviated drastically from accepted medical practice." The Court of Appeals, in affirming the conviction, disagreed, noting that the jury was instructed that the prosecution must prove not only that the defendant acted "outside the course of professional practice" but also that he acted "for other than a legitimate medical purpose."[42]

Federal criminal prosecutions of physicians concerning pain management do not always result in convictions. As part of the initiative to aggressively pursue "pill mill" operations in the state of Florida, a federal prosecutor indicted Debra Roggow, MD, who was board-certified in physical medicine and rehabilitation, on 10 counts of drug trafficking based on allegations that she was inappropriately prescribing opioids to some of her patients.[43] However, based on significant part on her meticulous patient records carefully documenting the justification for the prescribing of opioids in the case of each patient, the jury acquitted her of all charges.[44]

Before concluding the discussion of these federal prosecutions of physicians who were at the far liberal end of the prescribing

continuum, it may be helpful to delineate the parameters of that entire continuum, and perhaps even to suggest where, as a matter of law and public policy, the line should be drawn between "the bounds of medicine" and the realm of drug dealing and trafficking by health care professionals. The thrust of the argument goes something like this: Just as we do not criminally prosecute clinicians whose failure or refusal to provide pain relief subjects some of their patients to physical and mental anguish, neither ought we to criminally prosecute clinicians whose excessive prescribing creates or exacerbates some of their patients' addiction disorders or propensity to engage in drug dealing under the guise of being a pain patient. In the most egregious instances at both ends of the continuum, the appropriate public policy stance is to suspend or permanently revoke their professional licensure.

Currently, however, at least clinicians at the far liberal end of the prescribing continuum, such as Hurwitz and McIver, prosecutors, and judges (through approved jury instructions) invite juries to act as though no real physician–patient relationship existed. As suggested by the Kansas Court of Appeals in the Naramore case, whenever the criminally charged clinician is able to present expert testimony that what he or she did was within the "bounds of medicine," the mere fact that the prosecution can offer expert testimony maintaining that it was not should never be sufficient for a conviction. Such a conflict of testimony should necessarily create the reasonable doubt that precludes a jury verdict against a criminal defendant.

Constitutional Cases

Several decisions by the Supreme Court of the United States in the last two decades have addressed issues related to the treatment of pain. Each case also involved highly controversial ethical and political issues: physician-assisted suicide and medical marijuana. As is typical of the Supreme Court, the rulings in each case were not an effort to decide which side was correct on the ethics or the politics but rather to determine what was consistent with the Constitution and a reasonable interpretation and application of federal statutes.

The first of these, the companion cases of *Washington v Glucksberg*[45] and *Vacco v Quill*[46] decided in 1997 directly involved the question of whether there was a constitutional right on the part of dying patients to be able to acquire lethal doses of medication from willing physicians for purposes of hastening their death. In the process of unanimously ruling that there was no such constitutional right, five of the nine justices joined in two concurring opinions that have been interpreted as a recognition by a majority of the court of a constitutional right on the part of terminal patients to receive palliative care.[46] The language from these companion cases most consistently cited for this proposition include the following passage from the concurring opinion by Justice O'Connor:

> The parties and amici agree that in these states [Washington and New York] a patient who is suffering from a terminal illness and who is experiencing great pain has no legal barriers to obtaining medication from qualified physicians, to alleviate that suffering, even to the point of causing unconsciousness and hastening death.

Combined with language from a separate opinion by Justice Breyer:

> Were the legal circumstances different [than in Washington and New York]—for example were state law to prevent the provision of palliative care, including the provision of drugs as needed to avoid pain at the end of life—then the law's impact upon serious and otherwise unavoidable physical pain (accompanying death) would be more directly at issue. And as Justice O'Connor suggests, the Court might have to revisit its conclusions in these cases.[46]

The focus on pain and suffering at the end of life by the concurring justices may simply be a consequence of the fact that a right to lethal medication was asserted by the plaintiffs in these cases only as to patients with terminal illness. However, a right to appropriately aggressive palliative care as opposed to a lethal prescription, especially if defined quite broadly as the relief of pain and suffering, might be of even greater significance for a patient with severe chronic noncancer pain than for a terminally ill patient because it could persist for years or decades rather than merely weeks or months. Only future cases will illuminate whether there might be constitutional protection from unreasonable governmental barriers to pain relief for such patients.

The constitutionality of the Oregon Death with Dignity Act (ODWDA), pursuant to which the state of Oregon legalized and regulated physician-assisted suicide (referred to by its proponents as physician aid in dying) was not directly at issue in either *Washington v Glucksberg* or *Vacco v Quill*. However, those decisions by implication upheld the ODWDA because they determined that there is neither a constitutional right to nor a constitutional prohibition of such a practice. Consequently, it is a matter for each individual state to determine as part of its authority to regulate the practice of health care professionals.[47]

In 2001, Attorney General John Ashcroft issued an interpretive rule (IR) of the federal CSA, maintaining that prescribing a controlled substance for the purpose of assisting a patient in ending his or her life, even pursuant to a state statutory scheme such as the ODWDA, contravened the CSA and rendered the prescriber vulnerable to federal prosecution. Because all lethal prescriptions written pursuant to the ODWDA were federally controlled substances, the Ashcroft IR would essentially nullify the Oregon law. The State of Oregon immediately challenged the IR in federal court and obtained first a temporary restraining order and subsequently an injunction prohibiting enforcement of the IR pending resolution by the courts. When Ashcroft resigned as attorney general, his successor Alberto Gonzales decided to continue the legislation. By then, review of adverse rulings by the federal district and Ninth Circuit Court of Appeals had been sought and the case was pending before the US Supreme Court.

The central issue decided by the Supreme Court in *Gonzales v Oregon* was "who decides whether a particular activity is 'in the course of medical practice' or done for a 'legitimate medical purpose.'"[48] The attorney general claimed authority under the CSA to define standards of medical practice at least insofar as the prescribing of scheduled drugs. Taking into consideration the legislative history of the CSA, the Supreme Court majority ruled that the intent of Congress was to combat a national problem of recreational drug abuse by ensuring that scheduled narcotics were secured within the health care setting through the prescribing by licensed practitioners for legitimate medical purposes. Nothing in the language or the legislative history of the CSA suggests that Congress intended to confer on the attorney general, in his capacity of law enforcement, to usurp the usual authority of the individual states in regulating the practice of medicine, which includes the writing of prescriptions. For this and other reasons discussed at length by the Court, the IR was held to exceed the authority of the attorney general under the CSA.

The legalization of physician aid in dying has gained a great deal of momentum in the past decade. Following the lead of Oregon, the state of Washington passed a similar law through the referendum process. The Vermont and California legislatures have more recently enacted aid-in-dying legislation. In Montana, the state Supreme Court ruled that current law did not preclude physicians from providing such assistance to terminally ill patients with decisional capacity who requested it.[49]

The issue is also currently before the New Mexico Supreme Court.

In 2015, the Canadian Supreme Court ruled that sections of the criminal code violated the national Charter of Rights to the extent that they prohibited physician-assisted death for a competent adult who (1) clearly consents to the termination of life and (2) has a grievous and irremediable medical condition (including an illness, disease, or disability) that causes enduring suffering that is intolerable to the individual in the circumstances of his or her condition.[50] The decision was stayed in order to provide the government with time to enact legislation consistent with the ruling. In June of 2016, the Canadian House of Commons and Senate passed an aid in dying law.[51] However, because it limited the access to patients whose natural deaths were reasonably foreseeable, it is currently being challenged in court.[52]

The issue of the legitimate medical use of marijuana reached the Supreme Court in the case of *Gonzales v Raich*. The plaintiffs in this case, Angel Raich and Diane Monson, were California residents suffering from a variety of serious medical conditions. Raich carries at least 10 diagnoses, including an inoperable brain tumor, seizure disorder, and several chronic pain syndromes. Monson suffered from severe chronic back pain and muscle spasms related to a degenerative disease of the spine.

California was one of a growing number of states that enacted legislation insulating seriously ill patients or their physicians from prosecution under state law for cultivating or possessing cannabis for use by the patient pursuant to the physician's written recommendation or approval. The plaintiffs in this case argued that they were being treated by board-certified family practitioners who had determined after prescribing a wide variety of standard medications that marijuana is the only drug available that provides effective relief of their symptoms. As a Schedule I drug, the CSA recognizes no legitimate basis for patients such as Raich and Monson to possess or use marijuana, even though their physicians authorized it pursuant to the California statute. The plaintiffs filed suit against Attorney General Ashcroft and the administrator of the DEA in federal district court seeking declaratory and injunctive relief preventing the federal government from prosecuting them under the CSA. The crux of their argument was that enforcement of the CSA against them required that interstate commerce be implicated in their acquisition and use of medical marijuana. The district court ruled against the plaintiffs, finding that the Commerce Clause of the Constitution applied to them despite the fact that the marijuana they used was grown in California.

The Ninth Circuit Court of Appeals reversed the district court, holding that the plaintiffs' intrastate, noncommercial cultivation, possession, and use of marijuana for personal medical purposes on the advice of a physician does not constitute drug trafficking. Much of the court's discussion involved arcane legal principles and Supreme Court precedents. Ultimately, it was these very principles and precedents that provided the basis for the Supreme Court's reversal of the Ninth Circuit. Simply stated, the Court held that "Congress' power to regulate interstate markets for medicinal substances encompasses the portions of those markets that are supplied with drugs produced and consumed locally. . . . The CSA is a valid exercise of federal power, even as applied to the troubling facts of this case."[53] Thus, the Court's ruling in *Gonzales v Raich* cannot be understood as a pronouncement on the clinical question of whether the known risks and purported benefits of medical marijuana use ever justify a physician recommending it to patients when standard therapies are found to be inadequate.

Since this decision, not only have additional states permitted the use of "medical marijuana" but also some have legalized recreational marijuana and other states have this change on the ballot in November of 2016. Nevertheless, the DEA in August of 2016 reaffirmed its position that marijuana has no legitimate medical purpose and will remain a Schedule I drug that is illegal for any purpose.[54]

Lessons from the Litigation

Generalizations that meet minimal criteria of accuracy and practicality concerning the lessons one should learn from the varieties of litigation surveyed in this chapter are both difficult and dangerous. They are difficult because of the wide variation in cases; for example, state and federal courts, some patients who were dying, others facing chronic noncancer pain, still others who were addicted to prescription drugs or simply "planted" as a part of ongoing investigations by law enforcement. They are dangerous when they constitute gross oversimplifications of complex phenomena that have only superficial similarities. Nevertheless, some attempt at synthesis is both necessary and appropriate.

- Lesson 1: A new medical ethos has clearly emerged, grounded on the recognition that timely and effective assessment and management of all types of pain is essential to sound patient care. Nationally recognized clinical practice guidelines and organizational policies (such as The Joint Commission) affirm this basic proposition.
- Lesson 2. Evidence- or consensus-based guidelines and policies reinforce the proposition that there are recognized standards of care for the management of acute, chronic noncancer, and pain associated with terminal illness. These standards apply to all clinicians who care for patients with pain and not merely pain medicine or palliative care specialists.
- Lesson 3. Material departures from these standards render clinicians vulnerable to a variety of adverse legal consequences. Egregiously conservative approaches to opioid analgesia may result in civil liability for undertreatment of pain or professional licensing board sanctions. Excessively liberal approaches to the prescribing of opioids, particularly when a reasonable clinician would have recognized red flags or other warning signs, may result in criminal prosecution at the state or federal level.
- Lesson 4. Prudent practitioners should ensure that their knowledge, skills, and attitudes (at least insofar as they affect professional practice) are informed by the current authoritative clinical practice guidelines and policy statements. When that is the case, their approach to pain management will reflect a reasonable balance between effective pain management for their patients and due diligence to ensure that their prescribing practices are neither harming their patients nor contributing to the phenomena of prescription drug abuse and diversion.
- Lesson 5. As with any other aspect of patient care, timely, accurate, and thorough documentation in the medical record that reflects not only what was done but also what informed the decision on what to do and what alternatives were considered is absolutely essential. In every legal setting, incomplete, inaccurate, or untimely documentation of professional conduct is problematic, sometimes devastatingly so.
- Lesson 6. Clinicians who heed Lessons 1 to 5 earlier are not at any serious risk of adverse legal action arising out of their responsible efforts to relieve the pain of their patients.

References

1. Prosser WL, Keeton WP, Dobbs DB, et al. *Prosser and Keeton on Torts.* 5th ed. St. Paul, MN: West; 1984.
2. Brookoff D. Commentary on state medical boards and pain management. *J Pain Symptom Manage* 1998;15:381–382.
3. Gilson AM, Joranson DE. Controlled substances and pain management: changes in knowledge and attitudes of state medical regulators. *J Pain Symptom Manage* 2001;21:227–237.
4. Matter of DiLeo, 661 So2d 162 (1995).
5. *Hoover v Agency for Health Care Administration,* 676 So2d 1380 (1996).
6. Martino AM. In search of a new ethic for treating patients with chronic pain: what can medical boards do? *J Law Med Ethics* 1998;26:263, 332–349.
7. Federation of State Medical Boards. *Model Guidelines for the Use of Controlled Substances for the Treatment of Pain.* Euless, TX: Federation of State Medical Boards; 1998.
8. Hill CS. The negative influence of licensing and disciplinary boards and drug enforcement agencies on pain treatment with opioid analgesics. *J Pharm Care Pain Symptom Control* 1993;1:43–62.
9. Oregon Board of Medical Examiners. *Stipulated Order in the Matter of Paul A. Bilder, M.D.* Portland, OR: Oregon Board of Medical Examiners; 1999.
10. Oregon Board of Medical Examiners. Oregon medical board: board action report. Available at: http://www.oregon.gov/omb/BoardActions/October%2016,%202008%20-%20November%2015,%202008.pdf. Accessed October 10, 2016.
11. Medical Board of California. *In the Matter of the Accusation against Eugene B. Whitney, M.D.* Sacramento, CA: Medical Board of California; 2003.
12. Medical Board of California. *In the Matter of the Accusation against Eugene B. Whitney, M.D. Decision.* Sacramento, CA: Medical Board of California; 2003.
13. Federation of State Medical Boards. *Model Policy for the Use of Controlled Substances for the Treatment of Pain.* Euless, TX: Federation of State Medical Boards; 2013.
14. Federation of State Medical Boards. Pain management policies, board-by-board overview. Available at: http://www.fsmb.org/globalassets/advocacy/key-issues/pain-management-by-state.pdf. Accessed April 24, 2018.
15. Cushing M. Pain management on trial. *Am J Nurs* 1992;92:21–23.
16. *Estate of Henry James v Hillhaven Corporation,* 89 CVS 64 (NC Super Ct 1991)
17. Shapiro RS. Liability issues in the management of pain. *J Pain Symptom Manage* 1994;9(3):146–52.
18. North Carolina General Assembly General Statute §§10–15(b), 1D-25 (2003).
19. Rich BA. Moral conundrums in the courtroom: reflections on a decade in the culture of pain. *Camb Q Healthc Ethics* 2002;11:180–190.
20. California Welfare and Institutions Code, §15610 (2006).
21. *Bergman v Chin,* No. H205732-1 (Cal Super Ct, Alameda County 1999).
22. Agency for Health Care Policy and Research. *Management of Cancer Pain.* Washington, DC: U.S. Department of Health and Human Services; 1994. Clinical practice guideline no. 9.
23. Cassell EJ. The nature of suffering and the goals of medicine. *N Engl J Med* 1982;306:639–645.
24. *Tomlinson v Bayberry Care Center,* C 02-00120 (Cal Super Ct, Contra Costa County 2002).
25. Medical Board of California. *In the Matter of the Accusation against Eugene B. Whitney, M.D. No. 12 2002 133376. Stipulation for Public Reprimand. Filed January 14, 2004.* Sacramento, CA: Medical Board of California; 2004.
26. AHC Media. Pain cases settled: nursing home fined. Available at: https://www.ahcmedia.com/articles/26746-pain-cases-settled-nursing-home-fined. Accessed September 20, 2016.
27. *Tugg Valley Pharmacy LLC, et al. v All Plaintiffs Below in Mingo County,* 14-0144, WL 3401425 (West Va 2015).
28. Annas GW. Medicine, death and the criminal law. *N Engl J Med* 1995;333:527–530.
29. *State v Naramore,* 965 P2d 211 (Kan Ct App 1998), *cert denied.*
30. Alpers A. Criminal act or palliative care? Prosecutions involving the care of the dying. *J Law Med Ethics* 1998;26:308–331.
31. Federal Bureau of Investigation, Louisville Division. Cincinnati doctor sentenced for illegal distribution of prescription pills. Available at: https://archives.fbi.gov/archives/louisville/press-releases/2010/lo051410.htm. Accessed September 26, 2016.
32. Gerber M, Girion L, Queally J. California doctor convicted of murder in overdose deaths of patients. *Los Angeles Times.* October 30, 2015. Available at: http://www.latimes.com/local/lanow/la-me-ln-doctor-prescription-drugs-murder-overdose-verdict-20151030-story.html. Accessed October 3, 2016.
33. Gerber M. Doctor convicted of murder for patients' drug overdoses gets 30 years to life in prison. *Los Angeles Times.* February 5, 2016. Available at: http://www.latimes.com/local/lanow/la-me-ln-doctor-murder-overdose-drugs-sentencing-20160205-story.html. Accessed October 3, 2016.
34. Freeman M. Jury acquits former pain clinic doctor of murder, convicts him of minor drug charge. *SunSentinel.* September 16, 2015. Available at: http://www.sun-sentinel.com/local/palm-beach/fl-doctor-murder-trial-verdict-watch-20150915-story.html. Accessed October 3, 2016.
35. Associated Press. Kentucky settles lawsuit with OxyContin maker for $24 million. *CBS News.* December 23, 2015. Available at: http://www.cbsnews.com/news/kentucky-settles-lawsuit-with-oxycontin-maker-for-24-million/. Accessed October 3, 2016.
36. Bernstein L. Pfizer agrees to truth in opioid marketing. *The Washington Post.* July 5, 2016. Available at: https://www.washingtonpost.com/national/health-science/pfizer-agrees-to-truth-in-opioid-marketing/2016/07/05/784223cc-42c6-11e6-88d0-6adee48be8bc_story.html. Accessed October 3, 2016.

37. *United States v Rosen*, 582 F2d 1032, 1033 (1978).
38. United States Attorney's Office, Eastern District of Virginia. *News Release. April 14, 2005.* Newport News, VA: United States Attorney's Office, Eastern District of Virginia; 2005.
39. U.S. Drug Enforcement Administration. DEA administrator Karen Tandy's remarks on Hurwitz sentencing. Available at: http://www.dea.gov/pubs/pressrel/pr041405b.html. Accessed April 14, 2005.
40. *United States v Hurwitz*, 459 F3d 463 (4th Cir 2006).
41. *United States v McIver*, 470 F3d 550 (4th Cir 2006).
42. *McIver, DO v United States of America*, Petition for a Writ of Certiorari to the Supreme Court of the United States (2007).
43. *United States v Debra Roggow*. 2:11-CR-114-FTM-29SPC (MD Fla, Fort Myers 2012).
44. Bolen J. Board-certified doctor cleared of criminal charges for high-dose opioid prescribing. Available at: http://www.practicalpainmanagement.com/resources/ethics/board-certified-doctor-cleared-criminal-charges-high-dose-opioid-prescribing. Accessed September 26, 2016.
45. *Washington v Glucksberg*, 521 US 702 (1997).
46. *Vacco v Quill*, 521 US 793 (1997).
47. Burt Robert A. The Supreme Court speaks—not assisted suicide but a constitutional right to palliative care. *N Engl J Med* 1997;337:1234–1236.
48. *Gonzales v Oregon*, 546 US 243 (2006).
49. *Baxter v Montana*, 224 P3d 1211 (2009).
50. *Carter v Canada*, 1 SCR 331 (2015).
51. House of Commons of Canada. Bill C-14. Available at: http://www.parl.gc.ca/HousePublications/Publication.aspx?Language=E&Mode=1&DocId=8309978. Accessed October 8, 2016.
52. *Julia Lamb and British Columbia Civil Liberties Association v Attorney General of Canada*, Supreme Court of British Columbia. June 27, 2016. Available at: https://bccla.org/wp-content/uploads/2016/06/2016-06-27-Notice-of-Civil-Claim-1.pdf. Accessed October 8, 2016.
53. *Gonzales v Raich*, 545 US 1 (2005).
54. Downs D. The science behind the DEA's long war against marijuana. *Scientific American*. April 19, 2016. Available at: http://www.scientificamerican.com/article/the-science-behind-the-dea-s-long-war-on-marijuana/. Accessed October 3, 2016.

CHAPTER 16

International Access to Therapeutic Opioids

JAMES F. CLEARY, MARTHA A. MAURER, and **S. ASRA HUSAIN**

Over three decades ago, the World Health Organization (WHO) concluded that most pain due to cancer could be relieved if health professionals followed a simple medical treatment method called the *three-step analgesic ladder*, which recommends using various types of analgesics (including opioid analgesics), in combination with adjuvant drugs when needed, depending on the severity of the patient's pain.[1] This approach also has been recognized by the WHO as appropriate with HIV/AIDS patients experiencing pain throughout the disease.[2]

United Nations (UN) health and regulatory agencies have repeatedly appealed to governments and health professionals to cooperate in order to implement the WHO analgesic method and remove barriers that block patient access to opioid pain medications.[3-12] Although drug regulations and opioid availability have improved in some countries, the vast majority of cancer and HIV/AIDS patients in low- and middle-income countries (LMICs), and many in high-income countries (HICs), still lack access to these essential medications.[13,14] The inadequate access to opioids is further illustrated by the disparity in reported medical consumption of opioid medicines between HICs comprising a small proportion of the global population and the large and growing population of LMICs.[15] With the shifting burden of cancer to LMICs,[16] the public health problem of inadequate availability of pain medications and unrelieved pain is projected to become far worse.

The purpose of this chapter is to outline the body of knowledge and experience that is relevant to understanding and improving national opioid availability and patient access to controlled pain medicines. It is critically important for health care professionals and government drug regulators, as well as advocates involved in the area of palliative care and pain relief, to understand the policies that govern the use of opioid medicines and how they can impact medication availability and patient access to opioid medicines. This chapter begins with background about the importance of pain relief in cancer and HIV/AIDS control. Focusing on opioids indicated for the relief of moderate to severe pain (e.g., hydromorphone, fentanyl, morphine, oxycodone), this chapter discusses the designation of these opioid medicines as both essential and controlled by international authorities. The disparities in opioid consumption globally and regionally are detailed, followed by an overview of common barriers preventing the adequate availability and accessibility of opioid medicines. Lastly, the UN's recommendations to address the barriers to opioid availability are described followed by a summary of recent initiatives to improve the availability and access to opioid medications.

Pain Relief Is Part of Cancer and HIV/AIDS Control

The global incidence and prevalence of cancer and HIV/AIDS is a public health problem of great concern. The WHO estimates that in 2012, approximately 14.1 million individuals were newly diagnosed with cancer and more than 8 million died from this noncommunicable disease.[17] Experts predict that the cancer burden will increase by 70% in the next two decades, with major impacts on LMICs, where it is estimated that the majority of new cases and deaths from cancer, including children, will occur.[17] The global occurrence of HIV/AIDS is also a public health problem of great concern. The Joint United Nations Programme on HIV/AIDS (UNAIDS) indicated that in 2015, 36.7 million people were living with HIV, and 1.1 million people died from HIV/AIDS.[18]

People with HIV/AIDS[19,20] and/or cancer[21-25] experience pain and a variety of other symptoms during the course of their disease that have a negative impact on their quality of life. Patients who are approaching the end of life are likely to experience even more severe symptoms,[7,8,26,27] which include pain, anxiety, constipation, cough, depression, dyspnea, and nausea.[1,7,8] Although it is necessary to address all symptoms, this chapter focuses on the need for adequate pain relief and access to opioid pain medications. In LMICs, most cancers are diagnosed in late stages of the disease,[16,28,29] when people often experience severe pain.[7,8,26,27]

PAIN AND PALLIATIVE CARE

Palliative care, including the critically important component of pain management, is a model of care aimed at relieving symptoms of disease and its treatment and improving the patient and family's quality of life throughout the course of the disease. The WHO has long recognized that relieving pain and other symptoms in cancer[1] and HIV/AIDS[2,30] is a necessary part of palliative care, including for children.[31,32] In 2014, the Worldwide Hospice and Palliative Care Alliance and the WHO collaborated to produce the *Global Atlas of Palliative Care at the End of Life*, which examines the state of palliative care and hospice programs globally, quantifying the need for and availability of palliative care worldwide.[26] They found that over 20 million people require palliative care at the end of life every year, with the highest proportion of adults in need of palliative care (78%) living in LMICs.[26] Despite this great need, palliative care is underdeveloped in most of the world, and access to quality palliative care is very rare in LMICs.[26]

Palliative care and pain relief medicines should be available and accessible to all individuals who have pain and other symptoms.[8,26] There is a strong international imperative that palliative care, including pain management, should be included in national cancer and HIV/AIDS control efforts. The WHO has repeatedly reaffirmed the necessity of including palliative care as a critical component of cancer or HIV/AIDS control efforts in a country.[33,34] At the country level, national policies should provide a policy framework for developing and expanding health care services to reach patients who need disease treatment as well as relief of pain and other symptoms. Notably, in 2014, the World Health Assembly (WHA), for the first time in its history, adopted a palliative care resolution that urges member states to integrate palliative care into their health care systems, to improve training for health care workers, and to ensure that relevant medicines, including strong pain medicines, are available to patients.[11]

Opioids Are Essential Medicines and Controlled Substances

Guidance from the WHO dating back to 1986 acknowledges the need for a varied approach to managing pain, including nonpharmacologic therapies, and that not all types of pain will respond equally, if at all, to opioids.[1] Indeed, there are many useful pharmacologic and nonpharmacologic therapies for treating cancer pain.[7,27] And yet, opioid medicines, and in particular orally administered morphine, are regarded by international health experts as the first choice for relieving moderate to severe pain due to cancer.[35–37] Since 1977, the WHO Expert Committee on the Selection and Use of Essential Medicines has designated morphine as an *essential medicine* for the treatment of cancer pain.[38] According to WHO, *essential medicines* are those medicines that " . . . satisfy the priority health care needs of the population . . . are selected with due regard to public health relevance, evidence on efficacy and safety, and comparative cost-effectiveness."[39] By giving them this designation, the WHO is asserting that these medicines " . . . are intended to be available within the context of functioning health systems at all times in adequate amounts, in the appropriate dosage forms, with assured quality and adequate information, and at a price the individual and the community can afford."[39]

In 2012, at the request of the WHO, the International Association for Hospice and Palliative Care (IAHPC) led an expert group to develop a summary of the evidence available for essential medicines for palliative care. As a result of these recommendations, the WHO's 18th *Model List of Essential Medicines* published in April 2013 contained a new section specific to palliative care, which included both immediate- and sustained-release morphine for the treatment of pain and listed hydromorphone and oxycodone as alternatives to morphine.[40] The WHO's 20th *Model List of Essential Medicines* published in March 2017 expanded the opioid medicines indicated to treat cancer pain to include transdermal fentanyl and methadone.[41]

In addition to being medicines that are essential for relieving pain, opioids have a potential for being misused or abused, which can result in harms. Therefore, they are designated as controlled substances by an international treaty, the Single Convention on Narcotic Drugs, 1961, as amended by the 1972 Protocol Amending the Single Convention on Narcotic Drugs, 1961 (Single Convention) (Fig. 16.1).[42] The term *narcotic drugs* refers to a subset of controlled substances and is a legal term that will be used where the context requires. Nearly every government in the world has formally acceded to the Single Convention, thereby agreeing to adopt laws, regulations, and administrative procedures to carry out the dual aims of the Single Convention, which are to prevent the abuse and diversion of opioid medicines while making them available for medical purposes.

The Single Convention establishes an international framework of prohibitions and requirements for governments concerning the legitimate production, manufacture, and distribution of narcotic drugs that is intended to prevent illicit trafficking, nonmedical use of narcotic drugs, and diversion (the illegal movement of controlled medications from the licit distribution system into the illicit market). The principal *international* requirement is that the legitimate trade in narcotic drugs is regulated, including the cultivation of opium and manufacture of medicinal opioids such as codeine and morphine. To prevent diversion, an import–export system is established to limit trade to the amounts necessary for medical use; trade is regulated by the International Narcotics Control Board (INCB), an independent and quasi-judicial monitoring body to implement UN international drug control conventions.[43]

The Single Convention establishes several national obligations, among them that governments must regulate all entities

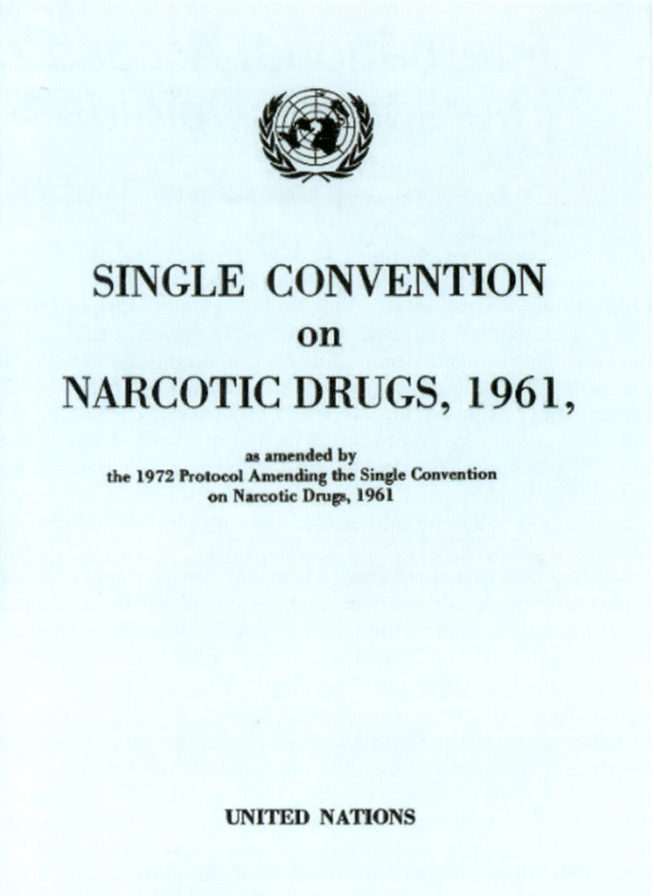

FIGURE 16.1 The United Nations Single Convention on Narcotic Drugs, 1961, as amended by the 1972 Protocol Amending the Single Convention on Narcotic Drugs, 1961.

that handle controlled substances. The goal is to create a closed distribution system, including security and record keeping. Only clinical professionals authorized under national law, using "medical prescriptions," may prescribe and dispense controlled substances to individuals and only for medical purposes. Distribution outside of the regulated system is prohibited in order to prevent diversion of controlled drugs from medical to nonmedical uses. Efforts to prevent diversion should be balanced so as not to interfere in medical practice and patient care.[4,10]

Examples of efforts to lessen the risks of abuse and diversion include clinical training of health care professionals and students regarding appropriate pain management as a means to reduce inappropriate use.[6,44–46] Some countries have provided informational sessions for health officials and drug regulators when policies were updated to facilitate their knowledge of the new legal requirements.[45,46] Some areas of India[47] and countries such as Sierra Leone[48] and Uganda[49] have successfully increased the availability of morphine without experiencing diversion and abuse of these medicines; such activities require sound security, record keeping, and prescriptive practices.

GOVERNMENTS MUST ENSURE ADEQUATE OPIOID AVAILABILITY

In addition to controlling drugs to prevent their diversion and nonmedical use, the Single Convention stipulates a second obligation to ensure adequate availability of narcotic drugs for medical and scientific purposes. The Single Convention clearly recognizes the importance of narcotic drugs as analgesic medications and asserts that medical access to opioids for relief of pain is to be assured by governments because they are obligated to conform their laws to the Single Convention, " . . . the medical use of narcotic drugs continues to be indispensable for the relief of pain and suffering and that adequate provision must be made to ensure the availability of narcotic drugs for such purposes."[42]

The availability obligation is no less important than the obligation to prevent diversion, but it is poorly understood and implemented by health professionals and governments. There is no indication that the medical value of controlled substances is lessened as a result of scheduling under the Single Convention. Scholars of international narcotic drug policy have concluded that the Single Convention, as amended, recognizes that the basic purpose of international drug control is to reduce the availability of drugs for nonmedical purposes but "that this should not affect or limit their therapeutic use."[50]

The Single Convention establishes a critically important policy framework, the *principle of balance*, which asserts that governments' obligation to control controlled medicines is not only to prevent drug abuse but also to ensure their availability for medical purposes.[10] Controls aimed at preventing drug abuse and diversion must not prevent the adequate availability of opioid medicines for patients' pain relief. Drug abuse controls that hinder opioid availability and patient access to effective pain treatment would be considered unbalanced and should be identified and corrected (Table 16.1).

To accomplish these dual objectives, the Single Convention requires that governments adopt laws, regulations, and administrative procedures to implement two specific mechanisms that are intended to ensure adequate availability of opioid medicines in countries while preventing nonmedical use. First, governments must annually establish an estimate of the amounts of opioids that will be required for all medical and scientific needs for the coming year.[51] Licit trade in narcotic drugs can be lawfully conducted only within this amount. If imports exceed a country's estimated requirements, exporters are obligated to refrain from further trade with the country, unless the INCB approves a supplementary estimate from the importing country that increases the estimated amount of the narcotic. Governments are encouraged to develop valid estimation methods, to establish estimates that take increasing demand into consideration, to cooperate with health professionals to obtain information about unmet needs, and to increase the estimate whenever necessary to always satisfy medical needs.[51] Second, governments must report the amounts of each narcotic drug consumed (i.e., distributed to the retail level) to allow identification of consumption that either exceeds or falls short of the estimate.[52]

Each Party to the Single Convention is expected to establish a drug control program not only to prevent illicit trafficking and diversion but also to ensure the adequate availability of narcotic drugs for medical and scientific purposes[4] and to designate an agency called the Competent National Authority (CNA) to implement the functions required by the Single Convention.[43] This office is usually located in the pharmaceutical department of the Ministry of Health, the national drug control, or public security agency, or the functions may be divided between agencies. The CNA is the principal national administrative authority for carrying out the estimation and statistical reporting procedures that are necessary for ensuring that opioid medicines are adequately available for medical and scientific purposes. Guidelines for estimating the amounts of opioids required for medical and scientific use and for reporting consumption statistics are useful for those who want to understand the administrative procedures to be followed by CNAs.[51-53] The INCB provides guidelines for CNAs to comply with the Single Convention, including the administration of effective mechanisms to ensure opioid availability.[54]

Disparities in Opioid Consumption

The Single Convention requirement that national governments report annual consumption statistics provides a unique source of data to describe global and national opioid consumption trends and to study disparities. Consumption means the amounts of opioid medicines distributed for medical purposes to the "retail" level in a country (i.e., to those institutions and programs that are licensed to dispense to patients, such as hospitals, nursing homes, pharmacies, hospices, and palliative care programs). The INCB uses consumption statistics to (1) monitor compliance of governments with the provisions of the Single Convention, (2) identify trade discrepancies between importing and exporting countries, (3) detect imbalances between quantities of medications available and disposed within a country, (4) identify trends in the worldwide availability of opioids and other drugs for medical needs, and (5) monitor and maintain a global balance of supply and demand of opioids for medical and scientific needs.[52]

Opioid consumption statistics have several useful applications for those who study and improve opioid availability to (1) identify whether a country has available opioids that can relieve moderate to severe pain, (2) learn whether the amounts indicate any substantial current consumption or progress over time,[27] and (3) evaluate the outcome of efforts to improve opioid availability.

Consumption statistics provided in INCB reports have several limitations that should be considered when using them as an indicator of opioid availability:

1. In any given year, the data may be incomplete or invalid as a result of some governments reporting late, not reporting for a particular year or period, or submitting inaccurate data. These deficiencies may be corrected in subsequent years. Each year, the INCB publishes updated statistics for the previous 4 years of data which reflect corrections to previous reports and data submitted after the deadline.
2. The INCB's published reports do not include the exact amounts of consumption for quantities less than 1 kg. Instead, the symbol "<<" is used to signify that a country reported between 0 and 0.499 kg, and consumption amounts between 0.5 and 0.999 kg are rounded up to 1 kg.[55] Knowing the exact amounts of small quantities of controlled medicines consumed is particularly important for countries with small populations or those which have recently initiated efforts to increase their consumption of controlled medicines for pain or other health care needs.

TABLE 16.1 **The Central Principle of "Balance"**
The central principle of "balance" represents a dual obligation of governments to establish a system of control that ensures the adequate availability of controlled substances for medical and scientific purposes, while simultaneously preventing abuse, diversion and trafficking. Many controlled medicines are essential medicines and are absolutely necessary for the relief of pain, treatment of illness and the prevention of premature death.
To ensure the rational use of these medicines, governments should both enable and empower healthcare professionals to prescribe, dispense and administer them according to the individual medical needs of patients, ensuring that a sufficient supply is available to meet those needs. While misuse of controlled substances poses a risk to society, the system of control is not intended to be a barrier to their availability for medical and scientific purposes, nor interfere in their legitimate medical use for patient care.[10(p11)]

Reprinted with permission from World Health Organization. *Ensuring Balance in National Policies on Controlled Substances: Guidance for Availability and Accessibility of Controlled Medicines.* 2nd ed, rev ed. Geneva, Switzerland: World Health Organization; 2011.

3. Consumption statistics are reported as one aggregate amount of controlled substance consumed. Therefore, they do not provide information about
   a. The proportion of the amount used for different clinical indications. For example, methadone is used to treat pain and dependence syndrome, and fentanyl is used for analgesia or anesthesia.
   b. The location where the controlled substances are being used, such as hospitals and hospices, or
   c. Which products or dosage forms of an opioid are available within a country (i.e., whether an opioid is in oral, parenteral, or transdermal form).
4. Consumption statistics are not a valid clinical indicator of the quality of pain control in a country.

Each year for nearly two decades, the Pain & Policy Studies Group/WHO Collaborating Center for Policy and Communications in Cancer Care (PPSG/WHOCC) has received from the INCB consumption data for six principal opioids used to treat moderate to severe pain (fentanyl, hydromorphone, methadone, morphine, oxycodone, and pethidine). The PPSG/WHOCC has developed an in-house global database of opioid consumption statistics and provides these data on its Web site (Table 16.2).

MORPHINE EQUIVALENCE METRIC

For decades, the WHO has considered a country's annual consumption of morphine to be an indicator of the extent that opioids are used to treat severe cancer pain and an index to evaluate improvements in the capacity for treating pain.[7,27] However, additional opioid analgesic medications and formulations such as fentanyl, hydromorphone, and oxycodone have been introduced in global and national markets over the past 30 years, which should also be taken into consideration when studying opioid consumption in a country, region, and globally.

In an effort to compare morphine consumption with the consumption of other opioids, the PPSG/WHOCC developed a morphine equivalence (ME) metric for five principal opioids used to treat moderate to severe pain: fentanyl, hydromorphone, morphine, oxycodone, and pethidine.[56–58] A total ME statistic combines consumption of those opioid medicines into one metric. The conversion values were based on standard units of measurement for presenting drug utilization statistics from the WHO Collaborating Centre for Drug Statistics Methodology in Oslo, Norway.[59] All ME statistics are adjusted for population, expressed in milligram per capita, allowing for cross-country or regional comparisons. These data are obtained directly from the INCB, thereby eliminating the small quantity limitation; however, the other limitations of opioid consumption statistics apply to the data expressed in the ME metric.

In a 2013 study, PPSG/WHOCC statistically examined the extent that morphine consumption reflected the aggregate consumption of all other opioids consumed on the global, regional and national levels, finding that over time, morphine has become less and less of a valid indicator of overall opioid consumption.[60] Most recently, in 2014, PPSG/WHOCC conducted a descriptive analysis of opioid consumption trends,[58] which is presented in the following section including the most recently available data from the INCB.

GLOBAL OPIOID CONSUMPTION TRENDS

The 35-year global opioid consumption trend ending in 2015 in Figure 16.2 shows that prior to 1986, morphine consumption was very low and stable throughout the world and was paralleled by total ME opioid consumption. After WHO announced its cancer pain relief *three-step analgesic ladder*[1] in 1986 and encouraged use of oral morphine, morphine consumption began to increase with total ME consumption increasing more rapidly and diverging from morphine use. With the emergence of additional opioid products and dosage forms in the mid-1990s, total ME opioid consumption increased even more so that morphine use became less and less of a valid indicator of global opioid consumption. In 1986, global morphine consumption was 33% of total ME opioid consumption, compared to 12% in 2015. And yet, morphine has continued, until recently, to be designated by WHO as the primary essential medicine for the treatment of severe cancer pain. IAHPC included both immediate-release and sustained-release oral morphine in their recommended list of essential medicines for palliative care. Furthermore, several notable clinical guidelines continue to recommend morphine as one option for first-line treatment of severe cancer pain.[36,61,62]

Since the late 1990s, fentanyl and oxycodone accounted for the greatest portion of opioid consumption, at least for the global aggregate data. The global total ME opioid consumption trend mirrors the trend lines for oxycodone and fentanyl, which have been increasingly consumed throughout the world. The increasing clinical use of opioids other than morphine is reflected in WHO's recent expansion of their *Model List of Essential Medicines* to include oxycodone and hydromorphone as alternative opioid medicines for treating cancer pain[40] and methadone and transdermal fentanyl for the treatment of cancer pain.[41] Fentanyl is commonly used intravenously in the perioperative period which may account for some of its increase.

Another noteworthy trend is the long-term decline in consumption of pethidine (meperidine), likely due to increasing recognition of the potential risks associated with accumulation of the toxic metabolite norpethidine. Pethidine has been used in many countries mainly by injection for postoperative pain because of a perception that its very short duration of action reduces the risk of dependence. Pethidine is no longer recommended by the WHO for the treatment of pain,[63,64] although it continues to be used. Programs that move away from pethidine should ensure that other suitable opioids are accessible; if pethidine is available, there should be no regulatory barrier to this

---

TABLE 16.2   Pain & Policy Studies Group/World Health Organization Collaborating Center for Policy and Communications in Cancer Care Opioid Consumption Data Resources

Global consumption of opioids: global opioid consumption data as reported to the INCB for fentanyl, hydromorphone, methadone, morphine, oxycodone and pethidine: http://www.painpolicy.wisc.edu/global

Regional consumption of opioids: consumption of fentanyl, hydromorphone, methadone, morphine, oxycodone and pethidine in each of the six WHO regions: http://www.painpolicy.wisc.edu/regional

Country level consumption of opioids: Opioid consumption trends for each country: http://www.painpolicy.wisc.edu/countryprofiles

Tools to interactively explore these data:

Interactive global map: users select the opioid medicine and year (1964 to most recent) to display, providing an immediate visual image of the variation in consumption of opioids throughout the world: https://ppsg.medicine.wisc.edu/

Interactive opioid consumption chart: users explore the relationship between opioid consumption trends for a particular country and other country characteristics such as the Human Development Index: https://ppsg.medicine.wisc.edu/chart

Chart tool: users select, customize and create charts of the opioid consumption data and download them as either an image file (png) or a PDF for use in presentations or publications: https://ppsg-chart.medicine.wisc.edu/

INCB, International Narcotics Control Board; WHO, World Health Organization.

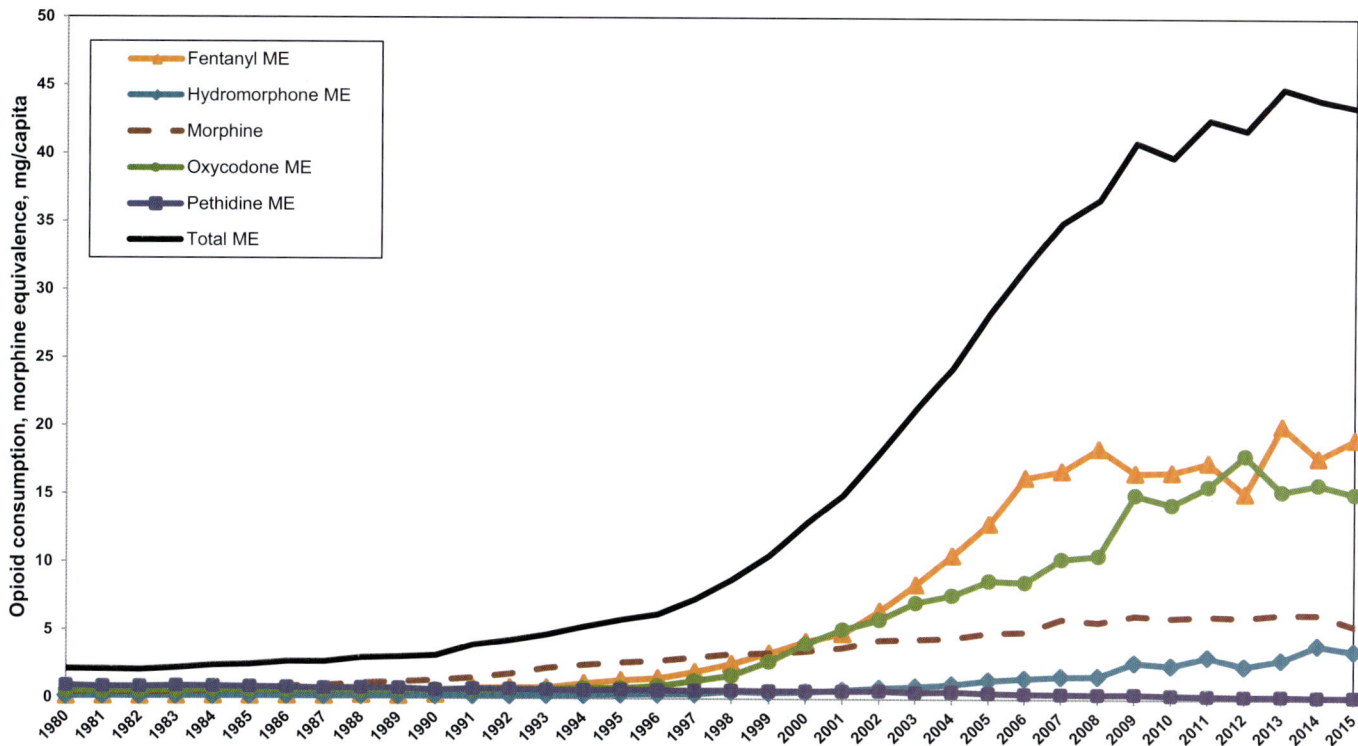

FIGURE 16.2 Global opioid consumption morphine equivalence (ME) (milligram per capita).

transition, as pethidine and other opioids such as morphine are controlled in the same schedule and are typically subject to the same international and national controls.

DISPARITIES IN CONSUMPTION BY INCOME LEVEL
At the national and regional level, there are great disparities in the amount of morphine consumed between HICs and LMICs. The INCB has consistently reported that a small number of HICs consume most of the morphine in the world, whereas the remaining countries, which are composed of over 80% of the world's population, consume a small fraction.[6] A recent statistical analysis of opioid consumption over an 11-year period by the INCB found substantial increases over time and confirmed that HICs in North America, Oceania, and Europe accounted for the large increase in consumption, whereas LMICs experienced very little change in consumption levels.[15]

Regional Opioid Consumption Trends

ME opioid consumption trends for each of the six WHO geographic regions (Table 16.3) illustrate great variability in consumption in different parts of the world (Fig. 16.3), notably that opioid consumption tends to be significantly lower in regions predominantly composed of LMICs and higher in regions with many HICs. Throughout the 35-year period, the WHO region of the Americas (AMRO) had the highest consumption of all regions and was substantially higher than the global ME consumption. In 2015, AMRO ME consumption was more than 4 times higher than the global mean consumption (43.5 mg per capita). The WHO region for Europe (EURO) had the next highest consumption, which also consistently exceeded the global ME consumption over the years, followed by the Western Pacific region (WPRO), whose ME opioid consumption was lower than EURO but considerably higher than the other three WHO regions (EMRO, AFRO, and SEARO), likely due to the influence of the HICs in the region. The remaining three WHO regions (EMRO, AFRO,

and SEARO) had substantially lower ME opioid consumption than the global mean throughout the period, and in 2015, their ME consumption represented 5%, 3%, and 1% of the global mean ME consumption, respectively.

Examining ME opioid consumption trends within each WHO region provides information about which opioids were available for the treatment of pain throughout the 35-year period.

WORLD HEALTH ORGANIZATION REGION FOR AFRICA (AFRO)
From the early 1980s to the late 2000s, the total ME consumption trend in the AFRO was largely composed of morphine and pethidine consumption with some minimal contributions of fentanyl and oxycodone (Fig. 16.4). Beginning in 2008, fentanyl ME consumption began to increase surpassing pethidine consumption. Following a spike in 2010, fentanyl ME consumption decreased but still remained higher than ME pethidine consumption.

WORLD HEALTH ORGANIZATION REGION FOR THE AMERICAS (AMRO)
Prior to the mid-1990s, the total ME opioid consumption in the AMRO was composed of a somewhat equivalent contribution of all the individual opioid consumption trends (Fig. 16.5). Beginning in the late 1990s, there was a notable and consistent increase in oxycodone and fentanyl consumption, while at the same time, morphine consumption increased steadily, and hydromorphone consumption rose notably beginning in the early 2000s. It is likely that opioid consumption in HICs in North America (e.g., Canada and the United States) primarily drives the regional consumption trend. Furthermore, as discussed earlier, the total ME consumption trend for the AMRO is the most similar to the global total ME opioid consumption trend. However, when considering the opioid medicines that individually contribute to the overall trend line, for AMRO, oxycodone consumption is the highest followed by fentanyl, and for the global trend, it is the opposite as fentanyl consumption is higher than oxycodone.

TABLE 16.3 World Health Organization Regions and Their Member Countries

Regional Office for Africa (AFRO)

Algeria	Comoros	Ghana	Mauritius	South Africa
Angola	Congo	Guinea	Mozambique	South Sudan
Benin	Cote d'Ivoire	Guinée-Bissau	Namibia	Swaziland
Botswana	Democratic Republic of	Kenya	Niger	Tanzania
Burkina Faso	Congo	Lesotho	Nigeria	Togo
Burundi	Equatorial Guinea	Liberia	Rwanda	Uganda
Cameroon	Ethiopia	Madagascar	São Tomé and Príncipe	Zambia
Cape Verde	Eritrea	Malawi	Senegal	Zimbabwe
Central African Republic	Gabon	Mali	Seychelles	
Chad	Gambia	Mauritania	Sierra Leone	

Regional Office for the Americas (AMRO)

Anguilla	British Virgin Islands	El Salvador	Mexico	Saint Vincent and the
Antigua and Barbuda	Canada	Grenada	Montserrat	Grenadines
Argentina	Cayman Islands	French Guiana	Netherlands Antilles	Suriname
Aruba	Chile	Guadeloupe	Nicaragua	Trinidad and Tobago
Bahamas	Colombia	Guatemala	Panama	Turks and Caicos
Barbados	Costa Rica	Guyana	Paraguay	United States of America
Belize	Cuba	Haiti	Peru	Uruguay
Bermuda	Dominica	Honduras	Puerto Rico	Venezuela
Bolivia	Dominican Republic	Jamaica	Saint Kitts and Nevis	
Brazil	Ecuador	Martinique	Saint Lucia	

Regional Office for the Eastern Mediterranean (EMRO)

Afghanistan	Iraq	Oman	Somalia	Yemen
Bahrain	Jordan	Pakistan	Sudan	
Djibouti	Kuwait	Palestine	Syrian Arab Republic	
Egypt	Lebanon	Qatar	Tunisia	
Iran	Libya	Saudi Arabia	United Arab Emirates	

Regional Office for Europe (EURO)

Albania	Czech Republic	Israel	Netherlands	Spain
Andorra	Denmark	Italy	Norway	Sweden
Armenia	Estonia	Kazakhstan	Poland	Switzerland
Austria	Finland	Kyrgyzstan	Portugal	Tajikistan
Azerbaijan	France	Latvia	Republic of Moldova	Turkey
Belarus	Georgia	Lithuania	Romania	Turkmenistan
Belgium	Germany	Luxembourg	Russian Federation	Ukraine
Bosnia and Herzegovina	Greece	Macedonia	San Marino	United Kingdom
Bulgaria	Hungary	Malta	Serbia	Uzbekistan
Croatia	Iceland	Monaco	Slovakia	
Cyprus	Ireland	Montenegro	Slovenia	

Regional Office for South East Asia (SEARO)

Bangladesh	India	Maldives	Nepal	Thailand
Bhutan	Indonesia	Myanmar	Sri Lanka	Timor-Leste
Democratic People's Republic of Korea				

Regional Office for the Western Pacific (WPRO)

American Samoa	Guam	Marshall Islands	Northern Mariana Islands	Solomon Islands
Australia	Hong Kong	Micronesia (Federal States	Palau	Tokelau
Brunei Darussalam	Japan	of)	Papua New Guinea	Tonga
Cambodia	Kiribati	Mongolia	Philippines	Tuvalu
China	Lao People's Democratic	Nauru	Pitcairn Islands	Vanuatu
Cook Islands	Republic	New Caledonia	Republic of Korea	Viet Nam
Fiji	Macau	New Zealand	Samoa	Wallis and Futuna
French Polynesia	Malaysia	Niue	Singapore	

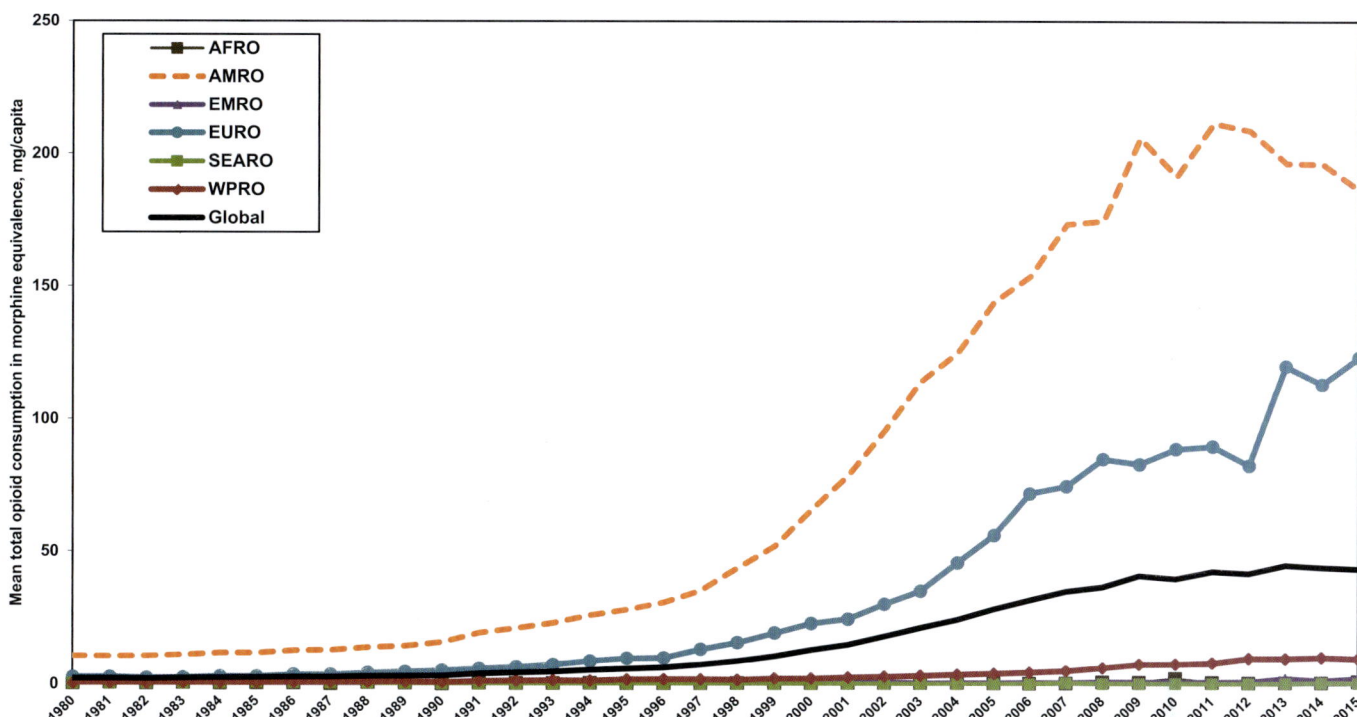

FIGURE 16.3 Global and World Health Organization regional annual total opioid consumption in morphine equivalence (ME) (milligram per capita). AFRO, Africa Regional Office; AMRO, America Regional Office; EMRO, Eastern Mediterranean Regional Office; EURO, Europe Regional Office; SEARO, Southeast Asia Regional Office; WPRO, Western Pacific Regional Office.

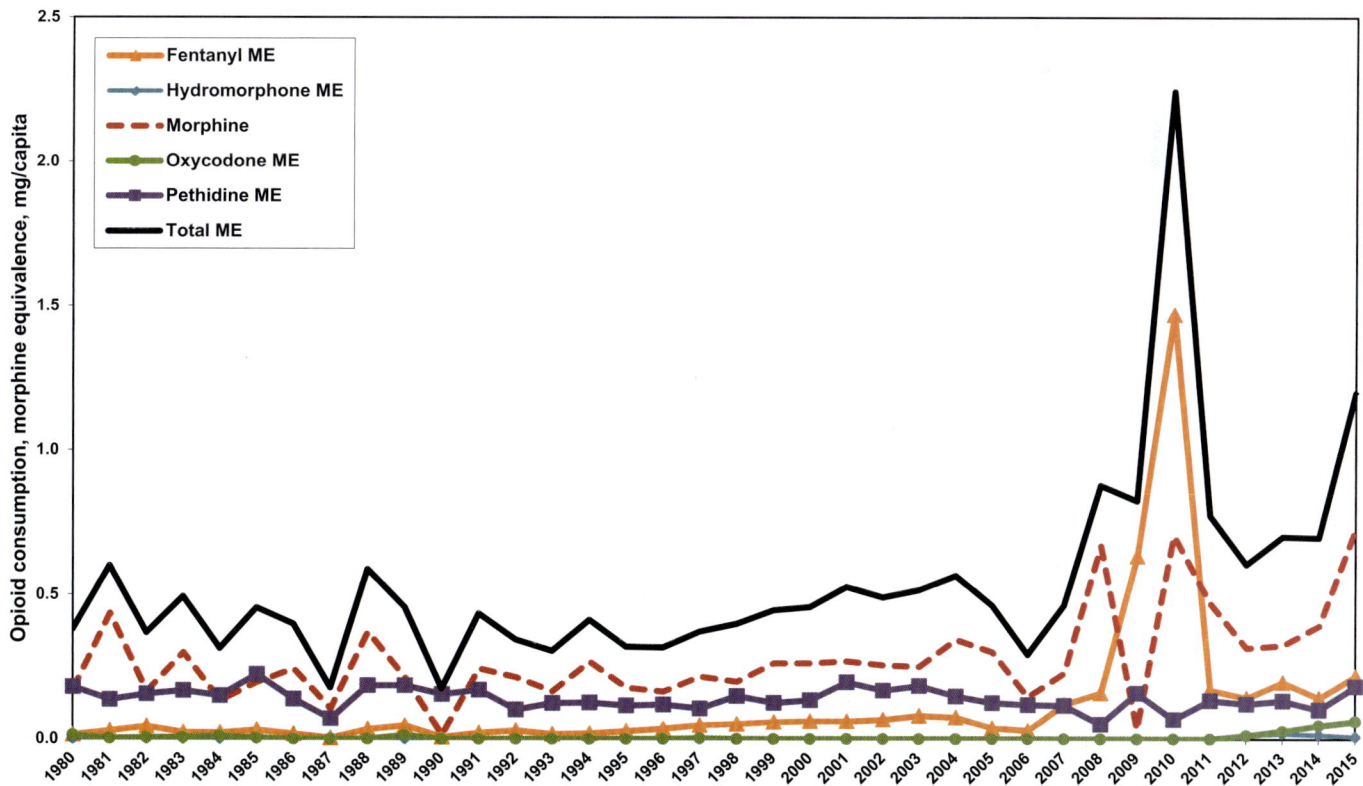

FIGURE 16.4 Opioid consumption in the World Health Organization Regional Office for Africa (AFRO), in morphine equivalence (ME) (milligram per capita).

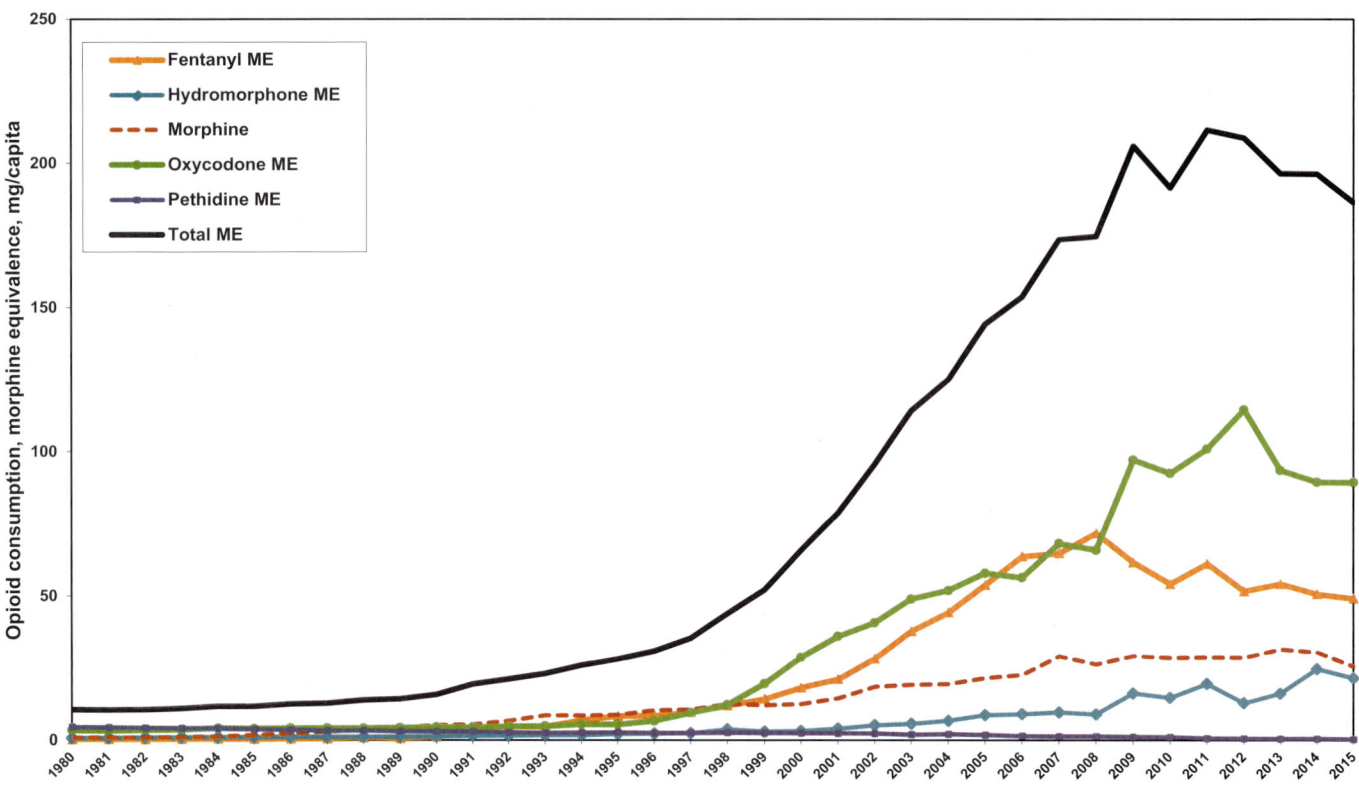

FIGURE 16.5   Opioid consumption in the World Health Organization Regional Office for the Americas (AMRO), in morphine equivalence (ME) (milligram per capita).

WORLD HEALTH ORGANIZATION REGION FOR THE EASTERN MEDITERRANEAN (EMRO)

For EMRO, the total ME opioid consumption has increased fairly consistently since the mid-1990s (Fig. 16.6). Of all the opioids included, fentanyl consumption has risen the most steadily, particularly since 2000 when it exceeded morphine consumption, whereas morphine consumption has seemingly leveled off for more than 20 years, with the exception of a temporary increase in 2014. Oxycodone consumption was low and stable but has slowly increased since 2000, with an upswing in use from 2008 to 2013. Prior to the 1990s, pethidine consumption represented the total ME trend line, but by 2003, fentanyl consumption surpassed it and generally continued to do so. Pethidine consumption, however, remained the second largest contributor to this region's overall ME opioid consumption until about 2010. Hydromorphone consumption was variable, but steady and relatively low, from 1980 to 1991, and then in recent years, it has begun to increase.

WORLD HEALTH ORGANIZATION REGION FOR EUROPE (EURO)

In the EURO, composed of mostly HICs, total ME opioid consumption increased by the largest percentage between 1980 and 2015 as compared with other regions (see Fig. 16.3). Fentanyl consumption has contributed the most to the region's total ME consumption since 2000 (Fig. 16.7). This substantial and steady increase in fentanyl consumption in EURO represented the highest consumption of that medicine for any region, accounting for 73% (90 mg per capita) of the total ME for EURO in 2015 with the next closest region of fentanyl use being AMRO at 26% (49 mg per capita) of that region's total ME for 2015. This strong role of fentanyl in EURO further substantiates the prominent contribution of these countries to the global aggregate consumption. Morphine consumption has been steady since the mid-1990s and has been a distant second in overall contribution to EURO's total ME consumption, until

2012 when oxycodone consumption surpassed it. Hydromorphone consumption has steadily increased during the 35-year period but seems to be leveling off in recent years, whereas pethidine consumption has been consistent and quite low in this region.

WORLD HEALTH ORGANIZATION REGION FOR SOUTHEAST ASIA (SEARO)

Unlike other regions for which the total ME consumption trend increased steadily throughout the 35-year period, the SEARO total ME trend (Fig. 16.8) has been quite irregular with many sharp temporary increases in consumption from the early 1980s until 1990, followed by a sharp decline in morphine and pethidine consumption (which had been the two largest contributors to total ME consumption). In 1990, morphine use dropped below pethidine and remained as such from 1990 to 2006, except for a few years when morphine and pethidine had relatively uniform usages. However, in 2007, morphine use increased substantially but returned to lower levels in 2008 and spiked again in 2014, sharply decreasing in 2015. Fentanyl use had been markedly stable since early 2000s when a very slow by steady increase was evidenced since 2009. As a result, fentanyl and morphine consumption equally contributed more to SEARO's consumption pattern than the other opioids, with fentanyl consumption substantially higher than morphine in 2015 and pethidine consumption slightly declining over the years. Oxycodone and hydromorphone consumption was very low and stable throughout the time period.

WORLD HEALTH ORGANIZATION REGIONS FOR THE WESTERN PACIFIC (WPRO)

As demonstrated in Figure 16.9, the total ME opioid consumption trend for WPRO has been generally increasing over time with a sharp increase beginning in the early 2000s, which appears to be leveling off in recent years. Since about 1999, the top contributor to the WPRO total ME has been

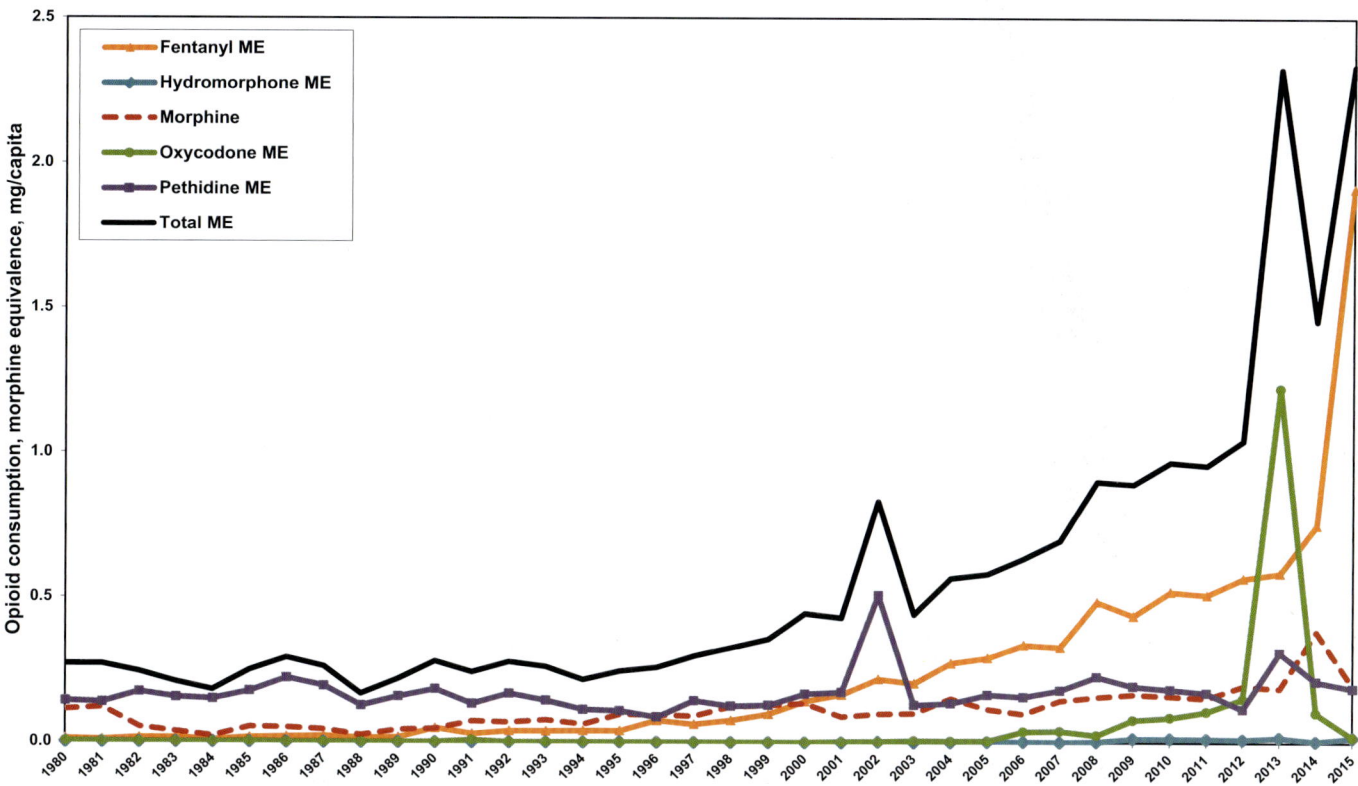

FIGURE 16.6 Opioid consumption in the World Health Organization Regional Office for the Eastern Mediterranean (EMRO), in morphine equivalence (ME) (milligram per capita).

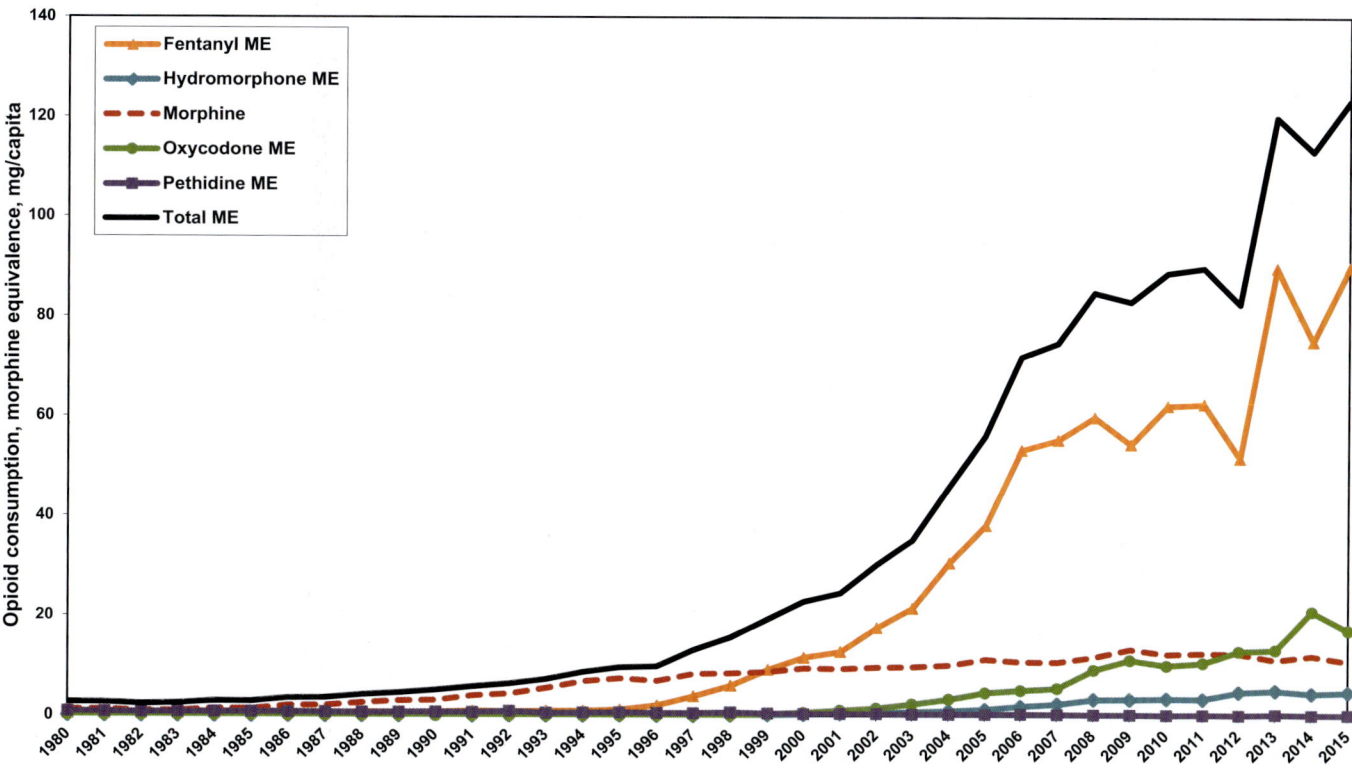

FIGURE 16.7 Opioid consumption in the World Health Organization Regional Office for Europe (EURO), in morphine equivalence (ME) (milligram per capita).

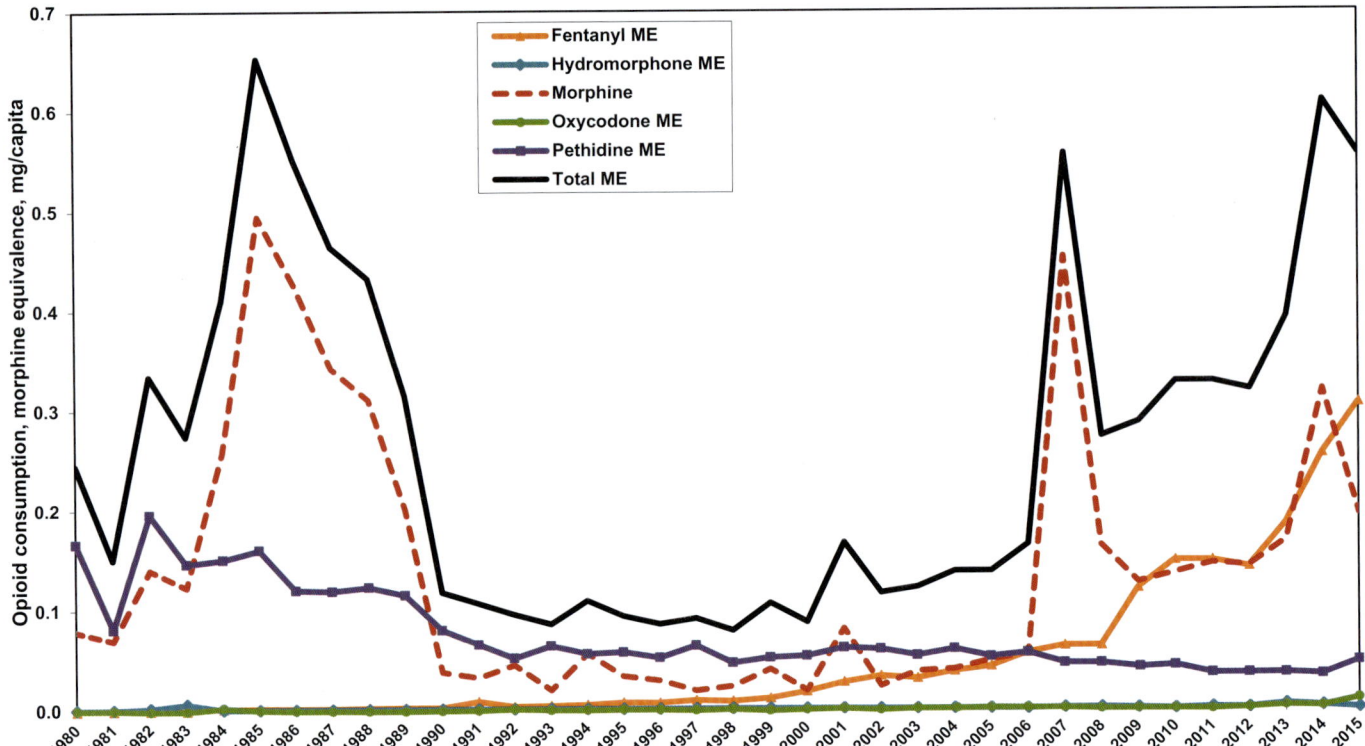

FIGURE 16.8   Opioid consumption in the World Health Organization Regional Office for Southeast Asia (SEARO), in morphine equivalence (ME) (milligram per capita).

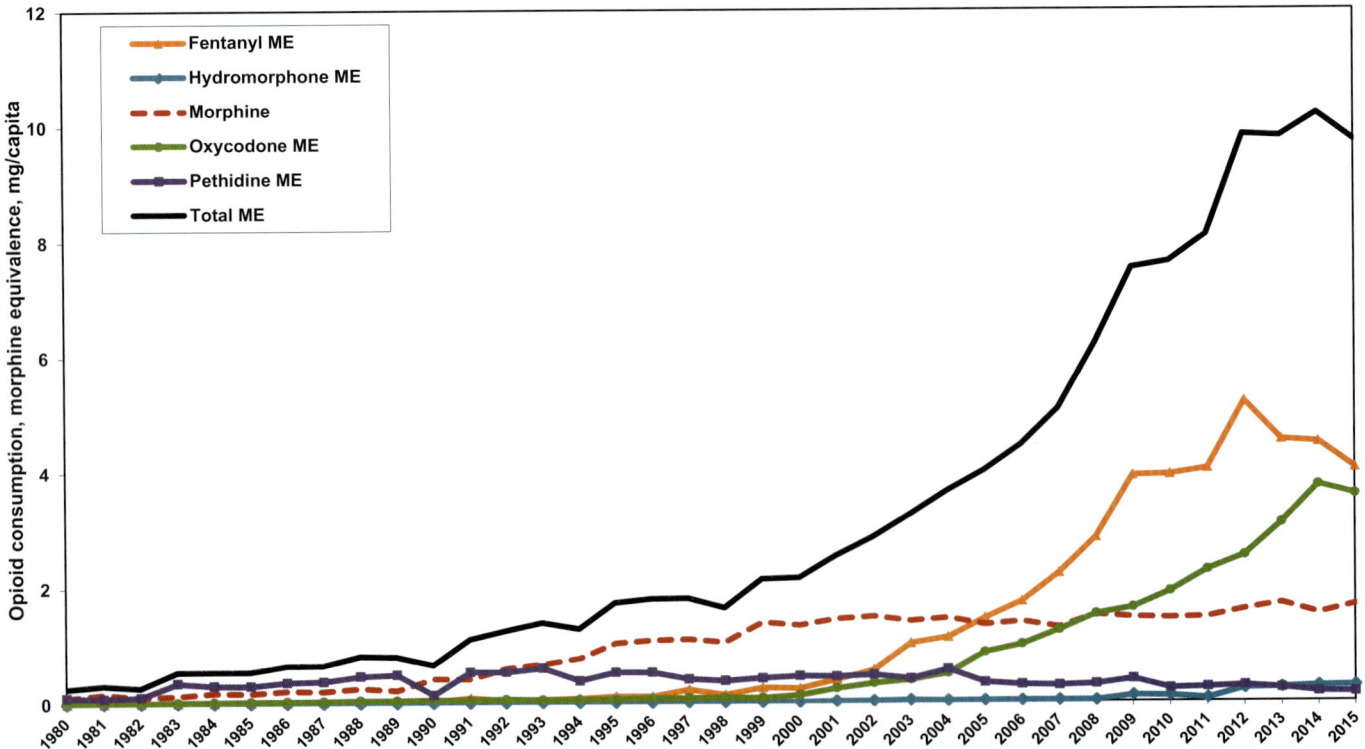

FIGURE 16.9   Opioid consumption in the World Health Organization Regional Office for the Western Pacific (WPRO), in morphine equivalence (ME) (milligram per capita).

fentanyl consumption. Morphine consumption was steadily increasing until the late 1990s but has been relatively constant since 2000. Both fentanyl and oxycodone consumption have exceeded morphine consumption around 2005 and 2009, respectively. Since 2000, fentanyl consumption has accounted for about half of the total ME, whereas in recent years, oxycodone has contributed to a quarter of the overall trend. Pethidine and hydromorphone consumption have been low and stable throughout the 35-year period.

Barriers to Opioid Availability and Accessibility

A number of factors, or barriers, contribute to the inadequate availability and accessibility of opioid medicines which is reflected in low consumption statistics in most of the world. The presence and severity of these barriers varies from country to country. Over the years, a number of barriers to opioid availability and accessibility have been identified through surveys of both government representatives and health care professionals. Because national laws govern the import, manufacture, and use of controlled substances, including controlled opioid medicines, it is critical to know how government drug regulators perceive the issues relating to opioid availability. In 1995, in consultation with the WHO, the INCB conducted their first survey of national governments about impediments to opioid availability in their countries.[4] In 2014, the INCB again surveyed governments about impediments to opioid availability and found that there were some changes since 1995 in the frequency that particular impediments to opioid availability were identified.[6,15] The barriers in Table 16.4 are listed in the order of how many governments identified them, with those listed first being the most frequently identified.

Surveys of health care professionals and, in particular, those with expertise in palliative care have identified very similar barriers as reported by governments to the INCB. A 2006 survey of health care professionals and hospice/palliative care staff from Asia, Africa, and Latin America identified the following barriers to accessing oral morphine: (1) excessively strict national laws and regulations; (2) fear of addiction, tolerance, or side effects; (3) poorly developed health care systems and supply of morphine; and (4) lack of knowledge about pain control and use of morphine on the part of health care professionals, the public, and policy makers.[65]

Another survey of palliative care professionals in 40 countries throughout the world found that there were very limited educational opportunities for health care professionals, 33 of the countries had restrictive regulations on morphine prescribing and nearly half of respondents said that health care professionals have fears of patients developing dependence syndrome or respiratory depression when taking opioids.[66]

The Global Opioid Policy Initiative (GOPI) conducted a survey of practicing palliative care or cancer clinicians in 2011 with responses from 104 countries and states,[67] identifying across-the-board insufficiencies in formulary availability of opioids and regulatory restrictions likely limiting appropriate medical opioid consumption in Africa,[68] Asia,[69] India,[70] Latin America and the Caribbean,[71] and the Middle East.[72]

In recent years, some analyses of the barriers have focused on legal and regulatory policies that have the potential to impede adequate access to opioid medicines. One initiative, the Access to Opioid Medication in Europe (ATOME) project,[73] reviewed relevant national legislation in 11 Eastern and Central European countries to identify legal and regulatory barriers to opioid access. Results of the review indicated that each of the study countries had several potential barriers in the evaluated policies, such as restrictions on controlled medicine prescribing, dispensing, usage, trade and distribution, manufacturing, affordability, and penalties.[74] Another project, led by the PPSG/WHOCC involved a systematic criteria-based evaluation of a selection of countries' policies in Latin America[75] identifying policy language that has the potential to impede opioid availability.

This chapter focuses on the opioid-related barriers involving health professionals, government drug regulatory policies, and medication distribution systems. The barriers are categorized into the following groups:
1. Knowledge and attitudes about pain, opioids, and dependence syndrome
2. Excessively strict laws or regulatory policies
3. Medication distribution system
4. Economic factors (including affordability)

Distinguishing one type of barrier from another is necessary to appropriately target efforts to address them. For example, it would be ineffective and a waste of resources to improve professional education as a solution to what in reality is a regulatory restriction or to work to change national law when its administration or the opioid medication distribution system are the root cause of the problem.

TABLE 16.4 Barriers to Availability of Opioid Medicines as Identified by the 1995 and 2014 International Narcotics Control Board Surveys

1995 Survey	2014 Survey
• Fear of addiction to opioids	• Lack of training of health care professionals about the use of opioids
• Lack of training of health care professionals about the use of opioids	• Fear of addiction to opioids
• Laws or regulations that restrict the manufacture, distribution, prescribing, or dispensing of opioids	• Limited resources
• Reluctance to prescribe or stock opioids stemming from fear of legal consequences	• Problems in sourcing
• Overly burdensome administrative requirements related to opioids	• Cultural/social attitudes
• Insufficient amount of opioids imported or manufactured in the country	• Fear of diversion
• Fear of diversion	• Control measures for international trade
• Cost of opioids	• Fear of prosecution/sanction
• Inadequate health care resources, such as facilities and health care professionals	• Onerous regulatory framework
• Lack of national policy or guidelines related to opioids[4(p5)]	• Overly burdensome administrative requirements related to opioids
	• Other
	• Action by the Board[6(p29)]

Adapted from International Narcotics Control Board. *Report of the International Narcotics Control Board for 1995: Availability of Opiates for Medical Needs.* New York: United Nations; 1996; International Narcotics Control Board. *Availability of Internationally Controlled Drugs: Ensuring Adequate Access for Medical and Scientific Purposes: Indispensable, Adequately Available and Not Unduly Restricted.* New York: United Nations; 2016.

KNOWLEDGE AND ATTITUDES ABOUT PAIN, OPIOIDS, AND DEPENDENCE SYNDROME

Incorrect or insufficient knowledge about pain, opioids, and addiction (i.e., now referred to as *dependence syndrome* in the 10th WHO International Classification of Diseases)[76] often underlies beliefs or attitudes that are reflected in policy and the opioid distribution system, potentially acting as barriers to adequate availability or accessibility.

Inadequate Education of Health Care Professionals

The inadequate education of health care professionals was identified by governments who responded to the INCB surveys[4,6] as well as two global surveys of palliative care professionals identified health care professionals' lack of knowledge about pain control and use of morphine and limited training opportunities as significant barriers to adequate opioid access.[65,66]

Many health care professionals do not have the necessary knowledge to appropriately assess and manage pain.[66,77–80] Professional education programs often do not include training in current pain management practices, and therefore, clinicians may either be unwilling to care for patients with pain or lack the self-confidence to prescribe medications like morphine. If health care professionals do not understand the importance of pain management, they may be reluctant to treat pain or lack the confidence to prescribe strictly controlled medications like morphine. In a 2016 report focused on the accessibility of controlled substances for medical purposes, the INCB added that physicians with insufficient education and training on pain management will likely underestimate the extent that pain can be relieved with appropriate treatment.[6] Indeed, given the major advances in knowledge regarding the treatment of pain, opioids, and dependence syndrome in the last few decades, it is likely that what health professionals and the public learned 30 years ago is now considered outdated and inaccurate.

Concerns about Dependence Syndrome (Addiction)

In 1995, the barrier identified most frequently by government authorities in the INCB survey was concern about opioid-related dependence syndrome (referred to as *addiction* in the report),[4] and in 2014, it was the second most identified impediment to opioid availability.[6] Likewise, surveys of health care professionals have identified similar fears of addiction.[65,66]

In the past, it was thought that mere exposure to morphine or other opioids would result in becoming addicted to it, and evidence of a withdrawal syndrome (a physiologic phenomenon expected from extended opioid use) was thought to be the primary characteristic of addiction.[81,82] However, more recent research about the biopsychosocial mechanisms of dependence syndrome has led to official recognition that its diagnosis depends on the primary characteristics of compulsive behavior and continued use despite harm and not only on the presence of a withdrawal syndrome or analgesic tolerance.[76,83] Evidence suggests that dependence syndrome, when defined correctly and diagnosed accurately, can occur but is not an expected result when opioids are used appropriately to relieve pain, especially when the patient has no history of substance abuse or is not experiencing psychosocial stressors.[10,84] Despite this reality, misperceptions about dependence syndrome contribute to some health care professionals refusing to prescribe opioids and other controlled medicines, which impedes adequate treatment for individuals experiencing severe pain. Continuous efforts are needed to not only increase health care professionals' awareness of the current definition of dependence syndrome but also appropriately apply the diagnostic criteria and, if necessary, treat or refer the patient.[32,61,85,86]

Misinformation among health care professionals about the use of opioid medicines, morphine in particular, appears to stem in part from continued use of outdated knowledge and concepts about opioids and dependence syndrome, coupled with a vivid history of legitimate international concerns about developing a dependence syndrome to illicit opioids (such as opium and heroin), which led to the control of opioids as narcotic drugs.

In some cases, opioids are also legally referred to as *dangerous drugs* and *toxic substances*, designations that do not communicate their important medical aspects. The WHO recommends that such stigmatizing terminology should be avoided.[10] Despite the WHO designating morphine and other opioids as essential medicines for the relief of pain, misunderstandings persist about the risks as well as the benefits of opioid medicines.

Concerns about Potential Side Effects

There are many concerns about the use of opioid medicines and potential side effects because of the long-standing, widespread stigma associated with these medicines. For example, patients and families sometimes fear that managing pain with opioid medicines will result in side effects (e.g., constipation, sedation). Some people assume that the use of opioid medicines for pain means that death is imminent, and for those patients who are near the end of life, frequently, they believe that opioids will hasten death. However, evidence suggests that opioid analgesics do not hasten death, when administered appropriately, and that adequate pain relief can actually improve quality of life and survival.[87–91]

And yet, health care professionals should be aware that there is a real possibility of side effects related to treatment with opioid medicines which should be continuously monitored and addressed when needed. Side effects include constipation, sedation, and nausea as well as the potential for transient cognitive impairment, hyperalgesia, sexual dysfunction, changes in hormone levels, and immune system changes.[35,36,85,92] Health care professionals should be knowledgeable about the potential for these side effects, discuss the benefits and risks of opioid analgesic treatment with the patient, and periodically assess for their possibility throughout treatment.[93]

Health Care Professionals' Fear of Prosecution or Sanction

The WHO has recognized that health care professionals may be reluctant to prescribe or stock opioid medications when they fear loss of their professional license, or even criminal prosecution, if governmental bodies misunderstand or do not recognize the legitimate medical use of opioids to relieve pain.[7] Such fears of prosecution or sanction were identified by the INCB surveys governments[4,6] and surveys of health care professionals and attributed to ambiguous legislation, a lack of legal knowledge, and harsh penalties, which sometimes were for unintentional violations.[66,74]

Some national drug regulations limit the patients who are eligible to receive prescription opioid medicines based on their diagnosis; restrict the dose or the amount that can be prescribed at one time to very low, subtherapeutic quantities; and establish heavy fines and prison sentences for violations. It should be noted that health professionals also may not have accurate information about regulatory requirements, which can contribute to exaggerated concerns and doubts about prescribing opioids. When policy changes are made to improve the regulatory environment for medical use of controlled medicines, it is important that health professionals, law enforcement, and regulatory personnel be educated about clinical aspects of modern pain management as well as the policy changes.

EXCESSIVELY STRICT LAWS OR REGULATORY POLICIES

Clearly, governments' main responsibility is to protect public health and safety, so it is reasonable and necessary for governments to take steps to prevent harms related to diversion and abuse of opioid medicines for nonmedical purposes. The WHO,[7,9,10,94] the INCB,[3–6] and UN member states through the Economic and Social Council (ECOSOC),[12,95] Commission on Narcotic Drugs (CND),[96,97] and the UN General Assembly[98] have repeatedly recognized, however, that that some legislators and administrators have attempted to minimize drug abuse by enacting laws, regulations, and administrative policies that ultimately impede the legitimate availability of opioid medicines. Inadequate knowledge and negative attitudes about opioids often underlie overly restrictive drug control policies.

It is clear that some countries have gone beyond the minimum control measures required by the Single Convention and have established very stringent controls, especially in relation to drug prescription and distribution.[1] These include complex prescription forms and prescription books that must be obtained from the government with considerable difficulty, restrictions that limit the diagnoses of eligible patients, limitations on prescription amount to a few days, limitations on daily dose, and elaborate licensing requirements for palliative care programs. In countries with states, as in India and the United States, some states have enacted restrictive laws and regulations that interfere with opioid distribution and patient access to opioid pain medications.[99–101]

The Single Convention clearly recognizes that governments have the right to regulate narcotic drugs more strictly than required by the Single Convention.[42] While recognizing that this is permissible, the 34th WHO Expert Committee on Drug Dependence (ECDD) said that governments should bear in mind that the aims of the Single Convention are to ensure availability for medical use as well as to prevent abuse. The ECDD called on national authorities to carefully consider whether " . . . any such measure currently in force could be modified to permit access for patients in need."[94]

Examples of regulatory barriers include the following:
- Complex prescription forms and prescription books that must be obtained from the government with considerable difficulty
- Restrictions that limit treatment based on the diagnoses of eligible patients
- Limitations on prescription amount to hours or a few days
- Severe limitations on the number of days that a prescription is valid until dispensed
- Elaborate licensing requirements for health care practitioners or palliative care programs

Table 16.5 provides specific country examples of regulatory requirements with the potential to impede pain management, many of which have since been amended.

MEDICATION DISTRIBUTION SYSTEM BARRIERS

In any country, opioid medications must first be approved and then procured by importation or domestic manufacture from narcotic raw materials or drugs seized by law enforcement. A system of government-regulated distributors then distributes to the retail level of pharmacies, hospitals, clinics, nursing homes, hospices, and palliative care programs, where registered health care professionals prescribe and dispense them to patients. The entire system of medication acquisition and disbursement is referred to as the medication distribution system. Figure 16.10 illustrates the key components of a medication distribution system. Common medication distribution system barriers that can interfere with patient access to opioid medicines include the following:
- Government has not made arrangements for the importation or domestic manufacture of procured opioids.
- There are delays in government decision making about procurement.
- Government's official estimate of type and quantity of opioids required is insufficient.

TABLE 16.5	Examples of Regulatory Requirements with the Potential to Impede Pain Management
Country	**Requirement**
Guatemala	There is an official form for the prescription of medicines that contain any of the substances included in Schedule I of the Single Convention on Narcotic Drugs of 1961. The forms are distributed to doctors by the Ministry of Health at cost, have a special format, and contain the information necessary for that organization. If pharmacies fill prescriptions that are not prescribed using the official prescription book and authorized by the Ministry of Health, this will be regarded as illegally supplying narcotic drugs and will be penalized as such.[75]
India	Prior to 1998 regulatory changes, the national government required all palliative care programs to have a drug license to possess morphine, which would require employment of a pharmacist. Several states have amended their regulations to eliminate the previous requirement of import, export, and transport licenses to move medical morphine from one state to another.[99] In 2014, India passed an amendment to the Narcotic Drugs and Psychotropic Substances Act, a central government policy, which streamlined the process of importing and exporting controlled medicines across state lines within India.[102]
Mexico	Prior to 2015 law changes, Mexico's general health law required that prescriptions for controlled medications carry barcoded stickers, which could only be issued by the health and sanitation authorities at one location in each state's capitals.[75]
Uganda	Prior to 2004, only physicians were allowed to prescribe morphine and other opioids. In 2004, the Ugandan government passed an amendment to the National Drug Policy and Authority Statute allowing specially trained palliative care nurses and clinical officers to prescribe morphine. This greatly expanded the number or health care professionals able to prescribe morphine and allowed Ugandans living in rural areas to have pain relief in their homes.[49]
Vietnam	Prior to a new opioid prescribing regulation in 2008, opioids, such as morphine, could only be prescribed only by doctors working at government hospitals. Opioid prescriptions were not allowed on an outpatient basis, requiring patients to obtain medications in person.[45]

- Government's method for estimating opioid requirements does not take into consideration the actual needs.
- Manufacturers and distributors do not distribute opioids in a timely way.
- Number and geographical distribution of health professionals, pharmacies, and patient care facilities authorized to procure and dispense opioids to patients who need them are insufficient.
- Governments do not have the systems in place to guarantee a safe and effective transfer of medications from wholesalers to retailers.

In some countries, opioid medicines are only available in certain locations, such as a cancer hospital or pharmacies in urban areas. Failure to distribute medications throughout the country can occur for a number of reasons: (1) low demand because of an insufficient number of prescribers and dispensers; (2) lack of reliable modes of transport; (3) lack of information about the need for opioid medicines, including in remote or rural areas; (4) lack of experience in making opioids available; and (5) high cost of medications, making them unaffordable.

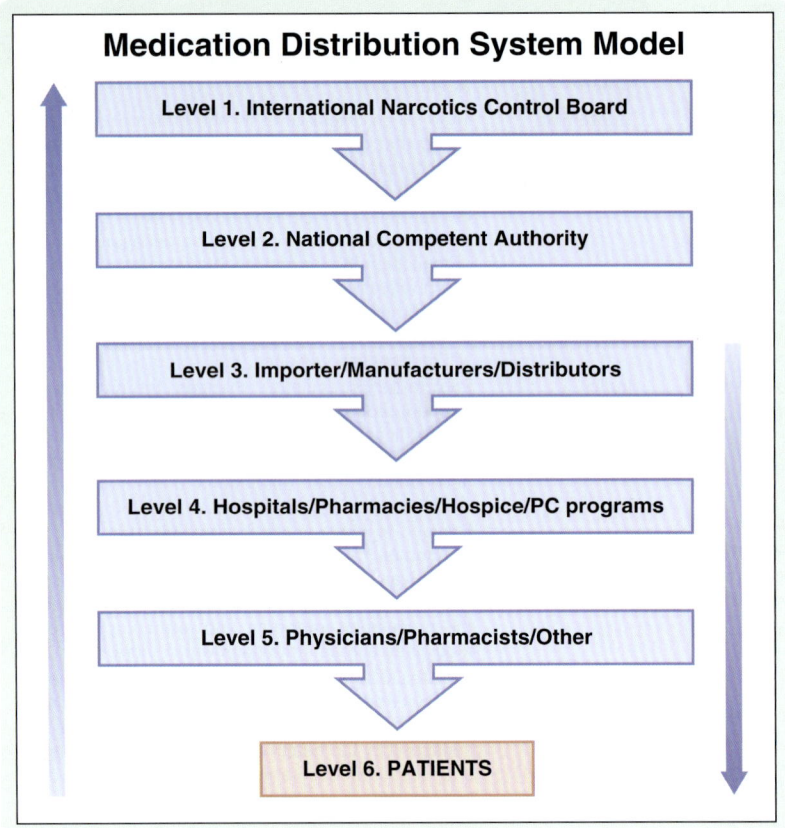

FIGURE 16.10 Controlled medication distribution system model. PC, palliative care.

In 1996, the WHO called on governments to ensure that opioids are available in locations that are accessible to as many cancer patients as possible.[4] In 2011, the WHO emphasized that having a well-functioning system of procurement and distribution is part of a government's obligation to ensure adequate availability and accessibility of controlled medicines.[10]

Restrictions on where opioid medicines can be dispensed can pose a significant barrier to the adequate distribution of opioid medicines throughout a country. The 2011 GOPI survey of palliative care experts in several regions,[67] found that restrictions on where opioids can be dispensed were common among reporting countries in Africa,[68] Asia,[69] the Middle East,[72] and India.[70] In most cases, opioids could only be dispensed at hospital pharmacies in urban areas, and often times, these pharmacies were very difficult to access for patients and families who live far away.

ECONOMIC FACTORS INCLUDING AFFORDABILITY

Economic factors can also be barriers to the availability and accessibility of opioid medicines. The price of opioid analgesic products can be prohibitive when procuring these medicines, as well as when distributing them to the retail level, where they are dispensed to patients. In particular, the dispensed price of opioid analgesic medicines has been identified by international organizations and researchers as a barrier to opioid access.[103–106] Comparative studies of HICs and LMICs have found that opioid costs relative to income was significantly higher in LMICs than in HICs.[103–107]

The GOPI study found that certain formulations of opioid medicines were only available at a high cost for patients.[108] Furthermore, the IAHPC Opioid Price Watch project identified that there is a disparity in the dispensed price between HICs and LMICs, finding that the dispensed price of immediate-release oral morphine (10 mg) was nearly 6 times higher and

less affordable for patients in LMICs than in HICs.[107] Similarly, 32% of the governments who responded to the 2014 INCB survey identified limited financial resources as a barrier to opioid availability,[6] which can be very problematic when the prices of opioids are high.

In some cases, overly restrictive measures limit the availability and accessibility of opioids for pain relief by affecting their affordability. Government-imposed controls and safety measures to minimize the potential for diversion can sometimes affect the dispensed price of opioids, making them more costly for patients.[107] For example, the WHO mentions licenses and registrations for opioids can be prohibitively costly and required safety measures for stocking opioids can be very expensive, preventing pharmacies from procuring them and stocking them.[10]

The cost of procuring opioid formulations can affect government procurement decisions. Immediate-release oral morphine is considered to be a better choice than sustained-release oral morphine as a first-line treatment for acute or cancer pain and is important for initial titration, especially for patients who have never had opioids.[109] At the same time, sustained-release formulations are more costly than immediate-release formulations. Despite this, immediate-release oral morphine is often not available in LMICs, whereas sustained-release oral morphine is typically more widely available. In fact, in some countries, sustained-release oral morphine is being made available prior to, or instead of, immediate-release oral morphine, which may act as a barrier to adequate pain relief.[67,108,110] In 2012, the global pain and palliative care community released the *Morphine Manifesto* calling for governments to ensure the affordable availability of immediate-release oral morphine in advance of sustained-release morphine and other more costly opioids.[111] It is important to consider what other opioid analgesic medicines and formulations are available, rather than considering efficacy or cost alone, to facilitate the best practice for pain management and palliative care.

Therefore, the WHO recommends that countries examine the extent that their control and safety measures are affecting the price of opioid medicines and consider whether the control measures are proportional to the actual risk of diversion. If necessary, countries should work to address any identified barriers.[10]

United Nations' Recommendations

A brief historical review of the recommendations of UN bodies shows they have made a number of useful observations and recommendations to governments and health professionals, including that they should cooperate with each other to ensure adequate availability of opioids for medical purposes including pain relief throughout the world. Indeed, representatives of national governments, acting through their membership in UN bodies, such as the ECOSOC and its CND, and the WHA, have for a number of years called attention to the inadequate availability of opioids and have requested governments to evaluate their national drug control policies for impediments and to improve the availability of opioid medicines for medical purposes.

Beginning in 1989, a consultation between the INCB and the WHO Cancer Unit produced an authoritative recognition of the opioid availability problem and a strong recommendation that governments should act to evaluate their national laws. The INCB requested governments throughout the world to "examine the extent to which their health-care systems and laws and regulations permit the use of opiates for medical purposes, identify possible impediments to such use and develop plans of action to facilitate the supply and availability of opiates for all appropriate indications."[3]

In 1990, the WHO Expert Committee on Cancer Pain Relief and Active Supportive Care made a recommendation similar to that of the INCB, requesting that national governments should conduct a "regular review [of legislation], with the aim of permitting importation, manufacture, prescribing, stocking, dispensing and administration of opioids for medical reasons, . . . [and] review of the controls governing opioid use, with a view to simplification, so that drugs are available in the necessary quantities for legitimate use."[112]

In 1995, the INCB returned to the subject of opioid availability for pain relief and conducted a survey[4] to determine whether governments had responded to its 1989 recommendations.[3] The responses of the 65 responding governments were analyzed and published along with several pointed conclusions and recommendations including that "governments that have not done so should determine whether there are undue restrictions in national narcotics laws, regulations or administrative policies that impede prescribing, dispensing or needed treatment of patients with narcotic drugs, or their availability and distribution for such purposes, and should make the necessary adjustments."[4] The INCB called specific attention to the role of health professionals, recommending that their organizations, including the International Association for the Study of Pain (IASP), teach students and practitioners about the medical use of opioids, their adequate control, and the correct use of terms related to dependence.[4] The INCB further recommended that IASP and other nongovernmental organizations establish ongoing communication about national requirements, unmet medical needs, and impediments to availability with the CNAs in their countries. Such recommendations are consistent with the ethical responsibilities of physicians not only to comply with all laws and regulations but also to work toward changing them if they interfere in the practice of medicine and patient care.[113]

One INCB recommendation in particular was to the WHO to develop "methods that can be used by government and nongovernment organizations to identify impediments to the appropriate medical availability of narcotic drugs."[4] Subsequently, the WHO revised its seminal publication *Cancer Pain Relief*[1] to include a Guide to Opioid Availability[7] and designated the PPSG as a WHO Collaborating Center (WHOCC), with terms of reference to develop methods to improve opioid availability.

In 2000, the WHO published a method for evaluating national policy, *Achieving Balance in National Opioids Control Policy: Guidelines for Assessment*.[9] In coordination with the WHO, PPSG/WHOCC led the development and review of these guidelines which were also endorsed by the INCB. They constituted a consensus at the highest level of international health policy and drug regulation. In 2011, the WHO updated the guidelines, publishing a second and revised version, *Ensuring Balance in National Policies on Controlled Substances: Guidance for Availability and Accessibility of Controlled Medicines*.[10,114] The updated guidelines are broader in scope than the first edition as they cover all controlled medicines, rather than solely focusing on opioid medicines. However, the focus of this chapter is on access to opioid medicines. The WHO guidelines are a central resource as they provide specific criteria to evaluate national policies, their administration, as well as the medication distribution system.

In 2005, the UN ECOSOC adopted a much more specific resolution about the treatment of pain using opioid medicines.[12] It recognized that medical use of narcotic drugs is indispensable for the relief of pain and suffering, that low national consumption of opioids is a matter of great concern, and that opioids such as morphine should be available at all times in adequate amounts and appropriate dosage forms to relieve severe pain. A resolution by the WHA,[115] *Cancer Prevention and Control*, in the same year called for the development of a funding mechanism to facilitate the actions necessary to improve the availability of opioids for the treatment of pain.

In 2010, the CND passed Resolution 53/4 entitled *Promoting Adequate Availability of Internationally Controlled Licit Drugs for Medical and Scientific Purposes While Preventing Their Diversion and Abuse*, calling on member states to take measures to establish a balanced drug control system through various measures including complying with INCB reporting requirements, removing overly restrictive barriers to medication availability, and educating and training health care professionals and patients on proper medication usage.[96]

The following year, the CND adopted Resolution 54/6, which reiterated the same desired outcomes and also requested the United Nations Office on Drugs and Crime (UNODC) to assist in updating the Model Law on controlled substances as well as create a technical guide for members in the regional offices to help member states implement the Single Convention requirements in the least restrictive manner.[97]

Also in 2011, the INCB again returned to the subject of opioid availability for pain relief making this the focus of a special report, entitled, *Report of the International Narcotics Control Board on the Availability of Internationally Controlled Drugs: Ensuring Adequate Access for Medical and Scientific Purposes*.[5] INCB again recommended that governments identify undue restrictions in national laws and regulations and address them as necessary. Notably, INCB also called on governments to determine whether the laws and regulations included important language supporting the availability of and accessibility of opioids such as statements recognizing that they are indispensable for the relief of pain and suffering and that it is the government's responsibility to ensure that they are adequately available.[5]

In 2014, the WHA again demonstrated a commitment to pain management by adopting a palliative care resolution entitled, *Strengthening of Palliative Care as a Component of Comprehensive Care Throughout the Life Course*.[11] Three of the

Resolution's seven recommendations for member states were to integrate palliative care into health care systems, to improve training for health care workers, and to ensure that relevant medicines, including strong pain medicines, are available to patients.

In 2016, the UN General Assembly held a Special Session on the World Drug Problem. At the conclusion of the General Assembly, UN member states adopted an outcome document that for the first time ever made a prominent and strong call for countries to ensure that controlled substances are adequately available for medical use.[98] Controlled medicines are discussed under their own heading in the Outcome Document, expressing concern about the lack of their availability and calling on countries to take a variety of steps to address the issue, including reviewing policies.

Prior to the 2016 UN General Assembly Special Session on the World Drug Problem, the INCB again published a supplementary annual report focusing access to controlled substances for medical and scientific purposes.[6] This report contained several recommendations from the INCB, reiterating the importance of evaluating policies and removing overly restrictive language when necessary.

Taken together, these findings and resolutions form an unmistakable and uncontroversial imperative from the highest level of international and national government health and regulatory authorities in the world that governments and health professionals should work together to identify and remove impediments to the adequate availability of opioids for medical purposes. Additionally, they represent significant momentum to raise the issue of medication availability at the global level and pave the way for concrete actions on the part of UN bodies and member states and other governments.

Efforts to Address Barriers and Improve Opioid Availability and Accessibility

Throughout this chapter, we have explored the relationship between government policy and pain relief, learning how policy and governmental administration is supposed to function to achieve balanced drug control so that opioid medicines are adequately available for medical needs and patient care.

Following the many high-level resolutions, reports and statements made in the last several years by the INCB, the UN ECOSOC, and the UNODC, these bodies have taken action and developed initiatives directed at improving the availability of opioids for pain relief. For example, in the mid-2000s, the WHO developed the Access to Controlled Medications Programme (ACMP)[116] in consultation with the INCB to improve legitimate access to all medications controlled under the international drug conventions. The ACMP's goal was to address all barriers to obtaining controlled medicines for medical treatment including legislative and administrative procedures, as well as knowledge among policy makers, health care workers, patients, and their families. The ACMP facilitated the ATOME project, a collaborative project for improving access to opioid medicines in 12 Eastern and Central European countries.[73] This project also included the revision and update of the WHO Guidelines on Balance in 2011.[10]

Another example of joint INCB and WHO cooperation is the joint 2012 publication, *Guide on Estimating Requirements for Substances Under International Control* (the *Estimate's Guide*), to assist governments in improving the methods and process used to calculate their national estimated requirements for controlled medicines.[53] In particular, the *Estimate's Guide* was designed to address the needs of countries with low consumption of controlled substances for medical purposes in an effort to improve their estimates to better reflect actual requirements. This publication, and the multiagency expert working group that drafted it, represent collaboration among international drug regulatory and health authorities. The INCB continues to offer support for governments in their use of the *Estimate's Guide* and has held a number of regional workshops to assist CNAs in improving their method to calculate their estimated requirements.[117]

Another collaborative effort between international drug and public health authorities, which also included civil society is the partnership between the UNODC, the WHO, and the Union for International Cancer Control (an international nongovernmental organization) to provide an organizing mechanism for a global response to improving access to controlled medicines while preventing the potential for abuse and diversion.[118] Ultimately, the goal of the joint global program is to increase the number of patients globally who are able to get the appropriate treatment for medical conditions, such as cancer pain. Supported by contributions from member states (e.g., Australia, Belgium, United States), this effort to date has included assistance to improve country-level activities such as data collection, regulatory revision and reform, training about estimates and statistics, procurement and distribution, and community-based health care.[118]

Global and regional nongovernmental organizations focused on improving pain and palliative care have also led efforts to improve opioid availability. Over the years, several regional workshops to improve opioid availability have been held drawing together government and nongovernment stakeholders to guide the identification of barriers and develop an action plan. Some of these workshops were organized cooperatively by the PPSG/WHOCC, the WHO, and national and/or regional nongovernmental organizations that had an interest in relieving pain due to cancer and HIV/AIDS,[119–122] whereas other workshops were organized and sponsored by other organizations, such as IAHPC[123] or the African Palliative Care Association.[124,125] These workshops typically have included carefully selected teams of health care and regulatory professionals from five or six countries, often including the CNA. Drawing together country teams from the same region has allowed for participants with cultural similarities and languages to learn together about the methods to improve opioid availability and the challenges and opportunities that often were similar in the region. These workshops culminated in the development of an action plan, which often has led to subsequent implementation of national projects to address barriers to opioid availability.

Similar to regional workshops, national or state workshops involving regulators, expert health care practitioners, and patient care programs have been held to initiate or continue the dialogue between government and health professionals to improve opioid availability for medical needs. Such workshops have been valuable opportunities to exchange information about pain management, palliative care, laws and regulations, and the need for opioids, which has led to increased awareness about the importance of opioid availability. Some national workshops have resulted in action plans that have led to significant changes.

Another important initiative to improve opioid availability at the national level is the International Pain Policy Fellowship (IPPF) program, developed by PPSG/WHOCC in the mid-2000s to expand leadership for improving opioid availability in more countries and increase the rate of positive changes.[126] The goal of the IPPF is to empower motivated health professionals and policy makers from LMICs with the knowledge and skills necessary to identify and overcome barriers to the use of opioids for pain control and palliative care in their country, without sacrificing the security of the existing drug control system. To date, there have been four cohorts of Fellows, comprising 30 individuals from 25 countries, which represents

TABLE 16.6 International Pain Policy Fellows
2006 Cohort
Jorge Eisenchlas (Argentina)
Marta Leon (Colombia)
Daisy Amanor-Boadu (Nigeria)
Rosa Buitrago (Panama)
Snezana Bosnjak (Serbia)
Gabriel Madiye (Sierra Leone)
Henry Ddungu (Uganda)
Nguyen Thi Phuong Cham (Vietnam)
2008 Cohort
Hrant Karapetyan (Armenia)
Irina Kazaryan (Armenia)
Pati Dzotsenidze (Georgia)
Eva Rossina Duarte (Guatemala)
Margaret Dingle Spence (Jamaica)
Verna Walker-Edwards (Jamaica)
Zipporah Ali (Kenya)
Bishnu Paudel (Nepal)
2012 Cohort
Kristo Huta (Albania)
Rumana Dowla (Bangladesh)
Farzana Khan (Bangladesh)
Priyadarshini Kulkarni (India)
Shalini Vallabhan (India)
Nandini Vallath (India)
Taalaigul Sabyrbekova (Kyrgyzstan)
Nadarajah Jeyakumaran (Sri Lanka)
Suraj Perera (Sri Lanka)
Nataliia Datsiuk (Ukraine)
2014 Cohort
Abraham Mengistu (Ethiopia)
Mawuli Gyakobo (Ghana)
Christian Ntizimira (Rwanda)
Nahla Gafer (Sudan)
Lewis Banda (Zambia)

about one-third of the world's population (Table 16.6). The IPPF program has four components including a training program which involves developing an action plan, an in-country project to implement the plan, continuous mentorship from global experts, and an update and review meeting to share progress and challenges with other Fellows.

There are numerous examples of positive outcomes that have resulted from the Fellows' efforts, working with government representatives, experts, PPSG/WHOCC staff, and colleagues both within and outside their countries. Several articles have been published describing Fellow's in-country efforts to improve opioid availability and accessibility.[44,45,48,102,127–129] These positive country-level outcomes, facilitated by the IPPF program, have likely contributed to increases in the very small amounts of opioids consumed prior to the IPPF. For example, in Serbia, total consumption of strong opioids increased more than twofold between 2006 and 2012, and from 2009 and 2014, the amount of immediate-release oral morphine sold to hospitals more than tripled.[127] Furthermore, a recent study found that Serbia's adequacy of opioid consumption increased by nearly 83% between 2006 and 2010.[14]

After completing the IPPF, several Fellows have served as mentors to subsequent Fellows. Many have developed as leaders and experts on access to opioid medicines, published articles about their work,[44,45,48,102,127–129] attended international meetings on forming policy, and successfully advocated for positive changes in the laws and regulations in their countries.

Conclusion

Deepening disparities between HICs and LMICs in the extent of availability of opioid pain medicines means that pain and suffering in the world is an increasing public health problem. This is cause for alarm and should precipitate concerted action by health professionals, their organizations, and their governments. Actions should be guided by an understanding not only of the need for pain medicines but also of the barriers, the drug control policy framework, and how to work with government drug regulators.

However, health care professionals from any country are not likely to know about these topics because they have not generally been included in basic professional education or continuing education about pain and palliative care. The purpose of this chapter is to outline the body of knowledge, methods, and experience that is relevant to understanding and improving national opioid availability and patient access to pain medicines.

Although the body of knowledge about the control and availability of opioid medicines may not be well known, the process of working with individual countries to improve opioid availability borrows from a method with which health professionals are very familiar. The elements of the medical model can be applied to solving problems in opioid availability: evaluation, diagnosis, and a treatment plan. Indeed, health care professionals and governments within countries have worked together to diagnose opioid availability barriers and implement action plans to remove the barriers. More recent efforts to diagnose and treat barriers have been led by International Pain Policy Fellows in LMICs.

There are hopeful signs of progress in some countries, but it is not likely that this progress—which is still in an early developmental phase—is sufficient to gain on the deepening global disparities in access to pain relief medications. Greater leadership and sustained efforts are needed to continue to make policy and regulatory improvements to ultimately relive patient suffering. The increasing prevalence of NCDs in LMICs and reduced funding opportunities will likely continue to be challenges for years to come. Now more than ever, there is a critical need for support and action on the part of UN agencies, governments, and palliative care nongovernmental organization to work collaboratively to relieve this suffering.

References

1. World Health Organization. *Cancer Pain Relief.* Geneva, Switzerland: World Health Organization; 1986.
2. World Health Organization. *A Community Health Approach to Palliative Care for HIV/AIDS and Cancer Patients in Sub-Saharan Africa.* Geneva, Switzerland: World Health Organization; 2004.
3. International Narcotics Control Board. *Report of the International Narcotics Control Board for 1989: Demand for and Supply of Opiates for Medical and Scientific Needs.* Vienna, Austria: United Nations; 1989.
4. International Narcotics Control Board. *Report of the International Narcotics Control Board for 1995: Availability of Opiates for Medical Needs.* New York: United Nations; 1996.
5. International Narcotics Control Board. *Report of the International Narcotics Control Board on the Availability of Internationally Controlled Drugs: Ensuring Adequate Access for Medical and Scientific Purposes.* New York: United Nations; 2011.
6. International Narcotics Control Board. *Availability of Internationally Controlled Drugs: Ensuring Adequate Access for Medical and Scientific Purposes: Indispensable, Adequately Available and Not Unduly Restricted.* New York: United Nations; 2016.
7. World Health Organization. *Cancer Pain Relief: With a Guide to Opioid Availability.* 2nd ed. Geneva, Switzerland: World Health Organization; 1996.
8. World Health Organization. *Symptom Relief in Terminal Illness.* Geneva, Switzerland: World Health Organization; 1998.
9. World Health Organization. *Achieving Balance in National Opioids Control Policy: Guidelines for Assessment.* Geneva, Switzerland: World Health Organization; 2000.
10. World Health Organization. *Ensuring Balance in National Policies on Controlled Substances: Guidance for Availability and Accessibility of Controlled Medicines.* 2nd ed, rev ed. Geneva, Switzerland: World Health Organization; 2011.

11. World Health Assembly. *Strengthening of Palliative Care as a Component of Comprehensive Care Throughout the Life Course.* Geneva, Switzerland: World Health Organization, 2014. WHA67.19.

12. United Nations Economic and Social Council. *Treatment of Pain Using Opioid Analgesics.* New York: United Nations; 2005. Resolution 2005/25.

13. Seya MJ, Gelders SF, Achara OU, et al. A first comparison between the consumption of and the need for opioid analgesics at country, regional and global level. *J Pain Palliat Care Pharmacother* 2011;25:6–18.

14. Duthey B, Scholten W. Adequacy of opioid analgesic consumption at country, global, and regional levels in 2010, its relationship with development level, and changes compared with 2006. *J Pain Symptom Manage* 2014;47:283–297.

15. Berterame S, Erthal J, Thomas J, et al. Use of and barriers to access to opioid analgesics: a worldwide, regional and national study. *Lancet* 2016;387:1644–1656.

16. Global Burden of Disease Cancer Collaboration. Global, regional and national cancer incidence, mortality, years of life lost, years lived with disability, and disability-adjusted life-years for 32 cancer groups, 1990 to 2015: a systematic analysis for the global burden of disease study. *JAMA Oncol* 2017;3:524–548.

17. World Health Organization. *World Cancer Report 2014.* Lyon, France: IARC Press; 2014.

18. Joint United Nations Programme on HIV/AIDS. *Global AIDS Update 2016.* Geneva, Switzerland: Joint United Nations Programme on HIV/AIDS; 2016.

19. Woodruff R, Cameron D. HIV/AIDS in adults. In: Hanks G, Cherny N, Christakis NA, et al, eds. *Oxford Textbook of Palliative Care.* 4th ed. New York: Oxford University Press; 2010:1195–1230.

20. Lohman D, Schleifer R, Amon JJ. Access to pain treatment as a human right. *BMC Med* 2010;8:8.

21. Portenoy RK, Thaler HT, Kornblith AB, et al. Symptom prevalence, characteristics and distress in a cancer population. *Qual Life Res* 1994;3:183–189.

22. Grond S, Zech DF, Diefenbach CF, et al. Prevalence and pattern of symptoms in patients with cancer pain: a prospective evaluation of 1635 cancer patients referred to a pain clinic. *J Pain Symptom Manage* 1994;9:372–382.

23. Vainio A, Auvinen A. Prevalence of symptoms among patients with advanced cancer: an international collaborative study. *J Pain Symptom Manage* 1996;12:3–10.

24. Burton AW, Fanciullo GJ, Beasley RD, et al. Chronic pain in the cancer survivor: a new frontier. *Pain Med* 2007;8:189–197.

25. Glare PA. Pain in cancer survivors. *J Clin Oncol* 2014;32:1739–1747.

26. Worldwide Hospice and Palliative Care Alliance. *Global Atlas of Palliative Care at the End of Life.* London: Worldwide Hospice and Palliative Care Alliance; 2014.

27. Foley KM, Wagner JL, Joranson DE, et al. Pain control for people with cancer and AIDS. In: Jamison DT, Breman JG, Measham AR, et al, eds. *Disease Control Priorities in Developing Countries.* New York: Oxford University Press; 2006:981–993.

28. Goudas LC, Bloch R, Gialeli-Goudas M, et al. The epidemiology of cancer pain. *Cancer Invest* 2005;23:182–190.

29. Davis MP, Walsh D. Epidemiology of cancer pain and factors influencing poor pain control. *Am J Hosp Palliat Care* 2004;21(2):137–142.

30. World Health Organization HIV-AIDS. *Palliative Care.* Geneva, Switzerland: World Health Organization; 2004.

31. World Health Organization. *Cancer Pain Relief and Palliative Care in Children.* Geneva, Switzerland: World Health Organization; 1998.

32. World Health Organization. *WHO Guidelines on the Pharmacological Treatment of Persisting Pain in Children with Medical Illnesses.* Geneva, Switzerland: World Health Organization; 2012.

33. World Health Organization. *National Cancer Control Programmes: Policies and Managerial Guidelines.* 2nd ed. Geneva, Switzerland: World Health Organization; 2002.

34. World Health Organization. *Cancer Control: Knowledge into Action: WHO Guides for Effective Programmes—Palliative Care.* Geneva, Switzerland: World Health Organization; 2007.

35. Hanks GW, Cherny N, Fallon M. Opioid analgesic therapy. In: Doyle D, Hanks GW, MacDonald N, et al, eds. *Oxford Textbook of Palliative Medicine.* New York: Oxford University Press; 2004:316–341.

36. Caraceni A, Hanks G, Kaasa S, et al. Use of opioid analgesics in the treatment of cancer pain: evidence-based recommendations from the EAPC. *Lancet Oncol* 2012;13:e58–e68.

37. Wiffen PJ, Wee B, Moore RA. Oral morphine for cancer pain. *Cochrane Database Syst Rev* 2016;(4):CD003868. Available at: http://cochranelibrary-wiley.com/doi/10.1002/14651858.CD003868.pub4/full. Accessed May 7, 2018.

38. World Health Organization. *Essential Medicines—WHO Model List.* Geneva, Switzerland: World Health Organization; 1977.

39. World Health Organization. Essential medicines. Available at: http://www.who.int/topics/essential_medicines/en/. Accessed May 7, 2018.

40. World Health Organization. *WHO Model List of Essential Medicines.* 18th ed. Geneva, Switzerland: World Health Organization; 2013.

41. World Health Organization. *WHO Model List of Essential Medicines.* 20th ed. Geneva, Switzerland: World Health Organization; 2017.

42. United Nations. *Single Convention on Narcotic Drugs, 1961, as Amended by the 1972 Protocol Amending the Single Convention on Narcotic Drugs, 1961.* New York: United Nations; 1972.

43. International Narcotics Control Board. *1961 Single Convention on Narcotic Drugs: Part 1: The International Control System for Narcotic Drugs.* Vienna, Austria: International Narcotics Control Board; 2005.

44. Paudel BD, Ryan KM, Skemp-Brown M, et al. Opioid availability and palliative care in Nepal: influence of an International Pain Policy Fellowship. *J Pain Symptom Manage* 2015;49:110–116.

45. Krakauer EL, Cham NTP, Husain SA, et al. Toward safe accessibility of opioid pain medicines in Vietnam and other developing countries: a balanced policy method. *J Pain Symptom Manage* 2015;49:916–922.

46. Pain & Policy Studies Group. *International Pain Policy Fellowship—Farzana Khan.* Madison, WI: University of Wisconsin; 2016. Available at: http://ppsg8.dom.wisc.edu/sites/default/files/2018-03/Khan.pdf. Accessed May 7, 2018.

47. Rajagopal MR, Joranson DE, Gilson AM. Medical use, misuse, and diversion of opioids in India. *Lancet* 2001;358:139–143.

48. Bosnjak S, Maurer MA, Ryan KM, et al. Improving the availability and accessibility of opioids for the treatment of pain: the International Pain Policy Fellowship. *Support Care Cancer* 2011;19:1239–1247.

49. Jagwe J, Merriman A. Uganda: delivering analgesia in rural Africa: opioid availability and nurse prescribing. *J Pain Symptom Manage* 2007;33:547–551.

50. Bayer I, Ghodse H. Evolution of international drug control, 1945-1995. *Bull Narc* 1999;51(1–2):1–17.

51. International Narcotics Control Board. *1961 Single Convention on Narcotic Drugs: Part 2: The Estimates System for Narcotic Drugs.* Vienna, Austria: International Narcotics Control Board; 2005.

52. International Narcotics Control Board. *1961 Single Convention on Narcotic Drugs: Part 3: The Statistical Returns System for Narcotic Drugs.* Vienna, Austria: International Narcotics Control Board; 2005.

53. International Narcotics Control Board, World Health Organization. *Guide on Estimating Requirements for Substances Under International Control.* Vienna, Austria: United Nations; 2012.

54. International Narcotics Control Board. *Guidelines for National Competent Authorities.* Vienna, Austria: International Narcotics Control Board; 2007.

55. International Narcotics Control Board. *Narcotic Drugs: Estimated World Requirements for 2017—Statistics for 2015.* New York: United Nations; 2017.

56. Joranson DE, Ryan KM, Maurer MA. Opioid policy, availability and access in developing and nonindustrialized countries. In: Fishman SM, Ballantyne JC, Rathmell JP, eds. *Bonica's Management of Pain.* 4th ed. Baltimore, MD: Lippincott Williams & Wilkins; 2010:194–208.

57. Joranson DE, Ryan KM. Ensuring opioid availability: methods and resources. *J Pain Symptom Manage* 2007;33:527–532.

58. Hastie BA, Gilson AM, Maurer MA, et al. An examination of global and regional consumption trends 1980-2011. *J Pain Palliat Care Pharmacother* 2014;28:259–275.

59. World Health Organization Collaborating Centre for Drug Statistics Methodology. *Anatomical Therapeutic Chemical/Defined Daily Dose.* Oslo, Norway: Norwegian Institute of Public Health; 2017. Available at: https://www.whocc.no/atc_ddd_index/. Accessed May 7, 2018.

60. Gilson AM, Maurer MA, Ryan KM, et al. Using a morphine equivalence metric to quantify opioid consumption: examining the capacity to provide effective treatment of debilitating pain at the global, regional, and country levels. *J Pain Symptom Manage* 2013;45:681–700.

61. National Institute for Health and Care Excellence. *Opioids in Palliative Care: Safe and Effective Prescribing of Strong Opioids for Pain in Palliative Care of Adults.* Manchester, United Kingdom: National Institute for Health and Care Excellence; 2012. NICE clinical guideline 140.

62. Miaskowski C, Cleary J, Burney R, et al. *Guideline for the Management of Cancer Pain in Adults and Children.* Glenview, IL: American Pain Society; 2005. APS clinical practice guidelines series no. 3.

63. Teoh N, Vainio A. The status of pethidine in the WHO Model List of Essential Drugs. *Palliat Med* 1991;5:185–186.

64. World Health Organization. *Essential Medicines—WHO Model List.* 15th ed. Geneva, Switzerland: World Health Organization; 2007.

65. Adams V. *Access to Pain Relief—An Essential Human Right: A Report for World Hospice and Palliative Care Day 2007.* London: Worldwide Palliative Care Alliance; 2007.

66. Human Rights Watch. *Global State of Pain Treatment: Access to Palliative Care as a Human Right.* New York: Human Rights Watch; 2011.

67. Cherny NI, Cleary J, Scholten W, et al. The Global Opioid Policy Initiative (GOPI) project to evaluate the availability and accessibility of opioids for the management of cancer pain in Africa, Asia, Latin America and the Caribbean, and the Middle East: introduction and methodology. *Ann Oncol* 2013;24:xi7–xi13.

68. Cleary J, Powell RA, Munene G, et al. Formulary availability and regulatory barriers to accessibility of opioids for cancer pain in Africa: a report from the Global Opioid Policy Initiative (GOPI). *Ann Oncol* 2013;24:xi14–xi23.

69. Cleary J, Radbruch L, Torode J, et al. Formulary availability and regulatory barriers to accessibility of opioids for cancer pain in Asia: a report from the Global Opioid Policy Initiative (GOPI). *Ann Oncol* 2013;24:xi24–xi32.

70. Cleary J, Simha N, Panieri A, et al. Formulary availability and regulatory barriers to accessibility of opioids for cancer pain in India: a report from the Global Opioid Policy Initiative (GOPI). *Ann Oncol* 2013;24:xi33–xi40.

71. Cleary J, De Lima L, Eisenchlas J, et al. Formulary availability and regulatory barriers to accessibility of opioids for cancer pain in Latin America and the Caribbean: a report from the Global Opioid Policy Initiative (GOPI). *Ann Oncol* 2013;24:xi41–xi50.

72. Cleary J, Silbermann M, Scholten W, et al. Formulary availability and regulatory barriers to accessibility of opioids for cancer pain in the Middle East: a report from the Global Opioid Policy Initiative (GOPI). *Ann Oncol* 2013;24:xi51–xi59.

73. Junger S, Larjow E, Linge-Dahl L, et al. *Access to Opioid Medication in Europe: Final Report and Recommendations to the Ministries of Health.* Bonn, Germany: Pallia Med Verlag; 2014.

74. Vranken MJM, Lisman JA, Mantel-Teeuwisse AK, et al. Barriers to access to opioid medicines: a review of national legislation and regulations of 11 central and eastern European countries. *Lancet Oncol* 2016;17:e13–e22.

75. Pain & Policy Studies Group. *Improving Global Opioid Availability for Pain & Palliative Care: A Guide to a Pilot Evaluation of National Policy.* Madison, WI: University of Wisconsin Carbone Cancer Center; 2013. Available at: http://www.painpolicy.wisc.edu/sites/default/files/sites /www.painpolicy.wisc.edu/files/Global%20evaluation%202013.pdf. Accessed May 7, 2018.

76. World Health Organization. *The ICD-10 Classification of Mental and Behavioural Disorders: Clinical Descriptions and Diagnostic Guidelines.* Geneva, Switzerland: World Health Organization; 2006.

77. Bistre S, Strauss Y. Errors in pain management: a Mexican perspective. *J Pain Palliat Care Pharmacother* 2012;26:266–270.

78. Bosnjak S, Susnjar S, Dimitrijevic J. Barriers relating to knowledge and attitudes about opioids among healthcare professionals in Serbia [abstract]. *Support Care Cancer* 2010;18:S67–S220.

79. Harding R, Powell RA, Kiyange F, et al. Provision of pain- and symptom-relieving drugs for HIV/AIDS in Sub-Saharan Africa. *J Pain Symptom Manage* 2010;40:405–415.

80. Zenz M, Zenz T, Tryba M, et al. Severe undertreatment of cancer pain: a 3-year survey of the German situation. *J Pain Symptom Manage* 1995;10:187–191.

81. World Health Organization. *WHO Expert Committee on Drugs Liable to Produce Addiction: Second Report.* Geneva, Switzerland: World Health Organization; 1950. Technical report series 21.

82. World Health Organization. *WHO Expert Committee on Drugs Liable to Produce Addiction: Third Report.* Geneva, Switzerland: World Health Organization; 1952. Technical report series 57.

83. World Health Organization. *The ICD-10 Classification of Mental and Behavioral Disorders: Clinical Descriptions and Diagnostic Guidelines.* Geneva, Switzerland: World Health Organization; 1992.

84. Minozzi S, Amato L, Davoli M. Development of dependence following treatment with opioid analgesics for pain relief: a systematic review. *Addiction* 2012;108:688–698.

85. Chou R, Fanciullo GJ, Fine PG, et al. Clinical guidelines for the use of chronic opioid therapy for chronic noncancer pain. *J Pain* 2009;10:113–130.

86. Kahan M, Mailis-Gagnon A, Wilson L, et al. Canadian guideline for safe and effective use of opioids for chronic noncancer pain. *Can Fam Physician* 2011;57:1257–1266.

87. Jolly M, Cornock M. Application of the doctrine of double effect in end stage disease. *Int J Palliat Nurs* 2003;9:240–244.

88. Meier DE, Brawley OW. Palliative care and the quality of life. *J Clin Oncol* 2011;29:2750–2752.

89. Rocque GB, Cleary JF. Palliative care reduces morbidity and mortality in cancer. *Nat Rev Clin Oncol* 2013;10:80–89.

90. Temel JS, Greer JA, Muzikansky A, et al. Early palliative care for patients with metastatic non-small-cell lung cancer. *N Engl J Med* 2010;363:733–742.

91. Van der Heide A, Deliens L, Faisst K, et al. End-of-life decision-making in six European countries: descriptive study. *Lancet* 2003;362:345–350.

92. Fallon M, Cherny NI, Hanks G. Opioid analgesic therapy. In: Hanks G, Cherny NI, Christakis NA, et al, eds. *Oxford Textbook of Palliative Medicine.* 4th ed. New York: Oxford University Press; 2010:661–698.

93. World Medical Association. WMA resolution on the access to adequate pain treatment. Paper presented at: 62nd World Medical Association General Assembly; October 2011; Montevideo, Uruguay.

94. World Health Organization. *WHO Expert Committee on Drug Dependence: Thirty-Fourth Report.* Geneva, Switzerland: World Health Organization; 2006.

95. United Nations Economic and Social Council. *Demand for and Supply of Opiates Used to Meet Medical and Scientific Needs.* New York: United Nations; 2005. Resolution 2005/26.

96. United Nations Economic and Social Council. *Promoting Adequate Availability of Internationally Controlled Licit Drugs for Medical and Scientific Purposes While Preventing Their Diversion and Abuse.* New York: United Nations; 2010. Resolution 53/4.

97. United Nations Economic and Social Council. *Promoting Adequate Availability of Internationally Controlled Narcotic Drugs and Psychotropic Substances for Medical and Scientific Purposes While Preventing Their Diversion and Abuse.* New York: United Nations; 2011. Resolution 54/6.

98. United Nations General Assembly. *S-30/1. Our Joint Commitment to Effectively Addressing and Countering the World Drug Problem.* New York: United Nations; 2016. Resolution S-30/1.

99. Joranson DE, Rajagopal MR, Gilson AM. Improving access to opioid analgesics for palliative care in India. *J Pain Symptom Manage* 2002;24:152–159.

100. Gilson AM, Rich BA. Legal and regulatory issues in pain management. In: Benzon HT, Raja SN, Liu SS, et al, eds. *Essentials of Pain Medicine.* 4th ed. Philadelphia: Elsevier Saunders; 2016.

101. Pain & Policy Studies Group. *Achieving Balance in State Pain Policy: A Progress Report Card (CY 2015).* Madison, WI: University of Wisconsin Carbone Cancer Center; 2016.

102. Vallath N, Tandon T, Pastrana T, et al. Civil society-driven drug policy reform for health and human welfare—India. *J Pain Symptom Manage* 2017;53:518–532.

103. De Conno F, Ripamonti C, Brunelli C. Opioid purchases and expenditure in nine western European countries: 'are we killing off morphine?' *Palliat Med* 2005;19:179–184.

104. De Lima L, Sweeney C, Palmer JL, et al. Potent analgesics are more expensive for patients in developing countries: a comparative study. *J Pain Palliat Care Pharmacother* 2004;18:59–70.

105. Mercadante S. Costs are a further barrier to cancer pain management. *J Pain Symptom Manage* 1999;18:3–4.

106. Moyano J, Ruiz F, Esser S, et al. Latin American survey on the treatment of cancer pain. *Eur J Palliat Care* 2006;13:236–240.

107. De Lima L, Pastrana T, Radbruch L, et al. Cross-sectional pilot study to monitor the availability, dispensed prices and affordability of opioids around the globe. *J Pain Symptom Manage* 2014;48:649–659.

108. Cleary J, Radbruch L, Torode J, et al. Next steps in access and availability of opioids for the treatment of cancer pain: reaching the tipping point? *Annals of Oncol* 2013;24:60–64.

109. Fitzgibbon DR. Cancer pain: principles of management and pharmacotherapy. In: Fishman SM, Ballantyne JC, Rathmell JP, eds. *Bonica's Management of Pain.* 4th ed. Philadelphia: Lippincott Williams & Wilkins; 2010:582–604.

110. Cherny NI, Baselga J, De Conno F, et al. Formulary availability and regulatory barriers to accessibility of opioids for cancer pain in Europe: a report from the ESMO/EAPC Opioid Policy Initiative. *Ann Oncol* 2010;21:615–626.

111. Pallium India, International Association for Hospice and Palliative Care, Pain & Policy Studies Group. *The Morphine Manifesto: A Call for Affordable Access to Immediate Release Oral Morphine.* Kerala, India: Pallium India; 2012.

112. World Health Organization. *Cancer Pain Relief and Palliative Care: Report of the WHO Expert Committee on Cancer Pain Relief and Active Supportive Care.* Geneva, Switzerland: World Health Organization; 1990. Technical report series 804.

113. American Academy of Pain Medicine Council on Ethics. *Ethics Charter.* Glenview, IL: American Academy of Pain Medicine; 2005.

114. Gilson AM, Maurer MA, Ryan KM, et al. Ensuring patient access to essential medicines while minimizing harmful use: a revised WHO tool to improve national drug control policy. *J Pain Palliat Care Pharmacother* 2011;25:246–251.

115. World Health Assembly. *Cancer Prevention and Control.* Geneva, Switzerland: World Health Organization; 2005. WHA 58.22.

116. World Health Organization. *Access to Controlled Medications Programme: Improving Access to Medications Controlled Under International Drug Conventions.* Geneva, Switzerland: World Health Organization; 2012.

117. International Narcotics Control Board. *INCB Learning Project Kicks Off Regional Training for Europe in Vienna.* Vienna, Austria: United Nations Information Service; 2017. Available at: https://www.incb.org/incb/en/news /press-releases/2017/press_release_20170704.html. Accessed May 7, 2018.

118. United Nations Office on Drugs and Crime. *Access to Controlled Drugs for Medical Purposes, While Preventing Diversion and Abuse.* Vienna, Austria: United Nations; 2017. Available at: https://www.unodc.org/unodc/en/drug -prevention-and-treatment/access-to-controlled-medicines/accessibility -medicines-availability-glok67.html. Accessed May 7, 2018.

119. World Health Organization Regional Office for the Eastern Mediterranean. *Summary Report on the Intercountry Meeting on controlled medicines.* Geneva, Switzerland: World Health Organization; 2016.

120. World Health Organization Regional Office for Europe. *Assuring Availability of Opioid Analgesics for Palliative Care. Report on a WHO Workshop.* Budapest, Hungary: World Health Organization Regional Office for Europe; 2002.

121. Pain & Policy Studies Group. Availability of opioid analgesics in the world and Asia with a special focus on: Indonesia, Philippines, Thailand. Paper presented at: Workshop on Assuring Availability and Accessibility of Opioid Analgesics for Pain and Palliative Care; April 2008; Madison, WI.

122. Pain & Policy Studies Group. Availability of opioid analgesics in the world and Europe, with a special focus on: Armenia, Republic of Moldova, Ukraine. Paper presented at: Workshop on Assuring Availability and Accessibility of Opioid Analgesics for Pain and Palliative Care; October 2008; Madison WI.

123. De Lima L, Pastrana T. Evaluation of the effectiveness of workshops on the availability and rational use of opioids in Latin America. *J Palliat Med* 2016;19:964–971.

124. African Palliative Care Association. *Advocacy Workshop for Palliative Care in Africa: A Focus on Essential Pain Medication Accessibility.* Kampala, Uganda: African Palliative Care Association; 2007.

125. African Palliative Care Association. *Advocacy Workshop for Palliative Care in Africa: A Focus on Essential Pain Medication Accessibility in Southern Africa.* Windhoek, Namibia: African Palliative Care Association; 2008.

126. Pain & Policy Studies Group. *International Pain Policy Fellowship.* Madison, WI: University of Wisconsin; 2016. Available at: http://www.painpolicy.wisc.edu/international-pain-policy-fellowship. Accessed May 7, 2018.

127. Bosnjak S, Maurer MA, Ryan KM, et al. A multifaceted approach to improve the availability and accessibility of opioids for the treatment of cancer pain in Serbia: results from the International Pain Policy Fellowship (2006-2012) and recommendations for action. *J Pain Symptom Manage* 2016;52:272–283.

128. Leon MX, De Lima L, Florez S, et al. Improving availability of and access to opioids in Colombia: description and preliminary results of an action plan for the country. *J Pain Symptom Manage* 2009;38:758–766.

129. Leon MX, Florez S, De Lima L, et al. Integrating palliative care in public health: the Colombian experience following an International Pain Policy Fellowship. *Palliat Med* 2011;25:365–369.

PART THREE

Evaluation of the Pain Patient

CHAPTER 17

Evaluation of the Chronic Pain Patient

GORDON IRVING and **PAMELA SQUIRE**

Introduction

Pain, as every textbook will report, is a warning system designed to protect our bodies from injury. To do this well, we must be able to determine the site of pain, its intensity, its meaning, and how much it should bother us.

All pain has four dimensions:

- The sensory experience (what it feels like)
- The cognitive experience (what it means)
- The affective experience (how much it bothers you)
- Autonomic activation (rapid heart rate, elevated blood pressure)

When we ask people to rate their pain, most patients will understand this as a rating for the first dimension alone. This is of course what most clinicians are after and document. But, how can patients separate these dimensions to rate only one part?

The role of a pain assessment is to sort out the different contributors to each dimension and their relative importance in affecting the functional impact of pain in each individual. This assessment should then direct treatment recommendations for each individual.

Consider this scenario. On a particularly bad Friday, a physician discovers that he has been suspended from practice following a college review. (He does not recall this review but opened the letter late on Friday, too late to call the college for details!) Distracted while driving home, he is involved in an accident and discovers his car insurance has lapsed. Distraught, he arrives home, in a taxi, and hears a family argument in the kitchen. Walking up the steps, he stubs his toe, and it bleeds. At that moment, his partner opens the door, notices the hopping behavior and the blood and asks, "Where would you rate your pain between 0 and 10?" The clinician, still hopping, shouts, "15 out of 10!!!!"

Later, in a calmer environment, he finds out his partner had renewed his auto insurance but had left the papers at home. On Monday, he finds out the college letter was meant to go another provider of the same name, and on Tuesday, he wins the local lottery, more than enough to retire on. That Friday, while walking up the steps of the theater to pick up the ceremonial lottery check, he again stubs his toe and it bleeds. His partner notices this and again asks, "Where would you rate your pain between 0 and 10?" The clinician, beaming, strides unbroken murmurs, "What pain?" and proceeds to center stage.

In both of these scenarios, the injury is both acute and identical, but the pain ratings are not. What then is the clinician rating?

He is rating primarily how much the pain bothered him, not what it meant or the stimulus intensity.

In a different scenario, a young women with a history of a slow growing tumor waits in the reception area for the results of her magnetic resonance imaging (MRI) to find out if her recent back pain is due to tumor recurrence. When completing the assessment forms that morning, she rated her back pain, then present for a month, at 8/10. One hour later, at the end of a consult which showed no recurrence of her tumor, she now rates her back pain at 4/10.

What was she rating? The sensory experience? Or perhaps the rating and the reduction more accurately reflected the cognitive component of the pain, what it meant to her.

Identifying each of these dimensions and the role they play in any individual's total pain forms the basic "layers" of an initial chronic pain assessment. Each layer will have important contributors, and this chapter attempts to provide an outline to assist the clinician or team perform an accurate and detailed assessment.

In addition to identifying each dimension of the pain experience, the clinician is expected to also identify the layers of each dimension. For example, with regard to the pain stimulus, research suggests that it is important not just to make a diagnosis but to identify individual pain mechanisms.

Is the pain of chronic knee arthritis nociceptive, neuropathic, centrally driven, or a combination?

Is the pain local, segmental, or regional or widespread?

Is the location of the pain due to abnormalities in the tissues, nerve terminals, nerve transmission, the dorsal root ganglion, dorsal horn, midbrain, cortex or forebrain, or several of these areas?

As a result of the location of the pain and the mechanisms involved, what does the patient report and what can we find on examination? Provoked or unprovoked pain? Muscle spasm, weakness, tremors, or reduced range of motion? Sensory changes of small fibers (changes to thermal stimuli or pinprick) or changes of central pain processing (widespread pain, light touch allodynia, cold hyperalgesia, or pressure allodynia.)?

Assessing for layers of the affective component of the pain means asking about adverse childhood events and current stressors and screening for anxiety, depression, posttraumatic stress disorder (PTSD), addiction, and others. Are patients having problems with motivation, insomnia, difficulties with memory, and focus?

Assessing for layers of the cognitive component means looking for pain beliefs. The two commonest beliefs to be assessed are the tendency to catastrophize and to experience fear of movement. Perceived injustice is another construct that seeks to look at the effect on an individual when he or she experiences chronic pain as a result of, or the perception of, another's error or negligence. If these "cognitive distortions" are present, how have they affected the patient? Do they have limited coping skills, deconditioning, or other problems?

225

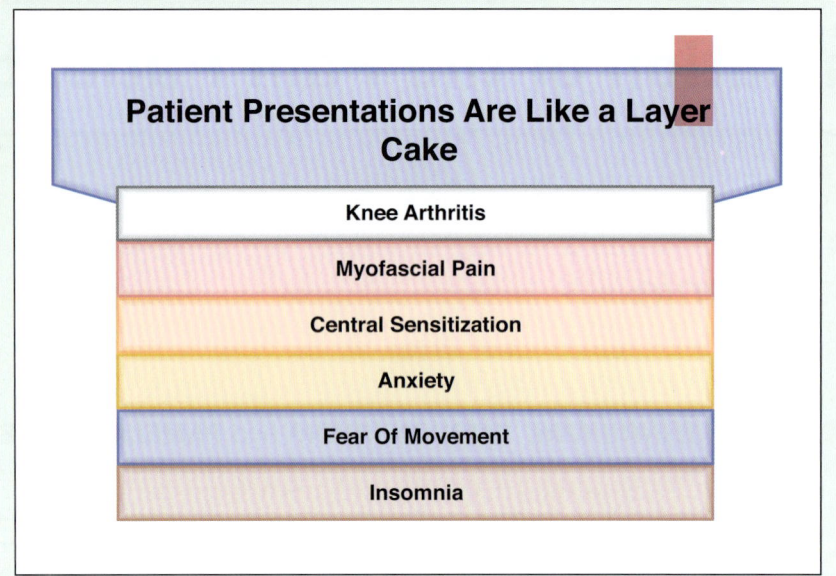

FIGURE 17.1 The multidimensional layers of chronic pain. Although this may identify the individual factors contributing to the overall pain experience, treatment will depend on the amount that each "layer" contributes to the loss of function. In certain patients, additional layers including the contribution of genetics or the role of additional diseases such as Parkinson will be relevant. *(Image courtesy of Dr. Atul Khullar, 2013.)*

Creating an individual "layer cake" for each patient fosters a very different approach that removes the focus from the pain and provides an image of potential treatment opportunities (Figs. 17.1 and 17.2).

In a traditional biologic model of pain, the pain is proportional to the tissue injury. In persistent pain, this linear relationship is often lost, and the patient may be labeled with pain out of proportion to physical findings. Under certain circumstances, this may be associated with malingering (a legal not a medical diagnosis) or secondary gain, but for most patients, this simply represents a clinician's inability to identify all of the layers contributing to the total pain.

The overall effect of persistent pain is a result of a complex interplay between the pain itself, other comorbidities, physical, psychiatric, and psychological as well as psychosocial factors such as support from significant others, financial factors, and job stability. Failure to identify and address these factors may lead to mutual frustration between the patient and the health care provider and poor therapeutic results.

For example, patients with kinesophobia fears moving because they believe the pain with movement is causing additional tissue damage. This leads to progressive physical deactivation and pain exacerbation with further loss of function. This can lead to feelings of unworthiness and poor self-esteem.[1] If this affects their ability to work and leads to financial stress, this can exacerbate anxiety and depression. Compounding these issues, the medications themselves may be a cause of fatigue and debility.

In today's health care environment, time to evaluate complex pain patients is limited. Where appropriate, this chapter suggests time-saving, self-assessment, nonproprietary questionnaires that can help a clinician to know where to perform a more detailed evaluation now or later.

Response to therapy should be gauged more by functional improvement than by a decrease in the pain score. The patient's trust in the health care provider is important. Patients should feel that they have been listened to, their fears have been acknowledged, and the provider is "there for them." People will forget what you said and forget what you did but never forget how you make them feel. This latter statement does not imply the practitioner has to feel the suffering of the patient. The practitioner should remain empathetic and compassionate to the patient's issues while trying to remain emotionally resilient.

The examination of the patient presenting with the various specific persistent pain syndromes is not addressed in this chapter. These are described in the chapters allotted to those problems. This chapter addresses some of the practical problems of assessing the patient with persistent pain so that treatment can be individualized. Some tools are provided that may assist the clinician and are included as appendices.

The appendices include the following:

1. Example of an initial history questionnaire to be completed by the patient
2. Colored pain diagram
3. Goal setting information for the patient
4. Example of a follow-up progress questionnaire to be completed by the patient

GENERAL GUIDELINES FOR ASSESSMENT OF PERSISTENT PAIN

Guidelines summary
- Consider using the term persistent pain.
- Persistent pain is complex and needs devoted time for the initial assessment and plan.

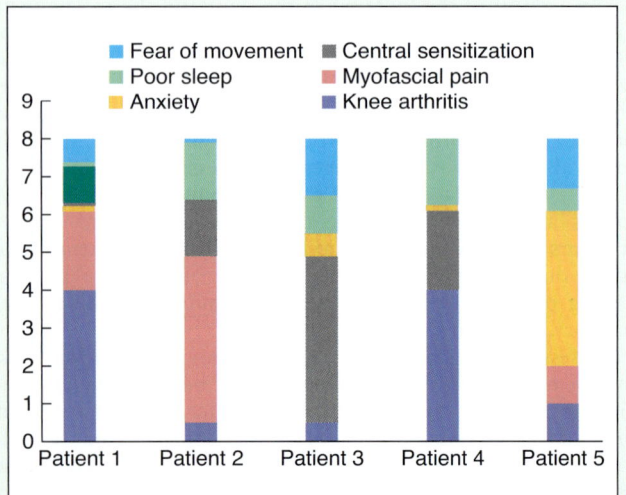

FIGURE 17.2 Five examples of patients with chronic knee pain and pain scores of 8/10. Determining the degree of contribution of each factor contributing to pain would dictate very different treatment recommendations for each of these patients. *(Image courtesy of Dr. Atul Khullar, 2013.)*

- Initial and follow-up pain questionnaires are important.
- Having a significant other accompanying the patient can be invaluable.
- Identifying goals of therapy is a difficult but important part of the assessment.

The assessment and treatment of a patient with ongoing chronic pain begins with the recognition that a complete pain cure is unlikely. Consider changing the name of the problem to persistent pain, which may have less of a pejorative meaning to the patient. The best long-term results are achieved by utilizing approaches that involve both the available community resources as well as the patient becoming more engaged in his or her own therapy. Involvement by the patient in decision-making and goal setting is important. Improving the patient's physical and mental functioning is the ultimate goal.

The time allotted to each patient depends on the type of practice. A pain specialist may allot 40 to 90 minutes to assess a new patient; the busy primary care practitioner may only have 15 to 20 minutes. Alternatively, the assessment can be divided, and information can be completed over several different visits.

An initial comprehensive questionnaire can be sent to the patient via the post or via an e-mail link prior to the consultation (see Appendix 17.1 as an example). If using an online questionnaire that is returned via e-mail, care should be taken to ensure it fulfills the health privacy regulations of the country.

Asking the patient to arrive 20 to 30 minutes early prior to the initial appointment enables any relevant paperwork and insurance verification, if necessary, to take place. It also gives time for the patient to complete the questionnaire, if not already done; have their blood pressure, etc., taken; and have a urine specimen collected for toxicology screening, if appropriate.

A companion, preferably a significant other, should accompany the patient when possible for the initial evaluation and when optimizing or initiating new therapies. By having this individual sit at the patient's side, much information can be gathered about the couple's relationship by body language as well as by visual and verbal expression. The companion may also contradict, or confirm, whether a therapy is working, either verbally or by gesture. As much of the therapeutic discussion is often missed by the patient, no matter how attentive he or she appears to be, having a second person there listening may help.

Outline of a Multidimensional Assessment Questionnaire for Persistent Pain History

It is important to assess the following:
- The pain history
- Medical and surgical history
- Mood
- Psychosocial comorbidities
- Sleep
- Cognitive impairment
- Vocational history and current disability
- Habits
- Risk of opioid misuse, abuse, or dependence
- Function
- Current and past treatments
- Current and past medications and supplements
- Allergies
- Previous investigations and consultations
- Goals
- Physical examination

Questionnaires used should ideally be
- Validated
- Simple and rapid to complete
- Valuable in identifying the problem and best therapy
- Allow functional outcomes to be followed
- Able to show health care benefits across a system and "follow" the patient between specialties

Davidson et al.[2] suggested that seven factors accounted for 59% of the total variance in outcomes of pain treatment. These were pain and disability, pain description, affective distress, support, positive coping strategies, negative coping strategies, and activity. A pain assessment should try to capture most of these factors.

Different practices will require different levels of questionnaire. Solo practitioners may differ in their need to validate their role in a health care organization. Other considerations are whether the questionnaire is proprietary, meaning its use for research in large organizations or in digital format on the web will need to be licensed. In the examples discussed in this chapter, most questionnaires are nonproprietary or available to be used freely. Most questionnaires may be used for individual practices and in paper format without licensing, as long as they are not going to be used in publications.

The Patient-Reported Outcomes Measurement Information System (PROMIS) initiative was a National Institutes of Health (NIH)-funded program to develop new ways to measure patient-reported outcomes (PROs), such as pain, fatigue, physical functioning, emotional distress, and social role participation. PROMIS has also created a psychometrically robust computer adaptive testing (CAT) system based on item response theory (IRT) to administer these items. Whether administered through the CAT system, or by paper version short forms, PROMIS questionnaires have been validated and have shown equal or even improved in efficiency and sensitivity in comparison with existing PROs (https://commonfund.nih.gov/promis/index).

SUMMARY OF SOME NONPROPRIETARY QUESTIONNAIRES

Depression: (Patient Health Questionnaire [PHQ] 2, PHQ 9, PROMIS Short Form Emotional Distress–Depression)
Anxiety: (General Anxiety Disorder [GAD] 7, GAD 2, PROMIS Short Form Emotional Distress–Anxiety)
Sleep: (STOP-Bang for sleep apnea, difficulty falling asleep, difficulty staying asleep; URGES for restless leg syndrome; PROMIS Short Form Sleep)
Mood: Interference with enjoyment of life, PROMIS Short Form
Function: Brief Pain Inventory, PEG, Interference with general activity, STarT Back, PROMIS Short Forms of Physical function, Pain Interference, Fatigue, Pain Behavior, Applied Cognition–Abilities, Global Health
Substance abuse: Alcohol Use Disorders Identification Test (AUDIT), PROMIS Short Form Alcohol Use
Opioid abuse: Opioid Risk Tool (ORT)

OTHER POTENTIALLY USEFUL QUESTIONS TO CONSIDER FOR GAUGING EFFECTIVENESS OF THERAPY

Difficulty with a specific activity, chosen by the patient
Goal identification and follow-up

SUMMARY OF PROPRIETARY QUESTIONNAIRES TO CONSIDER

Pain Catastrophization Scale—pain catastrophizing
Tampa Scale of Kinesiophobia (TSK)—fear of movement
Screener and Opioid Assessment for Patients with Pain (SOAPP14)
Current Opioid Misuse Measure (COMM)
Screening Instrument for Substance Abuse Potential (SISAP)[3]
CAGE-AID—screening tool to assess for risk of serious alcohol or drug problems

The following format for documentation of an initial multidimensional pain assessment is suggested. It encompasses the various dimensions of pain and should facilitate communication with other members of the health care team.

On the diagram below, shade in the areas where you feel pain. Put an "X" on the areas where it hurts the most. (BLACK =sharp/stabbing, RED=burning, BLUE=numbness, GREEN=pins and needles, YELLOW=aching, Arrows = shooting pain. Use colours if you have more than one type of pain)

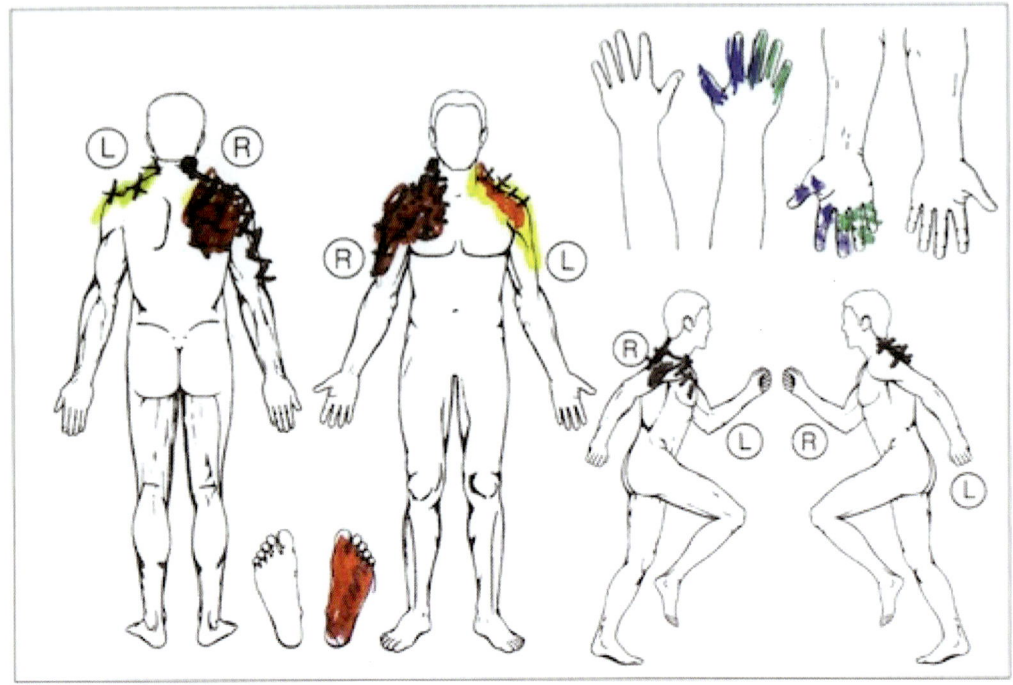

FIGURE 17.3 A pain diagram illustrates a patient with complex regional pain syndrome of the right shoulder and hand and myofascial pain in the left shoulder.

An excellent summary of measures to assess psychological, physical, emotional functioning, and disability as well as attitudes, beliefs, and coping are discussed by Turk et al.[4]

The Pain History

The history of each pain condition provides important clues to the underlying etiology and the chronicity of each condition. It is important to document the etiologies of all the patient's pain diagnoses. The mechanism, if known, date of onset, overall severity, and factors that worsen or improve pain should be noted. It can be formally done during an interview by having a patient-completed history form. For children, or patients with cognitive impairment, a caregiver should be present to provide additional information.

A pain diagram can often provide a "quick look" picture and, when colored ones are used, can help to determine potential areas of neuropathic pain (see Appendix 17.4 or Fig. 17.3 as examples).

Summary and suggested questionnaires
O = Onset
P = Provocative/palliative
Q = Quality/character (Does it have neuropathic features?)
Colored pain diagram
McGill Pain Questionnaire Short Form
R = Region/radiation
Body diagram with shading or colors
S = Severity/intensity
Numerical Rating Scale (NRS)
Graded Chronic Pain Rating Scale
T = Timing of pain (Continuous or intermittent?)

O: ONSET OF PAIN
How pain began is often informative. In many cases, the initial acute cause of the pain may identify an understandable etiology. In other cases, there may not be an obvious organic initiating cause. In these cases, the practitioner has to be careful not to automatically ascribe the pain to psychogenic causes but to accept the patient's description.

P: PROVOCATIVE/PALLIATIVE
Assessing what provokes or relieves the pain provides valuable clues to the diagnosis and treatment. Leg and back pain due to spinal stenosis has a characteristic pattern of worsening with walking or standing, with the pain being totally relieved with sitting or lying for a short time. Neuropathic pain can present with spontaneous pain or pain provoked by different stimuli such as cold, light touch, or the brushing of bedsheets. It is often improved with heat and worsened by cold, the opposite of inflammatory pain.

Q: QUALITY OR CHARACTER
Neuropathic pain is often described as burning, deep aching, shock-like, or shooting. Other associated sensations include numbness, tingling, pins, and needles. Patients may describe unusual sensations like cold water running down a leg or the feeling that they are walking on marbles. Patients with neuropathic pain may also have associated autonomic nervous symptoms including sweating, skin color, and temperature. Changes in hair and nail growth or swelling may also be present. The latter may be intermittent and not evident on the day of examination. They may be documented by photographs, as many patients now have a smartphone with a digital camera.

There are several neuropathic pain questionnaires which assess self-reported symptoms such as dysesthesias, electric shock-like qualities, numbness, temperature sensitivity, and allodynia. As many nonneuropathic pain syndromes may elicit positive responses, Mathieson et al. comment that these tools "should not replace a thorough clinical assessment."[7]

R: REGION/RADIATION
The different sites of pain and radiation patterns can be visually represented by having the patient draw the pain on a pain diagram. Neuropathic characteristics can be represented at the

Please color the areas where you experience pain. Use one of these five coloring pens to shade the specific type of pain that you are experiencing. Then circle with a pen all areas of pain and starting with the worst, number the areas in order of severity.

Red - burning   If you have other pain   Yellow - *feet feel too big for my skin*
Green - tingling   sensations name them
Blue - numbness   here and color as black   Black - *spasms*
                    or yellow

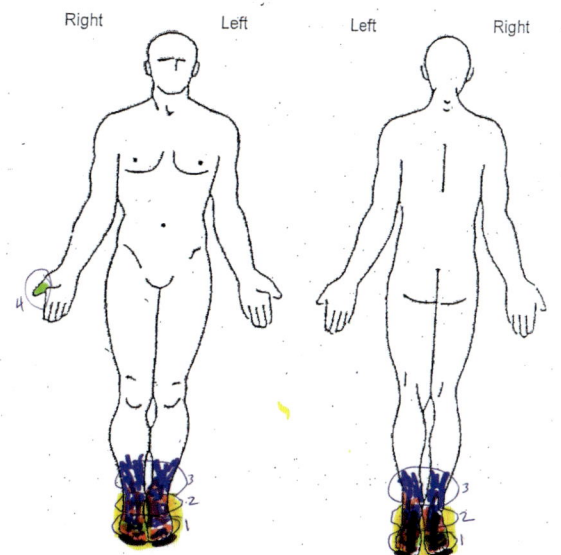

FIGURE 17.4 The pain diagram of a patient with bilateral peripheral neuropathy.

same time by using symbols or colors such as red for burning, green for tingling, and blue for numbness. Specific drawings for the head and face can be used to capture headache and orofacial pain (Fig. 17.4).

S: SEVERITY/INTENSITY OF PAIN

The NRS is the most commonly used method as it is easy to administer. It has been shown to have a higher compliance and ease of use than the Visual Analog Scale (VAS).[6] The scale is from 0 = no pain to 10 = worst pain imaginable or worst possible pain. In children and those with limited cognitive ability, the Faces Pain Scale should be considered. The time scale varies from the last 24 hours to the last week. The Graded Chronic Pain Scale which asks the worst, least, and average pain over the same period of time can give an idea of the patient's overall burden of pain.

Many physicians have difficulty when patients rate their pain score with a number that seems to be at odds with their demeanor and functionality. Acknowledging to the patient that you believe he or she must have significant pain and then offering further anchors to the scale often results in a different rating that may be more meaningful in follow-up. The following script may be helpful to consider in a patient who has rated the pain as 15/10:

> "I believe you have pain that is severe, and it is obviously very distressing to you, but I am not quite sure how to interpret your rating because I do need a number between 0 and 10. If I say 0 means absolutely no pain and 10 out of 10 pain would be severe burns to most of your body or the pain you would feel if your hand was caught in a meat grinder, where would you rate your pain?"

A patient who initially described the pain as 15/10 will often adjust the rating when belief, acknowledgment, and new anchors are provided. Remember, not all patients are able to separate the pain intensity from how much it bothers them and what it means.

T: TIMING OF PAIN

The timing of pain can provide diagnostic clues to pain etiology. Neuropathic pain is often spontaneous. Patients report episodes of severe pain without any provocation, although nociceptive pain, such as osteoarthritis of the hip, is usually not severe unless provoked by use. The typical timing of cluster headaches differentiates it from the ice-pick headache. The intermittent nature of trigeminal neuralgia would differentiate it from atypical facial pain.

ALTERED PERCEPTION

Many patients with persistent pain experience altered body perceptions. Hemi-attention (to both the affected, especially left-sided, body parts with associated mood change like depression) and hemi-neglect have been described in patients with some chronic musculoskeletal pain such as chronic low back pain and after limb amputation.[7]

Patients with complex regional pain syndrome (CRPS) may have subtle motor abnormalities. They may volunteer weakness but not mention tremor, dystonia, or motor incoordination unless specifically asked. They often have body perceptual distortions which are often not spontaneously reported. CRPS patients may feel like the affected limb does not belong to them and may want to amputate it because it feels alien. Ask how they feel emotionally about their limb, if it feels alien to them, and how aware they are of the physical position of the affected part. Consider asking them to close their eyes and describe how each affected part feels to them and draw it. In an affected foot, the calf may feel normal, but the foot feels larger and the toes may not be distinct compared to the other side.

Questionnaires to consider: Widely used multiple-item questionnaires with a high reliability and validity include the McGill Pain questionnaire which has two validated short forms. These yield subscales which can assist in distinguishing between different types of clinical pain.[8]

Past Medical and Surgical History

Past medical conditions should be noted that could be an important cause of current or potential pain conditions (multiple sclerosis, prior cancer diagnoses, diabetes). The past surgical history should be obtained when relevant. Visceral dysfunctions such as renal or hepatic compromise or short gut syndrome that could affect absorption or metabolic function have an important role when considering pharmacologic treatments.

Dementia, depending on the severity, may affect how the pain is assessed and is discussed in a different chapter.

MOOD ASSESSMENT

The psychological state of the individual with chronic pain is an important determinant of pain, disability, and coping. The pain itself can lead to an altered psychological state, but previous traumatic psychological events can also alter pain perception. The goal of the initial assessment is not to clearly define all psychological risk factors, mood disorders, or coping strategies but to get a sense of areas of concern, so that they can be more fully evaluated in the future.

Summary with potential questionnaires
- Anxiety
  - GAD 7, GAD 2
  - PROMIS Short Form
- Depression
  - PHQ 9, PHQ 2
  - PROMIS Short Form
- PTSD
  - PTSD Civilian
- Bipolar disorder
  - Mood Disorder Questionnaire (MDQ)

Anxiety and depression are common and may decrease the patient's tolerance to pain and reduce the coping ability. Major depression, anxiety disorders, PTSD, bipolar disorder, and suicidal ideation and plan should be identified and referred to the appropriate specialist.

A history of childhood traumatic events predicts an increased risk for the development of substance abuse, depressive disorders, and attempted suicides. Chronic pain creates an additional risk factor. Asking about childhood trauma can be difficult, especially in an initial interview, and the following question is suggested. "If you have a child, or imagine that you might, would you want them to have the same childhood you did?" Negative answers can be explored at a later time.

It is helpful to ask about current psychological states tactfully because many patients are sensitive to the idea that their pain, particularly pain that seems out of proportion to observable findings, is all in their head and become quite defensive when asked about how they are feeling. If the patient has completed a questionnaire, you should already know something about the mood and the way the patient thinks about the pain and coping strategies. You can use the patient's answers to gently probe for more information. For example, "I see on this one questionnaire that you feel down or depressed most of the days. Can you tell me about that?"

PSYCHOSOCIAL FACTORS

Psychosocial factors are important variables in the comprehensive assessment of persistent pain. Numerous relevant factors have been described, and there are multiple assessment tools and measures to evaluate them.

Summary with potential questionnaires
- Pain catastrophizing
  - Pain Catastrophizing Scale (PCS)
  - Modified STarT Back tool
- Fear avoidance
  - TSK
  - Fear-Avoidance Belief Questionnaire
- Perceived injustice
  - Injustice Experience Questionnaire (IEQ)

Two key ways of thinking about pain that impact functionality include pain catastrophizing and kinesophobia or health-related anxiety.

Pain catastrophizing is defined as "an exaggerated negative mental set, brought to bear during actual or anticipated painful experience."[9] Catastrophic thinking might contribute to the development or maintenance of anxiety, fear, or depression associated with pain. Life traumas such as major losses, severe accidents, and abuse experiences may sensitize individuals to distress reactions to future stressors.[10]

Those who catastrophically misinterpret innocuous bodily sensations, including pain, are more likely to become fearful of pain. This may result in avoidance behaviors and the avoidance of movement and physical activity in particular.

Kinesophobia is defined as "an irrational and debilitating fear of physical movement and activity resulting from a feeling of vulnerability to painful injury or re-injury."[1] The TSK measures the belief that painful activity will result in damage and/or will increase suffering and/or functional loss.[11] Avoidance also means withdrawal from rewarding activities such as work, leisure, and family.

Pain-related fear is associated with increased bodily awareness and pain hypervigilance. Hypervigilance, fear, and disuse are associated with increased pain levels and often interfere with successful completion of an active rehabilitation program and return to work programs.

Some patients who experience chronic pain as a result of, or the perception of, another's error or negligence may suffer from the perception of injustice. This has been described as an appraisal cognition comprising elements of the severity of loss consequent to injury, blame, a sense of unfairness, and irreparability of loss. In a prospective study of individuals with mixed musculoskeletal pain, Sullivan et al.[12] demonstrated that high scores on this measure predicted work disability at 1-year follow-up, even when controlled for depression, pain-related fear, catastrophizing, and pain severity.

Other psychosocial factors that may contribute to pain include the influence of others, for example, a spouse that is distant or even over solicitous; lack of family and/or community support; litigation issues; previous sexual or physical abuse; financial security; and status of health care coverage.

COPING STRATEGIES

Of the seven factors that predicted most of the pain-related disability, Davidson et al.[2] identified positive and negative coping strategies as being important.

Asking patients what coping strategies they use can help to identify their coping strengths and opportunities for future treatment strategies.

Some positive coping strategies include the following:
- Pacing
- Prioritizing and day planning
- Setting self-motivated goals and action plans
- Being patient and accepting small achievements over time
- Using relaxation skills such as reading, listening to music, meeting friends for coffee/tea or other social activity, practicing breathing, meditation skills, or walking
- Stretching and exercising regularly
- Keeping a diary to document progress
- Having a plan for when the pain flares

If available, a referral to a clinical psychologist specializing in pain should be made, especially if one or more of the following factors have been identified: pronounced emotional disturbance; pain behavior enabled by the family, possible secondary gain; failure to respond to several treatment modalities; reports of pain severity or functional impairment which seem inconsistent with disability; or excessive use of health care services.

SLEEP DISORDERS

The relationship between pain and sleep dysfunction can be complex, and up to 60% of patients with chronic pain report sleep disturbance.[13] Most patients report that sleep is interrupted due to pain, many develop unhealthy sleep patterns, and up to 70% of patients with insomnia have chronic pain.[14] A night continually interrupted by pain rather than reduced sleeping time may impair the endogenous pain-inhibitory function creating spontaneous pain.[15]

Summary with potential questionnaires
- PROMIS Sleep Disturbance (four-, six-, or eight-question version items)
- PROMIS Sleep-Related Impairment (nine items) (measures the effects of poor sleep on daily function)
- STOP-Bang (for obstructive sleep apnea)

A sleep history should identify the type of sleep difficulty (getting to sleep or staying asleep); document the patient's current sleep hygiene; and screen for possible sleep apnea, restless leg syndrome, and periodic limb movements. Patients may be unaware of either the leg jerking or apneic episodes but have associated partial awakenings that impair sleep and cause daytime fatigue. Bed partners may be able to give important information regarding leg jerking movements and apneic spells during the night. If they do not have a bed partner, overnight oximetry or a more formal sleep study may be necessary to make a diagnosis.

Patients with PTSD may have nightmares and flashbacks and often require specific therapies to ensure a restful sleep.

COGNITIVE IMPAIRMENT

Cognitive impairment in individuals with chronic pain has been widely described, and many patients report it has a marked effect on their quality of life. The relationship is not straightforward as pain can cause cognitive impairment, but increasing non–pain-related cognitive load (i.e., distraction) can reduce perceived pain.[16]

One study of a multidisciplinary pain center population demonstrated 20% of patients underperformed on tests measuring working memory, verbal learning and memory, psychomotor speed, and attention.[17]

Persistent pain moderately affects working memory in a consistent and significant manner and causes deficits in attentional control. Attention, which is linked closely with working memory, allows the brain to select the relevant inputs for storage and processing into working memory.[18] Many patients complain that pain is distracting.

Modeling the underlying causes of cognitive impairment in individuals with chronic pain has identified a few possibilities including pain competing for attention in a brain with limited resources, neuroplasticity, and dysregulated neurochemistry.[16] The effects of comorbid disease such as Parkinson and affective disorders such as anxiety or depression and the effects of age, sleep disturbance, and medication all play a role.

Medication has been shown to both increase and reduce cognitive impairment, the latter possibly due to the effects of tolerance to side effects and pain reduction.

Confirming cognitive impairment is an important element of the pain evaluation, but a detailed evaluation is better done by a qualified psychologist as there are many methodologic issues to consider including the exact nature of the deficits, comparison of objective and subjective complaints, control for effort, and covariates including pain severity, depression, and fatigue at the time of testing.[17]

VOCATIONAL HISTORY AND CURRENT VOCATIONAL DISABILITY

A brief history of the patient's schooling, vocational training, and recent employment or disability status should be obtained.

In 2009, a working group identified seven core factors affecting return to work in men with chronic low back pain where each of the core factors were at least supported by one review.[18] The seven core factors were (1) heavy physical demands, (2) ability to modify work, (3) job stress, (4) social support, (5) job satisfaction, (6) return to work expectation, and (7) fear of reinjury. Although job satisfaction is often assumed to be highly predictive, a study of 574 individuals with chronic low back pain reported that a high expectation of return to work was the strongest predictor of return to work and high levels of job satisfaction was not predictive.[19]

HABITS

Always ask about smoking history because this is something the patient has the choice to decide to quit, even though it is very difficult.

Also inquire about past attempts at quitting, alcohol use, diet, exercise, weight changes, the use of cannabis, and other nonprescribed or illicit drug use.

Risk of Opioid Misuse, Abuse, or Dependence

Opioid dependence exists as a spectrum disorder and can complicate the management of a patient with persistent pain. It is important to screen for opioid misuse and abuse and to re-evaluate for all of these problems in each follow-up visit for patients who take these and other controlled substances.

There are several questionnaires that can screen for the risk of aberrant behaviors that may occur with opioid use or assess the risk of addiction to alcohol or other substances or behaviors.[20]

Summary with potential questionnaires
- AUDIT
- SISAP
- PROMIS Short Form Alcohol Use
- CAGE-AID, screening tool to assess for risk of serious alcohol or drug problems
- ORT
- SOAPP14
- COMM

Urine toxicology testing can be done as a point-of-care test with the results available in as early as 5 minutes. This allows a discussion about potential aberrant results, either positive or negative, to be held at the time of the appointment. If no obvious explanation is forthcoming, without any accusation, the urine should be sent for more sensitive and specific laboratory confirmation. There are many medications that may give false positives on a clinic test, so laboratory confirmation and, if necessary, discussion with a forensic pathologist are important before potentially accusing the patient of aberrant behavior.

If available, a review of the local prescription monitoring program or pharmacy printout, to assess previous prescriptions of scheduled medications such as opioids and benzodiazepines, is important.

The prescription drug monitoring programs (PDMPs) are electronic databases run by all individual states in the United States except Missouri. They collect data entered by pharmacists on dispensed controlled medications. The data is housed by a specified statewide regulatory, administrative, or law enforcement agency.

The benefit is that they allow health care providers see patients' prescribing histories which may influence their prescribing decisions. Unfortunately, as yet, there is no conformity among states on the time to enter data after the prescription has been filled. This ranges from monthly to daily or even in "real time"; that is, under 5 minutes. Timely data should maximize the utility of the prescription history data, with significant implications for patient safety and public health.

Partly because of poor utilization, some states have implemented polices that require providers to check a state PDMP prior to prescribing certain controlled substances. PDMPs can also be used to send "proactive" reports to authorized users to protect patients at the highest risk and identify inappropriate prescribing trends. One study reported on sending prescribers unsolicited reports about individuals on opioids who fulfil certain criteria such as multiple prescribers. Compared to a comparison group whose prescribers were not sent a report, the interventional group had significant decreases in number and dosage of opioids prescribed, number of pharmacies used, and number of prescribers visited.[21]

States have taken a number of steps to make PDMPs easier to use and access. These include integrating PDMPs into electronic health record (EHR) systems, permitting physicians to delegate PDMP access to other allied health professionals in their office (e.g., physician assistants and nurse practitioners), and streamlining the process for providers to register with the PDMP. PDMPs are also used by state health departments to inform and evaluate interventions of perceived overprescribing of controlled substances. A 2017 study[21] reported that states with a strong PDMP program, calculated using legal data compiled by the Prescription Drug Abuse Policy System (PDAPS), together with other covariates such as laws that regulate pain clinics, access to naloxone, use of emergency services (Good Samaritan laws), and medical marijuana, had a significantly lower opioid overdose rate than states with a less robust program.[22]

PDMPs are playing an important role in evaluating the prescribing of controlled substances both for the prescriber and the regulatory authorities. Given the other general recommendations for careful charting of function and mood, opioid agreements, and random urine toxicology screens, PDMPs give the health care provider another objective way of assessing patients. The concern about opioid knowledge and too much regulation was addressed in a study by Hwang et al.[22] in 2016. Their conclusion was that "although physicians are unaware of some facets of prescription opioid-related morbidity, most support a variety of clinical and regulatory interventions to improve the risk-benefit balance of these therapies." Only a third of physicians contacted believed that interventions to reduce prescription opioid abuse would have a moderate or large effect on preventing patients' clinically appropriate access to pain treatment.[23]

Assessment and treatment of addiction is covered in a separate chapter.

Assessment of Function

It is important to assess the functional impact of persistent pain by trying to quantify an individual's ability to engage in a number of different activity domains. Function is one domain measured in quality-of-life assessments, so most questionnaires have overlapping questions that measure some aspects of both.

Three kinds of self-assessment questionnaires have been developed: general questionnaires applicable to all kinds of pain like the EuroQol, which is short, six questions but has complex scoring and weighting, or the four-, six-, or eight-item PROMIS Measures of Physical Function; disease-specific ones like the Fibromyalgia Impact Questionnaire; and regional ones, for example, the Oswestry Disability Index for back pain.

The questions should cover all of the relevant areas and usually include the impact of pain on domains such as employment, social, recreational, family, or home responsibilities. It should assess self-care and ideally evaluate the overall quality of life.

Summary of potential questionnaires
- General questionnaires
  - Brief Pain Inventory
  - PEG: measures three items, average pain, interference with enjoyment of life, and general activity
  - STarT Back: includes catastrophizing questions, useful to assess for potential chronicity
  - EuroQol
  - PROMIS Short Form Physical Function
  - PROMIS Global Health
  - Work Productivity and Activity Impairment Questionnaire
- Specific questionnaires (there are many—these are just a few)
  - Oswestry Disability Index: specific for back pain
  - Neck Disability Index: specific for the neck

It is not uncommon in clinical practice to see a patient in follow-up who declares the pain to be much better, yet a review of the functionality questionnaire indicates a higher score than the previous visit.

For instance, on the Brief Pain Inventory, patients may rate their leg pain at 8/10 and the pain interference for walking at 6/10 one week and a month later rate their leg pain less at 5/10 yet rate their pain interference for walking at 9/10.

This may be because they are walking less due to depression, are not paying attention to the weighing scale, or have forgotten how bad their pain used to be (recall bias).

But pain interference scales also suffer from something called response drift, which involves reprioritization, recalibration, and reconceptualization.

A patient can reprioritize his or her disabilities depending on the current circumstances. The main problem may have been headaches, and if the patient substantially improves, now the leg pain becomes the biggest issue and so not walking seems more impairing.

They may recalibrate it. In this case, a 5/10 one day is different than a 5/10 the next day. In the last month, the patient may have had a fracture dislocation of his left elbow and has now decided, that what he thought was 8/10 leg pain, he would now rate at 5/10.

When a patient reconceptualizes his or her disability, he or she has changed the internal concept of what disability due to leg function is. So, in this case, before, the patient felt disabled if he could not get to the bathroom, and now, he feels disabled if he can not get to the store.[24]

Current and Past Treatments

The initial questionnaire should allow the patient to list all the therapeutic modalities he or she is currently using and ones used in the past. This includes interventions such as biofeedback, physiotherapy, chiropractic, massage therapy, anesthetic pain blocks, or surgeries. It is important to determine which ones the patient felt were useful and how long they decreased the pain as well as which were ineffective or produced intolerable side effects.

CURRENT AND PAST MEDICATIONS INCLUDING OVER-THE-COUNTER MEDICATIONS

A complete list of the patient's present medication should be recorded and any changes documented at each follow-up. This is especially important if the patient is seeing other providers who are prescribing medications, as this poses an increased risk for unsuspected drug interactions. Inquire about other alternative therapists prescribing nonprescription medications, herbs, or supplements. These may interact with prescribed medications or create other side effects and should be documented (for more specific information, go to the Memorial Sloan-Kettering Cancer Centre Web site at http://www.mskcc.org/aboutherbs). A list of previous medications tried and the results should also be obtained.

ALLERGIES

Allergies or sensitivities to medications, contrast dye, or latex should be identified.

INVESTIGATIONS AND CONSULTATIONS

A list of previous investigations should be obtained with the relevant results. Prior or upcoming relevant consultations should be listed and the outcomes, if known.

Goals

Summary
- Should be patient-determined and patient-specific for time and activity
- Need to reassess treatment and comorbidities if the patient is not engaged

Goal setting seeks to determine which specific social, recreational, or occupational tasks or roles are important to the patient. Motivational interviewing is a skill that a provider can use to enable the patient identify a goal and set an expected date for change.

Examples of tasks in these categories include going out to see a movie (social), walking (recreational), decreasing or stopping smoking (health related), or being able to lift heavy objects (occupational).

Occupational task or roles could include active participation as a church volunteer, mentoring a student (social), or soccer or baseball coach (recreational).

Determining appropriate goals is an important part of the pain assessment as it will help to direct treatment. People resist coercion, so when getting the patient to identify achievable goals, it is important to influence and not control. (See Appendix 17.3 as an example.)

Goals need to be measurable, for example, "to walk three blocks," not "exercise more." They should reflect the patient's current abilities. Numbers can be used; if the patient states he or she is at a 3/10 on the way to stopping smoking, the question can be asked: "What would it take to get to a 6/10?" That answer can be used as a goal to discuss at the next visit. The patient should be encouraged to assess how confident he or she is in achieving the goal in the time line chosen.

If a patient cannot achieve his or her goals, the practitioner should reassess the goals made, find out what barriers prevented the patient from completing the goal, and assist in reframing the goal to something more achievable in the short term. The goal, however, should always be one that the patient identifies. Evaluation by a psychologist may provide some helpful insights when constructing or reevaluating goals.

If patient-identified goals are not met and the function does not improve, it is reasonable to assume the current treatment is not effective and should be changed. Documenting that a patient has achieved or exceeded goals, and has achieved an improvement in functional scores corroborates treatment efficacy and is rewarding to both patient and provider.

Physical Examination

The examination is usually a focused examination based on the patient's history. The goal is to determine the etiology of the pain (if possible) and to determine, if appropriate, the presence or absence of neuropathic pain and physical signs of substance abuse or misuse. The following evaluation outline for a comprehensive physical examination is suggested.

GENERAL EXAM: OBSERVE, IDENTIFY AND DOCUMENT

Mental status: Consider a mini-mental status exam if there are concerns about cognitive impairment; comment on mood, displays of emotion, or evidence of impairment (slurred speech, difficulty remaining alert) and any smell of substance of abuse on breath, body, or clothes
General appearance (whether it matches photo ID may be appropriate to comment on depending on the specific situation)
Blood pressure, heart rate, weight, and height
Stance and gait
Mobilization aids (what, how, and why they are used)
Signs of substance abuse including needle marks on lower arm, leg, or bottom of feet; rhinorrhea; red palms; spider veins on chest; and pupil diameter
Evidence of any tremors, muscle atrophy, trophic changes, or deformities

SITE OF PAIN
Perform a focused examination of the musculoskeletal system.

Observe

Positional relief postures (i.e., avoids weight bearing on one buttock, turns body instead of neck, prefers to stand and lean) or behaviors (wearing sunglasses inside in patients with chronic migraine and photosensitivity)
Pain distraction signs (i.e., permanent heating pad or ice burn marks, excessive teeth wear from clenching or grinding)
General posture (i.e., head forward posture, exaggerated lumbar lordosis)
Alignment of spine, shoulders, pelvis, and legs

Symmetry: deformities, visible muscle spasm, atrophy, hypertrophy, scars, tattoos and birthmarks
Leg length asymmetry
Evidence of damage to the local myotome segment which includes denervation sensitivity of the local spinal segment resulting in trophedema. Trophedema is nonpitting edema to digital pressure, but if the end of a matchstick is pushed into the skin, it will form a clear-cut indentation that persists for several minutes.

Palpate

Tenderness, swelling, crepitus, contour or bogginess of joint, muscle, ligament, bursa, or bone
Trigger points or taut bands

Test

Individual joints for swelling, crepitus, redness, warmth, and range of motion (active/passive)
Muscle tone
Muscle strength
Specific maneuvers (i.e., the impingement test to assess the shoulder, or the flexion adduction internal rotation [FAIR] test of the hip to assess for sciatic nerve impingement by the piriformis muscle)

NEUROLOGIC EXAM
Observe or Ask About

Signs of sensory avoidance (specific clothing to avoid clothes brushing, wearing dark glasses in the examination room, poor oral hygiene in patients with mouth pain)
Skin lesions (i.e., scarring from varicella zoster, foot ulcers with diabetic neuropathy)
Swelling of the painful area (neurogenic edema): Ask if this occurs as in many patients this can be an intermittent feature. Measure limb diameter or water displacement if in an area that is difficult to measure.
Changes in skin color: Ask if this occurs as in many patients this can be an intermittent feature. A photo by the patient can provide documentation of this signs.
Altered sweating: Ask about if not present.
Trophic changes: loss of hair, thinning skin, cracked dry skin, altered nails (Fig. 17.5)
Secondary changes associated with chronic peripheral neuropathy (e.g., Charcot neuropathic foot destruction with necrotic arthropathy and chronic ulcers on the plantar surface)

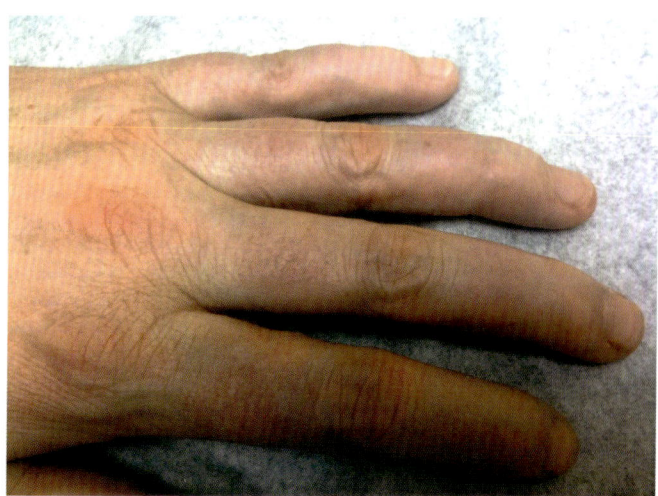

FIGURE 17.5 Late complex regional pain syndrome causing trophic changes in the left 4th and 5th fingers. *(Photo from the author's (PS) private collection. Used with permission from the patient.)*

TABLE 17.1   Key Sensory Areas Nerve Root

C5—lateral upper arm/lateral epicondyle
C6—thumb
C7—middle finger
C8—5th finger
T1—ulnar forearm/medial epicondyle
T3—3rd and 4th interspace
T4—nipple line/4th and 5th interspace
T6—xiphoid process
T10—navel
T12—pubis
L2—medial midthigh
L3—medial knee
L4—medial calf, just above medial malleolus and great toe
L5—lateral calf and dorsum of foot between great and second toe
S1—posterolateral foot and ankle (base of 5th toe)
S2—posteromedial thigh and popliteal fossa
S3–5—perianal area

Evidence of autonomic dysfunction, especially with CRPS or peripheral diabetic polyneuropathy
Involuntary movements: tremors, myoclonus, tics, dystonia, fasciculation, or others
Specific tests (i.e., upper limb tension test (ULTT) for "neurogenic" thoracic outlet syndrome, straight leg raise for lumbar radiculopathy)

Palpate

Temperature differences between affected and unaffected areas
Edema, swelling, tenderness

Test

Cranial nerves
Gait
Balance and coordination; finger tapping, rapid alternating movements; finger–nose and heel–shin testing; Romberg test
Tone

TABLE 17.2   Motor Power (Nerve Roots)

In the Arms, Test Resisted

Shoulder abduction C5
Elbow flexion C5–C6
Elbow extension C6–C7
Wrist extension C6–C7
Wrist flexion C7–C8
Finger flexion/extension C8
Finger abduction T1

In the Legs, Test Resisted

Hip flexion L3–L4
Hip extension L4–L5
Knee flexion L5–S1
Knee extension L3–L4
Ankle dorsiflexion L4–L5
Ankle plantar flexion S1–S2

Score Power By

0	No contraction
1	Visible muscle twitch but no movement of the joint
2	Weak contraction insufficient to overcome gravity
3	Weak contraction able to overcome gravity but no additional resistance
4	Weak contraction able to overcome some resistance but not full resistance
5	Normal; able to overcome full resistance

TABLE 17.3   Important Reflexes

Reflexes

- C5–C6 roots, the biceps and brachioradialis reflexes
- C6–C7 roots (mainly C7), the triceps reflex
- L3–L4 roots (mainly L4), the knee jerk
- S1 root, the ankle jerk

Score Reflexes By

0	No observable reflex
1	Trace reflex
2	Normal reflex
3	Brisk reflex
4	Nonsustained clonus (two or less beats of clonus)
5	Greater than three beats of clonus or sustained clonus. Anal "wink" reflex in a patient with suspected cauda equina syndrome (scratch the perianal skin about 2 cm away from the anus and look for muscle contraction to cause an "anal wink"). Patients with peripheral neuropathy may have diminished or absent reflexes. If they do not, look carefully for evidence of upper motor neuron dysfunction.

Spasticity: eliciting the "clasp knife phenomenon," which predominates in the upper limb flexors and the lower limb extensors
Rigidity: uniform resistance that worsened during the range of movement; usually worsens with distraction
Paratonia: increased resistance because the patient has difficulty consciously relaxing the muscle. This usually improves with distraction.
Hypotonia: decreased tone
Motor function (Tables 17.1 to 17.4)
Pronator drift: With the patient standing with both arms extended and palms up (supinated), look for one arm to drift downward and begin to turn palm down (pronate). A positive test is a subtle indicator of upper motor neuron weakness (in which supination is weaker than pronation)
Perceptual dysfunction: neglect
This may be detected by testing for extinction or double simultaneous stimulation. Patients may detect a stimulus on the affected side when presented alone, but when stimuli are presented simultaneously on both sides, only the stimulus on the unaffected side may be detected. In a patient with suspected motor neglect, normal strength or range of movement may be present, but the patient does not move the painful limb unless attention is strongly directed toward it. These individuals may benefit from specific physical therapy techniques.

TABLE 17.4   Upper and Lower Motor Neuron Dysfunction

Signs of Upper Motor Neuron Dysfunction

- Hyperreactive reflexes
- Spasticity
- Positive Babinski sign
- Positive pronator drift sign
- Weakness that is predominant in the arm extensors and leg flexors

Signs of Lower Motor Neuron Dysfunction

- Absent or hyporeactive reflexes
- Tone normal or reduced
- Negative Babinski sign
- Atrophy and fasciculations
- Weakness that is predominant in arm flexors and leg extensors. Mixed upper and lower motor neuron can present with hyperreflexia and spasticity mixed with depressed reflexes and weakness in patients with cervical myeloradiculopathy.

Perceptual distortions: Many patients with chronic pain experience perceptual disturbances of the affected body part. The body part may feel bigger, smaller, or just different than the normal body part. Different examination techniques to evaluate for these disturbances are now being reported in the literature, and the reader is referred to individual chapters in this book for more detailed information.

BEDSIDE METHOD FOR QUANTITATIVE SENSORY TESTING

In patients with suspected neuropathic pain, the Quantitative Sensory Testing (QST) can be used as part of a routine neurologic exam to define the extent and pattern of sensory abnormalities and to characterize the sensory changes.[25] QST does not seek to determine pain thresholds but to measure subjective experience (loss or gain of sensation) in response to particular thermal, mechanical, or vibratory stimuli. It also seeks to provide, indirectly, information used to evaluate underlying sensory function and abnormalities.[26]

1. Have the patient complete a pain diagram with pain descriptors to identify affected areas and direct the physical exam.
2. Begin by mapping out the area of abnormality. This is most rapidly done with a toothpick or a cotton swab starting in a normal area (based on the pain diagram) and progressing toward the abnormal area, marking the area of skin where the sensation changed and moving in a radial pattern from normal to abnormal until the area of sensory change has been identified.
3. Establish a control site where the patient has no sensory abnormalities or pain, preferably on the opposite side of the body in a similar position. Use this as a reference for normal sensation.
4. For each stimulus, start in the normal area and then move to the abnormal painful area and ask after applying the stimulus, "Do you feel this more, less, or the same as the normal side?" Patients may experience sensory gain to one kind of stimulus and loss to another in the same area.

Patients are examined for the following modalities.

Light Touch

Lightly brush the skin. This can be performed at the bedside with a cotton wisp, cotton wool tip, Q-tip, foam brush, or paint brush. Testing should start over the normal skin and move toward the affected area. Once the patient feels any change in sensation, the point on the skin is marked.

Drawing the area of abnormality on the skin can help to determine the pattern of loss (single nerve territory, polyneuropathy, or nondermatomal). If light touch is normal, it is still important to test for pinprick and temperature, as these tests evaluate different small fiber components of the nerve.

Vibration

Vibration sense is usually tested with a 128-Hz tuning fork. Test over the bony prominences moving from distal to proximal. In subjects with distal symmetric polyneuropathy, the tuning fork is placed over the interphalangeal joint of the big toe. If no vibration is noted, move to the medial malleolus and repeat the exam. If still unable to sense vibration, the test is repeated over the patella. For the hands, test over the second distal interphalangeal joint and move proximally to the ulnar styloid and lateral epicondyle, if no vibration is felt.

Punctate/Pinprick

This can be evaluated with a cocktail toothpick or a more standardized device such as a NeuroPEN. A safety pin should be avoided because with insensate skin, the skin may be damaged,

and the safety pin may be inadequately sterilized. The size and angle of the sharp tool can significantly affect the intensity of the stimulus. The NeuroPEN has a standardized probe tip and is designed to allow production of a consistent stimulus. Perform the testing in the area with the abnormal positive or negative sensations.

Warm and Noxious Heat

For bedside testing, thermal evaluation can be done by heating the round end of a tuning fork in warm or hot water. There are no commercially available small devices for standard bedside testing of warmth or heat pain. Unfortunately, it is difficult to get the tuning fork to the correct temperature for heat pain testing. This test is most useful to confirm the involvement of small fibers when evaluating small-fiber neuropathy. This most often occurs in a patient whose pain drawing suggests a peripheral neuropathy but in whom sensation to vibration and light touch is normal.

Cool and Noxious Cold

For cool testing, a tuning fork is held under cool water and applied to the area of altered skin sensation. For cold pain, the tuning fork is immersed in ice water. Comparison is made with the established control site. Have the patient report on the sensation. (Does it actually feel cool? In some patients, it feels paradoxically hot.)

Grading the Tests

Reduced sensation: Have the patient express the degree of loss by utilizing the simple 1-to-100 scale of a dollar. Ask, "If this is a dollar (stimulating the normal area), then how much is this worth? (stimulating the area of sensory loss)." A response of 90 cents reflects a very different degree of loss than a reply of 10 cents.

Increased sensation: In the case of a sensation that should have been painful (pinprick, noxious heat, or cold), have the patient grade the pain in the normal area first (0 to 100) and then grade the abnormal area.

Record dysesthesia if the nonpainful stimulus was felt as increased but not painful and write a description of the sensation (e.g., numb, pins, and needles).

Record hyperalgesia if the stimulus was a normally painful stimulus (pinprick, heat, or cold pain), but it produced more pain than the unaffected normal test site, and grade the intensity (0 to 100).

Record allodynia if the stimulus was nonpainful (brush, vibration, warm, cool) and either the threshold was normal or decreased (stimulus intensity reported as the same or more than the normal site) and the patient reported pain from the stimulus and grade the intensity (0 to 100).

Record hyperpathia if the stimulus threshold is increased (stimulus intensity reported as less than the normal site) and the patient reports it as painful. For example, you place a warm tuning fork on the affected area and the patient initially reports no warm sensation (because the threshold for feeling warm is increased) but then over the next 10 seconds gradually reports first a warm sensation and then reports it as painfully hot and grade the intensity (0 to 100).

The physical examination for central sensitization is not straightforward because *central sensitization* is a neurophysiologic term that can only be determined when both the input and output of the neural system are known.[27] Practically, this means being able to measure both the stimulus (easily done) and the neural event that occurs after the stimulus (not easily done). Central sensitization can therefore only be inferred (but not proven) from the following physical signs[28]:

Widened receptor field. Manifesting as an area of pain much larger than anticipated and affecting areas that do not have specific pathology

Wind-up. Manifested by repetitive activation of primary afferent C fibers leading to a synaptic strengthening of nociceptive transmission and measured by performing summation testing with a NeuroPEN or similar standardized device (see the following discussion)

Reduced thresholds. Caused by facilitation of non-nociceptive Ab fibers manifested as dynamic mechanical allodynia and nociceptive Ad fibers manifested as pinprick or cold hyperalgesia

After pain. Following pinprick testing or temporal summation, it is normal for the sharp sensation to linger for 1 to 2 seconds; however, patients with this condition often report that they can still feel the sensation for several seconds occasionally minutes, after the stimulus has ended.

Summation testing for the presence of central sensitization

With the NeuroPEN, apply 10 stimuli to a single location at a rate of 1 per second (rate is important).

Ask, "Does the sensation *change* as I continue to stimulate it?" If the patient answers

- Yes, ask if the sensation was *both* painful *and* increased with each stimulus:
  - Yes: Record as summation and rate the first and final stimulus and have the patient describe the sensation. It is normal for the stimulus to increase by 1 to 2 on a numerical pain score (i.e., the first stimulus is rated at 3 and the last is rated at 5/10). In patients with central sensitization, the first stimulus is often high at 6 to 7/10, and if the patient can tolerate all 10 stimuli, the last stimuli may be rated at 10/10.
  - No: Record as *nonpainful summation.*

Note: While testing, if the *first* stimulus was recorded as either decreased or absent but as the stimuli continue the sensation changes to painful, record as hyperpathia.

CAVEATS TO QUANTITATIVE SENSORY TESTING INTERPRETATION

Pain related to muscle overuse is often described as burning. Loss of sensation to touch and pinprick can be reported with nonneuropathic pain[29] (e.g., muscular pain). Patients with nociceptive pain may also report brush and warm allodynia and heat hyperalgesia, such as described with a sunburn. Pressure allodynia, in particular, is common in both nociceptive and neuropathic pain. Allodynia to brush, cold and heat, and temporal summation to tactile stimuli, although not pathognomonic, are observed in a much higher frequency in patients with neuropathic pain.[30] Bilateral sensory changes can occur in neuropathic pain conditions regarded as unilateral (e.g., postherpetic neuralgia), and cutaneous testing of deeper tissues (e.g., abdominal or pelvic tissues) has not been well validated in cases of nociceptive pain.

Although testing for hypoalgesia to pinprick, hypoesthesia to tactile stimuli, allodynia to brush and cold, and presence of temporal summation are highly reproducible, there is currently insufficient evidence for test–retest reliability and variance over time. Therefore, this examination cannot confidently be used as a monitoring tool to document changes over time.

Sensory testing is a psychophysical test, meaning a physical stimulus is applied, and the patient reports the elicited sensation. It is thus subject to reporting errors related to an individual's attention and reaction time.

FURTHER INVESTIGATIONS OR CONSULTS

Other investigations may include specific radiologic or electromyography testing, a sleep study, specific or baseline laboratory investigations, or urine toxicology screening. Referral to appropriate specialists for further assessments should be requested as needed.

Follow-up Visits

Ideally, the first follow-up visit should be within a few weeks to allow assessment of treatment efficacy and tolerability and to review any tests taken, consults, or goal achievement. An example of a follow-up form given to the patient to complete prior to being seen may be helpful (see Appendix 17.2 as an example). Ideally, the follow-up questionnaire should use some of the same questions as the initial questionnaire to allow outcomes to be collected on such items as mood, sleep, function, and quality of life as well as pain. This will enable appropriate changes to be made in care and recommendations to the patient.

The five *A*'s have been suggested as a useful acronym to document follow-up visits and evaluate the efficacy of opioid therapy. These are Adverse events (to treatment), Affect (mood), Activities (progress toward goals/functionality outcomes), Aberrant drug–related behavior if opioids are prescribed, and Action taken.[31]

Conclusion

Assessment and reassessment should be built into every treatment plan. Patients should leave each visit, whether an initial visit or a follow-up, with a definite and agreed plan. Ideally, this should be in a written/printed format the patients take with them. Patients should also be reminded that it will take engagement on their part to reach relevant goals

Nonadherence, or questioning an agreed treatment plan, occurs in up to 50% of patients. Merely repeating the original reasoning will often be ineffective. Patients need to be involved in a discussion about any concerns or objections they may have to the treatment plan as it evolves. Motivational interviewing plays an important role in developing any treatment plan. For any trial of treatment, a reasonable time to expected improvement must be defined early on (e.g., up to 3 to 4 weeks for an antidepressant to work but within 2 weeks before improvement in pain may be felt with the same drug). With physical therapy or chiropractic care, it may take three to four sessions for ongoing improvement. If there are no recognizable improvements after the agreed on trial time, consider changing or stopping that particular therapy.

Working with a chronic pain patient can be immensely satisfying if the practitioner sees a patient begin to engage more in treating the often disabling, all-encompassing pain and improve the quality of life and function. Having an organized way of getting the patient to give a comprehensive history and validating the pain but not being drawn into the "stories" is a skill that takes time to develop. Being prepared by using some of the suggestions outlined in this chapter and appendices should speed up the "learning curve." Equally important from the practitioner's point of view is to not do it alone, but involve the patients, their significant other, and other community resources. An integrative, multidisciplinary approach will provide the best possible outcome for patients with chronic pain.

Appendix 17.1: Initial Visit Questionnaire

Name:	Date of birth	Today's date

We realize that some of the questions might not address your exact situation, but we encourage you to answer them to your best ability.

Approximately how many years have you had your pain?
_____ years

How many areas of your body are now affected by chronic pain?

☐ 1	☐ 2 to 3	☐ 3 or more

Please indicate where your present pain is:

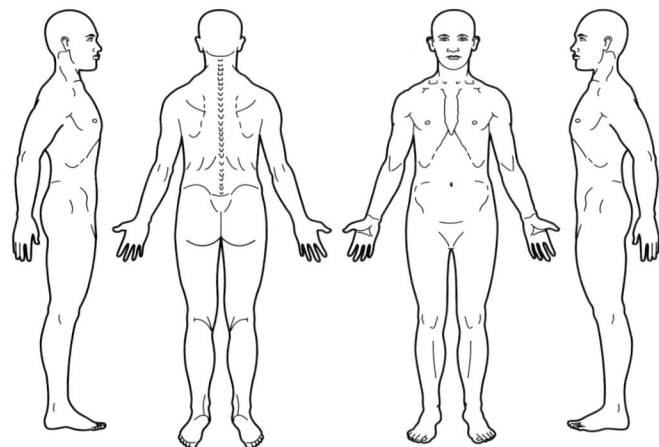

Please rate your level of pain *on average in the last week*:

No pain									Extreme pain
1	2	3	4	5	6	7	8	9	10
☐	☐	☐	☐	☐	☐	☐	☐	☐	☐

Please check the box of the number that best describes how, *during the last week*, pain has interfered with your:

	No interference									Complete interference
	1	2	3	4	5	6	7	8	9	10
General activity	☐	☐	☐	☐	☐	☐	☐	☐	☐	☐
Enjoyment of life	☐	☐	☐	☐	☐	☐	☐	☐	☐	☐
Falling asleep	☐	☐	☐	☐	☐	☐	☐	☐	☐	☐
Staying asleep	☐	☐	☐	☐	☐	☐	☐	☐	☐	☐

Activity difficulty: In order to monitor it during the course of your treatment, please list one important activity that is currently difficult for you to perform:

_____

How would you rate the difficulty you have performing this activity *over the past week*?

No difficulty										Extreme difficulty
0	1	2	3	4	5	6	7	8	9	10
☐	☐	☐	☐	☐	☐	☐	☐	☐	☐	☐

Pain Interference
In the past 7 days . . .

	Not at all	A little bit	Somewhat	Quite a bit	Very much
How much did pain interfere with your day-to-day activities?	☐	☐	☐	☐	☐
How much did pain interfere with work around the home?	☐	☐	☐	☐	☐
How much did pain interfere with your ability to participate in social activities?	☐	☐	☐	☐	☐
How much did pain interfere with your household chores?	☐	☐	☐	☐	☐

Anxiety
In the past 7 days . . .

	Never	Rarely	Sometimes	Often	Always
I felt fearful.	☐	☐	☐	☐	☐
I found it hard to focus on anything other than my anxiety.	☐	☐	☐	☐	☐
My worries overwhelmed me.	☐	☐	☐	☐	☐
I felt uneasy.	☐	☐	☐	☐	☐

Depression
In the past 7 days . . .

	Never	Rarely	Sometimes	Often	Always
I felt worthless.	☐	☐	☐	☐	☐
I felt helpless.	☐	☐	☐	☐	☐
I felt depressed.	☐	☐	☐	☐	☐
I felt hopeless.	☐	☐	☐	☐	☐

Global Health

	Excellent	Very good	Good	Fair	Poor
In general, would you say your health is:	☐	☐	☐	☐	☐
In general, would you say your quality of life is:	☐	☐	☐	☐	☐
In general, how would you rate your physical health?	☐	☐	☐	☐	☐
In general, how would you rate your mental health, including your mood and your ability to think?	☐	☐	☐	☐	☐
In general, how would you rate your satisfaction with your social activities and relationships?	☐	☐	☐	☐	☐
In general, please rate how well you carry out your usual social activities and roles. (This includes activities at home, at work, and in your community and responsibilities as a parent, child, spouse, employee, friend, etc.)	☐	☐	☐	☐	☐

Physical Function

	Without any difficulty	With a little difficulty	With some difficulty	With much difficulty	Unable to do
Are you able to do chores such as vacuuming or yard work?	☐	☐	☐	☐	☐
Are you able to go up and down stairs at a normal pace?	☐	☐	☐	☐	☐
Are you able to go for a walk of at least 15 minutes?	☐	☐	☐	☐	☐
Are you able to run errands and shop?	☐	☐	☐	☐	☐

	None	Mild	Severe	Very Severe
How would you rate your fatigue **on average**?	☐	☐	☐	☐

With the *last 2 weeks* in mind, please answer the following questions:

	Disagree	Agree
It's really not safe for a person with a condition like mine to be physically active.	☐	☐
I have experienced many worrying thoughts.	☐	☐
I feel that my problem is terrible and that it's never going to get any better.	☐	☐

Sleep Observation

	Yes	No
Has anyone observed you stop breathing during your sleep?	☐	☐
Have you ever had sleep study?	☐	☐
If yes, were you told you had sleep apnea?	☐	☐
If yes, do you use a CPAP or other sleep device to help you sleep?	☐	☐
Do you often have problems with restless legs (urge to move the legs, worse at rest, better with activity, worse at evening and night)?	☐	☐
Do your legs frequently jerk during sleep?	☐	☐

In your life, have you ever had any experience that was so frightening, horrible, or upsetting that *in the past month* you:

	Yes	No
Have had nightmares about it or thought about it when you did not want to?	☐	☐
Tried hard not to think about it or went out of your way to avoid situations that reminded you of it?	☐	☐
Were constantly on guard, watchful, or easily startled?	☐	☐
Felt numb or detached from others, activities, or your surroundings?	☐	☐

Do any of the following apply to you?

	Yes	No
Family history (parents and siblings) of alcohol abuse?	☐	☐
Family history (parents and siblings) of illegal drug use?	☐	☐
Family history (parents and siblings) of prescription drug abuse?	☐	☐
Personal history of alcohol abuse?	☐	☐
Personal history of illegal drug use?	☐	☐
Personal history of prescription drug abuse?	☐	☐
Diagnosis of ADD, OCD, bipolar, or schizophrenia?	☐	☐
Diagnosis of depression?	☐	☐
Age 16 to 45 years?	☐	☐
History of preadolescent sexual abuse?	☐	☐

	Yes	No
Have you ever seriously considered or attempted suicide?	☐	☐
Do you have a suicide plan at the moment?	☐	☐

Family Medical History

	Yes	No
Family history of arthritis	☐	☐
Family history of fibromyalgia	☐	☐
Family history of migraines	☐	☐
Family history of heart disease	☐	☐
Family history of similar pain	☐	☐

Past Medications Tried for Pain: (medications you are no longer taking)

Name of drug	Strength	Number per day	**Reason for stopping? (side effects, ineffective, other)**

Work History

What is your occupation? [＿＿＿＿＿＿＿＿]

Are you:

☐ Employed full-time	☐ Employed part-time
☐ Unemployed because of pain	☐ Unemployed because of other reasons
☐ Retired because of pain	☐ Retired but not because of pain
☐ In school or retraining	☐ Homemaker

Overall, on a scale of 0 to 10, how close are you to returning to work? (10 meaning ready to work full-time, 0 meaning you are not even close to work at any job.)

0	1	2	3	4	5	6	7	8	9	10
☐	☐	☐	☐	☐	☐	☐	☐	☐	☐	☐

Do you have an attorney working on your injury claim?

☐ Yes ☐ No

To the best of your recollection, how many different health care providers have you seen in the **LAST 6 MONTHS** for your pain?

	1	2	3	4	5	6	7	8	9	10+
General practice (i.e., family medicine, internal medicine)	☐	☐	☐	☐	☐	☐	☐	☐	☐	☐
Medical specialists	☐	☐	☐	☐	☐	☐	☐	☐	☐	☐
Pain specialists	☐	☐	☐	☐	☐	☐	☐	☐	☐	☐
Surgical specialists	☐	☐	☐	☐	☐	☐	☐	☐	☐	☐
Psychologists, psychiatrists, or other mental health professionals	☐	☐	☐	☐	☐	☐	☐	☐	☐	☐
Physical therapists	☐	☐	☐	☐	☐	☐	☐	☐	☐	☐
Complementary and alternative health care professionals (i.e., naturopath, massage, acupuncture)	☐	☐	☐	☐	☐	☐	☐	☐	☐	☐

Please identify 2 to 3 goals that you would want to achieve if, with therapy, your pain was 50% improved.

1.
2.
3.

Allergies: Are you allergic to any medication? ☐ Yes ☐ No
If YES, please list them.

Medication	Reaction

What over-the-counter (nonprescription) medications or herbal preparations are you taking for your pain or to help you sleep? (e.g., Advil, Aleve, Tylenol, Benadryl)

Name of drug	Strength	Number per day

What medications are you currently taking **for pain?**

Name of drug	Strength	Number per day

What other **non–pain**-related medications are you taking?

Name of drug	Strength	Number per day

Surgical History
Have you had surgeries? ☐ Yes ☐ No
IF YES, please list them.

Past Medical History: Have you had any of these conditions either now or in the past?

	Yes	No		Yes	No
Alcohol addiction	☐	☐	Heart disease	☐	☐
Anesthesia reaction	☐	☐	Heart failure	☐	☐
Arthritis	☐	☐	High blood pressure	☐	☐
Asthma	☐	☐	Kidney disease	☐	☐
Cancer	☐	☐	Mental health disease	☐	☐
COPD	☐	☐	No known problems	☐	☐
Diabetes	☐	☐	Stroke	☐	☐
Drug addiction	☐	☐	Thyroid disease	☐	☐
Acid reflux	☐	☐	Schizophrenia	☐	☐
Stomach ulcer	☐	☐	Panic disorder	☐	☐
Depression	☐	☐	Posttraumatic stress disorder	☐	☐
Bipolar	☐	☐	An unexplained weight loss of more than 10 lb in the last 6 months	☐	☐
Obsessive–compulsive disorder	☐	☐			

Social History
What is your marital status?

☐ Married	☐ Divorced	☐ Living with significant other

Do you have any children? ☐ Yes ☐ No

If yes, what are their ages?

Tobacco Use

☐ No - Never	☐ No - Former smoker	☐ Yes - Occasional smoker	☐ Yes - Smoke every day

If yes,

Ready to quit?	☐ Yes	☐ No			
Packs/day	☐ 0.25	☐ 0.5	☐ 1	☐ 1.5	☐ 2+
Start date			Quit date		

Alcohol Use   ☐ Yes ☐ No

Drinks per week: _____   Glasses of wine

_____   Cans or bottles of beers _____   Shots of liquor

Recreational Drug Use (not prescribed)

☐ Yes	☐ No

Use per week	☐ 1	☐ 2	☐ 5	☐ 10	☐ Other _____
Drug type?	☐ Benzodiaze-pines (Xanax, Ativan, Valium)		☐ Cannabis		☐ Cocaine
	☐ Methamphetamine				☐ Opiates

Appendix 17.2: Pain Diagram

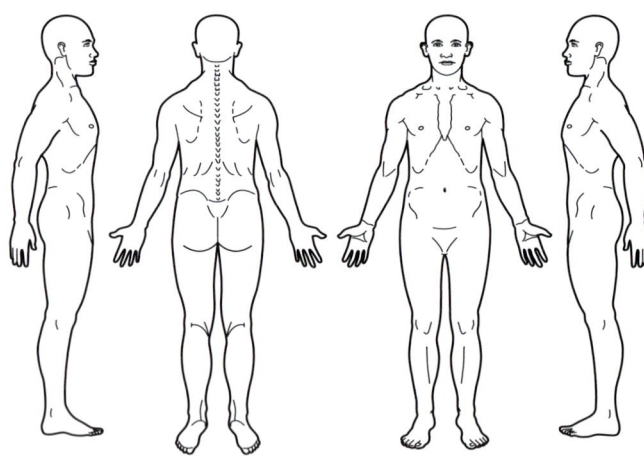

Name _____   Date _____

Please color the areas where you experience pain. Use one of these five coloring pens to shade the specific type of pain that you are experiencing. Then circle with a pen all areas of pain and, starting with the worst, number the areas in order of severity.

Blue—numbness
Red—burning
Green—tingling
If you have other pain sensations, name them here and color as black or yellow
Yellow—
Black—

Appendix 17.3: Goal Setting

GOALS

Your ability to make a change in your life or achieve a goal depends largely on your attitude, commitment, and motivation to do something about your situation. Taking full responsibility to do something about it is the most empowering step you can take.

Taking responsibility does not mean blaming yourself for the problem. And it does not mean you have to do it alone. The big question is "Are you willing to change and to incorporate new habits into your daily routine?"

Considering the Right Goal for You

- What are the most positive changes you would like to see in your life?
- How would these changes affect your feelings and relationships?
- What new opportunities could you gain from making these changes?
- Visualize your goals.
- Setbacks are inevitable and so is the fact that you can figure a way out to solve them.
- Use setbacks as an opportunity to learn; do not view them as a failure.
- Reach out to your social support system for a "reality check" for your goals.
- Do not expect change to be rapid or to do any goal to perfection.
- Enjoy the process of change; the journey is important.
- Reward yourself for making gradual changes and achieving small steps leading to the goal.
- Be fair and kind to yourself.

Setting SMART Goals

Setting realistic and achievable goals will help bring order, success, and accomplishment back to your life. The criteria for setting achievable goals are the following:

- *Specific.* Does it involve specific behavioral actions or steps?
- *Measurable.* How will you know when the goal has been reached?
- *Attainable.* You are the one engaging in the actions or behaviors. Do you want the results enough to make the effort?
- *Realistic.* Is it possible to achieve?
- *Timely.* What is the time frame in which you expect to reach this goal?

Consider your goal and determine what your progress will look like in 2 weeks from now. Imagine yourself looking back, what did you have to do in 1 week in order to get there?

Think about how many goals are reasonable for you to accomplish before your next meeting with your provider. Typically one to three goals is manageable.

Goal 1:

_____

Steps to take to reach this goal:

_____

_____

What could stop me from achieving this goal?

_____

What can I do to prevent it from stopping me?

_____

Goal 2:

_____

Steps to take to reach this goal:

_____

_____

What could stop me from achieving this goal?

_____

What can I do to prevent it from stopping me?

_____

Goal 3:

_____

Steps to take to reach this goal:

_____

_____

What could stop me from achieving this goal?

_____

What can I do to prevent it from stopping me?

_____

Appendix 17.4: Follow-up Questionnaire

Name: [   ]   Date of Birth: [   ]   Date: [   ]

Please indicate where your present pain is:

Please rate your level of pain *on average in the last week*:

No pain									Extreme pain
1	2	3	4	5	6	7	8	9	10
☐	☐	☐	☐	☐	☐	☐	☐	☐	☐

Please check the box of the number that best describes how, *during the last week*, pain has interfered with your:

	No interference									Complete interference
	1	2	3	4	5	6	7	8	9	10
General activity	☐	☐	☐	☐	☐	☐	☐	☐	☐	☐
Enjoyment of life	☐	☐	☐	☐	☐	☐	☐	☐	☐	☐

Please list the important activity **you chose at the last visit** that is currently difficult for you to perform:

[   ]

How would you rate the difficulty you have performing this activity *over the past week*?

No difficulty										Extreme difficulty
0	1	2	3	4	5	6	7	8	9	10
☐	☐	☐	☐	☐	☐	☐	☐	☐	☐	☐

In the past month, how many days have you had where you felt you needed to take more pain medication than your doctor is currently prescribing?

☐ None	☐ 1 to 2	☐ 3 to 4	☐ 5 or more

How would you rate your fatigue *on average*?

None	Mild	Severe	Very severe
☐	☐	☐	☐

Physical Function	Without any difficulty	With a little difficulty	With some difficulty	With much difficulty	Unable to do
Are you able to do chores such as vacuuming or yard work?	☐	☐	☐	☐	☐
Are you able to go up and down stairs at a normal pace?	☐	☐	☐	☐	☐
Are you able to go for a walk of at least 15 minutes?	☐	☐	☐	☐	☐
Are you able to run errands and shop?	☐	☐	☐	☐	☐

Sleep

In the past 7 days . . .	Very poor	Poor	Fair	Good	Very good
My sleep quality was . . .	☐	☐	☐	☐	☐
In the past 7 days . . .	Not at all	A little bit	Somewhat	Quite a bit	Very much
My sleep was refreshing.	☐	☐	☐	☐	☐
I had a problem with my sleep.	☐	☐	☐	☐	☐
I had difficulty falling asleep.	☐	☐	☐	☐	☐

Have you developed any new allergies recently?   ☐ Yes ☐ No

Have you had any changes to your medications since last seen?   ☐ Yes ☐ No

Are you getting side effects from your medications that you would like to discuss, for example, constipation, dry mouth, or drowsiness?   ☐ Yes ☐ No

Have you had any serious illness, hospitalization, or surgery since last visit?   ☐ Yes ☐ No

If yes, what was the event?   [   ]

Please list any concerns, in order of importance, which you would like to discuss today:

[   ]

How satisfied are you with your treatment at the Swedish Pain Services so far?

Very dissatisfied ☐ 1	☐ 2	☐ 3	☐ 4	☐ 5	☐ 6	Very satisfied ☐ 7

Did you achieve any of the goals you set for yourself at the last visit?

☐ Did not try   ☐ Almost achieved   ☐ Achieved   ☐ Achieved and more

New goal?   [   ]

References

1. Kori SH. Kinisophobia: a new view of chronic pain behaviour. *Pain Manage* 1990;3:35–43.
2. Davidson MA, Tripp DA, Fabrigar LR, et al. Chronic pain assessment: a seven-factor model. *Pain Res Manage* 2008;13:299–308.
3. Coambs RB, Jarry JL, Santhiapillai AC, et al. The SISAP: a new screening instrument for identifying potential opioid abusers in the management of chronic nonmalignant pain within general medical practice. *Pain Res Manage* 1996;1:155–162.
4. Turk DC, Fillingim RB, Ohrbach R, et al. Assessment of psychosocial and functional impact of chronic pain. *J Pain* 2016;17:T21–T49.
5. Mathieson S, Maher CG, Terwee CB, et al. Neuropathic pain screening questionnaires have limited measurement properties. A systematic review. *J Clin Epidemiol* 2015;68:957–966.
6. Hjermstad MJ, Fayers PM, Haugen DF, et al; and European Palliative Care Research Collaborative. Studies comparing numerical rating scales, verbal rating scales, and visual analogue scales for assessment of pain intensity in adults: a systematic literature review. *J Pain Symptom Manage* 2011;41:1073–1093.
7. Lewis JS, Kersten P, McPherson KM, et al. Wherever is my arm? Impaired upper limb position accuracy in complex regional pain syndrome. *Pain* 2016;149:463–469.
8. Dworkin RH, Turk DC, Revicki DA, et al. Development and initial validation of an expanded and revised version of the Short-Form McGill Pain Questionnaire (SF-MPQ-2). *Pain* 2009;144:35–42.
9. Sullivan MJL, Thorn B, Haythornthwaite JA, et al. Theoretical perspectives on the relation between catastrophizing and pain. *Clin J Pain* 2001;17:52–64.
10. Peterson C, Moon CH. Coping with catastrophes and catastrophizing. In: Snyder CR, ed. *Coping: The Psychology of What Works.* New York: Oxford University Press; 1999:252–278.
11. Bunzli S, Smith A, Watkins R, et al. What do people who score highly on the Tampa Scale of Kinesiophobia really believe? *Clin J Pain* 2015;31:621–632.
12. Sullivan MJ, Adams H, Horan S, et al. The role of perceived injustice in the experience of chronic pain and disability: scale development and validation. *J Occup Rehabil* 2008;18:249–261.
13. Meyer-Rosberg K, Kvarnström A, Kinnman E, et al. Peripheral neuropathic pain—a multidimensional burden for patients. *Eur J Pain* 2001;5:379–389.
14. Taylor DJ, Mallory LJ, Lichstein KL, et al. Comorbidity of chronic insomnia with medical problems. *Sleep* 2007;30:213–218.
15. Smith MT, Edwards RR, McCann UD, et al. The effects of sleep deprivation on pain inhibition and spontaneous pain in women. *Sleep* 2007;30:494–505.
16. Moriarty O, McGuire BE, Finn DP. The effect of pain on cognitive function: a review of clinical and preclinical research. *Prog Neurobiol* 2011;93:385–404.
17. Landrø NI, Fors EA, Våpenstad LL, et al. The extent of neurocognitive dysfunction in a multidisciplinary pain centre population. Is there a relation between reported and tested neuropsychological functioning? *Pain* 2013;154:972–977.
18. Glass JM. Review of cognitive dysfunction in fibromyalgia: a convergence on working memory and attentional control impairments. *Rheum Dis Clin North Am* 2009;35:299–311.
19. Kravitz HM, Katz RS. Fibrofog and fibromyalgia: a narrative review and implications for clinical practice. *Rheumatol Int* 2015;35:1115–1125.
20. Young LD, Kreiner PW, Panas L. Unsolicited reporting to prescribers of opioid analgesics by a state prescription drug monitoring program: an observational study with matched comparison group [published online ahead of print April 4, 2017]. *Pain Med.* doi:10.1093/pm/pnx044.
21. Pardo B. Do more robust prescription drug monitoring programs reduce prescription opioid overdose? *Addiction* 2017;112:1773–1783.
22. Hwang CS, Turner LW, Kruszewski SP, et al. Primary care physicians' knowledge and attitudes regarding prescription opioid abuse and diversion. *Clin J Pain* 2016;32:279–284.
23. Shaw WS, van der Windt DA, Main CJ, et al. Early patient screening and intervention to address individual-level occupational factors ("blue flags") in back disability. *J Occup Rehabil* 2009;19:64–80.
24. Opsahl J, Eriksen HR, Tveito TH. Do expectancies of return to work and Job satisfaction predict actual return to work in workers with long lasting LBP? *BMC Musculoskelet Disord* 2016;17:481.
25. Kuttikat A, Shaikh M, Oomatia A, et al. Novel signs and their clinical utility in diagnosing complex regional pain syndrome (CRPS): a prospective observational cohort study. *Clin J Pain* 2017;33:496–502.
26. Woolf CJ. Central sensitization: implications for the diagnosis and treatment of pain. *Pain* 2011;152:S2–S15.
27. Baron R, Hans G, Dickenson AH. Peripheral input and its importance for central sensitization. *Ann Neurol* 2013;74:630–636.
28. Leffler AS, Hansson P. Painful traumatic peripheral partial nerve injury-sensory dysfunction profiles comparing outcomes of bedside examination and quantitative sensory testing. *Eur J Pain* 2008;12:397–402.
29. Rasmussen PV, Sindrup SH, Jensen TS, et al. Symptoms and signs in patients with suspected neuropathic pain. *Pain* 2004;110:461–469.
30. Treede RD, Handwerker HO, Baumgärtner U, et al. Hyperalgesia and allodynia: taxonomy, assessment, and mechanisms. In: Brune K, Handwerker HO, eds. *Hyperalgesia: Molecular Mechanisms and Clinical Implications.* Seattle, WA: IASP Press; 2004:3–15. *Progress in Pain Research and Management*; vol 30.
31. Volkow NP, McLellan AT. Opioid abuse in chronic pain—misconceptions and mitigation strategies. *N Engl J Med* 2016;374:1253–1263.

CHAPTER 18

Electrodiagnosis in Pain Medicine

NATHAN J. RUDIN

To effectively treat acute and chronic pain, the clinician must understand its causes. Electrodiagnostic testing (EDX) can significantly improve that understanding. It complements the history, physical examination, laboratory testing, and imaging studies by providing quantitative assessments of the health, integrity, and function of muscle and nerve. Thoughtful electrodiagnostic studies can help narrow a differential or confirm a diagnosis. They can clearly identify the extent, severity, and location of nerve injury, muscle damage, or disease of the neuromuscular junction. Serial examinations can track disease progression, provide prognostic information, and measure recovery.

Clinicians should consider EDX whenever they suspect focal or diffuse neuromuscular disease. In these conditions, weakness, numbness, tingling, and pain are the most frequent complaints. The physical examination may include alterations in sensation, strength, reflexes, muscle bulk, muscle tone, and/or coordination. Imaging and laboratory studies may be normal or abnormal, depending on the condition. Common indications for EDX include nerve entrapment, radiculopathy, plexopathy, and traumatic injuries as well as metabolic disorders (e.g., diabetes mellitus), peripheral neuropathies, myopathies, and diseases of the neuromuscular junction. Special tests can assess disorders of cranial, pharyngeal, and perineal structures.

This chapter will familiarize the reader with the basic principles of EDX, provide guidance on interpretation of test reports, and help caregivers make optimal use of EDX when assessing patients in acute and chronic pain.

The Electrodiagnostic Laboratory

A reputable electrodiagnostic laboratory employs consistent techniques and norms to ensure accuracy and reliability. Test data should be interpreted by a trained and experienced physician, and electromyographers should be readily accessible for questions and case discussions from referring providers. To determine abnormal results, the laboratory should compare its results to documented and standardized normal values and should use the same norms consistently. Examiners within a laboratory should use the same techniques so that the same norms apply to all cases.

The laboratory should have good climate control set at a comfortable room temperature, as an excessively cold environment may adversely affect results. Electrical circuitry supplying the room should be properly shielded and grounded to ensure patient safety and to reduce line–current interference from equipment such as fluorescent light fixtures. Commercial electrodiagnostic units have been designed and rigorously tested to ensure safety and reliability.

The electrodiagnostic unit or "EMG machine" is primarily composed of a sensitive differential amplifier (high signal-to-noise ratio) and an electrical stimulator with precise control of stimulus duration and intensity, coupled to a computer for ease of data acquisition, analysis, and storage (Fig. 18.1). An active electrode (G1) is placed over the desired recording location, and a reference electrode (G2) is placed nearby. The amplifier subtracts the reference signal from the active signal to remove elements common to both, leaving only the information unique to the active electrode. The resulting signal (G1 to G2) is amplified, displayed, and stored.

Electrodiagnostic Tests

Most patients referred for EDX will undergo both nerve conduction studies (NCS) and needle electromyography (EMG). The entire procedure (both EMG and NCS) is often referred to as "EMG" when ordering the test or describing it to patients.

NERVE CONDUCTION STUDIES

NCS use electrical stimuli over a selected nerve to produce an action potential, which is recorded using electrodes placed further along the course of the stimulated nerve or the muscle it supplies. The resulting waveforms are analyzed and compared to normal values derived from a database of healthy individuals. The electrical stimulus is usually administered transcutaneously, with the stimulator probe (Fig. 18.2 shows an example)

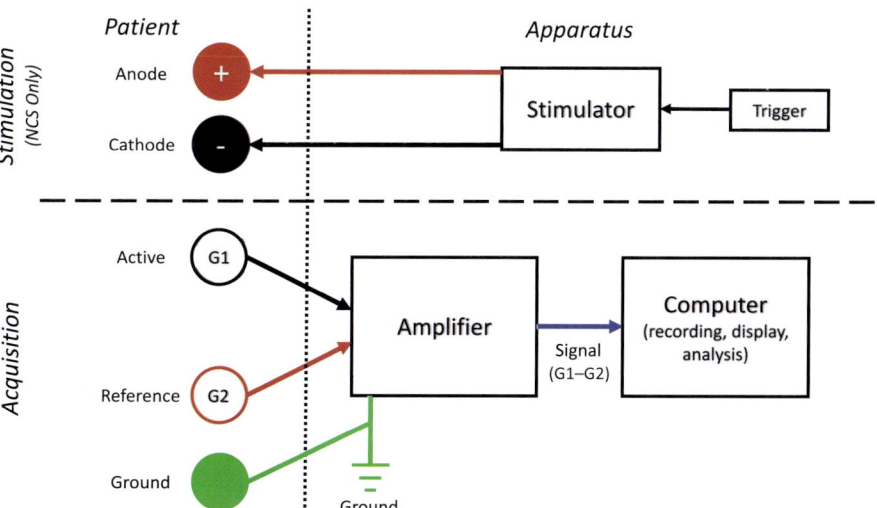

FIGURE 18.1 Typical electrodiagnostic setup. Connections to the patient are illustrated to the left of the *dotted line* and apparatus to the right; stimulation (during nerve conduction studies) is represented above the *dashed line* and data acquisition below it. Electrical stimulation produces a desired action potential (during nerve conduction studies; muscles produce their own potentials during needle electromyography). Potentials are recorded, amplified, displayed, and stored.

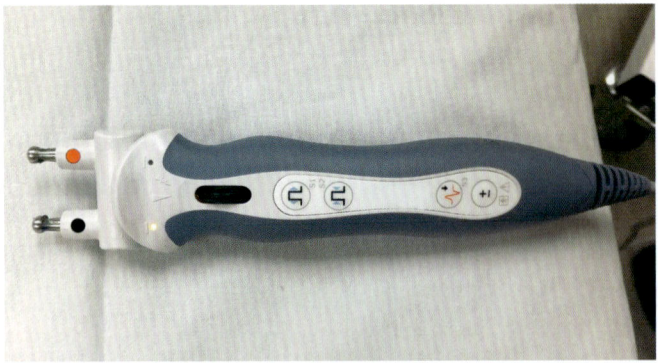

FIGURE 18.2 Example of a transcutaneous electrical stimulator probe. *Black dot* indicates the cathode; *red dot*, the anode. Some probe models, such as this one, permit the examiner to vary the stimulation intensity and trigger the stimulus from the probe itself; others require a separate control panel.

positioned on the skin overlying the desired nerve. Recording electrodes are generally placed on the skin. In special circumstances (e.g., deep nerves, obesity, edema), stimulation and/or recording may be accomplished using needle electrodes advanced through the skin and placed adjacent to the desired structures. Patients should be warned before testing that the stimulated limb may twitch when the shock is delivered.

Electrical stimulation should not be performed over or near pacemakers, implantable cardioverter-defibrillators, spinal cord stimulators, or other implanted medical electronics. In most patients, stimulation distant from the implant and its electrodes can be safely accomplished, but if there is any doubt, check with the device manufacturer before proceeding.

Electrical stimulation is generally perceived as a brief (0.1 to 0.2 ms), mildly uncomfortable "static" shock, repeated as stimulus amplitude is gradually increased. Once a maximal response is elicited from the nerve being studied, stimulation is terminated and the action potential is analyzed.

Parameters recorded during NCS include action potential latency (time between stimulation and initiation or peak of action potential), action potential amplitude, and nerve conduction velocity (NCV). Latency and NCV reflect myelin health; demyelination will prolong the latency and slow the NCV. Amplitude reflects axonal integrity; axonal loss or injury may produce decreased amplitude and temporal dispersion of the action potential. The distribution of abnormalities can distinguish focal, segmental, and diffuse neuropathic processes. Stimulation at multiple points along the nerve allows measurement of NCV across different nerve segments. Where abnormal results are seen, comparison to a contralateral asymptomatic structure, where available, provides a valuable intra-individual control.[1] Varieties of NCS are described in detail in the following text along with their specific applications.

Sensory nerve conduction studies (SNCS): SNCS provide detailed assessment of sensory nerve function. Nerve stimulation produces a sensory nerve action potential (SNAP), which is recorded over the same peripheral nerve at a distance from the stimulation point. Figure 18.3 illustrates a standard setup for a median SNCS (Fig. 18.3A) and the resulting normal SNAP (Fig. 18.3B). Because nerves conduct bidirectionally from the point of stimulation, SNCS may be performed *orthodromically* (in the physiologic direction, stimulating distally, and recording proximally) or, as in this case, *antidromically* (stimulating proximally and recording distally).

Figure 18.4 shows an orthodromic SNCS comparing distal conduction of the median and ulnar nerves across the wrist (Fig. 18.4A). This study is highly sensitive and specific for the

presence of carpal tunnel syndrome (median entrapment neuropathy at the wrist), which is demonstrated here (Fig. 18.4B). The two nerve segments are of equal lengths and should have approximately the same latency and NCV. In this case, the median SNAP latency is appreciably prolonged, indicating conduction delay. Median amplitude is also lower than the laboratory's norm of 51 μv. Values for the ulnar SNAP are normal.

SNCS results may be altered by cold skin temperatures, potentially leading to incorrect diagnoses. Warming the skin to ≥32°C will minimize this cause of error.

Like electrical cables, peripheral nerves are composed of numerous nerve fibers with varying functions, diameters, and degrees of myelination. The SNAP elicited during SNCS primarily reflects the response of faster conducting, more heavily myelinated afferent fibers. Responses from smaller diameter, less myelinated fibers (e.g., C and Aδ fibers transmitting pain and temperature signals) may not be detected. Standard SNCS therefore lack sensitivity for detecting small-fiber dysfunction in painful conditions.[2] Alternate techniques, such as quantitative sensory testing (see the following text) and skin punch biopsy with nerve fiber staining,[3] can augment the physical examination to help characterize small-fiber abnormalities.

Motor nerve conduction studies (MNCS): MNCS characterize the health of motor nerve fibers and the neuromuscular junction. Nerve stimulation produces a compound muscle action potential (CMAP), which is recorded over a muscle innervated by the stimulated nerve. Figure 18.5 shows the

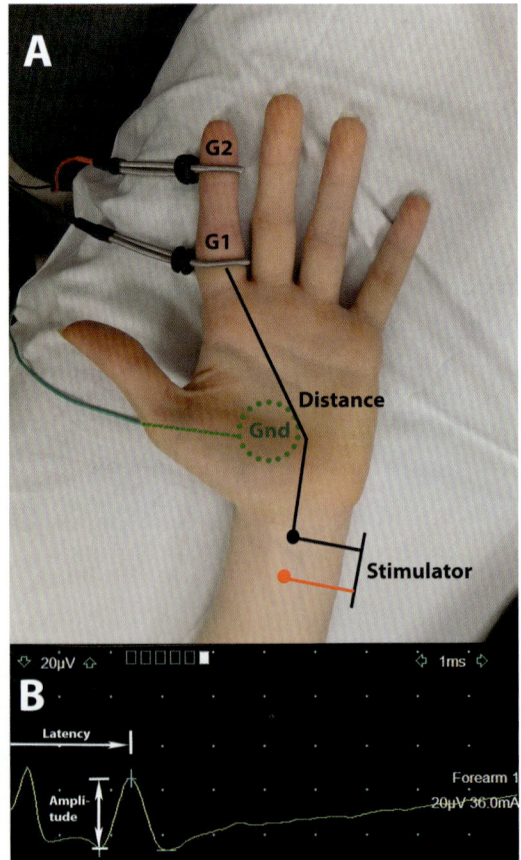

FIGURE 18.3 A: Setup for median nerve antidromic sensory nerve conduction studies (SNCS). Stimulation is applied at the wrist and recorded over the digital nerves to the index finger. **B:** Median sensory nerve action potential (SNAP). Graph measures amplitude (*y*-axis) versus time (*x*-axis). Left edge of the diagram corresponds to the moment of electrical stimulation. Peak latency and amplitude of the SNAP are illustrated. *GnD*, ground electrode.

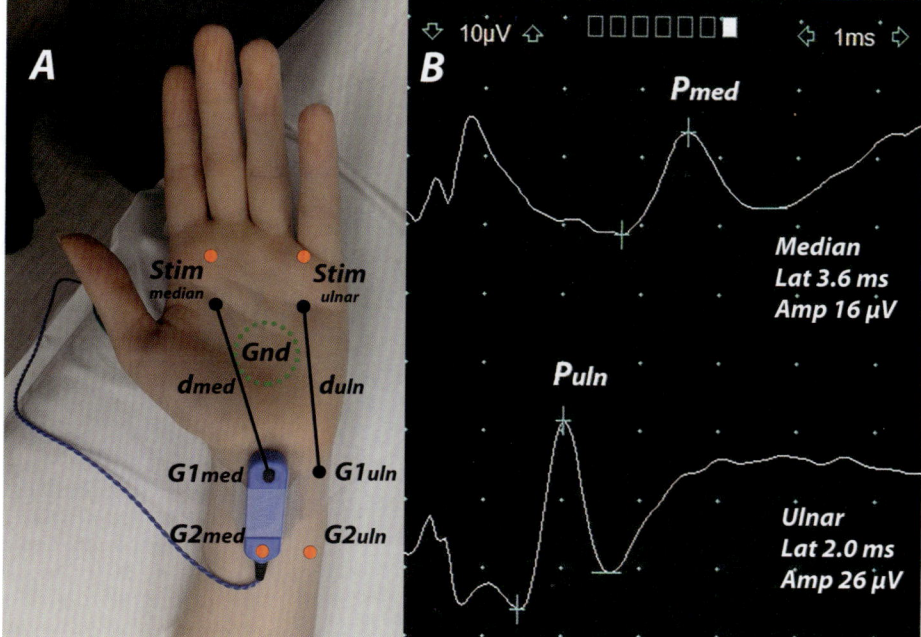

FIGURE 18.4 **A:** Setup for orthodromic median versus ulnar transcarpal sensory nerve conduction studies (SNCS). Palm is stimulated over median and then ulnar nerve. Sensory nerve action potentials (SNAPs) are recorded at the wrist. Distance (*d*) between G1 and the cathode is equal for median *(med)* and ulnar *(uln)* nerves. **B:** Results. In a normal study, median *(med)* and ulnar *(uln)* peak latencies are approximately equal. In this example, the ulnar SNAP is normal, but the median SNAP latency is prolonged and amplitude reduced, demonstrating conduction delay and axonal loss (or partial conduction block) from entrapment at the carpal tunnel. *Gnd*, ground electrode; *Stim*, stimulator position.

setup (Fig. 18.5A) and normal results (Fig. 18.5B) for an ulnar MNCS recording at abductor digiti minimi. The nerve is stimulated at multiple sites along its length; distances between stimulation points are measured and recorded. Onset latencies and CMAP amplitudes are measured. Motor NCV in meter per second (m/s) is calculated by dividing the distance between points (Δd, in millimeter) by the change in time between stimulation points (Δt, in millisecond).

Repetitive nerve stimulation studies (RNS): RNS are a variant of MNCS that can identify disorders of the neuromuscular junction. Rapid repetitive stimulation (usually 2 to 3 Hz) is performed, as illustrated in Figure 18.6A. A decrement in CMAP amplitude during RNS is abnormal and suggests a disorder of the neuromuscular junction. CMAP decrement with RNS is illustrated in Figure 18.6B. The response of CMAP amplitude to exercise can differentiate between neuromuscular disorders.

H-reflex studies: H-reflex studies are modified MNCS that help to identify some radiculopathies and peripheral neuropathies. The H-reflex is an analog of the muscle stretch reflex.

Most commonly, the tibial nerve is electrically stimulated at the popliteal region (analogous to an Achilles tendon tap) and the reflex response (H-reflex) in the soleus muscle is measured. A unilaterally absent or delayed tibial H-reflex may reflect an S1 radiculopathy, tibial neuropathy, or sciatic neuropathy. Bilateral abnormalities may be seen in peripheral neuropathies and in older individuals. H-reflexes may also be found by stimulating the median nerve at the elbow and recording at flexor carpi radialis. They are more widespread in hyperreflexic conditions (e.g., myelopathy) and in infants.[1]

Another modified MNCS, the *F-wave study,* allows indirect observation of nerve conduction between the dorsal root ganglion (DRG) and the spinal cord, permitting sensitive evaluation of polyneuropathies including Guillain-Barré syndrome (GBS), radiculopathies, and proximal nerve dysfunction.[4] Upon peripheral nerve stimulation, the stimulus travels bidirectionally, producing (1) a CMAP and (2) a small, later potential (F-wave) from antidromic activation of a small pool of alpha-motoneurons. Their appearance and latency are variable (Fig. 18.7).

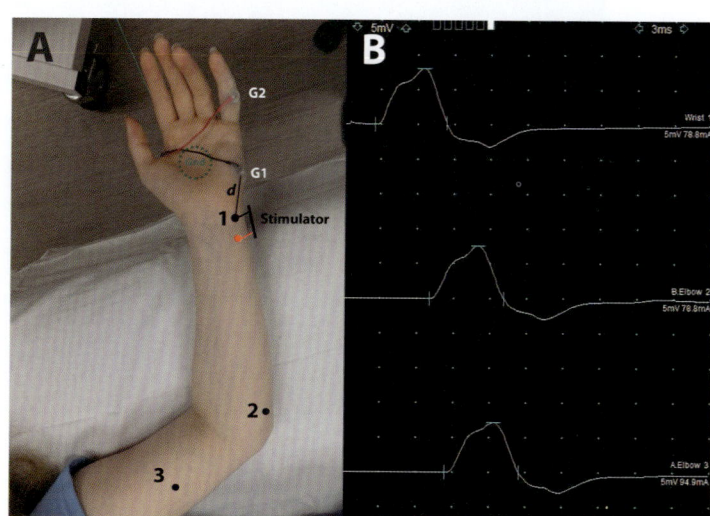

FIGURE 18.5 **A:** Setup for ulnar motor nerve condition studies (MNCS) recording at abductor digiti minimi. Stimulation is applied at the wrist *(1),* below the elbow *(2),* and above the elbow *(3).* **B:** Normal results, including onset latencies, amplitudes, and calculated motor NCV. *Gnd*, ground electrode; *d*, distance.

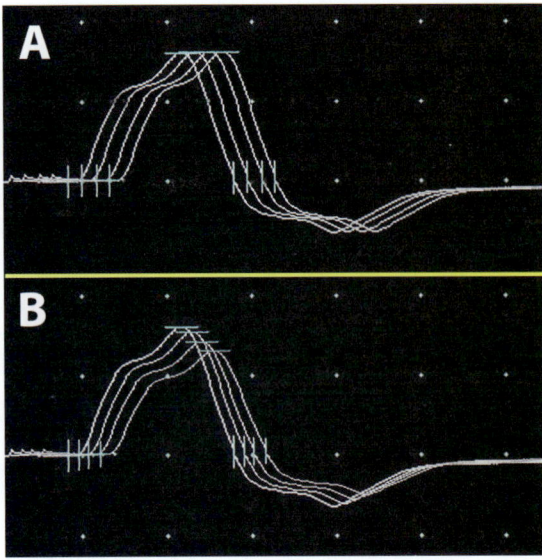

FIGURE 18.6 Motor nerve conduction studies (MNCS) (simulated) with repetitive nerve stimulation at ulnar nerve, recording at abductor digiti minimi, stimulation at wrist, frequency 2 Hz. **A:** Normal. Compound muscle action potential (CMAP) amplitude does not change with repetitive stimulation. **B:** Myasthenia gravis, preexercise. Decrement in CMAP amplitude with repetitive stimulation.

Cranial nerve studies: The trigeminal nerve reflexes (blink reflex, jaw jerk, and masseter inhibitory reflex) can be studied using special EDX,[5] providing valuable clues to lesions of cranial nerves and/or the brain stem.[6] The blink reflex (corneal reflex) is the most often studied and can provide information regarding the integrity of the ophthalmic division (V1) of the trigeminal nerve, the facial nerve (efferent limb), and the brain stem. In the normal blink reflex study, electrical stimulation of the supraorbital nerve unilaterally is followed by a facial nerve blink response bilaterally.

Sacral nerve studies: Special techniques are used to examine sacral sensory and motor innervation, including studies of the bulbocavernosus and clitorocavernosus reflexes (pudendal and perineal nerves). Along with EMG of pelvic floor muscles, these studies can help diagnose sacral nerve dysfunction due to cauda equina syndrome, peripheral neuropathy, focal neuropathies, pelvic pain syndromes, neurogenic erectile dysfunction,[7] and Tarlov cysts.[8] They may, however, be quite uncomfortable for the patient, so they are reserved for cases where the findings are crucial for treatment decisions.

NEEDLE ELECTROMYOGRAPHY

Needle EMG uses needle electrodes to directly assess the electrical activity of motor units, providing extensive information about their integrity, innervation, function, and recruitment. A skilled electromyographer can identify a broad range of disorders causing denervation, inflammation or other destruction, or failure of neuromuscular transmission.

EMG is indicated whenever muscular dysfunction is suspected. It can assist with the diagnosis of neuropathies, radiculopathies, or plexopathies; myopathies (inflammatory, congenital, or other); disorders of the neuromuscular junction; and motor neuron diseases. Where NCS has indicated abnormalities, EMG can help clarify their distribution and severity; also, EMG often detects significant abnormalities when NCS are normal (radiculopathy is a common example). Special electrodes and techniques permit the assessment of single muscle fibers, which can clarify diagnosis in some conditions, particularly neuromuscular junction disorders.[9]

The electromyographer chooses which nerves and muscles to examine, and which techniques to employ, based on the history and physical examination. A strong command of neuroanatomy is required. The electrodiagnostic exam will ideally screen for most conditions on the differential diagnosis. For example, when pathology in a nerve structure is suspected, the electromyographer will perform the appropriate NCS and then will use EMG to assess multiple muscles supplied by that structure. The choice of nerves and muscles will vary with suspicion of peripheral nerve, plexus, nerve root, muscle, or other neuromuscular pathology. Findings on earlier tests often change the choice of tests performed later as the differential is narrowed or widened.

Where it is important to diagnose a nerve lesion early, electrodiagnostic studies within 7 to 10 days of injury can localize

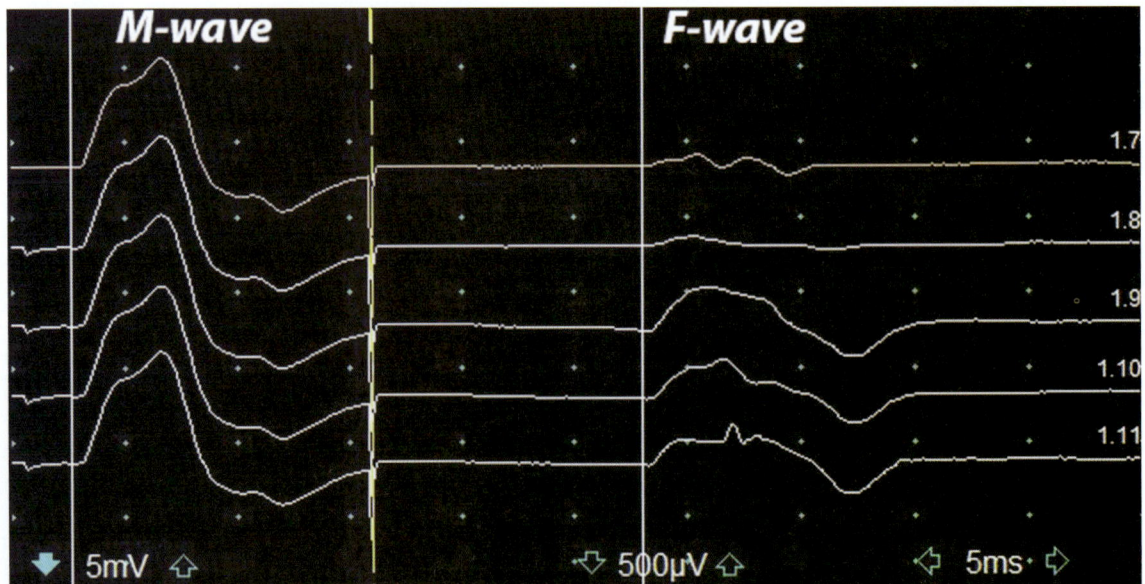

FIGURE 18.7 Ulnar motor F-wave study. The ulnar nerve is electrically stimulated, producing both orthodromic and antidromic action potentials. The orthodromic potential produces a compound muscle action potential (CMAP) (M-wave). The antidromic potential proceeds proximally via primary afferent neurons to the dorsal root ganglion, through the dorsal horn, and via reflex pathways activates a small pool of α-motor neurons in the ventral horn, producing a small motor response (F-wave).

FIGURE 18.8 Concentric electromyography (EMG) needle electrode. The angled electrode tip is the recording surface; the shaft of the needle is insulated with Teflon. The active electrode (center of the needle tip; see *insert*) is surrounded by the reference electrode. Thin needles (26G on average, usual range 23 to 30G) are used to minimize patient discomfort.

nerve lesions and quantify the severity of nerve injury. Studies performed 3 to 4 weeks after injury provide information on muscle denervation and can help with surgical planning. Studies done 2 to 6 months after injury can quantify healing and provide prognostic information.[10] In chronic illnesses such as motor neuron disease and peripheral neuropathies, serial studies document disease course, progression, and prognosis.

EMG should be performed with caution in patients with coagulopathies or who are taking anticoagulant agents. Bleeding with needle EMG is rare; anticoagulants should not routinely be discontinued, but caution is advised, particularly at higher levels of anticoagulation or where there are other reasons to suspect increased bleeding risk.[11] Antiplatelet agents do not appear to significantly increase the risk of bleeding.

Once postoperative healing is complete, needle examination at or near prosthetic joints does not usually require prophylactic antibiotics. In cases of lymphedema, needle puncture may increase the risk of cellulitis and/or lymph leakage, so caution is advised when choosing to perform EMG in such situations.[12] If a muscle may need to be biopsied, it should not be examined with needle electrodes, as the needle trauma may produce abnormalities in biopsy specimens.

Needle electrodes are most often monopolar (single conductor, requiring an external reference electrode) or concentric (active and reference electrodes within the same needle). As the distance between active and reference electrodes is much smaller using a concentric needle (Fig. 18.8), noise is minimized and signal clarity improves.

Needle EMG can be uncomfortable, but the examiner can minimize the pain by positioning the patient comfortably, moving the needle only when the muscle is relaxed, using the smallest gauge needle necessary, and warning the patient to prepare him or her before insertion occurs. More anxious individuals may wish to employ relaxation techniques, have a familiar person nearby, or take a mild prescribed anxiolytic before the procedure. As patients are asked to activate their muscles voluntarily during the procedure, it is important that they remain conscious and able to follow commands. Needle EMG can still be of value when conducted in heavily sedated or unconscious patients (such as in critical care situations), but analysis of voluntary motor unit activity is not possible in these circumstances.

The electromyographer chooses muscles for needle analysis according to the patient's specific clinical situation, the reported symptoms, and the findings on physical examination. By careful muscle selection and observation of abnormalities, the skilled examiner can distinguish among plexopathies, myopathies, radiculopathies, and numerous other conditions.

The needle is typically inserted through the skin into a relaxed muscle. Following insertion, the needle is moved short distances within the muscle at intervals of about once per second while the electromyographer studies the display and listens to muscle activity. Healthy muscles are electrically quiet at rest. They produce short bursts of noise (insertional activity, or IA) during needle movements and silence between movements. In cases of muscle scarring or fibrosis, IA may be decreased or muted.

Potentials present between insertions in a resting muscle are known as spontaneous activity (SA) and reflect abnormalities of the neuromuscular junction. SA may be caused by denervation (as in neuropathies or radiculopathies), muscle membrane injury (as in myopathies), or other abnormalities affecting neuromuscular function. Each type of SA has a distinct waveform and sound that skilled electromyographers rapidly recognize. Common types of SA include fibrillation potentials, positive sharp waves, and complex repetitive discharges, as illustrated in Figure 18.9. Fasciculations (spontaneous discharges of single motor units) may indicate motor neuron disease or other

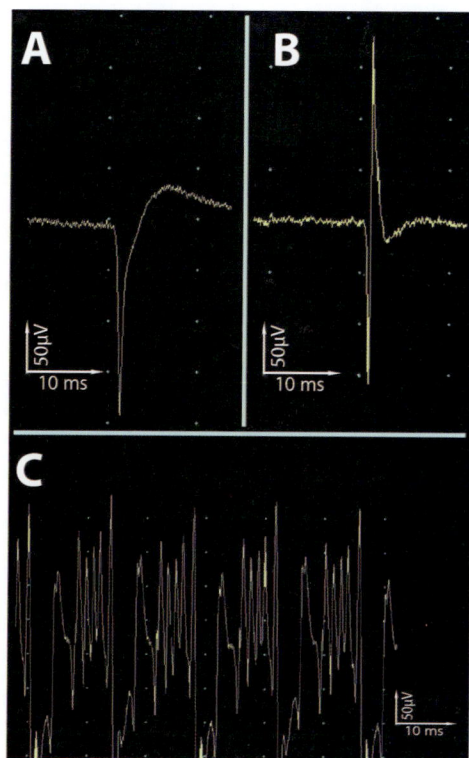

FIGURE 18.9 Spontaneous activity resulting from muscle membrane instability. **A:** Positive sharp wave. **B:** Fibrillation potential. **C:** Complex repetitive discharge.

TABLE 18.1   Scoring System for Abnormal Spontaneous Activity

0	None
1+	Transient but reproducible discharges after moving needle
2+	Occasional discharges at rest in more than two different sites
3+	Spontaneous activity at rest regardless of needle position
4+	Abundant, constant spontaneous activity

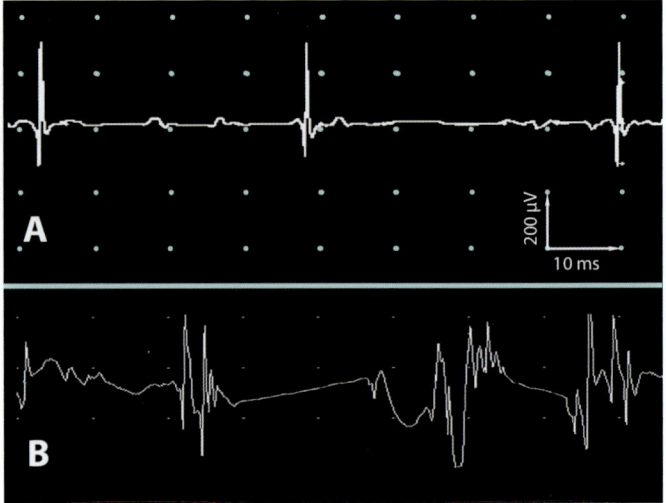

FIGURE 18.10 Motor unit potentials. **A:** Normal motor unit firing repeatedly. **B:** Polyphasic motor units in chronic lumbar radiculopathy, the result of reinnervation and motor unit reorganization following nerve injury.

neuromuscular disorders and may confirm a diagnosis of amyotrophic lateral sclerosis (ALS); distal limb muscles have the highest sensitivity for ALS-related abnormalities.[13] The amount and frequency of SA provide information about the acuity and/or severity of a disease process. SA are summarized in electrodiagnostic reports using the grading system in Table 18.1.

Once the resting muscle is analyzed, the patient is asked to voluntarily contract the muscle being studied, producing motor unit potentials (MUPs). Normal MUPs have a characteristic amplitude, duration, and number of phases (crossings of the signal baseline). Low-amplitude muscle contractions engage one or a few MUPs, but more are recruited in frequency-dependent fashion as the force of contraction increases. Abnormalities of MUP morphology and recruitment provide clues to the type and chronicity of neuromuscular disease. Figure 18.10 illustrates MUPs seen in normal muscle (Fig. 18.10A) and in chronic radiculopathy (Fig. 18.10B). Table 18.2 summarizes the significance of various EMG parameters mentioned in electrodiagnostic reports.

Somatosensory evoked potentials (SSEP): SSEP are employed to measure nerve conduction between a peripheral nerve and the spinal cord and/or cerebral cortex. Interruptions in peripheral or central conduction are manifest as delayed or absent responses. SSEP can be helpful diagnostically in multiple sclerosis, spinal cord injury, and other central nervous disorders. SSEP are particularly useful in the diagnosis of cervical myelopathy; responses from tibial nerve stimulation are recommended.[14] SSEP are frequently employed for intraoperative monitoring during neurosurgical procedures to assess continuity of nerve, root, and cord.[15]

Sympathetic skin response (SSR): SSR measures tonic changes in skin conductance caused by changing sweat output, providing a measure of sympathetic efferent innervation. Increased sympathetic tone normally causes increased sweating and a corresponding drop in skin conductance. SSR may be useful in the diagnosis of generalized and localized neuropathies where small-fiber dysfunction is suspected and can help characterize peripheral efferent dysfunction in complex regional pain syndrome (CRPS).[16–18]

SSR is generally performed using a 2- or 4-channel amplifier to record responses from multiple limbs simultaneously. A standardized stimulus, such as a small electrical shock, is delivered over a midline bodily structure, often the forehead. The SSR for each limb is recorded and differences between limbs are measured. Absence, delay, or decreased amplitude of SSR indicates abnormalities of sympathetic innervation.

Surface electromyography (sEMG): In sEMG, electrodes placed on the skin are used to detect skeletal muscle activity. sEMG acquisition is noninvasive and thus attractive. sEMG signals represent the summation of many CMAP. Although single motor units cannot be assessed, the technique is quite useful for specific applications. sEMG activity may reflect voluntary movement or hypertonic states such as muscle spasm. Trunk muscle sEMG activation patterns are altered in patients following low back injury, and these alterations may persist even after apparent recovery.[19]

When converted to an audible or visual signal, sEMG may be used clinically in biofeedback training to treat pain conditions. Once patients are made aware of the degree of activity in a muscle or muscles, they can learn to reduce activity in overused muscles, lowering muscle pain and promoting relaxation. Conversely, patients may learn to strengthen weakened or underused muscles. EMG biofeedback has been employed to treat low back pain with mixed results.[20–22] Somewhat better success

TABLE 18.2   Clinical Significance of Electromyography Parameters

Parameter	Increased	Decreased
Insertional activity	Denervation (as in neuropathy) or muscle membrane irritability (as in myopathy)	Fibrosis (as in scarring and/or muscle atrophy)
Spontaneous activity	Denervation (as in neuropathy) or muscle membrane irritability (as in myopathy)	No spontaneous activity is present in normal muscle.
MUP amplitude	Reinnervation after injury with spatial enlargement of motor units, as in recovery from neuropathy or myopathy	Loss or denervation of muscle fibers, as in myopathy, axonal neuropathy, motor neuron disease
MUP duration	Reinnervation after injury with spatially dispersed muscle fibers (neuropathy or myopathy)	Loss or denervation of muscle fibers, as in myopathy
MUP phases	Wider motor unit endplate zone (neuropathy); increased variability of fiber diameter (myopathy)	Normal MUPs have three to four phases; decreased phases are not seen
Recruitment	Muscle damage (fewer muscle fibers per motor unit); more units are needed to sustain a given force of contraction; usually seen in myopathies	Muscle denervation (loss of motor units); first unit fires more rapidly before the next is recruited; usually seen in neuropathies

MUP, motor unit potential.

has been seen with arthritic knee pain,[23] patellofemoral pain syndrome,[24,25] and tension-type headache.[26]

Spectral analysis of sEMG signals has led to additional applications; for example, the median frequency of sEMG signals from trunk muscles may be used as a real-time measure of muscle fatigue,[27,28] permitting analysis of abnormal muscle activation patterns and targeted muscle training.[29] sEMG biofeedback may be used to train computer users in maintenance of normal posture.[30] sEMG is commonly used as a proportional control signal for operating powered myoelectric prostheses.[31]

Application in Selected Conditions

Carpal tunnel syndrome (CTS): In this common neuropathy, the median nerve is entrapped by the transverse carpal ligament as it traverses the carpal tunnel. Pain, numbness, and tingling ensue, usually in a distribution corresponding to that of the median nerve. Weakness in median-innervated hand muscles may be present, especially in more severe cases. Nighttime exacerbations are common. The Tinel sign (percussion over the median nerve at the volar wrist) may be present but is neither sensitive nor specific for CTS. The Phalen sign (prolonged wrist flexion) is correlated with pain, paresthesia, and abnormal distal sensory and motor latencies.[32]

EDX is widely used to aid in the diagnosis of CTS and has been found to be valid, reliable, and reproducible for this application.[33] In their evidence-based clinical practice guideline, the American Academy of Orthopaedic Surgeons found moderate evidence for the use of EDX in diagnosing CTS.[34] One well-designed prospective study found that EDX results significantly influenced patient selection for surgical management.[35]

The sensitivity and specificity of EDX in CTS are difficult to determine precisely, as there are no firm criteria for diagnosing the syndrome. The diagnosis is best established by combining clinical symptoms and EDX findings.[36] Median SNCS are more likely to be abnormal than median MNCS in cases of CTS. Ten percent to 15% of patients with clinical symptoms of CTS will have normal NCS, so the sensitivity (true-positive rate) of NCS is 85% to 90%.[37] The specificity of NCS has been estimated at 82% to 85% (i.e., a 15% to 18% chance of a false positive).[33] Sensitivity and specificity may be improved by using multiple studies that compare median distal sensory latency to ulnar and radial distal sensory latencies.[37]

EDX may be complemented by ultrasonography of the carpal tunnel, which permits measurement of median nerve cross-sectional area; as yet, there is no standardized protocol for carpal tunnel ultrasound.[38] Ultrasonography may be most useful in patients with mild clinical CTS but negative EDX.[39]

The value of thenar muscle EMG in the carpal tunnel screen has been extensively debated, and recommendations vary regarding when and whether to perform this test. Thenar EMG is quite uncomfortable for patients, but thenar EMG abnormalities are useful indicators of median motor axonal loss (and therefore severity of median nerve entrapment),[40] and NCS results do not predict abnormal EMG on an individual basis.[41] Most practitioners perform thenar EMG during all CTS screens; others limit it to cases where the results are likely to change a treatment decision. Chang et al.[42] found that thenar EMG is most helpful when CMAP amplitude at abductor pollicis brevis is between 2.1 mV and normal; below 2.1 mV, SA is almost always present. SA is much less common when the CMAP is normal.[42]

Other entrapment neuropathies: NCS and EMG can be useful in the diagnosis of compressive ulnar neuropathy at the elbow, especially to precisely localize the site(s) of nerve compression.[43] EDX is effective and precise for the diagnosis of other ulnar and median neuropathies.[37] Lower limb neuropathies are also readily diagnosed, including lesions of the tibial,

peroneal, sciatic, saphenous, and other nerves.[40,44] Patients with piriformis syndrome demonstrate a delay in the tibial and peroneal H-reflexes when the affected hip is flexed, adducted and internally rotated[45]; needle EMG results in this disorder have been inconsistent.[46]

Painful polyneuropathies: EDX can provide unparalleled insights regarding the type, distribution, and severity of neuropathic processes. Most polyneuropathies are length-dependent (affecting the lower limbs first) and symmetric bilaterally, following the classic "stocking-glove" distribution of sensory disturbance. EDX can distinguish between axonal, demyelinating, and mixed polyneuropathies, each of which has its own potential causes. The distribution of abnormalities may suggest metabolic (e.g., diabetes mellitus, thyroid disease), toxic (alcoholic, chemotherapy, heavy metals), inflammatory (GBS, chronic inflammatory demyelinating polyneuropathy), hereditary (Charcot-Marie-Tooth disease), or other causes.[47,48] Characterization of polyneuropathy can help determine further diagnostic workup and, where possible, specific treatment.[49]

Guillain-Barré syndrome: Neuropathic pain is a common complaint of patients with this acute inflammatory demyelinating polyneuropathy. EDX is a valuable diagnostic and prognostic tool in GBS. Eighty percent of patients demonstrate conduction block and/or slowed NCVs during the illness. F-waves may be absent in cases of significant axonal involvement. Absence of the H-reflex is common. Proximal ulnar motor nerve conduction block (stimulating at Erb's point) is highly predictive of GBS.[50]

Radiculopathies: Needle EMG is the most useful test for diagnosing radiculopathy. MNCS are frequently normal, but more severe radiculopathies may result in temporally dispersed and/or low-amplitude CMAPs. SNCS are generally normal in radiculopathies because these studies assess the function of primary afferent neurons whose cell bodies reside in the DRG. Most radiculopathies are caused by compression within the spinal canal or neural foramen proximal to the DRG, sparing primary afferent neurons and thus causing no abnormality on SNCS.

Needle EMG is a highly specific but somewhat less sensitive measure for radiculopathy. Diagnostic yield is improved by careful selection of muscles for needle exam; a six-muscle screen (including paraspinal muscles) maximizes diagnostic yield.[51] Abnormalities should ideally be present in at least two muscles sharing a single nerve root innervation but supplied by different peripheral nerves. If only one muscle tested shows abnormalities suggesting radiculopathy, additional muscles should be studied.[51] SA is the primary clue to acute or subacute radiculopathy; positive waves and fibrillation potentials develop over the first few weeks following root injury. An examination performed too soon after injury may show little or no abnormality. SA may disappear within a few months of injury, but symptoms can persist. Abnormalities of motor unit recruitment and morphology (decreased recruitment, high-amplitude and/or polyphasic MUPs) indicate more chronic radiculopathy.

EDX and magnetic resonance imaging (MRI) are complementary tools for the diagnosis of radiculopathy. If radiculopathy is clinically suspected but MRI findings are nondiagnostic, or if the presentation is complex, adding EDX can significantly improve diagnostic precision.[52] EMG may also be useful prognostically. Abnormal needle EMG predicts long-term pain relief after lumbar interlaminar or translaminar epidural steroid injection in the treatment of lumbosacral radiculopathy.[53] Similarly, EMG-confirmed radiculopathy predicted >50% pain reduction and decreased opioid use following cervical and lumbar transforaminal epidural steroid injections.[54]

Complex regional pain syndrome: This severe neuropathic pain condition usually produces severe allodynia over multiple nerve root and peripheral nerve territories. EDX is not useful in the majority of CRPS patients. EDX is generally avoided in CRPS because patients find it too painful to tolerate. In cases where a specific nerve injury is suspected (i.e., CRPS "type 2" or causalgia) and intervention is being planned, EDX may help to isolate the site of nerve injury.

Conclusion

EDX provides a wealth of information about neuromuscular function, and every pain care practice should have ready access to a skilled electromyographer. Properly applied, EDX helps pain care providers diagnose painful conditions, localize nerve injuries, design treatment plans, target injections, measure treatment outcome, and monitor disease recovery. It increases our understanding of the patient, opening a clearer path to pain relief and improved function.

References

1. Liveson JA, Ma D. *Laboratory Reference for Clinical Neurophysiology.* New York: Oxford University Press; 1992.
2. Hovaguimian A, Gibbons CH. Diagnosis and treatment of pain in small-fiber neuropathy. *Curr Pain Headache Rep* 2011;15(3):193–200.
3. Lauria G, Hsieh ST, Johansson O, et al. European Federation of Neurological Societies/Peripheral Nerve Society guideline on the use of skin biopsy in the diagnosis of small fiber neuropathy. Report of a joint task force of the European Federation of Neurological Societies and the Peripheral Nerve Society. *Eur J Neurol* 2010;17(7):903–912, e44–e49.
4. Fisher MA. F-waves—physiology and clinical uses. *ScientificWorldJournal* 2007;7:144–160.
5. Kimura J. Electrodiagnosis of the cranial nerves. *Acta Neurol Taiwan* 2006;15(1):2–12.
6. Majoie CB, Aramideh M, Hulsmans FJ, et al. Correlation between electromyographic reflex and MR imaging examinations of the trigeminal nerve. *AJNR Am J Neuroradiol* 1999;20(6):1119–1125.
7. Podnar S. Utility of sphincter electromyography and sacral reflex studies in women with cauda equina lesions. *Neurourol Urodyn* 2014;33(4):426–430.
8. Hulens M, Bruyninckx F, Dankaerts W, et al. Electromyographic abnormalities associated with symptomatic sacral Tarlov cysts. *Pain Pract* 2016;16(5):E81–E88.
9. Tanhehco JL. Single-fiber electromyography. *Phys Med Rehabil Clin N Am* 2003;14(2):207–229.
10. Bergquist ER, Hammert WC. Timing and appropriate use of electrodiagnostic studies. *Hand Clin* 2013;29(3):363–370.
11. Gertken JT, Patel AT, Boon AJ. Electromyography and anticoagulation. *PM R* 2013;5(5)(suppl):S3–S7.
12. American Association of Neuromuscular and Electrodiagnostic Medicine. *Risks in Electrodiagnostic Medicine.* Rochester, MN: American Association of Neuromuscular and Electrodiagnostic Medicine; 2014.
13. Babu S, Pioro E, Li J, et al. Optimizing muscle selection for electromyography in amyotrophic lateral sclerosis. *Muscle Nerve* 2016;56(1):36–44.
14. Dvorak J, Sutter M, Herdmann J. Cervical myelopathy: clinical and neurophysiological evaluation. *Eur Spine J* 2003;12(suppl 2):S181–S187.
15. Park JH, Hyun SJ. Intraoperative neurophysiological monitoring in spinal surgery. *World J Clin Cases* 2015;3(9):765–773.
16. Kucera P, Goldenberg Z, Kurca E. Sympathetic skin response: review of the method and its clinical use. *Bratisl Lek Listy* 2004;105(3):108–116.
17. Clinchot D, Lorch F. Sympathetic skin response in patients with reflex sympathetic dystrophy. *Am J Phys Med Rehab* 1996;75:252–256.
18. Harden RN, Davis EL, Rudin NJ. Sympathetic skin response testing in sympathetically maintained pain. Paper presented at: 13th Annual Scientific Meeting of the American Pain Society; November 1994; Miami, FL.
19. Butler HL, Hubley-Kozey CL, Kozey JW. Changes in electromyographic activity of trunk muscles within the sub-acute phase for individuals deemed recovered from a low back injury. *J Electromyogr Kinesiol* 2013;23(2):369–377.
20. Bush C, Ditto B, Feuerstein M. A controlled evaluation of paraspinal EMG biofeedback in the treatment of chronic low back pain. *Health Psychol* 1985;4(4):307–321.
21. Flor H, Haag G, Turk DC. Long-term efficacy of EMG biofeedback for chronic rheumatic back pain. *Pain* 1986;27(2):195–202.
22. Stuckey SJ, Jacobs A, Goldfarb J. EMG biofeedback training, relaxation training, and placebo for the relief of chronic back pain. *Percept Mot Skills* 1986;63(3):1023–1036.
23. King AC, Ahles TA, Martin JE, et al. EMG biofeedback-controlled exercise in chronic arthritic knee pain. *Arch Phys Med Rehabil* 1984;65(6):341–353.
24. Ng GY, Zhang AQ, Li CK. Biofeedback exercise improved the EMG activity ratio of the medial and lateral vasti muscles in subjects with patellofemoral pain syndrome. *J Electromyogr Kinesiol* 2008;18(1):128–133.
25. Wise HH, Fiebert I, Kates JL. EMG biofeedback as treatment for patellofemoral pain syndrome. *J Orthop Sports Phys Ther* 1984;6(2):95–103.
26. Nestoriuc Y, Martin A, Andrasik F. Biofeedback treatment for headache disorders: a comprehensive efficacy review. *Appl Psychophysiol Biofeedback* 2008;33(3):125–140.
27. Gilmore LD, De Luca CJ. Muscle fatigue monitor (MFM): second generation. *IEEE Trans Biomed Eng* 1985;32(1):75–78.
28. Stulen FB, De Luca CJ. Muscle fatigue monitor: a noninvasive device for observing localized muscular fatigue. *IEEE Trans Biomed Eng* 1982;29(12):760–768.
29. Roy SH, De Luca CJ, Casavant DA. Lumbar muscle fatigue and chronic lower back pain. *Spine (Phila Pa 1976)* 1989;14(9):992–1001.
30. Gaffney BM, Maluf KS, Davidson BS. Evaluation of novel EMG biofeedback for postural correction during computer use. *Appl Psychophysiol Biofeedback* 2016;41(2):181–189.
31. Fougner A, Stavdahl O, Kyberd PJ, et al. Control of upper limb prostheses: terminology and proportional myoelectric control—a review. *IEEE Trans Neural Syst Rehabil Eng* 2012;20(5):663–677.
32. Ansari NN, Adelmanesh F, Naghdi S, et al. The relationship between symptoms, clinical tests and nerve conduction study findings in carpal tunnel syndrome. *Electromyogr Clin Neurophysiol* 2009;49(1):53–57.
33. Jablecki CK, Andary MT, So YT, et al. Literature review of the usefulness of nerve conduction studies and electromyography for the evaluation of patients with carpal tunnel syndrome: AAEM Quality Assurance Committee. *Muscle Nerve* 1993;16(12):1392–1414.
34. Graham B, Peljovich AE, Afra R, et al. The American Academy of Orthopaedic Surgeons evidence-based clinical practice guideline on: management of carpal tunnel syndrome. *J Bone Joint Surg Am* 2016;98(20):1750–1754.
35. Becker SJ, Makanji HS, Ring D. Changes in treatment plan for carpal tunnel syndrome based on electrodiagnostic test results. *J Hand Surg Eur Vol* 2014;39(2):187–193.
36. Rempel D, Evanoff B, Amadio PC. Consensus criteria for classification of carpal tunnel syndrome in epidemiologic studies. *Am J Public Health* 1998;88:1447–1451.
37. Werner RA. Electrodiagnostic evaluation of carpal tunnel syndrome and ulnar neuropathies. *PM R* 2013;5(5)(suppl):S14–S21.
38. Chen YT, Williams L, Zak MJ, et al. Review of ultrasonography in the diagnosis of carpal tunnel syndrome and a proposed scanning protocol. *J Ultrasound Med* 2016;35(11):2311–2324.
39. Roll SC, Case-Smith J, Evans KD. Diagnostic accuracy of ultrasonography vs. electromyography in carpal tunnel syndrome: a systematic review of literature. *Ultrasound Med Biol* 2011;37(10):1539–1553.
40. Jillapalli D, Shefner JM. Electrodiagnosis in common mononeuropathies and plexopathies. *Semin Neurol* 2005;25(2):196–203.
41. Werner RA, Albers JW. Relation between needle electromyography and nerve conduction studies in patients with carpal tunnel syndrome. *Arch Phys Med Rehabil* 1995;76(3):246–249.
42. Chang CW, Lee WJ, Liao YC, et al. Which nerve conduction parameters can predict spontaneous electromyographic activity in carpal tunnel syndrome? *Clin Neurophysiol* 2013;124(11):2264–2268.
43. Posner MA. Compressive ulnar neuropathies at the elbow: I. Etiology and diagnosis. *J Am Acad Orthop Surg* 1998;6(5):282–288.
44. Roy PC. Electrodiagnostic evaluation of lower extremity neurogenic problems. *Foot Ankle Clin* 2011;16(2):225–242.
45. Fishman LM, Dombi GW, Michaelsen C, et al. Piriformis syndrome: diagnosis, treatment, and outcome—a 10-year study. *Arch Phys Med Rehabil* 2002;83(3):295–301.
46. Halpin RJ, Ganju A. Piriformis syndrome: a real pain in the buttock? *Neurosurgery* 2009;65(4)(suppl):A197–A202.
47. Olney RK. AAEM minimonograph #38: neuropathies in connective tissue disease. *Muscle Nerve* 1992;15(5):531–542.
48. Bromberg M. *Electrodiagnosis of Primary Demyelinating Neuropathies.* Salt Lake City, UT: University of Utah Department of Neurology; 2005.
49. Callaghan BC, Burke JF, Feldman EL. Electrodiagnostic tests in polyneuropathy and radiculopathy. *JAMA* 2016;315(3):297–298.
50. Sudulagunta SR, Sodalagunta MB, Sepehrar M, et al. Guillain-Barré syndrome: clinical profile and management. *Ger Med Sci* 2015;13:16.
51. Dillingham TR. Evaluating the patient with suspected radiculopathy. *PMR* 2013;5(5)(suppl):S41–S49.
52. Reza Soltani Z, Sajadi S, Tavana B. A comparison of magnetic resonance imaging with electrodiagnostic findings in the evaluation of clinical radiculopathy: a cross-sectional study. *Eur Spine J* 2014;23(4):916–921.
53. Annaswamy TM, Bierner SM, Chouteau W, et al. Needle electromyography predicts outcome after lumbar epidural steroid injection. *Muscle Nerve* 2012;45(3):346–355.
54. McCormick Z, Cushman D, Caldwell M, et al. Does electrodiagnostic confirmation of radiculopathy predict pain reduction after transforaminal epidural steroid injection? A multicenter study. *J Nat Sci* 2015;1(8):e140.

CHAPTER 19

Diagnostic Imaging of Pain

RICHARD F. CODY Jr, ASAKO MIYAKOSHI, and **KENNETH R. MARAVILLA**

Pain is one of the most common indications for clinical imaging examinations. Pain could be an indicator of imminent tissue damage, such as ischemia, direct injury, malignancy, inflammation, and infection. It could also be due to peripheral or central nervous system diseases. Imaging protocols are tailored based on acuteness, character, and location of the pain and the working diagnosis. In case of acute pain, life-threatening and surgical emergency can be in the differential. Therefore, often imaging for acute pain is to confirm or exclude the presumed ominous diagnosis in doubt, such as acute fracture and associated tissue damage, intracranial hemorrhage, aortic dissection, pneumothorax, pneumoperitoneum, etc., based on history, labs, and physical exam findings. Even when the presumed urgent diagnosis is excluded, imaging exams are often useful in delineating the cause of pain.

For patients with recurrent or persistent pain whose diagnosis remains obscure after routine imaging workup, it might be challenging to make a diagnosis or find the cause of pain. Specialized imaging techniques such as magnetic resonance (MR) neurogram, discogram, and imaging-guided injection should be chosen depending on the careful review of the clinical scenarios. American College of Radiology (ACR) Appropriateness Criteria are a useful resource when the next imaging tool is uncertain. It consists of evidence-based guidelines to assist decision making for specific clinical conditions. In some institutions, it is incorporated into electronic medical records and ordering systems.

A comprehensive discussion of radiographs, computed tomography (CT), magnetic resonance imaging (MRI), ultrasound, and radionuclide examinations (such as bone scan) for evaluation of pain should include almost all radiologic subspecialties. This is beyond the scope of this chapter and can be found in most general diagnostic imaging textbooks.

This chapter is dedicated to the evaluation of pain related to the nervous system and reviews the imaging approach to several regional pain syndromes. It discusses imaging techniques that can be used to select surgical candidates among patients with back pain, tic douloureux, and peripheral nerve entrapment syndromes. Techniques and indications for MRI of the cranial nerves and posterior fossa vasculature, and high-resolution MRI of the brachial plexus and peripheral nerves are also discussed.

Headache

Headache is a common symptom. The lifetime prevalence of any form of headache is 93% in men and 99% in women.[1] Unless acute findings such as hemorrhage, tumor, and meningoencephalitis are of clinical concern, choosing the patient who should have a cranial imaging study can be challenging (see Chapter 62). The diagnostic yield of neuroimaging examinations in patients with headache and a normal neurologic examination, or in patients with typical migraine, is low (Table 19.1).[2] For example, in adult and pediatric patients with known migraine and no change in symptoms, routine neuroimaging is discouraged.[3]

Specific clinical features associated with significant intracranial abnormality, however, should prompt neuroimaging. Acute onset of an extremely severe headache (often described as "thunderclap" or "sudden worst headache of life") should be treated as an emergency, due to increased positive predictive value for subarachnoid hemorrhage (SAH) from intracranial aneurysms in adults, and arteriovenous malformation (AVM) or other vascular malformations in children.[2,4–7] Other imaging-appropriate clinical scenarios include worsening subacute headache, headache associated with focal neurologic signs or cognitive impairment (in patients without a history of migraine), new headache in patients older than age 50 years, and headache in immunocompromised patients or patients with known malignancy.[2,4,5,8] Patients over the age of 65 years with new onset of pathologic headache have a 15% incidence of serious intracranial disease, including temporal arteritis, tumor, and infarct. In contrast, patients younger than age 65 years (other than the acute SAH subset) have only a 1.5% incidence of detectable underlying pathology.[9]

ACUTE HEADACHE

Sudden onset of severe headache—especially if associated with neurologic abnormality or depressed sensorium—suggests possible acute SAH from an aneurysm or other vascular malformation. The devastating consequences of untreated, ruptured aneurysm require prompt exclusion of SAH in this setting: Patients who survive their initial hemorrhage have a 50% chance of a fatal rehemorrhage within 1 year, with the highest risk in the immediate postbleed period.[10,11] Rapid diagnosis with high sensitivity is best made by CT demonstration of hyperdense blood in the subarachnoid space.[12]

If SAH is found on initial noncontrast head CT, subsequent magnetic resonance angiography (MRA), computed tomography angiography (CTA), or catheter angiogram is directed at detecting and localizing an aneurysm (Fig. 19.1) or AVM (Fig. 19.2). Venous sinus thrombosis (Figs. 19.3 and 19.4),[13,14] benign perimesencephalic SAH,[15] and arterial dissection (Fig. 19.5)[16,17] may also result in SAH in the absence of an aneurysm or vascular malformation on CTA. In addition, migraine, and bacterial meningitis (in the proper clinical setting, e.g., stiff neck and fever) can also present as severe acute headache but without presence of SAH on acute CT.

TABLE 19.1	Neuroimaging Yield in Headache					
	Percentage of Patients with Underlying Condition					
Headache Type	**Tumor**	**AVM**	**Hydrocephalus**	**Aneurysm**	**SAH**	**Infarct**
Normal exam	0.8	0.2	0.3	0.1	0.2	1.2
Migraine	0.3	0.07	—	0.7	—	—

AVM, arteriovenous malformation; SAH, subarachnoid hemorrhage.
Adapted from Evans RW. Diagnostic testing for the evaluation of headaches. *Neurol Clin* 1996;14(1):1–26. Copyright © 1996 Elsevier. With permission.

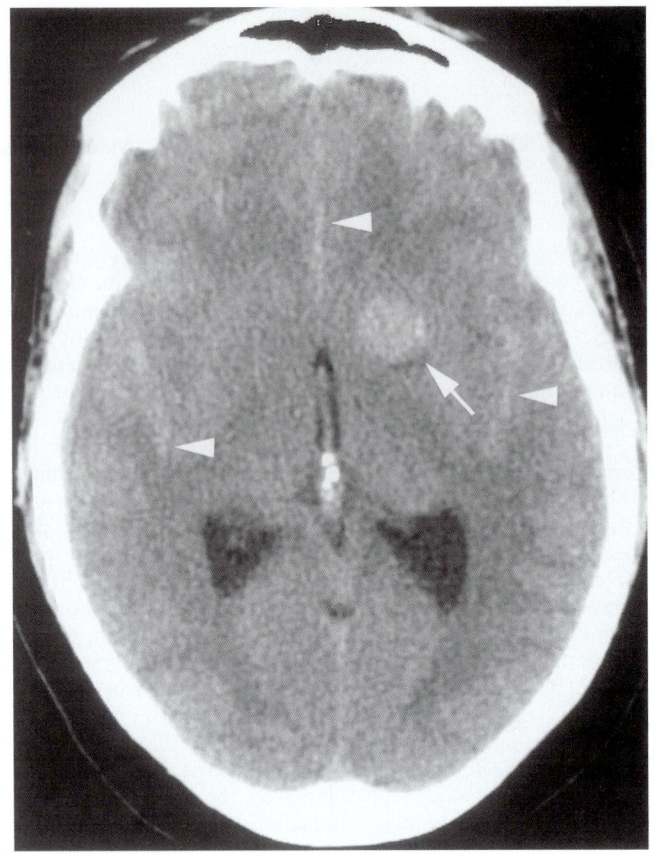

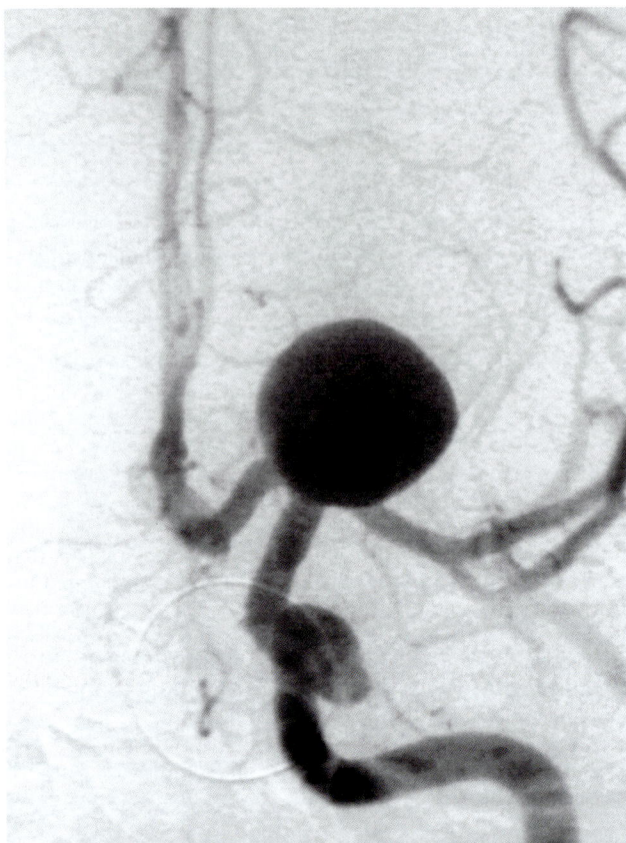

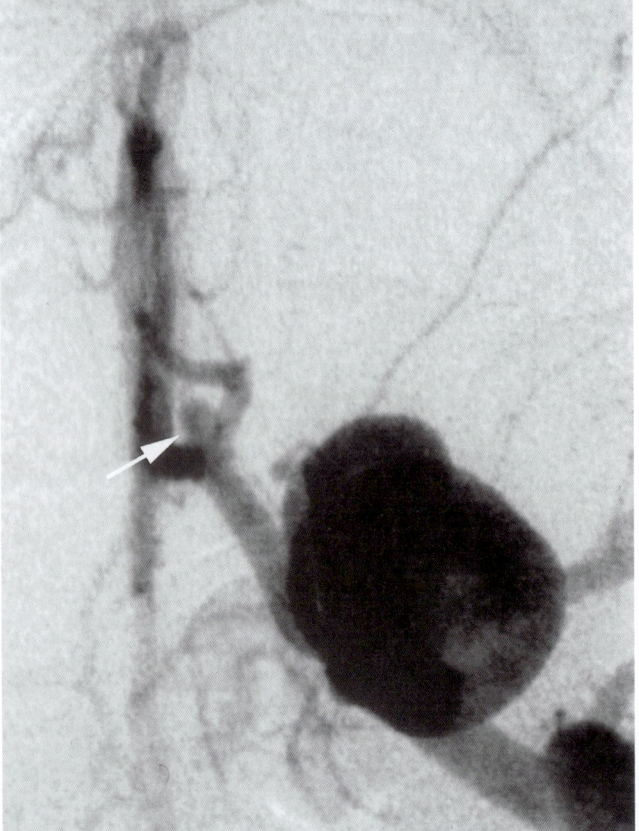

FIGURE 19.1 Subarachnoid hemorrhage caused by ruptured terminal internal carotid artery aneurysm. **A:** Nonenhanced computed tomography shows hyperdense aneurysm (*arrow*) and blood within interhemispheric and sylvian fissures (*arrowheads*). The ventricles are mildly enlarged and clot is present within the third ventricle. **B:** Left internal carotid artery arteriogram shows a 2-cm aneurysm arising from the termination of the internal carotid artery. **C:** A second, unruptured aneurysm is seen at the junction of the left anterior cerebral artery and the anterior communicating artery (*arrow*).

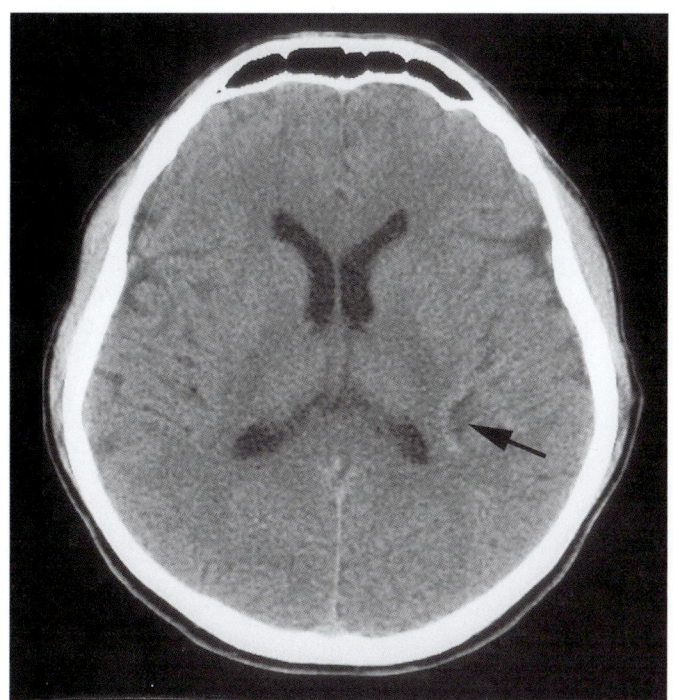

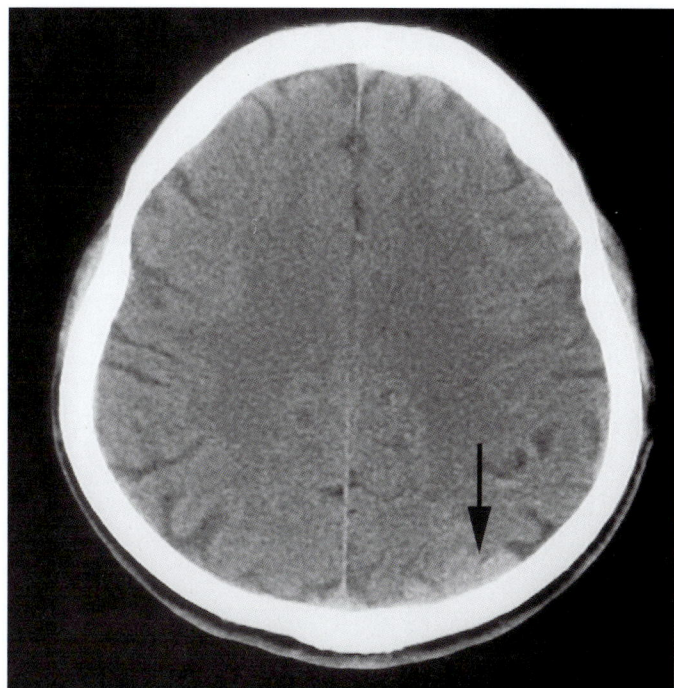

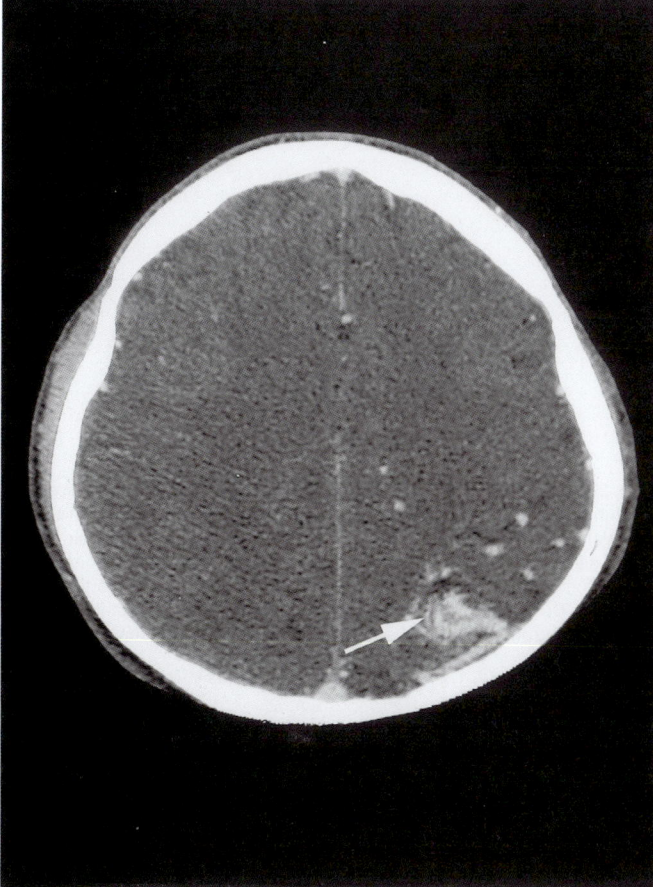

FIGURE 19.2 Arteriovenous malformation. A 39-year-old man with several days' headache. **A:** Noncontrast computed tomography shows enlarged, slightly hyperdense vessels in the sylvian fissure (*arrow*). **B:** Hyperdense, dilated veins at the parietal vertex (*arrow*). **C:** Computed tomographic angiography shows the arteriovenous malformation nidus (*arrow*), as well as dilated feeding arteries and peripheral draining veins.

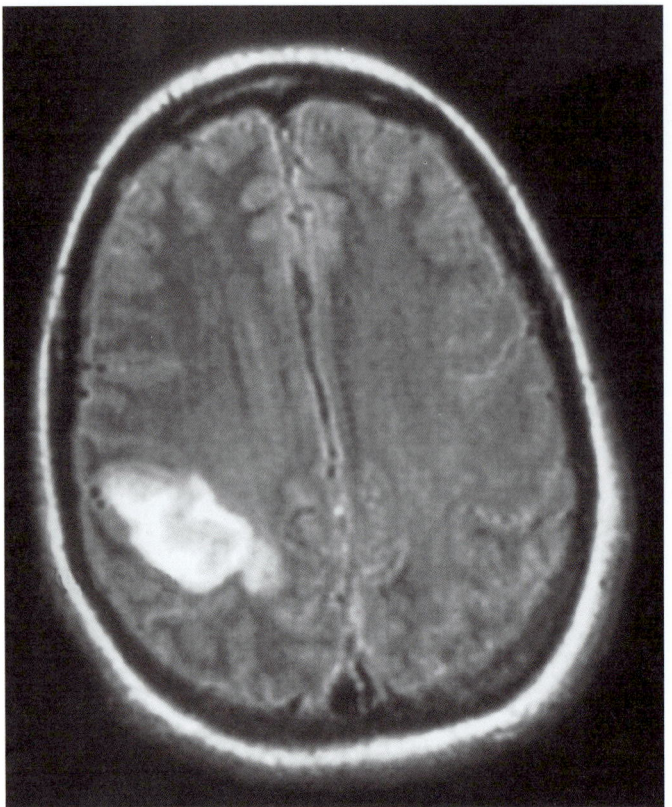

A

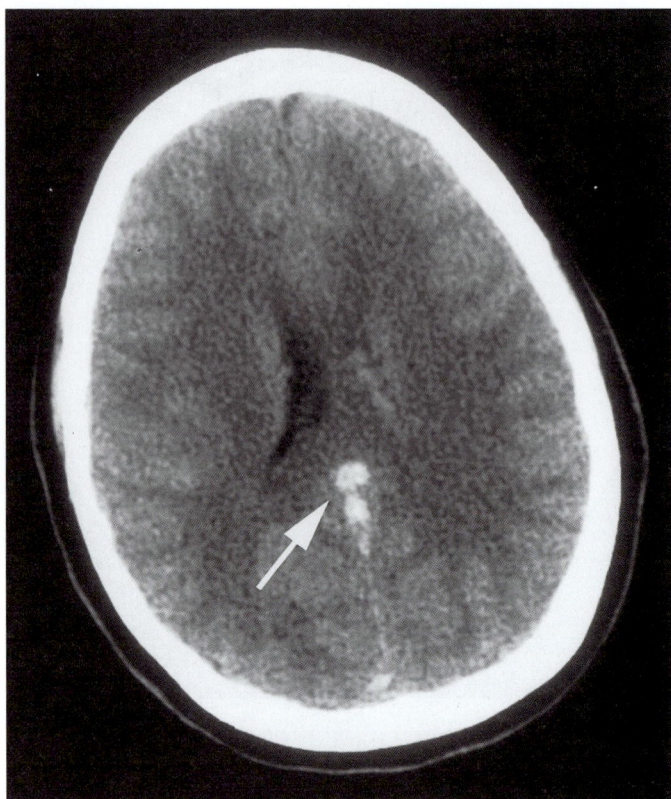

B

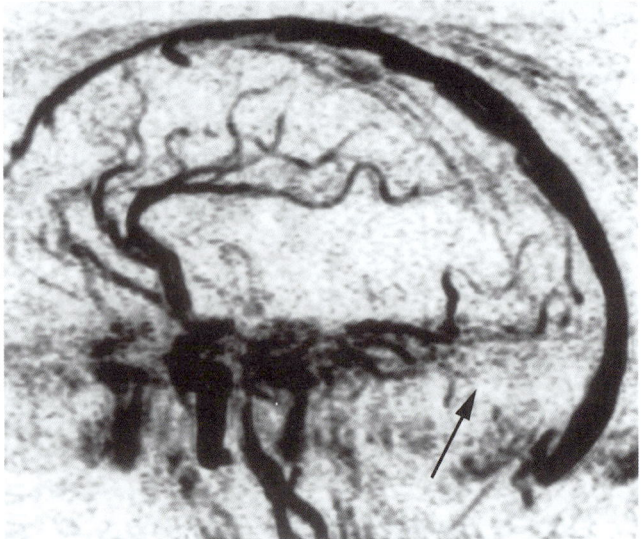

C

FIGURE 19.3 Venous sinus thrombosis with cortical infarct. A 26-year-old postpartum woman with headache and left hemiparesis. **A:** Axial fluid attenuation inversion recovery (FLAIR) image at level of centrum semiovale shows increased signal in precentral gyrus, indicating cortical infarct. **B:** Nonenhanced computed tomography shows high attenuation in vein of Galen and straight sinus (*arrow*). **C:** Magnetic resonance venogram shows absence of flow through straight sinus (*arrow*) with patent sagittal and transverse sinuses.

As noted earlier, imaging the patient with suspected SAH should begin with nonenhanced CT. Cisterns and sulci must be carefully examined for hyperdense acute blood, which can be subtle if the amount of hemorrhage is small, or if the study is performed more than 24 hours after the bleed occurred. Nonenhanced CT has a sensitivity of 98%[18] for detection of acute SAH within 12 hours of onset (in fact, 100% on emergency CTs has been reported).[19] CT sensitivity for detection of SAH is reduced as the time interval from hemorrhage increases.[2]

A lumbar puncture (LP) may be considered in the possible—but uncommon—scenario of a patient for whom there is a bona fide high clinical index of suspicion for acute SAH and a negative head CT.[18,20] Detection of xanthochromic cerebrospinal fluid (CSF) on LP remains the "gold standard" for sensitivity

in detecting SAH in this setting.[21,22] In patients for whom an LP is truly indicated to assess for occult SAH, care must be taken for pristine technique: ideally a one-pass, atraumatic tap, with small caliber (25G or 22G) spinal needle. No xanthochromia and red blood cell count <2000 × 10⁶/L reasonably excludes aneurysmal SAH.[23]

In the absence of SAH, nonenhanced CT can detect signs of other pathologies, including increased density within a thrombosed dural venous sinus, venous infarction, and edema associated with intracranial mass lesions. If subtle abnormalities are found on nonenhanced CT, further imaging evaluation may include contrast-enhanced CT or (preferably) MRI. In the absence of SAH, MRI is a more sensitive technique to evaluate the patient for other causes of headache, including dural venous sinus occlusion, infarct, mass lesion, or intracranial infection.

If SAH is detected, CTA and/or catheter angiography with digital subtraction angiography (DSA) is generally used to further evaluate the location and features of an aneurysm, pial AVM, dural arteriovenous fistula (DAVF), or other vascular malformation. Dural venous sinus thrombosis is better evaluated by computed tomography venogram (CTV) rather than magnetic resonance venogram (MRV) with contrast MRA/MRI because MRI and MRV may be affected by flow artifact resulting in false-positive appearance.

Computed Tomography Angiography and Magnetic Resonance Angiography

MRA and CTA are useful for rapid, noninvasive diagnosis of intracranial vascular lesions. CTA is a dynamic technique in which thin-slice, contiguous images are rapidly obtained during the first pass of an intravenous bolus injection of iodinated contrast. Through proper timing, the images are acquired as the bolus of contrast fills the intracranial arteries and provides high-resolution images of the intracranial vessels. This provides a sensitive, rapid, and relatively noninvasive means to detect aneurysms, AVMs and arteritis, which can be seen as vessel wall irregularities.

Using state-of-the-art multidetector CT, axial images covering the entire cerebral vasculature can be acquired in a few seconds. Using rapid computer processing, multiplanar and three-dimensional (3D) reconstructions can be created to display the enhanced blood vessels in a manner analogous to the projection images from catheter angiography. When indicated, CTA can be easily performed immediately following the initial noncontrast CT while the patient is still on the CT table. MRA is a possible alternative technique, but it is more time-consuming and may not be suitable in the setting of acute intracranial hemorrhage, when the patient may be unable to hold still and requires close monitoring. Whereas conventional MRA visualizes flow-related signal within the vascular lumen, CTA depicts the surrounding structures with better spatial resolution, such

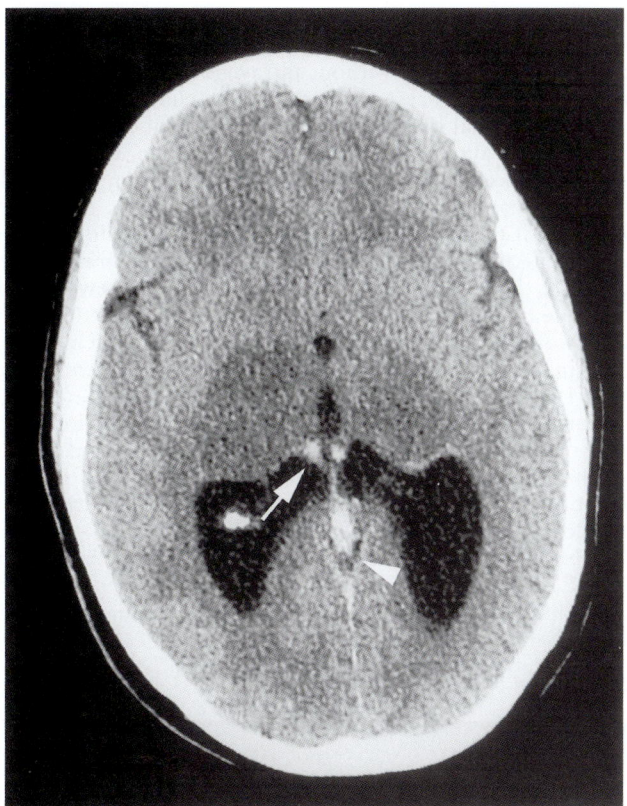

FIGURE 19.4 Venous sinus thrombosis with bilateral thalamic infarcts in a 24-year-old woman with 4 days of headache followed by several hours of nausea and depressed consciousness. Nonenhanced computed tomography shows low attenuation changes in both thalami, with increased attenuation in the internal cerebral veins (*arrow*) and straight sinus (*arrowhead*).

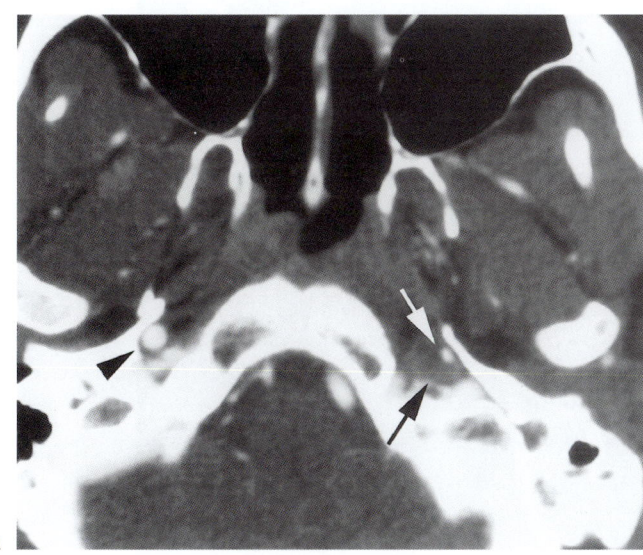

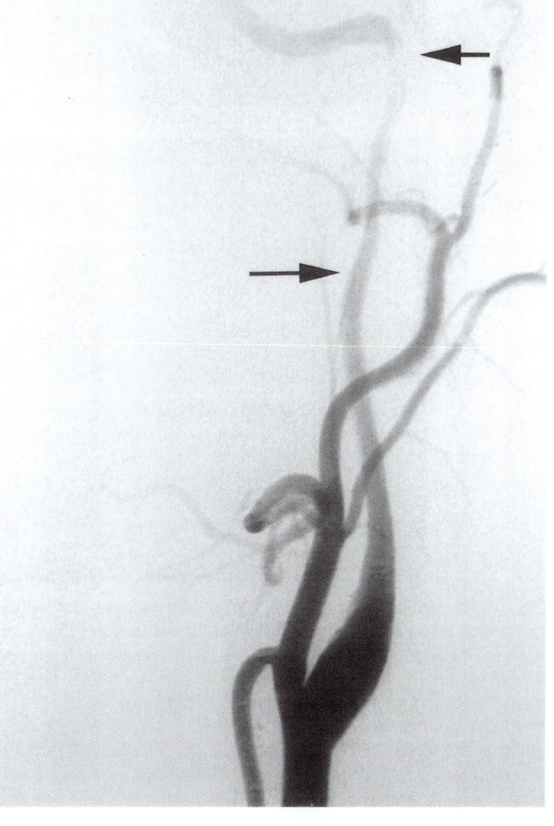

FIGURE 19.5 Internal carotid artery dissection in a 37-year-old man with headache and left pupillary constriction. **A:** Computed tomographic angiography at skull base shows decreased caliber of left internal carotid artery (*white arrow*) at the skull base. Intramural hematoma surrounds the narrowed lumen (*black arrow*). Normal right internal carotid artery (*arrowhead*). **B:** Left internal carotid arteriogram shows smooth narrowing of distal cervical internal carotid with near complete occlusion at the skull base (*arrows*).

as vascular calcification, plaque formation, and extrinsic compression. The quality of CTA in detecting aneurysms is comparable to DSA. However, DSA is still considered by many to be the "gold standard" for aneurysm assessment and may be superior to CTA for surgical treatment planning.[24–29]

CTA or MRA can provide rapid diagnosis or exclusion of aneurysms and AVMs in the patient with severe acute onset headache. These images are also used to clarify subtle findings in patients with questionable abnormalities on noncontrast CT. For example, carotid or vertebral artery dissection can be detected by imaging the upper cervical vasculature with the earlier described imaging techniques (see Fig. 19.5).[30,31] Supplemental MRI with axial fat-saturated T1-weighted sequences in addition to MRA is also highly sensitive for detection of small, focal mural thrombus seen in carotid or vertebral dissections.[32,33]

CHRONIC HEADACHE

Image findings are unrevealing in most cases of uncomplicated chronic headache. Intracranial lesions often present with headache but usually are associated with other neurologic signs or symptoms.[34] When headaches are caused by underlying pathologic disorders, the differential diagnosis is broad. Serious primary conditions include intraparenchymal, dural, or skull base

tumors[35]; unruptured aneurysms[36,37]; abscesses; arterial dissection[38,39]; venous sinus thrombosis; vasculitis[40]; and AVMs.[41] A normal CT or MRI without intravenous contrast excludes most intracranial masses to reassure the clinician and justify continued clinical observation and symptomatic treatment. If the clinical evaluation points toward neoplasm, abscess, or a vascular process, then contrast-enhanced CT or, preferably, contrast-enhanced MRI is appropriate next study. As already discussed, if there is a high clinical index of suspicion for vasculitis, CTA or MRA is useful technique to explore further.[42] So-called "black-blood" postcontrast MRA is a newer highly specialized MRI technique that may be used to better assess vessel wall abnormalities, such as vessel wall enhancement that occur in cases of inflammatory vasculitis or prior hemorrhage (Figs. 19.6 and 19.7).[43,44]

Noncontrast CT scanning of the craniofacial region is the study of choice for the imaging evaluation of acute and chronic inflammatory diseases of the sinonasal cavities. Conventional plain film radiography is no longer utilized for this purpose due to its low sensitivity and specificity.

Acute sinusitis is a common cause of headache or facial pain. Sinus CT is performed as a rapid, high-resolution, thin-section CT examination targeted to include the paranasal sinuses.

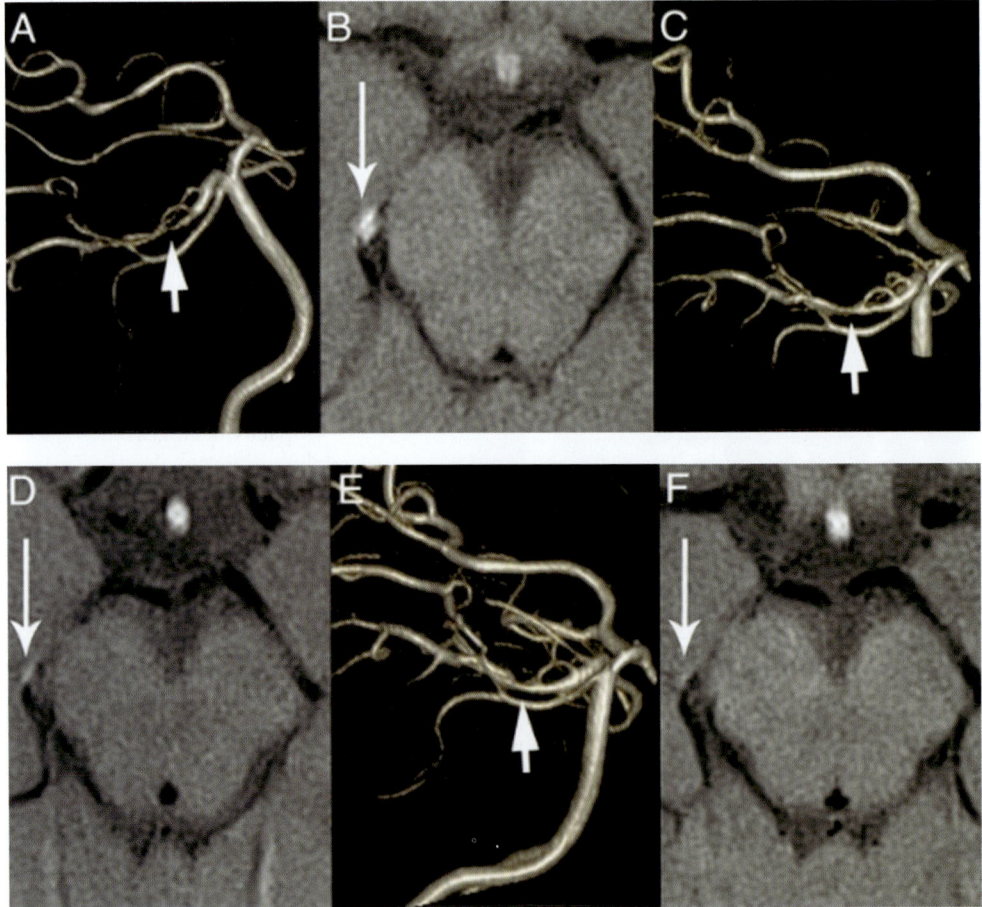

FIGURE 19.6 Vasculitis. Young patient who presented with aphasia and bilateral middle cerebral artery (MCA) territory infarcts. Cerebrospinal fluid analysis indicated the presence of anti-varicella zoster virus (anti-VZV) antibodies, confirming a diagnosis of VZV vasculitis. Three-dimensional reconstruction of the posterior circulation from time-of-flight (TOF) magnetic resonance angiography (MRA) **(A)** shows high-grade stenosis of the right P2 posterior cerebral artery (*short arrow*). There were additional stenoses involving the inferior division of the bilateral M1 MCA and bilateral A2 anterior cerebral artery (not shown). On T1 postcontrast intracranial vessel wall imaging (IVWI) **(B)**, there is a circumferential enhancing lesion involving the stenotic segment (*long arrow*), compatible with inflammatory vasculopathy. On follow-up IVWI and TOF MRA performed 2 months (**C** and **D**) and 4 months (**E** and **F**) later, there is progressive improved luminal patency (*short arrow*, **C** and **E**) and diminished wall enhancement (*long arrow*, **D** and **F**), which corresponded with clinical improvement. (*Reprinted from Mossa-Basha M, Alexander M, Gaddikeri S, et al. Vessel wall imaging for intracranial vascular disease evaluation. J Neurointerv Surg 2016;8[11]:1154–1159, with permission from BMJ Publishing Group Ltd.*)

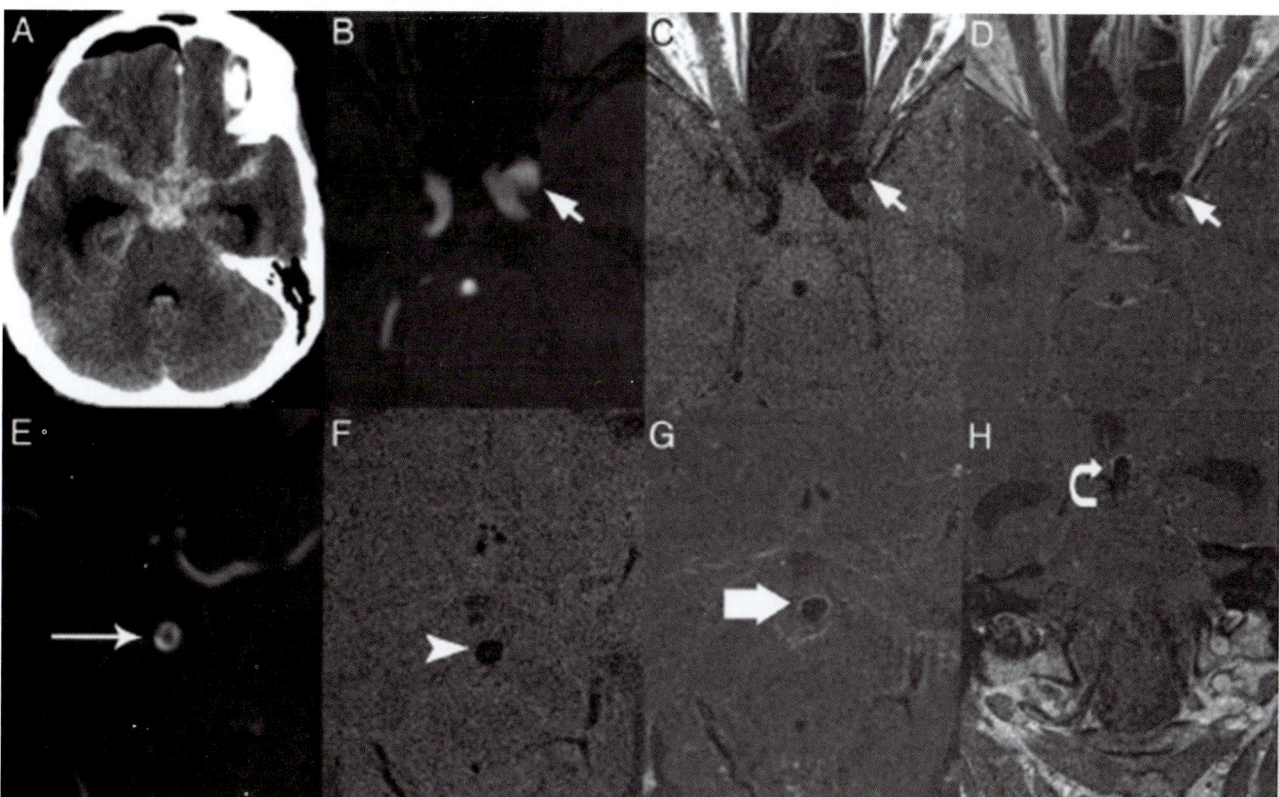

FIGURE 19.7 Black-blood magnetic resonance imaging to identify probable source of hemorrhage. Fifty-six-year-old female presenting with thunderclap headache. Axial noncontrast computed tomography (CT) head **(A)** shows diffuse basal cistern subarachnoid hemorrhage. On 3D time-of-flight (TOF) magnetic resonance angiography (MRA) **(B** and **E)**, there is a left supraclinoid internal carotid artery (ICA) aneurysm **(B**, *short white arrow*) and basilar tip aneurysm **(E**, *long white arrow*). There is no corresponding enhancement of the left supraclinoid aneurysm (*short white arrows*) on T1 pre- **(C)** and postcontrast **(D)** intracranial vessel wall imaging (IVWI), whereas the basilar tip aneurysm **(F**, *arrowhead*; **G**, *thick arrow*) shows circumferential wall enhancement when comparing T1 pre- **(F)** and postcontrast **(G)** IVWI. The basilar tip aneurysm was emergently treated endovascularly (*curved arrow*) as seen on coronal T1 postcontrast IVWI **(H)**. (*Reprinted from Alexander MD, Yuan C, Rutman A, et al. High-resolution intracranial vessel wall imaging: imaging beyond the lumen.* J Neurol Neurosurg Psychiatry *2016;87[6]:589–597, with permission from BMJ Publishing Group Ltd.*)

Because the information is primarily related to bone detail, these scans can be acquired with lower radiation dose levels. The axial thin-section, high-resolution data can be reformatted into coronal, sagittal, or any other desired imaging plane. CT has the additional advantage of enabling evaluation of the middle ear and mastoid air cells. Possible findings include observation of air–fluid levels that are associated with acute sinusitis. An additional finding suggestive of acute inflammatory sinusitis in the appropriate clinical setting is the presence of "frothy" material within one or more sinus cavities. Findings of mucosal thickening and subtle bony wall thickening reflect changes associated with chronic sinusitis and osteitis. When surgery is indicated for repetitive, recurrent, or intractable chronic sinusitis, thin-section, 3D CT technique with multiplanar viewing also assists in operative planning for endoscopic sinus surgery (Fig. 19.8).[45]

INTRACRANIAL HYPOTENSION

The syndrome of intracranial hypotension is often characterized by positional headache. Presenting signs and symptoms are variable and may include nausea/vomiting and visual, auditory, or vestibular disturbances. CSF hypotension can be caused by development of a CSF leak due to head or spinal trauma or secondary to skull base surgery. It can also develop spontaneously, likely arising from dural thinning/erosion from adjacent inflammation or infection.[46] Intracranial hypotension may also result from slow, persistent CSF leakage following a spinal puncture or from a spontaneous dural defect, or from overshunting of CSF after placement of a ventriculoperitoneal shunt.[47,48]

Findings associated with CSF hypotension are best demonstrated on cranial MRI with gadolinium enhancement. This demonstrates a "pachymeningeal" pattern of smooth, continuous, enhanced dural thickening. In some cases, this may be associated with small subdural effusions and/or downward vertical displacement of the brainstem and cerebellar tonsils (Fig. 19.9).

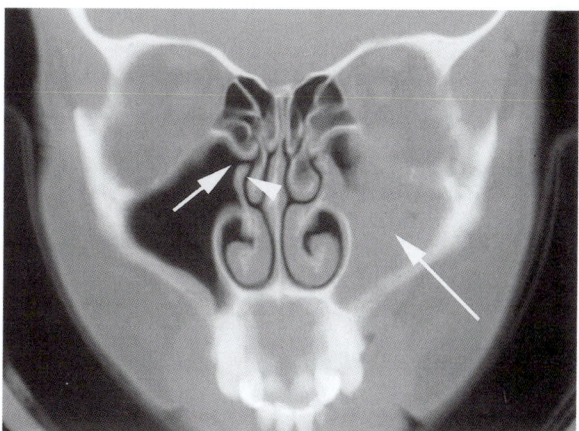

FIGURE 19.8 Chronic sinusitis. Coronal, nonenhanced screening sinus computed tomography through the face shows opacification of the left maxillary sinus caused by chronic inflammation (*long arrow*). The ostiomeatal unit (*short arrow*) and uncinate process (*arrowhead*) are clearly demonstrated on the opposite side.

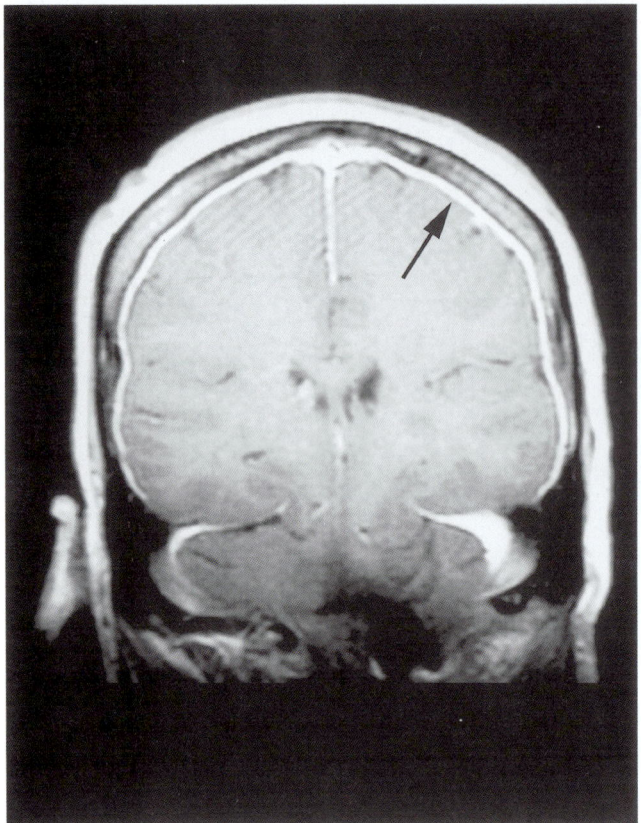

FIGURE 19.9 Cerebrospinal fluid hypotension caused by overshunting. A 54-year-old woman with ventriculoperitoneal shunt. Diffuse dural thickening and enhancement (*arrow*) caused by shunt valve with insufficient resistance. Similar findings may be seen in patients with postlumbar puncture, dural tears, or posttraumatic cerebrospinal fluid leaks.

These are generally reversible and disappear with resolution of CSF hypotension after successful treatment by blood patch, epidural saline injection, or surgical repair of the defect.[49-51] Headache with MR findings of diffuse enhanced dural thickening, not explained by prior surgery or infection, should prompt a diligent search for possible site of an occult CSF leak. This can be done with MRI using a heavily fluid-weighted 3D sequence such as Constructive Interference in Steady State (CISS, Siemens trade name), Balanced Fast Field Echo (BFFE, Philips) or Fast Imaging Employing STeady-state Acquisition (FIESTA, GE) to provide an MR cisternogram or MR myelogram type of image.[52-55]

INTRACRANIAL HYPERTENSION (PSEUDOTUMOR CEREBRI)

On the other hand, increased intracranial pressure could cause moderate to severe headache, vision change, nausea, and vomiting. Papilledema can be seen on funduscopic evaluation, which eventually leads to loss of vision if left untreated. After excluding secondary intracranial hypertension such as mass lesion, dural venous sinus thrombosis, systemic diseases, and medication, idiopathic intracranial hypertension should be considered. It is more common among overweight females. Increased intracranial pressure is confirmed by measuring opening pressure during LP. On imaging, prominent CSF in tortuous optic sheaths, empty sella turcica, and slit-like ventricles are supportive findings.

Facial Pain

Intractable trigeminal neuralgia (tic douloureux) can be caused from irritation of the nerve from a vascular loop that contacts the cisternal portion of the fifth cranial nerve near its exit from

the pons.[56] The vessels most responsible for this often arise from a branch of the superior, anterior-inferior, or posterior-inferior cerebellar arteries (see Chapter 67). Surgical intervention with placement of a small Teflon prosthetic "pad" or "spacer," to separate the offending vessel from the root entry zone of the cranial nerve, is often effective in relieving symptoms.[57] Diagnosis of vascular loops in the prepontine cistern and cerebellopontine angle was difficult before the development of high-resolution MRI. Thin-section heavily fluid-weighted steady-state, free precession, gradient echo techniques (BFFE, CISS, FIESTA) provide a cisternogram image of the basal cisterns that outline the cranial nerves and vessels in the area. This technique can effectively display the offending vascular loop in relation to the cranial nerve. The diagnosis of vascular loop syndrome is made by demonstration of a blood vessel contiguous with, or actually distorting, a cranial nerve close to its origin from the brainstem at the root entry zone in correlation with the appropriate clinical symptoms. This portion of the nerve lacks a full nerve sheath and thus is sensitive to irritation from pulsations from the contacting artery. The diagnosis must be based on appropriate correlation with clinical symptoms because up to 49% of asymptomatic patients may show similar vascular imaging findings.[58] These MR studies not only aid in identification of surgical candidates but also serve as a roadmap for surgical treatment planning (Fig. 19.10).[58-63]

Other structural causes of trigeminal nerve dysfunction include mass lesions near the trigeminal nerve such as meningioma, schwannoma, arachnoid cyst, cholesteatoma, and epidermoid cyst.[64,65] These can be diagnosed by conventional cranial MRI and CT studies.

In addition to trigeminal neuralgia, vascular loops can compromise other cranial nerves along the brainstem. Thus, chronic vertigo can be caused by posterior fossa vessels contacting the root entry zone of the eighth cranial nerve (Fig. 19.11) and compression of the intracisternal seventh nerve can result in hemifacial spasm. Similar high-resolution MRI techniques are used to identify potential vascular loop syndromes causing these symptoms. Of note, vascular loops contacting seventh and/or eighth cranial nerves are also common, and the finding of a vascular loop needs to be carefully interpreted.[66]

Spinal Pain

OVERVIEW

Technical advances in surgical fusion of lower lumbar vertebrae have resulted in safer, less invasive operations and have generated renewed interest in diagnostic tests that might predict a favorable surgical outcome for the back pain patient.[67-69] Conventional MRI, CT, and CT myelography can accurately evaluate central spinal canal or neuroforaminal stenosis. MR of the lumbar spine, in particular, is very sensitive for the detection of lumbar disk protrusion, extrusion, or sequestration in the patient with pain and radiculopathy. Also, facet arthropathy in patients with nonradicular back pain is readily assessed with CT or MRI (Fig. 19.12).[70] Gadolinium-enhanced MRI is useful in evaluation of patients with failed back surgery syndrome because it aids in distinguishing between postsurgical scar and recurrent disk herniation.[71] Postoperative scar tissue has a blood supply and thus demonstrates contrast enhancement, whereas a herniated disk fragment does not have a direct blood supply and does not exhibit significant enhancement on postcontrast MRI.[72]

CT and MRI are very sensitive imaging techniques that accurately depict spinal degenerative changes and disk pathology. However, it must be recognized that because of the prevalence of degenerative changes in the adult population, imaging findings such as annular tears, disk bulge, and even focal disk protrusion commonly occur in asymptomatic patients.

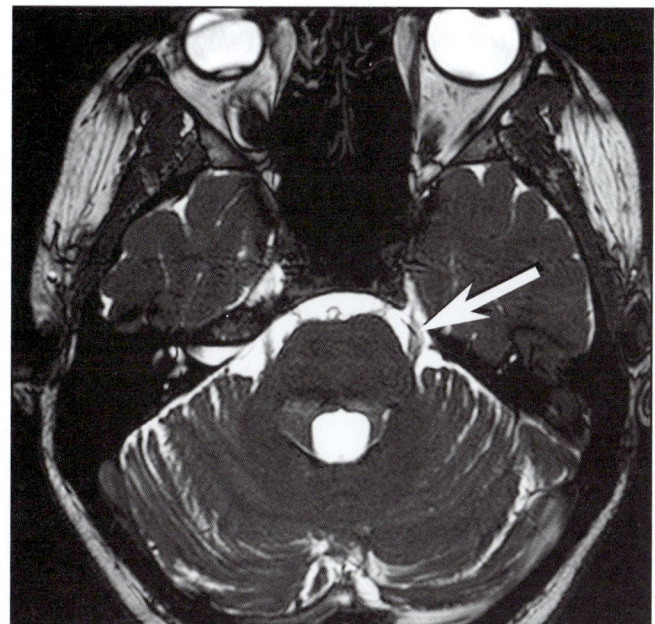

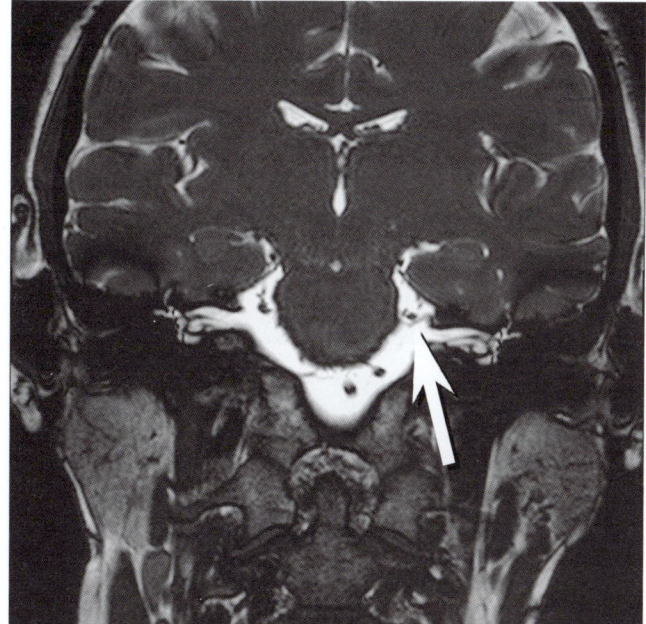

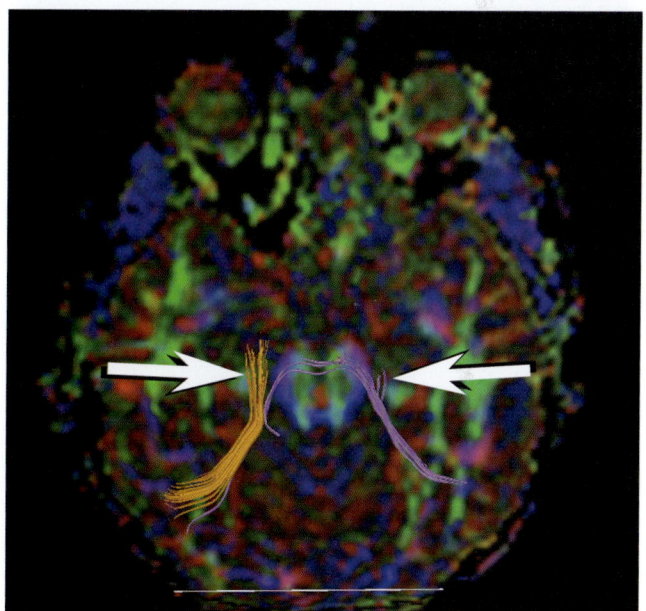

FIGURE 19.10 Vascular loop compression of the trigeminal nerve. Axial balanced fast field echo (BFFE) image **(A)** and coronal BFFE image **(B)** demonstrate the left superior cerebellar artery branch runs immediately inferior to the cisternal segment of the left trigeminal nerve (*arrows*) with possible compression. **C:** Diffusion tensor imaging (DTI) clearly delineates the asymmetry of the trigeminal nerves (*arrows*) with decreased anisotropy on the left (*right arrow*), which is suggestive of vascular compression.

Therefore, these imaging findings alone do not prove a causal effect in an individual patient with back pain.[73] Indeed, it is prudent to have a healthy (no pun intended) awareness of potential overreliance on using imaging findings alone to guide treatment decisions.[74] Rather, correlation of the patient's pain pattern and clinical findings with the imaging findings is needed to assess whether or not any observed abnormalities are likely to be the cause of a patient's pain. Only when such correlation is positive is it appropriate to proceed with invasive treatment planning. The natural history of acute back pain without fracture, infection, or malignancy is most often spontaneous resolution following primary conservative treatment (rest, physical therapy, exercise).[75] Indeed, in acute atraumatic low back pain without a "red flag" such as history of malignancy, weight loss, immunocompromise, etc., imaging is not indicated (ACR). Surgery should be reserved for cases with intractable pain, rapidly progressive symptoms, or patients with neurologic compromise.[76–79]

COMPRESSION FRACTURES

Workup of vertebral body compression deformity may include initial plain films, followed by MRI to assess for marrow edema if the acuteness of a lesion is in question. In cases of acute traumatic injury, CT can best assess extent of fracture planes and stability, along with presence and amount of posterior endplate retropulsion, whereas MR can best evaluate possible presence of associated intraspinal hemorrhage, nerve root/cauda equina compromise, and posterior ligamentous complex injury. If MRI is contraindicated, a nuclear medicine bone scan may also demonstrate marrow edema.

BENIGN VERSUS MALIGNANT; INFECTION/INFLAMMATION

Water/fat MR images obtained in-phase and opposed-phase (using gradient recalled-echo MRI sequences) are useful for differentiating pathologic compression fracture from benign compression fracture.[80] With this method, signal intensity ratio

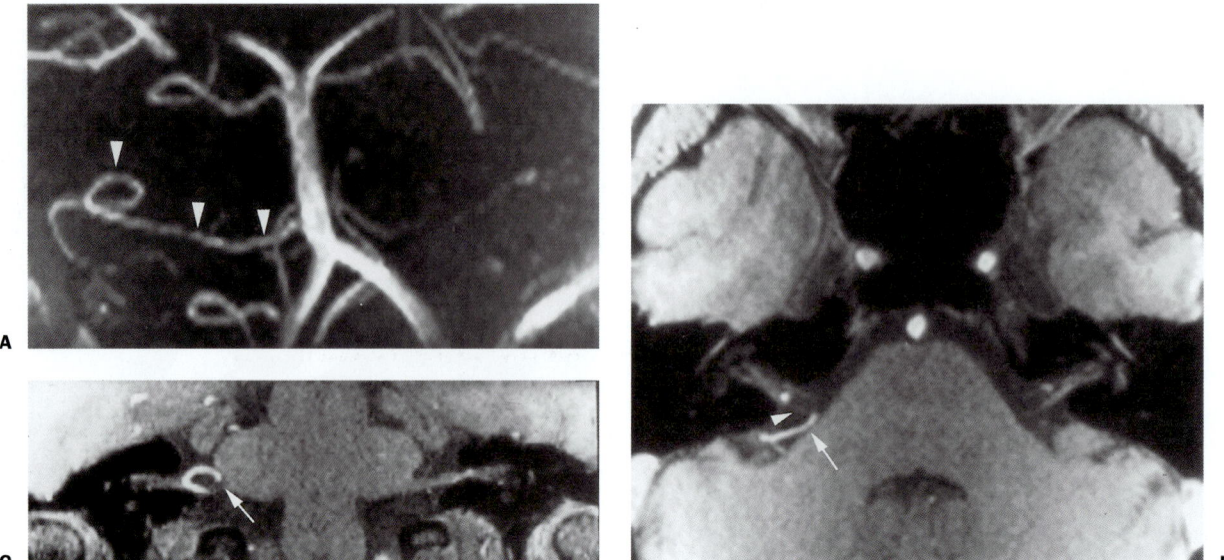

FIGURE 19.11   Vascular loop compression of the eighth nerve. **A:** Anteroposterior projection of a magnetic resonance angiography (MRA) of the vertebral basilar arterial system shows a good demonstration of a prominent right anterior inferior cerebellar artery (*arrowheads*). However, this standard MRA display does not allow one to determine the relationship of the looping portion of the vessel to the underlying neural structures. **B:** Axial source image of the MRA now shows a good demonstration of a vascular loop (*arrow*), which lies contiguous with the eighth nerve (*arrowhead*) near its origin from the brainstem. **C:** Coronal reformatted image from the MRA data set confirms the contiguous position of the vascular loop with the eighth nerve near its root entry zone (*arrow*).

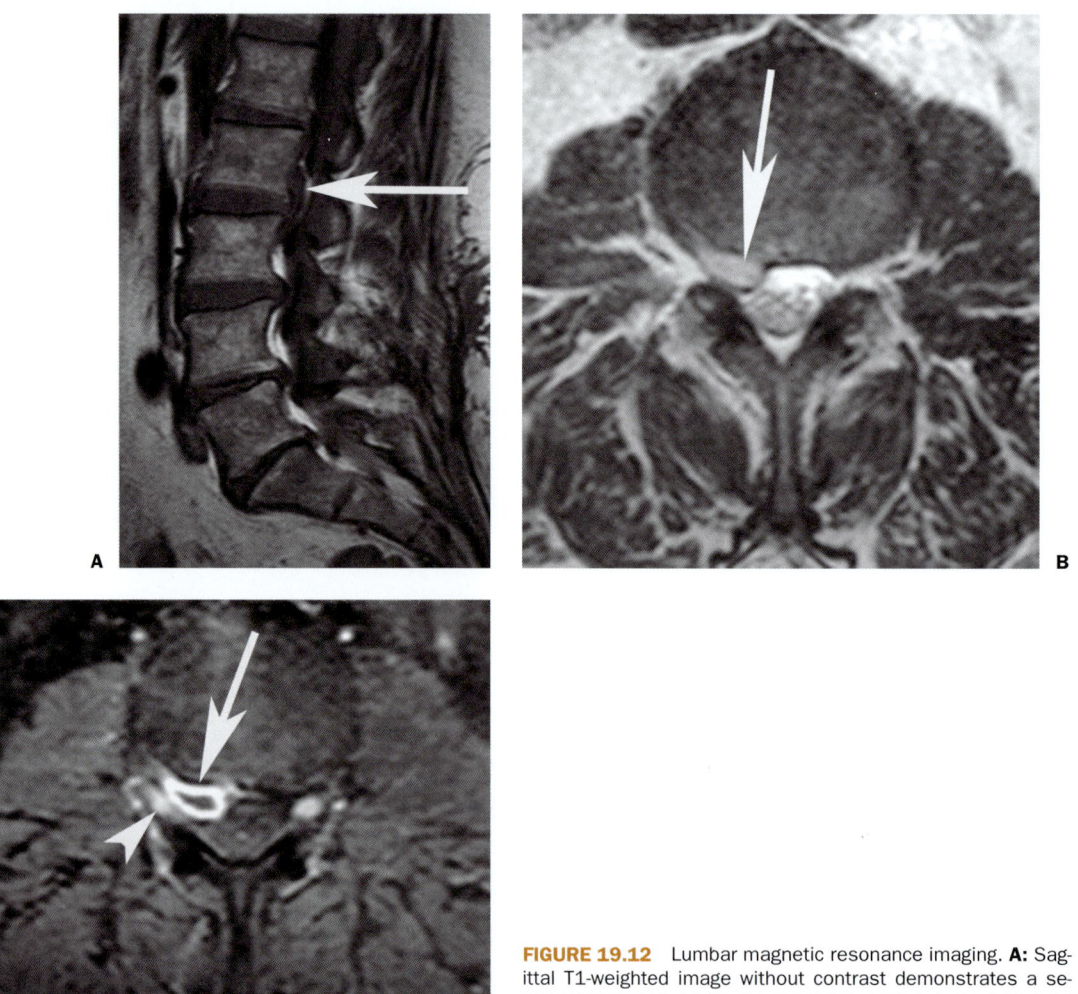

FIGURE 19.12   Lumbar magnetic resonance imaging. **A:** Sagittal T1-weighted image without contrast demonstrates a sequestration at L2–L3 level extending superiorly (*arrow*). **B:** Axial T2-weighted image demonstrates abnormal high signal in the sequestrum (*arrow*). The right lateral recess is compressed. **C:** Intense surrounding enhancement is present (*arrow*). The exiting right L2 nerve is compressed (*arrowhead*).

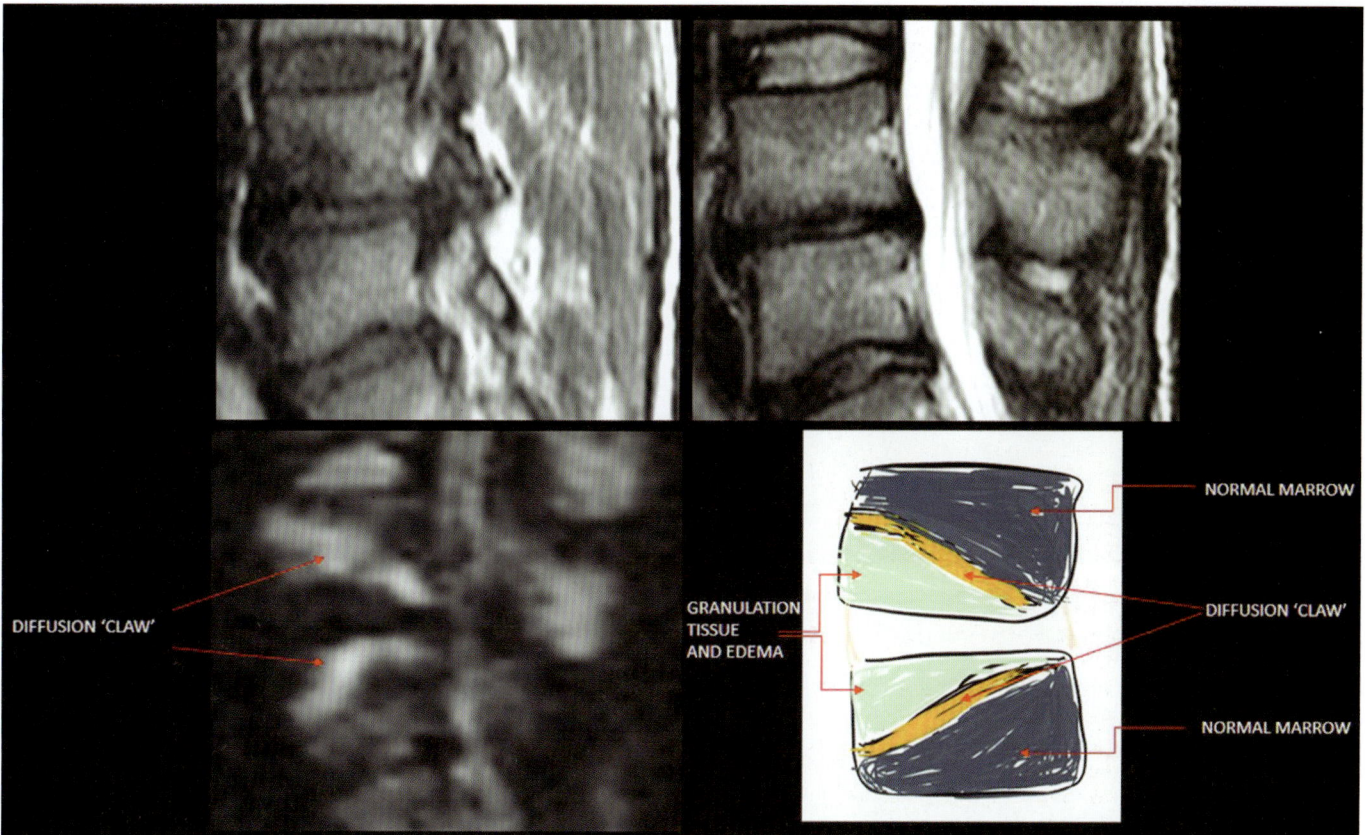

FIGURE 19.13 Diffusion magnetic resonance imaging "claw sign." The claw sign is identified on trace/combined diffusion-weighted imaging sequences (DWI) as well-marginated, linear, typically paired, regions of high signal situated within adjoined vertebral bodies at the boundaries between the normal bone marrow and vascularized bone marrow. *(Republished with permission of American Society of Neuroradiology from Patel KB, Poplawski MM, Pawha PS, et al. Diffusion-weighted MRI "claw sign" improves differentiation of infectious from degenerative modic type 1 signal changes of the spine. AJNR Am J Neuroradiol 2014;35[8]:1647–1652; permission conveyed through Copyright Clearance Center, Inc. Copyright © 2014 by American Journal of Neuroradiology.)*

on opposed-phase (water − fat) images compared to in-phase images (water + fat) of >0.8 suggests malignancy because malignant processes tend to infiltrate and replace normal fatty marrow, whereas benign compression fractures displace fat to a much lesser degree.

If an infectious or inflammatory process such as discitis/osteomyelitis is suspected, MRI with pre- and postcontrast fat-saturated T1-weighted sequences are most helpful. These show enhancement of bone and marrow space involvement accompanied by contiguous disk space inflammation (discitis) and uniform paraspinous enhancement of varying thickness. This complex of findings is generally absent with pathologic tumor or benign compression fractures.

Differentiating discitis/osteomyelitis from Modic type 1 degenerative edematous change can be challenging. Lack of paraspinal soft tissue abnormality and normal or dark signal of the intervening disk are suggestive findings for degenerative changes. Diffusion-weighted imaging sequences (DWI), if obtained, may demonstrate well-marginated linear high signal between normal and edematous marrow ("claw sign") which is highly indicative of degenerative changes; conversely, diffuse abnormal high signal on DWI in the edematous region (absence of claw sign) is highly suggestive of discitis/osteomyelitis (Figs. 19.13 and 19.14).[81]

Nuclear medicine gallium scan may also be considered for imaging in this setting, if MRI is contraindicated.

DISCOGENIC PAIN

Before the advent of spinal CT and MRI, discography was the only radiologic technique for directly assessing the anatomy and integrity of the intervertebral disk. Discography involves injection of radiographic contrast material into a suspected abnormal disk and one or two normal (control) disks while monitoring the patient's subjective reported pain (Fig. 19.15).[82] A positive test result is indicated by reproduction of the patient's symptoms during injection of the involved abnormal disk level, without similar symptoms on injection of control disk levels.[83]

Discography is a unique provocative test for discogenic pain, but its major limitation is the fact that it is highly subjective. Patient reliability in accurately reporting symptoms during disk injection can be affected by psychological factors as well as the interview technique.[84,85] The discographic identification of a painful disk also does not guarantee that the patient will respond to surgical fusion at that level.[86,87] Concordant pain could be present in patients with mild low back pain who do not seek treatment.[88]

Because ongoing controversy exists regarding the accuracy and reliability of discography[89–91] as well as the potential for sustained trauma to the disk by discography, its utilization has steeply declined in recent years coinciding with concurrent improvement in noninvasive MRI techniques. From an anatomic standpoint, CT and MRI have mostly replaced discography.[92] Currently, there is a limited role for discography as a provocative test in selected patients with persistent and presumed disk abnormalities but negative on imaging, with the aim of selecting patients with a greater likelihood of improvement after spinal fusion procedures.[93] Indeed, in many centers, it is no longer performed and has been supplanted by modern MRI spinal imaging techniques.

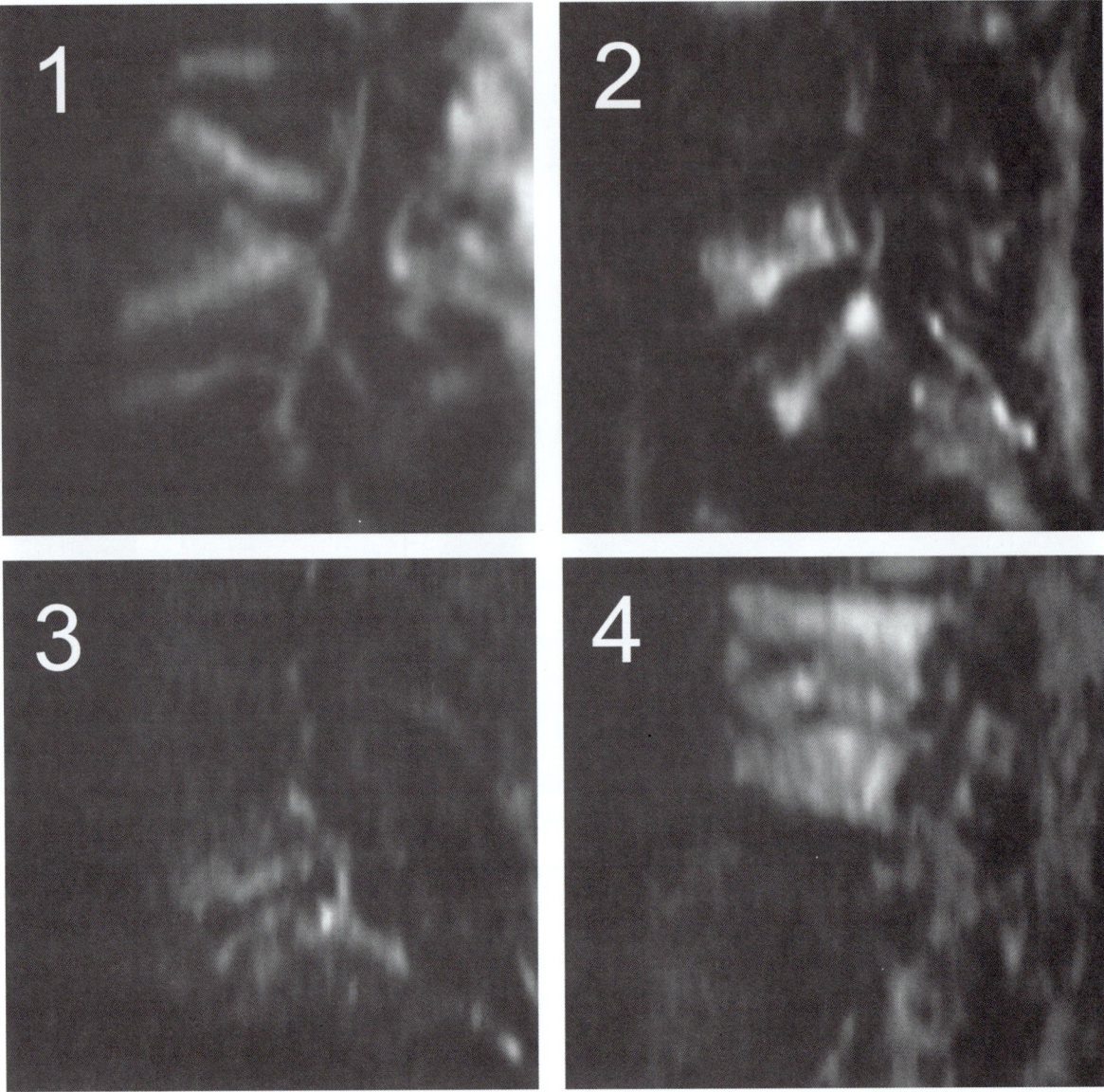

FIGURE 19.14   Gradation from positive to negative "claw signs." 1 = definite, 2 = probable, 3 = questionable, 4 = negative (diffuse signal). *(Republished with permission of American Society of Neuroradiology from Patel KB, Poplawski MM, Pawha PS, et al. Diffusion-weighted MRI "claw sign" improves differentiation of infectious from degenerative Modic type 1 signal changes of the spine. AJNR Am J Neuroradiol 2014;35[8]:1647–1652; permission conveyed through Copyright Clearance Center, Inc. Copyright © 2014 by American Journal of Neuroradiology.)*

Limb Pain and Magnetic Resonance Neurography

MAGNETIC RESONANCE NEUROGRAPHY

Magnetic resonance neurography (MRN) involves high-resolution imaging of peripheral nerves to confirm pathologic involvement of a nerve and to localize the site and extent of a pathologic process. It is targeted to specific peripheral nerves based on symptom pattern and neurologic exam. It should not be considered a screening technique and is ineffective as such. The primary purpose of MRN is to confirm presence of a suspected abnormality involving a specific nerve based on clinical neurologic signs and symptoms. It is also useful to localize the site and extent of pathology to help in assessing the need for surgical intervention and to aid in surgical treatment planning should intervention be indicated. MRN indications include evaluating a mass lesion, compressive neuropathy, nerve entrapment syndromes, unexplained focal neuropathy or plexopathy, and traumatic nerve injury. It is also useful in the posttreatment setting for evaluation of nerve response to invasive therapy.

With the advance of available surgical techniques, accurate presurgical evaluation of a nerve abnormality is becoming more and more important. MRN of the brachial or lumbosacral plexuses and major peripheral nerves permits direct visualization of the nervous structures and can visualize the presence of abnormalities associated with perineural irritation, edema, or compression.[94–98] Pathologic states caused by variant anatomy (such as compressive fibrous bands or offending bony spurs), prior trauma, scar tissue or mass lesion, and musculoskeletal causes of pain can be detected or excluded (Figs. 19.16 to 19.18). MRI of distal musculature can provide evidence of denervation in the distribution of a given peripheral nerve and provide further evidence of neuropathy (Figs. 19.19 and 19.20).[99–101] In rat models, increased T2 signal has been shown in the denervated muscles as soon as 48 hours following a denervation event and peaks at about 2 to 4 weeks. If there is nerve regeneration and reinnervation, the abnormal muscle signal resolves as reinnervation progresses in about 6 to 8 weeks in the rat model. But without regeneration of the nerve, denervation changes of the muscle progresses and eventually causes muscle atrophy with fatty infiltration several months later.[100,102–104]

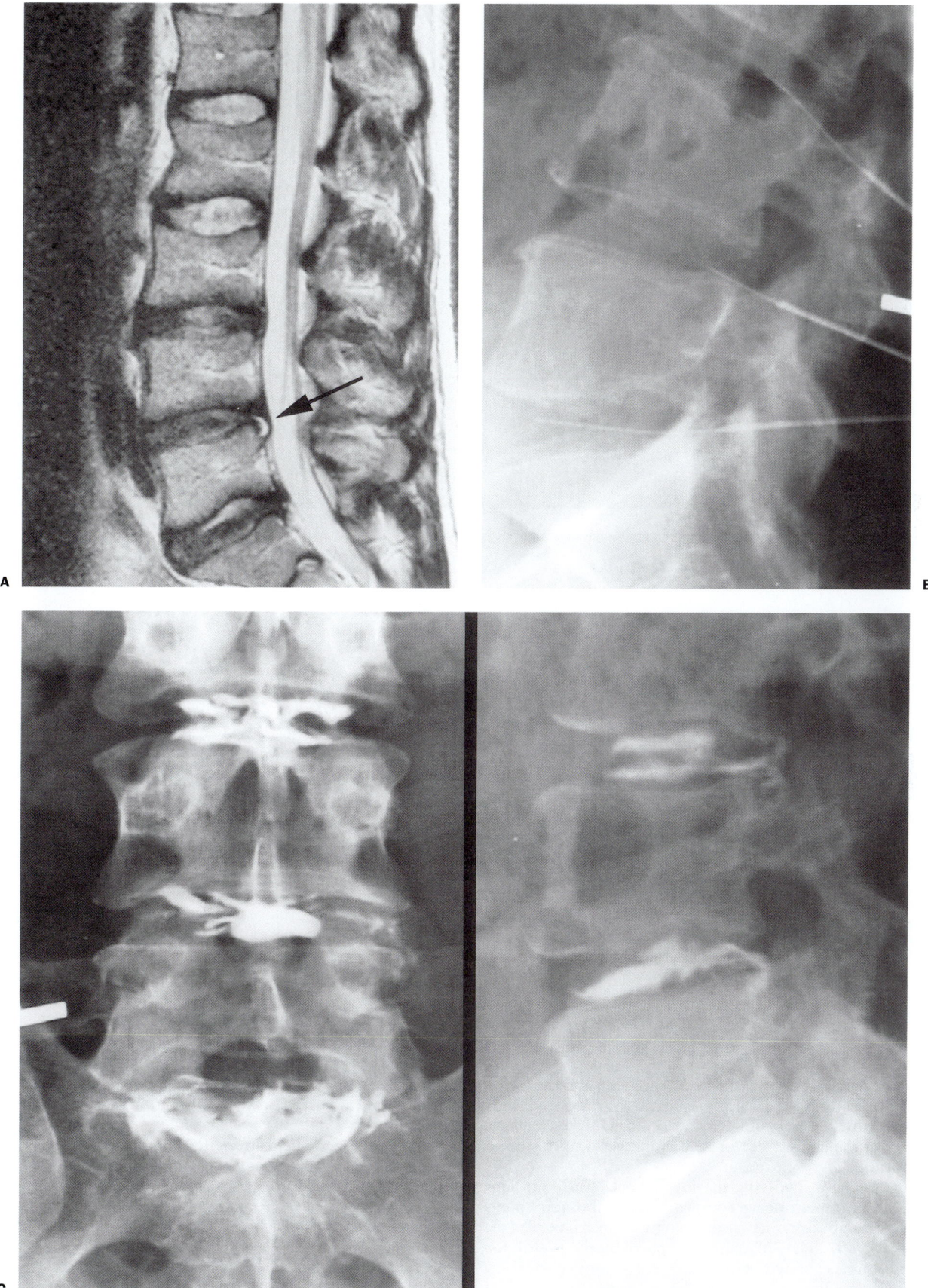

FIGURE 19.15 Discogram. A 34-year-old man with chronic lower back pain with radiation to left leg. **A:** Sagittal T2-weighted lumbar magnetic resonance imaging examination demonstrates an annular tear at L4–L5 as well as mild disk desiccation at L3–L4 and L5–S1. **B:** Lateral fluoroscopic spot film showing placement of 25G Chiba needles within the intervertebral disks at L3–L4, L4–L5, and L5–S1. **C:** Anteroposterior **(left)** and lateral **(right)** fluoroscopic images after injection of contrast material. During contrast injection, the patient reported no pain at L3–L4, mild (2/10) pain similar to clinical symptoms at L4–L5, and minimal (1/10) pain unlike clinical symptoms at L5–S1. *(continued)*

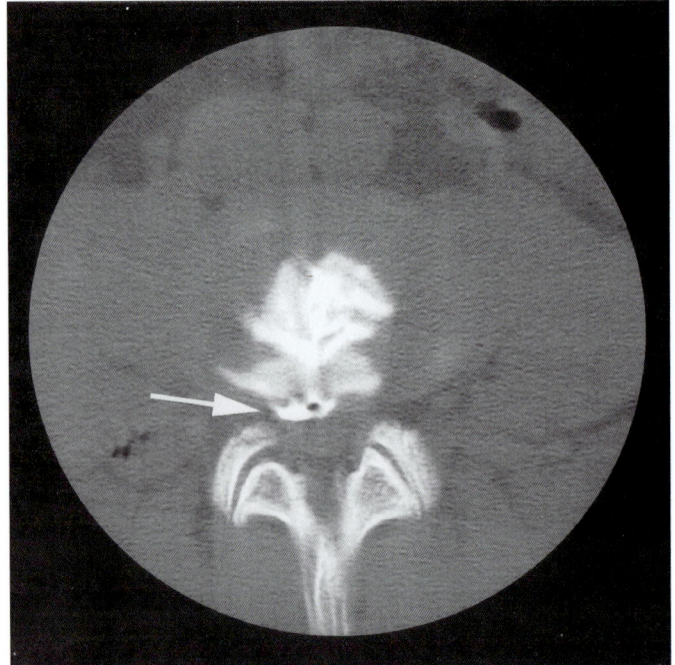

D

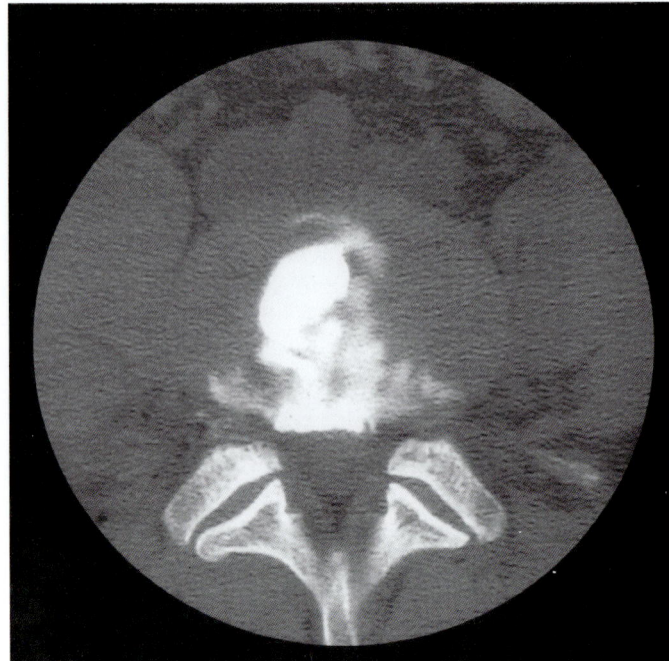

E

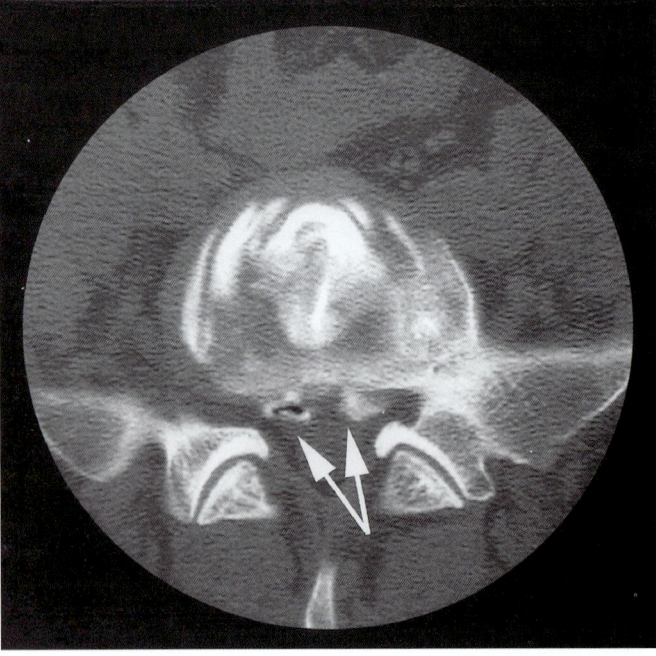

F

FIGURE 19.15 *(continued)* **D:** Postdiscography axial computed tomography (CT) through L3–L4. Internal fissures and small central annular tear (*arrow*). **E:** Axial CT through L4–L5. Internal fissures. **F:** Axial CT through L5–S1. Internal fissures and annular tear with focal herniation (*arrows*).

Neurogenic pain involving the neck, shoulder, and the upper extremity can result from cervical nerve root compression, brachial plexopathy, thoracic outlet syndrome (TOS), ulnar nerve entrapment at the elbow,[105,106] or median nerve compression at the carpal tunnel.

Neurogenic pain involving the lower back, hips, and legs can result from lumbar nerve compromise, lumbosacral plexopathy, and an abnormality in or along the sciatic nerve (see Chapters 40, 69, and 72). MRN is particularly useful for patients with unexplained neuropathy, for whom surgical intervention is considered, or when the exact anatomic site of abnormality remains unclear after clinical examination and electrodiagnostic studies. However, because only a relatively small field of view (FOV) can be imaged with high spatial resolution, it is necessary to clinically approximate the site of a suspected neuropathic lesion as closely as possible before

performing MRN. Imaging is then focused on the site of maximum clinical suspicion with optimal high-resolution imaging technique.

High magnetic field strength (3T) is preferred, although adequate studies can often be performed at 1.5T. T1-weighted images obtained parallel and perpendicular to the nerve of interest provide superb anatomic definition. Frequency selective fat saturation fast spin echo (FSE) T2 and/or short tau inversion recovery (STIR) sequences are sensitive to changes in normal signal intensity within a nerve. The roots, trunks, and cords of the brachial plexus can be shown for evaluation of possible pathology. Imaging of the lumbosacral plexus is done within the pelvis and upper thigh to follow the course of the sciatic or femoral nerves. In the case of bilateral nerve representation in the plexuses, it is often helpful to image both sides of the patient for comparison with the asymptomatic side.[107]

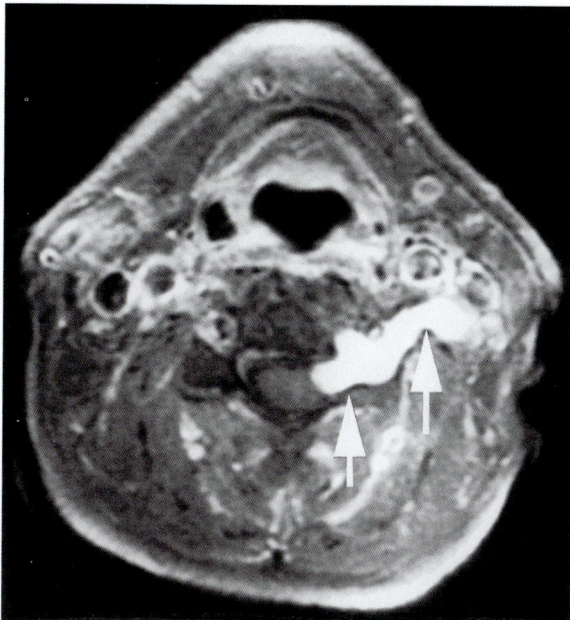

FIGURE 19.16 C5 schwannoma. An 81-year-old man with 4 years of left upper extremity pain and dysesthesia. Axial and coronal short tau inversion recovery images reveal a dumbbell-shaped high signal intensity extradural mass involving the left C4/C5 neural foramen (*arrows*).

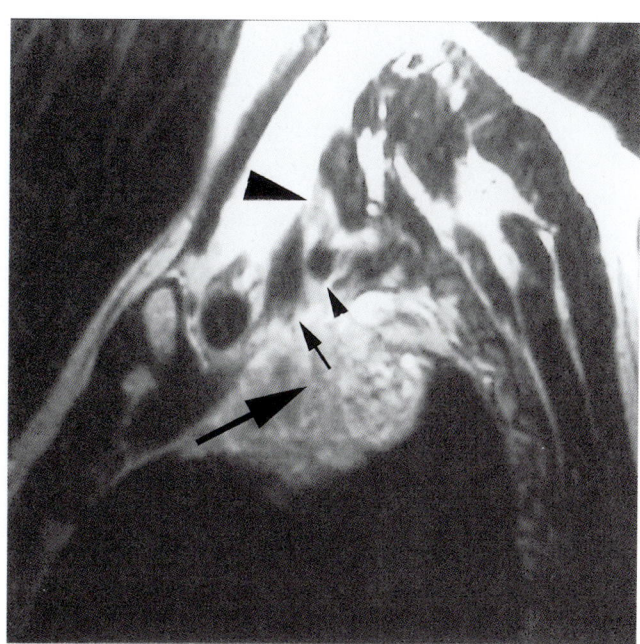

FIGURE 19.18 Pancoast tumor. A 42-year-old man with mild cough. Posterior superior mediastinal mass was identified on plain radiograph. Sagittal T2 images demonstrate the pulmonary apex mass (*long arrow*) that abuts but does not surround the subclavian artery (*small arrowhead*). At surgery, the mass was found to be a lung cancer. *Small arrow*, anterior scalene muscle; *large arrowhead*, brachial plexus.

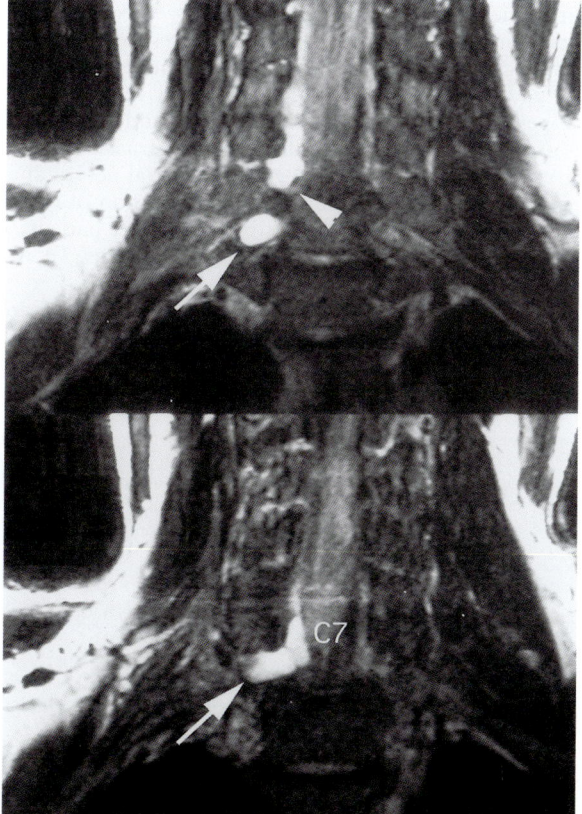

FIGURE 19.17 Nerve root avulsion. A 25-year-old man with traumatic injury to the right brachial plexus following a motorcycle accident that resulted in a flail upper extremity. After the accident, he suffered from daily, intermittent, lancinating pain. Electromyography demonstrated absent cortical and brainstem response to stimulation of median and ulnar nerves and upper trunk of brachial plexus (C6–C8 roots). Coronal T1 and short tau inversion recovery images show proximal meningeal diverticula at C6, C8, and T1 (*arrows, arrowhead*) as well as abnormal signal in the right brachial plexus.

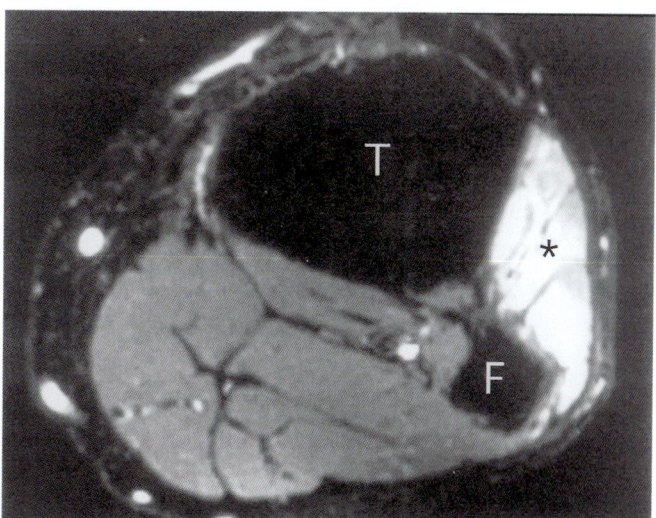

FIGURE 19.19 Subacute denervation in the distribution of the peroneal nerve. This axial short tau inversion recovery image of the proximal calf at the level of the fibular head (*F*) and the tibial metaphysis (*T*) demonstrates markedly hyperintense signal intensity within the anterior compartment muscles (*asterisk*). Note the muscles of the posterior calf for comparison, which show normal signal intensity. This illustrates the typical appearance of acute and subacute denervation that in this case followed severe injury to the left common perineal nerve.

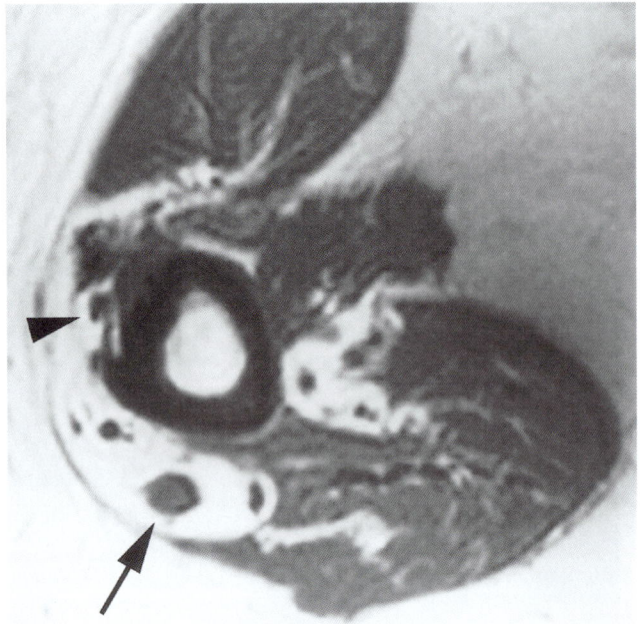
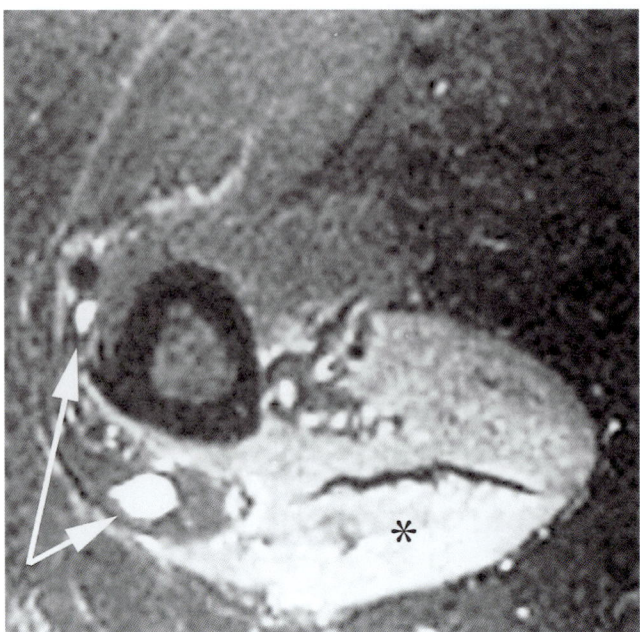

FIGURE 19.20 Ulnar and radial nerve injury. This patient suffered a severe left brachial plexus injury, with radial and ulnar neuropathy. **A:** T1-weighted axial image through the left upper arm showing location of the radial (*arrow*) and ulnar (*arrowhead*) nerves. T1 sequences generally demonstrate anatomic relationships better than corresponding short tau inversion recovery sequences. **B:** Short tau inversion recovery image showing increased signal in radial and ulnar nerves (*arrows*) as well as increased signal in triceps muscle (*asterisk*).

Optimal MR neurography at the elbow, wrist, and arm in the upper extremity and the thigh, knee, and ankle in the lower extremity requires even higher resolution imaging to enable visualization of these very small nerves that are of the order of 1.5 to 3 mm in cross-sectional size. However, similar T1, FSE T2, and STIR sequences are employed for imaging; in the extremities, these are generally conducted in the axial plane perpendicular to the nerve and in the coronal plane parallel to the nerve.

MRN appearance of normal nerves demonstrates iso- or slightly increased T2-weighted signal compared to muscles. Fascicles are easily seen within larger nerves such as the sciatic nerve but can often be seen even in smaller nerves including ulnar, median, and radial nerves in the upper extremity and the sciatic, tibial, and peroneal nerves in the lower extremity.

Abnormal changes in peripheral nerves identified by MR neurography include focal or generalized enlargement of the nerve, increased signal on T2 and STIR sequences, and swelling or loss of fascicular architecture. Enhancement after administration of gadolinium contrast is generally only seen with tumors of the peripheral nerves or with infection, and thus, for most MRN studies done for other indications, contrast enhancement is not used.[97,98,108] Direct imaging of peripheral nerves at common sites of entrapment can confirm the location of repetitive stress injury or tumor and help clinicians select patients who might benefit from decompressive surgery (see Figs. 19.20 and Figs. 19.21).[108]

A secondary sign of peripheral neuropathy may include acute and subacute denervation of musculature supplied by the involved peripheral nerve. This consists of increased signal on

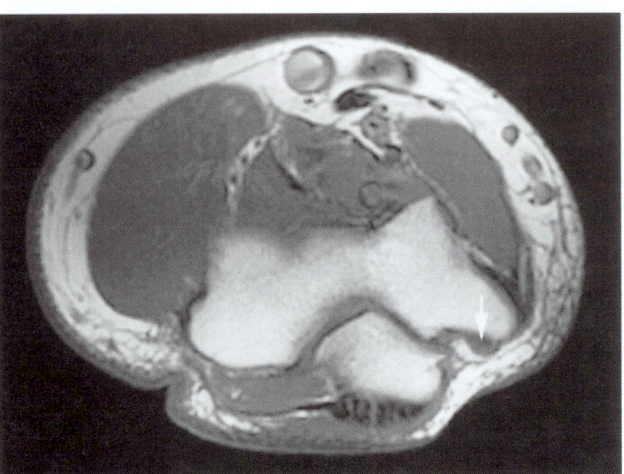
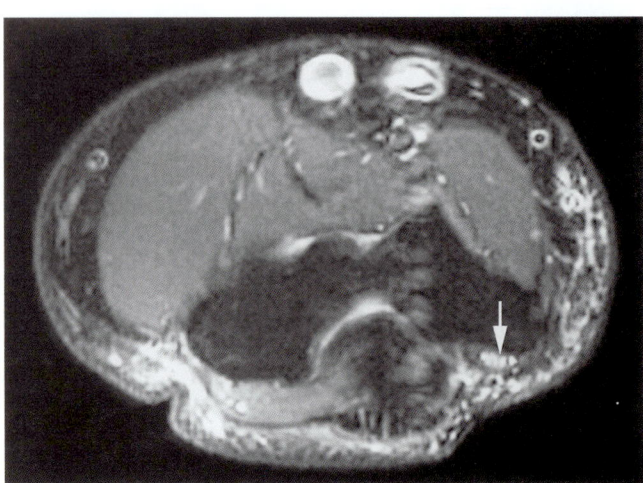

FIGURE 19.21 Ulnar entrapment. Axial T1 **(A)** and short tau inversion recovery (STIR) **(B)** images of the right elbow taken at the level in which the ulnar nerve passes through the cubital tunnel. **A:** On this T1-weighted image, a normal sized right ulnar nerve is nicely demonstrated surrounded by perineural fat (*arrow*). **B:** The STIR image, however, demonstrates abnormally increased hyperintensity within the nerve that is abnormal (*arrow*) and that, in the presence of appropriate symptoms, is an indication of ulnar nerve entrapment.

T2 and STIR sequences, sometimes accompanied by postcontrast enhancement of the denervated muscle in the acute phase. On the other hand, chronic denervation results in marked loss or atrophy of muscle mass, together with fatty infiltration. At the same time, the increased T2 signal seen in acute and subacute denervation disappears, and the muscle returns to a normal T2 signal intensity. Thus, the specific pattern of abnormal muscle denervation defines the involved peripheral nerve or nerves as well as providing a rough estimate of chronicity and is an effective means of confirming the affected nerve (see Figs. 19.19 and 19.20).[94,109]

THORACIC OUTLET SYNDROME

TOS is a group of disorders associated with impingement of the nervous or vascular structures during egress/ingress from the base of the neck to the axilla (see Chapter 40). Most patients have a controversial syndrome characterized by variable supraclavicular and upper extremity pain, dysesthesia, and weakness in the absence of a definitive etiology such as anomalous cervical rib.[110] Because musculoskeletal inflammatory conditions, complex regional pain syndromes, and distal compressive neuropathies can have similar symptoms, the diagnosis of TOS can be extremely difficult. Although decompression of the inferior brachial plexus and subclavian vessels by transaxillary resection of the first rib has been successful in management of some patients with intractable TOS after a failed trial of physical therapy, the decision to operate is rarely straightforward.

There are three forms of TOS: arterial, venous, and neurogenic. Neurogenic TOS is considered to be most common, consisting of more than 90% of all TOS cases.[111] Neurogenic TOS is difficult to diagnose. Patient symptoms are subtle and confusing but generally show chronic progression. It is usually considered to be associated with chronic compression and entrapment. Primary use of EMG is to exclude other peripheral neuropathies, rather than to rule in TOS.

A minority of patients (fewer than 10%) have a predominantly vascular form of TOS (arterial or venous). Arterial TOS symptoms result from subclavian or axillary artery compression, whereas venous TOS arises from venous insufficiency and/or thrombosis.[112] Arterial TOS typically presents with upper extremity arterial insufficiency symptoms or embolic episodes. Ultrasound and/or arteriography may help to demonstrate subclavian artery compression, arterial thrombosis, or distal emboli. Venous TOS (Paget-Schroetter syndrome) is due to thrombosis caused by compression of the subclavian or axillary vein and typically presents with upper limb swelling, pain, and cyanosis. It is significant in that it can result in pulmonary embolism.

The role of imaging in suspected TOS is not clearly established at present, and more investigation is required to evaluate the validity of imaging.[113] If cervical radiographs visualize the cervical ribs, the diagnosis is easily made. However, most cases of neurogenic TOS are not associated with cervical ribs. Neurogenic TOS may be imaged with MR neurography of the brachial plexus; the diagnosis may be made through identification of an angular deformity of the brachial plexus trunks as they pass through the scalene triangle (interscalene triangle), especially when there is abnormal insertion of the anterior scalene muscle. There may be accompanying increase in T2 signal of the affected nerve(s). Other potential compression sites are the costoclavicular space and the subpectoral space.

MRI is an emerging modality in evaluation of TOS.[114,115] It is noninvasive, does not require radiation, and demonstrates good soft tissue delineation. Panegyres and colleagues[114] reported sensitivity of 79% and specificity of 87.5% for the detection of distortion or displacement of the brachial plexus or subclavian vessels. Contrast-enhanced MRA is also useful to evaluate vascular compression,[116] especially with abducted arm position.[117–119] However, arterial compression can also be seen

in the normal population (0% to 1.39%), and venous compression is seen more frequently in normal populations (41.7% to 47%); therefore, clinical correlation is extremely important.

PIRIFORMIS SYNDROME

Piriformis syndrome is radiating leg pain from a non disk origin caused by compression or irritation of the sciatic nerve as it courses anterior/inferior to or through the piriformis muscle. On MR, abnormal high T2-weighted signal can be present in the affected sciatic nerve.[120,121] Filleret al.[121] reported that piriformis muscle asymmetry and sciatic nerve hyperintensity at the sciatic notch exhibited a 93% specificity and 64% sensitivity on MR, in distinguishing patients with piriformis syndrome from those who had similar symptoms but not attributable to pyriformis entrapment.

PERIPHERAL NERVE ENTRAPMENT SYNDROMES

Carpal tunnel syndrome is the most common form of nerve entrapment and is the result of median nerve compression at the carpal tunnel (see Chapter 72). Clinical features are usually sufficient for diagnosis. Frequent signs and symptoms include paresthesia and hyperesthesia in the median nerve distribution, radiation of pain along the volar aspect of the forearm, nocturnal pain, exacerbation with repetitive movements, and atrophy of the thenar muscles. Carpal tunnel syndrome is most often caused by repetitive injury of the median nerve within a tight carpal tunnel volume. Other possible etiologies include focal space-occupying lesions, local inflammatory processes, or metabolic derangements related to systemic illness.[122,123]

Proximal nerve entrapment can mimic carpal tunnel syndrome; potential sites of impingement are the cervical spine, thoracic outlet, and along the course of the median nerve. The pronator syndrome and the anterior interosseous syndrome are distal median nerve compression syndromes. In the former, the median nerve is compressed by the two heads of the pronator teres muscle. In the latter, the anterior osseous nerve is entrapped as it courses along the interosseous membrane. Both of these syndromes can produce symptoms identical to carpal tunnel syndrome.[97]

Although ultrasound and CT have been used to evaluate anatomy of the carpal tunnel and visualize the median nerve,[124] MR is superior to these technologies in confirming the diagnosis due to its sensitivity for detection of abnormal T2/STIR signal within a compressed median nerve. Axial T1 and STIR images are obtained from the distal radiocarpal joint to the metacarpal bases. High-resolution imaging with high field strength 3T MR systems are valuable in providing good image quality to optimally demonstrate these small structures (Fig. 19.22).[94]

Findings in carpal tunnel syndrome include increased cross-sectional size reflecting swelling of the median nerve proximal to the carpal tunnel, flattening of the nerve within the tunnel, increased palmer bowing of the flexor retinaculum, and increased median nerve T2 signal intensity on STIR sequences. Ganglion cysts, lipomas, and other soft tissue tumors and posttraumatic or degenerative bony deformities may result in similar symptoms. These abnormalities are easily identified and differentiated on MRI. Thickening or separation of tendons with increased signal changes on T2 or STIR sequences indicates tenosynovitis, often idiopathic. Amyloid, gout, acromegaly, hypothyroidism, and other systemic diseases associated with carpal tunnel syndrome are generally diagnosed on the basis of clinical, laboratory, and plain film findings.[125–128]

Additional entrapment syndromes are also found with ulnar nerve entrapment either in the cubital tunnel at the elbow or in Guyon's canal in the wrist.[129] Common symptoms include tingling sensation in the ring and little fingers. On MRN of the elbow or wrist, respectively, abnormal signal and enlargement of the ulnar nerve can be seen.[130] In the leg, common peroneal nerve entrapment may occur as it passes around the fibular

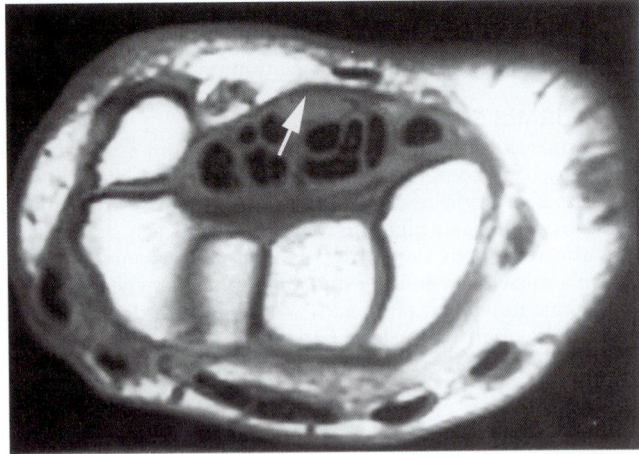
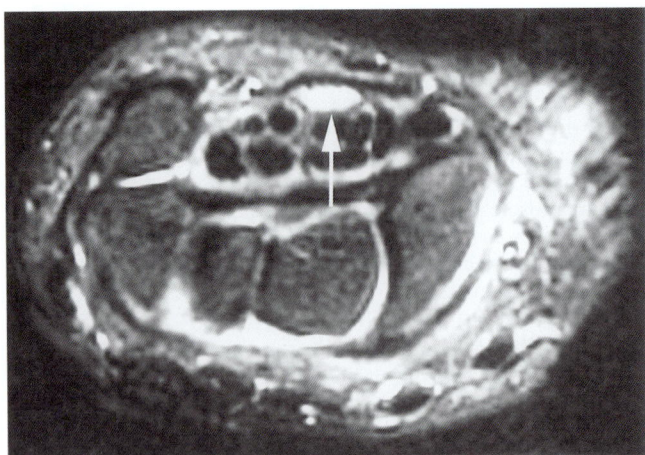

FIGURE 19.22   Carpal tunnel syndrome secondary to tenosynovitis. **A:** Axial T1 image through the carpal tunnel shows increased girth of the median nerve and bowing of the flexor retinaculum (*arrow*). **B:** Corresponding axial short tau inversion recovery image shows increased signal in the median nerve (*arrow*) as well as high signal fluid surrounding the tendon sheaths.

head and can be recognized by abnormal high T2 signal within the nerve.[101] MRN diagnosis of these various entrapment syndromes requires careful attention to the anatomy of the particular nerve involved.[94]

Imaging Guided Injection

Imaging studies play an important role in the facilitation of diagnostic and therapeutic nerve blocks, vertebroplasty, and kyphoplasty (see Chapters 100 to 104). Accurate placement of needles for the injection of local anesthetic or neurolytic substances is confirmed with image guidance that may utilize fluoroscopy, ultrasound, or CT scanning. These imaging techniques can assist with safe and accurate placement of a needle at the specific nerve, nerve root, or facet that is being blocked. The injection of a contrast agent with a local anesthetic solution can reveal the distribution of the agent used and confirm which nerve or facet has been exposed to the anesthetic solution. This is particularly important when a surgical decision is based on the responses to the blocks. These techniques are particularly useful in patients whose anatomy has been distorted by disease processes or prior surgical procedures.

Fluoroscopy is also used in the placement of epidural electrodes or catheters. Surgical procedures such as gangliolysis of the trigeminal nerve or radiofrequency rhizolysis of spinal nerves are performed with fluoroscopy or with intraoperative CT.[131] CT scans are commonly used for celiac plexus block.

These procedures are discussed in more detail in other chapters of this textbook.

Future Application of Pain Imaging

Pain is subjective and affected by emotional and psychological factors. Recent advances in functional and volumetric anatomic brain imaging have started to reveal the complex processes involved in central pain mechanisms. Patterns of brain activation with various pain syndromes are being explored, and the responses of individuals with chronic pain versus control subjects undergoing identical painful stimuli are beginning to reveal interesting findings (e.g., in evaluation of cluster headaches) (Fig. 19.23).[132–134]

Pain-related activity and the areas in the brain that subserve pain are complex and is termed the *pain matrix*. These evolving brain maps offer hope for understanding how pain relates to emotions, memory of pain, anticipation, personality, and other contributors. Imaging is used in investigating pain types, pursuing suppression mechanism of pain, and prevention of transition

from acute pain to chronic pain. Chronic pain is now known to be associated with reduction of gray matter density and altered network connectivity. How these will influence diagnosis and management of patients with chronic pain is yet to be defined but offer exciting possibilities and hope.

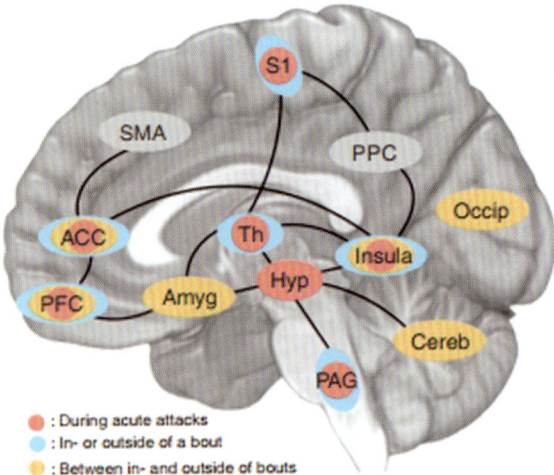

FIGURE 19.23   Neuroimaging of cluster headache. Schematic brain representation summarizing the findings of neuroimaging studies of cluster headache (CH): (1) CH appears to involve structural and functional changes in the pain matrix, especially in the descending pain modulation network; (2) disordered frontal top–down pain modulation is dynamically altered between in-bout and out-of-bout periods; (3) the anatomic and functional links between the hypothalamus and forebrain as well as cerebellar and occipital areas are altered in CH and may underlie its pathophysiology and clinical characteristics; and (4) the hypothalamus is likely involved in acute attacks, with a possible tendency to reverse outside acute attacks. The *blue circles* indicate the anatomic locations with structural and functional changes during in- or out-of-bout (without acute attacks) episodes. The *yellow circles* indicate the anatomic locations with structural and functional changes between in- and out-of-bouts. The *red circles* indicate the anatomic locations with structural and functional changes during acute attacks. ACC, anterior cingulate cortex; Amyg, amygdala; Cereb, cerebellum; Hyp, hypothalamus; Insula, insular cortex; PAG, periaqueductal gray; PFC, prefrontal cortex; PPC, posterior parietal cortex; SMA, supplementary motor area; S1, primary sensory cortex; Th, thalamus. (*Adapted and revised from May A. Structural brain imaging: a window into chronic pain.* Neuroscientist *2011;17[2]:209–220. Copyright © 2011 SAGE Publications; From Yang FC, Chou KH, Kuo CY, et al. The pathophysiology of episodic cluster headache: Insights from recent neuroimaging research.* Cephalalgia *2018;38[5]:970–983. Copyright © 2018 SAGE Publications.*)

Conclusion

Diagnostic imaging in patients with acute pain has a clearly defined role in establishing or confirming a pathologic diagnosis and directing medical, surgical, or radiologic intervention. Imaging for patients suffering from chronic or recurrent pain plays a significant role in detecting degenerative disease, anatomic variations, chronic inflammatory conditions, neoplasm, and postoperative or posttraumatic scarring. In selective cases, targeted and specialized imaging examinations may be of benefit for the determination of etiology, treatment planning, and prediction of the outcome of directed therapy.

References

1. Rasmussen BK, Jensen R, Schroll M, et al. Epidemiology of headache in a general population—a prevalence study. *J Clin Epidemiol* 1991;44(11):1147–1157.
2. Evans RW. Diagnostic testing for the evaluation of headaches. *Neurol Clin* 1996;14:1–26.
3. Sandrini G, Friberg L, Coppola G, et al. Neurophysiological tests and neuroimaging procedures in non-acute headache (2nd edition). *Eur J Neurol* 2011;18(3):373–381.
4. Perkins AT, Ondo W. When to worry about headache. Head pain as a clue to intracranial disease. *Postgrad Med* 1995;98:197–201, 204–208.
5. Silberstein SD. Evaluation and emergency treatment of headache. *Headache* 1992;32:396–407.
6. Young JY, Duhaime AC, Caruso PA, et al. Comparison of non-sedated brain MRI and CT for the detection of acute traumatic injury in children 6 years of age or less. *Emerg Radiol* 2016;23(4):325–331.
7. Roguski M, Morel B, Sweeney M, et al. Magnetic resonance imaging as an alternative to computed tomography in select patients with traumatic brain injury: a retrospective comparison. *J Neurosurg Pediatr* 2015;15(5):529–534.
8. Detsky ME, McDonald DR, Baerlocher MO, et al. Does this patient with headache have a migraine or need neuroimaging? *JAMA* 2006;296(10):1274–1283.
9. Pascual J, Berciano J. Experience in the diagnosis of headaches that start in elderly people. *J Neurol Neurosurg Psychiatry* 1994;57:1255–1257.
10. Tang C, Zhang TS, Zhou LF. Risk factors for rebleeding of aneurysmal subarachnoid hemorrhage: a meta-analysis. *PLoS One* 2014;9(6):e99536.
11. Naidech AM, Janjua N, Kreiter KT, et al. Predictors and impact of aneurysm rebleeding after subarachnoid hemorrhage. *Arch Neurol* 2005;62(3):410–416.
12. Dubosh NM, Bellolio MF, Rabinstein AA, et al. Sensitivity of early brain computed tomography to exclude aneurysmal subarachnoid hemorrhage: a systematic review and meta-analysis. *Stroke* 2016;47(3):750–755.
13. Pannke TS. Cerebral dural sinus thrombosis. *Ann Emerg Med* 1991;20:813–816.
14. de Bruijn SF, Stam J, Kappelle LJ. Thunderclap headache as first symptom of cerebral venous sinus thrombosis. CVST Study Group. *Lancet* 1996;348:1623–1625.
15. Wijdicks EF, Schievink WI, Miller GM. Pretruncal nonaneurysmal subarachnoid hemorrhage. *Mayo Clin Proc* 1998;73:745–752.
16. Guillon B, Biousse V, Massiou H, et al. Orbital pain as an isolated sign of internal carotid artery dissection. A diagnostic pitfall. *Cephalalgia* 1998;18:222–224.
17. Guillon B, Brunereau L, Biousse V, et al. Long-term follow-up of aneurysms developed during extracranial internal carotid artery dissection. *Neurology* 1999;53(1):117–122.
18. van der Wee N, Rinkel GJ, Hasan D, et al. Detection of subarachnoid haemorrhage on early CT: is lumbar puncture still needed after a negative scan? *J Neurol Neurosurg Psychiatry* 1995;58:357–359.
19. Boesiger BM, Shiber JR. Subarachnoid hemorrhage diagnosis by computed tomography and lumbar puncture: are fifth generation CT scanners better at identifying subarachnoid hemorrhage? *J Emerg Med* 2005;29(1):23–27.
20. Sidman R, Connolly E, Lemke T. Subarachnoid hemorrhage diagnosis: lumbar puncture is still needed when the computed tomography scan is normal [see comments in *Acad Emerg Med* 1996;3(9):823]. *Acad Emerg Med* 1996;3:827–831.
21. Horstman P, Linn FHH, Voorbij HAM, et al. Chance of aneurysm in patients suspected of SAH who have a "negative" CT scan but a "positive" lumbar puncture. *J Neurol* 2012;259(4):649–652.
22. Bakker NA, Groen RJ, Foumani M, et al. Appreciation of CT-negative, lumbar puncture-positive subarachnoid haemorrhage: risk factors for presence of aneurysms and diagnostic yield of imaging. *J Neurol Neurosurg Psychiatry* 2014;85(8):885–888.
23. Perry JJ, Alyahya B, Sivilotti ML, et al. Differentiation between traumatic tap and aneurysmal subarachnoid hemorrhage: prospective cohort study. *BMJ* 2015;350:h568.
24. Hoh BL, Cheung AC, Rabinov JD, et al. Results of a prospective protocol of computed tomographic angiography in place of catheter angiography as the only diagnostic and pretreatment planning study for cerebral aneurysms by a combined neurovascular team. *Neurosurgery* 2004;54(6):1329–1342.
25. Chen W, Wang J, Xin W, et al. Accuracy of 16-row multislice computed tomographic angiography for assessment of small cerebral aneurysms. *Neurosurgery* 2008;62(1):113–122.
26. McKinney AM, Palmer CS, Truwit CL, et al. Detection of aneurysms by 64-section multidetector CT angiography in patients acutely suspected of having an intracranial aneurysm and comparison with digital subtraction and 3D rotational angiography. *AJNR Am J Neuroradiol* 2008;29(3):594–602.
27. Pedersen HK, Bakke SJ, Hald JK, et al. CTA in patients with acute subarachnoid haemorrhage. A comparative study with selective, digital angiography and blinded, independent review. *Acta Radiol* 2001;42(1):43–49.
28. Romijn M, Gratama van Andel HA, van Walderveen MA, et al. Diagnostic accuracy of CT angiography with matched mask bone elimination for detection of intracranial aneurysms: comparison with digital subtraction angiography and 3D rotational angiography. *AJNR Am J Neuroradiol* 2008;29(1):134–139.
29. Dammert S, Krings T, Moller-Hartmann W, et al. Detection of intracranial aneurysms with multislice CT: comparison with conventional angiography. *Neuroradiology* 2004;46(6):427–434.
30. Anderson GB, Findlay JM, Steinke DE, et al. Experience with computed tomographic angiography for the detection of intracranial aneurysms in the setting of acute subarachnoid hemorrhage. *Neurosurgery* 1997;41:522–528.
31. Hope JK, Wilson JL, Thomson FJ. Three-dimensional CT angiography in the detection and characterization of intracranial berry aneurysms [see comments in *AJNR Am J Neuroradiol* 1997;18(4):790–792]. *AJNR Am J Neuroradiol* 1996;17:439–445.
32. Provenzale JM, Sarikaya B. Comparison of test performance characteristics of MRI, MR angiography, and CT angiography in the diagnosis of carotid and vertebral artery dissection: a review of the medical literature. *AJR Am J Roentgenol* 2009;193(4):1167–1174.
33. Sakurai K, Miura T, Sagisaka T, et al. Evaluation of luminal and vessel wall abnormalities in subacute and other stages of intracranial vertebrobasilar artery dissections using the volume isotropic turbo-spin-echo acquisition (VISTA) sequence: a preliminary study. *J Neuroradiol* 2013;40(1):19–28.
34. Weingarten S, Kleinman M, Elperin L, et al. The effectiveness of cerebral imaging in the diagnosis of chronic headache [see comments in *Arch Intern Med* 1993;153(13):1613–1614]. *Arch Intern Med* 1992;152:2457–2462.
35. Masson C, Lehericy S, Guillaume B, et al. Cluster-like headache in a patient with a trigeminal neurinoma. *Headache* 1995;35:48–49.
36. Smith WS, Messing RO. Cerebral aneurysm presenting as cough headache. *Headache* 1993;33:203–204.
37. Lehman VT, Brinjikji W, Mossa-Basha M, et al. Conventional and high-resolution vessel wall MRI of intracranial aneurysms: current concepts and new horizons. *J Neurosurg* 2017;9:1–13.
38. Guillon B, Levy C, Bousser MG. Internal carotid artery dissection: an update. *J Neurol Sci* 1998;153:146–158.
39. Ben Hassen W, Machet A, Edjlali-Goujon M, et al. Imaging of cervical artery dissection. *Diagn Interv Imaging* 2014;95(12):1151–1116.
40. Brinjikji W, Mossa-Basha M, Huston J, et al. Intracranial vessel wall imaging for evaluation of steno-occlusive disease and intracranial aneurysms. *J Neuroradiol* 2017;44(2):123–134.
41. Mossa-Bosha M, Alexander M, Gaddikeri S, et al. Vessel wall imaging for intracranial vascular disease evaluation. *J Neurointerv Surg* 2016;8(11):1154–1159.
42. Mossa-Bosha M, Hwang WD, De Havenon A, et al. Multicontrast high-resolution vessel wall magnetic resonance imaging and its value in differentiating intracranial vasculopathic processes. *Stroke* 2015;46(6):1567–1573.
43. Alexander MD, Yuan C, Rutman A, et al. High-resolution intracranial vessel wall imaging: imaging beyond the lumen. *J Neurol Neurosurg Psychiatry* 2016;87(6):589–597.
44. de Havenon A, Chung L, Park M, and Mossa-Bosha M. Intracranial vessel wall MRI: a review of current indications and future applications. *Neurovas Imaging* 2016;2:10. doi:10.1186/s40809-016-0021-6.
45. Mafee MF. Modern imaging of paranasal sinuses and the role of limited sinus computerized tomography; considerations of time, cost and radiation. *Ear Nose Throat J* 1994;73:532–534, 536–538, 540–542.
46. Blank SC, Shakir RA, Bindoff LA, et al. Spontaneous intracranial hypotension: clinical and magnetic resonance imaging characteristics. *Clin Neurol Neurosurg* 1997;99:199–204.
47. Ferrante E, Riva M, Gatti A, et al. Intracranial hypotension syndrome: neuroimaging in five spontaneous cases and etiopathogenetic correlations. *Clin Neurol Neurosurg* 2009;100:33–39.
48. Khurana RK. Intracranial hypotension. *Semin Neurol* 1996;16:5–10.
49. Bourekas EC, Lewin JS, Lanzieri CF. Postcontrast meningeal MR enhancement secondary to intracranial hypotension caused by lumbar puncture. *J Comput Assist Tomogr* 1995;19:299–301.
50. Pannullo SC, Reich JB, Krol G, et al. MRI changes in intracranial hypotension. *Neurology* 1993;43:919–926.
51. Fishman RA, Dillon WP. Dural enhancement and cerebral displacement secondary to intracranial hypotension. *Neurology* 1993;43:609–611.
52. el Gammal TA, Crews CE. MR myelography of the cervical spine. *Radiographics* 1996;16(1):77–88.
53. Matsumura A, Anno I, Kimura H, et al. Diagnosis of spontaneous intracranial hypotension by using magnetic resonance myelography. Case report. *J Neurosurg* 2000;92(5):873–876.

54. Chiapparini L, Ciceri E, Nappini S, et al. Headache and intracranial hypotension: neuroradiological findings. *Neurol Sci* 2004;25(suppl 3):S138–S141.

55. Tomoda Y, Korogi Y, Aoki T, et al. Detection of cerebrospinal fluid leakage: initial experience with three-dimensional fast spin-echo magnetic resonance myelography. *Acta Radiol* 2008;49(2):197–203.

56. Baldwin NG, Sahni KS, Jensen ME, et al. Association of vascular compression in trigeminal neuralgia versus other "facial pain syndromes" by magnetic resonance imaging. *Surg Neurol* 1991;36:447–452.

57. Brisman R. Surgical treatment of trigeminal neuralgia. *Semin Neurol* 1997;17:367–372.

58. Kakizawa Y, Seguchi T, Kodama K, et al. Anatomical study of the trigeminal and facial cranial nerves with the aid of 3.0-tesla magnetic resonance imaging. *J Neurosurg* 2008;108(3):483–490.

59. Kumon Y, Sakaki S, Kohno K, et al. Three-dimensional imaging for presentation of the causative vessels in patients with hemifacial spasm and trigeminal neuralgia. *Surg Neurol* 1997;47:178–184.

60. Majoie CB, Verbeeten B Jr, Dol JA, et al. Trigeminal neuropathy: evaluation with MR imaging. *Radiographics* 1995;15:795–811.

61. Majoie CB, Hulsmans FJ, Verbeeten B Jr, et al. Trigeminal neuralgia: comparison of two MR imaging techniques in the demonstration of neurovascular contact [see comments in *Radiology* 1998;208(2):550–552]. *Radiology* 1997;204:455–460.

62. Miller J, Acar F, Hamilton B, et al. Preoperative visualization of neurovascular anatomy in trigeminal neuralgia. *J Neurosurg* 2008;108(3):477–482.

63. Herweh C, Kress B, Rasche D, et al. Loss of anisotropy in trigeminal neuralgia revealed by diffusion tensor imaging. *Neurology* 2007;68(10):776–778.

64. Klieb HB, Freeman BV. Trigeminal neuralgia caused by intracranial epidermoid tumour: report of a case. *J Can Dent Assoc* 2008;74(1):63–65.

65. Ogütcen–Toller M, Uzun E, Incesu L. Clinical and magnetic resonance imaging evaluation of facial pain. *Oral Surg Oral Med Oral Pathol Oral Radiol Endod* 2004;97(5):652–658.

66. Gultekin S, Celik H, Akpek S, et al. Vascular loops at the cerebellopontine angle: is there a correlation with tinnitus? *AJNR Am J Neuroradiol* 2008;29(9):1746–1749.

67. Hacker RJ. Comparison of interbody fusion approaches for disabling low back pain. *Spine* 1997;22:660–666.

68. Ray CD. Threaded fusion cages for lumbar interbody fusions. An economic comparison with 360 degree fusions. *Spine* 1997;22:681–685.

69. Ray CD. Threaded titanium cages for lumbar interbody fusions. *Spine* 1997;22:667–680.

70. Bueff HU, Van der Reis W. Low back pain. *Prim Care* 1996;23:345–364.

71. Russo R, Cook P. Diagnosis of low back pain: role of imaging studies. *Occup Med* 1998;13:83–96.

72. Haughton V, Schreibman K, De Smet A. Contrast between scar and recurrent herniated disk on contrast-enhanced MR images [published correction appears in *AJNR Am J Neuroradiol* 2003;24(2):296]. *AJNR Am J Neuroradiol* 2002;23(10):1652–1656.

73. Stadnik TW, Lee RR, Coen HL, et al. Annular tears and disk herniation: prevalence and contrast enhancement on MR images in the absence of low back pain or sciatica. *Radiology* 1998;206:49–55.

74. Lurie JD, Birkmeyer NJ, Weinstein JN. Rates of advanced spinal imaging and spine surgery. *Spine (Phila Pa 1976)* 2003;28(6):616–620.

75. Hayden JA, Cartwright JL, Riley RD, et al. Exercise therapy for chronic low back pain: protocol for an individual participant data meta-analysis. *Systematic Reviews* 2012;1:64. doi:10.1186/2046-4053-1-64.

76. Willems PC, Staal JB, Walenkamp GH, et al. Spinal fusion for chronic low back pain: systematic review on the accuracy of tests for patient selection. *Spine J* 2013;13(2):99–109.

77. Mannion AF, Brox JI, Fairbank JC. Comparison of spinal fusion and non-operative treatment in patients with chronic low back pain: long-term follow-up of three randomized controlled trials. *Spine J* 2013;13(11):1438–1448.

78. Willems P. Decision making in surgical treatment of chronic low back pain: the performance of prognostic tests to select patients for lumbar spinal fusion. *Acta Orthop Suppl* 2013;84(349):1–35.

79. Jarvik JJ, Hollingworth W, Heagerty P, et al. The Longitudinal Assessment of Imaging and Disability of the Back (LAIDBack) study: baseline data. *Spine* 2001;26(10):1158–1166.

80. Erly WK, Oh ES, Outwater EK. The utility of in-phase/opposed-phase imaging in differentiating malignancy from acute benign compression fractures of the spine. *AJNR Am J Neuroradiol* 2006;27(6):1183–1188.

81. Patel KB, Poplawski MM, Pawha PS, et al. Diffusion-weighted MRI "claw sign" improves differentiation of infectious from degenerative Modic type 1 signal changes of the spine. *AJNR Am J Neuroradiol* 2014;35(8):1647–1652.

82. Kinard RE. Diagnostic spinal injection procedures. *Neurosurg Clin N Am* 1996;7:151–165.

83. Tehranzadeh J. Discography 2000. *Radiol Clin North Am* 1998;36:463–495.

84. Block AR, Vanharanta H, Ohnmeiss DD, et al. Discographic pain report. Influence of psychological factors. *Spine* 1996;21:334–338.

85. Ohnmeiss DD, Vanharanta H, Guyer RD. The association between pain drawings and computed tomographic/discographic pain responses. *Spine* 1995;20:729–733.

86. Parker LM, Murrell SE, Boden SD, et al. The outcome of posterolateral fusion in highly selected patients with discogenic low back pain [see comments in *Spine* 1997;22(12):1419–1420]. *Spine* 1996;21:1909–1917.

87. Carragee EJ, Lincoln T, Parmar VS, et al. A gold standard evaluation of the "discogenic pain" diagnosis as determined by provocative discography. *Spine* 2006;31(18):2115–2123.

88. Carragee EJ, Alamin TF, Miller J, et al. Provocative discography in volunteer subjects with mild persistent low back pain. *Spine J* 2002;2(1):25–34.

89. Bogduk N, Modic MT. Lumbar discography. *Spine* 1996;21:402–404.

90. Carragee EJ, Alamin TF, Carragee JM. Low-pressure positive discography in subjects asymptomatic of significant low back pain illness. *Spine* 2006;31(5):505–509.

91. Carragee EJ, Barcohana B, Alamin T, et al. Prospective controlled study of the development of lower back pain in previously asymptomatic subjects undergoing experimental discography. *Spine* 2004;29(10):1112–1117.

92. Schneiderman G, Flannigan B, Kingston S, et al. Magnetic resonance imaging in the diagnosis of disc degeneration: correlation with discography. *Spine* 1987;12:276–281.

93. Alamin TF, Kim MJ, Agarwal V. Provocative lumbar discography versus functional anesthetic discography: a comparison of the results of two different diagnostic techniques in 52 patients with chronic low back pain. *Spine J* 2011;11(8):756–765.

94. Aagaard BD, Maravilla KR, Kliot M. MR neurography. MR imaging of peripheral nerves [published correction appears in *Magn Reson Imaging Clin N Am* 1998;6(2):x]. *Magn Reson Imaging Clin N Am* 1998;6:179–194.

95. Dailey AT, Tsuruda JS, Goodkin R, et al. Magnetic resonance neurography for cervical radiculopathy: a preliminary report. *Neurosurgery* 1996;38:488–492.

96. Kuntz C IV, Blake L, Britz G, et al. Magnetic resonance neurography of peripheral nerve lesions in the lower extremity. *Neurosurgery* 1996;39:750–757.

97. Maravilla KR, Bowen BC. Imaging of the peripheral nervous system: evaluation of peripheral neuropathy and plexopathy [see comments in *AJNR Am J Neuroradiol* 1998;19(6):1001]. *AJNR Am J Neuroradiol* 1998;19:1011–1023.

98. Moore KR, Tsuruda JS, Dailey AT. The value of MR neurography for evaluating extraspinal neuropathic leg pain: a pictorial essay. *AJNR Am J Neuroradiol* 2001;22(4):786–794.

99. Polak JF, Jolesz FA, Adams DF. Magnetic resonance imaging of skeletal muscle. Prolongation of T1 and T2 subsequent to denervation. *Invest Radiol* 1988;23(5):365–369.

100. Wessig C, Koltzenburg M, Reiners K, et al. Muscle magnetic resonance imaging of denervation and reinnervation: correlation with electrophysiology and histology. *Exp Neurol* 2004;185(2):254–261.

101. Koltzenburg M, Bendszus M. Imaging of peripheral nerve lesions. *Curr Opin Neurol* 2004;17(5):621–626.

102. Aagaard BD, Lazar DA, Lankerovich L, et al. High-resolution magnetic resonance imaging is a noninvasive method of observing injury and recovery in the peripheral nervous system. *Neurosurgery* 2003;53(1):199–204.

103. Kikuchi Y, Nakamura T, Takayama S, et al. MR imaging in the diagnosis of denervated and reinnervated skeletal muscles: experimental study in rats [published correction appears in *Radiology* 2004;230(2):597]. *Radiology* 2003;229(3):861–867.

104. Bendszus M, Koltzenburg M, Wessig C, et al. Sequential MR imaging of denervated muscle: experimental study. *AJNR Am J Neuroradiol* 2002;23(8):1427–1431.

105. Rosenberg ZS, Beltran J, Cheung YY, et al. The elbow: MR features of nerve disorders. *Radiology* 1993;188:235–240.

106. Rosenberg ZS, Bencardino J, Beltran J. MR features of nerve disorders at the elbow. *Magn Reson Imaging Clin N Am* 1997;5:545–565.

107. Blake LC, Robertson WD, Hayes CE. Sacral plexus: optimal imaging planes for MR assessment. *Radiology* 1996;199:767–772.

108. Filler AG, Kliot M, Howe FA, et al. Application of magnetic resonance neurography in the evaluation of patients with peripheral nerve pathology. *J Neurosurg* 1996;85:299–309.

109. Freund W, Brinkmann A, Wagner F, et al. MR neurography with multiplanar reconstruction of 3D MRI datasets: an anatomical study and clinical applications. *Neuroradiology* 2007;49(4):335–341.

110. McGough EC, Pearce MB, Byrne JP. Management of thoracic outlet syndrome. *J Thorac Cardiovasc Surg* 1979;77:169–174.

111. Degeorges R, Reynaud C, Becquemin JP. Thoracic outlet syndrome surgery: long-term functional results. *Ann Vasc Surg* 2004;18(5):558–565.

112. Ohkawa Y, Isoda H, Hasegawa S, et al. MR angiography of thoracic outlet syndrome. *J Comput Assist Tomogr* 1992;16:475–477.

113. Estilaei SK, Byl NN. An evidence-based review of magnetic resonance angiography for diagnosing arterial thoracic outlet syndrome. *J Hand Ther* 2006;19(4):410–420.

114. Panegyres PK, Moore N, Gibson R, et al. Thoracic outlet syndromes and magnetic resonance imaging [see comments in *Brain* 1995;118(pt 3):819–821]. *Brain* 1993;116(pt 4):823–841.

115. Demondion X, Boutry N, Drizenko A, et al. Thoracic outlet: anatomic correlation with MR imaging. *AJR Am J Roentgenol* 2000;175(2):417–422.

116. Cosottini M, Zampa V, Petruzzi P, et al. Contrast-enhanced three-dimensional MR angiography in the assessment of subclavian artery diseases. *Eur Radiol* 2000;10(11):1737–1744.

117. Dymarkowski S, Bosmans H, Marchal G, et al. Three-dimensional MR angiography in the evaluation of thoracic outlet syndrome. *AJR Am J Roentgenol* 1999;173:1005–1008.

118. Hagspiel KD, Spinosa DJ, Angle JF, et al. Diagnosis of vascular compression at the thoracic outlet using gadolinium-enhanced high-resolution ultrafast MR angiography in abduction and adduction. *Cardiovasc Intervent Radiol* 2000;23(2):152–154.

119. Charon JP, Milne W, Sheppard DG, et al. Evaluation of MR angiographic technique in the assessment of thoracic outlet syndrome. *Clin Radiol* 2004;59(7):588–595.

120. Lewis AM, Layzer R, Engstrom JW, et al. Magnetic resonance neurography in extraspinal sciatica. *Arch Neurol* 2006;63(10):1469–1472.

121. Filler AG, Haynes J, Jordan SE, et al. Sciatica of nondisc origin and piriformis syndrome: diagnosis by magnetic resonance neurography and interventional magnetic resonance imaging with outcome study of resulting treatment. *J Neurosurg Spine* 2005;2(2):99–115.

122. Cantatore FP, Dell'Accio F, Lapadula G. Carpal tunnel syndrome: a review. *Clin Rheumatol* 1997;16:596–603.

123. Mesgarzadeh M, Triolo J, Schneck CD. Carpal tunnel syndrome. MR imaging diagnosis. *Magn Reson Imaging Clin N Am* 1995;3:249–264.

124. Buchberger W, Schön G, Strasser K, et al. High-resolution ultrasonography of the carpal tunnel. *J Ultrasound Med* 1991;10:531–537.

125. Allmann KH, Horch R, Uhl M, et al. MR imaging of the carpal tunnel. *Eur J Radiol* 1997;25:141–145.

126. Radack DM, Schweitzer ME, Taras J. Carpal tunnel syndrome: are the MR findings a result of population selection bias? [see comments in *AJR Am J Roentgenol* 1998;171(1):268–269]. *AJR Am J Roentgenol* 1997;169:1649–1653.

127. Mesgarzadeh M, Schneck CD, Bonakdarpour A. Carpal tunnel: MR imaging. Part I. Normal anatomy. *Radiology* 1989;171:743–748.

128. Mesgarzadeh M, Schneck CD, Bonakdarpour A, et al. Carpal tunnel: MR imaging. Part II. Carpal tunnel syndrome. *Radiology* 1989;171:749–754.

129. Zeiss J, Jakab E, Khimji T, et al. The ulnar tunnel at the wrist (Guyon's canal): normal MR anatomy and variants. *AJR Am J Roentgenol* 1992;158:1081–1085.

130. Grant GA, Britz GW, Goodkin R, et al. The utility of magnetic resonance imaging in evaluating peripheral nerve disorders. *Muscle Nerve* 2002;25(3):314–331.

131. Harrison C, Epton S, Bojanic S, et al. The efficacy and safety of dorsal root ganglion stimulation as a treatment for neuropathic pain: a literature review [published online ahead of print September 28, 2017]. *Neuromodulation*. doi:10.1111/ner.12685.

132. Yang FC, Chou KH, Kuo CY, et al. The pathophysiology of episodic cluster headache: Insights from recent neuroimaging research [published online ahead of print January 1, 2017]. *Cephalalgia*. doi:10.1177/0333102417716932.

133. Lai KL, Niddam D, Fuh JL, et al. Normalization of the resting-state network of ventral posteromedial nucleus in patients with chronic migraine is associated with good clinical outcome to prevention. Electronic poster EP-01-004. *Cephalalgia* 2017;37(15):25–51.

134. May A. Structural brain imaging: a window into chronic pain. *The Neuroscientist* 2011;17(2):209–220.

CHAPTER 20

Measurement of Pain

MARK P. JENSEN

Introduction

Valid and reliable pain assessment is essential for successful pain care. Adequate assessment is also necessary to determine the efficacy of pain treatments in clinical trials and for understanding the mechanisms of those effects. The clinician or researcher who wishes to use the most useful measures and strategies for pain assessment is faced with a large, and growing, number of options and decisions. The purpose of this chapter is to make those decisions easier.

Of course, in clinical settings, pain assessment in a broader sense should involve a detailed psychological and medical exam and often also involves the administration of general measures of physical and psychological function. These issues are addressed in detail in other chapters of this volume on different pain conditions. The focus of this chapter is on self-report and observational measures that are specific to the experience and impact of pain.

The chapter begins with a brief discussion of several important issues that clinicians and researchers need to consider when choosing from among pain measures and designing pain assessment procedures, including (1) evaluating the reliability, validity, and utility of pain measures; (2) determining the number of pain problems to assess; (3) choosing the pain domain(s) to assess; and (4) selecting the time period of assessment (e.g., current pain experience vs. recall of pain over the last day, week, or longer). The bulk of the chapter then reviews the available psychometric information regarding measures of six pain domains: pain intensity, pain affect, pain quality, pain site, pain's temporal characteristics, and pain interference. Next, the chapter briefly discusses strategies for assessing pain in special populations (e.g., infants and young children or other patients who might have difficulty expressing themselves verbally). It ends with a summary of recommendations.

VALIDITY, RELIABILITY, AND UTILITY IN THE CONTEXT OF PAIN ASSESSMENT

No measure is perfect. No one measure assesses all pain domains, nor is any single measure useful in all settings and with all populations. Moreover, because of the imperfection of available instruments, it is theoretically possible to modify any existing measure to improve it further or to develop new and better measures to replace existing ones. As a result, new pain assessment procedures and measures are constantly being developed and published. Thus, the clinician or researcher seeking to find the best measure for his or her needs should not only be aware of the existing pain assessment literature but should also know how to evaluate new measures as they are published.[1] The following section seeks to facilitate this task by briefly summarizing the three key issues that should be considered when evaluating any pain measure: *validity*, *reliability*, and *utility*.

Validity

Validity refers to the appropriateness, meaningfulness, and usefulness of a measure for a specific purpose. It is generally seen as the most important consideration in the evaluation of a measure.[2] Validity always needs to be evaluated with respect to the specific purpose a measure or instrument will be used for; measures are not inherently "valid" or "invalid" in and of themselves. For example, a hammer is not inherently valid. It is valid (useful) for driving nails into wood but invalid for washing dishes.

Rarely, if ever, can the validity of a measure be determined with a single study. Rather, support for the validity of a measure is usually established over time and with a series of studies. When evaluating the validity of a potential measure, the clinician or investigator should consider *content*, *construct*, and *criterion* validity.

Content Validity

Content validity concerns the degree to which the items of a measure represent a defined universe or domain of interest. For example, if a measure of a patient's *usual* pain or *average* pain over the last month is needed, then a single rating of current pain would not usually be considered to have content validity for assessing this construct because pain can vary so much from one moment to another. Similarly, if a measure of the impact of pain on a patient's life is needed, and a measure includes items that ask only about pain's impact on sleep and mobility (but not other important daily activities), the measure would not generally be viewed as adequately representing the domain of pain interference. Thus, a critical question that every test user should ask is whether or not a potential measure assesses or represents all of the key components of the domain of interest. If the measure does not meet this standard, it does not have content validity.

Construct Validity

Construct validity refers to how well the items of a measure perform as measures of the domain or construct of interest. Two measures can have similar content validity—that is, both may contain items that assess the critical components of some pain construct—but have different construct validity. For example, if two measures ask about pain interference with the same set of activities, yet respondents are asked to indicate the extent of interference with each activity using different response levels (e.g., yes/no response in one measure vs. 0-to-10 scales in the second), the latter measure may evidence more precision than the former. The more precise measure may represent the construct better and have more construct validity than the less precise one, despite the fact that the two measures have the same content validity.

Similarly, if the language used in the items of one measure is clear and succinct and the language used in another measure is confusing and complex, the former measure would likely contain less error than the latter measure, and the scores from the former measure would therefore be more likely to better represent the construct of interest. Thus, factors other than content validity will impact how the scores obtained from different measures behave, especially with respect to their associations with other important pain-related measures and the precision with which they represent the domain of interest. Evidence for the construct validity of a measure generally comes from studies that demonstrate strong associations between a measure's score and other measures of the same construct or related constructs and weak to moderate associations with measures of other constructs.

Criterion Validity

Criterion validity refers to a measure's associations with one or more key outcome criteria. Usually, the most important criterion of a pain measure is the responsivity of the measure to the effects of a pain treatment, or to changes in pain over time, because pain measures are most often used for detecting these differences and changes. Pain measures that are proposed to be used as outcome measures in clinical trials should therefore have evidence that they are able to detect treatment effects or show expected changes in pain over time.

But not all pain measures are designed to assess treatment efficacy. A number of measures of pain quality, for example, and as described later in this chapter, were designed to distinguish from among different types of pain (e.g., neuropathic vs. nociceptive). The validity of such measures should be determined by their ability to perform the task they were designed for or that they will be used for; their validity as measures of treatment efficacy need only be of concern when or if they are being considered for that specific purpose.

Reliability

Reliability refers to the extent to which the score from a test is free from errors of measurement. Many factors, other than a patient's experience of pain, could potentially influence his or her response to a pain measure or scale. Such factors could include the specific assessment setting (e.g., home vs. clinic), assessment burden (e.g., single assessment vs. a daily diary), the person administering the measure (e.g., research assistant, nurse, spouse, primary health care provider), other subjective experiences and feelings (e.g., being more or less fatigued or upset), motivational factors (e.g., desiring to appear stoic, wanting a prescription for a specific medication, ethnicity or culture, and previous learning experiences (e.g., the consequences of reporting of higher vs. lower pain levels), among many others. The variability in a pain score (the "variance") that is associated with these other factors, and that is not associated with the specific domain of interest, is considered error variance. Although no measure is 100% reliable, the best measures demonstrate relatively little influence of these other factors and potential sources of error.

Higher error variance means lower reliability. Unlike validity, which is considered with respect to the proposed use of the measure, and therefore varies depending on context, reliability is usually considered to exist within a measure. However, it is also possible for a measure to be more reliable in some settings or with some populations then in others. For example, as described in more detail later in this chapter, Visual Analogue Scales (VASs) of pain intensity (where the respondent is asked to make a mark on a line that represents the perceived magnitude of pain) have been found to be more difficult for patients with cognitive deficits than with patients who do not exhibit cognitive deficits. VAS measures, then, are now considered to be inadequately reliable in populations at risk for cognitive deficits, although evidence indicates that they may be adequately reliable in otherwise healthy adults. Thus, it is important that the reliability of any measure be established for the specific population with whom the measure will be used or at least in samples of individuals who are similar to the population with whom the measure will be used.

Utility

Finally, issues of reliability and validity need to be considered in light of a measures' utility, given that there is often a trade-off among these. For example, to maximize the content validity of a measure of pain interference, one would want the measure to assess the pain interference of all, or nearly all, of the possible (100s? 1,000s?) activities a person could engage in. Such a measure, although it would have clear content validity, would not be practical; no one would use it. Similarly, to maximize the content validity of a measure of a patient's usual pain over the course of the last month, one might ask the patient to report on his or her current pain every hour for 30 days and then average those responses into a single index of average pain. But few patients would be willing to perform this assessment task, and the costs of ensuring complete data for such a measure would be prohibitively expensive for most clinicians and many researchers. Deciding on which measure(s) to use for a particular application often comes down to selecting the measure that is both adequately valid and practical.

HOW MANY PAIN PROBLEMS SHOULD BE ASSESSED?

Patients often have more than one pain problem. For example, the majority of individuals with spinal cord injury have chronic pain, and the majority of these report pain at more than one site.[3] Clinicians and those researchers who do not limit their sample to the (few) patients with only one pain problem are faced with the difficult task of determining the number of pain problems to assess in any one patient or study participant. If only one "primary" pain problem is assessed at a clinic visit, but on the next visit, a different "primary" pain problem emerges as the most distressing, then it would be very difficult to track the effects of pain treatment from one clinic visit to the next.

Similarly, researchers who limit the number of pain problems assessed to just one primary problem run the risk of underestimating the magnitude of pain and its impact in their research findings. On the other hand, it is not practical to assess every pain problem in every patient seen in the clinic or in every participant of a research study. These considerations suggest that, in many situations, patients should have the opportunity to report on more than one pain problem but not necessarily be required or expected to report on every pain problem that they have at every assessment point.

But how many pain problems should be assessed? Two? Five? More? One approach to deal with this issue is to begin by assessing pain "in general"; for example, asking patients to consider all of their pain problems together when rating the overall average magnitude or intensity of their pain and the impact of pain on their lives. This is a practical solution, especially for assessing pain interference, because it may be very difficult for patients to identify the unique contribution of each different pain problem to interference with different activities. Moreover, assessing global pain intensity and interference allows the clinician or researcher to have a single primary measure of these two key pain domains, making analyses and tracking over time easier.

However, limiting assessment to only pain "in general" may oversimplify assessment and also interfere with determining the true effects of pain treatment. For example, if a pain treatment reduces the pain associated with one pain problem (e.g., headache) but not another (e.g., low back pain or a neuropathic pain condition), the specific effect of the treatment on headache pain might be less noticeable or even lost altogether if a measure of "general" pain intensity is used. So, in many situations, allowing for the assessment of more than one pain problem would be useful.

Unfortunately, however, there is not yet a clear consensus in the field concerning the best number of pain problems to assess. In the clinical setting, it probably makes sense to assess as many of the pain problems that are of concern to the patient. If the patient experiences eight unique pain problems and views each as a significant problem that contributes to dysfunction, then perhaps each of these should be assessed, at least at the initial evaluation, and then tracked at subsequent clinic visits as appropriate.

When determining how many pain problems to assess in a research study, the number of problems that should be assessed would vary as a function of the research question(s) being asked and the specific population being studied. One reasonable option would be to select the number of pain problems to assess that would capture the majority of patients in the population. For example, in persons with spinal cord injury, it has been recommended that investigators should consider assessing basic information (such as pain location and intensity) for up to three presenting pain problems.[4,5] In this instance, three was chosen as a way to balance the need for a thorough assessment against the need to minimize assessment burden, keeping in mind that the majority of persons with spinal cord injury and pain report three or fewer pain problems.[3] Although it is unlikely that a single upper limit of pain problems can be identified that should be assessed in every research project and with every patient population, each investigator would do well to consider this issue when developing assessment protocols.

WHICH PAIN DOMAIN(S) SHOULD BE ASSESSED?

Clinicians and researchers have long recognized that pain is a multidimensional experience that includes a number of measurable qualities such as intensity, affect (global bothersomeness of the pain experience as well as the impact of pain on emotional functioning), sensory quality, spatial quality (location), temporal quality, and impact on or interference with daily activities.[6,7] Although the focus of pain assessment in many clinical and research settings has often been, and continues to be, on pain intensity,[8] there is now a well-established recognition and interest in the assessment of pain's other domains.[9]

It is important that clinicians and investigators consider assessing more than just pain intensity for a number of important reasons. First, limiting assessment to only pain intensity leaves clinicians and researchers in the difficult position of having limited information about the presenting pain problem(s). In a clinical situation, changes in a pain domain not assessed might end up being critical for understanding the effects of a pain treatment (e.g., if pain qualities are not assessed, and a treatment reduces the "aching" and "deep" qualities of a pain problem, but perhaps not average pain intensity overall, or if a treatment produces a decrease in the impact of pain on sleep or other areas of functioning, even when there has been a minimal impact on pain intensity). For this reason, clinicians and researchers interested in assessing pain should at least *consider* all of the pain domains when determining which ones to assess and perhaps only avoid those domains they are certain will not be important to treatment (for clinicians) or understanding (for researchers).

One of the factors that might determine the selection of fewer domains and measures (e.g., perhaps choosing to assess just pain intensity and pain quality) over a more comprehensive assessment (e.g., including measures of pain site, pain interference, and the temporal qualities of pain as well as perhaps more general measures of psychological and physical functioning) is whether the pain problem being assessed is more acute or chronic. Acute pain, which may be defined as pain resulting from current or very recent damage to tissue, includes pain from medical procedures (e.g., injections, lumbar punctures, surgery) as well as both major and minor physical injuries. Because acute pain problems tend to resolve quickly in most individuals, their impact tends to be transitory. In this situation, and if the focus of treatment is on just one or two pain domains (e.g., pain intensity, mood), then it may be appropriate to assess only one or two pain domains.

Chronic pain, on the other hand, tends to be more complex than acute pain. It also tends to influence a large variety of quality of life domains (e.g., employment status, sleep quality, psychological status, social functioning). Patients' responses to chronic pain can also be quite variable, as can its impact. For chronic pain, then, in both clinical and research settings, and in order to ensure a thorough understanding of the pain problem, more pain domains, and perhaps more measures that assess these domains, are often required.

RECALL RATINGS VERSUS SUMMARY SCORES FROM MULTIPLE RATINGS USING DIARIES

Often, the clinician or researcher wishes to have a measure of a patient's usual pain during a specific period of time. A single measure or rating of current pain is not likely going to be an adequate index of usual pain, given that pain can vary from one moment to another. So what is the best way to assess usual pain? The three most common methods to assess pain intensity in clinical trials are (1) ask respondents to provide multiple ratings of current pain on pain diaries during the epoch of interest (e.g., four times per day for 7 days) and then compute the arithmetic mean of the ratings obtained, (2) assess pain once per day on several days, asking respondents to provide a *recall* rating of their average pain in the previous 24 hours and then computing the arithmetic mean of these 24-hour recalled average pain ratings to create a composite score representing usual pain, or (3) assess pain just once but ask respondents to provide recall ratings of their average pain over the entire epoch of interest. Each approach has strengths and weaknesses. In addition, pain assessment experts have not yet reached a clear consensus on which option should be recommended.

Support for the first approach, using multiple ratings of current pain from daily diary data (most often obtained electronically by asking patients to access a Web site to provide ratings or via automated telephone calls to patients) comes from studies that have demonstrated (1) a biasing impact of recent pain and worst pain (also known as "end" and "peak" effects) on recall ratings[10–12] and (2) access to computer-based and electronic diary technology which facilitates data collection.[13,14] When diaries are required, electronic, Web-based, or phone diaries are preferred over paper-and-pencil ones, given the common finding that respondents use paper-and-pencil diaries inappropriately.[15,16] Because of the strengths of diary approaches, there has been an increase over time in the use of this approach to collect data in clinical trials.[17–20]

However, there are also good reasons which make some investigators hesitant to embrace an approach that requires multiple daily diary entries to compute pain intensity scores, especially for use in clinical trials. First, as a practical issue, daily diary data can be expensive to collect. The financial cost of the hardware and software management associated with data collection via electronic diaries may be beyond the means of some investigators. Related to this, there is also a cost in terms of patient assessment burden. Some procedures ask respondents to provide only one assessment per day,[15,21–23] but it has been more common to ask patients to provide three[23] or even more (4 to 6 times[17,18,24]) ratings per day. This requires a significant effort on the part of patients, which may lower compliance with the task. To the extent that less costly recall ratings (that require just a few or even just one assessment) may be adequately valid, investigators may save substantial resources and significantly decrease the patient assessment burden if recall ratings are used instead of diary ratings.

A second problem with diary data requiring many ratings is that using this approach will result in missing data. The reported percentages of missing data points from electronic diary studies range from 6%[16] to 25%.[25] The reported rates of study participants who provide incomplete data (i.e., at least some missing data during the study period) can range from 17%[15] to 46%.[21] The primary reason reported for missing electronic data is that the patient did not hear the alarm or cue asking for the assessment.[26] Other reasons given include the alarm going off at an inconvenient time, the participant being too busy to respond, technical difficulties with a computer, emotional reasons, and pain being too severe at the time of assessment.[26] When data are missing, investigators need to either remove subjects from the analyses (which limits the generalizability of the findings and runs the risk of resulting in findings that overstate the impact of treatment) or use some approach to impute the missing data (i.e., estimate what the missing ratings might have been, had all subjects provided complete data). A variety of data imputation procedures can be used for clinical trial data, such as "last observation carried forward" which involves taking the most recent rating obtained and replacing all missing values with that rating.[17] A more conservative approach is to replace missing values with pretreatment ratings. However, if the treatment being examined is effective, this approach can underestimate the treatment effect size. Regardless of the approach used, however, data imputation adds error; imputed data are estimates only. In fact, the error added by the need to impute missing scores could potentially be greater than that associated with recall bias, so the use of diary data over recall ratings could potentially result in a more costly and effort-intensive assessment procedure that is ultimately also less accurate.

A third issue is that the use of electronic diaries limits the subjects who can participate in a study. For example, in one electronic diary study that approached 52 possible participants, 6 refused participation outright, 1 did not have the motor ability to hold the computer stylus, and 5 had visual problems that interfered with their ability to read the computer display.[21] By limiting the participants in clinical trials to those who are able and willing to use electronic diaries, their use in these trials limits the generalizability of the study findings.

Perhaps, the strongest argument against the strategy of computing average pain from multiple ratings of current pain over time is that research increasingly supports the conclusion that recall ratings of pain intensity are adequately valid for most research purposes. Although research does indicate that there can be both peak and end effects that bias recall ratings, these effects tend to be small.[10,12] Moreover, research indicates that the correlations between recalled average pain (in the previous 7 days) and actual average pain during that same period (as assessed by diaries) are strong (correlation coefficients range from 0.68 to 0.99[27-33])—well within a range that indicate they carry valid variance as measures of average or usual pain. In short, recall ratings reflect actual average pain and are therefore valid indicants of that pain. In addition, and perhaps most critically, the research finding that provides the most support for the validity of recalled pain ratings as outcome measures in pain clinical trials is indisputable: Recall ratings are responsive to the effects of pain treatments known to impact pain. Hundreds, if not thousands, of clinical trials have shown that effective treatments for chronic pain result in reductions in recall ratings of average pain. Thus, there is adequate evidence to support the use of recall ratings as valid measures of pain intensity in clinical and research settings.

That said, two important questions remain unresolved. First, if a researcher chooses to obtain multiple ratings of recalled pain over a relative small recall period (e.g., daily ratings of average pain in the past 24 hours) and compute the arithmetic mean of these ratings to create a composite score representing usual pain, how many of these recall ratings are needed to create an adequately valid measure of a patient's average pain? Second, might a single rating of recalled pain over a relatively larger recall period (e.g., a single rating of recalled average pain in the past week) be as adequately valid as a composite score made up of multiple 24-hour recall ratings?

Unfortunately, to date, relatively little research has been performed to address these two questions, despite the significant implications of the answers for designing and conducting pain clinical trials. Only three studies were identified which address the first question. In the first of these, investigators compared the reliability and sensitivity (i.e., ability to detect significant treatment effects) of pain intensity scores made up of one to nine 24-hour recall ratings of pain intensity using data from a clinical trial evaluating the efficacy of oxymorphone extended-release for the treatment of low back pain.[34] As would be expected based on psychometric theory, the reliability of the outcome measure reflecting average pain intensity increased as the number of ratings used to compute that measure increased from one to nine. However, and unexpectedly, this increase in reliability was not associated with improvements in the ability of the composite score to detect treatment effects. In fact, the first single 24-hour recall rating was about as sensitive for detecting treatments effects as the composite scores made up of 2 to 9 ratings.[34] In a commentary on this finding, other researchers noted that these results may have been due to the unusually strong test–retest reliability of the 24-hour recall ratings in the study sample.[35] To address this question further, these other investigators performed a similar set of analyses using data from a clinical trial evaluating the efficacy of a behavioral intervention for pain associated with osteoarthritis.[35] They found that the individual 24-hour recall ratings of average pain intensity evidenced a great deal of variability in their ability to detect treatment effects, with effect sizes ranging from medium ($d = .34$, $P = \text{NS}$) to large ($d = .88$, $P < .001$). Thus, had only a single 24-hour recall rating been used, the actual treatment effect might have been under- or overestimated and deemed either significant or nonsignificant, depending on the single rating used. On the other hand, the effect sizes for composite scores—which were .51, .55, and .66 for composites made up of two, three, and seven ratings—were more stable. Also, all of the composite scores were statistically significant ($Ps = .0005$ to $.007$).[35] The third study that addressed this question was a secondary analysis of a pilot study ($N = 10$ individuals with spinal cord injury and chronic pain) which examined the ability of pain intensity scores to detect changes in pain intensity from before to after 12 sessions of neurofeedback treatment.[36] In this study, the single-item ratings (of current pain and 24-hour recalled least, average, and worst pain) also evidenced a great deal of variability in effect sizes (ranging from 0.08 to 1.03). They also became more stable when two ratings were averaged (range, 0.16 to 0.38) and were not that much more stable than this when four ratings were averaged (range, 0.17 to 0.42). These investigators concluded that just two ratings (e.g., two ratings of 24-hour recalled average pain) may be adequate for assessing pain in outcome trials in clinical trials. However, they also noted that it is possible that in some populations—especially populations where pain can vary markedly from 1 day to the next, such as in individuals with chronic headache—more than two ratings might be needed to ensure adequate reliability and validity.

With respect to the second question, regarding the potential of a 7-day recall rating for providing valid ratings of average pain during the previous 7 days, although there are findings showing a tendency for people to overestimate recalled pain over the past week,[25,37] no study was identified which directly compared the validity of a single 7-day pain recall rating with composite scores made up of multiple diary ratings. Thus, this critical question remains unanswered at this point in time.

Given the current state of knowledge, what can or should researchers do with respect to assessing average or usual pain intensity? The answer probably depends on the resources available to the researcher. Certainly, there is evidence that a single 7-day recall rating of pain intensity can be sensitive to changes in pain with treatment (e.g., Hans et al.,[38] Branco et al.[39]). Therefore, 7-day recall ratings can be considered when resources are limited. However, given that psychometric theory predicts greater reliability (and therefore, ultimately, validity) when more measures are combined into composite scores, and until research is performed to compare single 7-day recall ratings with various combinations of 24-hour recall ratings, it would probably be wise for investigators to consider obtaining more than one rating (e.g., three or four 24-hour recall ratings obtained within a specified number of days) and combining these recall ratings into a single composite score.

Measuring Pain's Domains

MEASURING PAIN INTENSITY

The single pain domain assessed most often in clinical and research settings is pain intensity, or the magnitude of felt pain.[40] The three most commonly used scales to assess pain intensity are (1) the VAS, (2) the Numerical Rating Scale (NRS), and (3) the Verbal Rating Scale (VRS) (Fig. 20.1). The results from research across many different pain populations yield fairly consistent findings concerning the psychometric properties of these measures[6,9,41] and may be summarized as follows:

1. Each of these measures is adequately valid and reliable as a measure of pain intensity in most settings.
2. For both VAS and 0-to-10 NRSs, changes (decreases) between 30% and 35% appear to indicate a meaningful change in pain to patients across patient populations.
3. For 0-to-10 NRSs, the rating chosen has a specific meaning in terms of the impact of pain on function. In most samples, ratings in the 1 to 4 range have a minimal impact on function and can be viewed as representing "Mild" pain. Once ratings reach 5 or 6, patients report that pain has a greater impact on function; these ratings can be viewed as "Moderate" pain. Ratings ranging from 7 to 10 have the greatest impact on function and can be viewed as representing "Severe" pain.
4. When examined, single-item measures of pain intensity appear to have adequate test–retest stability (often, but not always, greater than 0.80) over short periods of time.

5. There are fairly consistent differences between available measures in terms of their failure rates. VASs usually show higher failure rates than NRSs and VRSs, and NRSs tend (when differences are found) to show slightly higher failure rates than VRSs, probably related to the increased complexity of matching a sensation to a line length versus a number or verbal descriptor.
6. In terms of preferences, patients in Western countries tend to prefer VRSs and NRSs over VASs. Patients from China prefer VRSs over NRS.[42] Whether this finding replicates to populations of patients in other non-Western countries remains to be seen.

Recommendations for Assessing Pain Intensity

Given the empirical support for the validity and reliability of VASs, NRSs, and VRSs as measures of pain intensity, any of these could reasonably be considered as options in most clinical settings or as outcome measures in clinical trials. Primarily because of (1) differences in failure rates between these measures in some populations (supporting NRSs and VRSs over VASs),[41] (2) the evidence that some people can differentiate between more than just four or five levels of pain between from "No pain" and "Extreme pain,"[43,44] and (3) the potential benefits of standardizing pain intensity assessment to allow for increased comparisons between studies, the field has recently moved toward recommending that clinicians and researchers consider first using the 0-to-10 NRS (see Fig. 20.1) over other pain intensity measures, at least in Western countries and cultures.[9]

Of course, there may be times when the 0-to-10 scale may not be appropriate. This scale requires the respondent to match his or her pain experience to a number, a task that may not be that easy for the very young, the extremely elderly, or individuals who are very ill. In these cases, and perhaps others, alternative pain intensity measures may be needed (see "Measuring Pain in Special Populations" section). Moreover, research suggests that 0-to-10 scales are not preferred by patients in China, as these individuals tend to describe their pain severity using verbal descriptions.[42] Additional research in non-Western countries regarding the utility and validity of the different pain intensity measures is needed to help determine which scale(s) might be most appropriate for cross-cultural research.

MEASURING PAIN AFFECT

The affective quality of pain includes both the general unpleasantness and/or bothersomeness of the pain sensation as well as the many varieties of affect (fear, anger, sadness, frustration, feelings of hopelessness) that pain can produce—especially as it becomes chronic. The most common measures of general, global pain unpleasantness are single-item rating scales (VASs, NRSs, and VRSs) that use endpoints that reflect extreme levels of unpleasantness (e.g., for a 0-to-10 NRS or 100 mm VAS, "not bad at all" for the 0 rating or 0-mm mark and "the most unpleasant feeling possible for me" for the 10 rating or 100-mm mark).[45] In general, these measures have proven useful in highly controlled laboratory studies that seek to differentiate intensity from affective components of pain.[45,46]

On the other hand, outside of the laboratory setting, patients appear to treat single-item VAS, NRS, and VRS measures of pain unpleasantness much like measures of pain intensity so that the two are often indistinguishable from one another in clinical populations.[47,48] Moreover, one might question the content validity of single-item measures of affect, given the complex and multidimensional nature of emotional experience.

Pain affect can also be assessed using multiple-item scales, the most common of which are the Affective subscale of the McGill Pain Questionnaire (MPQ)[49] and its associated short form, the Short-Form McGill Pain Questionnaire (SF-MPQ)[50] (Fig. 20.2). The original MPQ contains 78 descriptors that are

Visual Analogue Scale

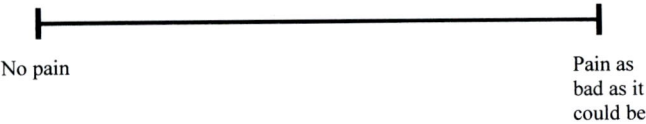

No pain   Pain as bad as it could be

Numerical Rating Scale

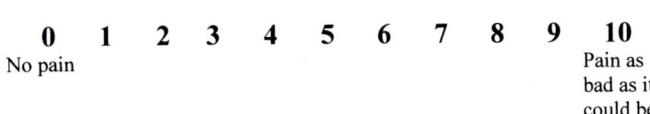

0   **1**   **2**   **3**   **4**   **5**   **6**   **7**   **8**   **9**   **10**
No pain   Pain as bad as it could be

Verbal (Categorical) Rating Scale

( ) No pain
( ) Mild pain
( ) Moderate pain
( ) Severe pain

FIGURE 20.1 The Visual Analogue Scale, Numerical Rating Scale, and Verbal Rating Scale.

Short-Form McGill Pain Questionnaire
(SF-MPQ)

A. PLEASE DESCRIBE YOUR PAIN DURING THE LAST WEEK. *(Check off one box per line.)*

	None	Mild	Moderate	Severe
1. Throbbing	0 ☐	1 ☐	2 ☐	3 ☐
2. Shooting	0 ☐	1 ☐	2 ☐	3 ☐
3. Stabbing	0 ☐	1 ☐	2 ☐	3 ☐
4. Sharp	0 ☐	1 ☐	2 ☐	3 ☐
5. Cramping	0 ☐	1 ☐	2 ☐	3 ☐
6. Gnawing	0 ☐	1 ☐	2 ☐	3 ☐
7. Hot-burning	0 ☐	1 ☐	2 ☐	3 ☐
8. Aching	0 ☐	1 ☐	2 ☐	3 ☐
9. Heavy (like a weight)	0 ☐	1 ☐	2 ☐	3 ☐
10. Tender	0 ☐	1 ☐	2 ☐	3 ☐
11. Splitting	0 ☐	1 ☐	2 ☐	3 ☐
12. Tiring-Exhausting	0 ☐	1 ☐	2 ☐	3 ☐
13. Sickening	0 ☐	1 ☐	2 ☐	3 ☐
14. Fear-causing	0 ☐	1 ☐	2 ☐	3 ☐
15. Punishing-Cruel	0 ☐	1 ☐	2 ☐	3 ☐

B. PLEASE RATE YOUR PAIN DURING THE LAST WEEK.

The following line represents pain of increasing intensity from "no pain" to "worst possible pain". Place a vertical mark (|) across the line in the position that best describes your pain **during the last week.**

No Pain   **Worst Possible Pain**

Score in mm
(Investigator's use only)

C. CURRENT PAIN INTENSITY

0 ☐ No pain
1 ☐ Mild
2 ☐ Discomforting
3 ☐ Distressing
4 ☐ Horrible
5 ☐ Excruciating

Questionnaire Developed by: Ronald Melzack

Copyright R. Melzack, 1984, 1987

FIGURE 20.2 The Short-Form McGill Pain Questionnaire. *(Reprinted with permission from Melzack R. The short-form McGill Pain Questionnaire. Pain 1987;30[2]:191–197.)*

categorized into 20 subgroups, 5 of which assess the impact of pain on affect. The five affective domains are tension (assessed using "tiring" and "exhausting" descriptors), autonomic (assessed using "sickening" and "suffocating" descriptors), fear (assessed using "fearful," "frightful," and "terrifying" descriptors), punishment (assessed using "punishing," "grueling," "cruel," "vicious," and "killing" descriptors), and affective miscellaneous (assessed using "wretched" and "blinding" descriptors).[49] Within each domain, when administered the MPQ, respondents are asked to circle or mark the single descriptor within each group that most accurately reflects or describes their pain. Descriptors are then ranked according to their position in the word set. The Pain Rating Index (PRI), which can be computed for each of the four primary MPQ subscales, including the Affective subscale, is the sum of the rank values of these descriptors.

The short form of the MPQ (SF-MPQ) contains 15 descriptors, four of which come from the MPQ Affective subscale ("tiring-exhausting," "sickening," "fearful," and "punishing-cruel").[50] However, unlike the MPQ, which requires respondents to select a single descriptor from each category list that best describes their pain, respondents to the SF-MPQ are allowed to rate the severity of each item individually on a 4-point Likert scale (0 = None to 3 = Severe). A severity or intensity score can then be calculated for the Affective subscale (as well as for Sensory and Total scale scores; see "Measuring Pain Quality" section). Research has shown that the correlations between the corresponding scales on the MPQ and SF-MPQ are high (rs range, 0.68 to 0.92).[50–52]

There is a substantial amount of data supporting the validity of the MPQ and SF-MPQ Affective subscales. First, like the other MPQ and SF-MPQ scales, the Affective subscale has been shown to be responsive to pain treatment.[53–56] Additional support for the validity of the MPQ Affective subscale as a measure of the affective component of pain, specifically, was reported by Ahles and colleagues,[57] who found that this scale was more strongly associated with measures of psychological distress than with measures of pain intensity. Also, Kremer and colleagues[58] reported that patients with cancer report a greater affective component of their pain on the MPQ Affective subscale than patients with low back pain, consistent with the hypothesis that cancer pain may be associated with higher levels of affect (e.g., be more worrisome and cause more fear) than low back pain.

Recommendations for Assessing Pain Affect

Although single-item measures of pain affect or pain bothersomeness have demonstrated validity in highly controlled laboratory studies, supporting their use in this setting, they have shown less discrimination (from single-item measures of pain intensity) in clinical populations. Thus, with clinical populations, when an index of pain affect is needed, clinicians and researchers should strongly consider administering the MPQ or SF-MPQ Affective items. The MPQ Affective subscale, having a longer history than the SF-MPQ, has more empirical support for its reliability and validity. However, given the strong associations between the MPQ and SF-MPQ scales, their high degree of item overlap, and the relative brevity and greater simplicity of the SF-MPQ for scoring, adequate evidence exists to support the use of the SF-MPQ as well.

MEASURING PAIN QUALITY

The experience of pain consists of much more than its magnitude or intensity and affective components. Pain is also often described using a number of different qualities, such as "burning," "aching," and "tender," among many others. Although historically, clinicians and researchers have focused on pain intensity as the single most important pain domain to assess,[40] there has been an upsurge of interest in the assessment of pain qualities. The two primary purposes of such measures are (1) to help diagnose the pain problem and (2) to more thoroughly describe the pain experience and determine the effects of pain treatments on that experience.

Using Pain Quality Measures as Diagnostic Aides

A growing body of research supports the conclusion that different pain qualities are associated with different causes, sources, or types of pain. In one study supporting this conclusion, Chang and colleagues[59] induced skin pain and muscle pain in human subjects through the use of intracutaneous and intramuscular injection of capsaicin into the left forearm, respectively. Although ratings of global pain intensity were very similar for both the skin and muscle pain, capsaicin injection into skin and muscle produced distinctly different pain qualities, as described

by the subjects. When capsaicin was injected into the skin, subjects described their pain as sharp, cutting, and burning; pain induced by intramuscular capsaicin injection was described as throbbing, pulsing, and tingling. The results of this study support the idea that different pain mechanisms or sources of pain produce different pain sensations and that these differences can be reliably assessed through the assessment of specific pain qualities. Also, it is generally thought that different nociceptors and fibers underlie different pain sensations, with the myelinated Aδ delta fibers responsible for localized "sharp," "stinging," and "shooting" pain, and the unmyelinated C fibers responsible for less localized dull pain sensations.[60–62]

The four most commonly used measures of pain quality that have been developed specifically to assist in the diagnosis or classification of pain include the (1) Leeds Assessment of Neuropathic Symptoms and Signs (LANSS),[63] (2) Self-Report Leeds Assessment of Neuropathic Symptoms and Signs (S-LANSS),[64] (3) Neuropathic Pain Diagnostic Questionnaire (DN4),[65] and (4) painDETECT.[66] Two of these measures (the LANSS and DN4) have both patient self-report and clinician examination items, and two (the S-LANSS and painDETECT) include only patient self-report items.

Leeds Assessment of Neuropathic Symptoms and Signs

The LANSS[63] was the first measure designed specifically to distinguish neuropathic from nociceptive pain. The self-report component of the measure consists of five items that ask respondents to indicate, yes or no, if their pain could be described as (1) "[consisting of] strange, unpleasant sensations . . . like pricking, tingling, pins and needles"; (2) "[making] . . . the skin in the painful area look different from normal . . . like mottled or looking more red . . ."; (3) "[making] . . . the affected skin abnormally sensitive to touch . . ."; (4) "[coming] . . . on suddenly and in bursts for no apparent reason . . . like electric shocks, jumping and bursting . . ."; and (5) "[feeling] . . . as if the skin temperature in the painful area has changed abnormally . . . like hot and burning. . . . " The sensory testing component asks a clinician to test for allodynia (by lightly stroking a nonpainful and the painful area with cotton wool) and to test for altered pinprick threshold (by comparing the patient response to a 23G needle mounted inside of a syringe barrel placed gently on the skin in a nonpainful area and then in the pain area). Each response is weighted, and the weights of all positive responses are summed to create a total score, with a score of less than 12 indicating an unlikelihood that neuropathic mechanisms are contributing to the patient's pain, and a score of 12 or greater (out of a total possible score of 24) indicating that neuropathic mechanisms are likely to be contributing to the patient's pain.

Self-report Leeds Assessment of Neuropathic Symptoms and Signs

One potential drawback to the LANSS, that could limit its use in some clinical and research settings, is that it requires a trained clinician to administer. To address this limitation, a self-report version of the LANSS (S-LANSS) has been developed.[64] The S-LANSS includes the same five pain quality items of the LANSS. However, the sensory items were modified to allow patients to self-administer them by gently rubbing the painful and a nonpainful area with their index finger for the allodynia item and gently pressing the painful and a nonpainful area with a fingertip to assess static allodynia.

Neuropathic Pain Diagnostic Questionnaire

The 7-item Neuropathic Pain Diagnostic Questionnaire (DN4)[65] was designed to discriminate between neuropathic and nonneuropathic pain. It is administered by a clinician and begins by asking patients if they do or do not experience their pain as having burning, painful cold, or electric shock qualities.

Patients are then asked to indicate if they do or do not experience tingling, pins and needles, numbness, or itching in the same area that they experience pain. Finally, and similar to the LANSS, the evaluating clinician determines if hypoesthesia (decreased sensitivity) to touch or to pinprick exists in the painful area, and whether lightly brushing the area elicits pain. The items are weighted to yield a score that can range from 0 to 10. A score of 4 or greater is used to classify the respondent as having possible neuropathic pain.

painDETECT

The painDETECT (PD)[66] consists of nine self-report items assessing seven sensory qualities (burning, tingling, sensitivity to light touch, electrical, sensitivity to temperature changes, numbness, sensitivity to light pressure), the temporal pattern of pain (e.g., persistent with slight fluctuations), and the spatial pattern of pain (i.e., if it does or does not radiate). The responses are scored and weighted to yield a score that can range from 0 to 38. Scores of 19 or more are used to classify the respondent as being likely to have a neuropathic component to their pain, scores of 12 or less as being indicative of being unlikely to have a neuropathic component to their pain, and scores from 13 to 18 are used to indicate an ambiguous result.

Strengths and Weaknesses of Pain Quality Measures as Diagnostic Aids

A growing body of research has examined the metrics of the LANSS, S-LANSS, DN4, and painDETECT, which has been summarized in review articles.[67,68] These reviews have noted that evidence supports the ability of each one of these measures to distinguish neuropathic from nonneuropathic pain in many patient groups, but that their accuracy (including sensitivity, or ability to identify someone as having neuropathic pain, and specificity, or ability to identify someone as not having neuropathic pain) can vary a great deal as a function of the clinical population being considered. Among the measures that include clinician's ratings, the DN4's overall accuracy has been shown to be the best on average (with sensitivity ranging 76% to 100% and specificity ranging from 45% to 92%) for many populations (see Canadian Agency for Drugs and Technologies in Health[67]). As indicated by these ranges, specificity tends to be lower than sensitivity with the DN4 and has been reported to be particularly low in individuals with leprosy (45%), patients with mixed chronic pain conditions (57%), and patients with a history of breast tumor resection (60%), even when sensitivity is good to excellent in these same conditions (100%, 87%, and 90%, respectively) (see Canadian Agency for Drugs and Technologies in Health[67]). In addition, the DN4 lacks accuracy for individuals with failed back syndrome (sensitivity: 62%; specificity: 44%; see Canadian Agency for Drugs and Technologies in Health[67]). On the other hand, the DN4 was reported to be superior to the LANSS and painDETECT for classifying patients with cancer and spinal cord injury as having neuropathic pain or not (see Canadian Agency for Drugs and Technologies in Health[67]). The tendency for the DN4 to be more accurate for classifying patients was also noted in a review by Mathieson and colleagues.[68]

The available research evidence does not provide strong support for the use of one of the self-report measures (i.e., S-LANSS or painDETECT) over the other, when a self-report measure is needed[67]; either could be selected and used. However, it is important to remember that all of these measures are screening questionnaires only and should not be used in an attempt to provide a definitive diagnosis of neuropathic pain.[69]

Pain Quality Scales as Descriptive and Outcome Measures

Pain quality measures may also be used to describe the pain associated with different pain conditions as well as to identify the effects of pain treatments on various qualities of the pain

experience. To the extent that different pain qualities are linked to different pain mechanisms, then understanding the effects of treatments on those qualities may be used to better understand the mechanisms of those treatments. In addition, given the evidence (reported later) that different pain treatments have different effects on various pain qualities, pain clinicians could potentially use pain quality assessment for helping to select from among different treatment options. For example, clinicians may offer patients reporting their pain as primarily "aching" those treatments shown to impact "aching" pain most effectively, while providing patients who describe their pain as "electrical" with treatments that have been shown to reduce "electrical" pain sensations.[70,71]

To date, six measures have been developed to assess pain quality and have been used as outcome measures in clinical trials. They include (1) the MPQ,[49] (2) the SF-MPQ,[50] (3) the Revised Short-Form McGill Pain Questionnaire (SF-MPQ-2),[72] (4) the Neuropathic Pain Symptom Inventory (NPSI),[73] (5) the Neuropathic Pain Scale (NPS),[74] and (6) the Pain Quality Assessment Scale (PQAS)[75] and its slight modification, the Revised Pain Quality Assessment Scale (PQAS-R).[76]

McGill Pain Questionnaire

The MPQ was introduced previously in the context of assessing pain affect. In addition to assessing the affective component of pain, the 78 MPQ descriptors can be scored to assess sensory pain (10 sensory categories, such as temporal, punctuate pressure, and thermal pain, assessed using 42 descriptors), evaluative pain (one category, assessed using 5 descriptors), and miscellaneous pain (four categories that do not clearly fall into sensory or affective components, assessed using 17 descriptors).[49]

As described previously, respondents are asked to select the single descriptor from each of the 20 categories (the number of descriptors listed per category varies from 2 to 6) that best describes his or her pain and the rank order of the descriptors in each category are summed to compute sensory, affective, evaluative, miscellaneous, and total scores.

Support for the usefulness of the MPQ comes from the fact that it has been used in hundreds of studies and has been translated into at least 20 languages.[77] Moreover, a three-factor (sensory, affective, and evaluative domains) structure of the MPQ has been confirmed in two studies,[78,79] although the high degree of association among these subscales suggests some limitations in discriminative validity of the different MPQ scales.[78] In support of the measure's validity, the MPQ scales have demonstrated validity as outcome measures given their responsivity to changes produced by pain treatments.[56,80,81]

A number of studies have examined the reliability of the MPQ. In populations of patients with cancer pain, studies have found that responses to the MPQ are generally consistent over the time span of several days.[82–84] In a study with patients with low back pain, Love and colleagues[83] found adequate test–retest stability for the MPQ scale scores (Total: $r = 0.83$; Sensory: $r = 0.76$; Affective: $r = 0.78$) over the course of several days.

Despite the many strengths of the MPQ, it also has some important limitations. First, although it has been reported to take only 5 minutes to complete by someone who is very familiar with the measure, the MPQ includes a large number of descriptors that are rarely used by individuals with pain; 78 descriptors suggests a very high degree of content validity, but so many descriptors may not be needed to adequately describe pain quality in many populations.

A second limitation of the MPQ concerns the way it is scored. Although it probably makes sense to combine multiple affective responses into a composite Affective subscale, there are limitations in combining a large number of different sensory descriptors into a composite Sensory subscale. Primary among these is the possibility that such a procedure does not allow investigators to detect the impact of treatments on specific unique pain quality domains or descriptors. Thus, a significant effect of a pain treatment on the MPQ Sensory subscale could have been due to its modest effects on many different pain qualities, or a large effect on just a few. One of the important reasons to assess pain quality in clinical trials is to determine the effects of treatment on specific pain qualities; scoring the MPQ descriptors into composite scales does not allow for this.

Also, because it is unlikely that pain treatments impact all pain qualities in the same way, the use of composite pain quality scores, based on many different items (recall that the MPQ Sensory subscale assesses 10 quality domains using 42 descriptors), runs the risk of reducing one's ability to detect significant effects. When using composite measures in clinical trials that include items that are not affected by treatment, or are affected only minimally, the effect size for the total scale is reduced. Indeed, when differences in responsivity to treatment are found, the MPQ scale scores tend to be less responsive to treatment effects than single-item pain intensity ratings.[85-87]

Short-Form McGill Pain Questionnaire

The SF-MPQ was developed in order to balance the need for pain quality data against the need to minimize assessment burden (see Fig. 20.2).[50] As previously mentioned in the "Measuring Pain Affect" section, the SF-MPQ consists of 15 descriptors, each of which can be rated on a 4-point severity scale from *none* to *severe*. Eleven of the descriptors assess sensory pain (throbbing, shooting, stabbing, sharp, cramping, gnawing, hot-burning, aching, heavy, tender, and splitting), and, as described previously, four items assess affective pain.

Evidence supporting the validity of both SF-MPQ scales includes data showing a strong association between the Sensory and Affective subscales scored from the SF-MPQ and the original MPQ Sensory and Affective subscales.[50-52] Also, a number of studies have demonstrated that the SF-MPQ is responsive to pain treatments, providing additional support for the validity of the SF-MPQ as an outcome measure.[88-90] Finally, because each of the SF-MPQ items is rated, SF-MPQ responses could theoretically be used in clinical trials to look at the specific effects of pain interventions on particular pain qualities, although this strength of the SF-MPQ has yet to be capitalized on.

Limitations of the SF-MPQ include the fact that some descriptors common to neuropathic pain (e.g., electrical, tingling) are not included in the measure, limiting its content validity for assessing neuropathic pain. An additional limitation of the SF-MPQ concerns scoring. As discussed previously with respect to the MPQ, if the sensory pain quality items are combined into composite scale scores, these scores may be less sensitive to treatment effects than are individual ratings of pain intensity or individual descriptor ratings. This makes the SF-MPQ scale scores, perhaps, less useful than global pain intensity ratings or even the individual SF-MPQ items as outcome measures.

Revised Short-Form McGill Pain Questionnaire

A revised version of the SF-MPQ (the SF-MPQ-2)[72] was developed with a goal of addressing the content validity problems of the SF-MPQ for assessing neuropathic pain and also to expand the severity response options for the items from 4 to 11 levels (i.e., to a 0 = "None" to 10 = "Worst possible" NRS) to increase measure responsiveness. The descriptor items that were added were "electric-shock pain," "cold-freezing pain," "piercing," "pain caused by light touch," "itching," "tingling or 'pins and needles,'" and "numbness." Exploratory and confirmative factor analyses indicated that the items can be scored into four reliable subscales assessing continuous pain, intermittent pain, predominantly neuropathic pain, and affective pain domains, all of which have been shown to be sensitive to the effects of a topical combination of amitriptyline and ketamine for painful diabetic peripheral neuropathy.[72] The reliability of

the SF-MPQ-2 scale scores has been replicated in a large sample of US veterans with chronic pain, although the very strong associations among the subscales in this sample, ranging from $r = 0.74$ to 0.91 and subsequent confirmatory factor analysis, supported the conclusion that although the SF-MPQ-2 items can be scored to assess four different domains, they also reliably assess a single global construct.[91] In addition, two studies have been published which have shown the SF-MPQ-2 subscales to be responsive to pain treatments.[92]

However, research suggests that even the SF-MPQ-2 may not be content valid in some samples of patients. Three different studies have sought to identify the most commonly used pain descriptors in patients with chronic pain.[93-95] Fourteen descriptors were found to be commonly used by patients with spinal cord injury and multiple sclerosis,[93] and 15 descriptors were found to be commonly used by patients with low back pain, fibromyalgia, and headache.[94] Both of these studies used participants with chronic pain from the United States. An additional study using individuals with chronic musculoskeletal pain problems from Nepal found that nine pain quality domains were used most often.[95] Based on the pain qualities spontaneously used by the participants in these studies, the SF-MPQ-2 might be considered to have mostly adequate content validity for assessing pain quality in patients with spinal cord injury or multiple sclerosis (assessing 13 of 14 descriptors identified).[93] However, it has somewhat less content validity for assessing pain quality in patients with musculoskeletal patients from Nepal (assessing 7 of 9 pain qualities)[95] and has marginal content validity for assessing pain in patients with low back pain, fibromyalgia, and headache (assessing only 12 of 15 descriptors).[94]

Neuropathic Pain Symptom Inventory

The NPSI[73] includes 12 items that were selected to assess four global domains of neuropathic pain (spontaneous ongoing pain, spontaneous paroxysmal pain, evoked pain, and paresthesias/dysesthesia). Respondents rate the severity or intensity of each descriptor item on 0-to-10 NRSs. Two additional items assess the temporal qualities of pain (number of hours of spontaneous pain in the past 24 hours, number of paroxysms during the last 24 hours).

As reported in the initial development study, short-term (3 hours) and longer term (1 month) test–retest stability of the NPSI items were shown to be very high (intraclass correlation coefficients range 0.78 to 0.98). Also, validity for the evoked pain items was evidenced through their significant associations (rs range 0.66 to 0.73) with related clinician scores of pain evoked by brushing, pressure, and cold stimuli. Changes in the NPSI total score have been found to be associated significantly with patient and provider ratings of global improvement over a 1-month period. The NPSI scales have also been shown to be sensitive to the effects of lidocaine medicated plaster and pregabalin[96] and ultramicronized palmitoylethanolamide[97] in samples of patients with postherpetic neuralgia. The evoked pain NPSI score, but not the total score, was shown to be sensitive to the effects of a thoracic sympathetic block in a sample of patients with complex regional pain syndrome, supporting the potential utility of the NPSI subscale scores for examining different pain qualities as distinct outcome domains.[98,99]

Crawford and colleagues[42] examined the cross-cultural content validity of the NPSI items by asking 132 individuals with neuropathic pain from six different countries to describe their pain on a written questionnaire and describe their pain in focus groups. Twenty descriptors were used by the participants to describe their pain in response to the questionnaires. As the NPSI only includes 12 items, then it clearly lacks content validity for assessing the descriptors used by these patients with neuropathic pain. This finding is consistent with the results of the studies, cited previously, which also evaluated the content validity of pain quality measures with respect to the descriptors patients actually use to describe their pain. Specifically, the NPSI only assesses 7 of 14 descriptors used by patients with chronic pain and spinal cord injury or multiple sclerosis,[93] and 5 of 15 descriptors used by patients with low back pain, fibromyalgia, or headache).[94]

In addition, questions remain regarding the number of underlying factors assessed by the NPSI items and how those items should be best scored. One factor analysis performed in 2008 in a large sample of patients with patients with neuropathic pain yielded five factors (assessing evoked, paraesthesia/dysesthesia, deep pain, paroxysmal pain and burning pain).[98] A factor analysis of the NPSI items in a different sample yielded three factors which the authors labeled pinpointed pain, deep pain, and provoked pain.[99] These differences in how the NPSI items should be scored into multi-item subscales have not yet been resolved.

One of the important strengths of pain quality measures, such as the NPSI, is that it is possible to evaluate the effects of treatment on specific pain quality items (also see how the NPS and PQAS/PQAS-R items have been used in this way later in this section). By analyzing the items individually, it is possible to identify the specific pain qualities that may be more or less responsive to different treatments. A study published by Cocito and colleagues[100] illustrated how the NPSI items could be used in this way. They found that an add-on treatment to patients with neuropathic pain (palmitoylethanolamide ultramicronized) was more effective for reducing paresthesia/dysesthesia pain qualities as measured by the NPSI than it was for reducing burning, pressing, paroxysmal, or evoked pain. Similarly, Freeman and colleagues found that combination therapy (duloxetine with pregabalin) was more effective than duloxetine alone for reducing pain described as squeezing and pressure and pain increased by brushing and pressure than other pain qualities.[99]

Neuropathic Pain Scale

The NPS, having been introduced in 1997, is the first measure developed to assess neuropathic pain qualities and probably for this reason has the most research supporting its reliability and validity for this purpose.[74] The NPS includes 10 items, 2 that assess global pain intensity and unpleasantness, and 8 that reflect specific pain domains (6 pain qualities and 2 spatial characteristics) likely to be reported by patients with neuropathic pain syndromes.

Respondents rate each item on a scale from 0 to 10, with 0 being "no ____" or "not ____" and 10 corresponding to "the most ____ sensation imaginable." An 11th item allows patients to report the temporal nature of their pain (constant with intermittent increases, intermittent, or constant with fluctuation). The NPS items were intended primarily to be used for assessing distinct pain qualities, which could then be used to create a profile of a person's pain quality experience. A large body of research supports the validity of the NPS for describing neuropathic pain conditions,[101-103] distinguishing between pain diagnoses,[64,101,104] predicting treatment outcome,[105] and other symptoms,[106] and detecting treatment effects.[76,107-114]

The NPS has also shown utility for identifying the pain qualities affected by different pain treatments.[104,107,110,114] For example, one study examined the effectiveness of the NPS for assessing changes in pain qualities in three groups (peripheral neuropathic pain, low back pain, and osteoarthritis) of patients treated with open label lidocaine patch 5%.[110] Although significant changes in almost all NPS pain qualities were found, significantly larger changes were seen for NPS items measuring sharp and deep pain than for items measuring cold, sensitive, or itching pain.[110] In another study, controlled-release oxycodone was found to be associated with decreases in sharp, dull, deep, and surface pain but had little impact on hot, cold, itchy, or sensitive pain in patients with painful diabetic neuropathy.[104]

In a sample of patients with mixed neuropathic pain conditions, intravenous lidocaine and phentolamine were found to have similar effects on 8 of 10 NPS items, although lidocaine had a greater effect on global pain unpleasantness and deep pain.[104] Finally, one study showed that tizanidine for neuropathic pain impacted the hot, cold, and sensitive NPS items (as well as global intensity and unpleasantness) after 2 weeks of treatment and then impacted sharp, dull, and deep pain NPS items after 8 weeks, indicating that the NPS may be used to show how treatments impact various pain qualities over time.[113]

Another strength of the NPS is its brevity, which makes it potentially useful in survey research and in settings where assessment burden may be a significant issue. Also, the NPS has been translated into 36 languages and so is useful for cross-cultural research comparing neuropathic pain conditions and treatments across cultures.

Although the NPS was originally designed to be scored to create a "profile" of sensation severity across different pain qualities, it is possible to combine the items into composite scores. Galer and colleagues,[108] for example, created four different NPS composite scores when examining the effects of a lidocaine patch 5% in a sample of patients with postherpetic neuralgia: an average of all 10 items (NPS10), an average of the 8 specific descriptors excluding the global ratings of pain intensity and unpleasantness (NPS8), an average of the 8 items that do not reflect allodynia (i.e., excluding the "sensitive" and "surface" items; NPS NA), and an average of 4 items thought to reflect nonperipheral pain mechanisms ("dull," "deep," "sharp," and "burning" items; NPS4). However, concerns about the use of composite scores from pain quality measures, raised earlier with respect to the MPQ and the NPSI, are also relevant here; use and interpretation of composite pain quality scores, regardless of the measure used for item selection, needs to proceed with caution.

The primary limitation of the NPS is associated with its brevity. Because it has only 10 items, the NPS has limited content validity for assessing pain across different diagnostic conditions. For example, the NPS items assess only 5 of 14 of the most commonly used pain descriptors in samples of patients with spinal cord injury and multiple sclerosis[93] and only 6 of the 15 most commonly used pain descriptors in samples of patients with low back pain, fibromyalgia, and headache.[94] Thus, although there is a great deal of research supporting the reliability and validity of the NPS for assessing treatment effects in patients with neuropathic pain, there is limited content validity for assessing pain quality in populations of individuals with nonneuropathic pain conditions.

Pain Quality Assessment Scale

The PQAS[75] was developed to make available a measure that had the strengths of the NPS but that would also be content valid for assessing both neuropathic and nonneuropathic pain. The PQAS used the original 10 NPS items as a starting point and then added 10 additional items to create a measure capable of assessing the most common pain qualities seen across a variety of chronic pain conditions.[75] Like the NPS, the PQAS also includes an item to differentiate between three primary temporal patterns of pain: intermittent (i.e., variable pain with some pain free periods), variable (variable pain without pain-free periods), and stable (i.e., constant pain with little variation). The PQAS instructions and items have also been cognitively tested to ensure that they were maximally clear and understandable to patients. This resulted in minor word modifications to the instructions and some of the items (but no changes in the specific pain quality domains assessed), creating the PQAS-R (Fig. 20.3).

All of the extensive data that support the validity of the NPS also support both versions of the PQAS because the NPS items are included in the PQAS. Research also provides support for the validity of the new items. For example, all of the new

PAIN QUALITY ASSESSMENT SCALE (PQAS)

<u>Instructions</u>: There are different aspects and types of pain that patients experience and that we are interested in measuring. Pain can feel sharp, hot, cold, dull, and achy. Some pains may feel like they are very superficial (at skin-level), or they may feel like they are from deep inside your body. Pain can also be described as unpleasant.

The Pain Quality Assessment Scale helps us measure these and other different aspects of your pain. For one patient, a pain might feel extremely hot and burning, but not at all dull, while another patient may not experience any burning pain, but feel like their pain is very dull and achy. Therefore, we expect you to rate very high on some of the scales below and very low on others.

Please use the 19 rating scales below to rate how much of each different pain quality and type you may or may not have felt ***OVER THE PAST WEEK, ON AVERAGE.***

Place an "X" through the number that best describes your pain. For example:

| 0 | 1 | 2 | ✗ | 4 | 5 | 6 | 7 | 8 | 9 | 10 |

---

1. Please use the scale below to tell us how **intense** your pain has been over the past week, on average.

No pain | 0 | 1 | 2 | 3 | 4 | 5 | 6 | 7 | 8 | 9 | 10 | The most **intense** pain sensation imaginable

---

2. Please use the scale below to tell us how **sharp** your pain has felt over the past week. Words used to describe sharp feelings include "<u>like a knife</u>," "<u>like a spike</u>," or "<u>piercing</u>."

Not sharp | 0 | 1 | 2 | 3 | 4 | 5 | 6 | 7 | 8 | 9 | 10 | The most **sharp** sensation imaginable ("like a knife")

---

3. Please use the scale below to tell us how **hot** your pain has felt over the past week. Words used to describe very hot pain include "<u>burning</u>" and "<u>on fire</u>."

Not hot | 0 | 1 | 2 | 3 | 4 | 5 | 6 | 7 | 8 | 9 | 10 | The most **hot** sensation imaginable ("burning")

---

4. Please use the scale below to tell us how **dull** your pain has felt over the past week.

Not dull | 0 | 1 | 2 | 3 | 4 | 5 | 6 | 7 | 8 | 9 | 10 | The most **dull** sensation imaginable

---

5. Please use the scale below to tell us how **cold** your pain has felt over the past week. Words used to describe very cold pain include "<u>like ice</u>" and "<u>freezing</u>."

Not cold | 0 | 1 | 2 | 3 | 4 | 5 | 6 | 7 | 8 | 9 | 10 | The most **cold** sensation imaginable ("freezing")

---

6. Please use the scale below to tell us how **sensitive** your skin has been to light touch or clothing rubbing against it over the past week. Words used to describe sensitive skin include "<u>like sunburned skin</u>" and "<u>raw skin</u>."

Not sensitive | 0 | 1 | 2 | 3 | 4 | 5 | 6 | 7 | 8 | 9 | 10 | The most **sensitive** sensation imaginable ("raw skin")

FIGURE 20.3 The Revised Pain Quality Assessment Scale. *(Copyright © Jensen, Galer, and Gammaitoni, 2010. Reproduced with permission. Clinicians and researchers interested in obtaining permission to use the PQAS-R can contact the MAPI Trust [https://eprovide.mapi-trust.org], and search the ePROVIDE database for "PQAS-R.")*

7. Please use the scale below to tell us how **tender** your pain is when something has pressed against it over the past week. Another word used to describe tender pain is "like a bruise."

Not tender | 0 | 1 | 2 | 3 | 4 | 5 | 6 | 7 | 8 | 9 | 10 | The most **tender** sensation imaginable ("like a bruise")

8. Please use the scale below to tell us how **itchy** your pain has felt over the past week. Words used to describe itchy pain include "like poison ivy" and "like a mosquito bite."

Not itchy | 0 | 1 | 2 | 3 | 4 | 5 | 6 | 7 | 8 | 9 | 10 | The most **itchy** sensation imaginable ("like poison ivy")

9. Please use the scale below to tell us how much your pain has felt like it has been **shooting** over the past week. Another word used to describe shooting pain is "zapping."

Not shooting | 0 | 1 | 2 | 3 | 4 | 5 | 6 | 7 | 8 | 9 | 10 | The most **shooting** sensation imaginable ("zapping")

10. Please use the scale below to tell us how **numb** your pain has felt over the past week. A phrase that can be used to describe numb pain is "like it is asleep."

Not numb | 0 | 1 | 2 | 3 | 4 | 5 | 6 | 7 | 8 | 9 | 10 | The most **numb** sensation imaginable ("asleep")

11. Please use the scale below to tell us how much your pain sensations have felt **electrical** over the past week. Words used to describe electrical pain include "shocks," "lightning," and "sparking."

Not electrical | 0 | 1 | 2 | 3 | 4 | 5 | 6 | 7 | 8 | 9 | 10 | The most **electrical** sensation imaginable ("shocks")

12. Please use the scale below to tell us how **tingling** your pain has felt over the past week. Words used to describe tingling pain include "like pins and needles" and "prickling."

Not tingling | 0 | 1 | 2 | 3 | 4 | 5 | 6 | 7 | 8 | 9 | 10 | The most **tingling** sensation imaginable ("pins and needles")

13. Please use the scale below to tell us how **cramping** your pain has felt over the past week. Words used to describe cramping pain include "squeezing" and "tight."

Not cramping | 0 | 1 | 2 | 3 | 4 | 5 | 6 | 7 | 8 | 9 | 10 | The most **cramping** sensation imaginable ("squeezing")

14. Please use the scale below to tell us how **radiating** your pain has felt over the past week. Another word used to describe radiating pain is "spreading."

Not radiating | 0 | 1 | 2 | 3 | 4 | 5 | 6 | 7 | 8 | 9 | 10 | The most **radiating** sensation imaginable ("spreading")

15. Please use the scale below to tell us how **throbbing** your pain has felt over the past week. Another word used to describe throbbing pain is "pounding."

Not throbbing | 0 | 1 | 2 | 3 | 4 | 5 | 6 | 7 | 8 | 9 | 10 | The most **throbbing** sensation imaginable ("pounding")

FIGURE 20.3 *(continued)*

16. Please use the scale below to tell us how **aching** your pain has felt over the past week. Another word used to describe aching pain is "like a toothache."

Not aching | 0 | 1 | 2 | 3 | 4 | 5 | 6 | 7 | 8 | 9 | 10 | The most **aching** sensation imaginable ("like a toothache")

17. Please use the scale below to tell us how **heavy** your pain has felt over the past week. Other words used to describe heavy pain are "pressure" and "weighted down."

Not heavy | 0 | 1 | 2 | 3 | 4 | 5 | 6 | 7 | 8 | 9 | 10 | The most **heavy** sensation imaginable ("weighted down")

18. Now that you have told us the different types of pain sensations you have felt, we want you to tell us overall how **unpleasant** your pain has been to you over the past week. Words used to describe very unpleasant pain include "annoying," "bothersome," "miserable," and "intolerable." Remember, pain can have a low intensity but still feel extremely unpleasant, and some kinds of pain can have a high intensity but be very tolerable. With this scale, please tell us how **unpleasant** your pain feels.

Not unpleasant | 0 | 1 | 2 | 3 | 4 | 5 | 6 | 7 | 8 | 9 | 10 | The most **unpleasant** sensation imaginable ("intolerable")

19. Finally, we want you to give us an estimate of the severity of your deep versus surface pain over the past week. We want you to rate each location of pain separately. We realize that it can be difficult to make these estimates, and most likely it will be a "best guess," but please give us your best estimate.

HOW INTENSE IS YOUR *DEEP* PAIN?

No **deep** pain | 0 | 1 | 2 | 3 | 4 | 5 | 6 | 7 | 8 | 9 | 10 | The most **intense deep** pain sensation imaginable

HOW INTENSE IS YOUR *SURFACE* PAIN?

No **surface** pain | 0 | 1 | 2 | 3 | 4 | 5 | 6 | 7 | 8 | 9 | 10 | The most **intense surface** pain sensation imaginable

20. Pain can also have different time qualities. For some people, the pain comes and goes and so they have some moments that are completely without pain; in other words the pain "comes and goes". This is called **intermittent** pain. Others are never pain free, but their pain types and pain severity can vary from one moment to the next. This is called **variable** pain. For these people, the increases can be severe, so that they feel they have moments of very intense pain ("breakthrough" pain), but at other times they can feel lower levels of pain ("background" pain). Still, they are never pain free. Other people have pain that really does not change that much from one moment to another. This is called **stable** pain. Which of these best describes the time pattern of your pain (please select only one):

( ) I have **intermittent** pain (I feel pain sometimes but I am pain-free at other times).
( ) I have **variable** pain ("background"pain all the time, but also moments of more
      pain, or even severe "breakthrough pain or varying types of pain).
( ) I have **stable** pain (constant pain that does not change very much from one moment to
      another, and no pain-free periods).

FIGURE 20.3 *(continued)*

items have been found to be responsive to the effects of both lidocaine patch 5% and a corticosteroid injection in a sample of patients with carpal tunnel syndrome.[75] A factor analysis of the PQAS items yielded three factors labeled paroxysmal sensations (shooting, sharp, electric, hot, radiating), superficial pain (itchy, cold, numb, sensitive, and tingling), and deep pain (aching, heavy, dull, cramping, and throbbing).[115] A large and growing body of research supports the sensitivity of the PQAS and PQAS-R scales and items for detecting treatment effects.[70,71,116–118]

The PQAS and PQAS-R items have also be shown to be useful for identify the "response profiles" of different pain treatments.[70,71,116,118] For example, oxymorphone was shown to have the larger effect on deep, aching, and sharp qualities than other pain qualities.[70] In addition, the PQAS/PQAS-R items and scales are able to predict who responds to pain treatments.[71,119] For example, in a sample of 50 patients with neuropathic pain, the PQAS-R items were able predict who did and did response to pregabalin with 85% sensitivity and 76% specificity.[119]

The PQAS and PQAS-R have been shown to be the most content valid of all of the available pain qualities measures. All of the most common pain qualities spontaneously used by individuals with spinal cord injury and multiple sclerosis and all of the most common pain qualities spontaneously used by individuals with low back pain, fibromyalgia, and headache are assessed by the PQAS.[93,94] Also, the PQAS assess eight of the nine most common pain qualities spontaneously used by individuals with musculoskeletal pain in patients from Nepal.[95]

Strengths and Weakness of Descriptive and Outcome Measures of Pain Quality

The original MPQ is the most established measure of pain quality and has been used in more research studies than any other pain quality measure combined. However, the length of the original MPQ—which includes a large number of items that are rarely endorsed—and its complicated scoring procedure has led researchers to develop new measures, including a short-form version of the MPQ (SF-MPQ). However, the SF-MPQ was subsequent found to have very limited content validity. Although the SF-MPQ-2 was developed to address the content validity problems of the SF-MPQ, recent research indicates that it too does not adequately assess some of the most common pain qualities reported by individuals with chronic pain.

The NPS was the first measure developed to assess neuropathic pain qualities specifically. It has a great deal of research supporting its validity for this purpose. It is particularly useful for assessing the effects of pain treatment on a variety of specific neuropathic pain quality domains. However, the NPS is not content validity for assessing pain quality in populations of patients with nonneuropathic pain.

The NPSI is the most recent addition to field. However, the NPSI has significant limitations with respect to its content validity (i.e., it does not measure many pain quality domains common to individuals with neuropathic and nonneuropathic pain conditions) and questions remain regarding how the items should be scored into composite scale scores.

The PQAS was developed to improve on the strengths and empirical foundation of the NPS by adding items to improve content validity for assessing pain in a variety of patient populations. The available research indicates that the PQAS—and by extension the PQAS-R—was successful in achieving this goal, having demonstrated 100% content validity for assessing pain in populations of patients with chronic pain in the United States[93,94] and demonstrating adequate content validity for assessing pain quality in a sample of patients with chronic pain from Nepal.[95]

Given the similarity between the existing measures (i.e., all of the viable measures, including those that were revised from earlier measures, emulate the format of the original NPS, by asking respondents to rate the severity of different pain qualities on 0-to-10 rating scales), the primary difference among them is their content validity. Based on this criterion, it would appear that the PQAS and PQAS-R would be the most valid for assessing pain quality in a variety of pain populations.

MEASURING PAIN'S SPATIAL CHARACTERISTICS

Pain can occur both at different body locations (e.g., head, leg) or at different depths (e.g., "surface" or "deep" pain). The two most common strategies used for assessing the body location of pain are the pain drawing and the pain site checklist. A pain drawing consists of an outline of a human form, and respondents are simply asked to mark or shade in the areas on the drawing which correspond to pain they are currently experiencing. Pain drawings are included in a number of standard pain questionnaires, such as the MPQ,[49] the LANSS,[63] and the original (non-short form) Brief Pain Inventory (BPI) scale.[120] One published pain drawing allows the assessor to use a template to score the patient's response, both for the specific area that has been shaded as well as for "pain extent" (which reflects the total number of areas that have been shaded).[121] Pain drawings can also be administered electronically, with respondents indicating the area(s) of pain on a computer or electronic tablet screen, and the specific body areas shaded (e.g., Barbero et al.[122]).

A site checklist is a simple list of possible sites for pain, and the respondent is asked to indicate which site(s) are currently painful.[123] Like pain drawings, site checklists can be scored for both the specific site(s) chosen as well as for "pain extent" (total number of sites chosen). The presence and severity of "deep" and "surface" pain can be determined by asking respondents to rate each (see the PQAS-R reflecting these in Fig. 20.3).

Research shows that pain drawings are reliable, regardless of the methods used to score them (e.g., Barbero et al.,[122] Ohnmeiss,[124] MacDowall et al.,[125] Hayashi et al.[126]). Research also shows that scores from pain drawings can be used as outcome measures in clinical trials, given evidence that they are sensitive to effective pain treatment (e.g., Voorhies et al.,[127] Marcus et al.[128]).

Scores derived from measures of pain site (i.e., "pain extent" as represented by the number or percent of body area involved) also predict, in some patients, important domains of patient function, including disability, pain interference, medication use, return to work, and psychological functioning. However, these associations are not consistent or strong enough to warrant the use of pain's spatial characteristic as proxy measures of psychopathology or disability.[129,130]

In addition, pain drawings, pain site checklists, and measures of the relative depth of pain are well suited for descriptive purposes. For example, research in patients with spinal cord injury has used pain drawings and pain site to describe the frequency of pain experienced at different body sites, as well as the relationship between pain location or number of pain sites and other related variables.[123,131]

Recommendations for Assessing Pain Site

Pain drawings, pain site checklists, and severity ratings of pain's perceived depth have all been used successfully to help patients describe their pain experience. These measures have also demonstrated responsivity as outcome measures in clinical trials. Decisions about which to use in any one setting or with any one population will largely depend on the preference of the assessor and practical issues concerning how the data will be used. Clinicians often prefer pain drawings, given that they provide a global overview of how patients experience the location(s) of their pain. However, when used in research, pain drawings require an additional step (usually with the aid of a template or software) to objectively determine the specific site(s) selected and the amount of body area with pain (i.e., pain extent). Pain site checklists may be more practical for the researcher, given that coding for the specific sites (e.g., legs, low back, head) is completed by the respondent once the checklist has been administered and completed.

MEASURING PAIN'S TEMPORAL CHARACTERISTICS

The temporal aspects of pain, such as its variability, frequency, and duration as well as its pattern across time (over minutes, hours, days, or months) can be assessed by asking patients to rate their pain on multiple occasions over time using pain diaries. The specific temporal domains of interest can then be operationalized by computing scores from the diary ratings. Based on diary data, *pain variability* can be operationalized as the standard deviation of pain intensity ratings during a specific epoch, *frequency* of "breakthrough" pain as the number of times pain reached and exceeded a specific cutoff (e.g., 7 or more on a 0-to-10 scale for severe breakthrough pain, or 5 or more for moderate to severe breakthrough pain),[102] and *pain duration* as the number of hours that pain was rated as being above a specific cutoff; for example, 5 or more on a 0-to-10 scale for duration of "moderate to severe" pain.[132]

Diary data can also be used to identify *temporal patterns*. Jamison and Brown,[133] for example, identified six different temporal pain pattern types (e.g., steady increase over the course of a day, steady decrease, curvilinear pattern, no consistent pattern) based on diary data. They found that the group of patients that showed no clear consistent pattern from one day to the next also reported the greatest emotional distress.[133] van Grootel and colleagues[134] identified two primary patterns of pain intensity from diary data in a sample of patients with temporomandibular disorders: (1) those reporting higher levels of pain later in the day and (2) those reporting higher levels of pain in the morning; with the former group reporting higher overall levels of pain intensity, more difficulty falling asleep at bedtime, more widespread pain, and greater endorsement about the role of a physician in managing their pain problem. These findings suggest the possibility that the time pattern of pain experience may play a role in how patients think about or manage their pain.

Pain diaries may be particularly important when assessing patients with pain problems that show marked variations in pain over time, such as patients with headaches.[135] The many strengths of diaries for this purpose include their utility in (1) identifying different headache diagnoses when they occur in the same patient, (2) identifying possible factors that trigger a patient's headaches, and (3) evaluating the efficacy of treatments used by patients over time.[135] Their ability to help identify triggers for pain flare-ups, in particular, makes diaries particularly useful clinically for enabling secondary prevention of the disabling effects of these flares (e.g., being unable to function, leaving work early, sleep interference) with appropriate behavioral, physical (e.g., ice and stretch), or pharmacologic (e.g., NSAIDs) interventions.

However, such diaries are not without limitations. They involve significant assessment burden and can be associated with low compliance rates and inaccurate reporting. They also carry the risk of sensitizing the patient to health problems and—at least temporarily—increasing the patient's focus on pain and its negative effects.[135]

Another way to assess pain pattern is to describe different temporal patterns to patients and allow them to select the description that best describes their pain. For example, an item from the PQAS-R (see Fig. 20.3) asks patients to indicate which of the following best describes their pain: (1) I have intermittent pain (I feel pain sometimes but I am pain-free at other times), (2) I have variable pain ("background" pain all the time, but also moments of more pain, or even severe "breakthrough" pain or varying types of pain), and (3) I have stable pain (constant pain that does not change very much from one moment to another, and no pain-free periods). One study found that these temporal characteristics differed as a function of neuropathic versus nonneuropathic pain, with patients rated by physicians as having "possible" neuropathic pain being more likely to endorse having variable pain then patients rating as being "unlikely" to have neuropathic pain.[136] The painDETECT also has a temporal item, which asks the respondent to select one from a selection of illustrations that depict four temporal patterns (i.e., persistent pain with slight fluctuations, persistent pain with pain attacks, pain attacks without pain in between, or pain attacks with pain between).[66]

Recommendations for Assessing Pain's Temporal Characteristics

Either diary-based measures or categorical scales may be used to assess pain's temporal characteristics. Categorical scales require less investigator and patient effort than diary-based measures, but diary-based measures allow for greater flexibility in coding different temporal patterns than categorical scales. Diary-based measures may be particularly useful for helping clinicians and researchers understand pain problems that are highly variable over time, such as headaches.

MEASURING PAIN INTERFERENCE

Pain interference refers to the extent to which pain interferes with day-to-day functioning. The two most commonly used measures of pain interference are the BPI Pain Interference scale (see Fig. 41.3)[120] and the Patient-Reported Outcomes Measurement Information System (PROMIS) Pain Interference item bank.[137]

Brief Pain Inventory Pain Interference Scale

The BPI Pain Interference scale includes seven items that assess the extent to which pain has interfered with: general activity, mood, walking ability, normal work (including both work outside the home and housework), relations with other people, sleep, and enjoyment of life. Respondents are asked to rate the degree of pain interference with each activity on 0 (does not interfere) to 10 (completely interferes) numerical scales. The responses to the seven items are then averaged to form the Pain Interference scale score.

Factor analyses of responses show that the seven interference items often but not always (see discussion of alternative scoring methods of the BPI Pain Interference scale items in the following paragraph)—load together onto a single factor[120,138-146] and that the scale has excellent internal consistency (with αs ranging from .78 to .91) when scored in this way.[132,139,140,143-145]

One early study used multidimensional scaling to determine the factors underlying the BPI Pain Interference scale items in a large sample of 1,843 persons with metastatic cancer.[147] These analyses yielded two underlying interference dimensions: interference with activity- (walking, work, general activity, sleep) and affectivity-related interference (relations, mood, enjoyment of life), suggesting the possibility of alternate scoring and use of the BPI Pain Interference scale. Support for scoring the BPI Pain Interference scale items into two distinct scales comes from a large-scale Rasch analysis study, using data from 1,000 patients from an ambulatory patient database.[148] These investigators found support for a two-factor model in which three of the activity interference items (walking, work, general activity) and the three affective items (relations, mood, enjoyment of life) were scored as distinct subscales. They recommended that the sleep item be removed or interpreted separately. However, findings from another study using four different samples of individuals with pain provided more support with a single-factor model for BPI Pain Interference scale items,[149] consistent with the many factor analyses, cited previously, that are also consistent with this model.

The BPI Pain Interference scale has been increasingly used as an outcome measure in clinical trials, and evidence demonstrating changes in the BPI Pain Interference scale score supports its validity for this purpose.[109,150–157]

The BPI Pain Interference scale has also been slightly modified (with permission from the copyright holder) to increase its utility for assessing pain interference in persons with physical disabilities.[158–160] Perhaps the most important modification was to change the wording of the interference with walking item to ask respondents to rate the degree of interference with "mobility (ability to get around)." This change makes it possible for individuals who have mobility restrictions unrelated to pain (i.e., who are wheelchair users) to rate the impact of pain on their mobility. Because many of these individuals would be unable to walk even if they had no pain, the original wording of this item would not be appropriate.

The other modification made was to increase the content validity of the scale by including items asking about pain interference with self-care, recreational activities, and social activities[159] as well as items asking about interference with communication and learning new information or skills.[158,160] These five activity domains are important to many individuals with disabilities and also reflect functioning domains defined as relevant and unique by the WHO's *International Classification of Functioning, Disability, and Health*.[161] Given the psychometric strength of the original BPI Pain Interference scale items, it is perhaps not surprising that the 10- and 12-item modified scales also have strong psychometric properties. First, the internal consistency of the modified scales are uniformly high (range, 0.89 to 0.96) in three samples of persons with disabilities, including individuals with cerebral palsy,[159] spinal cord injury,[160] and multiple sclerosis.[158] Second, like the original BPI Pain Interference scale, the modified and expanded scales show strong associations with measures of pain intensity (correlation coefficients range, 0.61 to 0.66), consistent with what would be expected if they measured the extent to which pain interfered with functioning.[159,160] Finally, factor analyses of the modified and expanded items show that new items all load strongly on a pain interference factor that is not only related to but also distinct from a pain intensity factor.[158]

However, although the modification of the original walking BPI item makes it possible for individuals who have difficulties walking for reasons other than pain to respond to that item, and the addition of items increases the content validity of the BPI, it is not clear that these modifications substantially improve other psychometric properties of the scale. For example, the internal consistency of a scale made up of 10 items (αs = 0.95 to 0.96)[158,160] is not that much larger than the original 7-item scale (α = 0.92 to 0.93)[158,160] in these same samples, suggesting that if scale brevity is important, the original 7-item BPI may provide as good a measure of pain impact as the expanded 10- or 12-item version. Indeed, if a single score representing the domain of pain interference is needed, more than three pain interference items may not be needed to detect significant changes with treatment.[155]

Patient-Reported Outcomes Measurement Information System Pain Interference Item Bank and Short Forms

A recent measure of pain interference introduced to the field is the 41 items from the PROMIS Pain Interference item bank.[137] Like all of the PROMIS measures (http://www.healthmeasures.net/explore-measurement-systems/promis), the PROMIS Pain Interference items were developed and calibrated using item response theory (IRT). The focus of an IRT-based item banking approach is on the final score rather than on the items that make up that score, which can be computed as a t-score from any number or any combination of items from the item bank. This score has mean of 50 and standard deviation of 10 in the normative sample. As a result, scores created from different items from the item bank can be directly and meaningfully compared.

PROMIS Pain Interference item scores have demonstrated validity through their associations with measures of other pain-related constructs (e.g., physical function, depression, anxiety, pain intensity, other measures of pain interference).[137,162,163] A PROMIS Pain Interference short form has also demonstrated responsivity to pain treatment.[163] In addition, a subset of items from the Pain Interference item bank have been identified as being appropriate for use with individuals with spinal cord injury and chronic pain.[164] Thus, there is not necessarily a need to "adapt" the items from the PROMIS scales for any one special population as there was with the BPI Pain Interference scale. Because PROMIS scores can be computed by using any one or more items from the item bank (of course, the more items used, the more precise the score) any "adaptation" needed can be performed by selecting the specific items most appropriate for the population to be studied. Also, the item bank approach allows for the administration of the PROMIS scales (including the PROMIS Pain Interference item bank items) using computer adaptive testing, in which a program selects the next item for the respondent based on the responses provided so far. With such an approach, it is possible to assess the domain of interest with very few items (e.g., often, with as few as four items) with as much precision that usually requires many more items.

Recommendations for Assessing Pain Interference

Both the BPI Pain Interference scale and PROMIS Pain Interference item bank items were developed using sound scale development strategies, and each has support for its reliability and validity as a measure of pain interference. Also, each measure is easy to administer and score. However, although both measures have been shown to be responsive to pain treatments, one study—the only one identified which compared the two measures directly—found that the BPI Pain Interference scale was more responsive as an outcome measure than the PROMIS Pain Interference short form was.[165]

Each measure also has its own unique strengths and weaknesses. The primary strength of the BPI Pain Interference scale is that it has a longer history and therefore has the most empirical support for its reliability and validity. Moreover, it has been translated into more languages that the PROMIS scale has (so far), making it more useful for comparing pain interference scores across different cultures. The BPI items can also be scored into two subscales (assessing interference with activity and social/affect interference domains), although in some populations, these two interference domains are strongly associated with one another and so may not always operate as distinct domains. Another strength of the BPI Pain Interference scale, as mentioned previously, is that one study found it to be more responsive to pain treatment than the PROMIS Pain Interference short form.

The strengths of the PROMIS item bank include those associated with item banking, which allows for a great deal of flexibility in administration (e.g., use of static short forms, use of computer adaptive testing, use of custom items most appropriate for the population, selection of items most appropriate for a specific population). In addition, the National Institutes of Health (NIH) in the United States is strongly advocating for the use of PROMIS measures in NIH research, which will result in a continued growth in their use and a likely explosion of additional knowledge regarding their psychometric properties over the next decade. Also, at least two consensus groups are recommending use of the PROMIS Pain Interference scales over other measures, including the BPI Pain Interference scale.[166,167]

Given the available data, and especially given the fact that algorithms exist for computing PROMIS Pain Interference scores from BPI Pain Interference scale scores,[168,169] an edge might be given to selecting the BPI over the PROMIS scales at this point in time, if the plan is to use the measure as an outcome in clinical trial. For other purposes (e.g., in research seeking to understand how pain interference is associated with other pain-related factors), either measure would appear adequate.

Measuring Pain in Special Populations

Although the measures described and recommended for use in this chapter can be used by many patients in most settings, there are special populations that may require different measures or approaches. These include patients that are at risk for cognitive deficits (e.g., patients with head injuries, the very elderly, the very ill) or who may not yet have reached an adequate developmental stage to understand the measure or the tasks that the measure requires (e.g., infants and toddlers). A detailed review of the many measures and procedures for assessing pain in special populations is beyond the scope of this chapter, and the interested reader is referred to other more detailed reviews to obtain information concerning the available options (for children,[170–172] for the elderly,[173–176] for individuals with limited communication abilities,[174,177] for individuals with cancer[178]). In general, when assessing pain in special populations who are unable to provide valid responses to standard measures, the clinician and researcher has two options: (1) to simplify the assessment strategy to a level that can be understood by the patient or (2) to depend on observation of behaviors known to reflect pain experience.

SIMPLIFIED MEASURES OF PAIN
Simple Pain Measures to Consider
Of the two options to consider when selecting a pain assessment approach for special populations, the first option, using a simplified measure of pain, may be considered a better option to select whenever possible and practical given the facts that (1) only patients have direct access to their pain experience and so are in the best position to describe this experience and (2) observational measures of pain behaviors show, at best, only moderate associations to patient reports of pain experience.[179,180]

Of the three primary pain intensity measures used most often in pain research and clinical settings, evidence indicates that VRSs tend to be easier for patients to understand and use than NRSs, and that NRSs are easier for patients to understand and use than VASs,[48,181–186] making simple VRSs (e.g., "None," "Mild," "Moderate," "Severe") a natural choice to consider when a simple measure of pain is needed.

Another measure to consider in this situation is a face scale. Face scales consist of line drawings of faces, each of which represent expressions that communicate different levels of pain and distress. Although a number of such scales have been developed, one that has many strengths is the Faces Pain Scale–Revised (FPS-R, Fig. 20.4).

There is ample evidence supporting the reliability and validity of the FPS-R as a measure of pain intensity (see review[174]). For example, the FPS-R of pain intensity is strongly associated with other measures of pain intensity[187,188] and shows adequate test–retest stability over a 2-week interval ($r = 0.76$).[187] Also, the FPS-R shows responsivity to treatments known to impact pain, including in a clinical trial involving children as young as 4 to 6 years old,[189] a trial involving children 5 to 12 years old,[188] and one that used the FPS-R in children aged 3 to 12 years old.[190]

An earlier version of the FPS-R[191] as well as the FPS-R have been shown to be easier to comprehend by older patients and patients with dementia than either a VRS or a VAS.[185,187,192,193] Interestingly, although the NRS tends to be preferred over other scales by older patients who are not cognitively impaired, in one study, the FPS-R was shown to be preferred over other pain measures by elderly patients who have cognitive impairments.[187] Thus, the FPS-R appears to be the best measure to when even simple VRSs are too complex for the patient or population being studied. Also, the instructions for the FPS-R are available in many languages (currently 64), and information about the FPS-R is readily available and kept updated on a Web site (https://www.iasp-pain.org/Education/Content.aspx?ItemNumber=1519).

However, one study reported that over half of a sample of 6-year-olds had difficulty understanding and using the FPS-R,[194] suggesting that when designing a pain trial with very young children, either (1) adequately large numbers of participants may be needed to overcome possible unreliability of the measure or (2) if limited numbers of possible participants are available, an alternative measure or procedure (such as a pain behavior observation procedure) may be needed.

Selecting the Best Measure for a Patient or Population
One way to determine which measure to use in any one patient in the clinical setting would be to begin by asking him or her to provide pain ratings using a number of different measures (e.g., a NRS, a VRS, or the FPS-R) for *six* domains of pain intensity: his or her own current pain; his or her own worst, least, and average pain during a specific period of time (e.g., the past 24 hours); the rating he or she would make on the scales that would represent mild pain; and the rating he or she

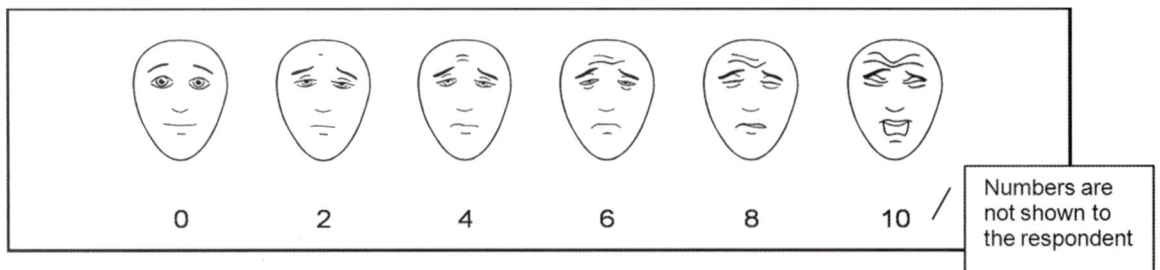

FIGURE 20.4   The Faces Pain Scale–Revised (FPS-R). Instructions to the respondent: "These faces show how much something can hurt. This face [point to left-most face] shows no pain [or hurt]. The faces show more and more pain [point to each from left to right] up to this one [point to right-most face]—it shows very much pain. Point to the face that shows how much you hurt [right now]." Do not use words like "happy" or "sad." This scale is intended to measure how the respondents feel inside, not how their face looks. Numbers are not shown to the respondent; they are shown here only for reference. The instructions for administration are currently available in over 31 languages from www.painsourcebook.ca. *(From Hicks CL, von Baeyer CL, Spafford PA, et al. The Faces Pain Scale–Revised. Toward a common metric in pediatric pain measurement. Pain 2001;93:173–183. This Faces Pain Scale-Revised has been reproduced with permission of the International Association for the Study of Pain® [IASP]. The figure may NOT be reproduced for any other purpose without permission.)*

would make on the scales that would represent severe pain. The patient's responses to the measures could then be examined to determine which scales show the most consistent responses; that is, the scales for which his or her own least pain is rated lower than worst pain, ratings of his or her own current and average pain ratings fall within the least-worst range, and the ratings they selected as representative of "mild" and "severe" pain fall within an expected range (e.g., severe pain is rated higher than mild pain, and both are rated higher than the lowest possible response on the scale). Evidence indicates that even among individuals with severe dementia, the majority can provide a valid response to at least one type of scale, although the scale that is most useful for any one patient may differ between individuals.[192] Thus, by first trying different scales with patients who are at risk for having difficulties with standard measures, the clinician can determine for each patient that measure or scale that provides the most consistent response and that the patient indicates is easiest for him or her to use. This is the scale that could then be used with that patient in future clinical encounters.

Selecting a measure to use in a clinical trial involving populations of patients who may have difficulty comprehending or using pain measures is more challenging, given that there is no single measure that will be universally valid for every individual. In this situation, it probably makes the most sense to (1) select the single measure that is most likely to be valid for the most study participants (e.g., either a simple VRS or the FPS-R), (2) ensure that the measure is adequately explained to all study participants, (3) ensure adequate power (e.g., large sample sizes) to deal with possible decreases in reliability of assessment due to possible difficulties with the measure in some study participants, and (4) consider using ability to comprehend and use the measure (as determined, e.g., by an ability to provide a consistent response when asked to rate current, least, average, most, "mild" and "moderate" pains, see previous discussion) as an eligibility criterion for participation in the study. If the study population of interest is known to include at least some participants who will not be able to provide a valid response on a self-report pain measure, and adequate sample sizes are not available to address possible increased unreliability in assessment because of this potential problem (or there is a need to determine the effects of the treatment even among those who are unable to validly describe their pain), then the use of pain behavior observation scales or procedures may be indicated.

BEHAVIOR OBSERVATION MEASURES

A large number of pain behavior observation scales and measures have been developed for use as proxy measures of pain when self-report scales cannot be used, for example, in preverbal children or in nonverbal adults. The field has not yet come to a consensus regarding which one of the available measures is the most valid and reliable in most populations. The interested reader is referred to the published reviews for the most up-to-date summary of the state of the science concerning these measures.[171,174,175,195–197]

Briefly, all of the available measures contain a list of behaviors commonly thought to be associated with the experience of pain, such as moaning, crying, furrowing one's brow, grimacing, and rubbing a body part, among many others. The scales often score the behaviors as being present or absent, but they sometimes ask the observer to rate the behaviors along a continuum of frequency or intensity. Item responses are then summed to create total pain behavior scores or subscales for specific classes of behaviors, such as vocal, social, and activity pain behavior subscales. One earlier review of pediatric measures[171] recommended two scales for assessing pain intensity associated with medical procedures: the Face, Legs, Activity, Cry, and Consolability, or FLACC scale[196] and

the Children's Hospital of Eastern Ontario Pain Scale, or CHEOPS,[197] one for assessing postoperative pain in the hospital (FLACC), one for assessing postoperative pain at home (Parents' Postoperative Pain Measure or PPPM),[198] one for assessing pain in critical care (the COMFORT scale),[199] and two for assessing pain-related fear or anxiety (the Procedure Behavior Checklist or PBCL[200] and the Procedure Behavior Rating Scale–Revised[201]). Consistent with this, a more recent paper noted that in 12 published reviews of behavioral observational scales, of 65 existing measures, the scales that were recommended most often were the FLACC or Revised FLACC (rFLACC),[202] CHEOPS, and COMFORT scales.[197] A review of pain behavior measures in elderly individuals with dementia[175] concluded that two scales appear most valid and useful in these populations: the Pain Assessment Checklist for Seniors with Limited Ability to Communicate (PACSLAC)[203] and the DOLOPLUS 2.[204] Finally, a review of pain observation measures for potential use in critical care patients who are otherwise unable to communicate about their pain[195] recommended the Critical-Care Pain Observation Tool.[205]

Measuring Pain in Busy Clinical Settings

Of course, in many busy clinical settings, it may only be possible to administer just a very few scales. Two newer very brief multidomain pain measures that have been developed for this situation are the Defense and Veterans Pain Rating Scale (DVPRS)[206] and the PEG (assessing pain intensity [P], interference with enjoyment of life [E], and interference with general activity [G]).[207] The DVPRS is a 5-item questionnaire assessing pain intensity and pain interference with usual activity and sleep, impact on mood, and contribution to stress, all using 0-to-10 scales with additional cues (e.g., color shading from yellow to red) to make understanding easier. The PEG items assess average pain intensity and pain interference with enjoyment of life and general activity, also using 0-to-10 NRSs. Not surprisingly, as these measures are based in large part on existing measures with proven reliability and validity, research findings support the validity and reliability of both the DVPRS (and the even more recent DVPRS-2) and PEG items.[206–210]

Summary and Conclusions

When considering which pain domains to assess for research or clinical purposes, investigators and clinicians must balance the need for a thorough assessment against the needs of the patient for minimal assessment burden. When determining this balance, all of the possible pain domains (intensity, affect, quality, temporal characteristics, and impact or interference) should at least be considered. Moreover, it is important to remember that many patients with pain often report more than one pain problem.

The ideal assessment, even when assessment needs to be brief, would probably involve assessing up to at least three "primary" or "most bothersome" pain problems, and include an evaluation of their intensities and locations. For assessing intensity of each pain problem or pain site, the data from a large number of studies in persons with chronic pain suggest that 0-to-10 Numerical Pain Scale of pain intensity (with 0 = "No pain" and 10 = "Pain as bad as you can imagine") have the most strengths and fewest weaknesses of the available measures in many populations. Four-point VRSs or the FPS-R would be most appropriate in populations who might struggle with the 0-to-10 NRS, such as the elderly or individuals who have cognitive impairment.

To assess pain site, pain drawings have been used more often than site checklists in published research. However, pain site checklists are easier to score, given that pain drawings require a second step of scoring to determine the location(s) and extent of pain, and there is no evidence to suggest that patients' responses to site checklists are any less valid than their responses to pain drawings. For these reasons, a site checklist, provided that the sites listed are adequately comprehensive, may be more practical in many research situations, although clinicians may prefer pain drawings for the overall gestalt that such measures can provide concerning how the patient views pain in his or her own body.

Whether or not to assess the temporal pattern(s) of the different pain problems would be important (1) if altering the temporal pattern of pain is a goal of treatment or (2) if knowledge about the temporal pattern is needed to help diagnose the pain problem. The available data indicate that pain's continuous versus intermittent nature can predict important functional outcomes, with continuous pain associated with poorer outcomes, suggesting that some assessment of this aspect of pain may be useful. A simple categorical question (e.g., such as that included on the PQAS-R or the painDETECT) appears to be adequate for assessing this characteristic of pain. More research is needed to determine the relative validity and utility of assessing other temporal characteristics of each pain problem.

Although pain does have an affective component, pain affect is not frequently measured in pain research. This may be due, in part, to the strong associations found between measures of pain intensity and pain affect; pain that is more severe usually bothers people more. There are, however, a number of situations in which it may be appropriate to assess pain affect in addition to pain intensity, for example, when evaluating the effects of treatments, such as cognitive-behavioral therapy or mindfulness-based interventions, that might have a greater impact on the affective or suffering component of pain than on pain intensity. In these situations, because of its brevity and demonstrated validity, the Affective subscale of the SF-MPQ would appear to be the best choice.

Although more research is needed to identify the pain quality scales (and items) that best classify pain types (e.g., neuropathic vs. nonneuropathic), at this point, the DN4 has the most empirical support for this purpose. When a self-report measure that can be used to classify patient pain is needed, both the S-LANSS and painDETECT could be used, with neither one evidencing stronger empirical support than the other at this point in time. To assess pain qualities for describing pain or determining the effects of treatment on pain qualities, the PQAS-R has the most empirical support for its content validity and ability to detect changes in distinct pain qualities with pain treatments.

Research has confirmed what many clinicians and patients with chronic pain already know; pain can have a significant negative impact on important activities. Assessing the critical domain of pain interference should be strongly considered by both clinicians and researchers. Clinicians can use this information to help target treatments (e.g., substantial impacts on mood might suggest the need for treatments that could address mood disturbances, whereas substantial impact on sleep would suggest the need for treatments that could help the patient sleep better) as well as track the efficacy of different pain treatments that are provided. Researchers could, and in many cases probably should, assess pain interference as a primary or secondary outcome in clinical trials in order to determine whether or not the treatment being examined has benefits on the patient's life beyond its effects on pain. For assessing this domain, the seven BPI Pain Interference scale items (with the "walking" item modified in samples of patients with physical disabilities so these patients can rate the interference of pain on "mobility [ability to get around]") and the PROMIS Pain Interference scales appear to have the most strengths of the available measures.

In populations of patients who might have limited ability to communicate or to use the measures recommended in the preceding text, clinicians can select from among the simpler measures, such as simple verbal categorical scales (i.e., "None," "Mild," "Moderate," or "Severe") or the FPS-R. Among patients who demonstrate an inability to understand or use these measures, then a very simple dichotomous question ("Do you have bothersome pain?") or some of the validated pain behavior observation scales may be needed.

One final point can be made concerning the pain assessment: In any setting, it is critical to remember that we are ultimately assessing individuals who have specific pain conditions as well as pain-related and non–pain-related comorbidities, which affect treatment choices and treatment outcomes. We are not only assessing their pain. Many of the measures that we use have extensive support for their reliability and validity and can provide numbers and ratings that can be used to help determine the efficacy of pain treatments, the need to continue or discontinue those treatments, and the possible need to provide additional treatments. But all of the numbers and ratings provided by patients and research subjects come from people, many of whom may be suffering a great deal. Measures, surveys, and questions can never replace the need to listen with compassion to the people we serve, in order to ensure the appropriate evaluation and treatment of their pain condition. The experience of a person reporting a pain level of "7" (out of 10) will rarely, if ever, be the same as the experience of another person reporting that same pain level. Much more important than obtaining a pain rating or score is an understanding of patients and their experience. We serve our patients best when we remember to take the time to listen.

References

1. Jensen MP. Questionnaire validation: a brief guide for readers of the research literature. *Clin J Pain* 2003;19:345–352.
2. American Educational Research Association, American Psychological Association, National Council on Measurement in Education. *Standards for Educational and Psychological Testing*. Washington, DC: American Educational Research Association; 2014.
3. Turner JA, Cardenas DD. Chronic pain problems in individuals with spinal cord injuries. *Semin Clin Neuropsychiatry* 1999;4:186–194.
4. Jensen MP, Stoelb BL, Molton IR. Measuring pain in persons with spinal cord injury. *Top Spinal Cord Inj Rehabil* 2007;13:20–34.
5. Widerström-Noga E, Biering-Sørensen F, Bryce TN, et al. The International Spinal Cord Injury Pain Basic Data Set (version 2.0). *Spinal Cord* 2014;52:282–286.
6. Jensen MP. Pain assessment in clinical trials. In: Wittink H, Carr D, eds. *Pain Management: Evidence, Outcomes, and Quality of Life in Pain Treatment*. Amsterdam, The Netherlands: Elsevier; 2008:57–88.
7. Melzack R, Torgerson WS. On the language of pain. *Anesthesiology* 1971;34:50–59.
8. Jensen MP. The validity and reliability of cancer pain measures. *J Pain* 2003;4:2–21.
9. Dworkin RH, Turk DC, Farrar JT, et al. Core outcome measures for chronic pain clinical trials: IMMPACT recommendations. *Pain* 2005;113:9–19.
10. Jensen MP, Mardekian J, Lakshminarayanan M, et al. Validity of 24-h recall ratings of pain severity: biasing effects of "peak" and "end" pain. *Pain* 2008;137:422–427.
11. Redelmeier DA, Katz J, Kahneman D. Memories of colonoscopy: a randomized trial. *Pain* 2003;104:187–194.
12. Schneider S, Stone AA, Schwartz JE, et al. Peak and end effects in patients' daily recall of pain and fatigue: a within-subjects analysis. *J Pain* 2011;12(2):228–235.
13. Jamison RN, Raymond SA, Levine JG, et al. Electronic diaries for monitoring chronic pain: 1-year validation study. *Pain* 2001;91:277–285.
14. Lewis B, Lewis D, Cumming G. Frequent measurement of chronic pain: an electronic diary and empirical findings. *Pain* 1995;60:341–347.
15. Krogh AB, Larsson B, Salvesen Ø, et al. A comparison between prospective Internet-based and paper diary recordings of headache among adolescents in the general population. *Cephalalgia* 2016;36:335–345.
16. Stone AA, Shiffman S, Schwartz JE, et al. Patient compliance with paper and electronic diaries. *Control Clin Trials* 2003;24:182–199.
17. Evans SR, Simpson DM, Kitch DW, et al; for Neurologic AIDS Research Consortium, AIDS Clinical Trials Group. A randomized trial evaluating prosaptide for HIV-associated sensory neuropathies: use of an electronic diary to record neuropathic pain. *PLoS One* 2007;25:551.
18. Roelofs J, Peters ML, Patijn J, et al. An electronic diary assessment of the effects of distraction and attentional focusing on pain intensity in chronic low back pain patients. *Br J Health Psychol* 2006;11:595–606.

19. Bigal ME, Edvinsson L, Rapoport AM, et al. Safety, tolerability, and efficacy of TEV-48125 for preventive treatment of chronic migraine: a multicentre, randomised, double-blind, placebo-controlled, phase 2b study. *Lancet Neurol* 2015;14:1091–1100.

20. Pedersen L, Borchgrevink PC, Breivik HP, et al. A randomized, double-blind, double-dummy comparison of short- and long-acting dihydrocodeine in chronic non-malignant pain. *Pain* 2014;155:881–888.

21. Gaertner J, Elsner F, Pollmann-Dahmen K, et al. Electronic pain diary: a randomized crossover study. *J Pain Symptom Manage* 2004;28:259–267.

22. Heiberg T, Kvien TK, Dale Ø, et al. Daily health status registration (patient diary) in patients with rheumatoid arthritis: a comparison between personal digital assistant and paper-pencil format. *Arthritis Rheum* 2007;57:454–460.

23. Stinson JN, Stevens BJ, Feldman BM, et al. Construct validity of a multidimensional electronic pain diary for adolescents with arthritis. *Pain* 2008;136:281–292.

24. Litcher-Kelly L, Kellerman Q, Hanauer SB, et al. Feasibility and utility of an electronic diary to assess self-report symptoms in patients with inflammatory bowel disease. *Ann Behav Med* 2007;33:207–212.

25. Lackner JM, Jaccard J, Keefer L, et al. The accuracy of patient-reported measures for GI symptoms: a comparison of real time and retrospective reports. *Neurogastroenterol Motil* 2014;26:1802–1811.

26. Aaron LA, Mancl L, Turner JA, et al. Reasons for missing interviews in the daily electronic assessment of pain, mood, and stress. *Pain* 2004;109:389–398.

27. Bolton JE. Accuracy of recall of usual pain intensity in back pain patients. *Pain* 1999;83:533–539.

28. Jamison RN, Sbrocco T, Parris WC. The influence of physical and psychosocial factors on accuracy of memory for pain in chronic pain patients. *Pain* 1989;37:289–294.

29. Jamison RN, Raymond SA, Slawsby EA, et al. Pain assessment in patients with low back pain: comparison of weekly recall and momentary electronic data. *J Pain* 2006;7:192–199.

30. Jensen MP, Turner LR, Turner JA, et al. The use of multiple-item scales for pain intensity measurement in chronic pain patients. *Pain* 1996;67:35–40.

31. Kikuchi H, Yoshiuchi K, Miyasaka N, et al. Reliability of recalled self-report on headache intensity: investigation using ecological momentary assessment technique. *Cephalalgia* 2006;26:1335–1343.

32. Stone AA, Broderick JE, Kaell AT, et al. Does the peak-end phenomenon observed in laboratory pain studies apply to real-world pain in rheumatoid arthritics? *J Pain* 2000;1:212–217.

33. Stone AA, Broderick JE, Shiffman SS, et al. Understanding recall of weekly pain from a momentary assessment perspective: absolute agreement, between- and within-person consistency, and judged change in weekly pain. *Pain* 2004;107:61–69.

34. Jensen MP, Hu X, Potts SL, et al. Single vs composite measures of pain intensity: relative sensitivity for detecting treatment effects. *Pain* 2013;154:534–538.

35. Stone AA, Schneider S, Broderick JE, et al. Single-day pain assessments as clinical outcomes: not so fast. *Clin J Pain* 2014;30:739–743.

36. Jensen MP, Tomé-Pires C, Solé E, et al. Assessment of pain intensity in clinical trials: individual ratings vs composite scores. *Pain Med* 2015;16:141–148.

37. Broderick JE, Schwartz JE, Vikingstad G, et al. The accuracy of pain and fatigue items across different reporting periods. *Pain* 2008;139:146–157.

38. Hans G, Sabatowski R, Binder A, et al. Efficacy and tolerability of a 5% lidocaine medicated plaster for the topical treatment of post-herpetic neuralgia: results of a long-term study. *Curr Med Res Opin* 2009;25:1295–1305.

39. Branco JC, Cherin P, Montagne A, et al. Longterm therapeutic response to milnacipran treatment for fibromyalgia. A European 1-year extension study following a 3-month study. *J Rheumatol* 2011;38:1402–1412.

40. Litcher-Kelly L, Martino SA, Broderick JE, et al. A systematic review of measures used to assess chronic musculoskeletal pain in clinical and randomized controlled clinical trials. *J Pain* 2007;8:906–913.

41. Jensen MP, Karoly P. Self-report scales and procedures for assessing pain in adults. In: Turk DC, Melzack R, eds. *Handbook of Pain Assessment.* 3rd ed. New York: Guilford; 2011:19–44.

42. Crawford B, Bouhassira D, Wong A, et al. Conceptual adequacy of the Neuropathic Pain Symptom Inventory in six countries. *Health Qual Life Outcomes* 2008;6:62.

43. Hardy JD, Wolff HG, Goodell H. *Pain Sensations and Reactions.* Baltimore, MD: Williams & Wilkins; 1952.

44. Jensen MP, Turner JA, Romano JM. What is the maximum number of levels needed in pain intensity measurement? *Pain* 1994;58:387–392.

45. Price DD, Barrell JJ, Gracely RH. A psychophysical analysis of experiential factors that selectively influence the affective dimension of pain. *Pain* 1980;8:137–149.

46. Price DD, Harkins SW, Baker C. Sensory-affective relationships among different types of clinical and experimental pain. *Pain* 1987;28:297–307.

47. Gaston-Johansson F, Franco T, Zimmerman L. Pain and psychological distress in patients undergoing autologous bone marrow transplantation. *Oncol Nurs Forum* 1992;19:41–48.

48. Jensen MP, Karoly P, O'Riordan EF, et al. The subjective experience of acute pain: an assessment of the utility of 10 indices. *Clin J Pain* 1989;5:153–159.

49. Melzack R. The McGill Pain Questionnaire: major properties and scoring methods. *Pain* 1975;1:277–299.

50. Melzack R. The Short-Form McGill Pain Questionnaire. *Pain* 1987;30:191–197.

51. Dudgeon D, Raubertas RF, Rosenthal SN. The Short-Form McGill Pain Questionnaire in chronic cancer pain. *J Pain Symptom Manage* 1993;8:191–195.

52. Putzke JD, Richards JS, Hicken BL, et al. Pain classification following spinal cord injury: the utility of verbal descriptors. *Spinal Cord* 2002;40:118–127.

53. Li G, Lv CA, Tian L, et al. A randomized controlled trial of botulinum toxin A for treating neuropathic pain in patients with spinal cord injury. *Medicine* 2017;96:e6919.

54. Picarelli H, Teixeira MJ, de Andrade DC, et al. Repetitive transcranial magnetic stimulation is efficacious as an add-on to pharmacological therapy in complex regional pain syndrome (CRPS) type I. *J Pain* 2010;11:1203–1210.

55. Rowbotham M, Harden N, Stacey B, et al. Gabapentin for the treatment of postherpetic neuralgia: a randomized controlled trial. *JAMA* 1998;280:1837–1842.

56. Viola V, Newnham HH, Simpson RW. Treatment of intractable painful diabetic neuropathy with intravenous lignocaine. *J Diabetes Complications* 2006;20:34–39.

57. Ahles TA, Blanchard EB, Ruckdeschel JC. The multidimensional nature of cancer-related pain. *Pain* 1983;17:277–288.

58. Kremer EF, Atkinson JH Jr, Ignelzi RJ. Pain measurement: the affective dimensional measure of the McGill Pain Questionnaire with a cancer pain population. *Pain* 1982;12:153–163.

59. Chang PF, Arendt-Nielsen L, Graven-Nielsen T, et al. Comparative EEG activation to skin pain and muscle pain induced by capsaicin injection. *Int J Psychophysiol* 2004;51:117–126.

60. Ahlquist ML, Franzén OG. Encoding of the subjective intensity of sharp dental pain. *Endod Dent Traumatol* 1994;10:153–166.

61. Beise RD, Carstens E, Kohllöffel LU. Psychophysical study of stinging pain evoked by brief freezing of superficial skin and ensuing short-lasting changes in sensations of cool and cold pain. *Pain* 1998;74:275–286.

62. Ngassapa DN. Comparison of functional characteristics of intradental A- and C-nerve fibres in dental pain. *East Afr Med J* 1996;73:207–209.

63. Bennett M. The LANSS Pain Scale: the Leeds Assessment of Neuropathic Symptoms and Signs. *Pain* 2001;92:147–157.

64. Bennett MI, Smith BH, Torrance N, et al. The S-LANSS score for identifying pain of predominantly neuropathic origin: validation for use in clinical and postal research. *J Pain* 2005;6:149–158.

65. Bouhassira D, Attal N, Alchaar H, et al. Comparison of pain syndromes associated with nervous or somatic lesions and development of a new neuropathic pain diagnostic questionnaire (DN4). *Pain* 2005;114:29–36.

66. Freynhagen R, Baron R, Gockel U, et al. painDETECT: a new screening questionnaire to identify neuropathic components in patients with back pain. *Curr Med Res Opin* 2006;22:1911–1920.

67. Canadian Agency for Drugs and Technologies in Health. *Diagnostic Methods for Neuropathic Pain: A Review of Diagnostic Accuracy.* Ontario, Canada; Canadian Agency for Drugs and Technologies in Health; 2015.

68. Mathieson S, Maher CG, Terwee CB, et al. Neuropathic pain screening questionnaires have limited measurement properties. A systematic review. *J Clin Epidemiol* 2015;68:957–966.

69. Bennett MI, Attal N, Backonja MM, et al. Using screening tools to identify neuropathic pain. *Pain* 2007;127:199–203.

70. Gould EM, Jensen MP, Victor TW, et al. The pain quality response profile of oxymorphone extended release in the treatment of low back pain. *Clin J Pain* 2009;25:116–122.

71. Gammaitoni AR, Smugar SS, Jensen MP, et al. Predicting response to pregabalin from pretreatment pain quality: clinical applications of the Pain Quality Assessment Scale. *Pain Med* 2013;14:526–532.

72. Dworkin RH, Turk DC, Revicki DA, et al. Development and initial validation of an expanded and revised version of the Short-Form McGill Pain Questionnaire (SF-MPQ-2). *Pain* 2009;144:35–42.

73. Bouhassira D, Attal N, Fermanian J, et al. Development and validation of the Neuropathic Pain Symptom Inventory. *Pain* 2004;108:248–257.

74. Galer BS, Jensen MP. Development and preliminary validation of a pain measure specific to neuropathic pain: the Neuropathic Pain Scale. *Neurology* 1997;48:332–338.

75. Jensen MP, Gammaitoni AR, Olaleye DO, et al. The Pain Quality Assessment Scale: assessment of pain quality in carpal tunnel syndrome. *J Pain* 2006;7:823–832.

76. Jensen MP, Lin CP, Kupper AE, et al. Cognitive testing and revision of the Pain Quality Assessment Scale. *Clin J Pain* 2013;29:400–410.

77. Katz J, Melzack R. The McGill Pain Questionnaire: development, psychometric properties, and usefulness of the long form, short form, and short-form-2 . In: Turk DC, Melzack R, eds. *Handbook of Pain Assessment.* 3rd ed. New York: Guilford; 2011:67–97.

78. Lowe NK, Walker SN, MacCallum RC. Confirming the theoretical structure of the McGill Pain Questionnaire in acute clinical pain. *Pain* 1991;46:53–60.

79. Turk DC, Rudy TE, Salovey P. The McGill Pain Questionnaire reconsidered: confirming the factor structure and examining appropriate uses. *Pain* 1985;21:385–397.

80. Tannock I, Gospodarowicz M, Meakin W, et al. Treatment of metastatic prostatic cancer with low-dose prednisone: evaluation of pain and quality of life as pragmatic indices of response. *J Clin Oncol* 1989;7:590–597.

81. Tesfaye S, Watt J, Benbow SJ, et al. Electrical spinal-cord stimulation for painful diabetic peripheral neuropathy. *Lancet* 1996;348:1698–1701.

82. Graham C, Bond S, Gerkovich M. Use of the McGill Pain Questionnaire in the assessment of cancer pain: reliability and consistency. *Pain* 1980;8:377–387.

83. Love A, Leboeuf C, Crisp TC. Chiropractic chronic low back pain sufferers and self-report assessment methods. Part I. A reliability study of the Visual Analogue Scale, the Pain Drawing and the McGill Pain Questionnaire. *J Manipulative Physiol Ther* 1989;12:21–25.

84. Walsh TD, Leber B. Measurement of chronic pain: Visual Analogue Scale and McGill Pain Questionnaire compared. *Adv Pain Res Ther* 1983; 5:897–899.

85. Jenkinson C, Carroll D, Egerton M, et al. Comparison of the sensitivity to change of long and short from pain measures. *Qual Life Res* 1995;4:353–357.

86. Bellamy N, Campbell J, Syrotuik J. Comparative study of self-rating pain scale in osteoarthritis patients. *Curr Med Res Opin* 1999;15:113–119.

87. Graff-Radford SB, Shaw LR, Naliboff BN. Amitriptyline and fluphenazine in the treatment of postherpetic neuralgia. *Clin J Pain* 2000;16:188–192.

88. Chandra K, Shafiq N, Pandhi P, et al. Gabapentin versus nortriptyline in post-herpetic neuralgia patients: a randomized, double-blind clinical trial—the GONIP Trial. *Int J Clin Pharmacol Ther* 2006;4:358–363.

89. Rosenstock J, Tuchman M, LaMoreaux L, et al. Pregabalin for the treatment of painful diabetic peripheral neuropathy: a double-blind, placebo-controlled trial. *Pain* 2004;110:628–638.

90. Siddall PJ, Cousins MJ, Otte A, et al. Pregabalin in central neuropathic pain associated with spinal cord injury: a placebo-controlled trial. *Neurology* 2006;67:1792–1800.

91. Lovejoy TI, Turk DC, Morasco BJ. Evaluation of the psychometric properties of the revised Short-Form McGill Pain Questionnaire. *J Pain* 2012;13:1250–1257.

92. Dworkin RH, Turk DC, Trudeau JJ, et al. Validation of the Short-Form McGill Pain Questionnaire-2 (SF-MPQ-2) in acute low back pain. *J Pain* 2015;16:357–366.

93. Lin CP, Kupper AE, Gammaitoni AR, et al. Frequency of chronic pain descriptors: implications for assessment of pain quality. *Eur J Pain* 2011;15(6):628–633.

94. Jensen MP, Johnson LE, Gertz KJ, et al. The words patients use to describe chronic pain: implications for measuring pain quality. *Pain* 2013;154:2722–2728.

95. Sharma S, Pathak A, Jensen MP. Words that describe chronic musculoskeletal pain: implications for assessing pain quality across cultures. *J Pain Res* 2016;9:1057–1066.

96. Rehm S, Binder A, Baron R. Post-herpetic neuralgia: 5% lidocaine medicated plaster, pregabalin, or a combination of both? A randomized, open, clinical effectiveness study. *Curr Med Res Opin* 2010;26:1607–1619.

97. Rocha Rde O, Teixeira MJ, Yeng LT, et al. Thoracic sympathetic block for the treatment of complex regional pain syndrome type I: a double-blind randomized controlled study. *Pain* 2014;155:2274–2281.

98. Attal N, Fermanian C, Fermanian J, et al. Neuropathic pain: are there distinct subtypes depending on the aetiology or anatomical lesion? *Pain* 2008;138:343–353.

99. Freeman R, Baron R, Bouhassira D, et al. Sensory profiles of patients with neuropathic pain based on the neuropathic pain symptoms and signs. *Pain* 2014;155:367–376.

100. Cocito D, Peci E, Ciaramitaro P, et al. Short-term efficacy of ultramicronized palmitoylethanolamide in peripheral neuropathic pain. *Pain Res Treat* 2014;2014:854560.

101. Carter GT, Jensen MP, Galer BS, et al. Neuropathic pain in Charcot-Marie-Tooth disease. *Arch Phys Med Rehabil* 1998;79:1560–1564.

102. Galer BS, Gianas A, Jensen MP. Painful diabetic polyneuropathy: epidemiology, pain description, and quality of life. *Diab Res Clin Prac* 2000; 47:123–128.

103. Galer BS, Henderson J, Perander J, et al. Course of symptoms and quality of life measurement in complex regional pain syndrome: a pilot survey. *J Pain Symptom Manage* 2000;20:286–292.

104. Jensen MP, Friedman M, Bonzo D, et al. The validity of the Neuropathic Pain Scale for assessing diabetic neuropathic pain in a clinical trial. *Clin J Pain* 2006;22:97–103.

105. Fishbain DA, Lewis J, Cole B, et al. Multidisciplinary pain facility treatment outcome for pain-associated fatigue. *Pain Med* 2005;6:299–304.

106. Fishbain DA, Lewis JE, Cole B, et al. Lidocaine 5% patch: an open-label naturalistic chronic pain treatment trial and prediction of response. *Pain Med* 2006;7:135–142.

107. Kalso E, Tasmuth T, Neuvonen PJ. Amitriptyline effectively relieves neuropathic pain following treatment of breast cancer. *Pain* 1996;4:293–302.

108. Galer BS, Jensen MP, Ma T, et al. The lidocaine patch 5% effectively treats all neuropathic pain qualities: results of a randomized, double-blind, vehicle-controlled, 3-week efficacy study with use of the neuropathic pain scale. *Clin J Pain* 2002;18:297–301.

109. Gammaitoni AR, Galer BS, Lacouture P, et al. Effectiveness and safety of new oxycodone/acetaminophen formulations with reduced acetaminophen for the treatment of low back pain. *Pain Med* 2003;4:21–30.

110. Jensen MP, Dworkin RH, Gammaitoni AR, et al. Assessment of pain quality in chronic neuropathic and nociceptive pain clinical trials with the Neuropathic Pain Scale. *J Pain* 2005;6:98–106.

111. Levendoglu F, Ogün CO, Ozerbil O, et al. Gabapentin is a first line drug for the treatment of neuropathic pain in spinal cord injury. *Spine* 2004;28:743–751.

112. Moseley GL. Graded motor imagery is effective for long-standing complex regional pain syndrome: a randomised controlled trial. *Pain* 2004;108:192–198.

113. Semenchuk MR, Sherman S. Effectiveness of tizanidine in neuropathic pain: an open-label study. *J Pain* 2000;1:285–292.

114. Tai Q, Kirshblum S, Chen B, et al. Gabapentin in the treatment of neuropathic pain after spinal cord injury: a prospective, randomized, double-blind, crossover trial. *J Spinal Cord Med* 2002;25:100–105.

115. Victor TW, Jensen MP, Gammaitoni AR, et al. The dimensions of pain quality: factor analysis of the Pain Quality Assessment Scale. *Clin J Pain* 2008;24:550–555.

116. Jensen MP, Gammaitoni AR, Bolognese JA, et al. The pain quality response profile of pregabalin in the treatment of neuropathic pain. *Clin J Pain* 2012;28:683–686.

117. Nalamachu S, Ruck D, Nalamasu R, et al. Open-label study to evaluate the efficacy and safety of extended-release hydromorphone in patients with chronic neuropathic pain. *J Opioid Manag* 2013;9:43–49.

118. Hsieh YL, Chou LW, Hong SF, et al. Laser acupuncture attenuates oxaliplatin-induced peripheral neuropathy in patients with gastrointestinal cancer: a pilot prospective cohort study. *Acupunct Med* 2016;34:398–405.

119. Jensen MP, Trudeau JJ, Radnovich R, et al. The pain quality response profile of a corticosteroid injections and heated lidocaine/tetracaine patch in the treatment of shoulder impingement syndrome. *Clin J Pain* 2015;31:342–348.

120. Cleeland CS, Ryan KM. Pain assessment: global use of the Brief Pain Inventory. *Ann Acad Med Singapore* 1994;23:129–138.

121. Margolis RB, Tait RC, Krause SJ. A rating system for use with patient pain drawings. *Pain* 1986;24:57–65.

122. Barbero M, Moresi F, Leoni D, et al. Test-retest reliability of pain extent and pain location using a novel method for pain drawing analysis. *Eur J Pain* 2015;19:1129–1138.

123. Jensen MP, Hoffman AJ, Cardenas DD. Chronic pain in individuals with spinal cord injury: a survey and longitudinal study. *Spinal Cord* 2005; 43:704–712.

124. Ohnmeiss DD. Repeatability of pain drawings in a low back pain population. *Spine* 2000;25:980–988.

125. MacDowall A, Robinson Y, Skeppholm M, et al. Pain drawings predict outcome of surgical treatment for degenerative disc disease in the cervical spine. *Ups J Med Sci* 2017;8:1–7.

126. Hayashi K, Arai YC, Morimoto A, et al. Associations between pain drawing and psychological characteristics of different body region pains. *Pain Pract* 2015;15:300–307.

127. Voorhies RM, Jiang X, Thomas N. Predicting outcome in the surgical treatment of lumbar radiculopathy using the Pain Drawing Score, McGill Short Form Pain Questionnaire, and risk factors including psychosocial issues and axial joint pain. *Spine J* 2007;7:516–524.

128. Marcus DA, Bernstein CD, Haq A, et al. Including a range of outcome targets offers a broader view of fibromyalgia treatment outcome: results from a retrospective review of multidisciplinary treatment. *Musculoskeletal Care* 2014;12:74–81.

129. Bertozzi L, Rosso A, Romeo A, et al. The accuracy of pain drawing in identifying psychological distress in low back pain-systematic review and meta-analysis of diagnostic studies. *J Phys Ther Sci* 2015;27:3319–3324.

130. Carnes D, Ashby D, Underwood M. A systematic review of pain drawing literature: should pain drawings be used for psychologic screening? *Clin J Pain* 2006;22:449–457.

131. Widerström-Noga EG, Duncan R, Turk DC. Psychosocial profiles of people with pain associated with spinal cord injury: identification and comparison with other chronic pain syndromes. *Clin J Pain* 2004;20:261–271.

132. Serlin RC, Mendoza TR, Nakamura Y, et al. When is cancer pain mild, moderate or severe? Grading pain severity by its interference with function. *Pain* 1995;61:277–284.

133. Jamison RN, Brown GK. Validation of hourly intensity profiles with chronic pain patients. *Pain* 1991;45:123–128.

134. van Grootel RJ, van der Glas HW, Buchner R, et al. Patterns of pain variation related to myogenous temporomandibular disorders. *Clin J Pain* 2005;21:154–165.

135. Nappi G, Jensen R, Nappi RE, et al. Diaries and calendars for migraine. A review. *Cephalalgia* 2006;26:905–916.

136. Bennett MI, Smith BH, Torrance N, et al. Can pain can be more or less neuropathic? Comparison of symptom assessment tools with ratings of certainty by clinicians. *Pain* 2006;122:289–294.

137. Amtmann D, Cook KF, Jensen MP, et al. Development of a PROMIS item bank to measure pain interference. *Pain* 2010;150:173–182.

138. Cleeland CS, Ladinsky JL, Serlin RC, et al. Multidimensional measurement of cancer pain: comparisons of US and Vietnamese patients. *J Pain Symptom Manage* 1998;3:23–27.

139. Caraceni A, Mendoza TR, Mencaglia E, et al. A validation study of an Italian version of the Brief Pain Inventory (Breve Questionario per la Valutazione del Dolore). *Pain* 1996;65:87–92.

140. Wang XS, Mendoza TR, Gao SZ, et al. The Chinese version of the Brief Pain Inventory (BPI-C): its development and use in a study of cancer pain. *Pain* 1996;67:407–416.

141. Uki J, Mendoza T, Cleeland CS, et al. A brief cancer pain assessment tool in Japanese: the utility of the Japanese Brief Pain Inventory—BPI-J. *J Pain Symptom Manage* 1998;16:364–373.

142. Ger LP, Ho ST, Sun WZ, et al. Validation of the Brief Pain Inventory in a Taiwanese population. *J Pain Symptom Manage* 1999;18:316–322.

143. Radbruch L, Loick G, Kiencke P, et al. Validation of the German Version of the Brief Pain Inventory. *J Pain Symptom Manage* 1999;18:180–187.

144. Saxena A, Mendoza T, Cleeland CS. The assessment of cancer pain in North India: the validation of the Hindi Brief Pain Inventory—BPI-H. *J Pain Symptom Manage* 1999;17:27–41.

145. Mystakidou K, Mendoza T, Tsilika E, et al. Greek Brief Pain Inventory: validation and utility in cancer pain. *Oncology* 2001;60:35–42.

146. Zelman DC, Gore M, Dukes E, et al. Validation of a modified version of the Brief Pain Inventory for painful diabetic peripheral neuropathy. *J Pain Symptom Manage* 2005;29:401–410.

147. Cleeland CS, Nakamura Y, Mendoza TR, et al. Dimensions of the impact of cancer pain in a four-country sample: new information from multidimensional scaling. *Pain* 1996;67:267–273.

148. Walton DM, Beattie T, Putos J, et al. A Rasch analysis of the Brief Pain Inventory Interference subscale reveals three dimensions and an age bias. *J Clin Epidemiol* 2016;74:218–226.

149. Lapane KL, Quilliam BJ, Benson C, et al. One, two, or three? Constructs of the Brief Pain Inventory among patients with non-cancer pain in the outpatient setting. *J Pain Symptom Manage* 2014;47:325–333.

150. Armstrong DG, Chappell AS, Le TK, et al. Duloxetine for the management of diabetic peripheral neuropathic pain: evaluation of functional outcomes. *Pain Med* 2007;8:410–418.

151. Arnold LM, Goldenberg DL, Stanford SB, et al. Gabapentin in the treatment of fibromyalgia: a randomized, double-blind, placebo-controlled, multicenter trial. *Arthritis Rheum* 2007;56:1336–1344.

152. Wardley A, Davidson N, Barrett-Lee P, et al. Zoledronic acid significantly improves pain scores and quality of life in breast cancer patients with bone metastases: a randomised, crossover study of community vs hospital bisphosphonate administration. *Br J Cancer* 2005;92:1869–1876.

153. White WT, Patel N, Drass M, et al. Lidocaine patch 5% with systemic analgesics such as gabapentin: a rational polypharmacy approach for the treatment of chronic pain. *Pain Med* 2003;4:321–330.

154. Skljarevski V, Zhang S, Desaiah D, et al. Duloxetine versus placebo in patients with chronic low back pain: a 12-week, fixed-dose, randomized, double-blind trial. *J Pain* 2010;11:1282–1290.

155. Kroenke K, Theobald D, Wu J, et al. Comparative responsiveness of pain measures in cancer patients. *J Pain* 2012;13:764–772.

156. Happich M, Schneider E, Boess FG, et al. Effectiveness of duloxetine compared with pregabalin and gabapentin in diabetic peripheral neuropathic pain: results from a German observational study. *Clin J Pain* 2014;30:875–885.

157. Silverman S, Raffa RB, Cataldo MJ, et al. Use of immediate-release opioids as supplemental analgesia during management of moderate-to-severe chronic pain with buprenorphine transdermal system. *J Pain Res* 2017;10:1255–1263.

158. Osborne TL, Raichle KA, Jensen MP, et al. The reliability and validity of pain interference measures in persons with multiple sclerosis. *J Pain Symptom Manage* 2006;32:217–229.

159. Tyler EJ, Jensen MP, Engel JM, et al. The reliability and validity of pain interference measures in persons with cerebral palsy. *Arch Phys Med Rehabil* 2002;83:236–239.

160. Raichle KA, Osborne TL, Jensen MP, et al. The reliability and validity of pain interference measures in persons with spinal cord injury. *J Pain* 2006;7:179–186.

161. World Health Organization. *International Classification of Functioning, Disability and Health*. Geneva, Switzerland: World Health Organization; 2001.

162. Bartlett SJ, Orbai AM, Duncan T, et al. Reliability and validity of selected PROMIS measures in people with rheumatoid arthritis. *PLoS One* 2015;10:e0138543.

163. Lee AC, Driban JB, Price LL, et al. Responsiveness and minimally important differences for 4 patient-reported outcomes measurement information system short forms: physical function, pain interference, depression, and anxiety in knee osteoarthritis. *J Pain* 2017;18:1096–1100.

164. Cohen ML, Kisala PA, Dyson-Hudson TA, et al. Measuring pain phenomena after spinal cord injury: development and psychometric properties of the SCI-QOL Pain Interference and Pain Behavior assessment tools [published online ahead of print February 10, 2017]. *J Spinal Cord Med*. doi:10.1080/10790268.2017.1279805.

165. Kean J, Monahan PO, Kroenke K, et al. Comparative responsiveness of the PROMIS Pain Interference Short Forms, Brief Pain Inventory, PEG, and SF-36 Bodily Pain Subscale. *Med Care* 2016;54:414–421.

166. Deyo RA, Dworkin SF, Amtmann D, et al. Report of the NIH task force on research standards for chronic low back pain. *J Pain* 2014;15:569–585.

167. Wolters PL, Martin S, Merker VL, et al. Patient-reported outcomes of pain and physical functioning in neurofibromatosis clinical trials. *Neurology* 2016;87(suppl 1):S4–S12.

168. Askew RL, Kim J, Chung H, et al. Development of a crosswalk for pain interference measured by the BPI and PROMIS pain interference short form. *Qual Life Res* 2013;22:2769–2776.

169. Cook KF, Schalet BD, Kallen MA, et al. Establishing a common metric for self-reported pain: linking BPI Pain Interference and SF-36 Bodily Pain Subscale scores to the PROMIS Pain Interference metric. *Qual Life Res* 2015;24:2305–2318.

170. Ruskin DA, Amaria KA, Warnock FF, et al. Assessment of pain in infants, children, and adolescents. In: Turk DC, Melzack R, eds. *Handbook of Pain Assessment*. 3rd ed. New York: Guilford; 2011:213–241.

171. von Baeyer CL, Spagrud LJ. Systematic review of observational (behavioral) measures of pain for children and adolescents aged 3 to 18 years. *Pain* 2007;127:140–150.

172. Kingsnorth S, Orava T, Provvidenza C, et al. Chronic pain assessment tools for cerebral palsy: a systematic review. *Pediatrics* 2015;136:e947–e960.

173. Gauthier LR, Gagliese L. Assessment of pain in older persons. In: Turk DC, Melzack R, eds. *Handbook of Pain Assessment*. 3rd ed. New York: Guilford; 2011:224–259.

174. Hadjistavropoulos T, Herr K, Turk DC, et al. An interdisciplinary expert consensus statement on assessment of pain in older persons. *Clin J Pain* 2007;23:S1–S43.

175. Zwakhalen SM, Hamers JP, Abu-Saad HH, et al. Pain in elderly people with severe dementia: a systematic review of behavioural pain assessment tools. *BMC Geriatr* 2006;6:3.

176. Hadjistavropoulos T, Herr K, Prkachin KM, et al. Pain assessment in elderly adults with dementia. *Lancet Neurol* 2014;13:1216–1227.

177. Hadjistavropoulos T, Breau LM, Craig KD. Pain assessment in persons with limited ability to communicate. In: Turk DC, Melzack R, eds. *Handbook of Pain Assessment*. 3rd ed. New York: Guilford; 2011:260–280.

178. Anderson KO. Assessments of patients with cancer-related pain. In: Turk DC, Melzack R, eds. *Handbook of Pain Assessment*. 3rd ed. New York: Guilford; 2011:376–395.

179. Labus JS, Keefe FJ, Jensen MP. Pain intensity and pain behavior: when are they correlated? *Pain* 2003;102:109–124.

180. McCahon S, Strong J, Sharry R, et al. Self-report and pain behavior among patients with chronic pain. *Clin J Pain* 2005;21:223–231.

181. Ferrell BA, Ferrell BR, Rivera L. Pain in cognitively impaired nursing home patients. *J Pain Symptom Manage* 1995;10:591–598.

182. Jensen MP, Karoly P, Braver S. The measurement of clinical pain intensity: a comparison of six methods. *Pain* 1986;27:117–126.

183. Herr KA, Spratt K, Mobily PR, et al. Pain intensity assessment in older adults: use of experimental pain to compare psychometric properties and usability of selected pain scales with younger adults. *Clin J Pain* 2004;20:207–219.

184. Littman GS, Walker BR, Schneider BE. Reassessment of verbal and visual analog ratings in analgesic studies. *Clin Pharmacol Ther* 1985;38:16–23.

185. Li L, Liu X, Herr K. Postoperative pain intensity assessment: a comparison of four scales in Chinese adults. *Pain Med* 2007;8:223–234.

186. Gagliese L, Weizblit N, Ellis W, et al. The measurement of postoperative pain: a comparison of intensity scales in younger and older surgical patients. *Pain* 2005;117:412–420.

187. Ware LJ, Epps CD, Herr K, et al. Evaluation of the Revised Faces Pain Scale, Verbal Descriptor Scale, Numeric Rating Scale, and Iowa Pain Thermometer in older minority adults. *Pain Manag Nurs* 2006;7:117–125.

188. Spafford PA, von Baeyer CL, Hicks CL. Expected and reported pain in children undergoing ear piercing: a randomized trial of preparation by parents. *Behav Res Ther* 2002;4:253–266.

189. Wood C, von Baeyer CL, Bourrillon A, et al. Self-assessment of immediate post-vaccination pain after two different MMR vaccines administered as a second dose in 4- to 6-year-old children. *Vaccine* 2004;23:127–131.

190. Migdal M, Chudzynska-Pomianowska E, Vause E, et al. Rapid, needle-free delivery of lidocaine for reducing the pain of venipuncture among pediatric subjects. *Pediatrics* 2005;115:393–398.

191. Bieri D, Reeve RA, Champion GD, et al. The Faces Pain Scale for the self-assessment of the severity of pain experienced by children: development, initial validation and preliminary investigation for ratio scale properties. *Pain* 1990;41:139–150.

192. Pautex S, Michon A, Guedira M, et al. Pain in severe dementia: self-assessment or observational scales? *J Am Geriatr Soc* 2006;54:1040–1045.

193. Taylor LJ, Herr K. Pain intensity assessment: a comparison of selected pain intensity scales for use in cognitively intact and cognitively impaired African American older adults. *Pain Manag Nurs* 2003;4:87–95.

194. Stanford EA, Chambers CT, Craig KD. The role of developmental factors in predicting young children's use of a self-report scale for pain. *Pain* 2006;120:16–23.

195. van Herk R, van Dijk M, Baar FP, et al. Observation scales for pain assessment in older adults with cognitive impairments or communication difficulties. *Nurs Res* 2007;56:34–43.

196. Merkel SI, Voepel-Lewis T, Shayevitz JR, et al. The FLACC: a behavioral scale for scoring postoperative pain in young children. *Pediatr Nurs* 1997;23:293–297.

197. McGrath PJ, Johnson G, Goodman JT, et al. CHEOPS: a behavioral scale for rating postoperative pain in children. In: Fields HL, Dubner R, Cervero F, eds. *Advances in Pain Research and Therapy*. Vol 9. New York, Raven Press; 1985:395–402.

198. Chambers CT, Reid GJ, McGrath PJ, et al. Development and preliminary validation of a postoperative pain measure for parents. *Pain* 1996;68:307–313.

199. Ambuel B, Hamlett KW, Marx CM, et al. Assessing distress in pediatric intensive care environments: the COMFORT scale. *J Pediatr Psychol* 1992;17:95–109.

200. LeBaron S, Zeltzer L. Assessment of acute pain and anxiety in children and adolescents by self-reports, observer reports, and a behavior checklist. *J Consult Clin Psychol* 1984;52:729–738.

201. Katz ER, Kellerman J, Siegel SE. Behavioral distress in children with cancer undergoing medical procedures: developmental considerations. *J Consult Clin Psychol* 1980;48:356–365.

202. Malviya S, Voepel-Lewis T, Burke C. et al. The revised FLACC observational pain tool: improved reliability and validity for pain assessment in children with cognitive impairment. *Paediatr Anaesth* 2006;16:258–265.

203. Fuchs-Lacelle S, Hadjistavropoulos T. Development and preliminary validation of the Pain Assessment Checklist for Seniors with Limited Ability to Communicate (PACSLAC). *Pain Manag Nurs* 2004;5:37–49.

204. Lefebre-Chapiro L; and Doloplus group. The Doloplus 2 scale—evaluating pain in the elderly. *Euro J Palliative Care* 2001;8:191–194.

205. Gélinas C, Fillion L, Puntillo KA, et al. Validation of the critical-care pain observation tool in adult in adult patients. *Am J Crit Care* 2006;15: 420–427.

206. Buckenmaier CC III, Galloway KT, Polomano RC, et al. Preliminary validation of the Defense and Veterans Pain Rating Scale (DVPRS) in a military population. *Pain Med* 2013;14:110–123.

207. Krebs EE, Lorenz KA, Bair MJ, et al. Development and initial validation of the PEG, a three-item scale assessing pain intensity and interference. *J Gen Intern Med* 2009;24:733–738.

208. Nassif TH, Hull A, Holliday SB, et al. Concurrent validity of the Defense and Veterans Pain Rating Scale in VA outpatients. *Pain Med* 2015;16:2152–2161.

209. de Waal MW, den Elzen WP, Achterberg WP, et al. A postal screener for pain and need for treatment in older persons in primary care. *J Am Geriatr Soc* 2014;62:1832–1837.

210. Polomano RC, Galloway KT, Kent ML, et al. Psychometric testing of the Defense and Veterans Pain Rating Scale (DVPRS): a new pain scale for military population. *Pain Med* 2016;17:1505–1519.

CHAPTER 21

Pain Psychology Evaluation

RAVI PRASAD, DESIREE AZIZODDIN, and **AMIR RAMEZANI**

Biopsychosocial approaches posit that biologic, psychological, and social factors interact to shape the overall experience of pain.[1] This relationship is exemplified by the negative impact on psychological well-being that results from the lack of definitive cure for many chronic pain conditions[2] and the ensuing development of a vicious cycle in which physical pain and emotional distress exacerbate each other. Psychosocial variables are also known to play a predictive role in medical intervention outcomes[3]; thus, assessing and addressing these risk factors can maximize treatment efficacy. Although the history and physical exam completed during a medical appointment may touch on psychosocial factors as they relate to pain, a full pain psychology evaluation provides a more comprehensive perspective regarding how past and current stressors, emotional functioning, sociocultural variables, and health behaviors may be influencing the etiology and maintenance of underlying pain conditions. The current chapter provides an overview of the various components of a psychological evaluation, the rationale for their inclusion, and briefly discusses several assessment devices that can be used to facilitate this process. A more thorough review of instruments that can be used to measure pain and its associated features can be found in the previous chapter. Just as the data from clinical interviews and objective assessment devices are used in a complementary fashion in pain evaluation, the information contained in the previous and current chapters should be used in a similarly integrative fashion.

Psychosocial History

Psychosocial factors evolve over the course of the life span have been associated with pain and pain outcomes.[4] A full psychosocial history should include information about early life experiences, academic history, and vocational functioning.

EARLY LIFE EXPERIENCES

Awareness the role that early life events play in the human experience—namely, adverse childhood experiences (ACE)—is fundamental to understanding how patients relate to their internal world and outside environment. ACE include verbal abuse, physical abuse, sexual abuse by an adult/or someone 5 years older, neglect, witnessing domestic violence, parental divorce, substance use in home, mental illness of someone in the home, and/or history of prison sentence of someone in the home. ACEs have been associated with a myriad of adverse health and behavior outcomes, including the development of pain conditions.[5-9] The negative impact of ACE is believed to occur through increased pituitary adrenal and autonomic nervous system reactivity, as evidenced by increased reactivity when compared to counterparts who have not experienced significant adverse events.[10-13] The relational strength seen between ACEs and the development of negative health outcomes can be mediated by a combination of psychological and physiologic factors such as negative schemas, decreased mood, decreased positive health behaviors, suppressed immunologic function, and increased stress reactivity.[3,14-16] Given the role that early life experiences can play in the development of pain conditions over time, it is important to assess this aspect of patients' personal history in the clinical interview. This process can be facilitated by use of the Adverse Childhood Experience

Questionnaire, a free, 10-item measure in which a score of 4 and above that indicates a higher likelihood of negative health outcomes.[5]

VOCATIONAL HISTORY

Past and current vocational functioning provides perspective regarding patients' activity patterns and is also predictive of the development of and prognosis for pain-related issues. A prospective study of 3,020 volunteers assessing risk factors associated with later back injury claims found that job dissatisfaction was the most predictive individual factor for reporting work-related low back pain over the course of time.[17] Subsequent studies of job satisfaction have further reinforced its predictive value in pain-related disability. It has been postulated that work satisfaction may serve as a protective factor for adverse pain outcomes across different work environments and socioeconomic groups.[18] The postinjury work environment itself also plays a role in pain outcomes. The lack of work place modifications to accommodate the limitations caused by the injury and the inability to modify the pace at which one completes job-related tasks are both predictive of chronic pain-related disability.[19]

All of the aforementioned underscores potential secondary gain variables that may influence response to treatment and should thus be explored in greater detail. It is imperative to note that these variables are not limited to the vocational environment: factors that can reinforce maintenance of impaired functioning should be assessed across all domains of patients' lives. If such influences are detected, it is useful for clinicians to delineate the mechanism by which they may be shaping response to treatment rather than merely identifying a clinical situation as having potential for secondary gain, as the latter can have negative ramifications for patients.[20] Finally, although it is important to assess for its presence, it is also incumbent on the clinician to ensure that a lack of response to treatment is not inappropriately attributed to secondary gain.

EDUCATIONAL HISTORY

Educational history is another patient variable that is known to influence chronic pain. A study examining correlates of back pain in German patients found that level of education significantly predicted low back pain and accounted for a large majority of the variance in the differences across age and gender.[21] Large-scale studies in other countries have also found links between education and pain. In a study of 17,543 adults from Australia, lower levels of completed education, unemployment benefits, and being unemployed for health reasons were all associated with having chronic pain.[22] A study of 8,970 individuals from Finland found an "educational gradient" for both chronic and disabling chronic pain, where lower levels of education were associated with a higher prevalence of chronic pain and disability.[23] Low educational attainment is strongly associated with low back pain, and this is believed to function primarily through psychological factors and health behaviors such as smoking, diet, exercise, and obesity.[24] An analysis targeting the link between education and pain found that individuals with lower levels of education achievement were more likely to report pain as a signal of harm and had increased self-reported disability, potentially explaining the mediating psychological factors between level of education and pain.[25] There is also evidence that the course of back pain is less successful for individuals with lower levels of education.[26] Level of education is of particular importance in understanding psychological and health literacy barriers that can impact pain treatment. Information related to education can be obtained by assessing level of academic preparation (e.g., less than high school, high school, college, and graduate school).

Current Functioning

An assessment of current status should delineate patients' daily activity patterns and the extent to which physical pain and pain-related beliefs affect functioning. Attention should focus on the presence or absence of adaptive coping skills and health behaviors such as time-based activity pacing, consistency in dietary and sleep habits, and engagement in activities that promote physical and psychological wellness (e.g., physical exercise, meditation).[27-29] Tension in interpersonal relationships, finances, and/or work should also be noted, as studies have found an association between stress and pain.[30,31] The pain experience and response to treatment is ultimately a product of the interaction among all of the aforementioned variables, belief structures, social relationships, and cultural factors.[32,33] As the latter three categories are more nuanced, they will be discussed in greater detail in the following text.

BELIEF STRUCTURES

Individuals' belief structures about their pain can influence their overall adjustment to the condition itself.[28] Pain catastrophization is characterized by maladaptive, exaggerated thoughts, and emotions about actual or anticipated pain. It is strongly associated with poor treatment outcomes across the life span and is predictive of function, opioid use, and pain intensity.[34,35] Individuals who engage in high levels of pain catastrophization are often somatically hypervigilant at baseline which can lead to both increased pain perception and affective distress. Activity reduction is frequently employed as a coping strategy to escape pain, but this approach can result in the development of a fear avoidance cycle. The latter construct refers to avoidance of activity secondary to fear of reinjury, pain, or worsening of the underlying condition. Over the course of time, the avoidance of activity contributes to emotional distress and declining physical functioning which further reinforces the fear. Fear avoidance beliefs are self-perpetuating in nature and are predictive of functional limitations and perceived disability.[36]

In addition to data gleaned from the clinical interview, there are a number of devices available to assist with the assessment of catastrophic and fear avoidance beliefs. The Pain Catastrophizing Scale (PCS)[37] is a commonly used device composed of 13 items rated on a Likert scale. In addition to general tendencies toward catastrophization, subscales indicate the extent to which the respondent's cognitions are characterized by magnification, rumination, and helplessness. The Fear-Avoidance Beliefs Questionnaire (FABQ)[38] and the Pain Anxiety Symptoms Scale (PASS-20)[39] assess various aspects of the fear-avoidance cycle. The FABQ was specifically developed to assess patients' beliefs as they relate to low back pain. It is composed of 16 items scored on a 7-point Likert scale and yields scores on two subscales: Scale 1 assesses fear-avoidance beliefs about work and Scale 2 assesses fear-avoidance beliefs about general physical activity. The PASS-20 is composed of 20 items on a 6-point Likert scale. It measures pain-related anxiety across four subscales: cognitive, escape/avoidance, fear, and physiologic anxiety.

Beyond interpretation of pain, it is also useful to assess patients' beliefs regarding the role that they play in their own care. There are differences in how treatment is approached in acute versus chronic pain: Patients often assume a more passive role in the former, whereas the latter requires active self-management.

Assessing patients' understanding of this process and providing appropriate education can facilitate their ability to become active participants in their treatment plan.[40]

Assessment for alignment in treatment expectations is also important. Clinicians and patients may have different perspectives regarding what constitutes a successful outcome: A clinician may perceive improvement in physical functioning despite the presence of pain as fitting in this category, whereas a patient may view this as unsuccessful due to the ongoing nature of the pain symptoms. The potential for such a discrepancy highlights the importance of ensuring that patients understand the treatments in which they will participate and that they have realistic expectations of outcomes they may experience.[41]

SOCIAL SUPPORT

Social support factors relate to chronic pain conditions in a bidirectional fashion. Experiencing pain and resulting disability can further stress one's family system and may create conflict, particularly if one is no longer able to complete their expected family responsibilities.[42-44] Supportive family systems can also reinforce disability as they may engage in overly solicitous behavior, which can lead to further disability and passivity in the patient.[45-47] This is evidenced through operant models of conditioning, where increased reinforcement of pain-related behavior translated to increased pain intensity and disability.[48] There is evidence to support further pain and disability with communal catastrophizing as well, where increased expression of distress can lead to exhaustion of social support.[49] At the same time, a dysfunctional family can further exacerbate patients' conditions. Studies show that individuals who felt invalidated by a partner experienced more marital conflict, which in itself is associated with increased negative pain outcomes.[50] A longitudinal study assessing the impact of social support on pain outcomes found that immediately after a motor vehicle accident, social support did not relate to perceived pain ratings; however, at 6-week follow-up, individuals with less perceived social support had higher pain ratings than those with elevated social support, and this relationship was more significant for men than women and for those with depression.[51] Assessing the level of social support is particularly relevant in chronic pain management, and evidence supports the need for assessment in acute instances as well. Depleted levels of support can predict negative outcomes; yet, overly solicitous social support can also be as deleterious. Evaluation in this arena should include information about the quantity, quality, and stability of the full range of past and present interpersonal connections, including marital, family, work, and other social relationships. The Social Provisions Scale is a free, 24-item, self-report questionnaire that has been validated across several samples that can provide useful data that complements information obtained from the clinical interview.[52]

CULTURAL FACTORS

In its seminal report *Relieving Pain in America*, Institute of Medicine[2] specifically highlighted the importance of addressing cultural factors in the delivery of pain care. The literature has demonstrated variability across gender, ethnicity, race, and age influences the pain experience and patients' responses to treatment.[53-55] Clinical interview questions should therefore focus on gathering information on the sociocultural background of patients, their families, and communities, including assessment for disparities that may affect access to care.

Substance Use

Substance use behaviors are consistently identified as factors that can influence pain and pain treatment.[56] The mere presence of substance use does not necessarily indicate the presence of a problem; however, continued use of a substance despite the presence of adverse outcomes, failed attempts at abstinence, and the experience of clinically significant impairment in daily functioning are hallmark characteristics of a substance use disorder (SUD).[57]

Concurrent diagnoses of pain and SUDs are of particular significance given the influence they can have on one another. Veterans who are diagnosed with hepatitis C and have a history of an SUD display an increased likelihood of having a pain diagnosis versus patients who have no SUD history.[56] One cross-sectional analysis of chronic pain prevalence among patients in current substance abuse treatment programs found that 37% to 60% reported experiencing chronic pain.[58] Within this sample, significant predictors of both pain and substance use included younger age, chronic illness, lifetime psychiatric illness, drug craving, and current psychiatric illness.[58] Persistent pain has also been associated with continued substance abuse after detoxification.[59]

There is a relative scarcity of randomized controlled trials assessing the variations in pain treatments for patients with chronic noncancerous pain (CNCP) and comorbid substance use; however, existing studies emphasize the effectiveness of psychological interventions in improving pain-related function while reducing the risk of relapse for patients with concurrent CNCP and SUDs.[60,61] Effective reduction of aberrant medication use behaviors among patients with comorbid CNCP and SUDs can be achieved through use of a multidisciplinary care framework, creating treatment plans with high levels of specificity, increasing visit frequency, utilizing urine drug screens, and limiting opioid supply.[62,63]

A large review of comorbid SUD in patients with CNCP found estimates of current SUD ranging between 3% and 43% and a lifetime prevalence ranging from 16% to 74%.[64] Of note, the highest rate of comorbid SUD with CNCP patients was found in those attending emergency rooms for opioid refills with 74% meeting criteria for lifetime SUD.[65] The data remains mixed on predictive value of demographic variables such as age, employment, race, gender, ethnicity, marital status, and years of education rates of comorbid SUD and CNCP.[64]

There is a wide array of evidence supporting the need to evaluate and consider previous and current substance use and SUDs as a means of improving outcomes and performing risk stratification.[66–70] The specific pathway to evaluate substance use risk in patients with chronic pain is often multimodal: More specifically, a combination of clinical evaluation, formal instruments, and review of adjunctive methods of evaluation (e.g., urine drug screens, prescription drug monitoring) is suggested. Assessment in this arena should include exploration of nicotine, alcohol, and prescribed and nonprescribed (e.g., medications obtained illegally, illicit substances) drug use patterns.

NICOTINE

The prevalence of nicotine use in individuals living with chronic pain is higher than what is found in the general population: The Centers for Disease Control and Prevention identifies approximately 15.6% of the US adult population as current smokers, whereas a recent analysis of 5,350 chronic pain patients found approximately 23.5% identify as active nicotine users.[71,72] Zvolensky and colleagues[73] found that individuals with a lifetime history of neck or back pain were significantly more likely to meet criteria for current or historical nicotine dependence. In their study of 9,282 participants, those with a lifetime history of medically unexplained chronic pain were more likely to be current smokers.[73] It has been proposed that these variables interact with one another in a feedback loop in which smoking behavior increases pain and the presence of pain motivates smoking behavior.[74] Pain-induced motivation to smoke is likely related to withdrawal-based learning and patients' expectations of the effects of smoking in improving mood.[75]

Nicotine's relationship with health outcomes is quite broad: It negatively impacts cardiovascular and pulmonary functioning, is associated with increased mortality, and can adversely influence the experience of pain.[76] The global negative effects of nicotine on health—particularly its impact on pain—highlight the importance of assessing for the use of this substance as a coping strategy.

ALCOHOL

Alcohol consumption can interfere with successful pain management and have adverse effects on psychological functioning.[77] Similar to other variables discussed in this chapter, pain and alcohol use have a bidirectional relationship. Pain has been identified as a situational factor that motivates alcohol use and excessive use of alcohol can complicate pain treatment.[78] Furthermore, alcohol can also play a causal role in the development of painful conditions such as peripheral neuropathy and pancreatitis. Individuals with lower socioeconomic status are more likely to report increased alcohol consumption and experience higher levels of alcohol use disorder.[79,80] Other factors have also been found to be related to increased likelihood of alcohol use disorder such as obesity, symptoms of anxiety and depression, family history of alcohol use disorder, other SUDs, and tobacco smoking.[79,81–85] The assessment of alcohol use among pain patients is particularly relevant given the potential dangers that exist when it is combined with prescribed pharmaceuticals (e.g., nonsteroidal anti-inflammatory medications, acetaminophen, opioids, and benzodiazepines).[78]

In addition to verbal inquiry, alcohol use can be assessed using the Alcohol Use Disorders Identification Test (AUDIT).[86] The AUDIT is a free, reliable, valid, self-administered, 10-item questionnaire, where scores above 8 are associated with negative health outcomes.[87] It has been validated in multiple languages within primary care, rural, and college populations.[88–93] A shortened version, the Alcohol Use Disorder Identification Test Consumption Questions (AUDIT-C), has been validated for use in screening for alcohol use disorder in primary care samples.[94]

PRESCRIBED AND NONPRESCRIBED DRUG USE

The rate of emergency department visits involving prescription drug misuse doubled from 2004 to 2011 and fatal prescription drug overdoses involving opioids roughly quadrupled from 1999 to 2011.[95–97] The sharp rise in opioid-related issues led to the development of clinical guidelines for opioid therapy in CNCP.[98] Included in the guidelines is the importance of assessing for aberrant drug-related behaviors as a part of ongoing treatment.

A large review study involving two large health plans found that prescribing of long-term used opioids for CNCP increased from 11.6% to 17% for those with SUD histories.[99] Additionally, those with prior substance use history received higher doses of opioids, were more likely to use other schedule II drugs, and were more often using sedative-hypnotic medications in conjunction with opioids.[99] Prior use of cocaine and cannabinoids, previous drug convictions including driving under the influence, and alcohol abuse histories are identified as predictors of opioid misuse above and beyond self-reported pain scores.[100]

A thorough assessment of prescribed and nonprescribed drug use includes current and previous use of such substances, personal and family histories of SUDs, and prior participation in substance abuse treatment programs. Social, legal, and/or occupational impairment secondary to use of these substances should be noted, as should lack of compliance with prescription instructions.

Prescription drug monitoring programs (PDMPs) are state-level databases that track prescribing and dispensing of controlled substances. They help characterize patients' use of such substances and are thus useful tools to use when planning pharmacologic treatment. Use of PDMPs has been associated with a reduction in drug-related deaths,[101] but the laws and guidelines surrounding their use vary across states. Although access to such databases is not readily available to nonprescribing clinicians such as psychologists, information from the medical record that comments on PDMP findings should be included in evaluations when available.

The Opioid Risk Tool (ORT) is a free, 10-item self-report measure that provides some identification around individuals who may develop aberrant behaviors when prescribed opioids for chronic pain symptoms.[102] It includes items related to personal and family history of substance use, age, history of preadolescent sexual abuse, and some psychological factors related to chronic pain and opioid use. Score interpretations include a score of 0 to 3 representing a low risk of aberrant behaviors, 4 to 7 representing a moderate risk, and greater than 8 representing a high risk of such aberrant behaviors. This assessment had previously been identified as having a high degree of sensitivity and specificity in identifying which patients are at greater risk of aberrant opioid use behavior.[102] More recent studies, however, have found that the ORT's utility has diminished.[103,104] It is mentioned here due to its high prevalence in clinical practice; however, caution should be exercised when using this or any other questionnaires that rely on self-report as they have a high risk of response bias. Use of self-report tools should thus be supplemented with collateral information from the clinical interview, medical record review, urine drug screens, and PDMPs.

Psychiatric Functioning

Evaluation of psychiatric functioning should include information about personal and family histories of psychiatric disturbances; lifetime history of involvement in formal mental health treatment (e.g., individual therapy, pharmacologic management of moods, and psychiatric hospitalization); and past, current, and imminent ideation, intent, or plan to harm self or others. Information regarding symptoms of psychosis, mania, panic, learning disabilities, obsessive-compulsive disorder, and other forms of psychopathology can initially be obtained through general queries as it is not practical to walk patients through the diagnostic criteria for all psychiatric disorders. Positive endorsement of any such inquiries should be followed by more thorough assessment. As depressive and anxious disorders have a higher societal prevalence,[105] their diagnostic criteria should be reviewed in more detail. Given the association between ACE and health and behavior outcomes,[5] trauma history also warrants more focused attention. Lastly, all of the aforementioned forms of psychological distress have the potential for somatic manifestations; thus, understanding somatic disorders and their associated symptoms is also a critical part of the evaluation. Psychiatric impressions and recommendations are based on a combination of information obtained through behavioral observations, the clinical interview, and objective assessment devices.

BEHAVIORAL OBSERVATIONS

Objective observations on cognitive, emotional, and behavioral domains characterize the disposition of patients during the evaluation itself. Cognitive functioning is assessed via orientation to time, person, place, and situation; content and linearity of thought processes; and speech and patterns. Mood, affect, insight, and judgment should be commented on, including their congruence with the situation. The presence of verbal (e.g., vocal complaints, moaning, sighing) and nonverbal (e.g., shifting position, wincing, taking medication) pain behaviors should also be noted, as they also play a role in the overall experience of pain.[106]

DEPRESSION

Depression is a mood disorder characterized by pervasive sadness and anhedonia that causes clinically significant impairment in daily functioning.[57] Associated symptoms may also include changes in sleep patterns, diet, weight, attention, concentration, energy, and motivation. Individuals with chronic pain are 3 times more likely to meet criteria for depression, and symptoms of pain and depression vary directly with each other.[107,108] Some prospective studies have shown that a history of depression may predispose a person to develop pain,[109,110] whereas others have postulated that the consequences of the pain experience result in the formation of depression.[111] Regardless of the causal direction of the relationship, 65% of individuals with depression report pain symptoms and depression is present in 5% to 85% (varies by setting) of patients with pain conditions.[112] More importantly, the presence of pain leads to decreased identification of depression, resulting in it being undertreated.[112] As untreated/undertreated psychological distress can impact pain, this underrecognition can trigger a self-perpetuating cycle in which pain and depression adversely impact each other.

Screening for depression can occur with use of the Patient Health Questionnaire-9 (PHQ-9). This brief assessment device is composed of 9 items plus a qualitative functional deficit item and helps to identify depressive symptoms and their severity.[113] Clinical interview questions should focus on *Diagnostic and Statistical Manual of Mental Disorders* (5th ed.; *DSM-5*)[57] diagnostic criteria for depression and must also include specific suicide risk assessment.

ANXIETY

Anxiety is characterized by excessive fear or worry that is intrusive and has a significant negative impact on a person's daily functioning.[57] Anxiety-related disorders and chronic pain can have reciprocating relationships that are similar to those observed between depression and pain. Anxious interpretations of pain stimuli can result in decreased functionality and increased pain. More specifically, novel pain symptoms can trigger fear of their underlying meaning resulting in pain being viewed as a threatening stimulus. This cognitive appraisal can then lead to decreased engagement of activities for fear of worsening pain or causing further damage, thereby completing a positive feedback loop by further increasing avoidance, inactivity, and disability. This process concurrently results in overstimulation of physiologic arousal leading to lower pain thresholds, increased pain sensitivity, and sustained pain.[114,115] Other studies have found that individuals with elevated trait anxiety report higher levels of pain intensity compared those who score lower on this construct.[116] Anxiety has also been found to negatively affect health outcomes, as it has been associated with increased surgical complications and prolonged hospital stays.[117,118]

The Generalized Anxiety Disorder-7 (GAD-7) assesses symptoms of generalized anxiety disorder.[119] Somatic, cognitive, and affective clusters of symptoms are assessed on a 4-point Likert scale with scores of 5 or greater considered mild elevation in symptoms. The GAD-7 can serve as an effective screen for anxiety, but further delineation of symptoms is necessary to assist with diagnosis and formulation of a specific treatment plan.

POSTTRAUMATIC STRESS DISORDER

Posttraumatic stress disorder (PTSD) may develop after experiencing or witnessing a traumatic event. It is often associated with reexperiencing the event, hypervigilance, avoidance, and emotional reactivity.[57] Approximately 30% to 80% of individuals with PTSD also report the presence of chronic pain.[120] It is believed that individuals with anxiety are more vulnerable to develop PTSD as a result of neurobiologic predispositions to negative reactivity to stimuli, maintenance of symptoms secondary to continued avoidance of associated stimuli, attentional biases to trauma-related cues, and reduction of pain thresholds and pain tolerance due to increased anxiety-related physiologic processes.[120] Although some degree of clinical specificity exists among symptoms of depression, anxiety, and PTSD, there seems to be overlap between neurobiologic processes underlying these disorders that explains their relationship with pain and pain-related outcomes.

The Primary Care-PTSD (PC-PTSD) scale is a 4-item screening instrument that assesses symptoms associated with traumatic stress conditions as defined by *DSM* diagnostic criteria.[121] There are four symptom cluster items that patients respond to in a dichotomous fashion. Although the original development of the scale identified the possibility of PTSD symptoms with 3 out of 4 items endorsed, later research has suggested that just 1 out of 4 items may indicate the presence of an underlying trauma condition. As with the GAD-7, this tool should be used as a screening device only and not as a tool to formally diagnose PTSD. Information gleaned from a throughout clinical interview is necessary for the latter.

SOMATIZATION

Psychological distress can often manifest in the form of physical symptoms, a process referred to as *somatization.*[57] The *DSM-5* identifies a number of somatic symptom disorders that are often seen in pain settings[57]: (1) Somatic symptom disorder is marked by ruminations of thoughts about the seriousness of the symptoms or excessive anxiety or time and energy spent related to symptoms; (2) illness anxiety is characterized by high level of anxiety, preoccupation, and behaviors associated with possibly getting or having a medical or physical health condition; (3) functional neurologic symptom disorder is marked by motor, cognitive, or sensory symptoms that are largely medically unexplained; (4) psychological factors affecting medical conditions centers around emotional, behavioral, cognitive, or psychiatric factors that impact treatment of medical condition or the course of medical treatment; (5) factitious disorder is the intentional exaggeration of injury or medical condition for the sake of maintaining a patient role; and (6) malingering disorder is also the exaggeration of injury or medical condition but specifically for the purpose of some sort of secondary gain. Understanding the mentioned disorders and the differences among them is fundamental for diagnostic accuracy.

Psychological Screening for Advanced Interventional Procedures

Some insurance carriers require a pain psychology evaluation prior to undergoing implantable therapy trials (e.g., neurostimulation, intrathecal pump). Although this is not always mandated, it is useful to include such screening to maximize the benefit that patients may receive from the intervention itself, as psychological factors have been demonstrated to impact treatment outcome.[122]

Preprocedure psychology evaluations do not merely provide dichotomous responses regarding whether or not a patient is a decent candidate for a particular medical intervention; rather, they help identify risk factors that may contraindicate a treatment pathway and provide recommendations for how to address them. In addition to obtaining information from all of the domains outlined in this chapter, evaluations in these situations also assess patients' understanding of the procedure including risks and benefits and establishes that they have appropriate treatment expectations and an ability to cope with an unsuccessful trial. They further assess for psychological stability, the presence of chemical dependency issues, social support, and historical compliance with medical care. If deficits are noted

in any of the aforementioned areas, recommendations may be made for behavioral preparation to optimize patients' overall pain management care.[123]

Conclusion

The pain psychology evaluation is a critical component of multidisciplinary approaches to pain treatment. It is rooted in biopsychosocial models of pain and provides useful information regarding psychosocial factors that can contribute to the onset, maintenance, and exacerbation of pain conditions. Most importantly, it helps inform the creation of comprehensive treatment pathways that can maximize patients' overall physical and emotional functioning.

References

1. Gatchel RJ, McGeary DD, McGeary CA, et al. Interdisciplinary chronic pain management: past, present, and future. *Am Psychol* 2014;69:119–130.
2. Institute of Medicine. *Relieving Pain in America: A Blueprint for Transforming Prevention, Care, Education, and Research.* Washington, DC: National Academies Press; 2011.
3. Bruns D, Disorbio JM. The psychological evaluation of patients with chronic pain: a review of BHI 2 clinical and forensic interpretive considerations. *Psychol Inj Law* 2014;7(4):335–361.
4. Nieto R, Raichle KA, Jensen MP, et al. Changes in pain-related beliefs, coping, and catastrophizing predict changes in pain intensity, pain interference, and psychological functioning in individuals with myotonic muscular dystrophy and facioscapulohumeral dystrophy. *Clin J Pain* 2012;28(1):47–54.
5. Felitti VJ, Anda RF, Nordenberg D, et al. Relationship of childhood abuse and household dysfunction to many of the leading causes of death in adults: the Adverse Childhood Experiences (ACE) Study. *Am J Prev Med* 1998;14(4):245–258.
6. Saariaho T, Saariaho A, Karila I, et al. Maladaptive schema factors, chronic pain, and depressiveness: a study with 271 chronic pain patients and 331 control participants. *Clin Psychol Psychother* 2012;19:214–223.
7. Davis DA, Luecken LJ, Zautra AJ. Are reports of childhood abuse related to the experience of chronic pain in adulthood? A meta-analytic review of the literature. *Clin J Pain* 2005;21(5):398–405.
8. Anda R, Tietjen G, Schulman E, et al. Adverse childhood experiences and frequent headaches in adults. *Headache* 2010;50(9):1473–1481.
9. Dube SR, Anda RF, Felitti VJ, et al. Childhood abuse, household dysfunction, and the risk of attempted suicide throughout the life span: findings from the Adverse Childhood Experiences Study. *JAMA* 2001;286(24):3089–3096.
10. De Bellis MD, Chrousos GP, Dorn LD, et al. Hypothalamic-pituitary-adrenal axis dysregulation in sexually abused girls. *J Clin Endocrinol Metab* 1994;78(2):249–255.
11. Heim C, Ehlert U, Hanker JP, et al. Abuse-related posttraumatic stress disorder and alterations of the hypothalamic-pituitary- adrenal axis in women with chronic pelvic pain. *Psychosom Med* 1998;60(3):309–318.
12. Heim C, Newport DJ, Bonsall R, et al. Altered pituitary-adrenal axis responses to provocative challenge tests in adult survivors of childhood abuse. *Am J Psychiatry* 2001;158(4):575–581.
13. Bremner JD, Vythilingam M, Anderson G, et al. Assessment of the hypothalamic-pituitary-adrenal axis over a 24-hour diurnal period and in response to neuroendocrine challenges in women with and without childhood sexual abuse and posttraumatic stress disorder. *Biol Psychiatry* 2003;54(7):710–718.
14. Kiecolt-Glaser JK, Glaser R. Psychoneuroimmunology and cancer: fact or fiction? *Eur J Cancer* 1999;35(11):1603–1607.
15. Miller GE, Dopp JM, Myers HF, et al. Psychosocial predictors of natural killer cell mobilization during marital conflict. *Health Psychol* 1999;18(3):262–271.
16. Jones GT, Power C, Macfarlane GJ. Adverse events in childhood and chronic widespread pain in adult life: results from the 1958 British Birth Cohort Study. *Pain* 2009;143(1–2):92–96.
17. Bigos SJ, Battie MC, Spengler DM, et al. A longitudinal, prospective study of industrial back injury reporting. *Clin Orthop Relat Res* 1992;279:21–34.
18. Williams RA, Pruitt SD, Doctor JN, et al. The contribution of job satisfaction to the transition from acute to chronic low back pain. *Arch Phys Med Rehabil* 1998;79(4):366–374.
19. Teasell RW, Bombardier C. Employment-related factors in chronic pain and chronic pain disability. *Clin J Pain* 2001;17(4):S39–S45.
20. Gatchel RJ. Psychosocial factors that can influence the self-assessment of function. *J Occup Rehab* 2004;14(3):197–206.
21. Schmidt CO, Raspe H, Pfingsten M, et al. Back pain in the German adult population: prevalence, severity, and sociodemographic correlates in a multiregional survey. *Spine* 2007;32(18):2005–2011.
22. Blyth FM, March LM, Brnabid AJM, et al. Chronic pain in Australia: a prevalence study. *Pain* 2001;89:127–134.
23. Pepplina S, Paivi LA, Mikko L, et al. Socio-economic differences in the prevalence of acute, chronic, and disabling chronic pain among ageing employees. *Pain* 2005;114(3):364–371.

24. Katz JN. Lumbar disc disorders and low-back pain: socioeconoemic factors and consequences. *J Bone Joint Surg* 2006;88-A(2):21–24.

25. Roth RS, Geisser ME. Educational achievement and chronic pain disability: mediating role of pain-related cognitions. *Clin J Pain* 2002;18(5):286–296. doi:10.1097/00002508-200209000-00003.

26. Dionne CE, Von Korff M, Koepsell TD, et al. Formal education and back pain: a review. *J Epidemiol Community Health* 2001;55(7):455–468.

27. Brown GK, Nicassio PM. Development of a questionnaire for the assessment of active and passive coping strategies in chronic pain patients. *Pain* 1987;31(1):53–64.

28. Jensen MP, Turner JA, Romano JM, et al. Coping with chronic pain: a critical review of the literature. *Pain* 1991;47(3):249–283.

29. Stayner SR, Ramezani A, Prasad R, et al. Chronic pain and psychiatric illness: managing comorbid conditions: pay close attention to risk and benefit when planning pain management. *Curr Psychiatr* 2016;15(2):26–33.

30. Andrasik F, Flor H, Turk DC. An expanded view of psychological aspects in head pain: the biopsychosocial model. *Neurol Sci* 2005;26(suppl 2):S87–S91.

31. Gil KM, Carson JW, Porter LS, et al. Daily mood and stress predict pain, health care use, and work activity in African American adults with sickle-cell disease. *Health Psychol* 2004;23(3):267–274.

32. Larkin KT, Klonoff EA. *Specialty Competencies in Clinical Health Psychology*. New York: Oxford University Press; 2014.

33. Turk DC, Melzak R. *Handbook of Pain Assessment*. 3rd ed. New York: Guilford Press; 2011.

34. Feinstein AB, Sturgeon JA, Bhandari RP, et al. The impact of pain catastrophizing on outcomes: a developmental perspective across children, adolescents and young adults with chronic pain. *J Pain* 2017;18(2):144–154.

35. Darnall BD. Pain psychology and pain catastrophizing in the perioperative setting. A review of impacts, interventions, and unmet needs. *Hand Clinics* 2016;32(1):33–39.

36. Gatchel RJ, Neblett R, Kishino N, Ray CT. Fear-avoidance beliefs and chronic pain. *J Orthop Sports Phys Ther* 2016;46:38–43.

37. Sullivan MJL, Bishop SR, Pivik J. The Pain Catastrophizing Scale: development and validation. *Psychol Assess* 1995;7:524–532.

38. Waddell G, Newton M, Henderson I, et al. A Fear-Avoidance Beliefs Questionnaire (FABQ) and the role of fear-avoidance beliefs in chronic low back pain and disability. *Pain* 1993;52:157–168.

39. McCracken LM, Dhingra L. A short version of the Pain Anxiety Symptoms Scale (PASS-20): preliminary development and validity. *Pain Res Manage* 2002;7(1):45–50.

40. Dorflinger LM, Kerns RD, Auerbach SM. Providers' roles in enhancing patients' adherence to pain self-management. *Transl Behav Med* 2013;3(1):39–46.

41. Noble PC, Fuller-Lafreniere S, Meftah M, et al. Challenges in outcome measurement: discrepancies between patient and provider definitions of success. *Clin Orthop Relat Res* 2013;471(11):3437–3445.

42. Hamberg K, Johansson E, Lindgren G, et al. The impact of marital relationship on the rehabilitation process in a group of women with long-term musculoskeletal disorders. *Scand J Soc Med* 1997;25(1):17–25.

43. MacGregor EA, Brandes J, Eikermann A, et al. Impact of migraine on patients and their families: the Migraine and Zolmitriptan Evaluation (MAZE) survey—phase III. *Curr Med Res Opin* 2004;20(7):1143–1150.

44. Kemler MA, Furnee CA. The impact of chronic pain on life in the household. *J Pain Symptom Manage* 2002;23(5):433–441.

45. Kerns RD, Haythornthwaite J, Southwick S, et al. The role of marital interaction in chronic pain and depressive symptom severity. *J Psychosom Res* 1990;34(4):401–408.

46. Block AR, Kremer EF, Gaylor M. Behavioral treatment of chronic pain: the spouse as a discriminative cue for pain behavior. *Pain* 1980;9(2):243–252.

47. Matos M, Bernardes SF, Goubert L. Why and when social support predicts older adults' pain-related disability: a longitudinal study. *Pain* 2017;158(10):1915–1924.

48. Prenevost MH, Reme SE. Couples coping with chronic pain: how to intercouple interaction relate to pain coping? *Scand J Pain* 2017;16:150–157.

49. Cano A. Pain catastrophizing and social support in married individuals with chronic pain: the moderating role of pain duration. *Pain* 2004;110:656–664.

50. Schwartz L, Slater MA, Birchler GR. The role of pain behaviors in the modulation of marital conflict in chronic pain couples. *Pain* 1996;65:227–233.

51. Richmond NL, Meyer ML, Hollowell AG, et al. Social support and pain outcomes after trauma exposure among older adults: a multicenter longitudinal study. *Clin J Pain* 2018;34:366–374.

52. Cutrona CE, Russell D. The provisions of social relationships and adaptation to stress. In: Jones WH, Perlman D, eds. *Advances in Personal Relationships*. Greenwich, CT: JAI Press; 1987:37–67.

53. Molton IR, Terrill AI. Overview of persistent pain in older adults. *Am Psychol* 2014;69(2):197–207. doi:10.1037/a0035794.

54. Robinson ME, Riley JL, Myers CD, et al. Gender role expectations of pain: relationship to sex differences in pain. *J Pain* 2001;2:251–257.

55. Tait RC, Chibnall JT. Racial/ethnic disparities in the assessment and treatment of pain. *Am Psychol* 2014;69(2):131–141.

56. Morasco BJ, Dobscha SK. Prescription medication misuse and substance use disorder in VA primary care patients with chronic pain. *Gen Hosp Psychiatr* 2008;30(2):93–99.

57. American Psychiatric Association. *Diagnostic and Statistical Manual of Mental Disorders*. 5th ed. Arlington, VA: American Psychiatric Publishing; 2013.

58. Rosenblum A, Joseph H, Fong C, et al. Prevalence and characteristics of chronic pain among chemically dependent patients in methadone maintenance and residential treatment facilities. *JAMA* 2003;289(18):2370–2379.

59. Larson MJ, Paasche-Orlow M, Cheng DM, et al. Persistent pain is associated with substance use after detoxification: a prospective cohort analysis. *Addiction* 2007;102(5):752–760.

60. Currie SR, Hodgins DC, Crabtree A, et al. Outcome from integrated pain management treatment for recovering substance abusers. *J Pain* 2003;4(2):91–100.

61. Khatami M, Woody G, O'Brien C. Chronic pain and narcotic addiction: a multitherapeutic approach—a pilot study. *Compr Psychiatry* 1979;20:55–60.

62. Wiedemer NL, Harden PS, Arndt IO, et al. The opioid renewal clinic: a primary care managed approach to opioid therapy in chronic pain patients at risk for substance abuse. *Pain Med* 2007;8:573–584.

63. Jamison RN, Ross EL, Michna E, et al. Substance misuse treatment for high-risk chronic pain patients on opioid therapy: a randomized trial. *Pain* 2010;150(3):390–400.

64. Morasco BJ, Gritzner S, Lewis L, et al. Systemic review of prevalence, correlates, and treatment outcomes for chronic non-cancer pain in patients with comorbid substance use disorder. *Pain* 2011;152(3):488–497.

65. Wilsey BL, Fishman SM, Tsodikov A, et al. Psychological comorbidities predicting prescription opioid abuse among patients in chronic pain presenting to the emergency department. *Pain Med* 2008;9:1107–1117.

66. Akbik H, Butler SF, Budman SH, et al. Validation and clinical application of the Screener and Opioid Assessment for Patients with Pain (SOAPP). *J Pain Symptom Manage* 2006;32:287–293.

67. Graziotti P, Goucke R. The use of oral opioids in patients with chronic nonmalignant pain: management strategies. *Med J Austr* 1997;167:30–34.

68. Jovey RD, Ennis J, Gardner-Nix J, et al. Use of opioid analgesics for the treatment of chronic noncancer pain: a consensus statement and guidelines from the Canadian Pain Society, 2002. *Pain Res Manag* 2003;8(suppl):3A–28A.

69. Kalso E, Allan L, Dellemijn PL, et al. European Federation of Chapters of the International Association for the Study of Pain. Recommendations for using opioids in chronic non-cancer pain. *Eur J Pain* 2003;7(5):381–386.

70. U.S. Department of Veteran Affairs. *VA/DoD Clinical Practical Guidelines: Management of Opioid Therapy for Chronic Pain*. Washington, DC: U.S. Department of Veteran Affairs; 2003.

71. Orhurhu VJ, Pittelkow TP, Hooten WM. Prevalence of smoking in adults with chronic pain. *Tob Induc Dis* 2015;13(1):17. doi:10.1186/s12971-015-0042-y.

72. Centers for Disease Control and Prevention. Current cigarette smoking among adults —United States, 2005–2015. *MMWR Morb Mortal Wkly Rep* 2016;65(44):1205–1211.

73. Zvolensky MJ, McMillan K, Gonzalez A, et al. Chronic pain and cigarette smoking and nicotine dependence among a representative sample of adults. *Nicotine Tob Res* 2009;11(12):1407–1414.

74. Ditre JW, Brandown TH, Zale EL, et al. Pain, nicotine, and smoking: research findings and mechanistic considerations. *Psychol Bull* 2011;137(6):1065–1093.

75. Pomerleau OF. Nicotine and the central nervous system: biobehavioral effects of cigarette smoking. *Am J Med* 1992;93(1A):2S–7S.

76. D'Silva J, Devadiga S, Dengody PK, et al. Smoking and chronic pain. *J Health* 2014;1(2):34–39.

77. Lawton J, Simpson J. Predictors of alcohol use among people experiencing chronic pain. *Psychol Health Med* 2009;14(4):487–501. doi:10.1080/13548500902923177.

78. Zale EL, Maisto SA, Ditre JW. Interrelations between pain and alcohol: an integrative review. *Clin Psychol Review* 2015;37:57–71.

79. Hasin DS, Stinson FS, Ogburn E, et al. Prevalence, correlates, disability, and comorbidity of DSM-IV alcohol abuse and dependence in the United States: results from the National Epidemiologic Survey on alcohol and related conditions. *Arch Gen Psychiatr* 2007;64(7):830–842.

80. Huckle T, You RQ, Casswell S. Socio-economic status predicts drinking patterns but not alcohol-related consequences independently. *Addiction* 2010;105(7):1192–1202.

81. Bien TH, Burge R. Smoking and drinking: a review of the literature. *Int J Addict* 1990;25(12):1429–1454.

82. Manchikanti L, Cash KA, Damron KS, et al. Controlled substance abuse and illicit drug use in chronic pain patients: an evaluation of multiple variables. *Pain Physician* 2006;9(3):215–225.

83. Grant BF. The impact of a family history of alcoholism on the relationship between age at onset of alcohol use and *DSM-IV* alcohol dependence: results from the National Longitudinal Alcohol Epidemiologic Survey. *Alcohol Health Res World* 1998;22(2):144–147.

84. Hoftun GB, Romundstad PR, Rygg M. Association of parental chronic pain with chronic pain in the adolescent and young adult: family linkage data from the HUNT Study. *JAMA Pediatrics* 2013;167(1):61–69.

85. Petry NM, Barry D, Pietrzak RH, et al. Overweight and obesity are associated with psychiatric disorders: results from the National Epidemiologic Survey on alcohol and related conditions. *Psychosom Med* 2008;70(3):288–297.

86. Conigrave KM, Saunders JB, Reznik RB. Predictive capacity of the AUDIT questionnaire for alcohol-related harm. *Addiction* 1995;90(11):1479–1485.

87. Hays RD, Merz JF, Nicholas R. Response burden, reliability, and validity of the CAGE, Short MAST, and AUDIT alcohol screening measures. *Behav Res Methods Instrum Comput* 1995;27(2):277–280.

88. Gache P, Michaud P, Landry U, et al. The Alcohol Use Disorders Identification Test (AUDIT) as a screening tool for excessive drinking in primary care: reliability and validity of a French version. *Alcoholism* 2005;29(11): 2001–2007.

89. Dybek I, Bischof G, Grothues J, et al. The reliability and validity of the Alcohol Use Disorders Identification Test (AUDIT) in a German general practice population sample. *J Stud Alcohol* 2006;67(3):473–481.

90. Moussas G, Dadouti G, Douzenis A, et al. The Alcohol Use Disorders Identification Test (AUDIT): reliability and validity of the Greek version. *Annal Gen Psychiatr* 2009;8(1):11.

91. Gompertz PH, Irwin P, Morris R, et al. Reliability and validity of the intercollegiate stroke audit package. *J Eval Clin Prac* 2001;7(1):1–11.

92. Barry KL, Fleming MF. The Alcohol Use Disorders Identification Test (AUDIT) and the SMAST-13: predictive validity in a rural primary care sample. *Alcohol Alcohol* 1993;28(1):33–42.

93. Reinert DF, Allen J. The Alcohol Use Disorders Identification Test (AUDIT): a review of recent research. *Alcoholism* 2002;26(2):272–279.

94. Bush K, Kivlahan DR, McDonell MB, et al. The AUDIT alcohol consumption questions (AUDIT-C): an effective brief screening test for problem drinking. Ambulatory Care Quality Improvement Project (ACQUIP). Alcohol Use Disorders Identification Test. *Arch Intern Med* 1998;158(16): 1789–1795.

95. Maxwell JC. The prescription drug epidemic in the United States: a perfect storm. *Drug Alcohol Rev* 2011;30(3):264–270.

96. Warner M, Hedegaard H, Chen LH. Trends in drug-poisoning deaths involving opioid analgesics and heroin: United States, 1999-2012. Available at: http://www.cdc.gov/nchs/data/hestat/drug_poisoning/drug_poisoning.htm. Accessed May 4, 2018.

97. Substance Abuse and Mental Health Services Administration, Center for Behavioral Health Statistics and Quality. The DAWN report. Available at: https://www.samhsa.gov/data/sites/default/files/DAWN2k11ED/DAWN 2k11ED/DAWN2k11ED.pdf. Accessed May 4, 2018 .

98. Chou R, Fanciullo GJ, Fine PG, et al. Clinical guidelines for the use of chronic opioid therapy in chronic noncancer pain. *J Pain* 2009;10(2):113–130.

99. Weisner CM, Campbell CI, Ray GT, et al. Trends in prescribed opioid therapy for non-cancer pain for individuals with prior substance use disorders. *Pain* 2009;145(3):287–293.

100. Ives TJ, Chelminski PR, Hammett-Stabler CA, et al. Predictors of opioid misuse in patients with chronic pain: a prospective cohort study. *BMC Health Serv Res* 2006;6(46):1–10.

101. Delcher C, Wagenaar AC, Goldberger BA, et al. Abrupt decline in oxycodone-caused mortality after implementation of Florida's prescription drug monitoring program. *Drug Alcohol Depend* 2015;150(1):63–68.

102. Webster LR, Webster RM. Predicting aberrant behaviors in opioid-treated patients: preliminary validation of the opioid risk tool. *Pain Med* 2005;6(6): 432–442.

103. Webster L. Loss of trust and empathy ends era of opioid self-assessment [published online ahead of print February 5]. *Pain Med*. doi:10.1093/pm /pny010.

104. Clark MR, Hurley RW, Adams MCB. Re-assessing the validity of the opioid risk tool in a tertiary academic pain management center population [published online ahead of print February 5]. *Pain Med*. doi:10.1093/pm /pnx332.

105. World Health Organization. Depression and Other Common Mental Disorders: Global Health Estimates. Available at: http://apps.who.int/iris /bitstream/10665/254610/1/WHO-MSD-MER-2017.2-eng.pdf. Accessed May 4, 2018.

106. Keefe F, Pryor R. Assessment of pain behaviors. In: Schmidt R, Willis W, eds. *Encyclopedia of Pain*. Heidelberg, Berlin: Springer.

107. Taloyan M, Lofvander M. Depression and gender differences among younger immigrant patients on sick leave due to chronic back pain: a primary care study. *Prim Health Care Res Dev* 2014;15(1):5–14.

108. Kroenke K, Wu J, Bair MJ, et al. Reciprocal relationship between pain and depression: a 12-month longitudinal analysis in primary care. *J Pain* 2001;12(9):964–973.

109. Larson S, Clark M, Eaton W. Depressive disorder as a long-term antecedent risk factor for incident back pain: a 13-year follow-up study from the Baltimore Epidemiological Catchment Area sample. *Psychol Med* 2004;34(2):211–219.

110. Currie SR, Wang J. More data on major depression as an antecedent risk factor for first onset of chronic back pain. *Psychol Med* 2005;35(9):1275–1282.

111. Turk DC, Okifuji A, Scharff L. Chronic pain and depression—role of perceived impact and perceived control in different age cohorts. *Pain* 1995;61:93–101.

112. Bair MJ, Robinson RL, Katon W, et al. Depression and pain comorbidity: a literature review. *Arch Intern Med* 2003;163:2433–2445.

113. Kroenke K, Spitzer RL, Williams JBW. The PHQ-9: validity of a brief depression severity measure. *J Gen Intern Med* 2001;16(9):606–613. doi:10.1046 /j.1525-1497.2001.016009606.x.

114. Gatchel RJ. *Clinical Essentials of Pain Management*. Washington, DC: American Psychological Association; 2005.

115. Robinson ME, Riley JL. The role of emotion in pain. In: Gatchel RJ, Turk DC, eds. *Psychosocial Factors in Pain: Critical Perspectives*. New York: Guilford; 1999:74–88.

116. Tang J, Gibson SJ. A psychophysical evaluation of the relationship between trait anxiety, pain perception, and induced state anxiety. *J Pain* 2005;6(9):612–619.

117. De Groot KI, Boeke S, van den Berge HJ, et al. Assessing short- and long-term recovery from lumbar surgery with pre-operative biographical, medical and psychological variables. *Br J Health Psychol* 1997;2:229–243.

118. Pavlin DJ, Rapp SE, Pollisar, N. Factors affecting discharge time in adult outpatients. *Anesth Analg* 1998;87(4):816–826.

119. Spitzer RL, Kroenke K, Williams JB, et al. A brief measure for assessing generalized anxiety disorder. *Arch Intern Med* 2006;166(10):1092–1097.

120. Asmundson GJG, Coons MJ, Taylor S, et al. PTSD and the experience of pain: research and clinical implications of shared vulnerability and mutual maintenance models. *Can J Psychiatr* 2002;47(10);930–937.

121. Prins A, Ouimette P, Kimerling R, et al. The Primary Care PTSD Screen (PC-PTSD): development and operating characteristics. *Prim Care Psychiatr* 2003;9:9–14.

122. Sparkes E, Duarte RV, Raphael JH, et al. Qualitative exploration of psychological factors associated with spinal cord stimulation outcome. *Chron Ill* 2012;8(4):239–251.

123. Powell R, Scott NW, Manyande A, et al. Psychological preparation and postoperative outcomes for adults undergoing surgery under general anesthesia. *Cochrane Database Syst Rev* 2016;(5):CD008646.

CHAPTER 22

Disability Evaluation of Patients with Chronic Pain

JAMES P. ROBINSON and **LEE GLASS**

Issues related to the evaluation of work disability claims by patients with chronic pain have been considered in the third and fourth editions of *Bonica's Management of Pain*. The purpose of this chapter is to build on the concepts and data provided in the earlier chapters. In particular, we hope to shed light on issues related to the evaluation of disability in chronic pain patients by contrasting the approaches to the problem taken by two disability agencies—the Social Security Administration (SSA) and the Washington State Department of Labor and Industries (DLI).

Basic Concepts

Many societies have programs of financial support for individuals with medical conditions that render them incapable of working. The agencies that administer these programs differ in many respects, but their broad mandate is to evaluate claims for disability benefits made by their constituents and decide whether to accept or reject the claims.

Agencies that administer disability benefits in the United States include the SSA, the Department of Veterans Affairs, the Department of Defense, the Office of Personnel Management, the Department of Labor, workers' compensation carriers, welfare programs, and private disability insurance companies. These agencies have somewhat different eligibility criteria, but they all must answer the following questions when evaluating someone who applies for work disability benefits.

1. Does the applicant have a medical condition that might interfere with his or her ability to work? If so, what is the diagnosis?
2. How severely impaired is the body part or organ due to the person's medical condition?
3. What kinds of activity limitations might the person reasonably be expected to have because of his or her impairment?
4. How do these expected activity limitations compare with the essential activities required by various jobs?

In addressing these issues, disability agencies generally emphasize the significance of objective medical evidence. They apply their conclusions regarding the facts of a case to the rules in their respective jurisdictions to determine whether a claimant is actually disabled. The basic challenge in the evaluation of chronic pain patients is that incapacitation that may be alleged is at least in part inherently subjective. This challenge was succinctly summarized in a monograph about the evaluation of pain for purposes of the SSA:

> The notion that all impairments should be verifiable by objective evidence is administratively necessary for an entitlement program. Yet this notion is fundamentally at odds with a realistic understanding of how disease and injury operate to incapacitate people. Except for a very few conditions, such as the loss of a limb, blindness, deafness, paralysis, or coma, most diseases and injuries do not prevent people from working by mechanical failure. Rather, people are incapacitated by a variety of unbearable sensations when they try to work.[1(p28)]

Thus, the challenge for disability agencies is to reliably and consistently determine the extent to which "unbearable sensations" affect individuals who apply for benefits. If they discount "unbearable sensations" completely, they are likely to deny benefits to applicants who are actually unable to maintain employment. If they rely too heavily on statements of "unbearable sensations," they might encounter two adverse outcomes: First, they might give preference to patients who communicate their struggles very effectively over more stoic patients who actually have more severe medical conditions. Second, because it is possible to feign severe pain, the agencies might award disability benefits to individuals with completely fraudulent claims.[2-5]

Conceptual and Empirical Issues

In order to study the role that chronic pain plays in work disability awards, observers and researchers must consider several issues. These were discussed in detail in the fourth edition of *Bonica's Management of Pain* and will be summarized only briefly here.

IMPAIRMENT AND DISABILITY

Two concepts that are central to the functioning of agencies that administer disability programs are "impairment" and "disability." Unfortunately, these terms do not have unique definitions because different disability agencies define them in slightly different ways.

Impairment

The definition of *impairment* given by the SSA is "anatomical, physiological, or psychological abnormalities that can be shown by medically acceptable clinical and laboratory diagnostic techniques."[6(p3)] This definition captures essential features of the concept. A key point is that impairments are construed as biomedical abnormalities that can be analyzed at the level of organs or body parts. In fact, a critical distinction between impairment and disability is that they address limitations at different levels of analysis. Impairment refers to a limitation in the function or structure of an organ or body part, whereas disability refers to a limitation in the behavior of a person. This distinction is reflected in the syntax used to describe impairments and disabilities. For example, one would say "Ms. Smith's right leg is weak because of her polio" to describe her impairment and "Ms. Smith is unable to walk up stairs" to describe her consequent disability. In summary, impairment can generally be considered to be a medical issue—typically, the presence of an abnormality that interferes with an individual's normal functional ability.

Disability

In its broadest meaning, *disability* refers to an inability to carry out necessary tasks in any important domain of life because of a medical condition. Several distinctions need to be made regarding it.

First, a distinction needs to be made between self-reported disability and disability as a social construct. In medical research, it is common for investigators to use self-reported disability as an outcome variable. For example, patients might be asked to complete the Roland-Morris scale, which assesses the extent to which they are limited in activities of daily living (ADLs) because of low back pain.[7] In this sense, disability is specific to the individual and is often closely linked to impairment: "Because of her knee injury, Ms. Smith is unable to walk up stairs." In contrast, "disability" for insurance purposes reflects a very different meaning. Government-regulated disability insurance systems, including workers' compensation and Social Security, all to a greater or lesser degree reflect a societal view of what benefits should be awarded to an individual: "Because she cannot walk up stairs, Ms. Smith should be awarded X dollars." This linkage of a term that refers at one level to something very specific to an individual, but at another level to a societal determination that is applied to all covered individuals, is often not fully recognized and is often the source of great consternation. Moreover, two different government systems, which may exist in the same geographical area, which offer benefits to the same covered populations, but whose benefits flow from decisions made by two separate and distinct legislative bodies, may offer greatly distinct benefits for what at the individual level may be the same disability.

If a disability agency determines that a patient is eligible for benefits, he or she is granted the social status of being disabled. As a consequence of this determination, he or she is exempted from selected customary societal obligations. If the type of disability in question is work disability, the individual may receive financial support to compensate for lost income.

An obvious but important point regarding disability as a social construct is that the process of disability evaluation starts when a person applies to an insurance company or disability agency. That is, the person alleges that he or she is disabled. The insurance company or disability agency then has the task of evaluating the claimant and deciding whether to accept or reject the allegation of disability.

A second distinction relates to the domain(s) in which activities are limited. For example, a C5 quadriplegic is disabled in the sense of being unable to carry out many basic ADLs. Such an individual might need an attendant to assist in the performance of ADLs. A person with early Alzheimer might be unable to manage financial affairs responsibly and thus might need a relative or friend to assume power of attorney. Individuals with a wide range of medical conditions might be disabled from work. Different disability agencies may include or exclude benefits for disability in these domains, depending on their legislative or contractual mandates.

Finally, there is a distinction between short-term and long-term disability. For example, injured workers who believe they are unable to work due to symptoms they consider to be work-related typically apply for benefits under a workers' compensation claim. Most of these "time loss" claims are resolved within a matter of a few weeks because most workers return to work after a short period of disability.[8] In contrast, some medical conditions produce limitations that continue for an individual's entire life, so that the disability agencies to which they apply must decide whether to grant permanent disability benefits.

This chapter focuses on long-term or permanent work disability as a social construct.

ASSOCIATIONS BETWEEN IMPAIRMENT AND DISABILITY

Disability agencies typically require objective medical data that demonstrate that an applicant has a medical condition that causes impairment. They develop schedules and procedures that allow adjudicators to create linkages between applicants' medical data and activity limitations that the applicants might reasonably be expected to have. In order to follow these procedures, they rely on the assumption of a strong linkage between impairment and disability. First, they construe impairment as

a necessary condition for disability. The logic underlying this requirement is straightforward, especially in relation to work disability. Disability programs are designed to assist individuals who are unable to compete in the workplace because of a medical condition. In essence, disability programs attempt to partition individuals who fail in the workplace into two large groups: those who fail because of a medical condition and those who fail for nonmedical reasons. The distinction is necessary because there are many potential nonmedical reasons that may restrict employment, including a lack of demand for an individual's skills or lack of motivation on the part of the individual. Disability programs require evidence that an applicant has a medical problem underlying his or her workplace failure. Impairment provides the needed evidence because it can be viewed as a marker that an individual has a medical problem, which diminishes his or her capability. Conversely, if an individual has no identifiable impairment, this implies that employment limitations are not due to a medical condition.

Second, disability agencies typically assume that the severity of a patient's impairment correlates with the degree and/or probability of his or her being disabled from work. Even when an agency compensates for work disability and not for impairment, it will often seek information about the severity of a patient's impairment to rationalize its decision about whether or not to award disability benefits.

Despite the administrative need of disability agencies to assume a tight relationship between impairment and disability, there is reason to doubt the strength of the relationship, at least when it comes to work disability. Observers over at least the past 75 years have noted that the ability of an individual to work depends on a host of factors, only some of which are medical.[9] The widely held belief that work disability is a product of both medical and nonmedical factors implies that statistical associations between results of medical evaluations and severity of work disability would be expected to be modest.

THE "EMBEDDEDNESS" PROBLEM

One conceptual problem in any discussion of pain-related impairment is that pain is not completely distinct from medical conditions that cause organ/body part dysfunction. Rather, it is usually most appropriate to construe pain as a "component" of a medical disorder. From this perspective, it is arbitrary to examine the significance of pain in isolation from the medical condition underlying the pain, just as it would be arbitrary to evaluate shortness of breath in isolation from congestive heart failure. It would be seem conceptually appropriate to evaluate a medical disorder as an entity with characteristic signs, symptoms (e.g., pain), and pathophysiology. An impairment rating based on such an evaluation would take into account all manifestations of the disorder, including pain. Many disability agencies follow this logic; that is, they construe pain as one of many manifestations of injuries or diseases. This conceptualization involves the implicit and, in some cases, explicit assumption that impairment ratings based on objective evidence of derangement of organs or body parts capture the burden of illness borne by an individual, including the burden imposed by pain.

Unfortunately, this apparently plausible approach to the assessment of pain in the context of impairment ratings can run into either of two complications. First, pain severity may not (and often does not) correlate well with objective indicators of organ/body part dysfunction. In fact, empirical evidence has consistently demonstrated a low concordance between self-reports of pain and behavioral functioning (such as ADLs) or physiologic indices.[10,11] In such situations, impairment ratings based strictly on objective findings are likely to fail to capture the burden of illness of the disorder.

A second and even more difficult situation involves conditions that are associated with severe pain but are not amenable to conventional impairment ratings because they are not associated with unequivocal objective findings. In these conditions, it is not possible to make impairment ratings on the basis of such findings. Common examples include headache disorders and fibromyalgia (FM).

PRACTICAL PROBLEMS IN IDENTIFYING THE ROLE OF PAIN IN DISABILITY DETERMINATIONS

In order for an investigator to determine the role that pain plays in the decisions that a disability agency makes, it is necessary to consider a few basic questions. First, what benefits does the disability agency offer and to what individuals? Second, what methods do adjudicators for the agency follow when they evaluate a disability claim? Third, what are the outcomes of the evaluations? That is, claimants with which types of medical conditions typically receive benefits? Some disability agencies treat both their evaluation methods and the results of the evaluations as proprietary, so that investigators do not have access to either kind of data. Other agencies publish information about their evaluation methods; those used by two disability agencies (DLI and SSA) are discussed in the following text.

Even when information about the methods adjudicators use is available, it is often difficult to obtain and interpret data regarding the results of the evaluations. As discussed earlier, the problem is that pain is embedded in medical disorders in complex ways. For example, a patient with a chronic lumbar radiculopathy might have atrophy and weakness in one lower extremity, along with severe pain. If such a patient were awarded disability, it might not be clear whether the award was made on the basis of the objective evidence of lower extremity dysfunction or on the basis of chronic pain.

In some medical conditions, incapacitation may occur primarily because of pain, so that if disability is attributed to the conditions, it is likely that pain, rather than objectively measurable organ impairment, is the basis for the calculation of the disability. Examples of such conditions include most spine disorders (unless there is evidence of spinal cord injury or cauda equina syndrome), most sprains and strains (unless there is clear evidence of major ligamentous or muscle injury), and complex regional pain syndrome. Moreover, there are at least a few disorders in which pain is the dominant feature, and there is no definable associated organ impairment. The most prominent example of this is FM. A disability agency that allows self-reported pain to serve as a basis for concluding that an impairment exists may conclude that, in a given case, the impairment is of sufficient magnitude to warrant a declaration of disability. The same patient in a system that mandates the presence of a condition that can be verified objectively as a foundation for a declaration of disability may, in the absence of such evidence, be denied such a declaration.

In the following discussion, the aforementioned conditions are considered proxies for disorders in which pain is the major driver of impairment. But seeking such proxies does not necessarily make the role of pain in disability awards fully apparent. Disability agencies may provide only very general information about the medical conditions of claimants who are awarded disability. For example, data from the SSA indicate that 31.7% of Social Security Disability Insurance (SSDI) awards were given for conditions labeled as "Diseases of the musculoskeletal system and connective tissue" (2015 Statistical Report, Table 21).[12] No details are given within this broad category, and it is virtually impossible to determine the role that claimants' pain played in the decisions that the SSA made. For example, a claimant with severe loss of function in both hands due to rheumatoid arthritis is lumped together with a claimant with chronic low back pain.

Somewhat more useful data are available from the Bureau of Labor Statistics (BLS). Data from 2015 reveal that 37% of all work injury claims leading to time off work were coded as "sprains, strains, or tears," and that an additional 16% were coded as "soreness, pain."[13] If we accept the premise that most of the patients diagnosed with "sprain" or "strain" receive the diagnosis when they present to health care providers with musculoskeletal pain but do not have clear-cut objective findings, it would appear that about 50% of the injuries that lead workers to take time off work involve pain as the major driver of incapacitation. The BLS also provides at least some data on the frequency with which spinal disorders lead to time off work. For example, in 2015, 31% of all time loss claims nationally were coded as musculoskeletal,[13] and at least in Arkansas, 46% of musculoskeletal conditions were coded as "back" conditions.[14] These data suggest that approximately 14% of claims leading to work disability are attributable to disorders of the spine. These figures are crude and address only short-term work disability. However, they strongly suggest that painful conditions are a major cause of time lost from work and may in many instances serve as the basis for declarations of disability.

Methods for Evaluating Chronic Pain in Applicants for Disability Benefits

The following discussion addresses the methods that adjudicators in two agencies use when evaluating pain in disability applicants—the SSA and the Washington State DLI.

EVALUATION METHODS IN THE SOCIAL SECURITY ADMINISTRATION

The U.S. SSA manages two disability programs—Social Security Disability Insurance (SSDI) and Supplemental Security Income (SSI). The programs use the same medical criteria when determining whether a claimant is in fact disabled from work but differ in their nonmedical eligibility requirements.

Adults who become disabled after working long enough to meet the SSA's "work credits" criteria[15(p4)] are eligible to apply to the SSDI program. The SSI program is available to individuals who do not meet the work credits criterion for SSDI eligibility and have very limited financial resources. It pays substantially less than the SSDI program. Many SSI recipients are children or adults who have been disabled since childhood.[16]

The present discussion focuses on adults applying for benefits under the SSDI program. For these claimants, disability is defined as "inability to engage in any substantial gainful activity by reason of any medically determinable physical or mental impairment which can be expected to result in death or which has lasted or can be expected to last for a continuous period of not less than 12 months."[15(p2)] "Substantial gainful activity (SGA)" is defined in terms of the amount of money the claimant is making or could make—in 2015, SGA was defined as making more than $1,090 per month.

The SSDI program is construed as a permanent (or at least long-term) disability program, and there is evidence that individuals who have been awarded SSDI rarely return to work.[17,18]

The SSDI and SSI programs represent the largest disability programs in the United States by a wide margin. More than 2.5 million Americans apply for benefits under one of the programs each year, and as of 2013, 12.71 million were receiving disability benefits.[19]

Adjudicators for SSA use the following five-step process in determining whether an applicant is to be awarded SSDI/SSI benefits (Fig. 22.1).[20,21]

1. Is the claimant currently engaged in SGA as defined earlier? If the claimant is engaged in SGA, he or she is not eligible for SSDI or SSI.
2. If not, does the claimant have a medically determinable impairment (or a combination of medically determinable impairments) that is severe and either has lasted for more

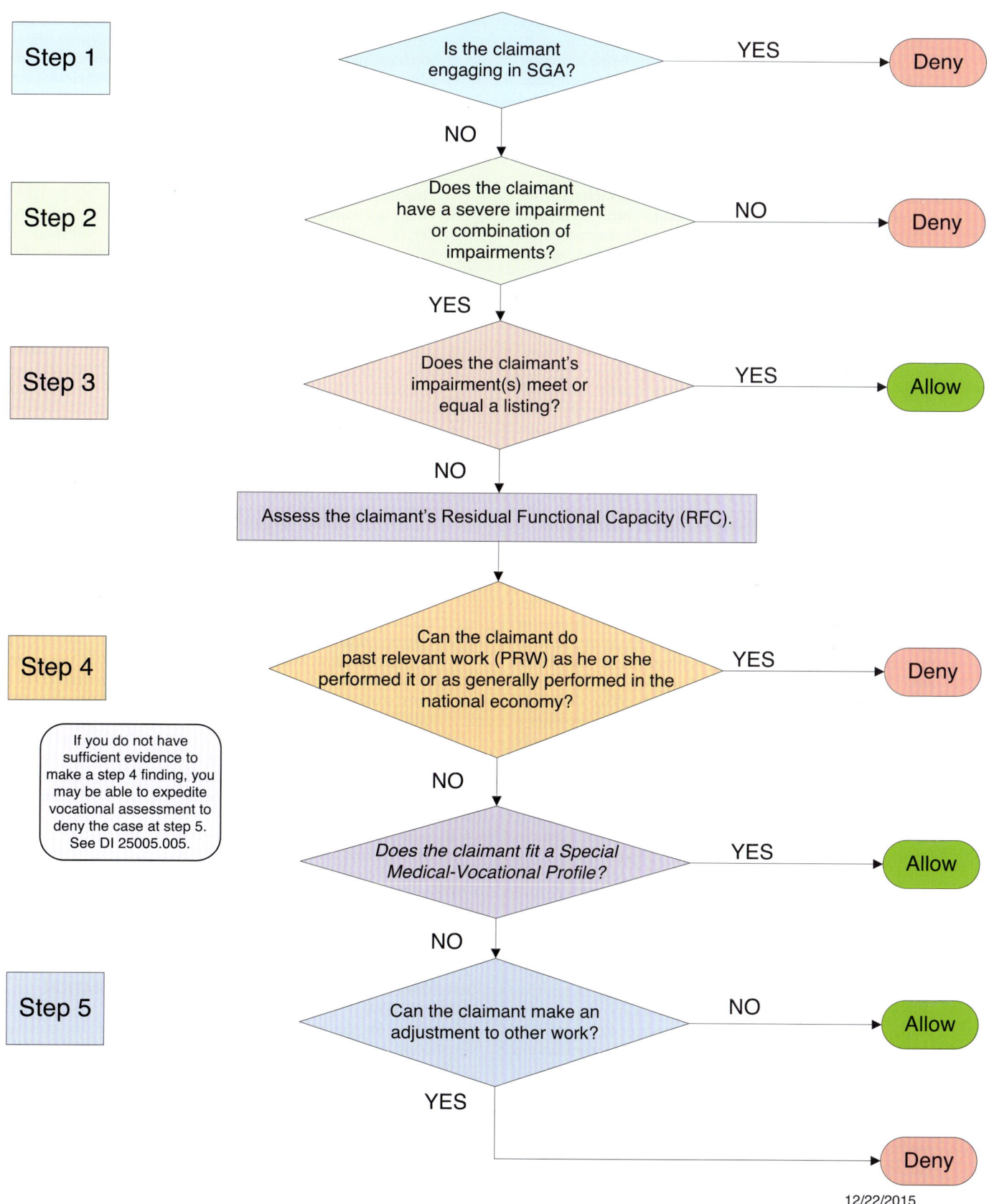

FIGURE 22.1 Social Security Disability Insurance steps.

than 12 months or is expected to last that long? If not, the claimant is not eligible.

3. If the criterion in step 2 is met, does the claimant's impairment meet a "listing," or is it medically equivalent to a listing? If yes, the claimant is awarded SSDI/SSI. If not, the evaluation proceeds to step 4.

4. Given the claimant's impairment, does he or she have sufficient residual functional capacity to perform work that he or she has actually performed in the past or that is similar to that work? If yes, the claimant is not eligible.

5. Given the claimant's residual functional capacity and other factors such as age, education, and work experience, does he or she have the ability to do any other kind of work? If yes, the claimant is not eligible.

The SSA provides detailed discussions of each of the steps.[20,21] For purposes of this chapter, several points need emphasis.

1. Adjudicators are instructed to consider both signs and symptoms of claimants. Pain is specifically mentioned as a symptom that should be considered. In theory, symptoms such as pain would make a claimant eligible for disability only if they were associated with signs and were considered secondary to a medically determinable impairment that is severe. The importance of signs is emphasized in "Disability evaluation under Social Security,"[6] which states that SSA regulations require "objective medical evidence" of impairment. Although this verbiage appears to require the presence of objective evidence of dysfunction of an organ or body part, a close examination reveals something more subtle. For example, SSA defines signs as "anatomical, physiological, or psychological abnormalities established by medically acceptable clinical diagnostic techniques that can be observed apart from individual's symptoms."[22] It is plausible to construe signs as akin to the objective medical findings mentioned earlier in this chapter. However, it appears that the SSA definition of "signs" basically acquiesces to the judgments of physicians regarding the findings that qualify as signs of a disease or injury. It does not specify that the findings must be ones that are not under the voluntary control of the claimant.[23] Essentially, the same logic applies to "medically determinable impairments." Again, the SSA defers to the opinions of physicians regarding what represents a medically determinable impairment—it does not require that such impairments be based on findings that cannot be influenced voluntarily by claimants. The evaluation of patients with FM highlights these issues. Because many patients with FM are awarded SSDI benefits,[24] it is clear that the SSA accepts either the diagnostic criteria articulated by the American College of Rheumatology in 1990 for diagnosing FM,[25] or the 2010, 2011, or 2016 modified criteria.[26-28] The latter three sets of criteria permit a diagnosis of FM without any clinical signs. The 1990 criteria include the responses of patients during tender point examinations, in which the examining practitioner palpates 18 designated sites on the body of a patient with approximately 4 kg of force and asks whether the palpation is painful. Patients are described as having positive tender point findings if they report pain in 11 or more of the 18 sites. The findings on a tender point examination could be viewed as a sign of FM, but it is obvious that a patient's responses during the examination are to some extent under voluntary control.

2. Step 2 of the evaluation protocol specifies that the medically determinable impairment must be severe. An impairment is described as severe if it has more than a minimal effect on an individual's physical or mental ability or abilities to do basic work activities.[29]

Text in "Disability Evaluation under Social Security"[6] states, "Once the existence of an impairment is established, SSA considers all evidence from all medical and nonmedical sources to assess the extent to which a claimant's impairment(s) affects his or her ability to function in a work setting; or in the case of a child, the ability to function compared to that of children the same age who do not have impairments. Nonmedical sources include, but are not limited to: the claimant, educational personnel, public and private social welfare agency personnel, family members, caregivers, friends, neighbors, employers, and clergy." Thus, symptoms reported by a claimant, as well as descriptions provided by her physician, friends, coworkers, etc., can influence an adjudicator to determine that a medically determinable impairment is severe.

3. Once a claimant has been found to have a medically determinable impairment that is severe, the subsequent steps in the decision-making algorithm center on the severity of the associated incapacitation. In evaluating severity, adjudicators are instructed to consider not only signs such as laboratory or imaging findings but also claimants' symptoms and their statements about the impact of their impairments on their ability to function. SSA specifies that pain and other symptoms should be considered when adjudicators determine whether an impairment is severe in step 2 of the evaluation process and also during steps 3 and 4 of the process.[30] Although SSA rulings indicate that adjudicators should look for consistency among medically determinable impairments, symptoms, signs, and various types of collateral data, the criteria for determining consistency are not well defined. The Program Operations Manual System (POMS) does specify that there should be qualitative congruence between a claimant's symptoms and his or her impairment.[30] Thus, for example, if a claimant were undergoing evaluation of a lumbar spine condition, her statement that she cannot raise her right arm above shoulder height would not be considered as evidence regarding the severity of her impairment. But the POMS is silent about the more difficult issue of how adjudicators might assess claimants' statements about the severity of limitations that are qualitatively congruent with their medical conditions. For example, it is not clear how an adjudicator evaluating a claimant with a lumbar spine condition would factor in the claimant's statement that she experiences unbearable pain if she sits for more than 15 minutes or walks more than one block.

In summary, the SSA considers pain and other symptoms throughout its five-step evaluation process. Although it nominally emphasizes signs at step 2, the fact that many FM patients receive SSDI or SSI awards strongly suggests that the SSA's requirements regarding signs include physical exam findings that are to some extent under the control of a patient.

OUTCOMES OF SOCIAL SECURITY ADMINISTRATION EVALUATIONS

Regardless of the procedures that SSA nominally follow when considering applicants for permanent disability, consideration of the types of claimants who actually receive disability awards could in principle provide important insights into the decision making of the agency. Unfortunately, data regarding the medical conditions of SSDI and SSI beneficiaries are difficult to obtain largely because the SSA classifies beneficiaries into very large diagnostic groups. For example, as noted earlier, 31.7% of SSDI beneficiaries in 2015 were classified as having "diseases of the musculoskeletal system and connective tissue." The problem with this broad category is that it does not differentiate between conditions that we consider proxies for chronic pain disorders from other musculoskeletal conditions.

There are a few publications from outside the SSA that do provide hints about chronic pain patients who are receiving SSDI or SSI benefits. For example, Meseguer[31] provided data indicating that about 11% of all SSDI awards are given to claimants with a diagnosis of "Disorders of the back (discogenic and degenerative)."

Walitt et al.[24] identified FM patients based on responses to the 2012 National Health Interview Survey. They found that 30% of individuals so identified reported that they had received "SS disability payments" during the previous years. The authors did not distinguish between SSDI and SSI recipients. These data are fragmentary but clearly support the conclusion that large numbers of people with at least two conditions which we consider proxies for chronic pain disorders—low back pain and FM—receive SSDI or SSI benefits.

DISABILITY EVALUATION AND DISABILITY MANAGEMENT IN THE WASHINGTON STATE DEPARTMENT OF LABOR AND INDUSTRIES

The Washington State DLI is the sole source of workers' compensation insurance for nonfederal employees in Washington State. (Companies of sufficient financial capability can elect to be self-insured, although they must provide the same benefits offered by DLI through its insurance program.) DLI serves as a funder of medical services and disability payments for injured workers. It provides additional services and has regulatory responsibilities that are not relevant to this chapter.

If a worker covered by DLI sustains an injury at work, he or she must file a claim in a timely manner in order to receive workers' compensation benefits. A health care professional typically files the claim on the worker's behalf. To be accepted by DLI, the claim must be supported by a licensed health care professional and submitted to DLI on a Report of Accident form. A claim for benefits will generally be allowed when the claim manager concludes that the worker has had an injury in the course of employment or has incurred an occupational disease in the course and scope of employment. The allowance determination is generally made by the claim manager based on the information provided by the worker and the health care professional on the Report of Accident. About 80% of claims do not involve more than 3 days of lost time from work. For these claims, DLI pays for medical services only. However, if the work injury or occupational disease causes the worker to miss more than 3 days from work, the worker is designated as being temporarily totally disabled from work and is eligible for wage replacement benefits from DLI. DLI proceeds on several fronts simultaneously in managing claims associated with wage replacement payments:

1. As described in the following discussion, DLI has instituted several programs to reduce the occurrence and duration of work disability associated with claims.
2. Repeated assessments of the worker's ability to work are made. Often, the attending provider for the worker's claim is asked to assess whether the worker has recovered well enough to return to work. DLI also has the option of referring the worker to an independent medical examination to get an opinion from physicians not involved in the injured worker's care.
3. Vocational rehabilitation services are often provided for the injured worker. Depending on the nature and extent of a worker's condition, the counselor who provides these services may help guide the injured worker back to the type of work that the worker did at the time of injury or

may provide guidance about other kinds of work that the worker might do.
4. Toward the end of a claim, DLI determines whether a worker's condition qualifies him or her for a permanent partial impairment award or a pension. A worker who is awarded permanent partial impairment receives a cash award from DLI that is determined by rules that relate to an assessment of the severity of the worker's impairment. Typically, the workers' compensation claim is closed following such an award. If it is determined that the worker is permanently disabled from reasonably consistent gainful employment and that the worker is not a candidate for vocational rehabilitation, the worker is deemed permanently totally disabled and is awarded a pension. In such cases, the claim is closed when the pension is awarded. Pensions in the DLI system are analogous to SSDI/SSI awards in the SSA system because they embody the premise that the worker is totally and permanently disabled and therefore eligible for wage replacement payments in perpetuity.

There are significant differences between the SSDI/SSI system and the DLI system. Some of the differences are the following:

1. As described earlier, and as more fully described in the following text, DLI interacts with injured workers in a variety of ways and over extended periods of time. In contrast, SSA makes only one determination regarding a claimant—whether he or she is eligible to SSDI/SSI benefits.*
2. DLI not only evaluates the impairment and disability status of injured workers but also utilizes multiple strategies to reduce the likelihood that injured workers will develop long-term disability (see the following discussion). In contrast, the mandate of SSA is strictly to make disability determinations.
3. Causation of a worker's inability to engage in employment is central to the DLI system. As a workers' compensation system, DLI is responsible only for injuries and occupational diseases that are proximately caused by workplace exposures. Therefore, when DLI adjudicators evaluate the reports of claimants' conditions, they consider both the severity of the workers' incapacitation and the causal relationship between the incapacitation and workplace exposures. In contrast, causation is irrelevant in the SSDI/SSI programs, so that the only task for adjudicators is to determine the severity of a claimant's incapacitation.
4. Information from nonmedical sources, such as friends of a claimant, is considered by adjudicators in the SSA system but generally not in the DLI system.

---

*In some instances, SSA makes a rapid decision to grant SSDI/SSI benefits to a claimant so that the claimant's interactions with SSA occur over only a short period of time. But if a claim for disability is rejected, the claimant has the option of going through a series of appeals leading up to a face-to-face hearing with an administrative law judge. Thus, an application for SSDI/SSI benefits can drag on for years. Also, if the applicant is finally denied SSDI/SSI, he or she can start the evaluation process all over again by filing another claim for disability benefits. Finally, although SSDI/SSI awards typically end up being permanent, SSA is required by law to review the eligibility of beneficiaries on a periodic basis.[32] This responsibility starts with a letter or similar communication to the beneficiary. It asks about the beneficiary's work status and medical treatment. This usually ends the reevaluation process, but in about 2.5% of instances, SSA officials refer the beneficiary's file for a more thorough evaluation after reviewing his or her responses to the mailing. This is carried out by agents of the Office of Continuing Disability Reviews and can lead to termination of the beneficiary's disability award.

WASHINGTON STATE DEPARTMENT OF LABOR AND INDUSTRIES PROGRAMS TO REDUCE DISABILITY

Pain that interferes with or prevents employment may have ramifications at many levels:

- It most obviously affects the individual, potentially adversely, in many ways.
- It will likely affect the individual's family—also adversely—in many ways.
- It may significantly impact the individual's employer through lost productivity and the need to hire and train a replacement worker. This is a special concern for small businesses for which the increased cost of DLI insurance because of an employee's work-related injury can force the closing of a business.
- It may affect coworkers through work redistribution and, potentially, in indirect ways secondary to financial impacts on the employer.
- It may affect society as a whole should its treatment be reflective of unsafe or ineffective practices, such as the use of high doses of opioids to treat chronic noncancer pain.

This section summarizes some of Washington State's efforts to minimize the potentially broad, adverse impact that pain can have on individuals, families, employers, coworkers, and society. Although this section focuses principally on workers' compensation matters, it will touch on Washington State's efforts to ensure that the pain-related health care services for which it pays are safe and effective.

Since 2006, it has been the intent of the Washington State legislature that health care programs for which state agencies pay will deliver care that is based "to the extent possible, upon the best available scientific and medical evidence."[33] The legislature has passed a number of bills over the years to facilitate the implementation of its intent. For example, it passed legislation that created the Health Technology Clinical Committee (HTCC) and gave that committee the authority to determine, after an evidence-based review, whether a given health technology will be included as a covered benefit in health care programs of the participating state agencies.[34] The HTCC has assessed, among others, technologies used to treat pain, such as spinal cord stimulation and spinal injections. Based on its evidence reviews, the committee has determined that certain pain-related technologies should be covered, others covered with conditions, and certain others not covered. Its determinations bind all state agencies that purchase health care services.

Separately, the legislature mandated that all state-purchased health care programs, with minor exceptions, implement evidence-based best practice guidelines or protocols applicable to advanced diagnostic imaging services.[35] Such imaging studies are commonly used by health care providers in the diagnosis and treatment of pain-related conditions.

The Washington legislature created the Robert Bree Collaborative[36] and gave the Collaborative the charge of identifying health care services in the state that meet the following criteria:

- The services are associated with substantial variation in practice patterns, or
- The services are associated with high utilization trends in Washington State, but
- The services do not produce "better care outcomes for patients, that are indicators of poor quality and potential waste in the health care system."

When the Collaborative identifies such a service, it is charged with several responsibilities that are intended to potentially lead to improved services. The Collaborative must, among other responsibilities,

- Analyze and identify evidence-based best practices and guidelines that are relevant to the issue,
- Identify data collection and reporting that is necessary to develop baseline health service utilization rates, and
- Identify strategies to increase the use of evidence-based best practice approaches among those providing the services.

The aforementioned, and other actions of the Washington State legislature with regard to evidence-based medicine, inform and give direction to the development of programs by which state agencies fund services that diagnose and treat pain and other conditions. Among others, these programs affect prisoners, Medicaid recipients, retirees covered by state pensions, and injured workers. The following paragraphs focus on the panoply of services potentially available to Washington State's injured workers who present with pain.

With the exception of employment that falls under federal jurisdiction, all workers' compensation insurance in Washington State is sold by the state's DLI. An employer with a sufficiently large economic base may be allowed to self-insure, but all other employers must purchase insurance through the state fund run by DLI. Self-insured employers are required to follow the same policies that DLI mandates in state fund claims.

DLI has sought to create an environment in which workers with pain can be successfully and efficiently diagnosed and treated. In significant part, DLI has endeavored to positively incentivize physicians (medical doctors, doctors of osteopathic medicine, physician assistants, advanced registered nurse practitioners, dental surgery doctors, and others who can serve as attending health care providers) to follow occupational medicine best practices and relevant evidence-based guidelines. These efforts on DLI's part have included the following:

- Modest financial incentives for following certain best occupational medicine practices. For example,
  - In Washington State, it is the physician who first sees the worker who files the Report of Accident. Because DLI cannot pay for benefits until a claim is filed, DLI has authorized an incentive payment for physicians to file the Report of Accident within two business days of its creation.
  - Similarly, because long-term disability can be minimized in many cases by an employer keeping an injured worker in the workplace, DLI created an incentive payment for physicians to telephone the employer if the worker is to be removed from employment or placed on restricted activities. Physicians are able to advise employers about restrictions and can help employers define work activities that will not adversely affect the injured worker.
  - A modest payment was created to incentivize the health care provider to see the patient at least every 2 weeks and to complete an Activity Prescription Form at each visit.
  - A payment was also created to incentivize disability assessment at 4 weeks' postinjury if the worker is not back to work, in the absence of a clear medical explanation for the worker's inability to engage in employment. An example of such an explanation might be a pending surgery.

  It is noteworthy that these four modest incentive payments, after 1 year of implementation, produced the following results, among others[37]:
  - There was a 30% reduction in disability claims for back injuries.
  - Disability days per claim were reduced by 4.1 days ($P = .004$).
  - Disability costs were reduced by $347 per claim, and medical costs were reduced $245 per claim, after subtracting the program costs (each $P \leq .001$).
  - There was a 20% reduction in the likelihood of 1-year disability.
- The creation of Centers for Occupational Health and Education (COHE). DLI contracts with organizations that provide health service coordinators (HSCs) who facilitate injured workers' medical needs by interfacing on the care providers' behalf with DLI. These coordinators

function as an aid to the providers and injured workers, not as an agent of the insurer. For example, should a patient be given return-to-work restrictions, which occurs in about 30% of industrial injury cases, an HSC can interface on the physician's behalf with both the claim manager and the employer to assure that the restrictions are understood and to explore their impact on the patient's return to work.

- The piloting of a three-question Functional Recovery Questionnaire (FRQ) to guide care coordination and treatment decision making. DLI has found that the answers to three questions in its FRQ can help predict long-term disability. With that understanding, DLI authorizes payments to COHE HSCs to assist workers' caregivers in devising treatment approaches that may reduce the risk of long-term disability.[38] Functional recovery interventions (FRIs) that follow FRQ-related disability concerns may include the following:
  - Addressing biopsychosocial considerations, including recovery expectations, activity avoidance, and concerns about work activities potentially aggravating the industrial condition;
  - Addressing returning to work, including speaking with the employer, assessing the availability of modified work, and using the services of an HSC, or DLI staff, to assist the patient in returning to work;
  - Incrementally increasing activity, potentially monitored by review of a weekly activity diary with appropriate follow-up and a physical therapy or occupational therapy referral if needed;
  - Emphasizing and tracking functional improvement, including setting specific functional improvement targets and timelines and potentially using a validated instrument to track functional progress;
  - Should an employer not be able to offer modified duty to an injured worker, involvement of an HSC to explore whether there are other return-to-work options that may be available;
  - If the patient is awaiting surgery or a specialty consultation, reinforcing the need for the patient to be an active participant in his or her recovery, addressing concerns that the patient about discomfort or aggravation while becoming or staying active; and
  - Offering a structured program in which a trained activity coach who combines skill development to address biopsychosocial factors with sessions that focus on progressive increases in activity.
- The creation of Centers of Excellence for Burns and Amputations. Not uncommonly, catastrophic injuries result in severe pain, at times from major burns, and not uncommonly associated with limb compromise. Such injuries require considerable expertise and multidisciplinary health care services. To assure that the risk of harm from such injuries is minimized and to facilitate the best possible outcomes from those injuries, DLI has contracted with a tertiary care facility to provide the health care services needed by such catastrophically injured workers.[39]
- The creation of a Center of Excellence for Chemically Related illnesses. DLI has contracted with a tertiary care facility to provide the necessary multidisciplinary care to address the needs of workers who have been chemically injured.
- Providing a process to assess return-to-work for workers who have been given restrictions. DLI's computer system flags claims in which restrictions have been placed and brings them to the attention of COHE-employed HSCs. Acting as resources for workers' providers, HSCs contact injured workers, answer (or find answers to)

questions that the workers may have, assess return-to-work issues, and have such discussions with employers and providers as may be helpful in assuring the safe and efficient return to the highest reasonably attainable functional level.

- Providing access to activity coaching resources. A treating provider may request that DLI provide funding for activity coaching. DLI can fund such coaching for workers who have not been able to return to work by 4 weeks following injury, who are not making progress with early interventions such as physical or occupational therapy, and who are not being considered for surgery. The coaching that is funded by DLI involves 10 weekly 1-hour sessions that may be in-person or telephonic.[40]
- Providing, in a pilot program, incentive payments to surgeons who demonstrate and document high-quality and efficient patient care. The performance of surgeons seeking such payments is measured against their compliance with six specified quality indicators. Payments are tiered. To receive Tier 1 pay, a surgeon must demonstrate compliance with three specified quality indicators. Surgeons who qualify for Tier 1 incentive payments will receive payments at the Tier 2 level if they are additionally in compliance with one or two of three other quality indicators. Surgeons who are in compliance with all six quality indicators receive payments that are at the Tier 3 level.[41]
- In collaboration with Washington State's Industrial Insurance Medical Advisory Committee (IIMAC), developing guidelines that are applicable to the diagnosis and treatment of industrial injuries and occupational diseases. In 2007, the legislature mandated that DLI establish an industrial insurance medical advisory committee, and it specified the duties and the composition of the committee.[42]† In collaboration with the IIMAC and subject matter experts selected by the IIMAC, in an open and transparent process that includes opportunities for public comment, DLI has developed guidelines related to the diagnosis and treatment of multiple body regions and conditions that commonly present as pain or paresthesia. The guidelines combine medical literature evidence as developed by a master's-level epidemiologist with input from subject matter experts from the medical and surgical communities. These guidelines serve as the basis for utilization review recommendations to claim managers.
- Making a best effort attempt to assure that injured workers are not further harmed by the treatment they receive for their industrial injuries and occupational diseases. In addition to the guideline development process described

---

†Revised Code of Washington 51.36.140 states, "(1) . . . The industrial insurance medical advisory committee shall advise the department on matters related to the provision of safe, effective, and cost-effective treatments for injured workers, including but not limited to the development of practice guidelines and coverage criteria, review of coverage decisions and technology assessments, review of medical programs, and review of rules pertaining to health care issues. . . . (2) The industrial insurance medical advisory committee is composed of up to fourteen members appointed by the director. The members must not include any department employees. The director shall select twelve members from the nominations provided by statewide clinical groups, specialties, and associations, including but not limited to the following: Family or general practice, orthopedics, neurology, neurosurgery, general surgery, physical medicine and rehabilitation, psychiatry, internal medicine, osteopathic, pain management, and occupational medicine. At least two members must be physicians who are recognized for expertise in evidence-based medicine. The director may choose up to two additional members, not necessarily from the nominations submitted, who have expertise in occupational medicine. . . ."

earlier, DLI has addressed the public health crisis of accidental deaths involving prescribed opioids in a variety of ways. These have included development of an online opioid dose calculator so prescribers can easily calculate the morphine equivalent dose (MED) of prescribed opioid medications and efforts to educate prescribing doctors in the potential harms that opioids can cause. Additionally, DLI has adopted stringent administrative regulations that include the following[43]:

- Mandatory prescriber checking of the prescription monitoring program database, if available
  - Before opioids are prescribed in the subacute phase of an injury
  - At risk-related intervals if chronic opioid therapy is prescribed
- Recommended prescriber checking of the prescription monitoring program database for first-time prescriptions and for preoperative evaluation for surgery
- Mandatory administration of a urine drug test, followed by appropriate documentation of the results, during the subacute phase of an injury, and at repeated risk-related intervals if prescribing chronic opioid therapy
- Mandatory use of validated instruments to track pain and function when prescribing opioids during the acute and subacute phase of an injury and regularly at not greater than 90-day intervals when chronic opioid therapy is prescribed
- For workers who were on opioid therapy prior to their work injury, nonpayment of opioids beyond the acute phase, except for catastrophic injuries, and for other severe injuries for which payment may extend to the subacute phase of the injury
- If opioids are to be prescribed during the acute phase of the injury (0 to 6 weeks)
  - Mandatory assessment and documentation of baseline pain and function measurements
- If opioids are to be prescribed during the subacute phase (6 to 12 weeks of the injury)
  - Mandatory verification of clinically meaningful improvement in function and pain with the use of opioids during the acute phase;
  - If indicated, mandatory use of a validated instrument to screen the worker for comorbid psychiatric conditions, such as depression or anxiety;
  - Verification of the absence of contraindications to the use of opioids;
  - Mandatory checking of the prescription monitoring program database, if it is available, to verify that the controlled substance history is consistent with the prescribing record and with the worker's report;
  - Mandatory use of a validated screening instrument to verify the absence of any current substance use disorder (except nicotine) or a history of opioid use disorder;
  - Mandatory administration of a baseline urine drug test to verify the absence of cocaine, amphetamines, alcohol, and nonprescribed opioids; and
  - Verification that the worker shows no evidence of, and is not at high risk for, serious adverse outcomes from opioid use.
- If opioids are to be prescribed during the chronic phase (beyond 12 weeks of the injury)
  - Documentation that clinically meaningful improvement in function has occurred with opioid therapy during the acute or subacute phases of the injury;
  - Reasonable alternatives to opioids have been tried and have failed;
  - A pain treatment agreement has been agreed on and signed by the worker and the prescribing physician;
  - Documentation of a consult with a pain management specialist if the opioid dose is to exceed 120 mg per day MED (with certain narrow exceptions);
  - Documentation of the absence to any contraindication to the use of opioids;
  - Documentation of the absence of the worker being at high risk of serious adverse outcomes from opioid use;
  - Documentation of the absence of more than one episode of aberrant behavior identified by the prescription monitoring program database, by urine drug testing, or by some other source; and
  - The creation of a time-limited treatment plan that documents how opioid therapy is predicted to improve the worker's work capacity, or the ability to progress in vocational rehabilitation.
- If chronic opioid therapy is to be prescribed
  - The prescribing doctor must, at risk-based intervals not to exceed 90 days, review the effects of opioid therapy and document the following best practices:
    - Clinically meaningful improvement in function is maintained with stable dosing;
    - If the opioid dose is increased, clinically meaningful improvement in function most be demonstrated in response to the dose change;
    - There must be a current signed pain treatment agreement;
    - The worker has no contraindication to opioid use, including substance use disorders (excluding nicotine), or a history of opioid use disorder;
    - The worker is not at high risk for serious adverse outcomes from opioid use;
    - There must be a consultation with a pain management specialist before the opioid dose is increased above 120 mg per day MED (with minor exceptions); and
    - The worker has not had more than one episode of aberrant behavior identified by the prescription monitoring program database, by urine drug testing, or by some other source.
- If opioids are to be prescribed to treat catastrophic injuries
  - There must be a current signed pain treatment agreement;
  - There must be a consultation with a pain management specialist before the opioid dose is increased above 120 mg per day MED (with minor exceptions);
  - The worker has not had more than one episode of aberrant behavior identified by the prescription monitoring program database, by urine drug testing, or by some other source;
  - The dose is stable; and
  - The worker is not at high risk for serious adverse outcomes from opioid use.
- Discontinuation of opioids
  - Opioid therapy must be discontinued if
    - The worker requests discontinuation; or
    - Out of concern for potential adverse outcomes the attending provider (who may not in all circumstances be the prescribing physician) requests opioid discontinuation; or
    - After 3 months of opioid maintenance therapy, there is no sustained clinically meaningful improvement in function, as measured by validated instruments; or

■ Risk of further treatment outweighs the potential benefits; or

■ The worker experienced an opioid overdose event related to

□ Aberrant behavior, or

□ Substance use disorder other than nicotine, or

□ A prescribing pattern that is not in compliance with applicable rules or guidelines, or

■ The worker has experienced any other severe adverse outcome; or

■ There has been more than one aberrant behavior, including, but not limited to

□ Inconsistent urine drug test results

□ Lost prescriptions

□ Multiple requests for early refills

□ Multiple prescribers

□ Unauthorized dose escalation

□ Apparent intoxication

● The use of opioids is not in compliance with applicable rules or guidelines.

○ Under certain circumstances, DLI may pay for weaning, detoxification, and/or addiction treatment.

In summary, DLI, acting as a state agency that administers a monopolistic workers' compensation insurance system, has used financial incentives, guidelines, and regulations that have the force of law in its efforts to assure that pain arising from industrial injuries is treated timely, safely and effectively.

METHODS USED BY WASHINGTON STATE DEPARTMENT OF LABOR AND INDUSTRIES TO EVALUATE INJURED WORKERS FOR PERMANENT DISABILITY BENEFITS

In determining whether an injured worker is entitled to a permanent disability award (also called a *pension*), the DLI adjudicator must determine, when the worker is at maximum medical improvement, whether a permanent impairment exists and, if so, its nature and extent. Whether a permanent impairment exists is determined by assessing information provided by health care professionals. Typically, treating providers or independent medical examiners identify the presence of any such impairment and describe its nature. If the adjudicator concludes that, on a more likely than not basis, a permanent impairment exists as the result of an industrial injury or occupational disease, the adjudicator must determine the extent of the impairment. Two principal inquiries are made; one relates to the extent of physical or mental impairment per se, and the other relates to the impact of the impairment on employability. To determine the extent of a physical or mental impairment for rating purposes, the adjudicator applies relevant medical information in the claim file to either the American Medical Association's *Guides to the Evaluation of Permanent Impairment* (5th edition) (AMA *Guides*)[44] or to a statutory rating system that applies to certain types of cases. The adjudicator must also determine whether the worker is employable given the worker's preinjury status and the effect that any impairment-related restrictions may have on his or her ability to return to employment. A discussion of the various factors that an adjudicator must take into consideration in making this determination is beyond the scope of this chapter, but the issue can be summarized as follows: If the worker can, given the restrictions that have been placed on him or her, return to a type of employment for which he or she is otherwise qualified, or if the worker has been successfully retrained for employment, the demands of which are consistent with his or her impairment-related restrictions, the worker is deemed employable. An employable worker receives a payment for the permanent impairment that has been calculated using the AMA *Guides* or the statutory rating system. A worker who is not employable due to the effects of an industrial injury or occupational disease may be awarded a pension. A pension from DLI is analogous to an SSDI/SSI award by SSA because they both require that a claimant be totally and permanently disabled from work.

The role that pain plays in DLI pension decisions can be seen by examining: (1) the AMA *Guides* handling of pain-related impairment and (2) policies that DLI has developed in relation to the evaluation of pain. The AMA *Guides* focuses on impairment rather than work disability. Thus, it addresses only some of the issues that SSA and DLI adjudicators address during disability evaluations. For the most part, the AMA *Guides* emphasizes objective assessment of organ/body part dysfunction and asserts that effects of pain can be assessed by determining the severity of organ/body part dysfunction with which the pain is associated. Thus, it states in Chapter 1, "Physicians recognize the local and distant pain that commonly accompanies many disorders. Impairment ratings in the AMA Guides 5th already have accounted for commonly associated pain, including that which may be experienced in areas distant to the specific site of pathology." Chapter 18 of the AMA *Guides*, which was coauthored by one of us (JPR), gives a very different message. It asserts that the impact of pain cannot always be determined by assessing objective indicators of organ/body part dysfunction and therefore needs to be directly assessed. However, Chapter 18 was written after all the other chapters of the AMA *Guides* had been completed, and the concepts outlined in it were never integrated into the rest of the book.

DLI's policies emphasize the importance of objective factors in its disability evaluations. DLI has determined that pain has been incorporated into both its statutory rating system for specified disabilities and into the ratings in the AMA *Guides*. Because pain is a subjective symptom and because a worker's report of pain cannot be objectively measured, DLI has determined that there is no valid, reliable, or consistent means to segregate the worker's subjective complains of pain from the pain already rated and compensated for in the conventional rating methods.[45] In providing self-insured employers with claims adjudication guidelines, DLI has written, "The AMA Guides to the Evaluation of PPD and the category system both incorporate subjective complaints. Subjective complaints, such as pain, cannot be objectively validated or measured. When rating PPD, reliance is primarily placed on objective findings."[46] Also, DLI has explicitly rejected the use of Chapter 18 of the AMA *Guides* in evaluations of injured workers in Washington State.[47]

OUTCOMES OF WASHINGTON STATE DEPARTMENT OF LABOR AND INDUSTRIES EVALUATIONS

DLI does not have fields in its claim-related databases that allow it to determine whether pain was a significant symptom leading to the filing of any given claim. Anecdotally, the great majority of injuries and most of the musculoskeletal occupational disease presentations involve pain or paresthesias. As discussed earlier, DLI generally does not accept liability for "pain" per se—accepted conditions typically are diagnoses that indicate the medical conditions that are thought to underlie workers' reports of pain.

In summary, DLI and SSA differ significantly in the ways they incorporate pain into disability awards. The differences in approach between the two systems to pain beg a question: Is it possible to determine which system is working better in distinguishing between chronic pain patients who are truly work disabled and ones who are capable of working? Unfortunately, we are not able to provide an answer to this question. We are not aware of any research that compares the outcomes of DLI versus SSA evaluations and believe such comparative research would be extremely difficult because of a host of methodologic problems.

Conclusion

This chapter has briefly discussed general conundrums related to disability awards for chronic pain and has discussed in detail the manner in which two disability systems that provide benefits in the same area, not uncommonly to the same individuals at the same time for the same medical condition have addressed these conundrums. The DLI and SSA systems were chosen in part for the practical reason that the authors are familiar with them. But there was another reason for choosing them: If chronic pain could easily be assessed and incorporated into disability evaluations, we would expect different disability agencies to use similar methods to evaluate it. In fact, though, the distinctly different legislative mandates under which DLI and SSA operate have resulted in very different approaches to the assessment of chronic pain. In our opinion, the differences between the two systems highlight differing societal views regarding disability in the context of chronic pain and also the challenge faced by any disability system in the evaluation of chronic pain.

References

1. Osterweis M, Kleinman A, Mechanic D, eds. *Pain and Disability*. Washington, DC: National Academy Press; 1987.
2. Bogdanich W. A disability epidemic among a railroad's retirees. *New York Times*. September 20, 2008: A1.
3. Railroaded [editorial]. *New York Times*. September 23, 2008: A28.
4. Wilson D. Insurers detail rail workers' path to disability pay. *New York Times*. November 14, 2008: A17.
5. Weiser B. Doctor gets eight years in L.I.R.R. fraud scheme. *New York Times*. May 24, 2013: A16.
6. Disability evaluation under Social Security. Available at: https://www.ssa.gov/disability/professionals/bluebook/general-info.htm. Accessed September 1, 2017.
7. Schiphorst Preuper HR, Reneman MF, Boonstra AM, et al. The relationship between psychosocial distress and disability assessed by the Symptom Checklist-90-Revised and Roland Morris Disability Questionnaire in patients with chronic low back pain. *Spine J* 2007;7(5):525–530.
8. Cheadle A, Franklin G, Wolfhagen C, et al. Factors influencing the duration of work-related disability: a population-based study of Washington State workers' compensation. *Am J Public Health* 1994;84(2):190–196.
9. International Labour Office. *The Evaluation of Permanent Incapacity for Work in Social Insurance* [Studies and Reports Series M #13]. Washington DC: The International Labour Office; 1937.
10. Flores L, Gatchel R, Polatin PB. Objectification of functional improvement after nonoperative care. *Spine* 1997;22:1622–1633.
11. Gatchel RJ. Comorbidity of chronic mental and physical health disorders: the biopsychosocial perspective. *Am Psychol* 2004;59:792–805.
12. Annual Statistical Report on the Social Security Disability Insurance Program, 2015. Available at: https://www.ssa.gov/policy/docs/statcomps/di_asr/2015/index.html. Accessed April 15, 2018.
13. Bureau of Labor Statistics. Nonfatal occupational injuries and illnesses requiring days away from work, 2015. *News Release*. November 10, 2016.
14. United States Department of Labor, Bureau of Labor Statistics. Number, incidence rate, and median days away from work for nonfatal occupational injuries and illnesses involving days away from work for musculoskeletal disorders by part of body and ownership, Arkansas, 2015. Available at: https://www.bls.gov/iif/oshwc/osh/case/ar2015_pob.pdf. Accessed September 1, 2017.
15. Social Security Administration. *Annual Statistical Report on the Social Security Disability Insurance Program, 2015*. Washington, DC: Social Security Administration. Available at: https://www.ssa.gov/policy/docs/statcomps/di_asr/2015/di_asr15.pdf. Accessed September 1, 2017.
16. Social Security Administration. *SSI Annual Statistical Report, 2015*. Washington, DC: Social Security Administration. Available at: https://www.ssa.gov/policy/docs/statcomps/ssi_asr/2015/index.html. Accessed September 1, 2017.
17. Muller LS. Disability beneficiaries who work and their experience under program work incentives. *Soc Secur Bull* 1992;55(2):2–19.
18. Stapleton D, Liu S, Phelps D, et al. *Work Activity and Use of Employment Supports under the Original Ticket to Work Regulations: Longitudinal Statistics for New Social Security Disability Insurance Beneficiaries*. Washington, DC: Social Security Administration; 2010.
19. Tatham SJ, Wiener ML. Evaluating subjective symptoms in disability claims. Available at: http://www.acus.gov/publication/evaluating-subjective-symptoms-disability-claims. Accessed September 1, 2017.
20. Johns T. SSA's sequential evaluation process for assessing disability. Available at: https://www.ssa.gov/oidap/Documents/Social%20Security%20Administration.%20%20SSAs%20Sequential%20Evaluation.pdf. Accessed September 1, 2017.
21. Social Security Administration. Program Operations Manual System. DI 22001.001. Sequential Evaluation of Title II and Title XVI Adult Disability Claims. Available at: https://secure.ssa.gov/poms.nsf/lnx/0422001001. Accessed September 1, 2017.
22. Social Security Administration. Program Operations Manual System. DI 24501.020. Establishing a medically determinable impairment (MDI). Available at: https://secure.ssa.gov/apps10/poms.nsf/lnx/0424501020. Accessed September 1, 2017.
23. Robinson JP, Turk DC, Loeser JD. Pain, impairment, and disability in the AMA Guides. *J Law Med Ethics* 2004;32(2):315–326.
24. Walitt B, Nahin RL, Katz RS, et al. The prevalence and characteristics of fibromyalgia in the 2012 National Health Interview Survey. *PLoS One* 2015;10(9):e0138024.
25. Wolfe F, Smythe HA, Yunus MB, et al. The American College of Rheumatology 1990 criteria for the classification of fibromyalgia. Report of the Multicenter Criteria Committee. *Arthritis Rheum* 1990;33:160–172.
26. Wolfe F, Clauw DJ, Fitzcharles MA, et al. The American College of Rheumatology preliminary diagnostic criteria for fibromyalgia and measurement of symptom severity. *Arthritis Care Res* 2010;62:600–610.
27. Wolfe F, Clauw DJ, Fitzcharles MA, et al. 2016 Revisions to the 2010/2011 fibromyalgia diagnostic criteria. *Semin Arthritis Rheum* 2016;46:319–329.
28. Wolfe F, Clauw DJ, Fitzcharles MA, et al. Fibromyalgia criteria and severity scales for clinical and epidemiological studies: a modification of the ACR preliminary diagnostic criteria for fibromyalgia. *J Rheumatol* 2011;38:1113–1122.
29. Social Security Administration. Program Operations Manual System. DI 24505.005. Evaluation of Medical Impairments that are Not Severe. Available at: https://secure.ssa.gov/poms.NSF/lnx/0424505005. Accessed September 1, 2017.
30. Social Security Administration. Program Operations Manual System. DI 24501.021. Evaluating Symptoms. Available at: https://secure.ssa.gov/poms.nsf/lnx/0424501021. Accessed September 1, 2017.
31. Meseguer J. Outcome variation in the Social Security Disability Insurance program: the role primary diagnoses. *Soc Secur Bull* 2013;73(2):39–75.
32. Social Security Administration. Program Operations Manual System. DI 28001.003 An Overview of Processing Continuing Disability Review (CDR) Mailer Forms SSA-455 and SSA-455-OCR-SM. Available at: https://secure.ssa.gov/poms.nsf/lnx/0428001003. Accessed September 1, 2017.
33. Wash Rev Code §41.05.013.
34. Wash Rev Code §70.14.110.
35. Wash Rev Code §70.250.030.
36. Wash Rev Code §70.250.050.
37. Wickhizer TM, Franklin G, Fulton-Kehoe D, et al. Improving quality, preventing disability and reducing costs in workers' compensation healthcare: a population-based intervention study. *Med Care* 2011;49:1105–1111.
38. Washington State Department of Labor and Industries (L&I). https://www.lni.wa.gov/ClaimsIns/Providers/Reforms/EmergingBP/FuncRecover.asp. Accessed April 21, 2018.
39. Washington State Department of Labor and Industries (L&I). http://lni.wa.gov/News/2016/pr160223a.asp 37. Accessed April 19, 2018.
40. Washington State Department of Labor and Industries (L&I). http://lni.wa.gov/ClaimsIns/Providers/Reforms/EmergingBP/Coaching.asp. Accessed April 18, 2018.
41. Washington State Department of Labor and Industries (L&I). http://lni.wa.gov/ClaimsIns/Providers/Reforms/SurgicalPilot/default.asp. Accessed 18, 2018.
42. Wash Rev Code §51.36.140.
43. Wash Admin Code §296-20-03035 through §296-20-03085.
44. Cocchiarella L, Andersson GBJ, eds. *Guides to the Evaluation of Permanent Impairment*. 5th ed. Chicago, IL: American Medical Association; 2001.
45. Wash Admin Code §296-20-19030.
46. Washington State Department of Labor and Industries. Permanent partial disabilities. Available at: http://www.lni.wa.gov/ClaimsIns/Files/SelfIns/ClaimMgt/PermanentPartialDisabilities.pdf. Accessed September 1, 2017.
47. *Rating Permanent Impairment* [Provider Bulletin 02-12]. Olympia, WA: Department of Labor and Industries, Health Services Analysis Section; 2002.

CHAPTER 23

Multidisciplinary Assessment of Patients with Chronic Pain

DENNIS C. TURK and **JAMES P. ROBINSON**

This chapter deals with the multidisciplinary assessment of patients with chronic noncancer pain. In order to be specific, especially with regard to the medical evaluation of chronic pain patients, we organize the discussion around a typical and common chronic pain problem (e.g., persistent cervical spine pain). We note, though, that many of the concepts in the chapter are relevant to the assessment of virtually any chronic pain patient. In particular, concepts related to the assessment of psychological factors, social factors, and functional limitations have wide applicability.

A key premise in this chapter is that multiple factors influence the symptoms and functional limitations of patients with chronic pain. As a consequence, we believe that evaluation along multiple dimensions, performed by professionals with a variety of skills, provides important insights into the factors governing the reports of these patients and assists in treatment planning.

Conceptual Issues

CONUNDRUMS IN THE ASSESSMENT OF PAIN

How we think about symptoms such as pain influences the way in which we go about evaluating patients. Physicians and the lay public alike tend to assume that some underlying pathology is both a necessary and a sufficient cause of the symptoms reported and experienced by patients. Consequently, medical assessment usually begins with taking a thorough history and performing a physical examination, followed by, when deemed appropriate, laboratory tests and diagnostic imaging procedures in an attempt to identify or confirm the presence of an underlying pathology that *causes* the symptom (see later). However, over the years, research has revealed puzzling observations that challenge the presumed isomorphism between pain and organic pathology. For example, the exact pathophysiology underlying some of the most common and recurring acute (e.g., primary headache) and chronic (e.g., back pain, fibromyalgia [FM]) pain problems is largely unknown. Thus, it is common for patients to have pain that cannot be attributed unambiguously to an organic pathologic process. Conversely, many people have abnormalities on diagnostic tests but no pain. For example, studies using plain radiography, computed tomography (CT), and magnetic resonance imaging (MRI) reveal that more than 30% of *asymptomatic* individuals have structural abnormalities such as herniated disks, spinal stenosis, joint space narrow in degenerative knees, and torn rotator cuffs that would be accepted as valid explanations of pain if the individuals had been symptomatic.[1-3] Thus, we are confronted with a rather strange set of circumstances: people with no identified organic pathology who report severe pain and, conversely, others with significant pathology who are apparently pain-free.

When health care providers are unable to identify organic pathology that reasonably accounts for a patient's reports of pain, they may assume that the reports reflect psychological factors such as personality characteristics, psychopathology, and malingering. A psychological evaluation may be requested to detect the psychological factors that underlie the patient's reports. Thus, there is a duality where the report of symptoms is attributed to *either* somatic *or* psychogenic mechanisms. This dualistic perspective dates back at least to the 17th century and the philosopher René Descartes. The assumption that symptoms that cannot be explained by medical findings must originate from psychological distress is, albeit unfortunately common, overly simplistic and inconsistent with current scientific understanding. The dichotomous view is incomplete and, as described throughout this chapter, is not compatible with available research evidence or the current understanding of chronic pain.[4]

A CONCEPTUAL MODEL FOR ASSESSING PAIN

The conundrums described suggest that multiple factors likely contribute to persistent pain and related disability. There is a growing consensus that these consist of (1) genetic composition[5]; (2) physical pathology associated with trauma or disease; (3) alterations in the peripheral and central nervous system (CNS) attributable to the initial insult (peripheral and central sensitization); (4) psychological contributors including various types of psychopathology, prior learning history, and available coping resources (e.g., emotional support, financial resources, acquired coping skills); and (5) environmental influences (e.g., response by significant others, disability compensation, features inherent in the workplace) that all likely interact. A comprehensive evaluation should provide information about each of these factors. Examination of unique genetic contributions is in its infancy at this time and is generally not performed in clinical settings, although it will likely be gaining attention in the coming years. Thus, in this chapter, we describe a general strategy for assessing factors 2 to 5.

Pain Behavior

It is useful to begin a discussion of assessment of patients with chronic pain with the concept of pain behaviors. Pain is a subjective perception, and there is currently no objective way to know about the experience of pain other than by patients' behavior. Pain behaviors include verbal behaviors (i.e., statements about pain). They also include nonverbal behaviors such as limping or wincing.[6] These pain behaviors are sources of communication; they convey to others the presence and severity of pain.

The challenge for an examiner is how to interpret patients' pain behaviors. Although these behaviors are sometimes determined entirely by an abnormal biologic process in the area of injury, they are typically also influenced by changes in nervous system encoding and processing of nociceptive signals; by a patient's beliefs and appraisals, emotional status, and coping strategies; and by the social environment.

Classes of Variables Underlying Pain Behavior

We will return to more formal assessment of pain behaviors later in this chapter. For now, a useful way to conceptualize this challenge is to think of a prediction equation with multiple unknowns: $PB = f(Xa_1, Xa_2 \ldots Xa_{an}; Xb_1, Xb_2 \ldots Xb_{bn}; Xc_1, Xc_2 \ldots Xc_{cn}; Xd_1, Xd_2 \ldots Xd_{dn})$.

Where PB = the pain behavior that a patient demonstrates, and predictor variables are organized into four categories, such that Xa_1, Xa_2 . . . Xa_{an} refer to biomedical factors at the end organ where the patient reports pain; Xb_1, Xb_2 . . . Xb_{bn} refer to alterations in nervous system function (especially CNS sensitization [CNSS]) that perpetuate pain after nociceptive impulses from the end organ have diminished or ceased; Xc_1, Xc_2 . . . Xc_{cn} refer to psychological variables; and Xd_1, Xd_2 . . . Xd_{dn} refer to social or contextual variables that influence pain behavior.[7]

The prediction equation emphasizes the multiplicity of factors that influence patients' expressions of pain and highlights the dilemma facing an evaluating clinician. The dilemma is that it is extremely difficult to determine the weights that should be assigned to various factors for an individual patient. To make matters even worse, there is no consensus about what the possible variables within various categories are (e.g., to specify the types of psychological factors that may affect a patient's pain behavior).

In accordance with the model, the discussion is organized around the assessment of medical factors, CNSS, psychological factors, and social factors in chronic pain patients. We also consider the assessment of the severity of functional incapacitation in these patients.

Assessment of Medical Factors

A careful medical evaluation is a basic element in a multidisciplinary evaluation of a patient with chronic pain. The general goals of such an evaluation are to (1) make a medical diagnosis, (2) determine whether additional diagnostic testing is needed, (3) make a judgment about the extent to which medical data regarding a patient adequately explain his or her symptoms and the severity of his or her apparent incapacitation, (4) determine

whether there is any medical or surgical treatment that has a reasonable chance of reversing the pathophysiologic processes underlying the patient's pain, (5) determine whether there are any symptomatic treatments that should be prescribed if a reversal of pathophysiology is not possible, and (6) establish the objectives of treatment.

The specific procedures that physicians perform and the differential diagnostic possibilities they entertain vary enormously with patients' symptoms and presumed medical disorders. For example, the medical evaluation of a patient with pelvic pain is entirely different from the evaluation of a patient with neck pain. Also, the medical evaluation of a pain patient depends on the chronicity of the patient's symptoms and the physical evaluations and diagnostic testing that the patient has already undergone.

In order to be reasonably specific, the discussion here focuses on the medical evaluation of patients with persistent neck pain, especially in the aftermath of a "whiplash" injury.

There is no uniformly accepted algorithm for evaluating neck pain patients. In fact, as will be discussed, clinicians differ sharply about some aspects of such evaluations. The approach discussed in the following section is summarized in Figure 23.1, which identifies key questions that should be asked in the evaluation of a patient with persistent neck pain.

ARE THERE RED FLAGS?

Although the assumption in this section is that the patient is undergoing evaluation for residuals of a neck injury, occasionally, the physician will find that the patient has misattributed his or her symptoms and is actually symptomatic because of a disease rather than because of any injury.

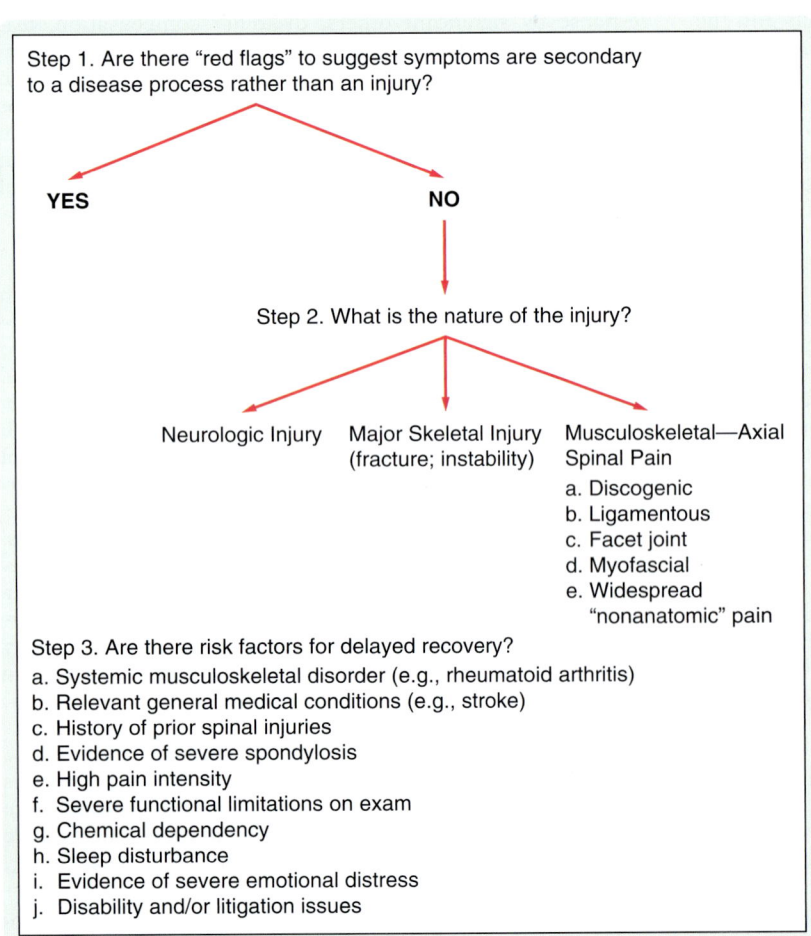

FIGURE 23.1 Key issues to address in the medical evaluation of chronic pain patients.

A general medical history that addresses issues such as weight loss or fevers should alert the physician to the possibility that a patient is symptomatic because of a disease such as an neoplasm or infection.[8,9]

If symptoms appear to be the result of injury, what is the nature of the injury?

1. Neurologic injuries. The physician needs to be alert to clinical evidence of a cervical radiculopathy or a myelopathy. Evidence for these possibilities is obtained from the patient's history (e.g., pain and paresthesias into an extremity in a segmental distribution) and a careful neurologic examination. Electrodiagnostic studies can provide additional evidence regarding the presence of a cervical radiculopathy[10]; MRI scans can provide evidence of anatomic compromise of nerve roots or the cervical spinal cord.[11–14]

2. Major skeletal injuries. When a history of significant trauma is elicited, radiologic studies are needed to rule out the possibility that a patient has a spinal fracture or a ligamentous injury severe enough to yield instability.[14–16] Although these major skeletal injuries are often accompanied by spinal cord injury or radiculopathy,[17] they may occur among individuals who are neurologically intact.[18]

3. Other musculoskeletal injuries (axial spinal pain). The overwhelming majority of patients with chronic neck pain do not have evidence of a neurologic injury or a major skeletal injury but present with localized axial cervical spine pain that suggests a musculoskeletal injury or with pain in a pattern suggesting referral from a joint in the cervical spine.[19,20] These patients are often very difficult to evaluate medically because there are no physical examination findings or diagnostic tests that unequivocally identify the structural basis of axial cervical spine pain. In this ambiguous situation, it is important for the examining physician to be aware of the structures that might underlie a patient's symptoms.

   a. Ligamentous injuries. Ligaments abound in the cervical spine, so pain felt to be ligamentous in origin could stem from various structures. The ligaments most often proposed as causes of axial cervical spine pain are the alar ligament, the posterior longitudinal ligament, and the facet joint capsular ligaments.[15,21,22] Because ligaments are critical to the stability of the cervical spine, severe damage to them is often assessed by looking for instability. Most commonly, this gross instability is associated with major skeletal injuries and is diagnosed in emergency room settings. A more subtle type of ligamentous abnormality has been postulated to be identifiable based on an abnormal MRI signal from ligaments, such as high signal intensity on proton attenuation–weighted high-resolution MRI. In principle, these signal abnormalities could reflect ligamentous injuries that cause pain but are not severe enough to cause instability. Some investigators have reported that ligamentous injuries identified by abnormal MRI signals play a significant role in whiplash injuries and that the severity of self-reported disability among people with these injuries correlates with the severity of the MRI signal abnormalities.[23–25] However, longitudinal studies on whiplash patients as well as research on asymptomatic people and ones with neck pain secondary to cervical degenerative conditions rather than injury suggest that the MRI signals that some investigators have interpreted as indicators of ligamentous injuries should actually be considered normal variants or indicators of cervical degenerative disk disease.[26–28]

   b. Disk pathology. It is widely accepted that cervical disk herniations can cause radiculopathies. But a more controversial issue is whether pathology of cervical disks can cause axial cervical spine pain and, if so, how such discogenic pain can be diagnosed and treated. Some investigators have proposed that cervical discogenic pain does occur and that it can be diagnosed via discography—a procedure in which imaging is performed after injection of contrast dye into a cervical disk and the pain response of the patient is assessed during injection of the dye and just after follow-up injection of a local anesthetic. The presence of an abnormal discogram, defined on the basis of some combination of the morphology of a disk and the pain responses of a patient during the procedure, is viewed as an indication that the disk accounts for the patient's pain and that a cervical spinal fusion is the appropriate definitive treatment.[29] The evidence supporting discography as a means of identifying cervical discogenic pain is weak, with some reviews concluding that there is no compelling evidence to support its use[30,31] and others specifically recommending against its use.[32] Skepticism regarding cervical spine discography is bolstered by research on lumbar spine discography. This research has demonstrated a high false-positive rate for discography, a tendency for psychosocially stressed people to have an especially high false-positive rate, and failure of spinal fusion based on discography results to produce satisfactory results.[29,33] Although dueling literature reviews make it somewhat difficult to reach any definite conclusions about cervical discogenic pain,[34] a reasonable conclusion is that although discogenic pain is biologically plausible,[31] no technology currently exists to demonstrate its presence in an individual patient or to provide treatment based on its suspected presence.

   c. Facet joint injury. Bogduk and colleagues[35–37] have asserted that facet joint injuries often underlie persistent cervical pain and have pioneered techniques for identifying painful facet joints on the basis of patients' reports of symptoms during injection procedures designed to provoke or palliate pain. Using these techniques, they have reported that approximately 70% of individuals with persistent neck pain following motor vehicle collisions have pain mediated by one or more of the cervical facet joints. Equally important, they have demonstrated that when patients diagnosed with facet joint–mediated pain receive injections (facet neurotomies) designed to denervate the affected facet joint, approximately 70% experience prolonged symptom relief.[37,38] More recent research has supported the importance of facet joint pathology in whiplash pain, although the frequency was reported as 29% rather than 70%.[39] As with discography, prominent teams of reviewers have reached opposite conclusions about the prevalence of facet joint–mediated pain, the validity of the diagnostic procedures used to diagnose this kind of pain, and the efficacy of invasive therapies to treat it.[30,32] It is beyond the scope of this chapter to try to resolve the discrepant assessments of facet joint–mediated whiplash pain, although we believe the evidence supporting it is more impressive than the evidence supporting discogenic pain.

   d. Muscle pain. Opinions about the prevalence and significance of muscle pain in chronic axial neck pain are, if anything, more divided than opinions about discogenic pain or pain associated with facet joint or ligamentous injury. Most investigators of muscle pain use the language and concepts developed by Travell and Simons,[40] who popularized the term *myofascial pain* and emphasized its importance as a cause of persistent musculoskeletal pain. Proponents of myofascial pain have argued that this is extremely common in patients with persistent neck pain. For example, one recent study found evidence of myofascial pain in 100% of a cohort 224 patients treated for chronic neck pain by primary care providers.[41] But the quality of the data supporting the importance of myofascial pain in spinal disorders is questionable,[42] and the term *myofascial pain* is not even mentioned in comprehensive reviews of neck pain (e.g., Côté et al.,[43] Hogg-Johnson et al.,[44] Holm et al.[45]). Again, it is beyond the scope of this chapter to resolve the conflicting views regarding the importance of myofascial problems among patients with chronic neck pain. But a few observations are worth making. First, there are no accepted diagnostic tests for myofascial pain. Clinicians rely on the history and physical examination to make the diagnosis. Second, clinicians should be aware that many neck pain patients will describe pain that suggests irritation of muscles and will report tenderness to palpation of neck and shoulder girdle muscles. Third, there is uncertainty about the appropriate interpretation of these symptoms and reports during physical exams. Because pain that seems to be muscular is typically widespread and because CNS hypersensitivity is now recognized as at

least one contributor to the pathophysiology of myofascial pain,[46] symptoms that some physicians construe as indicators of myofascial pain could instead be construed as widespread "nonanatomic" pain, or as pain secondary to CNSS rather than peripheral nociception.

4. Widespread "nonanatomic" pain. As described earlier, physicians who practice musculoskeletal medicine try to explain symptoms following a musculoskeletal injury in terms of some structural lesion in joints, periarticular tissues, muscles, and nerves in the body region where the patient is symptomatic.[47] The first step in this approach is to elicit a patient's symptoms and consider pathophysiologic processes that might reasonably account for them. But this approach founders when the symptoms of patients do not fit a pattern that suggests some discrete injury to a musculoskeletal structure. For example, Figure 23.2 is a pain drawing provided by a chronic pain patient who reported that she initially hurt her lower back pain when she lifted a heavy box on her job. Although the patient denied injuries other than her low back injury, the figure indicates that she was now experiencing widespread pain. In interpreting such figures, it is important to note that research has demonstrated that irritation of intervertebral disks and facet joints produces

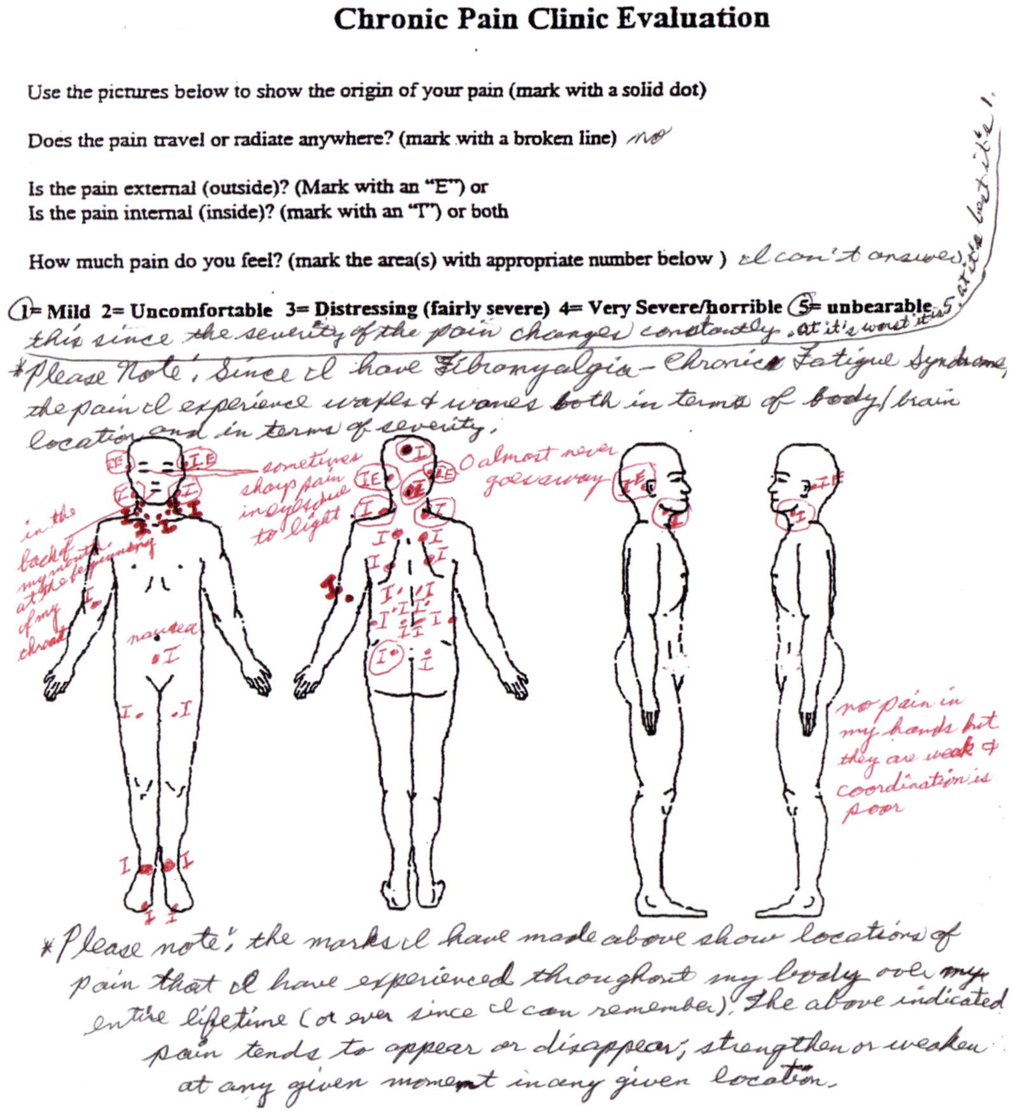

FIGURE 23.2   Patient indication of pain location.

characteristic patterns of referred pain[48,49] and that experts in myofascial pain have proposed characteristic patterns of referred pain from affected muscles. Thus, it is sometimes possible to explain widespread symptoms as indications of referred pain. However, the drawing shown in Figure 23.2 does not lend itself to such an interpretation because it does not conform to any known pattern of referred pain from an intervertebral disk, a facet joint, a ligament, or a muscle in the cervical region. The most plausible interpretation of such widespread pain is that it is a manifestation of altered perception based on CNSS (described later) or psychological factors.

ARE THERE RISK FACTORS FOR DELAYED RECOVERY?

It is important to evaluate risk factors for delayed recovery in a patient with chronic neck pain. Unfortunately, research on the validity of many potential indicators is lacking. Thus, the following list of indicators should be viewed as *plausible* candidates for consideration during the medical evaluation of a chronic pain patient rather than as proven predictors. Another caveat is that although some of the potential indicators refer to medical variables, others refer to psychosocial variables that might be evaluated better by a psychologist than by a physician.

- Presence of a systemic disorder of the musculoskeletal system, such as rheumatoid arthritis or one of the muscular dystrophies
  - Presence of general medical conditions that influence prognosis. For example, if a patient has severe cardiovascular disease, this may have implications for his or her ability to function in a physical therapy program. A patient who has had a stroke may have difficulty following medical directions.
  - History of prior spinal injuries or of significant prior symptoms in the absence of injury
  - Evidence of severe spondylosis
  - High pain intensity
  - Severe functional limitations on examination
- Chemical dependency. The patient's history in this domain is important because it may bear on the appropriateness of prescribing opioids or sedatives.
- Sleep disturbance. Disturbed sleep is a common symptom reported by chronic pain patients, and most clinicians who treat these patients accept the premise that disordered sleep plays a role in perpetuating symptoms and disability.[50] Thus, if a patient reports significantly disturbed sleep, a treatment plan for him or her should include interventions to promote normalization of sleep.
- Evidence of severe emotional distress
- Disability and litigation issues

SPECIFIC EVALUATION PROCEDURES

The physician should gather at least some information on most or all of the issues outlined earlier. For factors that are not biomedical, it is important for the physician to at least identify areas of concern, so that follow-up evaluations can be provided by the appropriate specialists. Broadly speaking, the information will come from three sources: the patient's history, the physical examination, and ancillary studies.

History

It is beyond the scope of this chapter to discuss the elements of a thorough history. It is worth noting, though, that in evaluating a chronic pain patient, the physician should pay careful attention to certain historical items that are considered only cursorily in other clinical settings. In particular, the physician should be careful to assess the patient's history with respect to

chemical dependency, sleep disturbance, apparent severity of incapacitation, and his or her status with respect to litigation and compensation.

Physical Examination

A neurologic and musculoskeletal examination should be performed on all patients with chronic cervical spine pain. In a patient with a normal neurologic examination, a musculoskeletal evaluation of the neck (including assessment of soft tissue hypersensitivity and range of motion) is often not especially revealing.[19] In particular, it is virtually impossible to identify a distinct pain generator on the basis of a physical examination of such patients. But some useful information can be gleaned from a musculoskeletal examination. First, the physician can determine the severity of the patient's functional limitations, especially restricted motion of the spine and pain-inhibited weakness of neck and extremity muscles. Second, the physician can check for hyperalgesia over muscles of the neck and shoulder girdle as well as more widespread hyperalgesia involving remote sites. Third, the physician can determine whether the patient demonstrates significant apprehension and "nonorganic signs."[51,52] Research indicates that patients with nonorganic signs usually have significant somatic anxiety. This emotional distress may impair their recoveries and may be a focus of treatment.

One caution about physical examination concerns the reliability of the assessment of factors such as range of motion. Evidence suggests that the interrater reliability of commonly performed physical examination tests is limited,[53,54] and thus, it is important to determine whether findings on a single examination are consistent with a patient's history, previous examination findings, and diagnostic tests.

Ancillary Studies

Although laboratory studies and electrodiagnostic evaluations are occasionally helpful in the assessment of patients with chronic neck pain, imaging studies are the procedures that are done the most frequently. There is significant controversy about how and when imaging should be done on chronic pain patients. When judged against guidelines, one-third to two-thirds of spinal CT and MRI imaging may be inappropriate.[55,56] High imaging rates can be problematic because irrelevant but alarming findings, including herniated disks, are common in asymptomatic people.[2,57] Without attempting to resolve these controversies in any systematic way, we suggest the following: (1) for pain involving a trauma, it is reasonable to check for the possibility of a fracture or significant spinal instability using plain x-rays of the spine; (2) additional imaging is generally not needed for such a patient, unless there is clinical evidence of a neurologic injury. In that case, an MRI scan is generally indicated; and (3) CT scans and bone scans usually have a limited role—they can be obtained to identify an occult fracture or an inflamed facet joint.

Another type of diagnostic test for patients with chronic neck pain is one that uses local anesthetic blocks of structures thought to be the pain generators. The logic underlying this approach is that if a patient reports dramatic relief following a local anesthetic injection of a structure in his or her neck, it is reasonable to assume that the structure is functioning as a pain generator for the patient. The most widely used procedures of this kind are nerve root blocks, medial branch blocks, and discography. As discussed earlier, there is controversy about how valuable local anesthetic blocks are in the diagnosis of patients with chronic neck pain. We believe that nerve root blocks can play an important role in identifying the structural basis of radicular symptoms and are often used to guide surgical decision making. We believe that medial branch blocks should be used selectively but can be helpful in the management of patients who do not have evidence of nervous system sensitization or psychological or social processes that might interfere with their recovery. We are skeptical of the value of discography in neck pain patients.

CONCLUSION

The previous discussion addresses the medical evaluation of chronic pain within the context of patients with cervical spinal pain. We have gone into some detail in order to make the point that medical decision making in relation to cervical spine pain is far from simple. It is our opinion that in order for pain patients to participate fully in evaluations of nonmedical factors contributing to their pain, they need to be confident that their problem has been evaluated thoroughly from a medical perspective. Thus, it is important for physicians participating in a multidisciplinary team either to have a lot of expertise in medical aspects of the problems that afflict their patients or to consult with colleagues who have this expertise.

Assessment of Central Nervous System Sensitization

During the past 35 years, CNSS has emerged as an important phenomenon in chronic pain.[58,59] Early research on nonhumans demonstrated that they predictably developed CNSS in response to tissue injury and that the CNSS was manifested by characteristic changes in the behavior of dorsal horn neurons in the spinal cord, including a lowered response threshold and an expansion of receptive fields.[59] Expansion of receptive fields was postulated to correlate with referral of pain and lowered response threshold with hyperalgesia.[60,61]

Several methods have been developed to assess CNSS in humans. Among them is quantitative sensory testing, which has shown that people with chronic pain demonstrate reduced thresholds to multiple modalities of sensory stimulation, including pressure, thermal, and electrical stimuli.[62,63] These abnormalities occur when stimuli are applied to the specific location of the reported pain and even to body regions where patients do not experience clinical pain.

Another approach has been to study withdrawal reflexes in response to potentially noxious stimuli. Relevant studies have shown that these reflexes can be elicited among chronic pain patients at lower stimulus intensities than the ones required to elicit the reflexes in healthy people.[64,65]

Still another promising method for assessing CNSS is functional MRI (fMRI). Several investigators have used fMRI methodology to identify brain areas associated with processing of noxious stimuli and have found that patients with chronic pain (e.g., FM, chronic low back pain, and chronic pelvic pain) demonstrate more dramatic activation of these areas than healthy controls.[66,67]

Findings from the aforementioned lines of inquiry have been interpreted by several researchers as evidence of CNSS among people with persistent pain[60] and as a central feature in the development of neuropathic pain.[68] Although these proposals have not been conclusively proven, the widespread belief among many neuroscientists and pain specialists that CNSS is a major factor in chronic pain has implications for the evaluation of the condition. At a conceptual level, CNSS challenges the simple dichotomy between organic pain and psychogenic pain that held sway in the orthopedic literature of a generation ago.[47] At the level of clinical evaluation of an individual patient, the absence of definitive tests to determine the presence of CNSS makes it difficult for a clinician to rule in or out the hypothesis that it is affecting symptoms. The ambiguity introduced by CNSS is increased by the fact that although it is usually identified during an examination by a physician, it is not a medical diagnosis in

the usual sense. For example, the *International Classification of Disease*, 10th edition, does not include any codes that can be used to designate that a patient's pain is a reflection of CNSS. Also, no clear delineation has been drawn between CNSS versus psychological factors as a cause of persistent symptoms. The evaluation of CNSS is given a separate section in this chapter because of its ambiguous middle ground status between traditional medical processes and psychological processes.

At a practical level, clinicians who treat chronic pain patients need to be aware that CNSS may be playing a role in the reports of their patients. One reason for this is that in the presence of CNSS, many of the inferential rules followed by clinicians when they interpret reports of pain are invalid because the rules are based on a simple model of an isomorphic correspondence between symptoms and dysfunction of tissues (nerves, joints, periarticular tissues, muscles) in the region where the patient indicates pain. The inferential rules are simply not valid when CNSS has occurred. For example, stocking glove numbness has long been considered a nonphysiologic complaint, but it can logically be interpreted as a result of CNSS.[69] Another practical issue is that clinicians should not expect to find a one-to-one relation between symptoms and a definable structural lesion in a patient whose pain is mediated by CNSS rather than by ongoing nociceptive input from specific body locations. Finally, clinicians need to be cautious about invasive therapies for patients whose pain is mediated by CNSS. The problem is that the pain of such patients may be generated primarily by spontaneous activity within the nervous system rather than by ongoing nociception from peripheral tissues, so that surgical alterations of tissues have little impact on it.

Given the potential importance of CNSS in the symptoms and functional limitations of pain patients, it would be highly desirable to have sensitive and specific tests to determine whether it is occurring in individual patients. Unfortunately, although the methods described earlier and several others have been examined in research on CNSS,[63,67] no definitive test for its presence is available for clinical use. In clinical settings, practitioners usually rely on various indirect indices to decide whether CNSS is playing a major role in their patients' symptoms.[70]

Assessment of Psychosocial Factors

A comprehensive psychological evaluation of a pain patient is a fundamental component of a multidisciplinary evaluation. It addresses the specific psychosocial, behavioral, cognitive, and contextual factors such as current mood (anxiety, depression, anger), interpretation of the symptoms, expectations about the meaning of symptoms, and the responses to the patient's symptoms by significant others (e.g., family members, coworkers), each of which contributes to the subjective experience of pain. This type of information should be included in the development of a comprehensive treatment plan.

PSYCHOLOGICAL FACTORS AS CAUSES VERSUS CONSEQUENCES OF CHRONIC PAIN
Psychological Factors as Causal Agents in Development of Chronic Pain

Patients often resist psychological evaluations because they intuitively sense that the outcome of such evaluations might be the conclusion that their pain is a result of psychological dysfunction rather than the injury to which they attribute their symptoms. Indeed, early reports suggested that preexisting psychopathology or neurotic traits might be the underlying mechanisms for unremitting chronic pain.[71,72] As early as 1953, Gay and Abbot[71] mentioned "neurotic reactions," noting that particular psychological factors predisposed an individual to chronic problems after an injury. In 1982, Blumer and Heilbronn[72] postulated that patients with chronic symptoms had a distinct personality type that predisposed them to developing chronic pain—"pain-prone personality." They specifically suggested that persistent symptoms offered a solution for their preexisting neurosis. There has been little empirical support indicating that the majority of chronic pain patients manifest character traits comprising a common and unique disposition.[73] However, some studies have noted the high lifetime prevalence of psychiatric diagnoses observed in chronic pain patients,[74] and prospective studies that followed healthy individuals who subsequently develop back pain[2] and from acute injuries to the presence of disabling pain[75] have observed that premorbid psychological factors were the best predictor of persistent pain chronicity.

Psychological Consequences of Chronic Pain

Psychological symptoms following the onset of pain have also been thoroughly documented. Acute and long-lasting psychological symptoms following symptom onset are prevalent.[76,77] Disabling emotional symptoms have been observed in as many as 59% of people following initial pain onset.[74]

A number of studies have implicated the role of the patient's idiosyncratic appraisals of his or her symptoms, expectations regarding the cause of the symptoms, and the meaning of the symptoms, in addition to organic factors, as essential in understanding the individual's report of pain and subsequent disability.[2,78] Moreover, the patient's current mood, ways of coping with symptoms, and responses by significant others including physicians may modulate the experience of pain, particularly chronic or recurrent pain.[79] Failure to address these factors can result in poor response to treatments that focus exclusively on somatic causes.

The results of many studies implicate psychological symptoms as *concomitants* rather than *precursors* to chronic symptoms after chronic pain.[80] Initial reaction to an injury, rather than the preexisting psychological status, has been shown to predict chronicity.[2,78] It seems reasonable that preexisting psychological status may predispose *some* individuals to chronic emotional disturbances following an injury. For example, acute emotional distress has been shown to be related to pain severity 1 month following a motor vehicle collision.[81] The correct answer is probably somewhere in the middle where preexisting psychological disturbances, immediate emotional reaction, coupled with medical complications contribute to chronicity of pain, at least for some people. In either case, these studies underscore the importance of evaluating psychological factors for all chronic pain patients.

ELEMENTS OF THE PSYCHOLOGICAL EVALUATION

Table 23.1 contains a brief set of salient issues with the acronym ACT-UP (Activity, Coping, Think, Upset, People's responses) that can be used as a guide for interviewing patients who report persistent or recurring symptoms. Generally, a referral for evaluation may be indicated where disability greatly exceeds what would be expected based on physical findings alone, when patients make excessive demands on the health care system, when the patient persists in seeking medical tests and treatments when these are not indicated, when patients display significant

emotional distress (e.g., depression or anxiety), or when the patient displays evidence of addictive behaviors or continual nonadherence to the prescribed regimen. Table 23.2 contains a detailed outline of the areas that should be addressed in a more extensive psychological interview for pain patients.

Interviews

A psychological interview with chronic pain patients is typically semi-structured. A structured format of psychiatric interview[82] can be incorporated as a tool to examine psychopathology. However, a psychological interview with pain patients' needs to go beyond an assessment of psychopathology because its main purpose is to assess a wide range of psychosocial factors (not just psychopathology) related to a patient's symptoms and disability.

When conducting an interview with chronic pain patients, the health care professional should focus not only on gathering information provided by the patient but also on observing patients' pain behaviors and the manner in which they convey information (e.g., facial expressions, movement patterns). We discuss some specific measures that have been proposed to systematically assess pain behaviors later.

Chronic pain patients' beliefs about the cause of symptoms, their trajectory, and beneficial treatments will have important influences on emotional adjustment and adherence to therapeutic interventions. A habitual pattern of maladaptive thoughts may contribute to a sense of hopelessness, dysphoria, and unwillingness to engage in activity. These reactions, in turn, deactivate the patient and severely limit his or her physical and emotional adaptation. The interviewer should also determine both the patient's and the significant other's expectancies and goals for treatment. An expectation that pain will be eliminated completely may be unrealistic and will have to be addressed to prevent discouragement when this outcome does not occur. Setting appropriate and realistic goals is an important process in pain rehabilitation as it requires the patient to attain better understanding of chronic pain and goes beyond the dualistic, traditional medical model—somatogenic versus psychogenic.

In order to help chronic pain patients understand the psychosocial aspects of pain, attention should focus on the patients' reports of specific thoughts, behaviors, emotions, and physiologic responses that precede, accompany, and follow pain episodes or exacerbation as well as the environmental conditions and consequences associated with their responses in these situations. During the interview, the clinician should attend to the temporal association of these cognitive, affective, and behavioral events; their specificity versus generality across situations; and the frequency of their occurrence to establish salient features of the target situations, including the controlling variables. The interviewer should seek information that will assist in the development of potential alternate responses, appropriate goals for the patient, and possible reinforcers for these alternatives.

Patients with chronic pain problems typically consume a variety of medications to alleviate their symptoms. It is important to discuss a patient's medications during the interview, as many pain medications (particularly opioids) are associated with side effects that may mimic emotional distress and can have deleterious adverse effects. A clinician, for example, should be familiar with side effects that result in fatigue, sleep difficulties, and mood changes to avoid misdiagnosis of depression. A general understanding of commonly used medications for chronic pain is important, as some patients also may use opioid analgesics to manage dysphoric mood that accompanies pain and its impact. During the interview, potential psychological dependence and aberrant drug-seeking behaviors on pain-relieving medications should be evaluated. In the majority of states in the United States, a physician is able to obtain a record of prescriptions of controlled substances. When in doubt, a psychologist

---

TABLE 23.1 Brief Psychosocial Screening: ACT-UP

Activities: How is your pain affecting your life (i.e., sleep, appetite, physical activities, relationships)?

Coping: How do you deal/cope with your pain (what makes it better/worse)?

Think: Do you think your pain will ever get better?

Upset: Have you been feeling worried (anxious)/depressed (down, blue)?

People: How do people respond when you have pain?

TABLE 23.2	Areas Addressed in Psychological Interviews

Experience of Pain and Related Symptoms
- Location and description of pain (e.g., "sharp," "burning")
- Onset and progression
- Perception of cause (e.g., trauma, virus, stress)
- What has the patient been told about the symptoms and condition? Does the patient believe that this information is accurate?
- Exacerbating and relieving factors (e.g., exercise, relaxation, stress, massage)
- Pattern of symptoms (e.g., worse certain times of day or following activity or stress)
- Sleep habits (e.g., difficulty falling to sleep or maintaining sleep, sleep hygiene)
- Thoughts, feelings, and behaviors that precede, accompany, and follow fluctuations in symptoms

Treatments Received and Currently Receiving
- Medication (prescribed and over-the-counter). How helpful have these been?
- Pattern of medication use (as needed, time-contingent), changes in quantity or schedule
- Physical modalities (e.g., physical therapy). How helpful have these been?
- Exercise (e.g., Do they participate in a regular exercise routine? Is there evidence of deactivation and avoidance of activity due to fear of pain or exacerbation of injury?). Has the pattern changed (increased, decreased)?
- Complementary and alternative (e.g., chiropractic manipulation, relaxation training). How helpful have these been?
- Which treatments have they found the most helpful?
- Compliance (adherence) with recommendations of health care providers
- Attitudes toward previous health care providers

Compensation and Litigation
- Current disability status (e.g., receiving or seeking disability, amount, percentage of former job income, expected duration of support)
- Current or planned litigation

Responses by Patient and Significant Others
- Typical daily routine
- Changes in activities and responsibilities (both voluntary and obligatory) due to symptoms
- Changes in significant other's activities and responsibilities due to patient's symptoms
- Patient's behavior when pain increases or flares up
- Significant others' responses to behavioral expressions of pain
- What does the patient do when pain is not bothering him or her (uptime activities)?
- Significant other's response when patient is active
- Impact of symptoms on interpersonal, family, marital, and sexual relations (e.g., changes in desire, frequency, or enjoyment)
- Activities that patient avoids because of symptoms
- Activities continued despite symptoms
- Pattern of activity and pacing of activity (can use activity diaries that ask patients to record their pattern of daily activities [e.g., sitting, standing, walking] for several days or weeks)

Coping
- How does the patient try to cope with his or her symptoms? Does patient view himself or herself as having any role in symptom management? If so, what role?
- Current life stresses
- Pleasant activities

Educational and Vocational History
- Level of education completed, including any special training
- Work history
- How long at most recent job?
- How satisfied with most recent job and supervisor?
- What like least about most recent job?
- Would the patient like to return to most recent job? If not, what type of work would the patient like?
- Current work status, including homemaking activities
- Vocational and avocational plans

Social History
- Relationships with family or origin
- History of pain or disability in family members
- History of substance abuse in family members
- History of or current, physical, emotional, and sexual abuse. Was the patient a witness to abuse of someone else?
- Marital history and current status
- Quality of current marital and family relations

Alcohol and Substance Use
- Current and history of alcohol use (quantity, frequency)
- History and current use of illicit psychoactive drugs
- History and current use of prescribed psychoactive medications
- Consider the CAGE questions as a quick screen for alcohol dependence.[a] Depending on response, consider other instruments for alcohol and substance abuse.[b]

Psychological Dysfunction
- Current psychological symptoms/diagnosis (depression including suicidal ideation, anxiety disorders, somatization, posttraumatic stress disorder). Depending on responses, consider conducting structured interview such as the Structured Clinical Interview for *Diagnostic and Statistical Manual of Mental Disorders* (4th ed., text rev.; DSM-IV-TR) (SCID).[c]
- Is the patient currently receiving treatment for psychological symptoms? If yes, what treatments (e.g., psychotherapy or psychiatric medications)? How helpful are the treatments?
- History of psychiatric disorders and treatment including family counseling
- Family history of psychiatric disorders

Concerns and Expectations
- Patient concerns/fears
- Explanatory models of pain held by the patient
- Expectations regarding the future and treatment (will get better, worse, never change)
- Attitude toward rehabilitation versus "cure"

Treatment Goals

[a]Adapted from Mayfield D, McLeod G, Hall P. The CAGE questionnaire: validation of a new alcoholism screening instrument. *Am J Psychiatry* 1974;131:1121–1123.
[b]Adapted from Allen JP, Litten RZ. Screening instruments and biochemical screening tests. In: Graham A, Schultz T, Wilford BB, eds. *Principles of Addiction Medicine*. Chevy Chase, MD: American Society of Addiction Medicine; 1998:263–278.
[c]Adapted from American Psychiatric Association. *User's Guide for the Structured Clinical Interview for DSM-IV Axis I: Clinician Version*. Washington, DC: American Psychiatric Press; 1997.

may recommend that such a record be obtained and request urine toxicology screening to rule out aberrant opioid-taking behaviors.[83]

Self-report Inventories
In addition to interviews, a number of standardized assessment instruments designed to evaluate patients' attitudes, beliefs, and expectancies about themselves, their symptoms, and the health care system have been developed and published. One survey[84]

of clinicians who treated pain indicated that the five most frequently used instruments in the assessment of pain, in order of frequency, were the McGill Pain Questionnaire,[85,86] Beck Depression Inventory (BDI),[87,88] Multidimensional Pain Inventory (MPI),[89] Coping Strategies Questionnaire (CSQ),[90] and the Oswestry Low Back Pain Disability Questionnaire.[91]

Standardized instruments have advantages over semi-structured and unstructured interviews. They are easy to administer, require less time, assess a wide range of behaviors, obtain information about behaviors that may be private (sexual relations) or unobservable (thoughts, emotional arousal), and, most importantly, have been submitted to analyses that permit demonstration of their psychometric properties (e.g., reliability and validity). These instruments should not be viewed as alternatives to interviews; rather, they are complements that may suggest issues to be addressed in more depth during an interview or investigated with other measures.

There is an important caveat when interpreting the results of patient self-report inventories. Studies of the psychometric properties of these inventories typically involve data collection from a large number of patients. As reliability estimates are influenced by sample size, it follows that the measurement error of questionnaire data from one person should be expected to be much greater than that found in reports based on group data.

PROBLEM AREAS TO ASSESS
Assessment of Pain
Pain Intensity
Self-report measures of pain often ask patients to quantify their pain by providing a single, general rating of pain: "Is your usual level of pain 'mild,' 'moderate,' or 'severe'?" or "Rate your typical pain on a scale from 0 to 10 where 0 equals no pain and 10 is the worst pain you can imagine." There are a number of simple methods that can be used to evaluate pain intensity—Numerical Rating Scale (NRS), Verbal Ratings Scale (VRS), and Visual Analog Scale (VAS) using different variation. For example, the Brief Pain Inventory (BPI) includes four individual questions using NRSs—right now, pain on average, pain at worst, and pain at least.[92,93]

Each of the commonly used methods of rating pain intensity, NRS, VRS, and VAS, appear sufficiently reliable and valid, and no one method consistently demonstrates greater responsiveness in detecting improvements associated with pain treatment.[94,95] However, there are important differences among NRS, VRS, and VAS measures of pain intensity with respect to missing data stemming from failure to complete the measure, patient preference, ease of data recording, and ability to administer the measure by telephone or with electronic diaries. NRS and VRS measures tend to be preferred over VAS measures by patients, and VAS measures usually demonstrate more missing data than do NRS measures. Greater difficulty completing VAS measures is associated with increased age and greater opioid intake, and cognitive impairment has been shown to be associated with inability to complete NRS ratings of pain intensity.[95] Patients who are unable to complete NRS ratings may be able to complete VRS pain ratings (e.g., none, mild, moderate, severe). Other measures are available to assess pain in children and those who are unable to verbally communicate (e.g., stroke patients, mentally impaired).[96,97]

There has been some concern expressed that retrospective reports may not be valid, as they may reflect current pain severity that serves as an anchor for recall of pain severity over some interval.[98,99] More valid information may be obtained by asking about current level of pain, pain over the past week, worst pain of the last week, and lowest level of severity over the last week (e.g., BPI). This has also led to the use of daily diaries that are believed to be more accurate as they are based on real time rather than recall. For example, patients are asked to maintain regular diaries of pain intensity with ratings recorded several times each day (e.g., at meals and bedtime) for several days or weeks. One problem noted with the use of paper-and-pencil diaries is that patients may not follow the instruction to provide ratings at specified intervals. Rather, patients may complete diaries in advance ("fill forward") or shortly before seeing a clinician ("fill backward").[99,100] These two reporting approaches undermine the putative validity of diaries. As an alternative to the paper-and-pencil diaries, a number of commentators have advocated for the use of electronic devices that can prompt patients for ratings and "time stamp" the actual ratings, thus facilitating real-time data capture.[100–102] Although there are numerous advantages to the use of advanced technology to improve the validity of patient ratings, they are not without potential problems, including hardware problems, software problems, and user problems.[103] These methods are also costly, and although they may be appropriate for research studies, their usefulness in clinical settings may be limited.

Pain Quality
Pain is known to have different sensory and affective qualities in addition to its intensity, and measures of these components of pain may be used to more fully describe an individual's pain experience. It is possible that the efficacy of pain treatments varies for different pain qualities, and measures of pain quality may therefore identify treatments that are efficacious for certain types of pain but not for overall pain intensity. Assessment of specific pain qualities at baseline also makes it possible to determine whether certain patterns of pain quality moderate the effects of treatment. The Short-Form McGill Pain Questionnaire (SF-MPQ)[86] assesses 15 sensory and affective pain descriptors, and its sensory and affective subscales have demonstrated responsivity to treatment in a number of clinical trials.[104] More recently, a revision of the SF-MPQ (SF-MPQ-2) was developed to increase the range of items (rated on a 0-to-10 scale) and items added to assess characteristics of neuropathic pain that have been not been adequately assessed in the SF-MPQ.[105]

Pain Modifiers
For the majority of people with chronic pain, pain severity varies. Thus, it is useful to inquire as to what the patient believes makes his or her pain worse. For example, are their specific activities that result in increase in symptoms? Are their certain circumstances that contribute to exacerbation of pain such as stress including interpersonal conflicts? Does pain vary with time of day? For example, does the patient notice that his or her pain is worse in the morning or later in the day? In the same way, it is important to identify factors that magnify or initiate pain episodes; it is important to ask about what factors result in reductions of pain. For example, does medication, rest, heat or cold, distraction, or exercise result in reductions of pain severity or even elimination of symptoms for some period? Pain may be influenced by the context or activities being undertaken. For example, pain intensity when an individual is at rest may differ substantially from pain experienced during movement. Thus, it is important to address what factors modify pain such as the nature of different activities.

Assessment of Overt Expressions of Pain
As noted previously, patients display a broad range of responses that *communicate* to others that they are experiencing pain, distress, and suffering. Some of these pain behaviors may be consciously controllable by the person, whereas others are not. Informally, a health care provider can observe patients' behaviors during their interviews and examinations. It is useful to observe patients in multiple contexts when possible (e.g., waiting room, ambulating to an exam room, during interview with clinician, during physical examination). When patients know they are being observed and are presenting information to a health care provider, they may use behavior to convey information in ways most likely to support the impact of their symptoms. They may feel a need to convince the health care provider of the severity of their symptoms, functional limitations, and distress. Thus, observation of the patient in the waiting room, when ambulating to the examination room, and when departing may allow the clinician to establish the stability and consistency of pain behaviors. We have also found it useful to observe patients in the presence of a significant other to note differences in behaviors when the significant other is present and absent and also how the significant other responds to the patient's pain behaviors.

A number of different observational procedures have been developed to identify and quantify pain behaviors. Structured methods that require patients to engage in a set of behaviors during which their behavior is observed and rated have been proposed by Keefe and colleagues.[106,107] Such structured approaches may be useful in research studies but can be cumbersome in clinical settings. Several investigators have developed observational Pain Behavior Checklists[108,109] that can be used in any setting. Although they have the advantage of efficiency, these methods may be less appropriate to compare among patients who are viewed in different contexts (e.g., during a physical examination or interview). As noted, the context may influence the behaviors observed. For example, the nature of pain behaviors observed might be quite different during a physically demanding examination compared to an interview. The number and nature of pain behaviors might be influenced by the presence of significant others during the observation period. At a minimum, it is important to note the context in which the behaviors were observed. Studies using Pain Behavior Checklists have found a significant association between these self-reports and behavioral observations. A variant of this observational procedure was developed by Kerns and colleagues[110] who developed a self-report version in which patients endorsed specific behaviors that they engaged in when they were experiencing pain.

Facial expressions and muscle patterns can provide objective, fine-grained analysis of the subjective experience of pain.[111] Formal assessment of facial expression has been found to be valuable in research but may be too complex for use in a clinical setting.

Uses of the health care system and analgesic medication are other ways to assess pain behaviors. Patients can record the times when they take medication over a specified interval such as a week. Despite the cautions regarding patient diaries noted, diaries can not only provide information about the frequency and quantity of medication but may also permit identification of the antecedent and consequent events of medication use. Antecedent events might include stress, boredom, or activity. Examination of antecedents is useful in identifying patterns of medication use that may be associated with factors other than pain per se. Similarly, patterns of response to the use of analgesic may be identified. Does the patient receive attention and sympathy whenever he or she is observed by significant others taking medication? That is, do significant others provide positive reinforcement for the taking of analgesic medication and thereby unwittingly increase medication use?

Assessment of Emotional Distress

The results of numerous studies suggest that chronic pain is frequently associated with emotional distress, particularly depression, anxiety, anger, and irritability. The presence of emotional distress in people with chronic pain presents a challenge when assessing symptoms such as fatigue, reduced activity level, decreased libido, appetite change, sleep disturbance, weight gain or loss, and memory and concentration deficits. These symptoms are often associated with pain and have also been considered "vegetative" symptoms of depressive disorders. Improvements or deterioration in such symptoms, therefore, can be a result of changes in either pain or emotional distress.

The BDI and BDI-2,[87,88] the Profile of Mood States (POMS),[112] the Hospital Anxiety and Depression Scale (HADS),[113,114] and Patient Health Questionnaire (PHQ-9)[115] have well-established reliability and validity in the assessment of symptoms of depression and emotional distress, and they have been used in numerous clinical trials in psychiatry and an increasing number of studies of patients with chronic pain.[116] In research in psychiatry and chronic pain, the BDI provides a well-accepted criterion of the level of psychological distress in a sample and its response to treatment. The POMS[112] assesses six mood states—tension–anxiety, depression–dejection, anger–hostility, vigor–activity,

fatigue–inertia, and confusion–bewilderment—and also provides a summary measure of total mood disturbance. Although the discriminant validity of the POMS scales in patients with chronic pain has not been adequately documented, it has scales for the three most important dimensions of emotional functioning in chronic pain patients (depression, anxiety, and anger) and also assesses three other dimensions that are very relevant to chronic pain and its treatment, including a positive mood scale of vigor–activity. Moreover, the POMS has demonstrated beneficial effects of treatment in some (but not all) chronic pain trials.[117,118] The HADS include seven items assessing anxiety and depression. One advantage of the HADS is that it was developed and standardized with medical patients rather than psychiatric patients. Shorter measures of anxiety (Generalized Anxiety Disorder [GAD]-7)[119] and depression (PHQ-9)[115] have been reported to provide reliable and valid assessments and might also be considered for research as well as clinical use. Any of these measures reasonable choices as brief measures of emotional distress.

As noted previously, various symptoms of depression—such as decreased libido, appetite or weight changes, fatigue, and memory and concentration deficits—are also common. It is unclear whether the presence of such symptoms in patients with chronic pain (and other medical disorders) should nevertheless be considered evidence of depressed mood or whether the assessment of mood in these patients should emphasize symptoms that are less likely to be secondary to physical disorders.[111,120]

Assessment of Fear

Many patients with chronic pain, especially those who attribute their symptoms to trauma, are fearful of engaging in activities that they believe may either contribute to further injury or exacerbate their symptoms. Avoidance of activities may, in the short term, lead to symptom reduction. But over time, restriction of activities is likely to lead to decreased functional capacities as a result of deconditioning. Also, avoidance of activity has the unfortunate consequence of preventing corrective feedback where patients can learn about their erroneous beliefs. Health care providers may inadvertently contribute to avoidance of activity by providing patients with cervical collars that restrict neck movements and advising them to avoid activities that hurt (i.e., hurt = harm). They may contribute to patients' anxiety that something is seriously wrong with their bodies by continuing to order sophisticated diagnostic tests in search of occult physical pathology. Self-report measures of fear of movement that might increase pain or physical damage are available (e.g., Tampa Scale of Kinesiophobia [TSK], Fear Avoidance and Beliefs Questionnaires [FABQ]).[121,122]

Assessment of Beliefs, Coping, and Psychosocial Adaptation to Pain

Historically, psychological measures designed to evaluate psychopathology have been used to identify specific individual differences associated with reports of pain, even though these measures were usually not developed for or standardized on samples of medical patients. Because disease status and medication can affect responses to such items, patients' scores may be elevated, thereby distorting the meaning of their responses. As a result, a number of measures have been developed for use specifically with pain patients. Instruments have been developed to assess psychological distress; the impact of pain on patients' lives, feeling of control, coping behaviors, and attitudes about disease, pain, and health care providers; and the patient's plight.[123,124]

Two particularly potent beliefs (i.e., self-efficacy and catastrophizing) held by patients have been demonstrated to play important roles in chronic pain. Self-efficacy is the conviction that one can successfully perform a certain task or produce a desirable outcome.[125] A major determinant of self-efficacy is prior mastery experience. In chronic pain patients, self-efficacy positively affects physical and psychological functioning,[126,127] and improvements in self-efficacy after self-management and cognitive-behavioral interventions are associated with improvements in pain, functional status, and psychological adjustment. Self-report instruments to assess self-efficacy with chronic pain patients have been developed and have been used in both clinical research and practice.[128,129]

Pain catastrophizing can be defined as an exaggerated negative orientation toward actual or anticipated pain experiences. Current conceptualizations most often describe it in terms of appraisal or as a set of maladaptive beliefs.[130] It is a cognitive and emotional process that involves magnification of pain-related stimuli, feelings of helplessness, and a negative orientation to pain and life circumstances. It includes obsessive rumination about pain, and its meaning and magnification of symptoms also are associated with decreases in pain severity ratings and functional disability. Catastrophizing has been shown to be an important predictor of response to both acute and chronic pain. Catastrophizing have been associated with increased perceptions of pain severity in both acute[131] and chronic pain severity[132] and disability among groups with diverse pain diagnosis.[132–134]

Several self-report measures of catastrophizing have been developed and shown to have good psychometric properties (Coping Strategies Questionnaire [CSQ],[90] Pain Catastrophizing Scale [PCS][135]). These measures have been used in both clinical research and contexts and have shown to have predictive validity for disability and response to various treatments. A brief, two-item measure of catastrophizing have been shown to have a high correlation with the longer form and may be useful as a screening device.[136]

Assessing Functional Impact

A major focus of the discussion earlier has been on the identification of factors underlying the symptoms of a chronic pain patient. It is important to note, though, that the identification of factors that qualitatively play a role in a patient's symptoms is not the same as an explanation of the severity of these symptoms or the extent to which the patient is disabled by them. Thus, we recommend that an evaluation of any chronic pain patient should include an assessment of the extent to which the patient is affected by his or her symptoms. When a multidisciplinary evaluation is conducted, physical therapists, vocational rehabilitation counselors, physicians, and psychologists may participate in the evaluation of function among pain patients. Conceptually, the impact of chronic pain on function can be subdivided into (1) the ability of patients to function in the sense of performing activities of daily living, (2) their physical capacities as demonstrated in a structured setting, and (3) their ability to function in adult roles such as work.[137]

Physical functioning and activity can be considered from three complementary perspectives, namely, the patient's perspective on his or her functioning (self-report), observation during performance on structure tasks in a clinical or laboratory setting (e.g., timed walking, gait pattern), and objective assessment of activity in the natural occurring environment (e.g., using technical instruments and devices such as accelerometry).[138,139] Each of these perspectives will provide different information about performance and are complementary. Objective assessment of physical functioning will depend to some extent on the nature of the physical capacity and diagnostic condition being assessed, and detailed discussions are beyond the scope of this chapter (see Taylor et al.[139] for a comprehensive review).

SELF-REPORT MEASURES OF FUNCTION

Self-report measures have been developed to assess people's reports of their abilities to engage in a range of functional activities such as the ability to walk up stairs, sit for specific periods of time, lift specific weights, and perform activities of daily living as well as the severity of the pain experienced upon the performance of these activities.[139] There are a number of well-established, psychometrically supported generic (e.g., Short-Form 36 [SF-36]),[140] pain-specific (e.g., BPI Interference Scale,[92] Pain Disability Index [PDI],[141] MPI Interference Scale), and diagnosis back pain–specific (Oswestry Low Back Pain Disability Questionnaire [OLBPQ],[91] Western Ontario McMaster Assessment of Knee and Hip Osteoarthritis [WOMAC])[142] measures of functional status (for a review, see Taylor et al.[139]).

The OLBPQ is a widely used, 10-item scale that asks patients about disability associated with back pain.[91] It has the advantage of being a disease-specific instrument. In general, disease-specific measures are designed to evaluate the specific effects of a disorder that may not be assessed by a generic measure.[138,139] In addition, responses on disease-specific measures will generally reflect the effects of comorbid conditions on physical functioning, which may confound the interpretation of change occurring over the course of a trial when generic measures are used. Disease-specific measures may be more sensitive to the effects of treatment on function, but generic measures provide information about physical functioning and treatment benefits that can be compared across different conditions and studies.[139,143] Each of these approaches has strengths. Decisions regarding whether to use a disease-specific or a generic measure, or some combination, will depend on the purpose of the assessment. For individual patients in clinical practice, it would be most appropriate to use measures developed on samples with comparable characteristics. If the clinician wishes to compare across a group of patients, then one of the broader based pain-specific measures should be considered. If the assessment is being performed as part of a research study, some combination might be appropriate to compare chronic pain samples with a larger population of people with diverse medical diseases (e.g., SF-36).

A particularly important aspect of physical functioning that is particularly important to those with chronic pain is sleep.[50] Pain is frequently reported as have a significant impact on sleep quality as well as duration.[144] Patients being evaluated should be asked about their sleep, and depending on the information acquired during an interview, more detailed methods are available to assess sleep objectively using formal sleep laboratory evaluation, accelerometry, and self-report measures (e.g., Medical Outcomes Study [MOS] Sleep Scale).[145]

Assessment of Physical Capacity

The physical capacities of pain patients are typically assessed by physical and occupational therapists. In some clinical settings, evaluation protocols are developed informally by individual therapists, sometimes in conjunction with a physician. In other settings, formal assessment protocols are used. Although the validity of such protocols has been questioned,[139] they are frequently used—particularly when injured workers are being evaluated. The purpose of such evaluations is to obtain objective information about the capabilities of patients. In clinical settings, this information is used in the planning of rehabilitative treatment. In more adversarial settings (e.g., workers' compensation), physical capacities data are used when adjudicative decisions about claims are made.

Ideally, a multidisciplinary evaluation would include having a vocational rehabilitation counselor perform a comprehensive evaluation of the work status of pain patients and their potential for vocational rehabilitation. In many situations, though, the job of assessing vocational disability falls on the physician or psychologist on the multidisciplinary team.

We are not aware of standardized instruments to assess the vocational status of pain patients. In the absence of a standard instrument, we recommend that clinicians assessing these patients address the following issues: (1) Is the patient currently working? (2) If the patient is not working, is this related to his or her health? (3) How long has the patient been out of the workforce? (4) Is he or she receiving any kind of work disability benefits? Which ones?

Assessment of Social Factors

Social factors are construed as factors in the social environment that influence people independent of their individual psychological characteristics. A good example is the receipt of workers' compensation benefits.

Social factors include demographic variables that influence the presentation and clinical course of people with painful conditions. In particular, research indicates that an individual's clinical presentation is associated with his or her age, sex, ethnicity,[146,147] and education level.[148,149]

The social factors that have attracted the most research attention in relation to chronic pain are participation in work (including household activities), interpersonal interactions, litigation, and participation in a workers' compensation system.[139,150]

Important social factors also include influences from an individual's immediate social environment. For example, there is good evidence that pain patients generally demonstrate more dramatic pain behaviors when they are in the presence of solicitous spouses.[151]

A significant proportion of individuals involved in injuries file personal injury claims. There is some evidence that injured workers with workers' compensation claims respond more poor to a variety of treatments compared to individuals with these same medical conditions but without workers' compensation claims.[150] Research on the relation between litigation and clinical course, however, has been contradictory. For example, whereas several studies have reported a negative effect of attorney involvement and litigation on recovery from whiplash disorders,[69,152] Others have not supported the prognostic role of these factors.[153] It is beyond the scope of this chapter to review the often contentious literature on the effect of litigation/attorney involvement on outcomes of chronic pain.[154-158]

Organization of Multidisciplinary Evaluations

As discussed previously, the clinicians who might participate in multidisciplinary evaluations include physicians, psychologists, vocational rehabilitation counselors, physical and occupations therapists, and perhaps other professionals. An obvious question is "How do these clinicians orchestrate their evaluations and communicate with each other?"

The model that has received the most attention in research literature has been multidisciplinary intensive pain rehabilitation.[159] In the United States, the multidisciplinary pain centers and functional restoration programs that provided intensive pain rehabilitation began in the late 1960s, flourished during the 1980s and early 1990s, and more recently have been in decline.[160]

Given the decline in intensive pain rehabilitation programs, it will probably be necessary in the future for professionals involved in the evaluation of patients with chronic pain to develop a number of informal strategies for working together. There are almost certainly a variety of models that can succeed. The key issue is for professionals to work together in acquiring data on the multiple dimensions that affect chronic pain patients and to communicate with each other so that the patients benefit from the data that are gathered.

Conclusion

Pain and associated symptoms are the results of a complex interplay of factors. Assessment and treatment of patients with chronic pain can be complicated by the web of influential factors that modulate the overall pain experience and associated disability. Furthermore, traditional biomedical approaches with diagnostic tests are often not helpful because structural damage and persistent pain reports do not necessarily coincide. Pain research in the last half century has repeatedly shown that pain is not just a physiologic phenomenon and that a range of "person variables," such as psychosocial, environmental, and behavioral factors, play a significant role in determining the occurrence, severity, and quality of pain. Given the multifactorial nature of chronic pain, adequate assessment requires an interdisciplinary team approach. In this chapter, we discussed the assessment of medical factors, altered CNS processing, psychological factors, and social factors in patients with chronic pain. We introduced a number of self-report inventories that can be used in conjunction with interviews and medical examinations. As we have repeatedly stressed, an adequate assessment of patients with chronic pain means the evaluation of the *person* with the symptoms. We must not just focus on the pathology or symptom report but must reach out to understand the person and his or her well-being. Although there is no shortcut in this, the delineation of relevant medical, psychosocial, and behavioral factors contributing to pain in a patient is critical in planning and executing a successful treatment plan.

A number of national and international efforts have recommended minimal data sets composed of standardized measures that should be considered for use in clinical practice as well as research on specific pain disorders.[161,162] These efforts include many of the multidimensional concepts and constructs reviewed in this chapter. The adoption of these recommendations would permit the aggregation of assessment information across studies and advance the understanding of individuals with chronic pain and the evaluation of treatments.

References

1. Dunn WR, Kuhn JE, Sanders R, et al; for MOON Shoulder Group. Symptoms of pain do not correlated with rotator cuff tear severity. A cross-sectional study of 393 patients with a symptomatic atraumatic full-thickness rotator cuff tear. *J Bone Joint Surg AM* 2014;96:793–800.
2. Jarvik JG, Hollingworth W, Heagerty PJ, et al. Three-year incidence of low back pain in an initially asymptomatic cohort: clinical and imaging risk factors. *Spine* 2005;30:1541–1548.
3. Wiesel BB, Sankar WN, Delahay JN, et al. *Orthopedic Surgery: Principles of Diagnosis and Treatment*. Philadelphia: Lippincott Williams & Wilkins; 2010.
4. Flor H, Turk DC. *Chronic Pain: An Integrated Biobehavioral Perspective*. Washington, DC: IASP Press; 2011.
5. Buskila D. Genetics of chronic pain states. *Best Pract Res Clin Rheumatol* 2007;21:535–547.
6. Fordyce WE. *Behavioral Methods for Chronic Pain and Illness*. St. Louis, MO: CV Mosby; 1976.
7. Turk DC, Robinson JP. Assessment of patients with whiplash associated disorders: a comprehensive approach. In: Duckworth MP, Iezzi A, O'Donohue W, eds. *Motor Vehicle Collisions: Medical, Psychosocial, and Legal Consequences*. New York: Elsevier; 2008:187–227.
8. Chou R, Qassem A, Snow V, et al. Diagnosis and treatment of low back pain: a joint clinical practice guideline from the American College of Physicians and the American Pain Society. *Ann Intern Med* 2007;147:478–491.
9. Henschke N, Maher CG, Refshauge KM, et al. Prevalence of and screening for serious spinal pathology in patients presenting to primary care settings with acute low back pain. *Arthritis Rheum* 2009;60:3072–3080.
10. Hakimi K, Spanier D. Electrodiagnosis of cervical radiculopathy. *Phys Med Rehabil Clin N Am* 2013;24:1–12.
11. Martin AR, Aleksanderek I, Cohen-Adad J, et al. Translating state-of-the-art spinal cord MRI techniques to clinical use: a systematic review of clinical studies utilizing DTI, MT, MWF, MRS, and fMRI. *Neuroimage Clin* 2015;10:192–238.
12. Nardone R, Höller Y, Brigo F, et al. The contribution of neurophysiology in the diagnosis and management of cervical spondylotic myelopathy: a review. *Spinal Cord* 2016;54:756–766.
13. Tan WQ, Wong BS. Clinics in diagnostic imaging. Cervical OPLL with cord compression. *Singapore Med J* 2015;56:373–377.

14. Li H, Huang Y, Cheng C, et al. Comparison of the technique of anterior cervical distraction and screw elevating-pulling reduction and conventional anterior cervical reduction technique for traumatic cervical spine fractures and dislocations. *Int J Surg* 2017;40:45–51.

15. Murphy JM, Park P, Patel RD. Cost-effectiveness of MRI to assess for post-traumatic ligamentous cervical spine injury. *Orthopedics* 2014;37:e148–e152.

16. Riascos R, Bonfante E, Cotes C, et al. Imaging of atlanto-occipital and atlantoaxial traumatic injuries: what the radiologist needs to know. *Radiographics* 2015;35:2121–2134.

17. Greg Anderson D, Voets C, Ropiak R, et al. Analysis of patient variables affecting neurologic outcome after traumatic cervical facet dislocation. *Spine J* 2004;4:506–512.

18. McLoughlin LC, Jadaan M, McCabe J. Severe sprains of the sub-axial cervical spine in adolescents: a diagnostic and therapeutic challenge: a report of three cases. *Eur Spine J* 2014;23(suppl 2):150–156.

19. Bodguk N, McGurik B. *Management of Acute and Chronic Neck Pain: An Evidence-Based Approach.* New York: Elsevier; 2006.

20. Hartling L, Brison RJ, Ardern C, et al. Prognostic value of the Quebec Classification of Whiplash-Associated Disorders. *Spine (Phila Pa 1976)* 2001;26:36–41.

21. Kwon SY, Shin JJ, Lee JH, et al. Prognostic factors for surgical outcome in spinal cord injury associated with ossification of the posterior longitudinal ligament (OPLL). *J Orthop Surg Res* 2015;10:94.

22. Oh JJ, Asha SE, Curtis K. Diagnostic accuracy of flexion-extension radiography for the detection of ligamentous cervical spine injury following a normal cervical spine computed tomography. *Emerg Med Aust* 2016;28:450–455.

23. Kaale BR, Krakenes J, Albrektsen G, et al. Clinical assessment techniques for detecting ligament and membrane injuries in the upper cervical spine region—a comparison with MRI results. *Man Ther* 2008;13:397–403.

24. Stemper BD, Yoganandan N, Pintar FA, et al. Anterior longitudinal ligament injuries in whiplash may lead to cervical instability. *Med Eng Phys* 2006;28:515–524.

25. Tominaga Y, Ndu AB, Coe MP, et al. Neck ligament strength is decreased following whiplash trauma. *BMC Musculoskelet Disord* 2006;7:103.

26. Myran R, Kvistad KA, Nygaard OP, et al. Magnetic resonance imaging assessment of the alar ligaments in whiplash injuries: a case-control study. *Spine (Phila Pa 1976)* 2008;33:2012–2016.

27. Vetti N, Kråkenes J, Ask T, et al. Follow-up MR imaging of the alar and transverse ligaments after whiplash injury: a prospective controlled study. *AJNR Am J Neuroradiol* 2011;32:1836–1841.

28. Vetti N, Kråkenes J, Damsgaard E, et al. Magnetic resonance imaging of the alar and transverse ligaments in acute whiplash-associated disorders 1 and 2: a cross-sectional controlled study. *Spine (Phila Pa 1976)* 2011;36:E434–E440.

29. Carragee EJ, Alamin TF, Carragee JM. Low-pressure positive discography in subjects asymptomatic of significant low back pain illness. *Spine* 2006;31:505–509.

30. Manchikanti L, Abdi S, Atluri S, et al. An update of comprehensive evidence-based guidelines for interventional techniques in chronic spinal pain. Part II: guidance and recommendations. *Pain Physician* 2013;16(2 suppl):S49–S283.

31. Curatolo M, Bogduk N, Ivancic PC, et al. The role of tissue damage in whiplash-associated disorders: discussion paper 1. *Spine (Phila Pa 1976)* 2011;36(25 suppl):S309–S315.

32. Nordin M, Carragee EJ, Hogg-Johnson S, et al. Assessment of neck pain and its associated disorders: results of the Bone and Joint Decade 2000-2010 Task Force on Neck Pain and Its Associated Disorders. *J Manipulative Physiol Ther* 2009;32(2 suppl):S117–S140.

33. Carragee EJ, Lincoln T, Parmar VS, et al. A gold standard evaluation of the "discogenic pain" diagnosis as determined by provocative discography. *Spine* 2006;31:2115–2123.

34. Chou R, Atlas SJ, Loeser JD, et al. Guideline warfare over interventional therapies for low back pain: can we raise the level of discourse? *J Pain* 2011;12:833–839.

35. Bogduk N. Diagnostic nerve blocks in chronic pain. *Best Pract Res Clin Anaesthesiol* 2002;16:565–578.

36. Gibson T, Bogduk N, Macpherson J, et al. Crash characteristics of whiplash associated chronic neck pain. *J Musculoskeletal Pain* 2000;8:87–95.

37. Lord S, Barnsley L, Wallis BJ, et al. Chronic cervical zygapophyseal joint pain after whiplash: a placebo-controlled prevalence study. *Spine* 1996;21:1737–1745.

38. McDonald G, Lord SM, Bogduk N. Long-term follow-up of patients treated with cervical radiofrequency neurotomy for chronic neck pain. *Neurosurgery* 1999;45:61–68.

39. Persson M, Sörensen J, Gerdle B. Chronic whiplash associated disorders (WAD): responses to nerve blocks of cervical zygapophyseal joints. *Pain Med* 2016;17:2162–2175.

40. Simons DG, Travell JG, Simons LS. *Travell & Simons' Myofascial Pain and Dysfunction: Upper Half of the Body.* Vol 1. 2nd ed. Philadelphia: Lippincott Williams & Wilkins; 1999.

41. Cerezo-Téllez E, Torres-Lacomba M, Mayoral-Del Moral O, et al. Prevalence of myofascial pain syndrome in chronic non-specific neck pain: a population-based cross-sectional descriptive study. *Pain Med* 2016;17:2369–2377.

42. Chiarotto A, Clijsen R, Fernandez-de-Las-Penas C, et al. Prevalence of myofascial trigger points in spinal disorders: a systematic review and meta-analysis. *Arch Phys Med Rehabil* 2016;97:316–337.

43. Côté P, van der Velde G, Cassidy JD, et al. The burden and determinants of neck pain in workers: results of the Bone and Joint Decade 2000-2010 Task Force on Neck Pain and Its Associated Disorders. *J Manipulative Physiol Ther* 2009;32(2 suppl):S70–S86.

44. Hogg-Johnson S, van der Velde G, Carroll LJ, et al. The burden and determinants of neck pain in the general population: results of the Bone and Joint Decade 2000-2010 Task Force on Neck Pain and Its Associated Disorders. *J Manipulative Physiol Ther* 2009;32(2 suppl):S46–S60.

45. Holm LW, Carroll LJ, Cassidy JD, et al. The burden and determinants of neck pain in whiplash-associated disorders after traffic collisions: results of the Bone and Joint Decade 2000-2010 Task Force on Neck Pain and Its Associated Disorders. *J Manipulative Physiol Ther* 2009;32(2 suppl):S61–S69.

46. Lluch Girbés E, Dueñas L, Barbero M, et al. Expanded distribution of pain as a sign of central sensitization in individuals with symptomatic knee osteoarthritis. *Phys Ther* 2016;96:1196–207.

47. Robinson JP, Ricketts D, Hanscom DA. Musculoskeletal pain. In: Merskey H, Loeser JD, Dubner R, eds. *The Paths of Pain.* Seattle, WA: IASP Press; 2005:1975–2005.

48. Dwyer A, Aprill C, Bogduk N. Cervical zygapophyseal joint pain patterns. I: a study in normal volunteers. *Spine* 1990;15:453–457.

49. Slipman CW, Plastaras C, Patel R, et al. Provocative cervical discography symptom mapping. *Spine J* 2005;5:381–388.

50. Turk DC, Dworkin RH, Revicki D, et al. Identifying important outcome domains for chronic pain clinical trials: an IMMPACT survey of people with pain. *Pain* 2008;137:276–285.

51. Main CJ, Waddell G. Behavioral responses to examination. A reappraisal of the interpretation of "nonorganic signs." *Spine* 1998;23:2367–2371.

52. Waddell G, McCulloch JA, Kummel E, et al. Nonorganic physical signs in low-back pain. *Spine* 1980;5:117–125.

53. Hunt DG, Zuberbier OA, Kozolowski AJ, et al. Reliability of the lumbar flexion, lumbar extension, and passive straight leg raise test in normal populations embedded within a complete physical examination. *Spine* 2001;26:2714–2718.

54. Nitschke JE, Nattrass CL, Disler PB, et al. Reliability of the American Medical Association guides' model for measuring spinal range of motion. Its implication for whole-person impairment rating. *Spine* 1999;24:262–268.

55. Rao JK, Kroenke K, Mihaliak KA, et al. Can guidelines impact the ordering of magnetic resonance imaging studies by primary care providers for low back pain? *Am J Manag Care* 2002;8:27–35.

56. Weiner DK, Kim YS, Bonino P, et al. Low back pain in older adults: are we utilizing healthcare resources wisely? *Pain Med* 2006;7:143–150.

57. Jensen MC, Brant–Zawadski MN, Obuchowski N, et al. Magnetic resonance imaging of the lumbar spine in people with back pain. *N Engl J Med* 1994;331:69–73.

58. Ji RR, Kohno T, Moore KA, et al. Central sensitization and LTP: do pain and memory share similar mechanisms? *Trends Neurosci* 2003;26:696–705.

59. Hoheisel U, Mense S. Long-term changes in discharge behaviour of cat dorsal horn neurons following noxious stimulation of deep tissues. *Pain* 1989;36:239–247.

60. Curatolo M, Arendt-Nielsen L, Petersen-Felix S. Evidence, mechanisms, and clinical implications of central hypersensitivity in chronic pain after whiplash injury. *Clin J Pain* 2004;20:469–476.

61. Robinson JP, Arendt-Nielsen L. Muscle pain syndromes. In: Braddom R, ed. *Physical Medicine and Rehabilitation.* 3rd ed. Edinburgh: Elsevier/Saunders; 2007:989–1020.

62. Nijs J, Malfliet A, Ickmans K, et al. Treatment of central sensitization in patients with 'unexplained' chronic pain: an update. *Expert Opin Pharmacother* 2014;15:1671–1683.

63. Woolf CJ. Central sensitization: implications for the diagnosis and treatment of pain. *Pain* 2011;152(3 suppl):S2–S15.

64. Hellman N, Barnoski K, Sturycz C, et al. Is history of traumatic events associated with nociceptive flexion reflex (NFR) threshold? *J Pain* 2016;17(4 suppl):S62.

65. Wallwork SB, Grabherr L, O'Connell NE, et al. Defensive reflexes in people with pain—a biomarker of the need to protect? A meta-analytical systematic review. *Rev Neurosci* 2017;28:381–396.

66. Kutch JJ, Yani MS, Asavasopon S, et al. Altered resting state neuromotor connectivity in men with chronic prostatitis/chronic pelvic pain syndrome: a MAPP: Research Network Neuroimaging Study. *Neuroimage Clin* 2015;8:493–502.

67. López-Solà M, Woo CW, Pujol J, et al. Towards a neurophysiological signature for fibromyalgia. *Pain* 2017;158:34–47.

68. Woolf CJ, Mannion RJ. Neuropathic pain: aetiology, symptoms, mechanisms, and management. *Lancet* 1999;353:1959–1964.

69. Gun RT, Osti OL, O'Riordan A, et al. Risk factors for prolonged disability after whiplash injury: a prospective study. *Spine* 2005;30:386–391.

70. Robinson JP, Apkarian AV. Low back pain. In: Mayer EA, Bushnell MC, eds. *Functional Pain Syndromes: Presentation and Pathophysiology.* Seattle: IASP Press; 2009:23–53.

71. Gay J, Abbot K. Common whiplash injuries of the neck. *JAMA* 1953:152:1698–1704.

72. Blumer D, Heilbronn M. Chronic pain as a variant of depressive disease: the pain-prone disorder. *J Nerv Ment Dis* 1982;170:381–406.

73. Turk DC, Salovey P. "Chronic pain as a variant of depressive disease": a critical reappraisal. *J Nerv Ment Dis* 1984;172:398–404.

74. Kroenke K, Price RK. Symptoms in the community. Prevalence, classification, and psychiatric comorbidity. *Arch Intern Med* 1993;153:2474–2480.

75. Lee H, Hubscher M, Moseley GL, et al. How does pain lead to disability? A systematic review and meta-analysis of mediation studies in people with back and neck pain. *Pain* 2015;156:988–997.

76. Bair MJ, Robinson RL, Katon W, et al. Depression and pain comorbidity. A literature review. *Arch Intern Med* 2003;63:2433–2445.

77. Kroenke K, Wu J, Bair MJ, et al. Reciprocal relationship between pain and depression: a 12-month longitudinal analysis in primary care. *J Pain* 2011;12:964–973.

78. Carragee EJ, Alamin TF, Miller JL, et al. Discographic, MRI and psychosocial determinants of low back pain disability and remission: a prospective study in subjects with benign persistent back pain. *Spine J* 2005;5:24–35.

79. Turk DC, Okifuji A, Scharff L. Chronic pain and depression: role of perceived impact and perceived control in different age cohorts. *Pain* 1995;61:93–101.

80. Rudy TE, Kerns RD, Turk DC. Chronic pain and depression: toward a cognitive–behavioral mediational model. *Pain* 1988;35:129–140.

81. Mayou R, Bryant B, Duthie R. Psychiatric consequences of road traffic accidents. *BMJ* 1993;307:647–651.

82. American Psychiatric Association. *User's Guide for the Structured Clinical Interview for DSM-IV Axis I Disorders SCID-1: Clinician version.* Washington, DC: American Psychiatric Press; 1997.

83. Turk DC, Swanson KS, Gatchel RJ. Predicting opioid misuse by chronic pain patients: a systematic review and literature synthesis. *Clin J Pain* 2008;24:497–808.

84. Piotrowski C. Review of the psychological literature on assessment instruments used with pain patients. *N Am J Psychol* 2007;9:303–306.

85. Melzack R. The McGill Pain Questionnaire: major properties and scoring methods. *Pain* 1975;1:277–299.

86. Melzack R. The short-form McGill Pain Questionnaire. *Pain* 1987;30:191–197.

87. Beck AT, Ward CH, Mendelson M, et al. An inventory for measuring depression. *Arch Gen Psychiatry* 1961;4:561–571.

88. Beck AT, Steer RA, Ball R, et al. Comparison of Beck Depression Inventories-IA and -II in psychiatric outpatients. *J Pers Assess* 1996;67:588–597.

89. Kerns RD, Turk DC, Rudy TE. The West Haven–Yale Multidimensional Pain Inventory (WHYMPI). *Pain* 1985;23:345–356.

90. Rosenstiel AK, Keefe FJ. The use of coping strategies in chronic low back pain patients. *Pain* 1983;17:33–44.

91. Fairbank JC, Couper J, Davies JB, et al. The Oswestry Low Back Pain Disability Questionnaire. *Physiotherapy* 1980;66:271–273.

92. Cleeland CS, Ryan KM. Pain assessment: global use of the Brief Pain Inventory. *Ann Acad Med Singapore* 1994;23:129–138.

93. Keller S, Bann CM, Dodd SL, et al. Validity of the Brief Pain Inventory for use in documenting the outcomes of patients with noncancer pain. *Clin J Pain* 2004;20:309–318.

94. Hjermstad MJ, Fayers PM, Haugen DF, et al; and European Palliative Care Research Collaborative. Studies comparing Numerical Rating Scales, Verbal Rating Scales, and Visual Analogue Scales for assessment of pain intensity in adults: a systematic literature review. *J Pain Symptom Manage* 2011;41:1073–1093.

95. Jensen MP, Karoly P. Self-report scales and procedures for assessing pain in adults. In: Turk DC, Melzack R, eds. *Handbook of Pain Assessment.* 3rd ed. New York: Guilford Press; 2011:19–44.

96. Hadjistavropoulos T, von Baeyer C, Craig KD. Pain assessment in persons with limited ability to communicate. In: Turk DC, Melzack R, eds. *Handbook of Pain Assessment.* 2nd ed. New York: Guilford; 2001:134–152.

97. McGrath PJ, Walco GA, Turk DC, et al. Core outcome domains and measures for pediatric acute and chronic/recurrent pain clinical trials: PedIMMPACT recommendations. *J Pain* 2008;9:771–783.

98. Gendreau M, Hufford MR, Stone AA. Measuring clinical pain in chronic widespread pain: selected methodological issues. *Best Pract Res Clin Rheumatol* 2003;17:575–592.

99. Stone AA, Shiffman S, Schwartz JE, et al. Patient compliance with paper and electronic diaries. *Control Clin Trials* 2003;24:182–199.

100. Shiffman S, Stone AA, Hufford MR. Ecological momentary assessment. *Annu Rev Clin Psychol* 2008;4:1–32.

101. Stone AA, Broderick JE, Schneider S, et al. Expanding options for developing outcome measures from momentary assessment data. *Psychosom Med* 2012;74:387–397.

102. Junker U, Freynhagen R, Langler K, et al. Paper versus electronic rating scales for pain assessment: a prospective, randomised, cross-over validation study with 200 chronic pain patients. *Curr Med Res Opin* 2008;4:1797–1806.

103. Turk DC, Burwinkle T, Showlund M. Assessing the impact of chronic pain in real-time. In: Stone A, Shiffman S, Atienza A, et al, eds. *The Science of Real-time Data Capture: Self-reports in Health Research.* New York: Oxford University Press; 2007:204–228.

104. Katz J, Melzack M. The McGill Pain Questionnaire: development, psychometric properties, and usefulness of the long form, short form, and short form-2. In: Turk DC, Melzack RJ, eds. *Handbook of Pain Assessment.* 3rd ed. New York: Guilford; 2011:45–66.

105. Dworkin RH, Turk DC, Trudeau JJ, et al. Validation of the Short-form McGill Pain Questionnaire-2 (SF-MPQ-2) in acute low back pain. *J Pain* 2015;16:357–366.

106. Keefe FJ, Block AR. Development of an observation method for assessing pain behavior in chronic low back pain. *Behav Ther* 1982;12:363–375.

107. Keefe FJ, Williams DA, Smith SJ. Assessment of pain behaviors. In: Turk DC, Melzack RJ, eds. *Handbook of Pain Assessment.* 2nd ed. New York: Guilford; 2001:170–190.

108. Richards JS, Nepomuceno C, Riles M, et al. Assessing pain behavior: the UAB Pain Behavior Scale. *Pain* 1992;14:313–338.

109. Turk DC, Wack JT, Kerns RD. An empirical examination of the "pain behavior" construct. *J Behav Med* 1985;9:119–130.

110. Kerns RD, Haythornthwaite J, Rosenberg R, et al. The Pain Behavior Checklist (PBCL): factor structure and psychometric properties. *J Behav Med* 1991;14:155–167.

111. Prkachin KM. Dissociating spontaneous and deliberate expressions of pain: signal detection analyses. *Pain* 1992;51:57–65.

112. McNair DM, Lorr M, Droppleman LF. *Profile of Mood States.* San Diego, CA: Educational and Industrial Testing Service; 1971.

113. Bjelland I, Dahl AA, Haug TT, et al. The validity of the Hospital Anxiety and Depression Scale. An updated literature review. *J Psychosom Res* 2002;52:69–77.

114. Zigmond AS, Snaith RP. The Hospital Anxiety and Depression Scale. *Acta Psychiatrica Scand* 1983;67:361–370.

115. Kroenke K, Spitzer RL, Williams JB. The PHQ-9: validity of a brief depression severity measure. *J Gen Intern Med* 2001;16:606–613.

116. Turk DC, Fillingim RB, Ohrbach R, et al. Assessment of psychosocial and functional Impact of chronic pain. *J Pain* 2016;17(9 suppl):T21–T49.

117. Dworkin RH, Corbin AE, Young JP, et al. Pregabalin for the treatment of postherpetic neuralgia: a randomized, placebo-controlled trial. *Neurology* 2003;60:1274–1283.

118. Rowbotham MC, Harden N, Stacey B, et al. Gabapentin Postherpetic Neuralgia Study Group. Gabapentin for the treatment postherpetic neuralgia: a randomized controlled trial. *JAMA* 1998;280:1837–1842.

119. Spitzer RL, Kroenke K, Williams JB, et al. A brief measure for assessing generalized anxiety disorder: the GAD-7. *Arch Intern Med* 2006;166:1092–1097.

120. Wilson KG, Mikail SF, D'Eon JL, et al. Alternative diagnostic criteria for major depressive disorder in patients with chronic pain. *Pain* 2001;91:227–234.

121. Kori SH, Miller RP, Todd DD. Kinesiophobia: a new view of chronic pain behaviour. *Pain Manage* 1990;3:35–42.

122. Waddell G, Newton M, Henderson I, et al. A Fear-Avoidance Beliefs Questionnaire (FABQ) and the role of fear-avoidance beliefs in chronic low back pain and disability. *Pain* 1993;52:157–168.

123. Danzie EJ, Turk DC. Assessment of patients with chronic pain. *Br J Anaesth* 2013:111:19–25.

124. DeGood DE, Cook AJ. Psychosocial assessment: comprehensive measures and measures specific to pain beliefs and coping. In: Turk DC, Melzack R, eds. *Handbook of Pain Assessment.* 3rd ed. New York: Guilford; 2011:67–97.

125. Bandura A. *Self-efficacy: The Exercise of Control.* New York: Freeman; 1997.

126. Benyon K, Hill S, Zadurian N, et al. Coping strategies and self-efficacy as predictors of outcome in osteoarthritis: a systematic review. *Musculoskeletal Care* 2010;8:224–236.

127. Sarda J Jr, Nicholas MK, Asghari A, et al. The contribution of self-efficacy and depression to disability and work status in chronic pain patients: a comparison between Australian and Brazilian samples. *Eur J Pain* 2009;13:189–195.

128. Anderson KO, Dowds BN, Pelletz RE, et al. Development and initial validation of a scale to measure self-efficacy beliefs in patients with chronic pain. *Pain* 1995;63:77–84.

129. Nicholas MK. The Pain Self-Efficacy Questionnaire: taking pain into account. *Eur J Pain* 2007;11:153–163.

130. Quartana PJ, Campbell CM, Edwards RR. Pain catastrophizing: a critical review. *Expert Rev Neurotherapy* 2009;9:745–758.

131. Kapoor SH, White J, Thorn BE, et al. Patients presenting to the emergency department with acute pain: the significant role of pain catastrophizing and state anxiety. *Pain Med* 2016;17:1069–1078.

132. Edwards RR, Smith MT, Stonerock G, et al. Pain related catastrophizing in healthy women is associated with greater temporal summation of and reduced habituation to thermal pain. *Clin J Pain* 2006;22:730–737.

133. Buitenhuis J, de Jong PJ, Jaspers JP, et al. Catastrophizing and causal beliefs in whiplash. *Spine* 2008;33:2427–2433.

134. Menendez ME, Baker DK, Oladeji LO, et al. Psychological distress is associated with perceived disability and pain in patients presenting to a shoulder clinic. *J Bone Joint Surg Am* 2015;97:1999–2003.

135. Sullivan MJL, Bishop S, Pivik J. The Pain Catastrophizing Scale: development and validation. *Psychol Assess* 1995;7:524–532.

136. Jensen MP, Keefe FJ, Lefebvre J, et al. One- and two-item measures of pain beliefs and coping strategies. *Pain* 2003;104:453–469.

137. World Health Organization. *International Classification of Functioning, Disability, and Health (ICF).* Geneva, Switzerland: World Health Organization; 2001.

138. Patel K, Dansie E, Turk DC. Impact of chronic musculoskeletal pain on objectively measured daily physical activity: current findings and applications in clinical practice. *Pain Manag* 2013;14:467–474.

139. Taylor AM, Phillips K, Patel KV, et al. Assessment of physical function and participation in chronic pain clinical trials: IMMPACT/OMERACT recommendations. *Pain* 2016;157:1836–1850.
140. Ware JE Jr, Sherbourne CD. The MOS 36-item short-form health survey (SF-36). *Med Care* 1992;30:473–483.
141. Pollard CA. Preliminary validity study of the Pain Disability Index. *Percept Mot Skills* 1984;59:974.
142. Bellamy N, Buchanan WW, Goldsmith CH, et al. Validation study of WOMAC: a health status instrument for measuring clinically important patient relevant outcomes to antirheumatic drug therapy in patients with osteoarthritis of the hip or knee. *J Rheumatol* 1988;15:1833–1840.
143. Guyatt GH, Feeney DH, Patrick DL. Measuring health-related quality of life. *Ann Intern Med* 1993;118:622–629.
144. Tang K, Boonen A, Verstappen SM, et al. Worker productivity outcome measures: OMERACT filter evidence and agenda for future research. *J Rheumatol* 2014;41:165–176.
145. Spitzer KL, Hays RD. *MOS Sleep Scale: A manual for use and scoring.* Version 1. Los Angeles, CA: RAND; 2003.
146. Hernandez A, Sachs–Ericsson N. Ethnic differences in pain reports and the moderating role of depression in a community sample of Hispanic and Caucasian participants with serious health problems. *Psychosom Med* 2006;68:121–128.
147. Watson PJ, Latif RK, Rowbotham DJ. Ethnic differences in thermal pain responses: a comparison of South Asian and White British healthy males. *Pain* 2005;118:194–200.
148. Berglund A, Bodin L, Jensen I, et al. The influence of prognostic factors on neck pain intensity, disability, anxiety and depression over a 2-year period in subjects with acute whiplash injury. *Pain* 2006;125:244–256.
149. Holm LW, Carroll LJ, Cassidy JD, et al. Factors influencing neck pain intensity in whiplash-associated disorders. *Spine* 2006;31:E98–E104.
150. Harris I, Mulford J, Solomon M, et al. Association between compensation status and outcome after surgery: a meta-analysis. *JAMA* 2005;293:1644–1652.
151. Thieme K, Spies C, Sinha P, et al. Predictors of pain behaviors in fibromyalgia syndrome patients. *Arthritis Care Res* 2005;53:343–350.
152. Dufton JA, Kopec JA, Wong H, et al. Prognostic factors associated with minimal improvement following acute whiplash-associated disorders. *Spine* 2006;31:E759–E766.
153. Scholten-Peeters GM, Verhagen AP, Bekkering GE, et al. Prognostic factors of whiplash associated disorders: a systematic review of prospective cohort studies. *Pain* 2003;104:303–322.
154. Cassidy JD, Carroll LJ, Cote P, et al. Effect of eliminating compensation for pain and suffering on the outcome of insurance claims for whiplash injury. *N Engl J Med* 2000;342:1179–1186.
155. Clionsky M. Effect of eliminating compensation for pain and suffering on the outcome of insurance claims. *N Engl J Med* 200;343:1119.
156. Freeman MD, Rossignol AM. Effect of eliminating compensation for pain and suffering on the outcome of insurance claims. *N Engl J Med* 2000;343:1118–1119.
157. Merskey H, Teasell RW. Effect of eliminating compensation for pain and suffering on the outcome of insurance claims. *N Engl J Med* 2000;343:1119.
158. Russell RS. Effect of eliminating compensation for pain and suffering on the outcome of insurance claims. *N Engl J Med* 2000;343:1119–1120.
159. Loeser JD, Turk DC. Multidisciplinary pain management. In: Loeser JD, Butler SH, Chapman CR, et al, eds. *Bonica's Management of Pain*. 3rd ed. Baltimore, MD: Lippincott Williams & Wilkins; 2001:2069–2080.
160. Schatman ME. The demise of multidisciplinary pain management clinics? *Practical Pain Manage* 2006;6:30–41.
161. Boers M, Kirwan JR, Wells G, et al. Developing core outcome measurement sets for clinical trials: OMERACT filter 2.0. *J Clin Epidemiol* 2014;67:745–753.
162. Deyo RA, Dworkin SF, Amtmann D, et al. Report of the NIH Task Force on Research Standards for Chronic Low Back Pain. *J Pain* 2014:15:569–585.

CHAPTER **24**

Painful Neuropathies

GEORGIOS MANOUSAKIS, MIROSLAV BACKONJA, and **DAVID WALK**

Pain as a Symptom of Neuropathy

Neuropathy is a common clinical problem. Pain merits attention in any discussion of neuropathy for several reasons. First, insofar as pain varies among neuropathy etiologies, the presence, absence, and type of pain when present can contribute to the diagnostic process. Second, for many people with neuropathy, pain is the chief complaint and the only cause of disability. The traditional neurologic focus on deficits rather than positive sensory phenomena does not serve these patients well. Finally, and perhaps most importantly, pain is a neurologic symptom. The study of pain due to nerve disorder or injury is providing essential insights into the function of the nervous system, as has the study of other neurologic symptoms in the past.

The Evaluation and Diagnosis of Neuropathy

NEUROPATHY CLASSIFICATION

The approach to the diagnosis of neuropathy is fully covered in textbooks devoted to this topic.[1,2] The present section is a conceptual overview to allow readers unfamiliar with neuromuscular practice to better understand the balance of this chapter. Throughout this section, specific neuropathies are named for the purpose of illustration only. More comprehensive and detailed information about specific types of neuropathy can be can be found later in this chapter under "Painful Neuropathies."

The four principal questions to address in the etiologic classification of neuropathy are the *time course* of symptoms, the *distribution* of neuropathy symptoms and signs, the *modalities* affected (motor, small fiber sensory, large fiber sensory, and autonomic), and the primary *locus of pathology* (axon or myelin). Answers to these four questions will narrow the differential diagnosis substantially.

Time course: Many common neuropathies, particularly those due to metabolic or genetic conditions, progress insidiously over years. Some, such as chronic inflammatory demyelinating polyradiculoneuropathy (CIDP), can progress over a period of weeks to months, often with unpredictable relapses or remissions. Relatively few neuropathies present acutely over days to weeks; among these are Guillain-Barré syndrome (GBS), toxic neuropathies, and peripheral nerve vasculitis.

Distribution: The distribution of neuropathy symptoms and signs can be identified by the history and confirmed by the examination and electrophysiologic studies. Most neuropathies conform to one of two patterns: symmetric, length-dependent versus asymmetric, multifocal, nonlength-dependent. The symmetric, length-dependent pattern begins with symptoms in both feet and progresses rostrally in a symmetric fashion. Symptoms usually do not appear in the hands until lower limb symptoms have progressed to the proximal calves or thighs. Symptoms appear last in the trunk and face. The term *length dependent* refers to the fact that nerve dysfunction in these patients begins in the longest axons and progresses rostrally. The implicated pathophysiology is that all nerves are exposed in equal measure to a systemic stressor and that the effect of this stressor on nerve function is closely correlated to the distance of the nerve terminal from the cell body. Many metabolic, toxic, and genetic disorders of nerve present in this fashion.

Asymmetric, nonlength-dependent neuropathies can affect proximal and distal nerve segments concomitantly in an unpredictable manner. Examples of those include CIDP, necrotizing vasculitis, granulomatous disorders such as sarcoidosis and leprosy, hereditary neuropathy with liability to pressure palsies (HNPP), and lymphomatous or carcinomatous infiltration of peripheral nerves.

Modality: The modalities affected refer to motor axons, large fiber (Aβ myelinated) sensory axons, small fiber (A∂ and C) sensory axons, and autonomic (cardiorespiratory, vasomotor, and visceromotor) axons. As with *distribution*, the involvement of these fiber classes can be identified by the history and confirmed by the neurologic examination and electrophysiologic studies; in addition, numerous clinical tools have been developed in recent decades to assist in the confirmation of small fiber sensory and autonomic involvement. Most symmetric, length-dependent metabolic or toxic neuropathies are clinically sensory-predominant until they are relatively advanced. The relative involvement of large and small sensory axons varies among, and in some cases within, etiologies. Patients with clinical findings isolated to small fiber modalities are often referred to as having small fiber neuropathy (SFN), although there is evidence that this progresses over time to involve large fibers as well. Etiologies of SFN are discussed in subsequent paragraphs. Large fiber sensory symptoms predominate in those neuropathies in which the primary pathology is a disorder of myelin, such as Charcot-Marie-Tooth (CMT) type I or CIDP. Necrotizing vasculitis, CMT, and CIDP demonstrate prominent motor and sensory involvement. Motor neuropathies without discernible sensory or autonomic involvement are uncommon in general clinical practice. They include multifocal motor neuropathy (MMN) and toxic neuropathy due to lead or dapsone exposure. Because pain is not a prominent feature of those, they are not discussed further. Diabetic, uremic, amyloid, paraneoplastic, and certain hereditary neuropathies can have clinically significant autonomic involvement.

Locus of pathology: The primary locus of pathology (axon or myelin) may be inferred by clinical examination. For example, demyelinating neuropathies are often characterized by early loss of stretch reflexes even before the development of substantial muscle weakness, and by relatively preserved muscle bulk, because demyelination alone does not result in denervation, and therefore, denervation atrophy does not develop unless or until there is secondary axonal injury. By contrast, axonal neuropathies result in relative preservation of reflexes and early atrophy of clinically affected muscles. Nevertheless, these clinical clues require confirmation by nerve conduction studies which, if interpreted correctly, provide reliable information about the primary pathologic substrate. For this reason, nerve biopsy is rarely needed to determine whether the primary pathology is axonal or demyelinating. The only common disorders of peripheral myelin are GBS, CIDP, and CMT type I.

Pain is common in some neuropathies and uncommon in others. Pain commonly manifests in neuropathies which have a predominance of small fiber involvement. There are pain descriptors that are common in painful neuropathies and less common in other painful conditions. This clinical observation has led to the development of several neuropathic pain questionnaires.[3-6] The process of validating such questionnaires has resulted in the identification of several symptoms that correlate well with the presence of neurologic pathophysiologic processes that lead to pain. These symptoms include paresthesias; spontaneous ongoing pain most frequently described as burning, numbness, and shooting; and tactile allodynia.[7]

The presence or absence of pain and characteristics of neuropathic pain can help the clinician identify the most likely type and etiology of a patient's neuropathy. For example, neuropathic pain is one of the defining characteristics of SFN. Allodynia is almost universally present in postherpetic neuralgia (PHN). Severe, aching, boring pain is an essential feature of neuralgic amyotrophy (NA) and a common complaint in necrotizing vasculitis. By contrast, CMT may be associated with musculoskeletal pain, but the presence of prominent neuropathic pain would put this diagnosis in doubt. One of the neuropathic pain symptom questionnaires, whether structured or unstructured, should be included in every diagnostic evaluation for neuropathy.

HISTORY, EXAMINATION, AND DIAGNOSTIC STUDIES

The medical history of a patient with neuropathy should include a systematic assessment of positive and negative sensory, motor, and autonomic symptoms. The neuropathy symptom profile instrument includes all of these.[8] As noted previously, neuropathic pain questionnaires allow systematic and comprehensive assessment of spontaneous and stimulus-evoked positive sensory symptoms, as well as pain descriptors, in patients with neuropathic pain.

The examination of the patient with neuropathy must include bedside assessments of both large and small fiber sensory modalities.

In addition to the standard neurologic examination, several laboratory investigations have proven valuable in the assessment of neuropathy in general and painful neuropathy in particular. These include psychophysical, neurophysiologic, and histopathologic investigations.

Psychophysical tests investigate the relationship between physical stimulus properties and corresponding perceptions of the stimulus.[9] The sensory component of the standard neurologic examination is a series of psychophysical tests. The term *quantitative sensory testing* (QST) is often used to describe one of several psychophysical testing paradigms for quantitative determination of perception of thermal or mechanical stimuli. In addition to threshold testing, QST can be used to obtain an intensity rating in response to application of a stimulus with fixed suprathreshold predetermined properties. For example, QST can be used to establish either a thermal pain threshold or the perceived intensity of pain evoked by a thermal stimulus of fixed intensity. Like the neurologic examination, QST can be used to determine whether a subject's sensory function is normal and, if not, the characteristics of those abnormalities. In addition, as a quantitative tool, QST can be used to monitor neuropathy and associated pain and as a tool in research.[10,11]

There is growing interest in developing a standardized assessment protocol for neuropathic pain to include tests of thermal, mechanical, and even chemical sensory function, including presence and intensity of allodynia and hyperalgesia. It is the expectation that comprehensive assessments of neuropathic pain features such as these would allow clinicians to identify patterns of pain phenotypes that would reveal underlying mechanisms irrespective of the etiology of neuropathy and point to the unique treatment options of neuropathic pain for individual patient groups. This type of development would complement now-standard neurologic examination which has proved critical for lesion localization and disease pattern recognition. Thermal hyperalgesia applying suprathreshold stimuli would be tested along with thermal sensory threshold testing, using commercially available devices. A comprehensive test of sensory thresholds, allodynia, and hyperalgesia has been designed and implemented by the German Neuropathic Pain study group.[12,13] A simpler test which combines mapping of areas of allodynia or hyperalgesia with fixed stimulus intensity rating and multimodality neuropathic pain assessment has been proposed by the Neuropathic Pain Research Consortium (NPRC) in the United States.[14] These efforts are still in their infancy and await further validation and large-scale implementation.

Neurophysiologic studies investigate the activity of electrically excitable tissues (nerve or muscle cells) either at rest, during normal activity, or in response to externally applied stimuli. The most commonly used neurophysiologic studies are nerve conduction studies and electromyography (NCS/EMG). NCS/EMG can provide objective evidence of dysfunction of large myelinated (Aβ) nerves, valuable evidence of whether the primary pathology is in the myelin or axon, and information about the distribution of disease.

One of the major limitations of NCS/EMG is that it provides no information about the functional status of small myelinated (Aδ) or unmyelinated (C) fibers. In the last two decades, the advent of immunohistochemical staining of skin biopsy tissue for evaluation of epidermal nerve fibers (ENFs) has allowed the identification of patients with normal nerve conduction studies but loss of cutaneous nerves.[15,16] In most cases, there are corresponding signs of abnormal nociception and thermal perception, consisting of both sensory loss and spontaneous or stimulus-evoked neuropathic pain,[17,18] although such patients likely lose large (Aβ) fibers over time as well.[19] This syndrome is known as SFN, and the ability to diagnose it through skin biopsy has spurred tremendous interest. Because small myelinated (Aδ) fibers also innervate sweat glands, neurophysiologic quantitative assessment of the stimulated sweat gland output, by quantitative sudomotor axon reflex testing (QSART) or other methods, is also valuable to diagnose SFN.[20,21] Currently, investigational approaches for the evaluation of small fiber function include microneurography,[22] laser-evoked potentials, and corneal confocal microscopy.[23]

Pathologic examination of peripheral nerve trunks also plays an important role to establish the specific cause of the neuropathy, especially when vasculitis, amyloidosis, granulomatous, or neoplastic disorders are suspected. Nerve biopsy can also be used to support a diagnosis of CIDP or other chronic demyelinating neuropathies.[24]

Painful Neuropathies

There is a higher incidence of pain among some etiologic categories of neuropathy than others. In this section, we describe those common neuropathies that are often painful.

DISTAL SYMMETRIC POLYNEUROPATHIES
Metabolic Causes
Diabetic Neuropathy
The most readily recognized cause of distal symmetric polyneuropathy (DSP) in the developed world is diabetes. Diabetic neuropathy is often but not always painful. The prevalence of painful neuropathy symptoms in one community study of diabetics was 25% to 50%.[25] All features of neuropathic pain, including mechanical allodynia, mechanical and thermal hyperalgesia, spontaneous shooting pains, and spontaneous burning, may occur. Like the sensory deficits of diabetic neuropathy, diabetic neuropathy pain presents in a length-dependent, symmetric pattern. Therefore, focal neuropathic pain in a diabetic should prompt consideration of an alternative etiology for the pain. Mononeuropathies in diabetes are discussed later under the heading "Painful Mononeuropathy Multiplex and Focal Neuropathic Syndromes."

There is no established metabolic or genetic distinction between diabetics whose neuropathy is or is not associated with neuropathic pain, although it has been suggested that neuropathic pain often develops early in the course of nerve injury and recedes when neuropathy becomes more severe. Experimental models of diabetic neuropathy have provided evidence that pain in diabetic neuropathy is probably mediated by pathophysiologic processes at peripheral or central nervous system (CNS) levels. Work in the streptozotocin model has demonstrated altered expression and kinetics of voltage-gated sodium; transient receptor potential cation channel, subfamily A, member I (TRPA-I); and T-type calcium channels at the axon terminals, or shaker-potassium channels in nodes of Ranvier, mediated by methylglyoxal or other metabolites. CNS mechanisms include altered descending inhibition of pain and aberrant neuroplasticity.[26] It remains to be determined whether these mechanisms apply in people with diabetic neuropathy.

Investigation of the syndrome of SFN has revealed a disproportionate number of patients with impaired glucose tolerance (IGT), suggesting that the etiology of neuropathy in such cases is incipient diabetes and the mechanism is the same as that of diabetic neuropathy. Although appealing, this remains a hypothesis only. Many such patients also have the metabolic syndrome.[27] Among disorders of lipids, hypertriglyceridemia in particular has been found to be prevalent in this syndrome.[28,29] Conversely, there is some evidence that, among diabetics, the prevalence or severity of neuropathy is greater if other components of the metabolic syndrome are present.[30,31] These observations suggest that microvascular disease exacerbates the nerve injury associated with hyperglycemia.

Infectious Causes
Both HIV infection and several of the commonly used highly active antiretroviral therapies (HAART) for HIV infection are associated with DSP.[32–34] The two etiologies may coexist, and the neuropathies associated with them are clinically indistinguishable; therefore, initial management for DSP in a patient on HAART usually consists of a therapeutic trial of medication change or discontinuation. DSP is most closely associated with the use of dideoxynucleoside analogues stavudine (D4T), zalcitabine (ddC), and didanosine (ddI). The mechanism of this effect is believed to be the inhibition of mitochondrial DNA polymerization, leading to mitochondrial dysfunction and, in turn, reduced energy availability. DSP in HIV infection commonly presents with symptoms of small fiber involvement, with prominent pain and paresthesias. The mechanism of HIV directly on development of pain and neuropathy is unknown, although there is some experimental evidence implicating inflammatory mechanisms triggered by infection of periaxonal Schwann cells.[32]

Chronic hepatitis C virus (HCV) infection is a well-recognized cause of polyneuropathy. DSP, SFN, mononeuropathy multiplex, and cranial neuropathy can all be seen in this context. Polyneuropathy due to HCV infection is usually, but not always, associated with secondary cryoglobulinemia, and nerve biopsy often demonstrates features suggestive or diagnostic of vasculitis. Depending on the severity and time course of the condition, as well as the pathologic findings, treatment can be supportive or may include antiviral therapy, immunomodulating therapy, or both.[35,36]

Lyme disease is a well-recognized cause of cranial neuropathy and polyradiculopathy. Less commonly, polyneuropathy and mononeuropathy multiplex have been described in the context of Lyme disease. Although direct infection is difficult to demonstrate, a diagnosis of peripheral nervous system Lyme disease can be inferred in the context of a subacute progressive neuropathy with clinical and serologic evidence of Lyme and clinical improvement with antibiotic therapy. Lyme radiculopathy, polyneuropathy, and mononeuropathy multiplex could all be associated with pain.[37,38]

Toxic Neuropathies
Neurotoxic substances impair a number of neural processes such as protein synthesis, axonal transport, and myelin maintenance. Exposure to several industrial toxins is well known to lead to polyneuropathy. These usually cause motor symptoms and signs, although painful and dysesthetic symptoms may ensue in a minority of patients. Very few pathologic studies have been conducted in humans. N-hexane, a common ingredient in household glue, and methyl-n-butyl ketone, an industrial solvent, are known to cause focal swelling of axons to 2 to 3 times their normal diameter and can result in painful neuropathy.[39,40]

Several pharmaceutical agents may cause painful polyneuropathy. Vincristine, taxanes, bortezomib, and the newer agents, ixabepilone and eribulin, all can cause painful polyneuropathy by interference with the function of microtubules.[41] Recent evidence also implicates mitochondrial dysfunction in chemotherapy-induced neuropathy, which will probably dictate treatment strategies for this type of painful polyneuropathy.[42] Of particular interest are the recent descriptions of immune-mediated neuropathies related to the use of immune checkpoint inhibitors for metastatic cancers, including the cytotoxic T-lymphocyte antigen 4 inhibitor, ipilimumab, and the PD-1 inhibitors nivolumab and pembrolizumab. Treatment of those neuropathies requires not only discontinuation of the offending agent but also immunosuppression.[41]

Many other drugs are known to cause polyneuropathies which are not always painful. Among these are isoniazid, gold, disulfiram, nitrofurantoin, amiodarone, and bezafibrate.

Nutritional Neuropathies
Pyridoxine Deficiency from Isoniazid Use
Isoniazid is an effective and inexpensive antituberculosis drug, but it is associated with distal neuropathy when administered in high doses. Patients with a genetic predisposition for slow metabolism of isoniazid are more susceptible to this adverse effect. Isoniazid interferes with essential metabolic functions of pyridoxine, leading to axonal damage. This axonopathy affects small and large fibers, causing motor deficits, sensory deficits, and pain. Pain is described as deep aching pain in calf muscles and burning paresthesias in upper and lower extremities.

Oral pyridoxine in doses of 30 to 100 mg per day can prevent or reverse isoniazid neuropathy. Excessive doses should be avoided because pyridoxine itself can cause neuropathy if given in excess.

Beriberi

Beriberi is the most widely recognized nutritional neuropathy and is a disease of the peripheral nerves and heart[43] caused by thiamine deficiency. If the heart is affected, it presents with heart failure (wet beriberi), but the majority of patients present with neuropathy alone (dry beriberi). Presenting symptoms are slowly progressive distal weakness, paresthesias, and pain. Rarely, beriberi develops acutely. There are multiple presentations of pain symptoms, including dull, constant ache, lancinating brief pain similar to tabes dorsalis, tightness, and burning. Unlike idiopathic distal symmetric SFN, in beriberi, burning usually involves the hands as well as the feet shortly after onset. Physical examination reveals symmetric sensory loss across all modalities as well as positive phenomena such as allodynia, hyperalgesia, and hyperpathia as well as distal weakness and areflexia. Large fiber involvement is demonstrated by nerve conduction studies.[44] Nutritional supplementation with thiamine is essential. With treatment, beriberi neuropathy improves slowly.

Pellagra Neuropathy

Pellagra is a nutritional disorder that when fully developed affects the skin, gastrointestinal, hematopoietic, and nervous systems. Nervous system manifestations include encephalopathy, myelopathy, and neuropathy. Neuropathy is infrequent but can be quite disabling.

Alcohol Neuropathy

It is well established that excessive and prolonged intake of alcohol is associated with a DSP which is often characterized by distal paresthesias, burning, and other features of neuropathic pain. The precise cause of alcohol polyneuropathy is unknown. For decades, the principal question has been whether alcohol polyneuropathy is due solely to deficiency of thiamine and, perhaps, other B vitamins or is due to a direct toxic effect of alcohol, its metabolites, or even other neurotoxins in alcoholic beverages. Support for a neurotoxic role of alcohol comes from an animal model of alcoholic neuropathy in which rats that are provided adequate nutritional supplementation along with alcohol develop polyneuropathy.[45] Some interesting clinical observations support this as well. For example, alcohol polyneuropathy is prevalent among Danish alcoholics despite the fact that beer, which is the alcoholic beverage of choice in that country, is supplemented with B vitamins.[46] In addition, an elegant series of studies of Japanese alcoholics has demonstrated that neuropathy is prevalent among alcoholics with normal serum thiamine levels and that sural nerve pathology differs between alcoholics with and without thiamine deficiency.[47]

Neuromuscular Manifestations of Intestinal Malabsorption after Bariatric Surgery and Other Gastrointestinal Surgical Procedures

The growing use of bariatric surgery has led to resurgence in awareness of neurologic disorders associated with malabsorption, some of which can be associated with neuropathic pain. Wernicke's encephalopathy, beriberi, and subacute combined degeneration due to vitamin B_{12} or copper deficiency are among the neurologic disorders attributable to known deficiency states that have been described after bariatric surgery. In some cases, a presumed nutritional myeloneuropathy has been ascribed to multiple nutritional deficiencies or deficiency of an unknown nutrient in such patients. Neuropathic pain can occur in beriberi, and in subacute combined degeneration, the latter most likely as a result of an associated sensory neuropathy.

Hereditary Neuropathies

CMT is the most common hereditary neuropathy, with an estimated prevalence of 40 per 100,000.[48] The clinical syndrome is a progressive symmetric length-dependent motor and sensory neuropathy. CMT differs from the length-dependent polyneuropathy seen in diabetes and most other metabolic, nutritional, and toxic disorders because, in CMT, weakness and atrophy are prominent early signs, and both upper and lower extremities are typically affected. Most forms of CMT are inherited in an autosomal dominant fashion, the exception being the X-linked form (CMTX). Neuropathic pain is uncommon in CMT, and when it occurs, it is usually not the most prominent symptom. Fatigue, neuromuscular discomfort, and aching pain from foot deformities and overuse syndromes do occur. Acute intermittent porphyria is an autosomal dominant disorder with neuropathy which may have pain as one of the presenting symptoms, but pain is always overshadowed by weakness.

Fabry's Disease

Fabry's disease is one of the few hereditary neuropathies in which neuropathic pain is the cardinal symptom. It is a multisystem disorder affecting peripheral nerves, kidneys, heart, and skin. It is inherited in X-linked recessive fashion, and its symptoms start in childhood or adolescence. The biochemical abnormality is a deficiency of α-galactosidase, a lysosomal enzyme. The estimated prevalence is about 2 per 100,000 males. The clinical features include red punctate skin lesions in the lower body and thighs, corneal opacifications, cardiac and renal failure, and polyneuropathy. Cardiac and renal failures are terminal events for these patients. The neuropathy of Fabry's disease is characterized by continuous burning pain in the hands and feet, with spontaneous paroxysms of more severe pain. On examination, there are surprisingly modest sensory deficits, and muscle stretch reflexes are preserved. Nerve conduction studies are usually normal. In addition to pain, patients with Fabry's disease have marked autonomic dysfunction manifesting with episodic diarrhea, vomiting, urinary retention, and diminished sweating. Gastrointestinal symptoms can be relieved with metoclopramide.[49]

Fabry's disease may be unique in that it appears to exclusively affect small myelinated and unmyelinated axons, at least until such time as renal insufficiency occurs and causes a superimposed mixed polyneuropathy. This has been demonstrated pathologically by comparison of ENF density with sural nerve morphometry in the same patients. Enzyme replacement therapy has been shown to have multiple benefits, including an improvement in the Brief Pain Inventory.[50,51] In a recent study of 120 patients, enzyme replacement improved proximal skin innervation only, and this effect was limited to men with preserved renal function. ENF densities and thermal thresholds remained otherwise unchanged.[52] Clearly, more needs to be learned about the effect of enzyme replacement therapy on the neuropathy of Fabry's disease.[51,52]

Hereditary Sodium Channelopathies

The SCN9A and SCN10A genes encode for the sodium channels Nav 1.7 and Nav 1.8, which are selectively expressed in sensory and autonomic neurons at the dorsal root ganglia. Dominant gain of function mutations in Nav 1.7 and 1.8 can lead to a number of effects including lower threshold for activation and slowed deactivation. As a result, the channel is kept open longer once activated, and normally, subthreshold stimuli can result in depolarization.[53] The ultimate result is hyperexcitability and degeneration of small nerve fibers, mediated by increased sodium load and reversal of sodium–calcium exchange. The prototypical disorders described in association with SCN9A mutations are inherited erythromelalgia and paroxysmal extreme pain disorder (PEPD).[54,55] Inherited erythromelalgia is characterized by episodic burning pain and red discoloration of hands and feet, with onset usually in the first two decades of life. The attacks can be triggered by mild warming stimuli, including exercise, and can often be ameliorated by cooling the affected limbs. PEPD is characterized by attacks of pain involving the rectum, eyes, and jaw, often associated with flushing and other autonomic disturbances. Recently, SCN9A, and more rarely SCN10A, variants were found in approximately one-third of patients labeled as having idiopathic SFN.[56,57] The penetrance of those variants is not fully understood, and for that reason, they may be considered major risk factors, as opposed to penetrant causative mutations for SFN. This important discovery has led to the targeted development of small molecules that inhibit Nav1.7 or Nav1.8 channels, many of which are currently in clinical trials for various conditions associated with neuropathic pain.[58]

Amyloid Neuropathy

Neuropathy is a common, early, and often prominent manifestation of amyloidosis. Neuropathy can occur in both familial and acquired amyloidosis. There are several distinct clinical groups of familial (transthyretin [TTR]) amyloidosis, but all of them have an autosomal dominant inheritance pattern. The prevalence varies greatly among ethnic groups. The initial symptoms are numbness, paresthesias, and pain in the feet and lower legs. Autonomic involvement is also common, manifesting with abnormal pupillary reflexes, miosis, anhidrosis, orthostatic hypotension, diarrhea alternating with constipation, and impotence. Cranial nerve involvement manifests late in the disease. About half of the patients have neuropathic symptoms at onset, whereas half present with cardiac, hematologic, or renal dysfunction.

Patients with familial amyloid polyneuropathy can benefit from liver transplantation[59] or newly developed small molecules that function as TTR tetramer kinetic stabilizers, including tafamidis,[60] which is approved in Europe. Experimental stabilization of TTR tetramer with diflunisal, and the antisense oligonucleotide patisiran, appear promising.[61]

OTHER WIDESPREAD BUT NONLENGTH-DEPENDENT NEUROPATHIES

Neuropathy with Paraproteinemia

Monoclonal gammopathy, defined as the presence of a single clone of immunoglobulin (Ig) identified via serum protein electrophoresis or immunofixation, is common in the elderly. Although sometimes due to myeloma or lymphoma, monoclonal gammopathy can present in the absence of a malignant lymphoproliferative disorder and, in such cases, is referred to as monoclonal gammopathy of undetermined significance (MGUS). There is an increased prevalence of neuropathy among individuals with MGUS and an increased prevalence of MGUS among individuals with otherwise unexplained neuropathy.[62] Despite this, with the exception of a few well-characterized specific antibody-mediated syndromes, such as the syndromes associated with IgM antibodies to the sulfated glucuronyl paragloboside epitope of myelin-associated glycoprotein (MAG-SGPG)[63] and disialosyl antibodies, there is no compelling evidence of a causal relationship between MGUS and neuropathy. Nonetheless, the association is sufficiently common that it is prudent to obtain a serum protein immunofixation as part of the evaluation of idiopathic neuropathy and to consider that MGUS in a patient with neuropathy may represent more than a chance association.

Several clinical phenotypes, both axonal and demyelinating, have been described in neuropathy with MGUS. CIDP, a chronic acquired demyelinating neuropathy that usually responds to immune manipulation, is occasionally associated with MGUS. Distal acquired demyelinating syndrome (DADS) is an indolent syndrome of sensory ataxia, often with distal weakness, with electrophysiologic evidence of distal predominant demyelination. DADS is usually associated with an IgM monoclonal gammopathy which, in about two-thirds of cases, is directed against MAG-SGPG.[64] Allodynia was recently reported as presenting manifestation of DADS, with good response to intravenous Ig (IVIg).[65]

Axonal pathology is also common in MGUS neuropathy, particularly among patients with IgG and IgA monoclonal proteins. Axonal MGUS neuropathy is usually an indolent condition with prominent negative and positive sensory symptoms.

Neuropathy can be associated with lymphoproliferative malignancies as well. Perhaps most notably, polyneuropathy is part of the POEMS syndrome, an acronym which refers to polyneuropathy, organomegaly, endocrinopathy, M-spike, and skin changes. POEMS syndrome most often occurs in the setting of osteosclerotic myeloma, multiple myeloma, or angiofollicular lymph node hyperplasia (Castleman's syndrome). The polyneuropathy in POEMS syndrome, unlike most polyneuropathies associated with MGUS, is usually progressive and disabling but does often respond to appropriate treatment of the associated lymphoproliferative syndrome. Electrophysiologic studies usually reveal a primary demyelinating pattern.[66]

Neuropathic pain can occur with all paraproteinemic polyneuropathies. Although negative sensory symptoms usually predominate in acquired demyelinating neuropathies, pain and paresthesias can occur and are occasionally severe. Although speculative, it is possible that this reflects dysfunction or ectopic discharge of small myelinated nociceptors, loss of collateral inhibition of afferent input from small myelinated and unmyelinated axons, or sensitization due to the expression of inflammatory cytokines in nerve.

Autoimmune Demyelinating Neuropathies
Guillain-Barré Syndrome

GBS is an inflammatory polyneuropathy with an estimated 100,000 people developing it annually, worldwide.[67] The syndrome is characterized by rapidly progressive, widespread, and often severe weakness of the limbs and cranial musculature with areflexia. Approximately 20% to 30% of patients require ventilatory support. Weakness reaches a nadir within 4 weeks, with substantial spontaneous recovery in the majority of patients. Nonetheless, despite a generally good prognosis for recovery of strength, many patients are left with considerable fatigue, and some with distal weakness and paresthesias.

Electrophysiologic investigations demonstrate features of demyelination, including focal motor conduction block, in most patients with GBS. This is concordant with pathologic investigations which demonstrate lymphocytic infiltration and macrophage-mediated demyelination of nerve roots and peripheral nerves.[68] Thus, until recently, the descriptive term *acute inflammatory demyelinating polyradiculoneuropathy* (AIDP) was considered synonymous with GBS. Occasional patients with evidence of axon loss were felt to have suffered secondary axonal injury in a fulminant demyelinating disease. In 1995, a seminal description of Chinese patients with an epidemic form of GBS without electrophysiologic or pathologic features of demyelination led to the elucidation of GBS subtypes, now referred to as acute motor axonal neuropathy (AMAN) and acute motor axonal sensory motor neuropathy (AMSAN),[69] which appear to reflect immunologically mediated disruption of paranodal sodium channels, leading to reversible conduction failure without myelin disruption.[70] Whether they are AIDP, AMAN, or AMSAN, all forms of GBS often develop several weeks following a systemic infection, suggesting molecular mimicry as a triggering event, but AMAN in particular is strongly associated with preceding gastrointestinal infection with *Campylobacter jejuni* and the subsequent development of serum IgG antibodies directed against ganglioside GM1, which are probably pathogenic.[70] Pain has been reported to be one of the presenting symptoms in more than three quarters of patients with GBS, and in many, it precedes weakness. Pain is present throughout the course of GBS, and in half of those patients, it is rated as severe. Pain intensity upon admission does not correlate with neurologic disability.[71] The major pain syndromes observed in GBS are back and leg pain, dysesthetic extremity pain, and myalgic extremity pain.[72]

About two-thirds of patients experience back and leg pain at sometime during the course of GBS. This pain is usually described as a deep, aching, or throbbing pain in the low back frequently radiating to the buttocks, thighs, and occasionally to the calves. This pain may reflect root inflammation or endoneurial edema. Dysesthetic extremity pain, described as burning, tingling, or shock-like, involves the legs more frequently than the arms, and is also common in GBS. This type of pain is present in a minority of patients upon admission, although about half experience dysesthetic pain sometime during the course of the illness. It may persist indefinitely in 5% to 10%.[71] It is postulated that neuropathic pain of this type is due to ectopic impulse formation at sites of demyelination and axonal degeneration or regeneration.[73] Myalgic extremity pain, described as aching or cramping pain, often with joint stiffness, is less frequent than radicular low back pain. This pain is most notable during the passive and active assisted exercises associated with physical therapy.[72]

A recent review of pain symptoms in GBS demonstrated that backache, interscapular pain, and myalgias are most common early in the course of the disease and generally resolve during the recovery phase, whereas dysesthesias and paresthesias are more likely to persist, sometimes for months or longer.[72] This is compatible with the theorized etiologies noted previously.

Pain Management in Guillain-Barré Syndrome
In a prospective study, 75% of patients required oral or parenteral opioids to provide adequate pain relief.[71] Epidural morphine has been used as an alternative to systemic opioids in ventilated patients with primarily low back and leg pain.[74] In nonventilated patients in the acute stage of illness, opioid analgesics must be titrated carefully because of increased risk of respiratory depression. During the recovery phase, when muscle and joint pain is routinely precipitated by passive and active exercises, immediate-release codeine or morphine can be given an hour or two prior to treatment to facilitate compliance with physical therapy. Most patients do not require opioid analgesics beyond the first 8 weeks of illness.

A wide variety of medications used to manage neuropathic pain in other settings can be used in GBS, although caution should be taken with medications that can exacerbate hypotension or precipitate cardiac arrhythmias because of the autonomic instability which is common in GBS.

There are no controlled studies on the efficacy of any treatment of pain associated with GBS.

Chronic Inflammatory Demyelinating Polyradiculoneuropathy
CIDP is a chronic peripheral nervous system disorder that can have progressive, relapsing-remitting, and monophasic courses. The prevalence of CIDP has been estimated at 0.8 to 1.9 per 100,000. In contrast to GBS, association with preceding viral illnesses is uncommon. Some autoimmune and infectious disorders, such as MGUS, lupus, and HIV infection, have been associated with CIDP, but most cases are unrelated to systemic illness. The presenting symptoms are numbness and/or weakness with hyporeflexia progressing over at least 8 weeks' time. Pain may or may not occur, but when it does, it can have any of the features of neuropathic pain. Therapy is aimed at treating the underlying disease process with immunotherapy, usually steroids or IVIg.[75,76] Pain management should follow the basic principles of neuropathic pain pharmacologic therapy.

PAINFUL MONONEUROPATHY MULTIPLEX AND FOCAL NEUROPATHIC SYNDROMES
The conditions discussed next are commonly associated with substantial pain. About 50% of vasculitic neuropathies are painful, and when present, the pain is usually severe, requiring treatment with multiple medications including narcotic analgesics. In addition to characteristic features of neuropathic pain, a deep, aching, boring pain is often present in peripheral nerve vasculitis. This has been attributed to infarction of vasa nervorum. Immunohistologic studies have demonstrated a correlation between neuropathic pain and the presence of cytokines in nerve biopsy specimens, and it is a common observation that the pain of vasculitic neuropathy is alleviated promptly by steroid therapy.

Like vasculitic neuropathy, the pain of NA and diabetic amyotrophy also often has a deep, aching quality and, if treated promptly, can improve with immunomodulating therapy.

Vasculitic Neuropathy
Vasculitis is an autoimmune disorder characterized by inflammation and necrosis of blood vessel walls. The principal primary systemic vasculitides affecting peripheral nerve include polyarteritis nodosa, Churg-Strauss syndrome, and Wegener's granulomatosis. Peripheral nerve vasculitis also occurs as a complication of systemic inflammatory and infectious disorders, including lupus, rheumatoid arthritis, Sjögren's syndrome (SS), progressive systemic sclerosis, chronic hepatitis C infection, and HIV infection. Peripheral nerve vasculitis can also occur in isolation. Although immunomodulation is almost always indicated, important differences exist in therapy and prognosis between the types of vasculitis, making accurate classification important.[77] Thus, a comprehensive general medical evaluation and serologic studies relevant to the aforementioned disorders are indicated if vasculitis is suspected. The diagnosis can only be confirmed by tissue biopsy; in cases of peripheral nerve involvement, the sural, superficial peroneal, and superficial radial nerves are most commonly studied. Ideally, a biopsy should be taken from a nerve that is affected, based on clinical and electrophysiologic criteria, but not one that has undergone severe and long-standing injury. The diagnostic histologic finding is transmural lymphocytic infiltration and fibrinoid degeneration of the medium-sized arteries in the epineurium and axonal degeneration that is nonuniform both within and between nerve fascicles.[24]

Most patients with neuropathy due to vasculitis experience sensory loss and weakness in a multifocal pattern, although in long-standing vasculitis, the deficits can become confluent and mimic a symmetric process. In about 20% of cases of peripheral nerve vasculitis, the presentation is of a DSP at onset. When present, as it is in about 50% of cases, pain has characteristics of acute neuropathic pain as well as a continuous deep, aching pain.

The primary treatment goal in vasculitic neuropathy is control of the underlying disease process. This usually requires prompt and aggressive immunotherapy with corticosteroids and, in some circumstances, other immunomodulatory agents such as cyclophosphamide. The pain associated with necrotizing vasculitis is different in character and pathogenesis than the neuropathic pain associated with nonvasculitic neuropathy. A combination of opioids and other medications indicated specifically for neuropathic pain is usually required in this setting.

Neuralgic Amyotrophy
NA usually manifests as sudden, severe, deep aching pain in the shoulder girdle and proximal upper limb, followed within days to weeks by marked atrophy and weakness and relatively modest sensory loss. Weakness can be isolated to the distribution of one or two nerve trunks only and can include nerves, such as the phrenic nerve, which involve the upper body but not the upper limb per se. Commonly affected nerves include

the long thoracic, suprascapular, phrenic, musculocutaneous, and anterior interosseous. NA can occur at any age and is more common in men than women. It is also known as idiopathic brachial neuritis and as Parsonage-Turner syndrome. The etiology of this syndrome is not established, although the following clinical observations suggest that it may be disimmune. First, NA often follows a viral infection, as is the case in GBS. Second, NA often begins with severe focal pain followed by atrophy and weakness, as is often the case in vasculitic neuropathy. Third, NA is a mononeuropathy multiplex, which is the most common pattern seen in peripheral nerve vasculitis. Careful clinical and electrodiagnostic examination often reveals differential fascicular involvement within a nerve trunk. The natural history of NA is of very gradual improvement over the course of 1 to 2 years, as axonal regeneration occurs. Empiric immunotherapy is occasionally used. It is our impression that steroid therapy accelerates recovery and pain relief, but this has not been evaluated systematically.[78,79]

Pain in NA is usually described as deep, aching, and severe. It is made worse with movements of the affected limb, and as a result, patients often avoid movement at the shoulder joint, resulting at times in a secondary adhesive capsulitis (frozen shoulder). Deep aching pain generally improves over a matter of weeks but can persist and can be followed by painful paresthesias and dysesthesias. Residual weakness and pain can occur. A hereditary form, known as hereditary neuralgic amyotrophy (HNA), has been identified and may represent a substantial proportion of cases.[80] HNA is inherited in an autosomal dominant fashion and has been linked to a mutation in the SEPT9 gene, which is responsible for the formation of a possible cytoskeletal protein.[81]

Diabetic Amyotrophy
Like NA, diabetic amyotrophy is a well-recognized syndrome characterized by sudden, severe pain, usually in the proximal segment of the limb, followed shortly thereafter by striking atrophy and weakness. Unlike NA, diabetic amyotrophy usually affects the lower limb, although similar presentations involving the upper limb have been described. Also unlike NA, and as indicated by the name, diabetic amyotrophy occurs almost exclusively in diabetics, although an identical syndrome has been described in patients with IGT. This syndrome is also known as the Bruns-Garland syndrome and as diabetic lumbosacral radiculoplexus neuropathy, which describes the postulated localization of the pathology. Biopsy of proximal cutaneous nerves has demonstrated features of microvasculitis.[82] In keeping with this, there is extensive anecdotal evidence of prompt resolution of pain, and possible acceleration of recovery, after immune manipulation with steroids or IVIg.

Other Diabetic Mononeuropathies
All health care providers should also be familiar with diabetic mononeuropathies because of their clinical management implications as well as the striking pain associated with these conditions. In addition to inducing a predisposition to entrapment neuropathies, diabetes is associated with several acute, painful mononeuropathies or focal neuropathic syndromes affecting cranial nerves (third, fourth, sixth, seventh), roots (thoracic radiculopathy), and root/plexus (diabetic amyotrophy). In addition, a multifocal polyneuropathy ("diabetic mononeuropathy multiplex") can occur in the setting of diabetes. There is published evidence, supported by biopsy material, that several of these diabetic mononeuropathy syndromes are vasculitic.[83] Recognizing clear risks associated with both treatments in this population, there is also anecdotal evidence that immunotherapy with steroids or Ig infusions may accelerate pain relief and possibly recovery of function in diabetic focal neuropathies.[84]

SENSORY NEURONOPATHIES
The following conditions are believed to reflect pathology in the cell bodies of sensory neurons. PHN follows reactivation of a viral infection, whereas the others are believed to represent primary disimmune processes. In all cases, neuropathic pain is often the principal symptom. The high prevalence of neuropathic pain in sensory neuronopathies may be attributable to the presence of an inflammatory process in relative proximity to the dorsal horn of the spinal cord.

Postherpetic Neuralgia
PHN is one of the most common and disabling neuropathic pain states. Epidemiologic surveys estimated the incidence of herpes zoster at 4.1 per 1,000 person-years, with PHN developing in 18% of cases.[85] Herpes zoster is due to a reactivation of varicella-zoster virus (VZV), which remains sequestered and clinically dormant in cells of sensory ganglia after an initial infection but becomes reactivated in the context of age-related or disease-related reduction in cell-mediated immunity to the virus. There is some evidence of persistent active infection in patients with PHN. PHN is presumed to be due to sensitization of nociceptors and central sensitization after herpes zoster. PHN is more likely to occur in patients with pain associated with acute zoster and patients with zoster affecting multiple dermatomes. There is a positive correlation between age at the time of developing herpes zoster and the likelihood of developing PHN.[86,87] Several studies have demonstrated that antiviral treatment of herpes zoster substantially reduces the risk of developing PHN and the duration of PHN if it develops.[88–90] PHN is described in greater detail in Chapter 27.

Sjögren's Syndrome
SS is a systemic autoimmune disorder. The cardinal features are sicca syndrome, supported by objective evidence of diminished tear production, salivary gland inflammation, and serologic evidence of antibodies highly correlated with this disorder.[91] SS is commonly associated with disease of both the peripheral system and CNS. The range of neurologic disorders that have been associated with SS is remarkably broad, including multiple sclerosis-like cerebral disorders, myelopathy, polyradiculoneuropathy, sensory neuronopathy, vasculitic mononeuropathy multiplex, and myositis.[92] The peripheral nervous system disorders for which the association with SS is clearest are sensory neuronopathy and vasculitic neuropathy. In patients with SS, sensory neuronopathy can present with sensory ataxia, neuropathic pain, or both, presumably reflecting the relative involvement of large and small sensory neurons. Sensory neuronopathy from SS is usually an indolent, progressive condition.[92–94] Evidence of response to immunotherapy is anecdotal. Disimmune sensory neuronopathy can occur as an idiopathic phenomenon as well.

As with other systemic autoimmune conditions, necrotizing peripheral nerve vasculitis from SS is a rapidly progressive, disabling, and commonly painful condition which nonetheless does respond to immunotherapy.

Paraneoplastic Sensory Neuronopathy
Paraneoplastic sensory neuronopathy is one of several paraneoplastic syndromes associated with the presence of anti-Hu antibodies which is encompassed under the rubric of paraneoplastic encephalomyelitis. The predominant clinical syndrome is a sensory ataxia rather than neuropathic pain. Paraneoplastic sensory neuronopathy may respond to treatment of the tumor and, occasionally, immunomodulating therapy, but the prognosis is nonetheless poor.[95]

Toxic Neuronopathy
Cisplatin is an antineoplastic agent known to cause sensory loss and neuropathic pain. The pathophysiology is felt to be disruption of mitochondrial DNA synthesis resulting in a sensory neuronopathy.[96]

Treatment of Painful Neuropathies

GENERAL PRINCIPLES OF THERAPY

Treatment of neuropathy and neuropathic pain is complementary. Treatment of neuropathy is targeted at the underlying disease process. Such therapy should be administered as soon as possible to control or even reverse the process responsible for neuropathy and neuropathic pain. Nevertheless, in the authors' experience, patients commonly report persistent neuropathic pain even after stabilization or reversal of neuropathy. This is particularly true in vasculitic neuropathy, where progressive weakness and sensory loss can be aborted with steroid therapy, but pain often persists even years after resolution of necrotizing vasculitis. Assuming that inflammation and injury in peripheral nerve terminals has stabilized or receded in these cases, this observation might be attributable to central sensitization.

ANALGESIA THERAPY: GUIDELINES FOR PHARMACOTHERAPY

Treatment of neuropathic pain should begin as soon as possible and in tandem with treatment of neuropathy. Postulated mechanisms of neuropathic pain and neuropathic pain pharmacotherapy are addressed in other chapters. Here, we address treatment of painful neuropathy in particular.

Diabetic neuropathy is the most prevalent painful neuropathy in developed countries and has therefore been most widely studied as a target for treatment of neuropathic pain from neuropathy. It follows, therefore, that most clinical trial data regarding efficacy of analgesic treatments in painful neuropathy were obtained in patients with diabetic neuropathy pain. There is little formal evidence that these data apply to neuropathic pain from other etiologies.

Primary outcome measures of most large clinical trials are overall change in pain severity and improvement in quality of life indicators. There is a growing recognition that clinical trial design in neuropathic pain should also include systematic evaluation of individual neuropathic pain symptoms and signs.[97] Thus, there is potential utility in the systematic evaluation of the effect of treatments on specific neuropathic pain symptoms, such as paresthesias, dysesthesias, and burning; neuropathic pain descriptors, such as sharp, dull, stabbing, or exhausting; and neuropathic pain signs, such as dynamic mechanical allodynia, punctate hyperalgesia, thermal allodynia, and thermal hyperalgesia. It is not clear at present whether it is better to ask the question "Which treatment is best for neuropathic pain from this disease?" or, rather, "Which treatment is best for this neuropathic pain symptom/sign complex?" Implied in the latter is the hypothesis that pain symptoms and signs inform us about the principal mechanisms of pain in a given individual, which in turn may match the mechanism of action of a particular treatment.

For now, however, evidence-based treatment of neuropathic pain from neuropathy is based largely on evidence of reduction in overall pain severity in diabetic neuropathy and few other conditions, and practitioners are obliged to extrapolate from these data.[98] Most large clinical trials in this arena are industry-supported pivotal trials of the agent in question against placebo. There is very little evidence comparing treatments against each other. One way to try to make such a comparison is by comparing the number needed to treat (NNT), defined as the average number of individuals that must be treated with a medication to obtain a defined degree of pain relief in one subject.[99] NNT takes into consideration treatment failures for any reason, both lack of efficacy and lack of tolerability. Although NNT is usually based on 50% improvement, it has been shown that 30% improvement in pain severity or a reduction in pain severity by at least 2 points on a 0-to-10 Likert scale is clinically meaningful.[100,101]

The medication classes with the best evidence for efficacy in the management of neuropathic pain are tricyclic agents (TCAs), $\alpha_2\delta$ ligands, serotonin and norepinephrine reuptake inhibitors (SNRIs), and opioids.[102] Tramadol and tapentadol, which are believed to both inhibit serotonin and norepinephrine reuptake and act as μ-opioid agonists, have demonstrated efficacy as well.

Tricyclic Agents

TCAs are believed to derive their analgesic effect from serotonin and norepinephrine reuptake inhibition as well as sodium channel blockade. The benefit is independent of an antidepressant effect. Most undesirable effects from this class derive from its anticholinergic properties. TCAs have been demonstrated to be beneficial in relieving neuropathic pain from diabetic neuropathy in several small series. A recent Cochrane review found an overall class NNT of 3.6 for moderate pain relief among 17 studies of TCAs for neuropathic pain.[103] TCAs should be used with caution in patients at risk for cardiac arrhythmias because they can prolong the QTc interval. The most common side effects of the tricyclics are due to their anticholinergic activity and include constipation, dry mouth, blurred vision, cognitive changes, tachycardia, and urinary hesitancy. Sedation and weight gain may occur from antihistaminergic activity. α-Adrenergic receptor blockade may result in orthostatic hypotension. All of these potential side effects can be minimized by slow titration. Nortriptyline and desipramine are better tolerated than their parent drugs, amitriptyline and imipramine. Contraindications to the tricyclics include closed-angle glaucoma, benign prostatic hypertrophy, and acute myocardial infarction.

Treatment with a tricyclic should be initiated with a dose of 10 or 25 mg a few hours before bedtime to minimize daytime sedation. The lower 10-mg dose should be prescribed for the elderly, frail, or side effect–prone patient. The dose is titrated by one tablet, 10 or 25 mg, every 7 days if the patient has poor pain relief and does not complain of intolerable side effects. The majority of patients will report significant pain relief or intolerable side effects within the dose range of 30 to 150 mg. The mean dose of amitriptyline that often results in pain reduction is 75 to 150 mg per day. Onset of the analgesic effect occurs within 1 to 2 weeks and peaks around 4 to 6 weeks.[104,105] Improvement in sleep, mood, and anxiety can augment the benefit of pain control.

$\alpha_2\delta$ Ligands

Mechanical allodynia in neuropathic pain is believed to be mediated in part by increased expression of N-type calcium channels in the central terminals of primary afferent neurons, resulting in pathologically enhanced neurotransmission in the dorsal horn. Gabapentin and pregabalin are chemically related compounds that have been shown to have a modulatory effect via binding to the $\alpha_2\delta$ subunit of the calcium channel. Several studies have demonstrated that gabapentin alleviates diabetic neuropathy pain at doses ranging from 900 to 3,600 mg per day, with a combined NNT for 50% pain relief of 2.9. Two small series comparing gabapentin with amitriptyline demonstrated improvement in pain ratings with both drugs, and no statistically significant difference in benefit between them.[106,107] It should be noted, however, that serious adverse events can occur with amitriptyline and are virtually unknown with gabapentin. Gabapentin can cause weight gain, reversible cognitive symptoms, and peripheral edema.

Gabapentin bioavailability is limited because absorption from the gastrointestinal tract is dependent on a single saturable active transport mechanism. Pregabalin shares gabapentin's presumed mechanism of action but demonstrates more linear kinetics than gabapentin. Presumably for this reason, pregabalin is absorbed more quickly and demonstrates more linear kinetics than gabapentin. Pregabalin has been shown to be effective in relieving the pain of diabetic neuropathy, with NNTs for 50% pain relief of 3.4 and 3.3 for the 300 mg per day and 600 mg per day doses, respectively.[108,109] Like gabapentin, pregabalin can cause cognitive side effects which are usually mild to moderate in severity as well as weight gain and peripheral edema.

Serotonin and Norepinephrine Reuptake Inhibitors

Serotonin and norepinephrine reuptake inhibition is believed to alleviate neuropathic pain by facilitating descending inhibition of afferent pain signaling. This descending inhibition is mediated by neurons of the rostroventral medulla. It is believed that both neurotransmitters are important in this pathway, which may explain the observation that selective serotonin reuptake inhibitors (SSRIs) alone are of little benefit in alleviating pain from neuropathy.[107] Duloxetine, an SNRI with relative balance between serotonergic and noradrenergic effects, has demonstrated efficacy in relieving pain from diabetic neuropathy, with an NNT for 50% pain relief of 4.3 at a dose of 60 mg per day and 3.8 at a dose of 120 mg per day.[110] Venlafaxine, an SNRI with balanced pharmacology at high doses, has also been shown to be beneficial, with an NNT of 4.5 for 50% pain relief in the 150- to 225-mg dose range.[111] SNRIs can cause nausea, hyperhidrosis, and sexual side effects in some patients. Although they do not have substantial anticholinergic properties, they can cause some symptoms of dry mouth and dizziness, possibly on a noradrenergic basis; however, these effects are probably less frequent or severe than with tricyclic medications. Combining SNRIs with other serotonergic agents, including other antidepressants, triptans, and tramadol, should be done with caution because of the risk of serotonin syndrome. SNRIs are also known to inhibit the metabolism of other antidepressants, thus substantially increasing blood levels of such drugs when they are used in combination. For these reasons, it is usually best to avoid the use of SNRIs with other antidepressants and to consider using one SNRI or TCA alone to treat both pain and depression if treatment of both conditions is indicated.

Opioids

Opioids strongly inhibit central nociceptive neurons mainly through interaction with μ-opioid receptors, producing neuronal membrane hyperpolarization. Although controlled-release oxycodone has been shown to reduce pain from diabetic neuropathy in two small randomized controlled trials, with an NNT for moderate pain relief of 2.6,[112,113] complications of chronic opioid use, including dependence, tolerance, and hyperalgesia, have led to substantial morbidity and mortality among users of opioids for noncancer pain in the last two decades. Systematic review of evidence does not support or refute long-term use of opioids for treatment of neuropathic pain.[114] However, a recently published large population study showed that patients using opioids for polyneuropathy pain had lower self-reported functional outcome scores compared to users of nonopioid medications.[115] These facts have led to a substantial reduction in opioid prescriptions for neuropathic pain in recent years, along with increased monitoring of prescriptions and stricter mandates for training of prescribing providers by federal agencies. Particular caution is required in patients with pulmonary disease. Prophylactic treatment of common side effects such as nausea or constipation can improve patient compliance.

Tramadol and Tapentadol

Tramadol and tapentadol are both inhibitors of serotonin and norepinephrine reuptake and μ-opioid agonists. Both have been shown to effectively alleviate pain in diabetic neuropathy.[116–118] They are available in immediate- and extended-release formulations.

Other Pharmacologic Agents

Several other agents approved for the treatment of epilepsy have demonstrated limited evidence of efficacy in the management of pain from neuropathy. These include oxcarbazepine, which has demonstrated benefit in one randomized controlled study in diabetic neuropathy pain, lamotrigine, and topiramate, both agents which have demonstrated conflicting results in randomized controlled trials for pain from diabetic neuropathy.[119–123] Despite limited evidence of efficacy, these have all been used on occasion as second- or third-line agents for patients who have not responded to or tolerated other treatments. Carbamazepine, which is approved for pain from trigeminal neuralgia, has been found to be effective in two double-blind, placebo-controlled studies for control of pain in diabetic neuropathy.[124,125] Prior to the availability of many of the aforementioned agents for neuropathic pain management, phenytoin was shown to be effective in controlled trials of pain from diabetic polyneuropathy[126] and pain in Fabry's disease.[127] Phenytoin is no longer commonly used to treat pain due to neuropathy.

Bupropion, a unique agent which inhibits norepinephrine and dopamine uptake, has shown benefit in one study involving pain from a variety of neuropathy etiologies.[128]

Acetyl-L-carnitine (ALC) is believed to have several potentially neuroprotective properties that have led to extensive study of this agent as a treatment for diabetic, HIV, and chemotherapy-induced neuropathy.[129–131] It also has analgesic properties. ALC has been administered at doses between 1 and 3 g per day. α-Lipoic acid, a potent antioxidant, has also been studied as a potential treatment of both diabetic neuropathy and diabetic neuropathy pain. The recently completed SYDNEY 2 trial showed that daily oral therapy at a dose of 600 mg per day, the lowest dose yet studied, reduced the neuropathy total symptom score by 50% or greater with an NNT of 2.8.[132,133]

Cannabinoids

In the last decade, the use of cannabis and selective cannabinoids (synthetic cannabinoids containing only tetrahydrocannabinol [THC] and cannabis-based medicinal extracts containing a combination of THC and cannabidiol [CBD]) has gained popularity for the treatment of neuropathic pain. Cannabinoid receptors, CB1 and CB2, are linked to pain modulation, whereby activity at these receptors causes inhibitory effects on pain responses.[134,135] Furthermore, endocannabinoids have been shown to interact with other receptor systems including γ-aminobutyric acid (GABA), serotonergic, adrenergic, and opioid receptors, many of which are involved in the analgesic mechanisms of neuropathic pain drugs. A recent elegant meta-analysis of 11 randomized controlled trials including a total 1,219 patients, showed that patients who received selective cannabinoids reported a significant, but clinically small, reduction in mean numerical rating scale pain scores compared with placebo groups (-0.65 points; $P = .002$). Use of selective cannabinoids was also associated with improvements in quality of life and sleep with no major adverse effects. Major limitations of the studies included variability in quality of reporting, etiology of neuropathic pain, and type and dose of selective cannabinoids.[136] Larger randomized controlled trials, with better control of the aforementioned variables, as well as regulatory changes, would be needed before cannabinoids can become standard of care for the management of painful neuropathies.

Topical Agents

Capsaicin stimulates the release of substance P from small-caliber primary afferent neurons and is believed to alleviate neuropathic pain with regular use by exhausting stores of substance P. Capsaicin also causes prompt epidermal denervation so reliably that capsaicin denervation has become an important human model of neuropathy. Although capsaicin can alleviate neuropathic pain with sustained use, it also causes considerable burning discomfort which limits its use. A high-potency capsaicin patch is presently undergoing clinical trials and demonstrated efficacy and safety for treatment of pain in DPN.[137]

Topical lidocaine, a local anesthetic which acts via sodium channel blockade, has been approved for the treatment of PHN. It is used on occasion to treat cutaneous pain from other neuropathic conditions as well. Systemically administered lidocaine, mexiletine, and tocainide have also been demonstrated to have analgesic effects for control of diabetic neuropathic pain and in PHN.[138–140] Systemically administered local anesthetics block ectopic discharges due to experimental peripheral nerve injury and in axotomized dorsal root ganglion cells of the peripheral nerves,[141] probably by blocking sodium channels.[142] In addition, there is evidence that lidocaine and similar local anesthetics have actions on G protein-coupled receptors that can result in long-lasting modulation of pain via effects both on sensitization and on the immune response to nerve injury.[143,144]

Principles of Pharmacotherapy for Pain from Neuropathy

Polypharmacy is common in the treatment of pain from neuropathy for several reasons. First, neuropathy pain can be treated with several classes of agents, with different postulated mechanisms of action. Second, on a more practical level, there is (fortuitously) relative compatibility among these medication classes. And finally, despite evidence that these treatments are generally efficacious, it is uncommon to achieve complete or even adequate pain relief with a single agent, although it is common to encounter significant adverse effects. Therefore, one usually begins with slow upward titration of one of the first-line drugs (SNRIs, $\alpha_2\delta$ ligands, or tricyclics), followed by the addition of another first-line agent (but generally *not* an SNRI *with* a tricyclic) if pain relief is inadequate at the highest tolerated dose of the first drug. Because these are generally chronic conditions, there is no need to titrate faster than tolerability will permit. Opioids or tramadol is often used as third-line agents or as rescue drugs and are particularly helpful for patients who can predict an increase in pain after a physically active day. Topical and nonpharmacologic treatments are particularly valuable as add-on therapy for patients who do not tolerate medication well. Cognitive-behavioral therapy, discussed in Chapter 84, can be very helpful because it is often the distress associated with pain, sometimes more than the pain itself, that causes pain-related disability.

Unresolved Questions

There are a number of unresolved questions in the evaluation and management of painful neuropathies. First, the pathophysiologic mechanisms responsible for the wide variety of painful neuropathy symptoms remain inadequately understood. Second, it is not known whether treatment of neuropathic pain influences the natural history of neuropathy or even whether successful treatment with an analgesic medication alters the natural history of pain. There is also insufficient evidence to guide duration of therapy. For example, do patients who report significant pain relief with a certain medication need to be treated with that particular medication at that dose indefinitely? Most pivotal clinical trials in this field run for about 12 weeks' duration, which is woefully inadequate in the context of conditions that usually persist for years.

Much of our understanding of mechanisms, such as ectopic and ephaptic transmission, neurogenic inflammation, descending modulation, and peripheral and central sensitization, comes from animal models that do not mimic human neuropathies. A better understanding of mechanism in humans will likely require systematic investigation of pain in people with neuropathy. Just as the diagnosis and management of conditions causing neurologic deficit rely on an ever more sophisticated clinical/laboratory/radiographic correlation, so too the management of pain from neuropathy must advance with the help of evidence gleaned in a systematic fashion from neuropathic pain questionnaires; neuropathic pain examinations; and relevant imaging, pathologic, and laboratory tools.

References

1. Dyck PJ, Thomas PK, eds. *Peripheral Neuropathy*. 4th ed. Philadelphia: Elsevier Saunders; 2005.
2. Donofrio P, eds. *Textbook of Peripheral Neuropathy*. New York: Demos Medical; 2012.
3. Bennett M. The LANSS pain scale: the Leeds assessment of neuropathic symptoms and signs. *Pain* 2001;92:147–157.
4. Galer BS, Jensen MP. Development and preliminary validation of a pain measure specific to neuropathic pain: the neuropathic pain scale. *Neurology* 1997;48:332–338.
5. Bouhassira D, Attal N, Fermanian J, et al. Development and validation of the neuropathic pain symptom inventory. *Pain* 2004;108:248–257.
6. Krause SJ, Backonja MM. Development of a neuropathic pain questionnaire. *Clin J Pain* 2003;19:306–314.
7. Bennett MI, Attal N, Backonja MM, et al. Using screening tools to identify neuropathic pain. *Pain* 2007;127:199–203.
8. Dyck PJ, Karnes J, O'Brien PC, et al. Neuropathy symptom profile in health, motor neuron disease, diabetic neuropathy, and amyloidosis. *Neurology* 1986;36:1300–1308.
9. Savage CW. *The Measurement of Sensation*. Berkeley: University of California Press; 1970.
10. Hansson P, Backonja M, Bouhassira D. Usefulness and limitations of quantitative sensory testing: clinical and research application in neuropathic pain states. *Pain* 2007;129(3):256–259.
11. Greenspan JD. Quantitative assessment of neuropathic pain. *Curr Pain Headache Rev* 2001;5:107–113.
12. Rolke R, Magerl W, Campbell KA, et al. Quantitative sensory testing: a comprehensive protocol for clinical trials. *Eur J Pain* 2006;10:77–88.
13. Vollert J, Maier C, Attal N, et al. Stratifying patients with peripheral neuropathic pain based on sensory profiles: algorithm and sample size recommendations. *Pain* 2017;158:1446–1455.
14. Walk D, Sehgal N, Moeller-Bertram T, et al. Quantitative sensory testing and mapping: a review of non-automated quantitative methods for examination of the patient with neuropathic pain. *Clin J Pain* 2009;25:632–640.
15. Hoitsma E, Reulen JP, de Baets M, et al. Small fiber neuropathy: a common and important clinical disorder. *J Neurol Sci* 2004;227:119–130.
16. Periquet MI, Novak V, Collins MP, et al. Painful sensory neuropathy: prospective evaluation using skin biopsy. *Neurology* 1999;53:1641–1647.
17. Lacomis D. Small-fiber neuropathy. *Muscle Nerve* 2002;26:173–188.
18. Walk D, Wendelschafer-Crabb G, Davey C, et al. Concordance between epidermal nerve fiber density and sensory examination in patients with symptoms of idiopathic small fiber neuropathy. *J Neurol Sci* 2007;255:23–26.
19. Walk D, Zaretskaya M, Parry GJ. Symptom duration and clinical features in painful sensory neuropathy with and without nerve conduction abnormalities. *J Neurol Sci* 2003;214:3–6.
20. Low VA, Sandroni P, Fealey RD, et al. Detection of small-fiber neuropathy by sudomotor testing. *Muscle Nerve* 2006;34(1):57–61.
21. Casellini CM, Parson HK, Richardson MS, et al. Sudoscan, a noninvasive tool for detecting diabetic small fiber neuropathy and autonomic dysfunction. *Diabetes Technol Ther* 2013;15(11):948–953.
22. Serra J, Bostock H, Solà R, et al. Microneurographic identification of spontaneous activity in C-nociceptors in neuropathic pain states in humans and rats. *Pain* 2011;153:42–55.
23. Hossain P, Sachdev A, Malik RA. Early detection of diabetic peripheral neuropathy with corneal confocal microscopy. *Lancet* 2005;366:1340–1343.
24. Said G. Indications and usefulness of nerve biopsy. *Arch Neurol* 2002;59:1532–1535.
25. Abbott CA, Malik RA, van Ross ER, et al. Prevalence and characteristics of painful diabetic neuropathy in a large community-based diabetic population in the U.K. *Diabetes Care* 2011;34:2220–2224.
26. Feldman EL, Nave KA, Jensen TS, et al. New horizons in diabetic neuropathy: mechanisms, bioenergetics, and pain. *Neuron* 2017;93(6):1296–1313.
27. Grundy SM, Cleeman JI, Daniels SR, et al. Diagnosis and management of the metabolic syndrome. *Circulation* 2005;112:2735–2752.
28. Hughes RA, Umapathi T, Gray IA, et al. A controlled investigation of the cause of chronic acquired idiopathic axonal polyneuropathy. *Brain* 2004;127:1723–1730.
29. McManis PG, Windebank AJ, Kiziltan M. Neuropathy associated with hyperlipidemia. *Neurology* 1994;44:2185–2186.
30. Isomaa B, Henricsson M, Almgren P, et al. The metabolic syndrome influences the risk of chronic complications in patients with type II diabetes. *Diabetologia* 2001;44:1148–1154.

31. Tesfaye S, Chaturvedi N, Eaton SE, et al. Vascular risk factors and diabetic neuropathy. *N Engl J Med* 2005;352:341–350.

32. Kamerman PR, Moss PJ, Weber J, et al. Pathogenesis of HIV-associated sensory neuropathy: evidence from in vivo and in vitro experimental models. *J Peripher Nerv Syst* 2012;17:19–31.

33. Wulff EA, Wang AK, Simpson DM. HIV-associated peripheral neuropathy: epidemiology, pathophysiology and treatment. *Drugs* 2000;59(6):1251–1260.

34. Morgello S, Estanislao L, Simpson D, et al. HIV-associated distal sensory polyneuropathy in the era of highly active antiretroviral therapy. *Arch Neurol* 2004;61:546–551.

35. Biasiotta A, Casato M, La Cesa S, et al. Clinical, neurophysiological, and skin biopsy findings in peripheral neuropathy associated with hepatitis C virus-related cryoglobulinemia. *J Neurol* 2014;261(4):725–731.

36. Yoon MS, Obermann M, Dockweiler C, et al. Sensory neuropathy in patients with cryoglobulin negative hepatitis-C infection. *J Neurol* 2011;258(1):80–88.

37. Halperin JJ. Lyme disease and the peripheral nervous system. *Muscle Nerve* 2003;28:133–143.

38. Said G. Infectious neuropathies. *Neurol Clin* 2007;25:115–137.

39. London Z, Albers JW. Toxic neuropathies associated with pharmaceutic and industrial agents. *Neurol Clin* 2007;25:257–276.

40. Umapathi T, Chaudhry V. Toxic neuropathy. *Curr Opin Neurol* 2005;18:574–580.

41. Staff NP, Grisold A, Grisold W, et al. Chemotherapy-induced peripheral neuropathy: a current review. *Ann Neurol* 2017;81:772–781.

42. Flatters SJ, Bennett GJ. Studies of peripheral sensory nerves in paclitaxel-induced painful peripheral neuropathy: evidence for mitochondrial dysfunction. *Pain* 2006;122(3):245–257.

43. Kril JJ. Neuropathology of thiamine deficiency disorders. *Metab Brain Dis* 1996;11(1):9–17.

44. Djoenaddi W, Notermans SL, Lilisantoso AH. Electrophysiologic examination of subclinical beriberi polyneuropathy. *Electromyogr Clin Neurophysiol* 1995;35:439–442.

45. Bosch EP, Pelham RW, Rasool CG, et al. Animal models of alcoholic neuropathy: morphologic, electrophysiologic, and biochemical findings. *Muscle Nerve* 1979;2(2):133–144.

46. Behse F, Buchtal F. Alcoholic neuropathy: clinical, electrophysiological, and biopsy findings. *Ann Neurol* 1977;2:95–110.

47. Koike H, Sobue G. Alcoholic neuropathy. *Curr Opin Neurobiol* 2006;19:481–486.

48. Laski JR, Garcia A. Charcot-Marie-Tooth peripheral neuropathies and related disorders. In: Scriver CR, Beaudet AL, Sly WS, et al, eds. *The Metabolic and Molecular Bases of Inherited Diseases.* 8th ed. New York: McGraw-Hill; 2001:5759–5788.

49. Desnick RJ, Ioannou YA, Eng CM. Alpha-galactosidase A deficiency: Fabry disease. In: Scriver CR, Beaudet AL, Sly WS, et al, eds. *The Metabolic and Molecular Bases of Inherited Diseases.* 8th ed. New York: McGraw-Hill; 2001:3733–3774.

50. Beck M, Ricci R, Widmer U, et al. Fabry disease: overall effects of agalsidase alfa treatment. *Eur J Clin Invest* 2004;34:838–844.

51. Hoffman B, Garcia de Lorenzo A, Mehta A, et al; for FOS European Investigators. Effects of enzyme replacement on pain and health-related quality of life in patients with Fabry disease: data from the FOS (Fabry outcome survey). *J Med Genet* 2005;42:247–252.

52. Üçeyler N, He L, Schönfeld D, et al. Small fibers in Fabry disease: baseline and follow-up data under enzyme replacement therapy. *J Periph Nerv Syst* 2011;16:304–314.

53. Dib-Hajj SD, Yang Y, Black JA, et al. The Na(V)1.7 sodium channel: from molecule to man. *Nat Rev Neurosci* 2013;14:49–62.

54. Yang Y, Wang Y, Li S, et al. Mutations in SCN9A, encoding a sodium channel alpha subunit, in patients with primary erythromelalgia. *J Med Genet* 2004;41:171–174.

55. Fertleman CR, Baker MD, Parker KA, et al. SCN9A mutations in paroxysmal extreme pain disorder: allelic variants underlie distinct channel defects and phenotypes. *Neuron* 2006;52:767–774.

56. Faber CG, Hoeijmakers JG, Ahn HS, et al. Gain of function Nav1.7 mutations in idiopathic small fiber neuropathy. *Ann Neurol* 2012;71:26–39.

57. Faber CG, Lauria G, Merkies IS, et al. Gain-of-function Nav.18 mutations in painful neuropathy. *Proc Natl Acad Sci USA* 2012;109:1944–1949.

58. Emery EC, Luiz AP, Wood JN. Nav1.7 and other voltage-gated sodium channels as drug targets for pain relief. *Expert Opin Ther Targets* 2016;20(8):975–983.

59. Bergethon PR, Sabin TD, Lewis D, et al. Improvement in the polyneuropathy associated with familial amyloid polyneuropathy after liver transplantation. *Neurology* 1996;47:944–951.

60. Coelho T, Merlini G, Bulawa CE, et al. Mechanism of action and clinical application of tafamidis in hereditary transthyretin amyloidosis. *Neurol Ther* 2016;5:1–25.

61. Adams D, Cauquil C, Labeyrie C, et al. TTR kinetic stabilizers and TTR gene silencing: a new era in therapy for familial amyloidotic polyneuropathies. *Expert Opin Pharmacother* 2016;17:791–802.

62. Kwan JY. Paraproteinemic neuropathy. *Neurol Clin* 2007;25:47–69.

63. Steck AJ, Stalder AK, Renaud S. Anti-myelin-associated glycoprotein neuropathy. *Curr Opin Neurol* 2006;19:458–463.

64. Katz JS, Saperstein DS, Gronseth G, et al. Distal acquired demyelinating symmetric neuropathy. *Neurology* 2000;54:615–620.

65. Liewluck T, Engelstad JK, Mauermann ML. Immunotherapy-responsive allodynia due to distal acquired demyelinating symmetric (DADS) neuropathy. *Muscle Nerve* 2016;54(5):973–977.

66. Sung JY, Kuwabara S, Ogawara K, et al. Patterns of nerve conduction abnormalities in POEMS syndrome. *Muscle Nerve* 2002;26:189–193.

67. Willison HJ, Jacobs BC, van Doorn PA. Guillain-Barré syndrome. *Lancet* 2016;388(10045):717–727.

68. Richardson EP Jr, De Girolami U. *Pathology of the Peripheral Nerve.* Philadelphia: W.B. Saunders; 1995.

69. Griffin JW, Li CY, Ho TW, et al. Guillain-Barré syndrome in northern China. The spectrum of neuropathological changes in clinically defined cases. *Brain* 1995;118:577–595.

70. Yuki N, Kuwabara S. Axonal Guillain-Barré syndrome: carbohydrate mimicry and pathophysiology. *J Peripher Nerv Syst* 2007;12:238–249.

71. Thakur S, Dworkin RH, Freeman R, et al. Pain in acquired inflammatory demyelinating polyneuropathies. *Pain* 2016;157:1887–1894.

72. Ruts L, van Koningsveld R, Jacobs BC, et al. Determination of pain and response to methylprednisolone in Guillain-Barré syndrome. *J Neurol* 2007;254:1318–1322.

73. Devor M. The pathophysiology of damaged peripheral nerves. In: Wall PD, ed. *Textbook of Pain.* New York: Churchill Livingstone; 1989:63–81.

74. Genis D, Busquets C, Manubens E, et al. Epidural morphine analgesia in Guillain-Barré syndrome. *J Neurol Neurosurg Psych* 1989;52:999–1001.

75. Hughes RA, Bouche P, Cornblath DR, et al. European Federation of Neurological Societies/Peripheral Nerve Society guideline on management of chronic inflammatory demyelinating polyradiculoneuropathy: report of a joint task force of the European Federation of Neurological Societies and the Peripheral Nerve Society. *Eur J Neurol* 2006;13(4):326–332.

76. Lewis RA. Chronic inflammatory demyelinating polyneuropathy. *Neurol Clin* 2007;25:71–87.

77. Kissel JT, Mendel JR. Vasculitic neuropathy. In: Johnson RT, ed. *Current Therapy in Neurology Disease.* 4th ed. St. Louis, MO: B.C. Decker; 1993:365–368.

78. van Alfen N, van Engelen BG. The clinical spectrum of neuralgic amyotrophy in 246 cases. *Brain* 2006;129:438–450.

79. Nakajima M, Fujioka S, Ohno H, et al. Partial but rapid recovery from paralysis after immunomodulation during early stage of neuralgic amyotrophy. *Eur Neurol* 2006;55:227–229.

80. van Alfen N, Gabreëls-Festen AA, Ter Laak HJ, et al. Histology of hereditary neuralgic amyotrophy. *J Neurol Neurosurg Psychiatry* 2005;76:445–447.

81. Kuhlenbäumer G, Hannibal MC, Nelis E, et al. Mutations in SEPT9 cause hereditary neuralgic amyotrophy. *Nat Genet* 2005;37(10):1044–1046.

82. Kelkar P, Masood M, Parry GJ. Distinctive pathologic findings in proximal diabetic neuropathy (diabetic amyotrophy). *Neurology* 2000;55(1):83–88.

83. Kelkar P, Parry GJ. Mononeuritis multiplex in diabetes mellitus: evidence for underlying immune pathogenesis. *J Neurol Neurosurg Psychiatry* 2003;74:803–806.

84. Tracy JA, Dyck PJ. The spectrum of diabetic neuropathies. *Phys Med Rehabil Clin N Am* 2008;19:1–26.

85. Yawn BP, Saddier P, Wollan PC, et al. A population-based study of the incidence and complication rates of herpes zoster before zoster vaccine introduction. *Mayo Clin Proc* 2007;82(11):1341–1349.

86. Niv D, Maltsman-Tseikhin A. Postherpetic neuralgia: the never-ending challenge. *Pain Pract* 2005;5(4):327–340.

87. Weinberg JM. Herpes zoster: epidemiology, natural history, and common complications. *J Am Acad Dermatol* 2007;57:S130–S135.

88. Tyring S, Barbarash RA, Nahlik JE, et al. Famciclovir for the treatment of acute herpes zoster: effects on acute disease and postherpetic neuralgia. A randomized, double-blind, placebo-controlled trial. *Ann Intern Med* 1995;123:89–96.

89. Quan D, Hammack BN, Kittelson J, et al. Improvement of postherpetic neuralgia after treatment with intravenous acyclovir followed by oral valacyclovir. *Arch Neurol* 2006;63:940–942.

90. Jackson JL, Gibbons R, Meyer G, et al. The effect of treating herpes zoster with oral acyclovir in preventing postherpetic neuralgia. A meta-analysis. *Arch Intern Med* 1997;157(8):909–912.

91. Vitali C, Bombardieri S, Jonsson R, et al. Classification criteria for Sjögren syndrome: a revised version of the European criteria proposed by the American-European Consensus Group. *Ann Rheum Dis* 2002;61:554–558.

92. Delalande S, de Seze J, Fauchais AL, et al. Neurologic manifestations in primary Sjögren syndrome: a study of 82 patients. *Medicine (Baltimore)* 2004;83(5):280–291.

93. Mori K, Iijima M, Koike H, et al. The wide spectrum of clinical manifestations in Sjögren's syndrome-associated neuropathy. *Brain* 2005;128:2518–2534.

94. Gorson KC, Herrmann DN, Thiagarajan R, et al. Non-length dependent small fibre neuropathy/ganglionopathy. *J Neurol Neurosurg Psychiatry* 2008;79(2):163–169.

95. Vedeler CA, Antoine JC, Giometto B. Management of paraneoplastic neurological syndromes: report of an EFNS task force. *Eur J Neurol* 2006;13:682–690.

96. Krarup-Hansen A, Helweg-Larsen S, Schmalbruch H, et al. Neuronal involvement in cisplatin neuropathy: prospective clinical and neurophysiological studies. *Brain* 2007;130:1076–1088.

97. Dworkin RH, Turk DC, Wyrwich KW, et al. Interpreting the clinical importance of treatment outcomes in chronic pain clinical trials: IMMPACT recommendations. *J Pain* 2008;9(2):105–121.

98. Gilron I, Baron R, Jensen T. Neuropathic pain: principles of diagnosis and treatment. *Mayo Clin Proc* 2015;90:532–545.

99. Cook RJ, Sackett DL. The number needed to treat: a clinically useful measure of treatment effect. *BMJ* 1995;310:452–454.

100. Farrar JT, Portenoy RK, Berlin JA, et al. Defining the clinically important difference in pain outcome measures. *Pain* 2000;88:287–294.

101. Farrar JT, Berlin JA, Strom BL. Clinically important changes in acute pain outcome measures: a validation study. *J Pain Symptom Manage* 2003;25(5):406–411.

102. Dworkin RH, O'Connor AB, Backonja M, et al. Pharmacologic management of neuropathic pain: evidence-based recommendations. *Pain* 2007;132(3):237–251.

103. Saarto T, Wiffen PJ. Antidepressants for neuropathic pain. *Cochrane Database Syst Rev* 2007;(4):CD005454.

104. Max MB, Culnane M, Schafer SC, et al. Amitriptyline relieves diabetic neuropathy pain in patients with normal or depressed mood. *Neurology* 1987;37:589–596.

105. Max MB, Schafer SC, Culnane M, et al. Amitriptyline, but not lorazepam, relieves postherpetic neuralgia. *Neurology* 1988;38:1427–1432.

106. Rao RD, Michalak JC, Sloan JA, et al. Efficacy of gabapentin in the management of chemotherapy-induced peripheral neuropathy: a phase 3 randomized, double-blind, placebo-controlled, crossover trial (N00C3). *Cancer* 2007;110(9):2110–2118.

107. Wiffen PJ, McQuay HJ, Edwards JE, et al. Gabapentin for acute and chronic pain. *Cochrane Database Syst Rev* 2005;(3):CD005452.

108. Rosenstock J, Tuchman M, LaMoreaux L, et al. Pregabalin for the treatment of painful diabetic peripheral neuropathy: a double-blind, placebo-controlled trial. *Pain* 2004;110:628–638.

109. Lesser H, Sharma U, LaMoreaux L, et al. Pregabalin relieves symptoms of painful diabetic neuropathy: a randomized controlled trial. *Neurology* 2004;63:2104–2110.

110. Goldstein DJ, Lu Y, Detke MJ, et al. Duloxetine vs. placebo in patients with painful diabetic neuropathy. *Pain* 2005;116:109–118.

111. Rowbotham MC, Goli V, Kunz NR, et al. Venlafaxine extended release in the treatment of painful diabetic neuropathy: a double-blind, placebo-controlled study. *Pain* 2004;110:697–706.

112. Watson CP, Moulin D, Watt-Watson J, et al. Controlled-release oxycodone relieves neuropathic pain: a randomized controlled trial in painful diabetic neuropathy. *Pain* 2003;105:71–78.

113. Gimbel JS, Richards P, Portenoy RK. Controlled-release oxycodone for pain in diabetic neuropathy: a randomized controlled trial. *Neurology* 2003;60:927–934.

114. Cooper T, Chen J, Wiffen PJ, et al. Morphine for chronic neuropathic pain in adults. *Cochrane Database Syst Rev* 2017;(5):CD011669.

115. Hoffman EM, Watson JC, St Sauver J, et al. Association of long-term opioid therapy with functional status, adverse outcomes, and mortality among patients with polyneuropathy. *JAMA Neurol* 2017;74(7):773–779.

116. Harati Y, Gooch C, Swenson M, et al. Double-blind randomized trial of tramadol for the treatment of the pain of diabetic neuropathy. *Neurology* 1998;50:1842–1846.

117. Sindrup SH, Andersen G, Madsen C, et al. Tramadol relieves pain and allodynia in polyneuropathy: a randomized, double-blind, controlled trial. *Pain* 1999;83:85–90.

118. Schwartz S, Etropolski M, Shapiro DY, et al. Safety and efficacy of tapentadol ER in patients with painful diabetic peripheral neuropathy: results of a randomized-withdrawal, placebo-controlled trial. *Curr Med Res Opin* 2011;27(1):151–162.

119. Beydoun A, Kobetz SA, Carrazana EJ. Efficacy of oxcarbazepine in the treatment of painful diabetic neuropathy. *Clin J Pain* 2004;20:174–178.

120. Eisenberg E, Lurie Y, Braker C, et al. Lamotrigine reduces painful diabetic neuropathy: a randomized, controlled study. *Neurology* 2001;57:505–509.

121. Vinik AI, Tuchman M, Safirstein B, et al. Lamotrigine for treatment of pain associated with diabetic neuropathy: results of two randomized, double-blind, placebo-controlled studies. *Pain* 2007;128:169–179.

122. Thienel U, Neto W, Schwabe SK, et al. Topiramate in painful diabetic polyneuropathy: findings from three double-blind placebo-controlled trials. *Acta Neurol Scand* 2004;110:221–231.

123. Raskin P, Donofrio PD, Rosenthal NR, et al. Topiramate vs. placebo in painful diabetic neuropathy: analgesic and metabolic effects. *Neurology* 2004;63:865–873.

124. Rull JA, Quibrera R, González-Millán H, et al. Symptomatic treatment of peripheral diabetic neuropathy with carbamazepine (Tegretol): double-blind crossover trial. *Diabetologia* 1969;5:215–218.

125. Wilton TD. Tegretol in the treatment of diabetic neuropathy. *S Afr Med J* 1974;48:869–872.

126. Chadda VS, Mathur MS. Double blind study of the effects of diphenylhydantoin sodium diabetic neuropathy. *J Assoc Physicians India* 1978;26:403–406.

127. Lockman LA, Hunninghake DB, Krivit W, et al. Relief of pain of Fabry's disease by diphenylhydantoin. *Neurology* 1973;23:871–875.

128. Semenchuk MR, Sherman S, Davis B. Double-blind, randomized trial of bupropion SR for the treatment of neuropathic pain. *Neurology* 2001;57:1583–1588.

129. De Grandis D. Acetyl-L-carnitine for the treatment of chemotherapy-induced peripheral neuropathy. *CNS Drugs* 2007;1(suppl 21):39–43.

130. Sima AA. Acetyl-L-carnitine in diabetic polyneuropathy: experimental and clinical data. *CNS Drugs* 2007;1(suppl 21):13–23.

131. Youle M. Acetyl-L-carnitine in HIV-associated antiretroviral toxic neuropathy. *CNS Drugs* 2007;1(suppl 1):25–30.

132. Foster TS. Efficacy and safety of alpha-lipoic acid supplementation in the treatment of symptomatic diabetic neuropathy. *Diabetes Educ* 2007;33(1):111–117.

133. Ziegler D, Ametov A, Barinov A, et al. Oral treatment with alpha-lipoic acid improves symptomatic diabetic polyneuropathy: the SYDNEY 2 trial. *Diabetes Care* 2006;29:2365–2370.

134. Kelly S, Jhaveri MD, Sagar DR, et al. Activation of peripheral cannabinoid CB1 receptors inhibits mechanically evoked responses of spinal neurons in noninflamed rats and rats with hindpaw inflammation. *Eur J Neurosci* 2003;18:2239–2243.

135. Ibrahim MM, Rude ML, Stagg NJ, et al. CB2 cannabinoid receptor mediation of antinociception. *Pain* 2006;122:36–42.

136. Meng H, Johnston B, Englesakis M, et al. Selective cannabinoids for chronic neuropathic pain: a systematic review and meta-analysis. *Anesth Analg* 2017;125:1638–1652.

137. Simpson DM, Robinson-Papp J, Van J, et al. Capsaicin 8% patch in painful diabetic peripheral neuropathy: a randomized, double-blind, placebo-controlled study. *J Pain* 2017;18(1):42–53.

138. Rowbotham MC, Reisner-Keller LA, Fields HL. Both intravenous lidocaine and morphine reduce the pain of postherpetic neuralgia. *Neurology* 1991;41:1024–1028.

139. Kastrup J, Petersen P, Dejgård A, et al. Intravenous lidocaine infusion—a new treatment of chronic painful diabetic neuropathy? *Pain* 1987;28:69–75.

140. Bach FW, Jensen TS, Kastrup J, et al. The effect of intravenous lidocaine on nociceptive processing in diabetic neuropathy [see comments]. *Pain* 1990;40:29–34.

141. Devor M, Wall PD, Catalan N. Systemic lidocaine silences ectopic neuroma and DRG discharge without blocking nerve conduction. *Pain* 1992;48:261–268.

142. Devor M, Matzner O. Sodium channel accumulation in the injured axons as a substrate for neuropathic pain. In: Boivie J, Hansson P, Lindblom U, eds. *Touch, Temperature, and Pain in Health and Disease: Mechanisms and Assessments.* Seattle, WA: IASP Press; 1994:207–230.

143. Amir R, Argoff CE, Bennett GJ, et al. The role of sodium channels in chronic inflammatory and neuropathic pain. *J Pain* 2006;7(suppl 3):S1–S29.

144. Wrzosek A, Woron J, Dobrogowski J, et al. Topical clonidine for neuropathic pain. *Cochrane Database Syst Rev* 2015;(8):CD010967.

CHAPTER 25

Complex Regional Pain Syndrome

MICHAEL T. MASSEY and ROBERT NORMAN HARDEN

Complex regional pain syndrome (CRPS) is the current taxonomy for the syndrome previously known by various names, including reflex sympathetic dystrophy (RSD), causalgia, Sudeck's atrophy, shoulder–hand syndrome, neuro-algodystrophy, and reflex neurovascular dystrophy, etc. It was originally recognized as a distinct pain syndrome seen among Union veterans of the War Between the States following traumatic nerve injury ("causalgia").[1] It is an extremely heterogeneous disease with inflammatory, autoimmune, sympathetic, and neuropathic features that change over time. It is usually a chronic disease that involves a full measure of biopsychosocial features, and it can be significantly disabling.

Epidemiology

Epidemiologic data regarding CRPS in the general population are limited, although three large-scale studies are available. Sandroni et al.[2] reported an incidence of 5.46 new cases of CRPS type I per 100,000 annually (see Table 25.1 for distinction between type I and type II).[2] A larger study reported an incidence as high as 26.2 new cases per 100,000 annually.[3] Based on this reported incidence, over 50,000 new cases of CRPS type I could be anticipated annually in the United States alone.[4] However, both of these studies used the 1994 International Association for the Study of Pain (IASP) diagnostic criteria.[5] These results may be inflated as the new 2012 IASP criteria, being more objective, have been demonstrated to reduce diagnostic rates by about 50% when compared to the old 1994 IASP criteria.[6] Most recently, a retrospective analysis from a Nationwide Inpatient Sample Database during 2007 to 2011 demonstrated 22,533 patients with a discharge diagnosis of CRPS type I sampled from 33,406,123 patients. Based on these data, the general prevalence of CRPS type I in an inpatient environment could be 67.4 cases per 100,000 patients. However, these numbers are limited to an inpatient environment and should not be generalized to patients or healthy individuals in an outpatient setting. Further, there was no relevant data indicating what criteria were used to make the diagnosis leaving validity of the diagnostic coding uncertain.[7] For physicians making pain diagnoses, the incidence of CRPS in relevant at-risk populations

(e.g., postfracture) may be more clinically relevant. Three recent large-scale prospective studies examine the incidence of CRPS postfracture.[8–10] Beerthuizen et al.[8] reported an incidence of 7.0% from 596 patients after acute fracture of the wrist or ankle and receiving conventional treatment. The highest rate of incidence occurred at about 3 months after the fracture.[8] Moseley et al.[9] reported an incidence of 3.8% within 4 months of a wrist fracture in 1,549 patients. Bullen et al.[10] reported an incidence of 0.3% within 3 months of ankle fracture or postoperative treatment of ankle fracture in 300 patients. Several smaller prospective studies suggest that acute CRPS type I may develop in up to 11% to 18% of patients following fracture or total knee arthroplasty, although most cases resolve relatively quickly with conservative care.[11–13]

Based on available epidemiologic data, fractures and sprains may be the most common events triggering CRPS. CRPS appears to be more common in the upper extremities, is more common in females, and is most likely to occur in the 50 to 70 years age range.[2,3]

Pathophysiology

CRPS remains one of the most enigmatic and difficult to treat of all pain conditions. Although good clinical characterizations started to appear in the literature in the late 1800s,[1] a definitive pathophysiology remains to be determined, and it may be that there are a collection of distinct pathophysiologies, early or late, that are currently grouped under the rubric of CRPS. This lack of a precise, singular mechanism partially explains the relative lack of clinical progress to date.[14] There is a great deal of discussion now of identification of clinically relevant subsets, both pathophysiologically and diagnostically. In the following section, animal and human models that have relevance to understanding CRPS are first described and then several pathophysiologic mechanisms that may contribute are reviewed.

ANIMAL MODELS

There are several animal models that may shed light on the mechanisms of CRPS, albeit indirectly. However, as always, one must be cautious extrapolating from animal models to human syndromes. The most useful animal model, best paralleling CRPS type II (causalgia) in which major nerve injury is a key feature, is the chronic constriction injury model in rat that was first described by Bennett and Xie.[15] This model produces some behavioral features (e.g., guarding, disuse, vasomotor disturbance) that mimic some of the features of human CRPS (e.g., allodynia, hyperpathia, spontaneous pain) as well as some of the sympathetic abnormalities.[15] This model has been utilized in the preclinical screening of pharmacologic interventions for CRPS. Another model that may be useful is the spinal nerve injury model,[16] although there is some controversy as to whether this model actually produces "sympathetically maintained pain" (SMP) and how similar the resulting pain syndrome is to human CRPS.[14,17] A third model, involving partial ligation of the sciatic nerve, may also have some relevance to human CRPS type II.[18] All three models likely generate ectopic activity at the site of injury and/or the dorsal root ganglion (DRG) which may (or may not) be responsive to sympathetic outflow and which may cause/maintain central sensitization.[19]

TABLE 25.1 1994 IASP Diagnostic Criteria for Complex Regional Pain Syndrome

1. The presence of an initiating noxious event or a cause of immobilization
2. Continuing pain, allodynia, or hyperalgesia with which the pain is disproportionate to any inciting event
3. Evidence at some time of edema, changes in skin blood flow, or abnormal sudomotor activity in the region of pain
4. This diagnosis is excluded by the existence of conditions that would otherwise account for the degree of pain and dysfunction.

Type I: without obvious nerve damage (aka "reflex sympathetic dystrophy")

Type II: with obvious nerve damage (aka "causalgia")

Modified from Merskey H, Bogduk N. *Classification of Chronic Pain: Descriptions of Chronic Pain Syndromes and Definitions of Pain Terms.* 2nd ed. Seattle, WA: IASP Press; 1994.

These models also result in various other phenomena putatively related to CRPS, such as sprouting of fibers in lamina II of the dorsal horn.[20,21] All of the aforementioned models appear most relevant to understanding CRPS type II, although two less widely used models may be relevant to understanding CRPS type I (no major nerve injury evident). Models using tetanic electrical stimulation[22] and an ischemic reperfusion injury[23] appear to produce a syndrome that mimics some of the features of CRPS type I in the absence of signs of major nerve injury.[22] These animal models may help somewhat in understanding mechanisms of CRPS, but their ultimate value may be in screening pharmaceutical interventions.

HUMAN MODELS

Intracutaneous injection of capsaicin induces burning pain and cutaneous mechanical hypersensitivity (allodynia) and as such may represent a useful model to study certain features of CRPS. The capsaicin model demonstrates the impact of intense nociceptive stimulation of normal skin with the rapid development of areas of primary and secondary hyperalgesia, allodynia, wheal, and flare peripheral sensitization.[24–26] This model results in hyperalgesia to suprathreshold heat within the capsaicin-induced secondary hyperalgesic skin despite the absence of changes in heat pain threshold.[27] Another interesting human model of CRPS-like pain is the controlled heat injury model, which also leads to a zone of secondary hyperalgesia to suprathreshold heat.[28] These models and other lines of evidence corroborate a primary role of central sensitization in CRPS[29–31]; however, the overlapping regions of flare/vasodilatation and hyperalgesia may also suggest peripheral sensitization.[32] Peripheral sensitization likely has a significant role in clinical CRPS. Polymodal C receptors may mediate the temperature allodynia,[27,33] polymodal A receptors the pinprick hyperalgesia,[34] and Aβ receptors the mechanical allodynia[26] in these models. Whole-body cooling (to induce sympathetic activation) and sympathetic block have shown no effects on features of either the capsaicin or heat injury models,[28,35] although phentolamine (an adrenergic antagonist) reduces the area of allodynia in the capsaicin model.[36] Given these mixed findings, the value of these models in understanding interactions between sympathetic nervous system (SNS) activity and pain in CRPS remains uncertain. Although some features of these models are concordant with signs and symptoms of CRPS, the usefulness of these normal nociception models in unraveling disease specific mechanisms in CRPS is limited to date. As with animal models, a primary use of these human models may be in the testing of certain interventions for CRPS.[27,37]

INFLAMMATION

Clinical evidence indicates that some features of acute/early CRPS often attributed exclusively to sympathetic hypofunction (i.e., vasodilatation, swelling, and edema) could perhaps be better explained by an exaggerated localized inflammatory process.[38] Sudeck[39] was the first to propose this, along with a "patchy inflammatory osteoporosis," and Goris[40] revitalized this idea. Consistent with inflammatory mechanisms, one experimental study demonstrated that 82% of "acute" CRPS patients exhibited a progressive accumulation of immunoglobulin in the affected extremity relative to the unaffected extremity compared to only 17% of "chronic" CRPS patients (in this study, Oyen et al.[41] defined chronic as 5 months or more since onset). Analyses of joint fluid and synovial biopsies in CRPS patients have shown an increase in protein concentration, synovial hypervascularity, and neutrophil infiltration.[42–44] Free radicals, suspected to play a prominent role in inflammation and ischemic damage, recreate acute CRPS symptomatology in a rat model (vasomotor abnormalities, edema, and pain behavior), and this is the partial rationale for some investigators recommending free radical scavengers in acute CRPS patients.[45] Eisenberg et al.[46] demonstrated an increase in antioxidant levels in saliva and serum for 31 CRPS type I patients compared to 21, and they suggest these lab markers could be utilized as a potential screening tool for CRPS. From these lines of evidence, it is logical to conclude that an inflammatory component is likely in CRPS type I, particularly in the early phase.[45,47] A shift toward a pro-inflammatory cytokine profile in patients with CRPS suggests a potential pathogenic role for these compounds in the generation of pain and other symptoms.[48] In plasma, no alterations in inflammatory mediators were observed in CRPS patients. However, in "blister fluid" obtained in the region of CRPS pain, significantly higher levels of interleukin (IL)-6 and tumor necrosis factor-α (TNF-α) were observed in the involved extremity relative to the uninvolved extremity.[49] Wesseldijk et al.[50] demonstrated the differences in levels of TNF-α and IL-6 of 12 CRPS type I patients are significantly decreased in blister fluid 6 years, compared to levels taken at 6 and 30 months, after their initial event. In addition, significantly elevated CSF levels of pro-inflammatory cytokines (IL-1β, IL-6) have been shown in CRPS patients compared to healthy controls and those with other types of pain.[48] Results to date do not support genetic factors as determinants of the cytokine profile that may contribute to CRPS.[51] Mast cells might also be involved in inflammatory reactions observed in CRPS type I and probably play a role in the production of proinflammatory cytokines such as TNF-α.[49]

Some evidence suggests that "neurogenic inflammation" is facilitated in CRPS patients. Transcutaneous electrical stimulation caused increased axon reflex vasodilatation and provoked protein extravasation only in CRPS patients, whereas it resulted in decreased axon reflex vasodilatation in healthy controls.[52] Animal studies demonstrate that the SNS can influence the intensity of an inflammatory process.[53–56] In human pain models, sympatholytic procedures can reduce pain, inflammation, and edema.[57,58]

IMMUNOLOGIC FACTORS

There has been a recent emphasis on immunologic factors being associated with the pathophysiology of CRPS.[59–61] A possible autoimmune etiology of CRPS in some cases has also been proposed, and autoantibodies against nervous system structures have been described in some patients.[62] Kohr et al.[63] demonstrated autoantibodies from the serum of CRPS patients binding to autonomic neurons including sympathetic and myenteric plexus neurons compared to controls. They subsequently reported CRPS autoantibody binding against β2-adrenergic receptors and muscarinic-2 receptors.[64] Dubuis et al.[65] conducted a study reporting binding of long-standing (at least 6 months) CRPS patient autoantibody binding to α-1A receptors compared to controls. Interestingly, they noted that CRPS patients who had pain relief from an earlier trial of immunoglobulin treatment all had the binding CRPS autoantibody.[65]

Autoantibodies from CRPS serum incubated with endothelial cells, smooth muscle cells, and osteoblasts have been demonstrated to produce changes that could explain the clinical signs of CRPS.[66] Tékus et al.[67] conducted a study where they injected mice with immunoglobulin G (IgG) from CRPS patients prior to making a hind limb muscle incision and reported the mice developing CRPS clinical signs including mechanical hyperalgesia and edema compared to mice injected with IgG from healthy subjects of saline. Reilly et al.[68] demonstrated CRPS IgG binding to DRGs when they are incubated with inflammatory mediators representing an "inflammatory soup." However, this did not occur without preincubation from inflammatory mediators.[68]

Other immunologic factors besides immunoglobulins have been demonstrated to possibly contribute to CRPS clinical signs.

Li et al.[69] conducted a study that demonstrated the depletion of CD20+ B cells from anti-CD20 antibodies reduces the amount of CRPS changes seen in mice in a fracture/cast CRPS model compared to controls. Further, pro-inflammatory monocytes CD14+ and CD16+ have been found to be elevated in CRPS patients compared to controls along with a decreased IL-10, an anti-inflammatory cytokine IL typically low in CRPS patients.[70]

Afferent Dysfunction

CRPS is characterized by "disproportionate" spontaneous and evoked pain (e.g., hyperalgesia, thermal and mechanical allodynia). Whether these sensory symptoms are due to peripheral and/or central sensitization is the subject of considerable debate and investigation. Sensory impairment occurs in more than 70% of CRPS patients.[71,72] Although traditionally these sensory changes were thought to occur in a distal, regional distribution along with characteristic autonomic disturbances, some data suggest that the afferent disturbances may be hemilateral or quadrantic.[73] Study observations corroborate that CRPS may be associated with more generalized sensory impairments.[74,75] The types of remote sensory abnormalities described include not only the allodynia and hyperalgesia typical of CRPS but also hypoesthesia and other dysesthesias. Psychophysical technologies such as temperature quantitative sensory testing reveal that ipsilateral "hypoalgesia" is common, and contralateral hypoesthesia may occur in some cases.[75] Patients found to have generalized sensory impairment were also found to have ipsilateral weakness.[74] Another study showed that patients with generalized sensory impairment had ipsilateral hemibody increases in thresholds for touch, thermal sensation, and heat pain, whereas those with sensory deficits limited to the distal affected limb showed touch threshold elevations only in the affected limb.[75] In this trial, 46% of patients showed abnormalities in nerve conduction testing, and 24% abnormalities in somatosensory evoked potentials, although these abnormalities did not correspond to the extent of sensory impairments observed on quantitative sensory testing.[75] These studies and others suggest that the sensory impairments in CRPS often extend beyond the area affected by pain, and up to 50% of subjects show hypoesthesia and hypoalgesia in a quadrantic or hemibody distribution ipsilateral to the pain. These effects are more likely to occur with greater CRPS chronicity, suggesting centralization of the pathology over time.

Skin biopsies have revealed decreased C-fiber and Aδ-fiber axonal densities in the affected limb of CRPS type I patients compared to the unaffected side.[76] It is not known whether such changes are primary to the disease or a consequence of nutritional changes and ischemia caused by chronic vasoconstriction and inflammation.[39] These changes could help account for some of the sensory alterations described earlier that may occur in CRPS type I (as well as CRPS type II).[77,78]

A recent study examined patterns of sensory signs for upper limb CRPS type I, CRPS type II, and peripheral nerve injury (PNI) patients.[79] Recruitment included 416 patients from the German Research Network on Neuropathic Pain. Quantitative sensory testing demonstrated several overlapping somatosensory abnormalities between CRPS and PNI patients. This suggests quantitative sensory testing cannot, alone, differentiate between CRPS and PNI patients. In all syndromes, most patients (66% to 69%) were determined to have a combination of sensory loss and hyperalgesia/allodynia. Increased pressure pain in CRPS patients was the only obvious differentiating sign between CRPS and PNI sensory abnormalities. Loss of mechanical detection was greater in CRPS type II than CRPS type I and was considered to be the greatest differentiator between these two syndromes in this study.

CENTRAL DYSFUNCTION

There is considerable evidence supporting centralization of the pathology in chronic CRPS.[73,80–82] Further support comes from evidence suggesting presence of sympathetic and motor dysfunction in the region of pain (see discussion in the following section). An acute "nociceptive barrage" from an inciting trauma, or due to peripheral sensitization and/or neurogenic inflammation, can cause rapid changes in the central nervous system (brain and spinal cord), a process commonly referred to as central sensitization.[83] As a corollary, it has been hypothesized that normalization of afferent activity will reset and/or dampen this sensitization (e.g., increased "functional" input on large fiber tracts may modulate or normalize activity of small fiber tracts or "shut the pain gate"[84]).

Evidence for supraspinal central mechanisms in CRPS also derives from studies using neuroimaging techniques that permit exploration of changes in information processing in the brains of CRPS patients. Studies using magnetoencephalography (MEG), quantitative electroencephalography (EEG), functional magnetic resonance imaging (fMRI), and positron emission tomography (PET) techniques all indicate that alterations of afferent input lead to cortical and thalamic plasticity and reorganization of sensory representations in patients with CRPS type I.[85–89] Increased brain responsiveness among CRPS patients in some imaging studies also supports the presence of central sensitization.[88] Some studies suggest a reduced size of the motor cortex devoted to the affected limb in unilateral CRPS type I patients compared to the unaffected side,[88] and the relevance of such brain changes to clinical symptoms is supported by the fact that degree of this "shrinkage" correlates with the degree of hyperalgesia to pinprick.[90] fMRI studies indicate different patterns of cortical activation to pinprick in the CRPS-affected side (S1, S2, insula, frontal, anterior cingulate cortex) compared to the unaffected side (S1, S2, insula only).[91] Moreover, prospective research using MEG indicates that stimulation of early, unilateral CRPS type I subjects leads initially only to contralateral activation, whereas after 3 years of CRPS, the same stimulation leads to bilateral activation.[88] Such results suggest one possible brain mechanism by which reported contralateral "spreading" of CRPS symptoms may occur. A meta-analysis that included six studies investigated S1 representation in upper extremity CRPS.[92] They determined, from these limited data, that S1 representation is smaller in the CRPS-affected upper limb compared to the unaffected limb. A follow-up study comparing 17 patients with upper extremity CRPS and 16 healthy controls determined that the S1 representation was the same size in the affected limb of CRPS subjects and controls.[93] Further, they found S1 representation in the unaffected limb of CRPS patients was larger than controls. This is consistent with the previous meta-analysis and provides interesting insight on the possible neuroplasticity changes that occur in CRPS pathology. Further studies are needed to explore these findings.

Imaging studies suggest that CRPS-related brain changes like those described earlier may reverse after successful treatment; thus, a reduction or resolution of CRPS pain may correlate with "resetting" of the cortical reorganization associated with the disorder.[90,94]

SYMPATHETIC DYSFUNCTION

Although autonomic dysfunction has long been implicated as a key mechanism involved with CRPS pathology, the actual role of the SNS is incompletely characterized.[95] A seminal role of the SNS in CRPS is pivotal in most diagnostic criteria, emphasizing signs and symptoms of autonomic disturbance (e.g., vasomotor, sudomotor, and fluid regulation changes[71,96,97]). The crucial role of the SNS in at least some cases of CRPS is also suggested by the fact that sympatholytic blocks cause substantial pain relief in a subset of patients (those with SMP; e.g., Wasner et al.,[98] and see following discussion). Because of the frequent beneficial response empirically seen to sympathetic blocks in chronic, cold, blue, sweaty CRPS, logically, sympathetic hyperactivity was originally thought to be a primary pathophysiologic mechanism.[99] However, an analysis of the current available data provides evidence that sympathetic vasoconstrictor activity is inhibited rather than enhanced, at least in early CRPS.[100,101] The clinical presentation of CRPS appears to take two distinct forms, which may be sequential. Acutely, vasodilatation and sudomotor dysfunction (hot, red, occasionally dry) is characteristically observed; in contrast, patients with chronic CRPS often exhibit signs of vasoconstriction and hyperhidrosis (cold, blue, sweaty).[102] This apparent temporal progression of vasomotor dysfunction from hypoactive to hyperactive is in accord with the sequential changes in rat paw temperature observed in the chronic constriction injury animal model of CRPS.[103] In a series of human studies examining thermoregulation and sympathetic reflexes in response to whole-body warming or cooling using a thermal suit, Wasner and colleagues[98,100] have corroborated the temporal progression from acute, relative sympathetic hypofunction, through an intermediate stage, to a chronic state of relative hyperfunction. Whole-body cooling, a very effective stimulus to tonically activate cutaneous vasoconstrictor pathways, induced a much lower level of vasoconstriction in the affected side as compared with the healthy side in acute CRPS patients.[98] Wasner et al.[100] also reported a significant negative correlation ($P < .001$) between the duration of the disease and the maximal temperature difference between the affected and unaffected sides achieved during this thermoregulatory testing. The "cold" symptom pattern often seen in chronic CRPS is most likely related to adrenergic receptor supersensitivity, perhaps resulting from early sympathetic hypofunction due to local sympathetic nerve damage,[104] decreased central drive, or both. This hypothesis is supported by studies examining plasma catecholamines in CRPS and studies using PET scanning techniques.[105–107] These mechanisms do not exclude processes at the capillary and venular site of the vascular bed that may involve the sympathetic and unmyelinated afferent neurons[108] that could contribute to neurogenic inflammation and edema.[58]

Results of thermoregulatory sweat tests and quantitative sudomotor axon tests often reveal increased sudomotor activity in acute CRPS; however, only results of the former are increased in chronic CRPS.[98,109] Although these sudomotor changes are not entirely in line with the pattern of reported vasomotor changes in CRPS, they do support a central sympathetic dysregulation in this acute period that is in accord with known thermoregulatory mechanisms.[98,109] The dysfunctional effectors of the SNS that are most prominent in CRPS (vasomotor and sudomotor) are thermoregulatory and thought to be primarily under hypothalamic control.[95,110] It is important to note that these sympathetic signs and symptoms are highly variable between patients and even within patients over time.[111,112]

During the 1980s and early 1990s, many clinicians and researchers considered the presence of SMP to be a central feature of CRPS. SMP was corroborated by reports of significant analgesia when the efferent sympathetic nerve supply to the affected area was blocked.[113–115] The concept of SMP remains potentially useful clinically, as it suggests an intervention that may provide a relatively pain-free window of opportunity so that responsive patients might begin a functional restoration course. Physiologically, it is well established that nociceptive afferents are not influenced by sympathetic fibers under normal conditions,[116,117] and the specific role of the SNS in perpetuating pain in pathologic states such as CRPS is not clear.[118] However, evidence from several studies suggests potential direct interactions between SNS activity and CRPS pain. Drummond[119] introduced

a small dose of norepinephrine into capsaicin-treated skin by iontophoresis and showed markedly increased thermal hyperalgesia. Moreover, injection of adrenergic agonists into the symptomatic limb of CRPS patients often provokes or enhances pain, even if the limb has been sympathectomized.[114,120,121] These findings are consistent with the clinical observation that CRPS pain often increases in cold weather or in response to psychological stress, when catecholamine secretion would be expected to increase.[98] Experimentally evoking the startle response also causes increased pain intensity in CRPS type I patients, presumably via sympathetic activation, and these pain changes are paralleled by significantly greater vasoconstriction on the affected side versus the unaffected side.[122] Many of the motor abnormalities of CRPS have also been reported to improve with sympatholytic blocks, implying that some of these motor symptoms may also be sympathetically maintained.[123] Despite the hyperalgesic impact of increased SNS activity on CRPS pain in experimental studies, and the common clinical assumption that SNS hyperactivity contributes directly to CRPS pain, unilateral fracture patients who later developed CRPS showed *impaired* SNS shortly after injury (recorded with laser Doppler fluxmetry).[124] In addition, presence of impaired SNS function shortly after fracture prospectively predicted which later developed acute CRPS type I.[124] In a small trial, 33.5% of CRPS patients exhibited asymmetric vasomotor responses compared to a homologous symmetric pattern of response in all healthy controls when both groups view ambiguous visual stimuli, which is meant to illicit an autonomic response.[125] Further, 61% of the CRPS patients had intense pain within seconds of viewing ambiguous visual stimuli.

A theoretical synthesis of this SNS data: There is acute damage to small efferent sympathetic fibers with the original trauma (such as a fracture or crush injury) resulting in relative sympathetic hypofunction (hot, red, dry). Soon thereafter, cholinergic receptor upregulation occurs in the target tissues (vessels, sweat glands), and importantly, adrenergic receptors may become activated/sensitized on afferent pain fibers as well. Ultimately, there may be regeneration of transformed sympathetic fibers into this pathologically altered region (or restitution/upregulation of central sympathetic drive), giving the clinical appearance of sympathetic hyperfunction (cold, blue, sweaty) and providing direct stimulation of noradrenergically sensitized nociceptors.[100,102,104,105]

TROPHIC, DYSTROPHIC, AND NUTRITIONAL ABNORMALITIES

Trophic/dystrophic changes to skin (thin and glossy, or thickened), nails (thickened, striated), and hair growth (increased or decreased) are ubiquitous in reports of chronic CRPS symptomatology but are of unknown etiology. These changes may simply be due to relative hypoxia with chronic vasoconstriction,[77,126,127] and a similar process could also lead to the observed nerve dropout[76] and osteopenia[39] reported in CRPS. There is evidence of cellular hypoxia or impaired oxygen utilization in the CRPS affected side compared to the unaffected side based on magnetic resonance spectroscopy.[128] Skin capillary hemoglobin oxygenation (HbO_2) has also been shown to be decreased on the affected side in CRPS patients as determined by microlight guide spectrophotometry.[127] Skin, but not venous lactate, was also reported to be increased on the affected side as measured by dermal microdialysis, suggesting decreased oxygenation.[126] The decreased range of motion often seen in CRPS could be due in part to trophic changes of joints, tendons, or ligaments. It is also possible that many of these changes could be caused by inflammation as originally suggested by Sudeck[39] or by hormonal changes.[129] Small-fiber dropout may be a nutritional/relative hypoxia type of "trophic" change or may be an essential etiologic factor in some cases.[76,130–132]

Since Sudeck[133] first described osteopenia in 1901, this bone loss has been shown to be a prominent feature of most chronic CRPS patients.[134] Whether this is due to disuse or is an elemental change in the osteoclast/osteoblast relationship is unclear, and elements of both may be present in most subjects. Certainly, the correction of these aberrations (e.g., bisphosphonates, graded exercise) may provide treatment targets.

MOTOR AND MOVEMENT DISORDERS

Although older diagnostic criteria do not mention motor or movement disorders,[5] the new empirically derived criteria and clinical experience feature motor system abnormalities prominently.[97,135] Most CRPS patients show weakness, spasm, tremor, bradykinesia, and/or range of motion abnormalities at some time in the disease,[123] whereas a minority (~10%) may show more dramatic aberrations such as dystonia.[136] Weakness of skeletal muscles of the affected distal extremity is common, being either true weakness (motor dysfunction) or weakness due to pain/kinesophobia.[136] Tremor may occur in as many as 70% of patients with upper extremity CRPS, with most represented by an apparent increase in physiologic tremor.[123,135] This tremor may decrease with sympathetic block or sympathectomy, suggesting that some motor features of CRPS may be sympathetically maintained.[123] Muscle spindles have extensive adrenergic innervation[137] and may become sensitized similar to the vasomotor system. Inflammatory mediators, especially cytokines, may also sensitize muscle spindles.[138] Bradykinesia is a common abnormality in CRPS and is likely a central abnormality at a spinal and/or cortical level.[123,135] Cerebral motor processing abnormalities have been shown in CRPS with kinematic and grip force analysis.[139] Increased reactivity of the motor cortex has been shown by MEG[88] and transcranial magnetic stimulation (TMS) studies.[140] In sum, numerous findings suggest clinically important motor abnormalities in CRPS that may be of central origin. A systematic review and meta-analysis attempted to examine the literature to determine the extent the motor cortex may be altered in CRPS.[141] There were 18 studies included in the systematic review that included 14 unique data sets using TMS, fMRI, MEG, and PET modalities with 8 studies included in the meta-analysis. The study determined there was limited evidence of bilateral M1 disinhibition in CRPS of the upper limb and better designed studies were needed to reexamine other claims about motor cortex involvement in CRPS. There is some evidence that there may be an incongruity between sensory input and motor output, and this hypothesis has been used as the rationale for a treatment that involves "normalizing" the sensory input with mirror therapy.[142] An apparent motor neglect syndrome could also contribute to significant motor dysfunction in some patients, further suggesting a central etiology of the motor dysfunction of CRPS.[143] CRPS-related motor dysfunction may worsen problems with disuse (see following discussion). An area of interest in motor dysfunction is the basal ganglia, as this is an area of somatosensory and motor processing physiologically positioned to explain motor aberrations in CRPS.[144] Chronic nociceptive input to the basal ganglia may lead to abnormal programming of motor tasks in CRPS patients.

IMMOBILIZATION AND DISUSE

Patients with prolonged casting/immobilization of a limb present with many signs and symptoms considered characteristic of CRPS (e.g., sensory disturbances, vasomotor and sudomotor asymmetry, atrophic and dystrophic changes including osteopenia[145]). In rats casting of hind paw for 4 weeks led to warmer limbs, edema, enhanced cellular extravasation, allodynia, and periarticular osteopenia that reversed after removing the casts, and rats casted after tibial fracture showed vasomotor and nociceptive abnormalities that persisted for several months longer than casting alone.[146] A follow-up study from Guo et al.[147] demonstrated glucocorticoid treatment had no effect on periarticular osteopenia. The potential contribution of disuse to CRPS symptomatology provides a primary rationale for functional restoration as treatment.[148,149]

Genetics

One of the unsolved questions in human pain is why only a minority of patients develop chronic pain after identical inciting events (e.g., nerve lesions).[150,151] In contrast, in animal models of nerve lesion, almost all animals develop neuropathic pain behavior (e.g., Bennet and Xie,[15] Kim and Chung,[16] Selzer et al.,[18] Blenk et al.,[152] Decosterd and Woolf[153]). In CRPS specifically, it is interesting to consider why some individuals who have frequent, sometimes severe injuries considered etiologic never develop CRPS (e.g., soccer players, American football players); yet in others, trivial injuries may lead to full-blown CRPS (e.g., intravenous starts, minor sprains).[150] As always, there may be environmental considerations that predispose, but genetic factors will likely ultimately prove to be important. The human leucocyte antigen (HLA) molecules encoded by genes of the major histocompatibility complex (MHC) may contribute to several neurologic disorders including CRPS.[154] A study evaluated 150 phenotypically homogenous CRPS patients with fixed dystonia and found a significant association with HLA alleles HLA-B62 and HLA-DQ8.[155] The same research group conducted a follow-up study to evaluate whether a phenotypically homogenous CRPS group without dystonia has the same associations, and they found HLA-DQ8 to be the only significantly associated allele.[156] However, these results were not replicated by another group that interrogated about 83% of common single-nucleotide polymorphisms in the human genome, finding they were not associated with CRPS phenotype in their cohort.[157] An early report described three families with two or more members in each affected by CRPS, suggesting the possibility that CRPS risk was heritable.[158] In small studies, the HLA loci A3, B7, DQ1(06), DR2(15), and DR13 are specifically implicated.[159–161] One Japanese study suggests an association between CRPS and the (non-MHC axis) angiotensin-converting enzyme gene and notes elevated angiotensin II in CRPS patients.[162] At present, data regarding possible genetic contributions to CRPS are rather limited but are sufficient to justify further exploration of this very plausible contribution to pathophysiology.

A Convergent Pathophysiologic Theory

These seemingly divergent factors that are proven, theorized, or hypothesized to be involved in the pathophysiology of CRPS can be synthesized.[14] The peripheral factors such as nerve and tissue damage and inflammation (regional and neurogenic) cause an afferent barrage that begins the process of peripheral and central sensitization. Central effects such as changes in the dorsal horn, brainstem, limbic areas, and cortex acutely and chronically occur. An efferent response evolves as feedback from all these areas along the motor (corticospinal) and sympathetic (limbic-hypothalamic-brainstem) systems. This efferent outflow may then substantially impact the peripheral dynamic by affecting the nutritional and inflammatory stasis in the damaged region. All of these sites interconnect, for instance, by ephapses and short loops in the CNS (e.g., the sensory to sympathetic ganglion, dorsal to lateral horn, brainstem). Overlying all of this is variance in response on the basis of genetics (nature) and psychosocial factors (nurture). Thus, nested feedback and feed forward loops and cascades within the neuraxis develop. Importantly, these feedback and feed forward loops can be self-maintaining and can "spread" (come to involve more and more elements of the central nervous) (Fig. 25.1).

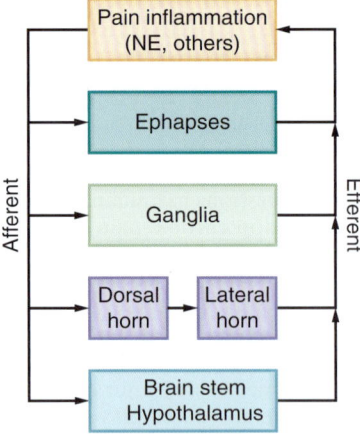

FIGURE 25.1 Complex regional pain syndrome maintained and reinforced by nested, reverberating, feed forward (afferent) and feedback (efferent) loops. Overlaying this are the vectors of genetics (endogenous) and sociologic operant paradigms (exogenous). NE, norepinephrine. *(Modified from Merskey H, Bogduk N. Classification of chronic pain: descriptions of chronic pain syndromes and definitions of pain terms. 2nd ed. Seattle: IASP Press; 1994. This table has been reproduced with permission of the International Association for the Study of Pain® [IASP]. The table may not be reproduced for any other purpose without permission.)*

Diagnosis

In the past, CRPS was diagnosed using a variety of nonstandardized and idiosyncratic diagnostic systems (e.g., Gibbons and Wilson,[96] Bonica,[163] Kozin et al.,[164] Wilson et al.[165]), each of which was derived from the authors' clinical experiences and none of which achieved wide acceptance. This lack of a common diagnostic criteria hindered clinical progress for decades.

THE INTERNATIONAL ASSOCIATION FOR THE STUDY OF PAIN CRITERIA

After much debate, the name for the syndrome was ultimately changed to complex regional pain syndrome (CRPS) at a consensus workshop in Orlando, Florida, in 1994,[54,166] with the new name and diagnostic criteria codified by the IASP taskforce on taxonomy (see Table 25.1).[5] This new diagnostic entity was meant to be descriptive, general, and not to imply any pathophysiology (including any direct role for the SNS). According to these criteria, CRPS can be diagnosed regardless of whether the pain is SMP (SNS block responsive) or sympathetically independent pain (SIP). These IASP-endorsed criteria had the potential to lead to improved clinical communication and greater generalizability across research samples.[54] However, realization of this potential has been somewhat limited by the fact that these rather vague criteria were derived solely by consensus. Also, since publication in 1994, utilization of the criteria has been sporadic (although increasing) in the literature,[167] and certain groups had resisted the change (especially certain advocacy groups and payors). As a consequence, the full benefits of common criteria have not been completely realized.

Experience gained in developing diagnostic criteria in headache and psychiatric disorders indicates that consensus-based criteria can be significantly improved by systematic empirical validation[168] and consensus-derived criteria that are not subsequently validated may lead to over- or underdiagnosis, thus reducing the ability to provide timely, optimal treatment. Results of validation studies to date suggest that the 1994 IASP criteria are adequately sensitive (i.e., rarely miss a case of actual CRPS); however, both internal and external validation research suggest potential problems with specificity (overdiagnosis).[97,169,170] The 1994 IASP criteria implicitly assume that signs and symptoms of vasomotor, sudomotor, and edema-related changes provide redundant diagnostic information; that is, presence of any one of these is sufficient to meet criterion 3 (see Table 25.1). This combination

of multiple distinct elements of the syndrome into the same diagnostic criterion and allowing patient-reported symptoms are likely elements contributing to overdiagnosis in the 1994 IASP scheme.[97,171] An additional weakness of these criteria was the failure to include motor/trophic signs and symptoms, which could lead to important information being ignored that may help discriminate CRPS from other syndromes.

These conclusions are supported by the results of factor analysis (a statistical pattern recognition technique) that was conducted in a series of 123 CRPS patients. These results indicated that signs and symptoms of CRPS clustered into four statistically distinct subgroups.[97] The first of these subgroups was a set of signs and symptoms indicating abnormalities in pain processing (e.g., allodynia, hyperalgesia). Skin color and temperature changes characterized the second subgroup, indicative of vasomotor dysfunction. Edema and sudomotor dysfunction (e.g., sweating changes) combined to form a third unique subgroup. The finding that vasomotor signs and symptoms were statistically distinct from those reflecting sudomotor changes/edema is in contrast to the 1994 IASP criteria, which treats all three of these as diagnostically equivalent. A fourth and final subgroup was identified that included motor and trophic signs and symptoms. Numerous studies have described various signs of motor dysfunction (e.g., dystonia, tremor) as important characteristics of this disorder,[143,165,172] and trophic changes have frequently been mentioned in historical clinical descriptions. The absence of both of these features from the 1994 IASP criteria is therefore notable, especially given factor analytic findings that this subgroup of signs and symptoms does not overlap significantly with other characteristics of CRPS currently used in diagnosis.

External validity, which addresses the ability of the diagnostic criteria to distinguish CRPS patients from those with other types of pain conditions, is also an important issue. In the absence of a definitive pathophysiology of CRPS and thus the absence of a definitive objective test to serve as a "gold standard," providing evidence for the external validity of diagnostic criteria is challenging.[173] However, the upper limit of external validity can be evaluated by using the original criteria themselves as a reference point.[97,169,173] In this methodology, a CRPS patient group is identified using a strict application of the 1994 IASP/CRPS criteria with a comparison group of non-CRPS neuropathic pain patients defined by independent diagnostic information (e.g., diabetic neuropathy diagnosed by presence of chronic diabetes with ascending symmetrical pain and corroborated by electrodiagnostic studies). Existing criteria and modifications to these criteria can then be evaluated with regard to their ability to distinguish between these two groups based on patterns of signs and symptoms. This model was used to test the utility of the 1994 IASP/CRPS criteria for discriminating between 117 patients meeting 1994 IASP criteria and 43 neuropathic pain patients with established non-CRPS etiology. The 1994 IASP/CRPS criteria and decision rules (e.g., "evidence at some time" of edema *or* color changes *or* sweating changes satisfy criterion 3) did discriminate significantly between the CRPS and non-CRPS groups. However, closer examination of the results indicated that although diagnostic sensitivity (i.e., being able to detect the disorder when it is present) was quite high (.98), specificity (i.e., minimizing false-positive diagnoses) was poor (.36), and a positive diagnosis of CRPS was likely to be correct in as few as 40% of cases.[97,170]

For clinical purposes, sensitivity is extremely important. On the other hand, the issue of specificity is quite important for selection of research samples as well as for minimizing unnecessary, potentially invasive treatments. The clinical implication of high sensitivity at the expense of specificity is that CRPS may be overdiagnosed and, ultimately, overtreated. It also has the very significant downside of identifying pathophysiologically heterogeneous groups for research, contributing potentially to negative results in clinical trials.[97]

THE BUDAPEST CRITERIA

A meeting of international researchers and clinicians with expertise in CRPS (the "Budapest Group") was held in Budapest, Hungary, in 2003 to make consensus recommendations on proposed revisions to the 1994 IASP diagnostic criteria. The criteria ultimately proposed by the Budapest group were consensus-based modifications of the criteria that were statistically derived from the validation studies, as in the earlier discussion.[97,170] These modified criteria assessed CRPS characteristics within each of the four statistically derived factors described earlier. Given evidence that objective signs on examination and patient-reported symptoms both provide useful but nonidentical information, the modified criteria required the presence of signs *and* symptoms of CRPS for diagnosis.[97,169,174] A test of these modified criteria regarding their ability to discriminate between the CRPS and non-CRPS neuropathic pain groups indicated that they could increase diagnostic accuracy.[97,173] Results indicated that a decision rule requiring that *two of four sign* categories and *three of four symptom* categories be positive for a diagnosis to be made resulted in a sensitivity of .85 and a specificity of .69. This decision rule represented a good compromise between identifying as many patients as possible in the clinical context while substantially reducing the high level of false-positive diagnoses associated with 1994 IASP criteria. This decision rule was therefore adopted in a set of proposed clinical diagnostic criteria endorsed by the Budapest group (summarized in Table 25.2).[97,174]

The proposed clinical diagnostic criteria described reflected an improvement over 1994 IASP criteria for clinical purposes but still suffered from less than optimal specificity for use in the research context.[174] Tests of the aforementioned modified CRPS criteria indicated that modifying the decision rules to require that *two of four sign* categories and *four of four symptom* categories be positive for diagnosis to be made resulted in a sensitivity of .70 and a specificity of .94. Of all the permutations tested, this decision rule resulted in the greatest probability of accurate diagnosis for both CRPS and non-CRPS patients (approximately 80% and 90% accuracy, respectively[97,170,171,174]). This high level of specificity was considered desirable in the research context by the Budapest consensus group and therefore was adopted as part of a set of proposed research diagnostic criteria.[171,174] Current distinctions between CRPS type I and CRPS type II subtypes, reflecting respectively the absence and presence of evidence of PNI, were ultimately retained despite ongoing questions by the consensus group as to whether such distinctions have clinical utility.[174] The Budapest criteria were adopted by the IASP in 2012 after they consistently demonstrated a better way to maintain sensitivity and specificity when diagnosing CRPS.[175]

Thus, CRPS is a clinical diagnosis made with simple bedside testing techniques known by all physicians. Technical testing procedures are sometimes used to corroborate or objectively document clinical impressions (e.g., thermography, bone scans[47]). Recently, there was a study that suggested osteoprotegerin, an inhibitor of osteoclastic function, may aid as a biomarker for diagnosis.[176] To date, none of these have been formally validated.

SEQUENTIAL STAGES AND SUBSETS OF COMPLEX REGIONAL PAIN SYNDROME

Although not part of clinical diagnosis per se, it is lore among clinicians that CRPS entails three sequential stages that differ in patterns of signs and symptoms. This traditional staging model is summarized by Bonica.[163] The early, acute stage of CRPS (stage I) was characterized by pain/sensory abnormalities (e.g., hyperalgesia, allodynia), vasomotor and sudomotor dysfunction, and prominent edema. Stage II (dystrophic stage) was proposed to occur 3 to 6 months after onset and to be

---

TABLE 25.2 Budapest Diagnostic Criteria for Complex Regional Pain Syndrome (Officially Adopted by IASP in 2012)

General Definition of the Syndrome

Complex regional pain syndrome describes an array of painful conditions that are characterized by a continuing (spontaneous and/or evoked) regional pain that is seemingly disproportionate in time or degree to the usual course of any known trauma or other lesion. The pain is regional (not in a specific nerve territory or dermatome) but may spread and usually has a distal predominance of abnormal sensory, motor, sudomotor, vasomotor, and/or trophic findings. The syndrome shows variable progression over time.

To make a clinical[a] diagnosis, the following criteria must be met:

1. Continuing pain, which is disproportionate to any inciting event

2. Must report at least one symptom in *three of the four* following categories:

    ____ **Sensory:** reports of hyperesthesia and/or allodynia

    ____ **Vasomotor:** reports of temperature asymmetry and/or skin color changes and/or skin color asymmetry

    ____ **Sudomotor/edema:** reports of edema and/or sweating changes and/or sweating asymmetry

    ____ **Motor/trophic:** reports of decreased range of motion and/or motor dysfunction (weakness, tremor, dystonia) and/or trophic changes (hair, nail, skin)

3. Must display at least one sign *at time of evaluation* in *two or more* of the following categories:

    ____ **Sensory:** evidence of hyperalgesia (to pinprick) and/or allodynia (to light touch and/or deep somatic pressure and/or joint movement)

    ____ **Vasomotor:** evidence of temperature asymmetry and/or skin color changes and/or asymmetry

    ____ **Sudomotor/edema:** evidence of edema and/or sweating changes and/or sweating asymmetry

    ____ **Motor/trophic:** evidence of decreased range of motion and/or motor dysfunction (weakness, tremor, dystonia) and/or trophic changes (hair, nail, skin)

4. There is no other diagnosis that better explains the signs and symptoms.

[a]For *research* purposes, diagnostic decision rule should be at least one symptom *in all four* symptom categories and at least one sign observed at evaluation in two or more sign categories.

Modified from Harden RN, Bruehl S, Stanton-Hicks M, et al. Proposed new diagnostic criteria for complex regional pain syndrome. *Pain Med* 2007;8(4):326–331. Reproduced by permission of American Academy of Pain Medicine.

---

characterized by more marked pain/sensory dysfunction, with continued evidence of vasomotor dysfunction and development of significant motor/trophic changes. Stage III (atrophic stage) was characterized by decreased pain/sensory disturbance, continued vasomotor disturbance, and markedly increased motor/trophic changes. Although until recently, there had been only limited empirical tests of this hypothesized staging of CRPS, the concept has frequently been accepted as fact in the CRPS literature.[163,177,178]

The limited available prospective research that followed patients who develop CRPS-like symptoms after surgery, fracture, or severe hand injury suggests that in many cases, the condition does not progress through increasingly problematic stages like those described earlier.[12,71,179,180] Retrospective surveys completed by CRPS patients with an average pain duration of over 3 years similarly indicate that CRPS symptoms often tend to remain stable or improve rather than progressively deteriorate.[169] More recently, the statistical technique of cluster analysis was used to test for evidence of sequential stages.[181,182] In one study, three unique subgroups were identified, with patients in each subgroup displaying statistically similar patterns of symptoms but that there were no significant pain duration differences between the three subgroups, and in contrast to the traditional staging model, the group with the most motor/trophic signs and symptoms had a slightly shorter mean pain duration.[181] The observation of pain duration having no statistical significance, or relevance, between subgroups was reported in a subsequent study that examined CRPS patients with an average prolonged disease duration of 5.8 years when using cluster analysis.[182] Findings such as these suggest the possibility that the presumed sequential "stages" often reported by clinicians may reflect CRPS subtypes rather than an actual staging that follows a progressive, deteriorating course. There is some evidence that "temperature staging" may occur; early CRPS may tend to present with increased temperature ("hot CRPS") and longer duration CRPS to present with decreased temperature ("cold CRPS").[101,183] A recent large prospective trial conducted by Bruehl et al.[184] used two-step cluster analysis with results identifying "warm CRPS" and "cold CRPS" subtypes. Analysis of the "warm CRPS" patient cluster was characterized as warm, red, edematous, and sweaty extremity and the "cold CRPS" patient cluster was characterized as cold, blue, and less edematous extremity. The inflammatory characteristics of the "warm CRPS" cluster were diminished over time during the trial.[184] This is consistent with other studies as inflammatory and immune biomarkers have been observed to be increased in patients with an early diagnosis of CRPS and diminish over time.[50,185] However, there would be greater power in future studies of CRPS temperature subtypes if they included inflammatory and immune biomarkers.

PSYCHOLOGICAL FACTORS IN COMPLEX REGIONAL PAIN SYNDROME

It is critical to properly deem CRPS (as all chronic pain conditions) a biopsychosocial disease; as such, it is crucial to clinical success that psychological and "sociologic" diagnoses be identified and targeted for intervention. Psychological factors could theoretically influence onset or maintenance of CRPS via adrenergic mechanisms believed to contribute to CRPS pathophysiology as described earlier.[104,105,108,115,183,186] The impact of catecholamine release in the pathophysiologic mechanisms described earlier may be important to recognize given that psychological factors such as life stress and dysphoric emotional states (e.g., anxiety, anger, depression) can be associated with increased catecholaminergic activity (e.g., Charney et al.,[187] Light[188]). For example, levels of plasma epinephrine were found to correlate significantly with depressive symptoms in a sample of 16 CRPS patients.[189] Similarly, plasma norepinephrine levels were significantly higher in a sample of 15 CRPS patients than in age- and gender-matched healthy controls, and these elevations were associated significantly with higher scores on a measure of posttraumatic stress symptoms.[190] It is plausible that stress and emotional distress could, through their impact on catecholamine release, interact with adrenergically mediated pathophysiologic mechanisms to contribute to onset or maintenance of CRPS. Interestingly, recent evidence suggests that elevated stress levels in CRPS patients may also be associated with altered immune response, which could potentially impact on CRPS as well.[190]

Examination of the historical CRPS literature frequently reveals the implicit assumption that psychological dysfunction (usually emotional disorders) contributes to CRPS in at least some patients. This assumption probably colored physicians' conceptualization of CRPS patients despite the absence until 10 years ago of a significant body of controlled studies examining this issue. In the existing research literature, most studies assessing the role of psychological factors in CRPS have been limited to case series descriptions or cross-sectional psychological comparisons between CRPS patients and non-CRPS chronic pain patients.[191]

The ability to make conclusions about psychological factors *contributing to onset* of CRPS depends on prospective research designs in the CRPS literature. One prospective study indicated that higher levels of anxiety symptoms prior to total knee arthroplasty were associated with greater likelihood of displaying CRPS-like symptoms at 1 month postsurgery.[12] These latter findings would be consistent with the psychophysiologic model proposed earlier. However, it is notable that neither anxiety nor depression predicted occurrence of CRPS-like symptoms at 6 months, so the long-term impact of psychological factors on development of chronic CRPS remains unclear. Even if the psychophysiologic model is accurate, this should not be taken to imply that the presence of psychological "risk factors" alone would be either necessary or sufficient to cause CRPS. For example, one prospective study indicated that among 88 consecutive patients assessed shortly after acute distal radius fracture, 14 had significantly elevated life stress but did not develop CRPS, and the 1 patient who did develop CRPS had no apparent psychological risk factors (i.e., no major life stressors, average emotional distress levels).[192] Another prospective study reported anxious personality as a risk factor for developing CRPS at a 2- to 4-month follow-up.[193] A large multicenter prospective trial of patients recruited from emergency rooms postfracture were evaluated and found that multiple psychological factors, including anxiety and depression, did not develop CRPS type I.[194] There is some disparity in the literature about whether psychological factors contribute, or predict, the onset of CRPS, but the majority supports that they do not.[195]

In the absence of other prospective studies, the question of whether psychological factors affect the development and maintenance of CRPS must be addressed solely on the basis of case reports and retrospective or cross-sectional research designs which do not allow causation to be inferred. Two uncontrolled retrospective case series reported a relationship between onset of CRPS and contemporaneous emotional loss or major life stressors,[196,197] although these can at best be considered anecdotal. The only controlled study regarding the role of life stress in CRPS onset found that 80% of patients in a CRPS sample recalled a stressful life event temporally concurrent with the initiating physical trauma, in contrast to only 20% of non-CRPS controls.[198] Although this suggests that stressful life events occurring concurrently with a physical trauma may contribute to development of CRPS, this study's findings still must be viewed with caution due to its retrospective design.

If psychological dysfunction is somehow uniquely involved in onset or maintenance of CRPS, one might expect an increased prevalence of psychiatric disorders or elevated levels of emotional distress in this population. Based on structured interviews, estimates for prevalence of Axis I psychiatric disorders (e.g., anxiety and depressive disorders) in CRPS patients indicate a prevalence ranging from 24% to as high as 65%.[75,199,200] It should be noted that only Monti et al.[199] included a non-CRPS chronic pain control group, and these authors reported that prevalence of Axis I disorders was not significantly higher in CRPS compared to non-CRPS pain patients.[199] None of the aforementioned studies documented psychiatric status *prior to* CRPS onset and therefore cannot address the issue of causality. At present, there is no evidence that CRPS patients suffer from diagnosable psychiatric disorders at a higher rate than do other chronic pain patients.

Controlled studies have also addressed the issue of whether CRPS patients are more emotionally distressed than other types of chronic pain patients. Several cross-sectional studies have found that CRPS patients report being more emotionally distressed than non-CRPS pain patients in terms of greater depression and/or anxiety levels.[198,201–204] These findings for depressed mood may be relevant when one considers that in a study using time series diary methodology, depression levels on a given day were a significant predictor of CRPS pain intensity on the following day.[205]

More recently, results of a prospective study indicated that patients displaying signs and symptoms of CRPS 6 months following total knee replacement reported significantly higher levels of anxiety than did patients not displaying CRPS despite the fact that both groups were continuing to experience at least some degree of pain.[12] However, *baseline* anxiety and depression did not predict CRPS status at 6 months, suggesting that the observed elevations in psychological distress were a result of CRPS pain rather than a cause. Follow-up of this dataset in a subsequent study demonstrated increased CRPS symptom severity at 6 months and 12 months if there were greater depressive symptoms presurgically and at 1 month postsurgery.[206] A recent prospective study evaluated a sample of patients diagnosed with CRPS according to the 1994 IASP to increase the sample size and found that patients with higher baselines of anxiety and pain-related fear had increased CRPS severity scores over 12 months.[207] In light of these findings, one possible explanation for elevated distress often reported in CRPS patients relative to non-CRPS chronic pain patients might be that the unusual and sometimes dramatic symptomatology of CRPS (e.g., allodynia, hyperalgesia, vasomotor changes, significant edema, motor changes) is more distressing than experiencing more common forms of chronic pain. Moreover, the validity of these symptoms is often questioned by health care providers, potentially adding to patient distress.

Some studies suggest CRPS patients are more distressed than comparable non-CRPS chronic pain patients, yet other studies have reported no such differences. For example, work by Ciccone and colleagues[204] provided only partial support for this hypothesis, finding that CRPS patients reported more somatic symptoms of depression than non-CRPS patients with local neuropathy yet displayed no emotional differences relative to low back pain patients. Other studies have found no evidence of elevated distress among CRPS patients compared to low back pain patients[208,209] or headache patients.[208] In the absence of additional well-controlled studies, it remains unclear whether the findings suggesting uniquely elevated distress in CRPS patients are an artifact of sample selection.

Two studies report that emotional distress, when present, may have a greater impact on pain intensity in CRPS than in other types of chronic pain.[203,210] For example, correlations between pain intensity and both anxiety and anger expressiveness are significantly stronger in CRPS patients than in non-CRPS chronic pain patients.[203,210] These results suggest that even if CRPS patients are not uniquely distressed, the impact of that distress may be unique, possibly due to the hypothesized adrenergic interactions described earlier. These findings could have significant treatment implications, as psychological interventions that reduce distress may directly contribute to reductions in CRPS symptoms (e.g., pain, vasomotor changes).

Another important operant mechanism that may contribute to CRPS is the sometimes dramatic disuse that patients develop in an effort to avoid stimuli that may trigger pain. Even in healthy individuals, prolonged disuse leads to temperature/color changes and hyperalgesia similar to those observed in CRPS.[145] Significant inverse correlations between CRPS pain intensity and ability to carry out activities of daily living suggest that pain avoidance is likely one of the common reasons for CRPS-related activity impairments.[198] Learned disuse, reinforced by either avoidance of actual pain or reduced anxiety subsequent to avoiding *anticipated* pain exacerbations (kinesophobia), may prevent desensitization and eliminate the normal tactile and proprioceptive input from the extremity that may be necessary to restore normal central signal processing.[211,212] Learned disuse may also inhibit the natural movement-related pumping action that helps prevent accumulation of catecholamines, tachykinins, and other nociceptive and inflammatory mediators in the affected extremity, which may impact negatively on

CRPS signs and symptoms.[52] A recent study utilized a rat tibia fracture model to demonstrate immobilization without fracture and immobilization with fracture had similar increases of inflammatory mediators and CRPS clinical features at 4-week follow-up.[213] Pain-related learned disuse might therefore interact with other pathophysiologic mechanisms to help maintain and exacerbate both the pain-related and autonomic features of CRPS (see following discussion).[191]

In summary, although the contribution of psychological factors to the development and maintenance of CRPS is largely speculative, it is theoretically consistent and highlights the importance of addressing psychological factors in the clinical management of CRPS.

Treatment

THE RATIONALE FOR FUNCTIONAL RESTORATION

CRPS can be a very challenging condition to successfully manage. It is biomedically heterogenous and should be treated as such.[214] The patient presentation often changes over time, and the natural history is variable and poorly characterized. Evidence for efficacy of various treatment modalities is scarce and has developed slowly,[148] due in large part to the vagaries of diagnosis. The only treatment methodology that can have a reasonable chance of successfully bridging the varied presentation and mechanisms of disease and the profound gaps in treatment evidence is a systematic and orderly interdisciplinary approach.[215] Interdisciplinary treatment is defined as a dedicated, coherent, coordinated, specially trained group of relevant professionals that meet regularly to plan, coordinate care, and adapt to treatment eventualities.[174] It is critical to identify and aggressively treat all spheres of the pain experience in CRPS; obsessing with the biomedical alone dooms the clinician and patient to failure, especially in CRPS in which pathophysiology is incompletely understood. Psychosocial targets that may impact pain and dysfunction are often readily and effectively treatable and should be embraced as important avenues of help.

Pain is a central component of CRPS diagnosis, and thus, appropriate analgesia must figure prominently in any treatment regimen. However, its subjective nature makes this symptom a "moving target" that can only be effectively addressed by addressing not only subjective pain but also learned pain behavior and dysfunction. Thus, it is critical to target both subjective and objective clinical benchmarks and outcomes. Ideally, the treatment of CRPS should rely on an intuitive, measurable, and stepwise functional restoration algorithm as the pivotal feature of treatment.[181,212,216] This line of reasoning has been codified by two large international consensus-building conferences.[212,217] The Initiative on Methods, Measurement, and Pain Assessment in Clinical Trials has concluded that physical functioning is a "core domain" in the assessment of pain treatment efficacy, second only to pain assessment.[218,219] Functional restoration emphasizes physical activity ("reanimation"), desensitization, and normalization of sympathetic tone in the affected limb and involves a steady progression from the most gentle, least invasive interventions to the ideal of complete rehabilitation in all aspects of the patient's life (Fig. 25.2).[174,212,217] Although the benefits of functional restoration are intuitive (and are becoming dogma), the evidence as to which modalities are optimal, when to use what and for how long, is currently unavailable.[173,217,220] In an early pivotal paper, Davidoff et al.[216] conducted a prospective uncontrolled study in RSD that supported the functional restoration approach with three key findings: (1) Objective functional components and biometric data could be quantified longitudinally, (2) these components were reactive enough to display change over time (e.g., in response to a functional restoration-based interdisciplinary program), and (3) they were associated with improvements in subjective

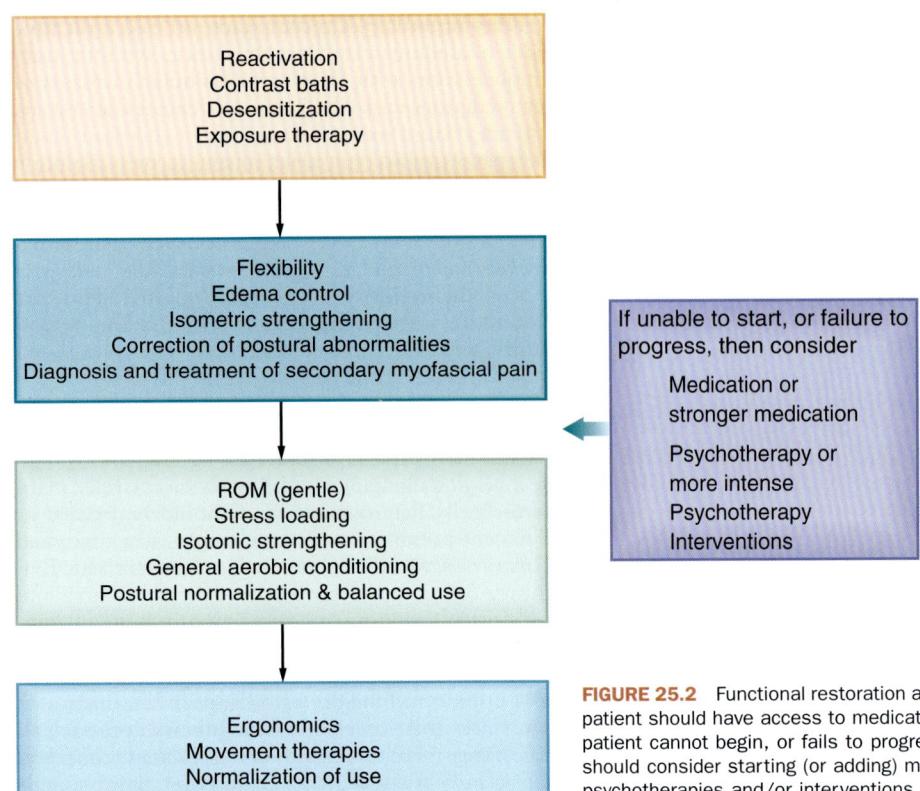

FIGURE 25.2 Functional restoration algorithm. From the outset, in appropriate cases, the patient should have access to medications and/or psychotherapy and/or injections. If the patient cannot begin, or fails to progress, at any step or in any regard, the clinical team should consider starting (or adding) more or stronger medications and/or more intensive psychotherapies and/or interventions. ROM, range of motion. *(Modified and with permission from Harden R. Complex Regional Pain Syndrome: Treatment Guidelines. Milford, CT: RSDSA Press; 2006.)*

outcomes (e.g., decreased pain).[216] This study supplied a primary rationale for a reliance on functional measures as the basis for assessing success in the treatment of CRPS. Various uncontrolled studies suggest that CRPS patients benefited from certain physiotherapeutic modalities, including stress loading and isometric techniques.[211] Oerlemans et al.[220,221] conducted a prospective controlled study of 135 CRPS patients with pain located in an upper extremity and reported that both physical therapy (PT) and occupational therapy proved valuable in managing pain, restoring mobility, and reducing impairment.[220,221] Birklein et al.[109] similarly found that pain reports were notably lower for patients undergoing PT.

Immobilization is recognized as a possible cause and/or perpetuating factor in the syndrome.[5] Patients (and animals) with prolonged casting of a limb often have many signs and symptoms considered part of the CRPS syndrome: vasomotor and sudomotor asymmetry, trophic/dystrophic changes including osteopenia, and occasionally sensory disturbances.[222] Diminished active range of motion is common in early CRPS,[223] and CRPS is associated with significantly reduced mobility and impaired ability to use the affected area normally.[224] Thus, normalized movement is a key objective in treating central changes linked with the syndrome, loosely categorized under the rubric of "altered central processing" and salient to this argument, "neglect."[225] "Pain-related fear is more disabling than pain itself," and this fear appears to be a dynamic clinical factor in CRPS.[226,227] The ability to impact this "kinesophobia" seen in most CRPS patients clinically provides a persuasive argument for functional restoration as fundamental. Meta-analyses have shown that an interdisciplinary approach like that used in comprehensive functional restoration programs for CRPS improves symptoms in patients with chronic pain.[228,229]

A recent observational study examined 49 CRPS patients who completed an interdisciplinary program. McCormick et al.[230]

assessed and tracked a variety of metrics, finding improvement in physical functioning and perceived disability, chronic pain acceptance, and emotional distress. Furthermore, initial medication use was significantly reduced, and 14 of the 16 worker's compensation patients were successfully released to work when discharged from the program. Patient report of pain was not significantly reduced. These results continue to demonstrate that the main utility of functional restoration programs is to improve a patient's life in multiple domains despite the pain[230] and to break the firm link between pain and disability.

REHABILITATION-BASED TREATMENT MODALITIES

Occupational therapists are the ideal therapeutic leaders in the functional restoration process, as they are trained in the biopsychosocial principles of disease and are primary in functional assessment and treatment.[231] An occupational therapist begins with an assessment of the patient's status and current function (e.g., range of motion, activities of daily living, edema). Occupational therapy treatment should aim to normalize sensation and posture, decrease muscle guarding, minimize edema, and increase normalized use.[232,233] Specialized garments, bandaging, and manual edema mobilization techniques can help manage edema.[234] Regular use of the affected limb during everyday tasks is promoted and strongly reinforced throughout the rehabilitation process. A stress-loading ("scrubbing" and "carrying") program should be implemented as soon as possible.[211,235] Later, treatments emphasizing active range of motion, coordination/dexterity, strengthening, and proprioceptive neuromuscular facilitation can be applied (see Fig. 25.2).[236] In extreme CRPS cases, functional splinting may be required to encourage improved circulation/nutrition to the affected area as well as to promote more normal tissue length/positioning during rehabilitation. Graded motor imagery (GMI) is a treatment modality that is employed by occupational therapists with CRPS patients in an effort to activate cortical networks to improve cortical abnormalities without limb movement before beginning mirror therapy.[237] The latest Cochrane review on physiotherapy and CRPS concluded GMI and mirror therapy may improve pain and function with CRPS patients, but the quality of the supporting evidence is low.[238] One study attempted to evaluate GMI in clinical practice using a "prospective audit" and failed to demonstrate significant efficacy.[239] Large high-quality studies are needed to determine the efficacy of GMI for CRPS patients.

PT plays an equally critical role in functional restoration.[240,241] PT emphasizes range of motion, flexibility, posture, and, later, weight bearing and strength through the use of gentle progressive exercise. PT must be executed within the bounds of the patients' tolerance[242] and never when the affected limb is insensate (such as immediately after a block[243]). Inappropriately aggressive PT can trigger extreme pain, edema, distress, and fatigue and may in turn exacerbate the inflammation and sympathetic symptoms of CRPS. However, there have been recent studies that examine pain exposure physical therapy (PEPT). This treatment consists of a progressive-loading exercise program and management of pain-avoidance behavior without the use of specific CRPS medications or analgesics.[244] One small randomized controlled trial (RCT) compared PEPT with "conventional" treatment of CRPS type I patients and found they had similar outcomes on multiple psychometrics, but PEPT had greater active range of motion compared to "conventional" treatment.[245] Another small RCT similarly exposed CRPS type I patients to performing regular daily activities compared with "treatment as usual" and found the patients with exposure to daily activities had reduced self-reported disability in daily life when they had at least moderate levels of pain-related fear.[246] The efficacy of this type of therapy has not been replicated.

Oerleman's group[220,221,247] has shown that PT (and to a lesser extent occupational therapy) improves pain scores and "active mobility" versus controls.[220,221,247] In children with CRPS, a single-blind, randomized trial of PT combined with cognitive-behavioral therapy demonstrated significant improvement on five measures of pain and function[248] and in a prospective review of 103 children with CRPS, "intensive PT" (aerobic, hydrotherapy, and desensitization) supplemented by psychological counseling was effective.[233] The therapy program should be primarily based on functional goals and achieved through active or active-assisted means or the use of low-tech devices (e.g., swiss balls, foam rolls). PT should encourage pacing and include rest breaks and relaxation techniques as well. Mat exercises provide strengthening of both the extremity and the postural muscles in a non–weight-bearing approach and may include movement therapies such as Feldenkrais or Pilates. Virtually all patients with advanced CRPS will present with myofascial pain syndrome of the supporting joint, and effective treatment of this is critical to optimize outcomes. Aquatic therapy can be quite valuable to CRPS patients because of its hydrostatic/compressive principles and its buoyancy effect.[233] Massage, electrostimulation, ultrasound, and contrast baths are empirical modalities administered by PT (see Fig. 25.2).[241]

The recreational therapist is often the first clinician to succeed in getting the CRPS patient to initiate increased movement. The incentive of returning to a favorite pastime is often the appropriate reinforcer to modify kinesophobia and bracing.[249] Through the use of modifications, adaptive equipment, and creative problem solving (e.g., large handled gardening equipment, bowling with the nondominant hand), a patient can enhance self-efficacy and develop confidence through previously lost recreational activities (see Fig. 25.2).[241] Unfortunately, poor reimbursement for recreational therapy has prevented development and research with this promising modality.

The vocational rehabilitation (VR) counselor helps prepare appropriate CRPS patients for return to work; the "ultimate" functional restoration. Consultation with employer, supervisor, employee health nurse, and work site visits are potential interactions initiated by VR. The VR counselor uses information from medical, occupational, educational, financial, and labor markets interfaced with the client's job description/analysis to attempt to reset negative operant paradigms and operationalize "the benefits of work."[241] The VR counselor should participate in the work capacity evaluation, transferable skills analysis, job-specific reconditioning, work hardening, and functional capacities evaluation and be central in the development and documentation of modifications, restrictions, return-to-work assessments, and work release documents.[241,250,251] VR counselor, occupational therapist, and responsible physician work closely together in these tasks, with an ideal goal of return to the original job with the original employer (see Fig. 25.2). The sociologic issues surrounding CRPS are pervasive but very poorly characterized. The best approach to managing these is to compassionately and firmly pursue the goals of optimal functional restoration while proactively providing tools for closure in the forensic and compensation arenas.

Because the symptoms of CRPS patients encompass all the biopsychosocial complexities of chronic pain, the best hope of helping patients is the adoption of a systematic, stable, empathic, and, above all, interdisciplinary approach that addresses those symptoms.[241] Pharmacotherapy, psychotherapy, and interventional techniques should be efficiently deployed for patients who either cannot begin or fail to progress using the interdisciplinary functional restoration approach outlined earlier. Most patients will require medication and psychotherapy from the beginning to be successful in the pivotal functional restoration algorithm (see Fig. 25.2).[241,252] That functional restoration can and should be the central intervention, and outcome standard in CRPS is a theory that must be tested. Until then, the interdisciplinary approach for treating patients with CRPS clearly remains the most pragmatic, helpful, and cost-effective therapeutic approach available today.

PHARMACOTHERAPY

In the 130 years since Weir-Mitchell recommended laudanum (tincture of opium) and the use of a new invention, the hypodermic syringe, to perform cocaine nerve blocks,[1] multiple pharmacotherapeutic interventions for CRPS have been described.[76,214,252] Unfortunately, there are very few RCTs in CRPS.[148,253] The best empirical approach must therefore employ the limited data available, extrapolate from better evidence that is available in related conditions (e.g., neuropathic pain),[254] and pragmatically utilize sequential informed drug trials in each unique case based on putative mechanisms, driven by close monitoring of outcome and risk (Fig. 25.3).

Pharmacotherapy in CRPS, as with most chronic pain syndromes, achieves the greatest benefit when used in conjunction with an interdisciplinary approach to treatment. In CRPS patients, the initial pain intensity is often sufficient that pharmacotherapy may be necessary to begin available nonpharmacologic treatments and "rational polypharmacy" is usually required to optimize analgesia.[214,252] In treating CRPS, the clinician must construct a drug regimen that draws from two basic classes of medications: prophylactic drugs (for maintenance, drugs used on a scheduled basis) to obtain baseline analgesia and abortive drugs (rescue agents, "as needed" [PRN]) for breakthrough pain or symptom flares. Although analgesia for its own sake has obvious value, a unifocal palliative strategy without concurrent functional restoration is useless in CRPS.[174,212,252]

A recent network meta-analysis evaluated multiple class drugs in the treatment of CRPS and rank ordered them according to efficacy.[255] In this study, 16 RCTs were utilized and

Mild to moderate pain	Simple analgesic and/or blocks
Excruciating, intractable pain	Opioids and/or blocks or later, more experimental interventions
Inflammation/swelling and edema	Steroids, systemic or targeted (acutely) or NSAIDs (chronically); immunomodulators
Depression, anxiety, insomnia	Sedative, analgesic antidepressant/anxiolytics and/or psychotherapy
Significant allodynia/hyperalgesia	Anticonvulsants and/or other sodium channel blockers and/or NMDA-receptor antagonists
Significant osteopenia, immobility and trophic changes	Calcitonin or bisphosphonates
Profound vasomotor disturbance	Calcium channel blockers, sympatholytics, and/or blocks

FIGURE 25.3 Pharmacotherapy considerations. These very general guidelines are overruled by individual patient presentation. It is also important to note that certain drugs, such as bisphosphonates, may be associated with analgesia as well as the more primary action. (*Modified with permission from Harden R.* Complex Regional Pain Syndrome: Treatment Guidelines. *Milford, CT: RSDSA Press; 2006.*)

determined the most efficacious treatment of CRPS based on duration of symptoms and results of follow-up at different time intervals. Bisphosphonates were the most effective drug class for the treatment of CRPS of short-term duration (i.e., less than 12 months of symptom duration) with continual relief after 2-month follow-up. Calcitonin had superior effects than bisphosphonates in more chronic stages of CRPS (i.e., 12 months or more) in the short term (i.e., less than 2 months). However, calcitonin was recommended to be limited to 6 weeks maximum due to a potential association with cancer incidence and limited efficacy after 2 months. It was also noted that, of all the medications evaluated, only bisphosphonates, N-methyl-D-aspartate (NMDA) analogs and vasodilators showed better long-term (i.e., 2 months or more) pain relief than placebo.

Nonsteroidal anti-inflammatory drugs (NSAIDs), corticosteroids, cyclooxygenase-2 (COX-2) inhibitors, and free radical scavengers are generally used to treat CRPS pain in the context of discernible inflammation. As described previously, there is evidence that inflammatory components are critical to the development or perpetuation of CRPS, especially early in the course.[49,256] Anti-inflammatory medications can be used for both rescue and prophylaxis. NSAIDs have shown mixed results in several clinical trials of neuropathic pain, including one trial that showed that NSAIDs had no value in treating CRPS type I.[257] Even though COX-2 selective inhibitors have not been properly assessed in CRPS, they have been used anecdotally.[258]

Oral corticosteroids are the only anti-inflammatory drugs with strong evidence in CRPS,[148,259] and there are three RCTs supporting their efficacy, at least in acute CRPS,[260–262] as there are numerous obvious contraindications to chronic steroid use. "Free radical" oxygen species are known to have a role in inflammatory processes and may be involved in CRPS; thus, specific antioxidants in theory might have a role in CRPS treatment.[40] One early RCT of the antioxidant vitamin C was found to reduce the incidence of RSD in patients with wrist fractures.[263] This was followed up by multiple RCTs that examined the role of vitamin C in preventing CRPS.[264–267] One large prospective, double-blind, randomized controlled multicenter study evaluated the dose response of vitamin C patients in three treatment groups (200, 500, and 1,500 mg daily for 50 days). The prevalence of CRPS after the trial was 2.4% in the vitamin C groups and 10.1% in the placebo group. This was not replicated with a large double-blind RCT of 336 patients with an acute fracture of the distal radius that used 500 mg daily for 50 days in the treatment arm. In fact, there was an increased incidence of CRPS at 6 weeks compared to placebo, and no significant difference in the development of CRPS between groups for the remainder of the 1-year trial.[264]

Further high-quality studies are needed to examine the role of vitamin C as a treatment to prevent the incidence of CRPS. Neuroimmune modulators affecting inflammation such as thalidomide have showed some efficacy in case reports and open some label support.[268–270] Lenalidomide, a derivative of thalidomide with a more favorable side effect profile, was studied in a randomized, double-blind, placebo-controlled study to evaluate its efficacy in CRPS patients.[253] Although lenalidomide was well tolerated, the efficacy of the treatment arm was no better than placebo. This high-quality study provides an excellent framework for the design of future CRPS trials.

There is mostly anecdotal support for anticonvulsant drugs in CRPS. There are meta-analytic and systematic reviews compiling evidence for the efficacy of certain anticonvulsant compounds as prophylactic agents in other forms of neuropathic pain[271–274] and the diverse mechanisms of action of some anticonvulsants theoretically should be useful in addressing some of the putative pathophysiologic mechanisms underlying CRPS.[214,275] Gabapentin, pregabalin, and carbamazepine have strong evidence supporting their use in neuropathic pain conditions and anecdotal support in CRPS.[276–282] One small RCT of gabapentin that was double-blinded and placebo-controlled demonstrated mild improvement in pain for the first half of the trial but was no better than placebo at the end of the trial. Interestingly, gabapentin was found to reduce the sensory deficits of the effected limb.[283]

There are also several meta-analyses of the analgesic efficacy of antidepressant/anxiolytics (ADs) in neuropathic conditions,[271,272,284,285] with some low-quality evidence supporting the use of ADs in CRPS.[148,286] These drugs have obvious use in managing some of the comorbidities in CRPS, such as major depression and anxiety.[149,285] Second-generation ADs have not been studied in CRPS, but the so-called serotonin/norepinephrine reuptake blockers show some promise.

The use of opioids for general chronic pain management is still the subject of some controversy,[148,287] but this class has anecdotal support for both abortive and prophylactic treatment in CRPS.[288] Only one RCT has been conducted specifically in CRPS, with negative results.[282] In general, neuropathic pain does not respond to opioids as well as nociceptive pain[289–292]; consequently, neuropathic pain may require higher doses (with an increase in the risk of side effects). Moreover, some animal data suggest that long-term opioid use may actually evoke symptoms characteristic of CRPS, such as allodynia and hyperpathia.[293,294] NMDA receptor antagonists (e.g., MK-801, ketamine, amantadine, and dextromethorphan), which theoretically should reduce central sensitization, have been considered for the treatment of neuropathic pain, but some of these have proven too toxic for regular clinical use in oral formulations.[295-299] Ketamine has shown favorable results in case reports of patients with CRPS.[300-302] There is some ongoing interest in high-dose anesthetic ketamine protocols,[303] although there are no well-controlled studies supporting this approach. There are multiple small RCTs that have evaluated the efficacy of subanesthetic ketamine infusions.[304-306] These treatment protocols demonstrated some utility, but larger well-designed RCTs are needed to better evaluate safety and efficacy. Amantadine has shown some benefit in neuropathic pain.[307,308] Dextromethorphan may augment the effect of other medications, especially opioids.[309]

Clonidine has been considered for the treatment of CRPS[310] but most often by the epidural route.[311] A case series showed that transdermal clonidine could reduce local CRPS-induced hyperalgesia and allodynia,[312] but results of a systematic review failed to support the efficacy of this treatment approach.[148] Nifedipine has demonstrated some benefit in uncontrolled trials, particularly for the management of vasoconstriction.[313,314] Phenoxybenzamine and phentolamine have some low-quality evidence supporting their use in CRPS.[113,313,315,316] Calcitonin is one of the best studied drugs in the treatment of CRPS.[317-320] A meta-analysis of a limited number of controlled calcitonin studies supported the therapeutic value of intranasal doses of 100 to 300 U per day for the management of CRPS.[319,321] However, one study reported no improvement after administration of 200 IU twice daily for 4 weeks.[317] A recent Cochrane review determined there is a lack of high-quality evidence for the effectiveness of calcitonin treating CRPS.[322]

There are multiple small positive randomized studies of bisphosphonates for the treatment of CRPS.[323-329] These trials demonstrate an improvement in pain and function. The impact of these drugs on the osteopenia (Sudeck's atrophy) that is often prominent in chronic CRPS is unknown. Large, definitive trials of bisphosphonates are planned.

Topical medications may also be of some use in management of CRPS. There is limited research endorsing the use of local anesthetic creams in neuropathic pain,[330] but RCTs have not been performed. A patch containing 5% lidocaine is U.S. Food and Drug Administration (FDA)-approved for the management of postherpetic neuralgia and is used anecdotally for CRPS.[331,332] A study of high-dose topical capsaicin with pretreatment with regional anesthesia demonstrated partial efficacy.[333] In one high-quality study, the topical free radical scavenger dimethyl sulfoxide (DMSO) (50% cream for 2 months) showed significant pain reduction when compared with placebo.[334] Topical clonidine has been mentioned, as discussed earlier.[312] Topical ketamine demonstrated a reduction in allodynia in a small RCT for patients with CRPS.[335]

In most cases, no single drug will provide sufficient analgesia long term, nor will it completely prevent the need for abortive/rescue agents. This clinical reality usually requires multiple medications to adequately manage the pain (see Fig. 25.3). There are numerous other medications that have been anecdotally mentioned as treatments for CRPS (e.g., case reports), but there is insufficient evidence to justify their inclusion in this chapter.

PSYCHOLOGICAL INTERVENTIONS

As psychological and sociologic factors often contribute to CRPS pain and dysfunction, and given the relative effectiveness of psychotherapeutic interventions, it is clear psychological and behavioral treatments must play an important role in CRPS management.[214,215,336] Such interventions are likely to be maximally effective if provided in the context of multidisciplinary care. Psychological interventions for CRPS, typically based on cognitive-behavioral therapy principles, should target learned disuse, fear of pain, cognitive responses to CRPS

(e.g., catastrophizing), life stress, and emotional distress that may contribute to maintenance or exacerbation of the disorder.[214,215] Training in relaxation techniques (progressive muscle relaxation, breathing relaxation, autogenics, imagery) is of anecdotal use in giving patients some degree of control over their symptoms, particularly if complemented with biofeedback (especially thermal and myogenic). Moreover, as in all types of chronic pain, better pain coping skills may lead to improved functioning and quality of life and increased ability to self-manage pain.[214] At minimum, such treatments are likely to enhance patients' sense of control over the condition and thereby reduce fears that may be a barrier to achieving success in functional therapies. Interventions that target a family's reinforcing responses to the patient's pain may also be helpful in addressing problems with learned disuse and dysfunction. It should be noted that the aforementioned psychological interventions will only be successful to the extent that patients are willing to accept some responsibility for managing their condition, as opposed to an exclusive focus on achieving a medical "cure." Facilitating this cognitive shift to a self-management approach is often the first step necessary to achieve successful outcomes in both functional and psychological therapies.[214]

A number of studies have addressed efficacy of psychological interventions for CRPS, although nearly all of these reflect uncontrolled designs that permit only limited conclusions to be drawn. An additional caveat regarding these studies is that the criteria used to diagnose CRPS were often not adequately described and in all likelihood varied substantially across studies. This lack of consistent or specified diagnostic criteria limits the ability to generalize these results to patients diagnosed according to current IASP criteria.

Only one randomized trial specifically testing psychological interventions in CRPS patients has been published to date. In this pilot study, Fialka et al.[337] randomized treatment for 18 CRPS patients to receive either home PT or home PT plus once-weekly autogenic relaxation training for 10 weeks. In this small trial, both groups showed similar improvements in pain, range of motion, and edema, although patients in the PT plus autogenics group could demonstrate significantly greater improvements in limb temperature.[337] The impact of this learned control over vasomotor tone and the probable improvement in self-efficacy are unknown.

Results of several published case studies and small case series in adult CRPS patients further support the potential utility of a variety of psychological techniques, including relaxation training, imagery, and thermal and muscular biofeedback. In all of these studies, 75% to 100% pain relief was reported despite the fact that these patients had chronic CRPS that had failed to improve with previous medical treatments.[336,338-341] It should be noted that the complete resolution of symptoms described in some of these cases using only psychological interventions may be atypical. Although the uncontrolled designs used in these studies prevent definitive conclusions from being drawn regarding the efficacy of psychological techniques for CRPS, they clearly support the recommendation that such techniques should play an important role in effective interdisciplinary treatment. Key to this analysis is the very favorable risk–benefit ratio.[214]

Other research has addressed psychotherapy in the context of multidisciplinary treatment, suggesting that integration of psychological methods with medical and PT may be helpful in managing CRPS.[220,233,248,342] Two RCTs examining efficacy of PT for CRPS have included components of psychological treatment in the therapy package. Oerlemans et al.[220,221] tested a PT protocol that included relaxation exercises and cognitive interventions (designed to increase perceived control over pain). This combined intervention was found to produce significantly greater improvements in pain, active range of motion, and impairment levels than were observed in the social work control group.[221,342] In another RCT of PT, Lee et al.[248] examined two different frequencies of PT treatment (once per week vs. three times per week) for child and adolescent CRPS patients, with both groups additionally receiving six sessions of cognitive-behavioral treatment. Although no attentional control group was available for comparison, both groups were found to improve significantly in terms of pain and function when compared to their pretreatment baselines.[248] Although the multicomponent interventions in both of these studies do not indicate the unique efficacy of psychological interventions, they do suggest that psychological treatment in combination with PT may prove effective in a rehabilitation-focused approach to management of CRPS.[214]

The efficacy of psychological interventions for CRPS would not be surprising, given the strong evidence of their utility in other types of chronic pain.[343–350]

INTERVENTIONAL THERAPIES

Multiple interventional therapies, including a variety of nerve blocks, infusions, stimulators, and implants, have been used over the years for management of CRPS.[217,351] Because the SNS is traditionally implicated in the symptomatology and perhaps the pathogenesis of the syndrome, it is logical (but unfortunately not evidence-based) that sympathetic nerve blocks (SNBs) and surgical sympathectomies have played a prominent role in the treatment (and diagnosis) of CRPS.[163,352] In fact, CRPS diagnosis at one time was determined primarily based on a positive response to a sympathetic block.[96] However, at present, analgesia to SNBs merely indicates the presence of SMP. SMP is a subset of CRPS, whereas some CRPS patients display sympathetically independent pain.[353] The presence of SMP provides a rationale for using SNBs to relive pain and to provide a "therapeutic window" to allow initiation of, or continued participation in, functional restoration.

Ideally, the pain relief following SNB should outlast the somatic effect of the local anesthetic and may be very long-lasting in some cases.[354,355] A systematic review of local anesthetic blocks included 19 retrospective reports, 5 prospective case series, 2 nonrandomized controlled studies, and 3 RCTS; unfortunately, due to the wide range of methodology in the studies, the results were inconclusive.[356,357] In the absence of better evidence, if an SNB provides good analgesia in a specific patient, then a short series of empiric blocks in conjunction with active reactivation-focused therapy is advocated based on consensus recommendations.[217,351]

The brachial plexus is anatomically well suited for continuous regional anesthesia in upper extremity CRPS because of its well-defined perivascular compartment and the close proximity to nerves supplying the upper extremity.[351,358,359] Axillary blocks and catheters have their advocates.[360] Epidural infusions of local anesthetics and sympatholytics (single or continuous infusions) are used empirically and have some research support.[311,361,362] Intrathecal analgesia has less support[363] with the exception of research using baclofen.[363,364] The complications of these interventions must be weighed versus the putative benefits and include bleeding, infection, intravascular injection, intrathecal injection, epidural abscess, pneumothorax, and others.[311,351,365]

Use of systemic infusions, especially of sympatholytics such as phentolamine, has been proposed for both treatment and diagnosis of CRPS. One early study showed positive results with guanethidine regional infusion.[366] A later study suggested that neither placebo, phentolamine, nor phenylephrine infusions conferred any benefit.[367] Phentolamine infusion is now seldom used therapeutically and principally used as a putative diagnostic tool to differentiate SIP from SMP. A small RCT reported reduced pain in refractory CRPS patients who received intravenous immunoglobulin treatment.[368] Intrathecal drug

delivery of baclofen demonstrated some benefit in a single-blind, placebo-run-in, dose escalation study of CRPS patients with dystonia.[369] However, there was a high complication rate insinuating whether this invasive procedure is worth the risk.

Intravenous regional anesthesia (IVRA) is a procedure that allows infusion of medications directly into the affected region, usually using a variety of sympatholytic agents.[370] IVRA with guanethidine, lidocaine, bretylium, clonidine, droperidol, ketanserin, or reserpine have been described.[148,259,321] Although three IVRA studies with active controls have shown positive results,[371–373] the majority of studies and results of meta-analysis suggest no significant benefits.[148,259,321,374,375] Some authors advocate combination drug IVRA therapy,[376,377] and the use of new agents with this technology may eventually establish the worth of this technique (e.g., anticytokine agents).

There is one prospective RCT comparing spinal cord stimulation (SCS) versus "conservative therapy" for upper extremity CRPS.[378] This trial showed a significant reduction in pain and a positive global perceived effect at 6 months, without functional improvement. Marginal improvement in these features, as well as in health-related quality of life, were maintained at 2 years.[378] At 5-year follow-up, the trial reported no difference between the SCS group and PT alone group.[379] It should be noted that the SCS technology used in this trial was low-frequency, and there has been a call for a new prospective trial to evaluate whether higher frequency or burst stimulation may provide better relief.[380] A recent prospective case series suggested DRGs stimulation may be a more specific neuromodulation technique to target pain in CRPS patients.[381] There are several case reports, predictably supportive of the procedure.[382,383] There are a variety of other interventions that have been mentioned, such as peripheral nerve stimulation or cortical stimulation, but there is no compelling evidence supporting such interventions to date.[384,385] Currently, neuromodulation through SCS is being promoted as a cost-effective treatment for CRPS that should be considered early rather than a last resort.[386,387] Larger prospective trials are needed with the latest technology to determine the efficacy of this treatment modality for patients with CRPS.

DRG stimulation is a new evolving form of neuromodulation for the treatment of CRPS. In a recent prospective case series, eight CRPS subjects with lower extremity pain were implanted with a neurostimulation system placed near lumbar DRGs and reported some degree of pain relief.[381] At 12 months, six of the eight subjects reported ≥50% pain relief in the foot. A prospective observational cohort study randomly compared traditional SCS with DRG stimulation as the preferred treatment of choice for CRPS patients with knee pain[388] after a 16-day trial period. After the trial period, 10 out of the 12 patients preferred DRG stimulation for their preferred treatment. Recently, a large prospective multicenter RCT evaluated the safety and efficacy of DRG stimulation compared to traditional SCS for the treatment of CRPS of the lower limbs.[389] In this trial, 152 subjects were initially randomized into a DRG stimulation group or an SCS (control) group. All subjects that received a trial stimulator (n = 139) and a fully implantable system (n = 114) were analyzed. The primary endpoint was ≥50% pain relief in the primary area of pain and freedom from stimulation-induced neurologic deficits. The percentage of subjects achieving the primary endpoint for DRG stimulation and SCS trial populations were 81.2% versus 55.7% at 3 months and 74.2% versus 53% at 12 months, respectively. The percentage of subjects achieving the primary endpoint for DRG stimulation and SCS implant populations were 93.3% versus 72.2% at 3 months and 86% versus 70% at 12 months, respectively.[389] These results demonstrate DRG stimulation to be potentially superior to SCS for the treatment of lower limb CRPS. DRG stimulation is a very promising treatment modality for

CRPS, and larger trials are needed to further explore its efficacy including duration of benefit.

In the face of this lack of evidence for most interventions in CRPS, it is incumbent on the clinician to carefully consider and fully educate patients as to the risks and cost of any intervention entertained and not overplay anecdotal benefits. One recommended strategy is to use interventional treatments for CRPS only in patients who are having difficulty either starting or progressing in a functional restoration/interdisciplinary program, starting with less invasive blocks, then infusions, and finally, if necessary, progressing to the more experimental neurostimulation techniques.[351]

As surgery is often mentioned as a *cause* of CRPS, it is somewhat illogical to consider surgery as an effective treatment. Nonetheless, surgical sympathectomy has a long anecdotal history in the treatment of RSD,[352,390] and more recently, endoscopic and radiofrequency sympathectomy have been tried.[391,392] There are no RCTs available, and the risks are significant.[390,393] There is also no strong evidence, and specifically no RCTs, supporting the efficacy of neurolytic procedures, either chemical or radiofrequency.[351]

OTHER THERAPEUTIC MODALITIES

Hyperbaric oxygen therapy has been assessed in one RCT and produced a significant decrease in pain and edema versus "normal air."[394] These results need replication, but cost–benefit considerations will also be important. Although acupuncture is mentioned in many treatment reviews, there is only one small RCT in CRPS, and this trial failed to show significance. The authors noted that a "definitive trial" was planned, but this has been pending since 1999.[395] There is no evidence supporting the use of chiropractic manipulation in CRPS.[396] There are many, many other interventions that have been mentioned in the literature but without experimental support. Discussion of the myriad anecdotes extant is far beyond the scope of this effort. Obviously, there is a critical need for well-designed, well-executed, randomized, and, if possible, placebo-controlled trials in CRPS.

In summary, because the symptoms of CRPS patients encompass all the biopsychosocial complexities of chronic pain, the best hope of helping our patients is the adoption of a systematic, stable, empathetic, and, above all, interdisciplinary approach that addresses those symptoms. Drugs, psychotherapy, and interventions should be efficiently deployed for patients who either cannot begin or fail to progress using the interdisciplinary approach outlined here. Many patients will require medication and psychotherapy from the beginning to be successful in the pivotal functional restoration algorithm. Treatment guidelines that center on progressive functional restoration delivered by an interdisciplinary team are traditional; have substantial empiric and anecdotal support; and have been assessed and ultimately codified by three large, expert, consensus-building conferences. Although high-level evidence supporting the rationale for interdisciplinary treatment of CRPS is fairly sparse (as it is for any treatment of CRPS), much stronger evidence exists for the efficacy of the interdisciplinary approach in other pain conditions, such as chronic low back pain. That functional restoration can and should be the central intervention and outcome standard in CRPS is a theory that must be tested (see Fig. 25.2). Until then, the interdisciplinary approach for treating patients with CRPS remains the most pragmatic, helpful, and cost-effective therapeutic approach available today.[149]

References

1. Mitchell SW. *Injuries of Nerves and Their Consequences.* Philadelphia: J.B. Lippincott; 1872.
2. Sandroni P, Benrud-Larson LM, McClelland RL, et al. Complex regional pain syndrome type I: incidence and prevalence in Olmsted county, a population-based study. *Pain* 2003;103(1–2):199–207.
3. de Mos M, de Bruijn AG, Huygen FJ, et al. The incidence of complex regional pain syndrome: a population-based study. *Pain* 2007;129(1–2):12–20.
4. Bruehl S, Chung OY. How common is complex regional pain syndrome-type I? *Pain* 2007;129(1–2):1–2.
5. Merskey H, Bogduk N. *Classification of Chronic Pain: Descriptions of Chronic Pain Syndromes and Definitions of Pain Terms.* 2nd ed. Seattle, WA: IASP Press; 1994.
6. Perez RS, Collins S, Marinus J, et al. Diagnostic criteria for CRPS I: differences between patient profiles using three different diagnostic sets. *Eur J Pain* 2007;11(8):895–902.
7. Elsharydah A, Loo NH, Minhajuddin A, et al. Complex regional pain syndrome type 1 predictors—epidemiological perspective from a national database analysis. *J Clin Anesth* 2017;39:34–37.
8. Beerthuizen A, Stronks DL, Van't Spijker A, et al. Demographic and medical parameters in the development of complex regional pain syndrome type 1 (CRPS1): prospective study on 596 patients with a fracture. *Pain* 2012;153(6):1187–1192.
9. Moseley GL, Herbert RD, Parsons T, et al. Intense pain soon after wrist fracture strongly predicts who will develop complex regional pain syndrome: prospective cohort study. *J Pain* 2014;15(1):16–23.
10. Bullen M, Lang C, Tran P. Incidence of complex regional pain syndrome I following foot and ankle fractures using the Budapest criteria. *Pain Med* 2016;17(12):2353–2359.
11. Gradl G, Gierer P, Ewert A, et al. Radio-radial external fixation in the treatment of distal radius fractures allows for free wrist motion [in German]. *Zentralbl Chir* 2003;128(12):1014–1019.
12. Harden RN, Bruehl S, Stanos S, et al. Prospective examination of pain-related and psychological predictors of CRPS-like phenomena following total knee arthroplasty: a preliminary study. *Pain* 2003;106(3):393–400.
13. Puchalski P, Zyluk A. Complex regional pain syndrome type 1 after fractures of the distal radius: a prospective study of the role of psychological factors. *J Hand Surg Br* 2005;30(6):574–580.
14. Harden R, Baron R, Jänig W. Preface. In: Harden R, Baron R, Jänig W, eds. *Complex Regional Pain Syndrome.* Seattle, WA: IASP Press; 2001:xi–xiii.
15. Bennett GJ, Xie YK. A peripheral mononeuropathy in rat that produces disorders of pain sensation like those seen in man. *Pain* 1988;33:87–107.
16. Kim SH, Chung JM. An experimental model for peripheral neuropathy produced by segmental spinal ligation in the rat. *Pain* 1992;50(3):355–363.
17. Jänig W. CRPS-I and CRPS-II: a strategic view. In: Harden RN, Baron R, Jänig W, eds. *Complex Regional Pain Syndrome.* Seattle, WA: IASP Press; 2001:3–19.
18. Seltzer Z, Dubner R, Shir Y. A novel behavioral model of neuropathic pain disorders produced in rats by partial sciatic nerve injury. *Pain* 1990;43(2):205–218.
19. Yoon YW, Na HS, Chung JM. Contributions of injured and intact afferents to neuropathic pain in an experimental rat model. *Pain* 1996;64(1):27–36.
20. Noguchi K, Kawai Y, Fukuoka T, et al. Substance P induced by peripheral nerve injury in primary afferent sensory neurons and its effect on dorsal column nucleus neurons. *J Neurosci* 1995;15(11):7633–7643.
21. Kohama I, Ishikawa K, Kocsis JD. Synaptic reorganization in the substantia gelatinosa after peripheral nerve neuroma formation: aberrant innervation of lamina II neurons by Abeta afferents. *J Neurosci* 2000;20(4):1538–1549.
22. Vatine JJ, Argov R, Seltzer Z. Brief electrical stimulation of c-fibers in rats produces thermal hyperalgesia lasting weeks. *Neuroscience Lett* 1998;246(3):125–128.
23. Coderre TJ, Xanthos DN, Francis L, et al. Chronic post-ischemia pain (CPIP): a novel animal model of complex regional pain syndrome-type I (CRPS-I; reflex sympathetic dystrophy) produced by prolonged hindpaw ischemia and reperfusion in the rat. *Pain* 2004;112(1–2):94–105.
24. Culp WJ, Ochoa J, Cline M, et al. Heat and mechanical hyperalgesia induced by capsaicin. Cross modality threshold modulation in human C nociceptors. *Brain* 1989;112(pt 5):1317–1331.
25. Simone DA, Baumann TK, LaMotte RH. Dose-dependent pain and mechanical hyperalgesia in humans after intradermal injection of capsaicin. *Pain* 1989;38(1):99–107.
26. Gracely RH, Lynch SA, Bennett GJ. Painful neuropathy: altered central processing maintained dynamically by peripheral input. *Pain* 1992;51(2):175–194.
27. Andersen OK, Yucel A, Arendt-Nielsen L. Human models of hyperalgesia induced by capsaicin—a discussion of secondary hyperalgesia to heat. In: Harden R, Baron R, Jänig W, eds. *Complex Regional Pain Syndrome Progress in Pain Research and Management.* Seattle, WA: IASP Press; 2001:165–181.
28. Pedersen JL, Kehlet H. Secondary hyperalgesia to heat stimuli after burn injury in man. *Pain* 1998;76(3):377–384.
29. LaMotte RH, Shain CN, Simone DA, et al. Neurogenic hyperalgesia: psychophysical studies of underlying mechanisms. *J Neurophysiol* 1991;66(1):190–211.
30. Torebjörk HE, Lundberg LE, LaMotte RH. Central changes in processing of mechanoreceptive input in capsaicin-induced secondary hyperalgesia in humans. *J Physiol* 1992;448:765–780.
31. Sang CN, Gracely RH, Max MB, et al. Capsaicin-evoked mechanical allodynia and hyperalgesia cross nerve territories. Evidence for a central mechanism. *Anesthesiology* 1996;85(3):491–496.

32. Serra J, Campero M, Ochoa J. Flare and hyperalgesia after intradermal capsaicin injection in human skin. *J Neurophysiol* 1998;80(6):2801–2810.

33. LaMotte R. Neurophysiological mechanisms of cutaneous sensory hyperalgesia in the primate. In: Willis WD, ed. *Hyperalgesia and Allodynia.* New York: Raven Press; 1992:175–185.

34. Ziegler EA, Magerl W, Meyer RA, et al. Secondary hyperalgesia to punctate mechanical stimuli. Central sensitization to A-fibre nociceptor input. *Brain* 1999;122(pt 12):2245–2257.

35. Baron R, Wasner G, Borgstedt R, et al. Effect of sympathetic activity on capsaicin-evoked pain, hyperalgesia, and vasodilatation. *Neurology* 1999;52(5):923–932.

36. Liu M, Max MB, Parada S, et al. The sympathetic nervous system contributes to capsaicin-evoked mechanical allodynia but not pinprick hyperalgesia in humans. *J Neurosci* 1996;16(22):7331–7335.

37. Petersen KL, Rowbotham MC. A new human experimental pain model: the heat/capsaicin sensitization model. *Neuroreport* 1999;10(7):1511–1516.

38. van der Laan L, Goris R. The role of an exaggerated regional inflammatory response in the pathophysiology of CRPS. In: Harden R, Baron R, Jänig W, eds. *Complex Regional Pain Syndrome Progress in Pain Research and Management.* Seattle, WA: IASP Press; 2001:183–191.

39. Sudeck P. Die sogen akute Knochenatrophie als ntzudndengsvorgang. *Der Chirurg* 1942;15:449–458.

40. Goris RJ. Treatment of reflex sympathetic dystrophy with hydroxyl radical scavengers. *Unfallchirurg* 1985;88(7):330–332.

41. Oyen WJ, Arntz IE, Claessens RM, et al. Reflex sympathetic dystrophy of the hand: an excessive inflammatory response? *Pain* 1993;55(2):151–157.

42. Kozin F, McCarty DJ, Sims J, et al. The reflex sympathetic dystrophy syndrome. I. Clinical and histologic studies: evidence for bilaterality, response to corticosteroids and articular involvement. *Am J Med* 1976;60:321–331.

43. Hannington-Kiff JG. Relief of Sudeck's atrophy by regional intravenous guanethidine. *Lancet* 1977;1(8022):1132–1133.

44. Renier JC, Arlet J, Bregeon C, et al. The joint in algodystrophy. Joint fluid, synovium, cartilage [in French]. *Rev Rhum Mal Osteoartic* 1983;50(4):255–260.

45. van der Laan L, Goris RJ. Reflex sympathetic dystrophy. An exaggerated regional inflammatory response? *Hand Clin* 1997;13(3):373–385.

46. Eisenberg E, Shtahl S, Geller R, et al. Serum and salivary oxidative analysis in complex regional pain syndrome. *Pain* 2008;138(1):226–232.

47. Leitha T, Korpan M, Staudenherz A, et al. Five phase bone scintigraphy supports the pathophysiological concept of a subclinical inflammatory process in reflex sympathetic dystrophy. *Q J Nucl Med* 1996;40(2):188–193.

48. Uçeyler N, Eberle T, Rolke R, et al. Differential expression patterns of cytokines in complex regional pain syndrome. *Pain* 2007;132(1–2):195–205.

49. Huygen FJ, De Bruijn AG, De Bruin MT, et al. Evidence for local inflammation in complex regional pain syndrome type 1. *Mediators Inflamm* 2002;11(1):47–51.

50. Wesseldijk F, Huygen FJ, Heijmans-Antonissen C, et al. Six years follow-up of the levels of TNF-alpha and IL-6 in patients with complex regional pain syndrome type 1. *Mediators Inflamm* 2008;2008:469439.

51. van de Beek WJ, Remarque EJ, Westendorp RG, et al. Innate cytokine profile in patients with complex regional pain syndrome is normal. *Pain* 2001;91(3):259–261.

52. Weber M, Birklein F, Neundörfer B, et al. Facilitated neurogenic inflammation in complex regional pain syndrome. *Pain* 2001;91(3):251–257.

53. Levine JD, Taiwo YO, Collins SD, et al. Noradrenaline hyperalgesia is mediated through interaction with sympathetic postganglionic neurone terminals rather than activation of primary afferent nociceptors. *Nature* 1986;323(6084):158–160.

54. Jänig W, Stanton-Hicks M. *Reflex Sympathetic Dystrophy: A Reappraisal.* Seattle, WA: IASP Press; 1996.

55. Perl ER. Cutaneous polymodal receptors: characteristics and plasticity. *Prog Brain Res* 1996;113:21–37.

56. Green PG, Luo J, Heller PH, et al. Further substantiation of a significant role for the sympathetic nervous system in inflammation. *Neuroscience* 1993;55(4):1037–1043.

57. Levine JD, Fye K, Heller P, et al. Clinical response to regional intravenous guanethidine in patients with rheumatoid arthritis. *J Rheumatol* 1986;13(6):1040–1043.

58. Blumberg H, Hoffmann U, Mohadjer M, et al. Clinical phenomenology and mechanisms of reflex sympathetic dystrophy: emphasis on edema. In: Gebhart GF, Hammond DL, Jensen TS, eds. *Proceedings of the 7th World Congress on Pain.* Seattle, WA: IASP Press; 1994:455–481.

59. Goebel A. Autoantibody pain. *Autoimmun Rev* 2016;15(6):552–557.

60. Bruehl S. Complex regional pain syndrome. *BMJ* 2015;351:h2730.

61. Goebel A, Blaes F. Complex regional pain syndrome, prototype of a novel kind of autoimmune disease. *Autoimmun Rev* 2013;12(6):682–686.

62. Blaes F, Tschernatsch M, Braeu ME, et al. Autoimmunity in complex-regional pain syndrome. *Ann NY Acad Sci* 2007;1107:168–173.

63. Kohr D, Tschernatsch M, Schmitz K, et al. Autoantibodies in complex regional pain syndrome bind to a differentiation-dependent neuronal surface autoantigen. *Pain* 2009;143(3):246–251.

64. Kohr D, Singh P, Tschernatsch M, et al. Autoimmunity against the β2 adrenergic receptor and muscarinic-2 receptor in complex regional pain syndrome. *Pain* 2011;152(12):2690–2700.

65. Dubuis E, Thompson V, Leite MI, et al. Longstanding complex regional pain syndrome is associated with activating autoantibodies against alpha-1a adrenoceptors. *Pain* 2014;155(11):2408–2417.

66. Dharmalingam B. *Immune Mediated Disturbances of Bone, Connective Tissue and Vascular Metabolism in Complex Regional Pain Syndrome (CRPS)—A New Pathogenic Mechanism of Therapeutic Relevance [dissertation].* Giessen, Germany: Justus Liebig University; 2014.

67. Tékus V, Hajna Z, Borbély É, et al. A CRPS-IgG-transfer-trauma model reproducing inflammatory and positive sensory signs associated with complex regional pain syndrome. *Pain* 2014;155(2):299–308.

68. Reilly JM, Dharmalingam B, Marsh SJ, et al. Effects of serum immunoglobulins from patients with complex regional pain syndrome (CRPS) on depolarisation-induced calcium transients in isolated dorsal root ganglion (DRG) neurons. *Exp Neurol* 2016;277:96–102.

69. Li WW, Guo TZ, Shi X, et al. Autoimmunity contributes to nociceptive sensitization in a mouse model of complex regional pain syndrome. *Pain* 2014;155(11):2377–2389.

70. Ritz BW, Alexander GM, Nogusa S, et al. Elevated blood levels of inflammatory monocytes (CD14+ CD16+) in patients with complex regional pain syndrome. *Clin Exp Immunol* 2011;164(1):108–117.

71. Veldman P, Reynen H, Arntz I, et al. Signs and symptoms of reflex sympathetic dystrophy: prospective study of 829 patients. *Lancet* 1993;342:1012–1016.

72. Boas R. Sympathetic nerve blocks: in search of a role. *Reg Anesth Pain Med* 1998;23(3):292–305.

73. Leriche R, Fontaine R. Sur la sensibilite de la chaine sympathique cervicale et des rameaux communicants chez l'homme. *Gaz Hop Civ Milit* 1925;36:581–583.

74. Thimineur M, Sood P, Kravitz E, et al. Central nervous system abnormalities in complex regional pain syndrome (CRPS): clinical and quantitative evidence of medullary dysfunction. *Clin J Pain* 1998;14(3):256–267.

75. Rommel O, Malin JP, Zenz M, et al. Quantitative sensory testing, neurophysiological and psychological examination in patients with complex regional pain syndrome and hemisensory deficits. *Pain* 2001;93(3):279–293.

76. Oaklander AL, Rissmiller JG, Gelman LB, et al. Evidence of focal small-fiber axonal degeneration in complex regional pain syndrome-I (reflex sympathetic dystrophy). *Pain* 2006;120(3):235–243.

77. Birklein F, Weber M, Ernst M, et al. Experimental tissue acidosis leads to increased pain in complex regional pain syndrome (CRPS). *Pain* 2000;87(2):227–234.

78. Harden R. Interdisciplinary management/functional restoration. *J Neuropathic Pain Symptom Palliation* 2006;2:57–67.

79. Gierthmühlen J, Maier C, Baron R, et al; and the German Research Network on Neuropathic Pain (DFNS) study group. Sensory signs in complex regional pain syndrome and peripheral nerve injury. *Pain* 2012;153(4):765–774.

80. Rommel O, Gehling M, Dertwinkel R, et al. Hemisensory impairment in patients with complex regional pain syndrome. *Pain* 1999;80(1–2):95–101.

81. Rommel O, Thimineur M. Clinical evidence of central sensory disturbances in CRPS. In: Harden RN, Baron R, Jänig W, eds. *Complex Regional Pain Syndrome Progress in Pain Research and Management.* Seattle, WA: IASP Press; 2001:193–208.

82. Sieweke N, Birklein F, Riedl B, et al. Patterns of hyperalgesia in complex regional pain syndrome. *Pain* 1999;80(1–2):171–177.

83. Ji RR, Kohno T, Moore KA, et al. Central sensitization and LTP: do pain and memory share similar mechanisms? *Trends Neurosci* 2003;26(12):696–705.

84. Melzack R, Wall PD. Pain mechanisms: a new theory. *Science* 1965;150:971–979.

85. Maihöfner C, Handwerker HO, Neundörfer B, et al. Patterns of cortical reorganization in complex regional pain syndrome. *Neurology* 2003;61(12):1707–1715.

86. Pleger B, Tegenthoff M, Schwenkreis P, et al. Mean sustained pain levels are linked to hemispherical side-to-side differences of primary somatosensory cortex in the complex regional pain syndrome I. *Exp Brain Res* 2004;155(1):115–119.

87. Maleki J, LeBel AA, Bennett GJ, et al. Patterns of spread in complex regional pain syndrome, type I (reflex sympathetic dystrophy). *Pain* 2000;88(3):259–266.

88. Juottonen K, Gockel M, Silén T, et al. Altered central sensorimotor processing in patients with complex regional pain syndrome. *Pain* 2002;98(3):315–323.

89. Fukumoto M, Ushida T, Zinchuk VS, et al. Contralateral thalamic perfusion in patients with reflex sympathetic dystrophy syndrome. *Lancet* 1999;354(9192):1790–1791.

90. Maihöfner C, Handwerker HO, Neundörfer B, et al. Cortical reorganization during recovery from complex regional pain syndrome. *Neurology* 2004;63(4):693–701.

91. Maihöfner C, Forster C, Birklein F, et al. Brain processing during mechanical hyperalgesia in complex regional pain syndrome: a functional MRI study. *Pain* 2005;114(1–2):93–103.

92. Di Pietro F, McAuley JH, Parkitny L, et al. Primary somatosensory cortex function in complex regional pain syndrome: a systematic review and meta-analysis. *J Pain* 2013;14(10):1001–1018.

93. Di Pietro F, Stanton TR, Moseley GL, et al. Interhemispheric somatosensory differences in chronic pain reflect abnormality of the healthy side. *Hum Brain Mapp* 2015;36(2):508–518.

94. Pleger B, Tegenthoff M, Ragert P, et al. Sensorimotor retuning [corrected] in complex regional pain syndrome parallels pain reduction. *Ann Neurol* 2005;57(3):425–429.

95. Jänig W, Häbler HJ. Organization of the autonomic nervous system: structure and function. In: Vinken PJ, Bruyn GW, eds. *The Autonomic Nervous System, Part I: Normal Functions, Handbook of Clinical Neurology.* Amsterdam, The Netherlands: Elsevier Science; 1999:1–52.

96. Gibbons JJ, Wilson PR. RSD score: criteria for the diagnosis of reflex sympathetic dystrophy and causalgia. *Clin J Pain* 1992;8:260–263.

97. Harden RN, Bruehl S, Galer B, et al. Complex regional pain syndrome: are the IASP diagnostic criteria valid and sufficiently comprehensive? *Pain* 1999;83:211–219.

98. Wasner G, Drummond PD, Birklein F, et al. The role of the sympathetic nervous system in autonomic disturbances and "sympathetically maintained pain" in CRPS. In: Harden RN, Baron R, Jänig W, eds. *Complex Regional Pain Syndrome.* Seattle, WA: IASP Press; 2001:89–118.

99. Bonica J. Causalgia and other reflex sympathetic dystrophies. In: Bonica JJ, Liebeskind JC, Albé-Fessard DG, eds. *Proceedings of the Second World Congress on Pain, Advances in Pain Research and Therapy.* New York: Raven Press; 1979:141–166.

100. Wasner G, Heckmann K, Maier C, et al. Vascular abnormalities in acute reflex sympathetic dystrophy (CRPS I): complete inhibition of sympathetic nerve activity with recovery. *Arch Neurol* 1999;56(5):613–620.

101. Wasner G, Schattschneider J, Heckmann K, et al. Vascular abnormalities in reflex sympathetic dystrophy (CRPS I): mechanisms and diagnostic value. *Brain* 2001;124(pt 3):587–599.

102. Birklein F, Riedl B, Claus D, et al. Pattern of autonomic dysfunction in time course of complex regional pain syndrome. *Clin Auton Res* 1998;8(2):79–85.

103. Wakisaka S, Kajander KC, Bennett GJ. Abnormal skin temperature and abnormal sympathetic vasomotor innervation in an experimental painful peripheral neuropathy. *Pain* 1991;46(3):299–313.

104. Kurvers H, Daemen M, Slaaf D, et al. Partial peripheral neuropathy and denervation induced adrenoceptor supersensitivity: functional studies in an experimental model. *Acta Orthop Belg* 1998;64(1):64–70.

105. Harden RN, Duc TA, Williams TR, et al. Norepinephrine and epinephrine levels in affected versus unaffected limbs in sympathetically maintained pain. *Clin J Pain* 1994;10(4):324–330.

106. Goldstein DS, Tack C, Li ST. Sympathetic innervation and function in reflex sympathetic dystrophy. *Ann Neurol* 2000;48(1):49–59.

107. Drummond PD, Finch PM, Smythe GA. Reflex sympathetic dystrophy: the significance of differing plasma catecholamine concentrations in affected and unaffected limbs. *Brain* 1991;114(pt 5):2025–2036.

108. Arnold JM, Teasell RW, MacLeod AP, et al. Increased venous alpha-adrenoceptor responsiveness in patients with reflex sympathetic dystrophy. *Ann Intern Med* 1993;118(8):619–621.

109. Birklein F, Riedl B, Sieweke N, et al. Neurological findings in complex regional pain syndromes—analysis of 145 cases. *Acta Neurol Scand* 2000;101(4):262–269.

110. Jänig W, McLachlan EM. Neurobiology of the autonomic nervous system. In: Mathias CJ, Bannister R, eds. *Autonomic Failure.* 4th ed. Oxford, United Kingdom: Oxford University Press; 1999:3–15.

111. Sherman RA, Karstetter KW, Damiano M, et al. Stability of temperature asymmetries in reflex sympathetic dystrophy over time and changes in pain. *Clin J Pain* 1994;10(1):71–77.

112. Tahmoush AJ, Malley J, Jennings JR. Skin conductance, temperature, and blood flow in causalgia. *Neurology* 1983;33(11):1483–1486.

113. Raja SN, Treede RD, Davis KD, et al. Systemic alpha-adrenergic blockade with phentolamine: a diagnostic test for sympathetically maintained pain. *Anesthesiology* 1991;74:691–698.

114. Torebjörk E, Wahren L, Wallin G, et al. Noradrenaline-evoked pain in neuralgia. *Pain* 1995;63(1):11–20.

115. Baron R, Maier C. Reflex sympathetic dystrophy: skin blood flow, sympathetic vasoconstrictor reflexes and pain before and after surgical sympathectomy. *Pain* 1996;67:317–326.

116. Jänig W, Koltzenburg M. What is the interaction between the sympathetic terminal and the primary afferent fiber? In: Basbaum AI, Besson JM, eds. *Towards a New Pharmacotherapy of Pain.* Chichester, United Kingdom: John Wiley & Sons; 1991:331–352.

117. Jänig W, Koltzenburg M. Possible ways of sympathetic afferent interaction. In: Jänig W, Schmidt RF, eds. *Reflex Sympathetic Dystrophy: Pathophysiological Mechanisms and Clinical Implications.* New York: VCH Verlagsgesellschaft; 1992:213–243.

118. Verdugo RJ, Campero M, Ochoa JL. Phentolamine sympathetic block in painful polyneuropathies. II. Further questioning of the concept of "sympathetically maintained pain." *Neurology* 1994;44:1010–1014.

119. Drummond PD. Noradrenaline increases hyperalgesia to heat in skin sensitized by capsaicin. *Pain* 1995;60(3):311–315.

120. Wallin G, Torebjörk E, Hallin RG. Preliminary observations on the pathophysiology of hyperalgesia in the causalgic pain syndrome. In: Zotterman Y, ed. *Sensory Functions of the Skin in Primates.* Oxford: Pergamon Press; 1976:489–502.

121. Ali Z, Raja SN, Wesselmann U, et al. Intradermal injection of norepinephrine evokes pain in patients with sympathetically maintained pain. *Pain* 2000; 88(2):161–168.

122. Drummond PD, Finch PM, Skipworth S, et al. Pain increases during sympathetic arousal in patients with complex regional pain syndrome. *Neurology* 2001;57(7):1296–1303.

123. Deuschl G, Blumberg H, Lücking CH. Tremor in reflex sympathetic dystrophy. *Arch Neurol* 1991;48(12):1247–1252.

124. Schürmann M, Gradl G, Zaspel J, et al. Peripheral sympathetic function as a predictor of complex regional pain syndrome type I (CRPS I) in patients with radial fracture. *Auton Neurosci* 2000;86(1–2):127–134.

125. Cohen HE, Hall J, Harris N, et al. Enhanced pain and autonomic responses to ambiguous visual stimuli in chronic complex regional pain syndrome (CRPS) type I. *Eur J Pain* 2012;16(2):182–195.

126. Birklein F, Weber M, Neundörfer B. Increased skin lactate in complex regional pain syndrome: evidence for tissue hypoxia? *Neurology* 2000;55(8): 1213–1215.

127. Koban M, Leis S, Schultze-Mosgau S, et al. Tissue hypoxia in complex regional pain syndrome. *Pain* 2003;104(1–2):149–157.

128. Heerschap A, den Hollander JA, Reynen H, et al. Metabolic changes in reflex sympathetic dystrophy: a 31P NMR spectroscopy study. *Muscle Nerve* 1993;16(4):367–373.

129. Sternberg WF, Mogil J. Genetic and hormonal basis of pain states. *Best Pract Res Clin Anaesthesiol* 2001;15(2):229–245.

130. Oaklander AL, Fields HL. Is reflex sympathetic dystrophy/complex regional pain syndrome type I a small-fiber neuropathy? *Ann Neurol* 2009; 65(6):629–638.

131. Albrecht PJ, Hines S, Eisenberg E, et al. Pathologic alterations of cutaneous innervation and vasculature in affected limbs from patients with complex regional pain syndrome. *Pain* 2006;120(3):244–266.

132. Albrecht PJ, Rice FL. Role of small-fiber afferents in pain mechanisms with implications on diagnosis and treatment. *Curr Pain Headache Rep* 2010;14(3):179–188.

133. Sudeck PHM. Uber die akute (reflektorische) Knochenatrophie nach Entzundungen und Verletzungen an den Extremitaten und ihre klinischen Erscheinungen. *Fortschr Geb Rontgenstr* 1901;5:277.

134. Iolascon G, de Sire A, Moretti A, et al. Complex regional pain syndrome (CRPS) type I: historical perspective and critical issues. *Clin Cases Miner Bone Metab* 2015;12(suppl 1):4–10.

135. Schwartzman RJ, Popescu A. Reflex sympathetic dystrophy. *Curr Rheumatol Rep* 2002;4(2):165–169.

136. Baron R, Jänig W. Human experimentation. In: Harden RN, Baron R, Jänig W, eds. *Complex Regional Pain Syndrome.* Seattle, WA: IASP Press; 2001:239–246.

137. Marsden CD, Meadows JC, Lange GW. Effect of speed of muscle contraction on physiological tremor in normal subjects and in patients with thyrotoxicosis and myxoedema. *J Neurol Neurosurg Psychiatry* 1970;33(6): 776–782.

138. Gazda LS, Milligan ED, Hansen MK, et al. Sciatic inflammatory neuritis (SIN): behavioral allodynia is paralleled by peri-sciatic proinflammatory cytokine and superoxide production. *J Peripher Nerv Syst* 2001;6(3):111–129.

139. Schattschneider P, Hébert C, Jouffrey B. Orientation dependence of ionization edges in EELS. *Ultramicroscopy* 2001;86(3–4):343–353.

140. Schwenkreis P, Janssen F, Rommel O, et al. Bilateral motor cortex disinhibition in complex regional pain syndrome (CRPS) type I of the hand. *Neurology* 2003;61(4):515–519.

141. Di Pietro F, McAuley JH, Parkitny L, et al. Primary motor cortex function in complex regional pain syndrome: a systematic review and meta-analysis. *J Pain* 2013;14(11):1270–1288.

142. McCabe C, Haigh R, Ring E, et al. A controlled pilot study of the utility of mirror visual feedback in the treatment of complex regional pain syndrome (type 1). *Rheumatology (Oxford)* 2003;42(1):97–101.

143. Galer BS, Butler S, Jensen MP. Case report and hypothesis: a neglect-like syndrome may be responsible for the motor disturbance in reflex sympathetic dystrophy (complex regional pain syndrome-1). *J Pain Sym Manage* 1995;10:385–391.

144. Jääskeläinen SK, Rinne JO, Forssell H, et al. Role of the dopaminergic system in chronic pain—a fluorodopa-PET study. *Pain* 2001;90(3):257–260.

145. Butler S. Disuse and CRPS. In: Harden RN, Baron R, Jänig W, eds. *Complex Regional Pain Syndrome.* Seattle, WA: IASP Press; 2001:141–150.

146. Guo T, Offley S, Boyd E, et al. Substance P signaling contributes to the vascular and nociceptive abnormalities observed in a tibial fracture and rat model of complex regional pain syndrome type I. *Pain* 2004;108(1–2):95–107.

147. Guo TZ, Wei T, Kingery WS. Glucocorticoid inhibition of vascular abnormalities in a tibia fracture rat model of complex regional pain syndrome type I. *Pain* 2006;121(1–2):158–167.

148. Kingery WS. A critical review of controlled clinical trials for peripheral neuropathic and pain complex regional pain syndromes. *Pain* 1997;73: 123–139.

149. Harden RN. Pharmacotherapy. In: Harden RN, ed. *Complex Regional Pain Syndrome: Treatment Guidelines.* Milford, CT: RSDSA Press; 2006:25–36.

150. Richards RL. Causalgia. A centennial review. *Arch Neurol* 1967;16:339–350.

151. Sunderland S. *Nerve Injuries and Their Repair.* Edinburgh: Churchill Livingstone; 1991.

152. Blenk KH, Häbler HJ, Jänig W. Neomycin and gadolinium applied to an L5 spinal nerve lesion prevent mechanical allodynia-like behaviour in rats. *Pain* 1997;70(2–3):155–165.

153. Decosterd I, Woolf CJ. Spared nerve injury: an animal model of persistent peripheral neuropathic pain. *Pain* 2000;87(2):149–158.

154. Mailis A, Wade JA. Genetic considerations in CRPS. In: Harden RN, Baron R, Jänig W, eds. *Complex Regional Pain Syndrome*. Seattle, WA: IASP Press; 2001:227–237.

155. de Rooij AM, Florencia Gosso M, Haasnoot GW, et al. HLA-B62 and HLA-DQ8 are associated with complex regional pain syndrome with fixed dystonia. *Pain* 2009;145(1–2):82–85.

156. van Rooijen DE, Roelen DL, Verduijn W, et al. Genetic HLA associations in complex regional pain syndrome with and without dystonia. *J Pain* 2012;13(8):784–789.

157. Janicki PK, Alexander GM, Eckert J, et al. Analysis of common single nucleotide polymorphisms in complex regional pain syndrome: genome wide association study approach and pooled DNA strategy. *Pain Med* 2016;17(12):2344–2352.

158. Greipp ME, Thomas AF. Familial occurrence of reflex sympathetic dystrophy. *Clin J Pain* 1991;7(1):48.

159. Mailis A, Wade J. Profile of Caucasian women with possible genetic predisposition to reflex sympathetic dystrophy: a pilot study. *Clin J Pain* 1994;10(3):210–217.

160. van de Beek WJ, Roep BO, van der Slik AR, et al. Susceptibility loci for complex regional pain syndrome. *Pain* 2003;103(1–2):93–97.

161. Kemler MA, van de Vusse AC, van den Berg-Loonen EM, et al. HLA-DQ1 associated with reflex sympathetic dystrophy. *Neurology* 1999;53(6):1350–1351.

162. Kimura T, Komatsu T, Hosoda R, et al. Angiotensin-converting enzyme gene polymorphism in patients with neuropathic pain. In: Devor M, Rowbotham MC, Wiesenfeld-Hallin D, eds. *Proceedings of the 9th World Congress on Pain, Progress in Pain Research and Management*. Seattle, WA: IASP Press; 2000:471–476.

163. Bonica JJ. *The Management of Pain*. Philadelphia: Lea and Feibiger; 1953.

164. Kozin F, Ryan LM, Carerra GF, et al. The reflex sympathetic dystrophy syndrome III: scintigraphic studies, further evidence for the therapeutic efficacy of systemic corticosteroids, and proposed diagnostic criteria. *Am J Med* 1981;70:23–30.

165. Wilson PR, Low PA, Bedder MD, et al. Diagnostic algorithm for complex regional pain syndromes. In: Jänig W, Stanton-Hicks M, eds. *Progress in Pain Research and Management*. Seattle, WA: IASP Press; 1996:93–106.

166. Stanton-Hicks M, Jänig W, Hassenbusch S, et al. Reflex sympathetic dystrophy: changing concepts and taxonomy. *Pain* 1995;63:127–133.

167. Reinders MF, Geertzen JH, Dijkstra PU. Complex regional pain syndrome type I: use of the International Association for the Study of Pain diagnostic criteria defined in 1994. *Clin J Pain* 2002;18(4):207–215.

168. Merikangas KR, Frances A. Development of diagnostic criteria for headache syndromes: lessons from psychiatry. *Cephalalgia* 1993;13(suppl 12):34–38.

169. Galer BS, Bruehl S, Harden RN. IASP diagnostic criteria for complex regional pain syndrome: a preliminary empirical validation study. *Clin J Pain* 1998;14:48–54.

170. Bruehl S, Lofland KR, Semenchuk EM, et al. Use of cluster analysis to validate IHS diagnostic criteria for migraine and tension-type headache. *Headache* 1999;39:181–189.

171. Harden R, Bruehl S. Diagnostic criteria: the statistical derivation of the four criterion factors. In: Wilson PR, Stanton-Hicks M, Harden RN, eds. *CRPS: Current Diagnosis and Therapy*. Seattle, WA: IASP Press; 2005:45–58.

172. Schwartzman RJ, Kerrigan J. The movement disorder of reflex sympathetic dystrophy. *Neurology* 1990;40:57–61.

173. Bruehl S, Harden RN, Galer BS, et al. External validation of IASP diagnostic criteria for complex regional pain syndrome and proposed research diagnostic criteria. *Pain* 1999;81:147–154.

174. Harden RN, Bruehl S, Stanton-Hicks M, et al. Proposed new diagnostic criteria for complex regional pain syndrome. *Pain Med* 2007;8(4):326–331.

175. International Association for the Study of Pain. *Classification of Chronic Pain*. 2nd rev ed. Seattle, WA: IASP Press; 2012. Available at: http://www.iasp-pain.org/files/Content/ContentFolders/Publications2/ClassificationofChronicPain/Part_II-A.pdf. Accessed July 30, 2017.

176. Krämer HH, Hofbauer LC, Szalay G, et al. Osteoprotegerin: a new biomarker for impaired bone metabolism in complex regional pain syndrome? *Pain* 2014;155(5):889–895.

177. DeTakats G. Reflex dystrophy of the extremities. *Arch Surg* 1937;34:939.

178. Schwartzman RJ, McLellan TL. Reflex sympathetic dystrophy: a review. *Arch Neurol* 1987;44:555–611.

179. Bickerstaff DR, Kanis JA. Algodystrophy: an under-recognized complication of minor trauma. *Br J Rheumatol* 1994;33(3):240–248.

180. Zyluk A. The natural history of post-traumatic reflex sympathetic dystrophy. *J Hand Surg (Br)* 1998;23(1):20–23.

181. Bruehl S, Harden R, Galer B, et al. Complex regional pain syndrome: are there distinct subtypes and sequential stages of this syndrome? *Pain* 2002;95:119–124.

182. de Mos M, Huygen FJ, van der Hoeven-Borgman M, et al. Outcome of the complex regional pain syndrome. *Clin J Pain* 2009;25(7):590–597.

183. Birklein F, Riedl B, Neundörfer B, et al. Sympathetic vasoconstrictor reflex pattern in patients with complex regional pain syndrome. *Pain* 1998;75(1):93–100.

184. Bruehl S, Maihöfner C, Stanton-Hicks M, et al. Complex regional pain syndrome: evidence for warm and cold subtypes in a large prospective clinical sample. *Pain* 2016;157(8):1674–1681.

185. Birklein F, Drummond PD, Li W, et al. Activation of cutaneous immune responses in complex regional pain syndrome. *J Pain* 2014;15(5):485–495.

186. Jänig W, Baron R. The role of the sympathetic nervous system in neuropathic pain: clinical observations and animal models. In: Hansson PT, Fields HL, Hill RG, et al, eds. *Neuropathic Pain: Pathophysiology and Treatment*. Seattle, WA: IASP Press; 2001:125–149.

187. Charney DS, Woods SW, Nagy LM, et al. Noradrenergic function in panic disorder. *J Clin Psychiatry* 1990;51(suppl A):5–11.

188. Light KC, Kothandapani RV, Allen MT. Enhanced cardiovascular and catecholamine responses in women with depressive symptoms. *Int J Psychophysiol* 1998;28(2):157–166.

189. Harden RN, Rudin NJ, Bruehl S, et al. Increased systemic catecholamines in complex regional pain syndrome and relationship to psychological factors: a pilot study. *Anesth Analg* 2004;99(5):1478–1485.

190. Kaufmann I, Eisner C, Richter P, et al. Psychoneuroendocrine stress response may impair neutrophil function in complex regional pain syndrome. *Clin Immunol* 2007;125(1):103–111.

191. Bruehl S. Do psychological factors play a role in the onset and maintenance of CRPS? In: Harden R, Baron R, Jänig W, eds. *Complex Regional Pain Syndrome*. Seattle, WA: IASP Press; 2001:279–290.

192. Dijkstra PU, Groothoff JW, ten Duis HJ, et al. Incidence of complex regional pain syndrome type I after fractures of the distal radius. *Eur J Pain* 2003;7(5):457–462.

193. Dilek B, Yemez B, Kizil R, et al. Anxious personality is a risk factor for developing complex regional pain syndrome type I. *Rheumatol Int* 2012;32(4):915–920.

194. Beerthuizen A, Stronks DL, Huygen FJ, et al. The association between psychological factors and the development of complex regional pain syndrome type 1 (CRPS1)—a prospective multicenter study. *Eur J Pain* 2011;15(9):971–975.

195. Lohnberg JA, Altmaier EM. A review of psychosocial factors in complex regional pain syndrome. *J Clin Psychol Med Settings* 2013;20(2):247–254.

196. Van Houdenhove B. Prevalence and psychodynamic interpretation of premorbid hyperactivity in patients with chronic pain. *Psychother Psychosom* 1986;45(4):195–200.

197. Egle UT, Hoffmann SO. Psychosomatic correlations of sympathetic reflex dystrophy (Sudeck's disease). Review of the literature and initial clinical results [in German]. *Psychother Psychosom Med Psychol* 1990;40(3–4):123–135.

198. Geertzen JH, de Bruijn-Kofman AT, de Bruijn HP, et al. Stressful life events and psychological dysfunction in complex regional pain syndrome type I. *Clin J Pain* 1998;14(2):143–147.

199. Monti DA, Herring CL, Schwartzman RJ, et al. Personality assessment of patients with complex regional pain syndrome type I. *Clin J Pain* 1998;14(4):295–302.

200. Rommel O, Willweber-Strumpf A, Wagner P, et al. Psychological abnormalities in patients with complex regional pain syndrome (CRPS) [in German]. *Schmerz* 2005;19(4):272–284.

201. Hardy M, Merritt W. Psychological evaluation and pain assessment in patients with reflex sympathetic dystrophy. *J Hand Ther* 1988;1:155–164.

202. Geertzen JHB, de Bruijn H, de Bruijn-Kofman AT, et al. Reflex sympathetic dystrophy: early treatment and psychological aspects. *Arch Phys Med Rehabil* 1994;75:442–446.

203. Bruehl S, Husfeldt B, Lubenow TR, et al. Psychological differences between reflex sympathetic dystrophy and non-RSD chronic pain patients. *Pain* 1996;67:107–114.

204. Ciccone DS, Bandilla EB, Wu W. Psychological dysfunction in patients with reflex sympathetic dystrophy. *Pain* 1997;71(3):323–333.

205. Feldman SI, Downey G, Schaffer-Neitz R. Pain, negative mood, and perceived support in chronic pain patients: a daily diary study of people with reflex sympathetic dystrophy syndrome. *J Consult Clin Psychol* 1999;67(5):776–785.

206. Harden RN, Bruehl S, Perez RS, et al. Development of a severity score for CRPS. *Pain* 2010;151(3):870–876.

207. Bean DJ, Johnson MH, Heiss-Dunlop W, et al. Do psychological factors influence recovery from complex regional pain syndrome type 1? A prospective study. *Pain* 2015;156(11):2310–2318.

208. Haddox JD, Abram SE, Hopwood MH. Comparison of psychometric data in RSD and radiculopathy. *Reg Anesth* 1988;13:27.

209. DeGood DE, Cundiff GW, Adams LE, et al. A psychosocial and behavioral comparison of reflex sympathetic dystrophy, low back pain, and headache patients. *Pain* 1993;54(3):317–322.

210. Bruehl S, Chung OY, Burns JW. Differential effects of expressive anger regulation on chronic pain intensity in CRPS and non-CRPS limb pain patients. *Pain* 2003;104(3):647–654.

211. Carlson LK, Watson HK. Treatment of reflex sympathetic dystrophy using the stress-loading program. *J Hand Ther* 1988;1:149–154.

212. Stanton-Hicks M, Baron R, Boas R, et al. Consensus report: complex regional pain syndromes: guidelines for therapy. *Clin J Pain* 1998;14:155–166.

213. Guo TZ, Wei T, Li WW, et al. Immobilization contributes to exaggerated neuropeptide signaling, inflammatory changes, and nociceptive sensitization after fracture in rats. *J Pain* 2014;15(10):1033–1045.

214. Harden R. *Complex Regional Pain Syndrome: Treatment Guidelines.* Milford, CT: RSDSA Press; 2006.

215. Harden R. The rationale for integrated functional restoration. In: Wilson P, Stanton-Hicks M, Harden R, eds. *CRPS: Current Diagnosis and Therapy.* Seattle, WA: IASP Press; 2005:163–172.

216. Davidoff G, Morey K, Amann M, et al. Pain measurement in reflex sympathetic dystrophy syndrome. *Pain* 1988;32(1):27–34.

217. Stanton-Hicks M, Burton A, Bruehl S, et al. An updated interdisciplinary clinical pathway for CRPS: report of an expert panel. *Pain Pract* 2002;2(1):1–16.

218. Turk D, Dworkin R, Allen R, et al. Core outcome domains for chronic pain clinical trials: IMMPACT recommendations. *Pain* 2003;106(3):337–345.

219. Revicki D, Ehreth J. Health-related quality of life assessment and planning for the pharmaceutical industry. *Clin Ther* 1997;19(5):1101–1115.

220. Oerlemans HM, Oostendorp RA, de Boo T, et al. Pain and reduced mobility in complex regional pain syndrome I: outcome of a prospective randomised controlled clinical trial of adjuvant physical therapy versus occupational therapy. *Pain* 1999;83(1):77–83.

221. Oerlemans H, Goris J, de Boo T, et al. Do physical therapy and occupational therapy reduce the impairment percentage in reflex sympathetic dystrophy? *Am J Phys Med Rehabil* 1999;78(6):533–539.

222. Butler S H, Nyman M, Gordth T. Immobility in volunteers produces signs and symptoms of CRPS I and a neglect-like state. In: *Abstracts: 9th World Congress on Pain.* Seattle, WA: IASP Press; 1999.

223. Schürmann M, Gradl G, Andress HJ, et al. Assessment of peripheral sympathetic nervous function for diagnosing early post-traumatic complex regional pain syndrome type I. *Pain* 1999;80(1–2):149–159.

224. Kemler MA, de Vet HC. Health-related quality of life in chronic refractory reflex sympathetic dystrophy (complex regional pain syndrome type I). *J Pain Symptom Manage* 2000;20(1):68–76.

225. Galer B, Jensen M. Neglect-like symptoms in complex regional pain syndrome: results of a self-administered survey. *J Pain Symptom Manage* 1999;18(3):213–217.

226. Crombez G, Vlaeyen J, Heuts P, et al. Pain-related fear is more disabling than pain itself: evidence on the role of pain-related fear in chronic back pain disability. *Pain* 1999;80:329–339.

227. Boersma K, Linton S, Overmeer T, et al. Lowering fear-avoidance and enhancing function through exposure in vivo: a multiple baseline study across six patients with back pain. *Pain* 2004;108(1–2):8–16.

228. Flor H, Fydrich T, Turk DC. Efficacy of multidisciplinary pain treatment centers: a meta-analytic review. *Pain* 1992;49:221–230.

229. Guzmán J, Esmail R, Karjalainen K, et al. Multidisciplinary rehabilitation for chronic low back pain: systematic review. *BMJ* 2001;322(7301):1511–1516.

230. McCormick ZL, Gagnon CM, Caldwell M, et al. Short-term functional, emotional, and pain outcomes of patients with complex regional pain syndrome treated in a comprehensive interdisciplinary pain management program. *Pain Med* 2015;16(12):2357–2367.

231. Severens JL, Oerlemans HM, Weegels A, et al. Cost-effectiveness analysis of adjuvant physical or occupational therapy for patients with reflex sympathetic dystrophy. *Arch Phys Med Rehabil* 1999;80:1038–1043.

232. Swan M. *Treating CRPS: A Guide for Therapy.* Milford, CT: RSDSA Press; 2004.

233. Sherry DD, Wallace CA, Kelley C, et al. Short- and long-term outcomes of children with complex regional pain syndrome type I treated with exercise therapy. *Clin J Pain* 1999;15(3):218–223.

234. Uher EM, Vacariu G, Schneider B, et al. Comparison of manual lymph drainage with physical therapy in complex regional pain syndrome, type I. A comparative randomized controlled therapy study [in German]. *Wien Klin Wochenschr* 2000;112(3):133–137.

235. Watson HK, Carlson L. Treatment of reflex sympathetic dystrophy of the hand with an active "stress loading" program. *J Hand Surg Am* 1987;12(5 pt 1):779–785.

236. Voss D, Ionta M, Myers B. Proprioceptive neuromuscular facilitation. In: Voss D, Ionta M, Myers B, eds. *Patterns and Techniques.* 3rd ed. New York: Harper & Row; 1985:xvii.

237. Moseley GL. Graded motor imagery is effective for long-standing complex regional pain syndrome: a randomised controlled trial. *Pain* 2004;108(1–2):192–198.

238. Smart KM, Wand BM, O'Connell NE. Physiotherapy for pain and disability in adults with complex regional pain syndrome (CRPS) types I and II. *Cochrane Database Syst Rev* 2016;(2):CD010853.

239. Johnson S, Hall J, Barnett S, et al. Using graded motor imagery for complex regional pain syndrome in clinical practice: failure to improve pain. *Eur J Pain* 2012;16(4):550–561.

240. Rho RH, Brewer RP, Lamer TJ, et al. Complex regional pain syndrome. *Mayo Clin Proc* 2002;77(2):174–180.

241. Harden RN, Swan M, King A, et al. Treatment of complex regional pain syndrome: functional restoration. *Clin J Pain* 2006;22(5):420–424.

242. Birklein F, Handwerker HO. Complex regional pain syndrome: how to resolve the complexity? *Pain* 2001;94(1):1–6.

243. Phillips M, Katz J, Harden R. The use of nerve block in conjunction with occupational therapy for complex regional pain syndrome type I. *Am J Occupat Ther* 2000;54:544–549.

244. van de Meent H, Oerlemans M, Bruggeman A, et al. Safety of "pain exposure" physical therapy in patients with complex regional pain syndrome type 1. *Pain* 2011;152(6):1431–1438.

245. Barnhoorn KJ, van de Meent H, van Dongen RT, et al. Pain exposure physical therapy (PEPT) compared to conventional treatment in complex regional pain syndrome type 1: a randomised controlled trial. *BMJ Open* 2015;5(12):e008283.

246. den Hollander M, Goossens M, de Jong J, et al. Expose or protect? A randomized controlled trial of exposure in vivo vs pain-contingent treatment as usual in patients with complex regional pain syndrome type 1. *Pain* 2016;157(10):2318–2329.

247. Vicdan K, Isik A, Oerlemans H, et al. Pain and reduced mobility in complex regional pain syndrome I: outcome of a prospective randomised controlled clinical trial of adjuvant physical therapy versus occupational therapy. *Pain* 1999;83(1):77–83.

248. Lee BH, Scharff L, Sethna NF, et al. Physical therapy and cognitive-behavioral treatment for complex regional pain syndromes. *J Pediatr* 2002;141(1):135–140.

249. Russ R. Pain, the disease. Available at: http://www.acofp.org/member%5Fpublications/canov_02.html. Accessed August 14, 2005.

250. Sanders S, Harden R, Benson S, et al. Clinical practice guidelines for chronic non-malignant pain syndrome patients II: an evidence-based approach. *J Back Musculoskel Rehabil* 1999;13:47–58.

251. State of Colorado Department of Labor and Employment. *Reflex Sympathetic Dystrophy/Complex Regional Pain Syndrome Medical Treatment Guidelines.* Denver, CO: State of Colorado Department of Labor and Employment; 1998.

252. Harden RN. Pharmacotherapy of complex regional pain syndrome. *Am J Phys Med Rehabil* 2005;84(3 suppl):S17–S28.

253. Manning DC, Alexander G, Arezzo JC, et al. Lenalidomide for complex regional pain syndrome type 1: lack of efficacy in a phase II randomized study. *J Pain* 2014;15(12):1366–1376.

254. Beydoun A. Neuropathic pain: from mechanisms to treatment strategies. *J Pain Symptom Manage* 2003;25(5 suppl):S1–S3.

255. Wertli MM, Kessels AG, Perez RS, et al. Rational pain management in complex regional pain syndrome 1 (CRPS 1)—a network meta-analysis. *Pain Med* 2014;15(9):1575–1589.

256. van der Laan L, Veldman P, Goris JA. Severe complications of reflex sympathetic dystrophy: infection, ulcers, chronic edema, dystonia, myoclonus. *Arch Phys Med Rehabil* 1998;79:424–429.

257. Rico H, Merono E, Gomez-Castresana F, et al. Scintigraphic evaluation of reflex sympathetic dystrophy: comparative study of the course of the disease under two therapeutic regimens. *Clin Rheumatol* 1987;6(2):233–237.

258. Pappagallo M, Rosenberg A. Epidemiology, pathophysiology, and management of complex regional pain syndrome. *Pain Pract* 2001;1(1):11–20.

259. Forouzanfar T, Köke A, van Kleef M, et al. Treatment of complex regional pain syndrome type 1. *Eur J Pain* 2002;6:105–122.

260. Christensen K, Jensen EM, Noer I. The reflex dystrophy syndrome response to treatment with systemic corticosteroids. *Acta Chir Scand* 1982;148(8):653–655.

261. Barbalinardo S, Loer SA, Goebel A, et al. The treatment of longstanding complex regional pain syndrome with oral steroids. *Pain Med* 2016;17(2):337–343.

262. Atalay NS, Ercidogan O, Akkaya N, et al. Prednisolone in complex regional pain syndrome. *Pain Physician* 2014;17(2):179–185.

263. Zollinger PE, Tuinebreijer WE, Kreis RW, et al. Effect of vitamin C on frequency of reflex sympathetic dystrophy in wrist fractures: a randomized trial. *Lancet* 1999;354(9195):2025–2028.

264. Ekrol I, Duckworth AD, Ralston SH, et al. The influence of vitamin C on the outcome of distal radial fractures: a double-blind, randomized controlled trial. *J Bone Joint Surg Am* 2014;96(17):1451–1459.

265. Zollinger PE, Tuinebreijer WE, Breederveld RS, et al. Can vitamin C prevent complex regional pain syndrome in patients with wrist fractures? A randomized, controlled, multicenter dose-response study. *J Bone Joint Surg Am* 2007;89(7):1424–1431.

266. Jaiman A, Lokesh M, Neogi DS. Effect of vitamin C on prevention of complex regional pain syndrome type I in foot and ankle surgery. *Foot Ankle Surg* 2011;17(3):207.

267. Cazeneuve JF, Leborgne JM, Kermad K, et al. Vitamin C and prevention of reflex sympathetic dystrophy following surgical management of distal radius fractures [in French]. *Acta Orthop Belg* 2002;68(5):481–484.

268. Schwartzman RJ, Chevlen E, Bengtson K. Thalidomide has activity in treating complex regional pain syndrome. *Arch Intern Med* 2003;163(12):1487–1488.

269. Prager J, Fleischman J, Lingua G. Open label clinical experience of thalidomide in the treatment of complex regional pain syndrome type I. Los Angeles, CA: California Pain Medicine Centers and Reflex Sympathetic Dystrophy Institute; 2003: Poster 868.

270. Ching DW, McClintock A, Beswick F. Successful treatment with low-dose thalidomide in a patient with both Behçet's disease and complex regional pain syndrome type I: case report. *J Clin Rheumatol* 2003;9(2):96–98.

271. Sindrup SH, Jensen TS. Efficacy of pharmacological treatments of neuropathic pain: an update and effect related to mechanism of drug action. *Pain* 1999;83(3):389–400.

272. Collins SL, Moore RA, McQuay HJ, et al. Antidepressants and anticonvulsants for diabetic neuropathy and postherpetic neuralgia: a quantitative systematic review. *J Pain Symptom Manage* 2000;20(6):449–458.

273. McQuay H, Carroll D, Jadad AR, et al. Anticonvulsant drugs for management of pain: a systematic review. *BMJ* 1995;311(7012):1047–1052.

274. Wiffen P, Collins S, McQuay H, et al. Anticonvulsant drugs for acute and chronic pain. *Cochrane Database Syst Rev* 2000;(3):CD001133.

275. Hord ED, Oaklander AL. Complex regional pain syndrome: a review of evidence-supported treatment options. *Curr Pain Headache Rep* 2003; 7(3):188–196.

276. Rowbotham M, Harden N, Stacey B, et al. Gabapentin for the treatment of postherpetic neuralgia: a randomized controlled trial. *JAMA* 1998; 280(21):1837–1842.

277. Backonja M, Beydoun A, Edwards KR, et al. Gabapentin for the symptomatic treatment of painful neuropathy in patients with diabetes mellitus. *JAMA* 1998;280(21):1831–1836.

278. Mellick GA, Mellick LB. Reflex sympathetic dystrophy treated with gabapentin. *Arch Phys Med Rehabil* 1997;78(1):98–105.

279. Wheeler DS, Vaux KK, Tam DA. Use of gabapentin in the treatment of childhood reflex sympathetic dystrophy. *Pediatr Neurol* 2000;22(3): 220–221.

280. Burchiel KJ. Carbamazepine inhibits spontaneous activity in experimental neuromas. *Exp Neurol* 1988;102:249–253.

281. Rull J, Quibrera R, Gonzalez-Millan H, et al. Symptomatic treatment of peripheral diabetic neuropathy with carbamazepine: double-blind crossover study. *Diabetologia* 1969;5:215–220.

282. Harke H, Gretenkort P, Ladleif HU, et al. The response of neuropathic pain and pain in complex regional pain syndrome I to carbamazepine and sustained-release morphine in patients pretreated with spinal cord stimulation: a double-blinded randomized study. *Anesth Analg* 2001;92(2):488–495.

283. van de Vusse AC, Stomp-van den Berg SG, Kessels AH, et al. Randomised controlled trial of gabapentin in complex regional pain syndrome type 1 [ISRCTN84121379]. *BMC Neurol* 2004;4:13.

284. McQuay HJ, Tramer M, Nye BA, et al. A systematic review of antidepressants in neuropathic pain. *Pain* 1996;68:217–227.

285. Sindrup SH, Jensen TS. Pharmacologic treatment of pain in polyneuropathy. *Neurology* 2000;55(7):915–920.

286. Watson CP, Vernich L, Chipman M, et al. Nortriptyline versus amitriptyline in postherpetic neuralgia: a randomized trial. *Neurology* 1998;51(4): 1166–1171.

287. Harden RN. Chronic opioid therapy: another reappraisal. *Am Pain Soc Bull* 2002;12(1):1,8–12.

288. Eisenberg E, McNicol ED, Carr DB. Efficacy and safety of opioid agonists in the treatment of neuropathic pain of nonmalignant origin: systematic review and meta-analysis of randomized controlled trials. *JAMA* 2005;294(24):3043–3052.

289. Dellemijn PL, van Duijn H, Vanneste JA. Prolonged treatment with transdermal fentanyl in neuropathic pain. *J Pain Symptom Manage* 1998; 16(4):220–229.

290. Cherny NI, Thaler HT, Friedlander-Klar H, et al. Opioid responsiveness of cancer pain syndromes caused by neuropathic or nociceptive mechanisms: a combined analysis of controlled, single-dose studies. *Neurology* 1994;44(5):857–861.

291. Portenoy R, Foley K, Inturrisi C. The nature of opioid responsiveness and its implications for neuropathic pain: new hypotheses derived from studies for opioid infusions. *Pain* 1990;43:273–286.

292. Dellemijn P. Are opioids effective in relieving neuropathic pain? *Pain* 1999;80(3):453–462.

293. Brush DE. Complications of long-term opioid therapy for management of chronic pain: the paradox of opioid-induced hyperalgesia. *J Med Toxicol* 2012;8(4):387–392.

294. Mao J, Price D, Caruso F, et al. Oral administration of dextromethorphan prevents the development of morphine tolerance and dependence in rats. *Pain* 1996;67:361–368.

295. Eide PK, Jørum E, Stubhaub A, et al. Relief of post-herpetic neuralgia with the N-methyl-D-aspartic acid receptor antagonist ketamine: a double-blind, cross-over comparison with morphine and placebo. *Pain* 1994;58:347–354.

296. Mao J, Price DD, Mayer DJ, et al. Intrathecal MK-801 and local nerve anesthesia synergistically reduce nociceptive behaviors in rats with experimental peripheral mononeuropathy. *Brain Res* 1992;576:254–262.

297. Nelson KA, Park KM, Robinovitz E, et al. High dose oral dextromethorphan versus placebo in painful diabetic neuropathy and postherpetic neuralgia. *Neurology* 1997;48:1212–1218.

298. Qian J, Brown SD, Carlton SM. Systemic ketamine attenuates nociceptive behaviors in a rat model of peripheral neuropathy. *Brain Res* 1996;715: 51–62.

299. Tal M, Bennett GJ. Dextrorphan relieves neuropathic heat-evoked hyperalgesia. *Neurosci Lett* 1993;151:107–110.

300. Takahashi H, Miyazaki M, Nanbu T, et al. The NMDA-receptor antagonist ketamine abolishes neuropathic pain after epidural administration in a clinical case. *Pain* 1998;75(2–3):391–394.

301. Harbut RE, Correll GE. Successful treatment of a nine-year case of complex regional pain syndrome type-I (reflex sympathetic dystrophy) with intravenous ketamine-infusion therapy in a warfarin-anticoagulated adult female patient. *Pain Med* 2002;3(2):147–155.

302. Gammaitoni A, Gallagher R, Welz-Bosna M. Topical ketamine gel: possible role in treating neuropathic pain. *Pain Med* 2000;1(1):97–100.

303. Kiefer R, Rohr P, Unertl K, et al. Recovery from intractable complex regional pain syndrome type I (RSD) under high-dose intravenous ketamine-midazolam sedation. *Neurology* 2002;suppl 3:A474.

304. Sigtermans MJ, van Hilten JJ, Bauer MC, et al. Ketamine produces effective and long-term pain relief in patients with complex regional pain syndrome type 1. *Pain* 2009;145(3):304–311.

305. Schwartzman RJ, Alexander GM, Grothusen JR, et al. Outpatient intravenous ketamine for the treatment of complex regional pain syndrome: a double-blind placebo controlled study. *Pain* 2009;147(1–3):107–115.

306. Connolly SB, Prager JP, Harden RN. A systematic review of ketamine for complex regional pain syndrome. *Pain Med* 2015;16(5):943–969.

307. Pud D, Eisenberg E, Spitzer A, et al. The NMDA receptor antagonist amantadine reduces surgical neuropathic pain in cancer patients: a double blind, randomized, placebo controlled trial. *Pain* 1998;75(2–3):349–354.

308. Eisenberg E, Pud D. Can patients with chronic neuropathic pain be cured by acute administration of the NMDA receptor antagonist amantadine? *Pain* 1998;74(2–3):337–339.

309. Sang CN. NMDA-receptor antagonists in neuropathic pain: experimental methods to clinical trials. *J Pain Symptom Manage* 2000 Jan;19(1 suppl): S21–S25.

310. Tracey DJ, Cunningham JE, Romm MA. Peripheral hyperalgesia in experimental neuropathy: mediation by alpha-2 and adrenoreceptors on post-ganglionic sympathetic terminals. *Pain* 1995;60:217–327.

311. Rauck R, Eisenach J, Jackson K, et al. Epidural clonidine for refractory reflex sympathetic dystrophy. *Anesthesiology* 1993;79:1163–1169.

312. Davis KD, Treede RD, Raja SN, et al. Topical application of clonidine relieves hyperalgesia in patients with sympathetically maintained pain. *Pain* 1991;47(3):309–317.

313. Muizelaar JP, Kleyer M, Hertogs IA, et al. Complex regional pain syndrome (reflex sympathetic dystrophy and causalgia): management with the calcium channel blocker nifedipine and/or the alpha-sympathetic blocker phenoxybenzamine in 59 patients. *Clin Neurol Neurosurg* 1997;99(1):26–30.

314. Prough DS, McLeskey CH, Poehling GG, et al. Efficacy of oral nifedipine in the treatment of reflex sympathetic dystrophy. *Anesthesiology* 1985;62(6):796–799.

315. Ghostine SY, Comair YG, Turner DM, et al. Phenoxybenzamine in the treatment of causalgia. Report of 40 cases. *J Neurosurg* 1984;60(6): 1263–1268.

316. Dellemijn PL, Fields HL, Allen RR, et al. The interpretation of pain relief and sensory changes following sympathetic blockade. *Brain* 1994;117(pt 6):1475–1487.

317. Bickerstaff DR, Kanis JA. The use of nasal calcitonin in the treatment of post-traumatic algodystrophy. *Br J Rheum* 1991;30:291–294.

318. Gobelet C, Meier JL, Schaffner W, et al. Calcitonin and reflex sympathetic dystrophy syndrome. *Clin Rheum* 1986;5:382–388.

319. Gobelet C, Waldburger M, Meier JL. The effect of adding calcitonin to physical treatment on reflex sympathetic dystrophy. *Pain* 1992;48: 171–175.

320. Braga PC. Calcitonin and its antinociceptive activity: animal and human investigations 1975-1992. *Agents Actions* 1994;41(3–4):121–131.

321. Perez R, Kwakkel G, Zuurmond W, et al. Treatment of reflex sympathetic dystrophy (CRPS type I): a research synthesis of 21 randomized clinical trials. *J Pain Symptom Manage* 2001;21(6):511–526.

322. O'Connell NE, Wand BM, McAuley J, et al. Interventions for treating pain and disability in adults with complex regional pain syndrome. *Cochrane Database Syst Rev* 2013;(4):CD009416.

323. Varenna M, Zucchi F, Ghiringhelli D, et al. Intravenous clodronate in the treatment of reflex sympathetic dystrophy syndrome. A randomized, double blind, placebo controlled study. *J Rheumatol* 2000;27(6):1477–1483.

324. Adami S, Fossaluzza V, Gatti D, et al. Bisphosphonate therapy of reflex sympathetic dystrophy syndrome. *Ann Rheum Dis* 1997;56(3):201–204.

325. Robinson JN, Sandom J, Chapman PT. Efficacy of pamidronate in complex regional pain syndrome type I. *Pain Med* 2004;5(3):276–280.

326. Kubalek I, Fain O, Paries J, et al. Treatment of reflex sympathetic dystrophy with pamidronate: 29 cases. *Rheumatology* 2001;40(12):1394–1397.

327. Manicourt DH, Brasseur JP, Boutsen Y, et al. Role of alendronate in therapy for posttraumatic complex regional pain syndrome type I of the lower extremity. *Arthritis Rheum* 2004;50(11):3690–3697.

328. Varenna M, Adami S, Rossini M, et al. Treatment of complex regional pain syndrome type I with neridronate: a randomized, double-blind, placebo-controlled study. *Rheumatology (Oxford)* 2013;52(3):534–542.

329. Giusti A, Bianchi G. Treatment of complex regional pain syndrome type I with bisphosphonates. *RMD Open* 2015;1(suppl 1):e000056.

330. Attal N, Brasseur L, Chauvin M, et al. Effects of single and repeated applications of a eutectic mixture of local anaesthetics (EMLA) cream on spontaneous and evoked pain in post-herpetic neuralgia. *Pain* 1999;81(1–2):203–209.

331. Galer BS, Rowbotham MC, Perander J, et al. Topical lidocaine patch relieves postherpetic neuralgia more effectively than a vehicle topical patch: results of an enriched enrollment study. *Pain* 1999;80(3):533–538.

332. Devers A, Galer BS. Topical lidocaine patch relieves a variety of neuropathic pain conditions: an open-label study. *Clin J Pain* 2000;16(3):205–208.

333. Robbins WR, Staats PS, Levine J, et al. Treatment of intractable pain with topical large-dose capsaicin: preliminary report. *Anesth Analg* 1998;86(3):579–583.

334. Zuurmond WW, Langendijk PN, Bezemer PD, et al. Treatment of acute reflex sympathetic dystrophy with DMSO 50% in a fatty cream. *Acta Anaesthesiol Scand* 1996;40(3):364–367.

335. Finch PM, Knudsen L, Drummond PD. Reduction of allodynia in patients with complex regional pain syndrome: a double-blind placebo-controlled trial of topical ketamine. *Pain* 2009;146(1–2):18–25.

336. Alioto JT. Behavioral treatment of reflex sympathetic dystrophy. *Psychosomatics* 1981;22(6):539–540.

337. Fialka V, Korpan M, Saradeth T, et al. Autogenic training for reflex sympathetic dystrophy: a pilot study. *Complement Ther Med* 1996;4:103–105.

338. Barowsky EI, Zweig JB, Moskowitz J. Thermal biofeedback in the treatment of symptoms associated with reflex sympathetic dystrophy. *J Child Neurol* 1987;2(3):229–232.

339. Blanchard EB. The use of temperature biofeedback in the treatment of chronic pain due to causalgia. *Biofeedback Self Regul* 1979;4(2):183–188.

340. Kawano M, Matsuoka M, Kurokawa T, et al. Autogenic training as an effective treatment for reflex neurovascular dystrophy: a case report. *Acta Paediatr Jpn* 1989;31(4):500–503.

341. Gainer MJ. Hypnotherapy for reflex sympathetic dystrophy. *Am J Clin Hypn* 1992;34(4):227–232.

342. Oerlemans HM, Oostendorp RA, de Boo T, et al. Adjuvant physical therapy versus occupational therapy in patients with reflex sympathetic dystrophy/complex regional pain syndrome type I. *Arch Phys Med Rehabil* 2000;81(1):49–56.

343. Carlson CR, Hoyle RH. Efficacy of abbreviated progressive muscle relaxation training: a quantitative review of behavioral medicine research. *J Consult Clin Psy* 1993;61:1059–1067.

344. Stetter F, Kupper S. Autogenic training: a meta-analysis of clinical outcome studies. *Appl Psychophysiol Biofeedback* 2002;27(1):45–98.

345. Eccleston C, Morley S, Williams A, et al. Systematic review of randomized controlled trials of psychological therapy for chronic pain in children and adolescents, with a subset meta-analysis of pain relief. *Pain* 2002;99(1–2):157–165.

346. Holroyd KA, Penzien DB. Pharmacological versus non-pharmacological prophylaxis of recurrent migraine headache: a meta-analytic review of clinical trials. *Pain* 1990;42(1):1–13.

347. Crider AB, Glaros AG. A meta-analysis of EMG biofeedback treatment of temporomandibular disorders. *J Orofac Pain* 1999;13(1):29–37.

348. Astin JA, Beckner W, Soeken K, et al. Psychological interventions for rheumatoid arthritis: a meta-analysis of randomized controlled trials. *Arthritis Rheum* 2002;47(3):291–302.

349. Sim J, Adams N. Systematic review of randomized controlled trials of nonpharmacological interventions for fibromyalgia. *Clin J Pain* 2002;18(5):324–336.

350. Devine EC. Meta-analysis of the effect of psychoeducational interventions on pain in adults with cancer. *Oncol Nurs Forum* 2003;30(1):75–89.

351. Burton AW. Interventional therapies. In: Harden RN, ed. *Complex Regional Pain Syndrome: Treatment Guidelines*. Milford, CT: RSDSA Press; 2006:51–61.

352. Evans J. Sympathectomy for reflex sympathetic dystrophy: report of 29 cases. *JAMA* 1946;132:620–623.

353. Jänig W, Habler H. Sympathetic nervous system: contribution to chronic pain. *Prog Brain Res* 2000;129:451–468.

354. Price D, Long S, Wilsey B, et al. Analysis of peak magnitude and duration of analgesia produced by local anesthetics injected into sympathetic ganglia of complex regional pain syndrome patients. *Clin J Pain* 1998;14:216–226.

355. Burton A, Conroy B, Sims S, et al. Complex regional pain syndrome type II as a complication of subclavian line insertion (letter). *Anesthesiology* 1998;89:804.

356. Cepeda M, Lau J, Carr D. Defining the therapeutic role of local anesthetic sympathetic blockade in complex regional pain syndrome: a narrative and systematic review. *Clin J Pain* 2002;18:216–233.

357. O'Connell NE, Wand BM, Gibson W, et al. Local anaesthetic sympathetic blockade for complex regional pain syndrome. *Cochrane Database Syst Rev* 2016;(7):CD004598.

358. Raj P. Nerve blocks: continuous regional analgesia. In: Raj P, ed. *Practical Management of Pain*. 3rd ed. St. Louis, MO: Mosby; 2000:710–722.

359. Raj PP, Montgomery SJ, Nettles D, et al. Infraclavicular brachial plexus block—a new approach. *Anesth Analg* 1973;52(6):897–904.

360. Wang J, Chen H, Chang P, et al. Axillary brachial plexus block with patient controlled analgesia for complex regional pain syndrome type I: a case report. *Reg Anesth Pain Med* 2001;26(1):68–71.

361. Cooper DE, DeLee JC, Ramamurthy S. Reflex sympathetic dystrophy of the knee. Treatment using continuous epidural anesthesia. *J Bone Joint Surg Am* 1989;71(3):365–369.

362. Koning H, Christiaans C, Overdijk G, et al. Cervical epidural blockade and reflex sympathetic dystrophy. *Pain Clinic* 1995;8:239–244.

363. Lundborg C, Dahm P, Nitescu P, et al. Clinical experience using intrathecal bupivacaine infusion in three patients with complex regional pain syndrome type I. *Acta Anaesthesiol Scand* 1999;43(6):667–678.

364. van Hilten R, van de Beek W, Hoff J, et al. Intrathecal baclofen for the treatment of dystonia in patients with reflex sympathetic dystrophy. *N Engl J Med* 2000;343:625–630.

365. Du Pen S, Peterson D, Williams A, et al. Infection during chronic catheter epidural catheterization: diagnosis and treatment. *Anesthesiology* 1990;73:905–909.

366. Arnér S. Intravenous phentolamine test: diagnostic and prognostic use in reflex sympathetic dystrophy. *Pain* 1991;46:17–22.

367. Verdugo R, Ochoa JL. 'Sympathetically maintained pain.' I. Phentolamine block questions the concept. *Neurology* 1994;44:1003–1010.

368. Goebel A, Baranowski A, Maurer K, et al. Intravenous immunoglobulin treatment of the complex regional pain syndrome: a randomized trial. *Ann Intern Med* 2010;152(3):152–158.

369. van Rijn MA, Munts AG, Marinus J, et al. Intrathecal baclofen for dystonia of complex regional pain syndrome. *Pain* 2009;143(1–2):41–47.

370. Hannington-Kiff JG. Intravenous regional sympathetic block with guanethidine. *Lancet* 1974;1(7865):1019–1020.

371. Hord AH, Rooks MD, Stephens BO, et al. Intravenous regional bretylium and lidocaine for treatment of reflex sympathetic dystrophy: a randomized, double-blind study. *Anesth Analg* 1992;74(6):818–821.

372. Bonelli S, Conoscente F, Movilia P, et al. Regional intravenous guanethidine versus stellate ganglion blocks in reflex sympathetic dystrophy: a randomized trial. *Pain* 1983;16(3):297–307.

373. Reuben S, Sklar J. Intravenous regional analgesia with clonidine in the management of complex regional pain syndrome of the knee. *J Clin Anesth* 2002;14:87–91.

374. Ramamurthy S, Hoffman J, Group GS. Intravenous regional guanethidine in the treatment of reflex sympathetic dystrophy/causalgia: a randomized double-blind study. *Anesth Analg* 1995;81:718–723.

375. Jadad AR, Carroll D, Glynn CJ, et al. Intravenous regional sympathetic dystrophy: a systemic review and a randomized, double-blind crossover study. *J Pain Symptom Manage* 1995;10:13–20.

376. Lubenow T, Dragisic B, Breuhl S, et al. Bretylium, lidocaine, phentolamine and hydrocortisone in combination for IV regional sympathetic blocks in the treatment of reflex sympathetic dystrophy. Paper presented at: American Academy of Pain Management Annual Meeting; 1996; Albuquerque, NM.

377. Suresh S, Wheeler M, Patel A. Case series: IV regional anesthesia with ketorolac and lidocaine: is it effective for the management of complex regional pain syndrome 1 in children and adolescents? *Anesth Analg* 2003;96:694–695.

378. Kemler MA, De Vet HC, Barendse GA, et al. The effect of spinal cord stimulation in patients with chronic reflex sympathetic dystrophy: two years' follow-up of the randomized controlled trial. *Ann Neurol* 2004;55(1):13–18.

379. Kemler MA, De Vet HC, Barendse GA, et al. Effect of spinal cord stimulation for chronic complex regional pain syndrome type I: five-year final follow-up of patients in a randomized controlled trial. *J Neurosurg* 2008;108(2):292–298.

380. Kriek N, Groeneweg JG, Stronks DL, et al. Comparison of tonic spinal cord stimulation, high-frequency and burst stimulation in patients with complex regional pain syndrome: a double-blind, randomised placebo controlled trial. *BMC Musculoskelet Disord* 2015;16:222.

381. Van Buyten JP, Smet I, Liem L, et al. Stimulation of dorsal root ganglia for the management of complex regional pain syndrome: a prospective case series. *Pain Pract* 2015;15(3):208–216.

382. Grabow T, Tella P, Raja S. Spinal cord stimulation for complex regional pain syndrome: an evidence-based review of the literature. *Clin J Pain* 2003;19(6):371–383.

383. Turner J, Loeser J, Deyo R, et al. Spinal cord stimulation for patients with failed back surgery syndrome or complex regional pain syndrome: a systematic review of effectiveness and complications. *Pain* 2004;108(1–2):137–147.

384. Burton AW, Hassenbusch SJ III, Warneke C, et al. Complex regional pain syndrome (CRPS): survey of current practices. *Pain Pract* 2004;4(2):74–83.

385. North RB, Levy RM. Consensus conference on the neurosurgical management of pain. *Neurosurgery* 1994;34(4):756–761.

386. Poree L, Krames E, Pope J, et al. Spinal cord stimulation as treatment for complex regional pain syndrome should be considered earlier than last resort therapy. *Neuromodulation* 2013;16(2):125–141.

387. Kemler MA, Raphael JH, Bentley A, et al. The cost-effectiveness of spinal cord stimulation for complex regional pain syndrome. *Value Health* 2010;13(6):735–742.

388. van Bussel CM, Stronks DL, Huygen FJPM. Dorsal column stimulation vs. dorsal root ganglion stimulation for complex regional pain syndrome

confined to the knee: patients' preference following the trial period. *Pain Pract* 2018;18:87–93.

389. Levy R, Deer T. A prospective, randomized, multi-center, controlled clinical trial to assess the safety and efficacy of the spinal modulation Axium™ neurostimulator system in the treatment of chronic pain. Paper presented at: Annual Meeting of the North American Neuromodulation Society Meeting; December 2015; Las Vegas, NV.

390. Kim K, DeSalles A, Johnson J, et al. Sympathectomy: open and thoracoscopic. In: Burchiel K, ed. *Surgical Management of Pain.* New York: Thieme; 2002:688–700.

391. Robertson D, Simpson R, Rose J. Video assisted endoscopic thoracic ganglionectomy. *J Neurosurg* 1993;79:238–240.

392. Wilkinson H. Percutaneous radiofrequency upper thoracic sympathectomy. *Neurosurgery* 1996;38:715–725.

393. Mockus MB, Rutherford RB, Rosales C, et al. Sympathectomy for causalgia. Patient selection and long-term results. *Arch Surg* 1987;122(6):668–672.

394. Kiralp MZ, Yildiz S, Vural D, et al. Effectiveness of hyperbaric oxygen therapy in the treatment of complex regional pain syndrome. *J Int Med Res* 2004;32(3):258–262.

395. Korpan MI, Dezu Y, Schneider B, et al. Acupuncture in the treatment of posttraumatic pain syndrome. *Acta Orthop Belg* 1999;65(2):197–201.

396. Muir JM, Vernon H. Complex regional pain syndrome and chiropractic. *J Manipulative Physiol Ther* 2000;23(7):490–497.

CHAPTER 26

Phantom Pain

KELLY A. BRUNO, HOWARD S. SMITH, IRFAN LALANI, and **CHARLES E. ARGOFF**

Ambrose Pare, a French military surgeon, is credited with first describing phantom limb pain (PLP) in the 16th century.[1] The concept of PLP was further popularized by Silas Weir Mitchell, a 19th century Civil War surgeon, who coined the term "phantom limb pain" in a publication of a long-term study on the fate of Civil War amputees.[2] PLP may occur in up to 85% of amputees and tends to be seen in the first 3 weeks after amputation,[3] although less commonly may develop 1 to 12 months following amputation.[4] Most phantom sensations resolve without treatment after 2 to 3 years.

Phantom pain refers to pain perceived in a missing body part and may occur in up to 50% to 80% of all amputees.[5] Pain may be related to certain positions or movements of the phantom and may be elicited or exacerbated by a range of physical factors (e.g., changes in weather or pressure on the residual limb) and psychological factors (e.g., emotional stress). It seems to be more intense in the distal portions of the phantom and can have several different qualities, such as stabbing, throbbing, burning, or cramping.[6]

Residual limb pain (RLP)—previously referred to in the literature as stump pain—refers to a regional pain restricted to the distal residual limb. Unlike phantom pain, it occurs in the area of the body that actually exists. Patients may also experience feelings of tingling, itching, cramping, or involuntary movements in the residuum.

Commonly, the phantom is exactly the same size and shape as the missing limb immediately after the amputation.[7] Over time, the phantom may gradually reduce in size and shorten into the residual limb (telescope) so that eventually only the foot, hand, or digits are left on the stump.[8–11] Hill[12] proposed that telescoping occurs in one-third of amputees.

The exteroceptive component describes the feelings within the phantom. Examples are "pins and needles," "tingling," "tickling," "itching," "numbness," and "like it is asleep."[8,12–17] Superadded sensations are the sensation of an object such as a ring, wristwatch, or shoe still being present on the phantom[18,19] or the return of a painful condition such as an ingrown toenail that existed some time before the amputation.[10,20] Superadded sensations were identified by 5 of 68 amputees (7%) in one study.[11,21] Exteroceptive sensations included pins and needles (50%) and itching (42.9%).[11] The high report of itching is interesting in terms of the mechanism of both PLP and itch. It has been found that similar areas of the brain, including the premotor areas, are involved in both sensations.[22,23]

Epidemiology

In 1983, Sherman and Sherman[24] published a survey of 590 war veteran amputees in which 85% reported phantom pain. A study with 2,694 amputees showed that 51% experienced PLP severe enough to hinder lifestyle on more than 6 days per month, 21% reported daily pain over a 10- to 14-hour period, and 27% for more than 15 hours per day.[25] The incidence of PLP increases with more proximal amputation. RLP is reported in up to 50% of amputees.[14,26–31]

PLP is also a major contributor to overall morbidity in veterans and service members after major limb amputation. Of 298 veterans who served in the Vietnam war and 283 service members and veterans who served in Operation Iraqi Freedom/Operation Enduring Freedom (OIF/OEF), 72.2% (Vietnam) and 76.0% (OIF/OEF) reported PLP, and 48.3% (Vietnam) and 62.9% (OIF/OEF) reported RLP.[32] Investigation of pain phenotypes in 124 active military service members after traumatic amputation injury found a significant association between neuropathic RLP and posttraumatic stress disorder (PTSD) and depression.[32]

Predisposing factors for developing PLP have been more challenging to discern. Most prospective studies report that increased pain before amputation is associated with increased PLP after amputation. However, other studies report no such association. Differences in these findings may be due, in part, to the fact that patients enrolled in prospective studies generally have a preexisting medical disease necessitating the amputation and often exclude patients who suffer traumatic amputation resulting in an overestimation of the association between preamputation pain and PLP.[33]

A retrospective study by Dijkstra et al.[34] of 536 amputees further characterized risk factors based on a logistic regression analysis, finding bilateral amputation and amputation of a lower limb to be the strongest risk factors for PLP. Anxiety as well as passive coping and catastrophizing personality traits were found in one study to be independent contributors to persistent postamputation pain.[35] In addition, there may be a sympathetic component to PLP triggered by stress, anxiety, depression, and other emotional states.[36]

PLP has been reported to occur as early as 1 week after amputation and as late as 40 years after amputation.[37,38] However, most studies report that the onset of PLP occurs within the first week for 75% of patients, with onset occurring within the initial 24 hours after amputation for nearly 50% of patients.[33] Phantom pain may diminish with time and eventually fade away. However, some prospective studies indicate that even 2 years after amputation, the incidence is not greatly diminished from that at onset.[31,39]

Modulation of Phantom Pain

Phantom pain may be modulated by multiple factors, both internal as well as external. Exacerbations of pain may be produced by trivial, physical, or emotional stimuli. Anxiety, depression, urination, cough, defecation, sexual activity, cold environment, or changes in the weather may worsen PLP.[24,39–45] It also has been reported that general, spinal, or regional anesthesia in amputees may cause appearance of phantom pain in otherwise pain-free subjects.[46–51]

Pathophysiology of Phantom Pain

The mechanisms underlying phantom pain are complex and multifactorial. Although incompletely understood, the pathophysiology likely involves peripheral, spinal, and supraspinal mechanisms as well as psychological factors.

After amputation, the distal end of axotomized afferent fibers initially undergoes retrograde degeneration with subsequent regenerative sprouting. These enlarged and disorganized endings of C fibers and demyelinated A fibers often form neuromas that show an increased rate of both spontaneous, ectopic activity, and abnormal, evoked activity in response to mechanical (e.g., pressure, Tinel sign) and chemical (e.g., norepinephrine) stimulation.[5] The proliferation of heterotopic sodium channels (Nav1.3, Nav1.7, Nav1.8) may also lower the stimulation threshold and provoke ectopic discharge.[52]

Clinically, peripheral causes of PLP is supported by the observation that RLP and phantom pain can be temporarily reduced in some (but not all) patients after injection of local anesthetics into stump neuromas. There have also been reports of alleviation of PLP after the removal of neuromas.[53] In contrast, two independent studies found that repetitive touching of the residual limb results in increased PLP.[33] Studies reporting the reduction of phantom pain with drugs blocking the sodium channels lend further support to this theory.[54,55]

Ectopic discharges can also occur at the level of the dorsal root ganglion (DRG), independently of stump neuromas. This can result in amplification of peripheral signals and recruitment of neighboring neurons. Electrophysiology studies by Nyström and Hagbarth[56] have shown that blocking stump neuromas eliminates the percussion-evoked Tinel sign and associated evoked activity, but does not block the ongoing spontaneous discharge recorded in the nerve. When compared to neuromas, the DRG has proved to be a more robust source of spontaneous firing than neuromas.[57]

The sympathetic nervous system may play a role in potentiating phantom pain. Sympathetic nerve blocks can temporarily relieve phantom pain in some patients, whereas injection of norepinephrine can exacerbate pain. Catecholamines can promote firing of peripheral mechanoreceptors, which in turn may activate sensitized dorsal horn neurons. Increased sympathetic tone can also promote ephaptic neuronal transmission in the periphery. Sympathetic tone is inversely related to skin temperature at the amputated stump.[6] Investigators have also shown an inverse relationship between phantom pain and skin temperature, suggesting that sympathetic tone promotes pain sensation.[6]

Peripheral nerve injury is also accompanied by reorganization of signal processing at the spinal cord level. Selective degeneration of unmyelinated C fibers results in functional denervation of lamina II neurons in the dorsal horn. A compensatory arborization of Aδ and Aβ fibers "sprouting" into lamina II can occur.[58,59] This change in innervation is accompanied by phenotypic switching, whereby Aβ-fiber terminals release substance P, a nociceptive peptide. These changes may form the anatomic and neurochemical substrate for the clinical phenomenon of allodynia, where a non-noxious mechanical stimulus is perceived as painful.

Increased excitatory input at the dorsal horn following nerve injury can cause apoptosis of inhibitory interneurons expressing γ-aminobutyric acid and glycine. Activation of microglia after neural injury can result in release of brain-derived neurotrophic factor, which promotes phenotypic switching of inhibitory interneurons, and may lead to release of excitatory neurotransmitters (e.g., glutamate). Opioid receptors are also downregulated along with upregulation of cholecystokinin, which is an endogenous opioid receptor antagonist.

Nikolajsen and Jensen[60] explained that the pharmacology of spinal sensitization involves increased activity in N-methyl-D-aspartate (NMDA) receptor complex,[61] and many aspects of the central sensitization can be reduced by NMDA receptor antagonists. This was supported in human amputees where the evoked stump or phantom pain produced by repetitive stimulation of the stump by nonnoxious pinprick was reduced by the NMDA receptor antagonist, ketamine.[60]

Waxman and Hains proposed that abnormal expression of Nav1.3 sodium channels in the second- and third-order neurons along nociceptive pathways after spinal cord injury may make these neurons hyperexcitable.[62] These neurons may then function as pain amplifiers/generators and conceivably contribute to phantom phenomena.

Peripheral injury after amputation is also accompanied by remapping of supraspinal synaptic networks, including those in the primary somatosensory cortex. Some patients with PLP exhibit "topographical remapping," where stimulation of an unaffected site (e.g., face) will result in a sensation perceived in the phantom limb. Functional imaging studies have shown activation of areas in the primary somatosensory cortex and are both adjacent and distant from the area normally subserving the affected limb. Topographical remapping appears to correlate with persistence of phantom pain, with data showing that upper extremity amputees with phantom pain have expansion of the mouth area into the hand area in the sensory homunculus (primary somatosensory cortex). These findings have also been described in the primary motor cortex of amputees, with good correlation between reorganization and presence of phantom pain symptoms.

Melzack[63] observed that a substantial number of children who are born without a limb feel a phantom of the missing part and suggested the existence of a neural network, or *neuromatrix*, that subserves body sensation and has a genetically determined substrate that is modified by sensory experience. Lotze et al.[64] revealed that functional magnetic resonance imaging (fMRI) data from amputees without pain and healthy volunteers during a lip pursing task were similar. In amputees with PLP, however, the cortical representation of the mouth extends into the region of the hand and arm. Giummarra et al.[65] proposed that phantom pain may reflect a maladaptive failure of the neuromatrix to maintain global bodily constructs. Cortical map reorganization may be facilitated via selective loss of C fibers, which occurs after amputations. C fibers appear to have an important role in the maintenance of cortical maps.

Psychological factors can also play a role in the pathogenesis of phantom pain. Although these factors may not play a causative role, they may certainly modulate the pain experience.

Longitudinal diary studies showed that there is a significant relation between stress and the onset and exacerbation of episodes of PLP, probably mediated by activity in the sympathetic nervous system and increases in muscle tension.[66] Patients who received less support before the amputation tend to report more PLP.[27]

Animal work on stimulation-induced plasticity suggests that extensive behaviorally relevant (but not passive) stimulation of a body part leads to an expansion of its representation zone.[67] Intensive use of a myoelectric prosthesis is positively correlated with reduced cortical reorganization and analgesic effects.[64] These effects could not be achieved with standard medical treatment and general psychological counseling because it is felt that in order to achieve analgesia, input into the amputation zone of the cortex is needed in order to "undo" the reorganizational changes induced by amputation. Similar beneficial effects on phantom pain and cortical activation were reported for imagined movement of the phantom and may also occur to some degree with mirror treatment (where a mirror is used to trick the brain into perceiving movement of the phantom when the intact limb is moved).[68]

Prevention of Phantom Pain

PLP cannot currently be completely prevented; however, perioperative epidural techniques, placement of peripheral nerve catheters, and other analgesic strategies utilized preoperatively, intraoperatively, and postoperatively may at least address postoperative pain control better than not employing any specific perioperative analgesic techniques.[69–75]

Madabhushi and colleagues[74] reported on a patient with a history of PLP from a below-knee amputation who then came for an above-knee amputation in the same extremity. Before transection, the sciatic nerve was infiltrated with 0.25% bupivacaine 5 mL and clonidine 50 µg. After the nerve was severed, a 20-gauge epidural catheter was inserted into the nerve sheath and externalized laterally through a separate skin incision. Before closure, 0.25% bupivacaine 10 mL and clonidine 50 µg was injected and then 0.1% bupivacaine and clonidine 2 µg/mL was infused perineurally for the first 96 hours postoperatively. The mean postoperative pain score (from 0 to 10) for 96 hours was 1.2 ± 0.7.[74] The patient required a total of 10 mg of oxycodone postoperatively. Over a 1-year follow-up period, the patient never reported stump or phantom pain.[74]

Treatment of Phantom Pain

Treatment for phantom pain often requires a multimodal approach. Treatment options range from behavioral techniques and pharmacologic treatments to invasive electrical brain and spinal cord stimulation (SCS) and surgical interventions. There remains a paucity of data from large randomized controlled trials to guide treatment options. As a general rule, initial treatments should be low-risk, low-cost, and noninvasive, with more expensive and invasive treatments reserved for patients who fail conservative care.

Pharmacologic Interventions

ANTIDEPRESSANTS

Antidepressants are commonly used for many painful conditions but especially for neuropathic pain. Although antidepressants are utilized for the treatment of postamputation pain, they have not been well studied for PAP. Wilder-Smith et al.[76] studied 94 treatment-naive posttraumatic limb amputees with phantom pain (intensity: mean Visual Analog Scale [VAS] score [0 to 100], 40 [95% confidence interval, 38 to 41]) who were randomly assigned to receive individually titrated doses of tramadol, placebo (double-blind comparison), or amitriptyline (open comparison) for 1 month. Wilder-Smith and colleagues[76] concluded that in treatment-naive patients, both amitriptyline and tramadol provided excellent and stable phantom limb and stump pain control with no major adverse events.

Alternatively, Robinson et al.[77] studied 39 persons with amputation-related pain lasting more than 6 months in a 6-week randomized controlled trial of amitriptyline (titrated up to 125 mg per day) or an active placebo (benztropine mesylate). No significant differences were found between the treatment groups in outcome variables when controlled for initial pain scores, thus not supporting the use of amitriptyline in the treatment of postamputation pain.[77]

Kuiken et al.[78] studied four individuals with PLP for at least 3 months after amputation. All subjects received oral mirtazapine between 7.5 and 30 mg per day.[78] An 11-point numeric rating scale (0 to 10) measured pain intensity and relief during monitored outpatient follow-up visits. Mirtazapine use improved the PLP experienced by these subjects by at least 50%, measured by an 11-point numerical rating scale (NRS-11).[78] Subjects with PLP-related sleeping difficulties reported the greatest pain relief concomitant with improved sleep quality.[78]

ANTIEPILEPTIC DRUGS

Carbamazepine, an anticonvulsant (and heterocyclic), has also been well documented for use in neuropathic pain syndromes and serves as a potent sodium channel blocker. Historically, it has also been the most commonly prescribed anticonvulsant for pain. Despite this, the results of its efficacy on PLP have been mixed. Patterson reported cases of phantom pain that were alleviated with the use of oral carbamazepine.[79,80] However, only brief, shock-like pain was assessed.[79] There are no studies that have shown its effectiveness in treating any of the other qualities of pain.

The effectiveness of gabapentin in postamputation PLP was studied in a randomized, double-blind, placebo-controlled, crossover study by Bone et al.[81] They evaluated analgesic efficacy of gabapentin in PLP in patients attending a multidisciplinary pain clinic. The daily dose of gabapentin was titrated in increments of 300 mg to a maximum dose of 2,400 mg or the maximum tolerated dose. Nineteen eligible patients were randomized, of which 14 completed both arms of the study. Both placebo and gabapentin treatments resulted in reduced VAS scores compared with baseline. However, the pain intensity difference was significantly greater than placebo for gabapentin therapy at the end of the treatment. Bone et al.[81] concluded that after 6 weeks, gabapentin monotherapy was better than placebo in relieving postamputation PLP.

In contrast, two other studies did not find an association between gabapentin therapy and relief of PLP. One study of 24 patients with chronic phantom limb and stump pain following amputation of various etiologies, found that the average phantom pain intensity differences on the NRS-11 (mean [standard deviation]) in the gabapentin phase did not differ significantly from placebo (0.94 [1.98] vs. 0.49 [2.20], t = 0.70).[82] The second study by Nikolajsen et al.[83] concluded that gabapentin administered in the first 30 postoperative days after amputation does not reduce the incidence or intensity of postamputation pain.[83] Pregabalin may exhibit analgesic effects on postamputation pain states but has not yet been evaluated.

Four PLP subjects[84] were treated during a larger prospective, double-blind, randomized, placebo-controlled pilot study conducted to test the efficacy of topiramate in managing various neuropathic pain conditions associated with rehabilitation.[84] Three of the four subjects who had experienced over 2 years of refractory PLP experienced significantly reduced pain after treatment with topiramate.[84]

OPIOIDS

Mishra et al.[85] reported a case of intractable PLP that did not respond to usual treatment, however, high dose of morphine made the patient totally pain-free.[85]

Wilder-Smith et al.[76] evaluated a recent study of 94 treatment-naive posttraumatic limb amputees with phantom pain who were randomly assigned to receive individually titrated doses of tramadol (mean dose 448 mg) or placebo (double-blind comparison) for 1 month. It was found that tramadol provided excellent and stable PLP and RLP control with no major adverse events.[76] A separate review found a 50% to 90% reduction in pain at 12 to 26 months with methadone 10 to 20 mg per day.[86]

Huse and colleagues[87] studied the efficacy of oral long-acting morphine sulfate (MS) against placebo in a double-blind crossover design in 12 patients with PLP after unilateral leg or arm amputation.[87] The dose of MS was titrated to at least 70 mg per day and at highest 300 mg per day.[87] Pain, reorganization of somatosensory cortex, and pain thresholds were assessed pre- and posttreatment.[87] A significant pain reduction was found during MS therapy but not during placebo. A clinically relevant response to MS (pain reduction of more than 50%) was evident in 42%, with a partial response (pain reduction of 25% to 50%) in 8% of the patients.[87] Neuromagnetic imaging utilizing magnetoencephalographic recordings of three patients showed initial evidence for reduced cortical reorganization with MS treatment concurrent with the reduction in pain intensity.[87] Huse et al.[87] concluded that opioids show efficacy in the treatment of PLP and may also potentially influence cortical reorganization.[87]

Intravenous lidocaine and morphine have also been evaluated for their therapeutic use in postamputation pain. Wu et al.[88] conducted a randomized double-blind trial to compare the analgesic effects of intravenous morphine and lidocaine on postamputation stump and phantom pains. A bolus of morphine, lidocaine, and an active placebo (diphenhydramine) were used over a span of 3 consecutive days. The results showed that 31 of 32 subjects enrolled completed the study. Eleven subjects had both stump and phantom pains; 11 and 9 subjects had stump and phantom pain alone, respectively. Compared with placebo, morphine reduced both RLP and phantom pains significantly. In contrast, lidocaine decreased RLP but not phantom pain. The authors concluded that the mechanisms of RLP and phantom pain are different.[88]

NMDA RECEPTOR ANTAGONISTS

To date, six studies have investigated the effectiveness of NMDA receptor antagonists in PLP: Maier et al., Schwenkreis et al., and Wiech et al. examined memantine versus placebo; Abraham et al. investigated dextromethorphan versus placebo; Nikolajsen et al. investigated ketamine versus placebo; and Eichenberger et al. examined ketamine versus calcitonin, combination ketamine and calcitonin, and placebo.[89]

Pain intensity was not significantly decreased with 30 mg per day of memantine for 3 to 4 weeks in traumatic amputees with chronic pain in three independent studies.[89] Another randomized, double-blind, controlled trial of 19 patients with acute traumatic amputation of the upper extremity found that memantine (20 to 30 mg daily) reduced the number of requested ropivacaine bolus injections during the first week after amputation and significantly decreased PLP prevalence and intensity at 4 weeks and 6 months but not at 12-month follow-up.

A double-blind, placebo-controlled, crossover study of three cancer patients with PLP who received oral dextromethorphan (120 to 180 mg daily) during a 3-week study followed by an additional 1-month continued treatment regimen reduced PLP compared to placebo.[90]

Stannard and Porter[91] described three cases in which PLP was successfully treated with ketamine hydrochloride. Nikolajsen et al.[92] administered ketamine intravenously to a patient with established stump pain in a double-blind saline-controlled fashion. Following infusion, stump pain was alleviated for 31 hours.[92] Ketamine reduced the allodynic area and wind-up–like pain and increased pressure pain thresholds.[92] Treatment was started with ketamine 50 mg taken four times daily dissolved in juice.[93] No side effects or development of tolerance were observed during a 3-month treatment period.[92]

Nikolajsen et al.[94] administered ketamine (bolus at 0.1 mg/kg/5 min followed by an infusion of 7 µg/kg/min) intravenously to 11 patients with established stump pain and PLP in a double-blind saline-controlled study.[94] All 11 patients responded with a decrease in the rating of RLP and PLP assessed by VAS and McGill Pain Questionnaire (MPQ).[94] Ketamine increased pressure pain thresholds significantly. Wind-up–like pain (pain evoked by repeatedly tapping the dysesthetic skin area) was reduced significantly by ketamine.[94] In contrast, no effect was seen on pain evoked by repeated thermal stimuli. Side effects were observed in nine patients.[94]

Eichenberger et al.[95] conducted a randomized, double-blind, crossover study in which 20 patients received four intravenous infusions of 200 IU calcitonin, ketamine 0.4 mg/kg (only 10 patients), 200 IU of calcitonin combined with ketamine 0.4 mg/kg, placebo, and 0.9% saline. Intensity of phantom pain (VAS) was recorded before, during, at the end, and the 48 hours after each infusion.[95] Ketamine, but not calcitonin, reduced PLP.[95] The combination was not superior to ketamine alone.[95]

CALCITONIN

Although calcitonin may have analgesic effects for amputation pain postoperatively,[96] it does not appear to be effective for chronic amputation pain conditions.[95]

Two studies have examined the effectiveness of S-calcitonin infusion in treating PLP. Jaeger et al.[96] compared calcitonin to saline placebo in a group of 21 patients with severe PLP developing

within a week after amputation. Eichenberger et al.[95] compared calcitonin to ketamine, combination ketamine and calcitonin, and placebo in 20 patients with chronic PLP. Neither study demonstrated significant improvement in pain scores compared to placebo, and both studies described adverse events including headache, vertigo, facial flushing, nausea, vomiting, sedation, dizziness, and increased phantom sensation.[89]

TRANSIENT RECEPTOR POTENTIAL CATION CHANNEL SUBFAMILY V MEMBER 1 (TRPV1) MODULATORS

Topical capsaicin has been utilized for the treatment of PLP. In a study performed in a double-blind fashion with 24 patients, the authors concluded that capsaicin may be used as an alternative treatment for PLP.[97] A 12-week prospective, observational study in 21 patients with PAP (10 with PLP, 4 with RLP, 7 with PLP and RLP) treated with a single 8% capsaicin transcutaneous patch significantly reduced the average pain intensity. After the observational period, 80% of patients with PLP and 50% with both RLP and PLP expressed the wish to receive retreatment with capsaicin 8% patches.[98] Future developments may produce higher strength capsaicin products, more potent capsaicin analogues, TRPV1 antagonists, and intravenous capsaicin formulations.

INTERVENTIONAL THERAPY

A wide range of neural blockade techniques have been utilized in the treatment of PLP, including trigger point injections, sympathetic blocks, stump injections, and peripheral nerve blocks as well as epidural and subarachnoid blocks.[24] Despite this, studies have shown that only 14% of patients report a significant temporary change and 5% report a prolonged change with these blocks.[24]

The use of neural blockade in the treatment of PLP is largely based on anecdotal reports in the literature.[99-101] Blankenbaker[99] reported that sympathetic blocks are successful if amputees are treated soon after the onset of PLP. However, Halbert et al.,[102] in a systematic review to evaluate evidence for the optimal management of acute and chronic phantom pain, were unable to find any trials that met criteria for inclusion. A crossover pilot study by Ilfeld et al.[103] suggests that ropivacaine 0.5% delivered via continuous peripheral nerve catheter may offer therapeutic relief for intractable PLP.

The use of botulinum toxin A injections in PLP patients has also been utilized for RLP control. It is possible that muscle tension, perhaps resulting from cortical reorganization, may contribute to phantom pain as a trigger of spinal reflexes. Botulinum toxin may work by initiating muscle relaxation in the stump or by modulating the release of neurotransmitters that cause analgesia. In a small pilot trial, researchers injected 100 IU botulinum toxin A in four muscle trigger points of a residual stump. It was found that the use of botulinum toxin A reduced phantom pain about 60% to 80%.[104] These findings were supported by another pilot study with targeted injection of 500 IU botulin toxin A via electromyography into the residual stump.[105]

Kern et al.[106] administered a total dose of 2,500–5,000 IU of botulinum toxin type B to the residual stump of upper and lower extremity amputees.[106] Two patients reported that the injection was very painful. All patients experienced a reduction in RLP, which lasted for many weeks.[106] Other reports included a reduction in the frequency of pain attacks, cessation of "balloon feelings," improvement in stump allodynia, and decreased occurrence of involuntary stump movements. In addition, quality of sleep at night significantly improved in one patient.[106]

Furthermore, Kern and colleagues[107] suggested that by diminishing muscle tone, pain, and hyperhidrosis, botulinum toxin may facilitate prosthesis use. Four postamputation patients (one with phantom pain, three with RLP) were each treated with 100 IU botulinum toxin A, divided between several trigger points in the distal stump musculature. In one female patient, in addition to pronounced reduction in phantom pain, the patient reported hyperhidrosis of the stump ceased completely, probably after diffusion of the drug into the dermal sweat glands, leading to longer and safer use of the prosthesis. Intentional intradermal injection for this purpose therefore could be potentially valuable. Another patient was able to use her prosthesis for the whole day again after botulinum toxin A treatment for substantial RLP, compared with only 4 hours a day before treatment. In two male patients, RLP while wearing the prosthesis subsided to a considerable extent, and one of the two reported an improvement in steadiness of gait. They suggested that stump treatment with botulinum toxin in rehabilitative medicine should be investigated in more detail.[107]

In a larger, randomized, double-blind pilot study, 14 amputees with intractable RLP and/or PLP who had failed conventional treatment received either one botulinum toxin injection or an injection of lidocaine and methylprednisolone (Depo Medrol). The study found that both botulinum toxin and lidocaine/methylprednisolone (Depo Medrol) injections resulted in immediate improvements of RLP and pain tolerance for the entire 6-month follow-up period. However, no immediate improvement of PLP and no change in posttreatment VAS-PLP were observed after botulinum toxin or lidocaine/methylprednisolone (Depo Medrol) injection.[108]

Dahl and Cohen[109] treated six soldiers with RLP and phantom pain with a series of perineural etanercept injections. Five of the six patients reported significant improvements in RLP at rest and with activity, PLP, functional capacity, and psychological well-being 3 months after injections.[109] The one soldier who failed therapy was the only patient who presented with pain greater than 1 year in duration. At the reduced doses administered, no adverse effects were observed. These results seem to warrant further large well-designed studies.[109]

NEUROMODULATION

Transcutaneous electrical nerve stimulation (TENS) has been used with some success in the treatment of phantom pain. Katz and Melzack[110] reported that 10 minutes after receiving low-frequency (4 Hz), high-intensity (10 to 30 V) auricular TENS, phantom pain patients demonstrated a modest yet statistically significant decrease in pain as measured by the MPQ.[110] Investigators have reported good to excellent results in roughly 25% of patients treated with TENS.[110,111]

A case series involving two patients with PLP showed a significant improvement in perception of PLP and sensations that was maintained at 1-year follow-up using TENS applied to the contralateral limb. The study author acknowledges that a randomized controlled trial to confirm these outcomes is necessary.[112] A systematic review of controlled clinical trials investigating the effectiveness of acupuncture/TENS for phantom limb syndrome found that there is some evidence for the use of acupuncture and TENS for the treatment of PLP/phantom limb sensation but insufficient high-quality evidence.[113]

Repetitive transcranial magnetic stimulation (rTMS) focused at the motor cortex has demonstrated therapeutic benefit in treating PLP in multiple studies.[114–116] The therapy is thought to target synaptic mechanisms linked to long-term potentiation and long-term depression phenomena.[117] A study of 27 patients with unilateral amputation found reduced PLP pain scores in patients who received real rTMS compared to sham after five treatments and at 1 and 2 months after stimulation.[115] A randomized, double-blind, placebo-controlled, parallel group study of 54 landmine victims found that active rTMS induced a significantly greater reduction in pain intensity 15 days after treatment compared with sham; however, this effect was not significant 30 days after treatment.[116] Similarly, transcranial direct current stimulation has

shown encouraging results in two independent small-scale, double-blind, sham-controlled studies.[118,119]

SCS has also been used for PLP since the 1970s. Early studies in patients with PLP implanted with subdural and epidural electrodes found 45% to 100% had greater than 50% pain relief at initial follow-up.[120–122] Seigfried and Zimmerman[123] reported that 51% of patients with SCS had a 50% or more decrease in pain but without long-term follow-up.[123] Viswanathan et al.[124] found that 100% of patients had >80% pain relief and McAuley et al.[125] found that 92% and 100% had >50% pain relief immediately and at long-term follow-up (median of 11 years), respectively. These studies propose that SCS for PLP may be an effective intervention for select patients who have not obtained adequate relief with other interventions.

Direct stimulation of the DRG is a relatively novel therapeutic treatment option that offers more targeted paresthesia stimulation. A pilot study of eight patients with PLP looked at percentage of pain relief and change in analgesic medication intake immediately after placement and at 5- to 24-month follow-up. The average immediate pain relief was 50%. Of the seven patients available for follow-up, three continued to have >50% pain relief.[126] The use of radiofrequency stimulation prior to DRG implantation has been proposed as a method to improve accurate coverage of the phantom limb by targeting the DRG.[127]

Peripheral nerve stimulation allows even more focused targeting of electrical stimulation. A few devices have been marketed specifically for PLP based on limited pilot data and case reports.[128–131] Larger studies are needed to evaluate long-term efficacy of these devices.

Bittar and colleagues[132] concluded that deep brain stimulation has been utilized successfully for the treatment of PLP resulting in decreased pain scores, decreased opiate intake, and improved quality of life. Bittar et al.[133] published a meta-analysis supporting this pain improvement as well, especially in the burning component—perhaps via a reorganization in the central nervous system.

Sol et al.[134] used chronic motor cortex stimulation in three patients with intractable PLP after upper limb amputation. fMRI correlated to anatomical MRI permitted frameless image guidance for electrode placement. Pain control was obtained for all the patients initially, and the relief was stable in two of the three patients at 2-year follow-up. fMRI data may be useful in assisting the neurosurgeon in electrode placement for this indication.[134]

SURGICAL INTERVENTIONS

PLP has generally been difficult to treat with surgical interventions. Part of the difficulty in addressing PLP and stump pain surgically lies in the postsurgical restriction or growth retardation of stump neuromas. Residual limb neuromas develop at the site of the severed end of peripheral nerves. Surgical management may involve implanting the end of severed nerves into a nearby/adjacent large muscle belly, which may alleviate stump pain somewhat, although it does not permanently cure patients.[93]

Sakai et al.[135] theorized that preventing neuroma formation might also significantly decrease the incidence of postamputation stump pain. Techniques to prevent neuroma formation include nerve transposition or ligation, embedding of the nerve end in bone or muscle, and capping of the nerve stump with a nerve graft, epineurium, or atelocollagen.[135,136]

Sehirlioglu et al.[137] retrospectively studied 75 patients who were treated for painful neuroma after lower limb amputation following landmine explosions between the years 2000 and 2006.[137] The average time period from use of prosthesis to start of symptoms suggesting neuroma was 9.6 months. The average time period from start of pain symptoms to neuroma surgery was 7.8 months. All clinically proven neuromas were surgically resected.[137] In the mean follow-up of 2.8 years, all patients were satisfied with the end results, and all were free of any pain symptoms.[137] In a painful residual limb with clinical diagnostic findings of neuroma, if conservative measures fail, surgery may be considered as a therapeutic option.[137]

Aggressive surgical techniques, such as anterolateral cordotomy and dorsal root entry zone lesions, have been attempted in PLP but do not have large multicenter studies supporting their use at all and have significant morbidity and some mortality.

BEHAVIORAL MEDICINE INTERVENTIONS

Many psychological modalities have been investigated for managing symptoms of PLP, including biofeedback, relaxation techniques, mirror therapy, virtual reality training, and eye movement desensitization and reprocessing.[138]

Biofeedback treatments resulting in vasodilatation or decreased muscle tension in the residual limb may help to reduce PLP and seem promising in patients in whom peripheral factors contribute to the pain.[139] Harden et al.[140] conducted a pilot study that examined the effectiveness of biofeedback in the treatment of nine individuals with PLP who received up to seven thermal/autogenic biofeedback sessions over the course of 4 to 6 weeks. Pain was assessed daily using the VAS, the sum of the sensory descriptors, and the sum of the affective descriptors of the McGill short form. Interrupted time series analytical models were created for each of the participants, allowing biofeedback sessions to be modeled as discrete interventions.[140] Analyses of the VAS revealed that a 20% pain reduction was seen in five of the nine patients in the weeks after session 4 and that at least 30% pain reduction (range: 25% to 66%) was seen in six of the seven patients in the weeks following session 6.[140]

Relaxation training has also been shown to provide significant benefit in many patients. One report noted that 12 of 14 patients with chronic PLP improved with muscular relaxation training.[138] Hypnotic imagery has been used alone and with relaxation training; however, further studies need to be done before any conclusions regarding this therapy can be made.[141]

Ramachandran and Rogers-Ramachandran[16] described another behaviorally oriented approach: A mirror was placed in a box, and the patient inserted his or her intact arm and the residual limb. The patient was then asked to look at the mirror image of the intact arm, which is perceived as an intact hand where the phantom used to be, and to make symmetrical movements with both hands, thus suggesting real movement from the lost arm to the brain. This procedure may reestablish control over the phantom limb and alleviate pain in some patients, although controlled data are lacking.

Graded motor imagery is a promising, nonpharmacologic means of treating PLP. A randomized controlled trial using graded motor imagery to treat complex regional pain syndrome type 1 and PLP showed number needed to treat of 3 at 6 months for a composite endpoint of 50% pain reduction and improvement in function.[142] Patients in the placebo arm of this study received standard physical therapy and usual medical care. Graded motor imagery involves training patients to improve right/left discrimination and imagine pain-free movements of affected and normal limbs followed by practicing pain-free movements with the aid of a mirror box.[142]

Murray et al.[143] reported three patients who experienced PLP (two with an upper limb amputation and one with a lower limb amputation) that took part in between two and five immersive virtual reality (IVR) sessions over a 3-week period. The movements of patients' anatomical limbs were transposed into the movements of a virtual limb.[143] All patients reported the transferal of sensations into the muscles and joints of the phantom limb, and all patients reported a decrease in phantom pain during

at least one of the sessions.[143] The authors suggested the need for further research studying IVR for PLP using controlled trials.

Schneider et al.[144] evaluated eye movement desensitization and reprocessing (EMDR) treatment with extensive follow-up. Five patients with PLP ranging from 1 to 16 years who were on extensive medication regimens underwent 3 to 15 sessions of EMDR, which was used to treat the pain and the psychological ramifications.[144] EMDR resulted in a significant decrease or elimination of phantom pain, reduction in depression and PTSD symptoms to subclinical levels, and significant reduction or elimination of medications related to the phantom pain and nociceptive pain at long-term follow-up.[144] Further research is needed to explore the theoretical and treatment implications of this information-processing approach.[144]

MISCELLANEOUS TREATMENTS FOR RESIDUAL LIMB PAIN

Chronic RLP may occur as a result of skin pathology, vascular insufficiency, infection, bone spurs, or neuromas.[12,39,40,136]

Fitting of a prosthetic socket is a critical stage in the process of rehabilitation of a transtibial amputation (TTA) patient because a misfit may cause pressure ulcers or a deep tissue injury (DTI; necrosis of the muscle flap under intact skin) in the residual limb.[145] To date, prosthetic fitting topically depends on the subjective skills of the prosthetist and is not supported by biomedical instrumentation that allows evaluation of the quality of fitting.[145] Portnoy et al.[145] concluded that real-time patient-specific finite element analysis of internal stresses in deep soft tissues of the residual limb in TTA patients is feasible. This method may be improving the fitting of prostheses in the clinical setting and protecting the residual limb from pressure ulcers and DTI.[145]

The use of a myoelectric prosthesis might be one way to influence PLP. Intensive use of a myoelectric prosthesis was positively associated with both less PLP and less cortical reorganization.[146] One study found that use of a forearm prosthesis with somatosensory feedback is effective in reducing PLP.[147]

Topical clonidine patches (and other topical therapies) have been utilized on the residuum but have not been studied. For relatively superficial neuromas, lidocaine via iontophoresis (e.g., LidoSite patch [developed and manufactured by Vyteris, Inc, Fair Lawn, NJ]) theoretically may be useful.

Gruber et al.[148] prospectively evaluated "neurosclerosis" of residual limb neuromas, present after amputation, on 82 patients by means of high-resolution sonographically guided injection with up to 0.8 mL of 80% phenol solution. During treatment, all patients had marked improvement in terms of reduction of pain measured with a VAS.[148] Twelve (15%) of the subjects were pain-free after one to three treatments, with 9 of the 12 achieving relief with the initial instillation.[148] After 6 months, patients had an overall decrease in median VAS score from 10.0 ± 1.5 (standard deviation) (range, 2 to 10) to 3.0 ± 2.6 (range, 1 to 10) after one (25 patients), two (12 patients), and three treatment sessions (15 patients). At the 6-month follow-up evaluation, 20 (38%) of the 52 patients reported almost unnoticeable pain, and 33 (64%) reported pain equal to the minimum pain they had reached during phenol injection therapy. In 18 (35%) of the 52 patients, the incidence of painful periods had markedly decreased.[148] The "neurosclerosis" procedure had a low complication rate (5% rate of minor complications, 1.3% rate of major complications).[148]

Pulsed radiofrequency treatment of the DRG at the L4 and L5 nerve root level was utilized as a therapeutic option for two patients with peripherally mediated intractable stump pain. A decrease in pain intensity and improved toleration of the limb prosthesis was appreciated in both patients.[136]

Anecdotes of other analgesic strategies such as acupuncture[149] and electroconvulsive therapy[117] for postamputation pain exist.

Summary

Phantom pain remains an incompletely understood, difficult to treat pain condition. It is present, at least in the early stages after amputation, in a majority of postamputation patients. It is a painful condition in which an obvious loss of sensory information coupled with a disruption of the nervous system leads to pain. Phantom pain also appears to be a painful condition in which the involvement of supraspinal mechanisms may be more intuitive than in the case of other painful conditions. Optimal treatment approaches involve the coordination of an interdisciplinary pain medicine team familiar with the therapy of postamputation pain syndromes. A combination of pharmacologic, physical medicine and rehabilitation, behavioral medicine, neuromodulation, and interventional treatments may be needed to achieve optimal outcomes. Further basic and clinical research is needed to better understand the pathophysiologic mechanisms, prevention strategies, and optimal treatment approaches for different patients and their varying phantom conditions.

References

1. Weinstein SM. Phantom limb pain and related disorders. *Neurol Clin* 1998;16(4):919–935. doi:10.1016/S0733-8619(05)70105-5.
2. Mitchell SW. *Injuries of Nerves and Their Consequences.* London: Smith Elder; 1872.
3. Parkes CM. Factors determining the persistence of phantom pain in the amputee. *J Psychosom Res* 1973;17:97–108.
4. Gillis L. The management of the painful amputation stump: a new theory for the phantom phenomena. *Br J Surg* 1964;51:87–95.
5. Jensen TS, Nikolajsen L. Phantom pain and other phenomena after amputation. In: Wall P, Melzack R, eds. *Textbook of Pain.* 4th ed. Edinburgh: Churchill Livingstone; 1999:799–814.
6. Flor H. Phantom-limb pain: characteristics, causes, and treatment. *Lancet Neurol* 2002;1:182–189.
7. Melzack R, Wall P. *The Challenge of Pain.* London: Penguin; 1984.
8. Montoya P, Larbig W, Grulke N, et al. The relationship of phantom limb pain to other phantom limb phenomena in upper extremity amputees. *Pain* 1997;72:87–93.
9. Jensen TS, Rasmussen P. Phantom pain and related phenomena after amputation. In: Melzack R, Wall P, eds. *Textbook of Pain.* London: Churchill Livingstone; 1989:651–665.
10. Katz J. Psychophysical correlates of phantom limb experience. *J Neurol Neurosurg Psychiatry* 1992;55:811–821.
11. Richardson C, Glenn S, Nurmikko T, et al. Incidence of phantom phenomena including phantom limb pain 6 months after major lower limb amputation in patients with peripheral vascular disease. *Clin J Pain* 2006;22:353–358.
12. Hill A. Phantom limb pain: a review of the literature on attributes and potential mechanisms. *J Pain Symptom Manage* 1999;17:125–142.
13. Vaida G, Friedmann LW. Postamputation phantoms: a review. *Phys Med Rehabil Clin North Am* 1991;2:325–353.
14. Wilkins KL, McGrath PJ, Finley GA, et al. Phantom limb sensations and phantom limb pain in child and adolescent amputees. *Pain* 1998;78:7–12.
15. Krane EJ, Heller LB. The prevalence of phantom sensation and pain in pediatric amputees. *J Pain Symptom Manage* 1995;10:21–29.
16. Ramachandran VS, Rogers-Ramachandran D. Synaesthesia in phantom limbs induced with mirrors. *Proc Biol Sci* 1996;263:377–386.
17. McGrath PA, Hillier LM. Phantom limb sensations in adolescents: a case study to illustrate the utility of sensation and pain logs in pediatric clinical practice. *J Pain Symptom Manage* 1992;7:46–53.
18. Katz J, Melzack R. Pain memories in phantom limbs: review and clinical observations. *Pain* 1990;43:319–336.
19. Wesolowski JA, Lema MJ. Phantom limb pain. *Reg Anaesth* 1993;18:121–127.
20. Melzack R. Phantom limbs. *Sci Am* 1992;266:120–126.
21. Pohjolainen T. A clinical evaluation of stumps in lower limb amputees. *Prosthet Orthot Int* 1991;15:178–184.
22. Hsieh JC, Hagermark O, Stahle-Backdahl M, et al. Urge to scratch represented in the human cerebral cortex during itch. *J Neurophysiol* 1994;72:3004–3008.
23. Drzezga A, Darsow U, Treede RD, et al. Central activation by histamine-induced itch: analogies to pain processing: a correlational analysis of O-15 H₂O positron emission tomography studies. *Pain* 2001;92:295–305.
24. Sherman RA, Sherman CJ. Prevalence and characteristics of chronic phantom limb pain among American veterans: results of a trial survey. *Am J Phys Med* 1983;62:227–238.
25. Sherman RA, Sherman CJ, Parker L. Chronic phantom and stump pain among American veterans: results of a survey. *Pain* 1984;18:83–95.
26. Alamo Tomillero F, Rodriguez de la Torre R, Caba Barrientos F, et al. Prospective study of prevalence and risk factors for painful phantom limb in the immediate postoperative period of patients undergoing amputation for chronic arterial ischemia. *Rev Esp Anestesiol Reanim* 2002;49:295–301.
27. Gallagher P, Allen D, Maclachlan M. Phantom limb pain and residual limb pain following lower limb amputation: a descriptive analysis. *Disabil Rehabil* 2001;23:522–530.
28. Ehde DM, Czerniecki JM, Smith DG, et al. Chronic phantom sensations, phantom pain, residual limb pain, and other regional pain after lower limb amputation. *Arch Phys Med Rehabil* 2000;81:1039–1044.
29. Sherman RA, Sherman CJ. A comparison of phantom sensations among amputees whose amputations were of civilian and military origins. *Pain* 1985;21:91–97.
30. Helm P, Engel T, Holm A, et al. Function after lower limb amputation. *Acta Orthop Scand* 1986;57:154–157.
31. Nikolajsen L, Illkjaer S, Kroner K, et al. The influence of preamputation pain on post amputation stump and phantom pain. *Pain* 1997;72:393–405.
32. Reiber GE, McFarland LV, Hubbard S, et al. Servicemembers and veterans with major traumatic limb loss from Vietnam war and OIF/OEF conflicts: survey methods, participants, and summary findings. *J Rehabil Res Dev* 2010;47(4):275–297. doi:10.1682/JRRD.2010.01.0009.
33. Weeks SR, Anderson-Barnes VC, Tsao JW. Phantom limb pain. *Neurologist* 2010;16(5):277–286. doi:10.1097/NRL.0b013e3181edf128.
34. Dijkstra PU, Geertzen JH, Stewart R. Phantom pain and risk factors: a multivariate analysis. *J Pain Symptom Manage* 2002;24(6):578–585.
35. Richardson C, Glenn S, Horgan M, et al. A prospective study of factors associated with the presence of phantom limb pain six months after major lower limb amputation in patients with peripheral vascular disease. *J Pain* 2007;8:793–801.
36. Hsu E, Cohen SP. Postamputation pain: epidemiology, mechanisms, and treatment. *J Pain Res* 2013;6:121–136.
37. Ribera H, Cano P, Dora A, et al. Phantom limb pain secondary to post-traumatic stump hematoma 40 years after amputation: description of one case. *Revista de la Sociedad Espanola del Dolor* 2001;8:217–220.
38. Rajbhandari SM, Jarett JA, Griffiths PD, et al. Diabetic neuropathic pain in a leg amputated 44 years previously. *Pain* 1999;83:627–629.
39. Jensen TS, Krebs B, Nielsen J, et al. Immediate and long-term phantom limb pain in amputees: incidence, clinical characteristics and relationship to pre-amputation limb pain. *Pain* 1985;21:267–278.
40. Jensen TS, Krebs B, Nielsen J, et al. Phantom limb, phantom pain and stump pain in amputees during the first 6 months following limb amputation. *Pain* 1983;17:243–256.
41. Bailey AA, Moersch FP. Phantom limb. *Can Med Assoc J* 1941;45:37–42.
42. Wall R, Novotny-Joseph P, MacNamara TE. Does preamputation pain influence phantom limb pain in cancer patients? *South Med J* 1985;78:34–36.
43. Frazier SH. Psychiatric aspects of causalgia, the phantom limb, and phantom pain. *Dis Nerv Syst* 1966;27:441–451.
44. Saris SC, Iacono RP, Nashold BS. Dorsal entry zone lesions for post amputation pain. *J Neurosurg* 1985;62:72–76.
45. Sherman RA, Barja RH, Bruno GM. Thermographic correlates of chronic pain: analysis of 125 patients incorporating evaluations by a blind panel. *Arch Phys Med Rehabil* 1987;68:273–279.
46. Miles JE. Phantom limb syndrome occurring during spinal anesthesia: relationship to etiology. *J Nerv Ment Dis* 1956;123:365–368.
47. Mackenzie N. Phantom limb pain during spinal anaesthesia. Recurrence in amputees. *Anaesthesia* 1983;38:886–887.
48. Martin G, Grant SA, MacLeod DB, et al. Severe phantom leg pain in an amputee after lumbar plexus block. *Reg Anesth Pain Med* 2003;28:475–478.
49. Murphy JP, Anandaciva SP. Phantom limb pain and spinal anaesthesia. *Anaesthesia* 1984;39:188.
50. Sellick BC. Phantom limb pain and spinal anesthesia. *Anesthesiology* 1985;62:801–802.
51. Lee ED, Donovan K. Reactivation of phantom limb pain after combined interscalene brachial plexus block and general anesthesia: successful treatment with intravenous lidocaine. *Anesthesiology* 1995;82:295–298.
52. Devor M, Govrin-Lippmann R, Angelides K. Na+ channel immunolocalization in peripheral mammalian axons and changes following nerve injury and neuroma formation. *J Neurosci* 1993;13(5):1976–1992.
53. Bek D, Demiralp B, Komurcu M, et al. The relationship between phantom limb pain and neuroma [in Turkish]. *Acta Orthop Traumatol Turc* 2006;40(1):44–48.
54. Karanikolas M, Aretha D, Tsolakis I, et al. Optimized perioperative analgesia reduces chronic phantom limb pain intensity, prevalence, and frequency: a prospective, randomized, clinical trial. *Anesthesiology* 2011;114(5):1144–1154. doi:10.1097/ALN.0b013e31820fc7d2.
55. Borghi B, D'Addabbo M, White PF, et al. The use of prolonged peripheral neural blockade after lower extremity amputation: the effect on symptoms associated with phantom limb syndrome. *Anesth Analg* 2010;111(5):1308–1315. doi:10.1213/ANE.0b013e3181f4e848.
56. Nyström B, Hagbarth KE. Microelectrode recordings from transected nerves in amputees with phantom limb pain. *Neurosci Lett* 1981;27(2):211–216. doi:10.1016/0304-3940(81)90270-6.
57. Vaso A, Adahan HM, Gjika A, et al. Peripheral nervous system origin of phantom limb pain. *Pain* 2014;155(7):1384–1391. doi:10.1016/j.pain.2014.04.018.

58. Mannion RJ, Doubell TP, Gill H, et al. Deafferentation is insufficient to induce sprouting of A-fibre central terminals in the rat dorsal horn. *J Comp Neurol* 1998;393:135–144.

59. Ma QP, Tian L, Wolff CJ. Resection of sciatic nerve retriggers central sprouting of A-fibre primary afferents in the rat. *Neurosci Lett* 2000;288:215–218.

60. Nikolajsen L, Jensen TS. Postamputation pain. In: Melzack R, Wall PD, eds. *Handbook of Pain Management*. Edinburgh: Churchill Livingstone. 2003;247–257.

61. Doubell TP, Mannion RJ, Woolf CJ. The dorsal horn: state-dependent sensory processing, plasticity and the generation of pain. In: Wall PD, Melzack R, eds. *Textbook of Pain*. 4th ed. Edinburgh: Churchill Livingstone. 1999;165–181.

62. Waxman SG, Hains BC. Fire and phantoms after spinal cord injury: Na+ channels and central pain. *Trends Neurosci* 2006;29:207–215.

63. Melzack R. Phantom limbs and the concept of a neuromatrix. *Trends Neurosci* 1990;13:88–92.

64. Lotze M, Grodd W, Birbaumer N, et al. Does use of a myoelectric prosthesis prevent cortical reorganization and phantom limb pain? *Nature Neurosci* 1999;2:501–502.

65. Giummarra MJ, Gibson SJ, Georgiou-Karistianus N, et al. Central mechanisms in phantom limb perception: the past, present and future. *Brain Res Rev* 2007;54:219–232.

66. Arena JG, Sherman RA, Bruno GM, et al. The relationship between situational stress and phantom limb pain: cross-lagged correlational data from six-month pain logs. *J Psychosom Med* 1990;34:71–77.

67. Jenkins WM, Merzenich MM, Ochs MT, et al. Functional reorganization of primary somatosensory cortex in adult owl monkeys after behaviorally controlled tactile stimulation. *J Neurophysiol* 1990;63:82–104.

68. Chan BL, Witt R, Charrow AP, et al. Mirror therapy for phantom pain. *N Engl J Med* 2007;357:2206–2207.

69. Gehling M, Tryba M. Prophylaxis of phantom pain: is regional analgesia ineffective? *Schmerz* 2003;17:11–19.

70. Jahangiri M, Jayatunga AP, Bradley JW, et al. Prevention of phantom pain after major lower limb amputation by epidural infusion of diamorphine, clonidine, and bupivacaine. *Ann R Coll Surg Engl* 1994;76:324–326.

71. Wilson JA, Nimmo AF, Fleetwood-Walker SM, et al. A randomized double blind trial of the effect of pre-emptive epidural ketamine on persistent pain after lower limb amputation. *Pain* 2008;135:108–118.

72. Malawer MM, Buch R, Khurana JS, et al. Postoperative infusion continuous regional analgesia. A technique for relief of postoperative pain following major extremity surgery. *Clin Orthop* 1991;266:227–237.

73. Pinzur MS, Garla PG, Pluth T, et al. Continuous postoperative infusion of a regional anesthetic after an amputation of the lower extremity: a randomized clinical trial. *J Bone Joint Surg Am* 1996;78:1501–1505.

74. Madabhushi L, Reuben SS, Steinberg RB, et al. The efficacy of postoperative perineural infusion of bupivacaine and clonidine after lower extremity amputation in preventing phantom limb and stump pain. *J Clin Anesth* 2007;19:226–229.

75. Grant AJ, Wood C. The effect of intra-neural local anaesthetic infusion on pain following major limb amputation. *Scott Med J* 2008;53:4–6.

76. Wilder-Smith CH, Hill LT, Laurent S. Postamputation pain and sensory changes in treatment-naive patients: characteristics and responses to treatment with tramadol, amitriptyline, and placebo. *Anesthesiology* 2005;103:619–628.

77. Robinson LR, Czerniecki JM, Ehde DM, et al. Trial of amitriptyline for relief of pain in amputees: results of a randomized controlled study. *Arch Phys Med Rehabil* 2004;85:1–6.

78. Kuiken TA, Schechtman L, Harden RN. Phantom limb pain treatment with mirtazapine: a case series. *Pain Pract* 2005;5:356–360.

79. Patterson JF. Carbamazepine in the treatment of phantom limb pain. *South Med J* 1988;81:1100–1102.

80. Elliott F, Little A, Milbrandt W. Carbamazepine for phantom-limb phenomena. *N Eng J Med* 1976;295:678.

81. Bone M, Critchley P, Buggy DJ. Gabapentin in postamputation phantom limb pain: a randomized, double-blind, placebo-controlled, cross-over study. *Reg Anesth Pain Med* 2002;27:481–486.

82. Smith D, Ehde D, Hanley M, et al. Efficacy of gabapentin in treating chronic phantom limb and residual limb pain. *J Rehabil Res Dev* 2005;42(5):645–654.

83. Nikolajsen L, Finnerup NB, Kramp S, et al. A randomized study of the effects of gabapentin on postamputation pain. *Anesthesiology* 2006;105:1008–1015.

84. Harden RN, Houle TT, Remble TA, et al. Topiramate for phantom limb pain: a time-series analysis. *Pain Med* 2005;6:375–378.

85. Mishra S, Bhatnagar S, Singhal AK. High-dose morphine for intractable phantom limb pain. *Clin J Pain* 2007;23:99–101.

86. Bergmans S, Snijdelaar DG, Katz J, et al. Methadone for phantom limb pain. *Clin J Pain* 2002;18:203–205.

87. Huse E, Larbig W, Flo H, et al. The effect of opioids on phantom limb pain and cortical reorganization. *Pain* 2001;90:47–55.

88. Wu CL, Tella P, Staats PS, et al. Analgesic effects of intravenous lidocaine and morphine on post amputation pain: a randomized double blind, active placebo controlled, crossover trial. *Anesthesiology* 2002;96:841–848.

89. Alviar M, Hale T, Dungca M. Pharmacologic interventions for treating phantom limb pain. *Cochrane Database Syst Rev* 2011;(1):CD006380. doi:10.1002/14651858.CD006380.pub3.

90. Abraham RB, Marouani N, Kollender Y, et al. Dextromethorphan for phantom pain attenuation in cancer amputees: a double-blind cross-over trial involving three patients. *Clin J Pain* 2002;18(5):282–285. doi:10.1097/00002508-200209000-00002.

91. Stannard CF, Porter GE. Ketamine hydrochloride in the treatment of phantom limb pain. *Pain* 1993;54:227–230

92. Nikolajsen L, Hansen PO, Jensen TS. Oral ketamine therapy in the treatment of postamputation stump pain. *Acta Anaesthesiol Scand* 1997;41:427–429.

93. Prantl L, Schremi S, Heine N, et al. Surgical treatment of chronic phantom limb sensation and limb pain after lower limb amputation. *Plast Reconstr Surg* 2006;118:1562–1572.

94. Nikolajsen L, Hansen CL, Nielsen J, et al. The effect of ketamine on phantom limb pain: a central neuropathic disorder maintained by peripheral input. *Pain* 1996;67:69–77.

95. Eichenberger U, Neff F, Sveticic G, et al. Chronic phantom limb pain: the effects of calcitonin, ketamine, and their combination on pain and sensory thresholds. *Anesth Anal* 2008;106:1265–1273.

96. Jaeger H, Maier C, Wawersik J. Postoperative treatment of phantom pain and causalgias with calcitonin [in German]. *Anaesthesist* 1988;37:71–76.

97. Atesalp AS, Ozkan Y, Komurcu M, et al. The effects of capsaicin in phantom limb pain. *Agri* 2000;12:30–33.

98. Kern KU, Baust H, Hofmann W, et al. Capsaicin 8% cutaneous patches for phantom limb pain. Results from everyday practice (non-interventional study) [in German]. *Schmerz* 2017;28(4):374–383.

99. Blankenbaker WL. The care of patients with phantom limb pain in a pain clinic. *Anesth Analg* 1977;56:842–846.

100. Wassef MR. Phantom pain with probable reflex sympathetic dystrophy: efficacy of fentanyl infiltration of the stellate ganglion. *Reg Anesth* 1997;22:287–290.

101. Lierz P, Schroegendorfer K, Choi S, et al. Continuous blockade of both brachial plexus with ropivacaine in phantom pain: a case report. *Pain* 1998;78:135–137.

102. Halbert J, Crotty M, Cameron ID. Evidence for the optimal management of acute and chronic phantom pain: a systematic review. *Clin J Pain* 2002;18:84–92.

103. Ilfeld BM, Moeller-Bertram T, Hanling S, et al. Treating intractable phantom limb pain with ambulatory continuous peripheral nerve blocks: a pilot study. *Pain Med* 2013;14(6):935–942. doi:10.1111/pme.12080.

104. Kern U, Martin C, Scheicher S, et al. Treatment of phantom pain with botulinum-toxin A. A pilot study. *Schmerz* 2003;17:117–124.

105. Jin L, Kollewe K, Krampfl K, et al. Treatment of phantom limb pain with botulinum toxin type A. *Pain Med* 2009;10(2):300–303. doi:10.1111/j.1526-4637.2008.00554.x.

106. Kern U, Martin C, Scheicher S, et al. Effects of botulinum toxin type B on stump pain and involuntary movements of the stump. *Am J Phys Med Rehabil* 2004;83:396–399.

107. Kern U, Martin C, Scheicher S, et al. Does botulinum toxin A make prosthesis use easier for amputees? *J Rehabil Med* 2004;36:238–239.

108. Wu H, Sultana R, Taylor K, et al. A prospective randomized double-blinded pilot study to examine the effect of botulinum toxin type A injection versus Lidocaine/Depomedrol injection on residual and phantom limb pain: initial report. *Clin J Pain* 2012;28(2):108–112. doi:10.1097/AJP.0b013e3182264fe9.A.

109. Dahl E, Cohen SP. Perineural injection of etanercept as a treatment for postamputation pain. *Clin J Pain* 2008;24:172–175.

110. Katz J, Melzack R. Auricular transcutaneous electrical nerve stimulation (TENS) reduces phantom limb pain. *J Pain Symptom Manage* 1991;6:73–83.

111. Katz J, France C, Melzack R. An association between phantom limb sensations and stump skin conductance during transcutaneous electrical nerve stimulation (TENS) applied to the contralateral leg; a case study. *Pain* 1989;36:367–377.

112. Giuffrida O, Simpson L, Cot D, Halligan PW. Contralateral stimulation, using TENS, of phantom limb pain: two confirmatory cases. *Pain Med* 2009;11:133–141. doi:10.1111/j.1526-4637.2009.00705.x.

113. Hu X, Trevelyan E, Yang G, et al. The effectiveness of acupuncture/TENS for phantom limb syndrome. I: a systematic review of controlled clinical trials. *Eur J Integr Med*. 2014;6(3):355–364. doi:10.1016/j.eujim.2014.01.003.

114. Di Rollo A, Pallanti S. Phantom limb pain: low frequency repetitive transcranial magnetic stimulation in unaffected hemisphere. *Case Rep Med* 2011;2011:130751. doi:10.1155/2011/130751.

115. Ahmed MA, Mohamed SA, Sayed D. Long-term antalgic effects of repetitive transcranial magnetic stimulation of motor cortex and serum beta-endorphin in patients with phantom pain. *Neurol Res* 2011;33:953–958. doi:10.1179/1743132811Y.0000000045.

116. Malavera A, Silva FA, Fregni F, et al. Repetitive transcranial magnetic stimulation for phantom limb pain in land mine victims: a double-blinded, randomized, sham-controlled trial. *J Pain* 2016;17(8):911–918. doi:10.1016/j.jpain.2016.05.003.

117. Morales-Quezada L. Noninvasive brain stimulation, maladaptive plasticity, and bayesian analysis in phantom limb pain. *Med Acupunct* 2017;29(4): 220–228. doi:10.1089/acu.2017.1240.

118. Bolognini N, Olgiati E, Maravita A, et al. Motor and parietal cortex stimulation for phantom limb pain and sensations. *Pain* 2013;154(8):1274–1280. doi:10.1016/j.pain.2013.03.040.

119. Bolognini N, Spandri V, Ferraro F, et al. Immediate and sustained effects of 5-day transcranial direct current stimulation of the motor cortex in phantom limb pain. *J Pain* 2015;16(7):657–665. doi:10.1016/j.jpain.2015.03.013.

120. Nielson K, Adams JE, Hosobuchi Y. Phantom limb pain. Treatment with dorsal column stimulation. *J Neurosurg* 1975;42:301–307. doi:10.3171/jns.1975.42.3.0301.

121. Miles J, Lipton S. Phantom limb pain treated by electrical stimulation. *Pain* 1978;5:373–382.

122. Krainick J, Thoden U, Riechert T. Pain reduction in amputees by long-term spinal cord stimulation. *J Neurosurg* 1980;52:346–350.

123. Seigfried J, Zimmerman M. *Phantom and Stump Pain*. Berlin: Springer Verlag; 1981:148–155.

124. Viswanathan A, Phan PC, Burton AW. Use of spinal cord stimulation in the treatment of phantom limb pain: case series and review of the literature. *Pain Pract* 2010;10(5):479–484.

125. McAuley J, van Gröningen R, Green C. Spinal cord stimulation for intractable pain following limb amputation. *Neuromodulation* 2013;18(6): 530–536. doi:10.1111/j.1525-1403.2012.00513.x.

126. Eldabe S, Burger K, Moser H, et al. Dorsal root ganglion (DRG) stimulation in the treatment of phantom limb pain (PLP). *Neuromodulation* 2015;18(7):610–616. doi:10.1111/ner.12338.

127. Hunter CW, Yang A, Davis T. Selective radiofrequency stimulation of the dorsal root ganglion (DRG) as a method for predicting targets for neuromodulation in patients with post amputation pain: a case series. *Neuromodulation* 2017;20(7):708–718. doi:10.1111/ner.12595.

128. Jensen W, Micera S, Navarro X, et al. Development of an implantable transverse intrafascicular multichannel electrode (TIME) system for relieving phantom limb pain. *Conf Proc IEEE Eng Med Biol Soc* 2010;2010: 6214–6217. doi:10.1109/IEMBS.2010.5627733.

129. Soin A, Shah NS, Fang Z. High-frequency electrical nerve block for postamputation pain: a pilot study. *Neuromodulation* 2015;18:197–206. doi:10.1111/ner.12266.

130. Cornish P, Wall C. Successful peripheral neuromodulation for successful peripheral phantom limb. *Pain Med* 2015;16:761–764.

131. Rauck RL, Cohen SP, Gilmore CA, et al. Treatment of post-amputation pain with peripheral nerve stimulation. *Neuromodulation* 2014;17:188–197. doi:10.1111/ner.12102.

132. Bittar RG, Otereo S, Carter H, et al. Deep brain stimulation for phantom limb pain. *J Clin Neuerosci* 2005;12:399–404.

133. Bittar RG, Kar-Purkayastha I, Owen SL, et al. Deep brain stimulation for pain relief: a meta-analysis. *J Clin Neurosci* 2005;12:515–519.

134. Sol JC, Casaux J, Roux FE, et al. Chronic motor cortex stimulation for phantom limb pain: correlation between pain relief and functional imaging studies. *Stereotact Funct Neurosurg* 2001;77:172–176.

135. Sakai Y, Ochi M, Uchio Y, et al. Prevention and treatment of amputation neuroma by an atelocollagen tube in rat sciatic nerves. *J Biomed Mater Res B Appl Biomater* 2005;73:355–360.

136. Ramanavarapu V, Simopoulos TT. Pulsed radiofrequency of lumbar dorsal root ganglia for chronic post-amputation stump pain. *Pain Physician* 2008;11:561–566.

137. Sehirlioglu A, Ozturk C, Yazicioglu K, et al. Painful neuroma requiring surgical excision after lower limb amputation caused by landmine explosions. *Int Orthop* 2009;33:533–536.

138. Sherman RA, Gall N, Gormley J. Treatment of phantom limb pain with muscular relaxation training to disrupt the pain-anxiety-tension cycle. *Pain* 1979;6:47–55.

139. Sherman RA. Stump and phantom limb pain. *Neurol Clin* 1989;7:249–264.

140. Harden RN, Houle TT, Green S, et al. Biofeedback in the treatment of phantom limb pain: a time-series analysis. *Applied Psycho Biofeed* 2005: 30:83–93.

141. Oakley DA, Whitman LG, Halligan PW. Hypnotic imagery as a treatment for phantom limb pain: two case reports and a review. *Clin Rehabil* 2002;16:368–377.

142. Moseley GL. Graded motor imagery for pathologic pain: a randomized controlled trial. *Neurology* 2006;67:2129–2134.

143. Murray CD, Pettifer S, Howard T, et al. The treatment of phantom limb pain using immersive virtual reality: three case studies. *Disabil Rehabil* 2007;29:1465–1469.

144. Schneider J, Hoffman A, Rost C, et al. EMDR in the treatment of chronic phantom limb pain. *Pain Med* 2008;9:76–82.

145. Portnoy S, Yarnitzky G, Yizhar Z, et al. Real-time patient-specific finite element analysis of internal stresses in the soft tissues of a residual limb: a new tool for prosthetic fitting. *Ann Biomed Eng* 2007;35:120–135.

146. Lotze M, Flor H, Grodd W, et al. Phantom movements and pain: an fMRI study in upper limb amputees. *Brain* 2001;124:2268–2277.

147. Dietrich C, Walter-Walsh K, Preissler S, et al. Sensory feedback prosthesis reduces phantom limb pain: proof of a principle. *Neurosci Lett.* 2012;507(2):97–100. doi:10.1016/j.neulet.2011.10.068.

148. Gruber H, Glodny B, Bodner G, et al. Practical experience with sonographically guided phenol instillation of stump neuroma: predictors of effects, success, and outcome. *AJR Am J Roentgenol* 2008;190: 1263–1269.

149. Bradbrook D. Acupuncture treatment of phantom limb pain and phantom limb sensation in amputees. *Acupunct Med* 2004;22:93–97.

CHAPTER 27

Herpes Zoster and Postherpetic Neuralgia

SIDDARTH THAKUR, ROBERT H. DWORKIN, and RAJBALA THAKUR

The objective of this chapter is to provide an overview of the clinical presentation and management of herpes zoster and its most common complication in immunocompetent patients, postherpetic neuralgia (PHN). Herpes zoster is a viral infection caused by the reactivation of the varicella-zoster virus (VZV). The primary varicella infection occurs when the patient contracts chicken pox. Following the resolution of chicken pox, the virus then remains dormant in dorsal sensory ganglia and cranial nerve ganglia for years to decades. Individuals are asymptomatic while the virus is dormant, and reactivation of VZV results in a characteristic and usually painful vesicular dermatomal rash. Some patients with herpes zoster develop PHN, and this persisting neuropathic pain can last for years.

Herpes zoster afflicts millions of older adults worldwide each year and causes significant suffering and disability because of both the acute pain that occurs in association with the rash and the chronic pain that is present in those patients who develop PHN. VZV-induced neuronal destruction and inflammation causes pain that interferes with activities of daily living and reduces quality of life. Contemporary advances have improved our ability to both diminish the incidence of these conditions as well was manage the remaining cases more effectively. These include the development of herpes zoster vaccines, consensus that antiviral therapy and aggressive pain management can reduce the burden of this disease, the identification of efficacious treatments for PHN, and the recognition of PHN as a study model for neuropathic pain research. An interesting ongoing development is recognition of phenotype-based identification of subsets of patients that may help clinicians make individualized therapeutic decisions.[1–4]

Clinical Picture and Natural History of Herpes Zoster

Herpes zoster is a neurodermatomal illness that does not cross the midline. Typically, a single dermatome is affected in immunocompetent patients, although in some cases, involvement of adjacent dermatomes can be seen due to normal variation of cutaneous innervation. In immunocompromised patients, there can be cutaneous dissemination and, rarely, visceral dissemination. The sequence of events described in the following sections is typically observed.

PRODROME
Herpes zoster may begin with fatigue, headache, or flu-like symptoms, including fever, neck stiffness, malaise, and nausea. This may be accompanied by unilateral dermatomal pain and abnormal sensations, including pruritus. The prodromal symptoms usually precede the appearance of a rash by 3 to 7 days, although longer periods have been reported. The prodrome probably occurs in association with the initiation of viral replication and the accompanying inflammatory response. This process results in ganglionitis as well as the destruction of neurons and supporting cells in the dorsal root ganglion (DRG) and accompanying dermatome.[5,6] In cases where patients experience a prolonged course of prodromal symptoms, diagnostic investigations are frequently undertaken to identify other medical conditions that may cause pain in the affected anatomic distribution. Common examples include pursuing the diagnosis of glaucoma in cases of herpes zoster ophthalmicus; sciatica in cases of sacral dermatomal involvement; and angina, renal colic, or cholecystitis in cases of truncal involvement. Diffuse or regional adenopathy is seen in a minority of cases and has not been correlated with any residual or long-term complications.

RASH
The reactivated virus replicates in the sensory ganglion and travels antidromically via the cutaneous nerves to the nerve endings at the dermoepidermal junction. Further replication in the skin results in tissue inflammation and necrosis which ultimately leads to the appearance of a rash in the same distribution as the prodrome. The rash is initially maculopapular and evolves into the classic appearance of grouped vesicle formations on an erythematous base. Regional lymphadenopathy may appear at this stage. Over the next 7 to 10 days, the lesions progress to a pustular rash. Open lesions will develop superficial crusting. Scabs are cleared within 2 to 3 weeks. Skin in the affected region may be left completely normal or may develop a patchwork of either hypo- or hyperpigmented scarring (Fig. 27.1).

PAIN
Pain often precedes or accompanies the herpes zoster rash.[7,8] Pain may be accompanied by other sensations such as itching, paraesthesias (i.e., nonpainful abnormal sensations that are not unpleasant), and dysesthesias (i.e., nonpainful abnormal sensations that are unpleasant). The timing of the pain may be constant or intermittent, and the quality of the pain is variously described as burning, throbbing, stabbing, electric shock-like, or various combinations of these. It is frequently associated with increased tactile sensitivity and allodynia (i.e., pain in response to a normally nonpainful stimulus). The pain may interfere with the patient's sleep and other aspects of physical and emotional functioning. The acute pain associated with herpes zoster gradually resolves in most patients around the time that the rash resolves. Pain that persists beyond the acute phase of the rash is considered subacute herpetic neuralgia or PHN, depending on its duration. A distinction between these three phases of pain associated with herpes zoster has been identified and is useful in both clinical and research settings.[9] Acute herpetic neuralgia has been defined as pain that occurs within 30 days of rash onset, subacute herpetic neuralgia as pain that persists beyond 30 days from rash onset but that resolves before the diagnosis of PHN can be made, and PHN as pain that persists for 120 days or more after rash onset (Fig. 27.2).

DISTRIBUTION OF HERPES ZOSTER
Thoracic dermatomes are the most commonly affected sites. These are followed, in order of incidence, by the ophthalmic division of the trigeminal nerve, other cranial nerves, and cervical, lumbar, and sacral dermatomes[10] (Table 27.1). The reason for this pattern is not understood, but it has been speculated that this may reflect the characteristic distribution of the chicken pox rash. The pattern of rash seen in herpes zoster follows the same centripetal distribution observed with the primary varicella infection. Patients can develop lesions in the adjoining dermatomes, and much

Order of Rash Progression

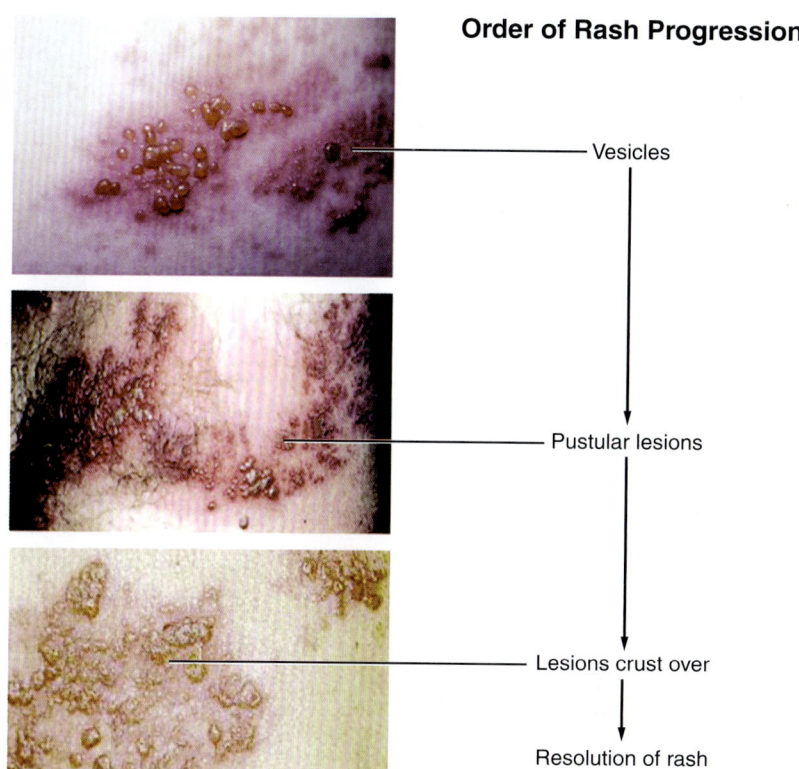

Vesicles

Pustular lesions

Lesions crust over

Resolution of rash

FIGURE 27.1 Herpes zoster rash progression. *(Reprinted from Weinberg JM. Herpes zoster: epidemiology, natural history, and common complications. J Am Acad Dermatol 2007;57(6 Suppl):S130–S135. Copyright © 2007 American Academy of Dermatology, Inc. With permission.)*

less commonly, a diffuse cutaneous or even visceral dissemination can occur, most often in immunocompromised individuals.

CLINICAL VARIANTS

Herpes Zoster Ophthalmicus
Herpes zoster ophthalmicus (HZO) occurs in approximately 10% to 20% of herpes zoster cases.[11] The involvement of the ophthalmic branch of the fifth cranial nerve is five times as common compared with cases involving the maxillary or mandibular branches. The predilection for the ophthalmic branch may be due to more frequent trauma to that area with subsequent virus reactivation.[12] It is easily recognized by the presence of vesicles and erythema of the ipsilateral forehead and upper eyelid. HZO requires particularly prompt treatment and careful follow-up monitoring because of the possibility of ocular involvement, which occurs in approximately one-half of patients with HZO (Fig. 27.3).

Herpes Zoster Oticus (Ramsay-Hunt Syndrome)
This presentation of herpes zoster is relatively rare, but this may reflect, at least in part, a failure to properly recognize and

diagnose cases. Classically, herpes zoster oticus begins with otalgia and the formation of herpetiform vesicles within the external ear canal. Associated findings that may be present include facial paralysis resulting from facial nerve (cranial nerve VII) involvement, auditory symptoms including unilateral deafness, and/or vestibular symptoms. This condition may also result from zoster of the 9th or 10th cranial nerves because the external ear has complex innervation by branches of several cranial nerves (V, VII, IX, and X) as well as vertebral nerves C2 and possibly C3.

Zoster Sine Herpete
Herpes zoster infections presenting with only dermatomal pain in the absence of rash have been described in the literature for many years.[13,14] The actual prevalence of this condition is unknown. Positive serology in the acute or convalescent phase is the only definitive way to establish the diagnosis in such patients. Given that it would be rare to perform the required serologic studies early in the disease course in most clinical settings, this diagnosis is rarely confirmed.

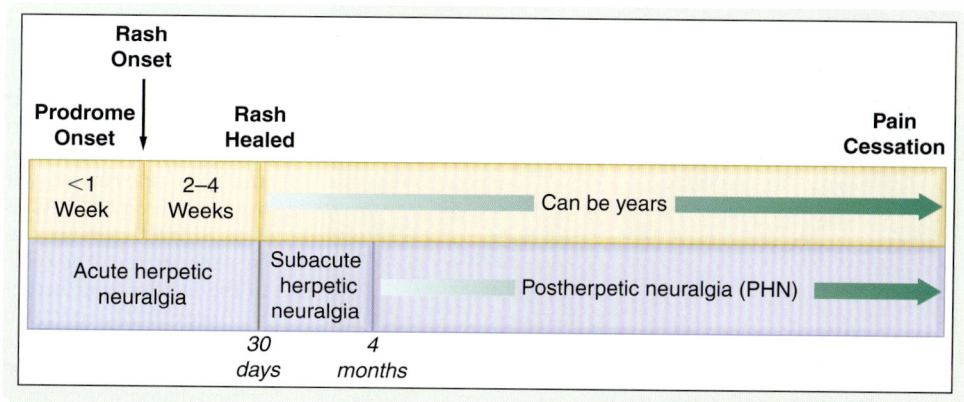

FIGURE 27.2 Natural history of herpes zoster and postherpetic neuralgia.

TABLE 27.1   Dermatomal Distribution of Herpes Zoster in Immunocompetent Patients

Thoracic: up to 50% of all cases
Cranial: 10%–20%
Cervical: 10%–20%
Lumbar: 10%–20%
Sacral: 2%–8%
Generalized: <1%

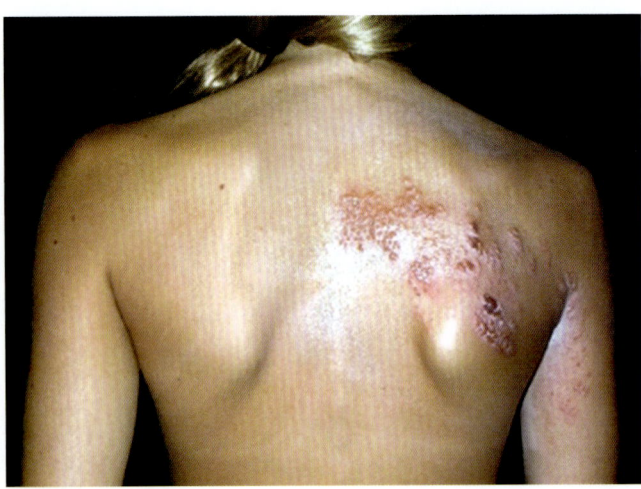

FIGURE 27.4   Herpes zoster rash in the T2 dermatomal distribution. *(Reproduced from Dworkin RH, Johnson RW, Breuer J, et al. Recommendations for the management of herpes zoster. Clin Infect Dis 2007;44[1]:S1–26. Reproduced by permission of Infectious Diseases Society of America.)*

Diagnosis of Herpes Zoster

The diagnosis of herpes zoster is usually established based on the clinical findings of a characteristic dermatomal rash (Fig. 27.4) and the presence of associated pain. The differential diagnosis frequently includes contact dermatitis. Herpes simplex virus (HSV) infection must also be considered, particularly if sacral dermatomes are involved. The main differentiating features of an HSV infection are that it tends to occur predominantly around the mouth or genitalia, is more prevalent in younger patients versus the predilection for herpes zoster to afflict more elderly patients, and HSV has a propensity for recurrent outbreaks which are relatively rare in herpes zoster. In cases of atypical presentations or when there is confusion as to whether VZV or HSV is the pathogen, diagnosis can be confirmed by laboratory testing.

LABORATORY TESTING
Viral Culture
Isolation of the virus in cell cultures can be done but takes 1 to 2 weeks to complete. The virus is also quite labile and may be difficult to recover from lesion swabs especially after the vesicular phase has resolved. This test has low sensitivity but high specificity. Treatment of presumed cases should not be delayed to await culture results given the prolonged turnaround time and low sensitivity (and thus high false-negative rate) of the test.

Direct Immunofluorescence Assay
Direct immunofluorescence assay is often preferable to viral culture due to its low cost and rapid turnaround time, which can be within 1.5 hours. Sensitivity is approximately 90% but decreases if the lesions are beyond the vesicular stage.

Viral DNA Testing
Viral DNA can be detected in the vesicle fluid and cutaneous tissue by polymerase chain reaction (PCR) technology. It has the advantage that it can be effective even on old and crusted lesions. It usually has a turnaround time of 1 day but can be completed in less than 5 hours with rapid real-time PCR.[15] It is generally more expensive than other approaches and has exceptional sensitivity and specificity of near 100%.

Biopsy
A biopsy is not typically needed in clinical practice and should be reserved for difficult to diagnose cases. Histologic findings of ballooning degeneration and acantholysis of keratinocytes resulting in intraepidermal vesicles are common to all herpes infections. Multinucleated giant cells with accentuation of nuclear material at the periphery of the nuclei are present. Underlying leukocytoclastic vasculitis is often a prominent finding and helps differentiate zoster from other herpesvirus infections.

Testing for Underlying Disorders
If clinically indicated, testing for HIV or occult malignancy may be advisable, but this is typically not necessary and is not recommended on a routine basis.

Epidemiology of Herpes Zoster

The epidemiology of herpes zoster is primarily affected by a combination of the incidence of primary varicella infections as well as age and level of immunosuppression in the population. Herpes zoster is among the most common of neurologic illnesses, affecting about 1 million people in the United States annually.[16] According to the Centers for Disease Control and Prevention (CDC), the lifetime incidence of herpes zoster in the United States is estimated to be 32%.[17] A systematic review of global herpes zoster incidence rates found between 3 and 5 cases per 1,000 person-years in North America, Europe, and the Asia Pacific, with a precipitous increase beyond that noted with aging.[18] At 60 years old, the incidence increases to 6 to 8/1,000 person-years and 8 to 12/1,000 person-years at 80 years of age. The findings were similar in a subsequent study of the incidence of herpes zoster in the United States.[19]

Accordingly, increasing age is the most potent risk factor for herpes zoster in both immunocompetent and immunocompromised individuals (Table 27.2). The decline in VZV-specific cell-mediated immunity is believed to drive the increase in herpes zoster observed in patients as they age.[20] There is a notable

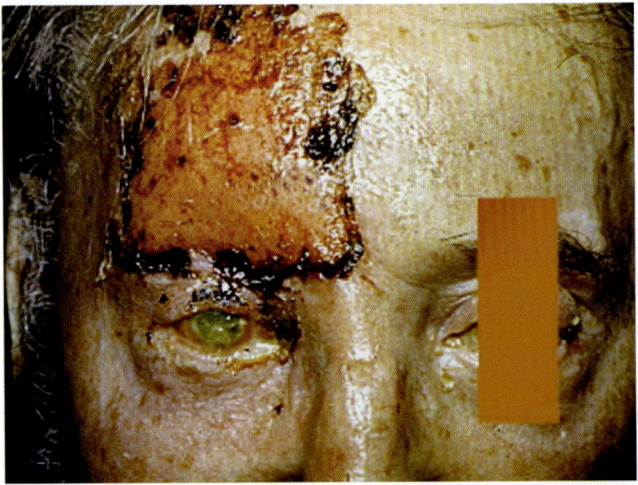

FIGURE 27.3   Ophthalmic zoster. *(Reproduced from Dworkin RH, Johnson RW, Breuer J, et al. Recommendations for the management of herpes zoster. Clin Infect Dis 2007;44[1]:S1–S26. Reproduced by permission of Infectious Diseases Society of America.)*

TABLE 27.2 Factors Associated with an Increased Incidence of Herpes Zoster

1. Increasing age
2. Disease states
   HIV
   Lymphoproliferative disorders
3. Immunosuppressive therapy
   After organ transplant
   Chemotherapy
   Steroid treatment
4. Possible association with
   Caucasian vs. African American racial group
   Psychological stress
   Physical trauma

increase in disease rates around 50 years of age,[16] and the lifetime prevalence reaches approximately 50% in individuals living to be 85 years of age.[21] There has also been a higher incidence in women, thought to be related to a combination of biologic factors (immunologic or hormonal) as well as differences in health seeking behaviors.[19,22–25]

Immunocompromised individuals have a relatively high risk for developing herpes zoster.[26,27] Patients with a history of HIV infection, solid organ and bone marrow or stem cell transplantation, immunosuppressive chemotherapy, or systemic lupus erythematosus are 2 to 10 times more likely to develop herpes zoster compared to immunocompetent individuals.[27] Immunocompromised individuals also experience higher recurrence rates of zoster compared to those who are immunocompetent.[28]

Other factors that appear to increase the risk for herpes zoster that are less well replicated include Caucasian versus African American racial group,[29] presence of elevated psychological stress,[30] physical trauma,[31] and diabetes mellitus.[32] Exposure to varicella antigen, either through contact with chicken pox or by vaccination, has a protective effect and reduces the incidence of herpes zoster.[33,34]

The epidemiology of varicella and herpes zoster is likely to change as childhood vaccination against the primary infection alters the long established relationships between humans and this viral infection. The incidence of primary varicella infections has declined dramatically in the United States since the implementation of routine childhood vaccination.[35]

It has been hypothesized that there will be an acceleration of incidence of herpes zoster beyond expectations in the future as the opportunities for subclinical immune boosting in aging adults, which result from exposure to VZV, will decline due to the decreased incidence of chicken pox.[36–38] To date, there is little

evidence to support this hypothesis, as multiple studies have demonstrated rates of herpes zoster increasing across all adult age groups before the implementation of the varicella vaccine in 1996,[39] and that have continued since.[25,28,40,41] Furthermore, the rates of herpes zoster are similar in areas with high levels of varicella vaccination and those without. One population-based study analyzed the incidence of herpes zoster over a 60-year period and noted an over fourfold increase was not likely related to introduction of the varicella vaccine.[42] Furthermore, a decrease in the number of herpes zoster cases in children less than 10 years of age has been reported, presumably due to vaccination.[25,43] It is possible that there has not been enough time since the implementation of the recommended childhood varicella vaccination for the acceleration in zoster incidence to be observed.

Eventually, as children immunized against VZV grow into adulthood, the number of adults infected with latent wild-type virus will decrease. Therefore, the incidence of herpes zoster is expected to decline as the live attenuated virus used in the varicella vaccine appears to be less likely to reactivate and cause herpes zoster.

Pathophysiology of Herpes Zoster and Mechanisms of Acute Pain

As noted earlier, herpes zoster most commonly manifests in the distribution of a single dorsal sensory or cranial nerve ganglion. Why the reactivation occurs in one ganglion when latent virus is present throughout the patient's sensory ganglia is not clear. Declining cellular immunity is a major risk factor for reactivation of the virus, which is thought to occur when cell-mediated immunity falls below a critical level.[21] This impression is supported by evidence that even individuals with adequate levels of serum antibodies to VZV antigen can, over time, exhibit T cells with reduced ability to proliferate and defend against VZV infections.[44] Hence, cell-mediated immunity appears to play a crucial role in preventing reactivation of latent VZV (Fig. 27.5). Common causes of decreased cellular immunity include increasing age, various diseases, and immune-suppressing medical interventions, all of which are known risk factors for herpes zoster.

During reactivation of the virus, newly synthesized viral particles are transported in a retrograde and anterograde fashion to the central and distal axons of the involved spinal or cranial sensory ganglion. Viral replication causes inflammatory and neural tissue injury in the affected dermatome,[5] which can ultimately result in infectious hemorrhagic necrosis and subsequent neuronal loss and scarring centered in the sensory ganglion of affected cranial and peripheral nerves.[4,45] Microscopic examination of the zoster affected ganglion shows significant hypocellularity and collagen scarring. The corresponding peripheral nerves may exhibit a long-lasting reduction in myelinated axons and increased numbers

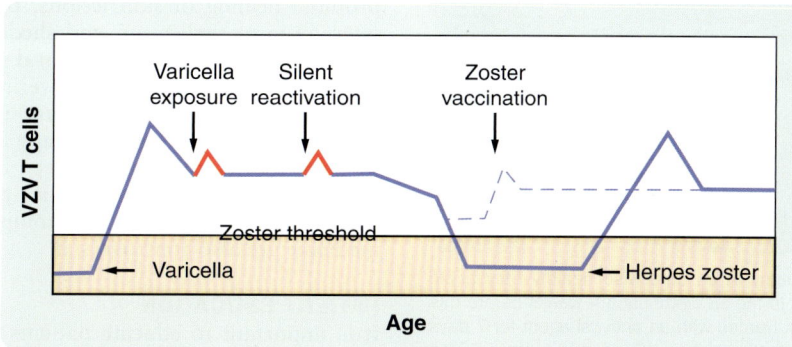

FIGURE 27.5 Host factors in varicella-zoster virus (VZV) latency and reactivation. Varicella is the primary infection caused by VZV, and its resolution is associated with the induction of VZV-specific memory T cells (*blue line*). Memory immunity to VZV may be boosted periodically by exposure to varicella or silent reactivation from latency (*red peaks*). VZV-specific memory T cells decline with age. The decline below a threshold (*black line* below zoster threshold) correlates with an increased risk of zoster. The occurrence of zoster, in turn, is associated with an increase in VZV-specific T cells. The administration of zoster vaccine to older persons may prevent VZV-specific T cells from dropping below the threshold for zoster occurrence (*dashed blue line*). (*Reprinted from Arvin A. Aging, immunity, and the varicella-zoster virus.* N Engl J Med *2005;352[22]:2266–2267. Copyright © 2005 Massachusetts Medical Society. Reprinted with permission from Massachusetts Medical Society.*)

of small unmyelinated axons. These structural changes contribute to the pain and other characteristic sensory findings along the corresponding sensory dermatomes of the involved ganglion. Excessive electrical activity in the damaged peripheral nociceptors is the major cause of pain in the acute herpes zoster infection. Although VZV is a sensory-specific virus, involvement of anterior horn cells, autonomic neurons, and leptomeninges can be observed as a result of a bystander effect,[46] with consequent muscle weakness, palsy, and/or pleocytosis of cerebral spinal fluid (CSF).

Complications Associated with Herpes Zoster

In general, the frequency and severity of complications are greater in older and immunocompromised individuals. The most common morbidity of herpes zoster in immunocompetent individuals is the development of PHN; this often severe pain can persist well beyond the resolution of herpes zoster. This complication is discussed in detail in the latter part of this chapter.

OPHTHALMIC COMPLICATIONS

The incidence of complications associated with HZO has been reported to be 2% to 6% of cases. A variety of complications have been described,[11] including retinitis, keratitis, iritis, scleritis, secondary glaucoma, and ptosis. These are obviously serious problems that can result in temporary or permanent deterioration in visual acuity or complete blindness. For these reasons, patients with ophthalmic zoster should be evaluated by an ophthalmologist as promptly as possible following diagnosis.

MOTOR NEUROPATHY

Motor nerve involvement is present in 5% to 15% of patients presenting with herpes zoster. Paresis in extraocular nerves, facial nerves, and a variety of other motor nerves has been described. Diaphragmatic paresis is not an uncommon occurrence with the involvement of the phrenic nerve, and intercostal nerve involvement may lead to paresis of intercostal muscles (Fig. 27.6). Involvement of cervical motor nerve roots may present as shoulder and arm weakness, and lower extremity weakness can occur when lumbosacral nerve roots are affected. In some cases, significant motor weakness may be the presenting symptom, and

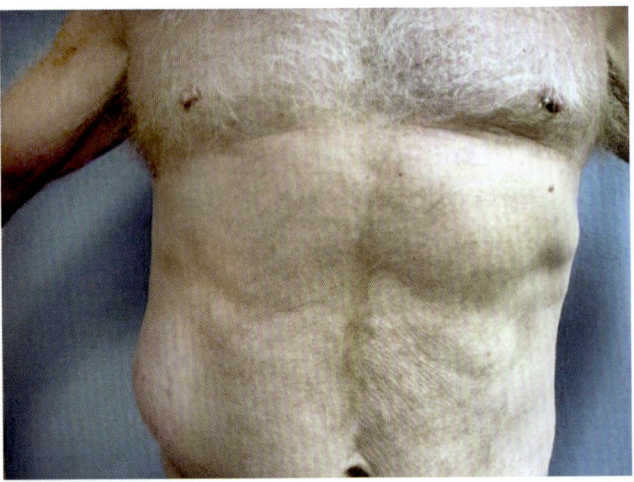

FIGURE 27.6 T8 motor neuropathy in an otherwise healthy 59-year-old man who presented with vesicles in the T8 distribution 4 weeks before this photo was taken. The patient was treated with an antiviral agent for 7 days and with analgesics as needed. As the rash resolved, this bulge became apparent; it is consistent with motor damage by varicella zoster virus to the muscles of the abdomen. *(Reproduced from Dworkin RH, Johnson RW, Breuer J, et al. Recommendations for the management of herpes zoster. Clin Infect Dis 2007;44[1]:S1–26. Reproduced by permission of Infectious Diseases Society of America)*

this can delay accurate diagnosis. In general, paresis improves with time and physical rehabilitation; however, the likelihood and completeness of muscle function recovery appears to decrease with older age and greater initial severity of the paralysis.

RARE NEUROLOGIC COMPLICATIONS

VZV is a common cause of aseptic meningitis with a sharp pleocytosis and elevated proteins evident on CSF studies. Most patients with VZV meningitis experience a complete resolution of the symptoms in 1 to 2 weeks,[47] although meningeal involvement can result in long-term sequelae from subsequent scarring of the involved neural structures. Myelitis and encephalitis are other rare central manifestations of reactivated VZV. VZV encephalitis can present as an acute delirium accompanied by few focal neurologic signs.[48] Factors that elevate the risk of central nervous system (CNS) involvement include the presence of altered immune function (e.g., HIV), cranial nerve or ophthalmic involvement, two or more prior zoster episodes, and evidence of cutaneous dissemination.[49] Although more common in immunocompromised patients, CNS involvement has also been reported in immunocompetent individuals[50] and in both children and adults.[51] Herpes zoster may be a risk factor for Guillain-Barré syndrome developing within the 2 months following the rash.[52]

VISCERAL COMPLICATIONS

Visceral involvement in herpes zoster is rare but may result in organ dysfunction as a consequence of scar formation around the involved structures. In such cases, the associated signs and symptoms would be related to the specific structures mechanically affected by scarring.

DECREASED QUALITY OF LIFE

The acute pain associated with herpes zoster can cause significant suffering and is often accompanied by interference in the patient's ability to carry out normal activities of daily living. In addition, acute pain is associated with the greater use of analgesic medications and their attendant side effects, most notably sedation and constipation.[53–58] The resultant impact of herpes zoster and related complications on health-related quality of life is at least as great as what has been found with other chronic diseases such as diabetes or congestive heart failure.[57]

Treatment of Herpes Zoster

All patients should have a thorough medical evaluation with added attention to factors related to the individual's immunocompetence. Patient education, reassurance, and supportive therapy are essential to allay fears and promote compliance with pharmacologic therapy. The primary goals of pharmacologic therapy are to reduce the severity and duration of pain, promote healing of skin lesions, prevent PHN, and decrease ongoing viral replication and shedding, thereby reducing the risk of transmission. Limiting viral replication has been shown to reduce the incidence and severity of acute pain associated with herpes zoster. The primary pharmacologic approaches include the use of antiviral therapy in conjunction with analgesic agents. Steroids have also been used, but their role is more controversial. The potential roles of neural blockade, neuroaugmentation strategies, and complementary and alternative medicine are also controversial.

PATIENT EDUCATION

It is important to educate patients and their family members about their disease. Patients and caretakers can be reassured that herpes zoster does not cause any illness in seropositive individuals who have contact with the patient. Herpes zoster does, however, pose a risk of viral transmission to individuals who do not have preexisting immunity to VZV. Given this, it is

TABLE 27.3 Benefits of Antiviral Therapy[17,59,62,63,65,66,67]

- Inhibition of viral replication
- Reduces duration of viral shedding
- Hastens rash healing
- Decrease in degree of neural damage
- Decreases severity and duration of acute pain
- Decreases duration of postherpetic neuralgia

important for patients with herpes zoster to avoid contact with individuals who are known to be seronegative for VZV or have known or suspected immune system impairment, especially if it is unclear whether they have a history of chicken pox. Patients should be counseled regarding maintaining appropriate nutrition and optimal levels of social and physical activities. In addition, patients should be told to keep the rash area clean and to avoid application of ointments or adhesive dressings because these can cause skin irritation and secondary infections. Patients should inform their physician if fever, confusion, or other significant constitutional symptoms develop and should return for further evaluation if rash healing appears delayed.

ANTIVIRAL THERAPY

Antiviral therapy has been shown to be efficacious in suppressing viral replication and also has beneficial effects on both acute and chronic pain (Table 27.3).[59–64] Antiviral medication is recommended for all herpes zoster patients who are older than 50 years, have moderate to severe pain, have a moderate to severe rash, have ophthalmic involvement, or are immunocompromised.[68] In current clinical practice, most physicians prescribe antiviral therapy to all patients with herpes zoster because of the very favorable risk–benefit ratio of these medications. Antiviral treatment should be started as soon as possible; this should ideally be within 72 hours of the onset of rash, the inclusion criterion for initiating treatment in the clinical trials of antiviral agents in herpes zoster patients. The early initiation of antiviral therapy is intuitively logical and an important treatment objective. However, viral replication may continue beyond the third day after rash onset, suggesting that even delayed antiviral

therapy may provide some benefit. Unfortunately, there are no well-designed clinical trials examining the efficacy of initiating antiviral therapy beyond 72 hours of rash onset. Two uncontrolled trials examined the effectiveness of antiviral treatment initiated at a later time, and the results suggested that such treatment may have beneficial effects.[65,69] In clinical practice, the diagnosis of herpes zoster is often not made within 72 hours of the onset of symptoms; nevertheless, it is important to identify patients who could still benefit from antiviral medication even when it is initiated relatively late in the disease course. One example of patients who warrant such later initiation of treatment is those with ophthalmic zoster. The duration of viral shedding from the ocular surface is highly variable[70] and may continue for a longer period of time. Immunocompromised patients, those with disseminated zoster, patients with neurologic complications, and possibly those with new lesions still forming should also be started on antiviral medication irrespective of whether they are beyond 72 hours of rash onset.

There are two main classes of antiviral medication, and these are differentiated by their reliance on viral phosphorylation to be activated. The first class of drugs is nucleoside analogues that require phosphorylation by viral thymidine kinase and includes acyclovir, brivudin, famciclovir, and valacyclovir (Table 27.4). These drugs are phosphorylated to a triphosphate form that impairs viral replication by inhibiting viral DNA polymerase. Acyclovir, famciclovir, and valacyclovir are all available in the United States and are approved by the U.S. Food and Drug Administration (FDA) for the treatment of herpes zoster. These medications are excreted renally, and dosages should therefore be adjusted in patients with renal insufficiency. Special dosing regimens are also needed in patients on dialysis. Although the dose necessary to treat HZV is higher than that for HSV, these medications have established safety and are generally well-tolerated. Acyclovir must be taken five times daily for 7 days, whereas famciclovir and valacyclovir are taken three times daily for 7 days. Thus, patient compliance with famciclovir and valacyclovir is likely to be considerably greater than with acyclovir, and this may translate to somewhat greater efficacy. Famciclovir and valacyclovir may also be somewhat better than acyclovir in reducing the incidence of prolonged pain.[66,67,71] Although brivudin is currently

TABLE 27.4 Antiviral Medications for Herpes Zoster

Medication	Oral Bioavailability	Dosage	Duration of Treatment (Days)	Uncommon Side Effects	Special Considerations
Acyclovir	15%–30%	800 mg 5 times daily (every 4–5 h)	7–10	Neurotoxicity and nephrotoxicity	Additive nephrotoxic effects with cyclosporine
Famciclovir	77%	500 mg 3 times daily (approved dosage in United States; in some other countries, 250 mg 3 times daily is approved)	7		Probenecid, theophylline increase levels of famciclovir. Digoxin levels increased
Valacyclovir	55%	1,000 mg 3 times daily	7		Thrombotic thrombocytopenic purpura/hemolytic uremic syndrome reported at dosages of 8,000 mg daily in immunocompromised patients
Foscarnet	NA	40–90 mg/kg IV for induction and 120 mg/kg/d for maintenance therapy	10–14 d for induction and variable duration for maintenance	Nephrotoxicity, neurotoxicity, neutropenia, anemia	Increased risk of nephrotoxicity with cyclosporine. Increased risk of seizures with ciprofloxacin
Brivudin[a]		125 mg once daily	7		Contraindicated for patients treated with 5-fluorouracil or other 5-fluoropyrimidines because of drug interaction associated with severe and potentially fatal bone marrow suppression

NOTE: All antivirals are renally excreted; hence, dosage needs to be adjusted in patients with renal insufficiency, including patients on dialysis. Nausea and headache are common side effects.
[a]Not available in the United States.

not available in the United States, it has been approved for the treatment of herpes zoster in several other countries; it is dosed once daily for 7 days.

The second class of antiviral medications is not dependent on viral phosphorylation. These agents noncompetitively inhibit viral DNA polymerase, and include vidarabine, foscarnet, and cidofovir. Foscarnet is useful in patients with known resistance to acyclovir due to lack of viral thymidine kinase, which can be seen in patients with AIDS or prolonged exposure to acyclovir (as in transplant patients). Hence, this agent plays an important role in treating infections in individuals with known resistance to acyclovir.

ANALGESIC TREATMENT

Antiviral therapy does not completely abolish the acute pain associated with herpes zoster, nor does it necessarily prevent PHN,[27] and supplemental analgesic medications are required in most patients. Effective analgesia improves patient comfort and may also reduce the risk of PHN beyond what is achieved by antiviral therapy alone.[72,73] These considerations argue for aggressive management of the acute pain associated with herpes zoster. A multimodal analgesic strategy should be used to balance efficacy, safety, and tolerability of the medication regimen. Unfortunately, well-designed studies to delineate which combinations of therapies are optimal have rarely been conducted. In lieu of focused studies, clinicians must use the available data, extrapolate available information, and individualize therapy based on patient-specific factors. The World Health Organization analgesic ladder can be applied as one useful analgesic strategy with well-proven efficacy and ease of application. Patients with mild pain can be started on acetaminophen alone or in combination with a mild opioid analgesic such as tramadol. Nonsteroidal anti-inflammatory drugs (NSAIDs) can also be used provided there are no contraindications to their use. Patients with moderate pain can be started on short-acting opioid medications and, if tolerated, can be converted to a timed-release preparation if clinically warranted. Opioids have not been well-studied in patients with herpes zoster, but one small clinical trial did show that controlled-release oxycodone was superior to placebo in relieving acute pain within the first 2 to 3 weeks of rash onset, although the small sample size precluded an evaluation of the effect of this treatment on the development of PHN.[74]

If acute pain in herpes zoster patients is not adequately controlled with the mentioned analgesics, other medications that have demonstrated efficacy in the treatment of chronic neuropathic pain can also be used in combination with antiviral therapy.[68] Gabapentin, pregabalin, and tricyclic antidepressants such as nortriptyline and desipramine can be considered in patients when conventional analgesic medications are not adequate in managing acute pain. Studies are limited, but a single-dose trial of 900 mg of gabapentin versus placebo did demonstrate a reduction in acute pain over 6 hours in patients with herpes zoster.[75] Both gabapentin and pregabalin would seem like reasonable alternatives because they not only have efficacy in the treatment of PHN but have also demonstrated efficacy in reducing pain and analgesic requirements in some acute pain conditions.[76,77]

Although tricyclic antidepressants have not been well-studied in patients with herpes zoster, they have proven efficacy in chronic neuropathic pain and are additional rational choices for treating acute pain associated with herpes zoster. Dual reuptake inhibitors (selective serotonin and norepinephrine reuptake inhibitors) can be considered in lieu of tricyclic antidepressants given their more favorable side effect profiles. Both duloxetine and venlafaxine have demonstrated efficacy in painful diabetic peripheral neuropathy[78,79] and could thus be considered a potential therapy for the treatment of acute pain in patients with herpes zoster.

A pragmatic approach is to start with a short-acting opioid in combination with acetaminophen or an NSAID. Gabapentin or pregabalin can then be added if conventional analgesics are not entirely effective. Many clinicians would use one of these medications rather than a tricyclic antidepressant because of their generally safer side effect profile. The analgesic regimen should be tailored based on the individual patient's needs and tolerances (Table 27.5). Frequent follow-up and reassessment are vital to assess efficacy and tolerability while titrating analgesic therapy.

CORTICOSTEROIDS

The use of corticosteroids in the treatment of herpes zoster has been controversial.[80,81] One placebo-controlled trial demonstrated a benefit in terms of significantly accelerated return of uninterrupted sleep, cessation of analgesic therapy, and return to normal activity in patients treated with the combination of a corticosteroid and acyclovir as compared to those treated with acyclovir alone.[81] The patients in this trial were 60 years of age on average and possessed no contraindications to corticosteroid treatment. Based on these results, the addition of oral corticosteroids can be considered in healthy older adults with moderate-to-severe pain unrelieved by antiviral therapy and analgesics, provided there are no contraindications to steroid use.

Oral steroids are empirically used in VZV-induced facial nerve palsy or other cases of cranial neuritis, although there is limited evidence supporting the effectiveness of such treatment. It must be emphasized that corticosteroids should not be used alone in herpes zoster and must be initiated in combination with antiviral therapy.

Lidocaine Patch

A 5% lidocaine patch is traditionally used for PHN pain and approved by the FDA for the same indication. A randomized placebo-controlled study showed that lidocaine patches reduced pain associated with herpes zoster[82]; based on this information and the excellent side effect profile of lidocaine patches, their use can be considered. The patch should only be applied to intact skin after the initial rash has completely healed.

NEURAL BLOCKADE

Although no conclusive and strong recommendations can be made for the use of any invasive interventions due to lack of consistent data, if pain is not controlled with medical management, referral to a pain specialist should be considered for possible interventions. These may include neuraxial injections of local anesthetics and steroids, neuraxial local anesthetic infusion, paravertebral blocks, or sympathetic blocks. All these interventions have been used for years in clinical practice, but few controlled studies have been conducted to systematically examine their effects on herpes zoster acute pain or the development of PHN. As per NeuPSIG recommendations, moderate quality of available evidence provided the basis for a weak recommendation for the use of epidural or paravertebral blocks with local anesthetic and steroids injections for herpes zoster pain.[83] These guidelines were based on three RCTs.[84–86] One of the RCTs[84] found significant reduction in acute pain following a single epidural injection of steroid and local anesthetic within the first month after rash onset as compared to standard therapy alone. The incidence of developing PHN, however, was not reduced in this study. A more recent systematic review and meta-analysis also showed a favorable outcome with the use of interventional procedures for the management of acute herpes zoster related pain; in addition, these authors also addressed the role of interventions in reducing the incidence of PHN.[87,88] The findings suggest that nerve blocks do shorten the duration of acute pain in

TABLE 27.5 Pharmacologic Options that Can Be Considered for Treatment of Acute Pain in Herpes Zoster

Medication	Initial Dose	Titration	Maximum Daily Dose	Side Effects
Acetaminophen	500–1,000 mg every 6 h as needed	Not needed	2.6 g in elderly; 4 g in younger patients	Liver toxicity with prolonged use; avoid alcohol use
NSAIDs (dosages given are for ibuprofen)	400 mg every 6 h as needed	Not needed	2,400 mg	Gastrointestinal side effects, CV and renal toxicity, and increased bleeding tendency
Opioid analgesics (dosages given are for oxycodone)	5 mg every 4 h as needed	Increase by 5 mg 4 times daily every 2 d as tolerated; dosage can be converted to extended-release opioid analgesic combined with short-acting medication as needed	No maximum dosage with careful titration	Nausea/vomiting, constipation, sedation, dizziness
Tramadol	50 mg once or twice daily	Increase by 50–100 mg daily in divided doses every 2 d as tolerated; dosage can be converted to extended release preparation combined with immediate release one as needed.	400 mg daily (100 mg 4 times daily); for patients >75 y of age, 300 mg daily in divided doses	Nausea/vomiting, constipation, sedation, dizziness, seizures, postural hypotension
Gabapentin	300 mg at bedtime or 100–300 mg 3 times daily	Increase by 100–300 mg 3 times daily every 2 days as tolerated	3,600 mg daily (1,200 mg 3 times daily; reduce if renal function is impaired)	Sedation, dizziness, peripheral edema
Pregabalin	75 mg at bedtime or 75 mg twice daily	Increase by 75 twice daily every 3 days as tolerated	600 mg daily (300 mg twice daily; reduce if renal function is impaired)	Sedation, dizziness, peripheral edema
Tricyclic antidepressants, especially nortriptyline	25 mg at bedtime	Increase by 25 mg daily every 2–3 days as tolerated	150 mg daily	Sedation, dry mouth, blurred vision, weight gain, urinary retention
Oral corticosteroid (dosages given for prednisone)	60 mg daily for 7 days	After 60 mg daily for 7 days, decrease to 30 mg daily for 7 days, then decrease to 15 mg daily for 7 days, and then discontinue.	60 mg daily	Gastrointestinal distress, nausea, changes in mood, edema

NOTE: Dose of opioids, pregabalin, and tricyclic antidepressants can be reduced in frail elderly individuals. Consider a screening electrocardiogram for patients with preexisting cardiac disease.

CV, cardiovascular; NSAID, nonsteroidal anti-inflammatory drugs.

Adapted from Dworkin RH, Johnson RW, Breuer J, et al. Recommendations for the management of herpes zoster. *Clin Infect Dis* 2007;44(1):S1–S26. Reproduced by permission of Infectious Diseases Society of America.

herpes zoster and repeat or continuous epidural blocks and paravertebral blocks reduce the likelihood of PHN. Single stellate ganglion blocks fail to decrease the incidence, but multiple blocks may have a beneficial effect in this regard.[87,88] The exact mechanism by which sympathetic or somatic blocks could prevent PHN or lessen its severity is poorly understood. The sympathetic nervous system is important in mediating pain in some neuropathic pain conditions. It has been hypothesized that in the acute phase of herpes zoster, inflammation induces intense stimulation of the sympathetic nervous system leading to reduced intraneural blood flow with resultant neuronal hypoxia and endoneural edema. Other putative mechanisms of sympathetic nervous system involvement include the formation of ephaptic connections between the sensory system and the sympathetic system as well as the upregulation of adrenoreceptors. These phenomena could result in inappropriate activation of primary nociceptive fibers in response to sympathetic nervous system activation. Blockade of sympathetic nerves with local anesthetics may reverse these effects. It is also hypothesized that these interventions may favorably affect the progression of herpes zoster acute pain to PHN because the effective treatment of acute pain may prevent the development of PHN or at least decrease the severity of subsequent PHN.

In conclusion, we do not make a strong recommendation for routine use of interventions for acute herpes zoster pain. Interventions can be considered if the pain is not well controlled, or if pharmacotherapy results in intolerable side effects. The use of local interventions should be carefully considered, and the type of intervention should be guided by the patient's condition and the provider's expertise.

COMPLEMENTARY AND ALTERNATIVE MEDICINE

Complementary and alternative medicine modalities are becoming increasingly popular in patients with acute as well as chronic pain conditions and herpes zoster, and related pain syndromes are no exception. Integrative (complementary) therapies include meditation, hypnosis, relaxation therapy, imagery, music therapy, magnet therapy, dietary and herbal supplements, and acupuncture. There are no reliable data available that will help make strong and specific recommendations in the treatment of zoster-related pain with these approaches.

Acupuncture has been examined in small studies for the treatment of herpes zoster pain. One of the mechanisms of action is thought to be associated with endorphin release at both the spinal and supraspinal levels. In a small randomized study, subjects were randomized to receive weekly acupuncture treatment versus standard therapy including pregabalin, local anesthetic injections for all patients and opioids for patients who had intractable pain.[89] Patients in the acupuncture arm were only allowed acetaminophen as a rescue analgesic. No significant differences were observed between the groups in terms of mean pain reduction, incidence of PHN or total pain burden, concluding that acupuncture could have similar efficacy as conventional analgesic therapies. Although this study alone does not provide high-quality evidence to support the routine use of acupuncture, it does provide some evidence as to the potential role of acupuncture in the treatment of acute herpes pain.

SPINAL CORD STIMULATION

Spinal cord stimulation (SCS) has been tried in a case series of four patients with active herpes zoster and reported to be effective.[90] It is difficult to extrapolate these results to routine clinical practice as the majority of patients with herpes zoster have resolution of their symptoms as part of the natural history of the disease; hence, authors do not recommend this modality of treatment for acute zoster.

Prevention of Herpes Zoster

CHILDHOOD VACCINATION

The propensity to develop herpes zoster and PHN can ultimately be traced back to an individual's primary varicella infection. Thus, one obvious prevention strategy would include the prevention of the primary VZV infection through the use of varicella vaccination in childhood. Two types of vaccines are approved by the FDA for vaccination in children from 12 months to 12 years of age; both are based on the Oka virus. The first agent is a single-antigen vaccine, and the more recent vaccine is a combination product and protects against multiple childhood infections (i.e., measles, mumps, rubella, and varicella). The current recommendations for routine immunization of immunocompetent children are two doses of varicella vaccine (either single antigen or combined product) with the first dose at 12 to 15 months, followed by a second dose at 4 to 6 years of age.[91] The live attenuated Oka vaccine virus establishes latency in sensory ganglia, like wild-type VZV, but it appears to cause herpes zoster much less frequently. Hence, childhood varicella vaccination should eventually result in an overall decrease in the incidence of herpes zoster and PHN.

VARICELLA-ZOSTER IMMUNOGLOBULIN

Temporary passive immunization may be required in specific circumstances. The CDC currently recommends administration of purified varicella-zoster immune globulin preparation, VariZIG (Cangene Corp, Winnipeg, Canada), to prevent or modify clinical illness in immunocompromised or pregnant seronegative persons and a select group of infants with recent exposure to patients with chicken pox or zoster. VariZIG should be administered as soon as possible, ideally within 96 hours of exposure to provide maximum benefit, but it may be used within 10 days.[92] Treatment with VariZIG should be followed by vaccination in eligible patients 5 months after administration.

HERPES ZOSTER VACCINATION FOR ADULTS

Herpes zoster is caused by reactivation of VZV from a single sensory ganglion. The precise mechanism of reactivation is not known but thought to be due to waning VZV specific cell-mediated immunity. Therefore, adult vaccination can confer the immunologic boost to prevent herpes zoster and the associated pain, suffering, and decreased quality of life.

In 2006, a live attenuated Oka virus–based varicella vaccine was approved by the FDA for adults 60 years of age or older. The approval was based on the results of the Shingles Prevention Study—a large, multicenter, randomized, placebo-controlled trial—that established efficacy and safety of a single-dose herpes zoster vaccination.[33] The results of the trial indicated that the herpes zoster vaccine reduces the likelihood of developing herpes zoster in immunocompetent individuals 60 years of age or older. Important results of this study included a decrease in the incidence of herpes zoster by 51.3%, a reduction in the overall burden of illness (BOI) by 61.1%, and a decrease in the incidence of PHN by 66.5%.[93] Subsequently, in order to investigate the durability of benefit from vaccination, the Short-Term Persistence Substudy (STPS) was performed by the same group of investigators.[94] The study

was designed to evaluate efficacy up to 7 years postvaccination. The major findings included a drop in efficacy in herpes zoster BOI by 11%, 6.4% for PHN incidence, and 11.7% for herpes zoster incidence. The results regarding incidence for BOI and incidence of herpes zoster were significant through 5 years postvaccination leading the authors to conclude the persistence of efficacy at 5 years but the benefit beyond that time point was unclear. To address this question, the same group performed the Long-Term Persistence Substudy (LTPS) evaluating patients 7 to 11 years postvaccination.[95] All participants in the prior two studies had been vaccinated, leaving no controls to use for comparison. Therefore, the authors used regression models to estimate incidences of herpes zoster and PHN, finding that efficacy of the vaccine continued to decline. Only for herpes zoster BOI was efficacy retained at 10 years, efficacy for incidence of herpes zoster persisted through year 8. The findings from the LTPS have been supported by an analysis of over 175,000 vaccinated individuals from an integrated health care organization, which found the effectiveness of the vaccine drops from 68.7% in the first year to 4.2% in the 8-year postvaccination.[96] In order to address the issue of waning efficacy the logical next step would be evaluation of a "booster" dose of vaccine. In fact, that work has been initiated and demonstrated enhanced VZV-specific cell-mediated immunity in individuals >70 years of age who received a second dose of varicella zoster vaccine.[97] The findings are promising and support further investigation of the use of booster doses to prevent herpes zoster.

Recently, a novel glycoprotein-based herpes zoster subunit vaccine has been developed, potentially for adults older than 50 years and immunocompromised hosts. It has been evaluated in two phase 3, large, international, multicenter, randomized, placebo-control trials. The first demonstrated an overall vaccine efficacy against herpes zoster of 97.9 % for those 70 years or older and 97.2% for all individuals greater than 50 years of age.[98] The second looked specifically at those 70 years of age or older and found an overall vaccine efficacy of 89.9%.[99] A pooled analysis from the two trials demonstrated an 88.8% vaccine efficacy against PHN for individuals greater than 70 years of age and 91.2% for those greater than 50 years of age. The results from these studies are very encouraging and the vaccine is currently under review by the FDA.

Clinical Picture of Postherpetic Neuralgia

PHN is the most common complication of herpes zoster in the immunocompetent patient. This condition can result in significant patient suffering and causes a large economic burden to society. Our ability to diagnose and treat PHN has benefited from consensus among researchers as to its definitions and guidelines for treatment of chronic neuropathic pain conditions. Currently, the term PHN is used to describe dermatomal pain that persists for more than 90 to 120 days after the onset of the herpes zoster rash.[9,33] Pain persisting for more than 180 days after the rash onset is less likely to resolve and hence can be considered "well-established PHN" to reflect its recalcitrant nature.[100] Following the same pattern as herpes zoster, PHN is most commonly found in the thoracic, cervical, and trigeminal dermatomes.

A variety of signs and symptoms are characteristic of patients with PHN, although none are pathognomonic. These include various types of stimulus-independent pain, for example, intermittent sharp, shooting, or electric shock-like pain and continuous burning or throbbing pain. Stimulus-evoked pain is also very common in patients with PHN and includes tactile allodynia, one of the most debilitating symptoms associated with this condition. Tactile allodynia can be so severe that patients with truncal PHN may not be able to tolerate the sensation of clothing against their skin and those with craniofacial PHN may not be able to wear hats, glasses, or tolerate even breezes or air conditioning on the affected site. Estimates of allodynia in PHN patients have ranged from 48.6% to over 90%, with differences likely due to varied quantitative sensory testing (QST) protocols and patient heterogeneity.[101–103] Hyperalgesia, which is an abnormally increased perception of pain in response to a painful stimulus, can occur with application of painful thermal or mechanical stimuli. These types of stimulus-independent and stimulus-evoked pain are caused by nerve damage (i.e., neuropathic pain), but musculoskeletal pain can also occur in patients with PHN as a result of excessive guarding of the affected area. Myofascial trigger points, atrophy, and reduced joint range of motion may be seen in severe cases where pain has resulted in excessive guarding.

Additional sensory abnormalities are also common in PHN. Involved areas may be hypoesthetic, which can occur even in regions that exhibit tactile allodynia. The areas of altered tactile sensitivity may become larger than the sites originally affected by the zoster rash. Alterations in temperature sensation have also been demonstrated. Furthermore, various paresthesias and dysesthesias (abnormal or unpleasant but not painful sensations) can occur. Chronic pruritus can persist or develop following herpes zoster and is particularly problematic for some individuals; it may be present with or without comorbid pain.

Areas of hyperpigmentation, hypopigmentation, or scarring may be present in the affected dermatomes following rash healing, and affected areas may also exhibit a persistent reddish or brownish hue. These cosmetic changes do not occur in all patients, and the skin in the affected dermatome is normal in appearance in many patients with PHN.

Although less well-studied and generally less disabling than pain, altered motor function occurs in herpes zoster and can persist after rash healing. Facial paralysis may be evident in the form of ptosis or loss of the nasolabial fold in cases of facial nerve involvement. In cases of thoracic involvement, a truncal bulge resulting from intercostal muscle weakness may be present (see Fig. 27.6).

DIAGNOSIS AND ASSESSMENT OF POSTHERPETIC NEURALGIA

PHN is diagnosed primarily based on clinical findings. A history of herpes zoster rash, followed by persistent pain in the same distribution, usually establishes the diagnosis. The presence of known risk factors (see the following text) on history and sensory abnormalities on physical exam such as allodynia or hyperalgesia also support the diagnosis. Occasionally, patients report having a quiescent period between the resolution of the initial herpes zoster–associated pain and the onset of the pain associated with PHN. In a study of 156 patients with PHN, Watson et al.[104] noted that 25% of patients with a poor outcome said that they could recall a time after the rash when they had little or no pain. This pain-free hiatus has been observed to last for a period of weeks to as much as 12 months. The recurrence of dermatomal pain is not associated with a recurrent episode of herpes zoster but may coincide with changes in the patient's emotional or physical status. As mentioned in the earlier discussion, a clear history of rash may not be present in all patients (i.e., zoster sine herpete). In these cases, a definitive diagnosis of VZV-related pain would require serial serologic assessments that are unlikely to be obtained in most clinical settings.

In addition to assessing the location, intensity, and characteristics of the pain, it is important to evaluate the overall impact that the pain has had on the patient. PHN can cause significant deleterious impacts on physical, emotional, and social functioning and therefore can have a widespread adverse effect on health-related quality of life.[105–108] In addition, PHN can lead to excess health care costs, albeit not as costly as painful diabetic peripheral neuropathy.[109,110] PHN can result in fatigue, insomnia, anxiety, depression, and suicidal ideation, and careful screening for the presence of any psychiatric comorbidities or any escalation of preexisting psychiatric symptoms should be performed.

Laboratory Diagnosis

Diagnostic tests have limited application in the clinical management of PHN patients. A variety of studies may be used but are predominately limited to clinical research settings. These include QST, skin biopsy, and nerve conduction studies. QST has been used to identify different phenotypic subtypes of PHN patients with distinct constellations of signs and symptoms, which are thought to reflect different pathophysiologic mechanisms. This is an especially interesting area of future research, and the hope is that such phenotypic subtypes will ultimately be used to guide mechanism-based treatment.[1,2]

Epidemiology and Natural History of Postherpetic Neuralgia

High-quality systematic studies of the epidemiology of specific chronic pain conditions are limited, including PHN. The large variation in definitions utilized, study design, and study population makes accurate estimates of incidence and prevalence of PHN difficult to obtain. Estimates of the prevalence of PHN have ranged from 500,000 to 1 million in the United States[111,112] but should decrease as herpes zoster vaccination becomes more widespread. One systematic review analyzed data from 49 studies and found the risk of developing PHN after herpes zoster varied from 5% to more than 30% worldwide.[18] Subsequent data from population-based studies[113–115] and large clinical trials[95,99] had similar findings; however, the precise figures differ greatly depending on whether patients in the community or in clinical trials were studied.

PHN is a chronic pain syndrome that can last for years. There is a relative paucity of data on its natural history due to the lack of population-based studies of zoster-related pain. Multiple studies consistently indicate that the majority of patients experience resolution of pain over weeks to months following rash onset.[62,104,105,107,116,117] The presence of persistent pain at 6 months after initial PHN diagnosis has been estimated to be 48% and 20% at 1 year.[10,118–120] There are few prospective studies that have followed and characterized patients for more than 6 months following the diagnosis of PHN. Hence, the exact number of patients who enjoy a complete resolution of PHN is unknown.

RISK FACTORS FOR POSTHERPETIC NEURALGIA

The most well-established risk factors for PHN in patients with herpes zoster include older age, presence of a painful prodrome, greater severity of acute pain, greater rash severity, and ophthalmic involvement.[105,121,122] Increasing age is a particularly potent risk factor for the development of PHN. The risk for PHN increases by 1.22 to 3.11 for every 10 year increase in age.[123] Approximately 20% of patients older than 50 years of age continue to have pain at 6 months after the onset of rash despite starting antiviral agents in a timely fashion.[62,67,121,124] Using a shorter duration of pain, patients 50 years of age or older were shown to have a 14.7-fold higher prevalence (95% confidence interval [CI], 6.8 to 32.0) of pain 30 days after rash onset compared with patients younger than 50 years.[125] Elderly patients also seem to be predisposed to developing particularly refractory cases of PHN that do not respond to currently available treatments.[104] Other risk factors for PHN are listed in Table 27.6.

TABLE 27.6   Risk Factors for Postherpetic Neuralgia[10,22,118,123,126]

Well Replicated
- Older age
- Severity of rash
- Severity of acute pain
- Prodromal pain

Less Well Replicated
- Ophthalmic distribution
- Female gender
- Greater sensory abnormalities in the affected dermatomes
- Polyneuropathy
- Psychosocial variables
- Severe immunosuppression
- Diabetes mellitus

Pathophysiology of Postherpetic Neuralgia

Viral replication is thought to result in a combination of neural and inflammatory damage, leading to sensitization of the peripheral and central sensory neural elements. There is evidence that various risk factors identified for the development of PHN make independent contributions to the likelihood of developing this chronic pain condition,[105,126] and these risk factors may reflect distinct underlying pathophysiologic mechanisms. For instance, elderly patients who are at high risk for PHN are more likely to have a subclinical polyneuropathy, which may reduce the amount of viral damage needed to cause PHN.[127,128] Other examples of the possible relationships between risk factors for PHN and underlying mechanisms include the presence of a prodrome, reflecting earlier and more extensive viral damage in the affected sensory ganglion[129]; greater rash severity, reflecting greater damage to and loss of epidermal nerve fibers[130–132]; and severe acute pain, reflecting the initiation of processes that ultimately result in central and peripheral sensitization.[133,134] These relatively independent processes may combine to cause more severe cases of PHN.

More severe zoster infections are accompanied by greater neural damage, and it has been proposed that this neural damage contributes prominently to the development of PHN.[133,135] However, knowledge of the pathophysiologic mechanisms of PHN remains limited. It is mainly derived from autopsy and skin biopsy neuroanatomic studies and research on patterns of sensory dysfunction and pharmacologic response. A variety of pathophysiologic mechanisms have been described and are hypothesized to be causally related to the qualitatively different types of pain associated with PHN. Different mechanisms may coexist in an individual patient, and there may be pathophysiologically distinct subgroups of patients.[136–138]

Modern anatomic understanding is based on data limited by the small number of patients studied to date. Watson and colleagues[129] compared autopsy tissue from patients with and without PHN following herpes zoster. They found that patients with PHN showed marked atrophy of the spinal cord dorsal horn on the ipsilateral versus contralateral side, a difference that was not present in the patients with a history of zoster but not PHN. Punch skin biopsy permits quantitative measurement of epidermal sensory nerve endings. Such studies have shown that PHN patients have reduced innervation density in the affected dermatome compared to the contralateral side (Fig. 27.7). In one murine study of PHN, the severity of dermal denervation correlated to the development of allodynia and hyperalgesia beyond the margins of the initial herpes zoster rash.[139] Notably, in both the postmortem and skin biopsy studies, pathologic features were only identified in PHN patients and were not found in patients with a history of zoster who did not go on to develop PHN.

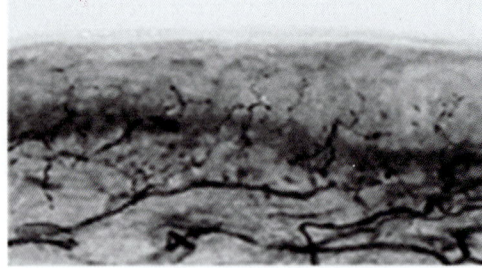

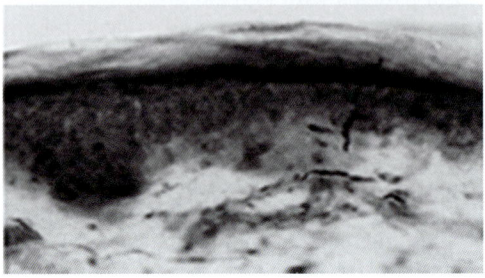

FIGURE 27.7 Representative, immunolabeled, dermal sensory nerve endings from skin biopsies of previously shingles-affected skin, with and without postherpetic neuralgia (PHN). **A:** Biopsy from the previously affected shingles site on the back of a 75-year-old woman without PHN (1,672 epidermal neuritis/mm²). **B:** Biopsy from the previous affected shingles site of a 72-year-old woman with PHN (145 neurites/mm²). The epidermis is at the **top of the image**, and the dermis is at the **bottom**. Individual neurites and neurite bundles are visible in the superficial dermis. *(Reprinted with permission from Oaklander AL. The density of remaining nerve endings in human skin with and without postherpetic neuralgia after shingles. Pain 2001;92[1]:139–145.)*

Sensory testing can be used to investigate the function of small afferent fibers including nociceptors. This type of testing helps create a detailed sensory profile of the affected area. Rowbotham and Fields have conducted a landmark series of studies of sensory dysfunction and pharmacologic response in an attempt to address the pathophysiology of PHN.[136,137] The results of this research, along with that of others, have emphasized the role of central processes in interpreting sensory dysfunction and its relationship to pain in patients with PHN[140–142] and have suggested that at least two different pathophysiologic mechanisms contribute to the development of PHN and other peripheral neuropathic pain conditions—sensitization and deafferentation.

Both peripheral and central sensitization appear to contribute to PHN. Peripheral sensitization occurs predominantly in small unmyelinated C-fiber nociceptors. Clinically, there can be minimal sensory loss in areas of marked allodynia.[132,136,141] However, thermal sensory thresholds can be decreased (heat hyperalgesia) by up to 2° to 4° C[95,105] in allodynic regions. Heat hyperalgesia is a well-known consequence of peripheral nociceptor sensitization.[130] These observations all suggest that sensitization of C nociceptors can be responsible for the spontaneous burning pain and heat hyperalgesia seen in some patients. In many PHN patients, the area of mechanical or tactile allodynia is much larger than the area originally affected during herpes zoster and the painful area may continue to change with time. Allodynia in a subset of PHN patients may be caused by ectopic discharges from damaged C nociceptors maintaining a state of central sensitization.[136,143] The major excitatory neurotransmitter involved in spinal cord pain processing is glutamate, and binding at the N-methyl-D-aspartic acid (NMDA) receptor has been thought to play a key role in central sensitization. The importance of persistent sensitization has been supported by the work of Petersen and Rowbotham,[135] who found patients with PHN were more likely to have a positive response to capsaicin application with expansion of allodynic area when compared to those with no pain at 6 months after having herpes zoster.

Dynamic and tactile allodynia may also result from sprouting of Aβ fibers into the superficial layers of the dorsal horn in response to partial loss of C-fiber input. This sprouting may lead to connections between these fibers, which normally do not transmit pain, and the ascending pain pathways that were formerly responsive to C-fiber input. This process would explain why nonpainful stimuli such as light touch or pressure can become painful in patient with PHN.

Deafferentation may also be playing a significant role in the maintenance of PHN. In a subset of patients, there is a loss of both large and small diameter sensory afferent fibers. This loss of peripheral input can result in the development of spontaneous discharge in deafferented central neurons. This may produce constant pain in the area of sensory loss.[136] Interestingly, these patients may still suffer from severe mechanical allodynia.[144] Assuming that the DRG and central connections are lost in such patients, the pain may be due to intrinsic CNS changes. However, there have been some studies that question the role of deafferentation in PHN due to the findings of persistent sensory abnormalities in patients with PHN and those without pain after HZ.[135,145]

The mentioned data suggest that there may be subsets of patients within the PHN population who have different underlying mechanisms responsible for the generation and maintenance of their chronic pain. These different mechanisms may account for the varied presentations of pain in patients with PHN. Unfortunately, these observations have yet to provide the foundation for a mechanism-based approach for selecting specific pharmacologic treatment options in clinical practice. This, of course, would be an extremely desirable goal to improve the therapeutic effects of existing treatments.

Treatment of Postherpetic Neuralgia

Tricyclic antidepressants, various anticonvulsants, opioid analgesics, and topical lidocaine are efficacious in the management of PHN (Table 27.7). There is a limited role of invasive interventions and alternative modalities, but these are utilized for patients who are refractory to conservative modalities. The choice of which therapy is used is often individualized based on the patient's comorbidities, concomitant medication use, and associated symptoms. Recent studies have evaluated the relative efficacy of these treatments.[146,147] Additionally, consensus recommendation and guidelines for the pharmacotherapeutic treatment of neuropathic pain, including PHN, have been published and serve as useful guides in selecting between the growing list of treatment options.[148–151] Despite the publication of treatment recommendations, many patients in the community with PHN do not receive evidence-based pharmacotherapy.[152] In clinical practice, certain anticonvulsants, topical lidocaine, and tramadol are often used as first-line medications, followed by serotonin norepinephrine reuptake inhibitors (SNRIs), tricyclic antidepressants, opioids, and high-dose capsaicin patch. Capsaicin patch as a second-line therapy is used in part because of better tolerance in elderly patients. Needless to say, all patients should have a thorough assessment, and treatment should be tailored to address their individual needs.

ANTICONVULSANTS: GABAPENTIN AND PREGABALIN
Although a number of anticonvulsants have been used for many years for the treatment of PHN and other neuropathic pain conditions, the greatest evidence of efficacy exists for gabapentin and pregabalin. Both are well-tolerated and much less toxic than the first-generation anticonvulsants previously used to treat neuropathic pain. There is good evidence to support the use of

gabapentin in PHN. In two large clinical trials,[153,154] its use was associated with a statistically significant reduction in daily pain ratings as well as improvements in sleep, mood, fatigue, and depression as well as other quality of life indicators like improved function and work at daily dosages of 1,800 to 3,600 mg. A meta-analysis of these trials indicated the number needed to treat (NNT) for gabapentin in the treatment of PHN is approximately 4.4 (95% CI, 3.3 to 6.1).[76] The precise mechanism of its analgesic action is not known, but evidence derived from rodent models suggests that gabapentin acts at the $\alpha_2\delta$ subunit of voltage-dependent calcium channels to decrease calcium influx. This effect inhibits the release of the excitatory neurotransmitters, including glutamate.[155,156] As noted in the earlier discussion, glutamate, via its effect at the NMDA receptor, is the primary neurotransmitter responsible for maintaining central sensitization.

Gabapentin is rapidly absorbed after oral administration. However, its absorption is mediated by a transport mechanism present only in the proximal part of small intestine that becomes saturated at higher doses. This phenomenon reduces the bioavailability of gabapentin as the dose is increased. For example, the bioavailability of gabapentin at a dose of 300 mg is about 60%, but the bioavailability falls to 40% with a 600-mg dose. Additionally, its half-life is 5 to 7 hours, necessitating three or four doses in a day. Peak serum concentrations are achieved approximately 3 hours after oral administration. Gabapentin does not exhibit significant protein binding, is eliminated unchanged via the kidneys, and is not metabolized by the liver.

The optimal dosing schedule for gabapentin has not been well characterized. One review suggested that dosing should be initiated at 300 mg on the first day, followed by 300 mg twice daily on the second day, and then increased to 300 mg three times daily on the third day.[157] At that point, the titration should be slowed down with a goal of reaching 600 mg three times daily over the ensuing 2 weeks. Daily dosages of up to 3,600 mg have been studied and shown efficacious.[153] The daily dosage should be divided into three or four doses per day as this drug has a relatively short half-life. In elderly patients, dosages should be reduced and titration should be executed more slowly. In frail patients, it is typical to start with 100 mg per day, increasing by 100 mg every 3 to 4 days. Once patients are tolerating a daily dose of 600 mg, the titration rate may be increased by 300 mg per day every 3 to 4 days to a target of 1,800 to 2,400 mg per day. The titration schedule may need to be modified if efficacy is achieved at lower dosages or unmanageable side effects are encountered. As gabapentin is excreted renally, dosages need to be adjusted in patients with renal insufficiency. Patients on dialysis should be started on a single dose of 100 mg given 1 hour after dialysis treatment on alternate days. This dose then can be titrated up slowly and cautiously. Of note, gabapentin is also available as an oral solution in 250 mg/5 mL preparation.

Side effects associated with gabapentin include somnolence, dizziness, peripheral edema, and gait or balance problems. In general, the side effects are short lived, but they can require monitoring and occasionally dosage adjustment.

Newer formulations of gabapentin have attempted to circumvent the issue of variable bioavailability of gabapentin. These include gastroretentive formulation of gabapentin (G-GR) and gabapentin enacarbil (GEn). The G-GR preparation is designed in a way that leads to a slow and steady release of gabapentin, resulting in a more efficient absorption, improved bioavailability, and possibly reduced side effects of somnolence and dizziness compared to regular gabapentin. Patients can titrate up an effective dose more quickly than regular gabapentin. An 11-week randomized, double-blind, placebo-controlled phase 3 clinical trial showed significant reduction in pain intensity and sleep interference in patients with PHN.[158] It is administered as a once-daily dosing of 1,200 to 1,800 mg with an evening meal. The dose should be adjusted

TABLE 27.7   Pharmacologic Options for the Treatment of Postherpetic Neuralgia

Medication	Starting Dose	Dose-Escalation Scheme	Common Side Effects	Contraindications/Caution	Comments
Gabapentin	100–300 mg	Start qhs and increase to tid dosing; increase by 100–300 mg every 3 d to total dose of 1,800–3,600 mg	Somnolence, dizziness, fatigue, ataxia, peripheral edema, and weight gain	Decrease dose in patients with renal impairment; qod dosing in dialysis patients	No clinically significant drug interactions, improved sleep; avoid sudden discontinuation. Gastroretentive or extended release enacarbil preparations can be used instead for better patient compliance and questionable improved tolerability.
Pregabalin	50 mg tid or 75 mg bid	300–600 mg/d in 1 wk	Somnolence, fatigue, dizziness, peripheral edema and weight gain, blurred vision, and euphoria	Decrease dose in patients with renal impairment by 50% or more based on CL creatinine	Caution with concomitant use of ACE inhibitors—angioedema; increased risk for weight gain and peripheral edema in patients on thiazolidinedione antidiabetic agents; extended release preparation available
SNRIs Duloxetine Venlafaxine	30 mg qd 37.5 mg qd	Increase by 30 mg weekly to a max dose of 60–120 mg/d Increase by 37.5–75 mg weekly to a max dose of 150–225 mg/d	Nausea Insomnia, somnolence, fatigue, dizziness Nervousness, sexual dysfunction Constipation Decreased appetite	Concomitant use of tramadol, MAO inhibitors, SSRI, or TCAs duloxetine is contraindicated in patients with liver disease. Caution in patients with close angle glaucoma especially with duloxetine and hypertension especially with venlafaxine	Be careful in patients with history of bipolar disorder; can precipitate mania. Venlafaxine has not been reported to cause additive liver toxicity.
TCAs Nortriptyline Desipramine Amitriptyline	10–25 mg qhs	Increase by 10–25 mg weekly with a target dose of 75–150 mg	Sedation, dry mouth, blurred vision, weight gain, urinary retention, constipation, sexual dysfunction	Cardiac arrhythmic disease, glaucoma, suicide risk, seizure disorder; concomitant use of tramadol, SSRI, or selective SNRIs	The lower starting dose may be more appropriate in the elderly. Amitriptyline has the most anticholinergic effects and hence less well tolerated by the elderly. Obtain baseline ECG in patients with history of cardiac disease.
Topical lidocaine	5%, 1–2 patches	Can use up to 3 patches 12 h/d	Local erythema, rash, blisters	Known hypersensitivity to amide local anesthetics	No significant systemic side effects Caution in patients receiving class 1 antiarrhythmic drugs (e.g., tocainide and mexiletine)

Medication			Side effects		
High-dose % capsaicin patch	Needs to be placed in a monitored setting	1–4 patches depending on the size of the affected area	Local irritation, erythema, and rash	Can lead to temporary increase in pain and discomfort	Need for systemic analgesics during and after the application for few days
Tramadol	50 mg every 6 h prn	Can titrate up to 100 mg every 6 h; max daily dose: 400 mg. Extended release dosing once a day	Nausea/vomiting, constipation, drowsiness, and dizziness	Seizure disorder, concomitant use of SSRI, selective SNRI, TCA medications. Decrease dose in patients with hepatic or renal disease.	Available as combination products with ibuprofen/acetaminophen. Extended release dose max is 300 mg/d.
Strong opioids Morphine	5–10 mg every 4–6 h prn	Titrate at weekly intervals balancing analgesia and side effects if patient tolerating the medications can titrate faster.	Nausea/vomiting, constipation, drowsiness, and itching	Driving impairment and cognitive dysfunction during treatment initiation. Be careful in patients with sleep apnea. Additive effects of sedation with neuromodulators	Gradual titration monitoring GI and CNS side effects; MME 50 per day in routine practice
Oxycodone	2.5–5 mg every 6 h prn				
Methadone	2.5 mg tid			Only should be prescribed by provider familiar with its titration and in opioid-tolerant patient	
Fentanyl patch	12 µg/h			Only should be prescribed by provider familiar with its titration and in opioid-tolerant patient	
Botulinum toxin A	Needs specialist services	50–200 units injected subcutaneously over multiple sites of the affected area in small aliquots.	Allergic reaction, rash, itching, headache, localized pain, muscle stiffness, shortness of breath, nausea, diarrhea, flulike symptoms	Be cautious if patient on medications that can affect the neuromuscular junction function like aminoglycosides	Contraindicated in patients with preexisting motor neuron diseases like myasthenia gravis, Lambert-Eaton syndrome, pregnancy, and lactation

NOTE: Must start a patient on short-acting opioid medications before changing over to a fentanyl patch. Differences in recommended dosages of medications between Tables 27.5 and 27.7 are in part because of the acuity of pain in herpetic neuralgia versus postherpetic neuralgia.

ACE, angiotensin-converting enzyme; CL, clearance; CNS, central nervous system; GI, gastrointestinal; MAO, monoamine oxidase; MME, morphine milligram equivalents; prn, when necessary; qd, every day; qhs, every night or at every bedtime; qod, every other day; SNRI, serotonin norepinephrine reuptake inhibitor; SSRI, selective serotonin reuptake inhibitor; TCA, tricyclic antidepressant; tid, three times a day.

Originally adapted from Wu CL, Raja SN. An update on the treatment of postherpetic neuralgia. *J Pain* 2008;9(1 Suppl):S19–S30. Copyright © 2008 American Pain Society. Modified based on our clinical practice and guidelines for neuropathic pain.: Finnerup NB, Attal N, Haroutounian S, et al. Pharmacotherapy for neuropathic pain in adults: a systematic review and meta-analysis. *Lancet Neurol* 2015;14(2):162–173. Copyright © 2015 Elsevier. With permission.

in patients with renal impairment and is contraindicated in patients on hemodialysis. Once-daily dosing could be a tremendous help in terms of patient compliance.

GEn is a prodrug of gabapentin that is actively transported and provides sustained, dose-proportional exposure to gabapentin. It is absorbed by a high-capacity transport system throughout the gut in comparison with the low-capacity transporter system in the upper intestine for regular gabapentin, hence, is said to provide a dose-proportional and extended exposure to gabapentin. It can be dosed in twice-daily dosing. Three different doses have been studied: 1,200, 1,800 and 3,600 mg total daily dose (divided into two dosages). All three daily dosages were efficacious in reducing pain intensity in patients with PHN, but the 1,200-mg dose demonstrated the most favorable balance between efficacy and adverse effects.[159]

G-GR or GEn are not as popular in clinical practice as the regular gabapentin despite significant advantages over the latter. The possible reasons could be provider familiarity and lower costs of standard generic gabapentin. Pregabalin appears to have a similar mechanism of action as gabapentin, and several large randomized clinical trials have demonstrated its efficacy in the treatment of PHN and other neuropathic pain conditions. Three double-blind trials comprising 776 patients with PHN showed that pregabalin resulted in superior pain relief and improved pain-related sleep interference compared to placebo. Dosages in these studies ranged between 150 and 600 mg per day,[160] and both fixed as well as flexible dosing schedules have been efficacious in clinical trials.[161,162] Pregabalin can be given in two divided doses each day. Frequently reported side effects are the same as with gabapentin: somnolence, dizziness, peripheral edema, and balance problems.

Pregabalin has also been demonstrated to possess an anxiolytic effect in patients with generalized anxiety disorder.[163,164] As patients with chronic pain often have comorbid anxiety disorders, it is possible that this anxiolytic effect may provide additional benefit in PHN patients. The analgesic efficacy and side effect profiles of gabapentin and pregabalin appear to be comparable. Pregabalin has greater convenience than gabapentin because of its twice-daily dosing and simpler titration, however, and an effective analgesic dosage can be reached more rapidly with pregabalin. Pregabalin CR is an extended release preparation in once-daily dosing. In a recent study, it was found to be more effective in decreasing weekly mean pain scores when compared with placebo as early as week 1 and the effect was maintained until the final end point.[165] Primary efficacy outcome was time to loss of therapeutic response (LTR) (<30% decrease in weekly mean pain score from single-blind baseline or discontinuation due to adverse event or lack of efficacy). Time to LTR was significantly longer with pregabalin CR than with placebo. Pregabalin CR was significant in improving several secondary measures such as patient global impression of change as well as other quality-of-life measures.

ANTIDEPRESSANT MEDICATIONS
Tricyclic Antidepressants
Tricyclic antidepressant medications have a number of proposed mechanisms that might explain their efficacy in the treatment of PHN. These include inhibition of the reuptake of norepinephrine and serotonin and sodium channel blockade.[166–168] There have been several clinical trials and meta-analyses of these agents demonstrating efficacy in the treatment of pain associated with PHN, with pooled data showing NNTs of 2.1 to 2.6.[76,169,170]

Amitriptyline has been the most widely studied antidepressant for PHN. Available evidence and clinical experience suggest that nortriptyline and desipramine[171] are equally effective[76] but are better tolerated than relatively more side effect prone amitriptyline. Thus, these secondary amine tricyclics

are generally preferred, especially in elderly and frail patients. Both amitriptyline and nortriptyline are often helpful in patients with insomnia because of their sedating properties. Desipramine has significantly less sedation than these two medications and is thus preferred in patients who may be intolerant to the sedative effects of this class of medication.

Both significant side effects and toxicities must be considered when using tricyclic antidepressants. Major side effects include tachyarrhythmias, prolongation of QT intervals with the potential for the precipitation of life-threatening arrhythmias, and the worsening of acute angle glaucoma. It would be prudent to review a baseline electrocardiogram (ECG) before starting these medications in elderly patients or those who possess other risk factors for increased cardiac toxicity.[172,173] Minor side effects include dryness of mouth, dizziness, weight gain, sedation, constipation, urinary retention, and orthostatic hypotension. These medications should be started at a low dose, typically 25 mg at night, and titrated slowly to a target dose of 75 to 100 mg per day in a single evening dose. In elderly or frail individuals, these agents can be started using a 10-mg evening dose. Concomitant use with selective serotonin reuptake inhibitor antidepressants should be monitored carefully as there is a risk of developing toxic tricyclic serum levels and serotonin syndrome with such combinations.

Selective Serotonin and Norepinephrine Reuptake Inhibitors (Dual Reuptake Inhibitors)
Two antidepressant medications, duloxetine and venlafaxine, are selective serotonin and norepinephrine reuptake inhibitors that have shown efficacy in patients with painful diabetic and other peripheral neuropathies but have not been studied in PHN. Milnacipran is another SNRI that is approved by FDA to treat pain due to fibromyalgia but has not been well studied or often used clinically for neuropathic pain. Duloxetine is approved by the FDA for the treatment of painful diabetic peripheral neuropathy and fibromyalgia as well as chronic musculoskeletal pain. Clinically, this medication seems to be better tolerated compared with tricyclic antidepressants and hence is being used in clinical practice for PHN. Randomized, double-blind, placebo-controlled clinical trials have found that duloxetine at 60-mg daily dose was superior to placebo in reducing pain scores and improving multiple quality of life measures in patients with diabetic neuropathy pain.[79,174] Two randomized clinical trials have shown that venlafaxine at higher dosages is also efficacious in painful diabetic and other peripheral neuropathies, but its value in treating patients with PHN is unknown.[149]

OPIOID ANALGESICS
Historically, the role of opioid analgesics in the treatment of chronic nonmalignant pain, and particularly neuropathic pain, has been controversial. Recent evidence, however, has shown that this class of drugs is efficacious in neuropathic pain conditions, including PHN. They are now recommended as second- or third-line analgesics by several respected sources.[148–150,175] These sources reserve them as second- and third-line agents based on concerns regarding their side effects, the potential for the development of tolerance, and concerns regarding misuse and abuse. The analgesic efficacy of oral oxycodone was evaluated in a double-blind, crossover trial in which treatment resulted in significant reductions in allodynia, steady pain, and spontaneous paroxysmal pain.[176] Oxycodone treatment also resulted in superior scores for global effectiveness, disability reduction, and patient preference compared to placebo. A quantitative review of pooled results for opioid therapy yielded an NNT of 2.67 (2.07 to 3.77).[76] It is noteworthy, however, that more frequent side effects were associated with the opioid therapy as compared to both tricyclics[176,177] and gabapentin[178] in head-to-head comparisons. Prescribers should carefully review

the CDC guidelines for prescribing opioids for chronic pain prior to making a decision about initiating opioid therapy.[179] If opioids are prescribed, the patients should be carefully counseled regarding common side effects such as nausea, sedation, urinary retention, pruritus, and constipation. Monitoring for immune suppression and hypogonadism is needed if opioid use is required chronically. Other adverse effects associated with chronic opioid use include tolerance, physical dependence, and possibly opioid-induced hyperalgesia, which also require appropriate patient counseling and monitoring. Lastly, opioids cannot be prescribed without some risk of developing misuse, abuse, or addiction, but this appears to be relatively rare in elderly patients with no prior history of addictive disorders.

Clinical recommendations based on the CDC guidelines[179] for the use of opioid analgesics in the treatment of PHN include the following: (1) clear and realistic treatment goals and expectations of reducing pain and improvement in function; (2) use of the lowest effective dose, initiating therapy with short-acting opioids, for example, 2.5 to 5 mg oxycodone or 5 to 10 mg morphine every 4 to 6 hours as needed with <50 morphine milligram equivalents (MME) per day; (3) if a patient needs more than 90 MME per day, a rigorous assessment of risks and benefits should be done and documented clearly; (4) once a patient demonstrates tolerability to the initial opioid therapy, conversion can be made to a long-acting opioid preparation (controlled release oxycodone or morphine), transdermal fentanyl patch, or methadone, this should only be done by providers who are familiar with using these opioid medications; (5) proactive effort should be made to anticipate and manage common side effects of nausea and constipation (with antiemetics and laxatives); and (6) regular assessment for efficacy and tolerability should be made. If the treatment is not effective, these medications should be tapered gradually to prevent the development of withdrawal symptoms.

TRAMADOL

Tramadol, a synthetic 4-phenyl piperidine analogue of codeine, is an analgesic medication with a unique mechanism of action. It has a μ-agonist effect like opioids, but in addition, it inhibits the reuptake of serotonin and norepinephrine like the antidepressants that are efficacious in neuropathic pain. Tramadol can be dosed 50 to 100 mg every 4 hours on an as-needed basis. The daily dose should not exceed 400 mg. Lower doses should be used in the elderly and in patients with impaired renal function. It has been shown to possess efficacy in the treatment of PHN in one randomized controlled trial in which a sustained-release preparation was compared to placebo. Superior pain relief and improved quality of life was seen with tramadol,[180] and the NNT was 4.8 (CI 95%, 3.5 to 6.0). However, these results have yet to be replicated, and overall, evidence for use of tramadol in neuropathic pain at best is low quality.[181] The most contemporary guidelines in the management of neuropathic pain recommend use of tramadol as a second-line drug.[150]

Adverse effects include nausea, vomiting, dizziness, constipation, urinary retention, somnolence, and headache. Concomitant use with medications that are inhibitors of CYP2D6, such as antidepressant medications, can lead to serotonin syndrome. Abuse of tramadol was thought to be rare but has recently been observed in increasing numbers.[182] In July 2014, tramadol was placed into schedule IV of the US Controlled Substances Act, a designation that indicates that tramadol has some potential for abuse. Furthermore, tramadol is associated with an increased risk of precipitating seizures in patients who have a history of seizures or who are also receiving drugs that can reduce the seizure threshold. These considerations usually result in clinicians avoiding tramadol in patients receiving CYP2D6 inhibitors or those patients at increased risk for seizures.

TAPENTADOL

Tapentadol is a centrally acting synthetic analgesic. Although its exact mechanism is unknown, analgesic efficacy is thought to be due to μ-opioid agonist activity and the inhibition of norepinephrine reuptake. It has structural similarities to tramadol but its μ-opioid agonist activity is stronger than tramadol. The usual adult dose is 50 to 100 mg every 4 to 6 hours, with a maximum daily dose is 600 mg per day. It is thought to have a lower incidence of gastrointestinal (GI)-related adverse events compared with equivalent doses of oxycodone. It is available in multiple strengths including 25-, 50-, 75-, and 100-mg tablets. It is also available as an extended-release product. Outpatient coverage by insurance carriers is variable due to the high cost of the drug. Dose adjustment is required in patients with renal and hepatic impairment. Side effects are similar to opioids but to a less severe degree. It may have drug interactions with antidepressant medications and use is contraindicated in patients with concomitant monoamine oxidase inhibitor use.

In our clinical experience, this medication is fairly well tolerated, especially when compared to strong opioids, and seems to be equally effective. However, due to the paucity of existing data for PHN, no conclusive recommendation can be made.

TOPICAL THERAPIES

An inherent advantage of topical therapies is that they are associated with few systemic effects due to minimal systemic absorption of the medication. The concept of establishing phenotypic subtypes to ultimately guide mechanism-based treatment is very attractive and may lead to development of novel topical therapies. For example, one trial of a topical sodium channel inhibitor (TV-45070) showed a preferential response to treatment in a subset of patients.[183] The postulated hypothesis was partially based on the thought that enhanced pain perception is mediated through an increased activity of the Nav1.7 sodium channel in patients with an R1150W polymorphism. Therefore, individuals with this genotype may render them more susceptible to pharmacologic intervention by specific sodium channel inhibitors such as TV-45070 compared with their wild-type counterparts. For now, high-dose capsaicin patch and 5% lidocaine patch are the only topical medications approved by the FDA for PHN. Lidocaine patches are the most commonly used topical modality for PHN in clinical practice because of ease of application and favorable side effect profile. High-dose capsaicin patch can be applied only by trained providers in an office setting. Over-the-counter capsaicin cream and other compounded mixtures are used less commonly.

Topical Lidocaine

Five percent lidocaine patches result in a local analgesic effect. Clinical trials have shown greater efficacy with the use of lidocaine patches as compared to vehicle-controlled patches in PHN patients presenting with allodynia.[184,185] There was no significant difference in the side effects between patients receiving lidocaine versus the control patches. The NNT is 4.4.[186] It is interesting to note that patients may respond well to topical lidocaine even if the skin at the targeted site appears to be completely devoid of nociceptors.[144] Lidocaine patches possess both excellent safety and tolerability profiles, making them an attractive treatment option for many older adults with PHN. Efficacy can be ascertained within 2 to 3 weeks of initiation of treatment; hence, there is no need for a prolonged trial period. The side effects are minimal because of the minimal systemic absorption of the lidocaine. Lidocaine patches are not approved for use in herpes zoster and should not be used in patients with active zoster lesions.

Clinical recommendations for use of lidocaine patches in the treatment of PHN include the following: (1) the patches can be cut to fit the affected area (unlike fentanyl patches);

(2) three patches can be applied with no additional risk of systemic side effects; (3) the recommendations are to keep the patches on for 12 hours and off for 12 hours, but the patches can be left on for 18 hours at a time to improve effectiveness[187]; (4) patches should be applied only on intact skin and directly over the area of maximum pain; and (5) lidocaine gel has also been shown to be efficacious in patients with PHN and allodynia,[188] and its use can therefore be considered if lidocaine patches are not available, affordable, or their application is problematic.

Topical Capsaicin

Capsaicin is an extract of hot chili peppers and an agonist for the vanilloid receptor (TRPV1), which is present on afferent nociceptor terminals. There are no systemic effects with a local application. In 2009, a high-concentration capsaicin patch (8%) was approved by the FDA for use in pain associated with PHN. Application is conducted in an office setting under medical supervision. To avoid discomfort, the affected area is prepared with topical local anesthetic cream for 45 to 60 minutes prior to application of patch. Depending on the area involved, up to four patches can be applied concurrently. Patients may also need additional analgesic before and after treatment. The transdermal patch releases capsaicin into the skin that act on the vanilloid receptor subtype 1 (TRPV1) receptors on nociceptor terminals. An initial phase of excitation is followed by dysfunction of these nociceptive fibers resulting in durable pain relief. Large clinical trials have evaluated its single application following a local anesthetic application. The results of these studies indicate that this approach can produce prolonged relief of pain in some PHN patients.[189] A recent review led to a conclusion that although more study participants with the high-dose capsaicin patch experienced significantly better pain relief and other quality of life measures than controls, still quality of evidence was moderate or low with an NNT as 7 to 8.8.[190] The patch is commonly used in clinical practice as a second- or third-line treatment.

Low-concentration capsaicin cream is also available over the counter in two concentrations, 0.025% and 0.075%. Pooled data from two placebo-controlled studies demonstrated superior pain relief following three to four times per day application of 0.075% capsaicin to the painful areas compared to an inert topical agent. The NNT was 3.3.[191,192] Blinding in these studies was problematic given that capsaicin produces a distinct burning sensation on initial application. In clinical practice, it is difficult to use, especially in patients who are experiencing significant allodynia, and many patients discontinue treatment too quickly for any beneficial effect to occur. Ironically, these are the very patients who would be expected to be most likely to benefit from this therapy. Low-concentration capsaicin is rarely used as a first-line agent in patients with PHN. Patients should be warned about the unpleasant burning sensation it causes with initial application and to avoid contact with their eyes.

Other Topical Treatments

Topical anti-inflammatory preparations have been studied in a few randomized, placebo-controlled trials.[193] There was significant heterogeneity in these studies, and definitive recommendations cannot be drawn from this literature. There have also been a few reports of other topical agents, including topical clonidine, cannabinoid, tricyclic antidepressants, gabapentin, ketamine, and vincristine as well as descriptions of novel delivery mechanisms, such as iontophoresis. The evidence for all these therapies is weak, and they are generally not used in clinical practice.

COMBINATION THERAPY

Although the use of combination therapy is common in clinical practice, few clinical trials have provided an evidence base for this approach. One study has demonstrated that the combination of gabapentin and morphine was superior to either of these medications used alone in relieving pain in patients with either painful diabetic neuropathy or PHN.[178] Another trial evaluated a nortriptyline–morphine combination compared with each monotherapy alone in neuropathic pain patients including patients with PHN.[194] The results suggest superior analgesia compared to monotherapy with either agent. According to a systematic review of available evidence for combination pharmacotherapy for neuropathic pain in adults, there are multiple, good-quality studies that demonstrate superior efficacy of two drug combinations; however, the low number of studies for any specific combination and other study factors prohibit any definitive recommendations to be made.[195] The goal of combination therapy is to arrive at a balanced, multimodal approach that improves the efficacy and tolerability of treatment while minimizing side effects of the individual medications. Disadvantages of combination therapy include an increased risk of side effects as the number of medications is increased. It may also be difficult to determine which medication is responsible for side effects. Ideally, medications that can cause similar side effects (e.g., sedation) should not be started simultaneously. There should be a judicious interval of time (e.g., at least a week or more) before a new medication is introduced to the regimen.

N-METHYL-D-ASPARTIC ACID ANTAGONISTS

The NMDA receptor is thought to play an important role in central sensitization and maintenance of chronic neuropathic pain states including PHN. Ketamine, an NMDA antagonist, is the most commonly utilized agent among this group that also includes dextromethorphan and memantine. Common side effects for this class of medications include hypertension, tachyarrhythmias, hallucinations, and other CNS side effects. In a small double-blind crossover comparison between ketamine (0.15 mg/kg), morphine (0.075 mg/kg), and saline for the treatment of PHN, intravenous (IV) ketamine effectively reduced pain and allodynia and decreased wind-up pain. Interestingly, wind-up pain was actually aggravated by morphine.[196] Dextromethorphan and memantine have been studied but did not show any benefit in decreasing pain due to PHN. Recommendations for use of this class of drugs are inconclusive as per the recent guidelines for the treatment of neuropathic pain.[150] In clinical practice, ketamine can be used as outpatient infusion therapy or as a component of the topical compounded creams or compounded oral preparations in patients with intractable symptoms.

OTHER PHARMACOLOGIC THERAPIES

A variety of other agents have been evaluated in the treatment of PHN and other neuropathic pain conditions. Several anticonvulsant and antidepressant medications besides those discussed earlier have shown evidence of efficacy in other neuropathic pain conditions in single clinical trials but lack convincing evidence of efficacy.[149,150] Cannabinoids have been studied in neuropathic pain, but there is little data to support their use in PHN. Similarly, the sodium channel blocker mexiletine has not demonstrated benefit in PHN, although there is some evidence of efficacy in painful diabetic peripheral neuropathy. However, this agent is usually avoided given its high toxicity profile. The use of all these medications can be considered in select circumstances, such as in cases where more conventional treatments have failed.

INVASIVE TREATMENTS FOR POSTHERPETIC NEURALGIA

A considerable percentage of PHN patients will not respond to currently available pharmacologic treatments. In these cases, a referral to a pain management center should be considered as early as possible. Invasive treatments may be considered for patients with refractory pain. A variety of interventional strategies have been described and examined as treatment options for PHN.

Unfortunately, the studies conducted to date have either been relatively poorly controlled or have not been replicated by independent investigators. Given the lack of objective evidence available to compare the efficacy of the various interventions available, the choice of specific therapy has been dependent on the treating physician's clinical experience. The lack of evidence demonstrating the efficacy of interventional treatments points more toward the lack of adequate research as opposed to the conclusion that these interventions are inherently ineffective. As per the recent guidelines for role of interventional techniques in neuropathic pain, authors concluded that due to the paucity of high-quality clinical trials, no strong recommendations can be made, but based on the available data, authors made a strong recommendations against use of sympathetic blocks for PHN pain.[83] Despite lack of strong evidence-based recommendation, a number of invasive interventions are used in clinical practice for patients with intractable symptoms.

Botulinum Toxin

Botulinum toxin has been traditionally used in the treatment of painful dystonias, headaches, and other spastic disorders. Multiple case reports and small studies have suggested that it may be efficacious in certain neuropathic pain conditions including PHN. There is a significant debate about its mechanism of action. Recent opinions on the mechanism responsible for antinociceptive effects of the toxin suggest that it inhibits the release of peripheral nociceptive neurotransmitters and inflammatory mediators responsible for pain generation and transmission from sensory nerves via TRPV1 receptors.[197] There are three well-designed studies showing a beneficial effect of botulinum toxin A injections in patients with PHN.[198–200] Injection of botulinum toxin is considered a third-line therapy in the management of PHN pain.[150] Recommended dose range from 50 to 200 units injected over multiple sites of the affected area in small aliquots.

Dorsal Root Ganglion Blocks

A number of procedures targeting the DRG may be utilized to treat patients suffering with PHN including steroid injections and pulsed radiofrequency ablation (RFA). Currently, an intervention that is infrequently used is the injection of steroid into the involved DRG. This approach is performed in a nearly identical manner as that used for performing a transforaminal epidural steroid injection. If an inflammatory process at the level of the DRG is considered to play a role in the pathophysiology of PHN, then this treatment would seem rational. There is, however, no convincing evidence to support the routine use of this treatment.

In terms of ablative procedures, lesioning of DRG using pulsed radiofrequency (PRF) has been studied in an open, nonrandomized study, and it was found that PRF lesioning of the DRG resulted in significant pain relief compared with the conventional treatments in patients with intractable PHN.[201] There has been another small, retrospective review published that reported good relief in all patients with zoster-related pain, but better pain relief was reported if procedure was performed within 90 days versus after 90 days of the rash onset.[202] As with other invasive interventions, there is no convincing, high-quality evidence available at this time to make a recommendation for the use of these procedures in routine clinical practice.

Peripheral Nerve Blocks

As PHN most commonly affects the thoracic dermatome, intercostal nerves are an attractive and relatively safer therapeutic target for interventions. Chemical neurolysis with 10% phenol in select patients has been used in clinical practice. A safer alternative would be pulsed RFA as it may lead to decreased incidence of deafferentation pain as well as other side effects associated with chemical neurolysis. In a randomized, double-blind clinical trial, PRF treatment of the intercostal nerves at a level above and below the level of the PHN was done weekly for 3 weeks and was found to result in improved pain, reduced dose of analgesic medication, and improvement in health-related quality of life domains compared to the sham group.[203] In addition, an older study found that intercostal nerve blocks provided long-lasting relief in PHN patients.[204] The quality of the evidence for intercostal nerve blocks or PRF treatment is limited, much as it is for the other neural blockade techniques described in the following text.

Neuroaugmentive Techniques

There has been an increasing role for neuromodulatory strategies in the management of chronic neuropathic pain conditions. Some encouraging data have been reported regarding the effects of SCS in patients suffering from PHN. In a case series of 28 patients (4 patients had herpes zoster and 24 patients had PHN), the effect of SCS was studied prospectively. Long-term relief was obtained in 82% of the patients with PHN.[90] Patients served as their own controls by intermittently switching their spinal cord stimulator off and then monitoring themselves for the reappearance of pain. This is an interesting case series, but confirmation of the benefit of SCS in PHN patients will require further studies with the inclusion of a formal control group. There have been case series supporting the use of temporary SCS for the treatment of subacute PHN in those who failed to respond to medication or other intervention techniques.[205,206] Also, SCS may be a viable option for those who cannot tolerate analgesics due to comorbidities such as chronic kidney disease.[207] Use of deep brain stimulation (DBS) has been studied in a series of 11 patients with PHN. Four out of 11 patients were considered responders.[208] Given the extent of resources, expertise needed and low quality of the available evidence, use of these therapies should be reserved for use only in patients with intractable symptoms.

An exciting development in this field could be the targeted DRG stimulation for the management of intractable PHN pain. A specially designed SCS system that has flexible small-diameter leads has been developed, allowing electrodes to be placed via standard percutaneous placement under fluoroscopic guidance in the vicinity of involved DRG. Potential benefits of DRG neuromodulation relative to traditional SCS include better pain-paraesthesia concordance and decreased side effects like paraesthesias with changing body positions compared to the conventional SCS. The new device has been studied in patients with chronic neuropathic pain, and 1 year outcomes demonstrate similar efficacy as tradition SCS with the added benefit of more targeted and precise coverage.[209] It is too early to draw any strong conclusions about its efficacy in PHN patients, but it is an exciting new development in the field of neuromodulation.

Sympathetic Nerve Blocks

Sympathetic nerve blocks have been used for the treatment of both the acute pain of herpes zoster and the chronic pain associated with PHN. Unfortunately, there is little high-quality evidence supporting the use of this treatment in patients with PHN. Retrospective data indicate that these blocks may provide temporary pain relief. These studies reported that 41% to 50% of patients with PHN noted short-term relief following the injection, but the effectiveness waned over time based on long-term follow-up.[210] Of note, the most recent guidelines make a strong recommendation against the use of sympathetic blocks in the management of PHN pain.[83] Based on these guidelines and our clinical experience, we no longer use sympathetic blocks for treatment of PHN.

Neuraxial Blocks

Similar to the literature regarding sympathetic blockade, there are inadequate data to convincingly demonstrate that neuraxial therapy is both safe and effective for the routine treatment of PHN. One study has yielded encouraging results with the use of subarachnoid methylprednisolone,[211] but concerns regarding the failure to replicate these results and the association between this therapy and the development of adhesive arachnoiditis have precluded its routine use.

In clinical practice, epidural injections of both local anesthetic and steroids are used in patients with pain that has been refractory to conservative treatment. The authors will occasionally use continuous thoracic epidural analgesia with a home infusion pump for a period of 1 to 2 weeks in patients with intractable PHN pain for symptom palliation. We have observed this approach to be helpful for severe cases, but objective evidence for this therapy is lacking. It does require home nursing care and significant coordination of care by the treating physician. In general, it is reserved for the most severe cases.

PSYCHOLOGICAL INTERVENTIONS

PHN has been demonstrated to adversely affect overall quality of life by impairing physical and emotional functioning. Studies have shown that the degree of catastrophizing predicts the level of pain in elderly patients with PHN,[212] and this has been shown to be independent of depressive symptoms. There also has been work that shows an association between anxiety and depression and severity of pain in PHN.[120,213] Although the effects of cognitive-behavioral therapy and other psychosocial treatments have not been specifically studied in patients with PHN, it would seem logical and prudent to utilize these treatments on an individualized patient basis. There are ample data to support the use of these therapies in other chronic pain conditions, and it is reasonable to extrapolate this evidence of efficacy to the treatment of patients with PHN.

ELECTROANALGESIA

Transcutaneous Electrical Nerve Stimulation

There have been conflicting responses reported to transcutaneous electrical nerve stimulation (TENS) therapy in patients with PHN. There are a few small case series[214,215] that showed beneficial effects with use of this treatment, but other similar reports failed to demonstrate any benefit. However, when used in combination with pregabalin, it was found to be more beneficial than pregabalin + TENS placebo in a blinded randomized placebo-controlled trial.[216] TENS is still clinically offered to many patients on a trial basis given its safety profile. Those patients who have a favorable response to the trial therapy can procure a TENS device for more long-term use.

Scrambler Therapy

Scrambler therapy is a relatively novel and noninvasive technique that utilizes electrocutaneous stimulation to relieve pain. In theory, it works through replacing painful afferent input associated with chronic pain with nonpainful information.[217] The nonpainful information is generated by 10 electrodes working through five channels which act as artificial neurons. The output from the artificial neurons is highly variable and difficult for the existing pain pathways to interpret, hence the name, scrambler. It is believed to accomplish this through activation of cutaneous nerves resulting in the synthetic nonpainful information enhancing neuroplasticity, retraining the brain to feel no pain in previously painful areas, although the exact mechanism is still unclear. The therapy has shown significant benefit in small trials of patients with chemotherapy-induced peripheral neuropathy and other neuropathic pain conditions. However, the data on PHN are less robust but nonetheless promising.[217–219] The authors have also had positive results

treating a limited number of PHN patients. In order to better gain an understanding of the therapy and its potential benefit, further study with larger clinical trials is warranted.

Surgical Approaches

Multiple surgical approaches are described in the literature for the treatment of PHN. In general, these are quite drastic procedures with no proven long-term benefit. Surgical treatments are largely avoided given the limited literature to support their use, their potential for serious sequelae (including pain exceeding presurgical levels)[220] and the expanding list of safer and more efficacious options.

Prevention of Postherpetic Neuralgia

The prevention of PHN is obviously closely tied to the prevention of herpes zoster. Thus, the salutary effects of vaccines in preventing herpes zoster described earlier in this chapter apply to the prevention of PHN as well. The beneficial effects of antiviral medication in decreasing the severity but not necessarily occurrence of PHN have also been reviewed in the earlier discussion. These approaches are the mainstays in our arsenal to prevent PHN. There are only scant data to suggest any other therapies are genuinely helpful in preventing PHN.

A small, placebo-controlled, randomized trial evaluated the effect of 25 mg daily of amitriptyline initiated within 48 hours of rash onset in herpes zoster patients older than 60 years of age.[221] Treatment with amitriptyline was associated with a 50% decrease in pain prevalence 6 months after rash onset. These results should be confirmed in a trial that controls for the presence of antiviral therapy. Although treatment with amitriptyline may have a beneficial effect in reducing the incidence of PHN, its use should be weighed carefully against potential side effects in elderly or otherwise frail patients.

Use of other medications that are efficacious in PHN, such as gabapentin and pregabalin, may decrease the severity of acute pain in herpes zoster and possibly reduce the incidence of PHN beyond what can be achieved by antiviral therapy alone. There are promising data in animal experiments to support this hypothesis, and results of a single-dose trial of gabapentin versus placebo demonstrated a reduction in acute pain in patients with herpes zoster.[75]

Two double-blind, randomized, controlled trials of corticosteroids given for a 21-day duration in herpes zoster did not show any effect on the incidence or duration of PHN.[80,81] The findings from these studies have been corroborated by a more contemporary Cochrane review which found moderate quality evidence that oral corticosteroids do not prevent PHN 6 months after herpes zoster.[222] Therefore, the currently available data do not support the routine use of corticosteroids as a strategy to prevent PHN.

The use of sympathetic blocks has been used for acute pain in herpes zoster, and uncontrolled studies have claimed a reduction in the development of PHN.[223,224] Other studies, however, failed to replicate this effect.[225] There may be some benefit in reducing PHN occurrence by applying local anesthetic and corticosteroids via the epidural route[85] and paravertebral route (in addition to antiviral treatment and analgesics) during acute zoster, either in a series of injections (every 48 hours for 1 week)[86] or as a single injection.[226]

However, these findings have yet to be replicated. Because the pain of herpes zoster and PHN improves over time as part of their natural history, a control group is critically important in any study of the effects of these and other treatments intended to reduce the incidence and duration of pain. Thus, currently available uncontrolled studies are inadequate to definitively support the routine use of blocks as a strategy for preventing PHN. In clinical practice, injections are still used for pain management in patients who are refractory to conservative therapy. This is empirically recommended by some authors with the rationale that better pain control in the acute phase of herpes zoster is an important clinical objective in its own right and may also favorably affect the likelihood of developing PHN.

Conclusions

Herpes zoster and its most common complication, PHN, affect millions of people annually. Their epidemiology is expected to change in complex and potentially unpredictable ways as a result of the implementation of varicella and zoster vaccination programs. Nevertheless, it is difficult to imagine a complete disappearance of these challenging conditions in the near future. Hence, there is a need to develop improved strategies for the treatment of both herpes zoster and PHN. Ongoing research into the underlying mechanisms of these conditions will shape the direction of future treatments. For instance, a better understanding of the biologic factors that contribute to the transition from acute to chronic pain may guide us toward therapies that will facilitate a more rapid and complete recovery of infected neurons. Genomic research also has the potential to guide us to new therapies.[227] Identification of patient subtypes by phenotyping may result in finding new mechanism-based treatment options in addition to identification of patients who have a better chance of responding to conventional therapies than others.[1-4]

For now, clinicians should treat herpes zoster with antiviral therapy and analgesic medications. Corticosteroids should not be routinely prescribed but can be considered in special circumstances, such as patients with ophthalmic involvement, associated motor deficits, or severe acute pain. Supplemental therapy with tricyclic antidepressants, gabapentin or pregabalin, and neural blockade can be considered in refractory cases where more conservative therapy has failed, although the evidence base for these treatments is weak.[68] The treatment of PHN is likely to be an ongoing challenge, at least into the near future. At the present time, there is good evidence to support the use of some pharmacologic therapies, including tricyclic antidepressants, gabapentin and pregabalin, topical lidocaine patches, and high-dose capsaicin patches as well as opioid analgesics. The potential merits of each of these agents needs to be carefully balanced against each patient's ability to tolerate their side effects. This is a particularly salient consideration given that many patients with PHN are older or otherwise frail. Invasive modalities such as SCS may play an important role in the future, especially in patients with intractable pain. Further controlled clinical trials will be needed before this treatment approach can be recommended for widespread use. Finally, the role of patient and family education and psychological support cannot be overemphasized given that the currently available treatments will not be effective for all patients.

Our major treatment recommendations may be summarized as follows:

1. Primary varicella vaccine in children is recommended to prevent chicken pox, and this is also expected to ultimately decrease the incidence of herpes zoster and PHN as vaccinated children become adults and replace those with wild-type virus in the population.

2. Herpes zoster vaccination is recommended for older immunocompetent adults >60 years of age to decrease the incidence of herpes zoster and PHN and to reduce the overall BOI. The utility of a second "booster" dose of the live attenuated herpes zoster vaccine is currently being debated.

3. In the future, new vaccine preparations with greater and potentially more durable efficacy and increased availability to immunocompromised individuals will likely become available.

4. Patients with herpes zoster should be treated with antiviral therapy as rapidly as possible to hasten the rate of healing, minimize neural damage, decrease the pain caused by the acute infection, and decrease the incidence and duration of PHN.

5. Acetaminophen, NSAIDs, tricyclic antidepressants, dual reuptake inhibitor antidepressants, gabapentin and pregabalin, and opioid analgesics can be used in patients with herpes zoster to treat acute pain, although it is important to recognize that few studies have investigated the efficacy of such treatments.

6. Topical treatments such as lidocaine patch and high-dose capsaicin patch may be considered as first-line treatments in frail elderly patients because of a better safety and tolerability profile compared to systemic therapies.

7. Gabapentin, pregabalin, tricyclic antidepressants, selective SNRIs, topical lidocaine patches, high-dose capsaicin patch, tramadol, and strong opioid analgesics can be used for the treatment of PHN given their well-established efficacy in this and other chronic neuropathic pain conditions.

8. Early referral to a pain specialist should be considered in case of intractable symptoms.

References

1. Baron R, Maier C, Attal N, et al. Peripheral neuropathic pain: a mechanism-related organizing principle based on sensory profiles. *Pain* 2017;158:261–272.
2. Vollert J, Maier C, Attal N, et al. Stratifying patients with peripheral neuropathic pain based on sensory profiles: algorithm and sample size recommendations. *Pain* 2017;158:1446–1455.
3. Demant DT, Lund K, Vollert J, et al. The effect of oxcarbazepine in peripheral neuropathic pain depends on pain phenotype: a randomised, double-blind, placebo-controlled phenotype-stratified study. *Pain* 2014;155:2263–2273.
4. Demant DT, Lund K, Finnerup NB, et al. Pain relief with lidocaine 5% patch in localized peripheral neuropathic pain in relation to pain phenotype: a randomised, double-blind, and placebo-controlled, phenotype panel study. *Pain* 2015;156:2234–2244.
5. Head H, Campbell AW, Kennedy PG. The pathology of herpes zoster and its bearing on sensory localisation. *Rev Med Virol* 1997;7:131–143.
6. Denny-Brown D, Adams R, Fitzgerald P. Pathologic features of herpes zoster: a note on geniculate herpes. *Arch Neurol Psychiatry* 1944;51:216–231.
7. Dworkin RH, Nagasako EM, Johnson RW, et al. Acute pain in herpes zoster: the famciclovir database project. *Pain* 2001;94:113–119.
8. Haanpää M, Laippala P, Nurmikko T. Allodynia and pinprick hypesthesia in acute herpes zoster, and the development of postherpetic neuralgia. *J Pain Symptom Manage* 2000;20:50–58.
9. Arani RB, Soong SJ, Weiss HL, et al. Phase specific analysis of herpes zoster associated pain data: a new statistical approach. *Stat Med* 2001;20:2429–2439.
10. Ragozzino M, Melton L III, Kurland L, et al. Population-based study of herpes zoster and its sequelae. *Medicine (Baltimore)* 1982;61:310–316.
11. Liesegang TJ. Herpes zoster ophthalmicus: natural history, risk factors, clinical presentation, and morbidity. *Ophthalmology* 2008;115:S3–S12.
12. Ostler HB, Thygeson P. The ocular manifestations of herpes zoster, varicella, infectious mononucleosis, and cytomegalovirus disease. *Surv Ophthalmol* 1976;21:148–159.
13. Gilden DH, Dueland AN, Devlin ME, et al. Varicella-zoster virus reactivation without rash. *J Infect Dis* 1992;166:S30–S34.
14. Lewis G. Zoster sine herpete. *Br Med J* 1958;2:418–421.
15. Loparev VN, McCaustland K, Holloway BP, et al. Rapid genotyping of varicella-zoster virus vaccine and wild-type strains with fluorophore-labeled hybridization probes. *J Clin Microbiol* 2000;38:4315–4319.
16. Yawn BP, Saddier P, Wollan PC, et al. A population-based study of the incidence and complication rates of herpes zoster before zoster vaccine introduction. *Mayo Clin Proc* 2007;82:1341–1349.
17. Harpaz R, Ortega-Sanchez IR, Seward JF. Prevention of herpes zoster: recommendations of the Advisory Committee on Immunization Practices (ACIP). *MMWR Recomm Rep* 2008;57:1–30.
18. Kawai K, Gebremeskel BG, Acosta CJ. Systematic review of incidence and complications of herpes zoster: towards a global perspective. *BMJ Open* 2014;4:e004833.
19. Johnson BH, Palmer L, Gatwood J, et al. Annual incidence rates of herpes zoster among an immunocompetent population in the United States. *BMC Infect Dis* 2015;15:502.
20. Weinberg A, Lazar AA, Zerbe GO, et al. Influence of age and nature of primary infection on varicella-zoster virus specific cell-mediated immune responses. *J Infect Dis* 2010;201:1024–1030.
21. Hope-Simpson RE. The nature of herpes zoster: a long-term study and a new hypothesis. *Proc R Soc Med* 1965;58:9–20.

22. Opstelten W, Van Essen GA, Schellevis F, et al. Gender as an independent risk factor for herpes zoster: a population-based prospective study. *Ann Epidemiol* 2006;16:692–695.
23. Leung J, Harpaz R, Baughman AL, et al. Evaluation of laboratory methods for diagnosis of varicella. *Clin Infect Dis* 2010;51:23–32.
24. Weitzman D, Shavit O, Stein M, et al. A population based study of the epidemiology of herpes zoster and its complications. *J Infect* 2013;67:463–469.
25. Russell ML, Dover DC, Simmonds KA, et al. Shingles in Alberta: before and after publicly funded varicella vaccination. *Vaccine* 2014;32:6319–6324.
26. Gnann JW, Whitley RJ. Clinical practice: herpes zoster. *N Engl J Med* 2002;347:340–346.
27. Chen SY, Suaya JA, Li Q, et al. Incidence of herpes zoster in patients with altered immune function. *Infection* 2014;42:325–334.
28. Yawn BP, Wollan PC, Kurland MJ, et al. Herpes zoster recurrences more frequent than previously reported. *Mayo Clin Proc* 2011;86:88–93.
29. Schmader K, George LK, Burchett BM, et al. Racial differences in the occurrence of herpes zoster. *J Infect Dis* 1995;171:701–704.
30. Thomas SL, Hall AJ. What does epidemiology tell us about risk factors for herpes zoster? *Lancet Infect Dis* 2004;4:26–33.
31. Zhang JX, Joesoef RM, Bialek S, et al. Association of physical trauma with risk of herpes zoster among medicare beneficiaries in United States. *J Infect Dis* 2013:1007–1011.
32. Heymann A, Chodick G, Karpati T, et al. Diabetes as a risk factor for herpes zoster infection: results of a population-based study in Israel. *Infection* 2008;36:226–230.
33. Oxman MN, Levin MJ, Johnson GR, et al. A vaccine to prevent herpes zoster and postherpetic neuralgia in older adults. *N Engl J Med* 2005;352:2271–2284.
34. Thomas SL, Wheeler JG, Hall AJ. Contacts with varicella or with children and protection against herpes zoster in adults: a case-control study. *Lancet* 2002;360:678–682.
35. Goldman GS. Universal varicella vaccination: efficacy trends and effect on herpes zoster. *Int J Toxicol* 2005;24:205–213.
36. Brisson M, Gay N, Edmunds W, et al. Exposure to varicella boosts immunity to herpes-zoster: implications for mass vaccination against chickenpox. *Vaccine* 2002;20:2500–2507.
37. Schuette MC, Hethcote HW. Modeling the effects of varicella vaccination programs on the incidence of chickenpox and shingles. *Bull Math Biol* 1999;61:1031–1064.
38. Edmunds W, Brisson M. The effect of vaccination on the epidemiology of varicella zoster virus. *J Infect* 2002;44:211–219.
39. Holmes SJ. Review of recommendations of the Advisory Committee on Immunization Practices, Centers for Disease Control and Prevention, on varicella vaccine. *J Infect Dis* 1996;174:S342–S344.
40. Leung J, Harpaz R, Molinari NA, et al. Herpes zoster incidence among insured persons in the United States, 1993–2006: evaluation of impact of varicella vaccination. *Clin Infect Dis* 2011;52:332–340.
41. Hales CM, Harpaz R, Joesoef MR, et al. Examination of links between herpes zoster incidence and childhood varicella vaccination. *Ann Intern Med* 2013;159:739–745.
42. Kawai K, Yawn BP, Wollan P, et al. Increasing incidence of herpes zoster over 60-year period from a population-based study. *Clin Infect Dis* 2016:221–226.
43. Civen R, Marin M, Zhang J, et al. Update on incidence of herpes zoster among children and adolescents after implementation of varicella vaccination, Antelope Valley, CA, 2000 to 2010. *Pediatr Infect Dis J* 2016;35:1132–1136.
44. Arvin A. Aging, immunity, and the varicella-zoster virus. *N Engl J Med* 2005;352:2266–2667.
45. Oaklander AL. The pathology of shingles: Head and Campbell's 1900 monograph. *Arch Neurol* 1999;56:1292–1294.
46. Haanpää M, Häkkinen V, Nurmikko T. Motor involvement in acute herpes zoster. *Muscle Nerve* 1997;20:1433–1438.
47. Echevarria JM, Casas I, Martinez-Martin P. Infections of the nervous system caused by varicella-zoster virus: a review. *Intervirology* 1997;40:72–84.
48. Jemsek J, Greenberg SB, Taber L, et al. Herpes zoster-associated encephalitis: clinicopathologic report of 12 cases and review of the literature. *Medicine (Baltimore)* 1983;62:81–97.
49. Elliott KJ. Other neurological complications of herpes zoster and their management. *Ann Neurol* 1994;35:S57–S61.
50. Verghese A, Sugar AM. Herpes zoster ophthalmicus and granulomatous angiitis: an ill-appreciated cause of stroke. *J Am Geriatr Soc* 1986;34:309–312.
51. Moriuchi H, Rodriguez W. Role of varicella-zoster virus in stroke syndromes. *Pediatr Infect Dis J* 2000;19:648–653.
52. Kang JH, Sheu JJ, Lin HC. Increased risk of Guillain-Barré syndrome following recent herpes zoster: a population-based study across Taiwan. *Clin Infect Dis* 2010;51:525–530.
53. Johnson RW, Bouhassira D, Kassianos G, et al. The impact of herpes zoster and post-herpetic neuralgia on quality-of-life. *BMC Med* 2010;8:37.
54. Chidiac C, Bruxelle J, Daures J-P, et al. Characteristics of patients with herpes zoster on presentation to practitioners in France. *Clin Infect Dis* 2001;33:62–69.
55. Coplan PM, Schmader K, Nikas A, et al. Development of a measure of the burden of pain due to herpes zoster and postherpetic neuralgia for prevention trials: adaptation of the brief pain inventory. *J Pain* 2004;5:344–356.
56. Katz J, Cooper EM, Walther RR, et al. Acute pain in herpes zoster and its impact on health-related quality of life. *Clin Infect Dis* 2004;39:342–348.
57. Lydick E, Epstein RS, Himmelberger D, et al. Herpes zoster and quality of life: a self-limited disease with severe impact. *Neurology* 1995;45:S52–S53.
58. Mauskopf J, Austin R, Dix L, et al. The Nottingham Health Profile as a measure of quality of life in zoster patients: convergent and discriminant validity. *Qual Life Res* 1994;3:431–435.
59. Levin MJ, Gershon AA, Dworkin RH, et al. Prevention strategies for herpes zoster and post-herpetic neuralgia. *J Clin Virol* 2010;48:S14–S19.
60. Parruti G, Tontodonati M, Rebuzzi C, et al. Predictors of pain intensity and persistence in a prospective Italian cohort of patients with herpes zoster: relevance of smoking, trauma and antiviral therapy. *BMC Med* 2010;11(8):58.
61. Pica F, Gatti A, Divizia M, et al. One-year follow-up of patients with long-lasting post-herpetic neuralgia. *BMC Infect Dis* 2014;14:556.
62. Wood M, Kay R, Dworkin R, et al. Oral acyclovir therapy accelerates pain resolution in patients with herpes zoster: a meta-analysis of placebo-controlled trials. *Clin Infect Dis* 1996;22:341–347.
63. Jackson JL, Gibbons R, Meyer G, et al. The effect of treating herpes zoster with oral acyclovir in preventing postherpetic neuralgia: a meta-analysis. *Arch Intern Med* 1997;157:909–912.
64. Crooks RJ, Jones DA, Fiddian AP. Zoster-associated chronic pain: an overview of clinical trials with acyclovir. *Scand J Infect Dis Suppl* 1991;80:62–68.
65. Dworkin RH, Johnson RW, Breuer J, et al. Recommendations for the management of herpes zoster. *Clin Infect Dis* 2007;44:S1–S26.
66. Decroix J, Partsch H, Gonzalez R, et al. Factors influencing pain outcome in herpes zoster: an observational study with valaciclovir. *J Eur Acad Dermatol Venereol* 2000;14:23–33.
67. Kurokawa I, Kumano K, Murakawa K, et al. Clinical correlates of prolonged pain in Japanese patients with acute herpes zoster. *J Int Med Res* 2002;30:56–65.
68. Zaal M, Völker-Dieben H, Wienesen M, et al. Longitudinal analysis of varicella-zoster virus DNA on the ocular surface associated with herpes zoster ophthalmicus. *Am J Ophthalmol* 2001;131:25–29.
69. Degreef H. Famciclovir, a new oral antiherpes drug: results of the first controlled clinical study demonstrating its efficacy and safety in the treatment of uncomplicated herpes zoster in immunocompetent patients. *Int J Antimicrob Agents* 1994;4:241–246.
70. Beutner KR, Friedman DJ, Forszpaniak C, et al. Valaciclovir compared with acyclovir for improved therapy for herpes zoster in immunocompetent adults. *Antimicrob Agents Chemother* 1995;39:1546–1553.
71. Wassilew SW, Wutzler P. Oral brivudin in comparison with acyclovir for herpes zoster: a survey study on postherpetic neuralgia. *Antiviral Res* 2003;59:57–60.
72. Dworkin RH, Perkins FM, Nagasako EM. Prospects for the prevention of postherpetic neuralgia in herpes zoster patients. *Clin J Pain* 2000;16:S90–S100.
73. Dworkin RH, Schmader KE, Goldstein EJ. Treatment and prevention of postherpetic neuralgia. *Clin Infect Dis* 2003;36:877–882.
74. Dworkin RH, Barbano RL, Tyring SK, et al. A randomized, placebo-controlled trial of oxycodone and of gabapentin for acute pain in herpes zoster. *Pain* 2009;142:209–217.
75. Berry JD, Petersen KL. A single dose of gabapentin reduces acute pain and allodynia in patients with herpes zoster. *Neurology* 2005;65:444–447.
76. Hempenstall K, Nurmikko TJ, Johnson RW, et al. Analgesic therapy in postherpetic neuralgia: a quantitative systematic review. *PLoS Med* 2005;2(7):e164.
77. Dahl JB, Mathiesen O, Møiniche S. Protective premedication: an option with gabapentin and related drugs? *Acta Anaesthesiol Scand* 2004;48:1130–1136.
78. Rowbotham MC, Goli V, Kunz NR, et al. Venlafaxine extended release in the treatment of painful diabetic neuropathy: a double-blind, placebo-controlled study. *Pain* 2004;110:697–706.
79. Goldstein DJ, Lu Y, Detke MJ, et al. Duloxetine vs. placebo in patients with painful diabetic neuropathy. *Pain* 2005;116:109–118.
80. Wood MJ, Johnson RW, McKendrick MW, et al. A randomized trial of acyclovir for 7 days or 21 days with and without prednisolone for treatment of acute herpes zoster. *N Engl J Med* 1994;330:896–900.
81. Whitley RJ, Weiss H, Gnann Jr JW, et al. Acyclovir with and without prednisone for the treatment of herpes zoster: a randomized, placebo-controlled trial. *Ann Intern Med* 1996;125:376–383.
82. Lin P-L, Fan S-Z, Huang C-H, et al. Analgesic effect of lidocaine patch 5% in the treatment of acute herpes zoster: a double-blind and vehicle-controlled study. *Reg Anesth Pain Med* 2008;33:320–325.
83. Dworkin RH, O'Connor AB, Kent J, et al. Interventional management of neuropathic pain: NeuPSIG recommendations. *Pain* 2013;154:2249–2261.
84. van Wijck AJ, Opstelten W, Moons KG, et al. The PINE study of epidural steroids and local anaesthetics to prevent postherpetic neuralgia: a randomised controlled trial. *Lancet* 2006;367:219–224.
85. Pasqualucci A, Pasqualucci V, Galla F, et al. Prevention of post-herpetic neuralgia: acyclovir and prednisolone versus epidural local anesthetic and methylprednisolone. *Acta Anaesthesiol Scand* 2000;44:910–918.
86. Ji G, Niu J, Shi Y, et al. The effectiveness of repetitive paravertebral injections with local anesthetics and steroids for the prevention of postherpetic neuralgia in patients with acute herpes zoster. *Anesth Analg* 2009;109:1651–1655.
87. Kim HJ, Ahn HS, Lee JY, et al. Effects of applying nerve blocks to prevent postherpetic neuralgia in patients with acute herpes zoster: a systematic review and meta-analysis. *Korean J Pain* 2017;30:3–17.
88. Jang YH, Lee JS, Kim SL, et al. Do interventional pain management procedures during the acute phase of herpes zoster prevent postherpetic neuralgia in the elderly?: a meta-analysis of randomized controlled trials. *Ann Dermatol* 2015;27:771–774.

89. Ursini T, Tontodonati M, Manzoli L, et al. Acupuncture for the treatment of severe acute pain in herpes zoster: results of a nested, open-label, randomized trial in the VZV Pain Study. *BMC Complement Altern Med* 2011;11:46.

90. Harke H, Gretenkort P, Ladleif HU, et al. Spinal cord stimulation in postherpetic neuralgia and in acute herpes zoster pain. *Anesth Analg* 2002; 94:694–700.

91. Marin M, Broder KR, Temte JL, et al. Use of combination measles, mumps, rubella, and varicella vaccine: recommendations of the Advisory Committee on Immunization Practices (ACIP). *MMWR Recomm Rep* 2010;59:1–12.

92. Bapat P, Koren G. The role of VariZIG in pregnancy. *Expert Rev Vaccines* 2013;12:1243–1248.

93. Gnann JW. Vaccination to prevent herpes zoster in older adults. *J Pain* 2008;9:31–36.

94. Schmader K, Oxman M, Levin M, et al. Persistence of the efficacy of zoster vaccine in the shingles prevention study and the short-term persistence substudy. *Clin Infect Dis* 2012;55:1320–1328.

95. Morrison VA, Johnson GR, Schmader KE, et al. Long-term persistence of zoster vaccine efficacy. *Clin Infect Dis* 2015;60:900–909.

96. Tseng HF, Harpaz R, Luo Y, et al. Declining effectiveness of herpes zoster vaccine in adults aged ≥ 60 years. *J Infect Dis* 2016;213:1872–1875.

97. Levin MJ, Schmader KE, Pang L, et al. Cellular and humoral responses to a second dose of herpes zoster vaccine administered 10 years after the first dose among older adults. *J Infect Dis* 2016;213:14–22.

98. Lal H, Cunningham AL, Godeaux O, et al. Efficacy of an adjuvanted herpes zoster subunit vaccine in older adults. *N Engl J Med* 2015;372:2087–2096.

99. Cunningham AL, Lal H, Kovac M, et al. Efficacy of the herpes zoster subunit vaccine in adults 70 years of age or older. *N Engl J Med* 2016;375:1019–1032.

100. Dworkin RH, Gnann JW, Oaklander AL, et al. Diagnosis and assessment of pain associated with herpes zoster and postherpetic neuralgia. *J Pain* 2008; 9:37–44.

101. Maier C, Baron R, Tölle TR, et al. Quantitative sensory testing in the German Research Network on Neuropathic Pain (DFNS): somatosensory abnormalities in 1236 patients with different neuropathic pain syndromes. *Pain* 2010;150:439–450.

102. Bowsher DM. Pathophysiology of postherpetic neuralgia towards a rational treatment. *Neurology* 1995;45:S56–S57.

103. Rowbotham MC, Fields HL. The relationship of pain, allodynia and thermal sensation in post-herpetic neuralgia. *Brain* 1996;119:347–354.

104. Watson CP, Watt VR, Chipman M, et al. The prognosis with postherpetic neuralgia. *Pain* 1991;46:195–199.

105. Dworkin RH, Schmader KE. Epidemiology and natural history of herpes zoster and postherpetic neuralgia. In: Watson CP, Gershon AA, eds. *Herpes Zoster and Postherpetic Neuralgia.* 2nd ed. New York: Elsevier; 2001:39–64.

106. Dworkin RH, Portenoy RK. Pain and its persistence in herpes zoster. *Pain* 1996;67:241–251.

107. Drolet M, Brisson M, Schmader KE, et al. The impact of herpes zoster and postherpetic neuralgia on health-related quality of life: a prospective study. *Can Med Assoc J* 2010;182:1731–1736.

108. Serpell M, Gater A, Carroll S, et al. Burden of post-herpetic neuralgia in a sample of UK residents aged 50 years or older: findings from the Zoster Quality of Life (ZQOL) study. *Health Qual Life Outcomes* 2014;12:92.

109. Dworkin RH, Malone DC, Panarites CJ, et al. Impact of postherpetic neuralgia and painful diabetic peripheral neuropathy on health care costs. *J Pain* 2010;11:360–368.

110. Meyers JL, Madhwani S, Rausch D, et al. Analysis of real-world health care costs among immunocompetent patients aged 50 years or older with herpes zoster in the United States. *Hum Vaccin Immunother* 2017;13:1861–1872.

111. Bennett G. Neuropathic pain: an overview. In: Borsook D, ed. *Molecular Neurobiology of Pain.* Seattle, WA: IASP Press; 1997:109–113.

112. Bowsher D. The lifetime occurrence of Herpes zoster and prevalence of post-herpetic neuralgia: a retrospective survey in an elderly population. *Eur J Pain* 1999;3:335–342.

113. Friesen KJ, Chateau D, Falk J, et al. Cost of shingles: population based burden of disease analysis of herpes zoster and postherpetic neuralgia. *BMC Infect Dis* 2017;17:69.

114. Rampakakis E, Pollock C, Vujacich C, et al. Economic burden of herpes zoster ("culebrilla") in Latin America. *Int J Infect Dis* 2017;58:22–26.

115. Yamada K, Iso H. Stressful life events are a risk factor for postherpetic neuralgia development but not for herpes zoster incidence: a population-based cohort study among Japanese older adults. *J Pain* 2016;17:S9–S10.

116. Helgason S, Petursson G, Gudmundsson S, et al. Prevalence of postherpetic neuralgia after a first episode of herpes zoster: prospective study with long term follow up. *BMJ* 2000;321:794.

117. Sato K, Adachi K, Nakamura H, et al. Burden of herpes zoster and postherpetic neuralgia in Japanese adults 60 years of age or older: results from an observational, prospective, physician practice-based cohort study. *J Dermatol* 2017;44:414–422.

118. De Moragas JM, Kierland RR. The outcome of patients with herpes zoster. *Arch Dermatol* 1957;75:193–196.

119. Kost RG, Straus SE. Postherpetic neuralgia—pathogenesis, treatment, and prevention. *N Engl J Med* 1996;335:32–42.

120. Drolet M, Brisson M, Schmader K, et al. Predictors of postherpetic neuralgia among patients with herpes zoster: a prospective study. *J Pain* 2010;11: 1211–1221.

121. Dworkin RH, Boon RJ, Griffin DR, et al. Postherpetic neuralgia: impact of famciclovir, age, rash severity, and acute pain in herpes zoster patients. *J Infect Dis* 1998;178:S76–S80.

122. McKendrick MW, Ogan P, Care CC. A 9 year follow up of post herpetic neuralgia and predisposing factors in elderly patients following herpes zoster. *J Infect* 2009;59:416–420.

123. Forbes HJ, Thomas SL, Smeeth L, et al. A systematic review and meta-analysis of risk factors for postherpetic neuralgia. *Pain* 2016;157:30–54.

124. Dworkin RH, Portenoy RK. Proposed classification of herpes zoster pain. *Lancet* 1994;343:1648.

125. Choo PW, Galil K, Donahue JG, et al. Risk factors for postherpetic neuralgia. *Arch Intern Med* 1997;157:1217–1224.

126. Jung BF, Johnson RW, Griffin DR, et al. Risk factors for postherpetic neuralgia in patients with herpes zoster. *Neurology* 2004;62:1545–1551.

127. Baron R, Haendler G, Schulte H. Afferent large fiber polyneuropathy predicts the development of postherpetic neuralgia. *Pain* 1997;73:231–238.

128. McCulloch D, Fraser D, Duncan L. Shingles in diabetes mellitus. *Practitioner* 1982;226:531–532.

129. Watson C, Deck J, Morshead C, et al. Post-herpetic neuralgia: further post-mortem studies of cases with and without pain. *Pain* 1991;44:105–117.

130. Rowbotham MC, Yosipovitch G, Connolly MK, et al. Cutaneous innervation density in the allodynic form of postherpetic neuralgia. *Neurobiol Dis* 1996;3:205–214.

131. Oaklander AL, Romans K, Horasek S, et al. Unilateral postherpetic neuralgia is associated with bilateral sensory neuron damage. *Ann Neurol* 1998;44:789–795.

132. Oaklander AL. The density of remaining nerve endings in human skin with and without postherpetic neuralgia after shingles. *Pain* 2001;92:139–145.

133. Bennett GJ. Hypotheses on the pathogenesis of herpes zoster associated pain. *Ann Neurol* 1994;35:S38–S41.

134. Scholz J, Broom DC, Kohno T, et al. Animal models of neuropathic pain induce apoptosis and a loss of GABAergic inhibition in the spinal dorsal horn. In: Dostrovsky JO, Carr DB, Koltzenburg M, eds. *Proceedings of the 10th World Congress on Pain.* Seattle, WA: IASP Press; 2003:387–395.

135. Petersen KL, Rowbotham MC. Natural history of sensory function after herpes zoster. *Pain* 2010;150:83–92.

136. Fields HL, Rowbotham M, Baron R. Postherpetic neuralgia: irritable nociceptors and deafferentation. *Neurobiol Dis* 1998;5:209–227.

137. Rowbotham MC, Petersen KL, Fields HL. Is postherpetic neuralgia more than one disorder? *Pain Forum* 1998;7:231–237.

138. Peng WW, Guo XL, Jin QQ, et al. Biological mechanism of postherpetic neuralgia: evidence from multiple patho-psychophysiological measures. *Eur J Pain* 2017;21:827–842.

139. Inomata Y, Gouda M, Kagaya K, et al. Association of denervation severity in the dermis with the development of mechanical allodynia and hyperalgesia in a murine model of postherpetic neuralgia. *Anesth Analg* 2013;116:722–729.

140. Bowsher D. Sensory change in postherpetic neuralgia. In: Watson CP, ed. *Herpes Zoster and Postherpetic Neuralgia.* Amsterdam, The Netherlands: Elsevier; 1993:97–103.

141. Baron R, Saguer M. Postherpetic neuralgia: are c-nociceptors involved in signalling and maintenance of tactile allodynia? *Brain* 1993;116: 1477–1496.

142. Baron R, Saguer M. Mechanical allodynia in postherpetic neuralgia: evidence for central mechanisms depending on nociceptive c-fiber degeneration. *Neurology* 1995;45:S63–S65.

143. Petersen KL, Fields HL, Brennum J, et al. Capsaicin evoked pain and allodynia in post-herpetic neuralgia. *Pain* 2000;88:125–133.

144. Wasner G, Kleinert A, Binder A, et al. Postherpetic neuralgia: topical lidocaine is effective in nociceptor–deprived skin. *J Neurol* 2005;252:677–686.

145. Reda H, Greene K, Rice FL, et al. Natural history of herpes zoster: late follow-up of 3.9 years (n = 43) and 7.7 years (n = 10). *Pain* 2013;154: 2227–2233.

146. Finnerup NB, Otto M, McQuay H, et al. Algorithm for neuropathic pain treatment: an evidence based proposal. *Pain* 2005;118:289–305.

147. Dworkin RH, Backonja M, Rowbotham MC, et al. Advances in neuropathic pain: diagnosis, mechanisms, and treatment recommendations. *Arch Neurol* 2003;60:1524–1534.

148. Attal N, Cruccu G, Haanpää M, et al. EFNS guidelines on pharmacological treatment of neuropathic pain. *Eur J Neurol* 2006;13:1153–1169.

149. Dworkin RH, O'Connor AB, Backonja M, et al. Pharmacologic management of neuropathic pain: evidence-based recommendations. *Pain* 2007;132:237–251.

150. Finnerup NB, Attal N, Haroutounian S, et al. Pharmacotherapy for neuropathic pain in adults: a systematic review and meta-analysis. *Lancet Neurol* 2015;14:162–173.

151. Dworkin RH, O'Connor AB, Audette J, et al. Recommendations for the pharmacological management of neuropathic pain: an overview and literature update. *Mayo Clin Proc* 2010;85:S3–S14.

152. Dworkin RH, Panarites CJ, Armstrong EP, et al. Is treatment of postherpetic neuralgia in the community consistent with evidence-based recommendations? *Pain* 2012;153:869–875.

153. Rowbotham M, Harden N, Stacey B, et al. Gabapentin for the treatment of postherpetic neuralgia: a randomized controlled trial. *JAMA* 1998;280: 1837–1842.

154. Rice AS, Maton S. Gabapentin in postherpetic neuralgia: a randomised, double blind, placebo controlled study. *Pain* 2001;94:215–224.

155. Bennett MI, Simpson KH. Gabapentin in the treatment of neuropathic pain. *Palliat Med* 2004;18:5–11.

156. Maneuf Y, Gonzalez M, Sutton K, et al. Cellular and molecular action of the putative GABA-mimetic, gabapentin. *Cell Mol Life Sci* 2003;60:742–750.

157. Backonja M, Glanzman RL. Gabapentin dosing for neuropathic pain: evidence from randomized, placebo-controlled clinical trials. *Clin Ther* 2003; 25:81–104.

158. Sang C, Sathyanarayana R, Sweeney M. Once-daily gabapentin for the treatment of postherpetic neuralgia. *Clin J Pain* 2013;29:281–288.

159. Zhang L, Rainka M, Freeman R, et al. A randomized, double-blind, placebo-controlled trial to assess the efficacy and safety of gabapentin enacarbil in subjects with neuropathic pain associated with postherpetic neuralgia (PXN110748). *J Pain* 2013;14:590–603.

160. Frampton JE, Foster RH. Pregabalin for the treatment of postherpetic neuralgia. *Drugs* 2005;65:111–118.

161. Dworkin RH, Corbin AE, Young JP, et al. Pregabalin for the treatment of postherpetic neuralgia: a randomized, placebo-controlled trial. *Neurology* 2003;60:1274–1283.

162. Freynhagen R, Strojek K, Griesing T, et al. Efficacy of pregabalin in neuropathic pain evaluated in a 12-week, randomised, double-blind, multicentre, placebo-controlled trial of flexible-and fixed-dose regimens. *Pain* 2005;115:254–263.

163. Montgomery SA, Tobias K, Zornberg GL, et al. Efficacy and safety of pregabalin in the treatment of generalized anxiety disorder: a 6-week, multicenter, randomized, double-blind, placebo-controlled comparison of pregabalin and venlafaxine. *J Clin Psychiatry* 2006;67:771–782.

164. Rickels K, Pollack MH, Feltner DE, et al. Pregabalin for treatment of generalized anxiety disorder: a 4-week, multicenter, double-blind, placebo-controlled trial of pregabalin and alprazolam. *Arch Gen Psychiatry* 2005; 62:1022–1030.

165. Huffman CL, Goldenberg JN, Weintraub J, et al. Efficacy and safety of once-daily controlled-release pregabalin for the treatment of patients with postherpetic neuralgia: a double-blind, enriched enrollment randomized withdrawal, placebo-controlled trial. *Clin J Pain* 2017;33:569–578.

166. Dick IE, Brochu RM, Purohit Y, et al. Sodium channel blockade may contribute to the analgesic efficacy of antidepressants. *J Pain* 2007;8:315–324.

167. Offenbaecher M, Ackenheil M. Current trends in neuropathic pain treatments with special reference to fibromyalgia. *CNS Spectr* 2005;10:285–297.

168. Guay DR. Adjunctive agents in the management of chronic pain. *Pharmacotherapy* 2001;21:1070–1081.

169. Watson CP, Vernich L, Chipman M, et al. Nortriptyline versus amitriptyline in postherpetic neuralgia: a randomized trial. *Neurology* 1998;51:1166–1171.

170. Sindrup SH, Jensen TS. Efficacy of pharmacological treatments of neuropathic pain: an update and effect related to mechanism of drug action. *Pain* 1999;83:389–400.

171. Rowbotham MC, Reisner LA, Davies PS, et al. Treatment response in antidepressant-naive postherpetic neuralgia patients: a double-blind, randomized trial. *J Pain* 2005;6:741–746.

172. Sansone RA, Todd T, Meier BP. Pretreatment ECGs and the prescription of amitriptyline in an internal medicine clinic. *Psychosomatics* 2002;43:250–251.

173. Vieweg WV, Wood MA. Tricyclic antidepressants, QT interval prolongation, and torsade de pointes. *Psychosomatics* 2004;45:371–377.

174. Yasuda H, Hotta N, Nakao K, et al. Superiority of duloxetine to placebo in improving diabetic neuropathic pain: results of a randomized controlled trial in Japan. *J Diabetes Res* 2011;2:132–139.

175. Moulin D, Boulanger A, Clark A, et al. Pharmacological management of chronic neuropathic pain: revised consensus statement from the Canadian Pain Society. *Pain Res Manag* 2014;19:328–335.

176. Watson CP, Babul N. Efficacy of oxycodone in neuropathic pain: a randomized trial in postherpetic neuralgia. *Neurology* 1998;50:1837–1841.

177. Khoromi S, Cui L, Nackers L, et al. Morphine, nortriptyline and their combination vs. placebo in patients with chronic lumbar root pain. *Pain* 2007;130:66–75.

178. Gilron I, Bailey JM, Tu D, et al. Morphine, gabapentin, or their combination for neuropathic pain. *N Engl J Med* 2005;352:1324–1334.

179. Dowell D, Haegerich TM, Chou R. CDC guideline for prescribing opioids for chronic pain—United States, 2016. *MMWR Recomm Rep* 2016;65(RR-1):1–49. doi:10.15585/mmwr.rr6501e1.

180. Boureau F, Legallicier P, Kabir-Ahmadi M. Tramadol in post-herpetic neuralgia: a randomized, double-blind, placebo-controlled trial. *Pain* 2003;104:323–331.

181. Duehmke RM, Derry S, Wiffen PJ, et al. Tramadol for neuropathic pain in adults. *Cochrane Database Syst Rev* 2017;(6):CD003726.

182. Bush D. *Emergency Department Visits for Drug Misuse or Abuse Involving the Pain Medication Tramadol.* Rockville, MD: Substance Abuse and Mental Health Services Administration; 2013.

183. Price N, Namdari R, Neville J, et al. Safety and efficacy of a topical sodium channel inhibitor (TV-45070) in patients with postherpetic neuralgia (PHN): a randomized, controlled, proof-of-concept, crossover study, with a subgroup analysis of the Nav1.7 R1150W genotype. *Clin J Pain* 2017;33:310–318.

184. Galer BS, Rowbotham MC, Perander J, et al. Topical lidocaine patch relieves postherpetic neuralgia more effectively than a vehicle topical patch: results of an enriched enrollment study. *Pain* 1999;80:533–538.

185. Rowbotham MC, Davies PS, Verkempinck C, et al. Lidocaine patch: a double-blind controlled study of a new treatment method for postherpetic neuralgia. *Pain* 1996;65:39–44.

186. Meier T, Wasner G, Faust M, et al. Efficacy of lidocaine patch 5% in the treatment of focal peripheral neuropathic pain syndromes: a randomized, double-blind, placebo-controlled study. *Pain* 2003;106:151–158.

187. Gammaitoni AR, Alvarez NA, Galer BS. Safety and tolerability of the lidocaine patch 5%, a targeted peripheral analgesic: a review of the literature. *J Clin Pharmacol* 2003;43:111–117.

188. Rowbotham MC, Davies PS, Fields HL. Topical lidocaine gel relieves postherpetic neuralgia. *Ann Neurol* 1995;37:246–253.

189. Backonja M. High-concentration capsaicin for treatment of PHN and HIV neuropathy pain. *Eur J Pain* 2007;11:S40.

190. Derry S, Sven-Rice A, Cole P, et al. Topical capsaicin (high concentration) for chronic neuropathic pain in adults. *Cochrane Database Syst Rev* 2017;(2):CD007393.

191. Bernstein JE, Korman NJ, Bickers DR, et al. Topical capsaicin treatment of chronic postherpetic neuralgia. *J Am Acad Dermatol* 1989;21:265–270.

192. Watson CPN, Tyler K, Bickers D, et al. A randomized vehicle-controlled trial of topical capsaicin in the treatment of postherpetic neuralgia. *Clin Ther* 1993;15:510–510.

193. De Benedittis G, Lorenzetti A. Topical aspirin/diethyl ether mixture versus indomethacin and diclofenac/diethyl ether mixtures for acute herpetic neuralgia and postherpetic neuralgia: a double-blind crossover placebo-controlled study. *Pain* 1996;65:45–51.

194. Gilron I, Tu D, Holden RR, et al. Combination of morphine with nortriptyline for neuropathic pain. *Pain* 2015;156:1440–1448.

195. Chaparro LE, Wiffen PJ, Moore RA, et al. Combination pharmacotherapy for the treatment of neuropathic pain in adults. *Cochrane Database Syst Rev* 2012;(7):CD008943.

196. Eide PK, Jørum E, Stubhaug A, et al. Relief of post-herpetic neuralgia with the N-methyl-D-aspartic acid receptor antagonist ketamine: a double-blind, cross-over comparison with morphine and placebo. *Pain* 1994; 58:347–354.

197. Oh HM, Chung ME. Botulinum toxin for neuropathic pain: a review of the literature. *Toxins (Basel)* 2015;7:3127–3154.

198. Xiao L, Mackey S, Hui H, et al. Subcutaneous injection of botulinum toxin a is beneficial in postherpetic neuralgia. *Pain Med* 2010;11:1827–1833.

199. Apalla Z, Sotiriou E, Lallas A, et al. Botulinum toxin A in postherpetic neuralgia: a parallel, randomized, double-blind, single-dose, placebo-controlled trial. *Clin J Pain* 2013;29:857–864.

200. Attal N, de Andrade DC, Adam F, et al. Safety and efficacy of repeated injections of botulinum toxin A in peripheral neuropathic pain (BOT-NEP): a randomised, double-blind, placebo-controlled trial. *Lancet Neurol* 2016;15:555–565.

201. Kim Y, Lee C, Lee S, et al. Effect of pulsed radiofrequency for postherpetic neuralgia. *Acta Anaesthesiol Scand* 2008;52:1140–1143.

202. Kim K, Jo D, Kim E. Pulsed radiofrequency to the dorsal root ganglion in acute herpes zoster and postherpetic neuralgia. *Pain Physician* 2017; 20:E411.

203. County C, Yingwei W, Jiaotong S. Efficacy of pulsed radiofrequency in the treatment of thoracic postherpetic neuralgia from the angulus costae: a randomized, double-blinded, controlled trial. *Pain Physician* 2013;16:15–25.

204. Doi K, Nikai T, Sakura S, et al. Intercostal nerve block with 5% tetracaine for chronic pain syndromes. *J Clin Anesth* 2002;14:39–41.

205. Moriyama K. Effect of temporary spinal cord stimulation on postherpetic neuralgia in the thoracic nerve area. *Neuromodulation* 2009;12:39–43.

206. Iseki M, Morita Y, Nakamura Y, et al. Efficacy of limited-duration spinal cord stimulation for subacute postherpetic neuralgia. *Ann Acad Med Singapore* 2009;38:1004–1006.

207. Baek IY, Park JY, Kim HJ, et al. Spinal cord stimulation in the treatment of postherpetic neuralgia in patients with chronic kidney disease: a case series and review of the literature. *Korean J Pain* 2011;24:154–157.

208. Cruccu G, Aziz T, Garcia-Larrea L, et al. EFNS guidelines on neurostimulation therapy for neuropathic pain. *Eur J Neurol* 2007;14:952–970.

209. Liem L, Russo M, Huygen FJ, et al. One-year outcomes of spinal cord stimulation of the dorsal root ganglion in the treatment of chronic neuropathic pain. *Neuromodulation* 2015;18:41–49.

210. Kumar V, Krone K, Mathieu A. Neuraxial and sympathetic blocks in herpes zoster and postherpetic neuralgia: an appraisal of current evidence. *Reg Anesth Pain Med* 2004;29:454–461.

211. Kotani N, Kushikata T, Hashimoto H, et al. Intrathecal methylprednisolone for intractable postherpetic neuralgia. *N Engl J Med* 2000;343:1514–1519.

212. Haythornthwaite JA, Clark MR, Pappagallo M, et al. Pain coping strategies play a role in the persistence of pain in post-herpetic neuralgia. *Pain* 2003;106:453–460.

213. Schlereth T, Heiland A, Breimhorst M, et al. Association between pain, central sensitization and anxiety in postherpetic neuralgia. *Eur J Pain* 2015; 19:193–201.

214. Nathan P, Wall P. Treatment of post-herpetic neuralgia by prolonged electric stimulation. *Br Med J* 1974;3:645–647.

215. Haas L. Post-herpetic neuralgia, treatment and prevention. *Trans Ophthalmol Soc N Z* 1977;29:133.

216. Barbarisi M, Pace MC, Passavanti MB, et al. Pregabalin and transcutaneous electrical nerve stimulation for postherpetic neuralgia treatment. *Clin J Pain* 2010;26:567–572.

217. Marineo G, Iorno V, Gandini C, et al. Scrambler therapy may relieve chronic neuropathic pain more effectively than guideline-based drug management: results of a pilot, randomized, controlled trial. *J Pain Symptom Manage* 2012;43:87–95.

218. Ko YK, Lee HY, Lee WY. Clinical experiences on the effect of scrambler therapy for patients with postherpetic neuralgia. *Korean J Pain* 2013;26:98–101.

219. Smith TJ, Marineo G. Treatment of postherpetic pain with scrambler therapy, a patient-specific neurocutaneous electrical stimulation device [published online ahead of print July 8, 2013]. *Am J Hosp Palliat Care.* doi:10.1177/1049909113494002.

220. Petersen KL, Rice FL, Suess F, et al. Relief of post-herpetic neuralgia by surgical removal of painful skin. *Pain* 2002;98:119–126.

221. Bowsher D. The effects of pre-emptive treatment of postherpetic neuralgia with amitriptyline: a randomized, double-blind, placebo-controlled trial. *J Pain Symptom Manage* 1997;13:327–331.

222. Han Y, Zhang J, Chen N, et al. Corticosteroids for preventing postherpetic neuralgia. *Cochrane Database Syst Rev* 2013;(3):CD005582.

223. Colding A. The effect of regional sympathetic blocks in the treatment of herpes zoster: a survey of 300 cases. *Acta Anaesthesiol Scand* 1969;13:133–141.

224. Dan K, Higa K, Noda B. Nerve block for herpetic pain. In: Fields HL, Dubner R, Cervero F, eds. *Advances in Pain Research and Therapy.* New York: Raven; 1985:831–838.

225. Yanagida H, Suwa K, Corssen G. No prophylactic effect of early sympathetic blockade on postherpetic neuralgia. *Anesthesiology* 1987;66:73–75.

226. Makharita MY, Amr YM, El-Bayoumy Y. Single paravertebral injection for acute thoracic herpes zoster: a randomized controlled trial. *Pain Pract* 2015;15:229–235.

227. Shir Y, Zeltser R, Vatine J-J, et al. Correlation of intact sensibility and neuropathic pain-related behaviors in eight inbred and outbred rat strains and selection lines. *Pain* 2001;90:75–82.

CHAPTER 28

Central Pain States

NANNA BRIX FINNERUP and **SHARONA BEN-HAIM**

Central neuropathic pain or central pain is defined as "pain caused by a lesion or disease of the central somatosensory nervous system."[1] Central pain is well described in stroke, multiple sclerosis (MS), and spinal cord injury (SCI), with the latter involving both traumatic and disease-related injuries. Other conditions associated with central pain include brain trauma, brain tumors, and possibly pain in epilepsy and Parkinson's disease. Central pain often becomes chronic and may be disabling with a negative impact on quality of life, mood, sleep, and functioning. Treatment of central pain remains challenging. This chapter describes the diagnosis, clinical characteristics, assessment, mechanisms, and treatment of central pain.

Diagnosis

A grading system for defining the level of certainty as to how likely a given pain condition is neuropathic in nature was first published in 2008[2] and updated in 2016.[3] It follows the classical clinical diagnostic methods used in neurology, in that history, clinical examination, and diagnostic test consecutively add to the level of diagnostic certainty.[3] The grading system adapted for central pain is illustrated in Figure 28.1.

Central pain is suspected when the history suggests that the pain is related to a central nervous system (CNS) disorder and not to other causes such as spasms, fractures, inflammation, etc. Different pain questionnaires have been developed as screening tools using clusters of descriptors to identify the presence of neuropathic pain. These include the Neuropathic Pain Questionnaire (NPQ),[4] the Leeds Assessment of Neuropathic Symptoms and Signs (LANSS),[5] the Douleur Neuropathique en 4 Questions (DN4) questionnaire,[6] the painDETECT questionnaire,[7] the ID-Pain questionnaire,[8] and the Spinal Cord Injury Pain Instrument (SCIPI) developed for patients with SCI.[9] These screening tools may be useful in epidemiologic research, but they cannot be used alone for identifying central pain in the individual patient.[10,11]

The first level of the grading system is *possible* central pain (see Fig. 28.1). Two criteria need to be fulfilled for possible neuropathic pain: (1) There should be a history of a relevant CNS disorder and pain development at or after the onset of the CNS disorder. Following stroke, SCI, and other acute onset CNS disorders, the pain typically develops within months after the onset, but the onset of central pain may be delayed up to about 1 year after the incident.[11-13] (2) The pain distribution should be neuroanatomically plausible, which means that the pain should be distributed within the area of the body that is affected by the CNS disorder—either the complete affected area or a smaller or larger proportion.

The next level is *probable* central pain (see Fig. 28.1). This involves a clinical sensory examination and confirmation of sensory abnormalities in the same neuroanatomical location. Demonstration of sensory loss to one or more sensory modalities such as touch, pinprick, cold, and warmth compatible with the CNS lesion is essential. Positive sensory signs (e.g., dynamic or cold allodynia) should also be compatible with the CNS lesion. Sensory abnormalities are often present on clinical examination, but a more thorough examination using quantitative sensory testing may be necessary.[3,14]

The final level is *definite* central pain (see Fig. 28.1). This requires a diagnostic test that confirms the CNS lesion. This often includes a computed tomography (CT) or magnetic resonance imaging (MRI) scan of the brain in patients with stroke, MS, SCI, or other CNS lesion. Heat- or laser-evoked potentials can also be used to demonstrate a lesion or disease of the spinothalamic tract (STT) pathways, and trigeminal reflex recordings may be useful in the diagnosis of secondary trigeminal neuralgia in MS. Reaching the level of definite central pain using these positive criteria in the grading system means that a CNS lesion *can* explain the pain but does not determine the cause of the pain.[3] This poses particular problems in CNS lesions where sensory abnormalities are common regardless of the presence of pain. Therefore, the exclusion of other causes of pain is critical when diagnosing central pain.

The exclusion of other types of pain is challenging given the lack of specific identifiers for distinguishing neuropathic pain from other pain types. Also, many patients experience more than one type of pain, and sometimes, different pain types occur in the same body location making diagnosis even more difficult.[15-17] A number of differential diagnoses should be considered when diagnosing central pain, including musculoskeletal pain, which is very common following CNS lesions

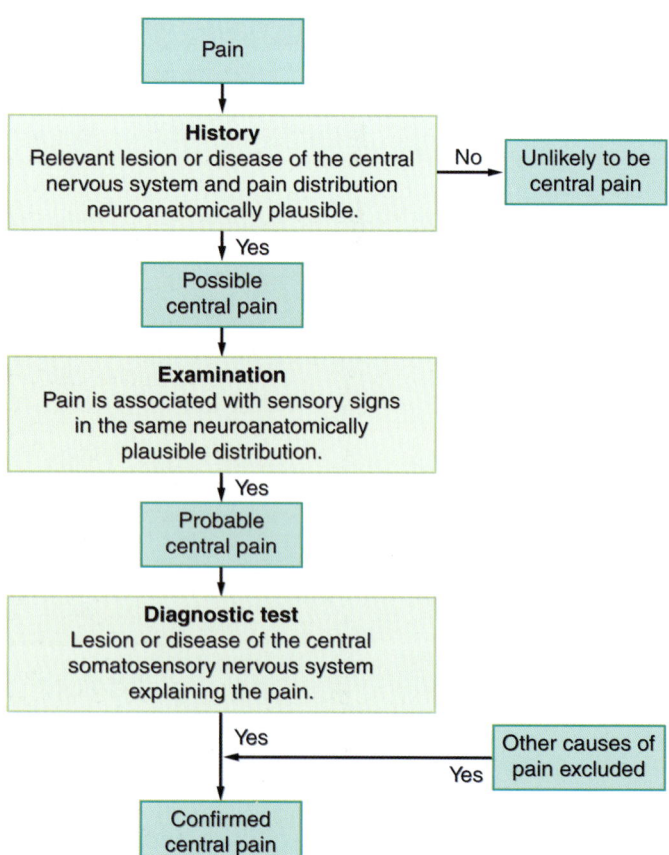

FIGURE 28.1 Grading system for central pain.

due to overuse, myofascial shoulder pain, stress fractures, spasticity, dystonia, etc., visceral pain, and peripheral neuropathic pain.[16,18–22]

Clinical Characteristics

Central pain is characterized by spontaneous and/or evoked pain in an area with partial or complete sensory loss to one or more modalities. Decreased sensation to thermal or painful stimuli is present in most patients with central pain, whereas decreased sensation to other modalities is less common.[23–26] The location of pain and sensory abnormalities is within an area compatible with the CNS lesion (Fig. 28.2). Spontaneous pain may be ongoing, intermittent, or paroxysmal. Studies in different central pain conditions show that pain descriptors such as hot/burning, shooting, pricking, pins and needles, cold, sharp, squeezing, and aching are common.[9–11,21,25,27–35] Evoked pain may be present as allodynia, which is pain due to a stimulus that does not normally provoke pain, and hyperalgesia, which is increased pain from a stimulus that normally provokes pain.[36,37] There may also be aftersensations, which is pain continuing after the stimulation has ceased. Cold allodynia and touch-evoked allodynia are particularly common in central pain.[24,27,31,32,34,38] Hyperpathia is an abnormal—often explosive—painful reaction to a stimulus in an area with increased sensory threshold when the stimulus exceeds the threshold. Due to aftersensations, the distinction between spontaneous and evoked pain may be difficult. Spontaneous pain may also be generated by central sensitization mechanisms by which decreased thresholds and temporal summation cause ongoing pain from stimuli common in daily life (e.g., movement, breathing, ambient temperature).[39] Nonpainful abnormal sensations are also common.[11,31,35,40] These include paresthesia, which are evoked or spontaneous abnormal sensations that are not unpleasant, and dysesthesia, which are unpleasant abnormal sensations.[36] Such sensations are described in terms of tingling, numb, cold, pressing, or warm.

Clinical Assessment

In the assessment of central pain, it is relevant to evaluate the intensity, impact, treatment, quality, and temporal aspects of pain as well as physical and emotional functioning and quality of life (Table 28.1).[41] The pain intensity of average and worst pain may be evaluated using a numerical rating scale, a visual analog scale (VAS), or a verbal rating scale.[42–44] Different scales have been developed to assess the multidimensional aspects of pain. One such scale is the Multidimensional Pain Inventory (MPI), which assesses pain and the impact of pain on physical and emotional functioning.[45] It has been adapted for use in SCI (MPI-SCI).[46] Other scales may be used to assess mood, sleep, resilience, pain catastrophizing, disability, and satisfaction with life.[44]

The quality of spontaneous and evoked pain may be assessed using open-ended questions or by providing the patients with a list of typical pain descriptors, for example, by using specific neuropathic pain scales such as the Neuropathic Pain Symptom Inventory (NPSI),[47] the NPQ,[4] and the painDETECT questionnaire.[7]

A sensory examination is important to identify sensory loss and gain by assessing decreased or increased sensation in the affected area compared with an area not affected by the CNS lesion. Simple bedside tests include assessment of static and dynamic touch using a brush or cotton ball; assessment of pinprick sensation using a stick, pin, or monofilament; assessment of vibration sense with a 128-Hz tuning fork; and assessment of cold and warm sensation using thermo rollers or cold and warm metal or glass objects (see Table 28.1).[14,37] Allodynia and hyperalgesia can be quantified by using a numeric rating scale

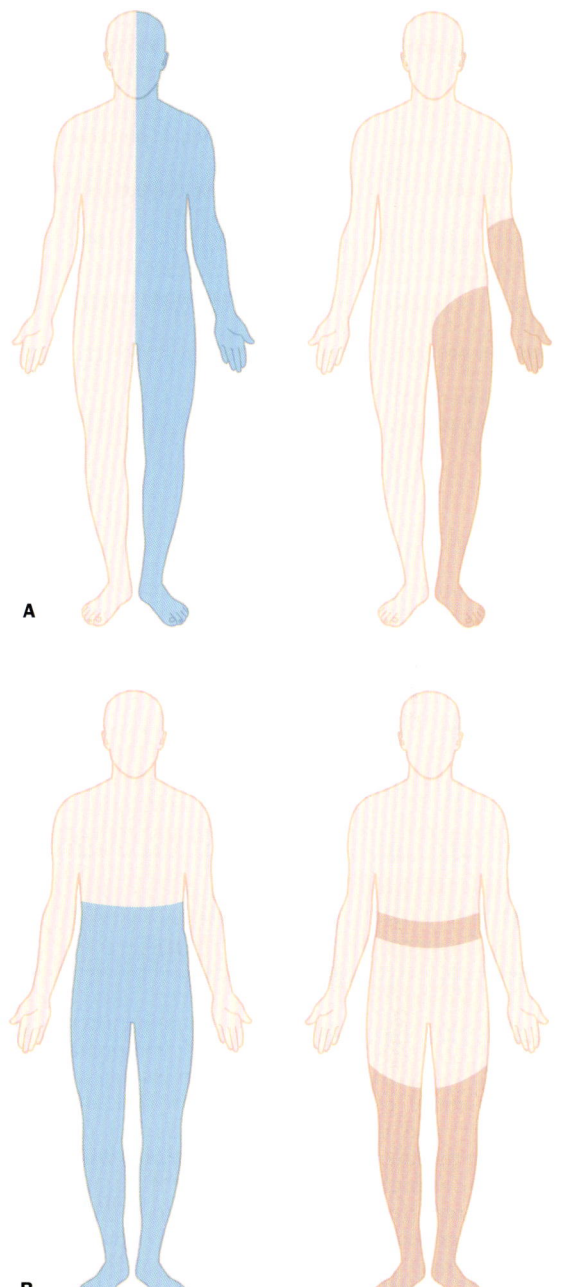

FIGURE 28.2 A: Distribution of sensory abnormalities (*blue*) and central pain (*red*) in a patient with central poststroke pain. A 64-year-old woman with a stroke affecting the left side of the body. Magnetic resonance imaging showed an infarct in the right internal capsule extending into part of the thalamus. A few months after the stroke, she complains of a burning, pricking pain in the left lower arm and left leg and touch-evoked allodynia in the hand and arm. The sensory examination showed abnormal sensation, particular to warmth and cold in the left side of the body and touch- and cold-evoked pain in the hand and lower arm. **B:** Distribution of sensory abnormalities (*blue*) and central pain (*red*) in a patient with central pain in spinal cord injury. A 55-year-old man with a spinal cord injury (SCI) after a motorbike accident. He has a complete SCI, a neurologic level Th5. Within the first months of his injury, he gradually developed two types of neuropathic pain. One pain was felt at the level of injury. It was described at an intermittent paroxysmal pain and pain evoked by light touch and cold. Another pain was felt diffusely in the legs and was described as a spontaneous, ongoing pain described as a squeezing, burning, and pricking pain. The sensory examination shows touch and cold allodynia in segments Th6 to Th7 and sensory loss to all modalities from Th8 and down.

TABLE 28.1 Clinical Assessment of Central Pain

Domain	Pain History and Clinical Assessment
Pain intensity	Numeric rating scale, visual analog scale
Pain quality	Pain questionnaires or interview
Pain location	Body map
Temporal aspects	Onset of pain, pain duration, pain frequency
Somatosensory function—sensory gain or loss	Thermal rollers
	Acetone droplet
	Pinprick
	Stroking the skin with brush
	Tuning fork
Psychological domains Pain impact Anxiety/depression Pain catastrophizing Participation	Questionnaires or interview

for evoked pain intensity. Mapping of sensory abnormalities and pain is a crucial part of the diagnosis of central pain to ensure that the distribution is compatible with a CNS lesion (see Fig. 28.2). Detailed quantitative sensory testing can supplement bedside sensory examination, but it is time-consuming and mainly used for research purposes.[14]

Laboratory tests can be used to confirm the diagnosis of a CNS lesion and specific abnormalities of the pain pathways, including the use of CT and MRI scans. Trigeminal reflexes are used in the diagnosis of trigeminal pain, and contact heat- and laser-evoked potentials are useful for assessing the function of the spinothalamic tract.[14]

Specific Central Pain Conditions

CENTRAL POSTSTROKE PAIN

Central poststroke pain (CPSP) is pain arising after a cerebrovascular lesion including ischemic and hemorrhagic lesions of the brainstem, thalamus, operculum-insula, and cerebral cortex.[48,49] Central pain occurs in 3% to 8% of stroke patients[11,18,28,35,50] and is particularly common in patients with infarctions in the lateral medullary infarctions, where the prevalence may be as high as 25%, and in the thalamus, where the prevalence is reported to be around 17% to 18%.[12,51,52]

CPSP is experienced contralateral to the side of the stroke. It may affect small areas such as the hand or the whole hemibody, which is common in thalamic infarctions.[23,27,35,51] In patients with lateral medullary infarctions, the pain distribution may be crossed, involving one side of the body contralateral to the lesion and the other side of the face ipsilateral to the lesion, and periorbital pain is commonly described.[12,53]

CENTRAL PAIN IN MULTIPLE SCLEROSIS

MS is a gradually progressing demyelinating disease with multiple sites of demyelination in the CNS. MS is an autoimmune disorder triggered by environmental factors in patients with a genetic predisposition. The inflammatory attacks give rise to plaques in the white matter of the brain and spinal cord and as the disease advances, the myelin loss is followed by damage to the axons and neurons with associated grey matter loss.[54,55] Central pain is present in about 25% of patients with MS.[56]

The distribution of central pain is compatible with spinal or brain lesions of the somatosensory nervous system.[57,58] It may be described as burning, tingling, pricking, and squeezing pain, sometimes associated with evoked pain.[34,56] In addition to this central pain type that is similar to central pain in other conditions, patients with MS may experience two specific types of central pain conditions, namely, secondary trigeminal neuralgia

and Lhermitte's phenomenon.[56,59–62] In patients with trigeminal neuralgia, the MRI scan should document a lesion in the ipsilateral side of the pons along the cause of trigeminal afferents or the recordings of trigeminal reflexes and trigeminal-evoked responses should show increased latency.[62] The pain is similar to classical trigeminal neuralgia with brief, severe, paroxysmal pain attacks restricted to one or more division of the trigeminal nerve. It is often unilateral but may be bilateral. The attacks may arise spontaneously or be triggered by movement or mechanical stimuli.[61,62] Lhermitte's phenomenon is an electric shock-like sensation that is transient and short lasting. It is typically provoked by neck movement and is felt spreading down in the back.[59,61] It is more common in younger patients and in patients with a progressive or progressive-relapsing cause and is assumed to be caused by ectopic discharges due to demyelination in the dorsal column.[60,61,63]

CENTRAL PAIN IN SPINAL CORD INJURY

SCI is a term that includes both traumatic and nontraumatic causes. The most common traumatic causes are traffic accidents and falls, and nontraumatic causes include syringomyelia, tumors, ischemia, hemorrhage, arteriovenous malformations, transverse myelitis, and infections.[64] Chronic pain is one of the most disabling consequences of an SCI—present in 70% to 80% of patients.[13,65–68] Neuropathic pain is present in about 50% of patients.[13,66,69] The onset of central pain may be immediately after the SCI or it may be delayed up to 1 year. A delayed onset and facial pain should alert the physician to the possibility of development of syringomyelia.[70] Neuropathic pain following SCI is divided into pain felt at and below the level of lesion.[16,66] At-level pain is located within the dermatome of the neurologic level of injury and three dermatomes below the neurologic level. This type of neuropathic pain may be caused by the SCI or a lesion of the nerve roots, and it is often not possible to determine whether it is a peripheral neuropathic pain caused by root lesion or a central pain caused by spinal cord lesion. Below-level pain is pain felt more than three dermatomes below the neurologic level and is a central pain caused by the spinal cord lesion. In patients with syringomyelia, the pain distribution is often segmental.[71,72] Different types of pain seen following SCI, including central pain, can be found in Chapter 40, and the readers are referred to that chapter for further details on SCI pain.

OTHER CENTRAL PAIN CONDITIONS

The diagnosis of central pain in brain trauma is often difficult and only few studies exist. The central pain is similar to that of other central pain patients.[73,74] The onset may be delayed for several months and often becomes persistent. The pain distribution is often unilateral, corresponding to the side with most severe sensory abnormalities and related to decreased thermal sensitivity. Ongoing pain described as pricking, cold, pressing, wretched, and burning is common, and some patients described touch- and cold-evoked allodynia.[73] There are very few reports in the literature on central pain in brain tumors, but it has been described in tumors affecting the thalamus and the parietal cortex.[75,76] Central pain following surgery such as dorsal root entry zone lesions, thalamic destructions, and mesencephalic and medullary tractotomies are only infrequently reported because these procedures are rarely done today.[77]

Pain is a common problem in Parkinson's disease. The pain is often located in the lower back and lower extremities, and musculoskeletal pain is the most common type.[78,79] It is also suggested that some pain conditions in Parkinson's disease are related to the CNS disease and has been termed *central pain*.[78–80] This type of pain is rare and is a poorly localized diffuse pain that is often associated with "off condition," autonomic symptoms, visceral pain, and improvement with levodopa administration.[78,79,81] This type of pain, however, does not entirely fulfill the criteria for central pain. Even though altered thermal and pain thresholds have been found in Parkinson's disease, suggesting altered responsiveness to painful stimuli,[81,82] lower laser N2/P2 amplitudes are also found in pain-free patients,[83] and one study found that the pain thresholds were not different in patients with and without pain.[84] However, there is increasing evidence that the basal ganglia and the dopaminergic system play an important role in the gating of nociceptive information and pain modulation,[85,86] and it is possible that some pain types in Parkinson's disease are related to altered sensory processing of nociceptive inputs.[80] Epileptic seizures may rarely be reported as pain.[87,88] One case report describes a patient with a dysplasia in the posterior insula.[89] Spontaneous high-frequency activity and spiking from this area propagated to other areas including the parietal operculum and the midcingulate gyrus. During the attack, the patients reported hemibody pain that started in the left hand and foot.[89]

Preclinical Models

Different models of SCI, stroke, brain trauma, and MS are used in preclinical pain research.[90–96] SCI models include hemisection, contusion, ischemic, electrolytic, and excitotoxic models.[97–100] The models mimic human CNS lesions reasonably well, but the assessment of pain and its translation into human central pain remains a challenge.[101]

One of the most obvious challenges for all preclinical models of pain is the difficulty in assessing the correlate of ongoing pain. Except for a very few studies that have used conditioned place preference paradigms[102] or overgrooming,[103] most preclinical studies of central pain exclusively use evoked responses to mechanical, cold, or warm stimuli. This may be valid because evoked pain is common and predicts the development of central pain,[31,38,104] but evoked pain-related responses do not always correlate with ongoing pain, and ongoing central pain may exist without evoked pain. A particular challenge in assessing pain-like behavior in models of CNS injury is the frequent coexistence of spasticity making the use of simple withdrawal reflexes unreliable as a pain-like behavioral outcome.[101,105–108] Because withdrawal reflexes are spinally mediated, persist after complete spinal transection, and may be increased as part of the spastic syndrome, methods that depend on brainstem or cortical processing (e.g., operant escape or place escape/avoidance paradigms) are needed.[109]

Mechanisms

Experimental animal models and studies in humans have provided insights into the pathophysiology of central pain, which involves plasticity in various areas and pathways of the CNS. Sensitization of the CNS plays a major role in central pain and involves neuronal hyperexcitability resulting in an increased response to synaptic inputs, decreased threshold, expansion of receptive fields, and access of low-threshold Aβ mechanoreceptors to pain pathways.[110,111] The clinical consequences are allodynia, hyperalgesia, and aftersensations. Central sensitization may also include spontaneous discharges.[112] Spontaneous discharges in damaged pain pathways or deafferented rostral neurons may be responsible for spontaneous ongoing or intermittent pain.[113] Seemingly, spontaneous pain may also be a result of decreased thresholds in nociceptor excitation and temporal summation of stimulus-evoked pain occurring at physiologic levels from stimuli caused by daily activity such as breathing, movement, and ambient temperature.[39] Recent studies have found that sensory hypersensitivity (mechanical and cold allodynia, hyperalgesia, and temporal summation of pain) precedes and predicts later development of central pain (CPSP and below-level SCI pain), supporting a role of neuronal hyperexcitability also for ongoing pain.[31,38,104]

The functional changes underlying central sensitization involve a range of anatomical, neurochemical, excitotoxic, and inflammatory mechanisms.[114–116] Changes in ion channels (sodium, calcium, potassium, acid-sensing) and phosphorylation of glutamate receptors may occur at various levels of the CNS,[117–121] and altered opioid receptor binding has also been demonstrated in patients with central pain.[122,123] Changes in the functions of microglia and astrocytes and release of inflammatory mediators also contribute to chronic pain following CNS injury.[90,119,124,125] Loss of inhibition, either through the altered balance of descending inhibitory and facilitatory pathways, loss of interneurons containing glycine or γ-aminobutyric acid (GABA), or via decreased GABAergic inhibitory function through downregulation of the potassium chloride exporter, may be additional mechanisms underlying central sensitization.[126,127]

Lesions of the STT and STT–thalamocortical pathways play an important but not well-understood role in the mechanisms of central pain. Impairment of pain and temperature sensation and STT injury are hallmarks of central pain,[48,128,129] but abnormal STT function is not a sufficient condition as STT lesions are also frequent in pain-free subjects. Approximately 50% of patients with a lesion of the STT after SCI or operculo-insular strokes develop central pain,[130] and the question is why STT lesions cause pain in some but not all individuals. Although central pain can occur in patients with complete lesions of the STT,[131] it is suggested that central pain is caused by sensitization of partially preserved residual STT neurons in some patients.[125,132–134] This is consistent with studies showing that microsimulation in the ventral caudal (Vc) sensory nucleus of the thalamus, which receives dense STT terminations, evokes pain in patients with central pain.[135,136] It is likely that the role of lesioned versus preserved ascending pathways in central pain depends on the pain phenotype. Patients with evoked pain are more likely to have preserved large- and small-fiber function than patients with spontaneous pain only, as shown in studies using quantitative sensory testing, somatosensory, and laser-evoked potentials and functional MRI (fMRI).[26,137–139]

The thalamus is implicated in central pain of spinal, brainstem, and brain origin. In addition to the Vc nucleus of thalamus, the medial and intralaminar nuclei, which receive STT input that further project to the anterior cingulate cortex (ACC), have also been implicated in central pain.[140,141] CPSP is particularly common in lesions of the ventral posterior and Vc thalamic nuclei, but the thalamus is also implicated in central pain following other CNS lesions.[142–147]

Various disinhibition hypotheses have been proposed—but also questioned—for central pain. These include an imbalance between the relative preservation of the dorsal column compared to the STT pathways[148] and an imbalance between spinothalamic and spinoreticulothalamic pathways following spinal cord and brainstem lesions.[149,150] In 1911, Head and Holmes[151] suggested that the pain in CPSP was due to a disinhibition of the medial thalamus caused by a lesion of the lateral thalamus. Later, Craig and colleagues suggested the thermosensory disinhibition theory.[152,153] This theory suggests that cold allodynia and burning pain occur in areas of cold sensitivity loss because lesions of a lateral cool-signaling STT pathway from lamina 1 of the dorsal horn through the lateral thalamus to the insula disinhibit a medial STT pain-signaling pathway. Loss of descending inhibitory pathways and deficient ability to conditioned pain modulation have been shown to be involved in central pain in SCI,[154,155] and injury to the periaqueductal gray (PAG), which plays an important role in descending pain modulation, was related to the degree of central pain in mild traumatic brain injury.[156]

Changes in spinal cord excitability are important for central pain following SCI. Spinal transection and dorsal root-entry zone (DREZ) lesions may relieve below-level pain in some patients, supporting a crucial role of changes in the rostral part of the spinal cord lesion for central SCI pain.[157–160] Also, sensory hypersensitivity and imbalance of pinprick and light touch sensation were more common at the level of injury in SCI patients with below-level pain,[161,162] supporting the role of this region for central pain in SCI. But several remote changes in the CNS—beside the thalamic changes mentioned earlier—may also play a role for SCI pain. Central pain in SCI has been associated with changes in spontaneous electroencephalogram (EEG), and in addition, imagining movement results in increased desynchronization in the θ, α, and β bands in pain versus pain-free patients.[163] Furthermore, reorganization of the primary somatosensory cortex has been linked to the intensity of neuropathic pain following SCI,[164] although results are conflicting,[165] and a recent systematic review suggested that there is only limited evidence for at relationship between pain due to deafferentation and cortical reorganization.[166] In addition, changes have been seen in anterior cingulate and prefrontal cortices following SCI.[167–171] Overall, more information is needed to understand the interaction of these different CNS regions in the generation, amplification, or modification of central pain.

Treatment of Central Pain

Treating central pain remains a great challenge, and a broad approach is essential. Patients with central pain may be elderly, and they may have concurrent medical problems and impairments such as paralysis, spasticity, gastrointestinal and autonomic dysfunctions, intellectual impairment, as well as depression, fatigue, sleep disturbances, or psychosocial problems. In addition, they may be treated with multiple drugs with unwanted CNS-related side effects. The diagnosis of central pain and the presumptive underlying mechanisms is the first important step and requires a thorough assessment. The treatment of central pain is often symptomatic, but in some cases, the underlying cause of neuropathic pain can be treated, for example, with the use of corticosteroids for the treatment of spinal cord compression. It is also important to be aware of factors that may exacerbate central pain (e.g., stress, depression, and urinary tract infections).[22] Realistic expectations for the treatment outcome should be discussed with the patient, explaining that often only partial pain relief from central pain can be expected. The approach is to start the treatment with complementary and pharmacologic therapies, and in refractory cases, consider interventional therapies such as neuromodulation.[116]

Treatment of neuropathic pain is often a "trial-and-error" process. In contrast to the disease-based classification of neuropathic pain, it is suggested that a mechanism-based classification will improve the treatment of the individual patient.[172] Because we do not have reliable tools to assess which pain mechanisms are important in which pain patients, a phenotype-based classification has been advocated. This approach suggests that the presence of specific clusters of pain descriptors or sensory profiles may reflect specific underlying pain mechanisms, and thus efficacy to specific drugs.[33,173,174] There is, however, still limited evidence for this approach, and in future clinical trials, it is important to obtain a well-characterized description of the patient's pain, including pain location, pain descriptors, sensory signs, and psychosocial factors, to gain more knowledge on phenotype-based pain classifications and treatments.

PHARMACOLOGIC TREATMENT

The drugs used for neuropathic pain have limited response rates, and typically, responders experience only partial pain reduction at tolerable doses. Because there is no evidence for a disease-based pharmacologic treatment of neuropathic pain, general treatment guidelines for neuropathic pain are also recommended for central pain—with the exception of topical treatments.[175] Overall, randomized, double-blind, placebo-controlled studies in central pain support the general treatment recommendations for neuropathic pain (Table 28.2).[175] A summary of pharmacologic treatments that are relevant for central pain is presented in the following discussion, and the reader is referred to Chapter 81 for a more detailed description of neuropathic pain pharmacotherapy. In the following, the NeuPSIG treatment recommendations will be used.[175] NeuPSIG is the Neuropathic Pain Special Interest group of the International Association for the Study of Pain (IASP). The NeuPSIG treatment recommendations are based on a systematic literature search of published and unpublished studies, a meta-analysis, and an evaluation of the quality of evidence and strength of recommendation using the Grading of Recommendations Assessment, Development, and Evaluation (GRADE).[175] Numbers needed to treat (NNTs) are used to describe effect sizes. The NNT is the number of patients needed to treat with a certain drug to obtain one patient with a defined degree of pain reduction (usually 50%) and is calculated as the reciprocal of the absolute risk reduction. As for neuropathic pain in general, there is a relatively large placebo response in clinical trials of central pain—sometimes making it difficult to show superiority of different treatments.[185]

First-line Pharmacologic Treatments

First-line pharmacologic treatments in central pain include tricyclic antidepressants (TCAs), serotonin-noradrenaline reuptake inhibitors (SNRIs), pregabalin, and gabapentin (Fig. 28.3).[175]

TCAs and SNRIs inhibit the presynaptic reuptake of serotonin and noradrenaline, and in addition, TCAs act on voltage-gated sodium channels and opioid and N-methyl-D-aspartate (NMDA) receptors.[186,187] The site of action is through descending aminergic pathways at spinal or supraspinal sites, but a peripheral site of action via sympathetic fiber sprouting in the dorsal root ganglia may also be involved.[186,187] The analgesic action of noradrenaline is likely to be mediated through both α2A and β2 adrenoceptors.[187]

The combined NNT for TCAs in neuropathic pain was 3.6 (95% CI, 3.0 to 4.4) with a moderate quality of evidence, and the combined NNT for SNRIs was 6.4 (5.2 to 8.4) with a high quality of evidence.[175] NNTs are not directly comparable due to differences in study design. The effect of antidepressants is independent of the antidepressant effect,[176] although in a study in SCI patients, the effect on pain was more pronounced in those with considerable depressive symptomatology.[178] Amitriptyline is the TCA most often studied in neuropathic pain, but there is no clinical evidence to suggest superior efficacy of one TCA, and imipramine and the TCAs with secondary amine structure (nortriptyline and desipramine) are often better tolerated.[188] The first study in central pain compared the effect of amitriptyline 75 mg per day with that of carbamazepine 800 mg per day and placebo in 15 patients with CPSP (see Table 28.2).[176] Amitriptyline, but not carbamazepine, significantly relieved central pain, and the effect size was highest if the total plasma concentrations of amitriptyline and its metabolite nortriptyline exceeded 300 nmol/L. Later studies also found an effect of amitriptyline in SCI- and MS-related pain,[178,179] whereas one study failed to show an effect of amitriptyline in SCI pain, but this study did not exclusively include neuropathic pain.[177] In one small study, duloxetine relieved CPSP and SCI pain, but the difference was not statistically significant.[180]

Side effects to TCAs include drowsiness, fatigue, weight gain, and effects related to anticholinergic actions such as dry mouth, constipation, urinary retention, and orthostatic hypotension. TCAs should not be used in patients with heart failure, and precautions should be taken in patients with cardiac conduction disturbances, seizures, and glaucoma. Tertiary amine TCAs (amitriptyline, imipramine, and clomipramine) and high TCA doses are not recommended in patients above 65 years of age due to the increased risk of falls or sudden cardiac

TABLE 28.2   Randomized Double-Blind Placebo-Controlled Trials of At Least 3 Weeks Duration in Central Pain[175]

Central Pain Condition	Authors and Publication Year	Patients Randomized	Active Drug and Max. Daily Dose	Study Outcome
Antidepressants				
CPSP	Leijon and Boivie 1989[176]	15	Amitriptyline 75 mg	Ami > pla
SCI	Cardenas et al. 2002[177,a]	84	Amitriptyline 125 mg	Ami = pla
SCI	Rintala et al. 2007[178]	38	Amitriptyline 150 mg	Ami > pla
MS	Österberg and Boivie 2005[179]	23	Amitriptyline 75 mg	Ami > pla
SCI/CPSP	Vranken et al. 2011[180]	48	Duloxetine 120 mg	Dul = pla
Pregabalin/gabapentin				
MS	Kim et al. 2011[253]	220	Pregabalin 600 mg	Pre = pla
SCI	Siddall et al. 2006[181]	137	Pregabalin 600 mg	Pre > pla
SCI	Cardenas et al. 2013[182]	220	Pregabalin 600 mg	Pre > pla
SCI/CPSP	Vranken et al. 2008[254]	40	Pregabalin 600 mg	Pre > pla
SCI	Levendoglu et al. 2004[255]	20	Gabapentin 3,600 mg	Gab > pla
SCI	Rintala et al. 2007[178]	38	Gabapentin 3,600 mg	Gab = pla
Other Anticonvulsants				
CPSP	Vestergaard et al. 2001[183]	30	Lamotrigine 200 mg	Lam > pla
SCI	Finnerup et al. 2002[184]	30	Lamotrigine 400 mg	Lam = pla
MS	Breuer et al. 2007[256]	17	Lamotrigine 400 mg	Lam = pla
CPSP	Leijon and Boivie 1989[176]	15	Carbamazepine 800 mg	Car = pla
MS	Österberg and Boivie, 2005[179]	23	Carbamazepine 600 mg	Car = pla
SCI	Drewes et al. 1994[257]	20	Valproate 2,400 mg	Val = pla
SCI	Finnerup et al. 2009[258]	36	Levetiracetam 3,000 mg	Lev = pla
CPSP	Jungehulsing et al. 2012[259]	42	Levetiracetam 3,000 mg	Lev = pla
CPSP	Falah et al. 2012[260]	30	Levetiracetam 3,000 mg	Lev = pla
Opioids				
SCI	Norrbrink and Lundeberg 2009[261]	36	Tramadol 400 mg	Tra > pla
Cannabinoids				
MS	Svendsen et al. 2004[262]	24	Dronabinol 10 mg	Can > pla
MS	Rog et al. 2005[263,a]	66	Sativex spray	Can > pla
MS	Langford et al. 2013[264]	339	Sativex spray	Can = pla
SCI	Clinicaltrials.gov (NCT01606202)	111	Sativex spray	Can = pla
Other				
SCI	Chiou-Tan et al. 1996[265]	11	Mexiletine 450 mg	Mex = pla
SCI	Han et al. 2016[266]	40	Botulinum toxin type A	BTX-A > pla
SCI	Andresen et al. 2016[267]	73	Palmitoylethanolamide 600 mg	PEA = pla

[a]Study includes nonneuropathic pain conditions.
Ami, amitriptyline; BTX-A, botulinum toxin type A; Can, cannabinoid; Car, carbamazepine; CPSP, central poststroke pain; Dul, duloxetine; Gab, gabapentin; Lam, lamotrigine; Lev, levetiracetam; Mex, mexiletine; MS, multiple sclerosis; PEA, palmitoylethanolamide; pla, placebo; Pre, pregabalin; SCI, spinal cord injury; Tra, tramadol; Val, valproate.

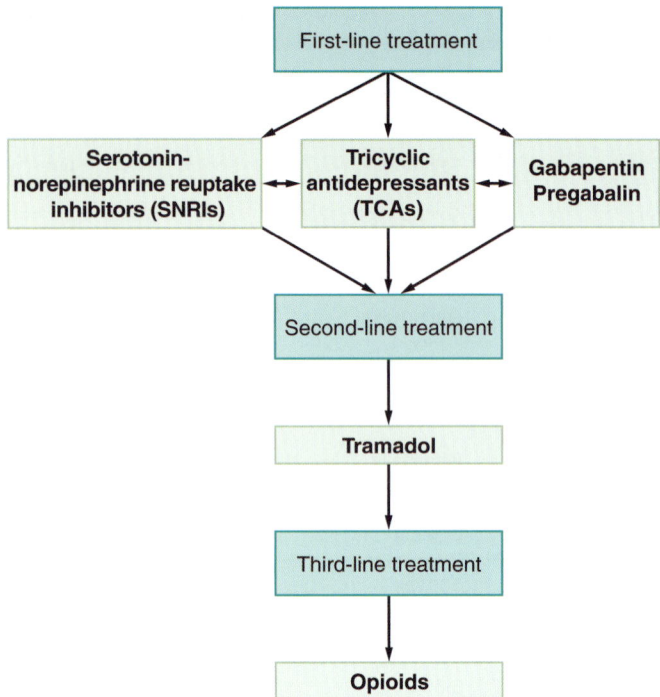

FIGURE 28.3 Treatment algorithm for the pharmacologic treatment of central pain.

death.[189,190] TCAs should be used with caution in combinations with other serotonergic agents due to the risk of serotonin syndrome. TCAs should be titrated slowly, starting at 10 to 25 mg daily and titrated up to 75 to 100 mg per day. TCAs are metabolized by the hepatic cytochrome P450 system, and genetic polymorphisms at CYP2D6 cause variability in pharmacokinetics. Titration is normally guided by the clinical response, but serum drug concentration measurements may improve the outcome.[186] SNRIs and selective serotonin reuptake inhibitors may cause nausea, abdominal pain, sedation, dizziness, sweating, and sexual dysfunction. They may also cause blood pressure elevation. Duloxetine is given at doses of 60 mg daily and should be avoided in patients with moderate liver disease and renal impairment with creatinine clearance below 30 mL per minute. Venlafaxine treatment should be titrated slowly up to 150 mg per day, with reduced dosage in patients with renal and liver impairment. For both drugs, drug–drug interactions concern serotonergic agents and drugs affecting coagulation.

Gabapentin and pregabalin are ligands of the $\alpha_2\delta$ subunit of voltage-gated calcium channels, and the analgesic effects is thought to be mediated through an attenuation of calcium channels influx into cells and a reduced release of neurotransmitters, although other actions such as an effect on glia cells and expression of proinflammatory cytokines may also be involved.[187] The expression of the $\alpha_2\delta$ calcium channel subunit can be increased in some neuropathic pain conditions, but the effect of gabapentin and pregabalin does not require increased $\alpha_2\delta$ subunits.[187] Gabapentin and pregabalin act at peripheral, spinal, and supraspinal levels.[187,191–193]

The combined NNT for gabapentin in neuropathic pain was 6.3 (95% CI, 5.0 to 8.3), and the NNT for pregabalin was 7.7 (95% CI, 6.5 to 9.4) with a high quality of evidence. Six studies have examined the effect of gabapentin or pregabalin in central pain, of which four were positive on the primary outcome (see Table 28.2). The two largest studies in SCI pain found an effect of pregabalin as add-on therapy on pain, pain-related sleep interference, and anxiety with a combined NNT of 7.0

(4.5 to 16.5).[181,182] Pregabalin showed an effect on anxiety scores on the Hospital Anxiety and Depression Scale (HADS) in one study[181] and on depression scores in another study,[182] although patients did not have clinically relevant levels of anxiety and depression. Pregabalin tended to be more effective in those with a high HADS score.[181,194]

Side effects include somnolence, dizziness, peripheral edema, and weight gain. The frequency of somnolence may be higher in patients with central pain,[181] possibly due to a high frequency of concomitant medication for pain and spasticity. Gabapentin is initiated at 100 to 300 mg per day and increased up to 1,800 to 3,600 mg daily in three divided doses, and pregabalin is increased from 75 mg twice daily to 300 to 600 mg per day. Doses should be decreased in patients with renal insufficiency.

Second- and Third-Line Pharmacologic Treatments
Tramadol is a weak agonist of μ-opioid receptors and a SNRI. The combined NNT for tramadol in neuropathic pain was 4.7 (95% CI, 3.6 to 6.7) with a moderate quality of evidence, and tramadol is recommended as a second-line drug.[175] Tramadol is particularly useful in the treatment of episodic exacerbations of pain.[195] The combined NNT for strong opioids, including morphine and oxycodone, in neuropathic pain was 4.3 (95% CI, 3.4 to 5.8) with a moderate quality of evidence.[175] Due to potential safety concerns with risk of abuse, cognitive impairment, and endocrine and immunologic changes,[196–199] the final strength of recommendation was weak, and opioids were recommended as third-line drugs.[175]

Other Drugs, Combination Therapy, and Intrathecal Drug Administration
The recommendations for other antiepileptics for neuropathic pain are inconclusive due to conflicting and overall negative results.[175] However, some patients do seem to respond to sodium channel blockers,[200] and there was an effect of lamotrigine in one study of CPSP,[183] and post hoc analyses suggested effect of lamotrigine in SCI subjects with incomplete lesions and evoked pain.[184] In addition, a recent study in peripheral neuropathic pain found that oxcarbazepine was effective in patients with preserved nociceptors and evoked pain but not in those without this pain phenotype.[201] Therefore, sodium channel blockers may be indicated in some patients, although further studies are needed to confirm the specific predictors for effects.[202] For neuropathic pain in general, there was an overall weak recommendation against the use of cannabinoids.[175] Also in central pain, the results are conflicting (see Table 28.2), and more studies on the long-term efficacy and safety are needed to establish whether there is a role for the use of cannabinoids in central pain.

When treatment with a single drug is only partly effective, combination with another drug of a complementary mechanism of action may be tried. Side effects should be carefully monitored, and normally sequential add-on therapy is recommended.

In refractory cases, spinal drug administration may be considered. There is, however, little evidence from randomized controlled trials. One study examined clonidine, morphine, and their combination in SCI pain.[203] Each drug alone did not provide significant pain relief, but the combination of clonidine and morphine provided effect on central pain. The effect size correlated with the concentration of morphine in the cervical cerebrospinal fluid, and it was suggested that if there is a pathology restricting the flow of cerebrospinal fluid, the drugs need to be administered above the level of injury.[203] Ziconotide—a drug that is given intrathecally—is recommended for moderate to severe chronic pain and can be combined with intrathecal morphine or baclofen, but there is limited experience with central pain, and the treatment is often associated with severe side effects.[204] Short-term side effects to spinal drug administration include nausea, sedation, hypotension, and respiratory depression. Lidocaine, ketamine, and opioids given intravenously have also been shown to relieve central pain, but these treatments have a limited role in chronic pain treatment.[205–209]

PSYCHOLOGICAL AND PHYSIOTHERAPY TREATMENT

The treatment of central pain often requires a multidisciplinary approach. A large proportion of patients use nonpharmacologic treatments, and patients with SCI reported that massage and heat were the nonpharmacologic treatments to result in the best pain alleviation.[210] Concomitant psychological distress, anxiety, and depression should be treated. Cognitive-behavioral therapy and other psychological interventions may be useful.[211] A Cochrane review evaluated the effects of psychological treatments on pain, disability, mood, and health care used in patients with neuropathic pain and found that there was insufficient evidence of psychological interventions with only two eligible studies.[212] Smaller studies have found some effect of hypnosis on the impact of MS-related pain,[213,214] personalized positive psychology exercises in different central pain conditions,[215] and multidimensional pain management programs comprising educational, cognitive, and behavioral intervention in SCI pain.[216,217] Another systematic review with less strict criteria concluded that virtual reality interventions and hypnosis are effective for pain related to MS and SCI.[218]

Physical therapy may be useful in alleviating musculoskeletal pain, spasticity, and other complications to a CNS disorder. Visual illusion, where patients see a movie of a lower body walking aligned with a mirror image of their own upper body, has been shown to decrease pain in SCI in small trials.[219,220] Other studies have found increased pain following movement imagery in patients with complete SCI,[168] and neurofeedback aimed at self-regulating abnormal brain activity during imaged movement has been suggested to be effective in central pain in SCI.[221] More information is needed on the methodology, long-term efficacy, and predictors of response of various techniques related to visual illusion and neurofeedback.

NEUROSURGICAL MANAGEMENT

The neurosurgical management of central pain can be utilized when noninvasive treatment options fail. A multitude of techniques have been employed with myriad anatomical targets in the peripheral nervous system and CNS with varying degrees of efficacy. Lack of consistent evidence secondary to the variability in techniques across centers as well as small sample sizes has led to difficulty in drawing definitive conclusions. Currently, evidence for the majority of neurosurgical treatment options lies within case reports or small case series that consistently find improvement in variable degree in a subset of patients. Central pain syndromes are notoriously recalcitrant to medical treatment, and consideration should be given to offering neurosurgical intervention depending on the type of pain, severity, and influence on quality of life in each individual case.

Targeted Drug Delivery

Targeted drug delivery into the subarachnoid space for the treatment of refractory central pain has been attempted through various techniques including most commonly via a catheter inserted into the intrathecal space in the spinal column or less commonly directly into the brain via an intraventricular catheter. The catheters are subsequently connected to a subcutaneously implanted drug delivery pump allowing the controlled infusion of a variety of medications. Infused drugs of choice have included GABAergic agonists like baclofen or midazolam, sometimes in combination with an adrenergic agent such as clonidine.[222,223] One randomized, double-blind study in 15 patients undergoing intrathecal drug delivery for the treatment of neuropathic pain after SCI found that the combination of morphine and clonidine produced significantly greater pain control than placebo or either medication given alone.[203] Much of the literature about pain reduction via subarachnoid infusion of medication in central pain states comes from patients with SCI and MS undergoing intrathecal therapy for the treatment of spasticity and suggests that there is direct additional suppression of neuropathic pain distinct from the suppression of spasm-related pain,[224] although no controlled studies have been published and there is general consensus that the effects are limited.

Neuroablation

Since the introduction of stereotactic surgery in the late 1940s, targeted neuroablative techniques have been utilized to intervene in central pain pathways in the most refractory patients suffering from pain syndromes. Some of the more successfully targeted regions include the sensory thalamus in patients undergoing stereotactic or radiosurgical thalamotomy and the spinothalamic and quintothalamic pathways in stereotactic mesencephalotomy[225] most commonly used for the treatment of CPSP. New techniques have largely replaced these ablative procedures with the capacity for reversible and titratable modulation of deep brain-stimulating electrodes. These are now most often used in the treatment of pain except in certain circumstances where ablative techniques are preferred, most notably in the palliative treatment of cancer-related pain. Technologic advancements in our ability to create lesions in the brain through incisionless techniques, including new technology such as MR-guided high-intensity focused ultrasound, as well as improvements in the use of focused radiation may forecast a resurgence in interest in the revival of these ablative techniques.

Neuromodulation

Motor Cortex Stimulation

Perhaps the most robust evidence in the neurosurgical treatment of central pain lies in epidural cortical stimulation (ECS), most commonly of the motor cortex. This treatment modality was first reported in 1991 by Tsukobawa et al.,[226] after investigating the cortical patterns associated with burst hyperactivity of thalamic neurons in an animal model of STT deafferentation. They found that stimulation of the motor cortex provided complete, long-term inhibition of this burst hyperreactivity and applied this model to a case series of patients with thalamic pain syndrome by inserting epidural electrode over the motor cortex, ultimately achieving "excellent or good" pain control in all cases. Indications for motor cortex stimulation (MCS) have expanded over the last decade to include refractory SCI pain, phantom limb pain, and neuropathic facial pain among many others.[227]

This procedure is performed via a small craniotomy or burr hole contralateral to the region of pain. The sensory and motor cortices are typically mapped intraoperatively using electrophysiology to identify the central sulcus. Typically, one or two 4-contact strip electrodes are then placed in the targeted region in either a longitudinal orientation over the motor cortex or perpendicular to the central sulcus in the epidural space. The electrodes are then sutured down, and extension wires are typically externalized for a 3- to 7-day trial during which pulse width, frequency, and amplitude are optimized. There is a considerable amount of variation in stimulation parameters, and typically, the stimulus intensity is increased to test the motor threshold and decreased subsequently as a percentage of this amplitude. Patients typically do not experience paresthesias or other stimulation-induced sensory phenomena. If patients are felt to achieve sufficient (typically 40% or more) pain relief, stage 2 of the trial involves removing the trial extension wires and tunneling the lead to an infraclavicular implantable pulse generator (IPG), most often placed in the infraclavicular space.[228] MCS has risks that are typical of most cranial procedures, including infection and the possibility of hemorrhage, as well as seizures and hardware problems; however, these complications are rare, and the procedure is considered overall to be safe.[229,230]

Although the mechanisms that underlie the effects of MCS have not been clearly identified, studies suggest that activity in the first- and second-order somatosensory pathways is affected,[231] and various patterns of cerebral blood flow changes have been noted in thalamus and other regions of the brain in successful cases.[232] In a critical review of the literature, greater than 40% improvement in pain scores were reported in 54% of 117 patients with central pain.[230] Good results have also been reported in isolated cases of patients with pain secondary to MS[233] and pain after posttraumatic brain injury[234]; however, CPSP has been the most comprehensively studied central pain indication. In a review of its efficacy, Nguyen et al.[235] reported that MCS showed a greater than 40% pain reduction on the VAS in 60% of patients with CPSP. Although these and other trials have demonstrated the efficacy of MCS in the treatment of various types of neuropathic pain, they include a limited number of patients and often patients with various etiologies of pain are analyzed concurrently. These findings thus need to be confirmed by larger, randomized controlled multicenter trials and include more methodical selection of patient cohorts.[235,236]

Deep Brain Stimulation

Deep brain stimulation has been used for the treatment of pain since the 1950s and became widely employed by the 1970s for the treatment of neuropathic pain of various origins.[236] Enthusiasm for using this treatment modality for chronic, refractory pain was dampened when two industry supported open-label studies failed to reach their clinical endpoints for success.[237] Critics of these trials contend that they were neither randomized nor case-controlled, had variability in patient selection, inconsistencies in neurosurgical technique, and lack of rigorous evaluation of individual pain etiologies which have been shown to have dramatically variable responses to invasive treatment.[236,238,239] Utilizing improvements in hardware, imaging modalities, and with attention to patient selection, specialized centers across the country continue to use deep brain stimulation effectively for the treatment of various types of pain syndromes on an "off label" basis.

Currently, there is no consensus for best anatomical target in the treatment of pain, and many regions of the brain have been trialed over past several decades. The most commonly utilized targets the sensory-discriminative sphere of pain circuitry and includes the PAG area/periventricular gray area (PVG)[240] and the Vc (ventral posterior lateral) nucleus of the sensory thalamus.[227,241] More recently, efficacy has been found in regions targeting the affective components of pain including ACC[242] and the anterior limb of the internal capsule (ALIC).[243] The surgical approach is similar in nature and risk to the technique widely used for implanting deep brain-stimulating leads for the treatment of movement disorders including Parkinson's disease and essential tremor. Risks are rare but potentially serious and include most commonly infection, hemorrhage, and hardware complications.

A variety of case reports and case series have demonstrated efficacy in the treatment of various central pain pathologies including MS,[244] pain from malignancy,[245] and pain after SCI[246,247] as well as CPSP.[239,243,245] One large series comprising a variety of pain etiologies found overall that 60% of patients gained benefit and that the degree of efficacy varied by pathophysiology.[239] In this cohort, 15 patients were treated with deep brain stimulation for CPSP with stimulators placed in the PVG, Vc, or both. VAS scores revealed a mean improvement of 48.8% with a wide variability between patients and was found to be an effective treatment overall in 70% of patients.[239,245]

In 2016, the European Academy of Neurology (EAN) published guidelines on the role of neurostimulation in the treatment of neuropathic pain and concluded that studies for deep brain stimulation were heterogeneous and imprecise and despite some clear demonstration of efficacy were inconsistent in their findings. This lead the committee to an "inconclusive" recommendation as to the efficacy of this treatment modality.[248] Although deep brain stimulation has proven to be a potentially effective tool for those patients with severe, refractory central pain who have failed all other less invasive treatment modalities, prospective, randomized controlled trials are needed to further delineate effective targets, reliable stimulation parameters, and to refine patient selection criteria.

Spinal Cord Stimulation

Spinal cord stimulation (SCS) therapy is used most often to treat peripheral neuropathic pain, pain from failed back surgery syndrome, or complex regional pain syndrome and is not commonly employed in the treatment of central pain,[249] with some claiming that it plays no role in the treatment of brain central pain.[223] Few case reports support its use in CPSP,[250,251] citing modest long-term improvement. Reports of SCS in the use of pain from SCI similarly vary in their efficacy and are generally lacking. In one seminal series from 1972 of 30 patients undergoing SCS, 5 were implanted for pain from traumatic SCI including spinal fractures, gunshot wounds to the spine, and cord contusions, none of whom had an "excellent" response to treatment.[252] Since then, further reports have corroborated a generally poor response in these patients when compared to traditional indications like failed back surgery syndrome and pain from peripheral neuropathy, potentially owing in part to primary damage of the circuitry being stimulated. In the treatment of central cord pain, however, some continue to contend that given its less invasive nature, SCS should be attempted in those patients with at least partially preserved somatosensory pathways but note that the effects may be transient.[222,223]

References

1. Jensen TS, Baron R, Haanpää M, et al. A new definition of neuropathic pain. *Pain* 2011;152:2204–2205.
2. Treede RD, Jensen TS, Campbell JN, et al. Neuropathic pain: redefinition and a grading system for clinical and research purposes. *Neurology* 2008; 70:1630–1635.
3. Finnerup NB, Haroutounian S, Kamerman P, et al. Neuropathic pain: an updated grading system for research and clinical practice. *Pain* 2016;157: 1599–1606.
4. Krause SJ, Backonja MM. Development of a neuropathic pain questionnaire. *Clin J Pain* 2003;19:306–314.
5. Bennett M. The LANSS Pain Scale: the Leeds assessment of neuropathic symptoms and signs. *Pain* 2001;92:147–157.
6. Bouhassira D, Attal N, Alchaar H, et al. Comparison of pain syndromes associated with nervous or somatic lesions and development of a new neuropathic pain diagnostic questionnaire (DN4). *Pain* 2005;114:29–36.
7. Freynhagen R, Baron R, Gockel U, et al. painDETECT: a new screening questionnaire to identify neuropathic components in patients with back pain. *Curr Med Res Opin* 2006;22:1911–1920.
8. Portenoy R. Development and testing of a neuropathic pain screening questionnaire: ID Pain. *Curr Med Res Opin* 2006;22:1555–1565.
9. Bryce TN, Richards JS, Bombardier CH, et al. Screening for neuropathic pain after spinal cord injury with the Spinal Cord Injury Pain Instrument (SCIPI): a preliminary validation study. *Spinal Cord* 2014;52:407–412.

10. Hallström H, Norrbrink C. Screening tools for neuropathic pain: can they be of use in individuals with spinal cord injury? *Pain* 2011;152:772–779.

11. Harno H, Haapaniemi E, Putaala J, et al. Central poststroke pain in young ischemic stroke survivors in the Helsinki Young Stroke Registry. *Neurology* 2014;83:1147–1154.

12. MacGowan DJ, Janal MN, Clark WC, et al. Central poststroke pain and Wallenberg's lateral medullary infarction: frequency, character, and determinants in 63 patients. *Neurology* 1997;49:120–125.

13. Finnerup NB, Jensen MP, Norrbrink C, et al. A prospective study of pain and psychological functioning following traumatic spinal cord injury. *Spinal Cord* 2016;54:816–821.

14. Haanpää M, Attal N, Backonja M, et al. NeuPSIG guidelines on neuropathic pain assessment. *Pain* 2011;152:14–27.

15. Maixner W, Fillingim RB, Williams DA, et al. Overlapping chronic pain conditions: implications for diagnosis and classification. *J Pain* 2016;17:T93–T107.

16. Bryce TN, Biering-Sørensen F, Finnerup NB, et al. International spinal cord injury pain (ISCIP) classification: part I. Background and description. March 6–7, 2009. *Spinal Cord* 2012;50:413–417.

17. Treede RD, Rief W, Barke A, et al. A classification of chronic pain for ICD-11. *Pain* 2015;156:1003–1007.

18. Hansen AP, Marcussen NS, Klit H, et al. Pain following stroke: a prospective study. *Eur J Pain* 2012;16:1128–1136.

19. Roosink M, Renzenbrink GJ, Geurts AC, et al. Towards a mechanism-based view on post-stroke shoulder pain: theoretical considerations and clinical implications. *NeuroRehabilitation* 2012;30:153–165.

20. Zeilig G, Rivel M, Weingarden H, et al. Hemiplegic shoulder pain: evidence of a neuropathic origin. *Pain* 2013;154:263–271.

21. de Oliveira RA, de Andrade DC, Machado AG, et al. Central poststroke pain: somatosensory abnormalities and the presence of associated myofascial pain syndrome. *BMC Neurol* 2012;12:89.

22. Mehta S, Guy SD, Bryce TN, et al. The CanPain SCI clinical practice guidelines for rehabilitation management of neuropathic pain after spinal cord: screening and diagnosis recommendations. *Spinal Cord* 2016;54(suppl 1):S7–S13.

23. Boivie J, Leijon G, Johansson I. Central post-stroke pain—a study of the mechanisms through analyses of the sensory abnormalities. *Pain* 1989;37:173–185.

24. Vestergaard K, Nielsen J, Andersen G, et al. Sensory abnormalities in consecutive, unselected patients with central post-stroke pain. *Pain* 1995;61:177–186.

25. Bowsher D. Central pain: clinical and physiological characteristics. *J Neurol Neurosurg Psychiatry* 1996;61:62–69.

26. Greenspan JD, Ohara S, Sarlani E, et al. Allodynia in patients with poststroke central pain (CPSP) studied by statistical quantitative sensory testing within individuals. *Pain* 2004;109:357–366.

27. Leijon G, Boivie J, Johansson I. Central post-stroke pain—neurological symptoms and pain characteristics. *Pain* 1989;36:13–25.

28. Andersen G, Vestergaard K, Ingeman-Nielsen M, et al. Incidence of central post-stroke pain. *Pain* 1995;61:187–193.

29. Cardenas DD, Turner JA, Warms CA, et al. Classification of chronic pain associated with spinal cord injuries. *Arch Phys Med Rehabil* 2002;83:1708–1714.

30. Dworkin RH, Turk DC, Revicki DA, et al. Development and initial validation of an expanded and revised version of the Short-form McGill Pain Questionnaire (SF-MPQ-2). *Pain* 2009;144:35–42.

31. Finnerup NB, Norrbrink C, Trok K, et al. Phenotypes and predictors of pain following traumatic spinal cord injury: a prospective study. *J Pain* 2014;15:40–48.

32. Freeman R, Baron R, Bouhassira D, et al. Sensory profiles of patients with neuropathic pain based on the neuropathic pain symptoms and signs. *Pain* 2014;155:367–376.

33. Attal N, Fermanian C, Fermanian J, et al. Neuropathic pain: are there distinct subtypes depending on the aetiology or anatomical lesion? *Pain* 2008;138:343–353.

34. Svendsen KB, Jensen TS, Hansen HJ, et al. Sensory function and quality of life in patients with multiple sclerosis and pain. *Pain* 2005;114:473–481.

35. Klit H, Finnerup NB, Andersen G, et al. Central poststroke pain: a population-based study. *Pain* 2011;152:818–824.

36. Merskey H, Bogduk N. *Classification of Chronic Pain: Descriptions of Chronic Pain Syndromes and Definitions of Pain Terms.* Seattle, WA: IASP Press; 1994. Available at: http://www.iasp-pain.org/AM/Template.cfm?Section=Pain_Definitions&Template=/CM/HTMLDisplay.cfm&ContentID=1728.

37. Jensen TS, Finnerup NB. Allodynia and hyperalgesia in neuropathic pain: clinical manifestations and mechanisms. *Lancet Neurol* 2014;13:924–935.

38. Klit H, Hansen AP, Marcussen NS, et al. Early evoked pain or dysesthesia is a predictor of central poststroke pain. *Pain* 2014;155:2699–2706.

39. Bennett GJ. What is spontaneous pain and who has it? *J Pain* 2012;13:921–929.

40. Siddall PJ, McClelland J. Non-painful sensory phenomena after spinal cord injury. *J Neurol Neurosurg Psychiatry* 1999;66:617–622.

41. Dworkin RH, Turk DC, Farrar JT, et al. Core outcome measures for chronic pain clinical trials: IMMPACT recommendations. *Pain* 2005;113:9–19.

42. Bryce TN, Budh CN, Cardenas DD, et al. Pain after spinal cord injury: an evidence-based review for clinical practice and research. Report of the National Institute on Disability and Rehabilitation Research Spinal Cord Injury Measures meeting. *J Spinal Cord Med* 2007;30:421–440.

43. Widerström-Nöga E, Biering-Sørensen F, Bryce TN, et al. The international spinal cord injury pain basic data set (version 2.0). *Spinal Cord* 2014;52:282–286.

44. Widerström-Noga E, Biering-Sørensen F, Bryce TN, et al. The international spinal cord injury pain extended data set (version 1.0). *Spinal Cord* 2016;54:1036–1046.

45. Kerns RD, Turk DC, Rudy TE. The West Haven-Yale Multidimensional Pain Inventory (WHYMPI). *Pain* 1985;23:345–356.

46. Widerström-Noga EG, Duncan R, Felipe-Cuervo E, et al. Assessment of the impact of pain and impairments associated with spinal cord injuries. *Arch Phys Med Rehabil* 2002;83:395–404.

47. Bouhassira D, Attal N, Fermanian J, et al. Development and validation of the Neuropathic Pain Symptom Inventory. *Pain* 2004;108:248–257.

48. Klit H, Finnerup NB, Jensen TS. Central post-stroke pain: clinical characteristics, pathophysiology, and management. *Lancet Neurol* 2009;8:857–868.

49. Garcia-Larrea L, Perchet C, Creac'h C, et al. Operculo-insular pain (parasylvian pain): a distinct central pain syndrome. *Brain* 2010;133:2528–2539.

50. O'Donnell MJ, Diener HC, Sacco RL, et al. Chronic pain syndromes after ischemic stroke: PRoFESS trial. *Stroke* 2013;44:1238–1243.

51. Bogousslavsky J, Regli F, Uske A. Thalamic infarcts: clinical syndromes, etiology, and prognosis. *Neurology* 1988;38:837–848.

52. Lampl C, Yazdi K, Röper C. Amitriptyline in the prophylaxis of central poststroke pain. Preliminary results of 39 patients in a placebo-controlled, long-term study. *Stroke* 2002;33:3030–3032.

53. Fitzek S, Baumgärtner U, Fitzek C, et al. Mechanisms and predictors of chronic facial pain in lateral medullary infarction. *Ann Neurol* 2001;49:493–500.

54. Ksiazek-Winiarek DJ, Szpakowski P, Glabinski A. Neural plasticity in multiple sclerosis: the functional and molecular background. *Neural Plast* 2015;2015:307175.

55. Mallucci G, Peruzzotti-Jametti L, Bernstock JD, et al. The role of immune cells, glia and neurons in white and gray matter pathology in multiple sclerosis. *Prog Neurobiol* 2015;127–128:1–22.

56. Osterberg A, Boivie J, Thuomas KA. Central pain in multiple sclerosis—prevalence and clinical characteristics. *Eur J Pain* 2005;9:531–542.

57. Svendsen KB, Sørensen L, Jensen TS, et al. MRI of the central nervous system in MS patients with and without pain. *Eur J Pain* 2011;15:395–401.

58. Okuda DT, Melmed K, Matsuwaki T, et al. Central neuropathic pain in MS is due to distinct thoracic spinal cord lesions. *Ann Clin Transl Neurol* 2014;1:554–561.

59. O'Connor AB, Schwid SR, Herrmann DN, et al. Pain associated with multiple sclerosis: systematic review and proposed classification. *Pain* 2008;137:96–111.

60. Nurmikko TJ, Gupta S, Maclver K. Multiple sclerosis-related central pain disorders. *Curr Pain Headache Rep* 2010;14:189–195.

61. Truini A, Barbanti P, Pozzilli C, et al. A mechanism-based classification of pain in multiple sclerosis. *J Neurol* 2013;260:351–367.

62. Cruccu G, Finnerup NB, Jensen TS, et al. Trigeminal neuralgia: new classification and diagnostic grading for practice and research. *Neurology* 2016;87:220–228.

63. Martinelli Boneschi F, Colombo B, Annovazzi P, et al. Lifetime and actual prevalence of pain and headache in multiple sclerosis. *Mult Scler* 2008;14:514–521.

64. New PW, Marshall R. International spinal cord injury data sets for nontraumatic spinal cord injury. *Spinal Cord* 2014;52:123–132.

65. Rubinelli S, Glässel A, Brach M. From the person's perspective: perceived problems in functioning among individuals with spinal cord injury in Switzerland. *J Rehabil Med* 2016;48:235–243.

66. Siddall PJ, McClelland JM, Rutkowski SB, et al. A longitudinal study of the prevalence and characteristics of pain in the first 5 years following spinal cord injury. *Pain* 2003;103:249–257.

67. Andresen SR, Biering-Sørensen F, Hagen EM, et al. Pain, spasticity and quality of life in individuals with traumatic spinal cord injury in Denmark. *Spinal Cord* 2016;54:973–979.

68. Tran J, Dorstyn DS, Burke AL. Psychosocial aspects of spinal cord injury pain: a meta-analysis. *Spinal Cord* 2016;54:640–648.

69. Burke D, Fullen BM, Stokes D, et al. Neuropathic pain prevalence following spinal cord injury: a systematic review and meta-analysis. *Eur J Pain* 2017;21:29–44.

70. Tasker RR, DeCarvalho GT, Dolan EJ. Intractable pain of spinal cord origin: clinical features and implications for surgery. *J Neurosurg* 1992;77:373–378.

71. Milhorat TH, Kotzen RM, Mu HT, et al. Dysesthetic pain in patients with syringomyelia. *Neurosurgery* 1996;38:940–947.

72. Attal N, Bouhassira D. Chapter 47 Pain in syringomyelia/bulbia. *Handb Clin Neurol* 2006;81:705–713.

73. Ofek H, Defrin R. The characteristics of chronic central pain after traumatic brain injury. *Pain* 2007;131:330–340.

74. Widerström-Noga E, Govind V, Adcock JP, et al. Subacute pain after traumatic brain injury is associated with lower insular N-acetylaspartate concentrations. *J Neurotrauma* 2016;33:1380–1389.

75. Amâncio EJ, Peluso CM, Santos AC, et al. Central pain due to parietal cortex compression by cerebral tumor: report of 2 cases [in Portuguese]. *Arq Neuropsiquiatr* 2002;60:487–489.

76. Silbergeld DL, Hebb AO, Loeser JD. Vaginal allodynia as the presentation of a thalamic tumor. *Pain* 2011;152:698–702.

77. Tasker RR. Central pain states. In: Loeser JD, ed. *Bonica's Management of Pain*. Philadelphia: Lipponcott Williams & Wilkins; 2001:433–457.

78. Young Blood MR, Ferro MM, Munhoz RP, et al. Classification and characteristics of pain associated with Parkinson's disease. *Parkinsons Dis* 2016; 2016:6067132.

79. Ha AD, Jankovic J. Pain in Parkinson's disease. *Mov Disord* 2012;27:485–491.

80. Truini A, Frontoni M, Cruccu G. Parkinson's disease related pain: a review of recent findings. *J Neurol* 2013;260:330–334.

81. Schestatsky P, Kumru H, Valls-Solé J, et al. Neurophysiologic study of central pain in patients with Parkinson disease. *Neurology* 2007;69:2162–2169.

82. Cury RG, Galhardoni R, Teixeira MJ, et al. Subthalamic deep brain stimulation modulates conscious perception of sensory function in Parkinson's disease. *Pain* 2016;157:2758–2765.

83. Tinazzi M, Del Vesco C, Defazio G, et al. Abnormal processing of the nociceptive input in Parkinson's disease: a study with CO2 laser evoked potentials. *Pain* 2008;136:117–124.

84. Zambito Marsala S, Tinazzi M, Vitaliani R, et al. Spontaneous pain, pain threshold, and pain tolerance in Parkinson's disease. *J Neurol* 2011;258:627–633.

85. Pertovaara A, Wei H. Dual influence of the striatum on neuropathic hypersensitivity. *Pain* 2008;137:50–59.

86. Borsook D, Upadhyay J, Chudler EH, et al. A key role of the basal ganglia in pain and analgesia—insights gained through human functional imaging. *Mol Pain* 2010;6:27.

87. Gates P, Nayernouri T, Sengupta RP. Epileptic pain: a temporal lobe focus. *J Neurol Neurosurg Psychiatry* 1984;47:319–320.

88. Young GB, Blume WT. Painful epileptic seizures. *Brain* 1983;106:537–554.

89. Isnard J, Magnin M, Jung J, et al. Does the insula tell our brain that we are in pain? *Pain* 2011;152:946–951.

90. Wasserman JK, Koeberle PD. Development and characterization of a hemorrhagic rat model of central post-stroke pain. *Neuroscience* 2009;161:173–183.

91. Macolino CM, Daiutolo BV, Albertson BK, et al. Mechanical allodynia induced by traumatic brain injury is independent of restraint stress. *J Neurosci Methods* 2014;226:139–146.

92. Grace PM, Loram LC, Christianson JP, et al. Behavioral assessment of neuropathic pain, fatigue, and anxiety in experimental autoimmune encephalomyelitis (EAE) and attenuation by interleukin-10 gene therapy. *Brain Behav Immun* 2017;59:49–54.

93. Begum F, Zhu W, Cortes C, et al. Elevation of tumor necrosis factor α in dorsal root ganglia and spinal cord is associated with neuroimmune modulation of pain in an animal model of multiple sclerosis. *J Neuroimmune Pharmacol* 2013;8:677–690.

94. Wang CC, Shih HC, Shyu BC, et al. Effects of thalamic hemorrhagic lesions on explicit and implicit learning during the acquisition and retrieval phases in an animal model of central post-stroke pain. *Behav Brain Res* 2017;317:251–262.

95. Moon JH, Na JY, Lee MC, et al. Neuroprotective effects of systemic cerebral endothelial cell transplantation in a rat model of cerebral ischemia. *Am J Transl Res* 2016;8:2343–2353.

96. Blasi F, Herisson F, Wang S, et al. Late-onset thermal hypersensitivity after focal ischemic thalamic infarcts as a model for central post-stroke pain in rats. *J Cereb Blood Flow Metab* 2015;35:1100–1103.

97. Christensen MD, Everhart AW, Pickelman JT, et al. Mechanical and thermal allodynia in chronic central pain following spinal cord injury. *Pain* 1996;68:97–107.

98. Yezierski RP, Liu S, Ruenes GL, et al. Excitotoxic spinal cord injury: behavioral and morphological characteristics of a central pain model. *Pain* 1998;75:141–155.

99. Hao JX, Xu XJ, Aldskogius H, et al. Allodynia-like effects in rat after ischaemic spinal cord injury photochemically induced by laser irradiation. *Pain* 1991;45:175–185.

100. Wang G, Thompson SM. Maladaptive homeostatic plasticity in a rodent model of central pain syndrome: thalamic hyperexcitability after spinothalamic tract lesions. *J Neurosci* 2008;28:11959–11969.

101. Kramer JL, Minhas NK, Jutzeler CR, et al. Neuropathic pain following traumatic spinal cord injury: models, measurement, and mechanisms. *J Neurosci Res* 2017;95:1295–1306.

102. Davoody L, Quiton RL, Lucas JM, et al. Conditioned place preference reveals tonic pain in an animal model of central pain. *J Pain* 2011;12:868–874.

103. Yezierski RP, Yu CG, Mantyh PW, et al. Spinal neurons involved in the generation of at-level pain following spinal injury in the rat. *Neurosci Lett* 2004;361:232–236.

104. Zeilig G, Enosh S, Rubin-Asher D, et al. The nature and course of sensory changes following spinal cord injury: predictive properties and implications on the mechanism of central pain. *Brain* 2012;135:418–430.

105. Vierck CJ, Light AR. Assessment of pain sensitivity in dermatomes caudal to spinal cord injury in rats. In: Yezierski RP, Burchiel KJ, eds. *Spinal Cord Injury Pain: Assessment, Mechanisms, Management. Progress in Pain Research and Management*. Seattle, WA: IASP Press; 2002:137–154.

106. Baastrup C, Maersk-Moller CC, Nyengaard JR, et al. Spinal-, brainstem- and cerebrally mediated responses at- and below-level of a spinal cord contusion in rats: evaluation of pain-like behavior. *Pain* 2010;151:670–679.

107. Yezierski RP, Vierck CJ. Reflex and pain behaviors are not equivalent: lessons from spinal cord injury. *Pain* 2010;151:569–570.

108. van GS, Deumens R, Leerink M, et al. Translation of the rat thoracic contusion model; part 1—supraspinally versus spinally mediated pain-like responses and spasticity. *Spinal Cord* 2014;52:524–528.

109. Vierck CJ, Yezierski RP. Comparison of operant escape and reflex tests of nociceptive sensitivity. *Neurosci Biobehav Rev* 2015;51:223–242.

110. Basbaum AI, Bautista DM, Scherrer G, et al. Cellular and molecular mechanisms of pain. *Cell* 2009;139:267–284.

111. Woolf CJ. Central sensitization: implications for the diagnosis and treatment of pain. *Pain* 2011;152:S2–S15.

112. Loeser JD, Treede RD. The Kyoto protocol of IASP basic pain terminology. *Pain* 2008;137:473–477.

113. Vardeh D, Mannion RJ, Woolf CJ. Toward a mechanism-based approach to pain diagnosis. *J Pain* 2016;17:T50–T69.

114. Yezierski RP. Pain following spinal cord injury: central mechanisms. In: Cervero F, Jensen TS, eds. *Handbook of Clinical Neurology: Pain*. Amsterdam, The Netherlands: Elsevier; 2006:293–307.

115. Brown A, Weaver LC. The dark side of neuroplasticity. *Exp Neurol* 2012;235:133–141.

116. Colloca L, Ludman T, Bouhassira D, et al. Neuropathic pain. *Nat Rev Dis Primers* 2017;3:17002.

117. Hains BC, Waxman SG. Sodium channel expression and the molecular pathophysiology of pain after SCI. *Prog Brain Res* 2007;161:195–203.

118. Boroujerdi A, Zeng J, Sharp K, et al. Calcium channel alpha-2-delta-1 protein upregulation in dorsal spinal cord mediates spinal cord injury-induced neuropathic pain states. *Pain* 2011;152:649–655.

119. Gwak YS, Hulsebosch CE. Neuronal hyperexcitability: a substrate for central neuropathic pain after spinal cord injury. *Curr Pain Headache Rep* 2011;15:215–222.

120. Eijkelkamp N, Linley JE, Baker MD, et al. Neurological perspectives on voltage-gated sodium channels. *Brain* 2012;135:2585–2612.

121. Radu BM, Banciu A, Banciu DD, et al. Acid-sensing ion channels as potential pharmacological targets in peripheral and central nervous system diseases. *Adv Protein Chem Struct Biol* 2016;103:137–167.

122. Jones AK, Watabe H, Cunningham VJ, et al. Cerebral decreases in opioid receptor binding in patients with central neuropathic pain measured by [11C]diprenorphine binding and PET. *Eur J Pain* 2004;8:479–485.

123. Willoch F, Schindler F, Wester HJ, et al. Central poststroke pain and reduced opioid receptor binding within pain processing circuitries: a [11C] diprenorphine PET study. *Pain* 2004;108:213–220.

124. Naseri K, Saghaei E, Abbaszadeh F, et al. Role of microglia and astrocyte in central pain syndrome following electrolytic lesion at the spinothalamic tract in rats. *J Mol Neurosci* 2013;49:470–479.

125. Widerström-Noga E, Cruz-Almeida Y, Felix ER, et al. Somatosensory phenotype is associated with thalamic metabolites and pain intensity after spinal cord injury. *Pain* 2015;156:166–174.

126. Wiesenfeld-Hallin Z, Hao JX, Xu XJ. Mechanisms of central pain. In: Jensen TS, Turner JA, Wiesenfeld-Hallin Z, eds. *Proceedings of the 8th World Congress on Pain*. Seattle, WA: IASP Press; 1997:575–589.

127. Grau JW, Huang YJ, Turtle JD, et al. When pain hurts: nociceptive stimulation induces a state of maladaptive plasticity and impairs recovery after spinal cord injury. *J Neurotrauma* 2017;34:1873–1890.

128. Boivie J. Central pain. In: Wall PD, Melzack R, eds. *Textbook of Pain*. Edinburgh: Churchill Livingstone; 1994:871–902.

129. Kim JH, Ahn SH, Cho YW, et al. The relation between injury of the spinothalamocortical tract and central pain in chronic patients with mild traumatic brain injury. *J Head Trauma Rehabil* 2015;30:E40–E46.

130. Garcia-Larrea L. Insights gained into pain processing from patients with focal brain lesions. *Neurosci Lett* 2012;520:188–191.

131. Melzack R, Loeser JD. Phantom body pain in paraplegics: evidence for a central "pattern generating mechanism" for pain. *Pain* 1978;4:195–210.

132. Finnerup NB, Sørensen L, Biering-Sørensen F, et al. Segmental hypersensitivity and spinothalamic function in spinal cord injury pain. *Exp Neurol* 2007;207:139–149.

133. Wasner G, Lee BB, Engel S, et al. Residual spinothalamic tract pathways predict development of central pain after spinal cord injury. *Brain* 2008;131:2387–2400.

134. Cruz-Almeida Y, Felix ER, Martinez-Arizala A, et al. Decreased spinothalamic and dorsal column medial lemniscus-mediated function is associated with neuropathic pain after spinal cord injury. *J Neurotrauma* 2012;29:2706–2715.

135. Tasker RR, Gorecki J, Lenz FA, et al. Thalamic microelectrode recording and microstimulation in central and deafferentation pain. *Appl Neurophysiol* 1987;50:414–417.

136. Lenz FA, Gracely RH, Baker FH, et al. Reorganization of sensory modalities evoked by microstimulation in region of the thalamic principal sensory nucleus in patients with pain due to nervous system injury. *J Comp Neurol* 1998;399:125–138.

137. Ducreux D, Attal N, Parker F, et al. Mechanisms of central neuropathic pain: a combined psychophysical and fMRI study in syringomyelia. *Brain* 2006;129:963–976.

138. Garcia-Larrea L, Convers P, Magnin M, et al. Laser-evoked potential abnormalities in central pain patients: the influence of spontaneous and provoked pain. *Brain* 2002;125:2766–2781.

139. Truini A, Galeotti F, La CS, et al. Mechanisms of pain in multiple sclerosis: a combined clinical and neurophysiological study. *Pain* 2012;153:2048–2054.

140. Tasker RR. Identification of pain processing systems by electrical stimulation of the brain. *Hum Neurobiol* 1982;1:261–272.

141. Jeanmonod D, Magnin M, Morel A. Thalamus and neurogenic pain: physiological, anatomical and clinical data. *Neuroreport* 1993;4:475–478.

142. Hirayama T, Dostrovsky JO, Gorecki J, et al. Recordings of abnormal activity in patients with deafferentation and central pain. *Stereotact Funct Neurosurg* 1989;52:120–126.

143. Dostrovsky JO. Role of thalamus in pain. *Prog Brain Res* 2000;129:245–257.

144. Pattany PM, Yezierski RP, Widerström-Noga EG, et al. Proton magnetic resonance spectroscopy of the thalamus in patients with chronic neuropathic pain after spinal cord injury. *AJNR Am J Neuroradiol* 2002;23:901–905.

145. Zhao P, Waxman SG, Hains BC. Modulation of thalamic nociceptive processing after spinal cord injury through remote activation of thalamic microglia by cysteine cysteine chemokine ligand 21. *J Neurosci* 2007;27:8893–8902.

146. Kim JH, Greenspan JD, Coghill RC, et al. Lesions limited to the human thalamic principal somatosensory nucleus (ventral caudal) are associated with loss of cold sensations and central pain. *J Neurosci* 2007;27:4995–5004.

147. Gustin SM, Wrigley PJ, Youssef AM, et al. Thalamic activity and biochemical changes in individuals with neuropathic pain after spinal cord injury. *Pain* 2014;155:1027–1036.

148. Berić A, Dimitrijević MR, Lindblom U. Central dysesthesia syndrome in spinal cord injury patients. *Pain* 1988;34:109–116.

149. Pagni CA. Central pain due to spinal cord and brain stem damage. In: Wall PD, Melzack R, eds. *Textbook of Pain*. Edinburgh: Churchill Livingstone; 1989:634–655.

150. Tasker R. Pain resulting from central nervous system pathology (central pain). In: Bonica JJ, ed. *The Management of Pain*. Philadelphia: Lea & Febiger; 1990:264–283.

151. Head H, Holmes G. Sensory disturbances from cerebral lesions. *Brain* 1911;34:102–254.

152. Craig AD, Reiman EM, Evans A, et al. Functional imaging of an illusion of pain. *Nature* 1996;384:258–260.

153. Craig AD. A new version of the thalamic disinhibition hypothesis of central pain. *Pain Forum* 1998;7:1–14.

154. Gruener H, Zeilig G, Laufer Y, et al. Differential pain modulation properties in central neuropathic pain after spinal cord injury. *Pain* 2016;157:1415–1424.

155. Albu S, Gómez-Soriano J, Avila-Martin G, et al. Deficient conditioned pain modulation after spinal cord injury correlates with clinical spontaneous pain measures. *Pain* 2015;156:260–272.

156. Jang SH, Park SM, Kwon HG. Relation between injury of the periaqueductal gray and central pain in patients with mild traumatic brain injury: observational study. *Medicine (Baltimore)* 2016;95:e4017.

157. Druckman R, Lende R. Central pain of spinal cord origin: pathogenesis and surgical relief in one patient. *Neurology* 1965;15:518–522.

158. Edgar RE, Best LG, Quail PA, et al. Computer-assisted DREZ microcoagulation: posttraumatic spinal deafferentation. *J Spinal Disord* 1993;6:48–56.

159. Falci S, Best L, Bayles R, et al. Dorsal root entry zone microcoagulation for spinal cord injury-related central pain: operative intramedullary electrophysiological guidance and clinical outcome. *J Neurosurg* 2002;97:193–200.

160. Chun HJ, Kim YS, Yi HJ. A modified microsurgical DREZotomy procedure for refractory neuropathic pain. *World Neurosurg* 2011;75:551–557.

161. Finnerup NB, Johannesen IL, Fuglsang-Frederiksen A, et al. Sensory function in spinal cord injury patients with and without central pain. *Brain* 2003;126:57–70.

162. Levitan Y, Zeilig G, Bondi M, et al. Predicting the risk for central pain using the sensory components of the international standards for neurological classification of spinal cord injury. *J Neurotrauma* 2015;32:1684–1692.

163. Vuckovic A, Hasan MA, Fraser M, et al. Dynamic oscillatory signatures of central neuropathic pain in spinal cord injury. *J Pain* 2014;15:645–655.

164. Wrigley PJ, Press SR, Gustin SM, et al. Neuropathic pain and primary somatosensory cortex reorganization following spinal cord injury. *Pain* 2009;141:52–59.

165. Jutzeler CR, Freund P, Huber E, et al. Neuropathic pain and functional reorganization in the primary sensorimotor cortex after spinal cord injury. *J Pain* 2015;16:1256–1267.

166. Jutzeler CR, Curt A, Kramer JL. Relationship between chronic pain and brain reorganization after deafferentation: a systematic review of functional MRI findings. *Neuroimage Clin* 2015;9:599–606.

167. Stanwell P, Siddall P, Keshava N, et al. Neuro magnetic resonance spectroscopy using wavelet decomposition and statistical testing identifies biochemical changes in people with spinal cord injury and pain. *Neuroimage* 2010;53:544–552.

168. Gustin SM, Wrigley PJ, Henderson LA, et al. Brain circuitry underlying pain in response to imagined movement in people with spinal cord injury. *Pain* 2010;148:438–445.

169. Yoon EJ, Kim YK, Shin HI, et al. Cortical and white matter alterations in patients with neuropathic pain after spinal cord injury. *Brain Res* 2013;1540:64–73.

170. Widerström-Noga E, Pattany PM, Cruz-Almeida Y, et al. Metabolite concentrations in the anterior cingulate cortex predict high neuropathic pain impact after spinal cord injury. *Pain* 2013;154:204–212.

171. Jutzeler CR, Huber E, Callaghan MF, et al. Association of pain and CNS structural changes after spinal cord injury. *Sci Rep* 2016;6:18534.

172. Max MB. Towards physiologically based treatment of patients with neuropathic pain. *Pain* 1990;42:131–137.

173. Attal N, Bouhassira D, Baron R, et al. Assessing symptom profiles in neuropathic pain clinical trials: can it improve outcome? *Eur J Pain* 2011;15:441–443.

174. Baron R, Maier C, Attal N, et al. Peripheral neuropathic pain: a mechanism-related organizing principle based on sensory profiles. *Pain* 2017;158:261–272.

175. Finnerup NB, Attal N, Haroutounian S, et al. Pharmacotherapy for neuropathic pain in adults: a systematic review and meta-analysis. *Lancet Neurol* 2015;14:162–173.

176. Leijon G, Boivie J. Central post-stroke pain—a controlled trial of amitriptyline and carbamazepine. *Pain* 1989;36:27–36.

177. Cardenas DD, Warms CA, Turner JA, et al. Efficacy of amitriptyline for relief of pain in spinal cord injury: results of a randomized controlled trial. *Pain* 2002;96:365–373.

178. Rintala DH, Holmes SA, Courtade D, et al. Comparison of the effectiveness of amitriptyline and gabapentin on chronic neuropathic pain in persons with spinal cord injury. *Arch Phys Med Rehabil* 2007;88:1547–1560.

179. Österberg A, Boivie J. Central pain in multiple sclerosis—a double-blind placebo-controlled trial of amitriptyline and carbamazepine. In: Österberg A, ed. *Central Pain in Multiple Sclerosis—Clinical Characteristics, Sensory Abnormalities, and Treatment* [thesis]. Linköping, Sweden: Linköping University; 2005:903.

180. Vranken JH, Hollmann MW, van der Vegt MH, et al. Duloxetine in patients with central neuropathic pain caused by spinal cord injury or stroke: a randomized, double-blind, placebo-controlled trial. *Pain* 2011;152:267–273.

181. Siddall PJ, Cousins MJ, Otte A, et al. Pregabalin in central neuropathic pain associated with spinal cord injury: a placebo-controlled trial. *Neurology* 2006;67:1792–1800.

182. Cardenas DD, Nieshoff EC, Suda K, et al. A randomized trial of pregabalin in patients with neuropathic pain due to spinal cord injury. *Neurology* 2013;80:533–539.

183. Vestergaard K, Andersen G, Gottrup H, et al. Lamotrigine for central post-stroke pain: a randomized controlled trial. *Neurology* 2001;56:184–190.

184. Finnerup NB, Sindrup SH, Bach FW, et al. Lamotrigine in spinal cord injury pain: a randomized controlled trial. *Pain* 2002;96:375–383.

185. Cragg JJ, Warner FM, Finnerup NB, et al. Meta-analysis of placebo responses in central neuropathic pain: impact of subject, study, and pain characteristics. *Pain* 2016;157:530–540.

186. Sindrup SH, Otto M, Finnerup NB, et al. Antidepressants in the treatment of neuropathic pain. *Basic Clin Pharmacol Toxicol* 2005;96:399–409.

187. Kremer M, Salvat E, Muller A, et al. Antidepressants and gabapentinoids in neuropathic pain: mechanistic insights. *Neuroscience* 2016;338:183–206.

188. McQuay HJ, Tramer M, Nye BA, et al. A systematic review of antidepressants in neuropathic pain. *Pain* 1996;68:217–227.

189. Ray WA, Meredith S, Thapa PB, et al. Cyclic antidepressants and the risk of sudden cardiac death. *Clin Pharmacol Ther* 2004;75:234–241.

190. American Geriatrics Society 2012 Beers Criteria Update Expert Panel. American Geriatrics Society updated Beers Criteria for potentially inappropriate medication use in older adults. *J Am Geriatr Soc* 2012;60:616–631.

191. Bee LA, Dickenson AH. Descending facilitation from the brainstem determines behavioural and neuronal hypersensitivity following nerve injury and efficacy of pregabalin. *Pain* 2008;140:209–223.

192. Morimoto S, Ito M, Oda S, et al. Spinal mechanism underlying the antiallodynic effect of gabapentin studied in the mouse spinal nerve ligation model. *J Pharmacol Sci* 2012;118:455–466.

193. Harris RE, Napadow V, Huggins JP, et al. Pregabalin rectifies aberrant brain chemistry, connectivity, and functional response in chronic pain patients. *Anesthesiology* 2013;119:1453–1464.

194. European Medicines Agency. Lyrica—scientific discussion. Available at: http://www.ema.europa.eu/docs/en_GB/document_library/EPAR_-_Scientific_Discussion_-_Variation/human/000546/WC500046606.pdf. Accessed April 10, 2017.

195. Attal N, Cruccu G, Baron R, et al. EFNS guidelines on the pharmacological treatment of neuropathic pain: 2010 revision. *Eur J Neurol* 2010;17:1113–1123, e68–e88.

196. Buss T, Leppert W. Opioid-induced endocrinopathy in cancer patients: an underestimated clinical problem. *Adv Ther* 2014;31:153–167.

197. Schiltenwolf M, Akbar M, Hug A, et al. Evidence of specific cognitive deficits in patients with chronic low back pain under long-term substitution treatment of opioids. *Pain Physician* 2014;17:9–20.

198. Edlund MJ, Martin BC, Russo JE, et al. The role of opioid prescription in incident opioid abuse and dependence among individuals with chronic noncancer pain: the role of opioid prescription. *Clin J Pain* 2014;30:557–564.

199. Bohnert AS, Ilgen MA, Trafton JA, et al. Trends and regional variation in opioid overdose mortality among Veterans Health Administration patients, fiscal year 2001 to 2009. *Clin J Pain* 2013;30:605–612.

200. Sindrup SH, Jensen TS. Are sodium channel blockers useless in peripheral neuropathic pain? *Pain* 2007;128:6–7.

201. Demant DT, Lund K, Vollert J, et al. The effect of oxcarbazepine in peripheral neuropathic pain depends on pain phenotype: a randomised, double-blind, placebo-controlled phenotype-stratified study. *Pain* 2014;155:2263–2273.

202. Guy SD, Mehta S, Casalino A, et al. The CanPain SCI clinical practice guidelines for rehabilitation management of neuropathic pain after spinal cord: recommendations for treatment. *Spinal Cord* 2016;54(suppl 1):S14–S23.

203. Siddall PJ, Molloy AR, Walker S, et al. The efficacy of intrathecal morphine and clonidine in the treatment of pain after spinal cord injury. *Anesth Analg* 2000;91:1493–1498.

204. Wallace MS, Rauck RL, Deer T. Ziconotide combination intrathecal therapy: rationale and evidence. *Clin J Pain* 2010;26:635–644.

205. Eide PK, Stubhaug A, Stenehjem AE. Central dysesthesia pain after traumatic spinal cord injury is dependent on N-methyl-D-aspartate receptor activation. *Neurosurgery* 1995;37:1080–1087.

206. Attal N, Guirimand F, Brasseur L, et al. Effects of IV morphine in central pain: a randomized placebo-controlled study. *Neurology* 2002;58:554–563.

207. Finnerup NB, Biering-Sørensen F, Johannesen IL, et al. Intravenous lidocaine relieves spinal cord injury pain: a randomized controlled trial. *Anesthesiology* 2005;102:1023–1030.

208. Amr YM. Multi-day low dose ketamine infusion as adjuvant to oral gabapentin in spinal cord injury related chronic pain: a prospective, randomized, double blind trial. *Pain Physician* 2010;13:245–249.

209. Attal N, Gaudé V, Brasseur L, et al. Intravenous lidocaine in central pain: a double-blind, placebo-controlled, psychophysical study. *Neurology* 2000;54:564–574.

210. Norrbrink BC, Lundeberg T. Non-pharmacological pain-relieving therapies in individuals with spinal cord injury: a patient perspective. *Complement Ther Med* 2004;12:189–197.

211. Turk DC, Flor H. The cognitive-behavioral approach to pain management. In: McMahon SB, Koltzenburg M, eds. *Textbook of Pain*. Philadelphia: Elsevier/Churchill Livingstone; 2006:339–348.

212. Eccleston C, Hearn L, Williams AC. Psychological therapies for the management of chronic neuropathic pain in adults. *Cochrane Database Syst Rev* 2015;(10):CD011259.

213. Jensen MP, Barber J, Romano JM, et al. Effects of self-hypnosis training and EMG biofeedback relaxation training on chronic pain in persons with spinal-cord injury. *Int J Clin Exp Hypn* 2009;57:239–268.

214. Jensen MP, Gianas A, George HR, et al. Use of neurofeedback to enhance response to hypnotic analgesia in individuals with multiple sclerosis. *Int J Clin Exp Hypn* 2016;64:1–23.

215. Müller R, Gertz KJ, Molton IR, et al. Effects of a tailored positive psychology intervention on well-being and pain in individuals with chronic pain and a physical disability: a feasibility trial. *Clin J Pain* 2016;32:32–44.

216. Norrbrink BC, Kowalski J, Lundeberg T. A comprehensive pain management programme comprising educational, cognitive and behavioural interventions for neuropathic pain following spinal cord injury. *J Rehabil Med* 2006;38:172–180.

217. Heutink M, Post MW, Luthart P, et al. Long-term outcomes of a multidisciplinary cognitive behavioural programme for coping with chronic neuropathic spinal cord injury pain. *J Rehabil Med* 2014;46:540–545.

218. Castelnuovo G, Giusti EM, Manzoni GM, et al. Psychological treatments and psychotherapies in the neurorehabilitation of pain: evidences and recommendations from the Italian Consensus Conference on Pain in Neurorehabilitation. *Front Psychol* 2016;7:115.

219. Moseley GL. Using visual illusion to reduce at-level neuropathic pain in paraplegia. *Pain* 2007;130:294–298.

220. Soler MD, Kumru H, Pelayo R, et al. Effectiveness of transcranial direct current stimulation and visual illusion on neuropathic pain in spinal cord injury. *Brain* 2010;133:2565–2577.

221. Hasan MA, Fraser M, Conway BA, et al. Reversed cortical over-activity during movement imagination following neurofeedback treatment for central neuropathic pain. *Clin Neurophysiol* 2016;127:3118–3127.

222. Canavero S, Bonicalzi V. Neuromodulation for central pain. *Expert Rev Neurother* 2003;3(5):591–607.

223. Canavero S, Bonicalzi V. Central pain syndrome: elucidation of genesis and treatment. *Expert Rev Neurother* 2007;7(11):1485–1497.

224. Herman RM, D'Luzansky SC, Ippolito R. Intrathecal baclofen suppresses central pain in patients with spinal lesions. A pilot study. *Clin J Pain* 1992;8(4):338–345.

225. Shieff C, Nashold BS Jr. Thalamic pain and stereotactic mesencephalotomy. *Acta Neurochir Suppl (Wien)* 1988;42:239–242.

226. Tsubokawa T, Katayama Y, Yamamoto T, et al. Treatment of thalamic pain by chronic motor cortex stimulation. *Pacing Clin Electrophysiol* 1991;14(1):131–134.

227. Sukul VV, Slavin KV. Deep brain and motor cortex stimulation. *Curr Pain Headache Rep* 2014;18(7):427.

228. Deer TR, Mekhail N, Petersen E, et al. The appropriate use of neurostimulation: stimulation of the intracranial and extracranial space and head for chronic pain. Neuromodulation Appropriateness Consensus Committee. *Neuromodulation* 2014;17(6):551–570.

229. Moore NZ, Lempka SF, Machado A. Central neuromodulation for refractory pain. *Neurosurg Clin N Am* 2014;25(1):77–83.

230. Fontaine D, Hamani C, Lozano A. Efficacy and safety of motor cortex stimulation for chronic neuropathic pain: critical review of the literature. *J Neurosurg* 2009;110(2):251–256.

231. Canavero S, Bonicalzi V. Extradural cortical stimulation for central pain. *Acta Neurochir Suppl* 2007;97(pt 2):27–36.

232. Saitoh Y, Osaki Y, Nishimura H, et al. Increased regional cerebral blood flow in the contralateral thalamus after successful motor cortex stimulation in a patient with poststroke pain. *J Neurosurg* 2004;100(5):935–939.

233. Tanei T, Kajita Y, Wakabayashi T. Motor cortex stimulation for intractable neuropathic facial pain related to multiple sclerosis. *Neurol Med Chir (Tokyo)* 2010;50(7):604–607.

234. Son BC, Lee SW, Choi ES, et al. Motor cortex stimulation for central pain following a traumatic brain injury. *Pain* 2006;123(1–2):210–216.

235. Nguyen JP, Nizard J, Keravel Y, et al. Invasive brain stimulation for the treatment of neuropathic pain. *Nat Rev Neurol* 2011;7(12):699–709.

236. Honey CM, Tronnier VM, Honey CR. Deep brain stimulation versus motor cortex stimulation for neuropathic pain: a minireview of the literature and proposal for future research. *Comput Struct Biotechnol J* 2016;14:234–237.

237. Coffey RJ. Deep brain stimulation for chronic pain: results of two multicenter trials and a structured review. *Pain Med* 2001;2(3):183–192.

238. Bittar RG, Kar-Purkayastha I, Owen SL, et al. Deep brain stimulation for pain relief: a meta-analysis. *J Clin Neurosci* 2005;12(5):515–519.

239. Boccard SG, Pereira EA, Moir L, et al. Long-term outcomes of deep brain stimulation for neuropathic pain. *Neurosurgery* 2013;72(2):221–231.

240. Levy R, Deer TR, Henderson J. Intracranial neurostimulation for pain control: a review. *Pain Physician* 2010;13(2):157–165.

241. Abreu V, Vaz R, Rebelo V, et al. Thalamic deep brain stimulation for neuropathic pain: efficacy at three years' follow-up. *Neuromodulation* 2017;20:504–513.

242. Russo JF, Sheth SA. Deep brain stimulation of the dorsal anterior cingulate cortex for the treatment of chronic neuropathic pain. *Neurosurg Focus* 2015;38(6):E11.

243. Lempka SF, Malone DA Jr, Hu B, et al. Randomized clinical trial of deep brain stimulation for poststroke pain. *Ann Neurol* 2017;81(5):653–663.

244. Hamani C, Schwalb JM, Rezai AR, et al. Deep brain stimulation for chronic neuropathic pain: long-term outcome and the incidence of insertional effect. *Pain* 2006;125(1–2):188–196.

245. Owen SL, Green AL, Stein JF, et al. Deep brain stimulation for the alleviation of post-stroke neuropathic pain. *Pain* 2006;120(1–2):202–206.

246. Jermakowicz WJ, Hentall ID, Jagid JR, et al. Deep brain stimulation improves the symptoms and sensory signs of persistent central neuropathic pain from spinal cord injury: a case report. *Front Hum Neurosci* 2017;11:177.

247. Chari A, Hentall ID, Papadopoulos MC, et al. Surgical neurostimulation for spinal cord injury. *Brain Sci* 2017;7(2):E18.

248. Cruccu G, Garcia-Larrea L, Hansson P, et al. EAN guidelines on central neurostimulation therapy in chronic pain conditions. *Eur J Neurol* 2016;23(10):1489–1499.

249. Burkey AR, Abla-Yao S. Successful treatment of central pain in a multiple sclerosis patient with epidural stimulation of the dorsal root entry zone. *Pain Med* 2010;11(1):127–132.

250. Aly MM, Saitoh Y, Hosomi K, et al. Spinal cord stimulation for central poststroke pain. *Neurosurgery* 2010;67(3):ons206–ons212.

251. Lopez JA, Torres LM, Gala F, et al. Spinal cord stimulation and thalamic pain: long-term results of eight cases. *Neuromodulation* 2009;12(3):240–243.

252. Nashold BS Jr, Friedman H. Dorsal column stimulation for control of pain. Preliminary report on 30 patients. *J Neurosurg* 1972;36(5):590–597.

253. Kim JS, Bashford G, Murphy TK, et al. Safety and efficacy of pregabalin in patients with central post-stroke pain. *Pain* 2011;152:1018–1023.

254. Vranken JH, Dijkgraaf MG, Kruis MR, et al. Pregabalin in patients with central neuropathic pain: a randomized, double-blind, placebo-controlled trial of a flexible-dose regimen. *Pain* 2008;136:150–157.

255. Levendoglu F, Ogün CO, Ozerbil O, et al. Gabapentin is a first line drug for the treatment of neuropathic pain in spinal cord injury. *Spine (Phila Pa 1976)* 2004;29:743–751.

256. Breuer B, Pappagallo M, Knotkova H, et al. A randomized, double-blind, placebo-controlled, two-period, crossover, pilot trial of lamotrigine in patients with central pain due to multiple sclerosis. *Clin Ther* 2007;29:2022–2030.

257. Drewes AM, Andreasen A, Poulsen LH. Valproate for treatment of chronic central pain after spinal cord injury. A double-blind cross-over study. *Paraplegia* 1994;32:565–569.

258. Finnerup NB, Grydehøj J, Bing J, et al. Levetiracetam in spinal cord injury pain: a randomized controlled trial. *Spinal Cord* 2009;47:861–867.

259. Jungehulsing GJ, Israel H, Safar N, et al. Levetiracetam in patients with central neuropathic post-stroke pain—a randomized, double-blind, placebo-controlled trial. *Eur J Neurol* 2013;20:331–337.

260. Falah M, Madsen C, Holbech JV, et al. A randomized, placebo-controlled trial of levetiracetam in central pain in multiple sclerosis. *Eur J Pain* 2012;16:860–869.

261. Norrbrink C, Lundeberg T. Tramadol in neuropathic pain after spinal cord injury: a randomized, double-blind, placebo-controlled trial. *Clin J Pain* 2009;25:177–184.

262. Svendsen KB, Jensen TS, Bach FW. Does the cannabinoid dronabinol reduce central pain in multiple sclerosis? Randomised double blind placebo controlled crossover trial. *BMJ* 2004;329:253.

263. Rog DJ, Nurmikko TJ, Friede T, et al. Randomized, controlled trial of cannabis-based medicine in central pain in multiple sclerosis. *Neurology* 2005;65:812–819.

264. Langford RM, Mares J, Novotna A, et al. A double-blind, randomized, placebo-controlled, parallel-group study of THC/CBD oromucosal spray in combination with the existing treatment regimen, in the relief of central neuropathic pain in patients with multiple sclerosis. *J Neurol* 2013;260:984–997.

265. Chiou-Tan FY, Tuel SM, Johnson JC, et al. Effect of mexiletine on spinal cord injury dysesthetic pain. *Am J Phys Med Rehabil* 1996;75:84–87.

266. Han ZA, Song DH, Oh HM, et al. Botulinum toxin type A for neuropathic pain in patients with spinal cord injury. *Ann Neurol* 2016;79:569–578.

267. Andresen SR, Bing J, Hansen RM, et al. Ultramicronized palmitoylethanolamide in spinal cord injury neuropathic pain: a randomized, double-blind, placebo-controlled trial. *Pain* 2016;157:2097–2103.

CHAPTER 29

The Psychophysiology of Pain

C. RICHARD CHAPMAN and **FADEL ZEIDAN**

Psychophysiology is a field of study that seeks to relate subjective awareness and behavior to physiologic events.[1-3] As a field of scientific inquiry, it concerns itself with central mechanisms of perception, cognition, and behavior, including learning, the emotions, and the relationship of brain activity to consciousness. As a clinical area, psychophysiology has classically addressed somatoform disorders, stress (most recently posttraumatic stress disorders), and affective disorders in general. As a domain, psychophysiology is an important resource for the pain field for two primary reasons. On one hand, it offers a framework for understanding how stress contributes to pain, including the persistence of chronic pain. On the other hand, it uncovers links between cognitive processes (attention, expectancy, meaning, belief) and pain as well as pain relief through psychological intervention.

Most physicians and pain researchers think of pain as an unpleasant sensation that originates in traumatized or inflamed tissues; however, pain is more than sensory information about the condition of the body. Affect is an intrinsic dimension of pain. Any reasonable and unbiased observer studying mammals, particularly humans, would have to conclude that pain's affective features rather than its sensory properties govern behavioral responses to injury. People who experience pain do not quietly report the fact; they express negative emotions.

Is the affective dimension of pain as important as its sensory aspect? The linguist, Elaine Scarry,[4] described pain's qualities as comprising extreme aversiveness, an ability to annihilate complex thoughts and other feelings, an ability to destroy language, and a strong resistance to objectification. Her perspective resonates with the lessons of everyday life: Although pain has sensory features and lends itself to sensory description, it is above all else a powerful negative feeling state. One cannot evaluate and address the suffering of a person in pain without an appreciation of its emotional nature.

The International Association for the Study of Pain (IASP) acknowledged the central role of emotion in its keystone definition: "Pain [is] an unpleasant sensory and *emotional* [emphasis added] experience associated with actual or potential tissue damage, or described in terms of such damage."[5] This definition clearly emphasizes the role of affect as an intrinsic component of pain. Emotion is not a consequence of pain sensation that occurs after a noxious sensory message arrives at sensory cortices. Rather, it is an integral part of the pain experience.

Psychophysiology has revealed that emotion and cognition are interdependent. Strong emotions can alter thought processes, perceptions, beliefs, attitudes, and expectancies. Conversely, thoughts can generate negative or positive emotional states, and the physiologic changes associated with such states can interact with tissue injury or inflammation and alter both the sensory and affective aspects of pain. Because pain states rarely exist in isolation, it is important to consider the psychophysiologic context of a pain problem. The cognitive, emotional, and physiologic state of the patient presenting with pain is potentially very important for both assessment and intervention.

We propose here that the best framework for characterizing this state is stress theory.

The purposes of this chapter are to describe the psychophysiologic mechanisms supporting the subjective experience of pain and to explore the importance of said mechanisms for the assessment and care of patients with pain. The psychophysiology of pain requires an incursion into mind–body issues, consideration of the nature of emotion and its interdependence with cognition, and the overarching influence of stress. In this chapter, we show that (1) pain (awareness of tissue trauma) has intrinsic affective properties, including negative emotional arousal; (2) the brain creates bodily states of arousal (negative emotions) in response to threat to biologic and psychological integrity; and (3) the affective dimension of pain is intrinsically linked to the related processes of defense and stress, and the physiologic mechanisms of these processes shapes the affective dimension of pain.

Historical Perspective: Mind–Body Issues

Through most of the 20th century, our understanding of the relationship between mental processes and the body stemmed directly from Cartesian notions of mind–body dualism. For Descartes, a 17th century philosopher and mathematician, human beings are dualistic: The mind and body are separate entities. Descartes described the life processes of the body as though they were clockwork mechanisms. The actions of the mind were, in his thinking, the workings of the soul.

Descartes believed that the awareness of pain, like awareness of other bodily sensations, must take place in a specific location where the mind observes the body. Dennett[6] termed this hypothetical seat of the mind the *Cartesian theater*. In this theater, the mind observes and interprets the array of multimodality signals that the body produces. The body is a passive environment; the mind is the nonphysical activity of the soul.

Today, most people will agree that such a theater of the mind cannot exist. Scientifically, the activity of the brain and the mind are inseparable; yet, Cartesian dualism is endemic in Western thought and culture. Classical approaches to psychophysiology stemmed from Cartesian thinking, as did psychophysics. Early work on psychosomatic disorders focused on mind–body relationships. Today, much of the popular movement favoring integrative medicine emphasizes the "mind–body connection," keeping one's self healthy through health-promoting cognitive approaches to better regulate immune responses. It is hard to avoid Cartesian thinking when the very fabric of our language carries it along as we reason and speak.

Cartesian assumptions are a subtle but powerful barrier for someone seeking to understand the affective dimension of pain. Relegating emotions to the realm of the mind and their physiologic consequences for the body is classical Descartes. It prevents us from appreciating the intricate interdependence of subjective feelings and physiology, and it detracts from our ability to comprehend how the efferent properties of autonomic nervous function can contribute causally to the realization of an emotional state. This chapter emphasizes the interdependence of mental processes and physiology. What we call the mind is consciousness, and consciousness is an emergent property of the activity of the brain. In a feedback-dependent manner, the brain regulates the physiologic arousal of the body, and emotion is a part of this process.

Emotions: Definition and Mechanisms

WHAT ARE EMOTIONS?

The first step in understanding the nociceptive experience as an affective response is by appreciating the origins and purposes of emotion. Many physicians regard emotions as epiphenomenal feeling states associated with mental activity, subjective in character, and largely irrelevant to the state of a patient's physical health. In fact, emotions are primarily physiologic and only secondarily subjective. Because they can strongly affect cardiovascular function, visceral motility, genitourinary function, and immune competence, patient emotions can have an important role in health overall and especially in pain management. Simple negative emotional arousal can exacerbate certain pain states such as sympathetically maintained pain, angina, headache, neuropathic pain, and fibromyalgia. It contributes significantly to musculoskeletal pain, pelvic pain, and other pain problems in some patients.

Emotions are complex states of physiologic arousal and awareness that impute positive or negative hedonic qualities to a stimulus (event) in the internal or external environment. The objective aspect of emotion is autonomically and hormonally mediated physiologic arousal. The subjective aspects of emotion, *feelings*, are phenomena of consciousness. Emotion represents in consciousness the biologic importance or meaning of an event to the perceiver.

Emotion as a whole has two defining features: valence and arousal. Valence refers to the hedonic quality associated with an emotion—the positive or negative feeling attached to perception. Arousal refers to the degree of heightened activity in the central nervous system and autonomic nervous system (ANS) associated with perception.

Although emotions as a whole can be either positive or negative in valence, pain research addresses only negative emotion. Viewed as an emotion, pain represents a threat to the biologic, psychological, or social integrity of the person. In this respect, the emotional aspect of pain is a protective response that normally contributes to adaptation and survival. If uncontrolled or poorly managed in patients with severe or prolonged pain, it produces suffering.

EMOTION IN A SOCIOBIOLOGIC PERSPECTIVE

Psychologists have many frameworks for studying emotion. Nature has equipped us with the capability of negative emotion for a purpose; bad feelings are not simply accidents of human consciousness. They are protective mechanisms that normally serve us well, but like uncontrolled pain, sustained and uncontrolled negative emotions can become pathologic states that can produce both maladaptive behavior and physiologic pathology.

By exploring the emotional dimension of pain from the sociobiologic perspective, the reader may gain some insight about how to prevent or control the negative affective aspect of pain, which fosters suffering. Unfortunately, implementing this perspective requires that we change conventional language habits that involve describing pain as a transient sensory event. *Pain is a compelling and emotionally negative state of the individual that has as its primary defining feature awareness of, and adaptive adjustment to, tissue trauma or disease.*

ADAPTIVE FUNCTIONS OF EMOTION

Emotions, including the emotional dimension of pain, characterize mammals exclusively, and they foster mammalian adaptation by making possible complex behaviors and adaptations. Importantly, they play a strong role in consciousness, producing and summarizing information that is important for selection among alternative behaviors. According to MacLean,[7] emotions "impart subjective information that is instrumental in guiding behavior required for self-preservation and preservation of the species. The subjective awareness that is an affect consists of a sense of bodily pervasiveness or by *feelings localized to certain parts of the body* [emphasis added]." Because negative emotions, such as fear, evolved to facilitate adaptation and survival, emotion plays an important defensive role. The ability to experience threat when encountering injurious events protects against life-threatening injury.

The strength of emotional arousal associated with an injury indicates and expresses the magnitude of perceived threat to the biologic integrity of the person. Within the contents of consciousness, threat is a strong negative feeling state and not a pure informational appraisal. In humans, threatening events, such as injury that are not immediately present, can exist as emotionally colored somatosensory images.

Phenomenal awareness consists largely of the production of images. Visual images are familiar to everyone: We can readily imagine seeing things. We can also produce auditory images by imaging a familiar tune, a bird song, or the sound of a friend's voice. Similarly, we can generate somatosensory images. We can, for example, imagine the feeling of a full bladder, the sensation of a particular shoe on a foot, or a familiar muscle tension or ache. Cognition operates largely on images and plays a strong role in the experience of symptoms.

Patients can react emotionally to the mental image of a painful event before it happens (e.g., venipuncture), or for that matter, they can respond emotionally to the sight of another person's injury. The emotional intensity of such a feeling marks the adaptive significance of the event that produced the experience for the perceiver. In general, the threat of a minor injury normally provokes less feeling than one that incurs a risk of death. *The emotional magnitude of a pain is the internal representation of the threat associated with the event that produced the pain.*

EMOTIONS AND BEHAVIOR

Negative emotions compel action, such as fight or flight, along with expression through vocalization, posture, variations in facial musculature patterns, and alterations of activity. This represents communication and often elicits social support, thus contributing to survival. Darwin,[8] observing animals, noted that emotions enable communication through vocalization, startle, posture, facial expression, and specific behaviors. He held that emotions must be inborn rather than learned tendencies. Darwin[8] pursued this issue by comparing the facial and other emotional expressions of children born blind with those of other children, reasoning that blind children would express emotion differently if emotion is primarily a learned behavior. As others have since confirmed,[9] Darwin[8] learned that the basic blueprints for human emotional expression are innate.

Contemporary investigators who study emotions and human or animal social behavior emphasize that communication is a fundamental adaptive function of emotional expression.[10,11] Social mammals, including humans, depend on one another or their social group as resources for adaptation and survival. The emotional expression of pain in the presence of supportive persons is socially powerful; it draws on a fundamental sociobiologic imperative: communicating threat and summoning assistance.

THE CENTRAL NEUROANATOMY OF EMOTION: LIMBIC STRUCTURES

The limbic brain represents an anatomical common denominator across mammalian species,[7] and emotion is a common feature of mammals. Consequently, investigators can learn much about human emotion by studying mammalian laboratory animals. Humans and animals differ in that the limbic brain is more developed in humans, the frontal lobes are unique to our species, and the interdependence of cognition and emotion is greatest in humans.

Early investigators focused on the role of olfaction in limbic function, and this led them to link the limbic brain to emotion. Emotion may have evolutionary roots in olfactory perception. MacLean[12] introduced the somewhat controversial term "limbic system" and characterized its functions. He identified three main subdivisions of the limbic brain: amygdala, septum, and thalamocingulate[7] that represent sources of afferents to parts of the limbic cortex. He also postulated that the limbic brain responds to two basic types of input: interoceptive and exteroceptive. These refer to sensory information from internal and external environments, respectively. Figure 29.1 summarizes and extends this concept. Noxious signaling can arise from an injurious event in the external environment or from a pathologic condition in the internal environment.

Over the last decade, numerous studies have employed functional brain imaging to investigate how the human brain responds to painful laboratory stimulation as well as how it behaves in chronic pain conditions. These studies reveal unequivocally that limbic structures involved in emotion and cognition are active during pain. In addition, related studies show that cognitive processes such as threat appraisal and perceived control are related to pain modulation. Early brain imaging studies have shown that the following brain structures are consistently active during states of pain: thalamus, primary and secondary somatosensory cortices, insular cortex, anterior cingulate, and the prefrontal cortices (PFC) as well as deactivation of the posterior cingulate cortex and medial prefrontal cortex,[13–15] which compose of the default mode network involved in self-referential processing.[16] Thalamus and the somatosensory cortices played a prominent role in early neurophysiologic models of pain and processing of ascending nociceptive information. Insular cortex may play a role in the somatosensory representation of the body, and it appears to integrate multimodal sensory information.[17] PFC control the executive functions of the brain and the sense of self. They are involved in threat appraisal, meaning, and the integration of information from the internal and external environment.

PERIPHERAL NEUROANATOMY OF EMOTION: THE AUTONOMIC NERVOUS SYSTEM

The ANS plays a major role in regulating the constancy of the internal environment, and it does so in a feedback regulated fashion under the direction of the hypothalamus, the solitary nucleus (nucleus tractus solitarius) and ventral lateral medulla, the amygdala, and other brain structures.[18,19] In general, it regulates activities that are not normally under voluntary control. The hypothalamus is the principal integrator of autonomic activity. Stimulation of the hypothalamus elicits highly integrated patterns of response that involve the limbic system and other structures.[20]

Many researchers hold that the ANS has three divisions: the sympathetic, the parasympathetic, and the enteric.[21,22] Others subsume the enteric under the other two divisions. Broadly, the sympathetic nervous system makes possible the arousal needed for fight and flight reactions, whereas the parasympathetic system governs basal heart rate, metabolism, and respiration. The enteric nervous system innervates the viscera via a complex network of interconnected plexuses.

The sympathetic and parasympathetic systems are largely mutual physiologic antagonists—if one system inhibits a function, the other typically augments it. There are, however, important exceptions to this rule that demonstrate complementary or integratory relationships. The mechanism most heavily involved in the affective response to tissue trauma is the sympathetic nervous system.

During emergency or injury to the body, the hypothalamus uses the sympathetic nervous system to increase cardiac output, respiration rate, and blood glucose. It also regulates body temperature, causes piloerection, alters muscle tone, provides compensatory responses to hemorrhage, and dilates pupils. These responses are part of a coordinated, well-orchestrated response pattern called the defense response.[23–25] It resembles the better known orienting response in some respects, but it can only occur following a strong stimulus that is noxious or frankly painful. It sets the stage for escape or confrontation, thus serving to protect the organism from danger. In an awake cat, both electrical stimulation of the hypothalamus and infusion of norepinephrine into the hypothalamus elicit a rage reaction with hissing, snarling, and attack posture with claw exposure, and a pattern of sympathetic nervous system arousal accompanies this.[26–28] Circulating epinephrine and norepinephrine produced by the adrenal medulla during activation of the sympathoadrenomedullary (SAM) axis accentuate the defense response, fear responses, and aversive emotional arousal in general.

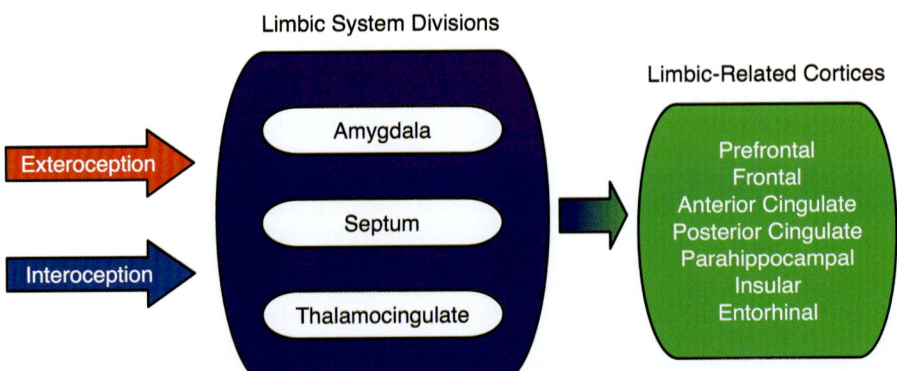

FIGURE 29.1 Three subdivisions of the limbic brain and their relationship to limbic cortices. MacLean[7] proposed a three-part grouping of limbic structures and functions: amygdalar, septal, and thalamocingulate subdivisions. These divisions receive information, including noxious signaling, from the external environment (exteroceptors) and the internal environment (interoceptors). Cortical areas related to limbic function include the prefrontal and frontal cortices (related to executive function and sense of self), the cingulate cortices (the anterior cingulate cortex is related to attentional states), the parahippocampal and entorhinal cortices, which are important in memory, and the insular cortex (emotional–motivational integration).

Autonomic Arousal and Subjective Experience

Because the defense response and related changes are involuntary in nature, we generally perceive them as something that the environment does to us. We typically describe such physiologic changes not as the bodily responses that they are but rather as feelings. We might describe a threatening and physiologically arousing event by saying that "It scared me" or that "It made me really mad."

Phenomenologically, feelings seem to happen to us; we do not "do" them in the sense that we think thoughts or choose actions. Emotions are who we are in a given circumstance rather than choices we make, and we commonly interpret events and circumstances in terms of the emotions that they elicit. ANS arousal, therefore, plays a major role in the complex psychological experience of injury and is a part of that experience.

Early views of the ANS followed the lead of Cannon[23] and held that emergency responses and all forms of intense aversive arousal are undifferentiated, diffuse patterns of sympathetic activation. Although this is broadly true, research has shown that definable patterns characterize emotional arousal and that these are related to the emotion involved, the motor activity required, and perhaps the context.[18,19] An investigator attempting to understand how humans experience emotions must remember that the brain not only recognizes patterns of arousal but also creates them.

The Role of Feedback

One of the primary mechanisms in the creation and management of emotion is feedback. Feedback means that information about the output of a system passes back to the input and thereby dynamically controls the level of the output. System self-regulation and self-organization depend on feedback, as does self-direction. Feedback loops can be negative or positive. Negative feedback permits stability, whereas positive feedback allows the organism to mount emergency responses. The regulatory processes of homeostasis and allostasis are negative feedback dependent. Negative feedback ensures system stability and maintains homeostasis. Feedback is positive when a variable changes and the system responds by changing that variable even more in the same direction, generating escalation and rapid acceleration.[29] This process abandons stability for instability. From an adaptation point of view, positive feedback loop capability is essential for meeting acute threat with defensive arousal. Each mode of operation has adaptive value as a short-range response in certain types of injurious events.

In general, defensive reactions involve a pattern of rapid arousal created through positive feedback that prepares the body and brain for emergency response, followed by a negative feedback-controlled transition to recovery and return to normalcy. Because smaller physiologic systems are nested within larger physiologic systems, higher order systems typically limit positive feedback processes in smaller systems. In some cases, top–down regulation of positive feedback fails, for example, in a panic attack. In other cases, the event that triggered the emotion terminates, and the positive feedback process then stops. Sustained periods of positive feedback have the potential for destructive consequences.

Feedback is the basis of neuroendocrine regulation, as we describe it in the following discussion. Neuroendocrine feedback depends on blood-borne messengers that are typically hormones or peptides. The ANS uses feedback for afferent and efferent functions. The afferent mechanisms signal changes in the viscera and other organs, whereas efferent activity conveys commands to those organs. Consequently, the ANS can maintain feedback loops related to viscera, muscle, blood flow, and other responses. The visceral feedback system exemplifies this process.

The feedback concept is central to the field of psychophysiology: Awareness of physiologic changes elicited by a stimulus is a primary mechanism of emotion. The patient presenting with panic attack, phobia, or anxiety in a mental health setting

is reporting a subjective state based on patterns of physiologic signals and not an existential crisis that exists somewhere in the domain of the mind, somehow apart from the body. Similarly, the patient in a medical context expressing emotional distress during a painful procedure, or during uncontrolled postoperative pain, is experiencing the sensory features of that pain against the background of a cacophony of sympathetic arousal and neuroendocrine stress response.

Relationship of Central and Peripheral Mechanisms

Figure 29.2 illustrates that noxious signaling undergoes parallel processing at the cognitive, affective, and sensory levels. An event representing a threat to biologic integrity elicits strong patterns of sympathetic and neuroendocrine response. These, in turn, contribute to the awareness of the perceiver. Sensory processing provides information about the environment, but this information exists in awareness against a background of emotional arousal, either positive or negative, and that arousal may vary from mild to extreme.

The transition from acute to chronic pain may involve complex changes in these pathways. The hypothalamo–pituitary–adrenocortical (HPA) and SAM axes are vulnerable to dysregulation with prolonged exposure to a stressor or series of stressors. This can include prolonged noxious signaling, as might occur with degenerative disease, or unrelenting noxious neuropathic signaling. Dysregulation in these systems may cause sensitization or impair normal inhibitory modulation. Moreover, neural networks associated with threat, dysphoria, or other

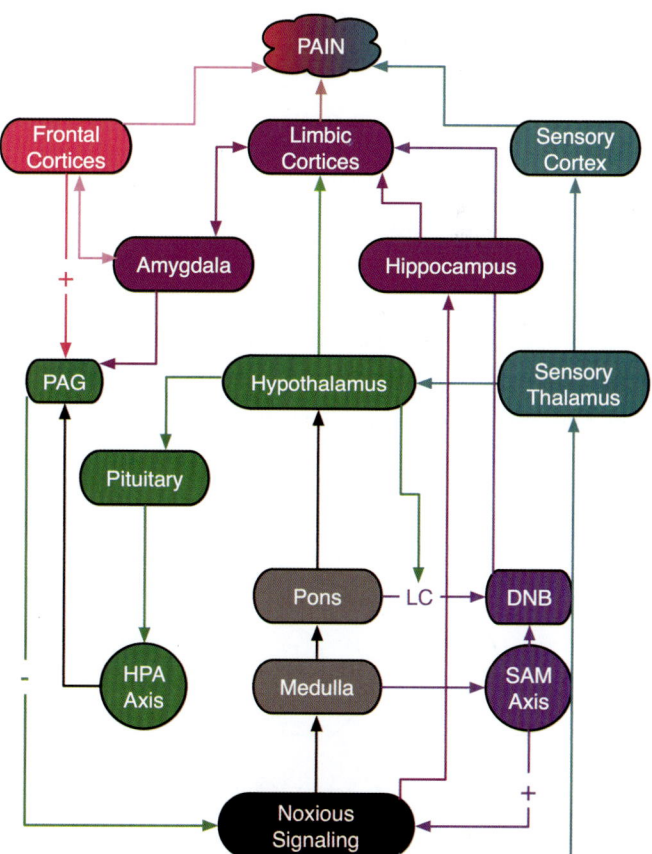

FIGURE 29.2 Parallel sensory, affective, and cognitive processing of noxious signaling arising from nociceptive or neuropathic sources. Parallel activation of sensory transmission and noradrenergic/limbic pathways leads to processing in somatosensory, limbic, and prefrontal/frontal cortical areas. In addition, noxious signaling triggers activity in the sympathoadrenomedullary (SAM) and the hypothalamo–pituitary–adrenocortical (HPA) axes. DNB, dorsal noradrenergic bundle; LC, locus coeruleus; PAG, periaqueductal gray.

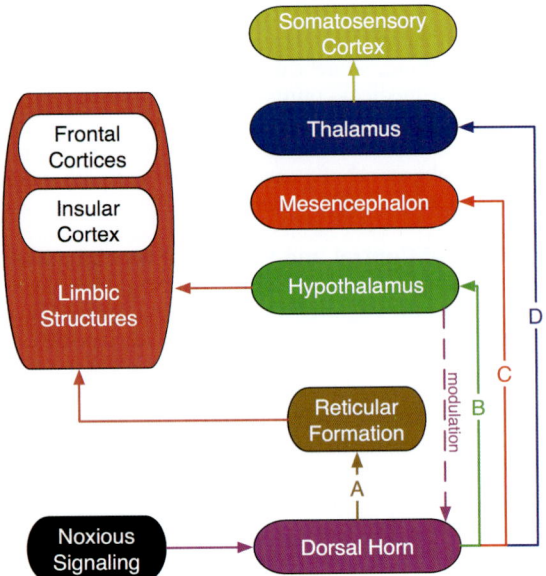

FIGURE 29.3 Multiple pathways of corticopetal noxious signal transmission. **A**, spinoreticular; **B**, spinohypothalamic; **C**, spinomesencephalic; **D**, spinothalamic.

the dorsal horn of the spinal cord. Sensory transmission follows spinothalamic pathways and transmission destined for affective processing takes place in spinoreticular pathways.

Noxious centripetal transmission engages multiple pathways: spinoreticular, spinomesencephalic, spinolimbic, spinocervical, and spinothalamic tracts,[31,32] as Figure 29.3 indicates. The spinoreticular tract contains somatosensory and viscerosensory afferent pathways that arrive at different levels of the brain stem. Spinoreticular axons possess receptive fields that resemble those of spinothalamic tract neurons projecting to medial thalamus, and, like their spinothalamic counterparts, they transmit tissue injury information.[33,34] Most spinoreticular neurons carry noxious signals, and many of them respond preferentially to noxious activity.[35,36] The spinomesencephalic tract comprises several projections that terminate in multiple midbrain nuclei, including the periaqueductal gray (PAG), the red nucleus, nucleus cuneiformis, and the Edinger-Westphal nucleus.[32] Spinolimbic tracts include the spinohypothalamic tract, which reaches both lateral and medial hypothalamus[37,38] and the spinoamygdalar tract that extends to the central nucleus of the amygdala.[39] The spinocervical tract, like the spinothalamic tract, conveys signals to the thalamus. All of these tracts transmit tissue trauma signals rostrally.

Central Neurotransmitter Systems

Central processing of noxious signals to produce affect undoubtedly involves multiple neurotransmitter systems. Four extrathalamic afferent pathways project to neocortex: the dorsal noradrenergic bundle (DNB) originating in the locus coeruleus (LC), the serotonergic fibers that arise in the dorsal and median raphe nuclei, the dopaminergic pathways of the ventral tegmental tract that arise from substantia nigra, and the acetylcholinergic (ACh) neurons that arise principally from the nucleus basalis of the substantia innominata.[40] Of these, the noradrenergic and serotonergic pathways link most closely to negative emotional states.[41–43] The set of structures receiving projections from this complex and extensive network corresponds to classic definition of the limbic brain.[7,43–45]

Although other processes governed predominantly by other neurotransmitters almost certainly play important roles in the complex experience of emotion during pain, we emphasize the role of central noradrenergic processing here. This limited perspective offers the advantage of simplicity, and the literature on the role of central noradrenergic pathways in anxiety, panic, stress, and posttraumatic stress disorder provides a strong basis.[41,46] This processing involves two central noradrenergic pathways: the dorsal and ventral noradrenergic bundles (VNBs) (Fig. 29.4).

negative emotions such as the frontal-amygdalar system may strengthen and become self-sustaining so that they can persist even in the absence of noxious signaling. Duric and McCarson[30] demonstrated that prolonged noxious signaling can produce stress-like damaging effects on the hippocampus, which is involved in the pathogenesis of depressive symptoms.

NOXIOUS SIGNALING AND CENTRAL LIMBIC PROCESSING

Central sensory and affective pain processes share common sensory mechanisms in the periphery. As other chapters in this book describe, Aδ and C fibers serve as tissue trauma transducers (nociceptors) for both, the chemical products of inflammation sensitize these nociceptors, and peripheral neuropathic mechanisms such as ectopic firing excite both processes. In some cases, neuropathic mechanisms may substitute for transduction as we classically define it, producing afferent signal volleys that appear, to the central nervous system, like signals originating in nociceptors. Differentiation of sensory and affective processing begins at

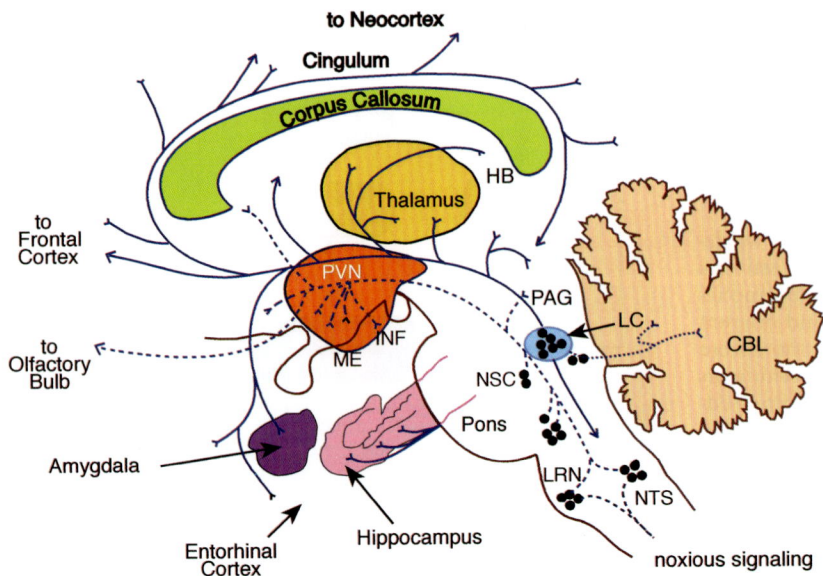

FIGURE 29.4 Central noradrenergic transmission. This parasagittal view identifies cell bodies of neurons that produce norepinephrine as *black circles*. The major projections of these cell bodies are the dorsal noradrenergic bundle (DNB) and the ventral noradrenergic bundle (VNB). The *solid blue lines* are DNB projections, whereas the *broken blue lines* are VNB. The projection from the locus coeruleus (LC) to the cerebellum appears as a *dotted line*. Hypothalamus is *orange*. Noxious signaling from spinoreticular pathways excites the primarily noradrenergic LC, activating the DNB, which extends throughout the limbic brain and to neocortex. CBL, cerebellum; HB, habenula; INF, infundibulum; LRN, lateral reticular nucleus; ME, median eminence; NSC, nucleus subcoeruleus; NTS, nucleus tractus solitaries; PAG, periaqueductal gray; PVN, paraventricular nucleus of the hypothalamus.

LOCUS COERULEUS AND THE DORSAL NORADRENERGIC BUNDLE

Substantial evidence supports the hypothesis that noradrenergic brain pathways are major mechanisms of anxiety and stress.[41] The majority of noradrenergic neurons originate in the LC. This pontine nucleus resides bilaterally near the wall of the fourth ventricle. The locus has three major projections: ascending, descending, and cerebellar. The ascending projection, the DNB, is the most extensive and important pathway for our purposes.[47] Projecting from the LC throughout limbic brain and to all of neocortex, the DNB accounts for about 70% of all brain norepinephrine.[48] The LC gives rise to most central noradrenergic fibers in spinal cord, hypothalamus, thalamus, and hippocampus,[49] and in addition, it projects to limbic cortex and neocortex. Consequently, the LC exerts a powerful influence on higher level brain activity.

The *noradrenergic stress response hypothesis* holds that any stimulus that threatens the biologic, psychological, or psychosocial integrity of the individual increases the firing rate of the LC, and this in turn results in increased release and turnover of norepinephrine in the brain areas involved in noradrenergic innervation. Studies show that the LC reacts to signaling from sensory stimuli that potentially threaten the biologic integrity of the individual or signal damage to that integrity.[48] Spinal cord lamina I cells terminate in the LC.[33] The major sources of LC afferent input are the paragigantocellularis and prepositus hypoglossi nuclei in the medulla, but destruction of these nuclei does not block LC response to somatosensory stimuli.[50,51] Other sources of afferent input to the locus include the lateral hypothalamus, the amygdala, and the solitary nucleus. Whether noxious signaling stimulates the LC directly or indirectly is still uncertain.

It is quite clear that noxious signaling inevitably and reliably increases activity in neurons of the LC, and LC excitation appears to be a consistent response to noxious signaling.[48,52-54] Notably, this does not require cognitively mediated attentional control because it occurs in anesthetized animals. Foote et al.[55] reported that slow, tonic spontaneous activity at the locus in rats changed under anesthesia in response to noxious stimulation. Experimentally induced phasic LC activation produces alarm and apparent fear in primates,[56,57] and lesions of the LC eliminate normal heart rate increases to threatening stimuli.[58] In a resting animal, LC neurons discharge in a slow, phasic manner.[59]

The LC reacts consistently, but not exclusively, to noxious signaling. LC firing rates increase following nonnoxious but threatening events, such as strong cardiovascular stimulation,[53,60] and certain visceral events, such as distention of the bladder, stomach, colon, or rectum.[48,61] Highly novel and sudden stimuli that could represent potential threat, such as loud clicks or light flashes, can also excite the LC in experimental animals.[59] Thus, the LC responds to biologically threatening or potentially threatening events, of which tissue injury is a significant subset. Amaral and Sinnamon[62] described the LC as a central analog of the sympathetic ganglia. Viewed in this way, it is an extension of the autonomic protective mechanism described earlier.

Invasive studies confirm the linkage between LC activity and threat. Direct activation of the DNB and associated limbic structures in laboratory animals produces sympathetic nervous system response and elicits emotional behaviors such as defensive threat, fright, enhanced startle, freezing, and vocalization.[63] This indicates that enhanced activity in these pathways corresponds to negative emotional arousal and behaviors appropriate to perceived threat. LC firing rates increase two- to threefold during the defense response elicited in a cat that has perceived a dog.[26] Moreover, infusion of norepinephrine into the hypothalamus of an awake cat elicits a defensive rage reaction that includes activation of the LC noradrenergic system. In general, the mammalian defense response involves increased regional turnover and release of norepinephrine in the brain

regions that the LC innervates. The LC response to threat, therefore, may be a component of the partly "prewired" patterns associated with the defense response.

Increased alertness is a key element in early stages of the defense response. Normally, activity in the LC increases alertness. Tonically enhanced LC and DNB discharge corresponds to hypervigilance and emotionality.[41,55,64] The DNB is the mechanism for vigilance and defensive orientation to affectively relevant and novel stimuli. It also regulates attentional processes and facilitates motor responses.[40,43,48,65] In this sense, the LC influences the stream of consciousness on an ongoing basis and readies the individual to respond quickly and effectively to threat when it occurs.

LC and DNB support biologic survival by making possible global vigilance for threatening and harmful stimuli. Siegel and Rogawski[66] hypothesized a link between the LC noradrenergic system and vigilance, focusing on rapid eye movement (REM) sleep. They noted that LC noradrenergic neurons maintain continuous activity in both normal waking state and non-REM sleep, but during REM sleep, these neurons virtually cease discharge activity. Moreover, an increase in REM sleep ensues after either lesion of the DNB or following administration of clonidine, an α_2 adrenoceptor agonist. Because LC inactivation during REM sleep permits rebuilding of noradrenergic stores, REM sleep may be necessary preparation for sustained periods of high alertness during subsequent waking. Siegel and Rogawski[66(p226)] contended that "a principal function of NE in the CNS is to facilitate the excitability of target neurons to specific high priority signals." Conversely, reduced LC activity periods (REM sleep) allow time for a suppression of sympathetic tone.

Both adaptation and sensitization can alter the LC response to threat. Abercrombie and Jacobs[67,68] demonstrated a noradrenergically mediated increase in heart rate in cats exposed to white noise. Elevated heart rate decreased with repeated exposure as did LC activation and circulating levels of norepinephrine. Libet and Gleason[69] found that stimulation via permanently implanted LC electrodes did not elicit indefinite anxiety. This indicates that the brain either adapts to locus excitation or engages a compensatory response to excessive LC activation under some circumstances. In addition, central noradrenergic responsiveness changes as a function of learning. In the cat, pairing a stimulus with a noxious air puff results in increased LC firing with subsequent presentations of the stimulus, but previous pairing of that stimulus with a food reward produces no alteration in LC firing rates with repeated presentation.[59] These studies show that, despite its apparently "prewired" behavioral subroutines, the noradrenergic brain shows substantial neuroplasticity. The emotional response of animals and people to a painful stimulus can adapt, and it can change as a function of experience.

From a different perspective, Bremner et al.[41] postulated that chronic stress can affect regional norepinephrine turnover and thus contribute to the *response sensitization* evident in panic disorder and posttraumatic stress disorder. Chronic exposure to a stressor (including perseverating noxious signaling) could create a situation in which noradrenergic synthesis cannot keep up with demand, thus depleting brain norepinephrine levels. Animals exposed to inescapable shock demonstrate greater LC responsiveness to an excitatory stimulus than animals who have experienced escapable shock.[70] In addition, such animals display "learned helplessness" behaviors—they cease trying to adapt to, or cope with, the source of shock.[71] From an evolutionary perspective, this is a failure of the defense response as adaptation; it represents surrender to suffering. Extrapolating this and related observations to patients, Bremner and colleagues[41] suggested that persons who have once encountered overwhelming stress and suffered exhaustion of central noradrenergic resources may respond excessively to similar stressors that they encounter at a later time.

THE VENTRAL NORADRENERGIC BUNDLE AND THE HYPOTHALAMO-PITUITARY-ADRENOCORTICAL AXIS

The VNB originates in the LC and enters the medial forebrain bundle. Neurons in the medullary reticular formation project to the hypothalamus via the VNB.[72] Sawchenko and Swanson[73] identified two VNB-linked noradrenergic and adrenergic pathways to paraventricular hypothalamus in the rat: the A1 region of the ventral medulla (lateral reticular nucleus [LRN]) and the A2 region of the dorsal vagal complex (the nucleus tractus solitarius, or solitary nucleus) which receives visceral afferents. These medullary neuronal complexes supply 90% of catecholaminergic innervation to the paraventricular hypothalamus via the VNB.[74] Regions A5 and A7 contribute in a comparatively minor way to the VNB.

The noradrenergic axons in the VNB respond to noxious stimulation[48] as does the hypothalamus itself.[75] Moreover, noxious-signaling neurons at all segmental levels of the spinal cord project to medial and lateral hypothalamus and several telencephalic regions.[32,37,38] These projections link tissue injury and the hypothalamic response, as do hormonal messengers in some circumstances.

The hypothalamic paraventricular nucleus (PVN) coordinates the HPA axis. Neurons of the PVN receive afferent information from several reticular areas including ventrolateral medulla, dorsal raphe nucleus, nucleus raphe magnus, LC, dorsomedial nucleus, and the nucleus tractus solitarius.[73,76,77] Still other afferents project to the PVN from the hippocampus, septum amygdala.[78] Nearly all hypothalamic and preoptic nuclei send projections to the PVN. This suggests that limbic connections mediate endocrine responses during stress. Feldman et al.[78] note that limbic stimulation always increases adrenocortical activity in rats.

In responding to potentially or frankly injurious stimuli, the PVN initiates a complex series of events regulated by negative feedback mechanisms, as Figure 29.5 indicates. These processes ready the organism for extraordinary behaviors that will maximize its chances to cope with the threat at hand,[79] but they must limit overshooting and return to recover when the stressor has passed. Although laboratory studies often involve highly controlled and specific noxious stimulation, real-life tissue trauma usually involves a spectrum of afferent activity, and the pattern of activity may be a greater determinant of the stress response than the specific receptor system involved.[80] Traumatic injury, for example, might involve complex signaling from the site of injury, including inflammatory mediators, baroreceptor signals from blood volume changes, and hypercapnia. Tissue trauma normally initiates much more than noxious signaling.

Diminished noxious signal transmission during stress or injury helps people and animals to cope with threat without the distraction of pain. The medullary mechanisms involved in this are complex and include the response of the solitary nucleus to baroreceptor stimulation.[81] Laboratory studies with rodents indicate that animals placed in restraint or subjected to cold water develop analgesia.[82–84] Lesioning the PVN attenuates such stress-induced analgesia.[85]

Some investigators[86,87] emphasize that neuroendocrine arousal mechanisms are not limited to emergency situations, even though most research emphasizes that such situations elicit them. In complex social contexts, submission, dominance, and other transactions can elicit neuroendocrine and autonomic responses, modified perhaps by learning and memory. This suggests that neuroendocrine processes accompany all sorts of emotion-eliciting situations.

The hypothalamic PVN supports stress-related autonomic arousal through neural as well as hormonal pathways. It sends direct projections to the sympathetic intermediolateral cell column in the thoracolumbar spinal cord and the parasympathetic vagal complex, both sources of preganglionic autonomic outflow.[88] In addition, it signals release of epinephrine and norepinephrine from the adrenal medulla. Adrenocorticotrophic hormone (ACTH) release, although not instantaneous, is quite rapid: It occurs within about 15 seconds.[89] These considerations

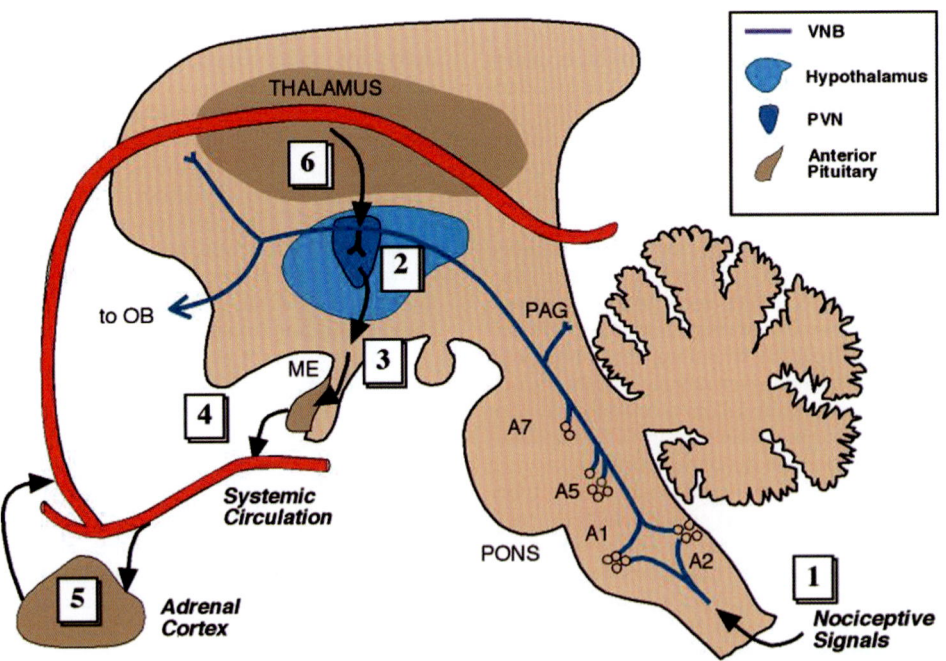

FIGURE 29.5 Response of the hypothalamo–pituitary–adrenocortical (HPA) axis to noxious signaling. The feedback modulated response involves six steps. In step 1, noxious signaling excites the ventral noradrenergic bundle (VNB), including several medullary and pontine nuclei (designated A1, A2, A5, and A7). When such signals reach hypothalamus, they stimulate the paraventricular nucleus (PVN); this is step 2. The PVN produces corticotropin-releasing hormone (CRH). CRH-producing neurons extend from the PVN to the median eminence (ME) where they release CRH into the portal circulation (step 3). At this point, the response becomes neurohumoral rather than neuronal. The anterior pituitary responds to CRH by releasing adrenocorticotropin (ACTH) into the systemic circulation (step 4). ACTH causes the adrenocortex to release corticosteroids into systemic circulation (step 5). In addition to their extensive metabolic effects, the corticosteroids bind to receptors at the PVN (step 6), thus closing the negative feedback loop. PAG, periaqueductal gray.

implicate the HPA axis in the neuroendocrinologic and autonomic manifestations of emotion associated with tissue trauma.

In addition to controlling neuroendocrine and ANS reactivity, the HPA axis coordinates emotional arousal with behavior.[90] As noted earlier, stimulation of the hypothalamus in animals can elicit well-organized action patterns, including defensive threat behaviors and autonomic arousal.[91] The existence of demonstrable behavioral subroutines in animals suggests that the hypothalamus plays a key role in matching behavioral reactions and bodily adjustments to challenging circumstances or biologically relevant stimuli. Moreover, stress hormones at high levels may affect central emotional arousal, lowering startle thresholds and influencing cognition.[89] Saphier[92] observed that cortisol altered the firing rate of neurons in limbic forebrain. Clearly, stress regulation is a complex, feedback dependent, and coordinated process. The hypothalamus appears to coordinate behavioral readiness with physiologic capability, awareness, and cognitive function.

PRIMARY AND SECONDARY FEATURES OF THE AFFECTIVE DIMENSION OF PAIN

The physiology of emotion suggests that the affective dimension of pain involves a two-stage mechanism. The primary mechanism generates an immediate experience akin to hypervigilance or fear. In nature, this rapid response to injury serves to disrupt ongoing attentional and behavioral patterns. At the same time, efferent messages from the hypothalamus, amygdala, and other limbic structures excite the ANS, and this in turn alters bodily states. Cardiac function, muscle tension, altered visceral function, respiration rate, and trembling all occur, and awareness of these reactions creates a strong negative subjective experience. This body state awareness is the second mechanism of the affective dimension of pain.

Damasio[93] contended that visceral and other event-related, autonomically mediated body state changes constitute "somatic markers." That is, they serve as messengers, delivering affective evaluations of perceptual experiences that either confirm or deny the potential threat inherent in an event. A somatic marker is essentially a somatic image. Perceptually, the brain operates on images that are symbolic representations of external and internal objects or events. Just as it is more efficient for a listener to work with words in language as opposed to phonemes, cognition is more efficient when it uses images rather than simple sensations. The somatic marker images associated with tissue trauma are often complex patterns of physiologic arousal. They serve as symbolic representations of threat to the biologic (and sometimes the psychological or social) integrity of the person. Like other images, they can enter into complex patterns of association. Because the secondary stage of the affective response involves images and symbols, it represents cognition as well as emotion.

SUMMARY OF THE CONSTRUCTION AND MODULATION OF PAIN

Pain is a complex and subjective conscious experience constructed and modulated by a constellation of sensory, cognitive, and affective factors including mood, psychological disposition, meaning-related cognitions (e.g., suffering), learning, desires, and pre-pain cognitive states (e.g., expectations, anxiety) to provide a continually changing experience. Feedback connections between low-level afferent and higher order neural processes foster the cultivation of a distributed, multidimensional network associated with the subjective experience of pain. Nociceptive sensory events are first *registered* by peripheral primary afferents (first pain = Aδ; second pain = C fibers) at the site of injury/tissue damage that then relay said nociceptive information to the dorsal horn of the spinal cord. From the spinal cord, nociceptive information ascends contralateral to the site of pain to the brain largely through the spinothalamic pathway. Nociceptive input is subsequently processed through feedback connections between lower level sensory regions including the parabrachial nucleus, PAG matter, thalamus, and primary and secondary somatosensory cortices.[13–15,94–97] Ascending nociceptive information is then transmitted to the posterior and anterior insular cortices where it is "fine-tuned" to foster the subsequent evaluation of pain.[98,99] The contextual meaning of pain is then facilitated through activation of higher order brain regions including the dorsal anterior cingulate cortex (dACC) and anterior cingulate cortex (ACC) and PFC.[99–101] Yet, the subjective experience of pain is highly influenced by the context in which it occurs. That is, previous experiences, expectations, mood, conditioning, desires, sensitization/habituation, and other cognitive factors can dramatically amplify and/or attenuate pain.[97,102–106]

Nonpharmacologic-based pain manipulations attenuate the subjective experience of pain through a common final pathway including overlapping endogenously driven and neural systems. Although the cognitive modulation of pain is mediated through a host of endogenous modulatory systems including cannabinoid, serotonergic, dopaminergic, cholecystokinin, adrenergic, and other neurochemical systems (i.e., vasopressin), the endogenous opioidergic system is the most understood (and studied) pain modulatory system.[107] Endogenous opioidergic mechanisms have been repeatedly demonstrated to mediate analgesia produced by placebo,[108–112] conditioned pain modulation,[113] acupuncture,[114] hypnosis,[115] and attentional control.[116] Pain relief produced by said cognitive techniques is associated with significant reductions in pain-related brain activation (i.e., primary and secondary somatosensory cortices, posterior insula, parietal operculum) and activation in higher order brain regions such as the ACC, PFC, and insula.[105,108,117–129] Importantly, the PFC, insula, and ACC contain high concentrations of opioid receptors and are associated with producing analgesia through descending inhibitory systems.[124,130–134] The ACC and PFC project to the PAG matter,[135] a structure that can be directly activated by opioids. The PAG projects to the rostral ventral medulla[136–138] that in turn projects to the spinal dorsal horn and can inhibit nociceptive processing through multiple neurotransmitter systems.[139]

Emotion and Cognition

Negative emotions and somatic markers are much more than reactions to undesirable events; in nature, they help an organism determine which things benefit and which things threaten survival, and they compel behavior consistent with such evaluations. Moreover, emotional expression communicates this judgment to others and thus sets up group approach or avoidance behaviors. MacLean[7] described emotion as a process that imparts subjective information. In these respects, our feelings approximate crude intelligence. How we feel about something is often as important, or more important, than what we know about it. If emotion is a proto-intelligence, then evolutionarily newer structures, namely, the later stages of cortical development, should have demonstrable links with limbic structures and functions.

Such interconnections exist. Parts of the frontal lobe (the dorsal trend) appear to have developed from rudimentary hippocampal formation, whereas other parts (the paleocortical trend) originated in olfactory cortex. Although these two areas interconnect anatomically, the former analyzes sensory information, whereas the latter contributes emotional tone to that sensory information.[68,69,140] Pribram,[141] noting that limbic function involves frontal and temporal cortex, offered a bottom–up concept for how cognition relates to feelings; that is, emotion determines cognition. However, the multimodal neocortical association areas project corticofugally to limbic structures,[142] which suggests that cognitions may drive emotions.

The debate on whether emotion or cognition is primary may never resolve. For immediate purposes, it seems best to conclude that knowing and feeling are closely interrelated. Still, these processes are not identical. We can know something about our feelings, and we can have emotional responses to what we know. The brain is a complex, dynamic organ, constantly constructing its internal model of reality from sensory input and memory storage. Feeling and thinking are major processes in this construction.

The Sense of Self

COGNITIVE PERSPECTIVE

Pain informs the brain of injury to bodily integrity, and its emotional aspect reflects the importance of that injury to the individual. An injury does not just cause objective harm, it harms "me." That is, it harms what I consider myself. Similarly, a social affront harms what I consider myself, and I might metaphorically describe the incident as something that "hurt" me. What constitutes the self? What would happen if an injured person had an altered or poorly developed sense of self? Clinical observations of schizophrenic patients and other psychiatric patients indicate that they sometimes mutilate themselves horribly and apparently with little or no pain.[143] This suggests that the sense of self may be an intrinsic part of the complex experience of pain because it is the focal point around which perceptions form and from which cognitions arise.

MULTIPLE PERSPECTIVES ON THE SELF

The *self* is a hierarchical construct that has different meanings at different levels of the neuraxis. Multiple levels of the self exist, and each level becomes a precondition for the existence of higher levels. At least two biologic definitions merit inclusion in the construct. At the level of the human genome, the self is the unique genetic code that makes each of us an individual. It sets the basic rules of life by defining sex, size and features, and basic abilities.

At a higher biologic level, the self is what the immune system recognizes as "me" versus "not me." The immunologic self is an enigma because "me" and my genetic code are not identical. Our bodies host elaborate microbial ecosystems, and disturbing or damaging these systems (e.g., via antibiotic use) compromises health. Various microorganisms in our digestive tracts, oropharyngeal passages, and on our skin qualify as self to our immune systems; we live comfortably with them in a symbiotic relationship. Our microbial floras are clearly us, even though they do not carry our genetic code. For the immune system, there is neither single chemical marker that defines individuality nor is the self-limited to certain biologic structures. Thus, even at this basic level, the boundaries of the self are fuzzy.

At a neurologic level, the self exists as a central representation of the body. Melzack termed this the *body neuromatrix*.[144–146] The brain maintains a detailed map of the body at several levels of the neuraxis. Study of phantom limb patients and patients born without limbs reveals that the brain has an elaborate internal representation of the body. If a person loses a leg, the brain maintains its representation of the leg, and the person experiences a phantom limb. Even patients born without limbs have an internal sense or representation of the absent body parts. Thus, humans and almost certainly higher order animals carry within them a phenomenal representation of a body self.

These biologic selves exist below the level of consciousness. They are very much a part of every person, but they normally play little or no part in what we think of as "me." Humans and animals do not differ with regard to self at this level.

Multiple psychological dimensions of the self also exist. At the most fundamental level, there is the self-as-agent, which engages in biologic adaptation and survival. From an evolutionary perspective, it is the agent that struggles to survive.

The self-as-agent sets goals, chooses among alternatives, and engages in behaviors. Animals and humans share self-as-agent, and this self is, in part, social. That is, it exists not alone but in relation to others of its kind. Animals, including humans, engage in social dominance and submission. In this respect, each organism defines its relationship to others, often via struggle or conflict. The defined relationship often determines the extent of one's opportunity to reproduce or one's access to the resources necessary for survival. The self-as-agent is primitive and does not require cognition. It is something that the individual does, not something that the individual experiences as a phenomenal reality. In other words, this is a self of behavior. It does not entail subjective awareness.

At a higher, and perhaps uniquely human, level, the psychological self is also a point of view (self-as-perspective). It is the center of experiential gravity about which the brain organizes present circumstances, past history, future goals, and expectations. This is an inevitable outcome of the higher order self-organizing processes of the brain. This aspect of the self stems from recognition of one's physical being as an entity in the environment, and it becomes a frame of reference for all that happens to the person.

On still another level, the self represents the individual's complex sense of identity, to which we have referred earlier as "me," *vide supra*. This self-as-identity resembles the self-as-agent in some respects, but it is an age-dependent, autobiographically based narrative and interpretation, modified by the immediate circumstances and surroundings. Unlike the self-as-agent, the self-as-identity is the product of a developmental process, and it changes over time.

Finally, every human has a sociologic self. That is, we have an identity defined by our relationships to social groups and to society and culture as a whole. Gender roles, social class, education level, age roles, and our culture constrain who we are. To some degree, we are the roles that we play in our families, vocational settings, recreational pursuits, and elsewhere.

Stress, Sickness, and Pain

BASIC DEFINITIONS: STRESS, HOMEOSTASIS, AND ALLOSTASIS

Human life entails repeated adverse physical and psychosocial events, and these challenges require an adaptive response. The brain mounts a coordinated, adaptive reaction characterized by physiologic arousal. This response is often associated psychologically with the experience of threat or other negative affect. The term for this arousal reaction is the *stress response*, and any event that triggers such a response is a *stressor*. Some stressors are singular events, such as traffic accidents or surgery. Other stressors are constellations of vexing problems that never end. Examples include dysfunctional family relationships and vocational problems. Stress and negative emotion feed one another, and the processes involved affect pain.

We have discussed the defense response earlier. It resembles the stress response and shares common mechanisms. The defense response and stress have historically different origins in science but seem to be different perspectives on a common adaptive mechanism. In order to integrate relevant information in these two fields, we consider the stress response to be a subset of the more general defense response. This position has the shortcoming of potentially obscuring an important distinction. Classically, the defense response pertained to threats appearing in the external environment and not the internal environment. However, the concept applies equally well to threatening internal events. The pain of a kidney stone, angina, or a migraine headache is threatening and can function as a stressor and elicit the physiologic changes common to the defense response and the stress response.

In everyday life, stress is the resource-intensive process of mounting adaptive coping responses to challenges that occur in the external or internal environment. A stressor may be a physical or social event, an invading microorganism, or, in the case of a chronic pain, patient pain itself. Selye[79] first described this response as a syndrome produced by "diverse nocuous agents." He eventually characterized the stress response as having three stages: alarm reaction, resistance, and, if the stressor does not relent, exhaustion. The normal stress responses of daily living consist of the alarm reaction, resistance, and recovery. Stressors have as their primary features intensity, duration, and frequency. The impact of a stressor is the magnitude of the response it elicits. This impact involves cognitive mediation (thought processes) because it is a function of both the predictability and the controllability of the stressor.

A stressor can threaten homeostasis,[147] which strictly means a limited set of systems concerned with maintaining the essentials of the internal milieu. Homeostasis represents the control of internal processes truly necessary for life, such as thermoregulation, blood gases, acid–base balance, fluid levels, metabolite levels, and blood pressure. Generic threats to homeostasis include environmental extremes, extreme exercise, depletion of essential resources, abnormal feedback processes, aging, and disease. Of course, various defensive processes must exist to protect homeostasis.

The term for the general adaptive process that protects against threats to homeostasis is *allostasis*. Allostatic processes dynamically adapt multiple internal systems to changes in the environment and coordinate their responses.[147,148] Allostasis exists when changes in the external or internal environment trigger physiologic coping mechanisms such as autonomic arousal. These mechanisms ensure that the processes sustaining homeostasis stay within normal range. Allostasis is the essence of the stress response because it mobilizes internal resources to meet the challenge that a stressor represents. When a stressor, such as neuropathic signaling, persists for a long period of time, or when repeated stressors occur in rapid succession, allostasis may burn resources faster than the body can replenish them. The cost to the body of allostatic adjustment, whether in response to extreme acute challenges or to lesser challenges over an extended period of time, is called *allostatic load*.

PHYSIOLOGIC MECHANISMS OF STRESS

The major mechanisms of the stress response are the HPA axis based in the hypothalamic PVN[149] and the SAM axis,[150] which includes the LC noradrenergic system (see Fig. 29.1). The peripheral effectors of these mechanisms are the ANS, the SAM circulating hormones, principally the catecholamines epinephrine and norepinephrine together with the sympathetic cotransmitter neuropeptide Y (NPY),[151] all of which originate in the chromaffin cells of the adrenal medulla. Circulating catecholamines increase blood pressure and heart rate, dilate pupils, and increase skin conductance, thereby initiating arousal for the fight or flight response. The stress response involves hypothalamically induced release of peptides derived from pro-opiomelanocortin (POMC) at the anterior pituitary. The POMC-related family of anterior pituitary hormones includes ACTH, β-lipotropin, β-melanocyte–stimulating hormone, and β-endorphin.

The hypothalamic PVN initiates the HPA stress response and controls it through negative feedback mechanisms. Corticotropin-releasing hormone (CRH) produced at the PVN initiates the stress response. CRH initializes and coordinates the stress response at many levels,[152] including the LC.[153] It is the key excitatory central neurotransmitter and regulator in the endocrine response to injury.

The PVN triggers another aspect of the stress response in the SAM axis by recruiting catecholaminergic cells in the rostral ventrolateral medulla. This structure is a cardiovascular regulatory area involved, along with the solitary nucleus, in the control of blood pressure. The rostral ventrolateral medulla activates the solitary nucleus and, together with it, provides tonic excitatory drive to sympathetic vasoconstrictor nerves that maintain resting blood pressure levels. A normal stress response involves a complex pattern of autonomic arousal that includes increased blood pressure followed by a period of recovery when blood pressure and other aspects of arousal return to normal.

Neural Substrates

Viewing stress as a mechanism of defense brings additional neural substrates into focus. Chief among them are the medial hypothalamus, amygdala, and dorsal PAG. These structures respond reliably but not exclusively to noxious signaling; interact with one another; and actively integrate cognitive, sensory, and emotional processes. Some pain researchers have begun to address the issue of integration. Tracey et al.[117] for example, employed functional brain imaging to study subjects attending to or distracting themselves from painful stimuli cued with colored lights. Distraction and pain reduction occurred in conjunction with activation of the PAG, linking cortical control and the PAG and the role of endogenous opioids to attenuate pain.

Frontal-amygdalar circuits are a well-studied aspect of the defense response.[154-156] Cognitive variables such as interpretation, attention, and anticipation can influence amygdalar response through the frontal-amygdalar circuit. The amygdala, in turn, can influence the HPA axis.[157-159] Frontal influences also affect patterns of activity at the LC, which is a part of the SAM axis.

An important implication of viewing stress within the defense response framework is that endogenous cognitive activity (thoughts) generated during anticipation or memory reconstruction can activate complex neural circuits that mobilize the stress response in the absence of tissue trauma. In other words, mental activity may have direct and deleterious physiologic consequences. Patients with chronic pain can stress themselves through negative thought processes, termed *catastrophizing*, and in so doing exacerbate and perpetuate their pain.[160]

The central nucleus of the amygdala projects to the PAG, which coordinates defensive behaviors.[161] In general, the amygdala is proving to be a key mechanism of conditioned fear.[162,163] It communicates with the hypothalamus via neural circuitry[164,165] as well as the frontal cortices.

A second, and underestimated, aspect of the defense response depends predominantly on the immune system. The brain controls the immune system via the actions of the sympathetic nervous system and the hypothalamic secretion of releasing factors into the bloodstream. These messenger substances activate the anterior pituitary via the HPA axis.[166] The pituitary body releases peptides related to POMC, such as ACTH and β-endorphin, and these in turn trigger the release of glucocorticoids. Because the cells and organs of the immune system express receptors for these hormones, they can respond to humoral messenger molecules of central origin. In this way, the brain enlists the immune system in the defense response.

Immune Mechanisms

Just as the nervous system is the primary agent for detecting and defending against threat arising in the external environment, the immune system is the primary agent of defense for the internal environment. Kohl[167] described the immune system as "a network of complex danger sensors and transmitters." This interactive network of lymphoid organs, cells, humoral factors, and cytokines works interdependently with the nervous and endocrine systems to protect homeostasis.

Physical trauma produces specific tissue breakdown, triggering release of nitric oxide (NO), bradykinin, histamine, and peptides, some of which are immunostimulatory. The neuropeptides substance P (SP) and neurokinin A (NKA) activate T cells and cause them to increase production of the proinflammatory cytokine interferon (IFN)-γ.[168] In addition, another proinflammatory cytokine, interleukin (IL)1-β, stimulates the release of SP from primary afferent neurons.[169] Thus, the neurogenic inflammatory response contributes to the immune defense response and at the same time is in part a product of that response.[170]

The immune system detects an injury event in at least three ways: (1) through bloodborne immune messengers originating at the site of injury, (2) through nociceptor-induced sympathetic activation and subsequent stimulation of immune tissues, and (3) through SAM endocrine signaling. Immune messaging begins with the acute phase reaction in the injured tissues.[171] Local macrophages, neutrophils, and granulocytes produce and release into intracellular space and circulation the proinflammatory cytokines IL-1, IL-6, IL-8, and tumor necrosis factor (TNF)-α. This alerts and activates other immune tissues and cells that have a complex systemic impact.

The acute phase reaction to tissue trauma is the immune counterpart to noxious signaling in the nervous system in that it encompasses transduction, transmission, and effector responses. This is a feedback-dependent process. Sympathetic outflow following tissue injury can directly modulate many aspects of immune activity and provide feedback. This can occur because all lymphoid organs have sympathetic nervous system innervation[172] and because many immune cells express adrenoceptors.[173-175]

In addition to the familiar acute phase reaction, the immune system manifests several complex response patterns to tissue injury. In a primitive world, microbial invasion normally accompanies any breach of the skin, and when the microorganisms reach the bloodstream, sepsis occurs. Resultant inflammation therefore assists the immune system in defense. Redness, pain, heat, and swelling are its cardinal signs. The inflammatory process creates a barrier against the invading microorganisms and activates a variety of cells, including macrophages and lymphocytes that find and destroy invaders. It also sensitizes the injured tissue and thereby minimizes the risk of further injury. Inflammation reduces function and increases pain by sensitizing nociceptors. Tracey[176] described the "inflammatory reflex" as an ACh-mediated process by which the nervous system recognizes the presence of, and exerts influence on, peripheral inflammation. Through vagal and glossopharyngeal bidirectional processes, the nervous system modulates circulating cytokine levels.[177] Put another way, the nervous system can sense the activities of the immune system.

The Sickness Response

The immune system can mount a system-wide defense response characterized by fatigue, fever, and sickness with associated pain.[178-183] This is the "sickness response," and although it is cytokine mediated, it depends on the central nervous system. Macrophages and other cells release proinflammatory cytokines including IL1-β, IL-6, IL-8, IL-12, IFN-γ, and TNF-α in response to tissue trauma. These substances act on the vagus nerve, the glossopharyngeal nerve, the hypothalamus, and elsewhere to trigger a cascade of unpleasant, activity-limiting symptoms.[180,184]

Subjectively, the sickness response is a vivid and dysphoric experience characterized by fever, malaise, fatigue, difficulty concentrating, excessive sleep, decreased appetite and libido, stimulation of the HPA axis, and hyperalgesia. The sickness-related hyperalgesia may reflect the contributions of spinal cord microglia and astrocytes.[182] Functionally, this state is adaptive; it minimizes risk by limiting normal behavior and social interactions and forces recuperation. Curiously, this response does not always resolve with physical healing.

The Sickness Response and Depression

Mounting evidence supports the hypothesis that the sickness response and depression are related immune response patterns. This hypothesis derives from evidence that proinflammatory cytokines are agents of depression. The specific mechanisms are still at issue,[185] but proinflammatory cytokines instigate the behavioral, neuroendocrine, and neurochemical features of depressive disorders.[186-189] The therapeutic use of proinflammatory cytokines INF-α and IL-2 for cancer treatment produces depression,[190,191] and their administration generates hyperactivity and dysregulation in the HPA axis. These are common features of severe depression. The sickness response and depression overlap in that many of the behavioral manifestations of sickness are also manifestations of a depressive disorder. Whether sickness and depression constitute separate states of the system is still uncertain. It is becoming clear, however, that the immune defense responses associated with tissue damage contribute to bodily awareness and the complex, multidimensional experience of pain.

SUMMARY OF THE PHYSIOLOGIC MECHANISMS OF STRESS

This review of mechanisms reveals that the emotional aspects of pain are the product of the defensive and stress responses that tissue trauma, a related stressor, or a constellation of stressors evokes. These responses comprise two forms of allostasis. At the neuroendocrine level, the defense response is an adaptive reaction characterized by sympathetic arousal, hypervigilance, and a sense of threat. However, a coordinated immune system adaptive defense response also occurs at the immune level. Mediated by proinflammatory cytokines, it produces a sense of sickness and curtails normal activity. The sickness response produces fatigue, general malaise, fever, and hyperalgesia typically experienced as musculoskeletal pain. Depression is apparently related to the sickness response in that both are the product of proinflammatory cytokines. Thus, the defensive responses generate negative emotions in the general domains of anxiety/threat, depression, and fatigue and sickness.

STRESS AND CHRONIC PAIN

Stress and related defensive responses can promote chronic pain and related disability in at least three ways.

- First, noxious somatic or neuropathic signaling or a central mechanism generating the perception of pain can function as stressors, thereby triggering a defense response and stress. As the mechanism discussion indicates, this can lead to negative emotional states, depressed mood, general sickness, and fatigue. If this is prolonged, patients typically undergo physical deconditioning that makes the pain worse.
- Second, psychosocial stressors such as dysfunctional family relationships or poor vocational adjustment can trigger the stress response and lead to all of the consequences noted earlier.
- Third, comorbid disorders and associated interventions are stressors and can contribute to pain by producing negative affective states, the sickness response, and, ultimately, physical deconditioning. Immunologic diseases, cancer, diabetes, neurologic disorders, and other disease states can increase patient vulnerability to chronic pain through these mechanisms.

The three mechanisms are not mutually exclusive; they can exist in any combination. The normal course of a stress response or defense response is immediate arousal with subsequent slow recovery to normalcy. When stressors confront a patient as a chain of events, the recovery process to the first mechanism may not finish before the second sets off another arousal pattern. A chain of stressors can dysregulate one or another feedback dependent aspect of the stress response system, such as the HPA axis. Hypercortisolemia, for example, characterizes almost half of severely depressed patients. Stress-induced chronobiologic dysregulation is perhaps more common. Patients with chronic pain often complain of disturbed sleep patterns.

Future Directions

Psychophysiology is a rapidly expanding domain of inquiry. We have been able to cover only a small fraction of the field in this review. Other relevant areas include sleep and sleep disorders, chronobiology, physiologic mechanisms of learning and memory, somatic representation, and psychoneuroimmunology. Painful conditions influence these various domains and in turn change in response to changes within these domains. Furthermore, functional brain imaging has opened new opportunities for pursing the relationship of brain activity to physical and psychological manipulations and also subjective experience. Building an interdisciplinary scientific evidence base in the domain of psychophysiology should be a priority in pain research because this field bridges psychological states and physiologic health.

Multisymptom syndromes such as fibromyalgia syndrome, irritable bowel syndrome, and temporomandibular disorder pose major challenges in pain medicine and other medical areas. It is clear that these problems are related to stress, but the causal mechanisms of such disorders and their resistance to treatment remain ill defined. These disorders are mind–body problems that refuse to yield to either purely physiologic or purely psychological intervention. Psychophysiology is the only approach formally organized to pursue such mechanisms from an integrated body–mind perspective. Future research on the nature of multisymptom disorders and the development of management strategies or curative interventions can benefit from a psychophysiologic approach.

Finally, psychophysiology as a field offers unique tools and methods for research that can address the mechanisms and benefits of interdisciplinary pain management. It is no surprise to experienced pain clinicians that psychological interventions and events have physiologic consequences, and conversely, physiologic events and interventions have psychological consequences. Psychophysiology as a field is well positioned to characterize such phenomena and also to optimize interdisciplinary intervention through the coordinated examination of subjective and objective outcomes.

References

1. Andreassi JL. *Psychophysiology: Human Behavior and Physiological Response.* 2nd ed. Hillsdale, NJ: Lawrence Erlbaum Associates; 1989.
2. Cacioppo JT, Tassinary LG. Psychophysiology and psychophysiological inference. In: Cacioppo JT, Tassinary LG, eds. *Principles of Psychophysiology: Physical, Social, and Inferential Elements.* New York: Cambridge University Press; 1990:3–33.
3. Hugdahl K. *Psychophysiology: The Mind-Body Perspective.* Cambridge, MA: Harvard University Press; 1995.
4. Scarry E. *The Body in Pain: The Making and Unmaking of the World.* New York: Oxford University Press; 1985.
5. Merskey H. Pain terms: a list with definitions and a note on usage. Recommended by the IASP Subcommittee on Taxonomy. *Pain* 1979;6:249–252.
6. Dennett D. *Consciousness Explained.* Boston, MA: Little Brown; 1991.
7. MacLean PD. Phenomenology of psychomotor epilepsy: basic and specific affects. In *The Triune Brain in Evolution: Role in Paleocerebral Functions.* New York: Plenum Press; 1990:425.
8. Darwin C. *The Expression of the Emotions in Man and Animals.* London: John Murray; 1872.
9. Thompson J. Development of facial expression of emotion in blind and seeing children. *Arch Psychol* 1941;37:264.
10. Ploog D. Biological foundations of the vocal expressions of emotions. In: Plutchik R, Kellerman H, eds. *Emotion: Theory, Research, and Experience.* New York: Academic Press; 1986:173–198.
11. Ploog D. Human neuroethology of emotion. *Prog Neuropsychopharmacol Biol Psychiatry* 1989;13(suppl):S15–S22.
12. MacLean PD. Some psychiatric implications of physiological studies on frontotemporal portion of limbic system (visceral brain). *Electroencephalogr Clin Neurophysiol* 1952;4:407–418.
13. Coghill RC, Sang CN, Maisog JM, et al. Pain intensity processing within the human brain: a bilateral, distributed mechanism. *J Neurophysiol* 1999;82(4):1934–1943.
14. Coghill RC, McHaffie JG, Yen YF. Neural correlates of interindividual differences in the subjective experience of pain. *Proc Natl Acad Sci U S A* 2003;100(14):8538–8542.
15. Derbyshire SW, Jones AK, Gyulai F, et al. Pain processing during three levels of noxious stimulation produces differential patterns of central activity. *Pain* 1997;73(3):431–445.
16. Raichle ME, MacLeod AM, Snyder AZ, et al. A default mode of brain function. *Proc Natl Acad Sci U S A* 2001;98(2):676–682.
17. Nagai M, Kishi K, Kato S. Insular cortex and neuropsychiatric disorders: a review of recent literature. *Eur Psychiatry* 2007;22(6):387–394.
18. Ledoux JE. The neurobiology of emotion. In: Ledoux JE, Hirst W, eds. *Mind and Brain: Dialogs in Cognitive Neuroscience.* Cambridge, MA: Cambridge University Press; 1986:301–354.
19. Ledoux JE. *The Emotional Brain: The Mysterious Underpinnings of Emotional Life.* New York: Simon and Shuster; 1996.
20. Morgane PJ. Historical and modern concepts of hypothalamic organization and function. In: Morgan PJ, Panksepp J, eds. *Handbook of the Hypothalamus.* New York: Marcel Dekker Inc; 1981:1–64.
21. Burnstock G, Hoyle CHV, eds. *Autonomic Neuroeffector Mechanisms.* Philadelphia: Harwood Academic Publishers; 1992.
22. Dodd J, Role LW. The anatomic nervous system. In: Kandel ER, Schwartz JH, Jessell TM, eds. *Principles of Neural Science.* 3rd ed. New York: Elsevier; 1991:761–775.
23. Cannon WB. *Bodily Changes in Pain, Hunger, Fear, and Rage.* New York: Appleton; 1929.
24. Sokolov EN. *Perception and The Conditioned Reflex.* Oxford, United Kingdom: Pergamon Press; 1963.
25. Sokolov EN. The orienting response, and future directions of its development. *Pavlov J Biol Sci* 1990;25(3):142–150.
26. Barrett JA, Shaikh MB, Edinger H, et al. The effects of intrahypothalamic injections of norepinephrine upon affective defense behavior in the cat. *Brain Res* 1987;426(2):381–384.
27. Hess WR. Hypothalamus und die zantren des autonomen nervensystems: physiologie. *Archiv Psychiatr Nervenkr* 1936;104(548–557).
28. Hilton SM. Hypothalamic regulation of the cardiovascular system. *Br Med Bull* 1966;22:243–248.
29. Ferrell JE Jr. Self-perpetuating states in signal transduction: positive feedback, double-negative feedback and bistability. *Curr Opin Cell Biol* 2002;14(2):140–148.
30. Duric V, McCarson KE. Persistent pain produces stress-like alterations in hippocampal neurogenesis and gene expression. *J Pain* 2006;7(8):544–555.
31. Villanueva L, Bing Z, Bouhassira D, et al. Encoding of electrical, thermal, and mechanical noxious stimuli by subnucleus reticularis dorsalis neurons in the rat medulla. *J Neurophysiol* 1989;61:391–402.
32. Willis WD, Westlund KN. Neuroanatomy of the pain system and of the pathways that modulate pain. *J Clin Neurophysiol* 1997;14(1):2–31.
33. Craig AD. Spinal and trigeminal lamina I input to the locus coeruleus anterogradely labeled with *Phaseolus vulgaris* leucoagglutinin (PHA-L) in the cat and the monkey. *Brain Res* 1992;584(1–2):325–328.
34. Villanueva L, Cliffer KD, Sorkin LS, et al. Convergence of heterotopic nociceptive information onto neurons of caudal medullary reticular formation in monkey (*Macaca fascicularis*). *J Neurophysiol* 1990;63:1118–1127.
35. Bing Z, Villanueva L, Le Bars D. Ascending pathways in the spinal cord involved in the activation of subnucleus reticularis dorsalis neurons in the medulla of the rat. *J Neurophysiol* 1990;63:424–438.
36. Bowsher D. Role of the reticular formation in responses to noxious stimulation. *Pain* 1976;2:361–378.
37. Burstein R, Cliffer KD, Giesler GJ. The spinohypothalamic and spinotelecephalic tracts: direct nociceptive projections from the spinal cord to the hypothalamus and telencephalon. In: Dubner R, Gebhart GF, Bond MR, eds. *Proceedings of the 5th World Congress on Pain.* New York: Elsevier; 1988:548–554.
38. Burstein R, Dado RJ, Cliffer KD, et al. Physiological characterization of spinohypothalamic tract neurons in the lumbar enlargement of rats. *J Neurophysiol* 1991;66(1):261–284.
39. Bernard JF, Besson JM. The spino(trigemino)pontoamygdaloid pathway: electrophysiological evidence for an involvement in pain processes. *J Neurophysiol* 1990;63(3):473–490.
40. Foote SL, Morrison JH. Extrathalamic modulation of corticofunction. *Annu Rev Neurosci* 1987;10:67–95.
41. Bremner JD, Krystal JH, Southwick SM, et al. Noradrenergic mechanisms in stress and anxiety: I. Preclinical studies. *Synapse* 1996;23(1):28–38.
42. Gray JA. *The Neuropsychology of Anxiety: An Enquiry into the Functions of the Septo-Hippocampal System.* New York: Oxford University Press; 1982.
43. Gray JA. *The Psychology of Fear and Stress.* 2nd ed. Cambridge, United Kingdom: Cambridge University Press; 1987.
44. Isaacson RL. *The Limbic System.* 2nd ed. New York: Plenum Press; 1982.
45. Papez JW. A proposed mechanism of emotion. *Arch Neurol Psych* 1937;38:725–743.
46. Charney DS, Deutch A. A functional neuroanatomy of anxiety and fear: implications for the pathophysiology and treatment of anxiety disorders. *Crit Rev Neurobiol* 1996;10(3–4):419–446.

47. Fillenz M. *Noradrenergic Neurons*. Cambridge, United Kingdom: Cambridge University Press; 1990.

48. Svensson TH. Peripheral, autonomic regulation of locus coeruleus noradrenergic neurons in brain: putative implications for psychiatry and psychopharmacology. *Psychopharmacology (Berl)* 1987;92:1–7.

49. Aston–Jones G, Foote SL, Segal M. Impulse conduction properties of noradrenergic locus coeruleus axons projecting to monkey cerebrocortex. *Neuroscience* 1985;15:765–777.

50. Rasmussen K, Aghajanian GK. Withdrawal-induced activation of locus coeruleus neurons in opiate-dependent rats: attenuation by lesions of the nucleus paragigantocellularis. *Brain Res* 1989;505(2):346–350.

51. Rasmussen K, Aghajanian GK. Failure to block responses of locus coeruleus neurons to somatosensory stimuli by destruction of two major afferent nuclei. *Synapse* 1989;4(2):162–164.

52. Korf J, Bunney BS, Aghajanian GK. Noradrenergic neurons: morphine inhibition of spontaneous activity. *Eur J Pharmacol* 1974;25:165–169.

53. Morilak DA, Fornal CA, Jacobs BL. Effects of physiological manipulations on locus coeruleus neuronal activity in freely moving cats. II. Cardiovascular challenge. *Brain Res* 1987;422:24–31.

54. Stone EA. Stress and catecholamines. In: Friedhoff AJ, ed. *Catecholamines and Behavior*. New York: Plenum Press; 1975:31–72.

55. Foote SL, Bloom FE, Aston-Jones G. Nucleus locus ceruleus: new evidence of anatomical and physiological specificity. *Physiol Rev* 1983;63:844–914.

56. Redmond DE Jr, Huang YH. Current concepts. II. New evidence for a locus coeruleus–norepinephrine connection with anxiety. *Life Sci* 1979;25:2149–2162.

57. Grant SJ, Aston-Jones G, Redmond DE Jr. Responses of primate locus coeruleus neurons to simple and complex sensory stimuli. *Brain Res Bull* 1988;21(3):401–410.

58. Redmond DE Jr. Alteration in the functions of the nucleus locus coeruleus: a possible model for studies of anxiety. In: Hannin I, Usdin E, eds. *Animal Models in Psychiatry and Neurology*. New York: Pergamon Press; 1977:293–306.

59. Rasmussen K, Morilak DA, Jacobs BL. Single unit activity of locus coeruleus neurons in the freely moving cat. I. During naturalistic behaviors and in response to simple and complex stimuli. *Brain Res* 1986;371(2):324–334.

60. Elam M, Svensson TH, Thoren P. Differentiated cardiovascular afferent regulation of locus coeruleus neurons and sympathetic nerves. *Brain Res* 1985;358:77–84.

61. Elam M, Thorén P, Svensson TH. Locus coeruleus neurons and sympathetic nerves: activation by visceral afferents. *Brain Res* 1986;375:117–125.

62. Amaral DB, Sinnamon HM. The locus coeruleus: neurobiology of a central noradrenergic nucleus. *Prog Neurobiol* 1977;9:147–196.

63. McNaughton N, Mason ST. The neuropsychology and neuropharmacology of the dorsal ascending noradrenergic bundle—a review. *Prog Neurobiol* 1980;14:157–219.

64. Butler PD, Weiss JM, Stout JC, et al. Corticotropin-releasing factor produces fear-enhancing and behavioral activating effects following infusion into the locus coeruleus. *J Neurosci* 1990;10:176–183.

65. Elam M, Svensson TH, Thorén P. Locus coeruleus neurons and sympathetic nerves: activation by cutaneous sensory afferents. *Brain Res* 1986;366:254–261.

66. Siegel JM, Rogawski MA. A function for REM sleep: regulation of noradrenergic receptor sensitivity. *Brain Res Rev* 1988;472:213–233.

67. Abercrombie ED, Jacobs BL. Single-unit response of noradrenergic neurons in the locus coeruleus of freely moving cats. I. Acutely presented stressful and nonstressful stimuli. *J Neurosci* 1987;7(9):2837–2843.

68. Abercrombie ED, Jacobs BL. Single-unit response of noradrenergic neurons in the locus coeruleus of freely moving cats. II. Adaptation to chronically presented stressful stimuli. *J Neurosci* 1987;7(9):2844–2848.

69. Libet B, Gleason CA. The human locus coeruleus and anxiogenesis. *Brain Res* 1994;634(1):178–180.

70. Weiss JM, Simson PG. Depression in an animal model: focus on the locus ceruleus. *Ciba Found Symp* 1986;123:191–215.

71. Seligman ME, Weiss J, Weinraub M, et al. Coping behavior: learned helplessness, physiological change and learned inactivity. *Behav Res Ther* 1980;18(5):459–512.

72. Sumal KK, Blessing WW, Joh TH, et al. Synaptic interaction of vagal afference and catecholaminergic neurons in the rat nucleus tractus solitarius. *J Brain Res* 1983;277:31–40.

73. Sawchenko PE, Swanson LW. The organization of noradrenergic pathways from the brain stem to the paraventricular and supraoptic nuclei in the rat. *Brain Res* 1982;257(3):275–325.

74. Assenmacher I, Szafarczyk A, Alonso G, et al. Physiology of neuropathways affecting CRH secretion. In: Ganong WF, Dallman MF, Roberts JL, eds. *The Hypothalamic–Pituitary–Adrenal Axis Revisited* 1987:149–161.

75. Kanosue K, Nakayama T, Ishikawa Y, et al. Responses of hypothalamic and thalamic neurons to noxious and scrotal thermal stimulation in rats. *J Thermobiol* 1984;9:11–13.

76. Peschanski M, Weil–Fugacza J. Aminergic and cholinergic afferents to the thalamus: experimental data with reference to pain pathways. In: Besson JM, Guilbaud G, Paschanski M, eds. *Thalamus and Pain*. Amsterdam, The Netherlands: Excerpta Medica; 1987:127–154.

77. Lopez JF, Young EA, Herman JP, et al. Regulatory biology of the HPA axis: an integrative approach. In: Risch SC, ed. *Central Nervous System Peptide Mechanisms in Stress and Depression*. Washington, DC: American Psychiatric Press; 1991:1–52.

78. Feldman S, Conforti N, Weidenfeld J. Limbic pathways and hypothalamic neurotransmitters mediating adrenocortical responses to neural stimuli. *Neurosci Biobehav Rev* 1995;19(2):235–240.

79. Selye H. *The Stress of Life*. New York: McGraw-Hill; 1978.

80. Lilly MP, Gann DS. The hypothalamic–pituitary–adrenal-immune axis. A critical assessment. *Arch Surg* 1992;127(12):1463–1474.

81. Ghione S. Hypertension-associated hypalgesia. Evidence in experimental animals and humans, pathophysiological mechanisms, and potential clinical consequences. *Hypertension* 1996;28(3):494–504.

82. Amir S, Amit Z. The pituitary gland mediates acute and chronic pain responsiveness in stressed and non-stressed rats. *Life Sci* 1979;24:439–448.

83. Kelly DD, Silverman AJ, Glusman M, et al. Characterization of pituitary mediation of stress-induced antinociception in rats. *Physiol Behav* 1993;53:769–775.

84. Bodnar RJ, Glusman M, Brutus M, et al. Analgesia induced by cold-water stress: attenuation following hypophysectomy. *Physiol Behav* 1979;23:53–62.

85. Truesdell LS, Bodner RJ. Reduction in cold-water swim analgesia following hypothalamic paraventricular nucleus lesions. *Physiol Behav* 1987;39:727–731.

86. Henry JP. Neuroendocrine patterns of emotional response. In: Plutchik R, Kellerman H, eds. *Emotion: Theory, Research and Practice*. Orlando, FL: Academic Press; 1986:37–60.

87. LeDoux JE, Iwata J, Cicchetti P, et al. Different projections of the central amygdaloid nucleus mediate autonomic and behavioral correlates of conditioned fear. *J Neurosci* 1988;8:2517–2529.

88. Krukoff TL. Neuropeptide regulation of autonomic outflow at the sympathetic preganglionic neuron. Anatomical and neurochemical specificity. *Ann N Y Acad Sci* 1990;579:160–167.

89. Sapolsky RM. *Stress, the Aging Brain, and the Mechanisms of Neuron Death*. Cambridge, MA: The MIT Press; 1992.

90. Panksepp J. The anatomy of emotions. In: Plutchik R, Kellerman H, eds. *Emotion: Theory, Research and Experience*. Orlando, FL: Academic Press; 1986:91–124.

91. Jänig W. Systemic and specific autonomic reactions in pain: efferent, afferent and endocrine components. *Eur J Anaesthesiol* 1985;2:319–346.

92. Saphier D. Cortisol alters firing rate and synaptic responses of limbic forebrain units. *Brain Res Bull* 1987;19:519–524.

93. Damasio AR. *Descartes' Error: Emotion and Reason in the Human Brain*. New York: Grosset/Putnam; 1994.

94. Basbaum AI, Fields HL. Endogenous pain control systems: brainstem spinal pathways and endorphin circuitry. *Annu Rev Neurosci* 1984;7:309–338.

95. Coghill RC, Talbot JD, Evans AC, et al. Distributed processing of pain and vibration by the human brain. *J Neurosci* 1994;14(7):4095–4108.

96. Tracey I, Mantyh PW. The cerebral signature for pain perception and its modulation. *Neuron* 2007;55(3):377–391.

97. Wiech K, Ploner M, Tracey I. Neurocognitive aspects of pain perception. *Trends Cogn Sci* 2008;12(8):306–313.

98. Oshiro Y, Quevedo AS, McHaffie JG, et al. Brain mechanisms supporting spatial discrimination of pain. *J Neurosci* 2007;27(13):3388–3394.

99. Oshiro Y, Quevedo AS, McHaffie JG, et al. Brain mechanisms supporting discrimination of sensory features of pain: a new model. *J Neurosci* 2009;29(47):14924–14931.

100. Lobanov OV, Quevado AS, Hadsel MS, et al. Frontoparietal mechanisms supporting attention to location and intensity of painful stimuli. *Pain* 2013;154(9):1758–1768.

101. Lobanov OV, Zeidan F, McHaffie JG, et al. From cue to meaning: brain mechanisms supporting the construction of expectations of pain. *Pain* 2014;155(1):129–136.

102. Bushnell MC, Ceko M, Low LA. Cognitive and emotional control of pain and its disruption in chronic pain. *Nat Rev Neurosci* 2013;14(7):502–511.

103. Kong J, White NS, Kwong KK, et al. Using fMRI to dissociate sensory encoding from cognitive evaluation of heat pain intensity. *Hum Brain Mapp* 2006;27(9):715–721.

104. Petrovic P, Ingvar M. Imaging cognitive modulation of pain processing. *Pain* 2002;95(1–2):1–5.

105. Seminowicz DA, Mikulis DJ, Davis KD. Cognitive modulation of pain-related brain responses depends on behavioral strategy. *Pain* 2004;112(1–2):48–58.

106. Villemure C, Bushnell MC. Cognitive modulation of pain: how do attention and emotion influence pain processing? *Pain* 2002;95(3):195–199.

107. Millan MJ. Descending control of pain. *Prog Neurobiol* 2002;66(6):355–474.

108. Eippert F, Bingel U, Schoell ED, et al. Activation of the opioidergic descending pain control system underlies placebo analgesia. *Neuron* 2009;63(4):533–543.

109. Grevert P, Albert LH, Goldstein A. Partial antagonism of placebo analgesia by naloxone. *Pain* 1983;16(2):129–143.

110. Levine JD, Gordon NC, Fields HL. The mechanism of placebo analgesia. *Lancet* 1978:2(8091):654–657.

111. Zubieta JK, Bueller JA, Jackson LR, et al. Placebo effects mediated by endogenous opioid activity on mu-opioid receptors. *J Neurosci* 2005;25(34):7754–7762.

112. Amanzio M, Benedetti F. Neuropharmacological dissection of placebo analgesia: expectation-activated opioid systems versus conditioning-activated specific subsystems. *J Neurosci* 1999;19(1):484–494.

113. King CD, Goodin B, Kinder LL, et al. Reduction of conditioned pain modulation in humans by naltrexone: an exploratory study of the effects of pain catastrophizing. *J Behav Med* 2013;36(3):315–327.

114. Harris RE, Zubieta JK, Scott DJ, et al. Traditional Chinese acupuncture and placebo (sham) acupuncture are differentiated by their effects on mu-opioid receptors (MORs). *Neuroimage* 2009;47(3):1077–1085.

115. Stephenson JB. Reversal of hypnosis-induced analgesia by naloxone. *Lancet* 1978;2(8097):991–992.

116. Sprenger C, Eippert F, Finsterbusch J, et al. Attention modulates spinal cord responses to pain. *Curr Biol* 2012;22(11):1019–1022.

117. Tracey I, Ploghaus A, Gati JS, et al. Imaging attentional modulation of pain in the periaqueductal gray in humans. *J Neurosci* 2002;22(7):2748–2752.

118. Valet M, Sprenger T, Boecker H, et al. Distraction modulates connectivity of the cingulo-frontal cortex and the midbrain during pain—an fMRI analysis. *Pain* 2004;109(3):399–408.

119. Koyama T, McHaffie JG, Laurienti PJ, et al. The subjective experience of pain: where expectations become reality. *Proc Natl Acad Sci U S A* 2005;102(36):12950–12955.

120. Zeidan F, Lobanov OV, Kraft RA, et al. Brain mechanisms supporting violated expectations of pain. *Pain* 2015;156(9):1772–1785.

121. Salomons TV, Johnstone T, Backonja MM, et al. Individual differences in the effects of perceived controllability on pain perception: critical role of the prefrontal cortex. *J Cogn Neurosci* 2007;19(6):993–1003.

122. Wager TD, Atlas LY, Leotti LA, et al. Predicting individual differences in placebo analgesia: contributions of brain activity during anticipation and pain experience. *J Neurosci* 2011;31(2):439–452.

123. Wager TD, Rilling JK, Smith EE, et al. Placebo-induced changes in FMRI in the anticipation and experience of pain. *Science* 2004;303(5661):1162–1167.

124. Wager TD, Scott DJ, Zubieta JK. Placebo effects on human mu-opioid activity during pain. *Proc Natl Acad Sci U S A* 2007;104(26):11056–11061.

125. Rainville P. Brain mechanisms of pain affect and pain modulation. *Curr Opin Neurobiol* 2002;12(2):195–204.

126. Rainville P, Carrier B, Hofbauer RK, et al. Dissociation of sensory and affective dimensions of pain using hypnotic modulation. *Pain* 1999;82(2):159–171.

127. Rainville P, Duncan GH, Price DD, et al. Pain affect encoded in human anterior cingulate but not somatosensory cortex. *Science* 1997;277(5328): 968–971.

128. Roy M, Lebuis A, Peretz I, et al. The modulation of pain by attention and emotion: a dissociation of perceptual and spinal nociceptive processes. *Eur J Pain* 2011;15(6):641.e10.

129. Roy M, Piché M, Chen JI, et al. Cerebral and spinal modulation of pain by emotions. *Proc Natl Acad Sci U S A* 2009;106(49):20900–20905.

130. Casey KL, Svensson P, Morrow TJ, et al. Selective opiate modulation of nociceptive processing in the human brain. *J Neurophysiol* 2000;84(1):525–533.

131. Willoch F, Schindler F, Wester HJ, et al. Central poststroke pain and reduced opioid receptor binding within pain processing circuitries: a [11C] diprenorphine PET study. *Pain* 2004 108(3):213–220.

132. Adler LJ, Gyulai FE, Diehl DJ, et al. Regional brain activity changes associated with fentanyl analgesia elucidated by positron emission tomography. *Anesth Analg* 1997;84(1):120–126.

133. Willoch F, Tölle TR, Wester HJ, et al. Central pain after pontine infarction is associated with changes in opioid receptor binding: a PET study with 11C-diprenorphine. *AJNR Am J Neuroradiol* 1999;20(4):686–690.

134. Jones AK, Qi LY, Fujiwara T, et al. In vivo distribution of opioid receptors in man in relation to the cortical projections of the medial and lateral pain systems measured with positron emission tomography. *Neurosci Lett* 1991;126(1):25–28.

135. Floyd NS, Price JL, Ferry AT, et al. Orbitomedial prefrontal cortical projections to distinct longitudinal columns of the periaqueductal gray in the rat. *J Comp Neurol* 2000;422(4):556–578.

136. Beitz AJ. The organization of afferent projections to the midbrain periaqueductal gray of the rat. *Neuroscience* 1982;7(1):133–159.

137. Mantyh PW. Connections of midbrain periaqueductal gray in the monkey. II. Descending efferent projections. *J Neurophysiol* 1983;49(3):582–594.

138. Mantyh PW. Connections of midbrain periaqueductal gray in the monkey. I. Ascending efferent projections. *J Neurophysiol* 1983;49(3):567–581.

139. Liebeskind JC, Guilbaud G, Besson JM, et al. Analgesia from electrical stimulation of the periaqueductal gray matter in the cat: behavioral observations and inhibitory effects on spinal cord interneurons. *Brain Res* 1973;50(2):441–446.

140. Pandya DN, Barnes CL, Panksepp J. Architecture and connections of the frontal lobe. In: Perecman E, ed. *The Frontal Lobes Revisited*. Hillsdale, NJ: Lawrence Erlbaum Associates; 1987:41–72.

141. Pribram KH. The biology of emotions and other feelings. In: Plutchik R, Kellerman H, eds. *Emotion: Theory, Research, and Experience*. New York: Academic Press; 1980:245–269.

142. Turner BH, Mishkin M, Knapp M. Organization of the amygdalopedal projections from modality-specific cortical association areas in the monkey. *J Comp Neurol* 1980;19:515–543.

143. Dworkin RH. Pain insensitivity in schizophrenia: a neglected phenomenon and some implications. *Schizophr Bull* 1994;20(2):235–248.

144. Melzack R. Phantom limbs and the concept of a neuromatrix. *Trends Neurosci* 1990;13:88–92.

145. Melzack R. Phantom limbs. *Sci Am* 1992;266(4):120–126.

146. Melzack R, Israel R, Lacroix R, et al. Phantom limbs in people with congenital limb deficiency or amputation in early childhood. *Brain* 1997;120(pt 9): 1603–1620.

147. McEwen BS. The neurobiology of stress: from serendipity to clinical relevance. *Brain Res* 2000;886(1–2):172–189.

148. Korte SM, Koolhaas JM, Wingfield JC, et al. The Darwinian concept of stress: benefits of allostasis and costs of allostatic load and the trade-offs in health and disease. *Neurosci Biobehav Rev* 2005;29(1):3–38.

149. Tsigos C, Chrousos GP. Hypothalamic–pituitary–adrenal axis, neuroendocrine factors and stress. *J Psychosom Res* 2002;53(4):865–871.

150. Padgett DA, Glaser R. How stress influences the immune response. *Trends Immunol* 2003;24(8):444–448.

151. Zukowska Z, Pons J, Lee EW, et al. Neuropeptide Y: a new mediator linking sympathetic nerves, blood vessels and immune system? *Can J Physiol Pharmacol* 2003;81(2):89–94.

152. Elenkov IJ. Glucocorticoids and the Th1/Th2 balance. *Ann N Y Acad Sci* 2004;1024:138–146.

153. Rassnick S, Sved AF, Rabin BS. Locus coeruleus stimulation by corticotropin-releasing hormone suppresses in vitro cellular immune responses. *J Neurosci* 1994;14(10):6033–6040.

154. Davidson RJ, Irwin W. The functional neuroanatomy of emotion and affective style. *Trends Cogn Sci* 1999;3(1):11–21.

155. Hariri AR, Mattay VS, Tessitore A, et al. Neocortical modulation of the amygdala response to fearful stimuli. *Biol Psychiatry* 2003;53(6):494–501.

156. Likhtik E, Pelletier JG, Paz R, et al. Prefrontal control of the amygdala. *J Neurosci* 2005;25(32):7429–7437.

157. Merali Z, Michaud D, McIntosh J, et al. Differential involvement of amygdaloid CRH system(s) in the salience and valence of the stimuli. *Prog Neuropsychopharmacol Biol Psychiatry* 2003;27(8):1201–1212.

158. Herman JP, Figueiredo H, Mueller NK, et al. Central mechanisms of stress integration: hierarchical circuitry controlling hypothalamo-pituitary-adrenocortical responsiveness. *Front Neuroendocrinol* 2003;24(3): 151–180.

159. Pessoa L, Padmala S, Morland T. Fate of unattended fearful faces in the amygdala is determined by both attentional resources and cognitive modulation. *Neuroimage* 2005;28(1):249–255.

160. Keefe FJ, Rumble ME, Scipio CD, et al. Psychological aspects of persistent pain: current state of the science. *J Pain* 2004;5(4):195–211.

161. Misslin R. The defense system of fear: behavior and neurocircuitry. *Neurophysiol Clin* 2003;33(2):55–66.

162. Rosen JB. The neurobiology of conditioned and unconditioned fear: a neurobehavioral system analysis of the amygdala. *Behav Cogn Neurosci Rev* 2004;3(1):23–41.

163. Pare D, Quirk GJ, Ledoux JE. New vistas on amygdala networks in conditioned fear. *J Neurophysiol* 2004;92(1):1–9.

164. Forray MI, Gysling K. Role of noradrenergic projections to the bed nucleus of the stria terminalis in the regulation of the hypothalamic–pituitary–adrenal axis. *Brain Res Rev* 2004;47(1–3):145–160.

165. Xu Y, Day TA, Buller KM. The central amygdala modulates hypothalamic-pituitary–adrenal axis responses to systemic interleukin-1beta administration. *Neuroscience* 1999;94(1):175–183.

166. Sternberg EM. Neuroendocrine factors in susceptibility to inflammatory disease: focus on the hypothalamic–pituitary–adrenal axis. *Horm Res* 1995; 43(4):159–161.

167. Kohl J. The role of complement in danger sensing and transmission. *Immunol Res* 2006;34(2):157–176.

168. Lambrecht BN. Immunologists getting nervous: neuropeptides, dendritic cells and T cell activation. *Respir Res* 2001;2(3):133–138.

169. Inoue A, Ikoma K, Morioka N, et al. Interleukin-1beta induces substance P release from primary afferent neurons through the cyclooxygenase-2 system. *J Neurochem* 1999;73(5):2206–2213.

170. Eskandari F, Webster JI, Sternberg EM. Neural immune pathways and their connection to inflammatory diseases. *Arthritis Res Ther* 2003;5(6): 251–265.

171. Gruys E, Toussaint M, Niewold T, et al. Acute phase reaction and acute phase proteins. *J Zhejiang Univ SCI* 2005;6(11):1045–1056.

172. Elenkov IJ, Wilder RL, Chrousos GP, et al. The sympathetic nerve—an integrative interface between two supersystems: the brain and the immune system. *Pharmacol Rev* 2000;52(4):595–638.

173. Vizi ES, Elenkov IJ. Nonsynaptic noradrenaline release in neuro-immune responses. *Acta Biol Hung* 2002;53(1–2):229–244.

174. Kin NW, Sanders VM. It takes nerve to tell T and B cells what to do. *J Leukoc Biol* 2006;79(6):1093–1104.

175. Oberbeck R. Catecholamines: physiological immunomodulators during health and illness. *Curr Med Chem* 2006;13(17):1979–1989.

176. Tracey KJ. The inflammatory reflex. *Nature* 2002;420(6917):853–859.

177. Maier SF, Goehler LE, Fleshner M, et al. The role of the vagus nerve in cytokine-to-brain communication. *Ann N Y Acad Sci* 1998;840: 289–300.

178. Dantzer R. Cytokine-induced sickness behavior: mechanisms and implications. *Ann N Y Acad Sci* 2001;933:222–234.

179. Elenkov IJ, Iezzoni DG, Daly A, et al. Cytokine dysregulation, inflammation and well-being. *Neuroimmunomodulation* 2005;12(5): 255–269.

180. Watkins LR, Maier SF. Immune regulation of central nervous system functions: from sickness responses to pathological pain. *J Intern Med* 2005;257(2):139–155.

181. Watkins LR, Maier SF. Implications of immune-to-brain communication for sickness and pain. *Proc Natl Acad Sci U S A* 1996;96(14): 7710–7713.

182. Wieseler–Frank J, Maier SF, Watkins LR. Immune-to-brain communication dynamically modulates pain: physiological and pathological consequences. *Brain Behav Immun* 2005;19(2):104–111.

183. Steinman L. Elaborate interactions between the immune and nervous systems. *Nat Immunol* 2004;5(6):575–581.

184. Romeo HE, Tio DL, Rahman SU, et al. The glossopharyngeal nerve as a novel pathway in immune-to-brain communication: relevance to neuroimmune surveillance of the oral cavity. *J Neuroimmunol* 2001;115(1–2): 91–100.

185. Reiche EM, Morimoto HK, Nunes SM. Stress and depression-induced immune dysfunction: implications for the development and progression of cancer. *Int Rev Psychiatry* 2005;17(6):515–527.

186. Wichers M, Maes M. The psychoneuroimmuno-pathophysiology of cytokine-induced depression in humans. *Int J Neuropsychopharmacol* 2002;5(4):375–388.

187. Anisman H, Merali Z. Cytokines, stress and depressive illness: brain-immune interactions. *Ann Med* 2003;35(1):2–11.

188. Pucak ML, Kaplin AI. Unkind cytokines: current evidence for the potential role of cytokines in immune-mediated depression. *Int Rev Psychiatry* 2005;17(6):477–483.

189. Schiepers OJ, Wichers MC, Maes M. Cytokines and major depression. *Prog Neuropsychopharmacol Biol Psychiatry* 2005;29(2):201–217.

190. Wood LJ, Nail LM, Gilster A, et al. Cancer chemotherapy-related symptoms: evidence to suggest a role for proinflammatory cytokines. *Oncol Nurs Forum* 2006;33(3):535–542.

191. Raison CL, Capuron L, Miller AH. Cytokines sing the blues: inflammation and the pathogenesis of depression. *Trends Immunol* 2006;27(1):24–31.

CHAPTER 30

Pain and Learning

ROBERT J. GATCHEL, BRIAN R. THEODORE, and **NANCY D. KISHINO**

One of the major contributions of the behavioral sciences to the area of medicine has been the application of learning principles to the development of effective illness management techniques. This has been especially true in the area of pain management. Before discussing these learning-based management techniques, an overview of the three major principles of learning will be provided.

Overview of the Three Major Principles of Learning

CLASSICAL CONDITIONING

Classical conditioning is one of the most basic forms of learning in which a learned association or connection develops between two stimuli or objects. As noted by Baum et al.,[1] the eminent Russian physiologist Ivan Pavlov (1849–1936) was the first to describe the process of classical conditioning with his work on the conditioned reflex. Reflexes are specific, automatic, unlearned reactions elicited by a specific stimulus. For example, if you have ever touched a surface that you did not know was hot (such as a hot stove), you showed a reflexive behavior—the immediate withdrawal of your hand from the stove. Similarly, if a piece of dust suddenly enters your eye, your eye will automatically blink and begin to secrete tears. These *unconditioned reflexes* are automatic and have a great deal of survival value for the organism. Pavlov demonstrated that such unconditioned reflexes could be *conditioned*, or learned. While studying dogs in order to understand more fully the digestive process, he began to notice that many of the dogs secreted saliva (an unconditioned reflex to the sight or smell of food) before food was delivered to them. He observed that this phenomenon occurred whenever the dogs either heard the approaching footsteps of the laboratory assistant who fed them or had a preliminary glimpse of the food. In order to investigate this phenomenon more systematically, Pavlov developed a procedure for producing a conditioned reflex. This procedure came to be called *classical conditioning*. It is one of the most basic forms of learning.

Pavlov conducted a series of well-known studies on the process of classical conditioning using dogs as experimental subjects (Fig. 30.1). In these studies, Pavlov studied situations in which a neutral stimulus or event (such as a bell) was presented to a dog just prior to the presentation of food (an unconditioned stimulus that normally elicits an automatic unconditioned reflex of salivation). After a number of such presentations, the bell (now a conditioned stimulus) would elicit a conditioned or learned salivation response when presented by itself in the absence of food. The conditioned reflex of salivation occurred to the bell alone. This represents the process of classical conditioning, and it is based on the learned association or connection between two stimuli, such that the bell is associated with food, that have occurred together at approximately the same point in time. An association is learned between a weak stimulus (such as the bell) and a strong stimulus (such as the sight of food) so that the weak stimulus comes to elicit the response originally controlled only by the stronger one (i.e., salivation).

Pavlov also subsequently demonstrated what would happen if the neutral stimulus, such as a bell, was presented just prior to the presentation of an aversive stimulus such as an electric shock or a pinprick. Normally, such aversive stimuli presented alone will produce a variety of negative responses such as whining/whimpering and fear-type reactions such as urination. When the bell preceded such an aversive stimulus, eventually, the formerly neutral bell stimulus would automatically produce the negative emotional responses.

In another variety of this design, Pavlov then evaluated what would happen if, instead of preceding food with the sound of the bell, it was preceded by the aversive stimulus such as electric shock. What Pavlov found in this situation was that, after this conditioning, the dogs subsequently failed to demonstrate any negative emotional responses to the aversive stimulus. Instead, these dogs began perceiving these painful stimuli as signals that food was on the way. The electric shock now actually elicited salivation and approach behaviors.

OPERANT CONDITIONING

Operant conditioning (also referred to as instrumental conditioning) is a different form of learning that was originally formulated by Edward Thorndike (1874–1949) and then more comprehensively developed by B. F. Skinner (1904–1990). Unlike classical conditioning, operant conditioning develops new behaviors that bring about positive consequences or remove negative events. In classical conditioning, a new stimulus (such as a bell) is conditioned to elicit the same responses that had previously occurred to the unconditioned stimulus, whereas in operant conditioning, a new response is learned. For example, new behaviors that produce food, social approval, or other positive consequences, or that reduce damaging or aversive events, illustrate operant behavior. The behavior "operates" on the environment to bring about changes in it. Thus, animal training, such as that involved in the learned performance of circus animals, involves basic principles of operant conditioning. Although operant training has existed for centuries, the behaviorist revolution in psychology provided the first carefully delineated methods and procedures

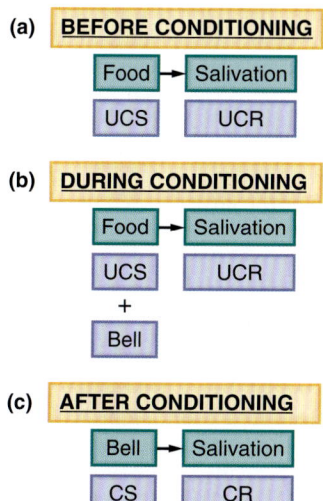

FIGURE 30.1 Pavlov's procedure of classical conditioning. CR, conditioned reflex; CS, conditioned stimulus; UCR, unconditioned reflex; UCS, unconditioned stimulus.

of operant conditioning so that such training could be accomplished most efficiently.[1] The key stimulus is *reinforcement*. Reinforcement refers to any consequence that increases the likelihood that a particular behavior will be repeated or that strengthens that behavior. *Extinction* involves the gradual decrease in the strength or tendency to perform a response due to the elimination of reinforcement. Based on these principles, what came to be known as the "Skinner box" was devised as an enclosed plexiglas box in which there was a light above a lever. The lever could be pressed down by the animal with its paws (rats were used in these early studies). Below the lever was a food tray into which food pellets could be dispensed. The task of the animal was to learn that pressing the lever (a certain number of times or at a certain rate, predetermined by the experimenter) resulted in food pellets being dispensed in the food tray. Thus, the animal learned to operate on the environment (the lever in the box) in order to receive reinforcement (food pellets).

Once the aforementioned response was learned, one could then introduce different *reinforcement schedules* in order to produce different patterns of responding. Reinforcement could now require variable numbers of bar presses or could be available every so often. Also, a *discriminative stimulus* could be introduced, so that the rat received reinforcement for pressing the bar only when the light was on in the box. The animal would soon learn not to respond when the light was off. In this manner, the rat's bar-pressing behavior came under *stimulus* (e.g., light) *control*.

This same shaping procedure is used in training circus and other animals to perform complicated acts. Dolphins can be shaped to leap out of the water, and lions can be taught to jump through flaming hoops in order to receive some reinforcement. These techniques are used in virtually every zoo and marine animal show.

OBSERVATIONAL LEARNING

Finally, the third major form of learning is called observational learning. There has been a great deal of research indicating that learning can occur through simple observation without the presence of any form of tangible direct reinforcement. Such learning, besides being called *observational learning*, is sometimes called imitation learning, cognitive learning, vicarious learning, or modeling. Observational learning is defined simply as that learning which occurs without any apparent direct reinforcement.[2] Many behaviors can be acquired if an individual sees the particular behavior performed or modeled by another person. In addition, behavior is often strongly guided by social norms, resulting in a given individual being motivated to adopt a set of behaviors that are consistent with these norms.[3,4] Observational learning is one such mechanism that transmits knowledge of these norms to the individual. These norms can be either explicit or implicit, and they can operate at the level of specific groups an individual may identify with, in addition to norms dictated at the larger societal level.

One of the earliest laboratory studies of observational learning[5] involved nursery school children. One group of children observed an adult perform a series of aggressive acts, both verbal and physical, toward a large toy Bobo doll. Another group watched a nonaggressive adult, who simply sat quietly and paid no attention to the doll. A third group of children was not exposed to a model. Later, after being mildly frustrated, all children were placed in a room alone with the Bobo doll and their behavior was observed. It was found that the behavior of the two model groups tended to be similar to that of their adult model. That is, children who had viewed the aggressive adult performed more aggressive acts toward the doll in the free-play situation than the other groups and also made more responses that were exact imitations of the model's aggressive behavior.

Those children who had observed a nonaggressive adult model performed significantly fewer aggressive responses than the aggressive model group.

Operant Conditioning and Pain

THE HALLMARK WORK OF WILBERT FORDYCE

As discussed earlier, and as reviewed by Gatchel,[6] operant conditioning refers to the strengthening of a response and behavior through reward or reinforcement. That is to say, the probability that a behavior will be performed again is increased if it is followed by some form of reinforcement. Behavior is controlled by its consequences. If a behavior is followed by a reward, it has a high probability of recurring; if it is ignored or punished, it has a low probability of recurring. Obviously, a great deal of our everyday behavior is learned and maintained through operant conditioning. For example, most of us work because of the rewards (both tangible, such as money, and intangible, such as a pleasant work environment) that it produces.

In terms of pain, many times a person in pain will elicit a great deal of sympathy and attention (both of which are rewarding). In addition, suggestions are usually made by others to rest and stay inactive, pain-relieving medications are usually administered, and often financial compensation is provided. The longer these reinforcing consequences continue, the longer the patient is likely to display the maladaptive pain behaviors such as inactivity and avoidance of work. Thus, this type of learning or conditioning can significantly contribute to the maintenance of pain behavior.

As pointed out by Baum et al.,[1] this operant conditioning conceptualization of pain was systematically employed in the operant pain treatment program originally developed at the University of Washington's Department of Rehabilitation Medicine by Fordyce and colleagues.[7] This program involved a 4- to 8-week inpatient period, designed to gradually increase the general activity level of the patient and to decrease medication usage. The program was based on the assumption that, although pain may initially result from some underlying organic pathologic condition, environmental reinforcement consequences (such as attention of the patient's family and the rehabilitation staff) can modify and further maintain various aspects of "pain behavior," such as complaining, grimacing, slow and cautious body movements, requesting pain medication, and so on. Viewing pain as an operantly conditioned behavior, Fordyce and colleagues[7] assumed that the potentially reinforcing consequences, such as the concern and attention from others, rest, medication, and avoiding unpleasant responsibilities and duties, as well as other events, frequently follow and reinforce the maladaptive pain behavior and, as a consequence, hinder the patient's progress in treatment.

In their treatment program, Fordyce and colleagues[7] systematically controlled environmental events (e.g., attention, rest, medication) and made them occur contingent on adaptive behaviors. A major goal of the program was to increase positive behaviors, such as participation in therapy and activity level, while simultaneously decreasing or eliminating negative pain behaviors. It should also be noted that members of the patient's family were actively involved in the treatment program and worked closely with the rehabilitation staff. They were taught how to react to the patient's behavior in a manner that would reduce pain and to maximize the patient's compliance with, and performance in, the rehabilitation program. Using this operant approach, the patient was basically taught to reinterpret the sensation of pain and tolerate it while performing more adaptive behaviors that would gain the attention and approval of others. Such a program was initially conducted in the hospital and would later be continued on an outpatient basis. These programs proved to be very successful at decreasing pain behaviors while increasing the levels of activities of daily living.

Of course, such examples do not imply that all pain is learned. The point being made is that our pain perceptions and responses often have a significant psychological learning component that directly and significantly contributes to these experiences of pain. Thus, psychological variables play a direct role in the pain experience. How one reacts to pain sensations is as important an issue as the specific physiologic mechanisms involved in transmitting and generating pain experiences. Pain is a complex behavior and not simply a sensory effect.

With the aforementioned view in mind, it is clear that one must conceptualize pain like any other form of complex behavior, consisting of multiple behavioral components. As Fordyce and Steger[8] have indicated, in order to describe pain, "there must be some form of pain behavior by which diagnostic inferences and treatment judgments can be made." A patient will signal the type of pain he or she is experiencing by describing the intensity, frequency, location, and type of pain experienced. In addition to these verbal cues available to the patient's environment as an indication of his or her pain, there is a myriad of nonverbal signs used to communicate pain experiences. These include grimaces, sighs, moans, limps, awkward or strained body positions, the use of a cane or crutch, and many other symbols associated in our society with discomfort or physical problems.

Traditionally, in attempts to describe pain, the focus was only on the physiologic or structural mechanisms underlying the report of pain and not on other components such as behavioral indices and self-report. The reliance on strictly one component, such as structural measures, does not yield a valid or precise measure of an individual's pain. Again, pain is a complex behavior and not purely a sensory event. One needs to consider multiple behavioral components in the assessment and treatment of this behavior.

OPERANT CONDITIONING AND CHRONIC PAIN: THE BASICS

Sanders[9] has provided an excellent overview of the key ingredients involved in the use of operant conditioning methods when managing chronic pain. Of course, as he appropriately points out, operant conditioning methods should not be viewed as the only technique to use in managing chronic pain. Rather, it is just one of a number of behavioral science methodologies that can be used in combination/unison with other methodologies. Operant techniques can be used to help significantly decrease many common overt pain behaviors, such as the following:

- Verbal pain behaviors, such as overt expressions of hurting (e.g., moaning, sighing, complaining)
- Nonverbal pain behaviors, such as limping, grimacing, overreliance on a cane or brace, rubbing the affected area, etc.
- Overly sedentary activities, such as decreased activity level, sitting, and lying down
- Overconsumption of medications and the sole reliance on other therapeutic devices to control pain

Rather than engagement in the aforementioned maladaptive pain behaviors, the patient is encouraged and reinforced to engage in "well behaviors" that involve more positive activity and alteration away from the overfocusing on pain. Through a comprehensive approach, health care professionals, family members, and others reinforce and encourage these well behaviors, whereas other effective pain management techniques are learned by the patient, such as biofeedback, stress management, coping skills, and appropriate pharmacotherapy, which is closely maintained. The overall goal is to increase function which will then be accompanied by a decrease in pain.[6]

Classical Conditioning and Pain

AVERSIVE CLASSICAL CONDITIONING AND PAIN

As discussed earlier in this chapter, Pavlov conducted studies demonstrating that when an initially neutral stimulus (such as a bell) was presented just prior to the presentation of an aversive, painful stimulus (such as electric shock) which will, in turn, produce negative emotional responses (such as whimpering, fear, avoidance, etc.), the bell itself will produce the negative emotional response when presented by itself. We then may generalize this to a patient who developed a sudden painful back problem at work, which does not go away after several days, after which just the act of going to work and anticipating lifting a heavy object may produce a negative emotional response such as fear of lifting and possible avoidance of the workplace because of pain.

CLASSICALLY CONDITIONED FEAR/AVOIDANCE AND PAIN

Figure 30.2 presents the conditioning sequence that a person may go through in the situation described earlier: (1) At first, before conditioning, there is no association between lifting an object at work and any avoidance of lifting because of fear of pain. (2) During conditioning, the individual now begins to experience some back pain while lifting objects at work. This pain becomes progressively worse over time, to the point that this person hesitates to lift anything because of fear of exacerbating the back pain he or she is already experiencing. (3) After conditioning, any prompting or requirement to lift an object automatically produces a fear response and active avoidance of any lifting to avoid pain. There is now a classically conditioned negative emotional response of lifting objects at work because of the fear of pain.

How can the aforementioned classically conditioned association between lifting and a fear of pain response be broken? As Pavlov's experiments have shown, just as a conditioned association can be learned, it can also be subsequently extinguished or broken under the right situations. One such method would be to initially teach patients how to correctly lift while keeping their back muscles relaxed. The weight they are then asked to lift is kept relatively light and then progressively made heavier as the individual is able to lift a certain weight while relaxed and not experiencing any pain. The person is also taught appropriate pacing skills so that enough time is given between

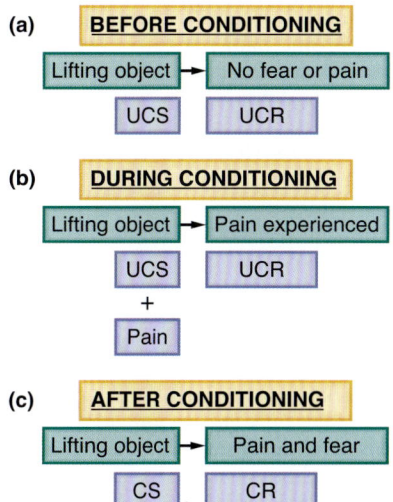

FIGURE 30.2 Classically conditioned fear and pain during a work task (lifting an object). CR, conditioned reflex; CS, conditioned stimulus; UCR, unconditioned reflex; UCS, unconditioned stimulus.

lifts for his or her back muscles to recuperate before performing the next lift. Thus, fear of lifting becomes "deconditioned" or extinguished in this work situation.

Observational Learning and Pain

Observational learning is defined simply as that learning which occurs without any apparent direct reinforcement.[2] Many behaviors can be acquired if an individual merely sees the particular behavior displayed or modeled by another person. Examples of behaviors acquired by observational learning abound. For example, investigations of dental fears in children have revealed that the attitudes and feelings of a child's family toward dental treatment are important in determining that child's own anxiety toward dental treatment. In one such study, it was found that children with anxious mothers showed significantly more emotionally negative behaviors during a tooth extraction than did children of mothers with low anxiety.[10]

In our society, there is a great deal of potential observational learning that can negatively influence comprehensive pain management effects. We are constantly being bombarded by advertisements that certain medications or pills will make us feel better. This, in turn, produces an unfortunate iatrogenic effect on patients who assume that there is some magic "silver bullet" pill or procedure that will automatically make them feel better and take away their pain. Unfortunately, such expectations are often not realized. Thus, patient education is often initially needed to dissuade patients of the notion that there is an immediate magical cure for their pain, especially as it becomes more chronic in nature.

Social norms can also influence an individual's response to pain, often through the mechanisms of observational learning. These normative influences play a role in behaviors associated with the reporting of pain, seeking treatment for pain, and level of pain tolerance. A study by Sternbach and Tursky[11] was among the earliest investigations that illuminated our further understanding of how normative factors influence responses to pain. In this study, the results implied that cultural differences associated with ethnicity played a role in an individual's tolerance of painful electrical stimulation. Parallel results in terms of ethnic differences were also demonstrated when physiologic indices (such as heart rate and palmar skin resistance levels) were measured in response to painful electrical stimulation despite relatively large intraethnic group variation.[12]

Recent studies have also demonstrated the role played by ethnic differences. For example, ethnicity has been reported to account for differences in self-reported levels of pain, as well as for tolerance of induced ischemic pain, during a study on a sample of chronic pain patients.[13,14] Cultural differences are also apparent in treatment preference and levels of health care utilization. A large population-based survey in the United States indicated that Caucasians had greater number of visits on average compared to African Americans and Hispanics and were more likely to have received complementary or alternative therapies for chronic pain.[15]

Early research on the association between gender and responses to pain also indicated that females had a lower tolerance level for experimentally induced pain[16] and were also more likely to report pain within clinical settings.[17] However, recent research has indicated that the extent of an individual's identification with his or her own gender group norms moderates his or her tolerance of pain. Gender differences in the tolerance of experimentally induced pain are present only among individuals strongly identifying with social norms that dictate that men should tolerate more pain than women.[18] Although it remains to be seen whether social norms also dictate gender differences in the probability of seeking treatment for pain, there is a demonstrable gender difference in health care utilization among chronic pain patients, with females being more likely to seek treatment for pain.[19]

Integrating Learning Principles in the Treatment of Pain

COGNITIVE-BEHAVIORAL THERAPY AND PAIN

As Turk[20] has highlighted in his discussion of the cognitive-behavioral therapy (CBT) approach to pain, there are important behavioral learning theory principles that are part of this overall therapeutic perspective. Certainly, classical conditioning (a focus on eliminating conditioned fear avoidance), operant conditioning (such as not reinforcing pain behavior), and observational learning (such as education about the negative iatrogenic expectation of immediate pain relief) are all important components. However, in addition, Turk[20] appropriately points out the fact that cognitive factors, in addition to behavioral factors, need to be considered: "The critical factor for the C–B model, therefore, is not that events occur together in time or are operantly reinforced but that people learn to predict them based on experiences and information processing. They filter information through their preexisting knowledge and organized representations of knowledge (e.g., cognitive scheme) . . . and react accordingly . . . Because interaction with the environment is not a static process, attention is given to the ongoing reciprocal relationships among physical, cognitive, affective, social, and behavioral factors" (p. 140). This perspective is in keeping with the biopsychosocial approach to pain,[6] to be discussed later.

With this aforementioned perspective in mind, there is no doubt that CBT is an effective treatment modality for the management of pain. Morley et al.,[21] on the basis of their systematic review of the scientific literature and a meta-analysis of randomized controlled trials, found that CBT produced significantly greater changes in self-reported pain and cognitive coping, as well as reduced behavioral expressions of pain, relative to waiting list control patients and alternative treatment control conditions. In a more recent comprehensive review, Gatchel and Okifuji[22] found comparable results. Table 30.1 provides a summary of some of the components of CBT, as delineated by Gatchel.[6]

TABLE 30.1 Summary of Some of the Major Components of Cognitive-Behavioral Therapy
• Educate patients about pain and their particular syndrome.
• Engender in patients a self-management and coping skills perspective to pain.
• Help patients focus on increasing physical functioning and management of their pain rather than expecting a sudden cure.
• Teach biofeedback, relaxation, and stress management techniques.
• Provide patients with coping skills in other areas, such as with interpersonal problems, work-related problems, marital problems, etc.
• Emphasize to patients the importance of identifying, and then eliminating, maladaptive thoughts about pain.
• Provide patients with guidance about increasing activities of daily living (in order to distract them from pain), with appropriate pacing activities.
• Provide help to improve sleep.
• Review the appropriate use of potential adjunctive modalities, such as medications, exercise, and physical methods (e.g., cold and heat packs).
• Assist patients with appropriate goal setting for the future (e.g., when to return to work or other activities).
• Provide relapse prevention strategies in order to help cope with potential future relapses.

Adapted from Gatchel RJ. *Clinical Essentials of Pain Management.* Washington, DC: American Psychological Association; 2005.

COGNITIVE-BEHAVIORAL THERAPY AS AN ESSENTIAL COMPONENT OF A COMPREHENSIVE INTERDISCIPLINARY APPROACH TO PAIN MANAGEMENT

The biopsychosocial perspective of pain is now accepted as the most heuristic approach to the understanding and treatment of pain disorders.[6,23] It views physical disorders, such as pain, as a result of a complex and dynamic interaction among physiologic, psychological, and social factors that perpetuate and may worsen the clinical presentation. Moreover, each individual experiences pain uniquely. Therefore, the range of psychological, social, and economic factors can interact with physical pathology to modulate a patient's report of symptoms and subsequent disability. As a consequence, a comprehensive biopsychosocial approach to assessment and treatment must be employed with each patient because of the unique interactions as well as to tailor the treatment to the specific needs of the patient. This is why comprehensive interdisciplinary pain management programs have proven to be more therapeutic and cost-effective than traditional unimodal treatment approaches.[22]

Within an interdisciplinary treatment program, there is a comprehensive treatment team that consists of the following: physician–nurse team to deal with medical issues, psychologist or psychiatrist to deal with the psychosocial issues of patients, a physical therapist to address any issues related to physiologic bases of pain as well as any issues related to physical progression toward recovery, and an occupational therapist who is involved in both physical and vocational aspects of the patient's treatment. For such a program to be effective, constant and efficient communication among all treatment personnel is imperative, during which patient progress can be discussed and evaluated. This is important so that patients hear the same treatment philosophy and message from each of the treatment team members. The overall goal is to produce an increase of functioning and the ability to manage pain and disability.

It is a major goal of the psychologist or psychiatrist to increase the patient's understanding of pain as well as their coping skills required to manage the pain. This is where CBT plays a major role. Of course, in keeping with the biopsychosocial perspective, it is not a standalone treatment but must be integrated with the other components of therapy in order to yield the best long-term outcomes.[6]

Conclusion

Pain is a complex behavior and is, therefore, subject to the general principles of learning and behavior change. The three major principles of learning include classical conditioning, operant conditioning, and observational learning. These principles play an important role in the development of pain behavior (e.g., social or environmental factors that can reinforce maladaptive pain behavior). However, these learning principles can also be effectively utilized in the treatment and management of pain. The biopsychosocial approach to the treatment and management of pain emphasizes interdisciplinary treatment modalities and eschews a "one-size-fits-all" approach in dealing with pain. Learning principles are therefore an important component in this approach due to its flexibility in addressing complex behavioral history at the individual level. CBT incorporates these learning principles and has been documented as an effective component of interdisciplinary pain management.

References

1. Baum A, Gatchel RJ, Krantz DS, eds. *An Introduction to Health Psychology.* 3rd ed. New York: McGraw-Hill; 1997.
2. Bandura A. *Principles of Behavior Modification.* New York: Holt, Rinehart & Winston; 1969.
3. Turner JC. *Social Influence.* New York: Brooks/Cole; 1991.
4. Cialdini RB, Trost MR. Social influence: social norms, conformity, and compliance. In: Gilbert D, Fiske S, Lindsey G, eds. *The Handbook of Social Psychology.* New York: McGraw-Hill; 1998:151–192.
5. Bandura A, Ross D, Ross SA. Imitation of film-mediated aggressive models. *J Abnorm Soc Psychol* 1963;66:3–11.
6. Gatchel RJ. *Clinical Essentials of Pain Management.* Washington, DC: American Psychological Association; 2005.
7. Fordyce WE, Fowler RS Jr, Lehmann JF, et al. Some implications of learning in problems of chronic pain. *J Chronic Dis* 1968;21:179–190.
8. Fordyce WE, Steger JC. Chronic pain. In: Pomerleau OF, Brady JP, eds. *Behavioral Medicine: Theory and Practice.* Baltimore, MD: Williams & Wilkins; 1979:125–154.
9. Sanders SH. Operant conditioning with chronic pain: back to basics. In: Turk DC, Gatchel RJ, eds. *Psychological Approaches to Pain Management: A Practitioner's Handbook.* New York: Guilford Press; 2002:128–137.
10. Weisenberg M. Cultural and racial reactions to pain. In: Weisenberg M, ed. *The Control of Pain.* New York: Psychological Dimensions; 1977:201–232.
11. Sternbach RA, Tursky B. Ethnic differences among housewives in psychophysical and skin potential responses to electric shock. *Psychophysiology* 1965;1(3):241–246.
12. Tursky B, Sternbach RA. Further physiological correlates of ethnic differences in responses to shock. *Psychophysiology* 1967;4:67–74.
13. Campbell CM, Edwards RR, Fillingim RB. Ethnic differences in responses to multiple experimental pain stimuli. *Pain* 2005;113(1–2):20–26.
14. Edwards RR, Doleys DM, Fillingim RB, et al. Ethnic differences in pain tolerance: clinical implications in a chronic pain population. *Psychosom Med* 2001;63(2):316–323.
15. Portenoy RK, Ugarte C, Fuller I, et al. Population-based survey of pain in the United States: differences among white, African American, and Hispanic subjects. *J Pain* 2004;5(6):317–328.
16. Riley JL III, Robinson ME, Wise EA, et al. Sex differences in the perception of noxious experimental stimuli: a meta-analysis. *Pain* 1998;74(2–3):181–187.
17. Unruh AM. Gender variations in clinical pain experience. *Pain* 1996; 65(2–3):123–167.
18. Pool GJ, Schwegler AF, Theodore BR, et al. Role of gender norms and group identification on hypothetical and experimental pain tolerance. *Pain* 2007;129:122–129.
19. McGeary DD, Mayer TG, Gatchel RJ, et al. Gender-related differences in treatment outcomes for patients with musculoskeletal disorders. *Spine J* 2003;3:197–203.
20. Turk DC. A cognitive-behavioral perspective on treatment of chronic pain patients. In: Turk DC, Gatchel RJ, eds. *Psychological Approaches to Pain Management: A Practitioner's Handbook.* 2nd ed. New York: Guilford Press; 2002:138–158.
21. Morley S, Eccleston C, Williams A. Systematic review and meta-analysis of randomized controlled trials of cognitive behaviour therapy and behaviour therapy for chronic pain in adults, excluding headache. *Pain* 1999;80:1–13.
22. Gatchel RJ, Okifuji A. Evidence-based scientific data documenting the treatment and cost-effectiveness of comprehensive pain programs for chronic nonmalignant pain. *J Pain* 2006;7(11):779–793.
23. Turk DC, Monarch ES. Biopsychosocial perspective on chronic pain. In: Turk DC, Gatchel RJ, eds. *Psychological Approaches to Pain Management: A Practitioner's Handbook.* 2nd ed. New York: Guilford Press; 2002:5–29.

CHAPTER 31

Psychiatric Illness, Depression, Anxiety, and Somatic Symptom Disorder

JOSEPH GREGORY HOBELMANN, MARK D. SULLIVAN,
MICHAEL R. CLARK, and AJAY D. WASAN

Chronic pain and psychiatric illness commonly occur together.[1] Yet the high rates of psychiatric illness in patients with chronic cancer and noncancer pain are still poorly understood. Diagnostic hierarchies taught to physicians in medical school and residency, impairment rating strategies used by compensation systems, and the natural scientific method used by medicine that looks for objective causes for clinical symptoms force us into a mind–body dualism. George Engel[2] helped develop our modern concept of "psychogenic pain." Psychogenic pain has been defined as pain due to psychological factors in the absence of an organic basis for pain.[3] If we cannot explain pain in terms of objective tissue pathology, Western biomedicine lures us to explain it in terms of patients' psychopathology.[4,5] This is not an evidence-based strategy but rather a reflection of what it means to explain a symptom in modern biomedicine.

The majority of patients with chronic pain and psychiatric illness have a physical basis for pain in the body, whose perception is made worse by overlying psychiatric illness.[6] Epidemiologic evidence supports the use of inclusive rather than exclusive models of psychiatric diagnoses in medical settings that allows for the presence of both medical disease and mental disorders (i.e., a comorbidity model). Medical illness in no way excludes the possibility of a clinically important psychiatric illness. Medically ill patients are much more likely to have psychiatric illness than patients without medical illness. Psychiatric illness in no way precludes the possibility of a clinically important medical illness. Psychiatric illness is, in fact, associated with health behaviors and psychophysiologic changes known to promote medical illness.

The structure of our clinical settings makes the integrated delivery of mental and physical health care difficult. Nowhere is this more important than in the care of the patient with chronic pain. Psychotherapeutic interventions for chronic pain are rarely effective in isolation from somatic treatments, and the success of somatic treatments is diminished by co-occurring mental illness. Distress, disuse, and disability are important facets of a chronic pain problem, and all require clinical attention by the pain practitioner. Neglect of one of these components can result in treatment failure even in the presence of excellent care for the other components. Research has indicated that psychiatric comorbidity has an adverse impact on treatments for chronic pain, such as rehabilitation, spinal cord stimulation, or opioid therapy.[3,7] Although the details of these interactions are quite relevant to understand, this chapter concentrates on the recognition and diagnosis of psychiatric illness in patients with chronic pain, a sizable task in and of itself. Similarly, psychiatric comorbidity has shown to be particularly prevalent in and salient to the outcomes of a range of noncancer pain disorders (e.g., chronic low back pain,[8] fibromyalgia,[9] temporomandibular joint disorder,[10] chronic daily headache,[11] and chronic pelvic pain[12]). However, the specific role that comorbid psychopathology plays in each of these disorders is beyond the scope of this chapter.

This chapter first outlines an approach to psychiatric diagnosis and to categorizing psychiatric symptoms in patients with chronic pain. Because of the breadth of psychiatric symptoms in pain patients, this section is substantial in order to provide a framework for organizing symptoms into diagnostic and treatment categories. Then, this chapter discusses the main illness categories of depression, anxiety, personality, and somatoform disorders. It is beyond this chapter to discuss to what extent a pain practitioner should evaluate and treat psychiatric problems and when to refer to a psychologist or psychiatrist.

Psychiatric Nosology and Diagnostic and Treatment Approaches

As noted, any discussion of psychiatric disorders in patients with chronic pain is haunted by the concept of psychogenic pain. We are drawn to the concept of psychogenic pain because it fills the gaps left when our attempts fail to explain clinical pain exclusively in terms of tissue pathology. Psychogenic pain, however, is often merely a diagnosis of exclusion made solely on the basis of the inability to identify an objective cause for pain. Positive criteria for the identification of psychogenic pain, mechanisms for the production of psychogenic pain, and specific therapies for psychogenic pain are lacking. Furthermore, neuroimaging studies indicate that anticipated pain, imagined pain, or empathizing with the pain of another are associated with activations of the same brain areas involved in processing a painful stimulus, such as applied noxious heat (the lateral and medial pain systems).[13,14] Thus, there is a dynamic interaction between our mental states (mind) and brain function. The dichotomy between mind and body (including brain) underlying the concept of psychogenic pain is hollow. As discussed later in this chapter, it may be more useful to frame the contributions of the mind to pain perception in terms of a process of central sensitization.

Psychiatric diagnosis of many disorders, such as depression, can be helpful to the clinician and patient by pointing to specific effective therapies. The *Diagnostic and Statistical Manual of Mental Disorders* (5th ed.; *DSM-5*) lists the current diagnoses treated by psychiatrists and the specific symptoms that serve as descriptive criteria for each condition.[15] However, *DSM* offers only consistency and reliability of symptoms and does not take into consideration course of illness, which is essential in recognizing mental illness.[16] This is particularly true of psychiatric disorders in those with medical illness. Most psychiatrists tend to use the *DSM* as a guide to the major diagnoses, not as a definitive diagnostic method. As a descriptive tool, many of the symptom lists for *DSM* diagnoses are quite complete and will be referred to throughout this chapter. However, when patients with chronic pain are in need of psychiatric care, they want to know the generative nature of their conditions and how to differentiate them for the sake of receiving prognoses and treatments.[17] Multidisciplinary pain treatment functions with the same limitations.[18,19] Without the method to determine a set of unique causes and direct specific treatments, the patient receives symptomatic treatments with the expected "partial" response. Despite the involvement of more disciplines, the approach is clearly dualistic—cures for "organic" problems and management for "functional" problems. Cartesian dualism lives.

The *DSM*, although it has limitations, provides a taxonomy that serves as the basis for psychiatrists and psychologists to communicate and further study disorders. This has been historically lacking for the classification of chronic pain conditions. However, the Analgesic, Anesthetic, and Addiction Clinical Trial Translations Innovations Opportunities and Networks (ACTTION) has partnered with the U.S. Food and Drug Administration and the American Pain Society (APS) to develop an evidence-based chronic pain classification system called the ACTTION-APS Pain Taxonomy (AAPT).[20] This classification incorporates available knowledge regarding both physiologic and biopsychosocial mechanisms contributing to pain conditions. It is important to recognize that psychological and social factors are not solely secondary consequences of chronic pain but rather play a complex role in the persistence and severity of pain conditions. These biopsychosocial factors can be risk factors, protective factors, and process variables within the dynamic system of forces that constitute a chronic pain condition.[21] The AAPT classification system provides a framework that incorporates these complicated factors and could be very useful clinically if validated in future outcome studies.

Patients with chronic pain come to or are referred to a psychiatrist because they are ill. In some way, they are considered a diagnostic dilemma.[22,23] Despite the utilization of extensive health care resources to perform an exhaustive evaluation, the patients remain ill. A temptation emerges to diagnose them with a psychogenic problem because no "good" cause can be found for their persistent pain and the accompanying disability and suffering.[24] The cause for their illness cannot be found until the investigation expands to include the domain of personal meaning.[25] This realm contains not only the diseases of the brain (cerebral faculties) but also the disruptions of the motivational rhythms of behavior, the psychological constitution of the individual, and the personal chronicle of desire and relationships. All mental disorders are expressions of life under altered circumstances that affect characteristic mental capacities and generate particular expressions.[26,27] These distinctions allow for independently informed perspectives about the nature of mental disorders and what may have happened to generate the disorder.

Four perspectives (diseases, behaviors, dimensions, and life stories) represent classes of disorders that each have a common essence and logical implications for causation and treatment.[28,29] In this approach to patient care, diseases are what people *have*, behaviors are what people *do*, dimensions are what people *are*, and life stories are what people *encounter*. The formulation of a patient with chronic pain should address the contributions from each perspective to the overall presentation and inform the design of a treatment plan that can address each component of the patient's illness. Although the basis for a mental illness may be dominated by one perspective (i.e., the disease perspective in schizophrenia), generally, each psychiatric diagnosis has contributions from each perspective that are responsible for the onset and maintenance of the disorder.

Diseases of the brain may manifest psychologically. The psychological faculties of the brain include, but are not limited to, consciousness, cognition, memory, language, affect, and executive functions. Abnormalities in the structures or their associated functions of these faculties are expressed in the symptoms typical of common diagnoses such as delirium, dementia, panic disorder, and major depression. However, the patient may describe deficits in these faculties with difficulty and rely on somatic symptoms (e.g., pain) as incomplete proxies for these criteria. The physical symptoms occur because the brain is malfunctioning and suggests pathology in the body.

The unifying feature of diseases is a broken part within the individual that is causing the characteristic signs and symptoms typically manifested by the affliction.[27] For the patient, only the symptoms and reduction of symptoms are of concern. Finding a cure may repair the broken part, prevent the initial damage from progressing, or compensate for the pathology through secondary compensatory measures.

The perspective of *behavior* encompasses a wide range of actions and activities. The complex behaviors of human beings are designed with purpose to achieve goals. Human consciousness is characterized by the regular, rhythmic alterations of attention and perception produced by internal drives that increase a person's motivation toward a particular activity.[29,30] The drive pushes the individual into action. Then, after the actions, the drive is satisfied and a state of satiety emerges. Over time, drives reemerge with subsequent effects on the individual's perceptual attitude toward his setting. In addition, personal assumptions or external opportunities increase the likelihood of certain behaviors. These present a choice to the person who must decide what action to take. After the choice is made and the behavior completed, external consequences emerge from the outcome and influence future actions. The person learns which choices are most effective. When aspects of choice and control over behavior become disrupted, physicians will be asked to address the distorted goals, excessive demands, damaging consequences, and a lack of responsiveness to negative feedback.[31,32] Eating disorders and opioid use disorders are examples. Treatment of behavioral disorders begins with regaining temporary control of the situation by stopping the behavior.[33] Restricting the patient's actions and preventing these problematic behaviors eventually limits the chaos of destructive actions. This stable foundation is required for the patient to gain insight about and motivation toward appropriate choices that will result in less distress and more satisfaction.[34] This is the basis for the effectiveness of behavioral approaches to chronic pain management as outlined in other chapters.

In contrast, many mental disorders emerge not from a disease of the brain or some form of abnormal illness behavior but a patient's personal affective or cognitive constitution.[29,30] Each individual possesses a set of personal *dimensions* such as intelligence, extraversion, and neuroticism. These traits describe who a person is, and they are carried into the world as a set of innate capabilities of their psychological makeup. Which traits are relied on and how much of them a person possesses will determine his potential to cope with different situations. Some circumstances are overwhelming and provoke a person's vulnerability to distress. The patient cannot manage the situation and what is required because of who he is. Borderline personality disorder is an example (Table 31.1). It is probably the most severe personality disorder and generally is evident prior to the onset of pain. Assessment of personality traits is discussed at greater length in the following text. Treatment for disorders of the dimensional type focuses on remediation of specific deficiencies and guidance about overcoming potential vulnerabilities through adaptations such as education about, assistance with, or modification of the particular stressors.[19,33]

The *life story* perspective utilizes a narrative composed of a series of events that a person encounters and determines to be personally meaningful.[29,30] These self-reflections are the means by which a person judges the value of his life as a whole. They impart a sense of self as the agent of a life plan unfolding in a social setting as well as the reflective subject experiencing and interpreting the outcome of such plans and commitments. If events are occurring as planned, then the person feels on track and successful. However, if the sequence of events results in an unexpected or disappointing outcome, the person will feel a sense of distress about this failure. Life story disorders are interpretive responses to life encounters such as grief from loss or anxiety due to expected threats.[31,35,36] In patients with chronic

TABLE 31.1 *Diagnostic and Statistical Manual of Mental Disorders*, Fifth Edition, Diagnostic Criteria for Borderline Personality Disorder

A pervasive pattern of instability of interpersonal relationships, self-image, and affects and marked impulsivity beginning by early adulthood and present in a variety of contexts, as indicated by five (or more) of the following:

1. Frantic efforts to avoid real or imagined abandonment (Note: Do not include suicidal or self-mutilating behavior covered in criterion 5.)
2. A pattern of unstable and intense interpersonal relationships characterized by alternating between extremes of idealization and devaluation
3. Identity disturbance: markedly and persistently unstable self-image or sense of self
4. Impulsivity in at least two areas that are potentially self-damaging (e.g., spending, sex, substance abuse, reckless driving, binge eating) (Note: Do not include suicidal or self-mutilating behavior covered in criterion 5.)
5. Recurrent suicidal behavior, gestures, or threats, or self-mutilating behavior
6. Affective instability caused by a marked reactivity of mood (e.g., intense episodic dysphoria, irritability, or anxiety usually lasting a few hours and only rarely more than a few days)
7. Chronic feelings of emptiness
8. Inappropriate, intense anger, or difficulty controlling anger (e.g., frequent displays of temper, constant anger, recurrent physical fights)
9. Transient, stress-related paranoid ideation, or severe dissociative symptoms

pain, the demoralization resulting from the inability to work or perform normal duties is a good example. Treatment begins with the expectation to forge a narrative of setting and sequence that suggests some role of the patient in his life, and that illuminates the troubled state of mind as the outcome of that role and course of events.[19,33] The effective treatment of life story disorders requires reframing and reinterpretation to remoralize the patient by transforming the story into one with the potential for success and fulfillment.

The four perspectives provide a comprehensive yet flexible approach to the evaluation of a patient in distress with chronic pain and other somatic symptoms.[29,37] The treatments prescribed are now designed from the individual formulation and relevant perspectives. If a patient's symptoms and distress continue, the physician must consider other factors that may have been overlooked. Usually, these factors are within one of

the perspectives initially thought to be less important. A new combination of therapies is then required to treat the patient successfully. Understanding the relevant contributions from each perspective is important to formulating treatment. In the discussion that follows, categories of psychiatric disorders as defined in the *DSM-5* (2013) of the American Psychiatric Association are used as an organizing strategy. The *DSM-5* is relatively new, and there are significant changes from the *DSM* (4th ed., *DSM-IV*), which was utilized for almost 20 years. As such, there is little research using the new criteria, so this chapter discusses concepts utilizing both *DSM-IV* and *DSM-5*.

Framework for Describing Psychiatric Symptoms

Figure 31.1 illustrates common psychiatric symptoms in patients with chronic pain. However, Figure 31.1 does omit substance use disorders, which are beyond the scope of this chapter. It is important to note that substance abuse or addiction in patients with chronic pain is estimated to range from 3% to 48% depending on the population sampled, with most estimates around 15%.[38] Psychiatry-based research and health psychology–based research have contributed important insights into characterizing the mental life of patients with chronic pain. The findings from these epistemologies overlap significantly, and although lacking until recently, the new AAPT classification system for pain is a model for integrating these results.[39] Common terms to describe the psychological condition in pain patients are heightened emotional distress, high negative affect, and elevated pain-related psychological symptoms (i.e., those that are a direct result of chronic pain, and when the pain is eliminated, the symptoms disappear). These can all be considered forms of psychopathology and psychiatric comorbidity because they represent impairments in mental health and involve maladaptive psychological responses to medical illness. This approach melds methods of classification from psychiatry and behavioral medicine to describe the scope of psychiatric disturbances in patients with chronic pain. *Psychiatry* is the field of medicine that is concerned with someone's mental life, such as their emotions, experiences, thoughts, and behaviors. It is focused particularly on disruptive, disordered, or pathologic psychological states. Thus, the constructs from pain psychology are situated in Figure 31.1 as psychiatric symptoms, which in themselves can be at pathologic levels, just as depression symptoms can rise to a level considered abnormal.

In pain patients, the most common manifestations of psychiatric comorbidity involve one or more core psychopathologies

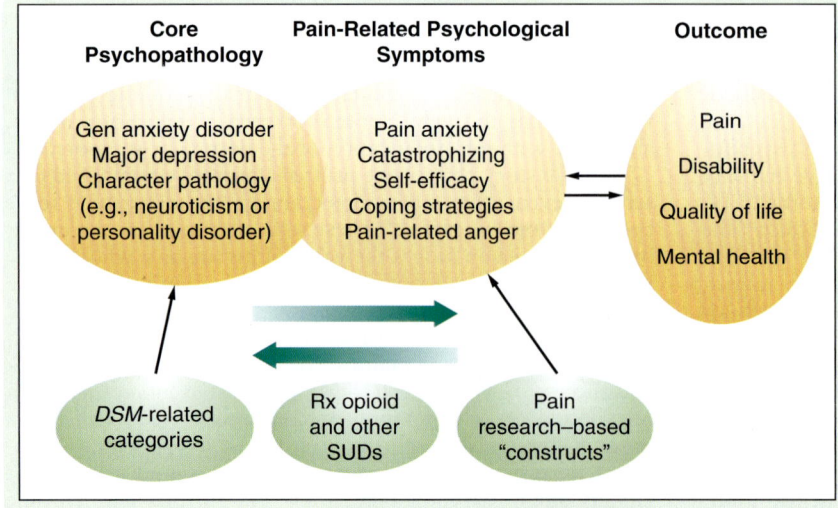

FIGURE 31.1 Common psychiatric symptoms in patients with chronic pain. *DSM, Diagnostic and Statistical Manual of Mental Disorders*; Gen, general; Rx, prescription; SUDs, substance use disorders. *(Adapted from Wasan AD, Alpay M. Pain and the psychiatric co-morbidities of pain. In: Stern T, ed. Comprehensive Clinical Psychiatry. Philadelphia: Elsevier; 2008:1067–1080.)*

in combination with pain-related psychological symptoms. For instance, poor pain self-efficacy or high levels of pain catastrophizing are most often found in conjunction with high levels of depression or anxiety symptoms.[40] These categories interact, and some component of each are part and parcel of other psychopathologies. In other words, "lumping" (a diagnostic approach) and "splitting" (a construct-based approach) are both valid approaches to psychiatric phenomenology. As described in the previous section, not all patients and their psychiatric symptoms fit neatly into DSM categories of illness. This is true not just of those with chronic pain, and hence, looking beyond DSM to broader and more specific methods of illness description and diagnosis is more prudent.

The pain-related psychological symptoms are described at length in other chapters, but it is important to understand how they interact with other psychiatric diagnoses. For example, pain-related anxiety (which includes state and trait anxiety-related to pain) is the form of anxiety most germane to pain.[41] Elevated levels of pain-related anxiety (such as fear of pain) also meet *DSM-5* criteria for an anxiety disorder due to a general medical condition. Because anxiety straddles both domains of core psychopathology and pain-related psychological symptoms, the assessment of anxiety in a patient with chronic pain (as detailed in the following discussion) must include a review of manifestations of generalized anxiety as well as pain-specific anxiety symptoms (e.g., physiologic changes associated with the anticipation of pain).

As indicated on Figure 31.1, elevated pain-related psychological symptoms have a clear, negative predictive relationship to many outcome areas. Poor coping skills often involve passive responses to chronic pain (e.g., remaining bed-bound and mistakenly assuming that chronic pain is indicative of ongoing tissue damage as a reason for inactivity). Poor copers employ few active self-management strategies (such as using ice, heat, or relaxation strategies for 10 to 20 minutes before resuming activities). Pain catastrophizing (cognitive distortions that are centered around pain) and low self-efficacy (a low estimate by the patient of what he/she is capable of doing) are linked with higher levels of pain and disability and worse quality of life.[39] A tendency to catastrophize predicts poor outcome and disability, often independent of other psychopathology, such as major depression. Duration of chronic pain and presence of psychiatric comorbidity are each independent predictors of pain intensity and disability. High levels of anger (which occur more often in men) can also explain significant variance in pain severity.[42]

Depression

One must begin by distinguishing between depressed mood and the clinical syndrome of major depression. It is important to note, especially when working with chronic pain patients, that depressed mood or dysphoria is not necessary for the diagnosis of major depression. Anhedonia, the inability to enjoy activities or experience pleasure, is an adequate substitute. It is common for patients with chronic pain to deny dysphoria but to acknowledge that enjoyment of all activities has ceased, even those without obvious relation to their pain problem (e.g., watching television for a patient with low back pain).

The *DSM-5* criteria for major depressive episodes are listed in Table 31.2. These include psychological symptoms, such as worthlessness, and somatic symptoms, such as insomnia. The three core symptoms of major depression in patients with pain (which also holds true in those without pain) are low mood, impaired self-attitude, and neurovegetative signs.[43] It is important to note that somatic symptoms count toward a diagnosis of major depression unless they are caused by "the direct physiologic effects of a general medical condition" or medication. The poor sleep, poor concentration, and lack of enjoyment often experienced by patients with chronic pain are frequently attributed to pain rather than depression. These should generally not be excluded

TABLE 31.2 *Diagnostic and Statistical Manual of Mental Disorders*, Fifth Edition, Criteria for Major Depressive Episode

A. Five (or more) of the following symptoms have been present during the same 2-wk period and represent a change from previous functioning; at least one of the symptoms is either (1) depressed mood or (2) loss of interest or pleasure.

Note: Do not include symptoms that are clearly attributable to another medical condition.

1. Depressed mood most of the day, nearly every day, as indicated by either subjective report (e.g., feels sad or empty) or observation made by others (e.g., appears tearful). Note: In children and adolescents, can be irritable mood.
2. Markedly diminished interest or pleasure in all, or almost all, activities most of the day, nearly every day (as indicated by either subjective account or observation)
3. Significant weight loss when not dieting or weight gain (e.g., a change of more than 5% of body weight in a month), or a decrease or increase in appetite nearly every day. Note: In children, consider failure to make expected weight gains.
4. Insomnia or hypersomnia nearly every day
5. Psychomotor agitation or retardation nearly every day (observable by others, not merely subjective feelings of restlessness or being slowed down)
6. Fatigue or loss of energy nearly every day
7. Feelings of worthlessness or excessive or inappropriate guilt (which may be delusional) nearly every day (not merely self-reproach or guilt about being sick)
8. Diminished ability to think or concentrate, or indecisiveness, nearly every day (either by subjective account or as observed by others)
9. Recurrent thoughts of death (not just fear of dying), recurrent suicidal ideation without a specific plan, or a suicide attempt or a specific plan for committing suicide

B. The symptoms cause clinically significant distress or impairment in social, occupational, or other important areas of functioning.

C. The symptoms are not caused by the direct physiologic effects of a substance (e.g., a drug of abuse, a medication) or a general medical condition (e.g., hypothyroidism).

D. The occurrence of the major depressive episode is not better explained by schizoaffective disorder, schizophrenia, schizophreniform disorder, delusional disorder, or other specified and unspecified schizophrenia spectrum and other psychotic disorders.

E. There has never been a manic episode or hypomanic episode.

as a direct physiologic effect of pain. Given the high rates of depression in chronic pain patients, in the context of low mood complaints, it is best to attribute these symptoms toward a diagnosis of depression. Indeed, studies of depression in medically ill populations have generally found greater sensitivity and reliability with "inclusive models" of depression diagnosis than with models that try to identify the cause of each symptom.[44] Similarly, just as in those without pain, those with depression and pain are very likely to also have high levels of anxiety.[45,46]

SUICIDAL IDEATION AND BEHAVIOR
Suicide accounts for 1.4% of all deaths in the world, making it the 15th leading cause of death.[47] In the United States, 4.6% of the population surveyed had made a suicide attempt, and 13.5% reported a history of suicidal ideation.[48] The majority of suicide attempts occur within a year of the onset of suicidal ideation. The risk of suicidality is greatest in patients with affective disorders (e.g., depression and anxiety), personality disorders, substance use disorders, and chronic debilitating physical illnesses.[49,50] Depression is the most consistent and strongest predictor of suicidal ideation.[51] In one study of patients with major depressive disorder, 58% reported suicidal ideation during a

current episode of illness.[52] Suicide was attempted by 15% of these patients with 95% preceded by suicidal ideation. Hopelessness, low levels of function, perceptions of poor social support, and disorders of alcohol use predicted suicidal ideation.

Medical illnesses and chronic pain particularly, increase the risk of suicide. In a study of suicide in the elderly, medical conditions such as congestive heart failure, chronic obstructive lung disease, seizure disorder, and urinary incontinence were significantly associated with suicide with treatment for multiple illnesses increasing the risk.[53] Yet, except for bipolar disorder, the highest risk of suicide was found in patients with severe pain (odds ratio [OR] = 7.52). Pain has been studied as a contributory factor in episodes of deliberate self-harm involving patients with medical problems admitted to a general hospital.[54] Multiple studies have shown that patients with chronic pain are at greater risk for suicidal ideation, suicide attempts, and suicide completions.[55]

Most clinical diagnoses of pain conditions have been associated with increased risk for suicide.[56] A recent comprehensive review notes that the likelihood of death by suicide in patients with chronic pain is 2 to 3 times the rate described in the general population.[50] The lifetime prevalence of suicide attempts in patients with chronic pain ranged from 5% to 14%, and the rate of suicide attempts is double that found in the general population. The lifetime prevalence of suicidal ideation associated with chronic pain is approximately 20%. The rate of suicidal ideation in patients with chronic pain is estimated between 5% and 24%. Although a number of methods are used to commit suicide, overdoses with medications are the most common. The relationship between chronic pain and suicidality is complex. Although the associations are consistent, the cause and effect pathways of transition from suicidal ideation to suicide attempt to suicide completion are more difficult to describe. At this time, no successful algorithm exists and only an in-depth and longitudinal evaluation of the patient with chronic pain offers the best strategy for detecting who is considering suicide as a personal option. Although understandable, it is not the norm to be suicidal even in those with severe pain. Most commonly, suicidality in a patient with chronic pain is indicative of an underlying psychiatric disorder.[57] Thinking one is better off dead (a passive death wish) is not the same as actively trying or wanting to kill oneself (suicidality). It is important to bear this distinction in mind in evaluating any patient with thoughts about death.

Part of the concern regarding the association between chronic pain and suicidality lies in whether chronic pain is an independent risk factor for suicidal behavior or the presence of depression completely explains this association. A thorough review described the evidence for eight pain-specific risk factors of suicidality, which is defined as suicidal ideation, suicide attempt, or suicide completion.[50] The studies available suffer from significant limitations including inadequate assessments, retrospective designs, limited control groups, and the failure to distinguish between the potential risk factors of pain versus pain-related disability. However, the existing pain literature coupled with the general knowledge of suicide supports the following as the strongest predictors of suicidality: family history of suicide, previous suicide attempts, and presence of comorbid depression. Evidence exists for other risk factors including pain characteristics (intensity, location, type, duration), female gender, comorbid insomnia, catastrophizing and avoidance, desire for escape, helplessness and hopelessness, and problem-solving deficits.[58-60] The prevention of suicide should remain a priority for the care of patients with chronic pain.

WHICH CAME FIRST, DEPRESSION OR PAIN?

Patients with chronic pain often dismiss a depression diagnosis, stating that their depression is a direct reaction to their pain problem. Psychiatry has long debated the value of distinguishing a *reactive* form of depression caused by adverse life events from an *endogenous* form of depression caused by biologic and genetic factors.[61] Life events are important in many depressive episodes, although they play a less important role in recurrent and severe or melancholic or psychotic depressions.[62] Determining whether a depression is a *reasonable response* to life's stress may be important to patients seeking to decrease the stigma of a depression diagnosis and has been of interest to pain investigators (for a review, see Fishbain and colleagues[6]). It is not, however, important in deciding that treatment is necessary and appropriate. Indeed, no clinical benefit is gained from debating whether the depression caused the pain or the pain caused the depression, although such information may be useful in psychotherapy. If patients meet the diagnostic criteria outlined previously, it is likely that they can benefit from appropriate treatment. There is evidence that subsyndromal depression—depression symptoms not quite satisfying the threshold for major depression but debilitating nonetheless—also benefits from treatment and should be treated.[63-65]

Prospective studies of patients with chronic musculoskeletal pain have suggested that chronic pain can cause depression,[66] that depression can cause chronic pain,[67] and that they exist in a mutually reinforcing relationship.[68] One fact raised to support the idea that pain causes depression is that the current depressive episode often began after the onset of the pain problem. The majority of studies appears to support this contention.[69] However, it has been documented that many patients with chronic pain (especially those disabled patients seen in pain clinics) have often had episodes of depression that predated their pain problem by years.[70] Among patients presenting to chronic pain clinics, one-third to more than one-half meet criteria for current major depression.[71] Depression in patients with chronic pain is associated with greater pain intensity, more pain persistence, application for early retirement, and greater interference from pain, including more pain behaviors observed by others.[72] This has led some investigators to propose that there may exist a common trait of susceptibility to dysphoric physical symptoms (including pain) and to negative psychological symptoms (including anxiety and depression).[73,74] They conclude that "pain and psychological illness should be viewed as having reciprocal psychological and behavioral effects involving both processes of illness expression and adaptation."

It may be useful when initiating depression treatment to accept that the pain caused the depression because it builds rapport and is consistent with epidemiologic evidence about the current depressive episode. And most frequently, depression follows the onset of chronic pain and is not preceded by it.[71]

DIFFERENTIAL DIAGNOSIS

When considering the diagnosis of depression in the patient with chronic pain, important alternatives include bipolar disorder, substance-induced mood disorder, and dysthymic disorder (particularly if accompanied by a severe personality disorder, such as borderline personality disorder). Patients with bipolar disorder have extended periods of abnormally elevated as well as abnormally depressed mood. These periods of elevated mood need to last more than one continuous day and include features such as inflated self-esteem, decreased need for sleep, and racing thoughts. A history of manic or hypomanic episodes predicts an atypical response to antidepressant medication and increases the risk of antidepressant-induced mania. Substance-induced mood disorders can also occur in those with pain. Patients with chronic pain may be taking medications such as opioids, corticosteroids, dopamine-blocking agents (including antiemetics), or sedatives (including muscle relaxants) that produce a depressive syndrome. Current medication lists should be scrutinized before additional medications are prescribed for any patient.

BIOLOGIC TESTS FOR DEPRESSION

A variety of biologic tests for depression have been investigated.[75] These tests have included the dexamethasone-suppression test, thyrotropin-releasing hormone stimulation test, clonidine-induced growth hormone secretion, and rates of imipramine binding to platelet membrane serotonin transporters. Forty percent to 50% of patients with major depression do not show normal suppression of morning plasma cortisol after receiving dexamethasone the night before. However, high false-positive rates for this dexamethasone-suppression test exist in patients who are pregnant; patients with dementia, alcoholism, anorexia nervosa, and other chronic debilitating diseases; and patients who are taking medications that induce microsomal enzymes, including barbiturates and opioids. This has limited the clinical value of this test.[76] The serotonin transport mechanism on platelet membranes is similar to that on serotonergic neurons. ^{3}H-imipramine binding to this platelet receptor is reduced in patients with major depression. It appears to be further reduced in patients who have both pain and depression.[77] Lower level of serotonin in the cerebral spinal fluid have found in depressed patients and have been linked to suicidal ideation.[78] Although patients show significant differences on these tests, when considered as a group, substantial variation between individual patients limits the usefulness of these tests in the clinical setting. In the future, they may be able to provide a better understanding of the biochemical links between pain and depression.

DYSTHYMIC DISORDER

Dysthymic disorder is a chronic form of depression lasting 2 years or longer. The symptoms are generally less severe than those during an episode of major depression. Individuals with dysthymia can develop major depression as well. This combined syndrome has often been called *double depression*.[79] It is important to note dysthymia because it is frequently invisible in medical settings, often being dismissed as "just the way that patient is." Dysthymia has been shown to respond to many antidepressants, including the selective serotonin reuptake inhibitors (SSRIs).[80] Treatment of double depression can be particularly challenging because of treatment resistance and concurrent personality disorders.[81] Psychiatric consultation should be considered when dysthymia or double depression is suspected.

EPIDEMIOLOGY OF DEPRESSION

The prevalence of depression is much higher in medical settings and in patients with chronic illnesses than in the general population. It has been shown in studies using structured psychiatric interviews that a linear increase occurs in the prevalence of major depressive disorder when comparing community, primary care, and inpatient medical populations. Although 2% to 4% have major depression in the community, 5% to 9% of ambulatory medical patients and 15% to 20% of medical inpatients meet diagnostic criteria.[82] Primary care patients with major depression have been found to have more severe medical illness than those who are not depressed.[83] Even among community samples, the risk for depression appears to increase with worse perceived health status, number of chronic medical conditions, and number of medications taken.[84]

Depression is the most prevalent mood disorder associated with comorbid chronic pain.[85] Prevalence rates of depression among patients in pain clinics have varied widely depending on the method of assessment and the population assessed. Rates as low as 10% and as high as 100% have been reported.[86] The reason for the wide variability may be attributable to a number of factors, including the methods used to diagnose depression (e.g., interview, self-report instruments), the criteria used (e.g., *DSM-5*, cutoff scores on self-report instruments), the set of disorders included in the diagnosis of depression

(e.g., presence of depressive symptoms, major depression), and referral bias (e.g., higher reported prevalence of depression in studies conducted in psychiatry clinics compared with rehabilitation clinics). The majority of studies report depression in more than 50% of chronic pain patients sampled.[87,88] There is a direct relationship between the duration of pain and the incidence of major depression. Certain chronic painful conditions are associated with higher rates of depression than others. For example, fibromyalgia, chronic daily headache, and chronic pelvic pain, each are associated with higher rates than arthritis.[45,89]

Studies of primary care populations (in which generalization is less problematic) have revealed a number of other factors that appear to increase the likelihood of depression in patients with chronic pain. Dworkin and colleagues[90] reported that patients with two or more pain complaints were much more likely to be depressed than those with a single pain complaint. Number of pain conditions reported was a better predictor of major depression than pain severity or pain persistence.[90] Von Korff and colleagues[91] developed a four-level scale for grading chronic pain severity based on pain disability and pain intensity: (1) low disability and low intensity; (2) low disability and high intensity; (3) high disability, moderately limiting; and (4) high disability, severely limiting. Depression, use of opioid analgesics, and doctor visits all increased as chronic pain grade increased. Engel and colleagues[92] showed that depression was associated with high total health care costs but not high back pain costs among health maintenance organization patients with back pain. When dysfunctional primary care back pain patients are studied for a year, those whose back pain improves also show improvement of depressive symptoms to normal levels.[93]

These epidemiologic studies provide solid evidence for a strong association between chronic pain and depression but do not address whether chronic pain causes depression or depression causes chronic pain. As indicated previously, this question has more importance in medicolegal contexts than clinical contexts. Overall, in most instances, depression follows the onset of pain.[93]

PAIN AND DEPRESSION: MECHANISMS OF ASSOCIATION

Beyond documenting the association of chronic pain and depression lies the question concerning mechanisms by which they may interact. Biologic, psychological, and social mechanisms have been proposed to explain the high co-occurrence of chronic pain and depression. There is also substantial evidence (beyond the scope of this chapter to recount) that the following mechanisms underlie the other psychiatric comorbidities of pain, such as anxiety disorders.

Biologic Theories
Pain Sensitivity
It is well documented that patients with major depression, or even depressive symptoms, have more pain complaints than those without depression. Studies have shown that 30% to 60% of depressed patients complain of pain.[94] These findings raise the possibility that depressed patients may have a greater sensitivity to noxious stimuli. In other words, depressed patients may have a reduced pain threshold. But many studies have shown that depressed patients and patients with other psychiatric disorders have an elevated, not reduced pain threshold.[95,96] Depression appears to elevate pain threshold more for exteroceptive (e.g., cutaneous) stimulation than interoceptive (e.g., ischemic) stimulation, but there is significant heterogeneity in findings among different patient populations and stimulus modalities.[97] Psychiatric patients with dissociation such as borderline personality disorder have reliably shown elevated pain thresholds to external noxious stimuli.[98,99] Patients with posttraumatic stress disorder (PTSD) show complex responses

with higher pain thresholds and higher pain ratings to noxious stimuli than controls. Elevated pain thresholds were associated with dissociation levels, whereas elevated experimental and clinical pain ratings were associated with anxiety and anxiety sensitivity.[100] Thus, there is an unexplained discrepancy between the higher experimental pain thresholds and the higher clinical pain complaints among patients with depression and other psychiatric disorders. But it is clear that the increased pain complaints of patients with psychiatric disorders cannot be explained by changes in pain thresholds.

Biogenic Amines, Cytokines, and Neural Pathways

The highly variable relationship between injury severity and pain severity has been known since Beecher's studies of the soldiers at Anzio beach in World War II. Since the 1970s, great strides have been made in identifying the central nervous system mechanisms of endogenous pain modulation. Opioid and nonopioid branches to this system have been identified. Stimulation of the rostral ventromedial medulla or the dorsolateral pontine tegmentum produces behavioral analgesia in animals and inhibition of spinal pain transmission. The rostral ventromedial medulla is the principal source of serotonergic neurons that project to the spinal dorsal horn. The dorsolateral pontine tegmentum is the major source of noradrenergic neurons that project to the dorsal horn. Both neurotransmitters (serotonin and norepinephrine) inhibit nociceptive dorsal horn neurons when locally applied.[101] The descending inhibitory system is modulated by serotonin and norepinephrine, which are also thought to modulate mood. This is perhaps best illustrated by the effects of selective serotonin norepinephrine reuptake inhibitors (SNRIs) on depression and pain. The two drugs approved for use in this class are duloxetine and venlafaxine. Both are FDA-approved antidepressants that have analgesic properties independent of their effects on mood.[102,103] These medications enhance serotonergic and noradrenergic neurotransmission. Additional studies indicate that opioid analgesia is enhanced in the presence of antidepressant treatment[104] and decreased after serotonin and norepinephrine depletion.[105] Therefore, it appears that biogenic amines play a critical role in endogenous pain modulation. To the extent that depletion or impaired function of amines such as serotonin and norepinephrine occurs in depression, this may contribute to the pain experienced and reported by those with major depression. Just as cytokine responses are important to the initiation and maintenance of chronic pain,[106] they have also been implicated in the pathogenesis of depression.[107] Depressed patients without pain have been found to have higher levels of proinflammatory cytokines and acute phase proteins. Administration of the cytokine interferon-α leads to depression in up to 50% of patients. Proinflammatory cytokines affect neurotransmitter metabolism, neuroendocrine function (particularly the hypothalamic-pituitary-adrenal axis), and synaptic plasticity.

Cortical Substrates for Pain and Affect

Advances in neuroimaging have linked the function of multiple areas in the brain which process pain and mood simultaneously, described at length in a previous chapter. This system is often termed the *medial pain system* or *spinolimbic pain system*.[108] These cortical areas (e.g., the anterior cingulate cortex [ACC], the insula, amygdala, and the dorsolateral prefrontal cortex [DLPFC]) form functional units through which psychiatric comorbidity may amplify pain and disability (Fig. 31.2). They are also laden with opioid receptors.[109] The ACC, insula, and DLPFC are less responsive to endogenous opioids in pain-free subjects with high negative affect (e.g., depression, anxiety, and anger symptoms).[110] Thus, high negative affect may diminish the effectiveness of endogenous and exogenous opioids through direct effects on supraspinal opioid binding. The medial pain system runs parallel to the spinothalamic tract and receives direct input from the dorsal horn of the spinal cord. The interactions among the function of these areas, pain perception, and psychiatric illness are still being investigated. But the spinolimbic pathway is involved in descending pain inhibition, whose function may be negatively affected by the presence of psychopathology. This, in turn, could lead to heightened pain perception. Coghill and colleagues[111] have shown that differences in pain sensitivity between patients can be correlated with differences in activation patterns in the ACC, the insula, and the DLPFC. The anticipation of pain—a form of anxiety for pain—is also modulated by these areas, suggesting a mechanism by which anxiety about pain can amplify pain perception. Ploghaus and colleagues[13] have demonstrated that anticipation for an acute painful stimulus in healthy volunteers is marked by brain activation patterns throughout the medial pain system.

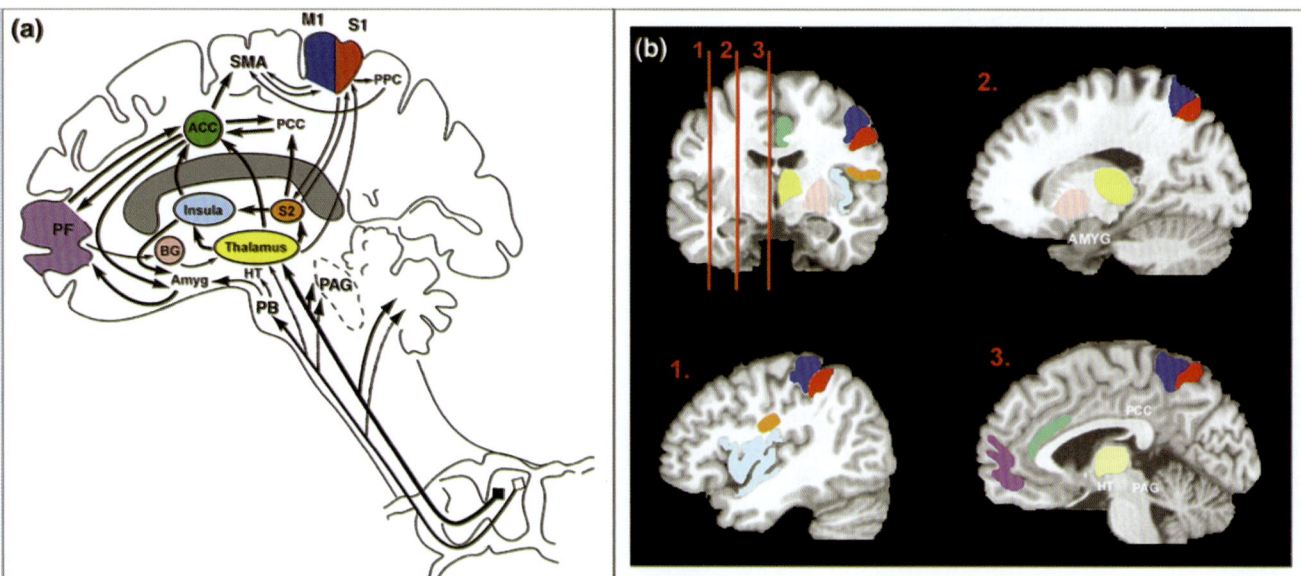

FIGURE 31.2 Supraspinal pathways of pain perception. ACC, anterior cingulate cortex; Amyg, amygdala; BG, basal ganglia; HT, hypothalamus; PAG, periaqueductal grayPB, parabrachial nucleus; PCC, posterior cingulate cortex; PF, prefrontal cortex; SMA, supplementary motor area. *(From Apkarian AV, Bushnell MC, Treede RD, et al. Human brain mechanisms of pain perception and regulation in health and disease. Eur J Pain 2005;9:463–484; Price DD. Psychological and neural mechanisms of the affective dimension of pain.* Science *2000;288[5472]:1769–1772.)*

Sleep Disturbance

Depression produces well-documented disturbances to sleep architecture. Polysomnographic recordings have documented reduced slow wave sleep, early onset of the first period of rapid eye movement (REM) sleep, and increased phasic REM sleep in patients with major depression.[112] Sleep continuity disturbances and increased phasic REM sleep tend to normalize with depression remission, even with psychotherapeutic treatment. However, reduction of REM latency and decreased slow wave sleep tend to persist despite clinical recovery. In sum, there appear to be *state* and *trait* elements to the sleep disturbance associated with depression. Studies have also demonstrated that sleep disturbance may be a result of chronic pain, which, in turn, can make it worse.[113] Fibromyalgia patients who were sleep deprived reported worsening pain and were found to be hyperalgesic (beyond their baseline pain) on pressure sensitivity testing.[114] Thus, whether depression or pain precipitated or worsened a sleep disturbance, its presence makes pain worse and is an important link between the two conditions.

Psychological Theories

Psychodynamic Theory

In classic psychoanalytic theory,[115] depression is postulated to be derived from anger unconsciously turned inward, excessive dependence on others for self-esteem, and feelings of helplessness in achieving one's goals. Some have suggested that the depression in some chronic pain patients is a manifestation of a personality style that draws from early developmental conflicts of guilt, anger, and masochism.[116,117] From this perspective, chronic pain may be a symptom of depressive disorder.[118]

Psychoanalytic theory stresses the fundamental parallelism between mental and physical pain and the possible displacement from the former to the latter. Intrapsychic links between pain and depression suggest that pain may function as a *hysterical* or conversion symptom that may prevent the breakthrough of more severe depression. These intrapsychic links largely correspond with the dynamics of *pain proneness* that were originally described by Engel[2] and, in a further elaboration, connected with the concept of *masked depression* by Blumer and Heilbronn.[116]

Blumer and Heilbronn[116] proposed a new psychological disorder, the "pain-prone" disorder, building on Engel's[2] notion of the pain-prone patient. In this view, pain should be considered as a variant of depressive disease. The central explanation is unconscious core conflicts. Core issues include "strong needs to be accepted and to depend on others as well as marked needs to receive affection and to be cared for."

Pain in the absence of organic pathology is considered by Blumer and Heilbronn[116] to be a *depressive spectrum disorder*. According to this model, pain and depression are viewed as manifestations of a single, common disease process. Specifically, the pain-prone disorder is viewed as a masked "depressive equivalent . . . the prime expression of a muted depressive state." No empiric research has supported the psychoanalytic formulation as presented by Blumer and Heilbronn.[116,119,120]

A more modern variant of this theory sees chronic pain as an expression of repressed anger and rage toward others. This was initially advanced by John Sarno, MD, a physiatrist practicing in New York City.[121,122] This theory has not been thoroughly investigated empirically, but there is preliminary evidence of a significant relationship between forgiveness and pain, anger, and psychological distress in patients with low back pain.[123]

Behavioral (Operant Conditioning) Theory

The behavioral model of depression concentrates on the most obvious symptom of depression, the motivational deficit characterized by a reduction in active behavior. A central feature of the behavioral model is response-contingent reinforcement (i.e., the responses from significant others to the individual's behavior). From this perspective, depressive behavior and depression are associated with low rates of positive reinforcement from the environment. Lack of positive reinforcement leads to a decrease in the frequency of the individual engaging in these behaviors, and ultimately, they may be extinguished completely. These low rates of reinforcement may occur because (1) positive reinforcers in the environment may become less available, or aversive events in the environment may have become more prevalent; (2) the positive effect of previous reinforcers may have declined, or the negative impact of aversive events may have increased; or (3) the individual may lack the skills either to attain the available positive reinforcers or to cope with aversive aspects of the environment. When individuals experience low rates of positive reinforcement, they reduce the performance of those behaviors, unless they are self-reinforcing. The reduction of behavior decreases further opportunities to receive positive reinforcement.

In the case of chronic pain, the individual may reduce his or her behavior because of physical impairments or because of fear of additional pain or further injury. Thus, by the restriction in behavior and social contacts, chronic pain patients may reduce the opportunity to achieve positive reinforcement and to engage in previously rewarding activities and consequently become depressed. The family can also reinforce maladaptive behavior. Although many families of patients with chronic pain are supportive with the best of intentions, excessive catering to the patient at the expense of maintaining function can perpetuate illness behavior, leading to depression. In other words, patients can occupy the sick role for reasons other than causal disease.

Cognitive Theory

According to Beck,[124] people may be vulnerable to depression because, from an early age, they have possessed negatively biased conceptualizations (schemas) of themselves and their experiences. When they are challenged by stressful life events, these schemas become activated, which, in turn, elicits negative thoughts about themselves, the world, and the future (the *negative cognitive triad*). These patients view themselves as hopeless, hapless, and helpless (i.e., "my life is not going to get better, no one can help me, and I can't help myself"). The latter can also be termed *poor self-efficacy*, or the belief that one is incapable of doing things to improve his or her life. Poor pain self-efficacy is the related belief that a patient cannot do anything to improve his or her pain or function.

In depressed patients, Beck[124] suggests that the cognitive triad serves as a filter for incoming information. This filter creates a negative bias that serves to put a pessimistic light on information and reinforces the depressed state. It also creates low expectations about their ability and thus may lead to lack of effort. Moreover, these people tend to discount their performance, underestimating their accomplishments.

Beck's[124] cognitive theory of depression emphasizes the importance of peoples' appraisal processes. In particular, it is believed that depressed persons show faulty information processing reflected by errors of logic. Through these cognitive errors (collectively referred to as *cognitive distortions*), depressed persons systematically misinterpret or distort the meaning of events so as to consistently construe themselves, their world, and their experiences in a negative way (the negative cognitive triad). According to this perspective, differences in cognitive errors and cognitive distortions, in general, should differentiate depressed and nondepressed patients. One of the most common cognitive distortions is *catastrophizing*, a tendency to view the most negative possible outcome as the only likely outcome. Pain catastrophizing (discussed at length in previous chapters) is the extension of this concept to patients viewing their pain as unbearable, uncontrollable, and leading to tissue damage. It has a significant co-occurrence and conceptual overlap with other depression and anxiety symptoms in pain patients. In other words, when pain patients with depression or anxiety catastrophize, they most often catastrophize over their pain.

Cognitive-Behavioral Perspective

The cognitive-behavioral perspective is based on five central assumptions: (1) People are active processors of information and not passive reactors. They attempt to make sense of information and determine what constitutes positive reinforcers. (2) Thoughts (e.g., appraisals, expectancies, beliefs) can elicit and influence mood, affect physiologic processes, have social consequences, and serve as impetuses for behavior; conversely, mood, physiology, environmental factors, and behavior can influence the nature and content of thought processes. (3) Behavior is reciprocally determined by both the individual and environmental factors. (4) People can learn more adaptive ways of thinking, feeling, and behaving. (5) Individuals should be active collaborative agents in changing their maladaptive thoughts, feelings, and behaviors.[125] From the cognitive-behavioral model, the way in which one thinks about pain and behaves in response to pain affects the extent of depression experienced. Like Beck's cognitive theory, its essential difference from the purely behavioral model is its view of patients as active interpreters of their environment.

Depression in chronic pain patients is postulated to result from patients' interpretations of the meaning and effect of their symptoms and their inability to exert any control over their symptoms. It is only when patients interpret their pain as interfering with important life activities and believe that they (or anyone) can do little to control the symptoms that they become depressed (i.e., they become depressed when they feel helpless and hopeless to exert any control, overwhelmed by the disruption of their lives, and unable to attain significant positive reinforcement from previous activities).[68] Thus, the cognitive-behavioral approach integrates the principles of operant conditioning and behavioral techniques with the emphasis of cognitive theory on the patients' appraisals, beliefs, and attributions.[126]

Diathesis-Stress Model

This is discussed at length in other chapters but should be restated here because it is the dominant model for understanding the interactions between pain and comorbid psychopathology, including depression.[3,127] This model frames the biologic and psychological mechanisms discussed earlier as diatheses or vulnerabilities. Under a condition of mental or physical stress, such as pain, the diatheses interact to produce the conditions of chronic pain and depression.[128,129] One can rephrase this notion such that in any given person, genetic susceptibilities to chronic pain and/or mental illness interact with the environment (e.g., physical experience of acute pain, reinforcement from the family, inability to work) leading to changes in the functioning of mental processes (mind, such as negative cognitive schema) and brain (such as neurotransmitter systems and endogenous opioid response), resulting in chronic pain and psychiatric comorbidity.[130]

Anthropologic Theories

Traditional and industrial societies appear to hold individuals less responsible for somatic symptoms than psychological symptoms. This difference may be especially prominent in modern Western biomedicine, in which symptom complexes are validated or invalidated through their correspondence with objective disease criteria.[131] A somatic "idiom of distress" may become the favored means for communicating distress of any origin that is overwhelming or disabling.[5,132] In other words, complaints about pain may be indicative of depression rather than a pain syndrome of a somatic origin. In many cultures including Western nations, pain is a more acceptable reason for disability than depression. Therefore, cultural incentives exist for translation of depression into pain. Because depressed patients have many physical symptoms, these can become the focus of clinical communication and concern. Giving patients with chronic pain permission to talk of distress in the clinical setting, using nonsomatic terms, can facilitate treatment as long as they do not feel that the somatic elements of their problem are being neglected or discounted.

This is one of the bedrock principles of narrative medicine,[133,134] which through the patient's description of their illness experience helps them to articulate the interrelationships between their physical symptoms, psychological states, and their roles among family, coworkers, and within society. The physical symptoms of chronic pain and the pathophysiology underlying them can be thought of as the *disease* of chronic pain. Although the constellation of disease, a patient's psychological state, and their experience of suffering can be termed, the *illness* of chronic pain.[133] Questions from the practitioner, such as "What have you lost as a result of your pain?" "How do you manage with your pain?" and "Is it a lot of work to stay well despite having pain?" are important to evoking an illness narrative and describing these interrelationships.[135]

DEPRESSION TREATMENT

Just as in the treatment of major depression in patients without chronic pain, the best quality treatment of depression in pain patients is to combine psychotherapy with medication management.[136,137] One of the most effective psychotherapy modalities in chronic pain patients is cognitive-behavioral therapy (CBT), discussed in the following text and in further detail in other chapters.

Pharmacologic Agents

In choosing an antidepressant agent in a patient with chronic pain, an important principle is that the medication should have independent analgesic properties. This means that the medication can be helpful for pain independent of its effect on mood (i.e., it works as an analgesic in those with and without depression). The two main classes with this property are the tricyclic antidepressants (TCAs) and the selective SNRIs. In the United States, duloxetine, venlafaxine, desvenlafaxine, and milnacipran are the SNRIs currently available. The monoamine oxidase inhibitors (MAOIs) (such as selegiline or tranylcypromine) are excellent antidepressants which do also have analgesic properties. But they are rarely used anymore except by psychiatrists (due to their side effect profile and medication interactions), and their use is confined to a third- or fourth-line agent in treatment resistant depression. Antidepressant medication can effectively treat depression in the presence of chronic pain, but there is some evidence that depression with comorbid pain is more resistant to treatment.[138] When depression accompanies chronic pain, as when it accompanies other chronic medical disorders, there may be some extra hurdles for depression treatment to overcome. These include aversive physical symptoms, severe deactivation, vocational dysfunction, marital conflict, social isolation, and concurrent medications. Comprehensive assessment of these issues and formulation of a treatment plan that takes them into account increase the likelihood of successful depression treatment in the chronic pain patient. If depression can be relieved, many other aspects of rehabilitation, such as physical therapy, are often much more easily accomplished. Pain often subsides with improvement in depressive symptoms.[139] Patients will typically report that they may still have pain but that "it doesn't bother me anymore." This statement is very telling that the affective component of pain has significantly improved.

All currently marketed antidepressants are equally effective for the initial treatment of depression. However, there is some evidence that medications with effects on dual neurotransmitter systems, such as serotonin and norepinephrine (the TCAs and SNRIs), are associated with a faster rate of improvement and lower rates of depression relapse.[140] Overall, whatever differences may exist among antidepressants in efficacy for neuropathic pain do not appear to affect their ability to treat depression.

The clinical art of depression treatment for those with chronic pain consists of establishing a solid therapeutic alliance around the problem of depression and finding a medication regimen with independent analgesic properties and a side effect profile that the patient can tolerate. Because patients with chronic pain can be vigilant and catastrophic in thinking about somatic symptoms, care must be taken to educate them about antidepressant side effects. Sometimes, it becomes necessary to initiate an antidepressant regimen at the lower doses used for geriatric patients to ease habituation to side effects. Because of their analgesic properties, the SNRIs and TCAs are the treatments of choice for patients with chronic pain and depression.

Although the TCAs are considered first line, their side effect profiles and the slower rate of titration needed to reach a therapeutic dose limit their usefulness compared to SNRIs. The TCAs have more side effects (anticholinergic) and more therapeutic effects (sleep continuity and anxiolysis) than the SNRIs. However, because the TCAs are used frequently in the management of neuropathic pain, it is very common to encounter a patient on lower doses of TCAs (10 to 75 mg). Typically, these patients have acclimated to many of the side effects, and gradual escalation of the dose to antidepressant ranges (approximately 100 to 300 mg, depending on the compound) can easily be performed in the pain management setting. In monitoring their use for depression, it is possible to obtain serum blood levels of TCAs to make sure that they are in the therapeutic range, but it is also appropriate to titrate to clinical effect. Disadvantages of TCAs include a wide range of adverse effects, including anticholinergic effects, orthostatic hypotension, effects on the cardiac conduction system, weight gain, sedation, sexual dysfunction, restlessness, "jitteriness," heightened anxiety on initial dosing, and cardiotoxicity in overdose. Before starting a TCA, in those over 45 years or in any patient with a history of cardiac disease, the QTc interval on an electrocardiogram (ECG) should be checked to see if it is <450 ms. Using TCAs in patients with QTc intervals >450 ms places them at a greater risk of developing torsades de pointes arrhythmia, even when lower doses of TCAs are used (10 to 75 mg), as is common in pain medicine. Of the TCAs, nortriptyline has the lowest incidence of side effects and thus is the preferred TCA for use in chronic pain patients, either for treatment of pain or depression. Although nortriptyline is more sedating than desipramine, it has a lower incidence of orthostatic hypotension and dizziness. Nortriptyline also has a comparable rate of analgesia to amitriptyline, despite the latter perhaps having broader effects on multiple analgesic mechanisms, such as sodium channel blockade. Nortriptyline is also twice as potent as amitriptyline, so it is much easier to get patients to therapeutic doses and to sustain use at these doses.

The SSRIs (those available in the United States include citalopram, escitalopram, fluoxetine, fluvoxamine, sertraline, and paroxetine) have become the most popular antidepressants because of their favorable side effect profiles but are more useful as second-line agents in a pain population because they do not have significant analgesic properties. Bupropion has effects on dopamine-norepinephrine reuptake inhibitors (DNRIs). Because of its energizing effects, it is very useful in those with chronic pain because many experience fatigue and poor concentration, either due to the pain itself or as side effects from pain medications. One study has shown that bupropion has analgesic properties in neuropathic pain.[141] Another study showed equivocal results in back pain.[142]

More detailed information on prescribing antidepressants is available in one of the standard psychopharmacology manuals.[143–145] In situations of treatment-resistant depression, studies have indicated that electroconvulsive therapy can be useful for treatment of depression and pain, across a variety of painful disorders.[146,147] However, no carefully controlled studies demonstrate the effectiveness of electroconvulsive therapy for treatment of chronic pain.

Chronic pain is frequently associated with insomnia and anxiety. It is, therefore, common that patients are treated with benzodiazepines or other sedatives (e.g., the muscle relaxers). Some patients begin taking these medications during the acute phase of the pain problem and then continue to take them for many months or years. Assessing chronic pain patients who take benzodiazepines for depression is important. These medications mask some symptoms of depression (e.g., initial insomnia, agitation), but they are not adequate treatments for depression. Indeed, dangerous levels of depression can develop under the cover of benzodiazepines. It has been suggested that benzodiazepines can induce depression with chronic use, but the evidence for this is not strong.[148] More important is the masking of depression by benzodiazepines.

Nearly, all patients with chronic pain should be tapered off benzodiazepines. Few conditions exist for which chronic benzodiazepines are the treatment of choice.[149] Many patients with chronic pain are treated with opioids, and the combination of opioid and benzodiazepine therapy is associated with large increases in mortality risk.[150,151] The Centers for Disease Control and Prevention (CDC) opioid guideline strongly recommends against simultaneous use of opioids and benzodiazepines in the treatment of patients with chronic pain.[152] The treatment of choice for chronic anxiety disorders, which are almost always accompanied by depressive symptoms, is antidepressant medication.[153] Buspirone (a 5-HT$_{1a}$ partial agonist) is marketed as an anxiolytic but is more similar to the antidepressants in its pharmacology and side effect profile. It is a reasonable alternative to the benzodiazepines for the treatment of breakthrough anxiety, particularly for those who experience agitation on the antidepressants.

PSYCHOTHERAPY
Psychodynamic Psychotherapy
In general, psychodynamic theory emphasizes the long-term predisposition to depression rather than the losses that occur in the short term. Treatment of depression from the classical psychoanalytic perspective tries to help the patient achieve insights into the repressed conflict and often encourages outward release of hostility turned inward. In the most general terms, the goal of therapy is to uncover latent motivations for the patient's depression. The psychodynamic approach to the depressed individual with chronic pain emphasizes the importance of individual differences in patients based on their developmental history, intrapsychic conflicts, interpersonal difficulties, and the subsequent failure to adapt to chronic illness. Patients' premorbid characteristics are hypothesized to color their adaptation to their current situation and affect their vulnerability to depression.

Psychodynamic therapy emphasizes the need for patients to address unconscious conflicts that may contribute to and maintain the depression and makes use of the therapeutic relationship, assuming that the patient will transfer or project his or her feelings onto the therapist.[154] This approach can be contrasted with treatment based on operant conditioning, in which it is assumed that the basic principles of learning apply to all individuals and the environmental contingencies of reinforcement can influence the reports of pain, distress, and suffering. As a treatment for depression, there is no good standardization of psychodynamic therapy, and thus, it is difficult to evaluate the studies of its effectiveness.

Behavioral Model

As noted, the behavioral model of depression concentrates on the reduction in active behavior that is a central feature of depression. Behavioral therapy for depression focuses on physical and social reactivation of patients.[155] As long as avoidance behaviors are targeted, it has efficacy equal to that of CBT, without any focus on cognitions.[156] The focus of treatment for depression is on the shaping of behavior through the use of graded task assignments and response-contingent reinforcement. Depressed individuals are encouraged to engage in more activities and to behave in ways that are likely to be regarded more positively by others. In some instances, it is believed that depressed patients are deficient in certain skills necessary to achieve positive reinforcement. Social skills training may also be included when the therapist determines that the patient is deficient in specific skills (e.g., communication skills). Attention may also be given to assisting the patient in planning pleasant events that the patient will find reinforcing.

Cognitive Model

From the cognitive perspective, therapy is based on the rationale that an individual's affect and behavior are largely determined by the ways in which he or she construes the world, and the therapeutic techniques were designed to identify, test, and correct distorted conceptualizations and the dysfunctional beliefs (schemas) underlying these cognitions. Beck's[124] therapy for depression is based on the assumption that the affected people engage in faulty information processing and reasoning and subscribe to schema that are self-defeating. In particular, depressed people are subject to the negative cognitive triad, in which they have feelings of pessimistic helplessness about themselves, the world, and their future. The aim of the cognitive therapist is to identify and then help patients to correct these distorted ideas and also to improve their information processing and reasoning. In contrast to psychodynamic therapy, the focus is on the here and now. Thus, attention to the origin of dysfunctional schemas in the cognitive model is limited.

The therapeutic procedures are highly structured and time limited and begin with the recognition of the connections between cognitions and affect, careful recording of these connections, collection of evidence for and against the ideas, followed by substitution of more adaptive and realistic interpretations. The cognitive approach is most frequently combined with behavioral techniques to treat patients with chronic pain, even though some debate exists about the compatibility of these approaches.[124,125]

Cognitive-Behavioral Model

No one cognitive-behavioral model exists but rather sets of models that share a perspective and incorporate some common features, namely (1) an interest in the nature and modification of patients' thoughts, feelings, and beliefs, as well as behaviors, and (2) some commitment to behavior therapy procedures in promoting change (e.g., graded practice, use of homework, training in relaxation, coping skills training, problem solving, and relapse prevention).[126]

Depressed people may focus attention selectively on and become preoccupied with somatic symptoms and their potentially ominous significance for their health and future. They may view themselves as helpless and their situation as hopeless and beyond their control. In depressed patients with chronic pain, the cognitive distortions often center around their pain, such as excessive fear of pain or fear of movement. To break this vicious circle, the cognitive-behavioral therapist applies a comprehensive approach to treatment that combines physical, psychological, behavioral, and social interventions. Coping skills training, problem-solving strategies, communications skills training, and directing patients to attend to their appraisals, interpretations, and beliefs surrounding pain are commonly used techniques. One of the most effective CBT methods in pain patients is to combine coping skills training focusing on fear of pain, reinjury, and movement with gradual activity and movement-based physical therapy.[157]

The cognitive-behavioral therapist attempts to assist patients to try new behaviors and to adopt more adaptive modes of thinking. Alterations in behavior become information that the patients are encouraged to use as the basis for changing their views of their situation and themselves from being helpless, hopeless, and out of their control to being resourceful and capable of exerting at least some control over their plights. Changing the cognitive schema by cognitive and behavioral means is designed to result in different interpretations of information about themselves and their futures. Thus, changing behaviors and thoughts may be reciprocally related and mutually reinforcing. Neither attending exclusively to behavior, as in the behavioral model, nor only attending to patients' thinking, as in the cognitive model, is adequate to alleviate depression.[125] The cognitive-behavioral approach has become a central component for treating depression in many multidisciplinary pain rehabilitation and functional restoration programs.

All of the psychological therapies emphasize patients' active role in alleviating depression. In contrast to the psychodynamic model, in which the therapist plays a relatively passive role, in behavioral, cognitive, and CBTs, the therapist takes an active, directive role, attempting to guide patients into changing their behavior and reorganizing their thinking and actions. The behavioral, cognitive, and CBTs are all centered in the present, compared with psychodynamic therapy, which focuses on the past.

Anxiety Disorders

It is not unusual for patients with symptoms of pain to be anxious and worried. Up to 30% of chronic pain patients meet criteria for an anxiety disorder such as generalized anxiety disorder (GAD), panic disorder, agoraphobia, and PTSD.[158] There may be stronger data for anxiety disorders preceding the onset of chronic pain than mood disorders.[159] This is especially true when the symptoms are unexplained, as is often the case for chronic pain syndromes. For example, in a large-scale, multicenter study of fibromyalgia patients, between 44% and 51% of patients indicated that they were anxious.[160] In other clinic samples, rates of an anxiety disorder ranged from 16% to 29% among pain patients.[161,162] Most researchers agree that the prevalence of anxiety disorders in patients with chronic pain is underestimated by these data.[1,55]

Anxiety and concern about symptoms are not synonymous with a psychiatric diagnosis of an anxiety disorder, necessarily. When anxiety is debilitating, it may meet criteria for an anxiety disorder. Anxiety disorders are a broad spectrum of disorders which include GAD, PTSD, obsessive-compulsive disorder, and panic disorder. As noted earlier in this chapter, pain anxiety is the most prevalent and salient form of anxiety in pain patients.[163] Although distinct in some respects, there is significant overlap of pain anxiety symptoms with the constructs of fear of pain, fear of movement, and pain catastrophizing.[164] High levels of pain anxiety (which are impairing, maladaptive, and predictive of higher pain levels[165]) also meet *DSM-5* criteria for anxiety due to a general medical condition.[15] Although this diagnosis was intended originally for anxiety secondary to chronic hypoxemia or steroid use, for example, chronic pain is a medical condition primarily and falls within the scope of this diagnostic category. Fears, worries, and preoccupations about pain are all secondary to having pain, and if the pain resolves, so do these psychological symptoms.

Anxiety disorders frequently accompany other affective disorders, such as major depression, so clinicians should remain alert to the possibility of a mood disorder when patients complain of severe anxiety.[1] In general, the approach is to diagnose and treat initially the most prominent mood disorder in a patient, whether it be depression or anxiety. For instance, in a patient with significant depression and anxiety symptoms, if the depression symptoms seem to be greater or more debilitating than the anxiety symptoms, the diagnosis is major depression with anxious features. In these situations, addressing the depression will also improve the anxiety symptoms. In a major depression with significant overlying anxiety, clinicians will often choose an antidepressant with significant antianxiety properties, such as the SNRIs or SSRIs.

GENERALIZED ANXIETY DISORDER

Table 31.3 outlines the criteria for GAD. GAD is characterized by excessive anxiety and worry (apprehensive expectation) and difficulty controlling the worry for at least 6 months, accompanied by at least three of the following symptoms: restlessness or feeling keyed up, being easily fatigued, difficulty concentrating, irritability, muscle tension, or sleep disturbance.[1] There is significant debate whether a 6-month duration of symptoms is necessary to make the diagnosis, and many psychiatrists contend that this is unnecessarily lengthy.[85] Often, there are significant associated depression symptoms, but they do not rise to the level of a major depressive disorder. It is very common for patients with GAD to also have panic attack symptoms or posttraumatic stress symptoms. There are trait and state (situational) components to anxiety disorder presentations in patients with pain. The trait components include excessive worry and concern, often about routine matters. The amount of worry and anxiety is out of proportion to the likelihood of the negative consequences occurring, and the patient has great difficulty controlling worry. In making a diagnosis of GAD, trait anxiety in this context does not imply that the symptoms or the tendency toward these symptoms have been present since the beginning of adulthood.

The situational (state) anxiety is often centered on the pain itself and its negative consequences (pain anxiety). Patients may have conditioned fear, believing that activities will cause uncontrollable pain, causing avoidance of those activities. Pain may also activate thoughts that a person is seriously ill.[41] Questions such as the following can be helpful: "Does the pain make you panic? If you think about your pain, do you feel your heart beating fast? Do you have an overwhelming feeling of dread or doom? Do you experience a sense of sudden anxiety that overwhelms you when you feel more pain?"

The best quality of treatment for GAD is CBT plus medications. The CBT is pain based as in major depression treatment. Psychotherapy alone is highly effective for anxiety disorders.[166] Successful CBT in patients with obsessive-compulsive disorder has been shown on neuroimaging studies to correlate to changes in the functioning of frontal lobe limbic areas.[167] As discussed, the most frequently chosen medication classes are the SNRIs or SSRIs. Unlike depression treatment and despite their lack of analgesic properties, in anxiety disorders, the SSRIs are considered first line because of their efficacy over most other antidepressant classes. The TCAs can be effective, but higher doses are often needed which are difficult for patients to tolerate. Benzodiazepines should almost always be avoided, especially in patients on opioid therapy. Breakthrough anxiety can be addressed with buspirone, hydroxyzine, or low-dose antipsychotics (which is beyond the scope of this discussion).

PANIC DISORDER

Panic disorder is a common, disabling psychiatric illness associated with high medical service use and multiple medically unexplained symptoms. The diagnosis of panic disorder requires recurrent, unexpected panic attacks (Table 31.4) followed by at least 1 month of worry about having another panic attack, the implications or consequences of the panic attacks, or behavioral changes related to the attacks. These attacks should not be the direct physiologic consequence of a substance or other medical condition. The panic attacks should not be better accounted for by another mental disorder, such as PTSD (see following discussion) or obsessive-compulsive disorder. At least two unexpected attacks are required for the diagnosis, although most patients have many more.

TABLE 31.3 _Diagnostic and Statistical Manual of Mental Disorders_, Fifth Edition, Criteria for Generalized Anxiety Disorder

A. Excessive anxiety and worry (apprehensive expectation), occurring more days than not for at least 6 mo, about a number of events or activities (such as work or school performance)

B. The person finds it difficult to control the worry.

C. The anxiety and worry are associated with three (or more) of the following six symptoms (with at least some symptoms present for more days than not for the past 6 mo). Note: Only one item is required in children.
1. Restlessness or feeling keyed up or on edge
2. Being easily fatigued
3. Difficulty concentrating or mind going blank
4. Irritability
5. Muscle tension
6. Sleep disturbance (difficulty falling or staying asleep, or restless unsatisfying sleep)

D. The anxiety, worry, or physical symptoms cause significant distress or impairment in social, occupational, or other important areas of functioning.

E. The disturbance is not attributable to the physiologic effects of a substance (e.g., a drug of abuse, a medication) or another medical condition (e.g., hyperthyroidism).

F. The disturbance is not better explained by another mental disorder (e.g., anxiety or worry about having panic attacks in panic disorder, negative evaluation in social anxiety disorder [social phobia], contamination or other obsessions in obsessive-compulsive disorder, reminders of traumatic events in posttraumatic stress disorder, gaining weight in anorexia nervosa, physical complaints in somatic symptom disorder, perceived appearance in flaws in body dysmorphic disorder, having a serious illness in illness anxiety disorder, or the content of delusional beliefs in schizophrenia or delusional disorder).

TABLE 31.4 _Diagnostic and Statistical Manual of Mental Disorders_, Fifth Edition, Criteria for Panic Attack Specifier

An abrupt surge of intense fear or intense discomfort that reaches a peak within minutes and during which time four (or more) of the following symptoms occur.

Note: The abrupt surge can occur from a calm state or an anxious state.
1. Palpitations, pounding heart, or accelerated heart rate
2. Sweating
3. Trembling or shaking
4. Sensations of shortness of breath or smothering
5. Feeling of choking
6. Chest pain or discomfort
7. Nausea or abdominal distress
8. Feeling dizzy, unsteady, lightheaded, or faint
9. Chills or heat sensations
10. Paresthesias (numbness or tingling sensations)
11. Derealization (feelings of unreality) or depersonalization (being detached from oneself)
12. Fear of losing control or "going crazy"
13. Fear of dying

One of the most common problems with panic disorder is the fear of an undiagnosed, life-threatening illness. Patients with panic disorder can receive extensive medical testing and treatment for their somatic symptoms before the diagnosis of panic disorder is made and appropriate treatment initiated.

EPIDEMIOLOGY

Lifetime prevalence of panic disorder throughout the world is estimated to be 1.5% to 3.5%. One-year prevalence rates are from 1% to 2%. Panic disorder is 2 to 3 times more common in women than in men. Age of onset is variable, but most patients typically start between late adolescence and the mid-30s. Of all common mental disorders in the primary care setting, panic disorder is most likely to produce moderate to severe occupational dysfunction and physical disability.[168] It was also associated with the greatest number of disability days in the past month. In some studies in pain patients, it has a prevalence of 5% to 8%, significantly higher than the general population.[1,169]

The most common complication of panic disorder is agoraphobia, or fear of public places. Patients with panic disorder learn to fear places where escape might be difficult or help not available in case they have an attack. One-half to two-thirds of patients with panic disorder also suffer from major depression. These patients are the most disabled panic disorder patients. The differential diagnosis of patients presenting with panic symptoms in the medical setting includes thyroid, parathyroid, adrenal, and vestibular dysfunction; seizure disorders; cardiac arrhythmias; and drug intoxication or withdrawal. Patients with panic disorder typically present in the medical setting with cardiologic, gastrointestinal, or neurologic complaints. These include chest pain, abdominal pain, and headaches.[170]

Chest pain is one of the most common complaints presented to primary care physicians, but a specific medical etiology is identified in only 10% to 20% of cases. From 43% to 61% of patients who have normal coronary arteries at angiography and 16% to 25% of patients presenting to emergency rooms with chest pain have panic disorder. A number of these patients eventually receive the diagnoses of vasospastic angina, costochondritis, esophageal dysmotility, or mitral valve prolapse. High rates of psychiatric disorders have been found in some of these groups as well.[171] Many of these patients remain symptomatic and disabled 1 year later despite reassurance concerning coronary artery disease.[172]

Patients with documented coronary disease also have elevated rates of panic disorder. A number of studies have found nearly identical rates of panic disorder in chest pain patients with and without coronary disease. Increased mortality has been noted in those with anxiety and coronary disease. These data point to the importance of remaining alert to both medical and psychiatric diagnoses in those presenting with chest pain. Patients with unexplained chest pain who were given low-dose imipramine (50 mg per day) reported significant reductions in pain regardless of whether they had increased anxiety symptoms or another psychiatric disorder. This has been postulated to be caused by a *visceral analgesic effect* of imipramine.[173] It is possible, however, that imipramine was treating subthreshold anxiety and depressive symptoms, because 63% of the sample had a history of these disorders at some point in their lives.

Approximately 11% of primary care patients present the problem of abdominal pain to their physician each year. Less than one-quarter of these complaints are associated with a definite physical diagnosis in the following year. Among the most common reasons for abdominal pain is irritable bowel syndrome. It is estimated that irritable bowel syndrome accounts for 20% to 52% of all referrals to gastroenterologists. Various studies have found that 54% to 74% of these patients with irritable bowel syndrome have associated psychiatric disorders. Walker and colleagues[174] determined that patients with irritable bowel syndrome have much higher current (28% vs. 3%) and

lifetime (41% vs. 25%) rates of panic disorder than a comparison group with inflammatory bowel disease. This suggests that the psychiatric disorder was not simply a reaction to the abdominal distress.

Among 10,000 persons assessed in a community survey who consulted their physicians for headache, 15% of female and 13% of male subjects had a history of panic disorder. Further studies have suggested that migraine headache is most strongly associated with panic attacks.[175] Often, anxiety symptoms precede the onset of the headaches, whereas depressive symptoms often have their onset after the headaches. Some authors have suggested that a common predisposition exists with headaches (especially migraines and chronic daily headache), anxiety disorders, and major depression.

TREATMENT

Psychopharmacologic and psychotherapeutic treatments for panic disorder have been proven effective. The American Psychiatric Association has released a "Practice Guideline for the Treatment of Patients with Panic Disorder."[176] Panic-focused CBT and four classes of medications (SSRIs, TCAs, MAOIs, and benzodiazepines) have demonstrated effectiveness. These drugs may be used in combination with CBT. Panic-specific CBT includes psychoeducation, continuous panic monitoring, development of anxiety management skills, cognitive restructuring, and in vivo exposure. As discussed previously with depression, the SSRIs likely are the easiest antidepressants to use for panic disorder. However, starting doses should be halved to avoid any initial exacerbation of agitation or anxiety. TCAs and MAOIs are now reserved for those patients who do not respond to the SSRIs. Benzodiazepines should be avoided. It is possible to use them for early symptom control in conjunction with one of the other classes of effective medication, but subsequent tapering can be difficult.

Posttraumatic Stress Disorder

DIAGNOSIS

At the time of initial physical trauma, patients who develop chronic pain may also experience overwhelming psychological trauma. George Crile, a surgeon and experimental physiologist, laid the foundation for our modern concept of psychological trauma. He suggested that fear is the memory of pain. This fear holds an adaptive advantage in directing individuals to anticipate and avoid injury. Freud added anxiety to our modern conceptualization. Anxiety is the capacity to imagine pain and not merely to remember it. In other words, anxiety is memory of pain set loose.[177]

After direct personal exposure to an extreme traumatic event, some individuals develop a syndrome that includes re-experiencing the event, avoidance of stimuli associated with the event, and persistent heightened arousal. PTSD was originally described after exposure to military combat but is now recognized to occur after sexual or physical assault, natural disasters, accidents, life-threatening illnesses, and other events that induce feelings of intense fear, hopelessness, or horror. Persons may develop the disorder after experiencing or just witnessing these events. *DSM-5* diagnostic criteria are shown in Table 31.5.

EPIDEMIOLOGY OF POSTTRAUMATIC STRESS DISORDER IN CHRONIC PAIN PATIENTS

Approximately 13% of all veterans returning from service in Iraq and Afghanistan receive diagnoses of PTSD. These constitute about half of all mental health diagnoses received.[178] Up to 80% of Vietnam veterans with PTSD report chronic pain in limbs, back, torso, or head.[179] Increased physical symptoms, including muscle aches and back pain, are also more common in Gulf War veterans with PTSD than in those without PTSD.[180] The prevalence of PTSD in medical populations has been shown

TABLE 31.5 *Diagnostic and Statistical Manual of Mental Disorders*, **Fifth Edition, Diagnostic Criteria for Posttraumatic Stress Disorder**

Note: The following criteria apply to adults, adolescents, and children older than 6 y.

A. Exposure to actual or threatened death, serious injury, or sexual violence in one (or more) of the following ways:
   1. Daily experiencing the traumatic event(s)
   2. Witnessing, in person, the event(s) as it occurred to others
   3. Learning the traumatic event(s) occurred to a close family member or close friend. In cases of actual or threatened death of a family member or friend, the event(s) must have been violent or accidental.
   4. Experiencing repeated or extreme exposure to aversive details of the traumatic event(s) (e.g., first responders collecting human remain, police officers repeatedly exposed to details of child abuse)
   Note: Criterion A4 does not apply to exposure through electronic media, television, movies, or pictures, unless this exposure is work related.

B. Presence of one (or more) of the following intrusive symptoms associated with the traumatic event(s), beginning after the traumatic event(s) occurred:
   1. Recurrent, involuntary, and intrusive memories of the traumatic event(s)
      Note: In children older than 6 y, repetitive play may occur in which themes or aspects of the traumatic event(s) are expressed.
   2. Recurrent distressing dreams in which the content and/or affect of the dream are related to the traumatic event(s)
      Note: In children, there may be frightening dreams without recognizable content.
   3. Dissociative reactions (e.g., flashbacks) in which the individual feels or acts as if the traumatic event(s) were recurring (Such reactions may occur on a continuum, with the most extreme expression being a complete loss of awareness of present surroundings.)
      Note: In children, trauma-specific reenactment may occur in play.
   4. Intense or prolonged psychological distress at exposure to internal or external cues that symbolize or resemble an aspect of the traumatic event(s)
   5. Marked physiologic reactions to internal or external cues that symbolize or resemble an aspect of the traumatic event(s)

C. Persistent avoidance of stimuli associated with the traumatic event(s), beginning after the event(s) occurred, as evidenced by one or both of the following:
   1. Avoidance of or efforts to avoid distressing memories, thoughts, or feelings about or closely associated with the traumatic event(s)
   2. Avoidance of or efforts to avoid external reminders (people, places, conversations, activities, objects, situations) that arouse distressing memories, thoughts, or feelings about or closely associated with the traumatic event(s)

D. Negative alterations in cognitions and mood associated with the traumatic event(s), beginning or worsening after the traumatic event(s) occurred, as evidenced by two (or more) of the following:
   1. Inability to remember an important aspect of the traumatic event(s) (typically due to dissociative amnesia and not to other factors such as head injury, alcohol, or drugs)
   2. Persistent and exaggerated negative beliefs or expectations about oneself, others, or the world (e.g., "I am bad," "no one can be trusted," "the world is completely dangerous," "my whole nervous system is permanently ruined")
   3. Persistent, distorted, cognitions about the cause or consequences of the traumatic event(s) that lead the individual to blame himself/herself or others
   4. Persistent negative emotional state (e.g., fear, horror, anger, guilt, shame)
   5. Markedly diminished interest or participation in significant activities
   6. Feelings of detachment or estrangement from others
   7. Persistent inability to experience positive emotions (e.g., inability to experience happiness, satisfaction, or loving feelings)

E. Marked alterations in arousal and reactivity associated with the traumatic event(s), beginning or worsening after the traumatic event(s) occurred, as evidenced by two (or more) of the following:
   1. Irritable behavior and angry outbursts (with little or no provocation) typically expressed as verbal or physical aggression toward people or objects
   2. Reckless or self-destructive behavior
   3. Hypervigilance
   4. Exaggerated startle response
   5. Problems with concentration
   6. Sleep disturbance (e.g., difficulty falling or staying asleep or restless sleep)

F. Duration of the disturbance (criteria A, B, C, D, and E) is more than 1 month.

G. The disturbance causes clinically significant distress or impairment in social, occupational, or other important areas of functioning.

H. The disturbance is not attributable to the physiologic effects of a substance (e.g., medication, alcohol) or another medical condition.

to be quite high. For example, a number of patients presenting at medical clinics with myocardial infarctions[181] and cancer[182,183] often meet the criteria for PTSD. Averaging the prevalence rates of PTSD across a number of studies reveals that after motor vehicle accidents sufficient to require medical attention, 29.5% of patients meet the criteria for PTSD.[184] For more than one-half of these patients, the symptoms resolve within 6 months. In one study, 15% of idiopathic facial pain patients seeking treatment were found to have PTSD.[185] In another study, 21% of fibromyalgia patients were found to have PTSD.[186] Case reports have associated reflex sympathetic dystrophy (complex regional pain syndrome) with PTSD. Other studies suggest that 50% to 100% of patients presenting at pain treatment centers meet the diagnostic criteria for PTSD.[186,187] Among adult urban primary care patients, 23% had PTSD, of whom 11%

had it noted in the medical record. The prevalence of PTSD, adjusted for demographic factors, was higher in participants with chronic pain, major depression, and anxiety disorders.[188]

Pain patients with PTSD have been shown to have more pain and affective distress than those without PTSD,[189] so it is not surprising that PTSD rates among pain patients increase as treatment settings become more specialized.

POSTTRAUMATIC STRESS DISORDER AND ASSOCIATIONS WITH PAIN

The relationship between pain and PTSD is multifaceted, as suggested by the early thinking by Crile and Freud discussed previously. Pain and PTSD may result from a traumatic event. Sometimes, acute pain can constitute the traumatic event, as described in a case of traumatic eye enucleation.[190] In a nationwide survey of patients admitted after trauma, 23% of injury survivors had symptoms consistent with a diagnosis of PTSD 12 months after their hospitalization.[191] PTSD symptoms have been significantly associated with greater levels of pain, emotional distress, interference, and disability.[192] Greater levels of early postinjury emotional distress and physical pain were associated with an increased risk of symptoms consistent with a PTSD diagnosis. Pain may also be a consequence of PTSD or a manifestation of it. In a sample of patients admitted to an orthopedic hospital, back pain after major trauma was not associated with measures of injury severity or demographic factors but was significantly associated with the presence of PTSD, the use of a lawyer, the presence of chronic illnesses, and lower education levels.[193] Compared with accident-related factors, PTSD symptoms and other psychological factors were the strongest predictors of the development of chronic pain in people who had severe accidents 3 years earlier.[194] Functional brain imaging studies suggest altered processing of noxious signaling in the brain of patients with PTSD. In one study, patients with PTSD revealed increased activation in the left hippocampus and decreased activation in the bilateral ventrolateral prefrontal cortex and the right amygdala.[195] Much research remains to be done on the relative contributions of physical trauma and psychological trauma to chronic pain problems.

TREATMENT

It is best to institute treatment for PTSD as close in time to the trauma as possible. Acute crisis intervention may reduce the development of chronic PTSD and other complications, including, possibly, chronic pain. This treatment should establish support, promote acceptance of what happened, provide education and information about symptoms, and attend to general health needs. Beyond the acute phase, the CBT treatment described for panic disorder earlier has been shown to be effective with PTSD as well. The most evidence-based therapies for PTSD are prolonged exposure (PE) and cognitive processing therapy (CPT).[196] Stress-inoculation training, implosive therapy, and systematic desensitization have also been reported to have some efficacy[185,197] as have complementary and alternative techniques such as recreational therapy, yoga, acupuncture, and alternative delivery methods of psychotherapy.[198]

Medications are rarely adequate as the sole treatment for PTSD. Controlled trials of TCAs, SSRIs, and MAOIs have demonstrated some benefit by 8 weeks at reducing core intrusive features. These benefits appear to be in addition to the antidepressant and antianxiety effects of these medications.[199] Recent PTSD treatment trials have demonstrated effectiveness of venlafaxine ER[200] and prazosin,[201] but these trials have not specifically monitored the effects on pain. Propranolol has been shown to attenuate traumatic memory in primary and tertiary use.[202]

Personality Disorders

EPIDEMIOLOGY

Several studies have reviewed the personality characteristics and disorders of patients with chronic pain.[161,162,203–205] The prevalence of personality disorders among clinic populations ranges from 31% to 81% and is greater than in the general population or in populations with either medical or psychiatric illnesses. The Minnesota Multiphasic Personality Inventory (MMPI) is the most widely used personality assessment tool of patients with chronic pain but is probably not purely a personality trait measure.[206–208] Previous studies have identified profiles defined by MMPI scale elevations that are proposed to be characteristic of chronic somatic symptoms such as pain.[209] The hypochondriacal reaction, conversion "V," and neurotic triad profiles exhibit different multivariate relationships between other constructs such as somatization, coping strategies, depression, pain severity, and activity level.[210] However, although patients with chronic pain differ from nonchronic pain controls in their scale profiles on the MMPI, there is no single personality trait or disorder associated with medically unexplained chronic pain or chronic pain from "organic" diseases.

OVERVIEW OF PERSONALITY DISORDERS

Personality pathology is best thought of along a continuum of traits present to greater or lesser degrees. Personality disorders described in the *DSM* represent the pathologic extreme of personality traits. Patients with personality disorders are one type of "difficult patient" characterized by an inflexible, pervasive, and maladaptive inner experience and set of behaviors.[15,135] Traits have been conceptualized as dimensional aspects of individual variation, whereas personality disorders are represented as categorical aberrations within the realm of psychopathology. This section presents an overview of personality pathology and not a discussion of the criteria for each specific personality disorder.

Analytic approaches undertaken to understand the features of temperament have described several core factors. The five-factor model is one of the most popular and characterized by the trait dimensions of neuroticism, extraversion, openness, agreeableness, and conscientiousness as described by the revised NEO Personality Inventory.[211–213] In contrast, the Temperament and Character Inventory (TCI) is composed of four heritable and stable dimensions of temperament (harm avoidance [HA], novelty seeking, reward dependence, persistence) that represent individual differences in associative learning and three dimensions of character (self-directedness [SD], cooperativeness [C], self-transcendence) that develop over time as a function of social learning and maturation of interpersonal behavior.[214] This psychobiologic model defines personality as the interaction of temperament and character. Studies have described three dimensions (HA, SD, C) as a core feature of all personality disorders.[215] However, this profile has also been associated with other constructs such as depressive and anxiety disorders.[216,217]

Only a portion of the variance in the factors or dimensions characterizing personality disorders is explained by core personality traits.[218] Personality traits are generally considered to be enduring features of an individual. The stability of personality after age 30 years has been consistently documented with long-term follow-up studies.[219] Longitudinal studies also demonstrate that dimensional models of personality disorders may represent a manifestation of personality traits interacting with life events or illness consistent with the diathesis-stress model.[220,221] Caution should be exercised in making the diagnosis of a personality disorder in the presence of any illness. Personality traits should be appreciated as sustaining or modifying factors that have the potential to complicate the treatment process rather than as causes of or the sole explanation for illnesses such as chronic pain.[203] Personality vulnerabilities contribute to the degree of potential disability that individuals experience by modifying their response to pain. Although these patients are more likely to be "difficult" because of their complexity, their prognosis should not be viewed as hopeless or unresponsive to treatment.

The diathesis-stress model may partly explain the high rates of personality pathology but also the decreases in these rates that have been observed with chronic pain treatment.[204,205] A comprehensive review of the effect of pain on the measurement of personality characteristics found substantial evidence that trait inventories are not pain state independent.[222] Pain treatment resulted in improvement in trait scores across the majority of studies that utilized the MMPI and measures of trait anxiety, coping/self-efficacy, and somatization/illness behavior. In a significant number of the studies reviewed, the trait changes could be attributed to improvements in pain. This state–trait interaction contradicts the notion that personality inventories catalog only enduring aspects of the individual. Instead, there is increasing evidence that a state disorder (psychiatric, medical, stress-related pain) may distort the measurement of traits and that treatment of that condition will decrease the presumed trait disorder.[223–226] Just as personality pathology may improve with adequate pain treatment, personality disorders may emerge in the context of chronic pain, even if prior to pain, there was no evidence of maladaptive personality traits. The explanation for this change may include several mechanisms or confounders including that trait measurements are being contaminated by state-specific questions; pain treatments (medications, CBT) directly alter traits; and pain treatments improve state disorders which were previously affecting trait measurement, test–retest-related problems; and that standardized tests are actually measuring both states and traits.

PERSONALITY AND PAIN TREATMENT OUTCOME

Current research has focused on how personality relates to treatment outcome, the transition from acute to chronic pain, and the persistence of pain-related disability. However, results have been inconsistent and more likely to detect emotional distress and psychopathology. Recently, a disability profile based on elevations of four or more clinical scales of the MMPI-II has been proposed as more common than those described earlier.[1] In a prospective investigation of almost 1,500 patients with chronic occupational spinal disorders, this disability profile was associated with 5 times the likelihood of having a personality disorder and 14 times the likelihood of having an Axis I disorder. Although associated with high levels of psychopathology, patients with the disability profile compared to those with neurotic triad, conversion V, and normal profiles showed no significant differences in response to treatment with an interdisciplinary rehabilitation program. In a 30-year longitudinal study of healthy college students, elevations on MMPI scales 1 and 3 were associated with increased reports of chronic pain conditions at midlife.[227] However, the magnitude of this association was small, and the clinical significance was unclear.

In a similar study, patients with chronic pain due to nonspecific musculoskeletal disorders exhibited higher levels of HA and lower levels of SD on the TCI.[228] This trait profile would characterize patients as cautious, insecure, pessimistic, lacking self-esteem and long-term goals, failing to accept responsibility, and struggling with their identity. Another study of patients with chronic pain of all types identified the same profile plus low levels of C.[162] Low levels of SD have been associated with learned helplessness, poor self-efficacy, and an external locus of control. High levels of HA overlap with the construct of fear-avoidance behavior, fearful cluster C personality disorders, and the development of pain-related disability. The fear-avoidance model and expectancy model of fear provide explanations for the initiation and maintenance of chronic pain disability, proposing that anxiety sensitivity amplifies reactions such as avoidance of specific activities.[229–232] Anxiety sensitivity is a significant predictor of fear of and anxiety about pain.[233] Fear of pain, movement, reinjury, and other negative consequences that result in the avoidance of activities promote the transition to and sustaining of chronic pain and its associated disabilities such as muscular reactivity, deconditioning, and guarded movement.[234]

Fear-avoidance beliefs have been found to be one of the most significant predictors of failure to return to work in patients with chronic low back pain.[235] Operant conditioning reinforces disability if the avoidance provides any short-term benefits such as reducing anticipatory anxiety or relieving the patient of unwanted responsibilities. In a study of patients with chronic low back pain, improvements in disability following physical therapy were associated with decreases in pain, psychological distress, and fear-avoidance beliefs but not specific physical deficits.[236,237] Decreasing work-specific fears was a more important outcome than addressing general fears of physical activity in predicting improved physical capability for work among patients participating in an interdisciplinary treatment program.[238] These studies suggest that certain personality traits or profiles should alert the clinician to the presence of psychological problems and psychiatric disorders that would benefit from more specific treatments as opposed to defining a group of patients with chronic pain who should be condemned to no treatment because of an expected poor outcome.

Somatic Symptom Disorders, Illness Behavior, and Sick Role

DEFINITIONS

Sickness is a complicated psychological and social state that has been understood from a variety of perspectives over the years. We consider those of sick role, illness behavior, and somatic symptom disorder (SSD).

The concept of the *sick role* was first introduced by Talcott Parsons[239] in 1951 and was formulated more concretely 12 years later.[240] The sick role is granted to an individual provided that he or she regards his or her condition as undesirable and is not held responsible for it (i.e., under his or her control and able to be reversed voluntarily). If granted, the individual is allowed exemption from his or her usual obligations to a greater or lesser extent and is considered to be deserving of care and attention. Associated with the sick role are the obligations of seeking the advice and assistance of a person regarded as competent to diagnose and treat the condition and of cooperating with that person.

The basic concept of *illness behavior* was introduced by Mechanic and Volkart[241] and later fully formulated by Mechanic.[242] Mechanic's[242] concept of illness behavior complements the sick role because it delineates the contribution of the patient to the role-granting process. Illness behavior was originally defined as the ways in which individuals differentially perceive, evaluate, and respond to their symptoms. This concept proved to be an extremely useful one because it has facilitated the empiric study of behaviors that are of considerable importance to clinicians and other health care providers as well as to the individual's family and society.

Although useful as it stands, health care providers find Mechanic's[242] definition restrictive because it refers to *symptoms* as the focus of behavior and consequently deemphasizes actions directed toward avoidance of the illness. A slightly modified definition describes illness behavior as "the ways in which individuals experience, perceive, evaluate, and respond to their own health status." This definition recognizes the possibility that a person may be concerned about illness in the absence of symptoms.

Illness behavior is a concept more easily applied to individual patients than sick role and has therefore seen more use in clinical settings. However, it is dependent on social definitions of what constitutes legitimate illness. Although medical science determines what qualifies as *disease* based on objective changes in anatomy and physiology, society determines what qualifies as illness. These often follow each other quite closely, but there can be interesting discrepancies. Essential hypertension is a disease usually without symptoms. It has taken a concerted educational effort on the part of the medical profession to convince the public that it is an illness that should be monitored and treated. Chronic fatigue syndrome and fibromyalgia are illnesses increasingly recognized and accepted by the public. Because the medical profession has not been able to identify objective changes in physiology with these illnesses, many physicians question whether they qualify as legitimate diseases. Physicians, insurance companies, and compensation systems can find themselves in disagreement with patients experiencing chronic pain about whether a legitimate disease or illness is causing the pain.

Pilowsky[243] introduced the concept of *abnormal illness behavior* for those situations in which physician and patient disagree about the applicability of the sick role to the patient's condition. He contends that patients with truly abnormal illness behavior have extreme difficulty accepting the advice of any physician if it does not agree with their own appraisal of their health status. He cautions that misdiagnoses of abnormal illness behavior can occur when physician and patient do no share a common culture. We might add that it is also important to keep in mind the limitations of current diagnostic tests and disease criteria when diagnosing the patient's disagreement with his or her physician as pathologic.

OVERVIEW OF SOMATOFORM DISORDERS AND SOMATIC SYMPTOM DISORDERS

Current psychiatric thinking frames the diagnoses of abnormal illness behavior or misuse of the sick role as SSDs. The categorization of these disorders has been significantly modified in the *DSM-5*. In the *DSM-5*, SSD appears in a new section, somatic symptoms, and related disorders. This section replaces the somatoform disorders of the *DSM-IV*. SSD is a single diagnostic entity that replaces three of the *DSM-IV* somatoform disorders: somatization disorder, pain disorder, and undifferentiated somatoform disorder. The *DSM-5* criteria for SSD are listed in Table 31.6. Currently, there is scant available research about SSD as it was fairly recently adopted.

The essential feature of the somatoform disorders is the presence of physical symptoms that suggest a general medical condition but are not fully explained by a general medical condition. The *DSM-5* diagnosis of SSD eliminated the requirement that somatic symptoms be medically unexplained. In either case, these symptoms must cause impairment in social and occupational functioning. These disorders are distinguished from factitious disorders and malingering in that the symptoms are not intentionally or voluntarily produced in the somatoform disorders or SSD. Malingering is the deliberate feigning of symptoms for a clear gain, often financial. In factitious disorder, although there is a feigning of symptoms, the patient is only partially aware that they are doing so, and their gain or benefit is much less clear. In factitious disorder, the maintenance of symptoms is for the psychological benefits of the sick role, similar to the gain in somatoform disorders.

In the majority of patients with pain and somatoform illness, there is a physical basis (including functional or structural pathology, such as neuropathic pain) for at least a portion of the pain complaints, in which symptom reporting is magnified by somatizing. Somatization is best thought of as a process (vs. somatization disorder, discussed in the following text). The spectrum of somatization includes amplification of symptoms, which entails "focusing on the symptoms, racking with intense alarm and worry, extreme disability, and a reluctance to relinquish them."[244] Pain-related psychological symptoms amplify pain perception and disability. Hence, there is a tremendous overlap between the somatoform component of a chronic pain syndrome and other psychiatric comorbidities. In other words, in a patient with pain and any psychiatric comorbidity, somatization is a ubiquitous, mediating process by which pain and disability are worsened. It has psychological and physiologic bases, which are still being elucidated. Similarly, pain complaints may become an "idiom of distress"[132] in which psychological distress or needs are communicated through the proxy of pain reporting.

In the *DSM-IV*, four somatoform disorders may involve pain: somatization disorder, conversion disorder, hypochondriasis, and pain disorder (with or without a physical basis for pain). In the *DSM-5*, three somatic symptoms and related disorders involve pain: SSD, illness anxiety disorder, and conversion disorder (functional neurologic symptom disorder). Somatoform disorders without any physical basis for pain are estimated to occur in 5% to 15% of patients with chronic pain who receive pain treatment.[245]

Somatic Symptom Disorder

The *DSM-IV* somatoform disorders were criticized for two main reasons: (1) the questionable importance of medically unexplained pain in pain disorder associated with psychological factors and (2) the lack of a definition of psychological factors or a description of when they are of sufficient importance to have a role in the experience of pain in the presence of a general medical condition, which made it a diagnosis of exclusion.[246] If a medical cause for pain is discovered, it means the SSD diagnosis is discarded regardless of the evidence previously considered supportive of it. However, somatic symptoms that are not attributable to a medical condition are a substantial problem in primary care and pain specialty practice. It is estimated that 20% of visits to medical doctors are for this type of complaint.[247] However, because somatoform disorders were restrictively defined, and many clinicians felt that giving patients a somatoform diagnosis could be interpreted as "everything is just in the mind," the diagnostic category was rarely used in the United States and Europe.[248]

The *DSM-5* Somatic Symptoms Disorders Work Group tried to address these issues when developing the criteria for the new diagnostic group. The new category was named Somatic Symptoms and Related Disorders with SSD as the prototype. The common feature of this category is that individuals have "somatic symptoms associated with significant distress and impairment." The major advance in the *DSM-5* is that it uses positive criterion, namely, maladaptive reaction to a somatic symptom, rather than the earlier negative criterion, namely, that the symptoms should be medically unexplained. The new diagnosis of SSD is designed to cover not only patients with somatization but also patients with chronic pain conditions, most patients with hypochondriasis, and many patients with medical conditions that

TABLE 31.6 *Diagnostic and Statistical Manual of Mental Disorders*, Fifth Edition, Diagnostic Criteria for Somatic Symptom Disorder

A. One or more somatic symptoms that are distressing or result in significant disruption of daily life

B. Excessive thoughts, feelings, or behaviors related to the somatic symptoms or associated health concerns as manifested by at least one of the following:
1. Disproportionate and persistent thoughts about the seriousness of one's symptoms
2. Persistently high level of anxiety about health or symptoms
3. Excessive time and energy devoted to these symptoms or health concerns

C. Although any one somatic symptom may not be continuously present, the state of being symptomatic is persistent (typically more than 6 mo).

Specify if:
With predominant pain (previously pain disorder): This specifier is for individuals whose somatic symptoms predominantly involve pain.

Specify if:
Persistent: A persistent course is characterized by severe symptoms, marked by impairment and long duration (more than 6 mo).

Specify current severity:
Mild: Only one of the symptoms specified in criterion B is fulfilled.
Moderate: Two or more of the symptoms specified in criterion B are fulfilled.
Severe: Two or more of the symptoms specified in criterion B are fulfilled, plus there are multiple somatic complaints (or one very severe symptom).

are accompanied by psychological features.[248] The diagnostic criteria for SSD includes one or more physical symptoms lasting 6 months or longer that are associated with excessive thoughts, feeling, or behaviors. There are three specifiers that describe the nature, duration, and severity of the symptoms.

Despite these advances in the *DSM-5*, criticisms have emerged. The main criticism is the high probability of misdiagnosing a medical illness, such as a chronic pain condition, as a mental illness.[249] The conditions that qualify for a diagnosis are highly variable and include patients with medically unexplained symptoms, medical patients with emotional stress, patients with typical chronic pain conditions, and patients with health-related anxiety.[248] This results in a classification with high sensitivity but low specificity. Several authors have proposed modified criteria that reduce the likelihood of diagnostic inflation and this misdiagnosis of a medical illness as a mental disorder and suggested that adjustment disorder may be a safer and more accurate diagnosis when one is needed for someone who is medically ill and troubled by symptoms.[246]

Conversion Disorder (Functional Neurologic Symptom Disorder)

The essential feature of conversion disorder is an alteration in voluntary motor or sensory function that suggests a neurologic or general medical disorder. Classic examples include hysterical paralysis, blindness, or mutism. Psychological factors must be associated with the initiation or exacerbation of this deficit. The name "conversion disorder" refers to a hypothesis based on a psychological etiology that has little supportive empirical evidence.[250] As such, the *DSM-5* has added the bracketed term, *functional neurologic symptom disorder*, to give a more proper and respectable definition to these symptoms. Diagnostic *DSM-5* criteria are displayed in Table 31.7. In the new criteria, there is less emphasis on psychological and emotional events prior to the development of symptoms and emphasis on the need for positive diagnostic signs and symptoms.[251] These changes may lead to a more collaborative approach between psychiatrists and neurologists and be more acceptable to patients.

Despite these changes, great caution must be exercised in making the diagnosis of conversion disorder because the presence of relevant psychological factors does not exclude the possibility of a concurrent organically caused condition.

In "Psychogenic Pain and the Pain-Prone Patient," George Engel[2] proposed that psychogenic pain arose from guilt and an intolerance of success. He indicated that it functioned as a substitute for loss or a replacement for aggression. He further stated that " . . . patients with conversion hysteria constitute the largest percentage of the pain-prone population." Others have also contended that pain is probably the most common conversion symptom encountered clinically.[252] However, only case reports exist to support this contention. Pain is not a classic conversion disorder symptom, and it is controversial whether chronic pain can ever qualify as a conversion disorder by itself. Some, for example, have contended that reflex sympathetic dystrophy (complex regional pain syndrome) can be understood as a conversion reaction; however, this is highly controversial.[253] Some elements of conversion disorders appear to be present in reflex sympathetic dystrophy/complex regional pain syndrome patients (e.g., indifference or neglect toward the affected body part), although it is highly unlikely that the condition is entirely psychogenic.

Rather than labeling some chronic pain problems as conversion reactions and others as not, it may be more useful to understand what components of conversion reaction may be present in chronic pain problems. Again, the emphasis should be on thinking about somatoform illnesses as a process. Being ill surely creates problems in living for those affected, but it can also solve problems in living. For example, being ill provides an excuse for not being at school or not meeting a deadline at work. These interpersonal advantages of illness were originally recognized by Freud and termed *secondary gain*.

The term *secondary gain* has been distorted and misunderstood in the care of chronic pain, probably because of medicolegal pressures. A number of corrections are in order. First, all illnesses are characterized by some secondary gain, not just illnesses considered to be psychogenic. Being sick always has advantages as well as disadvantages. Second, secondary gain includes all potential interpersonal benefits of illness, not just monetary advantages. Many of the advantages of illness are quite subtle and individualized. Third, secondary gain must be understood in the context of *primary gain*, the intrapersonal advantages of illness. For example, focusing on pain rather than depression may allow patients to avoid self-blame and thereby achieve primary gain. This is a common phenomenon in chronic pain. Indeed, blame avoidance has been hypothesized by some to be one of the main functions of somatization.[254] Thus, traditional elements of conversion disorder may be present in many chronic pain problems without many pain problems qualifying as conversion disorders per se.

Purely psychogenic or conversion models of chronic pain have some questionable implications for diagnosis and therapy of chronic pain disorders. Interview of the patient with a suspected conversion disorder with the aid of a sodium amobarbital (Amytal) infusion has been a standard tool in psychiatric diagnosis.[255] More recently, lorazepam interviews have been substituted. It is more common that motor and sensory deficits than pain resolve under sodium amobarbital (Amytal) or benzodiazepine sedation. Furthermore, some patients have had violent or suicidal reactions to abrupt resolution of their somatic symptoms under sodium amobarbital (Amytal), possibly caused by loss of face-saving primary gain aspects of the illness. Psychodynamic theories of the origin of conversion symptoms imply that psychological treatments alone will be effective.

Psychodynamic treatments for chronic pain, however, have little documented success. The most effective psychological treatments, such as CBT, include a reactivation component that addresses the profound disuse and deconditioning found in many patients with chronic pain.

ILLNESS ANXIETY DISORDER

Many patients with chronic pain resist their physician's reassurance that "nothing is wrong" or that the "tests reveal nothing." These patients know that they hurt and cannot accept that a bodily cause cannot be identified for their pain. This has been described as *disease conviction* in the chronic pain literature. Disease conviction has been measured with the Illness Behavior Questionnaire, and hypochondriasis is assessed with the MMPI. In *DSM-IV*, there also exists a disorder called *hypochondriasis*, which was changed to illness anxiety disorder

---

TABLE 31.7 *Diagnostic and Statistical Manual of Mental Disorders*, Fifth Edition, Diagnostic Criteria for Conversion Disorder (Functional Neurologic Symptom Disorder)

A. One or more symptoms of altered voluntary motor or sensory function

B. Clinical findings providing evidence of incompatibility between the symptom and recognized neurologic or medical conditions

C. The symptom or deficit is not better explained by another medical or mental disorder.

D. The symptom or deficit causes clinically significant distress or impairment in social, occupational, or other important areas of functioning or warrants medical evaluation.

in the *DSM-5*. The major change to the *DSM-5* criteria was the addition, in criterion B, that somatic symptoms should not be present, and if they are present, they are only mild in intensity. This will lead to some patients with previously diagnosed hypochondriasis now being diagnosed with SSD. Otherwise, hypochondriasis and illness anxiety disorder are essentially the same in concept, that is, a persistent fear in having a medical illness.

The prevalence of hypochondriasis in primary care has been reported to be 4% to 9%.[256] The prevalence of hypochondriasis in pain clinic populations is difficult to determine but is likely to be high if patients are not excluded by qualifying for pain disorder because of the likelihood of disagreement between patient and physician about the cause of the pain problem.

Treatments of hypochondriasis have attempted to shift patient focus from cure of the disease causing the symptoms to strategies of symptom management.[257] These strategies are common components of multidisciplinary pain treatment programs as well. It is indeed critical to achieve early in treatment some agreement with the patient about the cause of the pain that acknowledges the reality of the pain and yet points away from invasive attempts to cure disease or repair broken parts. The task is not to convince the patient that "nothing serious is wrong" because his or her pain may be severe and persistent. The task is to convince the patient that the appropriate treatment is different than the treatment he or she thought necessary.

Conclusion: Pain and Suffering and Psychiatry

Psychiatric diagnosis and treatment can add an essential and often neglected component to the conceptualization and treatment of chronic pain problems. The high rates of psychiatric comorbidity and the negative impact they have on chronic pain necessitate that a psychiatric assessment be part of any comprehensive pain evaluation. The expanse of psychiatric symptoms in patients with pain is broad and deep, and thus, a comprehensive framework for describing psychiatric symptoms and the relationships between them is essential to thorough diagnosis and treatment. Advances in neuroimaging have elucidated some of the interrelationships between pain perception and psychological states, underscoring that most painful conditions have an affective component to the pain experience.

It is this disordered affective experience of pain and, consequently, suffering that form a key interaction between pain and overlying psychiatric disorders. It is absolutely critical to avoid a dualistic model that postulates that pain is either physical or mental in origin. This model alienates patients who feel blamed for their pain. It is also inconsistent with modern models of pain causation. Since the gate control theory of pain, multiple lines of evidence suggest that pain is a product of efferent as well as afferent activity in the nervous system. Tissue damage and nociception are neither necessary nor sufficient for pain. Indeed, it is now widely recognized that the relationship between pain and nociception is highly complex and must be understood in terms of the situation of the organism as a whole.

We are only beginning to understand the complexities of the relationship between pain and suffering. Pain usually, but not always, produces suffering. Suffering can, through somatization, produce pain. We have traditionally understood this suffering, as we have understood nociception, as arising from a form of pathology intrinsic to the sufferer. Hence, the traditional view that pain is caused by either tissue pathology (nociception) or psychological states (suffering). Psychiatric comorbidity represents an additional layer of suffering, which also magnifies the perception on pain. Yet this is still somewhat dualistic; an alternative model is to think of pain as a *transdermal process* with causes outside as well as inside the body. For humans, social pathology can be as painful as tissue pathology. We can investigate the physiology and the psychology of this *sociogenic* pain without losing sight of its origins in relations *between* people.

Psychiatric care for patients with chronic pain should occur within the medical treatment setting whenever possible. This is the most effective way to reassure patients that the somatic elements of their problems are not neglected. It also allows integration of somatic and psychological treatments in the most effective manner.[1] The success of multidisciplinary approaches to pain underscores the value of psychiatric assessment and treatment by the pain medicine provider.

References

1. Dersh J, Gatchel DJ, Mayer T, et al. Prevalence of psychiatric disorders in patients with chronic disabling occupational spinal disorders. *Spine (Phila PA 1976)* 2006;31(10):1156–1162.
2. Engel GL. Psychogenic pain and the pain-prone patient. *Am J Med* 1959;26:899–918.
3. Dersh J, Polatin PB, Gatchel RJ. Chronic pain and psychopathology: research findings and theoretical considerations. *Psychosom Med* 2002;64:773–786.
4. Sternbach R. Psychological aspects of chronic pain. *Clin Orthop Relat Res* 1977;129:150–155.
5. Good MJ. *Pain as Human Experience: An Anthropological Perspective.* Berkeley: University of California Press; 1992.
6. Fishbain D, Cutler R, Rosomoff HL. Chronic pain associated depression: antecedent or consequence of chronic pain? A review. *Clin J Pain* 1997;13(2):116–137.
7. Wasan AD, Fernandez E, Jamison RN, et al. Association between anxiety and depression with reported disease severity in chronic rhinosinusitis. *Ann Otol Rhinol Laryngol* 2007;116(7):491–497.
8. Kinney RK, Gatchel RJ, Polatin PB, et al. Prevalence of psychopathology in acute and chronic low back pain patients. *J Occup Rehabil* 1993;3:95–103.
9. Epstein S, Kay G, Clauw D, et al. Psychiatric disorders in patients with fibromyalgia. A multicenter investigation. *Psychosomatics* 1999;40:57–63.
10. Kight M, Gatchel RJ, Wesley L. Temporomandibular disorders: evidence for significant overlap with psychopathology. *Health Psychol* 1999;18:177–182.
11. Okasha A, Ismail MK, Khalil AH, et al. A psychiatric study of nonorganic chronic headache patients. *Psychosomatics* 1999;40:233–238.
12. Savidge C, Slade P. Psychological aspects of chronic pelvic pain. *J Psychosom Res* 1997;42:443–444.
13. Ploghaus A, Tracey I, Gati S, et al. Dissociating pain from its anticipation in the human brain. *Science* 1999;284(5422):1979–1981.
14. Loggia ML, Mogil JS, Bushnell MC. Empathy hurts: compassion for another increases both sensory and affective components of pain perception. *Pain* 2008;136:168–176.
15. American Psychiatric Association. *Diagnostic and Statistical Manual of Mental Disorders.* 4th ed. Washington, DC: American Psychiatric Association; 1994.
16. Mayou R, Kirmayer LJ, Simon G, et al. Somatoform disorders: time for a new approach in DSM 5. *Am J Psychiatry* 2005;162:847–855.
17. McHugh PR, Slavney PR. Methods of reasoning in psychopathology: conflict and resolution. *Compr Psychiatry* 1982;23:197–215.
18. Clark MR, Chodynicki MP. Pain management. In: Levenson JL, ed. *Textbook of Psychosomatic Medicine.* Arlington, VA: American Psychiatric Publishing, Inc; 2005:827–867.
19. Clark M, Cox T. Refractory chronic pain. *Psychiatr Clin North Am* 2002;25(1):71–88.
20. Fillingim RB, Bruehl S, Dworkin RH, et al. The ACTTION-American Pain Society Pain Taxonomy (APTT): an evidence-based and multidimensional approach to classifying chronic pain conditions. *J Pain* 2014;15(3):241–249.
21. Edwards RR, Dworkin RH, Sullivan MD, et al. The role of psychosocial processes in the development and maintenance of chronic pain. *J Pain* 2016;9(suppl):T70–T92.
22. Barsky AJ. A comprehensive approach to the chronically somatizing patient. *J Psychosom Res* 1998;45:301–306.
23. McHugh PR, Clark MR. Diagnostic and classificatory dilemmas. In: Blumenfield M, Strain JJ, eds. *Psychosomatic Medicine in the 21st Century.* Baltimore, MD: Lippincott Williams & Wilkins; 2006:39–45.
24. Clark MR. Psychiatric conditions presenting as neurologic disease. Conversion disorder & hysteria. In: Johnson RT, Griffin JW, McArthur JC, eds. *Current Therapy in Neurological Diseases.* St. Louis, MO: Mosby; 2002:428–431.
25. Kirmayer LJ, Groleau D, Looper KJ, et al. Explaining medically unexplained symptoms. *Can J Psychiatry* 2004;49:663–672.
26. Brown RJ. Psychological mechanisms of medically unexplained symptoms: an integrative conceptual model. *Psychol Bull* 2004;130:793–812.
27. Rief W, Barsky AJ. Psychobiological perspectives on somatoform disorders. *Psychoneuroendocrinology* 2005;30:996–1002.
28. McHugh PR. A structure for psychiatry at the century's turn—the view from Johns Hopkins. *J R Soc Med* 1992;85:483–487.

29. McHugh PR, Slavney PR. *The Perspectives of Psychiatry.* 2nd ed. Baltimore, MD: The Johns Hopkins University Press; 1998.
30. Slavney PR. *Perspectives on "Hysteria."* Baltimore, MD: The Johns Hopkins University Press; 1990.
31. Ford CV. Somatization and fashionable diagnoses: illness as a way of life. *Scand J Work Environ Health* 1997;23(suppl 3): 7–16.
32. Reuber M, Mitchell AJ, Howlett SJ, et al. Functional symptoms in neurology: questions and answers. *J Neurol Neurosurg Psychiatry* 2005;76: 307–314.
33. Clark MR, Treisman GJ. Perspectives on pain and depression. *Adv Psychosom Med* 2004;25:1–27.
34. Stone JA, Carson A, Sharpe M. Functional symptoms and signs in neurology: assessment and diagnosis. *J Neurol Neurosurg Psychiatry* 2005;76(suppl 1): i13–i21.
35. Kirmayer LJ, Robbins JM. Three forms of somatization in primary care: prevalence, co-occurrence, and sociodemographic characteristics. *J Nerv Ment Dis* 1991;179:647–655.
36. Rief W, Nanke A. Somatoform disorders in primary care and inpatient settings. *Adv Psychosom Med* 2004;26:144–158.
37. Clark MR, Swartz KL. A conceptual structure and methodology for the systematic approach to the evaluation and treatment of patients with chronic dizziness. *J Anxiety Disord* 2001;15:95–106.
38. Strain EC. Assessment and treatment of comorbid psychiatric disorders in opioid-dependent patients. *Clin J Pain* 2002;18(suppl 4):S14–S27.
39. Keefe FJ, Rumble ME, Scipio CD, et al. Psychological aspects of persistent pain: current state of the science. *J Pain* 2004;5(4):195–211.
40. Wasan AD, Davar G, Jamison RN. The association between negative affect and opioid analgesia in patients with discogenic low back pain. *Pain* 2005;117:450–461.
41. McCracken L, Gross R, Aikens J, et al. The assessment of anxiety and fear in persons with chronic pain: a comparison of instruments. *Behav Res Ther* 1996;34(11–12):927–933.
42. Turk DC, Monarch ES. Biopsychosocial perspective on chronic pain. In: Turk DC, Gatchel R, eds. *Psychological Approaches to Pain Management.* New York: Guilford Press; 2002:3–29.
43. Novy DM, Nelson DV, Berry LA, et al. What does the Beck Depression Inventory measure in chronic pain?: a reappraisal. *Pain* 1995;61:261–270.
44. Koenig HG, George LK, Peterson BL, et al. Depression in medically ill hospitalized older adults: prevalence, characteristics, and course of symptoms according to six diagnostic schemes. *Am J Psychiatry* 1997;154: 1376–1383.
45. White K, Nielson W, Harth M, et al. Chronic widespread musculoskeletal pain with or without fibromyalgia: psychological distress in a representative community adult sample. *J Rheum* 2002;29(3):588–594.
46. BenDebba M, Torgerson W, Long D. Personality traits, pain duration and severity, functional impairment, and psychological distress in patients with persistent low back pain. *Pain* 1997;72:115–125.
47. World Health Organization. *The World Health Report 2004.* Geneva, Switzerland: World Health Organization; 2004.
48. Kessler RC, Borges G, Walters EE. Prevalence of and risk factors for lifetime suicide attempts in the National Comorbidity Survey. *Arch Gen Psychiatry* 1999;56:617–626.
49. Bernal M, Haro JM, Bernert S, et al. Risk factors for suicidality in Europe: results from the ESEMED study. *J Affect Disord* 2007;101:27–34.
50. Tang NK, Crane C. Suicidality in chronic pain: a review of the prevalence, risk factors and psychological links. *Psychol Med* 2006;36:575–586.
51. Möller HJ. Suicide, suicidality and suicide prevention in affective disorders. *Acta Psychiatr Scand Suppl* 2003;(418):73–80.
52. Sokero TP, Melartin TK, Rytsälä HJ, et al. Suicidal ideation and attempts among psychiatric patients with major depressive disorder. *J Clin Psychiatry* 2003;64:1094–1100.
53. Juurlink DN, Herrmann N, Szalai JP, et al. Medical illness and the risk of suicide in the elderly. *Arch Intern Med* 2004;164:1179–1184.
54. Theodoulou M, Harriss L, Hawton K, et al. Pain and deliberate self-harm: an important association. *J Psychosom Res* 2005;28:317–320.
55. Fishbain DA. Approaches to treatment decisions for psychiatric comorbidity in the management of the chronic pain patient. *Med Clin North Am* 1999;83(3):737–759.
56. Ilgen MA, Zivin K, McCammon RJ, et al. Pain and suicidal thoughts, plans and attempts in the United States. *Gen Hosp Psychiatry* 2008;30: 521–527.
57. Braden JB, Sullivan MD. Suicidal thoughts and behavior among adults with self-reported pain conditions in the national comorbidity survey replication. *J Pain* 2008;9:1106–1115.
58. Edwards RR, Smith MT, Kudel I, et al. Pain-related catastrophizing as a risk factor for suicidal ideation in chronic pain. *Pain* 2006;126:272–279.
59. Smith MT, Edwards RR, Robinson RC, et al. Suicidal ideation, plans, attempts in chronic pain patients: factors associated with increased risk. *Pain* 2004;111:201–208.
60. Smith MT, Perlis ML, Haythornthwaite JA. Suicidal ideation in outpatients with chronic musculoskeletal pain: an exploratory study of the role of sleep onset insomnia and pain intensity. *Clin J Pain* 2004;20:111–118.
61. Frank E, Anderson B, Reynolds CF III, et al. Life events and the research diagnostic criteria endogenous subtype. *Arch Gen Psychiatry* 1994;51:519–524.
62. Brown GW, Harris TO, Hepworth C. Life events and endogenous depression. *Arch Gen Psychiatry* 1994;51:525–534.
63. Mossey JM, Gallagher RM, Tirumalasetti F. The effects of pain and depression on physical functioning in elderly residents of a continuing care retirement community. *Pain Med* 2000;1:340–350.
64. Ackermann RT, Williams JW Jr. Rational treatment choices for non-major depressions in primary care: an evidence-based review. *J Gen Intern Med* 2002;17(4):293–301.
65. Lyness JM, Heo M, Datto CJ, et al. Outcomes of minor and subsyndromal depression among elderly patients in primary care settings. *Ann Intern Med* 2006;144(7):495–504.
66. Atkinson JH, Hampton MA, Slater TL, et al. Prevalence, onset, and risk of psychiatric disorders in men with chronic low back pain: a controlled study. *Pain* 1991;45(2):111–121.
67. Magni G, Moreschi C, Rigatti-Luchini S, et al. Prospective study on the relationship between depressive symptoms and chronic musculoskeletal pain. *Pain* 1994;56(3):289–297.
68. Rudy TE, Kerns RD, Turk DC. Chronic pain and depression: toward a cognitive-behavioral mediation model. *Pain* 1988;35(2):129–140.
69. Brown GK. A causal analysis of chronic pain and depression. *J Abnorm Psychol* 1990;99(2):127–137.
70. Katon W, Egan K, Miller D. Chronic pain: lifetime psychiatric diagnosis and family history. *Am J Psychiatry* 1985;142(10):1156–1160.
71. Dersh J, Mayer T, Theodore BR, et al. Do psychiatric disorders first appear preinjury or postinjury in chronic disabling occupational spinal disorders? *Spine (Phila PA 1976)* 2007;32:1045–1051.
72. Hasenbring M, Marienfeld G, Kuhlendahl D, et al. Risk factors of chronicity in lumbar disc patients. A prospective investigation of biologic, psychologic, and social predictors of therapy outcome. *Spine (Phila PA 1976)* 1994;19:2759–2765.
73. Blackburn-Munro G, Blackburn-Munro RE. Chronic pain, chronic stress, and depression: coincidence or consequence? *J Neuroendocrinol* 2001;13: 1009–1023.
74. Von Korff M, Simon G. The relationship between pain and depression. *Br J Psychiatry* 1996;168(suppl 30):101–108.
75. Nemeroff CB, Krishnan KR. Neuroendocrine alterations in psychiatric disorders. In: Nemeroff C, ed. *Neuroendocrinology.* Ann Arbor, MI: CRC Press; 1992.
76. American Psychiatric Association Taskforce on Laboratory Tests in Psychiatry. The dexamethasone suppression test: an overview of its current status in psychiatry. *Am J Psychiatry* 1987;144(10):1253–1262.
77. Mellerup ET, Dam H, Kim MY, et al. Imipramine binding in depressed patients with psychogenic pain. *Psychiatry Res* 1990;32(1):29–34.
78. Sullivan GM, Mann JJ, Oquendo MA, et al. Low cerebrospinal fluid transthyretin levels in depression: correlations with suicidal ideation and low serotonin function. *Biol Psychiatry* 2006;60:500–506.
79. Keller MB, Hirschfeld RM, Hanks D. Double depression: a distinctive subtype of unipolar depression. *J Affect Disord* 1997;45(1–2):65–73.
80. Thase ME, Fava M, Halbreich U, et al. A placebo-controlled, randomized clinical trial comparing sertraline and imipramine for the treatment of dysthymia. *Arch Gen Psychiatry* 1996;53(9):777–784.
81. Rush AJ, Thase ME. Strategies and tactics in the treatment of chronic depression. *J Clin Psychiatry* 1997;58(suppl 13):14–22.
82. Katon WJ, Sullivan MD. Depression and chronic medical illness. *J Clin Psychiatry* 1990;51(suppl):3–11.
83. Coulehan JL, Schulberg HC, Block MR, et al. Medical comorbidity of major depressive disorder in a primary medical practice. *Arch Intern Med* 1990;150:2363–2367.
84. Palinkas LA, Wingard DL, Barrett-Connor E. Chronic illness and depressive symptoms in the elderly: a population-based study. *J Clin Epidemiol* 1990;43(11):1131–1141.
85. Von Korff M, Crane P, Lane M, et al. Chronic spinal pain and physical-mental comorbidity in the United States: results from the national comorbidity study replication. *Pain* 2005;113(3):331–339.
86. Romano JM, Turner JA. Chronic pain and depression: does the evidence support a relationship? *Psychol Bull* 1985;97(1):18–34.
87. Fishbain DM, Goldberg BR, Meagher R, et al. Male and female chronic pain patients characterized by DSM-III psychiatric diagnostic criteria. *Pain* 1986;26:181–197.
88. Bair M, Robinson R, Katon W, et al. Depression and pain comorbidity: a literature review. *Arch Int Med* 2003;163:2433–2445.
89. McWilliams LA, Clara IP, Murphy PD, et al. Associations between arthritis and a broad range of psychiatric disorders: findings from a nationally representative sample. *J Pain* 2008;9(11):37–44.
90. Dworkin SF, Von Korff M, LeResche L. Multiple pains and psychiatric disturbance. An epidemiologic investigation. *Arch Gen Psychiatry* 1990; 47(3):239–244.
91. Von Korff MJ, Ormel J, Keefe FJ, et al. Grading the severity of chronic pain. *Pain* 1992;50(2):133–149.
92. Engel CC, Von Korff M, Katon WJ. Back pain in primary care: predictors of high health-care costs. *Pain* 1996;65(2–3):197–204.
93. Von Korff M, Deyo RA, Cherkin D, et al. Back pain in primary care. Outcomes at 1 year. *Spine* 1993;18:855–862.
94. Kroenke K, Price RK. Symptoms in the community. Prevalence, classification, and psychiatric comorbidity. *Arch Intern Med* 1993;153(21):2474–2480.

95. Adler G, Gattaz WF. Pain perception threshold in major depression. *Biol Psychiatry* 1993;34(10):687–689.

96. Dworkin RH, Clark WC, Lipsitz JD. Pain responsivity in major depression and bipolar disorder. *Psychiatry Res* 1995;56(2):173–181.

97. Thompson T, Correll CU, Gallop K, et al. Is pain perception altered in people with depression? A systematic review and meta-analysis of experimental pain research. *J Pain* 2016;17(12):1257–1272.

98. Ludäscher P, von Kalckreuth C, Parzer P, et al. Pain perception in female adolescents with borderline personality disorder. *Eur Child Adolesc Psychiatry* 2015;24(3):351–357.

99. Glenn JJ, Michel BD, Franklin JC, et al. Pain analgesia among adolescent self-injurers. *Psychiatry Res* 2014;220(3):921–926.

100. Defrin R, Schreiber S, Ginzburg K. Paradoxical pain perception in post-traumatic stress disorder: the unique role of anxiety and dissociation. *J Pain* 2015;16(10):961–970.

101. Fields HL. *Pain.* New York: McGraw-Hill; 1987.

102. Sindrup SH, Bach C, Madsen LF, et al. Venlafaxine versus imipramine in painful neuropathy: a randomized, controlled trial. *Neurology* 2003;60:1284–1289.

103. Raskin J, Pritchett YL, Wang F, et al. A double-blind, randomized multicenter trial comparing duloxetine with placebo in the management of diabetic peripheral neuropathic pain. *Pain Med* 2005;6:346–356.

104. Gordon NC, Heller PH, Gear RW, et al. Temporal factors in the enhancement of morphine analgesia by desipramine. *Pain* 1993;53(3):273–276.

105. Carruba MO, Nisoli E, Garosi V, et al. Catecholamine and serotonin depletion from rat spinal cord: effects on morphine and footshock induced analgesia. *Pharmacol Res* 1992;25(2):187–194.

106. Woolf CJ. Pain: moving from symptom control toward mechanism-specific pharmacologic management. *Ann Intern Med* 2004;140:441–451.

107. Raison CL, Capuron L, Miller AH. Cytokines sing the blues: inflammation and the pathogenesis of depression. *Trends Immunol* 2006;27(1):24–31.

108. Sprenger T, Valet M, Boecker H, et al. Opioidergic activation in the medial pain system after heat pain. *Pain* 2006;122:63–67.

109. Peyron R, Laurent B, Garcia-Larrea L. Functional imaging of brain responses to pain. A review and meta-analysis (2000). *Neurophysiol Clin* 2000;30:263–288.

110. Zubieta JK, Ketter TA, Bueller JA, et al. Regulation of human affective responses by anterior cingulate and limbic mu-opioid neurotransmission. *Arch Gen Psychiatry* 2003;60(11):1145–1153.

111. Coghill RC, McHaffie JG, Yen YF. Neural correlates of interindividual differences in the subjective experience of pain. *Proc Natl Acad Sci U S A* 2003;100(14):8538–8542.

112. Thase ME. Depression, sleep, and antidepressants. *J Clin Psychiatry* 1998;59(suppl 4):55–65.

113. Lautenbacher S, Kundermann B, Krieg J. Sleep deprivation and pain perception. *Sleep Med Rev* 2006;10:357–369.

114. Lentz MJ, Landis CA, Rothermel J, et al. Effects of selective slow wave sleep disruption on muscoskeletal pain and fatigue in middle aged women. *J Rheumatol* 1999;26:1586–1592.

115. Freud S. Mourning and melancholia. In: *Collected Papers.* London: Hogarth Press and the Institute of Psychoanalysis; 1917.

116. Blumer D, Heilbronn M. Chronic pain as a variant of depressive disease: the pain-prone disorder. *J Nerv Ment Dis* 1982;170(7):381–406.

117. Tinling DC, Klein RF. Psychogenic pain and aggression: the syndrome of the solitary hunger. *Psychosom Med* 1966;28:738–748.

118. von Knorring L, Perris C, Eisemann M, et al. Pain as a symptom in depressive disorders. II. Relationship to personality traits as assessed by means of KSP. *Pain* 1983;17(4):377–384.

119. Bouchoms AJ, Litman RE, Baer L. Denial in the depressive and pain-prone disorders of chronic pain. *Clin J Pain* 1985;1:165–169.

120. Gupta MA. Is chronic pain a variant of depressive illness? A critical review. *Can J Psychiatry* 1986;31(3):241–248.

121. Rashbaum IG, Sarno JE. Psychosomatic concepts in chronic pain. *Arch Phys Med Rehabil* 2003;84(3 suppl 1):S76–S82.

122. Sarno JE. *Healing Back Pain: The Mind-Body Connection.* New York: Warner Books; 1991.

123. Carson JW, Keefe FJ, Goli V, et al. Forgiveness and chronic low back pain: a preliminary study examining the relationship of forgiveness to pain, anger, and psychological distress. *J Pain* 2005;6(2):84–91.

124. Beck AT. *Depression: Causes and Treatment.* Philadelphia: University of Pennsylvania Press; 1967.

125. Turk DC, Meichenbaum D. A cognitive-behavioral approach to pain management. In: Wall PD, Melzack R, eds. *Textbook of Pain.* London: Churchill Livingstone; 1994:337–348.

126. Turk DC, Meichenbaum D, Genest M. *Pain and Behavioral Medicine: A Cognitive-Behavioral Perspective.* New York: Guilford; 1983.

127. Turk DC. Anxiety and related factors in chronic pain: a diathesis-stress model of chronic pain and disability following traumatic injury. *Pain Res Manag* 2002;7(1):9–19.

128. Gatchel RJ. Psychological disorders and chronic pain: cause and effect relationships. In: Gatchel RJ, Turk DC, eds. *Psychological Approaches to Pain Management: A Practitioner's Handbook.* New York: Guilford; 1996:33–54.

129. Banks SM, Kern RD. Explaining high rates of depression in chronic pain: a diathesis-stress framework. *Psychol Bull* 1996;119:95–110.

130. Caspi A, Mofitt TE. Gene-environment interactions in psychiatry: joining forces with neuroscience. *Nat Rev Neurosci* 2006;7:583–590.

131. Fabrega H Jr. The concept of somatization as a cultural and historical product of Western medicine. *Psychosom Med* 1990;52(6):653–672.

132. Nichter M. Idioms of distress: alternatives in the expression of psychosocial distress: a case study from South India. *Cult Med Psychiatry* 1981;5(4):379–408.

133. Kleinman A. *The Illness Narratives: Suffering, Healing, and the Human Condition.* New York: Basic Books; 1988.

134. Carr DB, Loeser JD, Morris DB. Why Narrative? In: Carr DB, Loeser JD, Morris DB, eds. *Narrative, Pain, and Suffering.* Seattle, WA: IASP Press; 2005:3–13.

135. Wasan AD, Wootton J, Jamison RN. Dealing with difficult patients in your pain practice. *Reg Anesth Pain Med* 2005;30:184–192.

136. Wasan AD, Alpay M. Pain and the psychiatric co-morbidities of pain. In: Stern T, ed. *Comprehensive Clinical Psychiatry.* Philadelphia: Elsevier; 2008:1067–1080.

137. Gilbody S, Bower P, Fletcher J, et al. Collaborative care for depression: a cumulative meta-analysis and review of longer-term outcomes. *Arch Int Med* 2006;166(21):2314–2321.

138. Kroenke K, Shen J, Oxman TE, et al. Impact of pain on the outcomes of depression treatment: results from the RESPECT trial. *Pain* 2008;134: 209–215.

139. Salerno SM, Browning R, Jackson JL. The effect of antidepressant treatment on chronic back pain: a meta-analysis. *Arch Int Med* 2002;162(1):19–24.

140. Rosenzweig-Lipson S, Beyer CE, Hughes ZA, et al. Differentiating antidepressants of the future: efficacy and safety. *Pharmacol Ther* 2007;113: 134–153.

141. Semenchuk MR, Sherman S, Davis B. Double-blind, randomized trial of bupropion SR for the treatment of neuropathic pain. *Neurology* 2001;57(9):1583–1588.

142. Katz J, Pennella-Vaughan J, Hetzel RD, et al. A randomized, placebo-controlled trial of bupropion sustained release in chronic low back pain. *J Pain* 2005;6(10):656–661.

143. Janicak PG, Davis JM, Preskorn SH, et al. Indications for antidepressants. In: Janicak PG, Davis JM, Preskorn SH, et al, eds. *Principles and Practice of Psychopharmacotherapy.* Philadelphia: Lippincott Williams & Wilkins; 2001:193–214.

144. Maxmen JS, Ward NG. *Psychotropic Drugs: Fast Facts.* 2nd ed. New York: Norton; 1995.

145. Hyman SE, Arana GW, Rosenbaum JF. *Handbook of Psychiatric Drug Therapy.* 3rd ed. Boston, MA: Little, Brown and Company; 1995.

146. Wasan AD, Artin K, Clark MR. A case-matching study of the analgesic properties of electroconvulsive therapy. *Pain Med* 2004;5(1):50–58.

147. Bloomstein JR, Rummans TA, Maruta T, et al. The use of electroconvulsive therapy in pain patients. *Psychosomatics* 1996;37:374–749.

148. Dellemijn PL, Fields HL. Do benzodiazepines have a role in chronic pain management? *Pain* 1994;57(2):137–152.

149. Salzman C. The APA task force report on benzodiazepine dependence, toxicity, and abuse. *Am J Psychiatry* 1991;148(2):151–152.

150. Nielsen S, Lintzeris N, Bruno R, et al. Benzodiazepine use among chronic pain patients prescribed opioids: associations with pain, physical and mental health, and health service utilization. *Pain Med* 2015;16(2): 356–366.

151. Larochelle MR, Zhang F, Ross-Degnan D, et al. Trends in opioid prescribing and co-prescribing of sedative hypnotics for acute and chronic musculoskeletal pain: 2001–2010. *Pharmacoepidemiol Drug Saf* 2015;24(8): 885–892.

152. Dowell D, Haegerich TM, Chou R. CDC guideline for prescribing opioids for chronic pain–United States, 2016. *JAMA* 2016;315(15):1624–1645.

153. Rickels K, Schweizer E. The treatment of generalized anxiety disorder in patients with depressive symptomatology. *J Clin Psychiatry* 1993;54(suppl): 20–23.

154. Grzesiak RC, Ury GM, Dworkin RH. Psychodynamic psychotherapy with chronic pain patients. In: Gatchel RJ, Turk DC, eds. *Psychological Approaches to Pain Management: A Practitioner's Handbook.* New York: Guilford Press; 1996:94–127.

155. Dimidjian S, Barrera M Jr, Martell C, et al. The origins and current status of behavioral activation treatments for depression. *Annu Rev Clin Psychol* 2011;7:1–38.

156. Dimidjian S, Hollon SD, Dobson KS, et al. Randomized trial of behavioral activation, cognitive therapy, and antidepressant medication in the acute treatment of adults with major depression. *J Consult Clin Psychol* 2006;74(4):658–670.

157. Brox JI, Reikeras O, Nygaard O, et al. Lumbar instrumented fusion compared with cognitive intervention and exercises in patients with chronic back pain after previous surgery for disc herniation: a prospective randomized controlled study. *Pain* 2006;122:145–155.

158. Outcalt SD, Kroenke K, Chambler NR, et al. Chronic pain and comorbid mental health conditions: independent associations of posttraumatic stress disorder and depression with pain, disability, and quality of life. *J Behav Med* 2015;38(3):535–543.

159. Tegethoff M, Belardi A, Stalujanis E, et al. Comorbidity of mental disorders and chronic pain: chronology of onset in adolescents of a national representative cohort. *J Pain* 2015;16(10):1054–1064.

160. Wolfe F, Smythe HA, Yunnus MB, et al. The American College of Rheumatology 1990 criteria for the classification of fibromyalgia. Report of the multicenter criteria committee. *Arthritis Rheum* 1990;33(2):160–172.

161. Dersh JR, Gatchel RJ, Polatin P, et al. Prevalence of psychiatric disorders in patients with chronic work-related musculoskeletal pain and disability. *J Occup Environ Med* 2002;44(5):459–468.

162. Conrad R, Schilling G, Bausch C, et al. Temperament and character personality profiles and personality disorders in chronic pain patients. *Pain* 2007;133:197–209.

163. McCracken L, Zayfert C, Gross R. The pain anxiety symptoms scale: development and validation of a scale to measure fear of pain. *Pain* 1992;50:67–73.

164. Vancleef LM, Peters ML, Roelofs J, et al. Do fundamental fears differentially contribute to pain-related fear and pain catastrophizing? An evaluation of the sensitivity index. *Eur J Pain* 2006;10:527–536.

165. McCracken L, Gross R, Sorg P, et al. Prediction of pain in patients with chronic low back pain: effects of inaccurate prediction and pain-related anxiety. *Behav Res Ther* 1993;31(7):647–652.

166. Hunot V, Churchill R, Silva de Lima M, et al. Psychological therapies for generalized anxiety disorder. *Cochrane Database Syst Rev* 2007;(1):CD001848.

167. Linden DE. How psychotherapy changes the brain—the contribution of functional neuroimaging. *Mol Psychiatry* 2006;11:528–538.

168. Ormel JM, VonKorff M, Ustun TB, et al. Common mental disorders and disability across cultures. Results from the WHO collaborative study on psychological problems in general health care. *JAMA* 1994;272(22):1741–1748.

169. Demyttenaere K, Bruffaerts R, Lee S, et al. Mental disorders among persons with chronic back or neck pain: results from the world mental health surveys. *Pain* 2007;129:332–342.

170. Zaubler TS, Katon W. Panic disorder and medical comorbidity: a review of the medical and psychiatric literature. *Bull Menninger Clin* 1996;60 (2 suppl A):A12–A38.

171. Carney RM, Freedland KE, Ludbrook PA, et al. Major depression, panic disorder, and mitral valve prolapse in patients who complain of chest pain. *Am J Med* 1990;89(6):757–760.

172. Beitman BD, Kushner MG, Basha I, et al. Follow-up status of patients with angiographically normal coronary arteries and panic disorder. *JAMA* 1991;265(12):1545–1549.

173. Cannon RO III, Quyyumi AA, Mincemoyer R, et al. Imipramine in patients with chest pain despite normal coronary angiograms. *N Engl J Med* 1994;330:1411–1417.

174. Walker EA, Gelfand AN, Gelfand MD, et al. Psychiatric diagnoses, sexual and physical victimization, and disability in patients with irritable bowel syndrome or inflammatory bowel disease. *Psychol Med* 1995;25(6):1259–1267.

175. Stewart W, Breslau N, Keck PE Jr. Comorbidity of migraine and panic disorder. *Neurology* 1994;44(suppl 7):S23–S27.

176. American Psychiatric Association. Practice guideline for treatment of patients with panic disorder. *Am J Psychiatry* 1998;155(5 suppl):1–34.

177. Kirmayer LJ, Young A, Hayton BC. The cultural context of anxiety disorders. *Psychiatr Clin North Am* 1995;18(3):503–521.

178. Seal KH, Bertenthal D, Miner CR, et al. Bringing the war back home: mental health disorders among 103,788 US veterans returning from Iraq and Afghanistan seen at Department of Veterans Affairs facilities. *Arch Intern Med* 2007;167(5):476–482.

179. Beckham JC, Crawford AL, Feldman ME, et al. Chronic posttraumatic stress disorder and chronic pain in Vietnam combat veterans. *J Psychosom Res* 1997;43(11):379–389.

180. Baker DG, Mendenhall CL, Simbartl LA, et al. Relationship between posttraumatic stress disorder and self-reported physical symptoms in Persian Gulf War veterans. *Arch Intern Med* 1997;157(18):2076–2078.

181. Doerfler LA, Pbert L, DeCosimo D. Symptoms of posttraumatic stress disorder following myocardial infarction and coronary artery bypass surgery. *Gen Hosp Psychiatry* 1997;16(3):193–199.

182. Alter CL, Pelcovitz D, Axelrod A, et al. Identification of PTSD in cancer survivors. *Psychosomatics* 1996;37:137–143.

183. Cordova MJ, Andrykowski MA, Kenady DE, et al. Frequency and correlates of posttraumatic-stress-disorder-like symptoms after treatment for breast cancer. *J Consult Clin Psychol* 1995;63(6):981–986.

184. Blanchard EB, Hickling EJ. *After the Crash: Assessment and Treatment of Motor Vehicle Accident Survivors.* Washington, DC: American Psychological Association; 1997.

185. Aghabeigi B, Feinmann C, Harris M. Prevalence of post-traumatic stress disorder in patients with chronic idiopathic facial pain. *Br J Oral Maxillofac Surg* 1992;30(6):360–364.

186. Amir M, Kaplan Z, Neumann L, et al. Posttraumatic stress disorder, tenderness and fibromyalgia. *J Psychosom Res* 1997;42(6):607–613.

187. Muse M. Stress-related, post-traumatic chronic pain syndrome: behavioral treatment approach. *Pain* 1986;25(3):389–394.

188. Liebschutz J, Saitz R, Browner V, et al. PTSD in urban primary care: high prevalence and low physician recognition. *J Gen Intern Med* 2007;22(6):719–726.

189. Geisser ME, Roth RS, Bachman JE, et al. The relationship between symptoms of post-traumatic stress disorder and pain, affective disturbance and disability among patients with accident and non-accident related pain. *Pain* 1996;66(2):207–214.

190. Schreiber S, Galai-Gat T. Uncontrolled pain following physical injury as the core-trauma in post-traumatic stress disorder. *Pain* 1993;54(1):107–110.

191. Zatick DF, Rivara FP, Nathens AB, et al. A nationwide US study of post-traumatic stress after hospitalization for physical injury. *Psychol Med* 2007;37(10):1469–1480.

192. Sherman JJ, Turk DC, Okifuji A. Prevalence and impact of posttraumatic stress disorder-like symptoms on patients with fibromyalgia syndrome. *Clin J Pain* 2000;16:127–134.

193. Harris IA, Young JM, Rae H, et al. Factors associated with back pain after physical injury: a survey of consecutive major trauma patients. *Spine (Phila PA 1976)* 2007;32(14):1561–1565.

194. Jenewein J, Moergeli H, Wittmann L, et al. Development of chronic pain following severe accidental injury. Results of a 3 year follow-up study. *J Psychosom Res* 2009;66:119–126.

195. Geuze E, Westenberg HG, Jochims A, et al. Altered pain processing in veterans with posttraumatic stress disorder. *Arch Gen Psychiatry* 2007;64(1):76–85.

196. Difede J, Olden M, Cukor J. Evidence-based treatment of post-traumatic stress disorder. *Annu Rev Med* 2014;65:319–332.

197. Solomon SD, Gerrity ET, Muff AM. Efficacy of treatments for posttraumatic stress disorder. An empirical review. *JAMA* 1992;268(2):633–636.

198. Wynn GH. Complementary and alternative medicine approaches in the treatment of PTSD. *Curr Psychiatry Rep* 2015;17(8):600.

199. Davidson JR. Biological therapies for posttraumatic stress disorder: an overview. *J Clin Psychiatry* 1997;58(suppl 9):29–32.

200. Davidson J, Baldwin D, Stein DJ, et al. Treatment of posttraumatic stress disorder with venlafaxine extended release: a 6-month randomized controlled trial. *Arch Gen Psych* 2006;63(10):1158–1165.

201. Raskind MA, Peskind ER, Hoff DJ, et al. A parallel group placebo controlled study of prazosin for trauma nightmares and sleep disturbance in combat veterans with post-traumatic stress disorder. *Biol Psychiatry* 2007;61(8):928–934.

202. Tawa J, Murphy S. Psychopharmacological treatment for military post-traumatic stress disorder: an integrative review. *J Am Assoc Nurse Pract* 2013;25(8):419–423.

203. Vendrig AA. The Minnesota Multiphasic Personality Inventory and chronic pain: a conceptual analysis of a long-standing but complicated relationship. *Clin Psychol Rev* 2000;20:533–559.

204. Weisberg JN. Personality and personality disorders in chronic pain. *Curr Rev Pain* 2000;4:60–70.

205. Weisberg JN, Vaillancourt PD. Personality factors and disorders in chronic pain. *Semin Clin Neuropsychiatry* 1999;4:155–166.

206. Hathaway SR, McKinley JC. *Minnesota Multiphasic Personality Inventory Manual.* Rev ed. New York: Psychological Corporation; 1967.

207. Turk DC, Fernandez E. Personality assessment and the Minnesota Multiphasic Personality Inventory in chronic pain: underdeveloped and overexposed. *Pain Forum* 1995;5:104–107.

208. Vendrig AA, Derksen JJ, de Mey HR. MMPI-2 Personality Psychopathology Five (PSY-5) and prediction of treatment outcome for patients with chronic back pain. *J Pers Assess* 2000;74:423–438.

209. Sternbach RA. Psychological aspects of pain and the selection of patients. *Clin Neurosurg* 1974(21):223–233.

210. Riley JL III, Robinson ME. Validity of MMPI-2 profiles in chronic back pain patients: differences in path models of coping and somatization. *Clin J Pain* 1998;14:324–335.

211. Norman WT. Toward an adequate taxonomy of personality attributes: replicated factors structure in peer nomination personality settings. *J Abnorm Soc Psychol* 1963;66:574–583.

212. Costa PT, McCrae RR. *The NEO Personality Inventory Manual.* Orlando, FL: Psychological Assessment Resources; 1985.

213. Widiger TA, Lowe JR. Five-factor model assessment of personality disorder. *J Pers Assess* 2007;89:16–29.

214. Cloninger CR, Svrakic DM, Przybeck TR. A psychobiological model of temperament and character. *Arch Gen Psychiatry* 1993;50:975–990.

215. Svrakic DM, Whitehead C, Przybeck TR, et al. Differential diagnosis of personality disorders by the seven-factor model of temperament and character. *Arch Gen Psychiatry* 1993;50:991–999.

216. Hirano S, Sato T, Narita T, et al. Evaluating the state dependency of the temperament and character inventory dimensions in patients with a major depression: a methodological contribution. *J Affect Disord* 2002;69:31–38.

217. Grucza RA, Przybeck TR, Spitznagel EL, et al. Personality and depressive symptoms: a multi-dimensional analysis. *J Affect Disord* 2003;74:123–130.

218. Nestadt G, Costa PT Jr, Hsu FC, et al. The relationship between the five-factor model and latent DSM-IV personality disorder dimensions. *Compr Psychiatry* 2008;49:98–105.

219. Terracciano A, Costa PT Jr, McCrae RR. Personality plasticity after age 30. *Pers Soc Psychol Bull* 2006;32:999–1009.

220. Skodol AE, Gunderson JG, Shea MT, et al. The Collaborative Longitudinal Personality Disorders Study (CLPS): overview and implications. *J Pers Disord* 2005;19:487–504.

221. Costa PT Jr, Patriciu NS, McCrae RR. Lessons from longitudinal studies for new approaches to the DSM-V: the FFM and FFT. *J Pers Disord* 2005;19:533–596.

222. Fishbain DA, Cole B, Cutler RB, et al. Chronic pain and the measurement of personality: do states influence traits? *Pain Med* 2006;7:509–529.

223. Loranger AW, Lenzenweger MF, Gartner AF, et al. Trait-state artifacts and the diagnosis of personality disorders. *Arch Gen Psychiatry* 1991;48:720–728.

224. Bronisch T, Klerman G. Personality functioning: change and stability in relationship to symptoms and psychopathology. *J Personal Disord* 1991;5: 307–317.

225. Stuart S, Simons AD, Thase ME. Are personality assessments valid in acute major depression? *J Affect Disord* 1992;24:281–290.

226. Hellerstein DJ, Kocsis JH, Chapman D, et al. Double-blind comparison of sertraline, imipramine, and placebo in the treatment of dysthymia: effects on personality. *Am J Psychiatry* 2000;157:1436–1444.

227. Applegate KL, Keefe FJ, Siegler IC, et al. Does personality at college entry predict number of reported pain conditions at mid-life? A longitudinal study. *J Pain* 2005;6:92–97.

228. Malmgren-Olsson EB, Bergdahl J. Temperament and character personality dimensions in patients with nonspecific musculoskeletal disorders. *Clin J Pain* 2006;22:625–631.

229. Greenberg J, Burns JW. Pain anxiety among chronic pain patients: specific phobia or manifestation of anxiety sensitivity? *Behav Res Ther* 2003;41:223–240.

230. Lethem J, Slade PD, Troup JD, et al. Outline of fear-avoidance model of exaggerated pain perceptions. *Behav Res Ther* 1983;21:401–408.

231. Reis S. Expectancy theory of fear, anxiety, and panic. *Clin Psychol Rev* 1991;11:141–153.

232. Vlaeyen JW, Linton SJ. Fear-avoidance and its consequences in chronic musculoskeletal pain: a state of the art. *Pain* 2000;85:317–332.

233. Zvolensky MJ, Goodie JL, McNeil DW, et al. Anxiety sensitivity in the prediction of pain-related fear and anxiety in a heterogeneous chronic pain population. *Behav Res Ther* 2001;39:683–696.

234. Asmundson GJ, Norton PJ, Norton GR. Beyond pain: the role of fear and avoidance in chronicity. *Clin Psychol Rev* 1999;19:97–119.

235. Waddell G, Newton M, Henderson I, et al. A Fear-Avoidance Beliefs Questionnaire (FABQ) and the role of fear-avoidance beliefs in chronic low back pain and disability. *Pain* 1993;52:157–168.

236. Mannion AF, Müntener M, Taimela S, et al. A randomized clinical trial of three active therapies for chronic low back pain. *Spine (Phila PA 1976)* 1999;24:2435–2448.

237. Mannion AF, Junge A, Taimela S, et al. Active therapy for chronic low back pain: part 3. Factors influencing self-rated disability and its change following therapy. *Spine* 2001;26:920–929.

238. Vowles KE, Gross RT. Work-related beliefs about injury and physical capability for work in individuals with chronic pain. *Pain* 2003;101:291–298.

239. Parsons T. *Social Systems.* London: Routledge and Kegan Paul; 1951.

240. Parsons T. *Social Structure and Personality.* New York: Free Press; 1964.

241. Mechanic D, Volkart EH. Stress, illness behavior, and the sick role. *Ann Soc Rev* 1961;26(1):51–58.

242. Mechanic D. The concept of illness behavior. *J Chron Dis* 1962;15: 189–194.

243. Pilowsky I. The diagnosis of abnormal illness behavior. *Aust NZ J Psychiatry* 1971;5:136–141.

244. Barsky AJ III. Patients who amplify bodily sensations. *Ann Intern Med* 1979;91(1):63–70.

245. Cloninger CR, Sigvardsson S, von Knorring AL, et al. An adoption study of somatoform disorders. II. Identification of two discrete somatoform disorders. *Arch Gen Psychiatry* 1984;41(9):853–859.

246. Katz J, Rosenbloom BN, Fashler S. Chronic pain, psychopathology, and DSM-5 somatic symptom disorder. *Can J Psychiatry* 2015;60(4): 160–167.

247. Steinbrecher N, Koerber S, Freiser D, et al. The prevalence of medically unexplained symptoms in primary care. *Psychosomatics* 2011;52: 263–271.

248. Rief W, Martin A. How to use the new DSM-5 somatic symptom disorder diagnosis in research and practice: a critical evaluation and proposal for modifications. *Annu Rev Clin Psychol* 2014;10:339–367.

249. Frances A. The new somatic symptom disorder in DSM-5 risks mislabeling many people as mentally ill. *BMJ* 2013;346:f1580.

250. Stone J, LaFrance WJ Jr, Levensen JL, et al. Issues for DSM-5: conversion disorder. *Am J Psychiatry* 2010;167(6):626–627.

251. Demartini B, D'Agostino A, Gambini O. From conversion disorder (DSM-IV-TR) to functional neurological symptom disorder (DSM-5): when a label changes the perspective for the neurologist, the psychiatrist and the patient. *J Neurol Sci* 2016;360:55–56.

252. Ziegler FJ, Imboden JB, Meyer E. Contemporary conversion reaction: a clinical study. *Am J Psychiatry* 1960;116:901–910.

253. Ochoa JL, Verdugo RJ. Reflex sympathetic dystrophy. A common clinical avenue for somatoform expression. *Neurol Clin* 1995;13(2):351–363.

254. Bridges K, Goldberg D, Evans B, et al. Determinants of somatization in primary care. *Psychol Med* 1991;21(2):473–483.

255. Fackler SM, Anfinson TJ, Rand JA. Serial sodium Amytal interviews in the clinical setting. *Psychosomatics* 1997;38:558–564.

256. Barsky AJ, Wyshak G, Klerman GL, et al. The prevalence of hypochondriasis in medical outpatients. *Soc Psychiatry Psychiatr Epidemiol* 1990;25: 89–94.

257. Barsky AJ. Hypochondriasis. Medical management and psychiatric treatment. *Psychosomatics* 1996;37:48–56.

CHAPTER 32

Treatment of Pain in Patients with Addiction

PEGGY COMPTON, FRIEDHELM SANDBRINK, and **MARTIN D. CHEATLE**

Substance use disorder (SUD), formerly called substance abuse, dependence, or addiction, is a prevalent chronic disease in our society, not only with implications for the health and quality of the life of the sufferers but also with often devastating consequences for the families and communities in which they live and for society. Perhaps unlike any other chronic illness, SUD has meaningful effects on all aspects of the pain experience, ranging from its perception to its management. Specifically, the neurologic and behavioral states associated with the disease tend to worsen the pain presentation and mitigate the efficacy of therapeutic interventions. These complications become particularly apparent in the case of opioid use disorder (OUD), where the abused substance is also a primary analgesic used to treat moderate to severe pain. The development of opioid tolerance, physical dependence, hyperalgesia, and/or relapse are all challenges clinicians face when attempting to manage the pain of persons with OUD.

This chapter provides a brief overview of SUD, conceptualizing it as a chronic, relapsing neurologic disease for which evidence-based treatments exist, however, with access to these treatments limited in part due to negative societal perceptions of the illness. The overlap in neurobiologic systems in pain and SUD is considered, and how the presence of an SUD in general, and OUD specifically, can affect the experience of pain is discussed. Finally, principles of acute and chronic pain management for the patient with SUD is outlined, differentiated by whether the patient is actively using, on medication-assisted therapy (MAT; i.e., methadone, buprenorphine, naltrexone), or in drug-free recovery. Evident in these recommendations is the understanding that effectively and thoughtfully treating pain in the patient with SUD concomitantly benefits the recovery process regardless of the state of disease progression.

Substance Use Disorder

Misusing and abusing drugs and alcohol is endemic in the United States. The most recent national surveys suggest that approximately 8% (or 20 million) of Americans older than 12 years met diagnostic criteria for an SUD in the past year.[1] Being legal and readily available, not surprisingly, three quarters of these individuals meet criteria for alcohol use disorder (AUD). Among those with an illicit drug use disorder, the most common drug is marijuana (4 million people), followed by an estimated 2.1 million people with an OUD, which includes 1.8 million people with a prescription pain reliever use disorder and 0.6 million people with a heroin use disorder.[1] There is good evidence to suggest that the prevalence of SUD is higher in patients seeking medical care secondary to the toxic effects of the drugs themselves and/or the risky behaviors associated with the disorder.[2-5]

Like chronic pain, addiction is an extremely complex human condition, with strong behavioral and social components, that cannot be entirely understood by analyzing its physiology. SUD is defined as a chronic, relapsing disorder that is characterized by (1) a compulsion to seek and take drugs, (2) loss of control over drug intake, and (3) emergence of strong negative emotional states (e.g., dysphoria, anxiety, and irritability) when access to the drug is prevented (Table 32.1).[6] The occasional, limited, recreational use of a drug is clinically distinct from the loss of control

over drug intake and the emergence of compulsive drug-seeking behavior that characterize SUD.[7] Because the disorder is primarily evident in behaviors, it is one of the few conditions in which the sufferer is the disease, as reflected in the pejorative labels ascribed to him or her (i.e., "drunk," "druggie," "addict," "lush").

Like all chronic disorders, SUD is never "cured," but it can be effectively managed with lifestyle changes and, in some cases, medication. Similar to other chronic conditions, there are demonstrable pathophysiologic changes underlying the disorder, which, in the case of addiction, reside in subcortical and cortical neural pathways underlying reward and memory and, ultimately, the prefrontal cortex, driving behavior (Fig. 32.1). Without treatment, the disease will predictably progress and result in disability and ultimately death. Known risk factors for SUD in both patients with pain and in those without pain include a prior history of alcohol and/or illicit drug abuse (including nicotine addiction), a family history of substance abuse or SUD, a history of mood or anxiety disorder, early onset (age <14 years) of alcohol or drug use, a history of child sexual abuse or child neglect, involvement in the legal system, and significant psychosocial stressors.[8,9] Furthermore, as with all chronic diseases, SUD is characterized by exacerbations (or relapses) over time, often at times of interpersonal or intrapersonal stress, and treatments are most effective when ongoing.

Adopting a chronic illness model for SUD provides the foundation for effective treatment; however, this model is inconsistent with societal perspectives. For example, SUD has been conceptualized as a moral failing, such that those who engage in problematic drug and alcohol use are often described as lacking honorable character or moral fortitude (i.e., "just say no"). Also, in the United States, illicit drug use is classified as a criminal behavior, with punishment, including incarceration, being the societal approach to treatment. Unfortunately, both the moral and criminal attributions to SUD result in significant shame and stigma for the sufferer, making them less likely to seek treatment and further isolating them from therapeutic supports. These negative perspectives

---

TABLE 32.1   Indicators of Substance Use Disorder

Indicators of Substance Use Disorder

- More substance (drug, alcohol) is used than intended or planned.
- Inability to cut down or control substance use
- Much of time obtaining, using, or recovering from substance
- Craving or a strong desire to use substance
- Inability to fulfill role obligations at work, school, or home
- Continued substance use despite accumulating consequences
- Reduced participation in social, occupational, or recreational activities due to substance use
- Substance use in situations in which it is physically hazardous
- Continued substance use despite health problems caused or exacerbated by substance
- Need for increased amounts of substance to achieve desired effect (tolerance)
- Characteristic withdrawal syndrome for substance when not used (physical dependence)

Adapted from the American Psychiatric Disorder. *Diagnostic and Statistical Manual of Mental Disorders.* 5th ed. Arlington, VA: American Psychiatric Publishing; 2013.

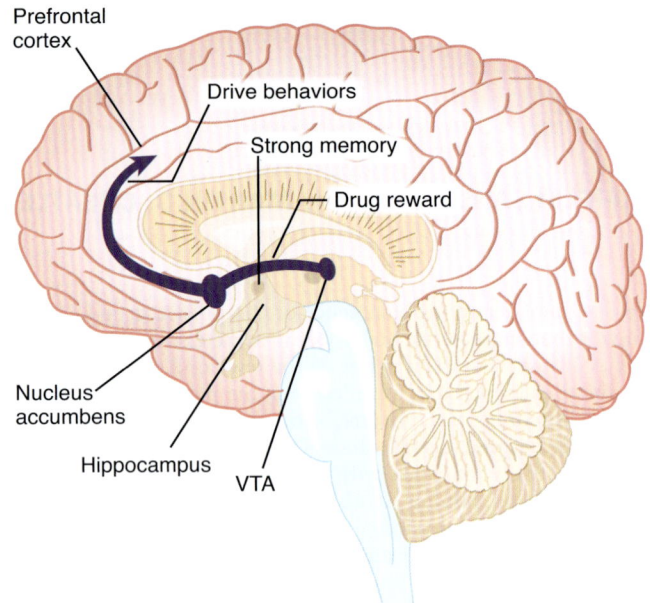

FIGURE 32.1 Neuroanatomy of substance use disorders. VTA, ventral tegmental area.

are reflected in the relative paucity and marginalization of SUD treatment services in the United States, such that in 2016, only about 1 in 10 people (10.6%) aged 12 years or older who needed substance use treatment were able to receive it.[1]

Fortunately, evidence-based treatments for SUD exist, and as a result of the current opioid abuse crisis, are becoming increasingly integrated into acute and primary care settings. For drugs of abuse with significant physiologic withdrawal syndromes (i.e., alcohol, opioids, benzodiazepines), treatment often begins with a taper or detoxification with a long-acting substitution agent. However, it is important to appreciate that detoxification in and of itself is not a treatment for SUD; it simply readies the patient for the cognitive, behavioral, and group support interventions necessary to mitigate disease progression. Opioid medications may be utilized as adjuncts to treatment in the case of AUD (naltrexone) and should be routinely offered to all patients with OUD (methadone, buprenorphine, naltrexone) to allay craving and withdrawal; in all cases, medications to treat underlying psychiatric disorders are indicated. Related to previous stressful or traumatic experiences, especially those occurring in childhood, individual or group psychotherapy can be highly beneficial for patients in whom adverse events are an issue, but access to and reimbursement for these services can be limited.

Clinical Implications of Substance Use Disorders on Pain

Pain and SUD are not unrelated phenomena, and this overlap becomes significant at the clinical level. Pain and drug reward share common neuroanatomical and neurochemical substrates, and the physiologic sequelae of SUD (i.e., tolerance, dependence, and altered stress response) have clear effects on pain management. Drugs of abuse often have inherent analgesic properties, yet SUD can bring with it mood states, behaviors, and social losses that worsen the pain experience. The clinical intersection of pain and SUD is particularly complex in the case of OUD, as opioids have rewarding, analgesic, and hyperalgesic activity. Furthermore, accumulating genetic data suggest that pain severity, opioid analgesia, and OUD may share similar patterns of gene expression, which become evident in the response of the individual patient to a painful stimulus.

NEUROBIOLOGIC OVERLAP BETWEEN PAIN AND ADDICTION SYSTEMS

It is not surprising that pain and SUD responses are related in that both are modulated by the activity of the same neuropeptide—the opioids at the opioid receptor. Whether administered endogenously or exogenously, opioids engender both pain relief and psychoactive reward, the latter of which provides the neurobiologic foundation for SUDs. All drugs of abuse, either directly or indirectly, activate opioid reward systems, which in individuals at risk can result in the compulsive behaviors diagnostic of SUD.

Of relevance to pain and pain treatment, the neurobiology of SUD is often characterized by two incompletely understood yet related allostatic states: tolerance and physical dependence. These neuroadaptations may be evident not only in those brain systems in which drugs of abuse exert direct actions but also in brain systems that oppose the actions of the drug.[10] Importantly, the simple presence of these adaptations in the nervous system does not infer meeting the diagnostic criteria for SUD. Any individual using alcohol or opioids on a regular basis will become tolerant to or physiologically dependent on the effects of the drug; it is simply a neurobiologic outcome of drug exposure. As noted earlier, SUD is identified by a cluster of aberrant patterns of behavior that, although partially motivated by these physiologic changes, is evident in much broader functional domains (see Table 32.1).

Tolerance

Ongoing use of substances of abuse often results in the development of drug tolerance, even when they are used for analgesic purposes, which is defined as a reduction in response to a given dose of drug after repeated administration.[10,11] The neuroadaptations associated with tolerance counter the acute drug effects to maintain system-level homeostasis. A theoretical explanation for the processes underlying tolerance is offered by the opponent process theory of acquired motivation.[12,13] Reflecting homeostatic assumptions, the theory describes how, over the course of repeated exposures to a stimulus, a counteracting or opposing emotional or physiologic response develops, which eventually accounts for habituation to the stimulus and becomes the predominant state in its absence. In the case of drug reward, the model predicts that in order to maintain a "normal" or homeostatic level of reward system activity, "antireward" systems are recruited to counteract drug effects, which become stronger with each exposure and extinguish more slowly than the original response.[14,15] Upon abrupt drug withdrawal, antireward or dysphoric processes are revealed. As described in the following discussion, analogous opponent processes are theorized to underlie the development of opioid-induced hyperalgesia (OIH).

Physiologic tolerance involves adaptations that occur both at the site of drug action and in systems distal to the site of drug action.[16–18] Because drugs typically act at selective receptors, tolerance has been conceptualized as a functional "uncoupling" of the receptor from its effector response (opening or closing an ion channel, initiating second messenger systems); in other words, a certain proportion of receptors are rendered less functional or nonfunctional, thus making the drug less effective.[18,19] Clinically, the resulting tolerance provides a certain amount of protection for the user, such as with the respiratory depressant effects of opioids or the anesthetic effects of ethanol. However, tolerance does not develop to all physiologic drug effects; for example, in the case of opioids, tolerance to opioid-induced constipation and opioid-induced androgen deficiency does not develop over time.[20,21]

Dependence

A related consequence of chronic drug use is physiologic dependence, defined as a physiologic adaptation to the continuous presence of a drug that results in symptoms of withdrawal when the drug effect significantly diminishes or stops.[22] Physical dependence occurs not only to drugs with reward potential, such as opioids and benzodiazepines, but also to those with little or no reward potential, such as α_2-adrenergic agonists (e.g., clonidine), β-blockers, and tricyclic antidepressants. It is associated with a drug class–specific withdrawal syndrome that can be produced in persons with prolonged exposure to the drug by abrupt cessation, rapid dose reduction, decreasing blood level of the drug (e.g., due to administration of an enzyme inducing medication resulting in accelerated metabolism to the drug), and/or administration of an antagonist. When a drug blood level falls below a critical point, the adaptive changes associated with tolerance predominate and become profoundly nonadaptive.[23] Suddenly unopposed by drug effects, the sources of tolerance become evident as the characteristic drug-specific withdrawal syndrome[22,23] and a more generalized negative emotional state. Such negative emotional states include malaise, anxiety, dysphoria, emotional pain, loss of interest in natural rewards, and depression. These are common to withdrawal from all drugs of abuse, underlie drug craving and relapse, and are particularly relevant to the interface of SUD and pain.

Analgesic Effects of Drugs of Abuse

As interactions between the neurobiology of pain and SUD are considered, it is notable that many classes of abused drugs have analgesic properties, recruiting ascending and descending pain pathways to diminish the perception of pain. The opioids are defined by their direct analgesic effects, and, at high doses, alcohol is a potent anesthetic and analgesic. The sedative hypnotics, particularly benzodiazepines, are used to treat painful muscle spasms and muscle spasticity secondary to upper motor neuron damage[24] and are a standard anxiolytic adjunct for procedural sedation and analgesia.[25,26] Central nervous system stimulants, such as cocaine and caffeine, produce and potentiate analgesia, presumably by increasing neurotransmitter activity in descending inhibitory pain pathways. Notably, all drugs of abuse provide reward via activation of subcortical opioid systems, and withdrawal from these substances increases sensitivity to pain.

Of current interest are the effects of cannabinoids on pain perception. Mao and colleagues[27] have provided good preclinical evidence for an independent tetrahydrocannabinol (THC)-responsive antinociceptive pathway that is particularly effective for pain of neuropathic origin. Interference with glutamate release at the level of the dorsal root ganglia or periaqueductal gray is a hypothesized mechanism by which cannabinoids provide analgesia.[28,29] Although clinical trials of cannabinoids in multiple sclerosis have suggested an analgesic benefit,[30,31] human studies of cannabinoid-mediated analgesia have been limited by study size, heterogeneous patient populations, subjective outcome measures, and variable drug pharmacokinetics.[32] Recent meta-analyses do not support that cannabinoids effectively treat acute,[33] fibromyalgia[34] or rheumatic pain.[35] There are reports of moderate efficacy to treat cancer pain,[36,37] although insufficient evidence for its use as an adjunct in this context.[38] It is identified as a fourth-line analgesic for the management of neuropathic pain, behind the more effective antiepileptics, tricyclic antidepressants, serotonin norepinephrine reuptake inhibitors (SNRIs), and lastly opioids.[39,40] However, all reviews note that the paucity of well-controlled clinical trials on the analgesic efficacy of cannabinoids limits comprehensive evaluation of benefit.

EFFECTS OF SUBSTANCE USE DISORDER ON PAIN

SUDs bring with them physical and psychological consequences which serve to worsen or facilitate the pain experience, including autonomic arousal and negative mood states. These changes are related to both the discrete effects of certain classes of drugs and the effects of all drugs of abuse

on reward-relevant systems. For example, important psychological sequelae characteristic of SUD, including sleep and psychiatric disorders, can contribute to the experience of pain and decrease the efficacy of analgesic interventions. SUD commonly co-occurs with mood and anxiety disorders[41–43] which—if not corrected—can increase the perception of pain. Depression has been demonstrated to increase the discomfort associated with pain and to impair function in studies of patients with chronic pain, and pain symptoms frequently improve with effective antidepressant treatment, in particular the selective SNRI antidepressants which appear to have direct effects on pain pathways.[44–46]

Drug use in those with SUD is characterized by frequent and often rapid fluctuations in blood levels of the drug. Abused substances tend to be ingested in short-acting formulations and via routes with rapid onset (i.e., inhalation, intravenous [IV]) to boost psychoactive effect. These use patterns result in rapidly alternating states of intoxication and subtle (or sometimes full-blown) withdrawal. As detailed earlier, strong and persistent negative affective states accompany withdrawal from many drugs of abuse, including anhedonia, prolonged dysphoria, and irritability.[47,48] Clearly, the negative feeling states associated with drug withdrawal can augment the subjective discomfort associated with pain.

Finally, and not insignificantly, the stress associated with interpersonal conflicts, role adjustments, and social support losses that characterize the lived experience of SUD can worsen the experience of pain, making the individual less able to manage or cope with discomfort, and to interfere with effective pain treatment engagement and implementation of active pain treatment modalities. The chaotic and drug-oriented lifestyle of the sufferer make it difficult to comply with prescribed pain management regimens and engage in pain reduction activities (i.e., exercise, mindfulness meditation). Empirical support for a worsened pain experience in individuals with active SUD has been demonstrated in the case of experimental pain; subjects currently using addictive drugs are significantly less tolerant of cold-pressor (CP) pain than matched drug-free ex-abusers regardless of whether the primary drug of abuse was a stimulant (cocaine) or an opioid.[49]

The development of SUD and chronic pain appear to share epigenetic mechanisms, underscoring the interrelated nature of these phenomena. In the case of alcoholism, epigenetic modifications in the amygdala have been demonstrated to contribute to the negative affective states characteristic of the allostatic changes associated with SUD,[50] whereas cocaine intake appears to alter gene expression in reward-relevant pathways in the nucleus accumbens.[51] Such epigenetic regulation may be especially significant during windows of neurodevelopmental vulnerability (prenatal, adolescence)[52] and explain the link between early substance abuse and SUD later in life. In the case of chronic pain, there is evidence that inflammation and tissue or neural injury can induce epigenetic modifications in the central nervous system resulting in pain hypersensitivity,[53] including allodynia and hyperalgesia. Portending overlap between epigenetic mechanisms that mediate both chronic pain and SUD, Descalzi and colleagues[54] describe chronic pain-induced modifications in brain reward systems which are analogous to those induced by exposure to drugs of abuse.

EFFECTS OF OPIOID USE DISORDER ON PAIN

Because the opioid class of drug abused is also a primary pharmacologic tool for the treatment of moderate to severe clinical pain, the effects of SUD on pain become particularly significant in the case of individuals addicted to opioid drugs. As noted earlier, OUD and opioid analgesia are dependent on agonist activity at the μ-opioid receptor; the reinforcing and analgesic effects of morphine, for example, can be blocked by the administration of μ-receptor antagonists and are absent in μ-opioid receptor gene knockout animal models. In that the same receptor is central to both SUD and pain systems, it is reasonable to expect that alterations related to the latter might be evident in individuals chronically exposed to opioids (agonists or antagonists) in the context of the former. Although drug reward and analgesia are distinct processes, opioids activate their shared anatomical substrate, inducing the previously described interrelated adaptations of tolerance and dependence. Individuals with OUD may seek psychoactive effects yet are not immune to the effects of these drugs on central and peripheral opioid-relevant pain systems.

Early research in both human and animal models indicated that opioids are less rewarding in the presence of pain,[55,56] suggesting that pain interfered with the reinforcing properties of the medication. This hypothesis is supported by reports from patients who say that opioids relieve their pain without psychoactive effects; furthermore, many patients experience dysphoria or other aversive feelings, rather than euphoria, when given opioids for their pain and often stop taking them for this reason alone. Nevertheless, based on our current understanding that a subgroup of patients treated with long-term opioids for chronic pain meet diagnostic criteria for OUD, the presence of pain cannot be considered a sufficiently protective factor against reward to occur and resulting OUD, particularly in those at risk.[57,58]

Genetics of Pain and Opioid Use Disorder

Individual differences in pain perception and opioid response have long been appreciated in the clinical setting, and genetic factors, which underlie these differences, are increasingly elucidated. For example, heritable differences in hepatic P450 isoenzyme activity affect both the amount of reward and analgesia received from an opioid. Individuals who are extensive "metabolizers" of opioids (i.e., those with high P450 activity) receive less analgesia and reward from a given opioid dose[59-61] theoretically putting them at decreased risk for SUD but increased risk for unrelieved pain.[62] Preliminary data suggest that these extensive metabolizers of opioids are less tolerant of experimental pain, possibly due to defects in the endogenous synthesis of opioids.[63]

The preclinical literature, primarily from the laboratories of Mogil et al.[64,65] and Elmer et al.,[66-68] shows that recombinant murine strains differ both in their baseline tolerance for pain and in the amount of reward or reinforcement they receive from opioids. Specifically, strains of animals with poor pain tolerance (i.e., C57, CXBK) find opioids to be highly reinforcing, whereas those with good pain tolerance (i.e., BALB/c, CXBH) receive little reinforcement from opioids.[69-71] Furthermore, pain-tolerant murine strains receive robust opioid analgesia and demonstrate increased opioid receptor binding activity as compared to pain-intolerant strains.[72]

Investigators in both the pain and SUD fields have been focusing on polymorphisms in the μ-opioid gene receptor (OPRM) as candidates underlying phenotypes for pain sensitivity,[73-75] opioid analgesic response,[76] and SUD.[77,78] Best characterized is the single nucleotide polymorphism A118G of the OPRM, such that normal human subjects with the variant allele have been shown to require almost twice as high as plasma level of morphine to achieve the analgesic response as those with the nonmutated allele.[79,80] Other genes that have been linked to pain and opioid responses include those that code for the δ-opioid receptor, the capsaicin-sensing vanilloid receptor,[81] the neurotransmitter enzyme catechol-O-methyltransferase,[82] and the melanocortin-1 receptor gene.[83]

Patients with OUD may present for pain care with untreated disease (actively using illicit opioids), on MAT (methadone, buprenorphine, naltrexone), or in drug-free recovery. Principles of pain treatment for each of these groups are presented in subsequent sections of this chapter. Outlined in the following discussion are the effects of illicit or prescribed opioid agonist use on pain responses of patients with OUD.

Tolerance

Tolerance occurs differentially to opioid analgesic and rewarding effects as well as to such adverse effects as respiratory depression, sedation, nausea, sleep disturbance, or constipation. As noted earlier, the presence of tolerance does not presuppose the presence of SUD and is simply an adaptive outcome secondary to opioid exposure. Opioid tolerance can be innate due to inherent biogenetic characteristics of the individual, or it can be acquired in response to ongoing opioid exposure. Acquired opioid tolerance may be due to both pharmacokinetic factors, such as changes in drug absorption and metabolism that reduce blood concentration, and to pharmacodynamic factors such as receptor desensitization or other density changes at the level of opioid receptors.[84,85] Changes in central immune signaling and in N-methyl-D-aspartate (NMDA) receptor activity have been demonstrated in the development of opioid tolerance.[86,87] As described earlier, behavioral opioid tolerance evident in mood and affect has been attributed to opponent adaptive processes in the mesocorticolimbic reward circuitry.[88]

The incidence of analgesic tolerance in clinical settings has not been well described. Animal studies suggest that tolerance to the analgesic effects of opioids occurs in some contexts but not in others.[84] Human studies of the management of acute pain document the development of progressive tolerance to the analgesic effects of opioids when they are administered on a continuous basis over a period of several days.[89] However, over longer periods of time (weeks to months), evidence for the continuing development of progressive opioid analgesic tolerance is mixed.[90-93] Interestingly, persons on MAT for OUD do not appear to develop tolerance to the opioids; patients can remain on the same dose of methadone or buprenorphine for years without a diminution of treatment effect. However, patients with OUD, whether actively using or on agonist MAT, do clinically present with notable opioid analgesic tolerance and in cases of acute obstetric, surgical, or traumatic pain require much larger doses of opioids to achieve relief than do opioid-naive individuals.[94-96]

Physical Dependence

As is the case of opioid tolerance, physical dependence on opioids does not presume the active presence of SUD; persons with SUD on MAT are physically dependent despite being in a state of recovery, and individuals taking opioid analgesics on a regular basis can become physically dependent on medications without meeting the diagnostic criteria of SUD.[97] Common symptoms of opioid withdrawal include autonomic signs and symptoms, such as diarrhea, piloerection, sweating, mydriasis, and mild increases in blood pressure and pulse, as well as signs of central nervous system arousal such as irritability, anxiety, and sleeplessness. The character and intensity of opioid withdrawal vary, depending on the dose and duration of opioid administration and a variety of host factors, including previous experience with withdrawal, prior long-term administration of opioids, and the patient's expectations regarding withdrawal.[98] These negative emotional states and stress-like responses during withdrawal have been ascribed to diminished function of the dopamine reward system as well as activation of certain brain stress neurotransmitters, such as corticotropin-releasing factor (CRF) and dynorphin.[99]

Craving for the medication is expected in the course of withdrawal, and pain—most often experienced as abdominal cramping, deep bone pain, or diffuse muscle aching—is common.[100] Providing evidence for opioid withdrawal hyperalgesia, patients with chronic pain report intensified levels of their usual pain syndrome during withdrawal.[101–103] In patients who are physically dependent on opioids, the use of short-acting opioids may result in intermittent withdrawal between doses, which may cause an increase in perceived pain.[104,105]

Opioid-Induced Hyperalgesia

Finally, it appears that OUD brings specific hyperalgesic changes to pain systems, which can further complicate the experience and management of pain. Extensive preclinical evidence demonstrates that at the same time opioids provide potent analgesia, they paradoxically set in motion molecular processes that eventually result in OIH. OIH is defined as increased sensitivity to pain resulting from opioid administration and characterized by increase in pain sensitivity to external stimuli over time and spreading of pain to locations beyond the initial pain site. Broadly conceptualized as an opponent process, the hyperalgesia induced by opioids is theorized to counter the analgesia these drugs provide. As with tolerance and physical dependence, OIH is not diagnostic of OUD; rather, it is an outcome of ongoing opioid exposure.

OIH has been best demonstrated in animal models, wherein pain-free rodents have significantly decreased nociceptive thresholds from baseline following single or repeated administration of opioids. These preclinical studies have shown that OIH generalizes across nociceptive stimuli (thermal chemical, electrical), opioid agent (heroin, fentanyl, morphine), and route of administration (IV, subcutaneous [SC], intrathecal [IT], intraperitoneal [IP], oral). The hyperalgesia is dose dependent (cumulative dose/cumulative exposure) and appears to resolve in a time course similar to its development, with increased magnitude of response correlated to its duration. It intensifies with antagonist precipitated withdrawal and worsens with repeated withdrawal episodes.[106–110]

Links have been hypothesized to exist between the neural mechanisms responsible for the hypersensitive negative emotional states associated with OUD and OIH.[47,48] For example, evidence suggests that the stress system neuroadaptations associated with SUD may overlap with substrates of emotional aspects of pain processing in the amygdala.[15,111,112] Supporting these links, opioid (and alcohol) withdrawal in animal models produce increased anxiety-like responses and hyperalgesia, both of which are blocked by CRF antagonists.[113,114]

Withdrawal Hyperalgesia

The phenomenon of hyperalgesia has long been recognized as a fundamental symptom of the opioid withdrawal syndrome in animal models of dependence,[115–119] and although not extensively studied, hyperalgesia and spontaneous muscle and bone pain have long been considered cardinal symptoms of opioid withdrawal in humans.[11,120] The time course, opioid dose-response relationship, and opioid pretreatment parameters of withdrawal hyperalgesia have been carefully characterized in preclinical models for over 30 years, such that it arises following single or chronic opioid exposure, can be detected up to 5 days following SC injection, and increases in intensity with pretreatment opioid dose or intrinsic efficacy.[121,122]

Heightened pain perception has been observed in persons during opioid withdrawal.[123] Individuals with OUD maintained on either methadone or buprenorphine showed increased sensitivity to CP pain.[124] Indeed, Ren et al.[125] found that a hyperalgesic state can persist for up to 5 months in abstinent individuals with a history of OUD, and those with more pain sensitivity

also displayed greater cue-induced craving at follow-up. Thus, OUD individuals with poor pain tolerance may suffer a more severe form of SUD, have difficulty tolerating the discomfort (pain) inherent in detoxification and early abstinence, and be more likely to relapse.

Opioid-Induced Hyperalgesia and Tolerance

The presence of hyperalgesia with ongoing opioid use provides an alternate conceptualization of analgesic tolerance. It is clear that similar systems are involved in the evolution of OIH and of opioid tolerance; however, the clinical and neurophysiologic relationships between opioid tolerance and OIH continue to be elucidated.[16–19] As eloquently hypothesized by Colpaert[126,127] and Célèrier et al.,[128–130] that which appears to be opioid analgesic tolerance, and therefore increased opioid need, may in fact be an organismic response to an opioid-induced hypersensitivity to pain or "apparent tolerance." Essentially, opioids lose their analgesic effectiveness in the face of decreased tolerance for pain. That OIH might contribute to the phenomenon of analgesic tolerance in the clinical setting is a paradigm-shifting idea; analgesic tolerance may reflect underlying neuroadaptive changes that reflect the development of hyperalgesia.

In an important series of early preclinical studies exploring the molecular mechanisms of hyperalgesia, Mao and colleagues[131–135] demonstrated many similarities between opioid analgesic tolerance and OIH. These investigators provide credible evidence that the development of opioid analgesic tolerance via intermittent morphine dosing induces hyperalgesia, whereas animals made hyperalgesic via neuropathic injury concomitantly exhibit opioid analgesic tolerance (results replicated with heroin by Célèrier et al.[129]).

Mechanisms of Opioid-Induced Hyperalgesia

Various explanations for the development of OIH have been offered and include spinal, supraspinal, and cortical (learned) sites of action (Fig. 32.2).[121,136–142] Mao and colleagues[131,132] have demonstrated that the shared pathway for the development of morphine tolerance/hyperalgesia is activation of excitatory NMDA receptors on dorsal horn neurons, with subsequent intracellular increases in protein kinase C and nitric oxide. Like the hyperalgesia associated with neuropathic pain,[132,141] OIH is conceptualized as a variant of central sensitization and thus prevented by NMDA receptor antagonism and calcium channel blockers.[131,143–147] The latter finding has spurred interest in the potential utility of NMDA receptor antagonists (i.e., ketamine) as a means to treat OIH[148–151] and complements the ongoing work of addiction scientists on the utility of these agents to reverse opioid tolerance and dependence.[152–156]

Alternatively, Vanderah and colleagues provide good preclinical evidence[142] that opioids activate descending pain facilitation systems arising in the rostral ventromedial medulla (RVM),[143] resulting in OIH.[142,145,157] Specifically implicated are opioid-induced increases in levels of cholecystokinin (CCK), a pronociceptive peptide, in the RVM; these increased CCK levels appear to play a role in the development of opioid analgesic tolerance as well.[158] It is suggested that CCK activity in the medulla drives descending pain facilitatory mechanisms, resulting in spinal hyperalgesic responses to nociceptive input[141,142]; notably, CCK is also involved in the opioid nocebo effect of hyperalgesia.[159]

Various spinal neuropeptides, distinct from excitatory amino acid systems, have also been implicated in the development of OIH. Over a decade ago, Simonnet's laboratory showed that a single dose of parenteral heroin resulted in significant release of the antiopioid neuropeptide FF from the spinal cord in rats, an effect blocked by the subsequent administration of the opioid antagonist naloxone. This induced a hyperalgesia 30% below

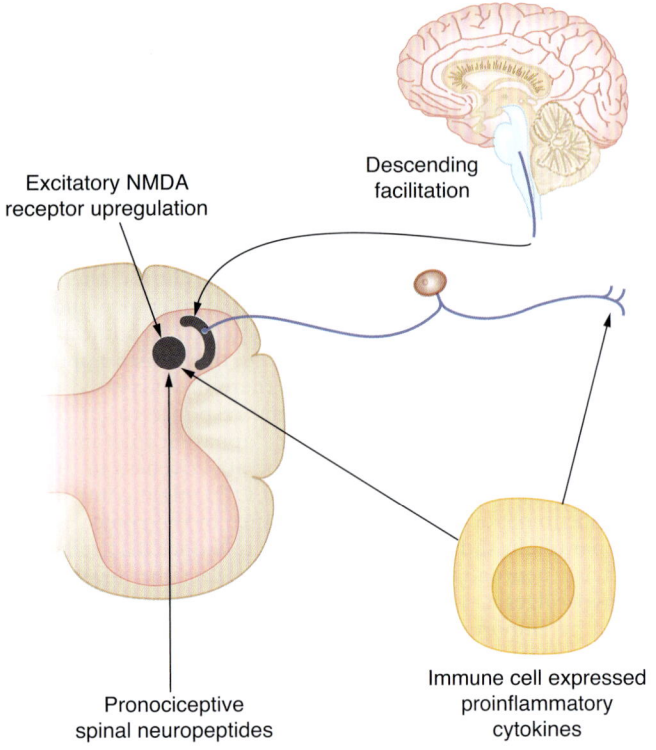

Excitatory NMDA receptor upregulation

Descending facilitation

Pronociceptive spinal neuropeptides

Immune cell expressed proinflammatory cytokines

FIGURE 32.2 Theorized mechanisms of opioid-induced hyperalgesia. *NMDA, N*-methyl-D-aspartate. *(Adapted from Angst MS, Clark JD.* Opioid-induced hyperalgesia: a qualitative systematic review. *Anesthesiology 2006; 104[3]:570–587.)*

threshold baseline.[160] More recent animal work in Porreca's laboratory has demonstrated increased levels of lumbar dynorphin, a κ-opioid agonist with pronociceptive activity, following sustained spinal opioid administration.[137,141] Interestingly, the hyperalgesic effects of opioids have been reversed by the administration of an antagonist to the neurokinin-1 receptor, which is the receptor mediating the nociceptive neuropeptide substance P. Particularly active in pain of inflammatory origin, substance P involvement suggests a neuroinflammatory component to the development of OIH.[161]

A related inflammatory mechanism mediated by neuro-immune processes has been hypothesized in the development OIH.[162] In this paradigm, peripheral immune cells activated in response to opioid administration are hypothesized to bind to astrocytes and induce specific classes of central proinflammatory (and therefore pronociceptive) cytokines, thus resulting in a state of heightened pain sensitivity.[163–168] For example, within hours of heroin or morphine administration, mice demonstrate increased serum levels of interleukin (IL)-6,[169] and splenocyte production of IL-1β, IFN-γ, IL-12, and TNF-α,[170] effects antagonized by naltrexone.[171] Proinflammatory consequences are suggested by parallel evidence for decreased expression of the anti-inflammatory cytokines, IL-10 and IL-4, following acute opioid exposure.[170,172,173] Via toll-like receptors, opioids induce proinflammatory effects on spinal glial cells, which is thought to lead to increases in cytokines in the plasma.[174,175] Reviewing the literature, Ossipov[157(p320)] commented that, "opioid-induced abnormal pain may share a molecular signature with pain of inflammatory origin."

Finally, a conditioned component to OIH was demonstrated by Siegel and colleagues more than 30 years ago.[176,177]

A robust hyperalgesia was observed in animals receiving saline in an environment previously paired with morphine administration.[176,177] This work showed that rats receiving acute morphine doses (3 to 9 doses separated by 48 hours) in a specific environment demonstrate significant hyperalgesia in the same setting as compared to rats receiving morphine unpaired with setting or saline control rats. Because conditioned responses to medications typically are opposite in direction to unconditioned drug effects, the learned responses were ascribed a causal role in the development of drug tolerance.

Clinical Evidence of Opioid-Induced Hyperalgesia

That hyperalgesic pain responses accompany OUD clinically is not a new idea. In an early essay describing his clinical observations on patients injecting morphine on a daily basis, physician and author Clifford Albutt[178] asked, "Does morphia [*sic*] tend to encourage the very pain it pretends to relieve?" He continues, "I have much reason to suspect that a reliance upon hypodermic morphia only ended in a curious state of perpetuated pain."[178] As noted, descriptions of OIH have been principally established in animal models, making it difficult to extrapolate to the clinical setting. Not only is pain a much more highly modulated experience in humans than in animals, but it is not entirely clear how pain tolerance in humans (point of subjective intolerance of pain, an indicator of hyperalgesia) maps onto putative pain threshold or perception (point at which animal withdraws tail, jumps, on hotplate) in animals. Furthermore, the development of OIH has been better characterized in animals without pain or with acute pain; thus, its effect and relevance in the common condition of chronic pain remain incompletely described.

Evidence for OIH in humans has primarily been demonstrated in three distinct populations: patients with OUD on MAT (methadone, buprenorphine), patients administered opioids during the surgical period, and healthy volunteers administered opioids acutely and then evaluated with experimental pain assays. Less common, but of increased interest in the era of the prescription opioid crisis, are data to support the presence of OIH in patients with chronic pain on opioid therapy; the degree to which prescribed opioids worsen outcomes in chronic pain patients is an important area of investigation (see Fig. 32.3 for differential diagnoses of requests for increase opioid medication).

Patients on Medication-Assisted Therapy. Over 50 years ago, Martin and Inglis[179] described significantly lower tolerance for CP-induced pain in a sample of incarcerated opioid-abusing women in comparison to matched nonaddicted controls. Ho and Dole[180] found that both methadone-maintained (MM) and drug-free opioid-addicted individuals had significantly lower thresholds for CP pain than did matched nonaddicted sibling controls. Subsequent work supports that, prior to methadone dosing, CP pain threshold (defined as time when cold sensation becomes painful) does not differ between MM and drug-free individuals with OUD but is significantly lower for MM patients in comparison to matched normal controls.[49,181,182] Under the same conditions, MM patients' CP pain tolerance (defined as time when pain becomes subjectively intolerable) is less than that in both matched drug-free patients with OUD[49] and matched controls.[181–183] With respect to perceived pain severity, Schall and colleagues[184] found no difference between MM and control subjects in their perception of pressure pain (measured on a scale of 1 to 10) immediately prior to methadone dosing.

Across nociceptive stimuli, methadone patients reliably demonstrate poor tolerance for experimental pain and are,

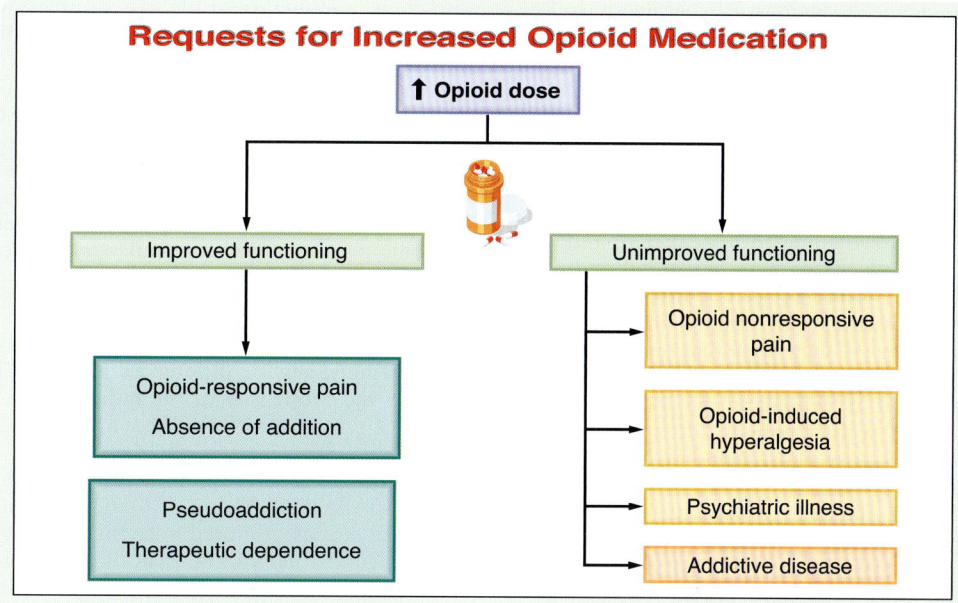

FIGURE 32.3 Differential diagnoses for patient requests for increased opioid. Pseudoaddiction refers to drug-seeking behaviors driven by unrelieved pain. Therapeutic dependence refers to drug-seeking/hoarding behaviors related to anxiety about being without.

on average, between 42% and 76%, less tolerant of CP pain than are normal controls matched on age, gender, and ethnicity.[124,181,182,185,186] Pilot data suggest that degree of hyperalgesia may vary with the intrinsic activity of the opioid maintenance agent, such that patients maintained on the partial agonist buprenorphine are less hyperalgesic than those maintained on methadone, a full agonist.[124] Note that all these data are correlational in nature, resulting in controversy as to whether or not the diminished tolerance in pain noted in persons on MAT for OUD is in fact "opioid induced" (Table 32.2). It is possible that patients prone to OUD are pain intolerant by nature, which is therefore present while on MAT.

Surgical Patients. Increasing evidence suggests that opioids administered in the intraoperative period induce postoperative hyperalgesia in patients without OUD undergoing

surgery[191–193] and perhaps in a dose-dependent manner. Data show that in patients undergoing various abdominal surgeries, postoperative reports of pain severity at rest and/or opioid consumption were significantly higher in those patients receiving IT or IV short-acting opioids (fentanyl and remifentanil) during surgery in comparison to those receiving placebo[192,193] or low-dose opioids.[191,194–196] The hyperalgesia is most pronounced early in the postoperative period (24 hours) and with high-dose remifentanil administration; patients receiving high-dose intraoperative opioids utilized approximately 18 mg more of morphine sulfate during the postoperative period and had larger margins of wound hyperalgesia than those in patients with lower intraoperative opioid exposure. The hyperalgesia was minimized if the cumulative intraoperative opioid dose was kept less than 40 µg/kg; if coadministered with ketamine,[197–199] magnesium,[200] dexmedetomidine,[201] pregabalin,[202] propofol,[203] nitrous oxide, and clonidine; or if tapered slowly. In that it is elicited with the abrupt offset of intraoperative remifentanil infusion suggests that rather than OIH, withdrawal hyperalgesia may be the source of increased sensitivity to pain. These findings have spurred current interest in evaluating opioid-sparing peri- and intraoperative procedures, such as preoperative administration of gabapentinoids; coadministration of nonopioid analgesics including nonsteroidal anti-inflammatory drugs (NSAIDs) and acetaminophen, ketamine, magnesium, propofol, nitrous oxide, and clonidine; and nonpharmacologic strategies to minimize postoperative OIH.[24,25]

Healthy Controls. Similarly, in healthy controls, remifentanil or fentanyl administered by bolus or slow (90 to 100 minutes) infusion has been shown to increase the perceived severity of experimental heat pain and CP pain 2 hours following administration and wound (electric burn or topical capsaicin) hyperalgesia from 30 minutes to 7 hours following administration. Again, in these instances, hyperalgesia was evaluated following offset of acute opioid effect; thus, it is unclear if withdrawal hyperalgesia accounted for the findings. In fact, healthy controls receiving a single dose of parenteral morphine

TABLE 32.2 Experimental Pain Responses by Opioid Use Disorder Status

	On Opioids		Drug-Free OUD	Matched Controls
Martin and Inglis[179]	—		×	< ×
Ho and Dole[180]	× <		×	= ×
Carcoba et al.[187]	—		×	< ×
Compton[49]	× <		×	—
Compton et al.[181]	× <		—	×
Liebmann et al.[188]	—		× >	×
Liebmann et al.[189]	—		× >	×
Prosser et al.[190]	—		× >	×
Pud et al.[186]	× <		—	×
Ren et al.[125]	—		×	< ×
Triester et al.[183]	× <		×	= ×

OUD, opioid use disorder; >, pain tolerance is greater than; <, pain tolerance is less than; =, pain tolerance is the same.

or hydromorphone evidenced significant hyperalgesia following an acute naloxone challenge.[123]

Patients with Chronic Pain. Reports of OIH in patients with chronic pain are much less common and are primarily limited to individuals with malignant pain. Across a number of case studies, the emergence of hyperalgesia and allodynia has been reported in cancer patients on large or rapidly escalating doses of morphine or fentanyl,[204-207] in at least one case resolving with discontinuation and switching to a weaker opioid.[208] A similar pattern of OIH induced with IT sufentanil and clearing with opioid discontinuation has been described in a single case report of a woman with chronic nonmalignant low back pain (failed back syndrome),[209] suggesting that regardless of the etiology of chronic pain (malignant vs. nonmalignant), OIH becomes evident in certain individuals in the context of high-dose opioid therapy. OIH in these patients often presents with constellation of neuroexcitatory signs, including agitation, myoclonus, and delirium.

In the case of chronic pain, few prospective studies exist. In this work, comparators typically include patients receiving low-dose opioids or placebo. As opioid dose increases (>100 mg morphine equivalent dose [MED]), hyperalgesia worsens, and "high-grade" tolerance is more likely to co-occur with OIH. There appears to be a negative correlation between OIH and opioid-derived analgesia,[210] and OIH is more robust in the presence of neuropathic, as opposed to nociceptive pain. Unknown is the degree to which the presence of chronic pain accounts for baseline hyperalgesia, which is reflected in OIH responses. Interestingly, those chronic pain patients screened at higher risk for OUD were also more likely to report increased pain sensitivity to punctuate mechanical stimuli, regardless of whether they were receiving no opioids or low- or high-dose opioids, suggesting that hyperalgesia may be less related to opioid prescription and more related to propensity for SUD.[211]

A single study by Chu and colleagues[212] demonstrated the development of OIH in a small sample of patients with chronic nonmalignant low back pain following 1 month of oral sustained-release morphine treatment (median dose 75 mg per day). In these six individuals, 30 days of morphine at therapeutic doses not only resulted in analgesic tolerance to challenge doses of remifentanil but also diminished tolerance to CP pain by almost 25% from baseline. Similarly, Suzan and colleagues[213] found that tolerance to heat pain diminished significantly following 4 weeks of oral hydromorphone therapy in patients with chronic pain, a finding that was not duplicated in matched healthy controls. In a sample of cancer patients with pain undergoing a standardized lidocaine injection, self-reported ratings of pain and unpleasantness as well as pain behaviors associated with the procedure increased by daily MED opioid dose.[214] When evaluating chronic pain patients on methadone for the treatment of OUD, Hay and colleagues[215] report diminished pain tolerance on the CP assay in both those with and without chronic pain. Most recently, a trend for increased pain severity in veterans with chronic pain assigned to receive opioid versus nonopioid therapy was reported.[216] Despite appreciating analgesia, the experimental and clinical pain responses of these patients suggest the presence of opioid-induced hyperalgesic changes.

Several structured evidence-based reviews conclude that there is insufficient evidence to determine whether clinically significant OIH occurs in the context of long-term opioid use in clinical settings.[217,218] Observational studies have long indicated that some individuals with pain who use opioids on a long-term basis experience improvement in pain after tapering or simple withdrawal of opioids,[219-222] including patients in both pain treatment and addiction treatment settings. A 2017 systematic review of patient outcomes in dose reduction or discontinuation of long-term opioid therapy suggests that pain, function, and quality of life may improve with opioid dose reduction,[223] but the degree to which these improvements can be attributed to decreased OIH is unknown.

Complicating isolating of the role of OIH in the maintenance of chronic pain is the understanding that there are many factors that may result in hyperalgesia and sensitization, including the long-term presence of pain itself and physiologic and psychological stressors such as sleep deprivation,[224] possibly mediated by aberrant glial activation.[225] In fact, some chronic pain disorders are understood as central sensitization syndromes, with hyperalgesia a typical or defining feature of these conditions (e.g., fibromyalgia).[226]

Genetics and Opioid-Induced Hyperalgesia

Interestingly, genetic differences in opioid response appear to predict the propensity of the individual to develop OIH. In a series of preclinical studies, Kest and colleagues[227] reported murine strain differences in the development of opioid tolerance and withdrawal severity,[228,229] both of which have been ascribed a role in the presentation of OIH. Liang et al.[230] evaluated 16 different strains of inbred mice for the development of thermal hyperalgesia following 4 days of morphine pretreatment and found significant variation among strains. Reduction percentage in nociceptive thresholds ranged from 4% (LP/J strain) to 36% (AJR/J strain) in these experiments, and interestingly, a strain found to be relatively pain intolerant (C57BL/6J) in previous work also developed a notable degree of hyperalgesia (24%) following chronic morphine administration.

In a related study, this investigative group evaluated the effects of chronic inflammatory pain on thermal pain perception and opioid responses across strains of mice.[231] Despite considerable variation, chronic pain induced thermal hyperalgesia and increased sensitivity to morphine analgesia across animals tested. Furthermore, following 4 days of opioid administration, those both with and without pain demonstrated dependence and tolerance, albeit with significant strain variation. Suggesting a shared mechanism for OIH, opioid tolerance, and physical dependence, haplotypic genetic analyses revealed that differential expression of a gene coding for the nonspecific P-glycoprotein transporter (Abcb1b gene) best accounted for strain-related differences in the development of thermal hyperalgesia following morphine administration.[231] Activity of this glycoprotein, which is a transporter for morphine, appears to play an important role in opioid response across domains.

Ongoing work provides evidence that OIH may arise from the epigenetic modifications associated with opioid tolerance. For example, He and Wang[232] suggest that microRNA activity regulates the expression of μ-opioid receptors, thereby interfering with both opioid analgesic and reward activity. Furthermore, to the degree that histone modification underlies the development of neuropathic pain, these mechanisms are likewise implicated in the initiation and maintenance of opioid tolerance and OIH.[109] Human studies of patients taking opioids for the treatment of OUD or chronic pain suggest that opioid-induced DNA methylation is related to increased chronic pain severity, which at the level of the patient is expressed as OIH.[54,233]

Pain Management in Persons with Substance Use Disorder

Consideration of the physiologic bases of pain and SUD, and how they overlap, provides direction for the management of pain in this population. Clearly, the human experiences of pain and SUD are not separate but interrelated; knowledgeable management of the former must reflect the extent to which, even at the physiologic level, its expression and response are affected by the latter.

Patients with SUD may present for pain management in different phases or states of the disorder; for example, they may be actively using drugs of abuse and not engaged in treatment; they may be in MAT taking an opioid agonist (methadone), partial agonist (buprenorphine), or antagonist (naltrexone) for the treatment of the disorder; or they may be in drug-free recovery with variable engagement in SUD treatment. The pain requiring management may be of acute, perioperative, cancer, or nonmalignant chronic origin. Each of these different situations requires slightly different pharmacologic and nonpharmacologic approaches to provide relief; however, the overall guiding principles remain the same. These include effective treatment of pain; avoiding potential withdrawal; utilization of opioid-sparing approaches; reinforcement or introduction of SUD treatment, including relapse prevention strategies; careful documentation of treatment plan; and active involvement of the patient and family in the plan of care.

PREVALENCE OF SUBSTANCE USE DISORDERS IN PATIENTS WITH PAIN

In light of the well-publicized links between opioids prescribed for chronic pain and the current opioid crisis, the true prevalence of SUD in patients with pain has received increased scrutiny. As noted earlier, current estimates indicate that the population prevalence of SUD is approximately 8%,[1] suggesting that 1 in every 12 patients encountered suffers from active disease. However, these data do not reflect the patients whose disease is in good control or remission, but at constant risk for relapse, especially in the face of the stressors associated with pain (loss of work and family roles, social isolation, depression). Furthermore, related to the toxic effects of abused substances on body tissues, the risky behaviors in which sufferers may engage, and the high rates of comorbid psychiatric disease, persons with SUD are highly likely to present to medical settings and therefore requiring pain care. Although one cannot state with certainty how many patients with pain have a history of SUD, these factors suggest that it should be assessed in all patients presenting with a need for pain management.

Most evaluations of SUD in pain patients have focused on those with chronic nonmalignant pain (CNMP) receiving opioid therapy. Early studies in the 1900s led to a perception that iatrogenic addiction through the medical use of opioids was a very frequent occurrence,[234,235] whereas a number of retrospective surveys in the 1980s of never-addicted medical patients suggested that the development OUD in the course of long-term opioid therapy for pain was negligible,[236,237] leading to an underappreciation of the risks and overprescribing of opioids. Albeit not evidence based, recent guidelines regarding long-term opioid therapy for chronic pain are based on the assumption that any exposure to opioid medication for pain may increase the risk of developing OUD,[92,93] which is an oversimplification of the complexity of pain and SUD.

Studies on the incidence and prevalence of SUD in the context of chronic pain treatment have generally examined a wide variety of "aberrant behaviors" rather than specifically assessing for SUD. In addition, many studies that assess opioid use and misuse in pain populations excluded the highest risk group, those with a prior history of SUD, or were sampled from pain clinics which tend to have a disproportion of patients engaging in aberrant drug-related behaviors (ADRB). A 2008 structured clinical review sought to estimate the risk of development of a clinically significant SUD in the course of long-term opioid therapy of pain and to distinguish these from misuse or ADRBs.[238] The review identified 67 scientifically acceptable studies of opioid use and misuse and divided them into those that excluded persons with history of SUD and those that identified "aberrant behaviors" versus those in which clinicians more formally identified *Diagnostic and Statistical Manual of Mental Disorders* (4th ed.; *DSM-IV*)–defined SUD. The review found that across these studies, in patients with no history of SUD, the risk of de novo opioid SUD was 0.19% and the risk of ADRBs was 0.59%. In studies

that included persons with a history of SUD, the risk of OUD was 3.27%, whereas the risk of ADRBs was 11.9%. The review also examined five studies that included urine drug screening and found that up to 20% of samples had unexpected findings, suggesting that actual rates of ADRBs and SUD may be higher than suggested based on behavioral observation and clinical assessment and supporting the value of urine drug screening in identifying misuse or addiction in the context of opioid therapy.

More recently, Boscarino and colleagues[57] assessed patients with CNMP receiving long-term opioid therapy within a large US health care system for diagnosis of OUD using the *DSM* (5th ed.; *DSM-5*) criteria. In their population, the lifetime prevalence of OUD by *DSM-5* was 41.3%, with 28.1% for mild symptoms, 9.7% for moderate symptoms, and 3.5% for severe symptoms. Campbell et al.[239] examined the prevalence of OUD in patients on opioid therapy for CNMP according to International Classification of Diseases , 11th revision (ICD-11), *DSM-5*, and the pain medicine concept of "addiction" (defined as behavior including one or more of the following: impaired control over drug use, compulsive use, continued use despite harm, and cravings).[240] Past 12-month prevalence was 19% for ICD-11, 18% for *DSM-5*, and 24% for "addiction," with "substantial" concordance between "addiction" and both *DSM-5* use disorder and ICD-11 dependence, noting that the definition of "addiction" captures a larger group of patients than other classification systems and includes people with fewer "risk" behaviors.[239] One could also argue that the criteria for establishing a diagnosis of OUD in both the *DSM-IV* and *DSM-5* are not completely applicable to patients receiving long-term opioid therapy. Well-conducted meta-analyses of the literature support that estimates of SUD in the chronic pain populations hover at 8% to 10%,[97] not unlike the past year rates of SUD in the US population in general (7.8%),[1] suggesting that the same factors that put an individual at risk for developing SUD (family history, psychiatric comorbidity, early onset of use) are also involved in the development of the same in persons with chronic pain and receiving opioid therapy.[8,241,242]

Conversely, the prevalence of pain among persons with SUDs may be significantly higher than that of the general population, with studies suggesting that up to 50% to 60% of patients on MAT report chronic pain, in which 25% to 35% of cases, the pain is rated as severe.[243,244] Higher severity of chronic pain in patients with SUD is associated with more chronic illness; poorer psychosocial, physical, and social functioning; and high rates of mental illness (primarily major depression).[245–251] The presence of chronic pain portends poorer OUD treatment outcomes, such that patients with pain are more likely to engage in continued polydrug use, require higher doses of methadone, experience higher ratings of opioid craving, and are more likely to relapse to opioid use.[252–254] Persons with alcohol and other SUDs are vulnerable to traumatic injury,[255] which may contribute to a relatively higher prevalence of chronic pain in persons with SUD.[256]

PRINCIPLES OF PAIN TREATMENT IN PATIENTS WITH SUBSTANCE USE DISORDERS

Principles of care for the patient with pain and a history of SUD include the provision of thoughtful and effective pain treatment, including the accommodation of opioid tolerance and avoidance of withdrawal when present and an emphasis on opioid-sparing approaches. In addition, directly addressing the presence or history of SUD is necessary to optimize pain outcomes. Finally, critical to effective pain management in this population is the development of a clearly documented pain treatment plan, including the involvement of the patient, family, and addiction treatment providers as possible.

Provide Effective Pain Relief

For acute, perioperative, and chronic pain, treatment approaches are increasingly utilizing effective multimodal nonopioid- or opioid-sparing regimens, which should be heavily relied on to provide pain relief for those with SUD. In general, these include utilization of nonpharmacologic interventions including heat, cold, massage, bracing and stretching, and behavioral interventions such as distraction, graded exercise, cognitive-behavioral therapy (CBT), and relaxation or mindfulness-based meditation. Nonopioid pharmacotherapies focus on around-the-clock use of acetaminophen or NSAIDs, with more specific medication adjuvants utilized for specific pain indications (described in the following discussion). In some cases, regional procedures with lidocaine or steroid injections can be an important component of the pain management plan. Increasingly, peripheral nerve blockade and regional anesthesia are temporarily continued during the initial phase of the postoperative period to reduce the need for systemic analgesia.[257,258]

It is important that patients with SUD who are experiencing pain receive adequate pain control in an effective and timely manner. Without adequate pain control, development of a therapeutic alliance is thwarted, and it is unlikely that the patient will be motivated or able to effectively engage in SUD or pain treatment. In addition, undertreated pain may create craving for pain-relieving medications as well as anxiety, frustration, anger, and other negative affect states that worsen pain and fuel drug seeking. Persons with a history of SUD have valid concerns that their reports of pain will not be believed; therefore, reassurance and actions to indicate otherwise are especially important with this patient population.

Acute Pain

As described in the following discussion, an acute painful event can provide a golden opportunity for motivational interviewing toward change. Hospitalization for a traumatic event or surgery can provide the patient respite from the drug-using lifestyle and an opportunity to connect with supportive others. Referral to treatment can be provided prior to discharge, and in some acute care settings, patients can be introduced to addiction specialists and interventions while hospitalized. For patients on MAT or in drug-free recovery, aggressive management of acute pain is likewise important to support treatment efforts and gains. Underscoring this need, acute pain exposure has been negatively correlated to SUD treatment retention related in part to insufficient pain relief.[242] Key strategies for managing acute pain in patients with SUD are outlined in Table 32.3.

Patients using opioids (prescribed or illicit) or on opioid agonist (methadone) or partial agonist (buprenorphine) MAT present with opioid tolerance and hyperalgesia, thus will require higher doses of opioids to provide anesthesia and analgesia than the opioid-naive patient. In that opioid withdrawal is likely to aggravate hyperalgesia, these patients must have their baseline opioid requirements met to avoid the emergence of withdrawal.[95,259,260] For those abusing prescribed or illicit opioids, the average baseline daily dose of opioid therapy should be determined or estimated and either the same drug provided at that dose or an alternative opioid provided at a lower than calculated equianalgesic dose. It is permissible under the US Controlled Substances Act to provide opioids to prevent withdrawal in a patient who is hospitalized for a diagnosis other than SUD. For example, if a patient with heroin use disorder is hospitalized for subacute bacterial endocarditis, the treating physician can legally provide opioid medications, including methadone, to prevent withdrawal, as well as additional medications for pain. Although opioids for pain treatment can be continued after discharge, opioids cannot be provided for treatment of SUD after discharge, except from a federally licensed methadone maintenance treatment program or from a federally certified/waivered buprenorphine provider.[261]

TABLE 32.3   Key Strategies for Managing Acute and Perioperative Pain in Patients with Substance Use Disorder

General Principles

Complete a thorough substance use history.
Consult state prescription drug monitoring program (PDMP) to determine use of controlled substances.
Believe and aggressively treat complaints of pain.
Consider effective pain management as an opportunity to introduce or support recovery.
Include patient and family in the pain management plan (from admission to discharge).
Initiate multidisciplinary liaisons (i.e., pain medicine, psychiatry, addiction medicine, nursing, social work).
If physically dependent on opioids, sedative hypnotics, or alcohol, utilize long-acting formulations as possible to avoid withdrawal.
Emphasize multimodal, opioid-sparing approaches.
   Ketamine, NSAIDs, acetaminophen, selective cyclooxygenase-2 (COX-2) inhibitors
   Local and regional analgesia techniques including wound infiltration, regional, or neuroaxial block
   Nonpharmacologic interventions including heat, cold, massage, bracing and stretching, and behavioral interventions such as distraction, graded exercise, cognitive-behavioral therapy, and relaxation or mindfulness-based meditation
When opioids are needed
   Utilize immediate release formulations.
   Utilize PCA to enable self-titration and minimize perceived drug-seeking behaviors or cues.
   As pain resolves, cautiously taper opioids with close observation.
If using opioids (licit or illicit) or on medication-assisted therapy (MAT; methadone, buprenorphine)
   Anticipate opioid tolerance or hyperalgesia, thus higher opioid dose requirements to appreciate analgesia.
   Avoid emergence of opioid withdrawal.
If on MAT (methadone, buprenorphine)
   Verify MAT dose with treatment clinic or provider.
   Avoid switching from MAT agent to another opioid to manage physical dependence.
When opioids are needed
   Titrate opioids to effect.
   Monitor closely for toxicity and have naloxone readily available.
   Use opioids other than MAT opioid to treat pain, *or*
   If plan to use MAT opioid to treat pain, split to BID or TID dosing.
   As pain resolves, bring the patient back to the usual MAT dose.
If on MAT (naltrexone)
   Expect no opioid analgesic effect until antagonist dissociates from receptor.
   Expect receptor supersensitivity to opioids following offset of naltrexone effect, thus increased risk for toxicity.
   For oral naltrexone, discontinue 72 h prior to planned procedures.
   For severe pain, regional or general anesthesia may be required.

BID, two times a day; NSAIDs, nonsteroidal anti-inflammatory drugs; PCA, patient-controlled analgesia; TID, three times a day.

Not uncommonly, the patient with SUD will be abusing more than one substance. A patient physically dependent on alcohol or sedative-hypnotic medications (either from long-term medically appropriate prescribing or alternatively from SUD) should have withdrawal symptoms treated when they occur in the course of pain treatment. Unrecognized alcohol or sedative-hypnotic withdrawal will make pain control difficult to achieve, and physical signs of withdrawal (such as hypertension and tachycardia) may be misinterpreted as reflecting acute pain. The short-term use of a long-acting benzodiazepine may be used for treatment of withdrawal symptoms; however, the combination of benzodiazepines with opioid medication greatly increases the risk of respiratory depression and fatal overdose, and the concurrent prescription should be avoided whenever possible.[92,93]

For patients with SUD, multimodal opioid-sparing techniques should be emphasized. In addition to acetaminophen or NSAIDs, ketamine administered in a low dose as a continuous IV or SC infusion has been demonstrated to treat acute pain for the hospitalized patient on MAT. Recommended dosing regimens include a starting dose of 100 to 200 mg over 24 hours, using a mixture of 200 mg ketamine and 5 mg midazolam made up to a total volume of 48 mL with normal saline and a rate of infusion of 1 to 2 ml per hour or 0.1 mg/kg/hour.[94,262] A regional anesthetic blockade should be implemented where possible.[263]

If opioids are required, immediate-release (IR) opioids can be utilized, titrated to analgesic effect and ideally administered via patient-controlled analgesia (PCA) to enable self-titration and minimize perceived drug-seeking behaviors or cues.[264] When used in addition to MAT (methadone, buprenorphine), it is important to remain vigilant for signs of toxicity with naloxone readily available should these emerge. Supplementation with a different opioid for acute pain has been recommended, as the use of the same medication for SUD and for acute pain management may confuse the issues of pain treatment and SUD treatment when the acute pain resolves, and it is time to taper the analgesic. If managed appropriately (see the following discussion), there is no evidence that opioids provided for acute pain exacerbate or worsen OUD outcomes, and as noted earlier, there is concern that untreated pain may precipitate relapse.

For those on opioid MAT (methadone or buprenorphine), it is important that the maintenance MAT dose be continued during pain treatment, which should be verified with the MAT provider; the state prescription drug monitoring program (PDMP) should also be consulted to determine if other opioids are being consumed. If the methadone dose cannot be confirmed, it is safest initially to give the patients reported dose in three or four divided doses of no greater than 30 mg total per day, so that doses can be modified according to patient response. Although both methadone and buprenorphine have intrinsic analgesic properties, the daily dosing regimen for OUD only treats the symptoms of withdrawal and craving, thus cannot be considered as providing any measurable pain relief. Patients on methadone should be continued on methadone rather than being switched to an alternative opioid; there is incomplete cross-tolerance of methadone with other μ-agonists, and methadone withdrawal has been observed in some patients despite calculated equianalgesic doses of alternative μ-agonists. In recognition of the significant risk of relapse in patients with OUD, in experienced hands, titration of methadone for acute pain can be effective, and dosage splitting to BID or TID dosing or an additional lower dose later in the day may be used as a strategy to provide analgesia around the clock.[265,266]

Strategies for managing acute pain in individuals with prescribed buprenorphine are emerging as experience accumulates. Buprenorphine binds tightly to the opioid receptor and thus tends to block the action of other opioids; thus, it is sometimes challenging to obtain analgesia by adding another opioid.[267] μ-Opioids can usually be titrated to higher doses to overcome the buprenorphine blockade; use of IV fentanyl or IV or oral hydromorphone, which bind with relatively high affinity to μ-opioid receptors, is often recommended, although morphine and others have been used effectively.[268] Opioid titration in this setting should be done by an experienced clinician with close monitoring of the patient with naloxone available. When acute pain can be predicted in persons on buprenorphine, such as after elective surgery, some experts suggest discontinuing buprenorphine a few days prior to surgery.[269–271] However, other experts note the challenges of reinducing patients on buprenorphine once acute pain has resolved and report good results with continuation of buprenorphine and titration of an alternative opioid to achieve analgesia in the same manner as for unanticipated acute pain.[272] Early recommendations that patients on

buprenorphine be rotated to methadone or other full agonists (fentanyl or morphine) to enable more predictable IR opioid-analgesic response appear unnecessary and may expose the patient to greater risk of withdrawal or relapse than continuing the usual buprenorphine dose. Alternatively, a patient on a low-dose buprenorphine (2 to 8 mg per day) may receive acceptable analgesia from a temporarily increased daily dose administered BID to achieve around-the-clock analgesia. Because of its partial agonist properties and its near full receptor occupancy at relatively low doses, buprenorphine has traditionally been thought to have a ceiling effect for analgesia[94]; however, this view has been challenged by recent studies and observations.[273,274]

Patients on naltrexone MAT present a particular challenge if opioid analgesia is required. There have been no clinical studies to guide opioid dosing or efficacy. It can be expected that patients will receive little to no opioid analgesia while opioid receptors are fully occupied; however, as the naltrexone formulation approaches half-life, case studies suggest that pain relief can be appreciated, and patients may even be supersensitive to opioid effects related to receptor resetting with antagonist treatment.[262] It has been demonstrated that the competitive blockade of naltrexone can be overcome with opioid agonists, but the required doses are on the order of 10 to 20 times the usual doses by weight.[94] This becomes particularly hazardous as naltrexone dissociates from the opioid receptor and subsequent receptor supersensitivity puts the patient at risk for opioid toxicity. Close monitoring and availability of naloxone become paramount when opioids are provided to those receiving naltrexone MAT. If IR opioid administration cannot override the receptor blockade, in cases of severe pain, patients on naltrexone therapy may require general or regional anesthesia.

For patients who were in drug-free recovery prior to the acute pain experience, it is critical that opioids provided for pain are tapered cautiously with close observation prior to discharge; nonopioid analgesics and strategies should be used early on and continued as clinically indicated after discontinuation of opioid analgesics. The emergence of withdrawal symptoms can precipitate relapse; thus, these should be assessed and managed aggressively. If the opioid taper is anticipated to continue after discharge, dosing should be highly structured on a scheduled basis with supervised dispensing of medication or issuing in short-term intervals. In addition, links to recovery resources, such as a sponsor or counselor, should be initiated to help the patient remain abstinent following discharge. It is important to note that tapering and discontinuation of opioids used for pain can be legally supervised by any clinician with a Drug Enforcement Administration (DEA) license; however, detoxification from opioids as a component of addiction treatment can only be done by a waivered buprenorphine provider or federally licensed methadone maintenance treatment center.

Perioperative Pain

Related to the general health consequences associated with addiction behaviors, patients with SUD are likely to suffer acute painful conditions (i.e., dental, infections, trauma), which may require surgical intervention. In that opioids have been a mainstay in the perioperative setting, utilized both intraoperatively and postoperatively to manage pain, providing pain care for patients with SUD undergoing surgical procedures requires mention. Although no specific practice guidelines exist to address surgical pain-relief interventions in this population, the general principles outlined earlier can be implemented.

Preoperative Management. Preoperative substance use assessment is critical to effective anesthesia and postoperative analgesia. Types and amounts of substances abused should be evaluated. If the patient is on MAT, the dose should be verified with the provider and the PDMP consulted. It is also important to determine if the patient is regularly using benzodiazepines or alcohol to avoid/manage associated withdrawal syndromes. The patient and family should be included in the management plan (admission to discharge) as well as other health care professionals (i.e., pain medicine, psychiatry, nursing, social work).[275]

If the patient on MAT will be NPO for greater than 24 hours postsurgery, plans to convert the patient from oral methadone or buprenorphine to IV equivalent should be instituted. Methadone can be administered parenterally; doses of half to two-thirds of the total daily oral dose can be given in three to four divided doses by intermittent intramuscular or SC injection or by continuous infusion.[265,276] Some clinicians opt to convert to morphine or another full agonist first, and when performing an opioid rotation, it is recommended to reduce the calculated equianalgesic dose by 30% to 50% due to the possibility of incomplete cross-tolerance.[277] Although it has been suggested that patients on buprenorphine be rotated to methadone prior to surgery,[278] there is no evidence that this improves pain management as opposed to keeping on their usual MAT. Others recommend that patients on higher dose buprenorphine maintenance (i.e., 16 mg to 32 mg per day) be titrated down to 12 mg per day prior to surgery to minimize potential dose-dependent opioid antagonism effects. If possible, it is recommended that oral naltrexone be discontinued 72 hours prior to surgery so that opioids can be utilized if necessary[276]; however, this becomes impractical for patients on naltrexone XR or with unplanned procedures. In these cases, nonopioid approaches that should be utilized in all patients become essential.

Intraoperative Management. As noted, baseline opioid, alcohol, or benzodiazepine requirements should be met, and if on methadone or buprenorphine, the usual prescribed MAT dose be taken on the day of surgery using a take-home dose provided by the MAT provider. Effective multimodal opioid-sparing anesthetic techniques, which differ across surgical procedures,[279] are highly recommended and may include preemptive administration of acetaminophen, celecoxib, or pregabalin; preloading the incision sites with local anesthetic before incision; and placement of an epidural catheter for intraoperative and postoperative use. Local and regional analgesia techniques are preferred when suitable. If opioids are used, higher opioid requirements can be anticipated due to tolerance and hyperalgesia; in spontaneously breathing patients, maintaining a respiratory rate of 12 to 14 can be used as a guide.[95] Instillation of long-acting lidocaine in the surgical wound prior to closure has been shown to significantly decrease pain and opioid requirement for several days following surgery. Local anesthetic techniques include wound infiltration or regional or neuroaxial block; local anesthetic catheters can prolong the benefits of regional anesthesia into the postoperative period.[278]

Postoperative Management. Postoperative pain management should proceed for acute pain as outlined above, with the goals of providing effective analgesia while maintaining opioid coverage as needed and relying on multimodal, opioid-sparing approaches as possible. Nonopioid analgesics, including around-the-clock NSAIDs, acetaminophen, and selective cyclooxygenase-2 (COX-2) inhibitors, as well as ketorolac administration,[263,276] can be utilized; these are available in parenteral and other forms of administration and associated with a reduction in postoperative opioid use and improved analgesia. Less well-tested agents include clonidine and dexmedetomidine, which elicit analgesia by agonism of the α-adrenergic receptor, and gabapentin and pregabalin, which inhibit pain transmission via binding to the $\alpha_2\delta$-1 subunit of voltage-gated calcium channels.[280] Regional blockade with local anesthetics can be useful in the early postoperative period because it theoretically

removes the need for additional systemic analgesia; although neuroaxial opioids allow for lower doses of opioid exposure, these may not prevent opioid withdrawal, and additional systemic opioids are often required[257]; furthermore, it may be difficult to estimate an appropriate or safe dose.

When regional analgesia is not applicable and/or IR opioids are indicated, an IV PCA administration system is highly recommended because it allows for individual dose titration and reduces workload for staff. Related to opioid tolerance and hyperalgesia, doses that are higher than those usually prescribed may be needed (including higher PCA bolus dose) for those on physically dependent on opioids. Similarly, it can be anticipated that their pain scores will be higher and decrease more slowly and that review and adjustment of dosing will be required more frequently. Several studies indicate that after a variety of surgical procedures, first 24-hour PCA morphine requirements were, on average, three times greater in the opioid-tolerant than opioid-naive patients. Determining the appropriate setting of bolus size and lockout interval may be challenging; one recommended method is to begin with the patient's usual 24-hour opioid requirement and base the size of the bolus dose at 50% of the hourly background infusion rate with a 5-minute lockout. Concerns that IR opioid provision may result in respiratory depression in patients with OUD are not supported by clinical experience, likely related to the development of cross-tolerance; however, evidence of opioid toxicity should be carefully monitored for and naloxone made readily available.

As postoperative pain subsides, it is important to bring the patient on methadone or buprenorphine therapy back to the usual MAT dose as soon as possible. Similarly, for those who were in drug-free recovery prior to the surgical experience, a gradual taper of opioids with recovery supports initiated or strengthened is critical to the maintenance of abstinence.[275]

Progressive Cancer-Related or Terminal Pain

Early studies reported low rates (5%) of SUD in oncology patients,[281–283] whereas more recent examination of Medicare data found that the prevalence of SUD in men with advanced prostate cancer to be 10.6%,[284] and another review found an OUD prevalence rate of 7.7% in patients with cancer pain of all types.[285] Increased rates of oncologic disease in patients with AUD are suspected due to the known injurious effects of abused substances on cells and body tissues. Inflammatory or other repair responses to cellular injury can result in DNA mutations that play a role in inducing neoplastic changes. A chart review of 598 patients with advanced cancers found that 17% were positive for *DSM-IV* (text revised; *DSM-VI-TR*)–defined AUD on the cut down, annoyed, guilty and eye-opener (CAGE) screening tool, and only 13% were identified as with the same diagnosis before their palliative care consultation.[286] They were also more likely to be taking potent opioids at the time of referral than patients who screened negative for SUD. Although not diagnostic, 39% to 43% of cancer patients on opioids scored as medium to high risk for *DSM-IV*–defined opioid abuse on standard opioid abuse screening tools.

Treatment of advanced cancer-related pain in the patient with addictive disease is usually similar to that in the person without addictive disease; the comfort of the patient should be the primary goal. Opioids generally should not be withheld in patients with terminal illness when they are needed and effective because of concerns regarding addiction. However, if SUD-related problems are diminishing the patient's quality of life, it can be necessary to maximize external controls (e.g., having medications dispensed daily by others) and to insist on concomitant SUD recovery work or to rely on nonopioid treatments.[287,288]

Cancer may be accompanied by significant distress arising from fear, grief over impending losses, depression, anger, and spiritual conflict, which patients may try to self-medicate with opioids. However, in the case of the patient with SUD, such use causes further declines in function and quality of life. Directed, evidence-based nonpharmacologic and pharmacologic means of addressing such stressors should be employed. For many individuals in SUD recovery, appropriate resources may provide meaningful support. Therefore, it is helpful for the clinician to assess the patient's experience with recovery and to help sustain participation in or reengaging with recovery groups, sponsors, and programs if these have been meaningful to the individual in the past.[5]

Chronic Nonmalignant Pain

As promulgated by the recent Centers for Disease Control and Prevention (CDC) guideline for prescribing opioids for chronic pain[92] and U.S. Department of Veterans Affairs/U.S. Department of Defense (VA/DoD) guidelines for opioid therapy in patients with chronic pain[93] and for low back pain,[289] it is increasingly appreciated that opioids are not first-line therapy for the management of CNMP, and that in some cases, functionality improves when opioids are tapered. The VA/DoD opioid guideline provides a strong recommendation against initiation of long-term opioid therapy; if opioids are prescribed for patients with CNMP, a short duration is recommended.[93] This is particularly pertinent in the case of patients with a history of SUD. Conceptualized as a chronic illness for which complete remission is not expected, nonpharmacologic approaches become central to the treatment of CNMP and include evidence-based interventions such as acupuncture, physical therapy, transcutaneous electrical nerve stimulation (TENS), graded exercise, weight loss, cognitive-behavioral/acceptance therapy, mindfulness mediation, and yoga. Non-opioid pharmacotherapies with demonstrated efficacy are the NSAIDs and acetaminophen; the anticonvulsants gabapentin and pregabalin; and the SNRIs, duloxetine and venlafaxine. Certain tricyclic antidepressants have also been recommended but are typically less useful due to associated adverse side effects. These same strategies are indicated for chronic pain patients with SUD; in fact, several of these (acupuncture, CBT, mindful meditation, antidepressants) are likely to provide support for recovery efforts.

However, there is a subpopulation of patients with chronic pain whose functionality and quality of life improve with opioid therapy, at least temporarily, which may include patients on MAT and in stable recovery (patients with active SUD are never candidates for opioid therapy as controlled use and functional improvements will not be realized). Although there is scant data supporting the efficacy of high-dose opioids in patients with CNMP, there is evidence that low-dose opioids in well-selected patients can be beneficial.[290] In veterans with chronic pain assigned to receive opioid versus nonopioid therapy over 1 year, there was no therapeutic advantage of opioids over those receiving NSAIDs or acetaminophen, although the opioid group reported a higher side effect burden.[216] In general, it is now believed that long-term opioid therapy likely carries greater risks than benefits in most patients and risks increase with duration and dosage, which may be particularly high in patients with SUD.[93] Risk mitigation strategies utilized for all patients with CNMP on opioid therapy, including the use of treatment agreements and/or written informed consents, random urine toxicology, and monitoring of PDMPs, should be implemented. Because patients with a history of SUD are at high risk for relapse, opioid provision to these patients requires expansion of the chronic pain treatment plan to include the integration of relapse prevention strategies, frequent assessment for evidence of misuse, and the expectation that they maintain good standing and engagement in addiction treatment.[291] Due to ongoing opioid blockade, opioid provision is not an option for patients on naltrexone MAT.

TABLE 32.4 Risk Mitigation Strategies for Opioid Prescription for Chronic Nonmalignant Pain[92,93]
• Comprehensive pain assessment
• Assessment of risk for opioid misuse
• Formulation of a differential diagnosis of contributing factors to pain
• Informed consent for treatment following risk–benefit discussion
• Documentation of a clear plan of treatment
• Initiation of opioid therapy as a trial with clear goals
• Reassessment of pain, level function, quality of life, and adherence to plan of care
• Urine drug testing (UDT) prior to opioid prescribing and routinely during opioid therapy at random intervals
• Querying state prescription drug monitoring programs (PDMP) prior to opioid prescribing and routinely during opioid therapy in concordance with state and federal guidelines
• Documentation of decision making and care
• Opioid overdose education and prescribing of naloxone rescue medication

Because the risk of opioid misuse for a given patient cannot be absolutely determined, it is prudent to view all patients who consume opioids as having some level of risk and to employ a set of universal precautions (Table 32.4).[92,93,292–294] With respect to assessment of risk for opioid misuse, it is important to be aware that no screening tools have been specifically validated for use in populations with identified SUDs. Although not a screen for risk per se, the Addiction Behaviors Checklist (ABC)[295] or Prescription Drug Use Questionnaire (PDUQ)[296] can be used to track behaviors of concern between clinic visits. Another promising tool to detect opioid misuse is the Current Opioid Misuse Measure (COMM), which has demonstrated 77% specificity and 77% sensitivity in identifying current prescription OUD in a primary care setting.[297] These tools assess risk of ADRB which is not necessarily a surrogate for SUD but can also reflect undertreatment of pain or self-treatment of concomitant mood, anxiety, or sleep disorders. Due to the limitations associated with the predictive and concurrent validity associated with these screeners, composite indices have also been described combining scores from tools with urine toxicology results. For example, Jamison and colleagues created the Aberrant Drug Behavior Index (ADBI) and the Drug Misuse Index (DMI) which combine PDUQ or ABC scores with urine toxicology to predict relative risk.[298] With respect to naloxone provision to persons using opioids for analgesia, a small survey study of veterans on opioids for chronic pain indicated that they underestimated their risk for opioid overdose.[299] Importantly, 21% reported having previously experienced an opioid overdose, and most desired a naloxone rescue kit to enhance their safety.[300]

Making opioids available in quantities that relieve pain, while not inviting misuse, may be a key factor in successful opioid therapy for pain in persons with SUD. The number of units of opioid medications available to the patient and the frequency with which they are dispensed are two variables that can be controlled. In persons with SUD, it is prudent to dispense smaller quantities more frequently, sometimes weekly, or even daily. Frequent dispensing of small doses can also preserve safety by ensuring that the patient does not have a potentially lethal supply of medications available. For patients at risk for OUD, transdermal buprenorphine for pain, which requires only weekly changes and may pose less risk of respiratory suppression if misused, may be a good option that allows close monitoring, even weekly dispensing of single patches. Also, oral buprenorphine with or without naloxone is effective in patients not currently using opioids in controlling acute pain[301,302] and thus may be advantageous to full μ-agonists in patients with history or at risk of OUD. Keeping the total dose dispensed sublethal may be an important strategy in some patients, but no method fully protects a patient who is at risk for major overuse. Frequent dispensing can be done by a pharmacy, a clinician's office, or a trusted other such as a family member, although care must be taken that this does not interfere with personal relationships that sustain the social support system needed by patients.

Several recent studies have suggested that, with the addition of structure and active programs to address substance misuse, opioid analgesia can be brought under control in some patients who demonstrate ADRBs and substance misuse. A US VA study utilized consultations with clinical pharmacists, signing of second-chance agreements, and simple limit-setting interventions (e.g., more frequent visits, limited supplies of opioids, urine toxicology screening) in patients manifesting ADRBs. Of those referred for this consultation, 45% were able to remain in pain management and had their behavior come under reasonable control, whereas about 38% self-discharged, indicating the likelihood of SUD among other issues (see Fig 32.3).[303] Another study of persons with active substance misuse and pain demonstrated that intensive psychological interventions, including adherence monitoring, motivational techniques, and cognitive-behavioral techniques added to a methadone-based pain management program led to a diminution in use of nonprescribed opioids and trends toward decreases in nonopioid drug use.[304] And a third study of patients with chronic pain and opioid misuse behaviors found that the addition of substance and motivational counseling, compliance checklists, and regular toxicology screening to standard care reduced the prevalence of drug misuse among high-risk, drug-misusing patients to that of low-risk patients receiving standard care.[298]

Reinforce or Introduce Substance Use Disorder Treatment

An open and nonjudgmental approach to the discussion of substance use concerns facilitates information exchange with patients; often, health professionals discuss concerns about a patient's substance use among themselves, without bringing the patient into the discussion. When SUD is understood as a medical disorder, it becomes easier to address it in the same manner as any other medical condition, with respectful and nonjudgmental, but matter-of-fact, concern. Patients with SUD often justifiably fear that awareness of their problem will negatively affect the manner in which their providers approach their care.[305] Therefore, they may not be immediately forthcoming about their problematic use. As noted earlier, it is important to allay the anxiety by reassuring the patient that the SUD diagnosis will not impede efforts to treat their pain.

As noted earlier, the patient who is hospitalized for an acute medical problem may be more receptive to intervention for SUD than would otherwise be as an outpatient. It is important to consider the hospitalization as a window of opportunity to bring patients into recovery. SUD treatment should be offered when the disorder is detected in the course of pain treatment. If the patient does not accept SUD intervention at the time it is offered, it may be helpful to use the acute pain problem to begin to explore the patient's motivation for recovery and to follow-up at future visits.

Critical to managing pain in patients with SUD is the understanding that the chronic nature of the disease requires continuous management; a single-mindedness focus on treating the former may allow the latter to progress unchecked. The presence of pain, be it acute or chronic, is a stressor, and even if opioids are not prescribed for its management, the associated anxiety, functional losses, sleep disturbances, and general discomfort can set the patient up for a relapse to use of the drug which in the past has reliably provided psychic relief. For the patient in recovery, most important to ensuring that an exacerbation of SUD does not occur is the establishment of a collaborative treatment relationship between the addiction treatment provider and the pain care provider, with regular communication about the patient's response to each.

Persons with SUD who require opioids for pain benefit from active cultivation of their recovery and implementation of relapse prevention interventions in the plan of care.[291] What constitutes meaningful recovery activities vary between individuals but may include attendance at self-help meetings, close interaction with a sponsor, work with a counselor, or active participation in a faith community, among others. SUD professionals may provide an important service to patients and their pain treatment providers by making recommendations on enriching recovery and by supervising the recovery plan while patients are using opioids for pain.[306] In persons with other conditions that put them at risk for misuse of medications, such as psychiatric disorders or cognitive impairment, engagement of appropriate professionals to assist in management of or accommodation to these disorders may be needed.

Although not addiction treatment providers, there are specific strategies the pain clinician can utilize to support the goals of SUD treatment. As noted earlier, continued and active engagement in addiction treatment should be encouraged; even if the patient is hospitalized, virtual 12-step meetings, visits from sponsors or the MAT provider, or access to readings or web-based programming can be facilitated. It is necessary to continuously evaluate the presence and severity of stressors that might precipitate relapse (such as unrelieved pain, sleep disturbance, withdrawal symptoms, psychiatric symptoms, interpersonal conflicts, craving) as well as identify protective factors against relapse and to support/strengthen these to the extent possible; the validated Defense and Veterans Pain Rating Scale (DVPRS) screening tool can be easily administered in the clinical setting to this end.[307] If it becomes apparent that a relapse has occurred, it is critical that recovery providers be notified as soon as possible to minimize the extent of the exacerbation and reinforce recovery efforts.

Document Pain Treatment Plan and Involve Patient and Family in the Plan of Care

It is important to achieve pain relief with methods that do not confuse, stress, or frustrate the staff or the patient. This requires clear communication regarding the pain treatment plan to all staff involved in caring for a patient with SUD. Stigma and misunderstanding are widespread among health care personnel and too often lead to inadequate pain management when the primary treating clinician is not available and the plan is not clearly documented. In the absence of a clear and consistent structure, the patient's behaviors may foster confusion of pain and addiction issues. Written documentation of the plan, displayed in a prominent and accessible location, may be necessary.

Shared decision making is based on the foundation of a patient-centered assessment of risks and benefits and a clinical synthesis performed by the provider.[92] To be effective, the patient (and often family) must be included in the decision-making process regarding the choice of treatment options including medication, dosing, and scheduling. This provides a sense of control and allays the anxiety and fear that worsens pain perception. It also may afford information that is useful in designing an effective treatment regimen. Patients with OUD often know the doses they require to meet their basic physical dependence needs as well as the additional levels required to treat their acute pain. If a patient becomes intoxicated or sedated at the prescribed dose, medications should be adjusted to avoid the observed side effects while continuing to provide analgesia.

Pain, Substance Use Disorder, and Suicide

There has been a great deal of scholarly activity devoted to the burgeoning rate of opioid misuse/abuse and opioid-related fatalities. State and federal policy makers have made a priority to develop risk mitigation strategies such as opioid prescribing guidelines, PDMPs, and educational programs to curb the rising rate of opioid abuse. However, these important efforts have overshadowed the equally devastating silent epidemic of suicidal ideation (SI) and suicidal behavior (SB), particularly in vulnerable populations. Suicide has become a global health crisis. The Word Health Organization published an executive summary, *Preventing Suicide: A Global Imperative.*[308] In this document, there were disturbing facts: Every 40 seconds someone in the world dies of suicide; an estimated 804,000 suicide deaths occurred worldwide in 2012; in the age group of 15 to 29 years, it is the second leading cause of death, and suicide constitutes 54% of the 1.5 million violent deaths per year globally.

Pain and Suicide

There is substantial literature indicating that there is a high prevalence of SI in patients suffering from CNMP, ranging from 18% to 50%.[309–324] A systematic review by Tang and Crane[321] revealed that the risk of successful suicide doubled in patients with CNMP as compared to nonpain controls. Ilgen and his colleagues[322] evaluated a large cohort from the VA database (n = 260,254) and discovered that veterans experiencing severe pain were more likely to end their life by suicide than veterans with no, mild, or moderate pain (hazard ratio [HR]: 1.33; 95% confidence interval [CI]: 1.15 to 1.54). Campbell et al.[323] examined data from a nationally representative household survey of 8,841 individuals. Results revealed that the odds ratio (OR) of lifetime and past 12-month SI and SB was two to three times greater in individuals with chronic pain than those without chronic pain.

Substance Use Disorders and Suicide

Individuals suffering from SUDs, like ones with pain, are at substantial risk for SI and SB. Greater than 40% of persons seeking treatment for their SUD endorse having a history of suicide attempts.[325–327] Individuals with an AUD are almost 10 times more likely to die by suicide and those who inject drugs are approximately 14 times more likely to commit suicide as compared to the general population.[328] These individuals tend to have multiple risk factors for SB including having depressive symptoms and significant numbers of severe stressors such as loss of relationships, jobs, health, and financial problems. Yuodelis-Flores and Ries[329] reviewed the literature examining the characteristics of SB in patients with SUDs and found that a history of attempted suicide was a strong predictor of future suicide which is very common in all populations, not just patients with an SUD. History of impulsiveness, aggression, pessimism, and hopelessness, along with acute stressors such as loss of relationships or income and a history of childhood sexual abuse all were important factors that contribute to the risk of suicide for patients with SUD. Certain mental disorders also strongly affected the risk for suicide attempts in patients with SUD, in particular, major depressive disorder, bipolar disorder, posttraumatic stress disorder (PTSD), and borderline personality disorder.

Pain, Substance Use Disorder, and Suicidal Ideation and Behavior

Pain and SUD are independent risk factors for SI and SB, putting patients with co-occurring pain and SUD at particularly at high risk for ending their lives by suicide.

Risk Factors. There are general, nonpain-specific risk factors and pain-specific risk factors for SI and SB. General, nonpain-specific risk factors include gender (female); age (>45 years old); having co-occurring mental disorders (especially depression and SUD); acute losses and stressors (relationships, job, finances); enduring chronic medical illnesses; sleep disturbance; experiencing conflict, disaster, and discrimination; past psychiatric hospitalizations; frequency of SI; severity of

psychiatric disorder; and poor social support; and the strongest predictor of suicide is a previous suicide attempt.[308,330] Although patients with pain and SUD commonly have a number of these risk factors (e.g., loss of vocational and home roles, isolation, depression),[331] pain-specific risk factors include pain type, pain duration, pain intensity, sleep disturbance, and opioid dosing.

Possible Mediators. Both catastrophizing and burdensomeness/social isolation have been identified as potential mediators for suicide in patients with chronic pain. Many patients with pain engage in a pain-related catastrophizing, which can be defined as magnified, exaggerated negative focus on pain that can contribute to depression and disability and in turn exacerbate an individual's experience of pain and suffering.[332] The association between SI and individual differences in the use of pain-related coping strategies and pain catastrophizing was assessed in a large cohort of 1,515 patients with CNMP. In this sample, 32% reported recent SI. It was revealed that the extent of depression and pain catastrophizing best predicted the occurrence and the degree of SI. Demographic variables, pain intensity, and pain duration were not particularly robust predictors of SI.[320]

With respect to burdensomeness and social isolation, the interpersonal theory of suicide by Joiner and colleagues[333,334] proposes that there are two primary factors that significantly contribute to the context that leads to SI and possible SB. These two factors are thwarted belongingness, which is defined as the unfulfilled need for social interaction and connectedness, and perceived burdensomeness, which perceives oneself as a burden or a liability to others, particularly family members. Kanzler and colleagues[335] evaluated 113 patients with CNMP, and a logistic regression model revealed that one question measuring perceived burdensomeness was the only predictor of SI. Cheatle et al.[319] discovered that social withdrawal and isolation were predictive of SI in a cohort of 466 patients referred to a pain center.

According to the interpersonal theory of suicide, whereas the confluence of burdensomeness and thwarted belongingness can lead to the desire for suicide, the capability for suicide attempts develops in response to repeated exposure to physically/emotionally painful and/or fear-inducing experiences. This theory of SI and SB is very relevant to patients with pain and those with an SUD because in both populations individuals tend to become isolated and often perceive that they are a burden on their friends and families and are often subjected to emotionally and, at times, physically painful events due to their disease and related disabilities.

Screening for Risk of Suicide

Screening for risk of suicide in patients with chronic pain and SUD should include general mental health screening, assessing sleep disturbance, and the use of specific tools to assess SI and SB.

Mental Health Screening. A number of well-validated screening tools for depression and anxiety have been used, both clinically and in research. The Beck Depression Inventory (BDI)[336] and the Profile of Mood States (POMS)[337] are the two measures recommended by Initiative on Methods, Measurement, and Pain Assessment in Clinical Trials (IMMPACT) consensus group to assess emotional function in chronic pain.[338] The BDI is a 21-item self-report measure of the severity of depressive symptoms over the past week, whereas the POMS assesses six distinct mood states including depression, anxiety, and anger, thought to be the most relevant factors in the pain population. A frequently employed depression screening tool for use in primary care is the Patient Health Questionnaire (PHQ-9),[339] which is a self-rating instrument derived from the Primary Care Evaluation of Mental Disorders (PRIME-MD) project[340] which includes nine symptoms of depression based on the *DSM-IV-TR* criteria, including one item specifically inquiring about self-harm (SI). The Patient Reported Outcome

Measurement Information System (PROMIS)-depression item is another brief instrument (five questions) to screen for and assess depression severity.[341] Finally, the PHQ-4 is a four-item screening tool for depression and anxiety that can be easily administered in a busy primary care practice.[342]

Screening Tools for Sleep Disturbance. Sleep disturbance is a risk factor for both increased pain and SI. Measures for insomnia predominantly include patient self-report in questionnaire and daily sleep diary to capture the subjective experience of sleep disturbance but may also include objective measures such as actigraphy and polysomnography to assess sleep patterns and possible concomitant sleep disorders (e.g., sleep apnea, restless leg syndrome/period limb movement disorder, narcolepsy). Self-report measures assess different aspects of sleep disturbance. Clinically useful tools typically assess sleep quality such as the Pittsburgh Sleep Quality Index,[343] Insomnia Severity Index,[344] PROMIS-sleep disturbance and sleep-related impairment item.[345] Moul and colleagues[346] provide a review of the various sleep assessment scales.

Screening Tools for Suicide. Although the majority of depression screening tools have a question assessing SI, there are a number of suicide screening tools that provide more granular information on risk of suicide and intentionality. For example, the P-4 Brief Assessment assesses **p**ast suicide attempts, a **p**lan for suicide, **p**robability of completing suicide, and **p**reventive factors.[347] The Columbia-Suicide Severity Rating Scale (C-SSRS) measures a number of suicide domains including ideation, intensity, behaviors, severity of self-injury, and potential lethality of suicide attempts.[348] The C-SSRS provides greater precision in the assessment of SB and SI but due to its length can be cumbersome with regards to clinical practice and is typically used in clinical trials during medication development.

The Suicide Assessment Five-Step Evaluation and Triage (SAFE-T) assessment tool was developed in collaboration with the Substance Abuse and Mental Health Services Administration (SAMHSA).[349] The SAFE-T includes assessment of risk factors including SB, current and past psychiatric disorders, key symptoms, family history, change in treatment, and access to firearms; protective factors, both internal, such as the ability to cope with stress, spiritual or religious beliefs, and frustration tolerance, and external, such as responsibility to children or others and having a positive therapeutic relationship and good social supports; suicidal inquiry with specific questions about thoughts, plans, behaviors, intents, risk level, and intervention; and the risk level based on the clinical judgment after completing the first three steps. Patients are stratified into low, moderate, and high risk, with specific interventions indicated for each risk level. The last step is documenting the risk level and rationale for the treatment plan to address or reduce the risk.

Suicide Risk Reduction and Interventions
Reducing the risk of developing SI and of engaging in SB possibly resulting in death by suicide relies in part on managing comorbidities commonly seen in patients with pain and SUD (mood disorders, sleep disturbance, catastrophizing). Patients who present with complaint of moderate to severe depression with or without acknowledging SI, if possible, should be co-managed with a mental health specialist. Patients who express active SI may require immediate inpatient treatment which is contingent on certain dynamics including severity of depression and SI, lack or presence of a specific plan for completing suicide, access to means (potentially lethal medications such as opioids and benzodiazepines or own a gun), and history of past SB or impulsivity.

Certain factors mitigate the need for inpatient care, such as patients having a robust social support system, having a history of demonstrating good impulse control, are willing to contract

that they will go to a local hospital or call emergency assistance if SI intensifies, and having a collaborative relationship with their health care provider. In these cases, patients may be able to be managed as an outpatient. During an acute suicidal phase, the patient will require both pharmacotherapy and intensive psychotherapy. The pharmacotherapy strategy should include managing depressive symptomatology, sleep disturbance, and pain. If opioid or benzodiazepine use is necessary, these medications should be prescribed judiciously, in small amounts and held and administered by a family member or close friend or sponsor. Patients determined to be high risk for engaging in SI and SB or have chronic SI should be involved in ongoing psychotherapy and remain under psychiatric care.[330]

Pharmacotherapy. There are no specific pharmacologic agents that have been identified to directly reduce SI, so the general strategy is to treat comorbid conditions that can contribute to increased risk of suicide, including depression, anxiety, sleep disorder, and poorly controlled pain. Typical pharmacologic agents might include a combination of antidepressants and antiepileptic drugs and sleep aids. There is, however, equivocal data that antidepressants and antiepileptics can actually increase the risk of SI/SB in a subgroup of patients. With this in mind, treating patients with pain, SUD, and comorbid suicidality, it is critical to closely monitor for ongoing suicide risk with any changes or additions to therapy. When treating sleep disturbance in this patient population, avoidance of benzodiazepines is advised especially if the patient is on opioid therapy and to rely on nonbenzodiazepine agents with low abuse potential and low risk of respiratory depression.

Nonpharmacologic Interventions. Individuals with pain and especially ones with both pain and concomitant SUD often experience co-occurring mood, anxiety, and sleep disorders, which can increase the risk of SI and SB. In a subgroup of patients, pharmacotherapy can improve mood, anxiety, and sleep which can in turn reduce the risk of SI/SB in a subgroup of patients, but the combination of appropriate pharmacotherapy and nonpharmacologic interventions, CBT in particular, is the most efficacious approach.

Cognitive-Behavioral Therapy for Pain. Patients experiencing persistent pain often engage in maladaptive behaviors for example kinesiophobia (or fear of movement) and dysfunctional thought patterns, most commonly catastrophizing. As noted previously, catastrophizing has been identified as a potential risk factor for SI/SB in patients with chronic pain. The goal of CBT is to assist and support the patient in identifying maladaptive behaviors and/or dysfunctional thought patterns that may reduce the patient's ability to adjust to and cope with their chronic pain, thus contributing to their related depression and anxiety.

The process of CBT typically involves the patient acquiring specific skills which can include mindfulness-based stress reduction, progressive muscle relaxation training, behavioral pacing, effective communication, cognitive restructuring, followed by skill consolidation, rehearsal, and relapse training.[350] There is persuasive research supporting the clinical efficacy and cost-effectiveness of CBT in improving mood, anxiety, and functionality in a number of chronic pain disorders, including chronic low back pain,[351,352] arthritis,[353] lupus,[354] fibromyalgia,[355] and sickle cell disease.[356]

Cognitive-Behavioral Therapy for Insomnia. CBT personalized to treat insomnia has been effective in improving sleep disturbance. Sleep disturbance is highly prevalent in patients with CNMP and patients with SUD. Pain and sleep are bidirectional with pain leading to sleep disturbance and sleep disturbance causing increased pain.[357,358] There is evidence that

CBT-insomnia (CBT-I) in patients with chronic primary insomnia is equally effective or even superior to pharmacotherapy in multiple outcomes.[359] A course of CBT-I typically includes psychoeducation about sleep and insomnia, stimulus control, sleep restriction, sleep hygiene, relaxation training, and cognitive restructuring. CBT-I can be delivered in an individual, group, and computer-assisted format with generally equal effectiveness.

Cognitive-Behavioral Therapy, Pain, and Substance Use Disorder. As noted, there has been a burgeoning rate of prescription opioid misuse/abuse and opioid-related fatalities. There is emerging evidence that CBT can reduce the risk of prescription opioid misuse and abuse in high-risk patients indirectly by improving mood, anxiety, sleep, and pain coping skills and also in improving outcomes in patients with pain who have a history of an SUD. In a recently published pilot study, patients with hepatitis C who also experienced chronic pain and had a history of SUD were enrolled in an eight-session integrated group CBT program for chronic pain and SUD. Results revealed improvement in key outcomes including pain-related interference, reduction in cravings for alcohol and other substances, and a decrease in past-month alcohol and substance use.[360]

Opioid Tapering and Suicide. Given the current concern over the opioid "epidemic' and the burgeoning rate of opioid misuse/abuse and opioid-related fatalities and fanned by the recent opioid prescribing guidelines, there is a trend to taper patients off opioids, even in the absence of evidence of ADRB. The findings of a recent opioid tapering study at a single pain clinic at a community hospital showed that a substantial fraction of patients on high-dose opioid therapy long-term wished to engage in voluntary opioid dosage reduction and was able to do so successfully without increase in pain intensity or pain interference. Combining patient education about the benefits of opioid reduction with a plan that reduces opioids slowly (in this study, over 4 months) with close clinician follow-up may help patients engage and succeed in voluntary outpatient tapering.[361]

However, tapering in patients with CNMP and SUD must be initiated cautiously. In a recent study,[362] 509 veterans with CNMP who were discontinued from opioid therapy were selected from a national cohort. The sample included patients with SUD and matched controls. Results indicated that in both groups, there was a high rate of SI (9.2%). These results underscore the importance of individualizing treatment, and being cognizant that those patients with pain receiving opioid therapy can be unnecessarily vilified, and increase the risk of SI and SB.

Future Directions
Predicting future SI and SB is a herculean endeavor even for seasoned mental health clinicians. There is emerging science on biomarkers of SI and SB. For example, there is evidence that patients with diminished central serotonin have a higher risk of SB. In particular, low concentration of 5-hydroxyindoleacetic acid (5-HIAA) in the cerebral spinal fluid was found to predict future SB and was discovered in depressed suicide attempters and in the brainstems of autopsied patients that committed suicide.[363–365] Further implicating the serotoninergic system is polymorphism of the gene coding for the serotonin transporter (5-HTTLPR) and brain-derived neurotropic factor.[366]

Conclusions

Patients with pain commonly present with comorbid disorders. Unlike other diseases or illnesses, comorbid SUD puts patients with pain at unique and increased risk of a worsened experience of pain and a limited response to pain management interventions. These poor outcomes are related not only to the behavioral manifestations of the disorder but also to the neurophysiologic processes which underlie its development.

SUDs disrupt motivational systems encoding reward; stimuli that are by nature stressful and unrewarding, such as pain, are likely to be preferentially affected by the presence of SUDs. These issues become particularly salient in the case of OUD, where tolerance, physical dependence, craving, and hyperalgesia complicate the provision of opioid analgesia.

Despite the challenges associated with managing their pain, it is critical that the pain suffered by patients with SUD be treated effectively, if not aggressively. Untreated pain puts them at risk for relapse or escalation of substance use, disengagement from treatment, and worsened morbidity, including overdose and suicide. The therapeutic alliance developed when pain reports are believed and relieved can be a powerful motivator or reinforcer of recovery. Fortunately, the current emphasis on, and growing evidence base for, multimodal pain treatment and opioid-sparing strategies provide tools for effective pain management in patients with SUD which do not engage addiction systems. Furthermore, with thoughtful and judicious oversight, opioids can be provided to individuals with acute and chronic pain of severity requiring their potent analgesic effects. Doing so requires vigilance on the part of the provider to monitor for withdrawal, relapse, and toxicity as well as ensuring that SUD treatment resources are included in the plan of care. By its very nature, effective pain care for the patient with SUD concomitantly benefits the recovery process, thus provision of such is critical in this vulnerable patient population.

References

1. Center for Behavioral Health Statistics and Quality. *2016 National Survey on Drug Use and Health: Detailed Tables.* Rockville, MD: Substance Abuse and Mental Health Services Administration; 2017.
2. Mehta AJ. Alcoholism and critical illness: a review. *World J Crit Care Med* 2016;5(1):27–35. doi:10.5492/wjccm.v5.i1.27.
3. Engler PA, Ramsey SE, Smith RJ. Alcohol use of diabetes patients: the need for assessment and intervention. *Acta Diabetol* 2013;50(2):93–99. doi:10.1007/s00592-010-0200-x.
4. Maldonado JR. An approach to the patient with substance use and abuse. *Med Clin North Am* 2010;94(6):1169–1205. doi:10.1016/j.mcna.2010.08.010.
5. Compton P, Chang YP. Substance abuse and addiction: implications for pain management in patients with cancer. *Clin J Oncol Nurs* 2017;21(2):203–209. doi:10.1188/17.CJON.203-209.
6. Koob GF, Le Moal M. Drug abuse: hedonic homeostatic dysregulation. *Science* 1997;278(5335):52–58.
7. American Psychiatric Association. *Diagnostic and Statistical Manual of Mental Disorders.* 5th ed. Arlington, VA: American Psychiatric Publishing; 2013.
8. Sehgal N, Manchikanti L, Smith HS. Prescription opioid abuse in chronic pain: a review of opioid abuse predictors and strategies to curb opioid abuse. *Pain Physician* 2012;15(suppl 3):ES67–ES92.
9. Jamison RN, Edwards RR. Risk factor assessment for problematic use of opioids for chronic pain. *Clin Neuropsychol* 2013;27(1):60–80.
10. Koob GF, Bloom FE. Cellular and molecular mechanisms of drug dependence. *Science* 1988;242(4879):715–723.
11. Basbaum AI. Insights into the development of opioid tolerance. *Pain* 1995;61(3):349–352.
12. Solomon RL. The opponent-process theory of acquired motivation: the costs of pleasure and the benefits of pain. *Am Psychol* 1980;35(8):691–712.
13. Koob GF, Stinus L, Le Moal M, et al. Opponent process theory of motivation: neurobiological evidence from studies of opiate dependence. *Neurosci Biobehav Rev* 1989;13(2–3):135–140.
14. Koob GF, Le Moal M. Drug addiction, dysregulation of reward, and allostasis. *Neuropsychopharmacology* 2001;24(2):97–129.
15. Koob GF, Le Moal M. Addiction and the brain antireward system. *Annu Rev Psychol* 2008;59:29–53.
16. Christie MJ. Cellular neuroadaptations to chronic opioids: tolerance, withdrawal and addiction. *Br J Pharmacol* 2008;154(2):384–396.
17. Koch T, Höllt V. Role of receptor internalization in opioid tolerance and dependence. *Pharmacol Ther* 2008;117(2):199–206.
18. Chao J, Nestler EJ. Molecular neurobiology of drug addiction. *Annu Rev Med* 2004;55:113–132.
19. Finn AK, Whistler JL. Endocytosis of the mu opioid receptor reduces tolerance and a cellular hallmark of opiate withdrawal. *Neuron* 2001;32(5):829–839.
20. Lugoboni F, Mirijello A, Zamboni L, et al. High prevalence of constipation and reduced quality of life in opioid-dependent patients treated with opioid substitution treatments. *Expert Opin Pharmacother* 2016;17(16):2135–2141.
21. Smith HS, Elliott JA. Opioid-induced androgen deficiency (OPIAD). *Pain Physician* 2012;15(suppl 3):ES145–ES156.

22. Bailey CP, Connor M. Opioids: cellular mechanisms of tolerance and physical dependence. *Curr Opin Pharmacol* 2005;5(1):60–68.

23. Redmond DE Jr, Krystal JH. Multiple mechanisms of withdrawal from opioid drugs. *Annu Rev Neurosci* 1984;7:443–478.

24. Taricco M, Pagliacci MC, Telaro E, et al. Pharmacological interventions for spasticity following spinal cord injury: results of a Cochrane systematic review. *Eura Medicophys* 2006;42(1):5–15.

25. Bahn EL, Holt KR. Procedural sedation and analgesia: a review and new concepts. *Emerg Med Clin North Am* 2005;23(2):503–517.

26. Mazurek MS. Sedation and analgesia for procedures outside the operating room. *Semin Pediatr Surg* 2004;13(3):166–173.

27. Mao J, Price DD, Lu J, et al. Two distinctive antinociceptive systems in rats with pathological pain. *Neurosci Lett* 2000;280(1):13–16.

28. Palazzo E, Marabese I, de Novellis V, et al. Metabotropic and NMDA glutamate receptors participate in the cannabinoid-induced antinociception. *Neuropharmacology* 2001;40(3):319–326.

29. Palazzos E, de Novellis V, Marabese I, et al. Metabotropic glutamate and cannabinoid receptor crosstalk in periaqueductal grey pain processing. *Curr Neuropharmacol* 2006;4(3):225–231.

30. Rog DJ, Nurmikko TJ, Young CA. Oromucosal delta9-tetrahydrocannabinol/cannabidiol for neuropathic pain associated with multiple sclerosis: an uncontrolled, open-label, 2-year extension trial. *Clin Ther* 2007;29(9):2068–2079.

31. Wade DT, Makela P, Robson P, et al. Do cannabis-based medicinal extracts have general or specific effects on symptoms in multiple sclerosis? A double-blind, randomized, placebo-controlled study on 160 patients. *Mult Scler* 2004;10(4):434–441.

32. Hosking RD, Zajicek JP. Therapeutic potential of cannabis in pain medicine. *Br J Anaesth* 2008;101(1):59–68.

33. Stevens AJ, Higgins MD. A systematic review of the analgesic efficacy of cannabinoid medications in the management of acute pain. *Acta Anaesthesiol Scand* 2017;61(3):268–280. doi:10.1111/aas.12851.

34. Walitt B, Klose P, Fitzcharles MA, et al. Cannabinoids for fibromyalgia. *Cochrane Database Syst Rev* 2016;7:CD011694. doi:10.1002/14651858.CD011694.pub2.

35. Fitzcharles MA, Häuser W. Cannabinoids in the management of musculoskeletal or rheumatic diseases. *Curr Rheumatol Rep* 2016;18(12):76.

36. Tateo S. State of the evidence: Cannabinoids and cancer pain—a systematic review. *J Am Assoc Nurse Pract* 2017;29(2):94–103. doi:10.1002/2327-6924.12422.

37. Tsang CC, Giudice MG. Nabilone for the management of pain. *Pharmacotherapy* 2016;36(3):273–286. doi:10.1002/phar.1709.

38. van den Beuken-van Everdingen MH, de Graeff A, Jongen JL, et al. Pharmacological treatment of pain in cancer patients: the role of adjuvant analgesics, a systematic review. *Pain Pract* 2017;17(3):409–419. doi:10.1111/papr.12459.

39. Deng Y, Luo L, Hu Y, et al. Clinical practice guidelines for the management of neuropathic pain: a systematic review. *BMC Anesthesiol* 2016;16:12. doi:10.1186/s12871-015-0150-5.

40. Beaulieu P, Boulanger A, Desroches J, et al. Medical cannabis: considerations for the anesthesiologist and pain physician. *Can J Anaesth* 2016;63(5):608–624. doi:10.1007/s12630-016-0598-x.

41. Nunes EV, Rounsaville BJ. Comorbidity of substance use with depression and other mental disorders: from Diagnostic and Statistical Manual of Mental Disorders, fourth edition (DSM-IV) to DSM-V. *Addiction* 2006;101(suppl 1):89–96.

42. Stein C. Opioids, sensory systems and chronic pain. *Eur J Pharmacol* 2013;716:179–187.

43. Schuckit MA. Comorbidity between substance use disorders and psychiatric conditions. *Addiction* 2006;101(suppl 1):76–88.

44. Begré S, Traber M, Gerber M, et al. Change in pain severity with open label venlafaxine use in patients with a depressive symptomatology: an observational study in primary care. *Eur Psychiatry* 2008;23(3):178–186.

45. Krebs EE, Gaynes BN, Gartlehner G, et al. Treating the physical symptoms of depression with second-generation antidepressants: a systematic review and metaanalysis. *Psychosomatics* 2008;49(3):191–198.

46. Perahia DG, Pritchett YL, Desaiah D, et al. Efficacy of duloxetine in painful symptoms: an analgesic or antidepressant effect? *Int Clin Psychopharmacol* 2006;21(6):311–317.

47. Koob GF. A role for brain stress systems in addiction. *Neuron* 2008;59(1):11–34.

48. Shurman J, Koob GF, Gutstein HB. Opioids, pain, the brain, and hyperkatifeia: a framework for the rational use of opioids for pain. *Pain Med* 2010;11(7):1092–1098.

49. Compton MA. Cold-pressor pain tolerance in opiate and cocaine abusers: correlates of drug type and use status. *J Pain Symptom Manage* 1994;9(7):462–473.

50. Pandey SC, Kyzar EJ, Zhang H. Epigenetic basis of the dark side of alcohol addiction. *Neuropharmacology* 2017;122:74–84. doi:10.1016/j.neuropharm.2017.02.002.

51. Cadet JL, McCoy MT, Jayanthi S. Epigenetics and addiction. *Clin Pharmacol Ther* 2016;99(5):502–511. doi:10.1002/cpt.345.

52. Cecil CA, Walton E, Viding E. Epigenetics of addiction: current knowledge, challenges, and future directions. *J Stud Alcohol Drugs* 2016;77(5):688–691.

53. Liang L, Lutz BM, Bekker A, et al. Epigenetic regulation of chronic pain. *Epigenomics* 2015;7(2):235–245. doi:10.2217/epi.14.75.

54. Descalzi G, Ikegami D, Ushijima T, et al. Epigenetic mechanisms of chronic pain. *Trends Neurosci* 2015;38(4):237–246. doi:10.1016/j.tins.2015.02.001.

55. Zacny JP, Klafta JM, Coalson DW, et al. The reinforcing effects of brief exposures to nitrous oxide in healthy volunteers. *Drug Alcohol Depend* 1996;42(3):197–200.

56. Martin TJ, Ewan E. Chronic pain alters drug self-administration: implications for addiction and pain mechanisms. *Exp Clin Psychopharmacol* 2008;16(5):357–366.

57. Boscarino JA, Hoffman SN, Han JJ. Opioid-use disorder among patients on long-term opioid therapy: impact of final DSM-5 diagnostic criteria on prevalence and correlates. *Subst Abuse Rehabil* 2015;6:83–91.

58. Degenhardt L, Bruno R, Lintzeris N. Agreement between definitions of pharmaceutical opioid use disorders and dependence in people taking opioids for chronic non-cancer pain (POINT): a cohort study. *Lancet Psychiatry* 2015;2(4):314–322.

59. Bertilsson L, Dahl ML, Dalén P, et al. Molecular genetics of CYP2D6: clinical relevance with focus on psychotropic drugs. *Br J Clin Pharmacol* 2002;53(2):111–122.

60. Ingelman-Sundberg M, Johansson I, Persson I, et al. Genetic polymorphism of cytochrome P450. Functional consequences and possible relationship to disease and alcohol toxicity. *EXS* 1994;71:197–207.

61. Otton SV, Schadel M, Cheung SW, et al. CYP2D6 phenotype determines the metabolic conversion of hydrocodone to hydromorphone. *Clin Pharmacol Ther* 1993;54(5):463–472.

62. Oertel B, Lötsch J. Genetic mutations that prevent pain: implications for future pain medication. *Pharmacogenomics* 2008;9(2):179–194.

63. Brøsen K, Hansen JG, Nielsen KK, et al. Inhibition by paroxetine of desipramine metabolism in extensive but not in poor metabolizers of sparteine. *Eur J Clin Pharmacol* 1993;44(4):349–355.

64. Mogil JS, Marek P, Flodman P, et al. One or two genetic loci mediate high opiate analgesia in selectively bred mice. *Pain* 1995;60(2):125–135.

65. Mogil JS, Wilson SG, Bon K, et al. Heritability of nociception I: responses of 11 inbred mouse strains on 12 measures of nociception. *Pain* 1999;80(1–2):67–82.

66. Elmer GI, Pieper JO, Goldberg SR, et al. Opioid operant self-administration, analgesia, stimulation and respiratory depression in mu-deficient mice. *Psychopharmacology (Berl)* 1995;117(1):23–31.

67. Sudakov SK, Goldberg SR, Borisova EV, et al. Differences in morphine reinforcement property in two inbred rat strains: associations with cortical receptors, behavioral activity, analgesia and the cataleptic effects of morphine. *Psychopharmacology (Berl)* 1993;112(2–3):183–188.

68. Elmer GI, Pieper JO, Negus SS, et al. Genetic variance in nociception and its relationship to the potency of morphine-induced analgesia in thermal and chemical tests. *Pain* 1998;75(1):129–140.

69. Belknap JK, Mogil JS, Helms ML, et al. Localization to chromosome 10 of a locus influencing morphine analgesia in crosses derived from C57BL/6 and DBA/2 strains. *Life Sci* 1995;57(10):PL117–PL124.

70. Semenova S, Kuzmin A, Zvartau E. Strain differences in the analgesic and reinforcing action of morphine in mice. *Pharmacol Biochem Behav* 1995;50(1):17–21.

71. Berrettini WH, Alexander R, Ferraro TN, et al. A study of oral morphine preference in inbred mouse strains. *Psychiatr Genet* 1994;4(2):81–86.

72. Petruzzi R, Ferraro TN, Kürschner VC, et al. The effects of repeated morphine exposure on mu opioid receptor number and affinity in C57BL/6J and DBA/2J mice. *Life Sci* 1997;61(20):2057–2064.

73. Edwards RR. Genetic predictors of acute and chronic pain. *Curr Rheumatol Rep* 2006;8(6):411–417.

74. Mogil JS, Yu L, Basbaum AI. Pain genes: natural variation and transgenic mutants. *Annu Rev Neurosci* 2000;23:777–811.

75. Stamer UM, Stüber F. Genetic factors in pain and its treatment. *Curr Opin Anaesthesiol* 2007;20(5):478–484.

76. Flores CM, Mogil JS. The pharmacogenetics of analgesia: toward a genetically-based approach to pain management. *Pharmacogenomics* 2001;2(3):177–194.

77. Mayer P, Höllt V. Pharmacogenetics of opioid receptors and addiction. *Pharmacogenet Genomics* 2006;16(1):1–7.

78. Ikeda K, Ogai Y, Nishizawa D, et al. Genetic analyses of morphine sensitivity [in Japanese]. *Nihon Rinsho* 2005;63(suppl 12):463–466.

79. Lötsch J, Geisslinger G. Relevance of frequent mu-opioid receptor polymorphisms for opioid activity in healthy volunteers. *Pharmacogenomics J* 2006;6(3):200–210.

80. Kim H, Neubert JK, San Miguel A, et al. Genetic influence on variability in human acute experimental pain sensitivity associated with gender, ethnicity and psychological temperament. *Pain* 2004;109(3):488–496.

81. Caterina MJ, Leffler A, Malmberg AB, et al. Impaired nociception and pain sensation in mice lacking the capsaicin receptor. *Science* 2000;288(5464):306–313.

82. McKemy DD, Neuhausser WM, Julius D. Identification of a cold receptor reveals a general role for TRP channels in thermosensation. *Nature* 2002;416(6876):52–58.

83. Mogil JS, Ritchie J, Smith SB, et al. Melanocortin-1 receptor gene variants affect pain and mu-opioid analgesia in mice and humans. *J Med Genet* 2005;42(7):583–587.

84. Taylor DA, Fleming WW. Unifying perspectives of the mechanisms underlying the development of tolerance and physical dependence to opioids. *J Pharmacol Exp Ther* 2001;297:11–18.

85. Williams JT, Ingram SL, Henderson G, et al. Regulation of μ-opioid receptors: desensitization, phosphorylation, internalization, and tolerance. *Pharmacol Rev* 2013;65:223–254.

86. Collin E, Cesselin F. Neurobiological mechanisms of opioid tolerance and dependence. *Clin Neuropharmacol* 1991;14:465–488.

87. Sánchez-Blázquez P, Rodríguez-Muñoz M, Berrocoso E, et al. The plasticity of the association between mu-opioid receptor and glutamate ionotropic receptor N in opioid analgesic tolerance and neuropathic pain. *Eur J Pharmacol* 2013;716(1–3):94–105.

88. Cahill CM, Walwyn W, Taylor AM, et al. Allostatic mechanisms of opioid tolerance beyond desensitization and downregulation. *Trends Pharmacol Sci* 2016;37(11):963–976.

89. Hutchinson MR, Shavit Y, Grace PM, et al. Exploring the neuroimmunopharmacology of opioids: an integrative review of mechanisms of central immune signaling and their implications for opioid analgesia. *Pharmacol Rev* 2011;63(3):772–810.

90. Foley K. Clinical tolerance to opioids. In: Basbaum A, Besson J, eds. *Towards a New Pharmacotherapy of Pain*. New York: John Wiley & Sons; 1991:181–203.

91. Roth SH, Fleischmann RM, Burch FX, et al. Around-the-clock, controlled-release oxycodone therapy for osteoarthritis-related pain: placebo-controlled trial and long-term evaluation. *Arch Intern Med* 2000;160:853–860.

92. Dowell D, Haegerich TM, Chou R. CDC guideline for prescribing opioids for chronic pain—United States, 2016. Available at: https://www.cdc.gov/mmwr/volumes/65/rr/rr6501e1.htm. Accessed October 30, 2017.

93. U.S. Department of Defense, U.S. Department of Veterans Affairs. VA/DoD clinical practice guideline: management of opioid therapy for chronic pain. Available at: https://www.healthquality.va.gov/guidelines/Pain/cot/. Accessed October 30, 2017.

94. Bryson EO. The perioperative management of patients maintained on medications used to manage opioid addiction. *Curr Opin Anaesthesiol* 2014;27:359–364.

95. Huxtable CA, Roberts LJ, Somogyi AA, et al. Acute pain management in opioid-tolerant patients: a growing challenge. *Anaesth Intensive Care* 2011;39(5):804–823.

96. Pan A, Zakowski M. Peripartum anesthetic management of the opioid-tolerant or buprenorphine/suboxone-dependent patient. *Clin Obstet Gynecol* 2017;60(2):447–458.

97. Volkow ND, McLellan AT. Opioid abuse in chronic pain—misconceptions and mitigation strategies. *N Engl J Med* 2016;374(13):1253–1263.

98. Evans CJ, Cahill CM. Neurobiology of opioid dependence in creating addiction vulnerability. *F1000Res* 2016;5.

99. Koob GF, Volkow ND. Neurobiology of addiction: a neurocircuitry analysis. *Lancet Psychiatry* 2016;3(8):760–773.

100. Lowinson J. Opiates: clinical aspects. In: Lowinson J, Ruiz P, Millman R, eds. *Substance Abuse: A Comprehensive Textbook*. Baltimore, MD: Williams & Wilkins; 1992:186–194.

101. Younger J, Barelka P, Carroll I, et al. Reduced cold pain tolerance in chronic pain patients following opioid detoxification. *Pain Med* 2008;9:1158–1163.

102. Hooten WM, Mantilla CB, Sandroni P, et al. Associations between heat pain perception and opioid dose among patients with chronic pain undergoing opioid tapering. *Pain Med* 2010;11:1587–1598.

103. Wang H, Akbar M, Weinsheimer N, et al. Longitudinal observation of changes in pain sensitivity during opioid tapering in patients with chronic low-back pain. *Pain Med* 2011;12:1720–1726.

104. Brodner RA, Taub A. Chronic pain exacerbated by long-term narcotic use in patients with nonmalignant disease: clinical syndrome and treatment. *Mt Sinai J Med* 1978;45:233–237.

105. Ballantyne JC, Sullivan MD, Kolodny A. Opioid dependence vs addiction: a distinction without a difference? *Arch Intern Med* 2012;172(17):1342–1343.

106. Angst MS, Clark JD. Opioid-induced hyperalgesia: a qualitative systematic review. *Anesthesiology* 2006;104(3):570–587.

107. Chu LF, Angst MS, Clark D. Opioid-induced hyperalgesia in humans: molecular mechanisms and clinical considerations. *Clin J Pain* 2008;24(6):479–496.

108. Koppert W, Angst M, Alsheimer M, et al. Naloxone provokes similar pain facilitation as observed after short-term infusion of remifentanil in humans. *Pain* 2003;106(1–2):91–99.

109. Li X, Angst MS, Clark JD. A murine model of opioid-induced hyperalgesia. *Brain Res Mol Brain Res* 2001;86(1–2):56–62.

110. Mao J. Opioid-induced abnormal pain sensitivity: implications in clinical opioid therapy. *Pain* 2002;100(3):213–217.

111. Koob GF. Neuroadaptive mechanisms of addiction: studies on the extended amygdala. *Eur Neuropsychopharmacol* 2003;13(6):442–452.

112. Aston-Jones G, Delfs JM, Druhan J, et al. The bed nucleus of the stria terminalis: a target site for noradrenergic actions in opiate withdrawal. In: McGinty JF, ed. *Advancing from the Ventral Striatum to the Extended Amygdala: Implications for Neuropsychiatry and Drug Abuse*. New York: New York Academy of Sciences; 1999:486–498. *Annals of the New York Academy of Sciences*; vol 877.

113. Funk C, O'Dell L, Crawford E, et al. Corticotropin-releasing factor within the central nucleus of the amygdala mediates enhanced ethanol self-administration in withdrawn, ethanol-dependent rats. *J Neurosci* 2006;26:11324–11332.

114. Edwards S, Vendruscolo LF, Schlosburg JE, et al. Development of mechanical hypersensitivity in rats during heroin and ethanol dependence: alleviation by CRF$_1$ receptor antagonism. *Neuropharmacology* 2012;62(2):1142–1151.

115. Kaplan H, Fields HL. Hyperalgesia during acute opioid abstinence: evidence for a nociceptive facilitating function of the rostral ventromedial medulla. *J Neurosci* 1991;11(5):1433–1439.

116. Martin WR, Gilbert PE, Jasinski DR, et al. An analysis of naltrexone precipitated abstinence in morphine-dependent chronic spinal dogs. *J Pharmacol Exp Ther* 1987;240(2):565–570.

117. Sweitzer SM, Allen CP, Zissen MH, et al. Mechanical allodynia and thermal hyperalgesia upon acute opioid withdrawal in the neonatal rat. *Pain* 2004;110(1–2):269–280.

118. Tilson HA, Rech RH, Stolman S. Hyperalgesia during withdrawal as a means of measuring the degree of dependence in morphine dependent rats. *Psychopharmacologia* 1973;28(3):287–300.

119. Bederson JB, Fields HL, Barbaro NM. Hyperalgesia during naloxone-precipitated withdrawal from morphine is associated with increased on-cell activity in the rostral ventromedial medulla. *Somatosens Mot Res* 1990;7(2):185–203.

120. Jasinski DS. Assessment of the abuse potentiality of the morphine-like drugs (methods used in man). In: Martin WR, ed. *Drug Addiction I*. New York: Springer-Verlag; 1997:197–258. *Handbook of Experimental Pharmacology*; vol 45.

121. Grilly DM, Gowans GC. Acute morphine dependence: effects observed in shock and light discrimination tasks. *Psychopharmacology (Berl)* 1986;88(4):500–504.

122. Kim DH, Fields HL, Barbaro NM. Morphine analgesia and acute physical dependence: rapid onset of two opposing, dose-related processes. *Brain Res* 1990;516(1):37–40.

123. Compton P, Athanasos P, Elashoff D. Withdrawal hyperalgesia after acute opioid physical dependence in nonaddicted humans: a preliminary study. *J Pain* 2003;4:511–519.

124. Compton P, Charuvastra VC, Ling W. Pain intolerance in opioid-maintained former opiate addicts: effect of long-acting maintenance agent. *Drug Alcohol Depend* 2001;63(2):139–146.

125. Ren ZY, Shi J, Epstein DH, et al. Abnormal pain response in pain-sensitive opiate addicts after prolonged abstinence predicts increased drug craving. *Psychopharmacology (Berl)* 2009;204:423–429.

126. Colpaert FC. System theory of pain and of opiate analgesia: no tolerance to opiates. *Pharmacol Rev* 1996;48(3):355–402.

127. Colpaert FC. Mechanisms of opioid-induced pain and antinociceptive tolerance: signal transduction. *Pain* 2002;95(3):287–288.

128. Célèrier E, Laulin J, Larcher A, et al. Evidence for opiate-activated NMDA processes masking opiate analgesia in rats. *Brain Res* 1999;847(1):18–25.

129. Célèrier E, Laulin JP, Corcuff JB, et al. Progressive enhancement of delayed hyperalgesia induced by repeated heroin administration: a sensitization process. *J Neurosci* 2001;21(11):4074–4080.

130. Laulin JP, Célèrier E, Larcher A, et al. Opiate tolerance to daily heroin administration: an apparent phenomenon associated with enhanced pain sensitivity. *Neuroscience* 1999;89(3):631–636.

131. Mao J, Price DD, Mayer DJ. Thermal hyperalgesia in association with the development of morphine tolerance in rats: roles of excitatory amino acid receptors and protein kinase C. *J Neurosci* 1994;14(4):2301–2312.

132. Mao J, Price DD, Mayer DJ. Experimental mononeuropathy reduces the antinociceptive effects of morphine: implications for common intracellular mechanisms involved in morphine tolerance and neuropathic pain. *Pain* 1995;61(3):353–364.

133. Mao J, Price DD, Mayer DJ. Mechanisms of hyperalgesia and morphine tolerance: a current view of their possible interactions. *Pain* 1995;62(3):259–274.

134. Mayer DJ, Mao J, Price DD. The association of neuropathic pain, morphine tolerance and dependence, and the translocation of protein kinase C. *NIDA Res Monogr* 1995;147:269–298.

135. Mayer DJ, Mao J, Price DD. The development of morphine tolerance and dependence is associated with translocation of protein kinase C. *Pain* 1995;61(3):365–374.

136. Dogrul A, Bilsky EJ, Ossipov MH, et al. Spinal L-type calcium channel blockade abolishes opioid-induced sensory hypersensitivity and antinociceptive tolerance. *Anesth Analg* 2005;101(6):1730–1735.

137. Gardell LR, Wang R, Burgess SE, et al. Sustained morphine exposure induces a spinal dynorphin-dependent enhancement of excitatory transmitter release from primary afferent fibers. *J Neurosci* 2002;22(15):6747–6755.

138. King T, Gardell LR, Wang R, et al. Role of NK-1 neurotransmission in opioid-induced hyperalgesia. *Pain* 2005;116(3):276–288.

139. Lim G, Wang S, Zeng Q, et al. Evidence for a long-term influence on morphine tolerance after previous morphine exposure: role of neuronal glucocorticoid receptors. *Pain* 2005;114(1–2):81–92.

140. Raghavendra V, Rutkowski MD, DeLeo JA. The role of spinal neuroimmune activation in morphine tolerance/hyperalgesia in neuropathic and sham-operated rats. *J Neurosci* 2002;22(22):9980–9989.

141. Vanderah TW, Gardell LR, Burgess SE, et al. Dynorphin promotes abnormal pain and spinal opioid antinociceptive tolerance. *J Neurosci* 2000;20(18):7074–7079.

142. Vanderah TW, Suenaga NM, Ossipov MH, et al. Tonic descending facilitation from the rostral ventromedial medulla mediates opioid-induced abnormal pain and antinociceptive tolerance. *J Neurosci* 2001;21(1):279–286.

143. Gardell LR, King T, Ossipov MH, et al. Opioid receptor-mediated hyperalgesia and antinociceptive tolerance induced by sustained opiate delivery. *Neurosci Lett* 2006;396(1):44–49.

144. Dunbar SA, Pulai IJ. Repetitive opioid abstinence causes progressive hyperalgesia sensitive to N-methyl-D-aspartate receptor blockade in the rat. *J Pharmacol Exp Ther* 1998;284(2):678–686.

145. Dunbar S, Yaksh TL. Concurrent spinal infusion of MK801 blocks spinal tolerance and dependence induced by chronic intrathecal morphine in the rat. *Anesthesiology* 1996;84(5):1177–1188.

146. Larcher A, Laulin JP, Celerier E, et al. Acute tolerance associated with a single opiate administration: involvement of N-methyl-D-aspartate-dependent pain facilitatory systems. *Neuroscience* 1998;84(2):583–589.

147. Richebé P, Rivat C, Creton C, et al. Nitrous oxide revisited: evidence for potent antihyperalgesic properties. *Anesthesiology* 2005;103(4):845–854.

148. Portenoy RK, Bennett GJ, Katz NP, et al. Enhancing opioid analgesia with NMDA-receptor antagonists: clarifying the clinical importance. A roundtable discussion. *J Pain Symptom Manage* 2000;19(suppl 1):S57–S64.

149. Price DD, Mayer DJ, Mao J, et al. NMDA-receptor antagonists and opioid receptor interactions as related to analgesia and tolerance. *J Pain Symptom Manage* 2000;19(suppl 1):S7–S11.

150. Sang CN. NMDA-receptor antagonists in neuropathic pain: experimental methods to clinical trials. *J Pain Symptom Manage* 2000;19(suppl 1): S21–S25.

151. Weinbroum AA, Rudick V, Paret G, et al. The role of dextromethorphan in pain control. *Can J Anaesth* 2000;47(6):585–596.

152. Bisaga A, Popik P. In search of a new pharmacological treatment for drug and alcohol addiction: N-methyl-D-aspartate (NMDA) antagonists. *Drug Alcohol Depend* 2000;59(1):1–15.

153. Elliott K, Hynansky A, Inturrisi CE. Dextromethorphan attenuates and reverses analgesic tolerance to morphine. *Pain* 1994;59(3):361–368.

154. Pasternak GW, Kolesnikov YA, Babey AM. Perspectives on the N-methyl-D-aspartate/nitric oxide cascade and opioid tolerance. *Neuropsychopharmacology* 1995;13(4):309–313.

155. Trujillo KA. Effects of noncompetitive N-methyl-D-aspartate receptor antagonists on opiate tolerance and physical dependence. *Neuropsychopharmacology* 1995;13(4):301–307.

156. Compton PA, Ling W, Torrington MA. Lack of effect of chronic dextromethorphan on experimental pain tolerance in methadone-maintained patients. *Addict Biol* 2008;13(3–4):393–402.

157. Ossipov MH, Lai J, King T, et al. Underlying mechanisms of pronociceptive consequences of prolonged morphine exposure. *Biopolymers* 2005; 80(2–3):319–324.

158. Xie JY, Herman DS, Stiller CO, et al. Cholecystokinin in the rostral ventromedial medulla mediates opioid-induced hyperalgesia and antinociceptive tolerance. *J Neurosci* 2005;25(2):409–416.

159. Benedetti F, Amanzio M, Vighetti S, et al. The biochemical and neuroendocrine bases of the hyperalgesic nocebo effect. *J Neurosci* 2006;26(46): 12014–12022.

160. Devillers JP, Boisserie F, Laulin JP, et al. Simultaneous activation of spinal antiopioid system (neuropeptide FF) and pain facilitatory circuitry by stimulation of opioid receptors in rats. *Brain Res* 1995;700(1–2):173–181.

161. Khasabov SG, Simone DA. Loss of neurons in rostral ventromedial medulla that express neurokinin-1 receptors decreases the development of hyperalgesia. *Neuroscience* 2013;250:151–165. doi:10.1016/j.neuroscience.2013.06.057.

162. DeLeo JA, Tanga FY, Tawfik VL. Neuroimmune activation and neuroinflammation in chronic pain and opioid tolerance/hyperalgesia. *Neuroscientist* 2004;10(1):40–52.

163. Watkins LR, Maier SF. The pain of being sick: implications of immune-to-brain communication for understanding pain. *Annu Rev Psychol* 2000; 51:29–57.

164. Wieseler-Frank J, Maier SF, Watkins LR. Immune-to-brain communication dynamically modulates pain: physiological and pathological consequences. *Brain Behav Immun* 2005;19(2):104–111.

165. Song P, Zhao ZQ. The involvement of glial cells in the development of morphine tolerance. *Neurosci Res* 2001;39(3):281–286.

166. Johnston IN, Westbrook RF. Inhibition of morphine analgesia by LPS: role of opioid and NMDA receptors and spinal glia. *Behav Brain Res* 2005;156(1):75–83.

167. Johnston IN, Milligan ED, Wieseler-Frank J, et al. A role for proinflammatory cytokines and fractalkine in analgesia, tolerance, and subsequent pain facilitation induced by chronic intrathecal morphine. *J Neurosci* 2004;24(33):7353–7365.

168. McNally GP. Pain facilitatory circuits in the mammalian central nervous system: their behavioral significance and role in morphine analgesic tolerance. *Neurosci Biobehav Rev* 1999;23(8):1059–1078.

169. Houghtling RA, Mellon RD, Tan RJ, et al. Acute effects of morphine on blood lymphocyte proliferation and plasma IL-6 levels. *Ann N Y Acad Sci* 2000;917:771–777.

170. Pacifici R, di Carlo S, Bacosi A, et al. Pharmacokinetics and cytokine production in heroin and morphine-treated mice. *Int J Immunopharmacol* 2000;22(8):603–614.

171. Holán V, Zajícová A, Krulova M, et al. Augmented production of proinflammatory cytokines and accelerated allotransplantation reactions in heroin-treated mice. *Clin Exp Immunol* 2003;132(1):40–45.

172. Sacerdote P. Effects of in vitro and in vivo opioids on the production of IL-12 and IL-10 by murine macrophages. *Ann N Y Acad Sci* 2003;992: 129–140.

173. Kelschenbach J, Barke RA, Roy S. Morphine withdrawal contributes to TH cell differentiation by biasing cells toward the TH2 lineage. *J Immunol* 2005;175:2655–2665.

174. Hutchinson MR, Coats BD, Lewis SS, et al. Proinflammatory cytokines oppose opioid-induced acute and chronic analgesia. *Brain Behav Immun* 2008;22(8):1178–1189.

175. Watkins LR, Hutchinson MR, Johnston IN, et al. Glia: novel counter-regulators of opioid analgesia. *Trends Neurosci* 2005;28(12):661–669.

176. Krank MD, Hinson RE, Siegel S. Conditional hyperalgesia is elicited by environmental signals of morphine. *Behav Neural Biol* 1981;32(2):148–157.

177. Siegel S, Hinson RE, Krank MD. The role of predrug signals in morphine analgesic tolerance: support for a Pavlovian conditioning model of tolerance. *J Exp Psychol Anim Behav Process* 1978;4(2):188–196.

178. Albutt C. On the abuse of hypodermic injections of morphia. *Practitioner* 1870;3:327–330.

179. Martin JE, Inglis J. Pain tolerance and narcotic addiction. *Br J Soc Clin Psychol* 1965;4(3):224–229.

180. Ho A, Dole VP. Pain perception in drug-free and in methadone-maintained human ex-addicts. *Proc Soc Exp Biol Med* 1979;162(3):392–395.

181. Compton P, Charuvastra VC, Kintaudi K, et al. Pain responses in methadone-maintained opioid abusers. *J Pain Symptom Manage* 2000;20(4): 237–245.

182. Doverty M, White JM, Somogyi AA, et al. Hyperalgesic responses in methadone maintenance patients. *Pain* 2001;90(1–2):91–96.

183. Treister R, Eisenberg E, Lawental E, et al. Is opioid-induced hyperalgesia reversible? A study on active and former opioid addicts and drug naïve controls. *J Opioid Manag* 2012;8(6):343–349. doi:10.5055/jom.2012.0134.

184. Schall U, Katta T, Pries E, et al. Pain perception of intravenous heroin users on maintenance therapy with levomethadone. *Pharmacopsychiatry* 1996;29(5):176–179.

185. Athanasos P, Smith CS, White JM, et al. Methadone maintenance patients are cross-tolerant to the antinociceptive effects of very high plasma morphine concentrations. *Pain* 2006;120(3):267–275.

186. Pud D, Cohen D, Lawental E, et al. Opioids and abnormal pain perception: new evidence from a study of chronic opioid addicts and healthy subjects. *Drug Alcohol Depend* 2006;82(3):218–223.

187. Carcoba LM, Contreras AE, Cepeda-Benito A, et al. Negative affect heightens opiate withdrawal-induced hyperalgesia in heroin dependent individuals. *J Addict Dis* 2011;30(3):258–270.

188. Liebmann PM, Lehofer M, Moser M, et al. Persistent analgesia in former opiate addicts is resistant to blockade of endogenous opioids. *Biol Psychiatry* 1997;42(10):962–964.

189. Liebmann PM, Lehofer M, Moser M, et al. Nervousness and pain sensitivity: II. Changed relation in ex-addicts as a predictor for early relapse. *Psychiatry Res* 1998;79(1):55–58.

190. Prosser JM, Steinfeld M, Cohen LJ, et al. Abnormal heat and pain perception in remitted heroin dependence months after detoxification from methadone-maintenance. *Drug Alcohol Depend* 2008;95(3):237–244.

191. Chia YY, Liu K, Wang JJ, et al. Intraoperative high dose fentanyl induces postoperative fentanyl tolerance. *Can J Anaesth* 1999;46(9):872–877.

192. Fletcher D, Martinez V. How can we prevent opioid induced hyperalgesia in surgical patients? *Br J Anaesth* 2016;116(4):447–449. doi:10.1093/bja/aew050.

193. Fletcher D, Martinez V. Opioid-induced hyperalgesia in patients after surgery: a systematic review and a meta-analysis. *Br J Anaesth* 2014;112(6): 991–1004. doi:10.1093/bja/aeu137.

194. Angst MS. Intraoperative use of remifentanil for tiva: postoperative pain, acute tolerance, and opioid-induced hyperalgesia. *J Cardiothorac Vasc Anesth* 2015;29(suppl 1):S16–S22. doi:10.1053/j.jvca.2015.01.026.

195. Lyons PJ, Rivosecchi RM, Nery JP, et al. Fentanyl-induced hyperalgesia in acute pain management. *J Pain Palliat Care Pharmacother* 2015;29(2): 153–160. doi:10.3109/15360288.2015.1035835.

196. Richebé P, Pouquet O, Jelacic S, et al. Target-controlled dosing of remifentanil during cardiac surgery reduces postoperative hyperalgesia. *J Cardiothorac Vasc Anesth* 2011;25(6):917–925. doi:10.1053/j.jvca.2011.03.185.

197. Leal PC, Salomão R, Brunialti MK, et al. Evaluation of the effect of ketamine on remifentanil-induced hyperalgesia: a double-blind, randomized study. *J Clin Anesth* 2015;27(4):331–337. doi:10.1016/j.jclinane.2015.02.002.

198. Loftus RW, Yeager MP, Clark JA, et al. Intraoperative ketamine reduces perioperative opiate consumption in opiate-dependent patients with chronic back pain undergoing back surgery. *Anesthesiology* 2010;113(3):639–646. doi:10.1097/ALN.0b013e3181e90914.

199. Tverskoy M, Oz Y, Isakson A, et al. Preemptive effect of fentanyl and ketamine on postoperative pain and wound hyperalgesia. *Anesth Analg* 1994;78(2):205–209.

200. Song JW, Lee YW, Yoon KB, et al. Magnesium sulfate prevents remifentanil-induced postoperative hyperalgesia in patients undergoing thyroidectomy. *Anesth Analg* 2011;113(2):390–397. doi:10.1213/ANE.0b013e31821d72bc.

201. Lee C, Kim YD, Kim JN. Antihyperalgesic effects of dexmedetomidine on high-dose remifentanil-induced hyperalgesia. *Korean J Anesthesiol* 2013;64(4):301–307. doi:10.4097/kjae.2013.64.4.301.

202. Lee C, Lee HW, Kim JN. Effect of oral pregabalin on opioid-induced hyperalgesia in patients undergoing laparo-endoscopic single-site urologic surgery. *Korean J Anesthesiol* 2013;64(1):19–24. doi:10.4097/kjae.2013.64.1.19.

203. Kaye AD, Chung KS, Vadivelu N, et al. Opioid induced hyperalgesia altered with propofol infusion. *Pain Physician* 2014;17(2):E225–E228.

204. Ali NM. Hyperalgesic response in a patient receiving high concentrations of spinal morphine. *Anesthesiology* 1986;65(4):449.

205. Mercadante S, Ferrera P, Villari P, et al. Hyperalgesia: an emerging iatrogenic syndrome. *J Pain Symptom Manage* 2003;26(2):769–775.

206. Mercadante S, Arcuri E. Hyperalgesia and opioid switching. *Am J Hosp Palliat Care* 2005;22(4):291–294.

207. Sjøgren P, Jonsson T, Jensen NH, et al. Hyperalgesia and myoclonus in terminal cancer patients treated with continuous intravenous morphine. *Pain* 1993;55(1):93–97.

208. Okon TR, George ML. Fentanyl-induced neurotoxicity and paradoxic pain. *J Pain Symptom Manage* 2008;35(3):327–333.

209. Devulder J. Hyperalgesia induced by high-dose intrathecal sufentanil in neuropathic pain. *J Neurosurg Anesthesiol* 1997;9(2):146–148.

210. Suzan E, Eisenberg E, Treister R, et al. A negative correlation between hyperalgesia and analgesia in patients with chronic radicular pain: is hydromorphone therapy a double-edged sword? *Pain Physician* 2013;16(1):65–76.

211. Edwards RR, Wasan AD, Michna E, et al. Elevated pain sensitivity in chronic pain patients at risk for opioid misuse. *J Pain* 2011;12(9):953–963. doi:10.1016/j.jpain.2011.02.357.

212. Chu LF, Clark DJ, Angst MS. Opioid tolerance and hyperalgesia in chronic pain patients after one month of oral morphine therapy: a preliminary prospective study. *J Pain* 2006;7:43–48.

213. Suzan E, Midbari A, Treister R, et al. Oxycodone alters temporal summation but not conditioned pain modulation: preclinical findings and possible relations to mechanisms of opioid analgesia. *Pain* 2013;154(8):1413–1418. doi:10.1016/j.pain.2013.04.036.

214. Kim SH, Yoon DM, Choi KW, et al. High-dose daily opioid administration and poor functional status intensify local anesthetic injection pain in cancer patients. *Pain Physician* 2013;16(3):E247–E256.

215. Hay JL, White JM, Bochner F, et al. Hyperalgesia in opioid-managed chronic pain and opioid-dependent patients. *J Pain* 2009;10(3):316–322. doi:10.1016/j.jpain.2008.10.003.

216. Krebs E, Gravely A, Nugent S, et al. Effect of opioid vs nonopioid medications on pain-related function in patients with chronic back pain or hip or knee osteoarthritis pain: the SPACE randomized clinical trial. *JAMA* 2018;319(9):872–882.

217. Fishbain DA, Cole B, Lewis JE, et al. Do opioids induce hyperalgesia in humans? An evidence-based structured review. *Pain Med* 2009;10(5):829–839.

218. Tompkins DA, Campbell CM. Opioid-induced hyperalgesia: clinically relevant or extraneous research phenomenon? *Curr Pain Headache Rep* 2011;15(2):129–136.

219. Baron MJ, McDonald PW. Significant pain reduction in chronic pain patients after detoxification from high-dose opioids. *J Opioid Manag* 2006;2: 277–282.

220. Krumova EK, Bennemann P, Kindler D, et al. Low pain intensity after opioid withdrawal as a first step of a comprehensive pain rehabilitation program predicts long-term nonuse of opioids in chronic noncancer pain. *Clin J Pain* 2013;29:760–769.

221. Darchuk KM, Townsend CO, Rome JD, et al. Longitudinal treatment outcomes for geriatric patients with chronic non-cancer pain at an interdisciplinary pain rehabilitation program. *Pain Med* 2010;11:1352–1364.

222. Hayhurst CJ, Durieux ME. Differential opioid tolerance and opioid-induced hyperalgesia: a clinical reality. *Anesthesiology* 2016;124(2):483–488.

223. Frank JW, Lovejoy TI, Becker WC, et al. Patient outcomes in dose reduction or discontinuation of long-term opioid therapy: a systematic review. *Ann Intern Med* 2017;167:181–191.

224. Schuh-Hofer S, Wodarski R, Pfau DB, et al. One night of total sleep deprivation promotes a state of generalized hyperalgesia: a surrogate pain model to study the relationship of insomnia and pain. *Pain* 2013;154(9):1613–1621.

225. Nijs J, Loggia ML, Polli A, et al. Sleep disturbances and severe stress as glial activators: key targets for treating central sensitization in chronic pain patients? *Expert Opin Ther Targets* 2017;21(8):817–826.

226. Sluka KA, Clauw DJ. Neurobiology of fibromyalgia and chronic widespread pain. *Neuroscience* 2016;338:114–129.

227. Kest B, Hopkins E, Palmese CA, et al. Genetic variation in morphine analgesic tolerance: a survey of 11 inbred mouse strains. *Pharmacol Biochem Behav* 2002;73(4):821–828.

228. Kest B, Palmese CA, Hopkins E, et al. Naloxone-precipitated withdrawal jumping in 11 inbred mouse strains: evidence for common genetic mechanisms in acute and chronic morphine physical dependence. *Neuroscience* 2002;115(2):463–469.

229. Kest B, Palmese CA, Juni A, et al. Mapping of a quantitative trait locus for morphine withdrawal severity. *Mamm Genome* 2004;15(8):610–617.

230. Liang DY, Liao G, Lighthall GK, et al. Genetic variants of the P-glycoprotein gene Abcb1b modulate opioid-induced hyperalgesia, tolerance and dependence. *Pharmacogenet Genomics* 2006;16(11):825–835.

231. Liang DY, Guo T, Liao G, et al. Chronic pain and genetic background interact and influence opioid analgesia, tolerance, and physical dependence. *Pain* 2006;121(3):232–240.

232. He Y, Wang ZJ. Let-7 microRNAs and opioid tolerance. *Front Genet* 2012;3:110. doi:10.3389/fgene.2012.00110.

233. Knothe C, Doehring A, Ultsch A, et al. Methadone induces hypermethylation of human DNA. *Epigenomics* 2016;8(2):167–179.

234. Kolb L. Types and characteristics of drug addicts. *Ment Hyg* 1925;9: 300–313.

235. Rayport M. Experience in the management of patients medically addicted to narcotics. *J Am Med Assoc* 1954;156:684–691.

236. Portenoy RK, Foley KM. Chronic use of opioid analgesics in non-malignant pain: report of 38 cases. *Pain* 1986;25(2):171–186.

237. Perry S, Heidrich G. Management of pain during debridement: a survey of U.S. burn units. *Pain* 1982;13:267–280.

238. Fishbain D, Cole B, Lewis J, et al. What percentage of chronic nonmalignant pain patients exposed to chronic opioid analgesic therapy develop abuse/addiction and/or aberrant drug-related behaviors? A structured evidence-based review. *Pain Med* 2008;9:444–459.

239. Campbell G, Bruno R, Lintzeris N, et al. Defining problematic pharmaceutical opioid use among people prescribed opioids for chronic noncancer pain: do different measures identify the same patients? *Pain* 2016;157(7): 1489–1498.

240. Smith SM, Dart RC, Katz NP, et al. Classification and definition of misuse, abuse, and related events in clinical trials: ACTTION systematic review and recommendations. *Pain* 2013;154:2287–2296.

241. Turk D, Swanson K, Gatchel R. Predicting opioid misuse by chronic pain patients: a systematic review and literature synthesis. *Clin J Pain* 2008;24: 497–508.

242. Chou R, Fanciullo G, Fine P, et al. Opioids for chronic noncancer pain: prediction and identification of aberrant drug-related behaviors: a review of the evidence for an American Pain Society and American Academy of Pain Medicine clinical practice guideline. *J Pain* 2009;10:131–146.

243. Cicero TJ, Lynskey M, Todorov A, et al. Co-morbid pain and psychopathology in males and females admitted to treatment for opioid analgesic abuse. *Pain* 2008;139(1):127–135.

244. Voon P, Hayashi K, Milloy MJ, et al. Pain among high-risk patients on methadone maintenance treatment. *J Pain* 2015;16(9):887–894.

245. Barry DT, Cutter CJ, Beitel M, et al. Psychiatric disorders among patients seeking treatment for co-occurring chronic pain and opioid use disorder. *J Clin Psychiatry* 2016;77(10):1413–1419.

246. Potter JS, Shiffman SJ, Weiss RD. Chronic pain severity in opioid-dependent patients. *Am J Drug Alcohol Abuse* 2008;34(1):101–107.

247. Rosenblum A, Joseph H, Fong C, et al. Prevalence and characteristics of chronic pain among chemically dependent patients in methadone maintenance and residential treatment facilities. *JAMA* 2003;289(18):2370–2378.

248. Jamison RN, Kauffman J, Katz NP. Characteristics of methadone maintenance patients with chronic pain. *J Pain Symptom Manage* 2000;19(1):53–62.

249. Peles E, Schreiber S, Gordon J, et al. Significantly higher methadone dose for methadone maintenance treatment (MMT) patients with chronic pain. *Pain* 2005;113(3):340–346.

250. Karasz A, Zallman L, Berg K, et al. The experience of chronic severe pain in patients undergoing methadone maintenance treatment. *J Pain Symptom Manage* 2004;28(5):517–525.

251. Ilgen MA, Trafton JA, Humphreys K. Response to methadone maintenance treatment of opiate dependent patients with and without significant pain. *Drug Alcohol Depend* 2006;82(3):187–193.

252. Novak SP, Herman-Stahl M, Flannery B, et al. Physical pain, common psychiatric and substance use disorders, and the non-medical use of prescription analgesics in the United States. *Drug Alcohol Depend* 2009;100(1–2):63–70.

253. Tsui JI, Lira MC, Cheng DM, et al. Chronic pain, craving, and illicit opioid use among patients receiving opioid agonist therapy. *Drug Alcohol Depend* 2016;166:26–31.

254. Griffin ML, McDermott KA, McHugh RK, et al. Longitudinal association between pain severity and subsequent opioid use in prescription opioid dependent patients with chronic pain. *Drug Alcohol Depend* 2016;163: 216–221.

255. West SL. Substance use among persons with traumatic brain injury: a review. *NeuroRehabilitation* 2011;29(1):1–8.

256. MacLeod JB, Hungerford DW. Alcohol-related injury visits: do we know the true prevalence in U.S. trauma centres? *Injury* 2011;42(9):922–926.

257. Chou R, Gordon DB, de Leon-Casasola OA, et al. Management of postoperative pain: a clinical practice guideline from the American Pain Society, the American Society of Regional Anesthesia and Pain Medicine, and the American Society of Anesthesiologists' Committee on Regional Anesthesia, Executive Committee, and Administrative Council. *J Pain* 2016;17(2):131–157.

258. Uskova A, O'Connor JE. Liposomal bupivacaine for regional anesthesia. *Curr Opin Anaesthesiol* 2015;28(5):593–597.

259. Bounes V, Palmaro A, Lapeyre-Mestre M, et al. Long-term consequences of acute pain for patients under methadone or buprenorphine maintenance treatment. *Pain Physician* 2013;16:E739–E747.

260. Sen S, Arulkumar S, Cornett EM, et al. New pain management options for the surgical patient on methadone and buprenorphine. *Curr Pain Headache Rep* 2016;20(3):16.

261. OpioidRisk. Government regulations on prescribing controlled substances. Available at: http://www.opioidrisk.com/book/export/html/555. Accessed May 23, 2013.

262. Simpson GK, Jackson M. Perioperative management of opioid-tolerant patients. *BJA Education* 2017;17(4):124–128.

263. Gevirtz C, Frost EA, Bryson EO. Perioperative implications of buprenorphine maintenance treatment for opioid addiction. *Int Anesthesiol Clin.* 2011;49(1):147–155.

264. Donroe JH, Holt SR, Tetrault JM. Caring for patients with opioid use disorder in the hospital. *CMAJ* 2016;188:17–18.

265. Taveros MC, Chuang EJ. Pain management strategies for patients on methadone maintenance therapy: a systematic review of the literature. *BMJ Support Palliat Care* 2017;7:383–389.

266. Eyler EC. Chronic and acute pain and pain management for patients in methadone maintenance treatment. *Am J Addict* 2013;22(1):75–83.

267. Harrington CJ, Zaydfudim V. Buprenorphine maintenance therapy hinders acute pain management in trauma. *Am Surg* 2010;76(4):397–399.

268. Tröster A, Ihmsen H, Singler B, et al. Interaction of fentanyl and buprenorphine in an experimental model of pain and central sensitization in human volunteers. *Clin J Pain* 2012;28(8):705–711.

269. Alford DP, Compton P, Samet JH. Acute pain management for patients receiving maintenance methadone or buprenorphine therapy. *Ann Intern Med* 2006;144:127–134.

270. Center for Substance Abuse Treatment. *Clinical Guidelines for the Use of Buprenorphine in the Treatment of Opioid Addiction.* Treatment Improvement Protocol (TIP) Series 40, DHHS Publication No. (SMA) 04-3939. Rockville, MD: Substance Abuse and Mental Health Services Administration; 2004.

271. Anderson TA, Quaye ANA, Ward EN, et al. To stop or not, that is the question: acute pain management for the patient on chronic buprenorphine. *Anesthesiology* 2017;126(6):1180–1186.

272. Kornfeld H, Manfredi L. Effectiveness of full agonist opioids in patients stabilized on buprenorphine undergoing major surgery: a case series. *Am J Ther* 2010;17(5):523–528.

273. Dahan A, Yassen A, Romberg R, et al. Buprenorphine induces ceiling in respiratory depression but not in analgesia. *Br J Anaesth* 2006;96(5):627–632.

274. Pergolizzi J, Aloisi AM, Dahan A, et al. Current knowledge of buprenorphine and its unique pharmacological profile. *Pain Pract* 2010;10(5):428–450.

275. Myers J, Compton P. Addressing the potential for perioperative relapse in those recovering from opioid use disorder [published online ahead of print November 22, 2017]. *Pain Med.* doi:10.1093/pm/pnx277.

276. Coluzzi F, Bifulco F, Cuomo A, et al. The challenge of perioperative pain management in opioid-tolerant patients. *Ther Clin Risk Manag* 2017;13:1163–1173.

277. Sasek C. Perioperative pain management in the chronic opioid user. *J Orthop Physician Assist* 2016;4(4):25–31.

278. Stromer W, Michaeli K, Sandner-Kiesling A. Perioperative pain therapy in opioid abuse. *Eur J Anaesthesiol* 2013;30:55–64.

279. Gritsenko K, Khelemsky Y, Kaye AD, et al. Multimodal therapy in perioperative analgesia. *Best Pract Res Clin Anaesthesiol* 2014;28(1):59–79.

280. Brill S, Ginosar Y, Davidson EM. Perioperative management of chronic pain patients with opioid dependency. *Curr Opin Anaesthesiol* 2006;19(3):325–331.

281. Bruera E, Moyano J, Seifert L, et al. The frequency of alcoholism among patients with pain due to terminal cancer. *J Pain Symptom Manage* 1995;10(8):599–603.

282. Derogatis LR, Morrow GR, Fetting J, et al. The prevalence of psychiatric disorders among cancer patients. *JAMA* 1983;249:751–757.

283. Passik SD, Portenoy RK, Ricketts PL. Substance abuse issues in cancer patients. Part 1: prevalence and diagnosis. *Oncology (Williston Park)* 1998;12(4):517–524.

284. Chhatre S, Metzger DS, Malkowicz SB, et al. Substance use disorder and its effects on outcomes in men with advanced-stage prostate cancer. *Cancer* 2014;120(21):3338–3345.

285. Ballantyne JC. Opioid misuse in oncology pain patients. *Curr Pain Headache Rep* 2007;11(4):276–282.

286. Dev R, Parsons HA, Palla S, et al. Undocumented alcoholism and its correlation with tobacco and illegal drug use in advanced cancer patients. *Cancer* 2011;117(19):4551–4556.

287. Kircher S, Zacny J, Apfelbaum SM, et al. Understanding and treating opioid addiction in a patient with cancer pain. *J Pain* 2011;12(10):1025–1031.

288. Modesto-Lowe V, Girard L, Chaplin M. Cancer pain in the opioid-addicted patient: can we treat it right? *J Opioid Manag* 2012;8(3):167–175.

289. U.S. Department of Defense, U.S. Department of Veterans Affairs. VA/DoD clinical practice guideline: diagnosis and treatment of low back pain (LBP) (2017). Available at: https://www.healthquality.va.gov/guidelines/Pain/lbp/. Accessed October 30, 2017.

290. Cheatle MD, Gallagher RM, O'Brien CP. Low risk of producing an opioid use disorder in primary care by prescribing opioids to prescreened patients with chronic noncancer pain. *Pain Med* 2018;19:764–773.

291. Chang YP, Compton P. Management of chronic pain with chronic opioid therapy in patients with substance use disorders. *Addict Sci Clin Pract* 2013;8:21. doi:10.1186/1940-0640-8-21.

292. McCarberg BH. Pain management in primary care: strategies to mitigate opioid misuse, abuse, and diversion. *Postgrad Med* 2011;123(2):119–130.

293. Gourlay DL, Heit HA, Almahrezi A. Universal precautions in pain medicine: a rational approach to the treatment of chronic pain. *Pain Med* 2005;6(2):107–112.

294. Oliver J, Coggins C, Compton P, et al. American Society for Pain Management nursing position statement: pain management in patients with substance use disorders. *Pain Manag Nurs* 2012;13(3):169–183.

295. Wu SM, Compton P, Bolus R, et al. The addiction behaviors checklist: validation of a new clinician-based measure of inappropriate opioid use in chronic pain. *J Pain Symptom Manage* 2006;32(4):342–351.

296. Compton P, Wu SM, Schieffer B, et al. Introduction of a self-report version of the Prescription Drug Use Questionnaire and relationship to medication agreement noncompliance. *J Pain Symptom Manage* 2008;36(4):383–395.

297. Meltzer EC, Rybin D, Saitz R, et al. Identifying prescription opioid use disorder in primary care: diagnostic characteristics of the Current Opioid Misuse Measure (COMM). *Pain* 2011;152(2):397–402.

298. Jamison RN, Ross EL, Michna E, et al. Substance misuse treatment for high-risk chronic pain patients on opioid therapy: a randomized trial. *Pain* 2010;150(3):390–400.

299. Wilder CM, Miller SC, Tiffany E, et al. Risk factors for opioid overdose and awareness of overdose risk among veterans prescribed chronic opioids for addiction or pain. *J Addict Dis* 2016;35(1):42–51. doi:10.1080/10550887.2016.1107264.

300. Tiffany E, Wilder CM, Miller SC, et al. Knowledge of and interest in opioid overdose education and naloxone distribution among US veterans on chronic opioids for addiction or pain. *Drug Educ Prev Policy* 2016;23(4):322–327.

301. Vadivelu N, Anwar M. Buprenorphine in postoperative pain management. *Anesthesiol Clin* 2010;28(4):601–609.

302. Jalili M, Fathi M, Moradi-Lakeh M, et al. Sublingual buprenorphine in acute pain management: a double-blind randomized clinical trial. *Ann Emerg Med* 2012;59(4):276–280.

303. Wiedemer NL, Harden PS, Arndt IO, et al. The opioid renewal clinic: a primary care, managed approach to opioid therapy in chronic pain patients at risk for substance abuse. *Pain Med* 2007;8(7):573–584.

304. Acosta M, Haller DL. Psychiatric and substance abuse comorbidity influences treatment outcomes in opioid-abusing patients. Paper presented at: College on Problems of Drug Dependence Annual Meeting; June 2006; Scottsdale, AZ.

305. Kelleher S. Health care professionals' knowledge and attitudes regarding substance use and substance users. *Accid Emerg Nurs* 2007;15(3):161–165.

306. Miotto K, Kaufman A, Kong A, et al. Managing co-occurring substance use and pain disorders. *Psychiatr Clin North Am* 2012;35(2):393–409.

307. Polomano RC, Galloway KT, Kent ML, et al. Psychometric testing of the Defense and Veterans Pain Rating Scale (DVPRS): a new pain scale for military population. *Pain Med* 2016;17(8):1505–1519. doi:10.1093/pm/pnw105.

308. World Health Organization. Preventing suicide: a global imperative. Available at: http://apps.who.int/iris/bitstream/10665/131056/1/9789241564779_eng.pdf?ua=1&ua=1. Accessed December 18, 2016.

309. Hitchcock L, Ferrell B, McCaffery M. The experience of chronic nonmalignant pain. *J Pain Symptom Manage* 1994;9:312–318.

310. Stenager EN, Stenager E, Jensen K. Attempted suicide, depression and physical diseases: a 1-year follow-up study. *Psychother Psychosom* 1994;61:65–73.

311. Fishbain DA, Goldberg M, Rosomoff RS, et al. Completed suicide in chronic pain. *Clin J Pain* 1991;7:29–36.

312. Fishbain DA. The association of chronic pain and suicide. *Semin Clin Neuropsychiatry* 1999;4:221–227.

313. Smith MT, Edwards RR, Robinson RC, et al. Suicidal ideation, plans, and attempts in chronic pain patients: factors associated with increased risk. *Pain* 2004;111:201–208.

314. Braden JB, Sullivan MD. Suicidal thoughts and behavior among adults with self-reported pain conditions in the national comorbidity survey replication. *J Pain* 2008;9:1106–1115.

315. Ilgen MA, Zivin K, McCammon RJ, et al. Pain and suicidal thoughts, plans and attempts in the United States. *Gen Hosp Psychiatry* 2008;30:521–527.

316. Ratcliffe GE, Enns MW, Belik SL, et al. Chronic pain conditions and suicidal ideation and suicide attempts: an epidemiologic perspective. *Clin J Pain* 2008;24:204–210.

317. Substance Abuse and Mental Health Services Administration. *Drug Abuse Warning Network, 2011: National Estimates of Drug-Related Emergency Department Visits.* Rockville, MD: Substance Abuse and Mental Health Services Administration; 2013. HHS publication (SMA) 13-4760, DAWN series D-39.

318. Racine M, Choinière M, Nielson WR. Predictors of suicidal ideation in chronic pain patients: an exploratory study. *Clin J Pain* 2014;30(5):371–378. doi:10.1097/AJP.0b013e31829e9d4d.

319. Cheatle M, Wasser T, Foster C, et al. Prevalence of suicidal ideation in patients with chronic non-cancer pain referred to a behaviorally based pain program. *Pain Physician* 2014;17(3):E359–E367.

320. Edwards RR, Smith MT, Kudel I, et al. Pain-related catastrophizing as a risk factor for suicidal ideation in chronic pain. *Pain* 2006;126:272–279.

321. Tang NK, Crane C. Suicidality in chronic pain: a review of the prevalence, risk factors and psychological links. *Psychol Med* 2006;36:575–586.

322. Ilgen MA, Zivin K, Austin KL, et al. Severe pain predicts greater likelihood of subsequent suicide. *Suicide Life Threat Behav* 2010;40(6):597–608.

323. Campbell G, Darke S, Bruno R, et al. The prevalence and correlates of chronic pain and suicidality in a nationally representative sample. *Aust N Z J Psychiatry* 2015;49(9):803–811.

324. Campbell G, Bruno R, Darke S, et al. Prevalence and correlates of suicidal thoughts and suicide attempts in people prescribed pharmaceutical opioids for chronic pain. *Clin J Pain* 2016;32(4):292–301.

325. Roy A, Janal MN. Risk factors for suicide attempts among alcohol dependent patients. *Arch Suicide Res* 2007;11:211–217.

326. Roy A. Characteristics of cocaine dependent patients who attempt suicide. *Arch Suicide Res* 2009;13:46–51.

327. Roy A. Risk factors for attempting suicide in heroin addicts. *Suicide Life Threat Behav* 2010;40:416–420.

328. Wilcox HC, Conner KR, Caine ED. Association of alcohol and drug use disorders and completed suicide: an empirical review of cohort studies. *Drug Alcohol Depend* 2004;76:S11–S19.

329. Yuodelis-Flores C, Ries RK. Addiction and suicide: a review. *Am J Addict* 2015;24(2):98–104.

330. Centers for Disease Control and Prevention, National Center for Injury Prevention and Control. National suicide statistics. Available at: https://www.cdc.gov/violenceprevention/suicide/statistics. Accessed December 18, 2016.

331. Cheatle MD. Depression, chronic pain, and suicide by overdose: on the edge. *Pain Med* 2011;12(suppl 2):S43–S48.

332. Turner JA, Aaron LA. Pain-related catastrophizing: what is it? *Clin J Pain* 2001;17(1):65–71.

333. Joiner T. *Why People Die by Suicide.* Cambridge, MA: Harvard University Press; 2005.

334. Van Orden KA, Witte TK, Cukrowicz KC, et al. The interpersonal theory of suicide. *Psychol Rev* 2010;117:575–600.

335. Kanzler KE, Bryan CJ, McGeary DD, et al. Suicidal ideation and perceived burdensomeness in patients with chronic pain. *Pain Pract* 2012;12: 602–609.

336. Beck A, Ward C, Mendelson M, et al. An inventory for measuring depression. *Arch Gen Psychiatry* 1961;4:561–571.

337. McNair D, Lorr M, Droppleman L. *EITS Manual for the Profile of Mood States.* San Diego, CA: Educational and Industrial Testing Service; 1971.

338. Dworkin RH, Turk DC, Farrar JT, et al. Core outcome measures for chronic pain clinical trials: IMMPACT recommendations. *Pain* 2005;113(1–2): 9–19.

339. Kroenke K, Spitzer RL, Williams JB. The PHQ-9: validity of a brief depression severity measure. *J Gen Intern Med* 2001;16(9):606–613.

340. Spitzer RL, Williams JB, Kroenke K, et al. Utility of a new procedure for diagnosing mental disorders in primary care. The PRIME-MD 1000 study. *JAMA* 1994;272(22):1749–1756.

341. Ader DN. Developing the Patient-Reported Outcomes Measurement Information System (PROMIS). *Med Care* 2007;45(5):S1–S2.

342. Kroenke K, Spitzer RL, Williams JB, et al. An ultra-brief screening scale for anxiety and depression: The PHQ-4. *Psychosomatics* 2009;50(6):613–621.

343. Buysse DJ, Reynolds CF III, Monk TH, et al. The Pittsburgh Sleep Quality Index: a new instrument for psychiatric practice and research. *Psychiatry Res* 1989;28(2):193–213.

344. Bastien CH, Vallières A, Morin CM. Validation of the Insomnia Severity Index as an outcome measure for insomnia research. *Sleep Med* 2001;2(4):297–307.

345. Buysse DJ, Yu L, Moul DE, et al. Development and validation of patient-reported outcome measures for sleep disturbance and sleep-related impairments. *Sleep* 2010;33(6):781–792.

346. Moul DE, Hall M, Pilkonis PA, et al. Self-report measures of insomnia in adults: rationales, choices, and needs. *Sleep Med Rev* 2004;8(3):177–198.

347. Dube P, Kurt K, Bair MJ, et al. The p4 screener: evaluation of a brief measure for assessing potential suicide risk in 2 randomized effectiveness trials of primary care and oncology patients. *Prim Care Companion J Clin Psychiatry* 2010;12(6):PCC.10m00978. doi:10.4088/PCC.10m00978blu.

348. Posner K, Brown GK, Stanley B, et al. The Columbia-Suicide Severity Rating Scale: initial validity and internal consistency findings from three multisite studies with adolescents and adults. *Am J Psychiatry* 2011;168(12): 1266–1277.

349. Jacobs D. *Screening for Mental Health: A Resource Guide for Implementing the Joint Commission 2007 Patient Safety Goals on Suicide.* Wellesley Hills, MA: Screening for Mental Health; 2007.

350. Turk DC, Flor H. Etiological theories and treatments for chronic back pain. II. Psychological models and interventions. *Pain* 1984;19(3):209–233.

351. Lamb SE, Hansen Z, Lall R, et al. Group cognitive behavioural treatment for low-back pain in primary care: a randomised controlled trial and cost-effectiveness analysis. *Lancet* 2010;375:916–923.

352. Linton SJ, Nordin E. A 5-year follow-up evaluation of the health and economic consequences of an early cognitive behavioral intervention for back pain: a randomized, controlled trial. *Spine (Phila Pa 1976)* 2006;31(8): 853–858.

353. Keefe FJ, Caldwell DS. Cognitive behavioral control of arthritis pain. *Med Clin North Am* 1997;81:277–290.

354. Greco CM, Rudy TE, Manzi S. Effects of a stress-reduction program on psychological function, pain, and physical function of systemic lupus erythematosus patients: a randomized controlled trial. *Arthritis Rheum* 2004;51(4):625–634.

355. Thieme K, Flor H, Turk D. Psychological pain treatment in fibromyalgia syndrome: efficacy of operant behavioural and cognitive behavioural treatments. *Arthritis Res Ther* 2006;8(4):R121.

356. Chen E, Cole SW, Kato PM. A review of empirically supported psychosocial interventions for pain and adherence outcomes in sickle cell disease. *J Pediatr Psychol* 2004;29:1997–2009.

357. Cheatle MD, Foster S, Pinkett A, et al. Assessing and managing sleep disturbance in patients with chronic pain. *Anesthesiol Clin* 2016;34(2): 379–393.

358. Smith MT, Perlis ML, Haythornthwaite JA. Suicidal ideation in outpatients with chronic musculoskeletal pain: an exploratory study of the role of sleep onset insomnia and pain intensity. *Clin J Pain* 2004;20(2):111–118.

359. Sivertsen B, Omvik S, Pallesen S, et al. Cognitive behavioral therapy vs zopiclone for treatment of chronic primary insomnia in older adults: a randomized controlled trial. *JAMA* 2006;295(24):2851–2858.

360. Morasco BJ, Greaves DW, Lovejoy TI, et al. Development and preliminary evaluation of an integrated cognitive-behavior treatment for chronic pain and substance use disorder in patients with the hepatitis c virus. *Pain Med* 2016;17(12):2280–2290.

361. Darnall BD, Ziadni MS, Stieg RL, et al. Patient-centered prescription opioid tapering in community outpatients with chronic pain. *JAMA Intern Med* 2018;178:707–708. doi:10.1001/jamainternmed.2017.8709.

362. Demidenko MI, Dobscha SK, Morasco BJ, et al. Suicidal ideation and suicidal self-directed violence following clinician-initiated prescription opioid discontinuation among long-term opioid users. *Gen Hosp Psychiatry* 2017;47:29–35.

363. Lester D. The concentration of neurotransmitter metabolites in the cerebrospinal fluid of suicidal individuals: a meta-analysis. *Pharmacopsychiatry* 1995;28:45–50.

364. Placidi GP, Oquendo MA, Malone KM, et al. Aggressivity, suicide attempts, and depression: relationship to cerebrospinal fluid monoamine metabolite levels. *Biol Psychiatry* 2001;50:783–791.

365. Boulougouris V, Malogiannis I, Lockwood G, et al. Serotonergic modulation of suicidal behaviour: integrating preclinical data with clinical practice and psychotherapy. *Exp Brain Res* 2013;230(4):605–624.

366. Costanza A, D'Orta I, Perroud N, et al. Neurobiology of suicide: do biomarkers exist? *Int J Legal Med* 2014;128(1):73–82.

CHAPTER 33

The Doctor–Patient Relationship in Pain Management: Dealing with Difficult Clinician–Patient Interactions

ROBERT N. JAMISON

Pain management physicians commonly have to deal with doctor–patient conflicts because of the nature of persons with chronic pain, the personalities of the pain practitioners who treat them, and added pressures stemming from the health care system. Persons with chronic pain frequently present with psychosocial stressors including sleep disturbances, loss of function, disability issues, and depression, which affect their ability to cope.[1] Medical conditions such as diabetes, hypertension, asthma, gastrointestinal distress, and other comorbidities such as substance abuse and psychiatric disorders make these patients challenging to manage.[2,3] Patients with chronic pain can be time-consuming when doctors are under increasing pressure to see more patients in a shorter amount of time. The need to provide detailed documentation and written justification of each treatment decision and to remain current with the latest treatments adds further time pressure for the pain practitioner. All of these conditions can add to difficulties that set up doctor–patient conflicts.[4,5]

Between 10% and 60% of patients treated in health care settings exhibit "difficult behavior,"[6–9] which can include extreme aggression, threats of homicide and suicide, and behavior related to substance abuse. Patients with chronic pain can be especially difficult because they have a tendency to be angry, mistrustful, anxious, and depressed.[10] Depression and anxiety disorders are 2 to 3 times more prevalent among patients with chronic pain than in the general population,[11,12] and patients with pain can frequently present with added behavioral symptoms of inflexibility, negativity, or entitled behavior.

The aim of this chapter is to describe difficult doctor–patient relationships in a pain center or primary care setting and focus on communication issues that may be useful in avoiding treatment dissatisfaction and possible legal reprisals. In this chapter, I first review the reasons that patients can be difficult and identify those patients who are prone to exhibit problems. Next, I discuss some of the major issues that lead to doctor–patient conflicts and review possible communication strategies to help the pain specialist successfully manage these patients. Finally, I outline common clinical scenarios leading to potential doctor–patient conflicts and give appropriate responses that may be beneficial in dealing with difficult patients. As implied in the title, this chapter focuses on the doctor–patient relationship, although it should be noted that this same information could easily be applied to any clinician and any person receiving treatment.

Difficult Patients and Difficult Doctor–Patient Relationships

In a study of over 500 adults presenting to a primary care clinic, Jackson and Kroenke[13] found that treating physicians rated over 15% of their patients to be difficult. In a comparable study of 750 subjects, Hinchey and Jackson[14] perceived 17.8% of patients to be difficult. These difficult patients tended to have a depression or anxiety disorder, poor functional status, unmet expectations, reduced satisfaction, and a greater use of health care services. These studies also showed that physicians who were less experienced and were less empathic were more likely to experience encounters with these patients as difficult. In another study, Jackson and Kroenke[15] found that patients' unmet expectations were common in those individuals experienced as difficult by the clinicians. These patients were also likely to have a mental disorder, with somatic symptoms, poorer function status, greater expectations for care, less satisfaction, and higher use of health services than patients who were not difficult ($P < .001$). Every clinician will encounter at least one extremely difficult patient who may require behavioral limit-setting and possible hospitalization and/or psychotropic medication.[3] Patients with chronic pain are known for being particularly difficult. In a recent survey study of 56 primary care physicians, 83.9% agreed that patients with chronic pain can be very stressful to deal with.[16]

Vegni and colleagues,[17] after analyzing difficult doctor–patient relationships, concluded that the doctor's personal and professional issues as well as changes in the health care system are the chief contributors to conflicts. Likewise, Haas and others[5] identified the fact that difficult doctor–patient relationships can be based on (1) patient factors (medical, psychiatric, personality, and substance abuse risk), (2) physician factors (workload, communication skills, personality, level of experience, quality of training and practice setting), and (3) the health care system (financial and productivity pressures, fragmentation of care, availability of outside resources, and documentation and treatment guidelines). In a survey of 750 patients and 200 physicians performed by Roper Starch Worldwide Inc,[18] the qualities of physicians that were most frustrating to patients were being too rushed (30%), hard to reach (19%), and not down to earth (11%). The qualities that described the most difficult patients were hostility or anger (49%), noncompliance (19%), and being too demanding or needy (19%).

Hahn and others[7] developed the Difficult Doctor–Patient Relationship Questionnaire (DDPRQ) and established its reliability and validity. The results of the DDPRQ, completed by physicians who had just concluded a patient encounter, showed that 10% to 21% of patient encounters were labeled as difficult. Most of these patients showed signs of psychosomatic symptoms and psychopathology. In subsequent studies by this same group conducted in four primary care clinics,[19,20] physicians rated 96 patients (15%) out of 627 to be difficult. Compared with patients who were described as not difficult, difficult patients had more functional impairment, higher health care utilization, lower satisfaction with care, and more psychiatric disorders of somatization, panic, dysthymia, anxiety, depression, and alcohol abuse or dependence.

PSYCHIATRIC AND PERSONALITY ISSUES

Difficult patients with pain can display destructive psychiatric behaviors such as suicidal ideation, self-mutilation, extreme noncompliance with treatment, or opioid misuse, and most pain specialists have little training in psychiatric assessment and treatment.[12] Many clinicians avoid pain medicine practice altogether because of the emotional challenge of working each day with demanding and draining patients. Patients with pain can be fearful of flare-ups and worry that their clinic will be unresponsive to the urgency of their condition. Their heightened anxiety adds to a need for frequent contact with their doctors, resulting in endless e-mails and phone messages. Patient–relations departments of hospitals and the state boards of registration and medical examiners are notified most often by patients who complain that their doctor is unresponsive to their care. As a result, physicians are watchful about the perception of inadequately treating or abandoning their patients.[21]

Epidemiologic studies indicate that 35% of chronic back and neck pain sufferers in the United States have a comorbid depression or anxiety disorder[22] and up to half of all patients with chronic pain can have a comorbid psychiatric condition.[11,23] Further studies also report that patients who are most difficult frequently have a personality disorder, which includes psychotic episodes, impulsivity, superficiality, problems with interpersonal relations, and affective disorders.[24] Surveys of chronic pain clinic populations as a whole indicate that 50% to 80% of patients with chronic pain have some signs of psychopathology, making this the most prevalent comorbidity in these patients.[25,26] Persons with fibromyalgia, chronic daily headache, and chronic pelvic pain have the highest rates of depression compared to patients with other chronic pain conditions.[27–29] Patients with two or more pain complaints are more likely to be depressed than those with a single pain complaint, and the number of pain conditions is a better predictor of major depression than pain severity or pain duration.[30] Patients with borderline and antisocial personality disorders can be commonly found in a pain management clinic. Taken together, these studies provide support for the association between chronic pain and having a mood disorder.[31] These patients often trigger the strongest negative reaction among their providers.[12]

Outcome studies highlight the poor response of patients with psychiatric comorbidity to many different treatments for chronic pain,[32] especially those patients with chronic low back pain.[33,34] Boersma and Linton[35] have shown that patients with chronic pain with a combination of anxiety and depression have a 62% worse return to work rate at 1 year than those with no psychopathology.

OPIOID THERAPY

Patients with chronic pain who have a mood disorder are likely to be prescribed opioids more often than those without a mood disorder, which can lead to doctor–patient conflicts. In a study of 50 Veterans Administration (VA) patients and 50 patients treated in outside primary care practices with opioids for non-cancer pain, Reid and colleagues[36] found a 50% prevalence of major depression and a 20% prevalence of an anxiety disorder. In a similar study, Breckenridge and Clark[37] determined a high prevalence of mood disorder among patients with pain who were prescribed opioids. In a study of 191 patients examining factors that led pain physicians to prescribe opioids for noncancer pain, Turk and Okifuji[38] concluded that neither pain severity nor objective physical pathology influenced the decision to prescribe. Rather, greater affective distress and pain behaviors drove the decisions. Thus, patients with chronic pain and psychopathology are likely to be prescribed opioids, and these patients report greater pain intensity, more pain-related disability, and a larger affective component to their pain than those without psychopathology.[39]

In terms of the impact of mood disorders on opioid response, a study examined the effects of intravenous (IV) opioid analgesia in patients with chronic pain with high and low levels of psychiatric comorbidity.[40] Sixty patients with low back pain stratified into three groups of severity of psychological symptoms (low, moderate, and high) were given IV morphine and placebo in random order on separate visits and completed pain ratings over 3 hours at each session. The low-psychopathology group had a 40% greater reduction in pain with IV morphine than the high-psychopathology group ($P < .01$). This study found that patients with chronic pain who had a high degree of negative affect benefited less from opioids in controlling their pain than those with a low degree of negative affect, a finding replicated by subsequent studies.[41]

DIFFICULT "NORMAL" PATIENTS

Not all patients with difficult behavior exhibit significant psychopathology, such as major depression or anxiety or a personality disorder. Patients who are otherwise "normal" can be perceived as difficult, for example, when they arrive at a pain center for treatment with unrealistic expectations about what should happen. They may have had problems with previous health care settings in which they were accused of exaggerating their pain. Lack of sleep, extreme fatigue, poor eating habits, and long travel to their appointments can also contribute to volatile and unstable behavior. They may experience their physicians as dismissive or skeptical of their pain rather than being understanding and sympathetic. Even comparatively well-adjusted patients can sometimes develop the idea that their pain physician should be able to eliminate all of their pain and that failure to do so is tantamount to withholding treatment. This becomes critical when medication regimens involving opioids are concerned. Patients may worry about being prescribed adequate amounts of medication or undergoing withdrawal if they are to be tapered off opioids.

Some patients with pain are entitled consumers who are no longer willing to be passive in their treatment but rather prefer to take control of their medical care. Medical information through the Internet is more accessible than ever, and patients frequently come to their appointments armed with information about a particular therapy. Patients are increasingly opinionated about their care. They look to have a mutually respectful relationship with their health care providers and want to take an active role in the decision-making process. They become dissatisfied with their treatment when their provider is unresponsive to their suggestions and not willing to hear their own ideas. Cultural and ethnic differences can also act as barriers to an effective doctor–patient relationship.[42]

COMORBID MEDICAL CONDITIONS

Most persons with chronic pain also have significant medical conditions that impact treatment decisions. Some are medically challenging as well as being interpersonally difficult. Patients with pain may report asthma, chronic obstructive pulmonary disease (COPD), diabetes, coronary artery disease, hypertension, ulcers, kidney, bladder and liver problems, and history of cancer. Persons with chronic pain often smoke cigarettes, have gained weight, and have lost bone density. Multiple providers can prescribe multiple medications including blood thinners, blood pressure and heart disease medications, inhalers, and antidepressants. These patients are also noted for allergies and reactions to certain medications. Occasionally, they have implanted medical devices (e.g., pacemakers, rods, stimulators) or wear prostheses. Some of the most challenging patients tend to be older, take many medications, have multiple psychosocial problems, have poor social support, limited education, and come from disadvantaged backgrounds.[3]

Kenny[43] points out in a survey study of 20 patients with chronic pain and 22 pain specialists that differences in communication interactions—especially when patients embrace a medical model to explain their pain and physicians perceive a psychogenic etiology of pain—can significantly negatively affect the doctor–patient relationship. In a study of how and why physicians dismiss patients from their practice, 25 general practitioners identified two types of patients who tend to be dismissed over others: (1) patients who break the rules of the doctor–patient relationship or clinic practice and (2) patients whose difficult personality makes it hard to care for them.[44]

SUBSTANCE USE DISORDERS

There are notable links between chronic pain and substance abuse.[45,46] Studies show that 10% to 16% of patients treated in a general practice and 25% to 40% of hospitalized patients have problems related to drug or alcohol addiction.[47,48] Other studies indicate that patients with pain and high rates of mood disorders are at high risk for alcohol or opioid abuse.[49–51] Hasin and Liu[52] found some patients abuse opioid pain medication in an attempt to alleviate their psychiatric symptoms. Thus, comorbid depression and/or anxiety disorders are associated with greater opioid misuse, even in those with no history of a substance use disorder. Wasan and colleagues[53] also found that increased craving for prescription opioids was associated with a greater urge to self-medicate the anxiety and depression that precede the sensations of craving. These individuals with a mood disorder who self-medicate negative affective symptoms are at increased risk for substance abuse.[51,54] Physicians are often in the difficult position of providing appropriate pain relief while minimizing the inappropriate use of pain medications by being ever watchful of substance use disorders.[55] Inappropriate use can include the following: selling and diverting prescription drugs, seeking additional prescriptions from multiple providers, concurrently using other illicit drugs, and manipulating the formulation to snort or inject the medications or use them in a manner in which they were not intended. It is important for the successful treatment of chronic noncancer pain to be able to frequently monitor patients on opioid regimens and to identify those patients who exhibit ongoing abuse behaviors, which can be an added burden to providers.[56,57]

Unfortunately, physicians can be deceived, which is all the more reason that steps are needed to perform a thorough evaluation for risk factors and to closely monitor patients on opioid therapy.[58] History of substance abuse further complicates treatment because it increases the potential for inadequate treatment of pain.[59] Thus, encounters with patients can be made difficult by underlying issues of substance abuse and addiction.

Physician Factors

Difficult doctor–patient relationships are not completely due to the patient. The attitudes and behavior of the physicians play an important role as well. Some doctors take patient behavior personally instead of realizing that this is how the patient responds and behaves in other situations as well. An understanding of the patient's situation helps in depersonalizing any reactions that they may experience. Doctors who show disrespect or have inward anger toward their patients transmit negative emotions that lead to distrust. Some physicians have hidden feelings of inadequacy or poor self-esteem, and others have an inability to listen to what the patient is saying.[60] Those personality and behavior qualities of doctors can lead to difficult relationships, including inward anger, impatience, lack of empathy, depression, poor self-esteem, and feelings of vulnerability.[61,62]

For health care providers, treating patients with chronic pain can also lead to reactive feelings of being manipulated, which, in turn, can lead to extreme dislike for certain patients.[63] Because physicians are frequently under pressure to see patients within a short period of time, pain patients who show vague symptoms and who are unresponsive to many different interventions can be particularly frustrating, especially when the burden of providing treatment is shouldered alone instead of being shared by an interdisciplinary team. More problematic patient issues, including verbal abuse or physical threats to the clinician and staff, stalking, criminal behavior, and gross noncompliance, can trigger negative reactive emotions in the provider.

Krebs et al.[64] interviewed 1,391 physicians to assess personal and practice characteristics associated with greater frustration with patients. Physicians who were younger, worked more hours, had symptoms of depression and anxiety, were under higher stress, and had more patients with psychosocial and substance abuse problems reported increased frustration with their jobs. In a qualitative study, Mathias and colleagues[65] interviewed 20 providers at a Veterans Affairs medical center. They concluded that the providers' needs should not be ignored and that improving the providers' patient-centered communication skills, including demonstrating empathy and encouraging shared decision making, would ultimately lead to improved patient care. Tam and Su[66] point out that pain clinicians may have extensive training in their area of expertise but have had little instruction in communication skills.

Health Care System Factors

Health care system factors also indirectly contribute to doctor–patient conflicts. Physicians frequently report being overworked and under constant pressure to be productive. The demands of the job include reading reports, meticulously documenting treatments and reconciling medications in the electronic medical records. Many have also witnessed changes in health care financing and fragmentation of care. Commercial insurance carriers and The Joint Commission Centers for Medicare & Medicaid Services frequently revise regulations in medical record documentation. Physicians are more than ever being asked to expand their role in the identification and management of psychiatric conditions and addictive disorders.[64] Keeping abreast of the latest pharmacologic therapies and screening devices can also be daunting.[67-70] Advances in information technology can radically transform decision-making and treatment processes, although there is no indication of whether they decrease the physician workload.[71,72] It has been suggested that the use of the Internet can have a negative effect on doctor–patient relationships by discrediting conventional therapies, misleading patients, and adding to consultation times.[71] Thus, productivity pressures from hospitals and medical centers, changes in health care financing, threats of legal repercussions related to treatment decisions, fragmentation of care, and the rising use of information technology can place burdens on the provider and add to additional external stress.

Patient Interaction Strategies

It is surprising to some outsiders when patients cherish their pain provider even though their treatment outcomes are not always successful. These patients may openly admit that their pain was made worse by a particular surgery or procedure but still feel that their doctor did all that could have been done without placing fault or blame on him or her. Conversely, other patients may hold their physician directly at fault for a negative outcome in what they perceive was inadequate or faulty treatment, even though the treatment technique was appropriate without evidence of complications. The differences may lie in the interpersonal skills that the physician used to help deal with the poor outcome, diffusing conflicts and building patient rapport. These same skills may have been lacking in another provider who was accused of causing further problems. Thus, the medical expertise and competence of the clinician is not the only quality needed for acceptance and satisfaction of treatment, regardless of the outcome, but rather the nonspecific effects of the doctor–patient relationship play an important role. Here, I review the components of positive doctor–patient relations, especially when dealing with challenging, difficult patients.

Much has been written on useful strategies in dealing with difficult patients, and an exhaustive review of the literature is beyond the scope of this chapter; however, a brief review of some studies will be useful. Elder and colleagues[73] interviewed 102 physicians who were identified as having excellent skills in interacting with difficult patients about how they identified, managed, and coped with these patients. The authors concluded that the key ingredients of changing a difficult encounter into a successful one included the use of empathy, appropriate use of power, and an understanding of the need for doctor–patient collaboration. Lown[74] also proposed strategies to deal with anger in the clinician–patient relationship, suggesting that clinicians who cultivate personal awareness, practice self-monitoring, understand the reasons for patient anger, demonstrate specific communication skills, set clear boundaries, and seek personal support are best at managing difficult patient encounters.

Halpern[63] also describes ways for physicians to manage difficult patients: recognize one's own emotions, attend to negative emotions, attune to patients' verbal and nonverbal emotional messages, and become receptive to negative feedback. These steps allow clinicians to reduce anger through increased empathy and ultimately increase therapeutic impact. Finally, Nisselle[75] felt that by considering the difficulties in the relationship, doctors would be less prone to labeling patients as difficult. Strategies in managing difficult patients included acknowledging the problem, setting boundaries, using communication skills, and including external resources when necessary.

PATIENT-FOCUSED CARE

In a study on physicians' communication style and perceptions of patients, Street et al.[76] audiotaped and coded interactions among 29 physicians and 207 patients. They concluded that more positive communication from one participant led to similar responses from the other and that reciprocity and mutual influence had a strong effect on quality of care. Klitzman[77] interviewed 50 doctors who had experienced a serious illness in which they were required to be hospitalized as patients. Because of their own experiences as a patient, these physicians acknowledged increased sensitivity to patients' experiences and the importance of empathy in the doctor–patient relationship. They included hospital practice recommendations of charting with the patient present, acknowledging whenever they keep a patient waiting, and being sensitive to nonverbal aspects of care. Their conclusions are in keeping with the differences described by Irwin and Richardson[78] between patient-focused care and a disease-centered model of care. They loosely define patient-focused care as care we would like those we care most about to receive. Having a disease-focused management approach does not exclude having a good bedside manner; however, patient-focused care takes in the whole person's experience in a way that suggests understanding and caring. This point is well illustrated in a study of 316 cancer patients among whom satisfaction with pain management was strongly related to the doctor–patient relationship and not related to the severity of the pain.[79] Likewise, studies of postoperative satisfaction with pain have been found to be more related to perception of care than actual report of pain.[80,81]

It has been suggested that poor communication style is the underlying problem in most medical–legal cases.[82] In a sample of 45 physician-related plaintiff dispositions, relationship issues appeared to be central to 71% of the lawsuits.[83] In fact, it has been suggested that the majority of negligence cases are not related to quality of care but are brought on by inadequate doctor–patient communication—often occurring before the incident that leads to a claim.[84] By concentrating more on the medical than the human needs of the patient, there is an increased chance of breakdown in communication and a greater perception of inadequate care. Those physicians who are less prone to legal action demonstrate skills in listening, empathy, and expressing understanding.[82] Gafaranga and Britten[85] believe that the opening statement made by the physician during the first patient encounter may have a lasting impression on the relationship. Roy and others[86] have also shown that doctors who inform their patients of changes that impact their care in person rather than by mail have greater patient satisfaction. Back et al.[87] identified some common pitfalls of doctor–patient communication that they label as blocking, lecturing, depending on a routine, collusion, and premature reassurance. They encourage instead employing open-ended communication skills they label as "ask-tell-ask" and "tell me more." Caregivers who show good patient communication skills are ones who speak in a caring way with an open body posture and do not transmit the impression of defensiveness or indifference when they engage in conversation with their patients. Thus, as pointed out in some training programs, the secret of caring for patients is really caring for patients.

Pomm, et al.[60] suggest that clinicians also need to understand the patient's perspective, attempt to actively listen to their patients, recognize what they can or cannot change, and get help from colleagues and friends for support if problems occur. They describe this as the CALMER (Catalyst for change, Alter thoughts to change feelings, Listen and then make a diagnosis, Make an agreement, Education and follow-up, Reach out and discuss feelings) approach to dealing with difficult patients. The literature on stages of change[88,89] also indicates that patients go through stages in which they are more prone to make positive behavioral changes than at other times. Physicians who recognize when a patient is not ready to change, despite the patient's giving lip service to what needs to be done, are less inclined to transmit disappointment when no changes are made.

Communication Framework: WIPS and E's

Different models have been promoted to improve doctor–patient communication. Kathleen Gordon (Connecting with Care, unpublished manual, 2006) identified what she believes are needs and expectations of all patients with pain and used the letters WIPS (welcome, important and informed, perspective, and secure) to help remember what all patients expect during each doctor–patient encounter (Table 33.1). First, patients want to feel welcome. They like to believe that their provider is happy to see them and is concerned about their condition. Second, patients want to feel important and to be informed about what is going on and what will take place. The impression that there is mutual respect and collaboration is key to meeting these needs. Third, patients need to believe that

TABLE 33.1 Four Expectations for Clinical Encounters (WIPS)
All patients want to
1. Feel **W**elcome
2. Feel **I**mportant and informed
3. Believe their **P**erspective was understood
4. Feel **S**ecure that their needs will be met

their perspective is understood, which necessitates listening skills and body posture that convey a sense of caring. Fourth, the patient wants to feel secure that his or her doctor is competent and knows what needs to be done. To this end, patients like to have the expectation that their needs will be met as well as possible.

The Bayer Institute for Health Care Communication adopted a consensus model for essential elements of physician–patient communication.[90] Even if the encounter is brief, those clinicians who follow particular interaction strategies are able to improve patient rapport. These strategies are remembered as the 4 E's: (1) Engage, (2) Empathize, (3) Educate, and (4) Enlist. A revised version is presented in Table 33.2. First, the clinician connects with the patient and builds rapport by greeting the patient warmly, having good eye contact, showing interest, and addressing any physical barriers by using nonverbal posturing that improves options for engagement (Engage). Second, the clinician listens to the patient and shows attentiveness by repeating the information back to the patient. The clinician acknowledges feelings and shows understanding. When appropriate, humor is also used (Empathize). Third, the clinician assesses the patient's understanding and informs the patient and answers any questions that might arise in order to address concerns and to alleviate anxiety (Educate). Fourth, the clinician seeks the patient's input about the treatment plan. Priorities are negotiated and different scenarios are discussed in order to address realistic expectations (Enlist). Finally, the clinician ends the encounter by summarizing the plan and outlining the next steps. Reassuring comments as well as positive concerns are expressed. The effective clinician will also be sure to follow through with what was discussed.

TABLE 33.2   Components of Every Patient Encounter

1. Engage (build rapport)
   a. Build rapport and professional partnership
   b. Greeting that is pleasant, warm, consistent
   c. Eye contact
   d. Consider barriers
   e. Nonverbal show of interest
   f. Be curious of how patient is doing
   g. Get patient's story with expectations and concerns
2. Empathize (patient feels seen, heard, accepted)
   a. Listen and feed back what you hear
   b. Be aware of feelings, values, and thoughts
   c. Note body language and demeanor
   d. Reflect understanding
   e. Acknowledge and legitimize feelings
   f. Employ humor when appropriate
3. Educate (inform and answer questions)
   a. Assess what the patient understands
   b. Address key concerns—let them know you reviewed their medical record
   c. Answer with compassion—what will happen, who will be there, what are the risks, what are some realistic expectations
4. Enlist (invite the patient's involvement)
   a. Seek the patient's input on the treatment plan
   b. Ask for patient's agreement and active participation
   c. Provide options
   d. Negotiate priorities
   e. Explain what will happen if a problem arises
5. End
   a. Anticipate and forecast close of visit
   b. Summarize the encounter
   c. Review the plan and next steps
   d. Express personal confidence, caring, and hope
   e. Follow through

Modified from Bayer Institute of Health Care Communication, 2001.

Clinical Scenarios

The following are some common scenarios encountered in a pain management clinic. How the clinician responds to these situations is important in preventing escalating problems and potential litigation. Although at times, patients present with a borderline personality disorder or have an underlying substance use disorder, employment of communication techniques can make clinicians more adept at managing these situations and improving outcomes. The following brief scenarios were chosen to address some of the points raised earlier. As you read them, try and picture what you might do in these situations.

SCENARIO 1

You are seeing a patient for the first time. You begin to ask questions about the patient's medical history. The patient becomes very angry.

PATIENT: "I sent you all of my records and medical notes. Didn't you even bother to read them? I keep having to repeat myself over and over again."
CLINICIAN: "I am sorry that I have to ask you the same questions as everyone else, but I want to make sure that we do not miss anything. It is also important that I get a fresh look at how you are doing and what the main issues are. The goal is to improve your quality of life as best as possible and your patience and cooperation are important."

Main issues: This interaction might happen with a patient who has had many previous problematic contacts with health care providers. The clinician's appearing impatient and demanding will not help the situation. Rather, maintaining an open empathic stance, acknowledging the patient's frustration that the first session may be repetitive and tedious, and showing caring will encourage the patient to cooperate.

As with any initial interview, listening and understanding are vital. It is important to summarize the major concerns and to help reconcile the issues. Many physicians choose to ignore anger for fear that addressing it will bring out more anger or for worry that it will lead to greater time involvement. However, addressing the situation early will pay dividends later on. Appearing impatient or demanding cooperation is an invitation for patient dissatisfaction and increased difficulties later on.

SCENARIO 2

It is late afternoon, and you have had several patients in the clinic with time-consuming complications. You are running 1 1/2 hours late. You enter the room to see your next patient, and you can tell this patient is very upset about having to wait so long.

CLINICIAN: "Hello Mrs. Black."
PATIENT: [noticeably upset] "I have been waiting a long time and I have to get back home. Can we hurry this up?"
CLINICIAN: "I recognize that you have been waiting a long time and I am sorry that you have had to wait so long. I hate it when anyone must be kept waiting. As with all my patients, I want to spend as much time with you as you need."

Main points: Apologizing ahead of time for any delay, even if it is for a short period, will acknowledge that you recognize that this person's time is valuable and he or she may be legitimately irritated. Validating the feelings of the patient first helps to defuse the situation. When running late, some clinicians make a point to quickly acknowledge that the patient is there and waiting and to let them know that they will be with them shortly.

SCENARIO 3

A patient is expecting to have a procedure, but the scheduler failed to put it in the schedule. You are running behind, and you can tell that this patient is very upset about the scheduling error.

CLINICIAN: [Sits down facing the patient with good eye contact and caring body posture.] "I need to apologize that there has been a mix-up about the schedule. I am afraid that we will not be able to do your procedure today."
PATIENT: "What? I have had this appointment for weeks and I brought a friend with me to drive me home. Why can't you just do it?"
CLINICIAN: "I can appreciate how upsetting this is especially when you have someone along with you. We simply can't do this today. Mistakes like this don't happen very often, and I am sorry that this happened to you. We will try and sort this out as best we can. I will have the scheduler set up another time as soon as possible."

Main issues: It is important to reflect the patient's perspective. If a mistake was made, it is always best to admit it and apologize without making excuses or directing the blame at others. Coming up with excuses or reasons for the problem right away without listening would not help to defuse the situation. It is important to use active listening techniques when patients are angry, including repetition, summary, validation, and empathy. Acknowledging that something will be done to help resolve the situation is important.

SCENARIO 4

A patient who calls and pages you often is pleasant when with you but is extremely disruptive while in the clinic. This patient is known to yell at the schedulers and the receptionist. Your receptionist insists that you speak to this patient.

CLINICIAN: "Mrs. Smith, I need to speak to you about your behavior in the clinic. I am aware that you get angry and raise your voice with staff at the front desk. We need to follow a protocol in our clinic, which means that everyone must respect each other. We cannot permit shouting or swearing in the waiting room."
PATIENT: "But your receptionist has been rude to me and has accused me of coming just to get drugs. I don't put up with that from anybody."
CLINICIAN: "The staff here has difficult jobs to do, but we try and treat others with respect by not raising our voice or causing a scene. We expect the same from everyone who is being served here, including you. I am afraid that if you persist in this behavior we will not be able to continue to see you."
PATIENT: "I don't have a problem with you, doctor. But I can't stand some members of your staff."
CLINICIAN: "Whether you like them or not, you cannot be disruptive while you are here."

Main issues: Some providers have difficulty in setting limits with difficult patients, but this is a case when firm limit setting is needed. Stating that it is difficult to work with anyone who is disruptive in the clinic and identifying the expected behaviors without showing anger or being demanding or blaming is best. For patients who are very disruptive in the waiting room, inviting them to come to a clinic room and to meet to discuss the issues privately would help to prevent further escalation of behavior.

SCENARIO 5

An elderly patient becomes combative and delusional following a procedure. This patient requires sedation and restraints. Family members see this patient in restraints and are very angry.

FAMILY MEMBER: "What are you doing to my mother? Is this a hospital or a prison? You should have notified us first. I want to transfer care to another facility."

CLINICIAN: "I can see why you would be upset seeing your mother in restraints. I want to reassure you that she is being cared for with her safety in mind."
FAMILY MEMBER: "But this can't be the way you are supposed to handle patients."
CLINICIAN: "I am sorry that you are upset, but we are doing this for her own safety. We try and take the greatest care with all our patients. Although your mother has been experiencing some of the effects of the medication, she will be fine."

Main issues: It is important to be reassuring and matter of fact without reacting in a negative way. By acknowledging how the person may be feeling and checking to see if this is accurate, you allow the person to share his or her feelings. Helping the person to get some understanding of what is happening and why things are done according to protocol can also be valuable.

SCENARIO 6

A middle-aged man develops an infection following the implantation of a device. His goal was to decrease his opioid medication. Now, he has more pain, is taking more opioids, and is very angry at the outcome. He returns with his wife and demands to know what will be done for his pain.

PATIENT: [Noticeably angry and upset] "I am a lot worse off now since that failed procedure. What are you going to do about my pain?"
CLINICIAN: "I know that you had hope that this would help your pain, and it must be frustrating that you are experiencing more pain. Having a set-back like this is difficult for all of us. We need to work together to get you back to a better state."
PATIENT: "But things are even worse now than ever."
CLINICIAN: "I wish we could be 100% successful every time, but unfortunately that is not the case. I am afraid that this did not work out as we expected, but we will keep working on this and hopefully we will be able to turn this around soon."

Main issues: In this case, underneath the anger, the patient is worried that he will be abandoned, and acknowledging this fear and worry as well as offering some reassurance is important. At first, allowing the patient to vent and express anger without becoming defensive or being angry in return can set the stage for greater partnership in the treatment process. It is important to speak slowly and calmly and to clarify expectations of treatment and limitations in the treatment process. Spending time with an angry patient despite levels of discomfort and helping to get the patient to commit to maintaining a mutual relationship in the treatment process are also important.

SCENARIO 7

A 42-year-old man was referred for treatment of his chronic back pain. He had two back surgeries following a work-related injury and has been taking opioids for his pain. His primary care provider has been prescribing his medication, and he was referred because he had been running out of his medication early and had an abnormal urine toxicology screen. This patient was seen on follow-up after having completed a comprehensive set of screening questionnaires, a structured interview with a psychologist, and a toxicology screen.

PATIENT: "My doctor referred me to you because she no longer wants to write for my pain medication. She thinks that you should take over writing for my pain medication since you are at a pain center."
CLINICIAN: "Your interview and questionnaire information suggest that you are at high risk for having problems with opioids. This means that we will need to be very cautious. So, if I manage your medication, I am going to have to require that you see me every 2 weeks, sign an opioid agreement, give a urine screen once a month, and participate in substance

compliance counseling. We may also find in the end that you are not a good candidate for opioids to treat your pain."
PATIENT: "You are just punishing me for being truthful about my drug history. Don't you realize that I have real pain and I need pain medication?"
CLINICIAN: "If you had heart problems, I would not be giving you treatments that would cause problems for your heart. Your test results suggest that these medications can be a problem for you, and as a result, we need to be very careful—for your sake and ours."

Main issues: The physician does not talk down to the patient or accuse him of being a drug abuser but instead educates him about the best course of treatment for someone with his risk factors. The suggestion is that there must be an up-front doctor–patient agreement and that cooperation will be needed. Ultimately, the physician is expressing the final authority to decide what will be the best course of treatment.

Summary and Conclusions

Many things can contribute to patient conflicts when treating chronic pain: Patients with personality disorders, a busy work schedule, and ever-demanding regulations all can create problematic encounters. Despite the many patient factors that contribute to doctor–patient conflicts, some clinicians know how to recover from difficult patient interactions without long-term repercussions. Much is due to their skills in interpersonal relations and the effects these skills have on patients' perception of their caregiver. Certain patients are difficult because of issues of psychiatric comorbidity and a substance use disorder, but the doctor's use of tested interpersonal communication skills can help to prevent the escalation of conflicts. It is important to have access to mental health professionals who can assist in working with the most difficult patients. Increased coordination and adequate communication among the other providers is also important. Ultimately, the employment of positive communication strategies can improve doctor–patient relations and minimize conflicts within a pain management practice.

ACKNOWLEDGMENT
Special thanks are extended to Kathleen Gordon and Edith Mariano from the Patient Family Relations Triaging Program, Brigham and Women's Hospital (BWH), for their invaluable assistance, and to the patients and staff of the Pain Management Center, BWH, Boston, for their inspiration and support.

References

1. Ross EL, Goldberg I, Scanlan E, et al. Dealing with difficult patients: do customer service initiatives improve patient satisfaction at an interdisciplinary pain center? *J App Biobehav Res* 2013;18:123–133.
2. Jamison RN, Scanlan E, Matthews ML, et al. Attitudes of primary care practitioners in managing chronic pain patients prescribed opioids for pain: a prospective longitudinal controlled trial. *Pain Med* 2016;17:99–113.
3. Anderson NK, Jamison RN, Wasan A. Management of difficult patients in the chronic pain setting. In: A Bajwa, RJ Wootton, CA Warfield, eds. *Principles and Practice of Pain Medicine*. 3rd ed. New York: McGraw-Hill; 2017:197–210.
4. Wasan AD, Wootton J, Jamison RN. Dealing with difficult patients in your pain practice. *Reg Anesth Pain Med* 2005;30:184–192.
5. Haas LJ, Leiser JP, Magill MK, et al. Management of the difficult patient. *Am Fam Physician* 2005;72:2063–2068.
6. Erb J. Assessment and management of the violent patient. In: Jacobson JL, Jacobson AM, eds. *Psychiatric Secrets*. 2nd ed. Philadelphia: Hanley & Belfus; 2001:440–447.
7. Hahn SR, Thompson KS, Wills TA, et al. The difficult doctor-patient relationship: somatization, personality and psychopathology. *J Clin Epidemiol* 1994;47:647–657.
8. Sellers RV, Salazar R, Martinez C, et al. Difficult encounters with psychiatric patients: a South Texas Psychiatry practice-based research network (PBRN) study. *J Am Board Fam Med* 2012;25:669–675.
9. Edgoose JY, Regner CJ, Zakletskaia LI. Difficult patients: exploring the patient perspective. *Fam Med* 2014;46:335–339.
10. Sansone RA, Whitecar P, Meier BP, et al. The prevalence of borderline personality among primary care patients with chronic pain. *Gen Hosp Psychiatr* 2001;23:193–197.
11. Wasan AD, Edwards RR, Edwards RR, et al. Psychiatric comorbidity is associated prospectively with diminished opioid analgesia and increased opioid misuse in patients with chronic low back pain. *Anesthesiology* 2015;123:861–872.
12. Jamison RN, Wasan AA. Depression in the patient with chronic pain. In: AJ Barsky, DA Sibersweig, eds. *Depression in Medical Illness*. New York: McGraw-Hill; 2017:287–298.
13. Jackson JL, Kroenke K. Difficult patients encounters in the ambulatory clinic: clinical predictors and outcomes. *Arch Intern Med* 1999;159:1069–1075.
14. Hinchey SA, Jackson JL. A cohort study assessing difficult patient encounters in a walk-in primary care clinic, predictors and outcomes. *J Gen Intern Med* 2011;26:588–594.
15. Jackson JL, Kroenke K. The effect of unmet expectations among adults presenting with physical symptoms. *Ann Intern Med* 2001;134:889–897.
16. Jamison RN, Sheehan KA, Scanlan E, et al. Beliefs and attitudes about opioid prescribing and chronic pain management: survey of primary care providers. *J Opioid Manage* 2014;10:375–382.
17. Vegni E, Visioli S, Moja EA. When talking to the patient is difficult: the physician's perspective. *Commun Med* 2005;2:69–76.
18. What Americans really want from their doctor: Roper Starch survey results reveals what patients want and how they feel about whey they're getting. Available at: http://findarticles.com. Accessed June 16, 2017.
19. Hahn SR. Physical symptoms and physician-experienced difficulty in the physician-patient relationship. *Ann Intern Med* 2001;134:897–904.
20. Hahn SR, Kroenke K, Spitzer RL, et al. The difficult patient: prevalence, psychopathology, and functional impairment. *J Gen Intern Med* 1996;11:1–8.
21. Hoffmann DE, Tarzian AJ. Achieving the right balance in oversight of physician opioid prescribing for pain: the role of state medical boards. *J Law Med Ethics* 2003;31:21–40.
22. Von Korff M, Crane P, Lane M, et al. Chronic spinal pain and physical-mental comorbidity in the United States: results from the National Comorbidity Survey Replication. *Pain* 2005;113:331–339.
23. Dersh J, Gatchel R, Polatin P, et al. Prevalence of psychiatric disorders in patients with chronic work-related musculoskeletal pain and disability. *J Occup Environ Med* 2002;44:459–468.
24. Koekkoek B, van Meijel B, Hutschemaekers G. "Difficult patients" in mental health care: a review. *Psychiatr Serv* 2006;57:795–802.
25. Fishbain DA. Approaches to treatment decisions for psychiatric comorbidity in the management of the chronic pain patients. *Med Clin North Am* 1999;83:737–760.
26. Bair MJ, Robinson RL, Katon W, et al. Depression and pain comorbidity: a literature review. *Arch Int Med* 2003;163:2433–2445.
27. White KP, Nielson WR, Harth M, et al. Chronic widespread musculoskeletal pain with or without fibromyalgia: psychological distress in a representative community adult sample. *J Rheum* 2002;29:588–594.
28. McWilliams LA, Goodwin RD, Cox BJ. Depression and anxiety associated with three pain conditions: results from a nationally representative sample. *Pain* 2004;111:77–83.
29. Ligthart LM, Gerrits M. Anxiety and depression are associated with migraine and pain in general: an investigation of the interrelationships. *J Pain* 2013;14:363–370.
30. Dworkin SF, Von Korff M. Multiple pains and psychiatric disturbance. An epidemiologic investigation. *Arch Gen Psychiatry* 1990;47:239–244.
31. Dersh J, Mayer T, Theodore BR, et al. Do psychiatric disorders first appear preinjury or postinjury in chronic disabling occupational spinal disorders? *Spine* 2007;32:1045–1051.
32. Nelson DV, Novy DM. Self-report differentiation of anxiety and depression in chronic pain. *J Pers Assess* 1997;69:392–407.
33. Evers AW, Kraaimaat FW, van Reil PL, et al. Cognitive, behavioral and physiological reactivity to pain as a predictor of long-term pain in rheumatoid arthritis patients. *Pain* 2001;9:139–146.
34. Harkins SW, Price DD, Braith J. Effects of extraversion and neuroticism on experimental pain, clinical pain, and illness behavior. *Pain* 1989;36:209–218.
35. Boersma K, Linton SJ. Screening to identify patients at risk: profiles of psychological risk factors for early intervention. *Clin J Pain* 2005;21:38–43.
36. Reid MC, Engles-Horton LL, Weber MB, et al. Use of opioid medications for chronic noncancer pain syndromes in primary care. *J Gen Intern Med* 2002;17:173–179.
37. Breckenridge J, Clark JD. Patient characteristics associated with opioid versus nonsteroidal anti-inflammatory drug management of chronic low back pain. *J Pain* 2003;4:344–350.
38. Turk DC, Okifuji A. What factors affect physicians' decisions to prescribe opioids for chronic noncancer pain? *Clin J Pain* 1997;13:330–336.
39. Passik SD, Kirsch KL, Whitcomb RK, et al. A new tool to assess and document pain outcomes in chronic pain patients receiving opioid therapy. *Clin Ther* 2004;26:552–561.
40. Wasan AD, Davar G, Jamison RN. The association between negative affect and opioid analgesia in patients with discogenic low back pain. *Pain* 2005;117:450–461.

41. Edwards RR, Wasan A, Michna E, et al. Elevated pain sensitivity in chronic pain patients at risk for opioid misuse. *J Pain* 2011;9:953–963.
42. Schouten BC, Meeuwesen L. Cultural differences in medical communication: a review of the literature. *Patient Educ Couns* 2006;64:21–34.
43. Kenny DT. Constructions of chronic pain in doctor-patient relationships: bridging the communication chasm. *Patient Educ Couns* 2004;52:297–305.
44. Stokes T, Dixon-Woods M, McKinley RK. Breaking up is never easy: GPs' accounts of removing patients from their lists. *Fam Pract* 2003;20:628–634.
45. Ballantyne JC, LaForge KS. Opioid dependence and addiction during opioid treatment of chronic pain. *Pain* 2007;129:235–255.
46. Jamison RN, Mao J. Opioid analgesics. *Mayo Clinic Proc* 2015;90:957–968.
47. Kissin B. Medical management of alcoholic patients. In: Kissin B, Begleiter H, eds. *Treatment and Rehabilitation of the Chronic Alcoholic.* New York: Plenum; 1977;53–103.
48. Brown RL, Leonard T, Saunders LA, et al. The prevalence and detection of substance use disorders among inpatients ages 18–49: an opportunity for prevention. *Prev Med* 1998;27:101–110.
49. Jamison RN, Kauffman J, Katz NP. Characteristics of methadone maintenance patients with chronic pain. *J Pain Symptom Manage* 2000;19:53–62.
50. Lazaridou A, Franceschelli O, Buliteanu A, et al. Influence of catastrophizing on pain intensity, disability, side effects, and opioid misuse among pain patients in primary care. *J Appl Behav Res* 2017;22:e12081.
51. Martel MO, Wasan AD, Jamison RN, et al. Catastrophic thinking and increased risk for prescription opioid misuse in patients with chronic pain. *Drug Alcohol Depend* 2013;132:335–341.
52. Hasin D, Liu X. Effects of major depression on remission and relapse of substance dependence. *Arch Gen Psychiatry* 2002;59:375–380.
53. Wasan AD, Ross EL, Michna E, et al. Characterizing craving of prescription opioids in patients with chronic pain: a longitudinal outcomes trial. *J Pain* 2012;13:146–154.
54. Quello S, Brady K. Mood disorders and substance use disorder: a complex comorbidity. *Sci Pract Perspect* 2005;3:13–24.
55. Hampton T. Physicians advised on how to offer pain relief while preventing opioid abuse. *JAMA* 2004;292:1164–1166.
56. Savage SR. Assessment for addiction in pain treatment settings. *Clin J Pain* 2002;18:S28–S38.
57. Michna E, Ross EL, Hynes WL, et al. Predicting aberrant drug behavior in patients treated for chronic pain: importance of abuse history. *J Pain Symptom Manage* 2004;28:250–258.
58. Jamison RN, Edwards RR. Risk factor assessment for problematic use of opioids for chronic pain. *Clin Neuropsychol* 2013;27:60–80.
59. Webster LR, Webster RM. Predicting aberrant behaviors in opioid-treated patients: preliminary validation of the Opioid Risk Tool. *Pain Med* 2005;6:432–442.
60. Pomm HA, Shahady E, Pomm RM. The CALMER approach: teaching learners six steps to serenity when dealing with difficult patients. *Fam Med* 2004;36:467–469.
61. Kristiansson MH, Brorsson A, Wachtler C, et al. Pain, power and patience—narrative study of general practitioners' relations with chronic pain patients. *BMC Fam Pract* 2011;12:31. doi:10.1186/1471-2296-12-31.
62. Homma M, Ishikawa H, Kiuch T. Association of physicians' illness perception of fibromyalgia with frustration and resistance to accepting patients: a cross-sectional study. *Clin Rheumatol* 2016;35:1019–1027.
63. Halpern J. Empathy and patient-physician conflicts. *J Gen Intern Med* 2007;22:696–700.
64. Krebs EE, Garrett JM, Konrad TR. The difficult doctor? Characteristics of physicians who report frustration with patients: an analysis of survey data. *BMC Health Serv Res* 2006;6:128.
65. Mathias MS, Parpart AL, Nyland KA, et al. The patient-provider relationship in chronic pain are: providers' perspectives. *Pain Med* 2010;11:1688–1697.
66. Tam M, Su M. How to manage difficult patients. 2006. Available at: http://vitualis.wordpress.com. Accessed June 15, 2017.
67. Hogan MF. The President's New Freedom Commission: recommendations to transform mental health care in America. *Psychiatr Serv* 2003;54:1467–1474.
68. Fiellin DA, O'Connor PG. Clinical practice. Office-based treatment of opioid-dependent patients. *N Engl J Med* 2002;347:817–823.
69. Weisner C, Mertens J, Tam T, et al. Factors affecting the initiation of substance abuse treatment in managed care. *Addiction* 2001;96:705–716.
70. Friedmann PD, Zhang Z, Hendrickson J, et al. Effect of primary medical care on addiction and medical severity in substance abuse treatment programs. *J Gen Intern Med* 2003;18:1–8.
71. Broom AF. The influence of the internet on patients' expectations. *Nature Clin Pract Urol* 2006;3:117.
72. Jamison RN, Fanciullo GJ, Baird JC. Computer and information technology in the assessment and management of patients with pain. *Pain Med* 2007;8:S83–S84.
73. Elder N, Ricer R, Tobias B. How respected family physicians manage difficult patient encounters. *J Am Board Fam Med* 2006;19:533–541.
74. Lown BA. Difficult conversations: anger in the clinician-patient/family relationship. *South Med J* 2007;100:40–42, 62.
75. Nisselle P. Difficult doctor-patient relationships. *Aust Fam Physician* 2000;29:47–49.
76. Street RL Jr, Gordon H, Haidet P. Physicians' communication and perceptions of patients: is it how they look, how they talk, or is it just the doctor? *Soc Sci Med* 2007;65:586–598.
77. Klitzman R. Improving education on doctor-patient relationships and communication: lessons from doctors who become patients. *Acad Med* 2006;81:447–453.
78. Irwin RS, Richardson ND. Patient-focused care: using the right tools. *Chest* 2006;130:73S–82S.
79. Dawson R, Spross JA, Jablonski ES, et al. Probing the paradox of patients' satisfaction with inadequate pain management. *J Pain Symptom Manage* 2002;23:211–220.
80. Jamison RN, Ross MJ, Hoopman P, et al. Assessment of postoperative pain management: patient satisfaction and perceived helpfulness. *Clin J Pain* 1997;13:229–236.
81. Kannan S, Jamison RN, Datta S. Maternal satisfaction and pain control in women electing natural childbirth. *Reg Anesth Pain Med* 2001;26:468–472.
82. Hegan T. The importance of effective communication in preventing litigation. *Med J Malaysia* 2003;58(suppl A):78–82.
83. Piasecki M. *Clinical Communication Handbook.* New York: Blackwell; 2002.
84. Levinson W, Roter DL, Mullooly JP, et al. Physician-patient communication. The relationship with malpractice claims among primary care physicians and surgeons. *JAMA* 1997;277:553–559.
85. Gafaranga J, Britten N. "Fire away": the opening sequence in general practice consultations. *Fam Pract* 2003;20:242–247.
86. Roy MJ, Herbers JE, Seidman A, et al. Improving patient satisfaction with the transfer of care. A randomized controlled trial. *J Gen Intern Med* 2003;18:364–369.
87. Back AL, Arnold RM, Baile WF, et al. Approaching difficult communication tasks in oncology. *CA Cancer J Clin* 2005;55:164–177.
88. Prochaska JO, DiClemente CC. *The Transtheoretical Approach: Towards a Systematic Eclectic Framework.* Homewood, IL: Dow Jones Irwin; 1984.
89. Kerns RD, Rosenberg R, Jamison RN, et al. Readiness to adopt a self-management approach to chronic pain: the Pain Stages of Change Questionnaire (PSOCQ). *Pain* 1997;72:227–234.
90. Makoul G. Essential elements of communication in medical encounters: the Kalamazoo consensus statement. *Acad Med* 2001;76:390–393.

CHAPTER **34**

Arthritis

GREGORY C. GARDNER

This chapter contains a discussion of the common causes of joint pain encountered in clinical practice. These include osteoarthritis (OA), rheumatoid arthritis, the spondyloarthropathies (ankylosing spondylitis, psoriatic arthritis, and reactive arthritis), and crystalline forms of arthritis (gout and pseudogout). In addition, there will be a brief discussion of two other rheumatologic conditions: septic arthritis and polymyalgia rheumatica.

Basic Considerations

PROBLEM IN PERSPECTIVE

In December 2012, a study on the Global Burden of Disease and the worldwide impact of all diseases and risk factors reported that musculoskeletal conditions, including arthritis and back pain, affect more than 1.7 billion people worldwide and are the second greatest cause of disability worldwide.[1] Musculoskeletal conditions have the fourth greatest impact on the overall health of the world population with regard to death and disability.

In the United States, the Bone and Joint Decade took place from 2002 to 2011, and data reported in 2012 found that 54% of adults (126 million) in the United States reported a chronic musculoskeletal condition that year. This is much higher than those reporting a circulatory problem (31%), respiratory problem (28%), diabetes (13%), or cancer (9%). Approximately 75 million Americans report neck or low back pain, 52 million arthritis, and 4.5 million Americans will have an activity-related musculoskeletal injury each year. In addition, it is expected that 1 in 2 women and 1 in 4 men over the age of 50 years will have an osteoporosis-related fracture during their remaining years. Rheumatoid arthritis, an autoimmune form of arthritis, affects over 1.5 million adults in the United States, whereas over 300,000 children are afflicted with juvenile inflammatory arthritis. Both of these conditions not only affect mobility and quality of life but can also shorten life expectancy.

The economic burden is significant with an estimated $874 billion being spent both for treatment of musculoskeletal condition and in lost wages of affected workers.

JOINT ANATOMY

Joints in the extremities are synovial (diarthrodial) joints that permit movement over a wide range (Fig. 34.1).[2] The joint is held together by a capsule of dense fibrous tissue and ligaments and gains further support from overlying muscle and tendons. The inner surface of the joint capsule is covered by synovium, which consists of an intimal layer of specialized cells called *synoviocytes*, and an outer layer of highly vascularized connective tissue. Synoviocytes comprise one to three cell layers and are of two basic types: A and B. Type A synoviocytes are active in phagocytosis, and type B cells synthesize hyaluronate, which is primarily responsible for the high viscosity of normal synovial fluid. Synovial fluid in a normal joint lubricates the surfaces of synovium and cartilage. The synovium is folded along the inside of the joint capsule and does not cover the load-bearing surface of articular cartilage. The connective tissue layer of synovium blends with periosteum, which does not cover the bone within the joint. The synovium has a rich network of capillaries, venules, and lymphatics, and it is innervated by sympathetic nerve fibers. The knee and the sternoclavicular and radiocarpal joints contain disks of fibrocartilage that help to stabilize these joints when they rotate. The fibrocartilage meniscus of the knee also helps improve joint congruity which is important in the normal distribution of weight with joint loading. The intervertebral facet joints are diarthrodial joints and are covered by synovium.

Amphiarthrodial joints are only slightly movable and include the symphysis pubis and the joints between vertebral bodies. The joint surfaces are separated by intervertebral disks. The sacroiliac joint has elements of both a diarthrodial and an amphiarthrodial joint.

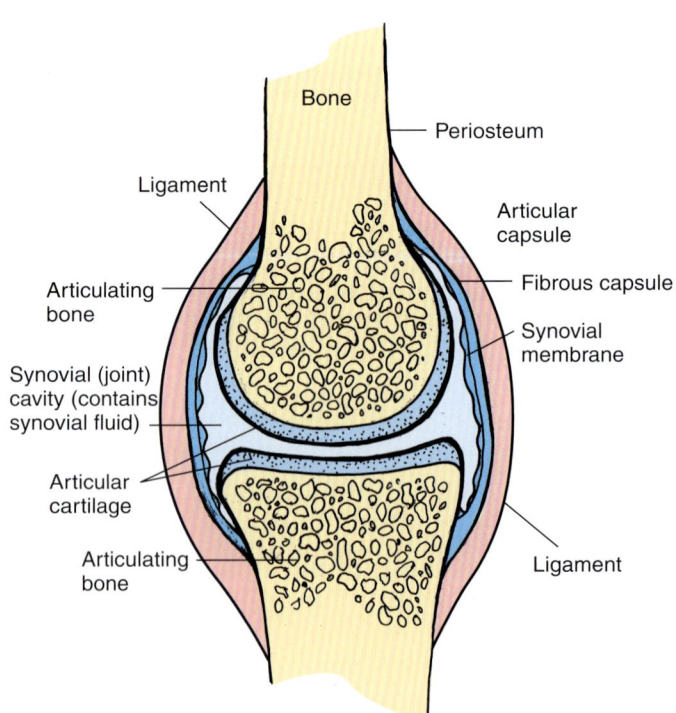

FIGURE 34.1 Schematic diagram of the anatomic features of a typical synovial joint seen in a section cut across the middle of the joint. (*Reprinted with permission from Oatis CA.* Kinesiology. The Mechanics and Pathomechanics of Human Movement. *3rd ed. Philadelphia, PA: Lippincott Williams & Wilkins; 2016. Figure 5-1.*)

Articular cartilage is composed of type 2 collagen and proteoglycans. Type 2 collagen is unique to joints and provides cartilage with form and tensile strength. Proteoglycan molecules are linked noncovalently to a long chain of hyaluronic acid and are interwoven within the network of collagen fibers. Proteoglycan molecules bind most of the water present in cartilage, which represents approximately 70% of the total weight of articular cartilage. The proteoglycan molecules are constrained within the meshwork of collagen fibers and are responsible for the resiliency of cartilage. Chondrocytes secrete collagen, proteoglycans, and enzymes that degrade the cartilaginous matrix. The process of remodeling and degradation is kept in balance unless the microenvironment of these cells is altered. Joints normally contain a small amount of synovial fluid, which is viscous and clear and does not clot spontaneously. Normal synovial fluid contains fewer than 200 white blood cells per cubic millimeter; most of these cells are mononuclear.

Nerve and Blood Supply

Joints are supplied partly by articular nerves, which are branches of major peripheral nerves, and partly by branches of nerves supplying adjacent muscles as well as vasomotor sympathetic fibers. Nerve endings are distributed in the interstitial and perivascular tissue located in the subsynovium fibrous capsule, in the articular fat pads, and in the adventitial sheaths of arteries and arterioles supplying the joints. The periosteum is innervated, but articular cartilage and subchondral bones are not and thus not a direct source of pain in arthritis.

There are four types of receptors that supply joints.[3] Type I receptors are ovoid corpuscles with a thin connective tissue capsule, and each is supplied by a small myelinated nerve fiber (5 to 8 mm in diameter) that arborizes within the capsule. The type I receptor occurs almost exclusively in the fibrous joint capsule, acts as a slowly adapting mechanoreceptor (stretch receptor), and resembles both structurally and functionally the Ruffini endings in the dermis. The type II receptor is approximately twice as large as the type I receptor and is supplied by a somewhat thicker myelinated fiber (8 to 12 mm in diameter) that usually ends as a single terminal within a rather thick laminated capsule. These receptors, which resemble the pacinian corpuscles, occur only in the fibrous joint capsule and have been shown to be rapidly adapting mechanoreceptors (acceleration receptors) that are sensitive to rapid movements. Type III receptors, which are the largest, are supplied by thick myelinated fibers that branch profusely. These receptors, which resemble the Golgi organs, are present in extrinsic and intrinsic ligaments (and not in the joint capsule) and adapt slowly and at high thresholds. Type IV receptors are represented by plexuses of fine unmyelinated fibers that occur in the fibrous joint capsules, ligaments, and subsynovial capsules and fat pads; they are considered to be the joint nociceptors.

An anastomotic plexus of blood vessels called the *periarticular anastomosis*, together with these nerves, surrounds the capsule, and its branches penetrate the capsule. The periarticular anastomosis is fed by branches of arteries passing the joint and is the source of blood to the capillary bed in the synovial membrane and also to the epiphysis.

Clinical Approach to Joint Pain

A variety of disorders, both systemic and local, can involve the joints. The process of arriving at a diagnosis begins with a thorough history which should initiate a differential diagnosis. The physical examination and subsequent laboratory and imaging testing continue the process of narrowing the differential.

HISTORY

The musculoskeletal history begins by determining the pattern or patterns of joint complaints. The rheumatologist often divides joint complaints into three different types: inflammatory, mechanical, and fibromyalgia-type discomfort. Inflammatory conditions, such as rheumatoid arthritis, are characterized by joint stiffness in the morning lasting at least 30 minutes but often several hours. Patients generally feel better after activity as the fluid accumulated during inactivity is pumped out of a swollen, stiff joint by the lymphatics, thus reducing the sensation of stiffness. The presence of inflammatory cytokines such as interleukin (IL)-1 or tumor necrosis factor (TNF) may cause fatigue, anorexia, or a loss of the sense of well-being. Joints may initially be stiff and painful but with time typically demonstrate swelling on examination. There is a subtype of inflammatory pain caused by the presence of microorganisms (usually bacteria), blood, or crystals. These conditions typically have an acute onset and cause severe joint pain. The affected person keeps the joint at 30 to 40 degrees of flexion and resists movement of the involved joint. This is the position of maximum joint volume and attempts to flex or extend the joint leads to decrease joint volume and thus an increase in joint fluid pressure leading to pain (Boyle's law). Joint contractures form in part because of this principle as chronic immobility can lead to capsular contraction even when the fluid in no longer present.

Mechanical joint pain, typified by OA, generally causes only 5 to 10 minutes of morning stiffness, but affected joints become progressively more painful with activity. There may be discomfort for some period of time following use as well. Swelling may or may not be present or only present following stress. There are no systemic symptoms in patients with mechanical forms of arthritis.

Fibromyalgia-associated pain is characterized by all over morning stiffness or pain, a period of loosening up late morning or early afternoon, followed by fatigue and increased pain as the afternoon progresses. Sleep is poor, memory may be reported to be poor, and activity and exercise are poorly tolerated, and in fact, patients will report being in bed for 1 or 2 days following a strenuous physical or even emotional event. The diagnosis of fibromyalgia should be considered when a patient reports that they have one or two days of feeling severe fatigue and pain after an episode of significant physical activity or emotional distress. Even doing household chores may exacerbate the discomfort. Patients often describe their pain in dramatic terms such as the sensation of hot pokers or ice picks being driven into a particularly painful area. Patients with fibromyalgia often have other somatic complaints such as chronic low back pain, temporal mandibular jaw pain, or chronic headaches.

With experience, the clinician can with some ease categorize a patient's joint complaints into one of these three major types. It is important to remember that Occam's razor (the simplest explanation is usually correct) is usually best to follow, but it is not uncommon for patients with inflammatory disease to have one, two, or all three patterns simultaneously (Hickam's dictum: the patients can have as many diseases as they darn well please). For example, a patient with rheumatoid arthritis can have active inflammatory arthritis (inflammatory pattern), have a rheumatoid arthritis associated damaged knee with secondary OA (mechanical pattern), and, because sleep and usual exercise activities may be disturbed by both former patterns, have fibromyalgia as well. With experience, a clinician can learn to distinguish the single-pattern from the multiple-pattern patient and help the patient understand that there is more than one cause to the pain. Patients generally adhere to Occam's razor until taught otherwise.

Number of Joints Affected

The next step in developing a differential diagnosis is determining the number of joints involved. There are three categories in joint number as well and include monoarthritis, pauciarthritis (two to five joints affected), and finally polyarthritis (six or

TABLE 34.1 Important Causes of Monoarthritis	
Inflammatory	**Mechanical**
Infection	Osteoarthritis
Bacterial arthritis	Osteonecrosis
Staphylococcus, Streptococcus, gram	Trauma
negatives, *Neisseria gonorrhoeae*	Tumor
Lyme arthritis	
Mycobacterial arthritis	
Fungal arthritis	
Crystals	
Monosodium urate	
Calcium pyrophosphate	
Hydroxyapatite	
Hemarthrosis	
Clotting disorder	
Anticoagulation therapy	
Trauma (ACL tear)	

ACL, anterior cruciate ligament.

TABLE 34.3 Important Causes of Polyarthritis (Six or More Joints)	
Inflammatory	**Mechanical**
Infection	Osteoarthritis
Poststreptococcal arthritis	Primary osteoarthritis
Viruses	Secondary osteoarthritis
Parvovirus	Hemochromatosis
Rubella	Acromegaly
Hepatitis B and C	Calcium pyrophosphate
Autoimmune disease	deposition
Rheumatoid arthritis	
Systemic lupus erythematosus	
Sjögren's syndrome	
Scleroderma	
Miscellaneous	
Serum sickness	

more joints). Tables 34.1, 34.2, and 34.3 give a general differential diagnosis inflammatory or mechanical joint pain pattern and number of joints involved. It is important to recognize that these are general guidelines because a polyarticular condition such as rheumatoid arthritis might initially present with less than six affected joint but progress over time to be polyarticular in character. Once a disease has been established for several weeks/months, these patterns tend to be more fixed.

Pattern Recognition

A helpful historical and examination finding is the pattern of joint involvement. For example, OA affects the spine, the hands, hips, knees, and first metatarsophalangeal (MTP) joints. In the hand, the distal interphalangeal (DIP) joints, proximal interphalangeal (PIP) joints, and base of the thumb joint (first carpometacarpal [CMC]) are affected. **The metacarpophalangeal (MCP) joints are spared in primary OA.** For rheumatoid arthritis, the pattern of involvement is cervical spine only, shoulders, elbows, wrists, hands, hips, knees, ankles, and MTP joints. In the hand, the PIP joints and MCP joints are affected, **but the DIP joints are spared.** Noting the distribution of affected joints is very helpful in developing a differential diagnosis. This will be discussed further when the individual conditions are presented.

Systemic Features of Arthritis

A variety of systemic or demographic features of illness also provides clues to the underlying diagnosis and is discussed with the individual conditions.

PHYSICAL EXAMINATION

When a patient reports that he or she has "joint pain," it may be the result of tendon, ligament, muscle, bone, joint, or nerve abnormalities. The clinician needs to keep this in mind during the examination. For example, "knee pain" may be caused by an L4 radiculopathy or hip pain may radiate to the area of the knee. Joints should be examined for evidence of synovial proliferation, fluid, and bony enlargement as well a range of motion. Tenderness, warmth, and any limitation of range of motion should be noted. Pain on passive motion of a joint suggests the possibility of inflammation or damage to the joint. Even though a patient may complain about a particular joint or joints, make sure to examine all joints. Milder abnormalities that may be present in nonpainful joints could add to the information on the number of joints involved and the pattern, thus helping with the differential diagnosis. Comparing an affected to a nonaffected joint often confirms the presence of swelling or deformity.

EXAMINATION OF SYNOVIAL FLUID

Examination of the joint fluid is helpful in patients who have undiagnosed arthritis. Diagnosis of infectious or crystal-induced arthritis is established by analysis of joint fluid. Characteristics of the joint fluid in various rheumatic conditions are shown in Table 34.4. Normal joint fluid usually contains fewer than 200 white blood cells per cubic millimeter, and these cells are predominantly mononuclear. In inflammatory effusions, the white blood cell count is usually elevated

TABLE 34.2 Important Causes of Pauciarthritis (Two to Five Joints)	
Inflammatory	**Mechanical**
Infection	Osteoarthritis
Bacterial arthritis	
Crystals	
Monosodium urate	
Spondyloarthropathies	
Ankylosing spondylitis	
Psoriatic arthritis	
Reactive arthritis	
Miscellaneous	
Sarcoidosis	

TABLE 34.4 Joint Fluid Characteristics in Various Forms of Arthritis			
Diagnosis	**Appearance**	**WBC/mm³**	**% PMNs**
Normal	Clear/ straw-colored	<200	<25
Osteoarthritis	Straw-colored	200–2,000	<25
Rheumatoid arthritis	Slightly opaque to cloudy	2,000–50,000	>50
Gout/ pseudogout	Slightly opaque to cloudy	2,000–100,000	>75
Spondylo- arthropathies	Slightly opaque to cloudy	2,000–100,000	>50
Bacterial arthritis	Cloudy to purulent	25,000–100,000	>75

WBC, white blood cell; PMN, polymorphonuclear leukocytes.

(typically over 2,000 white blood cells per cubic millimeter) with predominantly neutrophils present on cell count. Traditionally, cell counts greater than 75,000 per cubic millimeter suggest an infectious arthritis, but cell counts of this magnitude are also seen in noninfectious inflammatory joint diseases such as reactive arthritis or urate gout. Data suggested that a synovial fluid cell count over 25,000 cell per cubic millimeter should be evaluated for possible infection as the likelihood ratio of infection is greater than one; less than this level is unlikely to be related to a septic arthritis.

Clinical Considerations

OSTEOARTHRITIS

OA is characterized by progressive loss of articular cartilage leading to joint pain and limitation of movement. Weight-bearing and frequently used joints are most often affected. The disease is divided into a primary (idiopathic) form, in which no predisposing factors are apparent, and a secondary form, which is associated with trauma, sequela of an inflammatory joint disease, a metabolic disease such as hemochromatosis, or a congenital structural abnormality. Primary OA is the more common form, but pathologically, the two forms are indistinguishable.

Epidemiology and Pathophysiology

OA is the most common form of arthritis worldwide and is the leading cause of disability in seniors.[4,5] The disease occurs in all races and geographic areas. Prevalence and severity increase with age. Under age 55 years, the frequency and joint distribution of OA in men and women are approximately the same. After age 55 years, OA of the knee is more common in women and OA of the hip in men.[6] OA can be demonstrated radiographically in almost all persons over the age of 75 years. Weight-bearing joints such as the hips, knees, feet, and cervical and lumbosacral joints are most often affected. The DIP and PIP joints of the hands are also commonly involved. Certain occupations have been shown to predispose a person to OA. In coal miners, for example, OA of the shoulders and knees is more frequent, presumably because of the forces placed on these joints during work. Prizefighters are more likely to develop OA of their MCP joints, football players of their knees, and ballet dancers of their ankles. Hereditary factors also exist: Heberden's nodes are twice as frequent in mothers of affected persons and 3 times more frequent in sisters.[7] A single-point mutation in the complementary DNA (cDNA) coding for type II collagen was found in family members with an inherited form of OA associated with a mild chondrodysplasia.[8,9] Previous major trauma and repetitive use of a joint increase the risk of developing OA. Age alone is a risk factor, with the prevalence of OA increasing after age 45 years. Obesity has been shown to be a definite risk factor for developing OA of the hips and knees.[5]

The progressive change within the joint in OA is well known. The cartilage initially shows fissuring and pitting, which eventually progress to erosions and denuded areas. The proteoglycan content of cartilage and the number of chondrocytes decrease in proportion to the degree of disease. Subchondral bone becomes thickened and has an eburnated, or ivory-like, appearance. Cysts appear in the subchondral bone, and the formation of new bone at the joint margins produces osteophytes or spurs. The synovium is thickened and contains a modest infiltration of lymphocytes, plasma cells, and an occasional multinucleated giant cell. The joint capsule and ligaments are hypertrophied. Figure 34.2 shows the arthroscopic appearance progressive nature of OA in the knee.

Research in OA has identified a variety of factors associated with the development of OA. These include aging (older more at risk), gender (females have a higher prevalence and

severity than males), joint trauma, inflammation (inflammatory cytokines such as IL-1 are thought to contribute to joint damage), mechanical factors (weight/alignment issues), genetics (may account for as much as 60% of hip OA), and obesity (via a variety of factors including adipokines such as leptin).[5,10] An interesting observation is that obesity leads to OA of the weight-bearing joints as might be expected but also to an increase risk of OA of the hand joints. In individual patients, all these factors may be contributing to a greater or lesser degree. Ultimately, prevention and treatment approaches will require that these factors be addressed in a more holistic fashion.

Symptoms and Signs

OA may be limited to one or two joints or may occur in a generalized form involving many joints. Involved joints are stiff for 30 minutes or less in the morning and after periods of inactivity. Pain typically develops with use. The involved joints also can ache at night affecting the quality of sleep. Night pain is caused in part by increased intraosseous venous pressure.[11] As the disease progresses, pain becomes a constant feature of physical activity and can persist for several hours afterward. Eventually, restricted motion and joint deformities develop.

Primary OA most frequently affects the DIP joints, the first CMC joint, the scaphotrapezoid joint, the hips, knees, first MTP joint, and the cervical and lumbar spine.

Heberden's nodes usually develop after age 40 years and are associated with OA of the DIP joints. Similar nodes, called *Bouchard's nodes*, appear at the PIP joints (Fig. 34.3). At times, these nodes become red and painful to touch. Bony enlargement, small effusions, restricted motion, and angulation can be seen on physical examination. Radial subluxation of the first CMC joint gives a square appearance to this joint (shelf sign). A form of OA, referred to as *primary generalized OA*, appears most often in middle-aged women and affects the DIP and PIP joints of the hand, the first CMC joint, knees, hips, and the first MTP joint. Episodes of inflammation are characterized by warmth, pain, and swelling of these joints.

OA of the hip is usually unilateral, but the opposite side is also affected in approximately 20% of patients.[12] Congenital or developmental abnormalities such as slipped capital femoral epiphysis, Legg-Calvé-Perthes syndrome, or hip dysplasia underlie many of the cases. OA follows avascular necrosis, which can be related to deep-water diving, glucocorticosteroid therapy, alcohol, or sickle cell disease. Hip pain is experienced in the groin, over the greater trochanter, in the buttock, or down the anterior and inner thigh. Pain might be referred to the distal thigh and upper knee because the obturator nerve and its branches supply both hip and knee. As noted earlier, hip disease can be mistaken for knee arthritis or trochanteric bursitis because hip pain can be referred to those locations. The pain of hip disease is often described as dull and aching and is initially experienced with physical activity. Later, night pain is also experienced. Patients might limp and have difficulty rising from a sitting position. Functional shortening of the leg caused by adduction and flexion contractures causes the patient to walk with a shuffling gait. Examination of the hip shows initially decreased internal rotation that is followed later by decreased extension, abduction, and flexion as well as a flexion contracture.

Previous injury such as a torn meniscus or ligament predisposes the knee to secondary OA. The presence of an alignment abnormality such as genu varum (bow legs) or genu valgum (knock knees) increases the force directed through either the medial or lateral side of the knee and can lead to OA. These deformities are also acquired in OA as a result of destruction of either the medial or lateral articular cartilage. Obesity predisposes the knees to OA by the additional weight and by the thigh thickness, which places the legs in a genu varus position and increases the pressure on the medial compartment.

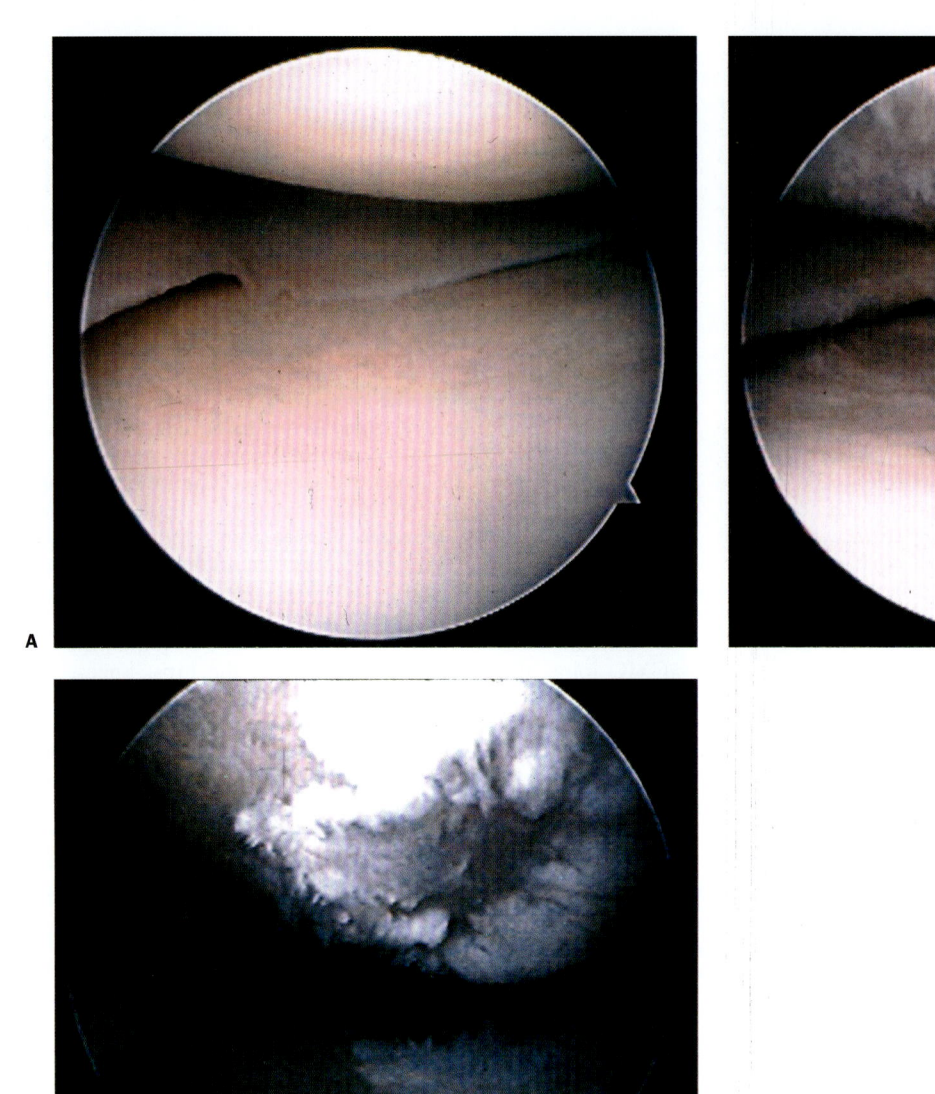

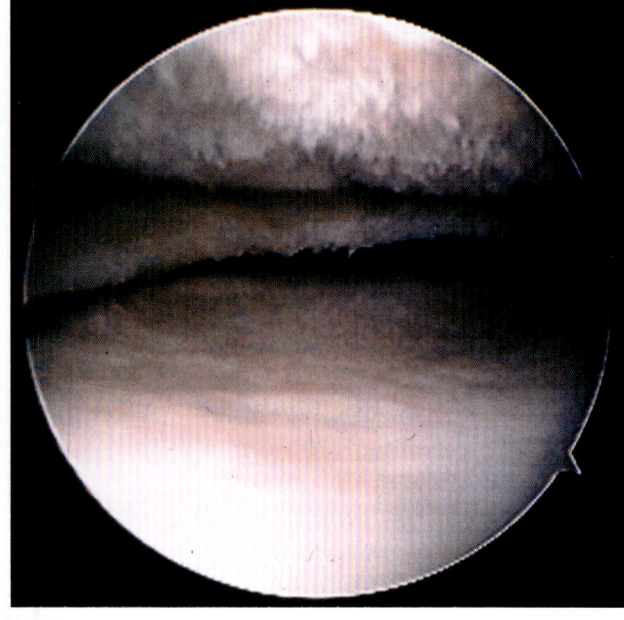

FIGURE 34.2 Progression of osteoarthritis of the knee via arthroscopy. **A:** Normal appearing knee. Note the smoothness of the articular cartilage of the femur as well as the meniscus. **B:** Thickening and fissuring of the cartilage and meniscus. **C:** Advanced osteoarthritis of the knee with bare areas devoid of cartilage and loss of meniscal tissue.

In addition, obesity leads to the production of a variety of cytokines and adipokines that may affect the quality or quantity of cartilage.[13] Pain also can be localized to either the medial or lateral aspect of the joint depending on which compartment is primarily involved. Atrophy and weakness of the quadriceps muscle develop with progression of the arthritis. Crepitus might be noted with bending of the knee as well as an effusion. With more severe disease, a contracture may be present which increases the energy required to stand upright. With loss of ligamentous and muscle support, the knee becomes unstable, and the patient may be hesitant to walk on uneven surfaces. The knee might suddenly give way because of a pain reflex. A loose cartilaginous fragment, sometimes referred to as a *loose body*, can prevent the joint from being fully extended.

Patellofemoral arthritis occurs alone or in conjunction with arthritis of the other knee compartments, especially in older patients. The term *chondromalacia patellae* is often used interchangeably with *patellofemoral arthritis*, although some restrict

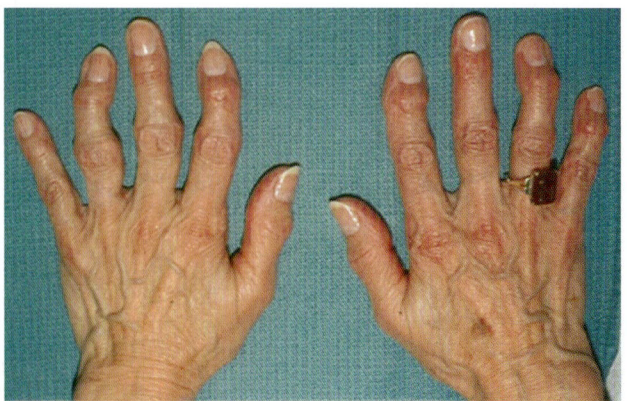

FIGURE 34.3 Osteoarthritis of the hands. Note Heberden's nodes (distal interphalangeal joints) and Bouchard's nodes (proximal interphalangeal joints) in this patient with classic hand osteoarthritis.

this term to a self-limiting disorder occurring in adolescents and young adults. Patellofemoral arthritis is caused in some patients by improper tracking of the patella through the patellofemoral groove (trochlea). The patella is pulled to the lateral margin of the groove by a tight lateral patellar retinaculum or a relative weakness of the vastus medialis compared with the vastus lateralis of the quadriceps muscle. Lateral subluxation of the patella can also be caused by an increased Q angle resulting from rotational misalignment of the femur and tibia.

In the spine, intervertebral disks and apophyseal (facet) joints are sites for OA. Involvement of intervertebral disks is referred to as *spondylosis*, whereas disease in the apophyseal joints is considered true OA. OA also affects the joints of Luschka (uncovertebral joints), which are located in the cervical spine between the superior process of one vertebral body and the inferior process of the vertebral body above it.

Symptoms of spine involvement are localized pain and stiffness, referred or dermatomal pain, and radicular pain from nerve root compression. Nerve root involvement produces paresthesias, decreased sensation, loss of muscle strength, and diminished or absent deep tendon reflexes. OA of the cervical spine causes either localized pain or pain referred to the occiput, shoulder, interscapular area, or arm, depending on the level affected. With upper cervical disease, the pain tends to be referred to the occiput, and with lower cervical involvement, it is referred to the shoulder, upper arm, or interscapular area. Neurologic manifestations are also caused by compression of the spinal cord by posteriorly directed osteophytes and by occlusion of the anterior spinal artery by a herniated disk. Cervical spine diseases are discussed in Chapter 67, and lumbar spine in Chapters 72 through 76.

SECONDARY OSTEOARTHRITIS

OA can develop in joints that have been damaged. A torn knee meniscus or ligament can lead to incongruity of the joint surfaces resulting in OA. In addition, ligaments contribute to proprioceptive input and injury to these structures may increase the risk of developing OA.[14] OA may follow joint damage produced by infectious arthritis or an inflammatory arthritis such as rheumatoid arthritis. Neuropathic joint disease is a severe form of OA resulting from the loss of pain sensation, proprioception, or both.[14,15] Without these protective mechanisms, joints are subjected to repeated trauma, leading to progressive cartilage damage. Diabetes is the most common cause of neuropathic joint disease. Other causes include tabes dorsalis, syringomyelia, amyloidosis, meningomyelocele in children, and leprosy.

OA occurs in patients with excessively hypermobile joints. Patients with Ehlers-Danlos syndrome, a hereditary disorder of connective tissue, develop OA of their hands, shoulders, knees, and ankles usually before age 40 years.[16] Debate exists regarding whether patients with idiopathic joint hypermobility are at risk of developing premature OA.

Several metabolic disorders are associated with the development of OA. These include hemochromatosis, ochronosis, and acromegaly. Arthritis occurs in 20% to 50% of patients with hemochromatosis and may appear before other overt clinical manifestations.[17,18] Hands, knees, and hips are most commonly affected. A particularly characteristic finding is involvement of the second and third MCP joints, which are rarely affected in primary OA. A person, especially a male with early onset OA or OA in unusual locations such as the MCP joints or the shoulder should be investigated for a metabolic disorder especially hemochromatosis. Look for >60% saturation of total iron binding capacity or a markedly elevated ferritin. Ochronosis is a rare disorder caused by a hereditary deficiency of homogentisic acid oxidase, leading to accumulation of homogentisic acid in connective tissue. Deposits of homogentisic acid impart a blue-black hue to the sclerae and external cartilage of the ears. Arthritis appears in middle age and involves most often the knees, shoulders, hips, and spine.[19] These patients frequently have calcified intervertebral disks. Approximately 60% of patients with acromegaly develop OA, which most often involves the spine, knees, hips, shoulders, and, occasionally, ankles.[20] The increased growth of articular cartilage causes joint surface incongruity and abnormal wear.

Laboratory Findings

Routine laboratory work is normal in patients with primary OA. The synovial fluid in OA is straw-colored and has good viscosity. The cell count is usually less than 2,000 white cells per cubic millimeter, and the cells are predominantly mononuclear. Radiographs in early OA are usually normal, but as the disease progresses joint space narrowing, subchondral bone sclerosis, subchondral cysts, and osteophytes are observed (Fig. 34.4). Erosive OA is characterized by erosions on the joint surface, sclerosis of subchondral bone, and later by bony ankylosis. Radiographic abnormalities do not always correlate with clinical symptoms.

Treatment

Think about the treatment of OA as a program especially when the weight-bearing joints are involved. Basically, the program consists of three parts: physical modalities, medications, and surgery. The goal in OA should not necessarily be 100% pain relief, as absence of pain in a biomechanically abnormal joint may not be a good thing. The goal should be to reduce pain to a level that promotes quality of life and activity.

Physical modalities include education, weight loss if needed, joint protective aerobic exercises, range of motion exercises especially focusing on reduction of contractures, muscle-strengthening exercises, assistive devices such as a cane, and attempts to affect alignment with off-loading knee braces or patellar taping, if needed. The Arthritis, Diet, and Activity Promotion Trial demonstrated the benefit of promoting both exercise and weight loss in an 18-month-long program that examined both together versus either one alone.[21] The control group was healthy lifestyle. The combination group lost more weight than the weight loss group alone (5.7% of body weight vs. 4.9%), and the combination group had a 24% improvement in physical functioning and a 30% decrease in knee pain over the study period. The exercise group only showed improvement in walk time while the weight loss group showed no significant improvement in any of the variables related to the arthritis. Correct use of a cane can off-load a joint by up to 24% and has been shown to reduce pain in OA of the hip

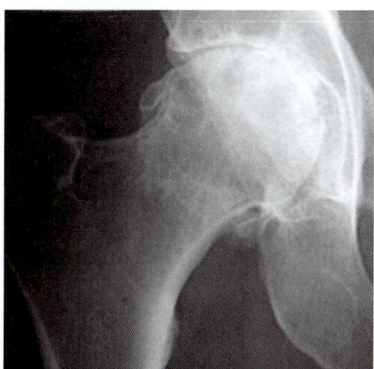

FIGURE 34.4 Osteoarthritis of the hip. The features of osteoarthritis are well illustrated in this x-ray including joint space narrowing, subchondral cysts, osteophytes, and subchondral sclerosis (thickening of the bone where cartilage has been lost).

or knee. There is evidence for a modest benefit with the use of an off-loading knee brace designed to realign either a varus or valgus knee misalignment.[22]

The first-line pharmacologic therapy for OA is over-the-counter analgesics (e.g., acetaminophen, 1,000 mg four times a day or even less if it is effective). If the patient remains symptomatic after 2 to 4 weeks, low-dose ibuprofen or nonacetylated salicylates are indicated. If the response is still inadequate after 2 to 4 weeks, the patient should be placed on a full dose of a nonsteroidal drug. In the patient with risk factors for upper gastrointestinal bleeding or ulcer disease, a proton pump inhibitor should also be provided. There is one cyclooxygenase-2 (COX-2) inhibitor currently on the market, celecoxib, which could be used for patients as significant risk of gastrointestinal bleeding if other options do not work. Because of a concern for cardiac toxicity from the COX-2 agents, use the recommended dose of no more than 200 mg per day. There was for a time some excitement about glucosamine based on a European trial (sponsored trial) published in the *Lancet* in 2001.[23] The data suggested not only a clinical benefit over placebo but also a possible disease modification of OA. A publicly funded U.S. five-arm trial (glucosamine, chondroitin, combination, nonsteroidal anti-inflammatory drug [NSAID], and placebo) did not demonstrate an impressive effect of either nutraceutical in OA, although the placebo response was impressive.[24,25] In the 2012, American College of Rheumatology (ACR) treatment guidelines for OA includes a recommendation that these not be used.[26]

Intra-articular corticosteroid injections are effective in OA and can be used as part of the overall program. How often can injections be given? For many years, these were limited due to the concern about the development of Charcot joints. Again, the comments about not being too effective in controlling pain should be remembered. Data suggested that corticosteroid injections can be given every 3 months for at least 2 years with clinic benefit without structural change. In the absence of data, injections should probably not be given more frequently than this.[27] Injectable hyaluronic acid is approved for use on OA of the knee. A meta-analysis of data on hyaluronic acid injections in knee OA suggests a small benefit especially for the higher molecular weight compounds.[28] Treatment with hyaluronic acid requires three to five injections and can be used in patients who fail more conservative therapy. Other options in the 2012 ACR guidelines include use of topical NSAIDs for hands and knees such as diclofenac and tramadol.

When a joint is severely damaged and painful, joint replacement should be considered. Total hip replacement has provided dramatic relief of pain and improvement of function. Placement of a knee or shoulder can also be quite helpful. Correction of a valgus or varus deformity by osteotomy of the knee improves weight distribution and extends the functional life of the joint. Rebuilding the first CMC joint and replacement of the PIP joint with a prothesis are now possible. Surgery is generally suggested for patients with a level of pain that is not controlled with physical modalities or medications and the patient is willing to endure a period of hospitalization and physical therapy.

RHEUMATOID ARTHRITIS
Rheumatoid arthritis is an inflammatory polyarthritis of unknown etiology that involves peripheral joints in a symmetric distribution. The worldwide prevalence varies from 0.097 to 2.900 per 1,000.[29,30] In the United States, the prevalence is 1% to 2%. Women are more commonly affected: The average ratio is 3:1. Certain Native American populations in the United States can have prevalence rates as high as 7%.[31]

Etiology and Pathophysiology
Even though the etiology of rheumatoid arthritis remains unknown, significant advancements have been made in the understanding of the inflammatory events leading to joint injury and extra-articular manifestations. It is a disease process where genes and environment interact in pathologic dance that leads to autoimmune disease. The genetic contribution is polygenic, and currently, there are 100 or so risk genes identified. It is estimated that 40% to 65% of the risk in rheumatoid arthritis is associated with genetic factors.[29] The strongest genetic association exists with the HLA-DR4 antigen that is present on the surface of cells of the immune system. The so-called shared epitope (SE), which is carried by the vast majority of people with rheumatoid arthritis, is a five-amino acid sequence found on the third allelic hypervariable region of the HLA-DRβ chain of the HLA DR4 molecule. The presence of the SE confers not only disease risk but also severity. One of the earliest events in the development of rheumatoid arthritis is the appearance of anti-citrullinated antibodies. These antibodies appear as a result of inflammation causing the deamination of the amino acid arginine and the formation of the amino acid citrulline. Citrulline is not a normally occurring amino acid in the human body and its appearance in human proteins constitutes neoantigen formation to which the immune system responds. The HLA-DR4 molecule with its HLA-DRβ on T cells interacts with processed antigen (i.e., proteins that contain citrulline) from antigen-presenting cells, and if the HLA-DRβ happens to contain the SE, it is perfectly shaped or charged to interact with citrullinated peptides. The active T cells then produce inflammatory cytokines and also interact with B cells to produce antibodies against the citrulline-containing peptides (anti-CCP antibodies). There is typically a period of time when only the anti-CCP antibodies are present with no articular symptoms. This may be as long as 14 years.[32] Then, at some point, the anti-CCP antibodies, joined often by rheumatoid factor, gain access to the joint and lead to inflammation. Rheumatoid factor is produced in the setting of immune complex disease and may serve as a protective mechanism to remove these from circulation. The hallmark of rheumatoid arthritis is the proliferation of synovium, which spreads over the articular surface as a pannus and damages cartilage, bone, and joint capsule. This process leads to eventual joint damage/destruction with the classic changes on examination.

The environmental exposure that may lead to lung inflammation and production of citrullinated peptides is smoking. An interesting piece of evidence in this light is the fact that rheumatoid arthritis was rare in the Old World before European exploration of the New World and seems to have appeared in Europe after this period.[33] Rheumatoid arthritis has been diagnosed via skeletal remains in certain Native American population antedating the age of exploration, leading some to speculate that the disease is a New World phenomenon that was transmitted back to the Old World. One of the New World products taken back to Europe was tobacco. There is a very strong relationship between smoking and the development of and severity of rheumatoid arthritis.[34]

Symptoms and Signs
The typical patient with rheumatoid arthritis is a young to middle-aged woman who presents to her physician with a history of 2 to 3 months of joint pain and stiffness in her hands. Constitutional symptoms of fatigue, weight loss, and low-grade fever might also be present. The hands and other involved joints are stiff on arising in the morning. Stiffness might last from 30 minutes to 2 hours or longer. In severe disease, the patient might remain stiff most of the day.

Patients with involvement of the hands and wrists might have difficulty performing tasks such as lifting pots, washing their hair, and opening jars or doors. A firm handshake can be quite painful. Tingling and numbness of the thumb and index and middle fingers, which often occur at night, indicate

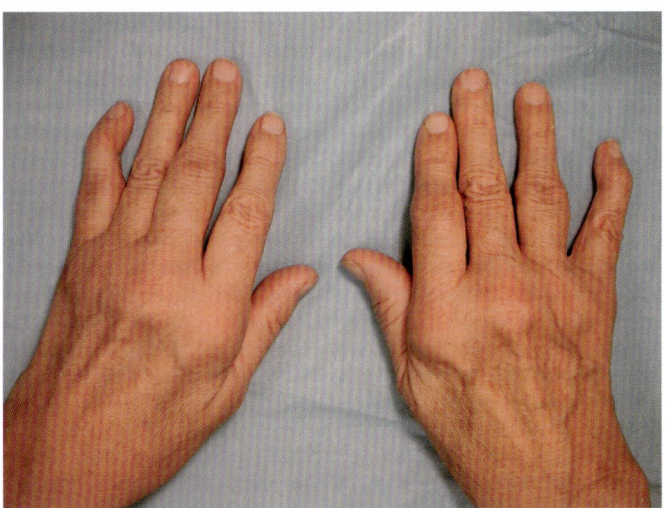

FIGURE 34.5 Example of rheumatoid arthritis of the hands. Distal interphalangeal joints are spared, whereas the metacarpophalangeal and proximal interphalangeal joints are swollen. There is beginning to be some early ulnar deviation on the left hand.

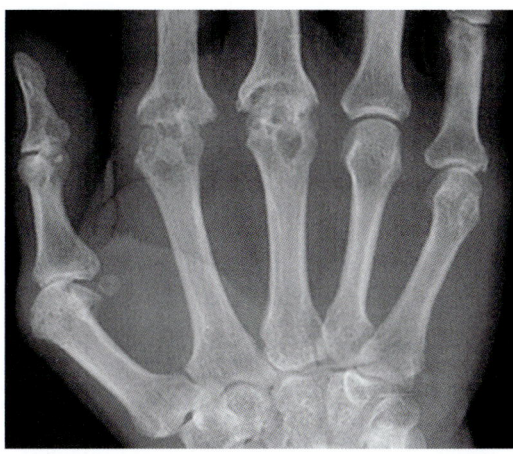

FIGURE 34.6 X-ray of rheumatoid arthritis of the right hand. Note the erosions and joint space narrowing at the second and third metacarpophalangeal joints.

compression of the median nerve by synovial tissue in the carpal tunnel (carpal tunnel syndrome). At times, the carpal tunnel syndrome produces pain radiating up the forearm and down into the hand. Rheumatoid arthritis can begin in the feet in the MTP joints. It is not unusual for a patient to attribute metatarsalgia to improperly fitting shoes before seeking medical attention.

On physical examination, the joints are swollen, tender to palpation, and warm but not hot. The combination of synovial proliferation and fluid gives the joint a boggy sensation on palpation (Fig. 34.5). Synovial proliferation in the flexor tendons of the fingers fills in the palm, giving it a flat appearance. The skin over the small joints often has a bluish discoloration resulting from venous engorgement. The hands may be cool and clammy. The range of joint motion is initially limited by pain and later by contractures. Ulnar deviation of the fingers at the MCP joint is a common deformity in established disease and results from radial deviation of the wrist and slippage of the extensor tendons to the ulnar side of the MCP joints. Another common deformity of the hand that develops in chronic disease is the swan-neck deformity. This appearance results from flexion of the DIP joint and MCP joint with hyperextension of the PIP joint. The boutonniere deformity is caused by avulsion of the extensor hood over the PIP joint, leading to a flexion deformity of this joint and hyperextension of the DIP joint. In advanced disease, subluxation and flexion deformities are common and involve the knees, ankles, elbows, wrists, shoulders, hands, and feet.

The natural history of rheumatoid arthritis is highly variable. Fifteen percent of patients may go into complete remission, whereas 10% or less go on to destructive disease that responds poorly to all forms of therapy. Most patients fall between these two groups with variable periods of remission and relapse. Some patients experience significant disability, whereas others respond to treatment and function quite well throughout their lifetimes. Prognostic factors for more severe disease include the presence of high titers of rheumatoid factor, elevated anti-CCP antibodies (see discussion later), presence of HLA-DR4, and more joints initially involved. Patients with seronegative rheumatoid arthritis (negative for anti-CCP and rheumatoid factor) are a different disease genetically and risk factor–wise and generally have a better prognosis that seropositive rheumatoid arthritis.

Laboratory Findings

Patients often have a normocytic normochromic anemia and an elevated erythrocyte sedimentation rate (ESR). Approximately 80% of patients have a positive rheumatoid factor test result. In the last several years, the anti-CCP has emerged as an important diagnostic and prognostic test. It detects the presence of antibodies to citrullinated peptides and is 75% sensitive and 96% specific for rheumatoid arthritis. The higher levels are correlated with more erosive disease and may appear before overt arthritis has appeared.[35] Radiography in early disease reveals only juxta-articular osteopenia and soft tissue swelling. In more advanced disease, one finds narrowing of joint spaces, erosions at the margins of the joint, and eventually subluxation (Fig. 34.6). The synovial fluid usually has a white blood cell count that varies from 5,000 to 25,000 cells per cubic millimeter (most of the cells are neutrophils), decreased viscosity, and a low glucose level, although this is rarely measured anymore (see Table 34.4).

Treatment Philosophy

The treatment of rheumatoid arthritis has undergone considerable rethinking over the years. The time-honored approach to the treatment of rheumatoid arthritis has been based on the *pyramid*, in large part because of the philosophy that rheumatoid arthritis was a disabling but otherwise benign disease. Following the treatment pyramid philosophy, patients would receive NSAIDs or salicylates along with education and physical and occupational therapy, and as the disease progressed, more aggressive therapy with immunomodulating drugs known as disease-modifying antirheumatic drugs (DMARDs) of increasing toxicity would be used. In 1965, up to 120 months would pass before a DMARD would be started.[36] Because a majority of patients with rheumatoid arthritis develop erosions by 2 years of disease and it has been found not to be the benign disease it was once thought to be, it has been suggested that we invert the pyramid; that is, begin with aggressive therapy up front to prevent erosive changes to joints that are generally not reversible and thus prevent the disability and potentially the mortality caused by unchecked rheumatoid arthritis.[37,38] There has been a dramatic change in the level of disability and prognosis of rheumatoid arthritis in the last 10 to 20 years with the philosophy of early aggressive therapy and treating to target to prevent joint damage.[29,39] Most patients who accept therapy will never know how sick they can be. Currently, rheumatologists start a DMARD as soon as the diagnosis of rheumatoid arthritis is made and medication-induced remission rates in rheumatoid arthritis are now approaching 50% with the combination of methotrexate and biologic agents that will be discussed later.

Current Management of Rheumatoid Arthritis
Disease-Modifying Agents
Current therapy of rheumatoid arthritis is early diagnosis and early aggressive therapy especially for patients who have factors indicative of a poor prognosis, namely, high titer rheumatoid factor or CCP and a high number of joints involved at presentation.[29,40–42] Disease activity scores are routinely monitored and therapy changed to lower rheumatoid arthritis disease activity into remission or low disease activity level. Patients with features that suggest more severe disease are typically started on methotrexate or even combination therapy from the outset, whereas patients with features or low disease activity may be started on less-potent DMARDs such as hydroxychloroquine or sulfasalazine. If after 3 to 6 months of therapy, if there is incomplete control of the disease, other agent(s) are added to the regimen. These can include triple therapy which is a combination of methotrexate, sulfasalazine, and hydroxychloroquine or methotrexate plus a biologic especially one of the anti-TNF agents.

Patients with early mild synovitis could be started on hydroxychloroquine. This agent takes 8 to 12 weeks before it begins to affect the synovitis. Its mechanism of action is thought to be on the basis of increasing the pH of the vacuoles in antigen-presenting cells and gently disrupting the interaction of the major histocompatibility complex with antigen, thus affecting the way antigen is presented to T cells.

Hydroxychloroquine is dosed by weight at 6.5 mg/kg/day in divided doses. Doses higher than this increase the risk for ocular toxicity. Common side effects include diarrhea, gastrointestinal upset, and rash. Serious side effects are listed in Table 34.5 as well as a monitoring schedule. Improvement in morning stiffness and pain, as well as a decrease in the number of tender and swollen joints, and a reduction in acute-phase reactants (i.e., ESR or C-reactive protein [CRP]) are measures of success. Patients with more significant synovitis may be candidates for either sulfasalazine or methotrexate as single agents.

Sulfasalazine is another DMARD used for less severe disease. It is a combination of sulfapyridine and 5-aminosalicylic acid, which is cleaved by gut bacteria into two compounds.

It is thought that the sulfapyridine moiety is the active one in rheumatoid arthritis. It is dosed generally at 2,000 mg in two divided doses. It takes 4 to 8 weeks for an effect to be apparent in most patients and in some may be up to 12 weeks. Common side effects include gastrointestinal upset, diarrhea, and rash. Severe agranulocytosis can occur and is idiosyncratic. Drug cessation resolves the cytopenias in most cases, but there have been a few cases requiring granulocyte colony-stimulating factor therapy. Glucose-6-phosphate dehydrogenase (G6PD) deficiency may lead to severe anemia in affected patients and should be checked before starting therapy if suspected.

Methotrexate is the current "workhorse" drug for rheumatoid arthritis. It is used by itself or more and more frequently in combination with other agents. In rheumatoid arthritis in particular, methotrexate plus something else seems to work better than either agent alone. The dose range and other characteristics are presented in Table 34.5. Methotrexate is a dihydrofolate reductase inhibitor. Its mode of action is uncertain but may be caused by an increase in adenosine, an anti-inflammatory compound.[42] Methotrexate has the advantage of being given once a week and can be given both orally and subcutaneously. Methotrexate begins to be effective generally in 3 to 8 weeks after initiation of therapy. Common side effects include stomatitis, nausea, gastrointestinal upset, and mild hair thinning. Stomatitis in particular might respond to the addition of 1 mg of folic acid daily without affecting its activity in rheumatoid arthritis.

Leflunomide is a newer DMARD. The usual dose is 10 to 20 mg per day. Data indicate that it is similar to methotrexate in efficacy as well as toxicity. It has had, if you would, the misfortune to come to market at the same time as the anti-TNF biologic agents and thus somewhat overshadowed by the impressive results of these agents.

Biologic Disease-Modifying Antirheumatic Drugs
There are currently five anti-TNF DMARD on the market. Etanercept, infliximab, adalimumab, certolizumab, and golimumab are anti-TNF agents that have been shown to be quite effective in not only controlling inflammation in rheumatoid arthritis but also preventing joint damage. In fact, data from the early anti-TNF studies for rheumatoid arthritis called the *TEMPO trial* indicated that the combination of methotrexate plus etanercept can prevent new erosion in 76% of patients over

TABLE 34.5 Immunomodulating Drugs Used in Rheumatology

Medications	Dosage Range	Route	Important Side Effects
Hydroxychloroquine	200–400 mg/d	PO	Retinopathy, neuromyopathy, skin discoloration
Sulfasalazine	1,000–3,000 mg/d	PO	Rash, hepatitis, bone marrow suppression
Methotrexate	5–25 mg/wk	PO, SC	Hepatitis, bone marrow suppression, pneumonitis
Leflunomide	10–20 mg/d	PO	Hepatitis, bone marrow suppression

TNF inhibitors
  Etanercept
  Infliximab
  Certolizumab
  Adalimumab
  Golimumab
	Several	SC, IV	Reactivation of TB and hepatitis B, serious infections, drug-induced lupus

Rituximab (anti–B cell)	1,000–2,000 mg every 6 mo	IV	Reactivation of hepatitis B, serious infection
Abatacept (anti–T cell)	125 mg SC weekly or 500–1,000 mg IV monthly	SC, IV	Reactivation of TB, serious infection, COPD exacerbation

Anti–IL-6 agents
  Tocilizumab
  Sarilumab
	Several	SC, IV	Reactivation of TB, serious infection, elevation of lipids

Tofacitinib (JAK inhibitor)	10 mg/d	PO	Reactivation of TB

COPD, chronic obstructive pulmonary disease; IL, interleukin; IV, intravenous; JAK, janus kinase; PO, by mouth; SC, subcutaneous; TB, tuberculosis; TNF, tumor necrosis factor.

3 years and even lead to filling in of previous erosions.[29,40,43] In addition to anti-TNF therapy, there is anti–T cell therapy with abatacept, anti–B cell therapy with rituximab, anti–IL-6 therapy with tocilizumab, and the first of likely many oral agents that affect cytokine activity, tofacitinib, a janus kinase inhibitor. Table 34.5 has a list of DMARD therapies, including name, mechanism of action, dose, and common side effects.

Glucocorticoids

The anti-inflammatory mechanisms of glucocorticoids include altering leukocyte traffic and function, stabilizing lysosomal membranes of neutrophils and monocytes, and inhibiting the secretion of destructive enzymes including collagenase and elastase.[44] They also inhibit the products of arachidonic acid metabolism including prostaglandins and leukotrienes.

A 2012 study of methotrexate plus 10 mg of prednisone compared to methotrexate alone for 2 years showed the combination therapy had less joint damage, needed less methotrexate to control disease activity, and needed to change therapy less often than those on methotrexate alone.[45] The study reported no more side effects in the combination group compared to the methotrexate alone group. Low-dose prednisone treatment can be especially beneficial during initiation of treatment with a DMARD. Glucocorticoids are often used as bridge agents for patients diagnosed with rheumatoid arthritis (i.e., 5 to 10 mg per day until the DMARD begins to work). In patients on corticosteroids, it is important to give calcium in the range of 1,000 to 1,500 mg per day and vitamin D 400 units a day. Patients should be monitored closely for evidence of hypercalcemia and hypercalcinuria. A bisphosphonate (e.g., alendronate) may also reduce the bone loss of calcium in patients on corticosteroids.

Judicious intra-articular administration of corticosteroids can be quite useful in the treatment of rheumatoid arthritis. In a badly damaged joint or one that is soon to be replaced by a prosthetic joint, corticosteroids should probably not be injected within 6 weeks of surgery.

Surgery

Indications for orthopedic surgery in rheumatoid arthritis are twofold: pain unresponsive to medical management and loss of function. Synovectomy of selected joints provides alleviation of symptoms and improvement of function in the first year after operation but may not provide a long-term effect. Removal of synovial tissue from the wrist and dorsal tendon sheath and resection of the ulnar head might prevent rupture of the extensor tendon. Patients with severely deformed hands can benefit from MCP arthroplasty. Patients with severe pain and loss of function can benefit from total joint replacement, especially the knee or hip. Metatarsal head resection can be of tremendous help in patients with painful metatarsal heads. Intermittent splinting of selected joints is beneficial.

Important Complications of Rheumatoid Arthritis Presenting with Pain

Carpal Tunnel Syndrome

Carpal tunnel syndrome is a common problem in rheumatoid arthritis caused by wrist synovitis that can lead to median nerve compression. Therapy is generally directed at the rheumatoid synovitis with DMARDs and anti-inflammatory agents. A wrist injection with corticosteroids may be helpful in many cases. Carpal tunnel release may be necessary in some cases.

Rheumatoid Vasculitis

This is a potentially life-threatening complication. Patients with long-standing, seropositive, erosive rheumatoid arthritis are generally at risk for this small to medium vessel vasculitis similar to polyarteritis nodosa.[46] Patients may present with digital gangrene or symptoms of mononeuritis multiplex (i.e., foot drop). More serious complications include intestinal perforation or cardiac involvement. Kidneys are less commonly involved than in polyarteritis nodosa. Treatment is traditionally with cyclophosphamide and high-dose prednisone, but even with aggressive therapy, historical survival rates were only 60% at 5 years. More recently, there has been some experience with rituximab in rheumatoid vasculitis with reported high rates of success in induction and maintenance, although the data is at the level of retrospective case series and case reports.[47] Fortunately, with the current approach to early aggressive treatment of rheumatoid arthritis, complications such as rheumatoid vasculitis are now relatively rare.

Cervical Spine Disease

The synovial portions of the cervical spine can be involved in rheumatoid arthritis. This can lead to C1–C2 instability or subaxial instability. Symptoms may be caused by cord or vascular compression and may include neck pain, shock-like sensation up or down the spine, and intermittent loss of consciousness when vertebral artery compression occurs. Before surgery, all patients with long-standing rheumatoid arthritis should have a set of lateral flexion and extension views of the cervical spine taken to evaluate the cervical spine for C1–C2 subluxation.

Septic Arthritis

Patients with rheumatoid arthritis are at increased risk of septic arthritis caused by abnormal joint architecture, use of immunosuppressive drugs, and skin breakdown over high-pressure, biomechanically abnormal sites such as the feet. Patients often present with one joint out of proportion to the others in terms of pain or swelling and may have a paucity of systemic symptoms typical in non–rheumatoid arthritis patients. Detection is imperative because of the high mortality in such patients (i.e., 20% mortality if a single joint is infected and over 50% in patients with multiple joints involved).[48]

THE SPONDYLOARTHROPATHIES
Ankylosing Spondylitis

Ankylosing spondylitis is an inflammatory arthritis involving sacroiliac joints and the spine. Inflammation also occurs at sites of tendon and ligament insertions (enthesitis). Hips and shoulders are the most common peripheral joints involved, but rarely, the joints of the hands and feet can be affected as well. Onset of disease is usually in the second or third decade, and men are predominantly affected. The histocompatibility antigen HLA-B27 is found in 90% or more of patients.[49] The normal frequency of HLA-B27 in the white population is approximately 7%.

Pathophysiology

Synovitis occurs in the apophyseal and costovertebral joints of the spine and peripheral joints and is characterized by synovial hyperplasia with focal accumulation of lymphoid and plasma cells. Inflammation also involves cartilaginous joints, which include the intervertebral disks, manubriosternal joint, and symphysis pubis. With progression, ossification of the outer layers of annulus fibrosus of the disk and the inner layers of the longitudinal ligaments forms syndesmophytes that eventually interconnect to give the spine the appearance of bamboo.

In recent years, the enthesis (insertion of tendons, ligaments, and joint capsule to bone) has become an important tissue in the understanding the pathophysiology of spondyloarthropathies.[50] These are common sites of inflammation, and it appears that inflammation may begin on the bone side at areas rich in fibrocartilage such as enthesis and extend to surrounding tissues. The knee has some 32 entheses alone, and the concept of enthesitis explains the clinic finding of dactylitis or sausage digits in the spondyloarthropathies (Fig. 34.7).

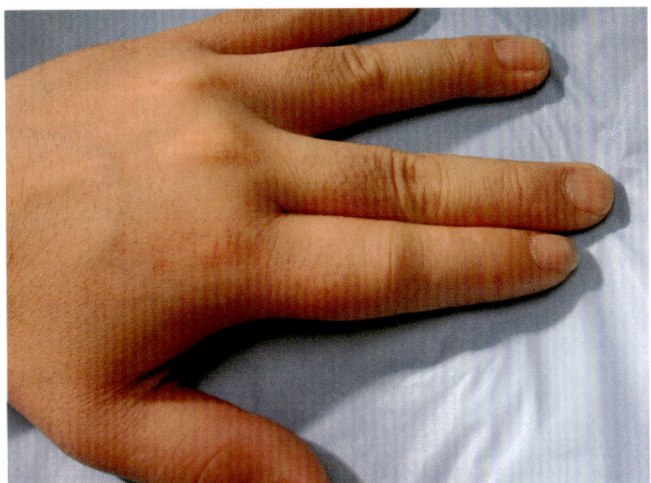

FIGURE 34.7 Classic example of dactylitis, a.k.a. "sausage digit," in a patient with a spondyloarthropathy (psoriatic arthritis in this case).

Symptoms and Signs

The patient initially notes low back pain and stiffness, especially at night when trying to sleep and on arising in the morning. The stiffness of the back lasts for several hours in the morning and occurs after periods of inactivity during the day. The pain might radiate into either buttock, extend down the back of the leg to the knee, and can be mistaken for the pain caused by herniated disk. The pain might alternate from side to side. The back symptoms can be continuous or may be episodic. Involvement of the hips and shoulders causes pain, stiffness, and decreased motion. Costovertebral joint arthritis can cause chest pain similar to that of angina pectoris or pleurisy. Spine ankylosis typically develops insidiously over 10 years or more of disease activity. The extent of involvement varies among patients and ranges from bilateral sacroiliitis to complete ankylosis of the spine. The spondylitis sometimes skips segments of the back. Atlantoaxial subluxation (with the potential danger of spinal cord compression) can occur, but this is observed less often in ankylosing spondylitis than in rheumatoid arthritis. The fused spine, especially the neck, is susceptible to fractures with even limited trauma.

Acute iritis occurs in approximately one-third of the patients. It is typically unilateral and episodic and can rarely lead to vision-altering changes. A rare manifestation of ankylosing spondylitis is fibrosis of the upper lobes of the lung, which occurs late in the course of the disease. Also with long-standing disease, dilatation of the proximal aorta may lead to insufficiency of the aortic valve and inflammation of the atrioventricular bundle can produce cardiac conduction abnormalities. Patients occasionally have significant constitutional symptoms of fever and weight loss.

On physical examination, sacroiliac tenderness is elicited by direct palpation or by maneuvers that stress the joint. A loss of normal lumbar lordosis occurs, giving the lumbar area an ironed-out appearance. Flexion is limited and can be documented by performing a modified Schober test. The test is performed marking the midpoint between the posterior superior iliac spines and measuring and marking 10 cm vertically. When the patient bends forward to touch toes with the knees straight the top, mark should move 5 cm or now measure 15 cm total. Tenderness can be present over costovertebral joints, iliac crests, greater trochanter, and heels. Chest expansion is limited. In advanced disease, the spine becomes rigid, fusing in varying degrees of flexion.

Laboratory Findings

The sedimentation rate or CRP can be elevated, and a mild hypoproliferative anemia can occur. The rheumatoid factor test result is negative, and one would rarely mistake rheumatoid arthritis and ankylosing spondylitis. The synovial fluid is inflammatory (see Table 34.4). Radiography of the sacroiliac joints in early disease shows blurring and irregularity of the joint margins, followed later by subchondral erosions, sclerosis, and eventually fusion (Fig. 34.8). Bony spurs appear at tendinous insertions such as the sites of attachment of the Achilles tendon and plantar fascia. Radiography shows a straight lumbar spine, squared vertebrae, and syndesmophytes. Syndesmophytes extend along the outer aspect of the intervertebral disk and eventually form a bridge between adjacent vertebrae (bamboo spine).

Treatment

Nonsteroidal Anti-inflammatory Drugs. NSAIDs are especially useful in reducing inflammation and relieving pain, and there is some evidence of mild disease-modifying behavior for high-dose NSAIDs.[51] It is speculated that NSAIDs may encourage the patient to be more mobile and possibly lessen the chance of spine fusion, but NSAIDs also influence bone metabolism. Preferred agents include indomethacin or a once-a-day agent such as piroxicam because of their anti-inflammatory activity. Any anti-inflammatory agent chosen usually needs to be dosed at an anti-inflammatory level (i.e., upper limit of dosing range) for benefit.

Disease-Modifying Antirheumatic Drugs. Sulfasalazine has been shown to be beneficial for the peripheral joint in ankylosing spondylitis but not the spine.[52] Methotrexate may also be helpful for peripheral joint disease. The anti-TNF agents have a significant impact on disease symptoms and also diminish both bone edema and enthesitis by serial magnetic resonance imaging (MRI) scan.[53,54] Anti-TNF agents may have disease-modifying activity if used early in the course of the illness. Once the patient has some degree of ossification, the anti-TNF agents may not halt further ossification. The newest agent for treatment of ankylosing spondylitis is secukinumab, an anti–IL-17 agent. It is given by subcutaneous injection every week for 1 month and then monthly thereafter. Anterior uveitis or iritis can be treated with topical or intraocular corticosteroids, and in severe cases, methotrexate or the monoclonal anti-TNF agents such as adalimumab (officially approved for treating uveitis) or infliximab can be used. Etanercept, a fusion protein, is not effective for uveitis.

Physical Therapy and Surgery. Physical therapy is directed at maintaining the erect posture of the patient. Patients should be

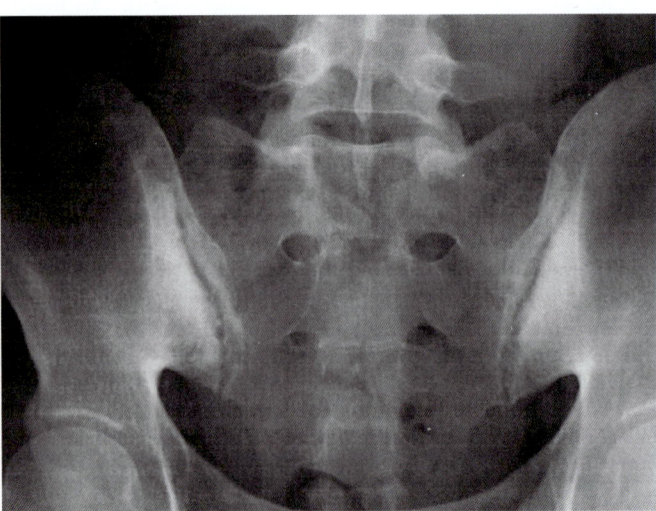

FIGURE 34.8 Ferguson view of the pelvis showing reactive bone changes around the sacroiliac joints as well as an indistinctness to the joints caused by erosions.

encouraged to sleep in the prone position and to avoid using a pillow when sleeping on their backs. Patients with severe hip or shoulder disease can benefit from total shoulder replacement, and in extreme cases, vertebral osteotomies with rod placement may change someone who can only look at the feet to someone in an upright forward looking position.

Important Complications of Ankylosing Spondylitis Presenting with Pain

Cauda Equina Syndrome. Patients with cauda equina syndrome generally have long-standing ankylosing spondylitis. The patient generally presents with progressive lower extremity weakness, pain, and loss of sensation in the lower extremities and perineum. Impotence and overflow incontinence are also frequently occurring problems. Radiographically, large dorsal diverticula are seen on myelography or MRI.[55] Electromyography demonstrates multi-root involvement. Neurosurgery needs to be involved with the treatment of these patients. Data regarding appropriate therapy is sparse.

Spondylodiskitis

Spondylodiskitis is a rare complication of long-standing ankylosing spondylitis. Patients have persistent mechanical-type back pain (pain with activity) rather than inflammatory low back pain (pain in the morning or with rest). It is caused by a mobile vertebral segment surrounded by fused segments. The focus of activity at the one segment may lead to significant inflammation and damage to the adjacent vertebral bodies, simulating infection. Infection generally needs to be ruled out, and treatment is directed to immobilizing the segment either via brace and allowing it to fuse or refuse; occasionally, it may need to be surgically fused.[56]

Vertebral Fracture

Vertebral segments connected by syndesmophytes are subject to fracture with even minor trauma.[56] The usual location for such fractures is the C5–C7 vertebral segments; the fractures are typically caused by a hyperextension injury. Patients suspected of fracture should be evaluated by computed tomographic scan or bone scan to try to identify a potential fracture site, as plain radiography may not be able to demonstrate the fracture. Patients with such fractures have a relatively high morbidity and mortality even if identified because of surgery or prolonged immobilization usually required for treatment. Only 40% of such patients return to their former level of activity.

Chronic Enthesitis

Enthesitis of the Achilles tendon, plantar fascia, and, occasionally, the ribs can be a chronic source of pain and may be more resistant than spondylitis to usual therapies. In such cases, indomethacin at maximum dose or use of a DMARD such as methotrexate, sulfasalazine, anti-TNF therapy, or anti–IL-17 agent may be warranted.

REACTIVE ARTHRITIS

Reactive arthritis (formally Reiter's syndrome) is defined as an asymmetric arthropathy involving predominantly joints of the lower extremities plus one or more of the following: urethritis or cervicitis, dysentery, mucocutaneous lesions, and inflammatory eye disease. It is also defined as an episode of arthritis lasting longer than 1 month that is associated with urethritis or cervicitis. The histocompatibility antigen HLA-B27 is present in approximately 80% of patients.[57] The reasons for the change in nomenclature for Reiter's to reactive arthritis is due to the involvement of Hans Reiter with the Nazi regime and the fact that the same syndrome had been described previously by others.

There appears to be a relationship between certain infections and a specific genetic background. Reactive arthritis can follow infections with *Shigella*, *Salmonella*, *Campylobacter*, or *Yersinia*.[58,59] An association also exists with urethritis associated with *Chlamydia* or *Mycoplasma* infections. In addition, reactive arthritis has been associated with HIV infection. Reactive arthritis develops in patients without these infections, however, and most patients with nonspecific urethritis do not develop this syndrome. The risk of an individual who has a positive result for HLA-B27 with nonspecific urethritis developing reactive arthritis is in the range of 20%. Up to 3% of individuals with nonspecific urethritis have been shown to develop a reactive arthritis. Reactive arthritis has a worldwide distribution and occurs more often in men. In post dysenteric reactive arthritis, the gender distribution is equal.

Symptoms and Signs

Arthritis affects several joints in an asymmetric fashion; knees and ankles are most often involved.[59] Patients also experience pain in the feet and ankles secondary to inflammation at the insertion of the Achilles tendon and plantar fascia. Joints can remain swollen for several months. Swelling of two adjacent interphalangeal joints and adjoining tendon sheath results in a sausage digit or dactylitis. In approximately 20% of patients, spinal involvement occurs. Sacroiliitis is usually unilateral, and spine involvement mild. Patients can also experience chest pain caused by inflammation at the tendinous insertions of the intercostal muscles.

The mucocutaneous lesions of reactive arthritis include oral ulcers, balanitis, and keratoderma blennorrhagica. The oral ulcers are shallow and irregular and have a slightly erythematous base. These lesions are only present for several days. Balanitis usually begins as small painless vesicles on the glans penis that become hyperkeratotic. These lesions are painless and remain crusted in the circumcised patient. In the uncircumcised patient, lesions are moist and can become secondarily infected. Keratoderma blennorrhagica consists of hyperkeratotic lesions/plaques that may coalesce and most commonly involves the feet soles of the feet. It can also involve the palms of the hands and rarely the trunk.

Conjunctivitis involves one or both eyes. Uveitis also occurs and again is unilateral and self-limited. Urethritis can precede or accompany the arthritis, and prostatitis may be an issue. As with ankylosing spondylitis, some patients may develop dilatation of the proximal aorta, leading to aortic valve insufficiency. The course of reactive arthritis is recurrent or persistent, with some patients experiencing a single transient, self-limited bout of disease.

Laboratory Findings

Routine laboratory test results are usually normal. The sedimentation rate is quite variable and does not correlate with disease activity. Synovial fluid shows an elevated white cell count ranging from 5,000 to 50,000 white blood cells per cubic millimeter, predominantly neutrophils. Radiography shows juxta-articular osteopenia, joint space narrowing, and bone erosions. Periostitis is present adjacent to the involved joints and at the insertion of tendons and fasciae. Erosions, sclerosis, and irregularity of the sacroiliac joint can be present and are usually unilateral. Changes of spondylitis are usually asymmetric, occur at various levels of the spine, and are similar to those seen in psoriatic arthritis. Testing for HLA-B27 is not necessary for diagnosis.[59] This test should be reserved for patients who have asymmetric arthritis without other evidence of reactive arthritis.

Treatment

Treatment of reactive arthritis is similar to that of ankylosing spondylitis. NSAIDs are first-line therapy followed by sulfasalazine in refractory cases. Methotrexate or azathioprine can be used in more severe disease. Intra-articular corticosteroid can also be useful. The anti-TNF agents are less well studied but are reported to be effective in case series and case reports. Combination antibiotic therapy with doxycycline, rifampin, and azithromycin was reported to be efficacious in patients with chronic reactive arthritis due to *Chlamydia*.[60]

Complications of Reactive Arthritis Associated with Chronic Pain

Rare patients may have more persistent inflammatory eye disease requiring continuous ophthalmology care. Enthesitis can be severe in some cases of reactive arthritis. Chronic foot involvement can lead to erosive disease at the MTP joints.

PSORIATIC ARTHRITIS

Arthritis appears in up to 30% of outpatients with psoriasis depending on the population studied.[61,62] Genetics play a role as an increased prevalence of psoriatic arthritis occurs in first-degree relatives with psoriasis. An association with HLA-B27 is seen in psoriatic arthritis with spondylitis but not in patients with peripheral arthritis. Onset of psoriatic arthritis is usually in the third or fourth decade, and the gender ratio is approximately equal. In most patients, psoriasis precedes the arthritis by several years, but arthritis may be the presenting manifestation. Most patients with psoriatic arthritis have oligoarthritis, and overall, the prognosis tends to be better than in rheumatoid arthritis.

Symptoms and Signs

Several patterns of arthritis are observed in patients with psoriasis. The majority of patients have an asymmetric oligoarthritis that can involve the proximal joints of the hands and feet, the knees, the wrist, and ankles. In approximately 10% of patients, arthritis affects predominantly the DIP joints and is usually accompanied by psoriatic changes of the adjacent nail. Other patients have a symmetric polyarthritis similar to that seen in rheumatoid arthritis. These patients usually have negative results for rheumatoid factor. If the rheumatoid factor test or the CCP result is positive, the patient may have both rheumatoid arthritis and psoriasis. Patients can also have sacroiliitis and variable degrees of spine involvement. A few patients have a severe, destructive, and deforming polyarthritis referred to as *arthritis mutilans*.

Joints are swollen, warm, and tender, and a digit may have the appearance of a sausage. Contractures and ankylosis of joints occur with long periods of persistent joint inflammation. In most cases, there appears to be no definite correlation between the degree of skin involvement and joint disease.

Laboratory Findings

Laboratory findings include an elevated sedimentation rate and a hypoproliferative anemia. The rheumatoid factor test result is negative. The synovial fluid shows evidence of inflammation with elevated white cell counts; the cells are predominantly polymorphonuclear. A somewhat characteristic radiographic finding is that of the pencil-in-cup deformity caused by osteolysis, or whittling of the distal end of the middle phalanx, which produces a pencil point that projects into a widened cup-like erosion in the adjacent surface of the distal phalanx (Fig. 34.9). Radiography shows joint space narrowing, erosions, osteolysis, and ankylosis, depending on the degree of clinical severity. The radiographic findings of the spine are similar to those found in patients with reactive arthritis.

Treatment

Initial treatment of psoriatic arthritis with one to two joints involved and little impairment may be an NSAID alone. In patients with progressive disease, methotrexate, cyclosporine, leflunomide, hydroxychloroquine, and sulfasalazine have been

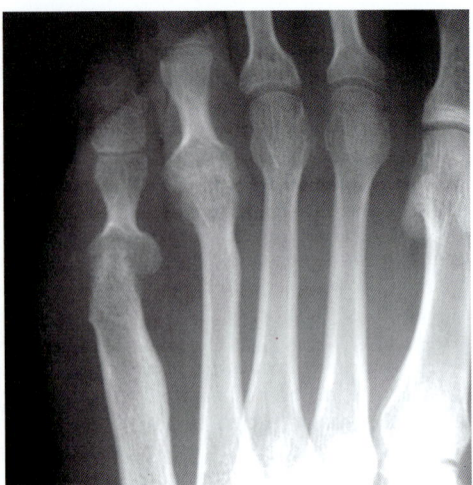

FIGURE 34.9 X-ray of the left foot in psoriatic arthritis demonstrating fusion of the fourth metatarsophalangeal joint and a developing pencil-in-a-cup deformity of the fifth metatarsophalangeal joint.

used successfully for peripheral arthritis.[61,62] Only methotrexate and cyclosporine are useful for the skin as well. None of these medications address spine involvement with present. Low-dose oral corticosteroids as well as intra-articular corticosteroids can also be used. Placing a patient on moderate- to high-dose prednisone and then tapering may exacerbate the skin disease. Prednisone doses if needed should be kept to 10 mg or less, if possible. There are a variety of biologic agents that are now available to use to treat psoriatic arthritis. The anti-TNF agents have an impressive effect on both skin and joints, including the spine.[62] Ustekinumab is an IL-12/IL-23 inhibitor that has effects on skin and joint disease as does secukinumab, a newer anti–IL-17 agent, and apremilast, an oral phosphodiesterase-4 inhibitor.

ARTHRITIS ASSOCIATED WITH INFLAMMATORY BOWEL DISEASE

Both ulcerative colitis and regional enteritis (Crohn's disease) are associated with peripheral arthritis spondylitis and enthesitis.[63] Peripheral arthritis occurs in approximately 10% to 20% of patients with inflammatory bowel disease. Type I peripheral arthritis affects one to five joints typically large weight-bearing joints and/or the MTP joints. This arthritis is present with active bowel disease and is acute, lasts several days to several weeks, and leaves no residual damage. In some cases, the arthritis may precede obvious bowel involvement. The knees and ankles are most frequently affected. Type II peripheral arthritis is a polyarthritis that affects the small joints, and MCP joints are commonly involved and may mimic rheumatoid arthritis.

Spondylitis is also associated with inflammatory bowel disease and is seen in 5% to 12% of patients with inflammatory bowel disease. The gender distribution is 3:1 male to female. The majority (70%) of patients with spondylitis associated with inflammatory bowel disease has positive results for HLA-B27. Asymptomatic bilateral sacroiliitis can be found in up to 15% of patients with inflammatory bowel disease. Frequency of HLA-B27 is not increased in patients with only peripheral arthritis.

Enthesitis typically occurs at the heel (plantar fasciitis, Achilles tendonitis) or the knee. Calcification may be seen at tendon insertions.

Treatment

Peripheral joint symptoms if mild can be managed with NSAIDs. NSAIDs, however, may lead to an exacerbation of the inflammatory bowel disease. Peripheral arthritis often in ulcerative colitis can disappear after colectomy. Many of the drugs used to treat inflammatory bowel disease also affect peripheral arthritis such as sulfasalazine, azathioprine, or methotrexate. The TNF agents, with the exception of etanercept, are useful for the bowel disease, peripheral arthritis, and spondylitis.

ARTHRITIS CAUSED BY CRYSTALS
Calcium Pyrophosphate Deposition Disease

Deposition of calcium pyrophosphate (CPP) dihydrate in the joint produces both an acute and chronic form of joint disease. The acute or subacute form is historically referred to as *pseudogout* because of its similarity to gout, but the suggested term for such arthritis is *acute CPP crystal arthritis*.[64] *Chondrocalcinosis* refers to CPP crystal deposits in articular tissue that are detectable radiographically. It is thought that the presence of the crystals can lead to low-grade inflammation and joint damage. If the crystals are recognized by the innate immune system, an attack of acute arthritis can occur. Acute CPP crystal arthritis affects persons over the age of 40 years and in men predominately. The knee is the most frequent site of acute arthritis, but the hip, shoulder, ankle, wrists, and bursae can be affected. It affects approximately 4% to 7% of the adult population in Europe and the United States.

Three forms of calcium pyrophosphate deposition disease (CPPD) are recognized: a hereditary form, CPPD associated with metabolic and other diseases, and an idiopathic form. The frequency of OA in CPPD varies from 40% to 70%. CPPD occurs in 41% of patients with hemochromatosis and in 5% to 15% with hyperparathyroidism.[65] An association is suspected in patients with diabetes mellitus, hypophosphatemia, Wilson's disease, ochronosis, and hypothyroidism.

Pathophysiology

The initial site of crystal formation is in articular cartilage. In idiopathic CPPD, it is not clear whether the primary event is deposition of crystals in cartilage or whether the crystals develop as a consequence of disturbed cartilage metabolism. Increased inorganic pyrophosphate is found in the synovial fluid and probably reflects a local disorder of pyrophosphate metabolism possibly due to overactivity of the ANKH membrane protein leading to deposition of CPP crystals in the joint.[64,66] Elevated levels are also found in patients with OA. Acute arthritis is brought on by shedding of crystals into the joint space. The mechanism for crystal shedding is the lowering of either calcium or pyrophosphate ions in synovial fluid. The decreased concentration of ionized calcium results in movement of crystals from cartilage into synovial fluid. Crystals can also be shed into the synovial fluid as a consequence of mechanical disruption of cartilage. Attacks can follow trauma. In addition, crystals can be released as a result of degradation of cartilage by enzymes from neutrophils during episodes of bacterial arthritis or other forms of inflammatory arthritis.

Symptoms and Signs

Several patterns of joint disease are recognized.[64] In approximately 25% of patients, CPPD presents as an acute arthritis (pseudogout) involving a single joint or a few joints at any given time. The clinical picture mimics that of acute gout in intensity. The onset of joint swelling and pain is abrupt and severe and usually reaches a peak within 24 to 36 hours. An attack can last up weeks to months as opposed to gout that typically last a few days to a week.[64] The joint is swollen, red, and tender. The most common site of involvement is the knee, but attacks can involve other large joints such as the ankles, wrists, elbows, or hips. Also, the lumbar and cervical spine can be involved. Trauma, surgery, or severe medical illness can precipitate an attack. The same joint is often involved in subsequent attacks. Radiographic evidence of chondrocalcinosis is usually present in affected joints.

Approximately 5% of patients with CPPD have a form of disease that mimics rheumatoid arthritis (*pseudorheumatoid disease*). Involvement of multiple joints, synovial proliferation, limitation of joint motion, and joint deformity can develop. Patients experience fatigue and morning stiffness. To further confuse the issue, CPP deposition can occur in rheumatoid arthritis.

CPPD also occurs in a chronic form that is similar to OA. Multiple joints are involved and include the knees, wrists, MCP joints, hips, shoulders, elbows, and ankles. The disease involves middle-aged to elderly patients, predominantly women. CPPD can mimic neuropathic arthropathy (pseudo-Charcot) with a more severe joint destructive pattern.

The diagnosis of CPP disease is established by identification of CPP crystals in synovial fluid, both free and in neutrophils. The crystals appear as short rods, rhomboids, and cuboids, and they have a sign of weakly positive birefringence under compensated polarized light. X-rays show calcification in articular hyaline cartilage that is parallel to and separated from the subchondral bone. Calcifications in fibrocartilage are thick and irregular densities and are found in the menisci of the knee, symphysis pubis, annulus fibrosus, and the triangular cartilage of the wrist. Calcifications also occur in the Achilles, supraspinatus, and triceps tendons but can involve any tendon. Changes in the joint are similar to those seen in OA with sclerosis of subchondral bone, joint space narrowing, and large subchondral cysts.

Treatment

The NSAIDs are effective in the treatment of acute and chronic joint disease. An NSAID is given for 10 to 14 days in patients with acute CPP crystal arthritis.[64] The drug can be continued indefinitely in patients with chronic CPP disease associated with OA. When an NSAID is contraindicated, another method of treatment for an acute attack is prednisone, starting with 40 mg the first day and gradually tapering over a 7-day period. Colchicine, 0.6 mg twice a day, is started on day 3 or 4 and continued for several weeks to avoid a flare of arthritis after prednisone is discontinued. An IL-1 inhibitor, anakinra, can be given subcutaneous for 1 to 3 days and will also treat an acute attack in patients who cannot use the aforementioned agents.[67] Anakinra is not approved for this indication yet but has been effective in case series and case reports. Colchicine, 0.6 mg twice a day, can also be given prophylactically to reduce the number and length of attacks (see colchicine in section on gout). Aspiration of the involved joint followed by an injection of glucocorticoids reduces pain and swelling.

URATE GOUT

Urate gout is characterized by elevated serum urate levels, recurrent attacks of acute arthritis involving a single joint or a few joints at any given time, and deposition of monosodium urate dihydrate (tophi) in and around joints, leading in some patients to a deforming and crippling arthritis. Monosodium urate can serve as a nidus for calcium oxalate to form renal stones or form renal stone in their own right.

Recognized since ancient times, gout has been depicted in caricatures as affecting well-fed aristocrats overindulging in rich foods and wines. The disease has been referred to as the *king of diseases* and the *disease of kings*.[68] Currently, it is estimated that 6.1 million adults in the United States have gout.[69]

The normal serum urate concentration depends on several factors including age (increases with maturity), gender (women generally have lower levels than men), body habitus (those with metabolic syndrome will generally have higher levels), and genetic background. As noted, the upper limit of urate level is 6.8 mg/dL, but with the "super size" of the population in the

United States, normative data which take the mean plus two standard deviations on either side has upper limit of normal as high in some labs as 8.5 mg/dL, which is above the level of urate solubility.

Both genetic and environmental factors play a role in the expression of hyperuricemia and gout. For example, higher serum urate levels are found in Filipinos living in the United States compared with racially identical persons living in the Philippines. These persons are unable to excrete the greater uric acid load resulting from the higher purine content of the diet eaten in the United States.[70]

Etiology and Pathophysiology

Uric acid is a product of purine metabolism.[68] The serum urate concentration depends on the rate of uric acid production and excretion. Approximately two-thirds of uric acid is excreted in the urine and one-third into the gastrointestinal tract. Normally, uric acid is completely filtered through the glomeruli and completely reabsorbed in the proximal tubule. Secretion of uric acid occurs in the proximal tubule, followed by a second reabsorption in the proximal tubule.

Primary gout is defined by the absence of other diseases or conditions such as drugs that lead to hyperuricemia and gout. Approximately 90% of patients with primary gout have decreased renal clearance of uric acid resulting from reduced glomerular filtration, increased tubular reabsorption, reduced tubular secretion, or combinations of these factors. Evidence for a molecular renal defect is still lacking in the majority of patients.

Approximately 10% of patients are overproducers of uric acid. Overproduction is defined as the urinary excretion of more than 800 to 1,000 mg of uric acid in 24 hours while the patient is on a regular purine diet.

Two inborn errors of purine metabolism make up a small number of primary gout patients who are overproducers of uric acid. The first disorder is caused by a partial deficiency of the enzyme hypoxanthine-guanine phosphoribosyltransferase, which catalyzes conversion of hypoxanthine to inosinic acid and guanine to guanylic acid.[68] The second disorder is caused by increased 5-phosphoribosyl-1-pyrophosphate synthetase activity leading to elevated levels of intracellular 5-phosphoribosyl-1-pyrophosphate and overproduction of uric acid. These patients usually experience the onset of gouty arthritis in the second or third decade and have a high frequency of uric acid stones. Both diseases are inherited as an X-linked disorder, therefore affecting male subjects, with women as carriers. Some of these patients also have dysarthria, hyperreflexia, lack of coordination, and mental retardation. A severe form of the first disorder with almost a complete deficiency of this enzyme, referred to as the Lesch-Nyhan syndrome, is characterized by self-mutilation, choreoathetosis, and mental retardation.[71] This disorder is classified under secondary hyperuricemia or gout because the neurologic disorder is predominant.

Secondary gout is defined as gout or hyperuricemia occurring in patients with other disorders. Overproduction of uric acid results in hyperuricemia in patients with disorders associated with increased cell proliferation and turnover of nucleic acids. These disorders include myeloproliferative and lymphoproliferative diseases, multiple myeloma, polycythemia, pernicious anemia, hemoglobinopathies, and some carcinomas. The hereditary disorder glucose 6-phosphatase deficiency (von Gierke's glycogen storage disease) is also manifested by overproduction of uric acid. Secondary hyperuricemia can also result from renal failure or the effects of drugs or toxins on renal clearance of uric acid. Diuretic agents, low doses of aspirin (less than 2 g per day), alcohol, ethambutol, cyclosporine, and lead are some of the agents that decrease the clearance of uric acid and thereby raise the serum urate level.

Pathophysiology of Acute Gouty Arthritis

Acute gouty arthritis results from the inflammatory reaction to urate crystals that form in the joint space or are released into the joint from synovium or articular cartilage. Plasma becomes supersaturated with urate at concentrations of approximately 6.8 mg/dL.[67] Factors in addition to supersaturation of plasma urate are necessary for crystal precipitation because most patients with hyperuricemia do not develop gout. The lower temperatures found in peripheral joints or tissues might contribute to urate precipitation at these sites. Urate is less soluble at 32° C, which is the temperature observed in a normal knee, compared with the core body temperature of 37° C.[72] Another mechanism for urate precipitation might be the faster reabsorption of extracellular fluid than urate from the joint space, resulting in a transient increased urate concentration and crystal formation.[73] Trauma or impact loading of a joint that breaks crystals loose from the joint surface is yet another possible mechanism and might explain the high frequency of gout at the base of the great toe, which is a joint subjected to great stress.

Urate crystals induce inflammation by several mechanisms.[68] Urate crystals activate Hageman's factor in joint fluid, leading to the formation of kinins that induce vasodilatation and increased vascular permeability. Urate crystals activate the complement system with the generation of leukocyte chemotactic factors and also stimulate the formation of leukotrienes from arachidonic acid. Furthermore, urate crystals can activate platelets, which secrete several inflammatory mediators including prostaglandins. Urate crystals can also stimulate synovial lining cells and macrophages that secrete prostaglandins and collagenase.

The key to urate-induced inflammation is the polymorphonuclear white cell. Urate crystals activate toll-like receptors on the surface of cells that lead to the activation of the inflammasome inside the cell which in turn leads to the release of inflammatory mediators such as IL-1.[74] Crystals also bind immunoglobulin G (IgG), leading to their attachment to and phagocytosis by polymorphonuclear white cells.[68] This process mediates the production of superoxide anions, which damage tissue. In addition, ingestion of crystals results in the release of chemotactic factors from the polymorphonuclear white cells, thus attracting more polymorphonuclear white cells. On ingestion by polymorphonuclear white cells, crystals are incorporated into phagosomes, which fuse with lysosomes. The rupture of phagolysosomes inside polymorphonuclear white cells damages these cells. Lysosomal and cytoplasmic enzymes are released into the joint space, resulting in tissue inflammation and injury.

Gouty arthritis often develops with fluctuation of serum urate levels. A rapid increase in serum uric acid results in precipitation of crystals in tissue or fluid. A rapid decrease in serum urate brings about release of urate from the joint surface into the joint space.

Drinking of alcohol is also associated with the precipitation of gouty attacks. Metabolism of ethanol results in an increased concentration of blood lactate, which blocks the renal excretion of uric acid by inhibiting tubular secretion and raising the serum urate level. Alcohol consumption also leads to accelerated degradation of adenosine triphosphate to adenosine monophosphate with accumulation of adenine nucleotides that are degraded to uric acid and other purine metabolites.[75] Beers and ales in particular increase the risk of gout due to the amount of purines these contain. The drinking of moonshine whiskey is associated with gouty arthritis and is referred to as *saturnine gout*.[76] Moonshine whiskey is often distilled in automobile radiators containing a lead core. Lead reduces the excretion of urate and decreases its solubility. In addition, lead may affect renal mechanisms for handling urate, leading to elevated levels.

Gout follows periods of fasting. During fasting, the increased plasma level of acetoacetate and hydroxybutyrate interferes with renal excretion of urate.[72] Overindulgence of food and wine has often been associated with gout. When a large protein- and purine-rich diet is ingested along with copious amounts of wine or other liquor, the uric acid serum concentration rises because of increased formation and decreased excretion of sodium urate. Acute gouty arthritis attacks occur when drugs increase or lower the serum uric acid level. Attacks are precipitated by allopurinol, which lowers the uric acid concentrations, and thiazides or low doses of aspirin, which raise the level. Cyclosporine interferes with the renal excretion of uric acid and induces hyperuricemia and gout.[73] An increased frequency of gout is seen in transplant recipients receiving cyclosporine and may affect atypical joints such as the hips, sacroiliac joints, or shoulders.

Signs and Symptoms

Gouty arthritis occurs mainly in middle-aged and older men and after menopause in women. Approximately one-fourth of the patients have a family history of gout. Nephrolithiasis precedes the first attack of arthritis in approximately 10% of patients. The first attack occurs most often in the MTP joint of the great toe (podagra) or ankles. Subsequent attacks might be separated by several months or even years. The involved joint usually returns to normal between attacks. In untreated cases, the attacks become more frequent and involve other joints, such as wrists, elbows, olecranon bursae, and the small joints of the hand. Gouty arthritis can occur in DIP joints already involved with OA and Heberden's nodes[77] (Figs. 34.10 and 34.11). Gout can be overlooked in these joints because acute inflammation can also occur with Heberden's nodes. Gouty arthritis of intervertebral joints, sacroiliac joints, and shoulders and hips is uncommon.

The typical attack of gout comes on acutely, often during the early hours of morning. Attacks also occur after surgery. Pain and swelling reach a peak within 24 hours. The joint is exquisitely tender, and overlying soft tissue is swollen and erythematous even to the degree that it could be mistaken for cellulitis. Pain is intense and throbbing. Patients are unable to tolerate even a light sheet touching the involved great toe. Jarring of the bed can make the patient wince with pain. The patient might even dread the landing of a fly on the involved toe. Both a low-grade fever and leukocytosis can accompany the attack, especially in polyarticular gout. An untreated attack of gout usually lasts for several days to 2 weeks.

Chronic tophaceous gout develops in patients if hyperuricemia is not corrected. Before the effective control of

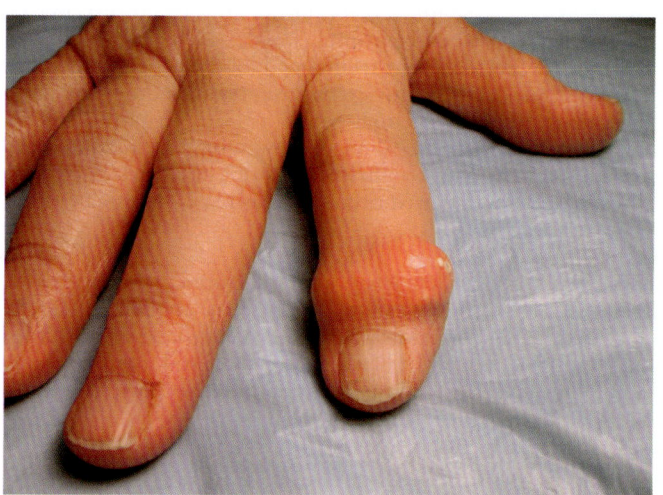

FIGURE 34.10 Tophaceous gout affecting the distal interphalangeal joint.

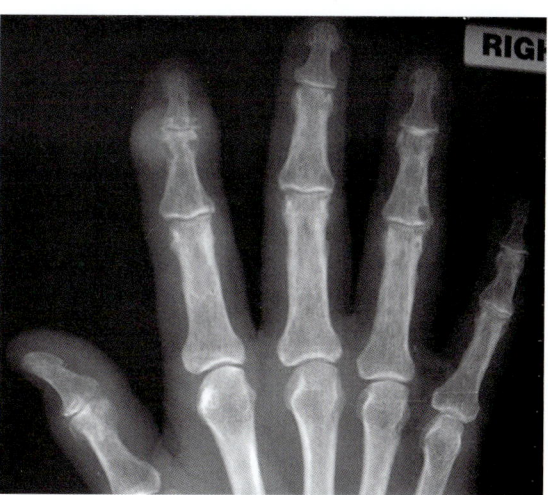

FIGURE 34.11 X-ray of same patient with tophaceous gout. Note erosions in the middle phalanx of the index finger caused by gout.

hyperuricemia, approximately one-half of the patients with episodes of gouty arthritis eventually developed deposits of monosodium urate dihydrate in and around joints as well as in other tissues. These deposits, referred to as *tophi*, usually become apparent at least 10 years after the onset of gouty arthritis. They develop in the olecranon, infrapatellar and prepatellar bursae, Achilles tendons, synovium, subchondral bone, and, infrequently, cartilage of the ear. Tophi can ulcerate and drain material that contains microscopic needle-shaped crystals of monosodium urate. Patients with tophaceous gout have frequent episodes of acute gouty arthritis or may have continuous joint inflammation. Joint deformity and destruction leading disability can be quite severe in the untreated patient.

There is recent data that suggests patients with hyperuricemia and chronic kidney disease may accelerate loss of kidney function more rapidly than those whose hyperuricemia is controlled.[78] Likewise, patients with coronary artery disease and hyperuricemia have an increased all-cause mortality compared to those without hyperuricemia.

Treatment of patients with underlying myeloproliferative or lymphoproliferative disorder results in extremely high levels of serum urate that can precipitate in the renal tubules, producing obstruction and oliguria. Patients should be treated with allopurinol and colchicine before treatment of the blood dyscrasia.

Renal calculi develop in approximately 20% of patients with gout. Hypertension, diabetes mellitus, and hypertriglyceridemia occur more frequently in patients with gout.

Laboratory Findings

Radiography of the affected joint in acute gouty arthritis is usually normal. When the first MTP joint is involved, radiography might show underlying changes of OA. The typical erosion caused by urate deposition is sharply defined and has a thin shell-like overhanging edge at the margins of the erosion. The diagnosis of gout is established by demonstration of the characteristic crystal of monosodium urate monohydrate in the synovial fluid or from tissue deposits. Crystals are found both in the polymorphonuclear white cells and free in fluid. The crystals in joint fluid are usually rod-shaped and 7 to 10 μm in length. They are identified by use of polarized microscopy. With use of a first-order red compensator, crystals have a sign of strongly negative birefringence.[79]

Treatment

Treatment of a patient with gout has two components: treatment of the acute gouty arthritis and treatment of hyperuricemia.[80,81]

Each is treated independently. Even though they are closely interrelated, the drugs used for each are different. In fact, the indiscriminate use of a drug to lower the uric acid can exacerbate or prolong an attack of gouty arthritis.

Anti-inflammatory Drugs

For the acute attack of gouty arthritis, the patient is given indomethacin 50 mg three times a day for 7 days, or naproxen 500 mg twice a day for 7 days has also been successful. NSAIDs for the treatment of acute gout should be avoided or used with caution in patients with symptomatic heart failure, renal failure, oliguria, or peptic ulcer disease.[69] Glucocorticoids are also quite effective in treatment of acute gout. Prednisone is given over a 7-day period with an initial dose of 40 mg as a single dose and then gradually tapered over a 7-day period or 35 mg daily for 5 to 7 days has also shown to be effective. Intra-articular corticosteroids can also be used to treat gout in a large joint such as the knee. Colchicine can be used if started within 24 hours of the initial symptoms with 1.2 mg given the first hour and 0.6 mg the second hour. Anakinra 100 mg subcutaneously for 1 to 3 days has also been shown to be very effective in patients who cannot tolerate these other therapies, but it is not yet approved for gout by the U.S. Food and Drug Administration.[82]

In patients who experience frequent attacks of acute gouty arthritis, colchicine, 0.6 mg once or twice a day, is effective in preventing attacks. Colchicine is also used to prevent flares of gout when hypouricemic therapy is initiated.

Myopathy and polyneuropathy may occur on maintenance doses of colchicine in patients who have renal insufficiency.[83] Myositis manifests as proximal muscle weakness, and serum creatine kinase becomes elevated. These abnormalities return to normal 3 to 4 weeks after stopping the drug. Polyneuropathy also disappears on discontinuing colchicine. In addition, agranulocytosis or aplastic anemia can occur in patients with renal insufficiency who are on regular doses of colchicine because the plasma drug levels in these patients greatly increase.

Hypouricemic Medications

Treatment of hyperuricemia in patients with gout is directed at lowering uric acid levels with a target serum level of 5 to 6 mg/dL in patients without tophi and 4 to 5 mg/dL in patients with tophi.[82] Lowering serum uric acid levels will prevent the formation of tophaceous deposits and eventually resolve existing tophi.

The uric acid concentration can be lowered by probenecid, which is a uricosuric agent.[84] In patients with normal renal function and no renal stones, probenecid is an effective agent. The dose of probenecid is 1 to 3 g per day given twice a day. It is given generally at mealtime to coincide with fluid intake and relative alkaline urine. Dumping uric acid in the urine when there is low urine flow and acidic urine will foster the development of renal stones.

Serum uric acid level is effectively reduced by allopurinol, which is a potent inhibitor of xanthine oxidase.[81] This drug blocks the conversion of hypoxanthine to xanthine and xanthine to uric acid. This leads to the accumulation of other oxypurines in the blood. The daily dose of allopurinol is 100 to 800 mg per day, which is regulated to reduce uric acid to a concentration below 6 mg/dL as noted. It is suggested that allopurinol be started at a low dose (i.e., 100 mg or even less in patients with chronic kidney disease) and slowly increased until serum uric acid levels are reached.[81] Allopurinol administration can precipitate an acute attack of gout, presumably because of fluctuation of sodium urate between tissue and blood. Colchicine, 0.6 mg once or twice a day, is given along with the allopurinol to prevent an acute attack. In general, current guidelines suggest the use of allopurinol over probenecid for ease of use and compliance.

Transient leukopenia and abnormalities of liver function are observed in some patients. In patients treated for many years, xanthine stones may occur. These tend to occur in patients who are overproducers and hyperexcretors of uric acid. A serious side effect of allopurinol is a rash that occasionally progresses to a severe life-threatening Stevens-Johnson syndrome/toxic epidermal necrolysis. This is particularly true in Asian patients who are HLA-B5801–positive. This allele is found in Han Chinese, Koreans, and Thai patients but low in Europeans and Japanese. These patients are also at risk for the most serious complication of allopurinol use which is the allopurinol hypersensitivity syndrome. This occurs in patients with chronic kidney disease and those on thiazide diuretics. The hallmarks of this hypersensitivity syndrome include fever, a serious rash, eosinophilia, hepatic abnormalities, and acute renal failure. The allopurinol hypersensitivity syndrome has a high mortality. It is thought to be avoided by starting with low doses of allopurinol and slowing increasing over time. Allopurinol potentiates the action of 6-mercaptopurine and azathioprine. The dose of the cytotoxic agent is usually reduced by at least one-third in patients on allopurinol.

There is another xanthine oxidase inhibitor available for use called *febuxostat* dosed 40 to 80 mg a day, and the advantage is that it is cleared by the liver and less so by the kidney. It can be used in patients with allopurinol associated rashes, but the use of febuxostat with 6-mercaptopurine or azathioprine still requires dose reduction of these agents as noted earlier.

Finally, a pegylated uricase inhibitor called *pegloticase* is available in intravenous (IV) form to treat patients with a significant tophaceous burden. Uricase metabolizes uric acid to the more soluble allantoin and will drop serum uric acid levels precipitously. It has a high immunogenicity but can be effective in selected patients.

INFECTIOUS ARTHRITIS
Nongonococcal Bacterial Arthritis

Acute bacterial or septic arthritis is a serious problem that requires prompt treatment to avoid joint damage.[84,85] Bacteria usually reach the joint by hematogenous spread from a primary infection elsewhere. Often, however, no primary source of infection is found. An infection in the adjacent bone or soft tissue can extend directly into the joint. Acute bacterial arthritis is most often caused by *Staphylococcus aureus*, *Streptococcus pneumoniae*, *Staphylococcus pyogenes*, or *Haemophilus influenzae*, with *Staphylococcus* spp. being the most common causative organisms. Gram-negative organisms include *Escherichia coli*, *Salmonella*, and *Pseudomonas* and are usually seen in patients who are immunosuppressed or use IV drugs. In the past, *Neisseria gonorrhoeae* was at the head of this list, but its importance has waned over time.

Patients with diabetes mellitus or blood dyscrasias or those receiving glucocorticoids or immunosuppressive drugs are more susceptible to joint infection. Septic arthritis is more likely to occur in joints previously damaged by trauma or inflammatory arthritis. Patients with rheumatoid arthritis in particular have an increased risk of septic arthritis and an increased mortality rate.[48]

Pathophysiology

The synovium is edematous and infiltrated by neutrophils. As the disease progresses, small abscesses are present in the synovium and subchondral bone. Proteolytic enzymes from neutrophils damage the cartilage, bone, and joint capsule. Healing is manifested by proliferation of fibroblasts, which can lead to ankylosis.

Symptoms and Signs

The onset of bacterial arthritis is usually abrupt and associated with severe pain and fever. A shaking chill occasionally accompanies the onset. Any motion of the joint causes excruciating pain. The overlying skin is usually erythematous. In elderly patients and those who are on glucocorticoids, the symptoms can be less severe.

The joint affected most frequently by septic arthritis is the knee, which is involved in at least one-half of the cases. Other commonly involved joints are hips, shoulders, wrists, ankles, elbows, and sternoclavicular and sacroiliac joints. Involvement of the latter two joints has been noted in IV drug users. The small joints of the hands and feet are rarely infected. In the spine, the intervertebral disk space and adjacent vertebral bodies are infected. Infection in the hip is more difficult to recognize because swelling is less evident. Patients with hip infection might hold the thigh in adduction, flexion, and internal rotation. Pain is felt in the groin or thigh and is also referred to the anterior surface of the knee.

An overlying infected bursa or cellulitis can be mistaken for septic arthritis. It is important in aspirating a joint not to insert the needle through an infected bursa or cellulitis and possibly infect a normal joint.

Laboratory Findings

Joint fluid usually shows increased numbers of neutrophils ranging from 10,000 to greater than 100,000 per cubic millimeter. The white cell count in infected bursa fluid is not as high as observed in the joint. Data from a study taking place in the emergency room suggests that a white count in the synovial fluid over 25,000 per cubic millimeter has a likelihood ration over one and should raise suspicion for an infected joint.[86] A peripheral blood leukocytosis might also be present. Gram stain performed on synovial fluid often shows bacteria except in gonococcal infections. Culture results of synovial fluid as well as blood are positive in over 90% of cases and are important to send if infection is suspected.

Radiography of the joint initially shows swelling as manifested by distension of the joint capsule, followed later by juxta-articular osteoporosis. As the process continues, destruction of articular cartilage leads to joint space narrowing followed by bony erosions. Juxta-articular bone destruction might indicate osteomyelitis. In the spine, the initial change consists of narrowing of the disk space and proliferation of bone at vertebral margins. Osteolytic lesions in adjacent vertebrae are seen later. MRI can be helpful in identifying infection in certain joints such as the hip, shoulder, spine, and sacroiliac joints.

Treatment

An infected joint requires immediate aspiration and rapid initiation of parenteral antibiotic therapy. It has been reported that joint outcome is best when patients are seen within 7 days of initial symptoms. Joint fluid should be immediately cultured and a Gram stain performed. Vancomycin is the current suggested antibiotic for gram-positive infections (especially where methicillin-resistant *S. aureus* [MRSA] infection is common) and generally a third-generation cephalosporin for gram-negative organisms. (The details of antibiotic therapy are beyond the scope of this text.) Antibiotics should be given intravenously for 2 to 4 weeks depending on the organism. Antibiotics do not need to be infused into the joint. The joint should be adequately drained to prevent damage. Usually, drainage can be accomplished with a large-gauge needle. Drainage reduces intra-articular pressure and removes white cells, which is a source of proteolytic enzymes. Repeated aspirations are only necessary during the first 5 days of treatment. Surgical drainage is required when the joint cannot be adequately aspirated and irrigated by needle or when the cell count in the synovial fluid does not decline in spite of what appears to be adequate drainage. Surgical drainage via arthroscopy should also be considered in patients with underlying arthritis and those with prolonged symptoms (i.e., longer than 7 days).[48] During the first

few days of treatment, splinting of the involved joint in extension makes the patient more comfortable and reduces the possibility of a flexion contracture. Daily physical therapy, once the acute process has resolved, improves the range of motion. In a severely damaged joint, bony fusion might be required.

Gonococcal Arthritis

Gonococcal arthritis was once considered the most frequent of bacterial arthritis in young adults. Women are more susceptible to gonococcal arthritis during menses and pregnancy. Persons who have a homozygous deficiency of complement component C5, C6, C7, or C8 are also susceptible to disseminated neisserial infections.[87] Patients with low complement levels caused by consumption of complement might also be more susceptible to disseminated neisserial infections.

Symptoms and Signs

Patients typically present with fever and migratory arthritis or arthralgias that evolve in several days into monoarticular arthritis. Patients also directly present with monoarticular arthritis. Wrists and knees are common sites of involvement, but any joint can be affected. Arthritis is manifested by swelling, erythema, and severe pain as in other bacterial arthritides. Skin lesions can accompany gonococcal arthritis. These lesions can be pustular, vesicular, or hemorrhagic and can ulcerate.

Laboratory Findings

Joint fluid shows increased numbers of polymorphonuclear white cells, but the white cell count might not be as high as in other bacterial infections. The joint fluid glucose is also not decreased to the low levels found in other bacterial joint infections.

Diagnosis

Gonococcal arthritis is suspected in a patient presenting with fever, typical skin lesions, and polyarthralgia or arthritis that evolves into monoarticular arthritis. Diagnosis is confirmed by positive culture results from synovial fluid or from blood, but culture results from these sites are positive in fewer than 50% of cases. Cultures from skin lesions are also usually negative. Gram stain or culture results from cervix, urethra, or rectum might be positive when joint, skin, and blood culture results are negative. Polymerase chain reaction (PCR) may be useful if patients with suspected gonococcal arthritis where the organism cannot be demonstrated by direct culture of the synovial fluid.

Treatment

The patient should be admitted to the hospital and receive parenteral antibiotics. Currently, the recommendation is to start a third-generation cephalosporin such as ceftriaxone because penicillin-resistant strains are now widespread. The dose of ceftriaxone is 1 g IV every 24 hours for daily for 2 to 4 days.[85] Most patients can be converted to oral antibiotic therapy in 48 hours. The patient is placed at bed rest for the first 2 days. Splinting of the affected joint provides pain relief. The infected joint should be immediately aspirated. The frequency of aspirations depends on the degree of inflammation. In most patients, residual joint damage does not occur.

POLYMYALGIA RHEUMATICA

Polymyalgia rheumatica (PMR) is an inflammatory disease affecting people over the age to 50 years and typically those of Northern European ethnic background. Patients can generally remember the day or the week the symptoms began and the symptoms include marked stiffness of the shoulders and hip girdle regions, fatigue, and low-grade fever.[88] A clue to PMR is a senior patient with bilateral "rotator cuff tendonitis." Patients may have rotator cuff signs and symptoms, but it is unusual to have bilateral rotator cuff tendonitis. PMR is a synovitis, and the tenosynovitis around the shoulder may lead to rotator cuff symptoms and signs. The general stiffness is often profound, and a patient will describe significant difficulty getting out of bed. Patients will relate that they had to roll out of bed in order to get up. A related illness, giant cell arteritis (GCA), can present with manifestations of PMR but also includes headache and may include visual changes, jaw pain with chewing, and more pronounced systemic symptoms. It is important to recognize the difference between isolated PMR versus PMR plus GCA. If GCA is untreated, it may lead to permanent visual loss in up to 50% or stroke in up to 10% of patients. More recently, modern imaging techniques have identified subclinical vascular inflammation in up to one-third of patients with isolated PMR.[89] Additional information will be necessary to determine if these patients are treated more aggressively than those with isolated PMR.

The laboratory hallmark of PMR is a markedly elevated ESR or CRP, with the CRP being more sensitive than the ESR in PMR.[88] A few patients though (10% to 15%) may have normal levels and still have PMR so that the history is the key as well and the response to prednisone. Patients can also have mild anemia typical of other inflammatory diseases.

Treatment is prednisone and has been for almost 50 years. If suspected, an initial of dose of 15 to 20 mg is sufficient in most patients with PMR especially if a small portion is given in the evening. The initial dose is maintained for 4 to 6 weeks and then slowly tapered. One taper regimen is to reduce the prednisone by 1 mg a week to 10 mg, 1 mg every 2 weeks to 5 mg, and then 1 mg every month until completely tapered off, but there are may be many small ups and downs on the prednisone dose. It must be recognized that the average length of disease duration is 24 months. If GCA is suspected, start the patients on high-dose prednisone (40 to 60 mg per day) and refer to a rheumatologist. The patient will need to have temporal artery biopsy scheduled as soon as possible and may need additional therapy. Methotrexate may offer steroid sparing therapy in patients who cannot reduce prednisone.

References

1. Bone and Joint Initiative. The big picture: burden of musculoskeletal disease (BMUS). Available at: http://www.boneandjointburden.org/2014-report/i0/big-picture. Accessed January 2, 2018.
2. Simkin PS, Gardner GC. Musculoskeletal system and joint physiology. In: Hochberg MC, Silman AJ, Smolen JS, et al, eds. *Textbook of Rheumatology*. Philadelphia: Mosby; 2003.
3. Brodal A. *Neurological Anatomy in Relation to Clinical Medicine*. 3rd ed. New York: Oxford University Press; 1981.
4. Zhang Y, Jordan JM. Epidemiology of osteoarthritis. *Clin Geriatr Med* 2010;26:335–369.
5. Johnson VL, Hunter DJ. The epidemiology of osteoarthritis. *Best Pract Res Clin Rheumatol* 2014;28:5–15.
6. Acheson RM, Collart AB. New Haven survey of joint diseases. *Ann Rheum Dis* 1975;34:379–387.
7. Stecher RM. Heberden's nodes. Heredity in hypertrophic arthritis of the finger joints. *Am J Med Sci* 1941;201:801–809.
8. Knowlton RG, Katzenstein PL, Moskowitz RW, et al. Genetic linkage of a polymorphism in the type II procollagen gene (COL2A1) to primary osteoarthritis associated with mild chondrodysplasia. *N Engl J Med* 1990;322:526–530.
9. Eyre DR, Weis MA, Moskowitz RW. Cartilage expression of a type II collagen mutation in an inherited form of osteoarthritis associated with a mild chondrodysplasia. *J Clin Invest* 1991;87:357–361.
10. Carman WJ, Sowers M, Hawthorne VM, et al. Obesity as a risk factor for osteoarthritis of the hand and wrist: a prospective study. *Am J Epidemiol* 1994;139:119–129.
11. Simkin PA. Bone pain and pressure in osteoarthritic joints. *Novartis Found Symp* 2004;260:179–186.
12. Lane NE. Osteoarthritis of the hip. *N Eng J Med* 2007;3587:1413–1421.
13. Wang X, Hunter D, Xu J, et al. Metabolic triggered inflammation in osteoarthritis. *Osteoarthritis Cartilage* 2015;23:22–30.
14. Sharma L, Pai YC. Impaired proprioception and osteoarthritis. *Curr Opin Rheumatol* 1997;9:253–258.
15. Bruckner FE, Howell A. Neuropathic joints. *Semin Arthritis Rheum* 1972;2:47–49.
16. Beighton P. Articular manifestations of the Ehlers-Danlos syndrome. *Semin Arthritis Rheum* 1972;1:246–261.
17. Askari AD, Muir WA, Rosner IA, et al. Arthritis of hemochromatosis. Clinical spectrum, relation to histocompatibility antigens, and effectiveness of early phlebotomy. *Am J Med* 1983;75:957–965.
18. Faraawi R, Harth M, Kertesz A, et al. Arthritis in haemochromatosis. *J Rheumatol* 1993;20:448.
19. Schumacher HR, Holdsworth DE. Ochronotic arthropathy. I. Clinicopathologic studies. *Semin Arthritis Rheum* 1977;6:207–246.
20. Bluestone R, Bywaters EG, Hartog M, et al. Acromegalic arthropathy. *Ann Rheum Dis* 1971;30:243–258.
21. Messier SP, Loeser RF, Miller GD, et al. Exercise and dietary weight loss in overweight and obese older adults with knee osteoarthritis: the Arthritis, Diet, and Activity Promotion Trial. *Arthritis Rheum* 2004;50:1501–1510.
22. Brouwer RW, van Raaij TM, Verhaar JA, et al. Brace treatment for osteoarthritis of the knee: a prospective randomized multi-centre trial. *Osteoarthritis Cartilage* 2006;14(8):777–783.
23. Reginster JY, Deroisy R, Rovati LC, et al. Long-term effects of glucosamine sulphate on osteoarthritis progression: a randomised, placebo-controlled clinical trial. *Lancet* 2001;357(9252):251–256.
24. Clegg DO, Reda DJ, Harris CL, et al. Glucosamine, chondroitin sulfate, and the two in combination for painful knee osteoarthritis. *N Engl J Med* 2006;354:795–808.
25. Vasiliadis HS, Tsikopoulos K. Glucosamine and chondroitin for the treatment of osteoarthritis. *World J Orthop* 2017;8:1–11.
26. Hochberg MC, Altman RD, April KT, et al. American College of Rheumatology 2012 recommendations for the use of nonpharmacologic and pharmacologic therapies in osteoarthritis of the hand, hip, and knee. *Arthritis Care Res* 2012;64:465–474.
27. Raynauld JP, Buckland-Wright C, Ward R, et al. Safety and efficacy of long-term intraarticular steroid injections in osteoarthritis of the knee: a randomized, double-blind, placebo-controlled trial. *Arthritis Rheum* 2003;48(2):370–377.
28. Lo GH, LaValley M, McAlindon T, et al. Intra-articular hyaluronic acid in treatment of knee osteoarthritis. *JAMA* 2003;290:3115–3121.
29. Smolen JS, Aletaha D, McInnes IB. Rheumatoid arthritis. *Lancet* 2016;388:1–16.
30. Kourilovitch M, Galarza-Maldonado C, Ortiz-Prado E. Diagnosis and classification of rheumatoid arthritis. *J Autoimmun* 2014;48–49:26–30.
31. Ferucci ED. Rheumatoid arthritis in American Indians and Alaska Natives: a review of the literature. *Semin Arthritis Rheum* 2005;34:662–667.
32. van Venrooij WJ, van Beers JJ, Pruijn GJ. Anti-CCP antibody, a marker for early detection of rheumatoid arthritis. *Ann NY Acad Sci* 2008;1143:268–285.
33. Rothschild BM, Woods RJ, Rothschild C, et al. Geographic distribution of rheumatoid arthritis in ancient North America: implications for pathogenesis. *Semin Arthritis Rheum* 1992;22:181–187.
34. Klareskog L, Malmstron V, Lunfberg K, et al. Smoking, citrullination, and genetic variability in the immunopathogenesis of rheumatoid arthritis. *Semin Immunol* 2011;23:92–98.
35. Avouac J, Gossec L, Dougados M. Diagnostic and predictive value of anti-citrullinated protein antibodies in rheumatoid arthritis: a systematic literature review. *Ann Rheum Dis* 2006;65;845–851.
36. Scott DL, Symmons DP, Coulton BL, et al. Long-term outcome of treating rheumatoid arthritis: results after 20 years. *Lancet* 1987;1:1108–1111.
37. Wilske KR, Healey LA. Remodeling the pyramid—a concept whose time has come. *J Rheumatol* 1989;16:565–567.
38. Fuchs HA, Kaye JJ, Callahan LF, et al. Evidence of significant radiographic damage in rheumatoid arthritis within the first 2 years of disease. *J Rheumatol* 1989;16:585–591.
39. Stoffer MA, Schoels MM, Smolen JS, et al. Evidence for treating rheumatoid arthritis to target: results of a systematic literature search update. *Ann Rheum Dis* 2015;75:16–22.
40. Zampeli E, Vlachoyiannopoulos PG, Tzioufas AG. Treatment of rheumatoid arthritis: unravelling the conundrum. *J Autoimm* 2015;65:1–18.
41. Singh JA, Saag KG, Bridges SL Jr, et al. 2015 American College of Rheumatology guidelines for the treatment of rheumatoid arthritis. 2016;68:1–26.
42. Cronstein BN. Low-dose methotrexate: a mainstay in the treatment of rheumatoid arthritis. *Pharmacol Rev* 2005;57:163–172.
43. van der Heijde D, Klareskog L, Landewé R, et al. Disease remission and sustained halting of radiographic progression with combination etanercept and methotrexate in patients with rheumatoid arthritis. *Arthritis Rheum* 2007;56:3928–3939.
44. Rhen T, Cidlowski JA. Anti-inflammatory actions of glucocorticoids: new mechanism for old drugs. *N Eng J Med* 2005;353:1711–1723.
45. Bakker MF, Jacobs JW, Welsing PM, et al. Low-dose prednisone inclusion in a methotrexate-based, tight control strategy for early rheumatoid arthritis. *Ann Int Med* 2012;156;329–339.
46. Turesson C, Matteson EL. Vasculitis in rheumatoid arthritis. *Curr Opin Rheumatol* 2009;21:35–40.
47. Puechal X, Gottenberg JE, Berthelot JM, et al. Investigators of the AutoImmunity Rituximab Registry. Rituximab therapy for systemic vasculitis associated with rheumatoid arthritis: results from the AutoImmunity and Rituximab Registry. *Arthritis Care Res (Hoboken)* 2012;64:331–339.

48. Gardner GC, Weisman MH. Pyarthrosis in patients with rheumatoid arthritis: a report of 13 cases and a review of the literature from the past 40 years. *Am J Med* 1990;88:503–511.
49. Brewerton DA, Hart FD, Nicholls A, et al. Ankylosing spondylitis and HLA27. *Lancet* 1973;1:904–907.
50. Benjamin M, McGonagle D. The anatomical basis for disease localisation in seronegative spondyloarthropathy at entheses and related sites. *J Anat* 2001;199:503–526.
51. Haroon N, Kim T, Inman RD. NSAIDs and radiographic progression in ankylosing spondylitis Bagging big game with small arms? *Ann Rheum Dis* 2012;71:1593–1595.
52. Dougados M, van der Linden S, Leirisalo-Repo M, et al. Sulfasalazine in the treatment of spondyloarthropathy. *Arthritis Rheum* 1995;5:618–627.
53. Calin A, Dijkmans BA, Emery P, et al. Outcomes of a multicentre randomized clinical trial of etanercept to treat ankylosing spondylitis. *Ann Rheum Dis* 2004;63:1594–1600.
54. Marzo-Ortega H, McGonagle D, O'Connor P, et al. Efficacy of etanercept in the treatment of the entheseal pathology in resistant spondyloarthropathy: a clinical and magnetic resonance imaging study. *Arthritis Rheum* 2001;44:2112–2117.
55. Mitchell MJ, Sartoris DJ, Moody D, et al. Cauda equina syndrome complicating ankylosing spondylitis. *Radiology* 1990;175:521–525.
56. Hunter T. The spinal complications of ankylosing spondylitis. *Semin Arthritis Rheum* 1989;19:172–182.
57. Brewerton DA, Caffrey M, Nicholls A, et al. Reiter's disease and HLA 27. *Lancet* 1973;2:996–998.
58. Calin A, Fries JF. An "experimental" epidemic of Reiter's syndrome, revisited: follow-up evidence on genetic and environmental factors. *Ann Intern Med* 1976;84:564–566.
59. Hannu T. Reactive arthritis. *Best Pract Res Clin Rheumatol* 2011;25:347–357.
60. Carter JD, Espinoza LR, Inman RD, et al. Combination antibiotics as a treatment for chronic Chlamydia induced reactive arthritis. *Arthritis Rheum* 2010;62:1298–1307.
61. Ritchlin C. Psoriatic disease—from skin to bone. *Nat Clin Pract Rheumatol* 2007;3:698–706.
62. Ritchlin CT, Colbert RA, Gladman DD. Psoriatic arthritis. *N Eng J Med* 2017;376:957–970.
63. Voulgari PV. Rheumatological manifestations of inflammatory bowel disease. *Ann Gastroenterol* 2011;24:173–180.
64. Rosenthal AK, Ryan LM. Calcium pyrophosphate deposition disease. *N Eng J Med* 2016;374:2575–2584.
65. Hamilton EBD. Diseases associated with CPPD deposition disease. *Arthritis Rheum* 1976;19:353–357.
66. Russell RG. Metabolism of inorganic pyrophosphate (PPi). *Arthritis Rheum* 1976;19:465–478.
67. McGonagle D, Tan AL, Madden J, et al. Successful treatment of resistant pseudogout with anakinra. *Arthritis Rheum* 2008;58:631–633.
68. Choi HK, Mount DB, Reginato AM. Pathogenesis of gout. *Ann Intern Med* 2005;143:499–516.
69. Neogi T. Gout. *N Eng J Med* 2011;364:443–452.
70. Healey LA, Bayani-Sioson PS. A defect in the renal excretion of uric acid in Filipinos. *Arthritis Rheum* 1971;14:721–726.
71. Lesch M, Nyhan WL. A familial disorder of uric acid metabolism and central nervous system function. *Am J Med* 1964;36:561–570.
72. Maclachlan MJ, Rodnan GP. Effects of food, fast, and alcohol on serum uric acid and acute attacks of gout. *Am J Med* 1967;42:38–57.
73. Lin HY, Rocher LL, McQuillan MA, et al. Cyclosporine-induced hyperuricemia and gout. *N Engl J Med* 1989;321:287–292.
74. Chruch LD. Primer: inflammasomes and interleukin 1 beta in inflammatory disorders. *Nat Clin Pract Rheumatol* 2008;4:34–42.
75. Faller J, Fox IH. Ethanol-induced hyperuricemia: evidence for increased urate production by activation of adenine nucleotide turnover. *N Engl J Med* 1982;307:1598–1602.
76. Halla JT, Ball GV. Saturnine gout: a review of 42 patients. *Semin Arthritis Rheum* 1982;11:307–314.
77. Simkin PA, Campbell PM, Larson EB. Gout in Heberden's nodes. *Arthritis Rheum* 1983;26:94–97.
78. Feig DI, Kang DH, Johnson RJ. Uric acid and cardiovascular risk. *N Eng J Med* 2008;359:1811–1821.
79. Gatter RA. The compensated polarized light microscope in clinical rheumatology [editorial]. *Arthritis Rheum* 1974;17:253–255.
80. Khanna D, Fitzgerald JD, Khanna P, et al. 2012 American College of Rheumatology guidelines for the management of gout part 2: therapy and antiinflammatory prophylaxis for acute gouty arthritis. *Arthritis Care Res* 2012;64:1447–1461.
81. Khanna D, Fitzgerald JD, Khanna P, et al. 2012 American College of Rheumatology guidelines for the management of gout part 1: systematic nonpharmacologic and pharmacologic therapeutic approaches to hyperuricemia. *Arthritis Care Res* 2012;64:1431–1446.
82. Ghosh P, Cho M, Rawat G, et al. Treatment of acute gouty arthritis in complex hospitalized patients with anakinra. *Arthritis Care Res (Hoboken)* 2013;65(8):1381–1384.
83. Kuncl RW, Duncan G, Watson D, et al. Colchicine myopathy and neuropathy. *N Engl J Med* 1987;316:1562–1568.
84. Tarkowski A. Infectious arthritis. *Best Pract Res Clin Rheumatol* 2006; 20:1029–1044.
85. Horowitz DL, Katzap E, Horowitz S, et al. Approach to septic arthritis. *Am Fam Physician* 2011;84:653–660.
86. Carpenter CR, Schur JD, Everett WW, et al. Evidenced-based diagnostics: adult septic arthritis. *Acad Emerg Med* 2011;18(8):781–796.
87. Petersen BH, Lee TJ, Snyderman R, et al. *Neisseria meningitidis* and *Neisseria gonorrhoea* bacteremia associated with C6, C7, or C8 deficiency. *Ann Intern Med* 1979;90:917–920.
88. Salvarani C, Pipitone N, Versari A, et al. Clinical features of polymyalgia rheumatica and giant cell arteritis. *Nat Rev Rheumatol* 2012;8: 509–521.
89. Dejaco C, Duftner C, Buttgereit F, et al. The spectrum of giant cell arteritis and polymyalgia rheumatica: revisiting the concept of disease. *Rheumatology (Oxford)* 2017;56(4):506–515.

CHAPTER 35

Myofascial Pain Syndrome

JAN DOMMERHOLT and **JAY P. SHAH**

Muscle pain is a common manifestation of many chronic pain conditions and is described as a diffuse, difficult to pinpoint, aching pain that may refer to deep somatic structures.[1] Muscle pain is common in all age groups, but chronic muscle pain is more frequent in the elderly than in younger populations.[2] Muscle-referred pain involves nociceptive-specific neurons in the spinal cord and in the brainstem. Wall and Woolf[3] have shown that muscle nociceptive afferents are especially effective in inducing neuroplastic changes in the spinal dorsal horn. Muscle pain activates specific cortical structures, such as the anterior cingulate gyrus, which is also involved in the emotional, affective component of pain.[4,5] Muscle pain is inhibited strongly by descending pain-modulating pathways, and under normal circumstances, there is a dynamic balance between the degree of activation of dorsal horn neurons and the descending inhibitory systems. Prolonged input from muscle nociceptors can be misinterpreted in the central nervous system and eventually can lead to allodynia, hyperalgesia, and an expansion of receptive fields.[6]

Although muscle pain is very common,[7] there is considerable controversy regarding its nature, existence, and relevance. Some clinicians consider muscle pain only secondary to other diagnoses, such as tendonitis, muscle strain, inflammation, degeneration, or injuries to joints and nerves.[8] Others view persistent muscle pain primarily as a manifestation of a presumed somatoform disorder.[9] Yet, others deny the existence of muscle pain all together as, in their view, all pain is produced by the brain, and focusing on peripheral tissues would be counterproductive.[10] With the development of orthopedic and manual medicine, many physicians, chiropractors, and physical therapists directed their attention mostly to articular dysfunction, although early manual medicine pioneers did include muscle dysfunction in their thinking.[11,12] In this context, it is noteworthy that although skeletal muscle comprises nearly half of the body's weight, it is the only organ in the human body that is not linked to a particular medical specialty. This led Simons[13] to suggest that muscle is an orphan organ, further evidenced by the fact that muscle research and the development of a knowledge base of muscle-specific ailments, pathophysiology, and diagnostic and treatment options have not evolved until fairly recently. The literature on myofascial pain is scattered among the literature of many different disciplines. One could wonder why persistent muscle pain and dysfunction have largely been ignored by the medical professions, but such contemplations are outside the scope of this chapter.

Brief Historical Overview

Muscle pain has been described by many different terms, including *fibrositis*, *interstitial myofibrositis*, *myogeloses*, *nonarticular rheumatism*, *myofascial pain*, *idiopathic myalgia*, *myofasciitis*, *perineuritis*, *myodysneuria*, and *fibromyalgia*.[14] Publications by Kellgren describing referred pain patterns from muscles and other soft tissues strongly influenced physicians James Cyriax in England and Janet Travell in the United States. At the time of Kellgren's first publications, Travell was a cardiologist and researcher. Initially, she was interested in the applicability of Kellgren's findings to cardiac pain, but soon, she became interested in musculoskeletal medicine.[15] In 1942,

she coauthored the first of many articles about the diagnosis and treatment of muscle pain.[16] In 1952, Travell and Rinzler[17] published an article of observed pain referral patterns of 32 muscles (Fig. 35.1).

At that time, there was virtually no research on muscle pain, and many of Travell's writings were based on her empirical observations and ability to establish clinical correlations. For example, Travell and Rinzler[17] observed that the fascia generated similar referred pain patterns as the contractile elements of the muscle; she subsequently modified her terminology to *myofascial pain* to encompass both the fibrous and contractile aspects. The similarities between referred pain patterns of fascia and muscle and the mechanical relationships between fascia and muscle were not further investigated until much later.[18]

Travell's work culminated in the publication of a two-volume textbook on myofascial pain, which she coauthored with Simons.[19,20] These books became known as the *Trigger Point Manuals*, and they have been translated in multiple languages. The term *trigger point* was introduced by Steindler in 1940 in a paper on muscle pain.[21] Travell and Rinzler[17] introduced the terms *myofascial trigger point* and *myofascial pain syndrome*, which are now intricately linked to a particular theoretical model, referred to as the "integrated trigger point hypothesis."[22] Although *muscle pain* and *myofascial pain* are sometimes used interchangeably, *muscle pain* is really a descriptive term, whereas *myofascial pain*, as introduced by Travell, is a more specific entity.[23]

In 1981, Simons and Travell[24] developed the "energy crisis hypothesis," which postulated that direct trauma and subsequent damage to the sarcoplasmic reticulum or the muscle cell membrane leads to an increase in intracellular calcium (Ca^{2+}) concentration, increased activation of actin and myosin, a relative shortage of adenosine triphosphate (ATP), and an impaired calcium pump, which in turn would increase the intracellular calcium concentration even more, perpetuating the cycle. Under normal physiologic conditions, the calcium pump is responsible for returning intracellular Ca^{2+} to the sarcoplasmic reticulum against a concentration gradient, which requires a functional energy supply. Eventually, the energy crisis hypothesis developed into the integrated trigger point hypothesis and more recently developed hypotheses, which incorporate newer electrodiagnostic, histopathologic, and pain science research.[25-27] It is now acknowledged that actual tissue damage is not required for the development of trigger points. This chapter provides an updated review of the etiology, mechanisms, pathophysiology, and clinical implications of myofascial trigger points.

Basic Myofascial Pain Concepts

Over time, research in the etiology, epidemiology, pathophysiology, diagnosis, and clinical management of myofascial pain has grown exponentially. Although the integrated trigger point hypothesis is not a perfect theoretical concept, it quickly became the most comprehensive evidence-informed model to explain the role of muscle tissue in acute and persistent pain conditions. Researchers around the world are conducting basic trigger point research, prevalence studies, and clinical outcome studies. Their findings show that trigger points are associated with virtually all painful musculoskeletal problems,

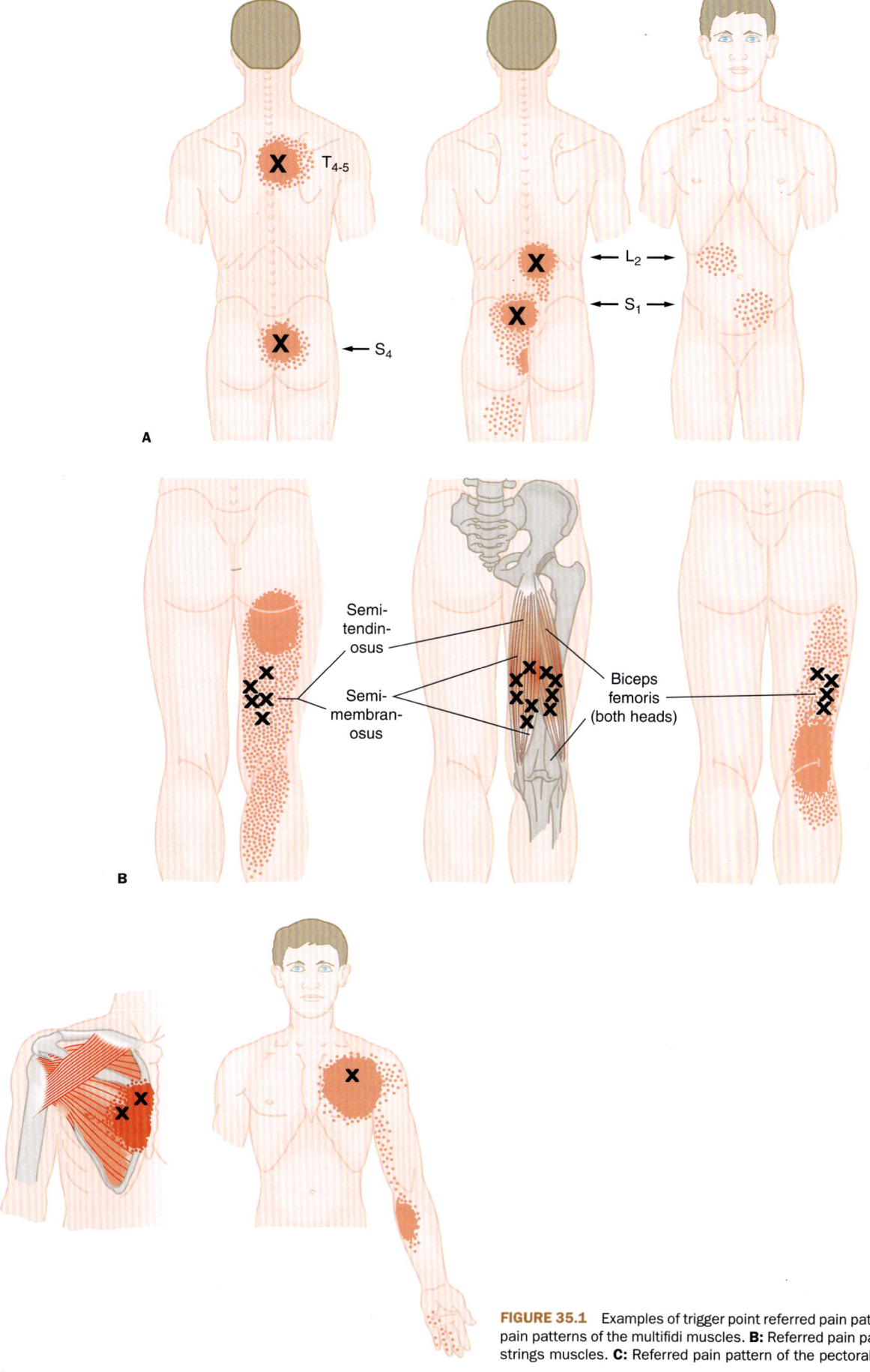

FIGURE 35.1 Examples of trigger point referred pain patterns. **A:** Referred pain patterns of the multifidi muscles. **B:** Referred pain patterns of the hamstrings muscles. **C:** Referred pain pattern of the pectoralis major muscle.

including migraines, tension-type headaches, craniomandibular dysfunction, epicondylalgia, low back pain, postlaminectomy syndrome, neck pain, disk pathology, carpal tunnel syndrome, osteoarthritis, radiculopathies, whiplash-associated disorders, fibromyalgia, postherpetic neuralgia, and complex regional pain syndrome, among others.[28] Trigger points have also been associated with visceral dysfunction, including endometriosis, interstitial cystitis, irritable bowel syndrome, urinary/renal and gallbladder calculosis, dysmenorrhea, and prostadynia.[29-33] Although trigger points are reportedly the most common diagnosis responsible for chronic pain and disability, they are frequently overlooked in the clinic.[34] Trigger points have been reported in all age groups except infants.[35-39]

A trigger point is defined as "a hyperirritable spot in skeletal muscle that is associated with a hypersensitive palpable nodule in a taut band".[19] Palpating for trigger points begins with identifying this taut band by palpating perpendicular to the fiber direction (Fig. 35.2). Taut bands are stiffer than relaxed muscle fibers, and the degree of stiffness can be assessed by phase-contrast analysis of vibration-induced cyclic shear waves.[40-46]

An active trigger point can spontaneously produce local tenderness and pain, referral of pain or other paresthesia to a distant site, and peripheral and central sensitization. A latent trigger point is only painful when stimulated. Motor phenomena associated with trigger points include disturbed motor function, muscle weakness as a result of motor inhibition, muscle stiffness, and restricted range of motion. Nociceptive input can perpetuate altered motor control strategies and lead to muscle overload or disuse.[47-49] Subjects with latent trigger points in several shoulder muscles featured altered shoulder abduction patterns when compared to healthy subjects.[50-52] Autonomic aspects may include, among others, vasoconstriction, vasodilatation, lacrimation, and piloerection.[53]

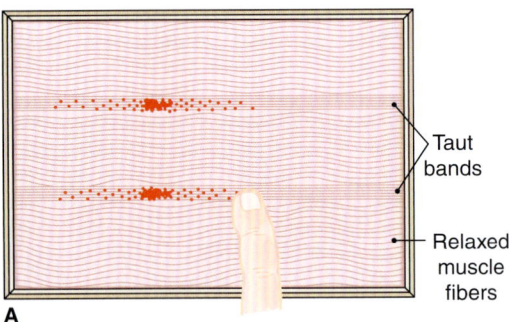

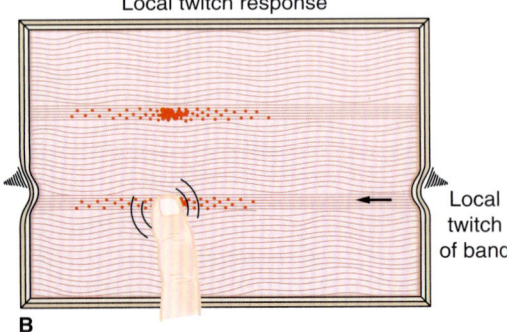

FIGURE 35.2 Palpation of trigger points. As the palpating finger of the examiner moves from normal areas of muscle **(A)** and encounters a painful trigger point **(B)**, a local twitch response often occurs within the muscle surrounding the trigger point. (Redrawn after Simons DG, Travell JG, Simons LS. *Upper Half of the Body.* 2nd ed. Baltimore, MD: Lippincott Williams & Wilkins; 1999. *Travell & Simons' Myofascial Pain and Dysfunction: The Trigger Point Manual;* vol 1.)

To discuss the current research and the clinical implications of myofascial trigger points and contemporary trigger point hypotheses, a brief review of muscle physiology, the role of the motor endplate, muscle pain, dorsal horn, and central sensitization is provided in the context of myofascial trigger points. The motor phenomena of trigger points are best explained by understanding the functions and structure of the motor endplate and the sarcomere assembly.

Muscle Physiology

Skeletal muscles consist of groups of fascicles, which are made of muscle fibers and myofibrils, accountable for contraction and relaxation of the fiber. The myofibril is approximately 1 to 2 μm in diameter and is separated from surrounding myofibrils by the mitochondria, the sarcoplasmic reticulum, and the transverse tubular systems or T-tubules.

The T-tubules lie perpendicular to the long axis of the muscle fiber with two zones of transverse tubules to each sarcomere. T-tubules conduct impulses from the exterior to the interior of the muscle fiber and activate voltage-dependent L-type calcium channels in the transverse tubular membrane, including type 1 sarcoplasmic reticulum calcium release ryanodine receptors and surface membrane calcium channel dihydropyridine receptors. Activation of these channels and receptors results in the release of Ca^{2+} into the myoplasm.[54] The sarcoplasmic reticulum is a store for the release and uptake of Ca^{2+}. Muscle contractions occur after actin and troponin are activated by Ca^{2+}. Calcium allows tropomyosin to shift its position and expose myosin-binding sites on actin, thus regulating the cross-bridge interactions between actin and myosin.[55] ATP-dependent processes are responsible for muscle force generation, which implies that both calcium and ATP are critical for the maintenance of the actin-myosin cross-bridges.[56] The organization of thin actin and thicker myosin filaments are responsible for the striated patterning observed when viewed under longitudinal electron micrograph scanning. In addition to actin and myosin, there are several other important proteins, such as titin, nebulin, desmin, tropomyosin, troponin, and tropomodulin, among others, which together maintain the architecture and stability of the sarcomere (Fig. 35.3).

Titin is the largest known vertebrate protein. It connects the Z-line with myosin filaments and cross-links with titin molecules of adjacent sarcomeres. Titin positions the myosin filaments at the center of the sarcomere as a spring.[57,58] One particular section of titin, referred to as the PEVK segment, is able to interact with actin filaments in close proximity to the Z-line, which may limit the degree of sarcomere contraction as the tip of the myosin filament may literally bounce back against a "viscous bumper" of the actin-titin interaction, comparable to a dragnet.[59,60] Titin filaments are responsible for passive tension generation when sarcomeres are stretched and provide muscle stiffness by virtue of their spring mechanism in the I-band. During sarcomere contractions, titin filaments are folded into a sticky gel-like structure at the Z-line,[57,58,61,62] which is an important contributor to the force generated by a contracting muscle.[63] It is conceivable that myofascial trigger points have a damaged sarcomere assembly; myosin filaments may have broken the actin–titin barrier and gotten stuck in the sticky titin substance at the Z-line.

Single molecules of nebulin span the full length of the actin filaments, and nebulin dictates the architecture of actin with direct involvement of titin and the Z-line protein myopalladin.[64] Titin and nebulin interact at many levels, especially during myofibrillogenesis.[65] Nebulin connects to the proteins myopalladin and desmin in the Z-line. Myopalladin binds to α-actinin, which in turn connects to actin and to titin.[66] Desmin filaments link adjacent Z-lines and interconnect the

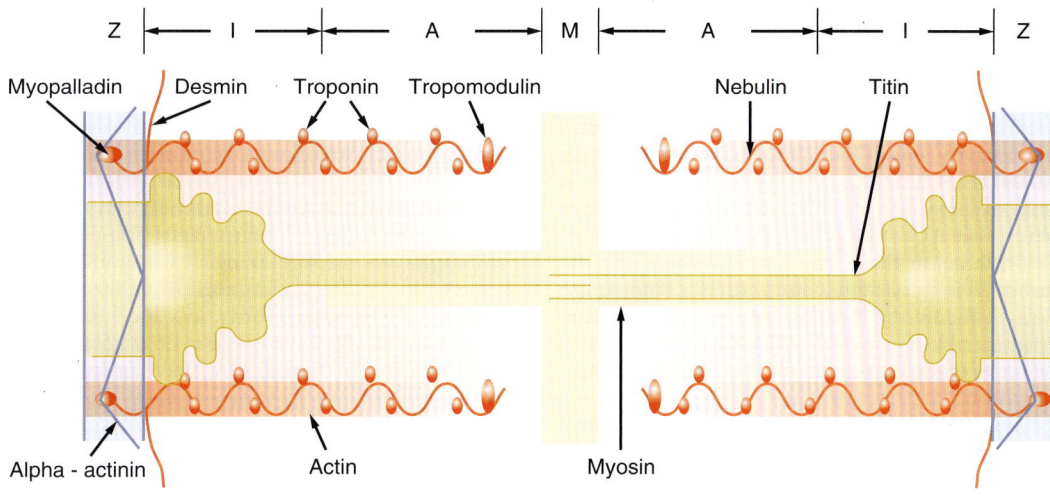

FIGURE 35.3 Sarcomere.

myofibrils with the sarcolemma, the nuclei, the T-tubules, the mitochondria, and possibly the microtubules.[55,67] Nebulin acts as a stabilizing structure through its specific binding sites at different places on actin, tropomyosin, troponin, and tropomodulin.[55,65,68–71] It regulates muscle contractions by inhibiting the cross-bridge formation until actin is activated by Ca^{2+}.[65] Troponin is a Ca^{2+}-receptive protein that sensitizes actomyosin to Ca^{2+} in association with tropomyosin, among other functions.[72] Of interest is that tropomyosin and tropomodulin can influence molecular processes related to synaptic signaling and modulate neuronal morphology.[73]

A key feature of the integrated trigger point hypothesis is the presence of excessive acetylcholine (ACh) at the neuromuscular junction, which stimulates voltage-gated sodium (Na^+) channels of the sarcoplasmic reticulum and ultimately results in a continuous increase of intracellular Ca^{2+} levels. This results in ongoing activation of nebulin, troponin, and tropomyosin and causes persistent muscle contractures consistent with taut bands and myofascial trigger points. The role of the motor endplate is reviewed in the next section.

The Motor Endplate

The terms *neuromuscular junction* and *motor endplate* are used interchangeably, although technically, the neuromuscular junction refers to function, whereas the motor endplate refers to structure. A motor endplate is the synapse between the terminal ends of motor neurons and skeletal muscle. The terminal branches of a single motor neuron terminate in multiple presynaptic boutons containing many ACh vesicles.[74]

When nerve impulses from a α-motor neuron reach the motor nerve terminal, voltage-gated Na^+ channels are opened, which trigger a Na^+ influx that depolarizes the terminal membrane. Voltage-gated Ca^{2+} channels are opened, which causes an influx of Ca^{2+} and a quantal release of ACh and other molecules, such as ATP, from the nerve terminal into the synaptic cleft (Fig. 35.4). When two ACh molecules bind to a nicotinic ACh receptor (nAChR) across the synaptic cleft, the nAChR opens a cation-specific pore, which facilitates a Na^+ influx and a potassium (K^+) efflux across the muscle cell membrane. Each single quantum of ACh will depolarize the postsynaptic cell and trigger a miniature endplate potential (MEPP). A sufficient number of MEPPs will produce a depolarization and an action potential, which travels along the T-tubules, triggers the ryanodine receptor in the sarcoplasmic reticulum, and causes a release of Ca^{2+} from the sarcoplasmic reticulum.

As stated, the release of Ca^{2+} triggers tropomyosin to shift its position and nebulin to allow cross-bridges to form between the actin and myosin filaments, resulting in a muscle contraction. The K^+ efflux restores the resting membrane potential. During the brief period before the actual muscle contraction, ACh is hydrolyzed by the enzyme acetylcholinesterase (AChE) into acetate and choline. Choline is reabsorbed into the nerve terminal, where it is synthesized into ACh by acetyltransferase by combining choline and acetyl coenzyme A from the mitochondria. ACh release is not only activated by motor nerve stimulation, but it is also modulated by the concentration of AChE. Inhibition of AChE will cause an accumulation of ACh in the synaptic cleft, which may stimulate motor nerve endings and tonically activate nAChRs.

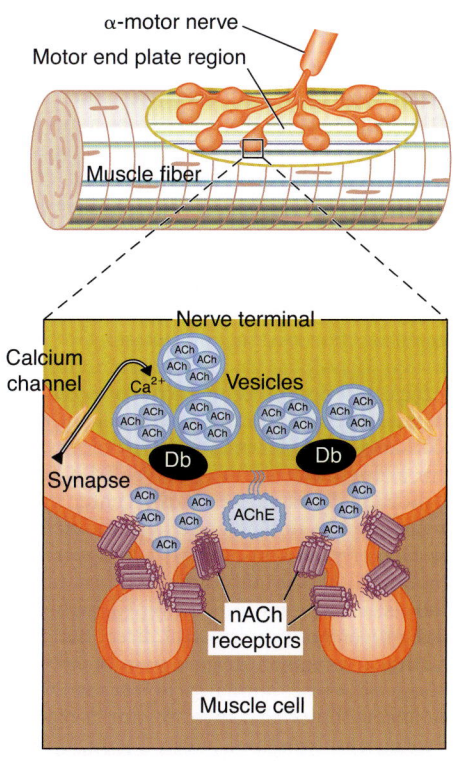

FIGURE 35.4 The motor endplate.

A 1993 publication illustrating spontaneous electrical activity in myofascial trigger points initiated a new line of research into the role of motor endplates.[75] Initially, the electrical activity was assumed to be the result of dysfunctional muscle spindles, but soon, multiple human, rabbit, and even equine studies confirmed that the activity was in fact abnormal endplate noise related to an excess of ACh at the motor endplate.[22,76–83] It is conceivable that in myofascial trigger points, the contractures resulting from excessive ACh may cause myosin filaments to get stuck in sticky titin gel at the Z-line, thereby damaging the sarcomere assembly. The persistent contractures compromise local blood vessels, reducing the local oxygen supply, resulting in hypoxia, a lowered pH, and hypoperfusion, which all contribute to muscle pain, tenderness, dysfunction, and peripheral nociceptor sensitization.[84]

The reduced oxygen levels in myofascial trigger points and an increased metabolic demand result in a local energy shortage and a local shortage of ATP.[25] Under normal physiologic circumstances, presynaptic ATP inhibits the release of ACh. Inversely, a decrease in ATP leads to an increased ACh release. Insufficient postsynaptic ATP results in a failure of the calcium pump, increased levels of Ca^{2+}, and a Ca^{2+}-induced Ca^{2+} release. An increase in the Ca^{2+} concentration will reinforce muscle contractures. The local energy crisis is likely related to the finding of abnormal mitochondria in the nerve terminal and ragged red fibers, which are an indication of structural damage to the cell membrane and the mitochondria.[85]

The presence of excessive ACh can be the result of AChE insufficiency, an acidic pH, hypoxia, a lack of ATP, certain genetic mutations, drugs and particular chemicals, such as calcitonin gene-related peptide (CGRP), diisopropyl fluorophosphate, or organophosphate pesticides, and increased sensitivity of the nAChRs.[26,86,87] Myofascial tension or muscle hypertonicity, as seen in trigger points, may also enhance the excessive release of ACh.[88,89] There are many possible vicious cycles capable of maintaining the resulting contractures and trigger points. For example, hypoxia leads to an acidic milieu, muscle damage, and an excessive local release of multiple nociceptive substances, including CGRP, bradykinin (BK), and substance P (SP).[90] Hypoxia may even trigger an immediate increased ACh release at the motor endplate.[87] CGRP stimulates the release of ACh from the motor endplate, decreases the effectiveness of AChE, and upregulates the nAChR. An acidic pH enhances the release of CGRP, downregulates AChE, and causes hyperalgesia.[26,91,92]

There are many similarities between the mechanisms and consequences of myofascial trigger points and eccentric loading or eccentric exercise. Eccentric training or exposure is frequently characterized by a certain degree of cytoskeletal muscle damage. Even very short bouts of eccentric exercise can result in a disorganization of the A-band, streaming of the Z-line, and a disruption of several cytoskeletal proteins, including titin, nebulin, vimentin, fibronectin, and desmin.[93–98] By comparison, postmortem histologic studies of myofascial trigger points show pathologic alterations of the mitochondria as well as an increased width of A-bands and decreased width of I-bands in muscle sarcomeres of trigger points.[99,100] A biopsy study of trigger points in a dog gracilis muscle revealed a similar pattern of severely shortened sarcomeres in the center and lengthened sarcomeres outside the immediate trigger point region.[101] The diagnosis of trigger points in animals is comparable to that in human subjects. Although an animal cannot verbalize recognition of pain, skilled palpation combined with an analysis of dysfunctional movement patterns will direct the investigator or clinician to clinically relevant trigger points.[102,103]

In addition to these similarities, eccentric loading and myofascial trigger points also involve local hypoxia, impaired local circulation, and local and referred pain.[104] Eccentric contractions in unconditioned muscle or unaccustomed eccentric contractions are likely sources of myofascial trigger point development.[26] Itoh and colleagues[105] confirmed that eccentric exercise triggers the formation of taut bands and myofascial trigger points in exercised muscle.

There are other possible causes of trigger points. Patients commonly report an onset of pain associated with trigger points following either acute, repetitive, prolonged, or chronic muscle overload. Piano students developed significantly decreased pressure thresholds over latent trigger points after only 20 minutes of continuous piano playing.[106] Computer operators developed trigger points after as little as 30 to 60 minutes of continuous typing.[107,108] In other words, low-level muscle contractions can contribute to the development of trigger points, which is best explained by the so-called Cinderella hypothesis.[109] According to the Cinderella hypothesis, low-level muscle contractions follow stereotypical patterns, where smaller motor units are recruited before and derecruited after larger motor units, which means that smaller type 1 fibers may be continuously activated during prolonged low-level contractions.[110,111] Low-level contractions have been shown to lead to muscle fiber degeneration, an increase in Ca^{2+} release, energy depletion, and the release of various cytokines, which all have been associated with the formation of trigger points.[112–115] During low-level contractions, the intramuscular pressure increases considerably especially near the muscle insertions, which may impair the local circulation, cause hypoxia, and eventually lead to trigger point formation.[28,116] As noted, motor phenomena associated with trigger points include disturbed motor function, muscle weakness as a result of motor inhibition, muscle stiffness, and restricted range of motion.

Sensitization and Activation of Muscle Nociceptors

To better understand the sensory aspects of myofascial trigger points, including local and referred tenderness, pain, and other paresthesia, as well as peripheral and central sensitization, a brief review of the current understanding of muscle nociceptors, spinal cord mechanisms, and sensitization is necessary.

Muscle nociceptors are dynamic structures that can be activated mechanically by deforming the axonal membrane of the nerve ending, as for example, following a blow to a muscle. Many receptors are susceptible to chemical activation by nociceptive substances released from the surrounding tissues and immune cells.[117] Matched receptors at the nociceptor exist for a variety of substances including BK, prostaglandins (PGs), serotonin (5-HT), protons (H^+), ATP, glutamate, and others, including the so-called purinergic and vanilloid receptors. Purinergic receptors bind ATP and stimulate nociceptors accordingly. Vanilloid receptors are especially sensitive under conditions of lowered tissue pH and muscle ischemia. Pain during tension-type headaches, tooth clenching, and bruxism is partially mediated by the vanilloid receptor molecule.[117] BK, 5-HT, and PG interact at many levels at the vanilloid receptors, potentially synergistically producing local muscle pain.[118] When injected together into the temporalis muscle of normal volunteers, BK and 5-HT produced more pain than when each stimulant was injected alone.[119]

The mechanism of chemical activation is of clinical interest, especially in evaluating chronic pain states where often there is little gross swelling evident. Endogenous substances such as BK, PG, and 5-HT not only are very effective at sensitizing or activating muscle nociceptors but also cause local vasodilation. Therefore, the release of these substances can lead to mechanoreceptor activation by distorting the normal tissue relationships. A sensitized muscle nociceptor has a lowered stimulation threshold into the innocuous range, such that it will respond to harmless stimuli like gentle pressure and muscle movement.[120]

The nociceptor terminals contain neuropeptides, such as SP and CGRP. When these substances are released, they stimulate local vasodilation, plasma extravasation, and liberation of sensitizing substances from the surrounding tissue. Upon activation by a noxious stimulus, the nociceptor releases the stored neuropeptides, which directly influence the local microcirculation by stimulating vasodilation and increasing the permeability of the microvasculature.[121,122] More importantly, the secretion of the neuropeptides in sufficient quantity leads to a cascade of events, including the release of histamine from mast cells, BK from kallidin, 5-HT from platelets, and PGs from endothelial cells.[123] The cumulative effect is the increased production and release of sensitized substances in a localized region of edema in the muscle tissue. Therefore, the muscle nociceptor is not merely a passive structure designed to record potentially noxious stimuli. Rather, muscle nociceptors play an active role in the maintenance of normal tissue homeostasis by sensing the peripheral biochemical milieu and mediating the vascular supply to peripheral tissue. With tissue injury, the secretion of SP and CGRP increases, leading to the response outlined earlier that can alter the responsiveness of the nociceptor. Muscle tenderness is mainly due to the sensitization of muscle nociceptors by BK, PG, and 5-HT, which may account for the exquisite tenderness found when firm pressure is applied over an active trigger point.[124,125]

As noted before, the activation of a nociceptive terminal is not primarily due to a nonspecific damage of the nerve ending by a strong stimulus but rather the binding of specific substances, including BK, PG, and 5-HT, to their paired receptors on muscle nociceptors. Receptor responsiveness is dynamic. For example, inflammation alters the population of BK G protein-coupled metabotropic receptors at the nociceptive terminal. In normal muscle tissue, the B2 receptor is more prevalent. With tissue inflammation, an additional BK receptor (B1) is synthesized in the cell body of the ending in the dorsal root ganglion and inserted into the nociceptor terminal membrane. Unlike the B2 receptor, which is constitutively expressed, the B1 receptor is inducible and is involved in sensitization of the peripheral nociceptor. The B2 and B1 receptors are mediators of several physiologic and pathologic responses via the kallikrein–kinin system.[126] Induction and binding of the B1 receptor can also lead to the production of pro-inflammatory mediators, including tumor necrosis factor-α (TNF-α) and interleukin-1 β (IL-1β). Stimulation of B2 receptors leads to only transient increases in the intracellular calcium concentration, making nociceptor sensitization unlikely; however, the B1 and B2 receptors do influence each other on many levels.[127]

Stimulation of the B1 receptor results in prolonged elevation of intracellular Ca^{2+} concentration, which can lead to sustained peripheral sensitization.[128] If the conformational change of the BK receptor persists after the inflammation subsides, this maladaptive change may herald the transition from acute to chronic pain. Therefore, the degree to which muscle nociceptors in a trigger point become sensitized or activated will vary according to the balance of sensitizing substances in the muscle tissue and the threshold of their respective receptors. There may be a spectrum of nociceptor irritability based on this balance that distinguishes a normal muscle from a muscle with a latent or active trigger point.

Central Sensitization

In addition to sensitization of the peripheral nociceptors, pain and dysfunction induced by trigger points may also be related to alterations in the responsiveness of the dorsal horn.[129,130] A chronic active trigger point may contribute to inflammatory exacerbation of the fascia and be a source of ongoing noxious input that sensitizes dorsal horn neurons and generates increased or referred pain to other spinal cord segments via central sensitization.[131] Conversely, a sensitized central nervous system may lead to a lowering of the activation threshold of the peripheral nociceptors in a trigger point, inducing the transition from latent to active. The latter may occur when trigger points develop secondary to referred pain from viscera or joints or as a result of psychological stress.[104,130] Giamberardino et al.[132] have established that visceral referred pain with hyperalgesia is usually associated with cutaneous hyperalgesia and trigger points.[132] Vecchiet et al.[133] measured significantly lower pain thresholds with electrical stimulation over active trigger points in the muscles and the overlying cutaneous and subcutaneous tissues. With latent trigger points, the sensory changes did not involve the cutaneous and subcutaneous tissues.[133,134]

Sensitization in the central nervous system can occur both segmentally and multisegmentally at the spinal level and also involve changes in activity of higher brain centers. Clinical characteristics of central sensitization include spontaneous pain, allodynia and hyperalgesia, and widespread pain.[129,130] Spontaneous pain is often related to increased background activity in nociceptive neurons in the spinal cord and higher brain centers. When background activity is great enough to elicit an action potential, pain may be sensed without specific visceral or peripheral nociception. The central mechanisms for allodynia, hyperalgesia, and widespread pain are discussed in more detail in the following text.

The primary peripheral sensing apparatus in muscle involves group III (thinly myelinated, low-threshold fibers) and group IV (unmyelinated, high-threshold fibers) afferent nerve fibers. These fibers cause aching, cramping pain when stimulated with microneural techniques. The central projections of these fibers share several important characteristics especially when compared to cutaneous nociception. First, a reduced spatial resolution, because of a lower innervation density of muscle tissue, makes it harder to localize muscle pain. Second, convergence of sensory input from skin, muscle, periosteum, bone, and viscera into lamina IV and V of the dorsal horn onto wide dynamic range neurons can blur the identification of the origin of the pain. Third, divergence of sensory input into the dorsal horn–sustained noxious stimulation as demonstrated, for example, in group IV fibers in animal models can open previously ineffective synaptic connections in the dorsal horn such that these fibers begin to respond to lower levels of stimulation, leading to mechanical allodynia, hyperalgesia, and secondary hyperalgesia.

Compared to normal muscle and muscle with latent trigger points, a muscle with active trigger points is more tender and mechanically sensitive, suggesting that peripheral nociceptors are already sensitized.[135] Once sensitized, the group IV afferent nerve fibers fire at lower thresholds, even though they are normally high-threshold nociceptors. For example, in animal models, injection of BK into muscle causes the group IV afferents to respond to much lower levels of stimulation, suggesting they have become sensitized.[136] Because muscle tenderness is mainly due to the sensitization of muscle nociceptors by BK, PGs, and 5-HT, peripheral sensitization by these substances presumably contributes to the tenderness seen in active trigger points and may contribute to the pain that individuals with active trigger points describe. Studies on the biochemical milieu of trigger points in the upper trapezius muscle have shown that active trigger points are associated with elevated levels of inflammatory mediators, neuropeptides, pro-inflammatory cytokines, and catecholamines.[137,138] These chemicals can act to sensitize and activate local nociceptors. It is important to note that active trigger points are associated with elevated levels of these biochemicals compared to both normal muscle tissue and that with latent trigger points, which suggests that the presence of these biochemicals is related to the pain experience.

Central sensitization is more readily induced as the activation threshold is lowered for peripheral muscle nociceptors. In animal models of pain, a nociceptive input from skeletal muscle is much more effective at inducing neuroplastic changes in the spinal cord than cutaneous input.[3] Experimentally induced myositis in animal models causes a marked expansion of the response of second-order neurons beyond the muscle's target area of the dorsal horn. Hoheisel et al.[139] found that after a localized inflammatory reaction was created, noxious input from the gastrocsoleus muscle (L5 segment) also activated second-order neurons in the L3 segment. This segment would not ordinarily be activated by noxious stimulation of the gastrocsoleus in noninflamed muscle. This study demonstrated an expansion of the receptive field in the dorsal horn as a result of a central sensitization. The L3 dorsal horn neurons became hyperexcitable after continuous nociceptive input from the inflamed L5 muscle. The sensitized surrounding segments caused the L3 segment to respond to previously ineffective afferent input. This model of referred pain combines peripheral input and central processing and is known as the central hyperexcitability theory.[140]

Several supraspinal mechanisms contribute to referred pain or secondary hyperalgesia.[4,5,141] Pain from myofascial trigger points is associated with increased activity in the somatosensory and limbic regions and suppressed hippocampal activity. The limbic regions of the brain are responsible for the emotional/affective component of pain, whereas the hippocampus modulates stress.[5] Increased cortical and subcortical activity spurred by disinhibition can disrupt function in descending pain-modulating pathways, which may lower pain thresholds peripherally.[142–144] Trigger points and myofascial pain are also associated with widespread microstructural changes concentrated in limbic system gray matter that may indicate damage.[145] A recent study showed that disinhibition of the motor cortex, consisting of either decreased intracortical inhibition or increased intracortical facilitation, is a marker of myofascial pain.[146]

Until recently, pain has been considered primarily related to neuronal activity; however, recent work has uncovered the contribution of microglia to the pain experience.[147–149] Microglia are not static cells; rather, they are capable of releasing a number of neuroexcitatory substances that modulate local neuronal activity.[150] Studies by Chacur and colleagues have helped characterize the role of microglia in spinal sensitization.[151] After experimentally induced myofascial inflammation, microglial cells evince morphologic changes both ipsilaterally and contralaterally to the inflamed tissue without activating the contralateral microglia cells to the point of inducing measurable effects of central sensitization. Inhibition of microglia through application of minocycline is sometimes effective at attenuating hypersensitivity in animals with muscle pain, which supports the role of microglia in mediating the pain experience.[152]

Expansion of the receptive field in the spinal cord with myositis-induced excitation is clinically relevant, helping to explain the unusual referral patterns seen in myofascial pain. For example, trigger points in the suboccipital muscles may refer to the frontal region of the head, and trigger points in the piriformis may cause pseudosciatica. Expansion of the receptive field may also explain the symptomatic hyperalgesia reported by many patients, as many of these neurons become hyperexcitable. It is likely that these myositis-induced changes in the spinal cord occur due to a rewiring of dorsal horn neurons in response to sustained peripheral drive from an irritable, sensitized muscle nociceptor, such as that found in an active trigger point.[153]

Visceral dysfunction can also manifest through central sensitization as trigger point development. For example, trigger points in the abdominal wall can be used for diagnostic purposes. Jarrell[154] found that the presence or absence of a trigger point in the abdominal wall helps to determine whether there is evidence of current or previously treated visceral disease. The presence of an abdominal wall trigger point predicted evidence of visceral disease in 90% of subjects. However, the absence of a trigger point was associated with no visceral disease in 64% of the subjects.[154,155] A cohort study of men with chronic pelvic pain syndrome found that abdominal pain or tenderness was present in 51% of patients, compared to only 7% of healthy controls.[156]

Trigger points may also be associated with joint dysfunction. Trigger points in the upper trapezius were found to correlate with cervical spine dysfunction at the C3 and C4 segmental levels, although a causal relationship was not established.[157] A single spinal manipulation induced changes in pressure pain sensitivity in latent trigger points in the upper trapezius muscle.[158] It is important to add that referred pain is not unique to muscle tissue or myofascial trigger points. All tissues, including fascia, intervertebral disks, internal organs, ligaments, and zygapophyseal joints are capable of referring pain.[132,159–162] Referred pain patterns from cervical zygapophyseal joints are very similar to those of trigger points in cervical muscles.[163] Clinically, referred pain phenomena can be rather confusing as patients frequently complain of pain in an area of the body where the pain did not originate.[164,165] For instance, pain in the elbow region, often considered a local problem due to epicondylitis, may in fact be referred pain from shoulder muscles.[166] Hsieh et al.[167] demonstrated that inactivating trigger points in the infraspinatus muscle using dry needling inactivated trigger points in the anterior deltoid muscle. Similarly, pain in the region of the masseter muscle can be resolved by treating trigger points in the trapezius muscle.[168] Headley[169] suggested that trigger points in a particular muscle can inhibit other muscles especially in the area of referred pain. For example, trigger points in the infraspinatus muscles may weaken the extensor carpi radialis muscles.[167,169] In other cases, muscle pain and trigger points may be secondary to other, nonmuscular disorders, such as internal organ, joint, or disk pathology. This finding underscores the necessity of an excellent and comprehensive differential diagnostic process to uncover the nuances of referred pain.[170] Patients with osteoarthritis of the hip or knee joint were found to have significantly higher numbers of trigger points in muscles crossing these joints than healthy controls.[171] The correlations between pathologic conditions and an increased number of trigger points may partially explain why localized painful conditions can become more widespread.[23]

There are several hypotheses of the causal relation between trigger points and central sensitization.[130] Hoheisel and colleagues studied central sensitization in the dorsal horn through histologic, electrophysiologic, and behavioral studies.[172] Experimentally induced fascial inflammation in animal models leads to an increase in input from the fascia to the dorsal horn, which may be due to the activation of ineffective or silent synapses. Increased input to the dorsal horn increases afferent bombardment and background activity leading to spinal sensitization. The synaptic changes observed at the dorsal horn after induced fascial inflammation make a clear connection between fascial dysfunction and central nervous system structure and function.

The integrated trigger point hypothesis is a popular model, but it is not without flaws.[27] Notably, it fails to account for trigger points observed with nonmusculoskeletal pathologies. The neurogenic hypothesis attempts to address the observation of trigger points in regions without local injury by suggesting a neurogenic incitement of trigger point formation after primary pathology, local or remote, within the common neurometric field.[173] According to Srbely, trigger points do not simply perpetuate central sensitization but are its neurogenic manifestations.[173] Central sensitization, spurred by the primary pathology, results in neurogenic inflammation and sensitization of peripheral nociceptors.[174] These in turn may lead to the formation of the characteristic discrete tender nodule or trigger point.[173] Hocking[175,176] maintained that an upregulation of L- or N-type voltage-dependent calcium channels and α_1-adrenergic receptors combined with a downregulation of calcium-activated K^+ channels would lead to an increase in the motor terminal cytosolic Ca^{2+} concentration. According to Hocking,[175,176] sympathetic activity would facilitate these phenomena because α_1-adrenergic receptors are linked to L-type voltage-dependent calcium channels.

Furthermore, the integrated trigger point hypothesis does not include other pertinent mechanisms, such as the role of reactive oxygen species (ROS).[27,154,173,174] Recently, Jafri[27] expanded the integrated trigger hypothesis by incorporating mechano-activation of ROS signaling to destabilized calcium signaling. Striated muscle generates ROS, especially superoxide that usually is produced by mitochondria. Under stressful or pathologic conditions, the enzyme xanthine oxidase and phospholipase A2-dependent processes have been shown to also produce ROS.[177,178] During repetitive contractions, nicotinamide adenine dinucleotide phosphate oxidase 2 (NOX2), located within the sarcoplasmic reticulum, the sarcolemma, and the transverse tubules,[179–181] is the major source of superoxide ROS.[182] In patients with Duchenne muscular dystrophy, the mechano-activation of NOX2-dependent ROS production plays a significant role in the pathogenic calcium and ROS signaling. Jafri[27] hypothesized that mechanical stress can trigger an excessive release of calcium in muscles through X-ROS signaling. According to Jafri,[27] mechanical deformation of the microtubule network can activate NOX2, which would produce ROS. The ROS oxidizes ryanodine receptors leading to increases in Ca^{2+} release from the sarcoplasmic reticulum. The Ca^{2+} mobilization resulting from mechanical stretch through this pathway is referred to as X-ROS signaling. In skeletal muscles, X-ROS sensitizes Ca^{2+}-permeable sarcolemmal transient receptor potential or TRP channels, which may be a source of nociceptive input and inflammatory pain.[27,183] Activating the transient receptor potential vanilloid 1 (TRPV1) leads to a quick increase in intracellular Ca^{2+} concentrations.[184,185] Jafri[27] suggested that myofascial pain is likely due to a combined activation of several ligand-gated ion channels, including the TRPV1 receptor, other acid-sensing ion channels (ASIC3), BK, and purinergic receptors, among others.

The Biochemical Milieu of Myofascial Trigger Points

Until recently, myofascial pain was characterized primarily by a physical finding and symptom cluster without demonstrable pathology. Research in the upper trapezius muscle has characterized the unique biochemical milieu of myofascial trigger points and has even identified quantitative differences between active and latent trigger points.[138,186] The presence and possible effects of these biochemicals are discussed in the following sections. It has not yet been determined whether the unique biochemical environment develops before and perhaps causes trigger points or is somehow a result of trigger point formation. Further study of the biochemical milieu of trigger points may not only lead to an improved biochemical characterization of trigger points but may also identify those who are at risk for developing persistent symptoms. Discovering if and which measurable substances are predictive of pain could lead to focused therapies in the future.

pH and Muscle Pain

A previous study demonstrated a positive correlation between pain and local acidity.[187] Sluka et al.[91] demonstrated that an acidic milieu without muscle damage is sufficient to cause profound changes in the properties of the pain matrix

such that alterations in pH would be sufficient to modify the threshold sensitivity of the nociceptor. An acidic pH stimulates the production of BK during local ischemia and inflammation; therefore, a local acidic milieu may explain some of the pain associated with an active trigger point. Mechanical hyperalgesia is a hallmark of a trigger point; however, ongoing nociceptive activity is not necessary to cause mechanical hyperalgesia. In a rat model, repeated injections of acidic saline boluses into one gastrocnemius muscle produced bilateral, long-lasting mechanical hyperalgesia of the paws.[91] Furthermore, the study showed that the persistent hyperalgesia does not require muscle tissue damage nor continued nociceptive input from the injection site, demonstrating that secondary mechanical hyperalgesia may be maintained by neuroplastic changes in the central nervous system, such as dorsal horn and thalamic neurons.[91]

Specific ASICs on muscle nociceptors can be sensitized and activated by acidic pH. For example, ASIC3 knockout mice do not develop hyperalgesia following repeated bolus injections of acidic saline.[92] Hong et al.[188,189] suggest that an integrative mechanism at the spinal cord level in response to sensitized nociceptors plays a role in the development of active trigger points and should be considered in any pathogenetic hypothesis. In an expansion of Simons's integrated hypothesis, Gerwin et al.[26] proposed that the acidic pH may also modulate the motor endplate by inhibiting AChE. This would result in increased concentration of ACh at the synaptic cleft, promoting sarcomere contraction and formation of the taut band characteristic of trigger points.[26]

Neuropeptides, Inflammatory Mediators, and Tissue Injury and Pain

Significantly elevated levels of SP and CGRP are found in the vicinity of active trigger points. The orthodromic and antidromic release of these substances is greatly increased in response to nociceptor activation, for example, by protons and BK binding to their matched receptors.[190] This may lead to neuroplastic changes in the dorsal horn and profound changes in neuronal activity and the perception of pain. In the studies by Shah et al.,[137,138] SP and CGRP were the only two analytes at active trigger points with concentrations significantly below their original baselines in the recovery period following a local twitch response. These biochemical changes correspond with the commonly observed decrease in pain and local tenderness after the inactivation of a trigger point by dry needling (Fig. 35.5).[191]

SP causes mast cell degranulation with the subsequent release of histamine, 5-HT, and upregulation of both pro-inflammatory cytokines, including TNF-α and IL-6, and anti-inflammatory cytokines, including IL-4 and IL-10. TNF-α is the only cytokine restored in the mast cell and is released immediately following mast cell degranulation.[192,193] The finding of elevated levels of 5-HT, BK, norepinephrine, and pro-inflammatory cytokines in active trigger points is consistent with biochemical pathways involved in tissue injury and inflammation.[137,138]

Catecholamines and the Autonomic Nervous System

Significantly elevated levels of 5-HT and norepinephrine are found in the vicinity of active trigger points, supporting the effect of the elevated TNF-α. The increased levels of norepinephrine may be associated with increased sympathetic activity in the motor endplate region of trigger points. In one study, sympathetic activity was recorded from rabbit myofascial trigger spots. Intra-arterial injection of phentolamine, an α-adrenergic antagonist, decreased the spontaneous electrical activity from a locus of a myofascial trigger spot in rabbit skeletal muscle.[79]

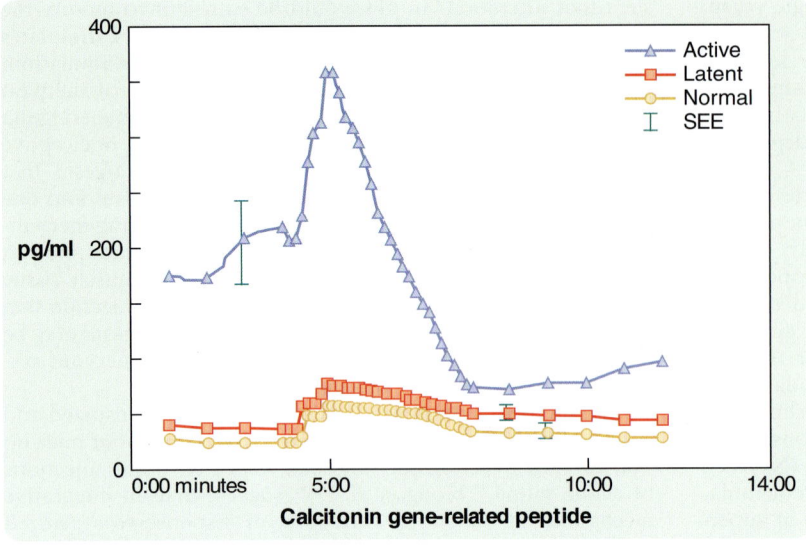

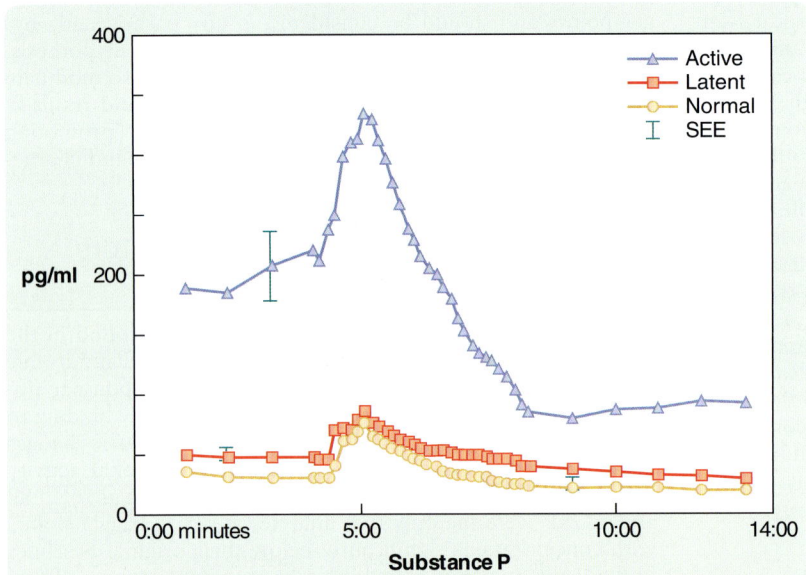

FIGURE 35.5 Concentrations of calcitonin gene-related peptide and substance P across time. A local twitch response was elicited at 5 minutes.

Conversely, the nAChR antagonist curare had no effect on the spontaneous electrical activity. Elevated levels of norepinephrine in the local milieu of active trigger points suggest that the autonomic nervous system is involved in the pathogenesis of spontaneously painful trigger points. A study by Ge et al.[53] provides evidence of sympathetic facilitation of mechanical sensitization of trigger points. The presence of α- and β-adrenergic receptors at the endplate may provide a possible mechanism for autonomic interaction,[26,84] for example, stimulation of the α- and β-adrenergic receptors stimulated the release of ACh in the phrenic nerve of rodents.[194]

Cytokines and Pain

A unique cascade of cytokines is released following tissue injury and inflammation. For example, BK stimulates the release of TNF-α, which leads to the release of IL-1β and IL-6. These two cytokines stimulate the cyclooxygenase (COX) nociceptive pathway, which leads to the production of PGs.[195,196] TNF-α also stimulates a separate nociceptive pathway via the release of IL-8, which mediates sympathetic pain by stimulating the liberation of sympathetic amines.[197]

TNF-α, IL-1β, IL-6, and IL-8 have been found at elevated levels at active trigger points in the upper trapezius.[138,186] TNF-α produces a time- and dose-dependent muscle hyperalgesia within several hours after injection into the gastrocnemius or biceps brachii of a rat. The hyperalgesia is completely reversed by systemic treatment with the nonopioid analgesic metamizol.[198] Furthermore, TNF-α does not cause histopathologic tissue damage or motor dysfunction. One day after injection of TNF-α, elevated levels of CGRP, nerve growth factor, and prostaglandin E2 are found in the muscle. According to Schafers et al.,[198] TNF-α and other pro-inflammatory cytokines such as IL-1β may play a role in the development of muscle hyperalgesia, and the targeting of pro-inflammatory cytokines might be beneficial for the treatment of muscle pain syndromes.

In rat model studies, Loram et al.[199] measured the tissue and plasma levels of cytokines following injection of carrageenan into the hind paw compared with intramuscular injection into the gastrocnemius muscle. They demonstrated, for the first time, that the initiation of primary muscle hyperalgesia is not associated with elevated levels in local muscle of TNF-α, IL-1β, or IL-6.[199] Loram et al.[199–201] also showed that IL-1β and IL-6 are elevated at a time interval when there is no hyperalgesia.

One possible explanation, they suggest, is that elevated intramuscular levels of IL-1β and IL-6 induce central sensitization but do not contribute to the initiation of hyperalgesia.[199]

Cytokines that lead to PG release via the COX pathway have been targeted for pharmacologic intervention because of their roles in the inflammatory response.[195,196] IL-1β is the major cytokine stimulus for central COX-2 expression during inflammation. Loram et al.[199] found that IL-1β was the only cytokine that reached a higher concentration in the muscle compared to the hind paw after carrageenan injection in the rat. Furthermore, IL-1β was significantly elevated 24 hours after inducing muscle inflammation at a time when secondary hyperalgesia was induced.[199] IL-1β also stimulates IL-6 production during muscle injury. Together, both cytokines are necessary for repair and regeneration of muscle.[202–204] In light of the importance of cytokines to muscle regeneration, Loram et al.[199] suggest that pharmacologic interventions preferentially target action of IL-1β and not IL-6 in order to reduce secondary muscle hyperalgesia and still conserve the cytokines' regenerative qualities.

Moreover, which cytokines and when to target them may depend on the time course of the muscle injury and inflammatory response. Whereas some groups have found that TNF-α produces a time- and dose-dependent muscle hyperalgesia within several hours after injection into rat muscle, others have found that injection of TNF-α into a rat's gastrocnemius muscle does not excite but rather has a short-term desensitizing action on group IV muscle afferents.[205] The data suggest that TNF-α has a dual action when released intramuscularly. Initially, it suppresses neuronal excitability, but in a later stage, it contributes to neuronal hyperexcitability.[205] Therefore, the elevated levels of TNF-α, IL-1β, and IL-6 found in active trigger points may mediate secondary hyperalgesia and central sensitization via the COX pathway.

A second distinct nociceptive pathway moderates the inflammatory hyper-nociception following tissue injury. Rat cytokine-induced neutrophil chemo-attractant 1 (CINC-1) and its homolog in humans, IL-8, coordinate the sympathetic components of hyper-nociception. Loram et al.[199] demonstrated that of the four cytokines—TNF-α, IL-1β, IL-6, and CINC-1—measured in muscle after carrageenan injection, only levels of CINC-1 were elevated at the time of primary hyperalgesia.[199] Moreover, CINC-1 and IL-8 induce a dose- and time-dependent mechanical hyper-nociception. Therefore, the elevated levels of IL-8 found in active myofascial trigger points may mediate inflammatory hyper-nociception, muscle tenderness, and pain via this pathway. Furthermore, this pathway is inhibited by β-adrenergic receptor antagonists, although not COX antagonists.[196]

Clinical Management

TRIGGER POINT DIAGNOSIS

The literature on the clinical management of patients with myofascial pain is scattered over multiple specialties and disciplines, including algology, physiatry, dentistry, otolaryngology, urology, neurology, osteopathy, orthopedics, gynecology, physical therapy, chiropractic, acupuncture, and massage therapy, among others. No medical specialty has claimed muscle as its organ of focus; therefore, the term *myofascial pain* may have different meanings among different disciplines, making understanding across disciplines challenging. In dentistry, for example, "myofascial pain dysfunction syndrome" is commonly used for nonspecific muscle pain with or without limited mouth opening.[206,207] The finding of trigger points should not preclude other aspects of the differential diagnosis, including neurologic examinations, biomechanical assessments of posture and movement patterns, and assessments of other possible contributing factors.

Trigger points may elicit symptoms similar to those of other conditions. Some trigger point–referred patterns are very similar to radicular pain patterns. For example, referred pain patterns of trigger points in the teres minor muscle or gluteus minimus muscle resemble a C8 or L5 radiculopathy, respectively.[208,209] However, the presence of myofascial trigger points does not rule out a radiculopathy and vice versa. Trigger points may also be associated with lumbar disk lesions or contribute to symptoms of thoracic outlet syndrome.[210–212] Even in fibromyalgia, which is considered a central sensitization disorder, myofascial trigger points play an important role in the perception of pain and sensitization.[213–215]

As part of the diagnostic process, clinicians should consider other diagnoses, which may feature widespread pain, including but not limited to hypothyroidism; systemic lupus erythematosus; Lyme disease; babesiosis; ehrlichiosis; *Candida albicans* infections; myoadenylate deaminase deficiency; herpes zoster; complex regional pain syndrome; hypoglycemia; parasitic diseases such as fascioliasis, amoebiasis, and giardia; systemic side effects of medications including any of the statin drugs or even glucosamine sulfate; and metabolic or nutritional deficiencies or insufficiencies of vitamin B_{12}, vitamin D, and ferritin.[216] Having patients complete standardized pain questionnaires at the time of the initial examination allows for objective outcome measurements. Because individual clinicians may not be familiar with discipline-specific differential diagnoses outside their own specialty, a multidisciplinary approach to assessment and treatment is preferred especially for more complex patients.[217] However, the underlying mechanisms and principles of muscle dysfunction, described earlier in this chapter, apply to all disciplines.

A significant problem in the myofascial pain literature is the inconsistent use of criteria to identify trigger points.[218] Palpation is the criterion standard for identifying myofascial trigger points in spite of the lack of research-validated definitional criteria. Simons et al.[19] defined empirically derived criteria, which have been applied to a number of interrater and intrarater reliability studies.[219–231] A recent Delphi study of 60 experts from 12 countries revealed that more than 70% of the experts considered only two palpatory findings and one symptom as essential criteria for the diagnosis of myofascial pain, namely, a taut band, a hypersensitive spot, and referred pain.[232] The presence of a taut band and spot tenderness has been shown to be a reliable indicator of myofascial trigger points in one comprehensive study, although in a more recent study, referred pain and a jump sign were the most reliable indicators.[219,221] The local twitch response is more difficult to elicit manually and has not been shown to be a reliable feature of trigger points. A systematic review in 2017 found that the overall interrater reliability of palpation for myofascial trigger points was moderate.[233] Experienced and inexperienced clinicians reached different levels of agreement when identifying trigger points.[234,235]

Occasionally, the concept of myofascial pain is challenged because acceptable interrater reliability is only achieved with experienced and well-trained clinicians.[234,236] However, the fact that trigger point palpation has to be learned is no different than most other clinical skills and procedures. Palpation and, more specifically, trigger point palpation is not taught in the vast majority of medical, physical therapy, and chiropractic schools, and it should come as no surprise that clinicians do not necessarily master trigger point palpation without specific training.[237] It is encouraging that several recent studies indicate that there has been much progress in the quality of myofascial pain studies, but there is always a need for better and higher quality research.[238,239]

PHYSICAL EXAMINATION AND DIAGNOSIS

The physical examination of myofascial trigger points is performed with either a flat or pincer palpation technique. With the flat palpation technique, the taut band and trigger point are

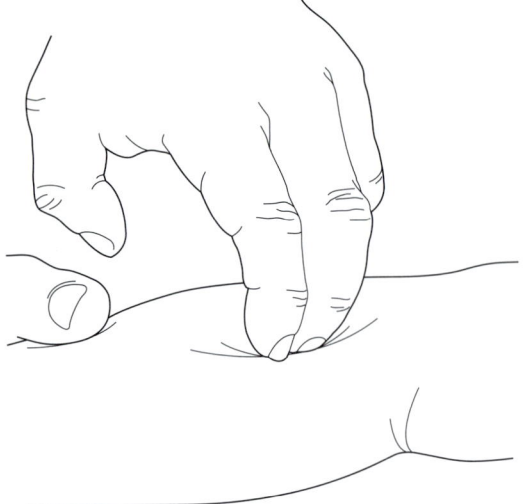

FIGURE 35.6   Flat palpation technique.

compressed in between a finger or thumb against the underlying tissue or bone (Fig. 35.6). With the pincer palpation technique, the taut band and trigger point are held in between the clinician's fingers and thumb (Fig. 35.7). The initial palpation focuses on the presence of taut bands as, by definition, trigger points are always located within a band of contracted muscle fibers. Palpation for trigger points is performed perpendicular to the fiber direction, which requires good anatomical knowledge of muscles and their fiber directions. Whether a muscle should be shortened, lengthened, or kept in a resting position depends entirely on the individual muscle, the tension in connective tissues and fascia, and available range of motion. The muscle needs to be placed in a position where the taut band can optimally be palpated. For patients with very tight and restricted muscles, the muscle may need to be placed in a relaxed position, whereas in hypermobile patients, the muscle may need to be prestretched to facilitate identification of taut bands.[28]

Familiarity with referred pain patterns of trigger points is essential in guiding clinicians to clinically relevant muscles and trigger points. Recent studies have established new and confirmed previously suggested referred pain patterns, especially in the head and neck region.[166,240–246] Prolonged pressure on trigger points for as long as 10 to 15 seconds may elicit referred

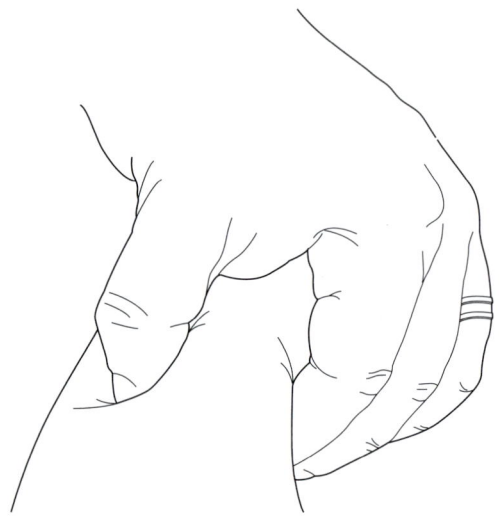

FIGURE 35.7   Pincer palpation technique.

pain patterns, and the patient's familiar pain complaint. Local twitch responses may be elicited by strumming the taut band, but this has little utility as part of the diagnostic process. The minimum criteria for identification of an active trigger point are the presence of a taut band with exquisite spot tenderness and patient-recognized pain. The physical examination for myofascial trigger points should be a standard component of the diagnostic process but does not preclude any other part of the standard examination process. In addition to trigger points, there are many other possible sources of nociception and pain. A detailed history is critical. There are also several predisposing or perpetuating factors that need to be assessed in addition to possible medical diagnoses.[170]

Mechanical perpetuating factors are relatively easy to identify by clinicians across disciplines and include forward head posture, which frequently contributes to migraines or tension-type headaches, neck pain, and upper thoracic pain,[247–249] decreased spinal mobility, structural misalignments, such as leg length discrepancies or pelvic torsions, or systemic or local hypermobility.[158,250–252] The combination of static and awkward postures, excessive force, and repetitive tasks predisposes a patient to the development of trigger points.[107,108] Ergonomic measures often play a vital role in correction and prevention of myofascial pain problems.[253]

Psychological arousal has a direct impact on the electrical activity of myofascial trigger points, although autogenic relaxation reduces the electrical activity.[254–256] Whether specific regions of the brain, such as the anterior cingulate gyrus and periaqueductal gray, which have been linked to nociceptive input from muscles and to depression, anxiety, and anger, can explain at least part of the association of psychological factors and trigger points remains to be seen.[4,257] In 2013, Gerber et al.[170] found that patients with cervical pain secondary to active myofascial trigger points had significantly poorer health status and quality of life compared to individuals with latent or no trigger points. Their poor health status was characterized by higher rates of depression, fatigue, tension, confusion, mood disturbances, and sleep disruption as well as greater disability. Adequate treatment of myofascial pain involves consideration not only of the physiologic cause of pain but also of the psychosocial deficiencies patients may experience. Depending on the severity of these symptoms, it may be prudent to include psychologists or social workers in a patient's long-term treatment plan.

Any nutritional or metabolic condition that interferes with the energy supply of muscle tissue can contribute to the development of myofascial trigger points.[216] Laboratory levels can be within the "normal" range yet be insufficient for a given individual. The connection between the insufficiency and an individual's pain may be difficult to appreciate, but it is no less important than in individuals with "abnormal" results. Empirically, common nutritional and metabolic deficiencies or insufficiencies include vitamins B_1, B_6, B_{12}, and D; iron, magnesium, and zinc insufficiency states; and thyroid deficiency states, among others. The importance of metabolic and nutritional perpetuating factors is illustrated for vitamin D.

Vitamin D deficiency is commonly observed with chronic, nonspecific musculoskeletal pain.[258] Nearly 90% of 150 subjects with musculoskeletal pain had vitamin D levels less than 20 ng/mL and 28% had less than 8 ng/mL, where levels above 30 ng/mL are considered optimal. Vitamin D deficiency in adults is defined as serum 25(OH)D levels below 20 ng/mL and vitamin D insufficiency as 25(OH)D levels between 20 and 30 ng/mL.[259,260] Vitamin D deficiencies are endemic in Northern Europe and America and are associated with muscle weakness, myofibrillar protein degradation, reduced muscle mass, osteoporosis, and decreased functional ability.[261–264] Low levels of magnesium and 25(OH)D have been linked not only to myofascial pain but also to cancer, adenomatous colon polyps, and tendon ruptures.[265]

Although palpation is truly the gold standard for trigger point identification, meaningful palpation takes time to learn and perfect.[237] This has driven researchers to seek ways to identify and characterize trigger points using more objective and quantitative techniques. Magnetic resonance and ultrasound elastography are increasingly used in research but are not yet common in clinical practice.[40,41,266] Piezoelectric and electrohydraulic shockwave emitters are common in Germany for the identification and treatment of trigger points and their specific referred pain patterns.[267,268] Both types of shockwave emitters are able to reproduce patients' familiar referred pain patterns. Although endplate noise was found to be characteristic of trigger points, in clinical practice, there is no advantage to using electromyography for the identification of trigger points.[269]

Recent advances in ultrasound technology have made it an especially appealing tool to try to bring into the clinical assessment of myofascial pain secondary to trigger points. Studies have focused on three modes of ultrasound imaging: two-dimensional (2D) grayscale (B-mode), Doppler, and vibration sonoelastography.[135,266,270–272] Under 2D grayscale ultrasound, healthy muscle appears uniform in fiber orientation and echotexture. Active and latent trigger points both appear as hypoechoic ellipses or bands, although no significant differences have been noted between them in terms of echogenicity or echotexture.[266,273] The underlying reason for the hypoechoic appearance is not known at this time. Color Doppler imaging of blood vessels in the vicinity of trigger points shows that although both active and latent trigger points have similar unique waveforms indicative of retrograde diastolic flow relative to normal muscle, more active than latent trigger points show abnormality (69% of active vs. 16.7% of latent).[45,273] Spectral Doppler imaging illustrates that both kinds of trigger points also have high pulsatile flow more frequently than normal muscle, further indicating that trigger points are associated with blood flow abnormality.[44,45,273] Under vibration sonoelastography, trigger points appear as regions of increased tissue stiffness corresponding to the localized hypoechoic regions in the 2D grayscale imaging. Although these results are promising, ultrasound is not a substitute for a comprehensive physical examination including palpation; however, it has the potential to be a useful supplemental clinical tool for the assessment of the heterogeneity and soft tissue properties of muscle and determination of treatment outcomes.[45]

TREATMENT OPTIONS

One of the first decisions to make after the initial examination is whether the patient's pain complaints have a significant myofascial component. Patients with chronic pain problems may present with a combination of possible contributing factors. If metabolic or nutritional insufficiencies are found, it is unlikely that therapy will be successful until such insufficiencies are adequately addressed. The choice of treatment modalities is partially based on a clinician's bias, preferences, experience, and skills. A dentist treating a patient with facial pain and trigger points in the masseter muscle may decide to improve the patient's occlusion assuming that the muscle pain is secondary to the malocclusion. An orthopedic surgeon may manage a patient's complaint of radiating pain down the leg with epidural injections to reduce radicular pain, whereas a physician familiar with referred pain patterns of myofascial trigger points may decide to treat trigger points in the gluteus medius muscle with trigger point injections or myofascial release techniques. Many patients with chronic myofascial pain may benefit from a comprehensive pharmacologic management strategy, which may include nonsteroidal anti-inflammatories, opiates, antidepressants, and anticonvulsants, although these are not specific for myofascial pain.[274]

Patient Education

Following the initial examination, patients need to be educated about the nature and complexity of their pain. Studies have shown that patients with chronic pain gain understanding and insight when the clinician explains the principles of peripheral and central sensitization rather than focuses on anatomical concepts such as spinal mechanics.[275–277] Excellent patient education can reduce disability and assist patients in making appropriate choices, overcoming counterproductive beliefs, and modifying dysfunctional behaviors by increasing physical activity and self-efficacy.[278,279] If the patient's pain complaint could easily be provoked by pressure on certain trigger points, it is likely that trigger point therapy will make significant improvements. However, clinicians should be cautious in promising complete relief, especially for chronic pain conditions with multiple interacting aspects.

Physical Therapy

The role of physical therapy in pain management centers is often limited to instructing patients in proper stretching and strengthening exercises, stabilization programs, and posture corrections as well as providing limited manual therapy interventions. Relatively few physical therapists receive adequate training in pain management, and physical therapists are poorly represented in professional pain management associations.[280] Few physical therapy schools have adopted a specific pain science curriculum,[281,282] which may explain why as many as 96% of orthopedic physical therapists preferred not to work with patients with chronic pain.[283] Patients need to learn self-pacing and setting appropriate and achievable goals, including physical, psychological, functional, and social goals.[284] An important variable is the degree of a patient's belief in their self-efficacy, which is defined as "the belief in one's capabilities to organize and execute the sources of action required to manage prospective situations."[278,285,286] Patients with a weak belief in their self-efficacy tend to avoid difficult tasks, have low aspirations, maintain a self-diagnostic focus, and emphasize personal deficiencies and adverse outcomes. They are more prone to depression and stress and give up quickly. Patients with a strong belief in their self-efficacy are more likely to set challenging goals, consider difficult tasks as challenges rather than as threats, and maintain a task-diagnostic focus. They usually are not depressed and increase their effort when faced with difficulties.

Needling Therapies

Invasive trigger point therapy usually involves either trigger point injections or dry needling. As Steinbrocker[287] already suggested in 1944, the mechanical stimulation of trigger points is an important mechanism to explain the effects of needling therapies. Trigger point injections are usually performed by medical doctors and their professional support staff. A growing number of physical therapists and physicians around the world utilize trigger point dry needling.[191]

The first comprehensive paper about dry needling was published in 1979 and reported that dry needling of various structures, including trigger points, ligaments, and fascia, caused immediate analgesia in almost 87% of the needle sites.[288] Lewit[288] referred to the immediate reduction of pain as "the needle effect." In 1980, a prospective dry needling study of injured workers with low back pain showed that dry needling was an effective treatment for low back pain.[289] A Cochrane review supported the use of dry needling as an adjunct for the treatment of patients with chronic low back pain.[290] Trigger point dry needling consists of superficial and deep dry needling based on the depth of needling.[191] The technique used with deep dry needling is similar to the technique of trigger point injections and usually aims to elicit local twitch responses (Fig. 35.8).

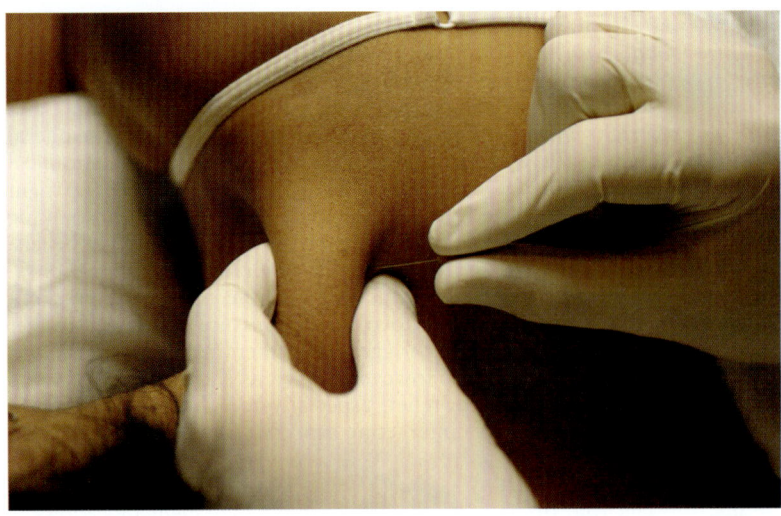

FIGURE 35.8   Trigger point dry needling of the trapezius muscle.

The mechanisms and effectiveness of deep dry needling are comparable to trigger point injections.[191,291–294] Earlier studies suggested that dry needling would cause more post-needling soreness, but there are no differences between injections and dry needling using solid filament needles. Post-needling soreness occurs in most patients and can vary in duration from just a few minutes to several 2 days.[295] Applying a cold application, using manual compression techniques, applying transcutaneous electrical stimulation, or performing low load exercises following needling procedures does reduce the post-needling soreness in the short term.[296–299] Psychological factors do impact the degree of post-needling soreness.[295,300] Vasovagal reactions can occur with any needling procedure, but they are relatively rare. To avoid unnecessary complications from possible vasovagal reactions, patients are needled preferably while lying down on a treatment table.

A local twitch response is an involuntary spinal cord reflex contraction of muscle fibers within a taut band, which can be elicited by manually strumming or needling of a taut band. Local twitch responses can be observed visually, recorded electromyographically, or visualized with diagnostic ultrasound.[301] When a trigger point is needled with a monopolar Teflon-coated electromyography needle, local twitch responses appear as high-amplitude polyphasic discharges.[302] Eliciting local twitch responses is helpful when using deep dry needling in clinical practice not only to accomplish optimal treatment results but also to confirm that the needle is placed into a taut band, which is critically important when needling close to peripheral nerves or internal organs, such as the lungs.[188,291,303,304] In a study of dry needling for low back pain, Koppenhaver et al.[305] noted that subjects who experienced a local twitch response reported a greater improvement in the function of the lumbar multifidus muscle compared to those who did not experience a twitch response; however, the difference was of short duration. Eliciting a local twitch response had no effect on levels of disability, nociceptive activity, or pain intensity.[305] Nevertheless, eliciting local twitch responses does normalize the chemical environment of active trigger points.[138,186,304] In clinical practice, patients commonly report never having experienced local twitch responses when they were treated with trigger point injections previously.

With superficial dry needling, a solid filament needle is placed into the tissues overlying active trigger points at a depth of approximately 5 to 10 mm for 30 seconds. If there is residual pain, the needle is inserted for another 2 or 3 minutes.[306,307] Local twitch responses are usually absent with superficial dry needling. The degree of available endogenous opioid peptide antagonists may determine how intensely a patient responds to the therapy. So-called weak responders may have excessive amounts of endogenous opioid peptide antagonists. A rodent model has shown that mice with deficient opioid peptide receptors did not respond well to needle-evoked nerve stimulation.[308]

The efficacy of dry needling may be monitored visually with ultrasound imaging. A 2015 study sought to characterize changes in ultrasound images taken before and after treatment while also recording changes in trigger point status from active to latent and resolution of pain symptoms.[45] Participants with at least one active trigger point received a 3-week course of dry needling at their most active trigger point. Grayscale 2D B-mode and color Doppler ultrasound images were taken at the trigger point and palpably normal muscle tissue at baseline and posttreatment. A significant reduction in the heterogeneity of muscle stiffness was observed at those trigger points that responded to treatment.[45] However, although ultrasound is a promising tool to objectively evaluate trigger points before and after treatment, further research is needed to improve reproducibility and standardize imaging methods and quantitative measures before it can be used reliably for diagnosis.

Trigger point injections are administered with a variety of injectables, including procaine and lidocaine, steroids, and vitamin B_{12} (Fig. 35.9). Travell preferred procaine hydrochloride, which is no longer available everywhere.[16,309] The current recommendation is to use 0.25% lidocaine, which was found to be more effective than stronger concentrations.[310,311] Other anesthetics used with trigger point injections include ropivacaine, levobupivacaine, and mepivacaine, among others.[312,313] Trigger point injections with the 5-HT antagonist tropisetron were found to be more effective than injections with lidocaine solution, but injectable 5-HT antagonists are not available in all countries.[314,315] Although widely used, there is no scientific evidence for injections with steroids, vitamin B_{12}, nonsteroidal anti-inflammatories, or bee venom. Bee venom has some potential based on its anti-nociceptive and anti-inflammatory effects through activation of brainstem catecholaminergic neurons and activation of the α_2 adrenergic and serotonergic pathways of the descending inhibitory system.[316–318] Melitin, an active ingredient of bee venom, can suppress lipopolysaccharide-induced nitric oxide and the transcription of COX-2 genes and pro-inflammatory cytokines, including TNF-α and IL-1β in microglia.[319,320] Injections of bee venom into specific acupuncture points in several animal and human studies of knee arthritis have been shown to be beneficial and reduced pain levels significantly, but there are no studies that demonstrate the effectiveness of trigger point injections with bee venom.[317,321,322]

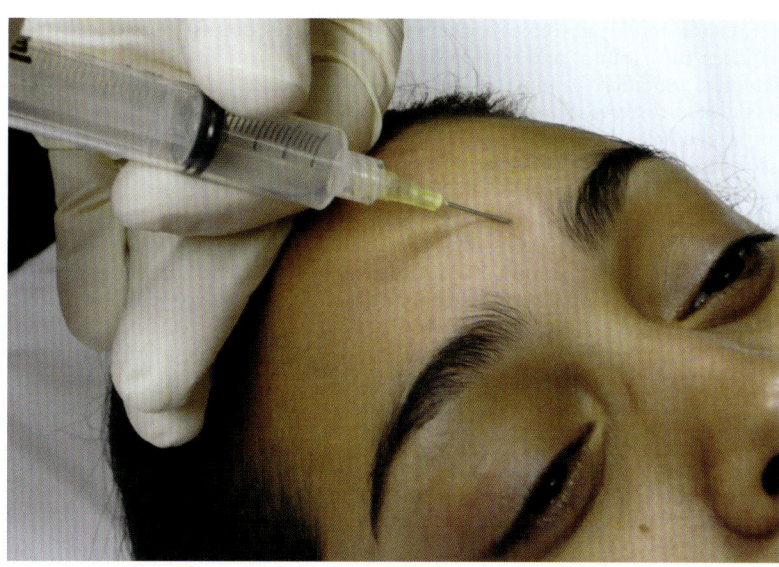

FIGURE 35.9 Trigger point injection to the frontalis muscle.

There is a growing body of literature supporting the use of botulinum toxin in the treatment of myofascial trigger points, although this remains a controversial issue. Many botulinum toxin studies fail to demonstrate superiority of botulinum toxin over placebo.[323] However, clinicians familiar with myofascial trigger points support its use based on the demonstrated mechanisms of botulinum toxin and empirical evidence.[324,325] Indeed, several studies have shown significant benefit of botulinum toxin injections in the treatment of myofascial trigger points and various pain states including migraine, tension-type headache, low back pain, and phantom pain.[326–335] Potential problems with these studies relate to the use of different dosages, varying injection sites, and the degree of familiarity with myofascial trigger points.[336] Botulinum toxin prevents the release of ACh from the presynpatic nerve terminal.[337] ACh is released in response to evoked stimulation of the nerve or spontaneously without axonal nerve activation.[87,338,339] Botulinum toxin also has an anti-nociceptive effect, which in part may be due to its ability to also block the release of CGRP from the nerve terminal.[340–342]

Extensive training is required to gain the necessary palpation skills and kinesthetic awareness, without which trigger point needling would become a random process. Anatomical knowledge is required prior to developing the sensory motor skills needed to visualize the tip of the needle and the pathway the needle follows inside patients' bodies.[191] Clinicians should be able to visualize a three-dimensional image of the exact location and depth of the trigger point and accurately elicit local twitch responses. The needle should not be used as a search tool except in muscles that cannot be palpated directly, such as the subscapularis or lateral pterygoid muscles.[343,344] Trained clinicians can almost always identify clinically relevant trigger points, except in obese patients where certain muscles may not be accessible to palpation.[191] Myofascial trigger point injections were the second most common procedure after epidural injections in a study of Canadian pain anesthesiologists, although the art of trigger point injections and trigger point palpation is not usually covered in medical schools, and there are no formal postgraduate training programs in Canada.[345]

Dry needling and injections can eliminate or reduce trigger point pain often in just a few sessions with a skilled clinician, allowing the patient to be more successful in the conditioning phase of the rehabilitation program.[51,131,346] There are many clinical outcome studies confirming that needling therapies are effective in inactivating trigger points, reducing pain levels, and improving function.[212,239,293,347–358]

In spite of a rapidly increasing number of clinical outcome studies, the exact mechanisms of trigger point injections and dry needling are still not known.[191] Deep dry needling and trigger point injections may destroy motor endplates and cause distal axon denervations,[359] which may trigger changes in the endplate cholinesterase and ACh receptors as part of the normal muscle regeneration process.[360,361] In a rodent study, dry needling caused a significant decrease of spontaneous electrical activity and ACh and AChR levels and a significant increase of AChE.[362]

It is likely that trigger point needling involves central pain mechanisms, including the limbic system, the subcortical gray structures, and the descending inhibitory system. Most deep needling procedures are painful, possibly stretch fibroblasts in connective tissues, and activate the enkephalinergic, serotonergic, and noradrenergic inhibitory systems associated with Aδ fibers through segmental inhibition.[363–365] Superficial dry needling is often explained in a similar fashion but is a painless procedure that would not activate Aδ fibers unless the needle is rotated after insertion.[191,306] Aδ nerve fibers are only activated by nociceptive mechanical stimulation for type I high-threshold Aδ fibers or by cold stimuli for type II Aδ fibers. It is conceivable that the light stimulus of superficial dry needling activates mechanoreceptors coupled to slow-conducting unmyelinated C-fiber afferents, stimulating the anterior cingulate cortex with emotional and hormonal reactions representing a sense of progress, reduction of pain, and well-being.[366–368]

NONINVASIVE TREATMENT OPTIONS

Rickards[369] and Fernández-de-las-Peñas et al.[370] published comprehensive systematic reviews of noninvasive treatment options for myofascial pain. A wide variety of manual therapies are being used in the treatment of myofascial trigger points, such as spray and stretch, trigger point compression, muscle energy techniques, and massage.[371–375] There is some evidence of the short-term effectiveness of manual therapies, but no conclusions can be made in relation to the medium- and long-term effectiveness.[370] Fernández-de-las-Peñas et al.[376] demonstrated that trigger point compression and transverse friction massage were equally effective in treating trigger points with a significant reduction in visual analogue scores and significant increase in the pressure pain threshold. Hou et al.[377] showed that trigger point compression reduced pain levels within minutes.

Several modalities have been applied to trigger points, such as laser, ultrasound, and electrotherapy. Laser proved to be an effective modality in most trials.[378-381] Therapeutic ultrasound has mixed reviews. Srbely and Dickey[382] demonstrated a short-term decrease of the sensitivity of trigger points following ultrasound. Another study of high-power static ultrasound was more beneficial than more traditionally applied ultrasound, whereas two other papers did not show any benefit of ultrasound.[383-386] Transcutaneous electrical stimulation is the most studied electrotherapy modality, but it remains difficult to draw any conclusions beyond short-term effects.[299,387-389] A prospective, randomized study of extracorporeal shockwave therapy in the treatment of athletes with acute or chronic shoulder pain showed significantly improved isokinetic force production, a reduction in pain, and overall performance.[390]

Summary

Myofascial trigger points are a very common cause of clinically observed local muscle pain, tenderness, and referred pain in patients with acute and chronic pain. However, they are also a common physical finding in asymptomatic individuals. This dichotomy challenges and behooves pain management practitioners to learn how to palpate the soft tissue and distinguish active from latent myofascial trigger points. Making this distinction is critical in order to adequately identify and treat a myofascial component of pain. Several independent and emerging lines of scientific inquiry, including histologic, neurophysiologic, biochemical, and somatosensory research into the nature of myofascial trigger points have revealed objective abnormalities. These findings suggest that myofascial pain consists of both motor and sensory abnormalities involving the peripheral and central nervous systems. Accordingly, active myofascial trigger points may be viewed as part of a complex series of changes in the peripheral tissue and central nervous system that occur with central sensitization, characteristic of a form of neuromuscular dysfunction. From this perspective, future clinical research studies should focus on identifying the mechanisms responsible for the pathogenesis, amplification, and perpetuation of myofascial pain syndrome. Successful treatment depends on identifying and targeting these mechanisms and addressing the perpetuating factors that sustain this common pain syndrome.

References

1. Chaiamnuay P, Darmawan J, Muirden KD, et al. Epidemiology of rheumatic disease in rural Thailand: a WHO-ILAR COPCORD study. Community Oriented Programme for the Control of Rheumatic Disease. *J Rheumatol* 1998;25(7):1382–1387.
2. McBeth J, Jones K. Epidemiology of chronic musculoskeletal pain. *Best Pract Res Clin Rheumatol* 2007;21(3):403–425.
3. Wall PD, Woolf CJ. Muscle but not cutaneous C-afferent input produces prolonged increases in the excitability of the flexion reflex in the rat. *J Physiol* 1984;356:443–458.
4. Niddam DM, Chan RC, Lee SH, et al. Central modulation of pain evoked from myofascial trigger point. *Clin J Pain* 2007;23(5):440–448.
5. Niddam DM, Chan RC, Lee SH, et al. Central representation of hyperalgesia from myofascial trigger point. *Neuroimage* 2008;39(3):1299–1306.
6. Mense S. Nociception from skeletal muscle in relation to clinical muscle pain. *Pain* 1993;54:241–289.
7. Handwerker HO, Arendt-Nielsen L. *Pain Models: Translational Relevance and Applications*. Washington, DC: IASP Press; 2013.
8. Cooper G, Bailey B, Bogduk N. Cervical zygapophysial joint pain maps. *Pain Med* 2007;8(4):344–353.
9. Kirmayer LJ, Looper KJ. Abnormal illness behaviour: physiological, psychological and social dimensions of coping with distress. *Curr Opin Psychiatry* 2006;19(1):54–60.
10. Sullivan MD, Cahana A, Derbyshire S, et al. What does it mean to call chronic pain a brain disease? *J Pain* 2013;14(4):317–322.
11. Mennell J. Spray-stretch for the relief of pain from muscle spasm and myofascial trigger points. *J Am Podiatry Assoc* 1976;66(11):873–876.
12. Mennell J. Myofascial trigger points as a cause of headaches. *J Manipulative Physiol Ther* 1989;12(4):308–313.
13. Simons DG. Orphan organ. *J Musculoskelet Pain* 2007;15(2):7–9.
14. Simons DG. Muscle pain syndromes—part 1. *Am J Phys Med* 1975;54:289–311.
15. Wilson VP. Janet G. Travell, MD: a daughter's recollection. *Tex Heart Inst J* 2003;30(1):8–12.
16. Travell JG, Rinzler S, Herman M. Pain and disability of the shoulder and arm: treatment by intramuscular infiltration with procaine hydrochloride. *JAMA* 1942;120:417–422.
17. Travell JG, Rinzler SH. The myofascial genesis of pain. *Postgrad Med* 1952;11(5):425–434.
18. Hoheisel U, Mense S. Inflammation of the thoracolumbar fascia excites and sensitizes rat dorsal horn neurons. *Eur J Pain* 2015;19(3):419–428.
19. Simons DG, Travell JG, Simons LS. *Upper Half of the Body*. 2nd ed. Baltimore, MD: Lippincott Williams & Wilkins; 1999. *Travell & Simons' Myofascial Pain and Dysfunction: The Trigger Point Manual*; vol 1.
20. Travell JG, Simons DG. *The Lower Extremities*. Baltimore, MD: Lippincott Williams & Wilkins; 1992. *Myofascial Pain and Dysfunction: The Trigger Point Manual*; vol 2.
21. Steindler A. The interpretation of sciatic radiation and the syndrome of low-back pain. *J Bone Joint Surg Am* 1940;22:28–34.
22. Simons DG. Review of enigmatic MTrPs as a common cause of enigmatic musculoskeletal pain and dysfunction. *J Electromyogr Kinesiol* 2004;14:95–107.
23. Robinson JP, Arendt-Nielsen L. Muscle pain syndromes. In: Braddom RL, ed. *Physical Medicine and Rehabilitation*. 3rd ed. Philadelphia: Elsevier; 2007:989–1020.
24. Simons DG, Travell JG. Myofascial trigger points, a possible explanation. *Pain* 1981;10(1):106–109.
25. McPartland JM, Simons DG. Myofascial trigger points: translating molecular theory into manual therapy. *J Man Manip Ther* 2006;14(4):232–239.
26. Gerwin RD, Dommerholt J, Shah JP. An expansion of Simons' integrated hypothesis of trigger point formation. *Curr Pain Headache Rep* 2004;8(6):468–475.
27. Jafri MS. Mechanisms of myofascial pain. *Int Sch Res Notices* 2014;2014.
28. Dommerholt J, Bron C, Franssen JLM. Myofascial trigger points: an evidence-informed review. *J Man Manip Ther* 2006;14(4):203–221.
29. Jarrell J. Myofascial pain in the adolescent. *Curr Opin Obstet Gynecol* 2010;22(5):393–398.
30. Jarrell J, Giamberardino MA, Robert M, et al. Bedside testing for chronic pelvic pain: discriminating visceral from somatic pain. *Pain Res Treat* 2011;2011:692102.
31. Zermann DH, Ishigooka M, Doggweiler R, et al. Chronic prostatitis: a myofascial pain syndrome? *Infect Urol* 1999;12(3):84–92.
32. Anderson RU, Sawyer T, Wise D, et al. Painful myofascial trigger points and pain sites in men with chronic prostatitis/chronic pelvic pain syndrome. *J Urol* 2009;182(6):2753–2758.
33. Weiss JM. Pelvic floor myofascial trigger points: manual therapy for interstitial cystitis and the urgency-frequency syndrome. *J Urol* 2001;166(6):2226–2231.
34. Hendler NH, Kozikowski JG. Overlooked physical diagnoses in chronic pain patients involved in litigation. *Psychosomatics* 1993;34(6):494–501.
35. Vecchiet L. Muscle pain and aging. *J Musculoskelet Pain* 2002;10(1/2):5–22.
36. Alfven G. The pressure pain threshold (PPT) of certain muscles in children suffering from recurrent abdominal pain of non-organic origin. An algometric study. *Acta Paediatr* 1993;82(5):481–483.
37. Zapata AL, Moraes AJ, Leone C, et al. Pain and musculoskeletal pain syndromes in adolescents. *J Adolesc Health* 2006;38(6):769–771.
38. Kao MJ, Han TI, Kuan TS, et al. Myofascial trigger points in early life. *Arch Phys Med Rehabil* 2007;88(2):251–254.
39. Cimbiz A, Beydemir F, Manisaligil U. Evaluation of trigger points in young subjects. *J Musculoskelet Pain* 2006;14(4):27–35.
40. Chen Q, Basford J, An KN. Ability of magnetic resonance elastography to assess taut bands. *Clin Biomech (Bristol, Avon)* 2008;23(5):623–629.
41. Chen Q, Bensamoun S, Basford JR, et al. Identification and quantification of myofascial taut bands with magnetic resonance elastography. *Arch Phys Med Rehabil* 2007;88(12):1658–1661.
42. Chen Q, Wang HJ, Gay RE, et al. Quantification of myofascial taut bands. *Arch Phys Med Rehabil* 2016;97(1):67–73.
43. Ringleb SI, Bensamoun SF, Chen Q, et al. Applications of magnetic resonance elastography to healthy and pathologic skeletal muscle. *J Magn Reson Imaging* 2007;25(2):301–309.
44. Sikdar S, Ortiz R, Gebreab T, et al. Understanding the vascular environment of myofascial trigger points using ultrasonic imaging and computational modeling. *Conf Proc IEEE Eng Med Biol Soc* 2010;1:5302–5305.
45. Turo D, Otto P, Hossain M, et al. Novel use of ultrasound elastography to quantify muscle tissue changes after dry needling of myofascial trigger points in patients with chronic myofascial pain. *J Ultrasound Med* 2015;34(12):2149–2161.
46. Turo D, Otto P, Shah JP, et al. Ultrasonic characterization of the upper trapezius muscle in patients with chronic neck pain. *Ultrason Imaging* 2013;35(2):173–187.

47. Gizzi L, Muceli S, Petzke F, et al. Experimental muscle pain impairs the synergistic modular control of neck muscles. *PLoS One* 2015;10(9):e0137844.

48. Hedayatpour N, Falla D. Physiological and neural adaptations to eccentric exercise: mechanisms and considerations for training. *Biomed Res Int* 2015;2015:193741.

49. Arendt-Nielsen L, Falla D. Motor control adjustments in musculoskeletal pain and the implications for pain recurrence. *Pain* 2009;142(3):171–172.

50. Bohlooli N, Ahmadi A, Maroufi N, et al. Differential activation of scapular muscles, during arm elevation, with and without trigger points. *J Bodyw Mov Ther* 2016;20:26–34.

51. Lucas KR, Polus BI, Rich PS. Latent myofascial trigger points: their effects on muscle activation and movement efficiency. *J Bodyw Mov Ther* 2004;8:160–166.

52. Lucas KR, Rich PA, Polus BI. Muscle activation patterns in the scapular positioning muscles during loaded scapular plane elevation: the effects of latent myofascial trigger points. *Clin Biomechanics* 2010;25(8):765–770.

53. Ge HY, Fernández-de-las-Peñas C, Arendt-Nielsen L. Sympathetic facilitation of hyperalgesia evoked from myofascial tender and trigger points in patients with unilateral shoulder pain. *Clin Neurophysiol* 2006;117(7):1545–1550.

54. Capes EM, Loaiza R, Valdivia HH. Ryanodine receptors. *Skelet Muscle* 2011;1(1):18.

55. Clark KA, McElhinny AS, Beckerle MC, et al. Striated muscle cytoarchitecture: an intricate web of form and function. *Annu Rev Cell Dev Biol* 2002;18:637–706.

56. Houdusse A, Sweeney HL. How myosin generates force on actin filaments. *Trends Biochem Sci* 2016;41(12):989–997.

57. Lindstedt SL, Reich TE, Keim P, et al. Do muscles function as adaptable locomotor springs? *J Exp Biol* 2002;205(pt 15):2211–2216.

58. Wang K, McCarter R, Wright J, et al. Viscoelasticity of the sarcomere matrix in skeletal muscles. The titin–myosin composite filament is a dual-stage molecular spring. *Biophys J* 1993;64:1161–1177.

59. Nagy A, Cacciafesta P, Grama L, et al. Differential actin binding along the PEVK domain of skeletal muscle titin. *J Cell Sci* 2004;117(pt 24):5781–5789.

60. Niederlander N, Raynaud F, Astier C, et al. Regulation of the actin-myosin interaction by titin. *Eur J Biochem* 2004;271(22):4572–4581.

61. Wang K. Titin/connectin and nebulin: giant protein rulers of muscle structure and function. *Adv Biophys* 1996;33:123–134.

62. Gregorio CC, Granzier H, Sorimachi H, et al. Muscle assembly: a titanic achievement? *Curr Opin Cell Biol* 1999;11(1):18–25.

63. Rivas-Pardo JA, Eckels EC, Popa I, et al. Work done by titin protein folding assists muscle contraction. *Cell Rep* 2016;14(6):1339–1347.

64. Ma K, Wang K. Interaction of nebulin SH3 domain with titin PEVK and myopalladin: implications for the signaling and assembly role of titin and nebulin. *FEBS Lett* 2002;532(3):273–278.

65. McElhinny AS, Kazmierski ST, Labeit S, et al. Nebulin: the nebulous, multifunctional giant of striated muscle. *Trends Cardiovasc Med* 2003;13(5):195–201.

66. Bang ML, Mudry RE, McElhinny AS, et al. Myopalladin, a novel 145-kilodalton sarcomeric protein with multiple roles in Z-disc and I-band protein assemblies. *J Cell Biol* 2001;153(2):413–427.

67. Bang ML, Gregorio C, Labeit S. Molecular dissection of the interaction of desmin with the C-terminal region of nebulin. *J Struct Biol* 2002;137(1–2):119–127.

68. McElhinny AS, Kolmerer B, Fowler VM, et al. The N-terminal end of nebulin interacts with tropomodulin at the pointed ends of the thin filaments. *J Biol Chem* 2001;276(1):583–592.

69. Jin JP, Wang K. Nebulin as a giant actin-binding template protein in skeletal muscle sarcomere. Interaction of actin and cloned human nebulin fragments. *FEBS Lett* 1991;281(1–2):93–96.

70. Chu M, Gregorio CC, Pappas CT. Nebulin, a multi-functional giant. *J Exp Biol* 2016;219(pt 2):146–152.

71. Pappas CT, Bliss KT, Zieseniss A, et al. The Nebulin family: an actin support group. *Trends Cell Biol* 2011;21(1):29–37.

72. Ohtsuki I, Morimoto S. Troponin: regulatory function and disorders. *Biochem Biophys Res Commun* 2008;369(1):62–73.

73. Gray KT, Kostyukova AS, Fath T. Actin regulation by tropomodulin and tropomyosin in neuronal morphogenesis and function. *Mol Cell Neurosci* 2017;84:48–57.

74. Arrowsmith JE. The neuromuscular junction. *Surgery (Oxford)* 2007;25(3):105–111.

75. Hubbard DR, Berkoff GM. Myofascial trigger points show spontaneous needle EMG activity. *Spine* 1993;18:1803–1807.

76. Hong CZ, Yu J. Spontaneous electrical activity of rabbit trigger spot after transection of spinal cord and peripheral nerve. *J Musculoskelet Pain* 1998;6(4):45–58.

77. Simons DG. Do endplate noise and spikes arise from normal motor endplates? *Am J Phys Med Rehabil* 2001;80:134–140.

78. Simons DG, Hong CZ, Simons LS. Endplate potentials are common to midfiber myofascial trigger points. *Am J Phys Med Rehabil* 2002;81(3):212–222.

79. Chen JT, Chen SM, Kuan TS, et al. Phentolamine effect on the spontaneous electrical activity of active loci in a myofascial trigger spot of rabbit skeletal muscle. *Arch Phys Med Rehabil* 1998;79(7):790–794.

80. Kuan TS, Chen JT, Chen SM, et al. Effect of botulinum toxin on endplate noise in myofascial trigger spots of rabbit skeletal muscle. *Am J Phys Med Rehabil* 2002;81(7):512–520.

81. Mense S, Simons DG, Hoheisel U, et al. Lesions of rat skeletal muscle after local block of acetylcholinesterase and neuromuscular stimulation. *J Appl Physiol* 2003;94(6):2494–2501.

82. Couppé C, Midttun A, Hilden J, et al. Spontaneous needle electromyographic activity in myofascial trigger points in the infraspinatus muscle: a blinded assessment. *J Musculoskelet Pain* 2001;9(3):7–17.

83. Macgregor J, Graf von Schweinitz D. Needle electromyographic activity of myofascial trigger points and control sites in equine cleidobrachialis muscle—an observational study. *Acupunct Med* 2006;24(2):61–70.

84. Maekawa K, Clark GT, Kuboki T. Intramuscular hypoperfusion, adrenergic receptors, and chronic muscle pain. *J Pain* 2002;3(4):251–260.

85. Henriksson KG, Bengtsson A, Lindman R, et al. Morphological changes in muscle in fibromyalgia and chronic shoulder myalgia. In: Værøy H, Merskey H, eds. *Progress in Fibromyalgia and Myofascial Pain*. Amsterdam, The Netherlands: Elsevier;1993:61–73.

86. McPartland JM. Travell trigger points—molecular and osteopathic perspectives. *J Am Osteopath Assoc* 2004;104(6):244–249.

87. Bukharaeva EA, Salakhutdinov RI, Vyskocil F, et al. Spontaneous quantal and non-quantal release of acetylcholine at mouse endplate during onset of hypoxia. *Physiol Res* 2005;54(2):251–255.

88. Chen BM, Grinnell AD. Kinetics, Ca2+ dependence, and biophysical properties of integrin-mediated mechanical modulation of transmitter release from frog motor nerve terminals. *J Neurosci* 1997;17(3):904–916.

89. Grinnell AD, Chen BM, Kashani A, et al. The role of integrins in the modulation of neurotransmitter release from motor nerve terminals by stretch and hypertonicity. *J Neurocytol* 2003;32(5–8):489–503.

90. Graven-Nielsen T, Arendt-Nielsen L. Induction and assessment of muscle pain, referred pain, and muscular hyperalgesia. *Curr Pain Headache Rep* 2003;7(6):443–451.

91. Sluka KA, Kalra A, Moore SA. Unilateral intramuscular injections of acidic saline produce a bilateral, long-lasting hyperalgesia. *Muscle Nerve* 2001;24(1):37–46.

92. Sluka KA, Price MP, Breese NM, et al. Chronic hyperalgesia induced by repeated acid injections in muscle is abolished by the loss of ASIC3, but not ASIC1. *Pain* 2003;106(3):229–239.

93. Barash IA, Peters D, Fridén J, et al. Desmin cytoskeletal modifications after a bout of eccentric exercise in the rat. *Am J Physiol Regul Integr Comp Physiol* 2002;283(4):R958–R963.

94. Peters D, Barash IA, Burdi M, et al. Asynchronous functional, cellular and transcriptional changes after a bout of eccentric exercise in the rat. *J Physiol* 2003;553(pt 3):947–957.

95. Fridén J, Lieber RL. Segmental muscle fiber lesions after repetitive eccentric contractions. *Cell Tissue Res* 1998;293(1):165–171.

96. Lieber RL, Shah S, Fridén J. Cytoskeletal disruption after eccentric contraction-induced muscle injury. *Clin Orthop Relat Res* 2002(403 suppl):S90–S99.

97. Stauber WT, Clarkson PM, Fritz VK, et al. Extracellular matrix disruption and pain after eccentric muscle action. *J Appl Physiol* 1990;69(3):868–874.

98. Thompson JL, Balog EM, Fitts RH, et al. Five myofibrillar lesion types in eccentrically challenged, unloaded rat adductor longus muscle—a test model. *Anat Rec* 1999;254(1):39–52.

99. Reitinger A, Radner H, Tilscher H, et al. Morphologische untersuchung an triggerpunkten. *Manuelle Medizin* 1996;34:256–262.

100. Windisch A, Reitinger A, Traxler H, et al. Morphology and histochemistry of myogelosis. *Clin Anat* 1999;12(4):266–271.

101. Simons DG, Stolov WC. Microscopic features and transient contraction of palpable bands in canine muscle. *Am J Phys Med* 1976;55(2):65–88.

102. Wall R. Introduction to myofascial trigger points in dogs. *Top Companion Anim Med* 2014;29(2):43–48.

103. Frank EM. Myofascial trigger point diagnostic criteria in the dog. *J Musculoskelet Pain* 1999;7(1–2):231–237.

104. Bron C, Dommerholt J. Etiology of myofascial trigger points. *Curr Pain Headache Rep* 2012;16(5):439–444.

105. Itoh K, Okada K, Kawakita K. A proposed experimental model of myofascial trigger points in human muscle after slow eccentric exercise. *Acupunct Med* 2004;22(1):2–13.

106. Chen SM, Chen JT, Kuan TS, et al. Decrease in pressure pain thresholds of latent myofascial trigger points in the middle finger extensors immediately after continuous piano practice. *J Musculoskelet Pain* 2000;8(3):83–92.

107. Hoyle JA, Marras WS, Sheedy JE, et al. Effects of postural and visual stressors on myofascial trigger point development and motor unit rotation during computer work. *J Electromyogr Kinesiol* 2011;21(1):41–48.

108. Treaster D, Marras WS, Burr D, et al. Myofascial trigger point development from visual and postural stressors during computer work. *J Electromyogr Kinesiol* 2006;16(2):115–124.

109. Hägg GM. The Cinderella hypothesis. In: Johansson H, Windhorst U, Djupsjöbacka M, et al, eds. *Chronic Work-Related Myalgia*. Gävle, Sweden: Gävle University Press; 2003:127–132.

110. Forsman M, Taoda K, Thorn S, et al. Motor-unit recruitment during long-term isometric and wrist motion contractions: a study concerning muscular pain development in computer operators. *Int J Ind Ergon* 2002;30:237–250.

111. Zennaro D, Laubli T, Krebs D, et al. Trapezius muscle motor unit activity in symptomatic participants during finger tapping using properly and improperly adjusted desks. *Hum Factors* 2004;46(2):252–266.

112. Febbraio MA, Pedersen BK. Contraction-induced myokine production and release: is skeletal muscle an endocrine organ? *Exerc Sport Sci Rev* 2005;33(3):114–119.

113. Gissel H. Ca2+ accumulation and cell damage in skeletal muscle during low frequency stimulation. *Eur J Appl Physiol* 2000;83(2–3):175–180.

114. Lexell J, Jarvis J, Downham D, et al. Stimulation-induced damage in rabbit fast-twitch skeletal muscles: a quantitative morphological study of the influence of pattern and frequency. *Cell Tissue Res* 1993;273(2):357–362.

115. Pedersen BK, Steensberg A, Keller P, et al. Muscle-derived interleukin-6: lipolytic, anti-inflammatory and immune regulatory effects. *Pflugers Arch* 2003;446(1):9–16.

116. Otten E. Concepts and models of functional architecture in skeletal muscle. *Exerc Sport Sci Rev* 1988;16:89–137.

117. Mense S. The pathogenesis of muscle pain. *Curr Pain Headache Rep* 2003;7(6):419–425.

118. Vyklicky L, Knotkova-Urbancova H, Vitaskova Z, et al. Inflammatory mediators at acid pH activate capsaicin receptors in cultured sensory neurons from newborn rats. *J Neurophysiol* 1998;79:670–676.

119. Jensen K, Tuxen C, Pedersen-Bjergaard U, et al. Pain and tenderness in human temporal muscle induced by bradykinin and 5-hydroxytryptamine. *Peptides* 1990;11(6):1127–1132.

120. Pinho-Ribeiro FA, Verri WA Jr, Chiu IM. Nociceptor sensory neuron-immune interactions in pain and inflammation. *Trends Immunol* 2017;38(1):5–19.

121. Ambalavanar R, Dessem D, Moutanni A, et al. Muscle inflammation induces a rapid increase in calcitonin gene-related peptide (CGRP) mRNA that temporally relates to CGRP immunoreactivity and nociceptive behavior. *Neuroscience* 2006;143(3):875–884.

122. Snijdelaar DG, Dirksen R, Slappendel R, et al. Substance. *Eur J Pain* 2000;4(2):121–131.

123. Massaad CA, Safieh-Garabedian B, Poole S, et al. Involvement of substance P, CGRP and histamine in the hyperalgesia and cytokine upregulation induced by intraplantar injection of capsaicin in rats. *J Neuroimmunol* 2004;153(1–2):171–82.

124. Mense S. Pathophysiologic basis of muscle pain syndromes. In: Fischer AA, ed. *Myofascial Pain: Update in Diagnosis and Treatment*. Philadelphia: W.B. Saunders Company; 1997:23–53.

125. Mense S. Muscle pain: mechanisms and clinical significance. *Dtsch Arztebl Int* 2008;105(12):214–219.

126. Leeb-Lundberg LM, Marceau F, Müller-Esterl W, et al. International union of pharmacology. XLV. Classification of the kinin receptor family: from molecular mechanisms to pathophysiological consequences. *Pharmacol Rev* 2005;57(1):27–77.

127. Zhang X, Brovkovych V, Zhang Y, et al. Downregulation of kinin B1 receptor function by B2 receptor heterodimerization and signaling. *Cell Signal* 2015;27(1):90–103.

128. Marceau F, Sabourin T, Houle S, et al. Kinin receptors: functional aspects. *Int Immunopharmacol* 2002;2(13–14):1729–1739.

129. Hoheisel U, Taguchi T, Treede RD, et al. Nociceptive input from the rat thoracolumbar fascia to lumbar dorsal horn neurones. *Eur J Pain* 2011;15(8):810–815.

130. Fernández-de-las-Peñas C, Dommerholt J. Myofascial trigger points: peripheral or central phenomenon? *Curr Rheumatol Rep* 2014;16(1):395.

131. Giamberardino MA, Tafuri E, Savini A, et al. Contribution of myofascial trigger points to migraine symptoms. *J Pain* 2007;8(11):869–878.

132. Giamberardino MA, Affaitati G, Iezzi S, et al. Referred muscle pain and hyperalgesia from viscera. *J Musculoskelet Pain* 1999;7(1/2):61–69.

133. Vecchiet L, Giamberardino MA, Dragani L. Latent myofascial trigger points: changes in muscular and subcutaneous pain thresholds at trigger point and target level. *J Manual Medicine* 1990;5:151–154.

134. Vecchiet L, Pizzigallo E, Iezzi S, et al. Differentiation of sensitivity in different tissues and its clinical significance. *J Musculoskelet Pain* 1998;6(1):33–45.

135. Calvo-Lobo C, Diez-Vega I, Martínez-Pascual B, et al. Tensiomyography, sonoelastography, and mechanosensitivity differences between active, latent, and control low back myofascial trigger points: a cross-sectional study. *Medicine (Baltimore)* 2017;96(10):e6287.

136. Hoheisel U, Mense S, Simons D, et al. Appearance of new receptive fields in rat dorsal horn neurons following noxious stimulation of skeletal muscle: a model for referral of muscle pain? *Neurosci Lett* 1993;153:9–12.

137. Shah JP, Danoff JV, Desai MJ, et al. Biochemicals associated with pain and inflammation are elevated in sites near to and remote from active myofascial trigger points. *Arch Phys Med Rehabil* 2008;89(1):16–23.

138. Shah JP, Phillips TM, Danoff JV, et al. An in vivo microanalytical technique for measuring the local biochemical milieu of human skeletal muscle. *J Appl Physiol* 2005;99:1977–1984.

139. Hoheisel U, Koch K, Mense S. Functional reorganization in the rat dorsal horn during an experimental myositis. *Pain* 1994;59(1):111–118.

140. Mense S. Referral of muscle pain: new aspects. *Amer Pain Soc J* 1994;3:1–9.

141. Caumo W, Deitos A, Carvalho S, et al. Motor cortex excitability and BDNF levels in chronic musculoskeletal pain according to structural pathology. *Front Hum Neurosci* 2016;10:357.

142. Botelho LM, Morales-Quezada L, Rozisky JR, et al. A framework for understanding the relationship between descending pain modulation, motor corticospinal, and neuroplasticity regulation systems in chronic myofascial pain. *Front Hum Neurosci* 2016;10:308.

143. Kwon M, Altin M, Duenas H, et al. The role of descending inhibitory pathways on chronic pain modulation and clinical implications. *Pain Pract* 2014;14(7):656–667.

144. Defrin R, Riabinin M, Feingold Y, et al. Deficient pain modulatory systems in patients with mild traumatic brain and chronic post-traumatic headache: implications for its mechanism. *J Neurotrauma* 2015;32(1):28–37.

145. Xie P, Qin B, Song G, et al. Microstructural abnormalities were found in brain gray matter from patients with chronic myofascial pain. *Front Neuroanat* 2016;10:122.

146. Thibaut A, Simis M, Battistella LR, et al. Using brain oscillations and corticospinal excitability to understand and predict post-stroke motor function. *Front Neurol* 2017;8:187.

147. Milligan ED, Watkins LR. Pathological and protective roles of glia in chronic pain. *Nat Rev Neurosci* 2009;10(1):23–36.

148. Watkins LR, Hutchinson MR, Milligan ED, et al. "Listening" and "talking" to neurons: implications of immune activation for pain control and increasing the efficacy of opioids. *Brain Res Rev* 2007;56(1):148–169.

149. Watkins LR, Milligan ED, Maier SF. Glial activation: a driving force for pathological pain. *Trends Neurosci* 2001;24(8):450–455.

150. Fields RD, Stevens-Graham B. New insights into neuron-glia communication. *Science* 2002;298(5593):556–562.

151. Chacur M, Lambertz D, Hoheisel U, et al. Role of spinal microglia in myositis-induced central sensitisation: an immunohistochemical and behavioural study in rats. *Eur J Pain* 2009;13(9):915–923.

152. Zhang J, Mense S, Treede RD, et al. Prevention and reversal of latent sensitization of dorsal horn neurons by glial blockers in a model of low back pain in male rats. *J Neurophysiol* 2017;118:2059–2069.

153. Fernández de las Peñas C, Cuadrado M, Arendt-Nielsen L, et al. Myofascial trigger points and sensitization: an updated pain model for tension-type headache. *Cephalalgia* 2007;27(5):383–393.

154. Jarrell J. Myofascial dysfunction in the pelvis. *Curr Pain Headache Rep* 2004;8(6):452–456.

155. Jarrell J, Robert M. Myofascial dysfunction and pelvic pain. *Can J CME* 2003:107–116.

156. Shoskes DA, Berger R, Elmi A, et al. Muscle tenderness in men with chronic prostatitis/chronic pelvic pain syndrome: the chronic prostatitis cohort study. *J Urol* 2008;179(2):556–560.

157. Fernández-de-las-Peñas C, Fernández Carnero J, Miangolarra-Page JC. Musculoskeletal disorders in mechanical neck pain: myofascial trigger points versus cervical joint dysfunction. *J Musculoskelet Pain* 2005;13(1):27–35.

158. Ruiz-Saez M, Fernández-de-las-Peñas C, Blanco CR, et al. Changes in pressure pain sensitivity in latent myofascial trigger points in the upper trapezius muscle after a cervical spine manipulation in pain-free subjects. *J Manipulative Physiol Ther* 2007;30(8):578–583.

159. Fukui S, Ohseto K, Shiotani M, et al. Referred pain distribution of the cervical zygapophyseal joints and cervical dorsal rami. *Pain* 1996;68:79–83.

160. O'Neill CW, Kurgansky ME, Derby R, et al. Disc stimulation and patterns of referred pain. *Spine* 2002;27(24):2776–2781.

161. Petros P, Bornstein J. Re: vulvar vestibulitis may be a referred pain arising from laxity in the uterosacral ligaments: a hypothesis based on three prospective case reports. *Aust N Z J Obstet Gynaecol* 2004;44(5):484–485.

162. Hackett GS. Referred pain from low back ligament disability. *AMA Arch Surg* 1956;73(5):878–883.

163. Bogduk N, Simons DG. Neck pain: joint pain or trigger points. In: Værøy H, Merskey H, eds. *Progress in Fibromyalgia and Myofascial Pain*. Amsterdam, The Netherlands: Elsevier; 1993:267–273.

164. Rubin TK, Gandevia SC, Henderson LA, et al. Effects of intramuscular anesthesia on the expression of primary and referred pain induced by intramuscular injection of hypertonic saline. *J Pain* 2009;10(8):829–835.

165. Rubin TK, Henderson LA, Macefield VG. Changes in the spatiotemporal expression of local and referred pain following repeated intramuscular injections of hypertonic saline: a longitudinal study. *J Pain* 2010;11(8):737–745.

166. Fernández-Carnero J, Fernández-de-las-Peñas CF, de la Llave-Rincon AI, et al. Prevalence of and referred pain from myofascial trigger points in the forearm muscles in patients with lateral epicondylalgia. *Clin J Pain* 2007;23(4):353–360.

167. Hsieh YL, Kao MJ, Kuan TS, et al. Dry needling to a key myofascial trigger point may reduce the irritability of satellite MTrPs. *Am J Phys Med Rehabil* 2007;86(5):397–403.

168. Carlson CR, Okeson JP, Falace DA, et al. Reduction of pain and EMG activity in the masseter region by trapezius trigger point injection. *Pain* 1993;55(3):397–400.

169. Headley BJ. Evaluation and treatment of myofascial pain syndrome utilizing biofeedback. In: Cram JR, ed. *Clinical Electromyography for Surface Recordings.* Nevada City, CA: Clinical Resources; 1990:235–254.

170. Gerber LH, Sikdar S, Armstrong K, et al. A systematic comparison between subjects with no pain and pain associated with active myofascial trigger points. *PM R* 2013;5(11):931–938.

171. Bajaj P, Bajaj P, Graven-Nielsen T, et al. Trigger points in patients with lower limb osteoarthritis. *J Musculoskelet Pain* 2001;9(3):17–33.

172. Hoheisel U, Reuter R, de Freitas MF, et al. Injection of nerve growth factor into a low back muscle induces long-lasting latent hypersensitivity in rat dorsal horn neurons. *Pain* 2013;154(10):1953–1960.

173. Srbely JZ. New trends in the treatment and management of myofascial pain syndrome. *Curr Pain Headache Rep* 2010;14(5):346–352.

174. Richardson JD, Vasko MR. Cellular mechanisms of neurogenic inflammation. *J Pharmacol Exp Ther* 2002;302(3):839–845.

175. Hocking MJ. Exploring the central modulation hypothesis: do ancient memory mechanisms underlie the pathophysiology of trigger points? *Curr Pain Headache Rep* 2013;17(7):347.

176. Hocking MJ. Trigger points and central modulation—a new hypothesis. *J Musculoskelet Pain* 2010;18(2):186–203.

177. Stofan DA, Callahan LA, DiMARCO AF, et al. Modulation of release of reactive oxygen species by the contracting diaphragm. *Am J Respir Crit Care Med* 2000;161(3 pt 1):891–898.

178. Powers SK, Radak Z, Ji LL. Exercise-induced oxidative stress: past, present and future. *J Physiol* 2016;594(18):5081–5092.

179. Santos CX, Anilkumar N, Zhang M, et al. Redox signaling in cardiac myocytes. *Free Radic Biol Med* 2011;50(7):777–793.

180. Sirker A, Murdoch CE, Protti A, et al. Cell-specific effects of Nox2 on the acute and chronic response to myocardial infarction. *J Mol Cell Cardiol* 2016;98:11–17.

181. Sirker A, Zhang M, Shah AM. NADPH oxidases in cardiovascular disease: insights from in vivo models and clinical studies. *Basic Res Cardiol* 2011;106(5):735–747.

182. Sakellariou GK, Vasilaki A, Palomero J, et al. Studies of mitochondrial and nonmitochondrial sources implicate nicotinamide adenine dinucleotide phosphate oxidase(s) in the increased skeletal muscle superoxide generation that occurs during contractile activity. *Antioxid Redox Signal* 2013;18(6):603–621.

183. Ibi M, Matsuno K, Shiba D, et al. Reactive oxygen species derived from NOX1/NADPH oxidase enhance inflammatory pain. *J Neurosci* 2008;28(38):9486–9494.

184. Cortright DN, Szallasi A. Biochemical pharmacology of the vanilloid receptor TRPV1. An update. *Eur J Biochem* 2004;271(10):1814–1819.

185. Cui M, Honore P, Zhong C, et al. TRPV1 receptors in the CNS play a key role in broad-spectrum analgesia of TRPV1 antagonists. *J Neurosci* 2006;26(37):9385–9393.

186. Shah J, Phillips T, Danoff JV, et al. A novel microanalytical technique for assaying soft tissue demonstrates significant quantitative biomechanical differences in 3 clinically distinct groups: normal, latent and active. *Arch Phys Med Rehabil* 2003;84:A4.

187. Issberner U, Reeh PW, Steen KH. Pain due to tissue acidosis: a mechanism for inflammatory and ischemic myalgia? *Neurosci Lett* 1996;208(3):191–194.

188. Hong CZ. Persistence of local twitch response with loss of conduction to and from the spinal cord. *Arch Phys Med Rehabil* 1994;75(1):12–16.

189. Hong CZ, Torigoe Y, Yu J. The localized twitch responses in responsive bands of rabbit skeletal muscle are related to the reflexes at spinal cord level. *J Musculoskelet Pain* 1995;3:15–33.

190. Willis WD. Retrograde signaling in the nervous system: dorsal root reflexes. In: Bradshaw RA, Dennis EA, eds. *Handbook of Cell Signaling.* San Diego, CA: Academic/Elsevier Press; 2004.

191. Dommerholt J, Mayoral O, Gröbli C. Trigger point dry needling. *J Man Manip Ther* 2006;14(4):E70–E87.

192. Gordon JR, Galli SJ. Mast cells as a source of both preformed and immunologically inducible TNF-alpha/cachectin. *Nature* 1990;346(6281):274–276.

193. Iuvone T, Den Bossche RV, D'Acquisto F, et al. Evidence that mast cell degranulation, histamine and tumour necrosis factor alpha release occur in LPS-induced plasma leakage in rat skin. *Br J Pharmacol* 1999;128(3):700–704.

194. Bowman WC, Marshall IG, Gibb AJ, et al. Feedback control of transmitter release at the neuromuscular junction. *Trends Pharmacol Sci* 1988;9(1):16–20.

195. Zeilhofer HU, Brune K. Analgesic strategies beyond the inhibition of cyclo-oxygenases. *Trends Pharmacol Sci* 2006;27(9):467–474.

196. Verri WA Jr, Cunha TM, Parada CA, et al. Hypernociceptive role of cytokines and chemokines: targets for analgesic drug development? *Pharmacol Ther* 2006;112(1):116–138.

197. Lund T, Østerud B. The effect of TNF-alpha, PMA, and LPS on plasma and cell-associated IL-8 in human leukocytes. *Thromb Res* 2004;113(1):75–83.

198. Schafers M, Sorkin LS, Sommer C. Intramuscular injection of tumor necrosis factor-alpha induces muscle hyperalgesia in rats. *Pain* 2003;104(3):579–588.

199. Loram LC, Fuller A, Fick LG, et al. Cytokine profiles during carrageenan-induced inflammatory hyperalgesia in rat muscle and hind paw. *J Pain* 2007;8(2):127–136.

200. Loram LC, Fuller A, Cartmell T, et al. Behavioural, histological and cytokine responses during hyperalgesia induced by carrageenan injection in the rat tail. *Physiol Behav* 2007;92(5):873–880.

201. Loram LC, Themistocleous AC, Fick LG, et al. The time course of inflammatory cytokine secretion in a rat model of postoperative pain does not coincide with the onset of mechanical hyperalgesia. *Can J Physiol Pharmacol* 2007;85(6):613–620.

202. Luo G, Hershko DD, Robb BW, et al. IL-1beta stimulates IL-6 production in cultured skeletal muscle cells through activation of MAP kinase signaling pathway and NF-kappa B. *Am J Physiol Regul Integr Comp Physiol* 2003;284(5):R1249–R1254.

203. Samad TA, Moore KA, Sapirstein A, et al. Interleukin-1beta-mediated induction of Cox-2 in the CNS contributes to inflammatory pain hypersensitivity. *Nature* 2001;410(6827):471–475.

204. Tidball JG. Inflammatory processes in muscle injury and repair. *Am J Physiol Regul Integr Comp Physiol* 2005;288(2):R345–R353.

205. Hoheisel U, Unger T, Mense S. Excitatory and modulatory effects of inflammatory cytokines and neurotrophins on mechanosensitive group IV muscle afferents in the rat. *Pain* 2005;114(1–2):168–176.

206. Dworkin SF, LeResche L. Research diagnostic criteria for temporomandibular disorders: review, criteria, examinations and specifications, critique. *J Craniomandib Disord Facial Oral Pain* 1992;6:301–355.

207. Schiffman E, Ohrbach R. Executive summary of the Diagnostic Criteria for Temporomandibular Disorders for clinical and research applications. *J Am Dent Assoc* 2016;147(6):438–445.

208. Escobar PL, Ballesteros J. Teres minor. Source of symptoms resembling ulnar neuropathy or C8 radiculopathy. *Am J Phys Med Rehabil* 1988;67(3):120–122.

209. Facco E, Ceccherelli F. Myofascial pain mimicking radicular syndromes. *Acta Neurochir Suppl* 2005;92:147–150.

210. Crotti FM, Carai A, Carai M, et al. Post-traumatic thoracic outlet syndrome (TOS). *Acta Neurochir Suppl* 2005;92:13–15.

211. Samuel AS, Peter AA, Ramanathan K. The association of active trigger points with lumbar disc lesions. *J Musculoskelet Pain* 2007;15(2):11–18.

212. Mahmoudzadeh A, Rezaeian ZS, Karimi A, et al. The effect of dry needling on the radiating pain in subjects with discogenic low-back pain: a randomized control trial. *J Res Med Sci* 2016;21:86.

213. Ge HY, Nie H, Madeleine P, et al. Contribution of the local and referred pain from active myofascial trigger points in fibromyalgia syndrome. *Pain* 2009;147(1–3):233–240.

214. Ge HY, Wang Y, Danneskiold-Samsøe B, et al. The predetermined sites of examination for tender points in fibromyalgia syndrome are frequently associated with myofascial trigger points. *J Pain* 2010;11(7):644–651.

215. Ge HY, Wang Y, Fernández-de-las-Peñas C, et al. Reproduction of overall spontaneous pain pattern by manual stimulation of active myofascial trigger points in fibromyalgia patients. *Arthritis Res Ther* 2011;13(2):R48.

216. Gerwin RD. A review of myofascial pain and fibromyalgia—factors that promote their persistence. *Acupunct Med* 2005;23(3):121–134.

217. Seal K, Becker W, Tighe J, et al. Managing chronic pain in primary care: it really does take a village. *J Gen Intern Med* 2017;32(8):931–934.

218. Myburgh C, Larsen AH, Hartvigsen J. A systematic, critical review of manual palpation for identifying myofascial trigger points: evidence and clinical significance. *Arch Phys Med Rehabil* 2008;89(6):1169–1176.

219. Gerwin RD, Shannon S, Hong CZ, et al. Interrater reliability in myofascial trigger point examination. *Pain* 1997;69(1–2):65–73.

220. Donnelly JM, Palubinskas L. Prevalence and inter-rater reliability of trigger points. *J Musculoskelet Pain* 2007;15(suppl 13):16.

221. Bron C, Franssen J, Wensing M, et al. Interrater reliability of palpation of myofascial trigger points in three shoulder muscles. *J Man Manip Ther* 2007;15(4):203–215.

222. Hsieh CY, Hong CZ, Adams AH, et al. Interexaminer reliability of the palpation of trigger points in the trunk and lower limb muscles. *Arch Phys Med Rehabil* 2000;81(3):258–264.

223. Lew PC, Lewis J, Story I. Inter-therapist reliability in locating latent myofascial trigger points using palpation. *Manual Ther* 1997;2(2):87–90.

224. Nice DA, Riddle DL, Lamb RL, et al. Intertester reliability of judgments of the presence of trigger points in patients with low back pain. *Arch Phys Med Rehabil* 1992;73(10):893–898.

225. Njoo KH, Van der Does E. The occurrence and inter-rater reliability of myofascial trigger points in the quadratus lumborum and gluteus medius: a prospective study in non-specific low back pain patients and controls in general practice. *Pain* 1994;58(3):317–323.

226. Barbero M, Bertoli P, Cescon C, et al. Intra-rater reliability of an experienced physiotherapist in locating myofascial trigger points in upper trapezius muscle. *J Man Manip Ther* 2012;20(4):171–177.

227. Sciotti VM, Mittak VL, DiMarco L, et al. Clinical precision of myofascial trigger point location in the trapezius muscle. *Pain* 2001;93(3):259–266.

228. Al-Shenqiti AM, Oldham JA. Test-retest reliability of myofascial trigger point detection in patients with rotator cuff tendonitis. *Clin Rehabil* 2005;19(5):482–487.

229. Zuil-Escobar JC, Martínez-Cepa CB, Martín-Urrialde JA, et al. Prevalence of myofascial trigger points and diagnostic criteria of different muscles in function of the medial longitudinal arch. *Arch Phys Med Rehabil* 2015;96(6):1123–1130.

230. Sanz DR, Lobo CC, López DL, et al. Interrater reliability in the clinical evaluation of myofascial trigger points in three ankle muscles. *J Manipulative Physiol Ther* 2016;39(9):623–634.

231. Rozenfeld E, Finestone AS, Moran U, et al. Test-retest reliability of myofascial trigger point detection in hip and thigh areas. *J Bodyw Move Ther* 2017;21:914–919.

232. Fernández-de-las-Peñas C, Dommerholt J. International consensus on diagnostic criteria and clinical considerations of myofascial trigger points: a Delphi study. *Pain Med* 2018;19:142–150.

233. Rathbone ATL, Grosman-Rimon L, Kumbhare DA. Interrater agreement of manual palpation for identification of myofascial trigger points: a systematic review and meta-analysis. *Clin J Pain* 2017;33(8):715–729.

234. Myburgh C, Lauridsen HH, Larsen AH, et al. Standardized manual palpation of myofascial trigger points in relation to neck/shoulder pain; the influence of clinical experience on inter-examiner reproducibility. *Man Ther* 2011;16(2):136–140.

235. Mora-Relucio R, Núñez-Nagy S, Gallego-Izquierdo T, et al. Experienced versus inexperienced interexaminer reliability on location and classification of myofascial trigger point palpation to diagnose lateral epicondylalgia: an observational cross-sectional study. *Evid Based Complement Alternat Med* 2016;2016:6059719.

236. Lucas N, Macaskill P, Irwig L, et al. Reliability of physical examination for diagnosis of myofascial trigger points: a systematic review of the literature. *Clin J Pain* 2009;25(1):80–89.

237. Anders HL, Corrie M, Jan H, et al. Standardized simulated palpation training—development of a palpation trainer and assessment of palpatory skills in experienced and inexperienced clinicians. *Man Ther* 2010;15(3):254–260.

238. Stoop R, Clijsen R, Leoni D, et al. Evolution of the methodological quality of controlled clinical trials for myofascial trigger point treatments for the period 1978-2015: a systematic review. *Musculoskelet Sci Pract* 2017;30:1–9.

239. Gattie E, Cleland JA, Snodgrass S. The effectiveness of trigger point dry needling for musculoskeletal conditions by physical therapists: a systematic review and meta-analysis. *J Orthop Sports Phys Ther* 2017;47(3):133–149.

240. Fernández-de-las-Peñas C, Alonso-Blanco C, Cuadrado ML, et al. Myofascial trigger points in the suboccipital muscles in episodic tension-type headache. *Man Ther* 2006;11:225–230.

241. Fernández-de-las-Peñas C, Alonso-Blanco C, Cuadrado ML, et al. Myofascial trigger points and their relationship to headache clinical parameters in chronic tension-type headache. *Headache* 2006;46(8):1264–1272.

242. Fernández-de-las-Peñas C, Ge HY, Arendt-Nielsen L, et al. Referred pain from trapezius muscle trigger points shares similar characteristics with chronic tension type headache. *Eur J Pain* 2007;11(4):475–482.

243. Cummings M. Referred knee pain treated with electroacupuncture to iliopsoas. *Acupunct Med* 2003;21(1–2):32–35.

244. Hwang M, Kang YK, Kim DH. Referred pain pattern of the pronator quadratus muscle. *Pain* 2005;116(3):238–242.

245. Hwang M, Kang YK, Shin JY, et al. Referred pain pattern of the abductor pollicis longus muscle. *Am J Phys Med Rehabil* 2005;84(8):593–597.

246. Minerbi A, Ratmansky M, Finestone A, et al. The local and referred pain patterns of the longus colli muscle. *J Bodyw Mov Ther* 2017;21(2):267–273.

247. Fernández-de-las-Peñas C, Cuadrado ML, Pareja JA. Myofascial trigger points, neck mobility and forward head posture in unilateral migraine. *Cephalalgia* 2006;26(9):1061–1070.

248. Fernández-de-las-Peñas C, Cuadrado ML, Pareja JA. Myofascial trigger points, neck mobility, and forward head posture in episodic tension-type headache. *Headache* 2007;47(5):662–672.

249. Fricton JR, Kroening R, Haley D, et al. Myofascial pain syndrome of the head and neck: a review of clinical characteristics of 164 patients. *Oral Surg Oral Med Oral Pathol* 1985;60(6):615–623.

250. Tewari S, Madabushi R, Agarwal A, et al. Chronic pain in a patient with Ehlers-Danlos syndrome (hypermobility type): the role of myofascial trigger point injections. *J Bodyw Mov Ther* 2017;21(1):194–196.

251. Fruth SJ. Differential diagnosis and treatment in a patient with posterior upper thoracic pain. *Phys Ther* 2006;86(2):254–268.

252. Hamada H, Moriwaki K, Shiroyama K, et al. Myofascial pain in patients with postthoracotomy pain syndrome. *Reg Anesth Pain Med* 2000;25(3):302–305.

253. Dommerholt J. Performing arts medicine—instrumentalist musicians: part III—case histories. *J Bodyw Mov Ther* 2010;14:127–138.

254. Banks SL, Jacobs DW, Gevirtz R, et al. Effects of autogenic relaxation training on electromyographic activity in active myofascial trigger points. *J Musculoskelet Pain* 1998;6(4):23–32.

255. Lewis C, Gevirtz R, Hubbard D, et al. Needle trigger point and surface frontal EMG measurements of psychophysiological responses in tension-type headache patients. *Biofeedback Self Regul* 1994;3:274–275.

256. McNulty WH, Gevirtz RN, Hubbard DR, et al. Needle electromyographic evaluation of trigger point response to a psychological stressor. *Psychophysiology* 1994;31(3):313–316.

257. Frewen PA, Dozois DJ, Lanius RA. Neuroimaging studies of psychological interventions for mood and anxiety disorders: empirical and methodological review. *Clin Psychol Rev* 2008;28(2):229–247.

258. Plotnikoff GA, Quigley JM. Prevalence of severe hypovitaminosis D in patients with persistent, nonspecific musculoskeletal pain. *Mayo Clin Proc* 2003;78(12):1463–1470.

259. Dawson-Hughes B, Heaney RP, Holick MF, et al. Estimates of optimal vitamin D status. *Osteoporos Int* 2005;16(7):713–716.

260. Vieth R, Bischoff-Ferrari H, Boucher BJ, et al. The urgent need to recommend an intake of vitamin D that is effective. *Am J Clin Nutr* 2007;85(3):649–650.

261. Gordon CM, DePeter KC, Feldman HA, et al. Prevalence of vitamin D deficiency among healthy adolescents. *Arch Pediatr Adolesc Med* 2004;158(6):531–537.

262. MacFarlane GD, Sackrison JL Jr, Body JJ, et al. Hypovitaminosis D in a normal, apparently healthy urban European population. *J Steroid Biochem Mol Biol* 2004;89–90(1–5):621–622.

263. Holick MF. High prevalence of vitamin D inadequacy and implications for health. *Mayo Clin Proc* 2006;81(3):353–373.

264. Bischoff HA, Stahelin HB, Tyndall A, et al. Relationship between muscle strength and vitamin D metabolites: are there therapeutic possibilities in the elderly? *J Rheumatol* 2000;59(suppl 1):39–41.

265. Hightower JM, Dalessandri KM, Pope K, et al. Low 25-hydroxyvitamin d and myofascial pain: association of cancer, colon polyps, and tendon rupture. *J Am Coll Nutr* 2017;36(6):455–461.

266. Sikdar S, Shah JP. Gilliams E, et al. Assessment of myofascial trigger points (MTrPs): a new application of ultrasound imaging and vibration sonoelastography. *Conf Proc IEEE Eng Med Biol Soc* 2008;2008:5585–5588.

267. Bauermeister W. Myofasziales triggerpunkt-syndrom; diagnose und therapie durch stoßwellen. *Extracta Orthopaedica* 2007;5:12–19.

268. Müller-Ehrenberg H, Licht G. Diagnosis and therapy of myofascial pain syndrome with focused shock waves (ESWT). *Medizinisch-Orthopädische Technik* 2005;5:1–6.

269. Kuan TS, Hsieh YL, Chen SM, et al. The myofascial trigger point region: correlation between the degree of irritability and the prevalence of endplate noise. *Am J Phys Med Rehabil* 2007;86(3):183–189.

270. Hafizah WM, Soh JZE, Supriyanto E, et al. Automatic classification of muscle condition based on ultrasound image morphological differences. *Int J Biol Biomed Eng* 2012;1(6):87–96.

271. Muller CE, Aranha MF, Gavião MB. Two-dimensional ultrasound and ultrasound elastography imaging of trigger points in women with myofascial pain syndrome treated by acupuncture and electroacupuncture: a double-blinded randomized controlled pilot study. *Ultrason Imaging* 2015;37(2):152–167.

272. Maher RM, Hayes DM, Shinohara M. Quantification of dry needling and posture effects on myofascial trigger points using ultrasound shear-wave elastography. *Arch Phys Med Rehabil* 2013;94(11):2146–2150.

273. Sikdar S, Shah JP, Gebreab T, et al. Novel applications of ultrasound technology to visualize and characterize myofascial trigger points and surrounding soft tissue. *Arch Phys Med Rehabil* 2009;90(11):1829–1838.

274. Cohen SP, Mullings R, Abdi S. The pharmacologic treatment of muscle pain. *Anesthesiology* 2004;101(2):495–526.

275. Moseley L. Unraveling the barriers to reconceptualization of the problem in chronic pain: the actual and perceived ability of patients and health professionals to understand the neurophysiology. *J Pain* 2003;4(4):184–189.

276. Burton AK, Waddell G, Tillotson KM, et al. Information and advice to patients with back pain can have a positive effect. A randomized controlled trial of a novel educational booklet in primary care. *Spine (Phila Pa 1976)* 1999;24(23):2484–2491.

277. Téllez-García M, de-la-Llave-Rincón AI, Salom-Moreno J, et al. Neuroscience education in addition to trigger point dry needling for the management of patients with mechanical chronic low back pain: a preliminary clinical trial. *J Bodywork Mov Ther* 2015;19:464–472.

278. Bandura A. Self-efficacy mechanism in physiological activation and health-promoting behavior. In: Madden JI, Matthysse S, Barchas S, eds. *Adaptation, Learning, and Affect*. New York: Raven Press; 1986:1169–1188.

279. Louw A. Treating the brain in chronic pain. In: Fernández-de-las-Peñas C, Cleland J, Dommerholt J, eds. *Manual Therapy for Musculoskeletal Pain Syndromes: An Evidenced and Clinical-Informed Approach*. Edinburgh: Elsevier; 2016:66–75.

280. Dommerholt J. Physical therapy in an interdisciplinary pain management center. *Pain Practitioner* 2005;14:32–36.

281. Scudds R, Solomon P. Pain and its management: a new pain curriculum for occupational therapists and physical therapists. *Physiother Can* 1995;47:77–78.

282. Hoeger Bement MK, Sluka KA. The current state of physical therapy pain curricula in the United States: a faculty survey. *J Pain* 2015;16(2):144–152.

283. Wolff MS, Michel TH, Krebs DE, et al. Chronic pain—assessment of orthopedic physical therapists' knowledge and attitudes. *Phys Ther* 1991;71(3):207–214.

284. Harding VR, Simmonds MJ, Watson PJ. Physical therapy for chronic pain. *Pain Clin Updates* 1998;6(3):1–7.

285. Bandura A, Cioffi D, Taylor CB, et al. Perceived self-efficacy in coping with cognitive stressors and opioid activation. *J Pers Soc Psychol* 1988;55(3):479–488.

286. Bandura A, O'Leary A, Taylor CB, et al. Perceived self-efficacy and pain control: opioid and nonopioid mechanisms. *J Pers Soc Psychol* 1987;53(3):563–571.
287. Steinbrocker O. Therapeutic injections in painful musculoskeletal disorders. *JAMA* 1944;125:397–401.
288. Lewit K. The needle effect in the relief of myofascial pain. *Pain* 1979;6:83–90.
289. Gunn CC, Milbrandt WE, Little AS, et al. Dry needling of muscle motor points for chronic low-back pain: a randomized clinical trial with long-term follow-up. *Spine* 1980;5(3):279–291.
290. Furlan A, Tulder M, Cherkin D, et al. Acupuncture and dry-needling for low back pain: an updated systematic review within the framework of the Cochrane Collaboration. *Spine* 2005;30(8):944–963.
291. Hong CZ. Lidocaine injection versus dry needling to myofascial trigger point. The importance of the local twitch response. *Am J Phys Med Rehabil* 1994;73(4):256–263.
292. Cummings TM, White AR. Needling therapies in the management of myofascial trigger point pain: a systematic review. *Arch Phys Med Rehabil* 2001;82(7):986–992.
293. Ga H, Choi JH, Park CH, et al. Acupuncture needling versus lidocaine injection of trigger points in myofascial pain syndrome in elderly patients—a randomised trial. *Acupunct Med* 2007;25(4):130–136.
294. Kamanli A, Kaya A, Ardicoglu O, et al. Comparison of lidocaine injection, botulinum toxin injection, and dry needling to trigger points in myofascial pain syndrome. *Rheumatol Int* 2005;25(8):604–611.
295. Martín-Pintado-Zugasti A, López-López A, González Gutiérrez JL, et al. The role of psychological factors in the perception of postneedling soreness and the influence of postneedling intervention. *PM R* 2017;9(4):348–355.
296. Martín-Pintado Zugasti A, Rodríguez-Fernández ÁL, García-Muro F, et al. Effects of spray and stretch on postneedling soreness and sensitivity after dry needling of a latent myofascial trigger point. *Arch Phys Med Rehabil* 2014;95(10):1925–1932.
297. Salom-Moreno J, Jiménez-Gómez L, Gómez-Ahufinger V, et al. Effects of low-load exercise on postneedling-induced pain after dry needling of active trigger point in individuals with subacromial pain syndrome. *PM R* 2017;9:1208–1216.
298. Martín-Pintado-Zugasti A, Pecos-Martin D, Rodríguez-Fernández ÁL, et al. Ischemic compression after dry needling of a latent myofascial trigger point reduces postneedling soreness intensity and duration. *PM R* 2015;7(10):1026–1034.
299. León-Hernández JV, Martín-Pintado-Zugasti A, Frutos LG, et al. Immediate and short-term effects of the combination of dry needling and percutaneous TENS on post-needling soreness in patients with chronic myofascial neck pain. *Braz J Phys Ther* 2016;20(5):422–431.
300. Martín-Pintado-Zugasti A, Rodríguez-Fernández ÁL, Fernandez-Carnero J. Postneedling soreness after deep dry needling of a latent myofascial trigger point in the upper trapezius muscle: characteristics, sex differences and associated factors. *J Back Musculoskelet Rehabil* 2016;29(2):301–308.
301. Gerwin RD, Duranleau D. Ultrasound identification of the myofascial trigger point. *Muscle Nerve* 1997;20(6):767–768.
302. Hong CZ, Torigoe Y. Electrophysiological characteristics of localized twitch responses in responsive taut bands of rabbit skeletal muscle. *J Musculoskelet Pain* 1994;2:17–43.
303. Gerber LH, Sikdar S, Aredo JV, et al. Beneficial effects of dry needling for treatment of chronic myofascial pain persist for 6 weeks after treatment completion. *PM R* 2017;9(2):105–112.
304. Hsieh YL, Yang SA, Yang CC, et al. Dry needling at myofascial trigger spots of rabbit skeletal muscles modulates the biochemicals associated with pain, inflammation, and hypoxia. *Evid Based Complement Alternat Med* 2012;2012:342165.
305. Koppenhaver SL, Walker MJ, Rettig C, et al. The association between dry needling-induced twitch response and change in pain and muscle function in patients with low back pain: a quasi-experimental study. *Physiotherapy* 2017;103(2):131–137.
306. Baldry P. Acupuncture treatment of fibromyalgia and myofascial pain. In: Chaitow L, ed. *Fibromyalgia Syndrome: A Practitioner's Guide to Practice.* Edinburgh: Churchill Livingstone; 2003:113–127.
307. Baldry P. Superficial versus deep dry needling. *Acupunct Med* 2002;20 (2–3):78–81.
308. Peets JM, Pomeranz B. CXBK mice deficient in opiate receptors show poor electroacupuncture analgesia. *Nature* 1978;273(5664):675–676.
309. Travell J. Basis for the multiple uses of local block of somatic trigger areas (procaine infiltration and ethyl chloride spray). *Miss Valley Med* 1949;71:13–22.
310. Iwama H, Akama Y. The superiority of water-diluted 0.25% to near 1% lidocaine for trigger-point injections in myofascial pain syndrome: a prospective, randomized, double-blinded trial. *Anesth Analg* 2000;91(2):408–409.
311. Iwama H, Ohmori S, Kaneko T, et al. Water-diluted local anesthetic for trigger-point injection in chronic myofascial pain syndrome: evaluation of types of local anesthetic and concentrations in water. *Reg Anesth Pain Med* 2001;26(4):333–336.
312. Garcia-Leiva JM, Hidalgo J, Rico-Villademoros F, et al. Effectiveness of ropivacaine trigger points inactivation in the prophylactic management of patients with severe migraine. *Pain Med* 2007;8(1):65–70.
313. Zaralidou AT, Amaniti EN, Maidatsi PG, et al. Comparison between newer local anesthetics for myofascial pain syndrome management. *Methods Find Exp Clin Pharmacol* 2007;29(5):353–357.
314. Ettlin T. Trigger point injection treatment with the 5-HT3 receptor antagonist tropisetron in patients with late whiplash-associated disorder. First results of a multiple case study. *Scand J Rheumatol Suppl* 2004;(119):49–50.
315. Müller W, Stratz T. Local treatment of tendinopathies and myofascial pain syndromes with the 5-HT3 receptor antagonist tropisetron. *Scand J Rheumatol Suppl* 2004;119:44–48.
316. Kim HW, Kwon YB, Han HJ, et al. Antinociceptive mechanisms associated with diluted bee venom acupuncture (apipuncture) in the rat formalin test: involvement of descending adrenergic and serotonergic pathways. *Pharmacol Res* 2005;51(2):183–188.
317. Kwon YB, Kim JH, Yoon JH, et al. The analgesic efficacy of bee venom acupuncture for knee osteoarthritis: a comparative study with needle acupuncture. *Am J Chin Med* 2001;29(2):187–199.
318. Kwon YB, Lee JD, Lee HJ, et al. Bee venom injection into an acupuncture point reduces arthritis associated edema and nociceptive responses. *Pain* 2001;90(3):271–280.
319. Son DJ, Kang J, Kim TJ, et al. Melittin, a major bioactive component of bee venom toxin, inhibits PDGF receptor beta-tyrosine phosphorylation and downstream intracellular signal transduction in rat aortic vascular smooth muscle cells. *J Toxicol Environ Health A* 2007;70(15–16):1350–1355.
320. Han S, Lee K, Yeo J, et al. Effect of honey bee venom on microglial cells nitric oxide and tumor necrosis factor-alpha production stimulated by LPS. *J Ethnopharmacol* 2007;111(1):176–181.
321. Lee JD, Park HJ, Chae Y, et al. An overview of bee venom acupuncture in the treatment of arthritis. *Evid Based Complement Alternat Med* 2005;2(1):79–84.
322. Son DJ, Lee JW, Lee YH, et al. Therapeutic application of anti-arthritis, pain-releasing, and anti-cancer effects of bee venom and its constituent compounds. *Pharmacol Ther* 2007;115(2):246–270.
323. Ho KY, Tan KH. Botulinum toxin A for myofascial trigger point injection: a qualitative systematic review. *Eur J Pain* 2007;11(5):519–527.
324. Silberstein N. More than a cosmetic fix. Combined with physical therapy, botulinum toxin type A can help provide relief for chronic muscle pain. *Rehab Manag* 2007;20(1):44, 46.
325. Ranoux D, Gury C, Fondarai J, et al. Respective potencies of Botox and Dysport: a double blind, randomised, crossover study in cervical dystonia. *J Neurol Neurosurg Psychiatry* 2002;72(4):459–462.
326. Dodick DW, Mauskop A, Elkind AH, et al. Botulinum toxin type A for the prophylaxis of chronic daily headache: subgroup analysis of patients not receiving other prophylactic medications: a randomized double-blind, placebo-controlled study. *Headache* 2005;45(4):315–324.
327. Benecke R, Heinze A, Reichel G, et al. Botulinum type A toxin complex for the relief of upper back myofascial pain syndrome: how do fixed-location injections compare with trigger point-focused injections? *Pain Med* 2011;12(11):1607–1614.
328. Göbel H. Botulinum toxin in migraine prophylaxis. *J Neurol* 2004;251 (suppl 1):I8–I11.
329. Göbel H, Heinze A, Heinze-Kuhn K, et al. Evidence-based medicine: botulinum toxin A in migraine and tension-type headache. *J Neurol* 2001;248(suppl 1):34–38.
330. Göbel H, Heinze A, Reichel G, et al. Efficacy and safety of a single botulinum type A toxin complex treatment (Dysport) for the relief of upper back myofascial pain syndrome: results from a randomized double-blind placebo-controlled multicentre study. *Pain* 2006;125(1–2):82–88.
331. Silberstein SD, Göbel H, Jensen R, et al. Botulinum toxin type A in the prophylactic treatment of chronic tension-type headache: a multicentre, double-blind, randomized, placebo-controlled, parallel-group study. *Cephalalgia* 2006;26(7):790–800.
332. Kern KU, Martin C, Scheicher S, et al. Auslosung von Phantomschmerzen und—sensationen durch muskulare Stumpftriggerpunkte nach Beinamputationen. *Schmerz* 2006;20(4):300–306.
333. Kern U, Martin C, Scheicher S, et al. Botulinum toxin type A influences stump pain after limb amputations. *J Pain Symptom Manage* 2003;26(6):1069–1070.
334. Halder GE, Scott L, Wyman A, et al. Botox combined with myofascial release physical therapy as a treatment for myofascial pelvic pain. *Investig Clin Urol* 2017;58(2):134–139.
335. Ranoux D, Martiné G, Espagne-Dubreuilh G, et al. OnabotulinumtoxinA injections in chronic migraine, targeted to sites of pericranial myofascial pain: an observational, open label, real-life cohort study. *J Headache Pain* 2017;18(1):75.
336. Gerwin R. Botulinum toxin treatment of myofascial pain: a critical review of the literature. *Curr Pain Headache Rep* 2012;16(5):413–422.
337. Silberstein S. Botulinum neurotoxins: origins and basic mechanisms of action. *Pain Pract* 2004;4(suppl 1):S19–S26.
338. Samigullin D, Bukharaeva EA, Vyskocil F, et al. Calcium dependence of uni-quantal release latencies and quantal content at mouse neuromuscular junction. *Physiol Res* 2005;54(1):129–132.
339. Wessler I. Acetylcholine release at motor endplates and autonomic neuroeffector junctions: a comparison. *Pharmacol Res* 1996;33(2):81–94.

340. Aoki KR. Review of a proposed mechanism for the antinociceptive action of botulinum toxin type A. *Neurotoxicology* 2005;26(5):785–793.

341. Bach-Rojecky L, Lackovic Z. Antinociceptive effect of botulinum toxin type a in rat model of carrageenan and capsaicin induced pain. *Croat Med J* 2005;46(2):201–208.

342. Mense S. Neurobiological basis for the use of botulinum toxin in pain therapy. *J Neurol* 2004;251(suppl 1):I1–I7.

343. Mesa-Jiménez JA, Sánchez-Gutiérrez J, de-la-Hoz-Aizpurua JL, et al. Cadaveric validation of dry needle placement in the lateral pterygoid muscle. *J Manipulative Physiol Ther* 2015;38(2):145–150.

344. Gonzalez-Perez LM, Infante-Cossio P, Granados-Nunez M, et al. Deep dry needling of trigger points located in the lateral pterygoid muscle: efficacy and safety of treatment for management of myofascial pain and temporomandibular dysfunction. *Med Oral Patol Oral Cir Bucal* 2015;20(3):e326–e333.

345. Peng PW, Castano ED. Survey of chronic pain practice by anesthesiologists in Canada. *Can J Anaesth* 2005;52(4):383–389.

346. Dilorenzo L, Traballesi M, Morelli D, et al. Hemiparetic shoulder pain syndrome treated with deep dry needling during early rehabilitation: a prospective, open-label, randomized investigation. *J Musculoskelet Pain* 2004;12(2):25–34.

347. Espí-López GV, Serra-Añó P, Vicent-Ferrando J, et al. Effectiveness of inclusion of dry needling in a multimodal therapy program for patellofemoral pain: a randomized parallel-group trial. *J Orthop Sports Phys Ther* 2017;47(6):392–401.

348. Ga H, Koh HJ, Choi JH, et al. Intramuscular and nerve root stimulation vs lidocaine injection to trigger points in myofascial pain syndrome. *J Rehabil Med* 2007;39(5):374–378.

349. He C, Ma H. Effectiveness of trigger point dry needling for plantar heel pain: a meta-analysis of seven randomized controlled trials. *J Pain Res* 2017;10:1933–1942.

350. Kietrys DM, Palombaro KM, Azzaretto E, et al. Effectiveness of dry needling for upper-quarter myofascial pain: a systematic review and meta-analysis. *J Orthop Sports Phys Ther* 2013;43(9):620–634.

351. Pérez-Palomares S, Oliván-Blázquez B, Pérez-Palomares A, et al. Contribution of dry needling to individualized physical therapy treatment of shoulder pain: a randomized clinical trial. *J Orthop Sports Phys Ther* 2017;47(1):11–20.

352. Castro-Sanchez AM, Garcia-Lopez H, Mataran-Penarrocha GA, et al. Effects of dry needling on spinal mobility and trigger points in patients with fibromyalgia syndrome. *Pain Physician* 2017;20(2):37–52.

353. Brennan KL, Allen BC, Maldonado YM. Dry needling versus cortisone injection in the treatment of greater trochanteric pain syndrome: a noninferiority randomized clinical trial. *J Orthop Sports Phys Ther* 2017;47(4):232–239.

354. Tadros NN, Shah AB, Shoskes DA. Utility of trigger point injection as an adjunct to physical therapy in men with chronic prostatitis/chronic pelvic pain syndrome. *Transl Androl Urol* 2017;6(3):534–537.

355. Shanmugam S, Mathias L. Immediate effects of paraspinal dry needling in patients with acute facet joint lock induced wry neck. *J Clin Diagn Res* 2017;11(6):YM01–YM03.

356. Calvo S, Quintero I, Herrero P. Effects of dry needling (DNHS technique) on the contractile properties of spastic muscles in a patient with stroke: a case report. *Int J Rehabil Res* 2016;39(4):372–376.

357. Arias-Buría JL, Fernández-de-Las-Peñas C, Palacios-Ceña M, et al. Exercises and dry needling for subacromial pain syndrome: a randomized parallel-group trial. *J Pain* 2017;18(1):11–18.

358. Arias-Buría JL, Valero-Alcaide R, Cleland JA, et al. Inclusion of trigger point dry needling in a multimodal physical therapy program for postoperative shoulder pain: a randomized clinical trial. *J Manipulative Physiol Ther* 2015;38(3):179–187.

359. Domingo A, Mayoral O, Monterde S, et al. Neuromuscular damage and repair after dry needling in mice. *Evid Based Complement Alternat Med* 2013;2013:260806.

360. Gaspersic R, Koritnik B, Erzen I, et al. Muscle activity-resistant acetylcholine receptor accumulation is induced in places of former motor endplates in ectopically innervated regenerating rat muscles. *Int J Dev Neurosci* 2001;19(3):339–346.

361. Sadeh M, Stern LZ, Czyzewski K. Changes in end-plate cholinesterase and axons during muscle degeneration and regeneration. *J Anat* 1985;140 (pt 1):165–176.

362. Liu QG, Liu L, Huang QM, et al. Decreased spontaneous electrical activity and acetylcholine at myofascial trigger spots after dry needling treatment: a pilot study. *Evid Based Complement Alternat Med* 2017;2017:3938191.

363. Langevin HM, Bouffard NA, Badger GJ, et al. Subcutaneous tissue fibroblast cytoskeletal remodeling induced by acupuncture: evidence for a mechanotransduction-based mechanism. *J Cell Physiol* 2006;207(3):767–774.

364. Langevin HM, Bouffard NA, Badger GJ, et al. Dynamic fibroblast cytoskeletal response to subcutaneous tissue stretch ex vivo and in vivo. *Am J Physiol Cell Physiol* 2005;288(3):C747–C756.

365. Sandkühler J. The organization and function of endogenous antinociceptive systems. *Prog Neurobiol* 1996;50(1):49–81.

366. Lund I, Lundeberg T. Are minimal, superficial or sham acupuncture procedures acceptable as inert placebo controls? *Acupunct Med* 2006;24(1):13–15.

367. Mohr C, Binkofski F, Erdmann C, et al. The anterior cingulate cortex contains distinct areas dissociating external from self-administered painful stimulation: a parametric fMRI study. *Pain* 2005;114(3):347–357.

368. Olausson H, Lamarre Y, Backlund H, et al. Unmyelinated tactile afferents signal touch and project to insular cortex. *Nat Neurosci* 2002;5(9):900–904.

369. Rickards LD. Effectiveness of noninvasive treatments for active myofascial trigger point pain: a systematic review. In: Dommerholt J, Huijbregts PA, eds. *Myofascial Trigger Points: Pathophysiology and Evidence-Informed Diagnosis and Management.* Sudbury, MA: Jones & Bartlett; 2011:129–158.

370. Fernández-de-las-Peñas C, Campo MS, Fernández-Carnero J. Manual therapies in myofascial trigger point treatment: a systematic review. *J Bodyw Mov Ther* 2005;9:27–34.

371. Lee M, Kim M, Oh S, et al. A self-determination theory-based self-myofascial release program in older adults with myofascial trigger points in the neck and back: a pilot study. *Physiother Theory Prac* 2017;33(9):681–694.

372. Morikawa Y, Takamoto K, Nishimaru H, et al. Compression at myofascial trigger point on chronic neck pain provides pain relief through the prefrontal cortex and autonomic nervous system: a pilot study. *Front Neurosci* 2017;11:186.

373. Behrangrad S, Kamali F. Comparison of ischemic compression and lumbopelvic manipulation as trigger point therapy for patellofemoral pain syndrome in young adults: a double-blind randomized clinical trial. *J Bodyw Mov Ther* 2017;21(3):554–564.

374. De Meulemeester KE, Castelein B, Coppieters I, et al. Comparing trigger point dry needling and manual pressure technique for the management of myofascial neck/shoulder pain: a randomized clinical trial. *J Manipulative Physiol Ther* 2017;40(1):11–20.

375. Mohammadi Kojidi M, Okhovatian F, Rahimi A, et al. The influence of Positional Release Therapy on the myofascial trigger points of the upper trapezius muscle in computer users. *J Bodyw Mov Ther* 2016;20(4):767–773.

376. Fernández-de-las-Peñas C, Alonso-Blanco C, Fernández-Carnero J, et al. The immediate effect of ischemic compression technique and transverse friction massage on tenderness of active and latent myofascial trigger points: a pilot study. *J Bodyw Mov Ther* 2006;10(1):3–9.

377. Hou CR, Tsai LC, Cheng KF, et al. Immediate effects of various physical therapeutic modalities on cervical myofascial pain and trigger-point sensitivity. *Arch Phys Med Rehabil* 2002;83(10):1406–1414.

378. Khalighi HR, Mortazavi H, Mojahedi SM, et al. Low level laser therapy versus pharmacotherapy in improving myofascial pain disorder syndrome. *J Lasers Med Sci* 2016;7(1):45–50.

379. De Carli BM, Magro AK, Souza-Silva BN, et al. The effect of laser and botulinum toxin in the treatment of myofascial pain and mouth opening: a randomized clinical trial. *J Photochem Photobiol B* 2016;159:120–123.

380. Altan L, Bingol U, Aykac M, et al. Investigation of the effect of GaAs laser therapy on cervical myofascial pain syndrome. *Rheumatol Int* 2005;25(1):23–27.

381. Gur A, Sarac AJ, Cevik R, et al. Efficacy of 904 nm gallium arsenide low level laser therapy in the management of chronic myofascial pain in the neck: a double-blind and randomize-controlled trial. *Lasers Surg Med* 2004;35(3):229–235.

382. Srbely JZ, Dickey JP. Randomized controlled study of the antinociceptive effect of ultrasound on trigger point sensitivity: novel applications in myofascial therapy? *Clin Rehabil* 2007;21(5):411–417.

383. Gam AN, Warming S, Larsen LH, et al. Treatment of myofascial trigger-points with ultrasound combined with massage and exercise—a randomised controlled trial. *Pain* 1998;77(1):73–79.

384. Lee JC, Lin DT, Hong CZ. The effectiveness of simultaneous thermotherapy with ultrasound and electrotherapy with combined AC and DC current on the immediate pain relief of myofascial trigger points. *J Musculoskelet Pain* 1997;5(1):81–90.

385. Majlesi J, Unalan H. High-power pain threshold ultrasound technique in the treatment of active myofascial trigger points: a randomized, double-blind, case-control study. *Arch Phys Med Rehabil* 2004;85(5):833–836.

386. Unalan H, Majlesi J, Aydin FY, et al. Comparison of high-power pain threshold ultrasound therapy with local injection in the treatment of active myofascial trigger points of the upper trapezius muscle. *Arch Phys Med Rehabil* 2011;92(4):657–662.

387. Ardiç F, Sarhus M, Topuz O. Comparison of two different techniques of electrotherapy on myofascial pain. *J Back Musculoskeletal Rehabil* 2002;16:11–16.

388. Graff-Radford SB, Reeves JL, Baker RL, et al. Effects of transcutaneous electrical nerve stimulation on myofascial pain and trigger point sensitivity. *Pain* 1989;37(1):1–5.

389. Hsueh TC, Cheng PT, Kuan TS, et al. The immediate effectiveness of electrical nerve stimulation and electrical muscle stimulation on myofascial trigger points. *Am J Phys Med Rehabil* 1997;76(6):471–476.

390. Müller-Ehrenberg H, Thorwesten L. Improvement of sports-related shoulder pain after treatment of trigger points using focused extracorporeal shock wave therapy regarding static and dynamic force development, pain relief, and sensomotoric performance. *J Musculoskelet Pain* 2007;15(suppl 13):33.

CHAPTER 36

Fibromyalgia: A Discrete Disease or the End of the Continuum

DANIEL J. CLAUW and **CHAD BRUMMETT**

Clinical practitioners commonly see patients with pain and other somatic symptoms that they cannot adequately explain based on the degree of damage or inflammation noted in peripheral tissues. In fact, this may be among the most common predicament for which patients seek medical attention.[1] Typically, an evaluation is performed looking for a "cause" for the pain. If none is found, these individuals are often given a diagnostic label that merely connotes that the patient has chronic pain in a region of the body, without an underlying mechanistic cause (e.g., chronic low back pain, headache, temporomandibular disorder [TMD]). In other cases, the label given alludes to an underlying mechanism that may or may not be responsible for the individual's pain (e.g., "knee osteoarthritis").

Fibromyalgia is merely the current term for individuals with chronic widespread musculoskeletal pain, for which no alternative cause can be identified. Gastroenterologists often see the exact same patients and focus on their gastroenterologic complaints and often use the terms *functional gastrointestinal disorder, irritable bowel syndrome* (IBS), *nonulcer dyspepsia, noncardiac chest pain,* or *esophageal dysmotility* to explain the patient's symptoms.[2] Neurologists see these patients for their headaches and/or unexplained facial pain; urologists for pelvic pain and urinary symptoms (and use labels such as interstitial cystitis, chronic prostatitis, vulvodynia, and vulvar vestibulitis); dentists for TMD, and so on.[3]

Until recently, these unexplained pain syndromes perplexed researchers, clinicians, and patients. However, it is now clear that

- Individuals will sometimes only have one of these "idiopathic" pain syndromes over the course of their lifetime. But more often, individuals with one of these entities, and their family members, are likely to have several of these conditions.[4,5] Many terms have been used to describe these coaggregating syndromes and symptoms, including *functional somatic syndromes, somatization disorders, allied spectrum conditions, sensory sensitivity syndromes, chronic multisymptom illnesses,* and *medically unexplained symptoms.* The most recent term coined by the National Institutes of Health in the United States is probably the best accepted at present: "chronic overlapping pain conditions" (COPCs).[6,7]
- Women are more likely to have these disorders than men, but the sex difference is much more apparent in clinical cohorts (especially tertiary care) when compared to population-based samples.[8,9]
- Groups of individuals with these conditions (e.g., fibromyalgia, IBS, headache, TMD) typically display diffuse hyperalgesia (increased pain to normally painful stimuli) and/or allodynia (pain to normally nonpainful stimuli) that is identifiable both via quantitative sensory testing and functional neuroimaging.[10–12] In addition, a number of other central nervous system (CNS) mechanisms are reproducibly seen in these conditions. This suggests that these individuals have a fundamental problem with augmented pain and/or sensory processing rather than simply a nociceptive focus confined to the region of the body where the person is currently experiencing pain.

- Similar types of therapies are efficacious for all of these conditions, including both pharmacologic (e.g., tricyclic compounds, serotonin norepinephrine reuptake inhibitors [SNRIs] and gabapentinoids) and nonpharmacologic treatments (e.g., education, exercise, cognitive-behavioral therapy). Conversely, individuals with these conditions typically do not respond to therapies that are typically more effective when pain is due to damage or inflammation of tissues (e.g., nonsteroidal anti-inflammatory drugs [NSAIDs], opioids, injections, surgical procedures).
- Subsets of individuals with any chronic pain condition (e.g., low back pain, osteoarthritis, autoimmune disorders, sickle cell disease) also have the same phenotypic features and underlying mechanisms as those seen in fibromyalgia.[3,13] These individuals with subthreshold fibromyalgia display the same pathologic features and differential responsiveness to peripherally directed versus centrally directed therapies. Thus, it is critical that clinicians seeing patients with chronic pain evaluate individuals for the presence of this phenotype as it can dramatically affect which treatments will work, or not work, for a given individual with chronic pain.

Until perhaps a decade ago, these conditions were all on somewhat equal (and tenuous) scientific ground. But within a relatively short period of time, research methods such as experimental pain testing, functional imaging, and genetics have led to tremendous advances in the understanding of several of these conditions, most notably fibromyalgia, IBS, and TMD. Many in the pain field now feel that much chronic pain itself is a neural disease and that many of the underlying mechanisms operative in these heretofore considered "idiopathic" or "functional" pain syndromes may be similar no matter whether that pain is present throughout the body (e.g., in fibromyalgia) or localized to the low back, the bowel, or the bladder. Because of this, the more contemporary terms used to describe conditions such as fibromyalgia, IBS, TMD, vulvodynia, and many other entities include "centralized pain" or "central sensitization" to imply that the CNS is playing a prominent role in amplifying or causing the pain in most individuals with these syndromes.[3,14] This review of fibromyalgia in the following discussion focuses on our current understanding of this disorder as the prototypical "centralized pain syndromes."

Historical Perspective

Although the term *fibromyalgia* is relatively new, this condition has been described in the medical literature since the early 1900s. Sir William Gowers coined the term "fibrositis" in 1904. During the next half century, fibrositis (as it was then called) was considered by some to be a common cause of muscular pain, by others to be a manifestation of "tension" or "psychogenic rheumatism," and by the rheumatology community in general to be a nonentity.

The current concept of fibromyalgia was established by Smythe and Moldofsky[15] in the mid-1970s. The name change reflected the fact that there was increasing evidence that there was no *-itis* (inflammation) in the connective tissues of individuals with this condition but instead -*algia* (pain). These authors characterized the most common tender points (regions of extreme tenderness in these individuals) and reported that patients with fibromyalgia had disturbances in deep and restorative sleep and that selective stage 4 interruptions induced the symptoms of fibromyalgia.[16] Yunus and colleagues[17] then reported on the major clinical manifestations of patients with fibromyalgia seen in rheumatology clinics.

The next advance in fibromyalgia was the development of the American College of Rheumatology (ACR) criteria for fibromyalgia, which were published in 1990.[18] These classification criteria required that an individual have both a history of chronic widespread pain (CWP) and the finding of ≥11 of a possible 18 tender points on examination. These ACR classification criteria were intended for research use to standardize definitions of fibromyalgia. In this regard, the criteria have been extremely valuable. Unfortunately, many practitioners use these criteria in routine clinical practice to diagnose individual patients, and this unintended use led to many of the current misconceptions regarding fibromyalgia that are discussed in the following text. New criteria that eliminate the need for the tender point exam were developed in 2010 and refined in 2011 and in 2016.[19–21] These criteria focus on identifying the cardinal symptoms seen in this condition including widespread pain, fatigue, sleep, memory, and mood disturbances.

Once structural damage to tissues or inflammation had been excluded as pathogenic factors in fibromyalgia, many groups of investigators began to explore neural mechanisms to explain the underlying pathogenesis of these disorders.[22,23] Fortuitously, newer neuroscience research techniques such as functional, chemical, and structural brain imaging were all becoming available tools to examine the CNS, in both healthy individuals and those with chronic pain.

Thus, the conditions we now mechanistically understand best within this spectrum include conditions where these central factors were first studied, including fibromyalgia, IBS (previously termed *spastic colitis* until the recognition that there was little -*itis* and that motility changes were not the major pathologic feature), and TMD (previously termed *temporomandibular joint syndrome* until it was recognized the problem was not largely within the joint[24–27]) and urinary chronic pelvic pain syndromes (where again, the condition previously called interstitial cystitis is now called bladder pain syndrome[28–31]). This is not to say peripheral factors, or low-grade inflammation that is not identifiable clinically, do not play some role in these entities. But it is relevant that clinicians who care for individuals with these conditions, and who are quite adept at identifying (with blood tests, imaging, or endoscopy) peripheral damage or inflammation, have generally concluded that these are not inflammatory or peripheral-based disorders.

Epidemiology

CHRONIC WIDESPREAD PAIN

Epidemiologic studies of the historical component of the ACR criteria for fibromyalgia, CWP, have been extremely instructive. CWP is typically operationalized as pain above and below the waist, involving the left and right sides of the body and also involving the axial skeleton. Population-based studies of CWP suggest that roughly 6% to 12% of the population has these features at any given point in time.[32,33] Chronic regional pain is found in 20% to 25% of the population. Both chronic widespread and regional pain occur about 1.5 times as commonly in women than men. These findings are very similar in different countries, ethnicities, and cultures, dispelling an early notion that this problem was somewhat unique to more developed countries.

FIBROMYALGIA

The original 1990 ACR criteria for fibromyalgia required that an individual has both a history of CWP and the finding of 11 or greater of 18 possible tender points on examination. Tender points represent nine paired predefined regions of the body, often over musculotendinous insertions.[18] If an individual reports pain when a region is palpated with 4 kg of pressure, this is considered a positive tender point. Between 25% and 50% of individuals who have CWP will also have 11 or greater tender points and thus meet the 1990 criteria for fibromyalgia.[34] Just as with CWP, the prevalence of fibromyalgia is just as high in rural or nonindustrialized societies as it is in countries such as the United States.[35]

SIGNIFICANCE OF TENDER POINTS

When the 1990 ACR criteria were published, it was thought that there may be some unique significance to the locations of tender points. In fact, a term "control points" was coined to describe areas of the body that should not be tender in fibromyalgia, and individuals were assumed to have a psychological cause for their pain is they were tender in these regions. Since then, we have learned that the tenderness in fibromyalgia extends throughout the entire body. Thus, relative to the pain threshold that a normal nonfibromyalgia patient would experience at the same points, "control" regions of the body such as the thumbnail and forehead are just as tender as in fibromyalgia tender points.[36]

The tender point requirement in the ACR criteria not only misrepresents the nature of the tenderness in this condition (i.e., local rather than widespread) but also strongly influences the demographic and psychological characteristics of fibromyalgia. Women are only 1.5 times more likely than men to experience CWP but are 11 times more likely than men to have 11 or more tender points.[37] Because of this, women are approximately 10 times as likely to meet the 1990 ACR criteria for fibromyalgia than men. Yet, most of the men in the population who have CWP but are not tender enough to meet criteria for fibromyalgia likely have the same fundamental underlying pathophysiologic problems as the women who meet the ACR criteria for fibromyalgia.

Another unintended consequence of requiring both CWP and at least 11 tender points to be diagnosed with fibromyalgia is that many individuals with fibromyalgia will have high levels of distress. Wolfe[38] has described tender points as a "sedimentation rate for distress" because of population-based studies showing that tender points are more common in distressed individuals. Until recently, many assumed that because *tender points* were associated with distress, that *tenderness* (an individual's sensitivity to mechanical pressure) was associated with distress. However, recent evidence suggests that this latter association is probably due to the standard tender point technique, which consists of applying steadily increasing pressure until reaching 4 kg. In this situation, individuals who are anxious or "expectant" have a tendency to "bail out" and report tenderness. Recently, more sophisticated measures of tenderness have been developed which give stimuli in a random, unpredictable fashion, and the results of these tests are independent of psychological status.[39,40] Because tender points are associated with high levels of distress, requiring 11 or greater tender points in order to diagnose someone with CWP with fibromyalgia dramatically increases the likelihood that these individuals will be female and/or and distressed, compared to individuals with CWP and <11 tender points. In fact, population-based studies suggest that the primary symptom of fibromyalgia, CWP, is only modestly associated with distress, and distress is only weakly associated with the subsequent development of CWP.[41,42] There are far more psychologically "normal" individuals who develop CWP than distressed or depressed people who do, and most individuals with CWP do not have or subsequently develop distress or depression.

In summary, although many clinicians uniquely associate fibromyalgia with women who display high levels of distress, much of this is an artifact of (1) the 1990 ACR criteria that require 11 tender points and (2) the fact that most studies of fibromyalgia have originated from clinical samples from tertiary care centers, where health care seeking behaviors lead to the fact that psychological and psychiatric comorbidities are much higher.[9] When all these biases are eliminated by examining CWP in population-based studies, a clearer picture of fibromyalgia can be gleamed, and CWP becomes much like chronic pain in any other region of the body.

OTHER FEATURES OF FIBROMYALGIA GLEANED FROM EPIDEMIOLOGIC OR OBSERVATIONAL STUDIES

Individuals who develop fibromyalgia nearly always have a lifelong history of chronic pain in various regions of the body as well as other CNS symptoms such as fatigue, sleep, memory, and mood difficulties. Most individuals who eventually develop fibromyalgia begin having pain in multiple body regions beginning earlier in life. The prevalence of any (regional or widespread) chronic musculoskeletal pain in the population is about 30%, so if a single individual has had chronic pain in multiple bodily regions early in his or her lifetime and he or she does not have an autoimmune or other disorder leading to widespread inflammation or damage, he or she is likely exhibiting a "chronic pain prone phenotype." Often beginning in childhood or adolescence, individuals who eventually go on to develop fibromyalgia are more likely to experience headaches, dysmenorrhea, TMD, chronic fatigue, IBS and other functional gastrointestinal disorders, interstitial cystitis/painful bladder syndrome, endometriosis, and other regional pain syndromes (especially back and neck pain).[43,44] In fact, what often looks to one health care provider as a new episode of acute or subacute pain is in fact simply the latest region of the body experiencing pain.[45] Because of this, many experts in the pain field have begun to feel that especially these "centralized" pain states are best thought of as a single lifelong disease that merely tends to manifest in different bodily regions over time.[14,46,47]

In addition to fibromyalgia patients having a high personal lifetime history of chronic pain, there is often a strong family history of chronic pain identifiable. The first-degree relatives of fibromyalgia patients are 8 times as likely to have this condition as the family members of controls and also have very high rates of other chronic pain states.[5] These studies also show that family members of individuals with fibromyalgia are much more tender than the family members of controls, regardless of whether they have pain or not. Family members of fibromyalgia patients are also much more likely to have IBS, TMD, headaches, and a host of other regional pain syndromes.[4,48,49] This familial and personal coaggregation of conditions which includes fibromyalgia was originally collectively termed *affective spectrum disorder*[50] and more recently *central sensitivity syndromes*,[51] *chronic multisymptom illnesses*,[51] and *chronic overlapping pain conditions*. In population-based studies, the key symptoms besides pain that typically coaggregate together are fatigue, memory difficulties, and mood disturbances.[7,52] Twin studies suggest that approximately 50% of the risk of developing fibromyalgia or related pain conditions such as IBS and headache is genetic, and 50% environmental.[53] The strong familial predisposition to fibromyalgia is shared by many chronic pain conditions, and there has been an explosion of knowledge recently regarding the role of specific genetic factors in chronic pain states, which is partially reviewed in the following text.[14,54]

The environmental factors that are most likely to trigger the development of fibromyalgia are various types of "stressors," typically that involve acute pain for at least a few weeks

TABLE 36.1 "Stressors" Capable of Triggering Fibromyalgia and Related Condition
• Ongoing inflammatory or nociceptive pain (e.g., autoimmune disorders, sickle cell disease, Ehlers-Danlos syndrome)
• Infections (e.g., parvovirus, EBV, Lyme disease, Q fever; not common upper respiratory infections)
• Physical trauma (e.g., automobile accidents)
• Psychological stress/distress (e.g., sexual assault, early childhood trauma)
• Hormonal alterations (e.g., hypothyroidism)
• Drugs
• Vaccines
• Certain catastrophic events (war but not natural disasters)

EBV, Epstein-Barr virus.

(Table 36.1). Psychological stress, including childhood trauma, is but one such stressor. Fibromyalgia or similar illnesses are found at much higher than expected rates in individuals who have experienced certain types of infections[55] (e.g., Epstein-Barr virus, Lyme disease, Q fever, viral hepatitis), trauma[56] (motor vehicle collisions), and deployment to war.[57] Of note, each of these stressors only leads to CWP or fibromyalgia in approximately 5% to 10% of individuals who are exposed; the overwhelming majority of individuals who experience these same infections or other stressful events regain their baseline state of health. This is a contentious legal issue, and not all would agree that all of these events can seemingly trigger or exacerbate fibromyalgia.[58] Certainly assessing "cause and effect" in any given individual is almost impossible because all individuals experience intermittent stressors of the variety that seemingly can trigger fibromyalgia. It is also likely that part of the reasons these different stressors can seemingly lead to worsening of fibromyalgia or fibromyalgia symptoms is because of how these stressors affect activity level, sleep, or overall distress, any of which then can lead to worsening of pain and other symptoms.[59–63]

Fibromyalgia also is very commonly seen as a comorbidity in other chronic pain conditions such as osteoarthritis, rheumatoid arthritis (RA), and lupus. The disorder is also associated with other regional pain conditions or autoimmune disorders.[64–67] This high rate of fibromyalgia in individuals with other chronic rheumatic or autoimmune disorders deserves special attention because of the relevance to practicing clinicians. As many as 25% of patients correctly diagnosed with generalized inflammatory disorders such as systemic lupus erythematosus (SLE), RA, and ankylosing spondylitis will also fulfill the clinical criteria for fibromyalgia.[68,69] However, in clinical practice, this coexpression may go unrecognized, especially when the fibromyalgia develops after the autoimmune disorder or regional pain syndrome. In this setting when comorbid fibromyalgia goes unrecognized, patients are often unnecessarily treated more aggressively with toxic immunosuppressive drugs leading to morbidity without the desired therapeutic effects.

This phenomenon had previously been termed *secondary fibromyalgia*, but because this is so common and might occur in a subset of nearly any chronic pain cohort, a more popular term we prefer to use for this phenomenon is that these individuals have "centralized" their pain. This simply connotes the fact that although peripheral nociceptive input might be responsible some or even much of that individual's pain, superimposed CNS factors are also likely amplifying pain and leading to other comorbid symptoms such as fatigue, memory problems, and disturbances of sleep and mood.[70] The term *central sensitization* is also sometimes used to describe this phenomenon, but many experts feel that this particular term should be reserved for the original spinal mechanism that was identified and called by this name rather than the more general phenomenon we now believe can result via a multitude of different spinal and supraspinal

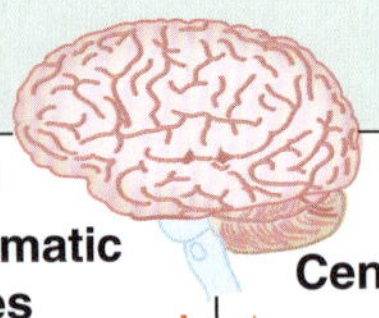

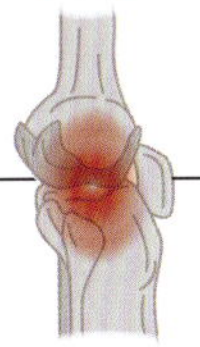

	Top-down **Functional Somatic Syndromes**	Bottom-up **Central Sensitization**
Resolves when nociceptive input removed	No	Yes
Sex ratio	Female > male	Female > male
Age of onset of pain	Young—typically following puberty	Any age when ongoing nociceptive input occurs
Family history of pain	Yes	No
Psych comorbidity	High	Moderate
Increased sensitivity to nonpain sensory stimuli	Yes	No
High number of functional somatic syndromes	Yes	No

FIGURE 36.1 There are (at least) two different forms of fibromyalgia, one (top-down) that occurs most commonly in younger individuals who have many other chronic overlapping pain conditions, and may be a primary brain disorder, and the other (bottom-up) that occurs in many individuals with other nociceptive or neuropathic pain conditions, and may be partially driven by ongoing peripheral nociceptive input (i.e., central sensitization).

mechanisms.[14,71] Regardless of what term an individual uses to describe this phenomenon, it is becoming increasingly important to identify it because emerging evidence suggests that therapies that work best for peripheral, nociceptive pain (e.g., NSAIDs, opioids, injections, surgical procedures) are less likely to be effective in these individuals.[72,73]

Most studies of fibromyalgia to date have excluded individuals with other conditions so nearly all studies to date have examined the pathophysiology of "primary" fibromyalgia. It is not yet clear if there are any key pathophysiologic differences between primary fibromyalgia (fibromyalgia as a stand-alone disorder, or accompanied by other COPCs, e.g., headache, IBS, TMD) and secondary fibromyalgia (i.e., central sensitization; Fig. 36.1). This latter group might be very responsive to peripherally directed therapies, if nociceptive input is driving central sensitization.

Fibromyalgia, especially the "primary" form, is also very comorbid with early life and current stress, and many if not most individuals will have a lifetime history of a psychiatric disorder such as depression or anxiety.[74] There is typically more psychiatric and psychological comorbidity seen in tertiary care settings or in individuals who are refractory to treatment. This bidirectional relationship between fibromyalgia and psychiatric conditions is likely due in part to the fact that there are common triggers to both sets of conditions (e.g., early life stress or trauma) as well as shared pathophysiology (i.e., most of the same neurotransmitters that affect pain transmission also affect mood, memory, fatigue, sleep). Other potentially modifiable risk factors for developing fibromyalgia include poor sleep, obesity, physical inactivity, and poor job or life satisfaction. Similarly, cognitive factors such as catastrophizing (the feeling that pain is very bad and associated with a poor prognosis for recovery) or fear of movement have been shown to be poor prognostic factors in fibromyalgia and other chronic pain states.

Etiology

ANIMAL MODELS OF FIBROMYALGIA

Although few would purport that there is an animal model that mimics all of the key clinical features of fibromyalgia, animal models can nonetheless be very helpful in understanding the pathogenesis of this condition. This topic has been covered in depth in a recent review.[75] For example, arguably the biggest controversy in the field of pain is what is the relative contribution of peripheral versus central factors in leading to chronic pain conditions. Some would argue that there must be some type of ongoing peripheral drive or input to cause chronic pain; however, this is almost certainly *not* the case. Animals develop the critical features of central sensitization or centralization of pain when exposed to swim stress,[76] neonatal separation from their mothers,[77] and many other nonpainful stimuli.[75] Features of central sensitization and animal pain behaviors consistent with diffuse pain are also seen when CNS neurotransmitters are purposefully altered in the direction found in fibromyalgia. For example, chronic reserpine administration which depletes bioamines leads to features consistent with fibromyalgia,[78,79] as does directly increasing glutamate levels in the insulae.[80] This latter model of increasing glutamate in the insulae was recently reverse translated to show that the findings of "small fiber neuropathy" could be induced simply by increasing CNS glutamate, as is known to occur in fibromyalgia.

GENETIC FACTORS

The strong familial predisposition to fibromyalgia and other chronic pain conditions has led many to study specific genetic polymorphisms that may be associated with a higher risk of developing fibromyalgia. First, candidate gene studies showed that genetic findings such as the serotonin 5-HT2A receptor polymorphism T/T phenotype, serotonin transporter, dopamine 4 receptor, and catechol-O-methyl transferase (COMT) polymorphisms all were noted in higher frequency in fibromyalgia patients than controls. Some subsequent studies confirmed some of these associations, whereas others did not.[81,82] Subsequent larger genome-wide linkage and candidate gene studies identified other putative targets.[83,84] The linkage studies confirmed the strong genetic contribution to fibromyalgia and suggested linkage of fibromyalgia to the chromosome 17p11.2-q11.2 region. The large candidate gene study identified significant differences in allele frequencies between cases and controls were observed for three genes: GABRB3 (rs4906902, $p = 3.65 \times 10^{-6}$), TAAR1 (rs8192619, $p = 1.11 \times 10^{-5}$) and GBP1 (rs7911, $p = 1.06 \times 10^{-4}$). These three genes, and seven other genes with suggestive evidence for association, were examined in a second, independent cohort of fibromyalgia patients and evidence of association in the replication cohort was observed for TAAR1, RGS4, CNR1, and GRIA4 genes. In light of the fact that classic genetic studies have not yet identified strong, reproducible polymorphisms or haplotypes associated with fibromyalgia, and because there is clear evidence of environmental factors such as stress playing a prominent role in the pathogenesis, other groups have postulated that epigenetic findings might be important in fibromyalgia.[85] This is a promising area that needs further research.

Many of the genes that have been identified to date in leading to increases or decreases in the frequency of chronic pain states, or of pain sensitivity, are involved in regulating the breakdown or binding of neurotransmitters that generally increase pain sensitivity (e.g., glutamate) or decrease pain sensitivity (serotonin, norepinephrine, γ-aminobutyric acid [GABA]). The fact that pain sensitivity is polygenic and that different individuals develop increased pain sensitivity because of imbalances or altered activity of many different neurotransmitters likely partly explains the "U-shaped curve" seen with many analgesics, wherein they either work fairly well or not at all.

EVIDENCE OF CENTRAL NERVOUS SYSTEM DISTURBANCES IN PAIN AND SENSORY PROCESSING

The physiologic hallmark of fibromyalgia, centralized pain, or central sensitization is augmented CNS pain processing. This was originally identified in fibromyalgia (and still can be clinically) by noting that an individual is diffusely tender to palpation. The scientific terms for this phenomenon are diffuse hyperalgesia (increased pain to normally painful stimuli) and/or allodynia (pain in response to normally nonpainful stimuli). In the absence of an identifiable diffuse "peripheral" inflammatory process involving the body tissues, this strongly suggests that the CNS (i.e., spinal cord and brain) is causing augmented pain processing. In 1990, when the original criteria for fibromyalgia were first published, this feature of diffuse tenderness was incorporated into the diagnostic criteria by requiring that an individual had a certain number of tender points (11 or greater) in addition to CWP order to qualify for this diagnosis.[18] Subsequent studies using more sophisticated measures of experimental pain testing showed that individuals with fibromyalgia are more tender everywhere in the body, not just in the 18 regions considered to be "tender points."[86,87] Subsequent experimental pain testing studies have identified multiple potential mechanisms that may be responsible for pain amplification in fibromyalgia, including a decrease in the activity of descending analgesic pathways.[88,89]

EVIDENCE OF A GLOBAL INCREASE IN SENSORY PROCESSING OF NONPAINFUL STIMULI

Individuals with fibromyalgia do not just display disturbances in pain processing, they also as display heightened sensitivity to any type of sensory stimuli (e.g., auditory, visual, olfactory). Gerster and colleagues[90] were the first to demonstrate that fibromyalgia patients display a low noxious threshold to auditory tones, and this finding was subsequently replicated.[91] However, both of these studies used ascending measures of auditory threshold, so these findings could theoretically be due to expectancy or hypervigilance. A study by Geisser and colleagues[92] used an identical random staircase paradigm to test fibromyalgia patients' threshold to the loudness of auditory tones and to pressure. This study found that fibromyalgia patients displayed low thresholds to both types of stimuli, and the correlation between the results of auditory and pressure pain threshold testing suggested that some of this was due to shared variance, and some unique to one stimulus or the other. The notion that fibromyalgia and related syndromes might represent biologic amplification of all sensory stimuli has significant support from functional imaging studies that suggest that the insula is the most consistently hyperactive region (see following text).

This region has been noted to play a critical role in sensory integration, with the posterior insula serving a purer sensory role, and the anterior insula being associated with the emotional processing of sensations.[93–96] This finding also strongly supports a crucial role of the CNS in the pathogenesis of fibromyalgia because the changes in pain processing that have been identified could theoretically be due to a diffuse, systemic process involving peripheral nociception. It is difficult to imagine what type of peripheral process could lead to aberrant processing of any type of sensory stimuli.

BRAIN IMAGING STUDIES

These initial observations that individuals with fibromyalgia were diffusely tender led to subsequent functional, chemical, and structural brain neuroimaging studies that have been among the best "objective" evidence that the pain in fibromyalgia and related pain amplification syndrome is "real."[10] These methods such as functional magnetic resonance imaging (fMRI) clearly demonstrate that when individuals with fibromyalgia are given a mild pressure or heat stimuli that most individuals would feel as "touch" rather than "pain," they experience pain, and similar brain activation patterns in brain areas involved in pain processing (Fig. 36.2).[97,98] fMRI has also proved useful in determining how comorbid psychological factors influence pain processing in fibromyalgia. For example, in fibromyalgia patients with variable degrees of comorbid depression, the authors found that the anterior insula and amygdala activations were correlated with depressive symptoms, consistent with these "medial" and prefrontal brain regions being involved with affective or motivational aspects of pain processing (and being more closely related to unpleasantness rather than the sensory intensity of pain).[99] However, the degree of neuronal activation in more lateral structures generally thought to be associated with the "sensory" processing of pain (i.e., where the pain is localized and how intense it is) were not associated with levels of depressive symptoms, or the presence or absence of major depression, consistent with a plethora of evidence in the pain field that pain and depression are largely independent but overlapping physiologic processes.

A more recent advance in the use of fMRI is to look at the extent brain regions are "connected" to each other, that is, simultaneously activated (or deactivated).[100] The advantage of resting state analysis is that it is a window into brain changes associated with chronic, ongoing spontaneous pain. Studies have shown that individuals with fibromyalgia have increased connectivity between brain regions involved in increasing pain transmission and neural networks not normally involved in pain such as the default mode network, and the degree of this hyperconnectedness is related to the severity of ongoing pain.[101,102] A different group has shown that during a painful stimulus, connectivity is decreased between key antinociceptive regions (e.g., the brainstem—the origin of descending analgesic pathways) and a region they had previously identified to be a potential source of dysfunctional pain inhibition in fibromyalgia.[103,104] Lopez-Sola et al.[12,105] have performed imaging studies confirming quantitative sensory testing (QST) studies that these individuals are more sensitive to a number of nonpainful sensory stimuli other than pain (e.g., auditory, visual) and that machine learning paradigms can accurately distinguish fibromyalgia from nonfibromyalgia patients with over 90% accuracy using these results. Similarly, Harte et al.[106] used fMRI to show that an aversive visual stimulus caused greater evoked insula activity in fibromyalgia patients when compared to a control population and that this stimulus (as well as painful stimuli) was significantly attenuated by pregabalin.

Other imaging techniques have been used to identify the neurotransmitter abnormalities that may be driving the pain amplification seen in fibromyalgia and other chronic pain disorders. Wood and colleagues[107] used positron emission

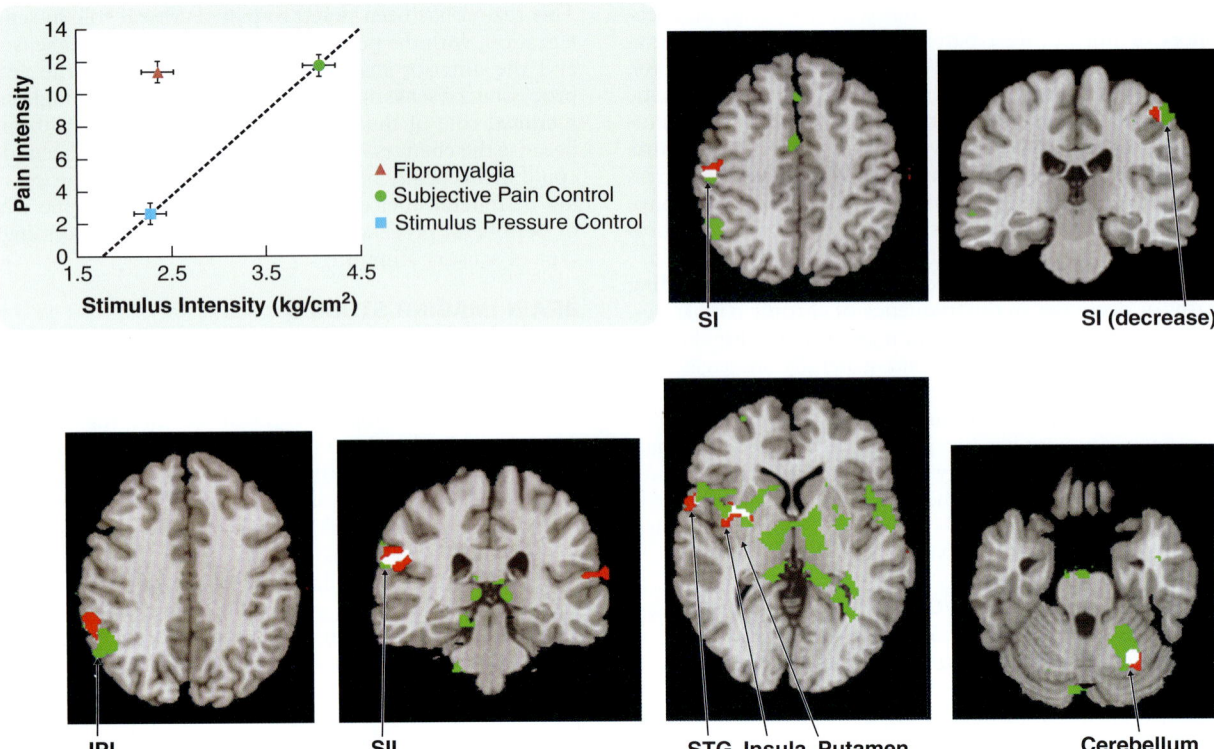

FIGURE 36.2 In top left panel, individuals with fibromyalgia (*red*) given a low-pressure stimulus have similar levels of pain and of neuronal activation in areas of the brain known to be involved in pain processing (*ends of arrows*) as controls given nearly twice as much pressure. Controls given the same low pressure that causes pain in fibromyalgia rate their pain as 2/20 instead of 12/20 and have no neuronal activation with this amount of pressure. IPL, inferior parietal lobule; SI, primary somatosensory cortex; SII, secondary somatosensory cortex; STG, superior temporal gyri. (*Gracely RH, Petzke F, Wolf JM, et al. Functional magnetic resonance imaging evidence of augmented pain processing in fibromyalgia.* Arthritis Rheum *2002;46[5]:1333–1343.*)

tomography (PET) to show that attenuated dopaminergic activity may be playing a role in pain transmission in fibromyalgia, whereas Harris and colleagues[108] showed evidence of decreased μ-opioid receptor availability (possibly due to increased release of endogenous μ-opioids) in fibromyalgia. This latter finding as well as previous studies showing increases in endogenous opioids in the cerebrospinal fluid (CSF) of fibromyalgia patients[109] has been suggested as evidence of why opioid analgesics appear to have poor efficacy in fibromyalgia.

Other groups have used proton magnetic resonance spectroscopy (H-MRS) to probe other neurotransmitters. Several groups have shown there are increases in brain concentrations of the body's major excitatory neurotransmitter, glutamate, in pain processing regions such as the insula in fibromyalgia.[110] This finding has also been noted in the CSF in fibromyalgia.[111] Drugs such as pregabalin and gabapentin are likely working in part in fibromyalgia by reducing glutamatergic activity.[112] This has been nicely demonstrated by Harris and colleagues[11] who showed that individuals with fibromyalgia that had the highest pretreatment levels of glutamate in the posterior insula were those most likely to respond to pregabalin. When pregabalin led to improvement in symptoms in these individuals, there was normalization of fMRI and connectivity findings, all suggesting that this neurotransmitter is playing a critical role in the pathogenesis of fibromyalgia in some individuals. An even more important finding from this study was the fact that individuals with fibromyalgia with normal or low baseline levels of glutamate in their posterior insula did not respond to pregabalin, even though this drug further lowered glutamate levels in these individuals as well. This helps us understand why no single class of CNS analgesic is likely to work in every patient with pain of CNS origin.

Conversely, H-MRS has recently been used to demonstrate low levels of one of the body's major inhibitory neurotransmitters, GABA.[113] This likely accounts for the efficacy of medications such as γ-hydroxybutyrate in fibromyalgia.[114] This finding may also suggest biologic plausibility for the associations between low alcohol consumption (compared to none or high) and improved symptomatology and functionality.[115] Alcohol is known to be a GABA agonist and analgesic, likely showing a U-shaped curve for analgesic effects just as for some beneficial cardiovascular effects. The fact that these imbalances between excitatory and inhibitory neurotransmitters are not diffusely noted in brain structures and seem to be somewhat confined to brain regions such as the insula that are known to be involved in polysensory processing[116,117] is concordant with the notion that there is a global problem with sensory hyperresponsiveness that is partly responsible for the pathophysiology of fibromyalgia and related conditions.[118,119] Figure 36.3 illustrates the neurotransmitters that have been demonstrated to influence pain transmission in the CNS.

THE ROLE OF NEUROENDOCRINE OR AUTONOMIC ABNORMALITIES

Because of the link between fibromyalgia and exposure to stress, and because both the neuroendocrine and autonomic nervous systems could cause many of the symptoms of fibromyalgia, these factors have been fairly extensively studied.[120–122] In fact, for several decades after it was understood that conditions such as fibromyalgia or chronic fatigue syndrome were not due to inflammation or infection, these areas were receiving considerable attention. The problem is that this research has generally yielded inconsistent findings, and treatment studies targeting these systems have failed, so these factors are now generally thought to play some role in some individuals but

Descending Influences on Nociceptive Processing

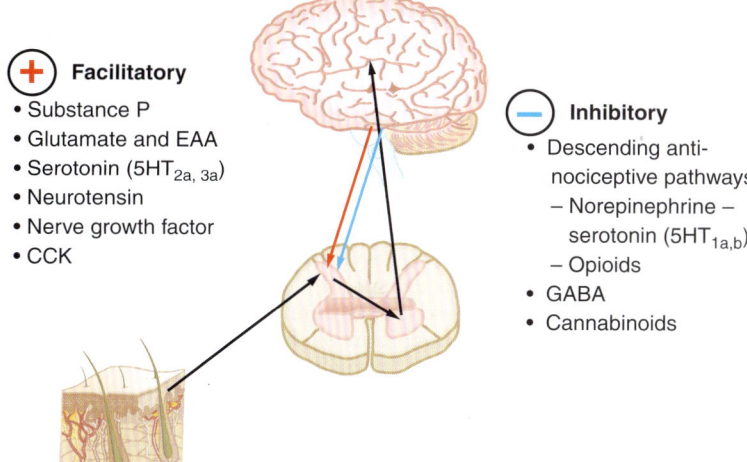

FIGURE 36.3 Neurotransmitters that are known to play either facilitatory (indicated in *red* and generally increase pain transmission in the spinal cord) or inhibitory (indicated in *blue* and decreasing pain transmission) roles in the central nervous system and the respective abnormality found in fibromyalgia (FM).

not central pathogenic factors in all with these conditions.[122–127] These studies note either hypo- or hyperactivity of both the hypothalamic-pituitary-adrenal (HPA) axis and sympathetic nervous system in individuals with fibromyalgia and related conditions and the precise abnormality varies from study to study. Moreover, these studies only find "abnormal" HPA or autonomic function in a very small percentage of patients, and there is tremendous overlap between patients and controls in any of these studies.

The inconsistency of these findings should not be surprising because nearly all of these studies were cross-sectional studies that assumed that if HPA and/or autonomic dysfunction was found in fibromyalgia, it must have *caused* the pain and other symptoms. Data now suggest the opposite. As noted earlier, there are better data suggesting that (especially HPA abnormalities) might represent a diathesis or be *due to* the pain or early life stress rather than causing it. In fact, in two recent studies examining HPA function in fibromyalgia, McLean showed that salivary cortisol levels covaried with pain levels, and that CSF levels of corticotropin-releasing hormone (CRH) were more closely related to an individual's pain level or a history of early life trauma than whether he or she were a fibromyalgia patient or control.[128,129] Because most previous studies of HPA and autonomic function in fibromyalgia failed to control for pain levels, a previous history of trauma, and posttraumatic stress disorder (PTSD) or other comorbid disorders that could affect HPA or autonomic dysfunction, it is not surprising for these inconsistencies.

THE ROLE OF PERIPHERAL FACTORS IN FIBROMYALGIA

Although most agree that the core symptoms of fibromyalgia are likely due to changes in the CNS, peripheral factors also play an important role in both the pathogenesis and treatment of fibromyalgia. For example, some elements of the processes of central sensitization can be worsened or driven by ongoing nociceptive input. Thus, it is possible or likely that the many individuals with fibromyalgia who also have comorbid conditions causing ongoing peripheral nociceptive input (e.g., myofascial pain, osteoarthritis, obesity[130]) would potentially benefit from therapies aimed at reducing peripheral drive of central sensitization. This was suggested in a short-term study by Affaitati[131] which showed that treating these common comorbid conditions could lead to improvement in the widespread pain and tenderness seen in fibromyalgia. In fact, one of the major areas of study needed into these conditions is to try to differentiate which individuals with these phenomena are being

driven from the CNS and which may be driven by ongoing peripheral nociceptive input and thus still benefit from these types of interventions.

EVIDENCE OF ABNORMAL CYTOKINES OR OF IMMUNE DYSFUNCTION IN FIBROMYALGIA

Although the prevailing view is that fibromyalgia is not an autoimmune disorder and that classic anti-inflammatory agents are not of benefit in this condition, there are some data suggesting that the immune system may be playing a role in the pathogenesis.[132] Perhaps, the most consistent finding noted to date is a mild elevation in interleukin 8 (IL-8), which is a cytokine associated with sympathetic function.[133,134] In other conditions closely linked to fibromyalgia such as interstitial cystitis, more sensitive assays of immune system function that can be gleaned by stimulating peripheral immune cells have been shown to be abnormal.[135] Some have speculated that diet or obesity could contribute to this low-grade inflammation in fibromyalgia and might be a potential target for therapy, whereas others have posited that this may provide evidence of microglia involvement in fibromyalgia. These are areas being actively explored.

THE ROLE OF "SMALL FIBER NEUROPATHY" IN FIBROMYALGIA

There is also a current ongoing controversy regarding the meaning of finding decreased intraepidermal nerve fiber density (i.e., small fiber neuropathy) in fibromyalgia. There is no question that this has been shown by many groups.[136–138] However, this is a very nonspecific finding that has now been noted in over 50 different pain and nonpain conditions.[137] Moreover, Harte et al.[106] recently demonstrated evidence that these findings could be induced in an animal model of central sensitization induced by increasing insular glutamate. We believe that this finding will eventually be shown to be a very nonspecific finding that might simply represent structural and functional reorganization of the peripheral nervous system (not unlike the changes in the CNS noted via voxel-based morphometry of the brain in chronic pain states[139]) in the context of chronic pain and other neurologic conditions. The hyperexcitable C nociceptors noted in fibromyalgia by Serra and colleagues[140] could also be secondary to CNS disinhibition of peripheral systems rather than indicating that there is primary pathology in the periphery. Regardless, the current evidence does not merit routine skin biopsies in suspected fibromyalgia patients and certainly does not yet suggest that this finding is of enough pathophysiologic significance to support the (noninvestigational) use of aggressive cytotoxic and anti-inflammatory regimens that some have proposed. When considering the available data regarding the pathophysiology of fibromyalgia, the data strongly favor CNS factors, and these findings should continue to drive clinical care.

Diagnosis

DIAGNOSIS OF FIBROMYALGIA

A careful musculoskeletal history and examination remains the most important diagnostic test for individuals with musculoskeletal pain. In other fields of medicine, advances in diagnostic testing have largely rendered a physical examination obsolete. However, in musculoskeletal medicine, technology confuses as much as it helps. For example, a high proportion of the healthy, asymptomatic population has a positive antinuclear antibody (ANA), positive rheumatoid factor, or abnormal results of imaging studies.[141-143] Worse yet, these diagnostic tests never tell us how severe the pain is because there is typically a significant discordance between the results of laboratory or imaging studies, and the severity of pain and other symptoms that the individual is experiencing. Therefore, the musculoskeletal history and examination must allow the clinician to arrive at the diagnosis (or at worst a very narrow differential diagnosis), and then if necessary, further diagnostic testing should be used to confirm these findings.

There are a number of diagnostic criteria that can be used for fibromyalgia. For reasons noted in the preceding text, the use of the original 1990 criteria is now being replaced by the more contemporary criteria proposed in 2010 and then modified in 2011 and 2016.[19-21] The advantages of these criteria are several-fold. These criteria acknowledge the nonpain symptoms of fibromyalgia and centralized pain and with the elimination of the tender point requirement appropriately diagnose the many men who have fibromyalgia or centralized pain. These criteria are also entirely symptom-based and thus are more likely to be embraced by primary care or other providers who never learned how to perform a tender point examination. Finally, perhaps the best advantage of these criteria is that instead of using a cut point to either declare that an individual does or does not meet criteria for fibromyalgia, these criteria can also be used to place a patient on a spectrum of central sensitivity, which has been termed "fibromyalgianess."

Wolfe[144] was the first to note the importance of the concept of fibromyalgianess, by showing the importance of "subsyndromic" or "subthreshold" fibromyalgia. In a series of studies, he showed that in individuals with conditions such as RA, low back pain, or osteoarthritis, an individual's fibromyalgia score, derived with measures very similar to the 2010/11/16 criteria, was typically more predictive of pain and disability than more objective measures of activity of these diseases, such as measures of inflammation or joint damage.[145,146]

The survey version of these criteria is entirely patient self-report and can be administered on a single piece of paper. Our group uses the Michigan Body Map to assess the Widespread Pain Index (up to 19 body areas each counted as one point)[147] as well as the Symptom Severity Index that asks about the presence and severity of fatigue, sleep disturbances, and memory difficulties (each scored 0 to 3 for the presence and severity) as well as irritable bowel, headaches, and mood problems (1 point each, total Symptom Severity Index Score is 0 to 12) (Fig. 36.4). The Widespread Pain Index and Symptom Severity Index are combined for a total score of 0 to 31. When used as a dichotomous measure with a variety of "cut points" that can be used, this measure will roughly identify most of the same individuals as the old criteria (except many more males).[19,20] However, when fibromyalgia is considered more as a physiologic construct to determine where on the continuum of pain sensitivity an individual is, then this can be used as a continuous measure (i.e., degree of fibromyalgianess or the degree to which pain is centralized) that can be useful in the diagnosis and treatment of virtually any patient with a rheumatic disorder that is experiencing pain.[144]

In several recent studies, this concept of fibromyalgianess or subsyndromal fibromyalgia has been shown to be very clinically important. In these studies by Brummett and colleagues,[147,148] individuals who were scheduled for either lower extremity joint replacement or hysterectomy completed a broad battery of validated self-report measures prior to their surgery. The group hypothesized that individuals with higher fibromyalgia scores on the 2011 Fibromyalgia Survey Criteria would predict increased opioid requirements in the inpatient admission following surgery as well as to long-term surgery pain outcomes. Again, this measure is scored from 0 to 31 with a level of 13 is typically used as being diagnostic cut point of fibromyalgia. These studies demonstrated that even after adjustment for each 1-point increase in this measure from 0 to 31, individuals needed an adjusted 7 to 9 mg more oral morphine equivalents to control their pain in the first 24 to 48 hours following surgery and were 15% to 20% less likely to improve following arthroplasty, all after adjustment for other patient

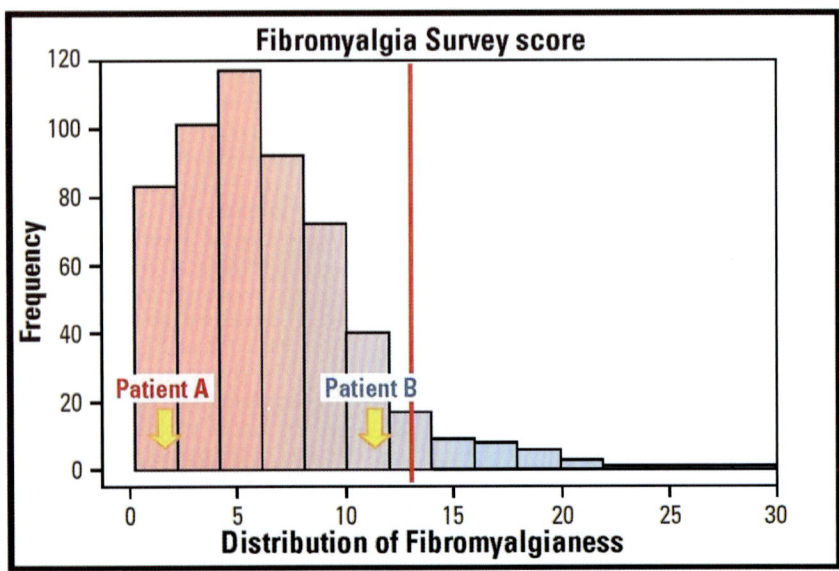

FIGURE 36.4 The histogram displays the distribution of fibromyalgia scores using the 2011 Fibromyalgia Survey Criteria from a cohort of patients undergoing total knee and hip arthroplasty. Both patient A (fibromyalgia score = 1) and patient B (fibromyalgia score = 11) have a fibromyalgia score below the threshold for being termed *fibromyalgia positive*. However, when compared to patient A, after adjustment for other covariates, patient B would consume 80 mg oral morphine equivalents more opioid during the postoperative inpatient admission and be five times less likely to achieve the threshold for meaningful pain improvement 6 months after surgery. *(Data from Brummett CM, Janda AM, Schueller CM, et al. Survey criteria for fibromyalgia independently predict increased postoperative opioid consumption after lower-extremity joint arthroplasty: a prospective, observational cohort study. Anesthesiology 2013;119[6]: 1434–1443.)*

and clinical care variables.[72,73,148] These findings were independent of a number of preoperative characteristics, including age, sex, anxiety, depression, catastrophizing, and opioid use. More importantly, these findings were linear and the same incremental increase in opioid and surgery nonresponsiveness was seen in individuals well below the threshold used to diagnose fibromyalgia and extending well into the range of individuals exceeding this threshold. Figure 36.5 shows two different individuals with osteoarthritis, neither of whom would meet criteria for fibromyalgia but who are at different points of the fibromyalgia continuum, and shows the marked difference in opioid responsiveness and improvement in pain following arthroplasty that these two individuals would experience. These data suggest that this measure of fibromyalgianess might serve as the degree of pain centralization an individual is experiencing and help identify individuals in perioperative or other settings who are less likely to respond to peripherally directed analgesics such as surgery, or opioids.

In clinical practice, one should suspect fibromyalgia in individuals with multifocal pain that cannot be explained on the basis of damage or inflammation in those regions of the body. In most cases, musculoskeletal pain is the most prominent feature, but because pain pathways throughout the body are amplified, pain can be perceived more generally. Thus, chronic headaches, sore throats, chest pain, abdominal pain, and pelvic pain are very common in individuals with fibromyalgia, and patients with chronic regional pain in any of these locations are more likely to have fibromyalgia.

Because pain is a defining feature of fibromyalgia, it is helpful to focus on the features of the pain that can help distinguish it from other disorders. The pain of fibromyalgia is typically diffuse or multifocal, is difficult to localize, often waxes and wanes, and is frequently migratory in nature. These characteristics of centralized pain are quite different from nociceptive pain, where both the location and severity of pain are typically more constant. Patients may complain of discomfort when they

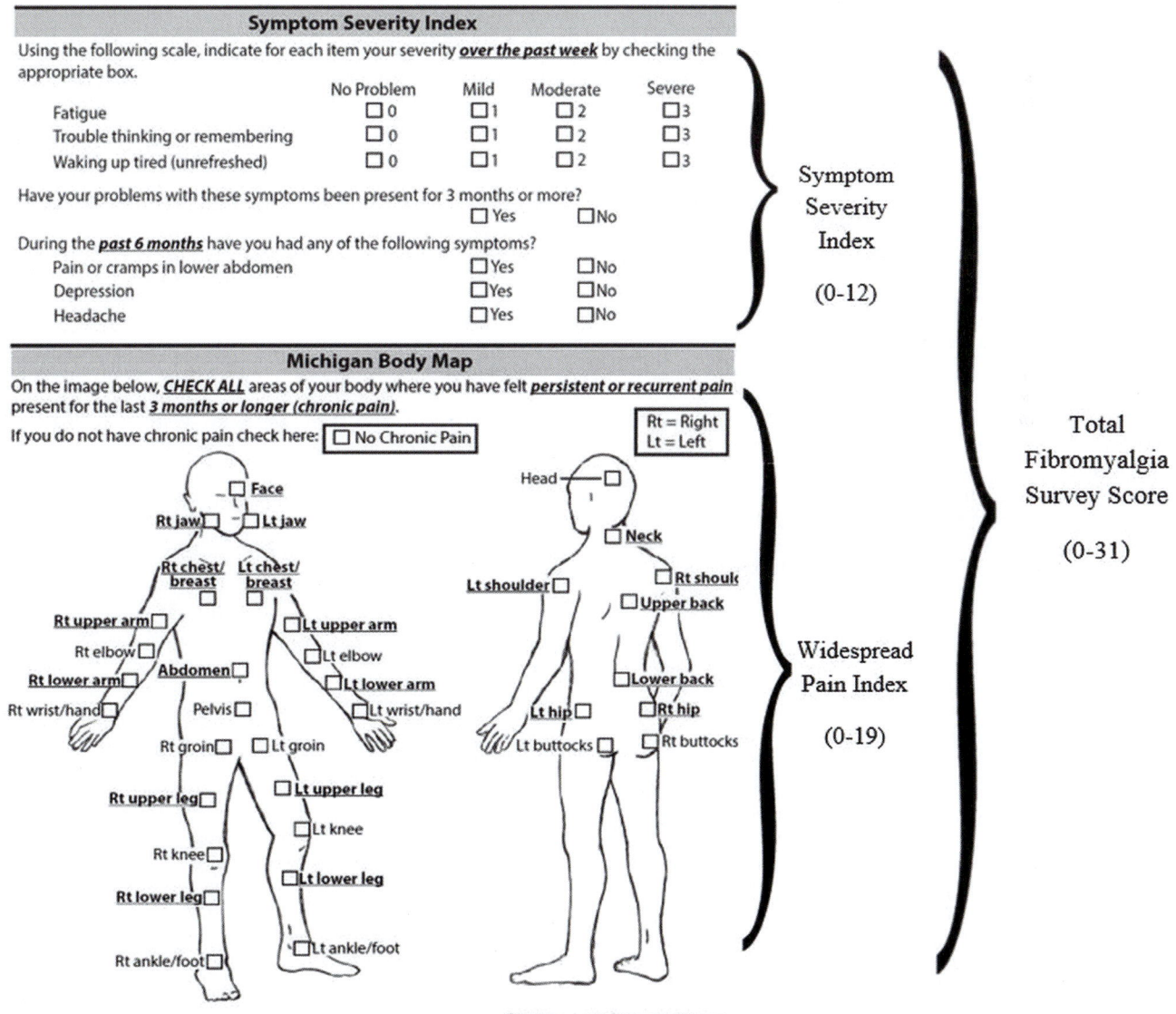

FIGURE 36.5 The 2011 Fibromyalgia Survey Criteria is a brief, simple self-report measure. It is made up of two components, the Symptom Severity Index (SSI) and the Widespread Pain Index (WPI). The SSI includes six questions about comorbid central nervous system symptoms with a score ranging from 0 to 12. Our group collects the WPI using the Michigan Body Map, which includes up to 31 body regions to allow patients to better describe their areas of pain. For the purposes of creating the fibromyalgia score, only the 19 body areas originally described are scored (original 19 areas are bolded and underlined). The total fibromyalgia score ranges from 0 to 31. *(Reprinted with permission from Dr. Chad Brummet and University of Michigan.*

are touched or when wearing tight clothing and may experience dysesthesias or paresthesias that accompany the pain.

Another defining characteristic of "centralized" pain is the company it keeps. In addition to pain, individuals typically experience a number of other somatic symptoms. These symptoms can generally be broken into two categories: (1) symptoms of CNS origin that are controlled by the same neurotransmitters that control pain processing and (2) symptoms due to generalized sensory hyperresponsiveness. In the first category, fatigue, memory difficulties, and sleep and mood disturbances are all very common in fibromyalgia and other centralized pain states. The reason it is thought that these symptoms are at least partially due to some of the same neurotransmitter abnormalities that contribute to the pathophysiology of fibromyalgia is that several of these symptoms will typically improve along with pain when an individual is successfully treated with drugs that alter these neurotransmitters. The second type of symptom due to generalized hyperresponsiveness often challenges clinicians to doubt the veracity of a fibromyalgia patient's complaints. This is often responsible for the "pan-positive review of symptoms" that has often characterized these individuals as "somatizers." As the biology of somatization is becoming increasingly understood as one of sensory hyperresponsiveness,[149] these sensory symptoms throughout the body can be better understood by clinicians if one realizes that all sensory experiences are interpreted by brain regions, such as the insula, that are known to be hyperactive in fibromyalgia and other centralized pain states.

The most common of these more systemic symptoms are fatigue, sleep difficulties, weakness, problems with attention or memory, unexplainable weight fluctuations, and heat and cold intolerance. "Allergies" are reported much more commonly in fibromyalgia patients, although these excess symptoms are better considered hypersensitivities rather than true IgE-mediated immunologic reactions. These patients are also more prone to nonallergic rhinitis, sinus and nasal congestion, and lower respiratory symptoms, all of which again may primarily attributable to neural mechanisms. Distortions in hearing, vision, and vestibular symptoms are often reported, as are sicca symptoms (dry eyes or dry mouth) sometimes so prominent that these individuals will overlap with those with Sjögren's syndrome.

Other COPCs, or sensory disturbances throughout the body, are more common in fibromyalgia. These include noncardiac chest pain, heartburn and palpitations, and the frequent comorbidity of IBS.[150] Syncope and neutrally mediated hypotension also occur more commonly in fibromyalgia, as does postural orthostatic tachycardia syndrome (POTS).[151] Pelvic complaints are common, including not only pain but also urinary frequency and urgency.[66] In females, the frequent comorbid diagnoses are dysmenorrhea, interstitial cystitis, endometriosis, and sensitivity disorders like vulvar vestibulitis and vulvodynia, whereas in males, these same symptoms are sometimes often diagnosed as having chronic or nonbacterial prostatitis.[152]

Laboratory testing is generally not useful, except for the purpose of differential diagnosis. One factor that can help guide the intensity of the diagnostic workup is the length of time the patient has had symptoms. If the patient's symptoms have persisted for several years, minimal testing is required, whereas a more aggressive strategy should be employed for acute or subacute onset of symptoms. Simple testing should be limited to complete blood count and routine serum chemistries, along with thyroid-stimulating hormone (TSH) and erythrocyte sedimentation rate (ESR). Serologic studies such as ANA and rheumatoid factor assays should generally be avoided unless there are historical features not seen in fibromyalgia or abnormalities on physical examination. This represents a problem in clinical practice because several autoimmune disorders share

TABLE 36.2	Conditions that Simulate Fibromyalgia
Common
Hypothyroidism
Polymyalgia rheumatica
Early in course of autoimmune disorders, for example, rheumatoid arthritis or SLE
Sjögren's syndrome
Less Common
Hepatitis C
Sleep apnea
Chiari malformation
Celiac sprue
Drug-induced myalgias (e.g., lipid-lowering drugs)

SLE, systemic lupus erythematosus.

overlapping symptomatology with fibromyalgia. These include not only fatigue, arthralgias, and myalgias but also such symptoms as morning stiffness and subjective swelling of the hands and feet. Certain dermatologic features commonly seen in fibromyalgia, including malar flushing, livedo reticularis, and Raynaud's disease–like reddening of the hands, also mimic symptoms of autoimmune disorders. This sometimes results in patients with fibromyalgia being misdiagnosed as having an autoimmune disorder such as SLE.

Aside from the many comorbid conditions already discussed, fibromyalgia may present similarly to a number of disorders or concurrently with other disorders that may confuse the diagnosis. Table 36.2 shows conditions that often mimic or present concurrently with fibromyalgia. Hypothyroidism and polymyalgia rheumatica can be differentiated from fibromyalgia by results of TSH and ESR. Sleep apnea and hepatitis C also simulate fibromyalgia and tend to present more often in men than women.

Although the physical examination is generally unremarkable in individuals with fibromyalgia, it is helpful to assess for diffuse tenderness, and there are many ways that this can be done clinically other than performing a tender point count. For example, individuals with fibromyalgia are more sensitive to the inflation of a blood pressure cuff.[153] Another way to assess overall pain threshold while also getting other valuable diagnostic information is to assess pain thresholds in the hands and arms of all chronic pain patients. A rapid examination by applying firm pressure over several interphalangeal (IP) joints of each hand and also over the adjacent phalanges and then more proximally to include firm palpation of the muscles of the forearm including the lateral epicondyle region. This is one way to assess overall pain threshold as well as get additional diagnostic information about the patient. If the individual is tender in many of these areas, or in just the muscles of the forearm, he or she are likely diffusely tender (i.e., have a low central pain threshold). However, if the individual is only tender over the IP joints and not the other regions, and especially if there is any swelling over these joints, one should be more concerned about a systemic autoimmune disorder, whereas if tenderness is confined to just the bones, one might suspect a metabolic bone disease or condition causing periostitis (e.g., hyperparathyroidism).

Once a clinician rules out other potential disorders, an important and at times controversial step in the management of fibromyalgia is asserting the diagnosis. Despite some assumptions that being "labeled" with fibromyalgia may adversely affect patients, all existing studies suggest that this is not the case and that the diagnosis of fibromyalgia is often a tremendous source of relief for the patient and leads to decreased health care utilization because of a reduction in referrals and diagnostic testing "looking for the cause of the pain."[154]

Treatment

GENERAL APPROACH

All individuals diagnosed with a condition such as fibromyalgia should first receive some basic education regarding this disorder. Clinicians can do this in the context of their practice (e.g., with nurse educators or other allied health professionals) or electronically using Web sites and videos (see the following text). This education should emphasize that it is important that the patient plays an active role in their management and that some of the most effective therapies are nondrug therapies, such as exercising, improving sleep, and reducing stress. Although recent treatment guidelines favor the use of nonpharmacologic versus pharmacologic therapies,[155] there are pragmatic factors in routine practice (lack of availability or reimbursement, patient is unwilling to use or try these therapies until his or her symptoms are somewhat better controlled) that often make this impractical.[156] Thus, most patients need some combination of pharmacologic and nonpharmacologic therapies to have meaningful improvement in symptoms and function. Education will be critical, however, to getting patients to consider nonpharmacologic options. Table 36.3 outlines all of the evidence-based treatments for individuals with fibromyalgia as well as practical suggestions for dosing and initiating therapy.

PHARMACOLOGIC THERAPY

There are a number of classes of drugs that can be of some benefit in fibromyalgia. Unfortunately, as in other chronic pain conditions, drugs only work well in a subset of patients, and the overall effect size of any of these therapies is modest, at best. However, it is a misconception that the drugs we use to treat fibromyalgia and centralized pain are less effective than drugs we use to treat other pain conditions, or nociceptive pain.[160] It is also of note that there have been very few negative clinical trials of new therapies in fibromyalgia (essentially all have targeted neurotransmitters in the CNS known to be abnormal in fibromyalgia) over the past two decades since drug development for this condition commenced. The majority of fibromyalgia clinical trials have involved CNS-acting drugs of one class or another. Trials studying the oldest class of agents, tricyclic antidepressants (TCAs), are perhaps most abundant but generally underpowered individually. More recently, larger trials have been performed of many other classes of drugs, especially SNRI and gabapentinoids.

Tricyclic Agents

The earliest studied pharmacologic therapy for fibromyalgia was low doses of tricyclic compounds. Most TCAs increase the concentrations of serotonin and/or norepinephrine (noradrenaline) by directly blocking their respective reuptake. The effectiveness of TCAs, particularly amitriptyline and cyclobenzaprine, in treating the symptoms of pain, poor sleep, and fatigue associated with fibromyalgia is supported by several randomized controlled trials.[157] Tolerability can be a problem but can be improved by beginning at very low doses (e.g., 10 mg of amitriptyline or 5 mg of cyclobenzaprine), giving the dose a few hours before bedtime, and very slowly escalating the dose. Very low dose cyclobenzaprine has recently shown to be quite effective in a subset of individuals with fibromyalgia with a specific sleep architecture, seemingly with less side effects than seen in some of the earlier studies of higher doses.[161]

Serotonin and Norepinephrine Reuptake Inhibitors

Because of a better side effect profile, newer antidepressants, that is, selective serotonin reuptake inhibitors (SSRIs), are frequently used in fibromyalgia. The SSRIs fluoxetine, citalopram, and paroxetine have each been evaluated in randomized, placebo-controlled trials.[162–166] In general, the results of studies of SSRIs in fibromyalgia have paralleled the experience in

other pain conditions. The newer "highly selective" serotonin reuptake inhibitors, for example, citalopram, seem to be less efficacious than the older SSRIs, which have some noradrenergic activity at higher doses.[167]

Because TCAs and high doses of certain "SSRIs" such as fluoxetine and sertraline that have the most balanced reuptake inhibition are the most effective analgesics, many have concluded that dual receptor inhibitors such as SNRIs and norepinephrine serotonin reuptake inhibitors (NSRIs) may be of more benefit than pure serotonergic drugs.[167] These drugs are pharmacologically similar to some TCAs in their ability to inhibit the reuptake of both serotonin and norepinephrine but differ from TCAs in being generally devoid of significant activity at other receptor systems, including acetylcholine. This selectivity results in diminished side effects and enhanced tolerability. The first available SNRI, venlafaxine, has data to support its use in the management of neuropathic pain, and retrospective trial data demonstrate that this compound is also effective in the prophylaxis of migraine and tension headaches.[168] Two studies in fibromyalgia have had conflicting results, with the one using a higher dose showing efficacy.[169]

Two newer SNRIs, duloxetine and milnacipran, have undergone more recent multicenter trials and were shown to be effective in a number of outcome variables and are both now approved in the United States for the treatment of fibromyalgia.[170,171] These drugs seem roughly comparable in the overall efficacy profile, with studies generally noting modest improvement (although not reaching statistical significance in all studies) in domains such as pain, overall improvement, physical functioning, level of fatigue, and degree of reported physical impairment. For both compounds, these effects seemed to be independent of the drug effect on mood, thus suggesting that the analgesic and other positive effects of this class of drugs in fibromyalgia is not simply due to their antidepressant effects. Both of these drugs are better tolerated if taken with food, and if patients are warned about likely initial nausea, and counseled that this typically resolves in a week or so, and if not then they should discontinue the drug. The maximum approved dose of duloxetine is 60 mg per day, but it was studied in trials at doses up to 120 mg and shown to be safe, and similarly, the initial dose of milnacipran is 100 mg, but some patients will benefit from increasing the dose as high as 200 mg. Hypertension is more likely to be a problem with milnacipran because it appears to have noradrenergic effects; for these same reasons, it might be slightly more likely to help with symptoms such as fatigue.

Es-reboxetine, a selective norepinephrine reuptake inhibitor, was also tested and shown to be efficacious in fibromyalgia.[172] This adds to emerging evidence suggesting that norepinephrine reuptake activity may be much more important than serotonergic reuptake for analgesic effects.

Anticonvulsants

A few classes of antiepileptic drugs have been shown to be effective in the treatment of various chronic pain conditions, including fibromyalgia, postherpetic neuralgia, and painful diabetic neuropathy.[173] Pregabalin and gabapentin have the same mechanism of action and bind to the $\alpha_2\delta$ subunit of calcium channels, and both are approved for the treatment of neuropathic pain as well as several other indications. Several studies have shown the efficacy of pregabalin against pain, sleep disturbances, and fatigue as compared to placebo in fibromyalgia, leading to this being the first drug approved in the United States for use in this condition.[174] Gabapentin has been shown to have very similar efficacy and side effect profile in fibromyalgia.[175] The tolerability of these drugs can be enhanced by beginning at a low dose and giving either two-thirds of the dose, or the entire dose, at bedtime. The maximally approved dose of pregabalin is 450 mg, but in trials, it was studied at doses as high as 600 mg and shown to be safe

TABLE 36.3 Evidence-Based Therapies for Fibromyalgia

Treatment	Cost	Specifics	Evidence Level	Side Effects	Clinical Pearls
General Recommendations					
Patient education[207]	Low	Incorporate principles of self-management including a multimodal approach	1, A		Following initial diagnosis, spend several visits (or use separate educational sessions) to explain the condition and set treatment expectations.
Nonpharmacologic Therapies					
Graded exercise[208]	Low	Aerobic exercise has been best studied, but strengthening and stretching have also been shown to be of value.	1, A	Worsening of symptoms when program is begun too rapidly	Counsel patients to "start low, go slow" For many patients, focusing first on increasing daily "activity" is more helpful before actually starting exercise.
Cognitive-behavioral therapy (CBT)[209]	Low or no cost for e-CBT but other forms can be costly and not reimbursed	Pain-based CBT programs have been shown to be effective in one-on-one settings, small groups, and via Internet.	1, A	No significant side effects of CBT per se, but patient acceptance is often poor when they view this as a "psychological" intervention. Some challenges to finding skilled providers Potential cost barriers if not covered by insurance	Internet-based programs are gaining acceptance and are more convenient for working patients.
Complementary and alternative medicine (CAM) therapies[210]	Variable	Most CAM therapies have not been rigorously studied	2, B	Generally safe Most are not covered by insurance leading to potential cost barriers.	There is emerging evidence that CAM treatments such as tai chi, yoga, balneotherapy, and acupuncture might be effective. Allowing patients to choose which CAM therapies to incorporate into an active treatment program can increase self-efficacy.
CNS neurostimulatory therapies[194]		Several different types of CNS neurostimulatory therapies have been shown to be effective in FM and other chronic pain states.	2, B	Headache	These treatments continue to be refined as we learn about optimal stimulation targets, "dosing," etc.
Pharmacologic Therapies		Pharmacologic therapy is best chosen based on the predominant symptoms and initiated in low dose with slow dose escalation.	5, Consensus		Some practitioners find that getting patients on a drug regimen that helps improve symptoms prior to initiating nonpharmacologic therapies can help improve compliance.
Tricyclic compounds[157,211]		Amitriptyline 10–70 mg qhs Cyclobenzaprine 5–20 mg qhs Nortriptyline 10–100 mg qhs	1, A	Dry mouth, weight gain, constipation, "groggy," or drugged feeling	When effective, can improve a wide range of symptoms including pain, sleep, bowel, and bladder symptoms Taking these drugs several hours prior to bedtime improves side effect profile.
Serotonin norepinephrine reuptake inhibitors[211]	Duloxetine is generic; milnacipran is not.	Duloxetine, 30–120 mg daily Milnacipran, 100–200 mg daily	1, A	Nausea, palpitations, headache, fatigue, tachycardia, hypertension	Warning patients about transient nausea, taking with food, and slowly increasing dose can increase tolerability. Milnacipran might be slightly more noradrenergic than duloxetine and thus potentially more helpful for fatigue, memory problems—but also more likely to cause HTN.

TABLE 36.3 (Continued)

Treatment	Cost	Specifics	Evidence Level	Side Effects	Clinical Pearls
Gabapentinoids[212]	Gabapentin is generic; pregabalin is not.	• Gabapentin, 800–3,200 mg/d in divided doses • Pregabalin up to 600 mg per day in divided doses	1, A	Sedation, weight gain, dizziness	• Giving most or all of the dose at bedtime can increase tolerability, especially during initiations and upward titration.
γ-Hydroxybutyrate[114]	Available for treating narcolepsy, cataplexy	γ-Hydroxybutyrate 4.5–6.0 g per night in divided doses	1, A	Sedation, respiratory depression, and death	• Shown to be efficacious but not approved by FDA because of safety concerns
Low-dose naltrexone[158]	Low	4.5 mg/d	2, B	Insomnia, vivid dreams	• Two small single-center RCTs; more data needed
Cannabinoids[159]	NA	Nabilone 0.5 mg po qhs to 1.0 mg bid	1, A	Sedation, dizziness, dry mouth	• No synthetic cannabinoid is approved in United States for treatment of pain.
Selective serotonin reuptake inhibitors (SSRIs)[211]	SSRIs that should be used in FM (see Clinical Pearls) are all generic.	Fluoxetine, sertraline, paroxetine	1, A	Nausea, sexual dysfunction, weight gain, sleep disturbance	• Older, less selective SSRIs may have some efficacy in improving pain, especially at higher doses that have more prominent noradrenergic effects. • Newer SSRIs (citalopram, escitalopram, des-venlafaxine) are less effective or ineffective as analgesics.
NSAIDs		• No evidence of efficacy • Can be helpful to treat comorbid "peripheral pain generators"	5, D	Gastrointestinal, renal, and cardiac side effects	• Use the lowest dose for the shortest period of time to reduce side effects
Opioids		• Tramadol with or without acetaminophen, 50–100 mg every 6 h • No evidence of efficacy for stronger opioids	5, D	Sedation, addiction, tolerance, opioid-induced hyperalgesia	• There is increasing evidence that opioids are less effective or ineffective for treating chronic pain, and this is especially true for FM. • Opioids may worsen hyperalgesia even in those patients who report short-term benefit after taking.

CNS, central nervous system; FDA, U.S. Food and Drug Administration; FM, fibromyalgia; HTN, hypertension; NA, not applicable; NSAIDs, nonsteroidal anti-inflammatory drugs; RCT, randomized controlled trial.

and efficacious. For most patients, the dose of gabapentin needed for analgesic is often 1,800 to 2,400 mg per day; however, some patients will derive benefit at lower doses. Another antiepileptic compound, clonazepam, has demonstrated efficacy in treating TMD and associated jaw pain and is useful in the treatment of restless legs syndrome.[173] Thus, clonazepam may be of value in subsets of fibromyalgia patients with these comorbidities; however, the risks associated with chronic benzodiazepine use likely outweigh the potential benefit. In addition, two other drugs that are likely working by counteracting the effects of increased glutamatergic activity in fibromyalgia are memantine and ketamine, both of which have some evidence of efficacy.[176,177]

Combination Drug Therapy

Combinations of multiple classes of adjunctive pain medications have been a common practice for many years. A recent study demonstrated that the combination of duloxetine and pregabalin was superior to either drug alone in treating fibromyalgia.[178] The combination improved pain, as well as Fibromyalgia Impact Questionnaire, 36-Item Short Form Health Survey (SF-36), and Medical Outcomes Study Sleep Scale scores. This is consistent with previous data demonstrating that combinations of therapies with differing mechanisms of action are effective in neuropathic pain.[179]

Other Central Nervous System–Acting Drugs

Sedative-hypnotic compounds are widely used by fibromyalgia patients. A handful of studies have been published on the use of certain nonbenzodiazepine hypnotics in fibromyalgia, such as zopiclone and zolpidem. These reports have suggested that these agents can improve the sleep and, perhaps, fatigue of fibromyalgia patients, although they had no significant effects upon pain.

On the other hand, γ-hydroxybutyrate (also known as sodium oxybate), a precursor of GABA with powerful sedative properties, was recently shown to be very efficacious in improving fatigue, pain, and sleep architecture in patients with fibromyalgia.[180] Note, however, that this agent is a scheduled substance due to its abuse potential and was not approved by the U.S. Food and Drug Administration (FDA) because of safety concerns. Nonetheless, these studies along with the H-MRS showing low GABA suggest that other less toxic GABA agonists may have an important role in treating fibromyalgia.

Cannabinoids are another class of drugs where there is renewed interest in chronic pain states. There have been two randomized controlled trials of synthetic cannabinoids in fibromyalgia (both with nabilone), and both studies concluded that the drug was efficacious (in one study for both pain and sleep, in the other study at lower dose for just sleep).[181,182] This is not surprising as there is increased recognition that this class of drugs may have utility in pain of neural origin.[159]

Pramipexole is a dopamine agonist indicated for Parkinson disease that has shown utility in the treatment of periodic leg movement disorder.[183] One study suggested that this compound may improve both pain and sleep in fibromyalgia patients, but these results have not been replicated with this or other dopamine agonists.[184] Because of this, this class of drug may be best reserved for individuals with other indications, such as comorbid restless legs syndrome.

Tizanidine is a centrally acting α_2-adrenergic agonist approved by the FDA for the treatment of muscle spasticity associated with multiple sclerosis and stroke. Literature suggests that this agent is a useful adjunct in treating several chronic pain conditions, including chronic daily headaches and low back pain. A recent trial reported significant improvements in several parameters in fibromyalgia, including sleep, pain, and measures of quality of life.[185]

Classic Analgesics

There have been no adequate, randomized controlled clinical trials of opiates in fibromyalgia, and most in the field (including the authors) have not found this class of compounds to be effective in anecdotal experience. Tramadol is a weak μ-agonist combined with serotonin/norepinephrine reuptake inhibition. This compound does appear to be somewhat efficacious in the management of fibromyalgia, as both an isolated compound and as fixed-dose combination with acetaminophen.[183]

In addition to the previously studied and cited mechanistic studies suggesting why opioids might not be effective in fibromyalgia (i.e., PET evidence of decrease opioid receptor availability, and high CSF levels of endorphins), recent functional and chemical imaging studies by this same group suggest an even more important potential problem. In these studies, the native state of fibromyalgia may be akin to that of opioid-induced hyperalgesia, in that the regions with the lowest receptor occupancy are the most hyperalgesic.[186] Thus, it is possible that at least in a subset of individuals, opioids may make these individuals' hyperalgesia worse rather than better. This notion is also supported by previously noted clinical studies suggesting that opioid *antagonists* such as naltrexone may be effective in fibromyalgia[158] (although the authors of these studies hypothesize these effects are due to glial cell inhibition). If opioids are used for refractory patients, it is possible that those opioids with mixed opioid antagonist effects (e.g., buprenorphine), norepinephrine reuptake inhibition (tapentadol), or NMDA receptor blockade (methadone) might be better than pure μ-agonists, but this is entirely conjecture. Another problem with opioid use in fibromyalgia is that this therapy appears to reduce patient motivation to pursue other approaches, particularly nonpharmacologic approaches.[187] Despite the fact that opioids are not recommended for the treatment of fibromyalgia, studies demonstrate that many fibromyalgia patients are prescribed opioids.[188]

A large number of fibromyalgia patients use NSAIDs and acetaminophen. Although numerous studies have failed to confirm their effectiveness as analgesics in fibromyalgia,[189] a recent study of the combination of celecoxib and acyclovir was shown to be effective in fibromyalgia.[190] It is not known whether the benefit came from one or both of these drugs, and future studies will be necessary to dissect out these findings. There is also limited evidence that patients may experience enhanced analgesia when treated with combinations of NSAIDs and other agents. This phenomenon may be a result of concurrent "peripheral" pain (i.e., due to damage or inflammation of tissues, e.g., osteoarthritis, RA) conditions that may be present and/or that these comorbid peripheral pain generators might lead to worsening of "central" pain.

NEUROSTIMULATORY THERAPIES

A variety of neurostimulatory therapies can be effective in treating musculoskeletal pain. For some time, transcutaneous electrical nerve stimulation (TENS) has been used to treat musculoskeletal pain.[191,192] Conventional TENS (C-TENS) is given at high stimulation frequency with low intensity. Pain relief is immediate, but short-lived, when it occurs. Acupuncture-like TENS (often abbreviated Al-TENS) is given at a lower frequency and higher intensity (which is sometimes uncomfortable) and when it works generally has a longer lasting effect than C-TENS. These neurostimulatory therapies would be expected to be most helpful for pain of peripheral/nociceptive origin.

A new set of neurostimulatory therapies is emerging that would be expected to be more effective for "centralized" pain because these therapies all aim to stimulate the CNS and, in doing so, modulate CNS pain transmission. Many such therapies have been developed and tested, with many showing some efficacy in several pain states. These include noninvasive techniques such as repetitive transcranial magnetic stimulation (rTMS), transcranial direct current stimulation (tDCS), and newer ways of noninvasively stimulating brain structures.[193,194] Although the studies to date with these therapies have yielded somewhat inconsistent results, a trend is emerging suggesting that these treatments might be most effective in centralized rather than purely peripheral pain states and with stimulation parameters that enable signals to travel into deeper cortical tissues than occurs with typical delivery of rTMS and tDCS. Other more invasive techniques have also shown promise in patients with more refractory pain states, such as spinal cord stimulation, deep brain stimulation, and vagal nerve stimulation.

NONPHARMACOLOGIC THERAPIES

The two best studied nonpharmacologic therapies are cognitive-behavioral therapy and exercise. Both of these therapies have been shown to be efficacious in the treatment of fibromyalgia as well as a plethora of other medical conditions.[195–197] Both of these treatments can lead to sustained (e.g., greater than 1 year) improvements and are very effective when an individual complies with therapy.

For exercise, it is important to "start low, go slow." Many fibromyalgia and other chronic pain patients are quite sedentary, and in these individuals, it is important to focus on becoming more active rather than classic "exercise." With respect to exercise, nearly any type (aerobic, stretching, strengthening) can be helpful. It is most important that patients understand that they must become more active and then eventually start very mild exercise (e.g., walking).

There are many elements to cognitive-behavioral therapy, but one that has had increased attention recently has been a focus on using behavioral measures to treat the sleep disorders seen in conditions such as fibromyalgia.[198] This increased focus on improving sleep is concordant with more and preclinical and clinical research showing how important sleep is in pain transmission. There is a free Web site for patients (http://www.fibroguide.com) that allows patients to access these behavioral interventions over the Internet rather than in person, and this Web site was tested in a randomized controlled trial and was shown to be effective.[199] "Lighter" options such as this will work well in many patients, whereas in other individuals with more severe psychological or psychiatric comorbidity will benefit from more intensive (i.e., group or one-on-one) treatments. A recent study suggested that adding emotional disclosure to standard cognitive-behavioral therapy may be of benefit to a subset of patients who will receive significant improvement.[200]

Complementary and alternative therapies have been explored by patients managing their own illness as well as health care providers. As with other diseases, there are few controlled trials to advocate their specific use in fibromyalgia, but there is general agreement that the evidence base for using these therapies across pain conditions is increasing dramatically.[201] Trigger-point injections, chiropractic manipulation, tai chi, yoga, acupuncture, and myofascial release therapy are among the more commonly used modalities, which achieve varying levels of success. There is some evidence that the use of alternative therapies gives patients a greater sense of control over their illness. In instances where this sense of control is accompanied by an improved clinical state (even in the absence of well-controlled studies showing efficacy), the decision to use these therapies is between physicians and patients themselves.

Prognosis

The prognosis of fibromyalgia depends largely on where the individual falls on a continuum. One end of the continuum are individuals in the population with CWP or individuals with fibromyalgia that are seen in primary care, with the prognosis in these individuals being quite good.[202,203] On the other hand, individuals with fibromyalgia seen in tertiary care settings do quite poorly.[204] In this latter study, there was little change in symptoms over time, and no significant change in health satisfaction, symptoms, or functional disability. With regard to function in fibromyalgia, studies have reported varying disability rates from 9% to 44%.[203,205,206] Disability has been most strongly associated with functional and work status, pain, mood disturbances, coping ability, depression, pending litigation, and educational background.

Conclusion

Fibromyalgia is one of several centralized pain disorders characterized by widespread body pain and comorbid symptoms, such as trouble thinking and headaches. Whereas the diagnosis has been controversial in the medical community for some time, it is now among the best studied chronic pain conditions, with overwhelming evidence demonstrating altered CNS function as a key contributor to symptomatology. Treatment should include patient education as well as a combination of behavioral therapies, lifestyle changes, medications, and complementary treatments, as appropriate.

Key Points

- Fibromyalgia is the prototypical centralized pain condition, which is characterized by widespread body pain and comorbid symptoms, such as fatigue, sleep, and memory problems.
- Fibromyalgia patients have higher levels of CNS neurotransmitters that upregulate pain (e.g., glutamate) and lower levels of those that downregulate pain (e.g., norepinephrine and GABA), with a paradoxical increase in endogenous opioids (which may explain why this condition does not appear to be responsive to opioids).
- Psychological comorbidities are more common in fibromyalgia patients but do not explain the sensory abnormalities or pain complaints.
- Rather than considering fibromyalgia as a binary diagnosis, one can consider the degree of "fibromyalgianess" as a means of placing patients on the continuum of more peripheral confined pain to more centralized or widespread pain. Individuals with higher degrees of fibromyalgianess are going to be less responsive to therapies that work well for acute or nociceptive pain (i.e., surgery, opioids) and more responsive to drug and nondrug therapies that work in the CNS.

- Opioids are not recommended in treating fibromyalgia.
- Medications that address the known CNS pathology are preferred, such as TCA, SNRIs, and gabapentinoids.
- Nonpharmacologic therapies should be the mainstay of therapy and can be very effective, especially promoting activity/exercise and improving sleep using sleep hygiene or cognitive-behavioral therapy.
- Although pain and comorbid symptoms may persistent, many patients appropriately treated for fibromyalgia can lead normal, functional lives.

References

1. Khan AA, Khan A, Harezlak J, Tu W, et al. Somatic symptoms in primary care: etiology and outcome. *Psychosomatics* 2003;44(6):471–478.
2. Mayer EA, Raybould HE. Role of visceral afferent mechanisms in functional bowel disorders. *Gastroenterology* 1990;99(6):1688–1704.
3. Clauw DJ. Fibromyalgia: a clinical review. *JAMA* 2014;311(15):1547–1555.
4. Hudson JI, Hudson MS, Pliner LF, et al. Fibromyalgia and major affective disorder: a controlled phenomenology and family history study. *Am J Psych* 1985;142(4):441–446.
5. Arnold LM, Hudson JI, Hess EV, et al. Family study of fibromyalgia. *Arthritis Rheum* 2004;50(3):944–952.
6. Barsky AJ, Borus JF. Functional somatic syndromes. *Ann Intern Med* 1999;130(11):910–921.
7. Fukuda K, Nisenbaum R, Stewart G, et al. Chronic multisymptom illness affecting Air Force veterans of the Gulf War. *JAMA* 1998;280(11):981–988.
8. Drossman DA, Li ZM, Andruzzi E, et al. U.S. householder survey of functional gastrointestinal disorders. Prevalence, sociodemography, and health impact. *Digestive Diseases and Sciences* 1993;38(9):1569–1580.
9. Aaron LA, Bradley LA, Alarcon GS, et al. Psychiatric diagnoses in patients with fibromyalgia are related to health care-seeking behavior rather than to illness. *Arthritis Rheum* 1996;39(3):436–445.
10. Harris RE, Clauw DJ. How do we know that the pain in fibromyalgia is "real"? *Curr Pain Headache Rep* 2006;10(6):403–407.
11. Harris RE, Napadow V, Huggins JP, et al. Pregabalin rectifies aberrant brain chemistry, connectivity, and functional response in chronic pain patients. *Anesthesiology* 2013;119(6):1453–1464.
12. Lopez-Sola M, Woo CW, Pujol J, et al. Towards a neurophysiological signature for fibromyalgia. *Pain* 2017;158(1):34–47.
13. Clauw DJ. Fibromyalgia: an overview. *Am J Med* 2009;122(12 suppl):S3–S13.
14. Woolf CJ. Central sensitization: implications for the diagnosis and treatment of pain. *Pain* 2011;152(3 suppl):S2–S15.
15. Smythe HA, Moldofsky H. Two contributions to understanding of the "fibrositis" syndrome. *Bull Rheum Dis* 1977;28(1):928–931.
16. Moldofsky H, Scarisbrick P, England R, et al. Musculoskeletal symptoms and non-REM sleep disturbance in patients with "fibrositis syndrome" and healthy subjects. *Psychosom Med* 1975;37(4):341–351.
17. Yunus M, Masi AT, Calabro JJ, et al. Primary fibromyalgia (fibrositis): clinical study of 50 patients with matched normal controls. *Semin Arthritis Rheum* 1981;11(1):151–171.
18. Wolfe F, Smythe HA, Yunus MB, et al. The American College of Rheumatology 1990 criteria for the classification of fibromyalgia. Report of the Multicenter Criteria Committee. *Arthritis Rheum* 1990;33(2):160–172.
19. Wolfe F, Clauw DJ, Fitzcharles MA, et al. Fibromyalgia criteria and severity scales for clinical and epidemiological studies: a modification of the ACR Preliminary Diagnostic Criteria for Fibromyalgia. *J Rheumatol* 2011;38(6):1113–1122.
20. Wolfe F, Clauw DJ, Fitzcharles MA, et al. The American College of Rheumatology preliminary diagnostic criteria for fibromyalgia and measurement of symptom severity. *Arthritis Care Res (Hoboken)* 2010;62(5):600–610.
21. Wolfe F, Clauw DJ, Fitzcharles MA, et al. 2016 Revisions to the 2010/2011 fibromyalgia diagnostic criteria. *Semin Arthritis Rheum* 2016;46(3):319–329.
22. Yunus MB. Towards a model of pathophysiology of fibromyalgia: aberrant central pain mechanisms with peripheral modulation. *J Rheum* 1992;19(6):846–850.
23. Clauw DJ, Chrousos GP. Chronic pain and fatigue syndromes: overlapping clinical and neuroendocrine features and potential pathogenic mechanisms. *Neuroimmunomodulation* 1997;4(3):134–153.
24. Bair E, Brownstein NC, Ohrbach R, et al. Study protocol, sample characteristics, and loss to follow-up: the OPPERA prospective cohort study. *J Pain* 2013;14(12 suppl):T2–T19.
25. Bair E, Ohrbach R, Fillingim RB, et al. Multivariable modeling of phenotypic risk factors for first-onset TMD: the OPPERA prospective cohort study. *J Pain* 2013;14(12 suppl):T102–T115.
26. Fillingim RB, Slade GD, Diatchenko L, et al. Summary of findings from the OPPERA baseline case-control study: implications and future directions. *J Pain* 2011;12(11)(suppl):T102–T107.
27. Greenspan JD, Slade GD, Bair E, et al. Pain sensitivity and autonomic factors associated with development of TMD: the OPPERA prospective cohort study. *J Pain* 2013;14(12)(suppl):T63–74.e1–6.

28. Alger JR, Ellingson BM, Ashe-McNalley C, et al. Multisite, multimodal neuroimaging of chronic urological pelvic pain: methodology of the MAPP Research Network. *Neuroimage Clin* 2016;12:65–77.

29. Bagarinao E, Johnson KA, Martucci KT, et al. Preliminary structural MRI based brain classification of chronic pelvic pain: a MAPP network study. *Pain* 2014;155(12):2502–2509.

30. Clemens JQ, Mullins C, Kusek JW, et al. The MAPP Research Network: a novel study of urologic chronic pelvic pain syndromes. *BMC Urol* 2014;14:57.

31. Farmer MA, Huang L, Martucci K, et al. Brain white matter abnormalities in female interstitial cystitis/bladder pain syndrome: a MAPP network neuroimaging study . *J Urol* 2015;194:118–126.

32. Mouraõ AF, Blyth FM, Branco JC. Generalised musculoskeletal pain syndromes. *Best Pract Res Clin Rheumatol* 2010;24(6):829–840.

33. McBeth J, Jones K. Epidemiology of chronic musculoskeletal pain. *Best Pract Res Clin Rheumatol* 2007;21(3):403–425.

34. Coster L, Kendall S, Gerdle B, et al. Chronic widespread musculoskeletal pain—a comparison of those who meet criteria for fibromyalgia and those who do not. *Eur J Pain* 2008;12(5):600–610.

35. Raspe H. Rheumatism epidemiology in Europe. *Soz Praventiv Med* 1992;37(4):168–178.

36. Petzke F, Khine A, Williams D, et al. Dolorimetry performed at 3 paired tender points highly predicts overall tenderness. *J Rheumatol* 2001;28(11):2568–2569.

37. Wolfe F, Ross K, Anderson J, et al. Aspects of fibromyalgia in the general population: sex, pain threshold, and fibromyalgia symptoms. *J Rheumatol* 1995;22(1):151–156.

38. Wolfe F. The relation between tender points and fibromyalgia symptom variables: evidence that fibromyalgia is not a discrete disorder in the clinic. *Ann Rheum Dis* 1997;56(4):268–271.

39. Petzke F, Ambrose K, Gracely RH, et al. What do tender points measure? *Arthritis Rheum* 1999;42(9 suppl):S342.

40. Clauw DJ, Petzke F, Ambrose K, et al. *Responses to Discrete Ascending and Random Pressure Stimuli in Healthy Controls (HC) and Patients with Fibromyalgia (FM)*. Bethesda, MD: National Institutes of Health; 1999.

41. Papageorgiou AC, Silman AJ, Macfarlane GJ. Chronic widespread pain in the population: a seven year follow up study. *Ann Rheum Dis* 2002;61(12):1071–1074.

42. Croft P, Burt J, Schollum J, et al. More pain, more tender points: is fibromyalgia just one end of a continuous spectrum? *Ann Rheum Dis* 1996;55(7):482–485.

43. Hudson JI, Pope HG. The concept of affective spectrum disorder: relationship to fibromyalgia and other syndromes of chronic fatigue and chronic muscle pain. *Baillieres Clin Rheumatol* 1994;8(4):839–856.

44. Aaron LA, Buchwald D. A review of the evidence for overlap among unexplained clinical conditions. *Ann Intern Med* 2001;134(9 pt 2):868–881.

45. Warren JW, Howard FM, Cross RK, et al. Antecedent nonbladder syndromes in case-control study of interstitial cystitis/painful bladder syndrome. *Urology* 2009;73(1):52–57.

46. Williams DA, Clauw DJ. Understanding fibromyalgia: lessons from the broader pain research community. *J Pain* 2009;10(8):777–791.

47. Tracey I, Bushnell MC. How neuroimaging studies have challenged us to rethink: is chronic pain a disease? *J Pain* 2009;10(11):1113–1120.

48. Kato K, Sullivan PF, Evengard B, et al. Importance of genetic influences on chronic widespread pain. *Arthritis Rheum* 2006;54(5):1682–1686.

49. Buskila D, Neumann L, Hazanov I, et al. Familial aggregation in the fibromyalgia syndrome. *Semin Arthritis Rheum* 1996;26(3):605–611.

50. Hudson JI, Goldenberg DL, Pope HG Jr, et al. Comorbidity of fibromyalgia with medical and psychiatric disorders. *Am J Med* 1992;92(4):363–367.

51. Yunus MB. Central sensitivity syndromes: a new paradigm and group nosology for fibromyalgia and overlapping conditions, and the related issue of disease versus illness. *Semin Arthritis Rheum* 2008;37(6):339–352.

52. Fukuda K, Dobbins JG, Wilson LJ, et al. An epidemiologic study of fatigue with relevance for the chronic fatigue syndrome. *J Psychiatr Res* 1997;31(1):19–29.

53. Kato K, Sullivan PF, Evengard B, et al. A population-based twin study of functional somatic syndromes. *Psychol Med* 2009;39(3):497–505.

54. Holliday KL, McBeth J. Recent advances in the understanding of genetic susceptibility to chronic pain and somatic symptoms. *Curr Rheum Rep* 2011;13(6):521–527.

55. Buskila D, Atzeni F, Sarzi-Puttini P. Etiology of fibromyalgia: the possible role of infection and vaccination. *Autoimmun Rev* 2008;8(1):41–43.

56. McLean SA, Diatchenko L, Lee YM, et al. Catechol O-methyltransferase haplotype predicts immediate musculoskeletal neck pain and psychological symptoms after motor vehicle collision. *J Pain* 2011;12(1):101–107.

57. Lewis JD, Wassermann EM, Chao W, et al. Central sensitization as a component of post-deployment syndrome. *Neuro Rehabilitation* 2012;31(4):367–372.

58. Wolfe F, Hauser W, Walitt BT, et al. Fibromyalgia and physical trauma: the concepts we invent. *J Rheumatol* 2014;41(9):1737–1745.

59. Moldofsky H, Saskin P, Lue FA. Sleep and symptoms in fibrositis syndrome after a febrile illness. *J Rheumatol* 1988;15(11):1701–1704.

60. Crook J, Moldofsky H, Shannon H. Determinants of disability after a work related musculoskeletal injury. *J Rheumatol* 1998;25(8):1570–1577.

61. Moldofsky H. Rheumatic manifestations of sleep disorders. *Curr Opin Rheumatol* 2010;22(1):59–63.

62. Ablin JN, Clauw DJ, Lyden AK, et al. Effects of sleep restriction and exercise deprivation on somatic symptoms and mood in healthy adults. *Clin Exp Rheumatol* 2013;31(6)(suppl 79):S53–S59.

63. Arnson Y, Amital D, Fostick L, et al. Physical activity protects male patients with post-traumatic stress disorder from developing severe fibromyalgia. *Clin Exp Rheumatol* 2007;25(4):529–533.

64. Buskila D, Neumann L, Vaisberg G, et al. Increased rates of fibromyalgia following cervical spine injury. A controlled study of 161 cases of traumatic injury. *Arthritis Rheum* 1997;40(3):446–452.

65. Buskila D, Shnaider A, Neumann L, et al. Fibromyalgia in hepatitis C virus infection. Another infectious disease relationship. *Arch Intern Med* 1997;157(21):2497–2500.

66. Clauw DJ, Schmidt M, Radulovic D, et al. The relationship between fibromyalgia and interstitial cystitis. *J Psychiatr Res* 1997;31(1):125–131.

67. McLean SA, Clauw DJ. Predicting chronic symptoms after an acute "stressor"—lessons learned from 3 medical conditions. *Med Hypotheses* 2004;63(4):653–658.

68. Clauw DJ. The pathogenesis of chronic pain and fatigue syndromes, with special reference to fibromyalgia. *Med Hypotheses* 1995;44(5):369–378.

69. Clauw DJ. Fibromyalgia: more than just a musculoskeletal disease. *Am Fam Physician* 1995;52(3):843–851, 853–854.

70. Phillips K, Clauw DJ. Central pain mechanisms in rheumatic diseases: future directions. *Arthritis Rheum* 2013;65:291–302.

71. Woolf CJ, Thompson SW. The induction and maintenance of central sensitization is dependent on N-methyl-D-aspartic acid receptor activation; implications for the treatment of post-injury pain hypersensitivity states. *Pain* 1991;44(3):293–299.

72. Brummett CM, Urquhart AG, Hassett AL, et al. Characteristics of fibromyalgia independently predict poorer long-term analgesic outcomes following total knee and hip arthroplasty. *Arthritis Rheumatol* 2015;67:1386–1394.

73. Janda AM, As-Sanie S, Rajala B, et al. Fibromyalgia Survey Criteria is associated with increased postoperative opioid consumption in women undergoing hysterectomy. *Anesthesiology* 2015;67:1386–1394.

74. Epstein SA, Kay GG, Clauw DJ, et al. Psychiatric disorders in patients with fibromyalgia. A multicenter investigation. *Psychosomatics* 1999;40(1):57–63.

75. Sluka KA, Clauw DJ. Neurobiology of fibromyalgia and chronic widespread pain. *Neuroscience* 2016;338:114–129.

76. Suarez-Roca H, Silva JA, Arcaya JL, et al. Role of mu-opioid and NMDA receptors in the development and maintenance of repeated swim stress-induced thermal hyperalgesia. *Behav Brain Research* 2006;167(2):205–211.

77. Pierce AN, Christianson JA. Stress and chronic pelvic pain. *Prog Mol Biol Transl Sci* 2015;131:509–535.

78. Sluka KA. Is it possible to develop an animal model of fibromyalgia? *Pain* 2009;146(1–2):3–4.

79. Taguchi T, Katanosaka K, Yasui M, et al. Peripheral and spinal mechanisms of nociception in a rat reserpine-induced pain model. *Pain* 2015;156(3):415–427.

80. Watson CJ. Insular balance of glutamatergic and GABAergic signaling modulates pain processing. *Pain* 2016;157(10):2194–2207.

81. Diatchenko L, Fillingim RB, Smith SB, et al. The phenotypic and genetic signatures of common musculoskeletal pain conditions. *Nat Rev Rheumatol* 2013;9(6):340–350.

82. Buskila D, Sarzi-Puttini P, Ablin JN. The genetics of fibromyalgia syndrome. *Pharmacogenomics* 2007;8(1):67–74.

83. Smith SB, Maixner DW, Fillingim RB, et al. Large candidate gene association study reveals genetic risk factors and therapeutic targets for fibromyalgia. *Arthritis Rheum* 2012;64:584–593.

84. Arnold LM, Fan J, Russell IJ, et al. The fibromyalgia family study: a genome-wide linkage scan study. *Arthritis Rheum* 2013;65(4):1122–1128.

85. Ciampi de Andrade D, Maschietto M, Galhardoni R, et al. Epigenetics insights into chronic pain: DNA hypomethylation in fibromyalgia—a controlled pilot-study. *Pain* 2017;158:1473–1480.

86. Petzke F, Gracely RH, Park KM, et al. What do tender points measure? Influence of distress on 4 measures of tenderness. *J Rheumatol* 2003;30(3):567–574.

87. Petzke F, Clauw DJ, Ambrose K, et al. Increased pain sensitivity in fibromyalgia: effects of stimulus type and mode of presentation. *Pain* 2003;105(3):403–413.

88. Kosek E, Hansson P. Modulatory influence on somatosensory perception from vibration and heterotopic noxious conditioning stimulation (HNCS) in fibromyalgia patients and healthy subjects. *Pain* 1997;70(1):41–51.

89. Julien N, Goffaux P, Arsenault P, et al. Widespread pain in fibromyalgia is related to a deficit of endogenous pain inhibition. *Pain* 2005;114(1–2):295–302.

90. Gerster JC, Hadj-Djilani A. Hearing and vestibular abnormalities in primary fibrositis syndrome. *J Rheumatol* 1984;11(5):678–680.

91. McDermid AJ, Rollman GB, McCain GA. Generalized hypervigilance in fibromyalgia: evidence of perceptual amplification. *Pain* 1996;66(2–3):133–144.

92. Geisser ME, Glass JM, Rajcevska LD, et al. A psychophysical study of auditory and pressure sensitivity in patients with fibromyalgia and healthy controls. *J Pain* 2008;9(5):417–422.

93. Tracey I. Neuroimaging of pain mechanisms. *Curr Opin Support Palliat Care* 2007;1(2):109–116.

94. Tracey I, Mantyh PW. The cerebral signature for pain perception and its modulation. *Neuron* 2007;55(3):377–391.

95. Craig AD. Human feelings: why are some more aware than others? *Trends Cogn Sci* 2004;8(6):239–241.

96. Craig AD. Interoception: the sense of the physiological condition of the body. *Curr Opin Neurobiol* 2003;13(4):500–505.

97. Gracely RH, Petzke F, Wolf JM, et al. Functional magnetic resonance imaging evidence of augmented pain processing in fibromyalgia. *Arthritis Rheum* 2002;46(5):1333–1343.

98. Cook DB, Lange G, Ciccone DS, et al. Functional imaging of pain in patients with primary fibromyalgia. *J Rheumatol* 2004;31(2):364–378.

99. Berna C, Leknes S, Holmes EA, et al. Induction of depressed mood disrupts emotion regulation neurocircuitry and enhances pain unpleasantness. *Biol Psychiatr* 2010;67(11):1083–1090.

100. Ploner M, Lee MC, Wiech K, et al. Prestimulus functional connectivity determines pain perception in humans. *Proc Natl Acad Sci USA* 2010;107(1):355–360.

101. Napadow V, Lacount L, Park K, et al. Intrinsic brain connectivity in fibromyalgia is associated with chronic pain intensity. *Arthritis Rheum* 2010;62:2545–2555.

102. Napadow V, Kim J, Clauw DJ, et al. Decreased intrinsic brain connectivity is associated with reduced clinical pain in fibromyalgia. *Arthritis Rheum* 2012;64:2698–2403.

103. Jensen KB, Loitoile R, Kosek E, et al. Patients with fibromyalgia display less functional connectivity in the brain's pain inhibitory network. *Mol Pain* 2012;8:32.

104. Jensen KB, Kosek E, Petzke F, et al. Evidence of dysfunctional pain inhibition in fibromyalgia reflected in rACC during provoked pain. *Pain* 2009;144(1–2):95–100.

105. Lopez-Sola M, Pujol J, Wager TD, et al. Altered functional magnetic resonance imaging responses to nonpainful sensory stimulation in fibromyalgia patients. *Arthritis Rheumatol* 2014;66(11):3200–3209.

106. Harte SE, Ichesco E, Hampson JP, et al. Pharmacologic attenuation of cross-modal sensory augmentation within the chronic pain insula. *Pain* 2016;157(9):1933–1945.

107. Wood PB, Schweinhardt P, Jaeger E, et al. Fibromyalgia patients show an abnormal dopamine response to pain. *Eur J Neurosci* 2007;25(12):3576–3582.

108. Harris RE, Clauw DJ, Scott DJ, et al. Decreased central mu-opioid receptor availability in fibromyalgia. *J Neurosci* 2007;27(37):10000–10006.

109. Baraniuk JN, Whalen G, Cunningham J, et al. Cerebrospinal fluid levels of opioid peptides in fibromyalgia and chronic low back pain. *BMC Musculoskelet Disord* 2004;5:48.

110. Harris RE. Elevated excitatory neurotransmitter levels in the fibromyalgia brain. *Arthritis Res Ther* 2010;12(5):141.

111. Sarchielli P, Di Filippo M, Nardi K, et al. Sensitization, glutamate, and the link between migraine and fibromyalgia. *Curr Pain Headache Rep* 2007;11(5):343–351.

112. Maneuf YP, Hughes J, McKnight AT. Gabapentin inhibits the substance P-facilitated K(+)-evoked release of [(3)H]glutamate from rat caudial trigeminal nucleus slices. *Pain* 2001;93(2):191–196.

113. Foerster BR, Petrou M, Edden RA, et al. Reduced insular gamma-aminobutyric acid in fibromyalgia. *Arthritis Rheumatism* 2012;64(2):579–583.

114. Russell IJ, Holman AJ, Swick TJ, et al. Sodium oxybate reduces pain, fatigue, and sleep disturbance and improves functionality in fibromyalgia: results from a 14-week, randomized, double-blind, placebo-controlled study. *Pain* 2011;152(5):1007–1017.

115. Kim CH, Vincent A, Clauw DJ, et al. Association between alcohol consumption and symptom severity and quality of life in patients with fibromyalgia. *Arthritis Res Ther* 2013;15(2):R42.

116. Craig AD. How do you feel? Interoception: the sense of the physiological condition of the body. *Nat Rev Neurosci* 2002;3(8):655–666.

117. Brooks JC, Tracey I. The insula: a multidimensional integration site for pain. *Pain* 2007;128(1–2):1–2.

118. Yunus MB. Fibromyalgia and overlapping disorders: the unifying concept of central sensitivity syndromes. *Semin Arthritis Rheum* 2007;36(6):339–356.

119. Ablin K, Clauw DJ. From fibrositis to functional somatic syndromes to a bell-shaped curve of pain and sensory sensitivity: evolution of a clinical construct. *Rheum Dis Clin North Am* 2009;35(2):233–251.

120. Crofford LJ. The hypothalamic-pituitary-adrenal stress axis in fibromyalgia and chronic fatigue syndrome. *Zeitschrift fur Rheumatologie* 1998;57 (suppl 2):67–71.

121. Clauw DJ, Crofford LJ. Chronic widespread pain and fibromyalgia: what we know, and what we need to know. *Best Pract Res Clin Rheumatol* 2003;17(4):685–701.

122. Demitrack MA, Crofford LJ. Evidence for and pathophysiologic implications of hypothalamic-pituitary-adrenal axis dysregulation in fibromyalgia and chronic fatigue syndrome. *Ann N Y Acad Sci* 1998;840:684–697.

123. Crofford LJ, Pillemer SR, Kalogeras KT, et al. Hypothalamic-pituitary-adrenal axis perturbations in patients with fibromyalgia. *Arthritis Rheum* 1994;37(11):1583–1592.

124. Qiao ZG, Vaeroy H, Morkrid L. Electrodermal and microcirculatory activity in patients with fibromyalgia during baseline, acoustic stimulation and cold pressor tests. *J Rheumatol* 1991;18(9):1383–1389.

125. Adler GK, Kinsley BT, Hurwitz S, et al. Reduced hypothalamic-pituitary and sympathoadrenal responses to hypoglycemia in women with fibromyalgia syndrome. *Am J Med* 1999;106(5):534–543.

126. Martinez-Lavin M, Hermosillo AG, Rosas M, et al. Circadian studies of autonomic nervous balance in patients with fibromyalgia: a heart rate variability analysis. *Arthritis Rheum* 1998;41(11):1966–1971.

127. Cohen H, Neumann L, Shore M, et al. Autonomic dysfunction in patients with fibromyalgia: application of power spectral analysis of heart rate variability. *Semin Arthritis Rheum* 2000;29(4):217–227.

128. McLean SA, Williams DA, Harris RE, et al. Momentary relationship between cortisol secretion and symptoms in patients with fibromyalgia. *Arthritis Rheum* 2005;52(11):3660–3669.

129. McLean SA, Williams DA, Stein PK, et al. Cerebrospinal fluid corticotropin-releasing factor concentration is associated with pain but not fatigue symptoms in patients with fibromyalgia. *Neuropsychopharmacology* 2006;31(12):2776–2782.

130. Dias DN, Marques MA, Bettini SC, et al. Prevalence of fibromyalgia in patients treated at the bariatric surgery outpatient clinic of Hospital de Clínicas do Paraná – Curitiba [published online ahead of print February 20, 2017]. *Rev Bras Reumatol*. doi:10.1016/j.rbr.2017.01.001.

131. Affaitati G, Costantini R, Fabrizio A, et al. Effects of treatment of peripheral pain generators in fibromyalgia patients. *Eur J Pain* 2011;15(1):61–69.

132. Gur A, Oktayoglu P. Status of immune mediators in fibromyalgia. *Curr Pain Headache Rep* 2008;12(3):175–181.

133. Wallace D, Bowman RL, Wormsley SB, et al. Cytokines and immune regulation in patients with fibrositis [letter] [published erratum appears in *Arthritis Rheum* 1989;32(12):1607]. *Arthritis Rheum* 1989;32(10):1334–1335.

134. Bazzichi L, Rossi A, Massimetti G, et al. Cytokine patterns in fibromyalgia and their correlation with clinical manifestations. *Clin Exp Rheumatol* 2007;25(2):225–230.

135. Schrepf A, Bradley CS, O'Donnell M, et al. Toll-like receptor 4 and comorbid pain in interstitial cystitis/bladder pain syndrome: a multidisciplinary approach to the study of chronic pelvic pain research network study. *Brain Behav Immun* 2015;49:66–74.

136. Kim SH, Kim DH, Oh DH, et al. Characteristic electron microscopic findings in the skin of patients with fibromyalgia: preliminary study. *Clin Rheumatol* 2008;27(2):219–223.

137. Clauw DJ. What is the meaning of "small fiber neuropathy" in fibromyalgia? *Pain* 2015;156(11):2115–2116.

138. Doppler K, Rittner HL, Deckart M, et al. Reduced dermal nerve fiber diameter in skin biopsies of patients with fibromyalgia. *Pain* 2015;156(11):2319–2325.

139. Smallwood RF, Laird AR, Ramage AE, et al. Structural brain anomalies and chronic pain: a quantitative meta-analysis of gray matter volume. *J Pain* 2013;14(7):663–675.

140. Serra J, Collado A, Sola R, et al. Hyperexcitable C nociceptors in fibromyalgia. *Ann Neurol* 2014;75(2):196–208.

141. Tan EM, Feltkamp TE, Smolen JS, et al. Range of antinuclear antibodies in "healthy" individuals. *Arthritis Rheumatism* 1997;40(9):1601–1611.

142. Pincus T. A pragmatic approach to cost-effective use of laboratory tests and imaging procedures in patients with musculoskeletal symptoms. *Primary Care* 1993;20(4):795–814.

143. Jensen MC, Brant-Zawadzki MN, Obuchowski N, et al. Magnetic resonance imaging of the lumbar spine in people without back pain. *N Engl J Med* 1994;331(2):69–73.

144. Wolfe F. Fibromyalgianess. *Arthritis Rheum* 2009;61(6):715–716.

145. Wolfe F, Michaud K, Busch RE, et al. Polysymptomatic distress in patients with rheumatoid arthritis: understanding disproportionate response and its spectrum. *Arthritis Care Res (Hoboken)* 2014;66:1465–1471.

146. Wolfe F, Michaud K, Li T, et al. Chronic conditions and health problems in rheumatic diseases: comparisons with rheumatoid arthritis, noninflammatory rheumatic disorders, systemic lupus erythematosus, and fibromyalgia. *J Rheumatol* 2010;37(2):305–315.

147. Brummett CM, Bakshi RR, Goesling J, et al. Preliminary validation of the Michigan Body Map (MBM). *Pain* 2016;157:1205–1212.

148. Brummett CM, Janda AM, Schueller CM, et al. Survey criteria for fibromyalgia independently predict increased postoperative opioid consumption after lower-extremity joint arthroplasty: a prospective, observational cohort study. *Anesthesiology* 2013;119(6):1434–1443.

149. Nakao M, Barsky AJ. Clinical application of somatosensory amplification in psychosomatic medicine. *Biopsychosoc Med* 2007;1:17.

150. Chang L. The association of functional gastrointestinal disorders and fibromyalgia. *Eur J Surg Suppl* 1998;583:32–36.

151. Staud R. Autonomic dysfunction in fibromyalgia syndrome: postural orthostatic tachycardia. *Curr Rheumatol Rep* 2008;10(6):463–466.

152. Naliboff BD, Stephens AJ, Lai HH, et al. Clinical and psychosocial predictors of urologic chronic pelvic pain symptom change over one year: a prospective study from the MAPP Research Network. *J Urol* 2017;198:848–857.

153. Chandran AB, Coon CD, Martin SA, et al. Sphygmomanometry-evoked allodynia in chronic pain patients with and without fibromyalgia. *Nurs Res* 2012;61(5):363–368.

154. Annemans L, Wessely S, Spaepen E, et al. Health economic consequences related to the diagnosis of fibromyalgia syndrome. *Arthritis Rheum* 2008;58(3):895–902.

155. Macfarlane GJ, Kronisch C, Atzeni F, et al. EULAR recommendations for management of fibromyalgia. *Ann Rheum Dis* 2017;76:e54.

156. Arnold LM, Clauw DJ. Challenges of implementing fibromyalgia treatment guidelines in current clinical practice. *Postgrad Med* 2017;129:709–714.

157. Arnold LM, Keck PE Jr, Welge JA. Antidepressant treatment of fibromyalgia. A meta-analysis and review. *Psychosomatics* 2000;41(2):104–113.

158. Younger J, Noor N, McCue R, et al. Low-dose naltrexone for the treatment of fibromyalgia: findings of a small, randomized, double-blind, placebo-controlled, counterbalanced, crossover trial assessing daily pain levels. *Arthritis Rheum* 2013;65(2):529–538.

159. Lynch ME, Campbell F. Cannabinoids for treatment of chronic non-cancer pain; a systematic review of randomized trials. *Br J Clin Pharmacol* 2011;72:735–744.

160. Clauw DJ. Pain management: fibromyalgia drugs are 'as good as it gets' in chronic pain. *Nat Rev Rheumatol* 2010;6(8):439–440.

161. Moldofsky H, Harris HW, Archambault WT, et al. Effects of bedtime very low dose cyclobenzaprine on symptoms and sleep physiology in patients with fibromyalgia syndrome: a double-blind randomized placebo-controlled study. *J Rheumatol* 2011;38(12):2653–2663.

162. Capaci K, Hepguler S. Comparison of the effects of amitriptyline and paroxetine in the treatment of fibromyalgia syndrome. *Pain Clin* 2002;14(3):223–228.

163. Goldenberg D, Mayskiy M, Mossey C, et al. A randomized, double-blind crossover trial of fluoxetine and amitriptyline in the treatment of fibromyalgia. *Arthritis Rheum* 1996;39(11):1852–1859.

164. Norregaard J, Volkmann H, Danneskiold-Samsoe B. A randomized controlled trial of citalopram in the treatment of fibromyalgia. *Pain* 1995;61(3):445–449.

165. Anderberg UM, Marteinsdottir I, Von Knorring L. Citalopram in patients with fibromyalgia—a randomized, double-blind, placebo-controlled study. *Eur J Pain* 2000;4(1):27–35.

166. Arnold LM, Hess EV, Hudson JI, et al. A randomized, placebo-controlled, double-blind, flexible-dose study of fluoxetine in the treatment of women with fibromyalgia. *Am J Med* 2002;112(3):191–197.

167. Fishbain D. Evidence-based data on pain relief with antidepressants. *Ann Med* 2000;32(5):305–316.

168. Adelman LC, Adelman JU, Von Seggern R, et al. Venlafaxine extended release (XR) for the prophylaxis of migraine and tension-type headache: a retrospective study in a clinical setting. *Headache* 2000;40(7):572–580.

169. Grothe DR, Scheckner B, Albano D. Treatment of pain syndromes with venlafaxine. *Pharmacotherapy* 2004;24(5):621–629.

170. Clauw DJ, Mease P, Palmer RH, et al. Milnacipran for the treatment of fibromyalgia in adults: a 15-week, multicenter, randomized, double-blind, placebo-controlled, multiple-dose clinical trial. *Clin Ther* 2008;30(11):1988–2004.

171. Arnold LM, Lu Y, Crofford LJ, et al. A double-blind, multicenter trial comparing duloxetine with placebo in the treatment of fibromyalgia patients with or without major depressive disorder. *Arthritis Rheum* 2004;50(9):2974–2984.

172. Arnold LM, Hirsch I, Sanders P, et al. Safety and efficacy of esreboxetine in patients with fibromyalgia: a fourteen-week, randomized, double-blind, placebo-controlled, multicenter clinical trial. *Arthritis Rheum* 2012;64(7):2387–2397.

173. Wiffen P, Collins S, McQuay H, et al. Anticonvulsant drugs for acute and chronic pain. *Cochrane Database Syst Rev* 2000;(3):CD001133.

174. Crofford LJ, Rowbotham MC, Mease PJ, et al. Pregabalin for the treatment of fibromyalgia syndrome: results of a randomized, double-blind, placebo-controlled trial. *Arthritis Rheum* 2005;52(4):1264–1273.

175. Arnold LM, Goldenberg DL, Stanford SB, et al. Gabapentin in the treatment of fibromyalgia: a randomized, double-blind, placebo-controlled, multicenter trial. *Arthritis Rheum* 2007;56(4):1336–1344.

176. Olivan-Blazquez B, Herrera-Mercadal P, Puebla-Guedea M, et al. Efficacy of memantine in the treatment of fibromyalgia: a double-blind, randomised, controlled trial with 6-month follow-up. *Pain* 2014;155(12):2517–2525.

177. Cohen SP, Verdolin MH, Chang AS, et al. The intravenous ketamine test predicts subsequent response to an oral dextromethorphan treatment regimen in fibromyalgia patients. *J Pain* 2006;7(6):391–398.

178. Gilron I, Chaparro LE, Tu D, et al. Combination of pregabalin with duloxetine for fibromyalgia: a randomized controlled trial. *Pain* 2016;157:1532–1540.

179. Finnerup NB, Attal N, Haroutounian S, et al. Pharmacotherapy for neuropathic pain in adults: a systematic review and meta-analysis. *Lancet Neurol* 2015;14:162–173.

180. Scharf MB, Baumann M, Berkowitz DV. The effects of sodium oxybate on clinical symptoms and sleep patterns in patients with fibromyalgia. *J Rheumatol* 2003;30(5):1070–1074.

181. Skrabek RQ, Galimova L, Ethans K, et al Nabilone for the treatment of pain in fibromyalgia. *J Pain* 2008;9(2):164–173.

182. Ware MA, Fitzcharles MA, Joseph L, et al. The effects of nabilone on sleep in fibromyalgia: results of a randomized controlled trial. *Anesth Analg* 2010;110(2):604–610.

183. Bennett RM. Pharmacological treatment of fibromyalgia. *J Func Syndr* 2001;1(1):79–92.

184. Holman AJ, Myers RR. A randomized, double-blind, placebo-controlled trial of pramipexole, a dopamine agonist, in patients with fibromyalgia receiving concomitant medications. *Arthritis Rheum* 2005;52(8):2495–2505.

185. Russell IJ, Michalek JE, Xiao Y, et al. Therapy with a central alpha 2-adrenergic agonist (tizanidine) decreases cerebrospinal fluid substance P, and may reduce serum hyaluronic acid as it improves the clinical symptoms of the fibromyalgia syndrome. *Arthritis Rheumatism* 2002;46(9):S614.

186. Schrepf A, Harper DE, Harte SE, et al. Endogenous opioidergic dysregulation of pain in fibromyalgia: a PET and fMRI study. *Pain* 2016;157(10):2217–2225.

187. Fitzcharles MA, Shir Y. Another nasty effect of opioids: attenuating the benefits of motivational interviewing in fibromyalgia? *J Rheumatol* 2017;44(4):407–409.

188. Fitzcharles MA, Ste-Marie PA, Gamsa A, et al. Opioid use, misuse, and abuse in patients labeled as fibromyalgia. *Am J Med* 2011;124(10):955–960.

189. Derry S, Wiffen PJ, Hauser W, et al. Oral nonsteroidal anti-inflammatory drugs for fibromyalgia in adults. *Cochrane Database Syst Rev* 2017;(3):CD012332.

190. Pridgen WL, Duffy C, Gendreau JF, et al. A famciclovir + celecoxib combination treatment is safe and efficacious in the treatment of fibromyalgia. *J Pain Res* 2017;10:451–460.

191. Brosseau L, Judd MG, Marchand S, et al. Transcutaneous electrical nerve stimulation (TENS) for the treatment of rheumatoid arthritis in the hand. *Cochrane Database Syst Rev* 2003;(3):CD004377.

192. Brosseau L, Milne S, Robinson V, et al. Efficacy of the transcutaneous electrical nerve stimulation for the treatment of chronic low back pain: a meta-analysis. *Spine (Phila Pa 1976)* 2002;27(6):596–603.

193. Williams JA, Imamura M, Fregni F. Updates on the use of non-invasive brain stimulation in physical and rehabilitation medicine. *J Rehab Med* 2009;41(5):305–311.

194. Hargrove JB, Bennett RM, Simons DG, et al. A randomized placebo-controlled study of noninvasive cortical electrostimulation in the treatment of fibromyalgia patients. *Pain Med* 2012;13:115–124.

195. Williams DA, Cary MA, Glazer LJ, et al. Randomized controlled trial of CBT to improve functional status in fibromyalgia. *Am Coll Rheum* 2000;43(9):S210.

196. Goldenberg DL, Burckhardt C, Crofford L. Management of fibromyalgia syndrome. *JAMA* 2004;292(19):2388–2395.

197. Bidonde J, Busch AJ, Schachter CL, et al. Aerobic exercise training for adults with fibromyalgia. *Cochrane Database Syst Rev* 2017;(6):CD012700.

198. Vitiello MV, McCurry SM, Shortreed SM, et al. Short-term improvement in insomnia symptoms predicts long-term improvements in sleep, pain, and fatigue in older adults with comorbid osteoarthritis and insomnia. *Pain* 2014;155(8):1547–1554.

199. Williams DA, Kuper D, Segar M, et al. Internet-enhanced management of fibromyalgia: a randomized controlled trial. *Pain* 2010;151(3):694–702.

200. Hsu MC, Schubiner H, Lumley MA, et al. Sustained pain reduction through affective self-awareness in fibromyalgia: a randomized controlled trial. *J Gen Intern Med* 2010;25:1064–1070.

201. Ablin J, Fitzcharles MA, Buskila D, et al. Treatment of fibromyalgia syndrome: recommendations of recent evidence-based interdisciplinary guidelines with special emphasis on complementary and alternative therapies. *Evid Based Complement Alternat Med* 2013;2013:485272.

202. Littlejohn G. The fibromyalgia syndrome. Outcome is good with minimal intervention [letter]. *BMJ* 1995;310(6991):1406.

203. Macfarlane GJ, Thomas E, Papageorgiou AC, et al. The natural history of chronic pain in the community: a better prognosis than in the clinic? *J Rheum* 1996;23(9):1617–1620.

204. Wolfe F, Anderson J, Harkness D, et al. A prospective, longitudinal, multicenter study of service utilization and costs in fibromyalgia. *Arthritis Rheum* 1997;40(9):1560–1570.

205. Dinerman H, Goldenberg DL, Felson DT. A prospective evaluation of 118 patients with the fibromyalgia syndrome: prevalence of Raynaud's phenomenon, sicca symptoms, ANA, low complement, and Ig deposition at the dermal-epidermal junction. *J Rheum* 1986;13(2):368–373.

206. Wolfe F, Anderson J, Harkness D, et al. Work and disability status of persons with fibromyalgia. *J Rheum* 1997;24(6):1171–1178.

207. Hauser W, Bernardy K, Arnold B, et al. Efficacy of multicomponent treatment in fibromyalgia syndrome: a meta-analysis of randomized controlled clinical trials. *Arthritis Rheum* 2009;61(2):216–224.

208. Hauser W, Klose P, Langhorst J, et al. Efficacy of different types of aerobic exercise in fibromyalgia syndrome: a systematic review and meta-analysis of randomised controlled trials. *Arthritis Res Ther* 2010;12(3):R79.

209. Bernardy K, Fuber N, Kollner V, et al. Efficacy of cognitive-behavioral therapies in fibromyalgia syndrome—a systematic review and metaanalysis of randomized controlled trials. *J Rheumatol* 2010;37(10):1991–2005.

210. Porter NS, Jason LA, Boulton A, et al. Alternative medical interventions used in the treatment and management of myalgic encephalomyelitis/chronic fatigue syndrome and fibromyalgia. *J Altern Complement Med* 2010;16(3):235–249.

211. Arnold LM. Duloxetine and other antidepressants in the treatment of patients with fibromyalgia. *Pain Med* 2007;8(suppl 2):S63–S74.

212. Hauser W, Bernardy K, Uceyler N, et al. Treatment of fibromyalgia syndrome with gabapentin and pregabalin—a meta-analysis of randomized controlled trials. *Pain* 2009;145(1–2):69–81.

CHAPTER 37

Pain of Dermatologic Disorders

SHELLEY YANG and **JOHN E. OLERUD**

Pain is not as distinctive a feature of dermatologic disorders as is the related disorder of itch, which is beyond the scope of this discussion. It is well known that itch appears to be so intolerable that the act of scratching inflicts a transient pain with attendant structural damage to the skin. It is generally considered that the induced pain is subjectively more tolerable than the itching. Nonetheless, pain is a distinctive feature of certain dermatologic disorders and merits attention simply because of the great prevalence of skin disorders.

In 2013, almost 85 million Americans (1 in 4 individuals) were seen by a physician for skin disease, resulting in direct health care costs of $75 billion and indirect lost opportunity costs of $11 billion. Of the 10 most prevalent skin diseases seen, viral diseases and wounds are potentially painful.[1] The prevalence of pain in dermatologic disorders is unknown and may be underreported. In one survey of patients with common skin conditions, pain was reported by 23% of all patients.[2] The effects of pain on the patient are best demonstrated by the impact of the persisting pain that sometimes follows herpes zoster or postherpetic neuralgia, which occasionally leads to suicide. This disease is discussed in Chapter 27, but this chapter focuses attention not only on the impact of pain but also on the need for appropriate diagnosis and on the value of appropriate treatment.

The diseases discussed in this chapter can be grouped into the categories of vasculitis, infections of viral and bacterial origin, inflammatory diseases of the subcutaneous space, and neoplasms. Some neoplasms, although benign, are specifically painful based on their neurovascular components. We discuss the causes and pathogenesis of the selected pain-related skin diseases, paying attention to symptoms and signs, methods of diagnosis, and preferred methods of treatment. For more comprehensive discussions of the individual diseases, refer to selected general textbooks of skin disease.[3–6] Vasculitides and tumors are described in Tables 37.1 and 37.2.

Basic Considerations: Anatomy and Physiology of the Skin

Human skin is a vast, sheet-like interface of the organism with its environment. It is adapted to the dryness of the atmosphere, resisting mechanical shearing and puncturing forces as well as the invasion of chemical and infective agents. This organ, which in aggregate covers an area of more than 2 m², has a mass greater than that of any other organ. It contains an extensive vascular and sweat gland system, essential for thermal regulation, and an even more extensive and finely attuned neuroreceptor network, including the varied transducers of pain and other sensations. It is also a major immune system interface.[7]

The skin is covered by a thin, stratified epithelium, the epidermis, which is only 75 to 100 μm thick except on the palms and soles, where it is 4 to 5 times thicker. The bulk of the skin is fibroelastic dense connective tissue known as the *dermis*, which supports the extensive network of vessels and nerves as well as the specialized glandular structure of the sweat apparatus and keratinizing appendages, such as hair and nail. The subcutaneous space is a variably fatty connective tissue perforated by collagenous septa, continuous on the outermost aspects with the fibers of the dermis and continuous beneath the skin with fascial or periosteal attachments to the skeleton. The immune system involves all layers of the skin.

It is generally believed that the peripheral pain receptors are the network of finely arborized free nerve endings that innervate the epidermis and superficial dermis[8–10] and has been referred to as the *cutaneous sensory nervous system*.[11] These fibers convey information from the skin to the central nervous system (CNS) and thus have a sensory role.

The primary sensory nerve fibers that innervate the skin are categorized based on diameter, conduction velocity, and myelination. The thickly myelinated Aβ fibers conduct tactile sensation. Thinly myelinated, fast-conducting Aδ fibers transmit noxious information and cold. Unmyelinated, slow-conducting C fibers transmit burning-quality pain, heat, and itch.

Pruritoception and nociception are physiologic sensations that prompt avoidance of the sensation-causing stimulus. The *labeled line theory* proposes the existence of itch-specific neuronal fibers that extend from the skin to the dorsal root ganglion. Nociceptive neurons express molecular pain transducers at their peripheral nerve terminals, such as transient receptor potential (TRP) ion channels, which sense heat, cold, and reactive chemicals. Pruriceptive neurons express G protein-coupled receptors and cytokine receptors that are activated by inflammatory mediators. Upon neuronal activation, signals are relayed via the dorsal horn of the spinal cord to the brain, where they are processed as pain or itch. Spinal interneurons may also play an important role in determining whether the brain interprets a signal as pain or itch.[12]

In the *selectivity theory*, overlapping populations of itch and pain fibers exist; although most fibers respond only to painful stimuli, some respond to both pain and itch. The larger population of pain-sensitive C fibers inhibits the smaller population of itch-related C fibers. If a stimulus activates both itch and pain, then the larger population of pain-sensitive C fibers will mask the itch. If the pain pathway is activated, it inhibits itch sensation.[12–14]

Sensory neurons also have an effector function in the skin and release molecular mediators from their peripheral nerve terminals, including the neuropeptides substance P, calcitonin gene-related peptide, somatostatin, and vasoactive intestinal peptide. The cutaneous sensory nervous system appears to play an important role in the "communication" between the nervous system and the immune system, the vascular system, and the cells of the epidermis. Neuropeptides appear to participate in vital functions such as neuroinflammation, tissue repair, and immunomodulation.[8,15,16] They have important biologic effects on a variety of cells in the skin, including keratinocytes, endothelial cells, fibroblasts, Langerhans cells, mast cells, macrophages, and smooth muscle cells.[11] It is easy to imagine how these effector functions may participate in the perpetuation of chronic skin conditions characterized by pain or itch.

The diagnosis of skin disease depends less on deductive logic than on direct observation. One should distinguish localized nodules resulting from small tumors of the skin from the large plaque-like swellings associated with acute edema and redness that mark inflammatory processes and umbilicated small vesicles occurring in clusters on inflammatory bases that are characteristic of the herpetic viral infections. Subtle or marked

TABLE 37.1　Characteristics of Cutaneous Vasculitides

Type	Clinical Signs	Pathologic Features	Immunofluorescence Findings	Granulomatous Changes	ANCA cANCA	ANCA pANCA	Allergic Rhinitis, Asthma, Eosinophilia	Pain	Comment	Treatment
Leukocytoclastic vasculitis	Palpable purpura on lower extremities	Infiltration and destruction of postcapillary venules by polymorphonuclear leukocytes with leukocytoclasis	Immunoglobulins and complement (C3) in small capillaries of the upper dermis (lesions <24 h old)	–	–	–		Small lesions are usually asymptomatic; larger papules, nodules, and ulcers are often painful.	Causative factors include infections, drugs, chemicals, serum, connective tissue diseases, and malignancy	No therapy for mild cases; antihistamines, nonsteroidal anti-inflammatory drugs, dapsone, colchicine, prednisone 7- to 10-d course starting with 60 mg/d
Polyarteritis nodosa	Tender nodules, livedo reticularis, ulcers, nodules along an artery	Segmental, transmural inflammation of medium-sized arteries	Immunoglobulins and complement in vessel walls	–	–	–	Eosinophilia sometimes	Aching pain is characteristic of the cutaneous form, aggravated by physical activity or edema.	Limited cutaneous form of polyarteritis nodosa rarely progresses to systemic polyarteritis nodosa.	NSAIDs, systemic corticosteroids for benign cutaneous PAN Prednisone and cyclophosphamide for moderate to severe systemic PAN
Granulomatosis with polyangiitis (Wegener's granulomatosis)	Papules, papulonecrotic lesions, nodules with ulceration, subcutaneous nodules, ulcers, petechiae, ecchymotic lesions, vesicles, pustules	Necrotizing vasculitis of small arteries and veins; necrotizing granulomas	Usually negative	+	44%–90%	12%–20%	Eosinophilia sometimes	Lesions can be tender.	Limited form does not have renal involvement.	Induction therapy with systemic corticosteroids and cyclophosphamide/rituximab, followed by maintenance with azathioprine or methotrexate

Disease	Cutaneous lesions	Histology	Immune deposits	+/−	ANCA	Associated features	Cutaneous pain	Systemic involvement	Treatment
Eosinophilic granulomatosis with polyangiitis (Churg-Strauss)	Cutaneous nodules usually on scalp and extremities Palpable purpura	Extravascular granulomas; necrotizing vasculitis of small- or medium-sized arteries and veins	Usually negative	+	30%–40%, mostly pANCA	Allergic rhinitis, asthma, eosinophilia (virtually all)	Cutaneous nodules are usually tender.	Serious renal involvement is infrequent; coronary arteritis and myocarditis are principal causes of death.	Prednisone Cytotoxic drug added if needed[236]
Microscopic polyangiitis	Palpable purpura, ulcers	Necrotizing vasculitis of small vessels; sometimes small- and medium-sized arteries	Immune deposits absent (pauci-immune)	−	38%–57% (60%–80% overall)	Eosinophilia sometimes	Similar to leukocytoclastic vasculitis	Renal involvement frequent; pulmonary involvement common	For patients with major organ damage, see GPA treatment.
Rheumatoid vasculitis	Petechiae, palpable purpura, leg ulcerations, nail fold and digital infarcts, gangrene	Vasculitis of small arteries, arterioles, capillaries, or venules	Immunoglobulins and complement in vessels reported in normal skin as well as in lesional skin in rheumatoid vasculitis	−	20% (rheumatoid arthritis) pANCA		Lesions are sometimes painful.	Associated with relatively severe rheumatoid arthritis	For patients with severe disease: steroids combined with cyclophosphamide/rituximab
Livedoid vasculitis	Livedo reticularis, purpuric macules, papules, ulcers, stellate scarring	Hyalinizing segmental vasculitis in middle and lower dermis, small vessel fibrin plugs	Immunoglobulins, complement and fibrin in vessel walls	−			Pain may be severe.		Treat coagulation defects; therapeutic ladder as proposed by Callen[69]

ANCA, antineutrophilic cytoplasmic antibodies; cANCA, ANCA of the cytoplasmic type; GPA, granulomatosis with polyangiitis; PAN, polyarteritis nodosa; pANCA, ANCA of the perinuclear type; +, present; −, absent.
Modified from Braverman IM. The angiitides. In: Braverman IM, ed. *Skin Signs of Systemic Disease.* 3rd ed. Philadelphia: WB Saunders, 1998:311.
Modified from Langlois JC, Olerud JE. Pain of dermatologic disorders. In: Loeser JD, Butler SH, Chapman CR, et al, eds. *Bonica's Management of Pain.* 3rd ed. Philadelphia: Lippincott Williams & Wilkins; 2001:575.

defects in the integrity of the protective epidermal sheet should be noted, as manifested by denuded sites of bullae (erosions). Also to be noted are deeper defects in the integrity of the protective barrier that involve loss of the epidermis as well as of some dermis, leading to ulcer formation. Such lesions are inevitably attended by pain, unless associated with a neuropathy, which can best be explained by exposure of free nerve endings.

Clinical Disorders

LEUKOCYTOCLASTIC VASCULITIS

Leukocytoclastic vasculitis (LCV), also known as cutaneous small vessel vasculitis, is a common form of vasculitis that may be confined to the skin[17] or related to systemic vasculitis, connective tissue diseases, or malignancy[18,19] (Fig. 37.1). LCV typically affects postcapillary venules producing palpable purpura which are the clinical hallmark of the disease.[17] Although palpable purpura occurring in dependent areas (e.g., the legs and ankles in ambulatory patients and the back and sacral area in bedridden patients) is typical, a spectrum of other cutaneous lesions may occur such as papules, nodules, vesicles, bullae, pustules, ulcers, urticarial lesions, and livedo reticularis.[20,21] Purpuric lesions may often be associated with tenderness, burning, stinging, or itch.[17] The presence of painful skin lesions has been reported to be associated with a lower risk of systemic involvement.[22]

Histologic changes seen with LCV consist primarily of infiltration of polymorphonuclear leukocytes within and/or around blood vessels and destruction of the vessel wall with fibrinoid necrosis, whereas hemorrhage, nuclear dust (leukocytoclasis), endothelial changes, ulceration, necrosis, and eccrine gland necrosis are considered secondary changes.[23] The differential diagnosis of LCV includes thrombocytopenia, coagulation, embolic phenomena, pigmented purpuric dermatoses, microvascular occlusion, and others.[24]

Etiology

Among the many reported etiologic factors associated with LCV are infectious agents (e.g., *Streptococcus*, hepatitis B and C, HIV, and influenza), medications (e.g., antibiotics and nonsteroidal anti-inflammatory drugs [NSAIDs]), connective tissue and inflammatory diseases (e.g., systemic lupus erythematosus (SLE), Sjögren's syndrome, rheumatoid arthritis, inflammatory bowel disease, and Behçet disease), and malignancy (both lymphoproliferative and solid tumors). Up to half of all cases of LCV do not reveal an identifiable cause and are considered to be idiopathic.[17,20,24]

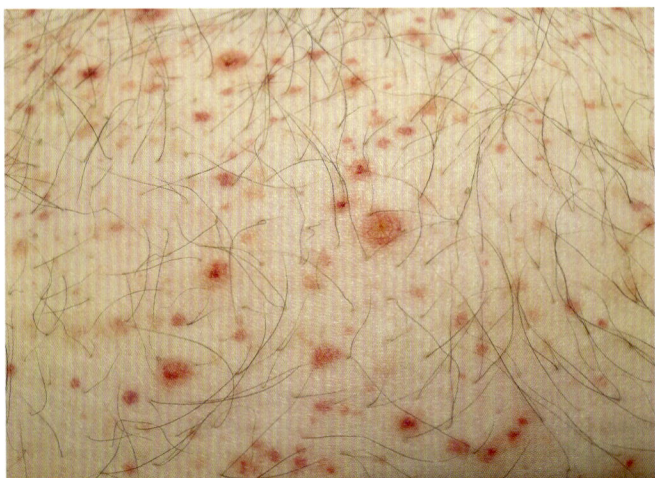

FIGURE 37.1 Leukocytoclastic vasculitis. *(Courtesy of Fan Liu, MD, University of Washington.)*

Pathogenesis

LCV is felt to be caused by deposition of circulating immune complexes within the vessel walls of postcapillary venules, activation of complement, infiltration by neutrophils, and release of lysosomal enzymes.[20] Immunoglobulins and complement can be detected in vessel walls by direct immunofluorescence in early lesions that are less than 24 hours old (preferably less than 4 hours), and the presence of immunoglobulin A (IgA) may support a diagnosis of IgA vasculitis.[21] Patients who present with LCV need to be evaluated for systemic involvement, particularly for involvement of kidneys, joints, gastrointestinal tract, and pulmonary and nervous systems. They may need to be reclassified depending on the type of systemic involvement according to the Chapel Hill Consensus Conference nomenclature.[25] Subsets or variants of LCV include urticarial vasculitis, Henoch-Schönlein purpura, and cryoglobulinemic vasculitis. Hepatitis C is an important cause of mixed cryoglobulinemic vasculitis and is responsible for the majority of cases that have an infectious etiology.[26,27]

Treatment

Any underlying infections should be treated, suspect medications stopped, and other potential etiologic agents avoided. Any associated connective tissue diseases should be treated, and the patient evaluated for underlying malignancy if another etiology is not found.

Specific treatment for the vasculitis should be tailored to the severity of the disease. For most patients, the condition is self-limited and spontaneously resolves within 2 to 4 weeks. Chronic or recurrent disease occurs in approximately 10% of patients.[28] For patients who are asymptomatic or have mild disease, options include conservative treatment with topical steroids, leg elevation, compression stockings, antihistamines, and NSAIDs. Dapsone and colchicine may be beneficial for more chronic disease. A short course of systemic corticosteroids may be useful for an acute exacerbation. For patients with more severe and recalcitrant disease, azathioprine, cyclosporine, mycophenolate mofetil, methotrexate, intravenous immunoglobulin (IVIg), and rituximab are considerations.[17]

POLYARTERITIS NODOSA

Polyarteritis nodosa (PAN) is an uncommon form of vasculitis affecting small- and medium-sized arteries. Two forms of cutaneous involvement can occur: benign cutaneous and systemic.

Symptoms and Signs

Cutaneous PAN characteristically manifests with tender nodules, livedo reticularis, and ulcers. It may also be associated with myalgias, arthralgias, neuropathy, and fever.[29,30] Patients may have periodic flares or exacerbations of their disease, but the long-term course of their disease is generally benign. Progression to systemic PAN is rare but has been reported. Patients need long-term follow-up to monitor for this possibility.[31]

Systemic PAN may have cutaneous involvement in up to 60% patients manifested most commonly as palpable purpura, bullae, and ulcerations and less commonly as nodules, livedo reticularis, and gangrene.[29,32,33] Nodules can sometimes be palpable along the course of an artery.[21]

In both forms of PAN, there is segmental, transmural inflammation of medium-sized arteries in the deep dermis or subcutaneous tissue[29,30] with immunoglobulin M (IgM), fibrin, or C3 demonstrable on direct immunofluorescence.[29] Although most cases are idiopathic, secondary PAN has been reported most commonly from hepatitis B and less commonly hepatitis C, streptococcal infection, cytomegalovirus, HIV, and others. In children, PAN has similar features as adenosine deaminase 2 (ADA2) deficiency, a newly described autosomal recessively inherited condition characterized by early onset vasculopathy with livedoid rash, strokes, and hematologic abnormalities.[34]

Treatment

First-line treatment of the benign cutaneous form of PAN is NSAIDs and systemic corticosteroids. A second, steroid-sparing immunosuppressant such as mycophenolate mofetil, azathioprine, or methotrexate may be added if patients do not respond or relapse. General supportive measures include rest, medications for pain, local wound care for ulcerated lesions, and antibiotics for secondary infection. Severe systemic PAN is treated with prednisone and cyclophosphamide to induce remission and then a safer immunosuppressive agent to maintain remission.[35]

ANTINEUTROPHILIC CYTOPLASMIC ANTIBODIES-ASSOCIATED VASCULITIDES: GRANULOMATOSIS WITH POLYANGIITIS (FORMERLY KNOWN AS WEGENER'S GRANULOMATOSIS)

Granulomatosis with polyangiitis (GPA) is an uncommon disease of unknown cause characterized by necrotizing vasculitis and granulomatous inflammation involving the upper and lower respiratory tracts, together with glomerulonephritis, although more limited forms of the disease without renal involvement may occur.[36,37] Approximately 90% of patients, when in the active stage of their disease, have antineutrophilic cytoplasmic antibodies (ANCA) of the cytoplasmic type (c-ANCA) directed at proteinase 3.[37] The pathogenesis of GPA remains poorly understood.

Symptoms and Signs

Cutaneous lesions occur in approximately 45% of patients and include palpable purpura, ulcers, vesicles, papules, nodules, necrotic papules, and pustules.[37,38] Pyoderma gangrenosum (PG)-like ulcerations may occur.[39] Papules, nodules, and ulcerative lesions may be tender or painful.[38,40,41] The upper airway is frequently affected and manifestations include oral ulcerations and gingival hyperplasia with petechiae.[38] Friable gingival hyperplasia with petechiae is said to be pathognomonic of GPA.[41-43] Saddle nose deformity occurs in some patients but is a rare manifestation.[39] On biopsy of cutaneous lesions, one may see small vessel vasculitis, granulomatous dermatitis, and least commonly granulomatous vasculitis. Not all changes may be seen in the same specimen.[44]

Treatment

Treatment of ANCA vasculitis is composed of two components: remission induction therapy and maintenance therapy. For induction, systemic corticosteroids are combined with cyclophosphamide or rituximab. Plasma exchange can be considered as adjunct therapy for severe vasculitis with active glomerulonephritis or alveolar hemorrhage. After remission is achieved, patients are switched to maintenance with a less toxic immunosuppressant, most commonly azathioprine or methotrexate.[45]

MICROSCOPIC POLYANGIITIS

Microscopic polyangiitis (MPA) is a systemic small vessel vasculitis commonly affecting the kidneys, lungs, and skin. The vasculitis affects arterioles, capillaries, venules, and sometimes small- and medium-sized arteries with few or no immune deposits evident on direct immunofluorescence (pauci-immune).[46] Positive ANCA, usually of the perinuclear type (p-ANCA), also referred to as myeloperoxidase-ANCA, has been reported in 60% to 80% patients. There is experimental evidence to suggest that myeloperoxidase-ANCA may be involved in the pathogenesis of vasculitis.[47]

Cutaneous involvement has been reported in 35% to 60% patients with MPA.[45] Purpura is commonly reported, but a variety of other cutaneous manifestations include vesicles, bullae, splinter hemorrhages, nodules, cutaneous necrosis, digital infarction, gangrene, PG-like ulcerations, livedo reticularis, facial edema, urticaria, orogenital ulceration, and erythema elevatum diutinum.[32,48-53] Although not focused on specifically in reports, ischemic pain would be expected as in other forms of vasculitis, particularly with ulcers, infarction, and gangrene.

Treatment

Serious major organ involvement, such as pulmonary or renal disease, is treated similarly to GPA.

EOSINOPHILIC GRANULOMATOSIS WITH POLYANGIITIS (FORMERLY KNOWN AS CHURG-STRAUSS SYNDROME)

Eosinophilic granulomatosis with polyangiitis (EGPA) is a rare syndrome characterized by allergic rhinitis, asthma, eosinophilia, granulomatous inflammation, and systemic vasculitis affecting small- to medium-sized arteries.[36,46] Pulmonary involvement and cardiac involvement are common with coronary arteritis and myocarditis being the principal cause of death, whereas renal involvement is relatively less common and tends to be mild.[32,36] Histologically, one sees a vasculitis affecting small vessels, extravascular granulomas, tissue infiltration with eosinophils, and an absence of vascular immune deposits on direct immunofluorescence.[44] Thirty percent to 40% of patients have positive ANCA, usually of the p-ANCA directed at myeloperoxidase.[45]

Symptoms and Signs

Cutaneous lesions occur in up to 50% to 70% of patients. The most common cutaneous findings are palpable purpura on the lower extremities and skin nodules.[54] Among the many other reported cutaneous manifestations are papules, plaques, petechiae, ulcers, infarcts, bullae, wheals, and livedo reticularis.[55] More recently described variations include severe digital gangrene associated with antiphospholipid antibodies[56] and purpura fulminans.[57] Pain or tenderness is characteristic of the skin nodules[58] and also likely occurs on an ischemic basis in some vasculitic lesions as well.

Treatment

The treatment of choice is systemic corticosteroids, which usually controls the disease. Severe EGPA requires aggressive treatment with corticosteroids and cyclophosphamide. More than 50% of patients may become steroid-dependent due to persistent asthma or sinusitis. Mepolizumab, an anti-interleukin (IL)-5 monoclonal antibody, is a potential steroid-sparing agent.[45]

RHEUMATOID VASCULITIS

Rheumatoid vasculitis is a systemic vasculitis that may affect vessels of different sizes including capillaries and small- and medium-sized arteries. It tends to occur in patients with more severe rheumatoid arthritis of long-standing duration and high titer rheumatoid factor.[59-61] The diagnostic criteria as originally proposed by Scott and Bacon[62] included rheumatoid arthritis (meeting American Rheumatism Association [ARA] criteria) plus one or more of the following: (1) mononeuritis multiplex, (2) peripheral gangrene, (3) biopsy evidence of acute necrotizing arteritis plus systemic illness such as fever or weight loss, and (4) deep cutaneous ulcers or active extra-articular disease (e.g., pleurisy, pericarditis, scleritis) if associated with typical digital infarcts or biopsy evidence of vasculitis.[62]

Histologically, one finds a vasculitis that may be leukocytoclastic, granulomatous, or lymphocytic.[63,64] Cutaneous manifestations are one of the most common features of the disease (up to 90% patients) and include Bywaters lesions (periungual infarctions), petechiae, palpable purpura, deep ulcers along medial or lateral malleoli, and erythema elevatum diutinum.[65] Ulcerations and gangrene may by painful on an ischemic basis.

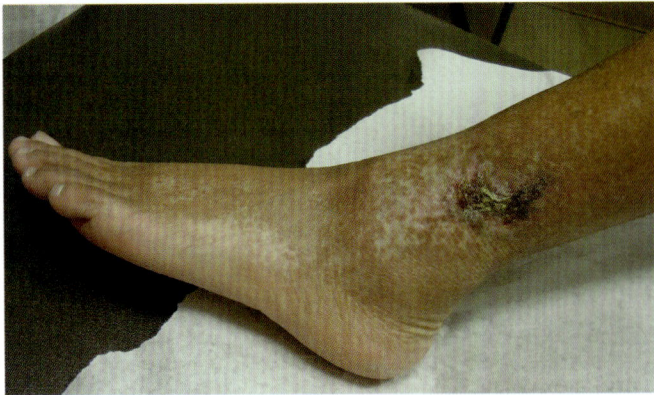

FIGURE 37.2 Livedoid vasculopathy. (*Courtesy of John Olerud, MD, University of Washington.*)

Treatment

Patients with isolated periungual infarcts have a low risk of progressing to systemic vasculitis and do not require treatment. Patients with more severe disease are treated with systemic agents, including systemic corticosteroids, cyclophosphamide, and rituximab.[66]

LIVEDOID VASCULOPATHY

Livedoid vasculopathy (livedoid vasculitis, see Fig. 37.2) is a recurrent, chronic disease that predominantly affects women. The distal lower legs, particularly the malleoli, are most commonly affected and may exhibit livedoid changes, painful purpuric papules and plaques on the bilateral lower extremities, porcelain-white stellate atrophic scars, and painful recurrent ulcerations. Approximately half of patients may have an underlying hypercoagulable disorder predisposing to thrombin formation.[67]

The histologic changes seen on biopsy are segmental and depend on the age of the lesion. In early stages, hyaline thrombi form in dermal blood vessels, and fibrinoid material is deposited in the vessel wall or surrounding stroma. Later stages show thickening/hyalinization of vessel walls and features of scarring. There are varying levels of inflammation but no leukocytoclasis. Direct immunofluorescence usually demonstrates fibrin, C3, and IgM in vessel walls.

A question arises as to how extensively to evaluate patients for underlying coagulation disorders. Laboratory evaluation for hypercoagulable states, collagen vascular disorders, fibrinolytic disorders, paraproteinemia, and infectious associations can be pursued.[67] Hairston et al.[68] recommend the following studies: complete blood count (CBC), cryoglobulins, cryofibrinogens, homocysteine, antinuclear antibody (ANA), anticardiolipin antibody, lupus anticoagulant, protein C and S levels, factor V Leiden gene mutation, prothrombin gene mutation [G20210A], and β2-glycoprotein-1 antibody.

Treatment

General supportive measures for livedoid vasculopathy include avoidance of smoking, rest, compression for associated venous insufficiency, local wound care for ulcerations, and pain control.

Any underlying coagulation disorders should be treated. In the absence of any specific defects, antiplatelet and antithrombotic agents may be beneficial. The literature on treatment of livedoid vasculopathy consists of case reports or small series with no controlled studies. The concept of a therapeutic ladder as proposed by Callen[69] with treatments with more potentially serious side effects higher on the ladder is a sound one and starts with low-dose aspirin, pentoxifylline, dipyridamole, folic acid/vitamin B complex in patients with homocysteinemia, hydroxychloroquine in patients with antiphospholipid syndrome (APS), stanozolol/danazol in patients with cryofibrinogenemia, warfarin, low molecular weight heparin, hyperbaric oxygen, and tissue plasminogen activator infusion and ends with IVIg.[69]

Other Vascular Disorders

ANTIPHOSPHOLIPID SYNDROME

APS is an uncommon syndrome characterized by thrombotic occlusion of arteries or veins, complications of pregnancy (miscarriage, spontaneous abortions, and prematurity), thrombocytopenia, and positive anticardiolipin and/or lupus anticoagulant antibodies.[70–72] The anticardiolipin and/or lupus anticoagulant tests should be positive on at least two occasions at least 12 weeks apart to exclude transiently positive tests. APS may occur as a primary disorder, as a secondary disorder in patients with lupus erythematosus, and also may occur in a subset of patients with Sneddon's syndrome (livedo reticularis and multiple cerebrovascular events). Antiphospholipid antibodies alone are not diagnostic of APS because they occur normally in a small percentage of the normal population and have been associated with multiple other conditions.[70,73] Histologically, skin biopsies demonstrate noninflammatory thrombosis of arteries and/or veins.

Symptoms and Signs

Cutaneous manifestations of APS are common, with livedo reticularis, digital necrosis, subungual splinter hemorrhages, and superficial venous thrombosis being the most common.[71] Other signs include cutaneous necrosis and gangrene, ulcers, painful skin nodules, lesions resembling vasculitis, necrotizing vasculitis, livedoid vasculitis, and anetoderma.[71,73,74] Livedo reticularis is the most common skin manifestation and reported to have irregular broken circles (livedo racemosa) as opposed to the unbroken circles of physiologic cutis marmorata.[71] The cutaneous lesions of APS may be painful on an ischemic basis, particularly areas of necrosis, ulcers, and gangrene.

Diagnosis is based on the presence of either a thrombotic vascular occlusive event or a qualifying complication of pregnancy, plus the presence of either anticardiolipin or lupus anticoagulant or anti-β2-glycoprotein-1 antibodies.[75]

Treatment

The patient should be treated for any risk factors for cardiovascular events including hypertension and hyperlipidemia and advised to avoid smoking and oral contraceptives.

APS patients with thrombosis should be anticoagulated indefinitely with an antithrombotic agent. Typically, heparin is used in the acute setting and then transitioned to warfarin. Low molecular weight heparin may also be used. Asymptomatic patients incidentally found to have antiphospholipid antibodies with no history of thrombosis or pregnancy complications may be offered no treatment or low-dose aspirin.[76] Multiple clinical studies have shown antimalarials to have an antithrombotic effect in patients with SLE.[77]

Catastrophic APS, an acute severe variant with widespread microvascular occlusive event, is treated with anticoagulation with heparin, high-dose systemic corticosteroids, plasma exchange, and IVIg. Rituximab and eculizumab has been used in more resistant cases. Careful monitoring to detect, treat, or prevent precipitating factors is also recommended, including infections, surgery, trauma, invasive procedures, underlying malignancy, SLE flares, and obstetric complications.[78]

WARFARIN (COUMADIN) SKIN NECROSIS

Warfarin-induced skin necrosis is a rare reaction to warfarin that causes painful skin necrosis.[79–81]

Pathophysiology

Warfarin-induced skin necrosis is believed to be caused by a temporary hypercoagulable state that occurs on initiation of warfarin treatment.[80] Protein C is a vitamin K–dependent natural anticoagulant, whereas factors II, VII, IX, and X are vitamin K–dependent clotting (procoagulant) factors. Because of shorter half-lives of protein C and factor VII, there is a relatively rapid fall in protein C and factor VII when warfarin is begun compared to factors II, IX, and X, leading to a transient hypercoagulable state.[82] Patients who have hereditary or acquired protein C deficiency, protein S deficiency, or antithrombin III deficiency are at greater risk.[80,83] Histologically, thrombi in capillaries and venules are considered to be the primary process, but other changes related to necrosis and hemorrhage can be seen.[80,84]

Symptoms and Signs

Symptoms usually begin within the first 3 to 6 days of starting warfarin but delayed onset of has been reported.[85] One or more erythematous edematous plaques appear that develop petechiae on their surface followed by blue-black discoloration, hemorrhage, bullous formation, gangrene or necrosis, and finally eschar formation.[86] The lesions are very painful and favor the areas of increased subcutaneous fat, such as the abdomen, buttock, thighs, and breasts.

Treatment

Warfarin therapy should be discontinued immediately and heparin substituted. Fresh frozen plasma and vitamin K may be used to restore levels of protein C and S. Avoidance of warfarin in the future is the most prudent approach. Restarting warfarin at low dosage under coverage of IV heparin has been done successfully; however, some patients have been reported to experience recurrences of skin necrosis.[87] Low molecular weight heparin has been recommended over chronic unfractionated heparin use if warfarin cannot be restarted because of less risk of osteoporosis, lower risk of thrombocytopenia, and there is no need to monitor partial thromboplastin time (PTT).[85] Meticulous wound care and pain management is necessary. More than 50% of patients require surgical intervention in the form of débridement, grafting, and amputation.[84]

COCAINE LEVAMISOLE TOXICITY

Since 2003, there have been increasing reports of vasculitis and vasculopathy due to levamisole-contaminated cocaine (Fig. 37.3). The Centers for Disease Control and Prevention (CDC) estimates about 70% of cocaine in the United States may be adulterated with levamisole, a veterinary antihelminthic agent used as a cutting agent to expand the volume of the drug and potentiate the effects of cocaine.

Levamisole-induced toxicity presents with a painful, purpuric rash that can be associated with agranulocytosis, neutropenia, arthralgias, fever, and oral pain. The purpura has a predilection for the external ears, nose, and cheeks and progresses to skin necrosis.[88] Retiform or stellate purpura can also affect the trunk and extremities.

As a diagnosis of exclusion, other causes of vasculitis should be investigated, including infection and autoimmune conditions. Many other types of vasculitis have also been described in cocaine abusers, including urticarial vasculitis, EGPA, thromboangiitis obliterans, and pseudovasculitis with nasal destruction mimicking GPA.[89] A positive urine toxicology test is contributory; however, the window of detection for cocaine is only 2 to 3 days. Levamisole testing is difficult, given its short half-life of 5.6 hours. ANCAs and antiphospholipid antibodies may be positive. On histology, LCV and fibrin thrombi may be present.

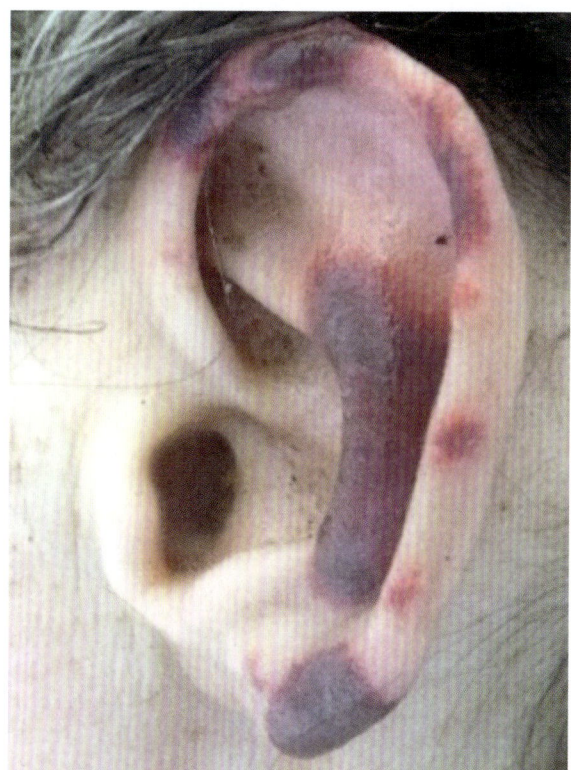

FIGURE 37.3 Cocaine levamisole toxicity. *(Courtesy of Cait May, MD, University of Washington.)*

Management is supportive and consists of discontinuing use of contaminated cocaine and appropriate wound care. The lesions typically resolve within 2 to 3 weeks.

CALCINOSIS CUTIS

Calcinosis cutis results from the deposition of calcium salts in the skin and can be categorized into four subtypes: dystrophic, metastatic, idiopathic, and iatrogenic. Dystrophic calcinosis cutis occurs when there is calcification in damaged tissue, such as in areas of trauma or inflammatory process, and is most commonly seen in autoimmune conditions such as dermatomyositis, systemic sclerosis, and CREST syndrome. Patients present with painful, firm nodules or plaques predominantly in periarticular areas and on fingertips and bony prominences. The lesions may ulcerate and extrude chalky, granular material through the skin. It is often painful and can be debilitating. In dermatomyositis, children diagnosed at a young age have a higher risk of calcinosis than adults, and anti-NXP2 autoantibodies are associated with a substantially increased risk of calcinosis in all age groups.[90]

The pathogenesis of calcinosis cutis remains poorly understood; chronic inflammation and vascular ischemia in the tissue injury has been implicated as well as macrophages, proinflammatory cytokines, and the impairment of calcium-regulating proteins.

Treatment of calcinosis cutis is challenging and should be individualized depending on the location and size of the deposits and the underlying condition. Surgical excision of localized lesions can help decrease discomfort. Results for medical therapies are mixed and inconsistent. Bisphosphonates, sodium thiosulfate, diltiazem, IVIg, tumor necrosis factor inhibitors, and colchicine have been beneficial in some.[91]

CALCIPHYLAXIS

Calciphylaxis (Fig. 37.4) is a potentially life-threatening cause of painful ulcerations of the skin that occurs most commonly in patients with chronic end-stage renal disease but also rarely

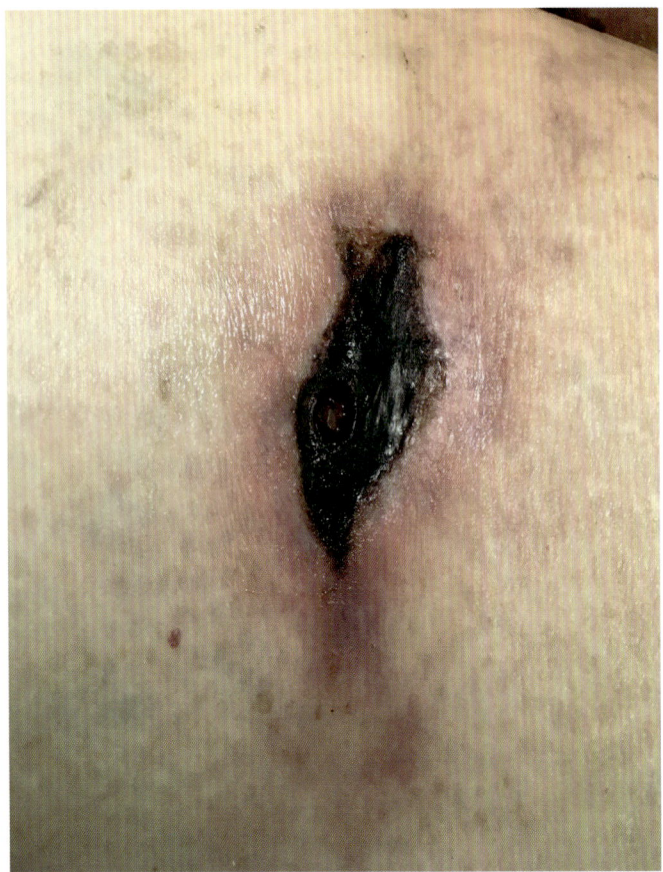

FIGURE 37.4   Calciphylaxis. *(Courtesy of Vanessa Pascoe, MD, University of Washington.)*

occurs in patients without renal failure.[92–94] It has a reported prevalence rate of 4.1% in patients undergoing hemodialysis.[95] Many patients have secondary hyperparathyroidism with elevated parathyroid hormone, increased alkaline phosphatase, increased calcium, phosphorous, or calcium × phosphate ion product.[95,96] Other potential risk factors include protein C deficiency, protein S deficiency, and warfarin therapy.[97]

Cutaneous manifestations may begin as very painful violaceous discoloration similar to livedo reticularis that evolves to indurated plaques, ulcerations, and eschar formation. Lesions favor adipose-rich areas such as the breast, buttocks, and thighs. The 1-year mortality is 45% to 80%, with ulcerated lesions associated with higher mortality and sepsis the principal cause of death.[98] Gangrene requiring amputation may also occur.[99] Diagnosis requires clinicopathologic correlation. Histologically, there is calcification of small arteries, intimal hyperplasia, and noninflammatory thrombosis of vessels.[100] Small vessel calcification, although nonspecific, can be identified on plain films and computed tomography (CT) scans and may aid in the diagnosis.[101] Preservation of pulses, proximal location of ulcers on extremities, and absence of neuropathy favors calciphylaxis over arteriosclerotic ulcers and diabetic ulcers, although patients may have concomitant disease and calciphylaxis ulcers may occur on acral locations.[95] Warfarin-associated nonuremic calciphylaxis appears to be a distinct entity, predominantly below the knees in females, and associated with better outcomes.[102]

Treatment

A multidisciplinary approach is necessary. Measures should be taken to lower the serum calcium, serum phosphate, and calcium × phosphate product when elevated. These measures may include low-calcium dialysate, noncalcium phosphate binders, and low-phosphate diet.[94,103] Sodium thiosulfate has emerged as a first-line treatment and may be given intravenously or injected intralesionally to isolated wounds. Possible adjunct therapies include pentoxifylline and bisphosphonates. Cinacalcet is preferred over vitamin D and parathyroidectomy to treat hyperparathyroidism.[98] Consideration should be given to switching from warfarin to one of the newer anticoagulants if appropriate. Local wound care, pain management, and antibiotics for secondary infection are also essential. Amputation may be needed in some patients.

Ulcers

ISCHEMIC ULCERS

Ischemic (arterial) ulcers are a cause of painful ulcerations on the lower extremities most often seen in patients with arteriosclerotic peripheral vascular disease. The ulcers typically have a dry punched out appearance and are located on the distal lower extremities at sites of trauma or pressure including the toes, feet, lateral malleoli, and pretibial areas.[104–106] There may be associated atrophic skin, loss of hair, delayed capillary filling pressure, and rubor with dependency (reactive hyperemia). The ulcer pain is worse at night and relieved by dependency. Patients also may have a history of intermittent claudication and rest pain if the obstruction is severe enough.

Histologically, arteriosclerosis affects medium and large arteries where one finds plaques with varying degrees of infiltrations with foam cells, smooth muscle cells, inflammatory cells, hemorrhage, platelets, thrombus formation, collagen deposition, and ulceration.[107] Patients may have ulcers with a mixture of venous and arterial disease. Diabetics may also have small vessel disease complicated by peripheral neuropathy leading to further trauma and injury at the site. Neuritis on an ischemic basis may also occur.

The patient should be examined for absent or diminished pulses and bruits over proximal arteries. The patient should be further evaluated with measurements to determine the ankle brachial index (ABI) (ratio of the systolic blood pressure in the ankle to the systolic blood pressure in the arm). A normal ABI is ≥ 1, <1 is abnormal, and ≤ 0.5 is severe disease.[108] Patients with calcification of arteries have a falsely elevated ABI because of noncompressibility of vessels.

Treatment

Measures should be taken to treat underlying causes of arteriosclerosis including cessation of smoking, control of blood pressure, hyperlipidemia, and control of diabetes.[106] Elevation of the extremity, compression, and débridement of ulcers are to be avoided. Protection of the extremities from trauma with sheepskin and foot cradling devices is helpful. Patients with claudication may benefit from an exercise program when the ulcer has healed. Adequate pain relief, local wound care, and treating any secondary infection are important. When conservative measures fail, there are a variety of nonoperative and operative revascularization procedures that may be used, including percutaneous transluminal angioplasty, stent placement, atherectomy, and bypass procedures depending on the individual patient.[108] Amputation may be necessary.

VENOUS ULCERS

Venous ulcers (Fig. 37.5) are a common cause of painful ulcerations on the ankles, typically over the medial malleoli in patients with chronic venous insufficiency.[106,109,110] Associated skin findings may include hyperpigmentation from hemosiderin deposition, varicosities, pitting edema, scars from prior ulcerations, and fibrosis and induration of tissues (lipodermatosclerosis). Lipodermatosclerosis itself may be very

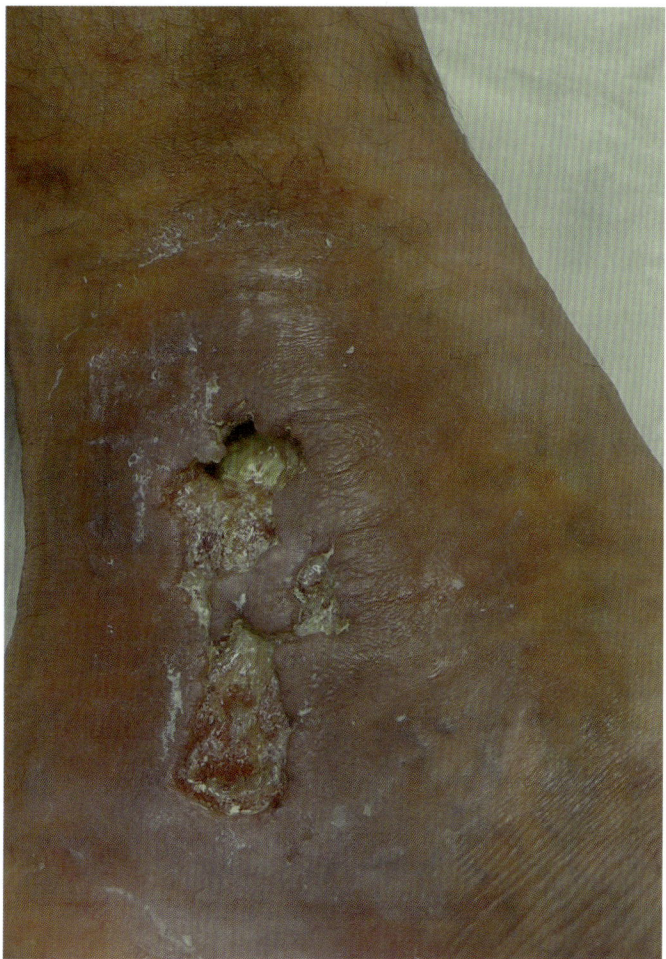

FIGURE 37.5 Venous ulcer on the medial malleolus. *(Courtesy of John Olerud, MD, University of Washington.)*

painful and resemble cellulitis. There may also be associated stasis dermatitis, contact dermatitis from topical medications, and secondary infection. The ulcer itself is typically shallow with irregular borders and sloping edge.[106,110]

Venous ulcers occur in the setting of chronic venous hypertension due to incompetent venous semi-lunar valves in superficial veins, communicating veins, or deep venous system or with disease of the calf muscles which act as a pump to empty the deep venous system.[104,110] The valves may be damaged by prior episodes of thrombophlebitis or be congenitally absent.[110] Obesity and peripheral edema from other causes such as pulmonary, cardiac, hepatic, or renal disease may be contributory or exacerbating factors. Pain in the ulcers is presumably on an ischemic basis.

Treatment

Elevation of the legs and support stockings help control peripheral edema. Unna boots and other compressive wraps speed wound healing. Compression should be used with care in patients with concomitant arterial disease. Bed rest with leg elevation for 1 to 2 weeks may be necessary for edema control when painful lipodermatosclerosis precludes the use of compression. Short stretch wraps applied before getting out of bed in the morning can prevent further leg swelling without being applied too tightly. They are usually well tolerated after the pain of lipodermatosclerosis subsides with bed rest.

Local wound care may include gauzes, films, hydrogels, hydrocolloid dressings, foams, alginates, hydrofibers, or antimicrobial dressings.[111] Occlusive dressings on the wound may also

relieve pain. Surgical débridement may sometimes be needed. Cultures should be taken if secondary infection is present and the patient treated with antibiotics effective for *Staphylococcus aureus* and *Streptococcus pyogenes*. Dermatitis from stasis dermatitis or contact dermatitis is treated with topical steroids and avoidance of responsible contactants. Surgical management with grafting may be necessary in refractory cases. Weight reduction and diuretics may be helpful in some obese patients. Optimization of therapy for any associated systemic conditions causing peripheral edema such as congestive heart failure or pulmonary insufficiency may also be helpful.

PYODERMA GANGRENOSUM

PG is a rare neutrophilic dermatosis characterized by painful skin ulcers (Fig. 37.6). The complex pathogenesis is multifactorial and incompletely understood, implicating neutrophil dysfunction, aberrant activation of inflammatory mediators, and genetic predisposition.[112] Lesions typically begin as an inflammatory pustule or nodule that enlarges and ulcerates with undermined, dusky violaceous margins. Peak incidence occurs in adults 20 to 30 years old without predilection for either sex; however, any age group can be affected. Pathergy (the appearance of lesions at sites of trauma) is present in 20% to 30% of patients. PG may be a component of autoinflammatory genetic syndromes such as PASH (PG, acne, hidradenitis suppurativa [HS]) and PAPA (pyogenic arthritis, PG, and acne).[113]

PG is a diagnosis of exclusion, as there are no diagnostic laboratory or histologic features, and it is important to exclude other more common etiologies for ulcer formation, including infection, venous, and arterial ulcers. The differential diagnosis also includes necrobiosis lipoidica, vasculitides, cutaneous Crohn's disease, spider bite, and factitial disease. Clinical variants of PG include pustular, bullous, vegetative, peristomal, postsurgical, and drug-induced.

Up to 75% of patients with PG have an associated underlying condition, most commonly inflammatory bowel disease, hematologic disorders, and inflammatory arthritis. Treatment can be challenging and requires multimodality management. After appropriate workup and treatment of any underlying

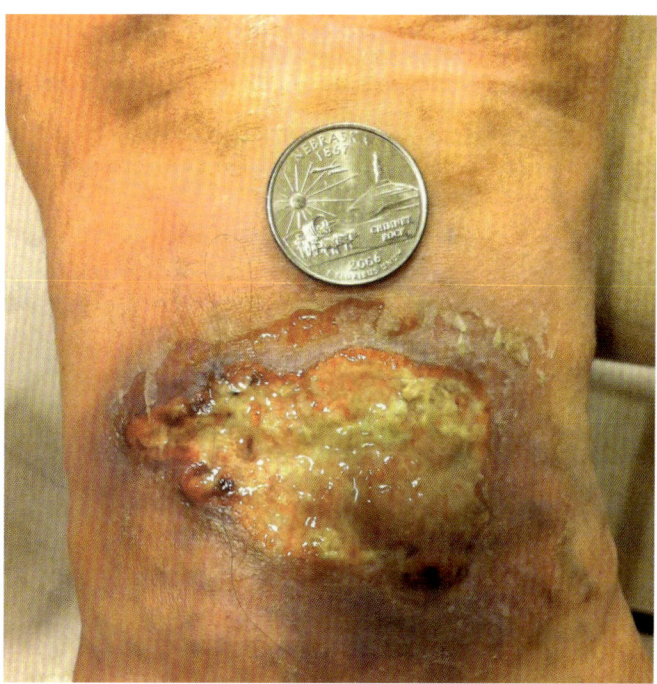

FIGURE 37.6 Pyoderma gangrenosum. *(Courtesy of John Olerud, MD, University of Washington.)*

diseases if present, early control with diligent wound care and anti-inflammatory medications are instituted. For limited disease, potent topical corticosteroids and intralesional steroid injection may be sufficient. For more widespread or progressive disease, systemic corticosteroids and immunosuppressive steroid-sparing agents such as cyclosporine and infliximab may be added. Due to pathergy, trauma including wound débridement should be avoided.[114]

Painful Infections

Many infections of the skin are painful. Common or selected skin infections are discussed here. For more comprehensive coverage of the topic, the reader is referred to a general textbook of dermatology.

NECROTIZING SOFT TISSUE INFECTION/ NECROTIZING FASCIITIS

Necrotizing fasciitis is an acute, life-threatening bacterial infection that spreads quickly along fascial planes and is characterized by high mortality, systemic toxicity, and tissue destruction. The pathogen is initially inoculated into the subcutaneous tissue, which may occur with any epithelial disruption. Risk factors include recent trauma, surgery, immunosuppression, diabetes, and alcohol abuse. Necrotizing infection localized to the perineum is termed *Fournier gangrene.*

The infection may be mono- or polymicrobial. Group A β-hemolytic streptococci is classically associated with necrotizing fasciitis; however, a wide spectrum of causative organisms have been reported, including *Staphylococcus aureus*, *Vibrio vulnificus*, Enterobacteriaceae, Pseudomonas, and Bacteroides spp.

Patients who are developing necrotizing fasciitis present with erythema, pain, and woody-feeling edema. They may initially be diagnosed with cellulitis; however, the infection progresses rapidly despite standard antibiotic therapy. Pain is out of proportion to visible skin signs, as the deeper tissues are affected and cutaneous manifestations may be minimal. The patient appears systemically ill and may meet sepsis criteria. Dusky-blue cyanotic discoloration appears, followed by bullae and frank gangrene. Crepitus, representing gas in the soft tissues, may be present. Pain progresses to anesthesia of the involved skin as superficial nerves are destroyed. The gold standard for diagnosis of necrotizing soft tissue infection (NSTI) is an operative exploration to assess the adherence of the fascia to other soft tissue layers.

Early detection and treatment with broad-spectrum IV antibiotics and surgical débridement is critical. Even with optimal treatment, mortality remains high, with rates of 25% to 35%.[115–117]

HERPES ZOSTER

Herpes zoster is a painful eruption caused by reactivation of the varicella virus in a dermatomal distribution.[118,119] The topic is presented and discussed in detail in Chapter 27.

HERPES SIMPLEX

Herpes simplex virus (HSV) infection is a common, often painful, DNA viral infection (Fig. 37.7). HSV presents as grouped vesicular lesions on an erythematous base and may be preceded by a 1- to 2-day prodrome of burning, tingling, or itching.[120–123] The early clear vesicular lesions progress through stages of clouding, central umbilication, crusting, and then healing.

Symptoms and Signs

Primary HSV infection (no antibodies to HSV in acute phase serum) may be painful and protracted. It is often accompanied by fever, malaise, tender regional adenopathy, and a higher rate of complications.[120] "First episode" HSV may be primary infection or may be recurrent HSV where the primary

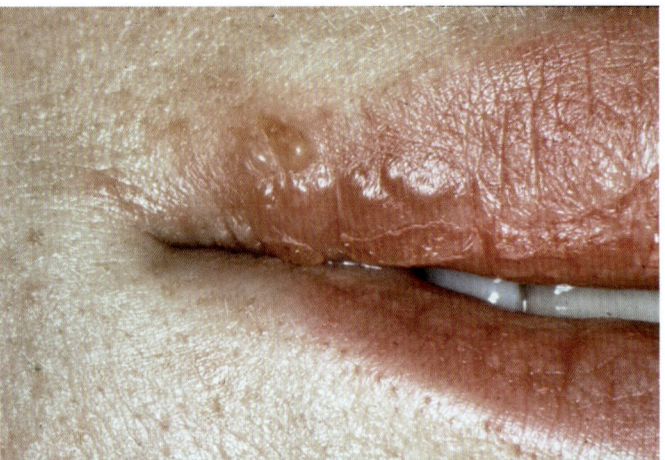

FIGURE 37.7   Herpes simplex virus. *(Courtesy of University of Washington Dermatology Division.)*

infection was asymptomatic.[121] Between episodes, the virus remains latent in sensory nerve ganglia and may periodically reactivate. Recurrent episodes are generally milder than the original episode and tend to become less frequent with time. Fever, stress, ultraviolet light, and certain surgical procedures may trigger reactivation of the virus (e.g., dermabrasion or laser resurfacing).

HSV infection may present in multiple clinical forms with orolabial (herpes labialis, typically caused by HSV type 1) and genital HSV (typically caused by HSV type 2) being the most common. Keratoconjunctivitis, herpetic sycosis (beard area), herpetic whitlow, herpes gladiatorum, eczema herpeticum, recurrent lumbosacral HSV, and neonatal HSV are other clinical forms of the disease. HSV may also trigger recurrent episodes of erythema multiforme where HSV DNA can be detected in the lesions of erythema multiforme by polymerase chain reaction (PCR).[124] Immunosuppressed patients tend to have more severe and slower healing HSV infections with atypical clinical appearance, such as persistent crusts, erosions, ulcerative, or vegetative lesions. Less commonly, visceral infection may occur affecting the esophagus, lungs, liver, and other organs.[120] Neonatal HSV may occur in utero, at the time of the delivery or in the immediate few weeks after delivery. Patients may have involvement of the skin, eyes, and mouth, CNS, or disseminated disease. Most patients with neonatal HSV have vesicular skin lesions, but a significant percentage of patients, especially with CNS or disseminated disease, have no skin lesions.[121]

Diagnosis

The diagnosis is most readily established by direct fluorescent antibody (DFA) testing of scrapings from early vesicular lesions. Cultures should also be taken when possible from early vesicular lesions and will usually grow out within 48 to 72 hours. PCR has a higher sensitivity and lower cost compared to DFA and is the preferred diagnostic method in suspected meningitis/ encephalitis.[125] Tzanck preparation has the advantage of obtaining immediate results but is dependent on the experience and skill of the interpreter and will not distinguish between HSV and herpes zoster virus. Skin biopsy will show ballooning degeneration of keratinocytes and multinucleate giant cells in the epidermis.

Treatment

The principal antiviral medications for treatment of HSV are acyclovir, valacyclovir, and famciclovir. Valacyclovir and famciclovir have an advantage of less frequent dosing and greater bioavailability but are more expensive than acyclovir.

Severe episodes of HSV are treated with IV acyclovir. The dosages of the medications need to be adjusted in patients with renal failure. Representative treatment schedules are available in the references.[120–123] In general, dosing schedules differ for primary infection, suppressive therapy, episodic therapy, severity of the infection, and immune status of the patient. Acyclovir resistance is more likely to be encountered in immunosuppressed patients, and treatment with foscarnet or cidofovir as alternative agents may be useful.[120] Treatment with analgesics for pain, damp compresses with Burow's solution, and antibiotics for secondary infection are helpful supportive measures.

ERYSIPELAS AND CELLULITIS

Both erysipelas and cellulitis (Fig. 37.8) are soft tissue infections that cause erythema, edema, warmth, and pain often on the lower extremities but other areas as well. Erysipelas is distinguished from cellulitis in being more superficial in the dermis and sharply demarcated from the surrounding normal skin, whereas cellulitis typically affects deeper tissues and is more indurated and poorly circumscribed.[126–129] Both may be associated with fever, chills, lymphangitis, and localized lymphadenopathy. Bullous formation may occur with erysipelas and rarely with cellulitis (e.g., vibrio vulnificus).[127,129] Group A *Streptococcus* (*S. pyogenes*) is the principal cause of erysipelas but may also cause cellulitis. Many other organisms may cause cellulitis as well. A break in the skin or portal of entry may sometimes be found (e.g., trauma or fissuring between the toes from tinea pedis).

The diagnosis is often made clinically before lab tests are available. Distinguishing erysipelas from cellulitis may be difficult at times. Culturing any breaks in the skin or ulcers may be helpful in recovering the organism but is not routinely recommended unless the patient is immunosuppressed or has an animal bite.[117] Culturing aspirates from the rash or skin biopsies are low-yield procedures and rarely performed. Blood cultures when positive provide a definitive diagnosis.

Treatment

Erysipelas responds to treatment with oral penicillin or amoxicillin. Because *S. aureus* may be difficult to exclude clinically, treatment with cephalexin or dicloxacillin pending culture results is prudent.

Cellulitis of the skin is often caused by *Staphylococcus aureus* and *Streptococcus pyogenes*, and coverage with oral cephalexin or dicloxacillin for milder cases of infection is usually sufficient. Initial therapy is highly dependent on the history of exposure to any unusual organisms, underlying illnesses of the patient, toxicity of the patient, clinical setting (e.g., diabetic foot ulcer), and likelihood of methicillin-resistant *Staphylococcus aureus* (MRSA), which would dictate other antibiotic coverage. Seriously ill patients may need hospitalization, IV antibiotics, and infectious diseases consult.

Elevation of the extremity if no arterial insufficiency is present, local wound care for any ulcers, and antifungal cream for tinea pedis are important adjunctive measures.

FURUNCULOSIS AND CARBUNCLE

Furuncles and carbuncles (Fig. 37.9) are painful staphylococcal infections in hair-bearing areas that begin as a folliculitis. A furuncle occurs when infection extends down the hair follicle to the subcutaneous tissue with abscess formation producing an erythematous, painful nodule with a superimposed follicular-centered pustule. A carbuncle occurs when infection spreads to multiple adjacent contiguous follicles by subcutaneous extension resulting in a larger, erythematous, painful mass with superimposed follicular pustules. Culture and sensitivity taken from the pustules should guide antibiotic therapy.[130]

Treatment

Fluctuant abscesses should be incised, drained, and cultured. Packing of abscesses less than 5 cm in diameter may be unnecessary.[131] Milder cases may respond to incision and drainage and moist heat alone, but careful follow-up is necessary if oral antibiotics are not given. If antibiotics are needed, dicloxacillin or cephalexin 500 mg four times per day for 7 days should be used to treat methicillin-sensitive *Staphylococcus aureus* (MSSA). If MRSA is suspected, treat with trimethoprim-sulfamethoxazole (TMP-SMX) one double-strength tablet twice daily or doxycycline 100 mg twice daily for 7 days, but it should be kept in mind that these agents will not treat group A *Streptococcus* infection. More seriously ill patients may need hospitalization and treatment with IV antibiotics.

In patients with recurrent furunculosis, elimination of nasal staphylococcal carriage and skin colonization may be helpful, although the information on efficacy is limited. Regimens include intranasal mupirocin ointment twice daily for 5 days per

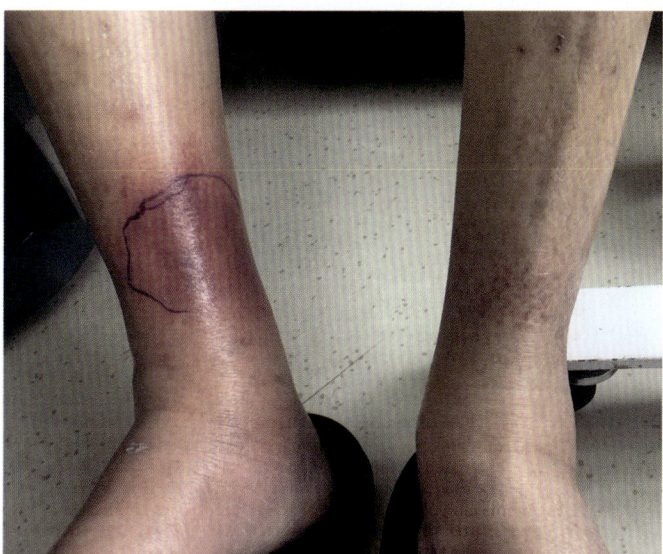

FIGURE 37.8 Cellulitis on the right lower extremity. *(Courtesy of Vanessa Pascoe, MD, University of Washington.)*

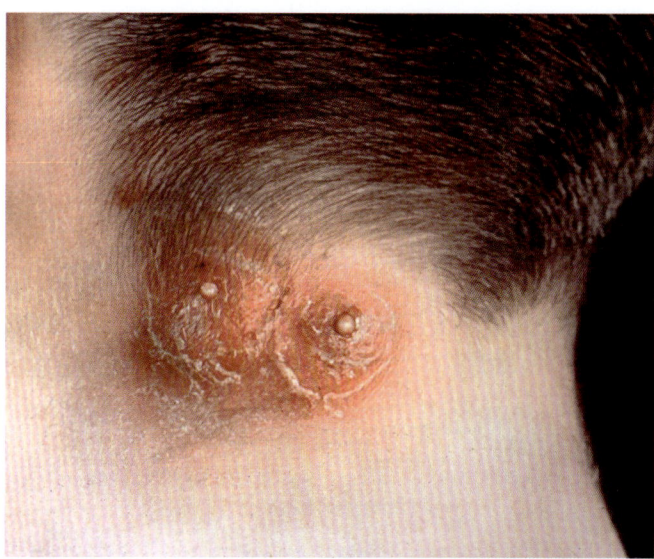

FIGURE 37.9 Carbuncle. *(Courtesy of University of Washington Dermatology Division.)*

month, chlorhexidine washes (away from eyes and ears), dilute bleach baths, and decontamination of personal items.[117,132,133]

Good hygienic measures may be helpful for patients in preventing recurrences and spread of infection to others such as frequent hand washing, keeping wounds cleanly bandaged, regular laundering of clothing in contact with the wound, regular bathing with soap, avoiding shared towels and other shared items, and cleansing of equipment and surfaces in contact with wound drainage.[134,135]

ERYSIPELOID

Erysipeloid is an acute painful infection of the skin caused by *Erysipelothrix rhusiopathiae*, a gram-positive rod. It is an occupational hazard of fishermen and butchers and occurs domestically in those who handle raw fish, poultry, and meat products.[136,137]

The organism gains entrance through a break in the skin to cause what has been referred to as an erysipeloid rash. A painful violaceous red, warm, raised, lesion develops usually on the hand or finger, spreads peripherally, and clears centrally. There is no ulceration or scaling. Usually, the infection remains localized, but systemic infection may occur.

The treatment of choice is penicillin or amoxicillin for 7 to 10 days. Higher doses are needed if systemic infection occurs.[117]

Inflammations

PANNICULITIS

The panniculitides are a heterogeneous group of inflammatory disorders of the subcutaneous fat, and all present as subcutaneous nodules that may be painful. They are conceptually classified by their histologic pattern into septal and lobular categories and are described well in a review by Requena and Yus.[138]

Erythema Nodosum

Erythema nodosum (EN) is the most common panniculitis (Fig. 37.10). It is a septal panniculitis that typically affects young adults between 20 and 30 years of age with male-to-female ratio of 1:6, although any age may be affected.[138,139] EN usually presents as bilateral tender, poorly circumscribed erythematous nodules, 1 to 10 cm in diameter, on the anterior tibial areas, but more widespread involvement may occur.[139] The lesions typically heal over a few weeks without scarring, although new lesions may continue to appear. Some patients have constitutional symptoms such as fever, malaise, arthralgias, headache, cough, abdominal pain, vomiting, or diarrhea.[138] Associated lab abnormalities may include leukocytosis and elevated erythrocyte sedimentation rate.[139]

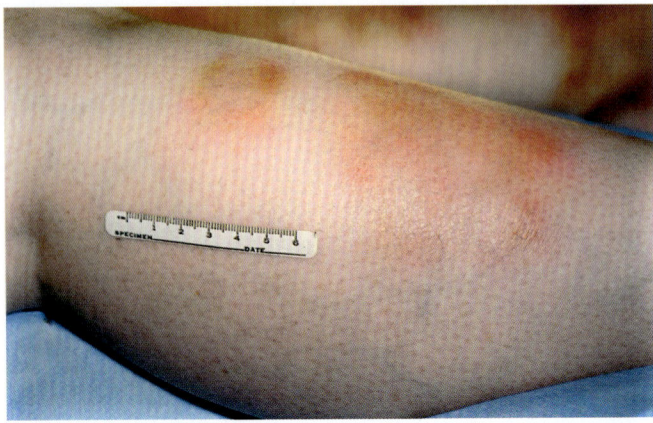

FIGURE 37.10 Erythema nodosum. *(Courtesy of University of Washington Dermatology Division.)*

There have been many reported causes of EN including infections (bacterial, viral, fungal, and protozoan), medications (e.g., penicillin, sulfonamides, oral contraceptives, iodides, and salicylates), malignancy, sarcoidosis, inflammatory bowel disease, and pregnancy.[138–141] Sarcoidosis and streptococcal infections are among the most frequent causes. *Streptococcus* infection is an important cause of EN in children, reported in 49% cases in one series.[142] In 35% to 55% cases, no etiology may be found.[140,141] Uncommon but important causes to exclude are *Mycobacterium tuberculosis*, deep fungal infections (histoplasmosis, coccidiomycosis, and blastomycosis), and malignancy (lymphoma, leukemia, and solid tumors).[138] EN is a feature of monocytopenia and mycobacterial infection (monoMAC) syndrome, caused by heterozygous mutations in GATA2 and characterized by monocytopenia and susceptibility to nontuberculous mycobacterial infections.[143]

The pathogenesis of EN is poorly understood and felt to be a hypersensitivity reaction to etiologic agents. Histologically, there is inflammation of the septae between fat lobules that evolves from acute inflammation to granulomatous change followed by fibrosis. The presence of Miescher's radial granulomas with aggregates of histiocytes and neutrophils around central clefts is a characteristic feature.[144]

Treatment

EN is typically self-limited and resolves within several weeks. Any underlying diseases or infections should be treated. Medications that are a potential cause should be discontinued. Bed rest and NSAIDs may be sufficient. In patients with more persistent or recalcitrant disease, potassium iodide may be helpful. Potassium iodide is contraindicated in pregnant women, should be avoided in renal insufficiency (risk of hyperkalemia), and used cautiously, if at all, in patients with thyroid disease (risk of hyperthyroidism or hypothyroidism).[145] It should be kept in mind that both aspirin and iodides have been reported as both causing and treating EN. A short course of systemic corticosteroids may be helpful if any underlying infectious diseases have been excluded.

DERCUM DISEASE (ADIPOSA DOLOROSA)

Dercum disease is a rare condition of painful lipomas of the skin on the trunk and extremities. It is seen most commonly in obese women between the ages of 35 and 50 years and may be associated with weakness, fatigue, depression, and anxiety. Most cases are sporadic, but familial cases with autosomal dominant inheritance pattern have also been reported. Histologically, one typically finds a lipoma with no distinguishing features from an ordinary lipoma.[146]

Treatment

Treatment is often ineffective and short-lasting. The pain in Dercum disease has been characterized as both nociceptive (localized pain in lipomas aggravated by palpation) and neuropathic with allodynia (light touch perceived as painful) so approaches to management similar to other chronic pain syndromes may be beneficial.[147]

Weight reduction and analgesics may be helpful. Excision of individual painful tumors may also be helpful, but new painful tumors may continue to appear.[148] Liposuction has also been reported to be of benefit.[149,150] IV lidocaine may provide pain relief lasting from hours to months.[151–153] Corticosteroids have been reported to both cause[154] and treat[155] Dercum disease. Other treatments with limited evidence include calcium-channel modulators, interferon α-2b, combined infliximab and methotrexate, and rapid cycling hypobaric pressure.[146]

HIDRADENITIS SUPPURATIVA

HS is a chronic inflammatory follicular-occlusive disease where recurrent painful nodules, abscesses, and sinus tracts involve

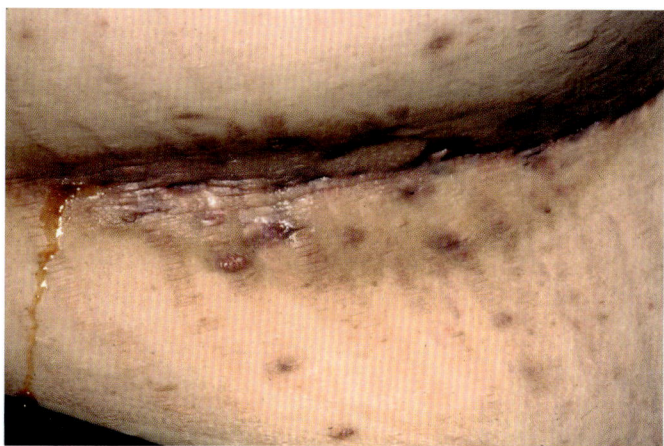

FIGURE 37.11 Hidradenitis suppurativa. *(Courtesy of University of Washington Dermatology Division.)*

the intertriginous skin (axillary, inframammary, inguinal, and gluteal folds) (acne inversa, see Fig. 37.11). The incidence has risen over the past decade and disproportionately affects women, young adults, and African Americans.[156] HS is associated with comorbidities, including metabolic syndrome, tobacco abuse, polycystic ovarian syndrome, and inflammatory bowel disease. HS may be part of a syndrome-like presentation, such as PAPASH syndrome (pyogenic arthritis, PG, acne, and suppurative hidradenitis) and PASH syndrome (PG, acne, and suppurative hidradenitis). It is also considered to part of the follicular occlusion tetrad, along with acne conglobata, pilonidal sinus, and dissecting cellulitis of the scalp.

Etiology
The etiology of HS is incompletely understood and is felt to be due in part to follicular hyperkeratosis and occlusion leading to rupture and acute suppurative inflammation. Keratinocyte activation and release of proinflammatory mediators also plays a role. The disease usually first appears at puberty, suggesting hormonal factors are contributory. Other factors include genetic susceptibility, mechanical stress, obesity, and smoking.[157] The role of bacteria in pathogenesis is controversial. Antibiotics can be an effective treatment modality; however, the most commonly isolated organisms are commensal bacteria.[158]

Symptoms and Signs
Early on, patients experience recurrent, painful, erythematous nodules that suppurate and eventually breakdown to form sinus tracts and scarring. The sinus tracts may form an extensive interconnecting network in the subcutaneous tissue with multiple openings. The disease process may be circumscribed or more diffuse. Secondary bacterial infection may occur. In addition to being physically painful, the disease may be psychologically debilitating and profoundly impair quality of life, especially in patients with long-standing disease.[159] Squamous cell cancer and amyloidosis are rare complications in patients with chronic HS.[160]

Diagnosis
Initially, the disease appears similar to furuncles or an inflamed epidermal cyst. However, when the erythematous nodules are recurrent and lead to sinus tracts and retracted scars, the diagnosis becomes clear.

Treatment
Treatment is individualized depending on the severity of the disease. Behavioral changes including weight reduction and smoking cessation is advised. Topical clindamycin and cleansing the

affected areas with antibacterial soaps such as chlorhexidine may be useful. The U.S. Food and Drug Administration (FDA) has recently issued a warning about rare, but serious, allergic reactions to chlorhexidine.[161]

For more limited nodules without sinus tracts, unroofing or intralesional corticosteroids may be beneficial. Incision and drainage is not an effective management strategy, as lesions tend to recur. Systemic antibiotics, such as doxycycline, are often used as initial treatment. The combination of clindamycin and rifampin may be used in patients who do not respond to other antibiotics. Antiandrogenic agents may provide additional benefit.[162]

Diffuse involvement with sinus tracts and extensive scarring may require the addition of a biologic agent, such as adalimumab or infliximab. A weekly adalimumab administration has the most robust efficacy data.[163]

Surgical interventions may provide relief for severe HS in a localized area that has failed to respond sufficiently to unroofing and medical therapies. Wide excision followed by a graft or healing by secondary intention can have good functional and cosmetic results, although recurrence of disease is possible.[164,165] Hair removal by 1064-nm Nd:YAG or intense pulsed light devices can reduce the disease activity in the affected area. Extensive disease has been removed by carbon dioxide (CO_2) laser.[166]

Pain management can be challenging. Topical analgesics, acetaminophen, and NSAIDs are first line. Additional agents may be required for the neuropathic component and has been reviewed by Horvath et al.[167]

INFLAMED EPIDERMAL CYST
Epidermal cysts (Fig. 37.12) are very common and typically present after puberty as whitish, sometimes pigmented, well-defined, partially compressible, subcutaneous nodules with a semisolid feel and often with a pore opening to the surface.[168,169] They may extrude a thick whitish material with a foul odor through the pore. The cyst wall is stratified squamous epithelium, and the contents are keratin. Most are asymptomatic, but when they are traumatized and rupture into the surrounding tissue, they incite an acute inflammatory reaction that mimics infection with pain, erythema, edema, warmth, and purulence. Initial management consists of hot compresses and incision and drainage. If secondary infection is suspected, culture and sensitivity should be done, and the patient treated an antibiotic

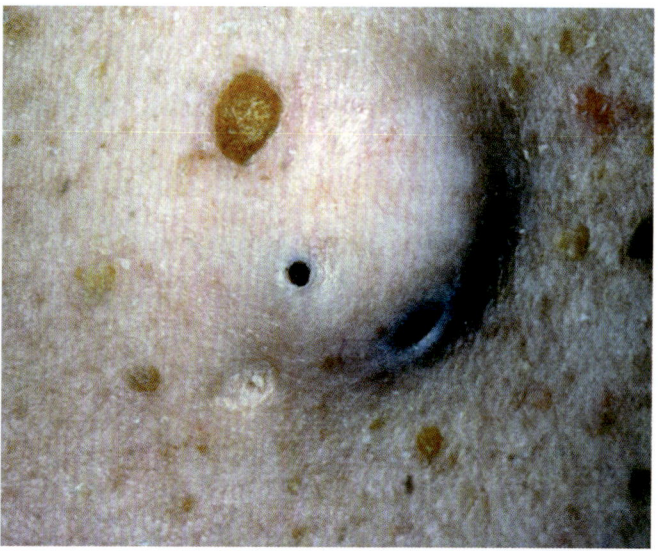

FIGURE 37.12 Epidermal cyst, noninflamed. *(Courtesy of University of Washington Dermatology Division.)*

effective for *Staphylococcus aureus* and *Streptococcus pyogenes* such as cephalexin or dicloxacillin pending culture results. Once inflammation subsides the residual cyst is excised. Some cysts are destroyed by the inflammation if severe enough.

Great care should be taken in excising previously inflamed cysts in certain locations because scar tissue may have entrapped important nerves or other structures, for example, the temporal branch of the facial nerve in the temple areas, the spinal accessory nerve in the posterior cervical triangle of the neck, or the parotid duct overlying the masseter muscle on the cheek. In these locations, it may be more prudent to open the cyst, evacuate the contents, and scrape the wall of the cyst with a curette if treatment is felt to be necessary.

Although epidermal cysts typically develop after puberty, an accurate history regarding a particular cyst may not always be available. Cysts that could possibly have been present since birth should be a cause of greater concern especially in certain locations such as the midline of the face, the midline of the scalp, or the midline of the back because they may communicate with the CNS. Should one of these cysts become inflamed or infected, surgery should not be attempted without prior imaging studies such as CT and magnetic resonance imaging (MRI). If a communication is found with the CNS, the surgery needs to be done by a neurosurgeon. Similarly, cysts present at birth on the lateral neck may be branchial cleft cysts that communicate with the pharynx. They may become infected in adult life simulating an inflamed epidermal cyst. Referral to an otolaryngologist is indicated for definitive treatment. Cysts presenting in childhood may be a sign of Gardner's syndrome, an autosomal dominant condition, associated with multiple benign tumors of the skin, osteomas, intestinal polyposis, and a high risk of colon cancer.[170] Ordinary epidermal cysts have a lining similar to normal epidermis with a granular layer, but cysts with Gardner's syndrome often have focal areas of pilomatrical differentiation.[170]

BULLOUS DERMATOSES WITH EROSIONS
Stevens-Johnson/Toxic Epidermal Necrolysis Syndrome

Adverse drug eruptions constitute a large percentage of inpatient hospital consultations for dermatologists. There are numerous types of drug eruptions beyond the scope of this chapter. When evaluating a drug eruption, a complete and thorough history of drug exposure is essential. Over-the-counter medications and dose adjustments should not be missed.

Stevens-Johnson/toxic epidermal necrolysis (SJS/TEN) is a severe, life-threatening mucocutaneous drug eruption that results in painful skin detachment (Fig. 37.13). The overall incidence is 1 to 2 cases per million, and mortality has been reported to be up to 30%. Clinically, SJS is defined as less than 10% body surface area (BSA) skin detachment; 10% to 30% BSA skin detachment is SJS/TEN overlap, and greater than 30% BSA is TEN.[171]

Over 100 medications have been reported to cause SJS/TEN. The most common inciting medications are TMP-SMX, allopurinol, nevirapine, lamotrigine, and carbamazepine. SJS/TEN is a delayed-type drug hypersensitivity reaction, with a latency of 4 to 28 days after exposure to the offending medication.

The eruption is preceded by fever and flu-like symptoms. Lesions are initially dusky, irregular, atypical targetoid with necrotic centers that form bullae and desquamate over the ensuing few days. Involvement of at least two mucous membrane sites is present in up to 90% of cases, most frequently the oral mucosa and conjunctiva, and can be very painful. Other mucosal surfaces that may be affected include the esophagus, respiratory tract, and genitourinary. Nikolsky sign (epidermal detachment with lateral pressure on an erythematous zone) may be positive but can be also present in other conditions such as pemphigus

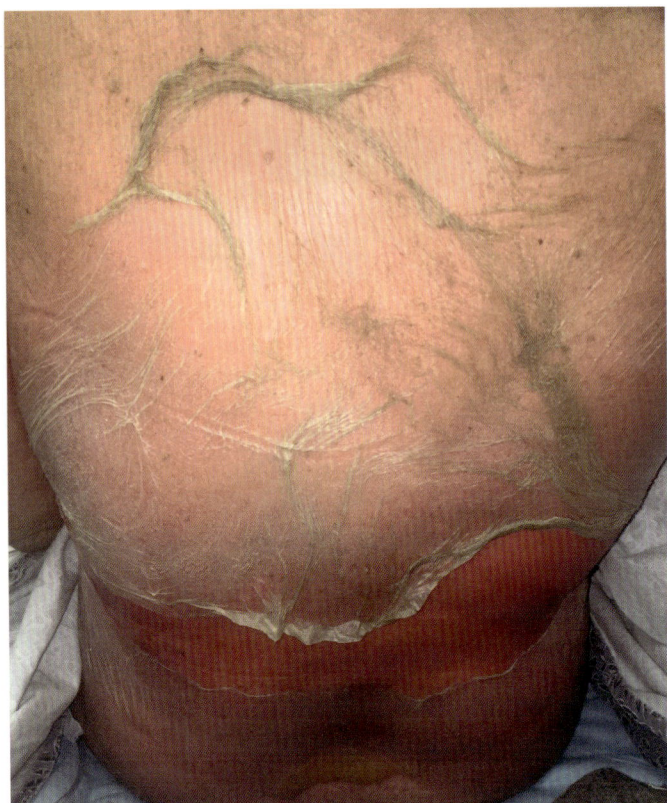

FIGURE 37.13 Toxic epidermal necrolysis. *(Courtesy of Vanessa Pascoe, MD, University of Washington.)*

vulgaris and staphylococcal scalded skin syndrome. Pain is a distinctive feature of SJS/TEN due to the skin detachment and may not be seen in other uncomplicated, exanthematous drug eruptions. The mean duration from the onset of symptoms to maximum detachment is 8 days.

The differential includes other blistering skin conditions, including bullous pemphigoid, pemphigus vulgaris, linear IgA bullous dermatosis, bullous erythema multiforme, and graft-versus-host disease. Histologically, there is a lymphocytic infiltrate at the dermoepidermal junction with epidermal necrosis that may be full thickness.

Pathogenesis: Keratinocyte necrosis occurs through multiple mechanisms. The culprit drug may act as a foreign antigen, recognized by T cell receptors to activate adaptive immune responses. Activated cytotoxic T cells and natural killer cells produce factors that induce keratinocyte death, including granulysin, perforin, and granzyme B. Apoptosis is induced by the soluble Fas ligand binding to the death receptor Fas/CD95. There is a strong association between HLA-B*1502 and the development of carbamazepine-induced SJS/TEN in the Han Chinese population but not in other races, and the FDA has recommended genotyping all Asian patients prior to initiation of carbamazepine therapy.[172]

Treatment: After prompt withdrawal of the offending drug, supportive care is paramount and management is similar to care for an extensive burn. Patients require burn critical care unit care, and coordination across multiple specialty services including ophthalmology, gynecology, and urology. Due to extensive cutaneous disruption, patients are at risk for fluid and electrolyte loss, increased caloric needs, and secondary bacterial infection. SCORTEN is a severity-of-illness score composed of seven variables that predict outcome, and its utility has been confirmed by several studies.[171]

The use of systemic medications is controversial, and the evidence is mixed. IVIg and systemic corticosteroids have been used; however, systematic reviews do not show a mortality benefit,[172] and use of systemic steroids can increase risk of sepsis. Re-epithelialization occurs over 3 weeks. The most common sequelae are visual impairment due to ocular scarring and skin dyspigmentation. Bronchiolitis obliterans, urogenital adhesions, and posttraumatic stress disorder are also reported.[173]

Pemphigus Vulgaris

Pemphigus vulgaris is a rare, autoimmune disorder and the most frequent member of a group of disorders referred to as pemphigus. Other members of the group include pemphigus foliaceous, pemphigus vegetans, pemphigus erythematosus, and paraneoplastic pemphigus.

Pemphigus vulgaris usually presents with painful blisters and nonhealing erosions in the mouth that eventually spread to the skin producing flaccid blisters and bullae followed by oozing, crusted, painful erosions.[174,175] Lateral pressure on the skin adjacent to a bullous lesion causes the epidermis to shear and detach (Nikolsky sign). Uncommonly, patients may have an associated thymoma or myasthenia gravis. Drug-induced pemphigus has been reported with a variety of medications including penicillamine, rifampicin, captopril, enalapril, penicillin, and other drugs.[174,176] The bullae and blisters are caused by autoantibodies to desmosomal cadherin adhesion molecules, either desmoglein 3 with isolated mucosal pemphigus vulgaris, or desmoglein 3 plus desmoglein 1 with mucocutaneous pemphigus vulgaris, whereas patients with pemphigus foliaceus have antibodies to desmoglein 1 only.[175] This leads to detachment of cells from one another (acantholysis) that is seen histologically as a suprabasilar split in the epidermis (suprabasilar acantholysis) in pemphigus vulgaris and subcorneal acantholysis in pemphigus foliaceus. The autoantibodies can be detected by direct immunofluorescence of perilesional skin producing a netlike pattern on the surface of keratinocytes. Circulating autoantibodies are commonly present and detected by indirect immunofluorescence or enzyme-linked immunosorbent assay (ELISA) for antibodies to desmoglein 3 and desmoglein 1. Titers of circulating autoantibodies may correlate with disease activity, and declining levels may predict progression from the active phase of disease to early remission.[177]

Treatment: The mainstay of treatment of pemphigus vulgaris are systemic corticosteroids.[174] A steroid-sparing agent is then typically added, usually azathioprine or mycophenolate mofetil. Pulse steroids and plasmapheresis with and without cyclophosphamide are other treatments that have been used. Rituximab has emerged as a treatment for recalcitrant cases and as a potential first-line adjuvant treatment. A combination of systemic corticosteroids and rituximab as first-line treatment was more effective than steroids alone in recent studies.[178,179] Patients need close monitoring for complications of therapy and preventive measures when possible (e.g., measures to prevent osteoporosis related to chronic corticosteroid use). Topical therapy and supportive measures for mucous membrane and cutaneous involvement are also needed.

Paraneoplastic Pemphigus

Paraneoplastic pemphigus is associated with benign and malignant neoplasms, most commonly lymphoproliferative disorders. It causes a painful stomatitis similar to pemphigus vulgaris but a more polymorphic eruption on the skin.[180] The skin eruption may have features resembling pemphigus vulgaris, bullous pemphigoid, erythema multiforme, or a lichen planus-like (lichenoid) appearance. The polymorphic clinical pattern is reflected in the histology where one sees suprabasilar acantholysis, keratinocyte necrosis, and interface dermatitis.

Direct immunofluorescence demonstrates IgG and C3 in a netlike pattern on keratinocytes similar to pemphigus vulgaris and less frequently a linear pattern along the basement membrane. Circulating autoantibodies detected by immunoprecipitation recognize desmoplakins, most commonly envoplakin and periplakin.[181] Paraneoplastic pemphigus is most frequently associated with non-Hodgkin lymphoma, followed by chronic lymphocytic leukemia, Castleman's disease, thymoma, Waldenström's macroglobulinemia, Hodgkin lymphoma, and monoclonal gammopathy. Mortality ranges from 51% to 90%, with most patients dying from sepsis, respiratory failure, or the underlying malignancy.[182,183]

Treatment: Treatment of paraneoplastic pemphigus involves treating the underlying tumor, which in some cases may clear the eruption but is less likely to if the tumor is malignant.[180] Variable response has been reported with prednisone alone or combined with other immunosuppressive agents.[182]

Bullous Pemphigoid

Bullous pemphigoid (Fig. 37.14) is the most common autoimmune subepidermal bullous disease and typically affects elderly patients. Other pemphigoids, including mucous membrane pemphigoid, pemphigoid gestationis, and anti-p200 pemphigoid, are beyond the scope of this chapter. Tense bullae develop on normal or erythematous skin, commonly distributed on the lower abdomen, axillae, groin, and flexor extremities. Transient oral lesions may also appear. Itch is common and may be severe, and erosions can be painful after of bullae. Peripheral blood eosinophilia is often an associated finding. Most cases of bullous pemphigoid are idiopathic, but exposure to certain systemic medications may play a role in the development of BP, including diuretics, antibiotics, analgesics, and others.

Histologically, one finds a subepidermal bullous lesion with varying degrees of cellular infiltrate, often with eosinophils. Direct immunofluorescence demonstrates IgG and C3 in a smooth linear pattern at the epidermal basement membrane. Two bullous pemphigoid antigens have been identified associated with the hemidesmosomal plaques at the dermal–epidermal junction. Bullous pemphigoid antigen 1 (230 kD) is an intracellular antigen, and bullous pemphigoid antigen 2 (180 kD) is a transmembrane protein.[184] ELISA detects BP180 autoantibodies in 72% to 93% of cases.[185]

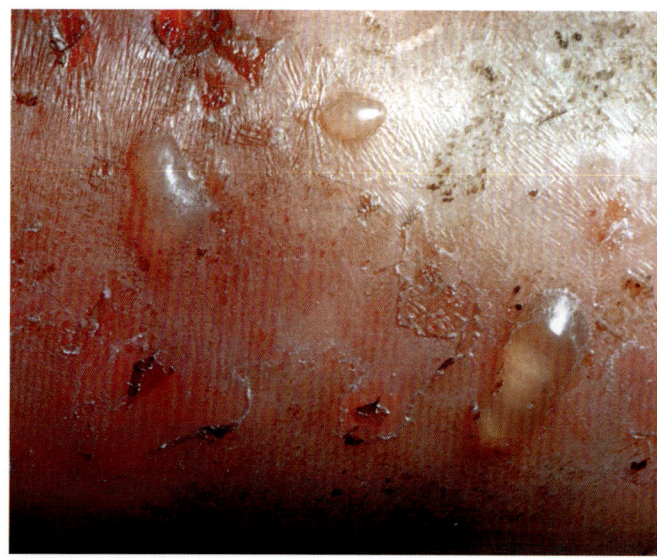

FIGURE 37.14 Bullous pemphigoid. *(Courtesy of University of Washington Dermatology Division.)*

Treatment: Milder cases of bullous pemphigoid or localized bullous disease may respond to high-potency topical steroids alone. Tetracycline or erythromycin 500 mg four times per day plus nicotinamide or dapsone may also be considered in patients with more severe disease who are not good candidates for treatment with systemic corticosteroids or as adjunctive treatment with systemic steroids.

Most patients with moderate to severe, generalized bullous pemphigoid are treated with prednisone, and a steroid-sparing agent is added if needed. Azathioprine or mycophenolate mofetil are used most commonly. For patient with severe or extensive disease, total body applications of clobetasol 0.05% cream twice daily was shown to be superior to prednisone 1 mg/kg/day in terms of effectiveness and survival in one study.[186] IVIg and rituximab has been used in refractory disease.[185]

Epidermolysis Bullosa

Epidermolysis bullosa refers to a group of rare disorders that may be inherited or acquired. They all exhibit abnormal skin and sometimes mucous membrane fragility with minor trauma leading to blister formation, painful erosions, and, in some cases, scarring.[187-191] Scarring may manifest as milia or dystrophic nails or, in more severe cases, as pseudosyndactyly, esophageal strictures, and conjunctival scarring.

The different types of epidermolysis bullosa are differentiated from one another on the basis of whether they are inherited or acquired; the inheritance pattern; level of split within, below, or at the junction of the epidermis and dermis; distribution and severity of skin and mucous membrane involvement; scarring or nonscarring; and the affected protein and mutated gene. Determining the level of the split within, below, or at the junction of the epidermis and dermis is an important part of the initial evaluation of the patient. This may be done with electron microscopy or immunofluorescent mapping with antibodies such as those to type VII collagen, laminin, or bullous pemphigoid antigen.[192] The inherited forms of epidermolysis bullosa demonstrate little if any inflammation on biopsy, whereas the acquired form, epidermolysis bullosa acquisita (EBA), may have an intense inflammatory infiltrate. In EBA, autoantibodies are bound in the basement membrane zone that is localized to the floor of the blister when detected by immunofluorescence on salt split skin. EBA can be associated with other diseases, such as malignancies, amyloidosis, diabetes, inflammatory bowel disease, SLE, and other autoimmune disorders; thus, workup of the patient for an underlying disease is indicated.[188,190,193]

Pathogenesis: Ultrastructural, immunohistochemical, and molecular biologic techniques have enabled the identification of affected proteins, point mutations, and corresponding ultrastructural findings in the inherited forms of epidermolysis bullosa.[192] For example, mutations in the keratins 5 and 14 are responsible for epidermolysis bullosa simplex, mutations in laminin 5 occur in junctional epidermolysis bullosa, and mutations in type VII collagen occur in dystrophic epidermolysis bullosa.[191] EBA is an autoimmune disease with autoantibodies against type VII collagen leading to loss of or diminution of anchoring fibrils in the papillary dermis similar to the dystrophic epidermolysis bullosa phenotype.[189]

Treatment: Avoidance of friction, pressure, trauma, and heat to skin and mucous membranes are important in the management of epidermolysis bullosa. Pain control, emollients, nutritional support, drainage of larger bullae, topical antibiotics, and nonadherent skin dressings are also important.[194] Some patients with the severest forms of the disease may need surgical correction of pseudosyndactyly, esophageal dilation for stricture, ophthalmologic care for scarring, dental care, and monitoring for renal complications and complicating squamous cell cancer of the skin.[194] Genetic counseling is also needed with the inherited forms of the disease.

Novel molecular and pharmacologic approaches are being investigated, such as cell-based therapies, bone marrow transplantation, and gene therapy.[195]

EBA is difficult to treat with no controlled studies and poor or variable response to a variety of agents. Dapsone and colchicine are usually first line, followed by systemic corticosteroids and steroid-sparing agents (azathioprine and mycophenolate mofetil). IVIg and rituximab have been used in refractory cases.[196,197]

Disorders of Connective Tissue Structure (Cartilage Disorders)

RELAPSING POLYCHONDRITIS

Relapsing polychondritis (RP) is a rare, potentially life-threatening, episodic systemic autoimmune inflammatory disease affecting cartilage containing structures (e.g., ears, nose, joints and respiratory tract) and proteoglycan-rich tissues (e.g., eyes, inner ear, cardiovascular system and kidneys). Recurrent episodes of pain, erythema, and swelling of the ears are the most common feature of the disease. The earlobe is spared, and eventually, the ears may become "floppy" or have a "cauliflower-like" appearance as the cartilage is destroyed. Nasal chondritis may lead to a saddle nose deformity over time, sometimes without clinically apparent inflammation. Ocular inflammation is common and may simulate cellulitis.[198] Other features of the disease include nonerosive polyarthritis, laryngotracheal and bronchial chondritis, cardiovascular disease, and renal disease. The most common cause of death is infection, usually pneumonia, in which airway collapse or steroid therapy may play a role. Associated diseases are not uncommon in RP, including myelodysplasia, Sweet's syndrome, and an underlying malignancy.[199] Autoantibodies to type II collagen, matrilin-I, and circulating immune complexes have been found in RP, suggesting an autoimmune pathogenesis. Trauma and the HLA-DR4 haplotype may also play a role.

Cutaneous manifestations have been reported in up to 37% of patients. Purpura, aphthosis, and EN-like nodules of the lower extremities were the most common manifestations. Other reported cutaneous features of RP include urticaria, livedo reticularis, superficial thrombophlebitis, ulcers, pustules, and distal necrosis. Cutaneous manifestations were noted in 91% of patients with associated myelodysplasia.[200] Different sets of revised diagnostic criteria are available in the references.[201,202]

Treatment

Milder cases of RP may respond to dapsone, colchicine, or NSAIDs.[199,203,204] Acute flares and more serious involvement of vital structures are usually treated with systemic corticosteroids and sometimes cyclophosphamide. Adjunctive steroid-sparing agents are added if needed, including azathioprine, methotrexate, or cyclosporine. Methotrexate was found to be the most effective in the series reported by Trentham and Le.[204] Other agents that have been used include tumor necrosis factor-α antagonists, tocilizumab, and abatacept.[205]

Surgery and other intervention may be needed for complications of the disease including tracheostomy, cardiac valve replacement, aortic aneurysm repair, and placement of a cardiac pacemaker for conduction disturbances.[198,199] Survival has improved over time with a 94% survival in patients who have had their disease on average 8 years.[204]

CHONDRODERMATITIS NODULARIS HELICIS

Chondrodermatitis nodularis helicis (CNH) is a common painful disorder where tender papules occur on the rim of the helix or the antihelix of the external ear. The papules may have scaling, crusting, or ulceration suggesting the diagnosis of squamous cell cancer or basal cell cancer. Biopsy should be performed if the diagnosis is in doubt. Histopathologic features may include ulceration with exudate, epidermal hyperplasia, fibrinoid dermal necrosis, mixed inflammatory cell infiltrate, thickening of the perichondrium, and degeneration of cartilage.[206] Neural hyperplasia has also been observed on occasion which has been suggested might explain the induction of pain by light pressure.[207] The pathogenesis remains unclear, but chronic pressure may lead to ischemia of the underlying cartilage.

Various treatments have been used employed with different degrees of success and recurrence rates. Pressure relief, surgical excision techniques, and topical nitroglycerin are among the most effective. If the patient sleeps habitually on one side, a pillow with a hole in it or self-adherent foam padding behind the ear may be helpful in relieving symptoms.[208]

Neurovascular Cutaneous Disease

SENSORY MONONEUROPATHIES

Further information on painful neuropathies can be found in Chapter 24. Sensory mononeuropathies are not uncommon and may affect the head, trunk, and extremities. They may manifest themselves as numbness, burning, itching, hyperesthesias, and frequently pain.[209] Among the more common are cheiralgia paresthetica (superficial branch of the radial nerve), meralgia paresthetica (lateral femoral cutaneous nerve), notalgia paresthetica (dorsal rami of T2–T6), and gonyalgia paresthetica (infrapatellar branch of the saphenous nerve). A less common but important neuropathy to be aware of is mental nerve neuropathy, which presents as unilateral numbness of the chin and lower lip (numb chin syndrome).[209–211] It is usually associated with malignancy, most commonly breast cancer or lymphoma, so thorough evaluation is needed.[210]

Notalgia paresthetica is a sensory neuropathy affecting the posterior rami of T2–T6. Patients usually complain of itch and less commonly pain, paresthesias, and hyperesthesia in a unilateral localized area on the upper back medial to the scapula.[212] Findings on examination may include hyperpigmentation and hypoesthesia.[209,213] Electromyographic evaluation may show evidence of paraspinal denervation in some cases.[214] In a study of 43 patients, 60.7% were found to have radiographic abnormalities of the spine corresponding to the nerves involved suggesting impingement of spinal nerves.[212] Massey[209] postulated the posterior rami of T2–T6 are subject to trauma because they traverse the multifidus spinal muscle at a right-angle course. A hereditary variant of notalgia paresthetica has been described and has also been reported in multiple endocrine neoplasia type 2 (MEN2A) syndrome.[213] Histologically, one may find postinflammatory hyperpigmentation, lichenification, and, in some cases, macular amyloidosis possibly related to excoriation.[215]

Treatment

Treatment of notalgia paresthetica and other sensory neuropathies has met with variable success with such agents as topical anesthetics, capsaicin, gabapentin, and amitriptyline.[216]

Oxcarbazepine (a derivative of the anticonvulsant carbamazepine with a better side effect profile) was reported to be partially effective in 3 of 5 patients treated with the medication.[217] A paravertebral block using a combination of bupivacaine and methylprednisolone led to complete resolution of symptoms for at least 1 year in one patient.[213] Gabapentin in a dose of 600 mg per day provided complete relief of symptoms in one patient with notalgia paresthetica.[218]

ERYTHROMELALGIA

Erythromelalgia is a rare acquired or hereditary (primary) condition characterized by hyperthermia, redness, and burning pain, usually of the extremities. The primary form is inherited in an autosomal dominant manner and is caused by a mutation in SCN9A, which encodes a sodium channel protein subunit in sympathetic and nociceptive sensory neurons of the dorsal root ganglion.

The feet are most frequently affected, followed by the upper extremities and face. The symptoms are usually symmetric, intermittent, and exacerbated by heat exposure and dependency and relieved by cold exposure and elevation. The pain can be debilitating and significantly impair quality of life. Erythromelalgia may be associated with an underlying myeloproliferative or autoimmune disorder. Acrocyanosis, ulcers, and even gangrene can develop, which is secondary to injury from excessive exposure to cold water in efforts to obtain relief.

The differential diagnosis includes reflex sympathetic dystrophy (also termed *complex regional pain syndrome type 1*, covered in Chapter 25), peripheral vascular disease, neuropathy, cellulitis, Fabry's disease (FD), Raynaud's phenomenon, and lipodermatosclerosis. Evaluation should include a CBC to exclude a myeloproliferative disorder.

Treatment is challenging, as erythromelalgia can often be refractory. Patients are advised to avoid excessive ambient heat, prolonged standing, and strenuous exercise. Cooling the affected area, such as with short, intermittent exposure to cool water, may be helpful; however, careful attention must be paid to avoiding prolonged exposure and subsequent cold injury. Topical therapy with compounded amitriptyline and ketamine cream has been reported to improve pain.[219] Systemic medications that have been used include aspirin (particularly for patients with underlying myeloproliferative disease), NSAIDs, gabapentin, β-blockers, sodium nitroprusside, misoprostol, topical or IV analgesics, carbamazepine, and antidepressants.[220–222]

FABRY'S DISEASE

FD (also known as Anderson-Fabry disease) is a rare X-linked recessive lysosomal storage disease caused by deficiency of the enzyme α-galactosidase A, leading to accumulation of globotriaosylceramide in lysosomes in the endothelium, vascular smooth muscle cells, autonomic and dorsal root ganglia, renal cells, cardiac conduction fibers, and other cell types. Deposition within these cells leads to its various symptoms, including vascular occlusions that lead to ischemia, infarction, and pain.

Symptoms and Signs

Angiokeratomas are the characteristic skin lesion of FD that occurs in a pattern referred to as angiokeratoma corporis diffusum (ACD) to distinguish them from other variants of angiokeratomas not associated with FD such as isolated angiokeratomas. Individual angiokeratomas are reddish-blue to black, 3- to 4-mm papules that may be scaly, hyperkeratotic, or verrucous. In ACD, they are usually distributed between the umbilicus and the knees but may be widespread and affect mucous membranes as well.

Hypohidrosis with heat intolerance, peripheral edema, and asymptomatic eye findings are other features of the disease. Female carriers in general may be asymptomatic, have mild disease, or rarely severe disease manifestations.[223] Episodic painful acroparesthesias, due to small fiber neuropathy of the hands and feet, may be the first manifestation of the disease. Acute attacks of abdominal pain may occur, simulating an acute abdomen. The most serious complications of the disease relate to involvement of the kidneys, heart, and CNS. Untreated patients typically develop end-stage renal disease by the fifth decade.

Histologically, ACD demonstrates dilated vessels in the papillary dermis with epidermal hyperplasia or acanthosis.[223] The abnormal lipid in the endothelial cells may be detected with a lipid stain or periodic acid-Schiff stain. Examination of the urine with polarized light may show birefringent glycosphingo-lipids in cells with a Maltese cross appearance.

Molecular genetic testing confirms the diagnosis, and genetic counseling should be offered to potentially affected family members.[224,225]

Treatment

Enzyme replacement therapy (ERT) with recombinant α-galactosidase A (agalsidase β, Fabrazyme, Genzyme Corp., Cambridge, MA) should be initiated as soon as possible in males with low levels of alpha-Gal-A, even if they are asymptomatic, and female carriers with clinical manifestations. ERT has been associated with improvement of neuropathic pain, relief of gastrointestinal symptoms, and stabilization of renal function and cardiomyopathy. Benefits are more limited in patients who already have advanced renal disease.[225,226]

There is no need to treat the angiokeratomas unless they are symptomatic, which can be done with a variety of local destructive methods such as laser or liquid nitrogen. The angiokeratomas have not been found to be a useful surrogate marker to follow disease activity with ERT.[227] There is some evidence for the efficacy of carbamazepine, phenytoin, and gabapentin for the treatment of neuropathic pain associated with FD.[228]

Other Painful Dermatologic Disorders

CUTANEOUS ENDOMETRIOSIS

Cutaneous endometriosis is a rare condition that may cause tender nodules in the skin.[229,230] They occur most frequently within surgical scars (e.g., cesarean section, episiotomy scars, or appendectomy scars) but also may occur as primary cutaneous endometriosis in which case they usually affect the umbilical area. Tenderness and bleeding may occur at times of menstruation. The histologic appearance may correspond to different stages in the menstrual cycle, but in general, there is a poor correlation between histologic appearance and the menstrual stage.[231] The range of histologic findings in cutaneous endometriosis has been reviewed.[232] Wide local excision usually suffices for treatment and recurrence is rare, but referral for gynecologic evaluation is also appropriate.[230,233]

PAINFUL NEOPLASMS

Both benign and malignant neoplasms may sometimes be painful because of ulceration, location on the body where they are repeatedly traumatized, or on pressure-bearing surfaces such as the soles of the feet. Certain benign neoplasms are characteristically painful and bring to mind a differential diagnosis that has been reported under the mnemonic acronym "ANGEL" for angiolipoma (also angioleiomyoma), neurilemmoma, glomus tumor (Fig. 37.15), eccrine spiradenoma, and leiomyoma (Fig. 37.16). These tumors are all true neoplasms where pain is a characteristic feature. They are listed in Table 37.2 with their comparative features. Treatment when needed consists of complete excision, which is usually curative.

Leiomyomas are deserving of further discussion because of their association with Reed's syndrome, characterized by hereditary leiomyomatosis and renal cell cancer.[234,235] This is an autosomal dominant condition due to mutations in the enzyme fumarate hydratase that is associated with cutaneous leiomyomas, leiomyosarcoma (rarely), uterine fibroids (leiomyomas), and renal cell cancer. Most patients have multiple cutaneous leiomyomas, but even a single leiomyoma may be a marker for the syndrome. When a patient with a cutaneous leiomyoma is encountered, a history should be taken for any personal or family history of cutaneous leiomyomas, uterine fibroids, early hysterectomy, and renal cell cancer.[235] If the history is suggestive, imaging studies of the kidneys and testing for fumarate hydratase mutations is indicated, along with lifetime surveillance and examination of relatives if studies confirm the diagnosis.

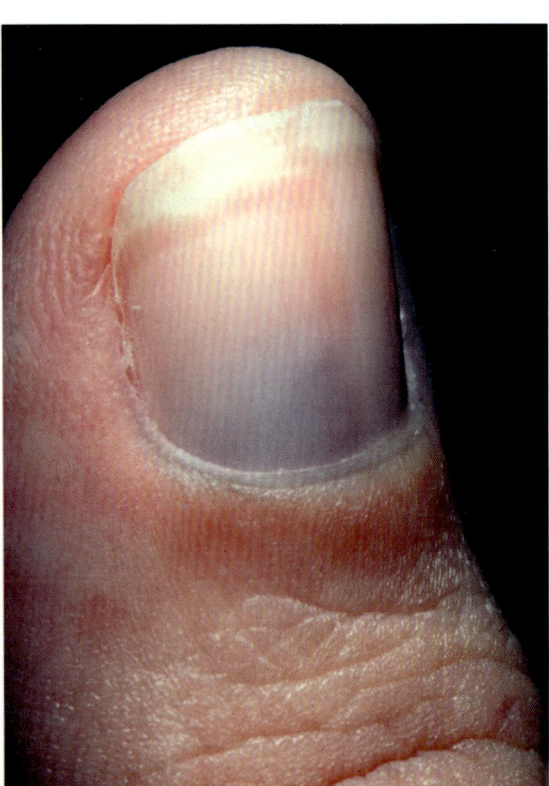

FIGURE 37.15 Subungual glomus tumor. *(Courtesy of University of Washington Dermatology Division.)*

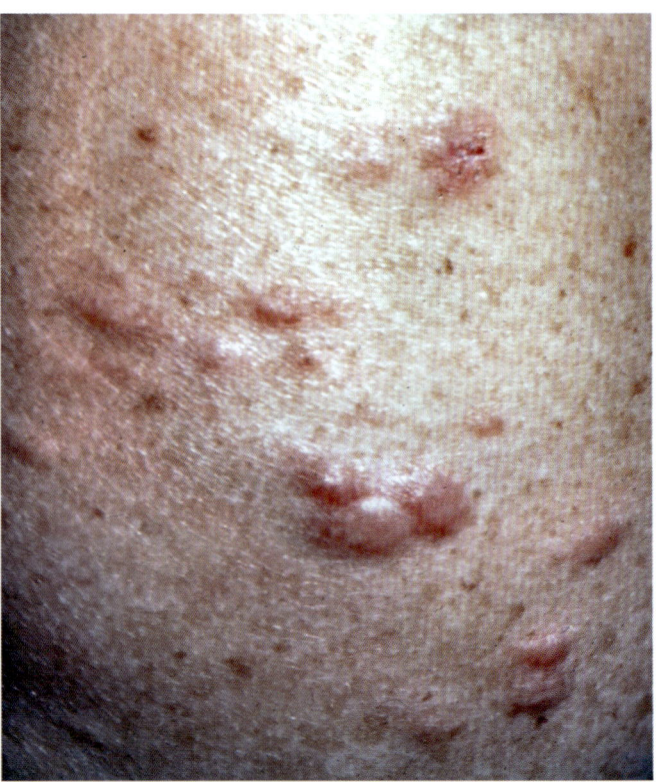

FIGURE 37.16 Leiomyomas. *(Courtesy of University of Washington Dermatology Division.)*

TABLE 37.2 Characteristic Features of Benign Painful Cutaneous Neoplasms

Tumor	Appearance	Usual Location	Pathologic Features	Comment
Angiolipoma[237,238]	Subcutaneous 0.5- to 4.0-cm nodule with normal, bluish or reddish overlying skin	Typically located on the forearm	Encapsulated tumor with mature adipocytes, many small-caliber blood vessels and microthrombi	Frequently painful with pressure or when moved
Angioleiomyoma[239,240]	Subcutaneous or deep dermal nodule or mass up to 4 cm in diameter	Lower extremities	Encapsulated tumor with interlacing bundles of smooth muscle cells and many small blood vessels	Pain or tenderness with pressure Some leiomyomas are associated with a hereditary syndrome with renal cancer.
Neurilemmoma (schwannoma)[241]	2- to 4-cm diameter flesh-colored tumor	Head and extremities (especially flexor) attached to a cranial or peripheral nerve	Intraneural proliferation of Schwann cells with Antoni type A or Antoni type B pattern	Pain may be localized or radiate along the course of the nerve.
Glomus tumor[242,243]	Reddish-blue papule or nodule usually <1 cm in diameter	Hands and fingers, especially subungually	Glomus cells with eosinophilic cytoplasm and round nuclei, blood vessels, and nerve fibers	Paroxysms of pain on exposure to cold or pressure; multiple glomus tumors (familial glomangiomas) are usually asymptomatic.
Eccrine spiradenoma[244,245]	0.3–5.0 cm firm intradermal nodule often with bluish overlying skin	Most often on ventral surface of the skin	Two populations of epithelial cells with eccrine differentiation; fibrous capsule and ductal differentiation often present	Usually tender or painful
Leiomyoma[240,246]	Firm erythematous to brown intradermal papules and nodules	Trunk and extremities	Interlacing bundles of smooth muscle cells with cigar-shaped nuclei	Pain on exposure to cold, pressure, trauma, emotion, or may occur spontaneously; may be associated with a hereditary syndrome with renal cell cancer

Modified from Langlois JC, Olerud JE. Pain of dermatologic disorders. In: Loeser JD, Butler SH, Chapman CR, et al, eds. *Bonica's Management of Pain.* 3rd ed. Philadelphia: Lippincott Williams & Wilkins; 2001:581.

ACKNOWLEDGMENTS

The authors wish to acknowledge the contributions of Dr. George F. Odland to this chapter. He was the original primary author, and many of his touches and words remain part of the fabric of the chapter.

References

1. Lim HW, Collins SA, Resneck JS Jr, et al. The burden of skin disease in the United States. *J Am Acad Dermatol* 2017;76:958.e2–972.e2.
2. Verhoeven EW, Kraaimaat FW, van de Kerkhof PC, et al. Prevalence of physical symptoms of itch, pain and fatigue in patients with skin diseases in general practice. *Br J Dermatol* 2007;156:1346–1349.
3. Wolff K, Goldsmith LA, Katz SI, et al. *Fitzpatrick's Dermatology in General Medicine.* 7th ed. New York: McGraw-Hill; 2008.
4. Kasper DL, Braunwald E, Fauci AS, eds. *Harrison's Principles of Internal Medicine.* 17th ed. New York: McGraw-Hill; 2008.
5. Braverman IM, ed. *Skin Signs of Systemic Disease.* 3rd ed. Philadelphia: WB Saunders; 1998.
6. Burns T, Breathnach S, Cox N, et al. *Rook's Textbook of Dermatology.* Vol 4. 7th ed. London: Blackwell Science; 2004.
7. Pasparakis M, Haase I, Nestle FO. Mechanisms regulating skin immunity and inflammation. *Nat Rev Immunol* 2014;14:289–301.
8. Steinhoff M, Luger TA. Neurobiology of the skin. In: Wolff K, Goldsmith LA, Katz SI, eds. *Fitzpatrick's Dermatology in General Medicine.* 7th ed. New York: McGraw-Hill; 2008:895–901.
9. Hilliges M, Wang L, Johansson O. Ultrastructural evidence for nerve fibers within all vital layers of the human epidermis. *J Invest Dermatol* 1995;104:134–137.
10. Reilly DM, Ferdinando D, Johnston C, et al. The epidermal nerve fibre network: characterization of nerve fibres in human skin by confocal microscopy and assessment of racial variations. *Br J Dermatol* 1997;137:163–170.
11. Ansel JC, Kaynard AH, Armstrong CA, et al. Skin-nervous system interactions. *J Invest Dermatol* 1996;106:198–204.
12. Garibyan L, Rheingold CG, Lerner EA. Understanding the pathophysiology of itch. *Dermatol Ther* 2013;26:84–91.
13. Yosipovitch G, Samuel LS. Neuropathic and psychogenic itch. *Dermatol Ther* 2008;21:32–41.
14. Ständer S, Steinhoff M, Schmelz M, et al. Neurophysiology of pruritus: cutaneous elicitation of itch. *Arch Dermatol* 2003;139:1463–1470.
15. Otsuka M, Yoshioka K. Neurotransmitter functions of mammalian tachykinins. *Physiol Rev* 1993;73:229–308.
16. Baral P, Mills K, Pinho-Ribeiro FA, et al. Pain and itch: beneficial or harmful to antimicrobial defense? *Cell Host Microbe* 2016;19:755–759.
17. Russell JP, Gibson LE. Primary cutaneous small vessel vasculitis: approach to diagnosis and treatment. *Int J Dermatol* 2006;45:3–13.
18. Langford CA. 15. Vasculitis. *J Allergy Clin Immunol* 2003;111:S602–S612.
19. Gibson LE. Cutaneous vasculitis update. *Dermatol Clin* 2001;19:603–615, vii.
20. Lotti T, Ghersetich I, Comacchi C, et al. Cutaneous small-vessel vasculitis. *J Am Acad Dermatol* 1998;39:667–687.
21. Braverman IM, ed. The angiitides. In: *Skin Signs of Systemic Disease.* 3rd ed. Philadelphia: WB Saunders; 1998:278–334.
22. Sais G, Vidaller A, Jucgla A, et al. Prognostic factors in leukocytoclastic vasculitis: a clinicopathologic study of 160 patients. *Arch Dermatol* 1998;134:309–315.
23. Carlson JA, Ng BT, Chen KR. Cutaneous vasculitis update: diagnostic criteria, classification, epidemiology, etiology, pathogenesis, evaluation and prognosis. *Am J Dermatopathol* 2005;27:504–528.
24. Goeser MR, Laniosz V, Wetter DA. A practical approach to the diagnosis, evaluation, and management of cutaneous small-vessel vasculitis. *Am J Clin Dermatol* 2014;15:299–306.
25. Jennette JC, Falk RJ, Bacon PA, et al. 2012 revised International Chapel Hill Consensus Conference Nomenclature of Vasculitides. *Arthritis Rheum* 2013;65:1–11.
26. Ferri C, La Civita L, Longombardo G, et al. Mixed cryoglobulinaemia: a cross-road between autoimmune and lymphoproliferative disorders. *Lupus* 1998;7:275–279.
27. Fiorentino DF. Cutaneous vasculitis. *J Am Acad Dermatol* 2003;48: 311–340.
28. Loricera J, Blanco R, Ortiz-Sanjuan F, et al. Single-organ cutaneous small-vessel vasculitis according to the 2012 revised International Chapel Hill Consensus Conference Nomenclature of Vasculitides: a study of 60 patients from a series of 766 cutaneous vasculitis cases. *Rheumatology (Oxford)* 2015;54:77–82.
29. Diaz-Perez JL, Winkelmann RK. Cutaneous periarteritis nodosa. *Arch Dermatol* 1974;110:407–414.
30. Daoud MS, Hutton KP, Gibson LE. Cutaneous periarteritis nodosa: a clinicopathological study of 79 cases. *Br J Dermatol* 1997;136:706–713.
31. Pak H, Montemarano AD, Berger T. Purpuric nodules and macules on the extremities of a young woman. Cutaneous polyarteritis nodosa. *Arch Dermatol* 1998;134:231–232, 234–235.
32. Lhote F, Cohen P, Guillevin L. Polyarteritis nodosa, microscopic polyangiitis and Churg-Strauss syndrome. *Lupus* 1998;7:238–258.
33. Cohen RD, Conn DL, Ilstrup DM. Clinical features, prognosis, and response to treatment in polyarteritis. *Mayo Clinic Proc* 1980;55:146–155.

34. Caorsi R, Penco F, Schena F, et al. Monogenic polyarteritis: the lesson of ADA2 deficiency. *Pediatr Rheumatol Online J* 2016;14:51.

35. De Virgilio A, Greco A, Magliulo G, et al. Polyarteritis nodosa: a contemporary overview. *Autoimmun Rev* 2016;15:564–570.

36. Jennette JC, Falk RJ. Small-vessel vasculitis. *N Engl J Med* 1997;337: 1512–1523.

37. Hoffman GS, Kerr GS, Leavitt RY, et al. Wegener granulomatosis: an analysis of 158 patients. *Ann Intern Med* 1992;116:488–498.

38. Francès C, Du LT, Piette JC, et al. Wegener's granulomatosis. Dermatological manifestations in 75 cases with clinicopathologic correlation. *Arch Dermatol* 1994;130:861–867.

39. Piette W. Primary systemic vasculitis. In: Sontheimer RD, Provost TT, eds. *Cutaneous Manifestations of Rheumatic Diseases*. 2nd ed. Philadelphia: Lippincott Williams & Wilkins; 2004:184–187.

40. Hu CH, O'Loughlin S, Winkelmann RK. Cutaneous manifestations of Wegener granulomatosis. *Arch Dermatol* 1977;113:175–182.

41. Patten SF, Tomecki KJ. Wegener's granulomatosis: cutaneous and oral mucosal disease. *J Am Acad Dermatol* 1993;28:710–718.

42. Manchanda Y, Tejasvi T, Handa R, et al. Strawberry gingiva: a distinctive sign in Wegener's granulomatosis. *J Am Acad Dermatol* 2003;49:335–337.

43. Knight JM, Hayduk MJ, Summerlin DJ, et al. "Strawberry" gingival hyperplasia: a pathognomonic mucocutaneous finding in Wegener granulomatosis. *Arch Dermatol* 2000;136:171–173.

44. Carlson JA, Chen KR. Cutaneous vasculitis update: small vessel neutrophilic vasculitis syndromes. *Am J Dermatopathol* 2006;28:486–506.

45. Pagnoux C. Updates in ANCA-associated vasculitis. *Eur J Rheumatol* 2016;3:122–133.

46. Jennette JC, Falk RJ, Andrassy K, et al. Nomenclature of systemic vasculitides. Proposal of an international consensus conference. *Arthritis Rheum* 1994;37:187–192.

47. Kallenberg CG. Antineutrophil cytoplasmic autoantibody-associated small-vessel vasculitis. *Curr Opin Rheumatol* 2007;19:17–24.

48. Peñas PF, Porras JI, Fraga J, et al. Microscopic polyangiitis. A systemic vasculitis with a positive P-ANCA. *Br J Dermatol* 1996;134:542–547.

49. Irvine AD, Bruce IN, Walsh M, et al. Dermatological presentation of disease associated with antineutrophil cytoplasmic antibodies: a report of two contrasting cases and a review of the literature. *Br J Dermatol* 1996;134: 924–928.

50. Irvine AD, Bruce IN, Walsh MY, et al. Microscopic polyangiitis. Delineation of a cutaneous-limited variant associated with antimyeloperoxidase autoantibody. *Arch Dermatol* 1997;133:474–477.

51. Guillevin L, Durand-Gasselin B, Cevallos R, et al. Microscopic polyangiitis: clinical and laboratory findings in eighty-five patients. *Arthritis Rheum* 1999;42:421–430.

52. Lauque D, Cadranel J, Lazor R, et al. Microscopic polyangiitis with alveolar hemorrhage. A study of 29 cases and review of the literature. *Medicine* 2000;79:222–233.

53. Peco-Antic A, Bonaci-Nikolic B, Basta-Jovanovic G, et al. Childhood microscopic polyangiitis associated with MPO-ANCA. *Pediatr Nephrol* 2006;21:46–53.

54. Guillevin L, Cohen P, Gayraud M, et al. Churg-Strauss syndrome. Clinical study and long-term follow-up of 96 patients. *Medicine* 1999;78:26–37.

55. Davis MD, Daoud MS, McEvoy MT, et al. Cutaneous manifestations of Churg-Strauss syndrome: a clinicopathologic correlation. *J Am Acad Dermatol* 1997;37:199–203.

56. Ferenczi K, Chang T, Camouse M, et al. A case of Churg-Strauss syndrome associated with antiphospholipid antibodies. *J Am Acad Dermatol* 2007;56:701–704.

57. Watson KM, Salisbury JR, Creamer D. Purpura fulminans—a novel presentation of Churg Strauss syndrome. *Clin Exp Dermatol* 2004;29:390–392.

58. Crotty CP, DeRemee RA, Winkelmann RK. Cutaneous clinicopathologic correlation of allergic granulomatosis. *J Am Acad Dermatol* 1981;5: 571–581.

59. Scott DG, Bacon PA, Tribe CR. Systemic rheumatoid vasculitis: a clinical and laboratory study of 50 cases. *Medicine* 1981;60:288–297.

60. Lipsky PE. Rheumatoid arthritis. In: Fauci AS, Kasper DL, Longo DL, et al, eds. *Harrison's Principles of Internal Medicine*. New York: McGraw-Hill; 2005:1968–1977.

61. Genta MS, Genta RM, Gabay C. Systemic rheumatoid vasculitis: a review. *Semin Arthritis Rheum* 2006;36:88–98.

62. Scott DG, Bacon PA. Intravenous cyclophosphamide plus methylprednisolone in treatment of systemic rheumatoid vasculitis. *Am J Med* 1984;76: 377–384.

63. Chen KR, Toyohara A, Suzuki A, et al. Clinical and histopathological spectrum of cutaneous vasculitis in rheumatoid arthritis. *Br J Dermatol* 2002;147:905–913.

64. Magro CM, Crowson AN. The spectrum of cutaneous lesions in rheumatoid arthritis: a clinical and pathological study of 43 patients. *J Cutan Pathol* 2003;30:1–10.

65. Xue Y, Cohen JM, Wright NA, et al. Skin signs of rheumatoid arthritis and its therapy-induced cutaneous side effects. *Am J Clin Dermatol* 2016;17:147–162.

66. Watts RA, Scott DG. Vasculitis and inflammatory arthritis. *Best Pract Res Clin Rheumatol* 2016;30:916–931.

67. Alavi A, Hafner J, Dutz JP, et al. Livedoid vasculopathy: an in-depth analysis using a modified Delphi approach. *J Am Acad Dermatol* 2013;69: 1033e1–1042e1.

68. Hairston BR, Davis MD, Pittelkow MR, et al. Livedoid vasculopathy: further evidence for procoagulant pathogenesis. *Arch Dermatol* 2006;142: 1413–1418.

69. Callen JP. Livedoid vasculopathy: what it is and how the patient should be evaluated and treated. *Arch Dermatol* 2006;142:1481–1482.

70. Levine JS, Branch DW, Rauch J. The antiphospholipid syndrome. *N Engl J Med* 2002;346:752–763.

71. Francès C, Niang S, Laffitte E, et al. Dermatologic manifestations of the antiphospholipid syndrome: two hundred consecutive cases. *Arthritis Rheum* 2005;52:1785–1793.

72. Kriseman YL, Nash JW, Hsu S. Criteria for the diagnosis of antiphospholipid syndrome in patients presenting with dermatologic symptoms. *J Am Acad Dermatol* 2007;57:112–115.

73. Asherson RA, Cervera R. Antiphospholipid syndrome. *J Invest Dermatol* 1993;100:21S–27S.

74. Gibson GE, Su WP, Pittelkow MR. Antiphospholipid syndrome and the skin. *J Am Acad Dermatol* 1997;36:970–982.

75. Arachchillage DR, Laffan M. Pathogenesis and management of antiphospholipid syndrome. *Br J Haematol* 2017;178:181–195.

76. Lim W, Crowther MA, Eikelboom JW. Management of antiphospholipid antibody syndrome: a systematic review. *JAMA* 2006;295:1050–1057.

77. Ruiz-Irastorza G, Khamashta MA. The treatment of antiphospholipid syndrome: a harmonic contrast. *Best Pract Res Clin Rheumatol* 2007;21: 1079–1092.

78. Rodriguez-Pintó I, Espinosa G, Cervera R. Catastrophic antiphospholipid syndrome: the current management approach. *Best Pract Res Clin Rheumatol* 2016;30:239–249.

79. Koch-Weser J. Coumarin necrosis. *Ann Intern Med* 1968;68:1365–1367.

80. Bauer KA. Coumarin-induced skin necrosis [editorial]. *Arch Dermatol* 1993;129:766–768.

81. Chan YC, Valenti D, Mansfield AO, et al. Warfarin induced skin necrosis. *Br J Surg* 2000;87:266–272.

82. Weiss P, Soff GA, Halkin H, et al. Decline of proteins C and S and factors II, VII, IX and X during the initiation of warfarin therapy. *Thromb Res* 1987;45:783–790.

83. Jillella AP, Lutcher CL. Reinstituting warfarin in patients who develop warfarin skin necrosis. *Am J Hematol* 1996;52:117–119.

84. Cole MS, Minifee PK, Wolma FJ. Coumarin necrosis—a review of the literature. *Surgery* 1988;103:271–277.

85. Essex DW, Wynn SS, Jin DK. Late-onset warfarin-induced skin necrosis: case report and review of the literature. *Am J Hematol* 1998;57:233–237.

86. DeFranzo AJ, Marasco P, Argenta LC. Warfarin-induced necrosis of the skin. *Ann Plast Surg* 1995;34:203–208.

87. Nazarian RM, Van Cott EM, Zembowicz A, et al. Warfarin-induced skin necrosis. *J Am Acad Dermatol* 2009;61:325–332.

88. Chung C, Tumeh PC, Birnbaum R, et al. Characteristic purpura of the ears, vasculitis, and neutropenia—a potential public health epidemic associated with levamisole-adulterated cocaine. *J Am Acad Dermatol* 2011;65: 722–725.

89. Hennings C, Miller J. Illicit drugs: what dermatologists need to know. *J Am Acad Dermatol* 2013;69:135–142.

90. Fujimoto M, Watanabe R, Ishitsuka Y, et al. Recent advances in dermatomyositis-specific autoantibodies. *Curr Opin Rheumatol* 2016;28: 636–644.

91. Valenzuela A, Chung L. Calcinosis: pathophysiology and management. *Curr Opin Rheumatol* 2015;27:542–548.

92. Khafif RA, DeLima C, Silverberg A, et al. Calciphylaxis and systemic calcinosis. Collective review. *Arch Intern Med* 1990;150:956–959.

93. Oh DH, Eulau D, Tokugawa DA, et al. Five cases of calciphylaxis and a review of the literature. *J Am Acad Dermatol* 1999;40:979–987.

94. Guldbakke KK, Khachemoune A. Calciphylaxis. *Int J Dermatol* 2007;46: 231–238.

95. Angelis M, Wong LL, Myers SA, et al. Calciphylaxis in patients on hemodialysis: a prevalence study. *Surgery* 1997;122:1083–1090.

96. Budisavljevic MN, Cheek D, Ploth DW. Calciphylaxis in chronic renal failure. *J Am Soc Nephrol* 1996;7:978–982.

97. Wilmer WA, Magro CM. Calciphylaxis: emerging concepts in prevention, diagnosis, and treatment. *Semin Dial* 2002;15:172–186.

98. Nigwekar SU, Kroshinsky D, Nazarian RM, et al. Calciphylaxis: risk factors, diagnosis, and treatment. *Am J Kidney Dis* 2015;66:133–146.

99. Ivker RA, Woosley J, Briggaman RA. Calciphylaxis in three patients with end-stage renal disease. *Arch Dermatol* 1995;131:63–68.

100. Hafner J, Keusch G, Wahl C, et al. Uremic small-artery disease with medial calcification and intimal hyperplasia (so-called calciphylaxis): a complication of chronic renal failure and benefit from parathyroidectomy. *J Am Acad Dermatol* 1995;33:954–962.

101. Halasz CL, Munger DP, Frimmer H, et al. Calciphylaxis: comparison of radiologic imaging and histopathology. *J Am Acad Dermatol* 2017;77: 241.e3–246.e3.

102. Yu WY, Bhutani T, Kornik R, et al. Warfarin-associated nonuremic calciphylaxis. *JAMA Dermatol* 2017;153:309–314.

103. Bazari H, Jaff MR, Mannstadt M, et al. Case records of the Massachusetts General Hospital. Case7-2007: a 59-year-old woman with diabetic renal disease and nonhealing skin ulcers. *N Engl J Med* 2007:1049–1057.

104. Ongenae KC, Phillips TJ. Leg ulcers and wound healing. In: Arndt KA, LeBoit PE, Robinson JK, et al, eds. *Cutaneous Medicine and Surgery: An Integrated Program in Dermatology.* Philadelphia: WB Saunders; 1996:558–573.

105. Miller OF III, Phillips TJ. Leg ulcers [bibliography]. *J Am Acad Dermatol* 2000;43:91–95.

106. Grey JE, Harding KG, Enoch S. Venous and arterial leg ulcers. *BMJ* 2006;332:347–350.

107. Ross R. Atherosclerosis—an inflammatory disease. *N Engl J Med* 1999; 340:115–126.

108. Creager MA, Dzau VJ. Vascular diseases of the extremities. In: Fauci AS, Kasper DL, Longo DL, et al, eds. *Harrison's Principles of Internal Medicine.* 16th ed. New York: McGraw-Hill; 2005:1486–1494.

109. Phillips TJ, Dover JS. Leg ulcers. *J Am Acad Dermatol* 1991;25:965–987.

110. Valencia IC, Falabella A, Kirsner RS, et al. Chronic venous insufficiency and venous leg ulceration. *J Am Acad Dermatol* 2001;44:401–424.

111. Fonder MA, Lazarus GS, Cowan DA, et al. Treating the chronic wound: a practical approach to the care of nonhealing wounds and wound care dressings. *J Am Acad Dermatol* 2008;58:185–206.

112. Braswell SF, Kostopoulos TC, Ortega-Loayza AG. Pathophysiology of pyoderma gangrenosum (PG): an updated review. *J Am Acad Dermatol* 2015;73:691–698.

113. Marzano AV, Borghi A, Meroni PL, et al. Pyoderma gangrenosum and its syndromic forms: evidence for a link with autoinflammation. *Br J Dermatol* 2016;175:882–891.

114. Alavi A, French LE, Davis MD, et al. Pyoderma gangrenosum: an update on pathophysiology, diagnosis and treatment. *Am J Clin Dermatol* 2017;18:355–372.

115. Hakkarainen TW, Kopari NM, Pham TN, et al. Necrotizing soft tissue infections: review and current concepts in treatment, systems of care, and outcomes. *Curr Probl Surg* 2014;51:344–362.

116. Burnham JP, Kirby JP, Kollef MH. Diagnosis and management of skin and soft tissue infections in the intensive care unit: a review. *Intensive Care Med* 2016;42:1899–1911.

117. Stevens DL, Bisno AL, Chambers HF, et al. Practice guidelines for the diagnosis and management of skin and soft tissue infections: 2014 update by the Infectious Diseases Society of America. *Clin Infect Dis* 2014;59: e10–e52.

118. Dworkin RH, Johnson RW, Breuer J, et al. Recommendations for the management of herpes zoster. *Clin Infect Dis* 2007;44(suppl 1):S1–S26.

119. James WD, Berger TG, Elston DM. Zoster (shingles, herpes zoster). In: James WD, Berger TG, Elston DM, eds. *Andrew's Diseases of the Skin Clinical Dermatology.* 10th ed. Philadelphia: Saunders Elsevier; 2006: 379–384.

120. Corey L. Herpes simplex viruses. In: Fauci AS, Kasper DL, Longo DL, et al, eds. *Harrison's Principles of Internal Medicine.* 16th ed. New York: McGraw-Hill; 2005:1035–1042.

121. James WD, Berger TG, Elston DM. Herpes simplex. In: James WD, Berger TG, Elston DM, eds. *Andrew's Diseases of the Skin Clinical Dermatology.* 10th ed. Philadelphia: Saunders Elsevier; 2006:367–376.

122. Paller AS, Mancini AJ. Herpes simplex viral infection. In: Paller AS, Mancini AJ, eds. *Hurwitz Clinical Pediatric Dermatology.* 3rd ed. Philadelphia: Elsevier Saunders; 2006:397–402.

123. Centers for Disease Control and Prevention, Workowski KA, Berman SM. Sexually transmitted diseases treatment guidelines, 2006. *MMWR Recomm Rep* 2006;55:1–94.

124. Weston WL, Brice SL. Atypical forms of herpes simplex-associated erythema multiforme. *J Am Acad Dermatol* 1998;39:124–126.

125. Patwardhan V, Bhalla P, Rawat D, et al. A comparative analysis of polymerase chain reaction and direct fluorescent antibody test for diagnosis of genital herpes. *J Lab Physicians* 2017;9:53–56.

126. Bisno AL, Stevens DL. Streptococcal infections of skin and soft tissues. *N Engl J Med* 1996;334:240–245.

127. Guberman D, Gilead LT, Zlotogorski A, et al. Bullous erysipelas: a retrospective study of 26 patients. *J Am Acad Dermatol* 1999;41:733–737.

128. Weinberg AN, Swartz MN, Tsao H. Soft tissue infections: erysipelas, cellulitis, gangrenous cellulitis, and myonecrosis. In: Freedberg IM, Eisen AZ, Wolff K, et al, eds. *Fitzpatrick's Dermatology in General Medicine.* 6th ed. New York: McGraw-Hill; 2003:1883–1895.

129. Swartz MN. Clinical practice. Cellulitis. *N Engl J Med* 2004;350:904–912.

130. Lee PK, Zipoli MT, Weinberg AN, et al. Pyodermas: staphylococcus aureus, streptococcus and other gram positive bacteria. In: Freedberg IM, Eisen AZ, Wolff K, et al, eds. *Fitzpatrick's Dermatology in General Medicine.* 6th ed. New York: McGraw-Hill; 2003:1856–1878.

131. O'Malley GF, Dominici P, Giraldo P, et al. Routine packing of simple cutaneous abscesses is painful and probably unnecessary. *Acad Emerg Med* 2009;16:470–473.

132. Fritz SA, Camins BC, Eisenstein KA, et al. Effectiveness of measures to eradicate *Staphylococcus aureus* carriage in patients with community-associated skin and soft-tissue infections: a randomized trial. *Infect Control Hosp Epidemiol* 2011;32:872–880.

133. Steinsapir KD, Woodward JA. Chlorhexidine keratitis: safety of chlorhexidine as a facial antiseptic. *Dermatol Surg* 2017;43:1–6.

134. Daum RS. Clinical practice. Skin and soft-tissue infections caused by methicillin-resistant *Staphylococcus aureus. N Engl J Med* 2007;357:380–390.

135. Gorwitz RJ, Jernigan DB, Powers JH, et al. *Strategies for Clinical Management of MRSA in the Community: Summary of an Experts' Meeting Convened by the Centers for Disease Control and Prevention.* Atlanta, GA: Centers for Disease Control and Prevention; 2006.

136. Swartz MN, Weinberg AN. Miscellaneous bacterial infections with cutaneous manifestations. In: Freedberg IM, Eisen AZ, Wolff K, et al, eds. *Fitzpatrick's Dermatology in General Medicine.* 6th ed. New York: McGraw-Hill; 2003:1918–1932.

137. Varella TC, Nico MM. Erysipeloid. *Int J Dermatol* 2005;44:497–498.

138. Requena L, Yus ES. Panniculitis. Part I. Mostly septal panniculitis. *J Am Acad Dermatol* 2001;45:163–186.

139. Schwartz RA, Nervi SJ. Erythema nodosum: a sign of systemic disease. *Am Fam Physician* 2007;75:695–700.

140. Cribier B, Caille A, Heid E, et al. Erythema nodosum and associated diseases. A study of 129 cases. *Int J Dermatol* 1998;37:667–672.

141. Psychos DN, Voulgari PV, Skopouli FN, et al. Erythema nodosum: the underlying conditions. *Clin Rheumatol* 2000;19:212–216.

142. Kakourou T, Drosatou P, Psychou F, et al. Erythema nodosum in children: a prospective study. *J Am Acad Dermatol* 2001;44:17–21.

143. Johnson JA, Yu SS, Elist M, et al. Rheumatologic manifestations of the "MonoMAC" syndrome. A systematic review. *Clin Rheumatol* 2015;34: 1643–1645.

144. McNutt NS, Moreno A, Contreras F. Inflammatory diseases of the subcutaneous fat. In: Elder DE, Elenitsas R, Johnson BL, et al, eds. *Lever's Histopathology of the Skin.* 9th ed. Philadelphia: Lippincott Williams & Wilkins; 2005:533–534.

145. Sterling JB, Heymann WR. Potassium iodide in dermatology: a 19th century drug for the 21st century-uses, pharmacology, adverse effects, and contraindications. *J Am Acad Dermatol* 2000;43:691–697.

146. Hansson E, Svensson H, Brorson H. Review of Dercum's disease and proposal of diagnostic criteria, diagnostic methods, classification and management. *Orphanet J Rare Dis* 2012;7:23.

147. Campen RB, Sang CN, Duncan LM. Case Records of the Massachusetts General Hospital. Case 25-2006. A 41-year old woman with painful subcutaneous nodules. *N Engl J Med;* 2006;355:714–722.

148. Held JL, Andrew JA, Kohn SR. Surgical amelioration of Dercum's disease: a report and review. *J Dermatol Surg Oncol* 1989;15:1294–1296.

149. DeFranzo AJ, Hall JH Jr, Herring SM. Adiposis dolorosa (Dercum's disease): liposuction as an effective form of treatment. *Plast Reconstr Surg* 1990;85:289–292.

150. De Silva M, Earley MJ. Liposuction in the treatment of juxta-articular adiposis dolorosa. *Ann Rheum Dis* 1990;49:403–404.

151. Iwane T, Maruyama M, Matsuki M, et al. Management of intractable pain in adiposis dolorosa with intravenous administration of lidocaine. *Anesth Analg* 1976;55:257–259.

152. Bonatus TJ, Alexander AH. Dercum's disease (adiposis dolorosa). A case report and review of the literature. *Clin Orthop Relat Res* 1986;(205):251–253.

153. Devillers AC, Oranje AP. Treatment of pain in adiposis dolorosa (Dercum's disease) with intravenous lidocaine: a case report with a 10-year follow-up. *Clin Exp Dermatol* 1999;24:240–241.

154. Greenbaum SS, Varga J. Corticosteroid-induced juxta-articular adiposis dolorosa. *Arch Dermatol* 1991;127:231–233.

155. Palmer ED. Dercum's disease: adiposis dolorosa. *Am Fam Physician* 1981;24:155–157.

156. Garg A, Lavian J, Lin G, et al. Incidence of hidradenitis suppurativa in the United States: a sex- and age-adjusted population analysis. *J Am Acad Dermatol* 2017;77:118–122.

157. Woodruff CM, Charlie AM, Leslie KS. Hidradenitis suppurativa: a guide for the practicing physician. *Mayo Clinic Proc* 2015;90:1679–1693.

158. Ring HC, Emtestam L. The microbiology of hidradenitis suppurativa. *Dermatol Clin* 2016;34:29–35.

159. Wolkenstein P, Loundou A, Barrau K, et al. Quality of life impairment in hidradenitis suppurativa: a study of 61 cases. *J Am Acad Dermatol* 2007;56:621–623.

160. James WD, Berger TG, Elston DM. Hidradenitis suppurativa (acne inverse). In: James WD, Berger TG, Elston DM, eds. *Andrew's Diseases of the Skin Clinical Dermatology.* 10th ed. Philadelphia: Saunders Elsevier; 2006:243–244.

161. FDA Drug Safety Communication: FDA warns about rare but serious allergic reactions with the skin antiseptic chlorhexidine gluconate. Available at: https://www.fda.gov/Drugs/DrugSafety/ucm530975.htm. Accessed April 25, 2017.

162. Alhusayen R, Shear NH. Scientific evidence for the use of current traditional systemic therapies in patients with hidradenitis suppurativa. *J Am Acad Dermatol* 2015;73:S42–S46.

163. Ingram JR, Woo PN, Chua SL, et al. Interventions for hidradenitis suppurativa: a Cochrane systematic review incorporating GRADE assessment of evidence quality. *Br J Dermatol* 2016;174:970–978.

164. Janse I, Bieniek A, Horvath B, et al. Surgical procedures in hidradenitis suppurativa. *Dermatol Clin* 2016;34:97–109.

165. Danby FW, Hazen PG, Boer J. New and traditional surgical approaches to hidradenitis suppurativa. *J Am Acad Dermatol* 2015;73:S62–S65.

166. Saunte DM, Lapins J. Lasers and intense pulsed light hidradenitis suppurativa. *Dermatol Clin* 2016;34:111–119.

167. Horvath B, Janse IC, Sibbald GR. Pain management in patients with hidradenitis suppurativa. *J Am Acad Dermatol* 2015;73:S47–S51.

168. Paller AS, Mancini AJ. Epidermal cyst. In: Paller AS, Mancini AJ, eds. *Hurwitz Clinical Pediatric Dermatology*. 3rd ed. Philadelphia: Elsevier Saunders; 2006:236.

169. James WD, Berger TG, Elston DM. Epidermal cyst (epidermal inclusion cyst, infundibular cyst). In: James WD, Berger TG, Elston DM, eds. *Andrew's Diseases of the Skin Clinical Dermatology*. 10th ed. Philadelphia: Saunders Elsevier; 2006:676–677.

170. James WD, Berger TG, Elston DM. Lipomas. In: James WD, Berger TG, Elston DM, eds. *Andrew's Diseases of the Skin Clinical Dermatology*. 10th ed. Philadelphia: Saunders Elsevier; 2006:624.

171. Bastuji-Garin S, Fouchard N, Bertocchi M, et al. SCORTEN: a severity-of-illness score for toxic epidermal necrolysis. *J Invest Dermatol* 2000;115:149–153.

172. Heng YK, Lee HY, Roujeau JC. Epidermal necrolysis: 60 years of errors and advances. *Br J Dermatol* 2015;173:1250–1254.

173. Lee HY, Walsh SA, Creamer D. Long-term complications of Stevens-Johnson syndrome / Toxic epidermal necrolysis: the spectrum of chronic problems in patients who survive an episode of SJS/TEN necessitates multi-disciplinary follow up. *Br J Dermatol* 2017;177:924–935.

174. James WD, Berger TG, Elston DM. Pemphigus vulgaris. In: James WD, Berger TG, Elston DM, eds. *Andrew's Diseases of the Skin Clinical Dermatology*. 10th ed. Philadelphia: Saunders Elsevier; 2006:459–463.

175. Stanley JR, Amagai M. Pemphigus, bullous impetigo, and the staphylococcal scalded-skin syndrome. *N Engl J Med* 2006;355:1800–1810.

176. Mutasim DF, Pelc NJ, Anhalt GJ. Drug-induced pemphigus. *Dematol Clin* 1993;11:463–471.

177. Abidi NY, Lainiotis I, Malikowski G, et al. Longitudinal tracking of autoantibody levels in a pemphigus vulgaris patient: support for a role of anti-desmoglein 1 autoantibodies as predictors of disease progression. *J Drugs Dermatol* 2017;16:135–139.

178. Joly P, Maho-Vaillant M, Prost-Squarcioni C, et al. First-line rituximab combined with short-term prednisone versus prednisone alone for the treatment of pemphigus (Ritux 3): a prospective, multicentre, parallel-group, open-label randomised trial. *Lancet* 2017;389:2031–2040.

179. Kim TH, Choi Y, Lee SE, et al. Adjuvant rituximab treatment for pemphigus: a retrospective study of 45 patients at a single center with long-term follow up. *J Dermatol* 2017;44:615–620.

180. Anhalt GJ. Paraneoplastic pemphigus. In: James WD, Cockerell CJ, Dzubow LM, eds. *Advances in Dermatology*. St. Louis, MO: Mosby; 1997:77–96.

181. Huang Y, Li J, Zhu X. Detection of anti-envoplakin and anti-periplakin autoantibodies by ELISA in patients with paraneoplastic pemphigus. *Arch Dermatol Res* 2009;301:703–709.

182. Kartan S, Shi VY, Clark AK, et al. Paraneoplastic pemphigus and autoimmune blistering diseases associated with neoplasm: characteristics, diagnosis, associated neoplasms, proposed pathogenesis, treatment. *Am J Clin Dermatol* 2017;18:105–126.

183. Leger S, Picard D, Ingen-Housz-Oro S, et al. Prognostic factors of paraneoplastic pemphigus. *Arch Dermatol* 2012;148:1165–1172.

184. Stern RS. Bullous pemphigoid therapy—think globally, act locally [editorial]. *N Engl J Med* 2002;346:364–367.

185. Bernard P, Antonicelli F. Bullous pemphigoid: a review of its diagnosis, associations and treatment. *Am J Clin Dermatol* 2017;18:513–528.

186. Joly P, Roujeau JC, Benichou J, et al. A comparison of oral and topical corticosteroids in patients with bullous pemphigoid. *N Engl J Med* 2002;346:321–327.

187. Fine JD. Epidermolysis bullosa. In: Arndt KA, LeBoit PE, Robinson JK, et al, eds. *Cutaneous Medicine and Surgery: An Integrated Program in Dermatology*. Philadelphia: WB Saunders; 1996:635–650.

188. Lapiere JC, Chan LS, Woodley DT. Epidermolysis bullosa acquisita. In: Arndt KA, LeBoit PE, Robinson JK, et al, eds. *Cutaneous Medicine and Surgery: An Integrated Program in Dermatology*. Philadelphia: WB Saunders; 1996:685–690.

189. Woodley DT, Chen M. Epidermolysis bullosa: then and now. *J Am Acad Dermatol* 2004;51:S55–S57.

190. James WD, Berger TG, Elston DM. Epidermolysis bullosa acquisita. In: James WD, Berger TG, Elston DM, eds. *Andrew's Diseases of the Skin Clinical Dermatology*. 10th ed. Philadelphia: Saunders Elsevier; 2006:473–474.

191. James WD, Berger TG, Elston DM. Epidermolysis bullosa. In: James WD, Berger TG, Elston DM, eds. *Andrew's Diseases of the Skin Clinical Dermatology*. 10th ed. Philadelphia: Saunders Elsevier; 2006:555–559.

192. Fine JD, Eady RA, Bauer EA, et al. Revised classification system for inherited epidermolysis bullosa: report of the Second International Consensus Meeting on diagnosis and classification of epidermolysis bullosa. *J Am Acad Dermatol* 2000;42:1051–1066.

193. Kasperkiewicz M, Sadik CD, Bieber K, et al. Epidermolysis bullosa acquisita: from pathophysiology to novel therapeutic options. *J Invest Dermatol* 2016;136:24–33.

194. McAllister JC, Peter Marinkovich M. Advances in inherited epidermolysis bullosa. *Adv Dermatol* 2005;21:303–334.

195. Uitto J, Bruckner-Tuderman L, Christiano AM, et al. Progress toward treatment and cure of epidermolysis bullosa: summary of the DEBRA International Research Symposium EB2015. *J Invest Dermatol* 2016;136:352–358.

196. Oktem A, Akay BN, Boyvat A, et al. Long-term results of rituximab-intravenous immunoglobulin combination therapy in patients with epidermolysis bullosa acquisita resistant to conventional therapy. *J Dermatolog Treat* 2017;28:50–54.

197. Gurcan HM, Ahmed AR. Current concepts in the treatment of epidermolysis bullosa acquisita. *Expert Opin Pharmacother* 2011;12:1259–1268.

198. Butterton JR, Collier DS, Romero JM, et al. Case records of the Massachusetts General Hospital. Case 14-2007. A 59-year-old man with fever and pain and swelling of both eyes and the right ear. *N Engl J Med* 2007;356:1980–1988.

199. Letko E, Zafirakis P, Baltatzis S, et al. Relapsing polychondritis: a clinical review. *Semin Arthritis Rheum* 2002;31:384–395.

200. Frances C, el Rassi R, Laporte JL, et al. Dermatologic manifestations of relapsing polychondritis. A study of 200 cases at a single center. *Medicine* 2001;80:173–179.

201. Damiani JM, Levine HL. Relapsing polychondritis—report of ten cases. *Laryngoscope* 1979;89:929–946.

202. McAdam LP, O'Hanlan MA, Bluestone R, et al. Relapsing polychondritis: prospective study of 23 patients and a review of the literature. *Medicine* 1976;55:193–215.

203. Mark KA, Franks AG Jr. Colchicine and indomethacin for the treatment of relapsing polychondritis. *J Am Acad Dermatol* 2002;46:S22–S24.

204. Trentham DE, Le CH. Relapsing polychondritis. *Ann Intern Med* 1998;129:114–122.

205. Smylie A, Malhotra N, Brassard A. Relapsing polychondritis: a review and guide for the dermatologist. *Am J Clin Dermatol* 2017;18:77–86.

206. Ioffreda MD. Inflammatory diseases of hair follicles, sweat glands and cartilage. In: Elder DE, Elenitsas R, Johnson BL, et al, eds. *Lever's Histopathology of the Skin*. 9th ed. Philadelphia: Lippincott Williams & Wilkins; 2005:500–501.

207. Cribier B, Scrivener Y, Peltre B. Neural hyperplasia in chondrodermatitis nodularis chronica helicis. *J Am Acad Dermatol* 2006;55:844–848.

208. Shah S, Fiala KH. Chondrodermatitis nodularis helicis: a review of current therapies. *Dermatol Ther* 2017;30.

209. Massey EW. Sensory mononeuropathies. *Semin Neurol* 1998;18:177–183.

210. Laurencet FM, Anchisi S, Tullen E, et al. Mental neuropathy: report of five cases and review of the literature. *Crit Rev Oncol Hematol* 2000;34:71–79.

211. Turner-Iannacci A, Mozaffari E, Stooler ET. Mental nerve neuropathy: case report and review. *CJEM* 2003;5:259–262.

212. Savk O, Savk E. Investigation of spinal pathology in notalgia paresthetica. *J Am Acad Dermatol* 2005;52:1085–1087.

213. Goulden V, Toomey PJ, Highet AS. Successful treatment of notalgia paresthetica with a paravertebral local anesthetic block. *J Am Acad Dermatol* 1998;38:114–116.

214. Massey EW, Pleet AB. Electromyographic evaluation of notalgia paresthetica. *Neurology* 1981;31:642.

215. Bernhard JD. Lichen simplex chronicus, prurigo nodularis, and notalgia paresthetica. In: Arndt KA, LeBoit PE, Robinson JK, et al, eds. *Cutaneous Medicine and Surgery: An Integrated Program in Dermatology*. Philadelphia: WB Saunders; 1996:208–210.

216. Shumway NK, Cole E, Fernandez KH. Neurocutaneous disease: neurocutaneous dysesthesias. *J Am Acad Dermatol* 2016;74:215–230.

217. Savk E, Bolukbasi O, Akyol A, et al. Open pilot study on oxcarbazepine for the treatment of notalgia paresthetica. *J Am Acad Dermatol* 2001;45:630–632.

218. Loosemore MP, Bordeaux JS, Bernhard JD. Gabapentin treatment for notalgia paresthetica, a common isolated peripheral sensory neuropathy. *J Eur Acad Dermatol Venereol* 2007;21:1440–1441.

219. Poterucha TJ, Weiss WT, Warndahl RA, et al. Topical amitriptyline combined with ketamine for the treatment of erythromelalgia: a retrospective study of 36 patients at Mayo Clinic. *J Drugs Dermatol* 2013;12:308–310.

220. Davis MD, O'Fallon WM, Rogers RS III, et al. Natural history of erythromelalgia: presentation and outcome in 168 patients. *Arch Dermatol* 2000;136:330–336.

221. Parker LK, Ponte C, Howell KJ, et al. Clinical features and management of erythromelalgia: long term follow-up of 46 cases. *Clin Exp Rheumatol* 2017;35:80–84.

222. Hisama FM, Dib-Hajj SD, Waxman SG. SCN9A-related inherited erythromelalgia. In: Pagon RA, Adam MP, Ardinger HH, et al, eds. *GeneReviews®*. Seattle, WA: University of Washington; 1993.

223. Larralde M, Boggio P, Amartino H, et al. Fabry disease: a study of 6 hemizygous men and 5 heterozygous women with emphasis on dermatologic manifestations. *Arch Dermatol* 2004;140:1440–1446.

224. Clarke JT. Narrative review: Fabry disease. *Ann Intern Med* 2007;146:425–433.

225. Mehta A, Hughes DA. Fabry disease. In: Pagon RA, Adam MP, Ardinger HH, et al, eds. *GeneReviews®*. Seattle, WA: University of Washington; 1993.

226. El Dib R, Gomaa H, Carvalho RP, et al. Enzyme replacement therapy for Anderson-Fabry disease. *Cochrane Database Syst Rev* 2016;(7): CD006663.

227. Ries M, Schiffmann R. Fabry disease: angiokeratoma, biomarker, and the effect of enzyme replacement therapy on kidney function. *Arch Dermatol* 2005;141:904–906.

228. Schuller Y, Linthorst GE, Hollak CE, et al. Pain management strategies for neuropathic pain in Fabry disease—a systematic review. *BMC Neurol* 2016;16:25.

229. James WD, Berger TG, Elston DM. Cutaneous endometriosis. In: James WD, Berger TG, Elston DM, eds. *Andrew's Diseases of the Skin Clinical Dermatology.* 10th ed. Philadelphia: Saunders Elsevier; 2006:628.

230. Muñoz H, Waxtein L, Vega ME, et al. An ulcerated umbilical nodule. *Arch Dermatol* 1999;135:1114–1115, 1117–1118.

231. Tidman MJ, MacDonald DM. Cutaneous endometriosis: a histopathologic study. *J Am Acad Dermatol* 1988;18:373–377.

232. Kazakov DV, Ondic O, Zamecnik M, et al. Morphological variations of scar-related and spontaneous endometriosis of the skin and superficial soft tissue: a study of 71 cases with emphasis on atypical features and types of müllerian differentiations. *J Am Acad Dermatol* 2007;57:134–146.

233. Din AH, Verjee LS, Griffiths MA. Cutaneous endometriosis: a plastic surgery perspective. *J Plast Reconstr Aesthet Surg* 2013;66:129–130.

234. Launonen V, Vierimaa O, Kiuru M, et al. Inherited susceptibility to uterine leiomyomas and renal cell cancer. *Proc Natl Acad Sci U S A* 2001;98: 3387–3392.

235. Rothman A, Glenn G, Choyke L, et al. Multiple painful cutaneous nodules and renal mass. *J Am Acad Dermatol* 2006;55:683–686.

236. Sneller MC, Langford CA, Fauci AS. The vasculitis syndromes. In: Fauci AS, Kasper DL, Longo DL, et al, eds. *Harrison's Principles of Internal Medicine.* 16th ed. New York: MacGraw-Hill; 2005:2002–2014.

237. McKee PH, Calonje E, Granter SR. Angiolipoma. In: McKee PH, Calonje E, Granter SR, eds. *Pathology of the Skin with Clinical Correlations.* 3rd ed. Philadelphia: Elsevier Mosby; 2005:1687–1688.

238. Ragsdale BD. Angiolipoma. In: Elder DE, Elenitsas R, Johnson BL, et al, eds. *Lever's Histopathology of the Skin.* 9th ed. Philadelphia: Lippincott Williams & Wilkins; 2005:1066–1068.

239. McKee PH, Calonje E, Granter SR. Angioleiomyoma. In: McKee PH, Calonje E, Granter SR, eds. *Pathology of the Skin with Clinical Correlations.* 3rd ed. Philadelphia: Elsevier Mosby; 2005:1799–1800.

240. Ragsdale BD. Leiomyoma. In: Elder DE, Elenitsas R, Johnson BL, et al, eds. *Lever's Histopathology of the Skin.* 9th ed. Philadelphia: Lippincott Williams & Wilkins; 2005:1078–1081.

241. Reed RJ, Argenyi Z. True neoplasms of Schwann cells. In: Elder DE, Elenitsas R, Johnson BL, et al, eds. *Lever's Histopathology of the Skin.* 9th ed. Philadelphia: Lippincott Williams & Wilkins; 2005:1116–1119.

242. Calonje E, Wilson-Jones E. Glomus tumor. In: Elder DE, Elenitsas R, Johnson BL, et al, eds. *Lever's Histopathology of the Skin.* 9th ed. Philadelphia: Lippincott Williams & Wilkins; 2005:1049–1051.

243. McKee PH, Calonje E, Granter SR. Glomus tumor. In: McKee PH, Calonje E, Granter SR, eds. *Pathology of the Skin with Clinical Correlations.* 3rd ed. Philadelphia: Elsevier Mosby; 2005:1848–1851.

244. McKee PH, Calonje E, Granter SR. Eccrine spiradenoma. In: McKee PH, Calonje E, Granter SR, eds. *Pathology of the Skin with Clinical Correlations.* 3rd ed. Philadelphia: Elsevier Mosby; 2005:1642–1644.

245. Klein W, Chan E, Seykora JT. Eccrine spiradenoma. In: Elder DE, Elenitsas R, Johnson BL, et al, eds. *Lever's Histopathology of the Skin.* 9th ed. Philadelphia: Lippincott Williams & Wilkins; 2005:903–904.

246. McKee PH, Calonje E, Granter SR. Pilar leiomyoma. In: McKee PH, Calonje E, Granter SR, eds. *Pathology of the Skin with Clinical Correlations.* 3rd ed: Philadelphia: Elsevier Mosby; 2005:1797–1799.

CHAPTER 38

Pain Due to Vascular Causes

KAJ JOHANSEN

Pain in one form or another is a frequent manifestation of arterial, venous, or lymphatic problems. The nature and location of pain complaints may be virtually diagnostic of the underlying vascular condition. On the other hand, pain arising from nonvascular conditions may mimic that associated with various vascular conditions, thereby delaying or complicating diagnosis and therapy. This chapter explores the mechanisms and pathophysiology of vascular pain and its relief; it emphasizes basic neuroanatomy and neurophysiology relevant to vascular pain and includes a compilation of different vascular pain syndromes.

Because pain is a frequent presenting feature of vascular disease and its therapy, topics covered herein necessarily share an interface with numerous other chapters in this text. Information provided in this chapter is, however, intended to be supplementary or expansive on material elsewhere rather than duplicative. For more detailed discussions of vascular pain, the reader is referred to comprehensive sources on this subject.[1-4]

Basic Neuroanatomic and Neurophysiologic Considerations

A review of the neuroanatomy and neurophysiology of vascular structures and the organs and parts they serve helps inform an understanding of the way vascular disease results in pain. This is further clarified by an understanding of how pain is stimulated peripherally and transmitted and experienced centrally.

The International Association for the Study of Pain defines pain as "an unpleasant sensory and emotional experience associated with actual or potential tissue damage, or described in terms of such damage."[5] The perception of pain is a consequence of many variables including past and current pain experiences, level of consciousness, and the patient's emotional state.

Nociceptive pain is an uncomfortable sensation associated with injurious stimulation, whereas *neuropathic* pain arises in the absence of such injury. From a teleologic perspective, pain's "purpose" is to signal the presence of (and presumably prevent) tissue damage and, thus, exists as one aspect of homeostasis. Only when it becomes chronic, or is a manifestation of the postoperative state, is pain unhelpful.

Pain can be characterized by its location, duration, quality, and severity or intensity. Qualities of pain include the descriptive terms "aching," "burning," "cramping," "radiating," "sharp," or "dull." Focal pain is noted at the site of injury, whereas diffuse pain is more characteristic of deep structures.

Radicular pain radiates along peripheral nerve pathways, not uncommonly in concert with motor or sensory neurologic deficits. Referred pain is perceived at a site remote from where the noxious stimulation is actually occurring and results from a misplaced cortical appreciation of pain. Referred pain generally follows spinal segmental innervation and must be differentiated from radicular pain, which generally follows specific dermatomal distributions. Visceral pain is dull, aching, and has an agonizing, "sickening" component.

Pain can result from numerous physical stimuli including pressure, puncture, squeeze, tension, and extreme heat or cold. Pain can also result from chemical effects such as those resulting from a marked change in pH or the presence of various mediators—histamine-like materials, serotonin, bradykinin, and other similar polypeptides. Endogenous prostanoids can lower the pain threshold as a consequence of certain stimuli; local acidosis can enhance perception of pain. Local mediators such as substance P are released at sites of injury and the neural stimulation which results can be interpreted as pain.

Nociceptive receptors are usually free nerve endings, and pain is transmitted from them in the small unmyelinated A-delta and C nerve fibers. These afferent nerves' cell bodies are located in the dorsal root ganglia, and their axons enter the spinal cord through the dorsal roots. These axons synapse in the dorsal grey of the cord with second-order neurons. Most pain is transmitted centrally via the crossed lateral spinothalamic tract up the cord to third-order neurons in the thalamus. The spinothalamic tract, including the periaqueductal grey region of the brainstem, is relevant to more diffuse, longer lasting pain and, probably, neuropathic pain. Interestingly, the precise central nervous system (CNS) location for pain perception remains obscure.

Large- and medium-sized *arteries* have two types of innervation: afferent (sensory) nerves and autonomic (sympathetic) nerves. Pain is the primary sensation transmitted via nociceptive afferents in arteries and veins; position, temperature, and other such sensations do not appear to be transmitted via the innervation of blood vessels. In large- and medium-sized arteries, these receptors appear to be stimulated by direct trauma (e.g., an arteriography needle), stretch (as noted with balloon dilatation or stent placement), or shear (as in arterial dissection).

Nociception in large- and medium-sized *veins* is due to pain receptors in the venous adventitia which appear to respond primarily to stretch (as in venous distention or engorgement, perhaps the consequence of downstream thrombosis or other obstruction).

Classic neuroanatomic investigations by Pick[6] demonstrated that sympathetic and sensory fibers enter the arterial (and venous) adventitia to form an intrinsic neural network ("adventitial plexus"), mostly composed of sensory afferents. From this plexus, bundles of nonmyelinated fibers (mostly sympathetic) approach the media ("border plexus"), and extensions of this network ramify within the media ("muscular plexus").

The basis for neuropathic pain, and how it is sustained, remain obscure. Neuropathic pain also appears to be transmitted by sensory afferents, but, unlike nociceptive pain, it has autonomic (sympathetic nerve) components as well. This results in the well-established (although poorly understood) role of sympathetic modulation for neuropathic pain by pharmacologic or anesthetic blockade or by sympathectomy. Recognition, diagnosis, and management of various forms of sympathetically mediated or sympathetically sustained pain (formerly termed *causalgia* or *reflex sympathetic dystrophy* [RSD] but now subsumed, by fiat of expert panels,[7] under the umbrella term *complex regional pain syndrome* [CRPS]) is discussed in detail in Chapter 25.

Most nociceptive pain is relieved when the underlying noxious stimulus is resolved. On occasion, the presence or severity of nociceptive pain warrants consideration of more invasive procedures to effect pain relief. Analysis of these procedures' results, both in the near term and chronically, has provided substantial insight into the way peripheral pain is transmitted and appreciated.

Vascular Pain Syndromes

Pain in one form or another is a common manifestation of various vascular disorders, and the location, quality, and natural history of such pain may be crucial to the diagnosis or treatment of the condition. For example, sudden tearing interscapular pain is virtually diagnostic of an acute type B thoracic aortic dissection; mitigation of this pain is a hallmark of satisfactory "medical" management of this condition by means of antihypertensive therapy with β-blockers. A compendium of the types of pain associated with various arterial, venous, and lymphatic conditions follows.

INTERMITTENT CLAUDICATION

Claudication is one of the most common pain complaints seen by vascular specialists. The pathophysiology of arterial claudication is based on a reduction of arterial perfusion to a degree that is inadequate to meet the needs of working muscles. The most common cause is arterial occlusive disease due to generalized atherosclerosis, and the most common sites are shown in Figure 38.1. The clinical phenomenon is not only seen most commonly in the gastrocnemius/soleus muscle group distal to atherosclerotic occlusion of the superficial femoral artery but can also be seen in more proximal thigh muscle groups

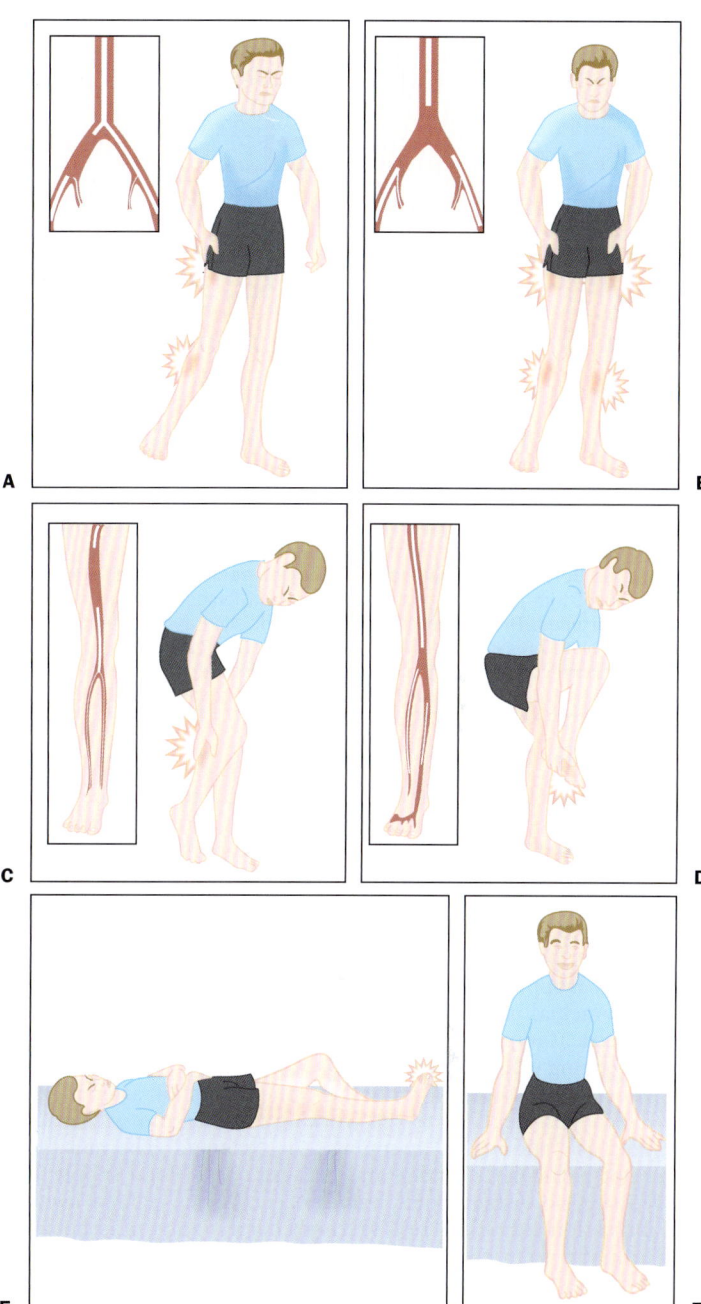

FIGURE 38.2 Sites of pain (radiating lines) caused by atherosclerotic occlusive arterial disease in different parts of the arteries of the lower limbs. **A:** Obstruction in the right common iliac artery, which produces pain in the right hip, buttock, thigh, and calf. **B:** Obstruction in both common iliac arteries and the lower aorta, which produces pain in both hips, buttocks, thighs, and calves—the so-called "Leriche syndrome." **C:** Obstruction of the superficial femoral artery, which produces severe and incapacitating intermittent pain in the calf. **D:** Obstruction of the popliteal and tibial arteries (and dorsal pedal arterial arch) produces pain in the foot. This foot pain can occur at rest in the distal part of the foot when the patient lies in bed (**E**) and the rest pain is often relieved when the limb is dependent (**F**).

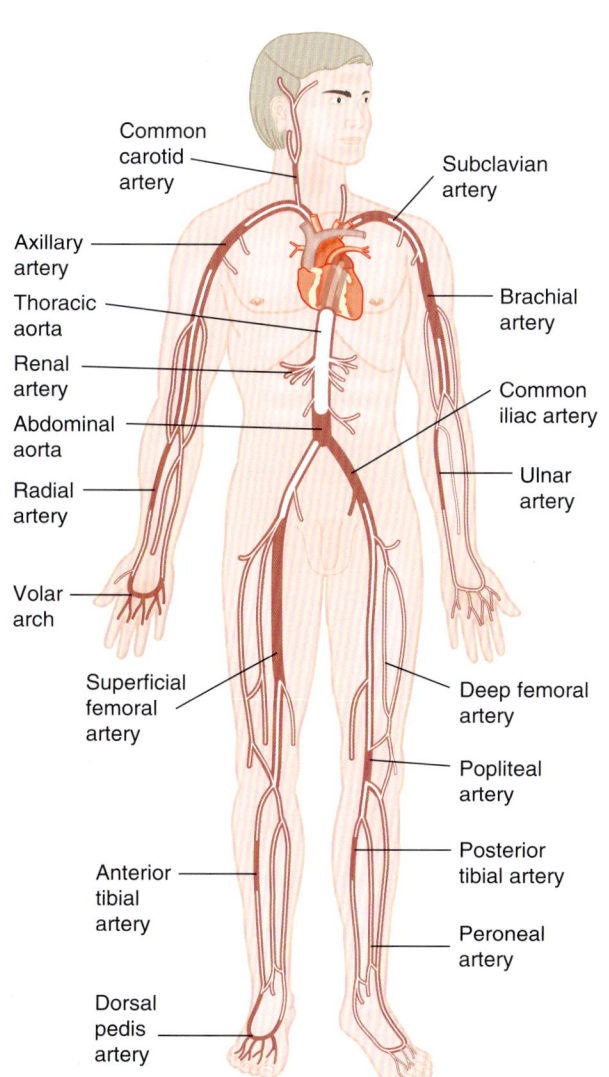

FIGURE 38.1 The most common sites for atherosclerotic occlusive arterial disease in peripheral arteries. The extent, degree, and pattern of the obstructive lesion vary considerably at each site.

with aortoiliac occlusive disease or in the upper extremities with chronic brachiocephalic arterial stenoses or occlusion (Fig. 38.2). Rarely, patients may note claudication of the gluteal or lumbar paraspinal muscles in association with pelvic arterial insufficiency. Claudication of the muscles of mastication is almost diagnostic of involvement of the external carotid artery by giant cell arteritis.[8]

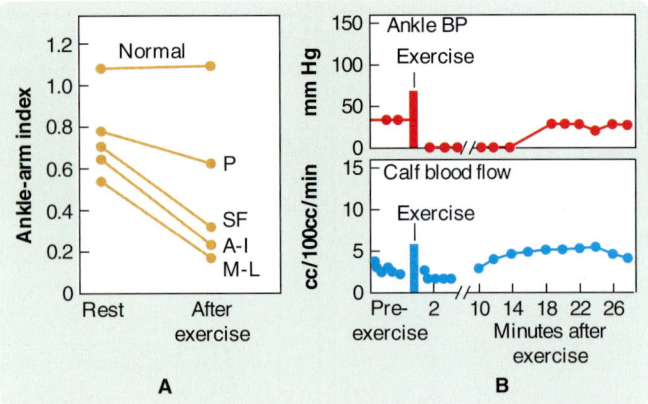

FIGURE 38.3 **A:** Mean ankle–arm indices (ankle systolic blood pressure divided by arm [brachial] systolic blood pressure) at rest and after exercise in normal subjects and subjects with atherosclerotic occlusive disease. The location of the occlusion is indicated by the letters: P, popliteal artery below the knee; SF, superficial femoral artery; AI, aorta and iliac arteries; ML, multilevel. **B:** Ankle pressure and calf blood flow before and after exercise in a patient with occlusion of the iliac, common femoral, and superficial femoral arteries. This patient had severe claudication and moderate rest pain. BP, blood pressure. *(Modified from Sumner DS. Practical approach to vascular laboratory testing in occlusive arterial disease. In: Rutherford RB, ed. Vascular Surgery. 2nd ed. Philadelphia: WB Saunders; 1984:45–56. Copyright © 1984 Elsevier. With permission.)*

The quality and pattern of the pain associated with intermittent claudication is stereotypical. It is absent at rest but appears following muscle exertion of a specific amount, disappearing quickly following cessation of exercise. That the phenomenon is a consequence of inadequate perfusion to working muscles is demonstrated by the parallel course of the development of symptoms and the decline in skeletal muscle perfusion as measured by Doppler arterial pressure ankle/arm indices (AAIs—or ankle/brachial indices, ABIs) during treadmill walking and by symmetrical improvement in symptoms and AAI when treadmill walking is halted (Fig. 38.3).

The pain associated with the claudication of arterial insufficiency is localized to the working muscles and is characterized as "burning," "cramping," or "aching." The muscles are not particularly tender, and because basal blood supply is adequate, no distal trophic lesions occur. At the cellular level, claudication pain likely results from a combination of ischemic neuropathy (particularly of small unmyelinated Aδ and C sensory fibers) and a localized lactic acidosis resulting from the anaerobic metabolism of ischemia, perhaps heightened by elaboration of substance P.

Several types of intermittent *pseudo*claudication exist and contribute to an important differential diagnosis among patients presenting with walking-related extremity pain. The most important and commonly seen of these alternative diagnoses is that of *neurogenic claudication*, resulting from one form or another of lumbosacral neurospinal compression syndrome—spinal stenosis, herniated disk, arachnoiditis, spondylolisthesis, and the like. Initially, such patients' complaints may appear to be very similar to those of subjects with arterial insufficiency, to the extent that they are occasionally subjected to surgical revascularization when they actually need a laminectomy (or vice versa).

Fortunately, a careful history will frequently solve this diagnostic conundrum. Because the basis for neurogenic claudication involves compression of nerve roots by a diffuse fibrotic or inflammatory process in the region of the lower spinal cord or the cauda equina, neurogenic claudication is more commonly bilateral than that associated with arterial insufficiency. Furthermore, the pain of neurogenic claudication is more diffuse, frequently extending from buttocks to feet, and often has a deeper, more aching or burning quality, not infrequently associated with distal paresthesias or numbness.

The subject with neurogenic claudication frequently finds relief from his or her steadily worsening symptoms by bending over while walking; when hip and leg pain forces the subject to halt, symptom relief commonly results only with sitting. Unlike the individual with arterial claudication who can walk the same distance on the level or on the treadmill over and over again with equal interspersed rest periods, the individual with neurogenic claudication who attempts to walk very far achieves shorter and shorter walking distances at the expense of longer and longer periods of sitting. Neurospinal compression may result in pain or numbness just with standing, once again and relieved by sitting.

The pain of neurogenic claudication is felt to result from both ischemia and reactive swelling of nerve roots at their site of compression, an impression confirmed by studies utilizing intrathecal fiber optic endoscopy during treadmill walking in patients with neurogenic claudication.[9] Temporary relief of the pain of neurogenic claudication by various postural changes such as sitting appears to result from the fact that flexion of the hip and back relieves lumbosacral nerve root "stretch" and allows decongestion of the epidural veins in the region.[9]

Substantial diagnostic confusion can result from the fact that older patients with lower extremity claudication may have *both* atherosclerotic arterial occlusive disease *and* degenerative lumbosacral spine disease. Minimal or no change in Doppler AAI in the presence of development of lower extremity symptoms during treadmill exercise excludes arterial occlusive disease as a cause of the patient's lower extremity symptoms.

Other much less common causes of intermittent claudication include the following: proximal venous occlusive disease of the lower extremities, resulting in a characteristic sense of "bursting" discomfort and engorgement of the exercising extremity ("venous claudication")[10] as well as various forms of myositis, the most common of which is an iatrogenic muscle inflammation and necrosis which results from the administration of various statin medications to treat hyperlipidemia.[11]

Lower extremity claudication in younger individuals should bring to mind two diagnoses—*popliteal entrapment syndrome* and (when exercise-induced pain is localized to the anterolateral aspect of the leg) *chronic compartment syndrome*. The intermittent claudication seen in young people (often athletes or military recruits) associated with popliteal artery entrapment syndrome (Fig. 38.4) has the same pathophysiologic mechanism

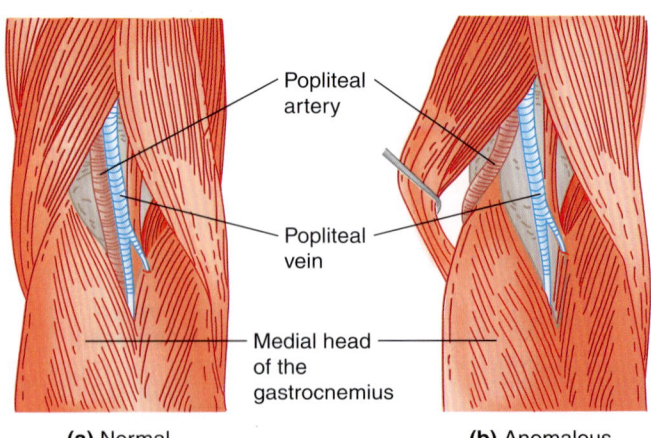

(a) Normal   **(b) Anomalous**

FIGURE 38.4 **A:** The normal relationship of the popliteal artery and the two heads of the gastrocnemius muscle. **B:** The most common anomaly, which causes popliteal artery entrapment syndrome. The popliteal artery is looped medially around and then under the medial head of the gastrocnemius. The medial hamstring muscles have been retracted for clarity. During strenuous exercise of the leg, the muscle compresses the artery, with consequent ischemia and intermittent claudication.

as that associated with atherosclerotic lower extremity arterial occlusive disease.[12] The cellular basis for the anterior muscle compartment pain associated with chronic compartment syndrome is ischemia resulting from diminution of the intramuscular arteriovenous pressure differential due to venous congestion and compartment tissue hypertension.[13]

AORTIC AND OTHER LARGE ARTERY PAIN

A substantial number of pain receptors populate the media of large- and medium-sized arteries. As noted previously, these receptors can respond to direct stimulation, for example by a needle or other penetrating instrument; they also may respond to stretch or shear. Sensory nerve fibers do not appear in or near the arterial intima, perhaps explaining why atherosclerosis, even when it is "inflammatory,"[14] is not painful. Chronic slow dilatation of arteries, such as occurs with abdominal aortic aneurysm (AAA), does not appear to stimulate intra-arterial pain fibers; although palpation of an AAA occasionally results in a diffuse deep sickening ache, in the author's experience, this occurs with equivalent frequency following deep palpation of normal nonaneurysmal aortas. Stimulation of periaortic autonomic fibers by such palpation may contribute to this characteristic sensation.

The pain associated with aortic aneurysmal rupture, usually into the peritoneal cavity, the retroperitoneum, or (rarely) the pleural space, is generally described as sudden, steady, burning, and penetrating in nature. Such pain likely arises as a consequence of nociception at several levels, including stimulation of pain fibers in the torn aorta, in the stretched or torn peritoneum or pleura and as a consequence of extravasation and hematoma expansion in an enclosed pleura or retroperitoneum (tellingly, free rupture of an AAA into the abdominal cavity is commonly characterized by transient pain only, followed by rapid loss of consciousness as the patient expires from hypovolemic shock).

Pain—characteristically "tearing," "ripping," or "boring" and located in a substernal or interscapular location—is a hallmark of aortic dissection. Similar burning pain in the lateral neck characterizes extracranial carotid arterial dissection. Shearing of nociceptive receptors in the aortic or carotid media by progression of the pulsatile hematoma within the media is the likely explanation for this pain. Except for patients with Marfan or Ehlers-Danlos syndromes, whose aortic or arterial dissections may occur asymptomatically, pain is a constant consequence of arterial dissection. As previously intimated, relief of such pain with hypotensive therapy is felt to indicate satisfactory control of an aortic dissection, whereas persistent pain suggests that such therapy is inadequate, obligating either that such therapy be augmented or be replaced by a more invasive intervention (operation or endovascular repair).

Vasculitic inflammatory involvement of large- and medium-sized arteries is uncommon but not rare. The most common such involvement of the aorta is the development of an inflammatory aneurysm, usually of the abdominal aorta. Although the pathophysiology of this process remains obscure, its presentation is stereotypically as a thickened "rind" of chronically inflamed fibrofatty perianeurysmal tissues, frequently with an adhesive involvement of the ureters or the duodenum which can significantly complicate open aneurysmal repair. Patients with inflammatory AAAs commonly complain of diffuse aching midback discomfort, and their aneurysms are dully tender to palpation.

Besides the jaw claudication often associated with giant cell arteritis,[8] such patients' inflammatory vasculitis can be associated with diffuse pain and tenderness over the affected arteries—especially the superficial temporal artery, biopsy (or duplex scanning)[15] of which may be diagnostic of the underlying condition. As for inflammatory AAA and other large- and medium-sized vessel arteritis, the diffuse and poorly localized pain seen in this condition is likely due to inflammatory involvement of nociceptors found both in the arterial media and adventitia as well as in periarterial connective tissue. That the pain associated with this condition is inflammatory is borne out by its resolution following administration of anti-inflammatory agents (particularly corticosteroids).

REST PAIN, ULCERS, AND GANGRENE

Advanced or critical arterial insufficiency—usually in the lower extremities—displays characteristic symptoms and signs which signal impending limb loss. Indeed, all patients with rest pain, ischemic ulcers, or gangrene will require an operative intervention—either a procedure to reestablish vascular supply to the affected area or an amputation. Such patients' arterial occlusive disease is severe and multilevel ("tandem"), and their mortality rate exceeds 50% over the next 5 years as a consequence of premature, aggressive coronary artery disease.

Rest pain is characterized by a diffuse, ill-localized aching or burning pain in the distal foot (occasionally the heel). It is generally initially present at night when the patient is recumbent or the leg and foot are elevated. Symptoms dissipate if the leg is hung over the edge of the bed or the subject arises and walks around. The pathophysiology of rest pain is likely that of an ischemic neuropathy, with positional malperfusion of small sensory nerves in the distal foot. The symptoms of rest pain (or other advanced arterial insufficiency) necessarily develop in the most distal small arteries, those farthest away from the heart. Thus, pain at rest does not occur proximal to the foot (with one cardinal exception: rest pain may develop with severe ischemia in the stump of a patient with a below- or above-knee amputation).

Arterial ulceration in the nondiabetic patient is characterized by a shallow, pallid, nonhealing erosion of the skin in the distal foot, in a similar location as that for rest pain. The pain of such ulcerations is unremitting and severe, occasionally refractory even to high-dose oral narcotic analgesic agents, and is treated only by urgent revascularization or by amputation. The pain of such ulcerations is described as aching or burning and arises not only from the same severe ischemic neuropathy, which gives rise to ischemic rest pain, but also to actual necrosis of sensory nerves in the skin at the site of the arterial ulcer.

Gangrenous changes of the toes or heel are indications that tissue death has occurred. Associated pain complaints are thus a summation not only of ischemic neuropathy but also of actual necrosis of sensory nerves as well as the consequences of skin and subcutaneous tissue infarction, osteomyelitis, and ascending infection. As for patients with arterial ulceration, such patients' pain may be severe and unremitting; on the other hand, in certain such patients, necrosis of sensory nerves may actually make such gangrenous distal feet insensate and anesthetic, paradoxically resulting in less pain than would be anticipated from the degree of tissue destruction present.

Atheroembolism, usually to the toes or distal foot ("blue toe syndrome")[16] occurs because of digital or distal branch artery occlusion from debris (clot, atheroma), which has embolized into the distal circulation from a proximal source (e.g., an aortoiliac or popliteal aneurysm or an ulcerated atherosclerotic plaque). The syndrome occurs only with patent proximal arteries, and the distal limb is usually not ischemic. Pain is therefore uncommon until digital ischemia is severe enough to result in sensory nerve damage.

The diabetic foot is a special circumstance in which chronic nonhealing lower extremity and foot ulceration and toe gangrene may occur; yet, the underlying pathogenesis revolves around not only ischemia but also diabetic neuropathy, foot structural changes, and diabetics' inability to combat bacterial infection. Indeed, most diabetic foot lesions are *not* ischemic,[17] and revascularization is not necessarily required as part of their management. Widespread loss of distal foot and even lower leg sensation in diabetics consequent to diabetic neuropathy makes pain due to ulceration, gangrene, or infection relatively uncommon. On the other hand, neuropathic pain is frequent (see later text).

PAIN SYNDROMES FOLLOWING STROKE

Pain is uncommon in association with cerebrovascular accident (CVA), except for patients whose cerebrovascular ischemia results from intracranial hemorrhage or tumor. Stroke survivors sometimes experience what appears to be a centrally mediated pain ipsilateral to the neurologic deficit.[18] Dejerine and Roussy first described excruciating pain involving the contralateral half of the body in a patient who had suffered a thalamic stroke and termed the condition *thalamic syndrome*.[19] Similar symptoms can arise following injury anywhere along the course of the spinothalamic tracts, and this syndrome has been termed *central poststroke pain* (CPSP).[20]

CPSP occurs after ischemic or hemorrhagic stroke. Patients report burning or lancinating pain associated with sensory abnormalities in the painful region. Sensory abnormalities include decreased perception of sharpness and temperature, often accompanied by allodynia and hyperalgesia.[21] The pain is often constant but may occur in paroxysms, and it is usually limited to an area that is smaller than the area affected by sensory deficits. The pain is often worsened by stress and relieved by relaxation, and the pain can present an enormous burden to the patient, causing severe depression.[22]

Following thalamic stroke, CPSP is not uncommon. In a series of 100 patients with thalamic hemorrhage, 9% developed CPSP.[23] In a prospective study of 267 consecutively admitted stroke patients, CPSP occurred in 8% of the patients during the first year, with more than half of those with pain reporting moderate to severe pain.[24] In 63% of the patients, pain onset was within 1 month after stroke.

CPSP is a difficult condition to treat, and pain reduction rather than pain relief has to be the goal of the treatment. Conventional analgesics and opioids have been noted to be ineffective.[25] Numerous other types of drugs have been tried in the treatment of CPSP, but large controlled trials are lacking, and the treatment is far from being standardized. Treatment of CPSP has been reviewed in detail elsewhere.[26]

PAIN ASSOCIATED WITH DISEASES INVOLVING SMALL ARTERIES

Numerous regional or systemic disorders include involvement of small arteries. In the extremities, such conditions commonly manifest coolness, pallor, numbness, cyanosis, and pain—manifestations of Raynaud's syndrome.[27] Often, such symptoms and signs result simply from abnormal arterial reactivity, such as occurs in its benign form, termed *Raynaud's disease* (seen primarily in young and middle-aged women or as a consequence of chronic vibratory tool use, primarily in young male laborers). Dull aching digit pain is noted by such patients during periods of extreme vasoconstriction; with the hyperemia of digital reperfusion, when vasoconstriction is replaced by vasodilatation, this dull aching pain is commonly replaced by a burning "fiery" pain as the digits are suffused via vasodilated digital arteries.

A more ominous form of small artery involvement associated with Raynaud's syndrome (termed *Raynaud phenomenon* in this setting) results from digital arterial occlusions resulting from one or another form of various rheumatoid conditions—especially scleroderma.[28] To these individuals' diffuse pain syndrome, resulting from digital vasoconstriction and then vasodilatation, is added intractably painful fingertip ulceration or necrosis. Such patients' distal digital pain is frequently severe and unremitting, not uncommonly refractory even to large doses of opiate analgesic medications, and may require amputation for relief. Pathophysiologically, these lesions are similar to those of advanced chronic lower extremity arterial insufficiency.

A rare form of small artery involvement resulting in severe pain is that associated with Buerger's disease (thromboangiitis obliterans [TAO]), a condition most commonly seen in young male tobacco addicts. TAO is a nonatherosclerotic necrotizing condition of smaller distal arteries, veins, and nerves, primarily in the extremities.[29] Because only the tibial arteries in the lower extremity, or the distal radial and ulnar arteries of the upper extremity, are commonly involved in Buerger's disease, these patients have excellent arterial inflow but inadequate collateralization (Fig. 38.5), and their ability to heal refractory ulcerations or areas of gangrene is poor. These patients' foot or hand pain is described as severe, unremitting, aching, burning, and agonizing; amputation is commonly the best management.

PAIN ASSOCIATED WITH VENOUS DISORDERS

Venous disease is common and is frequently undiagnosed. This occurs in part because one major component of venous disease—deep venous thrombosis (DVT)—commonly occurs in a relatively vegetative, bland fashion associated with only minimal inflammation. Such patients' first symptom may be painless lower extremity edema or, on occasion, chest pain and cardiorespiratory collapse associated with pulmonary embolus. Pain is only inconsistently associated with superficial venous disease. Patients with primary or secondary venous varicosities may note diffuse aching or burning pain associated with their venous varicosities, a discomfort likely secondary to stretch stimulation of nociceptors in and around the venous adventitia and media or in the surrounding soft tissue.

Patients who have suffered a prior lower extremity DVT often display symptoms and signs of the postphlebitic (postthrombotic) syndrome. This condition is characterized by chronic lower extremity edema, secondary venous varicosities, and characteristic skin changes including stasis pigmentation and eczema, subcutaneous atrophy, and, in advanced stages, skin breakdown and chronic nonhealing ulcerations around the medial and lateral malleoli. These stasis ulcerations, usually relatively small and shallow but occasionally circumferential and extending from ankle to midleg, are, in the author's experience, notably *nonpainful*, often manifesting only mild itching or burning. When significant pain occurs in a stasis ulcer, a secondary diagnosis should be entertained—invasive infection (usually streptococcal) or (rarely) malignant transformation, ischemia, or osteomyelitis.

Superficial phlebitis generally results from chemical irritation of the intima of peripheral veins as a consequence of intravenous infusions of various medications or agents of abuse, may be a manifestation of sterile inflammation secondary to indwelling catheters or other foreign bodies, or bacterial infection. Such phlebitis is characterized by marked localized tenderness with overlying cellulitis, demonstration of a palpable "cord" along the course of the vein and, rarely, systemic toxicity. Pain is characteristically well localized along the vein and is burning in nature, resulting from stimulation of vein-wall nociceptive receptors. In addition, perivenous inflammation results in elaboration of acidic inflammatory or infectious mediators which stimulates perivenous nociceptors.

PAIN ASSOCIATED WITH LYMPHATIC DISEASES

The most common lymphatic disorder is *lymphedema praecox*—idiopathic, bland nonvenous swelling, usually of a lower extremity. Other forms of lymphedema are either iatrogenic (consequent to lymphadenectomy or irradiation) or result from infections of various sorts. The lymphatics are not innervated so most forms of lymphedema are painful only when

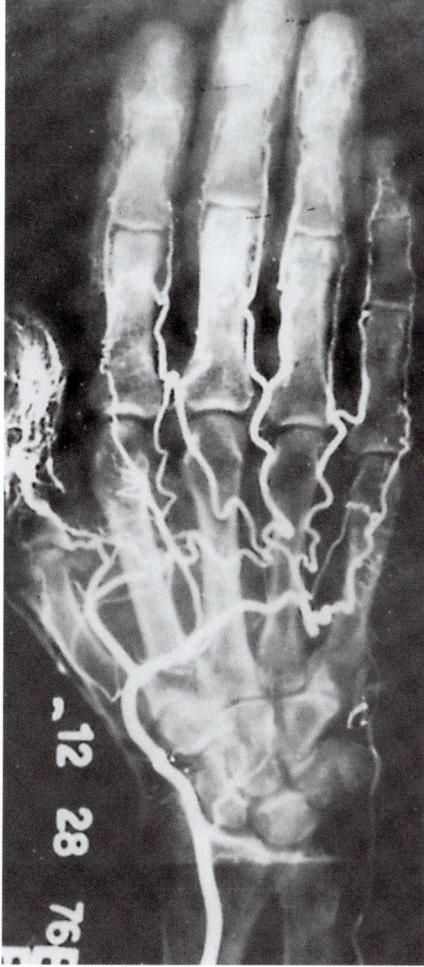 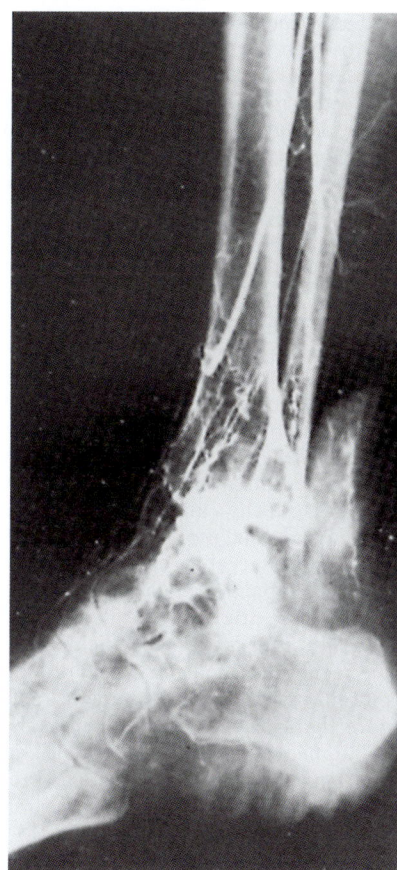

FIGURE 38.5 Angiograms of patients with thromboangiitis obliterans (Buerger's disease). **A:** Angiogram of the hand of a patient showing lack of filling of the ulnar artery, characteristic tortuous, corkscrew-like arteries in the hand, and "skipped" areas where no contrast enters the digital arteries. **B:** Angiogram of the distal part of the leg of a patient with thromboangiitis obliterans. The anterior and posterior tibial arteries appear normal until their abrupt occlusion at the ankle. (*From deWolfe VG. Chronic occlusive arterial disease of the lower extremities. In: Spittell JA Jr, ed.* Clinical Vascular Disease. *1st ed. Philadelphia: FA Davis; 1983:15–135. Reproduced with permission of F.A. Davis Co., in the format Republish in a book via Copyright Clearance Center.*)

cellulitis or lymphangitis—an unfortunately common complication of lymphedema—supervenes.

PAIN ASSOCIATED WITH AMPUTATION

Commonly performed because of intractable pain in a nonsalvageable limb, amputation itself sometimes results in pain of various types. These can be classified as being either acute—at the time of the amputation—or chronic—occurring weeks, months, or even (on occasion) years following the initial procedure.

Acute postamputation pain may be related to the surgical procedure itself or to incompletely understood central or neuraxial phenomena arising from the patient's preoperative pain status. Acute postamputation pain may result from the obligatory section of major nerves during limb amputation. The incisional and wound pain that results from transtibial or transfemoral amputation commonly resolves within a week or so following amputation—sooner in many surgeons' experience if a rigid dressing is applied to the residual limb.[30]

Other relatively straightforward amputation pain issues occurring early in the postoperative period include those related to stump hematoma or ischemia or actual muscle necrosis because the amputation was performed too far distally, resulting in thrombosis of the stump's residual arterial blood supply. The latter complication generally requires reamputation at a higher level.

Early postamputation pain problems unrelated to the wound itself include the development of diverse neuropathic phenomena, including phantom limb *sensation* or *pain*. Virtually all amputees experience the sense that the amputated

limb is still present, for example, that it itches and needs to be scratched. Phantom limb *sensation* is generally considered to be benign and self-limited. Phantom limb *pain*, on the other hand, can frequently be severe and, on occasion, even incapacitating, although patients can be reassured that the phenomenon generally diminishes or disappears within months to a year following amputation. Treatment with antiseizure medications, tricyclic antidepressants, regional sympathetic blockade with long-acting local anesthetic agents, cutaneous electrical stimulation units, sympathectomy, spinal cord stimulation (SCS),[31] or even rhizotomy or distal reentry zone sectioning[32] has been attempted for persistent or severe phantom limb pain.

Late postamputation pain most commonly results from a poorly fitted artificial limb, and an experienced prosthetist's opinion is invaluable in this setting. Other less common but important causes of late postamputation stump pain can include progressive stump ischemia, DVT, progressive autonomic dysfunction (e.g., CRPS), or neuroma formation—the last problem best prevented by assuring that large nerves sectioned at the time of the original amputation are buried in muscle, well away from cut bone ends and the skin flap.

Differentiating Vascular from Nonvascular Pain

It is clinically self-evident that a large overlap occurs between the pain syndromes arising from vascular and nonvascular diseases. The not infrequent misdiagnosis of a ruptured AAA as ureteral or biliary colic, of an aortic dissection as a myocardial infarction or gastroesophageal reflux, or of lower extremity ischemic pain as lumbar spinal stenosis all point to the importance of considering the entire constellation of diagnostic possibilities present in patients presenting with various forms of pain.

The scope of this chapter precludes an exhaustive discussion of those disease states in which the misdiagnosis of vascular for nonvascular disease (or, as important, the converse) can occur; the reader is referred to seminal general and vascular surgical texts for further details.[33–35] Those intent on formalizing the divergence of vascular surgery from general surgery,[36,37] both in the context of resident training and as a separate specialty, must make every effort to ensure that future vascular surgeons and their general surgery colleagues experience a shared body of clinical knowledge and judgment in this context.

The Relief of Vascular Pain

The relief (or at least the mitigation) of pain is the sine qua non of the rationale for many vascular interventions to the extent that an inability to achieve pain relief may be tantamount to failure—either of the original diagnosis or of the intervention itself. The patient who continues to experience calf claudication after a technically successful femoral–popliteal bypass may well have needed more preoperative attention paid to the status of his lumbosacral nerve roots. The return of claudication after a period of pain-free walking suggests the progressive deterioration of the original revascularization.

As in other areas of medicine and surgery, minimally invasive techniques and nanotechnology have grown increasingly to dominate therapeutic maneuvers. In industrialized countries more than 90% of aortic aneurysm patients are managed by percutaneous catheter-based stent graft means (Fig. 38.6). The initial approach to the management of lower extremity arterial occlusive disease is by means of similar transcatheter balloon angioplasty or stenting.

Relief of several types of aortic pain can take both "medical" and surgical forms. As previously intimated, the presence of tearing central truncal pain is a hallmark of aortic dissection. All type A aortic dissections require immediate referral to a cardiothoracic surgeon for urgent intervention. However, type B aortic dissections' natural history as well as their indications for operative or endovascular intervention are heavily dependent on the relief of this lesion's characteristic pain by pharmacologic therapy—specifically, the administration of β-blocker agents, whose effect is to halt the medial hematoma's dissection by lowering systolic and mean blood pressure as well as left ventricular dV/dt.[38]

The pain associated with an expanding, leaking, or ruptured abdominal or thoracic aortic or iliac aneurysm is relieved by successful graft interposition, either by open or stent-graft means. Graft repair of aneurysms eroding into the spine commonly relieves the pain from such bony erosion. Similarly, and for obscure reasons, graft repair of inflammatory AAAs tends to resolve the characteristic inflammatory "rind" around the aorta and, with it, the diffuse, poorly localized, boring mid-abdominal-to-mid-back ache these patients commonly note. Interestingly, the use of corticosteroids, administered systemically or by injection, can also diminish the pain associated with an inflammatory aneurysm,[39] although such therapy theoretically increases the risk of aneurysm expansion and rupture.[40]

A preponderance of pain resulting from vascular disease arises from inadequate tissue oxygenation, most commonly with exertion or other increased nutritive blood flow demands but also in basal blood flow states in which tissue viability itself is threatened. Many vascular interventions focus on restoring tissue perfusion to (or toward) normal—not only various revascularization procedures, either by open or endovascular means, but also pharmacologic or hygienic measures as simple as the encouragement of smoking cessation or aerobic exercise or the administration of hemorheologic medications.

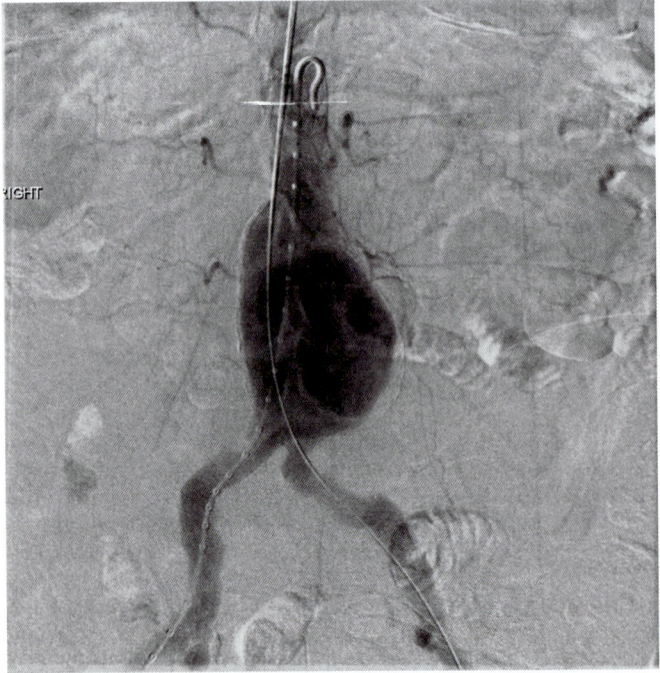

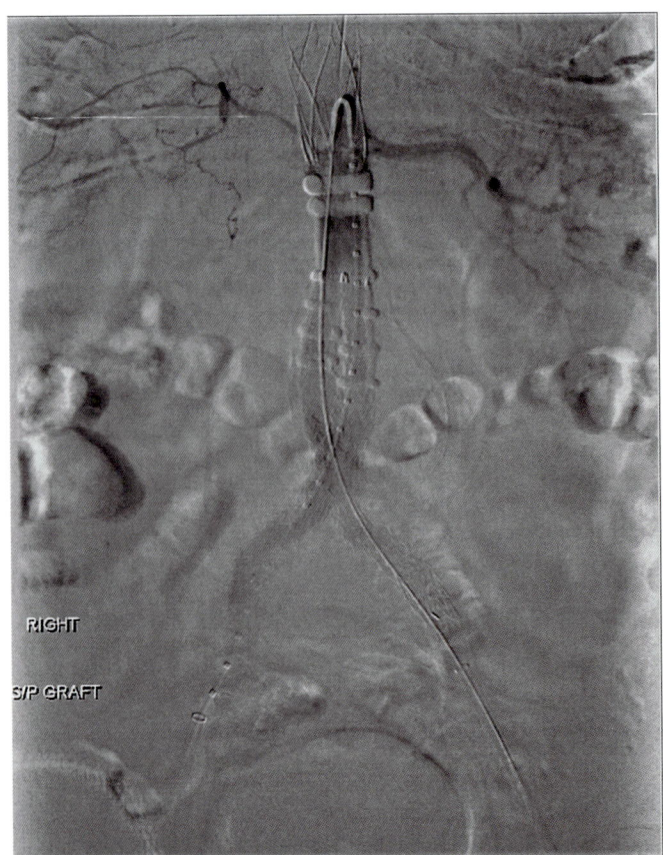

FIGURE 38.6 Contemporary percutaneous transcatheter management of aortic aneurysm. Such techniques have, to a great extent, assumed the therapeutic role previously occupied by open surgical graft interposition or bypass. Immediate postprocedure morbidity is vastly less but so is therapeutic durability, obliging an increased emphasis on postprocedural aneurysm or vessel surveillance and repeat interventions.

Although such interventions are most commonly carried out for the symptomatic consequences of lower extremity atherosclerotic occlusive disease, the principle of relieving vascular pain by improving tissue nutrition can be relevant for non-atherosclerotic diseases of the upper extremities as well—for example, the salubrious effects seen with the administration of cilostazol in patients with various small artery occlusive phenomena of the digits[41] or the relief of dialysis access-associated rest pain of the hand by the performance of distal revascularization/interval ligation.[42]

In unusual circumstances, revascularization by conventional operative or pharmacologic means may not be feasible or may not provide tissue reperfusion adequate to relieve pain or other ischemic manifestations. In certain limited circumstances, the observation, initially popularized by Leriche,[43] that sympathectomy can increase skin perfusion may offer a therapeutic alternative. Ipsilateral lumbar sympathectomy (most effectively by operative excision, although a therapeutic effect can result from phenol or absolute alcohol ablation) can heal shallow ischemic skin lesions and relieve associated ischemic rest pain, probably by the combined effects of increased skin blood flow and interruption of afferent pain fibers traveling within the lumbar sympathetic chain.[44,45] Patients subjected to such therapy have a 10% risk of developing a sometimes debilitating although transient burning pain termed *postsympathectomy neuralgia*.[46]

Revascularization to treat severe ischemia may not be possible or, even if technically feasible, may not be successful in relieving pain. When tissue loss—advanced ischemic ulceration or gangrene—supervenes, amputation is indicated. However, in that subset of patients with far-advanced, refractory ischemia in which significant tissue loss has not yet developed but in which pain is severe and unremitting, Jacobs and colleagues[47] have extensively investigated the possibility that SCS might relieve pain and forestall the need for amputation as a pain-relief measure. Initial enthusiasm for this approach, based on nonrandomized studies demonstrating improved microcirculatory blood flow in subjects with advanced nonreconstructible lower extremity arterial disease,[47] has waned with publication of less favorable results of more recent prospective trials of SCS.[48] At the current time, the role of SCS in the management of subjects with advanced chronic limb ischemia appears to be restricted to those with relatively preserved microcirculatory skin perfusion.[48]

Pain associated with venous disease of various sorts is ubiquitous although rarely severe or incapacitating. The central role of vein wall distention as the proximate cause of lower extremity venous symptoms associated with saphenous or deep venous insufficiency is perhaps best demonstrated by the almost universal symptomatic improvement associated with such "low-tech" maneuvers as limb elevation or the donning of elastic support stockings. The "swollen" or "bursting" sensations associated with significant large-vessel lower extremity venous obstruction ("venous claudication") may only be effectively treated by venous bypass or by endovascular relief of proximal venous occlusions.[49] The pain associated with acute venous thrombosis, either deep or superficial, is both congestive and inflammatory and is optimally treated with limb elevation and/or compression plus anti-inflammatory medications.

The management of acute pain is central to the cultural identity of most medical specialties. Unfortunately, published research has repeatedly documented that most medical professionals have inadequate training, experience, or understanding of the proper management of acute or chronic pain. Aronoff[50] has recently discussed this problem as well as recent research findings which could inform a more coherent approach to the medical management of pain. Pharmacologic (or other) management of chronic or severe pain of any origin is increasingly the domain of pain specialists, frequently with an anesthesiology background, in a multidisciplinary pain clinic setting.

Conclusion

How best to manage the manifold types of vascular pain is a vast and incompletely illuminated topic. Vascular pain's multifactorial nature confounds simple or stereotypical prescriptions for its relief. In a large majority of cases, restoration to (or toward) normalcy of the underlying arterial or venous condition will resolve or improve associated vascular pain. Chronic vascular pain is closely allied with neuritic or neuropathic abnormalities, the management of which warrants involvement of specialist consultants in chronic pain.[51]

References

1. Fishman S, Ballantyne J, Rathmell J, eds. *Bonica's Management of Pain*. 4th ed. Philadelphia: Lippincott Williams & Wilkins; 2010.
2. McMahon S, Koltzenburg M, Tracey I, et al, eds. *Wall and Melzack's Textbook of Pain*. 6th ed. Edinburgh: Churchill Livingstone; 2014.
3. Benzon H, Rathmell J, Wu CL, et al, eds. *Raj's Practical Management of Pain*. 5th ed. St. Louis, MO: Mosby; 2014.
4. Aronoff GM, ed. *Evaluation and Treatment of Chronic Pain*. 3rd ed. Baltimore, MD: Williams & Wilkins; 1998
5. Task Force on Taxonomy of the International Association for the Study of Pain. Classification of chronic pain: descriptions of chronic pain syndromes and definition of pain terms. *Pain Suppl* 1986;3:S1–S226.
6. Pick J. *The Autonomic Nervous System: Morphological, Comparative, Clinical and Surgical Aspects*. Philadelphia: Lippincott; 1970.
7. Harden RN, Bruehl S, Galer BS, et al. Complex regional pain syndrome: are the IASP diagnostic criteria valid and sufficiently comprehensive? *Pain* 1999;83:211–219.
8. Smetana GW, Shmerling RH. Does this patient have temporal arteritis? *JAMA* 2002;287:92–101.
9. Binder DK, Schmidt MH, Weinstein PR. Lumbar spinal stenosis. *Semin Neurol* 2002;22:157–166.
10. Delis KT, Bountouroglou D, Mansfield AO. Venous claudication in iliofemoral thrombosis: long-term effects on venous hemodynamics, clinical status, and quality of life. *Ann Surg* 2004;239:118–126.
11. Rosenson RS. Current overview of statin-induced myopathy. *Am J Med* 2004;116:408–416.
12. Levien LJ. Popliteal artery entrapment syndrome. *Semin Vasc Surg* 2003;16:223–231.
13. Turnipseed WD. Diagnosis and management of chronic compartment syndrome. *Surgery* 2002;132:613–619.
14. Danesh J, Whincup P, Walker M, et al. Low-grade inflammation and coronary heart disease: prospective study and updated meta-analyses. *BMJ* 2000;321:199–204.
15. LeSar CJ, Meier GH, DeMasi RJ, et al. The utility of color duplex ultrasonography in the diagnosis of temporal arteritis. *J Vasc Surg* 2002;36:1154–1160.
16. Renshaw A, McCowen T, Waltke EA, et al. Angioplasty with stenting is effective in treating blue toe syndrome. *Vasc Endovascular Surg* 2002;36:155–159.
17. Reiber GE, Vileikyte L, Boyko EJ, et al. Causal pathways for incident lower-extremity ulcers in patients with diabetes from two settings. *Diabetes Care* 1999;22:157–162.
18. Widar M, Ek AC, Ahlstrom G. Coping with long-term pain after a stroke. *J Pain Symptom Manage* 2004;27:215–225.
19. Bowsher D, Leijon G, Thuomas KA. Central poststroke pain: correlation of MRI with clinical pain characteristics and sensory abnormalities. *Neurology* 1998;51:1352–1358.
20. Boivie J, Leijon G, Johansson I. Central post-stroke pain: a study of the mechanisms through analysis of the sensory abnormalities. *Pain* 1989;36:173–185.
21. Vestergaard K, Nielsen J, Andersen G, et al. Sensory abnormalities in consecutive, unselected patients with central post-stroke pain. *Pain* 1995;61:177–186.
22. Leijon G, Boivie J, Johansson I. Central post-stroke pain: neurological symptoms and pain characteristics. *Pain* 1989;36:13–25.
23. Kumral E, Kocaer T, Ertübey N, et al. Thalamic hemorrhage: a prospective study of 100 patients. *Stroke* 1995;26:964–970.
24. Andersen G, Vestergaard K, Ingeman-Nielsen M, et al. Incidence of central post-stroke pain. *Pain* 1995;61:187–193.
25. Arnér S, Meyerson BA. Lack of analgesic effect of opioids on neuropathic and idiopathic forms of pain. *Pain* 1988;33:11–23.
26. Frese A, Husstedt IW, Ringelstein EB, et al. Pharmacologic treatment of central post-stroke pain. *Clin J Pain* 2006;22:252–260.
27. Wigley FM. Raynaud's phenomenon. *N Engl J Med* 2002;347:1001–1008.

28. Pope J, Fenlon D, Thompson A, et al. Iloprost and cisaprost for Raynaud's phenomenon in progressive systemic sclerosis. *Cochrane Database Syst Rev* 2000;(2):CD000953.

29. Ohta T, Ishioashi H, Hosaka M, et al. Clinical and social consequences of Buerger disease. *J Vasc Surg* 2004;29:176–180.

30. Smith DG, McFarland LV, Sangeorzan BJ, et al. Postoperative dressing and management strategies for transtibial amputation: critical review. *J Rehabil Res Dev* 2003;40:213–224.

31. Katayama Y, Yamamoto T, Kobayashi K, et al. Motor cortex stimulation for phantom limb pain: comprehensive therapy with spinal cord and thalamic stimulation. *Stereotact Funct Neurosurg* 2001;77:159–162.

32. Prestor B. Microsurgical junctional DREZ coagulation for treatment of de-afferentation syndromes. *Surg Neurol* 2001;56:259–265.

33. Mulholland M, Lillemoe KD, Doherty GM, et al, eds. *Greenfield's Surgery: Scientific Principles and Practice.* 5th ed. Philadelphia: Lippincott Williams & Wilkins; 2018.

34. Brunicardi FC, ed. *Schwartz's Principles of Surgery.* 9th ed. New York: McGraw-Hill; 2010.

35. Cronenwett J, Johnston KW, eds. *Rutherford's Vascular Surgery.* 8th ed. New York: Elsevier; 2014.

36. Veith FJ. The case for an independent American Board of Vascular Surgery. *J Vasc Surg* 2000;32:619–621.

37. Stanley JC. The discipline of vascular surgery at the close of the millennium, the American Board of Surgery Sub-Board for Vascular Surgery, and the wisdom of evolving a conjoint board of vascular surgery: one surgeon's perspective. *J Vasc Surg* 2000;31:831–835.

38. Westaby S. Management of aortic dissection. *Curr Opin Cardiol* 1995; 10:505–510.

39. Stotter AT, Grigg MJ, Mansfield AO. The response of peri-aneurysmal fibrosis—the "inflammatory" aneurysm—to surgery and steroid therapy. *Eur J Vasc Surg* 1990;4:201–205.

40. Reilly JM, Savage EB, Brophy CM, et al. Hydrocortisone rapidly induces aortic rupture in a genetically susceptible mouse. *Arch Surg* 1990;125: 707–709.

41. Rajagopalan S, Pfenninger D, Somers E, et al. Effects of cilostazol in patients with Raynaud's syndrome. *Am J Cardiol* 2003;92:1310–1315.

42. Diehl L, Johansen K, Watson J. Operative management of distal ischemia complicating upper extremity dialysis access. *Am J Surg* 2003;186:17–19.

43. Ewing M. The history of lumbar sympathectomy. *Surgery* 1971;70: 791–796.

44. Mailis A, Furlan A. Sympathectomy for neuropathic pain. *Cochrane Database Syst Rev* 2003;(2):CD002918.

45. AbuRahma AF, Robinson PA, Powell M, et al. Sympathectomy for reflex sympathetic dystrophy: factors affecting outcome. *Ann Vasc Surg* 1994;8:372–379.

46. Kramis RC, Roberts WJ, Gillette RG. Post-sympathectomy neuralgia: hypotheses on peripheral and central neuron mechanisms. *Pain* 1996;65:1–9.

47. Jacobs MJ, Jorning PJ, Beckers RC, et al. Post salvage and improvement of microvascular flow as a result of epidural spinal cord electrical stimulation. *J Vasc Surg* 1990;12:354–360.

48. Ubbink DT, Spincemaille GH, Prins MH, et al. Microcirculatory investigations to determine the effect of spinal cord stimulation for critical leg ischemia: the Dutch Multicenter randomized controlled trial. *J Vasc Surg* 1999;30:236–244.

49. Raju S, Owen S Jr, Neglen P. The clinical impact of iliac venous stents in the management of chronic venous insufficiency. *J Vasc Surg* 2002;35: 8–15.

50. Aronoff GM. What do we know about the pathophysiology of chronic pain? Implications for treatment considerations. *Med Clin N Am* 2016;100: 31–42.

51. Seretny M, Colvin LA. Pain management in patients with vascular disease. *Brit J Anaesth* 2016;117(suppl 2):ii95–ii106.

CHAPTER 39

Pain Due to Thoracic Outlet Syndrome

KAJ JOHANSEN, THOMAS TAI CHUNG, and **GEORGE I. THOMAS**

An important and incompletely understood cause of upper extremity pain is subsumed under the rubric of "thoracic outlet syndrome" (TOS). This condition arises from compression of neurovascular structures as they enter/exit the neuraxis and the mediastinum at the base of the neck. Particularly in cases involving chronic compression of the brachial plexus, TOS can be a complicated and frustrating condition to manage due to ongoing controversy about the underlying pathophysiology, how the diagnosis is best made, and differing views about proper and effective treatment. Many of the problems regarding TOS revolve around the uncertain natural history of the condition with and without intervention. In this chapter, we discuss the various types of TOS with a particular emphasis on the neurogenic type—by far the most common, the most disputed, and also the most likely to result in pain.

Anatomy and Pathophysiology

The thoracic outlet is the aperture through which the subclavian artery and trunks of the brachial plexus pass as they exit the neuraxis and the upper mediastinum at the base of the neck. In normal anatomic circumstances, the thoracic outlet is bound by several musculotendinous and bony structures including the anterior and middle scalene muscles and, inferiorly, the first rib (Fig. 39.1). In pathologic circumstances, compression of the neurovascular bundle at the thoracic outlet is most commonly the consequence of abnormalities of the scalene muscles and/or the first rib. However, neurovascular compression can also result from the presence of a cervical rib, abnormal fibrous bands, callus from a clavicular fracture, scarring from prior trauma or radiation therapy, or (rarely) a superior sulcus (Pancoast) tumor of the lunch.

Because the subclavian vein lies anterior to the anterior scalene muscles, it does not actually pass through the thoracic outlet. It is, however, located between the clavicle and the first rib in its course toward the mediastinum.

In normal circumstances, arm elevation or abduction results in a functional reduction in the caliber of the thoracic outlet aperture because of posterior rotation of the clavicle and contraction of the scalene muscles. The space between the clavicle and the first rib narrows, and below the shoulder, the pectoralis minor muscle contracts.

Trauma, particularly cervical hyperextension ("whiplash"), or chronic repetitive use of the upper extremities (particularly in an out-front or overhead position), may, over time, result in chronic spasm, inflammation, and contracture of the scalene muscles, producing both the thickening of the anterior and middle scalene muscles as well as microstructural changes in muscle fiber type.[1,2]

Provocative maneuvers of the arm may result in compression of the subclavian artery and vein in up to 30% of normal

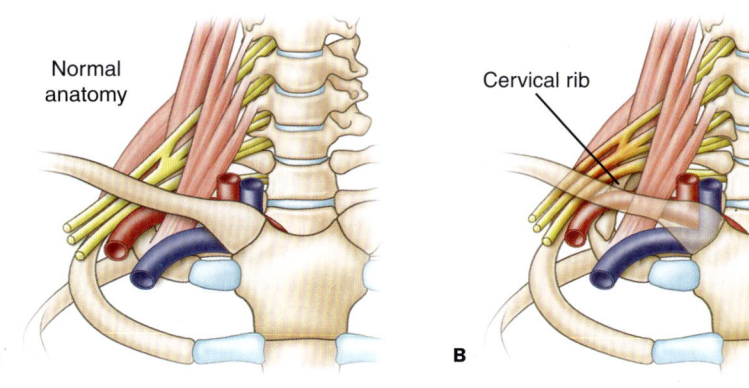

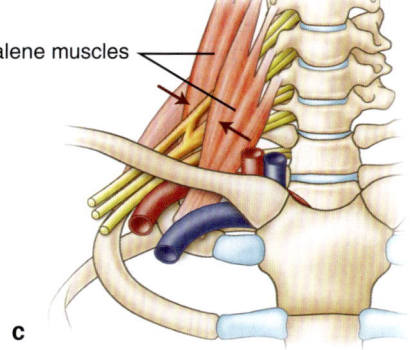

FIGURE 39.1 The anatomy of the normal thoracic outlet and abnormalities leading to thoracic outlet syndrome. **A:** Normal anatomy of the thoracic outlet. **B:** The presence of a first cervical rib can lead to compression of the subclavian artery and/or the brachial plexus (*red shaded region*) between the cervical rib and the clavicle. **C:** Hypertrophy of the anterior and middle scalene muscles following trauma can lead to compression (*arrows*) of the subclavian artery and/or the brachial plexus.

individuals.[3] Reduction in the caliber of the thoracic outlet by pathophysiologic circumstances can result in extrinsic compression of the subclavian artery or vein in more than 90% of patients with TOS.

A cervical rib, abnormal bands, or residua from a clavicular fracture can result in subclavian artery dilation or even aneurysm or mural thrombus formation, from which embolization into the arterial circulation of the wrist or hand may occur.

Extrinsic compression of the subclavian vein in the costoclavicular space, perhaps involving the tendon of the subclavius muscle, can, in concert with repetitive use of the upper extremity, result in axillosubclavian *venous* thrombosis, likely due to intimal damage and venous stasis.

Clinical Presentation: Symptoms and Signs

Arterial TOS is extremely uncommon, comprising less than 1% of the totality of any TOS practice, and almost always presents as forearm or hand "claudication" (or other upper extremity ischemic symptoms) or evidence for distal upper extremity embolization. Physical examination demonstrates diminished or absent wrist pulses; vascular laboratory examination may show occlusion of the radial and/or ulnar arteries or their palmar or digital branches. On occasion, patients may present with rest pain or gangrene of the fingers due to far-advanced ischemia from repetitive distal arterial embolic occlusion.

Physical findings in patients with arterial TOS are primarily those of absent or diminished pulses and/or manifestations of distal upper extremity ischemia.

Involvement of the upper extremity venous circulation by compression of the subclavian vein at the thoracic outlet comprises approximately 5% of a TOS practice. Patients with such venous TOS (also termed *Paget-Schroetter syndrome* or "effort" thrombosis of the axillosubclavian vein) may present with aching pain distributed diffusely throughout a swollen, ruborous upper extremity. In more chronic circumstances, pain and swelling may be less prominent.

On exam, patients with acute *venous* TOS manifest arm swelling and discoloration; in later stages, prominent veins can be seen over the upper arm and around the shoulder.

By far the most common presentation—the overwhelming majority of the patients seen in a TOS practice—results from compression of elements of the brachial plexus, that is, *neurogenic* TOS. Patients with neurogenic TOS almost always have a prior traumatic event—a cervical hyperextension ("whiplash") injury, a fall on an outstretched arm, an object falling on the head or the shoulder—or alternatively have a history for a repetitive stress injury, usually due to exigencies of their occupation. Workplace risk factors for neurogenic TOS include sustained effort with the upper extremity or extremities out-front or overhead and may be seen in drywall hangers, dental hygienists, beauticians or hairdressers, grocery checkers, shelf stockers, or clerical workers engaged in prolonged keyboarding.

Such injury or workplace-related postures and stresses have been demonstrated to result in chronic contracture and spasm of the suspensory muscles in and around the shoulder girdle—among them the anterior and middle scalene muscles. Obesity, sedentary lifestyles, and maladaptive postures—in neurogenic TOS, characterized by the head flexed on the neck and the shoulders down and forward—exacerbate chronic scalene muscle spasm.

Patients with neurogenic TOS may have few or no symptoms with the arms in a neutral position. However, they will quickly note the onset of pain and paresthesias with the arms placed in an out-front, overhead, or abducted posture. Indeed, this presentation is so stereotypic that we do not seriously entertain the diagnosis of neurogenic TOS in the absence of a subject's observation of worsened symptoms with the arms in such provocative postures.

Symptoms characteristically evoked in neurogenic TOS patients include elevational arm aching, particularly proximally around the shoulder, the axilla, and the upper arm, associated variably with numbness and tingling out the arm, distal weakness, and a limitation in range of motion of the affected upper extremity. Paresthesias are found predominantly in a lower trunk (C8–T1) distribution, appropriate to impingement on the lower aspects of the brachial plexus. Indeed, 80% of patients with neurogenic TOS demonstrate pain and paresthesias radiating along an ulnar nerve distribution, often into the small and ring finger as a consequence. This presumably results from upward traction on the first rib by the scalene muscles, thus selectively impacting the inferior aspects of the brachial plexus.

A significant proportion of patients with neurogenic TOS have significant headaches, primarily occipital.[4] They also may note symptoms of facial or jaw pain or pain around ear. Muscle pain is commonplace in neurogenic TOS, particularly around the neck and the shoulder, the scapula, and the upper arm. It is frequently difficult to discern whether such symptoms arose from neurogenic TOS itself or from concurrent soft-tissue injuries (e.g., the paraspinous or periscapular muscles: the rotator cuff in the shoulder) suffered at the same time as the injury causing the neurogenic TOS.

Patients with neurogenic TOS frequently display a series of symptoms associated with activities of daily living which, in the aggregate, strongly indicate the presence of neurogenic TOS. Elements of our clinical template are shown in Table 39.1.

In neurogenic TOS, objective physical examination findings are sparse. Such individuals have limited range of motion of the affected upper extremity and manifest diminished spontaneous (adventitial) movements of the extremity as well as an unwillingness to place or maintain the affected limb in various provocative postures. Muscle tenderness over the anterior and lateral neck is commonplace, as is neck muscle tightness or contracture. In the supraclavicular fossa, tenderness can be elicited with palpation over the brachial plexus at the scalene triangle, often resulting in radiation of neuritic sensations into the axilla or out the arm (a positive Tinel sign). Occasionally, a cervical rib can be palpated. Tenderness over the pectoralis minor tendon attachment at the coracoid process below the shoulder is commonplace.

More peripherally in the upper extremity, tenderness may be elicited with palpation deep in the axilla. Tenderness of the arm or forearm muscles or tendons, or evidence for peripheral nerve compression at the carpal or cubital tunnels, may be present but is not, however, a primary manifestation of neurogenic TOS. Instead, this may represent the concurrent upper extremity injury that may accompany neurogenic TOS ("double crush" syndrome).[5] Rarely, intrinsic hand muscle atrophy may be observed, a so-called Gilliatt-Sumner hand.[6]

A series of provocative tests are commonly performed which, individually or in the aggregate, are thought by many to demonstrate the presence of neurogenic TOS. The *Adson test* is carried out with the affected arm held downward and

TABLE 39.1 Clinical Elements that Suggest Neurogenic Thoracic Outlet Syndrome
Inability to drive with the hands elevated in the normal 10 o'clock/ 2 o'clock position on the steering wheel
Problems with grooming (shampooing the hair or use of a hairdryer)
Awakening at night with pain or numbness in the affected arm(s)
"Drop attacks": the tendency to drop things, often without recognizing that grip strength has diminished
Inability to carry out sustained overhead activities, for example, changing multiple light bulbs in the ceiling
Loss of handwriting legibility (with involvement of the dominant upper extremity)
Inability to remove a tight jar lid

backward: The ipsilateral wrist pulse is palpated as the head is turned toward this arm while the subject undertakes a sustained inspiration. A positive test, suggesting the presence of neurogenic TOS, results when the wrist pulse is obliterated.

The *military* or *shoulder brace position* involves retraction of the shoulders backward and downward, which may result in pulse obliteration at the wrist.

The Roos or *abduction/external rotation (AER)* ("hands-up") *test* involves, as described, the arms held at 90 degrees at the shoulders, the elbows flexed 90 degrees, and the hands then contracted repeatedly. A positive test involves rapid fatiguing and pain in the affected upper extremity.

Sanders and colleagues[7] have reported the high positive and negative predictive value of the *brachial plexus tension test*. Here, the arms are held horizontally with the elbows and wrists straight and the neck is laterally flexed *away* from the affected arm: Both wrists are then extended. A positive test is characterized by a sense of tightness and pain in the ipsilateral neck as well as neuritic symptoms radiating out the affected arm.

Although not a provocative test for neurogenic TOS, the *Spurling* test is important in the evaluation of this condition. Because an important alternative diagnosis in these patients may be cervical radiculopathy, development of characteristic symptoms with lateral flexion of the neck *toward* the affected extremity makes neuroforaminal compression due to herniated disk, scar, or arthritis more probable and neurogenic TOS less likely.

The aforementioned provocative tests are commonly performed as part of an evaluation for neurogenic TOS. Skeptics point out that, although the sensitivity of each of these tests may be high, their specificity is very low (e.g., more than 30% of the asymptomatic population may have a positive Adson test).[3] Similar results hold for the military (shoulder brace) position. The AER ("hands-up") test has a high sensitivity and much better specificity for neurogenic TOS. Experienced clinicians' view is that patients ultimately demonstrated to have neurogenic TOS will be strongly positive for many or most of these tests, individually or in the aggregate.

Diagnostic Tests

In patients with arterial TOS, chest roentgenography will frequently confirm the presence of a cervical rib or callus from a clavicular fracture. A noninvasive vascular laboratory examination of the upper extremity will confirm the absence of (or reduction in) arterial flow at the hand and wrist level, not uncommonly in a pattern consistent with thromboembolic occlusion. Duplex scanning of the subclavian artery may demonstrate stenosis with poststenotic dilation or aneurysm formation with mural thrombus within. Computed tomography (CT) scan or catheter-directed arteriography may demonstrate sharp angulation of the subclavian artery over a cervical rib or around a clavicular fracture callus (Fig. 39.2); such imaging studies may also document the specific distribution of distal forearm, wrist, or hand arterial occlusions.

In venous TOS, noninvasive vascular laboratory examination will demonstrate partial or complete axillosubclavian venous thrombosis.[8] Enlarged venous collaterals around the shoulder

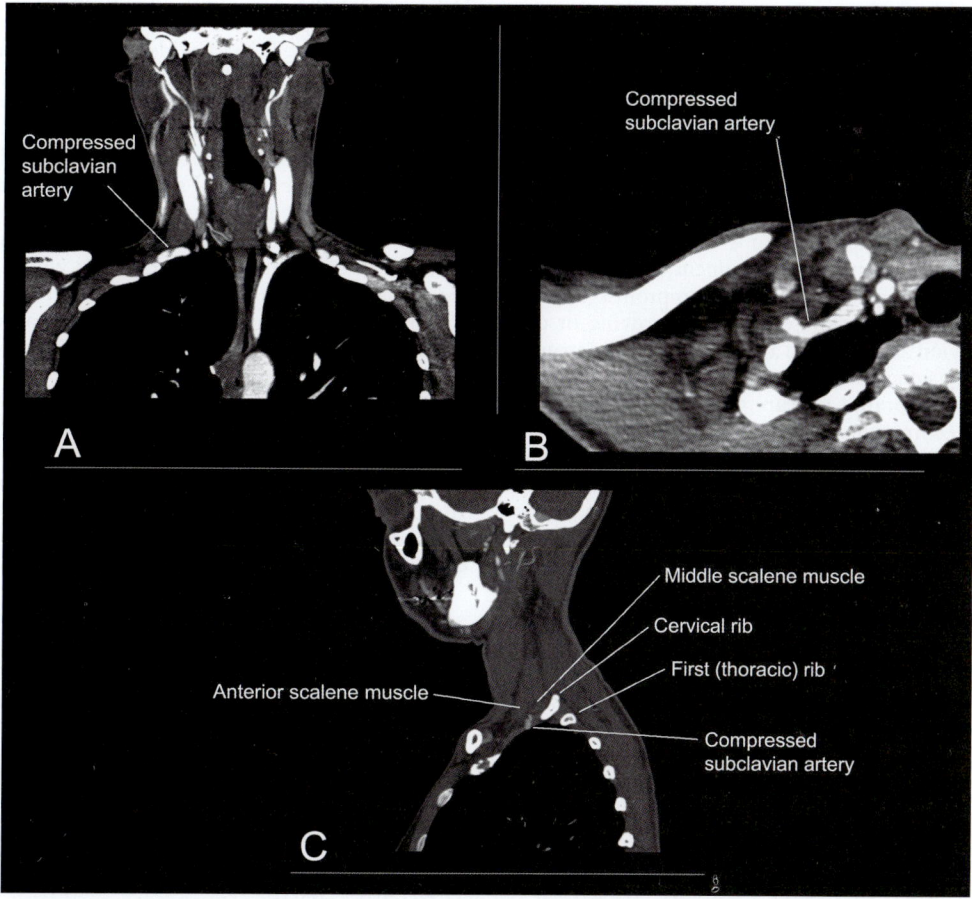

FIGURE 39.2 Computed tomography angiography with multiplanar reformatted images demonstrating compression of the subclavian artery between the insertions of the anterior and middle scalene muscles in a patient with a cervical rib. **A:** Coronal image demonstrating external compression of the subclavian artery as it passes cephalad to the cervical rib. **B:** Axial image demonstrating narrowing of the subclavian artery due to compression on the artery by the anterior scalene muscle. **C:** Sagittal, right paramedian image demonstrating compression of the subclavian artery as it passes between the insertion of the anterior and middle scalene muscles on the cervical rib. (*Images courtesy of Dean Donahue, MD, Division of Thoracic Surgery, Massachusetts General Hospital, Boston, MA.*)

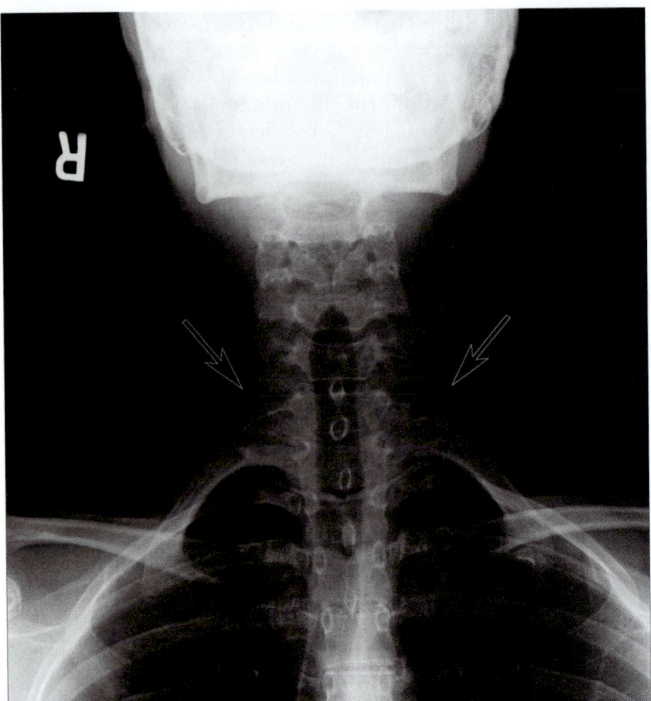

FIGURE 39.3   Chest x-ray demonstrating presence of cervical rib (*arrows*) in a patient with symptoms of thoracic outlet syndrome. (*Image courtesy of Dean Donahue, MD, Division of Thoracic Surgery, Massachusetts General Hospital, Boston, MA.*)

may be displayed. Not uncommonly, upstream venous tributaries of the arm such as the basilic vein may demonstrate partial or complete thrombosis as well.

In neurogenic TOS, chest roentgenography may demonstrate a cervical rib. We commonly perform an apical lordotic view because, with a standard chest roentgenogram, on occasion, a cervical rib may be hidden as it underlies the first rib (Fig. 39.3). A chest roentgenogram may also, as for arterial TOS, demonstrate a clavicular fracture; it may also document the presence of a superior sulcus tumor causing the patient's symptoms.

Arteriography may demonstrate extrinsic narrowing or occlusion of the subclavian artery by the aforementioned anatomic stricture, particularly when the affected arm is maintained in an abducted/externally rotated posture. Imaging studies such as magnetic resonance imaging (MRI) or CT may demonstrate hypertrophied or inflamed scalene muscles or edema or inflammation of the brachial plexus.[9,10]

Electrodiagnostic testing is commonly performed in patients thought to have neurogenic TOS. For patient with "true" neurogenic TOS (a rarely seen condition which results from direct brachial plexus trauma, e.g., a stab or gunshot wound), specific electrodiagnostic criteria have been established—primarily, reduction in median motor and ulnar sensory nerve amplitude. In patients with the much more common "nonspecific" or "disputed"[11] neurogenic TOS, standard electromyography (EMG) or nerve conduction velocity testing is almost always normal.[12] This is not because nerve compression is not present but, rather, as demonstrated by Tender et al.,[13] it is because such compression occurs much more centrally, at the level of the cervical nerve roots and proximal brachial plexus trunks—an area that is difficult to assess via nerve conduction testing.

More recent data have suggested the possibility that electrodiagnostic evaluation of the median antebrachial cutaneous nerve may provide useful diagnostic information in neurogenic TOS.[14]

Most significant in the diagnostic evaluation of neurogenic TOS in our practice has been the use of temporary scalene muscle

inactivation, carried out by EMG-guided intrascalene injection of either bupivacaine[15] or botulinum toxin A (Botox).[16] Scalene muscle block has been demonstrated to have a sensitivity *and* specificity exceeding 90% for the presence of neurogenic TOS.[15] After administration of one of these agents into the scalene muscle, the patient with neurogenic TOS commonly notes a reduction in pain and paresthesias as well as an improvement in flexibility and range of motion in the affected arm. Headache is frequently relieved and the dysautonomic symptoms (bluish discoloration, constant aching pain, moist skin) that accompany neurogenic TOS in up to 10% of patients are relieved.

On occasion, after a positive block, patients become emotional and burst into tears with such novel and unanticipated relief of their symptoms (sometimes having been told by prior examiners that they are delusional or are malingerers). The effects start within a few minutes with bupivacaine injection and last from 15 minutes to several hours; with botulinum toxin A administration (which we utilize both diagnostically and as a treatment maneuver), the onset of relief of symptoms, which occurs in more than 95% of patients who have had a positive bupivacaine block, occurs within 48 to 72 hours and last for 1 to 4 months.[16,17]

Differential Diagnosis

A number of alternative conditions present with symptoms and signs similar to those of various forms of TOS, thus complicating the diagnosis. This is most particularly true for neurogenic TOS, although on occasion, arterial TOS may be written off for a time as Raynaud syndrome (or phenomenon) or some sort of dysautonomic disorder such as complex regional pain syndrome (CRPS). Venous TOS may uncommonly be misdiagnosed as lymphedema or, again, some variety of sympathetic dystrophy.

In neurogenic TOS, a wide range of conditions in the central nervous system or the neuraxis, most particularly multiple sclerosis but also such exotic disorders as syringomyelia, have masqueraded for a time as neurogenic TOS. Impingement on the cervical spinal cord or its nerve roots by herniated disk, arthritis, or cervical spinal stenosis can commonly present with neck, supraclavicular, shoulder, axillary, or upper extremity symptoms. Involvement of the shoulder joint or the scapula is a common concomitant of the injury which may initially have led to the neurogenic TOS itself. Cubital tunnel compression of the ulnar nerve in the elbow, or even carpal tunnel compression of the median nerve at the wrist, may manifest upper extremity symptoms which, on occasion, may be difficult to distinguish from those of neurogenic TOS.

Migraineurs may sometimes experience facial, jaw, or neck pain. Generalized shoulder girdle pain is a commonplace manifestation of fibromyalgia. Polymyositis, temporal (cranial) arteritis, and polymyalgia rheumatic are connective tissue disorders which variably present with pain and tenderness of the muscles of the head, neck, and shoulder girdle.

The initial trauma (e.g., the "whiplash" injury suffered in a motor vehicle crash) commonly results in aches and pains and tenderness in the neck and out one or both upper extremities; it may even result in radicular symptoms which worsen with provocative postures of the arm. Such symptoms are not, however, those of neurogenic TOS, which we consider to be the consequence of *chronic* scarring and contracture of the scalene muscles. Indeed, we assert that the diagnosis of neurogenic TOS should not be invoked until at least 3 to 6 months after the initial traumatic event.

Management

In patients with arterial TOS, two separate treatment goals must be met: relief of distal limb ischemia and eradication of the more proximal embolic source that resulted in the distal extremity ischemia. Although repair of the proximal subclavian arterial lesion is relatively straightforward (usually aneurysmorrhaphy with a short segment of prosthetic graft material or of reversed saphenous vein), restoration of distal arterial flow is often difficult because the embolization that has occurred is chronic. The fact that the occlusion is long-standing often stymies efforts at catheter-directed thrombolysis or open arterial thrombectomy. Fortunately, if pulsatile flow can be restored to the level of the palmar arch, then more distal digital tissue loss is generally avoided.

Conventional management of venous TOS should include systemic anticoagulation (this is, after all, a form of deep venous thrombosis and pulmonary emboli have certainly occurred as a consequence[18]) and, particularly if the onset of symptoms is recent, an attempt at catheter-directed axillosubclavian vein thrombolysis. If venous thrombus is thus relieved, a stricture is often identified within the subclavian vein at the costoclavicular junction. Balloon angioplasty may frequently be carried out[19]; however, it is generally agreed that venous stenting should not be performed at this site because of the high likelihood of stent fracture between the "hammer" and "anvil" formed by the clavicle and first rib.[20]

Because of concerns about recurrent axillosubclavian venous thrombosis and chronic upper extremity postthrombotic symptoms, conventional management of venous TOS has also commonly included not only thrombolysis and anticoagulation but also staged operative thoracic outlet decompression.[21,22] Such an approach is designed to resolve the structural mechanism which led to the initial venous damage (also, by removing the costoclavicular "anvil," later stenting of the stenotic subclavian vein can be carried out if this is deemed necessary).

However, several recent natural history studies have suggested that recurrent axillosubclavian venous thrombosis is quite uncommon and that the natural history of this condition is benign—enough so that thoracic outlet decompression may only rarely be warranted.[23,24] These authors argue that, far from preventing further complications, the magnitude of the dissection required for first rib resection is such that collateral vein disruption around the damaged axillosubclavian vein might paradoxically lead to worsening of the patient's venous congestive symptoms.

Early and mild-to-moderate neurogenic TOS should be treated by aggressive physiotherapy emphasizing postural training, abdominal breathing, and emphasis on stretching and relaxing the scalene muscles. Unfortunately, physiotherapy attempted in the early stages of neurogenic TOS is frequently misdirected, emphasizing resistance exercises; these, of course, tend only to exacerbate further scalene muscle contracture. Soon, the scalene muscles are hypertrophied and scarred, such that it is difficult to imagine much benefit from physiotherapy. Histologic studies of scalene muscle removed at this stage further support this conclusion: The muscle fibers are found to have changed from type II to type I and are interwoven with abundant fibroblasts.[1,2]

For these and other reasons, we believe that, once established, neurogenic TOS is effectively managed only by thoracic outlet decompression. Two means—chemodenervation with botulinum toxin A[16,17] or open surgical decompression of the thoracic outlet—are practiced: Each has advantages and disadvantages.

Botulinum toxin, administered intramuscularly under EMG- or ultrasound-guided control, relieves symptoms of neurogenic TOS in the vast majority of subjects who have previously responded positively to a diagnostic scalene muscle block with local anesthetic. Such patients' symptoms are relieved for 1 to 4 months (mean 3 months).[17] A substantial proportion of such individuals can undergo repeat intrascalene botulinum toxin administration with attainment of another equivalent period of symptom relief.

However, scalene muscle chemodenervation, although temporarily affective at relieving symptoms of neurogenic TOS, does not appear to alter the underlying natural history of neurogenic TOS. Even when vigorous physiotherapy has been pursued during the period of time of scalene muscle denervation, durable improvement in the underlying condition is uncommon. Tachyphylaxis to botulinum toxin is demonstrable in a substantial number of patients. The use of botulinum toxin for the treatment of TOS is not approved by the U.S. Food and Drug Administration; thus, there is limited availability of this treatment. Insurance authorization is difficult to achieve, and botulinum toxin is costly. Although a few of our surgery-averse patients have continued to undertake repeat botulinum toxin chemodenervation, a majority have ultimately opted for operation.

Surgical decompression of the thoracic outlet has historically been based on partial or complete excision of the first rib. The operative rationale is transparent—because the first rib is located at the bottom of the anatomic "triangle" forming the thoracic outlet and serves as the site of insertion of the anterior and middle scalene muscles which comprise the remaining two sides of the "triangle," first rib removal should effectively open this orifice. Because the short, wide first rib plays no significant role in chest wall dynamics and the scalene muscles (developmentally archaic accessory muscles of respiration) serve no significant functional role, dismantling of the musculoskeletal bounds of the thoracic outlet should have minimal functional impact. Numerous patients undergoing first rib resection by transaxillary,[25,26] supraclavicular,[27] or posterior[28] approaches have demonstrated significant improvements in their prior neurocompressive symptoms 75% to 90% of the time.

Patients with symptoms of neurogenic TOS who have cervical ribs have generally done well simply with resection of the cervical rib as well as the tight adhesions ("bands of Roos"[29]) commonly associated with these extrathoracic ribs.

However, based in part on neurogenic TOS patients' stereotypic response to intrascalene bupivacaine or botulinum-mediated chemodenervation, we have rethought our operative strategy for neurogenic TOS. Because a positive response to scalene muscle block is an obligatory part of our indications for operative intervention for neurogenic TOS (a positive block has a >90% positive predictive value for a favorable outcome of operative intervention[15]), we have concluded that the pathophysiology of this condition resides in the scalene muscles and not the first rib. We now consider the rib a *victim* of the condition rather than its *cause*. Others[30,31] have reasoned similarly.

We have thus ceased performing resection of the first rib and now focus our operative efforts on radical excision of the anterior and middle scalene muscles. We have carried out more than 850 consecutive thoracic outlet decompression procedures without excising the first rib: Our results (90% "excellent" or "good" outcomes) are equivalent to those we recorded with rib excision plus total scalenectomy, but patients in whom rib preservation has been carried out appear to rehabilitate substantially more rapidly than those in whom subtotal first rib resection had taken place.

We have come to believe that a separate site of brachial plexus compression, in addition to the well-accepted interscalene and costoclavicular locations, occurs beneath the pectoralis minor tendon attachment to the coracoid process, a site where tendinous impingement on the upper aspect of the axillary nerve can occur. It has long been our practice to decompress this area by dividing the pectoralis minor tendon via a small vertical infraclavicular incision separate from the supraclavicular approach through which we decompress the brachial plexus. Sanders and Rao[32] had likewise recently adopted this approach.

Outcomes

Patients with *arterial* TOS are generally diagnosed and managed in timely fashion due to the importance of finger, hand, and upper extremity neurovascular function. Even when chronic thrombotic occlusion of distal vessels is present, upper extremity arterial collateralization is generally robust enough to maintain distal hand and finger tissue viability and function.

For *venous* TOS, the long-term outcome following first rib resection appears to be good.[21,22] However, the natural history of this condition *without* first rib resection also appears to be excellent,[23,24] leading to recent skepticism regarding whether excision of the first rib in such patients really is in fact an obligatory part of management of this condition.

Published data suggest that, although thoracic outlet decompression rarely completely resolves symptoms of *neurogenic* TOS, the vast majority of patients undergoing surgical thoracic outlet decompression appear to improve and to do well. Even among a high-risk group of workmen's compensation patients undergoing surgery for neurogenic TOS following prolonged administrative delays, the vast majority felt themselves to be improved and indicated they would undergo operation again if confronted by the problem.[33]

Approximately 5% to 10% of patients who have initially undergone decompressive surgery for neurogenic TOS will display persistent or recurrent neurogenic TOS symptoms. Such individuals may be found to have a missed cervical rib, a residual stub of first rib impinging on the brachial plexus, or, most frequently in our experience, adherence of scar and unresected residual scalene muscle to the brachial plexus.[34] In such circumstances, reoperative surgery, although associated with increased risk of peripheral nerve or brachial plexus damage, may be helpful in relieving symptoms. EMG-guided scalene muscle block may be highly useful in demonstrating the presence of adherent residual scalene muscle as the inciting problem in such patients.[34]

Recently, a 496-page, 70-author compendium on various forms of TOS has been published,[35] and reporting standards for TOS have been proposed by the Society for Vascular Surgery.[36]

References

1. Machleder HI, Moll F, Verity MA. The anterior scalene muscle in thoracic outlet compression syndrome: histochemical and morphometric studies. *Arch Surg* 1986;121:1141–1144.
2. Sanders RJ, Jackson CG, Banchero N, et al. Scalene muscle abnormalities in traumatic thoracic outlet syndrome. *Am J Surg* 1990;159:231–236.
3. Juvonen T, Satta J, Laitala P, et al. Anomalies at the thoracic outlet are frequent in the general population. *Am J Surg* 1995;170:33–37.
4. Raskin NH, Howard MW, Ehrenfeld WK. Headache as the leading symptom of the thoracic outlet syndrome. *Headache* 1985;25:208–210.
5. Wood VE, Biondi J. Double-crush nerve compression in thoracic-outlet syndrome. *J Bone Joint Surg Am* 1990;72:85–87.
6. Wulff CH, Gilliatt RW. F waves in patients with hand wasting caused by a single rib and band. *Muscle Nerve* 1979;2:452–457.
7. Sanders RJ, Hammond SL, Rao NM. Diagnosis of thoracic outlet syndrome. *J Vasc Surg* 2007;46:601–604.
8. Mustafa BO, Rathbun SW, Whitsett TL. Sensitivity and specificity of ultrasonography in the diagnosis of upper extremity deep vein thrombosis: a systemic review. *Arch Intern Med* 2002;162:401–404.
9. Demondion X, Boutry N, Drizenko A, et al. Thoracic outlet: anatomic correlation with MR imaging. *AJR Am J Roentgenol* 2000;175:417–422.
10. Hagspiel KD, Spinosa DJ, Angle JF, et al. Diagnosis of vascular compression at the thoracic outlet using gadolinium-enhanced high-resolution ultrafast MR angiography in abduction and adduction. *Cardiovasc Intervent Radiol* 2000;23:152–154.
11. Wilbourn AJ. The thoracic outlet syndrome is overdiagnosed. *Arch Neurol* 1990;47:328–330.
12. Komanetsky RM, Novak CB, Mackinnon SE, et al. Somatosensory evoked potentials fail to diagnose thoracic outlet syndrome. *J Hand Surg (AM)* 1996;21:662–666.
13. Tender GC, Thomas J, Thomas N, et al. Gilliatt-Sumner hand revisited: a 25-year experience. *Neurosurgery* 2004;55:883–890.
14. Machanic DI, Sanders RJ. Medial antebrachial cutaneous nerve measurements to diagnose neurogenic thoracic outlet syndrome. *Ann Vasc Surg* 2008;22:248–254.
15. Jordan SE, Machleder HI. Diagnosis of thoracic outlet syndrome using electrophysiologically guided anterior scalene blocks. *Ann Vasc Surg* 1998;12:260–264.
16. Jordan SE, Ahn SS, Freischlag JA, et al. Selective botulinum chemodenervation of the scalene muscles for treatment of neurogenic thoracic outlet syndrome. *Ann Vasc Surg* 2000;14:365–369.
17. Jordan SE, Ahn SS, Gelabert H. Combining ultrasonography and electromyography for botulinum denervation treatment of thoracic outlet syndrome: comparison with fluoroscopy and electromyography guidance. *Pain Physician* 2007;10:541–546.
18. Hingorani A, Ascher E, Lorenson E, et al. Upper extremity deep venous thrombosis and its impact on morbidity and mortality rates in a hospital-based population. *J Vasc Surg* 1997;26:853–860.
19. Sharafuddin MJ, Sun S, Hoballah JJ. Endovascular management of venous thrombotic diseases of the upper torso and extremities. *J Vasc Interv Radiol* 202;13:975–990.
20. Bjarnason H, Hunter DW, Drain MR, et al. Collapse of a Palmaz stent in the subclavian vein. *AJR Am J Roentgenol* 1993;160:1123–1124.
21. Lee MC, Grassi CJ, Belkin M, et al. Early operative intervention after thrombolytic therapy for primary subclavian vein thrombosis: an effective treatment approach. *J Vasc Surg* 1998;27:1101–1108.
22. Sanders RJ, Cooper MA. Surgical management of subclavian vein obstruction, including six cases of subclavian vein bypass. *Surgery* 1995;118:856–863.
23. Lee WA, Hill BB, Harris JJ, et al. Surgical intervention is not required for all patients with subclavian vein thrombosis. *J Vasc Surg* 2000;32:57–67.
24. Lokanathan R, Salvian AJ, Chen JC, et al. Outcome after thrombolysis and selective thoracic outlet decompression as primary axillary vein thrombosis. *J Vasc Surg* 2001;33:783–788.
25. Sanders RJ, Monsour JW, Baer SB. Transaxillary first rib resection for the thoracic outlet syndrome. *Arch Surg* 1968;97:1014–1023.
26. Roos DB. Transaxillary approach for first rib resection to relieve thoracic outlet syndrome. *Ann Surg* 1996;163:354–358.
27. Sanders RJ, Raymer S. The supraclavicular approach to scalenectomy and first rib resection: description of technique. *J Vasc Surg* 1985;2:751–756.
28. Tender GC, Kline DE. Posterior subscapular approach to the brachial plexus. *Neurosurgery* 2005;57(4 suppl):377–381.
29. Roos DB. Congenital anomalies associated with thoracic outlet syndrome. *Am J Surg* 1976;132:777–778.
30. Sanders RJ, Pearce WH. The treatment of thoracic outlet syndrome: a comparison of different operations. *J Vasc Surg* 1989;10:626–634.
31. Cheng SW, Reilly LM, Nelken NA, et al. Neurogenic thoracic outlet decompression: rationale for sparing the first rib. *Cardiovasc Surg* 1995;3:617–623.
32. Sanders RJ, Rao NM. Pectoralis minor obstruction of the axillary veins: report of six patients. *J Vasc Surg* 2007;45:1206–1211.
33. Franklin GM, Fulton-Kehoe D, Bradley C, et al. Outcome of surgery for thoracic outlet syndrome in Washington state workers' compensation. *Neurology* 2000;54:1252–1257.
34. Ambrad-Chelala E, Thomas GI, Johansen KH. Recurrent neurogenic thoracic outlet syndrome. *Am J Surg* 2004;187:505–510.
35. Illig K, Thompson R, Freischlag J, et al, eds. *Thoracic Outlet Syndrome.* London: Springer-Verlag; 2014.
36. Illig K, Donahue D, Duncan A, et al. Reporting standards of the Society for Vascular Surgery for thoracic outlet syndrome: executive summary. *J Vasc Surg* 2016;64:797–802.

CHAPTER 40

Pain Following Spinal Cord Injury

KEVIN N. ALSCHULER, MARIA REGINA REYES, and **THOMAS N. BRYCE**

Pain following spinal cord injury (SCI) is common and includes a spectrum of pain types which can impact function across the physical, psychological, and social domains. This chapter provides an overview of SCI-related pain, including the extent and impact, assessment and classification, psychosocial aspects, and treatment.

Extent and Impact of the Problem

Four out of five individuals with SCI report pain, defined as an unpleasant sensory and emotional experience associated with actual or potential tissue damage[1] as an ongoing problem.[2] Many individuals with SCI and pain do not have just one pain but experience at least two different distinct types of pain with many reporting three or more.[3,4] In the same person, this might, for example, include shoulder pain from overuse and neuropathic pain related to SCI or spinal cord disease.

In more than half of individuals who report ongoing pain, the ongoing pain interferes with activities of daily living and work,[2] whereas one out of every five individuals with SCI who is unemployed reports that it is pain rather than loss of function that prevents them from working.[5] One out of every four people with SCI and significant pain note they would be willing to trade a chance of recovery of bowel, bladder, or sexual function for relief from the pain.[6]

Pain prevalence does not differ among those with different levels of injury nor degree of completeness of injury.[7] The same holds for men and women with SCI with neither group being more likely to report pain.[7]

Assessment and Classification of Pain Following Spinal Cord Injury

Most pains after SCI are either nociceptive or neuropathic. Nociceptive pain occurs when intact peripheral nerve sensory receptors capable of transducing and encoding noxious stimuli (also known as nociceptors) are activated within an intact somatosensory nervous system, whereas neuropathic pain occurs when a lesion or disease of the somatosensory nervous system activates the somatosensory nervous system.[1,8]

The International Spinal Cord Injury Pain (ISCIP) Classification was developed to organize the different types of pain seen after SCI in to an easily understandable framework (Table 40.1).[9,10] Within this framework, in addition to the nociceptive and neuropathic pain types, there is a third type of pain, labeled as "other" pain, for which no identifiable noxious stimulus nor any inflammation or damage to the nervous system responsible for the pain can be identified. Pain syndromes of unknown etiology such as fibromyalgia and complex regional pain syndrome type I fall into this category.

The ISCIP Classification is an integral part of the International Spinal Cord Injury Pain Basic Data Set (ISCIPBDS) (Table 40.2),[11] one of more than 20 data sets which have been developed to standardize clinical data collection related to SCI throughout the world.[12]

In determining where a particular pain that a person describes fits within the ISCIP Classification, it is helpful for clinicians to elicit the seven cardinal pain attributes described in Table 40.3 through the completion of a thorough history and physical examination. This physical examination should include a neurologic examination which incorporates the International Standards for the Neurological Classification of SCI as a correct neurologic classification of the SCI and is essential in order to correctly differentiate between at-level and below-level SCI pain and to provide insight into the likelihood of nociceptive pains being perceived in relation to retained sensation.[13]

As it is clear that that there can be an enormous emotional, physical, and social impact of pain on a person's daily life, any assessment of pain is not complete without an assessment of the numerous psychosocial factors and conditions that have been associated with pain-related distress and pain-related functional disability after SCI. It is important to obtain a psychosocial history that includes an assessment of present and past mental health history, as well as a more general understanding of the patient's perception of pain, with specific focus on important coping strategies, such as pain catastrophizing. Furthermore, the assessment should seek to understand how environmental factors, such as the impact of the workplace or home environment, or social factors, such as interactions with family, friends, and coworkers when a person is in pain, contribute to the chronic pain experience. To aid in this assessment, clinicians may find it useful to use questionnaires to routinely screen for common difficulties, such as mood disorders. Measures like the Patient Health Questionnaire-9 (PHQ-9) or its 2-item form, the PHQ-2, are validated in SCI and can be quickly scored and interpreted.[14] All of these psychosocial factors and conditions also referred to as yellow flags (Table 40.4)[15] must be addressed if the treatment of pain is to be successful if they are contributing to ongoing or worsening pain. At an absolute minimum, pain interference with sleep, mood, and activities should always be evaluated and therefore are included in the ISCIPBDS (see Table 40.2).[11]

TABLE 40.1	The International Spinal Cord Injury Pain Classification[10]	
Tier 1: Pain Type	**Tier 2: Pain Subtype**	**Tier 3: Primary Pain Source and/or Pathology (Examples of)**
Nociceptive pain	Musculoskeletal pain	Lateral epicondylitis, comminuted femur fracture, muscle spasm
	Visceral pain	Abdominal pain owing to bowel impaction, cholecystitis
	Other nociceptive pain	Migraine headache, surgical skin incision
Neuropathic pain	At-level SCI pain	Spinal cord compression, nerve root compression
	Below-level SCI pain	Spinal cord ischemia, spinal cord compression
	Other neuropathic pain	Carpal tunnel syndrome
Other pain		Fibromyalgia, complex regional pain syndrome type I, interstitial cystitis, irritable bowel syndrome
Unknown pain		

SCI, spinal cord injury.

TABLE 40.2   International Spinal Cord Injury Pain Basic Data Set (Complete for Each Different Pain)[11]

Pain Locations/Sites (Can Be More than One, Check All that Apply): Right (R), Midline (M), or Left (L)	R	M	L	Type of Pain / Intensity and Duration of Pain / Treatment of Pain
Head				Type of pain (check one):
Neck/shoulders		▨		
Throat				**Nociceptive**
Neck				☐ Musculoskeletal
Shoulder		▨		☐ Visceral
Arms/hands		▨		☐ Other
Upper arm				
Elbow				**Neuropathic**
Forearm				☐ At-level SCI
Wrist				☐ Below-level SCI
Hand/fingers				☐ Other
Frontal torso/genitals		▨		
Chest				☐ **Other**
Abdomen				
Pelvis/genitalia				☐ **Unknown**
Back		▨		
Upper back				
Lower back				**Intensity and duration of pain:**
Buttocks/hips		▨		**Average pain intensity in the last week:** 0 = no pain; 10 = pain as bad as you can imagine
Buttocks				☐ 0; ☐ 1; ☐ 2; ☐ 3; ☐ 4; ☐ 5; ☐ 6; ☐ 7; ☐ 8; ☐ 9; ☐ 10
Hip				
Anus		▨		
Upper leg/thigh		▨		Date of onset: YYYY/MM/DD
Lower legs/feet		▨		
Knee				**Are you using or receiving any treatment for your pain problem?**
Shin				☐ No ☐ Yes
Calf				
Ankle				
Foot/toes		▨		

In general, how much has pain interfered with your day-to-day activities in the last week?
0 = no pain; 10 = pain as bad as you can imagine
☐ 0; ☐ 1; ☐ 2; ☐ 3; ☐ 4; ☐ 5; ☐ 6; ☐ 7; ☐ 8; ☐ 9; ☐ 10

In general, how much has pain interfered with your overall mood in the last week?
0 = no pain; 10 = pain as bad as you can imagine
☐ 0; ☐ 1; ☐ 2; ☐ 3; ☐ 4; ☐ 5; ☐ 6; ☐ 7; ☐ 8; ☐ 9; ☐ 10

In general, how much has pain interfered with your ability to get a good night's sleep?
0 = no pain; 10 = pain as bad as you can imagine
☐ 0; ☐ 1; ☐ 2; ☐ 3; ☐ 4; ☐ 5; ☐ 6; ☐ 7; ☐ 8; ☐ 9; ☐ 10

MUSCULOSKELETAL PAIN

Musculoskeletal pain is nociceptive pain resulting from activation of nociceptors within musculoskeletal structures including muscles, tendons, ligaments, and bones within areas of at least partially retained sensation. In areas of apparent complete loss of sensation, nociceptors may be activated and can exacerbate at-level and below-level neuropathic pain as well as trigger autonomic dysreflexia (AD) and AD headache (see "Other Nociceptive Pain" section). Musculoskeletal pain typically changes in intensity with movement or palpation of the responsible musculoskeletal structures in which the nociceptors are activated. Appropriate imaging (x-ray, magnetic resonance imaging [MRI], ultrasound) often shows musculoskeletal pathology consistent with the pain presentation. As might be expected after a traumatic SCI, musculoskeletal pain is common in the acute period related to acute fractures of the spine and other musculoskeletal trauma.[16,17] Subsequently, this acute injury–related pain resolves, and other pains then begin to appear as individuals begin to function in new ways which predispose them to develop overuse injuries.

If it is unclear if a particular pain is nociceptive or neuropathic, as musculoskeletal pain typically responds better than other types of pain to rest, joint protection, anti-inflammatory medications, and physical measures such as stretching and massage, treatment of the pain using these specific interventions may be diagnostic. The converse may also be true in that many of the adjuvant medications recommended for the treatment of neuropathic pain such as those within the gabapentinoid and antidepressant classes may also be effective in ameliorating nociceptive pain.

Shoulder Pain

Approximately one-half of individuals with SCI, including people with either paraplegia or tetraplegia and complete

TABLE 40.3 Cardinal Pain Attributes[210]

Pain Attribute	Examples of Usefulness for SCI Pain Classification
History of onset	• Links the SCI to a specific pain • Indicates a pain generator through the mechanism of inciting event
Pain location	• Indicates a neuropathic type when occurring at or below the level of injury in a specific pattern • Indicates pain generator through its specific location
Temporal pattern	• Differentiates between subtypes, as nociceptive pain often is present only when there is stimulation of offending nociceptors, whereas neuropathic pain often may be more persistent due to damage related neuronal ectopy
Pain quality	• Indicates subtype, especially if a few specific descriptors such as "burning," "electric shock-like," or "tender" are specified, as the first two descriptors are more commonly seen in neuropathic types, whereas the latter is commonly described for nociceptive pain
Ameliorating and exacerbating factors	• Differentiates nociceptive and neuropathic subtypes, especially if movement is involved, as a pain generator can often be localized by replicating exacerbating factors
Associated sensory disturbances	• Allodynia or hyperpathia, either noted on history or on physical examination, are highly suggestive of neuropathic subtypes.
Pain intensity	• Intensity is an accepted proxy for severity of pain and is the most commonly used measure of the effectiveness of treatment.

SCI, spinal cord injury.

or incomplete injuries who use all types of mobility devices ranging from wheelchairs to ambulatory assist devices, experience shoulder pain.[18] In the acute period after SCI, shoulder pain is thought to develop due to the high demand on unconditioned muscles, whereas in the chronic phase, shoulder pain is thought to be related to overuse from repetitive motions and secondary degeneration of affected musculoskeletal structures.

Either global shoulder muscle weakness related to a high level cervical SCI or an imbalance of specific stabilizing muscles of the shoulder and scapula can be a factor in the development of pain in both acute and chronic phases for individuals with paraplegia or tetraplegia. This imbalance can develop insidiously through relative strengthening of certain muscles (e.g., shoulder abductors and flexors) with everyday activities such as transfers and wheelchair propulsion or through substitution of different muscles in those with cervical SCI if some of the usual shoulder stabilizers are not fully innervated and are therefore weak. Different activities stress different muscles; for example, in propelling a wheelchair up a ramp, the greatest activation is found in the shoulder flexors followed by the external rotators. This is in contrast to the greatest activation in the sternal pectoralis major muscle followed by the infraspinatus and supraspinatus muscles during push-up lift maneuvers.[19,20] It has been shown that many individuals who develop shoulder pain have decreased muscle strength, particularly in the shoulder adductors, and lower levels of physical activity even before the onset of pain.[21]

TABLE 40.4 Yellow Flags: Psychosocial Factors and Conditions Associated with Pain-Related Distress and Functional Disability[15]

Psychosocial Factors and Conditions

Depression often manifesting with decreased appetite, poor sleep, and low energy and lack interest in activities

Anxiety

Poor motivation to complete daily activities or work because of pain

Decreased participation in valued activities

Avoidance of activities associated with pain

A history of preexisting pain problems

Poor coping especially with evidence of catastrophic thinking

Use and dependence on alcohol or illicit substances

Use and dependence on prescribed opioids, especially if there is evidence of misuse

Acquired tightness of the shoulder capsule and contracture of the scapular thoracic articulation caused by a lack of passive or active range of motion and underlying spasticity are also commonly associated with shoulder pain in individuals with tetraplegia, much less so in individuals with paraplegia. Individuals with tetraplegia are also more likely to have pain related to shoulder instability resulting from weakness of the muscles that stabilize the shoulder joint.

Specific etiologies of shoulder pain related to all of the mentioned mechanisms include the rotator cuff impingement syndrome, subacromial bursitis, bicipital tendonitis, adhesive capsulitis, and osteoarthritis.[22–24]

Elbow and Wrist Pain

Musculoskeletal causes of elbow pain in persons with SCI include medial and lateral epicondylitis, triceps tendonitis, osteoarthritis, and olecranon bursitis. The latter often occurs in individuals who lean on their elbows for balance support or in those who push off with their elbows to assist with positioning and bed mobility.

Common musculoskeletal causes of wrist pain in adults include de Quervain tenosynovitis, inflammation/arthritis of the carpometacarpophalangeal joint of the thumb, and arthritis of the wrist. These typically are overuse injuries caused, for example, by repetitive grasping of a wheelchair push rim during wheelchair propulsion.

Back Pain

Musculoskeletal back pain in persons with SCI is common for a number of reasons, including a high prevalence of spinal surgeries, trunk muscle imbalances owing to spasticity and/or trunk weakness, kyphoscoliosis, and frequent dependence on wheelchairs. Structures in which nociceptors may be activated in and near the spine include muscles, tendons, and ligaments; the facet joint; the intervertebral disk; and the sacroiliac joint. Pain caused by spinal instability or spinal hardware failure is typically primarily nociceptive. After a portion of the spine is fused, the spinal segments adjacent to (above or below) the fusion often compensate for the lost motion of the fused segments and, over time, develop secondary degeneration and often pain. Sitting in a wheelchair, especially sitting in a kyphotic posture, can induce back pain in individuals with or without SCI.[25]

When an individual with limited hip flexion range (usually less than 90 degrees) is positioned for an extended period in a wheelchair with a seatback angle of 90 degrees, he or she is at increased risk of acquiring back pain depending on the degree of at least partially preserved sensation. If the lack of hip flexion is unilateral, the individual will accommodate to leaning to the side opposite whenever sitting. If the lack of hip flexion is bilateral, the only way the individual will be able to "fit" within the chair is to have his or her ischial tuberosities (and sacrum) contact the seat more anteriorly than is optimal causing the lumbar spine to be unsupported and the thoracic spine to assume an exaggerated kyphotic posture.

Muscle Pain Related to Spasticity

Spasticity is a syndrome of different components, including a velocity-dependent increased resistance to passive motion, involuntary muscle contractions or spasms, and hyperreflexia. The involuntary muscle contractions result from different muscles acting synergistically, typically in a specific flexion or extension pattern. In someone with retained sensation, continuous or paroxysmal muscle spasms are often painful. Spasticity when significant and present to a greater degree on one side of the trunk as compared to the other often causes a coronal imbalance in spinal alignment (or a functional scoliosis) which can lead to musculoskeletal back pain especially in those with retained sensation in the spinal region of imbalance. Nociceptors activated through this coronal imbalance may arise not only from spastic muscles such as for instance the quadratus lumborum and thoracolumbar paraspinals but also from within the sacroiliac joint and lumbar facet joints on the side with more significant spasticity through the greater forces transmitted through these joints.

VISCERAL PAIN

Visceral pain refers to pain located in the thorax, abdomen, or pelvis, which is believed to be primarily generated in visceral structures.[10] Visceral pain of gastrointestinal system origin often is temporally related to food intake or bowel function and can be associated with symptoms of AD, anorexia, nausea, or vomiting as well, any of which can be more prominent than the pain itself. Tenderness to palpation of the abdomen is a common physical sign (in persons with some retained trunk sensation) as are the pain descriptors of "cramping," "dull," or "tender." The characteristics of chronic abdominal pain in SCI are very similar to those of chronic constipation,[26] and appropriate imaging often shows visceral pathology consistent with the pain presentation (e.g., colonic distension by stool). Abdominal visceral pain has a late onset being relatively uncommon during the first 5 years after SCI and increasing in prevalence afterward with approximately one-fifth of those at 10 years and one-third of those at 20 years reporting it; the prevalence does not seem to increase after 20 years, however.[27]

Other less common causes of visceral pain include bowel obstruction, bowel infarction, bowel perforation, cholecystitis, choledocholithiasis, pancreatitis, appendicitis, splenic rupture, bladder perforation, pyelonephritis, urinary tract infection, or superior mesenteric syndrome. As individuals with limited somatic sensation in the abdominal wall may experience only dull or aching pain, even with serious intra-abdominal emergencies such as acute appendicitis, cholecystitis, peritonitis, bowel obstruction, or mesenteric artery thrombosis, a degree of suspicion for these other causes should always be maintained.

OTHER NOCICEPTIVE PAIN

Other (nociceptive) pain refers to a nociceptive pain that does not fall into either the musculoskeletal or visceral categories.[10] These pains may be indirectly related to the SCI (e.g., pain from nociceptor activation within the disrupted integument due to pressure injury) or may be unrelated to SCI (e.g., migraine headache).[28]

One particular other nociceptive pain worthy of special mention is headache pain due to AD. It can be severe and usually is described as "pounding." It is most common in a person with a neurologic level of injury (NLI) at or above T6. AD headache is associated with an elevated blood pressure and often with diaphoresis, piloerection, cutaneous vasodilatation above the level of injury, bradycardia or tachycardia, nasal stuffiness, conjunctival congestion, and mydriasis. AD is usually triggered by a noxious stimulus caudal to the NLI, usually related to the bowel or bladder (e.g., bowel impaction or urinary tract infection).

An algorithm for the assessment of nociceptive pain developed by Siddall and Middleton[29] is outlined in Figure 40.1.

AT- AND BELOW-LEVEL SPINAL CORD INJURY PAIN

At-level SCI pain is neuropathic pain perceived within the dermatome of the NLI and/or a maximum of three dermatomes below this level. It must be attributed to damage to the spinal cord or nerve roots.[11] Pain thought due to injury to the cauda equina is always classified as at-level SCI pain. One-third of individuals with SCI report at-level SCI pain soon after injury, and its prevalence over time does not seem to change.[16,17] At-level SCI pain is suggested by altered sensation within the painful area, especially allodynia or hyperalgesia, and the descriptors of "hot," "burning," "tingling," "pricking," "pins and needles," "sharp," "shooting," "squeezing," "painful cold," or "electric shock-like."[10] It is usually difficult to distinguish between the two subcategories of at-level SCI pain, spinal cord pain and radicular pain, because both are typically involved in any traumatic SCI and may have the exact same clinical presentation. However, radicular pain is generally, although not always, unilateral and radiating in a dermatomal pattern. When at-level SCI pain is associated with spinal instability where spinal movement exacerbates the pain especially if there is evidence of nerve root traction or compression, the pain is presumably more likely to be radicular in etiology. Neuropathic pain in this location at or inferiorly adjacent to the NLI that is not attributed to either spinal cord or nerve root damage should be classified as other neuropathic pain and not as at-level SCI pain. One example of other neuropathic pain is focal peripheral nerve compression (e.g., symptomatic carpal tunnel syndrome in a person with a lower cervical SCI).

Below-level SCI pain refers to neuropathic pain perceived more than three dermatomes below the NLI, with or without extension up to the NLI, that is attributed to damage to the spinal cord.[10] If a pain that occurs within the NLI and the three dermatomes immediately below the NLI is considered by the individual experiencing it to be the same pain that is experienced distal to those three dermatomes adjacent to the NLI, this pain should be classified as a single below-level pain and not as at-level and below-level pain.

The pain distribution of below-level spinal cord pain should be thought of, not as dermatomal, but regional, enveloping large areas such as the anal region, the bladder, the genitals, the legs, or commonly the entire body below the NLI. It is usually continuous in presence, although the intensity of the pain can fluctuate in response to yellow flag factors and conditions (see Table 40.4), fatigue, smoking, noxious stimuli below the level of injury, and weather changes.

Less than one-fifth of individuals report below-level SCI pain in the first year after injury, but its prevalence increases to approximately one-third after the first year and beyond.[16,17,30] Below-level SCI pain can occur in persons with complete or incomplete SCI, and its descriptors are the same as those listed for at-level SCI pain.[10] Allodynia or hyperalgesia can be present within the pain distribution for persons with incomplete injuries. In fact, sensory hypersensitivity (particularly cold-evoked dysesthesia) at 1 month postinjury seems to be a predictor for

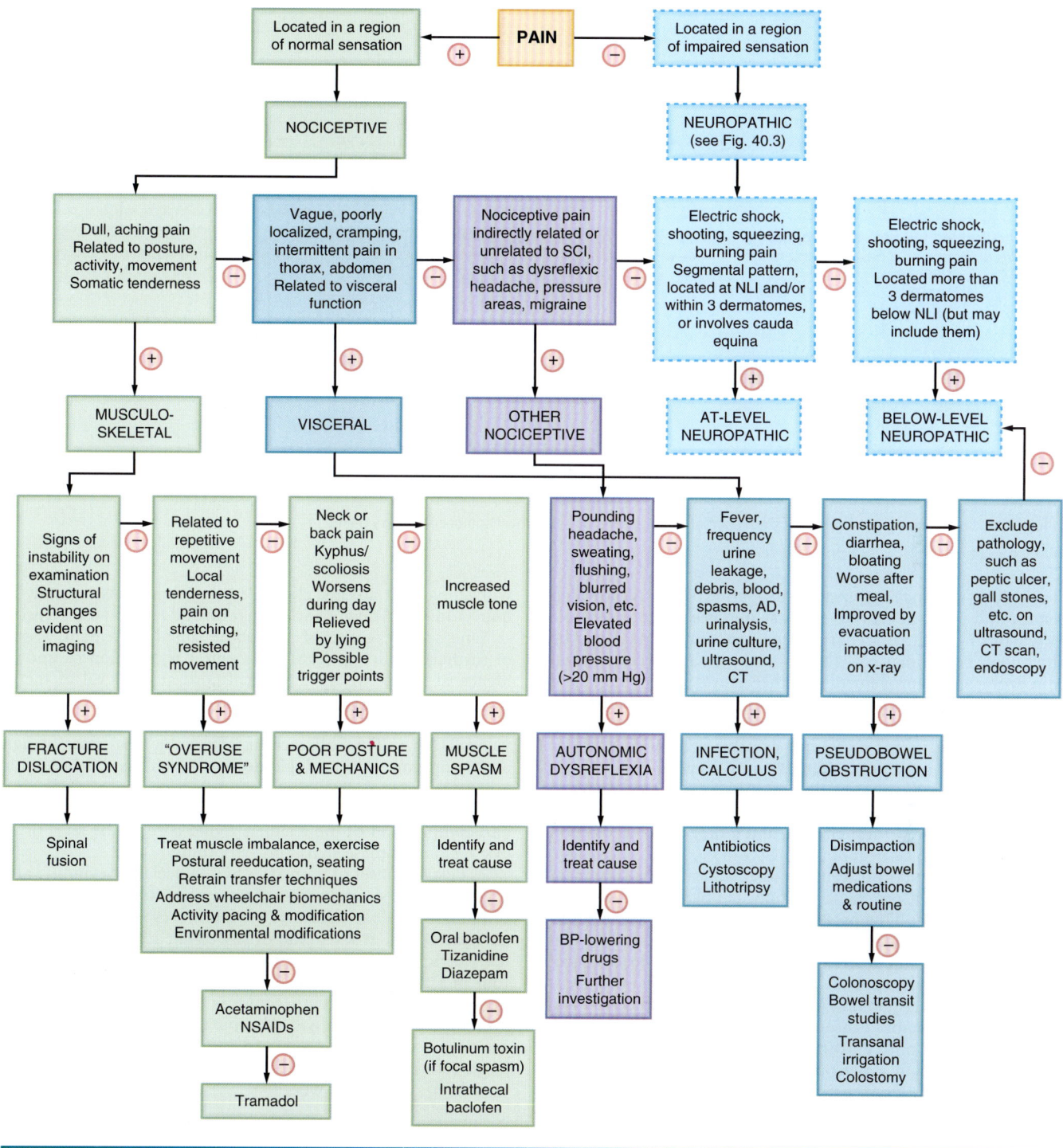

FIGURE 40.1 Algorithm for assessing and treating nociceptive pain after spinal cord injury. (*From Chhabra HS. ISCoS Text Book on Comprehensive Management of Spinal Cord Injuries. 1st ed. New Delhi: Wolters Kluwer; 2015. Figure 55.3.*)

the development of below-level SCI pain at 1 year.[16] Similar to at-level SCI pain, neuropathic pain that occurs in this distribution that cannot be attributed to spinal cord damage should be classified as other neuropathic pain and not as below-level SCI pain.

An evaluation including search for potentially treatable causes of neuropathic pain, such as nerve root or spinal cord compression, tethering, or posttraumatic syringomyelia (PTS), should be initiated when the cause is not clearly apparent.

There are three scenarios where worsening of already established neuropathic pain can be seen (Fig. 40.2). In the first, the worsening is due to the natural history of the pain related to ongoing neuroplastic changes occurring within the nervous system during that first year after SCI. In the second, there is progression of the neurologic injury (nerve root or spinal cord) due to changes in degree of nerve root or spinal cord compression, tethering, or PTS. In the third and probably most common scenario, there is the development of a red flag condition

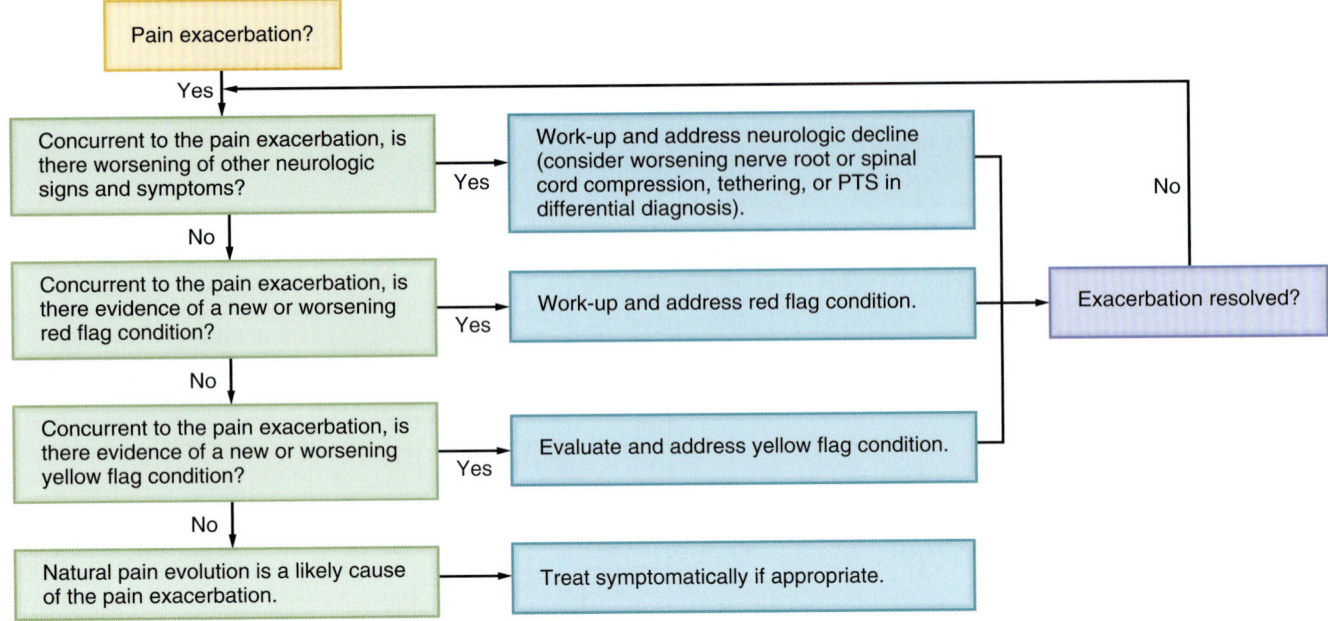

FIGURE 40.2 Algorithm for evaluating an exacerbation of at-level or below-level spinal cord injury pain.

(Table 40.5) that may aggravate neuropathic pain.[15] A thorough history and physical exam is the first step needed to determine to which of the three scenarios the worsening of pain can be attributed. For evidence of the first, which we can call natural pain evolution, improvements in other neurologic findings such as improved sensation and motor strength on examination (or at least no signs of neurologic deterioration) can be reassuring. In contrast, concurrent worsening of other neurologic findings such as loss of sensation, strength, and deep tendon reflexes indicates that the neurologic decline is likely due to changes in or development of nerve root or cord compression, tethering, or PTS or other structural change, and a diagnostic workup in most cases should be begun.

Evidence for the third scenario, aggravation of existing neuropathic pain by a red flag condition, is bolstered by a stable neurologic exam and the presence of signs and symptoms pointing to changes in other organ systems. It is not uncommon that associated changes in severity of at-level or below-level neuropathic pain can even be more prominent than those other signs and symptoms of a potential red flag condition. These red flag conditions presumably cause ascending noxious stimuli which provide feedback onto existing pain pathways (not necessarily perceived as such in a person with impaired or absent sensation), although the exact pathophysiologic mechanisms for the worsening pain are not clear. Red flag conditions typically require additional diagnostic evaluation and medical intervention.

One specific cause of late-onset spinal cord pain worthy of further mention is PTS. Although it is common to find evidence of a cyst within the spinal cord at the level of the injury using appropriate imaging (MRI or computed tomography [CT] myelogram), only 2% to 5% of all people with SCI develop PTS.[31–33] The hallmark of PTS is the new onset of signs and symptoms of neurologic decline which may include pain, sensory loss, weakness, altered muscle tone, and various autonomic symptoms presumably caused by expansion of the cyst and compression of the residual spinal cord at the level of the cyst leading to these signs and symptoms.

A delayed onset of pain after SCI, especially beginning after 1 year, should strongly raise the suspicion of PTS as the cause of pain.[32–35] Bulbar signs and symptoms, especially facial pain, associated with at-level pain of late onset, are rare but virtually diagnostic of PTS. The most commonly reported initial symptom of PTS is pain, either unilateral or bilateral,[32,36] whereas pain presenting only with cough is not an uncommon initial presentation historically.[34] "Burning," "dull," and "aching" are the most commonly reported descriptors reported in several large series, although "sharp," "electrical," and "stabbing" have been reported as well.[32,33,37]

TABLE 40.5   Red Flag Conditions that May Cause, Aggravate, or Mimic Neuropathic Pain and that Require Further Investigation and Prompt Medical Review[15]

System	Red Flag Indicators	Red Flag Conditions
Musculoskeletal	Recent trauma, new deformity, changes in range of motion, new-onset localized swelling, and warmth	Fracture or dislocation, heterotopic ossification
Dermatologic	Redness, ulceration	Pressure injury, ingrown nail
Cardiovascular	Chest pain, shortness of breath, fevers, chills or sweats, autonomic symptoms, new limb swelling	Abdominal aortic aneurysm, aortic dissection, myocardial infarction, deep vein thrombosis
Respiratory	Chest pain, shortness of breath	Pulmonary embolism, pneumonia
Genitourinary	Changes in urine appearance or smell, pain over kidneys, new incontinence, leakage between catheterizations, a history of renal or bladder calculi, scrotal or testicular swelling	Lower urinary tract infection, pyelonephritis, renal or bladder calculi, urinary retention, testicular torsion, epididymitis
Pelvic	Relation of pain to menstruation	Ovarian cysts, endometriosis and other genitourinary conditions
Gastrointestinal	Changes in bowel habit, distended abdomen	Stool impaction, constipation, volvulus, appendicitis, cholecystitis

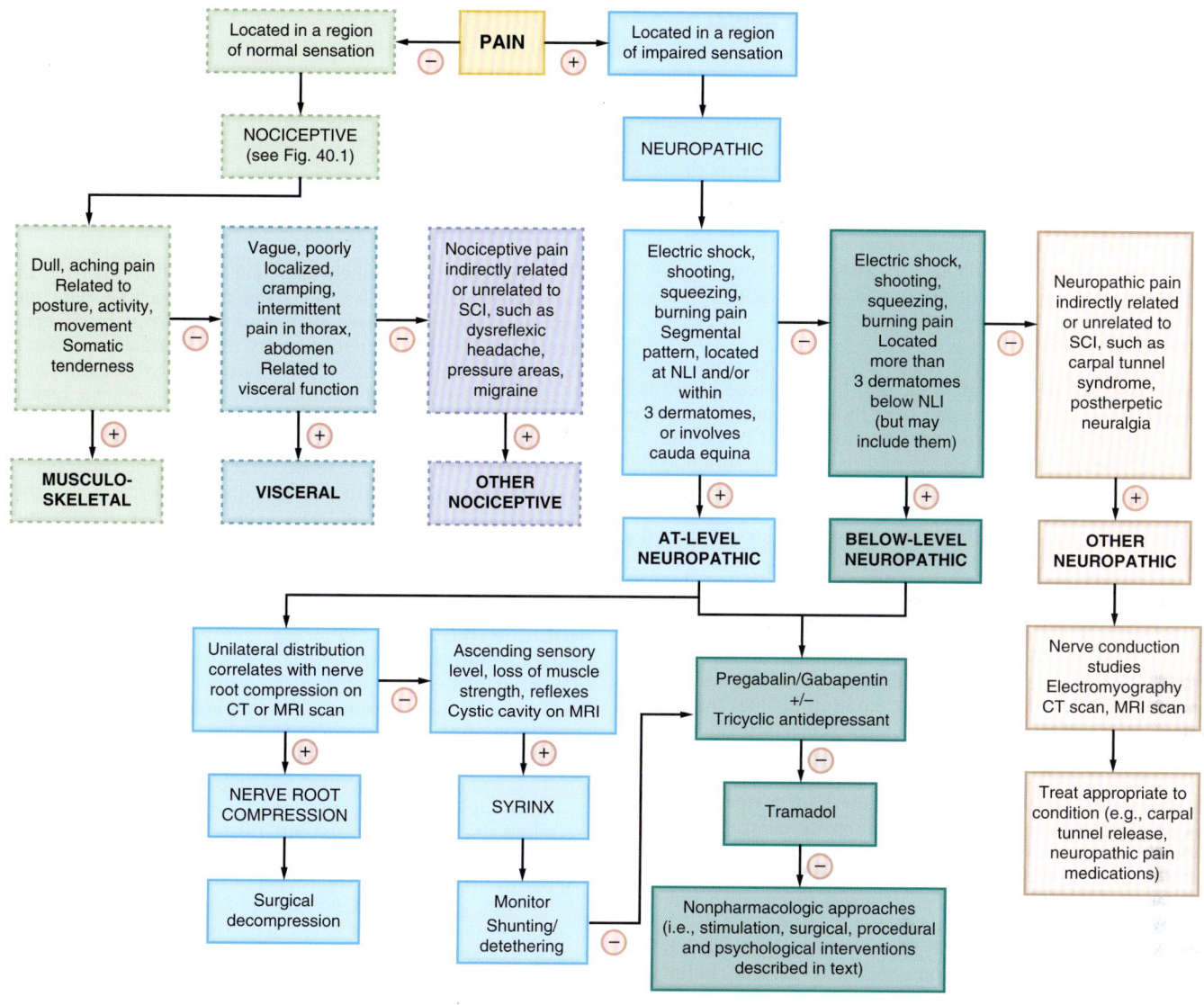

FIGURE 40.3 Algorithm for assessing and treating neuropathic pain. *(From Chhabra HS. ISCoS Text Book on Comprehensive Management of Spinal Cord Injuries. 1st ed. New Delhi: Wolters Kluwer; 2015. Figure 55.4.)*

MRI is the diagnostic study of choice in the evaluation of PTS, although a CT myelogram with up to 24-hour delayed imaging often will show contrast dye within a syrinx cavity in those for whom an MRI is unobtainable.

Another late cause of neuropathic pain is spinal cord or nerve root tethering. Tethering of the spinal cord is a result of meningeal or arachnoid scar formations that can occur after SCI and prevent normal rostrocaudal sliding of the cord within the spinal canal. Tethering of the cord in the cervical spine can generate enough cord traction with flexion of the neck to cause cord or brainstem displacement and neurologic symptoms, including pain, weakness, and sensory deficits. Tethering of the thoracic and lumbar spine often also includes changes in bowel and bladder function. MRI is the diagnostic study of choice for the evaluation of tethering.

At-level spinal cord and nerve root and below-level SCI can result from late compression of the spinal cord or nerve roots by progressive spondylosis, progressive spinal deformity caused by posttraumatic or surgical destabilization, intervertebral disk herniation, or hardware failure. Nociceptive musculoskeletal pain is typically experienced concurrently. X-rays, CTs, and MRIs are the diagnostic studies of choice.

An algorithm for the assessment of neuropathic pain developed by Siddall and Middleton[29] is outlined in Figure 40.3.

OTHER NEUROPATHIC PAIN

Other neuropathic pain refers to neuropathic pain that is present above, at, or below the NLI but is not directly related to the SCI.[10] Compressive neuropathy pain fits within this category and occurs in a specific peripheral nerve distribution distal to the root level and is attributed to compression of a specific peripheral nerve or plexus of nerves, most commonly affecting not only the median nerve at the wrist but also the ulnar, radial, and axillary nerves. The signs and symptoms of carpal tunnel syndrome include numbness or tingling of thumb, index, or middle fingers; abnormal sensation on testing; or numbness or tingling with provocative tests. This syndrome is thought to result from a combination of repetitive trauma, as occurs with propulsion of manual wheelchairs, and ischemia from repetitive marked increases in carpal canal pressures, as occurs with push-up pressure reliefs or transfers from one seating surface to another.[38] A higher risk for developing pain has been shown in those who are overweight or use improper wheelchair propulsion biomechanics.[39]

PSYCHOSOCIAL ASPECTS OF PAIN AFTER SPINAL CORD INJURY

Psychosocial factors are understood to play a significant role in the chronic pain experience. In contrast to past generations of medicine where the mind–body dualistic perspective resulted in medically unexplained pain being labeled *psychogenic*, the modern biopsychosocial approach suggests that few patients—if any—should be classified in such a manner. In addition to being inaccurate, the diagnosis is also often counterproductive to successful pain management.[40] However, one must always be attentive to the psychosocial factors that may have a significant impact on pain intensity, function, and quality of life.

Psychological Factors

A growing body of research suggests a strong relationship between pain and psychological factors. Indeed, some have suggested that psychosocial rather than biologic factors are more closely associated with the presence and severity of pain.[4,6] Broadly, research on psychology and pain can be summarized in two areas.

The first explores the association between pain (primarily pain intensity) and psychological factors (primarily mood), through cross-sectional research. These studies have consistently identified strong relationships between psychological symptoms (depression, anxiety, and/or posttraumatic stress disorder [PTSD]) and pain intensity.[41–47] The few longitudinal studies have highlighted potential causal relationships, with one study supporting a likely bidirectional relationship, such that the presence of either pain or mood difficulties may make higher levels of the other more likely[48]; in contrast, another study more specifically highlighted the ways in which chronic pain contributes to depressed mood.[49] Furthermore, a longitudinal study assessing mood trajectories in people with SCI suggested that having greater pain intensity is associated with a moderate to severe depression trajectory.[50] As with much of the chronic pain experience, though, it is important to note that stronger relationships may be present between pain interference and mood rather than pain intensity and mood.[51]

The second broad area of pain psychology research refers to the ways in which a person copes with pain, including his or her thoughts, beliefs, and pain-related behaviors. Although these are generally factors that emerge once a person already has pain, it is important to recognize that how individuals approach their pain at onset may influence the evolution of their pain and function over time. The most commonly studied pain coping construct is pain catastrophizing, a maladaptive and disproportionate worry about chronic pain, which has consistently been associated with greater pain intensity and pain interference in persons with SCI.[52,53] Important implications also exist for other coping strategies, with task persistence repeatedly demonstrated as an adaptive approach, but guarding (e.g., tensing muscles for self-protection or avoiding engaging affected muscles) and resting (e.g., avoiding activity) have been found to be maladaptive approaches.[53] More generally, active coping strategies (e.g., those that promote engagement with the world) have more positive impacts on outcomes relative to passive coping strategies (e.g., those that cause an individual to withdraw from the world around them).[53,54] Finally, more recent research has emphasized the relationship of pain acceptance with pain-related outcomes, such that being willing to experience pain and/or engaging with valued life activities despite pain is associated with greater function and quality of life.[55,56]

Social and Environmental Factors

Research also suggests a strong association of social and environmental factors with the pain experience. In general, greater social support is associated with greater function in persons with chronic pain and disabilities, including SCI.[57]

However, functioning is greater in individuals who receive social support without solicitous responses relative to those who receive solicitous support.[53] Furthermore, perceived negative responses from friends, caregivers, and relatives may have a negative effect. For example, punishing responses have been shown to have a negative impact on pain severity.[58]

Management of Pain in People with Spinal Cord Injury

Effective management of chronic pain after SCI remains a clinical challenge. Although some types of nociceptive pain may respond to commonly used interventions, neuropathic SCI pain has been a poorly understood entity that is largely resistant to a variety of interventions.[59,60] Treatment approaches attempt to address the growing but incomplete body of knowledge regarding the multiple potential mechanisms underlying the development of neuropathic pain. Variable responses are common, and many interventions found to be successful in the treatment of non-SCI neuropathic pain have had disappointing results when applied to SCI neuropathic pain. The experience of pain must be considered and treated in the context of psychosocial factors. This section reviews existing literature for available interventions for chronic SCI pain.

NOCICEPTIVE PAIN
Musculoskeletal Pain

The principles of care used in the general population to treat degenerative and inflammatory musculoskeletal conditions may be applied to people with SCI, although there are specific therapeutic considerations.[61] For example, complete or even relative rest of a painful overused upper extremity can be difficult to implement in a person who is reliant on the upper extremities for all mobility. Activity restrictions may result in the need for additional caregiver or transportation services, new equipment such as power mobility, or modifications to transfer techniques. Surgery may not always result in good functional long-term outcomes due to the overuse of the repaired structures necessitated by the intrinsic limitations in functional mobility caused by SCI. Because of this impact, knowledgeable and timely treatment of such pain is critical to preserving independence. Physical and occupational therapy play a key role in appropriately adapting musculoskeletal care principles to those with impaired mobility, or utilizing SCI-specific protocols for addressing common musculoskeletal problems, such as shoulder impingement and dysfunction.[62,63]

The primary treatment strategy to address chronic nociceptive musculoskeletal pain after SCI is focused on addressing the established or probable etiologic condition and its root cause. Short-term and occasional long-term pharmacologic management may be required if nonpharmacologic interventions fail to sufficiently improve function and quality of life.

Nonpharmacologic Management

Factors that may lead to chronic inflammatory musculoskeletal pain include abnormal posture, altered gait or upper limb biomechanics, and the cumulative effects of repeated transfers and wheelchair or assistive device use. Correcting or reducing excessive mechanical stresses is a fundamental and key principle in the treatment of musculoskeletal SCI pain and can be addressed by appropriate education, retraining, and equipment modifications. Seating in wheelchair users influences not only trunk position but also shoulder position and biomechanical forces during wheelchair propulsion, transfer activities, and activities of daily living. Optimizing seated position is the foundation for long-term protection of upper limbs in wheelchair users. Comprehensive guidelines to address the highly prevalent problem of upper limb musculoskeletal SCI pain are available.[62]

Pharmacologic Management

Pharmacologic interventions for inflammatory musculoskeletal pain are often indicated. Options include the use of simple analgesics, nonsteroidal anti-inflammatory drugs (NSAIDs), local corticosteroid injections, and antispasticity medications.

Acetaminophen is preferable over NSAIDs as the first-line analgesic for musculoskeletal pain, due to the risk for NSAID-related gastric erosion and the potential for poor clinical detection of gastrointestinal bleeding in people with high SCI levels. However, cautious use of NSAIDs may be considered as the next option, in the absence of other contraindications, and preferably outside the acute period following SCI when the risk for gastritis is at its peak. If NSAIDs and acetaminophen are not appropriate or effective, opioids with relatively weak opioid activity, such as tramadol, would be reasonable. Rarely, "stronger" opioids may be necessary for short-term management of severely limiting pain such as might occur after surgery. However, the use of "stronger" opioids, as a treatment in chronic, noncancer pain is discouraged due to inconclusive or weak evidence in support of this practice[64,65] and high rates of adverse effects including tolerance, dependence (both physical and psychological), and opioid-induced hyperalgesia.[66] Specific considerations for long-term use of opioids in people with SCI, if they are used at all, include the potential for these drugs to exacerbate bowel or bladder dysfunction, contribute to cardiovascular and respiratory compromise, osteoporosis, and hypogonadism.[67–69] Case-by-case consideration for long-term opioid therapy should strictly follow published clinical and regulatory guidelines.[70–73]

Extended-release venlafaxine is a serotonin-norepinephrine reuptake inhibitor that has been used effectively to manage non-SCI nociceptive pain and neuropathic pain from peripheral sources.[74,75] Research of individuals with SCI and major depressive disorder suggests that *extended-release* venlafaxine may be superior to placebo in reducing nociceptive pain intensity and interference, with half of the subjects in one study experiencing >50% improvement in nociceptive pain intensity, whereas the same effect was not present for neuropathic pain.[76] Interestingly, in the same study, treatment with a minimally effective dose of 150 mg daily resulted in improved benefit profiles for subjects with mixed SCI pain.

Surgical Management

Stabilization is the most effective treatment for pain arising from spinal instability. Charcot spine, or traumatic spinal arthropathy, is a potential late complication after traumatic SCI that leads to instability. The affected segments typically involve the thoracolumbar spine. Patients with Charcot spine can present with back pain, a change in spasticity or bladder function, audible noises with trunk motion, or otherwise unexplained AD.[77–80] Timely diagnosis and stabilization is critical to prevent further progression of pain, deformity, or possible neurologic decline. Concurrent infection should be excluded and appropriately addressed if present.

Management of Spasticity-Related Pain

Spasticity is a common neuromuscular complication of SCI, affecting the majority of individuals with chronic SCI.[81,82] Spasticity can interfere with safe mobility, seating, or sleep and may cause varying levels of pain in some individuals. It is important to note that spasticity may also be beneficial when individuals use it to aid function such as to facilitate transfers. Therefore, the decision to treat spasticity should include weighing the beneficial effects of treatment such as pain relief with potential adverse effects of treatment such as sedation or functional loss. Because the features and mechanisms underlying muscle hypertonia associated with SCI spasticity are distinct from muscle spasms that occur in people who are neurologically intact, a different treatment approach is warranted. SCI disrupts descending inhibitory neural control pathways, resulting in hyperreflexia and spasticity in muscle groups below the NLI. People with chronic SCI will frequently develop a baseline level of spasticity and may also have exacerbations due to noxious triggers that maintain a heightened reflex arc, such as urinary tract infections or skin breakdown. In the latter, appropriate treatment would eliminate the induced nociceptor activation allowing the spasticity to return to a baseline level.

The current collective quality of evidence for antispasticity treatment is varied due in part to the multifaceted nature of spasticity and small studied subject populations. Common nonpharmacologic management options include stretching, positioning, heat or cold modalities, static and dynamic orthotic treatment, vibratory, and electrical stimulation. These are frequently used in conjunction with pharmacologic management. More comprehensive reviews are available on this topic.[83–85] However, conventional practice and the strongest level of evidence support the use of oral *baclofen*, a γ-aminobutyric acid (GABA) B spinal receptor agonist, as the first-line agent for SCI-related spasticity.[82] The primary limiting side effect is somnolence, and slow and cautious uptitration is critical. Cautious use in people with seizure disorder is indicated, as baclofen use can lower the seizure threshold. *Tizanidine* is an imidazoline derivative with affinity for spinal and supraspinal α_2 receptors and has reasonably strong evidence for efficacy in reducing polysynaptic reflexes contributing to spasticity in SCI. The drug enhances presynaptic inhibition.[86] When combined with CYP1A2 inhibitors, including ciprofloxacin, tizanidine may lead to heightened tizanidine adverse effects. Common side effects may include sedation, dry mouth, dizziness, and hypotension. Aminotransferase level monitoring is recommended due to the risk for hepatotoxicity.[87]

Benzodiazepines used for spasticity treatment include the GABAergic medications *diazepam*, *clonazepam*, and *clorazepate*. Diazepam was historically a mainstay in the treatment of SCI spasticity but is currently considered as a second- or third-line agent, after baclofen or tizanidine, and is primarily used to control nocturnal spasms that interfere with sleep quality, or if a parenteral antispasticity medication is needed. Consideration must be given to the potential for developing drug tolerance, as well as side effects such as sedation that are associated with benzodiazepine use, particularly if used in combination with other sedating agents. *Dantrolene*, a peripherally acting muscle relaxant, decreases calcium release from the sarcoplasmic reticulum, resulting in a reduction in the strength of muscle contractions. Although dantrolene is an appealing and reasonable adjunct antispasticity treatment that would theoretically limit cognitive adverse effects, evidence specifically addressing the treatment of SCI-related spasticity is scarce, and concerns regarding potential hepatotoxicity have led to its infrequent use in persons with spasticity related to SCI.

Chemodenervation via injection of *botulinum toxin* is widely used as an effective treatment for focal muscle spasticity for 3 months or longer, although the body of evidence for its efficacy in SCI spasticity is limited.[84,88,89] Direct neurolysis with alcohol or phenol disrupts the reflex arc that mediates spasticity and effectively creates lower motor neuron dysfunction in a selected distribution to reduce focal muscle spasticity. Effects typically last for at least 3 months, possibly longer.[89] Because of the risk for dysesthesias, alcohol or phenol nerve blocks are conventionally used to target peripheral nerves innervating larger muscle groups with limited sensory innervation, such as the obturator nerve to decrease adductor spasticity. Targeted motor point blocks to individual muscle branches may also be considered. However, there is a paucity of SCI-specific controlled studies that assess efficacy and safety of alcohol or phenol neurolytic and motor point blocks for spasticity treatment. Factors currently limiting widespread use include the greater time intensity with motor point localization compared to botulinum toxin chemodenervation, and fewer practitioners with experience in the injection technique. Given the potential to manage spasticity with fewer limiting adverse side effects, it is very reasonable to consider chemodenervation and neurolytic blocks to address localized muscle spasticity, either alone or in combination with other agents.

If these interventions fail to provide sufficient pain relief or result in unacceptable side effects, there are some evidence to support consideration of *intrathecal baclofen* administration via an implantable, programmable drug delivery device or pump. As with other treatment interventions for SCI-related spasticity, higher quality evidence for use of intrathecal baclofen in SCI is limited, although there is widespread and anecdotally successful use of this intervention.[90–92]

There are many proposed nonpharmacologic strategies for managing spasticity.[84] Stretching results in short-term spasticity reduction. Transcutaneous electrical nerve stimulation (TENS) has evidence from a small randomized controlled trial (RCT) to support spasticity reduction in SCI, whereas variable benefit has been documented in studies using functional and spinal cord electrical stimulation.[93–95]

In general, the treatment of SCI spasticity is complex and multidimensional and often involves a range of pharmacologic and nonpharmacologic interventions used in combination. As such, a physiatric consultation for spasticity assessment and management can be helpful in navigating all the options.

VISCERAL PAIN

The primary treatment approach for visceral SCI pain is the identification and appropriate treatment of the underlying painful condition, with specific consideration given to medical conditions frequently associated with SCI, such as complications of neurogenic bowel and bladder, or an atypical presentation of visceral disease, such as acute abdomen in those with high neurologic levels of injury.

OTHER NOCICEPTIVE PAIN

Treatment should be targeted for the specific condition, such as incisional pain or headache due to AD or migraine headache.

OTHER NEUROPATHIC PAIN AND OTHER PAIN

Pain attributed to compression or disease involving nerve roots, plexus, or peripheral nerves may be treated with therapy, orthotics, local or systemic medications, interventional procedures, or surgical decompression following similar indications and principles as the general population. However, special consideration should be given to the impact of activity or postoperative restrictions on the function of people with SCI. Treatment of complex regional pain syndrome often requires a comprehensive treatment plan and is discussed elsewhere.[96,97]

AT- AND BELOW-LEVEL NEUROPATHIC PAIN
Anticonvulsants

The ability of anticonvulsant or antiepileptic drugs to modulate excessive neuronal discharge by decreasing excitability or augmenting inhibition has led to its widespread adoption as the preferred treatment for various neuropathic pain conditions, including SCI. Drugs in this category modulate neuronal firing through a wide variety of cellular-level mechanisms, including decreasing sodium channel conductance, binding to the $\alpha_2\delta$ subunit of dorsal horn voltage-gated calcium channels or NMDA receptors, attenuation of excitatory glutamate release, or facilitation of GABAergic inhibition.

Gabapentinoids: *Gabapentin* and *pregabalin* are distinguished by an apparent dichotomy of structure and action. Although they are structurally related to GABA, they do not seem to significantly bind to GABA receptors or affect sodium conductance. Instead, these drugs purportedly interact primarily with the $\alpha_2\delta$ ligand of voltage-gated calcium ion channels, and

secondarily with NMDA receptors. A meta-analysis concluded that both gabapentin and pregabalin are effective at reducing SCI neuropathic pain intensity as well as improving sleep interference, anxiety, and depression.[98]

Pregabalin currently has the highest quality of evidence supporting its tolerability and efficacy in reducing SCI neuropathic pain. This body of evidence includes two large, multisite RCTs of subjects with SCI[99,100] and one RCT of subjects with central neuropathic pain, including a subpopulation with SCI.[101] The studies reported significant improvement in pain intensity among subjects with at- or below-level SCI neuropathic pain treated with a flexible regimen of 150 to 600 mg pregabalin daily. A significantly greater percentage of subjects who received pregabalin as compared to placebo reported at least 30% or 50% reduction in pain intensity and the studies showed improvement in secondary outcome measures such as sleep-related pain interference and health status. Therapeutic benefit was usually seen within 1 week.[99,102] The average effective daily dose in the studies was generally more than 350 mg per day, and in one study, two-thirds of participants received a maximum daily dose ranging between 450 and 600 mg daily.[100] The primary adverse effects were noted to be mild to moderate somnolence, dizziness, lower limb edema, dry mouth, and fatigue.[99,100]

Gabapentin has long been the mainstay in the treatment of various neuropathic pain conditions, albeit with conflicting and less robust evidence than pregabalin to support its use in SCI. An unequivocal determination of efficacy in previous studies may have been limited by the small sample sizes, dosing regimens with low maximal doses, or withdrawal due to adverse effects from rapid dose escalation. A significant reduction in neuropathic pain and improvement in most neuropathic pain subtypes (but not "itching," "dull," "sensitive," and "cold" characterized pains) has been reported in various studies.[103–106] Statistically significant pain relief has been achieved by the second week of gabapentin administration when subjects receive 1,800 mg daily. Gabapentin doses of 3,600 mg per day are tolerated by most people, although a significantly higher rate of adverse side effects in one study was seen in the active treatment group as compared to placebo (65% vs. 25%) that was both reversible with dose adjustment and did not result in withdrawal from the study. Primary adverse side effects noted with gabapentin treatment include somnolence, dizziness, weakness, edema, and vertigo.[103,107,108] Two RCTs, however, failed to demonstrate significant difference in pain intensity between gabapentin and placebo.[107,108] One of these studies showed a significant reduction in "unpleasant feeling" and a trend toward improved pain intensity and decreased burning pain.[107] A small sample size may have limited achieving significance. Despite the conflicting evidence, a meta-analysis of gabapentinoid treatment studies suggest that gabapentin is effective at reducing neuropathic pain intensity.[98]

Lamotrigine which is primarily used to treat peripheral neuropathic pain is purported to inhibit voltage-gated sodium channels to decrease neuronal excitability and inhibit excitatory glutamine release.[109,110] Although a single RCT did not show significant reduction in overall pain from SCI, a subgroup analysis supported the effective use of 200 to 400 mg of lamotrigine daily to reduce at- and below-level neuropathic pain among subjects with incomplete SCI.[111] One randomized longitudinal comparative study demonstrated that lamotrigine was effective in reducing neuropathic pain intensity in participants with SCI.[112] Adverse side effects noted include dizziness, somnolence, headache, and rash. There is an U.S. Food and Drug Administration (FDA) black box warning regarding possible Stevens-Johnson syndrome with lamotrigine use.

Valproic acid has wide-ranging neuromodulation mechanisms which make this drug an appealing candidate for the treatment of neuropathic SCI pain. A single RCT evaluated the use of valproic acid in a small population of subjects with SCI-related central pain. Compared to placebo, use of valproic acid resulted in a nonsignificant trend toward SCI pain reduction.[113]

Levetiracetam may have several analgesic mechanisms, including binding to voltage-gated calcium channels and thru its GABAergic properties. One crossover RCT showed levetiracetam did not significantly reduce pain intensity versus placebo.[114]

Carbamazepine acts primarily on voltage-dependent sodium channels to dampen neuronal firing.[115] *Oxcarbazepine*, a structural analog, may share a similar mechanism of action. One RCT demonstrated limited protective benefit from early carbamazepine use on SCI neuropathic pain severity at 1 month but not at 3 or 6 months.[116]

Topiramate targets sodium and calcium channels, potentiates GABAergic inhibition, and inhibits glutamate receptors. There is currently scant evidence to support its efficacy in managing neuropathic SCI pain. One small RCT in people with neuropathic SCI pain showed positive results with topiramate at the highest doses tested, 800 mg, only after the subjects were treated with this dose for 4 weeks.[117]

Conclusion: anticonvulsants for management of neuropathic spinal cord injury pain: Gabapentinoid anticonvulsants are considered first-line treatment for neuropathic pain following an SCI. Gabapentin and pregabalin monotherapy are both effective at reducing SCI neuropathic pain intensity as well as potentially improving sleep interference, anxiety, and depression. However, the relatively increased risk for adverse side effects such as dizziness, edema, and somnolence warrants close monitoring for dose titration. Lamotrigine may be of benefit to reduce neuropathic pain in individuals with incomplete SCI, especially those with evoked pain, but has a risk of significant potential serious adverse effects that must be carefully weighed against the potential benefit before initiating treatment.

Antidepressants

Although the neuromodulatory actions of antidepressants are conventionally attributed to norepinephrine and serotonin reuptake inhibition, other actions including NMDA-receptor antagonism and sodium channel blockade may also play a role in analgesia. A meta-analysis of four antidepressant RCTs for neuropathic pain control after SCI (two studying amitriptyline, one studying trazodone, and one studying duloxetine) showed a small, but significant, benefit over placebo. The effect was greatest for amitriptyline, followed by duloxetine. Those treated with antidepressants experienced a higher rate of complications such as constipation and dry mouth, with side effects limiting adherence rates and potentially underestimating treatment effect.[118]

Tricyclic antidepressants: *Amitriptyline* is a tricyclic antidepressant found to be effective in treating other pain conditions such as diabetic and postherpetic neuropathy and headaches. Effective doses range from 25 to 150 mg daily.[108] As with many other pharmacologic interventions for SCI pain, there is scarce and conflicting direct evidence for the effectiveness of tricyclic antidepressants in the treatment of neuropathic SCI pain. For example, relative to controls, amitriptyline was found to be efficacious in treating neuropathic pain in patients with SCI and major depressive disorder, but no significant differences were found in a study that excluded individuals with major depressive disorder.[108,119] Furthermore, no significant differences were found when amitriptyline was compared to gabapentin[108] or lamotrigine.[112] The most common adverse effects of amitriptyline cited are dry mouth, dizziness, constipation, increased spasticity, and urinary retention.[119] Secondary and tertiary amine tricyclic antidepressants such as nortriptyline and desipramine have not been adequately studied in the treatment of neuropathic pain after SCI but are purported to have less intense anticholinergic effects which may improve tolerability. Some studies indicate benefit from combined therapy with amitriptyline and other pharmacologic and nonpharmacologic treatments.[120,121]

Trazodone: The selective serotonin reuptake inhibitor *trazodone*, at doses of 150 mg daily, has not been shown to be more effective than placebo in managing neuropathic pain in subjects with traumatic SCI.[122]

Duloxetine: *Duloxetine*, a dual serotonin and norepinephrine reuptake inhibitor, has been demonstrated to be safe and effective in the treatment of painful conditions such as diabetic peripheral polyneuropathy at doses of 60 to 120 mg daily[123–125] and with lower quality of evidence of effectiveness for fibromyalgia.[125,126] However, in neuropathic central pain due to SCI and stroke, one RCT noted only a nonsignificant trend toward pain intensity reduction. Duloxetine did appear to be superior to placebo in reducing cold-induced allodynia in this mixed patient population and in improving Patient Global Impression of Change scale scores.[127] Duloxetine merits further study in the treatment of pain conditions in SCI given the emerging broad applications for pain treatment. Although generally well tolerated, side effects are dose-dependent and most commonly include nausea, dry mouth, dizziness, fatigue, and constipation. Hypertension and serotonin syndrome is possible and due diligence is needed due to potential drug interactions.[128]

Venlafaxine: As previously addressed under treatment of nociceptive musculoskeletal pain, the serotonin-norepinephrine reuptake inhibitor venlafaxine XR did not significantly improve neuropathic SCI pain in the presence of major depressive disorder in one study. However, some benefit was noted with higher doses in subjects with mixed SCI pain.[76]

Conclusion: antidepressants for the management of chronic neuropathic spinal cord injury pain: A trial of tricyclic antidepressants appears to be reasonable in clinical practice given supportive evidence from other neuropathic pain conditions, particularly in the presence of concurrent depression. It may be beneficial as an adjunct treatment intervention. However, tricyclic antidepressants may have a number of side effects that should be considered in the population with SCI including sedation, constipation, dry mouth, orthostasis, headache, nausea, and urinary retention. Additional considerations include the potential for cardiac side effects and potential drug interactions.[118,129,130]

Local Anesthetics

Lidocaine, a sodium channel blocker, has been the most frequently studied local anesthetic for neuropathic pain conditions. Intravenous lidocaine infusion in a small population that included individuals with SCI neuropathic pain demonstrated reduction of spontaneous ongoing pain, brush-evoked allodynia, and static mechanical hyperalgesia but had no effect on thermal allodynia.[131–133] One RCT of intravenous lidocaine failed to demonstrate significant improvement in SCI neuropathic pain intensity.[134] Nevertheless, ongoing outpatient treatment with parenteral lidocaine administration is not practical. Several case reports for the use of topical lidocaine for at-level neuropathic pain after SCI exist, but no RCTs have been performed.[135–137] Mexiletine, an oral lidocaine analog, was not shown to be effective for neuropathic SCI pain at a dose of 450 mg per day in an RCT of 11 subjects.[138]

N-Methyl-ᴅ-Aspartate Receptor Antagonists

In support of the hypothesis that NMDA receptor activation is one mechanism for neuropathic pain, parenterally administered NMDA receptor antagonist ketamine was found to be more effective than placebo at managing below-level neuropathic SCI pain in three RCTs.[134,139,140] Ketamine was shown to have similar analgesic efficacy as fentanyl and was particularly beneficial for evoked, wind-up pain more than chronic ongoing pain. In general, the effective doses for treating mixed-diagnosis neuropathic pain were subanesthetic doses. Ketamine has typically been administered as a bolus or short-term infusion, with a similarly limited analgesic period.[141,142] In one study,[140] a multiday low-dose ketamine infusion combined with oral gabapentin was more effective at reducing neuropathic SCI pain intensity than intravenous placebo + gabapentin, and the effect was noted up to 2 weeks after cessation of the infusion. As with lidocaine, long-term and outpatient administration of ketamine remains problematic. Although there are reported extemporaneously formulated oral compounds, there are currently no effective commercially available oral alternatives. There are significant risks associated with its use, including hallucinations, panic attacks, cognitive impairment, somnolence, abuse potential, cardiovascular, and gastrointestinal side effects with rare hepatotoxicity. One uncontrolled, open-label study explored treatment of acute allodynia in 13 subjects with highly motor incomplete SCI using parenteral ketamine followed by variable periods of oral ketamine. All subjects had successful pretreatment single-dose ketamine challenges with dramatic neuropathic pain reduction. Pain improvement with ketamine treatment was seen in three quarters of participants at the study conclusion and in 97% at follow-up. Those treated acutely were reported not to experience recurrence, and five of the subjects experienced mild side effects that included a sensation of floating while receiving the infusion.[143] Parenteral ketamine may prove to be an option in treating severe, refractory neuropathic pain with in-hospital monitoring. Although the preliminary studies suggest ketamine has potent analgesic properties for neuropathic pain, further studies are needed to determine therapeutic indications and methods of administration and to better understand its toxicity profile.

Opioids

In general, the evidence to support opioid use across various chronic neuropathic pain conditions is limited or of low quality.[144,145] Although RCTs evaluating *intravenous morphine*[146] and *alfentanil*[139] in decreasing neuropathic SCI pain have shown statistically significant short-term benefit, there is very limited evidence for the use of oral or transdermal opioids for SCI neuropathic pain.

Tramadol, a low-affinity μ-receptor agonist and monoamine reuptake inhibitor, is a scheduled drug in the United States. One RCT demonstrated effective reduction in pain intensity and anxiety versus placebo and improved sleep quality and global satisfaction with life. However, nearly half of the subjects in the active treatment group withdrew from the study primarily due to the adverse effects experienced by over 90% of subjects in this group.[147] The most frequently cited adverse effects were fatigue, dry mouth, and dizziness. There is a risk for serotonin syndrome when tramadol is taken concurrently with tricyclic antidepressants and tramadol lowers the seizure threshold for those at risk for seizure activity.[148]

A multisite observational study of *oxycodone* in subjects with SCI showed significant reduction in neuropathic pain intensity at 3 months, with improvements in quality of life and impact on physical activity and sleep. The study did not exclude concurrent treatment with anticonvulsants, and the majority of subjects received such treatment.[149]

All opioid medications carry the risk for dependence and withdrawal, with additional considerations in the SCI population for sedation, constipation, cardiorespiratory, and endocrine suppression. The decision to use opioids in the treatment of chronic SCI pain is rarely indicated and the decision to initiate treatment should include a careful analysis of the risks and benefits and should comply with any state or federal regulatory requirements and available clinical practice guidelines as previously referenced.

Cannabinoids

Tetrahydrocannabinol (δ9-THC) is the active component in cannabis that binds to cannabinoid receptors to modulate pain, mood, and memory. The current direct evidence for use of cannabinoids for SCI pain is limited and conflicting, but increasingly widespread access and use has resulted in anecdotal reports of benefit and a strong expert panel recommendation for prioritization of targeted research in this area.[131] Common adverse effects included dry mouth, constipation, and drowsiness.

One small pilot study comparing dronabinol and diphenhydramine placebo showed no significant reduction in chronic below-level neuropathic pain.[150] Another open-label prospective study of chronic neuropathic pain in a mixed population, including four of eight participants who had SCI, failed to demonstrate reduction in pain, quality of life, and functional impact.[151] The majority of the participants exhibited adverse side effects, necessitating drug cessation. Of concern is the noted hyperalgesia in one quarter of participants in one study of δ9-THC in patients with SCI-related spasticity versus one-fifth who noted pain improvement.[152]

Drug Combinations

Combined drug therapy or concurrent drug and nonpharmacologic interventions may be beneficial when a single agent is ineffective. For example, combinations of anticonvulsants and tricyclic antidepressants may be more effective than either administered alone.[120,121] This approach requires cautious exploration of possible side effects of drug combinations, such as the potential for serotonin syndrome with the concurrent use of tramadol or duloxetine and a tricyclic antidepressant.

Spinal Drug Administration

Intrathecal (IT) drug administration has emerged as an alternative to systemic or parenteral drug delivery when the latter is ineffective or associated with unacceptable side effects. However, the body of evidence for its efficacy in reducing SCI pain is limited to case series and a small number of controlled trials, and the strength of evidence varies depending on the drug(s) infused.

In one case series, spinal administration of morphine and clonidine was found to be effective in some individuals.[153] IT clonidine or morphine alone was not found to be more effective than placebo in reducing the intensity of SCI-related pain. However, combined intrathecal morphine and clonidine administration was found to be superior to monotherapy with either drug. Although the combination was effective in the population with chronic at- and below-level neuropathic SCI pain, greater pain reduction was noted in the group with at-level neuropathic pain.[154] *Intrathecal ziconotide* has been used to treat neuropathic pain conditions,[155] but the evidence for its successful use to manage SCI-related at- and below-level neuropathic pain is currently limited to one case report of combination therapy with intrathecal hydromorphone.[156] Beneficial combinations of IT morphine, clonidine, or ziconotide with baclofen in those with neuropathic pain and spasticity from SCI have been described.[156,157] Although intrathecal baclofen can reduce pain related to spasticity in people with SCI, it has not been shown to significantly improve neuropathic pain.[158]

Any combination IT drug regimen requires very knowledgeable and cautious titration of each drug to prevent overdose or underdose. Use of nonapproved drugs in an intrathecal drug delivery system may lead to premature device failure.[159] The risks associated with surgical implantation and management of an implanted drug delivery system requires careful and often multidisciplinary assessment and screening for physical and cognitive candidacy, a drug trial, and a detailed discussion to ensure the candidate has full understanding of the potential risks and benefits and maintenance requirements and to manage expectations from the therapy. Sufficient cerebrospinal fluid flow through areas of potential scarring or blockage is also necessary for the drug to reach its local target.

PSYCHOLOGICAL AND ENVIRONMENTAL MANAGEMENT

There are multiple roles for psychological intervention in pain management. In terms of direct intervention, there are now numerous psychotherapeutic approaches focused directly on improving how individuals cope with chronic pain. Cognitive-behavioral therapy (CBT) represents a variety of therapeutic approaches targeting the improvement of cognitive content and behavioral engagement,[160] including modules such as cognitive restructuring and relaxation therapy. Preliminary research supports the use of CBT for the treatment of pain after SCI.[161–164] Acceptance and commitment therapy (ACT) is a newer therapeutic technique that focuses on psychological flexibility, being present-focused despite the presence of challenges, and focusing behavior on engagement with valued activities.[165] Although there are no studies evaluating the technique for the treatment of pain after SCI, a growing body of literature suggests that the intervention is effective for persons with chronic pain and there are no apparent reasons that the intervention would function differently for persons with SCI.[166–168] Furthermore, ACT targets the acceptance-based coping strategies that have been shown to be highly correlated with pain outcomes in persons with SCI, such as activity engagement and willingness.[55,56] Finally, hypnotic approaches have been effective in facilitating pre- to posttreatment improvements in pain intensity that are maintained at 3-month follow-up in persons with SCI.[169] Hypnotic analgesia involves an induction of a hypnotic (or suggestible) state, followed by the therapist giving suggestions of alternative interpretations of painful sensations, alternative responses in the setting of pain, and other similar opportunities for improving the way one experiences pain.

Given the association of mood and psychiatric disorders with pain outcomes, it is also important to consider whether psychological intervention is warranted focused more on the presence of those factors. Whereas pain management would be primary in the previously described interventions, here, pain management might be secondary to more traditional psychotherapies that focus on depression, anxiety, PTSD, or other mental health conditions. Moreover, given the significant adjustment inherent to experiencing SCI, therapy focused on adjustment to SCI may also be warranted. A myriad of interventions may be useful, but the majority of existing evidence again focuses on the use of CBT.[170]

Although psychological interventions can be delivered in a standalone format, such interventions may be best delivered in concert with other interventions. Psychologists routinely play a critical role within multidisciplinary teams that together address the totality of the biopsychosocial spectrum.[171]

OTHER NONPHARMACOLOGIC MANAGEMENT OF PAIN IN PEOPLE WITH SPINAL CORD INJURY

The impact and treatment challenge presented by chronic SCI pain, along with the desire to minimize drug adverse side effects, has engendered interest in exploring nonpharmacologic strategies for pain management.[60,172]

A Cochrane review of studies on nonpharmacologic treatment strategies for SCI pain found the body of evidence generally insufficient to support the efficacy of these interventions, underscoring the need for more high-quality studies of such treatments.[173]

Neurostimulation

The effect of *TENS* was evaluated in two studies, with one RCT that found significant reduction in SCI neuropathic pain with low-frequency stimulation.[174,175] One study of subjects with longer duration of SCI did not show benefit in reducing pain with either high- or low-frequency stimulation protocols.[176] The recommended electrode application site is a region with sensory preservation.[131]

Surgical neuromodulation strategies via spinal cord, deep brain, and motor cortex stimulation have also been studied. *Spinal cord.*[177,178] However, diminished pain relief is noted over time.[179] Sufficient dorsal column function is presumed necessary for effective treatment.[130] In general, response rates from spinal cord stimulation are felt to be less robust than seen in other pain populations.[180] These factors may limit its clinical utility in SCI, particularly in the setting of complete SCI.

The evidence for effectiveness of *deep brain stimulation* (*DBS*) in reducing SCI pain is conflicting and limited, and DBS is considered investigational for the treatment of pain.[180] Multiple targets have been reported, including the thalamic nuclei, periaqueductal grey, and internal capsule. One systematic review noted less than one-fifth of subjects had long-term improvement in subjects with SCI pain.[181] The surgical risks, investigational status for pain treatment, and lack of sufficient evidence currently limit the justification for the clinical use of DBS for SCI pain.

Motor cortex stimulation has primarily been studied to provide relief from central poststroke and facial pain. There are very few reports of its use to treat SCI pain, primarily case reports and series. These modalities had varying but generally inferior results in SCI when compared to other populations.[180,182,183]

The mechanism underlying pain relief from *transcranial direct current stimulation* (*tDCS*) is uncertain, although it is postulated to modulate central pathways.[184] The use of tDCS resulted in greater short-term reduction in pain intensity over sham control in three RCTs[185–188] but was not effective versus sham treatment in another trial.[189] A meta-analysis of the data suggests tDCS produces moderate effect in reducing neuropathic SCI pain, but the relief is not sustained at follow-up.[190] However, combination therapy using tDCS and visual illusion has been shown in one study to be highly effective at reducing pain intensity and the benefits are sustained for at least 12 weeks.[187] No serious adverse effects have been noted with conventional tDCS use.[191] tDCS is favored for neuromodulation because of ease of use, cost, and duration of benefit.[185] Preliminary results support the need for further investigation of tDCS, alone or in combination with other modalities.

Massage

Massage therapy was identified as one of the most frequently explored nonpharmacologic interventions among people with chronic SCI pain.[172] A recent RCT of 40 individuals with SCI who received 30 minutes of weekly massage therapy or guided imagery showed statistically significant reduction in both pain and fatigue from both interventions at 5 weeks. Massage therapy twice weekly for 6 weeks reduced pain interference measures at 6 weeks, but the result was not sustained at 2 months.[192]

Acupuncture

At present, the body of evidence for the use of acupuncture to treat neuropathic SCI pain is conflicting and varied, yielding overall inconclusive findings. However, a few small pilot trials showed promise in the treatment of SCI pain, including short-term significant reduction in neuropathic[192,193] and mixed SCI pain types.[194] One RCT showed a moderate but nonsignificant trend in the treatment of shoulder pain in SCI, but a large placebo effect may have blunted the treatment effect.[195] Potential practical limitations cited include finding a qualified provider and selecting stimulation sites.[130] Larger, randomized controlled studies of acupuncture for SCI pain are warranted.

Physical Therapy and Exercise

Physical therapy addresses factors contributing to chronic musculoskeletal pain in people with SCI as previously described, whereas regular physical activity and exercise routines have been shown to improve pain and mood.[196,197]

Evolving knowledge about neuroplasticity mechanisms for pain development, sensory pathway activation by exercise, and activity-dependent neuroplasticity has intensified research interest in the effects of exercise interventions on neuropathic pain.[198] Despite this, large, randomized studies in humans of the effects of exercise on neuropathic SCI pain are currently lacking. Two studies on small populations of people with SCI have shown beneficial effects of exercise on pain. One study of seated double-poling ergometry showed that four of seven subjects with neuropathic pain showed clinically meaningful reduction in pain intensity with over half noting improvement on patient global impression of change. More significant improvement was noted in nociceptive musculoskeletal pain.[199] Both neuropathic pain intensity and mood were significantly improved by a single 15-minute wheelchair propulsion exercise in 10 individuals with SCI. Electroencephalogram correlates showed exercise-related effects on peak α activity, felt to be a biomarker for neuropathic pain. Preexercise baseline peak α activity in the parietal and occipital lobes was lower in subjects with SCI than in healthy controls, and the central peak α activity increased after exercise.[200] Exercise intervention may address SCI pain by not only mitigating existing pain but also potentially as an intervention that seeks to modify the underlying mechanisms of pain evolution after SCI. Given the potential health and analgesic benefits of exercise for both neuropathic and musculoskeletal SCI pain, and relative safety of the intervention, further research into this area is encouraged.

SURGICAL INTERVENTIONS

Surgical care to address a neurologically significant structural lesion, such as decompression of a nerve root or peripheral nerve, detethering of roots, and treatment of progressive, symptomatic syrinx formation, may be performed to improve pain or prevent neurologic decline. However, the surgical correction may not always result in pain reduction and may at times exacerbate pain, highlighting the need for individualized surgical assessment and thorough discussion of potential and expected risks and benefits.

Surgical ablative approaches, including microsurgical techniques, address pain by abolishing or severing pathways to the site of abnormal neuronal activity. As with other interventions, variable outcomes have been described in SCI and only several uncontrolled studies are available due to the invasive nature of the interventions. *Cordotomy* or *cordomyelotomy* is rarely used due to the risk for neurologic loss and with variable reports of effectiveness and is not currently recommended.[201–203] *Dorsal root entry zone* (DREZ) *lesioning* aims to selectively deafferent hyperactive dorsal horn neurons close to the level of injury and may provide relief of neuropathic pain, particularly at-level neuropathic pain.[204,205] Extension of the DREZ lesion may improve outcomes in more diffuse SCI pain.[203] Use of intramedullary recordings of spontaneous and C fiber evoked electrical hyperactivity to guide DREZ lesioning also seems to boost effectiveness at relieving both at- and below-level neuropathic pain. One study reported 100% pain relief of pain in more than three quarters of subjects who received DREZ with intramedullary guidance.[206,207] Although additional study is warranted, DREZ shows promise as a valuable treatment option for refractory neuropathic SCI pain.

Conclusion

Pain represents a common and impactful challenge for individuals living with SCI. Consistent with chronic pain at large, individuals living with SCI and pain are understood to have poorer function, more physical and psychological comorbidities, and lower quality of life than their peers who live without pain. As described in this chapter, there is significant diversity in the types, causes, and treatments for SCI-related pain. The limited evidence and varied quality of literature to address the problem of pain in people with SCI speaks to the value of systematic reviews,[129,208] updated evidence-based expert panel consensus on management,[130,209] as well as further targeted and high-quality research to explore promising individual and combination regimens. To facilitate this inquiry, use of standardized systems of assessment and classification, such as the ISCIP Classification and the ISCIPBDS, as well as the selection of appropriate outcome measures are vital. Optimal management attends to not only the intensity of the pain but also, more importantly, improving patient function despite the challenge of pain. When effectively utilized, clinical intervention can aid patients in improving the function and quality of life that has been negatively impacted by this challenge.

References

1. Loeser JD, Treede RD. The Kyoto protocol of IASP Basic Pain Terminology. *Pain* 2008;137(3):473–477.
2. Cardenas DD, Bryce TN, Shem K, et al. Gender and minority differences in the pain experience of people with spinal cord injury. *Arch Phys Med Rehabil* 2004;85(11):1774–1781.
3. Felix ER, Cruz-Almeida Y, Widerström-Noga EG. Chronic pain after spinal cord injury: what characteristics make some pains more disturbing than others? *J Rehabil Res Dev* 2007;44(5):703–715.
4. Störmer S, Gerner HJ, Grüninger W, et al. Chronic pain/dysaesthesiae in spinal cord injury patients: results of a multicentre study. *Spinal Cord* 1997;35(7):446–455.
5. Rose M, Robinson JE, Ells P, et al. Pain following spinal cord injury: results from a postal survey. *Pain* 1988;34(1):101–102.
6. Nepomuceno C, Fine PR, Richards JS, et al. Pain in patients with spinal cord injury. *Arch Phys Med Rehabil* 1979;60(12):605–609.
7. Dijkers M, Bryce T, Zanca J. Prevalence of chronic pain after traumatic spinal cord injury: a systematic review. *J Rehabil Res Dev* 2009;46(1):13–29.
8. Jensen TS, Baron R, Haanpaa M, et al. A new definition of neuropathic pain. *Pain* 2011;152:2204–2205.
9. Bryce TN, Biering-Sørensen F, Finnerup NB, et al. International Spinal Cord Injury Pain (ISCIP) Classification: part 2. Initial validation using vignettes. *Spinal Cord* 2012;50(6):404–412.
10. Bryce TN, Biering-Sørensen F, Finnerup NB, et al. International Spinal Cord Injury Pain Classification: part I. Background and description. March 6-7, 2009. *Spinal Cord* 2012;50(6):413–417.
11. Widerstrom-Noga E, Biering-Sørensen F, Bryce TN, et al. The International Spinal Cord Injury Pain Basic Data Set (version 2.0). *Spinal Cord* 2014;52(4):282–286.
12. International Spinal Cord Society. *International SCI Data Sets.* Aylesbury, United Kingdom: International Spinal Cord Society; 2015.
13. Kirshblum SC, Burns SP, Biering-Sørensen F, et al. International standards for neurological classification of spinal cord injury (revised 2011). *J Spinal Cord Med* 2011;34(6):535–546.
14. Cook KF, Kallen MA, Bombardier C, et al. Do measures of depressive symptoms function differently in people with spinal cord injury versus primary care patients: the CES-D, PHQ-9, and PROMIS(R)-D. *Qual Life Res* 2017;26(1):139–148.
15. Mehta S, Guy SD, Bryce TN, et al. The CanPain SCI clinical practice guidelines for rehabilitation management of neuropathic pain after spinal cord: screening and diagnosis recommendations. *Spinal Cord* 2016;54(suppl 1):S7–S13.
16. Finnerup NB, Norrbrink C, Trok K, et al. Phenotypes and predictors of pain following traumatic spinal cord injury: a prospective study. *J Pain* 2014;15(1):40–48.
17. Siddall PJ, McClelland JM, Rutkowski SB, et al. A longitudinal study of the prevalence and characteristics of pain in the first 5 years following spinal cord injury. *Pain* 2003;103(3):249–257.
18. Dyson-Hudson TA, Kirshblum SC. Shoulder pain in chronic spinal cord injury, part I: epidemiology, etiology, and pathomechanics. *J Spinal Cord Med* 2004;27(1):4–17.
19. Perry J, Gronley JK, Newsam CJ, et al. Electromyographic analysis of the shoulder muscles during depression transfers in subjects with low-level paraplegia. *Arch Phys Med Rehabil* 1996;77(4):350–355.

20. Sabick MB, Kotajarvi BR, An KN. A new method to quantify demand on the upper extremity during manual wheelchair propulsion. *Arch Phys Med Rehabil* 2004;85(7):1151–1159.

21. Mulroy SJ, Hatchett P, Eberly VJ, et al. Shoulder strength and physical activity predictors of shoulder pain in people with paraplegia from spinal injury: prospective cohort study. *Phys Ther* 2015;95(7):1027–1038.

22. Bayley JC, Cochran TP, Sledge CB. The weight-bearing shoulder. The impingement syndrome in paraplegics. *J Bone Joint Surg Am* 1987;69(5):676–678.

23. Gellman H, Sie I, Waters RL. Late complications of the weight-bearing upper extremity in the paraplegic patient. *Clin Orthop Relat Res* 1988;233:132–135.

24. Sie IH, Waters RL, Adkins RH, et al. Upper extremity pain in the postrehabilitation spinal cord injured patient. *Arch Phys Med Rehabil* 1992;73(1):44–48.

25. Samuelsson K, Larsson J, Thyberg M, et al. Back pain and spinal deformity—common among wheelchair users with spinal cord injuries. *Scand J Occup Ther* 1996;3:28–32

26. Faaborg PM, Finnerup NB, Christensen P, et al. Abdominal pain: a comparison between neurogenic bowel dysfunction and chronic idiopathic constipation. *Gastroenterol Res Pract* 2013;2013:365037.

27. Nielsen SD, Faaborg PM, Christensen P, et al. Chronic abdominal pain in long-term spinal cord injury: a follow-up study. *Spinal Cord* 2017;55(3):290–293.

28. Bryce TN, Rangarsson KT. Epidemiology and classification of pain after spinal cord injury. *Top Spinal Cord Inj Rehabil* 2001;7:1–17.

29. Siddall PJ, Middleton JW. Pain following spinal cord injury. In: Chhabra HS, ed. *Comprehensive Management of Spinal Cord Injuries*. Lippincott Williams & Wilkins; 2015.

30. Finnerup NB, Jensen MP, Norrbrink C, et al. A prospective study of pain and psychological functioning following traumatic spinal cord injury. *Spinal Cord* 2016;54(10):816–821.

31. Griffiths ER, McCormick CC. Post-traumatic syringomyelia (cystic myelopathy). *Paraplegia* 1981;19(2):81–88.

32. Rossier AB, Foo D, Shillito J, et al. Posttraumatic cervical syringomyelia. Incidence, clinical presentation, electrophysiological studies, syrinx protein and results of conservative and operative treatment. *Brain J Neurol* 1985;108(pt 2):439–461.

33. Schurch B, Wichmann W, Rossier AB. Post-traumatic syringomyelia (cystic myelopathy): a prospective study of 449 patients with spinal cord injury. *J Neurol Neurosurg Psychiatry* 1996;60(1):61–67.

34. Barnett H, Jousse A. Syringomyelia as late sequel to traumatic paraplegia and quadriplegia: clinical features. In: Barnett H, ed. *Syringomyelia*. London: Saunders; 1973:129–152.

35. Williams B, Terry AF, Jones F, et al. Syringomyelia as a sequel to traumatic paraplegia. *Paraplegia* 1981;19(2):67–80.

36. Lee TT, Alameda GJ, Gromelski EB, et al. Outcome after surgical treatment of progressive posttraumatic cystic myelopathy. *J Neurosurg* 2000;92(2 suppl):149–154.

37. Frisbie JH, Aguilera EJ. Chronic pain after spinal cord injury: an expedient diagnostic approach. *Paraplegia* 1990;28(7):460–465.

38. Gellman H, Chandler DR, Petrasek J, et al. Carpal tunnel syndrome in paraplegic patients. *J Bone Joint Surg Am* 1988;70(4):517–519.

39. Boninger ML, Cooper RA, Baldwin MA, et al. Wheelchair pushrim kinetics: body weight and median nerve function. *Arch Phys Med Rehabil* 1999;80(8):910–915.

40. Katz J, Rosenbloom BN, Fashler S. Chronic pain, psychopathology, and DSM-5 somatic symptom disorder. *Can J Psychiatry* 2015;60(4):160–167.

41. Murray CB, Zebracki K, Chlan KM, et al. Medical and psychological factors related to pain in adults with pediatric-onset spinal cord injury: a biopsychosocial model. *Spinal Cord* 2017;55(4):405–410.

42. Tran J, Dorstyn DS, Burke AL. Psychosocial aspects of spinal cord injury pain: a meta-analysis. *Spinal Cord* 2016;54(9):640–648.

43. Hassanijirdehi M, Khak M, Afshari-Mirak S, et al. Evaluation of pain and its effect on quality of life and functioning in men with spinal cord injury. *Korean J Pain* 2015;28(2):129–136.

44. Alschuler KN, Jensen MP, Sullivan-Singh SJ, et al. The association of age, pain, and fatigue with physical functioning and depressive symptoms in persons with spinal cord injury. *J Spinal Cord Med* 2013;36(5):483–491.

45. Ullrich PM, Lincoln RK, Tackett MJ, et al. Pain, depression, and health care utilization over time after spinal cord injury. *Rehabil Psychol* 2013;58(2):158–165.

46. Ataoglu E, Tiftik T, Kara M, et al. Effects of chronic pain on quality of life and depression in patients with spinal cord injury. *Spinal Cord* 2013;51(1):23–26.

47. Ullrich PM, Smith BM, Poggensee L, et al. Pain and post-traumatic stress disorder symptoms during inpatient rehabilitation among operation enduring freedom/operation Iraqi freedom veterans with spinal cord injury. *Arch Phys Med Rehabil* 2013;94(1):80–85.

48. Kennedy P, Hasson L. The relationship between pain and mood following spinal cord injury. *J Spinal Cord Med* 2017;40(3):275–279.

49. Craig A, Tran Y, Siddall P, et al. Developing a model of associations between chronic pain, depressive mood, chronic fatigue, and self-efficacy in people with spinal cord injury. *J Pain* 2013;14(9):911–920.

50. Bombardier CH, Adams LM, Fann JR, et al. Depression trajectories during the first year after spinal cord injury. *Arch Phys Med Rehabil* 2016;97(2):196–203.

51. Cuff L, Fann JR, Bombardier CH, et al. Depression, pain intensity, and interference in acute spinal cord injury. *Top Spinal Cord Inj Rehabil* 2014;20(1):32–39.

52. Hirsh AT, Bockow TB, Jensen MP. Catastrophizing, pain, and pain interference in individuals with disabilities. *Am J Phys Med Rehabil* 2011;90(9):713–722.

53. Jensen MP, Moore MR, Bockow TB, et al. Psychosocial factors and adjustment to chronic pain in persons with physical disabilities: a systematic review. *Arch Phys Med Rehabil* 2011;92(1):146–160.

54. Molton IR, Stoelb BL, Jensen MP, et al. Psychosocial factors and adjustment to chronic pain in spinal cord injury: replication and cross-validation. *J Rehabil Res Dev* 2009;46(1):31–42.

55. Kratz AL, Ehde DM, Bombardier CH, et al. Pain acceptance decouples the momentary associations between pain, pain interference, and physical activity in the daily lives of people with chronic pain and spinal cord injury. *J Pain* 2017;18(3):319–331.

56. Kratz AL, Hirsh AT, Ehde DM, et al. Acceptance of pain in neurological disorders: associations with functioning and psychosocial well-being. *Rehabil Psychol* 2013;58(1):1–9.

57. Raichle KA, Hanley M, Jensen MP, et al. Cognitions, coping, and social environment predict adjustment to pain in spinal cord injury. *J Pain* 2007;8(9):718–729.

58. Summers JD, Rapoff MA, Varghese G, et al. Psychosocial factors in chronic spinal cord injury pain. *Pain* 1991;47(2):183–189.

59. Warms CA, Turner JA, Marshall HM, et al. Treatments for chronic pain associated with spinal cord injuries: many are tried, few are helpful. *Clin J Pain* 2002;18(3):154–163.

60. Widerstrom-Noga EG, Turk DC. Types and effectiveness of treatments used by people with chronic pain associated with spinal cord injuries: influence of pain and psychosocial characteristics. *Spinal Cord* 2003;41(11):600–609.

61. Goldstein B. Musculoskeletal conditions after spinal cord injury. *Phys Med Rehabil Clin N Am* 2000;11(1):91–108, viii–ix.

62. Paralyzed Veterans of America Consortium for Spinal Cord Medicine. Preservation of upper limb function following spinal cord injury: a clinical practice guideline for health-care professionals. *J Spinal Cord Med* 2005;28(5):434–470.

63. Mulroy SJ, Thompson L, Kemp B, et al. Strengthening and optimal movements for painful shoulders (STOMPS) in chronic spinal cord injury: a randomized controlled trial. *Phys Ther* 2011;91(3):305–324.

64. Large RG, Schug SA. Opioids for chronic pain of non-malignant origin—caring or crippling. *Health Care Anal* 1995;3(1):5–11.

65. Chou R, Turner JA, Devine EB, et al. The effectiveness and risks of long-term opioid therapy for chronic pain: a systematic review for a National Institutes of Health Pathways to Prevention Workshop. *Ann Intern Med* 2015;162(4):276–286.

66. Yi P, Pryzbylkowski P. Opioid induced hyperalgesia. *Pain Med* 2015;16(suppl 1):S32–S36.

67. Hartung DM, Middleton L, Haxby DG, et al. Rates of adverse events of long-acting opioids in a state Medicaid program. *Ann Pharmacother* 2007;41(6):921–928.

68. Kalso E, Edwards JE, Moore RA, et al. Opioids in chronic non-cancer pain: systematic review of efficacy and safety. *Pain* 2004;112(3):372–380.

69. Benyamin R, Trescot AM, Datta S, et al. Opioid complications and side effects. *Pain Physician* 2008;11(2 suppl):S105–S120.

70. Nicholas MK, Molloy AR, Brooker C. Using opioids with persisting non-cancer pain: a biopsychosocial perspective. *Clin J Pain* 2006;22(2):137–146.

71. Kirpalani D. How to maximize patient safety when prescribing opioids. *PM R* 2015;7(11 suppl):S225–S235.

72. Dowell D, Haegerich TM, Chou R. CDC guideline for prescribing opioids for chronic pain—United States, 2016. *MMWR Recomm Rep* 2016;65(1):1–49.

73. Manchikanti L, Kaye AM, Knezevic NN, et al. Responsible, safe, and effective prescription of opioids for chronic non-cancer pain: American Society of Interventional Pain Physicians (ASIPP) guidelines. *Pain Physician* 2017;20(2 suppl):S3–S92.

74. Rudroju N, Bansal D, Talakokkula ST, et al. Comparative efficacy and safety of six antidepressants and anticonvulsants in painful diabetic neuropathy: a network meta-analysis. *Pain Physician* 2013;16(6):E705–E714.

75. Aziz MT, Good BL, Lowe DK. Serotonin-norepinephrine reuptake inhibitors for the management of chemotherapy-induced peripheral neuropathy. *Ann Pharmacother* 2014;48(5):626–632.

76. Richards JS, Bombardier CH, Wilson CS, et al. Efficacy of venlafaxine XR for the treatment of pain in patients with spinal cord injury and major depression: a randomized, controlled trial. *Arch Phys Med Rehabil* 2015;96(4):680–689.

77. Standaert C, Cardenas DD, Anderson P. Charcot spine as a late complication of traumatic spinal cord injury. *Arch Phys Med Rehabil* 1997;78(2):221–225.

78. Selmi F, Frankel HL, Kumaraguru AP, et al. Charcot joint of the spine, a cause of autonomic dysreflexia in spinal cord injured patients. *Spinal Cord* 2002;40(9):481–483.

79. Mohit A, Mirza S, James J, et al. Charcot arthropathy in relation to autonomic dysreflexia in spinal cord injury: case report and review of the literature. *J Neurosurg Spine* 2005;2(4):476–480.

80. Morita M, Iwasaki M, Okuda S, et al. Autonomic dysreflexia associated with Charcot spine following spinal cord injury: a case report and literature review. *Eur Spine J* 2010;19(suppl 2):S179–S182.

81. Adams MM, Hicks AL. Spasticity after spinal cord injury. *Spinal Cord* 2005;43(10):577–586.

82. Chang E, Ghosh N, Yanni D, et al. A review of spasticity treatments: pharmacological and interventional approaches. *Crit Rev Phys Rehabil Med* 2013;25(1–2):11–22.

83. Taricco M, Adone R, Pagliacci C, et al. Pharmacological management for spasticity following spinal cord injury: results of a Cochrane systematic review. *Eura Medicophys* 2006;42:5–15.

84. Hsieh J, Wolfe D, Connolly S, et al. Spasticity after spinal cord injury: an evidence-based review of current interventions. *Top Spinal Cord Inj Rehabil* 2007;13(1):81–97.

85. Harrington A, Bockenek W. Spasticity. In: Kirshblum S, Campagnolo D, eds. *Spinal Cord Medicine*. 2nd ed. Philadelphia: Lippincott Williams & Wilkins; 2011:265–281.

86. Acorda Therapeutics. *ZANAFLEX Capsules® (Tizanidine Hydrochloride) Capsules, for Oral Use.* Ardsley, NY: Acorda Therapeutics; 2013.

87. Nance PW, Bugaresti J, Shellenberger K, et al. Efficacy and safety of tizanidine in the treatment of spasticity in patients with spinal cord injury. North American Tizanidine Study Group. *Neurology* 1994;44(11)(suppl 9): S44–S52.

88. Marciniak C, Rader L, Gagnon C. The use of botulinum toxin for spasticity after spinal cord injury. *Am J Phys Med Rehabil* 2008;87(4):312–320, 329.

89. Lui J, Sarai M, Mills PB. Chemodenervation for treatment of limb spasticity following spinal cord injury: a systematic review. *Spinal Cord* 2015;53(4):252–264.

90. McIntyre A, Mays R, Mehta S, et al. Examining the effectiveness of intrathecal baclofen on spasticity in individuals with chronic spinal cord injury: a systematic review. *J Spinal Cord Med* 2014;37(1):11–18.

91. Lewis KS, Mueller WM. Intrathecal baclofen for severe spasticity secondary to spinal cord injury. *Ann Pharmacother* 1993;27(6):767–774.

92. Herman RM, D'Luzansky SC, Ippolito R. Intrathecal baclofen suppresses central pain in patients with spinal lesions. A pilot study. *Clin J Pain* 1992;8(4):338–345.

93. Skold C, Lonn L, Harms-Ringdahl K, et al. Effects of functional electrical stimulation training for six months on body composition and spasticity in motor complete tetraplegic spinal cord-injured individuals. *J Rehabil Med* 2002;34(1):25–32.

94. Barolat G, Myklebust JB, Wenninger W. Effects of spinal cord stimulation on spasticity and spasms secondary to myelopathy. *Appl Neurophysiol* 1988;51(1):29–44.

95. Krause P, Szecsi J, Straube A. Changes in spastic muscle tone increase in patients with spinal cord injury using functional electrical stimulation and passive leg movements. *Clin Rehabil* 2008;22(7):627–634.

96. Kingery WS. A critical review of controlled clinical trials for peripheral neuropathic pain and complex regional pain syndromes. *Pain* 1997;73(2):123–139.

97. O'Connell NE, Wand BM, McAuley J, et al. Interventions for treating pain and disability in adults with complex regional pain syndrome. *Cochrane Database Syst Rev* 2013;(4):CD009416.

98. Mehta S, McIntyre A, Dijkers M, et al. Gabapentinoids are effective in decreasing neuropathic pain and other secondary outcomes after spinal cord injury: a meta-analysis. *Arch Phys Med Rehabil* 2014;95(11):2180–2186.

99. Siddall PJ, Cousins MJ, Otte A, et al. Pregabalin in central neuropathic pain associated with spinal cord injury: a placebo-controlled trial. *Neurology* 2006;67(10):1792–1800.

100. Cardenas DD, Nieshoff EC, Suda K, et al. A randomized trial of pregabalin in patients with neuropathic pain due to spinal cord injury. *Neurology* 2013;80(6):533–539.

101. Vranken JH, Dijkgraaf MG, Kruis MR, et al. Pregabalin in patients with central neuropathic pain: a randomized, double-blind, placebo-controlled trial of a flexible-dose regimen. *Pain* 2008;136(1–2):150–157.

102. Cardenas DD, Emir B, Parsons B. Examining the time to therapeutic effect of pregabalin in spinal cord injury patients with neuropathic pain. *Clin Ther* 2015;37(5):1081–1090.

103. Levendoglu F, Ogun CO, Ozerbil O, et al. Gabapentin is a first line drug for the treatment of neuropathic pain in spinal cord injury. *Spine (Phila Pa 1976)* 2004;29(7):743–751.

104. To TP, Lim TC, Hill ST, et al. Gabapentin for neuropathic pain following spinal cord injury. *Spinal Cord* 2002;40(6):282–285.

105. Putzke JD, Richards JS, Kezar L, et al. Long-term use of gabapentin for treatment of pain after traumatic spinal cord injury. *Clin J Pain* 2002;18(2):116–121.

106. Ahn SH, Park HW, Lee BS, et al. Gabapentin effect on neuropathic pain compared among patients with spinal cord injury and different durations of symptoms. *Spine (Phila Pa 1976)* 2003;28(4):341–347.

107. Tai Q, Kirshblum S, Chen B, et al. Gabapentin in the treatment of neuropathic pain after spinal cord injury: a prospective, randomized, double-blind, crossover trial. *J Spinal Cord Med* 2002;25(2):100–105.

108. Rintala DH, Holmes SA, Courtade D, et al. Comparison of the effectiveness of amitriptyline and gabapentin on chronic neuropathic pain in persons with spinal cord injury. *Arch Phys Med Rehabil* 2007;88(12):1547–1560.

109. Leach MJ, Marden CM, Miller AA. Pharmacological studies on lamotrigine, a novel potential antiepileptic drug: II. Neurochemical studies on the mechanism of action. *Epilepsia* 1986;27(5):490–497.

110. Teoh H, Fowler LJ, Bowery NG. Effect of lamotrigine on the electrically-evoked release of endogenous amino acids from slices of dorsal horn of the rat spinal cord. *Neuropharmacology* 1995;34(10):1273–1278.

111. Finnerup NB, Sindrup SH, Bach FW, et al. Lamotrigine in spinal cord injury pain: a randomized controlled trial. *Pain* 2002;96(3):375–383.

112. Agarwal N, Joshi M. Effectiveness of amitriptyline and lamotrigine in traumatic spinal cord injury-induced neuropathic pain: a randomized longitudinal comparative study. *Spinal Cord* 2017;55(2):126–130.

113. Drewes AM, Andreasen A, Poulsen LH. Valproate for treatment of chronic central pain after spinal cord injury. A double-blind cross-over study. *Paraplegia* 1994;32(8):565–569.

114. Finnerup NB, Grydehoj J, Bing J, et al. Levetiracetam in spinal cord injury pain: a randomized controlled trial. *Spinal Cord* 2009;47(12):861–867.

115. Macdonald RL, Kelly KM. Antiepileptic drug mechanisms of action. *Epilepsia* 1995;36(suppl 2):S2–S12.

116. Salinas FA, Lugo LH, Garcia HI. Efficacy of early treatment with carbamazepine in prevention of neuropathic pain in patients with spinal cord injury. *Am J Phys Med Rehabil* 2012;91(12):1020–1027.

117. Harden R, Brenman E, Saltz S, et al. Topiramate in the management of spinal cord injury pain: a double-blind, randomized, placebo-controlled pilot study. In: Yezierski R, Burchiel K, eds. *Spinal Cord Injury Pain: Assessment, Mechanisms, Management. Progress in Pain Research and Management.* Vol 23. Seattle, WA: IASP Press; 2002:393–407.

118. Mehta S, Guy S, Lam T, et al. Antidepressants are effective in decreasing neuropathic pain after SCI: a meta-analysis. *Top Spinal Cord Inj Rehabil* 2015;21(2):166–173.

119. Cardenas DD, Warms CA, Turner JA, et al. Efficacy of amitriptyline for relief of pain in spinal cord injury: results of a randomized controlled trial. *Pain* 2002;96(3):365–373.

120. Sandford PR, Lindblom LB, Haddox JD. Amitriptyline and carbamazepine in the treatment of dysesthetic pain in spinal cord injury. *Arch Phys Med Rehabil* 1992;73(3):300–301.

121. Erzurumulu A, Dursun H, Gunduz S. The management of chronic pain in spinal cord injured patients. The comparison of effectiveness of amitriptyline and carbamazepine combination and electroacupuncture application. *J Rheumatol Med Rehabil* 1996;7:176–180.

122. Davidoff G, Guarracini M, Roth E, et al. Trazodone hydrochloride in the treatment of dysesthetic pain in traumatic myelopathy: a randomized, double-blind, placebo-controlled study. *Pain* 1987;29(2):151–161.

123. Goldstein DJ, Lu Y, Detke MJ, et al. Duloxetine vs. placebo in patients with painful diabetic neuropathy. *Pain* 2005;116(1–2):109–118.

124. Wernicke JF, Raskin J, Rosen A, et al. Duloxetine in the long-term management of diabetic peripheral neuropathic pain: an open-label, 52-week extension of a randomized controlled clinical trial. *Curr Ther Res Clin Exp* 2006;67(5):283–304.

125. Lunn MP, Hughes RA, Wiffen PJ. Duloxetine for treating painful neuropathy, chronic pain or fibromyalgia. *Cochrane Database Syst Rev* 2014;(1):CD007115.

126. Russell IJ, Mease PJ, Smith TR, et al. Efficacy and safety of duloxetine for treatment of fibromyalgia in patients with or without major depressive disorder: results from a 6-month, randomized, double-blind, placebo-controlled, fixed-dose trial. *Pain* 2008;136(3):432–444.

127. Vranken JH, Hollmann MW, van der Vegt MH, et al. Duloxetine in patients with central neuropathic pain caused by spinal cord injury or stroke: a randomized, double-blind, placebo-controlled trial. *Pain* 2011;152(2):267–273.

128. Lilly E. *Prescribing information—Cymbalta.* Available at: https://www.accessdata.fda.gov/drugsatfda_docs/label/2010/022516lbl.pdf. Accessed August 3, 2017.

129. Felix ER. Chronic neuropathic pain in SCI: evaluation and treatment. *Phys Med Rehabil Clin N Am* 2014;25(3):545–571, viii.

130. Guy SD, Mehta S, Harvey D, et al. The CanPain SCI clinical practice guideline for rehabilitation management of neuropathic pain after spinal cord: recommendations for model systems of care. *Spinal Cord* 2016;54(suppl 1):S24–S27.

131. Backonja M, Gombar KA. Response of central pain syndromes to intravenous lidocaine. *J Pain Symptom Manage* 1992;7(3):172–178.

132. Attal N, Gaude V, Brasseur L, et al. Intravenous lidocaine in central pain: a double-blind, placebo-controlled, psychophysical study. *Neurology* 2000;54(3):564–574.

133. Finnerup NB, Biering-Sørensen F, Johannesen IL, et al. Intravenous lidocaine relieves spinal cord injury pain: a randomized controlled trial. *Anesthesiology* 2005;102(5):1023–1030.

134. Kvarnstrom A, Karlsten R, Quiding H, et al. The analgesic effect of intravenous ketamine and lidocaine on pain after spinal cord injury. *Acta Anaesthesiol Scand* 2004;48(4):498–506.

135. Wasner G, Naleschinski D, Baron R. A role for peripheral afferents in the pathophysiology and treatment of at-level neuropathic pain in spinal cord injury? A case report. *Pain* 2007;131(1–2):219–225.

136. Hans GH, Robert DN, Van Maldeghem KN. Treatment of an acute severe central neuropathic pain syndrome by topical application of lidocaine 5% patch: a case report. *Spinal Cord* 2008;46(4):311–313.

137. Freo U, Ambrosio F, Furnari M, et al. Lidocaine 5% medicated plaster for spinal neuropathic pain. *J Pain Palliat Care Pharmacother* 2016;30(2):111–113.

138. Chiou-Tan FY, Tuel SM, Johnson JC, et al. Effect of mexiletine on spinal cord injury dysesthetic pain. *Am J Phys Med Rehabil* 1996;75(2):84–87.

139. Eide PK, Stubhaug A, Stenehjem AE. Central dysesthesia pain after traumatic spinal cord injury is dependent on N-methyl-D-aspartate receptor activation. *Neurosurgery* 1995;37(6):1080–1087.

140. Amr YM. Multi-day low dose ketamine infusion as adjuvant to oral gabapentin in spinal cord injury related chronic pain: a prospective, randomized, double blind trial. *Pain Physician* 2010;13(3):245–249.

141. Backonja M, Arndt G, Gombar KA, et al. Response of chronic neuropathic pain syndromes to ketamine: a preliminary study. *Pain* 1994;56(1):51–57.

142. Niesters M, Dahan A. Pharmacokinetic and pharmacodynamic considerations for NMDA receptor antagonists in the treatment of chronic neuropathic pain. *Expert Opin Drug Metab Toxicol* 2012;8(11):1409–1417.

143. Kim K, Mishina M, Kokubo R, et al. Ketamine for acute neuropathic pain in patients with spinal cord injury. *J Clin Neurosci* 2013;20(6):804–807.

144. Gaskell H, Derry S, Stannard C, et al. Oxycodone for neuropathic pain in adults. *Cochrane Database Syst Rev* 2016;(7):CD010692.

145. Cooper TE, Chen J, Wiffen PJ, et al. Morphine for chronic neuropathic pain in adults. *Cochrane Database Syst Rev* 2017;(5):CD011669.

146. Attal N, Guirimand F, Brasseur L, et al. Effects of IV morphine in central pain: a randomized placebo-controlled study. *Neurology* 2002;58(4):554–563.

147. Norrbrink C, Lundeberg T. Tramadol in neuropathic pain after spinal cord injury: a randomized, double-blind, placebo-controlled trial. *Clin J Pain* 2009;25(3):177–184.

148. U.S. Food and Drug Administration. Ultram® (tramadol hydrochloride) tablets. Full prescribing information. Available at: https://www.accessdata.fda.gov/drugsatfda_docs/label/2009/020281s032s033lbl.pdf. Accessed August 3, 2017.

149. Barrera-Chacon JM, Mendez-Suarez JL, Jauregui-Abrisqueta ML, et al. Oxycodone improves pain control and quality of life in anticonvulsant-pretreated spinal cord-injured patients with neuropathic pain. *Spinal Cord* 2011;49(1):36–42.

150. Rintala DH, Fiess RN, Tan G, et al. Effect of dronabinol on central neuropathic pain after spinal cord injury: a pilot study. *Am J Phys Med Rehabil* 2010;89(10):840–848.

151. Attal N, Brasseur L, Guirimand D, et al. Are oral cannabinoids safe and effective in refractory neuropathic pain? *Eur J Pain* 2004;8(2):173–177.

152. Hagenbach U, Luz S, Ghafoor N, et al. The treatment of spasticity with Delta9-tetrahydrocannabinol in persons with spinal cord injury. *Spinal Cord* 2007;45(8):551–562.

153. Glynn CJ, Jamous MA, Teddy PJ, et al. Role of spinal noradrenergic system in transmission of pain in patients with spinal cord injury. *Lancet* 1986;2(8518):1249–1250.

154. Siddall PJ, Molloy AR, Walker S, et al. The efficacy of intrathecal morphine and clonidine in the treatment of pain after spinal cord injury. *Anesth Analg* 2000;91(6):1493–1498.

155. Rauck RL, Wallace MS, Burton AW, et al. Intrathecal ziconotide for neuropathic pain: a review. *Pain Pract* 2009;9(5):327–337.

156. Saulino M, Burton AW, Danyo DA, et al. Intrathecal ziconotide and baclofen provide pain relief in seven patients with neuropathic pain and spasticity: case reports. *Eur J Phys Rehabil Med* 2009;45(1):61–67.

157. Middleton JW, Siddall PJ, Walker S, et al. Intrathecal clonidine and baclofen in the management of spasticity and neuropathic pain following spinal cord injury: a case study. *Arch Phys Med Rehabil* 1996;77(8):824–826.

158. Loubser PG, Akman NM. Effects of intrathecal baclofen on chronic spinal cord injury pain. *J Pain Symptom Manage* 1996;12(4):241–247.

159. Medtronic. Increased risk of motor stall and loss of or change in therapy with unapproved drug formulations. Available at: http://www.medtronic.com/content/dam/medtronic-com/professional/documents/product-advisories/tdd/risk-motor-stall.pdf. Accessed August 3, 2017.

160. Ehde DM, Dillworth TM, Turner JA. Cognitive-behavioral therapy for individuals with chronic pain: efficacy, innovations, and directions for research. *Am Psychol* 2014;69(2):153–166.

161. Ehde DM, Jensen MP. Feasibility of a cognitive restructuring intervention for treatment of chronic pain in persons with disabilities. *Rehabil Psychol* 2004;49:254–258.

162. Heutink M, Post MW, Bongers-Janssen HM, et al. The CONECSI trial: results of a randomized controlled trial of a multidisciplinary cognitive behavioral program for coping with chronic neuropathic pain after spinal cord injury. *Pain* 2012;153(1):120–128.

163. Perry KN, Nicholas MK, Middleton JW. Comparison of a pain management program with usual care in a pain management center for people with spinal cord injury-related chronic pain. *Clin J Pain* 2010;26(3):206–216.

164. Perry KN, Nicholas MK, Middleton J. Multidisciplinary cognitive behavioural pain management programmes for people with a spinal cord injury: design and implementation. *Disabil Rehabil* 2011;33(13–14):1272–1280.

165. Castelnuovo G, Giusti EM, Manzoni GM, et al. Psychological treatments and psychotherapies in the neurorehabilitation of pain: evidences and recommendations from the Italian Consensus Conference on Pain in Neurorehabilitation. *Front Psychol* 2016;7:115.

166. McCracken LM, Vowles KE, Eccleston C. Acceptance-based treatment for persons with complex, long standing chronic pain: a preliminary analysis of treatment outcome in comparison to a waiting phase. *Behav Res Ther* 2005;43(10):1335–1346.

167. Vowles KE, McCracken LM. Acceptance and values-based action in chronic pain: a study of treatment effectiveness and process. *J Consult Clin Psychol* 2008;76(3):397–407.

168. McCracken LM, Vowles KE. Acceptance and commitment therapy and mindfulness for chronic pain: model, process, and progress. *Am Psychol* 2014;69(2):178–187.

169. Jensen MP, Barber J, Romano JM, et al. Effects of self-hypnosis training and EMG biofeedback relaxation training on chronic pain in persons with spinal-cord injury. *Int J Clin Exp Hypn* 2009;57(3):239–268.

170. Mehta S, Orenczuk S, Hansen KT, et al. An evidence-based review of the effectiveness of cognitive behavioral therapy for psychosocial issues post-spinal cord injury. *Rehabil Psychol* 2011;56(1):15–25.

171. Burns AS, Delparte JJ, Ballantyne EC, et al. Evaluation of an interdisciplinary program for chronic pain after spinal cord injury. *PM R* 2013;5(10):832–838.

172. Cardenas DD, Jensen MP. Treatments for chronic pain in persons with spinal cord injury: a survey study. *J Spinal Cord Med* 2006;29(2):109–117.

173. Boldt I, Eriks-Hoogland I, Brinkhof MW, et al. Non-pharmacological interventions for chronic pain in people with spinal cord injury. *Cochrane Database Syst Rev* 2014;(11):CD009177.

174. Celik EC, Erhan B, Gunduz B, et al. The effect of low-frequency TENS in the treatment of neuropathic pain in patients with spinal cord injury. *Spinal Cord* 2013;51(4):334–337.

175. Davis R, Lentini R. Transcutaneous nerve stimulation for treatment of pain in patients with spinal cord injury. *Surg Neurol* 1975;4(1):100–101.

176. Norrbrink C. Transcutaneous electrical nerve stimulation for treatment of spinal cord injury neuropathic pain. *J Rehabil Res Dev* 2009;46(1):85–93.

177. Cioni B, Meglio M, Pentimalli L, et al. Spinal cord stimulation in the treatment of paraplegic pain. *J Neurosurg* 1995;82(1):35–39.

178. Lang P. The treatment of chronic pain by epidural spinal cord stimulation—a 15 year follow up; present status. *Axone* 1997;18(4):71–73.

179. Richardson RR, Meyer PR, Cerullo LJ. Neurostimulation in the modulation of intractable paraplegic and traumatic neuroma pains. *Pain* 1980;8(1):75–84.

180. Chari A, Hentall ID, Papadopoulos MC, et al. Surgical neurostimulation for spinal cord injury. *Brain Sci* 2017;7(2):E18.

181. Previnaire JG, Nguyen JP, Perrouin-Verbe B, et al. Chronic neuropathic pain in spinal cord injury: efficiency of deep brain and motor cortex stimulation therapies for neuropathic pain in spinal cord injury patients. *Ann Phys Rehabil Med* 2009;52(2):188–193.

182. Im SH, Ha SW, Kim DR, et al. Long-term results of motor cortex stimulation in the treatment of chronic, intractable neuropathic pain. *Stereotact Funct Neurosurg* 2015;93(3):212–218.

183. Nguyen JP, Lefaucheur JP, Decq P, et al. Chronic motor cortex stimulation in the treatment of central and neuropathic pain. Correlations between clinical, electrophysiological and anatomical data. *Pain* 1999;82(3):245–251.

184. Knechtel L, Thienel R, Schall U. Transcranial direct current stimulation: neurophysiology and clinical applications. *Neuropsychiatry* 2013;3:89–96.

185. Fregni F, Boggio PS, Lima MC, et al. A sham-controlled, phase II trial of transcranial direct current stimulation for the treatment of central pain in traumatic spinal cord injury. *Pain* 2006;122(1–2):197–209.

186. Ngernyam N, Jensen MP, Arayawichanon P, et al. The effects of transcranial direct current stimulation in patients with neuropathic pain from spinal cord injury. *Clin Neurophysiol* 2015;126(2):382–390.

187. Soler MD, Kumru H, Pelayo R, et al. Effectiveness of transcranial direct current stimulation and visual illusion on neuropathic pain in spinal cord injury. *Brain* 2010;133(9):2565–2577.

188. Kumru H, Soler D, Vidal J, et al. The effects of transcranial direct current stimulation with visual illusion in neuropathic pain due to spinal cord injury: an evoked potentials and quantitative thermal testing study. *Eur J Pain* 2013;17(1):55–66.

189. Wrigley PJ, Gustin SM, McIndoe LN, et al. Longstanding neuropathic pain after spinal cord injury is refractory to transcranial direct current stimulation: a randomized controlled trial. *Pain* 2013;154(10):2178–2184.

190. Mehta S, McIntyre A, Guy S, et al. Effectiveness of transcranial direct current stimulation for the management of neuropathic pain after spinal cord injury: a meta-analysis. *Spinal Cord* 2015;53(11):780–785.

191. Bikson M, Grossman P, Thomas C, et al. Safety of transcranial direct current stimulation: evidence based update 2016. *Brain Stimul* 2016;9(5):641–661.

192. Norrbrink C, Lundeberg T. Acupuncture and massage therapy for neuropathic pain following spinal cord injury: an exploratory study. *Acupunct Med* 2011;29(2):108–115.

193. Estores I, Chen K, Jackson B, et al. Auricular acupuncture for spinal cord injury related neuropathic pain: a pilot controlled clinical trial. *J Spinal Cord Med* 2017;40(4):432–438.

194. Nayak S, Shiflett SC, Schoenberger NE, et al. Is acupuncture effective in treating chronic pain after spinal cord injury? *Arch Phys Med Rehabil* 2001;82(11):1578–1586.

195. Dyson-Hudson TA, Kadar P, LaFountaine M, et al. Acupuncture for chronic shoulder pain in persons with spinal cord injury: a small-scale clinical trial. *Arch Phys Med Rehabil* 2007;88(10):1276–1283.

196. Ginis K, Latimer A, McKechnie K, et al. Using exercise to enhance subjective well-being among people with spinal cord injury: the mediating influences of stress and pain. *Rehabil Psychol* 2003;48:157–164.

197. Latimer AE, Ginis KA, Hicks AL, et al. An examination of the mechanisms of exercise-induced change in psychological well-being among people with spinal cord injury. *J Rehabil Res Dev* 2004;41(5):643–652.

198. Cooper MA, Kluding PM, Wright DE. Emerging relationships between exercise, sensory nerves, and neuropathic pain. *Front Neurosci* 2016; 10:372.

199. Norrbrink C, Lindberg T, Wahman K, et al. Effects of an exercise programme on musculoskeletal and neuropathic pain after spinal cord injury—results from a seated double-poling ergometer study. *Spinal Cord* 2012;50(6):457–461.

200. Sato G, Osumi M, Morioka S. Effects of wheelchair propulsion on neuropathic pain and resting electroencephalography after spinal cord injury. *J Rehabil Med* 2017;49(2):136–143.

201. Tasker RR, DeCarvalho GT, Dolan EJ. Intractable pain of spinal cord origin: clinical features and implications for surgery. *J Neurosurg* 1992;77(3):373–378.

202. Pagni CA, Canavero S. Cordomyelotomy in the treatment of paraplegia pain. Experience in two cases with long-term results. *Acta Neurol Belg* 1995;95(1):33–36.

203. Konrad P. Dorsal root entry zone lesion, midline myelotomy and anterolateral cordotomy. *Neurosurg Clin N Am* 2014;25(4):699–722.

204. Mehta S, Orenczuk K, McIntyre A, et al. Neuropathic pain post spinal cord injury part 2: systematic review of dorsal root entry zone procedure. *Top Spinal Cord Inj Rehabil* 2013;19(1):78–86.

205. Sindou M, Mertens P, Wael M. Microsurgical DREZotomy for pain due to spinal cord and/or cauda equina injuries: long-term results in a series of 44 patients. *Pain* 2001;92(1–2):159–171.

206. Edgar RE, Best LG, Quail PA, et al. Computer-assisted DREZ microcoagulation: posttraumatic spinal deafferentation pain. *J Spinal Disord* 1993;6(1):48–56.

207. Falci S, Best L, Bayles R, et al. Dorsal root entry zone microcoagulation for spinal cord injury-related central pain: operative intramedullary electrophysiological guidance and clinical outcome. *J Neurosurg* 2002;97 (2 suppl):193–200.

208. Teasell RW, Mehta S, Aubut JA, et al. A systematic review of pharmacologic treatments of pain after spinal cord injury. *Arch Phys Med Rehabil* 2010;91(5):816–831.

209. Siddall PJ, Middleton JW. A proposed algorithm for the management of pain following spinal cord injury. *Spinal Cord* 2006;44(2):67–77.

210. Bryce TN, Gomez J. Management of pain after spinal cord injury. *Curr Phys Med Rehabil Rep* 2015;3:189–196.

CHAPTER 41

Epidemiology, Prevalence, and Cancer Pain Syndromes

NEIL A. HAGEN

Cancer is a highly prevalent and serious public health issue. It most commonly affects the elderly—*the average cancer patient in the Western world is aged 65 at first diagnosis*[1]—and cancer is more likely to occur in particular clinical settings, such as life-long smokers, in obesity, and with certain environmental and heritable risks. Specifically, the World Health Organization reports that about one-third of cancer deaths are attributed to the increased risk associated with five major behavioral and dietary risk factors: tobacco use, high body mass index, low fruit and vegetable intake, lack of physical activity, and alcohol use. Tobacco use itself is responsible for about 22% of cancer deaths around the world.[2] However, there is no one who is immune from the disease regardless of age. In North America, about 1 in 3 adults will develop cancer in their lifetime, with about a 50% fatality rate. Cancer is sufficiently prevalent that some individuals will develop more than one type of malignancy, either sequentially or concurrently. Cancer is often painful, and pain is a common heralding manifestation of the disease. For example, about two-thirds of women have pain at the onset or recurrence of ovarian cancer.[3] As cancer progresses, it is more likely to be associated with pain, and the pain is more likely to be severe. A range of epidemiologic studies in several countries and practice settings suggests that pain from a wide variety of cancers is present in about one-third of patients receiving cancer treatment and in 60% to 90% of patients with advanced illness.[4]

Cancer treatment can also cause pain, and cancer pain is commonly classified as being either due to the underlying disease or due to its treatment. In pediatric malignancies, pain due to treatment is more common than pain from the underlying disease.[5] Cancer patients can also have pain from non–cancer-related conditions, and the causes and prevalence are similar to pain in patients without a cancer diagnosis. Clinicians should be especially wary about missing a treatable cause of pain in cancer patients, whether the pain is due to cancer, cancer treatment, or due to a noncancer mechanism.

There is an array of factors that contribute to the likelihood of pain being present, its severity, and the best approach to its management. Thus, in order to understand the wisest approach to assessing and managing the cancer patient who presents with cancer pain, the situation is best appreciated within the perspective of where the patient is in the disease trajectory and what other clinical factors are likely to be at play.

The intention of this introductory chapter is to provide a clinical context of the individual patient and to bring into focus the extensive information that follows in subsequent chapters where more detailed approaches to assessment and management will be elaborated. This chapter is divided into six sections:

- Summary of the epidemiology of cancer pain
- How to perform a cancer pain history
- How to perform a physical examination of a cancer pain patient, including bedside provocative maneuvers to help identify potential underlying pain-sensitive structures
- Problem formulation
- Constructing an analgesic strategy
- Managing pain in specific clinical situations

Epidemiology of Cancer Pain

Epidemiology is "the study of disease as it affects groups of people. . . . [It] contributes to the control not only of infectious diseases but also of conditions such as heart disease and cancer. Their distributions in populations can provide important insight to possible causes. The relation between the environment and disease is an essential part of epidemiology."[6] The epidemiology of cancer pain refers to cancer pain within the overall population, and its characterization suggests plausible factors at play within an individual patient.

PAIN RELATED TO EXTENT OF DISEASE: THE CANCER DISEASE TRAJECTORY

Commonly, patients with solid tumor malignancies present with an asymptomatic mass; less than 15% of patients with nonmetastatic disease describe pain from their cancer.[4] Cancer can present clinically in a wide variety of ways, including dyspnea, nausea, urinary symptoms, weakness, numbness, weight loss, and other signs and symptoms. When pain is the first symptom of cancer, there is a tendency for the cancer to be more advanced, and perhaps for this reason, pain can be an independent predictor for poorer survival.

The clinician can use this information to suspect the underlying cause of pain. For example, imagine a patient with a diagnosis of melanoma who presents with a 3-day history of new onset of headache. Headache could be due to a benign cause (e.g., migraine) or due to malignancy (e.g., brain metastasis). Stage of cancer strongly predicts the risk of brain metastases from a solid tumor. In this example, the likelihood of central nervous system metastasis is much lower in a patient who has recently undergone resection of a primary melanoma in the leg, with regional lymph nodes negative, compared to the patient who has known liver and lung metastases from melanoma. About 90% of patients with advanced melanoma have central nervous system metastases at the time of autopsy, and the report of any headache in a patient with known metastatic melanoma is ominous. If imaging studies of the brain are negative in a patient with metastatic melanoma and a new headache, the possibility of meningeal disease should be considered, along with a diagnostic dural puncture for cerebrospinal fluid analysis.

SPECIAL NEEDS OF PARTICULAR AGE GROUPS: PEDIATRIC, YOUNG ADULT, ADULT, GERIATRIC

Pain is a subjective experience, and the pain of cancer can be foreign and puzzling for the patient. Pediatric patients can lack the language and the sophistication of adults in communicating their inner world. Although cancer can result in an overwhelming sense of threat at any age, the pediatric age group requires special skills and support. For instance, pediatric patients and their families become the "unit of care," far more so than with adult oncology, and specialized assessment tools must be used for this population (see Chapter 49).

Cancer pain is prevalent at all ages. However, there are several remarkable features of cancer pain within the pediatric population. Pain from cancer *treatment* is highly prevalent, in part related to the high prevalence of procedures to manage hematologic malignancies and other malignancies which are prevalent in this age group.[5] Particular attention needs to be taken to diminish the fear of pain from procedures and treatment. Painful procedures include placement of intravenous catheters, repeated spinal taps, bone marrow biopsies, extensive cancer surgery, and others. Importantly, young patients are often proficient at managing their pain once taught an appropriate technique. Patients as young as 5 years can safely and effectively use a patient-controlled analgesia device, with the overall outcome of good pain control and potentially less risk of nausea or respiratory depression compared to continuous opioid infusions.[7]

Sarcoma and hematologic malignancies are more common in the 16- to 21-year-old age group. Rarely, young adults can present with what looks clinically to be depression, but in fact, the patient has uncontrolled pain. Particular attention needs to be placed on supporting the patient to be as active and have as normal a life as possible despite the potentially disfiguring effects of cancer treatment, difficulty with cancer pain, and the many challenges of cancer treatment.

Working-age adults with cancer pain face their own challenges. A need to generate income or fulfill parenting roles despite illness, financial obligations, fear of addiction, and the difficulties of managing emotional distress are all issues that need to be directly addressed in order to provide comprehensive symptom control. Young adults often choose or have indications for more aggressive or prolonged cancer treatments. For example, aromatase inhibitors are commonly used in the adjuvant treatment of breast cancer over the course of several years; almost half of these patients describe joint pain or stiffness. Usually, symptoms are mild or moderate, but nearly one quarter of patients rate their symptoms from aromatase inhibitors as severe.[8]

The geriatric population often has medical comorbidity, such as underlying heart, lung, renal, or cognitive impairment, and may be on a variety of medications that interact with analgesic medications. Dosages of medications such as opioids may need to be lowered because the metabolism of medication can be much slower with advanced age or underlying organ impairment. An important, emerging concept within the geriatric population is that of frailty. Factors that promote return to health or maintenance of good health—resilience—are powerful in the pediatric and young adult population; with advancing years, the ability to maintain homeostasis becomes less. *Frailty* is a term that describes what has become an area of intense research in the geriatric health care community and is a key factor in analgesic care in the older cancer population.[9] Changes in medications in the geriatric population should generally be made more slowly and with smaller dosing increments. Attention needs to be paid to drug–drug interactions, and the clinician should be vigilant for the appearance of early signs of cognitive impairment. Because of the high prevalence of delirium in the medically ill geriatric oncology population and the difficulty in making an early diagnosis, some clinicians have advocated for the routine use of delirium screening tools.[10]

SPECIAL NEEDS OF PARTICULAR ETHNIC GROUPS: COMMUNICATION STYLES, COMMON PREFERENCES, AND MANAGING TABOOS

Some countries and certain ethnic groups are particularly vulnerable to specific health issues. Ineffective cervical cancer prevention programs, low rates of cervical cancer screening, and difficulty accessing cancer treatment services are associated with higher rates of cervical cancer and higher rates of cancer death. About 90% of cervical cancer deaths occur in low- to middle-income countries.[11] Nasopharyngeal cancers are highly prevalent in patients who originate from Pacific Rim countries, and the higher risk persists for decades after moving to a Western country.[12] There are some First Nations communities in North America where diabetes mellitus has reached epidemic proportions, with half or more of all adults being afflicted; cancer care can be greatly complicated by underlying diabetes. Every culture and ethnic group has a unique set of medical issues that are of particular concern.

Some countries, or parts of countries, have a lengthy history of violence and social upheaval in association with the licit or illicit drug trade, and the medical use of opioids is greatly frowned on. Some religious cultures are believed to hold the experience of suffering to be of spiritual value. Others are commonly believed to place a taboo on disclosure of a cancer diagnosis to the patient, relegating the burden of that knowledge and the decision making about cancer care to the eldest son.

There are approximately 6,900 discrete languages spoken in the world[13] and uncountable distinct ethnic, religious, and other cultures. How is the clinician to be alert to all possible areas where culture can have a major influence on patient preferences and on patient assessment?

Basic knowledge of common beliefs within certain cultures is inarguably important, such as the prevalence of modesty as a dominant value in the Muslim faith community. Beliefs common to many cultures are complicated by the tendency in Western society for a shift to occur within immigrant families, with increasing orientation toward secular values from one generation to the next. So when the patient who is thought to belong to a particular culture is in the physician's office along with his or her spouse and his or her adult children, which is likely to be the dominant culture? The clinician is wise to not make assumptions about what are the beliefs, values, and preferences of the patient or his or her family. Instead, it is far better to ask because these issues will all have an impact on the patient's pain experience and treatment. There are many variations of beliefs within broad cultural groups, and it has been recommended in the clinical realm to instead focus on the patient and the family unit as having their own culture. It is the task of the clinician to understand and respect that culture.

If there is a taboo against disclosing a life-threatening diagnosis to the patient, the family will almost invariably make this wish abundantly clear to the clinician at an early stage. This traditional practice can conflict with a patient's right to information.[14] There is an emerging ethical construct that supports the clinician to respect a family's request, if it is the explicit wish of the patient. If the patient indicates that another family member is to be the receiver of medical information and is to make all treatment and other decisions on the care of the patient, the patient has duly exercised his or her autonomy. The family, or a specific individual within the family, becomes the unit to which the authority of informed consent is conferred. It is legitimate for the clinician to periodically confirm what is the preferred communication style and to whom the patient has conferred decision-making authority. Fortunately, taboos in disclosure of diagnostic information rarely interfere with obtaining information directly from the patient regarding his or her experience of pain and the effect of analgesic interventions.

COMORBIDITIES ASSOCIATED WITH SPECIFIC CANCERS: LUNG DISEASE, LIVER DISEASE, RENAL DISEASE, AND NEUROLOGIC DISEASE

Lung cancer is about 30 times as prevalent in life-long smokers as life-long nonsmokers. Patients with lung cancer commonly have clinically significant chronic obstructive lung disease, ischemic heart disease, or symptomatic peripheral vascular disease. If patients have preexisting carbon dioxide retention, there is a risk the carbon dioxide retention will worsen with the use of opioids, especially if benzodiazepines are taken concurrently for anxiolysis, for example. Other than in the situation of life-threatening carbon dioxide retention, where very careful titration under monitored conditions may be indicated, opioids are generally not contraindicated by the presence of lung disease and should be carefully titrated to effect while monitoring for toxicity.

Premorbid liver disease is also prevalent in patients with specific cancer types, such as hepatoma and esophageal cancer. The major clinical features of liver disease relate to portal hypertension, with an elevated risk of episodes of gastrointestinal (GI) bleeding, ascites, and malnutrition. The capacity of the liver to metabolize medications is often less affected than other aspects of liver function, and the dose of medications commonly used in cancer pain such as opioids should not routinely be reduced. Instead, medications should be titrated to effect. Acetaminophen should be used with caution, however, particularly in the setting of cirrhosis. The clinical presentation of liver metastases is often pain and jaundice; it is rare to encounter metabolic liver failure until almost all of the liver is replaced by cancer.

Renal disease is becoming much more prevalent in Western society, and many cancer treatments, such as platinum-based chemotherapy, are nephrotoxic. Cancer patients are at risk to accumulate medications or their active metabolites in the presence of even mild underlying renal impairment. This has led to recommendations of some opioids over others, although the evidence for this approach is still emerging. Some authorities recommend morphine be used with caution in the presence of known renal impairment.[15] Doses of some medications used for neuropathic pain, such as gabapentin, are routinely reduced in the setting of renal impairment, but opioids are not. Instead, opioids should be titrated to effect, recognizing that a reduction in dose or increase in dosing interval may be required. In the face of end-stage disease with near-complete or total kidney failure, renally cleared opioids (or those with clinically active renally excreted metabolites such as morphine) should be avoided or administered on an as-needed basis rather than around-the-clock.

About half of cancer patients are aged 65 years and older, an age group that has a particularly high prevalence of comorbid neurologic illness. Also, cancer and its treatments are associated with neurologic illness, such as stroke, meningitis, and other conditions. Concurrent cancer and neurologic disease affects pain management in several ways, but two deserve particular mention. First, pain assessment largely depends on an intact cognition. The widespread use of pain assessment tools such as the numeric rating scale has helped to bring some quantification to what is otherwise a subjective and often silent experience. But what if the patient is confused and provides the wrong numbers? There is then a risk of overmedication or undermedication. The Brief Pain Inventory documents several discrete domains of the pain experience: average pain in the past 24 hours, worst pain in the past 24 hours, least pain in the past 24 hours, and others. Study of the psychometrics of pain tools has revealed that the *present pain intensity* is the most reliable domain in the setting of cognitive impairment and is the measure that should be used if there is any question of cognitive impairment. Also, the information should be confirmed by other direct questions by the clinician, such as "Is the pain bad, or not bad right now?" Furthermore, cognitive impairment in cancer patients generally arises because of many contributing factors. Families are often quick to blame the pain medications. Only uncommonly are analgesics the sole or the major cause. However, in the absence of other obvious causes for delirium, rotating to a different pain medication, along with hydration and other general supportive measures, can reverse an episode of delirium even when other contributing factors are not correctable.

CANCER PAIN AND SUBSTANCE ABUSE

"Abuse" is a somewhat pejorative word, but its use has been widely accepted. Substance abuse has been defined in a variety of ways but is generally taken to mean use of a recreational drug despite harm to self or others. "Addiction" is taken to be a far extreme in the spectrum of abuse, where there is an overwhelming focus on obtaining a supply, craving, and social disintegration.[16] About 15% of adult men in Western societies abuse alcohol, and only about half that proportion of adult women. A smaller proportion of the population abuses other substances, such as cocaine, methamphetamine, or cannabinoids. Some cancer patients are actively abusing psychoactive substances, and others have a past but not current history of abuse. Some active abusers are open about their lifestyle choices, and others keep it a secret.

Pain management is challenging in patients who have a prior history of substance abuse; they have more symptoms, have more interference of function from pain, have more distress, and have more problematic drug-related behaviors than cancer pain patients who do not have a history of substance abuse.[17] Pain is common in the street-connected opioid-abusing population, with about a third of patients in methadone maintenance programs describing moderate to severe, chronic noncancer pain.[18] Pain can be difficult to reliably assess in cancer patients who have preexisting chronic pain, a history of abuse of pain medications or other psychoactive compounds, or a coping strategy that has included the use of chemicals ostensibly to help them cope. There is a clash of cultures when the clinician, who believes that the pain is what the patient describes it to be, becomes aware that there may be reasons to not fully trust the patient's description. In the setting of possible or definite past or present substance abuse, the clinician should carefully document the patient's description of his or her pain experience and obtain collateral information from family, friends, or other members of the health care team, whenever possible. There is a role for greater reliance on diagnostic imaging to confirm clinical assessment. Furthermore, there is an emerging appreciation of the use of routine risk stratification tools to assess the potential for opioid misuse in *all* cancer pain patients.[19]

All patients deserve adequate pain control and to be treated with respect. However, the situation of a cancer patient with active substance abuse requires a distinct approach that will protect the patient and his or her environment from things that can get in the way of successful pain management. An overall strategy for managing cancer pain in the addict is described at the end of this chapter, along with a summary of safe prescribing practices and universal precautions that should be used when prescribing opioids whether or not there is a history of substance abuse.

CANCER PAIN IN INMATES

The incarcerated population has unique cancer risks, in part related to underlying demographics.[20] Most inmates are men, are from ethnic minorities, and are less likely to be in the geriatric age group compared to the general population. Certain cancer risk factors are known to be highly prevalent in inmates, including smoking, drug and alcohol use, and AIDS-related illnesses.

Rates of infection of inmates are higher for hepatitis C, and HIV infection rates are much higher than the national average.[21] High rates of human papillomavirus infection have been found in women inmates. The incidence of lung cancer, head and neck cancers, liver cancer, and cervical cancer are much higher in inmates than expected compared to age-matched controls. Survival from cancer is poorer in incarcerated cancer patients compared to controls: In one study, the standardized mortality ratio was 1.6 (95% confidence interval [CI], 1.4 to 1.7) in men and 1.4 (95% CI, 1.0 to 1.9) in women.[20] In brief, compared to the general population, inmates are more likely to be affected by certain cancers, more likely to have cancers that are characterized by difficult-to-manage symptoms, and more likely to have a past history of substance abuse or viral infection that can complicate pain management.

Not surprisingly, inmates with cancer have been found to have a high prevalence of pain and to be undermedicated for cancer pain.[22] Drug misuse, actual drug diversion, fears held by prescribers of potential drug diversion, and lack of patient credibility have been identified as barriers to cancer pain management.

Components of the Comprehensive Medical Evaluation of a Patient with Chronic Cancer Pain

An enormous amount of information is available to guide the clinician in assessing a patient with chronic cancer pain. Pain assessment tools have been extensively validated in a range of clinical settings, languages, and in different ages and disease states (see Chapter 20 referencing pain assessment).

However, cancer patients are often systemically ill. In addition to pain, they may have low energy and may have a range of other symptoms. Clinicians need to find a balance between the wish to complete a comprehensive assessment and yet respect the constraints of patients' abilities to tolerate such a comprehensive evaluation. Cancer patients and their families are not always able to endure lengthy clinic visits with use of extensive bedside assessment tools, detailed psychosocial evaluations, and evaluation of other important domains.

Furthermore, cancer patients and their families have many needs that compete for their time and attention. In addition to symptom control, they also are keen to learn about cancer treatment options, meet the needs of their family members such as children, and fulfill other social obligations related to their employment, completing required insurance forms and managing competing financial imperatives, such as purchasing food and prescriptions. Likewise, clinicians need to attend to their many professional roles despite the constraints of competing demands for their time: They must not only assess patients but also discuss treatment options and facilitate decision making, coordinate care, provide treatment, communicate with other team members, and attend to many other patients and other professional responsibilities. Time itself can be scarce: Health care professionals involved in symptom control can be predicted to have many calls on their time, which can have effects on patient care such as pushing palliative and supportive care issues into the background and also can result in professional stress and burnout.

How does a clinician decide on the most appropriate level of assessment of the cancer pain patient? Pragmatically, it is wisest to comprehensibly evaluate the patient at the first encounter, to the extent the patient is able to tolerate it. If necessary, the evaluation can be completed with more than one encounter to respect patient or family limitations. After that point, it should only be necessary to comprehensively reevaluate if there is a major change in the clinical presentation.

The complete bedside evaluation of the patient with cancer pain includes five major components: history, physical examination, bedside provocative maneuvers, diagnosis formulation, and construction of an overall analgesic strategy.

Pain History

DEFINITION OF PAIN

Pain is defined as "an unpleasant sensory and emotional experience associated with actual or potential tissue damage, or described in terms of such damage."[23] Pain is always a subjective experience. Most nociception is mediated by nociceptors (pain receptors) found within visceral and somatic tissues. Nociceptors are present in most tissues in the body. There are some striking exceptions including most parts of the parenchyma of the central nervous system. Also, certain modalities of nociception cannot be sensed in certain parts of the body; for example, the stomach can sense stretch as an unpleasant sensation, whereas when cauterized, there is no pain sensation that results.

Presumably, all receptors within more vulnerable body parts will have been activated many times during a person's lifetime, such as nociceptors found in the nondominant thumb: Pretty much everyone has hit their thumb with a hammer or some other blunt object many times. In contrast, the majority of nociceptors throughout the body will rarely or never actually be activated during the entire lifetime of the individual. It should come as no surprise that patients describe their pain experience in a way that reflects their own uniqueness as a person and often, reflects their unfamiliarity with the new pain experience.

Imagine, for example, the situation of a patient who has metastasis involving the left C3 facet. Most people will never experience left C3 facet pain in their entire life. The experience of nociceptors being discharged for the first time in a person's life can be puzzling, unpleasant, and difficult to describe. When experiencing a new, unfamiliar pain, patients may want to not use the word *pain* but instead use alternative descriptive words such as *discomfort*, *unpleasant*, *hurt*, and others. The clinician should recognize that any unpleasant sensation may in fact be pain and should at all times support and legitimize the patient's experience.

Furthermore, the pattern of pain referral may have gone unnoticed by the patient, particularly if the referred pain is less severe than the primary site of pain. If recognized, however, patterns of referral can greatly assist the identification of the underlying pain-sensitive structure. Studies have evaluated the referral pattern of pain in a range of tissues in many parts of the body, particularly nerves, connective tissues, ligaments, and muscles; mapping out the distribution of the resultant pain has resulted in construction of somatotopic maps. Clinicians are generally most familiar with the distribution of referred neuropathic pain along the corresponding dermatomes. *Sclerotomal pain* refers to the pattern of referred pain when the pain-sensitive structure arises in connective tissues and ligaments. Stimulation of various muscles has resulted in similar, although distinct, patterns of referred pain, known as *myotomal pain*. Going back to the previous example of left C3 facet pain, this is a kind of sclerotomal pain and has a characteristic pattern of referral, with pain felt draped laterally across the ipsilateral neck and projected rostrally toward the occipitonuchal junction.

DEFINITION OF SUFFERING

Suffering, as a human experience, needs to be distinguished from pain, per se, although the two are often interdependent: Suffering is commonly present with pain and often increases as pain increases. There have been many insightful approaches to understanding suffering within the medical domain. One of the most widely accepted approaches describes suffering as a perceived threat to an individual's sense of intactness as a complete person.[24] If suffering is in part caused by pain, this definition speaks to the meaning that the person attributes to their pain. For example, at childbirth, intensity of labor pains commonly reaches 8 out of 10 or greater and is often described as "horrible" on the McGill categorical scale. The sense of threat to a person's intactness as a human being during labor, however, is generally believed to be less than the situation of pain of a similarly high intensity caused by a life-threatening illness such as advanced cancer.

In Western countries, patients often conceptually link "pain" and "suffering" and may use the words interchangeably. In the comprehensive assessment of a patient with cancer pain, it is incumbent on the clinician to have an approach that is respectful of the patient's current circumstance. The clinician should not make assumptions about how much of the patient's distress is due to pain and how much is due to suffering. Remaining curious and empathic, the clinician works within the limitations of the comprehensive assessment in order to discover along with the patient as to how much of each of pain and suffering is present, and how they might be related. There may be early clues about exigent pain as a major component of suffering: Pain descriptors with a high affective component, such as "suffocating pain," have been found to predict the presence of suffering.[25]

Clinicians will encounter cancer patients with severe pain who are suffering enormously, particularly toward the end of life. This often results in clinicians being drawn into a strong awareness of their own sense of compassion. But what does "compassion" mean, within the health care setting? The nature of compassion within health care providers has been studied, as have cancer patients' preferences about compassionate care delivered by their health care providers.[26,27]

VALIDATED ASSESSMENT TOOLS

Many clinicians routinely use validated tools to support assessment of cancer patients, particularly to distinguish pain and suffering. There are several outstanding and widely used tools which are available. Some selected examples of the most largely used are as follows:

The Edmonton Symptom Assessment Scale—Revised Version (i.e., the ESAS-R, commonly referred to as "the ESAS"), includes 10 items: pain, tiredness, nausea, depression, anxiety, drowsiness, appetite, well-being, shortness of breath, and "other problem" (Fig. 41.1). Like many successfully applied clinical tools, it is short and has been extensively validated in a variety of countries and practice settings. The ESAS has several strengths: It is not overly burdensome to fill out, it is an effective screening tool to identify distress due to symptoms, and it identifies symptom clusters (see the following text) which, if present, can make pain more difficult to manage.

The Edmonton Classification System for Cancer Pain (ECS-CP) is a 5-item bedside tool that helps characterize prognosis for control of pain (Fig. 41.2).

The Brief Pain Inventory—Short Form (widely referred to as the BPI), delineates several aspects of the pain experience, including worst pain in the past 24 hours, average pain in the past 24 hours, least pain in the past 24 hours, physical functioning, and emotional functioning. The BPI holds several advantages: It has been extensively validated, it assesses several specific dimensions of the pain experience, and it has been used for both research outcomes and for clinical care (Fig. 41.3).

There are several other widely used screening tools to support assessment of cancer pain patients (see Chapter 20).

TYPES OF PAIN

Throughout the pain history, the clinician is looking for clues as to the underlying mechanism of pain. Because pain can be a foreign experience, it can be difficult to characterize in words.

Patients sometimes appreciate being offered choices of words that might help describe their pain, such as burning, achy, dull, sharp, deep, and so on. Broadly, pain can be thought of as somatic, visceral, or neuropathic. The words the patient uses to describe their pain experience can guide the clinician to make inferences regarding the underlying mechanism.

Somatic pain arises from bone, muscle, ligament, subcutaneous tissue, or skin. It is often experienced as sharp or dull and is typically well localized by the patient. Less commonly, it can be referred to cutaneous sites characteristic of the tissue of origin, such as sclerotomal (connective tissue in origin) or myotomal (muscle) referred pain, as described earlier.

Visceral pain arises from organs such as lung, liver, or bowel and is broadly understood to arise from tissue that is embryologically mesodermal in origin (see Chapters 47 and 61–65). It is characteristically described as dull and achy and is usually poorly localized; typically, the patients will use their entire hand to describe the location of the pain. Visceral pain is often also referred to distant sites, such as liver pain being experienced in the ipsilateral shoulder. Examination of the shoulder does not reproduce this pain.

Neuropathic pain is generally described as dull, achy, itchy, or burning. The skin can be sensitive to light touch ("allodynia": pain due to a stimulus that does not normally provoke pain—see Chapters 24–28),[23] and there may be brief stabbing episodes of neuralgic pain. The burning may be superficial as in the experience of scalded skin or can be deep, as if there is a feeling of having been burned deep inside. The spontaneous use of the word *burning* by the patient predicts the presence of neuropathic pain. However, the clinician should be cautious: Several other pains can also be experienced as an unpleasant, burning sensation, such as muscle spasm pain—a kind of somatic pain.[28] Combinations of words, such as *burning numbness*, and clinical findings such as hypesthesia, anesthesia, hyperalgesia, or allodynia in a segmental pattern within an area of pain, are of greater value in making the clinical diagnosis of neuropathic pain. For example, neuropathic pain should be diagnosed if there is significant clinical evidence such as a description of burning numbness along with tingling experienced in a distribution consistent with damage to a particular part of the nervous system; there may also be signs of motor dysfunction such as the loss of deep tendon reflexes (e.g., ankle or knee jerks) or muscle weakness; there may be bedside provocative maneuvers that reproduce the pain, such as the presence of a Tinel sign or a positive straight-leg raise maneuver. The clinician should be wary of making a diagnosis of neuropathic pain based solely on the patient's description of "burning pain," although this is an important clue to initiate further investigations.

Mixed pain is the clinical situation where there is both nociceptive (i.e., somatic and/or visceral) and neuropathic pain. A common example is chest wall pain from lung cancer; there may be poorly localized deep ache consistent with visceral (pleural) pain, sharp and well-localized somatic pain from contiguous rib invasion, and burning numbness of the overlying skin due to invasion of intercostal nerves. The term *mixed pain* has less commonly been applied to the situation of multiple mechanisms of somatic pain in the same patient—for example, painful metastasis to the humerus with contiguous muscle spasm and shoulder joint articular changes because of immobility of the painful limb. Mixed pain may benefit greatly from applying several modalities of analgesic intervention concurrently, such as simple analgesics (acetaminophen or anti-inflammatories); opioids; adjuvant analgesics in specific pain syndromes; non-drug interventions such as heat, cold, stretch, and massage; or orthotic interventions such as a joint-immobilizing splint.

Teasing out the many components of pain in the region of the body where the patient is experiencing pain will help the

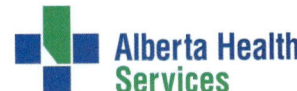 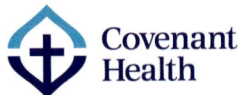

Edmonton Symptom Assessment System:
(revised version) (ESAS-R)

Please circle the number that best describes how you feel NOW:

No Pain	0	1	2	3	4	5	6	7	8	9	10	Worst Possible Pain
No Tiredness *(Tiredness = lack of energy)*	0	1	2	3	4	5	6	7	8	9	10	Worst Possible Tiredness
No Drowsiness *(Drowsiness = feeling sleepy)*	0	1	2	3	4	5	6	7	8	9	10	Worst Possible Drowsiness
No Nausea	0	1	2	3	4	5	6	7	8	9	10	Worst Possible Nausea
No Lack of Appetite	0	1	2	3	4	5	6	7	8	9	10	Worst Possible Lack of Appetite
No Shortness of Breath	0	1	2	3	4	5	6	7	8	9	10	Worst Possible Shortness of Breath
No Depression *(Depression = feeling sad)*	0	1	2	3	4	5	6	7	8	9	10	Worst Possible Depression
No Anxiety *(Anxiety = feeling nervous)*	0	1	2	3	4	5	6	7	8	9	10	Worst Possible Anxiety
Best Wellbeing *(Wellbeing = how you feel overall)*	0	1	2	3	4	5	6	7	8	9	10	Worst Possible Wellbeing
No _____ Other Problem *(for example constipation)*	0	1	2	3	4	5	6	7	8	9	10	Worst Possible _____

Patient's Name _____

Date _____   Time _____

Completed by (check one):
☐ Patient
☐ Family caregiver
☐ Health care professional caregiver
☐ Caregiver-assisted

BODY DIAGRAM ON REVERSE SIDE

ESAS-r
Revised: November 2010

FIGURE 41.1   Edmonton Symptom Assessment Scale—Revised Version. The Edmonton Symptom Assessment Scale (ESAS) along with guidelines for its use are available at http://www.palliative.org/tools.html. The ESAS is available in over 30 languages. *(From Watanabe SM, Nekolaichuk C, Beaumont C, et al. A multi-centre comparison of two numerical versions of the Edmonton Symptom Assessment System in palliative care patients. J Pain Symptom Manage 2011;41[2]:456–468; and Bruera E, Kuehn N, Miller MJ, et al. The Edmonton Symptom Assessment System (ESAS): a simple method for the assessment of palliative care patients. J Palliat Care 1991;7[2]:6–9.)*

Edmonton Classification System for Cancer Pain (ECS-CP)

Edmonton Classification System for Cancer Pain

Patient Name: _____

Patient ID No: _____

For each of the following features, circle the response that is most appropriate, based on your clinical assessment of the patient.

1.   Mechanism of Pain

No   No pain syndrome
Nc   Any nociceptive combination of visceral and/or bone or soft tissue pain
Ne   Neuropathic pain syndrome with or without any combination of nociceptive pain
Nx   Insufficient information to classify

2.   Incident Pain

Io   No incident pain
Ii   Incident pain present
Ix   Insufficient information to classify

3.   **Psychological Distress**

Po   No psychological distress
Pp   Psychological distress present
Px   Insufficient information to classify

4.   **Addictive Behavior**

Ao   No addictive behavior
Aa   Addictive behavior present
Ax   Insufficient information to classify

5.   Cognitive Function

Co   No impairment. Patient able to provide accurate present and past pain history unimpaired
Ci   Partial impairment. Sufficient impairment to affect patient's ability to provide accurate present and/or past pain history
Cu   Total impairment. Patient unresponsive, delirious or demented to the stage of being unable to provide any present and past pain history
Cx   Insufficient information to classify.

ECS-CP profile: N__ I__ P__ A__ C__   *(combination of the five responses, one for each category)*

Assessed by: _____   **Date:** _____

FIGURE 41.2 Edmonton Classification System for Cancer Pain (ECS-CP). The ECS-CP along with an administration manual are found at http://www.palliative.org/tools.html. *(From Fainsinger R, Nekolaichuk C, Lawlor P, et al. A multicentre validation study of the Revised Edmonton Staging System for classifying cancer pain in advanced cancer patients. J Pain Symptom Manage 2005;29[3]:224–237; and Nekolaichuk C, Fainsinger R, Lawlor P. A validation study of a pain classification system for advanced cancer patients using content experts: The Edmonton classification system for cancer pain. Palliat Med 2005;19[6]:466–476.)*

STUDY ID #:_ _ _ _ _ _ _ _ _   DO NOT WRITE ABOVE THIS LINE   HOSPITAL #:_ _ _ _ _ _ _ _ _

Brief Pain Inventory (Short Form)

Date:_ _ _ _ / _ _ _ _ / _ _ _ _   Time:_ _ _ _ _ _ _

Name:_ _ _ _ _ _ _ _ _ _ _ _ _ _ _ _ _ _   _ _ _ _ _ _ _ _ _ _ _ _ _ _ _ _ _ _   _ _ _ _ _ _ _ _ _ _ _ _ _ _ _

               Last   First   Middle Initial

1.   Throughout our lives, most of us have had pain from time to time (such as minor headaches, sprains, and toothaches). Have you had pain other than these every-day kinds of pain today?

                   1.   Yes   2.   No

2.   On the diagram, shade in the areas where you feel pain. Put an X on the area that hurts the most.

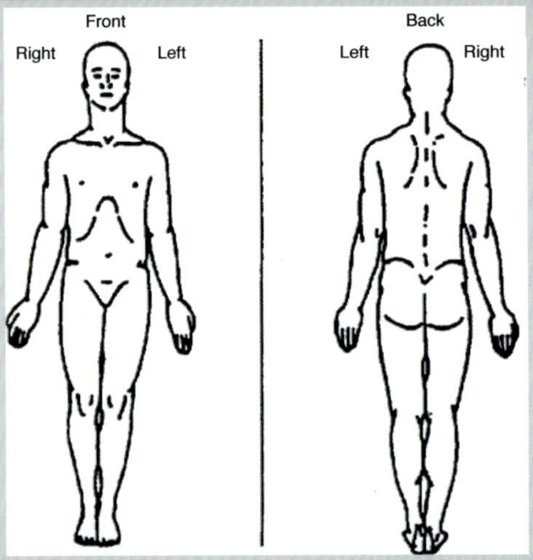

3.   Please rate your pain by circling the one number that best describes your pain at its worst in the last 24 hours.

0	1	2	3	4	5	6	7	8	9	10
No Pain										Pain as bad as you can imagine

4.   Please rate your pain by circling the one number that best describes your pain at its least in the last 24 hours.

0	1	2	3	4	5	6	7	8	9	10
No Pain										Pain as bad as you can imagine

5.   Please rate your pain by circling the one number that best describes your pain on the average.

0	1	2	3	4	5	6	7	8	9	10
No Pain										Pain as bad as you can imagine

6.   Please rate your pain by circling the one number that tells how much pain you have right now.

0	1	2	3	4	5	6	7	8	9	10
No Pain										Pain as bad as you can imagine

Page 1 of 2

FIGURE 41.3 Brief Pain Inventory. The Brief Pain Inventory is copyrighted. Permission to reproduce can be obtained from http://www.mdanderson.org/BPI. The tool is available in over 50 languages. *(Copyright © 1991 Dr. Charles S. Cleeland.)*

STUDY ID #:_ _ _ _ _ _ _ _ _ _   DO NOT WRITE ABOVE THIS LINE   HOSPITAL #:_ _ _ _ _ _ _ _ _ _

Date:_ _ _ _/_ _ _ _/_ _ _ _   Time:_ _ _ _ _ _ _ _

Name:_ _ _ _ _ _ _ _ _ _ _ _ _ _ _ _ _   _ _ _ _ _ _ _ _ _ _ _ _ _ _ _ _ _   _ _ _ _ _ _ _ _ _ _ _ _ _ _

   Last   First   Middle Initial

7.   What treatments or medications are you receiving for your pain?

8.   In the last 24 hours, how much relief have pain treatments or medications provided? Please circle the one percentage that most shows how much relief you have received.

0%   10%   20%   30%   40%   50%   60%   70%   80%   90%   100%

No   Complete
Relief   Relief

9.   Circle the one number that describes how, during the past 24 hours, pain has interfered with your:

A.   General Activity

0   1   2   3   4   5   6   7   8   9   10

Does not   Completely
Interfere   Interferes

B.   Mood

0   1   2   3   4   5   6   7   8   9   10

Does not   Completely
Interfere   Interferes

C.   Walking Ability

0   1   2   3   4   5   6   7   8   9   10

Does not   Completely
Interfere   Interferes

D.   Normal Work (includes both work outside the home and housework)

0   1   2   3   4   5   6   7   8   9   10

Does not   Completely
Interfere   Interferes

E.   Relations with other people

0   1   2   3   4   5   6   7   8   9   10

Does not   Completely
Interfere   Interferes

F.   Sleep

0   1   2   3   4   5   6   7   8   9   10

Does not   Completely
Interfere   Interferes

G.   Enjoyment of life

0   1   2   3   4   5   6   7   8   9   10

Does not   Completely
Interfere   Interferes

Page 2 of 2

FIGURE 41.3   *(continued)*

clinician to develop a more comprehensive approach to managing the pain and is therefore an essential part of the comprehensive pain assessment in a cancer patient.

PRESENTING COMPLAINT

The presenting complaint of the pain should contain four elements: onset, progression, focality, and accompaniments. Once the patient assessment has been completed, these four elements can be summarized in a single sentence and often represent a thumbprint of the underlying mechanism of pain.

Pain Onset

Patients are understandably often keen to tell you how long the pain has been severe. In order to characterize the nature of the underlying process, however, it is critical to also delineate the onset of pain: the time from when the pain first ever began until it became as bad as it was going to get (Table 41.1). Broadly, cancer pain unfolds in three different ways: It may have an onset of less than a day, days to weeks, or months in duration. Be wary of the tendency of pain to fluctuate, with good days and bad days, or good weeks or bad weeks; behind this background noise is the true onset of how the pain developed over time. As a guideline, pain that takes less than 1 day to become as bad as it is going to get is often vascular in origin. An example of this is an acute thigh hematoma from trauma to the leg or pain from hemorrhage into a site of metastasis. Pain that takes between a day and a month to reach its peak often has an inflammatory mechanism, such as a subcutaneous abscess, with each day being worse than the previous. Pain that is worse month after month, pain that is chronic, progressive, and focal, is most consistent with a diagnosis of cancer. These are only general guidelines, and there are many exceptions. However, delineating the onset of the pain, the time from when it first began until it reaches its peak, can be an important clue regarding the nature of the underlying diagnosis.

Pain Progression

There are only a few common patterns of how cancer pain progresses over time. Once it has commenced, cancer pain is typically *progressive*, and usually, this progression occurs over months. A second pattern of cancer pain is *fluctuating*, such as pain that is worse with standing because of metastasis

to weight-bearing bone, pain worse with bladder emptying due to cancer invading the detrusor muscle, and pain that is worse at night and relieved by pacing, a classical description of pain experienced with epidural spinal cord compression. Back pain that gets worse with lying down is especially concerning for the presence of neuraxial tumor. A third pattern of pain progression is pain that is *improving*: It began, peaked, and is now getting better or has resolved. This temporal profile is consistent with an underlying mechanism of pain that has been effectively treated, such as successful radiation treatment of an area of metastasis. A fourth temporal profile is *intermittent episodes* of pain. This temporal profile of pain can be incapacitating and can often be effectively managed with specific interventions. One example is a patient with neuropathic pain who has constant, deep, achy pain in the affected dermatome and also has superimposed spells of brief stabbing neuralgic pain. This pain is characteristically electrical in character, peaks instantly, and lasts seconds. Neuralgic pain commonly improves dramatically with anticonvulsant agents such as gabapentin, pregabalin, or carbamazepine. Another example of intermittent episodes of pain is the patient with baseline achy neuropathic pain with superimposed brief episodes of burning pain in the skin precipitated by light touch: allodynia.[23] Allodynia is a strong predictor of the presence of underlying neuropathic pain, and once the diagnosis is made, there are several analgesic interventions that can be effective.

Focality

In what region of the body is the pain being experienced? The medical approach to the cancer patient involves a systems approach, such as the respiratory system, the cardiac system, and so on, but it is also important to assess where pain is experienced because of referral sites remote from the organ involved or due to the presence of painful distant metastases. There are several ways to classify regional pains. A simple approach is to describe seven regions of the body: head and neck, chest, shoulder and arm, abdomen, pelvis, back, and the buttock and leg region. There is commonly overlap, such as the patient who has back pain, buttock pain, and leg pain. In considering the patient who has pain in a certain region of the body, it encourages the clinician to be mindful of all potential pain-sensitive structures that could result in the experience

TABLE 41.1	Formulating a Pain Presenting Complaint			
Domain	**Onset of Symptoms**	**Progression**	**Focality**	**Accompaniments**
Description	Time until peak of symptoms	Pattern of unfolding over time	Right or left; what region of the body	Symptoms that suggest what system is involved
Categories and examples	Less than a day • Typically a vascular process • Bleeding into a tumor • Arterial embolus Between 1 day and 1 month • Typically an inflammatory process • Infected cancer wound • Shingles pain More than 1 month • Chronic, progressive and focal: likely cancer. Example: progressive neck pain due to bone metastasis • Chronic, progressive and diffuse: likely toxic or degenerative. Example: peripheral neuropathy pain	Sudden and unchanging • Typical of trauma Began, peaked, and now improving or resolved • A typical monophasic course of a painful area successfully treated, such as following radiation therapy Relapsing and remitting • A relapsing and remitting condition such as multiple sclerosis or change in lymphoma pain with steroids Spells • Neuralgic pains are brief, electrical stabs of pain lasting seconds • Seizures	Head and neck Chest Shoulder and arm Abdomen Pelvis Back Buttock and leg	Cardiac (palpitations) Pulmonary (shortness of breath, cough) Upper gastrointestinal (nausea or pain on eating) Urinary (cardiac or pulmonary) Small or large bowel diarrhea or constipation Urinary (hematuria) Neurologic (confusion) Endocrine (hypoglycemia)

of pain in that part of the body. The following pain history exemplifies this phenomenon.

A 47-year-old premenopausal woman presented to her oncologist with a 3-month history of progressive back pain. Two months ago, the pain progressed down the right leg into the foot, in association with tingling and loss of sensation in a distribution similar to the pain. She had a prior history of breast cancer with 3 of 12 nodes positive, treated with surgery followed by radiation therapy, chemotherapy, and was currently on aromatase inhibitors.

The regional pain exam revealed marked local spine tenderness including paraspinal muscle spasm that reproduced her back pain. Also, there were signs of active right L5 radiculopathy, including an unequivocally positive ipsilateral straight-leg raise maneuver (neuropathic pain in the right leg below the knee). An MRI of the spine revealed evidence of a large right lateral herniated L4–L5 disk and no evidence of cancer.

The presenting complaint of this cancer patient helped focus the rest of the history and the regional pain examination toward diagnoses, both cancer and noncancer, that can potentially cause chronic, progressive back pain and unilateral neurologic trouble in a leg.

Symptoms That Accompany Pain

Are there other symptoms that accompany the pain? They can be a strong indicator of the underlying disease process. Consider a patient suspected of having cancer who presents with chest pain. Accompanying symptoms can provide helpful guidance about the underlying disease. Typical examples could be chest pain with breathlessness and cough from lung cancer; episodes of chest pain associated with palpitations from angina; or deep achy chest pain associated with nausea after eating, a 30-lb weight loss, and dysphagia over 3 months from esophageal cancer (see Table 41.1). The symptoms that accompany the pain are a clue as to the underlying system that is involved in the disease process. Often, these other symptoms will unfold in a similar temporal profile of the underlying pain.

Formulating the Presenting Complaint

Integrating these four elements of the pain presenting complaint together within a single sentence—pain onset, progression, focality, and accompaniments—can bring clarity to an otherwise complex clinical presentation, even if the clinician has never encountered the situation previously. Here is an example of such a presenting complaint, described by a patient who was encountered by the author:

A 68-year-old man presented with a 1-year history (onset) of progressive (progression) left lateral abdominal wall and flank (focality) deep ache, burning numbness of overlying skin, and a 30-lb weight loss (accompaniments).

This pain syndrome is neuropathic and potentially also visceral. This perplexing presenting complaint suggests cancer of the left flank area, as the pain is chronic, progressive, and focal. The differential diagnosis includes diabetic abdominal wall neuropathy, a rare diabetic neuropathy typically encountered in adults with early-onset, mild diabetes. There are other possible causes of this presenting complaint, but postherpetic neuralgia is not likely if the presenting complaint is accurate: Being inflammatory, shingles pain typically has a subacute onset, becoming maximal within days of its first appearance. This particular patient was not known to have active cancer (although there was a past cancer diagnosis), and all investigations at the time of presentation were negative. Pain was controlled with opioids and adjuvant analgesics, and he was given appointments for follow-up computed tomography (CT) scans

of the abdomen every 3 months for a year. At 9 months, the patient developed CT findings consistent with a left adrenal metastasis and retroperitoneal lymphadenopathy, and after a biopsy demonstrated metastatic adenocarcinoma, palliative radiation therapy was effective to relieve pain. This is an example of a presenting complaint that was strongly suggestive of the underlying mechanism of pain.

DETAILS OF THE PAIN HISTORY

Because pain is a subjective experience, it is essential to obtain from the patient a description of the experience of pain, including the amount of pain. There is evidence that estimates of a patient's pain by others are commonly inaccurate; health care providers tend to underestimate pain,[29] and family caregivers often overestimate pain.[30] The input of surrogates should take second place to direct input of the patient's own experience. Estimating how much pain a patient is in, based on their facial expression or other indicators, should be approached with great caution, although behavioral cues may be the only way to assess pain in a non–self-reporting patient.

Extensive research has found that there are ways to inquire of a patient which are more likely than others to get a response from the patient that is valid, reliable, and reproducible. A widely used approach is to ask the patient how much pain he or she is experiencing on a scale of 0 to 10, if 0 is "no pain" and 10 is the "worst pain possible." This approach has been broadly adopted as clinical policy within health care institutions. The clinician needs to be wary of the uncommon circumstance where the numeric rating scale turns out to be less reliable. One such situation is delirium, a syndrome of fluctuating encephalopathy commonly encountered in cancer patients before death or in association with concurrent acute illness. When delirium is known to be present, it is still appropriate to ask the patient how much pain he or she is experiencing using the 10-point numeric scale and to record his or her answer but also one should record that he or she have delirium. In this setting and any other settings where there is doubt about the reliability of the patient's description, an additional method to quantify pain intensity should be used to confirm their description. A highly reliable, valid, and reproducible scale is the McGill categorical scale.[25] One asks the patient if he or she would describe his or her pain as none, mild, discomforting, distressing, horrible, or excruciating. If there is any question to the reliability of the patient's description, it is best to keep the questions simple and dichotomous, for example, "Is your pain bad, or not bad?" The more ways one poses the question, the more confident the clinician can be about the interpretation of the patient's response.

A detailed description of the many facets of the pain experience is described in detail in Chapter 20. In cancer pain, clinicians often ask the patient about his or her present pain intensity (on a scale of 0 to 10), the worst pain experienced in the past 24 hours, the least pain experienced in the past 24 hours, and the average pain.

If the patient is struggling to find words to describe his or her pain, the clinician should be supportive and encouraging, offering words to the patient such as burning, sharp, or crushing. If the patient spontaneously offers a word with a strong affective component, such as "suffocating" pain, the clinician should not only inquire about comorbidities such as concurrent dyspnea but also recognize the possibility that such affectively loaded words may signal a more global sense of suffering. This requires further inquiry and evaluation.[25]

After delineating the intensity of the pain and the description of the pain, the clinician should find out, in detail, what part(s) of the body are affected and what the characteristics of the pain are throughout these locations. A differential description of discrete pains within the same region of the body

| TABLE 41.2 | List of Medications Taken for Pain | | | | | | |

Patient name _____
Today's date _____

Name of Medication	Start Date	End Date	Maximum Daily Dose (in milligrams)	What Benefit	Side Effects	Comments

can give a clue to as to the underlying mechanism. For example, patients with malignant brachial plexopathy often describe several different pains. There is often a deep, achy, poorly localized discomfort draped over the ipsilateral shoulder, with burning pain and tingling in the ipsilateral lateral hand. There can also be pain with light touching of the area of numbness in the affected arm (allodynia), and superimposed spontaneous episodes of brief stabbing electrical pain in the arm, experienced as single neuralgic jabs or brief trains (volleys) of pain. If present for several months, patients can develop pain from frozen shoulder or other articular or myofascial complications of immobility of the affected shoulder girdle region. All of these discrete pains can be elicited and described by the patient during the pain history.

The clinician then focuses on the experience of pain over time: what makes it better and what makes it worse. In particular, one seeks a description of the change of pain over time with medication (i.e., pharmacodynamics). Typically, one would expect there would be relief of pain beginning about one half hour after swallowing a short-acting opioid, peaking at approximately 60 to 90 minutes, and then it would wear out sometime thereafter. If the duration of analgesia is too brief (in this case, less than 4 hours after taking a short-acting opioid), the patient probably has end-of-dose failure. Identifying this phenomenon can guide the clinician to estimate the extent to which the patient is undermedicated.

Next, construct a detailed list of all prescription and nonprescription medications the patient has taken; the patient or family should be encouraged to look through the medication cabinet for all pills. The list should include the names of medications, the maximum dose that was taken, and the duration that the maximum dose was taken, with what effect and what toxicity (Table 41.2). The goal is to be as confident as possible that the patient has completed an adequate trial of each of these medications, and if they did not have an adequate trial, one then can consider reembarking on a trial of that medication in a more thorough manner. By the end of this description,

the clinician should have a clear understanding what sequential trials of analgesics and combinations of analgesics the patient has had over time.

Depending on the patient's past history and current social circumstances, it may be appropriate to apply certain chemical misuse/abuse/dependency risk tools, such as the CAGE (Table 41.3) or the Opioid Risk Tool (ORT). Stratifying risk allows for a structured approach to pharmacotherapy that is tailored to each patient's particular circumstances.

The clinician should also seek information about other risk factors for poor pain prognosis. This includes any history of psychiatric disorder, the presence of breakthrough pain, neuropathic pain, other psychosocial stressors, use of high-dose opioids without satisfactory pain control or excessive adverse effects, and the presence of significant interference of function by pain. Interference of function refers to pain interfering with physical functions, such as sleep, activities of daily living, and work; social functioning, such as a parenting role and sexual relations; and emotional functioning, such as ability to engage meaningfully with those around them and ability to cope.

The clinician then embarks on a detailed medical and psychosocial history. The medical history involves a review of systems such as respiratory, cardiovascular, GI, genitourinary, musculoskeletal, dermatologic, neurologic, and endocrine. There is a high risk of comorbidity with particular patterns of systems dysfunction in specific cancers. An example is the high prevalence of underlying respiratory disease in a patient who has a tobacco-related malignancy or a lengthy history of tobacco use.

The elements of a psychosocial history have been described elsewhere in this book (Chapter 21).

Physical Examination

The pain physical exam includes a general physical exam, more specific neurologic examination guided by history, a regional pain exam, and bedside provocative maneuvers.

GENERAL PHYSICAL EXAMINATION

The general examination of the cancer patient includes a brief screening physical exam including vital signs, head and neck, respiratory system, cardiovascular system, the abdominal exam, genitourinary exam including rectal exam (as appropriate to the clinical circumstance), musculoskeletal exam, peripheral vascular exam, neurologic exam and in particular detail as informed by the history, and dermatologic exam. Attention is paid to document the extent of underlying malignancy; patients presenting with cancer pain may have a greater extent of

| TABLE 41.3 | Cage Test to Screen for Alcoholism |

Please check the one response to each item that best describes how you have felt and behaved over your whole life.
1. Have you ever felt you should *cut* down on your drinking?
2. Have people *annoyed* you by criticizing your drinking?
3. Have you ever felt bad or *guilty* about your drinking?
4. Have you ever had a drink first thing in the morning to steady your nerves or get rid of a hangover (*eye-opener*)?

disease than was previously suspected, so the clinician needs to examine the patient with a view toward stigmata of underlying organ disease.

THE REGIONAL PAIN PHYSICAL EXAMINATION

The clinician approaches the regional pain examination as guided by the pain history. This approach complements but does not replace the more traditional systems approach to the physical examination described earlier. Seven regions of the body are head and neck, chest, shoulder girdle and arm, abdomen, back, pelvis, and buttock and leg (Table 41.4). For example, if the patient describes pain in the head and neck, a regional pain exam is done of that part of the body. The clinician pays particular attention to look for evidence of underlying disease in that region, which may be vascular, infectious, or neoplastic in origin. The clinician looks for evidence of degenerative neck disease, with reduced range of motion of the neck, neurologic disease with ptosis suggesting ipsilateral cancer in

TABLE 41.4	A Regional Approach to the Pain Physical Examination	
Region	**Syndrome**	**Examples of Pain-Sensitive Structures**
Head and neck	Somatic Visceral Neuropathic	Paraspinal muscles Focal neck myofascial pain Occipitonuchal junction Dentition Sinuses Periorbital area Bone: base of skull, facial Carotids Orbits Cervical radiculopathy
Shoulder and arm	Somatic Visceral Neuropathic	Shoulder joint Ligamentous Muscle Axilla Apex of lung Radicular pain referred from neck Brachial plexus
Chest	Somatic Visceral Neuropathic Mixed pain	Parietal pleura Vertebral body Visceral pleura Thoracic nerve root Chest wall: rib, muscle, nerve Intradural lesion
Abdomen and flank	Somatic Visceral Neuropathic	Flank muscle Rib Referred from vertebral body Intra-abdominal: liver, hollow viscus, Peritoneum Kidney, adrenals Retroperitoneal structure: pancreas Intercostals nerve Intradural lesion
Back and buttocks	Somatic Visceral Neuropathic	Bone: vertebral body, sacrum, bony pelvis Paraspinal muscle Cauda equina; nerve root; plexus Presacral region, peritoneum Cauda equina, nerve root, plexus, intercostals nerve
Pelvis	Somatic Visceral Neuropathic	Bony pelvis Introitus Ovaries, uterus Plexus, pudendal nerve
Leg and foot	Somatic Visceral Neuropathic	Bone: pelvis, femur, tibia Muscle: gluteus, obturator Ligament: insertion of biceps Joint: hip, sacroiliac Presacral area Cauda equina, nerve root, plexus, nerve

the low cervical spine, vascular disease such as carotid artery or vertebral artery bruit, palpable muscle spasm, and other signs of an underlying pathologic process.

BEDSIDE PROVOCATIVE MANEUVERS

The bedside provocative maneuvers are an important part of the pain physical exam. The goal is to gently reproduce the patient's pain complaint(s). If the clinician successfully reproduces the pain, the patient may be relieved, having their subjective complaints validated. As described earlier, because pain is a subjective experience, often, patients have the sense that others might not appreciate how serious their pain is. If the clinician is able to reproduce the pain, the patient may believe that the clinician has confirmed that it exists. Furthermore, if the clinician is able to localize, or "touch," the pain, the patient may have greater confidence the pain can be relieved. For the clinician, being able to reproduce the pain provides insight into the underlying mechanisms or pain-sensitive structures.

For each of the seven regions of the body, there is a list of regional bedside provocative maneuvers (Table 41.5). For example, in the situation of a patient who presents with head and neck pain, the clinician would first do a general physical exam and then a regional pain exam in order to look for underlying disease processes. After this time, the clinician would systematically embark on bedside provocative maneuvers. This would include neck range of motion in six directions, including an evaluation for meningismus, palpation of the skin, assessing for allodynia, and deep palpation of underlying tissues. One continues to palpate more deeply trying to identify areas of myofascial pain or muscle spasm. One looks at typical tender points[31,32] and also areas that commonly develop muscle spasm in response to disease, such as the paraspinal muscles. Muscle tenderness can be sought throughout the neck, the face, the jaw, and other areas. The clinician should put on a glove and palpate the masseter musculature as well as posterior pharyngeal examination of the pterygoid muscles. Following this, bone structures should be systematically examined by palpation and percussion, including the orbit, the skull, the occipital condyle, and then down the cervical spine. Next, palpate the carotid arteries (gently), the orbits, and the sinuses. Additional bedside provocative maneuvers can be performed based on the clinical situation. The clinician should approach bedside provocative maneuvers as a sleuth, looking for evidence that will rule in or rule out various pain-sensitive structures as being the source of the pain. Further detail on pain caused by cancer of the head and neck and oral mucositis is covered in Chapter 45.

SPECIFIC BEDSIDE PROVOCATIVE MANEUVERS AND THEIR ROLE IN PAIN DIAGNOSIS
Spurling's Test

Spurling's test of the cervical spine (also known as Spurling's maneuver) is performed if there is concern the patient might have active cervical nerve root compression.[33] It is analogous to the straight-leg raise maneuver that detects active lumbosacral radiculopathy (see the following text).[34] Spurling's test consists of gentle lateral flexion of the neck for about 1 minute toward the side of the pain, followed by lateral flexion of the neck for about 1 minute away from the side of the pain. A variation is lateral flexion plus lateral rotation of the neck ("throw your ear over your shoulder") for 1 minute to one side and then to the other. The test is positive if it results in neuropathic pain, tingling, or numbness below the elbow or loss of a previously present arm reflex such as a triceps reflex. The side and nerve root distribution of the arm pain or other neurologic impairment localizes the site of the mass that is pushing on the thecal space. Some reports have recommended axial loading be undertaken at the same time as lateral flexion and rotation (the examiner pushes down on the top of the head).[33] We do not recommend

TABLE 41.5 **Examples of Bedside Provocative Maneuvers**

Region	Structure	Provocative Maneuver	Finding
Head and neck	Skin	Wave hand over skin	Allodynia
	Paraspinal muscle	Pinprick	Hyperpathia
	Bone	Cold temperature	Cold allodynia
	Occipitonuchal junction	Gentle palpation	Palpable paraspinal spasm
	Neck range of motion	Gentle palpation of spinous processes; deeper palpation over vertebral bodies	Tenderness
	Spurling's maneuver	Gentle palpation	Tenderness
		Patient moves neck in six directions	Pain; limited range of motion
		Patient laterally flexes or laterally flexes and laterally rotates neck (see Fig. 41.4)	Neuropathic pain or other neuropathic symptoms or signs
Shoulder and arm	Shoulder girdle	Active range of motion of shoulder	Pain
	Brachial plexus	Passive range of motion of shoulder	Tenderness; reduced range of motion (e.g., frozen shoulder)
	Axilla	Examination for tender areas	Bicipital tendonitis
		Gentle percussion over Erb's point in the supra-clavicular fossa	Tinel's sign positive tenderness
		Palpation	
Chest	Subcutaneous tissue	Gently pinch skin	Unilateral lymphedema
	Spine	Palpation; percussion	Tenderness
Abdomen and flank	Organs	Gentle then deep palpation, at rest then with inspiration	Tenderness
	Abdominal wall	Carnett's maneuver	Worse with tension of abdominal muscles (see Fig. 41.6)
	Retroperitoneal structures (e.g., pancreas)	Retroperitoneal stretch maneuver (see Fig. 41.5)	Thoracic spine is not tender but back pain arises with retroperitoneal stretch
Back	Vertebral body	Spine palpation and percussion	Tenderness
	Sacroiliac joint	Gently press thumb into sacroiliac joint	Tenderness
	hips	Flexion, abduction, internal, and then external rotation; palpate hip joint; palpate trochanteric bursae	Tenderness; limited range of motion
Pelvis	Pelvic organs	Internal examination	Tenderness
	Rectum	Rectal examination	Tenderness
Buttock and leg	Low lumbar and sacral nerve roots	Straight-leg raise maneuver	Ipsilateral neuropathic pain below the knee with other neurologic symptoms
	Upper and midlumbar nerve roots	Crossed straight-leg maneuver	Ipsilateral neuropathic pain below the knee with other neurologic symptoms
		Reverse straight-leg raise maneuver	Ipsilateral neuropathic pain in the anterior thigh with other neurologic symptoms

that approach for cancer patients as there may be bone destruction and the test could be dangerous. Spurling's test can be particularly helpful to distinguish malignant brachial plexopathy (in which case the maneuver is almost invariably negative) from spinal cord compression in the cervical spine (in which case the maneuver is often but not always positive) (Fig. 41.4). The procedure should not be undertaken if baseline pain is severe, until radiographs or other imaging studies confirm that the neck is mechanically stable. Positive and negative predictive values for Spurling's test along with other bedside provocative maneuvers have been described for active cervical radiculopathy due to underlying benign disease but has not been well studied when due to cancer.[33]

Dermatomal Pain

At some point, the clinician is likely to encounter an area of primary tenderness with pain apparently referred to a distant site.

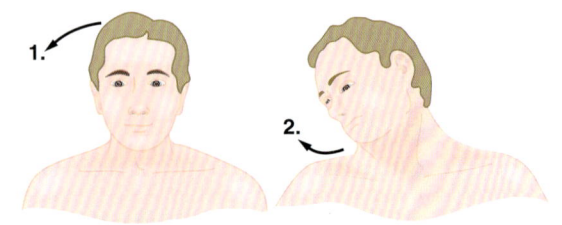

FIGURE 41.4 Spurling's test.

Clinicians are familiar with dermatomal pain or radicular pain, such as L5 nerve root pain caused by a herniation of the L5–S1 disk. The radicular pain can be provoked by a straight-leg raise maneuver. The straight-leg raise maneuver is a validated bedside provocative maneuver that has been carefully tested in a range of clinical situations, disease types, and ages and with a range of specific techniques to perform the test.[34] L5 radicular pain is felt down the ipsilateral buttock into the posterior part of the thigh and down the posterolateral leg into the dorsal or dorsolateral foot.

Sclerotomal Pain

There are other mechanisms for pain that may appear strikingly similar to dermatomal pain, including sclerotomal pain. A common example of sclerotomal referred pain is pain referred from the sacroiliac joint. The bedside provocative maneuver is to gently place the thumb in the sacroiliac joint and press with a few kilograms of pressure (see "Myofascial Pain: How Hard Should You Press?" section). The positive maneuver reproduces the ipsilateral paraspinal and low back pain the patient has been having. Referred sclerotomal pain goes down the ipsilateral posterior buttock and lateral leg into the lateral aspect of the ipsilateral ankle. L5 radicular pain and ipsilateral sacroiliac pain can occur in the same patient. This confusing clinical scenario may arise in a patient with active lumbosacral radiculopathy due to disk protrusion. Presumably, the sacroiliac pain is a consequence of biomechanical changes that occur in a patient who is limping because of pain from the active radiculopathy. Eventually, the stress on the ipsilateral sacroiliac joint is such that it too starts to hurt. The patient may ultimately have a surgical procedure to remove herniated disk material. However, the sacroiliac pain can persist, leaving the patient with a wrong impression that the surgery was a failure. This clinical situation raises the complexity of regional pain in cancer patients, whereby there can be several distinct but interdependent mechanisms of pain in the same region of the body. Teasing out the various components of that regional pain will allow the clinician to direct therapeutic interventions at each.

Myotomal Pain

A third kind of referred pain is myotomal pain: pain that arises from muscles. Referred myotomal pain does not generally extend far from the irritated muscle. In cancer patients, myotomal pain is generally not a major cause of referred pain, but it can occur in a manner similar to sclerotomal pain resulting from secondary mechanical dysfunction.

Myofascial Pain: How Hard Should You Press?

Myofascial pain is a term that can be used to describe specific myofascial tender point sites[31] or can be used as a more generic term for regional pain of muscular origin that is not due to primary pathology in the muscle. Myofascial pain is common in cancer pain patients, and it can mimic other types of pathology. Identifying its presence can lead to specific therapeutic interventions, such as heat, stretch, cold and massage, trigger point injections, or regional blockade, and it is therefore important to make the diagnosis when possible. Separate from regional myofascial pain, rheumatologists have characterized the systemic condition fibromyalgia (in part) by a series of bedside provocative maneuvers palpating for tenderness in specific areas, applying an amount of pressure that would not normally be uncomfortable. Whether in health or disease, muscle tenderness will result if the examiner presses hard enough. Research in muscle tenderness has identified that most commonly, muscles do not normally hurt when the examiner presses with up to 4 kg of pressure per square centimeter using the thumb. The clinician can use a baby weigh scale to become familiar with what represents 4 kg or can use a bedside dolorimeter, which is a bedside tool meant to gauge how hard one is pressing. Fibromyalgia can be diagnosed through the patient's history without performing a tender point exam.[32] However, the condition is usually associated with myofascial tenderness using a standardized methodology, with the finding of at least 11 of 18 typical tender point sites. The tender point exam in fibromyalgia has a diagnostic sensitivity of 88.4% and a specificity of 81.1%.[31] The bedside exam of the cancer patient, looking for regional myofascial pain unrelated to fibromyalgia, is best undertaken with a similar technique.

Back Pain

In approaching the bedside examination of the patient with back pain, the clinician needs to pay particular attention to be gentle. In examining the spine, one would first palpate in the area where the patient describes the worst pain. Push very gently, with less than a kilogram of pressure per square centimeter on the palpating finger on the area of the worst pain and then the broad area around it, looking for paraspinal muscle spasm. If negative, one can palpate with more pressure. There are some situations where a patient appears to have severe back pain and yet the regional pain exam demonstrates that the spine is completely aligned and there is neither spinal tenderness nor palpable paraspinal muscle spasm. How can there be severe back pain but not back tenderness? Retroperitoneal tumor can cause lumbar or thoracic regional pain where there is no tenderness with even deep percussion. There may be a suggestion that the patient has a retroperitoneal cause of back pain based on the patient's posture as you enter the examination room: The patient

may have adopted a so-called pain-relieving posture, such as sitting on the bed with the knees folded up into the chest. This posture results in lumbar kyphosis and, therein, relief of pain from a retroperitoneal pain-sensitive structure.

Retroperitoneal Pain Stretch Maneuver

In order to diagnose a retroperitoneal source of back pain, once the spine and paraspinal areas have been examined and have been found to not be tender, have the patient sit upright in the bed with the legs stretched out. This is best done in a bed in which the back of the bed can be elevated. Place a pillow into the small of the back so there is moderate thoracolumbar lordosis and have the patient lay back down in the bed. Gently lower the back of the bed so the patient goes toward a supine direction (Fig. 41.5). Retroperitoneal tumor can cause severe back pain and is reproduced with this maneuver. Oddly, it can take a few minutes for the pain to become fully apparent as the bed is lowered and the spine is extended. The history will commonly give a suggestion that this sign will be positive because the patient may describe back pain upon laying flat, with the patient having thereafter sought sleep in a recliner.

Abdominal Wall Pain

The abdominal *wall* is frequently a source of pain, and how to examine it has been less clearly defined than examination of underlying abdominal structures. Abdominal wall pain is a common mechanism of severe idiopathic abdominal pain.[35,36] It also can be a long-term sequela of abdominal surgery such as hernia repair, open cholecystectomy, etc.[37] The distinction between an underlying and medically serious intra-abdominal source of pain from a benign abdominal wall source of pain is made through a bedside provocative test, Carnett's maneuver.

Carnett's maneuver: The patient is found to be tender on gentle palpation, typically in the left or right lower quadrant (Fig. 41.6). If the patient tenses the abdominal wall, such as by lifting both legs a few centimeters in the air or lifting the shoulders off the bed, an inflamed visceral organ is protected from the palpating hand. Alternatively, if the pain-sensitive structure is within the abdominal wall, such as caused by a myofascial trigger point, a neuroma, a hematoma, or some other cause, pain becomes markedly worse with tensing of the abdominal wall during palpation.

Another cryptic cause of abdominal wall pain can be neuropathic pain. This can be caused by cancer invading intercostal muscles, by retroperitoneal tumor, by diabetic abdominal wall neuropathy, shingles, and by other mechanisms. There are several bedside provocative maneuvers that can diagnose abdominal wall neuropathic pain. First, gently touch the normal side and then the abnormal side with a cold object, then a piece of cotton, then a pin (see Table 41.5). If any of these normally nonnoxious stimuli results in pain, the patient likely has abdominal neuropathic wall pain. Sensitivity to temperature, touch, or pinprick can be one of the most dramatic bedside signs in the pain physical examination and is strong evidence of the presence of underlying neuropathic pain. The abnormal sensation can linger for up to a minute or longer, so called "after sensation." Abdominal wall neuropathic pain can be accompanied by numbness or loss of abdominal wall muscle tone.[38]

Formulating a Cancer Pain Diagnosis

SYNDROME DIAGNOSIS

Although it can be tempting for the clinician to make a specific diagnosis as to the underlying cause of the pain, it may be wiser to begin with a more general syndrome diagnosis. Broadly, pain can be classified into somatic, visceral, neuropathic, or mixed syndromes. Diagnosing the pain syndrome based on the characteristics, the pattern of referral, the accompaniment, and the

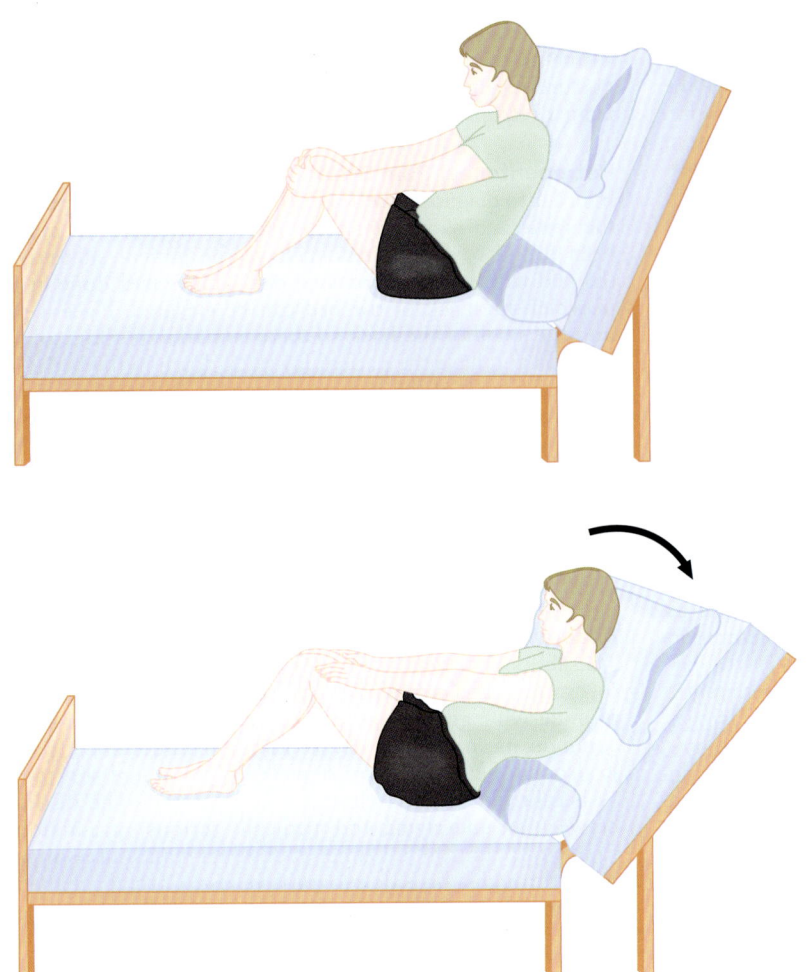

FIGURE 41.5 Retroperitoneal stretch maneuver.

provocative maneuvers can make it more likely that the clinician will consider a broad differential diagnosis.

The use of the taxonomy of somatic, visceral, and neuropathic pain syndromes can be challenged by closer scrutiny of their pathophysiologic basis. For example, some peripheral nerves are themselves pain-sensitive structures, being innervated by nociceptors. In addition, other aspects of neuropathic pain can be nonnociceptive, that is, pain generated by a damaged nervous system. Thus, when the peripheral nervous system is invaded by cancer, there can be both nociceptive and nonnociceptive pain. A common clinical scenario is malignant brachial plexopathy. The nociceptive component generated by nociceptors within the brachial plexus is pain draped over the ipsilateral shoulder; the nonnociceptive component of the pain is commonly burning pain in the ipsilateral, numb hand. An example of a central generator of neuropathic pain is poststroke thalamic pain. Central pain caused by brain metastases is extraordinarily uncommon and may relate to the long period of time it takes for central pain to develop. However, the taxonomy remains of clinical value, and a more complex version is described in Table 41.6.

There are other causes of pain which appear nociceptive in characteristic but have a nonnociceptive mechanism. Pain purely or mostly of psychological origin (often inappropriately termed *psychogenic pain*) is extraordinarily rare in the cancer population and must be used cautiously as it can either take the focus away from other equally or more important causes of pain or might stigmatize the patient as being less than genuine, truthful, or trustworthy. For this reason, the term *psychogenic pain* is usually avoided. An example of pain of psychological origin

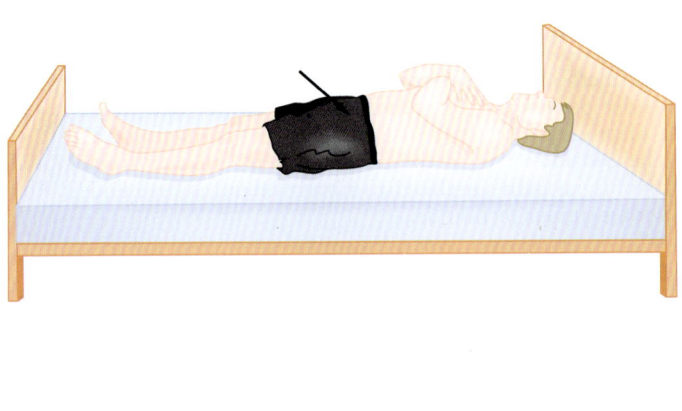

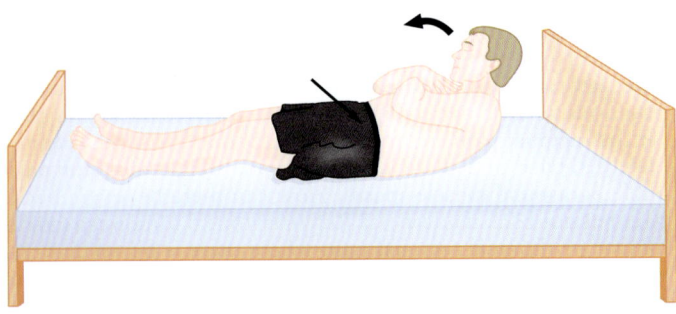

FIGURE 41.6 Carnett's maneuver.

TABLE 41.6 Pain Mechanisms

Nociceptive pain	Somatic	Bone metastasis
	Visceral	Liver pain
	Neuropathic	Brachial plexopathy
	Mixed	Pancoast tumor
Nonnociceptive pain	Neuropathic with peripheral generator	Neuroma
	Neuropathic with central generator	Thalamic pain
	Pain of psychological origin	Psychosis presenting as pain
	Factitious	Compulsive need for health care
	Idiopathic	Advanced but cryptic cancer

would be a patient who feels pain as part of a psychotic sensory hallucination. Likewise, factitious pain is uncommon and is due to a compulsive need for unwarranted health care (different than malingering). Idiopathic pain is pain for which the cause is not evident after a detailed history, physical exam including bedside provocative maneuvers, and referral for appropriate diagnostic imaging, laboratory tests, and consultation as needed. The pain clinician should be wary about the situation of idiopathic pain in a patient with known cancer. Commonly, idiopathic pain in a cancer patient turns out to be due to metastatic disease that was not evident despite extensive investigations. A wise approach to the cancer patient with idiopathic pain is to complete investigations and then see the patient in follow-up on a regularly scheduled basis such as every 3 months. Diagnostic imaging can be repeated at that time along with a repeat clinical assessment.

The role of bedside provocative maneuvers in formulating a cancer pain diagnosis has been described.[39] In this prospective study of 50 patients, all or much of the pain that brought the patient to the clinical venue was reproduced by a positive maneuver in 47 of 50 patients. Most commonly, pain was somatic, but it could also be visceral or neuropathic, and about half the time, it was mixed pain. Myopathic pain or muscle spasm pain was present in about half of all patients and allowed a broader approach to overall pain control strategies.

PATHOPHYSIOLOGIC DIAGNOSIS

The temporal profile of how the pain progressed over time will commonly reveal the underlying mechanism of pain (see Table 41.1). Vascular events are usually as bad as they are going to get within less than a day. An example of a vascular event is a spontaneous bleed within a tumor bed, exemplified by a patient with a vascular neoplasm, such as choriocarcinoma or melanoma, who develops a headache and accompanying neurologic symptoms that become fully established in less than a day. An inflammatory process typically takes between 1 and 30 days to be as bad as it is going to get. An example could be a tumor-related skin or deep tissue abscess. When pain takes more than a month to become as severe as it is going to get, is focal, and is progressive, it is usually due to a growing mass. Needless to say, in a patient with known cancer, severe pain should be considered to be progression of malignancy in that region of the body until proven otherwise.

Complementary Clinical Perspectives in the Care of Cancer Patients

Pain is a symptom and not a diagnosis. Chronic pain can be a symptom of ongoing tissue injury or a disease process in and of itself as previously discussed. The overall approach to a pain management strategy, therefore, is greatly shaped by the underlying pain mechanisms involved and the overall goals of care.

The *medical approach* focuses on disease diagnosis and disease cure; the *palliative approach* aims to relieve, suppress, or mask pain to the greatest extent possible; the *rehabilitative approach* (an approach widely employed by chronic noncancer pain clinics) focuses on improved function and adaptive coping; and the *anesthetic approach* has the objective to diagnose and block, such as a combination of "medical" and "palliative" approaches. With each of these perspectives, however, the goal is to relieve pain as quickly as possible, with the least toxicity possible. These various, but not mutually exclusive, approaches can be exemplified in a clinical case.

> A 53-year-old man, who was previously healthy, developed a gradual onset of epigastric pain. He began to develop nausea and heartburn; symptoms worsened after eating. He developed weight loss. He seeks care from his physician 4 months after the onset of these symptoms.

THE MEDICAL MODEL: PAIN IS A MANIFESTATION OF DISEASE

In the medical model, pain is seen as a manifestation of an underlying illness. The general orientation is that of a systems approach, whereby the clinician focuses on the affected system. Using a rule in/rule out method, the clinician considers GI disease such as erosive esophagitis, gastritis, duodenal ulcer, and upper GI malignancy; cardiovascular disease such as a descending aortic aneurysm and ischemic heart disease; and other neoplastic disease such as an intrathoracic malignancy with referred pain. Diagnostic tests are ordered to rule in or rule out each of these conditions. In this situation, pain is helpful in that it alerts the patient that something is wrong and needs to be investigated. This is discussed in Chapter 43.

PALLIATIVE MODEL: PAIN IS BOTH USELESS AND HARMFUL

In this model, the underlying mechanism for pain is almost always known. The extent of underlying disease is also known and pain is both physiologically useless and potentially harmful to patient health. Today, there is intense research and clinical interest whether better control of cancer symptoms, such as pain, results in prolonged survival.[40,41] "Palliative" is an invented word based on the Latin for mask or cloak. The approach of the palliative model is to comprehensibly assess the whole patient, including his or her underlying disease, his or her social situation, his or her emotional state, and his or her spirituality, and then to mask or suppress the pain as much as possible. Other symptoms, such as anorexia, low energy, or nausea, should also be assessed and suppressed with medications or other approaches. Another closely related term commonly used to describe a whole-person approach to care of the cancer patient is "supportive care." An example of a palliative approach to cancer treatment is palliative chemotherapy or radiation therapy and is discussed more fully in Chapter 48.

REHABILITATIVE ("CHRONIC NONMALIGNANT PAIN") MODEL: FOCUS ON DYSFUNCTIONAL PAIN BEHAVIOR AND PAIN-RELATED DECONDITIONING

A third model for pain diagnosis and treatment is the rehabilitation model for the management of the chronic pain syndrome and is applied in the setting of dysfunctional pain behaviors. In this scenario, pain has been investigated with findings of no underlying somatic, visceral, or neuropathic process to account for the pain or the underlying disease (e.g., arthritis) cannot be eradicated, so pain must be minimized in order to optimize quality of life. Either way, therapy is directed at reversing any chronic dysfunctional pain behaviors, and the client undergoes some form of behavior modification and functional restoration therapy. This is discussed in Chapter 88.

ANESTHETIC MODEL: DIAGNOSTIC AND THERAPEUTIC BLOCKS

A fourth approach is the anesthetic model. In this approach, the patient undergoes a diagnostic procedure whereby local anesthetic is injected into or around suspected pain generator sites or regional blockade of sensory or autonomic nerves is performed. If the pain goes away, the patient may also undergo a series of such interventions or, in selected cases, a more definitive therapeutic block with a neurolytic agent such as phenol or alcohol. A detailed description of interventional pain therapies is presented in Chapter 44.

All of the aforementioned are perspectives, and none should be adopted as the sole correct approach but applied and integrated, depending on clinical context. In the case history of the patient with epigastric pain in the earlier discussion, the patient may present to his or her physician for assessment and, through the medical model, will have several conditions ruled out until a definitive diagnosis, such as pancreatic cancer, is made, during which time analgesics should be used to treat pain. He or she may undergo cancer treatment, but at the same time, he or she may be started on long-acting opioids, with the plan of masking or suppressing the pain, or he or she may be referred for a celiac plexus block. If this patient is having difficulty coping, or if he or she develops dysfunctional pain behaviors or aberrant medication use, a rehabilitative approach that focuses on behavior modification should be employed. Thus, the sage clinician can fluently move between different models of pain treatment and care depending on the clinical context and may in fact consider more than one model at the same time (Fig. 41.7).

Management of Pain in Specific Clinical Presentations

BONE PAIN

Cancer-related bone pain is common. About 80% of patients who die from breast cancer will have bone metastases at the time of autopsy, and a similar prevalence has been observed in other kinds of cancer. Bone scintigraphy studies have revealed the surprising findings that bone metastases are far more numerous in any given patient than what would be expected by the pain history; about two-thirds of bone metastases are painless. Although the risk of pain correlates to an extent with the degree of bone destruction and whether or not the metastasis is

in a weight-bearing bone, it can be difficult to predict based on imaging studies as to whether a metastatic lesion is painful or not. Oddly, bone pain can be transient and migratory, that is, very painful for several days and then appears to not be painful but other bone metastases become painful.

Typically, pain from bone metastases become worse over the course of months. However, at a point in time, the pain may start to increase more quickly in a crescendo pattern, becoming worse each day. There is often severe muscle spasm in the contiguous muscles. This pattern of crescendo pain in bone metastasis predicts fracture. Crescendo back pain predicts collapse of a vertebral body; one should urgently investigate such patients for exigent or impending epidural cord compression to offer definitive treatment prior to developing their neurologic symptoms. Bone pain is described in more detail in Chapters 46 and 47.

PAIN AND DELIRIUM

Delirium is a transient and potentially reversible neuropsychiatric syndrome characterized by global cognitive dysfunction.[42] Tools have been developed to assist the clinician to make the diagnosis as it has been found that while delirium is common in cancer patients, the diagnosis is often delayed or missed. Because pain is a subjective symptom, there is a risk that the presence or severity of pain will be misunderstood if the diagnosis of delirium is not made.

Delirium can be caused by severe pain, pain medications, or can occur in a patient with advanced illness and organ failure who also happens to have pain. It can be challenging to distinguish between these different clinical scenarios. Almost invariably, delirium in the palliative setting is multifactorial in origin. In order to quantitate the pain, the patient's numeric rating of the pain should be dutifully recorded, if possible, using tools that are intended for cognitively impaired individuals. Behaviors suggestive of pain should be sought, such as the patient grabbing the painful part of the body, the patient using other words to describe the pain, or the presence of a known destructive process in that region of the body.

Pain patients who develop delirium commonly describe a worsening of their pain, but the pain is often generalized to the whole body. In this situation, if all other potential causes of delirium have been ruled out or treated and opioids are being used, a trial of opioid dose reduction or rotation to a different opioid may be employed. Potentially reversible causes of delirium should be identified and treated, including a very wide

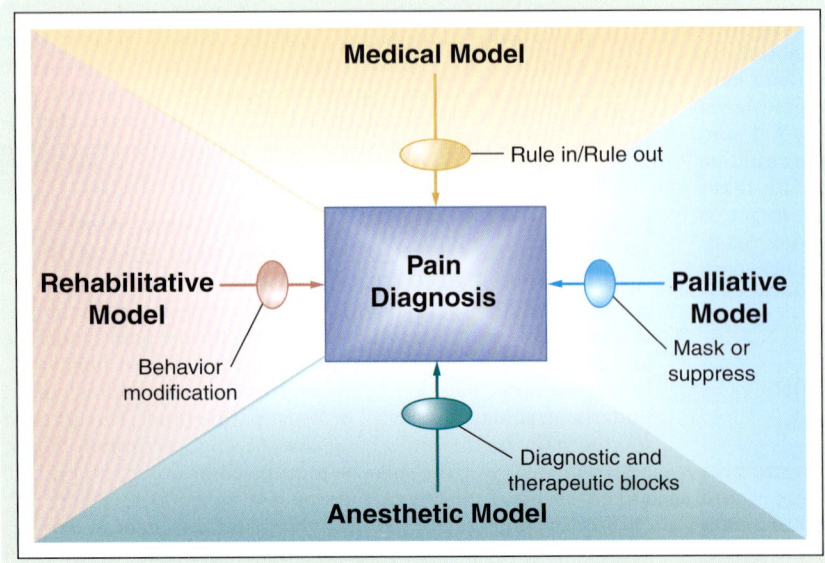

FIGURE 41.7 Complementary clinical perspectives in the care of cancer patients.

array of possibilities such as hypercalcemia, along with hydration and other supportive measures to manage the delirium.[43] If there is clinical suspicion that the delirium may be caused by uncontrolled pain, a short-acting opioid should be considered as a test dose.

PAIN AND NAUSEA

Chronic nausea is a prevalent symptom in cancer patients, and opioids themselves can be emetogenic. Complicating this situation is the experience of patients who have both pain and nausea and are unable to take oral medications.

A wise approach to the presence of both pain and nausea is to assess each of them individually and treat any underlying cause. If there is any possibility that the opioid is causing or contributing to the nausea, this symptom should be treated aggressively and/or the patient should be rotated to a different opioid or to a nonopioid pain treatment strategy. As common as opioid-related nausea is, it is fortunate that this symptom is usually self-limiting, only uncommonly necessitating discontinuation from opioid therapy. Alternative routes of administration, such as transdermal or injectable opioids, may need to be considered if the opioids are effective for pain but the patient cannot manage to take them by the oral route until habituation to this symptom occurs.

PAIN AND ANOREXIA/CACHEXIA/ASTHENIA

Anorexia/cachexia/asthenia is a common triad that accompanies many types of cancer, and when pain is also present, symptoms can be particularly difficult to manage. Although fatigue is the most common symptom in cancer patients, affecting about 70% of patients, a large minority fulfill diagnostic criteria of anorexia with cachexia. Such patients may have difficulty tolerating opioids, may have concurrent nausea, or may not be able to tolerate oral opioids because of upper GI malignancy. Such patients require alternative routes of drug administration or other pain treatment strategies. Furthermore, many interventions are available to support comprehensive assessment and management of anorexia, cachexia, and asthenia.

PAIN AND BOWEL DISEASE

Slow-release opioids are about 50% absorbed in the large colon. Patients who have had a partial or complete colectomy may malabsorb slow-release opioids, as a function of the more rapid transit time. The clinician may be suspicious of this by the presence of end-of-dose failure of the opioid, occurring several hours before the medication would be expected to wear off. Patients may report seeing the "ghost" of slow-release tablets in their stool. Most patients who have a low colostomy (in the left lower quadrant on abdominal exam) only uncommonly malabsorb slow-release opioids, whereas patients with a right-sided colostomy or ileostomy are at much higher risk. These patients should be considered for transdermal opioids or some other route of opioid administration.

Patients who have upper GI malignancy and pain are also at risk to develop concurrent nausea, obstruction, or other GI symptoms. At an early stage in their disease, they should be considered for another route of administration of analgesic medication.

MANAGING CANCER PAIN IN THE ADDICT

The overall strategy for pain management in the patient who carries an addiction diagnosis should be tempered according to whether the history is that of remote addiction, recent addiction, or active addiction. It must be stated that use of controlled substances for any legitimate medical purpose requires vigilance and a risk management approach that considers diversion and abuse, irrespective of the patient's diagnosis or history. However, medical judgment must be used to determine the extent of such

programs relative to the patient's individual circumstances. In all situations, the clinician will want to understand if the patient is in active recovery and/or maintenance therapy, communicate with the patient's addiction counselor/therapist, and look carefully for evidence of aberrant or problematic drug-taking behavior. The patient with a remote history of substance abuse and who currently has a stable social situation and a spouse or other close family member should be managed as any other cancer pain patient. However, these patients and their family members are oftentimes very concerned about rekindling addiction and may be highly opioid phobic. Long-acting oral opioids, transdermal opioids, or opioid preparations with abuse-deterrent technologies are the preference. The dose should be titrated upward to effect, with a structured management program (e.g., frequent follow-up visits, small or modest supplies of medicine dispensed at any given time, urine drug screens) to provide sufficient support for the patient and family. There should in most circumstances be only one prescribing physician, and once stable analgesia is achieved, there should be sufficient confidence and evidence of compliance and increasingly longer periods of time between prescribing visits. To the patient who is a recent user and in recovery, the discussion needs to be more frank and the plan of care more structured. The clinician should not only outline the goals of care (improved comfort and improved function) but also inquire the patient about his or her level of concern regarding opioids. The physician should warn the patient to not take the opioids for any reason other than relief of pain. Together, they should agree as to how often the medication prescriptions should be refilled and by whom. Comanagement with an addiction specialist is advised if the prescribing clinician is not well versed in addiction medicine. Unsanctioned dose escalation is not allowed, and if necessary, the medications may need to be controlled by the spouse or other family member.

Cancer patients who are actively abusing pose particular challenges. The patient and the clinician hope that the patient can achieve relief of pain, but the prescribing physician will be particularly wary of causing harm. Harm includes the risk of drug diversion or overdosing because the patient is accustomed to a less potent source of drug. Also, there is the risk that the pain medication may be stolen by those around the patient because of the social circumstances that often accompany addiction. There needs to be a firm, concrete framework to support clinical care. In these situations, daily dispensing of pain medication is often required, along with observed ingestion. If transdermal fentanyl patches are prescribed, which may be useful in these circumstances, the patch should be replaced under observation and then either disposed of properly or the used patch may be brought to the next prescribing visit and disposed under observation of clinicians. Liquid methadone may also be preferable over other analgesics or formulations in this circumstance.

A written agreement delineates expected behavior and the consequences of nonadherence. The agreement (sometimes referred to as an *opioid contract*) should include periodic unscheduled drug screening if the patient has committed to not use other drugs. In certain jurisdictions, the prescribing physician can benefit from a state or provincial computerized prescription network whereby it can be determined if the patient is obtaining prescription medications from another legitimate source. One should avoid high doses of opioids and should also consider nonpharmacologic interventions at an earlier stage (such as palliative radiotherapy or neural blockage).

SAFE PRESCRIBING PRACTICES: UNIVERSAL PRECAUTIONS

Beyond strategies applicable for the situation of cancer pain in a patient with a history of addiction is an emerging approach to safe prescribing opioid practice which is designed to guide care for all patients who are potentially candidates for opioids, whether or not there is a history of substance abuse. Recent years have seen heightened awareness of risk of misuse of opioids acquired through the health care system—awareness by the health care community, by patients and their families, by the public, and by regulatory bodies. Extensive guidance is available regarding safe prescribing practices[44] and universal precautions.[45] Although much attention has been paid to safe practices in *noncancer* pain management, increasingly, there is awareness that cancer pain, palliative care, and end-of-life care are situations which warrant similar high levels of caution.

Accurate use of words helps to delineate the landscape of substance abuse and the clinician's role in risk reduction. As described elsewhere in this book (see Chapter 32), addiction is on the far end of a spectrum of substance use disorders. Addiction is characterized by continued substance use despite demonstrable harm, craving, loss of control, and compulsive drug use such as gorging. Drug abuse is defined as drug use in a manner different than social norms. Evidence of drug abuse in the clinical setting can include aberrant drug behavior or nonadherence behavior.

A universal precautions strategy to prescribe opioids for cancer pain should be applied to all pain patients; it should include a specific focus on clinical assessment to stratify for risk, and a focus on elements of ongoing care:

Clinical assessment to stratify for risk
- Personal history of alcohol consumption
- Personal history of drug abuse
- Current heavy smoking/chronic unemployment
- Poor psychosocial support
- Family history of alcohol or drug abuse
- Establish treatment goals such as targets for pain reduction or improved function

Ongoing care
- Only one physician prescribes scheduled medications.
- Regularly review a patient's scheduled prescriptions using a state, provincial, or national prescription drug monitoring program.
- Monitor for and respond to aberrant behavior such as unsanctioned dose escalation, lost prescriptions, seeking medications from other physicians, or other aberrant activity.
- Continue opioid therapy only if meaningful benefits are present that outweigh the risks to patients.

Clinicians working in a cancer pain practice are often surprised at advice that they should consider instituting safe prescribing practices which are more commonly encountered in the chronic noncancer population. However, drug abuse touches almost all parts of society. Having a prospective, structured approach to safe prescribing equips the clinician to continue to have a prescribing relationship with a patient who subsequently develops what appears to be aberrant behavior. Commensurate with risk, the clinician should consider a range of approaches to respond to problematic behavior. These can include weekly, semiweekly, or daily carries of prescription refills for scheduled medications; random urine drug screens; blood levels of analgesics or of acetaminophen if it is present in breakthrough medications (record carefully when the last dose was taken in relation to timing of phlebotomy); home visits by physician or nurse, including medication reconciliation and direct interview of family members to explore their perspectives; or switch to opioid preparations considered to have a lower risk of diversion or abuse.

If drug diversion has occurred, stop prescribing or switch to a highly structured regimen such as witnessed ingestion of methadone.

SYMPTOM CLUSTERS

Cancer patients commonly have more than one symptom. A large survey of medical oncology inpatients and outpatients from a US Veterans Affairs medical center revealed that most had several symptoms, including low energy (62%), pain (59%), dry mouth (54%), shortness of breath (50%), and sleeping difficulty (45%).[46] Patients with "moderate" intensity pain had a median number of 11 symptoms, and as the performance status fell, the number of intense symptoms increased. Other studies have confirmed that cancer patients commonly have many distressing symptoms, and as the severity of disease increases, so does the number and severity of symptoms.[47]

The concept of symptom clusters has emerged as an area of intense research. Symptom clusters have been defined as three or more concurrent symptoms that are related to each other but do not necessarily share the same etiology.[48] There is evidence that the coexistence of several symptoms in the same patient is associated with worse quality of life and potentially will benefit from specific, targeted therapeutic approaches. For example, it has been suggested that release of cytokines may result in a range of symptoms related to cancer and its treatment.[49] A wide array of specific clusters has been reported. Examples posited to date include fatigue-anorexia-cachexia cluster (easy fatigue, weakness, anorexia, lack of energy, dry mouth, early satiety, weight loss, and taste changes), upper GI cluster (dizzy spells, dyspepsia, belching, bloating), neuropsychological cluster (sleep problems, depression, and anxiety), and others.[50] Further research is needed to confirm their existence as discrete nosologic entities, to delineate their underlying pathogenesis and connectedness, and to explore mechanism-based approaches to their management.[51,52] Cancer pain can be difficult to manage in the presence of other cancer-related symptoms, in part because opioids, nonopioids, and nondrug analgesic interventions can be more difficult for the patient to tolerate. Furthermore, even if pain is effectively managed, the patient may continue to have other severe symptoms and poor quality of life.

PAIN AT THE END OF LIFE

In the final hours of life, it may not be appropriate or there may not be sufficient time to obtain a detailed history, physical examination, and diagnostic studies in order to quickly obtain relief of distressing symptoms. The actual mechanism of pain becomes increasingly less relevant as death approaches. In the instance of severe pain, one would consider subcutaneous or intravenous opioids with rapid titration to effect. Severe regional pain such as abdominal, pelvic, or lower extremity pain can be managed with neuraxial (epidural, intrathecal) local anesthetics or opioids. In a pain crisis at the end of life, the patient may be a candidate for palliative sedation.[53] Palliative sedation is appropriate when the patient is aware that they are at the end of life, other interventions are not expected to relieve pain quickly enough, and the patient or family has requested this approach and given their informed consent. Assessment tools have been developed to guide the depth of sedation and must be used.[54] These issues are discussed further in Chapter 109.

CANCER PAIN EMERGENCIES

Occasionally, patients will present to their physician with persistent, horrible cancer pain. A cancer pain emergency has been defined as pain that is severe or excruciating (8 out of 10 on a 0 to 10 scale), for more than 6 hours.[55] Such patients typically come to an emergency room in great distress. The patient may already be on large doses of opioids and may be dehydrated due to limited oral intake during the previous days. Often, the patient will not have slept at all during that time. In such cases, the patient assessment is greatly truncated. The physician examines the patient quickly to determine whether there is evidence of a ruptured viscous, subarachnoid hemorrhage, ischemic crisis, pathologic fracture, spinal cord compression, or other catastrophe. Vital signs and cognitive status are monitored, and an intravenous access is secured. Opioid is administered with rapid upward titration using a mini-bolus technique until there is relief of pain. Intravenous protocols for cancer pain emergencies have been described for morphine[55] and fentanyl[56]; oral transmucosal and other routes of administration of opioids have also been described.[57] Unlike conscious sedation, rapid upward titration of opioid in the setting of unrelieved cancer pain almost never results in serious toxicity. After relief of pain is obtained, the physician reassesses the patient in detail for the underlying cause of the pain crisis. Some patients appear to be able to leave the emergency room an hour or few hours after obtaining relief of pain. Only uncommonly will the cause of the cancer pain emergency be apparent, such as a pathologic fracture. Typically, the flare of pain arises in a place of known metastatic disease, and the pain goes away as mysteriously as it came. Pain crises can occur in the palliative setting, and interventional approaches may be needed to obtain control of pain in a timely manner.[58]

OPIOID DIVERSION AT THE END OF LIFE

Cancer pain often increases as disease progresses and death approaches. As a result, opioid dose often also increases. Clinicians who have undertaken home visits in patients with advanced cancer have seen literally stacks of pill containers which have accumulated over time, covering bedroom furniture, filling bathroom cabinets, and overflowing onto the floor or stuffed into suit cases. After death, families often have custody of very large amounts of analgesic pills, injectable medications, and other drug preparations. What happens to these prescription medications?

Little is actually known. It is suspected, however, that some of this medication is diverted by family or friends and much of this may happen without it ever being discovered.

To prevent drug diversion at this most vulnerable of times, safe prescribing practice in end-of-life care should include identification of a medication custodian at an early time in this journey, usually the spouse or main caregiver. That individual should be asked to create an ongoing medication inventory and assure that scheduled medications are always secure. There should be a discussion about a formal plan for drug disposal after death, such as agreement with the dispensing pharmacy to dispose of this medication.

Conclusion

Cancer pain is common and, when present, is often severe. Fortunately, a great deal is known about its epidemiology, assessment, and management. An individualized approach to each patient offers the best opportunity to provide relief of pain and improve the quality of life at all stages of oncologic disease.

References

1. White MC, Holman DM, Boehm JE, et al. Age and cancer risk: a potentially modifiable relationship. *Am J Prev Med* 2014;46:S7–S15.
2. World Health Organization. Cancer fact sheet. Available at: http://www .who.int/mediacentre/factsheets/fs297/en/. Accessed February 22, 2018.
3. Portenoy RK, Kornblith AB, Wong G, et al. Pain in ovarian cancer patients. Prevalence, characteristics, and associated symptoms. *Cancer* 1994;74: 907–915.
4. Abernathy A, Foley KM. Management of cancer pain. In: Devita VT, Lawrence TS, Rosenberg SA, eds. *DeVita, Hellman, and Rosenberg's Cancer: Principles & Practice of Oncology*. 9th ed. New York: Lippincott Williams & Wilkins; 2011:2426–2447.
5. Mercadante S. Cancer pain management in children. *Palliat Med* 2004;18: 654–662.
6. Marcovitch H. *Black's Medical Dictionary*. 42nd ed. London: A&C Black; 2010. Available at: http://ezproxy.lib.ucalgary.ca/login?url=http://search.credo reference.com/content/entry/blackmed/epidemiology/0?institutionId=261. Accessed May 17, 2017.
7. McDonald AJ, Cooper MG. Patient-controlled analgesia: an appropriate method of pain control in children. *Paediatr Drugs* 2001;3:273–284.
8. Burstein HJ, Winer EP. Aromatase inhibitors and arthralgias: a new frontier in symptom management for breast cancer survivors. *J Clin Oncol* 2007;25:3797–3799.
9. Turner G, Clegg A. Best practice guidelines for the management of frailty: a British Geriatrics Society, Age UK and Royal College of General Practitioners report. *Age Ageing* 2014;43:744–747.
10. Karuturi M, Wong ML, Hsu T, et al. Understanding cognition in older patients with cancer. *J Geriatr Oncol* 2016;7:258–269.
11. World Health Organization. *Comprehensive Cervical Cancer Control. A Guide to Essential Practice*. 2nd ed. Geneva, Switzerland: World Health Organization. Available at: http://apps.who.int/iris/bitstream/10665/144785 /1/9789241548953_eng.pdf?ua=1. Accessed February 22, 2018.
12. Mousavi M, Sundquist J, Hemminki K. Nasopharyngeal and hypopharyngeal carcinoma risk among immigrants in Sweden. *Int J Cancer* 2010;127: 2888–2892.
13. Gordon RG Jr, ed. *Ethnologue: Languages of the World*. 15th ed. Dallas, TX: SIL International; 2005.
14. Wuensch A, Tang T, Goelz T, et al. Breaking bad news in China—the dilemma of patients' autonomy and traditional norms. A first communication skills training for Chinese oncologists and caretakers. *Psychooncology* 2013;22:1192–1195.
15. Sande TA, Laird BJ, Fallon MT. The use of opioids in cancer patients with renal impairment—a systematic review. *Support Care Cancer* 2017;25: 661–675.
16. West R, Farrell M. Behavioral science and addiction. In: Haber P, Day C, Farrell M, eds. *Addiction Medicine: Principles and Practice*. Melbourne, Australia: IP Communications; 2015:22–23.
17. Passik SD, Kirsh KL, Donaghy KB, et al. Pain and aberrant drug-related behaviors in medically ill patients with and without histories of substance abuse. *Clin J Pain* 2006;22:173–181.
18. Rosenblum A, Joseph H, Fong C, et al. Prevalence and characteristics of chronic pain among chemically dependent patients in methadone maintenance and residential treatment facilities. *JAMA* 2003;289:2370–2378.
19. Koyyalagunta D, Bruera E, Aigner C, et al. Risk stratification of opioid misuse among patients with cancer pain using the SOAPP-SF. *Pain Med* 2013;14:667–675.
20. Kouyoumdjian FG, Pivnick L, McIsaac KE, et al. Cancer prevalence, incidence and mortality in people who experience incarceration in Ontario, Canada: a population-based retrospective cohort study. *PLoS One* 2017;12(2):e0171131.
21. Bai JR, Befus M, Mukherjee DV, et al. Prevalence and predictors of chronic health conditions of inmates newly admitted to maximum security prisons. *J Correct Health Care* 2015;21:255–264.
22. Lin JT, Mathew P. Cancer pain management in prisons: a survey of primary care practitioners and inmates. *J Pain Symptom Manage* 2005;29:466–473.
23. International Association for the Study of Pain. IASP taxonomy. Available at: https://www.iasp-pain.org/Taxonomy?navItemNumber=576#Pain. Accessed May 23, 2017.
24. Cassel EJ. The nature of suffering and the goals of medicine. *N Engl J Med* 1982;306:639–645.
25. Melzack R. The McGill Pain Questionnaire: major properties and scoring methods. *Pain* 1975;1:277–299.
26. Sinclair S, Norris JM, McConnell SJ, et al. Compassion: a scoping review of the healthcare literature. *BMC Palliat Care* 2016;15:6.
27. Sinclair S, Beamer K, Hack TF, et al. Sympathy, empathy, and compassion: a grounded theory study of palliative care patients' understandings, experiences, and preferences. *Palliat Med* 2016;31:437–447.
28. Marchettini P. The burning of neuropathic pain wording. *Pain* 2005; 114:313–314.
29. Prkachin KM, Solomon PE, Ross J. Underestimation of pain by health-care providers: towards a model of the process of inferring pain in others. *Can J Nurs Res* 2007;39:88–106.
30. Ferrell BR, Rhiner M, Cohen MZ, et al. Pain as a metaphor for illness, part I: impact of cancer pain on family caregivers. *Oncol Nurs Forum* 1991;18: 1303–1309.
31. Wolfe F, Smythe HA, Yunus MB, et al. The American College of Rheumatology 1990 criteria for the classification of fibromyalgia. Report of the Multicenter Criteria Committee. *Arthritis Rheum* 1990;33:160–172.
32. Wolfe F, Clauw DJ, Fitzcharles MA, et al. The American College of Rheumatology preliminary diagnostic criteria for fibromyalgia and measurement of symptom severity. *Arthritis Care Res* 2010;62:600–610.
33. Rubinstein SM, Pool JJM, van Tulder MW, et al. A systematic review of the diagnostic accuracy of provocative tests of the neck for diagnosing cervical radiculopathy. *Eur Spine J* 2007;16:307–319.
34. van der Windt DA, Simons E, Riphagen II, et al. Physical examination for lumbar radiculopathy due to disc herniation in patients with low-back pain. *Cochrane Database Syst Rev* 2010;(2):CD007431.
35. Abdominal wall tenderness test: could Carnett cut costs? *Lancet* 1991; 337:p1134.
36. Hershfield NB. The abdominal wall. A frequently overlooked source of abdominal pain. *J Clin Gastroenterol* 1992;14:199–202.
37. Cunningham J, Temple WJ, Mitchell P, et al. Cooperative hernia study: pain in the postrepair patient. *Ann Surg* 1996;224:598–602.
38. Parry GJ, Floberg J. Diabetic truncal neuropathy presenting as abdominal hernia. *Neurology* 1989;39(11):1488–1490.
39. Hagen NA. Reproducing a cancer patient's pain on physical examination: bedside provocative maneuvers. *J Pain Symptom Manage* 1999;18:406–411.

40. Temel JS, Greer JA, Muzikansky A, et al. Early palliative care for patients with metastatic non–small-cell lung cancer. *N Engl J Med* 2010;363: 733–742.

41. Irwin KE, Greer JA, Khatib J, et al. Early palliative care and metastatic non-small cell lung cancer: potential mechanisms of prolonged survival. *Chron Respir Dis* 2013;10(1):35–47.

42. Hui D, Bruera E. A personalized approach to assessing and managing pain in patients with cancer. *J Clin Oncol* 2014;32:1640–1646.

43. Bush SH, Kanji S, Pereira JL, et al. Treating an established episode of delirium in palliative care: expert opinion and review of the current evidence base with recommendations for future development. *J Pain Symptom Manage* 2014;48:231–248.

44. Dowell D, Haegerich TM, Chou R. CDC guideline for prescribing opioids for chronic pain—United States, 2016. *MMWR Recomm Rep* 2016;65(RR-01): 1–49. doi:10.15585/mmwr.rr6501e1.

45. Gourlay DL, Heit HA, Almahrezi A. Universal precautions in pain medicine: a rational approach to the treatment of chronic pain. *Pain Med* 2005;6(2):107–112.

46. Chang VT, Hwang SS, Feuerman M, et al. Symptom and quality of life survey of medical oncology patients at a veterans affairs medical center: a role for symptom assessment. *Cancer* 2000;88:1175–1183.

47. Portenoy RK, Thaler HT, Kornblith AB, et al. Symptom prevalence, characteristics and distress in a cancer population. *Qual Life Res* 1994;3: 183–189.

48. Dodd MJ, Miaskowski C, Paul SM. Symptom clusters and their effect on the functional status of patients with cancer. *Oncol Nurs Forum* 2001;28: 465–470.

49. Cleeland CS, Bennett GJ, Dantzer R, et al. Are the symptoms of cancer and cancer treatment due to a shared biologic mechanism? A cytokine-immunologic model of cancer symptoms. *Cancer* 2003;97:2919–2925.

50. Miaskowski C, Aouizerat BE, Dodd M, et al. Conceptual issues in symptom clusters research and their implications for quality-of-life assessment in patients with cancer. *J Natl Cancer Inst Monogr* 2007;37:39–46.

51. Gilbertson-White S, Aouizerat BE, Jahan T, et al. A review of the literature on multiple symptoms, their predictors, and associated outcomes in patients with advanced cancer. *Palliat Support Care* 2011;9:81–102.

52. Chow E, Fan G, Hadi S, et al. Symptom clusters in cancer patients with brain metastases. *Clin Oncol (R Coll Radiol)* 2008;20:76–82.

53. Schildmann E, Schildmann J. Palliative sedation therapy: a systematic literature review and critical appraisal of available guidance on indication and decision making. *J Palliat Med* 2014;17:601–611.

54. Arevalo JJ, Brinkkemper T, van der Heide A, et al. Palliative sedation: reliability and validity of sedation scales. *J Pain Symptom Manage* 2012;44:704–714.

55. Hagen NA, Elwood T, Ernst S. Cancer pain emergencies: a protocol for management. *J Pain Symptom Manage* 1997;14:45–50.

56. Soares LG, Martins M, Uchoa R. Intravenous fentanyl for cancer pain: a "fast titration" protocol for the emergency room. *J Pain Symptom Manage* 2003;26:876–881.

57. Burton AW, Driver LC, Mendoza TR, et al. Oral transmucosal fentanyl citrate in the outpatient management of severe cancer pain crises: a retrospective case series. *Clin J Pain* 2004;20:195–197.

58. Friedmann Nauck F, Alt-Epping B. Crises in palliative care—a comprehensive approach. *Lancet Oncol* 2008;9:1086–1091.

CHAPTER 42

Assessment and Diagnosis of the Cancer Patient with Pain

DERMOT FITZGIBBON

Cancer is a major health problem in the United States and other countries and is the second leading cause of death in the United States and the most prominent cause of death in terms of years of potential life lost (Fig. 42.1).[1,2] In the United States, there was a total of 1,688,780 new cancer cases (or 4,600 new cancer diagnoses per day) and 600,920 deaths for cancers in 2017.[3] For all sites combined, the cancer incidence rate is 20% higher in men than in women, whereas the cancer death rate is 40% higher in men. From 1991 to 2014, the overall cancer death rate dropped 25%. Prostate, lung and bronchus, and colorectum account for 42% of cases in men, whereas in women, breast, lung and bronchus, and colorectum account for 50% (Fig. 42.2). Prostate cancer accounts for 1:5 new diagnoses in men, and breast cancer almost 1:3 of new diagnoses in women. Lung and bronchus cancers present approximately 1:4 cancer-related deaths in men and women (see Fig. 42.1). Cancer incidence patterns reflect trends in behaviors associated with cancer risk and changes in medical practice, such as the introduction of screening. Over the past decade of data, the overall cancer incidence rate in men declined by about 2% per year overall, whereas the incidence rate in women has remained generally stable since 1987 (Fig. 42.3).

Over the past three decades, the 5-year relative survival rate for all cancers combined has increased 20 percentage points among whites and 24 percentage points among blacks. The decline in cancer mortality over the past two decades is the result of steady reductions in smoking and advances in early detection and treatment, reflected in considerable decreases for the four major cancers (lung, breast, prostate, and colorectum) (Fig. 42.4).

In contrast to declining trends for the four major cancers, death rates rose from 2010 to 2014 by almost 3% per year for liver cancer and by about 2% per year for uterine cancer. Cancer survival, particularly for advanced-stage diseases, will likely improve because of advances in precision medicine and immunotherapy for late-stage cancers (e.g., melanoma, lung cancer).[4,5] Cancer incidence and death rates vary considerably between racial and ethnic groups, with rates generally highest among blacks and lowest among Asian/Pacific Islanders.[3] The major behavioral determinants of cancer, such as smoking, diet, alcohol use, obesity, physical inactivity, reproductive behavior, occupational and environmental exposures, and cancer screening, are substantially influenced by individual and area-level socioeconomic factors.[6] Health care inequalities have also risen in both absolute and relative terms and socioeconomic and racial/ethnic disparities in stage at diagnosis and survival from major cancers have persisted.[1]

Figures 42.2, 42.3, and 42.4 show estimated new cancer cases and deaths, trends in cancer incidence (1975 to 2013) and death rates (1975 to 2014) by sex and trends in death rates by sex overall and for select cancers, United States (1930 to 2014).

The number of cancer survivors has steadily increased since the 1970s with an estimated 13.7 million people in the United States in 2012 who had been diagnosed with cancer representing approximately a threefold increase compared to 1975 (Fig. 42.5). The number of cancer survivors is projected to increase by 31% to almost 18 million in 2018, which indicates an increase of more than 4 million survivors in 10 years[7]

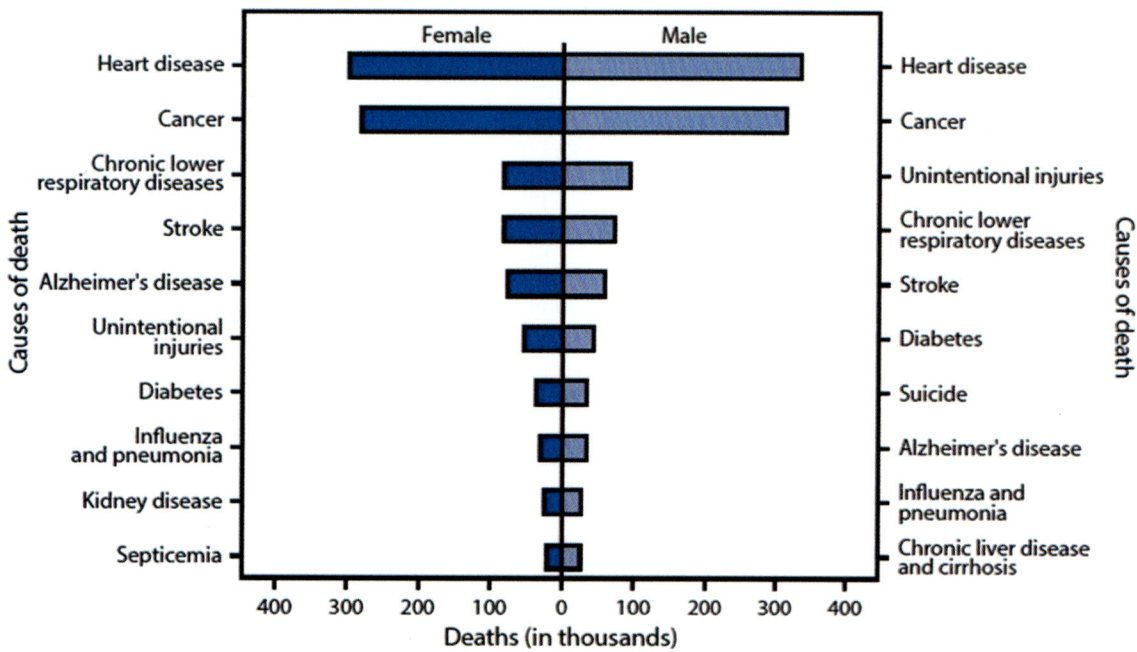

FIGURE 42.1 Number of deaths from 10 leading causes by sex—National Vital Statistics System, United States, 2015.

Estimated New Cases

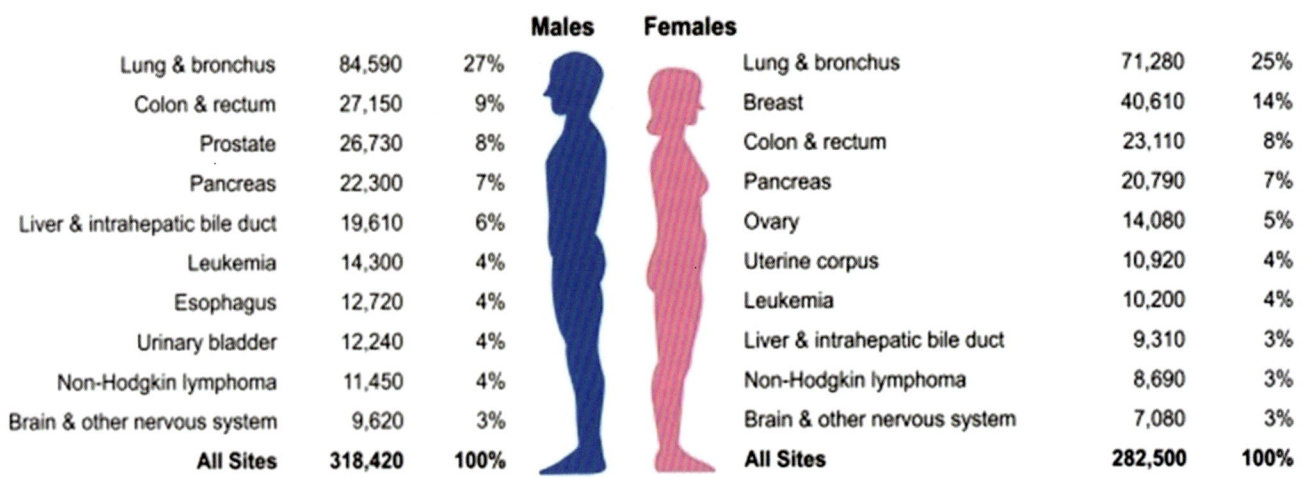

	Males				Females		
Prostate	161,360	19%		Breast	252,710	30%
Lung & bronchus	116,990	14%		Lung & bronchus	105,510	12%
Colon & rectum	71,420	9%		Colon & rectum	64,010	8%
Urinary bladder	60,490	7%		Uterine corpus	61,380	7%
Melanoma of the skin	52,170	6%		Thyroid	42,470	5%
Kidney & renal pelvis	40,610	5%		Melanoma of the skin	34,940	4%
Non-Hodgkin lymphoma	40,080	5%		Non-Hodgkin lymphoma	32,160	4%
Leukemia	36,290	4%		Leukemia	25,840	3%
Oral cavity & pharynx	35,720	4%		Pancreas	25,700	3%
Liver & intrahepatic bile duct	29,200	3%		Kidney & renal pelvis	23,380	3%
All Sites	**836,150**	**100%**		**All Sites**	**852,630**	**100%**

Estimated Deaths

	Males				Females		
Lung & bronchus	84,590	27%		Lung & bronchus	71,280	25%
Colon & rectum	27,150	9%		Breast	40,610	14%
Prostate	26,730	8%		Colon & rectum	23,110	8%
Pancreas	22,300	7%		Pancreas	20,790	7%
Liver & intrahepatic bile duct	19,610	6%		Ovary	14,080	5%
Leukemia	14,300	4%		Uterine corpus	10,920	4%
Esophagus	12,720	4%		Leukemia	10,200	4%
Urinary bladder	12,240	4%		Liver & intrahepatic bile duct	9,310	3%
Non-Hodgkin lymphoma	11,450	4%		Non-Hodgkin lymphoma	8,690	3%
Brain & other nervous system	9,620	3%		Brain & other nervous system	7,080	3%
All Sites	**318,420**	**100%**		**All Sites**	**282,500**	**100%**

FIGURE 42.2   Estimated new cancer cases and deaths. *(From Siegel RL, Miller KD, Jemal A. Cancer statistics, 2017. CA Cancer J Clin 2017;67[1]:7–30. Copyright © 2017 American Cancer Society. Reprinted by permission of John Wiley & Sons, Inc.)*

or more than 20 million in 2026[8] with 60% of cancer survivors aged 65 years or older by the year 2020.[9] Improvements in survival for the most common cancers have been similar by sex but are much more pronounced among patients aged 50 to 64 years than among those aged older than 65 years likely reflecting lower efficacy or use of new therapies in the elderly population.[10] Progress has been more rapid for the hematopoietic and lymphoid malignancies and less so for lung and pancreatic cancers for which the 5-year relative survival is 18% and 8%, respectively.[3] As the number of cancer survivors continue to grow, the need to address the effect of symptoms of cancer, including pain, on individuals' lives will become increasingly critical to efforts to reduce the burden of cancer and its treatment.

Despite advances in early detection and effective treatments, cancer is one of the medical conditions patients fear most.[11] The diagnosis often results in complex decisions at a time when patients may feel particularly vulnerable and distressed. Although clinical decisions previously followed one standard, many guidelines now outline several options and include explicit recognition of the need to incorporate patients' preferences to determine the most appropriate treatment.[12–14] Consequently, the demands and stresses imposed on patients during treatment

may be considerable.[15] In addition to anxiety about cancer as a potentially lethal disease, patient and family expectations that pain is an inevitable and untreatable consequence are additional major sources of distress.[16] Cancer pain elevates psychological distress,[17,18] alters social life,[19] disturbs sleep,[20] affects enjoyment of life,[21] and potentially compromises survival.[22] Fatigue, insomnia, neuropathy, and pain are among the most common troublesome symptoms experienced by cancer survivors[23] suggesting that pain rarely occurs in isolation. Furthermore, survivorship from cancer imposes its own issues including physical, psychosocial, and financial burdens with its associated impact on quality of life (QOL).

Differences exist between cancer pain patients and those that experience acute pain and/or chronic nonmalignant pain. The possibility of multiple complex and potentially painful oncology treatments (surgery, radiation therapy, chemotherapy, bone marrow transplantation, or other new treatments such as endocrine therapy for breast cancer) may result in a constant changing environment resulting in new pain complaints separate from the original tumor-related pain. For example, breast cancer is a major health burden and endocrine therapy with aromatase inhibitors (AIs) may be prescribed for up to

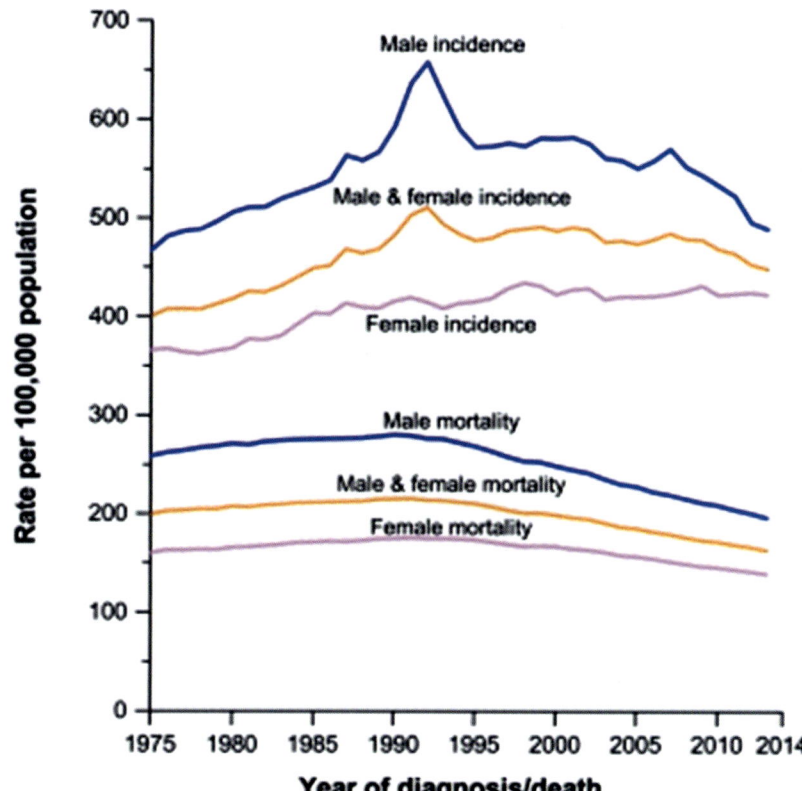

FIGURE 42.3 Trends in cancer incidence (1975 to 2013) and death rates (1975 to 2014) by sex. Rates are age adjusted to 2000 US standard population. *(From Siegel RL, Miller KD, Jemal A. Cancer statistics, 2017. CA Cancer J Clin 2017;67[1]:7–30. Copyright © 2017 American Cancer Society. Reprinted by permission of John Wiley & Sons, Inc.)*

10 years in patients with hormone receptor-positive tumors. Unfortunately, AI-associated arthralgia is an adverse event associated with low compliance with treatment.[24] Cancer patients also tend to have a higher symptom burden (especially psychological) compared to noncancer patients.[25] Patients may experience moderate-to-severe symptom distress (particularly pain, fatigue, and insomnia) after cancer treatment initiation.[15] End-of-life considerations and palliative care are rarely major issues for acute and chronic nonmalignant pain conditions, but these concerns become extremely important for the cancer pain patient with advanced disease (see Chapter 109). The complexities that emerge from the medical and psychosocial aspects of the situation necessitate a multi- and/or interdisciplinary approach for care. The changing nature of cancer pain, either in response to treatments directed at the tumor and/or progression of the tumor, mandates vigilance and potential frequent alteration of treatment strategies for pain. In addition, cancer survivors face ongoing surveillance for the possibility of disease recurrence, and new pain complaints in these patients require careful assessment. As cancer treatments continue to improve survival, many oncology patients face long-term pain management issues from aggressive treatment of their disease. As such, different treatment strategies may need to be considered. The effects of cancer diagnosis and subsequent treatment represent a continuum with an initial focus in early disease on health in survivorship and with advanced disease on QOL.[26] Comprehensive cancer care usually requires that many health care professionals become involved with the cancer pain patient at any one time. Successful pain management requires that the person or persons responsible for pain management adopt, or at least become familiar, an interdisciplinary approach. In addition, the humanitarian nature of cancer pain management, the focus on suffering and comfort, and the associated effects on patients' relatives all contribute to the uniqueness of this form of pain control.

Issues in Assessment and Diagnosis of Cancer Pain

Controlling pain associated with cancer is a major health care problem. Multiple studies from the 1990s documented inadequate treatment of pain in patients with cancer.[27–30] Despite the subsequent availability of effective pain treatments and various pain management guidelines, these deficiencies continued both in the United States and in other countries into the new millennium.[31–35] In 2008, approximately 1:2 patients with cancer pain was considered undertreated with geographic and economic trends in favor of the wealthiest countries.[36] A 2009 study suggested that 1:4 patients were untreated.[37] In a follow-up 2014 study from the 2008 study using similar methodology, 25% of patients were still considered untreated.[38] Ineffective pain management can have significant consequences. QOL for cancer patients and their families is profoundly affected by the presence of severe pain and other symptoms.[39] Health-related QOL parameters (physical functioning, appetite loss, and pain) provide significant prognostic value in addition to the sociodemographic variables (age and sex) and clinical variables (World Health Organization [WHO] performance status and distant metastases) and increase the predictive accuracy of the survival prognoses in patients with cancer.[40] Individual studies or those focusing on a particular cancer site generally reported a higher hazard ratio for pain,[41,42] appetite loss,[43] and physical functioning,[44] suggesting that the prognostic value of health-related QOL parameters scales might vary between different cancer sites.

Barriers to adequate pain management in cancer patients differ in low- versus high-resource environments.[45] Trainee physicians in the high resource group identified inadequate knowledge of cancer pain, assessment of pain etiology, concerns about opioid dependence, and drug-seeking behaviors as well as physicians' reluctance to prescribe opioids, as the major barriers. Trainee physicians in the low resource group reported less competence

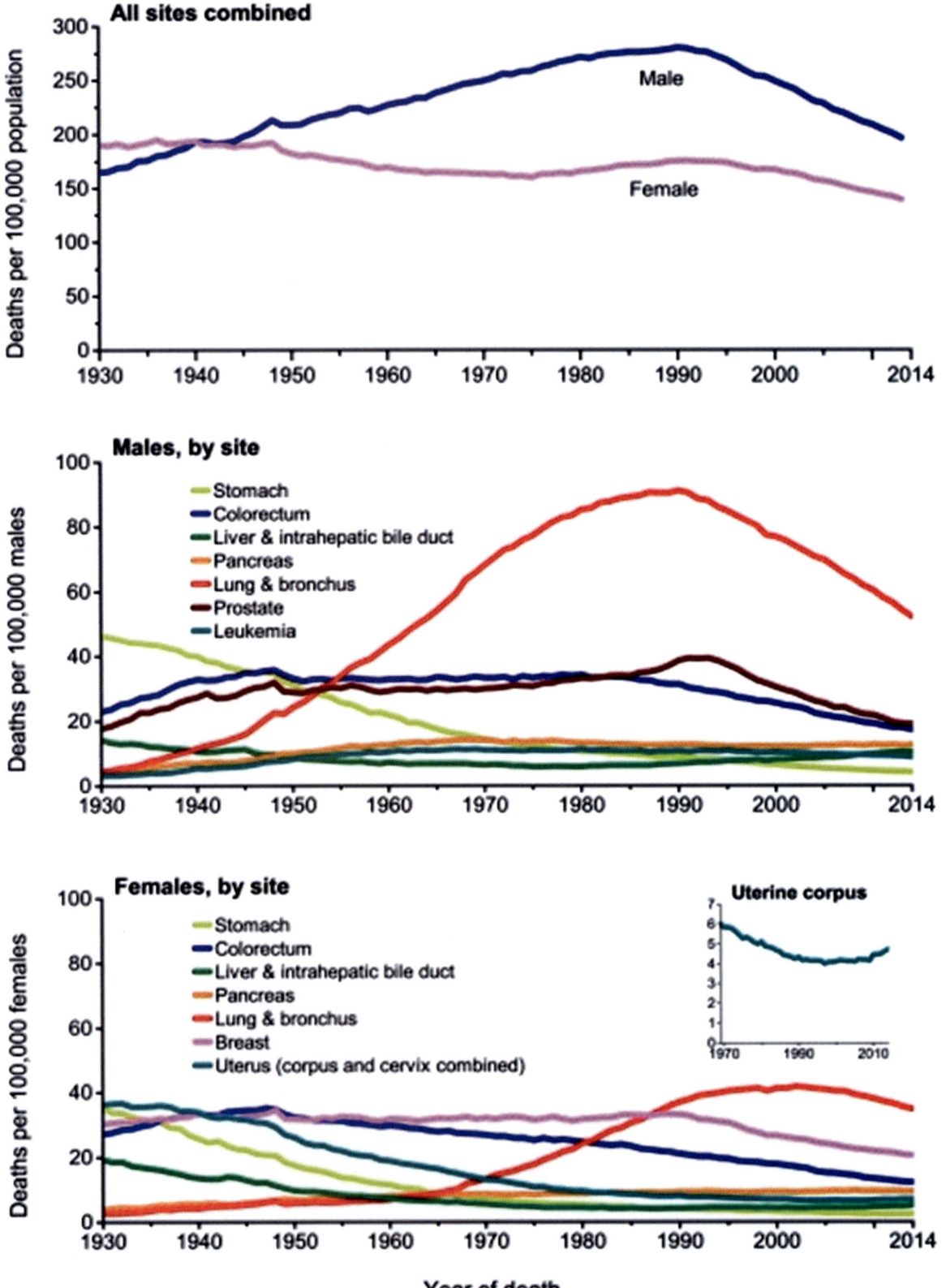

FIGURE 42.4   Trends in death rates by sex overall and for select cancers, United States, 1930 to 2014. *(From Siegel RL, Miller KD, Jemal A. Cancer statistics, 2017. CA Cancer J Clin 2017;67[1]:7–30. Copyright © 2017 American Cancer Society. Reprinted by permission of John Wiley & Sons, Inc.)*

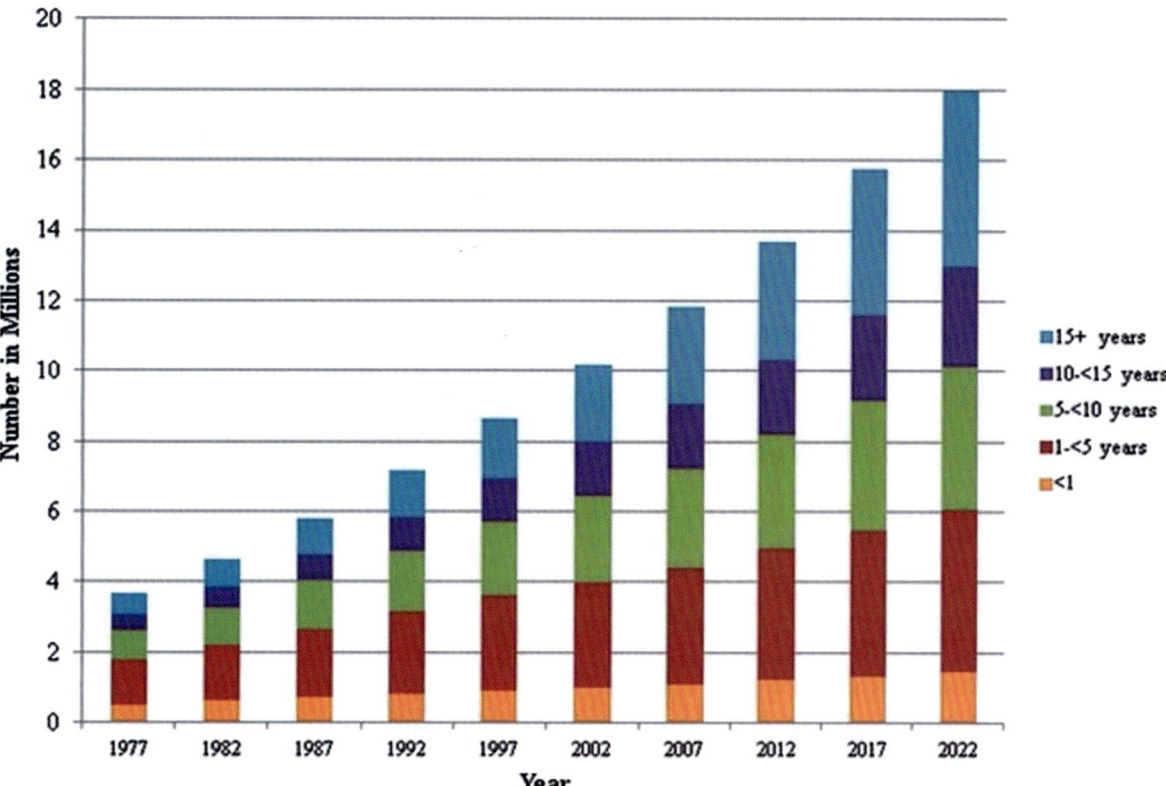

FIGURE 42.5 Estimated and projected number of cancer survivors in the United States from 1977 to 2022 by years since diagnosis. *(Data from Parry C, Kent EE, Mariotto AB, et al. Cancer survivors: a booming population.* Cancer Epidemiol Biomarkers Prev *2011;20[10]:1996–2005.)*

in cancer pain management despite having more cancer patients with advanced disease were less inclined to think that patients benefited from cancer pain management and less likely to consult another physician for cancer pain management and felt that patients poorly characterized their pain. Experienced physicians have also recognized a need for significant improvement in cancer pain assessment and treatment in their practice.[46,47] Lack of expertise by clinicians in assessing and managing cancer pain is an important cause of poor pain control.[30,48,49]

Pain management requires a variety of assessment skills and the integration of knowledge about pharmacology, pharmacokinetics and pharmacodynamics, patient characteristics like individual variability and compliance with medications, side effects and QOL determinants, and disease specifics. These skills must contribute to clinical judgment and decision making, often requiring substantial individual experience. Most studies concerning pain education of undergraduate medical students focus on knowledge, but relatively little is known about the interviewing skills and pain evaluation. Leila et al.[50] suggested that formative assessment of both knowledge and communication skills is essential for the development of a functional pain curriculum for training medical students in pain management of chronic pain patients. Core competencies in pain management include domains that define the multidimensional nature of pain, pain assessment and measurement, management of pain, and the context of pain management.[51] These serve as a foundation for developing, defining, and revising curricula and as a resource for the creation of learning activities across health care professions. Introducing pain education early in the training of health professionals offers the opportunity to reverse the disparity between what students are taught and what they confront in practice. Continuing education is needed across many disciplines but, in order to ensure the provision of quality pain management care, it is especially important to reach the following providers: oncologists, hematologists, urologists, surgeons, and radiation therapists who initially treat cancer patients; primary care physicians; nurses; and social workers and other providers of psychosocial services.

Pain and the Cancer Patient

Pain is an unpleasant sensory and emotional experience associated with actual or potential tissue damage or described in terms of such damage.[52] The sensory features and subjective qualities of pain vary, depending on its origin. Activity induced in the nociceptor and nociceptive pathways by a noxious stimulus is not pain, which is always a psychological state, even though one may well appreciate that pain most often has a proximate physical cause. Its emotional features depend in part on the social and physical context in which pain occurs, associated cognition, and the meaning of tissue trauma for the individual, but they are almost always negative.

It is important to recognize that the source of pain in the cancer patient is usually not a single entity but often has multiple sources that are dependent on different issues such as tumor staging, treatment phase, preexisting conditions that may cause chronic pain, and posttreatment complications.[53] As such, it is more accurate to use the term *pain in the cancer patient* than the more confusing term *cancer pain*. Many clinical trials in cancer pain do not differentiate the two and tend to use the latter descriptor resulting in difficulty in interpreting results.[54–59]

Tumor-related pain may be classified as nociceptive or neuropathic. Patients may present with different sources of tumor pain. Figure 42.6 shows a patient with extensive locally recurrent sacral chordoma presenting with tumor infiltration of somatic (sacrum, left sacroiliac [SI] joint, left iliac wing, left gluteal muscles) and neuropathic sources of pain (left S1 foramen with nerve root involvement, encasement of the left lumbosacral plexus). Pain is labeled nociceptive if the noxious stimulus is related to ongoing tissue injury and is subdivided into somatic

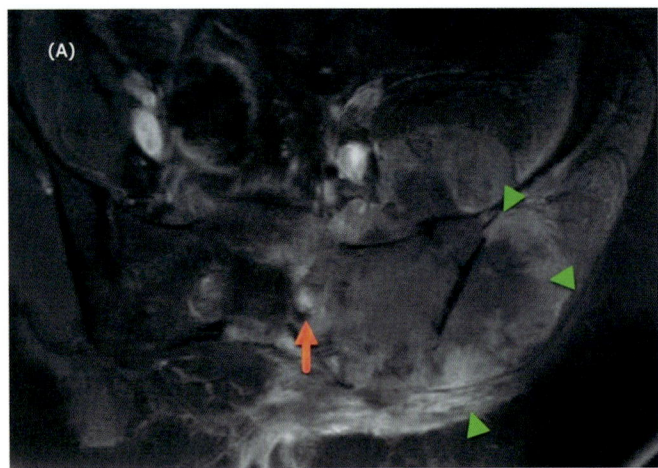 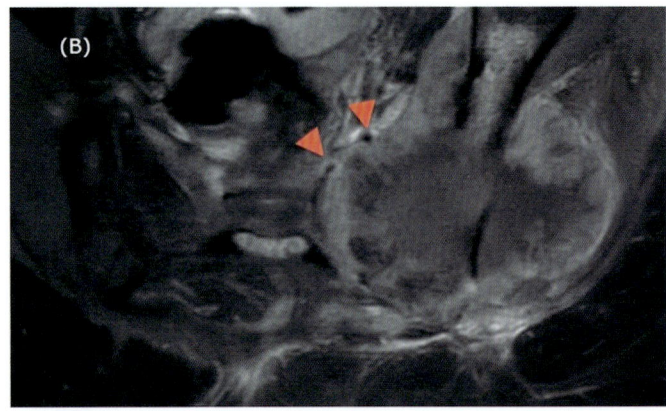

FIGURE 42.6 Magnetic resonance imaging image (axial T1 gadolinium-enhanced) of pelvis. Patient has extensive locally recurrent chordoma. **A:** A mass within the left sacrum and iliac wing spanning the left sacroiliac joint with large extraosseous soft tissue component extending into the left gluteal muscles (*green arrow heads*) and left iliopsoas muscle in addition to the left piriformis. The sacroiliac mass approaches the left S1 neural foramen (*red arrow*). **B:** The anterior margin of the left sacroiliac mass abuts and partly encases the left lumbosacral plexus at the level of S1 (*red arrow heads*).

and visceral types. Pain is neuropathic if there is evidence that the pain is associated with injury to neural tissues and is sustained by aberrant somatosensory processing in the peripheral or in the central nervous system (CNS). The International Association for the Study of Pain (IASP) defines neuropathic pain as pain caused by a lesion or disease of the somatosensory nervous system.[60] The restriction to the somatosensory nervous system is important because conditions such as musculoskeletal pain (e.g., due to spasticity) arising indirectly from disorders of the motor system should not be confused with neuropathic pain. Caraceni and Portenoy[53] defined tumor pain characteristics and syndromes and was nociceptive due to somatic injury in 71.6% of patients, nociceptive visceral in 34.7%, and neuropathic in 39.7%. Prevalence rates for tumor-related neuropathic pain are difficult to determine. Often, studies reporting on neuropathic pain in cancer patients tend to have mixed sources (Table 42.1).

The major pain syndromes comprised bone or joint lesions in 41.7% of patients, visceral lesions in 28.1%, soft tissue infiltration in 28.3%, and peripheral nerve injuries in 27.8%. Somatic nociceptive pain may be grouped into superficial (cutaneous) and deep. Most cutaneous pain is well localized, sharp, pricking, or burning. Deep tissue pain usually seems diffuse and dull or aching in quality. Visceral pain is very diffuse, often referred to the body surface, perseverating, and frequently associated with a queasy quality that patients describe as "sickening."

The mechanisms of tumor involvement of the nervous system are heterogeneous and include lesions within the cerebrospinal fluid (CSF) space, local invasion, compression, direct infiltration, perineural spread, and rarely intraneural metastasis.[62] Tumor involvement of the CNS occurs intracranially or within the spinal cord. Direct mechanisms for tumor involvement of the spinal cord occur in one of three anatomic compartments: parenchymal (intradural intramedullary), subarachnoid or CSF

(intradural extramedullary), or epidural (extradural).[63] Parenchymal (intradural intramedullary) spinal cord disease may be metastatic (intramedullary metastases from systemic cancer) or the consequence of a primary spinal cord tumor. Direct spinal cord disease may also result from disease of the subarachnoid/CSF compartment as in leptomeningeal metastasis (LM) or by extramedullary intradural primary spinal cord tumors. Direct spinal cord disease may also occur due to epidural metastases resulting in epidural spinal cord compression. Peripheral nerves consist of all the spinal nerves as well as the cranial nerves, with the exception of the optic nerve (cranial nerve II), which is a tract of the diencephalon rather than a peripheral nerve. Lymphoma, as well as breast, lung, prostate, colorectal, gynecologic, skin, and head and neck cancers, invade peripheral nerves through direct extrinsic involvement or perineural spread. Once the dense connective tissue of the epineurium is disrupted, malignant cells can travel both proximally and distally along the perineural and endoneural planes while remaining encased by the epineurium.[64] Compression and invasion of nerves by tumor results in the destruction of myelinated and unmyelinated fibers and of supporting tissue. Because peripheral nerves can usually evade pressure from a tumor on one side, infiltration by tumor tissue is the quintessential tissue trauma stimulus. In addition, indirect damage of unknown pathogenesis might also occur to peripheral nerves in the context of tumor conditions (e.g., paraneoplastic syndromes). Infiltration of tumor tissue into the perineural cleft is seen relatively often, and perineural tumor spread is more frequently associated with carcinoma arising in head and neck tumors with sources from minor or major salivary glands (more often adenoid cystic carcinoma), mucosal or cutaneous squamous cell carcinoma, basal cell carcinoma, melanoma, lymphoma, and sarcoma.[65] Neurolymphoma is a rare extranodal manifestation of lymphoma

TABLE 42.1	Etiology of Neuropathic Pain in Cancer Patients					
		Predominant Cause of Pain with Neuropathic Mechanism				
Study	Number of Pains with Neuropathic Mechanism	Cancer	Cancer Treatment	Associated with Cancer	Unrelated to Cancer	Unknown
Chua et al. 1999[503]	18	38.9%	27.8%	0%	11.1%	22.2%
García de Paredes et al. 2011[504]	477	52.8%	32.9%	0%	14.3%	0%
Grond et al. 1999[505]	254	72%	12%	4%	9%	3%
Grond et al. 1996[61]	925	68%	16%	5.3%	8.3%	2.4%
Total	1674	64%	20.3%	3.5%	10.2%	2%

Modified from Bennett MI, Rayment C, Hjermstad M, et al. Prevalence and aetiology of neuropathic pain in cancer patients: a systematic review. *Pain* 2012;153:359–365.

that reflects intraneural infiltration of malignant lymphocytes. Neurolymphoma has been encountered with both B-cell and T-cell lymphoma, yet it appears to occur most frequently in the context of large B-cell non-Hodgkin lymphoma (NHL).[66] A massive and subsequent painful entrapment of a nerve plexus or individual nerves may occur, especially in extensive breast carcinomas and their recurrences or in chest wall metastases of lung tumors.

MOLECULAR MECHANISM OF TUMOR PAIN

In addition to cancer cells, tumors consist of different cell types including inflammatory cells and blood vessels that are often adjacent to primary afferent nociceptors. These cells include immune system cells such as macrophages, neutrophils, and T cells. These secrete various factors that sensitize or directly excite primary afferent neurons and include prostaglandins (PGs), tumor necrosis factor (TNF), endothelin, interleukin (IL)-1 and IL-6, epidermal growth factor, transforming growth factor (TGF), and platelet-derived growth factor (PDGF). Receptors for many of these factors are expressed by primary afferent neurons. Endothelin (endothelin-1, endothelin-2, and endothelin-3) is a family of vasoactive peptides that are expressed at high levels by several types of tumor, including prostate cancer. Endothelin could contribute to cancer pain by directly sensitizing or exciting nociceptors, as a subset of small, unmyelinated primary afferent neurons expresses endothelin-A receptors.[67] Like PGs, endothelins that are produced by cancer cells are also thought to be involved in regulating angiogenesis and tumor growth.[68,69] Consequently, these factors and others from cancer and inflammatory cells, such as adenosine triphosphate (ATP), bradykinin (BK), H+, nerve growth factor (NGF), PGs, and vascular endothelial growth factor (VEGF) excite or sensitize adjacent nociceptors.[70] Tumor growth, spreading, and metastasis require the development of a local vasculature. One of the key signaling processes in the development of the tumor vasculature is the hypoxia-induced stimulation of VEGFs production, and the development of anti-VEGF therapy (e.g., bevacizumab) provides options for limiting tumor growth by targeting angiogenesis.[71] Adjacent nociceptors such as vanilloid receptor-1 (VR1) detect extracellular H+ and endothelin-A receptors detect endothelins released by cancer cells. NGF increases angiogenesis through its tropomyosin receptor kinase A (TrkA) on endothelial cells and by indirectly inducing VEGF expression.[72] Nociceptor activation results in the release of neurotransmitters, such as calcitonin gene-related peptide (CGRP), endothelin, histamine, glutamate, and substance P (SP). Nociceptor activation also causes the release of PGs from the peripheral terminals of sensory fibers, which can induce plasma extravasation, recruitment and activation of immune cells, and vasodilatation.

Other mechanisms, particularly tissue acidosis, may be involved in tumor-related pain. Tumors could cause a decrease in pH by several mechanisms. As inflammatory cells invade neoplastic tissue, they release protons that generate local acidosis. The large amount of apoptosis that occurs in the tumor environment also contributes to acidosis, as apoptotic cells release intracellular ions to create an acidic environment. This decrease in pH can activate signaling by acid-sensing channels (including VR1) that are expressed by nociceptors. Tumor-induced release of protons and acidosis might be particularly important in the generation of bone cancer pain.[73] Finally, tumor-induced distention of sensory fibers may also be involved in tumor-associated nociceptive processes.

SOMATIC PAIN

Somatic cancer pain can be caused by tumor invasion of bone, joint, muscle, or connective tissue. Somatic pain is the most common type of tumor pain with the most prevalent being tumor bone involvement. Nociceptive afferents are most concentrated

in the periosteum. Some of the mechanisms contributing to neoplastic bone pain include stretching of the periosteum by tumor expansion, local microfractures that cause bony distortion, nerve compression due to either collapsed vertebrae or direct tumor encroachment, and local release of algesic substances from the bone marrow. Because inactivity and deconditioning predisposes to muscle pain, the debilitated cancer patient may experience muscle pain that is likely to contribute to complaints of localized or generalized pain. Skeletal muscle accounts for approximately 50% of body weight and is a major cause of morbidity. Myofascial pain is often underdiagnosed and inappropriately treated. Myofascial pain should be considered separately from fibromyalgia. In 2010, the American College of Rheumatology abandoned the use of a tender point count in the diagnostic criteria of fibromyalgia with the definition now based on the number of painful body regions and the presence and severity of fatigue, unrefreshed sleep, cognitive difficulty, and the extent of somatic symptoms.[74] Myofascial pain syndrome (MPS) is a local or regional pain problem with tender areas that reproduce symptoms on palpation and may be primary or secondary to another condition.[75] There may be associated muscle stiffness and decreased range of motion with palpable taut bands or nodules. Trigger points may be defined as the presence of defined "exquisitely" painful trigger in a taut band of muscle that produce characteristic patterns of referred pain on palpation and a local twitch response to mechanical stimulation or needling. Proposed criteria for diagnosis of MPS are listed in Table 42.2. Sustained contractile activity leading to increased metabolic stress and reduced blood flow likely contributes to the persistence of a myofascial trigger point. In addition to the sustained contractile activity, metabolic alterations and cell stress trigger release of myokines, inflammatory cytokines, and neurotransmitters that contribute to myofascial trigger points and MPS.[76,77] Muscle pain is generally described as aching and cramp-like. It can be difficult to localize and may be referred to other deep somatic structures.

Muscle nociceptors are free nerve endings connected to the CNS by thin myelinated (group III) or unmyelinated (group IV) afferent fibers.[78] Muscle nociceptors can be sensitized to chemical and mechanical stimuli. Muscle nociceptors can be activated by BK, prostaglandin E_2 (PGE_2), serotonin (5-HT), and other endogenous substances.[79] SP, CGRP, and somatostatin are neuropeptides present in primary afferent fibers from muscle.[80] In muscle-free nerve endings, SP, CGRP, vasoactive intestinal polypeptide, NGF, and growth-associated protein 43 are present.[81] These neuropeptides are synthesized in the soma of the primary afferent neuron in the dorsal root ganglion and transported via axonal transport to the receptive ending in muscle and to the central terminals in the spinal cord. Molecular receptors for many algesic substances (BK, 5-HT, PGE_2, and ATP) are present in muscle tissue and are released during painful stimulation or pathologic conditions. Some of these receptors control ion channels that cause an ion flux across the membrane that can

---

TABLE 42.2 Proposed Criteria for Diagnosis of Myofascial Pain Syndrome

- A tender spot is found with palpation, with or without referral of pain ("trigger point").
- Recognition of symptoms by patient during palpation of tender spot *and* at least three of the following:
  - Muscle stiffness or spasm
  - Limited range of motion of an associated joint
  - Pain worsens with stress.
  - Palpation of taut band and/or nodule associated with tender spot

From Rivers WE, Garrigues D, Graciosa J, et al. Signs and symptoms of myofascial pain: an international survey of pain management providers and proposed preliminary set of diagnostic criteria. *Pain Med* 2015;16(9):1794–1805. Reproduced by permission of American Academy of Pain Medicine.

depolarize the ending. Purinergic receptors may be of particular importance for muscle pain because ATP, which is present in large amounts in muscle tissue and is released during muscle damage, could excite the nociceptor directly. Muscle nociceptors do not respond to everyday stimuli, such as normal contractions or weak deformation of muscle tissue.[82] Two chemical stimuli are particularly relevant as causes of muscle pain. The first is a drop in tissue pH, and a large number of painful alterations of muscle tissue are associated with an acidic interstitial pH. The second important cause of muscle pain is a release of ATP.[78,83]

VISCERAL PAIN

Visceral pain refers to pain resulting from noxious stimuli such as painful swelling, ischemia, and inflammation that act on visceral organs via peripheral and central pathways. Visceral pain is typically correlated with the excitation of spinal (thoracolumbar, sacral) visceral afferents. Spinal visceral afferents are polymodal and activated by adequate mechanical and chemical stimuli.[84] All groups of spinal visceral afferents can be sensitized (e.g., by inflammation). Spinal visceral afferent neurons project into the laminae I, II (outer part IIo), and V of the spinal dorsal horn over several segments; mediolateral over the whole width of the dorsal horn; and contralateral. Typically, patients complain of a vague sensation with an unclear location that may be referred to other nonvisceral somatic areas and associated with autonomic changes. The majority of thoracic and abdominal visceral organs, except the pancreas, are dually innervated by parasympathetic (craniosacral) and sympathetic (thoracolumbar) outflows. Thoracic viscera and upper abdominal viscera are primarily innervated by the vagus (cranial nerve X) and spinal thoracolumbar outflows. The lower abdominal viscera, including the small and the large intestine and the urogenital organs, are innervated by thoracolumbar (i.e., lumbar splanchnic nerve and hypogastric nerve) and sacral (i.e., pelvic nerve) outflows. Sensory afferents innervating the visceral organs are not just a homogeneous group of afferents signaling visceral pain to the CNS. Pain is primarily signaled by spinal afferents, whereas vagal afferents signal nonpainful sensations such as hunger, satiety, fullness, and nausea.[85] Transient receptor potential (TRP) channels are predominantly distributed in both somatic and visceral sensory nervous systems and play a crucial role in sensory transduction.[86] The majority of spinal afferents projecting to the gastrointestinal tract or pelvic organs are TRPV1, TRPA1, and/or TRPM8 positive and respond to mechanical stimulation[87–89] and are also sensitive to noxious stimuli from pungent compounds, temperature, acid, and inflammation.[90] Visceral nociceptive messages are conveyed to the spinal cord by relatively few visceral afferent fibers that activate many central neurons by extensive functional divergence through polysynaptic pathways.[84]

Pancreatic pain is perceived as a severe discomfort in the upper abdomen frequently radiating through to the back. Malignant pancreatic tumors, acute and chronic inflammation of the pancreas, and obstruction of the pancreatic duct can produce severe pain. Hepatic, biliary, and pancreatic pain appear to be mediated by afferent fibers in sympathetic nerves, and vagal innervation does not appear to contribute to nociceptive transmission.[91] Pain related to pancreatic cancer may occur in 50% to 70% of patients,[92] but only 30% of patients with early stage pancreatic cancer complain of abdominal pain, compared to 60% of patients with limited and 80% of patients with advanced pancreatic cancer.[93,94] Abdominal pain tends to occur regardless of tumor location, although it was reported by more patients with cancer in the body and tail of the pancreas (90%) compared with those with cancer in the head of the pancreas (70%).[95] Histopathologic and molecular changes have been observed in pancreatic cancer specimens which are associated with pain which include increased nerve density and nerve hypertrophy, peri- and endo-neural cancer cell invasion,

altered expression of nociceptors, parenchymal immune cell infiltration in the pancreas, and release of neurotrophic growth factors which are undetectable in the normal pancreas.[96] Others have proposed perineural spread or invasion by the tumor, capsular stretching, and pancreatic cancer ductal obstruction as mechanisms of pain.[97] Afferent signaling of pancreatic nociceptive processes is likely via the celiac plexus and thoracic splanchnic nerves as suggested by the efficacy of celiac plexus block in managing associated pain.[92]

NEUROPATHIC PAIN

Pain usually results from activation of nociceptive afferents by actual or potential tissue-damaging stimuli. Pain may also arise by activity generated within the nervous system without adequate stimulation of its peripheral sensory endings. Neuropathic pain arises as a direct consequence of a lesion or disease affecting the somatosensory system. The presence of symptoms or signs (e.g., touch-evoked pain) alone does not justify the use of the term *neuropathic* and as such neuropathic pain is a clinical description (and not a diagnosis) which requires a demonstrable lesion or a disease that satisfies established neurologic diagnostic criteria. As such, neuropathic pain should not be diagnosed by pain descriptors only. The process of tumor compression and invasion of nerves entails several degenerative, regenerative, and other pathophysiologic processes.[98] The whole afferent neuron is affected and goes through reactive, presumably reparative, biochemical changes. The neuron loses its neuropeptides,[99] atrophies, and may finally degenerate. Animal models indicate that axonal degeneration following peripheral nerve injury causes neuropathic pain,[100] and these effects are related to the production of proinflammatory cytokines such as TNF-α with upregulation in endoneurial macrophages and Schwann cells[101] with other cytokines such as IL-1β and IL-6 and of the anti-inflammatory cytokine IL-10 both in the peripheral (sciatic nerve, dorsal root ganglia [DRG]) and the central (spinal cord) nervous system.[102] Nerve injuries both proximal and distal to the DRG induce mechanical allodynia, which are likely related to DRG TNF-α expression and apoptosis.[103] Microglia and astrocytes within the CNS play a pivotal role in the development and maintenance of neuropathic pain. Microglia propagate neuroinflammation by recruiting other microglia and eventually activating nearby astrocytes, thus prolonging the inflammatory state and leading to chronic neuropathic pain.[104]

AFFECTIVE PROCESSING AND SUFFERING

Fear of pain in patients has cognitive and emotional variables in the experience of pain in patients with advanced cancer.[105] The aversive nature of pain elicits a powerful emotional reaction that feeds back to modulate pain perception. Negative emotions are associated with increased activation in the amygdala, anterior cingulate cortex, and anterior insula,[106] brain structures that not only mediate the processing of emotions but also are important nodes of the pain neuromatrix that tune attention toward pain, intensify pain unpleasantness, and amplify interoception.[107] Anger, sadness, and fear may result from pain and affect biobehavioral processes that influence pain perception to exacerbate anguish and suffering. The emotional mechanisms of cancer pain are the reasons that it generates suffering. Brain processing of pain in humans is based on multiple ascending pathways and brain regions that are involved in several pain components, such as sensory, immediate affective, and secondary affective dimensions.[108] Brain mechanisms supporting discrimination of sensory features of pain extend far beyond the somatosensory cortices and involve frontal regions traditionally associated with affective processing and the medial pain system. The level of psychological and emotional distress associated with a cancer diagnosis contributes to increased rates of comorbidities and mortality while reducing QOL and compliance to care.[109,110] Transient mood disturbances occur frequently among cancer patients during the disease trajectory, and depression often persists in these patients.[111] Lower QOL scores may be associated with variables related to a patient's premorbid psychological characteristics and with coping skills for the cancer than to cancer-related variables (e.g., treatment types and cancer severity).[112] Of course, most cancer patients suffer from a complex array of problems and not only pain. Nonetheless, sustained nociception in and of itself can produce suffering because of its ability to create negative emotional arousal and elicit associated stress responses.

Suffering is a complex, negative emotional and cognitive state characterized by perceived threat to the integrity of the self, perceived helplessness in the face of that threat, and exhaustion of psychosocial and personal resources for coping with that threat.[113] The perceived threat to the self may encompass the body, the psychosocial self, or both. Suffering related to cancer is inherently emotional, unpleasant, complex, and enduring. The clinician should recognize that, although suffering may be a consequence of pain, it is separate from pain and not a synonym for it. It differs from pain in that it entails additional cognitive affective states. For example, perceived helplessness (inability to cope; bankruptcy of physical, psychological, or social resources) is a key element in the suffering of most patients with incurable disease. Similarly, grief can ensue when a cancer patient perceives the loss of a psychological or social resource, a body part or desired personal appearance, a prized employment status, or a physical capability for a treasured activity. Loss often equates with perceived threat to self. In addition, suffering in the cancer patient sometimes involves a sense of separation from social support or alienation. These factors, combined with the emotional distress, fatigue, and stress associated with prolonged pain produce a complex state that differs from pain itself. Wilson et al.[114] in a study of 381 patients with advanced cancer found that 25% of patients were suffering at a moderate to extreme level and that suffering is a multidimensional experience related most strongly to physical symptoms but with contributions from psychological distress, existential concerns, and social-relational worries.

PSYCHOLOGICAL FACTORS AND THE COMPLEXITIES OF CANCER PAIN

Somatic symptoms are a feature of anxiety, depressive, somatoform, and other psychiatric disorders. Somatization refers to patients who transform distress and global suffering into pain and symptom expression, and health care providers frequently view pain reported by cancer patients as primarily somatogenic, whereas chronic nonmalignant pain in patients who lack adequate objective physical pathology is viewed as psychogenic.[115] Consequently, providers tend to treat cancer pain with pharmacologic, medical, or surgical modalities. Psychological factors tend to be considered of secondary importance.[116] Pain is a complex experience entailing physiologic, sensory, affective, cognitive, and behavioral components. The final individual perception of pain is dependent on nociceptive input and psychological modifiers such as fear, anxiety, anger, and depression (Fig. 42.7).

Turk et al.[115] classified the multidimensional nature of cancer pain and compared the adaptation of cancer patients and chronic noncancer patients to persisting pain. The majority of the cancer patients, both with (81%) and without (84%) metastatic disease as well as the noncancer chronic pain patients (85%) fit one of three psychosocial subgroups: dysfunctional (high levels of pain, perceived interference, affective distress, and low levels of perceived control and activity), interpersonally distressed (high levels of affective distress, negative responses from significant others, and low levels of perceived support), and adaptive copers (low levels of interference and affective distress, high levels of perceived control and activity).

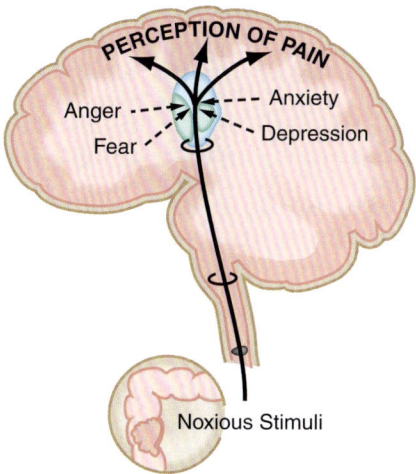

FIGURE 42.7 Individual perception of pain. Noxious stimuli are modified at supraspinal level by emotions such as anxiety, fear, and anger.

Substantial evidence suggests that psychological factors play an important role in exacerbating pain with clear origins of disease (see Chapters 29 to 33). For example, the belief that pain signifies disease, a commonly held belief among cancer patients,[117] is associated with elevated pain intensity.[118,119] Although pain is frequently associated with metastatic disease, it is by no means universal.[120,121] Spiegel and Bloom[119] reported on the affective states of cancer patients and the belief that pain is an indicator for disease progression and that medication use predicts pain severity. Patients who attribute their pain to a warning of underlying disease report greater pain intensity than patients with more non–tumor-associated interpretations, despite comparable levels of disease progression. In this study, the predictors of pain were use of analgesics, emotional distress, and pain beliefs, and that treatment of metastatic pain should include attention to the patient's mood and adjustment to illness.

Because of psychological factors, the relationship between pain severity and the extent of disease is rarely as linear as one might assume,[122] and there is a nonlinear relationship between cancer pain severity and interference with function.[123] Research investigating the relationships between physical pathology and pain in cancer has shown conflicting results. First, not all patients with advanced cancer report pain. Twycross and Fairfield[124] reported that only 41 of 100 terminal-stage cancer patients reported pain due to disease. Front et al.[120] demonstrated that for many cancer patients, pain reports did not correspond to the presence or location of bone metastases. Turk et al.[115] found that patients with cancer-related pain reported a significantly higher level of perceived disability and inactivity due to pain than did those with pain of nonmalignant origin. Because the level of pain severity was comparable for the two patient groups, elevated disability may have been a consequence of the meanings patients attributed to their pain. The progression of disease means further deterioration of health and impending death. Indeed, the patients with cancer-related pain appeared to be more fearful of pain and reported significantly higher levels of cognitive and behavioral fear responses than did the patients with chronic pain not associated with cancer. These patients appeared to think and worry more about pain, avoid activities in order to prevent initiation of pain, and they generally felt more hopeless than the patients with non–cancer-related pain.

Depression in Cancer Patients

The prevalence of major depressive episodes is increased with most chronic conditions but especially those characterized by inflammation and pain.[125] The prevalence of depression among cancer patients increases with disease severity and symptoms such as pain and fatigue.[126] Adjustment disorder, major depression, delirium, and anxiety disorders occur between 10% and 34% of cancer patients.[127–129] Major depression has been found to occur in approximately 16% of patients with cancer, with minor depression and dysthymia combined reported in almost 22% of patients.[130,131] Mood disturbance, sleep disturbance, fatigue, and pain either alone or in combination is also highly prevalent in patients receiving cancer therapy.[132] The overlap of physical illness and symptoms of major depression is widely recognized in physically healthy adults based on the presence of neurovegetative complaints, including insomnia, anorexia, fatigue, and weight loss in addition to depressed mood, hopelessness, guilt or worthlessness, and suicidal ideation. Major depressive disorder is a debilitating disease that is characterized by depressed mood, diminished interests, impaired cognitive function, and vegetative symptoms, such as disturbed sleep or appetite.[133,134] Similarly, vegetative symptoms such as appetite loss, insomnia, and fatigue are not uncommon in the cancer patient particularly with advanced disease or cancer treatment, and the diagnosis of depression in cancer patients can be difficult because of this overlap.[20,135] Levels of physical impairment, age (particularly younger patients), advanced stages of illness, inadequately controlled pain, prior history of depression, and the presence of other significant life stresses or losses are associated with a higher prevalence of depression in cancer patients. In addition, patients with certain cancer types such as pancreatic, head and neck, gastric, and lung cancers have higher rates of depression,[136,137] with the highest rates in lung, gynecologic, breast, colorectal, and genitourinary patients.[138] Within these disease states, a diagnosis of major depression was more likely in patients who were younger, had worse social deprivation scores, and, for lung cancer and colorectal cancer (CRC), female patients. Seventy three percent of 1,538 patients with depression were not receiving potentially effective treatment.[138] Various chemotherapy agents including alkylating agents (procarbazine, carmustine, busulfan), vinca alkaloids (vincristine, vinblastine), antimetabolites (pemetrexed, fludarabine), medications that interfere with DNA and RNA synthesis (doxorubicin, daunorubicin, L-asparaginase), and mitotic inhibitors (taxanes including paclitaxel, docetaxel) may cause depression. Biologic agents including IL-2, corticosteroids, tyrosine kinase inhibitors (imatinib, dasatinib, cetuximab, sorafenib, sunitinib), and hormonal agents (tamoxifen, anastrozole, gonadotropin-releasing hormone [GnRH] agonists) are associated with depression.[139]

Broadly speaking, depressed persons complain of a pervasive dysphoric mood, anhedonia, apathy and disinterest in normal activities, sleep problems, low energy, and in severe cases suicidal ideation. Approximately 20% to 30% of cancer patients meet the criteria for a psychiatric diagnosis, mainly depressive disorders, anxiety, and adjustment and stress-related disorders, across the trajectory of their disease,[130,140,141] whereas the prevalence of depression in primary care patients approximates 6% to 10% for outpatients and 10% to 14% for inpatients.[142–144] Depression is one of the strongest predictors of subsequent development of regular opioid use for treatment of chronic pain,[145] and multifocal pain is especially likely to be associated with depression and with opioid use.[146]

DETECTING AND ASSESSING DEPRESSION IN THE CANCER PATIENT

It is important for the physician treating cancer pain to recognize and address depression. Untreated depression has a significant impact on patient QOL, health care utilization, disease outcome, and influences care and participation in treatment.[147] Depression may go unnoticed or unaddressed in the cancer patient.[148–151] Few oncologists or supporting consultants feel qualified to address depression, and for those who do, time limits on patient contact time make it difficult to engage in extensive questioning about psychological well-being. Patients and family members may add to the problem by assuming that care providers concern themselves solely with controlling the disease and wish to avoid the distractions that psychological management entails.

Depressive disorders include disruptive mood dysregulation disorder, major depressive disorder (including major depressive episode), persistent depressive disorder (dysthymia), premenstrual dysphoric disorder, substance/medication-induced depressive disorder, and depressive disorder due to another medical condition. The common feature of all of these disorders is the presence of sad, empty, or irritable mood accompanied by somatic and cognitive changes that significantly affect the individual's capacity to function. Depression may have two components: the psychological or "cognitive" component (e.g., mood) and the physical or "somatic" component (e.g., loss of appetite). *Diagnostic and Statistical Manual of Mental Disorders* (5th edition; *DSM-5*) criteria requires either depressed mood or loss of interest or pleasure with four other depressive symptoms (changes in sleep, appetite or weight, activity, guilt/worthlessness, death/suicide, fatigue/loss of energy, decreased focus or concentration) for at least 2 weeks. Diagnosing depression in the cancer patient is not straightforward because there is symptom overlap between the psychiatric disorder, the toxicities of treatment, and the effects of the primary disease. Anxiety and depression may also mimic physical symptoms of cancer or treatments, and consequently, emotional distress may not be detected. Many clinicians tend to focus on somatic rather than psychological problems in patients with life-threatening illness, and some erroneously regard reactive depression in a patient who has received a diagnosis of cancer to be a normal response. Mitchell et al.[152] analyzed the diagnostic significance of somatic and nonsomatic symptoms indicative of depression in 279 patients within 9 months of first presentation with a diagnosis of cancer. No single symptom was a good proxy for depression. Emphasis on the presence of somatic symptoms (appetite loss, weight loss, insomnia, fatigue, loss of energy, and diminished ability to think or concentrate), feelings of worthlessness, and suicidal ideation may not be useful, among the *DSM* (4th ed.; *DSM-IV*) criteria, for diagnosing and/or judging the severity of depression among cancer patients.[153] Many of the traditional physical symptoms of depression such as fatigue, diminished appetite, and weight loss also occur in emotionally healthy cancer patients.[154]

The prevalence of depression in oncology varies widely by study and is often attributable to differences in assessment procedures.[155] Common assessment methods for depressive spectrum disorders in cancer settings are listed in Table 42.3. In practice, the diagnosis of depression is too complex for any screening tool, used in isolation, to be of diagnostic certainty. Structured clinical interviews have traditionally been considered the standard for identifying the prevalence, clinical significance, and potential treatment of depression because of their rigorous criteria. Common interview tools include the Structured Clinical Interview for *DSM* disorders (SCID) and Research Diagnostic Criteria. A disadvantage of such tools includes the lack of validation in a population without significant comorbid physical illness such as cancer. A variety of written self-report measures have been used to identify symptoms of depression in cancer patients. These include the Hospital Anxiety and Depression Scale (HADS), the Rotterdam Symptom Checklist (RSCL), the Beck Depression Inventory (BDI) (regular and short forms), the Brief Symptom Inventory-Depression scale, Center for Epidemiologic Studies Depression Scale (CES-D), and the Zung Self-Rating Depression Scale (both full and brief forms). The majority of research on depression in cancer patients has used the HADS, with much of this research focused on identifying the optimal cutoff scores for depressed patients with cancer.[111] The Patient Health Questionnaire-9 (PHQ-9)

TABLE 42.3 Common Assessment Methods for Depressive Spectrum Disorders in Cancer Settings

Tools	Characteristics	Clinical Use	Comments
Interviews			
Structured Clinical Interview for *DSM* disorders (SCID)	Clinician version and standard research version to be used in research and clinical settings	Designed to be administered by a clinician or trained mental health professional	Assessment of current psychiatric patients, lifetime psychiatric diagnoses in medical patients, family members, community samples
World Health Organization World Mental Health Composite International Diagnostic Interview (WHO WMH-CIDI)	Comprehensive, fully structured interview	Designed to be used by trained lay interviewers	Assessment of mental disorders according to the definitions and criteria of ICD-10 and *DSM-IV* in epidemiologic and cross-cultural studies and for clinical and research purposes
Diagnostic Criteria for Psychosomatic Research (DCPR)	Clinical interview	Set of 12 psychosocial syndromes demoralization, disease phobia, health anxiety thanatophobia, illness denial, persistent somatization, functional somatic symptoms secondary to a psychiatric disorder, conversion symptoms, anniversary reaction, irritable mood, type A behavior, and alexithymia	Research evidence accumulated in several clinical settings (cardiology, oncology, gastroenterology, endocrinology, primary care, consultation psychiatry, nutrition, and community)
Short Psychometric Questionnaires			
Hospital Anxiety Depression Scale (HADS)	14 items (7 for anxiety; 7 for depression) plus total score	Score HADS-D: 0–7 = normal; 8–10 = borderline case; 11–21 = case; HADS total ≥15 adjustment disorders; ≥19 MDD	In oncology, best thresholds for screening = 15 for the HADS total (sensitivity 0.87; specificity 0.88), 7 for the HADS-D subscale (sensitivity 0.86; specificity 0.81 disorders)
Center for Epidemiologic Studies Depression Scale (CES-D)	20 items 0–3 Likert scale	Scores ≥16: risk for clinical depression; ≥22: clinically relevant depression; ≥25: MDD	CESD-R (revised version) also available, reflecting *DSM-5* diagnosis of MDD
Beck Depression Inventory II (BDI-II)	21 questions, each answer being scored on a scale value of 0–3	Score 14–19: mild depression; 20–28: moderate depression; 29–63: severe depression. Sensitivity: 81%; specificity: 92%	
Profile of Mood States (POMS)	65 adjectives (5-point scale)	6 factors (Anger-Hostility; Confusion-Bewilderment; Depression-Dejection; Fatigue-Inertia; Tension-Anxiety; Vigor-Activity)	Short version available for cancer settings
Patient Health Questionnaire (PHQ-9)	9 items (scored 0–3, range 0–27) covering DSM criteria for MDD	Score 5–9: mild depression; 10–14: moderate depression; 15–19: moderately severe depression; 20–27: severe depression	Score ≥8: sensitivity 93%, specificity 81%, PPV 25%, NPV 99% in cancer settings
Demoralization Scale (DS) Demoralization Scale II (DS-II)	24 items on a 5-point Likert scale 16 items on a 3-point Likert scale	Scores ≥30: high demoralization Scores 0–3: low demoralization; 4–10: middle demoralization; ≥11: high demoralization	DS and DS-II validation studies in progress in cancer settings
Subjective Incompetence Scale (SI)	12 items on a 0–3 Likert scale	Studies on threshold scores in progress	SI validation studies in progress in cancer settings

DSM, Diagnostic and Statistical Manual of Mental Disorders; DSM-IV, DSM 4th edition; DSM-5, DSM 5th edition; ICD-10, International Statistical Classification of Diseases and Related Health Problems, 10th revision; MDD, major depressive disorder; NPV, negative predictive value; PPV, positive predictive value.
Modified from Caruso R, GiuliaNanni M, Riba MB, et al. Depressive spectrum disorders in cancer: diagnostic issues and intervention. A critical review. *Curr Psychiatry Rep* 2017;19:33.

and briefer versions, the PHQ-2 and PHQ-8, are easily administered, commonly used depression screening tools. In a study of 463 patients from 35 community-based radiation oncology sites and 2 academic radiation oncology sites, the PHQ-2 demonstrated good psychometric properties for screening for mood disorders, which were equivalent to the PHQ-9.[156] Some authors suggest that the CES-D and BDI-II may be most feasible given their time efficiency, administrative simplicity, and strong psychometric properties.[157] Others have suggested that the PHQ-9 with a cutoff score ≥8 is a good screening tool in cancer outpatients.[158,159]

Screening for depression should focus primarily on the cognitive/affective features of depression because these are not confounded with treatment-associated toxicities. In palliative care patients, several studies have found that the single question "Are you depressed?" was used as a screening tool with the high sensitivity, specificity, and positive predictive value.[160,161]

Cancer-Related Fatigue

Cancer-related fatigue (CRF) may be defined as a common, persistent, and subjective sense of tiredness related to cancer or to treatment for cancer that interferes with usual functioning.[162] It may be perceived as a feeling of extraordinary exhaustion associated with a high level of distress, disproportionate to activity, and is not relieved by sleep or rest. Patients may describe fatigue as feeling tired, weak, worn-out, heavy, slow, or that they have no energy or get-up-and-go. CRF and sleep disturbances may occur as distinct symptoms but are often comorbid.[163] Fatigue is also a nonspecific symptom that may be found in association with most mental and physical disorders. It is prevalent among all types of cancer, but breast, lung, and pancreatic are among the most frequently associated with persistent fatigue.[164] Abrahams et al.[165] estimated that 1:4 breast cancer survivors suffer from severe fatigue and identified higher disease stages, chemotherapy and receiving the combination of surgery, radiotherapy, and chemotherapy, both with and without hormone therapy, as risk factors.

Fatigue may be an issue during all phases of treatment and into survivorship for extended periods of time.[166] It is estimated that fatigue is present at the time of diagnosis in approximately 40% of cancer patients.[167] It occurs in up to 75% of patients if bone metastases already are present.[168] An estimated 60% to 96% of cancer patients in treatment experience fatigue, including 90% of patients on radiation treatment and 80% of patients on chemotherapy. Except for chemotherapy-induced anemia, the pathogenesis of fatigue in patients with cancer is understood poorly, but proposed mechanisms include the direct effects of cancer and the various modes of cancer treatment plus a wide variety of concomitant diseases (such as anemia, infections, dehydration, and electrolyte disorders), sleep disorders, chronic pain, immobility and lack of exercise, and a variety of psychosocial disorders. Because of the high prevalence of anemia in oncology patients, the association of anemia with fatigue has been extensively studied. Sobrero et al.[169] indicated that general scores for QOL, fatigue, and sensations of physical and functional well-being are significantly higher among patients with hemoglobin (Hb) levels >12 g/dL, but Bremberg et al.[170] found that physical and functional aspects may be more important to consider than increasing the Hb level to reduce the fatigue.

Screening for fatigue is an important issue in the overall care of the oncology patient.[171] Various tools for assessing CFR have been used (Table 42.4). The most widely used of these scales are the Functional Assessment of Cancer Therapy: Fatigue (FACT-F) and the European Organisation for Research and Treatment of Cancer Quality of Life Care Questionnaire (EORTC QLQ-C30) fatigue subscale which have data from over 10,000 patients between them and have been widely used in intervention studies to treat CRF. The FACT-F has the advantage of having a validated clinically significant score change—it also covers the social impact of CRF but takes longer to administer than the 3-item EORTC QLQ-C30 fatigue subscale.[172]

Once fatigue is identified, a detailed clinical evaluation should be performed. Components of the evaluation should include details of the cancer including the type and duration of the treatment and its capacity to induce fatigue. Other components include documenting the characteristics of the fatigue such as when it started, what factors aggravate it, etc. Emotional and psychological components should be identified, and the effect of the fatigue on the performance of normal, daily life activities should be determined. Then, various clinical organic conditions that can cause fatigue should be evaluated.

If a specific cause of CRF is identified (anemia, insomnia, depression, metabolic disorders, etc.), then this should be treated first. Antidepressants and analgesics should be prescribed for patients with depression and pain. After common causes of anemia have been excluded, patients with low levels of Hb should receive treatment with erythropoietic agents. Patients with sleep disorders should receive appropriate instructions for improving sleep quality or carefully prescribed drugs. Educating patients about fatigue is extremely useful.[173] Moderate exercise can be more effective than continuous rest.[174–176] Aerobic exercises can increase overall muscle tone, and it may be wiser to advise such exercise than rest.

Sleep Disturbance in Cancer

Sleep disturbances include reduced nocturnal sleep time, sleep fragmentation, nocturnal wandering, and daytime sleepiness. Acute insomnia is characterized as lasting up to a month and insomnia syndrome is defined as insomnia occurring more than three nights per week, difficulty falling asleep or nighttime awakenings (>30 minutes), ratio of sleep time to time spent in bed <85% (sleep efficiency), impaired daytime functioning, and marked distress. Insomnia syndrome is also called chronic insomnia, as it usually persists nightly for >4 weeks. A history of cancer increases the likelihood of having sleep disturbance.[177] Insomnia is a prominent problem for patients with cancer and 25% to 60% of patients may be affected[178–180] and a prevalence rate almost twice that of the general population.[181] The prevalence of sleep disturbance varies depending on the cancer type, cancer stage, treatment received, and time since completion of treatment. Compared with other types of cancer, breast cancer is associated with an exceptionally high rate of reduced sleep quality.[182,183] Insomnia in patients with lung cancer undergoing chemotherapy may be as high as 52%.[184] Sleep disturbance is one of the five most common symptoms reported as moderate to severe by primary brain tumor patients and occurs anywhere between 17% and 54% of patients.[185] Despite its prevalence and importance, insomnia is often unrecognized and poorly managed. Insomnia refers to difficulty falling or staying asleep, whereas sleep impairment refers to sleepiness, tiredness, and perceived functional impairments during wakefulness associated with sleep problems or impaired alertness. Insomnia typically occurs as a transient inability to initiate or maintain sleep or as hyperarousal, often in response to a situation or event. Daytime consequences of fatigue and insomnia are similar and include dysphoric states, such as irritability, impaired cognition (poor concentration and memory), and interference with usual activities.

TABLE 42.4	Fatigue Scales Used to Evaluate Cancer-Related Fatigue	
Instrument	**Dimensions of Measurement**	**Usefulness in Oncology**
Fatigue Symptom Inventory Scale	13-item, physical, cognitive, and psychosocial fatigue	Used in patients undergoing active treatment and survivors
Fatigue Severity Scale	9 questions, no clear dimensional separate	Not validated; limited use
Brief Fatigue Inventory	One dimension, 9-item VAS, cutoff scores for mild, medium, severe fatigue	Useful for screening purposes
Visual Analogue Scale for Fatigue	18-item, originally used in patients with sleep disorder	Very limited use in cancer patients
Multidimensional Fatigue Inventory	16-item, originally validated in rheumatoid arthritis, multidimensional	Relatively poorly validated
EORTC	Likert, 30-item, physical and mental fatigue, full tool used extensively as quality of life instrument	Ceiling effect in advanced cancer patients; not recommended as single measure in this group; used in cancer chemotherapy trials
FACT-F	Numerical, 13-item, physical functioning	Used in intervention studies to treat CRF
Cancer Fatigue Scale	15-item, 3 factors (physical, affective, cognitive) multidimensional	Designed for oncology use

CRF, cancer-related fatigue; EORTC, European Organisation for Research and Treatment of Cancer; FACT-F, Functional Assessment of Cancer Therapy: Fatigue; VAS, Visual Analogue Scale.
Modified from Gerber LH. Cancer-related fatigue: persistent, pervasive, and problematic. *Phys Med Rehabil Clin N Am* 2017;28(1):65–88. Copyright © 2016 Elsevier. With permission.

Identification of sleep disturbance typically involves screening for the problem followed by a comprehensive assessment for those who screen positive. The National Institutes of Health recommends that screening may include asking two questions: (1) Do you have problems with your sleep or sleep disturbance on average for three or more nights a week? If yes, (2) does the problem with your sleep negatively affect your daytime functioning? If the answer is yes to both questions, a more focused assessment of sleep disturbance is indicated.[186] Use of the Insomnia Severity Index (7-item, self-report questionnaire) was also recommended to screen for cases of insomnia in cancer patients and for assessing the effects of treatment (Table 42.5).[187] Once identified, the Pittsburgh Sleep Quality Index (PSQI) can be administered for a more detailed assessment. The PSQI is a 19-item questionnaire evaluating sleep quality and disturbances over the past month.[188] The first 4 items are open questions, whereas items 5 to 19 are rated on a 4-point Likert scale. Individual items scores yield 7 components (subjective sleep quality, sleep latency, sleep duration, habitual sleep efficiency, sleep disturbances, use of sleeping medication, and daytime dysfunction). A total score (global PSQI), ranging from 0 to 21, is obtained by adding the 7 component scores. A score >5 suggests poor sleep quality.

Treatment of insomnia favors the use of pharmacologic aids. The common hypnotics including barbiturates, benzodiazepines, the "Z" drugs (eszopiclone, zaleplon, zolpidem, zopiclone), and other benzodiazepine-receptor agonists bind to γ-aminobutyric acid (GABA) receptors. However, a European study demonstrated that publication bias exists for insomnia trials and that the positive trials are two times more likely to be published than the negative ones.[189] There is little controlled evidence that long-term uses of hypnotics produce benefits of any sort.[190] A study of almost 2,000 cancer patients found that 22.6% were taking hypnotic medication for sleep problems, and half of those were taking medication every night for periods longer than 6 months.[191] Use of hypnotic drugs is associated with a greatly increased risk of all-cause mortality. Some of this mortality has been documented as deaths caused by hypnotics by medical examiners, attributed to respiratory arrests resulting from "overdose." However, it is likely that many deaths from respiratory depression occur among patients never seen by coroners, especially when the death is caused by a combination of hypnotics with other contributing factors, so that the lethal hypnotic dosage may by itself have been within customary dosage ranges.[192] In addition to respiratory depression, hypnotics appear to be causally related to serious illnesses and premature deaths from cancer, serious infections, mood disorders, accidental injuries, suicides, and homicides.[193] Cognitive-behavior therapy for insomnia (CBT-I) includes components of sleep restriction (limiting time in bed), stimulus control (conditioning the bed for sleep by restricting behaviors incompatible with sleep in the bedroom), and cognitive restructuring (addressing maladaptive thoughts and beliefs about sleep) to reestablish a regular sleep pattern. CBT-I was superior to zopiclone both in short- and long-term management of insomnia in older adults.[194]

TABLE 42.5 Insomnia Severity Index

For each question, please CIRCLE the number that best describes your answer.
Please rate the *CURRENT (i.e., LAST 2 WEEKS) SEVERITY* of your insomnia problem(s).

Insomnia Problem	None	Mild	Moderate	Severe	Very Severe
1. Difficulty falling asleep	0	1	2	3	4
2. Difficulty staying asleep	0	1	2	3	4
3. Problem waking up too early	0	1	2	3	4

4. How SATISFIED/DISSATISFIED are you with your CURRENT sleep pattern?

Very Satisfied	Satisfied	Moderately Satisfied	Dissatisfied	Very Dissatisfied
0	1	2	3	4

5. How NOTICEABLE to others do you think your sleep problem is in terms of impairing the quality of your life?

Not at all Noticeable	A Little	Somewhat	Much	Very Much Noticeable
0	1	2	3	4

6. How WORRIED/DISTRESSED are you about your current sleep problem?

Not at all Worried	A Little	Somewhat	Much	Very Much Worried
0	1	2	3	4

7. To what extent do you consider your sleep problem to INTERFERE with your daily functioning (e.g., daytime fatigue, mood, ability to function at work/daily chores, concentration, memory, mood, etc.) CURRENTLY?

Not at all Interfering	A Little	Somewhat	Much	Very Much Interfering
0	1	2	3	4

Guidelines for Scoring/Interpretation:
Add the scores for all seven items (questions 1 + 2 + 3 + 4 + 5 + 6 + 7) = _____ your total score
Total score categories:
0–7 = No clinically significant insomnia
8–14 = Subthreshold insomnia
15–21 = Clinical insomnia (moderate severity)
22–28 = Clinical insomnia (severe)

From Charles M. Morin, PhD, Université Laval.

Sources of Pain in the Cancer Patient

Pain in the oncology patient can arise from different sources (Table 42.6):

- Direct or indirect tumor involvement
- Cancer-directed therapy
- Mechanisms unrelated to cancer or its treatment
- A combination of the above

Patients may present with complex patterns of pain that result from combinations of these categories, thus complicating the diagnosis. Factors influencing the pain complaint include the primary tumor type, stage of disease, tumor site, and mood factors (anxiety and depression). Although estimates vary, the prevalence of pain in cancer survivors has been reported to be as high as 40%[195–198] with variable durations of painful symptoms[199] and with disparities in race and sex.[200] The prevalence of pain in patients with cancer varies with tumor type, treatment phase, and stage of disease. Van den Beuken-van Everdingen et al.[196] estimated the pain prevalence rates were 39.3% after curative treatment; 55% during anticancer treatment; and 66.4% in advanced, metastatic, or terminal disease with 50.7% in all cancer stages. Moderate to severe intensity pain (numerical rating scale score ≥5) was reported by 38.0% of all patients. Of note, lower pain prevalence rates occurred in prostate cancer patient compared to head and neck, lung, and breast cancer patients. In 2007, the authors previously reported prevalence rates of 33% after curative treatment; 59% during treatment; 64% in advanced, metastatic, or terminal disease; and 64% in all cancer stages with approximately 33% grading pain intensity as moderate to severe and the highest prevalence in head/neck cancer patients.[201] High prevalence of pain has also been documented in hematologic tumor patients initially at diagnosis, during treatment, and in the last month of life.[202,203]

Many patients with advanced disease frequently have multiple pain complaints at different sites and were more common in patients with breast, lung, and prostate cancer compared with gastrointestinal cancers.[204] In a prospective study of 2,266 cancer patients, Grond et al.[61] assessed localization, etiology, and pathophysiologic mechanisms of pain syndromes associated with cancer. Thirty percent of the patients presented with one, 39% with two, and 31% with three or more distinct pain syndromes. The majority of patients had pain caused by cancer (85%) or antineoplastic treatment (17%); 9% had pain related to cancer disease and 9% due to etiologies unrelated to cancer. These investigations classified pain as originating from nociceptors in bone (35%), soft tissue (45%) or visceral

structures (33%), or of neuropathic origin (34%). Patients had localized pain syndromes in the lower back (36%), abdominal region (27%), thoracic region (23%), lower limbs (21%), head (17%), and pelvic region (15%). Regions and systems affected by the main pain syndrome varied widely depending on the site of cancer origin, whereas the cancer site did not markedly influence the pain's temporal characteristics, intensity, or etiology.

Many metastatic bone lesions cause few or no symptoms and are diagnosed incidentally during an initial staging workup or at follow-up restaging evaluations.[205] Bone cancer pain is the most common pain in patients with advanced cancer, and approximately two-thirds of patients with metastatic bone disease experience severe pain.[206] Many of the most common tumors (breast, prostate, thyroid, kidney, and lung) have a strong predilection for bone metastasis, and an estimated 70% of patients with breast and prostate cancers develop bone metastases compared with 20% to 30% of patients with lung or gastrointestinal cancers.[207] Although pain is frequently associated with the presence of metastases, certain tumor types are exceptions, notably breast and prostate cancers. Neither the prevalence nor the severity of pain among breast cancer patients varied directly as a function of metastatic sites of disease.[118,119] Palmer et al.[208] evaluated the sensitivity of pain as an indicator of bone metastases in patients with breast or prostate cancer. Pain was a common finding, whether or not metastatic disease was present, and it occurred in over half of the patients. Although most patients with bone metastases reported bone pain, some (21% of breast and 22% of prostate patients) were asymptomatic.

The majority of neoplasms are responsible for symptoms caused by mass effects to surrounding tissues and/or through the development of metastases. Paraneoplastic syndromes arise from tumor secretion of hormones, peptides, or cytokines or from immune cross-reactivity between malignant and normal tissues and may affect different organ systems, most notably the endocrine, neurologic, dermatologic, rheumatologic, and hematologic systems. The most commonly associated malignancies include small-cell lung cancer (SCLC), breast, gynecologic, and hematologic malignancies. Hypertrophic pulmonary osteoarthropathy (HPO) is characterized by periostosis and subperiosteal new bone formation along the shaft of long bones and the phalanges ("digital clubbing"), joint swelling, and pain and may be present in 1% to 10% of patients with lung tumors[209,210] and may also been seen in patients with mesothelioma and lymphoma. Classically, HPO is diagnosed based on clinical symptoms (severe pain, edema, and erythema in the extremities) and radiologic findings. Periostitis is the hallmark of HPO, and imaging shows periosteal membrane thickening and periosteal new bone formation particularly in the distal long bones (especially the tibia). Bone scan is also useful for the detection of HPO. Peripheral nerves are a common target in paraneoplastic syndromes.[211] Antibodies directed against neural antigens expressed by the tumor (onconeural antibodies) may occur in most of those affected by classical paraneoplastic syndromes, suggesting that an autoimmune process underlies these disorders. Subacute sensory neuronopathy (SSN) is a classical paraneoplastic syndrome.[212] The neuropathy generally develops subacutely accompanied by pain and rapidly progressive paresthesia. Involvement of the upper extremities may occur with asymmetric sensory deficit or multifocal with facial, thoracic, and abdominal involvement. Many patients with SSN also have signs and symptoms suggestive of multifocal involvement including areas of the CNS. Paraneoplastic vasculitis of the peripheral nervous system usually precedes the tumor diagnosis and presents as multineuritis or asymmetric distal sensory-motor neuropathy with pain as a commonly reported symptom. This form is generally associated with lymphoma or cancer at various sites (lung, prostate, uterus, kidney, or gastric).[213]

TABLE 42.6	Causes of Pain in Patients with Cancer
Cause	**Example**
As a direct consequence of tumor	Involvement of bones Obstruction of hollow organs Compression of nerves
As an indirect consequence of tumors	By infections By metabolic imbalances By venous/lymphatic occlusion By paraneoplastic syndromes
As a consequence of tumor therapy	Following surgical intervention Following chemotherapy Following radiation therapy
Without relation to cancer	Migraine Diabetic neuropathy Myofascial pain problems
A combination of the above	Metastatic lung cancer to bone with hypertrophic osteoarthropathy affecting tubular bones in a patient with painful peripheral diabetic neuropathy and chemotherapy-induced peripheral neuropathy

TABLE 42.7	NCI CTCAE v4.0 Neurotoxicity: National Cancer Institute Common Terminology Criteria for Adverse Events				
Adverse Event	Grade 1	Grade 2	Grade 3	Grade 4	Grade 5
Peripheral motor neuropathy	Asymptomatic, clinical or diagnostic observations only; intervention not indicated	Moderate symptoms; limiting instrumental ADL[a]	Severe symptoms; limiting self-care ADL[a]; assistive device indicated	Life-threatening consequences; urgent intervention indicated	Death
Peripheral sensory neuropathy	Asymptomatic; loss of deep tendon reflexes or paresthesia	Moderate symptoms; limiting instrumental ADL[a]	Severe symptoms; limiting self-care ADL[a]	Life-threatening consequences; urgent intervention indicated	Death
Paresthesia	Mild symptoms	Moderate symptoms; limiting instrumental ADL[a]	Severe symptoms; limiting self-care ADL[a]		

[a]Instrumental ADL include preparing meals, shopping, using the telephone, managing money. Self-care ADLs include bathing, dressing, using the toilet, and taking medications. Paresthesia is characterized by functional disturbances of sensory neurons resulting in abnormal cutaneous sensations of tingling, numbness, pressure, cold, and warmth that are experienced in the absence of a stimulus. Peripheral motor neuropathy is characterized by inflammation or degeneration of the peripheral motor nerves. Peripheral sensory neuropathy is characterized by inflammation or degeneration of the peripheral sensory nerves.
ADL, activities of daily living.

Cancer-directed therapy pain syndromes may result from chemotherapy, radiation therapy, or surgery. Chemotherapy-induced peripheral neuropathy (CIPN) is well described with a variety of agents.[214] Sensory symptoms tend to be greater than motor or autonomic, and the majority of signs and symptoms due to CIPN arise from damage to dorsal root ganglion neurons or their axons, leading to acral pain, sensory loss, and sometimes sensory ataxia. With platinum compounds, as many as 30% of patients experience worsening of neuropathy for a few months following completion of therapy, and a sizable cohort report persistent symptoms lasting years. Paclitaxel-associated CIPN usually improves in the months following treatment cessation but still has been associated with long-term persistence of some degree of neuropathy in up to 80% of patients, with roughly a third of these patients reporting severe symptoms.[215] Table 42.7 lists the National Cancer Institute Common Terminology Criteria for Adverse Events for neurotoxicity.

Chemotherapeutic toxicity may be attributable to steroids, which are coadministered in many chemotherapeutic protocols. In particular, avascular necrosis is a well-described complication of steroid use. Morbidity is related to progressive joint damage often leading to decreased range of motion, pain with movement, and arthritis. Weight-bearing joints are most commonly involved. The shoulder, elbow, wrist, hand, and vertebral bodies can also be involved. The total cumulative dose and daily dose of glucocorticoids, and likely the underlying condition, affect the risk of developing avascular necrosis.[216] Short-term, low-dose protocols are occasionally associated with necrosis.[217] It most commonly occurs in the femoral and humeral heads. Pain is usually the first symptom, but the clinical presentation is variable and depends on the site and size of the infarct. Persistent hip or shoulder pain, especially with joint movement, tenderness, or reduced range of motion, warrants magnetic resonance imaging (MRI) which can visualize aspects of the necrotic lesion (necrosis, reactive zone/granulation tissue, sclerotic changes, edema). Bone marrow signal abnormality, the double-line sign, and subchondral fracture are characteristic MRI findings of avascular necrosis.[218]

Combined medical and radiation therapies, both sequential and concurrent, are improving clinical outcomes for locoregional tumor control, with enhanced patient survival and delay of recurrence.[219] During the course of external radiation therapy, treatment generally influences normal tissue function in tissues that have more rapid self-renewing proliferative index (e.g., mucosal surfaces such as skin, head/neck, and esophagus) and other surface tissues that have more limited potential for self-renewal (e.g., hair, nails, and surface glands). Injuries to these tissues are often self-limited and heal without specific intervention secondary to stem cell renewal. Acute effects from radiation therapy do not uniformly predict for late effects from treatment. Late effects generally affect tissues that have limited potential for self-renewal, and injury is often more permanent, requiring surgical débridement and possibly resulting in functional damage.

Radiation-induced neural damage and pain may become apparent sometime after completion of radiation therapy confounding the diagnosis in some cases.[220–222] Postsurgical pain syndromes come in many varieties, including postmastectomy, postamputation, postthoracotomy, and other chronic pain states. Treatments for head and neck cancer have the potential to cause persistent pain and discomfort. Radical surgery, such as resection of portions of the tongue, palate, and mandible, and radical neck dissection (RND) cause major structural changes. Radiation therapy, which frequently is the primary therapy, may cause mucositis, xerostomia, loss of taste, and decreased QOL. Subsequent late fibrosis of skin and soft tissues may lead to temporomandibular joint dysfunction and MPSs. Eating difficulties and persistent pain are frequent issues in head and neck cancer survivors.[223,224]

Cancer patients and, in particular, cancer survivors may experience chronic non–tumor-related pain. The challenge for the treating clinician is to distinguish between tumor-associated and non–tumor-associated pain. Many of the same interdisciplinary treatment paradigms apply to cancer survivors as apply to all chronic pain patients, but an appreciation for the disabilities associated with treatments of cancer is essential. Long-term management of pain associated with cancer and its treatment poses a substantial challenge for the clinician. Pain complaints frequently change over time, involve multiple sites, stem from several origins including chronic disabilities, involve several causes simultaneously, and may relate loosely or not at all to the tumor.

Classification of Cancer Pain by Feature

Several schemata exist for classifying pain in the cancer patient and are potentially useful for diagnosis and management. One such scheme is presented in Table 42.8.

TABLE 42.8	Methods Used for Classifying Pain in the Cancer Patient
Chronicity	
Intensity/severity	
Pathophysiology/mechanism	
Individual type and stage of disease	
Pattern of pain	
Syndrome	

TABLE 42.9 Acute Pain Associated with Cancer Management

Procedure	Problem
Diagnostic procedures	Blood samples Lumbar puncture Biopsy
Chemotherapy	Mucositis GI distress including typhlitis, colitis, pancreatitis Cardiomyopathy Extravasation of drug into tissues
Radiation treatment	Skin burns Mucositis Pharyngitis Esophagitis Proctitis Itching
Interventional radiology procedures	Yttrium-90 radioembolization Chemoembolization Radiofrequency ablation
Surgical therapy	Postoperative pain

GI, gastrointestinal.

CHRONICITY

Acute pain is the normal, predicted physiologic response to a noxious stimulus and typically is associated with invasive procedures, trauma, and disease. Various anticancer therapies, particularly postoperative pain following surgical intervention and radiation therapy, can cause acute pain (Table 42.9). The course of acute pain is usually predictable and self-limiting, and the pain does not represent a difficult diagnostic problem. In contrast, assessment of patients with chronic pain tends to be much more difficult and complex. Chronic pain is best considered as persistent pain beyond the expected healing time. As healing times vary for different stimuli and trauma, conventional definitions of chronic pain based on arbitrary intervals between 3 months and 6 months are less useful. One exception to this is the development of postherpetic neuralgia (PHN) after the development of herpes zoster. Several cancers including oral, esophageal, stomach, colorectal, lung, breast, ovarian, prostate, kidney, bladder, and CNS cancers as well as lymphoma, myeloma, and leukemia were associated with an increased risk of zoster, particularly within the first 2 years after diagnosis and among younger individuals.[225] Some have proposed that only clinically relevant pain be defined as PHN to avoid overestimation of the problem and as pain ≥3 on a 10-point scale persisting 120 days after rash healing.[226-229]

INTENSITY/SEVERITY

Health care providers underestimate the severity of a patient's pain, particularly when relying on their own observations.[230-232] This tendency is problematic because pain is often undertreated when patients and physicians differ in their judgment of the pain's severity.[233] Patient self-report is always the primary source of information for the measurement of symptoms, and subjective reporting of pain is considered a key component of pain assessment.[234] Observer ratings of symptom severity correlate poorly with patient ratings and are generally inadequate substitutes for patient reporting. The discrepancies were most pronounced in those patients reporting severe pain.[233] Although clinicians can monitor some objective signs to clarify the manifestations and impact of certain symptoms, these signs only complement subjective assessment and self-reporting. An assessment of pain intensity should include an evaluation of not only the present or average pain intensity but also pain at its least and worst over a defined time period.

The three most commonly used instruments for assessing cancer pain intensity are the following:[235]

- Visual Analogue Scale (VAS): A slash mark corresponding to intensity of pain is placed on a 100 mm line ranging at one end from "No Pain," to the other end, "Pain as bad as it could possibly be."
- Numeric Rating Scale (NRS): A number is assigned to the intensity of pain on a scale of 0 to 10; 0 reflecting "No Pain" and 10 reflecting the "Worst Pain Possible."
- Verbal Rating Scale (VRS): The patient chooses one of the following words that best describes pain: "No Pain," "Mild Pain," "Moderate Pain," "Severe Pain," "Worst Possible Pain."

All three measures correlate highly with one another. For pain assessment in clinical settings, the VAS, VRS, and NRS approach equivalency[236] so that clarity, ease of administration, and simplicity of scoring become justifiable criteria in response scale selection. On the basis of relatively few studies in cancer, results or recommendations did not differ conclusively from those in other populations.[235] In clinical scenarios, the NRS or VRS has proven more popular than the VAS and scales has high correlations, especially with less educated patients.[237,238] Numerical scales as measures of QOL end points work well as cancer clinical trial instruments because they are easier to understand and easier to score.[239]

Several studies have shown that differences between categorical pain severity items are not linear.[240,241] For instance, when pain severity is rated at the midpoint or higher on numeric rating scales, patients report disproportionately more interference with daily function.[122] Many patients, both with and without cancer, function quite effectively with a background level of mild pain that does not seriously impair or distract them. As pain severity increases to moderate intensity, pain passes a threshold beyond which it is hard for the patient to ignore the pain. At this point, it disrupts many aspects of the patient's life. When pain is severe, it becomes a primary focus of attention and prohibits most activities. Pain severity and the degree to which the patient's function is impaired are highly associated. As a way of delineating different levels of cancer pain severity, Serlin et al.[122] explored the relationship between numerical ratings of pain *severity and ratings of pain's interference with such functions as activity, mood, and sleep*. Based on the degree of interference with function, ratings of 1 to 4 correspond to mild pain, 5 to 6 to moderate pain, and 7 to 10 to severe pain. In a follow-up study in categorizing the severity of cancer pain, Paul et al.[123] confirmed a nonlinear relationship between cancer pain severity and interference with function and that the boundary between a mild and a moderate level of cancer pain was at 4. However, they failed to confirm the boundary between moderate and severe cancer pain and reported that a rating of 7 was in the moderate category and ratings >7 being in the severe category.

PATHOPHYSIOLOGY/MECHANISMS

A general classification by pathophysiology distinguishes nociceptive (somatic and visceral) from neuropathic pain (see "Pain and the Cancer Patient" section). This distinction is fundamental in assessment because it may determine and guide therapy. In principle, pain results from stimulation of nociceptors or by lesions of afferent nerve fibers. Pain is nociceptive when the sustaining mechanisms are related to ongoing tissue pathology. Pain is neuropathic when there is evidence that the pain stems from injury to neural tissues and aberrant somatosensory processing in the periphery or in the CNS. Physical influences such as pressure, traction, compression, and tumor infiltration as well as metabolic or chemical disturbances produce pain. Obviously, classification by physiologic mechanism would be an improvement, but sufficient information to do this is not available.

Tumor Involvement of Encapsulated Organs

Primary or secondary tumors of the liver are the most frequent examples of tumors of encapsulated organs. These can enlarge the organ to several times the normal size. Because the organ capsule of connective tissue grows less rapidly than the tumor, the intracapsular pressure rises as capsular distention develops. In addition, tumor infiltrates the capsule locally, producing dull, and rarely also stabbing, pains. The massive growth of the organ not only stimulates intracapsular nociceptors, but it also irritates larger nerves by pressure or traction on the tissue suspending the organ. Similar organ-enlarging processes in the spleen and kidneys do not lead to pain to the same extent as in the liver, perhaps because of the more stable suspension or embedding of these organs, which are farther away from the midline with its abundant nerve pathways. The initial presentation of renal tumors can include pain, weight loss, and hematuria but typically occurs in only 9% of patients and is often indicative of advanced disease with approximately 30% of patients with renal carcinoma present with metastatic disease, 25% with locally advanced renal carcinoma, and 45% with localized disease.[242] The detection of kidney pain relies on input from sympathetic, parasympathetic, and sensory nerves. The sympathetic nerves supplying the kidneys originate in spinal cord segments T10–L1 and travel via white rami to the paravertebral ganglia. The sympathetic nerves travel via the lesser splanchnic nerves from the T10–T11 thoracic paravertebral ganglia to the synapse at the ipsilateral aorticorenal and celiac ganglia. From the 12th thoracic paravertebral ganglion, nerves travel via the least splanchnic nerve to the synapse either in the aorticorenal ganglion or in the renal plexus. The first lumbar splanchnic nerve and the postganglionic sympathetic nerves from the aorticorenal and celiac plexus synapse in the renal plexus. The parasympathetic innervation originates from the vagus nerve. These parasympathetic nerves traverse through the celiac plexus or pass directly to the renal plexus. Sensory renal nerves travel via the renal plexus, splanchnic nerves, thoracic sympathetic ganglia, T10–T12 spinal nerves, and spinal cord dorsal horn neurons. Patients may complain of abdominal, back, and flank pain in addition to the sensation of flank heaviness.

Pain-sensitive structures in the head include extracranial structures such as the skin, muscles, and blood vessels in the head and neck; mucosa of the sinuses and dental structures; and intracranial structures including the regions of the large arteries near the circle of Willis, the great intracranial venous sinuses, parts of the dura and dural arteries, and cranial nerves (particularly glossopharyngeal, vagus, and trigeminal). The cranium (except the periosteum), brain parenchyma, ependymal lining of the ventricles, and choroid plexus are all pain insensitive. The brain is also an encapsulated organ. Its special feature is that the bony skull capsule prevents any enlargement. Pain arises here, not by destruction of parenchyma, but by the increase of intracranial pressure with stimulation of the meningeal nociceptors. Such an increase of intracranial pressure occurs in space-occupying tumor growth or in focal or generalized brain edema. Focally, edema can develop around isolated tumors. Generalized edema develops in diffuse metastatic invasion of the meninges due to disturbance of the circulation of CSF. Such a tumor invasion of the leptomeninges is frequent in malignant lymphomas. However, metastatic invasion of the leptomeninges occurs in patients with solid tumors (e.g., bronchial carcinoma and malignant melanoma), with the predominant symptom being headache. In such cases, tumor infiltration of cranial nerves may also occur.

Tumor Infiltration of Peripheral Nerves

Because peripheral nerves can usually evade pressure from a tumor on one side, infiltration by tumor tissue is the quintessential tissue trauma stimulus. In addition, indirect damage of

unknown pathogenesis might also occur to peripheral nerves in the context of tumor conditions such as occur with paraneoplastic syndromes. Paraneoplastic syndromes may affect diverse organ systems, most notably the endocrine, neurologic, dermatologic, rheumatologic, and hematologic systems. The best described paraneoplastic syndromes are attributed to tumor secretion of functional peptides and hormones (endocrine paraneoplastic syndromes) or immune cross-reactivity between tumor and normal host tissues (neurologic paraneoplastic syndromes) and may affect up to 8% of cancer patients.[243] In paraneoplastic neurologic syndromes, tumor-directed onconeural antibodies are produced and may result in permanent damage to neural tissue.

Tumor tissue often infiltrates the perineural cleft; however, this does not regularly cause pain. A massive and then painful entrapment of the nerve plexus or individual nerves sometimes occurs, especially in extensive breast carcinomas and their recurrences or in chest wall metastases of bronchial carcinomas. The perineural cleft widens tumor infiltration, and infiltration of the tumor into the nerve itself is common. Degenerative changes of the axis cylinders are sometimes visible with conventional screening methods. Primary tumors of the peripheral nerves themselves lead to painful destruction. Tumor compression regularly elicits pain when the affected nerve cannot give way (e.g., a spinal nerve).

Tumor Infiltration of Soft Tissues

Tumor infiltration of soft tissues causes pain via the mechanisms described in the earlier discussion, as with massive infiltrations of the retroperitoneum. Infiltration and destruction of mobile structures (e.g., of the skeletal musculature) can lead to pain via disturbance of function. Here, the tumor spreads in the interstitium and destroys blood vessels, lymphatics, and nerves.

Tumor Infiltration of Bone

The most frequent cause of pain in tumor patients is infiltration of bone. This applies to primary and secondary neoplasias originating from the bone marrow as well as to neoplasias of the bone itself. Such tumors always cause pain when they lead to an elevation of the intraosseous pressure, to loss of stability, or to a lesion of the periosteum resulting in periosteal elevation, or with the release of chemical mediators of nociception. The neural structures that generate nociception reside in the bone marrow, in the bone, and in the periosteum.

In metastatic processes, the degree of bone destruction is often extensive. Vertebral spread of tumor may involve intervertebral foramina, where it can compress nerve roots. Further spread posteriorly leads to encroachment of the spinal cord and the spinal nerves. In the bone, metastases localized to the bone marrow result in osteolysis or osteosclerosis. Necroses and hemorrhages occur frequently in bone metastases and doubtless play a role in the etiology of pain. The hemorrhages probably result from microfractures. Metastatic bone disease is discussed in detail later.

Tumor Infiltration of Abdominal Hollow Organs

Tumor involvement in abdominal hollow organs causes pain. This applies to all primary and secondary intestinal tumors. However, their pain-eliciting potency differs widely from individual to individual. The pain results from ulcerations, motility disorders, dilatations, and disorders of blood flow. In accordance with the extent of the lymphatic tissue, large tumors with extensive ulceration and hemorrhage occur in malignant lymphomas of the gastrointestinal tract. Perineural tumor infiltration, arteritis, or perineural inflammatory reactions are common in tumors of the abdominal and urogenital hollow organs. Tumor infiltration of the urinary bladder can vary from a sense of uneasiness felt in the suprapubic region or a severe, constant agonizing deep pelvic pain. The pain may also radiate and extend into the thighs. Intolerable cystitis may occur with tumor infiltration of the bladder wall.

Tumor Infiltration and Inflammation of Serous Mucosa

The parietal pleura lines the inner chest wall, whereas the visceral pleura covers the lung surface including interlobar fissures. The peripheral part of the diaphragm and costal portion of the parietal pleura are innervated by somatic intercostal nerves with the central portion of the diaphragm innervated by the phrenic nerve. The visceral pleura are extensively innervated by pulmonary branches of the vagus nerve and the sympathetic trunk. Pleural carcinomatosis with infiltration of both parietal and visceral surfaces can be extremely painful and difficult to manage.[244] Somatic nerves innervate the parietal peritoneum. These nerves also supply the muscles and skin of the overlying body wall. Afferent nerves that travel with the autonomic supply of the underlying viscera innervate the visceral peritoneum. Nociceptive information from diseases that affect the parietal or visceral peritoneum reflects these different patterns of innervation. Animals with peritoneal carcinomatosis exhibit hypersensitivity to mechanical stimulation and visceral pain-like behavior.[245]

TUMOR TYPE AND STAGE OF DISEASE

Factors influencing the pain complaint include the primary tumor type, stage of disease, and tumor site. When metastatic disease appears, about one in three patients report significant pain. Vainio and Auvinen[246] reported that moderate to severe pain was present in 51% of patients with advanced cancer with severe pain more commonly seen in patients with prostate, esophageal, gynecologic, colorectal, head/neck, breast, and lung cancers. At least half of lung and breast cancer patients had at least moderate intensity pain. Although pain tends to reflect the presence of metastases, this may not always be the case for certain tumor types, particularly for patients with breast or prostate cancers. Although many patients with bone metastases report bone pain, a significant fraction (21% of breast and 22% of prostate patients) was asymptomatic.[208] Levren et al.[247] examined the relationship between pain and bone metastases in patients with prostate or breast cancer referred for bone scintigraphy. In patients with prostate cancer, metastases were found in 47% of the patients with pain but only in 12% of the patients without pain ($P = .01$). In patients with breast cancer, metastases were more common in patients without pain (71%) than in patients with pain (34%; $P = .02$).

Pain caused by tumor may occur at the onset of disease or at an advanced stage. Although rarely one of the early indicators of the onset of disease, pain is not a significant problem for the majority of patients in the early stages of disease, with 5% to 10% of patients with solid tumors reporting pain at a level that interferes with mood and activity. However, pain is obviously a major concern that often prompts the patient to seek medical consultation. Vuorinen[248] found that 28% of newly diagnosed unselected cancer patients reported pain. Cleeland[249] reported that the majority of patients with end-stage disease have pain of a severity that interferes with several aspects of the patient's QOL. Daut and Cleeland[118] found that pain was an early symptom of cancer in 40% to 50% of patients with cancer of the breast, ovary, prostate, colon, and rectum, and in about 20% of patients with cancer of the uterus and cervix.

Knowing the natural history of the disease facilitates an understanding of the pain process and is important in determining the nature and timing of treatment. Examples of the more common disease processes follow.

Pancreatic Cancer

Most pancreatic tumors are exocrine tumors, including ductal adenocarcinoma, acinar cell carcinoma, cystadenocarcinoma, adenosquamous carcinoma, signet ring cell carcinoma, hepatoid carcinoma, colloid carcinoma, undifferentiated carcinoma, pancreatoblastoma, and pancreatic mucinous cystic neoplasm. The most common form is ductal adenocarcinoma characterized by moderately to poorly differentiated glandular structures, comprising 80% to 90% of all pancreatic tumors. Endocrine pancreatic tumors are rare and account for only 1% to 2% of all pancreatic tumors. Pancreatic ductal adenocarcinoma is the fourth leading cause of cancer-related death in the United States.[3] Surgical resection is the only potentially curative treatment, but because of the late presentation, only 15% to 20% of patients are candidates for surgical intervention. Even after complete resection, prognosis is poor with only 6% of patients (ranges from 2% to 9%) surviving 5 years after diagnosis.[250,251] The highest incidence and mortality rates of pancreatic cancer are found in developed countries. Resectable cancers typically have no vascular or regional spread. Borderline cancers have regional spread into vessels (i.e., portal vein) or other organs (i.e., stomach), which would make surgery difficult, and locally invasive cancers have invasion into structures (e.g., celiac artery), which make curative surgery impossible. Up to 90% of patients with pancreatic cancer experience significant abdominal pain during the course of their illness.[250]

Incidence rates for pancreatic cancer in 2012 were highest in Northern America (7.4 per 100,000) and Western Europe (7.3 per 100,000), followed by other regions in Europe and Australia/New Zealand (equally about 6.5 per 100,000).[251] In the United States, whites and blacks experienced opposite trends in pancreatic cancer death rates between 1975 and 2013 with white men death rates decreased by 0.7% per year from 1970 to 1995 and then increased by 0.4% per year through 2009. Among white women, rates increased slightly from 1970 to 1984, stabilized until the late 1990s, then increased by 0.5% per year through 2009. In contrast, the rates among blacks increased between 1970 and the late 1980s (women) or early 1990s (men) and then decreased thereafter.[252] Pancreatic cancer is difficult to diagnose. The appearance of symptoms usually indicates an advanced stage and the most frequent presentations are progressive weight loss, anorexia, abdominal pain, and jaundice. These symptoms are nonspecific and varied in different regions of pancreas. Tumor in the head of the pancreas (75%) produces weight loss, painless jaundice, nausea, and vomiting. If cancer is located at the body/tail of the pancreas, patients usually present with abdominal pain that radiates to the sides or through to the back. Local tumor extension almost invariably involves the peripancreatic fat tissue through direct invasion of lymphatic channels and perineural spaces. Duodenum, stomach, gallbladder, and peritoneum are infiltrated by tumors located in the pancreatic head; body and tail tumors can invade liver, spleen, and left adrenal gland. Lymphatic spread to adjacent and distant lymph nodes seems to precede hematogenous spread, which affects, in descending order, liver, peritoneum, lungs, adrenals, kidneys, bones, and brain. At diagnosis, 30% to 40% of patients report abdominal pain, 80% develop pain with disease progression, and 44% of these describe the pain as severe. The presence of pain in newly diagnosed patients with potentially operable pancreatic cancer is an ominous predictor of resectability and of survival.[253]

A number of factors contribute to the generation and maintenance of pancreatic cancer pain. One of the most striking neural alterations in pancreatic cancer is neural invasion, which occurs in up to 100% of patients.[254,255] Pancreatic cancer is characterized by invasion of nerves by cancer cells (neural invasion), pancreatic nerve damage, pancreatic neuroinflammation (neuritis), and noticeable hypertrophy with sprouting of intrapancreatic nerves.[256] Cancer cells that invade nerves express a large set of neurotrophic factors such as NGF, artemin, neurturin that are similarly released by mast cells or other inflammatory cells and can strongly sensitize nociceptive

TABLE 42.10 Pancreatic Cancer Pain Syndromes	
Pain due to Tumor Involvement	**Pain due to Cancer Therapies**
Visceral pain: Pancreatic gland infiltration Gastric infiltration Duodenal infiltration Liver metastases: capsule disten- tion, diaphragmatic irritation Biliary tree distention Bowel obstruction (duodenal, peri- toneal carcinomatosis) Ischemic abdominal pain due to mesenteric vessel involvement	Postoperative pain syndromes: Delayed gastric emptying Wound dehiscence or non-healing
Somatic pain: Retroperitoneal involvement (direct, nodal) Parietal peritoneum and abdominal wall involvement Abdominal distention due to ascites Bone metastases	Biliary prosthesis complications
Neuropathic pain: Radiculopathy from retroperito- neal spread or bone metastatic involvement Lumbosacral plexopathy Epidural spinal cord compression	Post-chemotherapy pain syndromes: Liver chemoembolization Mucositis Post-radiation pain syndromes: Radiation enteritis

From Caraceni A, Portenoy RK. Pain management in patients with pancreatic carcinoma. *Cancer* 1996;78(3):639–653. Copyright © 1996 American Cancer Society. Reprinted by permission of John Wiley & Sons, Inc.

nerve endings. Intrapancreatic nerves increase in size (neural hypertrophy) and number (increased neural density). The proportion of autonomic and sensory fibers (neural remodeling) is switched and is invaded by pancreatic cancer cells (neural invasion).[257] These neuropathic alterations also correlate with neuropathic pain.

Pain due to pancreatic cancer is usually abdominal, typically referred to the epigastric region or the upper abdominal quadrants, but it can also involve the lower quadrants or be diffuse.[258] Back pain is associated with abdominal pain in 50% to 65% of cases, but only 5% to 10% of patients report it as their only complaint. In one series, 67% of patients could not describe their pain location better than as over the "diffuse abdomen."[259] Eating often aggravates the pain. Tumors of the head of the pancreas may cause epigastric pain with right flank radiation more often, whereas pain from tumors in the tail has left-sided radiation. Lying flat typically exacerbates it and sitting relieves it. This pain probably comes from retroperitoneal tumor involvement, and it may not respond to celiac plexus block. It often merges with similar syndromes caused by nodal or other soft-tissue tumor involvement in the retroperitoneal region (Table 42.10). The impact of pancreatic pain can be profound. It is commonly associated with depressed mood and contributes to the rapid decline in function that characterizes this disease.[259,260] In addition, severe pain can influence survival.[261–263]

Ovarian Cancer

Ovarian cancer may be subdivided into different histologic subtypes, which include epithelial cancer serous, endometrioid, clear-cell, and mucinous carcinomas. Of these types, high-grade serous carcinoma is the most commonly diagnosed. Histologically and clinically, low-grade endometrioid carcinoma and low-grade serous carcinoma are different compared with their high-grade counterparts. Other more rare pathology includes small-cell carcinoma (predominantly occurs in younger women) and carcinosarcoma. Nonepithelial ovarian cancers include germ cell tumors and sex cord stromal tumors, which account

for approximately 10% of ovarian cancers. Estimated new cancer cases in the United States for 2017 were 22,440 with 14,080 deaths (fifth most common cause of death from cancer in women).[3] Overall survival varies greatly based on stage at initial diagnosis with a 92% survival for stage I and 25% for stage IV.[264] Epithelial ovarian cancer can spread by intraperitoneal, lymphogenous, and hematogenous mechanisms.

The lifetime risk of ovarian cancer in women by the age 70 years is approximately 40% for BRCA1 and 18% for BRCA2.[265] Most of these cancers are high-grade serous cancers. Other inherited disorders, such as Lynch syndrome, can increase the risk of ovarian cancer. Lynch syndrome is associated with colorectal, endometrial, and ovarian cancers but is also associated with cancers of the urinary tract, stomach, small intestine, and biliary tract. The symptoms of ovarian cancer are relatively nonspecific and often occur when the disease has spread throughout the abdominal cavity or with the presence of ascites. Abdominal discomfort or vague pain, abdominal fullness, bowel habit changes, early satiety, dyspepsia, and bloating are frequent presenting symptoms. Occasionally, patients may present with bowel obstruction due to intra-abdominal masses or shortness of breath due to pleural effusion. Early-stage disease is usually asymptomatic, and the diagnosis is often incidental, although such patients may occasionally present with dyspareunia or pelvic pain due to ovarian torsion. Serum CA-125 level has been widely used as a marker for a possible epithelial ovarian cancer in the primary assessment of a pelvic mass. Although CA-125 is the best known serum ovarian cancer biomarker, it is not the only one: Carcinoembryonic antigen (CEA) (mucinous), lactate dehydrogenase (LDH) (dysgerminoma, mixed germ cell tumors), β-human chorionic gonadotropin (β-hCG) (choriocarcinoma, mixed germ cell tumors), inhibin B (granulosa cell tumors), α-fetoprotein (yolk sac tumors, embryonal cell tumors), and HE4 are also available.[266]

The prevalence of pain associated with ovarian cancer resembles the prevalence rates in populations with other solid tumors.[267] Ovarian cancer spreads by intraperitoneal, lymphatic, and locally invasive pathways. Lymphatic pathways may extend from the abdominal retroperitoneum to the groin via the inguinal/femoral canals or across the diaphragm to the pleural space. Intraperitoneal spread of tumor begins with extension of tumor through the ovarian capsule, allowing implantation of tumor throughout the abdomen. Intraperitoneal metastases show a predilection for the omentum and diaphragm, but no organ is spared, and concomitant ascites is frequent. Portenoy et al.[267] noted that pain, fatigue, and psychological distress were the most prevalent symptoms in patients with advanced (stage III or IV) ovarian cancer. Patients generally describe pain as occurring in the abdominopelvic or lower back region, as being frequent or almost constant and moderate to severe in intensity. Patients with advanced disease may experience pain in the lower extremities either from invasion of the lumbosacral plexus by tumor or by lymphedema secondary to iliac vessel occlusion.

Cervical Cancer

Cervical cancer is the fourth most common malignancy diagnosed in women worldwide. Nearly all cases result from infection with the human papillomavirus (HPV), and prevention includes screening and vaccination. Rates have declined in the United States with an estimated 12,820 new cases in 2017 and 4,210 deaths.[3] Disparities in incidence and mortality still occur, with black and Hispanic women continuing to have higher rates of cervical cancer than white women.[268] There are several histologic subtypes of cervical carcinoma, but the majority of cases tend to be HPV-associated malignancies including adenocarcinoma, squamous cell carcinoma, or adenosquamous carcinoma. Neuroendocrine (small-cell or large-cell) carcinomas are not associated with HPV exposure and clear cell carcinoma and are rare. Computed tomography (CT) or MRI is often used to define lymph node status and to assess extent of local disease. Combined positron emission tomography (PET) and CT imaging may be useful for detecting smaller nodal disease.[269] Cervical cancer usually spreads to regional lymph nodes, and parametrial invasion is common. The common sites of distant spread include the aortic (para-aortic, periaortic), lateral aortic and mediastinal nodes, lungs, and skeleton. Recurrent cervical cancer is almost always incurable.

Prostate Cancer

Prostate cancer is one of the most prevalent cancers in men worldwide. Estimated new cancer cases in the United States for 2017 were 161,360 with 26,730 deaths.[3] The majority of prostate cancer survivors (64%) tend to be older (aged 70 years or older) with less than 1% under the age of 50 years.[8] Prostate cancer varies widely in its intrinsic development, ranging from indolent to aggressive. Once clinically significant disease is established, surgery, radiation, and androgen deprivation therapy (ADT), which all carry substantial morbidities, are considered standard treatment options for localized disease. It is often insidious and asymptomatic even when advanced and for detection, MRI is currently the best imaging modality.[270] Prostate cancer is a heterogeneous group of malignant tumors and 95% are adenocarcinoma originating from the glands and ducts in the prostate. Most adenocarcinomas are of the acinar type, typically referred to as prostate carcinomas. More than 1% consist of other variants that often have a poor prognosis such as ductal carcinoma, mucinous carcinoma, signet ring cell carcinoma, and small cell carcinoma. Five percent of prostate cancer cases are of other types originating from transitional epithelial cells in the urethra or pars prostatic urethra (urothelial carcinoma), support tissue (sarcomas), or lymphoid tissue (lymphomas). Prostate adenocarcinoma may spread locally, by direct invasion of seminal vesicles, urinary bladder, or surrounding tissues or distantly. Distant metastases can derive from an initial lymphatic spread or from a direct hematogenous spreading, mainly to the bones. The Gleason system is the most widely used grading system for prostate cancer (adenocarcinoma only). Prostate cancers are stratified into five grades (1 to 5) on the basis of the glandular pattern and degree of differentiation. The Gleason score is derived from the sum of the most represented grade (primary grade) with the second most represented grade (secondary grade) (e.g., 3 + 4 = 7); this correlates better with prognosis than the single Gleason grade. The Gleason system can be applied to biopsy and surgical specimens, but not to fine needle biopsy (FNB), which lack architectural data. Most prostate cancers in the United States are diagnosed by prostate-specific antigen (PSA) testing, although many expert groups, including the American Cancer Society, have concluded that data on the efficacy of PSA screening are insufficient to recommend routine use of this test and recommend that for the average risk asymptomatic male over 50 years, a PSA with or without a digital rectal examination after receiving information about the benefits, risks, and uncertainties associated with prostate cancer screening is appropriate.[271] Digital rectal examination is recommended along with PSA for men with hypogonadism because of reduced sensitivity of PSA. Men at higher risk, including African American men and men with a family member (father or brother) diagnosed with prostate cancer before age 65 years, should receive this information beginning at age 45 years.

The clinical behavior of prostate cancer ranges from indolent, localized disease to aggressive, disseminated disease associated with significant morbidity and mortality. Although the majority of prostate cancer cases present while the disease is localized to the prostate, some patients have evidence of metastatic disease at diagnosis. Typically, metastases are found in the axial skeleton, pelvic lymph nodes, and the lungs. Because of the predilection of prostate cancer to spread to bony sites, a significant proportion of patients with metastatic disease will have bone pain. Metastases from prostate cancer, most of which are adenocarcinomas, nearly always form osteoblastic lesions in bone; in contrast, bone metastases from kidney, lung, or breast cancers more often are osteolytic. However, metastases from the relatively uncommon neuroendocrine tumors of the prostate also produce osteolytic lesions. Approximately 90% of patients who die from prostate cancer have evidence of bone metastases.[272] Radiographically, bone metastases are detected on technetium-99m (99mTc) bone scintigraphy scans. Newer modalities for detection include [18]sodium fluoride PET and [18]fluorodeoxyglucose PET (FDG-PET). Five-year relative survival varies with stage at diagnosis from 80% or more when malignancy is confined to the prostate to about 25% where bone metastases are present. Radium-223 (^{223}Ra) is an α emitter with a half-life of 11.4 days. It is a calcium mimetic and forms complexes with bone mineral hydroxyapatite in areas of active bone remodeling. The α particles cause double-strand DNA break of cells. With a range of penetration of <0.1 mm, ^{223}Ra is able to achieve localized killing of cancer cells with less collateral damage to the nearby bone marrow[273] and is the first radiopharmaceutical agent demonstrated to improve survival among patients with symptomatic bone-metastatic castrate-resistant prostate cancer with no known visceral disease.

Prostate cancer rarely spreads to vital organs, and the disease tends to progress slowly. Exceptions are spinal cord compression or ureteral obstruction secondary to retroperitoneal lymph node metastases. Tumors of the prostate gland may produce local rectal, urethral, suprapubic, and penile pain as a result of expansion and inflammation of the prostate, pain referred to the back, lower extremities, and abdominal area resulting from tumor growth within the pelvis, and distant bone pain with associated neurologic dysfunction associated with long bone, vertebral, and skull metastases (Table 42.11). The regional lymph nodes of the prostate are the nodes of the true pelvis, which are the pelvic nodes below the bifurcation of the common iliac arteries. Distant lymph nodes are outside the confines of the true pelvis. They are the aortic (para-aortic, periaortic, lumbar), common iliac, inguinal, superficial inguinal (femoral), supraclavicular, cervical, scalene, and retroperitoneal nodes.

Clinical syndromes may be identified by the site of bony involvement, the coexistence of mechanical instability secondary to fractures, and the neurologic dysfunction caused by tumor infiltration of contiguous neurologic structures. Bone metastases to the hip and pelvis often produce local pain that is exacerbated by movement, especially during weight bearing. Local invasion of tumor from the pelvis into the sacrum may produce the syndrome of perineal pain. Patients with this syndrome complain of local and perirectal pain that is accentuated by pressure on the perineal region, such as that caused by sitting

TABLE 42.11	Causes of Pain in Prostate Cancer
Causes of Pain	**Examples/Clinical Syndromes**
Bone metastasis	Single metastasis of pelvis or long bone
	Vertebral body metastasis, spinal cord compression
	Base-of-skull metastasis, cranial nerve palsies
	Perineal pain syndromes
Soft tissue metastasis	Lumbosacral plexopathy
	Pelvic tension "myalgia"
Pelvic visceral pain	"Prostatitis" pain

From Payne R. Pain management in the patient with prostate cancer. *Cancer* 1993; 71(suppl 3):1131–1137. Copyright © 1993 American Cancer Society. Reprinted by permission of John Wiley & Sons, Inc.

or lying prone. In its most extreme form, the patient cannot sit or lie flat. Dysfunction of the parasympathetic sacral innervation to bladder and bowel impairs continence early in the course of this syndrome. Local spread of tumor from the prostate into other pelvic and abdominal structures often produces visceral and neuropathic pain. Tumor invasion of the lumbosacral plexus may occur.

Breast Cancer

Breast cancer is the most commonly diagnosed cancer and the second leading cause of cancer-related mortality among North American women. Estimated new cancer cases for women in the United States for 2017 were 252,170 with 40,610 deaths.[3] Seventy-five percent of breast cancer survivors (more than 2.6 million women) are 60 years or older, whereas 7% are younger than 50 years.[8] Breast cancer tends to be diagnosed at a younger age than other common cancers, with a median age at diagnosis of 61 years with 19% of breast cancers are diagnosed in women ages 30 to 49 years, and 44% occur among women who are age 65 years or older. Lymphedema of the upper extremity occurs in 20% of women who undergo axillary lymph node dissection and in about 6% of women after sentinel lymph node biopsy.[274] Gene expression profiling of human tumors has provided a new paradigm for classifying breast carcinomas, predicting response to treatment, and risk of recurrence. Women diagnosed with breast cancer undergo receptor testing for estrogen (ER), human epidermal growth factor 2 (HER2) receptor tests, and progesterone (PR) status. Approximately 75% of breast cancers are hormone receptor positive and 15% to 25% are HER2 positive.[275] Approximately 15% to 20% of all breast cancers do not have hormone or HER2 receptors (triple negative) and are typically more aggressive and difficult to treat. Breast MRI has become a widely used second-line imaging modality with well-defined roles in assessing multifocal tumor and planning surgery and in monitoring local tumor response to neoadjuvant chemotherapy. MRI screening is used in high-risk young women such as those with a BRCA gene mutation or with previous mantle irradiation for lymphoma. PET scanning can be used to evaluate primary lesions, regionally metastatic and systemic metastases of breast cancer.

All breast cancers are adenocarcinomas arising from the terminal duct lobular units. Breast cancers are divided into two main categories, noninvasive and invasive. Infiltrating ductal carcinoma is the most common breast cancer histology, accounting for approximately 80% of all breast cancers. Lobular carcinoma constitutes 10% of the breast cancers. Ductal carcinoma in situ (DCIS) is the most common type of noninvasive breast cancer, accounting for about 15% of all newly diagnosed breast cancer cases. DCIS is classified into five histologic subtypes associated with varying prognostic implications. These include solid, papillary, cribriform, micropapillary, and comedo. Most lesions represent a combination of at least two of these subtypes. Comedocarcinoma is considered high grade and predictive of recurrence. Lobular carcinoma in situ (LCIS) is characterized as a benign-appearing proliferation of terminal ducts and ductules that is often multifocal and bilateral. LCIS is much less common and is associated with less risk of the development of invasive cancer than DCIS. Invasive ductal carcinoma (IDC) is the most common type of breast cancer. About 80% of invasive breast cancers are classified as IDC. Tubular carcinoma is a highly differentiated invasive carcinoma with limited metastatic potential and better than average prognosis. Medullary carcinoma is a relatively uncommon type of invasive carcinoma, accounting for less than 5% to 7% of all invasive breast cancers. Mucinous carcinoma is an invasive form of breast cancer characterized by large amounts of extracellular mucin production and is associated with a relatively favorable prognosis. Invasive cribriform carcinoma is a well-differentiated cancer that shares some features with tubular carcinoma and is also associated with better than average prognosis. Adenoid cystic carcinomas similarly rarely spread to the lymph nodes or distant areas and have a very good prognosis.

Breast cancer can metastasize to any organ in the body: Bone, lung, liver, and brain are frequent sites. Metastases usually appear within a few years but recurrence may occur, particularly in bone, many years later.

Approximately, 5% of women present with metastatic disease during breast cancer diagnosis,[276] and bone is the most frequent site of metastatic lesions.[206] In population-based cohort studies of patients with newly diagnosed breast cancer, 1% to 2% have bone metastases at diagnosis and another 5% to 6% are diagnosed to have bone metastases within the next 5 years.[277,278] In a Danish study of women with metastatic bone disease secondary to breast cancer, 1-year survival was just over 52%. Approximately, 13% survived 5 years after diagnosis of bone metastases, and shorter bone metastases free interval was independently associated with decreased survival among patients with breast cancer who were diagnosed with bone metastases ≥1 year following their breast cancer diagnosis. Survival among patients with metastatic breast cancer may vary according to the site of metastasis and receptor status. Risk of death within 1 year was highest for brain-only (62 %) and liver-only (43 %) involvement and nearly the same for patients with lung-only (32 %), bone-only (32 %) involvement, and other/combination of sites (34 %). Positive hormonal receptor status on the primary tumor was a favorable prognostic factor for all metastatic sites.[279]

Bone metastases are predominantly osteolytic (50%) or mixed osteolytic and osteoblastic (40%), with only a small proportion (about 10%) being osteoblastic alone.[280] Although metastatic disease may be asymptomatic, the most common site of metastases, bone, typically are painful. Between 40% and 60% of patients with metastatic breast cancer will have bony disease, and in many of these patients, the involved bones (vertebrae, femoral and humoral shafts, the acetabular area) are those that are involved with motion. Metastatic breast cancer is currently an incurable yet treatable disease. Although median survival is of the order of 18 to 24 months, survival ranges from a few weeks to several years.[281] This biologic variability means that for many women, metastatic breast cancer can be viewed as a chronic relapsing and remitting disease that may respond for a time to an array of cytotoxic and endocrine therapies.

The clinician will most likely have a long relationship with the patient with metastatic breast cancer and will have the opportunity to follow the course and progression of disease. The course of disease in patients with metastatic breast cancer fits one of two patterns: an indolent course or disease not immediately life threatening and that which is rapidly progressing or with extensive vital organ disease. Knowledge of the natural history of the disease is important in determining the nature and timing of treatment. Table 42.12 lists some of the common causes of pain in patients with breast cancer.

Lung Cancer

The two major forms of lung cancer are non–small-cell lung cancer (NSCLC) (85% of all lung cancers) and SCLC (15%). NSCLC can be divided into three major histologic subtypes: squamous cell carcinoma, adenocarcinoma, and large-cell lung cancer. Smoking causes all types of lung cancer but is most strongly linked with SCLC and squamous-cell carcinoma; adenocarcinoma is the most common type in patients who have never smoked. NSCLC is the leading cause of cancer death in the United States. Nearly 60% of NSCLC cases are metastatic at diagnosis, and the 5-year relative survival rate for metastatic disease is 4.2%.[282] SCLC is a very aggressive malignancy

TABLE 42.12 Causes of Pain in Patients with Breast Cancer

Etiology	Example	Example
Tumor related	Bone metastases	—
	Neural metastases	Brachial plexopathy
		Spinal cord compression
		Meningeal carcinomatosis
		Peripheral neuropathy secondary to tumor infiltration
	Visceral metastases	Pleural
		Liver
		Bowel
		Peritoneum
Anticancer therapy	Procedure-related pain in breast	—
	Postmastectomy syndrome	
	Lymphedema related	
	Postradiation treatment	
	Peripheral neuropathy	
	Phlebitis	
	Mucositis	
	Chemical cystitis (e.g., secondary to cyclophosphamide)	
	Osteoporosis or avascular necrosis	
Preexisting conditions	Chronic nonmalignant pain	—

characterized by high cellular proliferation and early metastatic spread. Most patients with SCLC receive chemotherapy. Unfortunately, SCLC initially exhibits a good response to chemotherapy and radiation therapy, but inevitably, relapses decrease patients' chance of survival. Metastases initially occur in the lymph nodes and thereafter in other organs such as the lung itself, liver, adrenal glands, brain, bone, and bone marrow. Histologically, SCLCs include small cell anaplastic carcinoma, which includes the oat cell type. Small cell anaplastic carcinoma is an aggressive and rapidly growing neoplasm and is limited to the thorax at presentation in only 25% of patients.

NSCLCs are a morphologically diverse group that includes squamous cell carcinoma, adenocarcinoma, and large cell anaplastic carcinoma. For stage I and II NSCLC, the majority of patients (69%) undergo surgery, and about 25% of surgical cases also receiving chemotherapy and/or radiation therapy. Most patients with stage III and IV NSCLC receive chemotherapy with or without radiation (53%). Squamous cell carcinoma is less likely to metastasize early. Adenocarcinoma metastasizes widely and frequently to the other lung, liver, bone, kidney, and the CNS. Large cell anaplastic carcinoma metastasizes in a pattern quite similar to adenocarcinoma with a predilection for mediastinal lymph nodes, pleura, adrenals, CNS, and bone. Lung cancers, particularly SCLC, often entail clinical paraneoplastic syndromes. Malignancy-associated hyponatremia is commonly associated with excessive production of arginine vasopressin (AVP) by tumor cells, and a large fraction of new cases of syndrome of inappropriate antidiuretic hormone secretion (SIADH) in elderly smokers are due to SCLC. Approximately, 10% of all lung cancer patients have hypercalcemia, and of these patients, 10% to 15% do not have evident bone metastases. Humoral hypercalcemia of malignancy is more common in NSCLC especially squamous cell carcinoma. The neurologic syndromes associated with lung cancer are rare disorders such as subacute cerebellar degeneration, optic neuritis and retinopathy, subacute necrotizing myelopathy, and peripheral

neuropathy. The 1-year relative survival for lung cancer increased from 34% during 1975 through 1977 to 45% during 2008 through 2011, largely because of improvements in surgical techniques and chemoradiation. The majority of lung cancers (57%) are diagnosed at a distant stage because early disease is typically asymptomatic; only 16% of cases are diagnosed at a local stage. The 5-year survival rate is 55% for cases detected when the disease is still localized, 27% for regional disease, and 4% for distant stage disease. The 5-year survival for SCLC (7%) is lower than NSCLC (21%).[8]

Pleural involvement by tumor can be a source of intractable severe pain. Diagnosis of pleural disease can be challenging and involve a variety of imaging modalities including CT, PET, MRI, and ultrasound. CT is widely used as the primary imaging modality with the most common CT findings being pleural thickening with or without pleural effusion, involvement of the interlobar fissures and/or mediastinal pleural involvement, volume reduction of the chest, mediastinal shift, and mediastinal lymph node invasion.

Pain is a major symptom in patients with all types of advanced lung cancer. Chest pain is the most common site of pain in patients with small cell cancer. The pain complaint is often poorly localized, dull in character, may radiate to the neck or back, and exacerbates with coughing. Mercadante et al.[283] reported that patients with advanced lung cancer commonly reported chest wall (including ribs and shoulder blade) pain, followed by lower extremities and lumbar regions, then abdomen and upper extremities, and the head area.

Renal Cell Cancers

Renal cell carcinoma (RCC) encompasses a heterogeneous group of cancers derived from renal tubular epithelial cells with the major subtypes being clear cell RCC (ccRCC), papillary RCC (pRCC), and chromophobe RCC (chRCC). The remaining subtypes are very rare (each with ≤1% total incidence), and in cases in which a tumor does not fit any subtype in the diagnostic criteria, it is designated as unclassified RCC. ccRCC is the most common subtype (75%) and accounts for the majority of deaths from kidney cancer. The majority of diagnoses result from incidental findings. Paraneoplastic syndromes—symptoms caused by hormones or cytokines excreted by tumor cells or by an immune response against the tumor—are not uncommon in RCC and symptoms include hypercalcemia, fever, and erythrocytosis. CT imaging with contrast enhancement of the chest, abdominal cavity, and pelvis is required for optimal staging.

Approximately 30% of people with RCC have already developed metastatic RCC at presentation,[284] and another 20% of people with clinically localized RCC eventually develop metastases during the course of the disease despite treatment.[285,286] Frequent sites include the lung (50% to 60%), bone (30% to 40%), liver (30% to 40%), and brain (5%). Unusual sites of metastases characterize renal cancer, however, and may involve virtually any organ site, including the thyroid, pancreas, skeletal muscle, and skin or underlying soft tissue. Regional and distant lymph nodes may be involved. The regional lymph nodes of the kidney are renal hilar, paracaval, aortic (para-aortic, periaortic, lateral aortic), and retroperitoneal. Metastatic bone disease is often highly osteolytic and particularly destructive causing substantial morbidity, including pain, pathologic fracture, spinal cord compression, and hypercalcemia. The presence of bone metastasis in RCC is associated with a poor prognosis.[287]

Colorectal Cancer

CRC is one of the most common malignancies in the Western world and is the third most commonly diagnosed cancer among men and women in the United States.[288] Incidence and mortality rates have been declining for several decades because of historical changes in risk factors (e.g., decreased smoking/red meat consumption, increased use of aspirin), the introduction and dissemination of screening tests, and improvements in treatment. The 5-year relative survival rate for patients diagnosed from 2006 to 2012 (all followed through 2013) was 65% declining to 58% at 10 years after diagnosis.[288] The median age at diagnosis for CRC is 66 years for males and 70 years for females. Patients with rectal cancer tend to be younger at diagnosis than those with colon cancer (median age, 63 years).

CRC often develops over more than 10 years, and dysplastic adenomas are the most common form of premalignant precursor lesions. The two most common forms of hereditary CRCs are hereditary nonpolyposis colon cancer (Lynch syndrome) and familial adenomatous polyposis coli. The vast majority of these tumors are adenocarcinoma (>90%) and, to a lesser degree, carcinoid tumors, leiomyosarcomas, and lymphoma. Spread to regional lymph nodes generally correlates to depth of invasion by the primary tumor and the grade of differentiation. Nodal spread occurs in 10% to 20% of tumors confined to the bowel wall. Hematogenous spread is usually to the liver via portal venous transmission.

The liver is the prime organ for metastatic spread (65%); extra-abdominal metastases in lung (25%) and brain and bone (10%) are much less common. Approximately, 15% to 20% of patients with CRC will present with metastatic liver disease, and half of all patient with CRC will develop liver metastases, with a median survival of 8 to 12 months in untreated patients.[289] Liver imaging should be done for all patients with CRC. MRI had a significantly higher sensitivity than did CT for lesions less than 10 mm. Surgical resection represents the only chance of long-term survival, but only 20% to 25% of patients may be eligible for resection.[290] Systemic chemotherapy and/or intra-arterial locoregional techniques may be options for patients not eligible for surgery. These techniques include hepatic arterial infusion, transarterial chemoembolization (TACE), embolization with drug-eluting beads (DEBTACE), selective internal radiation therapy with ^{90}Y (SIRT), and percutaneous ablation with radiofrequency or microwave ablation.

The majority of patients with stage I and II colon cancer undergo partial or total colectomy alone (84%), whereas about two-thirds of those with stage III disease (as well as some with stage II disease) receive chemotherapy in addition to colectomy to lower their risk of recurrence. For patients with rectal cancer, proctectomy or proctocolectomy is the most common treatment (61%) for stage I disease, and about one-half also receive radiation and/or chemotherapy. Stage II and III rectal cancers are often treated with neoadjuvant chemoradiation therapy.

Leukemias and Lymphomas

The majority of patients with leukemia (92%) are diagnosed aged 20 years or older. Acute myeloid leukemia (AML) and chronic lymphocytic leukemia (CLL) are the most common types in adults. Chemotherapy with or without stem cell transplantation (SCT) is the standard treatment for AML. Approximately 60% to 85% of adults aged 60 years and younger with AML can expect to attain complete remission status after the first phase of treatment, and 35% to 40% of patients in this age group will be cured. In contrast, 40% to 60% of patients aged older than 60 years will achieve complete remission, but only 5% to 15% will be cured.

The two types of lymphoma are Hodgkin lymphoma (HL) and NHL. NHLs may be indolent or aggressive and each include subtypes that progress and respond to treatment differently. Prognosis and treatment depend on the stage and type of lymphoma. The two major types of HL are classical HL (CHL) and nodular lymphocyte-predominant HL (NLPHL). CHL is the most common and is characterized by the presence of Reed-Sternberg cells. NLPHL comprises only about 5% of cases and is a more indolent disease with a generally favorable prognosis. The 5-year and 10-year survival rates for HL are 86% and 80%, respectively. The 5-year survival rate is 94% for NLPHL and 85% for CHL. The most common types of NHL are diffuse large B-cell lymphoma (DLBCL), representing 37% of cases, and follicular lymphoma, representing 20% of cases. DLBCLs grow quickly, but most patients with localized disease and about 50% of those with advanced-stage disease are cured. In contrast, follicular lymphomas tend to grow slowly and often do not require treatment until symptoms develop, but many are not curable. Some cases of follicular lymphoma transform into DLBCL. The 5-year survival rate is 86% for follicular lymphoma and 61% for DLBCL; 10-year survival declines to 77% and 53%, respectively.

Multiple Myeloma

Multiple myeloma (MM) is a clonal plasma cell malignancy that accounts for 10% of all hematologic malignancies. MM usually progresses from asymptomatic precursor stages, namely monoclonal gammopathy of undetermined significance (MGUS) and smoldering multiple myeloma (SMM) with possible progression to MM. Some patients experience rapid progression from MGUS/SMM to MM, whereas others may remain indolent with minimal progression during their lifetimes. The median age of diagnosis is 69 years. The 5-year survival rate of patients with MM is 48.5%, and despite the introduction of immunomodulatory drugs and proteasome inhibitors, many patients with high-risk features still have low progression-free survival rates and poor overall survival. CT imaging is useful for detecting early bone destruction but not for detecting myeloma activity in areas of prior destruction. MRI can detect early marrow infiltration. The first biomarker for MM was the Bence Jones protein. Other markers included M protein, plasmacytosis of the bone marrow, and β2 microglobulin. Serum free light chain (FLC) assays were developed to aid the diagnosis of MM and to monitor treatment response and disease progression. Treatment plans are guided by serially measuring serum FLC levels and the FLC ratio to define a complete response or progressive disease in oligosecretory myeloma.

Tumor Markers

A biomarker is a characteristic that is objectively measured and evaluated as an indicator of normal biologic processes, pathogenic processes, or pharmacologic responses to a therapeutic intervention and are important tools for diagnosis, prognosis, and management of malignancies.[291] Most tumor markers are produced by normal cells (tumor-associated) as well as by cancer cells (tumor-derived); however, they are produced at much higher levels in cancerous conditions. Markers include a variety of substances like cell surface antigens, cytoplasmic proteins, enzymes, hormones, oncofetal antigens, receptors, oncogenes, and their products. These substances can be found in the blood, urine, stool, tumor tissue, or other tissues or bodily fluids of some patients with cancer. Most tumor markers are proteins, but patterns of gene expression and changes to DNA are also used as tumor markers. Predictive biomarkers, which include somatic mutations in BRAF and EGFR genes where the presence of certain molecular targets helps identify the appropriate, targeted therapy and thus predict the response to these agents. They can also be beneficial to identify patients with high susceptibility to certain cancers through detection of germline mutations, such as BRCA or somatic mutations. DNA sequencing and gene expression studies have shown that at a molecular level, almost every case of breast cancer is unique and different from other breast cancers.[292] For optimal management, patients should receive treatment that is guided by the molecular composition of their tumor. Mandatory biomarkers for every newly diagnosed case of breast cancer are ER receptors and PR receptors in selecting patients for endocrine treatment and HER2 for identifying patients likely to benefit from anti-HER2 therapy.[293] Examples of tumor markers in malignancy are shown in Table 42.13.

TABLE 42.13 Tumor Markers in Malignancy

Marker	Tissue Analyzed	Cancer Type
α-Fetoprotein	Blood	Liver cancer, germ cell tumors
β-2-microglobulin	Blood, urine, CSF	MM, CLL, some lymphomas
β-human chorionic gonadotropin (β-hCG)	Urine, blood	Choriocarcinoma, germ cell tumors
BRCA1 and *BRCA2* gene mutations	Blood	Ovarian cancer
BRAF V600 mutations	Tumor	Melanoma, colorectal cancer
CA15-3/CA27.29	Blood	Breast cancer
CA19-9	Blood	Pancreatic cancer, gallbladder cancer, bile duct cancer, gastric cancer
CA-125	Blood	Ovarian cancer
Calcitonin	Blood	Medullary thyroid cancer
Carcinoembryonic antigen (CEA)	Blood	Colorectal cancer
Chromogranin A	Blood	Neuroendocrine tumors
EGFR gene mutation	Tumor	Non–small-cell lung cancer
Estrogen receptor (ER)/progesterone receptor (PR)	Tumor	Breast cancer
HER2/neu gene amplification or protein overexpression	Tumor	Breast cancer, gastric cancer, and gastroesophageal junction adenocarcinoma
Immunoglobulins	Blood, urine	Multiple myeloma and Waldenström macroglobulinemia
KRAS gene mutation analysis	Tumor	Colorectal cancer and non–small-cell lung cancer
Prostate-specific antigen (PSA)	Blood	Prostate cancer
Thyroglobulin	Blood	Thyroid cancer

NOTE: *Neu* is derived from a rodent glioblastoma cell line.
BRAF, gene that encodes protein B-Raf; BRCA1 and BRCA2, breast cancer gene and protein product; CA, cancer antigen; CLL, chronic lymphocytic leukemia; CSF, cerebrospinal fluid; EGRF, epidermal growth factor factor; HER2/neu, human epidermal growth factor receptor; KRAS, proto-oncogene for Kirsten rat sarcoma viral oncogene; MM, multiple myeloma.

PATTERNS OF CANCER PAIN

Cancer patients may have constant or intermittent pain. The term *breakthrough pain* (BTP) was popularized by Portenoy and Hagen[294] in 1990 and refers to sudden increases in the base level of pain or different but recurring pains. BTP was originally defined as "a transitory exacerbation of pain that occurs in addition to otherwise stable persistent pain or one that interrupts a tolerable background level of pain" or as "a transitory exacerbation of pain that occurs on a background of otherwise stable pain in a patient receiving chronic opioid therapy."[295] However, most definitions consider BTP only after the background pain is adequately controlled. BTP should be distinguished from crescendo pain, which largely results from poorly controlled baseline pain.[296] The estimated prevalence of BTP in cancer patients may be more than 50%,[297] but the prevalence is difficult to estimate because of difference between studies in the definitions and diagnostic criteria and the inclusion of patients with poorly controlled background pain.[298]

Different terms for BTP have been used in some studies including incident pain, incidental pain, episodic pain, and transitory pain.[295]

The cause and anatomical site of BTP is often, but not always, the same as that of the baseline persistent pain.[299] Typical features of BTP include rapid onset (the time from onset of BTP to peak severity is usually within 3 to 5 minutes), short duration (approximately 30 minutes), and of variable intensity.[300] There are three types of BTP:

1. *Incident pain*: pain that is precipitated, stimulus dependent, or triggered such as turning in bed, weight bearing, a bowel movement, coughing, swallowing meals, etc. Often, incident pain is well defined and predictable, so that clinicians can anticipate and treat the problem prophylactically. Incident pain may be volitional or nonvolitional.
2. *End of dose failure*: pain that emerges because of too much time between doses of medication. This pattern is predictable for the individual patient and readily preventable by using time-contingent dosing at an appropriate interval. The key is monitoring symptoms in relation to the dosing schedule.
3. *Spontaneous pain*: pain that occurs spontaneously without relationship to particular events or procedures. These pains are more difficult because of their unpredictable nature and often fleeting character.

Cancer-related BTP has high interference with activity, mood, ability to walk and work, social relations, sleep, and enjoyment of life.[300–302] Uncontrolled or poorly controlled pain of any etiology is strongly associated with impairment of sleep, walking, daily activities, enjoyment of life, and relationships with others. It also is correlated with worsening of anxiety and depression, dissatisfaction with opioid therapy, and poor medical outcomes.[303] In addition, patients with cancer-related BTP or uncontrolled pain are likely to use more health care resources, have more pain-related hospitalizations and emergency department visits, and have greater direct and indirect treatment costs than those without BTP.[304]

CANCER PAIN SYNDROMES

Tables 42.14 to 42.17 list the common pain syndromes in the patient with cancer.

Table 42.18 lists the prevalence of painful manifestations of cancer and their common etiologies. Bone, viscera, and nerve are the most common sites of metastases associated with chronic cancer pain. Each of these sites will be dealt with separately.

Bone Metastases

Common locations for metastasis are the lung, liver, brain, and bone. Bone is the third most common site for tumor cells to spread[305] and is most prevalent in advanced breast (70% to 80%), prostate (70% to 80%), thyroid (60%), lung (10% to 50%), and renal cancers (30%).[306] Prostate, lung, breast, kidney, and thyroid cancer account for 80% of skeletal metastases and MM favors involvement of the bone marrow. The most common sites of bone metastases are the spine, ribs, pelvis, proximal femur, and skull. Breast cancer preferentially metastasizes to the lungs and bones, whereas prostate cancer almost exclusively metastasizes to the bones.[307] Bone metastases may be classified according to the primary mechanism of interference with bone remodeling as osteolytic, osteoblastic, or mixed.[308] In osteolytic lesions, bone destruction is primarily mediated by osteoclasts and not a direct effect of tumor cells, whereas osteoblastic (or osteosclerotic) lesions are characterized by the deposition of new bone. Osteolytic bone metastases are presumed to be caused by the release of osteoclastogenic

TABLE 42.14 Pain Syndromes due to Tumor Involvement

Primary Etiology	Pathophysiology	Characteristics of Pain	Other Symptoms and Signs
Tumor Invasion of Bone			
Vertebral body metastases			
• Subluxation of atlas	Metastasis of odontoid process of axis → fracture of atlas → compression of spinal cord or brainstem	Severe neck pain radiating to back and top of skull, aggravated by flexion and other movements	Progressive sensory, somatomotor, and autonomic dysfunction beginning in upper extremity
• C7–T1 metastases	Cancer of breast and lung → hematogenous spread or more frequently tumor originating in brachial plexus or paravertebral space → spread to adjacent vertebra and epidural space	Constant, dull, aching pain in paraspinal area radiating to both shoulders; unilateral, radicular pain with radiation to shoulder and medial (ulnar) aspect of limb	Tenderness on percussion of spinous process; paresthesia and numbness in ulnar distribution of limb; progressive weakness of triceps and hand; Horner syndrome indicating sympathetic involvement
• L1 metastases	Frequent site of metastasis from breast, prostate, or other tumors	Dull, aching pain in midback with reference to regions of one or both sacroiliac joints and superior iliac crest; radicular pain with girdle-like distribution anteriorly or to both paraspinal areas in the sacroiliac region	Possible numbness and weakness in the back; pain exacerbated by lying or sitting and relieved by standing
• Sacral metastases	Another frequent site of metastasis from breast, prostate, or other tumors	Dull, aching pain in the low back and/or coccygeal region exacerbated by lying or sitting and relieved by walking	Perianal sensory loss and bowel and bladder dysfunction and impotence
Base of the skull metastases			
• Jugular foramen	Metastasis to jugular foramen with involvement of cranial nerves IX–XII	Occipital pain with reference to the vertex and one or both shoulders and arms, exacerbated by head movement	Tenderness of occipital condyle and often ptosis, hoarseness, dysarthria, dysphagia, and neck and shoulder weakness
• Clivus syndrome	Metastasis to clivus of sphenoid bone and basilar portion of occipital bone	Progressively severe vertex headache exacerbated by neck flexion	Dysfunction of lower cranial nerves (VII–XII), which begins unilaterally but extends bilaterally
• Sphenoid sinus	Metastasis to the sphenoid sinus on one or both sides	Severe bifrontal headache radiating to both temples with intermittent retro-orbital pain	Nasal stuffiness or sense of fullness in the head associated with diplopia
• Cavernous sinus	Metastasis to cavernous sinus syndrome from breast, prostate, and lung	Unilateral frontal headache and dull aching pain in supraorbital and facial region	Dysfunction of cranial nerves III–VI, diplopia, ophthalmoplegia, papilledema
• Occipital condyle	Metastasis from breast, lung, prostate	Severe localized continuous, unilateral occipital pain aggravated by neck flexion	Cranial nerve XII paralysis → paralysis of tongue; weakness of sternocleidomastoid, stiff neck
Other bone involvement			
• Pelvis	Metastasis from breast, prostate, or other tumors	Dull, aching pain in sacrum, hips, or pubis	Extension to sacral plexus with consequent motor, sensory, and/or autonomic changes
• Long bones	Metastasis from breast, prostate, or other tumors	Dull, aching, severe pain localized to site of tumor that may be referred (e.g., reference to knee from hip metastasis); pathologic fracture produces severe pain on movement	
Tumor Involvement of Nerves, Plexus, or Spinal Cord			
• Peripheral, cranial, or spinal neuropathy	Infiltration, compression, or damage to nerve	Dull, aching, burning pain associated with bouts of lancinating pain in distribution of affected nerve or nerves; hyperpathia	Hypesthesia, dysesthesia, motor, and/or autonomic dysfunction and reflex changes
• Brachial plexus	Compression, infiltration, or damage of brachial plexus by metastatic tumor or lower cervical and upper thoracic vertebra or Pancoast tumor	Progressively more severe, dull, aching pain which is first located in the shoulder and arm and vertebral border of scapula and later extends to medial part of arm, elbow, forearm, and hand	Paresthesia, dysesthesia, hypesthesia; subjective numbness and progressive muscle weakness in C7, C8, and T1 distribution, often Horner syndrome and anhidrosis of the ipsilateral face
• Lumbosacral plexus	Compression, infiltration, or damage of lumbar and sacral plexus by cancer of the prostate, bladder, uterus, cervix, or colon from extension of tumor into adjacent lymph nodes and bone	Radicular pain either in groin and anterior thigh (L1, L2, and L3 nerve involvement) or down the posterior aspect of leg to the heel (L5, S1, and S2 distribution) or dull, aching midline pain in the perianal area (S2, S3, S4 distribution)	Paresthesia followed by numbness and dysesthesia and progressive motor and sensory loss in the areas supplied by the involved nerves
• Reflex sympathetic dystrophy	Compression, infiltration, or damage of major nerve or plexuses	Severe burning pain not limited to a segmental or peripheral nerve distribution; aggravated by touch and emotional stress	Hyperalgesia, vasomotor, and sudomotor disturbances and other symptomatology of causalgia
• Leptomeningeal carcinomatosis	Tumor infiltration of the cerebrospinal leptomeninges with or without invasion of the meninges of the brain	Pain in 40% of patients of two types: headache, with or without neck stiffness and pain in the low back and buttock regions	Malignant cells in cerebrospinal fluid, elevated protein and low glucose levels
• Epidural spinal cord compression	Tumor compression of cervical, thoracic, or lumbosacral parts of spinal cord and involvement of vertebra or roots of spinal nerves	Local dull, aching pain, and tenderness in the region of involved vertebral body or radicular pain, which is unilateral with cervical or lumbosacral compression and bilateral with thoracic cord compression	Depends on site of epidural compression, includes motor weakness progressing to paraplegia, sensory loss, and loss of bowel and bladder function

(continued)

TABLE 42.14 (Continued)

Primary Etiology	Pathophysiology	Characteristics of Pain	Other Symptoms and Signs
Tumor Involvement of Viscera			
• Obstruction of hollow viscus or of ductal system of solid viscus	Contraction of smooth muscle under isometric conditions → intense distention of smooth muscles	Diffuse, poorly localized, dull, aching, or colicky pain referred to abdominal wall or chest wall	Dyspnea and cough with thoracic viscera; abdominal distention, nausea, vomiting with abdominal visceral pathology
• Rapid tumor growth in solid viscus	Rapid growth of hepatic, splenic, or kidney tumors → rapid distention and stretching of investing fascia → stimulation of mechanical nociceptors	Dull, aching, poorly localized pain referred to midline (liver) or in one side in lower thoracic and upper lumbar segments	Symptomatology of visceral dysfunction
Other Types of Tumor Involvement			
Tumor involvement of blood vessels			
• Infiltration	Perivascular lymphangitis and vasospasm	Burning pain in the areas supplied by the affected vessels	Signs of vasoconstriction or ischemia
• Obstruction of large vein	Venous engorgement → progressive edema → distention of fascial compartments and soft tissue	Severe headache with obstruction of veins to head; pain in limbs with obstruction in axilla or pelvis	Edema and cyanosis of affected part
• Obstruction of large artery	Ischemia in tissues with liberation of algesic substances	Progressively severe, burning pain	Paresthesia, pallor of affected part
• Necrosis or ulceration of mucous membrane	Necrosis, infection, and inflammation of mucous membrane → algesic substances → lowering of nociceptors' threshold	Excruciating local or referred pain depending on site of lesion	Signs of infection or inflammation

TABLE 42.15 Pain Syndromes Associated with Cancer Therapy

Primary Etiology	Pathophysiology	Characteristics of Pain	Other Symptoms and Signs
Postsurgical Syndromes			
• Postthoracotomy, postradical neck resection, postmastectomy	Partial injury or complete severance of nerves during operation → damage to nerve membrane or neuroma formation, which becomes hypersensitive to pressure and norepinephrine → abnormal sensory input to central nervous system (peripheral-central mechanisms)	Continuous, burning or dull, aching pain with occasional bout of lancinating pains in the areas supplied by affected nerves, aggravated by touch, movement, or emotional stress with catecholamine release	Dysesthesia, hyperesthesia in the scar area with hypesthesia in the surrounding zone
• Postamputation pain	Persistent nociception in stump and loss of sensory input to neuraxis → deafferentation (peripheral-central mechanism)	Constant aching or burning pain in stump or in phantom limb or cramping "proprioceptive" pain characterized by abnormal position of missing part of limb; also lancinating pain	Sudomotor and vasomotor changes in stump
Postchemotherapy Pain			
• Peripheral neuropathy	Symmetrical polyneuropathy caused by vinca alkaloids (peripheral mechanism)	Constant burning pain in the hand and/or feet	Dysesthesia and paresthesia
• Steroid	Diffuse myalgias and pseudorheumatism arthralgias caused by withdrawal of steroid medication (peripheral mechanism)	Diffuse pain and tenderness in affected muscles and joints	Fatigue and general malaise; these and the pain disappear with reinstitution of steroid medication
• Aseptic necrosis of bone	Aseptic necrosis of humoral head or femoral head as complication of chronic steroid therapy (peripheral mechanism)	Dull, aching pain in the shoulder or knee	Limitation of joint movement with inability to use arm or hip joint → frozen shoulder or impaired hip
• Mucositis	Drug produces biochemical changes in mucous membranes and other structures (peripheral mechanisms).	Severe, excruciating pain in mouth, throat, nasal passages, and gastrointestinal tract	Difficulty or inability to eat, drink, or even talk
Postradiation Therapy Pain			
• Radiation fibrosis of brachial or lumbosacral plexus	Radiation-induced fibrosis of connective tissue surrounding plexus and consequent injury to nerve structures develops 6 mo to 20 y following therapy → deafferentation (peripheral-central mechanisms)	Progressively increasing, severe, diffuse, burning pain in a part or the entire limb, which occurs after other symptomatology	Numbness, paresthesia, dysesthesia, and motor weakness in distribution of C5 and C6 in the upper limb or in lower limb
• Radiation myelopathy	Damage to spinal cord → Brown-Séquard syndrome progresses to complete transverse myelopathy (central pain)	Pain that is localized or referred to peripheral structures	Dysesthesia and other symptomatology of myelopathy
• Painful peripheral nerve tumors	Radiation induces nerve sheath tumors 4–20 y after therapy	Progressively severe, burning, aching pain in distribution of involved nerves	Progressive neurologic deficit
• Postherpetic neuralgia	Induced by radiation or after herpes zoster in the area of tumor pathology	Continuous burning pain associated with intermittent lancinating pain	Dysesthesia, hypesthesia, and hyperpathia

TABLE 42.16   Pain Syndromes Caused by Cancer-Induced Pathophysiologic Changes

Primary Etiology	Pathophysiology	Characteristics of Pain	Other Symptoms and Signs
Paraneoplastic syndromes	—	—	—
Myofascial pain syndromes	—	—	—
Debility, constipation, bed sores, rectal or bladder spasm, gastric distention	Related to specific lesions depending on involved site	Local or referred pain	Related to specific pathophysiology

agents by tumor cells in the bone microenvironment, whereas osteoblastic metastases are the result of the release of factors that stimulate osteoblast proliferation, differentiation, and uncontrolled bone formation by metastatic cancer cells. Accordingly, bone metastases are typically characterized as "lytic," "sclerotic," or "mixed," according to radiographic appearances. Metastasis to the bones is facilitated by the fenestrated structure of the bone marrow sinusoid capillaries, high blood flow in the areas of red marrow, and adhesive molecules on tumor cells that bind to the bone marrow stromal cells such as osteoblasts and osteoclasts as well as the bone matrix. Bone homeostasis is maintained by balanced production of osteoblasts and osteoclasts. Tumor cells influence bone cells in two predominant ways. Most often, cancer cells stimulate the osteoclast lineage to increase osteoclast differentiation and activity while simultaneously inhibiting osteoblasts. Osteoclastic bone resorption then exceeds osteoblastic bone formation resulting in bone degradation and the formation of osteolytic lesions (as may be seen in breast, lung, and MM). In some cases, instead of inhibiting osteoblasts, tumor cells release substances to stimulate the osteoblast lineage to increase osteoblast differentiation and new bone deposition causing osteoblastic lesions. Mechanistically, osteoclasts and osteoblasts play significant roles in the formation of both lesion types.

In osteolytic bone metastases, tumor cells secrete factors that stimulate osteoclast activity through the activation of the receptor activator of nuclear factor–κB ligand (RANKL)/RANK pathway, a primary mediator of osteoclast-mediated bone resorption.[309] Osteoblasts secrete receptor activator of RANKL which interacts with osteoclast precursors displaying RANK receptor on their surface, resulting in their activation and finally maturation into functional osteoclasts. Osteoblasts also produce osteoprotegerin (OPG), a soluble decoy receptor which can block RANK/RANKL signaling by scavenging of RANKL. The activation of osteoclasts is triggered by the balance between RANKL and OPG. RANKL also can induce factors involved in migration, invasion, and angiogenesis such as matrix metalloproteinases 1 and matrix metalloproteinases 9 (MMP1, MMP9), matrix metalloproteinase inducer EMMPRIN/CD147, intercellular adhesion molecule-1 (ICAM-1), IL-6 and IL-8, and VEGF and decrease the expression of metastasis suppressor serpin 5b/maspin. RANKL can also promote the function of regulatory T cells (Tregs) and macrophages. Osteolysis is based on a self-perpetuating signaling system (vicious cycle) that is maintained by mitogenic factors for tumor cells such as TGF-β, insulin-like growth factor-1 (IGF-1), fibroblast growth factors (FGFs), PDGFs, and Ca-ions released from demineralized bone as well as parathyroid hormone-related peptide (PTHrP) derived from tumor cells. PTHrP acts as a promotor of osteolysis by osteoclasts (Fig. 42.8).

Osteoblastic bone metastases are preferentially associated with prostate cancer but may also occur with breast, lung,

carcinoid, and medulloblastoma tumors and produce sclerotic lesions. Endothelin-1 has been implicated in osteoblastic metastasis from breast cancer. It stimulates the formation of bone and the proliferation of osteoblasts in bone organ cultures, and serum endothelin-1 levels are increased in patients with osteoblastic metastasis from prostate cancer.[310] Furthermore, in an animal model of osteoblastic metastasis, treatment with a selective endothelin-1A–receptor antagonist decreased both osteoblastic metastasis and the tumor burden. A vicious circle may also be involved in osteoblastic metastasis in which tumors induce osteoblast activity and thus the subsequent release from the osteoblasts of growth factors that increase tumor growth. In addition to endothelin-1, PDGF, a polypeptide produced by osteoblasts in the bone microenvironment, urokinase, and PSA may also be involved. Overproduction of urokinase-type plasminogen activator (u-PA) by prostate-cancer cells increases bone metastasis. Human PC3 prostate-cancer cells produce a factor that is homologous to u-PA. Prostate-cancer cells also release PSA, a kallikrein serine protease. PSA can cleave parathyroid hormone–related peptide at the N-terminal, which could block tumor-induced bone resorption. It may also activate osteoblastic growth factors released in the bone microenvironment during the development of bone metastases, such as IGF-I and IGF-II or TGF-β (Fig. 42.9).[310]

Imaging modalities available for diagnosing bone metastases are CT, MRI, bone scintigraphy, and PET imaging with tumor-specific or bone-specific tracers. Bone scintigraphy with 99mTc-labeled diphosphonates has limited sensitivity and poor specificity for identifying bone metastases particularly in the early stages of the disease when tumor is confined to the marrow. This is improved by the addition of single-photon emission computed tomography (SPECT), which has the advantage of providing anatomic localization of abnormal tracer uptake with better contrast resolution. An alternative strategy is PET-based radionuclide imaging. The commonly used radiopharmaceuticals are 18F-fluoro-2-deoxyglucose (FDG) and 18F/11C-choline as tumor-specific agents or sodium fluoride as a bone-specific tracer (NaF).

CHARACTERISTICS OF METASTATIC BONE PAIN

Adult bone receives a restricted and unique innervation as it is only innervated largely by thinly myelinated, TrkA+ sensory nerve fibers (Aδ) and TrkA+ C fibers, and receive little, if any, innervation by the larger more rapidly conducting Aβ fibers or the TrkA-negative, unmyelinated peptide poor C fibers. Most of the sensory nerves that innervate the bone appear to only be activated by injury or damage to the bone (i.e., silent nociceptors).[311] The initial sharp pain experienced from a fracture of any bone is probably detected by mechanotransducers expressed by the Aδ and C-sensory fibers. The dull aching pain following injury, bruising, or stabilization of the fractured bone is likely associated with activation of

TABLE 42.17   Pain Syndromes Unrelated to Cancer

Primary Etiology	Pathophysiology	Characteristics of Pain	Other Symptoms and Signs
Examples: arthritis, migraines, osteoporosis	Pathology of affected part	Local or referred pain	Related to specific pathophysiology

TABLE 42.18 Prevalence of Painful Manifestations of Cancer and Common Etiologies

Primary Site of Cancer	Approximate Incidence of Pain (%)	Common Pain Syndromes
Oropharynx	55–80	Post-radical neck dissection syndrome Infection
Colon–rectum	45–95	Bone metastasis Perineal pain syndrome Lumbosacral plexopathy Epidural spinal cord compression
Pancreas	70–100	Abdominal visceral pain
Liver/biliary tract	65–100	Abdominal visceral pain
Lung	55–90	Bone metastasis Epidural spinal cord compression Brachial plexopathy Postthoracotomy syndrome
Breast	55–100	Brachial plexopathy Postmastectomy syndrome Bone metastasis Epidural spinal cord compression Leptomeningeal carcinomatous
Uterus–cervix and ovary	40–100	Lumbosacral plexopathy
Prostate	55–100	Bone metastasis Base of skull syndromes Vertebral body syndromes Epidural spinal cord compression
Urinary tract	60–100	Lumbosacral plexopathy Epidural spinal cord compression
Lymphoma and leukemia	5–75	Leptomeningeal carcinomatosis Bone pain Mucositis
Sarcoma and primary bone tumors	75–90	Postamputation pain (stump, phantom limb) Epidural spinal cord compression

unmyelinated C fibers present in the periosteum. Cortical bone and bone marrow are also innervated by the same population of Aδ and C-sensory nerve fibers that innervate the periosteum, although the relative density of sensory nerve fibers per unit area is markedly lower.[311] Osteoclasts resorb bone by forming a highly acidic resorption area between the osteoclast and bone that stimulates the TRPV1 or ASIC3 channels expressed by a significant population of nerve fibers that drive bone cancer pain.[312] Tumor-associated bone pain is usually first described as dull in character and constant in nature with the pain gradually intensifying over time. Nociception from bony metastases can produce a variety of symptoms such as muscle spasms or paroxysms of stabbing pain. Hematologic malignancies (especially acute leukemias) may produce a syndrome of generalized and migrating bone pain as a result of marrow infiltration.[313] Limb pain is the most common presentation, and local bone tenderness (especially on long bone diaphyses) is a frequent finding. The vertebrae are the most common sites of bone metastases. The thoracic spine is affected in more than 66% of cases, the lumbosacral spine in 20%, and the cervical spine in 10%. Multiple vertebral lesions are common. Pain from metastases involving T12 and L1 often is referred to the iliac crest or SI joint unilaterally or bilaterally. Patients with tumor invasion of the upper cervical vertebrae may present with pain in the neck that is referred to the occipital region and skull vertex. Neck flexion typically exacerbates the pain.

Osteolytic bone metastases often present with bone pain, pathologic fractures, hypercalcemia, and, more rarely, swelling or neurologic complaints. The vertebrae, pelvis, ribs, femur, and skull are the sites most frequently involved.[314] Pain gradually develops during a period of weeks or months, becoming progressively more severe. The pain is usually well localized in a particular area and is often strongest at night or on weight bearing. Patients describe the pain as dull in character, constant in presentation, and gradually progressive in intensity. Pain increases with pressure on the involved area. Continuous pain may be moderate on resting and then increase with different movements or positions, such as standing, walking, or sitting. BTP can result from weight bearing or instability due to incipient or actual pathologic fractures. Although the locus of bone pain usually corresponds to the site of the underlying lesion, characteristic patterns of referral to noncontiguous cutaneous areas occurs. By way of example, hip pain due to a hip lesion may refer to the knee.

Fractures are common through lytic lesions in weight-bearing bones. Damage to both cortical and trabecular bone is structurally important. Radiologic features that may predict imminent fracture include large, predominantly lytic lesion that erode the cortex. The main complications of vertebral metastases are vertebral collapse, radiculopathy, and metastatic epidural spinal cord compression (MESCC). Collapse of vertebral bodies is particularly frequent in the thoracic spine metastases. Back pain is a frequent symptom in patients with advanced cancer and in 10% of cases is due to spinal instability. The pain, which can be severe, is mechanical in origin, and frequently, the patient is only comfortable when lying still. Radiculopathies can occur at any level; patients feel the pain in the spine, deep in the muscles innervated by the affected nerve root, and in the corresponding dermatome. Metastatic spinal cord compression is a serious complication of vertebral metastases (see section in the following text).

PROGNOSIS

A real estimate of the impact of bone metastases is difficult to assess because incidence is influenced by factors including the sensitivity of diagnostic tools and by the length of survival of the patients. In general, the prognosis for patients presenting with bone metastases is poor (Table 42.19).

Patients with fewer metastases or solitary lesions appear to have a better outlook than those with multiple metastatic deposits. Once tumor cells spread to the skeleton, the disease is usually incurable. Issues related to bone metastases include reduced survival, morbidity, and pain that negatively affect the patient's QOL as well as skeletal-related events (SREs). In prostate cancer, skeletal metastases are associated with overall survival ranging from 12 to 53 months.[315] In a Danish study of approximately 36,000 breast cancer patients, the 5-year survival was 75.8% for patients without bone metastases, 8.3% for patients with bone metastases, and 2.5% for those with both bone metastases and SREs. The adjusted mortality rate ratio (MRR) was 10.5 (95% confidence interval [CI] 9.5, 11.6) for breast cancer patients with bone metastases and 14.4 (95% CI 13.1, 15.8) for those with bone metastases and SREs, compared with breast cancer patients with no bone metastases but possibly other sites of metastases.[316] Bone metastases can be a major cause for morbidity, characterized by pain, impaired mobility, pathologic fractures, spinal cord compression, myelosuppression, and hypercalcemia with the most disability caused by long bone fracture or epidural extension of tumor into the spine. Both osteolytic and osteoblastic bone metastases are prone to fracture either because of increased bone resorption or because newly deposited bone is mostly immature is less mechanically competent than mature, lamellar bone.[317]

Factors that influence prognosis in patients with metastatic disease include the interval between primary diagnosis and the development of metastases and the Karnofsky performance status (Table 42.20). The Karnofsky score after palliative

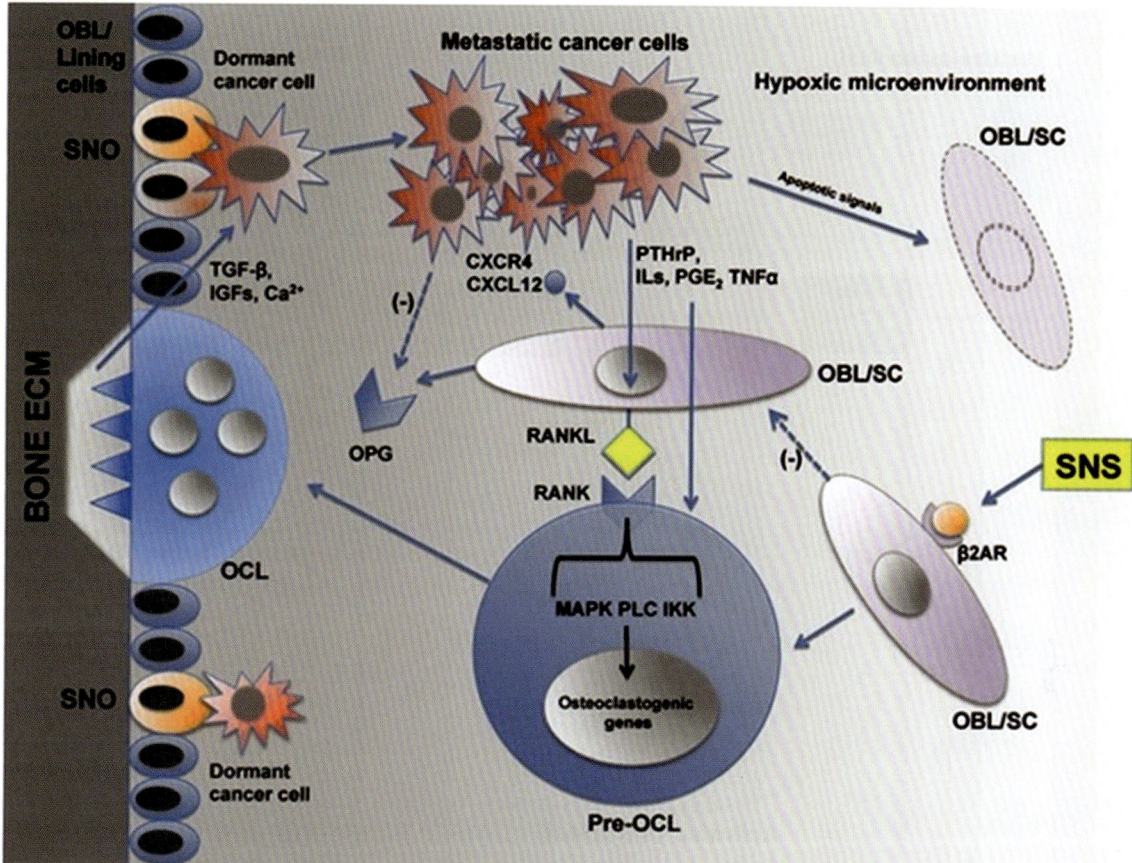

FIGURE 42.8 Mechanism of osteolytic bone metastases. Metastatic cancer cells are attracted to spindle-shaped N-cadherin positive osteoblasts (SNO) and remain dormant. Quiescent cells can become activated and grow giving rise to an overt metastasis. The metastatic cells produce factors, which include parathyroid hormone-related peptide (PTHrP), interleukins (ILs), PGEs, and CXCR4 that mediate their interaction with osteoblastic cells of the metastatic microenvironment. Osteoblasts, in turn, communicate with preosteoclasts, primarily via the receptor activator for nuclear factor κB (RANK)–receptor activator for nuclear factor κB ligand (RANKL) axis and promote osteoclastic morphologic and functional maturation. PTHrP can also induce osteoclastic maturation via non-RANK/RANKL-dependent pathways. Fully activated osteoclasts resorb bone causing osteolytic bone disease. Hypoxic conditions and factors that are released during the degradation of the bone extracellular matrix further stimulate cancer cells, feeding the "vicious circle" of lytic bone metastasis. β2AR, β2 adrenergic receptor; ECM, extracellular matrix; IGF, insulin-like growth factor; IKK, inhibitor of NF-κB kinase; MAPK, mitogen-activated protein kinase; OBL, osteoblast; OCL, osteoclast; OPG, osteoprotegerin; PGE, prostaglandin E; PLC, phospholipase C; SC, stromal cell; SNS, sympathetic nervous system; TGF-β, transforming growth factor-β; TNF-α, tumor necrosis factor-α. *(From Papachristou DJ, Basdra EK, Papavassiliou AG. Bone metastases: molecular mechanisms and novel therapeutic interventions. Med Res Rev 2012;32[3]:611–636. Copyright © 2010 Wiley Periodicals, Inc. Reprinted by permission of John Wiley & Sons, Inc.)*

irradiation reliably predicts survival.[318–320] Other factors that predict survival include the site of the primary disease and whether single or multiple bone metastases are present.[321,322] The distribution of metastases on bone scans also has prognostic significance. Bone involvement offers specific measurability criteria for tumor response assessment.[323] Patients with metastatic prostate carcinoma survive significantly longer if their metastases respond to therapy and do not spread beyond the pelvis or lumbar spine.[324] The use of [223]Ra dichloride for metastatic castration-resistant prostate cancer reduced symptomatic skeletal events[325] and significantly improved survival.[326]

SACRAL INSUFFICIENCY FRACTURES

Insufficiency fractures represent a special category of stress fractures that occur in bones with reduced mineral content and elastic resistance. They are often observed in osteoporosis, rheumatoid arthritis, prolonged glucocorticoid treatment, pelvic radiation therapy, and metabolic bone diseases. Pelvic radiation therapy has a reported prevalence of 21% to 34%[327–329] and may occur because of a direct effect on bone and an indirect effect associated with vascular changes.[330] Following radiation therapy, the reduction of the number of osteoblasts induces a reduction of collagen production and decreased alkaline phosphatase activity, key mechanisms involved in

bone mineralization. Radiation-induced occlusion of bone microvascularization also results in ischemia, which contributes to the formation of insufficiency fractures.[331] Osteoporosis is also a major risk factor because of a greater susceptibility to injury with normal repetitive activities and minor trauma. Trabecular bone is more affected by osteoporosis than cortical bone, but cortical bone is also significantly attenuated; hence, the vertebral bodies, pelvis, and sacrum are particularly susceptible to fractures as the ratio of trabecular to cortical bone is highest in the sacral alae and lower in the central portion of the sacrum.[332] Common areas for insufficiency fractures include weight-bearing areas such as the sacral ala, sacral body, and pubic limb. Typically, patients present with acute onset severe diffuse sacral pain and tenderness, frequently with radiation to the hips/buttocks and groin, and classically worsen with axial loading. Many patients have pain intense enough to render the patient nonambulatory. Physical examination may reveal low back or groin tenderness with restricted hip movement. Physical examination may reveal tenderness to palpation in the region of the sacral ala, but diagnosis is usually made radiologically in patients with a prior history of pelvic radiation treatment (Fig. 42.10). CT images should include coronal and sagittal reconstruction views. Patients with sacral insufficiency fractures may be misdiagnosed as having pathologic

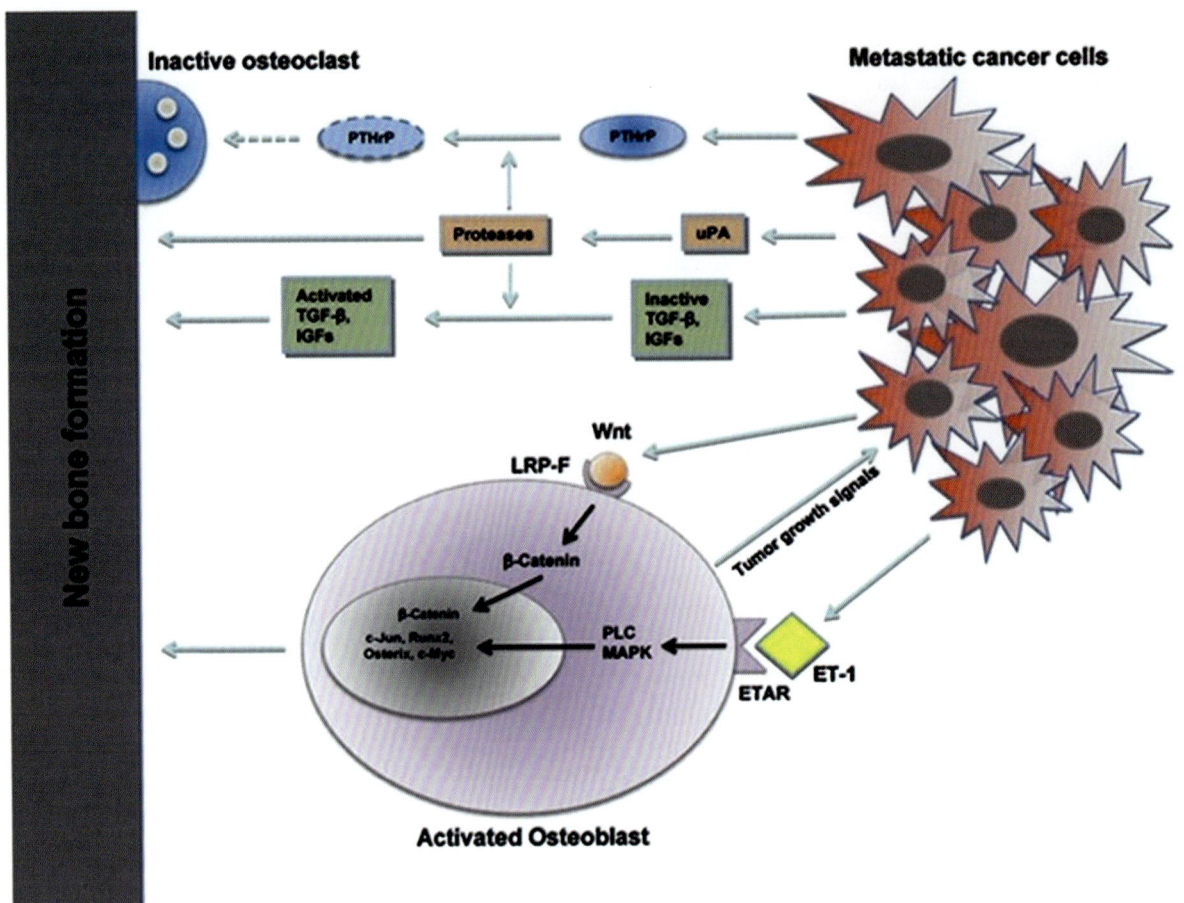

FIGURE 42.9 Mechanisms of osteoblastic bone metastases. Cancer cells secrete a series of factors that augment osteoblast activation and bone formation at the site of metastasis. Two of the major signaling cascades involved in this process are the endothelin-1A/endothelin-1A receptor and the Wnt/β-catenin, which target osteoblast-specific genes such as c-jun, runx2, osterix, and c-myc. In addition, cancer cells produce urokinase plasminogen activator (uPA) that activates proteases such as prostate-specific antigen, further enhancing the osteosclerotic process either via activation of the quiescent forms of TGF-β and IGF-1 or via degradation of parathyroid hormone-related peptide (PTHrP). ET-1, endothelin-1A; ETAR, endothelin-1A receptor; IGF, insulin-like growth factor; LRP-F, low-density lipoprotein receptor–related proteins-Frizzled complex; MAPK, mitogen-activated protein kinase; PLC, phospholipase C; TGF-β, transforming growth factor-β. *(From Papachristou DJ, Basdra EK, Papavassiliou AG. Bone metastases: molecular mechanisms and novel therapeutic interventions. Med Res Rev 2012;32[3]:611–636. Copyright © 2010 Wiley Periodicals, Inc. Reprinted by permission of John Wiley & Sons, Inc.)*

fractures from metastatic disease.[333,334] Biopsy of the lesion is not recommended because of low diagnostic yield. On MRI, stress fractures present an easily recognizable edema signal in contrast to metastases that disorganize the bone and form a real replacement tissue.[331] The most commonly used classification system for sacral fractures is the Denis classification and subclassification system (Fig. 42.11).[335] Zone I and II fractures can cause injury to the L5 nerve root in the lumbosacral tunnel (space between the lumbosacral ligament and the S1 ala).

Zone II and III fractures can cause injury to the S1 nerve root or pudendal nerve. S1 nerve injury in this setting is usually not isolated and tends to be associated with a lumbosacral plexus injury. Zone III fractures have the highest rate of neurologic deficit including bowel, bladder, and sexual dysfunction.

TABLE 42.19   Incidence and Prognosis of Bone Metastases

	Incidence of Bone Metastases in Patients with Advanced Disease (%)	Median Survival from Diagnosis of Bone Metastases (mo)
Breast	65–75	19–25
Prostate	65–75	12–53
Lung	30–40	6–7
Bladder	40	6–9
Renal cell	20–25	12
Thyroid	60	48
Melanoma	14–45	6

Reprinted from Selvaggi G, Scagliotti GV. Management of bone metastases in cancer: a review. *Crit Rev Oncol Hematol* 2005;56(3):365–378. Copyright © 2005 Elsevier Ireland Ltd. With permission.

TABLE 42.20   Karnofsky Performance Status

Grade	Performance Level
100	Normal, no complaints, no evidence of disease
90	Able to carry on normal activity; minor signs or symptoms of disease
80	Normal activity with effort; some signs or symptoms of disease
70	Cares for self; unable to carry on normal activity or to do active work
60	Requires occasional assistance, but is able to care for most of his or her needs
50	Requires considerable assistance and frequent medical care
40	Disabled, requires special care and assistance
30	Severely disabled, hospitalization indicated; death not imminent
20	Very sick, hospitalization necessary, active supportive treatment necessary
10	Moribund, fatal processes, progressing rapidly
0	Dead

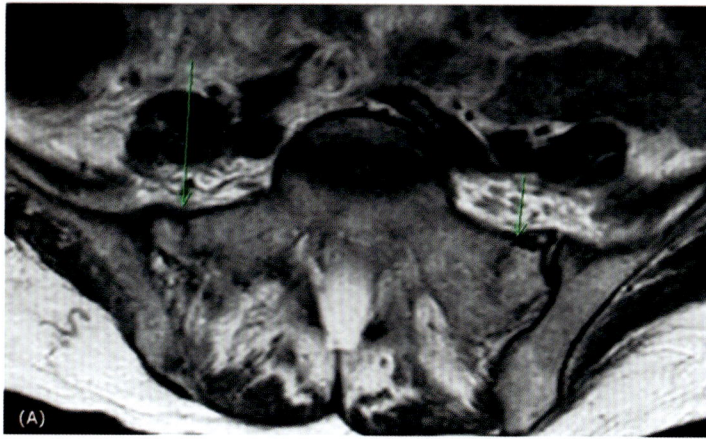
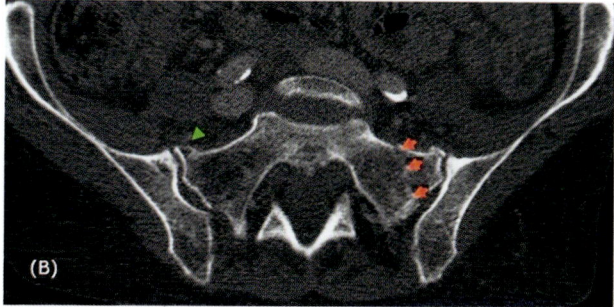

FIGURE 42.10 Magnetic resonance imaging (MRI) and computed tomography (CT) images of pelvis showing sacral insufficiency fracture. **A:** MRI axial T1 imaging shows H-shaped sacral fracture (type 1 transverse zone 3). *Green arrows* indicate fractures bilaterally. **B:** CT images of same fracture. Minimally displaced zone 1 sacral ala fractures. The fracture on the left is intra-articular and extends into the sacroiliac joint (*red arrow heads*). The fracture on the right is barely visible on this view with evidence of disruption of the cortex (*green arrow head*).

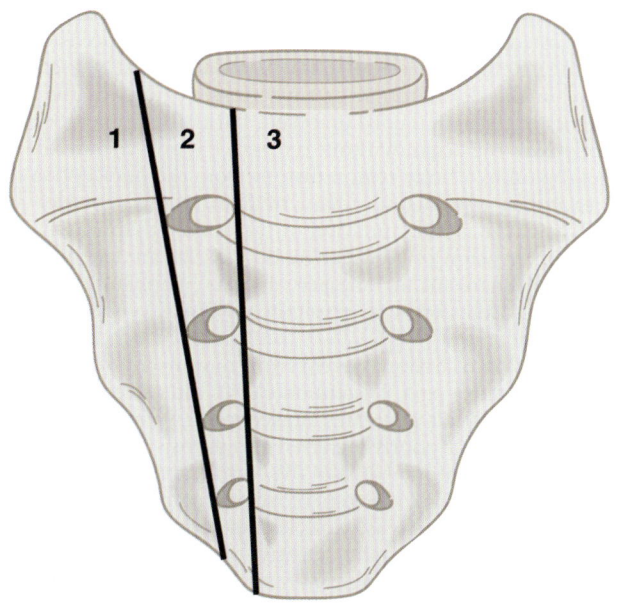

Zone 1: Fracture involves the sacral ala lateral to the neural foramina

Zone 2: Fracture involves the neural foramina, but does not involve the spinal canal

Zone 3: Fracture is medial to the neural foramen, involving the spinal canal; these may be transverse or longitudinal; This may be divided into the following types:
- Type 1: Only kyphotic angulation at the fracture site (no translation)
- Type 2: Kyphotic angulation with anterior translation of the distal sacrum
- Type 3: Kyphotic angulation with complete offset of the fracture fragments
- Type 4: Comminuted S1 segment, usually due to axial compression

FIGURE 42.11 Denis classification and subclassification system of sacral fractures. The classification is based on the direction, location, and level of sacral fractures. The fractures are based on the sacrum's division into three anatomic zones: zone I (alar region), zone II (foraminal region), and zone III (region of the central sacral canal). A zone II fracture can involve zone I but cannot extend into zone III, whereas a zone III fracture can involve zones I and II. Zone 3 fractures morphologically include "H"-, "U"-, "A"-, and "T"-shaped fractures.

GRANULOCYTE COLONY-STIMULATING FACTORS–ASSOCIATED BONE PAIN

Granulocyte colony-stimulating factor (G-CSF) agents act on the hematopoietic system to stimulate the proliferation and differentiation of neutrophil precursors and produce mature functional neutrophils. Agents such as filgrastim and pegfilgrastim are used as primary or secondary prophylaxis to reduce the risk of febrile neutropenia and allow the dose maintenance in patients receiving myelosuppressive chemotherapy. Pegfilgrastim is a long-acting, pegylated formulation of filgrastim that is given as a 6-mg dose subcutaneously on a once-per-cycle administration 24 to 72 hours after the administration of cytotoxic chemotherapy. Filgrastim is administered subcutaneously once daily. Pegfilgrastim causes proliferation of immature progenitor and mature myeloid cells within the bone marrow. Bone pain is the most commonly reported adverse event associated with pegfilgrastim occurring in approximately 26% of patients[336] with severe bone pain reported in 3% to 7% of patients with the highest incidence in the first cycle.[337] Although the exact mechanism of associated bone pain is unknown, inflammatory processes within the bone marrow, stimulation of osteoclasts and osteoblasts, and expansion of the bone marrow are potential sources of pain.[338] The incidence of bone pain between filgrastim and pegfilgrastim was similar between patients receiving either formulation of G-CSF when used as support with chemotherapy in breast cancer.[339]

Visceral Pain

Visceral infiltration is a common cause of pain in cancer patients. Table 42.21 lists the common pain syndromes associated with tumor infiltration.

MECHANISM

Visceral pain is defined as pain emanating from organs in the thorax, abdomen, or pelvis. The main factors capable of inducing pain in visceral structures include abnormal distention and contraction of hollow visceral walls, rapid stretching of the capsules of solid visceral organs, ischemia of visceral musculature, formation and accumulation of algogenic substances, direct action of chemical stimuli on compromised mucosa, and traction or compression of ligaments, vessels, or mesentery.[340–342] Gastric acid is a noxious stimulus that contributes to pain arising from the esophagus, stomach, and upper small intestine. Mechanical trauma to normal mucosa causes no pain, implying that preceding inflammation is necessary.

TABLE 42.21 Pain Syndromes Related to Tumor Infiltration of Viscera

Esophageal mediastinal pain

Shoulder pain from diaphragmatic infiltration

Epigastric pain from pancreatic or other upper abdominal tumor

Right upper quadrant pain from hepatic capsule distention

Left upper quadrant pain from splenomegaly

Diffuse abdominal pain from abdominal or peritoneal disease with or without obstruction

Pleural infiltration

Gastrointestinal perforation

Biliary obstruction

Ureteric obstruction

Suprapubic/pelvic pain from bladder infiltration

Perineal pain from infiltration of rectum or perirectal tissue

There are two distinct classes of nociceptive sensory receptors in viscera.[91] One population of afferents can code nonnoxious, as well as noxious stimuli, and a second population is not activated unless more intense and potentially damaging stimuli are encountered. These relatively insensitive fibers are normally silent and only become active following injury or in disease.[343] The first class is composed of "high-threshold" receptors that respond to mechanical stimuli within the noxious range. These have been identified within many viscera, including the heart, lungs, gastrointestinal tract, ureters, and urinary bladder. The second class is composed of receptors that have a low threshold to natural stimuli and encode the stimulus intensity in the magnitude of their discharges, the so-called "intensity-encoding" receptors. Both receptor types are mainly concerned with mechanical stimuli such as stretch and are involved in the peripheral encoding of noxious stimuli in viscera. In the presence of local inflammation or tissue injury, these afferents become sensitized and respond to previously innocuous natural stimuli. High-threshold afferents signal acute visceral pain. Local ischemia, hypoxia, and inflammation cause pain by sensitizing high-threshold receptors and these previously "silent" or unresponsive receptors. Pain in visceral structures is not necessarily linked to tissue injury but is more dependent on the nature of the provoking stimulus. Adequate stimuli that induce pain are distention, ischemia, and inflammation. Hollow organs such as the colon are very sensitive to luminal distention or inflammation but are totally insensitive to cutting or burning stimuli. Visceral structures from the esophagus to the transverse colon are innervated not only by DRG located in the cervical, thoracic, and upper lumbar regions but also by sensory neurons arising from the superior and inferior vagal ganglia.[343] Visceral structures located distal to the transverse colon, particularly the distal colon, rectum, and bladder, are also innervated by two populations of afferents; however, these are both of spinal origin arising from two different levels of the spinal cord (thoracolumbar and lumbosacral). Sensory neurons arising from these two spinal locations appear to convey different aspects of the complex sensation that humans identify as visceral pain.[343] Poorly localized visceral pain may be explained by the low density of visceral nociceptors, the functional divergence of visceral input with the CNS, and viscerovisceral convergence in the spinal cord.

Localization of visceral pain is difficult. Afferent nerves from viscera to the spinal cord are relatively few in number and comprise only 2% to 15% of all afferents to the spinal cord.[344,345] These visceral nociceptive afferents can excite many second-order neurons in the spinal cord which in turn generate extensive divergence within the CNS, sometimes involving supraspinal loops. Such a divergent input activates several systems—sensory, motor, and autonomic—and thus triggers the general reactions that are characteristic of visceral nociception: a diffuse and referred pain and prolonged autonomic and motor activity.[340] The dorsal column in the spinal cord contains an ascending excitatory pathway that plays a crucial role in the perception of visceral pain, especially under the conditions of peripheral inflammation.[346] Activation of thalamic neurons by the dorsal column pathway, through a relay in the dorsal column nuclei, may be an important element in this mechanism. The dorsal column pathway may contain an ascending part of an amplification loop that enhances the responsiveness of spinal cord neurons through a descending facilitatory pathway, possibly originating in the rostroventral medulla.[347] This amplification circuit could lead to potentiation of the responses of different projection neurons, including spinothalamic and postsynaptic dorsal column neurons. The effectiveness of the midline myelotomy in visceral pain patients could thus be explained by a direct reduction in the activation of thalamic neurons mediated by postsynaptic dorsal column neurons as well as by an interruption of the amplification loop, thereby preventing the potentiation of the visceral responses of other projection neurons such as spinothalamic tract cells.

The origin of nociceptive impulses determines the site and type of pain. Visceral pain is either true, referred, nonreferred parietal, or referred parietal. True parietal abdominal pain is dull and poorly localized; it occurs in the region of the epigastric, periumbilical, or lower mid-abdominal region. Patients may describe the pain as gnawing or cramping, and often, it is associated with nausea, sweating, pallor, and, occasionally, vomiting. Referred visceral pain is more precisely localized, usually in the dermatomal or myosomal regions of the same segments of the spinal cord involved. Parietal pain may localize directly over the organ without referral. Patients locate referred parietal pain in a body region distant from the nociceptive site. For example, patients complain of pain in the shoulder area when the cause is inflammation of the middle diaphragm.

Tumor invasion of adjacent blood vessels can generate nociception. Mechanisms include perivascular lymphangitis causing vasospasm, occlusion with resultant ischemia, venous engorgement, and edema.

Obstruction of hollow viscera from tumor with resultant distention may cause pain. Distention causes intense contraction of smooth muscle that generates nociception. Patients experience visceral pain that is poorly localized and diffuse but usually localized in same dermatomal area of the cord segments of the viscera.

Pain from tumor involvement of parenchymal viscera such as liver, spleen, pancreas, and kidney typically results from acute distention of the pain-sensitive fascia. These fascia contain many mechanical receptors, and nociception occurs when they are acutely stretched or placed under tension. This type of pain is poorly defined, dull, and generally located in the dermatomal region of the involved organ. The properties of visceral pain are discussed in Chapters 61–65.

VISCERAL PAIN DESCRIPTIONS BY SITE

Esophageal cancer usually elicits a history of heartburn: a burning or gnawing substernal discomfort. Patients usually describe the pain as being located in the epigastric or retrosternal areas, which often radiates to the back or interscapular region. The pain occurs often after eating and possibly relates to body position changes such as reclining or bending forward.

Gastric pain has a colicky quality associated with delayed emptying and slowed motility and digestive symptoms. The pain also localizes in the epigastrium, is usually sharply focused, and may radiate into the back.

Small intestine pain is usually crampy or colicky and localized in the periumbilical area. The cause of pain is usually a lesion causing distention with resultant abnormal mobility. Eating usually precipitates the pain, and defecation or fasting may afford relief. *Colon* pain tends to occur in the lower abdomen, varying according to which portion of the colon is affected. Change in bowel habits and occult blood in the stool often accompanies symptoms of discomfort. *Peritoneal* carcinomatosis is frequently found with abdominal tumors and advanced ovarian cancer. Pain may result from peritoneal irritation, mesenteric involvement, and abdominal distention with ascites. Bowel obstruction often complicates peritoneal carcinomatosis.

Liver parenchyma is insensitive to tumor distention and associated chemical changes. Right upper quadrant pain from liver pathology occurs only when there is acute distention of the liver capsule. It is usually a dull, aching sensation in the right upper abdominal quadrant and flank and is often referred to the right scapula and shoulder.

Perineal pain, worse when sitting and with aching and pressure-like quality is the first and, can be for a long time, the only symptom of pelvic tumors. The pain may be associated with tenesmus. Fistulas and recurrent infections can aggravate the pain syndrome. Ureteral obstruction is frequent. Direct invasion of the sacrum, sacral roots, plexus, or cauda equina are frequent complications. Pain from the *fundus of the uterus* typically occurs in the hypogastrium. Pain originating from the *uterine cervix* is commonly referred to the low back and sacral area as well as to the hypogastrium. *Ovarian* pain results from stretching of the surrounding peritoneum to which the ovaries adhere.

Neuropathic Pain

The following are among the most common cancer pain syndromes that present with a major neuropathic component.

NEUROPATHIC PAIN SECONDARY TO CANCER-RELATED PATHOLOGY IN CRANIAL NERVES

Painful cranial neuralgias may occur secondary to base of skull metastases, LMs, or head and neck cancers.[348] Base of skull metastases produce several well-described pain syndromes[349] and are often associated with primary tumors of the breast, lung, and prostate. Constant localized aching pain from bone destruction and neurologic deficits from progressive cranial nerve palsies are cardinal manifestations. Orbital and parasellar syndromes were characterized by frontal headache, diplopia, and first-division trigeminal sensory loss. Proptosis may occur with the orbital syndrome. The middle-fossa syndrome was characterized by facial pain or numbness or dysesthetic neuropathic pain in the distribution of the second or third divisions of the trigeminal nerve. Associated motor deficits include weakness in the masseter or temporalis muscles or abducens palsy. The jugular foramen syndrome was characterized by hoarseness and dysphagia, with paralysis of the 9th through 11th cranial nerves and may present as glossopharyngeal neuralgia.[349] This pain is distributed over the ear or mastoid region and may radiate to the neck or shoulder. Associated deficits include a Horner syndrome and paresis of the palate, vocal cords, sternocleidomastoid muscle, or trapezius muscle. It is sometimes associated with syncope.[350] The occipital condyle syndrome was characterized by unilateral occipital pain and unilateral tongue paralysis with patients complaining of a continuous, severe, unilateral, occipital pain which kept them with the head rotated to the side of the pain and held with their hands[351] and occipital region pain typically preceding the hypoglossal paresis by several days to 10 weeks.[352]

Occipital condyle syndrome, clinically mimics classical trigeminal neuralgia, can occur secondary to tumors in the middle or posterior fossa.[353–356] Middle fossa tumors may present as trigeminal neuralgia but usually cause severe pain of an atypical nature and a progressive neurologic deficit. Trigeminal neuralgia secondary to tumor usually presents as a constant, dull, well-localized pain related to the underlying pathology involving bone and other somatic structures associated with paroxysmal episodes of lancinating or throbbing pain. A higher incidence of hypesthesia in the trigeminal nerve regions as well as a reduced corneal reflex was noted in patients with a mass lesion compared to those with vascular compression.[355] Posterior fossa tumors are most likely to cause trigeminal neuralgia and are usually accompanied by subtle neurologic deficits.[353] This association between trigeminal neuralgia and tumor is uncommon, and cancer patients with a new onset of trigeminal neuralgia should have careful imaging of the base of skull.

Cervical Plexopathy

Tumor infiltration of the cervical plexus can produce several pain syndromes, depending on the pattern of nerve involvement.[357] The upper four cervical ventral rami join to form the cervical plexus, which has both cutaneous and muscular branches. The plexus lies close to C1–C4 vertebrae. Cutaneous branches include the lesser occipital nerve which innervates lateral part of the occipital region; the great auricular nerve (innervates skin near auricle and external acoustic meatus); the transverse cervical nerve which innervates anterior region of the neck; and the supraclavicular nerves which innervate shoulder, suprascapularis, and upper thoracic region. The main contributor among muscular branches is ansa cervicalis. Because sensory afferents from the cervical plexus enter the spinal tract of the trigeminal along with the sensory afferents from cranial nerves V, VII, IX, and X, nociceptive referral patterns from the face and neck overlap. Symptoms usually include local pain with lancinating or dysesthetic components referred to the retroauricular and nuchal areas (lesser and greater auricular nerves), preauricular area (greater auricular nerve), anterior neck and shoulder (transverse cutaneous and supraclavicular nerves), and the jaw.[348] Associated findings may include ipsilateral Horner syndrome or hemidiaphragmatic paralysis. Due to the proximity to the cervical spine, CT or MRI evaluation may be necessary to rule out associated epidural cord compression. Common clinical settings include local extension of a head and neck tumor or cervical lymph node metastases. In patients with head and neck tumors who have undergone RND followed by radiation treatment, new onset or worsening pain includes a differential diagnosis of post-RND syndrome or tumor recurrence.

Tumor-Related Mononeuropathy

The most commonly described tumor-related painful mononeuropathy is intercostal nerve injury secondary to rib metastases with local extension. Patients with tumor invasion of the sciatic notch may present with symptoms resembling sciatica. Isolated mononeuropathies particularly from lymphomas are reported.[358–360]

Radicular Pain/Radiculopathy

Radiculopathy is compression of a nerve root. Frequent signs and symptoms include varying degrees of sensory, motor, and reflex changes as well as pain, dysesthesias, and paresthesias related to nerve root(s) without evidence of spinal cord dysfunction (which is myelopathy). Patients with radiculopathy may not have pain. Evaluation includes history and physical examination. Imaging modalities commonly used for evaluation include MRI, CT, and myelography. For lower extremity issues, the most commonly used physical tests include Lasègue test* straight leg raising or crossed straight leg raising; tendon reflexes; and signs of weakness, atrophy, or sensory deficits.[361] For cervical/upper extremity radiculopathy, Spurling test† is

---

*Lasègue test (straight leg maneuver) is performed when the clinician lifts the extended leg of a patient in a supine position. A positive response occurs when the pain pattern of the lumbar radiculopathy is reproduced. The test should be stopped when the pain is reproduced or maximum flexion is achieved. The crossed straight leg maneuver is performed by raising the unaffected leg in a similar manner to the straight leg test. The examiner looks for the reproduction of radicular pain with elevation of the opposite leg.
†Spurling test requires the examiner to patient extends the neck and rotates and laterally bends the head toward the symptomatic side; an axial compression force is then applied by the examiner through the top of the patient's head; the test is considered positive when the maneuver elicits the typical radicular arm pain.

a provocative maneuver suggestive of radiculopathy. Patients with cancer-related radiculopathy may present with pain on either or both sides of the midline. The pain tends to be unilateral in the cervical and lumbosacral regions and bilateral in the thorax. Radiculopathy may result from epidural tumor mass effects with encroachment on exiting nerve roots or LMs. Coughing, sneezing, recumbency, and strain exacerbate the pain, which often has dysesthetic qualities. Radiculopathy may also develop secondary to LMs. Clinically, LMs may produce multifocal neurologic signs and symptoms at a variety of levels, including cranial neuralgias.[362]

Leptomeningeal Metastases

LM is defined as the appearance of tumor cells in the leptomeninges or CSF distant from the site of a primary tumor. It is also known as carcinomatous meningitis, neoplastic meningitis, neoplastic meningosis, leukemic meningitis (for leukemia), lymphomatous meningitis (for lymphoma), and meningeal carcinomatosis (for carcinoma). This complication occurs most commonly with cancers of the breast and lung, melanoma, lymphomas, and acute lymphocytic leukemia with an estimated survival at 1 year of approximately 10% that varies with the primary tumor.[363] Clinical evaluation, MRI, and CSF assessment including cytology are the most important diagnostic measures.

Neurologic dysfunction most commonly involves one or more segments of the neuraxis, including cerebral hemispheres, cranial nerves, spinal cord, or spinal roots.[364] Clinical manifestations that strongly suggest the diagnosis of LM include cauda equina symptoms or signs, communicating hydrocephalus, and cranial neuropathies. Early in the disease, neurologic involvement can be subtle, such as an isolated diplopia or radicular pain. Cerebral hemisphere symptoms such as altered mental status or seizures may predominate.[364] Symptoms may also include headache, back and radicular pain, and multiple cranial and spinal nerve involvement. Pain may occur in 30% to 76% of cases.[365,366] Table 42.22 lists the frequency of spinal cord symptoms and signs in patients with LMs. The most common symptom is pain (80%), and patients may report a diffuse headache (25%) or pain in a spinal, radicular, or meningeal pattern (>50%). Localizing symptoms include cranial neuropathies, mononeuritis, radiculopathy, urinary incontinence, and visual disturbance.

Solid tumors have the propensity to adhere to neural structures and form nodules that become visible on MRI.[367] MRI appearances include the presence of subarachnoid nodules, leptomeningeal enhancement, nerve root enhancement, parenchymal disease (intramedullary metastases), and epidural metastases.[368] These changes may occur intracranially and along the spinal canal. T1-weighted gadolinium-enhanced sequence of the entire neuraxis (brain and spine) plays an important role in supporting the diagnosis, demonstrating the involved sites, and guiding treatment. MRI images typically show enhancing nodular lesions.

Nearly all patients have some abnormality of CSF opening pressure, protein, glucose, or cell count. The finding of tumor cells in CSF establishes a definitive diagnosis. In patients with hematologic cancers, CSF flow cytometry is more sensitive than CSF cytology and additionally requires a comparatively smaller volume of CSF (<2 mL) for analysis.[364]

Myelopathies in Cancer

Spinal cord involvement may occur by direct or indirect mechanisms. Direct mechanisms can be parenchymal (intradural intramedullary), subarachnoid (intradural extramedullary), or epidural (extradural). Intradural intramedullary involvement can result from metastases or a primary spinal cord tumor, intradural extramedullary may occur from leptomeningeal disease or primary tumors such as peripheral nerve sheath tumors or meningiomas, and extradural disease is primarily related from MESCC. Indirect mechanisms may result from radiation therapy (radiation myelitis)[369,370] and intrathecally administered chemotherapy resulting in spinal cord injury.[371,372] Paraneoplastic neurologic disorders may also result in indirect injury.

Brachial Plexopathy

The brachial plexus is formed from the C5–T1 ventral rami; the nerve roots pass between the anterior and middle scalene muscles with the subclavian artery to form the trunks. Trunks then split into anterior and posterior divisions, form cords, and travel with the subclavian artery and vein within the infraclavicular region. The cords form terminal branches at the lateral margin of the pectoralis minor muscle and continue through the axilla. Most tumors involving the brachial plexus originate from the lung or breast (Fig. 42.12 and Table 42.23). Clinical features result from either compression or tumor infiltration of the brachial plexus from contiguous structures, such as axillary/supraclavicular nodes or vascular structures. Neuropathic pain due to tumor infiltration of the brachial plexus usually stems from lymph node metastases from breast carcinoma or lymphoma or direct extension from lung carcinoma (i.e., Pancoast tumor). Lung cancers that occur in the apex of the chest and invade chest wall structures are called superior sulcus tumors or Pancoast tumors. The classical description of such patients involves a syndrome of pain radiating down the arm as a manifestation of brachial plexus involvement. A Pancoast tumor occurs when it invades any of the structures at the apex of the chest, including the most superior ribs or periosteum, the lower nerve roots of the brachial plexus, the sympathetic chain near the apex of the chest, or the subclavian vessels. These tumors are divided into anterior, middle, and posterior compartment tumors depending on the location of the chest wall involvement in relation to the insertions of the anterior and middle scalene muscles on the first rib. A syndrome of pain radiating down the arm is not a prerequisite for an apical tumor to be designated a Pancoast tumor.[373] However, patients may complain of severe pain in the shoulder radiating toward the axilla and/or scapula and along the ulnar distribution of the upper arm and demonstrate atrophy of hand and arm muscles with obstruction of the subclavian vein resulting in edema of the upper arm.

The key features of malignant plexopathy are the neuropathic nature of the pain, with numbness, paresthesias, allodynia, and hyperesthesias. Typically, the pain begins in the shoulder girdle where it is often described as pressure-like or aching and may radiate to the elbow, medial forearm, and fourth and fifth fingers. It may also appear to localize at the posterior arm or elbow. The patient may report a burning quality to the pain, with hyperesthesia along the ulnar aspect of the forearm. Involvement of the lower plexus occurs when tumor arises from the lung apex; associated pain and dysesthesias involve the elbow, medial forearm, and fourth and fifth fingers (C7, C8,

TABLE 42.22 Frequency of Spinal Cord Symptoms and Signs in Patients with Carcinomatous Meningitis	
Symptoms or Signs	**%**
Weakness	33
Paresthesia	31
Back pain	25
Radicular pain	19
Bowel/bladder dysfunction	13
Reflex asymmetry	67
Weakness	4
Cauda equina syndrome	33
Sensory loss	31
Positive straight leg raise	13
Decreased tone of anal sphincter	12
Nuchal rigidity	11

From Zachariah B, Zachariah SB, Varghese R, et al. Carcinomatous meningitis: clinical manifestations and management. *Int J Clin Pharmacol Ther* 1995;33(1):7–12. Reprinted by permission of Dustri-Verlag Dr. Karl Feistle GmbH & Co. KG.

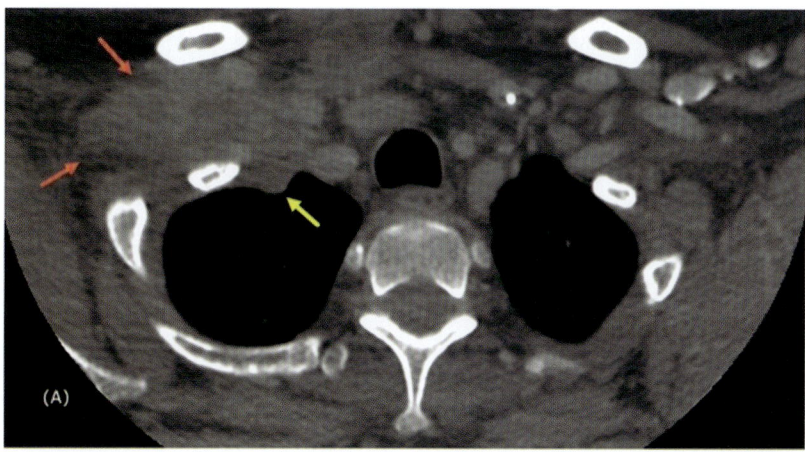

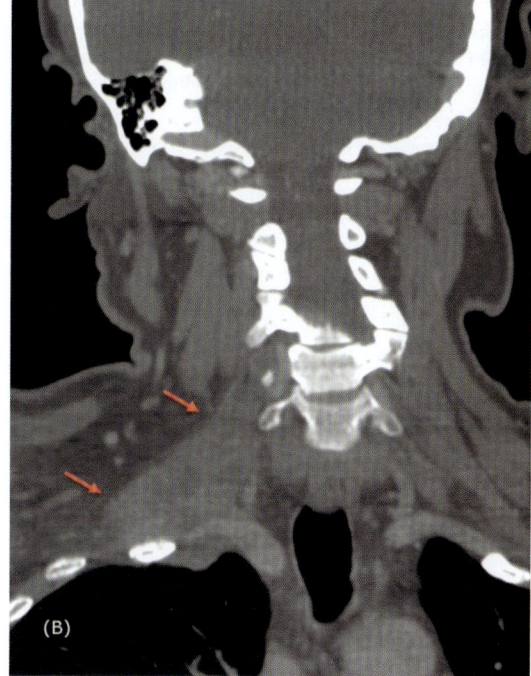

FIGURE 42.12 Computed tomography scan with contrast of patient with triple negative breast cancer involving the right brachial plexus. **A:** Axial view showing large mass encasing the brachial plexus at the infraclavicular level (*red arrows*). The mass also indents the lung (*yellow arrow*). **B:** Coronal view showing the mass the paraspinal muscles in proximity to transverse process from C5–T1 (*arrows*).

and T1). Upper plexus involvement (C5, C6), if it occurs alone, will usually develop into a panplexopathy. Upper plexus pain typically involves the shoulder girdle, with burning pain in the tips of both the index finger and thumb. Lung tumors can also present with pain involving the axilla and upper chest wall in the distribution of the intercostobrachial nerve.[374]

Neuroradiologic evaluations for brachial plexopathy are CT, PET/CT, and MRI. MRI is the preferred modality for imaging the brachial plexus. Most commonly, a combination of fat-suppressed T2-weighted (either frequency selective or short tau inversion recovery [STIR]) sequences and T1-weighted MR sequences are used.[375] FDG-PET scanning may also be useful in distinguishing between radiation-induced and metastatic plexopathy. Imaging the contiguous epidural space is recommended, particularly with paraspinal involvement. Electromyography (EMG) can also help distinguish malignant brachial plexopathy from radiation-induced brachial plexopathy (RBP) or cervical radiculopathy (Table 42.24). In patients with brachial plexopathy, EMG usually shows fibrillation potentials and positive waves (evidence of denervation) in affected muscles. RBP is discussed later.

Lumbosacral Plexopathy

The lumbosacral plexus is formed from the L1–L5 ventral rami with contributions from T12 and S1–S4. The lumbar roots emerge from the psoas major muscle, form anterior and posterior divisions, and finally form anterior and posterior

branches to innervate the muscles of the anterior and medial thigh. Anterior and posterior divisions also arise from the sacral roots and course over the sacral promontory posterolateral to the internal iliac vessels to form branches that innervate the muscles of the gluteal region, lateral and posterior thigh, and lower leg. The sciatic nerve exits the pelvis through the greater sciatic foramen usually below but sometimes dividing the piriformis muscle. Direct tumor infiltration from adjacent soft tissues or lymph nodes or by compression from metastases in the adjacent bony pelvis can damage the lumbosacral plexus. Most lumbosacral plexopathy reflects local extension or nodal metastases from colorectal and other pelvic tumors (cervix, uterus, bladder, prostate), sarcomas, and lymphomas, but it may also occur with metastases from breast or lung cancer.[376]

Complete plexopathy causes weakness, sensory loss, and flaccid loss of tendon reflexes in regions innervated by nerves in the L1–L4 distribution. Sacral plexopathy causes the same abnormalities in segments L5–S3, resulting in weakness and sensory loss in the gluteal (motor only), peroneal, and tibial nerve areas. The distribution of pain varies and may localize in the pelvis, low back or hip, or refer in a radicular or nonradicular pattern into the lower extremity. The local pain quality is pressure-like or aching. Referred pain varies with the site of plexus involvement and can be burning, cramping, or shooting. Sensory symptoms of numbness and paresthesias as well as weakness and leg edema usually develop. A "hot and dry foot" syndrome may result from lumbosacral plexopathy and may reflect sympathetic fiber dysfunction.[377] The most common clinical findings on examination include lower extremity weakness (86%), sensory loss (73%), reflex loss (64%), and leg edema (47%). Positive straight leg raising tests and sciatic notch tenderness are often present.[378]

Lumbosacral plexopathy may cause different clinical syndromes depending on the level of nerve involvement. Infiltration of the upper plexus occurs in approximately one-third of patients, who present with pain in the back, lower abdomen, flank, iliac crest, or anterolateral thigh. This syndrome has associated L1–L4 distribution neurologic deficits. Involvement of the lower plexus occurs in approximately one half of patients, and these present with pain in the buttocks and perineum, with referral to the posterolateral leg and thigh. Examination may reveal associated L4–S1 neurologic deficits, leg edema, and

TABLE 42.23 Frequency of Tumor-Associated Plexopathy by Location	
Brachial Plexus Tumors	**Lumbosacral Plexus Tumors**
Lung 37%	Colorectal 20%
Breast 32%	Sarcoma 16%
Lymphoma 8%	Breast 11%
Sarcoma 5%	Lymphoma 9%
All others 18%	Cervix 7%
	All others 37%

From Jaeckle KA. Neurologic manifestations of neoplastic and radiation-induced plexopathies. *Semin Neurol* 2010;30(3):254–262. Copyright © Georg Thieme Verlag KG.

TABLE 42.24 Differentiating Features of Brachial Plexopathy Induced by Tumor Infiltration, Radiation Fibrosis, and Reversible Radiation Injury

	Tumor Infiltration	Radiation Fibrosis	Reversible Radiation Injury
Incidence of pain	89%	18%	40%
Typical location of pain	Shoulder, upper arm, elbow, radiating to fourth and fifth fingers	Shoulder, wrist, hand	Hand, forearm
Nature of pain	Dull aching in shoulder; Lancinating pain in elbow and ulnar aspect of hand; Occasional dysesthesias, burning, or freezing sensations	Aching shoulder pain; Paresthesias in C5, C6 distribution in hand	Aching shoulder pain; Paresthesias in hand and forearm
Severity of pain	Moderate to severe (severe in 98% of patients)	Mild to moderate (severe in 35% of patients)	Mild
Course	Progressive neurologic dysfunction; atrophy and weakness with C7–T1 distribution; persistent pain; Horner syndrome	Progressive weakness with C5, C6 distribution; stabilizing pain with appearance of weakness	Transient weakness and atrophy affecting C6–C7, T1; complete resolution of motor findings
CT scan findings	Circumscribed mass with diffuse infiltration of tissue planes	Diffuse infiltration of tissue planes	Normal
EMG findings	Segmental slowing; no myokymia	Myokymia	Segmental slowing; no myokymia

CT, computed tomography; EMG, electromyography.
Modified from Foley KM. Brachial plexopathy in patients with breast cancer. In: Harris JR, Hellman S, Henderson IC, et al, eds. *Breast Diseases*. Philadelphia: JB Lippincott Co; 1987.

bowel or bladder dysfunction. Sacral plexopathy can signal direct bony extension of a bony sacral lesion or a presacral mass. Numbness of the dorsal medial foot and sole with associated weakness of knee flexion, ankle dorsiflexion, and inversion is typical of lumbosacral trunk extension. Involvement of the coccygeal plexus results in sphincter dysfunction and perineal sensory loss. Panplexopathy occurs in one-fifth of patients, and pain may refer anywhere in the territory of the plexus. Associated leg edema is relatively common.[377]

Jaeckle et al.[379] studied 85 cancer patients with lumbosacral plexopathy and documented pelvic tumor by CT or biopsy. They discerned three clinical syndromes: lower (L4–S1), 51%; upper (L1–L4), 31%; and panplexopathy (L1–S3), 18%. Seventy percent of patients had the insidious onset of pelvic or radicular leg pain, followed weeks to months later by sensory symptoms and weakness. The quintet of leg pain, weakness, edema, rectal mass, and hydronephrosis suggests plexopathy due to cancer. CT showed pelvic tumor in 96%. On myelography, epidural extension, usually below the conus medullaris, occurs in 45%. With treatment, only 28% of patients had objective responses on CT and 17% on examination.

In previously treated patients, the main differential diagnostic consideration is radiation-induced plexopathy (see in the following discussion). MRI is the choice for the diagnostic workup of patients with clinical and electrophysiologic evidence of plexopathy and suspected systemic cancer. Studies should include the L1 vertebral body through to the true pelvis. Neurologic findings include leg weakness, sensory loss, reflex asymmetry, focal tenderness (in the lumbar region in an upper plexopathy, sciatic notch and sacrum in a lower plexopathy, and lumbosacral region in panplexopathy), rectal mass, decreased sphincter tone, and positive direct and reverse straight leg raising signs.

Tumor Infiltration of the Sacrum and Sacral Nerves

Pain in a sacral distribution occurs usually as a result of the spread of bladder, gynecologic, or colonic cancer. There is dull aching midline pain and usually burning or throbbing pain in the soft tissues of the rectal or perineal region. Sitting or lying usually exacerbates the pain. With bilateral involvement, sphincter incontinence and impotence are common. There may be tenderness over the sacrum and in the regions of the sciatic notches. Sometimes there is limitation of both direct and reverse straight leg raise exam maneuvers. Involvement of S1 and S2 roots will produce weakness of ankle plantar flexion, and

the ankle jerks may be absent. There is usually sensory loss in the perianal region and in the genitalia, and this may be accompanied by hyperpathia.

Spinal and Radicular Pain

Patients perceive radicular pain as arising in a limb or trunk wall. The cause is ectopic activation of nociceptive afferent fibers in a spinal nerve or its roots or other neuropathic mechanisms. The pain is lancinating in quality and travels along a narrow band. It may be episodic, recurrent, or paroxysmal according to the causative lesion or any superimposed aggravating factors. Although patients may experience radicular pain as a deep tissue pain, it also has a cutaneous quality in proportion to the number of cutaneous afferent fibers ectopically activated. Radicular pain differs from nociception in the axons stimulated along their course; their peripheral terminals are not the sites of stimulation. Ectopic activation may occur as a result of mechanical deformation of a dorsal root ganglion, mechanical stimulation of previously damaged nerve roots, inflammation of a dorsal root ganglion, and possibly by ischemic damage to the DRG. Acute spine pain may be described as cramping or knifelike but may also be merely dull or aching. It is worse with movement. Chronic spine pain without a radicular component is generally aching, dull, or burning, or any combination of these three features. It also tends to be made worse with movement.

Central Pain Syndromes Caused by Cancer

Central pain syndromes are relatively infrequent in the cancer population. Although epidural spinal cord compression is almost always painful, central pain is not the predominant symptom; nociceptive input from progressive bony destruction by metastases is the usual cause of pain, with or without concurrent radicular pain from nerve root compression. Radiation myelopathy is also a possible cause of central pain syndrome.

Paraneoplastic Peripheral Neuropathy

Paraneoplastic syndrome refers to a group of disorders (caused by, or associated with, cancers) that are neither direct effects of the primary tumor mass nor metastatic to the involved organs. Various antibodies discovered in paraneoplastic syndromes target proteins shared by both the tumor cells and neurons.[380] Antibodies directed against neural antigens expressed by tumor (onconeural antibodies) may occur in most of those affected by classical paraneoplastic syndromes, suggesting that an autoimmune process underlies these disorders. In patients with anti-Hu antibodies, infiltration by T cells is seen in the peripheral and the CNS.[381] Clinically significant peripheral neuropathy in cancer patients is common, but only a small minority is paraneoplastic in origin. These disorders can affect virtually any portion of the nervous system. Peripheral nerves are a common target in paraneoplastic syndromes.[211] SSN is a classical paraneoplastic syndrome.[212] The neuropathy generally develops subacutely, accompanied by pain and rapidly progressive paresthesia. Involvement of the upper extremities may occur with asymmetric sensory deficit or multifocal with facial, thoracic, and abdominal involvement. Many patients with SSN also have signs and symptoms suggestive of multifocal involvement including areas of the CNS. Paraneoplastic vasculitis of the peripheral nervous system usually precedes the tumor diagnosis and presents as multineuritis or asymmetric distal sensory-motor neuropathy with pain as a commonly reported symptom. This form is generally associated with lymphoma or cancer at various sites (lung, prostate, uterus, kidney, or gastric).[213] Four types of polyneuropathy constitute most of the cases of paraneoplastic peripheral neuropathy: motor, sensory, sensorimotor, and autonomic. Most paraneoplastic peripheral neuropathies are sensorimotor and axonal. A pure sensory neuronopathy (i.e., pathology in the dorsal root ganglion) strongly suggests a paraneoplastic syndrome associated with the anti-Hu antibody. A pure motor neuropathy subacutely developing could be the Guillain-Barré syndrome associated with Hodgkin disease or a multifocal motor neuropathy with conduction block associated with plasma cell dyscrasias. An autonomic neuropathy is sometimes associated with the anti-Hu syndrome. Paraneoplastic disorders of the autonomic nervous system usually arise in the setting of encephalomyelitis. However, autonomic symptoms may predominate or rarely be the only symptoms or signs of a paraneoplastic neuropathy. The most common symptom is pseudo-obstruction of the bowel, but anhidrosis, orthostatic hypotension, hypoventilation, sleep apnea, and cardiac arrhythmias can also present either alone or, more commonly, as part of a more widespread autonomic neuropathy. Most autonomic neuropathies are associated with SCLC and the anti-Hu syndrome. Mononeuritis multiplex suggests a vasculitis, possibly paraneoplastic in origin. The classic paraneoplastic polyneuropathy is sensory neuronopathy. Typically, patients with this disorder initially have an asymmetrical and painful sensory neuropathy, which evolves into complete loss of proprioception. The pseudoathetotic movement of the hands and severe sensory ataxia is very severe in most cases. Motor neuropathies may be acute or chronic, progressive or remitting, demyelinating, axonal, or neuronal. Clinically, they are indistinguishable from the more common nonparaneoplastic motor neuropathies, unless they resolve after treatment of the cancer or are associated with a paraneoplastic antibody. These disorders include the Guillain-Barré syndrome, which occurs more frequently in patients with Hodgkin's disease than in the general population; a remitting and relapsing polyneuropathy resembling relapsing chronic inflammatory demyelinating polyneuropathy; and a subacute motor neuronopathy affecting patients with Hodgkin's disease or other lymphomas. The sensory neuropathies include a subacute pan-sensory neuropathy and a predominantly distal sensory neuropathy. Paraneoplastic vasculitis neuropathy may occur in malignancy (solid tumors including gastric cancer), and the presentation is similar to connective tissue-related vasculitic neuropathy with a painful, asymmetrical polyneuropathy or mononeuritis multiplex pattern.[380]

Paraneoplastic peripheral neuropathies are important because they may be the first sign of an otherwise occult cancer and/or because they may substantially disable the patient even when the cancer itself is asymptomatic. In about two-thirds of cases, patients with paraneoplastic neurologic disorders present to the neurologist without a known tumor.

Polyneuropathy, organomegaly, endocrinopathy, myeloma protein, and skin changes (POEMS) syndrome is a paraneoplastic syndrome due to an underlying plasma cell neoplasm. The major criteria for the syndrome are polyradiculoneuropathy, clonal plasma cell disorder (PCD), sclerotic bone lesions, elevated VEGF, and the presence of Castleman disease. Minor features include organomegaly, endocrinopathy, characteristic skin changes, papilledema, extravascular volume overload, and thrombocytosis. POEMS syndrome should be distinguished from the Castleman disease variant of POEMS syndrome, which has no clonal PCD and typically little to no peripheral neuropathy but has several of the minor diagnostic criteria for POEMS syndrome.[382]

NEUROPATHIC PAIN SECONDARY TO THERAPEUTIC INTERVENTIONS

Many pain syndromes occur in the course of or subsequent to treatment of cancer with surgery, chemotherapy, or radiation therapy. In most cases, there is injury to the peripheral nervous system or spinal cord, with pain as a major and often presenting complaint. In some cases, these syndromes occur long after the therapy is implemented, resulting in a difficult differential diagnosis between recurrent disease and a complication of therapy.

Postsurgical Neuropathic Pain

1. *Postmastectomy*: Pain can be a prominent postsurgical finding in breast cancer patients. It tends to appear in the postmastectomy period, a consequence of the disruption of normal neural pathways, or it may follow the development of lymphedema or the presence of metastases. In most situations, however, pain occurs primarily as a result of persistent restrictions in range of motion of the shoulder girdle in the region of surgery with findings of tender or trigger points in the associated muscle groups suggesting a nonneuropathic source that is misdiagnosed as neuropathic. The IASP defines postmastectomy pain syndrome as persistent pain soon after mastectomy/lumpectomy affecting the anterior thorax, axilla, and/or medial upper arm,[383] but patients may experience persistent postsurgical pain affecting one or more regions involving the scar, breast, chest wall, shoulder, and upper arm with an incidence ranging from 25% to 80%.[384] Chronic neuropathic pain with inherent sensory changes and somatosensory disturbances may overlap with persistent postsurgical pain, and definitive diagnosis can be challenging.

   Chronic pain after mastectomy may occur in patients whose surgery included axillary dissection, although the problem can occur in women who undergo any surgical procedure on the breast from lumpectomy to radical mastectomy. Postaxillary dissection pain is probably a more appropriate name than the usual postmastectomy pain for this syndrome. A neuropathic pain pattern typically involves paroxysms of lancinating pain against a background of burning, aching, tight constriction in the axilla, medial upper arm, and/or chest. Hyperesthesia, dysesthesia, hyperalgesia, allodynia, or hypoesthesia in the intercostobrachial nerve distribution may occur.[385] The exact cause is unclear, but various theories include dissection of the intercostobrachial nerve, intraoperative damage to axillary nerve pathways, and pain caused by neuroma formation. The intercostobrachial nerve is a cutaneous sensory branch of T1 and T2. The nerve is highly variable in size and distribution, making it difficult to avoid in these surgical procedures. Usually, the pain develops shortly after surgery, but it can emerge months after surgery. Late onset should prompt a search for other causes such as recurrent chest wall disease or bone metastases. Postmastectomy pain syndrome differs from metastatic or RBP in which there is a different pattern of sensory loss, lymphedema, and, usually, more severe pain.

2. *Neck dissection*: Head and neck cancer encompasses tumors of the upper aerodigestive tract and the skin of the region. Surgical management may include the removal of lymph nodes from the neck and is referred to as a neck dissection. A large spectrum of surgical procedures is available for treatment of cervical lymph nodes.[386] These may be classified as RND, extended RND, modified RND, and selective neck dissection. RND for head and neck cancers can result in an iatrogenic syndrome characterized by ipsilateral face and neck pain with associated paresthesias. Pain usually emerges weeks to months after surgery, consequent to injury to the cervical plexus or cervical nerves.[348] The most relevant functional sequel from RND is impairment of shoulder function due to sectioning the spinal accessory nerve and to the ensuing denervation of the upper trapezius muscle. Sacrifice of the spinal accessory nerve during RND is considered a critical factor in determining postoperative shoulder function. Injury to the nerve and subsequent denervation of the trapezius muscle reduces capacity to elevate the shoulder girdle (scapular dyskinesia) and has been associated with patient reported shoulder pain and functional loss.[387] Patients who undergo a nerve-sparing procedure (i.e., selective neck dissection or a modified RND) exhibit significantly better shoulder function than did patients who undergo RNDs.[388] In patients treated for head and neck cancer, neck dissection was considered a risk factor for the development of MPS.[389] Neck dissection was a predictive factor for reduced sensitivity in the neck, reduced range of motion of the neck, and MPS was strongly related to shoulder pain.[390]

Nahum et al.[391] coined the term "shoulder syndrome" to describe a clinical picture consisting of pain and limited abduction of the shoulder, full passive range of motion, and anatomic deformities such as scapular flaring, droop, and protraction. Pain is attributed to strain placed on other supporting muscles, such as the rhomboids and levator scapulae, as a consequence of shoulder drooping. A frequent ancillary sign of shoulder syndrome is sternoclavicular joint hypertrophy, due to the abnormal torque-like forces applied to the medial head of the clavicle, potentially complicated by stress fracture of the middle third of the clavicle. Recurrent tumor can also be a cause of pain that occurs or escalates after neck dissection.

3. *Postthoracotomy pain*: Most surgical procedures can potentially cause persistent pain which last months or years, and breast surgery (including interventions for breast cancer, augmentation, and reduction) and thoracic surgery (including open thoracotomies, video-assisted thoracoscopic surgery [VATS], sternotomies) are two with the highest reported prevalence (31% and 34%, respectively) with the prevalence of probable or definite neuropathic pain being approximately 66%.[392] Shortly following thoracotomy, a neuropathic pain can develop in the distribution of one or several intercostal nerves near the thoracotomy scar.[392,393] The pain may remain stable after onset and gradually decreases over a period of months or years. Hetmann et al.[394] noted in patients who underwent thoracotomies by an open posterolateral technique that the presence of preoperative pain was a predominant predictor for persistent pain 12 months after the procedure. Persistent postsurgical pain following anterior thoracotomy occurred in 19% of lung cancer patients for up to 10 years postoperatively.[395] Steegers et al.[396] noted the prevalence of chronic pain was 40% after thoracotomy and 47% after VATS. Definite chronic neuropathic pain was present in 23% of the patients with chronic pain, with an additional 30% having probable neuropathic pain. The probability of neuropathic pain correlated with more intense chronic pain and

predictive factors for chronic pain were younger age, radiation therapy, pleurectomy, and more extensive surgery. Pain is most profound around the scar, as 82% to 90% of pain patients relate their pain directly to the surgical site[397,398] and is primarily described as aching, tender, with numbness, and to a lesser degree burning.[399] Guastella et al.[400] noted in patient who underwent a lateral/posterolateral thoracotomy for cancer that the clinical picture in most patients with neuropathic pain included electric shocks and severe multimodal hypoesthesia in the sensory area of fifth/sixth intercostal nerves. Patients may also have higher depression and anxiety scores and lower self-rated health and demonstrate more evoked pain to mechanical stimuli and in particular to pinprick hyperalgesia.[401]

In my experience, many patients experience chronic pain in the shoulder girdle region following thoracic surgical procedures not primarily from intercostal nerve damage but from a persistent inability to normally range the shoulder girdle region. In effect, these patients demonstrate persistent myofascial tenderness in the muscles of the shoulder girdle region (pectorals, trapezius, rhomboids, and deltoid).

4. *Phantom pains*: After amputation, patients may experience phantom sensations (including temperature changes, itching, tingling) and/or phantom pain. Phantom pain is typically associated with amputation of limbs but may follow the amputation or loss of many body parts including the eyes,[402] teeth,[403] tongue,[404] nose,[405] breast,[406] genitals,[407] or parts of the gastrointestinal tract.[408,409] The onset is within 1 week after amputation in the majority of patients, with 50% of patients experiencing pain within 24 hours after amputation.[410,411] Phantom pain should be distinguished from residual limb pain that is localized to the residual limb. Patients may report that phantom sensations are present all the time and that phantom limb pain is intermittent with short episodes (lasting only seconds or minutes) of pain (often severe) which can occur several times a day. Patients may also report "telescoping" of their phantom which is a sensation in which the body of the limb shortens into the stump often completely, leaving the sensation of hands or feet very close to the stump.

Phantom pain disables a significant number of patients undergoing amputation of different body parts for malignancy.[412] Two years after mastectomy, the percentage of patients with phantom breast sensations was stable around 20%, and those with phantom breast pain reduced from 7% in the first year to 1%.[413] Phantom rectal sensation (including pain) occurs in up to 18% of patients after surgery for rectal carcinoma.[414] The reappearance or worsening of pain a long while after amputation can indicate tumor recurrence.

Radiation Myelopathy, Plexopathy, and Neuropathy

Tolerance of nervous system tissues to radiation therapy depends on several factors such as volume, total dose, dose per fraction, duration of irradiation, prior radiation, concomitant neurotoxic chemotherapy, and genetic susceptibility.[415] Radiation treatment may cause pain by damage to peripheral nerves or spinal cord by altering the microvascular of connective tissue surrounding peripheral nerves, via fibrosis and chronic inflammation in connective tissues, or bringing about demyelination and focal necrosis of the white and gray matter in the spinal cord. Typically, these changes occur late in the course of a patient's illness. The differential diagnosis should always include recurrent tumor. In most instances, pain is a component of the clinical picture, but it is rarely as severe as that associated with recurrent tumor. Myelopathy is a devastating late effect of radiation treatment and if the spinal cord dose does not exceed a total of 45 to 50 Gy in 1.8 to 2 Gy daily fractions, the risk of permanent injury is very low, estimated from 0.03% to 0.2%.[416] The pathologic findings of radiation-induced progressive myelopathy may include demyelination, focal necrosis and axonal loss, and vascular abnormalities such as telangiectasias, endothelial swelling with fibrin exudates, hyaline degeneration, thickening and fibrinoid necrosis of vessel walls with perivascular fibrosis, and sometimes vasculitis.[417] Early delayed radiation myelopathy occurs from 6 weeks to 6 months after treatment, and improvement follows in most cases within 2 to 9 months, although in some instances, symptoms may persist for prolonged periods. The cervical and thoracic spinal cord is the most commonly involved. Clinical signs are generally limited to a Lhermitte's sign.[‡] The spinal cord MRI is usually normal. Transient demyelination, probably resulting from radiation injury of oligodendrocytes, is likely the main pathogenic mechanism of early delayed myelopathy.[418] Late-delayed radiation-induced spinal cord disorders complications include progressive myelopathy and spinal hemorrhage. Progressive myelopathy or delayed radiation myelopathy may follow radiation treatment by 6 months to approximately 10 years. Risk factors include older age, previous irradiation (incidental or medical) particularly during childhood, large radiation port involving the dorsal or lumbar spinal cord, and large radiation dose and fractions. The clinical onset of delayed radiation myelopathy may be acute, but it is more often progressive. Patients can present with para- or tetraparesis with rapid development of sensory and/or motor deficits. The development of a Brown-Séquard syndrome[**] is a classic presentation. Another possible presentation is an ascending transverse myelopathy with bilateral leg weakness and sensory loss up to the level of irradiation. Patients may develop bladder or bowel dysfunction; pain has been occasionally reported. The involvement of the upper cervical spinal cord can cause diaphragm dysfunction. The course of symptoms is difficult to predict; some patients improve and others deteriorate. Despite its lack of specificity, MRI findings are important. Other potential causes of myelopathy should be carefully investigated.

Neuropathic syndromes associated with chest wall/axillary radiation therapy include brachial plexopathy, malignant peripheral nerve tumors, nerve entrapment in a lymphedematous shoulder, and ischemia. Both early onset and late-onset brachial plexopathy occur. Clinically, the plexopathy involves mixed sensory and motor deficits, with or without pain.

Most reports of radiation-induced plexopathy involve the brachial plexus and, although much less common, radiation-induced injury of the lumbosacral plexus has also been reported.[419] The risk of RBP from conventionally fractionated radiotherapy (i.e., 5,000 cGy in 200-Gy fractions) is <1% and when the dose per fraction increases to between 2,200 and 4,580 cGy with a total dose of 4,350 and 6,000 Gy, the risk of brachial plexus injury increases to 1.7% to 73%.[420] Olsen et al.[421] described the incidence and latency period of RBP in 79 patients with breast cancer. Thirty-five percent of patients developed RBP. Fifty percent had involvement of the entire plexus, 18% of the upper plexus alone, 4% of the lower plexus alone, and a definite level of involvement could not be determined in 28% of patients. RBP began in most patients either during or immediately after radiation treatment. RBP was more common in patients who received combination treatment with chemotherapy and radiation than with radiation alone. Clinically, plexopathy presents with subjective paresthesia or dysesthesia and progresses with the development of hypesthesia then anesthesia. Neuropathic pain is generally considered rare and moderate in intensity. Motor weakness is progressive, often delayed by several months, and then associated with fasciculations and amyotrophy.[221] Zeidman et al.[422] estimate that up to 20% of patients with radiation-induced plexopathy may report severe pain. Mondrup at al.[423] noted that the most prominent symptoms for RBP were numbness or paresthesia (71%) and pain (41%), whereas the most prominent objective signs were decreased or absent muscle stretch reflexes (93%) closely followed by sensory loss (82%) and weakness (71%). The neurologic deficits are relentlessly progressive and ultimately result in a useless limb. In contrast to malignant infiltration, patients with radiation injury to the plexus tend to have abnormal sensory and normal motor nerve conduction studies and characteristically manifest more fasciculations or myokymia on EMG than patients with neoplastic disease.[424]

Radiation induced of the lumbosacral plexus has been reported after intracavitary radium implants for carcinoma of the cervix.[425] Paresthesias, distal weakness progressing proximally, but rarely pain occur in the lower extremities 2 to 3 months after radiation of the sacral plexus.[426] Weakness commences distally in the L5–S1 segments and slowly progresses.[427] Painless, indolent leg weakness occurs early in radiation disease, whereas pain with or without unilateral weakness usually characterizes tumor plexopathy. Radiation disease often results in serious neurologic disability.

The diagnosis of radiation plexopathy can be supported by various studies. Approximately 60% of patients with radiation-induced plexopathy will show myokymia[††] on EMG.[428] MRI imaging of the plexus is also helpful. Enhancement of nerve roots and T2-weighted hyperintensity usually suggests tumor; generally, radiation plexopathy does not produce nerve enhancement, MRI appearances for RBP are isointense of hypointense relative to muscle on T2-weighted images and thus distinguishable from tumor infiltration which is usually hyperintense,[429] although increase in T2 signal may be present.[430] PET/CT scanning is also helpful in distinguishing tumor from radiation changes.[431] Features distinguishing radiation plexopathy from neoplastic plexopathy are listed in Table 42.24.

Chemotherapy-Induced Peripheral Neuropathy

Drug-induced neurotoxicity can affect nerve fibers or neuronal bodies (generally the DRG of the primary sensory neurons). Among the toxicities associated with chemotherapy, damage of the peripheral nervous system is particularly frequent and potentially severe. CIPN causes numerous debilitating symptoms, impairs functional capacity, and results in dose reductions or possible cessation of chemotherapy. CIPN is a predominantly sensory neuropathy that may be accompanied by motor and autonomic changes. The drugs most commonly reported to cause CIPN include the platinum-based drugs (particularly oxaliplatin and cisplatin), the vinca alkaloids (particularly vincristine and vinblastine), the epothilones (ixabepilone), the taxanes (paclitaxel, docetaxel), the proteasome inhibitors (bortezomib), and immunomodulatory drugs (thalidomide) (Table 42.25). The prevalence of CIPN is 68% in the first month after starting chemotherapy, 60% at 3 months, and 30% at 6 months or more with different drugs were associated with differences in CIPN prevalence.[432]

The clinical manifestations of CIPN are frequently predominantly subjective and manifest as pure sensory symptoms and are most commonly reported as progressive distal symmetrically distributed symptoms of numbness, tingling, pins and needles, burning, decreased or altered sensation, or increased sensitivity

---

[‡]Short, unpleasant sensation of numbness, tingling, and often electric-like discharge going down from the neck to the spine and extremities, triggered by neck flexion.

[**]Brown-Séquard syndrome results in ipsilateral pyramidal deficit and posterior column signs and, contralaterally, loss of spinothalamic function.

[††]Myokymia represents spontaneous discharges accompanied by wave-like muscle quivering.

TABLE 42.25 Summary of the Most Frequent Symptoms and Signs Associated with the Administration of Commonly Used Chemotherapy Drugs

Class	Drug	Symptoms/Signs
Platinum	Cisplatin (carboplatin)	• Distal, symmetric, upper and lower limb impairment/loss of all sensory modalities • Large myelinated fibers are more severely involved so that sensory ataxia and gait imbalance are frequent. • Early reduction/loss of DTR • Coasting phenomenon is frequent. • Carboplatin is generally much less neurotoxic than cisplatin.
	Oxaliplatin	*Acute* • Cold-induced transient paresthesias in mouth, throat, and limb extremities • Cramps/muscle spasm in throat muscle • Jaw spasm *Chronic* • Similar to cisplatin
Vinca alkaloids	Vincristine	• Distal, symmetric, upper and lower limb and impairment/loss of all sensory modalities • Reduction/loss of DTR • Neuropathic pain/paresthesia at limb extremities is relatively frequent. • Distal, symmetric weakness in lower limbs progressing to foot drop • Autonomic symptoms may be severe (e.g., orthostatic hypotension, constipation, paralytic ileus)
Epothilones	Ixabepilone, sagopilone	Similar to taxanes, but neuropathic pain is less frequent and recovery is reported to be faster
Antitubulin	Taxanes (paclitaxel, docetaxel)	• Distal, symmetric, upper and lower limb impairment/loss of all sensory modalities • Gait unsteadiness is possible due to proprioceptive loss. • Reduction/loss of DTR • Neuropathic pain/paresthesia at limb extremities is relatively frequent. • "Myalgia syndrome" is frequent, possible expression of atypical neuropathic pain. • Distal, symmetric weakness in lower limbs is generally mild.
Proteasome inhibitors	Bortezomib	• Mild to moderate, distal symmetric loss of all sensory modalities. Small myelinated and unmyelinated fibers are markedly affected leading to severe neuropathic pain. • Reduction/loss of DTR • Mild distal weakness in lower limbs is possible.
Immunomodulatory	Thalidomide	• Mild to moderate, distal symmetric loss of all sensory modalities • Reduction/loss of DTR • Relatively frequent neuropathic pain at limb extremities • Weakness is rare. • More neurotoxic than lenalidomide or pomalidomide

NOTE: Coasting is worsening of neuropathy signs/symptoms over months after drug withdrawal.
DTR, deep tendon reflex.
Modified from Cavaletti G. Chemotherapy-induced peripheral neurotoxicity (CIPN): what we need and what we know. *J Peripher Nerv Syst* 2014;19:66–76.

that may be painful in the feet and hands. The primary clinical objective in assessing patients is to determine the presence and severity of CIPN-associated symptoms that result in interference with activities of daily living because this finding is critical for treatment decisions. Symptoms of motor weakness due to CIPN are less commonly reported and when present are observed in patients with more persistent and severe sensory findings. If the patient has coexisting diabetes, it can be quite difficult to differentiate the onset or progression of diabetic neuropathy from CIPN, which may be mitigated in some instances if the physician has carefully evaluated and recorded the patient's baseline neurologic findings and symptoms prior to initiation of the neurotoxic chemotherapy. Diabetic neuropathy can be asymmetrical or symmetrical, focal or diffuse, or manifests as mononeuritis multiplex in its involvement and has many different clinical forms. The most common form of diabetic neuropathy, distal symmetrical polyneuropathic form, has clinical symptoms similar to CIPN.

The most commonly observed clinical findings of CIPN are symmetrical progressive onset of the following sensory symptoms and findings in a stocking-glove distribution: paresthesias, hyperesthesias, hypoesthesias, and dysesthesias, which more commonly appear earlier and with more pronounced symptoms in the toes and feet, with later involvement of the fingers and hands. Concurrent loss of deep tendon reflexes (loss of distal usually earlier than proximal) in the affected extremities with sensory deficits is an important diagnostic sign associated with greater neurosensory damage. Sensory findings, including diminished or absent proprioception, vibration, touch, two-point discrimination, sharp/dull discrimination, temperature,

and touch/pain are typically diminished in the stocking-glove distribution in symptomatic patients (Table 42.25).

CIPN has a high degree of similarity in the pattern and spectrum of clinical manifestations caused by different chemotherapeutic agents (e.g., vinca alkaloids, platinum agents, thalidomide, bortezomib, and taxanes), which includes the length-dependent, symmetrical stocking-glove distribution with predominantly sensory symptoms noted by the patient. CIPN generally arises as a consequence of the disruption of axoplasmic microtubule-mediated transport, distal axonal (wallerian) degeneration, and direct damage to the sensory nerve cell bodies of the DRG. Demyelination (diffuse or segmental) secondary to chemotherapy is an uncommon finding (but occasionally observed with cisplatin), and when observed, it is typically a secondary and isolated finding relative to the extent of axonal and DRG pathologic findings. It is important to recognize that CIPN commonly follows the administration of chemotherapeutic agents that cannot appreciably distribute across the blood–brain barrier (e.g., taxanes, platinum agents, vinca alkaloids, thalidomide, and bortezomib). CIPN is commonly characterized as a distal axonopathy,[‡‡] less commonly as a neuronopathy,[***] and may simultaneously manifest with both forms in some patients. To improve accurate and reliable reporting of chemotherapy-induced neuropathy, various grading systems have been developed.[433] Table 42.7 is an example of a grading scale for evaluation of CIPN.

[‡‡]An abnormality in peripheral nerve function resulting in degeneration of the terminal regions of sensory axons and also to motor axons.
[***]The result of direct toxic damage of neuronal cells in the DRG.

ORAL MUCOSITIS

Ulcerative lesions in the mucosa of patients undergoing chemo- or radiation therapy characterize oral mucositis. Oral lesions can result in dysphagia, dysarthria, and odynophagia. Patients may complain of oral burning or severe pain that may disrupt oral intake resulting in parenteral or enteral nutritional supplementation. The risk of oral mucositis increases as a function of the type of cancer therapy used, with the lowest risk occurring with "gentler" chemotherapeutics such as gemcitabine (Gemzar) and the higher risk occurring with more aggressive agents such as 5-fluorouracil (5-FU) and cisplatin and/or radiation therapy.[434] It may drastically affect cancer treatment as well as the patient's QOL. The incidence and severity of mucositis has both interpatient and treatment variability. It is estimated that there is 40% incidence of mucositis in patients treated with standard chemotherapy, and this will increase not only with the number of treatment cycles but also with previous episodes.[435] Oral mucositis is one of the most frequent adverse effects of allogenic or autologous hematopoietic stem cell transplant with 67% to 80% developing a severe grade of mucositis particularly with allogenic transplants.[436,437] The overall incidence of oral mucositis and xerostomia is approximately 80% in patients with squamous cell carcinoma of the head and neck who are treated with radiation therapy directed at the oral and pharyngeal regions[438] and is a frequent cause of treatment breaks.[439] Oral mucositis is typically diagnosed based on the clinical appearance, location, timing of oral lesions, and use of certain types of therapy known to be associated with mucositis. Other common conditions can have a similar clinical presentation to oral mucositis and may confuse the differential diagnosis. They include oral candidiasis, herpes simplex virus, and graft-versus-host disease (GVHD) in transplant patients.

Commonly used scales for the assessment of oral mucositis include National Cancer Institute Common Toxicity Criteria Stomatitis and WHO toxicity grading scale. The WHO oral toxicity scale is a relatively simple assessment for oral mucositis with grades 3 and 4 considered as evidence of severe mucositis (Table 42.26).

GRAFT-VERSUS-HOST DISEASE

Indications for SCT include the treatment of many different malignant and nonmalignant hematologic conditions, solid tumors, and metabolic and autoimmune diseases. SCT may be autologous, syngeneic, or allogeneic depending on whether the owner patient, another genetically identical or nonidentical individual, donates the hematopoietic stem cells (of bone marrow, peripheral blood, or cord blood origin) to reconstitute hematopoiesis. After transplantation, donor-derived T cells, GVHD can result in a range of issues from a mild skin rash to a life-threatening and, in some instances, life-ending complication. GVHD primarily occurs in many organs but most notably in the skin, lungs, gastrointestinal tract, liver, eyes, mucosa, and musculoskeletal system. GVHD is an immune-mediated reaction in which donor T cells recognize the host as antigenically foreign, causing donor T cells to expand and attack host tissues. GVHD may be acute or chronic based on the time of onset after SCT. Acute GVHD typically occurs within 100 days after transplantation and classically presents as erythema, maculopapular rash, nausea, vomiting, anorexia, profuse diarrhea, ileus, or cholestatic liver disease. Clinical manifestations of chronic GVHD nearly always present during the first year after transplantation, but some cases develop many years after transplant. Chronic GVHD may occur in 30% to 70% of allogenic hematopoietic cell transplantation patients.[440] Chronic GVHD is a syndrome of variable clinical features resembling autoimmune and other immunologic disorders, such as scleroderma, Sjögren's syndrome, primary biliary cirrhosis, wasting syndrome, bronchiolitis obliterans, immune cytopenias, and chronic immunodeficiency. All parts of the eye may be affected, and keratoconjunctivitis sicca is the most common presenting manifestation of chronic ocular GVHD. Manifestations of chronic GVHD may be restricted to a single organ or site or may be widespread, with profound impact on QOL. Unlike the acute form of the disease that is mediated by direct cytotoxic T-cell attack on host tissues, pathophysiology of chronic GVHD is significantly more complex and the mechanisms of dysregulated adaptive and innate immune responses are poorly understood.[441]

Metastatic Epidural Spinal Cord Compression

MESCC is compression of the dural sac and its contents, spinal cord or cauda equina, or both, by an extradural tumor mass. Because of a rich vascular supply of the bone marrow and extensive lymphatic drainage, the spine is a common site for metastatic disease and up to 40% of patient with cancer developing spinal metastases and 10% to 20% progressing to symptomatic cord compression.[442] The vast majority of spinal metastases in people with MESCC are found in the vertebral body with or without extension into the posterior elements and also into paravertebral regions and the epidural space; these metastases most commonly affect the thoracic spine (70%), followed by the lumbar spine (20%), multiple spinal regions (20% to 35%), and less commonly the cervical spine and sacrum.[443,444] MESCC is the most common neurologic complication of cancer after brain metastases. MESCC usually occurs in patients with disseminated disease but may present as an isolated finding in patients not diagnosed with cancer. Even though the progression of nearly all types of malignancies can be complicated by the occurrence of spinal cord compression, the most common tumors arise from breast, lung, or prostate cancer, followed by renal cell cancer, gastrointestinal, thyroid, sarcoma, and lymphoreticular malignancies.[445,446] Patients may present with malignant epidural spinal cord compression without a known history of a primary cancer.[447] If left untreated, virtually 100% of patients will become paraplegic. Although most patients with MESCC have limited survival, up to one-third will survive beyond 1 year.[448]

TABLE 42.26	Assessment Tools for Oral Mucositis

A. World Health Organization Oral Toxicity Scale

Grade	Assessment
0	Normal oral mucosa
1	Soreness, erythema
2	Erythema ulcers; patient can swallow solid food.
3	Ulcers with extensive erythema; patient cannot swallow solid food.
4	Extensive mucositis; alimentation is not possible.

B. NCI CTC Stomatitis

Grade	Assessment
0	No stomatitis
1	Painless ulcers, erythema, or mild soreness in the absence of lesions
2	Painful erythema, edema, or ulcers, but patient can swallow
3	Painful erythema, edema, or ulcers that prevent swallowing or necessitate hydration or parenteral (or enteral) nutritional support
4	Severe ulceration that requires prophylactic intubation or results in documented aspiration pneumonia

NCI CTC, National Cancer Institute Common Toxicity Criteria.
Modified from Cella D, Pulliam J, Fuchs H, et al. Evaluation of pain associated with oral mucositis during the acute period after administration of high-dose chemotherapy. *Cancer* 2003;98:406–412.

MECHANISM

Most epidural spinal cord compression comes from a solid tumor metastasis to the vertebral body, which spreads posteriorly to the epidural space (observed in 85% to 90% of cases) and presents as an osteolytic bony lesion in 70% of patients resulting in anterior compression of the spinal cord. Other tumors such as lymphoma, paragangliomas, and neuroblastomas invade the epidural space through the intervertebral foramina from the paravertebral tissues account for 10% to 15% of cases. The frequency of metastasis appears to correlate with the volume of bone in that region of the spine, presumably related to blood flow and blood-borne metastasis. As such, the thoracic spine is most likely to have a metastatic lesion due to its 12 vertebral bodies; the lumbosacral spine is the next most likely to have involvement due to the large size of the vertebral bodies, and the small cervical vertebral bodies are the least likely to be affected. MESCC damages the cord by direct compression, which causes demyelination and axonal damage, and by secondary vascular compromise. The most significant damage caused by MESCC appears to be vascular in nature. The epidural tumor causes epidural venous plexus compression, which leads to spinal cord edema. The increased vascular permeability and edema lead to increased pressure on the small arterioles. Capillary blood flow diminishes as the disease progresses, leading to white matter ischemia. Prolonged ischemia eventually results in infarction and permanent cord damage. The early mechanism of injury is vasogenic edema of white matter with direct involvement of cytokines, inflammatory mediators, and neurotransmitters.[449] Production of VEGF is associated with spinal cord hypoxia and has been implicated as a potential mechanism of damage after spinal cord injury.[450] The beneficial effects of dexamethasone in the CNS are at least partly mediated by its downregulation of VEGF expression.[451] In the later stages of MESCC, vasogenic edema is replaced by ischemic-hypoxic neuronal injury and by onset of cytotoxic edema, a transition associated with the glutamate system that is characterized by release of presynaptic glutamate, influx of calcium through N-methyl-D-aspartate (NMDA)-linked ion channels, excitotoxic neuronal injury, and neuronal disintegration.[452]

PATTERN OF PAIN

The pattern of pain associated with epidural metastases may be local, radicular, referred, or funicular. The majority of patients have local pain. *Local* pain over the involved vertebral body, which results from involvement of the vertebral periosteum, is dull and exacerbated by recumbency. The worsening of pain on recumbency is the most distinctive feature of the pain of epidural spinal cord compression. Many patients with cord compression find they must sleep in a sitting position. Even if pain is absent in the lying position, movements such as turning over in bed or rising from a lying position may be particularly painful.

Radicular pain from compressed or damaged nerve roots is usually unilateral in the cervical and lumbosacral regions and bilateral in the thorax, where patients often describe it as a tight band across the chest or abdomen. The pain is experienced in the overlying spine, deep in certain muscles supplied by the compressed root, and in the cutaneous distribution of the injured root. The pain is usually least severe when the patient is in a position that minimizes compression of the root and most severe in positions that compress or stretch the root. Increasing intraspinal/intracranial pressure, for example, coughing, sneezing, and straining, can also increase pain.

Referred pain in the midscapular region or in both shoulders may accompany cervicothoracic epidural disease, and bilateral SI and iliac crest pain occurs with L1 vertebral compression. The pain has a deep aching quality and is often associated with tenderness of subcutaneous tissues and muscles at the site of referral. Maneuvers that affect local pain usually have the same effect on referred pain. When pain is referred from pathologic processes in the low back, it is usually appreciated in the buttocks and posterior thighs. Pain from the upper lumbar spine is often referred to the flank, groin, and anterior thigh.

Funicular pain may be an early complaint in patients with cord compression and presumably results from compression of the ascending sensory tracts in the spinal cord. It usually occurs some distance below the site of compression and has hot or cold qualities in a poorly localized nondermatomal distribution. The pain is less sharp than radicular pain but like root pain is usually exacerbated by movements that stretch the compressed structure (neck flexion, straight leg raising) or that increase intraspinal pressure (coughing, sneezing, straining). Funicular pain may be experienced some distance from the site of compression. Patients with cervical cord compression may present with lower extremity pain only[453] or sciatica-type symptoms with cervical or thoracic cord compression.[454,455]

PRESENTATION AND PHYSICAL FINDINGS

The vast majority of patients have a known cancer diagnosis. Even without a prior cancer diagnosis, MESCC should be suspected in anyone who presents with progressively worsening back pain, incontinence, or paraplegia, especially in the high-risk population such as long-time smokers or women with a strong family history of breast cancer. The clinical picture of MESCC is uniformly reported as various combinations of pain, weakness, sensory loss, and autonomic dysfunction. Table 42.27 summarizes the signs of spinal cord compression.

Severe, local back pain that gradually increases in intensity over time is the earliest and most common symptom. In general, pain occurs an average of 7 weeks before other neurologic deficits.[456] As the bone marrow does not contain pain receptors, discomfort usually occurs only when the enlarging mass invades the periosteum, paravertebral soft tissues, or nerves. Pain may also be caused by the mass effect of the spinal cord compression itself, spinal instability, pathologic fracture, and the inflammatory and nociceptor stimulating substances that malignant cells secrete. Progressive pain occurs practically always in patients with MESCC. Weakness is the second most common symptom, which develops in approximately 60% to 80% of patients.[456] As the thoracic cord is the most common site of epidural metastases, weakness usually involves the lower limbs causing gait disorders. Gait difficulties may also be caused by sensory ataxia presumably due to posterior column compression. Certain spinal tracts appear to be more vulnerable to compression than others.[457] The corticospinal tracts and posterior columns are particularly vulnerable, the spinothalamic tracts and descending autonomic fibers less so.

TABLE 42.27	Signs of Spinal Compression		
Sign/Deficit	Spinal Cord	Conus Medullaris	Cauda Equina
Weakness	Symmetrical, profound	Symmetrical, variable	Decreased
Deep tendon reflexes	Increased or absent	Increased knee, decreased ankle	Decreased
Plantar response	Extensor	Extensor	Plantar
Sensory	Symmetric sensory level	Symmetric saddle	Asymmetric, radicular
Sphincters	Late onset	Early onset	Spared
Progression	Rapid	Variable	Variable

As a result, weakness, spasticity, and reflex hyperactivity tend to be the earliest signs of spinal cord compression, with paresthesias and vibratory and position sense loss occurring soon thereafter. Loss of pain and temperature sensation and of bladder and bowel function usually occur late in the course of spinal cord compression. The spinocerebellar pathways are also sensitive to compression, and at times, ataxia may be the only sign of spinal cord compression. Sensory symptoms are less common and may predate objective sensory signs. Patients may complain of paresthesias, decreased sensation, and numbness of the toes and fingers which may extend one to five dermatomes below the true level of cord compression. Cauda equina syndrome may occur when the site of the lesion is below the first lumbar vertebra. The main clinical signs are decreased sensation over the buttocks, posterior thighs, and perineal region in a saddle distribution, with most patients exhibiting decreased anal sphincter tone on examination. Urinary retention with overflow incontinence can be an important predictor.[458]

Ventafridda et al.[459] reported an association between Lhermitte's sign and epidural spinal cord compression. In their series, the sign appeared at an early stage of compression, particularly with thoracic lesions but may also be seen with cervical MESCC. Lhermitte's sign, however, lacks specificity and also occurs in patients with radiation myelopathy,[460] following cisplatin[461] or oxaliplatin[462] chemotherapy, and in noncancer-related problems such as multiple sclerosis[463] and subacute combined degeneration of the cord from vitamin B_{12} deficiency.[464]

Differential diagnosis for the individual patient with back pain includes intramedullary metastases, herniated disks, epidural hematoma or abscess, transverse myelopathy, and subluxation of the spine from pathologic fractures.

INVESTIGATIONS
Definitive diagnosis of MESCC is by radiographic investigation. Bone scan is an effective screening procedure of vertebral involvement, but definitive diagnosis is by MRI. MRI not only demonstrates the extent of epidural involvement but also allows visualization of the degree of involvement of bony structures and surrounding tissues. Epidural metastases are best visualized with postcontrast imaging, which allows clear delineation of the border of the metastasis in most cases.[465]

PROGNOSIS
MESCC is associated with reduced life expectancy and QOL.[452] Outcome of MESCC can be paraplegia or paraparesis. Without treatment, all patients would develop paraplegia and survival rates for nonambulatory patients are lower than for ambulatory patients.[466] Treatments for MESCC are intended to maintain or improve QOL by alleviating pain, preserving neurologic function, and assuring spinal stability. The most predictive factors for survival are primary tumor site and pretreatment neurologic and functional status.[467] The time lapse between diagnosis of the primary cancer and first symptoms of MESCC directly correlated with survival (e.g., a long interval denoted higher survival rate and vice versa). The most important prognostic indicator for the prediction of ambulatory outcome is a patient's pretreatment motor function.[467,468] The median survival time for patients with MESCC is 3 to 6 months.[469,470] Factors associated with longer survival times are the ability to walk before and after treatment,[467,469,471] radiosensitive tumor histologies,[469,472,473] no visceral or brain metastases,[469,474] and a single site of epidural cord compression rather than more than one site.[475] Survival is also related to the systemic spread of the neoplastic disease. The presence of multiple spinal epidural metastases (around 25% to 40% of patients) has been reported as an independent prognostic factor for poorer survival.[476]

TABLE 42.28	Goals of the Pain-Related History
Define the pain characteristics	
Outline the anatomical extent of the disease	
Determine responses to previous disease-modifying and analgesic therapies	
Anticipate response to planned disease therapies	
Clarify the impact of the pain on activity of daily living, psychological state, familial, vocational, and social function	
Determine the presence of associated symptoms that may modify the perception of pain	

Stepwise Approach to Pain Assessment

Assessing cancer pain is more than quantifying pain with a tool and recording it. A stepwise approach to cancer pain assessment begins with data collection and ends with a clinically relevant diagnosis, which will require a thorough understanding of the various components contributing to the pain complaint. At a minimum, this involves determining the etiology of the pain and forecasting its future trajectory. It also involves determining the number of sites from which pain originates and the probable mechanisms involved. Assessment must include evaluation of the impact of pain on sleep, functional capability, activity level, and psychological well-being. In addition, the clinician must determine the nature, course, and impact of the cancer on the patient. This is an imposing challenge because of the multiple causes of cancer and its impact on the patient. The clinician managing the patient's pain complaint must have an understanding of the disease process and the management strategy for that disease. A thorough evaluation will allow the clinician to obtain a basis for evaluating therapeutic intervention and determining the long-term goals of the patient and/or the patient's family.

The goals of the pain-related history are listed in Table 42.28. Optimal assessment includes a detailed description of these goals and classification by both pain syndrome and likely underlying mechanisms (see the following discussion).

FEATURES OF PAIN HISTORY
Table 42.29 lists the key components to assessing the characteristics of the pain complaint.

Onset
The onset of tumor-associated pain frequently correlates to the diagnosis of cancer. Preexisting chronic pain complaints need to be differentiated from tumor-associated pain and defined accurately. In cancer survivors, the onset of new pain may indicate the possibility of disease recurrence.[477]

Location
Many patients with advanced disease have multiple pains at different sites. Pain of tumor origin may be characterized by its

TABLE 42.29	Key Components of Pain Characteristics
Onset	
Location	
Intensity	
Character/quality	
Timing	
Exacerbating/relieving factors	
Response to previous analgesic and disease-modifying therapies	
Impact of pain	
Effect of pain on activities of daily living	
Psychological state	
Familial, vocational, social function	

location. For example, somatic pain resulting from bone metastases tends to be well localized, whereas visceral pain tends to be diffuse and is often referred. Neuropathic pain may be radicular in location.

Intensity

Numerous professional bodies recommend regular assessment of pain intensity in cancer patients.[478–482] These recommendations urge clinicians teach patients and families to use assessment tools in the home to promote continuity of pain management in all settings. Assessment tools for determining the intensity of pain are discussed previously.

Quality

Tumor-associated pain can be nociceptive (somatic or visceral structures) or neuropathic in origin. Each source of pain has distinguishing qualities. For example, patients tend to describe pain that is neuropathic in origin as burning, shock-like, or shooting in quality, whereas they often describe pain originating from somatic structures as aching, nagging, throbbing, or sharp.

Timing

Cancer patients may have constant or intermittent pain. Constant pain is present continuously and usually fluctuates in intensity. Intermittent pain implies that pain is present for definite periods of time and that the patient is relatively pain free between episodes of pain. Patients and their caregivers need to understand the concept of BTP, as should health care providers. BTP is discussed previously.

Exacerbating/Relieving Factors

Cancer patients with pain may experience a worsening of their pain over a wide range of activities. Commonly, patients with metastatic disease to weight-bearing bones experience an increase of their pain upon standing or sitting. Patients with breast cancer metastatic to the axillary nodes may have severe pain upon abduction of their upper extremity on positioning for external beam radiation therapy. Knowledge of these factors helps clinicians to design an appropriate pain treatment plan.

Responses to Previous Analgesic and Disease-Modifying Therapies

It is important to determine previous opioid use and benefits or side effects encountered during use. Previous unacceptable side effects to a particular opioid may limit successful future titration with the same opioid. Successful tumor shrinkage to chemotherapy or radiation therapy may indicate the need for further evaluation on tumor recurrence.

Impact of Pain

The initial pain assessment should elicit information about changes in activities of daily living, such as work and recreational activities, sleep patterns, mobility, appetite, sexual functioning, and mood. Numerous instruments, including symptom checklists and QOL measures may prove useful in this evaluation and are detailed in Chapter 22.

Effects of Pain on Activities of Daily Living

Many patients function quite effectively with a background level of mild pain that does not seriously impair or distract them.[122] As pain severity increases, the pain passes a threshold beyond which it is hard to ignore. At this point, it becomes disruptive to many aspects of the patient's life. Constant daily pain can significantly impact on a patient's daily activities. Williamson and Schulz[483] showed that as pain increased over time, restriction in activity occurred, which in turn predicted increases in depressed affect. General measures of functioning should include indicators of physical, psychological, social functional status, and, when appropriate, vocational status.

Some impact factors may include interference on general activity, mood, walking, ability to work, relations with others, and sleep. The Pain Disability Index was developed as a self-report measure of general and domain-specific, pain-related disability and is considered to be reliable and valid as a brief measure of pain-related disability (Table 42.30).[484]

Multiple clinical and physiologic factors influence prognosis for patients with advanced cancer. These include symptoms such as anorexia, dyspnea, and fatigue; disease characteristics such as cancer diagnosis, site of metastasis, and comorbidity; laboratory values such as hypoalbuminemia, leukocytosis, and anemia; the clinician's overall prediction of survival; and performance status.[485] Performance status represents a global assessment of the patient's level of function. Assessment of performance status is used routinely in oncology and may be used to assess eligibility for clinical trials, determine level of fitness to receive chemotherapy, and follow treatment response. Performance status tables (Tables 42.20 and 42.31) can help the physician assess physical activity levels.[486,487]

Psychological State

Psychological assessment of the cancer patient with pain is imperative and should reflect an understanding of the many factors that modulate distress, such as personality, coping, and both past and present psychiatric disorders. Knowing that the patient has received outpatient or inpatient psychiatric care helps to clarify the psychological risk. Information on how the patient handled previous painful events may provide insight into whether the patient has demonstrated chronic illness behavior.

Familial, Vocational, Social Function

The clinician must inquire about the patient's familial and social resources, financial situation, and the physical environment in which he or she lives. Knowledge of the patient's and family's previous experience with cancer, or other progressive medical disease, may provide useful insights into the response to physical illness or the genesis of psychological symptoms. Inquiry into a family history of addiction is helpful to define risk for pain management strategies.[488,489] Yellen and Cella[490] demonstrated that positive social well-being, as well as having children living at home, predicted patient willingness to accept aggressive treatment.

QUALITY OF LIFE ASSESSMENT

Prolongation of survival and maintenance or improvement of health-related QOL is the two important goals within the treatment of individual patients. Due to the severity of symptoms and the toxicity of treatment, QOL is a major area of concern when treating cancer patients in general and elderly patients in particular.[491–493] QOL is defined as the person's evaluation of his or her well-being and functioning in different life domains. It is a subjective, phenomenologic, multidimensional, dynamic, evaluative, and yet quantifiable construct. The routine assessment of QOL may have clinical uses at the individual patient level. These uses include fostering patient–provider communication, identifying frequently overlooked problems, prioritizing problems, and evaluating the impact of palliative and rehabilitative efforts. QOL is sensitive to the treatment of pain and treatment modalities, although pain is not synonymous with poor QOL and constitutes only one important factor determining QOL. In addition, pain reduction is not always attended by the expected improvement in QOL. The Functional Assessment of Cancer Therapy: General (FACT-G) was first developed in 1987 for adult cancer patients and has become one of the most widely used health-related QOL measures in clinical trials and other medical treatment evaluation studies. It has also been validated in thousands of patients of different cancer types.[494–496] FACT-G is self-reported and consists of questions on physical, functional, emotional, and social/family well-being. Patient responses are recorded on a 5-point Likert-type scale (Table 42.32).

TABLE 42.30 Pain Disability Index

The rating scales below are to measure the degree to which several aspects of your life are presently disrupted due to chronic pain. In other words, we would like to know how much your pain is preventing you from doing what you would normally do, or from doing it as well as you normally would. Respond to each category by indicating the *overall* impact of pain in your life, not just when the pain is at its worst.

For each of the seven categories of life activity listed, please circle the number on the scale, which describes the level of disability you typically experience. A score of 0 means no disability at all, and a score of 10 signifies that all of the activities in which you would normally be involved have been totally disrupted or prevented by your pain.

1. **Family/home responsibilities**
   This category refers to activities related to the home or family. It includes chores or duties performed around the house (e.g., yard work) and errands or favors for other family members (e.g., driving the children to school).

   0 1 2 3 4 5 6 7 8 9 10

   no disability   total disability

2. **Recreation**
   This category includes hobbies, sports, and other similar leisure time activities.

   0 1 2 3 4 5 6 7 8 9 10

   no disability   total disability

3. **Social activity**
   This category refers to activities which involve participation with friends and acquaintances other than family members. It includes parties, theater, concerts, dining out, and other social functions.

   0 1 2 3 4 5 6 7 8 9 10

   no disability   total disability

4. **Occupation**
   This category refers to activities that are a part of or directly related to one's job. This includes nonpaying jobs as well, such as that of a housewife or volunteer worker.

   0 1 2 3 4 5 6 7 8 9 10

   no disability   total disability

5. **Sexual behavior**
   This category refers to the frequency and quality of one's sex life.

   0 1 2 3 4 5 6 7 8 9 10

   no disability   total disability

6. **Self-care**
   This category includes activities which involve personal maintenance and independent daily living (e.g., taking a shower, driving, getting dressed, etc.).

   0 1 2 3 4 5 6 7 8 9 10

   no disability   total disability

7. **Life-support activity**
   This category refers to basic life-supporting behaviors such as eating, sleeping, and breathing.

   0 1 2 3 4 5 6 7 8 9 10

   no disability   total disability

Reprinted with permission from Tait RC, Chibnall JT, Krause S. The Pain Disability Index: psychometric properties. *Pain* 1990;40(2):171–182.

GENERAL ASSESSMENT

The initial step in the general assessment of the cancer patient is a complete medical history that reviews the cancer diagnosis; the chronology of significant cancer-related events; previous therapies; and all relevant medical, surgical, and psychiatric problems (Table 42.33). A detailed history of drug therapy should include current and prior use of prescription and nonprescription drugs, drug allergies/adverse drug reactions, including current side effects. The clinician should inquire about prior treatment modalities for pain. In the course of this assessment, the interviewer should document the patient's understanding of his or her current disease status. Discussion with other providers involved with the patient's care will also help determine disease status. Table 42.34 lists the different possible categories for a patient's clinical status. Because of the high use of opioids and other psychoactive substances in oncology care, a risk assessment for opioid use should be performed. Opioid use risk assessment tools generally are designed to detect opioid misuse prior to initiating long-term opioid therapy, detection of signs of misuse in patient currently using opioids, and general substance (e.g., alcohol) or illicit substance abuse (Table 42.35).

A physical examination, including a neurologic evaluation, is a necessary part of the initial pain assessment (see the following text). A careful review of previous laboratory and imaging studies can provide information about the cause of pain and the extent of the underlying disease (see the following text). Evaluation of concurrent concerns includes other symptoms and related psychosocial problems. Additional investigations are often needed to clarify uncertainties in the provisional assessment. The extent of these investigations must be appropriate to the patient's general status and the overall goals of care (Table 42.36). In the case of the patient illustrated in Table 42.36, monitoring of the patient's disease status required specialized testing over a period of time.

TABLE 42.31 Eastern Cooperative Oncology Group Performance Status

Grade	Performance Level
0	Fully active, able to carry on all predisease performance without restriction
1	Restricted in physically strenuous activity but ambulatory and able to carry out work of a light or sedentary nature (e.g., light housework, office work)
2	Ambulatory and capable of all self-care but unable to carry out any work activities; up and about more than 50% of waking hours
3	Capable of only limited self-care, confined to bed or chair more than 50% of waking hours
4	Completely disabled; cannot carry on any self-care; totally confined to bed or chair
5	Dead

TABLE 42.32 Functional Assessment Cancer Therapy: General Version 4

Below is a list of statements that other people with your illness have said are important.
Please circle or mark one number per line to indicate your response as it applies to the past 7 days.

Physical Well-being		Not at All	A Little Bit	Somewhat	Quite a Bit	Very Much
GP1	I have a lack of energy.	0	1	2	3	4
GP2	I have nausea.	0	1	2	3	4
GP3	Because of my physical condition, I have trouble meeting the needs of my family.	0	1	2	3	4
GP4	I have pain.	0	1	2	3	4
GP5	I am bothered by side effects of treatment.	0	1	2	3	4
GP6	I feel ill.	0	1	2	3	4
GP7	I am forced to spend time in bed.	0	1	2	3	4
Social/Family Well-being		**Not at All**	**A Little Bit**	**Somewhat**	**Quite a Bit**	**Very Much**
GS1	I feel close to my friends.	0	1	2	3	4
GS2	I get emotional support from my family.	0	1	2	3	4
GS3	I get support from my friends.	0	1	2	3	4
GS4	My family has accepted my illness.	0	1	2	3	4
GS5	I am satisfied with family communication about my illness.	0	1	2	3	4
GS6	I feel close to my partner (or the person who is my main support).	0	1	2	3	4
Q1	*Regardless of your current level of sexual activity, please answer the following question. If you prefer not to answer it, please mark this box and go to the next section.*					
GS7	I am satisfied with my sex life.	0	1	2	3	4
Emotional Well-being		**Not at All**	**A Little Bit**	**Somewhat**	**Quite a Bit**	**Very Much**
GE1	I feel sad.	0	1	2	3	4
GE2	I am satisfied with how I am coping with my illness.	0	1	2	3	4
GE3	I am losing hope in the fight against my illness.	0	1	2	3	4
GE4	I feel nervous.	0	1	2	3	4
GE5	I worry about dying.	0	1	2	3	4
GE6	I worry that my condition will get worse.	0	1	2	3	4
Functional Well-being		**Not at All**	**A Little Bit**	**Somewhat**	**Quite a Bit**	**Very Much**
GF1	I am able to work (include work at home).	0	1	2	3	4
GF2	My work (include work at home) is fulfilling.	0	1	2	3	4
GF3	I am able to enjoy life.	0	1	2	3	4
GF4	I have accepted my illness.	0	1	2	3	4
GF5	I am sleeping well.	0	1	2	3	4
GF6	I am enjoying the things I usually do for fun.	0	1	2	3	4
GF7	I am content with the quality of my life right now.	0	1	2	3	4

ASSOCIATED SYMPTOMS

Cancer patients may experience multiple symptoms with symptoms varying by type of treatment, gender, age, and cancer type. Cancer treatment and survivorship can result in multiple concurrent symptoms resulting in cognitive dysfunction, fatigue, insomnia, pain, dyspnea, appetite loss, constipation, diarrhea, nausea, and vomiting.[497,498] Some data suggest that fatigue, cognitive limitations, depression, anxiety, sleep problems, pain, and sexual difficulties persist, for up to 10 years after treatment, regardless of cancer type.[499] Not surprisingly, cancer patients have a much greater symptom burden completed to a noncan-

cer general medical population.[500] Symptoms can affect pain management, and it is important to clarify the degree to which each symptom induces or exacerbates other physical or psychological symptoms. The evaluation should determine whether symptoms are concurrent but unrelated in etiology, concurrent and related to the same pathologic process, concurrent with the one symptom directly or indirectly a consequence of a pathologic process initiated by another symptom, or concurrent with one symptom a consequence or side effect of therapy directed against the other. Fatigue may be the most prevalent symptom reported by cancer patients with one study suggesting that 45%

TABLE 42.33 Components of Medical History: Cancer History, Medications, Past Medical History, and Psychosocial Factors

Cancer History	Current Medications Medical History	Psychosocial/Addiction Issues
Diagnosis and time of diagnosis	Previous medical and surgical illness including illnesses that may complicate pain management (e.g., sleep apnea, pulmonary hypertension)	Family history of addiction; includes personal history or current use of substance abuse (with alcohol use)
Chronology of disease	Concurrent medical conditions	Social resources and support
Therapeutic interventions including surgeries and treatments (particularly chemotherapy and radiation therapy)	Drug allergies/adverse drug reactions	Impact of disease and symptoms on patient and family
Current clinical status including extent of disease (detailed imaging review)	Risk assessment for opioid use	Patient's and family's goals of care
Anticipated clinical course	Review of systems	Vocational status and issues

TABLE 42.34 Clinical Status of Patients Defined by Disease State and Treatment Strategy

Category	Status
I	Active disease; care—palliative and supportive only
II	Active disease; treatment (e.g., chemotherapy, radiation therapy) in progress
III	Active disease, no current treatment, surveillance of tumor status
IV	No active disease; treatment of tumor in progress
V	No active disease; no current treatment, surveillance of tumor status
VI	No active disease; no current treatment, specialized care (e.g., medical oncology) not required

TABLE 42.36 Patient with Chronic Myeloid Leukemia

Date	Abnormal Fluorescence In Situ Hybridization Result: BCR/ABL1 Rearrangement
January 19, 2016	82%
January 25, 2016	67%
February 15, 2016	62.5%
March 2, 2016	73%
March 30, 2016	32%
April 15, 2016	16.5%
May 11, 2016	2.1%
June 29, 2016	0.5%
July 25, 2016	No evidence
September 28, 2016	No evidence
October 4, 2016	No evidence
November 23, 2016	No evidence
January 27, 2017	No evidence

NOTE: Patients with chronic myeloid leukemia have BCR-ABL gene (a.k.a. the Philadelphia chromosome). The Philadelphia chromosome produces the BCR-ABL gene that signals the bone marrow to continue making abnormal white blood cells. Polymerase chain reaction (PCR) is used to detect and sometimes to quantify this gene. The clinical BCR-ABL assays for both p210 and p190 previously showed undetectable transcripts for both assays. The patient was then identified as having a rare e13/e14-a3 (also known as b2/b3-a3) transcript that is not detectable by. This transcript cannot be detected using commercially available quantitative PCR assays 9 standard P210 or P190 assays and requires a special qualitative assay to detect it. In this case, disease is monitored by BCR-ABL fluorescence in situ hybridization and qualitative PCR that detects rare variants. Over time, the patient went into complete remission after treatment with bosutinib.

of patients undergoing active treatment and 29% of survivors have moderate to severe levels of fatigue.[500] Disease progression increases the number of factors diminishing QOL as well as the prevalence and severity of physical and psychological symptoms. In addition to pain, patients with advanced cancer have fatigue, generalized weakness, dyspnea, delirium, nausea, and vomiting. These symptoms may have a major impact on both pain reporting and QOL. The Memorial Symptom Assessment Scale (MSAS) is a patient-rated instrument that was developed to provide multidimensional information about a diverse group of common symptoms.[501] The MSAS is a reliable and valid instrument for the assessment of symptom prevalence, characteristics, and distress.

LABORATORY AND IMAGING DATA
Careful review of previous laboratory and imaging studies can provide important additional information. Specific radiologic or laboratory tests may help the clinician understand the pathophysiology of symptoms and their relationships to the disease. This information provides the basis for a provisional pain diagnosis that clarifies both the status of the disease and the nature of other concurrent concerns that may require therapeutic focus.

Some patients require multiple studies to evaluate the pain problem, clarify extent of disease, or to assess other symptoms. Assistance from physicians in other disciplines, nurses, social workers, psychologists, or others may prove necessary to evaluate related physical or psychosocial problems identified during the initial assessment. It is appropriate and useful to review the findings of this evaluation with the patient, family, and other appropriate persons, so that they can prioritize problems according to their importance for the patient. It is also useful to identify potential outcomes that would benefit from contingency planning, including the need for advanced medical directives, the evaluation of home care resources, and prebereavement interventions with the family.

PHYSICAL EXAMINATION
A physical examination, including a neurologic and musculoskeletal examination, is a necessary part of the initial pain assessment. The need for a thorough neurologic assessment is justified by the high prevalence of painful neurologic conditions in the cancer population.[502] The physical examination should clarify the underlying causes of the pain problem, detail the extent of the underlying disease, and discern the relation of the pain complaint to the disease. The examination should also help define biomechanical problems that impair or impede function.

DIAGNOSIS
The provisional pain diagnosis includes inferences about the pathophysiology of the pain and an assessment of the pain syndrome. Evaluation of concurrent concerns includes other symptoms and related psychosocial problems. Additional investigations can often clarify uncertainties in the provisional assessment. Accuracy in pain diagnosis results in appropriate and disease-directed pain management.

Summary
Cancer is one of the medical conditions that patients fear the most. In addition to anxiety about cancer as a potentially lethal disease, patient and family expectancies that pain is an inevitable and untreatable consequence are major sources of distress. Controlling pain associated with cancer is a major health care problem. Lack of expertise by clinicians in assessing pain is an important cause of poor pain control. A stepwise approach to cancer pain assessment begins with a systematic clinical interview and ends with a clinically relevant diagnosis that outlines

TABLE 42.35 Examples of Screening Tools for Assessment of Opioid Risk

Tool	Time of Administration	Completed By
Opioid Risk Tool (ORT) (Webster and Webster, 2005[506])	Preinitiation of opioid therapy	Clinician
Screener and Opioid Assessment for Patients with Pain (SOAPP) (Butler et al., 2004[507])	Preinitiation of opioid therapy	Patient
Diagnosis, Intractability, Risk, and Efficacy Score (DIRE) (Belgrade et al., 2006[508])	Preinitiation of opioid therapy	Clinician
Current Opioid Misuse Measure (COMM) (Butler, 2007[509])	Monthly during opioid therapy	Patient
Alcohol Use Disorders Identification Test: Consumption (AUDIT-C) (Bush et al., 1998[510])	Preinitiation of opioid therapy	Patient
Cut Down, Annoyed, Guilty, Eye-Opener Tool (CAGE) (Brown and Rounds, 1995[511])	Preinitiation of opioid therapy	Clinician

the mechanisms and contributing factors to the pain complaint. It involves determining the etiology of the pain and forecasting its future trajectory. It also involves determining the number of sites from which pain originates and the probable mechanisms involved. Assessment must include evaluation of the impact of pain on sleep, functional capability, activity level, and psychological well-being. In addition, the clinician must determine the nature, course, and impact of the cancer on the patient. A thorough evaluation will allow the clinician to obtain a basis for evaluating therapeutic intervention and determining the long-term goals of the patient and/or the patient's family.

As many different health care professionals become involved with the cancer pain patient before, during, and after cancer care, successful pain management requires that the person or persons responsible for pain management adopt, or at least, become familiar with an interdisciplinary longitudinal approach to care. Pain management should never assume the primary focus of oncology care but should be an important supportive service throughout the care paradigm.

References

1. Singh GK, Williams SD, Siahpush M, et al. Socioeconomic, rural-urban, and racial inequalities in US cancer mortality: part I—all cancers and lung cancer and part II—colorectal, prostate, breast, and cervical cancers. *J Cancer Epidemiol* 2011;2011:107497.
2. Mandelblatt J, Andrews H, Kerner J, et al. Determinants of late stage diagnosis of breast and cervical cancer: the impact of age, race, social class, and hospital type. *Am J Public Health* 1991;81:646–649.
3. Siegel RL, Miller KD, Jemal A. Cancer statistics, 2017. *CA Cancer J Clin* 2017;67:7–30.
4. Chapman PB, Hauschild A, Robert C, et al. Improved survival with vemurafenib in melanoma with BRAF V600E mutation. *N Engl J Med* 2011;364:2507–2516.
5. Kwak EL, Bang YJ, Camidge DR, et al. Anaplastic lymphoma kinase inhibition in non-small-cell lung cancer. *N Engl J Med* 2010;363:1693–1703.
6. Singh GK, Jemal A. Socioeconomic and racial/ethnic disparities in cancer mortality, incidence, and survival in the United States, 1950–2014: over six decades of changing patterns and widening inequalities. *J Environ Public Health* 2017;2017:2819372.
7. de Moor JS, Mariotto AB, Parry C, et al. Cancer survivors in the United States: prevalence across the survivorship trajectory and implications for care. *Cancer Epidemiol Biomarkers Prev* 2013;22:561–570.
8. Miller KD, Siegel RL, Lin CC, et al. Cancer treatment and survivorship statistics, 2016. *CA Cancer J Clin* 2016;66:271–289.
9. Parry C, Kent EE, Mariotto AB, et al. Cancer survivors: a booming population. *Cancer Epidemiol Biomarkers Prev* 2011;20:1996–2005.
10. Zeng C, Wen W, Morgans AK, et al. Disparities by race, age, and sex in the improvement of survival for major cancers: results from the National Cancer Institute Surveillance, Epidemiology, and End Results (SEER) program in the United States, 1990 to 2010. *JAMA Oncol* 2015;1:88–96.
11. Patrick DL, Ferketich SL, Frame PS, et al. National Institutes of Health State-of-the-Science Conference statement: symptom management in cancer: pain, depression, and fatigue, July 15–17, 2002. *J Natl Cancer Inst* 2003;95:1110–1117.
12. Allen D, Gillen E, Rixson L. The effectiveness of integrated care pathways for adults and children in health care settings: a systematic review. *JBI Libr Syst Rev* 2009;7:80–129.
13. Brouwers MC, Vukmirovic M, Spithoff K, et al. Understanding optimal approaches to patient and caregiver engagement in the development of cancer practice guidelines: a mixed methods study. *BMC Health Serv Res* 2017;17:186.
14. Truglio-Londrigan M, Slyer JT, Singleton JK, et al. A qualitative systematic review of internal and external influences on shared decision-making in all health care settings. *JBI Libr Syst Rev* 2012;10:4633–4646.
15. Hong F, Blonquist TM, Halpenny B, et al. Patient-reported symptom distress, and most bothersome issues, before and during cancer treatment. *Patient Relat Outcome Meas* 2016;7:127–135.
16. Lee YH, Liao YC, Liao WY, et al. Anxiety, depression and related factors in family caregivers of newly diagnosed lung cancer patients before first treatment. *Psychooncology* 2013;22:2617–2623.
17. Li XM, Xiao WH, Yang P, et al. Psychological distress and cancer pain: results from a controlled cross-sectional survey in China. *Sci Rep* 2017;7:39397.
18. Baker TA, Krok-Schoen JL, McMillan SC. Identifying factors of psychological distress on the experience of pain and symptom management among cancer patients. *BMC Psychol* 2016;4:52.
19. Baker TA, Roker R, Collins HR, et al. Beyond race and gender: measuring behavioral and social indicators of pain treatment satisfaction in older black and white cancer patients. *Gerontol Geriatr Med* 2016;2:2333721415625688.
20. Davis MP, Goforth HW. Long-term and short-term effects of insomnia in cancer and effective interventions. *Cancer J* 2014;20:330–344.
21. Kelleher SA, Dorfman CS, Plumb Vilardaga JC, et al. Optimizing delivery of a behavioral pain intervention in cancer patients using a sequential multiple assignment randomized trial SMART. *Contemp Clin Trials* 2017;57:51–57.
22. Montazeri A. Quality of life data as prognostic indicators of survival in cancer patients: an overview of the literature from 1982 to 2008. *Health Qual Life Outcomes* 2009;7:102.
23. Pachman DR, Barton DL, Swetz KM, et al. Troublesome symptoms in cancer survivors: fatigue, insomnia, neuropathy, and pain. *J Clin Oncol* 2012;30:3687–3696.
24. Beckwee D, Leysen L, Meuwis K, et al. Prevalence of aromatase inhibitor-induced arthralgia in breast cancer: a systematic review and meta-analysis. *Support Care Cancer* 2017;25:1673–1686.
25. Deshields TL, Penalba V, Liu J, et al. Comparing the symptom experience of cancer patients and non-cancer patients. *Support Care Cancer* 2017;25:1103–1109.
26. Dulaney C, Wallace AS, Everett AS, et al. Defining health across the cancer continuum. *Cureus* 2017;9:e1029.
27. Larue F, Colleau SM, Brasseur L, et al. Multicentre study of cancer pain and its treatment in France. *Br Med J* 1995;310:1034–1037.
28. Cleeland CS, Gonin R, Hatfield AK, et al. Pain and its treatment in outpatients with metastatic cancer. *N Engl J Med* 1994;330:592–596.
29. Cleeland CS, Gonin R, Baez L, et al. Pain and treatment of pain in minority patients with cancer. The Eastern Cooperative Oncology Group Minority Outpatient Pain study. *Ann Intern Med* 1997;127:813–816.
30. Sloan PA, Donnelly MB, Schwartz RW, et al. Cancer pain assessment and management by housestaff. *Pain* 1996;67:475–481.
31. Dahl JL. Pain: impediments and suggestions for solutions. *J Natl Cancer Inst Monogr* 2004:124–126.
32. Cascinu S, Giordani P, Agostinelli R, et al. Pain and its treatment in hospitalized patients with metastatic cancer. *Support Care Cancer* 2003;11:587–592.
33. Gallagher R, Hawley P, Yeomans W. A survey of cancer pain management knowledge and attitudes of British Columbian physicians. *Pain Res Manag* 2004;9:188–194.
34. Jeon YS, Kim HK, Cleeland CS, et al. Clinicians' practice and attitudes toward cancer pain management in Korea. *Support Care Cancer* 2007;15:463–469.
35. Enting RH, Oldenmenger WH, Van Gool AR, et al. The effects of analgesic prescription and patient adherence on pain in a Dutch outpatient cancer population. *J Pain Symptom Manage* 2007;34:523–531.
36. Deandrea S, Montanari M, Moja L, et al. Prevalence of undertreatment in cancer pain. A review of published literature. *Ann Oncol* 2008;19:1985–1991.
37. Apolone G, Corli O, Caraceni A, et al. Pattern and quality of care of cancer pain management. Results from the Cancer Pain Outcome Research Study Group. *Br J Cancer* 2009;100:1566–1574.
38. Greco MT, Roberto A, Corli O, et al. Quality of cancer pain management: an update of a systematic review of undertreatment of patients with cancer. *J Clin Oncol* 2014;32:4149–4154.
39. Cleeland CS, Mendoza TR, Wang XS, et al. Assessing symptom distress in cancer patients: the M.D. Anderson Symptom Inventory. *Cancer* 2000;89:1634–1646.
40. Quinten C, Coens C, Mauer M, et al. Baseline quality of life as a prognostic indicator of survival: a meta-analysis of individual patient data from EORTC clinical trials. *Lancet Oncol* 2009;10:865–871.
41. Efficace F, Bottomley A, Smit EF, et al. Is a patient's self-reported health-related quality of life a prognostic factor for survival in non-small-cell lung cancer patients? A multivariate analysis of prognostic factors of EORTC study 08975. *Ann Oncol* 2006;17:1698–1704.
42. Herndon JE II, Fleishman S, Kornblith AB, et al. Is quality of life predictive of the survival of patients with advanced nonsmall cell lung carcinoma? *Cancer* 1999;85:333–340.
43. Yeo W, Mo FK, Koh J, et al. Quality of life is predictive of survival in patients with unresectable hepatocellular carcinoma. *Ann Oncol* 2006;17:1083–1089.
44. Chau I, Norman AR, Cunningham D, et al. Multivariate prognostic factor analysis in locally advanced and metastatic esophago-gastric cancer—pooled analysis from three multicenter, randomized, controlled trials using individual patient data. *J Clin Oncol* 2004;22:2395–2403.
45. Amoatey Odonkor C, Addison W, Smith S, et al. Connecting the dots: a comparative global multi-institutional study of prohibitive factors affecting cancer pain management. *Pain Med* 2017;18:363–373.
46. Payne R. Chronic pain: challenges in the assessment and management of cancer pain. *J Pain Symptom Manag* 2000;19(suppl 1):S12–S15.
47. Von Roenn JH, Cleeland CS, Gonin R, et al. Physician attitudes and practice in cancer pain management. A survey from the Eastern Cooperative Oncology Group. *Ann Intern Med* 1993;119:121–126.
48. Sun V, Borneman T, Piper B, et al. Barriers to pain assessment and management in cancer survivorship. *J Cancer Surviv* 2008;2:65–71.
49. Sloan PA, Donnelly MB, Vanderveer B, et al. Cancer pain education among family physicians. *J Pain Symptom Manage* 1997;14:74–81.
50. Leila NM, Pirkko H, Eeva P, et al. Training medical students to manage a chronic pain patient: both knowledge and communication skills are needed. *Eur J Pain* 2006;10:167–170.

51. Fishman SM, Young HM, Lucas Arwood E, et al. Core competencies for pain management: results of an interprofessional consensus summit. *Pain Med* 2013;14:971–981.

52. Merskey H, Bogduk N. *Classification of Chronic Pain. Descriptions of Chronic Pain Syndromes and Definitions of Pain Terms*. Seattle, WA: IASP Press; 1994.

53. Caraceni A, Portenoy RK. An international survey of cancer pain characteristics and syndromes. IASP Task Force on Cancer Pain. International Association for the Study of Pain. *Pain* 1999;82:263–274.

54. Caraceni A, Brunelli C, Martini C, et al. Cancer pain assessment in clinical trials. A review of the literature (1999–2002). *J Pain Symptom Manage* 2005;29:507–519.

55. Caraceni A. Evaluation and assessment of cancer pain and cancer pain treatment. *Acta Anaesthesiol Scand* 2001;45:1067–1075.

56. Turk DC, Monarch ES, Williams AD. Cancer patients in pain: considerations for assessing the whole person. *Hematol Oncol Clin North Am* 2002;16:511–525.

57. Anderson KO. Assessment tools for the evaluation of pain in the oncology patient. *Curr Pain Headache Rep* 2007;11:259–264.

58. Acquazzino MA, Igler EC, Dasgupta M, et al. Patient-reported neuropathic pain in adolescent and young adult cancer patients. *Pediatr Blood Cancer* 2017;64.

59. Kurita GP, Ulrich A, Jensen TS, et al. How is neuropathic cancer pain assessed in randomised controlled trials? *Pain* 2012;153:13–17.

60. Jensen TS, Baron R, Haanpaa M, et al. A new definition of neuropathic pain. *Pain* 2011;152:2204–2205.

61. Grond S, Zech D, Diefenbach C, et al. Assessment of cancer pain: a prospective evaluation in 2,266 cancer patients referred to a pain service. *Pain* 1996;64:107–114.

62. Grisold W, Piza-Katzer H, Jahn R, et al. Intraneural nerve metastasis with multiple mononeuropathies. *J Peripher Nerv Syst* 2000;5:163–167.

63. Chamberlain MC. Neoplastic myelopathies. *Continuum (Minneapolis, Minn)* 2015;21:132–145.

64. Crush AB, Howe BM, Spinner RJ, et al. Malignant involvement of the peripheral nervous system in patients with cancer: multimodality imaging and pathologic correlation. *Radiographics* 2014;34:1987–2007.

65. Maroldi R, Farina D, Borghesi A, et al. Perineural tumor spread. *Neuroimaging Clin N Am* 2008;18:413–429.

66. Hughes RA, Britton T, Richards M. Effects of lymphoma on the peripheral nervous system. *J R Soc Med* 1994;87:526–530.

67. Pomonis JD, Rogers SD, Peters CM, et al. Expression and localization of endothelin receptors: implications for the involvement of peripheral glia in nociception. *J Neurosci* 2001;21:999–1006.

68. Asham EH, Loizidou M, Taylor I. Endothelin-1 and tumour development. *Eur J Surg Oncol* 1998;24:57–60.

69. Knowles J, Loizidou M, Taylor I. Endothelin-1 and angiogenesis in cancer. *Curr Vasc Pharmacol* 2005;3:309–314.

70. Mantyh PW, Clohisy DR, Koltzenburg M, et al. Molecular mechanisms of cancer pain. *Nat Rev Cancer* 2002;2:201–209.

71. Bishop-Bailey D. Tumour vascularisation: a druggable target. *Curr Opin Pharmacol* 2009;9:96–101.

72. Retamales-Ortega R, Orostica L, Vera C, et al. Role of nerve growth factor (NGF) and miRNAs in epithelial ovarian cancer. *Int J Mol Sci* 2017;18.

73. Yoneda T, Hiasa M, Nagata Y, et al. Contribution of acidic extracellular microenvironment of cancer-colonized bone to bone pain. *Biochim Biophys Acta* 2015;1848:2677–2684.

74. Wolfe F, Clauw DJ, Fitzcharles MA, et al. The American College of Rheumatology preliminary diagnostic criteria for fibromyalgia and measurement of symptom severity. *Arthritis Care Res (Hoboken)* 2010;62:600–610.

75. Rivers WE, Garrigues D, Graciosa J, et al. Signs and symptoms of myofascial pain: an international survey of pain management providers and proposed preliminary set of diagnostic criteria. *Pain Med* 2015;16:1794–1805.

76. Jafri MS. Mechanisms of myofascial pain. *Int Sch Res Notices* 2014;2014.

77. Partanen JV, Ojala TA, Arokoski JP. Myofascial syndrome and pain: a neurophysiological approach. *Pathophysiology* 2010;17:19–28.

78. Mense S. Algesic agents exciting muscle nociceptors. *Exp Brain Res* 2009;196:89–100.

79. Babenko V, Graven-Nielsen T, Svensson P, et al. Experimental human muscle pain and muscular hyperalgesia induced by combinations of serotonin and bradykinin. *Pain* 1999;82:1–8.

80. Molander C, Ygge J, Dalsgaard CJ. Substance P-, somatostatin- and calcitonin gene-related peptide-like immunoreactivity and fluoride resistant acid phosphatase-activity in relation to retrogradely labeled cutaneous, muscular and visceral primary sensory neurons in the rat. *Neurosci Lett* 1987;74:37–42.

81. Reinert A, Kaske A, Mense S. Inflammation-induced increase in the density of neuropeptide-immunoreactive nerve endings in rat skeletal muscle. *Exp Brain Res* 1998;121:174–180.

82. Graven-Nielsen T, Mense S. The peripheral apparatus of muscle pain: evidence from animal and human studies. *Clin J Pain* 2001;17:2–10.

83. Hoheisel U, Reinohl J, Unger T, et al. Acidic pH and capsaicin activate mechanosensitive group IV muscle receptors in the rat. *Pain* 2004;110:149–157.

84. Cervero F. Visceral nociception: peripheral and central aspects of visceral nociceptive systems. *Philos Trans R Soc Lond B Biol Sci* 1985;308:325–337.

85. Sengupta JN. Visceral pain: the neurophysiological mechanism. *Handb Exp Pharmacol* 2009:31–74.

86. Yu X, Yu M, Liu Y, et al. TRP channel functions in the gastrointestinal tract. *Semin Immunopathol* 2016;38:385–396.

87. Christianson JA, McIlwrath SL, Koerber HR, et al. Transient receptor potential vanilloid 1-immunopositive neurons in the mouse are more prevalent within colon afferents compared to skin and muscle afferents. *Neuroscience* 2006;140:247–257.

88. Fasanella KE, Christianson JA, Chanthaphavong RS, et al. Distribution and neurochemical identification of pancreatic afferents in the mouse. *J Comp Neurol* 2008;509:42–52.

89. Balemans D, Boeckxstaens GE, Talavera K, et al. Transient receptor potential ion channel function in sensory transduction and cellular signaling cascades underlying visceral hypersensitivity. *Am J Physiol Gastrointest Liver Physiol* 2017;312:G635–G648.

90. Julius D. TRP channels and pain. *Annu Rev Cell Dev Biol* 2013;29:355–384.

91. Cervero F. Sensory innervation of the viscera: peripheral basis of visceral pain. *Physiol Rev* 1994;74:95–138.

92. Arcidiacono PG, Calori G, Carrara S, et al. Celiac plexus block for pancreatic cancer pain in adults. *Cochrane Database Syst Rev* 2011;(3):CD007519.

93. Greenwald HP, Bonica JJ, Bergner M. The prevalence of pain in four cancers. *Cancer* 1987;60:2563–2569.

94. Krech RL, Walsh D. Symptoms of pancreatic cancer. *J Pain Symptom Manage* 1991;6:360–367.

95. Furukawa H, Okada S, Saisho H, et al. Clinicopathologic features of small pancreatic adenocarcinoma. A collective study. *Cancer* 1996;78:986–990.

96. Barreto SG, Saccone GT. Pancreatic nociception—revisiting the physiology and pathophysiology. *Pancreatology* 2012;12:104–112.

97. Moossa AR, Gamagami RA. Diagnosis and staging of pancreatic neoplasms. *Surg Clin North Am* 1995;75:871–890.

98. Vega F, Davila L, Delattre JY, et al. Experimental carcinomatous plexopathy. *J Neurol* 1993;240:54–58.

99. Jessell T, Tsunoo A, Kanazawa I, et al. Substance P: depletion in the dorsal horn of rat spinal cord after section of the peripheral processes of primary sensory neurons. *Brain Res* 1979;168:247–259.

100. Wagner R, Myers RR. Endoneurial injection of TNF-alpha produces neuropathic pain behaviors. *Neuroreport* 1996;7:2897–2901.

101. Wagner R, Myers RR. Schwann cells produce tumor necrosis factor alpha: expression in injured and non-injured nerves. *Neuroscience* 1996;73:625–629.

102. Sacerdote P, Franchi S, Moretti S, et al. Cytokine modulation is necessary for efficacious treatment of experimental neuropathic pain. *J Neuroimmune Pharmacol* 2013;8:202–211.

103. Sekiguchi M, Sekiguchi Y, Konno S, et al. Comparison of neuropathic pain and neuronal apoptosis following nerve root or spinal nerve compression. *Eur Spine J* 2009;18:1978–1985.

104. Vallejo R, Tilley DM, Vogel L, et al. The role of glia and the immune system in the development and maintenance of neuropathic pain. *Pain Pract* 2010;10:167–184.

105. Lemay K, Wilson KG, Buenger U, et al. Fear of pain in patients with advanced cancer or in patients with chronic noncancer pain. *Clin J Pain* 2011;27:116–124.

106. Wiech K, Tracey I. The influence of negative emotions on pain: behavioral effects and neural mechanisms. *Neuroimage* 2009;47:987–994.

107. Garland EL. Pain processing in the human nervous system: a selective review of nociceptive and biobehavioral pathways. *Prim Care* 2012;39:561–571.

108. Price DD, Verne GN, Schwartz JM. Plasticity in brain processing and modulation of pain. *Prog Brain Res* 2006;157:333–352.

109. Linden W, Vodermaier A, Mackenzie R, et al. Anxiety and depression after cancer diagnosis: prevalence rates by cancer type, gender, and age. *J Affect Disord* 2012;141:343–351.

110. Thalen-Lindstrom A, Larsson G, Glimelius B, et al. Anxiety and depression in oncology patients; a longitudinal study of a screening, assessment and psychosocial support intervention. *Acta Oncol* 2013;52:118–127.

111. Vodermaier A, Linden W, Siu C. Screening for emotional distress in cancer patients: a systematic review of assessment instruments. *J Natl Cancer Inst* 2009;101:1464–1488.

112. Brunault P, Champagne AL, Huguet G, et al. Major depressive disorder, personality disorders, and coping strategies are independent risk factors for lower quality of life in non-metastatic breast cancer patients. *Psychooncology* 2016;25:513–520.

113. Chapman CR, Gavrin J. Suffering and its relationship to pain. *J Palliat Care* 1993;9:5–13.

114. Wilson KG, Chochinov HM, McPherson CJ, et al. Suffering with advanced cancer. *J Clin Oncol* 2007;25:1691–1697.

115. Turk DC, Sist TC, Okifuji A, et al. Adaptation to metastatic cancer pain, regional/local cancer pain and non-cancer pain: role of psychological and behavioral factors. *Pain* 1998;74:247–256.

116. Turk DC, Fernandez E. On the putative uniqueness of cancer pain: do psychological principles apply? *Behav Res Ther* 1990;28:1–13.

117. Potter VT, Wiseman CE, Dunn SM, et al. Patient barriers to optimal cancer pain control. *Psychooncology* 2003;12:153–160.

118. Daut RL, Cleeland CS. The prevalence and severity of pain in cancer. *Cancer* 1982;50:1913–1918.

119. Spiegel D, Bloom JR. Pain in metastatic breast cancer. *Cancer* 1983;52:341–345.
120. Front D, Schneck SO, Frankel A, et al. Bone metastases and bone pain in breast cancer. Are they closely associated? *JAMA* 1979;242:1747–1748.
121. Bond MR, Pilowsky I. Subjective assessment of pain and its relationship to the administration of analgesics in patients with advanced cancer. *J Psychosom Res* 1966;10:203–208.
122. Serlin RC, Mendoza TR, Nakamura Y, et al. When is cancer pain mild, moderate or severe? Grading pain severity by its interference with function. *Pain* 1995;61:277–284.
123. Paul SM, Zelman DC, Smith M, et al. Categorizing the severity of cancer pain: further exploration of the establishment of cutpoints. *Pain* 2005;113:37–44.
124. Twycross RG, Fairfield S. Pain in far-advanced cancer. *Pain* 1982;14:303–310.
125. Patten SB, Williams JV, Lavorato DH, et al. Patterns of association of chronic medical conditions and major depression. *Epidemiol Psychiatr Sci* 2016:1–9.
126. Spiegel D, Giese-Davis J. Depression and cancer: mechanisms and disease progression. *Biol Psychiatry* 2003;54:269–282.
127. Zabora J, BrintzenhofeSzoc K, Curbow B, et al. The prevalence of psychological distress by cancer site. *Psychooncology* 2001;10:19–28.
128. Traeger L, Greer JA, Fernandez-Robles C, et al. Evidence-based treatment of anxiety in patients with cancer. *J Clin Oncol* 2012;30:1197–1205.
129. Zabora JR, Macmurray L. The history of psychosocial screening among cancer patients. *J Psychosoc Oncol* 2012;30:625–635.
130. Mitchell AJ, Chan M, Bhatti H, et al. Prevalence of depression, anxiety, and adjustment disorder in oncological, haematological, and palliative-care settings: a meta-analysis of 94 interview-based studies. *Lancet Oncol* 2011;12:160–174.
131. Massie MJ. Prevalence of depression in patients with cancer. *J Natl Cancer Inst Monogr* 2004:57–71.
132. Cheng KK, Yeung RM. Impact of mood disturbance, sleep disturbance, fatigue and pain among patients receiving cancer therapy. *Eur J Cancer Care (Engl)* 2013;22:70–78.
133. Otte C, Gold SM, Penninx BW, et al. Major depressive disorder. *Nat Rev Dis Primers* 2016;2:16065.
134. Riepe MW, Gritzmann P, Brieden A. Preferences of psychiatric practitioners for core symptoms of major depressive disorder: a hidden conjoint analysis. *Int J Methods Psychiatr Res* 2017;26.
135. Inagaki M, Akechi T, Okuyama T, et al. Associations of interleukin-6 with vegetative but not affective depressive symptoms in terminally ill cancer patients. *Support Care Cancer* 2013;21:2097–2106.
136. Li M, Fitzgerald P, Rodin G. Evidence-based treatment of depression in patients with cancer. *J Clin Oncol* 2012;30:1187–1196.
137. Brintzenhofe-Szoc KM, Levin TT, Li Y, et al. Mixed anxiety/depression symptoms in a large cancer cohort: prevalence by cancer type. *Psychosomatics* 2009;50:383–391.
138. Walker J, Hansen CH, Martin P, et al. Prevalence, associations, and adequacy of treatment of major depression in patients with cancer: a cross-sectional analysis of routinely collected clinical data. *Lancet Psychiatry* 2014;1:343–350.
139. Celano CM, Freudenreich O, Fernandez-Robles C, et al. Depressogenic effects of medications: a review. *Dialogues Clin Neurosci* 2011;13:109–125.
140. Singer S, Das-Munshi J, Brahler E. Prevalence of mental health conditions in cancer patients in acute care—a meta-analysis. *Ann Oncol* 2010;21:925–930.
141. Hartung TJ, Brahler E, Faller H, et al. The risk of being depressed is significantly higher in cancer patients than in the general population: prevalence and severity of depressive symptoms across major cancer types. *Eur J Cancer* 2017;72:46–53.
142. Katon W, Sullivan MD. Depression and chronic medical illness. *J Clin Psychiatry* 1990;51(suppl):3–11.
143. Katon WJ. Epidemiology and treatment of depression in patients with chronic medical illness. *Dialogues Clin Neurosci* 2011;13:7–23.
144. Katon W, Schulberg H. Epidemiology of depression in primary care. *Gen Hosp Psychiatry* 1992;14:237–247.
145. Sullivan MD, Edlund MJ, Zhang L, et al. Association between mental health disorders, problem drug use, and regular prescription opioid use. *Arch Intern Med* 2006;166:2087–2093.
146. Sullivan MD. Who gets high-dose opioid therapy for chronic non-cancer pain? *Pain* 2010;151:567–568.
147. Steginga SK, Campbell A, Ferguson M, et al. Socio-demographic, psychosocial and attitudinal predictors of help seeking after cancer diagnosis. *Psychooncology* 2008;17:997–1005.
148. Passik SD, Dugan W, McDonald MV, et al. Oncologists' recognition of depression in their patients with cancer. *J Clin Oncol* 1998;16:1594–1600.
149. Somerset W, Stout SC, Miller AH, et al. Breast cancer and depression. *Oncology (Williston Park)* 2004;18:1021–1034.
150. Sharpe M, Strong V, Allen K, et al. Major depression in outpatients attending a regional cancer centre: screening and unmet treatment needs. *Br J Cancer* 2004;90:314–320.
151. Kissane DW. Unrecognised and untreated depression in cancer care. *Lancet Psychiatry* 2014;1:320–321.
152. Mitchell AJ, Lord K, Symonds P. Which symptoms are indicative of DSMIV depression in cancer settings? An analysis of the diagnostic significance of somatic and non-somatic symptoms. *J Affect Disord* 2012;138:137–148.
153. Akechi T, Ietsugu T, Sukigara M, et al. Symptom indicator of severity of depression in cancer patients: a comparison of the DSM-IV criteria with alternative diagnostic criteria. *Gen Hosp Psychiatry* 2009;31:225–232.
154. Endicott J. Measurement of depression in patients with cancer. *Cancer* 1984;53:2243–2249.
155. Trask PC. Assessment of depression in cancer patients. *J Natl Cancer Inst Monogr* 2004:80–92.
156. Wagner LI, Pugh SL, Small W Jr, et al. Screening for depression in cancer patients receiving radiotherapy: feasibility and identification of effective tools in the NRG Oncology RTOG 0841 trial. *Cancer* 2017;123:485–493.
157. Hopko DR, Bell JL, Armento ME, et al. The phenomenology and screening of clinical depression in cancer patients. *J Psychosoc Oncol* 2008;26:31–51.
158. Thekkumpurath P, Walker J, Butcher I, et al. Screening for major depression in cancer outpatients: the diagnostic accuracy of the 9-item patient health questionnaire. *Cancer* 2011;117:218–227.
159. Shinn EH, Valentine A, Baum G, et al. Comparison of four brief depression screening instruments in ovarian cancer patients: diagnostic accuracy using traditional versus alternative cutpoints. *Gynecol Oncol* 2017;145:562–568.
160. Chochinov HM, Wilson KG, Enns M, et al. "Are you depressed?" Screening for depression in the terminally ill. *Am J Psychiatry* 1997;154:674–676.
161. Lloyd-Williams M, Spiller J, Ward J. Which depression screening tools should be used in palliative care? *Palliat Med* 2003;17:40–43.
162. Mock V, Atkinson A, Barsevick A, et al. NCCN Practice Guidelines for cancer-related fatigue. *Oncology (Williston Park)* 2000;14:151–161.
163. Ancoli-Israel S, Moore PJ, Jones V. The relationship between fatigue and sleep in cancer patients: a review. *Eur J Cancer Care (Engl)* 2001;10:245–255.
164. Gerber LH. Cancer-related fatigue: persistent, pervasive, and problematic. *Phys Med Rehabil Clin N Am* 2017;28:65–88.
165. Abrahams HJ, Gielissen MF, Schmits IC, et al. Risk factors, prevalence, and course of severe fatigue after breast cancer treatment: a meta-analysis involving 12 327 breast cancer survivors. *Ann Oncol* 2016;27:965–974.
166. Minton O, Stone P. How common is fatigue in disease-free breast cancer survivors? A systematic review of the literature. *Breast Cancer Res Treat* 2008;112:5–13.
167. Hofman M, Ryan JL, Figueroa-Moseley CD, et al. Cancer-related fatigue: the scale of the problem. *Oncologist* 2007;12(suppl 1):4–10.
168. Stasi R, Abriani L, Beccaglia P, et al. Cancer-related fatigue: evolving concepts in evaluation and treatment. *Cancer* 2003;98:1786–1801.
169. Sobrero A, Puglisi F, Guglielmi A, et al. Fatigue: a main component of anemia symptomatology. *Semin Oncol* 2001;28(2 suppl 8):15–18.
170. Bremberg ER, Brandberg Y, Hising C, et al. Anemia and quality of life including anemia-related symptoms in patients with solid tumors in clinical practice. *Med Oncol* 2007;24:95–102.
171. Berger AM, Gerber LH, Mayer DK. Cancer-related fatigue: implications for breast cancer survivors. *Cancer* 2012;118:2261–2269.
172. Minton O, Stone P. A systematic review of the scales used for the measurement of cancer-related fatigue (CRF). *Ann Oncol* 2009;20:17–25.
173. Wilkie DJ, Huang HY, Berry DL, et al. Cancer symptom control: feasibility of a tailored, interactive computerized program for patients. *Fam Community Health* 2001;24:48–62.
174. Bennett S, Pigott A, Beller EM, et al. Educational interventions for the management of cancer-related fatigue in adults. *Cochrane Database Syst Rev* 2016;11:CD008144.
175. Larun L, Brurberg KG, Odgaard-Jensen J, et al. Exercise therapy for chronic fatigue syndrome. *Cochrane Database Syst Rev* 2017;4:CD003200.
176. Sandler CX, Goldstein D, Horsfield S, et al. Randomized evaluation of cognitive-behavioral therapy and graded exercise therapy for post-cancer fatigue. *J Pain Symptom Manage* 2017;54:74–84.
177. Mao JJ, Armstrong K, Bowman MA, et al. Symptom burden among cancer survivors: impact of age and comorbidity. *J Am Board Fam Med* 2007;20:434–443.
178. Otte JL, Carpenter JS, Manchanda S, et al. Systematic review of sleep disorders in cancer patients: can the prevalence of sleep disorders be ascertained? *Cancer Med* 2015;4:183–200.
179. Savard J, Villa J, Ivers H, et al. Prevalence, natural course, and risk factors of insomnia comorbid with cancer over a 2-month period. *J Clin Oncol* 2009;27:5233–5239.
180. Savard J, Ivers H, Villa J, et al. Natural course of insomnia comorbid with cancer: an 18-month longitudinal study. *J Clin Oncol* 2011;29:3580–3586.
181. Savard J, Morin CM. Insomnia in the context of cancer: a review of a neglected problem. *J Clin Oncol* 2001;19:895–908.
182. Savard J, Simard S, Blanchet J, et al. Prevalence, clinical characteristics, and risk factors for insomnia in the context of breast cancer. *Sleep* 2001;24:583–590.
183. Davidson JR, MacLean AW, Brundage MD, et al. Sleep disturbance in cancer patients. *Soc Sci Med* 2002;54:1309–1321.
184. Chen ML, Yu CT, Yang CH. Sleep disturbances and quality of life in lung cancer patients undergoing chemotherapy. *Lung Cancer* 2008;62:391–400.
185. Armstrong TS, Shade MY, Breton G, et al. Sleep-wake disturbance in patients with brain tumors. *Neuro Oncol* 2017;19:323–335.
186. Buysse DJ, Yu L, Moul DE, et al. Development and validation of patient-reported outcome measures for sleep disturbance and sleep-related impairments. *Sleep* 2010;33:781–792.

187. Morin CM, Belleville G, Belanger L, et al. The Insomnia Severity Index: psychometric indicators to detect insomnia cases and evaluate treatment response. *Sleep* 2011;34:601–608.

188. Buysse DJ, Reynolds CF III, Monk TH, et al. The Pittsburgh Sleep Quality Index: a new instrument for psychiatric practice and research. *Psychiatry Res* 1989;28:193–213.

189. Mattila T, Stoyanova V, Elferink A, et al. Insomnia medication: do published studies reflect the complete picture of efficacy and safety? *Eur Neuropsychopharmacol* 2011;21:500–507.

190. Kripke DF. Chronic hypnotic use: deadly risks, doubtful benefit. Review article. *Sleep Med Rev* 2000;4:5–20.

191. Casault L, Savard J, Ivers H, et al. Utilization of hypnotic medication in the context of cancer: predictors and frequency of use. *Support Care Cancer* 2012;20:1203–1210.

192. Kripke DF. Hypnotic drug risks of mortality, infection, depression, and cancer: but lack of benefit. *F1000Res* 2016;5:918.

193. Kripke DF. Mortality risk of hypnotics: strengths and limits of evidence. *Drug Saf* 2016;39:93–107.

194. Sivertsen B, Omvik S, Pallesen S, et al. Cognitive behavioral therapy vs zopiclone for treatment of chronic primary insomnia in older adults: a randomized controlled trial. *JAMA* 2006;295:2851–2858.

195. Jensen MP, Chang HY, Lai YH, et al. Pain in long-term breast cancer survivors: frequency, severity, and impact. *Pain Med* 2010;11:1099–1106.

196. van den Beuken-van Everdingen MH, Hochstenbach LM, Joosten EA, et al. Update on prevalence of pain in patients with cancer: systematic review and meta-analysis. *J Pain Symptom Manage* 2016;51:1070–1090.

197. Davidsen M, Kjoller M, Helweg-Larsen K. The Danish National Cohort Study (DANCOS). *Scand J Public Health* 2011;39:131–135.

198. van den Beuken-van Everdingen M. Chronic pain in cancer survivors: a growing issue. *J Pain Palliat Care Pharmacother* 2012;26:385–387.

199. Levy MH, Chwistek M, Mehta RS. Management of chronic pain in cancer survivors. *Cancer J* 2008;14:401–409.

200. Green CR, Hart-Johnson T, Loeffler DR. Cancer-related chronic pain: examining quality of life in diverse cancer survivors. *Cancer* 2011;117: 1994–2003.

201. van den Beuken-van Everdingen MH, de Rijke JM, Kessels AG, et al. Prevalence of pain in patients with cancer: a systematic review of the past 40 years. *Ann Oncol* 2007;18:1437–1449.

202. Morselli M, Bandieri E, Zanin R, et al. Pain and emotional distress in leukemia patients at diagnosis. *Leuk Res* 2010;34:e67–e68.

203. Stalfelt AM, Brodin H, Pettersson S, et al. The final phase in acute myeloid leukaemia (AML). A study on bleeding, infection and pain. *Leuk Res* 2003;27:481–488.

204. Twycross R, Harcourt J, Bergl S. A survey of pain in patients with advanced cancer. *J Pain Symptom Manage* 1996;12:273–282.

205. Yu HH, Tsai YY, Hoffe SE. Overview of diagnosis and management of metastatic disease to bone. *Cancer Control* 2012;19:84–91.

206. Coleman RE. Clinical features of metastatic bone disease and risk of skeletal morbidity. *Clin Cancer Res* 2006;12(20 pt 2):6243s–6249s.

207. Coleman RE, Rubens RD. The clinical course of bone metastases from breast cancer. *Br J Cancer* 1987;55:61–66.

208. Palmer E, Henrikson B, McKusick K, et al. Pain as an indicator of bone metastasis. *Acta Radiol* 1988;29:445–449.

209. Thiers BH, Sahn RE, Callen JP. Cutaneous manifestations of internal malignancy. *CA Cancer J Clin* 2009;59:73–98.

210. Ito T, Goto K, Yoh K, et al. Hypertrophic pulmonary osteoarthropathy as a paraneoplastic manifestation of lung cancer. *J Thorac Oncol* 2010;5: 976–980.

211. Koike H, Tanaka F, Sobue G. Paraneoplastic neuropathy: wide-ranging clinicopathological manifestations. *Curr Opin Neurol* 2011;24:504–510.

212. Graus F, Dalmau J. Paraneoplastic neuropathies. *Curr Opin Neurol* 2013; 26:489–495.

213. Loricera J, Calvo-Rio V, Ortiz-Sanjuan F, et al. The spectrum of paraneoplastic cutaneous vasculitis in a defined population: incidence and clinical features. *Medicine* 2013;92:331–343.

214. Staff NP, Grisold A, Grisold W, et al. Chemotherapy-induced peripheral neuropathy: a current review. *Ann Neurol* 2017;81:772–781.

215. Majithia N, Temkin SM, Ruddy KJ, et al. National Cancer Institute-supported chemotherapy-induced peripheral neuropathy trials: outcomes and lessons. *Support Care Cancer* 2016;24:1439–1447.

216. Weinstein RS. Glucocorticoid-induced osteoporosis and osteonecrosis. *Endocrinol Metab Clin North Am* 2012;41:595–611.

217. Powell C, Chang C, Naguwa SM, et al. Steroid induced osteonecrosis: an analysis of steroid dosing risk. *Autoimmun Rev* 2010;9:721–743.

218. Lee JA, Farooki S, Ashman CJ, et al. MR patterns of involvement of humeral head osteonecrosis. *J Comput Assist Tomogr* 2002;26:839–842.

219. Hegde JV, Chen AM, Chin RK. Advances in radiation oncology: what to consider. *Otolaryngol Clin North Am* 2017;50:755–764.

220. Cai Z, Li Y, Hu Z, et al. Radiation-induced brachial plexopathy in patients with nasopharyngeal carcinoma: a retrospective study. *Oncotarget* 2016;7:18887–18895.

221. Delanian S, Lefaix JL, Pradat PF. Radiation-induced neuropathy in cancer survivors. *Radiother Oncol* 2012;105:273–282.

222. Pradat PF, Delanian S. Late radiation injury to peripheral nerves. *Handb Clin Neurol* 2013;115:743–758.

223. Funk GF, Karnell LH, Christensen AJ. Long-term health-related quality of life in survivors of head and neck cancer. *Arch Otolaryngol Head Neck Surg* 2012;138:123–133.

224. Hoxbroe Michaelsen S, Gronhoj C, Hoxbroe Michaelsen J, et al. Quality of life in survivors of oropharyngeal cancer: a systematic review and meta-analysis of 1366 patients. *Eur J Cancer* 2017;78:91–102.

225. Hansson E, Forbes HJ, Langan SM, et al. Herpes zoster risk after 21 specific cancers: population-based case-control study. *Br J Cancer* 2017;116: 1643–1651.

226. Thyregod HG, Rowbotham MC, Peters M, et al. Natural history of pain following herpes zoster. *Pain* 2007;128:148–156.

227. Coplan PM, Schmader K, Nikas A, et al. Development of a measure of the burden of pain due to herpes zoster and postherpetic neuralgia for prevention trials: adaptation of the brief pain inventory. *J Pain* 2004;5:344–356.

228. Oxman MN, Levin MJ, Johnson GR, et al. A vaccine to prevent herpes zoster and postherpetic neuralgia in older adults. *N Engl J Med* 2005;352: 2271–2284.

229. Tontodonati M, Ursini T, Polilli E, et al. Post-herpetic neuralgia. *Int J Gen Med* 2012;5:861–871.

230. Solomon P. Congruence between health professionals' and patients' pain ratings: a review of the literature. *Scand J Caring Sci* 2001;15:174–180.

231. Kappesser J, Williams AC, Prkachin KM. Testing two accounts of pain underestimation. *Pain* 2006;124:109–116.

232. Prkachin KM, Solomon PE, Ross J. Underestimation of pain by health-care providers: towards a model of the process of inferring pain in others. *Can J Nurs Res* 2007;39:88–106.

233. Grossman SA. Undertreatment of cancer pain: barriers and remedies. *Support Care Cancer* 1993;1:74–78.

234. Baliki MN, Apkarian AV. Nociception, pain, negative moods, and behavior selection. *Neuron* 2015;87:474–491.

235. Hjermstad MJ, Fayers PM, Haugen DF, et al. Studies comparing Numerical Rating Scales, Verbal Rating Scales, and Visual Analogue Scales for assessment of pain intensity in adults: a systematic literature review. *J Pain Symptom Manage* 2011;41:1073–1093.

236. Jensen MP, Karoly P, Braver S. The measurement of clinical pain intensity: a comparison of six methods. *Pain* 1986;27:117–126.

237. Ferraz MB, Quaresma MR, Aquino LR, et al. Reliability of pain scales in the assessment of literate and illiterate patients with rheumatoid arthritis. *J Rheumatol* 1990;17:1022–1024.

238. Clark P, Lavielle P, Martinez H. Learning from pain scales: patient perspective. *J Rheumatol* 2003;30:1584–1588.

239. Moinpour CM, Feigl P, Metch B, et al. Quality of life end points in cancer clinical trials: review and recommendations. *J Natl Cancer Inst* 1989;81:485–495.

240. Wallenstein SL. Measurement of pain and analgesia in cancer patients. *Cancer* 1984;53:2260–2266.

241. Wallenstein SL, Heidrich G III, Kaiko R, et al. Clinical evaluation of mild analgesics: the measurement of clinical pain. *Br J Clin Pharmacol* 1980;10(suppl 2):319s–327s.

242. Corgna E, Betti M, Gatta G, et al. Renal cancer. *Crit Rev Oncol Hematol* 2007;64:247–262.

243. Pelosof LC, Gerber DE. Paraneoplastic syndromes: an approach to diagnosis and treatment. *Mayo Clin Proc* 2010;85:838–854.

244. Jackson MB, Pounder D, Price C, et al. Percutaneous cervical cordotomy for the control of pain in patients with pleural mesothelioma. *Thorax* 1999;54:238–241.

245. Suzuki M, Narita M, Hasegawa M, et al. Sensation of abdominal pain induced by peritoneal carcinomatosis is accompanied by changes in the expression of substance P and mu-opioid receptors in the spinal cord of mice. *Anesthesiology* 2012;117:847–856.

246. Vainio A, Auvinen A. Prevalence of symptoms among patients with advanced cancer: an international collaborative study. Symptom Prevalence Group. *J Pain Symptom Manage* 1996;12:3–10.

247. Levren G, Sadik M, Gjertsson P, et al. Relation between pain and skeletal metastasis in patients with prostate or breast cancer. *Clin Physiol Funct Imaging* 2011;31:193–195.

248. Vuorinen E. Pain as an early symptom in cancer. *Clin J Pain* 1993;9:272–278.

249. Cleeland CS. The impact of pain on the patient with cancer. *Cancer* 1984;54:2635–2641.

250. Fogel EL, Shahda S, Sandrasegaran K, et al. A multidisciplinary approach to pancreas cancer in 2016: a review. *Am J Gastroenterol* 2017;112: 537–554.

251. Ilic M, Ilic I. Epidemiology of pancreatic cancer. *World J Gastroenterol* 2016;22:9694–9705.

252. Ma J, Siegel R, Jemal A. Pancreatic cancer death rates by race among US men and women, 1970–2009. *J Natl Cancer Inst* 2013;105:1694–1700.

253. Kelsen DP, Portenoy R, Thaler H, et al. Pain as a predictor of outcome in patients with operable pancreatic carcinoma. *Surgery* 1997;122:53–59.

254. Demir IE, Ceyhan GO, Liebl F, et al. Neural invasion in pancreatic cancer: the past, present and future. *Cancers (Basel)* 2010;2:1513–1527.

255. Liu B, Lu KY. Neural invasion in pancreatic carcinoma. *Hepatobiliary Pancreat Dis Int* 2002;1:469–476.

256. Liebl F, Demir IE, Mayer K, et al. The impact of neural invasion severity in gastrointestinal malignancies: a clinicopathological study. *Ann Surg* 2014;260:900–907.

257. Demir IE, Friess H, Ceyhan GO. Neural plasticity in pancreatitis and pancreatic cancer. *Nat Rev Gastroenterol Hepatol* 2015;12:649–659.

258. Singh SM, Longmire WP Jr, Reber HA. Surgical palliation for pancreatic cancer. The UCLA experience. *Ann Surg* 1990;212:132–139.

259. Kelsen DP, Portenoy RK, Thaler HT, et al. Pain and depression in patients with newly diagnosed pancreas cancer. *J Clin Oncol* 1995;13:748–755.

260. Passik SD, Breitbart WS. Depression in patients with pancreatic carcinoma. Diagnostic and treatment issues. *Cancer* 1996;78:615–626.

261. Kim D, Zhu H, Nassri A, et al. Survival analysis of veteran patients with pancreatic cancer. *J Dig Dis* 2016;17:399–407.

262. D'Haese JG, Hartel M, Demir IE, et al. Pain sensation in pancreatic diseases is not uniform: the different facets of pancreatic pain. *World J Gastroenterol* 2014;20:9154–9161.

263. Takamori H, Hiraoka T, Kanemitsu K, et al. Identification of prognostic factors associated with early mortality after surgical resection for pancreatic cancer—under-analysis of cumulative survival curve. *World J Surg* 2006;30:213–218.

264. Matulonis UA, Sood AK, Fallowfield L, et al. Ovarian cancer. *Nat Rev Dis Primers* 2016;2:16061.

265. Andrews L, Mutch DG. Hereditary ovarian cancer and risk reduction. *Best Pract Res Clin Obstet Gynaecol* 2017;41:31–48.

266. Ueland FR. A perspective on ovarian cancer biomarkers: past, present and yet-to-come. *Diagnostics (Basel)* 2017;7.

267. Portenoy RK, Kornblith AB, Wong G, et al. Pain in ovarian cancer patients. Prevalence, characteristics, and associated symptoms. *Cancer* 1994;74:907–915.

268. Sawaya GF, Huchko MJ. Cervical cancer screening. *Med Clin North Am* 2017;101:743–753.

269. Sironi S, Buda A, Picchio M, et al. Lymph node metastasis in patients with clinical early-stage cervical cancer: detection with integrated FDG PET/CT. *Radiology* 2006;238:272–279.

270. Lindenberg ML, Turkbey B, Mena E, et al. Imaging locally advanced, recurrent, and metastatic prostate cancer: a review. *JAMA Oncol* 2017;3:1415–1422.

271. Smith RA, Andrews KS, Brooks D, et al. Cancer screening in the United States, 2017: a review of current American Cancer Society guidelines and current issues in cancer screening. *CA Cancer J Clin* 2017;67:100–121.

272. Larson SR, Zhang X, Dumpit R, et al. Characterization of osteoblastic and osteolytic proteins in prostate cancer bone metastases. *Prostate* 2013;73:932–940.

273. Wong WW, Anderson EM, Mohammadi H, et al. Factors associated with survival following radium-223 treatment for metastatic castration-resistant prostate cancer. *Clin Genitourin Cancer* 2017;15:e969–e975.

274. DiSipio T, Rye S, Newman B, et al. Incidence of unilateral arm lymphoedema after breast cancer: a systematic review and meta-analysis. *Lancet Oncol* 2013;14:500–515.

275. Keshtgar M, Davidson T, Pigott K, et al. Current status and advances in management of early breast cancer. *Int J Surg* 2010;8:199–202.

276. Cetin K, Christiansen CF, Svaerke C, et al. Survival in patients with breast cancer with bone metastasis: a Danish population-based cohort study on the prognostic impact of initial stage of disease at breast cancer diagnosis and length of the bone metastasis-free interval. *BMJ Open* 2015;5:e007702.

277. Jensen AO, Jacobsen JB, Norgaard M, et al. Incidence of bone metastases and skeletal-related events in breast cancer patients: a population-based cohort study in Denmark. *BMC Cancer* 2011;11:29.

278. Sathiakumar N, Delzell E, Morrisey MA, et al. Mortality following bone metastasis and skeletal-related events among women with breast cancer: a population-based analysis of U.S. Medicare beneficiaries, 1999–2006. *Breast Cancer Res Trea* 2012;131:231–238.

279. Ording AG, Heide-Jorgensen U, Christiansen CF, et al. Site of metastasis and breast cancer mortality: a Danish nationwide registry-based cohort study. *Clin Exp Metastasis* 2017;34:93–101.

280. Harvey HA. Issues concerning the role of chemotherapy and hormonal therapy of bone metastases from breast carcinoma. *Cancer* 1997;80:1646–1651.

281. Geiger S, Cnossen JA, Horster S, et al. Long-term follow-up of patients with metastatic breast cancer: results of a retrospective, single-center analysis from 2000 to 2005. *Anticancer Drugs* 2011;22:933–939.

282. Bradley CJ, Yabroff KR, Mariotto AB, et al. Antineoplastic treatment of advanced-stage non-small-cell lung cancer: treatment, survival, and spending (2000 to 2011). *J Clin Oncol* 2017;35:529–553.

283. Mercadante S, Armata M, Salvaggio L. Pain characteristics of advanced lung cancer patients referred to a palliative care service. *Pain* 1994;59:141–145.

284. Gupta K, Miller JD, Li JZ, et al. Epidemiologic and socioeconomic burden of metastatic renal cell carcinoma (mRCC): a literature review. *Cancer Treat Rev* 2008;34:193–205.

285. Athar U, Gentile TC. Treatment options for metastatic renal cell carcinoma: a review. *Can J Urol* 2008;15:3954–3966.

286. Zisman A, Pantuck AJ, Wieder J, et al. Risk group assessment and clinical outcome algorithm to predict the natural history of patients with surgically resected renal cell carcinoma. *J Clin Oncol* 2002;20:4559–4566.

287. Woodward E, Jagdev S, McParland L, et al. Skeletal complications and survival in renal cancer patients with bone metastases. *Bone* 2011;48:160–166.

288. Siegel RL, Miller KD, Fedewa SA, et al. Colorectal cancer statistics, 2017. *CA Cancer J Clin* 2017;67:177–193.

289. Collins D, Chua H. Contemporary surgical management of synchronous colorectal liver metastases. *F1000Res* 2017;6:598.

290. Akgul O, Cetinkaya E, Ersoz S, et al. Role of surgery in colorectal cancer liver metastases. *World J Gastroenterol* 2014;20:6113–6122.

291. Group BDW. Biomarkers and surrogate endpoints: preferred definitions and conceptual framework. *Clin Pharmacol Ther* 2001;69:89–95.

292. Duffy MJ, O'Donovan N, McDermott E, et al. Validated biomarkers: the key to precision treatment in patients with breast cancer. *Breast* 2016;29:192–201.

293. Harris LN, Ismaila N, McShane LM, et al. Use of biomarkers to guide decisions on adjuvant systemic therapy for women with early-stage invasive breast cancer: American Society of Clinical Oncology clinical practice guideline. *J Clin Oncol* 2016;34:1134–1150.

294. Portenoy RK, Hagen NA. Breakthrough pain: definition, prevalence and characteristics. *Pain* 1990;41:273–281.

295. Haugen DF, Hjermstad MJ, Hagen N, et al. Assessment and classification of cancer breakthrough pain: a systematic literature review. *Pain* 2010;149:476–482.

296. Patt RB, Ellison NM. Breakthrough pain in cancer patients: characteristics, prevalence, and treatment. *Oncology (Williston Park)* 1998;12:1035–1046.

297. Deandrea S, Corli O, Consonni D, et al. Prevalence of breakthrough cancer pain: a systematic review and a pooled analysis of published literature. *J Pain Symptom Manage* 2014;47:57–76.

298. Lohre ET, Klepstad P, Bennett MI, et al. From "breakthrough" to "episodic" cancer pain? A European Association for Palliative Care Research Network expert Delphi survey toward a common terminology and classification of transient cancer pain exacerbations. *J Pain Symptom Manage* 2016;51:1013–1019.

299. Svendsen KB, Andersen S, Arnason S, et al. Breakthrough pain in malignant and non-malignant diseases: a review of prevalence, characteristics and mechanisms. *Eur J Pain* 2005;9:195–206.

300. Katz NP, Gajria KL, Shillington AC, et al. Impact of breakthrough pain on community-dwelling cancer patients: results from the National Breakthrough Pain Study. *Postgrad Med* 2017;129:32–39.

301. Hjermstad MJ, Kaasa S, Caraceni A, et al. Characteristics of breakthrough cancer pain and its influence on quality of life in an international cohort of patients with cancer. *BMJ Support Palliat Care* 2016;6:344–352.

302. Montague L, Green CR. Cancer and breakthrough pain's impact on a diverse population. *Pain Med* 2009;10:549–561.

303. Gureje O, Von Korff M, Simon GE, et al. Persistent pain and well-being: a World Health Organization study in primary care. *JAMA* 1998;280:147–151.

304. Fortner BV, Okon TA, Portenoy RK. A survey of pain-related hospitalizations, emergency department visits, and physician office visits reported by cancer patients with and without history of breakthrough pain. *J Pain* 2002;3:38–44.

305. Ottewell PD. The role of osteoblasts in bone metastasis. *J Bone Oncol* 2016;5:124–127.

306. Fernandes R, Siegel P, Komarova S, et al. Future directions for bone metastasis research—highlights from the 2015 bone and the Oncologist new updates conference (BONUS). *J Bone Oncol* 2016;5:57–62.

307. Hess KR, Varadhachary GR, Taylor SH, et al. Metastatic patterns in adenocarcinoma. *Cancer* 2006;106:1624–1633.

308. Kraljevic Pavelic S, Sedic M, Bosnjak H, et al. Metastasis: new perspectives on an old problem. *Mol Cancer* 2011;10:22.

309. Weidle UH, Birzele F, Kollmorgen G, et al. Molecular mechanisms of bone metastasis. *Cancer Genomics Proteomics* 2016;13:1–12.

310. Roodman GD. Mechanisms of bone metastasis. *N Engl J Med* 2004;350:1655–1664.

311. Mantyh PW. The neurobiology of skeletal pain. *Eur J Neurosci* 2014;39:508–519.

312. Mantyh PW. Bone cancer pain: from mechanism to therapy. *Curr Opin Support Palliat Care* 2014;8:83–90.

313. Jonsson OG, Sartain P, Ducore JM, et al. Bone pain as an initial symptom of childhood acute lymphoblastic leukemia: association with nearly normal hematologic indexes. *J Pediatr* 1990;117:233–237.

314. Tubiana-Hulin M. Incidence, prevalence and distribution of bone metastases. *Bone* 1991;12(suppl 1):S9–S10.

315. Coleman RE. Metastatic bone disease: clinical features, pathophysiology and treatment strategies. *Cancer Treat Rev* 2001;27:165–176.

316. Yong M, Jensen AO, Jacobsen JB, et al. Survival in breast cancer patients with bone metastases and skeletal-related events: a population-based cohort study in Denmark (1999–2007). *Breast Cancer Res Trea* 2011;129:495–503.

317. Hensel J, Thalmann GN. Biology of bone metastases in prostate cancer. *Urology* 2016;92:6–13.

318. Jones PW, Bogardus CR, Anderson DW. Significance of initial "performance status" in patients receiving halfbody radiation. *Int J Radiat Oncol Biol Phys* 1984;10:1947–1950.

319. Angelo K, Dalhaug A, Pawinski A, et al. Survival prediction score: a simple but age-dependent method predicting prognosis in patients undergoing palliative radiotherapy. *ISRN Onco* 2014;2014:912865.

320. van der Linden YM, Steenland E, van Houwelingen HC, et al. Patients with a favourable prognosis are equally palliated with single and multiple fraction radiotherapy: results on survival in the Dutch Bone Metastasis Study. *Radiother Oncol* 2006;78:245–253.

321. Lai PP, Perez CA, Lockett MA. Prognostic significance of pelvic recurrence and distant metastasis in prostate carcinoma following definitive radiotherapy. *Int J Radiat Oncol Biol Phys* 1992;24:423–430.

322. Chow E, Fung K, Panzarella T, et al. A predictive model for survival in metastatic cancer patients attending an outpatient palliative radiotherapy clinic. *Int J Radiat Oncol Biol Phys* 2002;53:1291–1302.

323. De Giorgi U, Mego M, Rohren EM, et al. 18F-FDG PET/CT findings and circulating tumor cell counts in the monitoring of systemic therapies for bone metastases from breast cancer. *J Nucl Med* 2010;51:1213–1218.

324. Yamashita K, Denno K, Ueda T, et al. Prognostic significance of bone metastases in patients with metastatic prostate cancer. *Cancer* 1993;71: 1297–1302.

325. Sartor O, Coleman R, Nilsson S, et al. Effect of radium-223 dichloride on symptomatic skeletal events in patients with castration-resistant prostate cancer and bone metastases: results from a phase 3, double-blind, randomised trial. *Lancet Oncol* 2014;15:738–746.

326. Parker C, Nilsson S, Heinrich D, et al. Alpha emitter radium-223 and survival in metastatic prostate cancer. *N Engl J Med* 2013;369:213–223.

327. Peh WC, Khong PL, Sham JS, et al. Sacral and pubic insufficiency fractures after irradiation of gynaecological malignancies. *Clin Oncol (R Coll Radiol)* 1995;7:117–122.

328. Abe H, Nakamura M, Takahashi S, et al. Radiation-induced insufficiency fractures of the pelvis: evaluation with 99mTc-methylene diphosphonate scintigraphy. *AJR Am J Roentgenol* 1992;158:599–602.

329. Blomlie V, Rofstad EK, Talle K, et al. Incidence of radiation-induced insufficiency fractures of the female pelvis: evaluation with MR imaging. *AJR Am J Roentgenol* 1996;167:1205–1210.

330. Howland WJ, Loeffler RK, Starchman DE, et al. Postirradiation atrophic changes of bone and related complications. *Radiology* 1975;117:677–685.

331. Bazire L, Xu H, Foy JP, et al. Pelvic insufficiency fracture (PIF) incidence in patients treated with intensity-modulated radiation therapy (IMRT) for gynaecological or anal cancer: single-institution experience and review of the literature. *Br J Radiol* 2017;90:20160885.

332. Linstrom NJ, Heiserman JE, Kortman KE, et al. Anatomical and biomechanical analyses of the unique and consistent locations of sacral insufficiency fractures. *Spine (Phila Pa 1976)* 2009;34:309–315.

333. Salavati A, Shah V, Wang ZJ, et al. F-18 FDG PET/CT findings in postradiation pelvic insufficiency fracture. *Clin Imaging* 2011;35:139–142.

334. Halac M, Mut SS, Sonmezoglu K, et al. Avoidance of misinterpretation of an FDG positive sacral insufficiency fracture using PET/CT scans in a patient with endometrial cancer: a case report. *Clin Nucl Med* 2007;32:779–781.

335. Denis F, Davis S, Comfort T. Sacral fractures: an important problem. Retrospective analysis of 236 cases. *Clin Oral Implants Res* 1988;227:67–81.

336. Crawford J. Safety and efficacy of pegfilgrastim in patients receiving myelosuppressive chemotherapy. *Pharmacotherapy* 2003;23:15s–19s.

337. Xu H, Gong Q, Vogl FD, et al. Risk factors for bone pain among patients with cancer receiving myelosuppressive chemotherapy and pegfilgrastim. *Support Care Cancer* 2016;24:723–730.

338. Lambertini M, Del Mastro L, Bellodi A, et al. The five "Ws" for bone pain due to the administration of granulocyte-colony stimulating factors (G-CSFs). *Crit Rev Oncol Hematol* 2014;89:112–128.

339. Kubista E, Glaspy J, Holmes FA, et al. Bone pain associated with once-per-cycle pegfilgrastim is similar to daily filgrastim in patients with breast cancer. *Clin Breast Cancer* 2003;3:391–398.

340. Cervero F. Mechanisms of acute visceral pain. *Br Med Bull* 1991;47:549–560.

341. Cervero F. Visceral pain: mechanisms of peripheral and central sensitization. *Ann Med* 1995;27:235–239.

342. Gebhart GF, Ness TJ. Central mechanisms of visceral pain. *Can J Physiol Pharmacol* 1991;69:627–634.

343. Christianson JA, Davis BM. The role of visceral afferents in disease. In: Kruger L, Light AR, eds. *Translational Pain Research: From Mouse to Man.* Boca Raton, FL: CRC Press; 2010.

344. Cervero F, Connell LA, Lawson SN. Somatic and visceral primary afferents in the lower thoracic dorsal root ganglia of the cat. *J Comp Neurol* 1984;228:422–431.

345. Ness TJ, Gebhart GF. Visceral pain: a review of experimental studies. *Pain* 1990;41:167–234.

346. Palecek J, Willis WD. The dorsal column pathway facilitates visceromotor responses to colorectal distention after colon inflammation in rats. *Pain* 2003;104:501–507.

347. Palecek J. The role of dorsal columns pathway in visceral pain. *Physiol Res* 2004;53(suppl 1):S125–S130.

348. Vecht CJ, Hoff AM, Kansen PJ, et al. Types and causes of pain in cancer of the head and neck. *Cancer* 1992;70:178–184.

349. Greenberg HS, Deck MD, Vikram B, et al. Metastasis to the base of the skull: clinical findings in 43 patients. *Neurology* 1981;31:530–537.

350. Metheetrairut C, Brown DH. Glossopharyngeal neuralgia and syncope secondary to neck malignancy. *J Otolaryngol* 1993;22:18–20.

351. Moris G, Roig C, Misiego M, et al. The distinctive headache of the occipital condyle syndrome: a report of four cases. *Headache* 1998;38:308–311.

352. Capobianco DJ, Brazis PW, Rubino FA, et al. Occipital condyle syndrome. *Headache* 2002;42:142–146.

353. Bullitt E, Tew JM, Boyd J. Intracranial tumors in patients with facial pain. *J Neurosurg* 1986;64:865–871.

354. Cheng TM, Cascino TL, Onofrio BM. Comprehensive study of diagnosis and treatment of trigeminal neuralgia secondary to tumors. *Neurology* 1993;43:2298–2302.

355. Nomura T, Ikezaki K, Matsushima T, et al. Trigeminal neuralgia: differentiation between intracranial mass lesions and ordinary vascular compression as causative lesions. *Neurosurg Rev* 1994;17:51–57.

356. Puca A, Meglio M, Vari R, et al. Evaluation of fifth nerve dysfunction in 136 patients with middle and posterior cranial fossae tumors. *Eur Neurol* 1995;35:33–37.

357. Jaeckle KA. Nerve plexus metastases. *Neurol Clin* 1991;9:857–866.

358. He W, Wang W, Gustas C, et al. Isolated sciatic neuropathy as an initial manifestation of a high grade B-cell lymphoma: a case report and literature review. *Clin Neurol Neurosurg* 2016;149:147–153.

359. Gonzalvo A, McKenzie C, Harris M, et al. Primary non-Hodgkin's lymphoma of the radial nerve: case report. *Neurosurgery* 2010;67:E872–E873.

360. Misdraji J, Ino Y, Louis DN, et al. Primary lymphoma of peripheral nerve: report of four cases. *Am J Surg Pathol* 2000;24:1257–1265.

361. van der Windt DA, Simons E, Riphagen II, et al. Physical examination for lumbar radiculopathy due to disc herniation in patients with low-back pain. *Cochrane Database Syst Rev* 2010;(2):CD007431.

362. Chowdhary S, Chamberlain M. Leptomeningeal metastases: current concepts and management guidelines. *J Natl Compr Canc Netw* 2005;3:693–703.

363. Le Rhun E, Ruda R, Devos P, et al. Diagnosis and treatment patterns for patients with leptomeningeal metastasis from solid tumors across Europe. *J Neurooncol* 2017;133:419–427.

364. Chamberlain M, Soffietti R, Raizer J, et al. Leptomeningeal metastasis: a Response Assessment in Neuro-Oncology critical review of endpoints and response criteria of published randomized clinical trials. *Neuro Oncol* 2014;16:1176–1185.

365. Kaplan JG, Portenoy RK, Pack DR, et al. Polyradiculopathy in leptomeningeal metastasis: the role of EMG and late response studies. *J Neurooncol* 1990;9:219–224.

366. Wasserstrom WR, Glass JP, Posner JB. Diagnosis and treatment of leptomeningeal metastases from solid tumors: experience with 90 patients. *Cancer* 1982;49:759–772.

367. Clarke JL, Perez HR, Jacks LM, et al. Leptomeningeal metastases in the MRI era. *Neurology* 2010;74:1449–1454.

368. Chamberlain M, Junck L, Brandsma D, et al. Leptomeningeal metastases: a RANO proposal for response criteria. *Neuro Oncol* 2017;19:484–492.

369. Sahgal A, Ma L, Gibbs I, et al. Spinal cord tolerance for stereotactic body radiotherapy. *Int J Radiat Oncol Biol Phys* 2010;77:548–553.

370. Kirkpatrick JP, van der Kogel AJ, Schultheiss TE. Radiation dose-volume effects in the spinal cord. *Int J Radiat Oncol Biol Phys* 2010;76:S42–S49.

371. Counsel P, Khangure M. Myelopathy due to intrathecal chemotherapy: magnetic resonance imaging findings. *Clin Radiol* 2007;62:172–176.

372. Gosavi T, Diong CP, Lim SH. Methotrexate-induced myelopathy mimicking subacute combined degeneration of the spinal cord. *J Clin Neurosci* 2013;20:1025–1026.

373. Shen KR, Meyers BF, Larner JM, et al. Special treatment issues in lung cancer: ACCP evidence-based clinical practice guidelines (2nd edition). *Chest* 2007;132:290s–305s.

374. Marangoni C, Lacerenza M, Formaglio F, et al. Sensory disorder of the chest as presenting symptom of lung cancer. *J Neurol Neurosurg Psychiatry* 1993;56:1033–1034.

375. Andreou A, Sohaib A, Collins DJ, et al. Diffusion-weighted MR neurography for the assessment of brachial plexopathy in oncological practice. *Cancer Imaging* 2015;15:6.

376. Jaeckle KA. Neurologic manifestations of neoplastic and radiation-induced plexopathies. *Semin Neurol* 2010;30:254–262.

377. Dalmau J, Graus F, Marco M. "Hot and dry foot" as initial manifestation of neoplastic lumbosacral plexopathy. *Neurology* 1989;39:871–872.

378. Jaeckle KA. Neurological manifestations of neoplastic and radiation-induced plexopathies. *Semin Neurol* 2004;24:385–393.

379. Jaeckle KA, Young DF, Foley KM. The natural history of lumbosacral plexopathy in cancer. *Neurology* 1985;35:8–15.

380. Muppidi S, Vernino S. Paraneoplastic neuropathies. *Continuum (Minneap Minn)* 2014;20:1359–1372.

381. Tanaka M, Maruyama Y, Sugie M, et al. Cytotoxic T cell activity against peptides of Hu protein in anti-Hu syndrome. *J Neurol Sci* 2002;201:9–12.

382. Dispenzieri A. POEMS syndrome: update on diagnosis, risk-stratification, and management. *Am J Hematol* 2015;90:951–962.

383. Classification of chronic pain. Descriptions of chronic pain syndromes and definitions of pain terms. Prepared by the International Association for the Study of Pain, Subcommittee on Taxonomy. *Pain Suppl* 1986;3:S1–S226.

384. Abdallah FW, Morgan PJ, Cil T, et al. Comparing the DN4 tool with the IASP grading system for chronic neuropathic pain screening after breast tumor resection with and without paravertebral blocks: a prospective 6-month validation study. *Pain* 2015;156:740–749.

385. Henry BM, Graves MJ, Pekala JR, et al. Origin, branching, and communications of the intercostobrachial nerve: a meta-analysis with implications

for mastectomy and axillary lymph node dissection in breast cancer. *Cureus* 2017;9:e1101.

386. Cappiello J, Piazza C, Nicolai P. The spinal accessory nerve in head and neck surgery. *Curr Opin Otolaryngol Head Neck Surg* 2007;15:107–111.

387. Gane EM, Michaleff ZA, Cottrell MA, et al. Prevalence, incidence, and risk factors for shoulder and neck dysfunction after neck dissection: a systematic review. *Eur J Surg Oncol* 2017;43:1199–1218.

388. Sheikh A, Shallwani H, Ghaffar S. Postoperative shoulder function after different types of neck dissection in head and neck cancer. *Ear Nose Throat J* 2014;93:E21–E26.

389. Cardoso LR, Rizzo CC, de Oliveira CZ, et al. Myofascial pain syndrome after head and neck cancer treatment: prevalence, risk factors, and influence on quality of life. *Head Neck* 2015;37:1733–1737.

390. van Wilgen CP, Dijkstra PU, van der Laan BF, et al. Morbidity of the neck after head and neck cancer therapy. *Head Neck* 2004;26:785–791.

391. Nahum AM, Mullally W, Marmor L. A syndrome resulting from radical neck dissection. *Arch Otolaryngol* 1961;74:424–428.

392. Haroutiunian S, Nikolajsen L, Finnerup NB, et al. The neuropathic component in persistent postsurgical pain: a systematic literature review. *Pain* 2013;154:95–102.

393. Wildgaard K, Ravn J, Kehlet H. Chronic post-thoracotomy pain: a critical review of pathogenic mechanisms and strategies for prevention. *Eur J Cardiothorac Surg* 2009;36:170–180.

394. Hetmann F, Kongsgaard UE, Sandvik L, et al. Prevalence and predictors of persistent post-surgical pain 12 months after thoracotomy. *Acta Anaesthesiol Scand* 2015;59:740–748.

395. Grosen K, Laue Petersen G, Pfeiffer-Jensen M, et al. Persistent post-surgical pain following anterior thoracotomy for lung cancer: a cross-sectional study of prevalence, characteristics and interference with functioning. *Eur J Cardiothorac Surg* 2013;43:95–103.

396. Steegers MA, Snik DM, Verhagen AF, et al. Only half of the chronic pain after thoracic surgery shows a neuropathic component. *J Pain* 2008;9:955–961.

397. Kalso E, Perttunen K, Kaasinen S. Pain after thoracic surgery. *Acta Anaesthesiol Scand* 1992;36:96–100.

398. Perttunen K, Tasmuth T, Kalso E. Chronic pain after thoracic surgery: a follow-up study. *Acta Anaesthesiol Scand* 1999;43:563–567.

399. Maguire MF, Ravenscroft A, Beggs D, et al. A questionnaire study investigating the prevalence of the neuropathic component of chronic pain after thoracic surgery. *Eur J Cardiothorac Surg* 2006;29:800–805.

400. Guastella V, Mick G, Soriano C, et al. A prospective study of neuropathic pain induced by thoracotomy: incidence, clinical description, and diagnosis. *Pain* 2011;152:74–81.

401. Springer JS, Karlsson P, Madsen CS, et al. Functional and structural assessment of patients with and without persistent pain after thoracotomy. *Eur J Pain* 2017;21:238–249.

402. Hope-Stone L, Brown SL, Heimann H, et al. Phantom eye syndrome: patient experiences after enucleation for uveal melanoma. *Ophthalmology* 2015;122:1585–1590.

403. Marbach JJ. Phantom tooth pain: differential diagnosis and treatment. *J Mass Dent Soc* 1996;44:14–18.

404. Hanowell ST, Kennedy SF. Phantom tongue pain and causalgia: case presentation and treatment. *Anesth Analg* 1979;58:436–468.

405. Bowsher D. Human "autotomy." *Pain* 2002;95:187–189.

406. Guerreiro Godoy Mde F, Pereira de Godoy AC, de Matos MJ, et al. Phantom breast syndrome in women after mastectomy. *Breast J* 2013;19:349–350.

407. Ramachandran VS, McGeoch PD. Occurrence of phantom genitalia after gender reassignment surgery. *Med Hypotheses* 2007;69:1001–1003.

408. Gould CR, Branagan G. Phantom rectal sensations following abdominoperineal excision of the rectum (APER) and vertical rectus abdominis myocutaneous (VRAM) flap perineal reconstruction. *Int J Colorectal Dis* 2016;31:1799–1804.

409. Reategui C, Chiang FF, Rosen L, et al. Phantom rectum following abdominoperineal excision for rectal neoplasm: appearance and disappearance. *Colorectal Dis* 2013;15:1309–1312.

410. Weeks SR, Anderson-Barnes VC, Tsao JW. Phantom limb pain: theories and therapies. *Neurologist* 2010;16:277–286.

411. Woodhouse A. Phantom limb sensation. *Clin Exp Pharmacol Physiol* 2005;32:132–134.

412. Weinstein SM. Phantom pain. *Oncology (Williston Park)* 1994;8:65–74.

413. Dijkstra PU, Rietman JS, Geertzen JH. Phantom breast sensations and phantom breast pain: a 2-year prospective study and a methodological analysis of literature. *Eur J Pain* 2007;11:99–108.

414. Ovesen P, Kroner K, Ornsholt J, et al. Phantom-related phenomena after rectal amputation: prevalence and clinical characteristics. *Pain* 1991;44:289–291.

415. Stubblefield MD, Ibanez K, Riedel ER, et al. Peripheral nervous system injury after high-dose single-fraction image-guided stereotactic radiosurgery for spine tumors. *Neurosurg Focus* 2017;42:E12.

416. Schultheiss TE. The radiation dose-response of the human spinal cord. *Int J Radiat Oncol Biol Phys* 2008;71:1455–1459.

417. Behin A, Delattre JY. Complications of radiation therapy on the brain and spinal cord. *Semin Neurol* 2004;24:405–417.

418. Li YQ, Jay V, Wong CS. Oligodendrocytes in the adult rat spinal cord undergo radiation-induced apoptosis. *Cancer Res* 1996;56:5417–5422.

419. Georgiou A, Grigsby PW, Perez CA. Radiation induced lumbosacral plexopathy in gynecologic tumors: clinical findings and dosimetric analysis. *Int J Radiat Oncol Biol Phys* 1993;26:479–482.

420. Galecki J, Hicer-Grzenkowicz J, Grudzien-Kowalska M, et al. Radiation-induced brachial plexopathy and hypofractionated regimens in adjuvant irradiation of patients with breast cancer—a review. *Acta Oncol* 2006;45:280–284.

421. Olsen NK, Pfeiffer P, Mondrup K, et al. Radiation-induced brachial plexus neuropathy in breast cancer patients. *Acta Oncol* 1990;29:885–890.

422. Zeidman SM, Rossitch EJ, Nashold BS Jr. Dorsal root entry zone lesions in the treatment of pain related to radiation-induced brachial plexopathy. *J Spinal Disord* 1993;6:44–47.

423. Mondrup K, Olsen NK, Pfeiffer P, et al. Clinical and electrodiagnostic findings in breast cancer patients with radiation-induced brachial plexus neuropathy. *Acta Neurol Scand* 1990;81:153–158.

424. Esteban A, Traba A. Fasciculation-myokymic activity and prolonged nerve conduction block. A physiopathological relationship in radiation-induced brachial plexopathy. *Electroencephalogr Clin Neurophysiol* 1993;89:382–391.

425. Stryker JA, Sommerville K, Perez R, et al. Sacral plexus injury after radiotherapy for carcinoma of cervix. *Cancer* 1990;66:1488–1492.

426. Schiodt AV, Kristensen O. Neurologic complications after irradiation of malignant tumors of the testis. *Acta Radiol Oncol Radiat Phys Biol* 1978;17:369–378.

427. Thomas JE, Cascino TL, Earle JD. Differential diagnosis between radiation and tumor plexopathy of the pelvis. *Neurology* 1985;35:1–7.

428. Lederman RJ, Wilbourn AJ. Brachial plexopathy: recurrent cancer or radiation? *Neurology* 1984;34:1331–1335.

429. Bowen BC, Verma A, Brandon AH, et al. Radiation-induced brachial plexopathy: MR and clinical findings. *AJNR Am J Neuroradiol* 1996;17:1932–1936.

430. Qayyum A, MacVicar AD, Padhani AR, et al. Symptomatic brachial plexopathy following treatment for breast cancer: utility of MR imaging with surface-coil techniques. *Radiology* 2000;214:837–842.

431. Luthra K, Shah S, Purandare N, et al. F-18 FDG PET-CT appearance of metastatic brachial plexopathy in a case of carcinoma of the breast. *Clin Nucl Med* 2006;31:432–434.

432. Seretny M, Currie GL, Sena ES, et al. Incidence, prevalence, and predictors of chemotherapy-induced peripheral neuropathy: a systematic review and meta-analysis. *Pain* 2014;155:2461–2470.

433. Postma TJ, Heimans JJ. Grading of chemotherapy-induced peripheral neuropathy. *Ann Oncol* 2000;11:509–513.

434. Peterson DE, Keefe DM, Hutchins RD, et al. Alimentary tract mucositis in cancer patients: impact of terminology and assessment on research and clinical practice. *Support Care Cancer* 2006;14:499–504.

435. Naidu MU, Ramana GV, Rani PU, et al. Chemotherapy-induced and/or radiation therapy-induced oral mucositis—complicating the treatment of cancer. *Neoplasia* 2004;6:423–431.

436. Wardley AM, Jayson GC, Swindell R, et al. Prospective evaluation of oral mucositis in patients receiving myeloablative conditioning regimens and haemopoietic progenitor rescue. *Br J Haematol* 2000;110:292–299.

437. Chaudhry HM, Bruce AJ, Wolf RC, et al. The incidence and severity of oral mucositis among allogeneic hematopoietic stem cell transplantation patients: a systematic review. *Biol Blood Marrow Transplant* 2016;22:605–616.

438. Trotti A, Bellm LA, Epstein JB, et al. Mucositis incidence, severity and associated outcomes in patients with head and neck cancer receiving radiotherapy with or without chemotherapy: a systematic literature review. *Radiother Oncol* 2003;66:253–262.

439. Russo G, Haddad R, Posner M, et al. Radiation treatment breaks and ulcerative mucositis in head and neck cancer. *Oncologist* 2008;13:886–898.

440. Jagasia MH, Greinix HT, Arora M, et al. National Institutes of Health consensus development project on criteria for clinical trials in chronic graft-versus-host disease: I. The 2014 Diagnosis and Staging Working Group report. *Biol Blood Marrow Transplant* 2015;21:389.e1–401.e1.

441. Radojcic V, Pletneva MA, Couriel DR. The role of extracorporeal photopheresis in chronic graft-versus-host disease. *Transfus Apher Sci* 2015;52:157–161.

442. George R, Jeba J, Ramkumar G, et al. Interventions for the treatment of metastatic extradural spinal cord compression in adults. *Cochrane Database Syst Rev* 2015;(9):CD006716.

443. Sciubba DM, Petteys RJ, Dekutoski MB, et al. Diagnosis and management of metastatic spine disease. A review. *J Neurosurg Spine* 2010;13:94–108.

444. Yanez ML, Miller JJ, Batchelor TT. Diagnosis and treatment of epidural metastases. *Cancer* 2017;123:1106–1114.

445. Greenberg HS, Kim JH, Posner JB. Epidural spinal cord compression from metastatic tumor: results with a new treatment protocol. *Ann Neurol* 1980;8:361–366.

446. Schmidt MH, Klimo P Jr, Vrionis FD. Metastatic spinal cord compression. *J Natl Compr Canc Netw* 2005;3:711–719.

447. Klimo P Jr, Schmidt MH. Surgical management of spinal metastases. *Oncologist* 2004;9:188–196.

448. Maranzano E, Latini P, Checcaglini F, et al. Radiation therapy in metastatic spinal cord compression. A prospective analysis of 105 consecutive patients. *Cancer* 1991;67:1311–1317.

449. Siegal T. Spinal cord compression: from laboratory to clinic. *Eur J Cancer* 1995;31a:1748–1753.

450. Benton RL, Whittemore SR. VEGF165 therapy exacerbates secondary damage following spinal cord injury. *Neurochem Res* 2003;28:1693–1703.

451. Heiss JD, Papavassiliou E, Merrill MJ, et al. Mechanism of dexamethasone suppression of brain tumor-associated vascular permeability in rats. Involvement of the glucocorticoid receptor and vascular permeability factor. *J Clin Invest* 1996;98:1400–1408.

452. Prasad D, Schiff D. Malignant spinal-cord compression. *Lancet Oncol* 2005;6:15–24.

453. Langfitt TW, Elliott FA. Pain in the back and legs caused by cervical spinal cord compression. *JAMA* 1967;200:382–385.

454. Ito T, Homma T, Uchiyama S. Sciatica caused by cervical and thoracic spinal cord compression. *Spine (Phila Pa 1976)* 1999;24:1265–1267.

455. Chan CK, Lee HY, Choi WC, et al. Cervical cord compression presenting with sciatica-like leg pain. *Eur Spine J* 2011;20(suppl 2):S217–S221.

456. Al-Qurainy R, Collis E. Metastatic spinal cord compression: diagnosis and management. *Br Med J* 2016;353:i2539.

457. Tarlov IM. Acute spinal cord compression paralysis. *J Neurosurg* 1972;36:10–20.

458. Abrahm JL. Assessment and treatment of patients with malignant spinal cord compression. *J Support Oncol* 2004;2:377–388.

459. Ventafridda V, Caraceni A, Martini C, et al. On the significance of Lhermitte's sign in oncology. *J Neurooncol* 1991;10:133–137.

460. Lewanski CR, Sinclair JA, Stewart JS. Lhermitte's sign following head and neck radiotherapy. *Clin Oncol (R Coll Radiol)* 2000;12:98–103.

461. Inbar M, Merimsky O, Wigler N, et al. Cisplatin-related Lhermitte's sign. *Anticancer Drugs* 1992;3:375–377.

462. Park SB, Lin CS, Krishnan AV, et al. Oxaliplatin-induced Lhermitte's phenomenon as a manifestation of severe generalized neurotoxicity. *Oncology* 2009;77:342–348.

463. Solaro C, Brichetto G, Amato MP, et al. The prevalence of pain in multiple sclerosis: a multicenter cross-sectional study. *Neurology* 2004;63:919–921.

464. Butler WM, Taylor HG, Diehl LF. Lhermitte's sign in cobalamin (vitamin B12) deficiency. *JAMA* 1981;245:1059.

465. Switlyk MD, Hole KH, Skjeldal S, et al. MRI and neurological findings in patients with spinal metastases. *Acta Radiol* 2012;53:1164–1172.

466. Fattal C, Fabbro M, Gelis A, et al. Metastatic paraplegia and vital prognosis: perspectives and limitations for rehabilitation care. Part 1. *Arch Phys Med Rehabil* 2011;92:125–133.

467. Helweg-Larsen S, Sorensen PS, Kreiner S. Prognostic factors in metastatic spinal cord compression: a prospective study using multivariate analysis of variables influencing survival and gait function in 153 patients. *Int J Radiat Oncol Biol Phys* 2000;46:1163–1169.

468. Constans JP, de Divitiis E, Donzelli R, et al. Spinal metastases with neurological manifestations. Review of 600 cases. *J Neurosurg* 1983;59:111–118.

469. Rades D, Fehlauer F, Schulte R, et al. Prognostic factors for local control and survival after radiotherapy of metastatic spinal cord compression. *J Clin Oncol* 2006;24:3388–3393.

470. Loblaw DA, Laperriere NJ, Mackillop WJ. A population-based study of malignant spinal cord compression in Ontario. *Clin Oncol (R Coll Radiol)* 2003;15:211–217.

471. Rades D, Dunst J, Schild SE. The first score predicting overall survival in patients with metastatic spinal cord compression. *Cancer* 2008;112:157–161.

472. Sioutos PJ, Arbit E, Meshulam CF, et al. Spinal metastases from solid tumors. Analysis of factors affecting survival. *Cancer* 1995;76:1453–1459.

473. Maranzano E, Latini P. Effectiveness of radiation therapy without surgery in metastatic spinal cord compression: final results from a prospective trial. *Int J Radiat Oncol Biol Phys* 1995;32:959–967.

474. Tomita K, Kawahara N, Kobayashi T, et al. Surgical strategy for spinal metastases. *Spine (Phila Pa 1976)* 2001;26:298–306.

475. Tang SG, Byfield JE, Sharp TR, et al. Prognostic factors in the management of metastatic epidural spinal cord compression. *J Neurooncol* 1983;1:21–28.

476. Schiff D, O'Neill BP, Wang CH, et al. Neuroimaging and treatment implications of patients with multiple epidural spinal metastases. *Cancer* 1998;83:1593–1601.

477. Paice JA, Portenoy R, Lacchetti C, et al. Management of chronic pain in survivors of adult cancers: American Society of Clinical Oncology clinical practice guideline. *J Clin Oncol* 2016;34:3325–3345.

478. Swarm RA, Abernethy AP, Anghelescu DL, et al. Adult cancer pain. *J Natl Compr Canc Netw* 2013;11:992–1022.

479. Practice guidelines for cancer pain management. A report by the American Society of Anesthesiologists Task Force on Pain Management, Cancer Pain Section. *Anesthesiology* 1996;84:1243–1257.

480. Gordon DB, Dahl JL, Miaskowski C, et al. American Pain Society recommendations for improving the quality of acute and cancer pain management: American Pain Society Quality of Care Task Force. *Arch Intern Med* 2005;165:1574–1580.

481. Jost L, Roila F. Management of cancer pain: ESMO clinical recommendations. *Ann Oncol* 2009;20(suppl 4):170–173.

482. Management of cancer pain in older patients. AGS Clinical Practice Committee. *J Am Geriatr Soc* 1997;45:1273–1276.

483. Williamson GM, Schulz R. Activity restriction mediates the association between pain and depressed affect: a study of younger and older adult cancer patients. *Psychol Aging* 1995;10:369–378.

484. Tait RC, Chibnall JT, Krause S. The Pain Disability Index: psychometric properties. *Pain* 1990;40:171–182.

485. Jang RW, Caraiscos VB, Swami N, et al. Simple prognostic model for patients with advanced cancer based on performance status. *J Oncol Pract* 2014;10:e335–e341.

486. Oken MM, Creech RH, Tormey DC, et al. Toxicity and response criteria of the Eastern Cooperative Oncology Group. *Am J Clin Oncol* 1982;5:649–655.

487. Mor V, Laliberte L, Morris JN, et al. The Karnofsky Performance Status Scale. An examination of its reliability and validity in a research setting. *Cancer* 1984;53:2002–2007.

488. Liebschutz JM, Saitz R, Weiss RD, et al. Clinical factors associated with prescription drug use disorder in urban primary care patients with chronic pain. *J Pain* 2010;11:1047–1055.

489. Michna E, Ross EL, Hynes WL, et al. Predicting aberrant drug behavior in patients treated for chronic pain: importance of abuse history. *J Pain Symptom Manage* 2004;28:250–258.

490. Yellen SB, Cella DF. Someone to live for: social well-being, parenthood status, and decision-making in oncology. *J Clin Oncol* 1995;13:1255–1264.

491. Yellen SB, Cella DF, Leslie WT. Age and clinical decision making in oncology patients. *J Natl Cancer Inst* 1994;86:1766–1770.

492. Puts MT, Tapscott B, Fitch M, et al. A systematic review of factors influencing older adults' decision to accept or decline cancer treatment. *Cancer Treat Rev* 2015;41:197–215.

493. Puts MT, Tu HA, Tourangeau A, et al. Factors influencing adherence to cancer treatment in older adults with cancer: a systematic review. *Ann Oncol* 2014;25:564–577.

494. Cella DF, Tulsky DS, Gray G, et al. The Functional Assessment of Cancer Therapy scale: development and validation of the general measure. *J Clin Oncol* 1993;11:570–579.

495. Victorson D, Barocas J, Song J, et al. Reliability across studies from the functional assessment of cancer therapy-general (FACT-G) and its subscales: a reliability generalization. *Qual Life Res* 2008;17:1137–1146.

496. Brucker PS, Yost K, Cashy J, et al. General population and cancer patient norms for the Functional Assessment of Cancer Therapy-General (FACT-G). *Eval Health Prof* 2005;28:192–211.

497. Zucca AC, Boyes AW, Linden W, et al. All's well that ends well? Quality of life and physical symptom clusters in long-term cancer survivors across cancer types. *J Pain Symptom Manage* 2012;43:720–731.

498. Reilly CM, Bruner DW, Mitchell SA, et al. A literature synthesis of symptom prevalence and severity in persons receiving active cancer treatment. *Support Care Cancer* 2013;21:1525–1550.

499. Harrington CB, Hansen JA, Moskowitz M, et al. It's not over when it's over: long-term symptoms in cancer survivors—a systematic review. *Int J Psychiatry Med* 2010;40:163–181.

500. Wang XS, Zhao F, Fisch MJ, et al. Prevalence and characteristics of moderate to severe fatigue: a multicenter study in cancer patients and survivors. *Cancer* 2014;120:425–432.

501. Portenoy RK, Thaler HT, Kornblith AB, et al. The Memorial Symptom Assessment Scale: an instrument for the evaluation of symptom prevalence, characteristics and distress. *Eur J Cancer* 1994;30A:1326–1336.

502. Clouston PD, DeAngelis LM, Posner JB. The spectrum of neurological disease in patients with systemic cancer. *Ann Neurol* 1992;31:268–273.

503. Chua KS, Reddy SK, Lee MC, et al. Pain and loss of function in head and neck cancer survivors. *J Pain Symptom Manage* 1999;18:193–202.

504. García de Paredes ML, del Moral González F, Martínez del Prado P, et al. First evidence of oncologic neuropathic pain prevalence after screening 8615 cancer patients. Results of the On study. *Ann Oncol* 2011;22:924–930.

505. Grond S, Radbruch L, Meuser T, et al. Assessment and treatment of neuropathic cancer pain following WHO guidelines. *Pain* 1999;79:15–20.

506. Webster LR, Webster RM. Predicting aberrant behaviors in opioid-treated patients: preliminary validation of the Opioid Risk Tool. *Pain Med* 2005;6:432–442.

507. Butler SF, Budman SH, Fernandez K, et al. Validation of a screener and opioid assessment measure for patients with chronic pain. *Pain* 2004;112:65–75.

508. Belgrade MJ, Schamber CD, Lindgren BR. The DIRE score: predicting outcomes of opioid prescribing for chronic pain. *J Pain* 2006;7:671–681.

509. Butler SF, Budman SH, Fernandez KC, et al. Development and validation of the Current Opioid Misuse Measure. *Pain* 2007;130:144–156.

510. Bush K, Kivlahan DR, McDonell MB, et al. The AUDIT alcohol consumption questions (AUDIT-C): an effective brief screening test for problem drinking. Ambulatory Care Quality Improvement Project (ACQUIP). Alcohol Use Disorders Identification Test. *Arch Intern Med* 1998;158:1789–1795.

511. Brown RL, Rounds LA. Conjoint screening questionnaires for alcohol and other drug abuse: criterion validity in a primary care practice. *Wis Med J* 1995;94:135–140.

CHAPTER 43

Cancer Pain: Principles of Management and Pharmacotherapy

DERMOT FITZGIBBON

In 2008, the International Association for the Study of Pain (IASP) launched a global year against cancer pain to focus attention on the pain and suffering affecting patients with cancer. In 2011, the Institute of Medicine[1] recognized chronic noncancer pain management as a public health challenge. In spite of increased attention on assessment and management, pain continues to be a prevalent symptom in patients with cancer.[2] The consequences of unrelieved cancer pain can be devastating and include functional impairment, social isolation, and emotional distress. Inadequate treatment of cancer pain persists despite decades of efforts to provide clinicians with information about analgesics and pain-relieving techniques. The problems associated with undertreatment of cancer pain are outlined in Table 43.1. Although the reasons for inadequate treatment of cancer pain are complex, certain barriers to adequate pain relief are identified. These barriers primarily relate to health care professionals; patients, families, and the public; health care implementation and reimbursement; and drug regulatory systems.[3]

Cancer pain management guidelines typically incorporate pharmacologic, anesthetic, neurosurgical, and behavioral approaches. The World Health Organization (WHO) developed the most widely accepted approach for the treatment of cancer pain. The WHO algorithm largely focuses on pain intensity and the use of pharmacotherapy.[4] Some have questioned the current appropriateness of the WHO guidelines, which may be considered outdated and not specific to the pharmacologic and interventional options used in contemporary pain management practices.[5] Although the amount and quality of evidence regarding the use of opioids for treating cancer pain is low,[6] opioid therapy remains the cornerstone for pain management in oncology.[7–12] In the United States, physicians' concerns about

regulatory scrutiny and the possibility of unwarranted investigation by regulatory agencies negatively affect their prescribing of opioid analgesics to treat pain.[13] In addition, it is widely reported that the United States is experiencing an epidemic of drug overdose deaths particularly from the use of opioid medications.[14–17] The past two decades have been characterized by increasing abuse and diversion of prescription drugs, including opioid medications (see "Substance Abuse in Oncology" section).[18] In a study of malpractice claims associated with medication management for chronic pain, issues in care (including death) were noted when patients did not cooperate in their care and with inappropriate medication management by physicians.[19] Factors associated with death in this study included the use of long-acting opioids, additional concomitant psychoactive medications, and the presence of three or more factors commonly associated with medication misuse. In 2016, the U.S. Drug Enforcement Administration indicated that prescription drugs, heroin, and fentanyl were the most significant drug-related threats to the United States.[15] The misuse of prescription opioids is associated with misuse of illicit opioids and nonmedical use of prescription opioids is a significant risk factor for heroin use,[20] emphasizing the need for continued prevention efforts around prescription opioids. Regardless of age, gender, or type of user, the majority who misuse prescription pain relievers obtained the drugs from a friend or relative with the second most common source from a doctor.[21] Particularly for chronic noncancer pain, there is insufficient evidence to determine the effectiveness of long-term opioid therapy for improving pain and function, but there is increasing evidence to support the evidence for a dose-dependent risk for serious harm.[22] Higher opioid doses (50 mg per day or more of morphine) are associated with increased risk of opioid overdose death or adverse drug-related events.[23,24] Although the overall rate of overdose is lower among patients with cancer compared with other patients, there was a statistically significant association of prescribing patterns with overdose risk among patients with cancer receiving opioid therapy.[23] In response to persistent public health concerns regarding prescription opioids, the U.S. Food and Drug Administration (FDA) developed a multipart action plan in response to the opioid epidemic,[25] and many states and health care systems have implemented legislation and policies intended to regulate or guide opioid prescribing.[26] Unfortunately, data on state policy and systems-level interventions are limited and inconsistent.[27] Patients with cancer and other significant comorbidities have a higher prevalence for polypharmacy and greater risk for drug–drug interactions, adverse drug events, hospitalizations, and increased mortality.[28–31] Concurrent sedative-hypnotic use even at low opioid doses poses substantially greater risk of opioid overdose.[32,33] In spite of these concerns, clinicians have an ethical and professional responsibility for safe and appropriate pain management in cancer patients.

Pain management and relief can be achieved by several means (Table 43.2). Successful pain management requires an accurate diagnosis of the etiology of the pain complaint(s) and

TABLE 43.1	**Factors Contributing to Undertreatment of Cancer Pain in United States**
Factor	**Reason**

Patient-related	• Pain underreporting:
	  ○ Fear of disease progression
	  ○ Perceived lack of time or inadequate amount of time spent in physician's office discussing pain problems
	• Poor compliance with prescribed medications
	• Fear of addiction
	• Fatalistic beliefs about cancer pain

Physician-related	• Legal issues regarding overprescription or perceived overprescription of opioids • Difficulty/inadequate training for pain complaints assessment • Lack of information or lack of expertise on contemporary strategies for cancer pain management • Desire to provide the patient with the latest and greatest pain management strategies may pose difficulties with untried or unproven techniques or methods.

TABLE 43.2 Approaches to Pain Management in Cancer Patients	
Psychological approaches (Chapters 29, 75, 84, and 88)	Understanding
	Companionship
	Cognitive-behavioral therapies
Modification of pathologic process (Chapters 48 and 103–105)	Radiation therapy
	Hormone therapy
	Chemotherapy
	Surgery
Drugs (Chapters 77–81)	Analgesics
	Antidepressants
	Anxiolytics
	Neuroleptics
Interruption of pain pathways (Chapters 44, 98, 102–105)	Local anesthetics
	Neurolytic agents
	Neurosurgery
Modification of daily activities	Functional improvements/structure
Immobilization	Rest
	Surgical collar or corset
	Plastic splints or slings
	Orthopedic surgery

Modified with permission from World Health Organization. *Cancer Pain Relief with a Guide to Opioid Availability*. Geneva, Switzerland: World Health Organization; 1996.

tailoring treatment to the individual patient: matching drug treatment, anesthetic, neurosurgical, psychological, and behavioral approaches to the patient's needs. Successful management requires that the person or persons responsible for pain management be familiar with all these aspects of care and with the uniqueness and challenges of pain in oncology patients. Evidence-based medicine, systematic reviews, meta-analyses, and guidelines are increasingly incorporated into modern pain management. Scientific data and relevant evidence employing methodologic, rational judgments, analysis, and understanding of current knowledge can then be applied in clinical settings. In the areas of chronic noncancer and cancer-associated pain, evidence-based decision making for pharmacotherapy is lacking and decisions for pain management in oncology is frequently extrapolated or inferred from chronic pain situations. Often, practitioners must rely on clinical practice guidelines, limited clinical trial data, case reports, or anecdotal information for clinical decision making. Clinical practice guidelines are systematically developed statements that aim to help physicians and patients reach the best health care decisions. Guidelines and recommendations for management of cancer pain have largely focused on relieving acute pain or pain associated with advanced disease.[34–37] Not all patients with cancer experience tumor-related pain, and management principles differ depending on the source of pain and these recommendations are not appropriate for oncology patients with nonmalignant sources of pain or for pain management in cancer survivors.[38,39] However, pharmacotherapy remains the optimal and preferred modality for symptomatic pain management in oncology, but safe and effective drug prescribing practices must be observed and implemented. Since 1986, the focus of cancer pain treatment has been the use of strong opioids based on the WHO's analgesic ladder. Changing societal factors in the last 15 years suggest changes in the distribution of drug use disorders in the general US adult population. Prescriptions for opioid analgesics and other psychoactive medications with addiction potential have increased greatly, with consequences such as drug overdoses.[40] Comparisons of 12-month and lifetime *Diagnostic and Statistical Manual of Mental Disorders* (4th ed., *DSM-IV*) drug use disorder prevalence in the general adult population in 2001 to 2002 (2.0% and 10.3%, respectively)[41] and 2012 to 2013 (4.1% and 15.6%, respectively)[42] indicate that rates of 12-month drug use disorders more than doubled, whereas

rates of lifetime drug use disorders increased by 50%. Using *Diagnostic and Statistical Manual of Mental Disorders* (5th ed., *DSM-5*) criteria drug use in 2012 to 2013 disorder, prevalence of 12-month and lifetime drug use disorder were 3.9% and 9.9%, respectively.[43] Drug use disorder was generally greater among men, white and Native American individuals, younger and previously or never married adults, and those with lower education and income. A lower prevalence of drug abuse has been reported in the cancer population, with 3% of psychiatry consultations in a single cancer center in 1990 being requested for managing issues related to drug abuse.[44] Similarly, a low prevalence of drug abuse was reported by the Psychiatric Collaborative Oncology Group study in 1983, in which fewer than 5% of patients in ambulatory care met the criteria for a substance abuse disorder.[45] This low prevalence may not be an accurate reflection of the true prevalence because of underreporting. The prevalence of substance abuse in cancer patients is largely understudied and needs clarification. Patients with cancer are known to have an increased risk of psychiatric symptoms and disorders, cardiovascular diseases, and suicide.[46–48] Living or being diagnosed with cancer can induce severe psychological stress.[49] In a retrospective review of 204 supportive care clinic oncology patients (with the majority having active cancer) considered to be at risk for substance abuse based on history or behaviors, 46% had evidence of use of nonprescribed opioids, benzodiazepines, or illicit drugs such as heroin or cocaine, and 39% had inappropriately negative urine toxicology, raising concerns for diversion.[50]

Safe and appropriate medication prescribing practices are of paramount importance in the oncology pain population. The challenges presented to clinicians are numerous and include educational deficits, time restraints, and limited access to all types of care. New challenges to access are occurring as a result of interventions designed to combat the prescription drug abuse epidemic, with fewer clinicians willing to prescribe opioids, pharmacies reluctant to stock the medications, and payers placing strict limits on reimbursement.[39] In the era of personalized medicine, Hui and Bruera[51] suggested that pain management may be tailored to the individual need by use of a personalized pain goal, and this can be obtained by asking a patient to identify the maximal intensity of pain from 0 to 10 (0, no pain; 10, worst pain) that would still be considered comfortable. The concept is a personalized pain goal is attractive but managing pain by pain scores can be problematic,[52–54] and more appropriate goals may be to identify a pain management plan that results in a reduction in interference in activities of daily living and improvement in quality of life and overall functional ability.

Cancer Pain Management Overview

Successful management of the cancer patient with pain ultimately depends on the ability of the clinician to accurately assess problems, identify and evaluate the components that contribute to the pain complaint, and formulate a plan for continuing care that is responsible for the evolving goals and needs of the patient and the patient's family (see Chapter 42). In general, the goals of patient care in oncology are often complex, but they broadly include prolonged survival, and optimizing comfort and function with associated improved quality of life. Adoption of these goals logically leads to a multimodality treatment approach targeted to specific problems (Fig. 43.1).

Comprehensive cancer care encompasses a continuum that progresses from disease-oriented, curative, life-prolonging treatment through symptom-oriented, supportive, and palliative care extending to terminal-phase hospice care. Pain management is, and should be, an integral component of comprehensive cancer care.[55–59] Designing an effective pain control

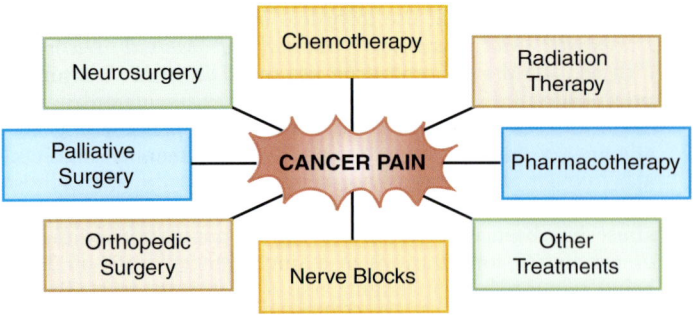

FIGURE 43.1 Multimodality therapeutic management of cancer pain. Others include psychosocial interventions, nursing care, alternative pain management strategies, and end-of-life issues.

strategy for the individual patient requires knowledge of the ways in which a patient's cancer, cancer therapy, and pain therapy can interact. Collaboration with different health care providers (such as medical oncologists and radiation oncologists) is essential to successful pain management.

Two important aspects of cancer affect management and include the oncologist's ability to treat the cancer and the ability to assess the components of the tumor pathophysiology that of themselves do not cause pain (the cancer's "nonpain" pathophysiology).[60] The ability to treat cancer modifies the need for pain management (successful treatment reduces the likelihood of persistent tumor-related pain) and the appropriateness of invasive pain procedures. Cancer nonpain pathophysiology can interfere with the oral administration of medications, narrow the patient's therapeutic window for analgesic drugs, limit the effectiveness of psychological pain therapies, and complicate or preclude invasive pain-reducing procedures. In addition, cancer therapy can interfere with, or enhance, pain therapy and vice versa. Antineoplastic treatment can interfere with pain therapy by causing additional pain or by producing other adverse effects such as fatigue and gastrointestinal (GI) disturbances. Cancer treatment can enhance pain therapy by reducing the extent of tumor burden, by acting as an adjuvant analgesic, and, often times, by providing intravenous access for parenteral drug administration to patients who require it. Pain therapy can sometimes interfere with cancer therapy by increasing or complicating the adverse effects of cancer therapy, for example, opioid-related bowel dysfunction. It can enhance cancer therapy by improving patient function or sense of well-being, and certain palliative surgical procedures may have the ancillary effect of improving organ function.

The basic principles of tumor-directed pain control include:

1. Modifying the source of pain by treating the cancer and the inflammatory effects of cancer
2. Altering the central perception of pain, for example, by the use of analgesics, antidepressants, anxiolytics, and psychotherapy
3. Interfering with nociceptive transmission outside of and within the central nervous system (CNS), for example, with anesthetic techniques (e.g., neurolytic celiac plexus block, neuraxial analgesia, and spinal neurolysis) or neurosurgery procedures (e.g., cordotomy and myelotomy)

The pain experienced by most cancer patients responds to direct and indirect modification of the source of the pain combined with pharmacologic and nonpharmacologic alteration of the central perception of pain.[37,61–63] The guiding principle in developing pain management goals is to individualize the approach to the patient's needs. Part of the process of developing treatment goals is to take into consideration the burdens (adverse effects; opportunity costs) and benefits of different treatment options.[63] Clinicians may find that patient treatment goals differ from their own, either because patients feel that pain is inevitable or because patients expect pain to be relieved with minimal effort on their part. Issues

that physicians should discuss with patients include expected lifestyle; cost and reimbursement issues; and concerns about opioid tolerance, addiction, and side effects. Discussing these issues in advance may uncover and address potential barriers to treatment. Moreover, treatment goals may change during the course of the patient's illness, and all health care providers interacting with the patient during the course of the illness need to keep abreast of such changes. Medication adherence has major implications for the effective treatments of different diseases.[64–67] Inadequate adherence with an analgesic regimen is problematic in oncology[68,69] and adherence rates for scheduled around-the-clock (ATC) regimens better than for as needed regimens.[70] Most interventions to improve cancer pain outcomes rely on psychoeducational approaches which focus on knowledge transfer to address attitudes and barriers to opioid use.[71–74] However Bennett et al.[75] found that patient-based educational interventions resulted in modest benefits in the management of cancer pain and did not have significant benefit on medication adherence or on reducing interference with daily activities. A large variety of approaches have been used with varying effect, and attempts to understand the reasons for heterogeneity between results have so far been unsuccessful.[76] A patient-centered approach that includes good communication between health providers and patients can promote adherence and improve outcomes.[74,77]

PRIMARY ANTICANCER TREATMENT

Pain produced by tumor infiltration may respond to antineoplastic treatment with radiation treatment and chemotherapy. These approaches to pain control are elaborated in Chapters 42 and 48.

Surgery

The surgeon treating a patient with newly diagnosed cancer must meet several responsibilities: biopsy for tissue diagnosis, adequate staging, consultation with medical and radiation oncologists for adjuvant therapy, and surgical resection. Surgery may also play a role in the relief of symptoms caused by specific problems, such as obstruction of a hollow viscus, unstable bone structures, and compression of neural tissues. A variety of surgical disciplines (e.g., general surgery, orthopedic, neurosurgical, plastic, and reconstructive) may participate in the care of the cancer patient.

Although the development of metastatic cancer usually indicates incurable disease, curative surgical resection is possible in rare instances. These instances must meet several criteria before the surgeon can operate: the primary lesion must be controlled, there must be the potential for complete resection of the metastases, there must be no other equally effective or better antitumor therapy available, metastases should involve only one organ, one should anticipate reasonable postoperative function, expected survival should be better than if left untreated, and the patient must be able to tolerate the surgical procedure. Sometimes, excision of the primary tumor is indicated in the presence of unresectable metastatic disease. Locally advanced

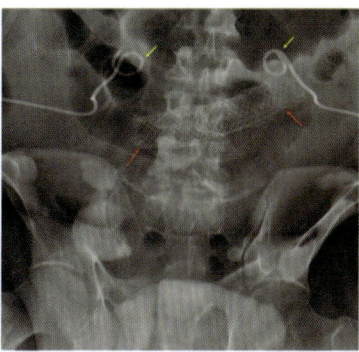

FIGURE 43.2 Patient with metastatic prostate cancer who presented with large bowel obstruction. Endoscopy revealed extrinsic tumor compression of the proximal sigmoid colon that required placement of a 10-cm metal stent *(red arrows)* with complete relief of obstruction. Patient has also bilateral percutaneous nephrostomies *(yellow arrows)* for relief of bilateral hydronephrosis.

tumor can be very painful and unsightly, can interfere with vital functions such as breathing and swallowing, and produce complications such as bleeding and local infection. Resection of isolated metastatic colorectal cancer, GI stromal tumors, neuroendocrine cancers, renal cell cancer, and sarcoma is associated with longer survival or even cure.[78] Most of the available information on metastasectomy relates to disease involving the liver, lung, and brain. Resection of primary renal cell cancer localized to the kidney has a 5-year survival rate approaching 95%.[79] However, the presence of metastasis reduces the median survival to only 10 months. At the time of diagnosis of primary renal cell cancer, about 20% of individuals will have metastases. The benefit of resection of isolated colorectal cancer metastases to the liver and lung and results in a 5-year survival reported in the range of 27% to 58%.[80–82] Surgical interventions for osseous (nonvertebral) disease depend on the severity of symptoms, location of tumor, expected associated morbidity if a fracture occurred, and availability of alternative or adjuvant treatments. The goal is primarily to decrease pain and to improve mobility and quality of life. The most obvious indication for surgery is the presence of a pathologic fracture in a weight-bearing long bone. Asymptomatic lesions may be followed clinically and radiographically. For metastatic spinal tumors, surgery can improve mechanical stability, cord compression, and pain. Complications may occur in up to 25% of patients who undergo surgery for spinal metastases, the most common being wound infection.[83,84] Life expectancy is usually determined by the overall extent of disease and, to be of benefit, surgery must improve quality of life.[85]

Stenting, Drainage Procedures, and Antibiotics

Common complications of advanced cancer include GI, hepatobiliary, and ureteric obstructions. Stents and laser treatment have a place in both upper GI and rectal obstruction due to advanced malignancy (Fig. 43.2).[86–89] Decompression for obstructive uropathy from advanced disease usually involves placement of nephrostomy tubes or ureteral stents. Malignant obstruction of the bile duct from cholangiocarcinoma, pancreatic adenocarcinoma, or other tumors may cause debilitating symptoms. Treatment of obstruction can be performed endoscopically, percutaneously, or surgically. Stents, nasobiliary drainage, or percutaneous drains may be used for liver hilar strictures. Endoscopic catheter-based therapies such as photodynamic therapy or radiofrequency ablation may prolong patient survival by achieving local tumor control.[90]

The goals of antibiotic use in terminally ill patients are sometimes to prolong life and always to relieve symptoms.[91] Treatment for cystitis, for instance, does not usually prolong life but may relieve the patient from painful dysuria and troublesome polyuria. Antibiotics may also have pain-relieving effects when the source of pain involves infection, as illustrated by the treatment of pyonephrosis or osteitis pubis.

Symptomatic Cancer Pain Management

Successful management strategies usually require a team approach focusing not only on the nociceptive processes but also on other factors that influence the final perception of pain. Figure 43.3 outlines an approach to tumor-related nociceptive and neuropathic pain.

Increasing severe pain and/or increasing and intractable side effects determine the appropriate treatment strategy. Most patients will respond satisfactorily to relatively simple oral pharmacotherapeutic strategies. When the patient requires drug treatment, therapy should comply with two basic principles: use oral analgesics and other noninvasive routes of administrations (e.g., transdermal and transmucosal) whenever possible and administer them in accordance with the principles in the WHO analgesic ladder (see later). Titrate opioid and adjuvant analgesics to maximally effective doses or to the appearance of dose-limiting side effects before considering alternative medications (e.g., opioid rotation) or more specialized (and usually) invasive approaches. As an adjunct—and occasionally as an alternative—to medication management, patients with certain pain syndromes will benefit from relatively simple anesthetic blocks, such as celiac and superior hypogastric plexus blocks, neurolytic subarachnoid and intercostal blocks, and selected peripheral nerve blocks (see Chapter 44).

Severe, uncontrolled pain and/or intractable side effects require interventional pain management to achieve rapid pain control.

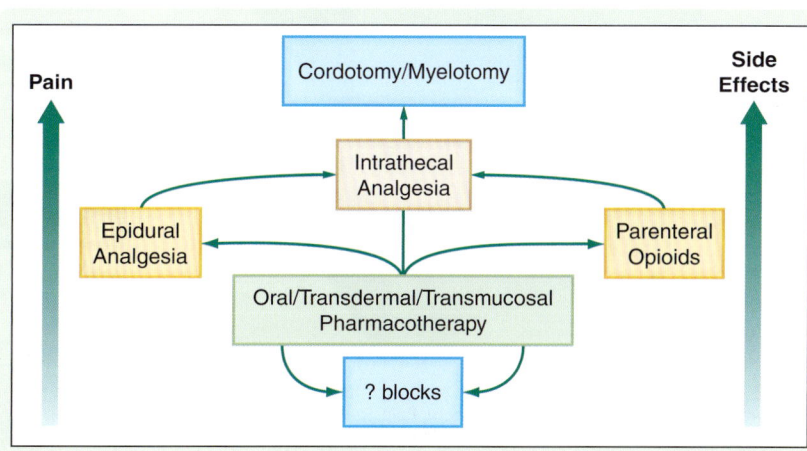

FIGURE 43.3 Tumor pain management algorithm.

Such interventions may include neuraxial (epidural or intrathecal) analgesia and/or parenteral opioid therapy (usually intravenous administration). As many of these patients have large systemic opioid requirements, it is not unusual to combine neuraxial and parenteral therapies. A small percentage of patients may fail these therapies and should then be treated with intrathecal drugs and/or cordotomy or myelotomy (see Chapter 44).

Occasionally, patients will have pain refractory to all interventional measures outlined, and palliative sedation should be considered (see Chapter 13).

WORLD HEALTH ORGANIZATION ANALGESIC LADDER

In 1986, WHO proposed a method for relief of cancer pain, based on a small number of relatively inexpensive drugs, including morphine.[92] Ten years later, a second edition[93] took into account many of the advances in understanding and practice that have occurred since the mid-1980s. The groundwork for this revision was started in 1989, in the context of the meeting of a WHO Expert Committee on Cancer Pain Relief and Active Supportive Care.[94]

The WHO "analgesic ladder" is a simple and effective method for controlling cancer pain (Fig. 43.4). The purpose was to make pain relief readily available to patients with cancer by using effective and inexpensive drugs. Opioid-based pharmacotherapy is the most important of these options. In many countries, access to opioid treatment is limited by governmental regulation intended to prevent misuse.[95–98] Advocacy for improved and affordable access to opioids for legitimate medical reasons must continue. At the same time, clinicians have to acknowledge the serious nature of drug misuse and addiction and the obligation to minimize these outcomes. This obligation is particularly pertinent in the United States because of the troubling increase in prescription drug misuse during recent decades. Codeine and morphine were selected for the original WHO analgesic ladder but have fallen from favor because of the genetically established variation in the effects of codeine and the potential effect of morphine metabolites in patients with renal impairment. The WHO analgesic ladder approach selects different opioids on the basis of pain intensity and any single-entity full μ-agonist opioid

TABLE 43.3 A Basic Drug List for Cancer Pain Relief

Category	Basic Drugs	Alternatives
Nonopioids	Acetylsalicylic acid (ASA)	Choline magnesium
	Acetaminophen	Trisalicylate
	Ibuprofen	Diflunisal
	Indomethacin	Naproxen
		Diclofenac
Opioids for mild to moderate pain	Codeine	Dihydrocodeine
		Standardized opium
		Tramadol
Opioids for moderate to severe pain	Morphine	Methadone
		Hydromorphone
		Oxycodone
		Levorphanol
		Buprenorphine
Opioid antagonist	Naloxone	Methylnaltrexone
Antidepressants	Amitriptyline	Imipramine
Anticonvulsants	Carbamazepine	Valproic acid
Corticosteroids	Prednisolone	Prednisone
	Dexamethasone	Betamethasone

Modified with permission from World Health Organization. *Cancer Pain Relief with a Guide to Opioid Availability.* Geneva, Switzerland: World Health Organization; 1996.

is appropriate. According to a Cochrane review, the amount and quality of evidence around the use of opioids for treating cancer pain is low, but 19 out of 20 people with moderate or severe pain who are given opioids and can tolerate them should have that pain reduced to mild or no pain within 14 days.[6] Because of opioid-related side effects, 1 to 2 in 10 patients treated with opioids will find adverse events intolerable resulting in a change in treatment. Somnolence, dry mouth, and anorexia were common adverse events in people with cancer pain treated with morphine, fentanyl, oxycodone, or codeine.[99] Historically, the proportion of cancer patients who report effective pain relief varies from 75% to 90%.[37,100,101]

Treatment for cancer pain should begin with a straightforward explanation to the patient of the causes of the pain or pains. Many pains respond best to a combination of drug and nondrug measures. Nevertheless, opioids, nonopioid analgesics and adjuvant agents, alone or in combination are the mainstay of cancer pain management (Table 43.3).

Pharmacologic strategies for the control of tumor pain appear in Table 43.4.

Table 43.5 lists the principles of pharmacotherapy endorsed by WHO.

These principles are as follows:

By Mouth

When possible, patients should take analgesic medications by mouth. However, alternative routes such as rectal, transdermal, transmucosal (buccal, intranasal, sublingual), and parenteral (subcutaneous and intravenous) administration may better serve patients with dysphagia, uncontrolled vomiting, or GI obstruction.

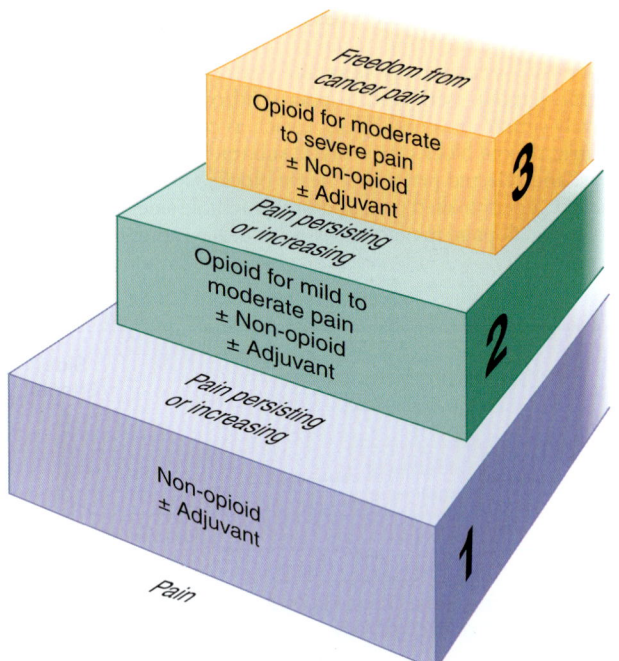

FIGURE 43.4 World Health Organization analgesic ladder. *(With permission from World Health Organization.* Cancer Pain Relief with a Guide to Opioid Availability. *Geneva, Switzerland: World Health Organization; 1996.)*

TABLE 43.4 Pharmacologic Strategies for the Control of Tumor Pain

Select the appropriate analgesic drug.
Prescribe the appropriate dose of that drug.
Administer the drug by the appropriate route.
Schedule the appropriate dosing interval.
Prevent persistent pain and treat breakthrough pain.
Titrate the dose of drug aggressively.
Prevent, anticipate, and manage drug side effects.

TABLE 43.5	The Principles of Drug Therapy for Cancer Pain
By the mouth	
By the clock	
By the ladder	
For the individual	
With attention to detail	

From World Health Organization. *Cancer Pain Relief with a Guide to Opioid Availability.* Geneva, Switzerland: World Health Organization; 1996.

By the Clock

After titration to optimal effect, patients with continuous pain should take analgesic medications on an ATC schedule. Once baseline pain is controlled, many patients will require breakthrough pain (BTP) therapy with immediate or rapid-onset opioids because BTP is a common occurrence in cancer patients.

By the Ladder

The WHO analgesic ladder[93] is based on the premise that most patients throughout the world will gain adequate pain relief if health care professionals learn how to use a few effective and relatively inexpensive drugs well (Fig. 43.4). Step 1 of the ladder involves the use of nonopioids. If this step does not relieve pain, add an opioid for mild to moderate pain (Step 2). When the opioid for mild to moderate pain in combination with a nonopioid fails to relieve the pain, substitute an opioid for moderate to severe pain (Step 3). Use only one drug from each of the groups at the same time. Give adjuvant drugs for specific indications (see later).

For the Individual

There are no standard doses for opioids. *The "right" dose is the dose that relieves the patient's pain with the minimum of side effects.* Adequate pain relief may be judged by patient satisfaction with pain management and/or meeting predefined functional goals. Combination opioid formulations (i.e., those with the nonopioid analgesic acetaminophen or a nonsteroidal anti-inflammatory drug [NSAID] are commonly used for mild-to moderate-intensity pain. These have a dose limit due to toxic effects of the coanalgesic.

With Attention to Detail

Carefully determine and monitor the patient's analgesic regimen. Follow-up regularly with the patient by monitoring adherence, drug efficacy, functional outcomes, side effects, and aberrant drug-related behaviors. Anticipate adverse effects, such as opioid-induced bowel dysfunction, and treat them prophylactically or as soon as they become problematic.

The WHO ladder advocates the use of three classes of analgesics—nonopioid, adjuvant, and opioid. Each of these classes will be considered separately.

Nonsteroidal Anti-Inflammatory Drugs

NSAIDs are essential drugs for the management of a wide variety of acute and chronic pain conditions. Clinicians should be familiar with the use, efficacy, and adverse effects of these agents. NSAIDs include a variety of drugs that differ in their clinical effects and pharmacokinetics. In general, they have high bioavailability, with peak concentrations occurring within the first 4 hours when administered orally. Intravenous forms of ibuprofen and ketorolac are available in the United States. NSAIDs may function to control pain independently (e.g., in the management of mild- to moderate-intensity bone or muscle pain) or may help reduce the dose of opioid required for pain control (opioid-sparing effect). A wide range of drugs with varying effects and side effects are available. These medications are discussed extensively in Chapter 78.

Cyclooxygenase (COX) is the pivotal enzyme in prostaglandin biosynthesis. It exists in two isoforms, constitutive COX-1 (responsible for physiologic functions) and inducible COX-2 (involved in inflammation and upregulated by cytokines, growth factors, and shear stress). Pharmacologic inhibition of COX explains both the therapeutic effects (inhibition of COX-2) and side effects (inhibition of COX-1) of NSAIDs. COX-1 and COX-2 both metabolize arachidonic acid to an unstable precursor, prostaglandin (PG) H_2. A variety of PG isomerases use PGH_2 as the substrate to form PGs, prostacyclin (PGI_2), and thromboxane (Tx) A_2. The analgesic and anti-inflammatory effects of NSAIDs are dependent on the extent and duration of COX-2 inhibition in the spinal cord and inflammatory sites. Aspirin differs from NSAIDs because aspirin irreversibly acetylates the enzyme. Most NSAIDs inhibit both COX isoenzymes with little selectivity, although some (coxibs, meloxicam) mainly block COX-2.

PGE_2 is the most physiologically abundant product of COX-2 as it exists at some level in nearly all cell types. Apart from biologic effects, such as induction of pain and inflammation, PGE_2 also participates in the mechanisms of cell proliferation, apoptosis, and metastasis, contributing to the progression of several human cancers, including colon cancer, breast cancer, and lung cancer, suggesting that NSAID use may be beneficial in these cancers.[102–105] COX-2 is markedly overexpressed in colorectal neoplasm and multiple epidemiologic studies clearly demonstrated that NSAID consumption prevents adenoma formation and decreases the incidence of, and mortality from, colorectal cancer.[106] COX-2 inhibition can reduce proliferation, induce apoptosis, suppress tumor angiogenesis, prevent immune suppression, and inhibit carcinogen conversion.[106,107] The efficacy of aspirin differs significantly according to COX-2 expression. Aspirin reduces the risk of colorectal cancer in COX-2–expressing cancers, but it is not an effective chemopreventive agent for cancers with weak or absent COX-2 expression.[108] In animal models, NSAIDs decrease the number and risk of metastasis[109] with some data now emerging of a reduced risk of metastasis development in humans.[110]

EFFICACY IN CANCER PAIN

Although many NSAIDs are available to treat various painful conditions, it is unclear which agent is most clinically efficacious for relieving cancer-related pain, and if there are clinical differences between these agents that justify their cost differences. In a Cochrane review of the use of NSAIDs either alone or in combination with opioids, the quality of evidence supporting the use of NSAIDs was poor and suggested that moderate to severe cancer pain was reduced to no worse than mild pain after 1 to 2 weeks in approximately 1 of 3 patients. One in 4 patients stopped taking NSAIDs because the drug did not work, and 1 of 20 stopped because of side effects.[61] In effect, there is no evidence to support or refute the use of NSAIDs alone or in combination with opioids for cancer pain. McNicol et al.[111] assessed and compared the efficacy of various NSAID and NSAID plus opioid combinations in the treatment of cancer pain. They concluded that most studies were of insufficient duration to demonstrate that the long-term use of NSAIDs is safe and effective in patients with cancer. They advised that clinicians should be as cautious in using NSAIDs in this population as they would any other population, especially given additional bleeding risks in cancer patients, and the probability that a patient with cancer may be on a broad regimen of medications, some of which may increase NSAID-related toxicity.

Acetaminophen

Acetaminophen (APAP) is one of the most popular antipyretic and analgesic medications worldwide. It is used either alone or in combination with other drugs. Its low cost and favorable side effect profile is attractive for use in a variety of painful conditions. The mechanism of action of the drug is not fully understood. However, it is known that acetaminophen is a weak inhibitor of the synthesis of PGs. It may have a selective COX-2 inhibitor effect[112] or a central effect, possibly due to activation of descending serotonergic pathways.[113] On average, APAP is considered a weaker analgesic than NSAIDs or COX-2 selective inhibitors but is often preferred because of its better tolerance. High use of APAP was associated with an almost twofold increased risk of incident hematologic malignancies such as myeloid neoplasms, non-Hodgkin lymphoma, and plasma cell disorders excluding chronic lymphocytic leukemia/small lymphocytic lymphoma[114] but not for other nonhematologic malignancies.[115] Severe liver injury can occur when acetaminophen use exceeds maximum dosage (currently 4,000 mg within a 24-hour period) or when an individual takes the drug and also consumes alcohol,[116] and with additional warnings that the drug may cause severe skin reactions including Stevens-Johnson syndrome, toxic epidermal necrolysis, and acute generalized exanthematous pustulosis.[117] Of note, the use of concentrated prescription APAP-containing medications (>500 mg) in combination with other sources of APAP can result in severe liver injury and death.[118] Acute liver failure secondary to APAP is most often associated with unintentional overdose, the use of a single product, an opioid-APAP combination, duration of use <7 days, and a median dose of 7.5 g per day.[119] Daily doses of APAP of 4 g for 10 days resulted in a maximum increase of serum alanine aminotransferase (ALT) more than 3 times normal in over 30% of patients,[120] and daily use of acetaminophen at half the maximum recommended daily dose for 12 weeks in a healthy adult population was associated with a small elevation in mean ALT of no probable clinical significance.[121] There is no high-quality evidence to support or refute the use of APAP alone or in combination with opioids for cancer-related pain[122] or with advanced disease.[123]

Opioid-Induced Bowel Dysfunction

Constipation is prevalent in oncology patients even among patients not on opioid therapy.[124] GI side effects such as nausea, vomiting, diarrhea, and constipation is associated with chemotherapy including alkylating agents, antimetabolites, immunomodulating agents, and mitotic inhibitors.[125] The prevalence of constipation after cytotoxic chemotherapy may be as high as 16% with 5% classified as severe.[126] Posttreatment constipation and diarrhea among cancer (particularly colorectal) survivors is prevalent with episodes persisting up to 10 years after treatment.[127,128] Opioid-induced constipation (OIC) and opioid-induced bowel dysfunction (OBD) are associated with opioid therapy. OBD is a distressing condition that may persist indefinitely in the clinical setting. Hard dry stool, gas distention, incomplete evacuation, and straining are common sequelae. OBD can affect quality of life significantly and result in hospitalization, pain, and frequent changes in opioid and laxative treatment.[129]

Clinical reviews on OIC indicate the lack of a common definition[130] and may be defined as a change when initiating opioid therapy from baseline bowel habits that is characterized by reduced bowel movement frequency, development or worsening of straining to pass bowel movements, a sense of incomplete rectal evacuation, or harder stool consistency.[131] OBD reflects the overall impact of opioids on the GI tract and include symptoms such as dry mouth, gastroesophageal reflux–related symptoms (heartburn), nausea, vomiting, chronic abdominal pain, bloating, constipation-related symptoms: straining, hard stools, painful, infrequent and incomplete bowel movements (BMs), and diarrhea-related symptoms: urgency, loose and frequent BMs.[132,133] OIC is the most common form of OBD.

Endogenous opioids and opioid receptors are widely distributed throughout the body, with strong expression in the CNS, peripheral nervous system, and enteric nervous system (ENS) and also within the endocrine and immune systems. The ENS has a network of small ganglia that can regulate GI motility and secretion independently of the CNS. Neurons in the ENS form plexuses between the circular and longitudinal muscle layers (the myenteric plexus) and between the mucosal and circular muscle layers (the submucosal plexus). The myenteric plexus innervates both the longitudinal and the circular muscle layers, and its primary role is to coordinate motility patterns. Submucosal plexuses are found in the small and large intestine and are primarily involved in the regulation of secretion and local blood flow. Opioids inhibit enteric neuronal activity in both the small intestine and the colon. The expression of μ-opioid receptors on myenteric and submucosal ganglia suggests that receptor agonists cause constipation by inhibiting peristaltic smooth muscle contractions by effects on the myenteric ganglia and also by inhibiting water and electrolyte movement across the lumen via effects on the submucosal ganglia. Opioid receptors and endogenous opioid agonists are altered in GI disease.[134] The mechanisms for OBD are associated with delays in gastric emptying, oral-cecal transit and colonic transit time, and inhibition of defecation, all of which are predominately mediated through peripheral μ receptors.[135–137] The effects of opioids on the gut also are partly a result of their ability to accumulate in the intestinal tissue and have a direct local effect on the bowel.[135] Centrally mediated antitransit effects are implicated in the pathophysiology of OBD. Opioids act centrally through alterations in autonomic outflow to the gut; however, their overall impact on GI motility appears to be correlated to their ability to penetrate the CNS.[138] Opioids mainly exert their action on the ENS where they bind to opioid receptors in the myenteric and submucosal plexuses and on immune cells in the lamina propria.[139] The coordination of the contractile and propulsive gut motility is determined by a balance between acetylcholine and nitric oxide/vasoactive intestinal peptide release.[140,141] Because opioids inhibit neurotransmitter release, administration will directly disrupt this balance, resulting in abnormal coordination of motility.[142]

The Bowel Function Index (BFI numerical analogue scale 0 to 100), calculated as the mean of three variables (ease of defecation, feeling of incomplete bowel evacuation, and personal judgment of constipation), was developed to evaluate bowel function in opioid-treated patients with pain.[143] This clinician-administered tool allows easy measurement of OIC from the patient's perspective.

Metoclopramide is commonly prescribed for patients with symptoms of gastroparesis.[144–146] It is a dopamine receptor antagonist, serotonin 5-hydroxytryptamine type 4 (5-HT$_4$) receptor agonist, and weak inhibitor of 5-hydroxytryptamine type 3 (5-HT$_3$) receptors. Activity appears to be by both peripheral (in the upper GI tract) and central mechanisms by inducing antidopaminergic effects. Recommended use of metoclopramide at the lowest effective dose for each patient beginning with 5 mg three times daily up to a maximum recommended dose of 40 mg per day.[147] Adverse events include restlessness, drowsiness, fatigue, and extrapyramidal effects, especially in younger patients and in children. Patients may experience extrapyramidal side effects at doses greater than 20 mg daily.[148] Metoclopramide is an inhibitor of CYP2D6 enzyme. Concurrent use of antidepressants such as tricyclics, selective serotonin reuptake inhibitors (SSRIs), and antidepressants acting as serotonin-norepinephrine reuptake inhibitors (SNRIs) (venlafaxine or duloxetine) may enhance adverse effects associated with metoclopramide.

The goals of therapy typically are threefold: keep stool volume maximized to trigger enterochromaffin cell serotonin release via mucosal stretch, keep stool softer and mechanically make it easier to move, and enhance peristalsis. Most treatment for constipation begins with encouraging exercise, activity, fluid intake, and dietary fiber and the use of stool softeners and laxatives. Fiber-bulking agents are organic polymers that retain water in stool. It is important that adequate water be taken concomitantly with fiber. Without sufficient fluid, fiber may worsen constipation. Many practitioners recommend a combination of a stool softener with a stimulant laxative for patients on chronic opioid therapy. Stool softeners, such as docusate sodium, are detergents that allow better water penetration into stool, making it softer and more voluminous. Stimulant laxatives, such as senna and bisacodyl, induce peristalsis via mechanisms that are not well understood. In vitro, applying senna to intestinal mucosa leads to immediate contraction. After optimal titration of these agents with persistent constipation, oral osmotics are commonly added to enhance laxation by pulling along water due to osmotic forces. Osmotics include sugars, such as lactulose or sorbitol; magnesium salts, such as magnesium citrate; or inert substances, such as polyethylene glycol. When unsuccessful, rescue oral and rectal interventions are also often needed. Rectal interventions include such agents as bisacodyl suppositories and phosphosoda enemas to soften, lubricate, and mobilize hard, dry distal stool. Often, synergism of multiple categories of agents is required for successful laxation. Another strategy has been the development of peripherally acting μ-opioid receptor antagonists (PAMORAs) that selectively target μ receptors in the GI tract. PAMORAs agents currently available include oral naloxegol and alvimopan and subcutaneously administered methylnaltrexone.

Naloxegol is a polymer conjugate of naloxone. The polyethylene glycol (PEG) moiety limits the ability to cross the blood–brain barrier. PEGs are also used as osmotic laxatives (e.g., macrogol 3,350/4,000), where they act as nonmetabolized, nonabsorbable, osmotic agents, forming hydrogen bonds with water in the intestinal lumen. PEGylation makes naloxegol a substrate for the P-glycoprotein (P-gp) transporter. Due to the reduced permeability and increased efflux of naloxegol across the blood–brain barrier, related to P-gp transporter, the CNS penetration of naloxegol is negligible and it reduces OIC in the GI tract without reversing the central analgesic effect.[149] administration of naloxegol with food is associated with increased bioavailability. The concentration and activity of naloxegol are increased by the concurrent use of CYP3A4 inhibitors and reduced by CYP3A4 inducers. Naloxegol is administered at a dose of 25 mg once daily on an empty stomach at least 1 hour before the first meal of the day or 2 hours after the first meal of the day. Cancer patients with symptoms of bowel obstruction and those with increased risk of GI perforation including GI or peritoneal tumors, recurrent or advanced ovarian cancer, and patients treated with vascular endothelial growth factor (VEGF) inhibitors should avoid the use of naloxegol.

Methylnaltrexone-bromide is a PAMORA and a quaternary methyl derivative of naltrexone. The addition of a methyl group to the nitrogen ring increases polarity and reduces lipophilicity such that the drug does not pass the blood–brain barrier. It is administered subcutaneously and is rapidly absorbed, with the peak plasma concentration attained within 30 minutes, and plasma elimination half-life ($t_{1/2}$) is approximately 8 hours.[150] It induces bowel movement in approximately 50% to 60% treated patients within 4 hours of its administration.[151,152] It is indicated for OIC patients with advanced disease who are receiving palliative care with inadequate response to laxative therapy.[153] Recommended dosing is 8 mg for patients weighing 38 to less than 62 kg and 12 mg for patients between 62 to 114 kg. Usual dosing is one dose every other day and not more

than one dose per day. Common side effects include abdominal pain, flatulence, and nausea. Contraindications include administration to patients with known or suspected mechanical bowel obstruction. Rare cases of GI perforation involving various regions of the GI tract have been reported in advanced illness patients.[154] Alvimopan is another orally administered PAMORA that does not cross the blood–brain barrier at clinically relevant doses and does not reverse analgesia or cause opioid withdrawal symptoms. The FDA approved alvimopan for postoperative ileus following partial small or large bowel resection with primary anastomosis in hospitalized patients.

Antiemetics

Nausea and vomiting is a common problem in oncology. Although opioids,[155] chemotherapy,[156] and radiation therapy[157] are commonly associated with nausea and vomiting, advanced disease is also frequently associated with nausea particularly in the last week of life.[158] Depending on the anatomic area irradiated, an estimated 50% to 80% of patients undergoing radiation therapy develop radiation therapy–induced nausea and vomiting (RINV).[159] Total body irradiation, half body irradiation, or abdominal radiotherapy are at a major risk of nausea and vomiting. The pathophysiology of nausea and vomiting is a complex process. The act of vomiting is coordinated by the vomiting center of the brain located in the lateral reticular formation of the medulla with efferent pathways through the vagus, phrenic, and spinal nerves. The vomiting center receives afferent input from various sources including the chemoreceptor trigger zone (CTZ) in the area postrema in the floor of the fourth ventricle, the vagus and sympathetic nerves, as well as impulses directly from the GI tract and other sources. The CTZ is also activated by mediators in the circulation, which may include hormones, peptides, medications, or toxins. The act of vomiting involves neurotransmitters (including serotonin, substance P, and dopamine found in the CTZ), the vomiting center, and enterochromaffin cells in the GI tract release efferent impulses that are transmitted to the abdominal musculature, salivation center, and respiratory center. CTZ effects are largely mediated through central dopamine type 2 (D2) receptors.

Opioids have emetogenic effects by central stimulation, vestibular effects and by inhibiting gut motility. The primary mechanism of opioid-induced nausea and emesis is central with direct stimulation of the CTZ.[160] Although opioid stimulation of the CTZ involve opioid receptors, signaling from the CTZ involves D2 and 5-HT$_3$ receptors and opioid stimulation of the vestibular apparatus and sensory input to the vomiting center may involve H1 and muscarinic acetylcholine pathways (Fig. 43.5).[161] The peripheral inhibitory effect of opioids on GI transit and stimulation of the pyloric sphincter delays gastric emptying or causes gastroparesis. Chemotherapy likely causes nausea and vomiting through stimulation of the CTZ mediated by 5-HT$_3$ and neurokinin type 1 (NK1) receptors. Because of these effects, 5-HT$_3$ and NK1 receptor antagonists are the most effective agents currently available. In most cases of chemotherapy-induced nausea and vomiting (CINV), these agents are used in conjunction with glucocorticoids.[162–165] Glucocorticoids are effective only for preventing nausea and vomiting and not for treating established nausea and vomiting.[166]

Typical strategies for management and minimization of opioid-induced nausea and vomiting include dose reduction, dose titration, opioid rotation, and the use of antiemetics. Commonly used antiemetics are listed in Table 43.6. It is not uncommon for patients to experience nausea and/or vomiting when starting opioid therapy, but these side effects tend to subside within days or weeks[167] unless opioid-induced bowel dysfunction develops. Until the late 1970s, dopamine-receptor antagonists,

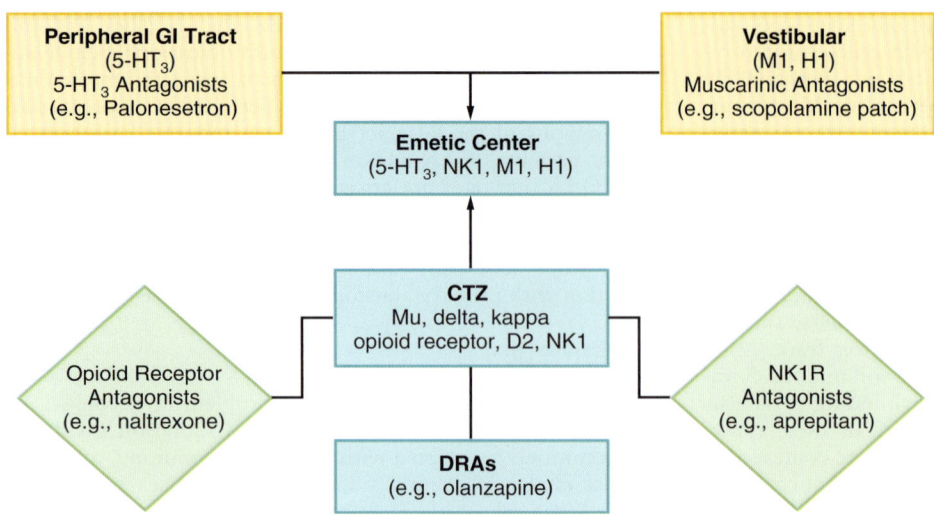

FIGURE 43.5 Opioid-induced nausea and vomiting pathophysiology and antiemetic therapy. 5-HT3, 5-hydroxytryptamine type 3; CTZ, chemoreceptor trigger zone; D2, dopamine type 2; DRA, dopamine receptor antagonist; GI, gastrointestinal; H1, histamine H1; M1, O-desmethyl tramadol; NK1, neurokinin type 1; NK1R, neurokinin type 1 receptor. *(Modified from Smith HS, Laufer A. Opioid induced nausea and vomiting.* Eur J Pharmacol *2014;722:67–78. Copyright © 2014 Elsevier. With permission.)*

such as metoclopramide, prochlorperazine, and haloperidol, formed the basis of antiemetic therapy. In 1991, the first 5-HT$_3$–receptor antagonist, ondansetron, was approved by the FDA for the treatment of chemotherapy-induced emesis followed by two additional 5-HT$_3$–receptor antagonists, granisetron and dolasetron, in 1997. Droperidol and ondansetron have an FDA black box warning after reports of prolonged rate-corrected QT (QTc) interval. Palonosetron is a second-generation 5-HT$_3$–receptor antagonist that has a prolonged t$_{1/2}$ with higher receptor binding affinity than other antiemetic agents. Aprepitant, the first NK1 receptor antagonist, was approved for chemotherapy-induced emesis in 2003. In 2008, fosaprepitant, a prodrug and intravenous form of aprepitant, was approved by the FDA. Dronabinol (Schedule III) and nabilone (Schedule II) are cannabis-derived pharmaceuticals indicated for the treatment of nausea and vomiting associated with cancer chemotherapy and of anorexia associated with weight loss in patients with acquired immune deficiency syndrome.[168]

Postoperatively, ondansetron is more effective than metoclopramide for the treatment of opioid-induced emesis.[169] Nausea and vomiting after acute administration of opioids may be partly related to serotonin receptor signaling.[170] Many consider dopamine receptor antagonists, including prochlorperazine and haloperidol

as the preferred drugs for managing opioid-induced nausea and vomiting.[171,172] Olanzapine, an atypical thienobenzodiazepine antipsychotic agent that is indicated for the treatment of schizophrenia and bipolar disorder, is also useful for the treatment of intractable nausea particularly at reducing during the delayed and overall phase of the CINV prevention.[173] It is also useful for the treatment of morphine-induced emesis and as an adjunct for the treatment of neuropathic pain associated with sleep disturbance.[161] It blocks multiple neurotransmitter receptors, including dopaminergic (D2), serotonergic (5-HT$_3$), adrenergic, histaminergic, and muscarinic receptors. Dose titration of olanzapine is over a period of 7 to 10 days (in the range of 2.5 to 7.5 mg) given at bedtime.

Many of the commonly prescribed antiemetic agents (e.g., phenothiazines, antihistamines, anticholinergic drugs, and metoclopramide) are generally effective but are often associated with undesirable side effects such as sedation, blurred vision, dysphoria, and extrapyramidal reactions. 5-HT$_3$ receptors are located centrally in the CTZ as well as peripherally on vagal nerve terminals. Ondansetron is effective for the control of opioid-induced nausea and vomiting.[174] The antiemetic actions noted from cannabinoids and endocannabinoids have been linked to CB1 effects, where antagonists can provoke acute emesis and agonists reduce acute nausea and vomiting.

TABLE 43.6	**Antiemetics**		
Agent	**Presumed Primary Receptor Site of Action**	**Dosage/Route**	**Major Adverse Effects**
Metoclopramide	D2 (primarily in GI tract) or 5-HT$_3$ (only at high doses)	5–20 mg orally or subcutaneously or IV	Dystonia, akathisia, esophageal spasm, and colic (in GI obstruction)
Haloperidol	D2 (primarily in CTZ)	0.5–4 mg orally or subcutaneously or IV q6h	Dystonia and akathisia
Prochlorperazine	D2 (primarily in CTZ)	5–10 mg orally or IV q6h or 25 mg rectally q6h	Dystonia, akathisia, and sedation
Chlorpromazine	D2 (primarily in CTZ)	10–250 mg orally q4h, 25–50 mg IV or IM q4h, or 50–100 mg rectally q6h	Dystonia, akathisia, sedation, postural hypotension
Promethazine	H1, muscarinic acetylcholine receptor, or D2 (primarily in CTZ)	12.5–25 mg orally or IV q6h or 25 mg rectally q6h	Dystonia, akathisia, and sedation
Diphenhydramine	H1	25–50 mg orally or IV or SQ q6h	Sedation, dry mouth, urinary retention
Scopolamine	Muscarinic acetylcholine receptor	1.5 mg transdermal patch q72h	Dry mouth, blurred vision, urinary retention, confusion
Hyoscyamine	Muscarinic acetylcholine receptor	0.125–0.25 mg SL or orally q4h or 0.25–0.5 mg SQ or IV q4h	Dry mouth, blurred vision, ileus, urinary retention, confusion
Ondansetron	5-HT$_3$	4–8 mg orally by pill or dissolvable tablet (ODT) or IV q4–8h	Headache, fatigue, constipation
Aprepitant	NK1	40 mg orally qd	

5-HT$_3$, 5-hydroxytryptamine type 3; CTZ, chemoreceptor trigger zone; D2, dopamine type 2; GI, gastrointestinal; H1, histamine H1; IM, intramuscular; IV, intravenous; NK1, neurokinin type 1; SL, sublingual; SQ, subcutaneous.

Adjuvant Analgesics

An adjuvant analgesic is a medication with a primary indication other than pain relief, but it may provide or enhance analgesia in certain circumstances. In the area of cancer pain, the common adjunctive analgesics are corticosteroids, anticonvulsants, and antidepressants. These drugs play an important role for some patients who cannot otherwise attain an acceptable balance between relief and opioid side effects. Adjuvant analgesics divide broadly into general purpose analgesics, adjuvants used for musculoskeletal pain, and those with specific use for neuropathic, bone, or visceral pain. Although ketamine has been used in the treatment of cancer pain refractory to opioid therapy, it is not licensed for this purpose and the evidence supporting its use is very low quality with potentially serious adverse events at higher doses[175] and will not be considered further.

GENERAL PURPOSE ADJUVANTS

Corticosteroids are the most widely used general purpose adjuvant analgesics and are available in a wide variety of formulations.[176] Various guidelines recommend the use of steroids as adjuvants for cancer pain but these guidelines are based on expert opinion.[177–181] Steroids are used to treat pain associated with increased intracranial pressure, acute spinal cord compression, superior vena cava syndrome, metastatic bone pain, neuropathic pain due to infiltration or compression, symptomatic lymphedema, and hepatic capsular distension. The mechanism for pain relief is unknown but the anti-inflammatory effect of steroids is often proposed as the putative mechanism.[182] The available data suggest that moderate doses of corticosteroids equivalent to methylprednisolone 32 mg or dexamethasone 8 mg daily are well tolerated for up to 7 days but that high doses equivalent to methylprednisolone 125 mg daily administered over 8 weeks have a significantly adverse impact and may even increase mortality.[183] Overall, data supporting the role of steroids for cancer pain control is weak and likely with only short-term benefit.[182]

Topical agents (see Chapter 80) may also be useful as an adjunctive form of pharmacotherapy, without increasing systemic toxicity. These agents are used for a variety of painful conditions such as strains or sprains, muscle aches, osteoarthritis of hand or knee, or neuropathic pain. Typical topical analgesic drugs include NSAIDs, salicylate rubefacients, capsaicin, and lidocaine. Agents such as diclofenac Emulgel, ketoprofen gel, piroxicam gel, and diclofenac plaster work reasonably well for strains and sprains. For hand and knee osteoarthritis, topical diclofenac and topical ketoprofen rubbed on the skin for at least 6 to 12 weeks help reduce pain by at least half in a modest number of people. For postherpetic neuralgia, topical high-concentration capsaicin can reduce pain by at least half in a small number of people.[184] There are a number of drugs in the area of pain management that have been formulated and compounded to treat conditions such as diabetic neuropathy, fibromyalgia, postherpetic neuralgia, joint pain, arthritis, and others. Significant portions of these compounded analgesic preparations are topical/transdermal dosage forms such as gels and creams. Although the efficacy and doses of these drugs in systemic dosage forms have been widely established, little is known about the permeation and efficacy of these compounds from these gels. A multicenter, phase III, randomized, double-blind, placebo-controlled trial was to investigate the efficacy of 2% ketamine plus 4% amitriptyline cream for reducing chemotherapy-induced peripheral neuropathy (CIPN) in 462 cancer survivors was ineffective for this problem.[185] A study examining topical 5% amitriptyline and 5% lidocaine in the treatment of mixed sources (noncancer) neuropathic pain showed that topical lidocaine reduced pain intensity but the clinical improvement was minimal and that topical 5% amitriptyline was not effective.[186] Although anecdotally, topical lidocaine may benefit some patient, there is no evidence from good quality randomized controlled studies to support the use of topical lidocaine to treat neuropathic pain.[187]

MUSCULOSKELETAL PAIN ADJUVANTS

The term *muscle relaxants* or *muscle relaxers* is broad and includes a wide range of drugs with different indications and mechanisms of action. Muscle relaxers are either antispasmodic or antispasticity medications. The antispasmodic agents are further subclassified into the benzodiazepines and the nonbenzodiazepines. Nonbenzodiazepines include a variety of drugs that can act at the brain stem or spinal cord level and include carisoprodol, chlorzoxazone, cyclobenzaprine, metaxalone, meprobamate, methocarbamol, tizanidine, zopiclone, and orphenadrine. Only three muscle relaxants—baclofen, dantrolene, and tizanidine—are FDA approved to treat spasticity. Tizanidine is an agonist at α_2-adrenergic receptor sites and presumably reduces spasticity by increasing presynaptic inhibition of motor neurons. It has linear pharmacokinetics over a dose of 1 to 20 mg.[188] In multiple dose, controlled clinical studies, 48% of patients receiving any dose of tizanidine reported sedation as an adverse event and sedation appears to be dose related.[189] A single dose of 8 mg of tizanidine reduces muscle tone in patients with spasticity for a period of several hours. The effect peaks at approximately 1 to 2 hours and dissipates between 3 and 6 hours.

The FDA-approved muscle relaxers for spasms (including carisoprodol, cyclobenzaprine, orphenadrine, metaxalone, chlorzoxazone, and methocarbamol) have only been approved for short-term use (up to 21 days), and their long-term efficacy is unknown. Evidence supporting the effectiveness of these drugs for muscle spasm is sparse; most trials are old and not of good quality. Much of the evidence from clinical trials regarding the use of these agents is limited because of poor methodologic design, insensitive assessment methods, and small numbers of patients.[190] These drugs are often used for treatment of musculoskeletal conditions, whether muscle spasm is present or not. Pharmacologic and nonpharmacologic approaches do not differ significantly from patients with musculoskeletal pain who do not have cancer (see Chapters 80 and 89), other than disease- or treatment-specific issues relevant to the cancer patient. Drug–drug and drug–disease interactions must always be considered and be an ongoing component of reassessment.

NEUROPATHIC PAIN ADJUVANTS

Neuropathic pain, caused by a lesion or disease affecting the somatosensory nervous system, is a common and oftentimes very debilitating source of distress in patients with cancer (see Chapters 24 to 28 and 42). In cancer and chronic noncancer pain, there is a large variety of causes. Most treatment strategies for cancer-related neuropathic pain are extrapolated from noncancer-related neuropathic pain (see Chapters 24 to 28).[191–194] Table 43.7 summarizes those agents that are used to treat neuropathic pain in noncancer patients. Of note, opioids are recommended as third line contrasting with previous recommendations.[195] This is largely because of the potential risk of abuse, particularly with high doses, and concerns about prescription opioid–associated overdose mortality, diversion, misuse, and other opioid-related morbidity. In addition, high-concentration capsaicin patches and cannabinoids are considered for the first time in therapeutic recommendations for neuropathic pain.

The causes of neuropathic pain in noncancer patients are diverse and generally can be considered as central or peripheral. Neuropathic pain has been extensively discussed in Chapters 24 to 28. Although chronic noncancer neuropathic pain occurs in oncology patients, unique sources of pain including disease infiltration of central and peripheral nervous tissue, paraneoplastic peripheral neuropathy, pain resulting

TABLE 43.7 Drugs or Drug Classes with Strong or Weak Recommendations for Management of Neuropathic Pain

	Total Daily Dose and Dose Regimen	Recommendations
Strong Recommendations for Use		
Gabapentin	1,200–3,600 mg, in three divided doses	First line
Gabapentin extended-release or enacarbil	1,200–3,600 mg, in two divided doses	First line
Pregabalin	300–600 mg, in two divided doses	First line
Serotonin-norepinephrine reuptake inhibitors duloxetine or venlafaxine[a]	60–120 mg, once a day (duloxetine); 150–225 mg, once a day (venlafaxine extended release)	First line
Tricyclic antidepressants	25–150 mg, once a day or in two divided doses	First line[b]
Weak Recommendations for Use		
Capsaicin 8% patches	One to four patches to the painful area for 30–60 min every 3 months	Second line (peripheral neuropathic pain)[c]
Lidocaine patches	One to three patches to the region of pain once a day for up to 12 h	Second line (peripheral neuropathic pain)
Tramadol	200–400 mg, in two (tramadol extended release) or three divided doses	Second line
Botulinum toxin A (subcutaneously)	50–200 units to the painful area every 3 months	Third line; specialist use (peripheral neuropathic pain)
Strong opioids	Individual titration	Third line[d]

[a]Duloxetine is the most studied, and therefore recommended, of the serotonin-norepinephrine reuptake inhibitors.
[b]Tricyclic antidepressants generally have similar efficacy; tertiary amine tricyclic antidepressants (amitriptyline, imipramine, and clomipramine) are not recommended at doses greater than 75 mg per day in adults aged 65 years and older because of major anticholinergic and sedative side effects and potential risk of falls; an increased risk of sudden cardiac death has been reported with tricyclic antidepressants at doses greater than 100 mg daily.
[c]The long-term safety of repeated applications of high-concentration capsaicin patches in patients has not been clearly established, particularly with respect to degeneration of epidermal nerve fibers, which might be a cause for concern in progressive neuropathy.
[d]Sustained-release oxycodone and morphine have been the most studied opioids (maximum doses of 120 mg per day and 240 mg per day, respectively, in clinical trials); long-term opioid use might be associated with abuse, particularly at high doses, cognitive impairment, and endocrine and immunologic changes.
Reprinted from Finnerup NB, Attal N, Haroutounian S, et al. Pharmacotherapy for neuropathic pain in adults: a systematic review and meta-analysis. *Lancet Neurol* 2015;14(2):162–173. Copyright © 2015 Elsevier. With permission.

from leptomeningeal metastases and neuropathic pain secondary to therapeutic interventions (postsurgical, radiation therapy, and CIPN) occur in cancer patients. Furthermore, combinations of different sources of pain may also occur. For example, a patient with persistent CIPN-associated pain may develop both central and peripheral sources of pain (brachial plexus tumor infiltration extending to the spinal canal causing cord compression). Management of such pain complaints may require multiple approaches including disease control (chemotherapy, radiation therapy) and symptomatic pharmacologic approaches. Extrapolation of treatment guidelines from noncancer pain patients are not appropriate for the management of oncology-associated neuropathic pain. Data relating to the use of neuropathic pain adjuvant medications for the management or prevention of CIPN-associated pain is inconsistent. Chemotherapeutic agents causing nerve dysfunction mainly target axons, dorsal root ganglia, and terminal trees of intraepidermal nerve fibers.[196] Purported chemoprotective agents (acetylcysteine, amifostine, calcium and magnesium, diethyldithiocarbamate, glutathione, Org 2766, oxcarbazepine, retinoic acid, or vitamin E) for platin drug toxicity were not beneficial.[197] Typical medications used for management of CIPN are antidepressants (tricyclics, SNRIs) or antiepileptic drugs (AEDs) (gabapentin, pregabalin). Venlafaxine is a reasonably well-tolerated antidepressant and is a serotonin reuptake inhibitor and weak norepinephrine reuptake inhibitor. Although some studies suggest benefit for use in acute oxaliplatin-induced[198] or acute taxane-oxaliplatin-related[199] neuropathy, others have found little compelling evidence to support the use of venlafaxine in neuropathic pain.[200] Because of the lack of effective management for CIPN, the National Cancer Institute sponsored a series of trials aimed at prevention and management.[201] A total of 15 studies were approved, evaluating use of various neuromodulatory agents (including nortriptyline, gabapentin, and lamotrigine) which have shown benefit in other neuropathic pain states. Gabapentin doses were targeted to 2,700 mg per day for a total of 6 weeks. Aside from duloxetine, none demonstrated therapeutic benefit for patients with CIPN. Smith et al.[202] studied the effect of duloxetine at initial doses of 30 mg for 1 week then 60 mg for 4 additional weeks for painful CIPN induced by paclitaxel, other taxane, or oxaliplatin. Fifty-nine percent of patients experienced some decrease in pain after 5 weeks of taking duloxetine, and more duloxetine-treated patients decreased their opioid analgesic intake. In a retrospective review on the use of duloxetine for paclitaxel-induced CIPN, some benefit was observed in younger patients, but elderly patients (>60 years) tended to be less responsive and experienced more drug-related adverse events.[203] It should also be noted, especially in breast cancer patients, that if duloxetine and tamoxifen are taken together, duloxetine-induced CYP P450 2D6 enzyme inhibition could inhibit tamoxifen conversion to its active metabolite, endoxifen.[204]

BONE PAIN ADJUVANTS

NSAIDs, corticosteroids, calcitonin, radiopharmaceuticals, and bisphosphonates all have a potential place in the treatment of cancer-related bone pain. The use of calcitonin has been disappointing in the management of painful bone metastases.[205,206] Dexamethasone is useful for the management of radiation-induced bone pain flares,[207] but there is no evidence of benefit for management of painful bone metastases. The risk of bone loss and fractures is increased with systemic glucocorticoid use with the highest rate of bone loss that occurs within the first 3 to 6 months of therapy.[208] More than 10% of patients who receive long-term steroid therapy are diagnosed with a fracture, and 30% to 40% have radiographic evidence of vertebral fractures.[209] Exposure to steroids is also a leading cause of osteonecrosis (avascular necrosis).[210,211]

VISCERAL PAIN ADJUVANTS

The literature offers little support for the potential efficacy of adjuvant agents for the management of bladder spasm, tenesmoid pain, and colicky intestinal pain. Although there is no well-established pharmacotherapy for painful rectal spasms, diltiazem can help in the management of proctalgia fugax.[212] Inhaled salbutamol also shortened the attack of severe pain in a randomized double-blind trial in 18 patients with proctalgia fugax.[213]

Most treatments for proctalgia fugax (e.g., oral diltiazem, topical glyceryl nitrate, nerve blocks) act by relaxing the anal sphincter spasm. The effectiveness of these treatments is supported only by case reports or case series.[214] For chronic proctitis associated with radiation therapy, anti-inflammatory agents such as sulfasalazine or 5-aminosalicylic acid (mesalamine) are usually first-line treatments, but they have low efficacy even in combination with other agents such as steroids and antibiotics.[215] Belladonna and opium suppositories have been used in the management of moderate to severe pain associated with ureteral spasm. The recommended adult dose of belladonna and opium rectal suppositories for the treatment of moderate to severe pain associated with ureteral spasm is 1 suppository (each suppository: belladonna 16.2 mg/opium 30 mg OR belladonna 16.2 mg/opium 60 mg) rectally once or twice a day; maximum of 4 doses per day. Belladonna and opium rectal suppositories have not been found by the FDA to be safe and effective and are not recommended for use.

Psychotropic Drugs

Psychoactive substances are substances that affect mental processes, for example, cognition or affect. This and its equivalent, psychotropic drug, are the most neutral and descriptive term for the whole class of substances, licit and illicit, of interest to drug policy. In a large population study in The Netherlands, cancer patients were often prescribed psychotropic drugs including benzodiazepines, antidepressants, and antipsychotics.[216] The pattern of use was more common soon after diagnosis with increases in the terminal stage of the disease. The presence of pain and (to a greater extent) poor pain control were associated with increased use of certain psychotropic drugs, such as anxiolytics and hypnotics.[217] Use of hypnotics or anxiolytics drugs is associated with increased mortality and should be used cautiously.[218–221] Among drugs most frequently involved in drug overdose deaths in the United States, alprazolam and diazepam are featured.[222] Concurrent benzodiazepine use was also associated with an increased risk of death from overdose in patients receiving opioids.[33] Cancer patients often require the use of a psychoactive drug. Some need it for pain relief (e.g., tricyclic antidepressants for nerve injury pain), whereas others need an antiemetic (e.g., lorazepam for CINV). Still, others require an anxiolytic, such as clonazepam or alprazolam. Some require a night sedative and others an antidepressant for identifiable depression. The concurrent use of two centrally acting drugs (e.g., opioid with psychotropic drug or two psychotropic drugs together) is more likely to produce sedation in ill and malnourished cancer patients than in others. A comprehensive review of psychotropic drugs in pain management appears in Chapters 31 and 81.

Cannabinoids

Cannabis sativa contains over 450 compounds, with at least 70 classified as phytocannabinoids. Of medical interest are delta 9-tetrahydrocannabinol (THC) and cannabidiol (CBD). THC is the main active constituent, with psychoactive and pain-relieving properties. CBD not only has lesser affinity for the cannabinoid (CB) receptors and the potential to counteract the negative effects of THC on memory, mood, and cognition but also has an effect on pain modulation. The discovery of the endocannabinoid system (cannabinoid receptors CB1 and CB2 and their endogenous ligands) resulted in studies concerning the pharmacologic activity of cannabinoids. Endocannabinoids act as ligands at cannabinoid receptors within the nervous system (primarily but not exclusively CB1 receptors) and in the periphery (primarily but not exclusively CB2 receptors). Cannabinoids have been recommended for the prevention of CINV[223] and may be effective in cancer patients who respond poorly to commonly used agents.[224] In a 2015 review, patients who received cannabinoids were 5 times as likely to report complete absence of vomiting, and three times as likely to report complete absence of nausea and vomiting but when compared with conventional antiemetic drugs, there was no evidence of a difference for nausea, vomiting, or nausea and vomiting.[225]

The DEA lists marijuana and its cannabinoids as Schedule I controlled substances, which means that they cannot legally be prescribed under federal law. Two cannabinoids (dronabinol, nabilone) are approved by the FDA and therefore can be legally prescribed in the United States. Dronabinol contains the trans isomer of THC within a gelatin capsule. Marijuana can be used to make hashish and hash oil, which contain concentrated cannabinoids. Both marijuana and hash oil can be consumed by inhalation (smoking and vaporizing) and by mouth (drinking it as a tea or eating after it is mixed into foods, such as baked goods). Smoked cannabis has been found to contain Aspergillosis, and immunosuppressed patients should not use it.[226] Vaporizing marijuana by heating it to temperatures between 180°C and 200°C releases substantial amounts of cannabinoids with only trace amounts of a few other chemicals. Maida et al.[227] assessed the effectiveness of nabilone in managing pain in advanced cancer patients which significantly improved pain, nausea, anxiety, and total distress. Johnson et al.[228] compared the efficacy of a THC:CBD extract (2.7 mg THC, 2.5 mg CBD delivered by oromucosal spray) and a THC extract (2.7 mg THC delivered by oromucosal spray), with placebo in 177 patients with refractory cancer pain to chronic opioid therapy (average daily oral morphine equivalent dose [MED] 271 mg) and reported that the THC:CBD extract was efficacious, but the number of THC responders was similar to placebo. In a pilot study of 18 patients with pain related to CIPN, nabiximols (THC/CBD oral mucosal spray) had an efficacy comparable to the use of gabapentin for this problem.[229] Both cannabis and cannabinoid pharmaceuticals can be helpful for a number of problems affecting patients with cancer.[230,231] Data supporting the use of these products for cancer-related pain is lacking.

Opioid Analgesics

Opioids are the mainstay of pharmacotherapy for patients with moderate or more intense pain resulting from virtually any cancer-related etiology. A detailed discussion of opioid pharmacology and principles of prescribing is found in Chapter 79.

SELECTION OF OPIOID THERAPY IN CANCER PAIN MANAGEMENT

As in all patients who may have pain-related indications for opioid therapy, the effective clinical use of opioid drugs requires familiarity with drug selection, routes of administration, dosage guidelines, and potential adverse effects. Several factors must be considered if opioids are to be used effectively. These include:

- Previous opioid exposure and preference
- Severity, nature, and stage of disease
- Age of patient
- Extent of cancer, particularly hepatic and renal involvement altering normal opioid pharmacokinetics
- Concurrent disease
- Available formulations
- Risk assessment for problematic opioid use (see "Substance Abuse in Oncology" section)

The presence of renal impairment or failure affects the pharmacokinetics of opioids (Table 43.8). Renal failure has different effects on individual opioids with some opioids having active or toxic metabolites. The effects from dialysis should also be considered with the likelihood of removal of any molecule in blood by dialysis dependent on the molecular weight, water solubility, degree of protein binding, and volume of distribution.

TABLE 43.8   Opioid Use in Renal Dysfunction[a] and Hemo/Peritoneal Dialysis

Drug	Recommendations for Safe Use	Comments	Removal by Hemo/Peritoneal Dialysis
Preferred Opioid			
HYDROmorphone (Dilaudid)	• Single dose safe • Consider a lower dose and less frequent dosing intervals with repeated use.	• Metabolized to active hydromorphone-3-glucuronide • Accumulation of this metabolite may cause neuroexcitatory effects: Monitor for agitation, confusion, hallucination.	• May be dialyzable to a certain extent • Monitor for rebound pain after dialysis.
Potentially Acceptable Opioids			
Fentanyl • Intravenous • Transmucosal (Actiq)	• Single dose safe • Consider a lower dose and less frequent dosing intervals with repeated use.	• No active metabolites • Appears to have no added risk of adverse effects in renal dysfunction except for drug accumulation	Poorly dialyzable
Hydrocodone (Vicodin, Norco)	• Single dose safe • Consider a lower dose and less frequent dosing intervals with repeated use.	• Metabolized to HYDROmorphone, which is metabolized to hydromorphone-3-glucuronide • Accumulation of this metabolite may cause neuroexcitatory effects: Monitor for agitation, confusion, hallucination.	• No data for parent drug, some removal of metabolites • Monitor for rebound pain after dialysis.
Methadone (Dolophine)	• Should only be used by prescribers with expertise in methadone management • Dose adjustment for renal impairment or failure unlikely to be needed	• No active metabolites • Minimal accumulation in renal failure or impairment due to elimination by hepatobiliary clearance • Variable pharmacokinetics, difficult to titrate dose	Not dialyzable
Oxycodone • Immediate-release (Roxicodone)	• Single dose safe • Consider a lower dose and less frequent dosing intervals with repeated use.	• Active metabolite oxymorphone AND parent drug can accumulate in renal failure • CNS toxicity and sedation have been reported with accumulation in renal failure	No data for oxycodone or metabolites
Oxycodone • Controlled release (OxyContin)	• Reduce dose until steady-state effects known (1–2 days) • Dialysis: lack of data in dialysis • _Avoid use (preferred)_ OR administer with caution and careful monitoring.		
Avoid Use			
Codeine	Do not use	Metabolites morphine-3-glucuronide and morphine-6-glucuronide can accumulate, causing unpredictable therapeutic and adverse effects.	Not extensively dialyzed
Fentanyl Transdermal (Duragesic)	Do not use	Long half-life and risk of drug accumulation	Poorly dialyzable
Meperidine (Demerol)	Do not use	Toxic metabolite normeperidine can accumulate which can decrease seizure threshold and may cause neuroexcitatory effects.	Limited data but appears minimally removed by dialysis
Morphine • Immediate release (MSIR)	• Avoid if possible • If used, reduce dose and extend frequency with repeated dosing	Active metabolites (morphine-3-glucuronide and morphine-6-glucuronide) can accumulate which may result in unpredictable therapeutic and adverse effects Morphine/metabolites are dialyzable and can be used with caution if patients adhere to scheduled dialysis and/or are on a stable regimen. However, there is significant risk of morphine/metabolite accumulation with missed dialysis sessions and should be used with caution.	• Parent drug and metabolites can both be removed with dialysis. • Monitor for rebound pain effect.

NOTE: 2 mg IV morphine = 0.4 mg IV HYDROmorphone = 20 µg IV fentanyl = 5 mg PO oxycodone (relative equivalency for opioid-naive patients).
[a]Estimated glomerular filtration rate for African or European American <50 mL per minute.
CNS, central nervous system.

Fentanyl, for example, has high protein binding and low water solubility, as well as a high volume of distribution, and a moderately high molecular weight suggesting poor removal by dialysis.[232,233] Glomerular filtration rate (GFR) approximates the renal excretion of many drugs, and some authors recommend adjustment of opioid dosage based on the GFR.[234] Unlike estimates of GFR in renal disease, adequate biomarkers relating to hepatic function and drug elimination capacity, are not available. The most commonly used systems to assess the severity of hepatic impairment are the Child-Pugh classification and the Model for End-Stage Liver Disease (MELD) system. Opioids used in patients with severe liver disease in patients with a history of hepatic encephalopathy may precipitate or aggravate encephalopathy.[235] Methadone is metabolized by oxidation,

TABLE 43.9	Opioid Pharmacokinetics in Patients with Severe Liver Disease (Unless Otherwise Stated)	
Drug	**Pharmacokinetic Changes**	**Recommendation and Dose Adjustments**
Codeine	Reduced metabolism to morphine	Avoid use.
Tramadol	3-fold ↑ AUC and 2.5-fold ↑ $t_{1/2}$	Prolong dosage intervals or reduce doses.
Tapentadol	1.7- to 4.2-fold ↑ AUC and 1.2- to 1.4-fold ↑ $t_{1/2}$ in mild and moderate liver disease	Moderate liver disease: reduce dose and prolong dosing interval. Severe liver disease: no data
Morphine	↑ Oral bioavailability; ↑ $t_{1/2}$; ↓ CL	2-fold prolongation in dosage intervals. Reduce oral doses.
Oxycodone	↑ AUC; ↑ $t_{1/2}$; ↓ CL	Lower doses with prolonged dosage intervals.
Hydromorphone	↑ Oral bioavailability; no change in $t_{1/2}$ in moderate liver disease.	Reduce doses; consider prolonged dosage intervals only in severe liver disease.
Meperidine	↑ Oral bioavailability; 2-fold ↑ $t_{1/2}$; 2-fold ↓ CL	Avoid repeated use; risk of neurotoxic metabolite accumulation
Methadone	↑ $t_{1/2}$; possible risk of accumulation	No dose changes in mild and moderate liver disease; careful titration in severe liver disease
Buprenorphine	No data	No recommendations
Fentanyl	No change after single IV dose in moderate liver disease	Dose adjustment usually not needed; consider dose adjustment with continuous infusion or with transdermal patch.

NOTE: Disease severity is classified as mild, moderate, or severe (Child-Pugh classes A, B, and C, respectively).
AUC, area under the plasma concentration-time curve; CL, total plasma clearance; $t_{1/2}$, elimination half-life.
Modified by permission from Springer: Bosilkovska M, Walder B, Besson M, et al. Analgesics in patients with hepatic impairment: pharmacology and clinical implications. *Drugs* 2012;72(12):1645–1669. Copyright © 2012 Springer International Publishing AG.

with principal involvement of CYP3A4 and CYP2B6. The elimination of methadone and its metabolites is urinary and fecal. The use of methadone was studied in 11 patients with severe liver disease and although the $t_{1/2}$ was longer, peak plasma levels were lower. None of the patients had signs or symptoms of overdose and six patients had flattened plasma methadone concentration-time curves (Table 43.9).[236]

The specific pathogenic mechanism that underlies a patient's cancer pain should not be a factor in deciding which opioid to use because the mechanism of pain does not reliably predict the response to opioid therapy.[237] This particularly applies to situations in which tumor-associated neuropathic mechanisms dominate the pain complaint. Opioids should be used as first-line therapy in such situations, particularly if the pain is considered moderate to severe in intensity. Haumann et al.[238] demonstrated a beneficial effect from methadone compared to fentanyl on head-and-neck cancer patients with neuropathic pain. Oxycodone/naloxone and pregabalin were also deemed effective in lung cancer patients with neuropathic pain.[239] Controlled-release oxycodone (average daily dose 28 mg with range 20 to 80 mg) was effective and well-tolerated in patients with bortezomib-associated painful CIPN.[240] There is limited data on the use of opioids for neuropathic nonmalignant pain. Extended-release oxycodone was used for the management of painful diabetic neuropathy and postherpetic neuralgia, but the data was considered very low quality.[241] Morphine was also studied for use in painful diabetic neuropathy, CIPN, postherpetic neuralgia, phantom limb or postamputation pain, and lumbar radiculopathy again with insufficient evidence to support or refute use.[242] Similarly, the data support the use of methadone[243] and fentanyl[244] for diverse neuropathic pain syndromes including postherpetic neuralgia is also inconclusive. Short-term studies provide only equivocal evidence regarding the efficacy of opioids in reducing the intensity of neuropathic pain. Intermediate-term studies demonstrated significant efficacy of opioids over placebo, but these results are likely to be subject to significant bias because of small size, short duration, and potentially inadequate handling of dropouts.[245]

Patients surviving cancer typically experience a shift in the use of opioids from the routine prescribing that occurred in the active treatment phase to an approach more consistent with prescribing patterns for chronic noncancer pain when pain is expected to persist for years.[246] However, the rate of opioid prescribing was significantly higher among survivors of cancer compared with age/sex-matched controls without a prior cancer diagnosis and higher prescribing rate persisted, even for survivors more than 10 or more years postdiagnosis. The rate of prescriptions was greater for survivors of lung, GI, genitourinary, or gynecologic cancer compared with their corresponding controls.[247]

There is little high-grade data on opioid use specifically in the elderly cancer patient. Elderly patients are more likely to have multiple comorbidities, the potential for drug interactions, and are physiologically more vulnerable to opioid use than younger patients. There are also age-related differences in the perception of, and response to, pain.[248] Because the elderly have a higher incidence of cognitive impairment, confusion, and memory loss, either from pathology or medication use, and confounded by sight and hearing impairment, problems with prescription adherence and medication-related adverse effects can occur. The tolerability profile of opioids is important in elderly patients, as adverse events such as drowsiness, dizziness, and motor imbalance can have serious consequences in patients who are already more prone to falls and fractures.[249] Daily use of three or more psychoactive medications was associated with recurrent falls in the elderly.[250] High-risk medications, in particular benzodiazepines and benzodiazepine-receptor agonists, often administered at higher-than-recommended geriatric daily doses, were associated with falls in elderly, hospitalized patients.[251]

In general, the clinical circumstance dictates the choice of a short- or long-acting opioid. For example, the treatment of acute or postoperative pain usually requires frequent titration, and short-acting opioids, with duration of action of 2 to 4 hours, are preferred. Short-acting agents may be favored initially for the management of mild- to moderate-intensity tumor pain as they are easier to titrate than long-acting or ATC opioids. Short-acting opioids are characterized by a rapid rise and fall in serum opioid levels, whereas serum levels of long-acting opioids increase slowly to therapeutic levels, remain there for an extended period, and then slowly decline.[252] Conversely, the treatment of cancer pain or chronic, moderate to severe nonmalignant pain usually can be treated with a long-acting oral agent, with a duration of action of 12 to 24 hours, with less need for daily titration. In patients treated with long-acting agents, short-acting opioids should be provided as rescue medication for breakthrough pain, which is very common in patients with cancer pain.[253,254] An ongoing opioid regimen should include provisions for rescue doses for the treatment of breakthrough pain. The rationale for providing rescue medication instead of increasing the dose of the ATC opioid is to prevent overmedication and associated adverse events. Often, there is a narrow therapeutic window between an opioid dose sufficient to achieve pain relief and one that is associated with unacceptable adverse events.[255] For patients treated with a long-acting opioid, an immediate-release (IR) or short-acting opioid formulation (often the same drug) may be used as the rescue medication. In general, the rescue drug should be started at a dose equivalent to approximately 10% of the 24-hour baseline dose and titrated upward to achieve adequate pain relief.[256] The dosing frequency of the rescue drug depends on the time to peak effect and the route of administration; in general, oral rescue doses can be administered as frequently as every 2 hours if needed but typically tend to be given every 3 to 4 hours as needed.[257] Generally, three types of breakthrough pain should be considered—spontaneous, incident, or end-of-dose failure.[258] A key principle in treating breakthrough pain is to optimize the background pain control by appropriately adjusting the ATC opioid regimen. With end-of-dose failure, the clinician can increase the dose or shorten the dosing interval of the ATC opioid or increase the dose of the rescue opioid. Similar strategies may be employed for spontaneous pain, but successful management of spontaneous or incident pain may require the use of short-acting, rapid-onset opioids ("Oral Transmucosal/Intranasal/Sublingual Fentanyl" section).

Because of the substantial interpatient variability in opioid responsiveness, clinicians who prescribe opioids for the treatment of cancer pain should be familiar with at least three different agents appropriate for the management of moderate to severe pain.[259] The pharmacology of these agents can be reviewed in Chapter 79.

The regimen for opioid medications should generally provide ATC analgesia with provision for rescue doses for the management of exacerbations of the pain not covered by the regular dosage. Various extended-release oral and transdermal opioids are listed in Table 43.10. At all times, causes of new or uncontrolled pain should be determined and addressed by disease-modifying treatments and a gradual increase in the opioid dose until either pain control is achieved or intolerable and unmanageable adverse effects supervene. The management of pain with opioid analgesics demands frequent patient

TABLE 43.10 Extended-Release Oral and Transdermal Opioids Used in the Treatment of Cancer Pain

Name	Trade Name	Generic
Morphine	MS contin	Various extended-release tablets and capsules
	Avinza	
	Kadian	
	Morphabond ER[a]	
	Arymo ER[a]	
Oxycodone	OxyContin[a]	
	Xtampza ER[a]	
	Troxyca ER[a] (oxycodone/naltrexone)	
	Targiniq[a] (oxycodone/naloxone)	
Hydrocodone	Hysingla ER[a]	
	Vantrela ER[a]	
Hydromorphone	Exalgo	
Oxymorphone	Opana ER	Various extended-release tablets
Fentanyl	Duragesic	Various extended-release transdermal patches
Buprenorphine	Butrans	
Tapentadol	Nucynta ER	

[a]Abuse-deterrent properties. Abuse-deterrent formulations target the known or expected routes of abuse, such as crushing in order to snort or dissolving in order to inject, for the specific opioid drug substance. Methadone is not included as it is not considered an extended-release (ER) product.

TABLE 43.11 Pharmacokinetics of Transdermal Fentanyl Following First 72-Hour Application

Dose	T_{max} (h) Mean (SD)	C_{max} (ng/mL) Mean (SD)
12 µg/h	28.8 (13.7)	0.38 (0.13)
25 µg/h	31.7 (16.5)	0.85 (0.26)
50 µg/h	32.8 (15.6)	1.72 (0.53)
75 µg/h	35.8 (14.1)	2.32 (0.86)
100 µg/h	29.9 (13.3)	3.36 (1.28)

T_{max}, time to maximal concentration; C_{max}, maximal concentration.
Janssen MD. *Duragesic (Fentanyl Transdermal System) for Transdermal Administration.* Titusville, NJ: Janssen MD; 2014.

assessment and a readiness to reevaluate the therapeutic plan in the setting of either inadequate relief or adverse effects. Predicting effectiveness of extended-release opioids requires knowledge of associated pharmacokinetics. In particular, the onset time and time to maximal concentration (T_{max}) is particularly helpful. Table 43.11 lists T_{max} for various doses of transdermal fentanyl. After initial application, the maximal concentration (peak analgesic effect or associated side effects) is not reached until approximately 32 hours. The dosing interval is determined by steady state. For the extended-release opioids, the $t_{1/2}$ is not particularly helpful because of altered absorption characteristics into the central compartment.

There is no single optimal or maximal dose of an opioid analgesic drug. In general, for progressive, tumor-related pain, the appropriate dose of an opioid is one that relieves a patient's pain throughout the dosing interval without causing unmanageable or intolerable adverse events.[260] The initial dose may be based on the severity of pain and known response to prior analgesic therapy, if any. Aggressive upward titration to a stable dose (i.e., one that provides adequate pain relief throughout the dosing interval) is predicated on continuing assessment of the effectiveness of therapy. Patients rarely benefit from combinations of different opioids given in suboptimal doses; ideally, clinicians should prescribe a single opioid analgesic and titrate to a stable dose.[261] However, it is important to recognize that there is significant interpatient variability with regard to responsiveness to different opioid drugs, and patients who respond poorly to one opioid may respond favorably to another.[262] In situations in which pain is not related to the tumor or its treatment, a dose limit should be considered.[263]

TOLERANCE AND HYPERALGESIA

Opioid tolerance is a phenomenon in which repeated exposure to an opioid results in decreased therapeutic effect of the drug or need for a higher dose to maintain the same effect. Tolerance can be overcome by increase the opioid dose. Opioid-induced hyperalgesia (OIH) is a state of nociceptive sensitization caused by opioid exposure and is characterized by a paradoxical response to opioid treatment where patients become more sensitive to pain. In contrast to tolerance, dose increases make the pain complaint worse. OIH is more commonly seen in patients receiving high opioid doses. The majority of reports not only involve the use of systemic (oral, intravenous, intramuscular) or intrathecal morphine[264,265] but may also occur with intrathecal sufentanil,[266] fentanyl,[267,268] remifentanil,[269] and hydromorphone.[270] In this setting, patients report increased pain as well as allodynia and myoclonus. OIH has been reported in various clinical settings including acute pain,[269] chronic non-cancer pain,[271] cancer pain,[272,273] and opioid addiction.[274] Very high intravenous and intrathecal opioid doses can cause OIH. OIH should be recognized as a syndrome of neuroexcitatory effects, which includes hyperalgesia, allodynia, myoclonus, and seizures. The predominant symptom of OIH is severe allodynia (touch-evoked pain) and is often accompanied by myoclonus.

Placing a blanket on or gently turning a bedridden patient can evoke excruciating pain. The diagnosis is confirmed if further dose escalation exacerbates pain complaints or symptoms and temporarily holding opioid therapy eliminates or reduces symptoms. Management strategies for hyperalgesia usually require a reduction in opioid dosage and/or switching to a different opioid, especially one that does not have known toxic metabolites. However, the occurrence of OIH with normal clinical doses is questionable.[275,276] In a study on the presence of OIH following oral administration of opioids (oxycodone and morphine in daily doses up to 200 mg) in both cancer and noncancer pain patients, OIH was not observed.[277] Not all patients develop OIH and the detection and occurrence of OIH poses a significant clinical challenge in acute, chronic, and cancer pain settings.

Theoretically, prolonged use of opioids is known to result in antinociceptive tolerance, in which higher doses of the opioid are required to elicit the same amount of pain relief or antinociception.[278–280] Chu et al.[281] showed that patients receiving sustained-release morphine to an end titration dose of 78 mg morphine per day developed tolerance after 1 month with an average 42% reduction in analgesic potency. Long-term exposure to one drug often results in the development of tolerance to the effects of other structurally similar drugs in the same pharmacologic class, a phenomenon termed *cross-tolerance*. Opioids exhibit cross-tolerance, but it is rarely complete, as evidenced by opioid rotation particularly in the treatment of cancer pain.[282–286] Clinically, opioid rotation is challenging because of a lack of evidence-based medicine to support the dose conversions with switching regimens largely based on anecdote or on observational and uncontrolled studies.[287] In practice, physical dependence and tolerance does not prevent the effective use of these drugs in patients with cancer pain. The evidence for the development of tolerance to the analgesic effects of opioids with chronic administration in oncology is mixed. Many of the studies were in cancer patients with severe pain and showed that they maintained a stable opioid dose (for weeks to years) even with different routes of administration.[279,288] Patients with stable disease often remain on a stable dose for weeks or months.[289] Collin et al.[290] demonstrated a relationship between tumor progression and escalation of opioid doses over time such that the development of opioid tolerance from chronic opioid use was unlikely in cancer patients with pain.

MORPHINE

Morphine is the oldest opioid and is generally considered to be the gold standard. In a Cochrane review, Wiffen et al.[12] reported that morphine was an effective analgesic for cancer pain and that pain relief did not differ between extended (modified) release and IR preparations. Modified-release morphine was effective for 12- or 24-hour dosing depending on the formulation. Daily doses in studies ranged from 25 to 2,000 mg with an average of between 100 and 250 mg. A small number of patients did not achieve adequate analgesia with morphine and although adverse events were common, they were predictable with approximately 6% stopping treatment because of intolerable adverse events. The main disadvantage of morphine in cancer patients who require high opioid doses, or who have reduced renal clearance, is the accumulation of active (morphine-6-glucuronide) and toxic (morphine-3-glucuronide), which may complicate the clinical picture with excessive sedation or neurotoxic adverse effects.[291] Early signs of these effects should trigger consideration for switching to a different opioid.

OXYCODONE

Oxycodone may exert its analgesic effects through μ-opioid receptor and κ receptors.[292] Modified-release oxycodone (OxyContin) reaches T_{max} at approximately 4.6 hours with an apparent $t_{1/2}$ of 4.5 hours. OxyContin was reformulated in 2010 with inactive ingredients intended to make the tablet more difficult to manipulate for misuse and abuse and has an oral bioavailability of 60% to 87%. With reformulation, the immediate component (estimated up to 30% of the total dose) was eliminated. Unlike morphine, the drug is not glucuronidated but metabolized primarily by CYP3A4. Concomitant use of with a CYP3A4 inhibitor, such as macrolide antibiotics (e.g., erythromycin), azole-antifungal agents (e.g., ketoconazole), and protease inhibitors (e.g., ritonavir), may increase plasma concentrations of oxycodone. Use with serotonergic drugs may result in serotonin syndrome. Oxycodone is extensively metabolized by multiple metabolic pathways to produce noroxycodone, oxymorphone, and noroxymorphone. Oxymorphone is present in the plasma only at low concentrations. Cancer cachexia can increase the plasma exposure of oxycodone through the reduction of CYP3A metabolic pathway.[293] Oxycodone offers similar levels of pain relief and adverse events to other opioids including morphine for cancer-related pain.[11,294] Like any opioid, the benefits of recommending oxycodone as an alternative opioid for moderate to severe cancer pain are in choice and flexibility.[295] Choice includes cost, perceptions, social or cultural factors, and availability. Flexibility is having the ability to offer an alternative should another opioid prove ineffective or poorly tolerated.

OXYMORPHONE

Oxymorphone is a semisynthetic μ-opioid agonist that exhibits greater specificity for the μ-opioid receptor than for the δ- or κ-opioid receptors.[296,297] In 2006, the FDA-approved extended-release oxymorphone HCl for the control of moderate to severe chronic pain. The pharmacokinetic profile is predictable, linear, and dose-proportional.[298] The $t_{1/2}$ is 9 to 11 hours. The T_{max} varies from 3 to 6 hours.[299] The absolute oral bioavailability is approximately 10%. Oxymorphone undergoes minimal CYP450 metabolism, and is metabolized primarily by UGT2B7 (and potentially UGT1A3) to the inactive metabolite noroxymorphone. Consequently, oxymorphone ER, along with morphine and hydromorphone, lacks significant potential for CYP-mediated drug interactions and is unaffected by genetic factors influencing these enzymes. In contrast, other opioids including methadone, oxycodone, buprenorphine, and others metabolized by CYP enzymes have the potential for clinically important pharmacokinetic interactions with other drugs that share this metabolic pathway. Slatkin et al.[300] evaluated the effectiveness and tolerability over 52 weeks of oxymorphone ER in patients with cancer and noted that the drug was well tolerated and provided long-term stable pain control. Oxymorphone IR has a $t_{1/2}$ longer than that of morphine, hydromorphone, and oxycodone and a T_{max} of 30 minutes. Food does not affect the shape of concentration time curve.[297]

HYDROMORPHONE

Hydromorphone is a semisynthetic derivative of morphine. It primarily acts on μ receptors and to a lesser degree on δ receptors.[301] Hydromorphone binds more specifically to μ receptors than structurally related morphine. The IR form is absorbed in the upper small intestine and is extensively metabolized by the liver. Approximately 60% of the oral dose is eliminated by the liver on first pass, partly accounting for oral bioavailability in the range of 1:2 to 1:8.[302] For orally administered, IR preparations, the onset of action is approximately 30 minutes, T_{max} 0.75 hours and duration of action is approximately 4 hours. Hydromorphone is glucuronidated into hydromorphone-3-glucuronide, a metabolite that may have neuroexcitatory effects.[291,303] Hydromorphone-3-glucuronide follows a similar time course to hydromorphone in plasma. Of note there is an extended-release hydromorphone product (Exalgo). Hydromorphone in clinically relevant concentrations has minimal potential to inhibit CYP enzymes. After oral intake, plasma concentrations gradually increase over 6 to 8 hours, with a T_{max} ranging from 12 to 16 hours and concentrations are sustained for 18 to 24 hours. Mean $t_{1/2}$ is approximately 11 hours, and linear pharmacokinetics occur over a dose range from 8 to 64 mg. Steady state is reached 3 to 4 days after once-daily dosing. The safety and tolerability of Exalgo has been reported in opioid-tolerant patient with moderate to severe chronic cancer and noncancer pain.[304] The mean duration of exposure was 43.1 days (range 1 to 396 days), and mean daily dose was 43.4 mg. Patients demonstrated a safety and tolerability profile consistent with the known safety profiles of opioids. Bao et al.[305] reported that in oncology pain, hydromorphone provides similar pain relief to morphine and oxycodone and has similar side effects.

METHADONE

Methadone is a synthetic opioid and is a potent agonist at the μ- and δ-opioid receptors. In animal studies, it has antagonist activity at the N-methyl-D-aspartate (NMDA) receptor, resulting in interest in the clinical application of the drug in neuropathic pain syndromes.[306–309] In most countries, it is available as a racemic mixture of two isomers, levorotatory (L) methadone and dextrorotatory (D) methadone. Following oral administration, the drug is rapidly absorbed with measurable plasma levels between 15 and 45 minutes. The peak plasma levels after an oral dose occur at four hours and begin to decline 24 hours after dosing.[310] Oral bioavailability is over 85%. The primary route of elimination is oxidative biotransformation. It is N-demethylated to 2-ethylidene-1,5-dimethyl-3, 3-diphenylpyrrolidine (EDDP). The major enzyme involved in N-demethylation is CYP3A4 and CYP2B6. CYP2D6 genetic status affects steady-state blood concentrations. The $t_{1/2}$ ranges from 5 to 130 hours with a mean of 20 to 35 hours.[310] Concomitant administration of CYP3A4 inducers will increase methadone metabolism potentially causing a reduction in methadone plasma concentrations. This may result in the need for larger doses of methadone during the period of interaction. In addition, doses of methadone may need to be reduced when a CYP3A4 inducer is discontinued. Known inducers of CYP3A4 include rifampin, rifabutin, carbamazepine, phenytoin, phenobarbital, and abacavir. The commonly used dietary supplement for depression, St. John's Wort, has also been shown to lower the plasma concentrations of methadone.[311] CYP2B6 plays a significant role in the stereoselective metabolism of (S)-methadone to 2-ethyl-1,5-dimethyl-3,3-diphenylpyrrolidine, an inactive methadone metabolite. Elevated (S)-methadone can cause cardiotoxicity by prolonging the QT interval. One or more single nucleotide polymorphisms (SNPs) located within the CYP2B6 gene can contribute to a poor metabolizer phenotype with higher than predicted methadone levels and can be associated with fatalities.[312,313]

Methadone is implicated in the prolongation of the QTc interval, which is considered a marker for arrhythmias such as torsade de pointes (TdP). Indications on the association between methadone, even at therapeutic dosages, and TdP or sudden cardiac death are reported.[314,315] A QTc of 500 milliseconds is generally accepted as a threshold of increased danger for TdP.[316] Evidence implicating the relationship between methadone and TdP is limited, and the contributions of other known risk factors (including other medications, drugs, electrolyte abnormalities, structural heart disease, and others) are also implicated.[317] In a pediatric oncology patient population, methadone dosage, and duration (mean dose was 27.0 mg per day with range, 5 to 125 mg per day; mean duration of therapy was 49 days) were not correlated with QTc prolongation, even in the presence of other risk factors at clinically effective analgesic doses.[318] In a pilot study on adult oncology patients

treated with oral methadone (median dose 23 mg, range 3 to 90 mg) over an 8 week period, 28% of patients had evidence of QTc prolongation prior to initiation of methadone and only 1 patient demonstrated a QTc >500 milliseconds without evidence of a clinically significant arrhythmia.[319] Of note, conventional chemotherapy and targeted therapies are associated with an increased risk of cardiac damage, including LV dysfunction and heart failure, treatment-induced hypertension, vasospastic and thromboembolic ischemia, as well as rhythm disturbances, including conduction system damage and potentially QTc prolongation that may be rarely life-threatening.[320] In addition, the use of some medications used in supportive care during cancer therapy (e.g., antiemetics, antidepressants) in combination with cancer treatments can lead to QT prolongation.[321]

Methadone is a versatile and potentially useful analgesic for cancer pain control. It has no known active metabolites, and it is relatively inexpensive compared with other modified-release opioid formulations. Because of a highly variable $t_{1/2}$, the use of methadone is complicated with potential for accidental overdose if not titrated appropriately. Because steady state is not attained for 3 to 5 days, dose changes need to be slow and situations that require frequent dose changes (e.g., rapidly escalating tumor pain) are not ideal for methadone use. Prescribers should be experienced with the use of methadone in oncology, and patients need to be carefully counseled and cautioned to use methadone only as directed in order to prevent unintended dose accumulation. Based on very limited amounts of data, there were no clear differences in participant-reported pain intensity or pain relief between methadone and morphine or transdermal fentanyl.[322] In a relatively small number of patients (146 patients) with cancer-related pain, methadone was considered effective as a second-line alternative opioid for patients with a lack of efficacy or intolerance issues with their previous opioid.[323]

LEVORPHANOL

Levorphanol is considered a full μ-opioid agonist and is relatively selective for μ-opioid receptors although it also has multiple receptor activity including δ, $κ_1$, and $κ_3$, with NMDA receptor antagonism and reuptake inhibition of both norepinephrine and serotonin.[324] It is well absorbed after PO administration with peak plasma concentrations occurring approximately 1 hour after dosing. Levorphanol has a $t_{1/2}$ of 11 to 16 hours with a duration of analgesic effect between 6 and 15 hours.[325] Expected steady-state plasma concentrations for a 6-hour dosing interval can reach 2 to 5 times those following a single dose, depending on the patient's individual clearance of the drug. It has no known effect on QTc interval or drug–drug interactions involving CYP450 enzymes. It is metabolized to levorphanol-3-glucuronide which is inactive. From a relative potency perspective at steady state, 2 mg oral dose of levorphanol is approximately equivalent to 10 mg oral oxycodone. Dose conversion suggestions for levorphanol are listed in Table 43.12. Typical initial doses are 1 to 2 mg every 6 to 8 hours and are available as a 2-mg tablet. Information on the use of levorphanol in cancer pain is limited. McNulty[326] reported on its use in a case series of 31 patients, 20 with chronic

TABLE 43.12 Conversion Ratios to Levorphanol

Oral Morphine Equivalent	Morphine–Levorphanol Ratio
<100 mg	12:1
100–299 mg	15:1
300–599	20:1
600–799	25:1
>800 mg	No data

From McNulty JP. Can levorphanol be used like methadone for intractable refractory pain? *J Palliat Med* 2007;10(2):293–296. The publisher for this copyrighted material is Mary Ann Liebert, Inc. publishers.

nonmalignant pain in a palliative care clinic and 11 terminally ill patients enrolled in hospice care whose severe chronic pain was not relieved by treatment with other opioids, were treated with oral levorphanol. Of those 31 patients, 16 (52%) reported excellent relief of pain and 7 (22%) reported fair relief.

FENTANYL

Fentanyl is a synthetic full agonist at μ-opioid receptors and has a high lipophilicity allowing rapid transfer from the plasma to cerebrospinal fluid (CSF). Nonparenteral fentanyl products first became available in the last 1980s as a transdermal patch and then as a transmucosal product in 1993. Nonintravenous formulations deliver fentanyl by transmucosal, intranasal, or by transdermal routes. The main advantage of the patch was maintenance of a steady-state plasma concentration ideal for the treatment of background cancer pain. The main advantage of the transmucosal product was its associated rapid absorption is ideal for the management of breakthrough cancer pain. The pharmacokinetic and clinical parameters of nonparenteral fentanyl formulations are listed in Table 43.13.

Transdermal Fentanyl

Transdermal therapeutic system fentanyl (fentanyl-TTS) patches are rectangular transparent units each comprising a protective liner and four functional layers. These layers consist of a backing layer of polyester film, a drug reservoir of fentanyl and alcohol USP gelled with hydroxyethyl cellulose, an ethylene-vinyl acetate copolymer membrane that controls the rate of fentanyl delivery to the skin surface, and a fentanyl-containing silicone adhesive. The amount of fentanyl released from each system per hour is proportional to the surface area (25 μg per hour per 10 cm²). Each patch contains a proportional fentanyl content, for example, the 12 μg per hour patch has a total fentanyl content of 1.25 mg and the 25 μg per hour patch 2.5 mg fentanyl content. The Duragesic patch has a protective liner and four functional layers consisting of a backing layer of polyester film, a drug reservoir of fentanyl and alcohol USP gelled with hydroxyethyl cellulose, an ethylene-vinyl acetate copolymer membrane that controls the rate of fentanyl delivery to the

skin surface, and a fentanyl-containing silicone adhesive. The initial formulation consisted of a liquid fentanyl drug reservoir separated from the adhesive layer by a rate-limiting membrane, and ethanol as coabsorbent to provide controlled drug release. This formulation was problematic because of the high concentration of fentanyl present, which could be easily syphoned off.[327–330] Newer transdermal fentanyl formulations exclusively use the matrix technique, with the drug dissolved in an inert polymer matrix that diminishes the risk of incidental drug leakage and complicates the extraction of the drug for abuse.[331]

The transdermal system releases fentanyl from the reservoir at a nearly constant amount per unit time. The concentration gradient existing between the saturated solution of drug in the reservoir and the lower concentration in the skin drives drug release. Fentanyl moves in the direction of the lower concentration at a rate determined by the copolymer release membrane and the diffusion of fentanyl through the skin layers. A cutaneous depot of fentanyl forms in the upper layers of the skin, the stratum corneum, from where it passively diffuses to the dermis and ultimately removed by the cutaneous microcirculation. Although the actual rate of fentanyl delivery to the skin varies over the application period, each system is labeled with a nominal flux, which represents the average amount of drug delivered to the systemic circulation per hour across average skin. Although there is variation in dose delivered among patients, the nominal flux of the systems is sufficiently accurate to allow individual titration of dosage for a given patient. Following patch application, the skin under the system absorbs fentanyl, and a depot of fentanyl concentrates in the upper skin layers. Fentanyl then becomes available to the systemic circulation. There is a lag time of approximately 2 hours before plasma levels of fentanyl are detected with therapeutic levels after 12 to 16 hours postapplication.[332] T_{max} for the patch is approximately 34 hours (see Table 43.13). The system delivers fentanyl continuously for up to 72 hours with a bioavailability of approximately 92%. After sequential 48- or 72-hour applications, patients reach and maintain steady-state serum concentrations that are determined by individual variation in skin permeability and body clearance of fentanyl. A number of

| Parameter | Oral Transmucosal | | | | | Intranasal | Transdermal |
	Lozenge	SL Tablet	SL Spray	Buccal Tablet	Buccal Film	Nasal Spray	Sustained-Release Patch
Product and fentanyl dosages (μg)	Actiq (200, 400, 600, 800, 1,200, 1,600)	Abstral (100, 200, 300, 400, 600, 800)	Subsys (200, 400, 600, 800)	Fentora (100, 200, 400, 600, 800)	Onsolis (200, 400, 600, 800, 1,200, 1,600)	Lazanda (100, 400)	Duragesic (12.5, 25, 50, 75, 100 μg/h every 72 h)
Bioavailability (%)	50	~70	76	65	71	120, relative to Actiq	92
T_{max}	40 min	40 min	40 min	45 min	60 min	20 min	Constant from 14–24 h based on venous blood samples
$t_{1/2}$	7.6 h	11.5–25 h	5.25 (100 μg) 8.45 (200 μg) 11.03 (400 μg) 10.64 (600 μg) 11.99 (800 μg)	13.3 h	19.03 h	15–24.9 h	17 h after patch removal
Onset of pain relief	4.2 min (for both 200, 800 μg)	15 min for 400 μg	5 min	10 min	15 min	10 min	12–24 h
Duration of pain relief	145 min (200 μg) 215 min (800 μg)	60 min for 100–800 μg	At least 60 min	At least 60 min	At least 60 min	At least 60 min	Up to 12 h after patch removal

SL, sublingual; $t_{1/2}$, elimination half-life; T_{max}, time to maximal concentration.
Modified by permission from Springer: Lotsch J, Walter C, Parnham MJ, et al. Pharmacokinetics of non-intravenous formulations of fentanyl. *Clin Pharmacokinet* 2013;52(1):23–36.
Copyright © 2012 Springer International Publishing Switzerland.

studies demonstrate that constant serum levels are maintained with the second transdermal system and that fluctuations of serum levels are small after the first 72 hours.[333,334] After system removal, serum fentanyl concentrations decline gradually and has an apparent $t_{1/2}$ of 17 hours. Because of the possibility of temperature-dependent increases in fentanyl release from the system, it is important to advise patients to avoid exposing the application site to direct external heat sources, such as heating pads, heat lamps, and heated waterbeds. Prolonged exposure to heat or use in patients who are febrile can cause a toxic overdose.[335,336] Fentanyl is metabolized primarily via cytochrome P450 3A4 isoenzyme system. Concomitant use of CYP3A4 inhibitors may increase fentanyl plasma concentrations. Fentanyl undergoes rapid and extensive first-pass metabolism that accounts for its poor oral bioavailability (less than 30%) and the lack of oral products. The patch should not be used in patients who are not opioid-tolerant, for acute pain issues, for postoperative pain management and in the management of intermittent pain.

The transdermal patch is widely used in the treatment of both malignant and nonmalignant chronic pain. Clinically, cachectic cancer patients may require higher transdermal doses for adequate pain relief than normal weight or obese patients. Heiskanen et al.[337] studied the pharmacokinetic profile in 10 cachectic (mean body mass index [BMI] 16 kg/m²) and noted that plasma fentanyl concentrations adjusted to dose were significantly lower at 48 and 72 hours in cachectic patients than normal weight patients suggesting that the absorption was impaired in cachectic patients. The cachectic patients had a significantly thinner upper arm skin fold, but no differences were found in local blood flow, sweating, or skin temperature. Hypoalbuminemia (albumin <3.5 g/dL) is also associated with poor absorption from fentanyl-TTS.[338] Although fentanyl-TTS is widely used in palliative care settings, there are relatively few studies in its use in cancer pain making judgment on efficacy difficult.[339] Rash and pruritus, commonly a concern with transdermal preparations, were infrequent and improved with time. A number of studies compared the impact of constipation between fentanyl-TTS and slow-release morphine.[340–342] Fewer study participants experienced constipation with fentanyl (28%) than with oral morphine (46%). Tassinari et al.[343] assessed the role of transdermal fentanyl as a first-line approach for moderate to severe cancer pain bases on the GRADE approach and concluded that the risk/benefit ratio was uncertain and that the quality of evidence was low. Finally, there is insufficient evidence to support or refute the suggestion that fentanyl has any efficacy in any neuropathic pain condition.[244] In the absence of any supporting evidence, it should probably not be recommended, except at the discretion of a pain specialist with particular expertise in opioid use.

Oral Transmucosal/Intranasal/Sublingual Fentanyl

IR fentanyl is available in oral transmucosal and intranasal preparations (see Table 43.13). The oral products include lozenge (Actiq), sublingual tablet (Abstral), sublingual spray (Subsys), buccal tablet (Fentora), and buccal film (Onsolis). The intranasal product is a metered nasal spray (Lazanda). The first IR fentanyl was the lozenge. Compared to IR morphine, this drug with its rapid onset of action (5 minutes) and relatively short duration of effect was significantly better in treating breakthrough cancer pain.[344] There are no head-to-head trials comparing any of the newer transmucosal formulations with each other.[345] Oral and nasal transmucosal fentanyl formulations were an effective treatment for breakthrough pain. When compared with placebo or oral morphine, study participants reported lower pain intensity and higher pain relief scores for transmucosal fentanyl formulations at all time points. Global assessment scores also favored transmucosal fentanyl preparations.[253]

In 2011, the FDA approved a single shared-system risk evaluation and mitigation strategy (REMS) for the entire class of transmucosal immediate-release fentanyl (TIRF) medications. TIRF medicines include Abstral (fentanyl) sublingual tablet, Actiq (fentanyl citrate) oral transmucosal lozenge and its generic equivalents, Fentora (fentanyl citrate) buccal tablet, Lazanda (fentanyl) nasal spray, and Onsolis (fentanyl) buccal soluble film. The TIRF REMS program required prescribers, pharmacies, distributors, and outpatients to enroll in order to prescribe, dispense, or receive all drugs in the category. In outpatient settings, all health care providers must complete and sign a TIRF REMS Access Patient-Prescriber Agreement Form with each new patient before writing the patient's first TIRF prescription. Health care providers must also provide patients with a copy of the Medication Guide during counseling about the proper use of their TIRF medicine. Health care providers who prescribe TIRF medicines for inpatient use only (e.g., hospitals, hospices, or long-term care facilities) are not required to enroll in the TIRF REMS Access program. TIRF medications are approved only to manage breakthrough pain in adults with cancer who are routinely taking and are tolerant to other opioid pain medicines ATC for pain. Opioid tolerance is the use of an opioid for one week or longer in doses equivalent to 60 mg oral morphine per day or an equianalgesic dose of another oral opioid. TIRF medications are contraindicated in the management of acute or postoperative pain, including headache/migraine and dental pain. Of note, TIRF medications are not interchangeable with each other nor equivalent to any other fentanyl product including another TIRF medication on an μg-per-μg basis. The only exception is the substitution of a generic equivalent for a branded TIRF medication. Dose conversions with initial dosing and titration schedules are listed in Table 43.14.

Fentanyl-Associated Deaths

Drug overdose is an important, yet an inadequately understood, public health problem with substantial increase in incidence and prevalence in several countries worldwide over the past decade, contributing to both increased costs and mortality.[346] The increase of fentanyl abuse (both legally and illegally produced) is a growing public health problem with multiple states reporting increases in fentanyl-involved overdose deaths.[16] One hundred and twelve fentanyl-related deaths were identified in Canada between 2002 and 2004.[347] Routes of administration included transdermal application of patches, intravenous injection of patch contents or fentanyl citrate solution, oral/transmucosal administration, and volatilization and inhalation of Duragesic systems. The high potency and narrow therapeutic range of fentanyl compounds and patches available may explain the potential of fentanyl abuse and associated deaths.[348] In the United States, between 2013 and 2014, the age-adjusted rate of deaths involving synthetic opioids increased by 80%[14] and by 250% among younger people.[349] Several fentanyl derivatives (initially sufentanil, alfentanil, remifentanil, carfentanil, and, more recently, acetylfentanyl, 6-butyrfentanyl, 4-MeO-butyrfentanyl, isobutyrylfentanyl, furanylfentanyl, α-methylfentanyl, 3-methylfentanyl or TMF, p-methylfentanyl, methylacetylfentanyl, acrylfentanyl, 2-fluorofentanyl, fluoroacetylfentanyl, ocfentanyl, and many others) are illegally manufactured.[350] The catastrophic emergence of potent fentanyl analogs mixed with street heroin is a major public safety concern. Concerns about legally prescribed fentanyl have also been expressed for some time. In July 2005, FDA issued a *Public Health Advisory* and *Information for Healthcare Professionals* that emphasized the appropriate and safe use of the fentanyl transdermal system (fentanyl patch), marketed as Duragesic and generics.[351] Despite these efforts, FDA has continued to receive reports of death and life-threatening adverse events related to fentanyl overdose that have occurred when the fentanyl patch was used

TABLE 43.14 Dose Conversions for Transmucosal Immediate-Release Fentanyl Medications

Drug	Initial Dose	Max Dose per Treatment Event	Frequency	Titration
Actiq	200 μg	Repeat same dose after 30 min if BTP not adequately relieved. Max doses per event = 2.	Wait >4 h for additional treatment.	Follow over time and plan dose with single unit.
Abstral	100 μg (unless being converted from Actiq ≥400 μg)	Repeat same dose after 30 min if BTP not adequately relieved. Max doses per event = 2.	Wait >2 h for additional treatment.	May use multiples of 100 μg tabs and/or 200 μg tabs for any single dose; no more than 4 tabs at one time
Fentora	100 μg (unless being converted from Actiq ≥600 μg)	Repeat same dose after 30 min if BTP not adequately relieved. Max doses per event = 2.	Wait >4 h for additional treatment.	Follow over time and plan dose with single unit. May use multiple tablets (one on each side of mouth in upper/lower buccal cavity) until maintenance dose achieved
Lazanda	100 μg	Only 1 dose per episode	Wait >2 h for additional treatment.	Follow over time and plan dose with single unit. Patients should confirm dose that is adequate with second episode of BTP
Onsolis	200 μg	Single episode treatment only; no redosing	Wait >2 h for additional treatment	Titrate with 200 μg increments. No more than 4 films at once. If inadequate pain relief after 800 μg (×4 200 μg films) and patient tolerates 800 μg dose, next episode may be treated with 1,200 μg.
Subsys	100 μg (unless being converted from Actiq ≥600 μg)	Repeat same dose after 30 min if BTP not adequately relieved. Max doses per event = 2.	Wait >4 h for additional treatment.	Follow over time and plan dose with single unit.

BTP, breakthrough pain.

to treat pain in opioid-naive patients and when opioid-tolerant patients have applied more patches than prescribed, changed the patch too frequently, and exposed the patch to a heat source. There is also a variety of methods associated with intentional abuse of fentanyl patches including attempts to extract the drug from the patch and inject intravenously, chewing or swallowing patches, inserting patches into the rectum, and inhaling fentanyl gel.[330,352–355] Aberrant behaviors have been associated with the use of transmucosal fentanyl in chronic pain patients.[356] Concerns about abuse and death have also been expressed with transmucosal fentanyl even among cancer patients with active disease.[357,358]

BUPRENORPHINE

Buprenorphine is a semisynthetic derivative of thebaine. It is available in the United States for the treatment of addiction and for the treatment of chronic pain. It is a potent partial agonist of the μ-opioid receptor with high affinity but low intrinsic activity. The slow dissociation ($t_{1/2}$ association/dissociation is 2 to 5 hours) accounts for its prolonged therapeutic effect. It is metabolized in the liver through CYP3A4 N-dealkylation. The relative bioavailability of the sublingual tablet is 29% with a $t_{1/2}$ of 20 to 73 hours. The transdermal buprenorphine product Butrans is available in strength of 5, 7.5, 10, 15, and 20 μg per hour delivering 7-day dosing and is indicated for pain severe enough to require daily, ATC opioid therapy. The 10 μg per hour patch corresponds to approximately 30 to 80 mg per day of oral morphine equivalents. The maximum recommended dose is 20 μg per hour. The median time for the 10 μg per hour patch to deliver quantifiable buprenorphine concentrations (≥25 pg/mL) was approximately 17 hours. After removal of the patch, mean buprenorphine concentrations decrease approximately 50% within 10 to 24 hours, followed by decline with an apparent terminal $t_{1/2}$ of approximately 26 hours. Sublingual formulations of buprenorphine are available in the United States market as monotherapy (generic tablet) and a combination therapy of buprenorphine with naloxone (Suboxone, Zubsolv as a tablet or film) for opioid addiction. One Zubsolv 5.7 mg/1.4 mg sublingual tablet provides equivalent buprenorphine exposure to one Suboxone 8 mg/2 mg sublingual tablet.

Buprenorphine should not be used for acute pain management, for example, when there is a need for rapid dose titration

for severe pain in cancer and palliative care settings. One potential issue is that because of the high affinity for μ-opioid receptors with a slow dissociation profile, buprenorphine may potentially displace or prevent the binding of competing μ-opioid receptor agonists, including IR opioids, in a dose-dependent manner. This may be less of an issue with the relatively lower doses of transdermal buprenorphine used in the United States.[359,360] There is insufficient evidence to make buprenorphine a valid first-line choice for the management of cancer-related pain with no clear dose-response relationship for transdermal buprenorphine.[361,362]

HYDROCODONE

Hydrocodone is a prodrug opioid, and the parent compound is a full μ-opioid receptor agonist and can interact with other opioid receptors at higher doses. It is metabolized into its active moiety, hydromorphone, by CYP2D6 and also by CYP3A to the inactive metabolite, norhydrocodone, although the extent of CYP3A metabolism of hydrocodone is unclear.

In 2013, the FDA approved the use of extended-release hydrocodone (Zohydro ER). Hydrocodone ER is a hard gelatin capsule. Measurable drug levels are obtained within 30 minutes after oral intake. The T_{max} is between 6 and 8 hours, and mean $t_{1/2}$ was 4.9 and 6.5 hours.[363] IR hydrocodone exists in various combinations with acetaminophen or ibuprofen. The most common forms of hydrocodone-acetaminophen preparations are 5/325 mg, 7.5/325 mg, and 10/325 mg. The common hydrocodone-ibuprofen preparations are 2.5/200 mg, 5/200 mg, 7.5/200 mg, and 10/200 mg. In oncology patients, hydrocodone at higher doses (≥40 mg per day) is equipotent to morphine and at lower doses (<40 mg per day) may be twice as potent as morphine and just as potent as oxycodone.[364] There are relatively few studies on the use of hydrocodone for cancer pain. Hydrocodone/acetaminophen at starting doses of 25 mg/2,500 mg per day was not more effective than tramadol 200 mg per day on patients with chronic cancer pain.[365]

CODEINE

Codeine is a synthetic opiate alkaloid. It is considered a prodrug that lacks intrinsic antinociceptive activity and must be metabolically converted to active forms. Eighty percent of codeine is conjugated with glucuronic acid to codeine-6-glucuronide with only 5% O-demethylated by CYP2D6 to morphine suggesting that the majority of its analgesic effect is from codeine-6-glucuronide.[366,367]

The value of codeine is limited in cancer pain management by the increasing incidence of side effects at doses above 1.5 mg per kilogram of body weight.[62,368] Codeine is rapidly absorbed from the GI tract reaching a peak level within 1 hour with a clinical duration of 4 to 6 hours.[369] The available evidence (which is of low quality) indicates that codeine is more effective against cancer pain than placebo but with increased risk of nausea, vomiting, and constipation.[370] The principal adverse effect associated with chronic dosing is constipation.

Dihydrocodeine is an equianalgesic semisynthetic analogue of codeine. It is used as an analgesic, antitussive, and antidiarrheal agent. The analgesic effect is probably twice as potent as that of codeine for the parenteral and slightly stronger for an oral route.[371] Dihydrocodeine has active metabolites (dihydromorphine and dihydromorphine-6-glucuronide).[372] The most common side effect that occurs in patients treated with dihydrocodeine is constipation.[373] Duration of effect is approximately 6 hours. In the United States, it is available only in combination with acetaminophen, caffeine, or aspirin.

TRAMADOL

Tramadol is a centrally acting analgesic with a μ-opioid receptor activity and also has weak effects on serotonin and norepinephrine reuptake inhibition. Opioid activity of tramadol is due to both low affinity binding of the parent compound and higher affinity binding of the O-desmethyl tramadol metabolite (M1) to μ-opioid receptors. The analgesic activity is due to both parent drug and the M1 metabolite. Oral formulations include those designed for immediate release and for modified release. Side effects associated with tramadol include typical opioid adverse events of nausea, dizziness, and dry mouth, although vomiting and constipation are considered to be less of a problem than with traditional opioids. Tramadol may also cause orthostatic hypotension. Use of tramadol with concurrent serotonergic therapy poses a risk of serotonin syndrome.[374] Seizures can occur with the recommended dosage range, and the risk is increased with concomitant use of SSRIs and tricyclic antidepressants. The daily maximum recommended dose of tramadol IR is 400 mg and 300 mg per day for tramadol ER. Tramadol ER should not be used concomitantly with other tramadol products. The IR preparation has a bioavailability of 75%, T_{max} 2.3 hours, and $t_{1/2}$ of 7 hours. The bioavailability of tramadol ER 200 mg tablet administered once daily relative to a 50 mg IR tramadol hydrochloride administered every 6 hours is approximately 85% to 90%. T_{max} of tramadol ER and M1 is 12 hours and 15 hours, respectively. Steady state is achieved within 4 days of once-daily dosing. The mean terminal plasma elimination half-lives of racemic tramadol and racemic M1 after administration of extended-release tablets are approximately 7.9 and 8.8 hours, respectively. The metabolic pathways are N-demethylation (mediated by CYP3A4 and CYP2D6), O-demethylation (mediated by CYP2D6), and glucuronidation or sulfation in the liver. Concomitant administration of CYP2D6 and/or CYP3A4 inhibitors may reduce metabolic clearance of tramadol increasing the risk for serious adverse events including seizures and serotonin syndrome.

Although advocated for the management of neuropathic pain,[193,375] the information supporting use is modest from small largely inadequate studies with potential for risk bias.[376] Overall, patients with cancer who are most likely to benefit from tramadol appear to be those with mild to moderate pain not relieved by acetaminophen, who cannot tolerate NSAIDs, and wish to avoid taking opioids that are more potent.

TAPENTADOL

Tapentadol is a centrally acting opioid agonist. The exact mechanism of action is unknown, but it has both μ-opioid receptor activity and is a norepinephrine reuptake inhibitor. It is available in both immediate- and extended-release formulations.

FDA-approved indications are for pain severe enough to require daily ATC opioid use and also pain diabetic peripheral neuropathy. The T_{max} for tapentadol IR is approximately 1.25 hours with a $t_{1/2}$ of 4 hours. It is available in both tablet form and solution. The mean absolute bioavailability after single-dose administration of Nucynta ER is approximately 32% due to extensive first-pass metabolism with a T_{max} between 3 and 6 hours. Steady-state exposure of tapentadol is achieved after the third dose (i.e., 24 hours after first twice-daily multiple-dose administration). The oral equivalent dose of tapentadol to morphine is approximately 2.5:1.[377,378] The major pathway of tapentadol metabolism is conjugation with glucuronic acid to produce glucuronides. Drug metabolism mediated by CYP450 system is of less importance than phase 2 conjugation. Initial dosing for patients who are not opioid-tolerant is 50 mg bid. Doses greater than 600 mg daily are not recommended. In a small study of 22 patients with CIPN-associated pain, patients initially were treated with tapentadol 50 mg bid and then titrated as tolerated over a 3-month period.[379] Nineteen patients showed a response to treatment (30% reduction in pain intensity) with 15 patients showing a 50% reduction in pain intensity over the study period, but 7 patients stopped therapy during the first week because of side effects (drowsiness, nausea, dizziness, dry mouth). In a Cochrane review of four studies with 1,029 patients with chronic tumor-related pain with twice-daily dosing varying from 50 mg to 500 mg, effects were comparable to those of equivalent doses of morphine or oxycodone.[380] The most common events were GI including nausea, vomiting, or constipation, and there was no advantage of tapentadol over morphine or oxycodone in terms of serious adverse events.

OPIOIDS NOT RECOMMENDED FOR ROUTINE USE IN CANCER PAIN CONTROL

There are several opioids that should be avoided in cancer pain management, including meperidine, pentazocine, butorphanol, dezocine, and nalbuphine. Meperidine has a short $t_{1/2}$, and its metabolite, normeperidine, is toxic.[381] Mixed agonist-antagonists such as pentazocine, butorphanol, dezocine, and nalbuphine present other problems. Although these agonist-antagonists are often classified as a κ receptor agonist and a μ-receptor antagonist, they are more accurately described as a partial agonist at both κ and μ receptors. These agents have a low maximal efficacy and have the potential to reverse μ-receptor analgesia and even precipitate a physical withdrawal syndrome when taken by patients already receiving full agonists such as morphine.[382] In addition, agonist-antagonist opioids have a ceiling effect.[382,383]

OPIOID-RELATED SIDE EFFECTS
Prevention or Minimizing Opioid-Related Side Effects

Appropriate dosing of opioids requires minimizing or preventing opioid-related side effects. For patients with constant pain, the early use of a long-acting opioid in preference to short-acting opioids as soon as dose titration permits may help attenuate side effects. If side effects are significant, the clinician should allow time for tolerance to develop. This may require a period of 3 to 7 days. Minimizing severe side effects during this period is appropriate. For example, a patient with nausea could benefit from a 1-week course of antiemetic medication at the outset of opioid therapy.

If side effects do not diminish satisfactorily over time, there are two alternatives: changing drugs and introducing supplementary medications that control the side effects. Changing from one opioid to another may enhance pain relief and reduce opioid-related side effects, particularly if incomplete cross-tolerance to opioid effect is experienced.[384–386] In some cases, changing the route of administration for a particular drug may eliminate certain difficult side effects. It is possible to alleviate many of the most difficult

TABLE 43.15 Pharmacologic Treatments for Opioid-Related Side Effects

Side Effect	Treatment
Constipation	Stool softener, laxative, PAMORA, ? opioid rotation
Sedation	Methylphenidate, modafinil
Pruritus	Diphenhydramine, hydroxyzine
Nausea	Prochlorperazine, haloperidol, metoclopramide, ondansetron, antihistamine, olanzapine
Dysphoria	Haloperidol, opioid rotation
Hypnogogic imagery	Haloperidol
Cognitive impairment	Methylphenidate, modafinil, opioid rotation
Respiratory depression	Naloxone
Myoclonus	Clonazepam, dose reduction, opioid rotation

PAMORA, peripherally acting μ-opioid receptor antagonist.

side effects pharmacologically when necessary. For example, prudent administration of methylphenidate to the cancer patient can help protect the cognitive functioning of patients using high doses of opioids.[387] Table 43.15 lists opioid-related side effects and their treatments. In cancer patients, certain pathophysiologic conditions commonly contribute to side effect problems or masquerade as side effect problems. For example, renal insufficiency in patients using morphine can lead to accumulation of morphine-6-glucuronide, which in turn can exacerbate side effects. Nausea is a frequent opioid toxicity, but it has other potential causes: gastric irritation, constipation or other changes in gut motility, chemotherapy, or hypercalcemia induced by bone metastases. Similarly, opioid-induced changes in mental status become less probable when the patient has been on a stable dose without recent significant dose escalation.

Opioid-induced bowel dysfunction is addressed earlier.

OPIOID EFFECTS ON COGNITION, MOTOR SKILLS, AND DRIVING ABILITY

Patients with advanced cancer may develop a wide range of symptoms, including cognitive dysfunction, which interfere with their daily life, compliance to treatment, social interactions, and quality of life. Causes for development of cognitive alterations are multiple and may be attributed to the cancer disease itself, comorbidities, and treatments including opioid therapy.[388] The spectrum of cognitive dysfunction attributed to opioid use can vary from subtle evidence of cognitive impairment, largely related to initial dosing or dose increases to delirium.[389] Opioids can interfere with acquirement, processing, storage, retrieval of information, altering cognitive processes associated with memory, psychomotor function, mood, concentration, and other mental capabilities.[390] Patients receiving daily opioid doses of 400 mg or more (oral morphine equivalents) had 1.75 (95% confidence interval [CI], 1.25 to 2.46) times higher odds of having lower Mini-Mental State Examination (MMSE) scores compared with those receiving daily doses less than 80 mg.[391] In addition, patient with lung cancer, older age, lower performance status, time since diagnosis (<15 months), and absence of breakthrough pain were more at risk of developing opioid-induced cognitive dysfunction. Opioids may cause measurable cognitive impairment, even at low doses (especially during initial or occasional use), and equianalgesic doses of different opioids may have nonequivalent adverse cognitive effects.[392] Although sedation and confusion may accompany opioid use, other potential causes in the cancer patient such as raised intracranial pressure, metabolic disturbances (e.g., hypercalcemia), sepsis, or concomitant psychoactive medication can merit consideration and should be excluded. Cognitive dysfunction can be associated with opioid dose increases and use of supplemental doses of short-acting opioids. However, the use of benzodiazepines has substantial more effects on cognitive and psychomotor function compared to opioid use.[393,394] In cancer survivorship, the evidence is mixed regarding long-term cog-

nitive deficits associated with the use of chemotherapy. Studies in patients with breast cancer previously treated with chemotherapy suggest observed cognitive deficits are small in magnitude and limited to the domains of verbal ability and visuospatial ability.[395] The presence of chronic pain can also be a factor in cognitive dysfunction. Basic neurocognitive function is impaired in a substantial portion of patients with persistent severe pain.[396] Use of psychostimulants (e.g., methylphenidate, modafinil) has been reported to be helpful in overcoming daytime drowsiness and mental clouding, but their use must be monitored carefully, both for adverse effects and overuse.[397] Modafinil in a single-dose regimen was beneficial for improving psychomotor speed and attention and for improving subjective scores of depression and drowsiness in patients with advanced cancer.[398]

An additional major concern that has arisen from long-term opioid therapy is the effect of long-term opioid use on motor skills such as driving.[399,400] Driving is considered an important activity affecting quality of life for many patients. Often, both prescribing clinicians and patients are unaware of the legal risk associated with driving and the use of legally prescribed opioids. Driving under the influence of drugs other than alcohol (DUID) is of concern to the medical and legal communities. "Under the influence" typically describes a level of impairment that interferes with driving abilities and is therefore considered criminal; however, this level of impairment is interpreted differently among various states.[401] Of the prescribed psychoactive medications, benzodiazepine use is associated with a significant increase in the risk of traffic accidents with the association being more pronounced in the younger driver. The motor vehicle accident risk is markedly increased with the coingestion of alcohol.[402,403] The prevalence of prescription opioids detected in fatally injured drivers has increased in the past two decades but of the drivers testing positive for prescription opioids, 30% had elevated blood alcohol concentrations (≥0.01 g/dL), and 66.9% tested positive for other drugs.[404] Results have been inconsistent regarding decrements in cognitive performance. Patients with chronic pain who have been using opioids for more than 3 days exhibit relatively few differences when cognitive performance is compared with performance before taking opioids or with that of a comparable patient population not taking opioids.[405] The majority of research has revealed that the greatest potential impairment in cognitive function from opioids occurs during the first several days of use. During longer periods, impairment has been demonstrated primarily in studies that have compared patients with significant pain with healthy volunteers. Twenty chronic pain patients using long-term stable doses of opioids, and 19 healthy controls were studied using standardized on-the-road driving tests in normal traffic.[406] Performance of controls with a blood alcohol concentration of 0.5 g/L was used as a reference to define clinically relevant changes in driving performance. Driving performance of the chronic pain patients did not significantly differ from that of controls suggesting that in clinical practice determination of fitness to drive in patients who receive opioids should be based on an individual assessment. Gomes et al.[407] found among drivers prescribed opioids that a significant relationship existed between opioid dose and risk of road trauma. Compared with patients prescribed very low opioid doses (MED <20 mg), those prescribed low (20 to 49 mg MED) and moderate (50 to 99 mg MED) doses had a 21% and 29% increased odds of road trauma, and patients prescribed high (100 to 199 mg MED) and very high (≥200 mg MED) doses of opioids had a 42% and 23% increased odds of road trauma, respectively, when compared with patients prescribed very low doses. The effects of opioid use specifically on driving ability has become a contentious issue, predictably because a growing number of patients are taking opioids and driving, and also because insurers may seek to assign liability in cases of motor vehicle accidents involving drivers who use opioids. Vainio et al.[408] examined the effects of continuous morphine medication on the

TABLE 43.16   Driving Instructions for Patients Taking Opioids

Opioid medications can cause side effects that impair your ability to drive. Driving while taking opioid medication is controversial. The final decision on whether you should drive while taking them is a legal issue and should be addressed with your automobile insurance carrier. Out of concern for your safety and the safety of others, please observe the following guidelines:

- Do not drive for 4–5 d after beginning opioid treatment or following a dose increase.
- Never drive if you feel sedated or if you feel your thinking is impaired. Take any concerns that others express regarding your ability to drive safely seriously.
- Report sedation, unsteadiness, or unclear thinking to our office as soon as possible.
- Please remember that the use of alcohol or other drugs such as cannabis ("marijuana") can increase the effects of opioid medications.
- Avoid taking over-the-counter medications that may cause drowsiness such as cold and allergy medications.

Nurse: _____ Date: _____

I have reviewed these follow-up instructions and understand and accept them before starting the procedure.

Patient/Guardian Signature: _____ Date: _____

TABLE 43.17   Reasons for Undertaking Opioid Rotations

1. Reduced ability to control pain due to:
   a. Worsening of existing pain or underlying disease process
   b. Pharmacodynamic factors
      Development of opioid analgesic tolerance
   c. Pharmacokinetic factors
      Drug absorption (inability to swallow oral medications/poor vascular status or edema limiting transdermal delivery)
      Interaction with other drugs
      Changes in protein binding
      Biotransformation and metabolism (accumulation of metabolites)
      Reduced clearance—renal failure
2. Development of intolerable side effects/opioid toxicity
   a. Gastrointestinal (i.e., constipation, nausea, vomiting)
   b. CNS (i.e., sedation, somnolence, dysphoria, hallucinations, myoclonus)
   c. Cardiovascular (i.e., orthostatic hypotension due to histamine release)
3. Practical concerns
   a. Dose required to produce analgesia exceeds maximum daily dose (patients taking combination products, e.g., acetaminophen)
   b. Cost of drugs
   c. Drug availability
   d. Need for large doses of drug to be delivered
   e. Changes in route of administration

CNS, central nervous system.

driving ability of cancer patients. They conducted psychological and neurologic tests, originally designed for professional motor vehicle drivers, in two groups of cancer patients who were similar apart from their experience of pain. Twenty-four patients received continuous morphine (mean 209-mg oral morphine daily) for cancer pain, and 25 were pain-free without regular analgesics. Although the results were a little worse in the patients taking morphine, there were no significant differences between the groups in intelligence, vigilance, concentration, fluency of motor reactions, or division of attention. Of the neural function tests, reaction times (auditory, visual, associative), thermal discrimination, and body sway with eyes open were similar in the two groups; only balancing ability with closed eyes was worse in the morphine group. These results indicate that in cancer patients receiving long-term morphine treatment with stable doses, morphine has only a slight and selective effect on functions related to driving. Galski et al.[409] published a structured, evidence-based review on the issue of opioids and driving. Overall, the majority of studies in the evidence-based review appeared to indicate that patients who use opioids are not impaired by the opioids with regard to driving ability. Byas-Smith et al. reported that many patients with chronic pain, even if treated with potent analgesics such as morphine and hydromorphone at equivalent average daily morphine doses of 118 mg, showed comparable driving ability as normal subjects.[409]

Clearly, opioids may affect cognitive function and impair driving ability in patients who are opioid-naive or in patients who are not on stable opioid regimens. Whether some degree of "cognitive tolerance" develops with chronic opioid use is unknown. Other unresolved questions include the effects of different types of opioids, dose effects, and interactions with other medications on driving ability. Each of these areas deserves further study, and clinicians need to counsel patients about potentially dangerous activities on a case-by-case basis. Guidelines are provided regarding opioid medications and driving (Table 43.16).

OPIOID ROTATION IN CANCER PAIN

Opioid rotation refers to the practice of converting from one opioid to a second when the opioid analgesic response is inadequate and/or if opioid-related adverse events are intolerable or unmanageable.[410,411] Reasons for initiating opioid rotation are listed in Table 43.17. In cancer patients, the most common

reasons for opioid rotation are intolerable side effects such as, cognitive failure, hallucinations, myoclonus, nausea, and uncontrollable pain.[282,283,412] In all cases of opioid rotation, patients must be followed closely to assess the adequacy of pain relief and the effect on opioid-related adverse events. As with any opioid regimen, subsequent dose adjustments will probably be necessary. Use of opioid rotation requires familiarity with a range of opioids and with the use of equianalgesic dose tables (see Chapter 79). However, it is also important to consider that the evidence to support dose ratios in standard equianalgesic tables refers largely to the context of single-dose administration; they do not necessarily reflect the clinical realities of chronic opioid administration in the treatment of cancer pain with repeated dosing of opioids at steady state. Thus, the doses listed in most standard equianalgesic dose tables may not be accurate in patients who have developed tolerance or have been taking opioids for long periods of time. In addition, the phenomenon of incomplete cross-tolerance can lead to unexpected potency in the newly introduced agent.[262,384,385,413]

Special care is required with methadone rotations. The process of switching from a high-dose opioid agonist to methadone is complex and should and should only be attempted by experienced physicians.[414–416] Even among experienced physicians, serious toxicity can occur during the administration of methadone.[417,418] Various studies provide guidelines for opioid dose conversions in cancer pain.[284,386,419–422]

PARENTERAL OPIOID THERAPY

Parenteral routes (subcutaneous or intravenous) should be considered for patients who require rapid onset of analgesia and for highly tolerant patients who require doses that cannot otherwise be conveniently administered.[423] Intravenous opioids allow for rapid control of pain. Ideally, patients with severe, uncontrolled pain who require intravenous therapy should start treatment in a monitored in-patient setting. High doses of intravenous opioids via patient-controlled analgesia (PCA) and/or by continuous infusion offers a means of rapidly controlling increasing severe pain. Intravenous therapy can employ any of several opioids: morphine, hydromorphone, fentanyl, and, less commonly, methadone. A brief hospitalization for stabilization of the intravenous regimen is preferable.

Continuous subcutaneous infusion of opioids is both an efficacious and safe method to control the chronic pain of the homebound and hospitalized patient.[424,425] Administration of opioids by continuous infusion via intravenous or subcutaneous routes have equal effects in similar doses.[426] In a pilot study in cancer patients comparing the efficacy of hydromorphone administered subcutaneously by continuous infusion only versus basal rate infusion with PCA, both methods provided adequate overall pain control in most patients, but a large interindividual variation was noted with some patients reporting marked discomfort during hydromorphone administration by PCA and few patients preferring the PCA modality.[427] Stuart-Harris et al.[428] studied the pharmacokinetics of 5 mg of morphine (and its metabolites) given intravenously, by subcutaneous bolus, and by subcutaneous infusion over 4 hours. After a single intravenous bolus, plasma morphine was typically detected up to 6 hours with a maximal concentration (C_{max}) of 283 ± 74 nmol/L with a T_{max} of 0.08 hour. After subcutaneous bolusing, plasma morphine was typically detected up to 8 hours, the C_{max} was similar to intravenous bolus, but the T_{max} was significantly longer (0.25 vs. 0.08 hour). Morphine administered by subcutaneous infusion was first detected in all subjects after 2 hours and was still detectable at 12 hours in some subjects at end of sampling. The median T_{max} was longer at 4 hours, and C_{max} was lower at 46 ± 8 nmol/L. The authors concluded that although intravenous and subcutaneous bolusing is bioequivalent with regard to their pharmacodynamic effects, it was likely that circulating morphine concentrations would have been higher immediately after the intravenous bolus was completed than at the first sampling point at 0.08 hour, and these early high concentrations may influence penetration into the brain. In contrast, the bioavailability of morphine was less after subcutaneous infusion versus bolusing by either method. Moulin et al.[429] noted that mean bioavailability from subcutaneous infusion of hydromorphone was 78% of that with intravenous infusion. This in combination with its solubility and the availability of a high-concentration preparation (10 mg/mL) makes hydromorphone a good choice for subcutaneous infusion. Parenteral hydromorphone is six times as soluble in aqueous solutions as morphine and five times as potent, allowing for smaller injection or infusion volumes in patients who require parenteral opioids.[430] Moulin et al.[429] compared the safety and efficacy of subcutaneous versus intravenous infusion of hydromorphone in cancer patients. Pain intensity, pain relief, mood, and sedation did not differ between the two techniques. Paix et al.[431] described the successful substitution of subcutaneous fentanyl and sufentanil for morphine, noting the benefits of sufentanil when the patient needs a very high dose of opioid that can be infused in a relatively small volume. Nelson et al.[426] compared continuous intravenous and subcutaneous morphine for chronic cancer pain and concluded that both routes were equianalgesic for most patients when administered as a continuous infusion.

Most patients will require a weekly change of the site of subcutaneous infusion.[424] The usual initial concentrations of morphine and hydromorphone are 5 mg/mL and 1 mg/mL, respectively, calculated according to the hourly infusion rate. Ideally, the subcutaneous rate should not exceed 2 mL per hour, although some have established considerably higher rates (rates of 20 to 80 mL per hour by adding hyaluronidase to the infusion to promote hypodermoclysis).[432] Due to a longer time to peak plasma levels after bolus injection with subcutaneous use than with intravenous use, the subcutaneous route requires a longer lockout interval (10 to 15 minutes compared to 6 to 8 minutes for the intravenous). PCA doses may equal 25% to 50% of the hourly infusion rate every 10 to 15 minutes as needed. Subcutaneous administration of opioids may prove impractical in patients with generalized edema, who develop erythema, soreness, or sterile abscesses with subcutaneous administration; in patients with coagulation disorders; and in patients with very poor peripheral circulation.

INTRACEREBROVENTRICULAR OPIOIDS

Intracerebroventricular (ICV) opioid delivery may be beneficial for highly selected cancer patients who are not obtaining adequate relief or experiencing intolerable side effects via other routes. The site of action of opioids via the ICV route appears to be predominantly supraspinal[433] although spinal effects are also observed. After ICV administration of morphine 0.28 to 0.61 mg, peak lumbar CSF morphine levels were observed after 4.5 ± 1.3 hours.[434] Ventricular morphine was approximately 20,000 ng/mL and declined to approximately 10 ng/mL at 24 hours. Lumbar morphine reached approximately 200 ng/mL at about 4 hours and declined to about 10 ng/mL at 24 hours. A short latency to onset of pain relief (20 minutes) corresponds to high levels of morphine in periventricular tissues and the duration of effect is enhanced by the morphine at the spinal level. With neurosurgical consultation, it is possible to deliver opioids directly into cerebral ventricles through ICV catheters from subcutaneous reservoirs. Morphine sulfate, the usual drug, gains a marked increase in potency when delivered ICV as compared to intrathecal or epidural infusion routes, and the ICV route appears to affect supraspinal pathways for analgesia.[435] Daily morphine doses for ICV delivery range from 0.3 to 2.5 mg per day[436] with an average daily dose of 1 mg per day[437] although higher doses have also been reported.[438] For administration, an Ommaya reservoir is placed subcutaneously and connected to the ventricular catheter placed into the lateral ventricle. The duration of pain relief after ICV injections appears to be significantly longer than with intraspinal delivery, and some patients gain adequate relief via an implanted ventricular catheter connected to a subcutaneous Ommaya reservoir–type device with 1 to 2 injections per day. This form of drug delivery is indicated for head and neck cancer pain, or, rarely, for patients with a good initial response to intraspinal infusions of opioids and subsequent development of apparent tolerance, but with limited (1 to 3 months) remaining survival time. The safety and side effects of ICV injections or infusions resemble those for intraspinal infusions with reservoir infection being the most common.[438] In a meta-analysis of 2,402 cancer patients, Ballantyne and Carwood[439] compared ICV (337 patients) with the more common epidural (1,343 patients) and intrathecal (722 patients) opioid treatments in an attempt to establish the utility and safety of ICV therapy. All patients considered had intractable cancer pain that proved resistant to systemic treatment. Persistent nausea, urinary retention, and pruritus occurred more frequently with the two spinal treatments than with ICV therapy but respiratory depression (4.3%), sedation (11%), and confusion (13% protracted, 20% transient) were most common with ICV. Data from these uncontrolled studies reported excellent pain relief among 73% of ICV patients compared with 72% epidural and 62% subarachnoid catheters. Unsatisfactory pain relief was low in all treatment groups. The incidence of major infection when pumps were used with epidural and subarachnoid catheters was zero. There was a lower incidence of other complications with ICV therapy than with epidural or subarachnoid catheters.

Substance Abuse in Oncology

The misuse or abuse of prescription medications should be of particular concern to oncology care providers, opioid therapy is central to the management of cancer-related pain, and benzodiazepines are frequently prescribed for a variety of issues (predominantly sleep disturbance, anxiety disorders, and nausea control). Although substance use disorders may be diagnosed via detection of aberrant behaviors displayed by patients,[440,441] patient reporting and documentation of issues in the medical record are inadequate to screen for these issues.[442–444] In a retrospective review of 82 oncology patients at high risk for substance misuse, 46% had evidence of nonprescribed opioids, benzodiazepines or potent illicit drugs such as heroin or cocaine, and 39% had inappropriately

TABLE 43.18 Risk Factors for Opioid Misuse
History of substance abuse—personal, family
Young age
History of criminal activity and/or legal problems including DUIs
Regular contact with high-risk individuals or high-risk environments
Significant psychiatric comorbidities (e.g., severe depression, anxiety) including ongoing issues with family members, and friends
Risk taking or thrill seeking behavior.
Continued tobacco use
Persistent psychosocial stressors including lack of support system
Prior drug and/or alcohol rehabilitation

DUI, driving under the influence.
Modified from Jamison RN, Serraillier J, Michna E. Assessment and treatment of abuse risk in opioid prescribing for chronic pain. *Pain Res Treat* 2011:941808. http://dx.doi.org/10.1155/2011/941808. Copyright © 2011 Robert N. Jamison et al.

negative urine drug screening, raising concerns for diversion.[50] In a study of urine drug testing in over 900,000 test samples in patients on chronic opioid therapy for chronic pain, 75% of patients were unlikely to be taking their medications in a manner consistent with their prescribed pain regimen. Thirty-eight percent of patients were found to have no detectable level of their prescribed medication, 29% had a nonprescribed medication present, 27% had a drug level higher than expected, 15% had a drug level lower than expected, and 11% had illicit drugs detected in their urine.[445] In a study to determine the frequency of undiagnosed alcoholism among patients with advanced cancer referred to palliative care and to explore its correlation with alcoholism, tobacco abuse, and use of illegal drugs, alcoholism was highly prevalent and frequently underdiagnosed. Using the CAGE questionnaire as a screening tool, CAGE-positive patients were more likely to have a history of, or to actively engage in, smoking and illegal recreational drug use.[446] Passik et al.[447] indicated in oncology and HIV patients seldom reported current aberrant drug-related behaviors and that many cancer patients would consider behaving aberrantly if pain or symptom management was suboptimal.

One hundred and eleven patients were randomly selected from a group of 215 patients who underwent urine toxicology screening in a cancer center.[448] Fifty-six of the 111 patients had evidence of one or more illicit drug use, a prescription medication that had not been ordered, or alcohol use.

Opioid abuse and misuse may manifest as self-medication, use for reward, compulsive use because of addiction, and diversion for profit. Risk factors for opioid misuse are listed in Table 43.18. There is a clear association between opioid prescription and opioid overdose, abuse, and death. Among opioid-related deaths, approximately half involved a prescription opioid.[449] Prescription opioid-related overdose deaths and admissions for treatment of opioid use disorder have increased in parallel with increases in opioids prescribed in the United States, which quadrupled from 1999 to 2010.[450] Because of these associations, health care providers are advised to carefully weigh the benefits and risks when prescribing opioids, follow evidence-based guidelines, and consider nonopioid therapy for chronic pain treatment.[449] Safe prescribing practice guidelines for noncancer patients suggest screening for the risk of substance abuse, the use of prescription monitoring programs, and monitoring with urine drug screens.[451-456] In addition, clinicians are advised to avoid concurrent opioids and benzodiazepines whenever possible, prescribe the lowest effective dose, and carefully reassess benefits and risks when considering increasing dosage to 50 morphine milligram equivalents or more per day.[457] There are relatively few guidelines in this area for cancer patients, and standard screening tools are not validated in oncology populations. Anghelescu et al.[451] suggest patients undergo evaluation through clinical psychological interview and/or Revised Screener and Opioid Assessment for Patients with Pain (SOAPP-R) assessment at the initiation of chronic opioid therapy for chronic cancer pain, and follow-up risk evaluation with Current Opioid Misuse Measure (COMM) assessment. Urine drug testing is recommended at the initiation of chronic opioid therapy and periodically throughout treatment to augment objective data about the patient's behaviors. Table 43.19 suggests establishment of policies for all patients being considered for chronic opioid therapy.

TABLE 43.19 Policies for Risk Evaluation and Monitoring for Continued Opioid Therapy in Oncology Patients	
Category	**Policy**
Universal risk stratification—all patients	• Screening tool such as Opioid Risk Tool (ORT) • Personal history of substance abuse including prescription opioids, psychoactive medications, illicit substances, alcohol • Family history of substance abuse including prescription opioids, psychoactive medications, illicit substances, alcohol • Review of support system (family, friends, social, etc.)
Universal education opioid use and safety—patient and support system	• Risk versus benefit • Consent for opioid therapy • Safe medication keeping • Adherence to prescription instructions
Screening and monitoring—ongoing	• Regular telephone follow-up with pill counts/opioid reconciliation • Prescription monitoring program review at each refill • Current Opioid Misuse Measure (COMM) at each clinic visit • Presence of aberrant drug behaviors • Urine toxicology screening (to include alcohol, illicit drug, comprehensive panel for opioids) at minimum yearly or as clinically indicated
High-risk patients—no evidence of current substance use	• Review of medical indication for opioid use • Referral for addiction specialist assessment (as indicated) • Frequent random urine drug screening (to include alcohol, illicit drug, comprehensive panel for opioids) based on aberrant behaviors • Elimination of other psychoactive medications when possible • Consequences for unsanctioned substance/nonprescribed medication use including alcohol
High-risk patients—evidence of current substance use	• No initiation of controlled substance prescriptions with ongoing illicit substance use including alcohol • Referral for addiction assessment and management • Frequent urine drug screening (to include alcohol, illicit drug, comprehensive panel for opioids) • Elimination of other psychoactive medications when possible • Consequences for unsanctioned substance/nonprescribed medication use including alcohol.

NOTE: The use of an opioid contract is not considered mandatory in oncology care. High-risk patients include patients with ORT score >7, history of chemical coping, or issues with prescription adherence. Aberrant drug-related behavior is behavior suggestive of a substance abuse and/or addiction disorder. Examples include diversion, prescription forgery, stealing or "borrowing" drugs from others, obtaining prescription drugs from nonmedical sources, multiple episodes of prescription "loss," repeatedly seeking prescriptions from other clinicians, evidence of deterioration in function not explained by illness (work, home, and family), and repeated resistance to changing therapy despite evidence of physical and psychological problems.

Home Infusion Therapy

Advances in pain management technology, such as ambulatory PCAs and the use of silicone subcutaneously tunneled neuraxial catheters, have expanded the scope and success of interventional pain management beyond the hospital to the home. Potential benefits of home infusion therapy include decreased health care costs, patient/caregiver convenience, less time spent in hospital with the ability to extend interventional pain management strategies into the patient's home. A possible disadvantage to home infusion therapy may include the additional burden placed on the patient/caregiver in terms of role responsibilities and schedules. Home care agencies must have explicitly defined policies and procedures consistent with regulatory bodies and national and regional standards of practice.

A provider of infusion therapy must be a licensed pharmacy or work in conjunction with a licensed pharmacy. Skilled and qualified home nursing services are an essential component of home-based care, necessary to educate patients and their caregivers regarding administering the drug therapy, complying with the prescribed dosing schedule, understanding the drug delivery device being used (an infusion pump or other device), and other important information regarding the treatment regimen. Additional roles include monitoring for adverse effects, infection, displacement of catheters, and equipment malfunction.

Drug therapies commonly administered via infusion at home include antibiotics, chemotherapy, analgesics, parenteral nutrition, and immune globulin. Diagnoses commonly requiring infusion therapy include infections that are unresponsive to oral antibiotics; cancer and cancer-related pain; GI diseases or disorders, which prevent normal functioning of the GI system; congestive heart failure; immune disorders; growth hormone deficiencies; and more.

Ambulatory infusion pumps are either designed to be therapy-specific, or are multipurpose, enabling treatments such as chemotherapy, systemic antibiotics, total parenteral nutrition, hydration therapy, and opioid pain control. Recent developments in pump design include remote access capability by modem with the ability to change pump settings and download data.

Home-based PCA therapy provides select patients with the ability to deliver analgesia based on their own perception of need. PCA therapy may be superior to oral analgesia, especially in the treatment of severe oscillating pain. Patient selection criteria include intact cognition and proper supervision from a family member or health professional. A collaborative interdisciplinary approach is necessary for effective pain control for the cancer patient receiving interventional pain management at home. Collaboration between the patient, the patient's family, the home care nurse and home care agency, and the patient's physician is necessary. The physician remains responsible for determining the appropriate drug, bolus dose, background infusion rate, and lockout interval.

PCA is increasingly more common in the home setting as an effective option in pain management. As discussed in the preceding text, the subcutaneous and intravenous routes are the primary methods of administration. The availability of a central vascular access device such as a tunneled or peripherally inserted central catheter (PICC) offers advantages over peripheral access to ensure safe and consistent administration of intravenous analgesia.

The safety and efficacy of home-based PCA opioid therapy has not been extensively reported as in-hospital use. One study reported on the use of morphine PCA in the home environment of 143 preterminally and terminally ill tumor patients suffering either from excruciating chronic pain or severe chronic/acute complex pain that could not be relieved adequately by oral analgesia.[458] After initial dose adjustment, which lasted 2 to 3 days, the median morphine dose was 93 mg per day (range 12 to 464 mg per day). This median was 28% lower than the median dose administered orally prior to PCA therapy. During the course of treatment, morphine requirements increased by a median of 2.3 mg per day (range 29–52 mg per day). Most patients were treated continuously in the home care setting until death; the median duration of treatment was 27 days (range 1 to 437 days). Terminal morphine demands reached a median of 188 mg per day (range 15 to 1,008 mg per day). The authors concluded that PCA was both safe and effective in the home environment, attaining excellent results in 95 (66%) patients and satisfactory pain relief in 43 (30%). PCA was considered insufficient in five (4%) cases. Side effects, in general, were considered mild: the most common being constipation, fatigue, and nausea. PCA use has also been reported in outpatients with cancer during the last week of life and deemed to be effective.[459]

Integrative Oncology

Integrative oncology, the diagnosis-specific field of integrative medicine, addresses symptom control with nonpharmacologic therapies.[460] Known commonly as complementary and alternative medicine (CAM), these therapies are used widely among cancer patients,[461] but patients frequently do not discuss CAM therapies with physicians.[462–464] These therapies have been used as an alternative to conventional medicine (alternative medicine) and complementary to conventional medicine (complementary medicine). Most cancer patients use CAM with the hope of boosting the immune system, relieving pain, and controlling side effects related to disease or treatment. Only a minority of patients include CAM in the treatment plan with curative intent. Integrative therapies have been used during and after breast cancer treatment and include indications for managing anxiety/stress, depression/mood disorders, fatigue, quality of life/physical functioning, CINV, lymphedema, CIPN, pain, and sleep disturbance.[465] For example, music therapy, meditation, stress management, and yoga are recommended for anxiety/stress reduction. Meditation, relaxation, yoga, massage, and music therapy are recommended for depression/mood disorders. Meditation and yoga are recommended to improve quality of life. Acupressure and acupuncture are recommended for reducing CINV. The CAM domains of mind–body medicine, CAM botanicals, manipulative practices, and energy medicine are widely used as complementary approaches to palliative cancer care and cancer symptom management.[466] Psychoeducational interventions, music interventions, acupuncture plus drug therapy, Chinese herbal medicine plus cancer therapy, compound Kushen injection, reflexology, lycopene, transcutaneous electrical nerve stimulation (TENS), qigong, cupping, cannabis, Reiki, homeopathy, and creative arts therapies might have beneficial effects on cancer pain,[467] but there is a lack of multi-institutional randomized controlled trials evaluating CAM therapies for cancer pain.[468,469] In a systematic review of CAM therapies for cancer-related pain, Bardia et al.[468] demonstrated a paucity of well-designed, multi-institutional trials with most being of short duration, with small numbers, without sample size justification, and inadequate reporting of adverse effects of CAM intervention. A National Institutes Health (NIH) consensus conference on the use of acupuncture for pain concluded that although there have been many studies of its potential usefulness, many of these studies provide equivocal results because of design, sample size, and other factors.[470] However, promising results have emerged, for example, showing efficacy of acupuncture in adult postoperative and chemotherapy nausea and vomiting and in postoperative dental pain. There are other situations such as addiction, stroke rehabilitation, headache, menstrual cramps, tennis elbow, fibromyalgia, myofascial pain, osteoarthritis, low back pain, carpal tunnel syndrome, and asthma, in which acupuncture may be useful as an adjunct treatment or an acceptable alternative or be included in a comprehensive management program. Guidelines have been proposed to assist clinicians in making decisions about acupuncture treatment for cancer pain patients and to promote best practice.[471] Three systematic reviews[472-474] and two meta-analyses[475,476] on the use of acupuncture on cancer-related pain have generated equivocal results. Because patients use acupuncture for other benefits and it is considered an intervention with few side effects, it can be used provided patients are aware of its limitations.

Summary

Although pain control is a high-priority goal of cancer care, the ultimate goal of most cancer patients is cure from disease and in most situations pain is often an undesirable by-product of treatment or disease. Pain management should be integrated into oncology care, but it should not become the focus of care. As a very common and debilitating component of disease or treatment, aggressive treatment of pain to maximize both quality and quantity of the patient's life with functional improvement is imperative. The ability to integrate this requires a detailed assessment of the pain compliant with accurate diagnosis of the cause or causes of pain and other quality-of-life concerns. Typically, the pain experience is multidimensional, and treatment must address physical, psychological, social, and existential components and not focus on a single component. Failure to sufficiently understand the etiology of the pain complaint will invariably result in poor pain management. Interdisciplinary collaboration is essential for comprehensive care of the cancer patient. Disciplines and specialties involved in care commonly include pain management specialists, oncologists, surgeons, psychiatrists, psychologists, physical therapists, pharmacists, nurses, and social workers. Aggressive therapy of both cancer and pain are mutually beneficial and are best done by skilled, interdisciplinary teams that understand and respond to the changing demands of oncology care.

Most patients can attain adequate symptomatic relief of cancer pain using appropriate oral pharmacotherapy. Comparatively, opioids are very effective for pain management compared to other agents, and the focus on pharmacotherapy should be safe, appropriate, and effective opioid use irrespective of the source of pain. Long-term use of opioid therapy is controversial and continued use of opioids requires a system that can assess, monitor, modify, and, if appropriate, reduce or taper opioid therapy as required. Modern guidelines on long-term opioid therapy commonly suggest upper limits of opioid therapy that are useful reminders of the potential hazards and risks that can occur with inappropriately high-dose opioid therapy particularly in the setting of failure to meet anticipated functional gains from therapy. The concurrent use of adjunctive or specialized therapies or complementary therapies is sometimes necessary, however, and referral for specialized surgical, anesthetic, or psychological intervention benefit a significant number of patients. However, the introduction of multiple psychoactive medications can be hazardous, and frequent efforts should be made to eliminate all unnecessary or ineffective medications. The continued growth of the home care industry and hospice and emphasis away from inpatient care has broadened the possibilities of extending basic and sophisticated pain management strategies into the home.

References

1. Institute of Medicine Committee on Advancing Pain Research, Care, Education. *Relieving Pain in America: A Blueprint for Transforming Prevention, Care, Education, and Research.* Washington, DC: National Academies Press; 2011.
2. van den Beuken-van Everdingen MH, Hochstenbach LM, Joosten EA, et al. Update on prevalence of pain in patients with cancer: systematic review and meta-analysis. *J Pain Symptom Manage* 2016;51:1070–1090.
3. Gunnarsdottir S, Sigurdardottir V, Kloke M, et al. A multicenter study of attitudinal barriers to cancer pain management. *Support Care Cancer* 2017;25(11):3595–3602.
4. Ventafridda V, Stjernsward J. Pain control and the World Health Organization analgesic ladder. *JAMA* 1996;275:835–836.
5. Carlson CL. Effectiveness of the World Health Organization cancer pain relief guidelines: an integrative review. *J Pain Res* 2016;9:515–534.
6. Wiffen PJ, Wee B, Derry S, et al. Opioids for cancer pain—an overview of Cochrane reviews. *Cochrane Database Syst Rev* 2017;(7):CD012592.
7. Caraceni A, Hanks G, Kaasa S, et al. Use of opioid analgesics in the treatment of cancer pain: evidence-based recommendations from the EAPC. *Lancet Oncol* 2012;13:e58–e68.
8. Gordon DB, Dahl JL, Miaskowski C, et al. American Pain Society recommendations for improving the quality of acute and cancer pain management: American Pain Society Quality of Care Task Force. *Arch Intern Med* 2005;165:1574–1580.
9. Ripamonti CI, Santini D, Maranzano E, et al. Management of cancer pain: ESMO Clinical Practice Guidelines. *Ann Oncol* 2012;23(suppl 7):vii139–vii54.
10. National Institute for Health and Clinical Excellence. *Opioids in Palliative Care: Safe and Effective Prescribing of Strong Opioids for Pain in Palliative Care of Adults.* Cardiff, United Kingdom: National Collaborating Centre for Cancer; 2012.
11. Schmidt-Hansen M, Bennett MI, Arnold S, et al. Oxycodone for cancer-related pain. *Cochrane Database Syst Rev* 2015;(2):CD003870.
12. Wiffen PJ, Wee B, Moore RA. Oral morphine for cancer pain. *Cochrane Database Syst Rev* 2016;(4):CD003868.
13. Reidenberg MM, Willis O. Prosecution of physicians for prescribing opioids to patients. *Clin Pharmacol Ther* 2007;81:903–906.
14. Rudd RA, Aleshire N, Zibbell JE, et al. Increases in drug and opioid overdose deaths—United States, 2000-2014. *MMWR Morb Mortal Wkly Rep* 2016;64:1378–1382.
15. Rudd RA, Seth P, David F, et al. Increases in drug and opioid-involved overdose deaths—United States, 2010-2015. *MMWR Morb Mortal Wkly Rep* 2016;65:1445–1452.
16. Gladden RM, Martinez P, Seth P. Fentanyl law enforcement submissions and increases in synthetic opioid-involved overdose deaths—27 States, 2013-2014. *MMWR Morb Mortal Wkly Rep* 2016;65:837–843.
17. Burke DS. Forecasting the opioid epidemic. *Science* 2016;354:529.
18. Dart RC, Severtson SG, Bucher-Bartelson B. Trends in opioid analgesic abuse and mortality in the United States. *N Engl J Med* 2015;372:1573–1574.
19. Fitzgibbon DR, Rathmell JP, Michna E, et al. Malpractice claims associated with medication management for chronic pain. *Anesthesiology* 2010;112:948–956.
20. Compton WM, Jones CM, Baldwin GT. Relationship between nonmedical prescription opioid use and heroin use and Heroin Use. *N Engl J Med* 2016;374:154–163.
21. Lipari RN, Hughes A. *How People Obtain the Prescription Pain Relievers They Misuse.* Rockville, MD: Substance Abuse and Mental Health Services Administration; 2013.
22. Chou R, Turner JA, Devine EB, et al. The effectiveness and risks of long-term opioid therapy for chronic pain: a systematic review for a National Institutes of Health Pathways to Prevention Workshop. *Ann Intern Med* 2015;162:276–286.
23. Bohnert AS, Valenstein M, Bair MJ, et al. Association between opioid prescribing patterns and opioid overdose-related deaths. *JAMA* 2011;305:1315–1321.
24. Dunn KM, Saunders KW, Rutter CM, et al. Opioid prescriptions for chronic pain and overdose: a cohort study. *Ann Intern Med* 2010;152:85–92.
25. Califf RM, Woodcock J, Ostroff S. A proactive response to prescription opioid abuse. *N Engl J Med* 2016;374:1480–1485.
26. Beaudoin FL, Banerjee GN, Mello MJ. State-level and system-level opioid prescribing policies: the impact on provider practices and overdose deaths, a systematic review. *J Opioid Manag* 2016;12:109–118.
27. Haegerich TM, Paulozzi LJ, Manns BJ, et al. What we know, and don't know, about the impact of state policy and systems-level interventions on prescription drug overdose. *Drug Alcohol Depend* 2014;145:34–47.
28. Prithviraj GK, Koroukian S, Margevicius S, et al. Patient characteristics associated with polypharmacy and inappropriate prescribing of medications among older adults with cancer. *J Geriatr Oncol* 2012;3:228–237.
29. Nightingale G, Hajjar E, Swartz K, et al. Evaluation of a pharmacist-led medication assessment used to identify prevalence of and associations with polypharmacy and potentially inappropriate medication use among ambulatory senior adults with cancer. *J Clin Oncol* 2015;33:1453–1459.
30. Tam-McDevitt J. Polypharmacy, aging, and cancer. *Oncology* 2008;22:1052–1055.

31. Flood KL, Carroll MB, Le CV, et al. Polypharmacy in hospitalized older adult cancer patients: experience from a prospective, observational study of an oncology-acute care for elders unit. *Am J Geriatr Pharmacother* 2009;7:151–158.

32. Garg RK, Fulton-Kehoe D, Franklin GM. Patterns of opioid use and risk of opioid overdose death among Medicaid patients. *Med Care* 2017;55: 661–668.

33. Park TW, Saitz R, Ganoczy D, et al. Benzodiazepine prescribing patterns and deaths from drug overdose among US veterans receiving opioid analgesics: case-cohort study. *BMJ* 2015;350:h2698.

34. Practice guidelines for cancer pain management. A report by the American Society of Anesthesiologists Task Force on Pain Management, Cancer Pain Section. *Anesthesiology* 1996;84:1243–1257.

35. Janjan N. Improving cancer pain control with NCCN guideline-based analgesic administration: a patient-centered outcome. *J Natl Compr Canc Netw* 2014;12:1243–1249.

36. Swarm RA, Abernethy AP, Anghelescu DL, et al. Adult cancer pain. *J Natl Compr Canc Netw* 2013;11:992–1022.

37. Zech DF, Grond S, Lynch J, et al. Validation of World Health Organization guidelines for cancer pain relief: a 10-year prospective study. *Pain* 1995;63:65–76.

38. Paice JA, Portenoy R, Lacchetti C, et al. Management of chronic pain in survivors of adult cancers: American Society of Clinical Oncology Clinical Practice Guideline. *J Clin Oncol* 2016;34:3325–3345.

39. Bennett M, Paice JA, Wallace M. Pain and opioids in cancer care: benefits, risks, and alternatives. *Am Soc Clin Oncol Educ Book* 2017;37:705–713.

40. Hedegaard H, Chen LH, Warner M. Drug-poisoning deaths involving heroin: United States, 2000-2013. *NCHS Data Brief* 2015;2015:1–8.

41. Compton WM, Thomas YF, Stinson FS, et al. Prevalence, correlates, disability, and comorbidity of DSM-IV drug abuse and dependence in the United States: results from the National Epidemiologic Survey on Alcohol and Related Conditions. *Arch Gen Psychiatry* 2007;64:566–576.

42. Compton WM, Dawson DA, Goldstein RB, et al. Crosswalk between DSM-IV dependence and DSM-5 substance use disorders for opioids, cannabis, cocaine and alcohol. *Drug Alcohol Depend* 2013;132: 387–390.

43. Grant BF, Saha TD, Ruan WJ, et al. Epidemiology of DSM-5 drug use disorder: results from the National Epidemiologic Survey on Alcohol and Related Conditions-III. *JAMA Psychiatry* 2016;73:39–47.

44. Passik SD, Portenoy RK, Ricketts PL. Substance abuse issues in cancer patients. Part 1: prevalence and diagnosis. *Oncology* 1998;12:517–521, 524.

45. Derogatis LR, Morrow GR, Fetting J, et al. The prevalence of psychiatric disorders among cancer patients. *JAMA* 1983;249:751–757.

46. Mitchell AJ, Chan M, Bhatti H, et al. Prevalence of depression, anxiety, and adjustment disorder in oncological, haematological, and palliative-care settings: a meta-analysis of 94 interview-based studies. *Lancet Oncol* 2011;12: 160–174.

47. Vasiliadis I, Kolovou G, Mikhailidis DP. Cardiotoxicity and cancer therapy. *Angiology* 2014;65:369–371.

48. Mehnert A, Brahler E, Faller H, et al. Four-week prevalence of mental disorders in patients with cancer across major tumor entities. *J Clin Oncol* 2014;32:3540–3546.

49. Lu D, Andersson TM, Fall K, et al. Clinical diagnosis of mental disorders immediately before and after cancer diagnosis: a nationwide matched cohort study in Sweden. *JAMA Oncol* 2016;2:1188–1196.

50. Rauenzahn S, Sima A, Cassel B, et al. Urine drug screen findings among ambulatory oncology patients in a supportive care clinic. *Support Care Cancer* 2017;25:1859–1864.

51. Hui D, Bruera E. A personalized approach to assessing and managing pain in patients with cancer. *J Clin Oncol* 2014;32:1640–1646.

52. Mularski RA, White-Chu F, Overbay D, et al. Measuring pain as the 5th vital sign does not improve quality of pain management. *J Gen Intern Med* 2006;21:607–612.

53. Lucas CE, Vlahos AL, Ledgerwood AM. Kindness kills: the negative impact of pain as the fifth vital sign. *J Am Coll Surg* 2007;205:101–107.

54. Vila H Jr, Smith RA, Augustyniak MJ, et al. The efficacy and safety of pain management before and after implementation of hospital-wide pain management standards: is patient safety compromised by treatment based solely on numerical pain ratings? *Anesth Analg* 2005;101:474–480.

55. Hammer KJ, Segal EM, Alwan L, et al. Collaborative practice model for management of pain in patients with cancer. *Am J Health Syst Pharm* 2016;73: 1434–1441.

56. Smith TJ, Saiki CB. Cancer pain management. *Mayo Clin Proc* 2015;90: 1428–1439.

57. Kwon JH. Overcoming barriers in cancer pain management. *J Clin Oncol* 2014;32:1727–1733.

58. Patrick DL, Ferketich SL, Frame PS, et al. National Institutes of Health State-of-the-Science Conference Statement: symptom management in cancer: pain, depression, and fatigue, July 15-17, 2002. *J Natl Cancer Inst* 2004;95: 1110–1117.

59. Kedziera P, Levy MH. Collaborative practice in oncology. *Semin Oncol* 1994;21:705–711.

60. Levy MH. Integration of pain management into comprehensive cancer care. *Cancer* 1989;63:2328–2335.

61. Derry S, Wiffen PJ, Moore RA, et al. Oral nonsteroidal anti-inflammatory drugs (NSAIDs) for cancer pain in adults. *Cochrane Database Syst Rev* 2017;(7):CD012638.

62. Jacox A, Carr DB, Payne R. New clinical-practice guidelines for the management of pain in patients with cancer. *N Engl J Med* 1994;330:651–655.

63. Meuser T, Pietruck C, Radbruch L, et al. Symptoms during cancer pain treatment following WHO guidelines: a longitudinal follow-up study of symptom prevalence, severity and etiology. *Pain* 2001;93:247–257.

64. Haynes RB, Ackloo E, Sahota N, et al. Interventions for enhancing medication adherence. *Cochrane Database Syst Rev* 2008;(2):CD000011.

65. Munro SA, Lewin SA, Smith HJ, et al. Patient adherence to tuberculosis treatment: a systematic review of qualitative research. *PLoS Med* 2007;4:e238.

66. van Dulmen S, Sluijs E, van Dijk L, et al. Patient adherence to medical treatment: a review of reviews. *BMC Health Serv Res* 2007;7:55.

67. Ryan R, Santesso N, Lowe D, et al. Interventions to improve safe and effective medicines use by consumers: an overview of systematic reviews. *Cochrane Database Syst Rev* 2014;(4):CD007768.

68. Valeberg BT, Miaskowski C, Hanestad BR, et al. Prevalence rates for and predictors of self-reported adherence of oncology outpatients with analgesic medications. *Clin J Pain* 2008;24:627–636.

69. Du Pen SL, Du Pen AR, Polissar N, et al. Implementing guidelines for cancer pain management: results of a randomized controlled clinical trial. *J Clin Oncol* 1999;17:361–370.

70. Miaskowski C, Dodd MJ, West C, et al. Lack of adherence with the analgesic regimen: a significant barrier to effective cancer pain management. *J Clin Oncol* 2001;19:4275–4279.

71. Kravitz RL, Tancredi DJ, Grennan T, et al. Cancer Health Empowerment for Living without Pain (Ca-HELP): effects of a tailored education and coaching intervention on pain and impairment. *Pain* 2011;152:1572–1582.

72. Rustoen T, Valeberg BT, Kolstad E, et al. The PRO-SELF© Pain Control Program improves patients' knowledge of cancer pain management. *J Pain Symptom Manage* 2012;44:321–330.

73. Street RL Jr, Tancredi DJ, Slee C, et al. A pathway linking patient participation in cancer consultations to pain control. *Psychooncology* 2014;23:1111–1117.

74. Butow P, Sharpe L. The impact of communication on adherence in pain management. *Pain* 2013;154(suppl 1):S101–S107.

75. Bennett MI, Bagnall AM, Jose Closs S. How effective are patient-based educational interventions in the management of cancer pain? Systematic review and meta-analysis. *Pain* 2009;143:192–199.

76. Lovell MR, Luckett T, Boyle FM, et al. Patient education, coaching, and self-management for cancer pain. *J Clin Oncol* 2014;32:1712–1720.

77. Dwamena F, Holmes-Rovner M, Gaulden CM, et al. Interventions for providers to promote a patient-centred approach in clinical consultations. *Cochrane Database Syst Rev* 2012;(12):CD003267.

78. Reddy S, Wolfgang CL. The role of surgery in the management of isolated metastases to the pancreas. *Lancet Oncol* 2009;10:287–293.

79. Zisman A, Pantuck AJ, Chao D, et al. Reevaluation of the 1997 TNM classification for renal cell carcinoma: T1 and T2 cutoff point at 4.5 rather than 7 cm. Better correlates with clinical outcome. *J Urol* 2001;166:54–58.

80. Jamison RL, Donohue JH, Nagorney DM, et al. Hepatic resection for metastatic colorectal cancer results in cure for some patients. *Arch Surg* 1997;132:505–510.

81. Choti MA, Sitzmann JV, Tiburi MF, et al. Trends in long-term survival following liver resection for hepatic colorectal metastases. *Ann Surg* 2002;235:759–766.

82. Fernandez FG, Drebin JA, Linehan DC, et al. Five-year survival after resection of hepatic metastases from colorectal cancer in patients screened by positron emission tomography with F-18 fluorodeoxyglucose (FDG-PET). *Ann Surg* 2004;240:438–447.

83. Wise JJ, Fischgrund JS, Herkowitz HN, et al. Complication, survival rates, and risk factors of surgery for metastatic disease of the spine. *Spine (Phila Pa 1976)* 1999;24:1943–1951.

84. Weigel B, Maghsudi M, Neumann C, et al. Surgical management of symptomatic spinal metastases. Postoperative outcome and quality of life. *Spine (Phila Pa 1976)* 1999;24:2240–2246.

85. Choi D, Crockard A, Bunger C, et al. Review of metastatic spine tumour classification and indications for surgery: the consensus statement of the Global Spine Tumour Study Group. *Eur Spine J* 2010;19:215–222.

86. Siersema PD, Marcon N, Vakil N. Metal stents for tumors of the distal esophagus and gastric cardia. *Endoscopy* 2003;35:79–85.

87. Courtney ED, Raja A, Leicester RJ. Eight years experience of high-powered endoscopic diode laser therapy for palliation of colorectal carcinoma. *Dis Colon Rectum* 2005;48:845–850.

88. Frech EJ, Adler DG. Endoscopic therapy for malignant bowel obstruction. *J Support Oncol* 2007;5:303–310, 319.

89. Fugazza A, Galtieri PA, Repici A. Using stents in the management of malignant bowel obstruction: the current situation and future progress. *Expert Rev Gastroenterol Hepatol* 2017;11:633–641.

90. Boulay BR, Birg A. Malignant biliary obstruction: from palliation to treatment. *World J Gastrointest Oncol* 2016;8:498–508.

91. Mirhosseini M, Oneschuk D, Hunter B, et al. The role of antibiotics in the management of infection-related symptoms in advanced cancer patients. *J Palliat Care* 2006;22:69–74.

92. World Health Organization. *Cancer Pain Relief.* Geneva, Switzerland: World Health Organization; 1986.

93. World Health Organization. *Cancer Pain Relief with a Guide to Opioid Availability.* Geneva, Switzerland: World Health Organization; 1996.

94. WHO Expert Committee on Cancer Pain Relief and Active Supportive Care. *Cancer Pain Relief and Palliative Care: Report of a WHO Expert Committee.* Geneva, Switzerland: World Health Organization; 1990.

95. Cherny NI, Baselga J, de Conno F, et al. Formulary availability and regulatory barriers to accessibility of opioids for cancer pain in Europe: a report from the ESMO/EAPC Opioid Policy Initiative. *Ann Oncol* 2010;21: 615–626.

96. Cleary J, Simha N, Panieri A, et al. Formulary availability and regulatory barriers to accessibility of opioids for cancer pain in India: a report from the Global Opioid Policy Initiative (GOPI). *Ann Oncol* 2013;24(suppl 11):xi33–xi40.

97. Cleary J, Radbruch L, Torode J, et al. Formulary availability and regulatory barriers to accessibility of opioids for cancer pain in Asia: a report from the Global Opioid Policy Initiative (GOPI). *Ann Oncol* 2013;24(suppl 11): xi24–xi32.

98. Cleary J, Silbermann M, Scholten W, et al. Formulary availability and regulatory barriers to accessibility of opioids for cancer pain in the Middle East: a report from the Global Opioid Policy Initiative (GOPI). *Ann Oncol* 2013;24(suppl 11):xi51–xi59.

99. Wiffen PJ, Derry S, Moore RA. Impact of morphine, fentanyl, oxycodone or codeine on patient consciousness, appetite and thirst when used to treat cancer pain. *Cochrane Database Syst Rev* 2014;(5):CD011056.

100. Hanks GW, Justins DM. Cancer pain: management. *Lancet* 1992;339: 1031–1036.

101. Schug SA, Zech D, Dorr U. Cancer pain management according to WHO analgesic guidelines. *J Pain Symptom Manage* 1990;5:27–32.

102. Sobolewski C, Cerella C, Dicato M, et al. The role of cyclooxygenase-2 in cell proliferation and cell death in human malignancies. *Int J Cell Biol* 2010;2010:215158.

103. Regulski M, Regulska K, Prukala W, et al. COX-2 inhibitors: a novel strategy in the management of breast cancer. *Drug Discov Today* 2016;21: 598–615.

104. Piazuelo E, Lanas A. NSAIDS and gastrointestinal cancer. *Prostaglandins Other Lipid Mediat* 2015;120:91–96.

105. Bittoni MA, Carbone DP, Harris RE. Ibuprofen and fatal lung cancer: a brief report of the prospective results from the Third National Health and Nutrition Examination Survey (NHANES III). *Mol Clin Oncol* 2017;6:917–920.

106. Hahn E, Kraus S, Arber N. Role of cyclooxygenase-2 in pathogenesis and prevention of colorectal cancer. *Dig Dis* 2010;28:585–589.

107. Sarkar FH, Adsule S, Li Y, et al. Back to the future: COX-2 inhibitors for chemoprevention and cancer therapy. *Mini Rev Med Chem* 2007;7: 599–608.

108. Chan AT, Ogino S, Fuchs CS. Aspirin and the risk of colorectal cancer in relation to the expression of COX-2. *N Engl J Med* 2007;356:2131–2142.

109. Hooijmans CR, Geessink FJ, Ritskes-Hoitinga M, et al. A systematic review and meta-analysis of the ability of analgesic drugs to reduce metastasis in experimental cancer models. *Pain* 2015;156:1835–1844.

110. Zhao X, Xu Z, Li H. NSAIDs use and reduced metastasis in cancer patients: results from a meta-analysis. *Sci Rep* 2017;7:1875.

111. McNicol E, Strassels SA, Goudas L, et al. NSAIDS or paracetamol, alone or combined with opioids, for cancer pain. *Cochrane Database Syst Rev* 2005;(1):CD005180.

112. Hinz B, Cheremina O, Brune K. Acetaminophen (paracetamol) is a selective cyclooxygenase-2 inhibitor in man. *FASEB J* 2008;22:383–390.

113. Graham GG, Scott KF. Mechanism of action of paracetamol. *Am J Ther* 2005;12:46–55.

114. Walter RB, Milano F, Brasky TM, et al. Long-term use of acetaminophen, aspirin, and other nonsteroidal anti-inflammatory drugs and risk of hematologic malignancies: results from the prospective VITamins and Lifestyle (VITAL) study. *J Clin Oncol* 2011;29:2424–2431.

115. Walter RB, Brasky TM, White E. Cancer risk associated with long-term use of acetaminophen in the prospective VITamins and Lifestyle (VITAL) study. *Cancer Epidemiol Biomarkers Prev* 2011;20:2637–2641.

116. Mitka M. FDA asks physicians to stop prescribing high-dose acetaminophen products. *JAMA* 2014;311:563.

117. Kuehn BM. FDA: acetaminophen may trigger serious skin problems. *JAMA* 2013;310:785.

118. Martinez RM, Nordt SP, Cantrell FL. Prescription acetaminophen ingestions associated with hepatic injury and death. *J Community Health* 2012;37:1249–1252.

119. Larson AM, Polson J, Fontana RJ, et al. Acetaminophen-induced acute liver failure: results of a United States multicenter, prospective study. *Hepatology* 2005;42:1364–1372.

120. Watkins PB, Kaplowitz N, Slattery JT, et al. Aminotransferase elevations in healthy adults receiving 4 grams of acetaminophen daily: a randomized controlled trial. *JAMA* 2006;296:87–93.

121. Ioannides SJ, Siebers R, Perrin K, et al. The effect of 1g of acetaminophen twice daily for 12 weeks on alanine transaminase levels—a randomized placebo-controlled trial. *Clin Biochem* 2015;48:713–715.

122. Wiffen PJ, Derry S, Moore RA, et al. Oral paracetamol (acetaminophen) for cancer pain. *Cochrane Database Syst Rev* 2017;(7):CD012637.

123. Israel FJ, Parker G, Charles M, et al. Lack of benefit from paracetamol (acetaminophen) for palliative cancer patients requiring high-dose strong opioids: a randomized, double-blind, placebo-controlled, crossover trial. *J Pain Symptom Manage* 2010;39:548–554.

124. Fallon MT, Hanks GW. Morphine, constipation and performance status in advanced cancer patients. *Palliat Med* 1999;13:159–160.

125. McQuade RM, Stojanovska V, Abalo R, et al. Chemotherapy-induced constipation and diarrhea: pathophysiology, current and emerging treatments. *Front Pharmacol* 2016;7:414.

126. Yamagishi A, Morita T, Miyashita M, et al. Symptom prevalence and longitudinal follow-up in cancer outpatients receiving chemotherapy. *J Pain Symptom Manage* 2009;37:823–830.

127. Schneider EC, Malin JL, Kahn KL, et al. Surviving colorectal cancer: patient-reported symptoms 4 years after diagnosis. *Cancer* 2007;110:2075–2082.

128. Denlinger CS, Barsevick AM. The challenges of colorectal cancer survivorship. *J Natl Compr Canc Netw* 2009;7:883–893.

129. Abramowitz L, Beziaud N, Labreze L, et al. Prevalence and impact of constipation and bowel dysfunction induced by strong opioids: a cross-sectional survey of 520 patients with cancer pain: DYONISOS study. *J Med Econ* 2013;16:1423–1433.

130. Gaertner J, Siemens W, Camilleri M, et al. Definitions and outcome measures of clinical trials regarding opioid-induced constipation: a systematic review. *J Clin Gastroenterol* 2015;49:9–16.

131. Camilleri M, Drossman DA, Becker G, et al. Emerging treatments in neurogastroenterology: a multidisciplinary working group consensus statement on opioid-induced constipation. *Neurogastroenterol Motil* 2014;26: 1386–1395.

132. Brock C, Olesen SS, Olesen AE, et al. Opioid-induced bowel dysfunction: pathophysiology and management. *Drugs* 2012;72:1847–1865.

133. Pappagallo M. Incidence, prevalence, and management of opioid bowel dysfunction. *Am J Surg* 2001;182:11s–18s.

134. Hughes PA, Costello SP, Bryant RV, et al. Opioidergic effects on enteric and sensory nerves in the lower GI tract: basic mechanisms and clinical implications. *Am J Physiol Gastrointest Liver Physiol* 2016;311:G501–G513.

135. De Luca A, Coupar IM. Insights into opioid action in the intestinal tract. *Pharmacol Ther* 1996;69:103–115.

136. Kaufman PN, Krevsky B, Malmud LS, et al. Role of opiate receptors in the regulation of colonic transit. *Gastroenterology* 1988;94:1351–1356.

137. Krevsky B, Libster B, Maurer AH, et al. Effects of morphine and naloxone on feline colonic transit. *Life Sci* 1989;44:873–879.

138. Manara L, Bianchetti A. The central and peripheral influences of opioids on gastrointestinal propulsion. *Annu Rev Pharmacol Toxicol* 1985;25: 249–273.

139. Sternini C, Patierno S, Selmer IS, et al. The opioid system in the gastrointestinal tract. *Neurogastroenterol Motil* 2004;16(suppl 2):3–16.

140. Wood JD, Galligan JJ. Function of opioids in the enteric nervous system. *Neurogastroenterol Motil* 2004;16(suppl 2):17–28.

141. Sarna SK, Otterson MF. Small intestinal amyogenesia and dysmyogenesia induced by morphine and loperamide. *Am J Physiol* 1990;258:G282–G289.

142. Thomas J. Opioid-induced bowel dysfunction. *J Pain Symptom Manage* 2008;35:103–113.

143. Rentz AM, Yu R, Muller-Lissner S, et al. Validation of the Bowel Function Index to detect clinically meaningful changes in opioid-induced constipation. *J Med Econ* 2009;12:371–383.

144. Snape WJ Jr, Battle WM, Schwartz SS, et al. Metoclopramide to treat gastroparesis due to diabetes mellitus: a double-blind, controlled trial. *Ann Intern Med* 1982;96:444–446.

145. Perkel MS, Moore C, Hersh T, et al. Metoclopramide therapy in patients with delayed gastric emptying: a randomized, double-blind study. *Dig Dis Sci* 1979;24:662–666.

146. McCallum RW, Ricci DA, Rakatansky H, et al. A multicenter placebo-controlled clinical trial of oral metoclopramide in diabetic gastroparesis. *Diabetes Care* 1983;6:463–467.

147. Camilleri M, Parkman HP, Shafi MA, et al. Clinical guideline: management of gastroparesis. *Am J Gastroenterol* 2013;108:18–37.

148. Roe NA, Sakaan S, Swanson H, et al. Evaluation of prokinetic agents used in the treatment of gastroparesis. *J Drug Assess* 2017;6:6–9.

149. Leppert W, Woron J. The role of naloxegol in the management of opioid-induced bowel dysfunction. *Therap Adv Gastroenterol* 2016;9:736–746.

150. Yuan CS. Clinical status of methylnaltrexone, a new agent to prevent and manage opioid-induced side effects. *J Support Oncol* 2004;2:111–117.

151. Thomas J, Karver S, Cooney GA, et al. Methylnaltrexone for opioid-induced constipation in advanced illness. *N Engl J Med* 2008;358: 2332–2343.

152. Slatkin N, Thomas J, Lipman AG, et al. Methylnaltrexone for treatment of opioid-induced constipation in advanced illness patients. *J Support Oncol* 2009;7:39–46.

153. Diego L, Atayee R, Helmons P, et al. Methylnaltrexone: a novel approach for the management of opioid-induced constipation in patients with advanced illness. *Expert Rev Gastroenterol Hepatol* 2009;3:473–485.

154. Mackey AC, Green L, Greene P, et al. Methylnaltrexone and gastrointestinal perforation. *J Pain Symptom Manage* 2010;40:e1–e3.

155. Wirz S, Wittmann M, Schenk M, et al. Gastrointestinal symptoms under opioid therapy: a prospective comparison of oral sustained-release hydromorphone, transdermal fentanyl, and transdermal buprenorphine. *Eur J Pain* 2009;13:737–743.

156. Kottschade L, Novotny P, Lyss A, et al. Chemotherapy-induced nausea and vomiting: incidence and characteristics of persistent symptoms and future directions NCCTG N08C3 (Alliance). *Support Care Cancer* 2016;24: 2661–2667.

157. Dennis K, Maranzano E, De Angelis C, et al. Radiotherapy-induced nausea and vomiting. *Expert Rev Pharmacoecon Outcomes Res* 2011;11: 685–692.

158. Walsh D, Davis M, Ripamonti C, et al. 2016 Updated MASCC/ESMO consensus recommendations: management of nausea and vomiting in advanced cancer. *Support Care Cancer* 2017;25:333–340.

159. Feyer PC, Maranzano E, Molassiotis A, et al. Radiotherapy-induced nausea and vomiting (RINV): MASCC/ESMO guideline for antiemetics in radiotherapy: update 2009. *Support Care Cancer* 2011;19(suppl 1):S5–S14.

160. Camilleri M, Lembo A, Katzka DA. Opioids in gastroenterology: treating adverse effects and creating therapeutic benefits. *Clin Gastroenterol Hepatol* 2017;15:1338–1349.

161. Torigoe K, Nakahara K, Rahmadi M, et al. Usefulness of olanzapine as an adjunct to opioid treatment and for the treatment of neuropathic pain. *Anesthesiology* 2012;116:159–169.

162. Trigg ME, Higa GM. Chemotherapy-induced nausea and vomiting: antiemetic trials that impacted clinical practice. *J Oncol Pharm Pract* 2010;16: 233–244.

163. dos Santos LV, Souza FH, Brunetto AT, et al. Neurokinin-1 receptor antagonists for chemotherapy-induced nausea and vomiting: a systematic review. *J Natl Cancer Inst* 2012;104:1280–1292.

164. Hesketh PJ, Warr DG, Street JC, et al. Differential time course of action of 5-HT3 and NK1 receptor antagonists when used with highly and moderately emetogenic chemotherapy (HEC and MEC). *Support Care Cancer* 2011;19:1297–1302.

165. Kaito D, Iihara H, Funaguchi N, et al. Efficacy of single-dose first-generation 5-HT3 receptor antagonist and dexamethasone for preventing nausea and vomiting induced by low-dose carboplatin-based chemotherapy. *Anticancer Res* 2017;37:1965–1970.

166. Kazemi-Kjellberg F, Henzi I, Tramer MR. Treatment of established postoperative nausea and vomiting: a quantitative systematic review. *BMC Anesthesiol* 2001;1:2.

167. Coluzzi F, Pappagallo M. Opioid therapy for chronic noncancer pain: practice guidelines for initiation and maintenance of therapy. *Minerva Anestesiol* 2005;71:425–433.

168. Borgelt LM, Franson KL, Nussbaum AM, et al. The pharmacologic and clinical effects of medical cannabis. *Pharmacotherapy* 2013;33:195–209.

169. Chung F, Lane R, Spraggs C, et al. Ondansetron is more effective than metoclopramide for the treatment of opioid-induced emesis in post-surgical adult patients. Ondansetron OIE Post-Surgical Study Group. *Eur J Anaesthesiol* 1999;16:669–677.

170. Smith HS, Laufer A. Opioid induced nausea and vomiting. *Eur J Pharmacol* 2014;722:67–78.

171. Aparasu R, McCoy RA, Weber C, et al. Opioid-induced emesis among hospitalized nonsurgical patients: effect on pain and quality of life. *J Pain Symptom Manage* 1999;18:280–288.

172. McNicol E, Horowicz-Mehler N, Fisk RA, et al. Management of opioid side effects in cancer-related and chronic noncancer pain: a systematic review. *J Pain* 2003;4:231–256.

173. Yoodee J, Permsuwan U, Nimworapan M. Efficacy and safety of olanzapine for the prevention of chemotherapy-induced nausea and vomiting: a systematic review and meta-analysis. *Crit Rev Oncol Hematol* 2017;112:113–125.

174. Sussman G, Shurman J, Creed MR, et al. Intravenous ondansetron for the control of opioid-induced nausea and vomiting. International S3AA3013 Study Group. *Clin Ther* 1999;21:1216–1227.

175. Bell RF, Eccleston C, Kalso EA. Ketamine as an adjuvant to opioids for cancer pain. *Cochrane Database Syst Rev* 2017;(6):CD003351.

176. Watanabe S, Bruera E. Corticosteroids as adjuvant analgesics. *J Pain Symptom Manage* 1994;(9):442–445.

177. Knotkova H, Pappagallo M. Adjuvant analgesics. *Med Clin North Am* 2007;91:113–124.

178. Fallon M, Hanks G, Cherny N. Principles of control of cancer pain. *BMJ* 2006;332:1022–1024.

179. Leppert W, Buss T. The role of corticosteroids in the treatment of pain in cancer patients. *Curr Pain Headache Rep* 2012;16:307–313.

180. Mitra R, Jones S. Adjuvant analgesics in cancer pain: a review. *Am J Hosp Palliat Care* 2012;29:70–79.

181. Mercadante S, Portenoy RK. Opioid poorly-responsive cancer pain. Part 3. Clinical strategies to improve opioid responsiveness. *J Pain Symptom Manage* 2001;21:338–354.

182. Haywood A, Good P, Khan S, et al. Corticosteroids for the management of cancer-related pain in adults. *Cochrane Database Syst Rev* 2015;(4): CD010756.

183. Paulsen O, Aass N, Kaasa S, et al. Do corticosteroids provide analgesic effects in cancer patients? A systematic literature review. *J Pain Symptom Manage* 2013;46:96–105.

184. Derry S, Wiffen PJ, Kalso EA, et al. Topical analgesics for acute and chronic pain in adults—an overview of Cochrane Reviews. *Cochrane Database Syst Rev* 2017;(5):CD008609.

185. Gewandter JS, Mohile SG, Heckler CE, et al. A phase III randomized, placebo-controlled study of topical menthol for chemotherapy-induced peripheral neuropathy (CIPN): a University of Rochester CCOP study of 462 cancer survivors. *Support Care Cancer* 2014;22:1807–1814.

186. Ho KY, Huh BK, White WD, et al. Topical amitriptyline versus lidocaine in the treatment of neuropathic pain. *Clin J Pain* 2008;24:51–55.

187. Derry S, Wiffen PJ, Moore RA, et al. Topical lidocaine for neuropathic pain in adults. *Cochrane Database Syst Rev* 2014;(7):CD010958.

188. Roberts RC, Part NJ, Pokorny R, et al. Pharmacokinetics and pharmacodynamics of tizanidine. *Neurology* 1994;44:S29–S31.

189. Kamen L, Henney HR III, Runyan JD. A practical overview of tizanidine use for spasticity secondary to multiple sclerosis, stroke, and spinal cord injury. *Curr Med Res Opin* 2008;24:425–439.

190. See S, Ginzburg R. Skeletal muscle relaxants. *Pharmacotherapy* 2008;28: 207–213.

191. Attal N, Cruccu G, Baron R, et al. EFNS guidelines on the pharmacological treatment of neuropathic pain: 2010 revision. *Eur J Neurol* 2010;17: 1113–e88.

192. Chaparro LE, Wiffen PJ, Moore RA, et al. Combination pharmacotherapy for the treatment of neuropathic pain in adults. *Cochrane Database Syst Rev* 2012;(7):CD008943.

193. Finnerup NB, Attal N, Haroutounian S, et al. Pharmacotherapy for neuropathic pain in adults: a systematic review and meta-analysis. *Lancet Neurol* 2015;14:162–173.

194. Moulin D, Boulanger A, Clark AJ, et al. Pharmacological management of chronic neuropathic pain: revised consensus statement from the Canadian Pain Society. *Pain Res Manag* 2014;19:328–335.

195. Dworkin RH, O'Connor AB, Backonja M, et al. Pharmacologic management of neuropathic pain: evidence-based recommendations. *Pain* 2007;132:237–251.

196. Saad M, Tafani C, Psimaras D, et al. Chemotherapy-induced peripheral neuropathy in the adult. *Curr Opin Oncol* 2014;26:634–641.

197. Albers JW, Chaudhry V, Cavaletti G, et al. Interventions for preventing neuropathy caused by cisplatin and related compounds. *Cochrane Database Syst Rev* 2014;(3):CD005228.

198. Durand JP, Deplanque G, Montheil V, et al. Efficacy of venlafaxine for the prevention and relief of oxaliplatin-induced acute neurotoxicity: results of EFFOX, a randomized, double-blind, placebo-controlled phase III trial. *Ann Oncol* 2012;23:200–205.

199. Kus T, Aktas G, Alpak G, et al. Efficacy of venlafaxine for the relief of taxane and oxaliplatin-induced acute neurotoxicity: a single-center retrospective case-control study. *Support Care Cancer* 2016;24:2085–2091.

200. Gallagher HC, Gallagher RM, Butler M, et al. Venlafaxine for neuropathic pain in adults. *Cochrane Database Syst Rev* 2015;(8):CD011091.

201. Majithia N, Temkin SM, Ruddy KJ, et al. National Cancer Institute-supported chemotherapy-induced peripheral neuropathy trials: outcomes and lessons. *Support Care Cancer* 2016;24:1439–1447.

202. Smith EM, Pang H, Cirrincione C, et al. Effect of duloxetine on pain, function, and quality of life among patients with chemotherapy-induced painful peripheral neuropathy: a randomized clinical trial. *JAMA* 2013;309: 1359–1367.

203. Otake A, Yoshino K, Ueda Y, et al. Usefulness of duloxetine for Paclitaxel-induced peripheral neuropathy treatment in gynecological cancer patients. *Anticancer Res* 2015;35:359–363.

204. Caraci F, Crupi R, Drago F, et al. Metabolic drug interactions between antidepressants and anticancer drugs: focus on selective serotonin reuptake inhibitors and hypericum extract. *Curr Drug Metab* 2011;12:570–577.

205. Tsavaris N, Kopterides P, Kosmas C, et al. Analgesic activity of high-dose intravenous calcitonin in cancer patients with bone metastases. *Oncol Rep* 2006;16:871–875.

206. Martinez-Zapata MJ, Roque M, Alonso-Coello P, et al. Calcitonin for metastatic bone pain. *Cochrane Database Syst Rev* 2006;(3):CD003223.

207. Chow E, Meyer RM, Ding K, et al. Dexamethasone in the prophylaxis of radiation-induced pain flare after palliative radiotherapy for bone metastases: a double-blind, randomised placebo-controlled, phase 3 trial. *Lancet Oncol* 2015;16:1463–1472.

208. Buckley L, Guyatt G, Fink HA, et al. 2017 American College of Rheumatology guideline for the prevention and treatment of glucocorticoid-induced osteoporosis. *Arthritis Rheumatol* 2017;69:1521–1537.

209. Angeli A, Guglielmi G, Dovio A, et al. High prevalence of asymptomatic vertebral fractures in post-menopausal women receiving chronic glucocorticoid therapy: a cross-sectional outpatient study. *Bone* 2006;39:253–259.

210. Jones LC, Hungerford DS. Osteonecrosis: etiology, diagnosis, and treatment. *Curr Opin Rheumatol* 2004;16:443–449.

211. Symptomatic multifocal osteonecrosis. A multicenter study. Collaborative Osteonecrosis Group. *Clin Orthop Relat Res* 1999;369:312–326.

212. Boquet J, Moore N, Lhuintre JP, et al. Diltiazem for proctalgia fugax. *Lancet* 1986;1:1493.

213. Eckardt VF, Dodt O, Kanzler G, et al. Treatment of proctalgia fugax with salbutamol inhalation. *Am J Gastroenterol* 1996;91:686–689.

214. Jeyarajah S, Purkayastha S. Proctalgia fugax. *CMAJ* 2013;185:417.
215. Do NL, Nagle D, Poylin VY. Radiation proctitis: current strategies in management. *Gastroenterol Res Pract* 2011;2011:917941.
216. Ng CG, Boks MP, Smeets HM, et al. Prescription patterns for psychotropic drugs in cancer patients; a large population study in The Netherlands. *Psychooncology* 2013;22:762–767.
217. Paras-Bravo P, Paz-Zulueta M, Alonso-Blanco MC, et al. Association among presence of cancer pain, inadequate pain control, and psychotropic drug use. *PLoS One* 2017;12:e0178742.
218. Parsaik AK, Mascarenhas SS, Khosh-Chashm D, et al. Mortality associated with anxiolytic and hypnotic drugs—a systematic review and meta-analysis. *Aust N Z J Psychiatry* 2016;50:520–533.
219. Weich S, Pearce HL, Croft P, et al. Effect of anxiolytic and hypnotic drug prescriptions on mortality hazards: retrospective cohort study. *BMJ* 2014;348:g1996.
220. Kripke DF. Mortality risk of hypnotics: strengths and limits of evidence. *Drug Saf* 2016;39:93–107.
221. Palmaro A, Dupouy J, Lapeyre-Mestre M. Benzodiazepines and risk of death: results from two large cohort studies in France and UK. *Eur Neuropsychopharmacol* 2015;25:1566–1577.
222. Warner M, Trinidad JP, Bastian BA, et al. Drugs most frequently involved in drug overdose deaths: United States, 2010-2014. *Natl Vital Stat Rep* 2016;65:1–15.
223. Gralla RJ, Osoba D, Kris MG, et al. Recommendations for the use of antiemetics: evidence-based, clinical practice guidelines. American Society of Clinical Oncology. *J Clin Oncol* 1999;17:2971–2994.
224. Machado Rocha FC, Stefano SC, De Cassia Haiek R, et al. Therapeutic use of Cannabis sativa on chemotherapy-induced nausea and vomiting among cancer patients: systematic review and meta-analysis. *Eur J Cancer Care (Engl)* 2008;17:431–443.
225. Smith LA, Azariah F, Lavender VT, et al. Cannabinoids for nausea and vomiting in adults with cancer receiving chemotherapy. *Cochrane Database Syst Rev* 2015;(11):CD009464.
226. Davis MP. Cannabinoids for symptom management and cancer therapy: the evidence. *J Natl Compr Canc Netw* 2016;14:915–922.
227. Maida V, Ennis M, Irani S, et al. Adjunctive nabilone in cancer pain and symptom management: a prospective observational study using propensity scoring. *J Support Oncol* 2008;6:119–124.
228. Johnson JR, Burnell-Nugent M, Lossignol D, et al. Multicenter, double-blind, randomized, placebo-controlled, parallel-group study of the efficacy, safety, and tolerability of THC:CBD extract and THC extract in patients with intractable cancer-related pain. *J Pain Symptom Manage* 2010;39:167–179.
229. Lynch ME, Cesar-Rittenberg P, Hohmann AG. A double-blind, placebo-controlled, crossover pilot trial with extension using an oral mucosal cannabinoid extract for treatment of chemotherapy-induced neuropathic pain. *J Pain Symptom Manage* 2014;47:166–73.
230. Kramer JL. Medical marijuana for cancer. *CA Cancer J Clin* 2015;65:109–122.
231. Birdsall SM, Birdsall TC, Tims LA. The use of medical marijuana in cancer. *Curr Oncol Rep* 2016;18:40.
232. Bastani B, Jamal JA. Removal of morphine but not fentanyl during haemodialysis. *Nephrol Dial Transplant* 1997;12:2802–2804.
233. Joh J, Sila MK, Bastani B. Nondialyzability of fentanyl with high-efficiency and high-flux membranes. *Anesth Analg* 1998;86:447.
234. Dean M. Opioids in renal failure and dialysis patients. *J Pain Symptom Manage* 2004;28:497–504.
235. Bosilkovska M, Walder B, Besson M, et al. Analgesics in patients with hepatic impairment: pharmacology and clinical implications. *Drugs* 2012;72:1645–1669.
236. Novick DM, Kreek MJ, Arns PA, et al. Effect of severe alcoholic liver disease on the disposition of methadone in maintenance patients. *Alcohol Clin Exp Res* 1985;9:349–354.
237. Cherny NI. Opioid analgesics: comparative features and prescribing guidelines. *Drugs* 1996;51:713–737.
238. Haumann J, Geurts JW, van Kuijk SM, et al. Methadone is superior to fentanyl in treating neuropathic pain in patients with head-and-neck cancer. *Eur J Cancer* 2016;65:121–129.
239. De Santis S, Borghesi C, Ricciardi S, et al. Analgesic effectiveness and tolerability of oral oxycodone/naloxone and pregabalin in patients with lung cancer and neuropathic pain: an observational analysis. *Onco Targets Ther* 2016;9:4043–4052.
240. Cartoni C, Brunetti GA, Federico V, et al. Controlled-release oxycodone for the treatment of bortezomib-induced neuropathic pain in patients with multiple myeloma. *Support Care Cancer* 2012;20:2621–2626.
241. Gaskell H, Derry S, Stannard C, et al. Oxycodone for neuropathic pain in adults. *Cochrane Database Syst Rev* 2016;(7):CD010692.
242. Cooper TE, Chen J, Wiffen PJ, et al. Morphine for chronic neuropathic pain in adults. *Cochrane Database Syst Rev* 2017;(5):CD011669.
243. McNicol ED, Ferguson MC, Schumann R. Methadone for neuropathic pain in adults. *Cochrane Database Syst Rev* 2017;(5):CD012499.
244. Derry S, Stannard C, Cole P, et al. Fentanyl for neuropathic pain in adults. *Cochrane Database Syst Rev* 2016;(10):CD011605.
245. McNicol ED, Midbari A, Eisenberg E. Opioids for neuropathic pain. *Cochrane Database Syst Rev* 2013;(8):CD006146.
246. Glare PA, Davies PS, Finlay E, et al. Pain in cancer survivors. *J Clin Oncol* 2014;32:1739–1747.
247. Sutradhar R, Lokku A, Barbera L. Cancer survivorship and opioid prescribing rates: a population-based matched cohort study among individuals with and without a history of cancer. *Cancer* 2017;123:4286–4293.
248. Gibson SJ, Farrell M. A review of age differences in the neurophysiology of nociception and the perceptual experience of pain. *Clin J Pain* 2004;20:227–239.
249. Saunders KW, Dunn KM, Merrill JO, et al. Relationship of opioid use and dosage levels to fractures in older chronic pain patients. *J Gen Intern Med* 2010;25:310–315.
250. Hanlon JT, Boudreau RM, Roumani YF, et al. Number and dosage of central nervous system medications on recurrent falls in community elders: the Health, Aging and Body Composition study. *J Gerontol A Biol Sci Med Sci* 2009;64:492–498.
251. Blachman NL, Leipzig RM, Mazumdar M, et al. High-risk medications in hospitalized elderly adults: are we making it easy to do the wrong thing? *J Am Geriatr Soc* 2017;65:603–607.
252. McCarberg BH, Barkin RL. Long-acting opioids for chronic pain: pharmacotherapeutic opportunities to enhance compliance, quality of life, and analgesia. *Am J Ther* 2001;8:181–186.
253. Zeppetella G, Davies AN. Opioids for the management of breakthrough pain in cancer patients. *Cochrane Database Syst Rev* 2013;(10):CD004311.
254. Mercadante S, Portenoy RK. Breakthrough cancer pain: twenty-five years of study. *Pain* 2016;157:2657–2663.
255. Coluzzi PH. Oral patient-controlled analgesia. *Semin Oncol* 1997;24:S16–S42.
256. Pappagallo M, Dickerson ED, Hulka S. Palliative care and hospice opioid dosing guidelines with breakthrough pain (BP) doses. *Am J Hosp Palliat Care* 2000;17:407–413.
257. Cherny N, Ripamonti C, Pereira J, et al. Strategies to manage the adverse effects of oral morphine: an evidence-based report. *J Clin Oncol* 2001;19:2542–2554.
258. Portenoy RK, Payne D, Jacobsen P. Breakthrough pain: characteristics and impact in patients with cancer pain. *Pain* 1999;81:129–134.
259. Cherny NJ, Chang V, Frager G, et al. Opioid pharmacotherapy in the management of cancer pain: a survey of strategies used by pain physicians for the selection of analgesic drugs and routes of administration. *Cancer* 1995;76:1283–1293.
260. Levy MH. Pharmacologic treatment of cancer pain. *N Engl J Med* 1996;335:1124–1132.
261. Hanks GW, Conno F, Cherny N, et al. Morphine and alternative opioids in cancer pain: the EAPC recommendations. *Br J Cancer* 2001;84:587–593.
262. Galer BS, Coyle N, Pasternak GW, et al. Individual variability in the response to different opioids: report of five cases. *Pain* 1992;49:87–91.
263. Fitzgibbon DR, Galer BS. The efficacy of opioids in cancer pain syndromes. *Pain* 1994;58:429–431.
264. Sjogren P, Jonsson T, Jensen NH, et al. Hyperalgesia and myoclonus in terminal cancer patients treated with continuous intravenous morphine. *Pain* 1993;55:93–97.
265. De Conno F, Caraceni A, Martini C, et al. Hyperalgesia and myoclonus with intrathecal infusion of high-dose morphine. *Pain* 1991;47:337–339.
266. Devulder J. Hyperalgesia induced by high-dose intrathecal sufentanil in neuropathic pain. *J Neurosurg Anesthesiol* 1997;9:146–158.
267. Mauermann E, Filitz J, Dolder P, et al. Does fentanyl lead to opioid-induced hyperalgesia in healthy volunteers?: a double-blind, randomized, crossover trial. *Anesthesiology* 2016;124:453–463.
268. Yildirim V, Doganci S, Cinar S, et al. Acute high dose-fentanyl exposure produces hyperalgesia and tactile allodynia after coronary artery bypass surgery. *Eur Rev Med Pharmacol Sci* 2014;18:3425–3434.
269. Fletcher D, Martinez V. Opioid-induced hyperalgesia in patients after surgery: a systematic review and a meta-analysis. *Br J Anaesth* 2014;112:991–1004.
270. Chung KS, Carson S, Glassman D, et al. Successful treatment of hydromorphone-induced neurotoxicity and hyperalgesia. *Conn Med* 2004;68:547–549.
271. Hooten WM, Lamer TJ, Twyner C. Opioid-induced hyperalgesia in community-dwelling adults with chronic pain. *Pain* 2015;156:1145–1152.
272. Juba KM, Wahler RG, Daron SM. Morphine and hydromorphone-induced hyperalgesia in a hospice patient. *J Palliat Med* 2013;16:809–812.
273. Wilson GR, Reisfield GM. Morphine hyperalgesia: a case report. *Am J Hosp Palliat Care* 2003;20:459–461.
274. Compton P, Charuvastra V, Ling W. Pain intolerance in opioid-maintained former opiate addicts: effect of long-acting maintenance agent. *Drug Alcohol Depend* 2001;63:139–146.
275. Fishbain DA, Cole B, Lewis JE, et al. Do opioids induce hyperalgesia in humans? An evidence-based structured review. *Pain Med* 2009;10:829–839.
276. Eisenberg E, Suzan E, Pud D. Opioid-induced hyperalgesia (OIH): a real clinical problem or just an experimental phenomenon? *J Pain Symptom Manage* 2015;49:632–636.
277. Reznikov I, Pud D, Eisenberg E. Oral opioid administration and hyperalgesia in patients with cancer or chronic nonmalignant pain. *Br J Clin Pharmacol* 2005;60:311–318.
278. Chu LF, Clark DJ, Angst MS. Opioid tolerance and hyperalgesia in chronic pain patients after one month of oral morphine therapy: a preliminary prospective study. *J Pain* 2006;7:43–48.

279. Collett BJ. Opioid tolerance: the clinical perspective. *Br J Anaesth* 1998;81:58–68.

280. Ossipov MH, Lai J, Vanderah TW, et al. Induction of pain facilitation by sustained opioid exposure: relationship to opioid antinociceptive tolerance. *Life Sci* 2003;73:783–800.

281. Chu LF, D'Arcy N, Brady C, et al. Analgesic tolerance without demonstrable opioid-induced hyperalgesia: a double-blinded, randomized, placebo-controlled trial of sustained-release morphine for treatment of chronic nonradicular low-back pain. *Pain* 2012;153:1583–1592.

282. de Stoutz ND, Bruera E, Suarez-Almazor M. Opioid rotation for toxicity reduction in terminal cancer patients. *J Pain Symptom Manage* 1995;10: 378–384.

283. Mercadante S. Opioid rotation for cancer pain: rationale and clinical aspects. *Cancer* 1999;86:1856–1866.

284. Benitez-Rosario MA, Feria M, Salinas-Martin A, et al. Opioid switching from transdermal fentanyl to oral methadone in patients with cancer pain. *Cancer* 2004;101:2866–2873.

285. Mercadante S, Ferrera P, Villari P, et al. Rapid switching between transdermal fentanyl and methadone in cancer patients. *J Clin Oncol* 2005;23: 5229–5234.

286. Reddy A, Tayjasanant S, Haider A, et al. The opioid rotation ratio of strong opioids to transdermal fentanyl in cancer patients. *Cancer* 2016;122:149–156.

287. Quigley C. Opioid switching to improve pain relief and drug tolerability. *Cochrane Database Syst Rev* 2004;(3):CD004847.

288. Arner S, Rawal N, Gustafsson LL. Clinical experience of long-term treatment with epidural and intrathecal opioids—a nationwide survey. *Acta Anaesthesiol Scand* 1988;32:253–259.

289. Foley KM. Controversies in cancer pain. Medical perspectives. *Cancer* 1989;63:2257–2265.

290. Collin E, Poulain P, Gauvain-Piquard A, et al. Is disease progression the major factor in morphine 'tolerance' in cancer pain treatment? *Pain* 1993;55:319–326.

291. Smith MT. Neuroexcitatory effects of morphine and hydromorphone: evidence implicating the 3-glucuronide metabolites. *Clin Exp Pharmacol Physiol* 2000;27:524–528.

292. Kalso E. How different is oxycodone from morphine? *Pain* 2007;132:227–228.

293. Sato H, Naito T, Ishida T, et al. Relationships between oxycodone pharmacokinetics, central symptoms, and serum interleukin-6 in cachectic cancer patients. *Eur J Clin Pharmacol* 2016;72:1463–1470.

294. Reid CM, Martin RM, Sterne JA, et al. Oxycodone for cancer-related pain: meta-analysis of randomized controlled trials. *Arch Intern Med* 2006;166:837–843.

295. King SJ, Reid C, Forbes K, et al. A systematic review of oxycodone in the management of cancer pain. *Palliat Med* 2011;25:454–470.

296. Matsumoto AK. Oral extended-release oxymorphone: a new choice for chronic pain relief. *Expert Opin Pharmacother* 2007;8:1515–1527.

297. Prommer E. Oxymorphone: a review. *Support Care Cancer* 2006;14: 109–115.

298. Adams MP, Ahdieh H. Pharmacokinetics and dose-proportionality of oxymorphone extended release and its metabolites: results of a randomized crossover study. *Pharmacotherapy* 2004;24:468–476.

299. Benedek IH, Jobes J, Xiang Q, et al. Bioequivalence of oxymorphone extended release and crush-resistant oxymorphone extended release. *Drug Des Devel Ther* 2011;5:455–463.

300. Slatkin NE, Rhiner MI, Gould EM, et al. Long-term tolerability and effectiveness of oxymorphone extended release in patients with cancer. *J Opioid Manag* 2010;6:181–191.

301. Murray A, Hagen NA. Hydromorphone. *J Pain Symptom Manage* 2005;29:S57–S66.

302. Vallner JJ, Stewart JT, Kotzan JA, et al. Pharmacokinetics and bioavailability of hydromorphone following intravenous and oral administration to human subjects. *J Clin Pharmacol* 1981;21:152–156.

303. Wright AW, Nocente ML, Smith MT. Hydromorphone-3-glucuronide: biochemical synthesis and preliminary pharmacological evaluation. *Life Sci* 1998;63:401–411.

304. Nalamachu SR, Kutch M, Hale ME. Safety and tolerability of once-daily OROS® hydromorphone extended-release in opioid-tolerant adults with moderate-to-severe chronic cancer and noncancer pain: pooled analysis of 11 clinical studies. *J Pain Symptom Manage* 2012;44:852–865.

305. Bao YJ, Hou W, Kong XY, et al. Hydromorphone for cancer pain. *Cochrane Database Syst Rev* 2016;(10):CD011108.

306. Mannino R, Coyne P, Swainey C, et al. Methadone for cancer-related neuropathic pain: a review of the literature. *J Opioid Manag* 2006;2:269–276.

307. Chizh BA, Schlutz H, Scheede M, et al. The N-methyl-D-aspartate antagonistic and opioid components of d-methadone antinociception in the rat spinal cord. *Neurosci Lett* 2000;296:117–120.

308. Sang CN. NMDA-receptor antagonists in neuropathic pain: experimental methods to clinical trials. *J Pain Symptom Manage* 2000;19:S21–S25.

309. Gorman AL, Elliott KJ, Inturrisi CE. The d- and l-isomers of methadone bind to the non-competitive site on the N-methyl-D-aspartate (NMDA) receptor in rat forebrain and spinal cord. *Neurosci Lett* 1997;223:5–8.

310. Eap CB, Buclin T, Baumann P. Interindividual variability of the clinical pharmacokinetics of methadone: implications for the treatment of opioid dependence. *Clin Pharmacokinet* 2002;41:1153–1193.

311. Izzo AA. Drug interactions with St. John's Wort (hypericum perforatum): a review of the clinical evidence. *Int J Clin Pharmacol Ther* 2004;42:139–148.

312. Ahmad T, Sabet S, Primerano DA, et al. Tell-tale SNPs: the role of CYP2B6 in methadone fatalities. *J Anal Toxicol* 2017;41:325–333.

313. Bunten H, Liang WJ, Pounder D, et al. CYP2B6 and OPRM1 gene variations predict methadone-related deaths. *Addict Biol* 2011;16:142–144.

314. Ehret GB, Desmeules JA, Broers B. Methadone-associated long QT syndrome: improving pharmacotherapy for dependence on illegal opioids and lessons learned for pharmacology. *Expert Opin Drug Saf* 2007;6:289–303.

315. Krantz MJ, Kutinsky IB, Robertson AD, et al. Dose-related effects of methadone on QT prolongation in a series of patients with torsade de pointes. *Pharmacotherapy* 2003;23:802–805.

316. Bednar MM, Harrigan EP, Ruskin JN. Torsades de pointes associated with nonantiarrhythmic drugs and observations on gender and QTc. *Am J Cardiol* 2002;89:1316–1319.

317. Justo D. Methadone-induced long QT syndrome vs methadone-induced torsades de pointes. *Arch Intern Med* 2006;166:2288.

318. Anghelescu DL, Patel RM, Mahoney DP, et al. Methadone prolongs cardiac conduction in young patients with cancer-related pain. *J Opioid Manag* 2016;12:131–198.

319. Reddy S, Hui D, El Osta B, et al. The effect of oral methadone on the QTc interval in advanced cancer patients: a prospective pilot study. *J Palliat Med* 2010;13:33–38.

320. Curigliano G, Cardinale D, Dent S, et al. Cardiotoxicity of anticancer treatments: epidemiology, detection, and management. *CA Cancer J Clin* 2016;66:309–325.

321. Brell JM. Prolonged QTc interval in cancer therapeutic drug development: defining arrhythmic risk in malignancy. *Prog Cardiovasc Dis* 2010;53: 164–172.

322. Nicholson AB, Watson GR, Derry S, et al. Methadone for cancer pain. *Cochrane Database Syst Rev* 2017;(2):CD003971.

323. Poulain P, Berleur MP, Lefki S, et al. Efficacy and safety of two methadone titration methods for the treatment of cancer-related pain: the EQUIMETH2 trial (methadone for cancer-related pain). *J Pain Symptom Manage* 2016;52:626–636.e1.

324. Gudin J, Fudin J, Nalamachu S. Levorphanol use: past, present and future. *Postgrad Med* 2016;128:46–53.

325. Dixon R, Crews T, Inturrisi C, et al. Levorphanol: pharmacokinetics and steady-state plasma concentrations in patients with pain. *Res Commun Chem Pathol Pharmacol* 1983;41:3–17.

326. McNulty JP. Can levorphanol be used like methadone for intractable refractory pain? *J Palliat Med* 2007;10:293–296.

327. Lilleng PK, Mehlum LI, Bachs L, et al. Deaths after intravenous misuse of transdermal fentanyl. *J Forensic Sci* 2004;49:1364–1366.

328. Kuhlman JJ Jr, McCaulley R, Valouch TJ, et al. Fentanyl use, misuse, and abuse: a summary of 23 postmortem cases. *J Anal Toxicol* 2003;27:499–504.

329. Reeves MD, Ginifer CJ. Fatal intravenous misuse of transdermal fentanyl. *Med J Aust* 2002;177:552–553.

330. Tharp AM, Winecker RE, Winston DC. Fatal intravenous fentanyl abuse: four cases involving extraction of fentanyl from transdermal patches. *Am J Forensic Med Pathol* 2004;25:178–181.

331. Marier JF, Lor M, Potvin D, et al. Pharmacokinetics, tolerability, and performance of a novel matrix transdermal delivery system of fentanyl relative to the commercially available reservoir formulation in healthy subjects. *J Clin Pharmacol* 2006;46:642–653.

332. Plezia PM, Kramer TH, Linford J, et al. Transdermal fentanyl: pharmacokinetics and preliminary clinical evaluation. *Pharmacotherapy* 1989;9:2–9.

333. Varvel JR, Shafer SL, Hwang SS, et al. Absorption characteristics of transdermally administered fentanyl. *Anesthesiology* 1989;70:928–934.

334. Portenoy RK, Southam MA, Gupta SK, et al. Transdermal fentanyl for cancer pain. Repeated dose pharmacokinetics. *Anesthesiology* 1993;78:36–43.

335. Frolich MA, Giannotti A, Modell JH. Opioid overdose in a patient using a fentanyl patch during treatment with a warming blanket. *Anesth Analg* 2001;93:647–648.

336. Ashburn MA, Ogden LL, Zhang J, et al. The pharmacokinetics of transdermal fentanyl delivered with and without controlled heat. *J Pain* 2003;4: 291–297.

337. Heiskanen T, Matzke S, Haakana S, et al. Transdermal fentanyl in cachectic cancer patients. *Pain* 2009;144:218–22.

338. Nomura M, Inoue K, Matsushita S, et al. Serum concentration of fentanyl during conversion from intravenous to transdermal administration to patients with chronic cancer pain. *Clin J Pain* 2013;29:487–491.

339. Hadley G, Derry S, Moore RA, et al. Transdermal fentanyl for cancer pain. *Cochrane Database Syst Rev* 2013;(10):CD010270.

340. Ahmedzai S, Brooks D. Transdermal fentanyl versus sustained-release oral morphine in cancer pain: preference, efficacy, and quality of life. The TTS-Fentanyl Comparative Trial Group. *J Pain Symptom Manage* 1997;13: 254–261.

341. van Seventer R, Smit JM, Schipper RM, et al. Comparison of TTS-fentanyl with sustained-release oral morphine in the treatment of patients not using opioids for mild-to-moderate pain. *Curr Med Res Opin* 2003;19:457–469.

342. Wong JO, Chiu GL, Tsao CJ, et al. Comparison of oral controlled-release morphine with transdermal fentanyl in terminal cancer pain. *Acta Anaesthesiol Sin* 1997;35:25–32.

343. Tassinari D, Drudi F, Rosati M, et al. Transdermal opioids as front line treatment of moderate to severe cancer pain: a systemic review. *Palliat Med* 2011;25:478–487.

344. Coluzzi PH, Schwartzberg L, Conroy JD, et al. Breakthrough cancer pain: a randomized trial comparing oral transmucosal fentanyl citrate (OTFC) and morphine sulfate immediate release (MSIR). *Pain* 2001;91:123–130.

345. Elsner F, Zeppetella G, Porta-Sales J, et al. Newer generation fentanyl transmucosal products for breakthrough pain in opioid-tolerant cancer patients. *Clin Drug Investig* 2011;31:605–618.

346. Martins SS, Sampson L, Cerda M, et al. Worldwide prevalence and trends in unintentional drug overdose: a systematic review of the literature. *Am J Public Health* 2015;105:2373.

347. Martin TL, Woodall KL, McLellan BA. Fentanyl-related deaths in Ontario, Canada: toxicological findings and circumstances of death in 112 cases (2002-2004). *J Anal Toxicol* 2006;30:603–610.

348. Fodale V, Mafrica F, Santamaria LB, et al. Killer fentanyl: is the fear justified? *Expert Opin Drug Saf* 2008;7:213–217.

349. Peterson AB, Gladden RM, Delcher C, et al. Increases in fentanyl-related overdose deaths—Florida and Ohio, 2013-2015. *MMWR Morb Mortal Wkly Rep* 2016;65:844–849.

350. Giorgetti A, Centola C, Giorgetti R. Fentanyl novel derivative-related deaths. *Hum Psychopharmacol* 2017;32:e2605.

351. U.S. Food and Drug Administration. *Safety Warnings Regarding Use of Fentanyl Transdermal (Skin) Patches.* Silver Spring, MD: U.S. Food and Drug Administration; 2005.

352. Jumbelic MI. Deaths with transdermal fentanyl patches. *Am J Forensic Med Pathol* 2010;31:18–21.

353. Schauer CK, Shand JA, Reynolds TM. The fentanyl patch boil-up—a novel method of opioid abuse. *Basic Clin Pharmacol Toxicol* 2015;117:358–359.

354. Moore PW, Palmer RB, Donovan JW. Fatal fentanyl patch misuse in a hospitalized patient with a postmortem increase in fentanyl blood concentration. *J Forensic Sci* 2015;60:243–246.

355. Coon TP, Miller M, Kaylor D, et al. Rectal insertion of fentanyl patches: a new route of toxicity. *Ann Emerg Med* 2005;46:473.

356. Passik SD, Messina J, Golsorkhi A, et al. Aberrant drug-related behavior observed during clinical studies involving patients taking chronic opioid therapy for persistent pain and fentanyl buccal tablet for breakthrough pain. *J Pain Symptom Manage* 2011;41:116–125.

357. Granata R, Bossi P, Bertulli R, et al. Rapid-onset opioids for the treatment of breakthrough cancer pain: two cases of drug abuse. *Pain Med* 2014;15:758–761.

358. Nunez-Olarte JM, Alvarez-Jimenez P. Emerging opioid abuse in terminal cancer patients taking oral transmucosal fentanyl citrate for breakthrough pain. *J Pain Symptom Manage* 2011;42:e6–e8.

359. Silverman S, Raffa RB, Cataldo MJ, et al. Use of immediate-release opioids as supplemental analgesia during management of moderate-to-severe chronic pain with buprenorphine transdermal system. *J Pain Res* 2017;10:1255–1263.

360. Mercadante S, Villari P, Ferrera P, et al. Safety and effectiveness of intravenous morphine for episodic breakthrough pain in patients receiving transdermal buprenorphine. *J Pain Symptom Manage* 2006;32:175–179.

361. Schmidt-Hansen M, Bromham N, Taubert M, et al. Buprenorphine for treating cancer pain. *Cochrane Database Syst Rev* 2015;(3):CD009596.

362. Naing C, Yeoh PN, Aung K. A meta-analysis of efficacy and tolerability of buprenorphine for the relief of cancer pain. *Springerplus* 2014;3:87.

363. Farr SJ, Robinson CY, Rubino CM. Effects of food and alcohol on the pharmacokinetics of an oral, extended-release formulation of hydrocodone in healthy volunteers. *Clin Pharmacol* 2015;7:1–9.

364. Reddy A, Yennurajalingam S, Desai H, et al. The opioid rotation ratio of hydrocodone to strong opioids in cancer patients. *Oncologist* 2014;19:1186–1193.

365. Rodriguez RF, Castillo JM, Castillo MP, et al. Hydrocodone/acetaminophen and tramadol chlorhydrate combination tablets for the management of chronic cancer pain: a double-blind comparative trial. *Clin J Pain* 2008;24:1–4.

366. Vree TB, van Dongen RT, Koopman-Kimenai PM. Codeine analgesia is due to codeine-6-glucuronide, not morphine. *Int J Clin Pract* 2000;54:395–398.

367. Lotsch J, Skarke C, Schmidt H, et al. Evidence for morphine-independent central nervous opioid effects after administration of codeine: contribution of other codeine metabolites. *Clin Pharmacol Ther* 2006;79:35–48.

368. Levy MH. Pharmacologic management of cancer pain. *Semin Oncol* 1994;21:718–739.

369. Andrzejowski P, Carroll W. Codeine in paediatrics: pharmacology, prescribing and controversies. *Arch Dis Child Educ Pract Ed* 2016;101:148–151.

370. Straube C, Derry S, Jackson KC, et al. Codeine, alone and with paracetamol (acetaminophen), for cancer pain. *Cochrane Database Syst Rev* 2014;(9):CD006601.

371. Leppert W. Dihydrocodeine as an opioid analgesic for the treatment of moderate to severe chronic pain. *Curr Drug Metab* 2010;11:494–506.

372. Schmidt H, Vormfelde SV, Walchner-Bonjean M, et al. The role of active metabolites in dihydrocodeine effects. *Int J Clin Pharmacol Ther* 2003;41:95–106.

373. Leppert W, Woron J. Dihydrocodeine: safety concerns. *Expert Rev Clin Pharmacol* 2016;9:9–12.

374. Beakley BD, Kaye AM, Kaye AD. Tramadol, pharmacology, side effects, and serotonin syndrome: a review. *Pain Physician* 2015;18:395–400.

375. Hollingshead J, Duhmke RM, Cornblath DR. Tramadol for neuropathic pain. *Cochrane Database Syst Rev* 2006;(3):CD003726.

376. Duehmke RM, Derry S, Wiffen PJ, et al. Tramadol for neuropathic pain in adults. *Cochrane Database Syst Rev* 2017;(6):CD003726.

377. Imanaka K, Tominaga Y, Etropolski M, et al. Ready conversion of patients with well-controlled, moderate to severe, chronic malignant tumor-related pain on other opioids to tapentadol extended release. *Clin Drug Investig* 2014;34:501–511.

378. Mercadante S, Porzio G, Aielli F, et al. Opioid switching from and to tapentadol extended release in cancer patients: conversion ratio with other opioids. *Curr Med Res Opin* 2013;29:661–666.

379. Galie E, Villani V, Terrenato I, et al. Tapentadol in neuropathic pain cancer patients: a prospective open label study. *Neurol Sci* 2017;38:1747–1752.

380. Wiffen PJ, Derry S, Naessens K, et al. Oral tapentadol for cancer pain. *Cochrane Database Syst Rev* 2015;(9):CD011460.

381. Kaiko RF, Foley KM, Grabinski PY, et al. Central nervous system excitatory effects of meperidine in cancer patients. *Ann Neurol* 1983;13:180–185.

382. Hoskin PJ, Hanks GW. Opioid agonist-antagonist drugs in acute and chronic pain states. *Drugs* 1991;41:326–344.

383. Goldstein DJ, Meador-Woodruff JH. Opiate receptors: opioid agonist-antagonist effects. *Pharmacotherapy* 1991;11:164–167.

384. Pasternak GW. Incomplete cross tolerance and multiple mu opioid peptide receptors. *Trends Pharmacol Sci* 2001;22:67–70.

385. Crews JC, Sweeney NJ, Denson DD. Clinical efficacy of methadone in patients refractory to other mu-opioid receptor agonist analgesics for management of terminal cancer pain. Case presentations and discussion of incomplete cross-tolerance among opioid agonist analgesics. *Cancer* 1993;72:2266–2272.

386. Bruera E, Pereira J, Watanabe S, et al. Opioid rotation in patients with cancer pain. A retrospective comparison of dose ratios between methadone, hydromorphone, and morphine. *Cancer* 1996;78:852–857.

387. Bruera E, Miller MJ, Macmillan K, et al. Neuropsychological effects of methylphenidate in patients receiving a continuous infusion of narcotics for cancer pain. *Pain* 1992;48:163–166.

388. Kurita GP, Ekholm O, Kaasa S, et al. Genetic variation and cognitive dysfunction in opioid-treated patients with cancer. *Brain Behav* 2016;6:e00471.

389. Lawlor PG. The panorama of opioid-related cognitive dysfunction in patients with cancer: a critical literature appraisal. *Cancer* 2002;94:1836–1853.

390. Kurita GP, Lundorff L, Pimenta CA, et al. The cognitive effects of opioids in cancer: a systematic review. *Support Care Cancer* 2009;17:11–21.

391. Kurita GP, Sjogren P, Ekholm O, et al. Prevalence and predictors of cognitive dysfunction in opioid-treated patients with cancer: a multinational study. *J Clin Oncol* 2011;29:1297–1303.

392. Schoedel KA, McMorn S, Chakraborty B, et al. Reduced cognitive and psychomotor impairment with extended-release oxymorphone versus controlled-release oxycodone. *Pain Physician* 2010;13:561–573.

393. O'Neill WM, Hanks GW, Simpson P, et al. The cognitive and psychomotor effects of morphine in healthy subjects: a randomized controlled trial of repeated (four) oral doses of dextropropoxyphene, morphine, lorazepam and placebo. *Pain* 2000;85:209–215.

394. Stewart SA. The effects of benzodiazepines on cognition. *J Clin Psychiatry* 2005;66(suppl 2):9–13.

395. Jim HS, Phillips KM, Chait S, et al. Meta-analysis of cognitive functioning in breast cancer survivors previously treated with standard-dose chemotherapy. *J Clin Oncol* 2012;30:3578–3587.

396. Landro NI, Fors EA, Vapenstad LL, et al. The extent of neurocognitive dysfunction in a multidisciplinary pain centre population. Is there a relation between reported and tested neuropsychological functioning? *Pain* 2013;154:972–977.

397. Fine PG, Portenoy RK. Management of adverse effects. In: Fine PG, Portenoy RK, eds. *Clinical Guide to Opioid Analgesia.* 2nd ed. New York: Vendome Press; 2007:53–70.

398. Lundorff LE, Jonsson BH, Sjogren P. Modafinil for attentional and psychomotor dysfunction in advanced cancer: a double-blind, randomised, crossover trial. *Palliat Med* 2009;23:731–738.

399. Fishbain DA, Cutler RB, Rosomoff HL, et al. Can patients taking opioids drive safely? A structured evidence-based review. *J Pain Palliat Care Pharmacother* 2002;16:9–28.

400. Fishbain DA, Cutler RB, Rosomoff HL, et al. Are opioid-dependent/tolerant patients impaired in driving-related skills? A structured evidence-based review. *J Pain Symptom Manage* 2003;25:559–577.

401. Nagpal A, Xu R, Pangarkar S, et al. Driving under the influence of opioids. *PMR* 2016;8:698–705.

402. Dassanayake T, Michie P, Carter G, et al. Effects of benzodiazepines, antidepressants and opioids on driving: a systematic review and meta-analysis of epidemiological and experimental evidence. *Drug Saf* 2011;34:125–156.

403. Barbone F, McMahon AD, Davey PG, et al. Association of road-traffic accidents with benzodiazepine use. *Lancet* 1998;352:1331–1336.

404. Chihuri S, Li G. Trends in prescription opioids detected in fatally injured drivers in 6 US states: 1995-2015. *Am J Public Health* 2017;107:1487–1492.

405. Chapman SL, Byas-Smith MG, Reed BA. Effects of intermediate- and long-term use of opioids on cognition in patients with chronic pain. *Clin J Pain* 2002;18:S83–S90.

406. Schumacher MB, Jongen S, Knoche A, et al. Effect of chronic opioid therapy on actual driving performance in non-cancer pain patients. *Psychopharmacology (Berl)* 2017;234:989–999.

407. Gomes T, Redelmeier DA, Juurlink DN, et al. Opioid dose and risk of road trauma in Canada: a population-based study. *JAMA Intern Med* 2013;173:196–201.

408. Vainio A, Ollila J, Matikainen E, et al. Driving ability in cancer patients receiving long-term morphine analgesia. *Lancet* 1995;346:667–670.

409. Galski T, Williams JB, Ehle HT. Effects of opioids on driving ability. *J Pain Symptom Manage* 2000;19:200–208.

410. Mercadante S, Casuccio A, Fulfaro F, et al. Switching from morphine to methadone to improve analgesia and tolerability in cancer patients: a prospective study. *J Clin Oncol* 2001;19:2898–2904.

411. Indelicato RA, Portenoy RK. Opioid rotation in the management of refractory cancer pain. *J Clin Oncol* 2002;20:348–352.

412. Ashby MA, Martin P, Jackson KA. Opioid substitution to reduce adverse effects in cancer pain management. *Med J Aust* 1999;170:68–71.

413. Smith HS, Peppin JF. Toward a systematic approach to opioid rotation. *J Pain Res* 2014;7:589–608.

414. Moryl N, Santiago-Palma J, Kornick C, et al. Pitfalls of opioid rotation: substituting another opioid for methadone in patients with cancer pain. *Pain* 2002;96:325–328.

415. Mercadante S, Porzio G, Ferrera P, et al. Sustained-release oral morphine versus transdermal fentanyl and oral methadone in cancer pain management. *Eur J Pain* 2008;12:1040–1046.

416. Kilonzo I, Twomey F. Rotating to oral methadone in advanced cancer patients: a case series. *J Palliat Med* 2013;16:1154–1157.

417. Hunt G, Bruera E. Respiratory depression in a patient receiving oral methadone for cancer pain. *J Pain Symptom Manage* 1995;10:401–404.

418. Hagen NA, Wasylenko E. Methadone: outpatient titration and monitoring strategies in cancer patients. *J Pain Symptom Manage* 1999;18:369–375.

419. Mercadante S, Caraceni A. Conversion ratios for opioid switching in the treatment of cancer pain: a systematic review. *Palliat Med* 2011;25:504–515.

420. Benitez-Rosario MA, Salinas-Martin A, Aguirre-Jaime A, et al. Morphine-methadone opioid rotation in cancer patients: analysis of dose ratio predicting factors. *J Pain Symptom Manage* 2009;37:1061–1068.

421. O'Bryant CL, Linnebur SA, Yamashita TE, et al. Inconsistencies in opioid equianalgesic ratios: clinical and research implications. *J Pain Palliat Care Pharmacother* 2008;22:282–290.

422. Gabrail NY, Dvergsten C, Ahdieh H. Establishing the dosage equivalency of oxymorphone extended release and oxycodone controlled release in patients with cancer pain: a randomized controlled study. *Curr Med Res Opin* 2004;20:911–918.

423. Cherny NI, Portenoy RK. Cancer pain management. Current strategy. *Cancer* 1993;72:3393–3415.

424. Bruera E, Brenneis C, Michaud M, et al. Use of the subcutaneous route for the administration of narcotics in patients with cancer pain. *Cancer* 1988;62:407–411.

425. Moulin DE, Johnson NG, Murray-Parsons N, et al. Subcutaneous narcotic infusions for cancer pain: treatment outcome and guidelines for use. *CMAJ* 1992;146:891–897.

426. Nelson KA, Glare PA, Walsh D, et al. A prospective, within-patient, crossover study of continuous intravenous and subcutaneous morphine for chronic cancer pain. *J Pain Symptom Manage* 1997;13:262–267.

427. Vanier MC, Labrecque G, Lepage-Savary D, et al. Comparison of hydromorphone continuous subcutaneous infusion and basal rate subcutaneous infusion plus PCA in cancer pain: a pilot study. *Pain* 1993;53:27–32.

428. Stuart-Harris R, Joel SP, McDonald P, et al. The pharmacokinetics of morphine and morphine glucuronide metabolites after subcutaneous bolus injection and subcutaneous infusion of morphine. *Br J Clin Pharmacol* 2000;49:207–214.

429. Moulin DE, Kreeft JH, Murray-Parsons N, et al. Comparison of continuous subcutaneous and intravenous hydromorphone infusions for management of cancer pain. *Lancet* 1991;337:465–468.

430. Roy SD, Flynn GL. Solubility and related physicochemical properties of narcotic analgesics. *Pharm Res* 1988;5:580–586.

431. Paix A, Coleman A, Lees J, et al. Subcutaneous fentanyl and sufentanil infusion substitution for morphine intolerance in cancer pain management. *Pain* 1995;63:263–269.

432. Hays H. Hypodermoclysis for symptom control in terminal care. *Can Fam Physician* 1985;31:1253–1256.

433. Tafani JA, Lazorthes Y, Danet B, et al. Human brain and spinal cord scan after intracerebroventricular administration of iodine-123 morphine. *Int J Rad Appl Instrum B* 1989;16:505–509.

434. Sandouk P, Serrie A, Urtizberea M, et al. Morphine pharmacokinetics and pain assessment after intracerebroventricular administration in patients with terminal cancer. *Clin Pharmacol Ther* 1991;49:442–448.

435. Tseng LF, Fujimoto JM. Differential actions of intrathecal naloxone on blocking the tail-flick inhibition induced by intraventricular beta-endorphin and morphine in rats. *J Pharmacol Exp Ther* 1985;232:74–79.

436. Lazorthes YR, Sallerin BA, Verdie JC. Intracerebroventricular administration of morphine for control of irreducible cancer pain. *Neurosurgery* 1995;37:422–428.

437. Karavelis A, Foroglou G, Selviaridis P, et al. Intraventricular administration of morphine for control of intractable cancer pain in 90 patients. *Neurosurgery* 1996;39:57–61.

438. Obbens EA, Hill CS, Leavens ME, et al. Intraventricular morphine administration for control of chronic cancer pain. *Pain* 1987;28:61–68.

439. Ballantyne JC, Carwood CM. Comparative efficacy of epidural, subarachnoid, and intracerebroventricular opioids in patients with pain due to cancer. *Cochrane Database Syst Rev* 2005;(1):CD005178.

440. Layton D, Osborne V, Al-Shukri M, et al. Indicators of drug-seeking aberrant behaviours: the feasibility of use in observational post-marketing cohort studies for risk management. *Drug Saf* 2014;37:639–50.

441. Chabal C, Erjavec MK, Jacobson L, et al. Prescription opiate abuse in chronic pain patients: clinical criteria, incidence, and predictors. *Clin J Pain* 1997;13:150–155.

442. Hamill-Ruth RJ, Larriviere K, McMasters MG. Addition of objective data to identify risk for medication misuse and abuse: the inconsistency score. *Pain Med* 2013;14:1900–1907.

443. Ready LB, Sarkis E, Turner JA. Self-reported vs. actual use of medications in chronic pain patients. *Pain* 1982;12:285–294.

444. Fishbain DA, Cutler RB, Rosomoff HL, et al. Validity of self-reported drug use in chronic pain patients. *Clin J Pain* 1999;15:184–191.

445. Couto JE, Romney MC, Leider HL, et al. High rates of inappropriate drug use in the chronic pain population. *Popul Health Manag* 2009;12:185–190.

446. Dev R, Parsons HA, Palla S, et al. Undocumented alcoholism and its correlation with tobacco and illegal drug use in advanced cancer patients. *Cancer* 2011;117:4551–4556.

447. Passik SD, Kirsh KL, McDonald MV, et al. A pilot survey of aberrant drug-taking attitudes and behaviors in samples of cancer and AIDS patients. *J Pain Symptom Manage* 2000;19:274–286.

448. Passik SD, Schreiber J, Kirsh KL, et al. A chart review of the ordering and documentation of urine toxicology screens in a cancer center: do they influence patient management? *J Pain Symptom Manage* 2000;19:40–44.

449. Guy GP Jr, Zhang K, Bohm MK, et al. Vital signs: changes in opioid prescribing in the United States, 2006-2015. *MMWR Morb Mortal Wkly Rep* 2017;66:697–704.

450. Centers for Disease Control and Prevention. Vital signs: overdoses of prescription opioid pain relievers—United States, 1999–2008. *MMWR Morb Mortal Wkly Rep* 2011;60:1487–1492.

451. Anghelescu DL, Ehrentraut JH, Faughnan LG. Opioid misuse and abuse: risk assessment and management in patients with cancer pain. *J Natl Compr Canc Netw* 2013;11:1023–1031.

452. Chou R, Fanciullo GJ, Fine PG, et al. Clinical guidelines for the use of chronic opioid therapy in chronic noncancer pain. *J Pain* 2009;10:113–130.

453. Manchikanti L, Abdi S, Atluri S, et al. American Society of Interventional Pain Physicians (ASIPP) guidelines for responsible opioid prescribing in chronic non-cancer pain: part 2—guidance. *Pain Physician* 2012;15:S67–S116.

454. Busse JW, Craigie S, Juurlink DN, et al. Guideline for opioid therapy and chronic noncancer pain. *CMAJ* 2017;189:E659–E666.

455. Bailey RW, Vowles KE. Using screening tests to predict aberrant use of opioids in chronic pain patients: caveat emptor. *J Pain* 2017;18:1427–1436.

456. Manchikanti L, Kaye AM, Knezevic NN, et al. Responsible, safe, and effective prescription of opioids for chronic non-cancer pain: American Society of Interventional Pain Physicians (ASIPP) guidelines. *Pain Physician* 2017;20:S3–S92.

457. Dowell D, Haegerich TM, Chou R. CDC guideline for prescribing opioids for chronic pain—United States, 2016. *JAMA* 2016;315:1624–1645.

458. Meuret G, Jocham H. Patient-controlled analgesia (PCA) in the domiciliary care of tumour patients. *Cancer Treat Rev* 1996;22(suppl A):137–140.

459. Schiessl C, Sittl R, Griessinger N, et al. Intravenous morphine consumption in outpatients with cancer during their last week of life—an analysis based on patient-controlled analgesia data. *Support Care Cancer* 2008;16:917–923.

460. Deng G, Cassileth B. Integrative oncology: an overview. *Am Soc Clin Oncol Educ Book* 2014:233–242.

461. Cassileth B, Trevisan C, Gubili J. Complementary therapies for cancer pain. *Curr Pain Headache Rep* 2007;11:265–269.

462. Adler SR, Fosket JR. Disclosing complementary and alternative medicine use in the medical encounter: a qualitative study in women with breast cancer. *J Fam Pract* 1999;48:453–458.

463. Robinson A, McGrail MR. Disclosure of CAM use to medical practitioners: a review of qualitative and quantitative studies. *Complement Ther Med* 2004;12:90–98.

464. Tasaki K, Maskarinec G, Shumay DM, et al. Communication between physicians and cancer patients about complementary and alternative medicine: exploring patients' perspectives. *Psychooncology* 2002;11:212–220.

465. Greenlee H, DuPont-Reyes MJ, Balneaves LG, et al. Clinical practice guidelines on the evidence-based use of integrative therapies during and after breast cancer treatment. *CA Cancer J Clin* 2017;67:194–232.

466. Mansky PJ, Wallerstedt DB. Complementary medicine in palliative care and cancer symptom management. *Cancer J* 2006;12:425–431.

467. Bao Y, Kong X, Yang L, et al. Complementary and alternative medicine for cancer pain: an overview of systematic reviews. *Evid Based Complement Alternat Med* 2014;2014:170396.

468. Bardia A, Barton DL, Prokop LJ, et al. Efficacy of complementary and alternative medicine therapies in relieving cancer pain: a systematic review. *J Clin Oncol* 2006;24:5457–5464.

469. Gorski DH. Integrative oncology: really the best of both worlds? *Nat Rev Cancer* 2014;14:e3822.

470. National Institutes of Health Consensus Conference. Acupuncture. *JAMA* 1998;280:1518–1524.

471. Filshie J, Hester J. Guidelines for providing acupuncture treatment for cancer patients—a peer-reviewed sample policy document. *Acupunct Med* 2006;24:172–182.

472. Lee H, Schmidt K, Ernst E. Acupuncture for the relief of cancer-related pain—a systematic review. *Eur J Pain* 2005;9:437–444.

473. Lian WL, Pan MQ, Zhou DH, et al. Effectiveness of acupuncture for palliative care in cancer patients: a systematic review. *Chin J Integr Med* 2014;20:136–147.

474. Chiu HY, Hsieh YJ, Tsai PS. Systematic review and meta-analysis of acupuncture to reduce cancer-related pain. *Eur J Cancer Care (Engl)* 2017;26:e12457.

475. Choi TY, Lee MS, Kim TH, et al. Acupuncture for the treatment of cancer pain: a systematic review of randomised clinical trials. *Support Care Cancer* 2012;20:1147–1158.

476. Paley CA, Johnson MI, Tashani OA, et al. Acupuncture for cancer pain in adults. *Cochrane Database Syst Rev* 2015;(10):CD007753.

CHAPTER 44

Interventional Pain Therapies

SHANE E. BROGAN, JILL SINDT, and **ASHWIN VISWANATHAN**

The World Health Organization (WHO) analgesic ladder, as described in the previous chapters on cancer pain management, is practical, easy to implement, and has been taught extensively to health professionals. However, even when the WHO approach is implemented appropriately and aggressively, 10% to 20% of patients do not attain acceptable pain control. Traditionally, it has been this refractory group of patients that has been considered for interventional pain management, but the approach of reserving interventional management as a last resort has been called into question.[1-4] This is particularly true in relation to intrathecal (IT) therapy, where a multicenter study suggests that early implementation of treatment leads to improved outcomes.[5] Another type of interventional therapy, namely, neurolytic celiac plexus block (NCPB), may be useful as an early intervention in controlling pancreatic cancer pain and other gastrointestinal system pain-producing malignancies.[6] Furthermore, there has been a recent resurgence in interest in neurosurgical techniques in refractory pain due to the precision afforded by recent advances in image-guided surgical approaches. Two interventions, in particular, cordotomy and myelotomy, are being increasingly considered for refractory somatic and visceral pain, respectively.

Impediments to the appropriate use of interventional and neurosurgical techniques include inaccessibility to suitably trained physicians and absence of up-to-date knowledge among cancer care providers of the various techniques available, including indications and timing, benefits, risks, and costs (Table 44.1).

The primary purpose of this chapter is to target this latter group of individuals. It is anticipated that a general understanding of interventional approaches to cancer pain control will lead to more appropriate and timely consideration of all potential therapeutic options.

Intrathecal Drug Therapy

IT drug delivery involves drug administration into the cerebrospinal fluid (CSF) through a small catheter. This route allows the medication to circulate in the CSF and adsorb directly onto central nervous system (CNS) effector sites. This direct delivery to the CNS reduces the systemic toxicity of medication administered via enteral, parenteral, or transdermal routes. Opioids, N-type calcium channel blockers, among other pain modulating agents, have been successfully infused intrathecally in the treatment of cancer pain. Effective analgesia using IT opioids is typically obtained using a small fraction (i.e., 1/100th) of the systemic dose. The addition of adjunctive IT agents that have specific activity within the neuraxis, such as local anesthetics and α_2 agonists, may be used to improve overall effectiveness of IT opioid therapy in refractory cases.[7]

TABLE 44.1	Overview of the More Commonly Performed Interventional Cancer Pain Therapies		
Intervention	**Indications**	**Major Adverse Effects and Risks**	**Comments**
Intrathecal (IT) therapy (lumbar region catheter placement; see Chapter 41 for a discussion of intracerebroventricular therapy)	1. Cancer pain refractory to usual pharmacotherapeutic approaches 2. The presence of unacceptable medication side effects	Infection, postdural puncture headache, and spinal cord injury are rare complications. Long-term use of IT opioids may be associated with suppression of the pituitary-gonadal axis.	Various delivery methods available depending on the prognosis. Cost of implanted programmable delivery system may be comparable to conventional medical therapy after several months of ongoing treatment, barring surgical complications.
Neurolytic celiac plexus block	Visceral abdominal (epigastric and referred) pain, originating from disease involving the distal stomach through the transverse colon; pancreatic cancer pain is the most typical indication.	Transient hypotension, diarrhea; very rarely, spinal cord injury	Efficacy of up to 90% and good safety profile
Neurolytic superior hypogastric plexus block	Visceral pain originating from the pelvic organs	Serious adverse effects are rare.	
Ganglion impar block	Anal, perineal pain	Serious adverse effects are rare.	
Intercostal block	Somatic pain of the chest or abdominal wall	Low risk of pneumothorax if ultrasound is used	
Spinal neurolysis	Pain refractory to other forms of therapy, particularly when IT therapy is contraindicated or inefficacious	Dependent on level blocked. Cervical or lumbar neurolysis carries the risk of extremity motor weakness. Lumbosacral neurolysis risks are bowel and bladder dysfunction, which are usually transient; deafferentation pain at any level	Alcohol or phenol is the typical agents used.
Vertebral augmentation	Painful compression fracture of the vertebral body without involvement of the spinal canal	Cement spread to the spinal canal causing neurologic injury; allergy to cement; pulmonary embolus	Better outcomes are noted with fractures <6 mo of age.
Image-guided tumor ablation	Painful bony metastases	Bone instability and fracture	Still not in widespread use but preliminary studies are promising

INDICATIONS

IT therapy is usually indicated in the small proportion of cancer patients for whom comprehensive medical management (CMM) has produced suboptimal pain control or unacceptable, dose-limiting, analgesic-related toxicity. Other factors may make IT therapy an attractive option, including inability to adhere to a more conventional analgesic regimen. Furthermore, cancer pain with a strong neuropathic component (e.g., plexopathy, complex regional pain syndrome) may respond better to IT therapy, particularly when adjunctive agents such as local anesthetics and clonidine are used.[8] In the setting of severe pain and the prospect of a very aggressive chemotherapy regimen, when the oral route will likely be an unreliable means of administering analgesics, strong consideration should be given to adopting an IT approach to pain management.

INTRATHECAL DRUG DELIVERY SYSTEMS

Simple Percutaneous Intrathecal Catheter

This is a minimally invasive technique that can be done at the bedside for short-term use. It may be implemented as a trial method (i.e., to assess efficacy of IT opioids, with the intent of placing an implantable system if the trial is deemed a success) or it can be used as a definitive method of delivering IT drug when life expectancy is extremely short (i.e., days rather than weeks to months). In the setting of a patient with severe pain and only several days of expected life, this method will allow

for rapid control of pain. Because the catheter is not tunneled, infection risk and mechanical failure is higher, markedly reducing successful longer term use.

Tunneled Intrathecal Catheter

Tunneled IT catheters are typically placed in the operating room under sterile conditions. A dorsally placed catheter is tunneled subcutaneously for a variable distance and usually exits from the lateral abdominal wall. With appropriate infection control measures, including the use of antimicrobial filters and meticulous exit site care, tunneled IT or epidural catheters can be used for months to years.[9,10] The catheter is usually not sutured internally, so it can be readily removed in the office if necessary. An advantage of the exteriorized system is that nonpain specialist palliative care clinicians, including those in-home hospice settings, may become proficient in its management with minimal training. Toward the end of life, when analgesic requirements may be rapidly escalating, hospice registered nurses can easily give IT boluses or increase the infusion rate as indicated and alter the drug(s) used with relative ease. With an implanted system (see the following discussion), drug changes are more complex than intravenous (IV) or oral dosing, and rapid dose titration is not as easily accomplished because of the need for pump reprogramming by trained specialists. Disadvantages of a tunneled system versus a self-contained implanted device are the need for an externalized pump apparatus, increased risk of infection, decreased patient mobility, and the possibility of inadvertent catheter dislodgment or removal.

Implantable Drug Delivery Systems

The implanted drug delivery system (IDDS) uses a small, programmable, computerized electronic pump to deliver drug to the IT space through a catheter (Figs. 44.1 and 44.2). The pump is placed subcutaneously in the anterior abdominal wall or buttock and has a reservoir that can be refilled via a port accessed by a specialized needle through the skin. The pump is programmed by an external handheld device that can alter the rate of infusion and deliver boluses and also allows for a patient-controlled analgesia function. The battery life is typically 5 to 7 years, so it

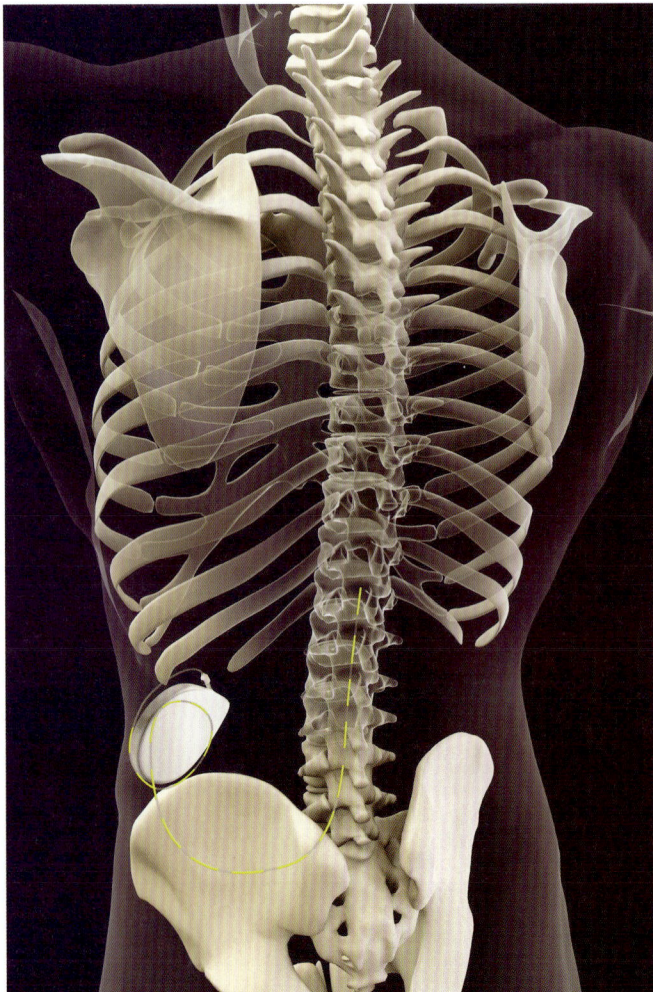

FIGURE 44.1 Schematic of an intrathecal (IT) drug delivery system showing the pump in the anterior abdominal wall and the catheter tunneled to the dorsal spine and into the IT space. *(Courtesy of Medtronic, Inc.)*

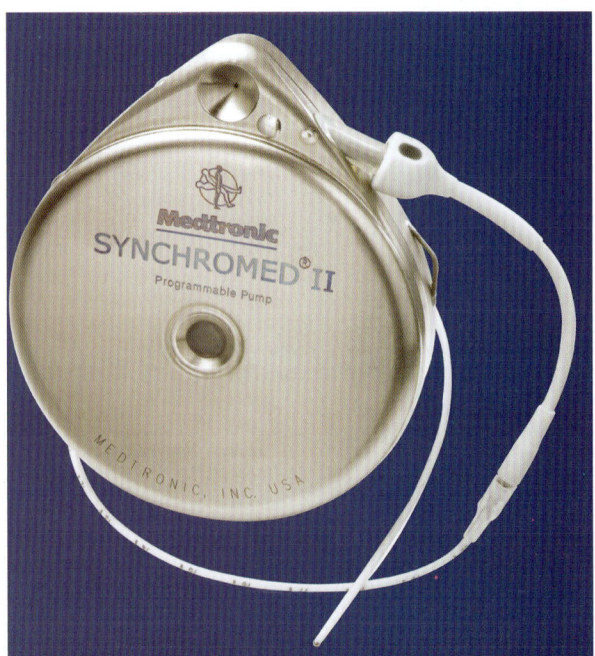

FIGURE 44.2 Intrathecal pump and catheter system. The pump is refilled percutaneously with a needle through the orifice in the center of the device. *(Courtesy of Medtronic, Inc.)*

TABLE 44.2 Comparison of Intrathecal Drug Delivery Systems

	IDDS	Exteriorized Intrathecal Delivery System
Cost	High initial cost but more cost-effective after 3 months	Lower cost for short-term use
Indications	Refractory cancer pain and prognosis >3 mo	Refractory cancer pain with prognosis <3 mo; pain crisis requiring rapid control
Infection risk	Early infection risk; low-risk longer term	Higher
Advantages	Patient freedom; low maintenance	Easier to change infusate; easier to give boluses for aggressive symptom control; can be removed in the office
Disadvantages	More invasive; requires more operator expertise in tertiary care setting	Risk of dislodgment and failure

IDDS, implantable drug delivery system.

is unlikely that a replacement would be necessary during the average lifetime of the cancer patient with advanced disease. Drug refills are office-based and minimally uncomfortable. Refills are needed every 1 to 6 months depending on the drug concentration and infusion rate.

Contraindications to an IDDS are generally related to difficulties forming a suitable subcutaneous pocket for the pump, as would be the case in severe ascites, emaciation, skin infection, or other abdominal wall pathology. Patients with systemic infection, concurrent bleeding diathesis, or clotting abnormalities are poor candidates until these abnormalities are corrected or stabilized. Advantages of this system, compared to an exteriorized system, include increased patient freedom of mobility, low maintenance, and lower infection risk. Disadvantages are the need for an initially more invasive surgery, high upfront costs, and the logistical problems concerning pump refills and programming. See Table 44.2 for a comparison of exteriorized versus implanted pump delivery systems.

INTRATHECAL VERSUS EPIDURAL DRUG DELIVERY

IT drug delivery has largely replaced the epidural route as the preferred neuraxial route of administration for various reasons. With all neuraxial administration of opioids, the target sites are opioid receptors of the dorsal horn of the spinal cord, which requires either direct CSF delivery or absorption of drug from the epidural space. Compared to IT delivery, epidural infusions require a 10-fold greater volume and dose of opioid in order to diffuse passively across the dura and enter the subarachnoid (IT) space. This large difference in infusion volumes and doses has a major impact both on cost and the frequency of drug reservoir changes, which necessitates breaking the system's sterility more frequently and likely results in a higher infection rate. Furthermore, treatment failure is more frequent with the epidural route due to inadvertent catheter dislodgment and the development of epidural fibrosis which impedes diffusion of drug to the subarachnoid space.[11] Technical complication rates have been shown to be higher with long-term epidural (55%) compared to IT (5%) infusions.[12] Finally, ziconotide, an increasingly used agent in refractory cancer pain, is not approved for epidural use.

Notwithstanding these considerations, there remain some specific indications for epidural analgesia. Pain in a pattern involving specific, consecutive dermatomes may be blocked with local anesthetics with an appropriately positioned epidural catheter. An example of this would be a thoracic epidural catheter for isolated thoracic pain caused by rib metastases, in the setting of a short life expectancy. This technique may allow for complete analgesia using local anesthetics alone without the use of epidural opioids.

IMPLANTABLE OR EXTERIORIZED INTRATHECAL DRUG DELIVERY: COST ANALYSIS

With an IDDS, the initial costs are relatively high ($15,000 to $20,000). Over time, the accruing and total care costs may be less in patients with an IDDS compared to those with an exteriorized system due to greater labor-related costs (including managing mechanical failures) with externalized systems. An older study suggested that, compared to an externalized system, an IDDS will be more cost-effective after approximately 3 months of therapy.[13] There are no recent cost comparisons available.

OUTCOME STUDIES

A 2002 study by Smith et al.[5] randomized 202 patients with advanced cancer to CMM or an IDDS plus CMM. Patients were eligible if they had a Visual Analog Scale (VAS) pain intensity rating of ≥5 at two measurements within a week of randomization, despite 200 mg per day or more of oral morphine or its equivalent. Patients on lower doses of opioids were also permitted entry if opioid side effects refractory to conservative management prohibited further escalation of total opioid dose. All patients were ≥18 years of age, had life expectancy ≥3 months, and were suitable for IDDS (no active infection, obstruction of CSF flow, or mechanical barriers). The primary outcome measure was pain control (VAS improvement ≥20%) combined with an improved toxicity profile, as measured by the National Cancer Institute Common Toxicity Criteria, 4 weeks after randomization. Clinical success was defined as a ≥20% reduction in VAS scores or equal scores with a ≥20% reduction in toxicity.

At 4 weeks, both groups had an improvement in pain scores and toxicity. Sixty of 71 IDDS patients (84.5%) achieved clinical success compared with 51 of 72 CMM patients (70.8%, $P = .05$). IDDS patients more often achieved ≥20% reduction in both pain VAS and toxicity (57.7% [41 of 71] vs. 37.5% [27 of 72], $P = .02$). The mean CMM VAS score fell from 7.81 to 4.76 (39% reduction); for the IDDS group, the scores fell from 7.57 to 3.67 (52% reduction, $P = .055$). The mean CMM toxicity scores fell from 6.36 to 5.27 (17% reduction); for the IDDS group, the toxicity scores fell from 7.22 to 3.59 (50% reduction, $P = .004$). The IDDS group had significant reductions in fatigue and depressed level of consciousness ($P < .05$). IDDS patients also had improved survival, with 53.9% alive at 6 months compared with 37.2% of the CMM group ($P = .06$). The authors concluded that IT therapy, compared to CMM alone, improved clinical success by reducing drug toxicity, trended toward improving pain reduction, and possibly improved survival. It should be noted that the data were analyzed on an intent-to-treat basis, but that some crossover (five patients) from CMM to the IDDS group did occur. When the data are interpreted on the basis of the actual treatment received, there was a significant difference between the VAS scores between groups, in favor of IT therapy.

In 2005, the same group of authors published a second paper examining the 6-month follow-up of the patients in the aforementioned trial.[14] The approach in this paper was to compare outcomes in terms of the actual treatment received (i.e., an IDDS vs. CMM alone) rather than the intent to treat at randomization approach used in the 2002 study. Outcome measures were the same as in the initial study but were also assessed in patients alive at 12 weeks after the initial randomization. At 4 weeks, 88.5% of IDDS patients achieved clinical success compared with 71.4% ($P = .02$) of non-IDDS patients and more often achieved a ≥20% reduction in both pain VAS and toxicity (67.3% vs. 36.3%; $P = .0003$). At 12 weeks, of the 56 patients remaining in the CMM group, 19 had received an IDDS. By 12 weeks, 82.5% of IDDS patients had clinical success compared with 77.8% ($P = .55$) of non-IDDS patients and more often had a ≥20% reduction in both pain VAS and toxicity (57.9 vs. 33.3%; $P = .01$). At 12 weeks, the IDDS VAS pain scores decreased from 7.81 to 3.89 (47% reduction) compared with 7.21 to 4.53 for non-IDDS patients (42% reduction; $P = .23$). The 12-week drug toxicity scores for IDDS patients decreased from 6.68 to 2.30 (66% reduction) and for non-IDDS patients from 6.73 to 4.13 (37% reduction; $P = .01$). All individual drug toxicities improved with IDDS at both 4 and 12 weeks. At 6 months, only 32% of the group randomized to CMM and who did not crossover to IDDS were alive, compared with 52% to 59% for patients in those groups who received IDDS. This study concluded that an IDDS improved clinical success, reduced pain scores, relieved most toxicity of pain control drugs, and was associated with increased survival for the duration of the 6-month trial.

PATIENT-CONTROLLED INTRATHECAL ANALGESIA

A shortcoming of the studies mentioned in the previous section is that patients relied only on basal infusions of morphine, without the ability to self-administer IT boluses.

Consequently, breakthrough medications were continued, and although drug toxicities were much improved, ongoing opioid-related side effects were likely observed. Several years after the completion of the original studies, the technology to self-administer IT opioid (and adjuncts) with a "remote control" device became available. A retrospective analysis of 43 patients with refractory cancer pain treated with intrathecal therapy (ITT) with the ability to self-administer IT boluses showed that, 1 month after implant, 50% stopped all conventional opioids, with the mean oral morphine equivalence decreasing from 796 mg.[15]

A follow-up prospective observational study of 98 refractory cancer pain patients performed satisfaction and symptom surveys, including a breakthrough pain survey, before and after ITT. Average "worst" pain scores decreased from 8.32 (SD, 1.73) pre-ITT to 4.98 (SD, 2.92) post-ITT ($P < .001$). The prevalence of severe pain (numerical rating score ≥7) decreased from 84% to 35% ($P < .001$). Mean daily morphine equivalent dosing decreased from 805 mg per day to 128 mg per day, with 65.5% of discontinuing all non-IT opioids. The mean M. D. Anderson Symptom Inventory symptom severity score decreased from 4.98 to 3.72 ($P < .0001$) and the symptom interference score from 6.53 to 4.37 ($P < .001$). When assessing breakthrough pain pharmacotherapy, pain intensity reduction was 46.8% with pre-ITT breakthrough medications and 65.2% with patient-controlled intrathecal analgesia (PCIA; $P < .001$). Median time to onset was 30 minutes with pre-ITT breakthrough medications and 10 minutes with PCIA ($P < .001$). Patient satisfaction was also higher with PCIA compared with conventional breakthrough pain medications: "a lot better" in 60.7% and "a little better" in 28.6%. Overall pain control satisfaction was also improved, with 78.2% "a lot better" and 10.9% reporting no pain.[16]

PHARMACOLOGY

Over a dozen different agents have been reported to be used intrathecally in the management of cancer pain, and most of these have never been approved by the U.S. Food and Drug Administration (FDA) for IT use (Table 44.3). Morphine sulphate, one of the few agents the FDA approved for IT use, is the standard first-line drug used in IT pain therapy. Additional agents are usually then added in a stepwise fashion depending on the response to morphine alone; it is not uncommon that one to three adjunctive agents are added to the infused solution. Consensus documents have attempted to standardize the therapeutic approach to IT drug selection and dosing in the cancer patient (see Table 44.3).[7,17]

Opioids

IT μ-opioid agonists directly activate dorsal horn and brainstem opioid receptors. Morphine sulphate is FDA-approved for IT use, and it remains the first-line agent for IT analgesia. Numerous other IT opioids have been used successfully including hydromorphone, fentanyl, sufentanil, meperidine, and methadone. The choice of agent is largely idiosyncratic. Many practitioners purport that hydromorphone causes less nausea than morphine, although there are no comparative trial data to support this view.

TABLE 44.3 Intrathecal Drugs Used in Cancer Pain Management

Drug	Receptor	Indication	Adverse Effects	Notes
Opioids Morphine Sulphate Hydromorphone Fentanyl Sufentanil	μ-Opioid receptors	Nociceptive and mixed pain, first-line therapy; neuropathic pain second-line therapy	Sedation, respiratory depression, urinary retention, nausea, pruritus, cognitive impairment	The lipophilic opioids like fentanyl and sufentanil are generally added when first-line treatments have failed.
Ziconotide	N-type calcium channels	First- or second-line therapy	Ataxia, auditory hallucinations, psychosis	With careful titration, adverse effects are minimized; no withdrawal phenomenon
Local anesthetics Bupivacaine	Neural sodium channels	Neuropathic and mixed pain, first-line therapy; nociceptive pain, second line	Motor weakness, hypotension, urinary retention	The chemical sympathectomy caused by intrathecal bupivacaine may promote gastrointestinal motility.
Clonidine	α₂ Adrenoceptor	Adjunct in neuropathic pain states	Orthostatic hypotension, sedation, edema	
Baclofen	γ-Aminobutyric acid (GABA)	Coexisting spasticity; third line for neuropathic pain	Ataxia, sedation, auditory disturbance	Abrupt discontinuation may cause a serious withdrawal syndrome.
Ketamine	N-methyl-D-aspartate (NMDA)	Used only at end of life when other IT agents have failed	Anxiety, agitation, facial flushing, delusions; neurotoxicity	Ketamine, given intravenously at subanesthetic doses has also been used effectively for refractory pain syndromes, especially in terminal care.[117]

Based on the practice guidelines published by Deer TR, Pope JE, Hayek SM, et al. The Polyanalgesic Consensus Conference (PACC): recommendations on intrathecal drug infusion systems best practices and guidelines. *Neuromodulation* 2017;20(2):96–132.

The comparatively greater lipophilicity of fentanyl and sufentanil leads to relatively rapid absorption into proximate neural structures with less CSF recirculation and migration to the brainstem. This has some theoretical advantages when a more regional analgesic effect is desired, with less risk of opioid activity (respiratory depression) at the brainstem level.

Ziconotide

Ziconotide (formally SNX-111) is a novel marine snail peptide that is an N-type voltage-sensitive calcium channel blocker. Ziconotide can only be given intrathecally and appears to act at the dorsal horn to decrease afferent sensory input by mechanisms different from those of other IT drugs.[18] Ziconotide has emerged as an indispensable tool in the management of advanced cancer pain, either as a first-line agent or as adjunct when IT opioids have failed either due to toxicity or inefficacy.[7] An advantage of ziconotide is the lack of any respiratory depressant effect as well as the absence of any withdrawal phenomenon. A randomized, placebo-controlled trial including cancer patients demonstrated improved mean visual analog scores of 53% in the ziconotide group compared with 18% in the placebo group (P < .001); 53% of patients in the ziconotide group reported moderate to complete pain relief compared with 18% in the placebo group (P < .001).[19]

Ziconotide has a distinct set of side effects that can hamper its use, including ataxia, auditory hallucinations, and psychosis. However, with more measured guidelines, including careful and slow titration, most of these side effects can be limited to mild events and major side effects are now rare.[7,20]

Local Anesthetics

Local anesthetics, such as bupivacaine and lidocaine, are sodium channel blockers which interrupt neural action potentials along sensory and motor nerves. When given intrathecally, local anesthetics can block incoming sensory nerves and produce complete analgesia. However, this comes at the price of motor blockade resulting in weakness and sympathetic nervous system blockade which may result in hypotension. High doses of local anesthetics may also result in neuro- or cardiotoxicity (seizure or arrhythmia).

Bupivacaine, given in doses less than 30 to 60 mg per day, is an excellent adjunct to IT opioids and generally causes minimal motor block. In the terminally ill patient who is bedbound and does not object to lower extremity weakness, higher doses of local anesthetics may be used to provide profound analgesia with no cognitive side effects. Supportive means to evacuate the bowels and void urine must be anticipated.

Clonidine

Clonidine is an α_2-adrenergic agonist that acts at the dorsal horn by modulating the transmission of noxious sensory signals. This modulation is accomplished by mimicking the activation of descending noradrenergic pathways and inhibiting neurotransmitter release.[21] Epidural and IT clonidine has been studied extensively in postoperative pain settings and in obstetric care for labor analgesia, but little data exist from cancer pain treatment studies. It is generally considered a very useful adjunct to opioids and local anesthetics when there is a predominant neuropathic pain component. Dosing is limited by side effects including sedation and hypotension. The consensus guideline by Deer et al.[7] now includes clonidine as a possible second-line adjunct (with an opioid) for both nociceptive and neuropathic pain.

Other Drugs

A diverse group of drugs have been reported to be useful IT adjuncts, including baclofen, ketamine, neostigmine, midazolam, ketorolac, and droperidol.

CONTRAINDICATIONS AND RISK MANAGEMENT

Absolute contraindications to IT analgesia are rare. Skin infection over the intended catheter site, bacteremia/sepsis, and uncorrectable coagulopathy represent absolute contraindications to IT catheter placement, given the respective risks of CNS infection and spinal hematoma. Coumadin needs to be held until the international normalized ratio is 1.5 or less. If indicated, a low molecular weight heparin (LMWH) may be used, provided it is held for 24 hours before the catheter placement. Given the plethora of novel anticoagulants on the market, specific guidelines have been created.[7] Hematologic relative contraindications include a lowered white cell count $\leq 2 \times 10^9/L$, an absolute neutrophil count $\leq 1,000/\mu L$, or a platelet count $\leq 20 \times 10^3/\mu L$.[17] Depending on the patient circumstances, thrombocytopenia may be treated with a platelet transfusion prior to implantation. Special consideration must be given to the feasibility of implanting available pump devices in the anterior abdominal wall, particularly in emaciated patients or children. A smaller 20-mL capacity pump is available and may be more practical in these instances.

COMPLICATIONS AND SIDE EFFECTS

In general, most of the commonly reported drug-related adverse effects are well tolerated or readily managed with palliative or supportive interventions. The usual IT-opioid side effects are similar to those experienced with the oral or transdermal route but usually much less pronounced and include sedation, nausea, pruritus, and urinary retention. The serious complication of respiratory depression is rare, especially in opioid-tolerant patients. Local anesthetics may cause lower extremity weakness, hypotension, and bowel or bladder dysfunction. Clonidine may cause hypotension and sedation.

Meningitis is the most feared complication of IT drug delivery, but it occurs infrequently when standard infection control measures are followed. Localized skin infection is more common and can usually be managed by oral antibiotics and close observation.

Occasionally, catheter or pump explantation will be necessary. Guidelines about the prevention and treatment of IT drug delivery system infection have been published.[22,23] Typical surgical complications may develop, including seroma formation and pump pocket hematoma. These are usually self-limiting, but ongoing assessment for infection is required, and they may add to postimplant discomfort. The best prophylaxis is an appropriately sized surgical pocket with fastidious hemostasis, and this is achieved through experience.

Catheter tip inflammatory masses (granuloma) are now a well-recognized complication of IT drug delivery. These granulomatous masses can present with new onset lower extremity neurologic symptoms and are associated with high doses and high concentrations of opioid infusate. Clinicians must have a high index of suspicion for this complication; to ignore it may result in permanent neurologic damage, whereas with early recognition and minimally invasive treatment, there are seldom any long-term sequelae.[24]

Postdural puncture headache can result from persistent CSF leak around the catheter. This uncomfortable and often distressing experience is usually self-limiting, resolving spontaneously over days to weeks. Conservative management includes rest, fluids, additional analgesia, and caffeine. A headache that persists may be treated with a fluoroscopically guided epidural blood patch, provided that there are no contraindications related to bleeding risk or leukopenia.

INTRATHECAL THERAPY AND ONGOING ONCOLOGIC CARE

The initiation or continuation of IT therapy need not interfere with chemotherapy or radiotherapy regimens. The superior symptom control offered by IT therapy may in fact allow patients to tolerate aggressive treatment more comfortably and increase the efficiency of the oncology suite by decreasing the amount of time spent managing complicated cancer-related symptoms. Particularly aggressive chemotherapy protocols may require that the implantation of an IT drug delivery system be strategically timed to avoid a white cell count or platelet count nadir. Radiation therapy may affect the battery life of IDDS and may result in electrical failure. The pump may be protected by lead shielding and, if possible, radiation field avoidance.

Spinal Chemoneurolysis

Spinal chemoneurolysis involves the destruction of nerve root axons or other spinal cord elements by chemical means, using alcohol or phenol. The destruction of selected nerve roots interrupts nociceptive pathways and can potentially create excellent analgesia in a relatively selective body area. Alcohol or phenol ablation of central neural structures has largely fallen out of favor in recent decades, mostly because of advances in the pharmacologic treatment of pain, including via the IT route as previously described.

Nevertheless, it remains a useful and effective technique in developing countries with limited opioid access and where a rapidly effective therapy, requiring little or no follow-up, is required. Like other interventional pain management techniques, intraspinal neurolysis offers the advantage of localized pain control while minimizing the burden of systemic side effects. However, the potential adverse effects of the procedure are significant, including motor nerve root dysfunction, bowel or bladder dysfunction, and dysesthesias in the denervated dermatomes.[25,26] In experienced hands, these adverse effects may be minimized, but the potentially high morbidity of these problems has generally placed intraspinal neurolysis toward the end of the treatment spectrum in modern day practice.[27]

SPINAL CHEMONEUROLYSIS TECHNIQUE

Spinal chemoneurolysis, or simply neurolysis, notwithstanding its value in appropriately selected patients, is rapidly becoming a forgotten technique, and therefore, physicians with experience with this treatment modality, and the ability to teach it to trainees, are becoming relatively scarce. Neurolysis is targeted at the sensory nerve root and dorsal root ganglion within the subarachnoid space while attempting to spare the more anteriorly located motor nerve roots. Neurolysis may be performed at the cervical, thoracic, or lumbosacral levels, with the last being the most common site of intervention. Neurolysis in the epidural space has also been described but is less favored because of pain on injection and disappointing outcomes.[28] Knowledge of the chemical properties of alcohol and phenol is essential to the safe and effective use of each agent. The disposition of alcohol and phenol are distinctly different when deposited in the IT space (Figs. 44.3 and 44.4). Alcohol is hypobaric relative to CSF and therefore will "float" upward, whereas phenol is hyperbaric and will "sink" within the subarachnoid space relative to the position of the needle tip. These properties allow for reasonably selective targeting of nerve roots using careful patient positioning and needle placement. The patient is placed in the lateral decubitus position, with the painful side uppermost for alcohol neurolysis, and dependent for phenol neurolysis. Because it is most common for patients to be intolerant of having the painful side down (dependent), alcohol ablation is the preferred technique. For alcohol neurolysis, the patient is rolled 45 degrees away from the operator who is on the dorsal side of the patient, so that the hypobaric alcohol preferentially floats to the dorsolateral subarachnoid space where the sensory dorsal roots reside. To treat this same anatomic location with phenol, the patient needs to be rolled toward the operator. A small-bore spinal needle is advanced into the IT space at the appropriate nerve root level for the affected pain site to be treated. Recall

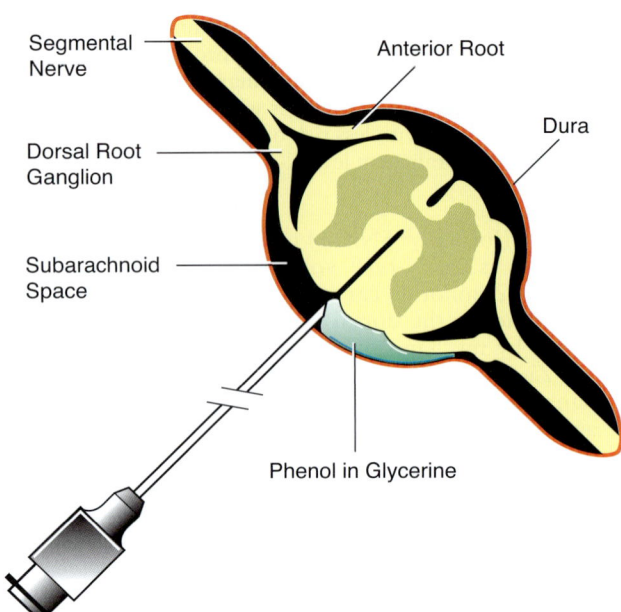

FIGURE 44.3 Lateral supine position used for injection of intrathecal phenol, with the hyperbaric solution falling toward the sensory dorsal roots.

that nerve roots and their respective dermatomal, myotomal, and sclerotomal levels do not necessarily line up anatomically.

Very small aliquots (0.1 to 0.2 mL) of the neurolytic agent are then injected incrementally with careful monitoring of sensory changes and dermatomal spread until the desired region is blocked. A detailed description of spinal neurolysis technique is contained within the text *Neural Blockade in Clinical Anesthesia and Management of Pain.*[25]

Lumbosacral Neurolysis

Lumbosacral spinal neurolysis can provide excellent pain relief of the pelvis, perineum, rectum, and genital area in patients who have been refractory or intolerant of aggressive conventional management. Patients, who are confined to bed due to their symptom burden or who have already had urinary and

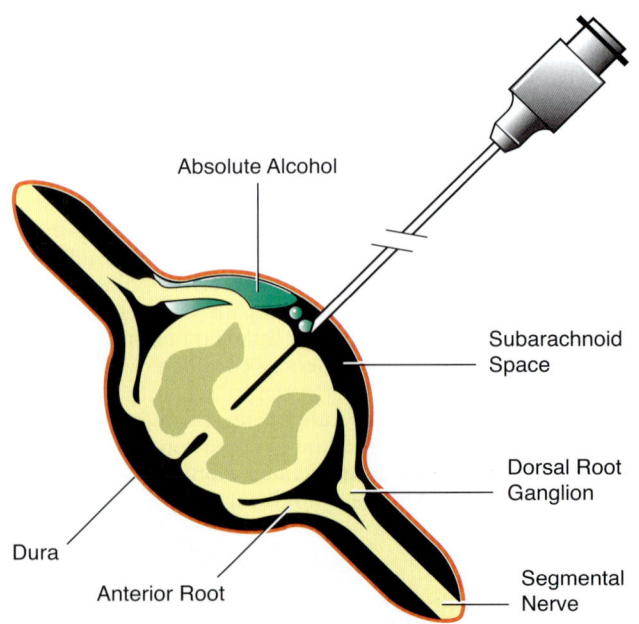

FIGURE 44.4 Lateral prone position used for injection of intrathecal alcohol, with the hypobaric solution rising toward the sensory dorsal roots.

bowel diversion procedures, can expect good pain relief with an acceptable risk of complication. Prior to proceeding with lumbosacral subarachnoid neurolysis, consideration should be given instead to performing a superior hypogastric plexus block (SHPB) because this procedure may be equally effective yet considerably safer.

Cervical and Thoracic Neurolysis

Cervical neurolysis is seldom performed due to the technical difficulty of subarachnoid access at this level, the compactness of anatomy in this region making selective neurolysis more difficult, as well as the inherent risk of causing injury to the cervical spinal cord with consequent neurologic deficits and adverse symptoms (including pain). Thoracic neurolysis for thoracic wall pain is also technically difficult, but the consequences of motor root dysfunction are less pronounced, in that the loss of several levels of intercostal muscle function is usually well tolerated. Thoracic neurolysis does have the advantage of not placing the innervation of the bowel, bladder, and lower extremities at risk and consequently has less risk of significant morbidity.

ADVERSE EFFECTS

Studies reporting on bladder and bowel dysfunction after lumbosacral neurolysis report that about one quarter of patients develop urinary incontinence, with most resolving within 10 days.[29–31] Bowel dysfunction and lower extremity weakness was relatively less frequent. Yet, it should be noted that some of these patients may already have had urinary and bowel diversion for surgical reasons, making the decision to proceed with neurolysis somewhat easier. Other adverse effects of IT neurolysis include deafferentation pain and headache. Rare complications include infection, spinal cord damage, and posterior spinal artery thrombosis causing paraplegia.

CONTRAINDICATIONS

IT neurolysis is contraindicated when (1) the patient has spinal cord tumor or tumor obliteration of the subarachnoid space at the selected level; (2) skin infection is present at the needle puncture site; (3) the patient is unable to tolerate appropriate positioning; and (4) there is a primary pain source, such as a bone metastasis or fracture, that is amenable to more definitive procedural treatment.

Celiac Plexus Block

Chemical neurolysis of the components of the celiac plexus can be a highly effective treatment for visceral pain of the upper abdomen and is the most commonly performed interventional cancer pain technique.

INDICATIONS

NCPB is typically performed for cancer-related visceral pain originating in the upper abdomen. Pain originating from the somatic nerve fibers emanating from the upper abdominal wall will not be blocked by NCPB, and therefore, it is very important to distinguish between visceral versus somatic pain before contemplating this procedure. The celiac plexus carries afferent fibers from the upper abdominal organs from the stomach to the mid transverse colon, including pancreas and gallbladder. Deep visceral pain related to pancreatic adenocarcinoma and cholangiocarcinoma are typical indications for NCPB. As will be discussed later, this is a highly efficacious and safe procedure, so it should be considered early in the treatment of upper abdominal cancer pain.[32]

ANATOMY OF THE CELIAC PLEXUS

Understanding the path of the needle and the position of its tip in relation to the local anatomy is crucial to the safe and effective performance of any interventional procedure. The celiac plexus is a complex grouping of one to five ganglia of various sizes interconnected by a dense network of neural fibers. The plexus is located in the upper abdomen typically anterolateral to the aorta at the L1 vertebral level, just caudal to the takeoff of the celiac artery; however, some variability has been noted, and the plexus can be found anywhere from the level of T12–L1 disk space to the level of the L2 vertebral body.[33] Just lateral to the celiac plexus are the adrenal glands and inferiorly are the renal arteries. The celiac plexus is formed by the convergence of sympathetic preganglionic and afferent fibers from the greater (originating from the T5–T10 spinal level), lesser (T10–T11), and least (T12) splanchnic nerves. The splanchnic nerves are composed of preganglionic autonomic efferent fibers to the upper abdominal viscera that synapse in the celiac ganglia and ascending afferent fibers capable of carrying nociceptive signals from abdominal viscera including the distal portion of the stomach; pancreas; gallbladder; and other hepatobiliary structures, the duodenum, the small intestine, and the large intestine, as far distal as the transverse colon. The splanchnic nerves travel from the spine in the posterior mediastinum, anterolateral to the thoracic vertebral bodies, and pierce the diaphragmatic crus to enter the retroperitoneal abdominal cavity. Parasympathetic preganglionic and afferent fibers originating from the vagus nerves also contribute to the celiac plexus.

GENERAL CONSIDERATIONS

Preparation of patients should include counseling regarding the potential adverse effects and complications of the procedure. Anticoagulants should be discontinued long enough to allow normalization of coagulation profiles. IV access is mandatory so that sedation may be administered, adverse effects can be treated, and prehydration can be accomplished. The latter point is important because celiac plexus blockade will cause splanchnic vasodilation potentially leading to systemic hypotension, particularly in the cancer patient who may already be dehydrated and hypovolemic. An important factor to consider is whether the patient will be able to tolerate lying in the prone position; a patient with gross ascites, even with sedation, will be unable to assume the appropriate position and may be a better candidate for an anterior or endoscopic approach.

Tumor location within the pancreas and the degree of local tumor burden has been shown to impact NCPB outcome, with pain related to head of pancreas lesions having a more favorable outcome compared to lesions of the body and tail of the pancreas.[34] Computed tomography (CT)-guided celiac plexus studies using a radiopaque injectate have shown that outcome may also be affected by local anatomic distortion caused by tumor infiltration.[35,36]

ADVERSE EFFECTS

NCPB is a relatively safe and well-tolerated procedure. Serious complications include transient or permanent spinal cord damage and paraplegia due to spread of the lytic injectate to the nerve roots, epidural, or IT space. Neurologic damage may also ensue after damage to an anterior spinal artery, such as the artery of Adamkiewicz, disrupting the vulnerable arterial supply of the spinal cord.[37,38] Fortunately, serious neurologic complications are very rare, with an incidence of less than 0.2% in one series of 2,730 NCPBs.[39] Side effects are common and generally mild and well tolerated. NCPB will predictably cause a disruption of the sympathetic nervous supply to the proximal bowel resulting in unopposed parasympathetic (vagal) tone. This excessive parasympathetic tone will typically result in transient gastrointestinal hypermotility and diarrhea in approximately 44% of patients, side effects that are seldom considered a problem by the patient who has been constipated due to opioid consumption and debilitation. The loss of sympathetic tone also results in splanchnic vasodilation, intravascular fluid shift to the bowel, and hypotension in approximately 38% of patients.[6]

This should be anticipated and prevented with preprocedural volume enhancement and sufficient means to monitor and treat hypotension.

CELIAC PLEXUS BLOCK TECHNIQUES

Numerous approaches to the celiac plexus have been described, ranging from traditional blind landmark techniques, sophisticated CT-guided methods, and endoscopic ultrasound (EUS) techniques. A 1992 study by Ischia et al.[40] compared the outcomes of the retrocrural technique, a transaortic approach, and neurolysis of the splanchnic nerves at the T12 level. No statistically significant differences ($P > .05$) were found among the three techniques in terms of either immediate or up-to-death results. Procedure mortality was zero with the three techniques and morbidity negligible. NCPB provided excellent pain relief in 70% to 80% of patients immediately after the block and in 60% to 75% until death. Celiac plexus neurolysis may also be achieved intraoperatively at the time of diagnostic or therapeutic laparotomy, with reported good success.[41]

Posterior Approach to the Splanchnic Nerves and Celiac Plexus

The most common celiac plexus block technique is the posterior approach using a needle on either side of midline. This was first described as a blind technique but is now performed with the help of fluoroscopy or CT. The L1 vertebral body is identified with fluoroscopy and then the C-arm is rotated obliquely so that a skin puncture site 6 to 8 cm (6 cm for smaller, cachectic individuals; more toward 8 cm for obese patients) lateral to the midline will allow for coaxial needle advancement to the anterolateral aspect of the upper half of L1 vertebral body. A 15 cm or longer 20-gauge needle is then advanced toward the anterolateral shadow of the L1 vertebral body. The intention is to just miss contact with the vertebral body because this can be quite uncomfortable for the patient. Care should be taken not to touch the L1 transverse process because this can be mistaken for the vertebral body, giving an incorrect, and potentially dangerous, estimate of depth. This author typically performs the left side first, so if an inadvertent aortic puncture is obtained, a transaortic approach can be completed, assuring good placement anterior to the aorta and avoiding the need for a second needle placement (the transaortic approach has been advocated as a safe,[42] alternative technique and involves intentionally piercing the aorta in order to provide direct chemoneurolysis to the celiac ganglia anterior to the aorta). The second needle is placed in identical manner from the right side, aiming for the space anterolateral to the right side of the L1 vertebral body. Final needle advancements should be done under lateral fluoroscopic guidance: The left needle tip should be advanced 0.5 cm ventral to the anterior edge of the L1 vertebral body

(further advancement may result in aortic puncture); the right needle tip is advanced 1 cm beyond the anterior edge of the vertebral body (Fig. 44.5). As the aorta is approached, transmitted arterial pulsations may be appreciable at the needle hub, but this is unreliable. The anatomic location of these needle tips is likely to be retrocrural and in good position to block the splanchnic nerves as they pierce the diaphragm. Note that the celiac plexus itself is not the primary target when using the retrocrural technique, but this appears to be of little clinical significance.[40]

If an anterocrural needle position is desired, with direct lysis of the celiac plexus itself, the needles need to be further advanced through the crus of the diaphragm. The final anatomic position of the needle can only be determined by injecting several milliliters of a radiopaque contrast agent through each needle in an anteroposterior (AP) and lateral projection. Retrocrural contrast will spread cephalad along the anterolateral aspect of the T12 and L1 vertebral bodies, whereas anterocrural spread will be noted in a more anterior and caudal plane. In either case, spread toward the midline should be present. While injecting the radiopaque contrast, meticulous attention should also be given to avoid (1) vascular uptake which might result in neurolytic being delivered to the spinal cord or other organs; (2) posterior spread toward the neuroforamina, the nerve roots, and the epidural space; and (3) contrast uptake into the intima of the aorta (this is seen, under real-time fluoroscopy, as a pulsating "streaking" outlining the assumed position of the aorta). Once the needles are in a radiographically satisfactory position, 5 to 10 mL of lidocaine 2% is injected through each needle after attempting aspiration of blood, CSF, or urine and confirming proper needle placement. After several minutes, the patient is questioned about the presence of any unwanted lower extremity weakness or other neurologic symptoms. A reduction in abdominal pain should also be noted, although this may be unreliable if the patient has received IV analgesics or sedatives.

Finally, neurolysis is achieved by injecting 10 to 12 mL of ethyl alcohol (60% or higher concentration) or phenol (6% or higher concentration) through each needle.

Anterior Approaches

Numerous anterior approaches to the celiac plexus have been described with efficacy and safety profiles comparable to those of the posterior approaches. A single needle may be placed through the anterior abdominal wall under CT guidance, potentially traversing the bowel, stomach, and pancreas, to the preaortic region where the celiac plexus elements reside.[35,43] An increasingly popular approach to the celiac plexus is via EUS endoscopy. A needle is advanced through the endoscope under ultrasound guidance through the posterior wall of the stomach into the preaortic area in the vicinity of the celiac plexus.[44–46] This technique requires that the patient can

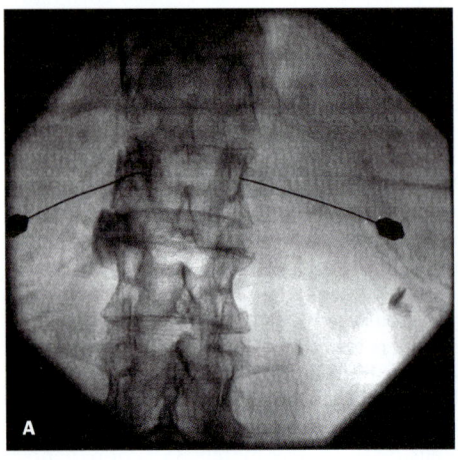 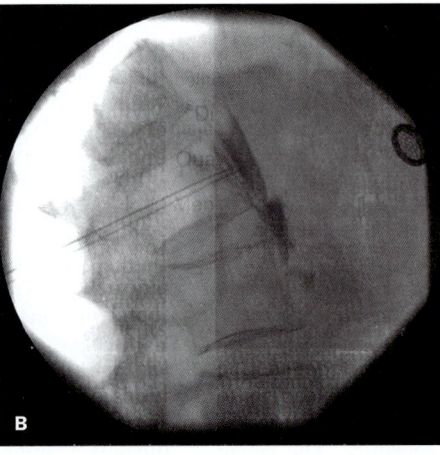

FIGURE 44.5 Fluoroscopic images of a retrocrural celiac plexus block. **A:** Anteroposterior view with the needie tips anterolateral to the L1 vertebral body. Contrast has been injected through the left needle with spread cephalad along the course of the splanchnic nerves. **B:** Lateral fluoroscopic view showing the needle tips advanced anterior to the anterior shadow of the L1 vertebral body and contrast spreading in the retrocrural fascial plane.

tolerate esophagogastroscopy and typically require deeper sedation or general anesthesia. However, if a patient is having EUS for diagnostic purposes, it is very expedient to complete a celiac neurolysis simultaneously.

OUTCOME STUDIES

Numerous case reports, uncontrolled case series, and several randomized controlled trials[40,41,47–49] report a preponderance of favorable outcomes with NCPB. A 1995 meta-analysis by Eisenberg et al.[6] revealed 24 papers (with 1,145 patients) suitable for inclusion. Included were 2 randomized controlled trials, 1 prospective case series, and 21 uncontrolled retrospective case series. When analyzed, good to excellent pain relief was reported in 89% during the first 2 weeks after NCPB. This effect persisted after 2 weeks, with partial or complete pain relief reported in 90% of living patients at 3 months and in 70% to 80% until death. The most frequent indication was unresectable pancreatic cancer (63%), with the balance being a variety of nonpancreatic pain sites including the stomach and esophagus. The pancreatic and nonpancreatic cases did not appear to have a significantly different outcome. The bilateral posterior approach with 15 to 50 mL of 50% to 100% ethyl alcohol was the most common technique used. No procedure-related mortality was reported, and adverse effects were minimal. The most common adverse effects reported were transient hypotension, diarrhea, and transient pain at the site of injection.

A controlled trial by Wong et al.[48] randomized 100 patients with unresectable pancreatic adenocarcinoma to either NCPB or systemic analgesia therapy (SAT) and a sham injection. A blinded observer recorded patient pain intensity, quality of life (QOL) measures, opioid consumption and related side effects, and survival time for 1 year.

Baseline pain scores were relatively low, but comparable, in both groups (VAS 4.4 ± 1.7 vs. 4.1 ± 1.8, respectively). The first week after randomization, pain intensity and QOL scores were improved (pain intensity, $P \leq .01$ for both groups; QOL, $P < .001$ for both groups), with a more significant decrease in pain for the NCPB group ($P = .005$). Using repeated measures analysis, pain was found to be lower for NCPB over time ($P = .01$). However, opioid consumption ($P = .93$), frequency of opioid adverse effects (all $P > .10$), and QOL ($P = .46$) were not significantly different between groups.

In the first 6 weeks, fewer NCPB patients reported moderate or severe pain (pain intensity rating of $\geq 5/10$) compared to opioid-only patients (14% vs. 40%, $P = .005$). At 1 year, 16% of NCPB patients and 6% of opioid-only patients were alive, but this was not a statistically significant difference.

Although the previous study did not show a difference in life expectancy, a randomized, placebo-controlled study by Lillemoe et al.[41] in patients with abdominal pain and unresectable pancreatic cancer demonstrated longer survival when an intraoperative chemical splanchnicectomy was performed compared to patients who received saline. A subsequent study by Staats et al.[49] involved additional follow-up and analysis of this same group of patients. Data on visual analog pain scores, mood, and interference with activity were collected preoperatively and every 2 months postoperatively until death. Univariate and multivariate analyses of variance showed that neurolysis, compared to the medical management, had a significant positive effect on mood scores, pain interference with activity, and had an associated increase in life expectancy (9.15 ± 9.04 vs. 6.75 ± 4.65 months, $P < .05$).

Superior Hypogastric Plexus Block

Pelvic pain is common in advanced cervical, uterine, ovarian, bladder, rectal, and prostate cancers. When pain is primarily visceral in origin, the use of SHPB can be a safe and effective treatment to reduce pain and opioid needs.

INDICATIONS

The primary indication for superior hypogastric plexus nerve block is visceral pelvic pain that has been refractory to medical management. A local anesthetic block is sometimes performed first; however, in the setting of severe pain and advanced cancer, proceeding directly to neurolytic block may be preferred.

ANATOMY OF THE SUPERIOR HYPOGASTRIC PLEXUS

The superior hypogastric plexus spans the anterior surfaces of the lower L4 and L5 vertebral bodies and upper sacrum, posterior to the psoas fascia and peritoneum, and bounded laterally by the iliac vessels. This plexus innervates the pelvic viscera through the hypogastric nerves and inferior hypogastric plexus.

GENERAL CONSIDERATIONS

Prior to SHPB, normal coagulation studies should be confirmed, and anticoagulants should be discontinued for a period of time sufficient to allow normal coagulation. A discussion of the potential risks and benefits of SHPB should be undertaken and IV access obtained prior to the procedure to allow appropriate sedation and to allow the patient to comfortably lay in the prone position during the procedure. In the setting of severe ascites that precludes the prone position, the patient may be better treated with an anterior ultrasound or CT-guided approach. Of note, in contrast to celiac plexus neurolysis, there are no hemodynamic effects associated with SHPB.

ADVERSE EFFECTS

There have not been any reports of serious complication related to superior hypogastric plexus diagnostic block or neurolytic procedure. Given its location, potential adverse effects include neuraxial injection of neurolytic substance with resulting damage to the cauda equina, discitis, bladder injury, iliac vessel injury, intravascular injection, and retroperitoneal hematoma.

TECHNIQUES

SHPB is most commonly performed using fluoroscopy and a bilateral posterior approach, with appropriate needle placement confirmed with radiographic contrast (Figs. 44.6 and 44.7). A single needle technique, traversing the L5–S1 intervertebral disk, has also been described in patients with difficult anatomy compromising the bilateral approach, with good outcomes and

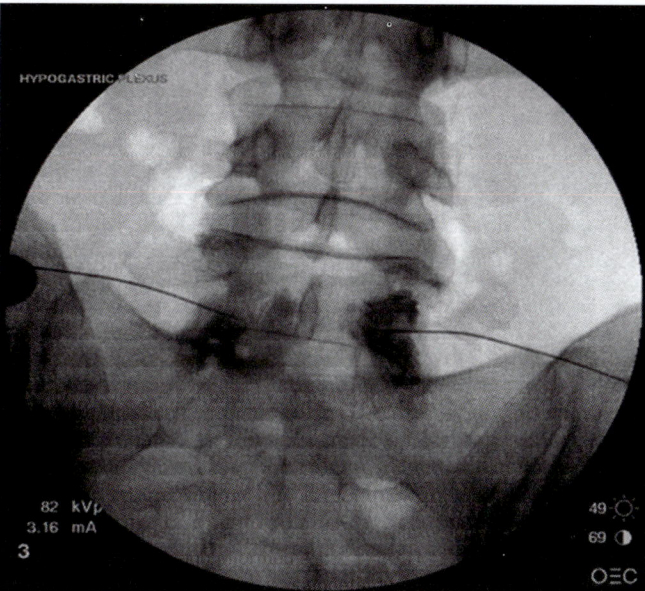

FIGURE 44.6 Fluoroscopic anteroposterior image of superior hypogastric plexus neurolysis.

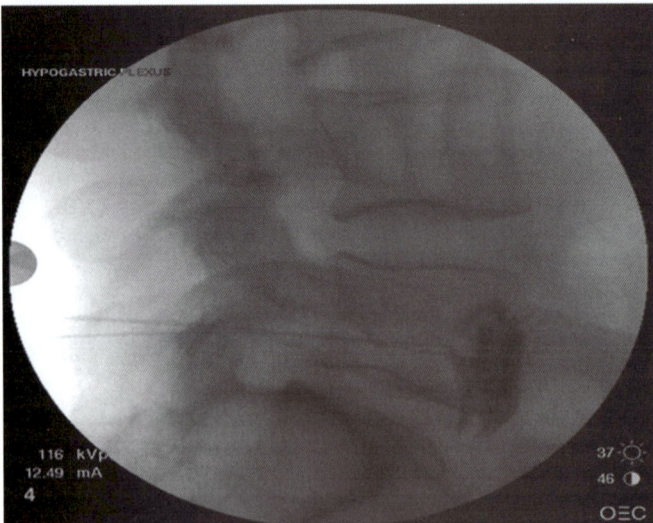

FIGURE 44.7 Fluoroscopic lateral image of superior hypogastric plexus neurolysis.

a favorable safety profile in a case series of eight patients.[50] Additionally, CT-guided and ultrasound-guided approaches have also been reported that has success using radiofrequency ablation rather than chemical neurolysis.[51-53]

OUTCOME STUDIES

Evidence supporting the use of superior hypogastric plexus neurolysis is limited to case reports, several prospective case series, and one randomized controlled trial. These studies have consistently demonstrated good to excellent pain relief in a majority of patients, reduced opioid consumption, and no significant adverse effects or complications.[32,54-58]

The largest study was published in 1997 by Plancarte and colleagues and reported on 227 patients with gynecologic, colorectal, or genitourinary cancer and cancer-related pelvic pain with poor pain control despite the use of oral opioids. All patients reported a VAS pain score of 7/10 or greater before a diagnostic block with 0.25% bupivacaine was performed. A positive response to the diagnostic block was obtained in 79% of patients, and these patients then went on to receive a neurolytic SHPB utilizing a bilateral percutaneous approach with 10% phenol. A second neurolytic block was offered in the event of suboptimal response to initial neurolytic block. SHPB reduced the VAS to <4/10 in 72% of patients, and the remaining 28% of patients had moderate reduction of VAS to 4 to 7/10. Oral opioid therapy was reduced 43% following neurolysis, no complications related to the procedure were reported, and no additional neurolytic blocks were required during the 3-month follow-up period.[56]

In the randomized controlled trial by Mishra et al.[57] 50 patients were randomized to anterior ultrasound-guided neurolytic SHPB plus oral morphine or oral morphine alone for severe pelvic pain associated with gynecologic malignancy. Patients treated with SHPB had a greater reduction in pain, lower total morphine consumption, greater patient satisfaction, and no increased incidence of adverse effects.[57]

A 2008 review of the literature applied evidence grades to 10 articles, including 4 case reports and 5 case series which received a grade of 1c and 1 prospective, randomized trial which received a grade of 1b in support of SHPB.[59] The European Association for Palliative Care (EAPC) conducted a systematic review in 2015 which lead to a weak recommendation for superior hypogastric plexus neurolysis for cancer-associated pelvic pain.[60]

Ganglion of Impar Block

The ganglion of impar, also known as the ganglion of Walther, is the terminal sympathetic ganglion in the body and neurolytic blockade of this ganglion that can aid in pain relief from visceral perineal pain as a result of neoplastic disease.

INDICATIONS

Ganglion of impar neurolysis is indicated for the treatment of visceral perineal pain as a result of primary or metastatic lesions of the distal rectum, anus, vulva, or perineum.

ANATOMY OF THE GANGLION OF IMPAR

The ganglion of impar is a solitary sympathetic ganglion located on the anterior inferior surface of the sacrum near the sacrococcygeal junction and supplies visceral innervation to the perineum and distal rectum/anus.

GENERAL CONSIDERATIONS

Normal coagulation profile should be confirmed and a discussion of the risks and benefits of ganglion impar neurolysis undertaken prior to the procedure. There are no hemodynamic effects of ganglion impar neurolysis, and the procedure often does not require sedation.

ADVERSE EFFECTS

Ganglion of impar neurolysis is a safe and technically straightforward procedure to perform. Reports in the literature of complications are rare. Given its location in close approximation to the rectum, care should be taken to avoid rectal perforation. Other potential risks include local infection or bleeding as well as intravascular injection.

TECHNIQUE

Neurolytic block of the ganglion of impar is most commonly performed using a percutaneous transcoccygeal approach with fluoroscopic guidance (Fig. 44.8).[61] A lateral view of the sacrum is obtained, and a needle inserted midline through the sacrococcygeal ligament until the tip lies just anterior to the sacrum, taking care to avoid perforating the rectum. Appropriate position is confirmed with contrast and a small amount of

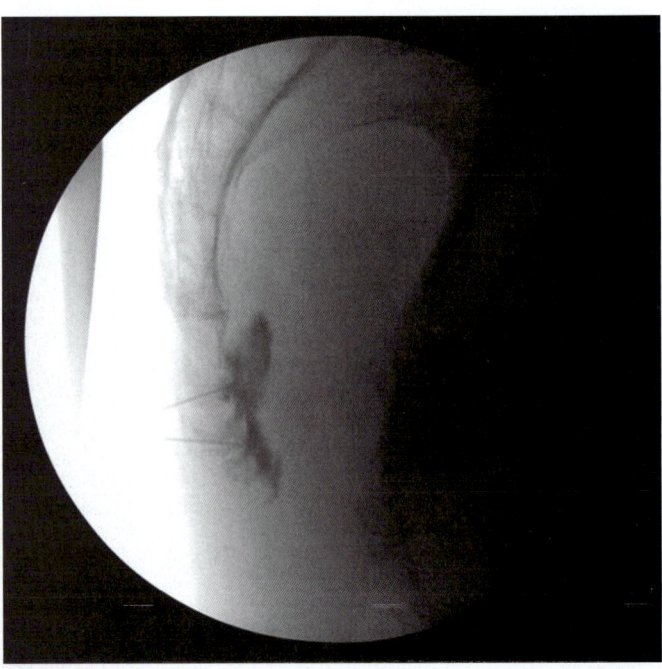

FIGURE 44.8 Fluoroscopic lateral view of ganglion of impar neurolysis.

local anesthetic is administered, followed by phenol or alcohol as a neurolytic agent. Approaching the ganglion of impar using an anococcygeal approach has also been described as having CT-guided approaches.[62]

Data regarding the efficacy of neurolytic ganglion of impar block for cancer-associated perineal pain are limited to case reports and case series. However, these studies consistently report significantly improved pain with no significant adverse effects.[59,61–64] In its 2017 Clinical Practice Guidelines in Oncology for Adult Cancer Pain, the National Comprehensive Cancer Network (NCCN) recommends consideration of ganglion impar block in the setting of cancer-associated rectal or perineal pain.[65]

Intercostal Nerve Block

Chest wall pain is a common symptom accompanying many cancers due to local tumor invasion as well as metastatic lesions to the area. Breast, lung, melanoma, and renal cell carcinomas are often associated with chest wall involvement and associated pain.

Oncologic chest wall pain often has both somatic and neuropathic components, making it potentially difficult to treat with conventional medications. Intercostal nerve block (ICNB) can be a useful adjunct in this setting.

INDICATIONS

ICNB is indicated in patients with cancer-associated chest wall pain recalcitrant to conservative medical treatment and palliative therapies such as radiation therapy.

ANATOMY OF THE INTERCOSTAL NERVES

The intercostal nerves and branches innervate the thoracic chest wall and parietal pleura. They arise from the ventral primary rami of T1–T12, which traverse the paravertebral space and then divide into anterior and posterior branches. The anterior branch forms the intercostal nerve and is initially located deep to the innermost intercostal muscle and superficial to the pleura. At approximately the midscapular line, the nerve pierces the innermost intercostal muscle and travels in a facial plane between the innermost intercostal and inner intercostal muscles until it terminates at the sternum. The intercostal nerve is reliably accessed at each level at the inferior aspect of the rib in close approximation but inferior to the intercostal artery and intercostal vein.

GENERAL CONSIDERATIONS

ICNB can be conducted as a diagnostic block with local anesthetic only or with therapeutic intention using either local anesthetic plus steroid or neurolytic agent. In many cases, a diagnostic block is first performed and if this provides short-term pain relief, neurolysis is then performed. Phenol is most commonly used; however, successful use of alcohol has also been described. Neurolysis will result in denervation of the associated intercostal muscles; however, this is rarely clinically significant unless multiple levels and/or bilateral blockade are performed in a patient with significantly compromised pulmonary function.

ADVERSE EFFECTS

There is a noteworthy risk of pneumothorax with ICNB due to the nerve's location in relation to the pleura. The ability to directly visualize the pleura and its relationship to the needle tip increasingly favors the use of ultrasound guidance with ICNB. Bleeding from intercostal vein or artery puncture can be a dangerous complication in patients who are anticoagulated.

As a result of the communication between the fascial planes of the intercostal muscles and the paravertebral space, there is also risk for neuraxial spread of medication. A 2016 study by Matchett[66] reported paravertebral extension of contrast dye

in 11/11 patients, and epidural extension in 1/11 patient, who underwent diagnostic ICNB. In the setting of local anesthetic, this results in a temporary unilateral paravertebral block or thoracic epidural block; however, there are two published case reports of permanent spinal cord injury resulting from intercostal neurolysis with phenol.[67,68] There is also a risk of deafferentation pain with neurolytic procedures using phenol or alcohol. Nevertheless, intercostal neurolysis is generally a safe and well-tolerated procedure with few reports of complications in the literature.

TECHNIQUE

Prior to the procedure, any available imaging should be reviewed to ensure correlation between the chest wall pathology and the patient's reported symptoms, with identification of the most likely rib level(s) affected. ICNB can be accomplished using either fluoroscopic or ultrasound guidance. In the case of fluoroscopic guidance, the appropriate rib is identified, and at a point 8 to 12 cm lateral to midline, the needle is inserted and advanced to contact bone, at which point it is carefully "walked off" the inferior aspect of the rib and advanced several millimeters. Contrast is then used to confirm spread along the inferior rib and rule out vascular uptake or neuraxial spread. Next, 2 to 3 mL of local anesthetic, local anesthetic plus steroid, or neurolytic substance is then injected slowly (Fig. 44.9).

For ultrasound-guided procedures, the appropriate level is identified, often by counting up from the 12th rib. The needle is inserted in an out-of-plane or in-plane approach, and hydrodissection is used to visualize the needle tip advancing into the fascial plane between the internal intercostal and innermost intercostal muscles, pushing pleura downward with medication administration, taking care to remain superficial to the pleura at all times (Fig. 44.10).

In addition to intercostal chemical neurolysis, a 2017 report detailed the successful use of thermal radiofrequency ablation of the intercostal nerves in 25 patients with uncontrolled cancer-related breakthrough pain arising from rib metastasis. More than half of patients experienced a 50% reduction in intensity and frequency of breakthrough pain episodes with minimal adverse effects.[69]

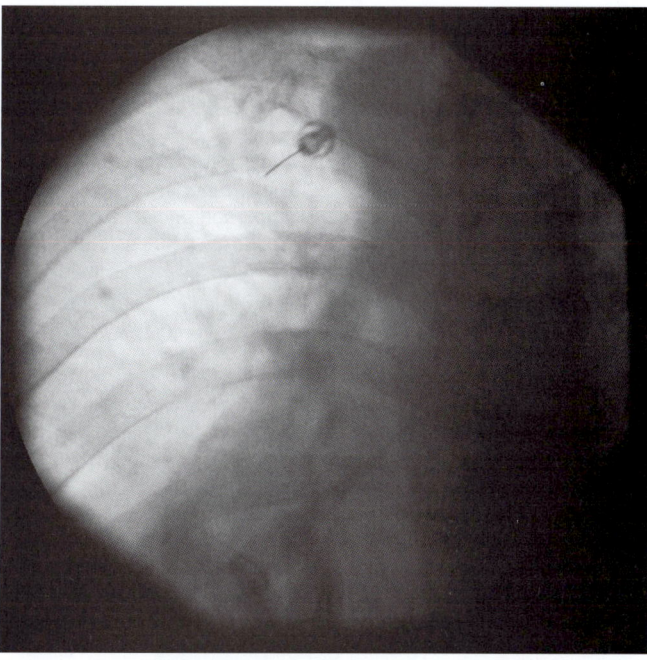

FIGURE 44.9 Fluoroscopic view of intercostal neurolysis with the needle tip inferior to the rib.

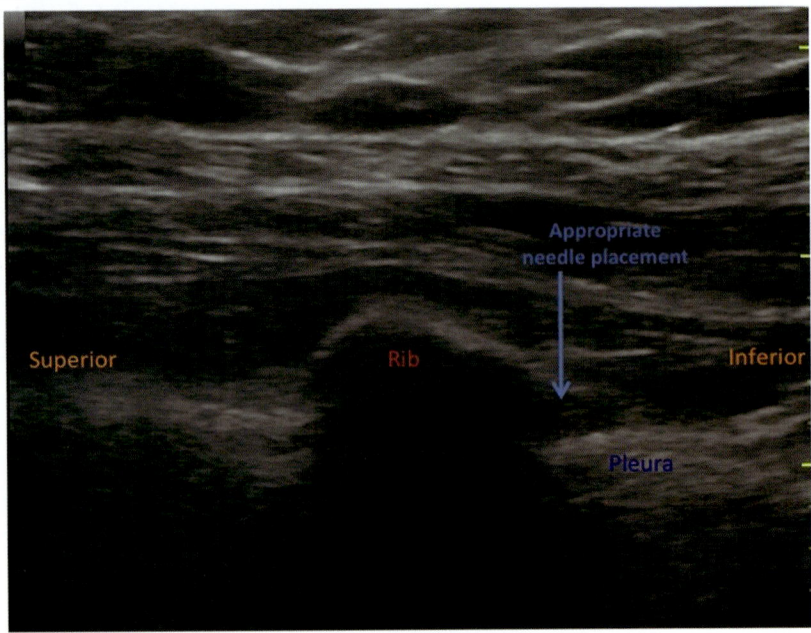

FIGURE 44.10 Ultrasound view of intercostal neurolysis with appropriate needle position indicated.

OUTCOME STUDIES

Published reports are limited to case reports and case series.[70] A 2007 publication detailed 25 patients with metastatic rib lesions who underwent neurolytic intercostal block. Optimal local pain control was reported in 80% of patients, and 56% reduced their analgesic use after the procedure.[71]

In 2015, Gulati et al.[72] reported on their experience with thoracic chest wall pain in the oncologic population between 2004 and 2014. Among 146 patients who underwent a diagnostic ICNB with local anesthetic and steroid, 79% had improvement in pain (defined as a reduction in VAS >1 point). Interestingly, 22% of patients had prolonged improvement in pain with an average duration of 21.5 days. However, only 32% of patients overall who responded to diagnostic blockade chose to undergo neurolytic ICNB with alcohol ablation, with a success rate of 62%. Additionally, the authors present an interventional treatment paradigm based on their review and clinical experience to guide the appropriate interventional modality for oncologic chest wall pain. In patients with peripheral tumor or anterior chest wall pain, they recommend diagnostic ICNB followed by neurolysis with good response to the diagnostic injection. However, with a more central location of tumor in the paravertebral area and posterior chest wall pain, they advocate for diagnostic paravertebral nerve block followed by paravertebral neurolysis as indicated if the tumor is not encroaching the thoracic nerve root and pulsed radiofrequency ablation of the thoracic nerve root in the setting of tumor encroachment on the neuroforamen (Fig. 44.11).

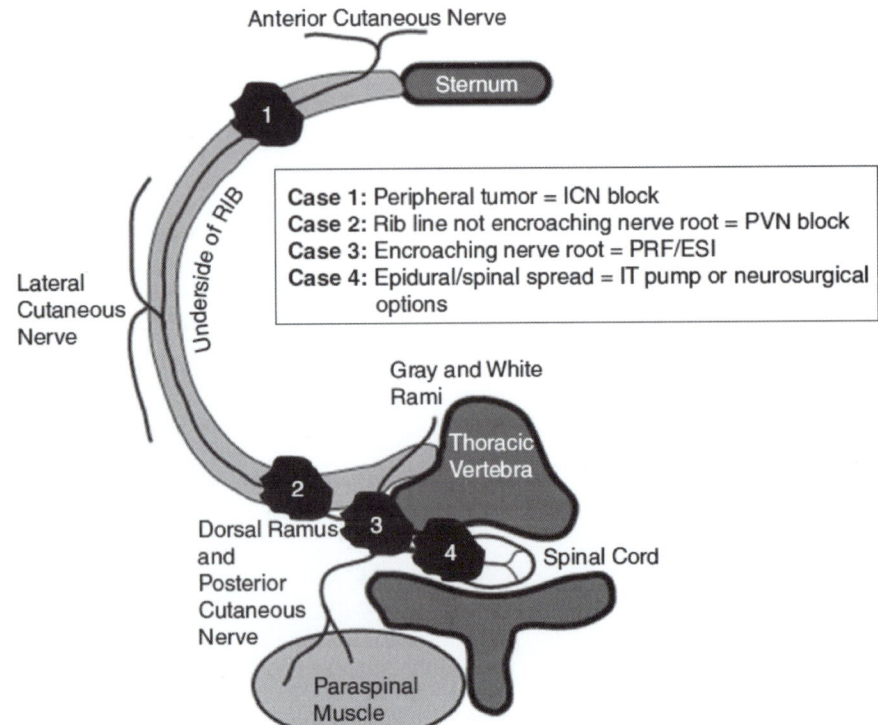

Case 1: Peripheral tumor = ICN block
Case 2: Rib line not encroaching nerve root = PVN block
Case 3: Encroaching nerve root = PRF/ESI
Case 4: Epidural/spinal spread = IT pump or neurosurgical options

FIGURE 44.11 Interventional procedure based on location of tumor for oncologic chest wall pain. ICN, intercostal nerve block; IT, intrathecal; PRF/ESI, pulsed radiofrequency/epidural steroid injection; PVN, paraventricular nucleus. *(Reprinted with permission from Gulati A, Shah R, Puttanniah V, et al. A retrospective review and treatment paradigm of interventional therapies for patients suffering from intractable thoracic chest wall pain in the oncologic population. Pain Med 2015;16[4]:802–810. Reproduced by permission of American Academy of Pain Medicine. Published online 2014 Sep 19. doi: 10.1111/pme.12558.)*

Blocks of the Head and Neck

Head and neck cancers have among the highest rates of cancer-associated pain, and these patients rate pain control just behind treatment outcome and life expectancy among their priorities after diagnosis.[73] Interventional targets for managing cancer-associated head and neck pain most commonly include the trigeminal ganglion and its branches; however, the autonomic sphenopalatine and stellate ganglia have also been successfully targeted.

Nerve Blocks of the Trigeminal Nerve and Its Branches

INDICATIONS

The trigeminal nerve is the fifth cranial nerve and has both motor and sensory function. In addition to innervating the muscles of mastication, it is responsible for sensation over most of the face. Neurolytic blockade of the trigeminal ganglion and its branches is indicated for patients with primary or metastatic head and neck cancer and associated severe pain. In the setting of cancer-associated pain, neurolytic blocks are most common, although local anesthetic block with indwelling catheter, thermal and pulsed radiofrequency ablation, and cryoablative techniques have all been described.[74–77]

ANATOMY OF THE TRIGEMINAL NERVE AND ITS BRANCHES

The trigeminal, or gasserian, ganglion arises from the brainstem and divides into its three primary branches, the ophthalmic nerve (V1), maxillary nerve (V2), and mandibular nerve (V3), just prior to exiting the skull via the superior orbital fissure, foramen rotundum, and foramen ovale respectively (Fig. 44.12).

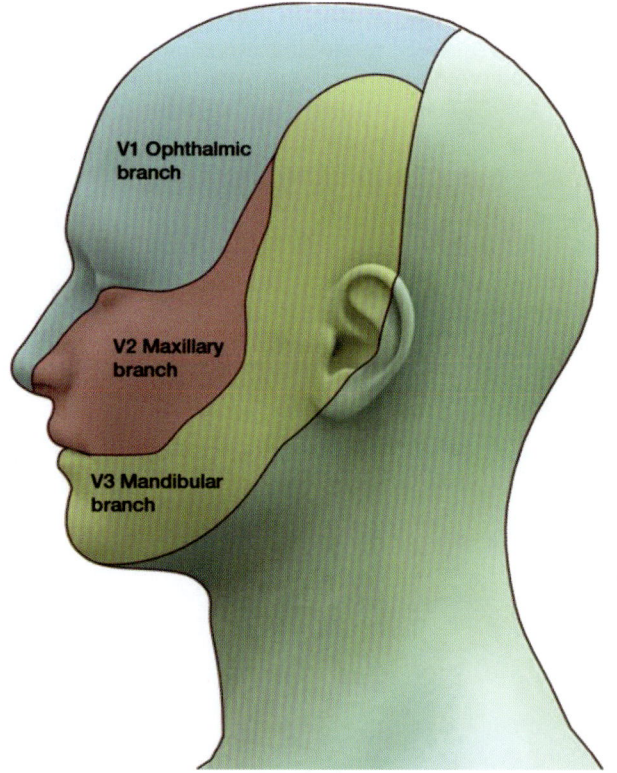

V1 Ophthalmic branch

V2 Maxillary branch

V3 Mandibular branch

FIGURE 44.12 Trigeminal nerve distribution. *(Reprinted with permission from Hoppenfeld JD. Fundamentals of Pain Medicine. 1st ed. Baltimore, MD: Lippincott Williams & Wilkins; 2014:20. Figure 2.1.)*

The ophthalmic nerve supplies sensory innervation to the skin of the scalp, forehead, upper eyelid, and tip of the nose via its terminal branches, the supraorbital and supratrochlear nerves. The maxillary nerve innervates the skin of the cheek, lower eyelid, nares, upper lip, upper teeth and gums, palate and roof, and the pharynx via its infraorbital and superior alveolar branches. In addition to supplying motor function to the muscles of mastication, the mandibular nerve innervates the skin of the chin, jaw, lower lip, external ear, and lower teeth and gums via its branches, the auriculotemporal, lingual, buccal, and inferior alveolar and mental nerves, all of which may be affected by direct tissue invasion, anatomic distortion, or metastatic lesions.[78]

GENERAL CONSIDERATIONS

Nerve blocks in the setting of head and neck cancer may present technical challenges owing to significant anatomic distortion from direct tumor invasion as well as prior surgical intervention. Both fluoroscopic and CT-guided approaches have been described for neurolytic blocks of the head and neck. The most common trigeminal nerve targets are summarized in Table 44.4.

ADVERSE EFFECTS

The trigeminal ganglion lies in close proximity to both the dura as well as the middle meningeal and carotid arteries, and care must be taken to avoid dural puncture, intrathecal injection, bleeding, or intravascular injection. Neuritis or deafferentation pain is a possible complication of neurolysis of the trigeminal ganglion or its branches. In the case of the ophthalmic (V1) branch, neurolysis can result in impaired corneal reflex and corneal anesthesia, whereas neurolysis of the mandibular branch may denervate the ipsilateral muscles of mastication. However, this is typically not clinically significant unless bilateral neurolysis blockade is performed, which can result in significant difficulties in chewing and swallowing.

TECHNIQUES

The trigeminal ganglion is most commonly accessed via the foramen ovale. A submental fluoroscopic view is used to identify the foramen and a needle is inserted 2.5 cm lateral to the corner of mouth. The needle is advanced in a trajectory in line with the ipsilateral pupil and an AP plane bisecting an imaginary line bisecting the angle between the external auditory meatus and the lateral canthus of the eye. Needle advancement should be discontinued when a lateral view shows appropriate placement in the foramen ovale, directly inferior to the sella turcica (Figs. 44.13 and 44.14). Iodinated contrast 0.1 to 0.5 mL is used to verify correct placement of the needle followed by neurolysis with 0.3 to 0.5 mL of neurolytic agent, mostly commonly phenol.

TABLE 44.4	Summary of Trigeminal Nerve Targets
Anatomic Target	**Innervation**
Trigeminal ganglion	Sensory innervation of face Motor innervation of muscles of mastication
Maxillary nerve	Sensory innervation of middle 1/3 of face
Mandibular nerve	Sensory innervation of lower 1/3 of face Motor innervation of muscles of mastication
Supraorbital nerve	Sensory innervation of forehead, upper eyelid, and anterior scalp
Supratrochlear nerve	Sensory innervation of medial forehead, bridge of nose, medial upper eyelid
Infraorbital nerve	Sensory innervation of lower eyelid, medial cheek, lateral naris, upper lip
Mental nerve	Sensory innervation of lower lip and chin

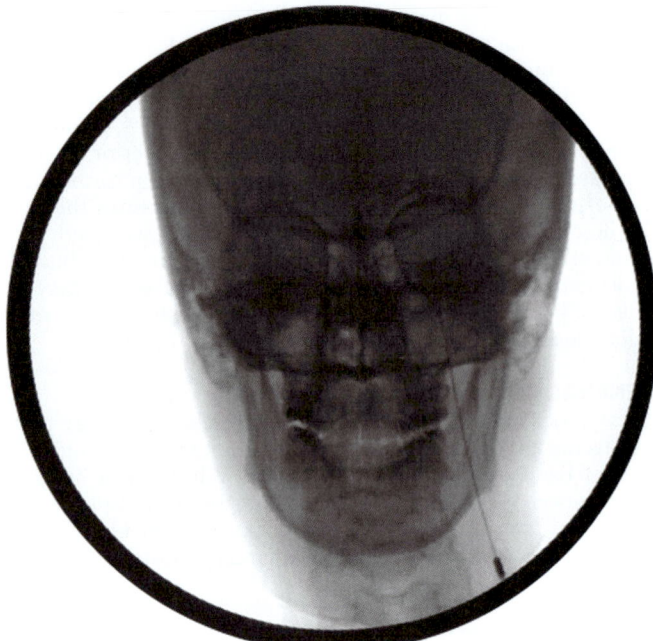

FIGURE 44.13 Fluoroscopic view of foramen ovale with needle in place—anteroposterior view.

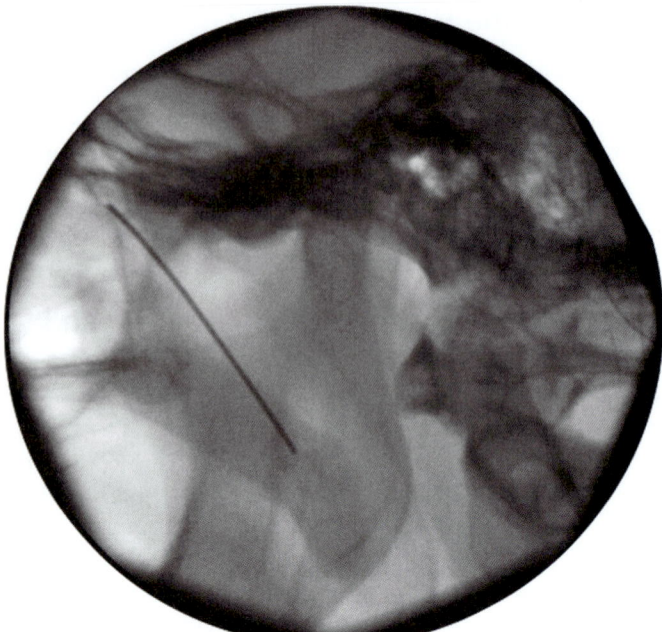

FIGURE 44.15 Lateral view of maxillary nerve block with needle in the superior anterior part of the pterygopalatine fossa.

To access the maxillary or mandibular nerve selectively, the coronoid notch is palpated just anterior to the external auditory meatus and inferior to the zygomatic arch, with the patient in a "slack jaw" position. Lateral fluoroscopy is used to identify the pterygopalatine fossa as a V-shaped structure superior to the upper molars and inferior to the orbit. The needle is inserted and directed in a plane perpendicular to the skull toward to pterygopalatine fossa. Once the lateral pterygopalatine plate is encountered, the needle is then be redirected anteriorly and superiorly for the maxillary nerve, or posteriorly and inferiorly for the mandibular nerve, and advanced approximately 0.5 to 1 cm to enter the pterygopalatine fossa. The position is

confirmed with AP fluoroscopic view showing the needle tip lateral to the middle nasal turbinate as well as with appropriate contrast spread (Figs. 44.15 and 44.16). In this location, chemical neurolysis has been reported anecdotally using phenol or alcohol, but no case reports or studies have been published. More commonly, local anesthetic and steroid or pulsed radiofrequency ablation is utilized.

The terminal branches of the maxillary and mandibular nerves are also interventional targets for cancer-related facial pain. Given their more superficial positions, chemical neurolysis is used infrequently, and local anesthetic and steroid as well as pulsed radiofrequency ablation are preferred.

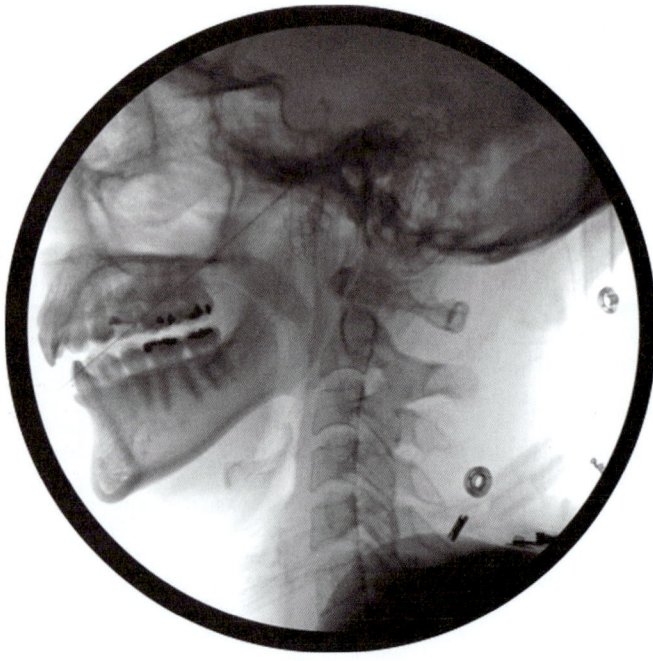

FIGURE 44.14 Fluoroscopic view of foramen ovale with needle in place—lateral view.

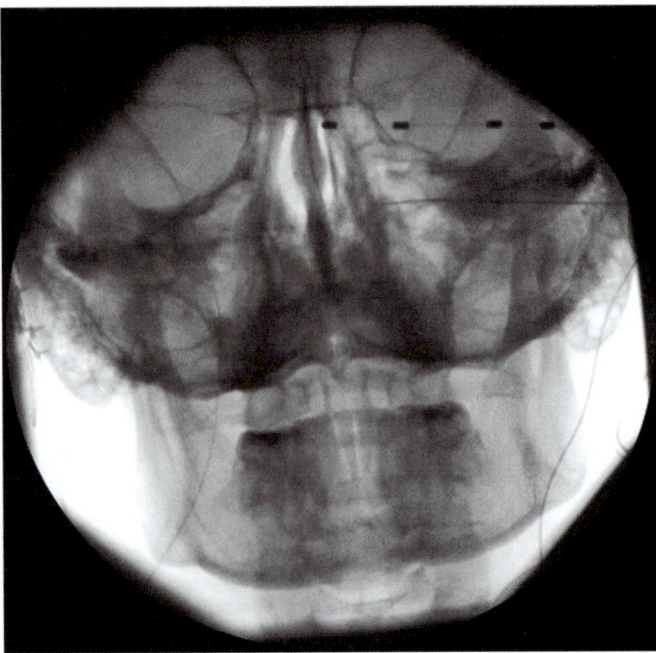

FIGURE 44.16 Anteroposterior view of maxillary nerve block.

The supraorbital nerve, innervating the skin of the ipsilateral forehead, is accessed by identifying the supraorbital foramen using fluoroscopy or palpating the supraorbital notch above the pupil along the orbital rim. The needle is then advanced toward the notch in a slight medial direction, taking care not to enter the foramen itself. The supratrochlear nerve, innervating the medial aspect of the forehead, is found by palpating the supratrochlear notch along the medial aspect of the supraorbital ridge just lateral to the junction of the supraorbital ridge and the bridge of the nose. The needle is advanced toward the notch until bone is contacted and then withdrawn slightly.

In the case of the infraorbital nerve, which innervates the lower eyelid, medial cheek, and lateral nares and upper lip, the infraorbital notch is identified using AP fluoroscopy and a needle is inserted 1 cm inferior and lateral to this. The needle is in an upward lateral trajectory toward the foramen. Finally, the mental nerve can be found by identifying the mental foramen using fluoroscopy or with palpation slightly superior to the mandible approximately 1 cm medial to the angle of the lip. A needle is directed toward the foramen in a slightly medial direction until bone is contacted.

OUTCOME STUDIES

Most published reports on trigeminal nerve interventions address its use for trigeminal neuralgia, with a reported success rate of 80% to 90%.[76] The literature in cancer pain is limited to case reports.[74,75,77] However, given the high burden of pain in the head and neck cancer population, the use of interventional treatment targeting the trigeminal ganglion and its distal branches should be considered for pain refractory to conservative treatment.

OTHER HEAD AND NECK INTERVENTIONAL TARGETS

The sphenopalatine ganglion (SPG) is a mixed parasympathetic and sympathetic ganglion that lies in close approximation to the maxillary nerve in the pterygopalatine fossa and has multiple connections to trigeminal and facial nerve fibers. It has been implicated in many facial pain and headache conditions and can be targeted in a similar fashion to the maxillary nerve block detailed previously, with the needle positioned slightly more inferiorly in the pterygopalatine fossa.[79,80] Varghese and Koshy[81], in 2001, reported good results with endoscopic neurolytic block of the SPG with phenol, but data on percutaneous approaches has been limited. In 2017, Sanghavi et al.[82] published a report of 33 patients with severe pain related to advanced head and neck cancer who underwent thermal radiofrequency ablation of the SPG following successful diagnostic block. Pain was reduced from an average VAS 8.4 to 1.4 after the procedure, and morphine consumption decreased to one-third the preprocedural level, with relief persisting for an average of 18 weeks.[82] Similarly, Rana[83] published a report of 20 patients with cancer-related orofacial pain, half of whom underwent pulsed radiofrequency ablation of the SPG and half who underwent SPG neurolytic block with alcohol. The authors did not report their technique for the procedures, but both groups experienced improved pain, with the radiofrequency ablation group having slightly better pain control at 1 month.[83]

Similar to SPG, the stellate ganglion is a sympathetic ganglion implicated in headache and neuropathic facial pain syndromes. It is formed from fusion of the inferior cervical first thoracic ganglia and overlies the anterolateral T1 and T2 vertebral bodies. It can be accessed under fluoroscopic or ultrasound guidance at Chassaignac tubercle at the C6 level. Ghai et al.[84] reported in 2016 on the use of stellate ganglion block with phenol and corticosteroid for intractable cancer-related facial pain and edema not amenable to trigeminal or sphenopalatine approaches due to anatomic distortion.

Spinal Cord Stimulation

The need for frequent magnetic resonance imaging (MRI) studies in cancer patients has previously limited the use of spinal cord stimulation in treating cancer-related pain. However, there are now multiple spinal cord stimulator systems that have MRI-conditional labeling, indicating these devices pose no known hazards in the specified MRI environment under specified conditions.

The use of spinal cord stimulation for cancer pain has expanded in recent years with this change, although data are limited to case reports and small case series. Spinal cord stimulation has been used successfully for multiple types and locations of cancer pain, including pain directly resulting from anal cancer, metastatic colon cancer, testicular cancer, and angiosarcoma.[85–88] There are also reports of its use for pain related to cancer treatment, including chronic chest wall pain following thoracotomy and radiation, chemotherapy-induced peripheral neuropathy, phantom limb pain following amputation, and failed back surgery syndrome related to resection of spinal tumors.[85,89,90]

Vertebral Augmentation

The percutaneous treatment of painful vertebral collapse secondary to metastatic tumor has emerged as a very promising therapy in recent years. Metastatic spread to the skeleton is common, and 30% to 80% of bony metastases involve the vertebrae (see Chapter 46).[91] Vertebroplasty is a minimally invasive outpatient procedure whereby painful vertebral compression fractures are stabilized by the injection of the bone cement polymethyl methacrylate (PMMA). Access to the vertebral body is typically achieved by passing a specialized needle under fluoroscopic guidance through the pedicles bilaterally.

Kyphoplasty differs in that the injection of cement is preceded by the creation of a cavity with a percutaneously placed intravertebral balloon, as demonstrated in Figure 44.17. Traditionally, the balloon inflation was intended to restore vertebral height loss, but this often requires very high pressures which may have been responsible for morbidity.

Vertebral height restoration is now considered less important, and the emphasis is now on creating a cavity so the cement injection can be performed under lower hydrostatic pressures with more predictable filling of the fractured vertebrae. A meta-analysis comparing vertebroplasty and kyphoplasty studies showed that vertebroplasty produced more significant pain relief but had a higher risk of cement extravasation into the spinal canal.[92]

INDICATIONS

Vertebroplasty or kyphoplasty are indicated in an acute or subacute (<6 months) painful vertebral body pathologic (secondary to osteoporosis or tumor) fracture without the involvement of the spinal canal and its elements.[92,93] Careful clinical correlation between the pain symptoms and the radiographic findings should be established because not all radiographically evident fractures are symptomatic. If there is doubt about the significance of a fracture, or in the presence of fractures at multiple levels, clinical correlation is often best achieved by examining the spine with the aid of fluoroscopy while palpating or percussing the spinous process of the vertebrae in question to see if concordant pain can be elicited. In the case of a fracture involving the spinal canal, actual or impending neurologic deficits are best treated by a surgical approach with decompression and probable spinal fusion.

CONTRAINDICATIONS

Absolute contraindications to vertebroplasty and kyphoplasty include asymptomatic stable fractures, clinically effective medical

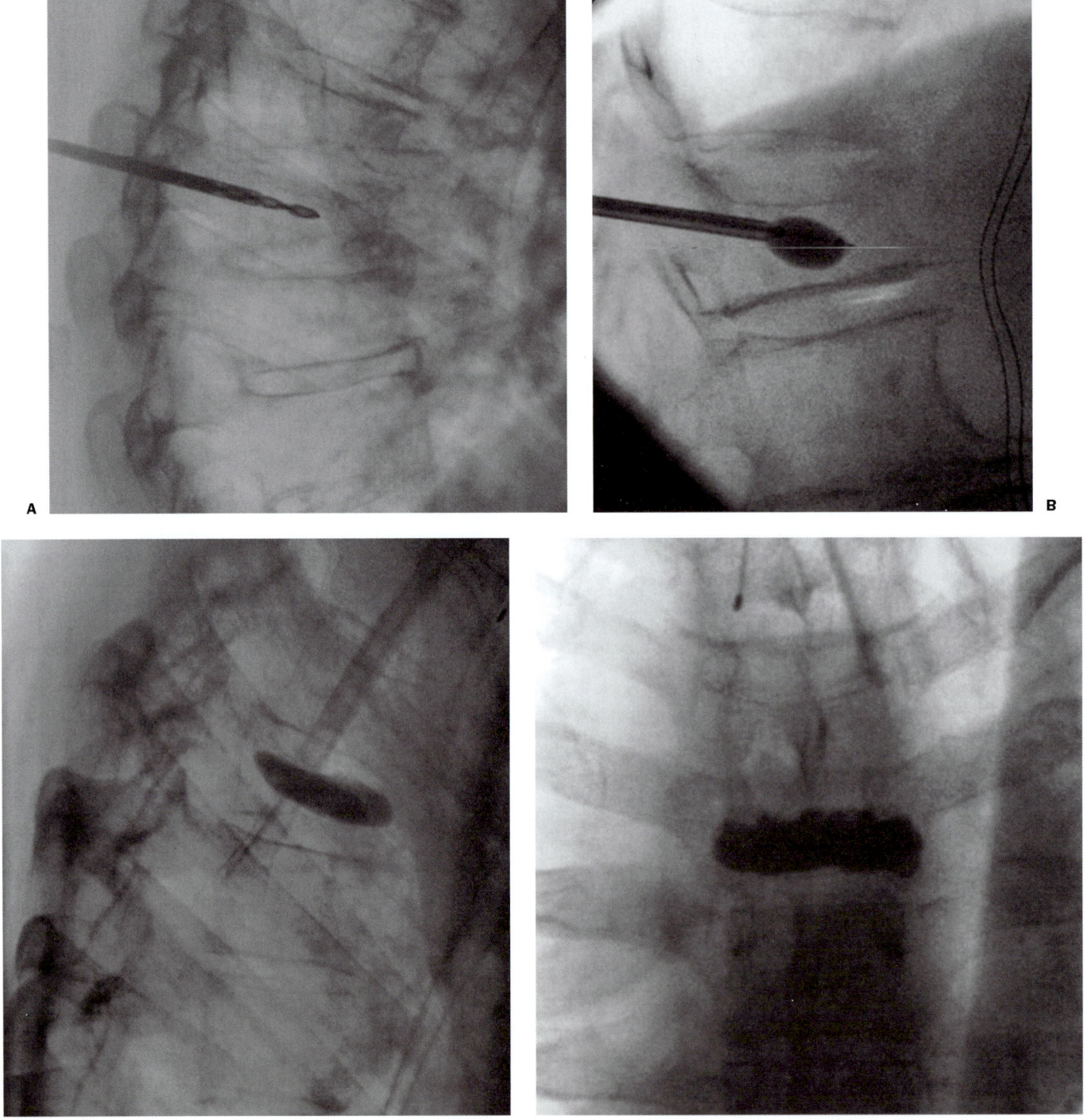

FIGURE 44.17 Kyphoplasty. **A:** Lateral projection of a thoracic vertebra with cannula in an appropriate position to traverse the pedicle and enter the vertebral body. **B:** Lateral projection demonstrating inflation of the balloon. **C:** Lateral projection demonstrating completed kyphoplasty following injection of cement. **D:** Anteroposterior projection of the completed kyphoplasty with the deposition of cement into the fracture site.

therapy, osteomyelitis of target vertebra, uncorrected coagulation disorders, allergy to any required component, and local or systemic infection. Relative contraindications include radicular pain or radiculopathy caused by a compressive syndrome unrelated to vertebral body collapse, a retropulsed fragment with >20% spinal canal compromise, tumor extension into epidural space, and severe vertebral body collapse (vertebra plana). The need for subsequent radiation to the area is not a contraindication because PMMA has been shown to be resilient to radiation at therapeutic doses.

OUTCOMES

Both vertebroplasty and kyphoplasty have consistently shown a significant improvement in postprocedure pain scores. In a meta-analysis by Eck et al.,[92] 168 eligible studies on vertebroplasty and kyphoplasty were assessed for their comparative analgesic efficacy and rates of complication. The mean pre- and postoperative VAS scores for vertebroplasty were 8.36 and 2.68, respectively, with a mean change of 5.68 ($P < .001$). The mean pre- and postoperative VAS scores for kyphoplasty were 8.06 and 3.46, respectively, with a mean change of 4.60 ($P < .001$).

The pain reduction for vertebroplasty was noted to be statistically greater ($P < .001$) compared with kyphoplasty. However, the risk of new vertebral fracture was 17.9% with vertebroplasty versus 14.1% with kyphoplasty ($P < .01$), and the risk of cement leak was 19.7% with vertebroplasty versus 7.0% with kyphoplasty ($P < .001$).

An important 2011 study by Berenson et al.[94] looked at balloon kyphoplasty versus conservative management in cancer-related vertebral compression fractures. There were 134 patients randomly assigned to either group, with the primary follow-up at 1 month. The kyphoplasty group, compared to conservative management group, demonstrated improved function relating to back pain as measured by the Roland-Morris Disability Questionnaire (RDQ), with the mean score in the kyphoplasty group changing from 17.6 at baseline to 9.1 (mean change −8.3 points, 95% CI −6.4 to −10.2; $P < .0001$) and the mean score in the control group changing from 18.2 to 18.0 (mean change 0.1 points; 95% CI −0.8 to 1.0; $P = .83$). At 1 month, the kyphoplasty treatment effect for RDQ was −8.4 points (95% CI −7.6 to −9.2; $P < .0001$). The most common adverse events were back pain (4 of 70 in the kyphoplasty group and 5 of 64 in the control group) and symptomatic vertebral fracture (two and three, respectively). One patient in the kyphoplasty group had an intraoperative non–Q-wave myocardial infarction, which was not directly related to the procedure.

A possible, emerging adjunct to vertebral augmentation for cancer of the spine is radiofrequency ablation followed by cementoplasty, although there is presently no data to support this therapy over vertebral augmentation alone.[95]

Spinal Cord Ablation

Spinal ablation remains a relevant and important technique for the treatment of medically refractory cancer pain. Interruption of the spinothalamic tract (cordotomy) or the dorsal column's visceral pain pathway (myelotomy) can be achieved either through open surgical techniques including laminectomy or percutaneously. Advantages of these techniques as compared with IT drug delivery include immediate onset pain relief, no ongoing medical visits for maintenance of therapy, and cost-effectiveness.

Cordotomy

INDICATIONS

Cordotomy, a lesion of the spinothalamic tract, is highly effective for the treatment nociceptive pain due to cancer. Cordotomy is safest when performed unilaterally, so as to avoid the well-documented complication of inducing sleep apnea by disrupting the bilateral interruption of reticulospinal fibers.[96,97] Due to the decussation of spinothalamic fibers, cordotomy is effective for pain arising two to five segments below the targeted spinal level. Because cordotomy is usually performed percutaneously at the C1–C2 level, it can usually have an effect on pain arising from the C5 or C6 dermatomes and below (Fig. 44.18).

SURGICAL TECHNIQUES

Although fluoroscopy can be used as the primary imaging modality for cordotomy, the additional safety and accuracy afforded by intraoperative CT imaging has improved outcomes for this procedure. Cordotomy may be performed either in an operating room equipped with a CT scanner or in the diagnostic radiology suite.

On the day of the procedure, the patient is transported to the diagnostic CT scanning area. A lumbar puncture is performed and IT contrast is administered to obtain an adequate

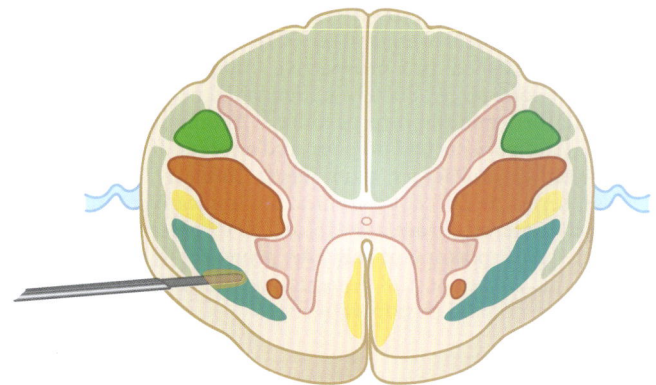

FIGURE 44.18 Cordotomy. Axial section of the cervical spine showing the spinothalamic tract ascending in the anterolateral quadrant of the spinal cord. A radiofrequency electrode is used to create a thermal lesion.

cervical myelogram. The patient is placed in the Trendelenburg position for 15 to 20 minutes to allow adequate dispersion of the contrast. IV sedation is provided, and local anesthetic is infiltrated in the skin approximately 1 cm inferior and posterior to the tip of the mastoid. A CT scan of the cervical spine is obtained, focusing on the C1–C2 region. A disposable percutaneous cordotomy electrode (LCED; Cosman Medical, Burlington, Massachusetts) kit may be used for this procedure. A 20-gauge spinal needle is advanced toward the C1–C2 interspace, and intermittent short-segment CT scans spanning 15 mm are used to direct the needle toward the dura. For lower extremity pain, the target for the spinal needle is just anterior to the AP midpoint of the spinal cord; for pain in the chest or upper extremities, the target is 1 to 2 mm more anterior to this. The tip of the spinal needle is advanced further until it is adjacent to the spinal cord. At this point the stylet was replaced with the electrode.

Electrical impedance measurement along with tactile feedback is used to determine the location of the electrode. When the electrode is in CSF, the impedance will measure a few hundred ohms ($<300\ \Omega$). As the electrode abuts and presses into the pia of the spinal cord, the impedance will increase significantly into the range of several hundred ohms (300 to 500 Ω). Entrance of the electrode into the spinal cord is met with a clear popping sensation, and the impedance will increase dramatically to greater than 700 Ω. At this point, another CT scan is obtained to confirm the position of the radiofrequency electrode.

Intraoperative physiologic testing is then performed to test for both sensory and motor effects. Sensory testing is performed at 100 hertz (Hz) and a 0.1-msec pulse width, whereas motor testing is performed at 2 Hz. At this point in the procedure, the patient's cooperation is needed, and hence, the sedation is adjusted until the patient can intelligibly answer questions. Sensory testing is performed to physiologically confirm the electrode tip's presence within the spinothalamic tract. Testing for motor contractions is also performed up to 1 V stimulation, indicating a safe distance from the corticospinal tract.

When the radiofrequency electrode is in the appropriate radiologic and physiologic location, lesioning is performed using increasing levels of temperature starting at 60° C for 60 seconds and proceeding up to 80° C for 60 seconds. Because lesioning the spinothalamic tract is not painful, additional sedation is not required for the ablation. Between lesions, testing for the development of hyperesthesia is helpful, because an additional lesion may be required if the patient has no decreased pinprick sensation. The goal of the cordotomy is to create a moderate hypoalgesia.

OUTCOMES

Two important neurosurgical series of CT-guided cordotomy have been published. In a prospective study of 41 patients who underwent cordotomy, 80% of patients had no pain postoperatively and for 1 month postprocedure.[98] At 6 months postprocedure, 32% of patients had no pain, and another 48% of patients had partially satisfactory pain relief. Similarly, in Kanpolat et al.'s[99] series of 207 cordotomies, a significant improvement in the pain intensity from a mean of 7.6/10 preoperatively to a mean of 1.3/10 postoperatively was achieved. When Kanpolat reported his subset of 108 patients with lung cancer, 89% of patients had no pain postoperatively.

COMPLICATIONS

Cordotomy has become a much safer procedure in the era of CT guidance. The risk associated with spinal needle insertion and penetration of the radiofrequency electrode into the pia of the spinal cord appears to be negligible. The radiofrequency ablation itself can be a source of complication for cordotomy. Hence, the art of cordotomy is determining the appropriate balance between an aggressive lesion to optimize a durable pain outcome and a safe lesion to avoid undesired side effects.

In 2008, Raslan[98] reported his series of 41 patients who underwent cordotomy, and no patients were found to have new neurologic deficits. In Kanpolat et al.'s[99] series of 207 cordotomies, 5 patients (2.4%) developed temporary weakness and 5 patients (2.4%) developed temporary ataxia. These symptoms resolved within 3 weeks after the procedure. In the 251 CT-guided cordotomies reported in the literature, four patients (1.6%) had dysesthetic pains. Respiratory complications or serious neurologic injury has not been reported using a CT-guided approach.

Myelotomy

INDICATIONS

Preclinical studies have augmented our understanding of the midline dorsal columns visceral pain pathway. The primary afferents for this dorsal column visceral pain pathway travel to cell bodies situated in the nucleus proprius and in the region of the spinal grey matter dorsal to the central canal of the spinal cord. From here, the axons ascend ipsilaterally along the midline portion of the dorsal columns prior to synapsing in the nucleus gracilis.[100–102]

Midline myelotomy seeks to interrupt this dorsal column visceral pain pathway. Candidates for midline myelotomy include patients with intractable visceral pain associated with malignancy in the abdominal or pelvic region.

SURGICAL TECHNIQUE

Myelotomy can be performed percutaneously or with a limited open surgical technique.

PERCUTANEOUS RADIOFREQUENCY LESIONING

Kanpolat et al.'s[103] first reported the technique for performing percutaneous radiofrequency myelotomy. This procedure can be performed either at the occiput-C1 level or in the thoracic spine. As Kanpolat et al.[103] has reported better experience using a larger diameter electrode for myelotomy, a custom 26-gauge radiofrequency electrode of diameter 0.46 mm (Cosman Medical, Burlington, Massachusetts) is the electrode of choice. This compares with the cordotomy electrode of 0.33 mm in diameter which has also been explored for myelotomy.

A spinal myelogram is performed prior to the procedure to visualize the spinal cord, and the patient is positioned prone with head flexed under monitored anesthesia care.

Intraoperative CT guidance is used to target the space between the occiput and C1 level or the relevant thoracic

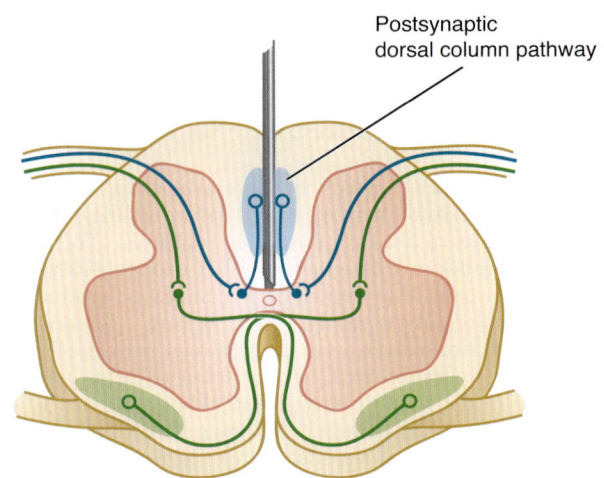

FIGURE 44.19   Myelotomy. Axial section of the thoracic spine showing the dorsal columns visceral pain pathway ascending bilaterally at the medial extent of the dorsal columns. A spinal needle is used to create a mechanical lesion during myelotomy.

level. The spinal needle is advanced toward the midline of the spinal cord from a posterior approach. The radiofrequency electrode is introduced into the spinal cord parenchyma with the goal of advancing the electrode to the AP midpoint of the spinal cord (Fig. 44.19). Impedance measurements are used to confirm the presence of electrode in the spinal cord parenchyma, and sensory stimulation (100 Hz, 100 μs) is performed, which can elicit lower limb paresthesias, usually at voltages less than 0.2 V. Two radiofrequency ablations at 70° C to 80° C for 60 seconds are performed.

OPEN LIMITED MYELOTOMY

A technique initially described by Nauta and others can be used to perform an open punctate myelotomy.[104–108] Under general anesthesia, patients are placed in the prone position and the surgical level is confirmed using fluoroscopy. With the understanding that the goal of surgery is the interruption of an ascending pain pathway, a spinal level is chosen which is rostral to the source of pain. Based on previous reports, the T3 or T4 level is chosen for upper abdominal pain, and the T6 to T8 level is chosen for perineal pain. A single-level thoracic laminectomy is performed at the intended level of lesioning. As the procedure is performed in the thoracic spine which is stabilized by the rib cage, a wide laminectomy is performed to allow visualization of the root entry zone bilaterally. Visualization of the root entry zone bilaterally helps to confirm the midpoint of the spinal cord. A midline dural incision is made, and dural retention sutures are placed. Preservation of the midline dorsal vein is attempted in all cases by mobilization of the vein if it obscured the dorsal median sulcus. Once the midline is confirmed, the pia is coagulated with a microbipolar. A 16-gauge angiocatheter is used to create the lesion. The catheter portion of the angiocatheter assembly is cut to allow an exposed tip of 5 mm, the desired lesion depth. Four lesions are made in one location by rotating the angiocatheter 90 degrees between lesions. The goal is to create a lesion that extends 0.5 mm from the midline bilaterally, with a lesion depth of 5 mm. The dura is closed with running sutures without the use of dural sealants, relaying on meticulous fascial closure to prevent CSF leak. The patient is mobilized on the evening of surgery.

OUTCOMES

Clinical studies for patients undergoing limited midline myelotomy have shown satisfactory pain relief in the majority of patients, lasting a few weeks to over 30 months.[106,109] The long-term durability of pain relief is difficult to assess given the short survival times due to the malignancy. Gildenberg and Hirshberg[110] reported excellent outcomes in 12 patients undergoing open limited myelotomy as compared to 2 patients undergoing percutaneous mechanical myelotomy. Kanpolat et al.'s[103] observed poorer outcomes in patients undergoing radiofrequency lesioning with smaller electrodes (0.25 mm diameter and 1 mm tip). Many reports, however, have not used a standardized outcome scale to evaluate pain relief, and therefore, a detailed comparison between open and percutaneous approaches is difficult to perform.

COMPLICATIONS

Motor complications when using image-guided percutaneous techniques are rare, given the opportunity for intraoperative motor stimulation and the relative distance of the corticospinal tract from the midline of the spinal cord. Using an open surgical technique is similarly safe, provided that care is taken to ensure the lesion is made in the midline.

We have found spinal cord motor and sensory monitoring to be a valuable adjunct to open punctate myelotomy.

As the lesion in myelotomy is between the dorsal columns, transient dysfunction of the dorsal columns can occur. This may manifest as decreased proprioception, sensations of coolness, or tingling. These side effects are generally mild and well tolerated.

Dorsal Root Entry Zone Lesioning

Dorsal root entry zone (DREZ) lesioning, an effective intervention for brachial plexus avulsion, has also been applied to the care of patients with cancer pain. DREZ may be considered for conditions such as radiation-induced brachial plexopathy and Pancoast tumors. However, in routine care of cancer patients, DREZ is not commonly used because it is a relatively large intradural operation which involves a multilevel laminectomy. The interested reader is directed to Gadgil and Viswanathan.[111]

IMAGE-GUIDED ABLATION OF PAINFUL BONE METASTASES

Isolated bone pain secondary to metastatic tumor activity is typically treated with external beam radiation, analgesics (opioids and nonsteroidal anti-inflammatory agents), and systemic therapies including bisphosphonates, radiopharmaceuticals, corticosteroids, and chemotherapy (see Chapters 43, 46, and 48). A recent advance has been the use of radiologically guided needle placement into selected painful metastases to provide thermal destruction using radiofrequency energy,[112] laser, and cryoablative[113,114] techniques. Another technique is percutaneous alcohol injection using selective arterial embolization[115] or direct tumor infiltration.[116]

A multicenter study by Goetz et al.[112] treated 43 patients who had failed standard therapy for painful osteolytic metastases with image-guided radiofrequency ablation. Ninety-five percent of patients had a clinically significant reduction in pain (VAS decrease of ≥ 2 on a 10-point scale). Before treatment, the mean worst pain score was 7.9; after treatment, the average worst pain score was 4.5 ($P < .0001$) at 4 weeks, 3.0 ($P < .0001$) at 12 weeks, and 1.2 ($P < .0005$) at 24 weeks. Pain interference scores and opioid consumption also improved during the 24 weeks of reported follow-up. Complications were seen in three patients: Two were not serious, whereas one involved an acetabular fracture following radiofrequency ablation to this area.

Summary

Interventional therapies have a well-defined and beneficial role in the treatment of appropriately selected patients with various cancer pain syndromes. Optimizing outcomes depends on timely referral with adequate assessment and patient selection; managing expectations of referring physicians, patients, and family members; assuring adequacy of postinterventional care; and an experienced, skilled interventionalist who will assume full responsibility for pre- and postintervention evaluation and follow-up care as indicated by the dictates of each patient's circumstances.

References

1. Cleeland CS, Gonin R, Hatfield AK, et al. Pain and its treatment in outpatients with metastatic cancer. *N Engl J Med* 1994;330(9):592–596.
2. Vainio A, Auvinen A. Prevalence of symptoms among patients with advanced cancer: an international collaborative study. Symptom Prevalence Group. *J Pain Symptom Manage* 1996;12(1):3–10.
3. Meuser T, Pietruck C, Radbruch L, et al. Symptoms during cancer pain treatment following WHO-guidelines: a longitudinal follow-up study of symptom prevalence, severity and etiology. *Pain* 2001;93(3):247–257.
4. van den Beuken-van Everdingen MH, de Rijke JM, Kessels AG, et al. Prevalence of pain in patients with cancer: a systematic review of the past 40 years. *Ann Oncol* 2007;18(9):1437–1449.
5. Smith TJ, Staats PS, Deer T, et al. Randomized clinical trial of an implantable drug delivery system compared with comprehensive medical management for refractory cancer pain: impact on pain, drug-related toxicity, and survival. *J Clin Oncol* 2002;20(19):4040–4049.
6. Eisenberg E, Carr DB, Chalmers TC. Neurolytic celiac plexus block for treatment of cancer pain: a meta-analysis. *Anesth Analg* 1995;80(2):290–295.
7. Deer TR, Pope JE, Hayek SM, et al. The Polyanalgesic Consensus Conference (PACC): recommendations on intrathecal drug infusion systems best practices and guidelines. *Neuromodulation* 2017;20(2):96–132.
8. Ackerman LL, Follett KA, Rosenquist RW. Long-term outcomes during treatment of chronic pain with intrathecal clonidine or clonidine/opioid combinations. *J Pain Symptom Manage* 2003;26(1):668–677.
9. Baker L, Lee M, Regnard C, et al. Evolving spinal analgesia practice in palliative care. *Palliat Med* 2004;18(6):507–515.
10. Nitescu P, Hultman E, Appelgren L, et al. Bacteriology, drug stability and exchange of percutaneous delivery systems and antibacterial filters in long-term intrathecal infusion of opioid drugs and bupivacaine in "refractory" pain. *Clin J Pain* 1992;8(4):324–337.
11. Bahar M, Rosen M, Vickers MD. Chronic cannulation of the intradural or extradural space in the rat. *Br J Anaesth* 1984;56(4):405–410.
12. Crul BJ, Delhaas EM. Technical complications during long-term subarachnoid or epidural administration of morphine in terminally ill cancer patients: a review of 140 cases. *Reg Anesth* 1991;16(4):209–213.
13. Bedder MD, Burchiel K, Larson A. Cost analysis of two implantable narcotic delivery systems. *J Pain Symptom Manage* 1991;6(6):368–373.
14. Smith TJ, Coyne PJ, Staats PS, et al. An implantable drug delivery system (IDDS) for refractory cancer pain provides sustained pain control, less drug-related toxicity, and possibly better survival compared with comprehensive medical management (CMM). *Ann Oncol* 2005;16(5):825–833.
15. Brogan SE, Winter NB. Patient-controlled intrathecal analgesia for the management of breakthrough cancer pain: a retrospective review and commentary. *Pain Med* 2011;12(12):1758–1768.
16. Brogan SE, Winter NB, Okifuji A. Prospective observational study of patient-controlled intrathecal analgesia: impact on cancer-associated symptoms, breakthrough pain control, and patient satisfaction. *Reg Anesth Pain Med* 2015;40(4):369–375.
17. Stearns L, Boortz-Marx R, Du Pen S, et al. Intrathecal drug delivery for the management of cancer pain: a multidisciplinary consensus of best clinical practices. *J Support Oncol* 2005;3(6):399–408.
18. Schmidtko A, Lötsch J, Freynhagen R, et al. Ziconotide for treatment of severe chronic pain. *Lancet* 2010;375(9725):1569–1577.
19. Staats PS, Yearwood T, Charapata SG, et al. Intrathecal ziconotide in the treatment of refractory pain in patients with cancer or AIDS: a randomized controlled trial. *JAMA* 2004;291(1):63–70.
20. Dupoiron D, Bore F, Lefebvre-Kuntz D, et al. Ziconotide adverse events in patients with cancer pain: a multicenter observational study of a slow titration, multidrug protocol. *Pain Physician* 2012;15(5):395–403.
21. Eisenach J, Detweiler D, Hood D. Hemodynamic and analgesic actions of epidurally administered clonidine. *Anesthesiology* 1993;78(2):277–287.
22. Follett KA, Boortz-Marx RL, Drake JM, et al. Prevention and management of intrathecal drug delivery and spinal cord stimulation system infections. *Anesthesiology* 2004;100(6):1582–1594.
23. Engle MP, Vinh BP, Harun N, et al. Infectious complications related to intrathecal drug delivery system and spinal cord stimulator system implantations at a comprehensive cancer pain center. *Pain Physician* 2013;16(3):251–257.
24. Coffey RJ, Burchiel K. Inflammatory mass lesions associated with intrathecal drug infusion catheters: report and observations on 41 patients. *Neurosurgery* 2002;50(1):78–87.
25. Cousins M. In: Cousins MJ, Bridenbaugh PO, eds. *Neural Blockade in Clinical Anesthesia and Management of Pain: Percutaneous Neural Destructive Techniques.* 3rd ed. Philadelphia: Lippincott Williams & Wilkins; 1998:1022–1033.
26. Swerdlow M. Intrathecal neurolysis. *Anaesthesia* 1978;33(8):733–740.

27. Candido K, Stevens RA. Intrathecal neurolytic blocks for the relief of cancer pain. *Best Pract Res Clin Anaesthesiol* 2003;17(3):407–428.

28. Swerdlow M. Subarachnoid and extradural blocks. *Adv Pain Res Ther* 1979;2:325.

29. Ischia A, Luzzani A, Pacini L, et al. Lytic saddle block: clinical comparison of the results, using phenol at 5, 10, and 15 percent. *Adv Pain Res Ther* 1984;7:339.

30. Ischia S, Luzzani A, Ischia A, et al. Subarachnoid neurolytic block (L5–S1) and unilateral percutaneous cervical cordotomy in the treatment of pain secondary to pelvic malignant disease. *Pain* 1984;20(2):139–149.

31. Lifshitz S, Debacker LJ, Buchsbaum HJ. Subarachnoid phenol block for pain relief in gynecologic malignancy. *Obstet Gynecol* 1976;48(3):316–320.

32. de Oliveira R, dos Reis MP, Prado WA. The effects of early or late neurolytic sympathetic plexus block on the management of abdominal or pelvic cancer pain. *Pain* 2004;110(1–2):400–408.

33. Ward EM, Rorie DK, Nauss LA, et al. The celiac ganglia in man: normal anatomic variations. *Anesth Analg* 1979;58(6):461–465.

34. Rykowski JJ, Hilgier M. Efficacy of neurolytic celiac plexus block in varying locations of pancreatic cancer: influence on pain relief. *Anesthesiology* 2000;92(2):347–354.

35. De Cicco M, Matovic M, Balestreri L, et al. Single-needle celiac plexus block: is needle tip position critical in patients with no regional anatomic distortions? *Anesthesiology* 1997;87(6):1301–1308.

36. De Cicco M, Matovic M, Bortolussi R, et al. Celiac plexus block: injectate spread and pain relief in patients with regional anatomic distortions. *Anesthesiology* 2001;94(4):561–565.

37. De Conno F, Caraceni A, Aldrighetti L, et al. Paraplegia following coeliac plexus block. *Pain* 1993;55(3):383–385.

38. Woodham MJ, Hanna MH. Paraplegia after coeliac plexus block. *Anaesthesia* 1989;44(6):487–489.

39. Davies DD. Incidence of major complications of neurolytic coeliac plexus block. *J R Soc Med* 1993;86(5):264–266.

40. Ischia S, Ischia A, Polati E, et al. Three posterior percutaneous celiac plexus block techniques. A prospective, randomized study in 61 patients with pancreatic cancer pain. *Anesthesiology* 1992;76(4):534–540.

41. Lillemoe KD, Cameron JL, Kaufman HS, et al. Chemical splanchnicectomy in patients with unresectable pancreatic cancer. A prospective randomized trial. *Ann Surg* 1993;217(5):447–457.

42. Ischia S, Luzzani A, Ischia A, et al. A new approach to the neurolytic block of the coeliac plexus: the transaortic technique. *Pain* 1983;16(4):333–341.

43. Montero Matamala A, Vidal Lopez F, Inaraja Martinez L. The percutaneous anterior approach to the celiac plexus using CT guidance. *Pain* 1988;34(3):285–288.

44. Wiersema MJ, Wiersema LM. Endosonography-guided celiac plexus neurolysis. *Gastrointest Endosc* 1996;44(6):656–662.

45. Abedi M, Zfass AM. Endoscopic ultrasound-guided (neurolytic) celiac plexus block. *J Clin Gastroenterol* 2001;32(5):390–393.

46. Levy MJ, Topazian MD, Wiersema MJ, et al. Initial evaluation of the efficacy and safety of endoscopic ultrasound-guided direct ganglia neurolysis and block. *Am J Gastroenterol* 2008;103(1):98–103.

47. Mercadante S. Celiac plexus block versus analgesics in pancreatic cancer pain. *Pain* 1993;52(2):187–192.

48. Wong GY, Schroeder DR, Carns PE, et al. Effect of neurolytic celiac plexus block on pain relief, quality of life, and survival in patients with unresectable pancreatic cancer: a randomized controlled trial. *JAMA* 2004;291(9):1092–1099.

49. Staats PS, Hekmat H, Sauter P, et al. The effects of alcohol celiac plexus block, pain, and mood on longevity in patients with unresectable pancreatic cancer: a double-blind, randomized, placebo-controlled study. *Pain Med* 2001;2(1):28–34.

50. Ina H, Kobyashi MD, Imai S, et al. A new approach to the superior hypogastric plexus block: transvertebral disc (L5–S1) technique. *Reg Anesth* 1992;17(suppl 3):123.

51. De Leon-Casasola OA, Plancarte-Sanchez R, Patt RB, et al. Superior hypogastric plexus block using a single needle and computed tomography guidance. *Reg Anesth* 1993;18(1):63.

52. Bosscher H. Blockade of the superior hypogastric plexus block for visceral pelvic pain. *Pain Pract* 2001;1(2):162–170.

53. Bharti N, Singla N, Batra Y. Radiofrequency ablation of superior hypogastric plexus for the management of pelvic cancer pain. *Indian J Pain* 2016;30(1):58–60.

54. Plancarte R, Amescua C, Patt RB, et al. Superior hypogastric plexus block for pelvic cancer pain. *Anesthesiology* 1990;73(2):236–239.

55. de Leon-Casasola OA, Kent E, Lema MJ. Neurolytic superior hypogastric plexus block for chronic pelvic pain associated with cancer. *Pain* 1993;54(2):145–151.

56. Plancarte R, de Leon-Casasola OA, El-Helaly M, et al. Neurolytic superior hypogastric plexus block for chronic pelvic pain associated with cancer. *Reg Anesth* 1997;22(6):562–568.

57. Mishra S, Bhatnagar S, Rana SP, et al., Efficacy of the anterior ultrasound-guided superior hypogastric plexus neurolysis in pelvic cancer pain in advanced gynecological cancer patients. *Pain Med* 2013;14(6):837–842.

58. Ahmed DG, Mohamed MF, Mohamed SA. Superior hypogastric plexus combined with ganglion impar neurolytic blocks for pelvic and/or perineal cancer pain relief. *Pain Physician* 2015;18(1):E49–E56.

59. Day M. Sympathetic blocks: the evidence. *Pain Pract* 2008;8(2):98–109.

60. Mercadante S, Klepstad P, Kurita GP, et al. Sympathetic blocks for visceral cancer pain management: a systematic review and EAPC recommendations. *Crit Rev Oncol Hematol* 2015;96(3):577–583.

61. Eker HE, Cok OY, Kocum A, et al. Transsacrococcygeal approach to ganglion impar for pelvic cancer pain: a report of 3 cases. *Reg Anesth Pain Med* 2008;33(4):381–382.

62. Agarwal-Kozlowski K, Lorke DE, Habermann CR, et al. CT-guided blocks and neuroablation of the ganglion impar (Walther) in perineal pain: anatomy, technique, safety, and efficacy. *Clin J Pain* 2009;25(7):570–576.

63. Plancarte-Sánchez R, Guajardo-Rosas J, Guillén Núñez M. Superior hypogastric plexus block and ganglion impar (Walther). *Tech Reg Anesth Pain Manag* 2005;9(2):86–90.

64. Toshniwal GR, Dureja GP, Prashanth SM. Transsacrococcygeal approach to ganglion impar block for management of chronic perineal pain: a prospective observational study. *Pain Physician* 2007;10(5):661–666.

65. National Comprehensive Cancer Network. *NCCN Clinical Practice Guidelines in Oncology: Adult Cancer Pain.* Fort Washington, PA: National Comprehensive Cancer Network; 2017:1.

66. Matchett G. Intercostal nerve block and neurolysis for intractable cancer pain. *J Pain Palliat Care Pharmacother* 2016;30(2):114–117.

67. Kowalewski R, Schurch B, Hodler J, et al. Persistent paraplegia after an aqueous 7.5% phenol solution to the anterior motor root for intercostal neurolysis: a case report. *Arch Phys Med Rehabil* 2002;83(2):283–285.

68. Kissoon NR, Graff-Radford J, Watson JC, et al. Spinal cord injury from fluoroscopically guided intercostal blocks with phenol. *Pain Physician* 2014;17(2):E219–E224.

69. Ahmed A, Bhatnagar S, Khurana D, et al. Ultrasound-guided radiofrequency treatment of intercostal nerves for the prevention of incidental pain arising due to rib metastasis. *Am J Hosp Palliat Care* 2017;34(2):115–124.

70. Koyyalagunta D, Burton AW. The role of chemical neurolysis in cancer pain. *Curr Pain Headache Rep* 2010;14(4):261–267.

71. Wong FC, Lee TW, Yuen KK, et al. Intercostal nerve blockade for cancer pain: effectiveness and selection of patients. *Hong Kong Med J* 2007;13(4):266–270.

72. Gulati A, Shah R, Puttanniah V, et al. A retrospective review and treatment paradigm of interventional therapies for patients suffering from intractable thoracic chest wall pain in the oncologic population. *Pain Med* 2015;16(4):802–810.

73. List MA, Stracks J, Colangelo L, et al. How do head and neck cancer patients prioritize treatment outcomes before initiating treatment? *J Clin Oncol* 2000;18(4):877–884.

74. Mendelsohn D, Ranjan M, Hawley P, et al. Percutaneous trigeminal rhizotomy for facial pain secondary to head and neck malignancy. *Clin J Pain* 2013;29(10):e4–e5.

75. Koyyalagunta D, Mazloomdoost D. Radiofrequency and cryoablation for cancer pain. *Tech Reg Anesth Pain Manag* 2010;14(1):3–9.

76. Day M. Neurolysis of the trigeminal and sphenopalatine ganglions. *Pain Pract* 2001;1(2):171–182.

77. Kohase H, Umino M, Shibaji T, et al. Application of a mandibular nerve block using an indwelling catheter for intractable cancer pain. *Acta Anaesthesiol Scand* 2004;48(3):382–383.

78. Faltas B, Phatak P, Sham R. Mental nerve neuropathy: frequently overlooked clinical sign of hematologic malignancies. *Am J Med* 2011;124(1):e1–e2.

79. Piagkou M, Demesticha T, Troupis T, et al. The pterygopalatine ganglion and its role in various pain syndromes: from anatomy to clinical practice. *Pain Pract* 2012;12(5):399–412.

80. Narouze SN. Role of sphenopalatine ganglion neuroablation in the management of cluster headache. *Curr Pain Headache Rep* 2010;14(2):160–163.

81. Varghese BT, Koshy RC. Endoscopic transnasal neurolytic sphenopalatine ganglion block for head and neck cancer pain. *J Laryngol Otol* 2001;115(5):385–387.

82. Sanghavi P, Patel D, Joshi G. Radiofrequency ablation of sphenopalatine ganglion for head and neck cancer pain management. *Indian Journal of Pain* 2017;31(1):13–17.

83. Rana SPS. Pulsed RFA of sphenopalatine ganglion vs. alcohol neurolysis for facial pain in cancer-related pain: a prospective study. *J Pain Symptom Manage* 2017;53(2):467.

84. Ghai A, Kaushik T, Kumar R, et al. Chemical ablation of stellate ganglion for head and neck cancer pain. *Acta Anaesthesiol Belg* 2016;67(1):6–8.

85. Yakovlev AE, Resch BE, Karasev SA. Treatment of cancer-related chest wall pain using spinal cord stimulation. *Am J Hosp Palliat Care* 2010;27(8):552–556.

86. Yakovlev AE, Ellias Y. Spinal cord stimulation as a treatment option for intractable neuropathic cancer pain. *Clin Med Res* 2008;6(3–4):103–106.

87. Yakovlev AE, Resch BE. Spinal cord stimulation for cancer-related low back pain. *Am J Hosp Palliat Care* 2012;29(2):93–97.

88. Nouri KH, Brish EL. Spinal cord stimulation for testicular pain. *Pain Med* 2011;12(9):1435–1438.

89. Cata JP, Cordella JV, Burton AW, et al. Spinal cord stimulation relieves chemotherapy-induced pain: a clinical case report. *J Pain Symptom Manage* 2004;27(1):72–78.

90. Viswanathan A, Phan PC, Burton AW. Use of spinal cord stimulation in the treatment of phantom limb pain: case series and review of the literature. *Pain Pract* 2010;10(5):479–484.

91. Mercadante S. Malignant bone pain: pathophysiology and treatment. *Pain* 1997;69(1–2):1–18.
92. Eck JC, Nachtigall D, Humphreys SC, et al. Comparison of vertebroplasty and balloon kyphoplasty for treatment of vertebral compression fractures: a meta-analysis of the literature. *Spine J* 2008;8:488–497.
93. Heary RF, Bono CM. Metastatic spinal tumors. *Neurosurg Focus* 2001;11(6):e1.
94. Berenson J, Pflugmacher R, Jarzem P, et al. Balloon kyphoplasty versus non-surgical fracture management for treatment of painful vertebral body compression fractures in patients with cancer: a multicentre, randomised controlled trial. *Lancet Oncol* 2011;12(3):225–235.
95. Anchala PR, Irving WD, Hillen TJ, et al. Treatment of metastatic spinal lesions with a navigational bipolar radiofrequency ablation device: a multicenter retrospective study. *Pain Physician* 2014;17(4):317–327.
96. Krieger AJ, Rosomoff HL. Sleep-induced apnea. 1. A respiratory and autonomic dysfunction syndrome following bilateral percutaneous cervical cordotomy. *J Neurosurg* 1974;40(2):168–180.
97. Nannapaneni R, Behari S, Todd NV, et al. Retracing "Ondine's curse." *Neurosurgery* 2005;57(2):354–363.
98. Raslan AM. Percutaneous computed tomography-guided radiofrequency ablation of upper spinal cord pain pathways for cancer-related pain. *Neurosurgery* 2008;62(3 suppl 1) 226–234.
99. Kanpolat Y, Ugur HC, Ayten M, et al. Computed tomography-guided percutaneous cordotomy for intractable pain in malignancy. *Neurosurgery* 2009;64(suppl 3):ons187–194.
100. Wang Y, Wu J, Lin Q, et al. Effects of general anesthetics on visceral pain transmission in the spinal cord. *Mol Pain* 2008;4:50.
101. Al-Chaer ED, Lawand NB, Westlund KN, et al. Pelvic visceral input into the nucleus gracilis is largely mediated by the postsynaptic dorsal column pathway. *J Neurophysiol* 1996;76(4):2675–2690.
102. Willis WD, Al-Chaer ED, Quast MJ, et al. A visceral pain pathway in the dorsal column of the spinal cord. *Proc Natl Acad Sci U S A* 1999;96(14):7675–7679.
103. Kanpolat Y, Savas A, Caglar S, et al. Computerized tomography-guided percutaneous extralemniscal myelotomy. *Neurosurg Focus* 1997;2(1):e5.
104. Nauta HJ, Hewitt E, Westlund KN, et al. Surgical interruption of a midline dorsal column visceral pain pathway. Case report and review of the literature. *J Neurosurg* 1997;86(3):538–542.
105. Nauta HJ, Soukup VM, Fabian RH, et al. Punctate midline myelotomy for the relief of visceral cancer pain. *J Neurosurg* 2000;92(suppl 2):125–130.
106. Hong D, Andrén-Sandberg A. Punctate midline myelotomy: a minimally invasive procedure for the treatment of pain in inextirpable abdominal and pelvic cancer. *J Pain Symptom Manage* 2007;33(1):99–109.
107. Hwang SL, Lin CL, Lieu AS, et al. Punctate midline myelotomy for intractable visceral pain caused by hepatobiliary or pancreatic cancer. *J Pain Symptom Manage* 2004;27(1):79–84.
108. Kim YS, Kwon SJ. High thoracic midline dorsal column myelotomy for severe visceral pain due to advanced stomach cancer. *Neurosurgery* 2000;46(1):85–92.
109. Sindou M, Jeanmonod D, Mertens P. Ablative neurosurgical procedures for the treatment of chronic pain. *Neurophysiol Clin* 1990;20(5):399–423.
110. Gildenberg PL, Hirshberg RM. Limited myelotomy for the treatment of intractable cancer pain. *J Neurol Neurosurg Psychiatry* 1984;47(1):94–96.
111. Gadgil N, Viswanathan A. DREZotomy in the treatment of cancer pain: a review. *Stereotact Funct Neurosurg* 2012;90(6):356–360.
112. Goetz MP, Callstrom MR, Charboneau JW, et al. Percutaneous image-guided radiofrequency ablation of painful metastases involving bone: a multicenter study. *J Clin Oncol* 2004;22(2):300–306.
113. Tuncali K, Morrison PR, Winalski CS, et al. MRI-guided percutaneous cryotherapy for soft-tissue and bone metastases: initial experience. *AJR Am J Roentgenol* 2007;189(1):232–239.
114. Callstrom MR, Atwell TD, Charboneau JW, et al. Painful metastases involving bone: percutaneous image-guided cryoablation—prospective trial interim analysis. *Radiology* 2006;241(2):572–580.
115. Chiras J, Adem C, Vallée JN, et al. Selective intra-arterial chemoembolization of pelvic and spine bone metastases. *Eur Radiol* 2004;14(10):1774–1780.
116. Gangi A, Kastler B, Klinkert A, et al. Injection of alcohol into bone metastases under CT guidance. *J Comput Assist Tomogr* 1994;18(6):932–935.
117. Lossignol DA, Obiols-Portis M, Body JJ. Successful use of ketamine for intractable cancer pain. *Support Care Cancer* 2005;13(3):188–193.

CHAPTER 45

Pain Caused by Cancer of the Head and Neck and Oral and Oropharynx

ANDREI BARASCH and **JOEL BRIAN EPSTEIN**

Malignant diseases are generally associated with high morbidity, as both the disease and therapy tend to be invasive and may be life-threatening. Head and neck pain in cancer patients has various etiologies, including the tumor and/or metastases, surgical and cytotoxic therapies, or conditions unrelated to the cancer or its treatment (Table 45.1). Reportedly, pain is present in head and neck cancer (HNC) in 50% or more of patients before diagnosis, 80% during treatment, and 70% posttherapy.[1] In one-third of treated patients, pain continues for longer than 6 month, and its severity is higher than in the pretherapy period.

One of the most common cancer-related pain-producing conditions affecting the head and neck region is ulcerative upper aerodigestive tract mucositis. Mucositis can be a dose- and rate-limiting toxicity of cancer therapy. Furthermore, mucositis can lead to new admission to hospital or extend admission to hospital and is the most debilitating patient-reported complication due to pain and effect on oropharyngeal function. This chapter reviews the pathogenesis of mucositis, mechanisms of pain in HNC, and current strategies for preventing and managing these algesic conditions. Pain due to HNC and/or mucositis includes multiple mechanisms that affect soft tissues, vascular, bone, and nervous system structures, including molecular mechanisms associated with reactive oxygen species (ROS), inflammatory mediators, neuropeptide release, and stimulation of sensory receptors.[2-4] Phenotypic changes may occur, involving all levels of the sensory and autonomic nervous system, and are impacted by individual variables including genetic and psychosocial features. Understanding these mechanisms may lead to additional approaches for prevention and management of pain.

TABLE 45.1	Orofacial Pain in Cancer Patients

I. Acute
1. Caused by disease: invasion of bone, nerve, muscle, mucosal damage; tumor pressure
2. Caused by cancer therapy: surgery, radiation therapy, and chemotherapy
   a. Oral/dental pain: mucositis, infection (e.g., *Candida*, dental, HSV), neuropathy
3. Unrelated conditions causing pain (e.g., myofascial pain, trauma)

II. Chronic
1. Caused by persisting/progressive disease
2. Caused by cancer therapy: surgery, radiation therapy, and chemotherapy
   a. Mucosal atrophy/xerostomia
   b. Mucosal infection
   c. Neuropathy
   d. Temporomandibular (myofascial) disorders
   e. Dental caries
   f. Osteonecrosis/mucosal necrosis
   g. Postherpetic neuralgia
3. Unrelated conditions causing pain

HSV, herpes simplex virus.

Pain Mechanisms Due to Local and Regional Cancer of the Head and Neck

TUMOR-INDUCED ALGESIA

A tumor may compress and/or invade adjacent tissues, affecting afferent nerves directly or through production of inflammatory cytokines. For example, potential mechanisms of musculoskeletal pain due to malignancy include periosteal pressure, invasion of nerves, vascular damage, microfractures of bone, and muscle spasm. Inflammatory mechanisms can be activated by both tumor cells and cancer therapies and include release of cytokines and other algesic molecules that induce pain in the tumor environment of hypoxia and low pH. Tumors and tumor necrosis release growth factors and cytokines that activate inflammation and nociceptive pathways. In HNC, inflammation is a major cause of pain,[3,4] initiated by ROS, and release of mediators from tumor cells, leukocytes, platelets, endothelial cells, and immune cells resident in the affected tissue and sensory fiber stimulation (sensory and sympathetic). ROS may cause endothelial cell damage and increase vascular permeability, whereas nitric oxide (NO) may induce second messenger mechanisms within neurons that may cause neuropathic pain. Oxidative stress activates transcription factors that cause upregulation of proinflammatory cytokines and may trigger apoptosis that release cell contents leading to increased inflammation and sensory stimulation.

Tissue inflammation increases circulating kallikreins leading to production of bradykinin (BK) that produces and amplifies pain induced by serotonin (5-HT). Glutamate is upregulated at sites of inflammation and affects amino-3-hydroxy-5-methyl-4-isoazolepropionic acid (AMPA), N-methyl-D-aspartate (NMDA), stimulating pain receptors. Furthermore, inflammation increases the expression and sensitivity of ion channels (such as sodium channels) on nociceptors, which may be stimulated, increasing pain sensation.

The low pH in solid tumors appears to be due to inflammation, tumor cell metabolism, and apoptosis. The release of cellular contents may cause pain due to activation of sensory neurons through acid-sensing ion channels (ASICs). In addition, cancer-induced activation of osteoclasts results in lower pH and dissolution of bone mineral.

Tumor necrosis factor (TNF) may activate cytokines and growth factors that play a significant role in inflammation and neuropathic pain. TNF is also a key mediator in mucositis. Nerve growth factor (NGF) production is mediated by interleukin (IL)-1β and is upregulated by TNF-α. NGF activates cutaneous mast cells, leading to release of inflammatory mediators that induce pain and may also activate the sympathetic nervous system. Norepinephrine (NE) causes hyperalgesia at sites of tissue injury.

Prostaglandins (PGs) synthesized by cyclooxygenase pathways (COX-1 and COX-2) are induced by inflammatory cytokines and growth factors. Increased levels of PGs are seen in locoregional tumors and in metastases. PGs cause sensitization of afferent nerve fiber including C-fiber and Aδ high-threshold mechanonociceptors and mediate hyperalgesia induced by BK and NE. COX-2 pathways are also upregulated in HNC and in mucositis.[5]

Modulation of sensory transmission involves presynaptic upregulation of the primary signal by excitatory and inhibitory input from adjacent neurons and from descending pathways. In addition to local modulation, second-order neurons and central pathways are also subject to modulation from higher centers. Modulation may be mediated by interactions with receptors including AMPA, NMDA, and by neurotransmitters including substance P (SP), 5-HT, NE-A, opioid, cholecystokinin (CCK), and γ-aminobutyric acid (GABA). Modulation of pain signaling is impacted by stress, learned behavior, social/cultural background, and acute pain. Perception of pain is impacted by attention, expectation, anxiety, and depression. Mucosal changes, hyposalivation, chronic infection, neurovascular changes, musculoskeletal changes, persisting/recurrent cancer, and secondary complications of cancer or therapy may result in chronic pain.

Neuropathic pain may result from insult to the peripheral nervous system (PNS) and/or the central nervous system (CNS), including alteration in sensory and autonomic function, and may result in peripheral and/or central sensitization. Surgery or cytotoxic and targeted agents may lead to neuropathy due to nerve damage due to surgery or inflammation, resulting in ectopic firing and changes in receptive field leading to neuronal excitability and spontaneous activity or "wind-up." Neuronal hyperexcitability may be due to overexpression of sodium channels and activation of the NMDA receptor, which develops at voltage-gated sodium channels. Persistent input may also result in increased receptive fields in second-order neurons and centrally.

Interactions between the sympathetic nervous system and nociceptors are thought to be associated with neuropathic pain. Injured C-fiber terminals may atrophy and be replaced by Aβ fibers that may contribute to sensory abnormalities following peripheral nerve injuries. SP in Aβ fibers may be increased and lead to pain.

In addition to neuronal sensitization, TNF-α, IL-6, and IL-11 promote osteoclast formation, which may play a role in malignant bone pain. The effects of IL-1 are probably mediated by induction of NO, BK,[6] and PGs and endothelin-1 (ET-1) that may cause pain in cancer involving bone. Prevention and treatment of pain based on increased understanding of cellular and molecular mechanisms may lead to novel approaches and improved pain prevention and management.

Pain Mechanisms Due to Chemotherapy and/or Radiotherapy

Peripheral neurotoxicity is associated with a number of chemotherapeutic agents, including vinca alkaloids, and platinum agents may lead to damage or loss of large myelinated sensory fibers. NGF and induction of lysosomal storage defects occur in the dorsal root ganglion (DRG) following the use of these agents. The taxanes (paclitaxel, docetaxel) cause microtubular aggregation leading to neuropathy and increase the risk of neurotoxicity when combined with platinum agents. Other agents including noncytostatic drugs used in cancer treatment (e.g., interferon, thalidomide) or in supportive care (e.g., amphotericin-B) may also induce sensory neuropathy. Drug-induced neurotoxicity is typically dose dependent and has an idiosyncratic tendency. Additive effects may occur from combinations of drugs.

Treatment of neuropathy focuses on use of centrally acting medications.[7,8] Unfortunately, strategies for prevention of neuropathy are not well documented. Amifostine and lipoic acid have been assessed in the prevention of neurotoxicity caused by platinum agents.[9,10] Melatonin was shown in one clinical trial to reduce chemotherapy-induced neurotoxicity,[11] and the potential role of glutamine has been examined.[12,13] Continuing study of approaches to prevent and manage cancer therapy-induced neurotoxicity are urgently needed.

Bisphosphonates are key medications used in the treatment of malignant disease involving bone and are commonly used in patients with multiple myeloma and metastatic breast, prostate, lung, and colon cancers. Benefits of bisphosphonate therapy include prevention of skeletal-related events, hypercalcemia of cancer, and reducing bone pain associated with malignancy. One of the acute side effects associated with bisphosphonate administration can be bone pain, including mandible pain that may present with vague symptoms, but can occasionally mimic dental pain. Since late 2002, bisphosphonates have been associated with avascular necrosis involving dentoalveolar bone. In cancer patients on bisphosphonates, the most frequent risk factor for bisphosphonate-associated osteonecrosis (BON) is dental extractions, but other dental procedures appear to be safe.[14–20] Prevalence of BON is also associated with type and duration of bisphosphonate treatment. Pain associated with BON, when present, is usually associated with secondary infection of the soft and hard tissues surrounding the areas of exposed bone.[21,22] Chronic BON can spread to involve nerve bundles (e.g., the inferior alveolar nerve) and produce nerve pain and/or numbness.

Pain Due to Surgery

Pain is common at the time of diagnosis for those patients with HNC[23] but is typically of mild severity (Visual Analog Scale [VAS] 3/10).[24] Surgical extirpation may alleviate pain, but more often, following treatment for HNC, pain increases due to the procedure and generally improves with healing of the surgical site.[25] Furthermore, surgery on the neck is associated with fibrosis that may be increased with postoperative radiation therapy, leading to shoulder and arm pain.[23]

Wittekindt et al. showed that subcutaneous botulinum toxin A may reduce chronic neuropathic pain following neck dissection.[26,27] Botulinum toxin A achieves pain relief by preventing acetylcholine release at the neuromuscular junction. Further investigation of the potential effects on posttreatment fibrosis in the neck is warranted to guide clinical care.

Spread of disease to regional lymph nodes is a prognostic factor in HNC.[28] Treatment for cervical metastasis traditionally includes resection of lymph nodes from levels I through V, the sternocleidomastoid (SCM) muscle, internal jugular vein (IJV), and spinal accessory nerve (SAN), known as *radical neck dissection*, originally described by Crile[29] in 1906.

Recent studies show that neck dissection has a negative impact on quality of life (QOL) and health status.[30–34] It has been demonstrated that more extensive neck dissections are associated with higher shoulder-related disability.[32,33,35,36] Fortunately, over the latter half of the 20th century, neck dissection has evolved to more conservative surgical approaches that has led to improved QOL; however, shoulder and neck pain after neck dissection continues to be a common cause of postoperative morbidity in HNC patients.[37] It has been postulated that mechanical overload of the shoulder secondary to postsurgical change leads to shoulder pain.[38] However, even with preservation of the SAN, patients may have shoulder pain.[39,40] Dissection of level V lymph nodes (the posterior triangle of the neck) is associated with neck pain and shoulder pain.[41]

Attention to the preservation of cervical sensory nerves and effect on QOL has been assessed. Roh et al.,[41] in a retrospective cohort study of 53 patients treated with selective or modified radical neck dissection, suggest that cervical sensory root branch preservation reduces postoperative sensory deficits.

Pain Due to Mucositis

Oral mucositis is a frequent complication of cancer chemotherapy and radiotherapy. A five-stage model for oral mucositis has been proposed where ROS are generated during the initial phase,[5,42–44] leading to cell damage and upregulation of secondary mediators by activation of nuclear factor-κB (NFκB) in the epithelium and connective tissue. NFκB increases proinflammatory cytokines such as TNF-α, IL-1β, and IL-6, which increases inflammation-causing algesia. NO may also be a key factor causing pain. The ceramide pathway has been implicated in amplification of oral mucositis and may modulate pain. Ulceration of the mucosa exposes nerve fiber endings, thus sensitizing the entire surface. Additionally, these ulcerations can become secondarily colonized/infected and further increase cytokine release and mucosal pain.

In addition to mucosal damage, radiation therapy affects bone by damage to osteocytes, osteoclasts, and osteoblasts. Further radiation irreversibly damages endothelial cells in the vasculature throughout the high-dose radiated volume, which may result in hypocellular, hypovascular, and hypoxic oral soft tissue. These changes increase the risk of soft tissue necrosis and osteonecrosis.

EPIDEMIOLOGY

Mucositis is the most common cause of oral pain during intensive treatment of cancer involving chemotherapy, radiation, or chemoradiotherapy[45–73] (Table 45.2). Oral mucositis affects a majority of patients on myeloablative conditioning regimens used in hematopoietic cell transplantation (HCT) and is essentially universal in patients treated with tumoricidal radiation therapy in the oropharynx. The increasing use of combined chemotherapy and radiation treatment modalities and generally more aggressive therapy protocols to improve cancer cure rates have increased the frequency, severity, and duration of oral complications.[45,47,48,50,53,56,58,61,66,73]

Recent advances in cancer therapy have produced a significant increase in the use of targeted therapies. These typically consist of disease- and cell-specific inhibition of enzymes or receptors that interferes with tumor growth or its microenvironment. The potential impact of targeted monoclonal antibodies and other tumor-specific targeting molecules on mucositis has not been fully documented. Prospective studies that assess mucositis as a primary or secondary outcome with targeted agents have not been conducted,[74,75] although the pattern of oral mucosal involvement and dermatologic involvement appears different than that seen in traditional chemotherapy, suggesting that different mechanisms are involved. Targeted therapy adverse events are generally assumed to be milder than those of cytotoxic agents. Nevertheless, these adverse events can be severe or even dose limiting. Most of these effects are cutaneous and commonly affect the oral mucosa.[76] The oral effects generally consist of aphthous-like or, in the case of immune checkpoint inhibitors, lichenoid or bullous lesions and tend to be mild to moderate. However, lesions may become severe, particularly with the recently approved combination of immune checkpoint inhibitors.[77,78]

Advances in cancer pain management and supportive care now include the use of antimicrobial prophylaxis/therapy and the use of growth factors to speed hematopoietic recovery; these therapies have increased the focus on oral mucositis as a significant and treatment-limiting complication.[79–81] Oral mucositis is often coincident with therapy-related toxicity at other sites, including veno-occlusive disease in HCT[73] and gastrointestinal toxicity.[82] The potential for systemic infection caused by oral opportunistic and acquired flora associated with oral mucositis has been documented in studies of leukemia and HCT patients.[83–86]

PATHOGENESIS

Intensive cytotoxic chemotherapy and radiation therapy directly affect the proliferation of epithelial cells leading to damage of the epithelium and submucosal tissues and potentially to loss of integrity of the mucosal barrier (Fig. 45.1 and Table 45.3). Epidermal growth factor (EGF) secretion may increase the risk of mucositis,[87] and conversely, cytokines that reduce epithelial cell proliferation during cytotoxic therapy have the potential to decrease the severity of tissue damage. Interaction with cytokines produced in the connective tissue such as granulocyte-macrophage colony-stimulating factor (GM-CSF), TNF, IL-6, IL-11, and others may affect the extent tissue damage.[79,82,88,89] The oral microflora may play a role in progression of mucosal damage, as suggested in studies of gram-negative bacterial flora in radiation-induced mucositis. The outcomes of microflora-associated mucosal damage are influenced by the potential effect of cancer therapies on the hematopoietic system and damage to local and systemic immune function. Resolution of mucositis may be dependent on production of pluripotential growth factors affecting epithelial and connective tissues.[56,79–82] During resolution, cytokines inducing epithelial cell proliferation and migration as well as angiogenesis also play a role.[56,90–96] Pain associated

TABLE 45.2 Frequencies of Oral Pain Associated with Cancer Therapy	
Acute Pain during Treatment	
Oropharyngeal mucositis	
Chemotherapy	15% to 70%
Bone marrow transplant	50% to 85%
Radiation therapy	Up to 100%
Postsurgical therapy	Up to 100%
Chronic Pain following Cancer Therapy	
Mucosal pain	Up to 33%
Pain associated with mucosal infection	
Candidiasis	
After stem cell transplant	Up to 50%
After radiation therapy	20% to 33%
Herpes simplex in seropositive stem cell transplant patients	Up to 90%
Neuropathy	16%
TMD/myofascial (patients with head and neck squamous cell carcinoma)	25% to 30%

TMD, temporomandibular disorder.

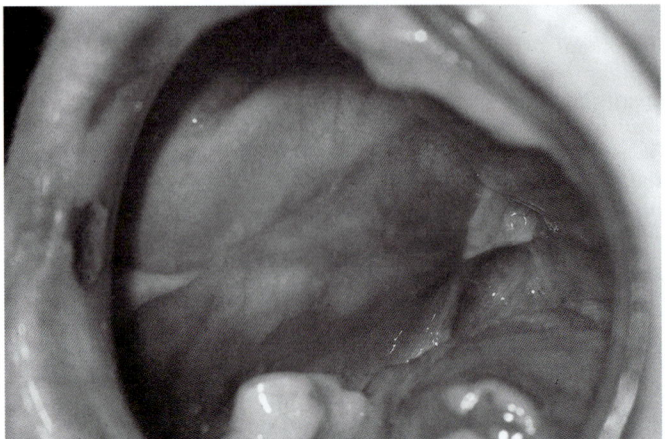

FIGURE 45.1 Mild mucositis with erythema and minor erosion of the cheek mucosa in a patient following autologous bone marrow transplant (at day +14). Mild mouth discomfort was reported.

TABLE 45.3 Factors Contributing to Oropharyngeal Mucositis	
Direct Factors	**Indirect Factors**
Radiation therapy	Myelosuppression
Dose/fraction	Immunosuppression
Total dose/days	T-cell loss/dysfunction
Chemotherapy	B-cell loss/dysfunction
Drug/dose/schedule	Reduced secretory
Bone marrow transplant	immunoglobulin A
Chemotherapy	Infections
Irradiation	Bacterial
Salivary gland dysfunction	Plaque control
Mucosal trauma	Viral
Physical	Herpes simplex
Chemical	Varicella zoster
Thermal	Cytomegalovirus
Microbial flora	Other
Graft-versus-host disease	Fungal
Manifestations	
Prophylaxis	
Therapy	
Patient susceptibility	

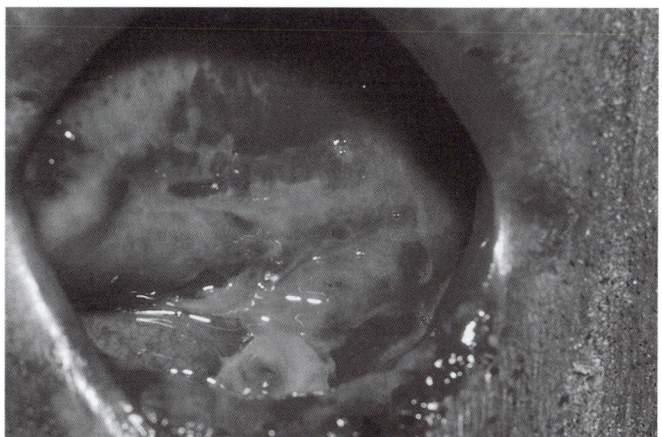

FIGURE 45.2 Severe ulcerated mucositis in a patient receiving an unrelated donor bone marrow transplant (day +14) requiring systemic opioid analgesic.

with mucositis is dependent on the degree of tissue damage, sensitization of nociceptors, and secretion of inflammatory and pain mediators.

In patients with HNC treated with radiation, pain intensity and pain interference scores directly correlate with mucositis severity. Symptoms increase at week 3, often peak at week 5, and persist for 4 to 6 weeks following the end of treatment. Concurrent chemoradiotherapy and intensified radiation protocols increase the severity and duration of oral mucositis.[97–99] However, marked improvement may take up to 12 months posttreatment, with general functional and physical appearance slowly returning toward baseline level. Follow-up of oropharyngeal cancer patients (up to 1 year) treated with radiation showed that mouth pain is common (58.4%) and interfered with daily activities in approximately one-third of subjects.[100]

HEMATOPOIETIC CELL TRANSPLANTATION

Ulcerative mucositis is the most debilitating patient-reported toxicity of HCT protocols and other treatments for hematologic cancer.[58,59,64,66] Mucositis is compounded in patients with herpes simplex virus (HSV) reactivation and in those with poor oral hygiene.[57,64,69,70,101] HSV prophylaxis has altered the frequency and severity of mucosal ulceration in HCT patients; however, even when acyclovir prophylaxis is used, oral ulcerative mucositis occurs in up to 75% of patients.[59]

Mucositis symptoms can be increased in HCT patients with hyposalivation,[67] and the related oral microflora and dental plaque changes may influence its severity.[101–107] Intensive oral hygiene has been documented to reduce the severity and duration of oral mucositis.[101] Studies have demonstrated that approximately 48% of the bacteremia cases in the early period post-HCT are associated with oral flora. Concerns about the risk of bacteremia secondary to gingival bleeding due to brushing and flossing in the first 3 weeks post-HCT are not supported by evidence. Septicemia was not increased in patients who continued intensive oral care.[101] Immunoglobulins and other antimicrobial proteins in saliva are decreased after HCT conditioning, which may be an additional factor in the increased risk of mucosal infection.[82]

Clinically, oral mucositis in autologous HCT patients becomes evident approximately 2 to 5 days after marrow infusion (day +2 to 5) with resolution in more than 90% of patients by day +15.[59] Allogeneic HCT patients generally show a slightly slower onset and slower resolution of mucositis. Damage to the mucosa typically presents in a bilateral pattern, primarily involving the nonkeratinized mucosa of the cheeks, lateral and ventral surfaces of the tongue, floor of the mouth, soft palate, and labial mucosa. The mucosal reaction may begin shortly after exposure to the conditioning regimen and progress to erythema and ulceration (Fig. 45.2; also see Fig. 45.1). Increased mucosal toxicity is usually seen in patients additionally conditioned for HCT with total body irradiation.[66,68,79]

Oral pain (including odynophagia/dysphagia and trismus) closely parallels development and severity of mucositis. Ulcerative lesions usually result in moderate to severe discomfort, leading to difficult or impossible oral nutrition and loss of oral function. Grades 3 and 4 mucositis typically require parenteral feeding and topical and systemic analgesics, usually opiates. Medications for the neuropathic components of pain are typically administered in the setting of mucositis. Symptoms recede as oral lesions heal but may be persistent in cases of mucosal atrophy and neuronal sensitization.

HEAD AND NECK RADIATION THERAPY

Tumor-related pain is commonly present at the time of diagnosis of head and neck/oral cancer (85%), although the intensity is usually not severe.[62,108] The presence and severity of pain are related to tumor stage and bone involvement.[62] All treatment methods for HNC can result in pain. Surgical resection of tumor is followed by postoperative algesia, which is related to the extent of tissue removed and whether bone was involved. Chemoradiation therapy affects tissue in the field of radiation producing pain that increases gradually as the treatment advances.[45,62,71,72] Radiotherapy-related mucositis is the most frequent complication in patients during radiation for HNCs (see Table 45.1; Figs. 45.3 and 45.4). Mucositis-related pain increases during radiation treatment and typically resolves within 1 to 2 months, or longer with combined radiation and chemotherapy. However, mucosal discomfort often continues for 6 to 12 months or longer, although the severity of pain decreases over time after treatment.[62] Chronic complaints include mucosal sensitivity attributed to mucosal atrophy (33%), musculoskeletal syndromes (temporomandibular disorder, fibrosis) (25%), and neurologic syndromes attributed to deafferentation (16%) and neuropathy.[62] The most common persisting complaints after radiation treatment include xerostomia (57%), pain involving the muscles of the jaw or joint (27%), and a 10% increased rate of dental caries.[109] Chronic complications of radiation therapy were assessed in 676 HNC patients treated in a multicenter

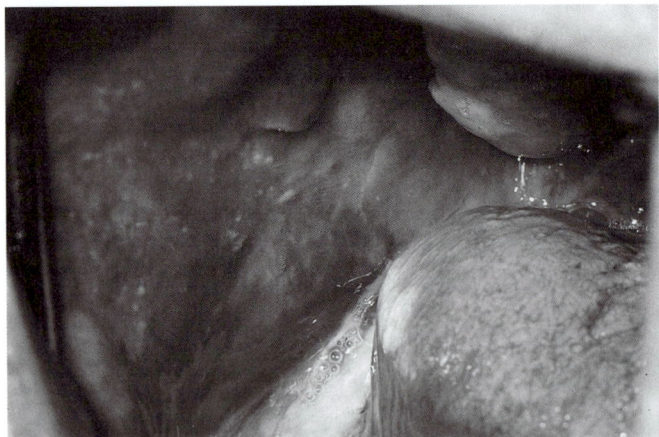

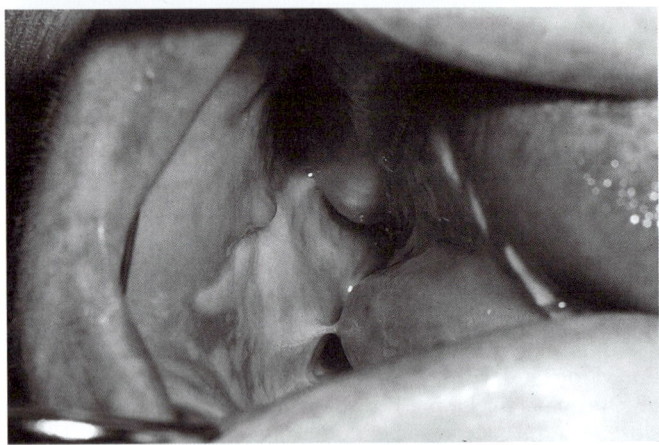

FIGURE 45.3   A: Initial tissue reaction in a patient receiving radiation therapy (dose received 1,400 cGy of planned 6,000 cGy) resulting in erythema and sensitivity of the right buccal mucosa. **B:** Late tissue reaction in the same patient receiving radiation therapy (total dose received 6,000 cGy) resulting in oral pain and mucosal ulceration within the radiation field.

study, and 11% were reported to have severe complications (grade 3 or 4) involving the oral mucosa, bone, or muscle.[110] These late complications were related to total radiation dose; complications in bone were more common with large radiation fields, and complications in bone and muscle were related to radiation fraction size. The severity of chronic mucosal damage may relate to severity of acute mucosal reaction.

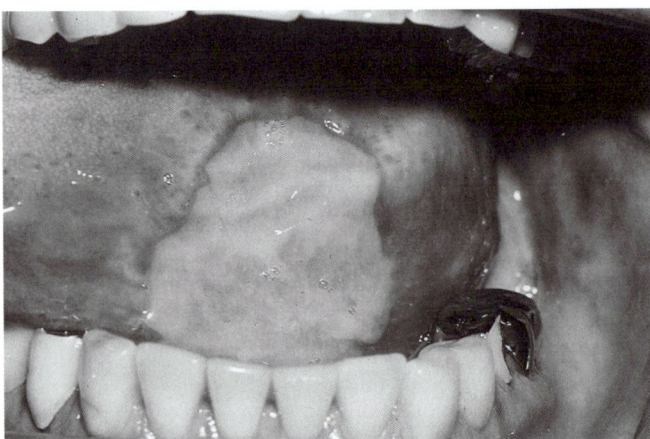

FIGURE 45.4 Localized ulcerative mucositis following brachytherapy for a squamous cell carcinoma of the middle portion of the lateral border of the tongue.

COMBINED RADIATION THERAPY, SURGERY, AND/OR CHEMOTHERAPY

Treatment of locally advanced head and neck carcinoma is associated with significant complications affecting oral function. Hyperfractionated radiotherapy and chemotherapy may improve survival, but treatment is frequently limited by the severity of oral toxicity.[45,48,50,61,111,112] Severe oral mucositis occurs in essentially all patients treated with accelerated fractionated irradiation for supraglottic cancer[2] and in those treated with combined chemo radiation.[111,112] Severe mucositis may cause considerable pain, limit or prevent oral intake, and may lead to suspension of cancer therapy.[45,112] Intensity-modulated radiation therapy (IMRT) may be associated with less skin and mucosal damage[113] but still results in significant ulcerative mucositis and symptoms.[99] Helical IMRT is a newer technique for radiation delivery, which unfortunately does not appear to provide a better profile of side effects.[114] Mucosal reactions in patients receiving radiation treatment for HNC are currently regarded as unavoidable side effects, but advances in knowledge of pathogenesis and new therapeutic models are expected to change this view, with prophylaxis, intervention, and improved symptom management.

The importance of fungal colonization and infection in radiation mucositis has not been clearly defined.[115–117] One study showed fewer cases of candidiasis in patients on prophylactic fluconazole and a 50% reduction in the number of breaks in radiation therapy than those not provided prophylaxis with fluconazole.[115] However, others have not found an association between candidiasis or oral colonization and mucositis during cancer therapy.[115,117]

Targeted chemotherapy with monoclonal antibodies and small molecules is becoming part of current HNC protocols. The impact on mucositis has not been well defined, as mucositis has only been recorded with multiple toxicities and no studies have assessed mucositis using a validated scale as a primary or secondary endpoint. However, the available data suggest that oral mucositis is not more common than that seen with standard therapy, although it may occur less frequently and be less severe.[74,75,118–124]

Pain Assessment

Most studies use a VAS or various Likert scales to assess oral pain; some use the more extensive McGill Pain Questionnaire.[60,125] The latter was compared with two different factor models in patients with oral mucositis pain after HCT, and it was recommended that a single pain rating may provide a better practical measurement.[125] Patients may be unable or unwilling to complete lengthy questionnaires, particularly when their overall condition including pain is at its worst. Notwithstanding analgesic use, most of the variance in pain reports is explained by the severity of the mucositis rather than psychosocial variables.[55]

Management of Oral Mucositis

Wide variation exists in quality of mucositis prevention and management studies. Many enroll a small number of patients, using outcome measures that are not validated, and may lack sensitivity. This makes assessment of outcomes difficult, mandating careful review of the methods employed in every study before generalizable conclusions can be drawn. Guidelines for the use of outcome measures and more refined study design and protocols in the management of mucositis are improving the value of more recent studies. Evidence-based guidelines[126–128] have been developed and will continue to evolve as new approaches to prevention and management are studied.

Development of strategies for the prevention and management of oral mucositis has been enhanced by an improved understanding of the multifactorial nature of the condition (Table 45.4). Radiation shields are recommended during standard radiation therapy. The use of midline mucosa-sparing blocks for protection of the mucosa during radiation therapy, thereby reducing mucositis, resulted in less weight loss, fewer hospitalizations for nutritional support, and a trend toward fewer treatment interruptions ($P = .07$) than in control patients.[52] The impact of IMRT on oral mucositis pain is not well understood, with reduced area of severe tissue damage but broader areas of low-dose radiation exposure.[99]

Palifermin (Kepivance; Biovitrum Inc, Stockholm, Sweden) is the only approved agent for prevention of oral mucositis in HCT.[17,129] Further study of patients with metastatic colon cancer treated with fluorouracil-based chemotherapy showed benefit of palifermin in reducing mucositis,[130] suggesting broader potential application than currently indicated. Benzydamine (not available in the United States) is recommended for use in patients receiving radiotherapy (>220 cGY per day). Oral cryotherapy is recommended for prevention of mucositis in those receiving bolus 5-fluorouracil (FU) or edatrexate treatments, or high-dose melphalan conditioning regimens for HCT. Low level laser therapy (LLLT), also called low-energy lasers have been studied in the prevention and management of mucositis associated with HCT and head and neck radiation with consistent positive findings across studies.[131-134] LLLT, also known as photobiomodulation (PBM), affects the cellular redox status by changes in the mitochondrial metabolism and influences cytokine release and vascularization.[135,136]

TABLE 45.4 Prevention and Management of Oral Mucositis

Pretreatment Oral/Dental Stabilization
Eliminate sites of infection, trauma
Dental cleaning
Good oral hygiene
    Saline mouth rinses

Antimicrobial Approaches
Systemic antimicrobials
    Antibiotics
    Antivirals acyclovir, valacyclovir, ganciclovir
    Antifungal fluconazole
Topical antimicrobials
    Chlorhexidine
    Antimicrobial lozenges (polymyxin, tobramycin, amphotericin)

Anti-inflammatory Approaches
Topical agents
    Prostaglandins
    Benzydamine
    Corticosteroids

Biologic Response Modifiers
Granulocyte-macrophage colony-stimulating factor
Granulocyte colony-stimulating factor
Epidermal growth factor
Transforming growth factor, interleukin-11

Miscellaneous Approaches
Good oral hygiene
Saline/bicarbonate mouth rinses
Low-energy lasers
Mucosal coating agents
Vitamin supplements
Anticholinergic agents (xerogenergic agents)
Modification in cancer treatment protocols

Pain Management

With only a small number of approaches documented to prevent the incidence or shorten the duration of oral mucositis, current clinical management depends on palliative approaches. The use of a *stepped protocol* for pain management is currently the most appropriate approach. The elements of this protocol include the progressive utilization of (1) basic oral care, (2) bland rinses, (3) topical anesthetic and mucosal coating agents, and (4) systemic analgesics.

BASIC ORAL CARE

A growing body of evidence is being accrued that supports the importance of maintaining oral care protocols to remove bacterial dental plaque from teeth and periodontal tissues during intensive cancer therapies.[126,127] Patients should maintain good oral hygiene by brushing, flossing, and possibly using antimicrobial rinses.

BLAND ORAL RINSES

Although there are no studies demonstrating the effectiveness of normal saline or bicarbonate rinses in decreasing mucositis, they have been shown to reduce mucosal pain.[137,138] Frequent use of bland rinses can provide relief for mild mucositis, help remove debris, and moisturize mucosal surfaces. However, some rinses may have the opposite effect. In a study of 40 patients undergoing radiotherapy to more than 50% of the oral cavity, half were randomized to an oral care protocol using either saline or hydrogen peroxide rinses, and the latter was associated with increased mucosal sensitivity.[139]

TOPICAL ANESTHETICS AND ANALGESICS

Topical anesthetics represent the next step in the strategy to manage mucositis pain. Although there are no studies specifically examining efficacy of various topical anesthetics, any agent that can be safely applied to oral mucosa to induce numbness and is tolerated by the patient can be used.[65] Lidocaine viscous solution is frequently recommended, but other useful agents include benzocaine, dyclonine, and diphenhydramine. Topical anesthetics can cause mild initial irritation, obtund taste, and diminish the gag reflex if gargled or swallowed. Hence, swallowing of these agents to control pharyngeal pain is not generally recommended also due to possible systemic side effects and toxicities. Benzydamine has been shown to reduce mucositis and associated oral pain in radiation-induced mucositis by initially producing an anesthetic effect, which is also longer acting.[65,72] Local applications of topical anesthetic creams or gels may be especially useful for localized painful mucosal ulcerations.

Topical analgesics have also shown effect in mucositis pain. Initial studies of topical morphine have shown analgesic effects,[140] and doxepin in single and multidose studies has shown extended duration pain relief without burning sensation when applied to ulcerated tissue.[141,142]

Coating agents used as oral rinses such as milk of magnesia and loperamide have been recommended frequently but have not been subjected to controlled studies.[65,126] Sucralfate suspension has been studied in mucositis, but results have been inconsistent and its use for radiation or chemotherapy mucositis is not supported.[71,143-145]

A number of mucosal coating agents or rinses have been licensed by the U.S. Food and Drug Administration (FDA) for the management of oral mucositis, including Gelclair (EKR Therapeutics, Bedminster, NJ), MuGard (Access Pharmaceuticals Inc, Dallas, TX), and Caphosol (EUSA Pharma Inc, Langhorne, PA). However, there is insufficient evidence to recommend their use for prevention or treatment of mucositis.[146,147]

TOPICAL ANTIMICROBIALS

Early studies suggested that topical antimicrobials may have utility in preventing oral mucositis, but follow-up research has failed to provide evidence to support their use.[126] Chlorhexidine has been assessed in HCT patients in a number of studies, but conflicting results with its use in mucositis have been seen and the majority of follow-up studies do not demonstrate a prophylactic effect on mucositis.[148] It is important to note that the effectiveness of chlorhexidine rinsing on plaque levels, gingival inflammation, and caries risk have not been endpoints in these studies, and the use of chlorhexidine for bacterial plaque control during cancer therapy may still be useful.

Studies of antimicrobial lozenges combining agents such as polymyxin, tobramycin, and amphotericin B in head and neck radiation therapy were shown in a single-center trial to be effective.[103] However, follow-up studies to duplicate the benefit of using either topical antimicrobials or β-defensin, while reducing oral microbial colonization, did not significantly impact on mucositis.[149–152]

SYSTEMIC ANALGESICS

Symptom management for oral mucositis often requires the use of systemic analgesics. Mucositis is the most common condition requiring the use of systemic opioid analgesics during cancer therapy.[49] A wide range of agents can be used, including acetaminophen, nonsteroidal anti-inflammatory agents (NSAIDs), and opiates/opioids.

Systemic analgesics should be prescribed following the World Health Organization (WHO) analgesic ladder.[65] These recommendations include the use of nonopioid analgesics alone, or in combination with opioids and adjunctive medications, based on pain severity and effectiveness of therapy (see Chapter 39). In patients with oral mucositis pain, topical approaches should be used initially and should continue to be used in combination with systemic analgesics in order that the best pain management can be achieved with the least potent and lowest doses of systemic pain medications. Studies have shown that optimum pain control may be achieved by moving directly from WHO ladder level I analgesics to titrated doses of WHO ladder level III analgesics. Improvement in pain control is achieved by combining level III analgesics with adjuvants at lower total doses of analgesics, and therefore, modification of the analgesic ladder has been discussed.[153]

A number of different delivery methods can be used for delivery of systemic analgesics. Oral, transmucosal, transdermal (patches), intravenous, and suppository routes can be used. Patient-controlled analgesia (PCA) is recommended in pain management for hospitalized cancer patients with severe mucositis.[154] A study of preteen children receiving HCT assessed morphine or hydromorphone PCA for mucositis or other painful conditions and found that children successfully mastered PCA to control pain associated with HCT.[49] No instance of drug overdose or difficulty stopping the opioid was noted.[49] As has been previously voiced, addiction is not a significant risk in these patients with severe and debilitating pain as is underuse and underdosing of analgesics.[65]

Persisting high levels of pain are common even with controlled opiate dosing due to mucositis pain, and it has been suggested that the neuropathic component of pain must be addressed to provide improved pain control, with gabapentin showing additional effect.[155]

ANTI-INFECTIVE APPROACHES

Infection may result in direct mucosal damage, initiating or complicating mucosal pain. Acyclovir prophylaxis in HSV-seropositive HCT patients is strongly supported in the literature as it prevents both viral reactivation and shedding (seen in 2.9% of patients) in most cases.[156] Oral ulcerations may also be due to reactivation of cytomegalovirus (CMV) in HCT,[157] and shedding of CMV was detected in 13.3% of CMV-seropositive patients. No correlation between severity of mucositis and serologic status of HSV or CMV was seen in patients provided acyclovir prophylaxis.[156] Ganciclovir after stem cell transplantation has been shown effective in suppressing CMV infection,[158] and acyclovir prophylaxis has also been shown to lower shedding of CMV by approximately half in these patients.[159]

Bacterial infections are also common in the setting of immune suppression. Consecutive HCT patients at risk of streptococcal bacteremia were treated for 5 days with clindamycin and ceftazidime for the initial management of fever associated with severe oral mucositis.[86] Bacteremia caused by viridans streptococci occurred in 70% of patients with severe mucositis, and blood culture results were positive a day prior to fever in approximately one-third of cases, showing that mucosal ulceration predisposes to systemic infection by oral flora. Approaches to reduce mucosal damage will also reduce pain and infection risk and have been suggested as a better means of minimizing systemic infection as compared to antimicrobial approaches.[86]

In a series of patients with leukemia receiving HCT, fluconazole prophylaxis was compared with no prophylaxis,[117] and a trend toward reduction in oropharyngeal colonization by *Candida albicans* was seen ($P = .07$). However, the clinical implications are unclear because no relationship was seen between *Candida* spp., antifungal prophylaxis, and mucositis, suggesting that *Candida* spp. was not involved in the etiology of mucosal damage in these patients.[116] In a randomized controlled trial, fluconazole prevented systemic fungal infections (7% of fluconazole versus 18% of placebo patients)[160] and the incidence of mucosal infection and oropharyngeal colonization by *C. albicans* was reduced.[161,162] Therefore, although *Candida* may complicate oral mucositis and cause mucosal sensitivity and systemic infection, it does not appear to be a risk factor of mucositis.[163]

Hyposalivation

Preventing mucosal toxicity also reduces the pain of oral mucositis. Mucosal toxicity is a dose-limiting toxicity for patients on etoposide and may be related to direct effects of myeloablative doses of etoposide secreted in saliva.[63] Twelve patients received propantheline, an anticholinergic agent, or placebo, and mucositis was less frequent and less severe ($P = .05$) in the propantheline arm. Another study investigated the effect of drug-induced hyposalivation on mucositis during HCT by comparing patients with historic controls.[164] Propantheline was found to significantly reduce oral mucositis due to high-dose etoposide, although no effect was seen on esophagitis and enteritis. These findings suggest that for chemotherapeutics that are secreted in saliva, pharmacologically induced hyposalivation may decrease the exposure to the mucosa to the cytotoxic drug and thereby reduce local tissue damage. It is unclear whether this strategy may apply to other regimens. These studies were small, and results must be interpreted cautiously.

BIOLOGIC RESPONSE MODIFIERS AND CYTOKINES

The effects of KGF-1 (palifermin) on mucositis are discussed above. Studies on KGF-20 (velafermin) have been terminated early due to the drug's association with Parkinson disease.[165]

A study on the effect of radiation on EGF in the oral cavity determined that the quantity decreased because of decreased volume of saliva and also decreased in concentration per milliliter of saliva as mucositis increased throughout the course of therapy.[87] These findings suggested that EGF may represent a marker of mucosal damage and has the potential to promote resolution of radiation-induced mucositis. Further studies on this topic are necessary.

Mixed results on prevention of mucositis have been seen with GM-CSF in several human trials.[79–82,89,90] Studies assessing granulocyte colony-stimulating factor (G-CSF) have also presented mixed outcomes. These results may be due to mucositis being a secondary endpoint in these studies that evaluated mainly the effects on white blood cells.[56,90,91] Overall, these conflicting results do not provide sufficient information to recommend use of white blood cell growth factors for the treatment of mucositis.

COGNITIVE AND BEHAVIORAL INTERVENTIONS

Relaxation, imagery, biofeedback, hypnosis, and transcutaneous electrical nerve stimulation have been employed in the management of cancer pain with varying patient acceptance and efficacy.[65,166,167] Cognitive-behavioral interventions in pediatric oncology and HCT included providing information before procedures and positive reinforcement after procedures and, less commonly, behavioral interventions such as rhythmic breathing, distraction, and imagery.[168] Psychological services were primarily available on an as-needed basis, and support groups were not generally offered. Increasing emphasis on psychological support and techniques for pain management may be useful for patients during HCT.

A controlled clinical trial of psychological interventions in cancer-related pain was conducted in 94 HCT patients with oral mucositis divided in four groups, and relaxation and imagery training was shown to reduce pain associated with oral mucositis. However, adding cognitive-behavioral skills to relaxation and imagery did not improve pain relief.[169] The reader is referred to other chapters in this text for more detail with regard to psychological approaches to pain and an in-depth review of treatment of bone pain, use of nonopioid and opioid pharmacotherapy for cancer pain, radiopharmaceuticals, and interventional approaches to pain control in cancer.

Conclusion

Pain in the oropharynx of cancer patients has a significant impact upon treatment implementation, prognosis and QOL, and needs to be dealt with aggressively in order to prevent other comorbidities. Cancer and cancer therapy result in release of ROS, growth factors, cytokines, and enzymes that may cause nerve irritation or damage that may result in neurogenic acute and chronic pain. Anxiety and depression compound the pain experience. Mucosal damage, particularly in the presence of immunosuppression and neutropenia, may significantly increase the risk of systemic infection (Fig. 45.5). Oropharyngeal pain in cancer patients frequently requires systemic analgesics, adjunctive medications, and physical and psychological therapy, in addition to oral care and topical treatments (see Table 45.4). Good oral hygiene including tooth brushing and dental flossing reduces the severity of oral mucositis and does not increase the risk of bacteremia.

Clinically apparent mucositis is the result of drug toxicities, tissue damage, and inflammation. The primary event is cell damage from chemotherapy, radiotherapy, or both. Secondary influences include indirect toxicities resulting in immunosuppression, neutropenia, reactivation of latent viruses (herpes viruses), and opportunistic microbial (bacterial and fungal) infections. Salivary gland dysfunction caused by dehydration and direct effects of the cancer therapy on gland function may alter the local mucosal defenses. Because the etiology is multifactorial (see Table 45.3), approaches to prevention and treatment also have been multifactorial (see Table 45.4). Effective prevention and management of mucositis affect the pain experienced during cancer treatment, and when mucositis is present, symptomatic management is needed (Table 45.5).

Systemic analgesics remain an important mainstay in pain treatment along with topical analgesics and anesthetics. Pain management including adjunctive analgesics are often underutilized in HNC-related pain syndromes. Novel approaches of potential interest are agents that affect neurotransmitters that modulate pain such as SP and potentially ROS, cytokine production, PGs, and other neurotransmitters.

Biologic response modifiers offer the potential for prevention and to speed healing. Oral care and continuing good oral hygiene are recommended prior to and during cancer therapy.

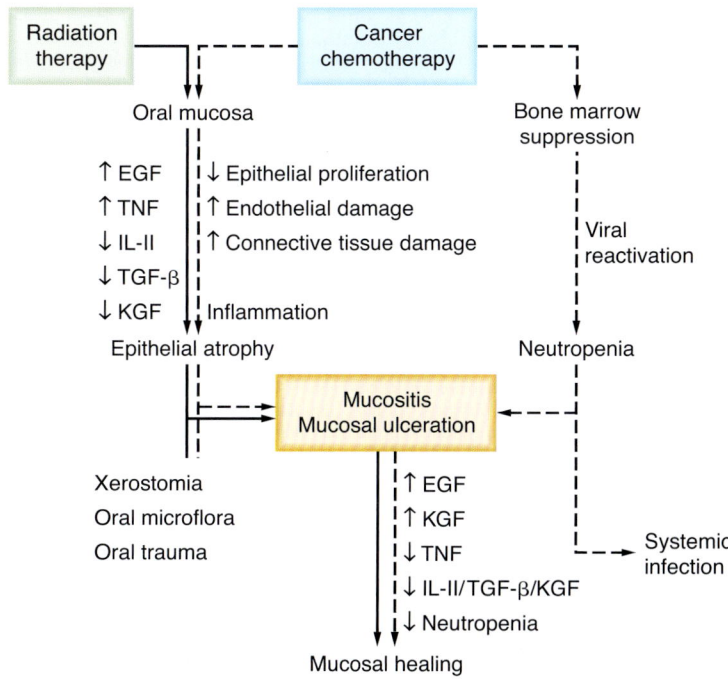

FIGURE 45.5 A model of the pathogenesis of oral mucositis.

EGF - Epidermal growth factor
TNF - Tumor necrosis factor
IL-II - Interleukin II
TGF-β - Transforming growth factor-beta
KGF - Keratinocyte growth factor

TABLE 45.5 Symptomatic Management of Pain of Oral Mucositis
Maintain good oral hygiene.
Prevent mucosal damage (see Table 45.4).
Coating agents (e.g., milk of magnesia, aluminum hydroxide gel [Amphojel], sucralfate, loperamide [Kaopectate], Gelclair, Caphosol)
Topical analgesic/anti-inflammatory (benzydamine)
Topical anesthetics/analgesics
Systemic analgesics
Adjuvant systemic medications
Adjuvant cognitive/psychological support
Physical therapy (rinsing, ice chips)
Miscellaneous agents

Keratinocyte growth factor (Kepivance) is the only approved and recommended medication for prophylaxis of mucositis in HCT. Benzydamine is recommended in head and neck radiation therapy, but it is not available in the United States. Oral cooling (cryotherapy) with ice chips is recommended for patients receiving bolus infusion, short half-life systemic chemotherapy. Available local agents of uncertain value include a coating agent (Gelclair) and a mineralizing oral solution (Caphosol), with MuGard, the best documented of these devices in mucositis.[170] Meanwhile, a number of agents with different mechanisms of action are undergoing investigation. Of potential value is the use of PBM (LLLT), which has been shown in several studies to mitigate prevalence, severity, and duration of both chemotherapy and radiotherapy-induced mucositis.[171]

Whereas antimicrobial approaches have been shown to not prevent mucositis, there may be a positive effect on dental and gingival health and on mucosal candidiasis. Other approaches that require further study include low-energy lasers and anti-inflammatory medications.

References

1. Mirabile A, Airoldi M, Ripamonti C, et al. Pain management in head and neck cancer patients undergoing chemo-radiotherapy: clinical practical recommendations. *Crit Rev Oncol Hematol* 2016;99:100–106.
2. Benoliel R, Epstein J, Eliav E, et al. Orofacial pain in cancer: part I—mechanisms. *J Dent Res* 2007;86(6):491–505.
3. Eliav E, Teich S, Benoliel R, et al. Large myelinated nerve fiber hypersensitivity in oral malignancy. *Oral Surg Oral Med Oral Pathol Oral Radiol Endod* 2002;94(1):45–50.
4. Eliav E, Tal M, Benoliel R. Experimental malignancy in the rat induces early hypersensitivity indicative of neuritis. *Pain* 2004;110(3):727–737.
5. Sonis ST, O'Donnell KE, Popat R, et al. The relationship between mucosal cyclooxygenase-2 (COX-2) expression and experimental radiation-induced mucositis. *Oral Oncol* 2004;40:170–176.
6. Möller T. Skeletal metastases. *Acta Oncol* 1996;35(suppl 7):125–136.
7. van Deventer H, Bernard S. Use of gabapentin to treat taxane-induced myalgias. *J Clin Oncol* 1999;17(1):434–435.
8. Wilson RH, Lehky T, Thomas RR, et al. Acute oxaliplatin-induced peripheral nerve hyperexcitability. *J Clin Oncol* 2002;20(7):1767–1774.
9. Bergstrom P, Johnsson A, Bergenheim T, et al. Effects of amifostine on cisplatin induced DNA adduct formation and toxicity in malignant glioma and normal tissues in rat. *J Neurooncol* 1999;42(1):13–21.
10. Rybak LP, Husain K, Whitworth C, et al. Dose dependent protection by lipoic acid against cisplatin-induced ototoxicity in rats: antioxidant defense system. *Toxicol Sci* 1999;47(2):195–202.
11. Lissoni P, Tancini G, Barni S, et al. Treatment of cancer chemotherapy-induced toxicity with the pineal hormone melatonin. *Support Care Cancer* 1997;5(2):126–129.
12. Jackson DV, Wells HB, Atkins JN, et al. Amelioration of vincristine neurotoxicity by glutamic acid. *Am J Med* 1988;84(6):1016–1022.
13. Jacobson SD, Loprinzi CL, Sloan JA, et al. Glutamine does not prevent paclitaxel-associated myalgias and arthralgias. *J Support Oncol* 2003;1(4):274–278.
14. Barasch A, Cunha-Cruz J, Curro F, et al. Dental risk factors for osteonecrosis of the jaws: a CONDOR case–control study. *Clin Oral Investig* 2013;17(8):1839–1845.
15. Ott SM. Long-term safety of bisphosphonates. *J Clin Endocrinol Metab* 2005;90(3):1897–1899.
16. Xing L, Boyce BF. Regulation of apoptosis in osteoclasts and osteoblastic cells. *Biochem Biophys Res Commun* 2005;328(3):709–720.
17. Nasilowska-Adamska B, Rzepecki P, Manko J, et al. The influence of palifermin (Kepivance) on oral mucositis and acute graft versus host disease in patients with hematological diseases undergoing hematopoietic stem cell transplant. *Bone Marrow Transplant* 2007;40(10):983–988.
18. Ensrud KE, Barrett-Connor EL, Schwartz A, et al. Randomized trial of effect of alendronate continuation versus discontinuation in women with low BMD: results from the Fracture Intervention Trial long-term extension. *J Bone Miner Res* 2004;19(8):1259–1269.
19. Ensrud KE, Fullman RL, Barrett-Connor E, et al. Voluntary weight reduction in older men increases hip bone loss: the osteoporotic fractures in men study. *J Clin Endocrinal Metab* 2005;90(4):1998–2004.
20. Mehrotra B, Ruggiero S. Bisphosphonate complications including osteonecrosis of the jaw. *Hematology Am Soc Hematol Educ Program* 2006; 356–360.
21. Fulfaro F, Casuccio A, Ticozzi C, et al. The role of bisphosphonates in the treatment of painful metastatic bone disease: a review of phase III trials. *Pain* 1998;78(3):157–169.
22. Mannix K, Ahmedzai SH, Anderson H, et al. Using bisphosphonates to control the pain of bone metastases: evidence-based guidelines for palliative care. *Palliat Med* 2000;14(6):455–461.
23. Chaplin J, Morton R. A prospective, longitudinal study of pain in head and neck cancer patients. *Head Neck* 1999;21(6):531–537.
24. Epstein J, Stewart K. Radiation therapy and pain in patients with head and neck cancer. *Eur J Cancer B Oral Oncol* 1993;29B(3):191–199.
25. Goodwin WJ. Salvage surgery for patients with recurrent squamous cell carcinoma of the upper aerodigestive tract: when do the ends justify the means? *Laryngoscope* 2000;110(3, pt 2 suppl 93):1–18.
26. Wittekindt C, Liu W, Preuss S, et al. Botulinum toxin A for neuropathic pain after neck dissection: a dose-finding study. *Laryngoscope* 2006;116(7):1168–1171.
27. Simons D, Hong C, Simons L. Endplate potentials are common to midfiber myofacial trigger points. *Am J Phys Med Rehabil* 2002;81(3):212–222.
28. Schuller D, McGuirt W, McCabe B, et al. The prognostic significance of metastatic cervical lymph nodes. *Laryngoscope* 1980;90(4):557–570.
29. Crile G III. On the technique of operations upon the head and neck. *Ann Surg* 1906;44(6):842–850.
30. Terrell J, Ronis D, Fowler K, et al. Clinical predictors of quality of life in patients with head and neck cancer. *Arch Otolaryngol Head Neck Surg* 2004;130(4):401–408.
31. Chandu A, Sun K, DeSilva R, et al. The assessment of quality of life in patients who have undergone surgery for oral cancer: a preliminary report. *J Oral Maxillofac Surg* 2005;63(11):1606–1612.
32. Kuntz A, Weymuller EJ. Impact of neck dissection on quality of life. *Laryngoscope* 1999;109(8):1334–1338.
33. Terrell J, Welsh D, Bradford C, et al. Pain, quality of life, and spinal accessory nerve status after neck dissection. *Laryngoscope* 2000;110(4):620–626.
34. Chepeha D, Taylor R, Chepeha J, et al. Functional assessment using Constant's Shoulder Scale after modified radical and selective neck dissection. *Head Neck* 2002;24(5):432–643.
35. Rogers S, Ferlito A, Pellitteri P, et al. Quality of life following neck dissections. *Acta Otolaryngol* 2004;124(3):231–236.
36. Taylor R, Chepeha J, Teknos T, et al. Development and validation of the neck dissection impairment index: a quality of life measure. *Arch Otolaryngol Head Neck Surg* 2002;128(1):44–49.
37. van Wilgen C, Dijkstra P, van der Laan B, et al. Morbidity of the neck after head and neck cancer therapy. *Head Neck* 2004;26(9):785–791.
38. Krause H. Shoulder-arm-syndrome after radical neck dissection: its relation with the innervation of the trapezius muscle. *Int J Oral Maxillofac Surg* 1992;21(5):276–279.
39. Cheng P, Hao S, Lin Y, et al. Objective comparison of shoulder dysfunction after three neck dissection techniques. *Ann Otol Rhinol Laryngol* 2000;109 (8, pt 1):761–766.
40. Townsend CM, Sabiston DC. *Sabiston Textbook of Surgery: The Biological Basis of Modern Surgical Practice.* Vol 1. 17th ed. Philadelphia: Saunders; 2004.
41. Roh J, Yoon Y, Kim S, et al. Cervical sensory preservation during neck dissection. *Oral Oncol* 2007;43(5):491–498.
42. Sonis ST. The pathobiology of mucositis. *Nat Rev Cancer* 2004;4(4):277–284.
43. Sonis ST, Elting LS, Keefe D, et al. Perspectives on cancer therapy-induced mucosal injury: pathogenesis, measurement, epidemiology, and consequences for patients. *Cancer* 2004;100(suppl 9):1995–2025.
44. Sonis ST, Scherer J, Phelan S, et al. The gene expression sequence of radiated mucosa in an animal mucositis model. *Cell Prolif* 2002;35(suppl 1):93–102.
45. Wang CC, Nakfoor BM, Spiro IJ, et al. Role of accelerated fractionated irradiation for supraglottic carcinoma: assessment of results. *Cancer J Sci Am* 1997;3:88–91.
46. DeCosse JJ, Cennerazzo WJ. Quality-of-life management of patients with colorectal cancer. *CA Cancer J Clin* 1997;47:198–206.
47. McIlroy P. Radiation mucositis: a new approach to prevention and treatment. *Eur J Cancer Care (Engl)* 1996;5:153–158.
48. International Nasopharynx Cancer Study Group, VUMCA I Trial. Preliminary results of a randomized trial comparing neoadjuvant chemotherapy (cisplatin, epirubicin, bleomycin) plus radiotherapy vs. radiotherapy alone in stage IV (> or = N2, M0) undifferentiated nasopharyngeal carcinoma: a positive effect on progression-free survival. *Int J Radiat Oncol Biol Phys* 1996;35:463–469.

49. Dunbar PJ, Buckley P, Gavrin JR, et al. Use of patient-controlled analgesia for pain control for children receiving bone marrow transplant. *J Pain Symptom Manage* 1995;10:604–611.

50. Ausili-Cefaro G, Marmiroli L, Nardone L, et al. Prolonged continuous infusion of carboplatin and concomitant radiotherapy in advanced head and neck cancer. A phase I study. *Am J Clin Oncol* 1995;18:273–276.

51. Pascual MJ, Maldonado J. Extramedullary toxicity in bone marrow transplantation using busulfan and cyclophosphamide conditioning. *Sangre (Barc)* 1995;40:191–197.

52. Perch SJ, Machtay M, Markiewicz DA, et al. Decreased acute toxicity by using midline mucosa-sparing blocks during radiation therapy for carcinoma of the oral cavity, oropharynx, and nasopharynx. *Radiology* 1995;197:863–866.

53. Broun ER, Sridhara R, Sledge GW, et al. Tandem autotransplantation for the treatment of metastatic breast cancer. *J Clin Oncol* 1995;13:2050–2055.

54. Berger A, Henderson M, Nadoolman W, et al. Oral capsaicin provides temporary relief for oral mucositis pain secondary to chemotherapy/radiation therapy. *J Pain Symptom Manage* 1995;10:243–248.

55. Syrjala KL, Chapko ME. Evidence for a biopsychosocial model of cancer treatment-related pain. *Pain* 1995;61:69–79.

56. Rosenthal MA, Grigg AP, Sheridan WP. High dose busulphan/cyclophosphamide for autologous bone marrow transplantation is associated with minimal non-hemopoietic toxicity. *Leuk Lymphoma* 1994;14:279–283.

57. Carrega G, Castagnola E, Canessa A, et al. Herpes simplex virus and oral mucositis in children with cancer. *Support Care Cancer* 1994;2:266–269.

58. Cole CH, Pritchard S, Rogers PC, et al. Intensive conditioning regimen for bone marrow transplantation in children with high-risk haematological malignancies. *Med Pediatr Oncol* 1994;23:464–469.

59. Woo SB, Sonis ST, Monopoli MM, et al. A longitudinal study of oral ulcerative mucositis in bone marrow transplant recipients. *Cancer* 1993;72:1612–1617.

60. McGuire DB, Altomonte V, Peterson DE, et al. Patterns of mucositis and pain in patients receiving preparative chemotherapy and bone marrow transplantation. *Oncol Nurs Forum* 1993;20:1493–1502.

61. Tomio L, Zorat PL, Paccagnella A, et al. A pilot study of concomitant radiation and chemotherapy in patients with locally advanced head and neck cancer. *Am J Clin Oncol* 1995;16:264–267.

62. Epstein JB, Stewart KH. Radiation therapy and pain in patients with head and neck cancer. *Eur J Cancer B Oral Oncol* 1993;29B:191–199.

63. Ahmed T, Engelking C, Szalyga J, et al. Propantheline prevention of mucositis from etoposide. *Bone Marrow Transplant* 1993;12:131–132.

64. Seto BG, Kim M, Wolinsky L, et al. Oral mucositis in patients undergoing bone marrow transplantation. *Oral Surg Oral Med Oral Pathol* 1985;60:493–497.

65. Epstein JB, Schubert MM. Management of orofacial pain in cancer patients. *Oral Oncol Eur J Cancer* 1993;29B:243–250.

66. Chapko MK, Syrjala KL, Schilter L, et al. Chemoradiotherapy toxicity during bone marrow transplantation: time course and variation in pain and nausea. *Bone Marrow Transplant* 1989;4:181–186.

67. Schubert MM, Izutsu KT. Iatrogenic salivary gland dysfunction. *J Dent Res* 1987;66:680–688.

68. Bearman SI, Appelbaum FR, Buckner CD, et al. Regimen-related toxicity in patients undergoing bone marrow transplantation. *J Clin Oncol* 1988;6:1562–1568.

69. Schubert MM, Peterson DE, Flournoy N, et al. Oral and pharyngeal herpes simplex virus infection after allogeneic bone marrow transplantation: analysis of factors associated with infection. *Oral Surg Oral Med Oral Pathol* 1990;70:286–293.

70. Epstein JB, Sherlock C, Page JL, et al. Clinical study of herpes simplex virus infection in leukemia. *Oral Surg Oral Med Oral Pathol* 1990;70:38–43.

71. Epstein JB, Wong FLW. The efficacy of sucralfate suspension in the prevention of oral mucositis due to radiation therapy. *Int J Radiat Oncol Biol Phys* 1994;28:693–698.

72. Epstein JB, Steveson-Moore P, Jackson S, et al. Prevention of oral mucositis in radiation therapy: a controlled study with benzydamine hydrochloride rinse. *Int J Radiat Oncol Biol Phys* 1989;16:1571–1575.

73. Wingard JR, Niehaus CS, Peterson DE, et al. Oral mucositis after bone marrow transplantation. A marker of treatment toxicity and predictor of hepatic veno-occlusive disease. *Oral Surg Oral Med Oral Pathol* 1991;72:419–424.

74. Bonner JA, Harari PM, Giralt J, et al. Radiotherapy plus cetuximab for squamous-cell carcinoma of the head and neck. *N Engl J Med* 2006;354(6):567–578.

75. Bonner JA, Keene KS. Is cetuximab active in patients with cisplatin-refractory squamous cell carcinoma of the head and neck? *Nat Clin Pract Oncol* 2007;4(12):690–691.

76. Hartl DM, Morel D, Saavedra E, et al. Otorhinolaryngologic toxicities of new drugs in oncology. *Adv Ther* 2017;34:866–894.

77. Collins LK, Chapman MS, Carter JB, et al. Cutaneous adverse effects of the immune checkpoint inhibitors. *Curr Probl Cancer* 2017;41:125–128.

78. Sibaud V, Eid C, Belum VR, et al. Oral lichenoid reactions associated with anti-PD-1/PD-L1 therapies: clinicopathological findings. *J Eur Acad Dermatol Venereol* 2017;31:e464–e469.

79. Gordon B, Spadinger A, Hodges E, et al. Effect of granulocyte-macrophage colony stimulating factor on oral mucositis after hematopoietic stem-cell transplantation. *J Clin Oncol* 1994;12:1917–1922.

80. Linch DC, Scarffe H, Proctor S, et al. Randomised vehicle-controlled dose-finding study of glycosylated recombinant human granulocyte colony-stimulating factor for bone marrow transplantation. *Bone Marrow Transplant* 1993;11:307–311.

81. Reynoso EE, Calderon E, Miranda E. GM-CSF mouthwashes to attenuate severe mucositis after high dose chemotherapy and allogeneic bone marrow transplantation (BMT) or autologous peripheral blood stem cell transplantation (APBSCT). *Ann Oncol* 1994;5(suppl 8):1062.

82. Garfunkel AA, Tager N, Chausu S, et al. Oral complications in bone marrow transplantation patients: recent advances. *Isr J Med Sci* 1994;30:120–124.

83. Epstein JB, Gangbar SJ. Oral mucosal lesions in patients undergoing treatment for leukemia. *J Oral Med* 1987;3:205–209.

84. Schubert MM, Peterson DE, Hamilton D, et al. Changes I oral microflora following marrow transplantation. *J Dent Res* 1988;67:249.

85. Valteau D, Hartmann O, Brugieres L, et al. Streptococcal septicemia following autologous bone marrow transplantation in children treated with high-dose chemotherapy. *Bone Marrow Transplant* 1991;7:415–419.

86. Donnelly JP, Muus P, Horrevorts AM, et al. Failure of clindamycin to influence the course of severe oromucositis associated with streptococcal bacteraemia in allogeneic bone marrow transplant recipients. *Scand J Infect Dis* 1993;25:43–50.

87. Epstein JB, Emerton S, Guglietta A, et al. Assessment of epidermal growth factor in oral secretions of patients receiving radiation therapy for cancer. *Oral Oncol* 1997;33:359–363.

88. Chi KH, Chen CH, Chan WK, et al. Effect of granulocyte-macrophage colony-stimulating factor on oral mucositis in head and neck cancer patients after cisplatin, fluorouracil and leucovorin chemotherapy. *J Clin Oncol* 1995;13:2620–2628.

89. Masucci G. New clinical applications of granulocyte-macrophage colony-stimulating factor. *Med Oncol* 1996;13:149–154.

90. Bültzingslöwen IV, Brennan MT, Spijkervet FK, et al. Growth factors and cytokines in the prevention and treatment of oral and gastrointestinal mucositis. *Support Care Cancer* 2006;14(6):519–527.

91. Cho SA, Park JH, Seok SH, et al. Effect of granulocyte macrophage-colony stimulating factor (GM-CSF) on FU-induced ulcerative mucositis in hamster buccal pouches. *Exp Toxicol Pathol* 2006;57(4):321–328.

92. Sonis S, Muska A, O'Brien J, et al. Alteration in the frequency, severity and duration of chemotherapy-induced mucositis in hamsters by interleukin-11. *Eur J Cancer Oral Oncol* 1995;31B:261–266.

93. Sonis ST, Van Vugt AG, McDonald J, et al. Mitigating effects of interleukin-11 on consecutive courses of 5-fluorouracil-induced ulcerative mucositis in hamsters. *Cytokine* 1997;9:605–612.

94. Sonis ST, Van Vugt AG, Brien JP, et al. Transforming growth factor-beta 3 mediated modulation of cell cycling and attenuation of 5-fluorouracil induced oral mucositis. *Oral Oncol* 1997;33:47–54.

95. Sonis ST, Lindquist L, Van Vugt A, et al. Prevention of chemotherapy-induced ulcerative mucositis by transforming growth factor beta 3. *Cancer Res* 1994;54:1135–1138.

96. Keith JC Jr, Albert L, Sonis ST, et al. IL-11, a pleiotropic cytokine: exciting new effects of IL-11 on gastrointestinal mucosal biology. *Stem Cells* 1994;12(suppl 1):89–90.

97. Bernier J, Domenge C, Ozsahin M, et al. Postoperative irradiation with or without concomitant chemotherapy for locally advanced head and neck cancer. *N Engl J Med* 2004;350(19):1945–1952.

98. List MA, Siston A, Haraf D, et al. Quality of life and performance in advanced head and neck cancer patients on concomitant chemoradiotherapy: a prospective examination. *J Clin Oncol* 1999;17(3):1020–1028.

99. Epstein JB, Beaumont JL, Gwede CK, et al. Longitudinal evaluation of the oral mucositis weekly questionnaire-head and neck cancer, a patient-reported outcomes questionnaire. *Cancer* 2007;109(9):1914–1922.

100. Epstein JB, Emerton S, Kolbinson DA, et al. Quality of life and oral function following radiotherapy for head and neck cancer. *Head Neck* 1999;21(1):1–11.

101. Borowski B, Benhamou E, Pico JL, et al. Prevention of oral mucositis in patients treated with high-dose chemotherapy and bone marrow transplantation: a randomised controlled trial comparing two protocols of dental care. *Eur J Cancer B Oral Oncol* 1994;30B:93–97.

102. Ferretti GA, Ash RC, Brown AT, et al. Chlorhexidine for prophylaxis against oral infections and associated complications in bone marrow transplant patients. *J Am Dent Assoc* 1987;114:461–467.

103. Spijkervet FKL, van Saene HK, van Saene JJ, et al. Effect of selective elimination of the oral flora on mucositis in irradiated head and neck cancer patients. *J Surg Oncol* 1991;46:167–173.

104. Samaranayake LP, Robertson AG, MacFarlane TW, et al. The effect of chlorhexidine and benzydamine mouthwashes on mucositis induced by therapeutic irradiation. *Clin Radiol* 1998;39:291–294.

105. Raether D, Walker PO, Bostrum B, et al. Effectiveness of oral chlorhexidine for reducing stomatitis. *Pediadtr Dent* 1989;11:37–42.

106. Wahlin YB, Granstrom S, Persson S, et al. Multivariate study of enterobacteria and *Pseudomonas* in saliva of patients with acute leukemia. 1991;72:300–308.

107. Dodd MJ, Larson PJ, Dibble SL, et al. Randomized clinical trial of chlorhexidine versus placebo for prevention of oral mucositis in patients receiving chemotherapy. *Oncol Nurs Forum* 1996;23:921–927.

108. Epstein JB, Jones CK. Presenting signs and symptoms of nasopharyngeal carcinoma. *Oral Surg Oral Med Oral Pathol* 1993;75:32–36.

109. Cacchillo D, Barker GJ, Barker BF. Late effects of head and neck radiation therapy and patient/dentist compliance with recommended dental care. *Spec Care Dent* 1993;13:159–162.

110. Withers HR, Peters LJ, Taylor JM, et al. Late normal tissue sequelae from radiation therapy for carcinoma of the tonsil: patterns of fractionation study of radiobiology. *Int J Radiat Oncol Biol Phys* 1995;33:563–568.

111. Hinohira Y, Yumoto E, Takahashi H, et al. Radiotherapy combined with daily administration of low dose cisplatin for head and neck cancer. *Gan To Kagaku Ryoho* 1996;23:561–565.

112. Leyvraz S, Pasche P, Bauer J, et al. Rapidly alternating chemotherapy and hyperfractionated radiotherapy in the management of locally advanced head and neck carcinoma: four-year results of a phase I/II study. *J Clin Oncol* 1994;12:1876–1885.

113. Gosh G, Tallari R, Malviya A. Toxicity profile of IMRT vs. 3D-CRT in head and neck cancer: a retrospective study. *J Clin Diagn Res* 2016;10: XC01–XC03.

114. Moroney LB, Helios J, Ward EC, et al. Patterns of dysphagia and acute toxicities in patients with head and neck cancer undergoing helical IMRT±concurrent chemotherapy. *Oral Oncol* 2017;64:1–8.

115. Gava A, Ferrarese F, Tonetto V, et al. Can the prophylactic treatment of mycotic mucositis improve the time of performing radiotherapy in head and neck tumors? *Radiol Med (Torino)* 1996;91:452–455.

116. Epstein JB, Ransier A, Lunn R, et al. Prophylaxis of candidiasis in patients with leukemia and bone marrow transplants. *Oral Surg Oral Med Oral Pathol Oral Radiol Endodosc* 1996;81:291–296.

117. Epstein JB, Frelich MM, Le ND. Risk factors for oropharyngeal candidiasis in patients who receive radiation therapy for malignant conditions of the head and neck. *Oral Surg Oral Med Oral Pathol* 1993;76:169–174.

118. Robert F, Ezekiel MP, Spencer SA, et al. Phase I study of anti-epidermal growth factor receptor antibody cetuximab in combination with radiation therapy in patients with advanced head and neck cancer. *J Clin Oncol* 2001;19(13):3234–3243.

119. Manegold C, Gatzemeier U, Buchholz E, et al. A pilot trial of gefitinib in combination with docetaxel in patients with locally advanced or metastatic non–small-cell lung cancer. *Clin Lung Cancer* 2005;6(6):343–349.

120. Wyatt AJ, Leonard GD, Sachs DL. Cutaneous reactions to chemotherapy and their management. *Am J Clin Dermatol* 2006;7(1):46–63.

121. Koyama N, Jinn Y, Takabe K, et al. The characterization of gefitinib sensitivity and adverse events in patients with non–small-cell lung cancer. *Anticancer Res* 2006;26:4519–4526.

122. Agero LA, Dusza ST, Benvenuto-Andrade C, et al. Dermatologic side effects associated with epidermal growth factor receptor inhibitors. *J Am Acad Dermatol* 2006;55:657–670.

123. Robert F, Blumenschein G, Herbst RX, et al. PhaseI/IIa study of cetuximab with gemcitabine plus carboplatin in patients with chemotherapy-naïve advanced non–small-cell lung cancer. *J Clin Oncol* 2005;23(36):9089–9096.

124. Pinto C, Di Fabio F, Siena S, et al. Phase II study of cetuximab in combination with FOLFIRI in patients with untreated advanced gastric or gastroesophageal junction adenocarcinoma (FOLCETUX study). *Ann Oncol* 2007;18:510–517.

125. Donaldson GW. The factorial structure and stability of the McGill Pain Questionnaire in patients experiencing oral mucositis following bone marrow transplantation. *Pain* 1995;62:101–109.

126. Keefe DM, Schubert MM, Elting LS. Updated clinical practice guidelines for the prevention and treatment of mucositis. *Cancer* 2007;109(5): 820–831.

127. Worthington H, Clarkson J, Eden O. Interventions for preventing oral mucositis for patients with cancer receiving treatment. *Cochrane Database Syst Rev* 2007;(4):CD000978.

128. Clarkson JE, Worthington HV, Eden OB. Interventions for treating oral mucositis for patients with cancer receiving treatment. *Cochrane Database Syst Rev* 2007;(2):CD001973.

129. Stiff PJ, Emmanouilides C, Bensinger WL, et al. Palifermin reduces patient-reported mouth and throat soreness and improves patient functioning in the hematopoietic stem-cell transplantation setting. *J Clin Oncol* 2006;24(33):5186–5193.

130. Rosen LS, Abdi E, Daivs ID, et al. Palifermin reduces the incidence of oral mucositis in patients with metastatic colorectal cancer treated with fluorouracil-based chemotherapy. *J Clin Oncol* 2006;24(33):5194–5200.

131. Schubert MM, Eduardo FP, Guthrie KA, et al. A phase III randomized double-blind placebo-controlled clinical trial to determine the efficacy of low level laser therapy for the prevention of oral mucositis in patients undergoing hematopoietic cell transplantation. *Support Care Cancer* 2007;15(10):1145–1154.

132. Eduardo FP, Mahnert DU, Monezi TA, et al. Cultured epithelial cells response to phototherapy with low intensity laser. *Lasers Surg Med* 2007;39(4): 365–372.

133. Corti L, Chiarion-Sileni V, Aversa S, et al. Treatment of chemotherapy-induced oral mucositis with light-emitting diode. *Photomed Laser Surg* 2006;24(2): 207–213.

134. Oberoi S, Zamperlini-Netto G, Beyene J, et al. Effect of prophylactic low level laser therapy on oral mucositis: a systematic review and meta-analysis. *PLoS One* 2014;9:e107418.

135. Wagner VP, Curra M, Webber LP, et al. Photobiomodulation regulates cytokine release and new blood vessel formation during oral wound healing in rats. *Lasers Med Sci* 2016;31:665–671.

136. Hamblin MR, Demidova TN. Mechanisms of low level light therapy. *Proc SPIE* 2006;6140:614001–614012.

137. Dodd MJ, Dibble SL, Miaskowski C, et al. Randomized clinical trial of the effectiveness of 34 commonly used mouthwashes to treat chemotherapy-induced mucositis. *Oral Surg Oral Med Oral Pathol Oral Radiol Endod* 2000;90:39–47.

138. Dodd MJ, Miaskowski C, Greenspan D, et al. Radiation-induced mucositis: a randomized clinical trial of micronized sucralfate versus salt and soda mouthwashes. *Cancer Invest* 2003;21:21–33.

139. Feber T. Management of mucositis in oral irradiation. *Clin Oncol (R Coll Radiol)* 1996;8:106–111.

140. Cerchietti LC, Navigante AH, Korte MW, et al. Potential utility of the peripheral analgesic properties of morphine in stomatitis-related pain: a pilot study. *Pain* 2003;105(1–2):265–273.

141. Epstein JB, Epstein JD, Epstein MS, et al. Management of pain in cancer patients with oral mucositis: follow-up of multiple doses of doxepin oral rinse. *J Pain Symptom Manage* 2007;33(2):111–114.

142. Leenstra JL, Miller RX, Qin R, et al. Doxepin rinse versus placebo in the treatment of acute oral mucositis pain in patients receiving head and neck radiotherapy with or without chemotherapy: a phase III, randomized, double-blind trial (NCCTG-N09C6 [Alliance]). *J Clin Oncol* 2014;32(15):1571–1577.

143. Adams S, Toth B, Dudley BS. Evaluation of sucralfate as a compounded oral suspension for the treatment of stomatitis. *Clin Pharmacol Ther* 1985;2:178.

144. Pfeiffer P, Madsen EL, Hansen OM, et al. Effect of prophylactic sucralfate suspension on stomatitis induced by cancer chemotherapy. *Acta Oncol* 1990;29:171–173.

145. Shenep JL, Kalwinsky DK, Hutson DK, et al. Efficacy of oral sucralfate suspension in prevention and treatment of chemotherapy-induced mucositis. *J Pediatr* 1988;113:758–763.

146. Innocenti M, Moscatelli G, Lopez S. Efficacy of Gelclair in reducing pain in palliative care patients with oral lesions: preliminary findings from an open pilot study. *J Pain Symptom Manage* 2002;24(5):456–457.

147. Papas AS, Clark RE, Martuscelli G, et al. A prospective, randomized trial for the prevention of mucositis in patients undergoing hematopoietic stem cell transplantation. *Bone Marrow Transplant* 2003;31(8):705–712.

148. Epstein JB, Vickers L, Spinelli J, et al. Efficacy of chlorhexidine and nystatin rinses in prevention of oral complications in leukemia and bone marrow transplantation. *Oral Surg Oral Med Oral Pathol* 1992;73: 692–699.

149. Stockman MA, Spijkervet FK, Burlage FR, et al. Oral mucositis and selective elimination of oral flora in head and neck cancer patients receiving radiotherapy: a double-blind randomised clinical trial. *Br J Cancer* 2003;88(7):1012–1016.

150. El-Sayed S, Babid A, Shelley W, et al. Prophylaxis of radiation-associated mucositis in conventionally treated patients with head and neck cancer: a double-blind, phase III, randomized, controlled trial evaluating the clinical efficacy of an antimicrobial lozenge using a validated mucositis scoring system. *J Clin Oncol* 2002;20:3956–3963.

151. Trotti A, Garden A, Warde P, et al. A multinational, randomized phase III trial of iseganan HCl oral solution for reducing the severity of oral mucositis in patients receiving radiotherapy for head-and-neck malignancy. *Int J Radiat Oncol Biol Phys* 2004;58(3):674–681.

152. Giles FJ, Rodriguez R, Weisdorf D, et al. A phase III, randomized, double-blind, placebo-controlled, study of iseganan for prevention of stomatitis in patients receiving stomatotoxic chemotherapy. *Leuk Res* 2004;28(6): 559–565.

153. Epstein JB, Elad S, Eliav E, et al. Orofacial pain in cancer: part II—clinical perspectives and management. *J Dent Res* 2007;86(6):506–518.

154. Dunbar PJ, Chapman CR, Buckley FP, et al. Clinical analgesic equivalence for morphine and hydromorphone with prolonged PCA. *Pain* 1996;68: 265–270.

155. Bar Ad V, Weinstein G, Dutta PR, et al. Gabapentin for the treatment of pain syndrome related to radiation-induced mucositis in patients with head and neck cancer treated with concurrent chemoradiotherapy. *Cancer* 2010;116(17):4206–4213.

156. Epstein JB, Ransier A, Sherlock CH, et al. Acyclovir prophylaxis of oral herpes virus during bone marrow transplantation. *Oral Oncol Eur J Cancer* 1996;32(B):158–162.

157. Lloid ME, Schubert MM, Myerson D, et al. Cytomegalovirus infection of the tongue following marrow transplantation. *Bone Marrow Transplant* 1994;14:99–104.

158. Goodrich JM, Bowden RA, Fisher L, et al. Ganciclovir prophylaxis to prevent cytomegalovirus disease after allogeneic marrow transplant. *Ann Intern Med* 1993;118:173–178.

159. Meyers JD. Prevention of cytomegalovirus infection after marrow transplantation. *Rev Infect Dis* 1989;11(suppl 7):S1691–S1705.

160. Slavin MA, Osborne B, Adams R, et al. Efficacy and safety of fluconazole prophylaxis for fungal infections after marrow transplantation—a prospective, randomized, double-blind study. *J Infect Dis* 1995;171:1545–1552.

161. Epstein JB, Truelove EL, Hanson-Huggins K, et al. Topical polyene antifungals in hematopoietic cell transplant patients: tolerability and efficacy. *Support Care Cancer* 2004;12(7):517–525.

162. Worthington HV, Eden OB, Clarkson JE. Interventions for preventing oral candidiasis for patients with cancer receiving treatment. *Cochrane Library* 2005;2:1–68.

163. Belazi M, Velegraki A, Koussidou-Eremondi T, et al. Oral candida isolates in patients undergoing radiotherapy for head and neck cancer: prevalence, azole susceptibility profiles and response to antifungal treatment. *Oral Microbiol Immunol* 2004;19(6):347–351.

164. Oblon DJ, Paul SR, Oblon MB, et al. Propantheline protects the oral mucosa after high-dose ifosfamide, carboplatin, etoposide and autologous stem cell transplantation. *Bone Marrow Transplant* 1997;20:961–963.

165. Wang X, Sun X, Zhang X, et al. Quantitative assessment of the effect of FGF20 rs12720208 variant on the risk of Parkinson's disease: a meta-analysis. *Neurol Res.* 2017;39:374–380.

166. Koerner ME. Using hypnosis to relieve pain of terminal cancer. *Hypnosis* 1977;20:39–46.

167. Barber J, Gritelson J. Cancer pain: psychological management using hypnosis. *Cancer* 1980;30:130–135.

168. McCarthy AM, Cool VA, Petersen M, et al. Cognitive behavioral pain and anxiety interventions in pediatric oncology centers and bone marrow transplant units. *J Pediatr Oncol Nurs* 1996;13:3–12.

169. Syrjala KL, Donaldson GW, Davis MW, et al. Relaxation and imagery and cognitive-behavioral training reduce pain during cancer treatment: a controlled clinical trial. *Pain* 1995;63:189–198.

170. Allison RR, Ambrad AA, Arshoun Y, et al. Multi-institutional, randomized, double-blind, placebo-controlled trial to assess the efficacy of a mucoadhesive hydrogel (MuGard) in mitigating oral mucositis symptoms in patients being treated with chemoradiation therapy for cancers of the head and neck. *Cancer* 2014;120(9):1433–1440.

171. Bjordal JM, Bensadoun RJ, Tunèr J, et al. A systematic review with meta-analysis of the effect of low-level laser therapy (LLLT) in cancer therapy-induced oral mucositis. *Support Care Cancer.* 2011;19:1069–1077.

CHAPTER 46

Cancer-Related Bone Pain

EDGAR ROSS, LALITHA SUNDARARAMAN, and **MARY ALICE VIJJESWARAPU**

Epidemiology Review

Bone pain due to cancer is caused by primary bone tumors and those malignant diseases that commonly metastasize to the bones. Bone is the third most common site of metastasis after lung and liver.[1] Metastatic bone pain most commonly results from cancers of the breast, prostate, and lung.[2] Other malignancies involving bone are renal cell carcinoma, thyroid cancer, lymphoma, and multiple myeloma.[3] The longer these malignancies persist, the higher the probability of finding bone metastases. Current therapies have increased survival time of patients suffering from many of these malignancies. This has resulted in an increasing prevalence of metastatic bone disease. Li et al.[4] estimated that 279,679 (95% confidence interval: 274,579 to 284,780) US adults alive on December 31, 2008, had evidence of metastatic bone disease in the previous 5 years (Table 46.1). Breast, prostate, and lung cancers accounted for 68% of these cases.

Prostate cancer is very likely to metastasize to bone rather than other organs. Because patients are living longer than other patients with metastatic diseases, prostate cancer patients are at increased risk of having prolonged periods of pain secondary to bony invasion.[5]

Vertebral involvement is the most common site of bony metastases. The incidence ranges from 30% to 70%.[6] Most patients with metastatic disease of the vertebrae experience back pain.[7]

Bony metastases compromise both the bone's integrity and strength. In the vertebrae, this leads to the increased risk of a pathologic fracture, found most commonly in the elderly. Compression fractures affect between 8% and 30% of cancer patients with vertebral body involvement.[8,9] In many cases, the fracture occurs without an initial traumatic event suggesting that vertebral load is an independent factor in the etiology of a pathologic fracture.[10] Other factors that can lead to pathologic fractures include iatrogenic causes such as steroids, malnutrition-induced osteoporosis, bone mineral loss as a result of inactivity, and destruction of bone secondary to radiation therapy.[11]

Complications from vertebral fracture include a redistribution of load across affected vertebral bodies creating the increased risk of fractures at adjacent levels, increased risk of embolic phenomena as a result of inactivity and pain, kyphosis-induced restriction of vital capacity,[12] predisposition to atelectasis, and early satiety-induced anorexia.[13] Because of this, bony metastases contribute significantly morbidity and decreased life span.[3,14]

PATHOPHYSIOLOGY

Over the past 10 years, animal models for bone tumor growth, bone remodeling, and bone pain have demonstrated a correlation with many features found in human bony metastatic pain. Mouse studies using murine sarcoma cells injected into the intramedullary space of the femur demonstrate mechanical as well as movement-related pain behaviors. These behaviors[15] increase with time and with increasing tumor-induced bone destruction offering a model that appears to replicate the human experience of how metastatic bone cancer contributes to bone pain. In normal mice, a nonnoxious stimulus to the femur does not elicit the synthesis of any tissue factors, whereas in mice with bone cancer, a nonnoxious stimulus elicits the synthesis of substance P, which binds to the neurokinin-1 receptor expressed in the spinal cord. Likewise, *c-fos* is not expressed at the level of the spinal cord in normal mice, but this protein is found in a population of mice with bony tumors.[16]

Both osteolytic and osteoblastic changes in bone occur in some tumor types such as lung, breast, and renal tumors. A predominance of osteolysis is found in multiple myeloma and sarcomas, leading to increased destruction of bone with time. The predominant lesion in men with bone metastases from prostate cancer is osteoblastic which leads to increased numbers of irregular bone trabeculae weakening bone.[17]

In the prostate model, colonies of malignant prostate tissue exist along the length of the intramedullary canal divided by newly formed bone.[18] In the sarcoma model, there is no new bone formation, only destruction, which is greatest at the proximal and distal head with little to no destruction at the midshaft of the bone. The prostate model also demonstrates the formation of new bone along the length of the long bone involving diaphysis and proximal and distal endpoints with an increase of osteoclasts throughout the length of the intramedullary canal. These cells stimulate osteolytic remodeling inducing an inflammatory reaction mediated by macrophages. It is suspected that this macrophage-induced inflammatory activity may be the basis for neuropathic type of pain found in malignancies of the bone.[19]

TABLE 46.1 Estimated Number of Prevalent Cases of Metastatic Bone Disease in the National Commercially Insured Population Aged 18–64 Years, The National Fee-for-Service Medicare Population Aged ≥65 Years, and the US Adult Population on December 31, 2008, All Cancers and by Specific Cancer Types

Cancer Type	Commercially Insured, Ages 18–64 years (*n* = 120,694,145)	Fee-for-Service Medicare, Ages ≥65 years (*n* = 25,950,760)	US adult population[a] (*n* = 230,118,000)
All cancers	60,411 (59,134–61,689)	128,540 (125,485–131,595)	279,679 (274,579–284,780)
Female breast	25,754 (24,911–26,596)	35,960 (34,341–37,579)	90,904 (88,095–93,714)
Prostate	4,969 (4,609–5,329)	37,240 (35,593–38,887)	62,841 (60,253–65,429)
Lung	7,879 (7,421–8,337)	15,900 (14,823–16,977)	35,222 (33,415–37,030)
Other	21,809 (21,046–22,573)	39,440 (37,745–41,135)	90,712 (87,843–93,580)

NOTES: Data presented as estimated number of patients with metastatic bone disease (95% confidence interval).
[a]US Census 2008.
From Li S, Peng Y, Weinhandl ED, et al. Estimated number of prevalent cases of metastatic bone disease in the US adult population. *Clin Epidemiol* 2012;4(1):87–93. Reproduced with permission of Dove Medical Press in the format Republish in a book via Copyright Clearance Center.

Multiple studies have demonstrated that the periosteum is richly innervated by both sympathetic and sensory nerve fibers.[20,21] The periosteum receives the greatest amount of afferent sensory fibers per unit area in bone. In addition, the periosteum, bone marrow, and mineralized bone are also innervated by both sensory and sympathetic fibers.

Osteolytic animal models demonstrate microscopic fragmentation and disruption of the bony matrix secondary to tumor growth. In the osteoblastic model, there is evidence of destructive injury as well as an increase in the density of sensory fibers compared to normal bone. An increase in specific transcription factors has also been demonstrated, including activating transcription factor-3 (ATF-3). Expression of ATF-3 is usually detectable in peripheral nerve injury models. It is also expressed in the nucleus of sensory neurons damaged by osteolytic tumor cells. However, this transcription factor is not detectable in normal sensory neuron nuclei or in sensory neurons affected by peripheral inflammation. Animal models with increased ATF-3 demonstrate an increase in movement-related pain behavior. Gabapentin improved pain-related behavior in this model[22] but did not change tumor growth, bone destruction, or changes in peripheral sensory fibers that were impacted by tumor infiltration. These changes suggest that pain experienced secondary to tumor infiltration is neuropathic.[23]

Osteolytic metastases in breast cancer secrete parathyroid hormone-related peptide (PTHrP) which, in turn, binds to the parathyroid hormone-related peptide receptor (PTHR1) on marrow stromal cells, resulting in the production of receptor activator of nuclear factor-κB ligand (RANKL). RANKL stimulates osteoclast differentiation which then demineralizes bone, leading to increased levels of insulin-like growth factor 1 (IGF-1) and TGF-β from bony matrix, supporting neoplastic proliferation increased PTHrP supporting growth of metastatic disease. This is exploited in the advent of the new antibody to RANKL denosumab that is used to combat bony metastatic proliferation and complications caused by it.[24]

Osteoclastic-induced changes in pH also play a role in bone pain. Tumor cell growth can exceed its vascular supply leading to tumor cell death and further decrease in tissue pH and more pain. Additionally, as tumors grow, associated inflammatory cells which may comprise as much as 80% of the tumor mass reduce local pH. This localized decrease of pH in the bony matrix will lead to an increased absorption of bone as manifested by osteoclastic activity.[25] The administration of a transient receptor potential vanilloid (TRPV) antagonist within the mouse model correlates with a decrease in pain behaviors in all stages of tumor growth, suggesting a new potential therapeutic target to reduce cancer-related bone pain.[25] Tumor cells also produce formaldehyde through a demethylation process by serine hydroxymethyltransferase and lysine-specific histone demethylase 1. When the cancer cells migrate into the bone marrow, formaldehyde leads to upregulation of the transient receptor potential vanilloid subfamily member 1 (TRPV1) in the peripheral nerve fibers. IGF-1 produced by osteoblasts also increases TRPV1 receptors that contribute to neuropathic pain associated with cancer spread.

Osteoprotegerin (OPG) is a secreted soluble receptor, which is a tumor necrosis factor receptor (TNFR). This receptor prevents the activation of osteoclasts via a binding–sequestering of the OPG ligand. This has been shown to decrease the amount of pain-related behavior in the mouse sarcoma model. The monoclonal antibody (AMG-162) can inhibit bone destruction by reducing osteoclast function leading to a reduction in inflammatory-mediated changes in the dorsal root ganglion (DRG) which has been correlated with bony metastatic pain.[26]

Inflammatory cells associated with tumor stroma secrete a variety of compounds that sensitize or excite afferent neurons. Compounds include prostaglandins, tumor necrosis factor-α, endothelins, interleukin-1 and interleukin-6, epidermal growth factor, transforming growth factor-β, and platelet-derived growth factor. Receptors for these factors are directly expressed by afferent neurons. All may play a role in bone pain suggesting new targets. In clinical practice, only prostaglandin and agents targeting endothelin have been used to control metastatic bone pain. Prostaglandins play a role in both sensitization and excitation of nociceptors via direct binding to the prostanoid receptor.[26]

Nerve growth factor (NGF) is a neurotrophic factor expressed in tissue following nerve injury by both the nerves injured as well as surrounding tissues. Upregulation of NGF is thought to be a component in the hyperalgesia following nerve injury. Anti-NGF therapy could be effective in the control of pain related to bone cancer.[27] In the osteolytic sarcoma mouse model, anti-NGF antibody demonstrated effectiveness in attenuation of pain behaviors and was found to be more effective than acute administration of 10 and 30 mg/kg doses of morphine sulfate.[28]

EVALUATION OF THE PATIENT WITH BONE CANCER

The two most important imaging modalities in the evaluation of malignancy of the bone are plain radiography and radioisotope bone scans.

Radiography

Radiographic studies should be ordered first in the evaluation of patients with complaints of bone pain in the context of malignancy. Radiographic patterns fall into osteolytic, osteoblastic, or mixed presentation. Osteoblastic lesions appear opaque and sclerotic. Osteolytic lesions appear more radiolucent compared to surrounding bone. Risk of fracture is greatest if more than 50% of long bone is involved.[7,29]

Bone Scan

Radioisotope bone scans are very good at identification of multifocal lesions.[30] Radioisotopes accumulate in areas of new bone growth and are diminished in areas of metastasis secondary to decreased blood flow to the area. Cancers such as melanoma and multiple myeloma may have false negatives when reviewed on bone scan secondary due to their lack of reactive bone activity.

Computed Tomography

Computed tomography (CT) offers improved spatial resolution in the evaluation of cortical bone destruction.[31] CT is beneficial in evaluation of the three-dimensional characteristics of diseased bone identified by plain radiographs and isotope scans. CT scan evaluations are optimal to study the pelvic and shoulder girdles and spinal lesions. Additionally, CT-guided needle biopsies can be used to identify cell types.

18F-FDG-PET-CT

The visualization of glucose metabolism by positron-emission tomography with 18F-fluorodeoxyglucose, coupled with a simultaneously obtained CT (18F-FDG-PET-CT), is now a standard diagnostic technique in oncology. In patients with highly metabolically active cancers such as lung cancer or malignant melanoma, PET-CT with FDG has replaced other techniques for the detection of bone metastases. In highly active tumors, bony metastases can be detected with high sensitivity and specificity.[32]

Magnetic Resonance Imaging

Magnetic resonance imaging (MRI) provides better contrast resolution in defining soft tissue and marrow involvement. Also, it can define vascular relationships without contrast enhancement.[31] MRI is very beneficial in the evaluation of tumor infiltration of muscle and bone marrow, spinal cord compression, and lesions which are otherwise insufficiently imaged by the previously listed approaches.

TREATMENT

The site and distribution of bone metastases and the skeletal sequelae, such as pathologic fracture and spinal cord compression, can impact the patient's prognosis. The focus of treatment should be directed at tumor regression, relief of cancer-related symptoms, and preservation of functional capacity. In some cases, metastatic disease is so advanced that it is resistant to both chemotherapy and radiotherapy. When metastatic involvement cannot be completely treated, the best way forward is to focus on symptom management. Impaired neurologic function, pathologic fractures, and debilitating pain are the most important reasons for aggressive treatment. Palliation may employ radiotherapy, radiopharmaceuticals, chemotherapy, hormone therapy, bisphosphonates, calcitonin, analgesics (opioids and antiinflammatory drugs), adjuvant analgesics (e.g., corticosteroids), and surgery.[33] Details for these interventions are found elsewhere.

Analgesic medications provide pain relief during therapy with more definitive modalities (e.g., surgical fixation, radiation therapy) as well as when malignant bone pain is resistant to other modalities of treatment. Conventional administration of opioids and nonsteroidal anti-inflammatory drugs (NSAIDs) may not produce adequate analgesia because of the incidental and intermittent nature of pain a patient might experience. These medications also have dose-limiting side effects. NSAID use is often limited by the risks of gastrointestinal (GI) bleeding and inhibition of platelet function, especially in patients with low platelet counts and taking steroids. In these latter patients, a cyclooxygenase-2 (COX-2) inhibitor may be preferred (see the following section). Patients can have renal and cardiovascular complications with both selective and nonselective NSAIDs. These patients are also prone to having comorbidities that may place them at increased risk of complications, particularly patients undergoing cancer chemotherapy and with advanced disease. Targeted pharmacotherapeutic and interventional approaches can be used to improve these risk–benefit ratios. The remainder of this chapter focuses on those therapies that have been studied specifically for the treatment of cancer-related bone pain to supplement material presented elsewhere in this text.

CYCLOOXYGENASE-2-SPECIFIC INHIBITORS

COX-2-specific inhibitors (coxibs) have demonstrated efficacy in the treatment of chronic and acute pain comparable to traditional (nonselective) NSAIDs without the severity of GI complication during short-term use or platelet inhibition effects.[34] The superior safety profile of coxibs in conjunction with similar efficacy of conventional NSAIDs supports their use in analgesic regimens for bone cancer. Many tumors express the COX-2 isoenzyme, which is involved in the synthesis of prostaglandins.[35] In the murine sarcoma model, acute administration of a selective COX-2 inhibitor attenuated both ongoing and movement-evoked bone cancer pain, whereas chronic inhibition of COX-2 significantly reduced ongoing and movement-evoked pain behaviors and reduced tumor burden, osteoclastogenesis, and bone destruction by >50%. COX-2 is expressed in 40% of human invasive breast cancers, and bone is the primary site of metastasis in cases of breast cancer.[36,37] COX-2 inhibition also inhibited bone metastasis in both a prevention and treatment regimen. This suggests COX-2 produced in breast cancer cells are significant in supporting progression of osteolytic bone metastases in patients with breast cancer, and that COX-2 inhibition may halt this process. Furthermore, COX-2 inhibition may benefit iatrogenically caused tumor progression.[38] COX-2 inhibitors, such as celecoxib, have also been shown to increase apoptosis and decreased progression of osteosarcoma cell lines.[39]

Morphine has been shown to stimulate angiogenesis supporting tumor growth in mice. COX-2 inhibition can prevent tumor growth without compromising opioid-dependent analgesia in a murine breast cancer model. Chronic morphine treatment alone stimulated angiogenesis in breast cancer with a corresponding increase in metastasis and reduced survival, whereas coadministration of a coxib prevented these morphine-induced effects and improved analgesia over either agent independently.[40]

CORTICOSTEROIDS

Corticosteroids are established analgesics in the treatment of pain secondary to metastatic bone pain. This analgesia is thought to occur through the blockade of cytokine synthesis that contributes to both inflammation and nociception.[41,42] The analgesic benefits of corticosteroids are dose-dependent and limited in their duration of activity. In a small uncontrolled study, approximately 40% of patients with metastatic prostate cancer were found to have analgesic benefit with the administration of oral corticosteroids. This was speculated to be secondary to suppression of hormone-sensitive disease that was stimulated by weak androgens of adrenal origin by negative feedback on secretion of adrenocorticotropic hormone.[43] Dexamethasone is the most commonly used agent because it has the least effect on mineralocorticoid activity.

BISPHOSPHONATES

Bisphosphonates are pyrophosphate analogues which bind to hydroxyapatite bone mineral surfaces acting to inhibit osteoclasts and thus bone resorption.[44] The optimal dose for this class is a function of the disease stage.[45]

Oral clodronate given to patients with breast cancer metastatic to bone reduced the frequency of skeletal events by more than one-fourth.[46] In two randomized placebo-controlled trials comparing monthly pamidronate infusions to placebo infusions showed that skeletal morbidity rate could be reduced by 30% to 40%.

A large, randomized, multicenter trial using intravenous (IV) zoledronic acid demonstrated a reduction of 20% in the risk of developing skeletal-related events compared with pamidronate for patients with breast cancer.[47] Moreover, these trials demonstrated for the first time that a bisphosphonate significantly reduces the occurrence of skeletal events in hormone-refractory prostate cancer, non–small-cell lung cancer, and a large range of solid tumors. Evidence from *in vitro* studies have shown that bisphosphonates are able to directly affect tumor cell growth.[46]

Of the available bisphosphonates, IV zoledronic acid has demonstrated the broadest clinical activity and is approved in many countries for the treatment of bone metastases from all solid tumors.[48,49] The indications for bisphosphonate therapy in breast cancer patients include correction of hypercalcemia and the prevention of cancer treatment-induced bone loss.[50]

In phase III clinical trials, denosumab, a human antibody to RANKL, is highly effective for preventing complications in patients with bone metastasis from prostate cancer, breast cancer, and other solid tumors. In addition, it decreased treatment-related bone loss in patients treated with androgen deprivation therapy for prostate cancer and women with breast cancer who are treated with aromatase inhibitors.[51,52] Limited postmarketing analysis has raised concerns regarding denosumab because of the potential for osteonecrosis of the jaw.[53]

Bisphosphonates, although effective in decreasing bony complications due to bone metastases in prostate cancer, breast cancer, and other solid tumors, can cause extensive side effects.[54]

Highly selective matrix metalloproteinase inhibitors inhibit osteoclastic and bone tumor cell lines but not osteoblasts. They are also more effective in promoting tumor apoptosis compared with the standard-of-care bisphosphonate, zoledronate.[55]

Bisphosphonates are now a routine part of therapeutic regimen for metastatic bone pain, and at least 50% of patients report clinically relevant analgesic effect. Placebo-controlled trials with oral or IV bisphosphonates have shown that prolonged administration can reduce the frequency of skeletal-related events by 30% to 40%. The superiority of zoledronic acid compared with pamidronate has been shown by a multiple-event analysis in a large randomized trial. The short infusion time of zoledronic acid also constitutes a convenient therapy. Flu-like symptoms, which are manageable with standard treatment, do occur. Renal monitoring is recommended, with dose reductions for patients with renal dysfunction. Osteonecrosis of the mandible has been reported in patients receiving bisphosphonates and might be avoidable with appropriate dental care.[56]

CALCITONIN

The hormone calcitonin has the potential to relieve pain and also retain bone density, leading to a decreased risk of fractures. However, there is limited evidence to support the routine use of calcitonin for pain secondary to bony metastases.[57] Data suggests that calcitonin offers adjuvant analgesia in the treatment of bone pain related to metastatic disease.[58,59]

A human clinical trial prospectively entered 22 patients to evaluate the efficacy of salmon calcitonin in controlling pain related to bone metastasis.[60] Other controlled clinical trials of salmon calcitonin in the treatment of cancer-related bone pain have shown equivocal analgesic results without evidence of reducing complications due to bone metastasis or improving quality of life or survival.[57,61] Like many pain-relieving strategies, there is considerable interpatient variability in responses. In those patients who are not responding well to other first-line approaches, a trial of calcitonin may be reasonable, but close follow-up should ensure that benefits outweigh risks.

OPIOIDS/OPIATE ANTAGONISTS

Opioids continue to be an important means of treating metastatic bone pain, but new research offers a challenge as to which treatment plan may be most appropriate. In a murine sarcoma model of bone cancer pain, the effects of sustained morphine found that morphine-enhanced, rather than diminished, spontaneous and evoked pain, and that the effects were dose dependent and naloxone sensitive.[62] Morphine increased ATF-3 expression only in DRG cells of sarcoma mice. Morphine did not alter tumor growth in vitro or tumor burden in vivo but accelerated sarcoma-induced bone destruction and doubled the incidence of spontaneous fracture in a dose- and naloxone-sensitive manner. Furthermore, morphine increased osteoclast activity and upregulated interleukin-1β within the femurs of sarcoma-treated mice suggesting enhancement of sarcoma-induced osteolysis.

These results suggest morphine may increase pain, osteolysis, bone loss, and spontaneous fracture as well as markers of neuronal damage and expression of proinflammatory cytokines. The data from this study suggest the need to understand the long-term effects of chronic opioid therapy for cancer pain.

ADJUVANT ANALGESICS

The pain of bone cancer can be refractory to traditional treatment modalities. This may be the result of neuropathic changes in involved bone tissues. In animal models of bone-invading malignancies, evidence for peripheral nerve injury provides the pathophysiologic rationale for the use of agents typically used to control neuropathic pain in the control of bone cancer pain.[63]

N-METHYL-D-ASPARTATE ANTAGONISM AND α_2 AGONISTS

Administration of α_2 agonists (dexmedetomidine and clonidine), *N*-methyl-D-aspartate (NMDA) antagonists (MK-801 and ketamine), and morphine were examined in a mouse sarcoma bone cancer pain model.[64] As expected, morphine produced a significant analgesic effect, and the α_2 agonists produced analgesic effects with an efficacy similar to that of morphine but only at doses that produced severe sedation. MK-801 demonstrated little analgesic effects, whereas ketamine yielded an analgesic effect with the same efficacy as morphine. The authors concluded that α_2 agonists produce an analgesic effect only at a sedative dose. Ketamine, but not MK-801, is associated with an analgesic response without overt side effects, suggesting that non-NMDA effects may be responsible for ketamine's analgesic efficacy in this model. Applicability of these findings to humans remains untested.

HORMONAL THERAPY

Progression of metastasis from breast, prostate, and uterine malignancies is hormone dependent.[65,66] Antihormonal treatment reduces an important stimulus for growth and is a common form of adjunctive therapy in breast, prostate, and endometrial cancers.[67]

Estrogen and estrogen analogue therapy in patients with breast cancer controls symptoms in 25% to 50% of patients temporarily.[68] Antihormonal therapy improved pain in 70% of patients with widespread bone metastases from prostate cancer.[69] Therapy with estrogens is efficacious but may take 30 to 60 days before complete palliation. However, serious adverse effects may exceed overall benefits. Although hormone therapy with androgen receptor antagonists (e.g., flutamide) or anti-growth factor agents (e.g., luteinizing hormone-releasing hormone analogs of somatostatin and 5-reductase inhibitor) can be used to induce tumor regression, the palliative effect may not offer long-term benefit as hormone-refractory elements continue to proliferate.[70]

RADIONUCLEOTIDES

Analgesic effects from radionucleotides are not dependent on tumor destruction per se but are thought to result from inhibition of pain mediators from normal bone cells. Therapeutic responsiveness is greatest in osteoblastic lesions. Multiple different agents have been used for palliative treatment of cancer-related bone pain, including phosphorus-32, strontium-89, yttrium-90, samarium-153, and rhenium-186.

Phosphorus-32 has been used for more than 30 years and relieves the pain from osteoblastic metastases in approximately 80% of treated patients.[71] Myelosuppression caused by this agent has led to the development of newer agents. Strontium-89 is a bone-seeking radionuclide, whereas samarium-153 is a bone-seeking tetraphosphonate. Both agents have been shown to have efficacy in the treatment of painful osseous metastases from prostate cancer, breast cancer, and, perhaps, from non–small-cell lung cancer. As many as 80% of selected patients[72] with painful osteoblastic bony metastases from prostate or breast cancer experience some pain relief following strontium-89 administration.[73] Additionally, 10% or more may become pain free, and the average duration of clinical response typically ranges from 3 to 6 months with minimal myelosuppression as compared to phosphorus-32.[74]

PROCEDURAL INTERVENTIONS

In addition to pharmacotherapy, interventional therapies can be used to relieve the pain associated with bone cancer. Examples include procedures such as intralesional injections, nerve blocks, intraarticular injections, radiofrequency rhizotomy, and vertebroplasty.

Intralesional Injection

In a study of patients with rib metastases or involvement of the ribs by multiple myeloma, infiltration of tender areas with methylprednisolone provided significant reduction in pain-related symptoms in over half the cases.[75] Of 20 assessable patients,

11 became pain free within 10 days with recurrence of pain in only 1 of these patients; in 8 others, the pain was considerably improved. The procedure was well tolerated, and there were no complications.[75] This technique has also been used to treat mandibular lesions in which surgical excision of tumor would risk destabilizing the affected bone.[76] This technique may be applicable to other areas of metastasis.[77] Additionally, localized injection of corticosteroid, local anesthetic, and even baclofen have been reported to offer clinically meaningful relief in areas of secondary muscular spasm.[78]

Percutaneous Vertebroplasty/Kyphoplasty

Vertebral bony metastases are seen in 30% to 70% of all bony lesions. These metastases compromise the strength of involved bone leading to pathologic vertebral fractures even in the absence of trauma. Additional causes of fractures include osteoporosis, malnutrition, radiation, and steroid administration. Vertebroplasty offers the potential of pain relief. In comparison, patients who have a nonmalignant basis for pathology of the bone such as osteoporosis, reports of analgesic benefit in cancer patients are not as high but are still significant with ranges reported between 50% and 80%.[79] This may be explained by the widespread nature of metastatic disease and the multifactorial origins of pain. The mechanism by which vertebroplasty provides pain relief is not completely understood but could be secondary to fixation of mobile bone fragments and/or thermal neurolysis secondary to the exothermic reaction of methylmethacrylate cement yielding temperatures in excess of 70° C.[80]

Rhizotomy

Minimally invasive neurodestructive techniques have been demonstrated to be effective in a number of malignancies, specifically of visceral and neuropathic nature. Techniques involve radiofrequency lesioning, cryotherapy, and chemical neurolysis using phenol, alcohol, and hypertonic saline. Because pain from bony metastasis has a neuropathic component, these techniques offer an option in the control of cancer-related bone pain. Other diagnoses where this approached can be applied to include chordoma, osteoid osteoma, and osseous metastasis. Studies of radiofrequency lesioning of bony and soft tissue malignancy have reported significant palliation of pain.[81–84]

ASSOCIATED PROCESSES
Avascular Necrosis

Avascular necrosis can be found in survivors of cancer who have been exposed to corticosteroid therapy. Pain is the result of weight bearing on the affected joint. In an MRI study of patients having survived childhood cancer, 67% of patients demonstrated osteonecrosis at the ankle.[85]

Postoperative Frozen Shoulder

In postthoracotomy or postmastectomy patients, pain leads to an increased risk for the development of frozen shoulder. The site may become an independent locus of pain and can be complicated by complex regional pain syndrome. Adequate mobilization of the joint with sufficient analgesia should be implemented soon following surgery to prevent this chronic, painful, and debilitating complication.[86]

GRANULOCYTE COLONY-STIMULATING FACTOR RELATED PAIN

Granulocyte colony-stimulating factor (G-CSF) is used to stimulate the production of granulocytes in immunocompromised patients following chemotherapy and radiation. Bone and generalized muscle pain is a common complication, which can last for 10 or more days.[87] Effective analgesia can require opioids.[88] G-CSF also induces an inflammatory reaction through undefined cellular signaling and histamine release.[89] Increased histamine levels cause nociceptive C-fiber–mediated pain and edema formation within bone leading to pain.[90] Antihistamines such as terfenadine and astemizole have anti-inflammatory properties in addition to their potency as histamine-1 antagonist and can be used to treat bone pain secondary to G-CSF therapy.

Conclusion

The bony skeleton is the most common location for metastatic cancer and leads to a very high incidence of morbidity including severe pain (spontaneous and provoked), hypercalcemia, pathologic fracture, and spinal cord and or nerve root compression. Bone pain is frequently undertreated. Approximately 80% of patients experienced pain before palliative therapy. Progress in understanding the prevention and treatment of cancer-related bone pain is being made. There are many therapies available to treat pain caused by infiltration of cancer into bone.[91]

Major skeletal-related events occur in cancer patients on average every 3 to 6 months. The prognosis of metastatic bone disease is dependent on the primary site. Breast and prostate cancer survival is measured in years; in lung cancer, survival may be measured in months. Severity and duration of tumor involvement in bone cancer are predictors of outcome and can be measured by bone-specific markers. Studies have demonstrated a significant correlation between the rate of bone resorption, clinical outcomes, skeletal morbidity, and overall life expectancy. Improved understanding and treatment will not only improve the quality of life of cancer patients but also improve long-term outcomes.[7]

References

1. Vigorita V. *Orthopaedic Pathology*. 2nd ed. Philadelphia: Lippincott Williams & Wilkins; 2008.
2. Coleman RE. Bisphosphonates: clinical experience. *Oncologist* 2004;9(suppl 4):14–27.
3. Buijs JT, van der Pluijm G. Osteotropic cancers: from primary tumor to bone. *Cancer Lett* 2009;273:177–193.
4. Li S, Peng Y, Weinhandl ED, et al. Estimated number of prevalent cases of metastatic bone disease in the US adult population. *Clin Epidemiol* 2012;4:87–93.
5. Halvorsan K, Sullivan L, Mantyh P. Bone pain. In: Fisch M, Burton A, eds. *Cancer Pain Management*. New York: McGraw-Hill; 2007:75–86.
6. Jajan N, Krishnan S, Das P, et al. Palliative radiation therapy techniques. In: Fisch M, Burton A, eds. *Cancer Pain Management*. New York: McGraw-Hill; 2007:271–296.
7. Coleman RE. Clinical features of metastatic bone disease and risk of skeletal morbidity. *Clin Cancer Res* 2006;12(20 pt 2):6243s–6249s.
8. Patel B, DeGroot H. Evaluation of the risk of pathological fractures secondary to metastatic bone disease. *Orthopedics* 2001;24:612–617.
9. Bunting R, Lamont-Havers W, Schweon D, et al. Pathological fracture risk in rehabilitation of patients with bony metastases. *Clin Orthop Relat Res* 1985;192:222–227.
10. Alberico R, Ahmed AH, Husain SH. Neuroradiologic evaluation of the patient with cancer pain. In: de Leon Casseola O, ed. *Cancer Pain Management: Pharmacologic, Interventional, and Palliative Approaches*. Philadelphia: Elsevier; 2006:141–147.
11. Mont'Alverne F, Vallee JN, Cormier E, et al. Percutaneous vertebroplasty for metastatic involvement of the axis. *Am J Neuroradiol* 2005;26:1641–1645.
12. Schlaich C, Minne HW, Brucker T, et al. Reduced pulmonary function in patients with spinal osteoporotic fractures. *Osteoporos Int* 1998;8(3):261–267.
13. Mazanec D, Podichetty VK, Mompoint A, et al. Vertebral compression fractures: manage aggressively to prevent sequelae. *Cleve Clin J Med* 2003;70(2):147–156.
14. Kado D, Browner WS, Palermo L, et al. Vertebral fractures and mortality in older women: a prospective study. Study of Osteoporotic Fractures Research Group. *Arch Intern Med* 1999;159(11):1215–1220.
15. Yoneda T, Hiraga T. Crosstalk between cancer cells and bone microenvironment in bone metastasis. *Biochem Biophys Res Commun* 2005;328(3):679–687.
16. Sohara Y, Shimada H, DeClerck YA. Mechanisms of bone invasion and metastasis in human neuroblastoma. *Cancer Lett* 2005;228(1–2):203–209.

17. Roudier MP, Vesselle H, True LD, et al. Bone histology at autopsy and matched bone scintigraphy findings in patients with hormone refractory prostate cancer: the effect of bisphosphonate therapy on bone scintigraphy results. *Clin Exp Metastasis* 2003;20(2):171–180.

18. Clines GA, Guise TA. Mechanisms and treatment for bone metastases. *Clin Adv Hematol Oncol* 2004;2(5):295–302.

19. Chung LW, Baseman A, Assikis V, et al. Molecular insights into prostate cancer progression: the missing link of tumor microenvironment. *J Urol* 2005;173(1):10–20.

20. Asmus SE, Parsons S, Landis SC. Developmental changes in the transmitter properties of sympathetic neurons that innervate the periosteum. *J Neurosci* 2000;20:1495–1504.

21. Bjurholm A. Neuroendocrine peptides in bone. *Int Orthop* 1991;15:325–329.

22. Lipton A. Management of bone metastases in breast cancer. *Curr Treat Options Oncol* 2005;6(2):161–171.

23. Peters CM, Ghilardi JR, Keyser CP, et al. Tumor-induced injury of primary afferent sensory nerve fibers in bone cancer pain. *Exp Neurol* 2005;193(1):85–100.

24. Yin JJ, Pollock CB, Kelly K. Mechanisms of cancer metastasis to the bone. *Cell Res* 2005;15(1):57–62.

25. Lipton A. Pathophysiology of bone metastases: how this knowledge may lead to therapeutic intervention. *J Support Oncol* 2004;2(3):205–220.

26. Eaton CL, Coleman RE. Pathophysiology of bone metastases from prostate cancer and the role of bisphosphonates in treatment. *Cancer Treat Rev* 2003;29(3):189–198.

27. Mantyh P. Pain due to bone metastases: new research issues and their clinical implications. In: de Leon Casseola O, ed. *Cancer Pain Management: Pharmacologic, Interventional, and Palliative Approaches.* Philadelphia: Elsevier; 2006:75–84.

28. Riccio AI, Wodajo FM, Malawer M. Metastatic carcinoma of the long bones. *Am Fam Physician* 2007;76(10):1489–1494.

29. Mentzel H, Kentouche K, Sauner D, et al. Comparison of whole-body STIR-MRI and 99mTc-methylene-diphosphonate scintigraphy in children with suspected multifocal bone lesions. *Eur Radiol* 2004;14(12):2297–2302.

30. Edeiken J, Karasick D. Imaging in bone cancer. *CA Cancer J Clin* 1987;37:239–245.

31. Beheshti M, Vali R, Waldenberger P, et al. The use of F-18 choline PET in the assessment of bone metastases in prostate cancer: correlation with morphological changes on CT. *Mol Imaging Biol* 2010;12:98–107

32. James SL, Davies AM. Post-operative imaging of soft tissue sarcomas. *Cancer Imaging* 2008;8:8–18.

33. Jayr C. Analgesic effects of cyclooxygenase 2 inhibitors. *Bull Cancer* 2004;91(suppl 2):S125–S131.

34. Sabino MA, Ghilardi JR, Jongen JL, et al. Simultaneous reduction in cancer pain, bone destruction, and tumor growth by selective inhibition of cyclooxygenase-2. *Cancer Res* 2002;62(24):7343–7349.

35. Singh B, Berry JA, Shoher A, et al. COX-2 involvement in breast cancer metastasis to bone. *Oncogene* 2007;26(26):3789–3796.

36. Singh B, Berry JA, Shoher A, et al. COX-2 induces IL-11 production in human breast cancer cells. *J Surg Res* 2006;131(2):267–275.

37. Farooqui M, Li Y, Rogers T, et al. COX-2 inhibitor celecoxib prevents chronic morphine-induced promotion of angiogenesis, tumour growth, metastasis and mortality, without compromising analgesia. *Br J Cancer* 2007;97(11):1523–1531.

38. Zhou X, Shi X, Ren K, et al. Celecoxib inhibits cell growth and modulates the expression of matrix metalloproteinases in human osteosarcoma MG-63 cell line. *Eur Rev Med Pharmacol Sci* 2015;19(21):4087–4097.

39. Clezardin P, Teti A. Bone metastasis: pathogenesis and therapeutic implications. *Clin Exp Metastasis* 2007;24(8):599–608.

40. Mercadante S. Malignant bone pain: pathophysiology and treatment. *Pain* 1997;69:1–18.

41. MacDonald N. Principles governing the use of cancer chemotherapy in palliative medicine. In: Doyle D, Hanks GW, MacDonald N, eds. *Oxford Textbook of Palliative Medicine.* Oxford, United Kingdom: Oxford Medical Publications; 1993:105–111.

42. Tannock I, Gospodarowicz M, Meakin W, et al. Treatment of metastatic prostatic cancer with low dose prednisone: evaluation of pain and quality of life as pragmatic indices of response. *J Clin Oncol* 1989;7:590–597.

43. Vitté C, Fleisch H, Guenther HL. Bisphosphonates induce osteoblasts to secrete an inhibitor of osteoclast-mediated resorption. *Endocrinology* 1996;137:2324–2333.

44. Body JJ, Mancini I. Bisphosphonates for cancer patients: why, how, and when? *Support Care Cancer* 2002;10(5):399–407.

45. Costa L. Biphosphonates: reducing the risk of skeletal complications from bone metastasis. *Breast* 2007;16(suppl 3):S16–S20.

46. Coleman RE. Optimising treatment of bone metastases by Aredia™ and Zometa™. *Breast Cancer* 2000;7(4):361–369.

47. Santini D, Fratto ME, Vincenzi B, et al. Zoledronic acid in the management of metastatic bone disease. *Expert Opin Biol Ther* 2006;6(12):1333–1348.

48. Rosen L, Gordon D, Kaminski M. Zoledronic acid versus pamidronate in the treatment of skeletal metastases in patients with breast cancer or osteolytic lesions of multiple myeloma: a phase III, double-blind, comparative trial. *Cancer J* 2001;7(5):377–387.

49. Pavlakis N, Stockler M. Bisphosphonates for breast cancer. *Cochrane Database Syst Rev* 2002;(1):CD003474.

50. Ellis GK, Bone HG, Chlebowski R, et al. Effect of denosumab on bone mineral density in women receiving adjuvant aromatase inhibitors for non-metastatic breast cancer: subgroup analyses of a phase 3 study. *Breast Cancer Res Treat* 2009;118(1):81–87.

51. Gnant M, Pfeiler G, Dubsky PC, et al. Adjuvant denosumab in breast cancer (ABCSG-18): a multicentre, randomised, double-blind, placebo-controlled trial. *Lancet* 2015;386(9992):433–443.

52. McGreevy C, Williams D. Safety of drugs used in the treatment of osteoporosis. *Ther Adv Drug Saf* 2011;2(4):159–172.

53. Saad D, Saad P. Report of a jaw osteonecrosis possibly caused by denosumab. *Eur J Oral Implantol* 2017;10(2):213–222.

54. Smith MR, McGovern FJ, Zietman AL, et al. Pamidronate to prevent bone loss during androgen-deprivation therapy for prostate cancer. *N Engl J Med* 2001;345(13):948–955.

55. Tauro M, Shay G, Sansil SS, et al. Bone-seeking matrix metalloproteinase-2 inhibitors prevent bone metastatic breast cancer growth. *Mol Cancer Ther* 2017;16(3):494–505.

56. Lipton A. Efficacy and safety of intravenous bisphosphonates in patients with bone metastases caused by metastatic breast cancer. *Clin Breast Cancer* 2007;7(suppl 1):S14–S20.

57. Martinez-Sapata MJ, Roqué M, Alonso-Coello P, et al. Calcitonin for metastatic bone pain. *Cochrane Database Syst Rev* 2006;19(3):CD003223.

58. Gennari C. Analgesic effect of calcitonin in osteoporosis. *Bone* 2002;30(suppl 5):67S–70S.

59. Visser E. A review of calcitonin and its use in the treatment of acute pain. *Acute Pain* 2005;7(4):185–189.

60. Mystakidou K, Befon S, Hondros K, et al. Continuous subcutaneous administration of high-dose salmon calcitonin in bone metastasis: pain control and beta-endorphin plasma levels. *J Pain Symptom Manage* 1999;18(5):323–330.

61. Tsavaris N, Kopterides P, Kosmas C, et al. Analgesic activity of high-dose intravenous calcitonin in cancer patients with bone metastases. *Oncol Rep* 2006;16(4):871–875.

62. King T, Vardanyan A, Majuta L, et al. Morphine treatment accelerates sarcoma-induced bone pain, bone loss, and spontaneous fracture in a murine model of bone cancer. *Pain* 2007;132(1–2):154–168.

63. Donovan-Rodriguez T, Dickenson AH, Urch CE. Gabapentin normalizes spinal neuronal responses that correlate with behavior in a rat model of cancer-induced bone pain. *Anesthesiology* 2005;102(1):132–140.

64. Saito O, Aoe T, Kozikowski A, et al. Ketamine and N-acetylaspartylglutamate peptidase inhibitor exert analgesia in bone cancer pain. *Can J Anaesth* 2006;53(9):891–898.

65. Sant'Agnese PA. The prostatic endocrine-paracrine regulation system and neuroendocrine differentiation in prostatic carcinoma: a review and future direction in basic research. *J Urol* 1992;152:2.

66. Wood BC. Hormone treatments in the common hormone-dependent carcinomas. *Palliat Med* 1993;7:257–272.

67. Mike S, Harrison C, Coles B, et al. Chemotherapy for hormone-refractory prostate cancer. *Cochrane Database Syst Rev* 2006;(4):CD00524.

68. Reale C, Turkiewicz AM, Reale CA. Antalgic treatment of pain associated with bone metastases. *Crit Rev Oncol Hematol* 2001;37:1–11.

69. Lattouf JB, Saad F. Preservation of bone health in prostate cancer. *Curr Opin Support Palliat Care* 2007;1(3):192–197.

70. Pelger RC, Soerdjbalie-Maikoe V, Hamdy NA. Strategies for management of prostate cancer-related bone pain. *Drugs Aging* 2001;18(12):899–911.

71. Silberstein EB. The treatment of painful osseous metastases with phosphorus-32-labeled phosphates. *Semin Oncol* 1993;20(3 suppl 2):10–21.

72. Oosterhof GO, Roberts JT, de Reijke SA, et al. Strontium(89) chloride versus palliative local field radiotherapy in patients with hormonal escaped prostate cancer: a phase III study of the European Organisation for Research and Treatment of Cancer, Genitourinary Group. *Eur Urol* 2003;44(5):519–526.

73. Robinson K. Strontium 89 therapy for the palliation of pain due to osseous metastases. *JAMA* 1995;274(5):420–424.

74. Kraeber-Bodéré F, Campion L, Rousseau, et al. Treatment of bone metastases of prostate cancer with strontium-89 chloride: efficacy in relation to the degree of bone involvement. *Eur J Nucl Med* 2000;27(10):1487–1493.

75. Rowell NP. Intralesional methylprednisolone for rib metastases: an alternative to radiotherapy? *Palliat Med* 1988;2(2):153–155.

76. Adornato M, Paticoff KA. Intralesional corticosteroid injection for treatment of central giant-cell granuloma. *J Am Dent Assoc* 2001;132(2):186–190.

77. Lin P, Frink SJ. Intralesional treatment of bone tumors. *Operative Techniques in Orthopaedics* 2004;14(4):251–258.

78. Sis T, Wong C. Difficult problems and their solutions in patients with cancer pain of the head and neck areas. *Curr Rev Pain* 2000;4(3):206–214.

79. Alberico R, Ahmed AH, Husain SH. Vertebroplasty and kyphoplasty. In: de Leon Casseola O, ed. *Cancer Pain Management: Pharmacologic, Interventional, and Palliative Approaches.* Philadelphia: Elsevier; 2006:439–448.

80. Fourney D, Schomer DF, Nader R, et al. Percutaneous vertebroplasty and kyphoplasty for painful vertebral body fractures in cancer patients. *J Neurosurg* 2003;98(suppl 1):21–30.

81. Dupuy D, Ahmed M, Rodrigues B, et al. Percutaneous radiofrequency ablation of painful osseous metastases: a phase II trial. *Proc Am Soc Clin Oncol* 2001;20:385a.

82. Locklin MA, Mannes A, Berger A, et al. Palliation of soft tissue cancer pain with radiofrequency ablation. *J Support Oncol* 2004;2:439–445.

83. Wood B, Fojo A, Levy EB, et al. Radiofrequency ablation of painful neoplasms as a palliative therapy: early experience. *J Vasc Interv Radiol* 2000;11S:207.

84. Goetz M, Callstrom MR, Charboneau JW, et al. Percutaneous image-guided radiofrequency ablation of painful metastases involving bone: a multicenter study. *J Clin Oncol* 2004;22(2):300–306.

85. Larkin K. Practical aspects of cancer pain and symptom management and pediatric palliative care. In: Fisch M, Burton A, eds. *Cancer Pain Management*. New York: McGraw-Hill; 2007:209–242.

86. Cherny N. The assessment of cancer pain. In: McMahon S, Koltzenburg M, eds. *Wall and Melzack's Textbook of Pain*. 6th ed. London: Elsevier; 2006:1039–1060.

87. Kubista E, Glaspy J, Holmes FA, et al. Bone pain associated with once-per-cycle pegfilgrastim is similar to daily filgrastim in patients with breast cancer. *Clin Breast Cancer* 2003;6:391–398.

88. Gudi R, Krishnamurthy M, Patcher BR. Astemizole in the treatment of granulocyte colony-stimulating factor-induced bone pain. *Ann Intern Med* 1995;123(3):236–237.

89. König B, König W. Effect of growth factors on Escherichia coli-hemolysin-induced mediator release from human inflammatory cells: involvement of the signal transduction pathway. *Infect Immun* 1994;62:2085–2093.

90. Bennett A. The role of biochemical mediators in peripheral nociception and bone pain. *Cancer Surv* 1988;7:55–67.

91. Slatkin N. Cancer-related pain and its pharmacologic management in the patient with bone metastasis. *J Support Oncol* 2006;4(2 suppl 1):15–21.

CHAPTER 47

Cancer-Related Visceral Pain

MARY ALICE VIJJESWARAPU, LALITHA SUNDARARAMAN, and **EDGAR ROSS**

Epidemiology Review

In 2004, 1.4 million Americans were diagnosed with cancer. This number equals approximately 4,000 new diagnoses per day. In the same year, over 500,000 American deaths were attributed to cancer, accounting for 22% overall mortality.[1] Currently, more than 10 million individuals in the United States carry the burden of a cancer diagnosis, which is 3% of the population.[2] Approximately 50% of patients who carry a diagnosis of cancer report pain as a symptom of the disease process. This percentage increases to 75% of patients reporting pain in the advanced stages of disease.[3,4]

In 2016, it is estimated that there are 1,685,210 new cases of cancer in the United States, and 595,690 people will die from the disease. The number of people living beyond a cancer diagnosis reached nearly 14.5 million in 2014 and is expected to rise to almost 19 million by 2024. Approximately 39.6% of men and women will be diagnosed with cancer at some point during their lifetimes (based on 2010 to 2012 data).[5] The prevalence of pain in cancer varies widely depending on the stage of cancer, type of cancer, and treatment received. The pooled prevalence is about 50% with the highest prevalence in head and neck cancer patients (70% 95% CI, 55% to 80%).[6]

With competent management, cancer pain can be eliminated or well controlled in 80% to 90% of cases, but nearly 1 in 2 patients in the developed world receives less than optimal care. Worldwide, nearly 80% of people with cancer receive little or no pain medication.[7] Trends in death rates for all cancer sites combined from 2000 to 2014 showed a decrease. Death rates decreased statistically, significantly from 2000 to 2014 by 1.8% (95% CI = −1.8% to −1.8%) on average per year among men and by 1.4% (95% CI = −1.4% to −1.3%) per year among women.[8]

After patients come to terms with the diagnosis of cancer and the implications of their disease, most patients and their families will express concern about the pain and suffering they will experience as their disease progresses. Commonly asked questions include how much pain will there be and can it be controlled?[4] Unfortunately, despite evidence that cancer pain can be controlled, it is managed poorly in many cases. Multiple factors limit adequate treatment of cancer pain, including misperceptions of disease processes, misconceptions regarding pain medications and procedures, professionals inadequately trained in pain management, failure to consult specialists trained in contemporary pain management methods, and social stigma around opioid use, including fears of addiction by patients, family members, and professional health care providers.[9] Also, many common cancers in the advanced stages of disease when pain is highly prevalent are incurable, and survival may be measured in months, not years. Whereas health care professionals may only measure survival duration as a meaningful treatment outcome, patients and families may measure outcomes in terms of improvement in quality of life, alleviation of pain, and relief of other associated symptoms related to cancer and treatment.[10]

Because pain syndromes arise from cancer therapies (including chemotherapy, radiation therapy, or surgery), patients who survive their primary malignancy may be left with pain secondary to an iatrogenic process. Chemotherapy may induce a painful peripheral neuropathy. Neuropathy is well described with vincristine, platinum, taxanes, thalidomide, bortezomib, and other agents. Pain secondary to radiation may appear years to decades after completion of radiotherapy. Pain syndromes following surgery may present after mastectomy, amputation, thoracotomy, or other surgical approaches to malignancies (see Chapters 41, 42, 45, and 48).[11]

Characteristics of Visceral Pain

ANATOMY AND PHYSIOLOGY

Visceral pain is caused by disorders of internal organs such as the stomach, kidney, gallbladder, urinary bladder, and intestines as well as changes in the central nervous system. Pain can result from distension, impaction, ischemia, inflammation, or traction on the mesentery and can be associated with symptoms such as nausea, fever, malaise, and pain.[12] Growth of visceral tumors disrupts normal physiologic processes secondary to compression and invasion of adjacent structures. Progression of disease may be asymptomatic until a critical event manifests (e.g., obstruction of a hollow viscus). Under these conditions, the first symptom a patient may experience is pain.[13-15]

Visceral pain is unique in quality of presentation when compared to pain that arises from musculoskeletal structures of the body. Visceral pain is usually vague in its presentation and may be confused by referral to a variety of somatic locations secondary to viscerosomatic convergence.[16] The phenomenon of viscerosomatic convergence refers to the diffuse nature of visceral pain and its referral to superficial structures due to the convergence of visceral and somatic afferents on the same dorsal horn neurons and secondary hyperalgesia. Symptoms may seem out of proportion to physical examination and imaging.[17] Additionally, visceral pain may be attributable both to the malignancy itself and to chemotherapeutic and radiation therapies. Increased pain following symptomatic relief may suggest the local recurrence of disease or a new locus of disease requiring repeat evaluation of the patient.[18]

Some features of visceral nociception may offer a better understanding of the experience of patients with visceral pain. Visceral pain is more frequently accompanied by an autonomic response than is somatic pain or pain from skin injury, unless the pain is referred visceral pain mimicking somatic pain.[16] There is a poor correlation between the extent of visceral tissue damage and the severity of pain experienced. Visceral pain is poorly localized because of poor representation within the primary somatosensory cortex. The majority of visceral afferents are specific to motor or reflex responses with few neural afferents that are specialized for pain transmission. Those afferents that are specialized for pain are sparsely distributed throughout the viscera; both high-threshold nociceptors and low-threshold "silent" nociceptors are invoked in the pain experience.[15]

Studies have demonstrated multiple visceral pain mechanisms as well as the mechanisms by which one class of visceral pain may relate to other sources of malignant pain. There are four primary classes of visceral pain:

1. Mechanical: caused by stretch of visceral structures (bowel lumen or hepatic capsule)
2. Ischemic: caused by tumor invasion or compression of visceral blood supply
3. Inflammatory: humoral mediators of inflammation released secondary to tumor infiltration of visceral structures
4. Neuropathic: compression or invasion of neural structures supplying the viscera[18]

Surgery, chemotherapy, or radiation therapy of cancer can also be responsible for iatrogenic damage of the viscera, associated visceral structures, or nerves. Applying a stimulus that causes tissue damage (e.g., cutting, burning, or pinching) to skin or muscle reliably produces the perception of pain, but these stimuli do not reliably evoke reports of pain when applied to visceral structures. Pain secondary to distension of a hollow viscous, such as in the case of bowel obstruction, does not necessarily produce a similar perception when applied to surface structures. In controlled studies, visceral pain can be consistently demonstrated by mechanical distension of hollow organs using distending fluids or balloon devices.[19] These modalities of inducing pain most closely reproduce the natural or pathophysiologic processes causing pain. Mechanical distension can be specifically applied to a given organ structure in isolation of other structures, mimicking processes involving the gastrointestinal, biliary, and urinary tracts which may occur from tumor obstruction (or adhesions) in these sites. Distension of organ capsules, such as the splenic, renal, or hepatic capsule, has also been demonstrated to produce profound pain. On the other hand, gentle or slow but progressive distension or obstruction may not produce pain until a critical point in which ischemia or rupture results. Torsion or stretch on mesenteric structures or omentum may produce states of ischemia, infarct, and inflammatory response producing reports of severe pain.[20]

Inflammatory processes in visceral structures may produce pain as a result of ischemic response, but some tumors may produce inflammatory mediators with no inciting ischemic event. Both prostaglandin E_2 and serotonin have been demonstrated as independent chemical stimuli in the production of pain as malignancy invades adjacent structures.[21–23] Experimental studies have demonstrated that the application of inflammatory chemical stimuli can evoke pain behaviors, yet specific mechanical means of eliciting pain have been limited in their translation to studies of other visceral structures.[24]

Ischemic pain has also been described as occurring secondary to occlusion of visceral vasculature or by compression of visceral structures by tumor growth. When tumor growth exceeds vascular supply, necrosis may result, inducing a variety of inflammatory processes.[23] Inflammatory mediators, such as hydrogen ions, kinins, prostanoids, leukotrienes, or other cytokines, are initiators of visceral pain. These chemical agents also sensitize neurologic afferents of organ structures amplifying nociception associated with mechanical stimuli. In general, healthy viscera are typically insensate to pain, whereas superficial structures are continually sensate.[24] When diseased, however, visceral organs produce pain severe enough to be incapacitating to other physical activity. Pain from surface structures of the body evokes reflexive motion in the classic "fight or flight" response, whereas the sensation of visceral pain discourages motion or physical activity. Anecdotal evidence supports an association between pain of visceral origin and emotional response and is commonly held to be more anxiety-provoking than pain from somatic structures. Some argue that this anxiety comes from a patient's inability to visualize the cause of the pain.[25] Anxiety scales are reported higher in patients with visceral pain ratings of 2 on a scale of 10 when compared to a higher rated pain experience with visible cause on a superficial structure.[26] Furthermore, some symptomatology is more common in patients with visceral pain. Perception of both nausea and dyspnea are more commonly associated with pain of a visceral organ. An autonomic response to visceral pain is far more common than to pain of superficial structures.[27,28]

Psychological processing of visceral pain is distinct from that related to somatic pain. There are a low number of visceral nociceptors compared with somatic nociceptors. There is a lack of specialization of visceral afferents. Many visceral afferents are polymodal nociceptors. Viscera have unique ascending tracts through the dorsal column and poor representation within the primary somatosensory cortex.[29,30] Viscera have significant input through the medial thalamus to the limbic cortex, amygdala, anterior cingulate, and insular cortex, which influence the affective aspect of pain perception.[31] Viscera also have a close association with autonomic nerves. The perception of visceral pain may be disproportionate to pathology exhibited by physical examination or imaging. As an example, a small nephrolith may offer some of the most severe pain states, whereas extensive cancer metastasis may evoke little or no discomfort. Disorders such as chronic pancreatitis demonstrate very little correlation between laboratory studies and flares in pain perception. Disorders such as irritable bowel syndrome and noncardiac chest pain syndrome appear to lack a definitive histopathologic basis for the discomfort and pain.[32,33]

Many models exist for visceral pain including intraperitoneal injection of a chemical, distension of hollow organs (cecum, colon, rectum), distension of the gallbladder and associated biliary system, and distention or chemical stimulation of the bladder and other urinary tract structures, as well as distension, compression, or traction on reproductive organs. However, lesions studied in one organ are limited in that they are specific to a given stimulus and do not necessarily translate to application in other visceral structures.[34]

SENSITIZATION

Sensitization occurring secondary to the repeated presentation of visceral stimuli has been noted in human psychophysical studies as well as in animal studies. Repeated presentation of the same visceral stimuli produces increasing strength of response in neuronal, cardiovascular, and visceromotor reflex responses. Inflammation of visceral structures increases the magnitude of response to a given mechanical stimulus and decreases the stimulation thresholds for the evocation of nociceptive responses.[35] Inflammation of visceral structures significantly modifies behavioral, neuronal, autonomic, and motor responses to visceral stimulation in experimental models. This model mirrors clinical circumstances because inflammation in visceral structures frequently leads to reports of pain.[36]

Painful conditions such as mucositis, esophagitis, gastritis, pancreatitis, and colitis all exhibit mucosal inflammatory changes. The inflammatory sensitization may take place at primary afferents. These afferents are normally nonreactive to most stimuli and have been described as "silent" in nonpathologic states. However, in the context of an inflammatory tissue response, they become spontaneously active and highly reactive to mechanical stimuli. Silent afferents may comprise 50% of the neuronal sample in a visceral organ but are infrequently noted in superficial or cutaneous structures. Lack of baseline sensitivity in normal viscera may be secondary to sparsity of visceral afferentation. There are fewer afferents per unit area than similar measures of cutaneous afferents. Because of this sparse innervation, increased activity may be necessary to cross a threshold for perception. Spinal neurons responsive to visceral stimuli also change their responsiveness to visceral stimuli in the presence of inflammation. The cause of this behavior is unknown, although voltage-gated sensitization by the transient receptor potential vanilloid 1 (TRPV-1) and tetrodotoxin-resistant (TTX-R) receptors may play a role.[37,38] Increased afferent activity, altered intrinsic properties of dorsal horn neurons, and altered modulatory influences or some combination may all serve a role in the process. Dorsal column pathways have been demonstrated to play a role in visceral nociception but not in cutaneous nociception. The results of multiple studies suggest that visceral pain requires a sensitization process both in the periphery and the spinal cord.[39]

LOCALIZATION

Visceral pain is classically thought of as deep and diffuse in presentation. Localization of the pain generator can be difficult to identify by physical examination. Superficial pain, in contrast, can be elicited by examination with precise localization and with consideration to the site of the body examined; pain locus can be identified within millimeters. Moreover, surface pain loci reliably localize to the same site, never migrating to other body areas, in the absence of neural injury.

Visceral pain is characterized as migratory in its presentation, often perceived in several loci simultaneously or migrating regionally in spite of localization of pathology. This is evident in the presentation of appendicitis. Furthermore, the perception of pain associated with visceral pathology is not normally localized to the organ itself but to somatic structures that receive afferent inputs at the same spinal segments as the visceral afferent entry. For this reason, visceral pain is classically described as either unlocalized pain or as referred pain that may have two separate features. Sensation of the diseased viscera is transferred to a surface site (e.g., an ischemic myocardium can be felt in neck and arms) or additional sites may become hypersensitive to inputs applied directly to those other sites (e.g., flank muscle becomes sensitive to palpation with urolithiasis). This latter phenomenon is referred to as secondary somatic hyperalgesia.

Psychophysical studies of internal organ sensation have focused on a given organ using simple stimuli, correlating the given stimuli to a given organ with perception at the respective site of stimulus. Other psychophysical studies using visceral stimuli have examined the referred sensations described by subjects. These studies have often failed to contrast referred pain to a body surface with cutaneous sensations at the same surface. Patient illustrations of referred sensations tend to extend over large surface areas, whereas studies using cutaneous stimuli generate pinpoint localization to highly precise sites.

The phenomenon of secondary somatic hyperalgesia produced by visceral pathology has been compared to sites of sensitivity with lesions produced by herpes zoster. These initial studies were fundamental to the development of dermatomal mapping. In visceral disease processes, multiple dermatomes have been identified suggesting that secondary somatic hyperalgesia is widely distributed (i.e., poorly localized).

Recent psychophysical studies have attempted to compare visceral with nonvisceral pain. In one study, the sensation produced with balloon distension of the esophagus was compared to thermal stimulation of the mid-chest skin. Subjects perceived larger areas of sensation for esophageal distension than for intensity-matched, heat-evoked sensation on body maps. Temporally, there was also a difference. A rapid response was noted with heat stimulus, whereas there was poor correlation with the esophageal stimulus and the perception of the sensation. Intense visceral discomfort remained after discontinuation of the distending apparatus but not after discontinuation of the cutaneous stimulation. Visceral sensation was concluded to be diffuse both spatially and temporally. Corollary observation of cerebral blood flow identified that similar cerebral areas were activated by both stimuli.

When evaluating the patient in visceral pain with malignancy, the early presentation may be misleading with vague midline discomfort. It may be poorly localized and accompanied by both an emotional response and autonomic event. Later in the evolution of disease process, patients may complain of somatic or referred pain hypersensitivity at the spinal level of the visceral nociceptor terminus. Referred pain is sharp and localized. It is often associated with allodynia and muscle spasm. Furthermore, visceral hypersensitivity may induce the perception of pain in another organ receiving innervation from the same spinal segment.

VISCERAL AFFERENTATION

Visceral primary afferents differ significantly from cutaneous primary afferents in both number and pattern of distribution. Visceral sensory pathways are organized into nerve fascicles and cell body groupings extending from prevertebral regions to contact viscera predominately via perivascular pathways. Cell bodies of visceral primary afferent nerve fibers are located in the visceral dorsal root ganglia of the thoracic and upper lumbar spine, but the peripheral axons of these neurons follow a circuitous path to visceral organs passing via the paravertebral sympathetic chain and ganglia as well as nerve fascicles that are termed the *cardiac* and *splanchnic nerves*. The splanchnic nerves are divided into the greater, lesser, least, thoracic, and lumbar divisions. The pelvic nerves arise from dorsal root ganglia at sacral levels, accepting sympathetic chain input before innervating urogenital structures.

Visceral sensory processing also differs from cutaneous sensory processing because visceral neuronal synapses exist at cell bodies of prevertebral ganglia such as the celiac ganglion, superior mesenteric ganglion, and pelvic ganglion, producing changes in local visceral function outside central control. The gastrointestinal tract is also supplied by an independent enteric nervous system relating to functions of digestion and absorption. In the pelvis, structures receive dual innervation with afferents from lower thoracic to upper lumbar segments and from sacral segments. Testicle and ovary embryologically originate in the superior aspect of the abdomen and, therefore, receive thoracic innervation. The urinary bladder has a similar thoracolumbar innervation with sensory inputs extending up to the T10 level but also receives sacral inputs (the pelvic nerve) with other tissues originating from sacral dermatomes (rectum, genital structures).

Pelvic organs also receive efferent and afferent connections from the vagus nerve and local ganglionic circuitry, resulting in a complex and diffuse neuroanatomy. Afferents with endings in a focal visceral site may have cell bodies in the dorsal root ganglia of 10 or more spinal levels in a bilaterally distributed fashion. In contrast, cutaneous afferents from a particular body surface arise from only 3 to 5 unilaterally located dorsal root ganglia.

Visceral receptors are located in mucosa, serosa, and muscle of hollow organs as well as visceral mesentery. They are not reported in parenchyma of solid organs. The specialized receptors that discriminate a variety of stimuli in somatic structures are absent in viscera. The mesentery, however, does contain Pacinian corpuscles. Hollow organs contain specialized low-threshold and high-threshold mechanoreceptors. Low-threshold receptors serve a basic regulatory function, whereas high-threshold receptors are activated only with noxious mechanical stimuli. Visceral nociception results from summation of nociceptive input to regulatory low-threshold receptors and noxious high-threshold and silent nociceptors rather than activation of stimulus-specific nociceptors.[40]

ASCENDING PATHWAYS

Visceral afferent fiber activation causes an increase in nitric oxide synthase in the dorsal horn of the spinal cord, causing expression of the oncogene c-Fos in laminae I, V, VII, X of the dorsal horn within the thoracolumbar spine. Similar upregulation is seen in the amygdala and paraventricular hypothalamic nuclei and consequent elevation in norepinephrine production within the locus ceruleus.

Features of visceral pain processing differing from somatic processing include dorsal column ascending secondary sensory afferents, the spinal trigeminal to parabrachioamygdaloid tract, and the spinohypothalamic pathway. In the visceral system, both ventrolateral and dorsal column postsynaptic neurons have a role in nociception. Ascending tracts synapse at the lateral thalamus first, then limbic centers, and then somatosensory cortex.

Whereas somatic nociception is represented somatotopically within the primary somatosensory cortex, visceral pain is represented in the secondary somatosensory cortex and poorly represented within the primary somatosensory cortex. Visceral pain is well represented in the limbic system, including anterior cingulate gyrus, insular cortex, and amygdala, suggesting a basis for the strong emotional component of visceral pain. Whereas visceral pain elicits decreased patient activity, nausea, and hypotension, somatic pain elicits agitation, reactive activity, and hypertension. Nociceptive activity within the gastrointestinal tract induces inhibition of dorsal motor neurons of the vagus within the medulla leading to gastroparesis and nausea.

Visceral Pain Syndromes

Although most pain associated with malignancy is diffuse and chronic, most acute pain syndromes in cancer are secondary to diagnostic or therapeutic interventions. Some tumors generate an acute onset of pain, which may be the result of a perforation of a hollow viscus or rupture of a visceral capsule. Any sudden onset of pain warrants a comprehensive pain assessment. Following is a list of possible pain syndromes that may be encountered by the health care provider.

ORAL MUCOSA
Paraneoplastic Pemphigus
Paraneoplastic pemphigus is a mucocutaneous disorder accompanying non-Hodgkin lymphoma and chronic lymphocytic leukemia. It is characterized by widespread shallow ulcers, hemorrhagic crusting of the lips, conjunctival bullae, and may be accompanied by pulmonary lesions, occurring secondary to autoantibodies directed against desmoplakins and desmogleins.[41]

Oropharyngeal Mucositis and Stomatitis
Mucositis and stomatitis should be distinguished as two separate processes (also see Chapter 45). Oral mucositis is an inflammation of oral mucosa resulting from chemotherapeutic agents or ionizing radiation, manifesting as erythema or ulcerations. Stomatitis is any inflammatory condition of oral tissue, including mucosa, dentition, periapices, and periodontium, including inflammation secondary to infection of oral tissues. Mucositis appears 7 to 10 days after initiation of high-dose cancer therapy and is generally self-limited when uncomplicated by infection, resolving 2 to 4 weeks after completion of chemotherapy. In order to standardize assessment, a variety of scales have been created to grade the level of stomatitis by characterizing alterations in lips, tongue, mucous membranes, gingiva, teeth, pharynx, quality of saliva, and voice. The clinical syndrome usually involves the oropharynx but may involve other gastrointestinal mucosal surfaces such as the esophagus, stomach, or intestine, producing such symptoms as odynophagia, dyspepsia, or diarrhea. Any mucosal damage may become superinfected with microorganisms, most commonly *Candida albicans* and herpes simplex.[42]

Radiotherapy may also induce mucositis. Doses of radiation in excess of 4,000 cGy frequently cause ulceration with pain lasting several weeks following treatment.[43] Acute pain associated with radiotherapy can be caused by acute radiation toxicity causing inflammation and ulceration of skin or mucous membranes. The syndrome produced is dependent on the exposed field.[44,45]

MEDIASTINUM
5-Fluorouracil-Induced Anginal Chest Pain
In patients receiving 5-fluorouracil (5-FU) infusions, ischemic chest pain may develop. Painful events are more common in patients with a history of coronary artery disease and are likely secondary to coronary vasospasm.

Pleura
Lung tumors, with or without chest wall involvement, may produce visceral pain. In a large case series of patients with lung malignancies, pain was found to be unilateral in 80% of patients and bilateral in 20% of patients. Patients with hilar tumors reported sternal or scapular pain. Patients with tumors involving the upper and lower lobe experienced referral of pain into the shoulder and lower chest, respectively.[46,47] Additionally, some lung malignancies generate ipsilateral facial pain, thought to be secondary to noxious stimulation of vagal afferent neurons.[48–51]

Pancoast Syndrome
Pancoast syndrome is caused by malignant neoplasms of the superior sulcus of the lung with destructive lesions of the thoracic inlet and involvement of the brachial plexus and cervical sympathetic nerves (stellate ganglion).[52,53] Patients report severe pain in the shoulder region radiating toward the axilla and scapula along the ulnar aspect of the muscles of the hand, and patients may also develop atrophy of hand and arm muscles, Horner syndrome (ptosis, miosis, hemianhidrosis, enophthalmos), and compression of the blood vessels with edema.[54] Ninety-five percent of patients have either squamous cell or adenocarcinomas. Small cell carcinoma is found in fewer than 5% of cases in most series. Along with these symptoms and signs, additional predictors of poor prognosis are weight loss, supraclavicular fossa or vertebral body involvement, disease stage, and surgical treatment.[55,56]

These bronchopulmonary tumors may invade the bony structures of the chest. The first or second thoracic vertebra or the first, second, or third ribs may be invaded. One review has described rib erosion in 50% of patients. The tumor may invade the first or second thoracic vertebral bodies or intervertebral foramina, extending to the spinal cord, and resulting in cord compression. The subclavian vein or artery may also be invaded. Advanced tumors may involve the recurrent laryngeal nerve, phrenic nerve, or superior vena cava (SVC).

PANCREAS
Midline Retroperitoneal Syndrome
The most common cancer-related causes of upper abdominal retroperitoneal pain are pancreatic cancer and retroperitoneal lymphadenopathy, particularly celiac lymphadenopathy. These disease processes elicit afferent activity via injury to deep somatic structures of the posterior abdominal wall, distortion of pain-sensitive connective tissue, vascular and ductal structures, as well as local inflammation and direct infiltration of the celiac plexus. Patients report pain in the epigastrium, in the low thoracic region of the back, or both. Pain is described as diffuse and dull, exacerbated with recumbency, and improved by sitting forward. Computed tomography (CT), magnetic resonance imaging, or ultrasound scanning of the abdomen may reveal the disease process.

Pancreatic Cancer
Patients with pain secondary to unresectable pancreatic cancer report severe abdominal pain radiating into the back. This pain is often refractory to analgesics, even strong opioids. Pain may be accompanied by obstructive jaundice (yellowing of the skin and eyes, itching, dark urine, clay-colored stool) and occurs more frequently when the cancer is located at the head of the pancreas. Other associated symptoms may include weight loss, anorexia, fatigue, and a change in bowel habits (constipation or diarrhea). Controlled trials support the use of neurolytic celiac plexus block with superior results in terms of pain relief over analgesics alone (see Chapter 44 and discussion of celiac plexus block in the following discussion).[57]

LIVER PAIN

Hepatic Distension Syndrome

The liver has many nociceptive structures including the liver capsule, blood vessels, and biliary tract. Afferents from these structures travel via the celiac plexus, the phrenic nerve, and the lower right intercostal nerves. Hepatic metastasis typically causes pain when the tumor stretches the capsule. Patients with intrahepatic metastases or hepatomegaly secondary to cholestasis may report discomfort in the right subcostal region or right midback or flank.[58] Patients may experience referred pain to the right neck, shoulder, or scapula.[59] Patients describe the pain as a dull ache exacerbated by movement, pressure in the abdomen, and deep inspiration. Associated symptoms include anorexia and nausea. Physical examination reveals a hard, irregular subcostal mass, which is dull to percussion, and descends with inspiration. Diagnostic ultrasound or CT may reveal a space-occupying lesion.

Analgesics are the first line of therapy for pain control with drug selection and titration a function of the extent of hepatic compromise. Corticosteroids reduce hepatic edema and liver pain. If a tumor is chemosensitive, chemotherapy may be the treatment of choice. Hormone therapy may decrease hepatomegaly from liver metastasis but may take several months to accomplish a goal of pain relief. As with pancreatic cancer, celiac plexus block may provide definitive relief. Two randomized controlled trials (RCTs) have demonstrated hepatic irradiation to be effective in palliation of hepatic pain in 80% of patients with a reduction of systemic symptoms in half as many patients.[60]

INTESTINAL PAIN

Chronic Intestinal Obstruction

In patients with abdominal or pelvic cancers, intestinal obstruction causes diffuse abdominal pain. Pain may be secondary to smooth muscle contraction, mesenteric tension, and ischemia of the bowel wall. Obstruction may be due to tumor, autonomic neuropathy, ileus, metabolic abnormality, or medication. Pain may be continuous or intermittent (colicky) and may be associated with vomiting, anorexia, and constipation.

Peritoneal Carcinomatosis

The peritoneal cavity, enclosed by visceral and parietal peritoneum, is the largest potential space in the body. Any pathologic process involving the peritoneal cavity can easily disseminate throughout this space by means of unrestricted movement of fluid and cells. Primary malignant diseases arising from the peritoneal cavity include malignant mesothelioma, cystic mesothelioma, and primary peritoneal carcinoma. Carcinomatosis can cause peritoneal inflammation, mesenteric tethering, and malignant adhesions and ascites, all of which can trigger nociceptive activity. Patients most commonly report abdominal pain and distension. Mesenteric tethering and tension appear to cause a diffuse abdominal or low back pain. Tense malignant ascites can produce diffuse abdominal discomfort and a distinct stretching pain in the anterior abdominal wall. Adhesions can also cause obstruction of a hollow viscus, with intermittent colicky pain.[61] CT scanning may demonstrate evidence of ascites, omental infiltration, and peritoneal nodules.

Radiation Enteritis

Acute radiation enteritis may develop in as many as 50% of patients receiving pelvic or abdominal radiotherapy. Patients with small intestinal involvement complain of cramping abdominal pain and have associated nausea and diarrhea. Patients receiving pelvic radiotherapy may develop proctocolitis, associated with pain, tenesmus, diarrhea, mucous discharge, and bleeding. These symptoms may resolve shortly after completion of therapy or may last as long as 6 months.

Intraperitoneal Chemotherapy Pain

Approximately 25% of patients receiving intraperitoneal chemotherapy may develop transient mild to moderate abdominal pain and complain of fullness or bloating.[62] A second group of patients (approximately 25%) may experience pain severe enough to require opioid analgesia or discontinuation of therapy. Pain is secondary to chemical serositis or infection. Infectious peritonitis is accompanied by fever and leukocytosis in blood and peritoneal fluid.

PELVIC PAIN

Malignancy-related pelvic pain not due to bone metastases is most often secondary to presacral recurrence of rectal carcinoma or secondary to pelvic recurrence of cervical cancer. Lumbosacral plexus infiltration is common, resulting in severe pain with a significant neuropathic contribution. Analgesics or interventional therapies should be implemented according to protocols and guidelines (see Chapter 43).

Malignant Perineal Pain

Perineal pain may be secondary to tumors of the colon or rectum, female reproductive tract, and distal genitourinary system. A report of perineal pain following therapeutic resolution of malignancy may be a precursor of recurrence and should prompt complete evaluation.[63] Pain preceding evidence of disease may be secondary to microscopic perineural invasion of an insidious malignant process. Patients report pain to be constant and aching, exacerbated with sitting or standing. Associated symptoms may include tenesmus or bladder spasm.[64] If tumor invades musculature of the pelvis, patients may complain of a constant aching in the pelvis, which is exacerbated with standing. Examination of the pelvic floor may demonstrate tumor.

Ureteral Obstruction

Patients with tumor involving the pelvis may have pain due to tumor compression or infiltration of the distal ureter.[10] Obstruction of the proximal ureter is less common and is associated with retroperitoneal lymphadenopathy, an isolated retroperitoneal metastasis, mural metastases, or intraluminal metastases. Cancers of the cervix, ovary, prostate, and rectum are most commonly associated with this complication. Other rare causes of ureteral obstruction include retroperitoneal fibrosis resulting from radiotherapy or graft-versus-host disease. Pain is described as dull, chronic discomfort in the flank often with associated radiation into the inguinal region or genitalia.[10] However, patients may have obstruction without evidence of pain.

Ovarian Cancer Pain

Patients experiencing severe chronic abdominal or pelvic pain may be experiencing the harbinger of ovarian cancer. It is the most common presenting symptom and most common symptom of recurrence.[10] Two-thirds of patients experience pain in the 2 weeks prior to the onset or recurrence of the disease. In patients who have been previously treated, it is an important symptom of potential recurrence.[10]

Tumor-Related Gynecomastia

In patients complaining of breast pain or tenderness, there is a risk of occult tumor of the testes or lung. Human chorionic gonadotrophin (HCG)-secreting tumors of testis, including malignant and benign types as well as other HCG-secreting tumors, may produce breast tenderness or gynecomastia.[65] Approximately 10% of patients diagnosed with testicular cancer complain of gynecomastia or breast tenderness.[66]

Intravesical Chemotherapy or Immunotherapy

Patients receiving intravesical Bacillus Calmette-Guérin (BCG) therapy for urinary bladder transitional cell carcinoma experience a syndrome of bladder irritability. Patients report urinary frequency and painful micturition. In rare cases, patients receiving BCG therapy may develop a painful polyarthritis.[67] Other intravesical chemotherapies, such as doxorubicin, may also cause a painful chemical cystitis.[68]

Corticosteroid-Induced Perineal Discomfort

In patients receiving high-dose corticosteroid therapy, some may report an uncomfortable sensation of burning perineal pain.[69]

ADRENAL PAIN SYNDROME

Patients with adrenal metastases of considerable size, common in lung cancer, may develop unilateral flank pain or abdominal pain. Patients report pain from this condition as highly variable, describing it as dull and aching to severe in presentation.[70]

Vascular Obstruction

Hypercoagulability with thrombosis is the most frequent complication associated with malignancy and the second most frequent cause of mortality in malignant disease. A thrombotic event may occur in advance of the diagnosis of cancer by months or years; therefore, thrombosis should be considered as a marker for occult malignancy. Chemotherapy and hormone therapy are associated with an increased thrombotic risk. Additionally, deep vein thrombosis (DVT) is a more common postoperative complication in patients with malignancies than in other postoperative populations.

Hypercoagulability in malignancy is secondary to tumor cell expression of tissue factor and cancer procoagulant. Apoptosis of malignant cells or penumbra of nonmalignant cells affected by invading malignant tissue activates normally dormant tissue factor, initiating a coagulation cascade and formation of thrombus. Tumor proliferation, chemotherapy, hormonal therapy, radiation therapy, and hematopoietic growth factors all increase apoptotic activity and increase the risk of thrombus. Factors contributing to the formation of thrombus include cytokine release, acute phase reaction, and neovascularization. Tumors associated with higher risk of hypercoagulability include tumors of the pelvis, pancreas, stomach, breast, and brain.

Venous Thrombosis

Patients with DVT most often present with pain and swelling of the lower extremity. Patients often report that pain is mild, dull and crampy, or a diffuse perception of pressure or heaviness. The calf is most often involved, but the sole of the foot, heel, thigh, groin, or pelvis may be the site of thrombus and pain. Exacerbating factors include standing or walking. Physical examination may reveal signs of DVT, including swelling, warmth, dilation of superficial veins, tenderness along venous tracts, and pain with stretching of the affected limb. Rarely, a patient may present with ischemia of the lower extremity or in worse cases, a gangrenous limb. This presentation may occur in the absence of arterial or capillary occlusion (phlegmasia cerulea dolens). Signs include severe pain, extensive edema, and cyanosis of the affected leg. Mortality varies but may be as high as 40% secondary to ischemia of the affected extremity or progression of thrombus to cause pulmonary emboli.

Only 2% of DVT cases involve the upper extremity with a low rate of associated pulmonary embolism. On physical examination, upper extremity DVT most often presents with edema, dilated collateral circulation, and pain.[69] In patients with malignancy, central venous catheterization is the most frequent cause along with extrinsic compression by tumor.[71,72]

Superior Vena Cava Obstruction

For patients with lung cancer and lymphoma, SVC obstruction develops with extrinsic compression of the SVC by tumor expansion or by enlarged mediastinal lymph nodes.[71] Intravascular catheters are an iatrogenic cause, especially with left-sided ports where the catheter tip rests in the upper portion of the vessel.[73] Physical examination reveals facial swelling, dilated neck veins, and dilated chest wall veins. Less common patient reports of symptoms associated with SVC obstruction include chest pain, headache, and mastalgia.[74]

Acute Mesenteric Vein Thrombosis

Acute thrombosis of the mesenteric veins is most commonly associated with hypercoagulability secondary to malignancy and more rarely secondary to venous compression by lymphadenopathy, extension of venous thrombosis, or iatrogenic hypercoagulable states.

PAIN SYNDROMES RELATED TO INTRAVENOUS CHEMOTHERAPEUTIC AGENTS

Chemotherapeutic agents may cause vascular pain secondary to venous spasm, chemical phlebitis, vesicant extravasation, and anthracycline-associated flare. Venospasm pain is not secondary to inflammation or phlebitis. Attenuation of symptoms may come from application of a warm compress or reduction of chemotherapeutic infusion rate.

Agents causing chemical phlebitis include amsacrine, dacarbazine, carmustine and vinorelbine, potassium chloride, and hyperosmolar solutions. The pain and erythema associated with chemical phlebitis should be monitored closely because it shares many of the early features of vesicant cytotoxic extravasation that in later stages presents as desquamation and ulceration of cutaneous structures. Venous flare reaction is often associated with the use of anthracycline or doxorubicin and presents with local urticaria, pain, or stinging.

Hepatic Artery Infusion Pain

Patients receiving cytotoxic infusions directly into the hepatic artery often report diffuse abdominal pain.[73] Pain is attributed to gastric ulceration, gastric erosion, or cholangitis. With no persistence of complications, resolution of pain occurs with completion of therapy.

COMPLEX VISCERAL PAIN SYNDROMES

Nontraumatic rupture of a visceral tumor may cause sudden, severe abdominal or pelvic pain and is most commonly associated with hepatocellular carcinoma.[75] Metastases from other tumors also cause visceral ruptures (e.g., kidney rupture from a metastasis from adenocarcinoma of the colon or metastasis-induced perforated appendicitis).[76,77] Torsion of pedunculated visceral tumors may cause cramping abdominal pain.[78]

POSTRADIATION VISCERAL PAIN

Postradiation therapy pain syndromes often involve both somatic and visceral structures, regardless of the target organ. Late effects, including connective tissue fibrosis, neural damage, and secondary malignancies, can occur long after completion of radiotherapy. A recent large retrospective cohort study revealed an association between previous pelvic radiation and hip fractures, with an increase in lifetime fracture rate from 17% (control) to 27% (radiation group). Pelvic pain after radiotherapy may be due to pelvic insufficiency fracture, enteritis, visceral dysfunction, or neural damage. Chronic pelvic pain has been reported as a consequence of prostate brachytherapy. Twenty percent of patients receiving brachytherapy have been reported to complain of dysuria 1 year after treatment.

Radiation Enteritis and Proctitis

In 2% to 10% of patients receiving pelvic or abdominal radiation therapy, chronic enteritis and proctocolitis may occur.[79] The rectum and distal colon are more frequently sites of involvement. Onset may be as early as 3 months or as late as 30 years.[80] Presentations may include proctitis (bloody diarrhea, tenesmus, and cramping pain), obstruction due to stricture formation, or fistulae to the bladder or vagina.[10] Small bowel radiation damage typically causes colicky abdominal pain, which can be associated with chronic nausea or malabsorption. Barium studies may demonstrate a narrow tubular bowel segment resembling Crohn's disease or ischemic colitis. Endoscopy and biopsy may be needed to identify recurrent cancer.

Burning Perineum Syndrome
Perineal discomfort may develop 6 to 18 months following pelvic radiotherapy. Patients complain of burning pain in the perianal region and may involve the vagina or scrotum. For those patients with postabdominoperineal resection, phantom anus pain and recurrent tumor should be considered.

Radiation Cystitis
Radiation therapy used in the treatment of tumors of the pelvic organs (prostate, bladder, colon/rectum, uterus, ovary, and vagina/vulva) may produce chronic radiation cystitis.[10] Symptoms of radiation injury to the bladder may be as minor as temporary irritation with voiding or asymptomatic hematuria, or as severe as gross hematuria, a contracted nonfunctional bladder, persistent incontinence, and fistula formation. Other signs and symptoms may include frequency, urgency, dysuria, hematuria, incontinence, hydronephrosis, pneumaturia, and fecaluria.[10]

POSTCHEMOTHERAPY VISCERAL PAIN
Painful peripheral neuropathy is frequently a dose-limiting side effect of some chemotherapeutic regimens. Once the therapy is stopped, the neuropathic pain will resolve with or without symptomatic treatment. However, in a small number of patients, the neuropathy does not resolve and may continue to be intensely painful. Prevalence during treatment varies from agent to agent, with the intensity of treatment (dose intensity and cumulative dose), with other concurrent therapies such as surgery and radiotherapy, and with the use of combination chemotherapy. Estimates of prevalence range from 4% to 76% during chemotherapy treatment.

Treatment

In general, treatment for cancer-related visceral pain syndromes should adhere to standard cancer pain treatment guidelines (e.g., World Health Organization (WHO) Analgesic Ladder; American Pain Society Guidelines). The reader is referred to Chapters 43, 44, and 48 for details of various pharmacotherapeutic, radiotherapeutic, and interventional treatment modalities. Therapies that target visceral pain mechanisms with some specificity that are not covered in detail in other chapters are elaborated in the following discussion.

N-METHYL-D-ASPARTATE RECEPTOR ANTAGONISTS
Ketamine, which blocks N-methyl-D-aspartate (NMDA) receptors, can influence visceral hypersensitivity. Primary visceral hypersensitivity is attributed to a reduction in peripheral nociceptive thresholds. Two central processes mediate secondary visceral hypersensitivity: (1) plasticity of activated C fibers and (2) convergence of afferents at multiple levels and maintained by glutamate release that binds to NMDA receptors. NMDA receptor activation results in nitric oxide synthase expression, nitric oxide production, and prostaglandin production.

Through these mechanisms (and perhaps others), ketamine has been found to be useful in the management of pain states that are either poorly responsive to opioids and other analgesics or when there are dose-limiting adverse effects to other pain treatments. Ketamine use has been described, with variable success, in adults, pediatric patients, via intrathecal, parenteral, and oral routes, and in inpatient as well as outpatient settings.[81–90]

CORTICOSTEROIDS
Dexamethasone inhibits neuronal nitric oxide synthase gene expression. It has been effective in treating visceral pain and bowel obstruction.[91]

GABAPENTIN
Gabapentin has been demonstrated to reduce glutamate levels and reduces hypersensitivity associated with celiac pain.[92]

SHORT INTERFERING RNA THERAPEUTICS
The discovery that short double-stranded RNA molecules can be used to induce RNA interference (RNAi) in mammalian systems has opened up several possible new avenues in treatment of pain. Gene silencing by small interfering RNAs (siRNAs) has been demonstrated in neurons, and several targets involved in pain perception have been identified can be modulated by these siRNAs. In the past decade, hundreds of molecular targets have been identified for their roles in pain modulation, but most molecular targets are not readily amenable to drugs with small molecules. In the past years, RNAi has become the most widely used technology to suppress gene expression. Effective delivery of nucleic acid-based therapeutic molecules to the central nervous system remains a limiting step for RNAi, and currently, transfection agents are being used via the intrathecal route to deliver siRNA into spinal cord cells as well as dorsal root ganglion cells and hence act on many possible targets for gene expression and modulation including nerves and spinal cord regions affected by cancer pain.[93–95]

T-TYPE CALCIUM CHANNEL ANTAGONISTS
T-type calcium channels are expressed in many diverse tissues, including neuronal, cardiovascular, and endocrine. T-type calcium channels are known to play roles in the development, maintenance, and repair of these tissues but have also been implicated in disease when not properly regulated. T-type calcium channels found on peripheral and central endings of primary afferent neurons are involved in nociception. Voltage-gated calcium channels can be divided into two groups: high-voltage activated calcium channels (L, N, P/Q, and R types) and low-voltage activated calcium channels (T types).[96] Li et al.[97] showed that paclitaxel-induced neuropathy causes hyperexcitability in dorsal root ganglion neurons that is paralleled by increased expression of low voltage–activated calcium channels or namely the T-type channels. Hence, there was great excitement that antagonism of these channels could be of great promise in the treatment of neuropathic pain. Additionally, Le Blanc et al.[98] proved that these T-type calcium channel blocker (CCB) antagonists restore synchrony in thalamic burst firing and possibly alter the affective pathway of pain.

Preclinical studies with ABT-639, a peripherally acting highly selective T-type $Ca_v3.2$ CCB, showed dose-dependent reduction of pain in multiple pain models including arthritic, neuropathic, cancer- and capsaicin-induced pain. However, the initial study results are still to be validated through repeat studies. Wallace et al.[99] compared the pharmacodynamic effects of a single 100-mg dose of ABT-639, a peripherally active, selective T-type $Ca_v3.2$ channel blocker, with pregabalin. They used an intradermal capsaicin model to assess drug efficacy and demonstrated that a single 100-mg dose of ABT-639 had no effect on experimental pain induced by intradermal capsaicin injection. Hence, the jury remains out on T-type calcium channel antagonists.

AMPA/KAINATE ANTAGONISTS
Glutamate activates three subtypes of ligand-gated ion channel: the NMDA, (S)-2-amino-3-(3-hydroxy-5-methyl-4-isoxazolyl) propionic acid (AMPA), and kainate receptors. Animal studies

suggest that AMPA and kainate receptors are involved in epilepsy, pain, and psychiatric disorders. Kainic acid activates nociceptors, and consequently, kainate receptor antagonists have a potential as analgesics. Receptors for AMPA (GluR1-4) are found throughout all superficial laminae of the dorsal horn pre- and postsynaptically. AMPA agonists augment responses of spinal neurons to noxious and nonnoxious stimuli. Kainate receptors (Glu 5-7; KA2) are expressed diffusely in the dorsal horn, mostly in lamina.[100,101]

Gormsen et al.[102] investigated the efficacy of NS1209, a test AMPA receptor antagonist and lidocaine in nerve injury pain. In a three-way RCT involving 13 patients comparing lidocaine, NS1209, and placebo, the authors found that like lidocaine, NS1209 was superior to placebo in alleviating some key symptoms of neuropathic pain (i.e., evoked types of pain, including mechanical and cold allodynia but not superior in alleviating spontaneous current pain). Possibly, more work is needed to delineate the disease mechanisms influenced by AMPA/kainate receptors before antagonists can be developed for the treatment of pain.

P38 KINASE INHIBITORS

p38 mitogen-activated protein kinases (MAPK) are serine/threonine protein kinases involved in the regulation and synthesis of inflammatory mediators and show great potential for the development of cytokine-targeted anti-inflammatory drugs. p38 inhibitors have been shown in preclinical models to decrease neuropathic pain, particularly where there is a substantial inflammatory component.[103]

In a randomized control trial involving 43 patients with carpal tunnel syndrome, radiculopathy or other causes of nerve trauma, Anand et al.[104] demonstrated lower pain scores with acceptable side effects for the new drug dilmapimod. However, other clinical trials of these medications have found prolongation of QT intervals by these agents and have largely been unsuccessful. Further studies require results to be ratified for use in cancer neurogenic pain.

CHEMOKINE RECEPTOR TYPE 2 ANTAGONISTS

Chemokine receptor type 2 (CCR2) is a chemokine receptor that mediates monocyte chemotaxis and hence is thought to play a crucial role in inflammatory and neuropathic pain states. Abbadie et al.[105] proved that mice with chronic pain showed activated CCR2-positive microglia in the spinal cord. They suggested that the recruitment and activation of macrophages and microglia peripherally and in neural tissue may contribute to both inflammatory and neuropathic pain states. Accordingly, blockade of the CCR2 receptor may provide a novel therapeutic modality for the treatment of chronic pain.

However, many trials including a recent one by AstraZeneca have failed. Newer emerging evidence suggests that alternate applications for CCR2 antagonists are possible. It has been shown that spinal CCR2 is upregulated in several neuropathic pain models and expressed by neuronal and glial cells in the spinal cord. Hu et al.[106] investigated the expression changes and cellular localization of spinal CCR2 in a rat model of bone cancer induced by Walker 256 cell inoculation. The results indicated that mechanical allodynia progressively increased in bone cancer pain rats with increased CCR2 expressed by both microglia and neurons in the spinal cord. These results suggest that CCR2 may be involved in the development of cancer pain, and that targeting CCR2 may be a new strategy for the treatment of cancer pain.

P2X PURINOCEPTOR 3 ANTAGONISTS

P2X purinoceptor 3 (P2X3) receptor subunits are expressed prominently and relatively selectively in so-called C- and Aδ-fiber primary afferent neurons in most tissues and organ systems, including skin, joints, and hollow organs, suggesting a high degree of specificity to the pain sensing system in the human body. P2X3 antagonists block the activation of these fibers by adenosine triphosphate (ATP) and reduce ATP sensitization of peripheral pain neurons. In addition, P2X3 is expressed presynaptically at the central terminals of C-fiber afferent neurons, where upregulation and sensitization of pain signals by ATP occurs. This is also potentially blocked by P2X3 receptor antagonists. Another exciting prospect offered by these agents is the potential of decreased side effects due to the selective expression of P2X3, with a lesser risk of affecting the gastrointestinal and renal systems that remain limiting factors for many other existing medications.[107] Gilchrist et al.[108] also suggested in their murine model study that there is increased expression of P2X3 receptors in tumor growth in rats with hence increased potential for ATP activation and bone cancer pain. This study opens avenues for possible use of P2X3 antagonists in bone cancer pain.

Newer research has suggested that a potentially significant pathway for the transmission of cancer visceral pain would be the highly specific postsynaptic dorsal column, which have been shown to express neurokinin receptors (neurokinin-1 [NK-1]) in the event of visceral stimulation that help propagate cancer visceral pain. Surgical lesioning of the dorsal column is potentially difficult, and hence, pharmacologic lesion of the pathway may be an alternate choice. Evidence has shown that spinal dorsal column neurons start to express NK-1 receptors after visceral stimulation, suggesting new targets for the development of pharmacologic strategies for the control of visceral pain. Wang et al.[109] suggested that targeted cytoxin composed of substance P coupled to the cytotoxic ribosome inactivating protein, saporin, might selectively destroy spinal postsynaptic dorsal column neurons expressing NK-1 receptors, to help improve intractable visceral pain of cancer origin.

Gillespie et al.[110] also demonstrated that there is increased NK-1 receptor signaling in colitis associated with cancer further suggesting that there is potential in antagonizing this transmission in the treatment of visceral cancer pain. However, this therapeutics is still in its infancy, and many more studies are needed for further ratification before this group of drugs can be of clinical significance.

NEWER OPIOID DERIVATIVES FOR THE TREATMENT OF CHRONIC PAIN

Opioid agonists act on the μ, κ, and δ receptors. Of the μ, δ, and κ subtypes of opioid receptors, most analgesia is thought to derive from mu activation.

Cebranopadol

Cebranopadol is a new opioid agonist that is under development by the Grünenthal company in collaboration with Depomed of United States. It is a full agonist at the nociceptin/orphanin pathway (NOP) and at μ and δ receptors, whereas being a partial agonist at the κ receptor. Conventional opioids are currently the mainstay of visceral cancer pain treatment. However, their efficacy is limited by potential side effects due to effects on the gastrointestinal, respiratory, and central nervous systems as well as the potential of addiction and tolerance.[111,112]

In animal studies, drugs acting at the nociceptin/orphanin receptors do not generate typical opioid-like side effects and may even ameliorate supraspinal opioid-related side effects when administered concurrently with an opioid. Hence, an agonist at the NOP and the opioid receptors would be particularly useful in the treatment of visceral pain with a more favorable side effect profile.[113]

In a bone cancer pain murine model, Linz et al.[114] demonstrated that cebranopadol caused dose-dependent increased pain withdrawal thresholds that reached statistical significance after 30- and 60-minute intervals.

However, there is evidence to suggest that cebranopadol is more effective in neuropathic rather than nociceptive bone cancer pain. Animal studies indicate that cebranopadol is more effective in experimental models of chronic neuropathic pain (e.g., streptozotocin-induced diabetic polyneuropathy and spinal nerve ligation models) compared to acute nociceptive pain (bone cancer pain and tail-flick test).[115] In the rat, there are strong indications that cebranopadol shows limited depression of breathing also which has been shown to be significant in comparison to conventional opioids.[116] Moreover, tolerance and addiction are less likely with cebranopadol than with conventional opioids due to slower metabolism and pharmacokinetic profile.[117]

In the rat, tolerance to morphine develops quickly, and in a study by Lambert et al.,[117] rats were completely tolerant to morphine (8.8 mg/kg intraperitoneal [IP] daily) in 11 days. In contrast, an equianalgesic dose of cebranopadol (only 0.8 μg/kg IP daily) was still effective for a further 15 days, or 26 days in total.[118] Hence, cebranopadol presents great potential in the treatment of cancer pain with a better side effect, tolerance, and dependence profile.

PROCEDURAL INTERVENTIONS
Ganglion Impar Block

The ganglion impar is a solitary retroperitoneal structure located at the level of the sacrococcygeal junction. This unpaired ganglion marks the end of two sympathetic chains. The ganglion receives sympathetic and parasympathetic fibers at the lumbar and sacral levels, providing sympathetic innervation to portions of the pelvic viscera and genitalia.[119] Visceral pain in the perineal area associated with malignancies may be effectively treated with neurolysis of the ganglion impar (also known as Walther ganglion).[120] Patients who will benefit from this block frequently present with a vague poorly localized pain that is frequently accompanied by sensations of burning and urgency. The ganglion impar block is useful to the management of sympathetically mediated pain in the perineum, rectum, and genitalia. It has been primarily used for malignancy; however, it has been used for treatment of associated syndromes such as radiation enteritis, proctalgia fugax, and reflex sympathetic dystrophy.

The ganglion impar is close in proximity to the rectum. There is increased risk of contamination through the needle track as the needle is removed. Infection and fistula are possible complications in patients who are already immunocompromised or have received radiation to the perineum.

Thoracic Sympathetic Ganglion Block

Preganglionic fibers of the thoracic sympathetics exit with respective thoracic paravertebral nerves from the intervertebral foramen. After exiting the intervertebral foramen, thoracic paravertebral nerves branch looping dorsal through the same foramen to provide innervation to the spinal ligaments, meninges, and respective vertebra. The paravertebral nerve at this level also affects the thoracic sympathetic chain through myelinated preganglionic fibers of the white rami communicantes. Preganglionic and postganglionic fibers synapse at the level of thoracic sympathetic ganglia. Postganglionic fibers provide sympathetic innervation to the vasculature, sweat glands, and pilomotor muscles of the skin as well as the cardiac plexus and terminate in distal ganglia as they course up and down the thoracic sympathetic trunk.[121]

Block of the thoracic sympathetic ganglion is useful for evaluation of sympathetically mediated pain to the thoracic and upper abdominal viscera, the thorax, and the chest wall. Differential blockade may serve as a prognostic indicator of the benefit to be expected from lesioning of the thoracic sympathetic ganglion. The block has been used in the past to treat intractable abdominal pain as well as intractable cardiac pain. It has also been demonstrated to be effective in the treatment of acute herpes zoster, postherpetic neuralgia, and phantom breast pain following mastectomy. Thoracic sympathetic chain destruction may be used to relieve pain in pain syndromes that have been improved by local anesthetic block.[122]

Because of the close proximity to the pleural space of the exiting nerve roots at the thoracic level from sympathetic ganglion, pneumothorax is a possible complication. The pleural space lies lateral and anterior to the thoracic sympathetic chain. The lower cervical ganglion fuses with the first thoracic ganglion to make the stellate ganglion. Caudad in the thoracic chain, thoracic ganglia move further anterior resting along the posterolateral surface of the vertebral body. Other possible complications include accidental injection of the epidural, subdural, and subarachnoid space. Infection is of greater concern in patients with malignancy because of their immunocompromised state.

Interpleural Catheters

The role of interpleural analgesia (IPA) in both acute and chronic pain management is still undergoing clinical scrutiny. Original work with this technique showed that IPA could provide analgesia in patients with subcostal incisions and fractured ribs.

The technique for insertion of an interpleural catheter is relatively easy, and an epidural tray can be utilized. Local anesthetics (0.5% bupivacaine or 2% lidocaine) have been traditionally utilized via intermittent bolus or a continuous infusion. Interpleural phenol has been described as an alternative for the treatment of visceral pain associated with esophageal cancer. This may be an effective technique to treat visceral pain associated with cancer of the esophagus, liver, biliary tree, stomach, and pancreas.

For analgesia associated with cancer, continuous infusions of bupivacaine or intermittent bolus doses of bupivacaine may also provide adequate analgesia. Higher concentrations of bupivacaine increase the risk of toxicity.

Complications are secondary to needle or catheter injury or are secondary to the neurolytic agent injected in the interpleural space. Pneumothorax may occur in 2% of patients, and lung injury has been reported when a rigid catheter is used. Phrenic nerve palsy may occur following this block resulting in respiratory failure. Thus, bilateral blocks should be avoided. Doses of phenol should be limited; systemic effects from drug absorption may occur because the pleural membranes are highly vascularized.

Surgery

Referral for surgical options should be pursued with diagnosis and treatment of pain in malignancy at any time during the course of care. Surgical objectives in the palliation of cancer include staging of disease, control of disease, control of pain and associated symptoms, reconstruction, and rehabilitation.[123] Patients interested in and capable of tolerating surgical options should be referred to a surgeon for consideration of options, even if there are nonsurgical options available. If no intervention is recommended, the patient will have an understanding for the surgical referral and have a sense of closure with regard to the variety of options available for palliation. Surgical consult is particularly valuable in the areas of wound management, complicated issues with regard to nutrition, and discussion of progression of disease.[122]

There is no standard set of procedures for the palliation of malignant visceral pain. The operations available are a reflection of the subjective pain experience of the patient, the specific stage of the disease, and the anatomic effects of the disease. Often, other distressing symptoms may be the reason for surgical management as well as the complaints of pain. The given surgical option should palliate as many symptoms as possible without altering benefit–risk ratios.[122] The most important preoperative measure involves reassurance to the patient that preparation is complete and that postoperative analgesia has been considered. This is best achieved with close coordination with the partnering anesthesia team and preoperative consultation regarding analgesic options. Furthermore, the operative encounter may be the foundation for continued postoperative pain management options.

Malignancy presenting with pain is likely to be advanced in nature. Resection of an organ or portion of an organ for management of pain is reasonable even in the case of uncontrollable disease, especially if the disease is resectable or partially resectable. There is little data, however, comparing the efficacy of resection with nonoperative approaches.

In visceral disease, surgical resection has proven effective for the relief of dysphagia, odynophagia, and chest pain in patients with esophageal carcinoma; the relief of painful ulceration in those with gastric carcinoma; and the preemptive control of jaundice, pain, and duodenal obstruction in those with pancreatic carcinoma.[122]

Surgery can promote comfort as well as eliminate pain. Mechanical bowel obstruction may be expected in as many as 15% of cancer patients. Pain is a reflection of the severity of the distension, the nature of the primary neoplasm, and the level of obstruction. Resection has also been offered on occasion for relief of pain associated with carcinoma of the kidney. In some situations, nephrectomy may be considered to prevent pain, hematuria, and constitutional effects of the disease. In patients with large bladder masses, total or partial organ resection may be a consideration in cases where more conservative options have been considered. Stent placement may relieve severe pain secondary to malignant ureteral obstruction by tumors of the prostate, cervix, bladder, and colon. If stent placement is not an option, percutaneous nephrostomy may be effective.[122]

Debulking of functional tumors of the liver may be beneficial in patients with carcinoid to decrease such symptoms as flushing and diarrhea. Debulking has also been used in patients with metastatic gastrinoma, ovarian cancer, and large and small bowel malignancies.

Finally, drainage of ascites, which may develop in as many as half of cancer patients, may relieve associated symptoms such as bloating, diffuse abdominal pain, dyspnea, nausea, early satiety, and gastric reflux.

Dorsal Myelotomy for Treatment of Intractable Visceral Cancer Pain

Neurosurgical interruption of midline visceral pain pathway can help control severe visceral pain without causing significant adverse neurologic sequelae in patients with advanced visceral cancer. However, surgery is not without side effects, and often, this approach is used when conventional pharmacologic treatment has failed. Hwang et al.[122] demonstrated a technique of punctate midline myelotomy (PMM) for the treatment of cancer pain refractory to opioids. In their study, a PMM at the T3 level was performed in six patients who experienced severe visceral pain caused by hepatobiliary or pancreatic cancer. In a small study involving six patients, follow-up periods ranged from 2 to 18 weeks after operation. All six patients had immediate pain relief after operation. Although the pain recurred from 2 to 12 weeks later in three patients, the severity of recurrent cancer pain was markedly decreased.[122]

Kim et al.[124] also attempted a high thoracic myelotomy in their palliation attempt in the treatment of severe pain due to stomach cancer. Under general anesthesia, patients received high thoracic midline dorsal column myelotomies after T1 or T2 laminectomy. In their study, they demonstrated clinically significant decrease in pain scores after the procedure, although one patient developed paresthesia and posterior column signs below the level of myelotomy without analgesia and another paresthesia responsive to corticosteroids. They concluded that dorsal column myelotomy at a high thoracic cord level effectively controls severe abdominal pain and should be considered as a new palliative operation for patients with severe visceral pain.[125]

Hypophysectomy and Cancer Pain

Destruction of the pituitary stalk has been a long established palliative approach to the treatment of severe refractory cancer pain especially due to widespread metastases and also in bone cancer pain in breast cancer. Surgical, stereotactic instillation of alcohol in to the sella turcica and other methods of chemical hypophysectomy have been long established in cancer pain treatment. A proposed mechanism is that or its associated neurophysins act as central pain transmitters. The production of these transmitters is decreased or abolished by chemical or surgical hypophysectomy through the destruction of hypothalamic nuclei.[126–128]

Conclusion

Failure to assess and treat cancer pain, whether of somatic, visceral, neuropathic, or mixed types, is still a common problem among patients in all stages of malignant disease. Barriers to adequate care have been discussed in previous chapters. Notwithstanding needed improvements in clinician education, access to pain and supportive care specialists, among other needed systems improvements, and similar to other causes of cancer pain, relief of pain in patients with visceral malignancies or treatment-related visceral pain syndromes should be organized as part of a comprehensive interdisciplinary approach to care. Visceral pain cannot be exclusively managed with pharmacotherapy, and the resources of several medical and supportive care disciplines should be considered with each patient so that pain management can be tailored to the individual requirements of each patient according to his or her unique constellation of clinical and social circumstances.

References

1. Goudas LC, Bloch R, Gialeli-Goudas M, et al. The epidemiology of cancer pain. *Cancer Invest* 2005;23(2):182–190.
2. Burton AW, Cleeland CS. Cancer pain: progress since the WHO guidelines. *Pain Pract* 2001;1(3):236–242.
3. Miguel R. Cultural and family issues. In: de Leon Casseola O, ed. *Cancer Pain Management: Pharmacologic, Interventional, and Palliative Approaches.* Philadelphia: Elsevier; 2006:25–32.
4. Mantyh P. Cancer pain: causes, consequences and therapeutic opportunities. In: McMahon S, Koltzenburg M, eds. *Wall and Melzack's Textbook of Pain.* 5th ed. London: Elsevier; 2006:1029–1038.
5. National Institutes of Health. *NIH National Cancer Institute SEER Cancer Statistics Review.* Available at: https://www.cancer.gov/about-cancer/understanding/statistics. Accessed September 14, 2016.
6. van den Beuken-van Everdingen MH, de Rijke JM, Kessels G, et al. Prevalence of pain in patients with cancer: a systematic review of the past 40 years. *Ann Oncol* 2007;18(9):1437–1449.
7. Hanna M, Zylicz Z. *Cancer Pain.* New York: Springer; 2013.
8. Jemal A, Ward EM, Johnson CJ, et al. Annual report to the nation on the status of cancer, 1975–2014, featuring survival. *J Natl Cancer Inst* 2017;109(9):djx030.
9. Passik S, Gibson C, Brietbart W, et al. Psychiatric issues in cancer pain management. In: Fisch M, Burton A, eds. *Cancer Pain Management.* New York: McGraw-Hill; 2007:137–154.
10. Paice J. Cancer pain. In: Von Roenn J, ed. *Current Diagnosis and Treatment Pain.* New York: Lange Medical Books; 2006:85–101.
11. Cherny N. The assessment of cancer pain. In: McMahon S, Koltzenburg M, eds. *Wall and Melzack's Textbook of Pain.* 5th ed. London: Elsevier; 2006:1069–1074.
12. Al-Chaer ER, Traub RJ. Biological basis of visceral pain: recent developments. *Pain* 2002;96(3):221–225.
13. Bielefeldt K. Visceral pain: basic mechanisms. In: McMahon S, Koltzenburg M, eds. *Wall and Melzack's Textbook of Pain.* 5th ed. London: Elsevier; 2006:703–717.

14. Ness T. Visceral pain. In: de Leon Casseola O, ed. *Cancer Pain Management: Pharmacologic, Interventional, and Palliative Approaches.* Philadelphia: Elsevier; 2006:85–94.
15. Gebhart G. Visceral pain mechanisms. *Pain* 1990;41S260.
16. Mackenzie, J. Remarks on the meaning and mechanism of visceral pain as shown by the study of visceral and other sympathetic (autonomic) reflexes. *Br Med J* 1906;1(2374):1523–1528.
17. Breivik H, Borchgrevink PC, Allen SM, et al. Assessment of pain. Br J Anaesth 2008;101:17–24. doi:10.1093/bja/aen103.
18. Reddy S. Pain following mastectomy, thoracotomy, and radical neck dissection. In: de Leon Casseola O, ed. *Cancer Pain Management: Pharmacologic, Interventional, and Palliative Approaches.* Philadelphia: Elsevier; 2006:97–101.
19. Ness T. Visceral pain. In: Von Roenn J, ed. *Current Diagnosis and Treatment Pain.* New York: Lange Medical Books; 2006:136–149.
20. Davis M, Hinshaw D. Management of visceral pain due to cancer-related intestinal obstruction. In: *Cancer Pain.* Philadelphia: Elsevier; 2006: 481–495.
21. Cervero F. Visceral hyperalgesia revisited. *Lancet* 2000;356(9236):1127–1128.
22. Sarkar S, Hobson AR, Hughes A, et al. The prostaglandin E2 receptor-1 (EP-1) mediates acid-induced visceral pain hypersensitivity in humans. *Gastroenterology* 2003;124(1):18–25.
23. Gebhart GF. Pathobiology of visceral pain: molecular mechanisms and therapeutic implications. IV. Visceral afferent contributions to the pathobiology of visceral pain. *Am J Physiol Gastrointest Liver Physiol* 2000;278(6): G834–G838.
24. Helmlinger G, Sckell A, Dellian M, et al. Acid production in glycolysis-impaired tumors provides new insights into tumor metabolism. *Clin Cancer Res* 2000;8(4):1284–1291.
25. Bueno L, Fioramonti J. Visceral perception: inflammatory and non-inflammatory mediators. *Gut* 2002;51:i19–i23.
26. Houghton LA, Calvert EL, Jackson NA, et al. Visceral sensation and emotion: a study using hypnosis. *Gut* 2002;51(5):701–704.
27. Strigo IA, Bushnell MC, Boivin M, et al. Psychophysical analysis of visceral and cutaneous pain in human subjects. *Pain* 2002;97(3):235–246.
28. Nishino T, Shimoyama N, Ide T, et al. Experimental pain augments experimental dyspnea, but not vice versa in human volunteers. *Anesthesiology* 1999;91(6):1633–1638.
29. Gebhart GF, Bielefeldt K. Physiology of visceral pain. *Compr Physiol* 2016; 6(4):1609–1633.
30. Lémann M, Dederding JP, Flourié B, et al. Abnormal perception of visceral pain in response to gastric distension in chronic idiopathic dyspepsia. *Dig Dis Sci* 1991;36(1):1249–1254.
31. Yamada T, Alpers DH, Laine L, et al, eds. *Textbook of Gastroenterology.* 3rd ed. Philadelphia: Lippincott Williams & Wilkins; 1999.
32. Honoré P, Kamp EH, Rogers SD, et al. Activation of lamina I spinal cord neurons that express the substance P receptor in visceral nociception and hyperalgesia. *J Pain* 2002;3(1):3–11.
33. Chadwick VS, Chen W, Shu D, et al. Activation of the mucosal immune system in irritable bowel syndrome. *Gastroenterology* 2002;122(7):1778–1783.
34. Ouatu-Lascar R, Fitzgerald RC, Triadafilipoulos G. Differentiation and proliferation in Barrett's esophagus and the effects of acid suppression. *Gastroenterology* 1999;117(2):327–335.
35. Marchand F, Perretti M, McMahon SB. Role of the immune system in chronic pain. *Nat Rev Neurosci* 2005;6(7):521–532.
36. McMahon S, Dmitrieva N, Koltzenburg M. Visceral pain. *Br J Anaesth* 1995;75(2):132–144.
37. Hillsley K, Lin JH, Stanisz A, et al. Dissecting the role of sodium currents in visceral sensory neurons in a model of chronic hyperexcitability using Nav1.8 and Nav1.9 null mice. *J Physiol* 2006;576(pt 1):257–267.
38. Ravnefjord A, Brusberg M, Kang D, et al. Involvement of the transient receptor potential vanilloid 1 (TRPV1) in the development of acute visceral hyperalgesia during colorectal distension in rats. *Eur J Pharmacol* 2009;611(1–3): 85–91. doi:10.1016/j.ejphar.2009.03.058.
39. Anand P, Aziz Q, Willert R, et al. Peripheral and central mechanisms of visceral sensitization in man. *Neurogastroenterol Motil* 2007;19(suppl 1): 29–46.
40. Eide PK. Wind-up and the NMDA receptor complex from a clinical perspective. *Eur J Pain* 2000;4(1):5–15.
41. Ménétrey D, De Pommer J. Origins of spinal ascending pathways that reach central areas involved in visceroception and visceronociception in the rat. *Eur J Neurosci* 1991;3(3):249–255.
42. Burton A, Fanciullow G, Beasley R. Chronic pain in the cured cancer patient. In: Fisch M, Burton A, eds. *Cancer Pain Management.* New York: McGraw-Hill; 2007:155–162.
43. Worthington H, Clarkson JE, Eden OB. Interventions for preventing oral mucositis for patients with cancer receiving treatment. *Cochrane Database Syst Rev* 2007;(4):CD000978.
44. Epstein J, Stewart K. Radiation therapy and pain in patients with head and neck cancer. *Eur J Cancer B Oral Oncol* 1993;29B(3):191–199.
45. Rider CA. Oral mucositis: a complication of radiotherapy. *J Colo Dent Assoc* 1991;69(3):23–25.
46. Worthington HV, Clarkson JE, Eden OB. Interventions for treating oral mucositis for patients with cancer receiving treatment. *Cochrane Database Syst Rev* 2001;(1):CD001973.

47. Marangoni C, Lacerenza M, Formaglio F, et al. Sensory disorder of the chest as presenting symptom of lung cancer. *J Neurol Neurosurg Psychiatry* 1993;56(9):1033–1034.
48. Marino C, Zoppi M, Morelli F, et al. Pain in early cancer of the lungs. *Pain* 1986;27(1):57–62.
49. Capobianco DJ. Facial pain as a symptom of nonmetastatic lung cancer. *Headache* 1995;35(10):581–585.
50. Des Prez RD, Freemon FR. Facial pain associated with lung cancer: a case report. *Headache* 1983;23(1):43–44.
51. Schoenen J, Broux R, Moonen G. Unilateral facial pain as the first symptom of lung cancer: are there diagnostic clues? *Cephalalgia* 1992;12(3): 178–179.
52. Shakespeare TP, Stevens M. Unilateral facial pain and lung cancer. *Australas Radiol* 1996;40(1):45–46.
53. Komaki R, Putnam JB Jr, Walsh G, et al. The management of superior sulcus tumors. *Semin Surg Oncol* 2000;18(2):152–164.
54. D'Silva K. Pancoast syndrome. Available at: http://www.emedicine.com /med/topic3418.htm. Accessed January 26, 2007.
55. Kori SH, Foley KM, Posner JB. Brachial plexus lesions in patients with cancer: 100 cases. *Neurology* 1981;31(1):45–50.
56. Kori SH. Diagnosis and management of brachial plexus lesions in cancer patients. *Oncology (Williston Park)* 1995;9(8):756–765.
57. Wong G, Wiersema M, Sarr MG. Palliation of pain in adenocarcinoma of the pancreas. In: Cameron JL, ed. *American Cancer Society Atlas of Clinical Oncology: Pancreatic Cancer.* Ontario, Canada: BC Decker Inc; 2001:231–246.
58. Warshaw A, Fernández-del Castillo C. Pancreatic carcinoma. *N Engl J Med* 1992;326(7):455–465.
59. Borgelt B, Gelber R, Brady LW, et al. The palliation of hepatic metastases: results of the Radiation Therapy Oncology Group pilot study. *Int J Radiat Oncol Biol Phys* 1981;7:587–591.
60. Mulholland MW, Debas H, Bonica JJ. Diseases of the liver, biliary system and pancreas. In: Bonica JJ, ed. *The Management of Pain.* 2nd ed. Philadelphia: Lea and Febiger; 1990:1214–1223.
61. Dawson LA. Radiation therapy for liver metastases. *Am Soc Clin Oncol Educ Book* 2008;1:161–164.
62. Averbach AM, Sugarbaker PH. Recurrent intra-abdominal cancer with intestinal obstruction. *Int Surg* 1995;80(2):141–146.
63. Almadrones L, Yerys C. Problems associated with the administration of intraperitoneal therapy using the Port-A-Cath system. *Oncol Nurs Forum* 1990;17(1):75–76.
64. Boas RA, Schug SA, Acland RH. Perineal pain after rectal amputation: a 5-year follow-up. *Pain* 1993;52(1):67–70.
65. Rigor BM Sr. Pelvic cancer pain. *J Surg Oncol* 2000;75(4):280–300.
66. Cantwell BM, Richardson PG, Campbell SJ. Gynaecomastia and extragonadal symptoms leading to diagnosis delay of germ cell tumours in young men. *Postgrad Med J* 1991;67(789):675–677.
67. Tseng A Jr, Horning SJ, Freiha FS, et al. Gynecomastia in testicular cancer patients. Prognostic and therapeutic implications. *Cancer* 1985;56(10): 2534–2538.
68. Kudo S, Tsushima N, Sawada Y, et al. Serious complications of intravesical bacillus Calmette–Guerin therapy in patients with bladder cancer [in Japanese]. *Nippon Hinyokika Gakkai Zasshi* 1991;82(10):1594–1602.
69. Perron G, Dolbec P, Germain J, et al. Perineal pruritus after I.V. dexamethasone administration. *Can J Anaesth* 2003;50(7):749–750.
70. Berger MS, Cooley ME, Abrahm J. A pain syndrome associated with large adrenal metastases in patients with lung cancer. *J Pain Symptom Manage* 1995;10(2):161–166.
71. Burihan E, de Figueiredo LF, Francisco Júnior J, et al. Upper-extremity deep venous thrombosis: analysis of 52 cases. *Cardiovasc Surg* 1993;1(1):19–22.
72. Bona RD. Central line thrombosis in patients with cancer. *Curr Opin Pulm Med* 2003;9(5):362–366.
73. Wudel LJ Jr, Nesbitt JC. Superior vena cava syndrome. *Curr Treat Options Oncol* 2001;2(1):77–91.
74. Morales M, Llanos M, Dorta J. Superior vena cava thrombosis secondary to Hickman catheter and complete resolution after fibrinolytic therapy. *Support Care Cancer* 1997;5(1):67–69.
75. Kemeny MM. Continuous hepatic artery infusion (CHAI) as treatment of liver metastases. Are the complications worth it? *Drug Saf* 1991;6(3):159–165.
76. Miyamoto M, Sudo T, Kuyama T. Spontaneous rupture of hepatocellular carcinoma: a review of 172 Japanese cases. *Am J Gastroenterol* 1991;86(1):67–71.
77. Wolff JM, Boeckmann W, Jakse G. Spontaneous kidney rupture due to a metastatic renal tumour. Case report. *Scand J Urol Nephrol* 1994;28(4): 415–417.
78. Ende DA, Robinson G, Moulton J. Metastasis-induced perforated appendicitis: an acute abdomen of rare aetiology. *Aust N Z J Surg* 1995;65(1): 62–63.
79. Andreasen DA, Poulsen J. Intra-abdominal torsion of the testis with seminoma [in Danish]. *Ugeskrift Laeger* 1997;159(14):2103–2104.
80. Saltz L. *Colorectal Cancer: Multimodality Management.* New York: Humana Press; 2002.
81. Nussbaum ML, Campana TJ, Weese JL. Radiation-induced intestinal injury. *Clin Plast Surg* 1993;20(3):573–580.

82. Finkel JC, Pestieau SR, Quezado ZM. Ketamine as an adjuvant for treatment of cancer pain in children and adolescents. *J Pain* 2007;8(6): 515–521.

83. Bell RF, Eccleston C, Kalso E. Ketamine as adjuvant to opioids for cancer pain. A qualitative systematic review. *J Pain Symptom Manage* 2003;26(3): 867–875.

84. Chung WJ, Pharo GH. Successful use of ketamine infusion in the treatment of intractable cancer pain in an outpatient. *J Pain Symptom Manage* 2007;33(1):2–5.

85. Fitzgibbon EJ, Viola R. Parenteral ketamine as an analgesic adjuvant for severe pain: development and retrospective audit of a protocol for a palliative care unit. *J Palliat Med* 2005;8(1):49–57.

86. Fitzgibbon EJ, Hall P, Schroder C, et al. Low dose ketamine as an analgesic adjuvant in difficult pain syndromes: a strategy for conversion from parenteral to oral ketamine. *J Pain Symptom Manage* 2002;23(2):165–170.

87. Mannion S, O'Brien T. Ketamine in the management of chronic pancreatic pain. *J Pain Symptom Manage* 2003;26(6):1071–1072.

88. Prommer E. Ketamine to control pain. *J Palliat Med* 2003;6(3):443–446.

89. Mercadante S, Arcuri E, Tirelli W, et al. Analgesic effect of intravenous ketamine in cancer patients on morphine therapy: a randomized, controlled, double-blind, crossover, double-dose study. *J Pain Symptom Manage* 2000; 20(4):246–252.

90. Gordon DB, Sehgal N, Schroeder ME, et al. Treatment of pain crisis at end of life from severe lower extremity venous outflow obstruction with hyperalgesia and allodynia. *J Pain* 2002;3(3):244–248.

91. Kotlińska–Lemieszek A, Luczak J. Subanesthetic ketamine: an essential adjuvant for intractable cancer pain. *J Pain Symptom Manage* 2004;28(2): 100–102.

92. Warr DG. Chemotherapy- and cancer-related nausea and vomiting. *Curr Oncol* 2008;15(suppl 1):S4–S9.

93. Tan PH, Yang LC, Shih HC, et al. Gene knockdown with intrathecal siRNA of NMDA receptor NR2B subunit reduces formalin-induced nociception in the rat. *Gene Ther* 2005;12(1):59–66.

94. Luo MC, Zhang DQ, Ma SW, et al. An efficient intrathecal delivery of small interfering RNA to the spinal cord and peripheral neurons. *Mol Pain* 2005;1:29.

95. Tan PH, Yang LC, Ji RR. Therapeutic potential of RNA interference in pain medicine. *Open Pain J* 2009;2:57–63.

96. Kopecky BJ, Liang R, Bao J. T-type calcium channel blockers as neuroprotective agents. *Pflugers Arch* 2014;466(4):757–765.

97. Li Y, Tatsui CE, Rhines LD, et al. Dorsal root ganglion neurons become hyperexcitable and increase expression of voltage-gated T-type calcium channels (Cav3.2) in paclitaxel-induced peripheral neuropathy. *Pain* 2017;158(3):417–429.

98. LeBlanc BW, Lii TR, Huang JJ, et al. T-type calcium channel blocker Z944 restores cortical synchrony and thalamocortical connectivity in a rat model of neuropathic pain. *Pain* 2016;157(1):255–263.

99. Wallace M, Duan R, Liu W, et al. A randomized, double-blind, placebo-controlled, crossover study of the T-type calcium channel blocker ABT-639 in an intradermal capsaicin experimental pain model in healthy adults. *Pain Med* 2016;17(3):551–560.

100. Tölle TR, Berthele A, Schadrack J, et al. Involvement of glutamatergic neurotransmission and protein kinase C in spinal plasticity and the development of chronic pain. *Prog Brain Res* 1996;110:193–206.

101. Furuyama T, Kiyama H, Sato K, et al. Region-specific expression of subunits of ionotropic glutamate receptors (AMPA-type, KA-type, and NMDA receptors) in the rat spinal cord with special reference to nociception. *Brain Res Mol Brain Res* 1993;18:141–151.

102. Gormsen L, Finnerup NB, Almqvist PM, et al. The efficacy of the AMPA receptor antagonist NS1209 and lidocaine in nerve injury pain: a randomized, double-blind, placebo-controlled, three-way crossover study. *Anesth Analg* 2009;108(4):1311–1319.

103. Gangwal RP, Bhadauriya A, Damre MV, et al. p38 Mitogen-activated protein kinase inhibitors: a review on pharmacophore mapping and QSAR studies. *Curr Top Med Chem* 2013;13(9):1015–1035.

104. Anand P, Shenoy R, Palmer JE, et al.Clinical trial of the p38 MAP kinase inhibitor dilmapimod in neuropathic pain following nerve injury. *Eur J Pain* 2011;15(10):1040–1048.

105. Abbadie C, Lindia JA, Cumiskey AM, et al. Impaired neuropathic pain responses in mice lacking the chemokine receptor CCR2. *Proc Natl Acad Sci U S A* 2003;100(13):7947–7952.

106. Hu J, Wu M, Tao M, et al. Changes in protein expression and distribution of spinal CCR2 in a rat model of bone cancer pain. *Brain Res* 2013;1509:1–7.

107. Ford AP. In pursuit of P2X3 antagonists: novel therapeutics for chronic pain and afferent sensitization. *Purinergic Signal* 2012;8(suppl 1):S3–S26.

108. Gilchrist LS, Cain DM, Harding-Rose C. Re-organization of P2X 3 receptor localization on epidermal nerve fibers in a murine model of cancer pain. *Brain Res* 2005;1044(2):197–205.

109. Wang Y, Mu X, Liu Y, et al. NK-1-receptor-mediated lesion of spinal post-synaptic dorsal column neurons might improve intractable visceral pain of cancer origin. *Med Hypotheses* 2011;76(1):102–104.

110. Gillespie E, Leeman SE, Watts LA, et al. Truncated neurokinin-1 receptor is increased in colonic epithelial cells from patients with colitis-associated cancer. *Proc Natl Acad Sci U S A* 2011;108(42):17420–17425.

111. Zöllner C, Stein C. Opioids. *Hand Exp Pharmacol* 2007;(177):31–63.

112. Sukhtankar D, Zaveri N, Ko MC. Pharmacological investigation of NOP-related ligands as analgesics without abuse liability. In: Ko M, Husbands SM. *Research and Development of Opioid-Related Ligands.* Oxford, United Kingdom: Oxford University Press; 2014:393–416.

113. Rutten K, De Vry J, Bruckmann W, et al. Effects of the NOP receptor agonist Ro65-6570 on the acquisition of opiate- and psychostimulant-induced conditioned place preference in rats. *Eur J Pharmacol* 2010;645:119–126.

114. Linz K, Christoph T, Tzschentke TM, et al. Cebranopadol: a novel potent analgesic nociceptin/orphanin FQ peptide and opioid receptor agonist. *J Pharmacol Exp Ther* 2014;349(3):535–548.

115. Linz K, Schröder W, Frosch S, et al. Opioid-type respiratory depressant side effects of cebranopadol in rats are limited by its nociceptin/orphanin FQ peptide receptor agonist activity. *Anesthesiology* 2017;126:708–715.

116. Kest B, Hopkins E, Palmese CA. Morphine tolerance and dependence in nociceptin/orphanin FQ transgenic knock-out mice. *Neuroscience* 2001;104(1):217–222.

117. Lambert DG, Bird MF, Rowbotham DJ. Cebranopadol: a first-in-class example of a nociceptin/orphanin FQ receptor and opioid receptor agonist. *Br J Anaesth* 2015;114(3):364–366.

118. Pelham A, Lee MA, Regnard CB. Gabapentin for coeliac plexus pain. *Palliat Med* 2002;16(4):355–356.

119. Waldman S. *Ganglion of Walther (Impar) Block. Atlas of Interventional Pain Management.* Philadelphia: Saunders; 2003.

120. Plancarte R, de Leon Casasola OA, El-Helaly M, et al. Presacral blockade of the ganglion of Walther. *Anesthesiology* 1990;73:A751.

121. Dunn, G. Selected surgical approaches. In: Simpson K, Budd K, eds. *Cancer Pain Management: A Comprehensive Approach.* Oxford, United Kingdom: Oxford University Press; 2000:175–187.

122. Hwang SL, Lin CL, Lieu AS, et al. Punctate midline myelotomy for intractable visceral pain caused by hepatobiliary or pancreatic cancer. *J Pain Symptom Manage* 2004;27(1):79–84.

123. Dunn GP. Surgical palliative care: an enduring framework for surgical care. *Surg Clin North Am* 2005;85(2):169–190.

124. Kim YS, Kwon SJ. High thoracic midline dorsal column myelotomy for severe visceral pain due to advanced stomach cancer. *Neurosurgery* 2000;46(1):85–90.

125. Carbonin G. Hypophysectomy and pain relief in cancer. *J Neurosurg* 1978;48(4):666–667.

126. Brodkey JS, Pearson OH, Manni A. Hypophysectomy for relief of bone pain in breast cancer. *N Engl J Med* 1978;299(18):1016.

127. Levin AB, Katz J, Benson RC, et al. Treatment of pain of diffuse metastatic cancer by stereotactic chemical hypophysectomy: long term results and observations on mechanism of action. *Neurosurgery* 1980;6(3):258–262.

128. Waldman S. Thoracic sympathetic ganglion block. In: Atlas of Interventional Pain Management. 4th ed. Philadelphia: Saunders; 2015:332–335.

CHAPTER 48

Radiotherapy and Chemotherapy in Cancer Pain Management

NORA JANJAN

Introduction

"Cancer pain is best controlled by removing the cancer or causing it to regress."[1] This succinct principle stated by palliative medicine specialist Dr. Neil MacDonald is a useful framework from which to consider the role of palliative chemotherapy and radiotherapy in the management of symptomatic disease. In the year 2016, 1,685,210 new cancer cases were diagnosed, and about 595,690 cancer-related deaths occurred. National expenditures for cancer care in the United States totaled nearly $125 billion in 2010 and are projected to reach $156 billion in 2020.[2]

There has been substantial progress in cancer incidence and mortality. The incidence of cancer from 2009 to 2013 was stable in women but decreased by 2.3% per year in men. An overall 13% decrease in cancer deaths occurred between the years 2004 and 2013.[2,3] Death rates decreased for 11 of the 16 most common cancer types in men and for 13 of the 18 most common cancer types in women; this decline in cancer death rates included lung, colorectal, female breast, and prostate cancer. The 5-year survival rate for breast cancer increased from 18.7% between 1975 and 1977 to 33.6% between 2006 and 2012. The improvements in 5-year survival rates also included meaningful increases in survival with distant-stage disease.[3] Deaths due to breast cancer declined almost 40% between 1989 and 2015, averting 322,600 deaths.[4,5] This trend can be attributed to the persistent efforts in research, early detection of disease, and treatment advances. Cancer and its treatment, however, still result in a significant burden of symptoms like pain.

Cancer has a negative impact on almost all cancer patients' domains of daily living. Quality-of-life measurements have been shown to predict survival and add to the prognostic information derived from the Karnofsky performance status (KPS) and extent of disease. Physical symptoms including pain, dry mouth, constipation, change in taste, lack of appetite and energy, feeling bloated, nausea, vomiting, weight loss, and feeling drowsy or dizzy often portend a poorer prognosis.[6] Palliative care is an integral component of cancer treatment with a goal to effectively and efficiently relieve symptoms and maintain the maximum functional and emotional well-being for the duration of the patient's life.[7–13]

Recognizing the value of the early integration of palliative care, an American Society of Clinical Oncology clinical practice guideline states that the standard for oncology care includes the control of the symptoms of cancer and its treatment from diagnosis to death. Data supporting this guideline includes nine randomized controlled trials and five secondary analyses from these trials that demonstrate the effectiveness of dedicated palliative care services early in the treatment of cancer. Essential components of palliative care may include symptom management, education about the cancer and its prognosis, clarification of treatment goals and assistance with medical decision making, coping needs, and coordination of care.[14]

Applying these principles, a prospective trial in 171 newly diagnosed advanced lung or noncolorectal gastrointestinal cancer patients evaluated the key elements of early palliative care from 2,921 clinic visits. The initial cancer therapy was chemotherapy (80.7%) or radiotherapy (19.3%). Patients randomly assigned to at least monthly visits in the palliative care clinic had assessments performed at baseline and at 24 weeks. Most of these palliative care visits addressed symptom management (74.5%) and coping (64.2%). By 24 weeks, patients who more frequently addressed treatment decisions were less likely to initiate chemotherapy ($P = .02$) or be hospitalized ($P = .005$) in the 60 days before death. With a higher proportion of visits addressing advanced care planning, hospice care was more frequently used ($P = .03$) (Fig. 48.1).[15]

Application of palliative care principles has a profound impact on the physical and psychological comfort of the patient and their caregivers. These palliative care principles also have a profound socioeconomic impact given that the highest costs incurred in health care are at the end of life. Referral to a specialty palliative care service only occurred in 298 (30%) of 978 patients. Of these 298 patients, only 94 (9.6% of the total) had an early referral, whereas the remaining 204 patients (21% of the total) had a late referral to the palliative care service. Early delivery of palliative care resulted in lower rates of inpatient admission in the last month of life (33% vs. 66%), lower rates of intensive care unit (ICU) stay in the last month of life (5% vs. 20%), fewer emergency department visits in the last month (34% vs. 54%), fewer instances of hospice service less than 3 days (7% vs. 20%), and lower rate of inpatient death (15% vs. 34%). The direct cost of inpatient medical care in the last 6 months of life with early palliative care was less than among those with late palliative care ($19,000 vs. $25,700).[16]

At the Johns Hopkins Medical Institutions, the palliative care unit and palliative care consults had a positive financial impact of $3,488,863.10. Palliative care consultations alone, with 60% of these involving cancer patients, saved $2,765,218.00. The 30-day readmission rate was cut from 15% to 10%. Hospice care was arranged in 57% of palliative care consultation patients as compared to only 27% if a palliative care consult was not requested.[17]

The early integration of palliative care services significantly reduces health care utilization during end-of-life care. Insurance claims during the last month of life from 6,568 cancer patients from a Surveillance, Epidemiology, and End Results (SEER) database between 2007 and 2015 were reviewed. At baseline, at least one imaging scan was performed in 48.9%, and 56.3% of patients were hospitalized; only 31.4% of patients younger than 65 years were enrolled in hospice. With changes in health care and reimbursement policies over this time frame, the administration of chemotherapy and/or radiotherapy, diagnostic imaging, and hospitalization rates declined (Fig. 48.2).[18]

Palliative chemotherapy has been an ambiguous term and mostly refers to chemotherapy given when the likelihood of cure was minimal. In the true sense, palliative chemotherapy means that systemic therapy is delivered to relieve symptoms and improve quality of life regardless of stage of disease or the likelihood of remission or cure. The primary outcomes of most studies involving disease-modifying systemic agents, however, do not have symptom relief as a major endpoint. Although virtually all systemic agents used in cancer have been surveyed

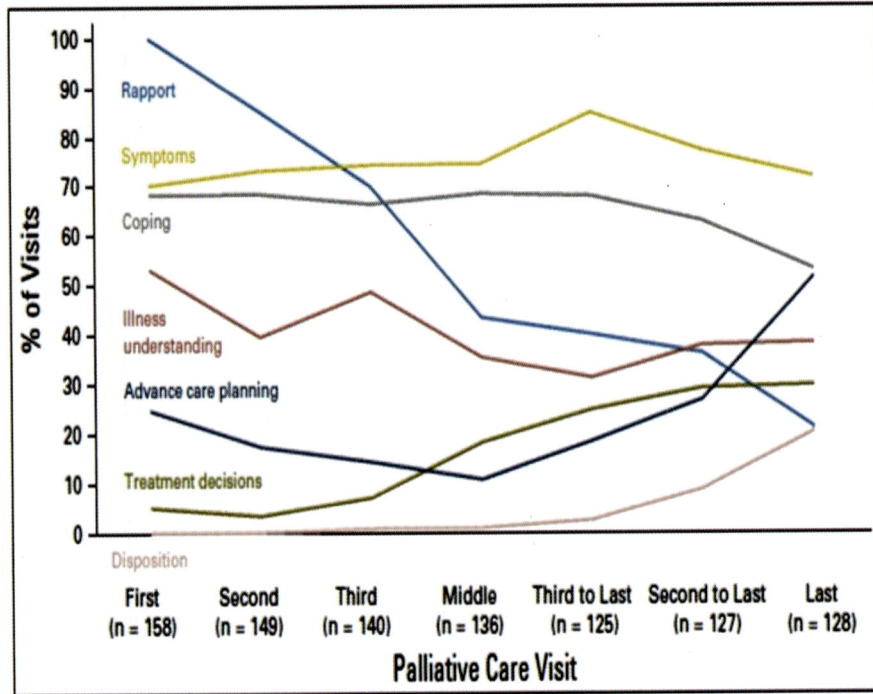

FIGURE 48.1 Content of palliative care (PC) visits across the illness trajectory. PC clinicians recorded the content they addressed after each visit. Reported proportions for the final three visits are restricted to decedents. Reported proportions for the initial three visits exclude visits that were also among the final three visits. Reported proportions for middle visits represent averages across all available middle visits. Relative to the initial three visits, the final three visits increasingly addressed treatment decisions ($P < .001$), advance care planning ($P < .001$), and disposition ($P < .001$) but decreasingly addressed rapport ($P < .001$) and illness understanding ($P < .001$). *(From Hoerger M, Greer JA, Jackson VA, et al. Defining the elements of early palliative care that are associated with patient-reported outcomes and the delivery of end-of-life care. J Clin Oncol 2018;36[11]:1096–1102. Reprinted with permission. Copyright © 2018 American Society of Clinical Oncology. All rights reserved.)*

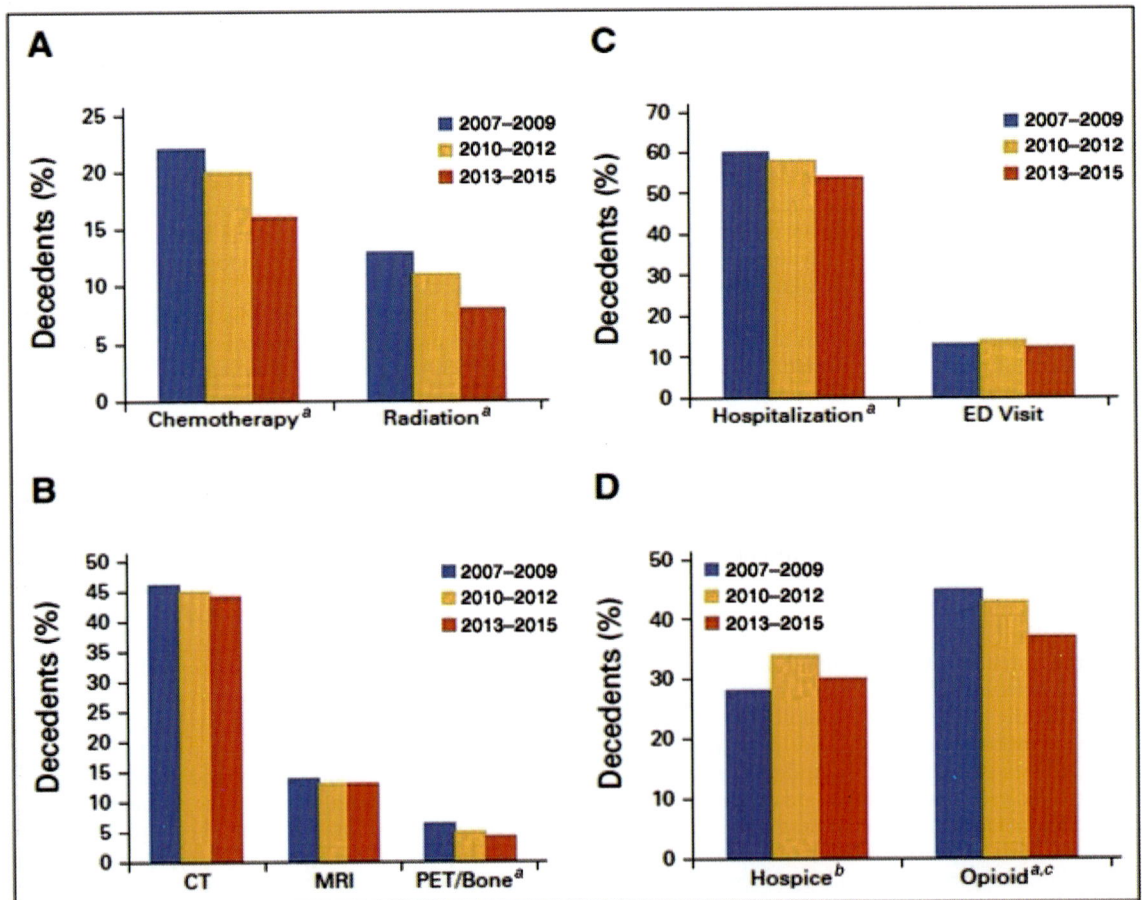

FIGURE 48.2 Trends in health care use in the last 30 days of life by year of death and percentage of decedents. **A:** Chemotherapy or radiation use. **B:** Imaging use. **C:** Hospitalization and emergency department (ED) visits. **D:** Hospice and opioid use. Overall, 963 patients died between 2007 and 2009, 2,628 between 2010 and 2012, and 2,977 between 2013 and 2015. [a]Statistically significant trend over time. [b]For people under 65 years of age: 426 died between 2007 and 2009, 1,088 died between 2010 and 2012, and 1,064 died between 2013 and 2015. [c]Under 65 years, not enrolled in hospice. CT, computed tomography; MRI, magnetic resonance imaging; PET, positron emission tomography. *(From McDermott CL, Fedorenko C, Kreizenbeck K, et al. End-of-life services among patients with cancer: evidence from cancer registry records linked with commercial health insurance claims. J Oncol Pract 2017;13[11]:e889–e899. Reprinted with permission. Copyright © 2017 American Society of Clinical Oncology. All rights reserved.)*

for impact on quality-of-life, the results of these quality-of-life surveys are rarely reported. Reduction in the size of the tumor, which is the intended goal of chemotherapy, should intuitively decrease cancer pain. However, because the therapeutic benefits of chemotherapy are limited by their own toxicities, the risks versus benefits need to be weighed as part of treatment planning and decision making on a case-by-case basis.

Palliative radiation often is used near the end of life to relieve pain and obstruction from tumor. To achieve the most benefit, palliative radiation should be administered to prevent or relieve symptoms before they become severe. If referral for palliative radiation is delayed until the patient becomes extremely debilitated and/or the lesion has progressed significantly, often the possibility of any benefit from palliative radiation is lost. Demonstrating this, a retrospective study of 1,424 patients with metastatic cancer was conducted between 2010 and 2015 found that 11.3% had received palliative radiation therapy before ICU admission. The in-hospital mortality rate was 36.7% for palliative radiation patients compared to 16.6% of other patients with metastatic cancer. After ICU admission, only 21.1% of patients previously treated with palliative radiation received additional cancer treatment.[19]

The median length of survival is critical to evaluating response to and determining the appropriate recommendations for palliative therapy. The most common application of palliative radiation is in management of pain related to bone metastasis. Seventy percent of metastatic bone lesions are painful and debilitating. The goal of treatment is to relieve pain, restore functional ability, and prevent pathologic fractures. In prostate cancer, the distribution of bone metastases has prognostic significance. Survival is longer when the metastases are restricted to the pelvis and lumbar spine or if there is a response to salvage hormone therapy, but lower if metastatic involvement is outside the pelvis and lumbar spine irrespective of response to salvage hormone therapy.[20–22] Survival rapidly declines once visceral metastases develop.[23–25]

The location of the metastasis can also be a limitation in the effectiveness of a palliative radiation. Metastatic involvement of weight-bearing bones and those used in functional activities are often less likely to respond completely to palliative interventions due to applied mechanical forces put on them. Pain relief is achieved in 73% of spine metastases, 88% of limb lesions, 67% of pelvic metastases, and 75% of metastases to other parts of the skeleton.[26–28]

Palliative therapy has become a recognized subspecialty within radiation oncology.[29] Despite the establishment of multiple palliative medicine programs in the country and the proven efficacy of palliative radiotherapy for symptoms, radiotherapy is often underutilized due to long radiation treatment schedules.[26] Even with a relatively short life expectancy, palliative radiotherapy may be helpful, but less than 3% of the patients in hospice care received radiation in one survey.[30]

Conducting randomized trials among large patient cohorts, shorter radiation treatment regimens have enhanced quality of care by achieving equivalent symptom reduction when compared to longer radiation regimens and have significantly reduced the lengths of hospitalization ($P = .01$).[31] Among 181 patients hospitalized for bone metastases between 2010 and 2016, a palliative care radiation oncology consult service recommended shorter palliative radiation schedules, increased palliative care utilization, and reduced hospital stays by 8.5 days. Median total hospitalization costs were $76,792 for patients with bone metastases before a palliative radiation oncology consult service was available and were reduced to $50,582 after the palliative radiation oncology consult service was formed.[32] Cost of outpatient radiation therapy was evaluated from claims-linked data from 207 breast and 233 prostate cancer patients in 98 cancer treatment centers in 16 US states between 2008 and 2010. The mean total cost of radiation for

bone metastases was $7,457 for breast cancer and $7,553 for prostate cancer patients.[33]

More sophisticated and costly radiation techniques, like stereotactic and proton radiation, are available to treat patients expected to have a longer survival or those with complicated clinical presentations, like those near critical structures and in/near previously irradiated sites. Stereotactic radiation is not cost-effective for routine cases having an incremental cost-effectiveness ratio of $124,552 per quality-adjusted life years. However, stereotactic radiation does become cost-effective, with an incremental cost-effectiveness ratio of less than $100,000 per quality-adjusted life years, among patients with a median survival of over 10 months.[34] More abbreviated radiation courses result in cost savings for less complicated clinical presentations. Ineffective therapy, however, incurs more personal and economic cost resulting from the continued need for analgesics and the functional limitations caused by unrelieved pain and disability.[35,36]

The most common barriers to radiotherapy still relate to the costs of radiation therapy and transportation difficulties. The selection of a radiation course or technique, like that for a systemic therapy, is dependent on the patient wishes, prognosis, and comorbidities.

BONE DISEASE

The annual prevalence of bone metastasis was determined to be 256,137 in the years 2000 to 2004. The direct cost for patients with bone metastasis was $75,329, and the incremental cost was $44,442 compared to patients with cancer without bone metastasis. The national cost burden for patients with skeletal metastasis was estimated at $12.6 billion which is 17% of the $74 billion total direct medical cost estimated by National Institutes of Health (NIH).[37] The prevalence of metastatic bone disease totaled 279,679 as determined by claims-based data from 2004 to 2008, with breast, prostate, and lung cancer accounting for 68% of these cases.[38]

Multidisciplinary evaluation of patients with metastatic disease to the bone allows comprehensive management of the associated symptoms, determines the risk for pathologic fracture, and helps coordinate administration of a wide range of available antineoplastic therapies (also see Chapter 46).[39,40] Bone metastases can be treated with localized, systemic, or both kinds of therapies. Because localized treatments, like radiation and surgery, provide treatment only to a localized symptomatic site of disease, it is frequently used in coordination with systemic therapies such as chemotherapy, hormonal therapy, and bisphosphonates. Radiopharmaceuticals provide another systemic option that treats diffuse symptomatic bone metastases.[39,41] Because the radiation is deposited directly at the involved area in the bone, radiopharmaceuticals, such as strontium 89 or samarium 153, can also be used to treat diffuse bone metastases or when symptoms recur in a previously irradiated site. Radiopharmaceuticals can also act as an adjuvant to localized external beam irradiation and reduce the development of other symptomatic sites of disease. A study was conducted among patients referred to a multidisciplinary bone metastases clinic between 2007 and 2015. Independent of age, 62% of patients received palliative radiation, whereas surgical stabilization was required in 30% over the age of 66 years and in 39% of patients 65 years of age or younger.[42]

Control of cancer-related pain with the use of analgesics is imperative to allow comfort during and while awaiting response to therapeutic interventions. Pain represents a sensitive measure of disease activity. Close follow-up should be performed to ensure control of cancer and treatment-related pain and to initiate diagnostic studies to identify progressive or recurrent disease. Pain, risk for pathologic fracture, and spinal cord compression are the most common indications to treat bone metastases with localized therapy including radiation and surgery.

CLINICAL APPLICATIONS OF RADIATION THERAPY

Radiotherapy can be delivered with curative or palliative intent. Curative treatment attempts to render the patient disease free of either primary or metastatic disease. Treatment with palliative intent is intended to control the symptoms of disease when the disease cannot be eradicated. A number of clinical, prognostic, and therapeutic factors must be considered to determine the most optimal treatment regimen for a course of palliative radiotherapy. Although any site of disease can be effectively palliated, treatment of bone metastases is one of the most common indications for palliative irradiation with external beam therapy. During the last year of life, one-third of patients receive radiation therapy, which decreased to 24.3% in the last 3 months of life and 8.5% during the last month of life. Although radiation with curative intent was delivered at a constant rate in 25% of patients, palliative radiation was administered at a supralinear rate over the last year of life in which the treatment of bone metastases and use of single-fraction radiation increased closer to death.[43]

The limited radiation tolerances of normal tissues, such as the spinal cord, make it impossible to administer a large enough dose of radiation to completely eradicate most tumors. Palliative radiation should result in sufficient tumor regression to relieve symptoms for the duration of the patient's life. Palliative radiotherapy is often combined with chemotherapy and/or surgery to optimize therapeutic outcomes from tumor-related pain, bleeding, visceral obstruction, or lymphatic and vascular obstruction. Common sites include respiratory system structures, pelvis, skin and subcutaneous tissues, brain, and all bony structures. Potential relief of symptoms is a more important determinant for palliative radiation than whether lesions result from locally advanced or metastatic disease. Symptoms that recur after palliative radiation most commonly result from localized regrowth of tumor in the radiation field.[44]

The palliative interventions recommended depend on the patient's clinical status, burden of disease, and location of the symptomatic site. For either locally advanced or metastatic disease, these factors are indexed to the relative effectiveness, durability, and morbidity of each palliative intervention. Each patient's prognosis represents the single most important factor in deciding the approach to palliative therapy.[45]

Because patients with metastatic disease have a limited life expectancy, the number of radiation fractions prescribed for treatment with palliative intent depends on prognosis and not primary histology, so a lower total dose is given with palliative radiation over 1 to 2 weeks (hypofractionated radiation schedule). Based on the radiation tolerance of normal tissues, a low daily radiation dose (1.8 to 2.0 Gy) is given with conventional radiation; in contrast, large daily radiation fractions are given with hypofractionated radiation schedules. Hypofractionated radiation schedules for palliative therapy can range from 2.5 Gy per fraction administered over 3 weeks for a total dose of 35 Gy to a single 8-Gy dose of radiation. Most frequently, 30 Gy is administered in 10 fractions over 2 weeks. Especially among patients with short life expectancies, many centers administer 20 Gy in 1 week or a single fraction of radiation because the rates of pain relief, mobility, and frequency of pathologic fractures are similar to more protracted radiation schedules.[46,47]

Palliative interventions not only should be limited in time relative to the patient's life expectancy but should also be focused to limit toxicity. Available radiation techniques that focus the radiation to the symptomatic site should be applied to limit toxicity. Although the relative cost of more advanced radiation planning and treatment may be higher, the tolerance to palliative radiation is better, avoiding the costs of treating toxicities, especially for radiation portals that include mucosal surfaces. Among the radiation techniques that more precisely focus the delivery of radiation to the tumor are intensity-modulated radiation therapy (IMRT), proton radiation therapy, and stereotactic radiation therapy (SRT).[48]

Response of Tumors to Radiotherapy

TRACHEA, BRONCHI, AND LUNGS

Locally advanced primary or metastatic involvement of the lung often requires palliative intervention because cure is possible in only a few of these cases. A variety of symptoms, some of them emergent, can manifest because of tumor involvement of the lung. Pain can result from tumor invasion of the ribs and nerve roots of the chest wall. Vertebral involvement can be associated with spinal cord compression. Lower respiratory tract obstruction, bleeding, and pneumonitis can result from tracheobronchial tumor growth. Mediastinal infiltration can cause superior vena cava syndrome.

All of these clinical presentations can be palliated with external beam radiation that encompasses the disease that is evident on diagnostic images and that treats pain referred along involved nerve roots. Radiation schedules that administer 30 Gy in 10 fractions over 2 weeks, 20 Gy in 5 fractions, 2 fractions of 8.5 Gy 1 week apart, or 1 fraction of 10 Gy (depending on the patient's life expectancy and ability to tolerate multifraction therapy) are typically prescribed to previously unirradiated sites.[48]

Optimal palliation of patients with incurable lung cancer requires coordinated interdisciplinary care. For patients with stage III non–small-cell lung cancer who have a life expectancy of at least 3 months, have a good performance status, and no comorbidities excluding the administration of chemotherapy, administration of a platinum-containing chemotherapy concurrent with hypofractionated palliative thoracic radiation therapy is recommended over treatment with either modality alone.[49]

Hemoptysis and chest pain can be effectively palliated with external beam radiation, although dyspnea and dysphagia are not as effectively relieved. If the area has been previously irradiated, techniques that exclude critical anatomic structures, such as the spinal cord, are applied. Other approaches, like brachytherapy, stereotactic radiation, and proton therapy, can be used when the symptomatic site is well localized and accessible. Brachytherapy can be used to treat bronchial obstruction and bleeding by placing a radioactive source directly against the tumor under bronchoscopic guidance. In these cases, large doses of radiation can be delivered over a few minutes by a high-dose rate brachytherapy unit.[48,49]

PANCREATIC CANCER

Palliative doses of radiation for unresectable pancreatic cancer have minimal to no impact on survival. Randomized trials have not shown any significant survival benefit when conventional radiation is used after chemotherapy for unresectable pancreatic cancer. Results from nonrandomized studies of 3 to 5 fractions that deliver a biologic equivalent dose (BED) of 53 Gy of stereotactic radiation (SRT) not only have less toxicity and a shorter treatment time but also a minimal impact on survival. However, when 15 to 25 fractions of SRT, which deliver a BED of 100 Gy, longer survival can be achieved with low toxicity. Based on the anatomic disease extension and the patient's performance status and wishes, SRT can be tailored to effectively relieve cancer-related symptoms, and in specific circumstances, extend life.[50]

PELVIS

Hemorrhage with or without obstruction or compression of viscera, lymphatics, vascular structures, and nerves commonly occurs with locally advanced or metastatic disease in the pelvis.

Treatment may require emergent radiotherapeutic, surgical interventions, or both. Hemorrhage is commonly associated with tumors involving the rectum and genitourinary tracts. As with tumors in the lung, radiation is an effective means of stopping active bleeding. Colorectal cancers are often diagnosed among patients with unexplained bleeding. In patients who have locally advanced tumors with months to years of life expectancy, 40 Gy in 2.5 Gy fractions to 50 Gy in 2 Gy fractions have been used with the intent to stop bleeding, render the patient operable, and provide a chance for cure. With extensive metastatic disease, 30 Gy in 10 fractions or 20 Gy in 5 fractions is used to palliate symptoms of bleeding and obstruction. Colorectal tumor involvement may also result in obstruction requiring stent placement to maintain the integrity of the visceral lumen while administering radiation. Diverting colostomy is occasionally required but is reported to have been avoided after chemohypofractionated irradiation.[51]

Tumors involving the cervix can hemorrhage and require emergent radiotherapeutic intervention. Superficial radiographs are applied directly to the bleeding cervix through a cone to treat the bleeding site and do not compromise later radiation of other pelvic structures. Usually, radiation doses between 5 and 10 Gy are administered in one to three applications of cone therapy. Brachytherapy also can be used to treat gynecologic tumors, especially in the vagina, cervix, and endometrium.[51]

Bladder cancers or tumors that secondarily invade the bladder can also result in significant bleeding that can be palliated by external beam radiation. Urinary obstruction commonly occurs with locally advanced pelvic cancers, especially with bladder, rectum, prostate, and cervical cancers. Occasionally, placement of a urinary stent, urostomy, or nephrostomy is required until sufficient tumor regression can be accomplished by radiation to reestablish integrity of the urinary tract. As with the bowel and gynecologic tracts, a bladder fistula, resulting from either the tumor itself or from tumor regression, is a concern.

The pelvic lymph nodes and major blood vessels may become obstructed by tumor. This is most frequently seen when tumors arise in pelvic structures but can also occur with pelvic metastases from breast and other cancers. Lymph-vascular obstruction results in painful edema that is refractory to diuretic and other therapies. Other than pain and functional interference, when severe, fluid and electrolyte imbalances can occur. Pelvic radiation can relieve lymph-vascular obstruction through tumor regression.[51]

Pelvic tumors can also invade the sacral plexus and result in intractable pain. Tumor can track along nerve roots and can be associated with bony invasion of the sacrum. Pain caused by visceral, lymph-vascular, or both kinds of obstructions often respond more rapidly to palliative radiation than the more refractory neuropathic pain seen with sacral plexus involvement. Other radiotherapeutic approaches, such as brachytherapy, are extremely limited when the cancer persists or recurs after external beam radiation. Interventional pain management techniques are frequently required to control pain associated with sacral plexus involvement (see Chapter 44).

The use of palliative radiation in colorectal, prostate, and breast cancer is common. Using SEER data of 39,619 patients between 2004 and 2011, half of the patients received radiation in the last 6 months of life, defined as the last 6 months of life. Of the patients who received radiation during the end of life (19,586), only 46% had not previously been treated with radiation. Surgery was performed at the end of life in 35% of the patients, with proportionately more patients undergoing both surgery and radiation. Radiation was administered during the last 14 days of life, in 5,723 patients (14%). Administration of radiation during the end of life strongly correlated with end-of-life chemotherapy use, including the last 14 days of life

(36% of chemotherapy patients); by comparison, only 15% of patients were treated with radiation in the group that did not receive chemotherapy during the last 14 days of life. Especially during the last 14 days of life, treatment may cause increased burden without improving quality of life.[52]

SKIN AND SUBCUTANEOUS TISSUES

Tumors can cause ulceration of the skin and subcutaneous tissues that are often painful and distressing because of constant drainage. Representing a source for the development of sepsis in immunocompromised patients, localized radiation can be applied to destroy tumor and allow reepithelialization of the skin. Radiation that treats only the skin and subcutaneous tissues (electron beam therapy) is generally used to avoid radiation side effects to underlying uninvolved normal structures. Although usually 10 radiation treatments are given, the course of radiation can be abbreviated further, ranging from 1 to 5 days. Occasionally, these lesions are treated with brachytherapy. The radioactive sources can be placed in a mold that sits on top of the tumor and delivers treatment over a few minutes (high-dose rate) or a few days (low-dose rate).

BRAIN METASTASES

Radiation is used to relieve the symptoms of headache, seizure, nausea and vomiting, and neurologic dysfunction associated with brain metastases. In patients with good performance status, surgery or radiosurgery followed by postoperative whole brain radiation is commonly administered. Radiation is generally with a total of 30 Gy in 10 fractions or 20 Gy in 5 fractions.[53]

Management of newly diagnosed single or multiple brain metastases, however, depends on the estimated prognosis and the aims of treatment, including survival, local treated lesion control, distant brain control, and neurocognitive preservation. Prognostic systems, such as recursive partitioning analysis and diagnosis-specific graded prognostic assessment, may assist in predicting prognosis. Single brain metastasis greater than 3 to 4 cm in size with a good prognosis (expected survival of 3 months or more), the lesion should be surgically resected followed by whole brain radiotherapy (WBRT) or surgical resection followed by intraoperative radiation or an SRT boost to the resection cavity. For a single metastasis less than 3 to 4 cm in size, multiple options exist including SRT alone, WBRT and SRT, WBRT and surgery, surgical resection, and SRT or intraoperative radiation boost. For anatomically unresectable or incompletely resected single brain metastases less than 3 to 4 cm in size, WBRT and SRT or SRT alone should be considered. With an unresected brain metastasis larger than 3 to 4 cm, WBRT should be considered.[54]

Multiple brain metastases, all of which are less than 3 to 4 cm in size with a good prognosis SRT alone if the multiple lesions are limited in number and location, WBRT and SRT, or WBRT alone are options. Other alternatives include WBRT alone or resection of large brain metastasis or metastases if it can be accomplished without causing significant mass effect or morbidity followed by postoperative WBRT.

With poor prognosis, patients with either a single or multiple brain metastases should be considered for palliative care with or without WBRT.

Bone Metastases

There are two major historical sets of experience with palliative radiation for bone metastases. The Radiation Therapy Oncology Group (RTOG) conducted a prospective trial that included a variety of treatment schedules (Table 48.1). To account for prognosis, patients were stratified on the basis of whether they had a solitary or multiple sites of bony metastases. The initial

TABLE 48.1   Dose–Response Evaluation from the Reanalysis of the Radiation Therapy Oncology Group Bone Metastases Protocol[55]

Dose per Fraction (Gy)	Total Dose (Gy)	Tumor Dose at 2 Gy per Fraction[a]	Complete Response Rate (%)[b]	P Value
Solitary Bone Metastases				P < .0003
2.7	40.5	42.9	55	
4	20	23.3	37	
Multiple Bone Metastases				P < .0003
3	30	32.5	46	
3	15	16.2	36	
4	20	23.3	40	
5	25	31.25	28	

[a]The radiobiologic equivalent dose if administered at 2 Gy per fraction.
[b]The complete response rate using the definition that excludes the use of analgesics and that accounts for retreatment.

TABLE 48.2   Percentage of Patients Who Responded to Radiation Relative to Time, Designated in Weeks after Completion of Radiation Therapy

Total Dose (Gy)	Dose per Fraction (Gy)	Tumor Dose at 2 Gy per Fraction	Weeks after Radiation <2 (%)	2–4 (%)	4–12 (%)	12–20 (%)
Solitary Metastases						
40.5	2.7	42.9	7	29	53	77
20	4	23.3	16	50	66	82
Multiple Metastases						
30	3	32.5	19	48	73	84
15	3	16.2	34	70	84	93
20	4	23.3	28	53	75	88
25	5	31.25	22	41	72	80

NOTE: This prospective trial, conducted by the Radiation Therapy Oncology Group, randomized radiation dose and number of fractions and stratified the randomization on the basis of solitary or multiple bone metastases.[58,59] Also listed is the radiobiologic equivalent dose if administered at 2 Gy per fraction.

analysis of the study concluded that low-dose, short-course treatment schedules were as effective as high-dose protracted treatment programs.[55] For solitary bone metastases, no difference existed in the relief of pain when 20 Gy using 4-Gy fractions was compared with 40.5 Gy delivered as 2.7 Gy fractions. Relapse of pain occurred in 57% of patients at a median of 15 weeks after completion of therapy for each dose level. In patients with multiple bone metastases, the following dose schedules were compared: 30 Gy at 3 Gy per fraction, 15 Gy given as 3 Gy per fraction, 20 Gy using 4 Gy per fraction, and 25 Gy using 5 Gy per fraction. No difference was identified in the rates of pain relief among these treatment schedules. Partial relief of pain was achieved in 83%, and complete relief occurred in 53% of the patients studied. More than 50% of these patients developed recurrent pain, the fracture rate equaled 8%, and the median duration of pain control was 12 weeks for all the radiation schedules used for multiple bony metastases. Prognostic factors for response included the initial pain score and site of the primary cancer.

In a reanalysis of the data, a different definition for complete pain relief was used and excluded the continued administration of analgesics. Using this definition, the relief of pain was significantly related to the number of fractions and the total dose of radiation that was administered.[56] Complete relief of pain was achieved in 55% of patients with solitary bone metastases who received 40.5 Gy at 2.7 Gy per fraction as compared with 37% of patients who received a total dose of 20 Gy given as 4 Gy per fraction. A similar relationship was observed in the reanalysis of patients who had multiple bone metastases. Complete relief of pain was achieved in 46% of patients who received 30 Gy at 3 Gy per fraction versus 28% of patients treated to 25 Gy using 5-Gy fractions. In most cases, the interval to response was 4 weeks for both complete and minimal relief of symptoms.

Three important issues are identified from the RTOG experience. First, the results of the reanalysis demonstrate the importance of defining what represents a response to therapy. Second, this revised definition of response showed that the total radiation dose did influence the degree that pain was relieved.[55,56] The response rates and the radiobiologically equivalent doses are listed from the reanalysis in Figure 48.1 for each of the treatment schedules used. Patients treated with total doses of 40 Gy or more had a 75% rate of complete pain relief versus a 62% rate of complete pain relief for patients treated with total doses of less than 40 Gy.[27,57] Third, the RTOG experience identified the amount of time that was needed to experience relief of pain after radiation for bone metastases (Table 48.2). It is important to note that only one-half of the patients who were going to respond had relief of symptoms at

2 to 4 weeks after radiation.[55,56] This underscores the need for continued analgesic support after completing radiation. Consistently, it took 12 to 20 weeks after radiation to accomplish the maximal level of relief. That period of time may reflect the time needed for reossification. Radiographic evidence of recalcification is observed in approximately one-fourth of cases, and in 70% of cases, recalcification is seen within 6 months of completing radiation treatments.[60–63] Recalcification is the basis of stabilization and prevention of fractures in the future. For pain relief, a short course of radiation is adequate; however, a longer schedule is recommended for adequate recalcification.[58,59] Again, clinical context, with a focus on life expectancy, is a key determinant of radiation type, dose, and fractionation schedule.

Single-Fraction Radiation

A single large radiation fraction has demonstrated, in large multiple prospective randomized clinical trials, as effective in relieving pain as other radiation schedules that have more treatments. Radiobiologically, a single 8-Gy fraction would give the same side effects to late reacting tissues (i.e., tissues such as the spinal cord that do not regenerate) as if 18 Gy were given over nine treatments at 2 Gy per fraction.[64] Because tumors and acute reacting tissues, such as the esophagus and other mucosal structures, respond differently than the late-reacting tissues, the radiobiologically equivalent dose to the tumor for a single 8-Gy fraction would be 12 Gy if 2 Gy fractions were used. The most common dose fractionation schedule used for palliative radiation in the United States is 30 Gy over 10 fractions. Radiobiologically, this is equivalent to 36 Gy at 2 Gy per fraction for late-reacting tissues and 32.5 Gy to the tumor. When a single dose of radiation was compared with a radiation schedule with multiple radiation fractions, no difference was reported in either how quickly symptoms resolved or the duration of pain relief.[57,65–77] Pain relief was achieved in 80% after treatment and 50% of patients at 6 months irrespective of the number of fractions. Complete response (CR) rates after a single 8-Gy fraction total 15% at 2 weeks, 23% at 4 weeks, 28% at 8 weeks, and 9% at 12 weeks postradiation.

Despite the radiobiologic differences in the dose administered, the similarities in response may be caused by tumor regression and reossification that occurs at 3 months. The RTOG experience showed that the maximum response to therapy was seen consistently at 3 months and was independent of dose administered.[55,56] The disparity in the relationship between radiation dose and clinical response may also be attributed to limited follow-up in the single-fraction study because a significant proportion of patients in the study were lost to follow-up after 3 months.[67–70] With longer follow-up, the response to a single radiation fraction may not prove to be as durable as multiple fractions that give high total radiation doses.[76–78] These data demonstrate that prognosis needs to be linked to variables such as site irradiated, total radiation dose, and reirradiation.[79]

A shorter radiation schedule, such as a single fraction, is advantageous for patients with poor prognostic factors. First, it is easier for patients with a poor KPS to complete therapy. Second, response rates are equal to single and multifraction therapy at 3 months because median survival is less than 6 months among patients with poor prognostic factors.[67–75] The option of retreatment after a single fraction of radiation may also provide an advantage among patients with good prognostic factors as a means to periodically reduce tumor burden and control symptoms in noncritical anatomic sites. Higher radiation doses that provide more durable pain relief are considered warranted for patients with good prognostic factors who require treatment over the spine and other critical sites.[80–86]

The projected length of survival is the critical issue to determine the optimal radiation dose and schedule for palliative radiation. In one study, only 12 of 243 patients were alive at the time of analysis, with approximately 50% alive at 6 months, 25% at 1 year, 8% at 2 years, and 3% at 3 years after palliative radiation. For breast cancer patients, the survival rates at these time points after palliative radiation were 60%, 44%, 20%, and 7%, respectively. For prostate cancer, the survival rates were 60% at 6 months and 24% at 1 year, and there were no patients who survived 2 years.[87] This survival difference may be an important observation because unrelieved pain and the resultant sequelae of immobility may contribute to mortality as well as morbidity.

The number of fractions used during a course of palliative radiation was found to correlate directly with survival in a cohort of 1,292 patients. Median survival was 13.4 months, 9.8 months, 7.0 months, and 6.9 months for 15, 10, 5, and single-fraction palliative radiation regimens, respectively. Performance status and insurance status also directly correlated with median survival in this study. From this retrospective study, radiation oncologists appropriately selected palliative treatment schedules based on prognostic factors.[88]

These findings were confirmed in a retrospective analysis of 297 patients who began palliative radiotherapy. Of this patient cohort, factors associated with 60 of these patients discontinuing palliative radiotherapy included low KPS, high number of fractions prescribed, and treatment site other than bone metastasis. However, the odds of discontinuing palliative radiotherapy decreased for every 10-point increase in KPS. Independent of all other factors, patients who discontinued treatment were more likely to die. Factors associated with a shorter survival also included low KPS, community practice location, multiple comorbidities, and treatment of brain metastasis (Fig. 48.3).[89]

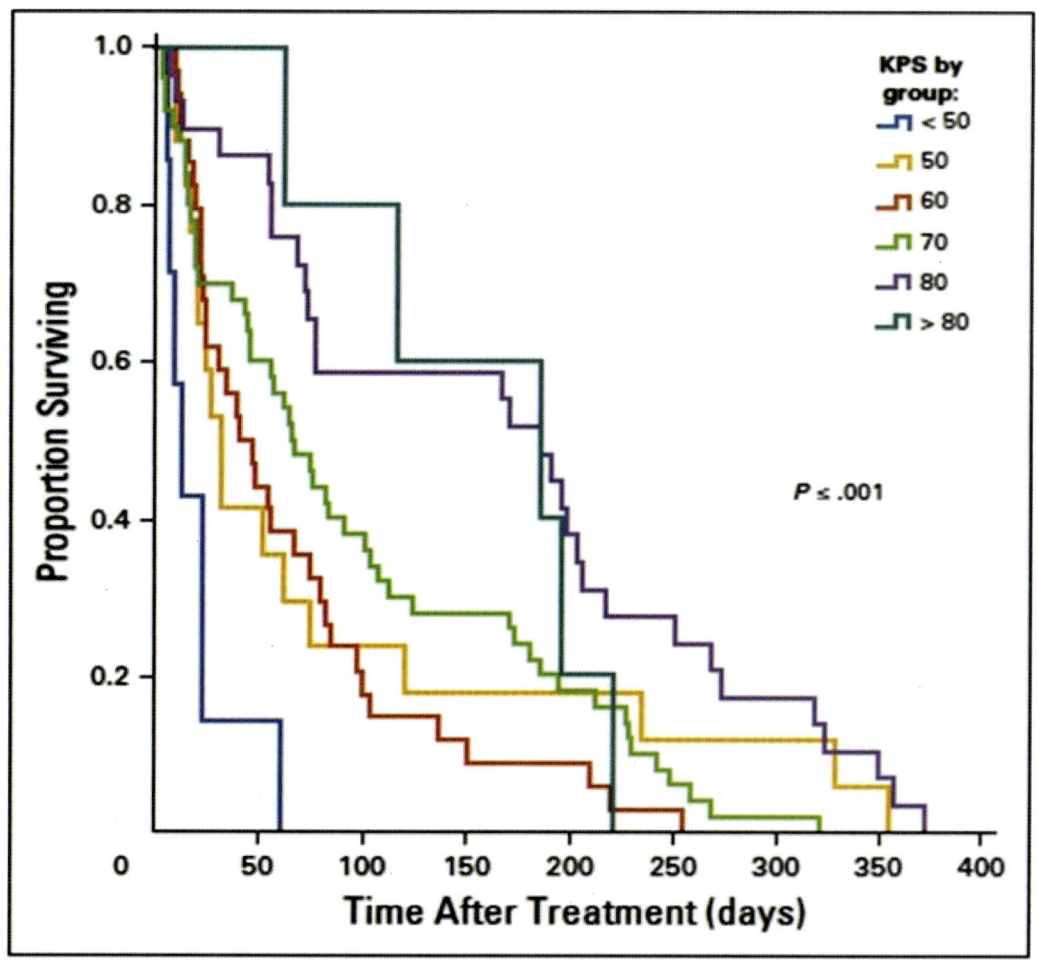

FIGURE 48.3 Association of Karnofsky performance status (KPS) with overall survival. *(From Puckett LL, Luitweiler E, Potters L, et al. Preventing discontinuation of radiation therapy: predictive factors to improve patient selection for palliative treatment. J Oncol Practice 2017;13[9]:e782–e791.)*

Between 2004 and 2007, only 17% of external beam palliative radiation courses were given in one to five radiation fractions, whereas from 2012 to 2016, 80% of patients received one to five radiation fractions. SRT was administered in 9.7% of patients and 5.8% with radiopharmaceutical therapy.[90] At another institution between 2007 and 2012, less than 10 radiation fractions were administered in 83% of 339 patients during their final course of radiation.[91]

With expanding evidence from multicenter prospective randomized clinical trials and changes in insurance reimbursement policies, the paradigm of palliative radiation for bone metastases has shifted.

Stereotactic Radiation for Nonspine Bone Metastases

Despite changes in insurance reimbursement policies, bone metastases located in anatomic areas other than the spine also have been treated with SRT. The indications for SRT over conventional palliative radiation included an oligometastasis (63%), progression of an oligometastasis (17.3%), retreatment (2.4%), and other reasons such as anatomic location (17.3%). The most common prescriptions were 30 Gy per five fractions (30.2%) and 35 Gy per five fractions (42.5%). The median age of the patients was 66.4 years (range 36 to 86 years); most of the patients were male (60.5%), and prostate cancer was the predominant primary tumor. Bone metastases were most commonly located in the pelvis (41.5%), and almost half of the metastases were sclerotic. With a 13-month mean follow-up, an association was found between local recurrence and the tumor volume. Local recurrence rates were 4.7% at 6 months, 8.3% at 18 months, and 13.3% at 24 months. Radiographic evidence of a pathologic fracture was documented in 8.5% of treated metastases, with lytic lesions and female gender being a predictor for pathologic fracture.[92]

Reirradiation

Many factors influence response to palliative radiation for bone metastases. Primary tumor site, performance status, and baseline pain score are among the factors predictive for pain response. The predicted response rates to palliative radiation range from 37.5% for patients with multiple adverse factors to 79.8% for patients with the fewest adverse factors.[93] Genetic factors may also help to identify the patients who will respond to palliative radiation and improve resource utilization. Single-nucleotide variants involved in DNA repair, inflammation, cellular adhesion, and cell signaling have significant association with radiation response.[94]

The radiation schedule used for palliative radiation is influenced by the radiation tolerance of adjacent normal tissues as well as prognosis. Acute radiation toxicities are a function of the dose per fraction, total dose, and the area and volume of tissue irradiated. If mucosal surfaces, such as the upper respiratory and digestive tract, bowel, and bladder, can be excluded from the radiation portals, acute radiation side effects can be significantly reduced. This principle of minimizing radiation to uninvolved adjacent tissues applies to the radiation given with curative intent (multiple small radiation doses over multiple weeks), palliative radiation, and reirradiation (few to one large radiation dose). Reirradiation is generally possible because the radiobiologic dose is relatively low after a single fraction of radiation, especially to a previously unirradiation site remote from critical structures like the small bowel or spinal cord.[57,64–70,77–79] If high total radiation doses had been previously administered, reirradiation for persistent or recurrent pain is often challenging or precluded based on the limitations of normal tissue tolerance, especially near the spinal cord.

For bone metastases, reirradiation was necessary in 25% of patients who initially received a single 8-Gy radiation fraction, but all of these patients responded to the second dose of radiation for bone metastases. Pain relief in reirradiated patients was better in patients who had a longer pain-free interval after the initial single 8-Gy dose of radiation (≥4 months), a better performance status, and a single bone metastasis.[95] There also was no significant difference in pain relief at 2 months or overall survival based on gender or age.[96] Using an intention-to-treat analysis for the treatment of bone metastases with palliative radiation, similar response rates were found for single fraction (61%; 1,867/3,059 patients) and multiple fractions (62%; 1,890/3,040 patients). Ten randomized trials were reported since 2010, resulting in a total of 29 trials for analysis. Retreatment was more frequent in the single-fraction arm with 20% receiving additional treatment to the same site versus 8% in the multiple fraction arm. However, no significant difference was seen in the risk for pathologic fracture, the rate of spinal cord compression or acute toxicity rates at the treatment site.[97]

Using SRT, reirradiation to a vertebral body can be safely accomplished with palliation of symptoms. When SRT is given at least 5 months after conventional palliative radiotherapy, and if the radiation dose to the thecal sac does not exceed a biologically equivalent radiation dose of 70 Gy normalized to a 2 Gy equivalent dose. Reirradiation with SRT can achieve favorable response rates if spinal cord radiation dose restraints (10 Gy to 10% of the spinal cord) are followed.[98]

The results of reirradiation of vertebral metastases are favorable. Having no other therapeutic option, tumor recurrence in the spinal and paraspinal areas in 372 spinal lesions were reirradiated using SRT. The time between the initial radiation course and the reirradiated course was a median of 9.8 months. The median survival was 6.9 months after the last radiation treatment (reirradiation), and median follow-up was 3.4 months (average of 21 months). Relief of pain and neurologic improvement was accomplished in 81%, and radiographic tumor control was evident in 71%. Adverse effects occurred in 11 patients, with radionecrosis and myelomalacia each occurring in 1 patient; 6% of patients had radiation associated vertebral compression fractures.[99]

The specimens of 30 patients who underwent surgery after salvage SRT (sSRT) and primary SRT (pSRT) to the spine were compared. This 30 patient cohort (69.6% sSRT, 30.4% pSRT) were identified from 704 patients treated with SRT for vertebral metastases between 2006 and 2012. The mean time to surgery was 8.3 months for sSRT and 10.3 months for pSRT. The most common reasons for surgery were pain (12.5% sSRT, 71.4% pSRT), fracture (37.5% sSRT, 28.6% pSRT), and neurologic symptoms (68.8% sSRT, 42.9% pSRT). Neurologic symptoms were common with radiologic tumor progression but not with fractures. Radiologic tumor progression was seen in 71.4% sSRT and 42.9% pSRT, and it significantly correlated with pathologic evidence of viable tumor and tumor bed necrosis. Viable tumor was pathologically documented in 62.5% sSRT and 71.4% pSRT, although tumor bed necrosis was more common after sSRT (81.3% in sSRT, 42.9% pSRT). Sequelae of radiation included soft tissue necrosis (20.0% in sSRT, 28.6% pSRT), osteonecrosis (14.3% in sSRT, 16.7% pSRT), or bone marrow fibrosis (42.9% in sSRT, 33.3% pSRT). Pathologic fractures were increased with bone marrow fibrosis but not with either soft tissue necrosis or osteonecrosis.[100]

Pathologic Fracture

The most significant complications of bone metastases relate to pathologic fracture and spinal cord compression. Pain that persists or that recurs after palliative radiation should be evaluated to exclude progression of disease, possible extension of disease outside the radiation portal that results in referred pain, and bone fracture. Although pure osteolytic metastases are more likely to fracture than osteoblastic lesions, osteoblastic lesions, by definition, have an osteolytic component so that new bone can be formed.[93] Reduced cortical strength can result in compression, stress, or microfractures associated with reduced cortical strength.

Serial radiography is useful in following postradiation disease progression and fractures. Pathologic fractures occur in 8% to 30% of patients with bone metastases.[101] Proximal long bones are more commonly involved than distal bones. Consequently, pathologic fractures occur 50% of the time in the femur and 15% in the humerus (Fig. 48.4). The femoral neck and head are the most frequent locations for pathologic fracture because of the propensity for metastases to involve

proximal bones and the stress of weight placed on this part of the femur. More than 80% of pathologic fractures occur in breast (50%), kidney, lung, and thyroid cancers.

Computed tomography (CT) was performed in femurs with bone metastases to determine risk for pathologic fracture. No difference in the CT scan was identified between femurs that fractured and did not fracture. However, when only the cortical bone was evaluated, the pathologic fracture group had a lower cumulative Hounsfield value compared to the no fracture and no fixation groups.[102]

Approximately 10% to 30% of metastatic lesions in long bones develop a pathologic fracture that requires surgical intervention. Patients with pathologic fracture caused by bone metastases have clinical outcomes after surgical repair that are comparable with patients sustaining a traumatic fracture.[103–106]

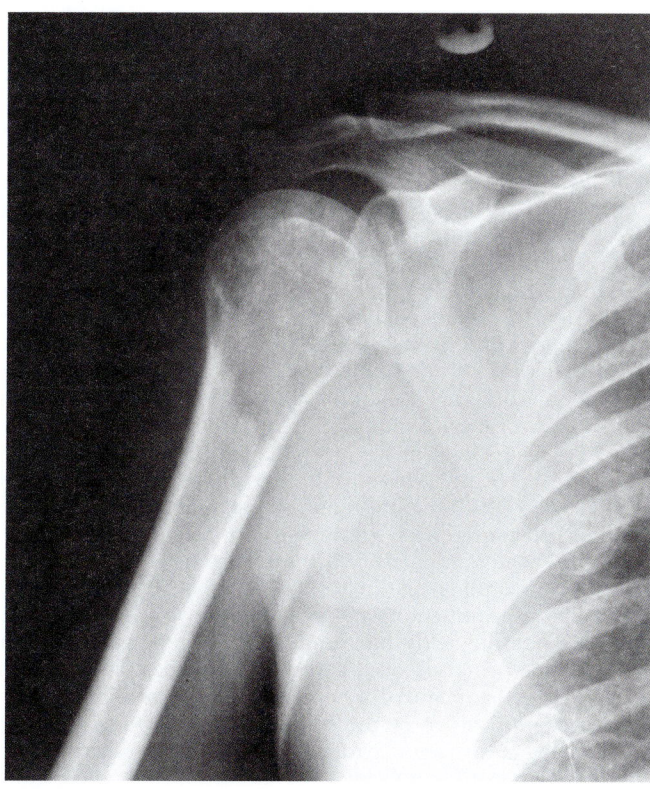

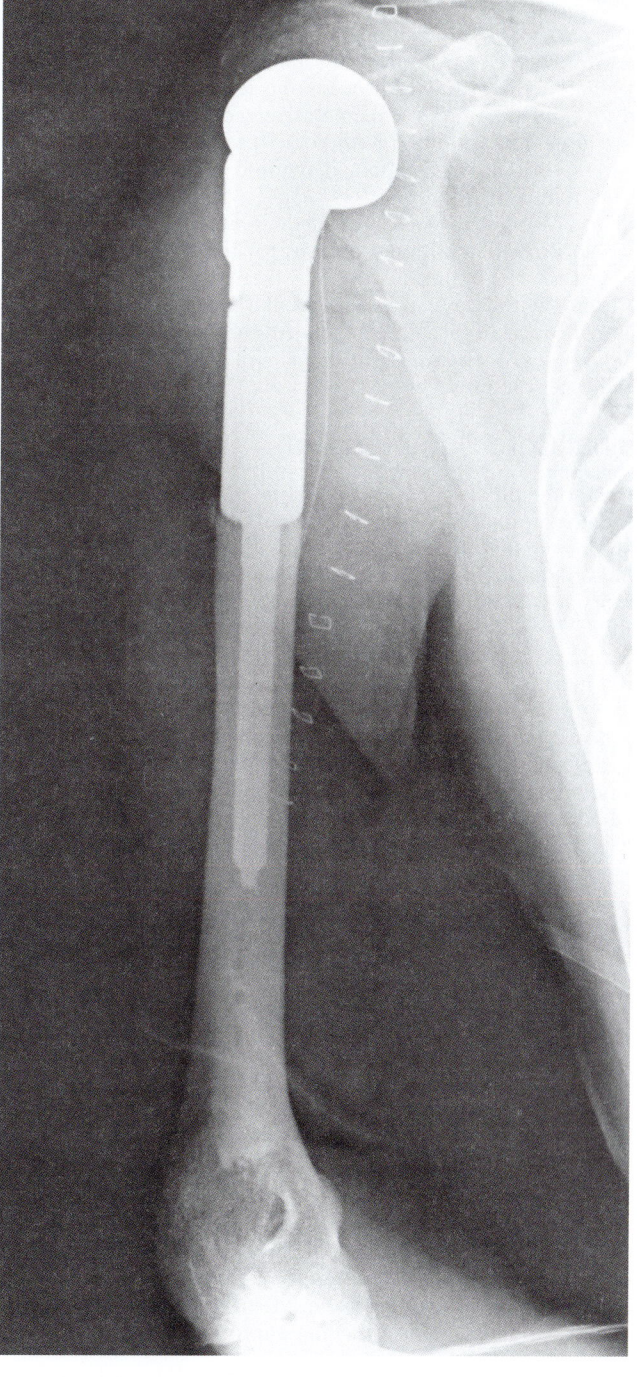

FIGURE 48.4 **A:** An extensive lytic lesion in the proximal humerus. **B:** Prophylactic internal fixation performed to prevent pathologic fracture. This patient, who complained primarily of pain in the hip, would have been placed on crutches to reduce stress on the involved femur. A bone scan and radiography, obtained to exclude other sites of metastatic involvement, identified this lesion in the humerus. The humerus would have certainly fractured if all the patient's weight had been displaced to the upper extremities with crutches.

Surgical management was performed in 184 patients with bone metastases to relieve severe pain, avoid impending or stabilize pathologic fractures between 2008 and 2016. Radiotherapy was previously administered in 77% of the patients. Surgical management substantially improved functional outcomes and relieved pain as early as 2 weeks after surgery.[107] However, poor prognosis is associated with hypercalcemia and ongoing severe pain from other metastatic bone lesions. Therefore, in those cases, the decision for surgical intervention should be weighed carefully based on a relative benefit to burden analysis.[103]

Treatment of pathologic fracture or impending fracture depends on the bone involved and the clinical status of the patient. Indications for surgical intervention of pathologic fracture or impending fracture include these factors: (1) an expected survival of more than 6 weeks, (2) an ability to accomplish internal stability of the fracture site, (3) no coexistent medical conditions that preclude early mobilization, (4) metastases involving weight-bearing bones, and (5) lytic lesions more than 2 to 3 cm in size or metastases that destroy more than 50% of the cortex.[103–106] Intramedullary stabilization without resection of metastases using locking nails meets the requirements of palliative therapy. This procedure is less invasive and allows early weight bearing.[106] Postoperative radiation is often given after surgical fixation of a pathologic fracture to reduce risk of progressive disease in the bone that could result in instability of the internal fixation.[104]

Significant technologic advances in interventional radiology also provide additional options for the treatment of bone metastases. These options include thermal ablation (destroy the tumor with heat) and endovascular therapies (destroy the tumor through devascularization). Additionally, interventional radiology can stabilize pathologic fractures or impending pathologic fractures.[108]

Spinal Cord Compression

Metastatic spinal cord compression (MSCC) is the most dreaded complication of cancer. Pain is the initial symptom in approximately 90% of patients with spinal cord compression.[109] Paraparesis or paraplegia occurs in more than 60%; sensory loss is noted in 70% to 80%; and 14% to 77% have bladder, bowel, or both kinds of disturbances.[80,81,110] Six predictive risk factors are associated with MSCC: the inability to walk, increased deep tendon reflexes, compression fractures on radiographs of spine, bone metastases present, bone metastases diagnosed more than 1 year earlier, and age less than 60 years. Patients with no risk factors had a 4% chance of developing cord compressions, and a patient with all six risk factors present had an 87% chance of developing cord compression.[103,104] Breast, lung, and prostate cancer comprised 21% to 24% risk of developing cord compression.[111–113]

The clinical course of spinal cord compression resulting from malignant melanoma is similar to that resulting from breast or prostate cancer. The time from the original diagnosis of melanoma to the development of metastatic spinal disease averages 32 months, and the average time is reported to be 27 months from diagnosis of skeletal metastases to spinal cord compression. The extent of the epidural mass influences prognosis because a complete spinal block results in greater residual neurologic impairment than a partial block. Median survival among patients with spinal cord compression is 7 months, with a 36% probability for a 1-year survival. For specific types of cancers, the mean survival time is 14 months for breast cancer, 12 months in prostate cancer, 6 months in malignant melanoma, and 3 months in lung cancer once epidural spinal cord compression is diagnosed.[14,82,94] After the diagnosis of epidural spinal cord compression, the overall survival time averages 12 months, with a median survival time of 5 months.

The vertebral column is involved by metastatic tumor in 40% of patients who die of cancer. Approximately 70% of vertebral metastases involve the thoracic spine, 20% the lumbosacral region, and 10% the cervical spine.

Using the Tokuhashi prognostic scoring system, 119 patients with epidural spinal cord compression were evaluated. Survival was 49 days in group 1, compared to 108 days in group 2. On multivariate analysis, better survival was also associated with breast, prostate cancer or lung cancers, nonvisceral metastases, and subsequent systemic chemotherapy.[114,115] A total of 43 different prognostic factors were investigated in 142 articles to determine whether models could be develop to predict survival in patients with vertebral metastases. Only two prognostic factors, primary tumor and performance status, were found to be associated with survival. Survival was not influenced by age, gender, pathologic fracture, or the number and location of the vertebral metastases.[116]

Weakness can signal the rapid progression of symptoms, and 30% of patients with weakness become paraplegic within 1 week. Rapid development of weakness, defined as occurring in less than 2 months, most commonly occurs in lung cancer, whereas breast and prostate cancers can progress more slowly. Neurologic deficits can develop within a few hours in up to 20% of patients with spinal cord compression.[80–86,117,118] The severity of weakness at presentation is the most significant factor for recovery of function. The slower the rate of development of motor deficits, the better the functional outcome.[110,119] If no neurologic deficits are present in a magnetic resonance imaging (MRI) scan proven spinal carcinoma, then radiation can preserve function. Patients with neurologic symptoms should be treated within 24 hours.[120,121] Ninety percent of patients who are ambulatory at presentation are ambulatory after treatment. Only 13% of paraplegic patients regain function, particularly if paraplegia is present for more than 24 hours before the initiation of therapy. Notwithstanding the high mortality associated with MSCC, more than 30% of patients who develop spinal cord compression are alive 1 year later, and 50% of these patients remain ambulatory if the syndrome is recognized and treated appropriately.

Pain can be present for months to just days prior to the onset of other neurologic dysfunction. Unlike degenerative joint disease, which primarily occurs in the low cervical and low lumbar regions, pain caused by epidural spinal cord compression can occur anywhere in the spinal axis and is aggravated by recumbency. Any cancer patient with back pain, especially with known metastatic involvement of the vertebral bodies, should be assessed for spinal cord compression. The risk of spinal cord compression exceeds 60% among patients with back pain and plain film evidence of vertebral collapse caused by metastatic cancer.[122–126]

Radiographic determination of the involved spinal levels is critical to radiation treatment planning. Plain film radiography shows involvement of more than one spinal level in approximately one-third of patients. If the results of MRI, tomographic studies, and surgical findings are included, more than 85% of patients have multiple sites of vertebral involvement.[80,81,122–126] For patients with known malignancy, a whole spine MRI is recommended as the preferred diagnostic modality.[110,127,128] With plain radiography, the destruction of the pedicles is the most common finding that identifies spine metastases. In contrast, CT shows that the initial anatomic location of metastases is in the posterior portion of the vertebral body and that destruction of the pedicles occurs only in combination with involvement of the vertebral body (Fig. 48.5).[125] Symptomatic patients with a normal vertebral contour and osteoblastic changes on plain film and bone scan should also be evaluated for spinal cord compression (Fig. 48.6). Osteoblastic bony expansion, commonly seen in both prostate and breast cancers, can result in

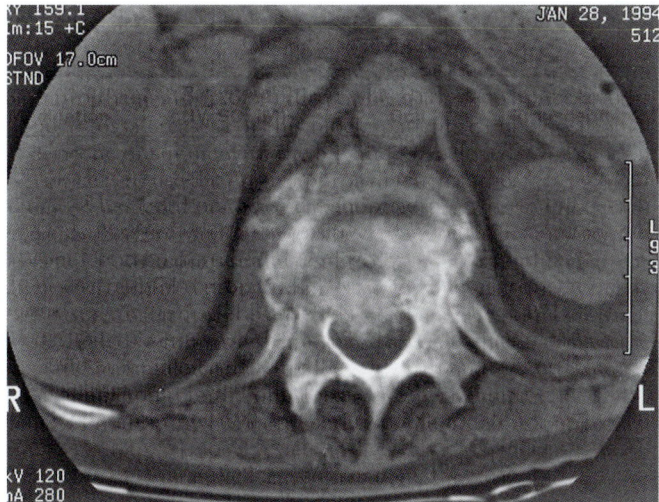

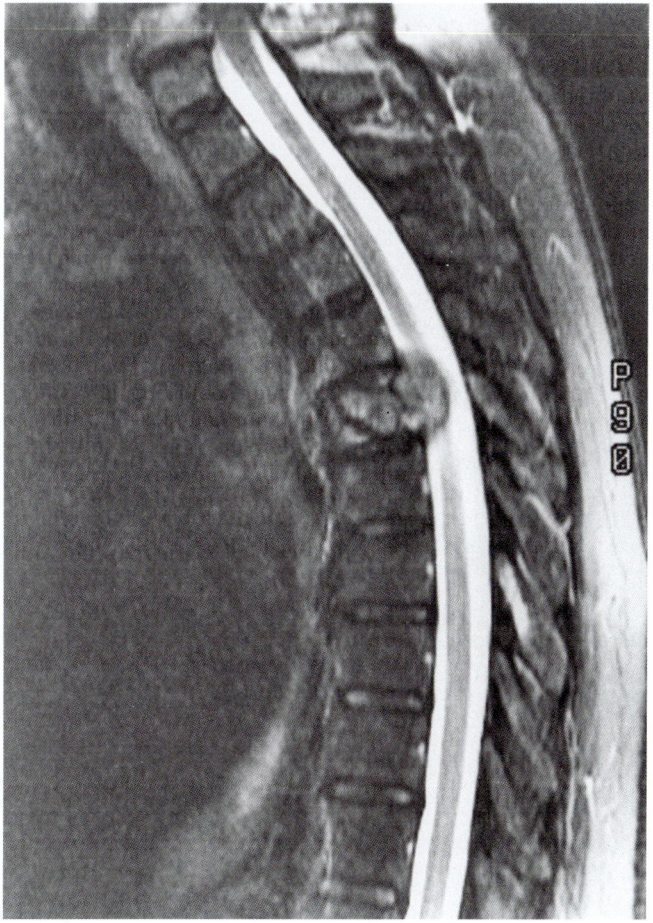

FIGURE 48.5 **A:** Computed tomographic scan showing involvement of the posterior aspect of the vertebral body resulting in partial spinal cord compression. **B:** Magnetic resonance imaging showing involvement of the posterior aspect of the vertebral body resulting in partial spinal cord compression.

spinal cord compromise as well as osteolytic vertebral compression fractures.[124]

Treatment of vertebral metastases has benefitted from less invasive surgical strategies, systemic therapy with checkpoint inhibitors, and advances in radiation therapy. Administered alone or postoperatively, SRT has allowed the delivery of tumoricidal radiation doses while sparing adjacent critical structures. A high-dose single (16 to 24 Gy) or hypofractionated (24 to 30 Gy in two to three fractions) SRT administers a significantly higher biologic effective dose over a shorter period of time than traditional external beam radiation. Radiation-induced spinal cord injury from SRT is rare, with only 6 cases of radiation-induced myelopathy out of 1,075 cases in one study.[129]

Emergency treatment of spinal cord compression includes corticosteroids, radiotherapy, neurosurgical intervention, or combinations of these three therapies. Radiotherapy is the treatment of choice for most cases of spinal cord compression and is a radiotherapeutic emergency (Fig. 48.7). Spinal cord compression resulting from metastatic tumor can be prevented or effectively treated when diagnosed early.[80,81,122–126] Radiotherapy with shorter courses (e.g., 1 fraction with 8 Gy or 5 fractions with 4 Gy) is as effective as a longer course (e.g., 30 Gy in 10 fractions), but the longer courses have lower recurrence rates. A scoring system for survival based on prognostic factors can guide the type of radiation course.[130] Patients with longer estimated survival time may benefit from the longer course of radiation. Pretreatment of lytic vertebral body disease, independent of the blastic component, predicts for subsequent SRT-induced vertebral compression fracture.[131]

Neurosurgical intervention for MSCC involves spinal cord decompression accomplished by a laminectomy and is indicated

in a variety of clinical presentations.[80,81,121–128,132,133] These situations include rapid neurologic deterioration in the setting of tumor progression in a previously irradiated area in order to provide stabilization of the spine, tumor-induced paraplegia in patients with otherwise limited disease and good probability of survival, and to establish a diagnosis.

Prognostic factors for survival after surgery for spine metastases were evaluated in over 1,266 patients. Patients who survived less than 3 months after surgery for spine metastases were in significantly worse condition preoperatively with more emergency cases and lower performance status, more severe neurologic deficits, worse American Society of Anesthesiologists (ASA) scores, unfavorable tumor histology, and extraspinal and visceral metastases. By comparison, patients who survived more than 2 years after surgery had a better performance status, less severe neurologic deficits, better ASA scores, a more favorable tumor histology and less extraspinal extension, and fewer visceral metastases. Patients with one spinal level involved had a 34.9% 2-year survival compared to a 22.7% survival when two or more spinal levels were involved.[134]

Adjuvant radiotherapy is often given to treat microscopic residual disease after neurosurgical intervention. A statistically significant improvement in functional outcome has been reported with laminectomy and radiotherapy in treatment of epidural spinal cord compression over either modality alone. In paraparetic patients who undergo laminectomy and radiation, 82% regain the ability to walk, 68% have improved sphincter function, and 88% have relief of pain. With radiation alone, 65% regained ambulation, 26% had improved sphincter function, and 70% had improvement of pain.[121,132,134–136] Laminectomy, however, carries risks associated with surgery

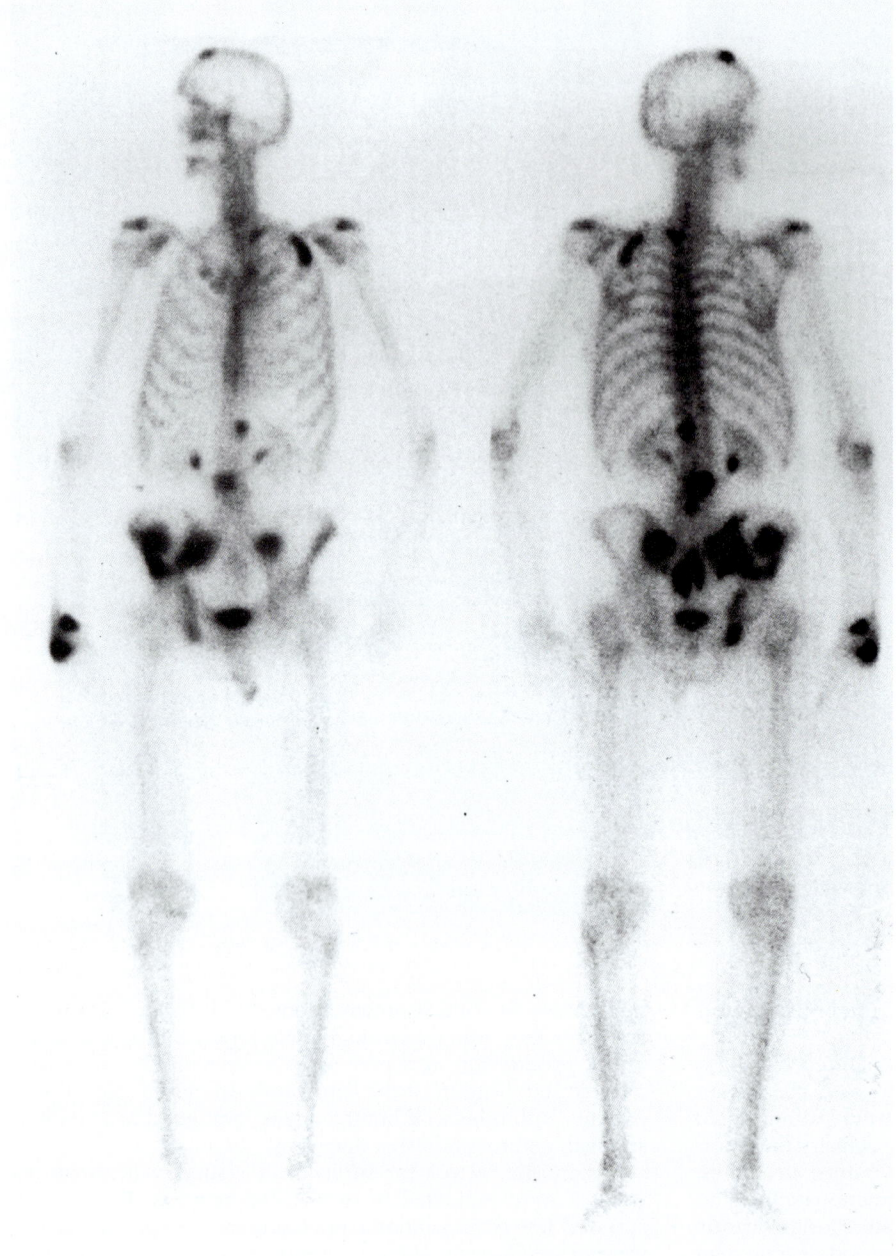

FIGURE 48.6 Bone scan that demonstrates multifocal disease involvement. Metastatic involvement in weight-bearing areas such as the pelvis and lower lumbar area significantly affects mobility.

and anesthesia. Pain may worsen after laminectomy if operative procedures fail to stabilize the spine. Vertebral collapse may occur because of cancer or vertebral instability after cancer therapy (Fig. 48.8).

A total of 6,651 courses of radiation were prescribed to 3,782 patients with a median age of 66 years. The most commonly treated skeletal sites were the spine (56.8%) followed by the pelvis (18.2%). The primary sites of most bone metastases were genitourinary (26.5%), lung (23.8%), and breast cancers (21.9%). However, complicated bone metastases were associated with hematolymphoid malignancies (39.1%), lung cancer (34.2%), gastrointestinal (32.5%), breast (28.4%), and genitourinary (28.4%) cancers. Factors that complicated 32.1% bone metastases were neurologic compromise (18.7%), soft tissue mass (18.3%), and pathologic fracture (6.5%). The most common sites of bone metastases with complicating factors included the extremity (43.6%), skull (42.7%), and spine

(39.2%). Although single-fraction radiation may be effective for uncomplicated bone metastases, more aggressive therapy is usually warranted for bone metastases with complicating factors.[137,138]

Paravertebral masses are most commonly associated with lung cancer and are rare in prostate cancer. Overall, approximately 20% of patients with epidural cord compression have an associated paravertebral mass. Surgical resection combined with radiation therapy has been suggested to improve functional outcome when a paravertebral mass is associated with spinal cord compression. The overall survival is worse with lung cancer and sarcoma than with breast and renal cancer.[136,139,140]

RADIATION TOLERANCE OF THE SPINAL CORD

Radiation tolerance is based on the dose per fraction, total dose, and the volume of tissue treated. The dose per fraction is the most important factor in the tolerance of tissues

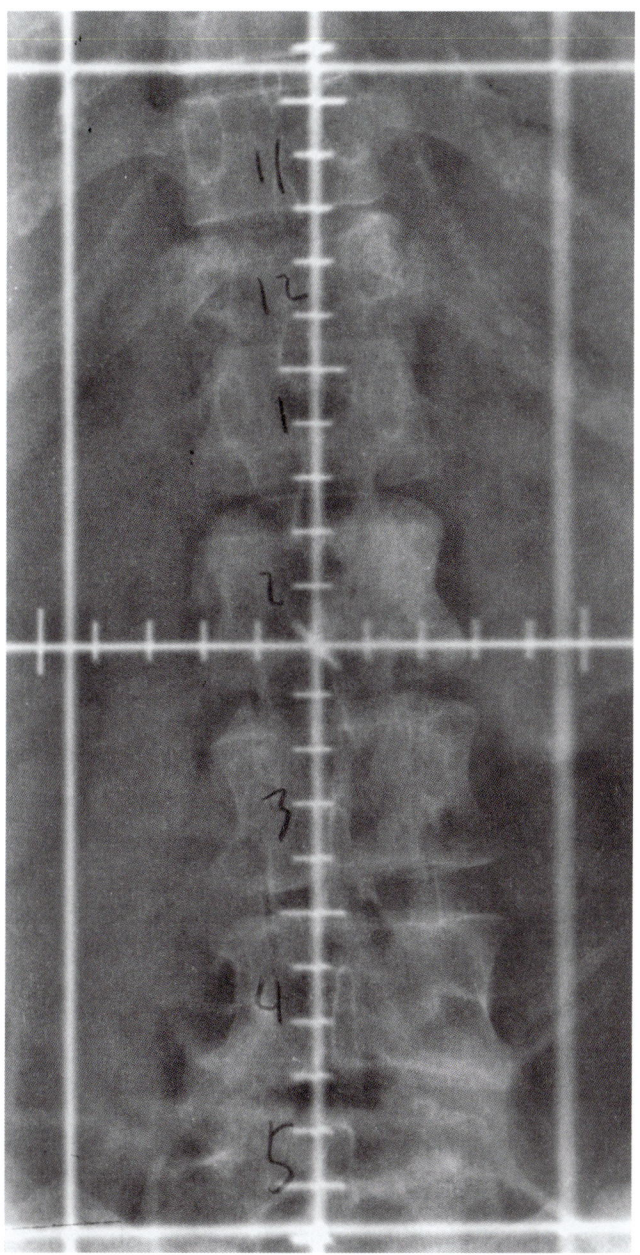

FIGURE 48.7 Typical radiation portal to treat multifocal areas of disease involvement in the vertebral bodies and epidural region.

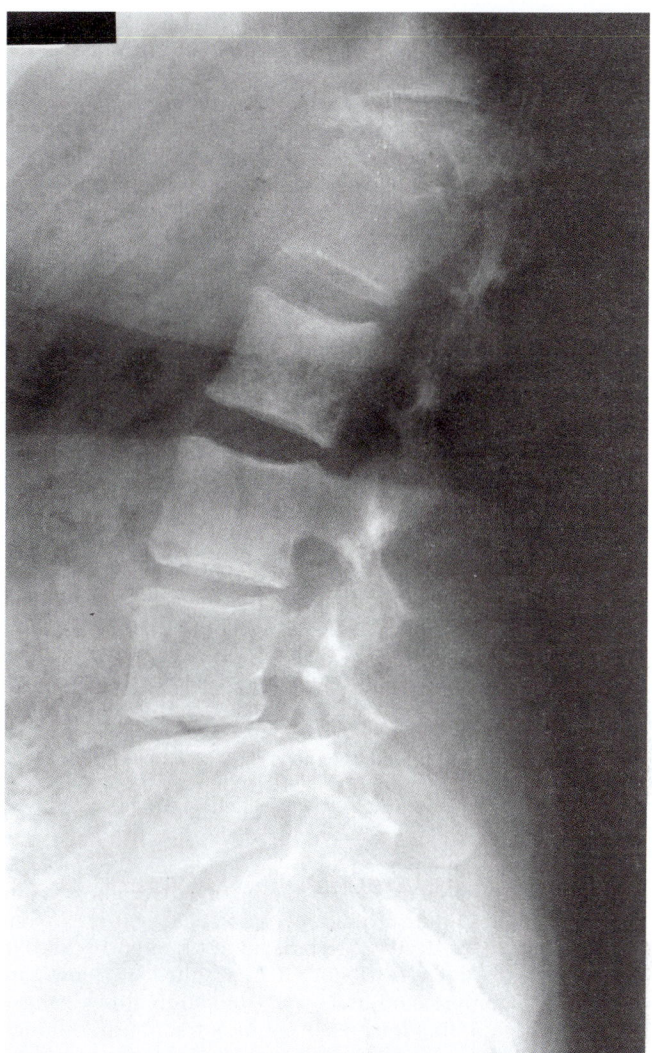

FIGURE 48.8 Compression fracture of the 12th thoracic vertebral body following an initial pain-free interval after palliative radiation. Vertebral weakness with rapid tumor regression resulted in a compression fracture that caused recurrent back pain because of spinal instability.

to radiation. Clinical and experimental experience has failed to demonstrate any difference in radiosensitivity in different segments of the spinal cord.[141] The risk of radiation myelitis in the cervicothoracic spine is less than 5% when 6,000 cGy is administered at 172 cGy per fraction or 5,000 cGy is given with daily fractions of 200 cGy per fraction. Especially among patients who have received chemotherapy, the total dose to the spinal cord is generally limited to 4,000 cGy administered at 200 cGy per fraction to minimize any risk of irreversible radiation injury to the spinal cord. The total dose is also an extremely important factor defining the radiation tolerance of the spinal cord. A steep curve based on total radiation dose predicts the risk of developing radiation myelopathy; a small increase in total radiation dose can result in a large increased risk for radiation myelopathy.[141–143] Retreatment of a previously irradiated segment of spinal cord results in high risk for

radiation-induced myelopathy because other neurologic pathways cannot compensate for an injury to a specific level of the spinal cord.

The radiation tolerance of the spinal cord can be compromised by prior injury. Difficulty arises in differentiating pathologic and radiotherapeutic injury when there has been spinal cord compression. Vasogenic edema of the spinal cord and nerve roots can be caused by compression injury. Metastatic epidural compression results in vasogenic spinal cord edema, venous hemorrhage, loss of myelin, and ischemia. Vasogenic edema results in an increased synthesis of prostaglandin E, which can be myelotoxic. Inhibition of this inflammatory pathway is one of the putative benefits of corticosteroids or nonsteroidal anti-inflammatory therapy. Other consequences of pathologic compression include hemorrhage, loss of myelin, and ischemia.[141–143]

Two separate mechanisms of radiation injury result from white matter damage and vasculopathies. White matter damage is associated with diffuse demyelination and swollen axons that can be focally necrotic and have associated glial reaction. Vascular damage has been shown experimentally to be age dependent and can result in hemorrhage, telangiectasia, and vascular necrosis.[141–143] Six major types of injuries have been shown experimentally to result from radiation to the spinal column. Five of these occur in the spinal cord and one in the dorsal root ganglia. The most severe spinal lesions, all of which are caused by vascular damage and result in neurologic dysfunction, include white matter necrosis, hemorrhage, and segmental parenchymal atrophy. The two less severe spinal lesions included focal fiber loss and scattered white matter vacuolization caused by damage to glial cells, axons, the vasculature, or all three; these less severe sequelae are seen with lower total doses of radiation and are less likely to result in neurologic dysfunction. In dorsal root ganglia, radiation damage included intracytoplasmic vacuoles and loss of neurons and satellite cells that could affect sensory function. These findings are distinct from the demyelination of the posterior columns associated with the self-limiting Lhermitte's syndrome.[144] Meningeal thickening and fibrosis can also be observed after radiation, but the clinical significance of this is unknown. Ependymal and nerve root damage from radiation is rare.

CLINICAL MANAGEMENT

Persistent pain after radiotherapy for vertebral metastases should be investigated to exclude the possibility of progressive disease inside or outside the radiation portal or mechanical spinal instability because of a vertebral compression fracture. Changes seen in the bone marrow on MRI after palliative radiotherapy initially include decreased cellularity, edema, and hemorrhage, followed by fatty replacement and fibrosis. These well-defined changes on MRI after radiotherapy can be distinguished from those seen with progressive malignant disease.[145–150]

SRT is increasingly used to treat vertebral metastases as it provides focused radiation to the involved vertebrae while limiting radiation injury to nearby mucosal structures. A retrospective study of 1,905 vertebral bodies treated by SRT in 791 patients between 2001 and 2013 resulted in a low rate of vertebral compression fractures. Radiation doses ranged from 10 Gy in 1 fraction to 60 Gy in 5 fractions. Although lytic lesions had a significantly increased risk for vertebral compression fractions, the overall rate was 8.4% including a single-fraction dose of 16 to 18 Gy.[151]

The outcomes of spine SRT were evaluated in 127 patients with 148 metastatic lesions between 2003 and 2013. The 1- and 2-year actuarial rates for local control were 82.6% and 75.8%, respectively; for overall survival, these rates were 72.9% and 51.5%, respectively. When evaluated by histology, the 1-year local failure rates were 8.7% for thyroid cancer, 7.0% for breast, 26.6% for lung, and 39.6% for colon cancer. Non–small-cell lung cancer and colorectal cancer was a significant predictor of local failure when SRT was used to treat spine metastases.[152]

Prior radiation portals may affect the ability to radiate spine metastases, especially in breast and lung cancer patients. Standard radiation portals currently used for breast cancer therapy infrequently treat the spinal axis. The upper thoracic and lower cervical region, however, may be irradiated in a field encompassing the supraclavicular nodes and axillary apex if significant axillary node involvement is documented. With techniques used in the past for breast cancer, the thoracic spine would receive a significant dose of radiation from a field that treated the internal mammary lymph nodes. Treatment of the mediastinum in lung cancer generally includes the majority of the thoracic spine treated to the maximum dose tolerated by the spinal cord.[136] Unfortunately, previous radiation of the spine as part of definitive therapy does not reduce the risk for subsequent spinal cord compression as a consequence of persistent or recurrent disease. As spinal metastases occur in up to 40% of cancer patients, and

median survival is less than 1 year, other options are available in previously irradiated patients. In select patients, including those with disease recurrence in a previously radiated area, interventional radiology techniques such as vertebral augmentation and radiofrequency ablation have been effective in relieving debilitating pain and providing mechanical stability.[153]

Surgical decompression is often the only available option for therapy because previously administered radiation may preclude further radiotherapy in the region of the malignant spinal cord compression. This is often the case in lung cancer because metastases are located in the thoracic spine in over 70% of cases, and many of these patients have received mediastinal irradiation.[140] Early involvement by the radiotherapist in the management of patients with suspected spinal cord involvement is important to allow time to obtain prior radiotherapy records; determine if further radiation is possible; and expedite the safest, most efficacious clinical decision-making process.

Based on clinical and radiographic grounds, leptomeningeal carcinomatosis must also be considered in the diagnostic evaluation. Leptomeningeal carcinomatosis occurs more commonly than clinically diagnosed. For example, only one-half of breast cancer patients with leptomeningeal carcinomatosis are diagnosed before death.[154,155] Performing a lumbar puncture is a relative barrier to the diagnosis; at least three cerebrospinal fluid samples are necessary to cytologically exclude the diagnosis of leptomeningeal disease because in 10% to 40% of patients, the initial cerebrospinal fluid sample fails to document tumor cells.[154] MRI can identify leptomeningeal disease among patients with normal cerebrospinal fluid cytology and is sensitive and specific in locating regions of nodular leptomeningeal involvement. Except in the case of nodular leptomeningeal involvement, in which localized radiotherapy may be of benefit as an adjuvant, intrathecal chemotherapy is generally the treatment of choice.[155]

Treatment of Diffuse Bone Metastases

Wide-field radiotherapy, systemic radionuclides, and bisphosphonates have been used to treat patients with disseminated bone metastases. These approaches are useful in augmenting the therapeutic effect of localized radiation and in preventing asymptomatic bony lesions from progressing. Although usually not a significant consideration in localized irradiation, adequate bone marrow reserve is required for wide-field radiotherapy and systemic radionuclides. Bone marrow scans can be performed to determine the volume of functioning marrow and assess the feasibility of delivering wide-field radiotherapy or radionuclides.

WIDE-FIELD RADIOTHERAPY

Hemibody irradiation was previously used to treat diffuse bone metastases by administering one fraction of about 6 to 10 Gy or fractions of 3 Gy for 2 to 5 consecutive days to the upper, mid, or lower body. Fractionation reduces the need for premedication and allows for higher total doses to be delivered, but the effect on pain is equivalent to single-dose radiation.[156–158] Response rates are consistently reported to be greater than 70%, and more than 20% of patients have complete relief of pain. In prostate and breast cancer patients, the overall response rate is 80%, and complete relief of pain is 30%, respectively.[156–161] Approximately one-half of patients experience relief of pain within 48 hours of treatment, and the overall response rates equal 80% for all types of primary tumors. About 70% of the patients treated did not require further palliative irradiation for recurrent bone pain over the duration of their lives.[157]

An RTOG study demonstrated that hemibody radiation reduced the time to disease progression and decreased the need for subsequent palliative radiation of bone metastases at 1 year of follow-up when compared with local field irradiation alone. These results from the RTOG study are consistent with other reported experience using hemibody irradiation.[159–161] Median survival after hemibody irradiation was significantly better among patients who present with a good performance status. Approximately 90% of patients with a CR and 70% of patients with a partial response (PR) had a good to excellent performance status before radiotherapy. Prior systemic therapy does not influence response to wide-field radiotherapy. Symptomatic bone metastases that are refractory to chemotherapy or hormonal therapy are reported to have CR rates of 70% and PR rates of 24% with hemibody radiation. Symptoms are palliated in 88% of cases when a previously treated area is reirradiated. Premedication prevents nausea, and partial shielding minimizes lung dose and the risk for radiation pneumonitis. Hematologic depression is limited. Toxicity is observed in less than 10% of patients, whereas 50% experience stabilization of disease at 1 year.

Hemibody radiation is currently rarely used for the treatment of metastases due to the potential toxicity to the visceral structures and the difficulties in treatment setup. Concerns regarding the permanent effects on bone marrow reserve also exist relative to the subsequent need for chemotherapy.

RADIOPHARMACEUTICALS

An alternative to hemibody irradiation for the treatment of widely disseminated bone metastases is the use of systemic radioisotopes. The most commonly used radiopharmaceutical in the treatment of bone metastases is strontium 89. Strontium 89 combines with the calcium component of hydroxyapatite in osteoblastic lesions. Many studies report effective palliation of pain lasting more than 6 months in 60% to 80% of patients with breast and prostate cancers.[162–176] Improvements in functional status and quality of life have been observed, and approximately 20% of patients have complete resolution of pain. Pain control has been reported to be superior among patients with disseminated prostate cancer treated both with strontium 89 and local radiotherapy as compared with localized irradiation alone.[165] Myelotoxicity resulting in 25% reduction of platelet and white blood cell counts represents the only significant toxicity associated with strontium 89, which is usually transient and reversible within 12 weeks.[177,178] Hematotoxicity is more pronounced in patients with pretreatment platelet counts of less than or equal to 60×10^3, white blood cell counts of less than or equal to 2.5×10^3, or greater than or equal to 30% involvement of the red marrow–bearing bone. The radiation dose absorbed by the bone marrow is 2 to 50 times less than the dose administered by strontium 89 to the osteoblastic lesion. Radiation doses to metastatic bony lesions with strontium 89 can range from 3 to more than 300 Gy.

Clinical response to strontium 89 is comparable with wide-field radiotherapy. Response to strontium 89 therapy has been documented both subjectively and objectively. Subjective response, manifested as symptomatic improvement, was reported by more than 80% of prostate cancer patients using a validated self-reporting tool. Objective evidence of response was documented by reductions in alkaline and acid phosphatase levels that corresponded with a decrease in evidence of active metastatic disease on sequential bone scans.[179] Prior therapies for prostate cancer, including local radiation therapy and systemic chemotherapy or hormone therapy, do not influence toxicity or affect clinical response to strontium 89. Administered as an adjuvant to localized external beam radiotherapy in metastatic prostate cancer, strontium 89 has been shown to improve pain relief, reduce analgesic requirements, and delay progression of disease in prospective randomized clinical trials. Quality-of-life assessments demonstrated increased physical activity along with improved pain relief after strontium 89 was administered in conjunction with localized external beam radiation therapy.[180,181] Cost–benefit analysis has also suggested an advantage to the administration of strontium 89 with reductions in costs of hospitalization for tertiary care.

Several other radiopharmaceuticals are available for clinical application including samarium 153, gallium nitrate, phosphorus 32, and rhenium 186.[182–184] The therapeutic mechanism of action relates to the physical and biologic half-life in the bony lesion, the mean energy, and the delivered dose of the radiopharmaceutical. Table 48.3 summarizes some of the physical characteristics and clinical data for various radionuclides. Phosphorus 32 and strontium 89 emit pure β-rays (little penetration in tissue), whereas rhenium 186 and samarium 153 emit both β-rays and relatively high-energy γ-ray photons that penetrate tissue for some distance (103 to 159 keV).

Because samarium 153 has a γ-ray component, it is possible to directly image the distribution of the radiation dose. The scans after injection of samarium 153 are comparable to diagnostic scans obtained with technetium 99m. The mean skeletal uptake is over 50% of the dose.[175] Nonskeletal sites receive negligible radiation doses, and complete clearance of radionuclide other than that absorbed by bone occurs within 6 to 8 hours of administration.[174] In a double-blind placebo-controlled clinical trial, samarium 153 has been shown to be an effective agent in palliating painful bone metastases in breast cancer patients. Pain relief occurred within 1 week and lasted at least 16 weeks after administration.[181,184] Approximately 65% of patients responded within the first 4 weeks, and 43% to 72% had relief of pain of at least 16 weeks' duration. No significant bone

TABLE 48.3 Physical Characteristics and Clinical Data for Radionuclides

Radionuclide	Half-life (Days)	β-Energy (MeV)	γ-Energy (keV)	Response Rate (%)	Duration of Response (mo)	Toxicity
[32]P	14.26	1.7	0	77	5.1	Moderate
[89]Sr	50.53	1.5	0	80	3–6	Low
[117m]Sn	13.61	0.16	159	NR	NR	NR
		1.1			1.3	
[186]Re	3.78	0.9	137	77	—	Low
		0.8				
[153]Sm	1.95	0.7	103	65	4	Low
		0.6				

[32]P, phosphorus 32; [83]Sr, strontium-89 chloride; [117m]Sn, [117m]Sn(4+)diethylenetriaminepentaacetic acid; [186]Re, rhenium 186; [153]Sm, samarium 153; NR, no response.
Data from Lam MG, de Klerk JM, van Rijk PP, et al. Bone seeking radiopharmaceuticals for palliation of pain in cancer patients with osseous metastases. *Anticancer Agents Med Chem* 2007;7(4):381–397; Liepe K, Kotzerke J. A comparative study of 188Re-HEDP, 186Re-HEDP, 153Sm-EDTMP, and 89Sr in the treatment of painful skeletal metastases. *Nucl Med Commun* 2007;28(8):623–630; and Bouchet LG, Bolch WE, Goddu SM, et al. Considerations in the selection of radiopharmaceuticals for palliation of bone pain from metastatic osseous lesions. *J Nucl Med* 2000;41(4):682–687.

marrow toxicities have been observed. Recommended doses range between 1.0 and 1.5 mCi/kg. In more than one-third of patients, multiple administrations are possible.[182] These observations suggest potential suitability of this form of palliative therapy for patients with both intermediate and limited life expectancies who are not tolerating or responding favorably to other pain-relieving treatments.

Selectively concentrating in bone, the mechanism of action of rhenium 186 is similar to that of technetium diphosphonate 99m, which is used in diagnostic bone scans. This characteristic allows direct imaging of the deposition of rhenium 186 in bony metastases. The metastatic lesion receives a highly concentrated dose of radiation after the administration of rhenium 186, whereas the radiation dose to the marrow is limited to 0.75 Gy. Thrombocytopenia appears to be the dose-limiting toxicity but is mild, allowing therapy to be repeated.[177] Phosphorus 32 has 77% of patients experiencing significant relief of pain.[179] The response rates and duration of response with phosphorus 32 are similar to wide-field radiation and strontium 89. However, the main disadvantage of phosphorus 32 is severe hematologic toxicity.

Clinical trials are ongoing to compare the conventional radiopharmaceuticals with newer radiopharmaceuticals and their effect in combination with bisphosphonates and chemotherapy. There is prolonged survival benefit in patients with hormone refractory prostate cancer if radiopharmaceuticals and chemotherapy are used in combination.[185] Although bone marrow toxicity is relatively limited in the doses of radiopharmaceuticals currently administered either alone or in combination with other agents, future dose intensity studies may require hematologic support with colony-stimulating factors.

Sequential radiography and bone scans after hormonal and radiopharmaceutical therapy for breast and prostate cancers demonstrate an osteoblastic response that reflects remodeling of the bone in osteolytic osseous metastases.[61,62] Approximately one-third of patients have evidence of increased tracer uptake on bone scans (flare) obtained 8 to 16 weeks after treatment. Of these patients with a flare response on bone scan, 72% experience a response to the treatment. By comparison, only 36% have a response to treatment when a limited response or no flare response is observed.

Relapse of disease has been associated with an increase in the osteolytic component. Osteoclast resorption in bone metastases is associated with the release of acid and acid-dependent proteases that dissolve the organic matrix of the bone. Gallium nitrate has been shown to inhibit accelerated bone turnover among patients with widespread bone metastases and has been clinically applied in the treatment of hypercalcemia. Preferentially accumulating in the cortical surface, which is the most metabolically active region of the bone, gallium nitrate acts to inhibit osteoclast resorption. Additionally, gallium nitrate increases the absorption of calcium and phosphorus and the incorporation of collagen into the bone.

Role of Palliative Chemotherapy

Chemotherapy can be used as an adjuvant to radiotherapy and/or surgery or as part of a combined antineoplastic regimen for primary treatment. Systemic chemotherapy has the advantage of ubiquitous distribution throughout the body, wherever the bloodstream might take a cancer cell. Thus, adjuvant chemotherapy is used in patients who appear cured after surgery but are suspected of having residual disease or micrometastasis. Adjuvant chemotherapy has proven effective in node-positive breast cancer, Dukes' B2 and C colorectal carcinoma, stage III ovarian carcinoma, testicular carcinoma, non–small-cell lung cancer, Wilms' tumor, osteogenic sarcoma, and anaplastic astrocytoma.[186]

Neoadjunct chemotherapy is used as initial chemotherapy in cancers that would be only partially curable by surgery or radiation. It is often administered with anal cancer, bladder cancer, esophageal cancer, laryngeal cancer, locally advanced non–small-cell lung cancer, and osteogenic sarcoma. The goals of this therapy are to (1) decrease the size of the tumor to be removed or radiated, (2) increase the likelihood that the tumor will be surgically extricable, and (3) decrease the likelihood of micrometastatic spread/seeding at the time of surgery.[186] Systemic chemotherapy is the primary treatment for disseminated/metastatic malignant disease.

Based on the mechanisms mentioned earlier, the goal of systemic chemotherapy is to interrupt the division of rapidly dividing cancer cells. It is usually administered in multiple (usually 4 to 6) cycles every 3 to 4 weeks. The timing and dosing of chemotherapy are established to maximize malignant cell kill while at the same time not exceeding the body's ability to regenerate the normally rapidly dividing cells that are "innocent bystanders" of the cytotoxic effects of chemotherapy, namely, the bone marrow progenitors, gastrointestinal epithelial cells, and hair follicles. The predominant effect of chemotherapy on the intestinal tract occurs in the first few days to a week after administration, whereas the peak effect on the blood progenitor cells occurs 10 to 14 days posttherapy. Thus, patients only require prophylactic antiemetics for the days around therapy, but they "nadir" their blood counts, with variable risks of infection and bleeding, approximately 2 weeks after receiving treatment.

Regardless of the setting of administration (primary, adjuvant, neoadjuvant, or combined modality), substantial evidence suggests that combination chemotherapy with agents that have different mechanisms of action as well as different (noncumulative) toxicities yields significantly higher efficacy than single-agent chemotherapy. On the basis of an extensive review of in vivo and in vitro laboratory research and clinical experiences acquired during the 1950s and 1960s, DeVita and Schein[187] developed a set of basic principles of combination chemotherapy for cancer patients, and these are still the guiding principles today. Among the most important of these principles are the following: (1) All of the component drugs in a combination must have activity against the neoplasm being treated; (2) drugs must be administered at dosages close to the minimum effective dosage for each drug as a single agent or beyond, if possible; (3) drugs that interrupt the synthesis of cellular macromolecules at several sites can be combined for additive or synergistic effects on the various synthetic pathways; (4) drugs in combination should have as little cross-toxicity as possible; and (5) mechanisms of tumor cell resistance to two agents in combination must not be similar.

Since 2006, the U.S. Food and Drug Administration (FDA) has approved more than 110 new cancer drugs. Advances in therapeutic regimens include a reduction in the risk of breast cancer recurrence with more prolonged hormonal therapy and a regimen that significantly extends survival in recurrent ovarian cancer. Other strategies have focused on reducing adverse effects from cancer therapy without compromising cancer control. Among these are shortening the duration of adjuvant chemotherapy for stage III colorectal cancer. With improvements in cancer therapy, a 25% decline in cancer death rate has been achieved since its peak in 1991.[188–190]

For all tumor sites, a high prevalence of moderate to severe symptoms was experienced by 120,745 cancer patients during the first year after cancer diagnosis. In the 729,861 symptom surveys conducted between 2007 and 2014 in patients who survived at least 1 full year after cancer diagnosis, the most symptoms were documented in the first month, whereas elevated scores for nausea persisted up to 6 months after diagnosis. On multivariable analysis, cancer site, younger age, higher comorbidities, female gender, lower income, and urban residence were significantly associated with a higher symptom burden. Consistent with other studies, greater symptom burden occurred in patients with respiratory and oropharyngeal cancers. Younger patients have a greater likelihood of receiving more aggressive therapies, an increased prevalence of advanced-stage cancers, and/or higher expectations for functioning and the resumption of their roles prior to the cancer diagnosis.[191]

Also in the first year after diagnosis, a 71% hospitalization rate was documented for 25,032 patients who were treated for advanced cancer between 2009 and 2012. Hospital admission was prompted through the emergency department in 64% of cases, and 16% of patients were hospitalized three or more times during the first year after cancer diagnosis. Readmission rates were significantly associated with minority status (race/ethnicity); public or no insurance; lower socioeconomic status; comorbidities; and pancreatic, non–small-cell lung, or colorectal cancers.[192]

The goal of personalized medicine is to have systemic therapies selectively target tumor cells located in any site while sparing normal tissues/organs from the toxicity of antineoplastic therapy. Significant advances have been accomplished in systemic therapies within the realm of precision medicine. These advances have resulted in two out of three cancer patients living at least 5 years after diagnosis, and an increased 10-year cancer survival rates to 64% in 2005 from 35% in 1975. From November 2016 through October 2017, the FDA approved 31 new therapies for more than 16 types of cancer. Adoptive cell immunotherapy allows genetic reprogramming of a patient's own immune cells to find and attack cancer cells throughout the body. Chimeric antigen receptor (CAR) T-cell therapy has resulted in significant advances in pediatric acute lymphoblastic leukemia (ALL), and adult lymphoma and multiple myeloma.[188–190]

The FDA approved the first adoptive cell immunotherapy in August 2017 for ALL. In May 2016, the FDA gave accelerated approval to a second CAR T-cell therapy, an immune checkpoint inhibitor for previously treated urothelial cancer that progressed despite platinum-based chemotherapy. Throughout 2017, the FDA approved four other immune checkpoint inhibitors. One checkpoint inhibitor, pembrolizumab, resulted in a 3-month survival improvement while the adverse effects were three times lower for pembrolizumab than the chemotherapy group (15% vs. 49%) in a major clinical trial. Based on these results, especially because two-thirds of patients are not eligible for cisplatin-based chemotherapy due to physical frailty, immunotherapy is now being considered as an initial treatment for advanced bladder cancer. In October 2017, an immune checkpoint inhibitor became the first cancer treatment to receive a tumor-agnostic indication. This accelerated FDA approval allows treatment of any type of solid tumor that has mismatch repair deficiency a defect that undermines the cell's ability to repair DNA damage.[188–190] Biomarkers ideally should temper the socioeconomic cost for administration of checkpoint inhibitors and other adoptive cell immunotherapies. Tumors with a large number of mutations are generally more susceptible to checkpoint inhibitors as mutations make more abnormal proteins (antigens) that the immune system recognizes as foreign.[193]

Although more traditional systemic therapies continue to be routinely administered, advances continue within personalized medicine. More traditional chemotherapy administered for palliative effect is then displaced by a novel agent that not only may be less toxic but also offers hope to reverse the course of disease from palliative back to curative intent. The two issues that exist in palliative chemotherapy involve whether a meaningful improvement in quality and the length of life can be achieved and the socioeconomic cost.

Breakthrough designated cancer drugs receive faster FDA approval. Between 2012 and 2017, the FDA approved 58 new cancer drugs; 25 (43%) of these drugs were approved through breakthrough therapy designation. Breakthrough therapy-designated drugs were not more likely to act via a novel mechanism of action. The median time to first FDA approval was 5.2 years for breakthrough designation versus 7.1 years for the routine approval process. Rates of death and serious adverse events were also similar in FDA approval through breakthrough designation and routine process. Additionally, no statistically significant difference in median progression free survival was found between drugs approved through the routine and the breakthrough designation (4 months vs. 8.6 months; $P = .11$).[194]

The issues of survival and quality of life will be borne out of expanded clinical experience with these novel agents. Although greater clinical experience may better define the indications for the agent, the same unwillingness to abandon hope for a cure will invariably be encountered. As was the experience when novel chemotherapeutic agents became available, patients would seek the hope offered by a newer chemotherapeutic regimen. The American Society of Clinical Oncology Value Framework and the European Society of Medical Oncology Magnitude of Clinical Benefit Scale evaluated the clinical benefits of novel anticancer drugs relative to increasing costs. Anticancer drugs from 42 phase III randomized controlled trials cited for clinical efficacy evidence in drug approvals between January 2006 and December 2015 were scored according to this value framework. Both monthly prices and incremental anticancer drug costs increased and were significantly associated with the year of approval, 9% and 21%, respectively. The mean incremental anticancer drug cost increased fivefold from $30,447 in 2006 to $161,141 in 2015; however, the clinical benefits of these drugs did not correlate with a proportional positive change.[195]

There are many factors responsible for the limited efficacy of chemotherapy in these tumors. First, the cellular biology of these solid tumors that often produce pain is such that they have limited response to current drug regimens. Second, the size of the tumor is inversely related to the incidence of satisfactory drug penetration into the mass. As a general principle, the larger the mass, the poorer the cytotoxic response. Furthermore, given that these tumors generally do not exhibit long-term responses to first-line therapy, additional therapy with second- or third-line drug treatments often yields a minimal (usually less than primary therapy) response rate. Finally, in certain target sites (e.g., head and neck, pelvis), prior radical surgery and/or prior radiation therapy impair the vascular supply to the tumor bed, thus interfering with delivery of an effective drug concentration to the target site.

Because this group represents the most challenging to demonstrate objective response rates to chemotherapy, it is the ideal patient population in which to demonstrate a purely palliative benefit of chemotherapy, represented by decreases in pain, dyspnea, and fatigue and increases in performance status, appetite, and weight gain. A few investigators have pursued these outcome measures with meaningful results. The initial FDA approval of gemcitabine was granted not by data showing its benefits on overall survival or objective response rate, but by improvements in pain control, weight gain, and performance status in patients with pancreatic cancer.

CLINICAL APPLICATIONS

Conventionally, efficacy of chemotherapy is defined by an objective decrease in the radiographic size of the tumor (usually by CT). A CR represents total disappearance of all observable disease for a minimum of 1 to 3 months, depending on the criteria used, whereas a PR represents a decrease in measurable tumor size by at least 50%. Overall response rate for a given regimen is the combination of CR + PR, and a significant response rate translates into an improved survival of responders compared with nonresponders. It also translates into relief of pain related to the tumor mass—although pain relief from chemotherapy has rarely been the endpoint of clinical trials.

PALLIATIVE CHEMOTHERAPY

The category that falls between an objective response and progressive disease, in which the tumor neither shrinks nor grows in the face of active anticancer therapy, is referred to as *stable disease*. Whether or not there is any pain-relieving benefit to the administration of chemotherapy in the setting of stable disease is undetermined. Although there is speculation about the role of chemotherapy in altering peripheral sensory nerve function, thereby producing analgesia as well as relieving pain by altering the "tumor-host milieu," these hypotheses have been tested in limited trials.[196-199] In the absence of empirically proven outcomes, clinical observations suggest that "systemically administered cytotoxic drugs do not relieve cancer pain in the absence of tumor regression."[196] Tumor regression is a function of responsiveness to a given chemotherapeutic regimen. Tumor variables that determine the course of chemotherapy and prognosis for response rate include histologic type (squamous cell carcinoma, adenocarcinoma, germ cell, lymphoma, etc.), grade (high, intermediate, low), and the degree of differentiation (well differentiated, poorly differentiated).

In general, the more rapidly growing the tumor, the more frequent its cellular division; therefore, the cells are more *potentially* responsive to cytotoxic therapy: In these cases, intervention can lead to increased pain control, long-term survival, and, potentially, cure. Those rapidly growing tumors that are chemotherapy-resistant tend to be imminently fatal.

LYMPHOMA

Compared with other solid tumor types, Hodgkin and non-Hodgkin lymphomas (NHLs) tend to respond better than most to combination chemotherapy. For Hodgkin lymphoma, there are several active regimens, but the preferred treatment regimen of doxorubicin, bleomycin, vinblastine, and dacarbazine is highly active and produces a complete remission rate that varies from 98% for early-stage disease (overall survival of more than 93% at 6 years) to 82% for advanced stage disease (overall survival of 73% at 6 years).[200] The therapeutic effect of this combination regimen is rapid, even in advanced cases, providing prompt pain relief in those patients who have pain (although this has never been a primary endpoint of clinical trials), with observed resolution of other symptoms and signs as well. In NHL, there is a larger variability based on histology, with high-grade NHL being significantly more responsive to therapy than low-grade types. For high-grade NHL, treatment with a variety of combination chemotherapy regimens (e.g., bleomycin, doxorubicin, cyclophosphamide, vincristine, and prednisone; cyclophosphamide, doxorubicin, vincristine, and prednisone; or others with antibody therapies with rituximab) produces a 79% event-free survival.[201-203] Again, no studies of NHL have examined pain as a primary endpoint, although pain remits in concert with active disease.

BREAST CANCER

In moderately chemosensitive tumors, the results obtained with the various chemotherapeutic combinations are less favorable (30% to 60% response rates), and in general, the therapeutic effect is slower in onset. Small-cell lung cancer, for example, tends to be quite aggressive, and combination chemotherapy regimens with cisplatin and etoposide or cyclophosphamide, doxorubicin, and vincristine can induce an objective response in approximately 60% of cases, with CR occurring in approximately 10%. Again, this and other studies have not attempted to quantify relief from pain or dyspnea in small-cell lung cancer.

The course of recurrent or metastatic breast cancer follows two dominant pathways. The hormone receptor–positive tumors tend to occur in older (postmenopausal) women and follow a more indolent course when treated with hormone therapy, with bone as the most common metastatic site. The hormone receptor–negative tumors tend to occur in younger (premenopausal) women and follow a more aggressive course, with visceral and soft tissue involvement that is usually responsive to chemotherapy. Conventional chemotherapy includes cyclophosphamide, methotrexate, and prednisone and has been shown to improve quality of life. Anthracycline-containing regimens have been shown to be superior to cyclophosphamide, methotrexate, and prednisone. Single agents that contain taxanes (docetaxel, paclitaxel, and protein-bound paclitaxel), capecitabine, gemcitabine, or vinorelbine have been shown to be as effective in improving survival and quality of life as combination chemotherapy in metastatic breast cancer.[204-206] Trastuzumab, alone or in combination in human epidermal growth factor receptor 2 (HER2)/neu–positive patients, has been shown to increase survival. Yet again, it is noteworthy that given the prevalence of recurrent breast cancer, few studies have specifically addressed quality-of-life issues and that even fewer address symptomatic benefits of therapy.

A British study evaluating patients with advanced breast cancer who received first-line palliative chemotherapy (a variety of regimens) did have primary palliative (subjective patient-centered) outcomes that were assessed by using the Rotterdam Symptom Checklist. In this study, one-fourth of the patients (26%) felt better after having received chemotherapy, with statistically significant decreases in psychological distress, pain, and improvement in lack of energy and sense of tiredness. As might be expected, feeling better correlated with disease response ($P = .03$).[206]

HEAD AND NECK CANCER

Head and neck cancer is one of the most challenging disease sites to treat. Cisplatin and 5-fluorouracil (5-FU) make the tumor more responsive to radiotherapy, and this is the standard accepted multimodal regimen that has been shown to increase survival. In fact, studies have shown that combination chemotherapy with cisplatin and 5-FU, hydroxyurea and 5-FU, and taxanes like pacletaxel and cisplatin followed by radiation have all increased survival by 50% to 60%.[207,208] Chemotherapy with a single agent like cisplatin or carboplatin followed by radiation is also being investigated.[209] These aggressive regimens have potential toxicities and twice-a-day radiotherapy with concomitant chemotherapy have shown improved regional control, survival, and improved quality of life.[210]

OVARIAN CANCER

Finally, ovarian cancer is one of the more sensitive malignancies to cytotoxic chemotherapy. Combination regimens in which a platinum-based agent (cisplatin or carboplatin) is used achieve overall response rates of 60% to 80%. Newer agents, most notably the taxanes, also have significant activity in ovarian cancer, with overall response rates of 20% to 40%. The combination of carboplatin and paclitaxel has demonstrated superior response rates and has become the standard of care for ovarian cancer amenable to chemotherapy.[211-212] Doyle et al.[213] showed that although objective responses are low with palliative chemotherapy, active palliation with chemotherapy is associated with substantive improvement in patients' emotional function and global quality of life.

In 2016, the FDA approved a regimen of bevacizumab to standard platinum-based chemotherapy when the addition of bevacizumab significantly extended median time to progression of disease to 13.8 months from 10.4 months with chemotherapy alone. Although not statistically significant, overall survival was also longer with bevacizumab being 42 months versus 37 months, respectively. Severe adverse effects occurred in 96% of bevacizumab compared to 86% of the chemotherapy-alone group.[188–190] The FDA approved a maintenance treatment in 2017 for ovarian cancer based on a clinical trial in which olaparib, a poly (adenosine diphosphate [ADP]-ribose) polymerase (PARP) inhibitor, markedly slowed ovarian cancer progression of disease (19.1 months vs. 5.1 months).

LUNG CANCER

Non–small-cell lung cancer is the most prevalent cancer type, and combinations of chemotherapeutic drugs like vinorelbine, gemcitabine, docetaxel, and paclitaxel provide modest survival and probable quality-of-life benefit in a significant number of patients when contrasted with best supportive care.[214–217] These agents show response rates in the 11% to 25% range when combined with platinum-based therapy. No study has examined the effects of therapy on pain or dyspnea, although a few have evaluated improvements in performance status and weight gain.[217] However, oral topotecan has been shown to improve pain, dyspnea, sleep, and fatigue, as well as increased survival, in patients with recurrent small-cell lung cancer compared with best supportive care. Even when early palliative care is performed, patients with metastatic non–small-cell lung cancer receive similar number of chemotherapy regimens. The early palliative care group, however, had half the odds of receiving chemotherapy within 60 days of death. There was also a longer interval between the last dose of intravenous chemotherapy and death in the early palliative care group (median 64 days vs. 40.5 days) and a higher hospice care enrollments for more than 1 week (60% vs. 33.3%; $P = .004$).[218]

GASTROINTESTINAL CANCERS

For gastrointestinal malignancies, the role of palliative chemotherapy is limited. The fluoropyrimidines (5-FU and its derivatives) are the conventional agents with demonstrated efficacy in gastrointestinal malignancies. 5-FU has resulted in disappointingly low response rates of approximately 20%.[219] In a large study of more than 400 patients conducted by the North Central Cancer Treatment Group,[220] 70% of patients who received 5-FU/low-dose leucovorin had improvements in performance status and weight gain; there was no assessment of pain as a primary endpoint. The combination of 5-FU and leucovorin with agents like oxaliplatin (FOLFOX) and irinotecan (FLOFIRI) have shown improvement in quality of life.[219–223]

In pancreatic cancer, the approval of gemcitabine for pancreatic cancer was based on the palliative endpoint of "clinical benefit" over the conventional 5-FU therapy. In this study, clinical benefit was defined by a composite of pain, performance status, and weight gain.[177] This was one of the first studies to directly assess the primary endpoint of pain via patient report of pain intensity together with analgesic consumption. Several recent systematic reviews have shown that gemcitabine-based combinations have shown improved survival as well as quality of life.[224,225]

PROSTATE CANCER

Prostate cancer is yet another prevalent disease that is poorly responsive to conventional chemotherapy. There is more palliative endpoint evidence supporting the use of chemotherapy in prostate cancer than any other disease in part because it is a slow-growing tumor that tends to cause significant pain and disability for a prolonged period of time. The most widely discussed study is Tannock's Canadian study that used mitoxantrone and prednisone for hormone-refractory metastatic prostate cancer where the primary endpoint was pain relief.[226] In this study, pain relief was again defined differently from previous studies as a "2-point decrease in pain as assessed by a

six-point pain scale . . . without an increase in analgesic medication and maintained for two consecutive evaluations at least 3 weeks apart." They found that this chemotherapy combination produced a positive effect above the benefit of prednisone alone in 29% of patients, with a 50% decrease in analgesic requirements. Other studies suggest the positive impact of docetaxel-based chemotherapy in providing relief of pain in hormone-refractory metastatic prostate cancer.[227,228] Androgen deprivation therapy (ADT) for metastatic prostate cancer plus docetaxel or abiraterone in newly diagnosed metastatic noncastrate prostate cancer offers a survival benefit as compared to ADT alone. The strongest evidence of benefit for docetaxel was for men with de novo metastatic disease or high-volume disease (defined as four or more bone metastases, one of more of which were outside the spine or pelvis and/or the presence of any visceral disease).[188–190,229]

DECISION MAKING ABOUT CHEMOTHERAPY

The diagnosis of cancer is often quite traumatic for both the patient and the family. On the one hand, the administration of chemotherapy is, by definition, cytotoxic—to malignant cells as well as normal host cells. On the other hand, the risks of not treating the disease are also quite significant. Given the fact that pain is a prevalent feature of both early- and advanced-stage cancer—present in nearly 50% of patients with early-stage disease and in 70% to 90% of cases of advanced cancer—the challenge is to strike a balance between therapeutic and toxic (including fatal) effects of chemotherapy. Thus, it is imperative that an interdisciplinary team of clinicians with expertise in oncologic surgery, radiation therapy and medical oncology, nursing, palliative medicine, and pharmacology evaluate patients to determine the treatment plan that is likely to provide the greatest cumulative benefit for the patient. If, as ought to be the ideal, the patient is always to be kept at the center of the decision-making process, then studies that assess patient-centered outcomes (pain, dyspnea, fatigue, appetite, weight loss, performance status, anxiety, well-being, and other quality-of-life measures) for chemotherapy merit a higher priority. Newer targeted therapies need to be evaluated for benefits related to reduction of symptom burden from neoplastic disease. Although it is generally accepted that patients with a poor performance status do not usually benefit from systemic chemotherapy, it is not known whether the response to newer targeted agents will shift this paradigm.

An additional challenge for the medical oncologist is decision making if first-line chemotherapy fails to control the tumor. For some disease types, there is clear objective benefit from second-line therapy. For many, however, second-line therapy is more likely to lead to enhanced cumulative toxicities rather than objective tumor response.

Oncology patients have among the highest rates of hospitalization, especially near the end of life. Changes in reimbursement policies result in losses to hospital systems with unplanned readmissions within 60 days of hospital discharge. In one cancer institute, 6% of all discharged patients accounted for more than 40% of unplanned readmissions. The use of hospital resources included ICU stay, emergency department visits, overuse of chemotherapy, and under use of hospice care. Instituting an interdisciplinary care team (ICT) was created to evaluate patients, on a bimonthly basis, with at least two unplanned hospital readmissions over the last 60 days. Over a 6-month period, 36 patients had 226 hospitalizations and 163 emergency department visits, resulting in an average number of hospitalizations of 1.08 per patient month (ppm); hospitalizations dropped to 0.23 ppm after implementation of the ICT. After the creation of the ICT, the average length of stay decreased from 7.17 to 4.06 days per admission, the average emergency department visits decreased from 0.58 to 0.34 ppm, and the average number of unplanned readmissions decreased from 0.43 to 0.13 ppm. Average time to death was 72 days, and time to death from the last exposure to chemotherapy was 58 days after institution of the ICT. Financial incentives for hospital systems have made a major impact on the aggressiveness of care at the end of life.[230]

A retrospective analysis of the hospital stay, lasting at least 3 days, was conducted in 695 adult cancer patients who died in the hospital. Prior to hospital admission, 21% had received outpatient palliative care (OPC), 46% inpatient palliative care (IPC), and 33% no palliative care (NPC). Despite the differences in the care prior to hospital admission, no differences were identified in the care administered during the final admission; 11.2% of patients received radiation therapy, and 12.5% received antineoplastic therapy. In the last 3 days of life, imaging tests occurred in 50.1% patients; imaging tests were obtained in fewer palliative care patients (43.5% OPC; 47.3% IPC) than the 58.1% who received NPC. Radiation therapy was administered in 11.2%, and approximately 16% of all patients received chemotherapy within 14 days of death among the study groups. All patients received pain medications. Do-not-resuscitate orders were in place within 6 months before the final admission at a greater rate for OPC patients (22%) than for IPC (8%) and those with NPC (12%).[231]

A sensitive and thoughtful discussion with the patient and the family regarding the goals and priorities of care is needed. Emphasis must be placed on the ability to successfully manage the symptoms of progressive advanced disease with nonchemotherapeutic modalities when burdens are likely to outweigh benefits.

SIDE EFFECTS AND COMPLICATIONS

The toxicities and side effects of chemotherapeutic agents, such as nausea, are commonly known. Perhaps the most common painful sequela of chemotherapy administration is a toxic peripheral neuropathy manifested as painful paresthesias, hyporeflexia, and, less frequently, sensory or motor loss or autonomic dysfunction. The drugs most commonly associated with this complication are the plant alkaloids, especially vincristine; antimetabolites; the taxanes, especially paclitaxel; and platinum-based compounds like cisplatin; vinorelbine, procarbazine, and interferon.[196–198,232,233] In some cases, the painful peripheral neuropathy not only limits the dosing of anticancer therapy but also significantly affects quality of life and can be more difficult to treat than the more common nociceptive pain syndromes associated with the disease.

Dermatologic complications can occur from extravasation of chemotherapeutic agents into the subcutaneous tissues. This is especially problematic with drugs like vinca alkaloids, anthracyclines, and taxanes that cause severe local pain and ulceration with progressive tissue destruction.[197]

Another painful complication of cancer and its therapy is acute herpes zoster and postherpetic neuralgia, which occur with increased frequency in patients with cancer—especially in those receiving chemotherapy or immunosuppressive drugs. Lastly, although the palliative benefits of glucocorticoids on mood, pain (as an anti-inflammatory coanalgesic), and appetite are well-known, chronic steroid therapy can cause myopathy, as well as necrosis of the femoral and humeral heads.[234] Furthermore, one should be aware of the fact that withdrawal of glucocorticoids can cause a sense of decreased well-being, with increased pain, decreased energy, and apathy.[235]

Endocrine Therapy

Many types of tumors have been shown to respond to hormonal manipulation, which is achieved either by ablating endocrine glands or by administration of an exogenous hormone or hormone antagonist. The mechanism of action of these agents has been clarified by the demonstration that receptors that bind with estrogen exist in the cytosol of normal and malignant cells. Hormones bind to receptors in the cytoplasm and sterically alter the shape of the receptive protein itself, which, after transport to the cell nucleus, interacts with DNA, and results in altered messenger RNA production and protein synthesis. After this interaction, cytoplasmic receptor concentration is restored and the cycle can be repeated. Estrogen receptors can be quantitated as 8S and 4S proteins. Primary tumors in humans have estrogen receptor values that range from 0 to almost 1,000 fmol/mg cytosol protein. Receptors also exist for progesterones and androgens, and receptors for corticosteroids have been identified in the cytosol of leukemic cells.

Hormonal ablation can be achieved by surgical means, as occurs with oophorectomy, adrenalectomy, and hypophysectomy; by irradiation of the ovaries or ablating the pituitary gland with the various radioactive compounds; by injecting alcohol; or by surgical extirpation. Medical adrenalectomy can be achieved by administering aminoglutethimide, a potent inhibitor of the conversion of cholesterol to pregnenolone in the adrenal gland. Hormone additive therapy is achieved by the administration of estrogens, progestins, androgens, antiestrogens, corticosteroids, and thyroid hormones. Such hormone changes can cause complex endocrine effects, such as pituitary inhibition of luteinizing hormone, follicle-stimulating hormone, and prolactin, as well as changes in endogenous steroid hormone production.[199]

ENDOCRINE THERAPY FOR RELIEF OF CANCER PAIN

The first reports of the efficacy of hormonal therapy on relieving cancer pain were correlated with tumor regression. A significant number of other studies only reported the reduction in tumor volume without also assessing pain relief.

Two large clinical trials were conducted in 2016 in hormone receptor–positive early breast cancer patients with the aromatase inhibitor letrozole. Compared to the recommended standard length of therapy was 5 years, the clinical trials found that 10 years of letrozole reduced breast cancer recurrences or a new cancer in the opposite breast by one-third. Despite these improvements in outcomes, longer hormonal therapy did not improve overall or disease-free survival in these trials. In 2017, the 5-year disease-free survival was improved to 83% when anastrozole was prescribed for 6 years after tamoxifen therapy.[188–190]

Bisphosphonates

Bisphosphonates have significantly reduced skeletal-related events (SREs) such as pathologic fracture, spinal cord compression, or the necessity of radiation or surgery to reduce the morbidity of bone metastases. Zoledronic acid (ZA), a third-generation aminobisphosphonate, reduces the risk of SREs by 40%; after an initial 9 to 12 monthly doses, ZA is then administered every 3 months. Denosumab, a human monoclonal antibody that inhibits osteoclasts by binding to the receptor activator of kappa B ligand, delays the onset of first and subsequent SREs more than ZA.[236]

The American Society of Clinical Oncology and Cancer Care Ontario guidelines indicate that breast cancer patients with bone metastases should be treated with bone modifying agents. Options include denosumab (120 mg subcutaneously every 4 weeks), pamidronate (90 mg intravenously every 3 to 4 weeks), or ZA (4 mg intravenously every 12 weeks or every 3 to 4 weeks). These agents are most effective in reducing the incidence of SRE and should not be used alone for bone pain.[237]

Summary

Sophisticated local and novel systemic therapeutic approaches are being developed to better localize or personalize treatment. In palliative radiotherapy, SRT (and to a lesser degree proton therapy) localizes radiation to the tumor, often allowing for repeat radiation near critical structures like the spinal cord. Novel systemic therapeutic approaches include adoptive cell immunotherapy. Using few high-dose radiation fractions, SRT is an accepted tool in palliative radiation therapy for specific indications, and single-fraction radiation therapy is now an accepted alternative to longer courses of palliative radiation. Although a sophisticated radiation technique is used to address a difficult clinical presentation, the palliative goals remain aligned. In contrast, novel systemic therapies, like adoptive cell immunotherapy, continue to provide hope for curative intent even in advanced disease. Although the therapeutic mechanisms of adoptive cell immunotherapy are novel, the paradigm of curative intent for the patient, despite advanced disease, remains unchanged. Furthermore, these therapeutic innovations have substantial socioeconomic costs.

Despite the development of palliative care teams that become involved early in the course of cancer care, much futile therapy continues to be administered. Palliative care teams have had some success in reducing chemotherapy administration in the last 14 days of life, increasing hospice placement, and reducing hospital admissions and readmissions in the last 60 days of life. However, palliative care teams are not available within all health systems, and decisions regarding antineoplastic therapy remain largely unchanged.

Therapeutic decisions for cancer care become more difficult as the stage of cancer advances. These therapeutic decisions are largely based on the patient's preferences and performance status, availability of novel therapies, and the availability of supportive care.

References

1. MacDonald N. The role of medical and surgical oncology in the management of cancer pain. In: Foley KM, Bonica JJ, Ventafridda V, eds. *Advances in Pain Research and Therapy*. Vol 16. New York: Raven Press; 1990:27–39.
2. Cancer Statistics. National Cancer Institute. Available at: https://www.cancer.gov/about-cancer/understanding/statistics. Accessed August 3, 2018.
3. Jemal A, Ward EM, Johnson CJ, et al. Annual report to the nation on the status of cancer, 1975 to 2014, featuring survival. *J Natl Cancer Inst* 2017;109(9):1–22. doi:10.1093/jnci/djx030.
4. McGinley L. Breast-cancer death rate drops almost 40 percent saving, 322,000 lives, study says. *Washington Post*. October 3, 2017. Available at: https://www.washingtonpost.com/news/to-your-health/wp/2017/10/03/breast-cancer-death-rate-drops-almost-40-percent-saving-32200-lives-study-says/?utm_term=.28c3afee5f41. Accessed August 3, 2018.
5. American Cancer Society. *Breast Cancer Facts & Figures 2017–2018*. Atlanta, GA: American Cancer Society Inc; 2017.
6. Chang VT, Thaler HT, Polyak TA, et al. Quality of life and survival: the role of multidimensional symptom assessment. *Cancer* 1998;83(1):173–179.
7. Jacox A, Carr DB, Payne R. New clinical-practice guidelines for the management of pain in patients with cancer. *N Engl J Med* 1994;330(9):651–655.
8. Brescia FJ, Portenoy RK, Ryan M, et al. Pain, opioid use, and survival in hospitalized patients with advanced cancer. *J Clin Oncol* 1992;10(1):149–155.
9. Porzsolt F. Goals of palliative cancer therapy: scope of the problem. *Cancer Treat Rev* 1993;19(suppl A):3–14.
10. Rubens RD. Approaches to palliation and its evaluation. *Cancer Treat Rev* 1993;19(suppl A):67–71.
11. Porzsolt F, Tannock I. Goals of palliative cancer therapy. *J Clin Oncol* 1993; 11(2):378–381.
12. Cella DF, Tulsky DS. Quality of life in cancer: definition, purpose, and method of measurement. *Cancer Invest* 1993;11(3):327–336.
13. Janjan NA. Radiation for bone metastases—conventional techniques and the role of systemic radiopharmaceuticals. *Cancer* 1997;80(suppl 8):1628–1645.
14. Ferrell BR, Temel JS, Temin S, et al. Integration of palliative care into standard oncology care: American Society of Clinical Oncology clinical practice guideline update. *J Clin Oncol* 2017;35:96–112.
15. Hoerger M, Greer JA, Jackson VA, et al. Defining the elements of early palliative care that are associated with patient-reported outcomes and the delivery of end-of-life care. *J Clin Oncol* 2018;36:1096–1102.
16. Scibetta C, Rabow MW, Kerr K. Early integration of palliative care in cancer care: care, quality, and cost implications of the timing of palliative care consultation among patients with advanced cancer. *J Clin Oncol* 2014; 32(31 suppl):8. doi:10.1200/jco.2014.32.31_suppl.8.
17. Isenberg SR, Lu C, McQuade J, et al. Impact of a new palliative care program on health system finances: an analysis of the palliative care program inpatient unit and consultations at Johns Hopkins Medical Institutions. *J Oncol Pract* 2017;13(5):e422–e430. doi:10.1200/JOP.2016.014860.
18. McDermott CL, Fedorenko C, Kreizenbeck K, et al. End-of-life services among patients with cancer: evidence from cancer registry records linked with commercial health insurance claims. *J Oncol Pract* 2017;13(11): e889–e899. doi:10.1200/JOP.2017.021683.
19. Kruser JM, Rakhra SS, Sacotte RM, et al. Intensive care unit outcomes among patients with cancer after palliative radiation therapy. *Int J Radiat Oncol Biol Phys* 2017;99(4):854–858. doi:10.1016/j.ijrobp.2017.06.2463.
20. Lai PP, Perez CA, Lockett MA. Prognostic significance of pelvic recurrence and distant metastases in prostate carcinoma following definitive radiotherapy. *Int J Radiat Oncol Biol Phys* 1992;24(3):423–430.
21. Yamashita K, Denno K, Ueda T, et al. Prognostic significance of bone metastases in patients with metastatic prostate cancer. *Cancer* 1993;71(4): 1297–1302.
22. Knudson G, Grinis G, Lopez-Majano V, et al. Bone scan as a stratification variable in advanced prostate cancer. *Cancer* 1991;68(2):316–320.
23. Greenwald HP, Bonica JJ, Bergner M. The prevalence of pain in four cancers. *Cancer* 1987;60(10):2563–2569.
24. Sherry MM, Greco FA, Johnson DH, et al. Breast cancer with skeletal metastases at initial diagnosis. Distinctive clinical characteristics and favorable prognosis. *Cancer* 1986;58(1):178–182.
25. Sherry MM, Greco FA, Johnson DH, et al. Metastatic breast cancer confined to the skeletal system. An indolent disease. *Am J Med* 1986;81(3): 381–386.
26. McCloskey SA, Tao ML, Rose CM, et al. National survey of perspectives of palliative radiation therapy: role, barriers, and needs. *Cancer J* 2007; 13(2):130–137.
27. Arcangeli G, Micheli A, Arcangeli F, et al. The responsiveness of bone metastases to radiotherapy: the effect of site, histology, and radiation dose on pain relief. *Radiother Oncol* 1989;14(2):95–101.
28. Cohen HJ. Cancer and the functional status of the elderly. *Cancer* 1997; 80(10):1883–1886.
29. Tseng Y, Krishnan MS, Jones JA, et al. Supportive and palliative radiation oncology service: impact of a dedicated service on palliative cancer care. *Pract Radiat Oncol* 2014;4(4):247–253. doi:10.1016/j.prro.2013.09.005.
30. Lutz S, Spence C, Chow E, et al. Survey on use of palliative radiotherapy in hospice care. *J Clin Oncol* 2004;22(17):3581–3586.
31. Chang S, May P, Goldstein NE, et al. A palliative radiation oncology consult service's impact on care of advanced cancer patients. *J Palliat Med* 2018;21(4):438–444. doi:10.1089/jpm.2017.0372.
32. Chang S, May P, Goldstein NE, et al. A palliative radiation oncology consult service reduces total costs during hospitalization. *J Pain Symptom Manage* 2018;55(6):1452–1458. doi:10.1016/j.jpainsymman.2018.03.005.
33. Hess G, Barlev A, Chung K, et al. Cost of palliative radiation to the bone for patients with bone metastases secondary to breast or prostate cancer. *Radiat Oncol* 2012;7:168–175.
34. Kim H, Rajagopalan MS, Beriwal S, et al. Cost-effectiveness analysis of a single fraction of stereotactic body radiation therapy compared with single fraction of external beam radiation therapy for palliation of vertebral bone metastases. *Int J Radiat Oncol Biol Phys* 2015;91(3):556–563. doi:10.1016/j.ijrobp.2014.10.055.
35. Dale RG, Jones B. Radiobiologically based assessments of the net costs of fractionated radiotherapy. *Int J Radiat Oncol Biol Phys* 1996;36(3):739–746.
36. Janjan NA. Radiotherapeutic approaches to cancer pain management. *Highlights Oncol Pract* 1997;14(4 suppl 11):103–113.
37. Schulman KL, Kohles J. Economic burden of metastatic bone disease in the U.S. *Cancer* 2007;109(11):2334–2342.
38. Li S, Peng Y, Weinhandl ED, et al. Estimated number of prevalent cases of metastatic bone disease in the US adult population. *Clin Epidemiol* 2012;4:87–93.
39. Janjan NA. Radiation for bone metastases: conventional techniques and the role of systemic radiopharmaceuticals. *Cancer* 1997;80(suppl 8):1628–1645.
40. Simone CB II. Palliative radiotherapy, bone metastases, and global assessments in palliative care. *Ann Palliat Med* 2017;6(suppl 1):S1–S3. doi:10.21037/apm.2017.08.14.
41. Pandit-Taskar N, Batraki M, Divgi CR. Radiopharmaceutical therapy for palliation of bone pain from osseous metastases. *J Nucl Med* 2004;45: 1358–1365.
42. Drost L, Ganesh V, Wan A, et al. Attendance of older patients with bone metastases at a multidisciplinary bone metastases clinic: an 8-year experience. *Ann Palliat Med* 2017;6(suppl 1):S47–S51. doi:10.21037/apm.2017.06.06.
43. Tseng YD, Gouwens NW, Lo SS, et al. Use of radiation therapy within the last year of life among cancer patients. *Int J Radiat Oncol Biol Phys* 2018;101(1):21–29. doi:10.1016/j.ijrobp.2018.01.056.
44. Kwok Y, Regine WF, Patchell RA. Radiation therapy alone for spinal cord compression: time to improve upon a relatively ineffective status quo. *J Clin Oncol* 2005;23(15):3308–3010.

45. Lutz ST, Jones J, Chow E. Role of radiation therapy in palliative care of the patient with cancer. *J Clin Oncol* 2014;32(26):2913–2919. doi:10.1200/JCO.2014.55.1143.

46. Wu JS, Wong RK, Lloyd NS, et al; and the Supportive Care Guidelines Group of Cancer Care Ontario. Radiotherapy fractionation for the palliation of uncomplicated painful bone metastases—an evidence-based practice guideline. *BMC Cancer* 2004;4:71–78. doi:10.1186/1471-2407-4-71.

47. Lutz S, Balboni T, Jones J, et al. Palliative radiation therapy for bone metastases: update of an ASTRO evidence-based guideline. *Pract Radiat Oncol* 2017;7:4–12. doi:10.1016/j.prro.2016.08.001.

48. Rodrigues G, Videtic GMM, Sur R, et al. Palliative thoracic radiotherapy in lung cancer: an American Society for Radiation Oncology evidence-based clinical practice guideline. *Pract Radiat Oncol* 2011;1(2):60–71. doi:10.1016/j.prro.2011.01.005.

49. Moeller B, Balagamwala EH, Chen A, et al. Palliative thoracic radiation therapy for non-small cell lung cancer: 2018 update of an American Society for Radiation Oncology (ASTRO) evidence-based guideline. *Pract Radiat Oncol* 2018;8(4):245–250. doi:10.1016/j.prro.2018.02.009.

50. Crane CH, O'Reilly EM. Ablative radiotherapy doses for locally advanced pancreatic cancer (LAPC). *Cancer J* 2017;23(6):350–354. doi:10.1097/PPO.0000000000000292.

51. Kagan AR. Palliation of visceral recurrences and metastases. In: Perez CA, Brady LW, eds. *Principles and Practice of Radiation Oncology*. 3rd ed. Philadelphia: Lippincott-Raven; 2004:2405–2411.

52. Kress MAS, Jensen RE, Tsai HT, et al. Radiation therapy at the end of life: a population-based study examining palliative treatment intensity. *Radiat Oncol* 2015;10:15–24. doi:10.1186/s13014-014-0305-4.

53. Kagan AR. Palliation of brain and spinal cord metastases. In: Perez CA, Brady LW, eds. *Principles and Practice of Radiation Oncology*. 4th ed. Philadelphia: Lippincott-Raven; 2004:2373–2384.

54. Tsao MN, Rades D, Wirth A, et al. Radiotherapeutic and surgical management for newly diagnosed brain metastasis(es): an American Society for Radiation Oncology evidence-based guideline. *Pract Radiat Oncol* 2012;2(3):210–225. doi:10.1016/j.prro.2011.12.004.

55. Tong D, Gillick L, Hendrickson FR. The palliation of symptomatic osseous metastases: final results of the study by the Radiation Therapy Oncology Group. *Cancer* 1982;50(5):893–899.

56. Blitzer PH. Reanalysis of the RTOG study of the palliation of symptomatic osseous metastasis. *Cancer* 1985;55(7):1468–1472.

57. Arcangeli G, Giovinazzo G, Saracino B, et al. Radiation therapy in the management of symptomatic bone metastases: the effect of total dose and histology on pain relief and response duration. *Int J Radiat Oncol Biol Phys* 1998;42(5):1119–1126.

58. Koswig S, Budach V. Remineralization and pain relief in bone metastases after different radiotherapy fractions (10 times 3 Gy vs. 1 time 8 Gy): a prospective study [in German]. *Strahlenther Onkol* 1999;175(10):500–508.

59. Koswig S, Buchali A, Böhmer D, et al. Palliative radiotherapy of bone metastases. A retrospective analysis of 176 patients [in German]. *Strahlenther Onkol* 1999;175(10):509–514.

60. Mercadante S. Malignant bone pain: pathophysiology and treatment. *Pain* 1997;69(1–2):1–18.

61. Hortobagyi GN, Libshitz HI, Seabold JE. Osseous metastases of breast cancer. Clinical, biochemical, radiographic, and scintigraphic evaluation of response to therapy. *Cancer* 1984;53(3):577–582.

62. Vogel CL, Schoenfelder J, Shemano I, et al. Worsening bone scan in the evaluation of antitumor response during hormonal therapy of breast cancer. *J Clin Oncol* 1995;13(5):1123–1128.

63. Ford HT, Yarnold JR. Radiation therapy: pain relief and recalcification. In: Stoll BA, Parbhoo S, eds. *Bone Metastases: Monitoring and Treatment*. New York: Raven; 1983:343–354.

64. Barton M. Tables of equivalent dose in 2 Gy fractions: a simple application of the linear quadratic formula. *Int J Radiat Oncol Biol Phys* 1995;31(2):371–378.

65. Bates T, Yarnold JR, Blitzer P, et al. Bone metastasis consensus statement. *Int J Radiat Oncol Biol Phys* 1992;23(1):215–216.

66. Niewald M, Tkocz HJ, Abel U, et al. Rapid course radiation therapy vs. more standard treatment: a randomized trial for bone metastases. *Int J Radiat Oncol Biol Phys* 1996;36(5):1085–1089.

67. Barak F, Werner A, Walach N, et al. The palliative efficacy of a single high dose of radiation in treatment of symptomatic osseous metastases. *Int J Radiat Oncol Biol Phys* 1987;13(8):1233–1235.

68. Cole DJ. A randomized trial of a single treatment versus conventional fractionation in the palliative radiotherapy of painful bone metastases. *Clin Oncol* 1989;1(2):59–62.

69. Hoskin PJ, Price P, Easton D, et al. A prospective randomised trial of 4 Gy or 8 Gy single doses in the treatment of metastatic bone pain. *Radiother Oncol* 1992;23(2):74–78.

70. Price P, Hoskin PJ, Easton D, et al. Prospective randomised trial of single and multifraction radiotherapy schedules in the treatment of painful bone metastases. *Radiother Oncol* 1986;6(4):247–255.

71. Amichetti M, Orrù P, Madeddu A, et al. Comparative evaluation of two hypofractionated radiotherapy regimens for painful bone metastases. *Tumori* 2004;90(1):91–95.

72. Wu JS, Wong R, Johnston M, et al. Meta-analysis of dose-fractionation radiotherapy trials for the palliation of painful bone metastases. *Int J Radiat Oncol Biol Phys* 2003;55(3):594–605.

73. Steenland E, Leer JW, van Houwelingen H, et al. The effect of a single fraction compared to multiple fractions on painful bone metastases: a global analysis of the Dutch Bone Metastasis Study. *Radiother Oncol* 1999;52(2):101–109.

74. Nielsen OS, Bentzen SM, Sandberg E, et al. Randomized trial of single dose versus fractionated palliative radiotherapy of bone metastases. *Radiother Oncol* 1998;47(3):233–240.

75. Hartsell WF, Scott CB, Bruner DW, et al. Randomized trial of short- versus long-course radiotherapy for palliation of painful bone metastases. *J Natl Cancer Inst* 2005;97(11):798–804.

76. Chow E, Harris K, Fan G, et al. Palliative radiotherapy trials for bone metastases: a systematic review. *J Clin Oncol* 2007;25(11):1423–1436.

77. Sze WM, Shelley M, Held I, et al. Palliation of metastatic bone pain: single fraction versus multifraction radiotherapy—a systematic review of the randomised trials. *Cochrane Database Syst Rev* 2004;(2):CD004721.

78. Sze WM, Shelley MD, Held I, et al. Palliation of metastatic bone pain: single fraction versus multifraction radiotherapy—a systematic review of randomised trials. *Clin Oncol (R Coll Radiol)* 2003;15(6):345–352.

79. Mithal NP, Needham PR, Hoskin PJ. Retreatment with radiotherapy for painful bone metastases. *Int J Radiat Oncol Biol Phys* 1994;29(5):1011–1014.

80. Boogerd W, van der Sande JJ. Diagnosis and treatment of spinal cord compression in malignant disease. *Cancer Treat Rev* 1993;19(2):129–150.

81. Byrne TN. Spinal cord compression from epidural metastases. *N Engl J Med* 1992;327(9):614–619.

82. Grant R, Papadopoulos SM, Greenberg HS. Metastatic epidural spinal cord compression. *Neurol Clin* 1991;9(4):825–841.

83. Maranzano E, Latini P, Checcaglini F, et al. Radiation therapy in metastatic spinal cord compression. A prospective analysis of 105 consecutive patients. *Cancer* 1991;67(5):1311–1317.

84. Janjan NA. Radiotherapeutic management of spinal metastases. *J Pain Symptom Manage* 1996;11(1):47–56.

85. Loblaw DA, Laperriere NJ. Emergency treatment of malignant extradural spinal cord compression: an evidence-based guideline. *J Clin Oncol* 1998;16(4):1613–1624.

86. Boogerd W. Central nervous system metastasis in breast cancer. *Radiother Oncol* 1996;40(1):5–22.

87. Gaze MN, Kelly CG, Kerr GR, et al. Pain relief and quality of life following radiotherapy for bone metastases: a randomised trial of two fractionation schedules. *Radiother Oncol* 1997;45(2):109–116.

88. Dudley SA, Aggarwal S, Qian Y, et al. (Po89) Comparison of survival by different palliative radiation therapy fractionation schedules. *Int J Radiat Oncol Biol Phys* 2017;98(2 suppl):e39. doi:10.1016/j.ijrobp.2017.02.185.

89. Puckett LL, Luitweiler E, Potters L, et al. Preventing discontinuation of radiation therapy: predictive factors to improve patient selection for palliative treatment. *J Oncol Practice* 2017;13(9):e782–e791. doi:10.1200/JOP.2017.021220.

90. Puckett L, Zhang I, Potters L, et al. Shifting paradigms in the treatment of bone metastases: an eye toward the future. *Int J Radiat Oncol Biol Phys* 2016;96(2 suppl):S196. doi:10.1016/j.ijrobp.2016.06.488.

91. Ellsworth SG, Alcorn SR, Hales RK, et al. Patterns of care among patients receiving therapy for bone metastases at a large academic institution. *Int J Radiat Oncol Biol Phys* 2014;89(5):1100–1105. doi:10.1016/j.ijrobp.2014.04.028.

92. Erler D, Brotherston D, Sahgal A, et al. Local control and fracture risk following stereotactic body radiation therapy for non-spine bone metastases. *Radiother Oncol* 2018;127(2):304–309. doi:10.1016/j.radonc.2018.03.030.

93. van der Velden JM, Peters M, Verlaan JJ, et al. Development and internal validation of a clinical risk score to predict pain response after palliative radiation therapy in patients with bone metastases. *Int J Radiat Oncol Biol Phys* 2017;99(4):859–866. doi:10.1016/j.ijrobp.2017.07.029.

94. Furfari A, Wan BA, Ding K, et al. Genetic biomarkers associated with response to palliative radiotherapy in patients with painful bone metastases. *Ann Palliat Med* 2017;1–9. doi:10.21037/apm.2017.09.03.

95. Hayashi S, Hoshi H, Iida T. Reirradiation with local-field radiotherapy for painful bone metastases. *Radiat Med* 2002;20(5):231–236.

96. Chow R, Ding K, Ganesh V, et al. Gender and age make no difference in the re-irradiation of painful bone metastases: a secondary analysis of the NCIC CTG SC.20 randomized trial. *Radiother Oncol* 2018;126(3):541–546. doi:10.1016/j.radonc.2017.10.006.

97. Rich SE, Chow R, Raman S, et al. Update of the systemic review of palliative radiation therapy fractionation for bone metastases. *Radiother Oncol* 2018;126(3):547–557. doi:10.1016/j.radonc.2018.01.003.

98. Sahgal A, Ma L, Weinberg V, et al. Reirradiation human spinal cord tolerance for stereotactic body radiotherapy. *Int J Radiat Oncol Biol Phys* 2012;82(1):107–116. doi:10.1016/j.ijrobp.2010.08.021.

99. Siddiqui F, Elibe E, Boyce-Fappiano D, et al. Reirradiation of the spinal cord: efficacy and toxicity. *Int J Radiat Oncol Biol Phys* 2015;93(3 suppl):S176. doi:10.1016/j.ijrobp.2015.07.423.

100. Foerster R, Cho BCJ, Fahim DK, et al. Histopathological findings after reirradiation compared to first irradiation of spinal bone metastases with stereotactic body radiotherapy: a cohort study [published online ahead of print March 14, 2018]. *Neurosurgery*. doi:10.1093/neuros/nyy059.

101. Huber S, Ulsperger E, Gomar C, et al. Osseous metastases in breast cancer: radiographic monitoring of therapeutic response. *Anticancer Res* 2002; 22(2B):1279–1288.

102. Janssen SJ, Paulino Pereira NR, Meijs TA, et al. Predicting pathological fracture in femoral metastases using a clinical CT scan based algorithm: a case control study. *J Orthop Sci* 2018;23(2):394–402. doi:10.1016/j.jos.2017.10.004.

103. Bunting RW, Boublik M, Blevins FT, et al. Functional outcome of pathologic fracture secondary to malignant disease in a rehabilitation hospital. *Cancer* 1992;69(1):98–102.

104. Townsend PW, Smalley SR, Cozad SC, et al. Role of postoperative radiation therapy after stabilization of fractures caused by metastatic disease. *Int J Radiat Oncol Biol Phys* 1995;31(1):43–49.

105. Heisterberg L, Johansen TS. Treatment of pathologic fractures. *Acta Orthop Scand* 1979;50(6 pt 2):787–790.

106. Piatek S, Westphal T, Bischoff J, et al. Intramedullary stabilisation of metastatic fractures of long bones [in German]. *Zentralbl Chir* 2003;128(2):131–138.

107. Nooh A, Goulding K, Isler MH, et al. Early improvement in pain and functional outcome but not quality of life after surgery for metastatic long bone disease. *Clin Orthop Relat Res* 2018;476(3):535–545. doi:10.1007/s11999.0000000000000065.

108. Arrigoni F, Bruno F, Zugaro L, et al. Developments in the management of bone metastases with interventional radiology. *Acta Biomed* 2018; 89(1–S):166–174. doi:10.10.23750/abm.v89i1-S.7020.

109. Helweg-Larsen S, Sørensen PS. Symptoms and signs in metastatic spinal cord compression: a study of progression from first symptom until diagnosis in 153 patients. *Eur J Cancer* 1994;30A(3):396–398.

110. Loblaw DA, Perry J, Chambers A, et al. Systematic review of the diagnosis and management of malignant extradural spinal cord compression: the Cancer Care Ontario Practice Guidelines Initiative's Neuro-Oncology Disease Site Group. *J Clin Oncol* 2005;23(9):2028–2037.

111. Talcott JA, Stomper PC, Drislane FW, et al. Assessing suspected spinal cord compression: a multidisciplinary outcomes analysis of 342 episodes. *Support Care Cancer* 1999;7(1):31–38.

112. Loblaw DA, Smith K, Lockwood G, et al. The Princess Margaret Hospital experience of malignant spinal cord compression. *Proc Am Soc Clin Oncol* 2003;22:119.

113. Loblaw DA, Laperriere NJ, Mackillop WJ. A population-based study of malignant spinal cord compression in Ontario. *Clin Oncol (R Coll Radiol)* 2003;15(4):211–217.

114. Mui WH, Lam TC, Wong FCS, et al. Survival analysis of malignant epidural spinal cord compression after palliative radiation therapy using Tokuhashi Scoring System and the impact of systemic therapy. *Int J Radiat Oncol Biol Phys* 2016;96(2):E81. doi:10.1016/j.ijrobp.2016.06.794.

115. Mui WH, Lam TC, Wong FCS, et al. Survival analysis of malignant epidural spinal cord compression after palliative radiation therapy using Tokuhashi scoring system and the impact of systemic therapy. *Ann Palliat Med* 2017;6(suppl 2):S132–S139. doi:10.21037/apm.2017.07.06.

116. Bollen L, Jacobs WCH, Van der Linden YM, et al. A systemic review of prognostic factors predicting survival in patients with spinal bone metastases. *Eur Spine J* 2018;27(4):799–805. doi:10.1007/s00586-017-5320-3.

117. Boogerd W, van der Sande JJ, Kröger R. Early diagnosis and treatment of spinal metastases in breast cancer: a prospective study. *J Neurol Neurosurg Psychiatry* 1992;55(12):1188–1193.

118. Rades D, Stalpers LJ, Veninga T, et al. Evaluation of functional outcome and local control after radiotherapy for metastatic spinal cord compression in patients with prostate cancer. *J Urol* 2006;175(2):552–556.

119. Rades D, Heidenreich F, Karstens JH. Final results of a prospective study of the prognostic value of the time to develop motor deficits before irradiation in metastatic spinal cord compression. *Int J Radiat Oncol Biol Phys* 2002;53(4):975–979.

120. Lövey G, Koch K, Gademann G. Metastatic epidural spinal compression: prognostic factors and results of radiotherapy [in German]. *Strahlenther Onkol* 2001;177(12):676–679.

121. Nagata M, Ueda T, Komiya A, et al. Treatment and prognosis of patients with paraplegia or quadriplegia because of metastatic spinal cord compression in prostate cancer. *Prostate Cancer Prostatic Dis* 2003;6(2):169–173.

122. Turner S, Marosszeky B, Timms I, et al. Malignant spinal cord compression: a prospective evaluation. *Int J Radiat Oncol Biol Phys* 1993;26(1):141–146.

123. Peteet J, Tay V, Cohen G, et al. Pain characteristics and treatment in an outpatient cancer population. *Cancer* 1985;57(6):1259–1265.

124. Wada E, Yamamoto T, Furuno M, et al. Spinal cord compression secondary to osteoblastic metastasis. *Spine (Phila Pa 1976)* 1993;18(10):1380–1381.

125. Algra PR, Heimans JJ, Valk J, et al. Do metastases in vertebrae begin in the body or the pedicles? Imaging study in 45 patients. *AJR Am J Roentgenol* 1992;158(6):1275–1279.

126. Landmann C, Hünig R, Gratzl O. The role of laminectomy in the combined treatment of metastatic spinal cord compression. *Int J Radiat Oncol Biol Phys* 1992;24(4):627–631.

127. Husband DJ, Grant KA, Romaniuk CS. MRI in the diagnosis and treatment of suspected malignant spinal cord compression. *Br J Radiol* 2001; 74(877):15–23.

128. Loughrey GJ, Collins CD, Todd SM, et al. Magnetic resonance imaging in the management of suspected spinal canal disease in patients with known malignancy. *Clin Radiol* 2000;55(11):849–855.

129. Barzilai O, Laufer I, Yamada Y, et al. Integrating evidence-based medicine for treatment of spinal metastases into a decision framework: neurologic, oncologic, mechanical stability, and systemic disease. *J Clin Oncol* 2017;35(21):2419–2427. doi:10.1200/JCO.2017.72.7362.

130. Rades D, Dunst J, Schild SE. The first score predicting overall survival in patients with metastatic spinal cord compression. *Cancer* 2008;112(1): 157–161.

131. Thibault I, Whyne CM, Zhou S, et al. Volume of lytic vertebral body metastatic disease quantified using computed tomography-based image segmentation predicts fracture risk after spine stereotactic body radiation therapy. *Int J Radiat Oncol Biol Phys* 2017;97(1):75–81.

132. Lövey G, Koch K, Gademann G. Metastatic epidural spinal compression: prognostic factors and results of radiotherapy. *Strahlenther Onkol* 2001;177(12):676–679.

133. Peteet J, Tay V, Cohen G, et al. Pain characteristics and treatment in an outpatient cancer population. *Cancer* 1986;57(6):1259–1265.

134. Verlaan JJ, Choi D, Versteeg A, et al. Characteristics of patients who survived <3 months or >2 years after surgery for spinal metastases: can we avoid inappropriate patient selection? *J Clin Oncol* 2016;34(25): 3054–3061.

135. Patchell RA, Tibbs PA, Regine WF, et al. Direct decompressive surgical resection in the treatment of spinal cord compression caused by metastatic cancer: a randomised trial. *Lancet* 2005;366(9486):643–648.

136. Klimo P Jr, Thompson CJ, Kestle JR, et al. A meta-analysis of surgery versus conventional radiotherapy for the treatment of metastatic spinal epidural disease. *Neuro Oncol* 2005;7(1):64–76.

137. Tiwana MS, Barnes M, Yurkowski E, et al. Incidence and treatment patterns of complicated bone metastases in a population-based radiation therapy program. *Radiother Oncol* 2016;118(3):552–556. doi:10.1016/j.radonc.2015.10.015.

138. Tiwana MS, Barnes M, Yurkowski E, et al. Incidence and treatment patterns of complicated bone metastases in a population-based radiation therapy program. *Int J Radiat Oncol Biol Phys* 2015;93(3 suppl):E471. doi:10.1016/j.ijrobp.2015.07.1750.

139. Kim RY, Smith JW, Spencer SA, et al. Malignant epidural spinal cord compression associated with a paravertebral mass: its radiotherapeutic outcome on radiosensitivity. *Int J Radiat Oncol Biol Phys* 1993;27(5): 1079–1083.

140. Bach F, Agerlin N, Sørensen JB, et al. Metastatic spinal cord compression secondary to lung cancer. *J Clin Oncol* 1992;10(11):1781–1787.

141. Jeremic B, Djuric L, Mijatovic L. Incidence of radiation myelitis of the cervical spinal cord at doses of 5500 cGy or greater. *Cancer* 1991;68(10): 2138–2141.

142. Powers BE, Thames HD, Gillette SM, et al. Volume effects in the irradiated canine spinal cord: do they exist when the probability of injury is low? *Radiother Oncol* 1998;46(3):297–306.

143. Tong XQ, Sugimura H, Kisanuki A, et al. Multiple fractionated and single-dose irradiation of bone marrow. Evaluation by MR and correlation with histopathological findings. *Acta Radiol* 1998;39(6):620–624.

144. Wen PY, Blanchard KL, Block CC, et al. Development of Lhermitte's sign after bone marrow transplantation. *Cancer* 1992;69(9):2262–2266.

145. Steiner RM, Mitchell DG, Rao VM, et al. Magnetic resonance imaging of diffuse bone marrow disease. *Radiol Clin North Am* 1993;31(2):383–409.

146. Algra PR, Bloem JL, Tissing H, et al. Detection of vertebral metastases: comparison between MR imaging and bone scintigraphy. *Radiographics* 1991;11(2):219–232.

147. Le Bihan DJ. Differentiation of benign versus pathologic compression fractures with diffusion-weighted MR imaging: a closer step toward the "holy grail" of tissue characterization? *Radiology* 1998;207(2):305–307.

148. Sugimura H, Kisanuki A, Tamura S, et al. Magnetic resonance imaging of bone marrow changes after irradiation. *Invest Radiol* 1994;29(1):35–41.

149. Yankelevitz DF, Henschke C, Knapp PH, et al. Effect of radiation therapy on thoracic and lumbar bone marrow: evaluation with MR imaging. *AJR Am J Roentgenol* 1991;157(1):87–92.

150. Paice JA, Portenoy R, Lacchetti C, et al. Management of chronic pain in survivors of adult cancers: American Society of Clinical Oncology clinical practice guideline. *J Clin Oncol* 2016;34(27):3325–3345.

151. Boyce-Fappiano D, Elibe E, Schultz L, et al. Analysis of the factors contributing to vertebral compression fractures after spine stereotactic radiosurgery. *Int J Radiat Oncol Biol Phys* 2017;97(2):236–245.

152. Bernard V, Bishop AJ, Allen PK, et al. Heterogeneity in treatment response of spine metastases to spine stereotactic radiosurgery within "radiosensitive" subtypes. *Int J Radiat Oncol Biol Phys* 2017;99(5):1207–1215. doi:10.1016/j.ijrobp.2017.08.028.

153. Kam NM, Maingard J, Kok HK, et al. Combined vertebral augmentation and radiofrequency ablation in the management of spinal metastases: an update. *Curr Treat Options Oncol* 2017;18(12):74. doi:10.1007/s11864-017-0516-7.

154. Bach F, Bjerregaard B, Sölétormos G, et al. Diagnostic value of cerebrospinal fluid cytology in comparison with tumor marker activity in central nervous system metastases secondary to breast cancer. *Cancer* 1993;72(8): 2376–2382.

155. Russi EG, Pergolizzi S, Gaeta M, et al. Palliative radiotherapy in lumbosacral carcinomatous neuropathy. *Radiother Oncol* 1993;26(2):172–173.

156. Salazar OM, DaMotta NW, Bridgman SM, et al. Fractionated half-body irradiation for pain palliation in widely metastatic cancers: comparison with single dose. *Int J Radiat Oncol Biol Phys* 1996;36(1):49–60.

157. Salazar OM, Sandhu T, da Motta NW, et al. Fractionated half-body irradiation (HBI) for the rapid palliation of widespread, symptomatic, metastatic bone disease: a randomized phase III trial of the International Atomic Energy Agency (IAEA). *Int J Radiat Oncol Biol Phys* 2001;50(3):765–775.

158. Scarantino CW, Caplan R, Rotman M, et al. A phase I/II study to evaluate the effect of fractionated hemibody irradiation in the treatment of osseous metastases—RTOG 88-22. *Int J Radiat Oncol Biol Phys* 1996;36(1):37–48.

159. Salazar OM, Rubin P, Hendrickson FR, et al. Single dose half-body irradiation for palliation of multiple bone metastases from solid tumors. Final Radiation Therapy Oncology Group report. *Cancer* 1986;58(1):29–36.

160. Poulter CA, Cosmatos D, Rubin P, et al. A report of RTOG 8206: a phase III study of whether the addition of single dose hemibody irradiation to standard fractionated local field irradiation is more effective than local field irradiation alone in the treatment of symptomatic osseous metastases. *Int J Radiat Oncol Biol Phys* 1992;23(1):207–214.

161. Skolyszewski J, Sas-Korczynska B, Korzeniowski S, et al. The efficiency and tolerance of half-body irradiation (HBI) in patients with multiple metastases: the Krakow experience. *Strahlenther Onkol* 2001;177(9):482–486.

162. Holmes RA. Radiopharmaceuticals in clinical trials. *Semin Oncol* 1993; 20(3 suppl 2):22–26.

163. Manoso MW, Healey JH. Metastatic cancer to the bone. In: DeVita VT, Hellman S, Rosenberg SA, eds. *Cancer: Principles and Practice of Oncology*. Philadelphia: Lippincott Williams & Wilkins; 2005:2373–2374.

164. Porter AT, McEwan AJ, Powe JE, et al. Results of a randomized phase-III trial to evaluate the efficacy of strontium-89 adjuvant to local field external beam irradiation in the management of endocrine resistant metastatic prostate cancer. *Int J Radiat Oncol Biol Phys* 1993;25(5):805–813.

165. Porter AT, McEwan AJB. Strontium-89 as an adjuvant to external beam radiation improves pain relief and delays in disease progression in advanced prostate cancer: results of a randomized controlled trial. *Semin Oncol* 1993;20(3 suppl 2):38–43.

166. Robinson RG, Preston DF, Baxter KG, et al. Clinical experience with strontium-89 in prostatic and breast cancer patients. *Semin Oncol* 1993; 20(3 suppl 2):44–48.

167. Robinson RG, Preston DF, Schiefelbein M, et al. Strontium 89 therapy for the palliation of pain due to osseous metastases. *JAMA* 1995;274(5): 420–424.

168. Krishnamurthy GT, Swailem FM, Srivastava SC, et al. Tin-117m(4+) DTPA: pharmacokinetics and imaging characteristics in patients with metastatic bone pain. *J Nucl Med* 1997;38(2):230–237.

169. Serafini AN, Houston SJ, Resche I, et al. Palliation of pain associated with metastatic bone cancer using samarium-153 lexidronam: a double-blind placebo-controlled clinical trial. *J Clin Oncol* 1998;16(4):1574–1581.

170. Rogers CL, Speiser BL, Ram PC, et al. Efficacy and toxicity of intravenous strontium-89 for symptomatic osseous metastases. *Brachyther Int* 1998;14:133–142.

171. de Klerk JMH, Zonnenberg BA, van het Schip AD, et al. Dose escalation study of rhenium-186 hydroxyethylidene bisphosphonate in patients with metastatic prostate cancer. *Eur J Nucl Med* 1994;21(10):1114–1120.

172. Sciuto R, Maini CL, Tofani A, et al. Radiosensitization with low-dose carboplatin enhances pain palliation in radioisotope therapy with strontium-89. *Nucl Med Commun* 1996;17(9):799–804.

173. Bolger JJ, Dearnaley DP, Kirk D, et al. Strontium-89 (metastron) versus external beam radiotherapy in patient with painful bone metastases secondary to prostatic cancer: preliminary report of a multicenter trial. *Semin Oncol* 1993;20(suppl 2):32–33.

174. Eary JF, Collins C, Stabin M, et al. Samarium-153-EDTMP biodistribution and dosimetry estimation. *J Nucl Med* 1993;34(7):1031–1036.

175. Bayouth JE, Macey DJ, Kasi LP, et al. Dosimetry and toxicity of samarium-153-EDTMP administered for bone pain due to skeletal metastases. *J Nucl Med* 1994;35(1):63–69.

176. McEwan AJB, Amyotte GA, McGowan DG, et al. A retrospective analysis of the cost-effectiveness of treatment with metastron in patients with prostate cancer metastatic to bone. *Eur Urol* 1994;26(suppl 1):26–31.

177. Liepe K, Runge R, Kotzerke J. Systemic radionuclide therapy in pain palliation. *Am J Hosp Palliat Care* 2005;22(6):457–464.

178. Liepe K, Kotzerke J. A comparative study of 188Re-HEDP, 186Re-HEDP, 153Sm-EDTMP, and 89Sr in the treatment of painful skeletal metastases. *Nucl Med Commun* 2007;28(8):623–630.

179. Bauman G, Charette M, Reid R, et al. Radiopharmaceuticals for the palliation of painful bone metastasis: a systemic review. *Radiother Oncol* 2005;75(3):258–270.

180. Baczyk M, Milecki P, Baczyk E, et al. The effectiveness of strontium 89 in palliative therapy of painful prostate cancer bone metastases. *Ortop Traumatol Rehabil* 2003;5(3):364–368.

181. Lam MG, de Klerk JM, van Rijk PP, et al. Bone seeking radiopharmaceuticals for palliation of pain in cancer patients with osseous metastases. *Anticancer Agents Med Chem* 2007;7(4):381–397.

182. Sartor O, Reid RH, Hoskin PJ, et al. Samarium-153-Lexidronam complex for treatment of painful bone metastases in hormone-refractory prostate cancer. *Urology* 2004;63(5):940–945.

183. Dolezal J, Vizda J, Odrazka K. Prospective evaluation of samarium-153-EDTMP radionuclide treatment for bone metastases in patients with hormone-refractory prostate cancer. *Urol Int* 2007;78(1):50–57.

184. Sartor O, Reid RH, Bushnell DL, et al. Safety and efficacy of repeat administration of samarium Sm-153 lexidronam to patients with metastatic bone pain. *Cancer* 2007;109(3):637–643.

185. Ricci S, Boni G, Pastina I, et al. Clinical benefit of bone-targeted radiometabolic therapy with 153Sm-EDTMP combined with chemotherapy in patients with metastatic hormone-refractory prostate cancer. *Eur J Nucl Med Mol Imaging* 2007;34(7):1023–1030.

186. Chu E, DeVita VT. Principles of medical oncology. In: DeVita VT, Rosenberg SA, eds. *Cancer: Principles and Practice of Oncology*. 7th ed. Philadelphia: Lippincott Williams & Wilkins; 2006:296–306.

187. DeVita VT, Schein PS. The use of drugs in combination for the treatment of cancer: rationale and results. *N Engl J Med* 1973;288(19):998–1006.

188. Hagen T. FDA approves bevacizumab for platinum-sensitive ovarian cancer. Available at: https://www.onclive.com/web-exclusives/fda-approves-bevacizumab-for-platinumsensitive-ovarian-cancer. Accessed August 4, 2018.

189. Aghajanian C, Blank SV, Goff BA, et al. OCEANS: a randomized, double-blind, placebo-controlled phase III trial of chemotherapy with or without bevacizumab in patients with platinum-sensitive recurrent epithelial ovarian, primary peritoneal, or fallopian tube cancer. *J Clin Oncol* 2012;30(17):2039–2045.

190. Coleman RL, Brady MF, Herzog TJ, et al. Bevacizumab and paclitaxel-carboplatin chemotherapy and secondary cytoreduction in recurrent, platinum-sensitive ovarian cancer (NRG Oncology/Gynecologic Oncology Group study GOG-0213): a multicentre, open-label, randomised, phase 3 trial. *Lancet Oncol* 2017;18(6):779–791.

191. Bubis LD, Davis L, Mahar A, et al. Symptom burden in the first year after cancer diagnosis: an analysis of patient-reported outcomes. *J Clin Oncol* 2018;36:1103–1111.

192. Whitney RL, Bell JF, Tancredi DJ, et al. Hospitalization rates and predictors of rehospitalization among individuals with advanced cancer in the year after diagnosis. *J Clin Oncol* 2017;35(31):3610–3617.

193. Burstein HJ, Krilov L, Aragon-Ching JB, et al. Clinical cancer advances 2017: annual report on progress against cancer from the American Society of Clinical Oncology. *J Clin Oncol* 2017;35(12):1341–1367. doi:10.1200/JCO.2016.71.5292.

194. Hwang TJ, Franklin JM, Chen CT, et al. Efficacy, safety, and regulatory approval of food and drug administration-designated breakthrough and non-breakthrough cancer medicines. *J Clin Oncol* 2018;36:1–10. doi:10.1200/JCO.2017.77.1592.

195. Saluja R, Arciero VS, Cheng S, et al. Examining trends in cost and clinical benefit of novel anticancer drugs over time. *J Oncol Pract* 2018;14(5):e280–e294. doi:10.1200/JOP.17.00058.

196. Verstappen CC, Heimans JJ, Hoekman K, et al. Neurotoxic complications of chemotherapy in patients with cancer: clinical signs and optimal management. *Drugs* 2003;63(15):1549–1563.

197. Nakane M. Neurotoxicity and dermatologic toxicity of cancer chemotherapy [in Japanese]. *Gan To Kagaku Ryoho* 2006;33(1):29–33.

198. Visovsky C. Chemotherapy-induced peripheral neuropathy. *Cancer Invest* 2003;21(3):439–451.

199. Goetz MP, Erlichman C, Loprinzi CL. Pharmacology of endocrine manipulation. In: DeVita VT, Rosenberg SA, eds. *Cancer: Principles and Practice of Oncology*. 7th ed. Philadelphia: Lippincott Williams & Wilkins; 2006:457–466.

200. Hoppe RT, Advani RH, Bierman PJ, et al. Hodgkin disease/lymphoma. Clinical practice guidelines in oncology. *J Natl Compr Canc Netw* 2006; 4(3):210–230.

201. Hennessy BT, Hanrahan EO, Daly PA. Non-Hodgkin lymphoma: an update. *Lancet Oncol* 2004;5(6):341–353.

202. Maloney DG. Immunotherapy for non-Hodgkin's lymphoma: monoclonal antibodies and vaccines. *J Clin Oncol* 2005;23(26):6421–6428.

203. Weingart O, Rehan FA, Schulz H, et al. Sixth biannual report of the Cochrane Haematological Malignancies Group—focus on non-Hodgkin lymphoma. *J Natl Cancer Inst* 2007;99(17):E1.

204. Muss HB. Breast cancer and differential diagnosis of benign lesions. In: Golgman L, Ausiello D, eds. *Cecil Textbook of Medicine*. 23rd ed. Philadelphia: WB Saunders; 2008:1501–1510.

205. Guarneri V, Conte PF. The curability of breast cancer and the treatment of advanced disease. *Eur J Nucl Med Mol Imaging* 2004;31(suppl 1): S149–S161.

206. Ramirez AJ, Towlson KE, Leaning MS, et al. Do patients with advanced breast cancer benefit from chemotherapy? *Br J Cancer* 1998;78(11): 1488–1494.

207. Noronha V, Joshi A, Patil VM, et al. One-a-week versus once-every 3-weeks cisplatin chemoradiation for locally advanced head and neck cancer: a phase III randomized noninferiority trial. *J Clin Oncol* 2017;36:1064–1072. doi:10.1200/JCO.2017.74.9457.

208. Garden AS, Harris J, Vokes EE, et al. Preliminary results of Radiation Therapy Oncology Group 97-03: a randomized phase ii trial of concurrent radiation and chemotherapy for advanced squamous cell carcinomas of the head and neck. *J Clin Oncol* 2004;22(14):2856–2864.

209. Robbins KT, Kumar P, Harris J, et al. Supradose intra-arterial cisplatin and concurrent radiation therapy for the treatment of stage IV head and neck

squamous cell carcinoma is feasible and efficacious in a multi-institutional setting: results of Radiation Therapy Oncology Group Trial 9615. *J Clin Oncol* 2005;23(7):1447–1454.

210. Magné N, Marcy PY, Chamorey E, et al. Concomitant twice-a-day radiotherapy and chemotherapy in unresectable head and neck cancer patients: a long-term quality of life analysis. *Head Neck* 2001;23(8):678–682.

211. Markman M. The use of chemotherapy as palliative treatment for patients with advanced ovarian cancer. *Semin Oncol* 1995;22(suppl 3):25–29.

212. Fung-Kee-Fung M, Oliver T, Elit L, et al. Optimal chemotherapy treatment for women with recurrent ovarian cancer. *Curr Oncol* 2007;14(5): 195–208.

213. Doyle C, Crump M, Pintilie M, et al. Does palliative chemotherapy palliate? Evaluation of expectations, outcomes, and costs in women receiving chemotherapy for advanced ovarian cancer. *J Clin Oncol* 2001;19(5): 1266–1274.

214. Bunn PA, Kelly K. New chemotherapeutic agents prolong survival and improve quality of life in non-small cell lung cancer: a review of the literature and future directions. *Clin Cancer Res* 1998;5:1087–1100.

215. Clegg A, Scott DA, Sidhu M, et al. A rapid and systematic review of the clinical effectiveness and cost-effectiveness of paclitaxel, docetaxel, gemcitabine, and vinorelbine in non-small-cell lung cancer. *Health Technol Assess* 2001;5(32):1–195.

216. Khuri FR. Docetaxel for locally advanced or metastatic non-small-cell lung cancer: current data and future directions as front-line therapy. *Oncology (Williston Park)* 2002;16(suppl 6):53–62.

217. Adelstein DJ. Palliative chemotherapy for non-small cell lung cancer. *Semin Oncol* 1995;22(suppl 3):35–39.

218. Greer JA, Pirl WF, Jackson VA, et al. Effect of early palliative care on chemotherapy use and end-of-life care in patients with metastatic non-small-cell lung cancer. *J Clin Oncol* 2011;30:394–400.

219. Pelley RJ. Role of chemotherapy in the palliation of gastrointestinal malignancies. *Semin Oncol* 1995;22(suppl 3):45–52.

220. Poon MA, O'Connell MJ, Moertel CG, et al. Biochemical modulation of fluorouracil: evidence of significant improvement of survival and quality of life in patients with advanced colorectal carcinoma. *J Clin Oncol* 1989;7(10):1407–1417.

221. Ajani JA, Moiseyenko VM, Tjulandin S, et al. Quality of life with docetaxel plus cisplatin and fluorouracil compared with cisplatin and fluorouracil from a phase III trial for advanced gastric or gastroesophageal adenocarcinoma: the V-325 Study Group. *J Clin Oncol* 2007;25(22):3210–3216.

222. Michael M, Hedley D, Oza A, et al. The palliative benefit of irinotecan in 5-fluorouracil-refractory colorectal cancer: its prospective evaluation by a Multicenter Canadian Trial. *Clin Colorectal Cancer* 2002;2(2):93–101.

223. Smith JJ, Garcia-Aguilar J. Advances and challenges in treatment of locally advanced rectal cancer. *J Clin Oncol* 2015;33(16):1797–1808 doi:10.1200 /JCO.2014.60.1054.

224. Yip D, Karapetis C, Strickland A, et al. Chemotherapy and radiotherapy for inoperable advanced pancreatic cancer. *Cochrane Database Syst Rev* 2006;(3):CD002093.

225. Sultana A, Smith CT, Cunningham D, et al. Meta-analyses of chemotherapy for locally advanced and metastatic pancreatic cancer. *J Clin Oncol* 2007;25(18):2607–2615.

226. Tannock IF, Osoba D, Stockler MR, et al. Chemotherapy with mitoxantrone plus prednisone or prednisone alone for symptomatic hormone-resistant prostate cancer: a Canadian randomized trial with palliative endpoints. *J Clin Oncol* 1996;14(6):1756–1764.

227. Tannock IF, de Wit R, Berry WR, et al. Docetaxel plus prednisone or mitoxantrone plus prednisone for advanced prostate cancer. *N Engl J Med* 2004;351(15):1502–1512.

228. Shelley M, Harrison C, Coles B, et al. Chemotherapy for hormone-refractory prostate cancer. *Cochrane Database Syst Rev* 2006;(4):CD005247.

229. Morris MJ, Rumble RB, Basch E, et al. Optimizing anticancer therapy in metastatic non-castrate prostate cancer: American Society of Clinical Oncology clinical practice guideline. *J Clin Oncol* 2018;36:1–21. doi:10.1200 /JCO.2018.78.0619.

230. Kunapareddy GC, Hooley J, Varella L, et al. Implementation of an interdisciplinary care team to create individualized care plans for high risk oncology patients: a model to decrease aggressiveness of care at the end of life and improve cost effectiveness of care. *J Clin Oncol* 2017;35 (31_suppl):171. doi:10.1200/JCO.2017.35.31_suppl.171.

231. Wiesenthal A, Goldman DA, Korenstein D. Impact of palliative medicine involvement on end-of-life services for patients with cancer with in-hospital deaths. *J Oncol Pract* 2017;13(9):e749–e759. doi:10.1200 /JOP.2016.019356.

232. Overmoyer BA. Chemotherapeutic palliative approaches in the treatment of breast cancer. *Semin Oncol* 1995;22(suppl 3):2–9.

233. Young DF, Posner JD. Nervous system toxicity of chemotherapeutic agents. In: Vinken TJ, Bruyn GW, eds. *Handbook of Clinical Neurology*. Amsterdam, The Netherlands: North Holland Publishing Company; 1980:91–129.

234. Solomon L. Drug-induced arthropathy and necrosis of the femoral head. *J Bone Joint Surg Br* 1973;55(2):246–261.

235. Rotstein J, Good RA. Steroid pseudorheumatism. *AMA Arch Intern Med* 1957;99(4):545–555.

236. Shapiro CL, Moriarty JP, Dusetzina S, et al. Cost-effectiveness analysis of monthly zoledronic acid, zoledronic acid every 3 months, and monthly denosumab in women with breast cancer and skeletal metastases: CALGB 70604 (Alliance). *J Clin Oncol* 2017;35(35):3949–3955. doi:10.1200 /JCO.2017.73.7437.

237. Van Poznak C, Somerfield MR, Barlow WE, et al. Role of bone-modifying agents in metastatic breast cancer: an American Society of Clinical Oncology—Cancer Care Ontario Focused Guideline Update. *J Clin Oncol* 2017;35(35):3978–3986.

CHAPTER 49

Cancer Pain in Children

ROY L. KAO, LONNIE ZELTZER, and **JACQUELINE CASILLAS**

Overview of Childhood Cancer

EPIDEMIOLOGY

Worldwide, cancer is diagnosed in approximately 300,000 children under age 20 years each year, and childhood cancer contributes to 80,000 deaths per year.[1] In the United States, almost 16,000 cases of cancer are diagnosed each year in children aged birth to 19 years, contributing to almost 2,000 deaths per year.[2] As recently as the 1970s, a diagnosis of cancer during childhood was considered a uniformly fatal disease. However, through enrollment in clinical trials available through cooperative pediatric oncology groups, as well as advances in supportive care, 5-year overall survival rates in childhood cancer are now over 80% in the United States.[3] The 12 major diagnostic categories of childhood cancer in The International Classification of Childhood Cancers, third edition (ICCC-3) include (1) leukemias and myeloproliferative and myelodysplastic diseases, (2) lymphomas, (3) central nervous system (CNS) neoplasms, (4) neuroblastoma and other peripheral nervous cell tumors, (5) retinoblastoma, (6) renal tumors, (7) hepatic tumors, (8) malignant bone tumors, (9) soft tissue and other extraosseous sarcomas (e.g., rhabdomyosarcoma), (10) germ cell tumors, (11) other malignant epithelial neoplasms and malignant melanomas (e.g., thyroid and nasopharyngeal carcinomas), and (12) other unspecified malignant neoplasms.[4] Certain types of cancer are more common in specific age groups of children. For example, acute leukemias, neuroblastoma, and renal tumors are more common in the younger age groups (ages 2 to 6 years), whereas the malignant bone tumors and lymphomas are more common during the adolescent years.

TREATMENT

The dramatic improvements in overall survival in childhood cancer are due to better supportive care and use of aggressive, multimodal treatment strategies combining chemotherapy, radiation, surgery, and/or hematopoietic stem cell transplant (HSCT). In addition, protein kinase inhibitors, monoclonal antibodies, and other targeted therapies have become part of standard therapy in some diseases.[5] Because the majority of pediatric cancer centers are participants in cooperative group clinical trials, children with cancer are often treated uniformly through the use of internationally available, standardized treatment protocols. There are "roadmaps" that are followed by the treating pediatric oncologists and communicated to the family and patient so that they know when to expect the next cycle of chemotherapy, including when the next invasive procedure can be anticipated to occur. As a result, there may be certain periods of higher anxiety, resulting in greater pain for pediatric cancer patients during the cancer treatment continuum as they anticipate the upcoming procedures. However, with careful planning, an effective pain management regimen can be developed and implemented.

SURVIVORSHIP

The end result of these aggressive treatment regimens for pediatric cancer patients is a success story for the 21st century. The current estimated survival rate for a pediatric cancer patient is 80%. The current number of survivors within the United States is over 370,000.[2,3] However, despite these advances, there continues to be a high risk for the development of chronic health conditions (late effects) years after the cancer treatment is completed. Complications of treatment include risk for second malignant neoplasms, cardiac and/or pulmonary dysfunction, skeletal problems, and neurocognitive deficits.[6] There is nearly a 75% risk of childhood cancer patients having a chronic health problem by 30 years postdiagnosis.[7] As the population of childhood cancer survivors continues to grow, it is important to be familiar with the unique challenges faced both during and after completion of treatment for cancer during childhood.

Pain in Children: How Does This Differ from That in Adults?

The model of pain for the adult population is a comprehensive one consisting not only of a physical domain but also psychological and social domains—the biopsychosocial model. In children, the biopsychosocial model of pain is more complex because the developmental level of the child needs to be considered. Childhood is a period in which there are complex and rapid neurodevelopmental changes occurring from birth to young adulthood. Children grow and develop through five stages of development: (1) infancy, (2) toddlerhood, (3) preschool period, (4) school-age period, and (5) adolescence. These levels of development are important because they directly impact the assessment and management of pain in children. For example, it was previously believed that newborns and infants could not experience pain because of immature neurologic systems and only as the child developed could pain be experienced. However, ongoing basic research has dispelled this myth, and newborns and infants can experience pain and mount a stress response to noxious stimuli. Furthermore, a noxious stimulus transmitted through neural afferent systems to a newborn brain may even be experienced as more painful than for an adult because the pain inhibitory system is not fully developed at birth.

INFANTS–PRESCHOOL

From birth through early childhood, a normal developmental assessment evaluates five main areas: gross motor skills, fine motor skills, language skills, personal/social skills, and cognitive skills. Changes occurring in these areas impact the pain assessment and emotional response of the child to the painful stimuli. For example, the language skills of a 2-year-old include a 50-word vocabulary and 2-word sentences. During this period, if the child is unable to effectively communicate his or her pain sensation and his or her pain is inadequately treated, there can be more fear and anxiety with each subsequent painful procedure. One year later, at 3 years of age, there is an expected 250-word vocabulary, 3-word sentences, and speech is intelligible to strangers 75% of the time. This child may be able to more effectively communicate with his or her parents and doctors and have a treatment for the pain initiated more promptly, a factor related to these enhanced communication skills that can serve to decrease anxiety for future procedures.

SCHOOL AGE–ADOLESCENCE

A school-age child will have a progressive ability to effectively communicate with the health care team. In turn, the providers must clearly communicate with the child about their treatment plan in order to minimize the anxiety children can experience from medical interventions. During adolescence, normal development of increasing desire for autonomy necessitates direct communication by the health care team, not only with parents but also directly with the adolescent based on the adolescent's desire for independent decision making (when possible). However, in all levels of normal development, the impact of illness can cause a pediatric patient to regress and become more dependent on his or her parents to support physical and emotional needs, with parents often providing the primary input to the health care team about children's pain and effectiveness of pain management. When possible, it is always helpful for the health care team to also attempt to get the child or adolescent's self-report of pain.

Pediatric Cancer Pain

The vast majority of children with cancer do not have a chronic medical condition at the time of diagnosis and therefore have not experienced chronic or recurrent episodic pain. Instead, they have mainly interfaced with the health care system for well-child checks with the associated immunization schedules and for acute, intermittent self-limiting infections or minor injuries. Thus, it is not surprising that the diagnosis and rapid initiation of treatment of cancer can overwhelm a child with fear and anxiety because of the number of invasive, painful medical procedures that are required, but for which the child is not psychologically prepared. In addition, acute pain associated with the first medical procedure at the time of diagnosis can set expectations of pain to be experienced by the child for all future procedures. Studies have demonstrated that even posttraumatic stress symptoms can be experienced by childhood cancer survivors due to memory recall of invasive procedures during treatment and that these painful memories continue beyond the treatment into the survivorship period.[8]

EPIDEMIOLOGY OF PEDIATRIC CANCER PAIN

Pain is a prevalent symptom accompanying pediatric cancer. Many patients (49% to 62%) with pediatric cancer have pain as a presenting symptom at diagnosis, with many of these patients having pain as the sole presenting symptom of their cancer.[9–11] Pain is often present for several months prior to diagnosis.[9] Using surveys during treatment, Miser et al.[12] found nonprocedural pain was prevalent for 54% of inpatients and 26% of outpatients in a single center. A national study in Germany by Zernikow et al.[13] found 15%, 28%, 50%, and 58% of patients diagnosed with cancer to be in pain at time of, within 24 hours, within 7 days, or within 28 days of interview, respectively. This is corroborated by Fortier et al.[14] who used a daily diary to show that 53.3% of children diagnosed with cancer had chronic or recurrent pain, with 40% of children requiring at least one dose of analgesic over the 14-day study period. Pain is more prevalent in pediatric inpatients with cancer versus outpatients (84% vs. 35%) and most prevalent in children with solid tumors (63%) versus leukemia (44%), lymphoma (27%), or CNS tumors (50%).[15]

In contrast to findings in adults, pain in children undergoing treatment for cancer was predominantly caused by antineoplastic treatments and procedures, rather than from the disease itself.[10,11,13,16–18] In one study, 49% of children stated that treatment-related pain was the most severe problem, followed by 38% of children for procedure-related pain, and finally 13% for disease-related pain.[10] Disease-related pain generally becomes less prevalent over time.[9,11,12] The difference in etiology between adult and pediatric cancer pain reflects differing cancer diagnoses and treatment strategies for adult and pediatric cancers. Although pediatric cancers are often rapidly proliferating mesenchymal tumors or leukemia and thus cause

pain at diagnosis, many are also responsive to an aggressive combination of intravenous and intrathecal chemotherapeutic agents, surgery, and/or radiation, which all can lead to painful therapy-related pain. In contrast, adult cancers are often slow-growing epithelial tumors which are often treated with less aggressive therapies.[13]

Increased pain prevalence is reported for certain groups of patients. Among children with acute lymphoblastic leukemia (ALL), pain is reported by the majority of patients throughout the first year of treatment, improving somewhat over time.[19,20] In children with progressive, recurrent, or nonresponsive cancer, pain prevalence is 49%, rising to 62% in the last 12 weeks of life. Furthermore, high-distress pain prevalence in the same group of children is 39%, rising to 58% in the last 12 weeks of life.[21] By the last month of life, other studies show pain prevalence at 82%, with about half of all patients suffering "a great deal" or "a lot" from the pain.[22]

UNDERTREATMENT AND IMPACT OF PEDIATRIC CANCER PAIN

Undertreatment of pain continues to be a concern in pediatric cancer, both in the inpatient setting[23–25] and in the outpatient and home settings.[14,19] Pain in these settings continues to be common, underrecognized, and undertreated. At the end of life, treatment of pain is often unsuccessful.[22]

Barriers to adequate pain control in pediatrics include lack of pain documentation and assessment[18,25,26] and clinical staff reluctance to prescribe or administer analgesics[25] whether because of fear of addiction[27] or inadequate pain management knowledge.[27,28] Some clinicians hold the mistaken belief that infants and children are less sensitive to pain.[27] Physicians have been found to underestimate children's pain as reported by the patient or the parent.[29] Other common misconceptions include beliefs that a significant percentage of children overreport pain, that increases in morphine dose beyond a certain amount will not produce increased pain relief, and that respiratory depression is likely to happen in patients who have received opioids for months.[30–32] Breakthrough pain, defined as episodes of medium to severe pain on a background of otherwise controlled pain, can occur suddenly. It can last seconds to minutes, often too fast for many "as-needed" medications to work effectively.[23]

In the home setting, barriers to adequate analgesia may include caregiver misconceptions regarding children's pain, fears of side effects of analgesic use, as well as avoidance of analgesic use.[33,34] Two studies in different cultural contexts have found that many parents reported believing that a child always tells his or her parent when he or she is in pain.[32,35]

In adolescents, patient attitudes may also act as barriers to effective treatment of pain. Similarly to adults, adolescents are concerned about addiction, development of tolerance, and analgesic side effects as well as losing their ability to monitor health-related bodily changes. Some also hold the fatalistic belief that cancer pain is unavoidable. Some attitudes are more uniquely seen in this age group and stem from developmental needs for autonomy and control, including concerns about how reporting pain may lead to undesirable tests and restrictions in social activities. They are also concerned about not being involved in treatment decisions. Thus, active listening is important when reviewing adolescents' pain symptoms.[36,37]

Finally, system-based barriers exist, including limits to access to opioids and accessibility of pain and palliative care specialists, especially for pediatric populations and resource-poor areas.[38–40]

Pain, especially from medical procedures, leads to fear and anxiety.[41] Younger children receiving medications to control pain prior to a procedure experienced not only less pain with each procedure but also had consistently lower pain scores for subsequent medical procedures.[42] Procedure-related pain contributes to posttraumatic stress symptoms in survivorship.[43] Pain with moderate to severe distress was associated with a significant worsening in total health-related quality of life (HRQOL) scores as well as scores in specific domains related to physical, emotional, and school HRQOL.[44] Adolescents with cancer, especially those experiencing severe pain, were significantly hindered in pursuing their personal goals, which are important to adolescent needs and their normal developmental trajectories.[45]

Evaluation of Pediatric Cancer Pain

Pain is a complex and subjective experience. Multiple components of the nervous system are involved in pain transmission, processing, and modulation, including sensory neurons, spinal cord, somatosensory cortex, prefrontal cortex, insula, and anterior cingulate cortex.[46] This is mirrored by the multidimensional nature of pain associated with cancer, where the cancer pain experience is affected by the complex interplay of biologic, psychological, and sociocultural domains of illness.[47] For example, many children with oral mucositis experience mouth and throat pain. This results in severe emotional turmoil for the children, psychological distress for the parents, cognitive dilemmas balancing eating and pain, oral care and discomfort, and an increased need for distraction and psychological support.[48] Thus, we advocate for a biopsychosocial approach to the evaluation of pain in children with cancer. In addition, because of the complexities of the physical, psychological, sociocultural, and spiritual contributors to pain in any one patient, a comprehensive pain evaluation is ideally accomplished by a holistic evaluation and discussion among a multidisciplinary team including a pediatric pain specialist, pediatric oncologist, bedside nurse, social worker, psychologist, chaplain, child life specialists, and other rehabilitative and expressive art therapists, with the patient and family unit at the center.

HISTORY AND PHYSICAL EXAM

The importance of eliciting and listening to all details of the pain narrative of the pediatric patient with cancer is critical. Again, what is asked of the child and expected of the child is dependent on his or her developmental level. For the school-age child or adolescent, the pain assessment should occur early on, where there is the support of family, and in a nonthreatening environment. At tertiary care centers that care for large numbers of pediatric cancer patients, child life services are available and can serve as another resource to help elucidate a clear description of the pain narrative. For the infant or toddler, the health care provider is dependent on the parents' narratives of the painful experience because they are the source of safety and communication for the young child.

Across the entire developmental continuum of pediatrics, the physical examination, including close observation of the child and the family dynamic, is critical to provide additional information about physical factors that contribute to the experience of pain. During the history and physical examination, it is also critical for the clinician to recognize and identify psychosocial factors, such as parental fear or anxiety, which can also increase the suffering associated with pain for the pediatric patient with cancer.

SENSORY EXPERIENCE—SELF-REPORT

The evaluation of pain often begins with assessment of its sensory experience. The PQRST method is a useful method of assessing the dimensions of the pain sensory experience in many children.[49,50] PQRST includes asking about *Palliating/provoking* factors, *Quality* descriptors of the pain, *Radiation* of the pain to other parts of the body, *Site/symptoms/severity* of the pain, and *Timing/triggers*. Different characteristics may suggest

neuropathic pain versus nociceptive pain and may help narrow down sources of pain or may suggest different treatment modalities.

The most commonly evaluated sensory dimension is pain intensity, and several one-dimensional self-report scales are available. The Pieces of Hurt/Poker Chip Tool,[51] Oucher,[52] Faces Pain Scale–Revised,[53] and the Visual Analogue Scale[54] have been extensively validated and have been recommended by several systematic reviews[55–57] as the best measures for clinical practice and research. These tools have been validated for a wide range of pediatric age groups—Pieces of Hurt for 3 to 18 years, Oucher for 3 to 12 years, Faces Pain Scale–Revised for 4 to 16 years, and the Visual Analogue Scale for at least 7 years and older. For children 8 years and older, the 11-point numerical rating (0 to 10) is recommended, when possible.[58] Specific one-dimensional self-report tools are also available for pain location[59,60] and to describe the temporal dimension of pain.[61]

SENSORY EXPERIENCE—OBSERVATION

Observing a patient's behaviors can be useful when self-report is not available or unreliable. In young children, facial expressions, body posture, cries, and inconsolability are commonly associated with acute pain. Observations of physiologic indices such as heart rate, oxygen saturation, or sweating can also be useful in acute pain and are sometimes used in behavior scales for critically ill patients.

These observations are reflected in observational pain intensity scales which can be employed in lieu or in addition to self-report scales. Patients whose pain might need to be measured with an observational (i.e., behavioral) scale might be too young (e.g., below 4 years of age); too distressed; impaired in their cognitive or communication abilities; very restricted by bandages, surgical tape, mechanical ventilation, or paralyzing drugs; or whose self-report ratings are considered to be exaggerated, minimized, or unrealistic due to cognitive, emotional, or situational factors. A systematic review by von Baeyer and Spagrud[62] recommends two scales for brief pain events and procedural pain (Face, Legs, Arms, Cry, and Consolability [FLACC][63] and Children's Hospital of Eastern Ontario Pain Scale [CHEOPS][64]), one scale for postoperative pain in the hospital (FLACC), one scale for postoperative pain at home (Parents' Postoperative Pain Measure [PPPM][65]), and one scale for critical care and ventilator patients (COMFORT Scale[66]).

However, many of these behaviors and observations normalize as the body adapts to persistent pain, and thus, different tools and observations may need to be utilized for persistent pain. Verbal expressions of pain continue to be an important indicator; however, lack of interest in surroundings, assuming pain-relieving postures, slowness and paucity of movement, and wariness at being moved become more prominent with persisting pain in young toddlers.[62] Recently, an observational scale incorporating the aforementioned observations was developed and validated specifically for persistent cancer pain in 2- to 6-year-olds (Hétero Evaluation Douleur Enfant [HEDEN]).[67]

In adolescents, nonverbal cues to persistent pain can be more subtle. In addition to decreased activity, adolescents with chronic pain have been described as exhibiting irritability and moodiness, social withdrawal, and sometimes uncooperativeness with treatments and medications, especially as a way to rebel and exert some bodily control when in pain.[50]

EMOTIONAL AND COGNITIVE EXPERIENCE

It is important to include emotional (affective) and cognitive (evaluative) measures when assessing children for pain. Affective measures reflect the emotional experience of pain. Evaluative measures reflect the child's ability to cope with his or her pain.

Toddlers with cancer who experience pain display specific pain behaviors but can also display psychomotor inertia and anxiety behaviors.[68,69] Anxiety behaviors include tenseness, hostility, crying easily, and wariness at being moved. On the opposite end of pain expression is withdrawal or psychomotor inertia. Behaviors that suggest this include resignation (lack of resistance), withdrawal, lack of expression, lack of interest in surroundings, and slowness and paucity of movement. This behavioral pattern is sometimes labeled "learned helplessness," "passive coping behavior," and "sickness behavior, such as fatigue and malaise." These depressive symptoms can be confused with actual depression, both for the observer as well as for the patient but may improve once pain is addressed.[69]

There are several multidimensional tools that bring together both questions about pain sensory experience as well as affective or evaluative measures. One of these, the Adolescent and Pediatric Pain Tool (APPT),[70,71] itself derived from the McGill Pain Questionnaire, has been validated in children 8 years and over and has been used in several studies of children with cancer.[18,19] It measures pain intensity, location, quality descriptors, temporal descriptors, and the evaluative and affective dimensions of pain. Affective words include words such as *awful*, *frightening*, and *suffocating*. Evaluative words include words such as *uncontrollable*, *horrible*, and *annoying*.

FUNCTIONAL AND QUALITY OF LIFE ASSESSMENT

Pain is but one of the symptoms that children experience while going through cancer. Fatigue, nausea/vomiting, poor appetite, and depression and anxiety are some of the most common, besides pain.[15] Symptoms often cluster and contribute toward overall decreases in HRQOL. For example, pain in children with cancer can often lead to decreased functioning and quality of life.[72,73] As physical activity or play activities can be exacerbated by pain from cancer, many patients instinctively avoid activities, a factor that leads to deconditioning and loss of function. This and the presence of pain itself can lead to depressive symptoms. Sleep is also intuitively affected by pain, leading to fatigue.

The National Institutes of Health (NIH)-sponsored Patient-Reported Outcomes Measurement Information System (PROMIS) initiative has developed a pain interference tool, evaluating the presence of psychological, social, and physical dysfunction secondary to pain.[74] The questionnaire asks patients if pain has hindered their function in regard to sleeping, attention, doing schoolwork, standing, walking, running, being happy, or being angry. Data from PROMIS shows strong positive correlations between pain interference and fatigue and pain interference and depressive symptoms and a strong negative correlation between pain interference and physical functioning-mobility.[75] Symptom cluster analyses show that pain in adolescents with cancer often co-occurs in the same patients as fatigue, sleep disturbance, and depression[76] or with nausea and vomiting.[77] Another cluster analysis study using PROMIS data in children with cancer showed that patients with high pain interference scores are more likely to also have high anxiety, depression, and fatigue scores.[78]

Based on these data, clinicians should assess the effect of the child's pain on their function in several different domains, including physical functioning and health; mood, coping, and psychological well-being; social and family relationships; and fatigue and sleep.

PAST PAIN-DIRECTED THERAPIES

Treatments for pain along with patient pain relief, functional improvement, and adverse effects should be noted in initial and ongoing evaluations of the patient. Past pain treatments, especially when associated with less than optimal control of pain, should be critically evaluated for appropriate medication or modality, dosing, route of administration, and both beneficial

and adverse effects on pain and function. Common reasons for pain treatment failure include intolerable adverse effects, too long of a dosing interval, too small of a dose, or inappropriate route of administration. In addition, not all pain treatments are equally effective for each patient, and thus, it is helpful to know the history of what has been attempted in the past.

CANCER HISTORY—DIAGNOSIS

Understanding the patient's cancer diagnosis, extent of disease, treatments, and prognosis is crucial to understanding the nature of pain that a patient with cancer might experience. Cancer, even in children, is a diverse set of diagnoses affecting almost any organ system or part of the body, and even each tumor type can present differently in each child. A cancer history for the pain clinician should start with understanding the patient's initial presentation and diagnosis. Some patients present asymptomatically, perhaps with a routine blood test, whereas some patients go for months or years with symptoms, often painful, while undergoing different blood tests, imaging studies, and even different surgical interventions before a diagnosis of cancer is finally made. Some patients carry congenital syndrome diagnoses or have undergone procedures, such as organ transplant, which predispose to the development of different cancers. Each of these situations brings a different set of pain experiences and pain expectations for patients undergoing cancer treatments and survivors.

The location and extent of neoplastic disease is an important consideration. Common solid tumor sites in children and adolescents include the brain and spinal cord, peripheral nervous system, abdominal organs (e.g., Wilms tumor, neuroblastoma, hepatoblastoma, germ cell tumors, some rhabdomyosarcomas), the genitourinary systems (testicular and ovarian germ cell tumors, rhabdomyosarcoma), the extremities (bone and soft tissue sarcomas, Langerhans cell histiocytosis), mediastinum (lymphomas, leukemia, teratoma), and the head and neck (rhabdomyosarcoma, lymphomas, retinoblastoma, neuroblastoma, Langerhans cell histiocytosis). By no means is this a comprehensive list, and other rare diagnoses have been known to present in any organ system.

Although some patients will have been diagnosed with a tumor which is localized to a specific organ or body part, other patients will have tumors which have locally extended to adjacent organs and body regions. Some common pediatric cancers are disseminated by nature, such as the leukemias and many lymphomas. These hematologic malignancies can involve not only bone marrow, lymph nodes, spleen, and mediastinum but also extramedullary sites such as the brain and CNS, testes, bones, and even skin. Other patients will have metastatic disease. Sites of metastasis vary for each diagnosis, but common sites of metastasis include adjacent lymph nodes, brain and CNS, lungs, liver, and bones. Each site of involvement can result in a potentially different set of pain symptoms for the patient.

CANCER HISTORY—TREATMENTS

Treatments vary considerably depending on the cancer diagnosis, location, extent, and other factors and bring along with them their own sets of pain and symptom experiences for each patient. The most common treatment plans for cancer in children include chemotherapy, surgery, and radiation. Radiation therapy, including external beam radiation, brachytherapy, and radioisotope therapy, and surgical resection have been mainstays of treatment for various pediatric tumors. Chemotherapy, in common usage, is often defined as any drug which works through the inhibition of mitosis and cell division to induce tumor cell death. Chemotherapy is commonly given orally, intravenously, intramuscularly, or intrathecally depending on the agent and treatment regimen.

Other drugs have also become part of the cancer armamentarium but work in other ways. Hormonal therapies, which are more common in adult cancers such as breast and prostate cancer, are less often used in pediatric cancers. Targeted therapies including monoclonal antibodies, small molecule inhibitors, and other immunotherapy agents, which have largely been developed for adult tumors, are becoming more and more frequently used in pediatric cancers as well. In addition, autologous or allogeneic hematopoietic stem cell infusions, sourced from bone marrow ("bone marrow transplant"), peripheral blood, or umbilical cord blood, can be used in different ways to replace a diseased hematopoietic system, rescue it from high-dose chemotherapy, and/or induce an immune response to a tumor (e.g., graft-versus-leukemia effect). Cellular therapies such as chimeric antigen receptor–T cell therapy build on the concept of graft-versus-tumor effect and have recently gained U.S. Food and Drug Administration (FDA) approval.[79]

Besides cancer-directed treatments, different supportive therapies are employed which can lead to pain. Stem cell factors such as granulocyte and granulocyte/monocyte colony-stimulating factors are used to decrease rates of febrile neutropenia and sepsis but can cause bone marrow expansion leading to pain. Medical devices and catheters are often placed to facilitate treatments. The most common of these include central venous access catheters such as tunneled catheters, peripherally inserted central catheters, and implanted port catheters; feeding tubes such as nasogastric tubes and percutaneous gastrostomy tubes; and intraventricular devices such as ventriculoperitoneal shunts and Ommaya reservoirs. Even in the presence of a central venous access catheter, peripheral intravenous catheter placements are sometimes necessary for certain imaging procedures and treatments.

Additionally, adverse effects of different cancer therapies are common and important to help understand the patient's cancer experience and identify possible sources of pain. Because of the cyclical nature of many treatment regimens, this knowledge can help the clinician anticipate possible pain for the patient in later cycles and plan appropriate pain preventive measures and treatments.

The patient's prognosis and—critically—the patient and family's understanding of prognosis and goals of treatment are also important considerations in evaluating pain in a patient with cancer. Treatment plans can be curative or palliative in intent, and it is important to elicit this intent in anticipating a patient's pain experience. Whereas curative treatments weigh the promise of long-term cure against possible short-term symptoms and other adverse effects, palliative treatments prioritize the preservation of a patient's quality of life.

PAST MEDICAL, PSYCHIATRIC, SOCIAL, AND SPIRITUAL HISTORY

Preexisting medical and psychiatric conditions are less common in children but play a role in their ability to cope, physically or psychologically, with cancer treatments. A patient and family's social situation and spirituality may also play a role in the support systems available in coping with both disease diagnosis and pain and symptom experience.

PROXY REPORTS

Whether or not a pediatric patient is able to provide a good history of his or her pain, it can be helpful to elicit observations and history from parents and other caretakers. Often, proxy report is the only source of information when patients are too young developmentally, in distress, or unwilling to provide this history. In addition, pediatric oncology patients are sometimes in the hospital so frequently, or for such an extended period of time, bedside nurses in oncology units and infusion centers will also have a longitudinal perspective on the patients and their current pain. On the other hand, the clinician needs to be mindful that proxy reports from parents sometimes differ from patient self-reports, especially when it comes to internalizing symptoms such as pain, fatigue, and emotional distress.[77,78] Parental anxiety can also affect their report of their child's pain.[79]

INTEGRATING DATA IN EVALUATION OF THE WHOLE CHILD

Some of the literature of pain evaluation focuses on pain intensity scales, which have been necessary for quantitating pain for the purposes of research and quality improvement efforts. In reality, however, each clinician faced with a patient experiencing pain integrates multiple data points from various sources in evaluating each patient. As an example, although self-report pain scores have classically been the gold standard in pain intensity assessment, recent observations and criticisms have led to a reevaluation of this dogma.[80] An isolated self-report pain score can have wide variability in meaning from patient to patient and can even be biased depending on situation, age, cognitive development, or experience. This leads to difficulty in translating overly simplistic pain scores directly into clinical decisions.

Instead, although pain is inherently a subjective experience and thus self-report is an important piece of information, bundled[81] or hierarchical[82] pain assessment approaches hint at ways to include other factors to inform clinical judgment. A bundled approach takes self-report, observation, proxy report, and other factors into account before making a global assessment of pain. One bundled approach, "CARES," uses the following factors: Context (evaluating for likely sources of pain), Assess pain expression (including self-report and observation of pain behaviors and functional limitations from pain), Risk (balancing adverse effects of treatment with the clinical situation of the patient), Emotional factors (considering developmental and psychological factors), and Sociocultural factors (understanding patient and family preferences).[81]

Hierarchical assessments take the bundled approach a step further, by arranging pain-modifying factors into a specified order. An example of this is a pain assessment guideline by Herr et al.,[82] developed for patients who cannot self-report pain reliably, including several groups which are often encountered in pediatric oncology—preverbal infants and toddlers, critically ill or unconscious patients, patients with intellectual disabilities, and some patients at the end of life. This particular hierarchical approach takes the following steps in order: (1) (attempt to) obtain self-report, (2) search for potential causes of pain, (3) observe patient behavior, (4) obtain proxy report, and (5) attempt an analgesic trial if pain behaviors continue despite providing for basic needs and comfort.

After consideration of all these factors, and a discussion with the child, caretakers, bedside providers, as well as the multidisciplinary team, a targeted treatment plan can then be developed. Reassessment after any analgesic trial is mandatory to further adjust the treatment plan to the patients' needs.

INCORPORATING TECHNOLOGY INTO ASSESSMENT

Finally, it is worth mentioning that there has been work done to develop technologies to address barriers of inadequate assessment and documentation of pain and patient reluctance to report pain. Phone text messaging has been used to improve patient compliance with reporting pain intensity, duration, and pain-related disability.[83] A smartphone application similarly has been shown to be feasible and perform consistently compared to traditional interviewer-administered questionnaires.[81,82] The NIH PROMIS can be used on multiple platforms. Studies have shown its feasibility and cross-cultural validity for measuring functional mobility, pain interference, fatigue, depression, anxiety, peer relationships, and anger.[84,85] Tablet applications not only improve patient reporting of pain and symptoms but can also incorporate basic cognitive and behavioral skills training through electronic games.[86]

Etiologies of Cancer Pain

Pain in children with cancer is often classified into one of four etiologies: (1) cancer- or disease-related pain, (2) treatment-related pain, (3) procedure-related pain, and (4) pain from other etiologies.[87]

DISEASE-RELATED PAIN
Bone Marrow Infiltration

The acute leukemias—ALL and acute myelogenous leukemia (AML)—are the most common diagnostic category of pediatric cancer.[88] The rapid proliferation of leukemic blasts within the bone marrow commonly results in the experience of diffuse bone pain. The clinical presentation of the bone pain, however, is variable depending on the age of the patient. Toddlers may present with a limp or inability to walk. A school-age child who is able to provide a pain narrative may report diffuse, poorly localized, total-body pain. An adolescent patient may have back pain that he or she associates with a sports injury and may localize the pain to a specific area in a long bone. Other pediatric leukemias include chronic myeloid leukemia (CML) and juvenile myelomonocytic leukemia (JMML) and in some situations can also present with bone pain. Some solid tumors, such as neuroblastoma, can metastasize to the bone marrow and can also present as a limp or, alternatively, as localized pain to a specific bony area.

Primary treatment of the underlying oncologic process is usually the most effective way to alleviate the pain, sometimes working within days of starting treatment. In the interim, standing or sometimes continuous opioids may sometimes need to be used for pain control. Nonsteroidal anti-inflammatory drugs (NSAIDs) should be avoided as they can exacerbate the risk of bleeding in a patient whose bone marrow may not be able to produce as many platelets, a condition which will soon be exacerbated by undergoing myelosuppressive chemotherapy. Acetaminophen can be helpful but may sometimes mask fever, which in a neutropenic or functionally neutropenic child may signal septicemia.

Brain and Spinal Tumors

CNS tumors are the second most common cancer in children and the most common group of solid tumors diagnosed during childhood. Headache is one of the most common initial presenting signs of brain tumor in children. In recent studies, 31% to 40% of children with a brain tumor had headache at symptom onset.[89,90] At diagnosis, headache is a prominent feature in 33% to 62%.[91,92] Headache is less common in children under the age of 3 years, likely because of both communication and expansile skull of the infant, and sometimes is noted as ear, face, or neck pain. Most commonly, headache is a result of mass effect of the brain tumor causing increased intracranial pressure. Other times, headache may be the result of a trigeminal or glossopharyngeal neuralgia caused by tumor compression of cranial nerves. To decrease the intracranial pressure and thereby treat the pain/headache for the child, different therapeutic approaches can be used.

For some brain tumors that are locally invasive without metastatic potential, such as low-grade gliomas (astrocytomas), complete surgical removal is the treatment of choice. For malignant brain tumors with metastatic potential, such as medulloblastoma, chemotherapy and radiation therapy are included in addition to the surgical treatment regimen. Not all primary resections of malignant brain tumors result in complete surgical removal of the tumor, so pain may persist due to residual disease. Often, the child will be started on a corticosteroid pulse pre- or postoperatively to decrease tumor- and surgery-associated cerebral edema. Temporary or permanent ventricular shunts or ventriculostomies are often used to alleviate intracranial pressure from the tumor and/or postoperative edema. If the child continues to have headache after surgical intervention, NSAIDs, such as ibuprofen, can be considered if there is no plan for chemotherapy and/or radiation therapy. A histamine H_2-receptor antagonist is used to inhibit gastric acid production, especially with concurrent corticosteroids. Otherwise, strong opioid therapy is the treatment of choice.

Benzodiazepines, such as midazolam, can also be used indirectly for the treatment of pain due to CNS tumors even though this class of medications does not have direct analgesic effect. Their mechanism of action for the treatment of pain in children includes decrease in anxiety, decrease in muscle spasm that may occur postoperatively, and facilitation of night sleep.[93] Postoperatively after the resection of the CNS tumor, the child may remain within the intensive care unit (ICU) because of the need for monitoring intracranial pressure. In this setting, benzodiazepines may be used as a continuous infusion or with frequent bolus dosing so that agitation is minimized.[94] Benzodiazepines are often used concomitantly with opioid analgesics in the ICU setting when significant postoperative pain is reported, observed, or expected. Antipsychotics, such as quetiapine, are also commonly used for agitation as are α-adrenergic agents such as clonidine.

Visceral Pain

The four major etiologies of visceral pain include (1) organ invasion with capsular wall stretching, (2) organ compression, (3) hollow organ obstruction (e.g., ureter or bowel), and (4) tumor regrowth within the organ or peritoneal cavity bleeding. In children, the abdominal tumors which are most commonly implicated in visceral pain are Wilms tumor (and other kidney tumors), neuroblastoma, abdominal germ cell tumors, rhabdomyosarcoma and other soft tissue sarcomas, lymphoma, and hepatic tumors (hepatoblastoma, hepatocellular carcinoma, sarcomas of the liver, and metastatic lesions of the liver). Although pain is a common complaint, many of these tumors may also present asymptomatically after incidental palpation of a mass by the parent or pediatrician, or through other symptoms, such as with Wilms tumor. As with bone pain in leukemia, treatment with chemotherapy, radiation, or resection of the diseased organ or part of the organ can eventually lead to a decrease in the child's pain. In the interim and in the postoperative period, opioids are the mainstay of treatment.

Bone Tumors

Primary malignant bone tumors, such as osteosarcoma or Ewing sarcoma, bone metastases from other malignancies, and Langerhans cell histiocytosis, and some benign tumors, such as giant cell tumor of the bone, can result in significant pain for the childhood cancer patient. Bone pain in cancer is a complex pain state involving nociceptive, neuropathic, and inflammatory elements.[95] Bone pain from osteosarcoma, for example, is due to both destruction of normal trabecular bone pattern from direct tumor invasion in combination with intense soft tissue inflammation from the periosteal new bone formation. Thus, the pain can often be very severe and often requires the use of opioids. NSAIDs could also be considered in the prechemotherapy setting. After the start of chemotherapy, however, NSAIDs should be used with caution as chemotherapy-related myelosuppression, and resultant thrombocytopenia may put the patient at a higher risk for bleeding.

Primary treatment of the tumor often provides the longest lasting effects on tumor-related pain from bone tumors. For osteosarcoma and Ewing sarcoma, neoadjuvant chemotherapy, followed by surgical resection and/or radiation, are the common treatment approaches. A small reduction in the size of the tumor may be enough to bring relief to the patient. Metastatic bone lesions may sometimes be treated symptomatically with radiation therapy, surgical decompression, or systemic chemotherapy depending on the disease.

In adults, osteoclast inhibition—using a bisphosphonate[96] or a receptor activator of nuclear factor kappa B (RANK)-ligand inhibitor[97]—has been shown to decrease fractures, spinal cord compression, and need for surgery or radiation therapy in the setting of bone metastasis from solid tumors such as breast and prostate cancer. Symptomatically, both treatments can delay the progression of moderate-to-severe pain in these adult patients.

Studies in children are lacking. There are encouraging results for bisphosphonates in pain control for benign cartilage tumors,[98] unresectable symptomatic benign bone tumors,[99] and Langerhans cell histiocytosis.[100] Newer agents, such as denosumab, a RANK-ligand inhibitor, have been shown to be useful for treatment of bone pain in giant cell tumor of the bone.[101] Children's Oncology Group studies on both zoledronic acid[102] and denosumab (ClinicalTrials.gov identifier NCT20470091) in metastatic or recurrent osteosarcoma have been undertaken, although effect on pain was not an aim of either study. Bisphosphonates have also been well tolerated in the treatment of children with hypercalcemia of malignancy.[103]

PROCEDURE-RELATED PAIN

A child undergoing cancer treatment will undergo many invasive, painful procedures. These include diagnostic or therapeutic procedures such as bone marrow biopsies, lumbar punctures (LPs), and surgery for tissue biopsy or tumor removal; venipunctures and subcutaneous port access (puncture) for diagnostic testing and/or treatment administration; placement of feeding tubes and urinary catheters; and placement of tunneled, peripherally inserted, or subcutaneous implanted "port" central venous access catheters. Even dressing changes (for central lines, surgical wounds) and suture and staple removal are a source of pain and distress for patients.[104]

Not only does a child newly diagnosed with cancer face many repeated painful stimuli but these pain-evoking procedures can also occur in a relatively short period of time (within a few days, weeks, or months). In addition to the physical pain that invasive procedures cause related to tissue damage by insertion of a needle or device through the skin and/or bone, the procedures themselves produce a great deal of psychological distress, including fear and anxiety.[105] This anxiety can result in a quick recall of the procedure that will impact future pain management for all future painful procedures. Children with ALL on current treatment protocols, for example, undergo LPs on a regular basis ranging from once or twice weekly during induction therapy to once every 3 months during maintenance therapy. The initial LPs that are done at time of diagnosis and for the initial induction treatment therefore set the stage for the pain anticipated and experienced for children during their 2 to 3 years of ongoing chemotherapy. Studies in leukemia patients have clearly demonstrated that children have accurate memories of their painful procedures. The more negative a memory a child had about a previous LP, the higher the likelihood of increasing distress related to future LPs.[106] Similar findings have been found for children undergoing other repeated painful procedures.[107,108]

There may also be specific groups of pediatric cancer patients that are at higher risk for distress due to painful, invasive procedures. Early studies have suggested that differences in reactions to painful stimuli can be attributed, at least in part, to a child's temperament, including the dimensions of distractibility and persistence.[109–112] Having a higher level of pain sensitivity (i.e., *pain perception*) is associated with greater anxiety and pain both prior to and during an LP procedure.[113] In addition, the psychological stress and corresponding coping experienced by the parent can affect the child's coping responses to the painful stressor. It has been shown that mothers of childhood cancer survivors do experience posttraumatic stress symptoms well into the survivorship period years after their child was treated for cancer.[114] Thus, given that a child is dependent on parents for both physical and emotional support throughout the cancer care continuum, a child can be at increased risk for distress due to pain if his or her caretaker is not able to soothe or provide a safe, consistent environment because of his or her own stress and maladaptive coping.

Topical and local therapies for pain control are important. More than 50% of children report pain during venipunctures or intravenous cannulation,[115] making these procedures an important target for pain prevention and control. Topical anesthetics are attractive because of the effectiveness without need for intravenous access and relative lack of systemic side effects. Eutectic mixture of lidocaine and prilocaine (eutectic mixture of local anesthetics [EMLA]) has been standard practice for decreasing procedural pain in children, available both in cream[116] and patch[117] forms. A warm lidocaine and tetracaine patch has also been shown to be effective for facilitating first-time needle procedure success.[118] If insufficient time is available to allow topical anesthetic creams to take effect, vapocoolant sprays may be helpful in decreasing pain and decreasing intravenous cannulation failures in children.[119] If anxiety is a major factor, low-dose oral midazolam has been useful in reducing fear and distress in younger children undergoing needle procedures such as subcutaneous port access.[120] High-dose acetaminophen[121] or morphine[122] did not have the same effect.

EMLA may also be useful by itself for LPs but only with those patients who undergo successful LP on their first attempt.[123] When used along with sedation, EMLA is useful in decreasing propofol use during LP.[124] When sedation is contraindicated, such as for patients with a large mediastinal mass with risk for airway compromise, topical and local anesthetic may be the only safe pain prevention strategy for these patients undergoing LP or bone marrow biopsy.

More and more pediatric oncology centers have instituted sedation and analgesia protocols for pediatric oncology procedures such as LPs and bone marrow biopsies and aspirations. Guidelines for pediatric procedural sedation have been published.[125,126] The desired level of sedation (e.g., anxiolysis vs. deep sedation vs. general anesthesia) depends on patient age and cognitive development and painfulness of the procedure, balanced with the risks of sedation (e.g., in setting of airway compression from a mediastinal mass).[127] Level of sedation also depends on the need for immobility, as there is a risk of introducing leukemic cells from blood into the spinal fluid with traumatic LP during induction therapy for ALL.[128]

The addition of intravenous fentanyl to intravenous propofol reduces movement, propofol dose, recovery time, and hypotension[129,130] and was preferred by families.[131] Intravenous ketamine had a superior effect on procedural pain and hemodynamic stability in comparison with an opioid alone[132]; however, ketamine/midazolam compared with propofol was associated with a longer recovery period.[133] Adding low-dose oral midazolam does not affect pain, fear, or distress levels whether given with or without intravenous ketamine prior to procedures for hematologic disease.[134]

A combination of these two approaches may be considered. Two studies showed the addition of ketamine (0.5 to 1 mg/kg) to fentanyl (1 μg/kg) and propofol (0.5 to 2 mg/kg induction followed by 0.5 to 1 mg/kg as needed) decreased propofol dose, rates of hypotension and hypoxia, and recovery time.[135,136] Ketamine may indeed replace the opioid, as a combination of ketamine, and propofol may decrease incidence of respiratory compression compared to propofol and alfentanil.[137]

Nitrous oxide (NO) may also be useful for pediatric procedural sedation, especially in children who might be willing to accept a mask, and for procedures which are not extremely painful. Delivery systems are being improved and are more available for procedural applications. Randomized controlled trials comparing other agents to NO are lacking,[138] but a recent study showed utility of NO in an outpatient setting for LPs.[139]

Postlumbar Puncture Headache

Even with adequate analgesia and sedation, LPs can sometimes be associated with postlumbar puncture headaches (PLPHA). These are characteristically postural headaches—worse with upright posture and improved in the supine position—occur within 6 to 72 hours of a LP, and last 3 to 15 days.[140] The mechanism is thought to be from ongoing leak of cerebrospinal fluid through the puncture site resulting in low cerebrospinal fluid pressure and volume. The incidence of PLPHA is rare in younger children and peaks in the fourth or fifth decade of life.[140,141] Preventive measures are mandatory. The most well-studied and recommended preventive measures include (1) using a needle no larger than 22 gauge,[142] (2) using a pencil point rather than a cutting point needle, and (3) orienting the needle bevel to be parallel, rather than perpendicular, to the long axis of the spinal column. Position of the patient in bed rest for 6 to 24 hours after LP does not appear to reduce the incidence of PLPHA compared to lifting of activity limitations after 0 to 1 hour.[143] Replacement of the stylette before withdrawal of the needle has also been recommended,[144] but application to pediatric cancer is limited because of the administration of intrathecal chemotherapy.

Placement of an epidural blood patch is one of the few therapies for PLPHA which has enough evidence to support its benefit.[145] Autologous blood is collected intravenously from the patient and injected into the epidural space near the site of the prior LP, working to tamponade the area of the previous dural puncture and facilitate sealing of the leak. Because autologous blood is used, this should be avoided if the patient has leukemia which is not yet in remission. Other therapies, such as intravenous or oral caffeine, intravenous or oral hydration, tramadol, acetaminophen, and ibuprofen, had either weak or no evidence supporting their use or lack of pediatric data.[143]

Postoperative Pain

Surgical biopsy is often necessary for diagnosis, and resection of tumors is a mainstay of therapy for most solid tumors. In addition, tunneled and subcutaneous "port" central venous access catheters are often placed surgically. These procedures, and the pain associated with them, are a commonly distressing part of the cancer experience in children. For abdominal surgery, an oncologic approach often precludes laparoscopic resection, and this also increases pain and recovery time. Joint guidelines from the American Pain Society, American Society of Regional Anesthesia and Pain Medicine, and several committees within the American Society of Anesthesiologists are available.[146] Recommendations include the consideration of using multimodal analgesia, using medications which target multiple mechanisms of action in the peripheral and CNS; physical modalities such as transcutaneous electrical nerve stimulation; cognitive behavioral modalities; nonopioid analgesics and gabapentin, intravenous ketamine, and opioids including patient-controlled analgesia (PCA); peripheral regional anesthesia; and neuraxial analgesia for major thoracic and abdominal procedures. More about pediatric postoperative pain management can be found in Chapter 50.

Phantom Limb Pain

Amputation and limb-salvage procedures may be used as surgical approaches to achieve local control of a bone tumor, and each can result in a chronic pain syndrome coined *phantom limb pain*. Phantom limb pain is experienced when the pediatric patient continues to have pain appearing to come from where the affected amputated limb used to be. There are multiple possible etiologies for the occurrence of phantom limb pain that include possible damage to the nerve endings in the surgical residual limb with abnormal regrowth postoperatively leading to abnormal painful discharges to spinal cord and brain. There may also be abnormalities in the CNS response to the loss of limb in which there may be loss of inhibitory sensory input from the amputated limb. Phantom limb pain is often severe and very challenging to treat.

Systematic analyses of studies to effectively treat chronic postoperative phantom limb pain have not clearly demonstrated an effective treatment option in randomized controlled trials.[147,148] Gabapentin and pregabalin, amitriptyline, ketamine infusion, and lidocaine infusion are some of the more commonly tested treatments. Central strategies, such as hypnotherapy, biofeedback, and acupuncture, aimed at altering metabolic activity in pain perception areas of the brain, such as the anterior cingulate cortical area, may be more effective than peripheral strategies or opioids (see Chapters 26 and 54). Mirror therapy, a nonpharmacologic therapy which aims to reverse postamputation maladaptive reorganization of the sensorimotor cortex, has been used to beneficial effect in the pediatric oncology population[149]; however, systematic reviews including a broader population of adults and children with different reasons for amputation show insufficient evidence of benefit for either mirror therapy or movement representation techniques.[150,151]

TREATMENT-RELATED PAIN

Bone Marrow Expansion

Filgrastim and pegfilgrastim (versions of granulocyte colony-stimulating factor), and sargramostim (granulocyte-macrophage colony-stimulating factor) are often used subcutaneously during chemotherapy treatment to raise neutrophil counts and reduce the number of episodes of febrile neutropenia in between cycles of myelosuppressive chemotherapy or during bone marrow engraftment after an HSCT. Alternatively, higher doses can be used in patients to mobilize and boost recovery of hematopoietic stem and progenitor cells for use later in autologous stem cell rescue after high-dose chemotherapy. One major adverse effect of these agents is bone pain secondary to a combination of bone marrow expansion, peripheral nociceptor sensitization to nociceptive stimuli, modulation of immune function, and a direct effect on bone metabolism.[152] A meta-analysis showed bone pain rates for filgrastim and its long-acting version, pegfilgrastim, to be similar, at around 25% to 50%.[153] As patients receiving colony-stimulating factors to prevent febrile neutropenia are by definition at risk for neutropenia and thrombocytopenia, NSAIDs should be avoided as well as around-the-clock acetaminophen to prevent masking of fever. As-needed acetaminophen and low-dose oral opioids are sometimes necessary to help patients manage this pain.

Mucositis

Mucositis may occur when chemotherapy is given alone, but certain treatments such as head and neck radiation, as well as high-dose chemotherapy in the setting of HSCT, can worsen and prolong mucositis.[154] After HSCT, there is often a longer period for stem cell recovery extending beyond the 7- to 10-day nadir occurring after chemotherapy exposure. The grading scale for describing the severity of oral mucositis established by the World Health Organization (WHO) ranges from mild, grade I mucositis, in which the oral mucosa is red and tender, to severe, grade IV mucositis in which the patient is unable to eat and maintain his or her own nutrition.[155] The severity of the mucositis often corresponds to the description of the severity of the pain by the patient. Grade I mucositis may only require bolus dosing of an opioid analgesic. In the high-dose chemotherapy and HSCT setting, however, mucositis pain often requires use of an opioid PCA given the chronicity of the pain (over a several week period) and the extensive tissue injury involving the entire gastrointestinal tract. This often precludes enteral analgesic therapies. An effective approach to PCA delivery of the opioid analgesic is to have a low basal rate that is augmented with demand dosing for breakthrough pain.[23] If demand dosing usage is frequent, resulting in a lockout of demand dose administration, then an increase in the basal rate is warranted. These patients may require several weeks' use of an opioid PCA because the pain from mucositis can be severe and occur over a prolonged time period while awaiting engraftment. However, when engraftment occurs and counts recover, the PCA can often be weaned off quickly. The caveat to this is that there may be withdrawal symptoms, including agitation and/or diarrhea, and a methadone taper should be considered.

Patients with head and neck cancers often will be treated with radiation to the head and neck area or concurrent chemoradiation and are thus at higher risk for severe oral mucositis in addition to other oral toxicities such as trismus, xerostomia, and taste loss caused by inclusion of the jaw, salivary glands, and tongue in radiation fields. These often present a major challenge to oromotor function, enteral nutrition management, and maintenance of quality of life. Mucosal erythema appears at around 10 Gy of radiation, with associated burning sensation and sensitivity to spicy foods. At 30 Gy, ulcers develop leading to opioid requirement and feeding difficulties, and then mucositis remains at its peak for at least 2 weeks following completion of radiation. Pain and symptoms of mucositis can persist for 8 weeks.[156]

Guidelines for the prevention of mucositis in children have been developed by the Pediatric Oncology Group of Ontario.[157] A similar guideline is available for adults and includes treatment options for mucositis.[158] Preventive measures with sufficient supportive evidence for both panel recommendations include oral cryotherapy, low-level light therapy (LLLT), and keratinocyte growth factor. Oral cryotherapy involves placing ice cubes or chips in the mouth continuously during a period of cytotoxic treatment, typically 30 to 60 minutes at a time, resulting in vasoconstriction in the oral mucosal surface and thus decreased exposure to chemotherapy. Cryotherapy significantly reduced severe oral mucositis in a pooled analysis of eight studies which reported on this outcome (RR 0.46, 95% confidence interval [CI] 0.30 to 0.71). There is, however, a lack of positive studies in children, and feasibility is limited to only chemotherapeutic agents with a short half-life given in a short infusion, as well as by the concern that ice may pose a risk of choking hazard in young children.

LLLT involves exposing oral mucosal tissues to a low-energy light source, which may have anti-inflammatory, wound-healing, and analgesic effects. Advantages include two studies which included children with positive results. Limitations for hospitals include acquiring LLLT machines and training. Overall severe mucositis was reduced (RR 0.37, 95% CI 0.20 to 0.67), as was severe pain (RR 0.26, 95% CI 0.18 to 0.37).[157] Finally, keratinocyte growth factor (e.g., palifermin) is an epithelial growth factor that works partly by thickening the oral mucosa. Severe oral mucositis was reduced with keratinocyte growth factor as well (RR 0.81, 95% CI 0.67 to 0.97), which is given for several days before and after mucositis-inducing chemotherapy.[157]

Other interventions, including filgrastim, glutamine, Traumeel S, topical vitamin E, chewing gum, oral chlorhexidine, sucralfate, and a preventive oral care protocol, were not effective in reducing mucositis. Additional recommendations from the adult guideline panel include PCA opioids for oral mucositis and benzydamine mouthwash in patients with head and neck cancer receiving moderate dose radiation therapy (up to 50 Gy) without concomitant chemotherapy. They also suggest transdermal fentanyl for oral mucositis due to high-dose chemotherapy, 2% morphine mouthwash for mucositis in patients receiving head and neck chemoradiation, 0.5% doxepin mouthwash for any oral mucositis, as well as systemic zinc supplementation for prevention of mucositis.[158] Again, studies in children are lacking

so their use should be limited to selected children and under expert guidance. Other topical treatments that have been used include honey[159] and aloe vera.[160] Honey has been used in other wound care settings to promote healing but requires irradiation to neutralize botulinum toxin spores and other microbes which may otherwise contraindicate their use in immunocompromised and very young children,[161] and further clinical trials would be needed to clarify its safety in these populations.

Neuropathic Pain
Pediatric cancer patients can experience neuropathic pain for a variety of reasons, including nerve invasion, inflammation of a nerve root due to the malignancy or infectious process, and/or from cancer treatment side effects. These etiologies include (1) chemotherapy-related peripheral neuropathies, such as with vincristine neurotoxicity; (2) neural compression or invasion by tumors, such as pelvic Ewing sarcomas; and (3) infection related, such as herpes zoster reactivation due to immune suppression. One common cause of chemotherapy-related peripheral neuropathy is vincristine, a vinca alkaloid used as an effective cytotoxic agent for many types of pediatric malignancies including leukemias, lymphomas, and various solid tumors. Vincristine binds to tubulin and inhibits microtubule formation and disrupts the formation of the mitotic spindle, which is thought to be one of the mechanisms by which it causes peripheral neuropathies, including jaw pain, leg pain, and abdominal pain.[162] In addition, direct injury of the nerve can occur with soft tissue sarcomas arising in the pelvis, such as Ewing sarcoma or rhabdomyosarcoma, and the child may present with complaints of abdominal pain, lower extremity weakness, and/or bladder and bowel dysfunction.

Assessment of chemotherapy-induced peripheral neuropathy is informed not just by the painful aspect, or even the sensory symptoms, but also by motor and autonomic symptoms; pin, vibration, and light touch sensation by exam; motor exam; and deep tendon reflexes. These are included in the pediatric Total Neuropathy Scale (TNS) and this can be included in the pain assessment.[163–165]

Besides vincristine, peripheral neuropathy is also associated with bortezomib, cisplatin, paclitaxel and other taxanes, and thalidomide.[166] Calcineurin inhibitors, such as tacrolimus and cyclosporine, often used after allogeneic HSCT, may also be associated with peripheral neuropathy. Newer agents including dinutuximab (aka ch14.18), a chimeric, monoclonal anti-GD2 antibody approved in the immunotherapy of neuroblastoma, can also be associated with neuropathic pain, specifically allodynia. In the phase 3 trial which led to its approval, grade 3 or 4 neuropathic pain was reported in 52% of patients receiving the drug,[167] typically occurring during the infusion and reported as abdominal pain, generalized pain, extremity pain, back pain, neuralgia, musculoskeletal chest pain, and/or arthralgia. Opioid analgesic premedication is usually given prior to start of the infusion, followed by continuous opioid infusion until 2 hours following the completion of the medication.[168] One study describes the use of dexmedetomidine in combination with hydromorphone for pain management during dinutuximab.[169] The pain is thought to be due to antibody binding to GD2 expressed on normal nerve cells. Another immunotherapy agent against neuroblastoma is being developed to avoid this adverse effect.[170]

PAIN FROM OTHER ETIOLOGIES
Infection
Patients undergoing immunosuppressive therapies such as chemotherapy, or those with decreased immunologic reserve, such as patients with leukemia, are susceptible to a myriad of infectious complications, many of which can be painful and involve almost any part of the body. An evaluation of pain in a patient with cancer must include evaluation for bacterial, fungal, or viral infections based on the patient's current level

of immunosuppression. Treatment of the primary infection and resolution of neutropenia lead to improvement in pain. In the meantime, analgesic therapy may be needed.

Of particular interest are herpes simplex viruses (HSV-1 and HSV-2) and varicella zoster virus (VZV). Primary HSV-1 infection is often asymptomatic in immunocompetent hosts but can commonly manifest as painful vesicles in the mouth, throat, or other parts of the body. HSV-2 has a tropism for the genital area. After primary infection, these viruses become latent in nerve cell nuclei. In immunocompromised hosts, however, primary infection can be disseminated, and reactivation of HSV and VZV infections is common and more severe, leading to substantial morbidity and in some cases mortality. HSV-1 seropositivity is also a strong risk factor for oral mucositis,[171] with reactivation contributing to as much as half of oral mucositis episodes[172] and greater mucositis severity[173] in HSV-1–seropositive children undergoing myelosuppressive chemotherapy.

VZV reactivation, also known as (herpes) zoster, often presents with painful lesions within a dermatomal distribution and severe postherpetic neuralgia, but immunocompromised patients are also at risk for cutaneous or visceral dissemination, retinal necrosis, and mortality. Zoster affects children with cancer at much higher rates than the general population, but this is improving with varicella immunization.[174,175]

HSV infections, and thus, a proportion of oral mucositis, can be treated and prevented with acyclovir.[176] VZV reactivation in a patient with cancer should also be treated with antivirals (e.g., acyclovir); however, additional analgesic therapy with acetaminophen and/or opioids is often needed for the acute neuritis associated with zoster, depending on severity. Postherpetic neuralgia can nevertheless develop despite antiviral therapy,[177] and persistent pain despite healed lesions can be treated with topical lidocaine or capsaicin on intact skin. Systemic therapy with gabapentinoids and tricyclic antidepressants may be considered to treat or attempt to prevent severe pain.[178]

Graft-versus-host Disease

Because of the intensity of treatment involved, pediatric cancer patients requiring HSCT as part of their treatment are considered a high-risk group of patients for the development of acute and chronic pain. Cancer diagnoses that may require HSCT, either allogeneic or autologous, for curative therapy include ALL, AML, myelodysplastic syndrome, and neuroblastoma. Pediatric cancer patients who have received HSCT have unique risk factors for the development of acute pain, including mucositis, graft-versus-host disease (GVHD), and tissue erosive infectious complications.[179] Thus, pain management is critical in the care of the HSCT patient and, if not treated adequately, can result in decreased quality of life.

GVHD is a unique complication of childhood cancer patients who undergo HSCT. GVHD occurs due to the host (recipient) cells appearing foreign to the engrafted hematopoietic stem cells. There are two forms of GVHD, consisting of acute and chronic GVHD. Acute GVHD occurs within the first 100 days of the HSCT, causing dermatitis, enteritis, and/or hepatitis. Acute GVHD can be clinically manifested by skin rash, right upper quadrant pain, and/or diarrhea and abdominal pain. The skin rash can range from mild erythema of the palms and soles of the feet to bullous desquamation in the severe form. Chronic GVHD typically occurs 100 days beyond the hematopoietic stem cell infusion and is thought to be an autoimmune process. Chronic GVHD primarily has skin manifestations that include scleroderma-type changes often accompanied by joint stiffness and immobility.

Bone Complications of Therapy

Pediatric cancer patients are at risk for decreased bone mineral density and painful and debilitating bone complications such as fractures and osteonecrosis. Risk factors which are commonly seen in patients treated for pediatric cancer include exposure to corticosteroids, methotrexate, skeletal radiation, hypogonadism and growth hormone deficiency from pituitary tumor or treatment, as well as long-term inactivity and suboptimal nutrition during treatment.[180,181] Severe osteonecrosis and most fractures are treated with surgical intervention, but nonsurgical treatments under investigation for osteonecrosis have included bisphosphonates and hyperbaric oxygen therapy.[182,183]

PAIN IN SURVIVORSHIP

As more children, adolescents, and young adults become long-term survivors of pediatric cancers, more is becoming known about their physical and mental health. Adult survivors of pediatric cancers are more likely to have chronic health conditions, some of them life threatening or painful.[7] A significant percentage of adult survivors of pediatric cancer also report poor physical or mental HRQOL.[184] Thus, it is not surprising that survivors of childhood cancers are much more likely to report pain than their siblings[185] and more likely to use prescription analgesics.[186] Cancer-related or cancer treatment–related pain still affected 21% of cancer survivors in the study. Predictors of recent pain attributed to pediatric cancer or its treatment in these studies include lower household income, divorced/separated/widowed status, lower educational attainment, and primary cancer diagnosis of bone cancer or soft tissue sarcoma. Risk factors for having been diagnosed with any pain condition, including headache, included age less than 3 years at diagnosis, female gender, minority race, single marital status, lower income, and unemployment.[185] Pain contributes negatively to quality of life in survivors. Survivors with pain were more likely to have comorbid internalizing and externalizing symptoms.[187] Thus, it is important to screen for and address pain in childhood cancer survivors and also important to take measures during initial treatment to prevent or moderate development of pain sensitization.

Management of Pain

Just as the assessment of pain in a pediatric patient with cancer ideally involves a multidisciplinary team, a multidisciplinary approach is also ideally employed in the management of pain in these patients. Anticipation of expected painful effects of cancer and its treatment, education of the parent and child, and prevention of procedural and therapy-related pain are paramount to improving the patient's cancer experience. A pain prevention plan could involve critically evaluating potentially painful procedures for their necessity.[104] It is also important to consider procedural sedation if indicated and consolidating painful procedures under one sedation if possible. Similarly to the strategy of antiemetic prophylaxis for emetogenic cancer treatments, the different interventions detailed in the following text can also be used for prevention of pain when pain is expected. A comprehensive approach incorporates this anticipatory guidance and prevention as well as physical, psychological, and pharmacologic approaches to treatment of the various pain syndromes in children with cancer. Prevention of or minimizing pain will reduce the likelihood of distressing pain memories that can impact future pain experiences.[188]

Pharmacologic Management of Cancer-Related Pain in Children

In 2012, the WHO[189] expanded guidelines on *Cancer Pain Relief and Palliative Care in Children*, now covering pharmacologic treatment of persisting pain in all children with medical illness with ongoing tissue damage or inflammation. The WHO now recommends a two-step approach to pharmacologic management of pain in this population. In this approach, acetaminophen (paracetamol) or an NSAID, such as ibuprofen, is given for mild pain, and strong opioids are given for moderate to severe pain. In previous guidelines, the WHO had recommended an intermediate step with weak opioids such as tramadol and codeine. However, because tramadol is generally not labeled for patients under 12 years, and codeine presents significant variability in response and toxicity related to CYP2D6 polymorphisms, this intermediate step has been removed from the pediatric recommendation. Several studies in adults[190,191] and the European Association for Palliative Care guidelines for treatment of cancer pain[192] are also supportive of this strategy.

Treatment of cancer-related pain in children should follow this two-step approach but with certain considerations. NSAIDs are known to cause temporary platelet dysfunction which can lead to an increased risk for bleeding. This may not be acceptable in the setting of bone marrow infiltration (such as with newly diagnosed leukemia) nor in the setting of bone marrow myelosuppression and resulting thrombocytopenia (such as with ongoing chemotherapy). In addition, prolonged NSAID use can result in renal injury, which can exacerbate cumulative renal insults from other chemotherapy and supportive care medications such as aminoglycosides. NSAIDs can also decrease renal clearance of toxic chemotherapy agents such as methotrexate.[193] Finally, NSAIDs are associated with gastric and duodenal ulcers, especially in combination with corticosteroids.[194] If given in combination with corticosteroids, a histamine H_2 receptor antagonist or proton pump inhibitor may be required to prevent gastroduodenal ulcerations and stomach discomfort.

For these reasons, acetaminophen is more commonly used than NSAIDs as a first-line treatment for mild pain in a child who has or is at risk of thrombocytopenia. This includes patients newly diagnosed with leukemia or other bone marrow infiltrating tumor as well as children undergoing chemotherapy. Acetaminophen is most effective at doses of 15 mg/kg every 6 hours.[195] It is also now available in the intravenous formulation for children not able to tolerate oral medications, but it can be costly. Acetaminophen, however, has its own limits, especially in the setting of liver dysfunction or failure.

Moreover, acetaminophen and ibuprofen are both used for their antipyretic effects as well. This can complicate the treatment of pain in patients with neutropenia (absolute neutrophil count <500 cells/μL). Because fever may be the earliest and only sign of a severe infection in a neutropenic patient, scheduled acetaminophen or NSAIDs may theoretically pose a risk for delayed recognition of an infection which can lead to sepsis or death. For this reason, these medications are usually dosed as needed ("PRN"), and persisting pain is treated with scheduled opioids.

Lastly, it should be emphasized that the two-step strategy does not necessarily preclude use of strong opioids as first-line therapy for moderate to severe pain. A randomized trial testing nonopioid analgesics against strong opioids as first-line therapy for moderate to severe pain in "terminal" adult cancer patients showed that patients started on strong opioids had better pain relief, fewer changes in therapy, greater reduction in pain, and greater satisfaction with treatment, without serious adverse events.[196]

The other principles advocated by WHO[189] guidelines are to treat pain "at regular intervals," "by the appropriate route," and "to the individual child."

- *At regular intervals*: Unless pain is truly intermittent or unpredictable, persisting pain should be treated at regular intervals, while monitoring for adverse effects, with the addition of "rescue doses" for intermittent and breakthrough pain.
- *By appropriate route*: Analgesia should be administered by the simplest, most effective, and least painful route. For most children, oral analgesics are the route of choice; however, intravenous, rectal, and subcutaneous routes

may be needed depending on the clinical situation. Of note, the rectal route is usually avoided in potentially immunocompromised children, including those receiving chemotherapy.
- *To the individual child*: Opioid analgesics should be titrated in collaboration with the patient to achieve the best possible analgesic effect with side effects acceptable to the patient.

Overview of Opioid Analgesia in Children

Strong opioids with the most evidence and clinical experience for pain in pediatric patients with cancer include morphine,[197] hydromorphone,[198] and fentanyl.[199] Other important strong opioids with less data in pediatric cancer patients include oxycodone, methadone, and buprenorphine.[200,201] PCA with morphine, hydromorphone, or fentanyl is also an effective option for pediatric patients as young as 5 years of age, depending on their level of cognitive development.[202–204]

There are several unique delivery systems of opioid analgesics which might prove useful in the pediatric cancer population to avoid the fear and pain associated with injections. Options for oral transmucosal delivery of fentanyl now include a lozenge/troche (Actiq), sublingual tablet (Abstral), buccal tablet (Fentora), soluble film (Onsolis), and a sublingual spray (Subsys). These preparations may even be more efficacious than oral morphine for breakthrough cancer pain.[205] Labeling, at this time, is limited to opioid-tolerant adult patients.

Another noninvasive method of opioid drug delivery includes the use of fentanyl or buprenorphine transdermal therapeutic systems (TTS). One practical advantage is that when the oral route of tablet, capsule, or liquid administration is contraindicated or not well tolerated by a child, the transdermal drug delivery method allows for an alternative route. There are emerging numbers of pharmacokinetic studies on the use of TTS in children.[206] The data supporting the transdermal route over traditional morphine is minimal, but there are studies that demonstrate child and parent satisfaction with the TTS delivery system of fentanyl and buprenorphine in both pain relief and quality of life in the pediatric palliative care setting.[207,208]

It has been shown that in the pediatric cancer population, opioid monotherapy is the *most* effective method for treating moderate to severe pain.[209] It is not effective, however, for all pediatric cancer patients due to various etiologies including opioid-induced tolerance and opioid-induced hyperalgesia.[210] The analgesic response to any given opioid dose depends on the tolerance of the patient. An opioid-tolerant patient will require a higher dose for the same analgesic response when compared to the opioid-naive patient.

ADVERSE EFFECTS

Adverse effects of opioid analgesics, for both the opioid-naive as well as the opioid-tolerant patient, include somnolence, constipation, pruritus, nausea, vomiting, urinary retention, and sweating. Management of opioid-induced adverse effects is critical in pediatric patients with cancer. Constipation may already be a significant problem for the child prior to the use of opioids as certain types of chemotherapeutic agents, such as vincristine, can cause severe impaired gut peristalsis. This, combined with mucosal breakdown in an immunocompromised host, can lead to severe infectious complications and sepsis. When using high dose or prolonged courses of opioids for the treatment of CNS pain, the treatment plan must also include a bowel regimen to reduce the likelihood of constipation. There are several different classes of medications that can be used to treat or prevent constipation including polyethylene glycol 3350 (often preferable because it is a tasteless and odorless powder that can be mixed with any liquid), senna (a stimulant laxative), docusate (a lubricating laxative), milk of magnesia (which contains magnesium hydroxide, an osmotic laxative), and/or mineral oil (a lubricant). Peripherally acting μ-opioid receptor antagonists such as subcutaneous methylnaltrexone and oral naloxegol[211] are approved for opioid-induced constipation not responsive to usual laxatives in adult noncancer patients, but they are often used off-label for cancer patients without known or suspected lesions in the intestinal wall.

Urinary retention may lead to hemorrhagic cystitis when combined with oxazaphosphorines such as ifosfamide and cyclophosphamide, and strict intake and output parameters must be monitored while receiving these medications. Patients with cancer are also at higher risk for nausea and vomiting with concurrent chemotherapy. They are also at higher risk for somnolence because of polypharmacy with potentially sedating medications such as diphenhydramine and lorazepam used as antiemetic therapy.

Opioid rotation is commonly used as a means of optimizing analgesia while minimizing opioid-related adverse effects.

DEPENDENCE AND ADDICTION

There can also be barriers to the use of high dose or long-term use of opioid analgesia in children due to parents' and health care providers' concerns regarding the risk of dependence or addiction.[212] Some of the more common symptoms of withdrawal in a child with physiologic opioid dependence include severe dysphoria, diarrhea, anxiety, restlessness, and chills and usually occur when the opioid analgesic is stopped abruptly. The symptoms observed in pediatric patients can vary from those observed in adults. For example, an infant can have a high-pitched cry and inability to be soothed with a pacifier, bottle, or swaddling. A toddler's signs of withdrawal may include only diarrhea and temperature instability. Conversely, addiction is a complex behavior characterized by the compulsive use of a drug and psychological craving. Addiction is not commonly seen in the pediatric population but may be observed in the older adolescent who has complex psychosocial issues resulting in maladaptive coping to pain.

TOLERANCE TO OPIOIDS

Given that tolerance to opioid analgesics can limit their clinical effectiveness, various approaches can be used to prevent or reverse tolerance in children who require prolonged exposure to high-dose opioids. One proposed approach to prevent tolerance includes the use of N-methyl-D-aspartate (NMDA) antagonists concomitantly with the opioid. Methadone is a synthetic, long-acting opioid that has often been used for both its μ-opioid effect as well as its NMDA receptor antagonist effect, which is thought to help prevent opioid tolerance. When managed by experienced clinicians, opioid rotation from other opioids to methadone in the face of opioid tolerance or unacceptable side effects can be safe and effective in cancer pain.[213]

Ketamine has been studied and shown to have a role in mitigating opioid-induced tolerance in children and adolescents who experience cancer pain.[214] Finkel et al.[215] have used ketamine at lower doses than used for anesthetic purposes. Specifically, they used ketamine from 0.1 to 1.0 mg/kg/hour in patients who had signs of opioid tolerance or had severe side effects such as profound sedation. With this regimen, they found that adjuvant ketamine infusions used in combination with opioid analgesics (including morphine, methadone, and hydromorphone) resulted in improved pain control.

"WEAK" OPIOID

Tramadol is an atypical opioid that has a weak affinity for the μ-opioid receptor as well as being a weak inhibitor of serotonin and noradrenaline reuptake. The advantage of tramadol is that it has negligible respiratory depression.[216] It is hepatically metabolized and renally excreted, factors that must be taken into consideration when using this medication in the pediatric cancer patient because chemotherapy can result in both renal and hepatotoxicity. The active metabolite is O-desmethyltramadol (M1), and recent pharmacokinetic studies in children have demonstrated that it is possible to produce enough of the active metabolite to achieve adequate pain relief.[217] Safe dosing regimens for children ≥12 months of age include 1 to 2 mg/kg per oral route of administration every 4 to 6 hours with a maximum dose of 8 mg/kg/day.[218]

ADJUVANT THERAPIES FOR NEUROPATHIC PAIN

A review by Friedrichsdorf and Nugent[219] acknowledges a lack of randomized clinical trial data about the management of neuropathic pain in children. There is evidence that NSAIDs (when not contraindicated), weak opioids, and strong opioids may be helpful in adults, and the authors suggest a stepwise approach including treatment of the underlying disease process, integrative/nonpharmacologic therapies, NSAIDs, and weak or strong opioids before considering a tricyclic antidepressant (such as amitriptyline), a gabapentinoid (gabapentin or pregabalin), or a combination of a tricyclic and gabapentinoid. Because these medications often take time to reach therapeutic effect, the addition of ketamine or methadone for NMDA-receptor-channel blockade may be considered, or low-dose benzodiazepine, α-agonists such as dexmedetomidine or clonidine, and/or intravenous lidocaine. Localized pain can also be treated with a lidocaine 5% patch. Regional anesthesia can also be considered. Duloxetine is also a consideration in some patients based on its modest effectiveness in adult chemotherapy-induced peripheral neuropathic pain.[220]

Physical and Psychological Therapies for Pain in the Pediatric Cancer Patient

There are multiple nonpharmacologic therapies that can be employed for pain management in the pediatric cancer patient (Table 49.1). These include massage therapy, yoga, hypnotherapy, meditation, biofeedback, relaxation, spirituality, acupuncture, botanicals, physical therapy (PT), and energy therapies including the use of magnets. The definition of complementary and alternative medicine (CAM) was those interventions that are neither generally provided by US hospital clinics nor widely taught in medical school.[221] More recently, there has been a concerted effort by the NIH and clinicians alike to consider these options as "integrative therapy."[222-224]

Thus, although these nontraditional pain treatments may not be familiar territory for physicians trained within the United States, there is an emerging body of literature discussing the state of the science of integrative therapy use in both adult and pediatric populations.[225] In addition, the latest literature in medical education has documented a clear trend of higher usage rates of integrative therapies by anesthesia

---

TABLE 49.1 Complementary and Alternative Medicine Therapies to Be Considered in the Treatment of Pediatric Cancer Pain

- Acupuncture
- Hypnotherapy
- Massage
- Biofeedback
- Botanicals
- Magnets
- Spirituality/religiosity
- Therapeutic yoga

training programs across the United States.[226] Thus, integrative interventions, including pharmacologic, psychologic, physical, and other therapies, should be considered in the treatment of pediatric cancer pain.

ACUPUNCTURE

Acupuncture consists of inserting fine needles into the skin's surface, or using heat, pressure, or other stimulation in areas that correspond to specific points along "meridians" (i.e., energy channels within the body). These meridians in which the body's life forces (spiritual, emotional, mental, and physical) flow can be out of balance and cause the physical sensations of pain, imbalance, and sickness. Insertion of the needles into specific points along meridians through the practice of acupuncture helps to restore the balance of forces within the body and thereby eliminate the pain by achieving a flow of energy or Qi (pronounced "chi"). Although the practice of acupuncture is more widely accepted within East Asian societies, the use of acupuncture for treatment of pain has been increasing across the United States.[227,228] Currently, 46 US states and the District of Columbia require licensure for the practice of acupuncture. For those states that do not regulate the practice, the health care provider should ask for certification by the National Certification Commission for Acupuncture and Oriental Medicine (see Chapter 94).

There is a growing body of literature evaluating its effectiveness for alleviating pain.[229,230] The available literature on the use and effectiveness of acupuncture in the treatment of pain in the pediatric population suggests it is an acceptable treatment modality for adolescents with chronic pain, as well as an effective modality for other common symptoms experienced by the childhood cancer patient, including headache, nausea, and vomiting.[231–233] Nonetheless, acupuncture has not been widely disseminated into pain treatment regimens for the pediatric population. One reason is preexisting beliefs by health care practitioners in the United States that children are afraid of needles, and thus, they do not make referrals for acupuncture. On the contrary, it has been shown that for those children who have been referred to acupuncture for various chronic pain syndromes, over two-thirds report that it was a positive experience and an effective modality for treatment of their pain.[234] Acupuncture, therefore, can be considered as a possible adjuvant treatment modality for neuropathic pain in the pediatric cancer patient.

BEHAVIORAL INTERVENTIONS

A Cochrane review on psychological interventions in needle-related procedural pain supports distraction as an effective modality for decreasing self-reported pain.[235] Distraction techniques include listening to music, watching cartoons, playing with a toy, nonprocedural talk, squeezing a rubber ball, using cards with questions on them, listening to stories via earphones, parental soothing, or a combination. Virtual reality is a specific type of distraction technique involving immersing the child in a virtual world using visual and auditory stimuli, with some positive results.[236–238]

Cognitive-behavior therapies (CBTs) have also been extensively studied needle-related procedural pain and distress in children. Specific therapies included procedural preparation and information, relaxation, guided imagery, modeling, procedural rehearsal, coping skills teaching, parent coaching, and memory alteration techniques. A Cochrane review in 2006[239] found sufficient evidence supporting combined CBT; however, an update in 2013[235] had stricter inclusion criteria for included studies and no longer had sufficient data to support the benefit of CBT.

HYPNOTHERAPY

Hypnosis is a cognitive strategy that helps the child achieve a narrowed focus of attention, relax, and learn how to dissociate from the current sensory environment. Several groups in randomized controlled studies of children with cancer undergoing medical procedures have shown hypnotherapy to be effective in reducing procedure-related pain and anxiety.[240–242] These are summarized in numerous reviews.[243,244] Wood and Bioy[245] provide a succinct review on the effectiveness of this technique, an understanding of the physiologic effect of hypnosis, and the practical application of its use to treat pain in children. For example, Rainville and colleagues[246] have demonstrated, through the use of positive emission tomography (PET), changes in regional cerebral blood flow when hypnosis is used. In hypnotic states, there is increased blood flow to the occipital cortical areas. This increase in blood flow to the occipital region is thought to result in a reduction of inhibitory processes that occur normally during high levels of attention.[247] Thus, hypnosis results in an acceptance of specific, altered sensations, thereby mediating changes in perception of the painful experience.

Several studies on the effect of hypnosis for symptom management in children, including the effect on pain perception, anxiety, and nausea/vomiting have been completed. Early studies demonstrated the feasibility of being able to hypnotize children.[248] Subsequent studies by Zeltzer et al.[249] have demonstrated the effectiveness of hypnosis in decreasing other symptoms experienced by pediatric cancer patients, including nausea. Studies have also demonstrated the effectiveness of hypnosis in decreasing pain and anxiety in children undergoing the invasive painful procedures of LPs and bone marrow biopsies.[250] Thus, there continues to be increasing evidence of both the feasibility of administration and the effectiveness of hypnosis in the pediatric population, and it should be considered when a pediatric cancer patient is undergoing invasive, painful procedures. As the review paper by Wood and Bioy[245] discusses, practical considerations of using hypnosis include the child's age (as younger children are more responsive to the hypnosis when compared to adolescents), cognitive development, and therapeutic relationship with his or her provider.

EXPRESSIVE ARTS THERAPIES

Expressive or creative arts therapies include such disciplines as art therapy, music therapy, dance/movement therapy, drama therapy, and poetry therapy. Expressive arts therapists are trained, credentialed specialists who use an expressive art form in the context of psychotherapy, medicine, or rehabilitation. The therapist systematically assesses the patient and tailors an interactive expressive art experience to the patient's psychological needs through a therapeutic process. The expressive arts not only help to distract from the patient's current illness and normalize the hospital or clinic environment but also use theoretical concepts to improve coping and manage distress. For example, Robb et al.[251] studied a therapeutic music video intervention in adolescents and young adults which was grounded in motivational and developmental coping therapy to (1) provide predictability through clearly defined goals and structured, preferred music; (2) autonomy support through patient-directed choices about music, lyric writing, video content, and involvement of others; and (3) relationship building through a nonthreatening, creative activity to help patients explore, identify, and express what is important to them.

Expressive arts therapies, especially music therapy, have been shown to improve symptoms, such as anxiety, pain, and need for analgesics; lower heart rate, respiratory rate, and blood pressure; and improve quality of life and perceived social support.[252] A small art therapy study using different techniques such as visual imagination, structured and free drawing, and medical play to promote coping behaviors helped improve patient cooperation with painful procedures.[253] Integrating different creative arts therapies together may also be beneficial.

A randomized study in pediatric brain tumor patients showed that creative arts therapies can help improve pain as well as nausea, anxiety, and mood.[254]

MASSAGE

Massage is the practice of light body stroking or deep tissue stroking that is thought to work by increasing serotonin and reducing cortisol. The basic principle of massage is that when muscles are overworked, there is a release of waste products that accumulate in the area that can be relieved using the hands of the therapist to manipulate muscles and surrounding tissues. Massage therapy has been used as an adjuvant therapy in pain management with a number of studies demonstrating its effectiveness. For example, it has been shown that when massage therapy was used in addition to a standard pharmacologic regimen for postoperative pain management, the experimental group demonstrated decreased pain intensity, pain unpleasantness, and anxiety when compared to the control group.[255] Massage therapy is also a CAM modality that can be easily instituted at the bedside for the cancer patient.[256] There are a few studies to date completed in the pediatric population on the use and effectiveness of massage therapy for cancer-related pain. For example, oncology and hematology inpatients who received a standardized massage therapy protocol experienced significant improvements in anxiety, emotional state, muscle soreness, discomfort, respiratory rate, and overall progress compared with a control group.[257] Children assigned to massage therapy for 20 minutes prior to an LP or bone marrow procedure, in addition to topical EMLA and intravenous midazolam, had significantly decreased levels of pain and anxiety after the massage therapy compared to patients in a control group.[258] In a study of children with ALL, a daily massage over a 1-month period was found to have an impact on the immune system as demonstrated by an increased white blood cell count as well as an improvement in children's negative affect.[259] Given the promising application of massage therapy to decrease pain in children, future research is warranted to evaluate the effectiveness of the healing powers of touch (i.e., massage) in a randomized controlled trial for pediatric cancer patients.

BIOFEEDBACK

Biofeedback involves measuring physiologic parameters, including blood pressure, heart rate, skin temperature, sweating, and muscle tension, and conveying the changes that occur while the child is learning breathing and imagery strategies to alter these bodily processes. This bodily feedback information can be provided through the use of computer-generated, audio-generated, or other forms of visual-generated systems with skin temperature or muscle contraction being the most commonly measured parameter. The basic concept of biofeedback is that by providing physiologic information to a patient who is usually unaware of these bodily processes, while also teaching the child cognitive and breathing strategies that alter these processes, the child can learn to reduce muscle tension and autonomic arousal, thereby reducing pain. For children, it provides proof that the mind can affect the body by being able to gain physiologic control of the part of the nervous system that is activated by pain or stress.

Studies on the use of biofeedback have primarily been focused on adult patients, particularly those with headaches. Meta-analysis of this mind–body approach for the treatment of headache pain indicates that it is effective when used alone or in combination with other CAM modalities.[260] Studies completed in pediatric patients again are limited in number, but those that have been completed also have focused on the treatment of pediatric migraine headache. Similar to the adult literature, meta-analysis on the use of biofeedback, as well as other behavioral methodologies to treat headache in children,

demonstrates that it can be considered as an important adjunct to the pain treatment regimen.[261] Given that there are minimal side effects and there is data suggesting its effectiveness, biofeedback can also be considered as another adjunctive therapy to pain management in the pediatric cancer patient. There is no license to practice biofeedback, although the majority of practitioners have other medical licensures, such as registered nursing (RN), PT, or marriage and family therapy (MFT). Hospitals and clinics with pediatric pain programs can often provide referral lists of biofeedback therapists.

BOTANICALS

The use of herbal or alternative medicines requires discussion in the treatment of cancer pain given the increasing frequency of use within the US population with or without data suggesting its effectiveness.[262] The studies that have evaluated the use of herbal medicine in pediatric patients have been for the treatment of otalgia and have been completed outside the United States.[263] One such study evaluating the use of the naturopathic ear drop, Otikon, concluded that it was as effective as anesthetic ear drops for acute otitis media associated with ear pain.[264] Thus, given the paucity of studies documenting effectiveness of botanicals, this CAM option cannot be recommended in the treatment of pediatric cancer pain. The lesson that must be taken away, however, is that it is important for practitioners to ask if botanicals (including megavitamins and herbs) are being used by the parent to help treat their child's pain because there may be drug interactions that may interfere with the cancer treatment regimen.

CANNABIS

Because of legalization efforts in several US states, Canada, and other countries, "medical" cannabis is becoming more available and in many different forms. Cannabis, including marijuana, is a psychoactive substance produced from the cannabis plant and often comprising multiple compounds, including plant-derived cannabinoids like tetrahydrocannabinol (THC) and cannabidiol (CBD). Synthetic cannabinoids have also been produced such as dronabinol, nabilone, and nabiximols spray. The use of cannabis, especially for pain, nausea, or even antitumor effects has generated significant interest in the public and among some patients with cancer and their families.[265] In humans, cannabinoids bind endocannabinoid receptors CB_1, found in the brain and nervous system, and CB_2, found in the immune system. Some reviews have found improvement in cancer-related or other pain with certain preparations of cannabis.[266,267] A review of medical cannabis in pediatric populations in many ways parallels the findings in adults in regard to chemotherapy-induced nausea/vomiting, seizures, and spasticity; however, data on pain, even neuropathic pain, in children is lacking. [268] Short-term side effects such as increased heart rate and blood pressure are common and may limit its use in patients with heart disease. Side effects of THC include drowsiness and dizziness. Side effects of CBD include somnolence, diarrhea, and decreased appetite. Prolonged use in recreational users has been associated with mood, anxiety, and psychotic symptoms and disorders.

Because of the heterogeneity of its composition and the lack of regulation, a great deal of caution must be used in extrapolating results from controlled studies to what is available on the market. Immunocompromised patients should be warned against use of unregulated marijuana, especially smoked and vaporized forms, because of potential infectious complications such as invasive pulmonary aspergillosis.[269] Data on effectiveness on pain in children with cancer are lacking, and effects of chronic cannabis use on the developing brain are concerning.[270,271] Because of a lack of efficacy data and these safety concerns, pediatric societies have advocated for further research and urged caution in recommending cannabis to pediatric patients, acknowledging that there may be a role in certain exceptional cases such as for children with life-limiting or severely debilitating conditions.[272,273] Comprehensive discussion of potential benefits and risks and robust monitoring of safety and efficacy during treatment is necessary.

MAGNETS

The use of magnets to treat chronic pain is another modality that has been under investigation in adult populations. Interestingly, despite the lack of clear data documenting the effectiveness, one study documented that magnet use was the second most common nontraditional modality used by adult patients with arthritis, second only to the use of a chiropractor.[274] The basic mechanism of magnet use is that they produce a type of energy—a magnetic field—that can affect pain sensation, although the exact mechanism by which pain reduction occurs has not been identified. There are various magnet products for use in health care including shoe insoles, shoe inserts, mattress pads, bandages, belts, pillows, bracelets, and headwear. Despite all of these various health care products, there are limited data documenting the effectiveness of this modality. A recent systematic review and meta-analysis of randomized trials demonstrated no significant difference in pain reduction.[275] There may be a placebo effect for the patient who places a magnet on the body in the form of a bracelet or bandage.[276] The only reports in the literature of magnets in pediatric populations refer to the dangers of magnet ingestions resulting in gastrointestinal injuries.[277] Thus, the use of magnets to treat young pediatric cancer patients is another treatment modality that cannot be recommended at this point in time and may be associated with risk of ingestion by a young child.

SPIRITUALITY/RELIGIOSITY

Spirituality (i.e., religiosity) is an important domain that must be considered when conceptualizing the model of palliative care for children with pain.[278] Spirituality is commonly used by cancer patients to cope with their diagnosis, aggressive treatment plans, and associated painful experiences. Spirituality has been shown to be an important coping mechanism for adult cancer patients. For example, it has been shown that breast cancer patients who rate their spirituality as high have lower rates of depression, although no effect on pain ratings.[279] Similarly, when mothers of childhood cancer patients were asked to rate their religiosity concomitantly with the measurement of depression using the Beck Depression Inventory-II, it was shown that those mothers who reported lower levels of religious beliefs and behaviors had higher rates of depressive symptoms.[280] It has therefore been recommended that health care providers consider—when they have patients practicing prayer or prayer-like behaviors—to include a discussion on the benefit of this behavior at improving health through the mind–body connection.[281] In addition, given that most major medical centers caring for children with cancer have access to a chaplain or spiritual support, consulting this service should be considered (where appropriate) when developing a pain management plan for the pediatric cancer patient.

THERAPEUTIC YOGA

Therapeutic yoga, including Iyengar yoga, has been used in children to reduce pain, anxiety, and correct health problems. Iyengar yoga, for example, uses poses (asanas) and breathing to correct body structure, enhance internal organ function, facilitate mindful awareness, and achieve a sense of mind–body–spiritual well-being. Studies conducted in adolescents have demonstrated the practice of yoga results in improvement of mood, a decrease in the stress hormones, and decreased pain and disability.[282,283] There are no published randomized controlled trials of yoga therapy in pediatric oncology; however,

several single-arm pilot studies suggest improvement in physical function, quality of life, functional mobility, flexibility, physical activity, energy, sleep, and mood and decreases in anxiety, nausea, and pain medication, as summarized in a recent review.[284] In the practice of Iyengar yoga, a teacher who has studied for a minimum of 5 years teaches various poses to a child that can be beneficial in decreasing pain. For the pediatric cancer patient with unique needs, including an impaired immune system, private yoga lessons are preferred over group lessons, with therapeutic Iyengar yoga our preferred method of yoga because of extensive teacher training, the use of supportive props, and selection of specific poses based on the needs of the child.

Palliative Care for Children with Cancer

A chapter on pain management for children with cancer is not complete without highlighting the important topic of palliative care given that overall 20% of children will not be cured of their disease. The WHO's definition of palliative care is "the active total care of patients whose disease is not responsive to curative treatment. Control of pain, other symptoms, and psychological, social, and spiritual problems is of paramount concern. The goal of palliative care is achievement of the best possible quality of life for patients and their families."[285] The "other symptoms" in addition to pain that can be experienced by the child without the option of curative therapy include fatigue, dyspnea, poor appetite, nausea, vomiting, constipation, and/or diarrhea.[23] Thus, symptom control for children facing end of life is imperative. Studies have demonstrated that when the multidisciplinary approach of palliative care is employed, families and patients report improved satisfaction with their care, improved informed decision making, and a decrease in the number of emergency room visits and inpatient admissions.[286]

The American Academy of Pediatrics (AAP) has put forth a policy statement promoting the use of palliative care at the end of life for children with life-limiting disease. Their statement highlights that palliative care can improve the quality of life for terminal patients and their families through the treatment of symptoms and by addressing the psychological, social, or spiritual aspects of facing a noncurable disease.[287] Despite this policy statement on the importance of the provision of palliative care services for children with life-threatening disease, there are barriers that currently exist and thereby impede its implementation across the US health care system. First, there can be differences in parents' understanding of prognosis of their child's illness when compared to their health care providers' knowledge, a discrepancy that in turn can impact a parental-informed decision for end-of-life care, including pain management.[288] Secondly, parents whose children have an incurable cancer diagnosis rate doctor–patient communication as the principal determinant of high-quality physician care. Conversely, physicians' care ratings depend on biomedical rather than doctor–patient relationship aspects of care.[289] It is, therefore, critical for physicians caring for the dying child to listen to the concerns of the patient and the parent particularly for those related to descriptions of pain. By listening to a patient's description of pain and thereby classifying the etiology of the pain one can determine the best therapeutic approach. By being aggressive with symptom management, the pain and suffering at the end of life for a terminal pediatric cancer can be minimized.[290]

Pediatric palliative care requires evaluation and reevaluation of symptoms. In addition to the assessment of pain, the provider needs to assess for symptoms of fatigue, dyspnea, anxiety, nausea, and sleep patterns. There should also be the assessment of caretaker function and support because fatigue or anxiety in the primary caretaker can in turn affect the symptoms associated with pain manifested by the child.

Treatment of other end-of-life symptoms, such as dyspnea, can require the use of opioids, especially morphine, to decrease the sensation of air hunger. If the child is heavily sedated and the family or caretaker has minimal awake time with the child, psychostimulants (e.g., methylphenidate, modafinil) can be used in the mornings to override some of the sedative side effects of high-dose opioids needed for pain. In addition, nondrug therapies, such as music therapy or hypnotherapy, can be used concurrently with pain medications. The pediatric palliative care model as described earlier can be delivered both in the inpatient setting as well as in the home if pediatric hospice services are available. In either setting, the goal of maximizing quality of life for the quantity of time that remains for a child without curative therapy should be emphasized. It should be noted that many clinicians now consider palliative care to begin with a serious diagnosis, such as cancer, even if the likelihood for cure is high, because even some children with lower risk cancers, like ALL in the young child, will die. Thus, a focus on maximizing quality of life and reducing distressing symptoms should be as important a focus in the child with cancer as is the aim for cure.[291,292]

Summary

Although pediatric cancer statistics are currently at an all time high with an overall survival rate of 80%, cancer-related morbidity, including the risk for the development of significant acute and chronic pain, persists. Thus, a comprehensive approach to pain management in the pediatric cancer patient, especially through empowerment of the child through a mind–body therapeutic approach to their pain management, is critical. There are several pharmacologic treatments that can be used to treat the various types of pediatric cancer pain including opioid analgesia, NMDA antagonist agents, atypical opioid medications, tricyclic antidepressants, and anticonvulsants. Integration of nonpharmacologic modalities as an adjuvant or alternative to pharmacologic interventions is also important because there can be limitations in the traditional pharmacologic approach to pain, particularly for chronic pain syndromes. Although not all nonpharmacologic therapies have a long track record in the scientific literature regarding their effectiveness, it does not mean these options should be excluded from pain management consideration, but rather, a discussion with families of the strengths and limitations of such approaches is warranted.

In summary, the foundation to the pain evaluation and treatment plans for children with cancer is a focus on the whole child. The importance of eliciting and listening to all details of the pain narrative of the pediatric cancer patient is critical. Child self-report will be dependent on the developmental level of the child and child pain evaluation encompasses the parental role in the pain experience, a proxy reporter of the pain narrative. For both the child and the parents, the pain assessment should occur early on, in a nonthreatening environment, where the strong triad relationship between the pediatric cancer patient, the parent, and the health care provider can be an effective one. In this family-centered care approach, the common goal of alleviating the child's pain can be achieved through education, empowerment, and the provision of mind–body therapeutics.

References

1. Steliarova-Foucher E, Colombet M, Ries LAG, et al, eds. International Incidence of Childhood Cancer, Volume III (electronic version). Lyon, France: International Agency for Research on Cancer. Available at: http://iicc.iarc.fr/results/. Accessed June 26, 2017.
2. Ward E, DeSantis C, Robbins A, et al. Childhood and adolescent cancer statistics, 2014. *CA Cancer J Clin* 2014;64(2):83–103.
3. Phillips SM, Padgett LS, Leisenring WM, et al. Survivors of childhood cancer in the United States: prevalence and burden of morbidity. *Cancer Epidemiol Biomarkers Prev* 2015;24(4):653–663.
4. Steliarova-Foucher E, Stiller C, Lacour B, et al. International Classification of Childhood Cancer, Third Edition. *Cancer* 2005;103:1457–1467.
5. Chandra HS, Heistekamp NC, Hungerford A, et al. Philadelphia Chromosome Symposium: commemoration of the 50th anniversary of the discovery of the Ph chromosome. *Cancer Genet* 2011;204(4):171–179.
6. Hudson MM, Mertens AC, Yasui Y, et al. Health status of adult long-term survivors of childhood cancer: a report from the Childhood Cancer Survivor Study. *JAMA* 2003;290:1583–1592.
7. Oeffinger KC, Mertens AC, Sklar CA, et al. Chronic health conditions in adult survivors of childhood cancer. *N Engl J Med* 2006;355:1572–1582.
8. Stuber Ml, Kazak AE, Meeske K, et al. Predictors of posttraumatic stress symptoms in childhood cancer survivors. *Pediatrics* 1997;100;958–964.
9. Miser AW, McCalla J, Dothage JA, et al. Pain as a presenting symptom in children and young adults with newly diagnosed malignancy. *Pain* 1987;29:85–90.
10. Ljungman G, Gordh T, Sörensen S, et al. Pain in paediatric oncology: interviews with children, adolescents, and their parents. *Acta Paediatr* 1999;88:623–630.
11. Ljungman G, Gordh T, Sörensen S, et al. Pain variations during cancer treatment in children: a descriptive survey. *Pediatr Hematol Oncol* 2000;17:211–221.
12. Miser AW, Dothage JA, Wesley RA, et al. The prevalence of pain in a pediatric and young adult cancer population. *Pain* 1987;29:73–83.
13. Zernikow B, Meyerhoff U, Michel E, et al. Pain in pediatric oncology—children's and patient's perspectives. *Eur J Pain* 2005;9:395–406.
14. Fortier MA, Wahi A, Bruce C, et al. Pain management at home in children with cancer: a daily diary study. *Pediatric Blood Cancer* 2014;61:1029–1033.
15. Collins JJ, Byrnes ME, Dunkel IJ, et al. The measurement of symptoms in children with cancer. *J Pain Symptom Manage* 2000;19:363–377.
16. Elliott SC, Miser AW, Dose AM, et al. Epidemiologic features of pain in pediatric cancer patients: a co-operative community-based study. North Central Cancer Treatment Group and Mayo Clinic. *Clin J Pain* 1991;7:263–268.
17. McGrath PJ, Hsu E, Cappelli M, et al. Pain from pediatric cancer: a survey of an outpatient oncology clinic. *J Psychosoc Onc* 1990;8:109–124.
18. Jacob E, Hesselgrave J, Sambuco G, et al. Variations in pain, sleep, and activity during hospitalization in children with cancer. *J Pediatr Oncol Nurs* 2007;24:208–219.
19. Van Cleve L, Bossert E, Beecroft P, et al. The pain experience of children with leukemia during the first year after diagnosis. *Nurs Res* 2004;53:1–10.
20. Dupuis LL, Lu X, Mitchell HR, et al. Anxiety, pain, and nausea during the treatment of standard-risk childhood acute lymphoblastic leukemia: a prospective longitudinal study from the children's oncology group. *Cancer* 2016;122:1116–1125.
21. Wolfe J, Orellana L, Ullrich C, et al. Symptoms and distress in children with advanced cancer: prospective patient-reported outcomes from the PediQUEST Study. *J Clin Oncol* 2015;33:1928–1935.
22. Wolfe J, Grier HE, Klar N, et al. Symptoms and suffering at the end of life in children with cancer. *N Engl J Med* 2000;342:326–333.
23. Friedrichsdorf SJ, Finney D, Bergin M, et al. Breakthrough pain in children with cancer. *J Pain Symptom Manage* 2007;34:209–216.
24. Bimie KA, Chambers CT, Fernandez CV, et al. Hospitalized children continue to report undertreated and preventable pain. *Pain Res Manag* 2014;19:198–204.
25. Friedrichsdorf SJ, Postier A, Eull D, et al. Pain outcomes in a US children's hospital: a prospective cross-sectional study. *Hosp Pediatr* 2015;5:18–26.
26. Van Cleve L, Muñoz CE, Riggs ML, et al. Pain experience in children with advanced cancer. *J Pediatr Oncol Nurs* 2012;29:28–36.
27. Wang XS, Tang JY, Zhao M, et al. Pediatric cancer pain management practices and attitudes in China. *J Pain Sympt Manag* 2003;26:748–759.
28. Van Hulle Vincent C, Denyes MJ. Relieving children's pain: nurses' abilities and analgesic administration practices. *J Pediatr Nurs* 2004;19:40–50.
29. Janse AJ, Sinnema G, Uiterwaal CSPM, et al. Quality of life in chronic illness: children, parents, and paediatricians have different, but stable perceptions. *Acta Paediatr* 2008;97:1118–1124.
30. Manworren RC. Pediatric nurses' knowledge and attitudes survey regarding pain. *Pediatr Nurs* 2000;26:610–614.
31. Rieman MT, Gordon M. Pain management competency evidenced by a survey of pediatric nurses' knowledge and attitudes. *Pediatr Nurs* 2007;33:307–312.
32. Stanley M, Pollard D. Relationship between knowledge, attitudes, and self-efficacy of nurses in the management of pediatric pain. *Pediatr Nurs* 2013;39:165–171.
33. Fortier MA, Wahi A, Maurer EL, et al. Attitudes regarding analgesic use and pain expression in parents of children with cancer. *J Pediatr Hematol Oncol* 2012;34:257–262.
34. Rosales A, Fortier MA, Campos B, et al. Postoperative pain management in Latino families: parent beliefs about analgesics predict analgesic doses provided to children. *Paediatr Anaesth* 2016;26:307–314.
35. Forgeron PA, Finley GA, Arnaout M. Pediatric pain prevalence and parents' attitudes at a cancer hospital in Jordan. *J Pain Symptom Manage* 2005;31:440–448.
36. Ameringer S, Serlin RC, Hughes SH, et al. Concerns about pain management among adolescents with cancer: developing the Adolescent Barriers Questionnaire. *J Pediatr Oncol Nurs* 2006;23:220–232.

37. Ameringer S. Barriers to pain management among adolescents with cancer. *Pain Manag Nurs* 2010;11:224–233.

38. Kwon JH. Overcoming barriers to cancer pain management. *J Clin Oncol* 2014;32:1727–1733.

39. Nelson KL, Yaster M, Kost-Byerly S. A national survey of American Pediatric Anesthesiologists: patient-controlled analgesia and other intravenous opioid therapies in pediatric acute pain management. *Anesth Analg* 2010;110:754–760.

40. Johnston DL, Nagel K, Friedman DL, et al. Availability and use of palliative care and end-of-life services for pediatric oncology patients. *J Clin Oncol* 2008;26:4646–4650.

41. Enskär K, Carlsson M, Golsäter M, et al. Life situation and problems as reported by children with cancer and their parents. *J Pediatr Oncol Nurs* 1997;14:18–26.

42. Weisman S, Bernstein B, Schechter N. Consequences of inadequate analgesia during painful procedures in children. *Arch Pediatr Adolesc Med* 1998;152:147–149.

43. Stuber ML, Christakis DA, Houskamp B, et al. Posttrauma symptoms in childhood leukemia survivors and their parents. *Psychosomatics* 1996; 37:254–261.

44. Rosenberg AR, Orellana L, Ullrich C, et al. Quality of life in children with advanced cancer: a report from the PediQUEST study. *J Pain Sympt Manag* 2016;52:243–253.

45. Schwartz LA, Brumley LD. What a pain: the impact of physical symptoms and health management on pursuit of personal goals among adolescents with cancer. *J Adolesc Young Adult Oncol* 2017;6:142–149.

46. Bushnell MC, Ceko M, Low LA. Cognitive and emotional control of pain and its disruption in chronic pain. *Nature Rev Neurosci* 2013;14:502–511.

47. Wool MS, Mor V. A multidimensional model for understanding cancer pain. *J Cancer Investigation* 2005;23:727–734.

48. Cheng KK. Oral mucositis: a phenomenological study of pediatric patients' and their parents' perspectives and experiences. *Support Care Cancer* 2009;17:829–837.

49. Brady MA. Introduction to disease and pain management. In: Burns CE, Brady MA, Dunn AM, et al, eds. *Pediatric Primary Care.* 4th ed. St Louis, MO: Saunders Elsevier; 2009:453–476.

50. Neale KL. The fifth vital sign: chronic pain assessment of the adolescent oncology patient. *J Pediatr Oncol Nurs* 2012;29:185–199.

51. Hester N, Foster R, Kristensen K. Measurement of pain in children: generalizability and validity of the pain ladder and Pieces of Hurt tool. *Adv Pain Res Ther* 1990;15:79–84.

52. Beyer JE, Denyes MJ, Villlarruel AM. The creation, validation, and continuing development of the Oucher: a measure of pain intensity in children. *J Pediatr Nurs* 1992;7:335–346.

53. Hicks CL, von Baeyer CL, Spafford PA, et al. The Faces Pain Scale–Revised: toward a common metric in pediatric pain measurement. *Pain* 2001;93: 173–183.

54. McGrath PA, Seifert CE, Speechley KN, et al. A new analogue scale for assessing children's pain: an initial validation study. *Pain* 1996;64:435–443.

55. Cohen LL, Lemanek K, Blount RL, et al. Evidence-based assessment of pediatric pain. *J Pediatr Psychol* 2008;33:939–955.

56. Stinson JN, Kavanagh T, Yamada J, et al. Systematic review of the psychometric properties, interpretability and feasibility of self-report pain intensity measures for use in clinical trials in children and adolescents. *Pain* 2006;125:143–145.

57. Huguet A, Stinson JN, McGrath PJ. Measurement of self-reported pain intensity in children and adolescents. *J Psychosom Res* 2010;68:329–336.

58. Tsze DS, von Baeyer CL, Bulloch B, et al. Validation of self-report pain scales in children. *Pediatrics.* 2013;132(4):e971–e979.

59. Hamill JK, Lyndon M, Liley A, et al. Where it hurts: a systematic review of pain-location tools for children. *Pain* 2014;155:851–858.

60. von Baeyer CL, Lin V, Seidman LC. Pain charts (body maps or manikins) in assessment of the location of pediatric pain. *Pain Manag* 2011;1:61–68.

61. Savedra MC, Tesler MD, Holzemer WL, et al. A strategy to assess the temporal dimension of pain in children and adolescents. *Nurs Res* 1995;44: 272–276.

62. von Baeyer CL, Spagrud LJ. Systematic review of observational (behavioral) measures of pain for children and adolescents aged 3 to 18 years. *Pain* 2007;127:140–150.

63. Merkel SI, Voepel-Lewis T, Shayevitz JR, et al. The FLACC: a behavioral scale for scoring postoperative pain in young children. *Pediatr Nurs* 1997; 23:293–297.

64. McGrath PJ, Johnson G, Goodman JT, et al. CHEOPS: a behavioral scale for rating postoperative pain in children. In: Fields HL, Dubner R, Cervero F, eds. *Advances in Pain Research and Therapy.* Vol 9. New York: Raven Press; 1985:395–402.

65. Chambers CT, Reid GJ, McGrath PJ, et al. Development and preliminary validation of a postoperative pain measure for parents. *Pain* 1996;68:307–313.

66. Ambuel B, Hamlett KW, Marx CM, et al. Assessing distress in pediatric intensive care environments: the COMFORT scale. *J Pediatr Psychol* 1992;17:95–109.

67. Marec-Berard P, Gomez F, Combet S, et al. HEDEN pain scale: a shortened behavioral scale for assessment of prolonged cancer or postsurgical pain in children aged 2 to 6 years. *Pediatr Hematol Oncol* 2015;32:291–303.

68. Gauvin-Piquard A, Rodary C, Rezvani A, et al. Pain in children aged 2–6 years: a new observational rating scale elaborated in a pediatric oncology unit—preliminary report. *Pain* 1987;31:177–188.

69. Gauvin-Piquard A, Rodary C, Rezvani A, et al. The development of the DEGR(R): a scale to assess pain in young children with cancer. *Eur J Pain* 1999;3:165–176.

70. Savedra M, Holzemer WL, Tesler M, et al. Assessment of postoperation pain in children and adolescents using the adolescent pediatric pain tool. *Nurs Res* 1993;42:5–9.

71. Jacob E, Mack AK, Savedra M, et al. Adolescent pediatric pain tool for multidimensional measurement of pain in children and adolescents. *Pain Manag Nurs* 2014;15(3):694–706.

72. Calissendorff-Selder M, Ljungman G. Quality of life varies with pain during treatment in adolescents with cancer. *Ups J Med Sci* 2006;111:109–116.

73. Dobrozsi S, Yan K, Hoffman R, et al. Patient-reported health status during pediatric cancer treatment. *Pediatr Blood Cancer* 2017;64:e26295.

74. Varni JW, Stucky BD, Thissen D, et al. PROMIS Pediatric Pain Interference Scale: an item response theory analysis of the pediatric pain item bank. *J Pain* 2010;11:1109–1119.

75. DeWalt DA, Gross HE, Gipson DS, et al. PROMIS pediatric self-report scales distinguish subgroups of children within and across six common pediatric chronic health conditions. *Qual Life Res* 2015;24:2195–2208.

76. Baggott C, Cooper BA, Marina N, et al. Symptom cluster analysis based on symptom occurrence and severity ratings among pediatric oncology patients during myelosuppressive chemotherapy. *Cancer Nurs* 2012;35:19–28.

77. Yeh CH, Chiang YC, Chien LC, et al. Symptom clustering in older Taiwanese children with cancer. *Oncol Nurs Forum* 2008;35:273–281.

78. Buckner TW, Wang J, DeWalt DA, et al. Patterns of symptoms and functional impairments in children with cancer. *Pediatr Blood Cancer* 2014;61: 1282–1288.

79. Dai H, Wang Y, Lu X, et al. Chimeric antigen receptors modified T-cells for cancer therapy. *J Natl Cancer Inst* 2016;108:djv439.

80. Eiser C, Morse R. Can parents rate their child's health-related quality of life? Results from a systematic review. *Qual Life Res* 2001;10:347–357.

81. Twycross A, Voepel-Lewis T, Vincent C, et al. A debate on the proposition that self-report is the gold standard in assessment of pediatric pain intensity. *Clin J Pain* 2015;31:707–712.

82. Herr K, Coyne PJ, McCaffery M, et al. Pain assessment in the patient unable to self-report: position statement with clinical practice recommendations. *Pain Manag Nurs* 2011;12:230–250.

83. Link CJ, Fortier MA. The relationship between parent trait anxiety and parent-reported pain, solicitous behaviors, and quality of life impairment in children with cancer. *J Pediatr Hematol Oncol* 2016;38:58–62.

84. Alfvén G. SMS pain diary: a method for real-time data capture of recurrent pain in childhood. *Acta Paediatr* 2010;99:1047–1053.

85. Stinson JN, Jibb LA, Nguyen C, et al. Development and testing of a multidimensional iPhone pain assessment application for adolescents with cancer. *J Med Internet Res* 2013;15:e51.

86. Stinson JN, Jibb LA, Nguyen C, et al. Construct validity and reliability of a real-time multidimensional smartphone app to assess pain in children and adolescents with cancer. *Pain* 2015;156:2607–2615.

87. Miser AW, Miser JS. The treatment of cancer pain in children. *Pediatr Clin North Am* 1989;36:979–999.

88. Reaman GH. Pediatric cancer research from past successes through collaboration to future transdisciplinary research. *J Pediatr Oncol Nurs* 2004; 21:123–127.

89. Wilne S, Collier J, Kennedy C, et al. Progression from first symptom to diagnosis in childhood brain tumors. *Eur J Pediatr* 2012;171(1):87–93.

90. Stocco C, Pilotto C, Passone E, et al. Presentation and symptom interval in children with central nervous system tumors. A single-center experience. *Childs Nerv Syst.* 2017;33(12):2109–2116.

91. Gilles FH; and Childhood Brain Tumor Consortium. The epidemiology of headache among children with brain tumor. *J Neurooncol* 1991;10: 31–46.

92. Wilne S, Collier J, Kennedy C, et al. Presentation of childhood CNS tumors: a systematic review and meta-analysis. *Lancet Oncol* 2007;8(8):685–695.

93. Richtsmeier AJ, Barkin RL, Alexander M. Benzodiazepines for acute pain in children. *J Pain Symptom Manage* 1992;7:492–495.

94. Tobias JD, Rasmussen GE. Pain management and sedation in the pediatric intensive care unit. *Pediatr Clin North Am* 1994;41:1269–1292.

95. Falk S, Dickenson AH. Pain and nociception: mechanisms of cancer-induced bone pain. *J Clin Oncol* 2014;32:1647–1654.

96. Zhu M, Liang R, Pan LH, et al. Zoledronate for metastatic bone disease and pain: a meta-analysis of randomized controlled trials. *Pain Med* 2013;14(2):257–264.

97. Vadhan-Raj S, von Moos R, Fallowfield LJ, et al. Clinical benefit in patients with metastatic bone disease: results of a phase 3 study of denosumab versus zoledronic acid. *Ann Oncol* 2012;23(12):3045–3051.

98. Winston MJ, Srivastava T, Jarka D, et al. Bisphosphonates for pain management in children with benign cartilage tumors. *Clin J Pain* 2012;28(3): 268–272.

99. Cornellis F, Truchetet ME, Amoretti N, et al. Bisphosphonate therapy for unresectable symptomatic benign bone tumors: a long-term prospective study of tolerance and efficacy. *Bone* 2014;58:11–16.

100. Chellapandian D, Makras P, Kaltsas G, et al. Bisphosphonates in Langerhans cell histiocytosis: an international retrospective case series. *Mediterr J Hematol Infect Dis* 2016;8(1):e2016033.

101. Martin-Broto J, Cleeland CS, Glare PA, et al. Effects of denosumab on pain and analgesic use in giant cell tumor of bone: interim results from a phase II study. *Acta Oncol* 2014;53:1173–1179.

102. Goldsby RE, Fan TM, Villaluna D, et al. Feasibility and dose discovery analysis of zoledronic acid with concurrent chemotherapy in the treatment of newly diagnosed metastatic osteosarcoma: a report from the Children's Oncology Group. *Eur J Cancer* 2013;49(10):2384–2391.

103. Ltief AN, Zimmerman D. Bisphosphonates for treatment of childhood hypercalcemia. *Pediatrics* 1998;102(4 pt 1):990–993.

104. Benhamou E, Fessard E, Com-Nougué, et al. Less frequent catheter dressing changes decrease local cutaneous toxicity of high-dose chemotherapy in children, without increasing the rate of catheter-related infections: results of a randomised trial. *Bone Marrow Transplant* 2002;29:653–658.

105. Jay SM, Elliot CH, Ozolins M, et al. Behavioral management of children's distress during painful medical procedures. *Behav Res Ther* 1985;23: 513–520.

106. Chen E, Zeltzer LK, Craske MG, et al. Children's memories for painful cancer treatment procedures: implications for distress. *Child Dev* 2000;71:933–947.

107. Frank NC, Blount RL, Smith AJ, et al. Parent and staff behavior, previous child medical experience, and maternal anxiety as they relate to child procedural distress and coping. *J Pediatr Psychol* 1995;20(3):277–289.

108. Noel M, McMurtry CM, Chambers CT, et al. Children's memory for painful procedures: the relationship of pain intensity, anxiety, and adult behaviors to subsequent recall. *J Pediatr Psychol* 2010;35(6):626–636.

109. Schechter NL, Bernstein BA, Beck A, et al. Individual differences in children's response to pain: role of temperament and parental characteristics. *Pediatrics* 1991;87:171–177.

110. Goldsmith HH, Buss AH, Plomin R, et al. Roundtable: what is temperament? Four approaches. *Child Dev* 1987;58:505–529.

111. Broom ME, Rehwaldt M, Fogg L. Relationships between cognitive behavioral techniques, temperament, observed distress, and pain reports in children and adolescents during lumbar puncture. *J Pediatr Nurs* 1998;13: 48–54.

112. Helgadóttir HL, Wilson ME. Temperament and pain in 3 to 7-year-old children undergoing tonsillectomy. *J Pediatr Nurs* 2004;19:204–213.

113. Chen E, Craske MG, Katz ER, et al. Pain-sensitive temperament: does it predict procedural distress and response to psychological treatment among children with cancer? *J Pediatr Psychol* 2000;25:269–278.

114. Stuber ML, Kazak AE, Meeske K, et al. Is posttraumatic stress a viable model for understanding responses to childhood cancer? *Child Adolesc Psychiatr Clin N Am* 1998;7:169–182.

115. Fradet C, McGrath PJ, Kay J, et al. A prospective survey of reactions to blood tests by children and adolescents. *Pain* 1990;40:53–60.

116. Rogers TL, Ostrow CL. The use of EMLA cream to decrease venipuncture pain in children. *J Pediatr Nurs* 2004;19:33–39.

117. Lüllman B, Leonhardt J, Metzelder M, et al. Pain reduction in children during port-à-cath catheter puncture using local anesthesia with EMLA. *Eur J Pediatr* 2010;169:1465–1469.

118. Cozzi G, Borrometi F, Bernini F, et al. First-time success with needle procedures was higher with a warm lidocaine and tetracaine patch than with an eutectic mixture of lidocaine and prilocaine cream. *Acta Paediatr* 2017;106:773–778.

119. Farion KJ, Splinter KL, Newhook K, et al. The effect of vapocoolant spray on pain due to intravenous cannulation in children: a randomized controlled trial. *CMAJ* 2008;179(1):31–36.

120. Heden L, von Essen L, Frykholm P, et al. Low-dose oral midazolam reduces fear and distress during needle procedures in children with cancer. *Pediatr Blood Cancer* 2009;53:1200–1204.

121. Hedén L, von Essen L, Ljungman G. Effect of high-dose paracetamol on needle procedures in children with cancer—an RCT. *Acta Paediatr* 2014;103:314–319.

122. Hedén L, von Essen L, Ljungman G. Effect of morphine in needle procedures in children with cancer. *Eur J Pain* 2011;15:1056–1060.

123. Juárez Gimenez JC, Oliveras M, Hidalgo E, et al. Anesthetic efficacy of eutectic prilocaine-lidocaine cream in pediatric oncology patients undergoing lumbar puncture. *Ann Pharmacother* 1996;30:1235–1237.

124. Whitlow PG, Saboda K, Roe D, et al. Topical analgesia treats pain and decreases propofol use during lumbar punctures in a randomized pediatric leukemia trial. *Pediatr Blood Cancer* 2015;62:85–90.

125. American Society of Anesthesiologists Task Force on Sedation and Analgesia by Non-Anesthesiologists. Practice guidelines for sedation and analgesia by non-anesthesiologists. *Anesthesiology* 2002;96:1004–1017.

126. Coté CJ, Wilson S. Guidelines for monitoring and management of pediatric patients before, during, and after sedation for diagnostic and therapeutic procedures: update 2016. *Pediatrics* 2016;38(4):13–39.

127. Krauss B, Green SM. Procedural sedation and analgesia in children. *Lancet* 2006;367(9512):766–780.

128. Bürger B, Zimmerman M, Mann G, et al. Diagnostic cerebrospinal fluid examination in children with acute lymphoblastic leukemia: significance of low leukocyte counts with blasts or traumatic lumbar puncture. *J Clin Oncol* 2003;21(2):184–188.

129. Anghelescu DL, Burgoyne LL, Faughan LG, et al. Prospective randomized crossover evaluation of three anesthetic regimens for painful procedures in children with cancer. *J Pediatr* 2013;162:137–141.

130. Hollmann GA, Schulz MM, Eickhoff JC, et al. Propofol-fentanyl versus propofol alone for lumbar puncture sedation in children with acute hematologic malignancies: propofol dosing and adverse events. *Pediatr Crit Care Med* 2008;9:616–622.

131. Cechvala MM, Christenson D, Eickhoff JC, et al. Sedative preference of families for lumbar punctures in children with acute leukemia: propofol alone or propofol and fentanyl. *J Pediatr Hematol Oncol* 2008;30(2):142–147.

132. Abdolkarimi B, Zareifar S, Eraghi MG, et al. Comparison effect of intravenous ketamine with pethidine for analgesia and sedation during bone marrow procedures in oncologic children: a randomized, double-blinded, cross-over trial. *Int J Hematol Oncol Stem Cell Res* 2016;10(4):206–211.

133. Seigler RS, Avant MG, Gwyn DR, et al. A comparison of propofol and ketamine/midazolam for intravenous sedation of children. *Pediatr Crit Care Med* 2001;2:20–23.

134. Belen FB, Kocak U, Kayillioglu H, et al. Use of low dose oral midazolam during invasive procedures in pediatric hematology patients. *Gazi Med J* 2015;26:177–179.

135. Aouad MT, Dagher CM, Muwakkit SA, et al. Addition of ketamine to propofol for initiation of procedural anesthesia in children reduces propofol consumption and preserves hemodynamic stability. *Acta Anaesthesiol Scand* 2008;52:561–565.

136. Chiaretti A, Ruggiero A, Barbi E, et al. Comparison of propofol versus propofol-ketamine combination in pediatric oncologic procedures performed by non-anesthesiologists. *Pediatr Blood Cancer* 2011;57:1163–1167.

137. Chiaretti A, Ruggiero A, Barone G, et al. Propofol/alfentanil and propofol/ketamine procedural sedation in children with acute lymphoblastic leukaemia: safety, efficacy and their correlation with pain neuromediator expression. *Eur J Cancer Care (Engl)* 2010;19:212–220.

138. Tobias JD. Applications of nitrous oxide for procedural sedation in the pediatric population. *Pediatr Emerg Care* 2013;29:245–265.

139. Livingston M, Lawell M, McAllister N. Successful use of nitrous oxide during lumbar punctures: a call for nitrous oxide in pediatric oncology clinics. *Pediatr Blood Cancer* 2017;64:e26610.

140. Amorim JA, Gomes de Barros MV, Valença MM. Post-dural (post-lumbar) puncture headache: risk factors and clinical features. *Cephalalgia* 2012; 32(12):916–923.

141. Bolder PM. Postlumbar puncture headache in pediatric oncology patients. *Anesthesiology* 1986;65:696–698.

142. Crock C, Orsini F, Lee KJ, et al. Headache after lumbar puncture: randomized crossover trial of 22-gauge versus 25-gauge needles. *Arch Dis Child* 2014;99:203–207.

143. Rusch R, Schulta C, Hughes L, et al. Evidence-based recommendations to prevent/manage post-lumbar puncture headaches in pediatric patients receiving intrathecal chemotherapy. *J Pediatr Oncol Nurs* 2014;31(4): 230–238.

144. Evans RW, Armon C, Frohman EM, et al. Assessment: prevention of post-lumbar puncture headaches: report of the Therapeutics and Technology Assessment Subcommittee of the American Academy of Neurology. *Neurology* 2010;55(7):909–914.

145. Boonmak P, Boonmak S. Epidural blood patching for preventing and treating post-dural puncture headache. *Cochrane Database Syst Rev* 2010;(1):CD001791.

146. Chou R, Gordon DB, de Leon-Casasola OA, et al. Management of postoperative pain: a clinical practice guideline from the American Pain Society, the American Society of Regional Anesthesia and Pain Medicine, and the American Society of Anesthesiologists' Committee on Regional Anesthesia, Executive Committee, and Administrative Council. *J Pain* 2016;17(2): 131–157.

147. Halbert J, Crotty M, Cameron ID. Evidence for the optimal management of acute and chronic phantom pain: a systematic review. *Clin J Pain* 2002;18:84–92.

148. Richardson C, Kulkarni J. A review of the management of phantom limb pain: challenges and solutions. *J Pain Res* 2017;10:1861–1870.

149. Anghelescu DL, Kelley CN, Steen BD, et al. Mirror therapy for phantom limb pain at a pediatric oncology institution. *Rehabil Oncol* 2016;34(3):104–110.

150. Barbin J, Seetha V, Casillas JM, et al. The effects of mirror therapy on pain and motor control of phantom limb pain in amputees: a systematic review. *Ann Phys Rehabil Med* 2016;59(4):270–275.

151. Thieme H, Morkisch N, Rietz C, et al. The efficacy of movement representation techniques for treatment of limb pain—a systematic review and meta-analysis. *J Pain* 2016;17(2):167–180.

152. Lambertini M, Del Mastro L, Bellodi A, et al. The five "W"s for bone pain due to the administration of granulocyte-colony stimulating factors (G-CSFs). *Crit Rev Oncol Hematol* 2014;89(1):112–128.

153. Pinto L, Liu Z, Doan Q, et al. Comparison of pegfilgrastim with filgrastim on febrile neutropenia, grade IV neutropenia and bone pain: a meta-analysis of randomized controlled trials. *Curr Med Res Opin* 2007;23(9): 2283–2295.

154. Silverman S Jr. Diagnosis and management of oral mucositis. *J Support Oncol* 2007;5(suppl 1):13–21.

155. Stiff PJ. Coding for mucositis. Available at: https://www.cdc.gov/nchs/ppt/icd9/att_mucositis_sep05.ppt. Accessed July 22, 2018.

156. Moslemi D, Nokhandani AM, Otaghsaraei MT, et al. Management of chemo/radiation-induced oral mucositis in patients with head and neck cancer: a review of the current literature. *Radiother Oncol* 2016;120:13–20.

157. Sung L, Robinson P, Treister N, et al. Guideline for the prevention of oral and oropharyngeal mucositis in children receiving treatment for cancer or undergoing haematopoietic stem cell transplantation. *BMJ Support Palliat Care* 2017;7(1):7–16.

158. Lalla RV, Bowen J, Barasch A, et al. MASCC/ISOO clinical practice guidelines for the management of mucositis secondary to cancer therapy. *Cancer* 2014;120(10):1453–1461.

159. Al Jaouni SK, Al Muhayawi MS, Hussein A, et al. Effects of honey on oral mucositis amont pediatric cancer patients undergoing chemo/radiotherapy treatment at King Abdulaziz University Hospital in Jeddah, Kingdom of Saudi Arabia. *Evid Based Complement Alternat Med* 2017;2017:5861024.

160. Mansouri P, Haghighi M, Besheshtipour N, et al. The effect of aloe vera solution on chemotherapy-induced stomatitis in clients with lymphoma and leukemia: a randomized controlled clinical trial. *Int J Community Based Nurs Midwifery* 2016;4(2):119–126.

161. Postmes T, van den Bogaard AE, Hazen M. The sterilization of honey with cobalt 60 gamma radiation: a study of honey spiked with spores of *Clostridium botulinum* and *Bacillus subtilis. Experientia* 1995;51:986–989.

162. Ozyurek H, Turker H, Akbalik M, et al. Pyridoxine and pyridostigmine treatment in vincristine-induced neuropathy. *Pediatr Hematol Oncol* 2007; 24:447–452.

163. Gilchrist LS, Marais L, Tanner L. Comparison of two chemotherapy-induced peripheral neuropathy measurement approaches in children. *Support Care Cancer* 2014;22:359–366.

164. Gilchrist LS, Tanner L. The pediatric-modified total neuropathy score: a reliable and valid measure of chemotherapy-induced peripheral neuropathy in children with non-CNS cancers. *Support Care Cancer* 2013;21: 847–856.

165. Lavoie Smith EM, Li L, Hutchinson RJ, et al. Measuring vincristine-induced peripheral neuropathy in children with acute lymphoblastic leukemia. *Cancer Nurs* 2013;36:E49–E60.

166. Gilchrist L. Chemotherapy-induced peripheral neuropathy in pediatric cancer patients. *Semin Pediatr Neurol* 2012;19:9–17.

167. Yu AL, Gilman AL, Ozkaynak MF, et al. Anti-GD2 antibody with GM-CSF, interleukin-2, and isotretinoin for neuroblastoma. *New Engl J Med* 2010;363:1324–1334.

168. United Therapeutics Corp. Package insert for dinutuximab. Available at: https://www.accessdata.fda.gov/drugsatfda_docs/label/2015/125516s000 lbl.pdf. Accessed July 22, 2018.

169. Görges M, West N, Deyell R, et al. Dexmedetomidine and hydromorphone: a novel pain management strategy for the oncology ward setting during anti-GD2 immunotherapy for high-risk neuroblastoma in children. *Pediatr Blood Cancer* 2015;62:29–34.

170. Terme M, Dorvillus M, Cochonneau D, et al. Chimeric antibody c.8B6 to O-acetyl-GD2 mediates the same efficient anti-neuroblastoma effects as therapeutic ch14.18 antibody to GD2 without antibody induced allodynia. *PLoS One* 2014;9:e87210.

171. Carrega G, Castagnola E, Canessa A, et al. Herpes simplex virus and oral mucositis in children with cancer. *Support Care Cancer* 1994;2(4): 266–269.

172. Righini-Grunder F, Hurni M, Warschkow R, et al. Frequency of oral mucositis and local virus reactivation in herpes simplex virus seropositive children with myelosuppressive therapy. *Klin Padiatr* 2015; 227:335–338.

173. de Mendonca RM, de Araujo M, Levy CE, et al. Oral mucositis in pediatric acute lymphoblastic leukemia patients: evaluation of microbiological and hematologic factors. *Pediatr Hematol Oncol* 2015;32(5):322–330.

174. Hardy I, Gershon AA, Steinberg SP, et al. The incidence of zoster after immunization with live attenuated varicella vaccine. A study in children with leukemia. Varicella Vaccine Collaborative Study Group. *N Engl J Med* 1991;325(22):1545–1550.

175. Lin HC, Chao YH, Wu KH. Increased risk of herpes zoster in children with cancer: a nationwide population-based cohort study. *Medicine (Baltimore)* 2016;95(30):e4037.

176. Glenny AM, Fernandez Mauleffinch LM, Pavitt S, et al. Interventions for the prevention and treatment of herpes simplex virus in patients being treated for cancer. *Cochrane Database Syst Rev* 2009;1:CD006706.

177. Chen N, Li Q, Yang J, et al. Antiviral treatment for preventing postherpetic neuralgia. *Cochrane Database Syst Rev* 2014;(2):CD006866.

178. Gan EY, Tian EA, Tey HL. Management of herpes zoster and post-herpetic neuralgia. *Am J Clin Dermatol* 2013;14(2):77–85.

179. Niscola P, Romani C, Scaramucci L, et al. Pain syndromes in the setting of haematopoietic stem cell transplantation for haematological malignancies. *Bone Marrow Transpl* 2008;41:757–764.

180. Wasilewski-Masker K, Kaste SC, Hudson MM, et al. Bone mineral density deficits in survivors of childhood cancer: long-term follow-up guidelines and review of the literature. *Pediatrics* 2008;121:e705–e713.

181. Cummings EA, Ma J, Fernandez CV, et al. Incident vertebral fractures in children with leukemia during the four years following diagnosis. *J Clin Endocrinol Metab* 2015;100(9):3408–3417.

182. Leblicq C, Laverdière C, Décarie JC, et al. Effectiveness of pamidronate as treatment of symptomatic osteonecrosis occurring in children treated for acute lymphoblastic leukemia. *Pediatr Blood Cancer* 2013;60:741–747.

183. Te Winkel ML, Pieters R, Wind EJ, et al. Management and treatment of osteonecrosis in children and adolescents with acute lymphoblastic leukemia. *Haematologica* 2014;99(3):430–436.

184. Nolan VG, Krull KR, Gurney JG, et al. Predictors of future health-related quality of life in survivors of adolescent cancer. *Pediatr Blood Cancer* 2014;61:1891–1894.

185. Lu Q, Krull KR, Leisenring W, et al. Pain in long-term adult survivors of childhood cancers and their siblings: a report from the Childhood Cancer Survivor Study. *Pain* 2011;152:2616–2624.

186. Brinkman TM, Ullrich NJ, Zhang N, et al. Prevalence and predictors of prescription psychoactive medication use in adult survivors of childhood cancer: a report from the Childhood Cancer Survivor Study. *J Cancer Surviv* 2013;7:104–114.

187. Brinkman TM, Li C, Vannatta K, et al. Behavioral, social, and emotional symptom comorbidities and profiles in adolescent survivors of childhood cancer: a report from the childhood cancer survivor study. *J Clin Oncol* 2016;34:3417–3425.

188. Marche TA, Briere JL, von Baeyer CL. Children's forgetting of pain-related memories. *J Pediatr Psychol.* 2016;41(2):220–231.

189. World Health Organization. *WHO Guidelines on the Pharmacological Treatment of Persisting Pain in Children with Medical Illnesses.* Geneva, Switzerland: WHO Press; 2012:172.

190. Maltoni M, Scarpi E, Modonesi C, et al. A validation study of the WHO analgesic ladder: a two-step vs three-step strategy. *Support Care Cancer* 2005;13(11):888–894.

191. Bandieri E, Romero M, Ripamonti C, et al. A randomized trial of low-dose morphine versus weak opioids in moderate cancer pain. *J Clin Oncol* 2016;34:436–442.

192. Caraceni A, Hanks G, Kaasa S, et al. Use of opioid analgesics in the treatment of cancer pain: evidence-based recommendations from the EAPC. *Lancet Oncol* 2012;13(2):e58–e68.

193. Kremer JM, Hamilton RA. The effects of nonsteroidal anti-inflammatory drugs on methotrexate (MTX) pharmacokinetics: impairment of renal clearance of MTX at weekly maintenance doses but not at 7.5 mg. *J Rheumatol* 1995;22(11):2072–2077.

194. Piper JM, Ray WA, Daugherty JR, et al. Corticosteroid use and peptic ulcer disease: role of nonsteroidal anti-inflammatory drugs. *Ann Intern Med* 1991;114(9):735–740.

195. de Martino M, Chiarugi A. Recent advances in pediatric use of oral paracetamol in fever and pain management. *Pain Ther* 2015;4:149–168.

196. Marinangeli F, Ciccozzi A, Leonardis M, et al. Use of strong opioids in advanced cancer pain: a randomized trial. *J Pain Symptom Manage* 2004; 27:409–416.

197. Wiffen PJ, Wee B, Moore RA. Oral morphine for cancer pain. *Cochrane Database Syst Rev* 2016;(4):CD003868.

198. Quigley C, Wiffen P. A systematic review of hydromorphone in acute and chronic pain. *J Pain Symptom Manage* 2003;25:169–178.

199. Hadley G, Derry S, Moore RA, et al. Transdermal fentanyl for cancer pain. *Cochrane Database Syst Rev* 2013;(10):CD010270.

200. Mercadente S. Cancer pain management in children. *Palliat Med* 2004; 18(7):654–662.

201. Mercadante S, Giarratano A. Pharmacological management of cancer pain in children. *Crit Rev Oncol Hematol* 2014;91:93–97.

202. Lehmann KA. Recent developments in patient-controlled analgesia. *J Pain Symptom Manage* 2005;29:S72–S89.

203. Dunbar PJ, Buckley P, Gavrin JR, et al. Use of patient-controlled analgesia for pain control for children receiving bone marrow transplant. *J Pain Symptom Manage* 1995;10:604–611.

204. Ruggiero A, Barone G, Liotti L, et al. Safety and efficacy of fentanyl administered by patient controlled analgesia in children with cancer pain. *Support Care Cancer* 2007;15:569–573.

205. Jandhyala R, Fullarton JR, Bennett MI. Efficacy of rapid-onset oral fentanyl formulations vs. oral morphine for cancer-related breakthrough pain: a meta-analysis of comparative trials. *J Pain Symptom Manage* 2013; 46(4):573–580.

206. Zernikow B, Michel E, Anderson B. Transdermal fentanyl in childhood and adolescence: a comprehensive literature review. *J Pain* 2007;8(3):187–207.

207. Noyes M, Irving H. The use of transdermal fentanyl in pediatric oncology palliative care. *Am J Hosp Palliat Care* 2001;18:411–416.

208. Ruggiero A, Coccia P, Arena R, et al. Efficacy and safety of transdermal buprenorphine in the management of children with cancer-related pain. *Pediatr Blood Cancer* 2013;60(3):433–437.

209. Zernikow B, Smale H, Michel E, et al. Paediatric cancer pain management using the WHO analgesic ladder—results of a prospective analysis from 2265 treatment days during a quality improvement study. *Eur J Pain* 2006;10:587–595.

210. Angst MS, Clark JD. Opioid-induced hyperalgesia: a qualitative systematic review. *Anesthesiology* 2006;104:570–587.

211. Jones R, Prommer E, Backstedt D. Naloxegol: a novel therapy in the management of opioid-induced constipation. *Am J Hosp Palliat Care* 2016; 33(9):875–880.

212. Von Roenn JH, Cleeland CS, Gonin R, et al. Physician attitudes and practice in cancer pain management. A survey from the Eastern Cooperative Oncology Group. *Ann Intern Med* 1993;119:121–126.
213. Davies D, De Vlaming D, Haines C. Methadone analgesia for children with advanced cancer. *Pediatr Blood Cancer* 2008;51:393–397.
214. Bredlau AL, Thakur R, Korones DN, et al. Ketamine for pain in adults and children with cancer: a systematic review and synthesis of the literature. *Pain Med* 2013;14:1505–1517.
215. Finkel JC, Pestieau SR, Quezado ZM. Ketamine as an adjuvant for treatment of cancer pain in children and adolescents. *J Pain* 2007;8:515–521.
216. Payne KA, Roelofse JA. Tramadol drops in children: analgesic efficacy, lack of respiratory effects, and normal recovery times. *Anesth Prog* 1999;46: 91–96.
217. Garrido MJ, Habre W, Rombout F, et al. Population pharmacokinetic/pharmacodynamic modelling of the analgesic effects of tramadol in pediatrics. *Pharm Res* 2006;23:2014–2023.
218. Payne KA, Roelofse JA, Shipton EA. Pharmacokinetics of oral tramadol drops for postoperative pain relief in children aged 4 to 7 years—a pilot study. *Anesth Prog* 2002;49:109–112.
219. Friedrichsdorf SJ, Nugent AP. Management of neuropathic pain in children with cancer. *Curr Opin Support Palliat Care* 2013;7:131–138.
220. Smith EM, Pang H, Cirrincione C, et al. Effect of duloxetine on pain, function, and quality of life among patients with chemotherapy-induced painful peripheral neuropathy: a randomized clinical trial. *JAMA* 2013; 309(13):1359–1367.
221. Eisenberg DM, Kessler RC, Foster C, et al. Unconventional medicine in the United States: prevalence, costs, and patterns of use. *N Engl J Med* 1993;328:246–252.
222. Cotton S, Luberto CM, Bogenschutz LH, et al. Integrative care therapies and pain in hospitalized children and adolescents: a retrospective database review. *J Altern Complement Med* 2014;20(2):98–102.
223. Young L, Kemper KJ. Integrative care for pediatric patients with pain. *J Altern Complement Med* 2013;19(7):627–632.
224. Section on Integrative Medicine. Mind-body therapies in children and youth. *Pediatrics* 2016;138(3):e20161896.
225. Tsao JC, Zeltzer LK. Complementary and alternative medicine approaches for pediatric pain: a review of the state-of-the-science. *Evid Based Complement Alternat Med* 2005;2:149–159.
226. Lin YC, Lee AC, Kemper KJ, et al. Use of complementary and alternative medicine in pediatric pain management service: a survey. *Pain Med* 2005;6:452–458.
227. Itoh K, Kitakoji H. Acupuncture for chronic pain in Japan: a review. *Evid Based Complement Alternat Med* 2007;4:431–438.
228. Kundu A, Berman B. Acupuncture for pediatric pain and symptom management. *Pediatr Clin North Am* 2007;54:885–889.
229. Golianu B, Yeh AM, Brooks M. Acupuncture for pediatric pain. *Children (Basel)* 2014;1(2):134–148.
230. Wang SM, Kain ZN, White PF. Acupuncture analgesia: II. Clinical considerations. *Anesth Analg* 2008;106:611–621.
231. Tsao JC, Meldrum M, Kim SC, et al. Treatment preferences for CAM in children with chronic pain. *Evid Based Complement Alternat Med* 2007;4:367–374.
232. Gottschling S, Meyer S, Gribova I, et al. Laser acupuncture in children with headache: a double-blind, randomized, bicenter, placebo-controlled trial. *Pain* 2008;137:405–412.
233. Reindl TK, Geilen W, Hartmann R, et al. Acupuncture against chemotherapy-induced nausea and vomiting in pediatric oncology. Interim results of a multi-center crossover study. *Support Care Cancer* 2006;14(2):172–176.
234. Kemper KJ, Sarah R, Silver-Highfield E, et al. On pins and needles? Pediatric pain patients' experience with acupuncture. *Pediatrics* 2000;105:941–947.
235. Uman LS, Birnie KA, Noel M, et al. Psychological interventions for needle-related procedural pain and distress in children and adolescents. *Cochrane Database Syst Rev* 2013;(10):CD005179.
236. Schneider SM, Workman ML. Effects of virtual reality on symptom distress in children receiving chemotherapy. *Cyberpsych Behav* 1999;2:124–134.
237. Wolitzky K, Fivush R, Zimand E, et al. Effectiveness of virtual reality distraction during a painful medical procedure in pediatric oncology patients. *Psychol Health* 2005;20:817–824.
238. Nilsson S, Finnström B, Kokinsky E, et al. The use of virtual reality for needle-related procedural pain and distress in children and adolescents in a paediatric oncology unit. *Eur J Oncol Nurs* 2009;13:102–109.
239. Uman LS, Chambers CT, McGrath PJ, et al. Psychological interventions for needle-related procedural pain and distress in children and adolescents. *Cochrane Database Syst Rev* 2006;(4):CD005179.
240. Liossi C, Hatira P. Clinical hypnosis in the alleviation of procedure-related pain in pediatric oncology patients. *Int J Clin Exp Hypn* 2003;51:4–28.
241. Liossi C, White P, Hatira P. Randomized clinical trial of local anesthetic versus a combination of local anesthetic with self-hypnosis in the management of pediatric procedure-related pain. *Health Psychol* 2006;25:307–315.
242. Liossi C, White P, Hatira P. A randomized clinical trial of a brief hypnosis intervention to control venipuncture-related pain of paediatric cancer patients. *Pain* 2009;142:255–263.
243. Tomé-Pires C, Miró J. Hypnosis for the management of chronic and cancer procedure-related pain in children. *Int J Clin Exp Hypn* 2012;60:432–457.
244. Birnie KA, Noel M, Parker JA, et al. Systematic review and meta-analysis of distraction and hypnosis for needle-related pain and distress in children and adolescents. *J Pediatr Psychol* 2014;39(8):783–808.
245. Wood C, Bioy A. Hypnosis and pain in children. *J Pain Symptom Manage* 2008;35(4):437–446.
246. Rainville P, Hofbauer RK, Paus T, et al. Cerebral mechanisms of hypnotic induction and suggestion. *J Cogn Neurosci* 1999;11:110–125.
247. Rainville P, Hofbauer RK, Bushnell MC, et al. Hypnosis modulates activity in brain structures involved in the regulation of consciousness. *J Cogn Neurosci* 2002;14:887–901.
248. LeBaron S, Zeltzer LK, Fanurik D. Imaginative involvement and hypnotizability in childhood. *Int J Clin Exp Hypn* 1988;36:284–295.
249. Zeltzer LK, Dolgin MJ, LeBaron S, et al. A randomized, controlled study of behavioral intervention for chemotherapy distress in children with cancer. *Pediatrics* 1991;88:34–42.
250. Butler LD, Symons BK, Henderson SL, et al. Hypnosis reduces distress and duration of an invasive medical procedure for children. *Pediatrics* 2005;115:e77–e85.
251. Robb SL, Burns DS, Stegenga KA, et al. Randomized clinical trial of therapeutic music video intervention for resilience outcomes in adolescents/young adults undergoing hematopoietic stem cell transplant. *Cancer* 2014; 120:909–917.
252. Bradt J, Dileo C, Magill L, et al. Music interventions for improving psychological and physical outcomes in cancer patients. *Cochrane Database Syst Rev* 2016;(8):CD006911.
253. Favara-Scacco C, Smirne G, Schilirò G, et al. Art therapy as support for children with leukemia during painful procedures. *Med Pediatr Oncol* 2001;36:474–480.
254. Madden JR, Mowry P, Gao D, et al. Creative arts therapy improves quality of life for pediatric brain tumor patients receiving outpatient chemotherapy. *J Pediatr Oncol Nurs* 2010;27(3):133–145.
255. Mitchinson AR, Kim HM, Rosenberg JM, et al. Acute postoperative pain management using massage as an adjuvant therapy: a randomized trial. *Arch Surg* 2007;142:1158–1167.
256. Gatlin CG, Schulmeister L. When medication is not enough: nonpharmacologic management of pain. *Clin J Oncol Nurs* 2007;11:699–704.
257. Haun JN, Graham-Pole J, Shortley B. Children with cancer and blood diseases experience positive physical and psychological effects from massage therapy. *Int J Ther Massage Bodywork* 2009;2:7–14.
258. Çelebioğlu A, Gürol A, Yildirim ZK, et al. Effects of massage therapy on pain and anxiety arising from intrathecal therapy or bone marrow aspiration in children with cancer. *Int J Nurs Pract* 2015;21:797–804.
259. Field T, Cullen C, Diego M, et al. Leukemia immune changes following massage therapy. *J Bodyw Mov Ther* 2001;5:271–274.
260. Sierpina V, Astin J, Giordano J. Mind-body therapies for headache. *Am Fam Physician* 2007;76:1518–1522.
261. Andrasik F. Behavioral treatment of migraine: current status and future directions. *Expert Rev Neurother* 2004;4:403–413.
262. Eisenberg DM, Davis RB, Ettner SL, et al. Trends in alternative medicine use in the United States, 1990–1997: results of a follow-up national survey. *JAMA* 1998;280:1569–1575.
263. Sarrell EM, Cohen HA, Kahan E. Naturopathic treatment for ear pain in children. *Pediatrics* 2003;111:e574–e579.
264. Sarrell EM, Mandelberg A, Cohen HA. Efficacy of naturopathic extracts in the management of ear pain associated with acute otitis media. *Arch Pediatr Adolesc Med* 2001;155:796–799.
265. National Academies of Sciences, Engineering, and Medicine, Health and Medicine Division, Board on Population Health and Public Health Practice, et al. *The Health Effects of Cannabis and Cannabinoids: The Current State of Evidence and Recommendations for Research*. Washington, DC: National Academies Press; 2017.
266. Whiting PF, Wolff RF, Deshpande S, et al. Cannabinoids for medical use: a systematic review and meta-analysis. *JAMA* 2015;313:2456–2473.
267. Blake A, Wan BA, Malek L, et al. A selective review of medical cannabis in cancer pain management. *Ann Palliat Med* 2017;6:S215–S222.
268. Wong SS, Wilens TE. Medical cannabinoids in children and adolescents: a systematic review. *Pediatrics* 2017;140:e20171818.
269. Szyper-Kravitz M, Lang R, Manor Y, et al. Early invasive pulmonary aspergillosis in a leukemia patient linked to aspergillus contaminated marijuana smoking. *Leuk Lymphoma* 2001;42(6):1433–1437.
270. Meier MH, Caspi A, Ambler A, et al. Persistent cannabis users show neuropsychological decline from childhood to midlife. *Proc Natl Acad Sci U S A.* 2012;109:E2657–E2664.
271. Meruelo AD, Castro N, Cota CI, et al. Cannabis and alcohol use, and the developing brain. *Behav Brain Res* 2017;325(pt A):44–50.
272. Ammerman S, Ryan S, Adelman WP. The impact of marijuana policies on youth: clinical, research, and legal update. *Pediatrics* 2015;135: 584–587.
273. Rieder MJ; and Canadian Paediatric Society, Drug Therapy and Hazardous Substances Committee. Is the medical use of cannabis a therapeutic option for children? *Paediatr Child Health* 2016;21:31–34.
274. Rao JK, Mihaliak K, Kroenke K, et al. Use of complementary therapies for arthritis among patients of rheumatologists. *Ann Intern Med* 1999;131:409–416.

275. Pittler MH, Brown EM, Ernst E. Static magnets for reducing pain: systematic review and meta-analysis of randomized trials. *CMAJ* 2007;177:736–742.

276. Carter R, Aspy CB, Mold J. The effectiveness of magnet therapy for treatment of wrist pain attributed to carpal tunnel syndrome. *J Fam Pract* 2002;51:38–40.

277. Centers for Disease Control and Prevention. Gastrointestinal injuries from magnet ingestion in children—United States, 2003–2006. *MMWR Morb Mortal Wkly Rep* 2006;55:1296–1300.

278. Donnelly JP, Huff SM, Lindsey ML, et al. The needs of children with life-limiting conditions: a health care-provider-based model. *Am J Hosp Palliat Care* 2005;22:259–267.

279. Aukst-Margetić B, Jakovljević M, Margetić B, et al. Religiosity, depression, and pain in patients with breast cancer. *Gen Hosp Psychiatry* 2005;27:250–255.

280. Elkin TD, Jensen SA, McNeil L, et al. Religiosity and coping in mothers of children diagnosed with cancer: an exploratory analysis. *J Pediatr Oncol Nurs* 2007;24:274–278.

281. Krebs K. The spiritual aspect of caring—an integral part of health and healing. *Nurs Adm Q* 2001;25:55–60.

282. Woolery A, Myers H, Sternlieb B, et al. A yoga intervention for young adults with elevated symptoms of depression. *Altern Ther Health Med* 2004;10:60–63.

283. Kuttner L, Chambers CT, Hardial J, et al. A randomized trial of yoga for adolescents with irritable bowel syndrome. *Pain Res Manag* 2006;11:217–223.

284. Danhauer SC, Addington EL, Sohl SJ, et al. Review of yoga therapy during cancer treatment. *Support Care Cancer* 2017;25:1357–1372.

285. World Health Organization. WHO definition of palliative care. Available at: http://www.who.int/cancer/palliative/definition/en/. Accessed July 22, 2018.

286. Jennings PD. Providing pediatric palliative care through a pediatric supportive care team. *Pediatr Nurs* 2005;31:195–200.

287. Bioethics CO, Committee on Hospital Care. Palliative care for children. *Pediatrics* 2000;106(2):351–357.

288. Wolfe J, Klar N, Grier HE, et al. Understanding of prognosis among parents of children who died of cancer: impact on treatment goals and integration of palliative care. *JAMA* 2000;284:2469–2475.

289. Mack JW, Hilden JM, Watterson J, et al. Parent and physician perspectives on quality of care at the end of life in children with cancer. *J Clin Oncol* 2005;23:9155–9161.

290. Calabrese CL. ACT—for pediatric palliative care. *Pediatr Nurs* 2007;33:532–534.

291. Levine D, Lam CG, Cunningham MJ, et al. Best practices for pediatric palliative cancer care: a primer for clinical providers. *J Support Oncol* 2013;11(3):114–125.

292. Downing J, Jassal SS, Mathews L, et al. Pediatric pain management in palliative care. *Pain Manag* 2015;5(1):23–35.

CHAPTER 50

Acute Pain Management in Children

STACY J. PETERSON, KRISTEN LYNN LABOVSKY, and **STEVEN J. WEISMAN**

Nociception alerts the organism to potential or actual sources of harm. Nociceptive functions are active at birth, even in preterm neonates, and the experience of pain or pleasure has a powerful impact on learning and neurologic development.[1] Fitzgerald and Walker,[1] using neurobiologic studies in infant rats and psychophysical studies in infant humans, showed that the infant nervous system is in many respects hyperresponsive to noxious stimuli compared to the mature nervous system. Infant rats and humans withdraw their limbs from milder mechanical or thermal stimuli compared to older rats or humans. Infant rats and humans develop hyperalgesia following tissue injury, with evidence for spinal sensitization even in preterm neonates.

In the 1980s, there was a growing acceptance that peripheral and spinal mechanisms of nociception are active in preterm and term neonates. Controversy persisted regarding maturation of supraspinal mechanisms and regarding how to view pain as a conscious experience or suffering in neonates. Recent studies have examined correlates of brain activation using near-infrared spectroscopy, which is sensitive to regional changes in blood flow. A noxious stimulus to the heel (performed for clinically indicated blood sampling) evoked increased signal overlying the contralateral, but not ipsilateral, cerebral cortex, which has been interpreted as a specific pattern of activation not solely dependent on global changes in autonomic arousal and blood pressure. These and other lines of evidence suggest that "painful stimulation reaches the brain" in neonates, although they do not per se establish the nature of pain viewed as conscious experience or suffering in neonates. Additional discussion follows later in the chapter regarding potential consequences of either untreated pain or pain treatment in critically ill neonates.[1]

Care of infants and children with acute pain has changed considerably over the past several decades, and available evidence suggests that undertreatment of acute pain has become less prevalent in economically developed countries over this time period.[2] Changes in practice appear to be the combined result of a series of developments in basic research, clinical trials, and advocacy by parents as well as by clinicians, as listed in Table 50.1.

Pain Assessment in Infants and Children

Assessing pain in infants and children is a fundamental but challenging aspect of pediatric care. Uniform assessment of pain should be part of the standard of care for hospitals and clinics caring for children. Typical adult pain measures are not applicable to preverbal and young children. Infants and very young children are dependent on adult caregivers to adequately interpret their behavior and other signs in determining whether they have pain. Methods of measuring pain in preverbal patients and toddlers (ages 2 and 3 years) generally involve combinations of behavioral observation, such as facial expression, crying, and physiologic parameters. Preschool-age and early school-age children (ages 3 years or 4 to 8 years) are generally

able to give some degree of self-report and pain scales in this age group incorporate self-report measures. In the younger group (ages 3 to 4 years), pain may be only be expressed in a binary way (i.e., either present or not present), but by early school age (ages 5 to 6 years), children are generally able to communicate a variety of pain levels.[3] Fear and anxiety in children may complicate pain assessment and, in some cases, leads them to either overrate or underrate pain. For this reason, many behavioral scales are taken to be measures of "distress," which combines pain, fear, and anxiety. For example, a 2-year-old child fearful of having a relatively painless ear examination may appear to have extreme pain based on behavioral measures. A 7-year-old child may deny pain because of the fear of having to receive a "shot" if he admits to having pain. Valid and reliable pain measures have been developed for children based on developmental levels reflecting a child's ability to communicate and understand concepts of pain. In general, behavioral measures tend to underrate persistent pain relative to self-report.

Pain assessment in infants, neonates, and premature infants is especially challenging. Previously, infants were not thought to be fully capable of experiencing pain, which led in part to inadequate efforts to treat pain in infants. Numerous studies have examined the response of neonates and preterm infants to pain and have shown various response patterns including changes in stress hormones levels; observed behavioral responses; and alterations in heart rate, heart rate variability, oxygen saturation, and other physiologic responses.[4-7] Studies have shown that neonates who are subjected to heel lancing for blood sampling consistently swipe the foot being lanced with the unaffected foot, indicating that neonates have the ability to localize to the site of pain.[8,9] Other data have shown that hospitalized infants display graded responses of heart rate, oxygen saturation, mean arterial pressure, and behavioral state with varying degrees of pain intensity, indicating that infants have the ability to distinguish severity of pain.[10] Pain assessment scales for infants are

TABLE 50.1 Factors Possibly Contributing to Increased Awareness of and Treatment of Pain in Infants and Children

1. Studies demonstrating maturation of nociceptive pathways in infant animals and in infant humans
2. Clinical trials demonstrating improved outcomes of neonates undergoing surgery under adequate anesthesia
3. Studies of pain assessment in infants, children, and adolescents
4. Pharmacologic studies examining pharmacokinetic, pharmacodynamic, and clinical outcomes of analgesics in infants and children
5. Development of acute pain services in pediatric tertiary centers
6. Development of regional anesthesia skills and service for infants and children
7. Advocacy by parents

typically composite pain scores consisting of behavioral parameters such as facial grimacing, posture, and crying combined with more objective data such as heart rate, blood pressure, and oxygen saturation. Pain ratings may be erroneous in critically ill infants because sepsis, hypotension, respiratory failure, and other conditions will change many of the physiologic and behavioral parameters in composite pain scales. The CRIES; Face, Legs, Activity, Cry, and Consolability (FLACC) scales; and the Premature Infant Pain Profile have been validated for infants and premature infants.[11-13]

Concrete thinking and stages of cognitive and language development of preschool-age children can present difficulties in pain assessment. Many toddlers when ill, hospitalized, or confronted with strangers refuse to cooperate with self-report or formal testing of pain. Involving parents or other familiar caregivers in the assessment of pain for toddlers can provide useful information. Studies comparing parents' to clinicians' pain ratings are inconsistent with some showing good agreement but others showing disparities.[14]

The Children's Hospital of Eastern Ontario Pain Scale (CHEOPS) and the Behavioral Observational Pain Scale (BOPS) have been validated for assessing postoperative pain in toddlers and young children.[15,16] The FLACC scale is a very widely used scale involving five items, each scored from 0 to 2 to give a composite score ranging from 0 to 10.[17] The FLACC scale has become widely used because it is quick and versatile and its components appear reasonable for a wide range of patient groups, including infants and older patients with developmental disabilities.[13,17-21] A recent review does find evidence to support its use in children aged 2 months to 7 years for postoperative pain as well as in children from ages 4 to 10 years who have cognitive impairment.[21]

Several validated self-report pain scores have been developed for children 4 years and older, including photos or drawings of faces where numerical anchors signify gradations of pain and a slide rule device where increasing color intensity indicates increasing pain intensity.[22] Young children are able to differentiate pain intensity when presented with facial expressions, although more than five choices of facial expressions interfere with the child's ability to reliably indicate pain.[23] Most older school-age children and adolescents have the cognitive and emotional maturity to use adult numerical visual analogue scales; nevertheless, pain, illness, hospitalization, and separation from parents cause some older children and teenagers to regress emotionally, making scales used for younger children, such as faces scale, more applicable. There has been considerable dispute regarding relative merits of different presentations of face-type scales; however, the most widely accepted and validated face-based scale is the Bieri Faces Pain Scale-Revised.[23,24]

Analgesic Pharmacology in Infants and Children

Age-related differences in analgesic pharmacology are explained by a combination of pharmacokinetic and pharmacodynamics factors that vary with development. Neonates and young children have delayed maturation of hepatic enzymes involved in the metabolism of analgesics such as opioids and amide local anesthetics, increasing the risk of drug accumulation and toxicity.[25] For example, ester-type local anesthetics are metabolized by pseudocholinesterase. Young infants have significantly less of this enzyme compared to the adult population; therefore, clearance can be decreased and the effect of the local anesthetic is prolonged. Most neonates and young infants will have considerable maturation of the hepatic enzyme systems involved in biotransformation and conjugation by the age of 6 months, although enzyme maturation rates can vary considerably.[26] Neonates and young infants have decreased plasma concentrations of albumin and α_1 acid glycoprotein, which leads to decreased

protein binding and greater concentrations of unbound, pharmacologically active drug.[27] Neonates also have reduced glomerular filtration rates in the first few weeks of life resulting in slower elimination of many drugs and many active metabolites of drugs that have undergone hepatic metabolism which are excreted via the kidneys. A number of specific age-related differences in pharmacokinetics and in drug actions and risks are detailed with each drug class in the following text.

Nonopioid Analgesics

Nonopioid analgesics traditionally refer to aspirin, acetaminophen, nonsteroidal anti-inflammatory drugs (NSAIDs), and selective cyclo-oxygenase (COX) inhibitors. More recently, evidence of analgesic efficacy in adjuvant medications such as gabapentin and pregabalin have expanded the choices of nonopioid analgesics. Several new entities, such as the G protein-related receptor agonists, will provide other nontraditional opioid receptor mediated analgesic choices. Many of the NSAID analgesics were thought of as primarily peripherally active agents; however, analgesia does occur from a combination of peripheral as well as central actions, involving mechanisms in the spinal cord and brain, especially with activation of microglia. Nonopioid analgesics are often first-line drugs used for mild to moderate pain in infants and children because they do not produce respiratory effects and are generally nonsedating.

ONTOGENY OF PROSTANOID BIOSYNTHESIS AND CYCLO-OXYGENASES

A variety of prostanoids are produced during fetal life, and COX inhibition can alter essential functions, including patency of the ductus arteriosus. Recent studies by Ririe and coworkers[28] in infant rats suggest that COX-mediated processes in spinal microglia are quite immature at birth. These studies raise the question of whether commonly used analgesics acting on COX isoforms might be ineffective in infants due to this delayed maturation of a prominent site of action.

ASPIRIN AND OTHER SALICYLATES

The use of aspirin in children has diminished significantly, largely due to its association with Reye syndrome. The elimination of aspirin is greatly reduced in infants. In our practice, aspirin is almost never prescribed as an analgesic; its use is confined to situations in which antiplatelet actions are required.

ACETAMINOPHEN

Acetaminophen is the most commonly used analgesic in pediatrics and has been safely used in children of all ages. It is typically used for mild to moderate pain, fever, and can be combined with opioids to provide additional analgesic effect and decreased opioid use. The mechanisms underlying acetaminophen's analgesic and antipyretic actions remain controversial. Multiple central targets of acetaminophen's actions have been described, including COX isoenzyme (type 3 as well as type 2) inhibition, endogenous cannabinoid receptors, and nitric oxide pathways.[29] Clinically, acetaminophen, by itself, appears to produce minimal gastropathy, minimal effect on platelet function, and much milder anti-inflammatory actions compared to NSAIDs. Acetaminophen, combined with NSAIDs, can produce additional analgesic benefits, with synergism in some models.[30] The elimination of acetaminophen is primarily through glucuronidation and sulfation and elimination rates are similar among infants, children, and adults.[31,32] Various formulations are available with different concentrations in the United States, although there has been a recent attempt at standardization of dose formulations.[33] Inadvertent dosing errors have led to reports of fulminant hepatic failure among infants and children.[34] Typical oral dosing is 10 to 15 mg/kg per dose. The maximum daily dosing is 40 mg/kg/day for premature infants and 75 mg/kg/day for term infants and children. Rectal dosing can be used for children who are unable to tolerate oral dosing, although absorption of rectal dosing can be variable.[35] Maximal concentration after rectal dosing occurs at approximately 2 to 3 hours. Typical rectal dosing is 30 to 45 mg/kg initially, followed by 20 mg/kg every 6 hours.[32,34] In 2010, the U.S. Food and Drug Administration (FDA) approved the use of intravenous acetaminophen. Peak plasma concentration is reached in 15 minutes following infusion and data show improved pain control with use of the intravenous, with opioid sparing effect.[36–38] There is a role for use of the intravenous form in children who are both nothing by mouth (NPO) and nothing by rectum (NPR), as well as situations where children are NPO alone, given that rectal dosing can lead to discomfort, fear, or anxiety in children beyond infancy.

NONSTEROIDAL ANTI-INFLAMMATORY DRUGS

NSAIDs are commonly used for mild to moderate pain and for fever control in children. They are often combined with opioids to augment analgesic efficacy and potentially reduce opioid use and opioid side effects. The use of several NSAIDs in postsurgical patients has been shown to reduce opioid use by approximately 30% to 40%.[39]

NSAIDs produce their anti-inflammatory effect by reversibly inhibiting COX-1 and COX-2 isoforms and inhibiting the conversion of arachidonic acid to prostanoids.[40] The clearance of ibuprofen, ketorolac, and several other NSAIDs is more rapid in toddlers and preschool children compared to adults.[41]

Based on epidemiologic studies and pooled data from clinical trials, NSAIDs have a generally good safety margin in children and infants from roughly age 6 months onward, particularly with short-term use. There are limited safety data on the use of NSAIDs among neonates and young infants. In certain situations, one can consider NSAID use, such as ketorolac, in infants under 6 months, if the risk of using alternate analgesics is felt to be greater than use of an NSAID.[42,43] Indomethacin has been used for closure of patent ductus arteriosus in neonates. Elimination of indomethacin is slower in neonates and has the associated risk of hyponatremia and renal toxicity in this age group.[44] The incidence of NSAID side effects is quite low in children, when administered for postoperative pain relief. A large-scale study in children administered short-term use of ibuprofen showed a very low overall risk of severe side effects.[45] The risks of renal and hepatic toxicities are increased in states of decreased renal and hepatic blood flow, such as with significant surgical blood loss or shock. Much of the safety data for long-term use of NSAIDs in children is based on experience in treating juvenile rheumatoid arthritis (JRA).[46] Long-term use is associated with a higher incidence of mild gastrointestinal distress, but significant gastropathy and gastrointestinal bleeding in children is less common when compared to adults.

Although NSAIDs inhibit platelet aggregation and can prolong bleeding time, clinically significant bleeding is uncommon in healthy children. The use of NSAIDS after tonsillectomy procedures remains somewhat controversial. Children requiring tonsillectomy often have obstructive sleep apnea and are at increased risk of hypoventilation and apnea with opioids, making nonopioid analgesics an attractive alternative. Nausea and vomiting are also common after tonsillectomy, and opioids exacerbate these problems. Life-threatening bleeding can occur after tonsillectomy in the immediate postoperative period and approximately 7 days postoperatively after the patient has been discharged from the hospital.

Two meta-analyses came to different conclusions about the safety of NSAIDs in tonsillectomy. One found no significant increase in bleeding, whereas the other reported a threefold increase in bleeding episodes of sufficient severity to require reoperation.[47,48] A more recent retrospective chart review did support the findings that postoperative use of ibuprofen did increase posttonsillectomy bleeding.[49] It is less clear if single dosing of ketorolac during the

perioperative period increases the risk of postoperative bleeding in this population. A recent meta-analysis does not show increased risk of posttonsillectomy hemorrhage in children with perioperative ketorolac use.[50] Despite these concerns, NSAIDs remain commonly used in the posttonsillectomy population worldwide at many institutions both perioperatively and in the postoperative healing period.

An additional concern with NSAID use is impaired bone healing after orthopedic surgeries that involve osteoclast activation and new bone formation.[51] In vitro studies, animal models, and some case-control studies in adults suggest a higher incidence of impaired bone healing and nonunion with NSAID use. However, compared to adults, children are less likely to have impairment of bone formation with similar orthopedic procedures. Even in major procedures such as posterior spinal fusion for scoliosis, perioperative use of NSAIDS appears to be safe and not to result in a higher incidence of nonunion.[52] For surgeries with lower risk of nonunion, or for selected patients with greater than average risks or side effects from opioids, judicious use of NSAIDs for brief time periods should be considered.

Selective COX-2 inhibitors have the advantage of lower incidence of gastrointestinal symptoms and decreased effect on platelet function compared to traditional NSAIDs in adult patients. The risk of nephropathy with selective COX-2 inhibitors is similar to that of traditional NSAIDs.[53] Anti-inflammatory and analgesic effects of COX-2 inhibitors are also similar to those of traditional NSAIDs. COX-2 inhibitors have been associated with cardiovascular complications in adults, with both short- and long-term use. Rofecoxib and valdecoxib have been withdrawn from the market in response to these reports of cardiovascular complications in adults. The cardiovascular risk of COX-2 inhibitors in infants and children remains unclear. The use of COX-2 inhibitors may be considered in children with JRA who experience good analgesia with traditional NSAIDs, but who have significant gastrointestinal symptoms, or in children with bleeding disorders, such as hemophilia or thrombocytopenia, to achieve analgesia with less risk of bleeding than with traditional NSAIDs. Studies of COX-2 inhibitors for analgesia after tonsillectomy are mixed. One study found better analgesia with ibuprofen compared to placebo.[54] One double-blind randomized controlled trial (RCT) found benefit to use of celecoxib in the posttonsillectomy population with a modest decrease in pain scores in addition to decreased use of acetaminophen.[55] Some studies suggest that COX-2 inhibitors might be less likely to interfere with active bone formation. Please see Table 50.2 for dosing guidelines of common nonopioid analgesics.

KETAMINE

Ketamine is increasingly used in both acute and chronic pain, especially in the postoperative period. Ketamine has anti-N-methyl-D-aspartate (NMDA) activity, which acts to decrease wind-up, central sensitization, opioid-induced hyperalgesia, and opioid tolerance. Multiple studies in the adult population have shown that ketamine has not only opioid-sparing effects but also analgesic and antihyperalgesic effects.[56] Literature supporting the use of ketamine in the perioperative period in children is not as clear. A 2016 meta-analysis of perioperative ketamine use in children did not find that ketamine beneficial in decreasing the amount of opioids used postoperatively.[57] Although the meta-analysis was not favorable, individual studies favor the use of ketamine in the postoperative period. This study showed decreased opioid use and lower pain scores following Nuss procedure in the group that received ketamine in addition to fentanyl.[58] One study published in 2016 did not find that low-dose ketamine postoperatively in posterior fusion spine surgery in children decreased opioid use postoperatively.[59] This particular study also did not find benefit in

TABLE 50.2   Dosing Guidelines for Nonopioid Analgesics

	Dose <60 kg	Dose >60 kg
Acetaminophen	10–15 mg/kg q4h PO	650–1,000 mg q4h PO
Acetaminophen	15 mg/kg q6h IV	15 mg/kg q6h IV
Naproxen	5 mg/kg q12h PO	250–500 mg q12h PO
Ibuprofen	6–10 mg/kg q6–8h PO	400–600 mg q6h PO
Celecoxib	2–4 mg/kg q1h PO	100–200 mg q12h PO
Ketorolac	0.3–5 mg/kg q6–8h IV, not for >5 d	15–30 mg q6–8h IV, not for >5 d
Ketamine	0.1 mg/kg/h IV infusion with titration	0.1 mg/kg/h IV infusion with titration
Gabapentin	15 mg/kg PO preoperative	1 g PO preoperative

NOTE: Dosing guidelines listed herein refer to children > 1 year of age. Maximum dose acetaminophen: 75 mg/kg/day. Further modifications in dosing are required for use of these agents in term and preterm neonates and in infants. Modifications are detailed in the text.
IV, intravenous; PO, orally.

preventing long-term postoperative pain, although the incidence of persistent postoperative pain in this demographic is not clearly known. It is reasonable to consider use of ketamine in children, particularly in those with difficult to control pain or a history of chronic opioid use. The data for use in adults is well-established and thus is an area that can be further explored in pediatrics.

ANTICONVULSANTS

The use of anticonvulsants in chronic pain is well established; however, their use in acute pain, especially in children, is not as well established. There is evidence to support perioperative use of gabapentin for spine surgery in children. A study published in 2010 did show benefit to perioperative use of gabapentin 15 mg/kg prior to posterior spine fusion.[60] Gabapentin (continued at 5 mg/kg three times a day for a total of 5 days) decreased opioid requirements and postoperative pain scores only in the first 48 hours after surgery. Therefore, some clinicians only provide a preoperative oral loading dose. Valproic acid is another anticonvulsant that finds limited use in the acute treatment of pediatric migraine with one study finding approximately 50% of patients receiving significant relief from their headache.[61] There is some evidence to support its efficacy in the treatment of acute migraine; however, the studies are few and also complicated by the fact that valproic acid was not the first-line treatment; thus, other medications, treatments, and factors likely played a role in the reported relief.[62]

Opioids

Opioids are among the most widely used analgesics for treating moderate to severe pain in infants and children. As with adults, they are extremely useful but require careful patient selection, titrated dosing, and active treatment of side effects.

ONTOGENY OF OPIOID ACTIONS

The ontogeny of opioid actions has been studied in human clinical trials, in case series, and in a number of infant animal models. Infant animal models have provided useful information, although there are marked differences among species in opioid actions. There are age-related differences in analgesia and side effects involving pharmacokinetic and pharmacodynamics differences. Opioids (except for remifentanil) have prolonged actions in neonates and infants due to immature hepatic enzyme systems and immature renal excretion of active metabolites. Effects of hepatic and renal dysfunction on opioid clearance are discussed in a separate section in the following text.

Additional factors that influence opioid pharmacokinetics include developmental changes in expression of P-glycoproteins, both in the gastrointestinal tract and in the blood–brain barrier, and changes in protein binding.

Pharmacodynamic studies of opioids in neonates and younger infants have examined analgesia and side effects, with a major emphasis on measures of respiratory depression. These studies are made difficult by a number of factors, including the imprecision inherent in observational pain measures in neonates, on the state dependence of behavioral responses, on the confounding effects of critical illness on measures, and on the variability of painful stimuli. Major sites of opioid actions, including the periaqueductal grey matter and descending pathways of the dorsolateral funiculus, appear immature in infant rats. Conversely, opioids administered systemically or via the epidural route show strong analgesic responses in infant rats at developmental stages corresponding to preterm neonates. In human studies, there are mixed results with use of opioids in studies of procedural pain in neonates, and studies randomly assigning ventilated neonates to receive morphine infusions versus placebo infusions (with both groups receiving morphine for painful procedures) have not shown clear advantages in the morphine infusion groups.[63,64]

Children who are at particular risk for respiratory depressant effects of opioids include those with tonsillar hypertrophy, obstructive sleep apnea, certain neurologic conditions, and craniofacial abnormalities as well as neonates and young infants. Neonates and infants, particularly premature infants, have an increased risk of apnea and hypoventilation in response to opioids on a pharmacodynamic as well as pharmacokinetic basis. Careful dosing, cardiorespiratory monitoring, and close nursing observation are warranted for neonates and younger infants receiving opioids.

CODEINE

Codeine is an opioid previously used widely to treat mild to moderate pain. It is available as an elixir in pill and parenteral forms. Although it has seen a declining use for pain, it remains commonly used in cough suppressant formulations. For reasons to be detailed in the following text, our opinion is that codeine is in general a suboptimal choice as an analgesic in children in most settings, and we recommend against its use.[65] Codeine is a prodrug extensively metabolized in the liver. It is demethylated to morphine, which accounts for the analgesic effect.[66] A study of children undergoing surgery, receiving a fairly large dose of codeine, found that roughly one-third of the subjects generated undetectable blood concentrations of morphine, which would result in no discernible analgesic effect. Conversely, there are genotypes associated with ultrarapid metabolism of codeine to morphine.[67,68] In these subjects, standard recommended codeine doses can produce apnea. Standard dosing is 0.5 to 1 mg/kg every 4 hours. Dose escalation beyond this range appears to generate a higher incidence of side effects, particularly nausea and vomiting. In standard doses, codeine is a very weak analgesic. Studies in adult patients comparing efficacy of codeine to ibuprofen have shown that 30 to 45 mg codeine has less analgesic effect than 600 mg of ibuprofen. Because of the relatively high incidence of the impaired inability to demethylate codeine and higher incidence of side effects, other oral opioids such as oxycodone, morphine, hydromorphone, and hydrocodone are preferred. Intramuscular (IM) codeine has the double disadvantage of being a weak and inconsistent analgesic delivered by a noxious route.

Codeine is often dispensed in combination with acetaminophen to increase efficacy. When prescribing codeine combined with acetaminophen, care is required to avoid inadvertent administration of toxic doses of acetaminophen, particularly when increased dosages are prescribed for pain or when patients are taking other over-the-counter preparations containing acetaminophen. Codeine is also commonly prescribed as an antitussive.

As of 2013, the FDA has issued a new contraindication for the use of codeine to treat pain or cough in children younger than 12 years as well as a warning against its use the 12- to 18-year-old age group of children who have sleep apnea and/or are obese.[69]

TRAMADOL

Tramadol has both opioid and nonopioid properties. It exists in a racemic mixture where the positive enantiomer has opioid and serotoninergic properties and its negative enantiomer exerts noradrenergic reuptake properties.[70] Like codeine, it is metabolized to O-desmethyltramadol by the P450 isoenzyme CYP2D6. It exerts its analgesic effect via the μ-opioid as well as acting as a serotonin and norepinephrine reuptake inhibitor. In the United States, it is available only in the oral form. In other countries, it is also available in an intravenous preparation. Although not approved for use in children under the age of 12 years, it is widely used for postoperative pain as well as acute pain in children.[71]

Tramadol is also associated with many reports of toxicity in children. Overall, the incidence of these adverse reactions is low, but they do occur. Toxicity for tramadol, like opioids, not only can result in respiratory depression but can also result in seizures.

As of 2017, the FDA has issued new black box contraindication for the use of tramadol to treat pain or cough in children less than 12 years of age. They have also included a contraindication to the use of tramadol in children undergoing tonsillectomy and/or adenoidectomy in patients under the age of 18 years. In addition to these contraindications, a new warning against the of tramadol in the 12- to 18-year-old age group in children with sleep apnea or who are obese is also in place. These were put in place after the recognition of the implications of genetic variability in P450 2D6 metabolism and the potential for life-threatening reactions.[72]

OXYCODONE

Oxycodone can be used for moderate pain in doses of 0.05 to 0.1 mg/kg every 4 hours and for moderate to severe pain in starting doses of 0.1 to 0.2 mg/kg every 4 hours in infants and children >1 year of age. Less information regarding the use of oxycodone in neonates and small infants is available. Recent review and modeling suggests the use of lower doses in preterm neonate and small infants starting as low as 0.035 mg/kg and increasing to 0.065 mg/kg in term neonates.[73,74] Although historically prescribed in smaller doses, oxycodone dosing can be escalated as needed much like any of the so-called *strong opioids*. Oxycodone is generally well tolerated by children either alone or in combination with acetaminophen. Our impression is that it is associated with fewer side effects than codeine when used to treat moderate to severe pain. Oxycodone is metabolized in the liver to oxymorphone, which is metabolically active.[75] Because oxymorphone is eliminated by the kidneys, it can accumulate in patients with renal failure. Oxycodone is commonly used in children postoperatively when transitioning from parenteral opioids to oral opioids in preparation for discharge.

A sustained-release preparation of oxycodone (OxyContin) is available for use in the treatment of chronic pain and was approved use in children age 11 to 16 years in 2015. Recently, the trend at our institution is away from the use of long-acting oxycodone for postoperative pain. It has a bioavailability of approximately 60% and reaches peak analgesic effect after 60 to 90 minutes.[76]

MORPHINE

Morphine is often the first-line opioid chosen for parenteral use in children. It has a long track record in pediatrics; it has received extensive pharmacologic study at all age groups; it is inexpensive; and it can be administered via oral, sublingual, intravenous, subcutaneous, rectal, and neuraxial routes.

The duration of morphine's clinical effects are related in a complex manner to distribution into and out of the central nervous system, hepatic metabolism, and excretion of active metabolites, including morphine 6-glucuronide. Morphine primarily undergoes glucuronidation by the UDP glucuronosyltransferase (UGT) pathway in the liver to morphine-3-glucuronide, which has predominantly excitatory actions, and morphine-6-glucuronide, which has analgesic, sedative, and respiratory depressant actions more potent than morphine.[77] Because morphine-6-glucuronide is renally eliminated, it can accumulate in patients with renal failure, producing delayed sedation and hypoventilation. In addition, accumulation of morphine 3-glucuronide can contribute to delirium, agitation, and seizures. The elimination half-life of morphine in older children and adults is approximately 3 to 4 hours. The elimination half-life is approximately 7 hours in full-term newborns and even longer in premature infants.[78,79] Long-acting preparations of morphine, such as MS Contin or KADIAN, are typically used for children with sickle cell pain, cancer pain, and other types of chronic pain.

Dosing of morphine in children, as with all opioids, should be titrated to effect and individualized based on severity of pain, underlying medical conditions, age, side effects, and weight. See Table 50.3 for dosing guidelines for oral and parenteral morphine.

HYDROMORPHONE

Hydromorphone is a commonly used opioid for acute pain management in children for both parenteral and oral use. Like morphine, it is used in children for patient-controlled analgesia (PCA), continuous infusions, oral dosing, intermittent intravenous boluses, and epidural analgesia. Hydromorphone can provide effective analgesia in children with cancer pain and mucositis. In steady-state dosing, hydromorphone is 5 to 6 times more potent than morphine when given intravenously in children.[80]

Although hydromorphone is commonly prescribed to patients with renal insufficiency, this practice is not evidence-based. Hydromorphone is metabolized primarily to hydromorphone-3-glucuronide (H3G) and, to a much lesser extent, hydromorphone-6-glucuronide (H6G) through UGT pathways.[81] These glucuronides can also accumulate in patients with renal insufficiency. Information on metabolism of hydromorphone in neonates and young infants is very sparse.

METHADONE

Methadone is a long-acting opioid with a slow elimination and prolonged duration of analgesia.[82,83] The elimination half-life is highly variable, ranging from 6 to 30 hours. Methadone has a high oral bioavailability of 70% to 100%. Due to these unique properties, methadone is convenient to use as a prolonged duration opioid. Intermittent intravenous dosing at prolonged intervals (e.g., every 4, 6, or 8 hours) can provide a basal level of analgesia similar to that achieved by continuous infusions or frequent intravenous boluses of other opioids.[84]

Methadone is available as an elixir and is often used in place of sustained-release opioid preparations to treat chronic pain in young children or in children unable to swallow pills. Conversely, methadone requires careful titration and vigilance to avoid overdosage, both because of extreme pharmacokinetic variability and for pharmacodynamic reasons detailed in the following text.

Methadone is prepared as a racemic mixture of levo (l-) and dextro (d-) isomers. The l-isomer acts as a μ-receptor agonist; the d-isomer acts as an antagonist at the NMDA receptor in the brain and spinal cord. Antagonism at the NMDA receptors

TABLE 50.3	Initial Dosing Guidelines for Opioids						
	Equianalgesic Doses and Intervals		Parenteral Dosing			Oral Dosing	
			Usual Starting Intravenous or Subcutaneous Doses			Usual Starting Oral Doses and Intervals	
Drug	Parenteral	Oral	Child <50 kg	Child >50 kg	Ratio Parenteral to Oral	Child <50 kg	Child >50 kg
Codeine	120 mg	200 mg	NR	NR	1:2	NR	NR
Morphine	10 mg	30 mg (long term)	Bolus: 0.1 mg/kg every 2–4 h	Bolus: 5–8 mg every 2–4 h	1:3 (long term)	Immediate-release: 0.3 mg/kg every 3–4 h	Immediate-release: 15–20 mg every 3–4 h
			Infusion: 0.03 mg/kg/h	Infusion: 1.5 mg/h	1:6 (single dose)	Sustained-release: 20–35 kg, 10–15 mg every 12 h; 35–50 kg, 15–30 mg every 12 h	Sustained-release: 30–45 mg every 12 h
Oxycodone	NA	15–20 mg	NA	NA	NA	0.1–0.2 mg/kg every 3–4 h	5–10 mg every 3–4 h
Methadone[a]	10 mg	10–20 mg	0.1 mg/kg every 4–8 h	5–8 mg every 4–8 h	1:2	0.1–0.2 mg/kg every 4–8 h	5–10 mg every 4–8 h
Fentanyl	100 mg (0.1 mg)	NA			NA	NA	NA
			Bolus: 0.5–1.0 mg/kg every 1–2 h	Bolus: 25–50 mg every 1–2 h			
			Infusion: 0.5–2.0 mg/kg/h	Infusion: 25–100 mg/h			
Hydromorphone	1.5–2 mg	7.5–10 mg	Bolus: 0.02 mg every 2–4 h	Bolus: 1 mg every 2–4 h	1:5	0.05–0.1 mg/kg every 3–4 h	2–4 mg every 3–4 h
			Infusion: 0.006 mg/kg/h	Infusion: 0.3 mg/h			
Meperidine[b]	75–100 mg	300 mg	NR	NR	1:4	NR	NR

NOTE: Doses are for patients over 6 months of age. In infants under 6 months, initial per kilogram doses should begin at roughly 25% of the per kilogram doses recommended here. Higher doses are often required for patients receiving mechanical ventilation. All doses are approximate and should be adjusted according to clinical circumstances. Recommendations are adapted from previous summary tables, including those of a consensus statement from the World Health Organization and the International Association for the Study of Pain.

[a]Methadone requires additional vigilance because it can accumulate and produce delayed sedation. If sedation occurs, doses should be withheld until sedation resolves. Thereafter, doses should be substantially reduced, the interval between doses should be extended to 3 to 12 hours, or both. Electrocardiogram (ECG) for QT interval required.

[b]The use of meperidine should generally be avoided. Can consider use for postoperative shivering.

NA, not applicable; NR, not recommended.

Adapted from Berder CB, Sethna NF. Analgesics for the treatment of pain in children. *N Engl J Med* 2002;347(14):1094–1103. Copyright © 2002 Massachusetts Medical Society. Reprinted with permission from Massachusetts Medical Society.

results in analgesia and reduced hyperalgesia as well as partially reversing tolerance to opioids.[85]

The NMDA antagonism of methadone is also a rationale for its use in the treatment of neuropathic pain. The combined μ-agonist and NMDA antagonist actions of methadone result in incomplete cross tolerance. Thus, the dose conversion ratios between methadone and morphine and other μ-opioids are different for opioid-naive versus opioid-tolerant patients. For opioid-naive patients, the average daily intravenous methadone requirement is roughly one-third of the corresponding intravenous morphine requirement; however, average daily methadone requirements for opioid-tolerant patients may be a little as 10% to 15% of the total daily morphine dosing.[86] This is particularly relevant when converting morphine to methadone for children with advanced cancer and when weaning nonventilated infants and children following prolonged opioid therapy, especially following intensive care. Careful titration and frequent patient assessment for respiratory depression is warranted in dosing methadone. When anticipating long-term methadone use, either when weaning from a long-term opioid infusion, the opioid-dependent infant, or in cancer-related pain, care should be taken during initial titration of methadone given its long and variable half-life. It is generally our practice to increase methadone no more frequently than every 2 to 3 days. For patients showing signs of oversedation or respiratory depression, it is often necessary to hold multiple doses of methadone because of its prolonged duration of action. In our practice, we also use methadone intraoperatively during certain procedures such as posterior-spinal fusion or Nuss bar placement.[87,88] We do not routinely manage acute pain with methadone given other available alternatives.

FENTANYL

Fentanyl has a rapid onset and brief duration of action after single-dose administration, and it is often used for brief painful procedures in children, such as lumbar punctures, bone marrow aspirations, fracture reductions, and dressing changes. Fentanyl is also used for PCA in children with acute and chronic pain and in highly selected situations as a transdermal patch for children with cancer-related chronic pain.[89]

Fentanyl primarily undergoes glucuronidation in the liver to inactive metabolites, making it a preferred opioid for patients with renal or liver failure. Fentanyl is 50 to 100 times more potent than morphine with single-dose administration and roughly 20 to 50 times more potent with continuous infusions. The action of fentanyl after single-dose administration is terminated by rapid redistribution; however, after prolonged infusion or repeated boluses, the termination of fentanyl effect is determined more by elimination than redistribution and results in a prolonged duration of action. In addition, pharmacokinetics of fentanyl are easily altered in small infants, as hepatic blood flow is affected during surgery.[90] Continuous infusions or repeated boluses in neonates can cause a particularly prolonged effect. Rapid administration is associated with glottic and chest wall rigidity, which can be especially pronounced in neonates and young infants. Neuromuscular blockade and assisted ventilation are usually necessary for treatment, particularly in neonates and young infants. Naloxone may sometimes be effective in reversing fentanyl-induced rigidity, but this action is not reliable.

For brief painful procedures, incremental doses of fentanyl at 0.5 to 1 µg/kg every 1 to 3 minutes usually provide effective analgesia. Cardiorespiratory monitoring and immediate availability of airway equipment and personal skilled in airway management are necessary. Oral transmucosal fentanyl has also been used for brief painful procedures in children and for breakthrough cancer pain.[91] The oral transmucosal dose is partially absorbed across the buccal mucosa and partially swallowed; overall, the bioavailability is approximately 50%. It is generally well tolerated by children, although almost 90% of children experience facial pruritus. Additionally, the peak analgesic effect after a standard 15 µg/kg dose is 20 minutes, which may be limiting for some procedures. Another option is the use of intranasal fentanyl, which is particularly beneficial in patients who do not have established intravenous access.[92] Dosing of intranasal fentanyl is higher than intravenous, at 1.5 µg/kg. Intranasal fentanyl may be used in a variety of acute pain situations including sickle cell crisis, limb injuries, and during general anesthesia for myringotomy.[93]

Transdermal fentanyl is used in children with cancer pain and other forms of chronic pain requiring regular opioid dosing. It is indicated in a small subgroup of children who are unable to swallow pills, who have limited intravenous access, or who have experienced side effects with a number of other opioids. Approximately 12 to 24 hours are necessary to achieve steady-state plasma levels after applying the transdermal fentanyl patch, and it is therefore not indicated for acute fluctuations in pain intensity. Additional short-acting opioids are necessary to treat breakthrough pain. Transdermal fentanyl is indicated for opioid-tolerant patients who have relatively constant pain. Serious and lethal adverse events have been reported among opioid-naive patients who were treated with transdermal fentanyl for acute postsurgical pain.[94] There has been a series of manufacturing problems that have led to inconsistent delivery for some batches of transdermal fentanyl. We emphasize here that transdermal fentanyl is not recommended for opioid-naive patients under any circumstances.

MEPERIDINE

Meperidine is a synthetic opioid roughly one-tenth the potency of morphine when administered intravenously. It has some anticholinergic actions and is metabolized to normeperidine, which can cause seizures, hallucinations, and agitation, particularly with repeated dosing. Metabolism in infants is quite variable.[95] Life-threatening reactions can occur with the use of meperidine in patients taking monoamine oxidase inhibitors, leading to hyperreflexia, seizures, hemodynamic instability, and death.

Meperidine does have the unique property in subanalgesic doses of treating rigors associated with blood product transfusions or shivering following general anesthesia. Because of the serious adverse effects of meperidine and because it offers no particular advantage for pain control, its use should be limited to the treatment of rigors or shivering.

Opioid Administration in Infants and Children

As in adult patients, there are several means for systemic opioid delivery in pediatric patients. The choice of which method depends to a certain extent on available resources, coexisting medical conditions, types of pain, patients' mobility, and other factors.

Regardless of method of opioid delivery, protocols for safe opioid administration should be in place to detect excess sedation, signs of respiratory depression, and impending respiratory failure. Protocols should include regular nursing assessments, documentation of vital signs and levels sedation, and, where appropriate, use of electronic cardiorespiratory monitoring that should include pulse oximetry. Patients who should be considered for cardiorespiratory monitoring include infants who are younger than 6 months, infants who have a history of apnea and bradycardia, or prematurity, and opioid-naive children who require a continuous opioid infusion. Children at increased risk for airway obstruction while receiving opioids such as those with tonsillar hypertrophy and obstructive sleep apnea or children with craniofacial abnormalities should also be considered for cardiorespiratory monitoring. There is considerable variation in practices regarding methods to detect and prevent opioid-induced respiratory depression. It is our general practice to use continuous pulse oximetry for children who are utilizing continuous opioids, PCA, or parent-/nurse-controlled analgesia (PNCA). Many recommendations are based on reasonable extrapolation from physiologic considerations. Nevertheless, evidence to quantify the risk reduction from specific forms of monitoring is quite sparse.

INTERMITTENT INTRAVENOUS BOLUS DOSING

In clinical care areas other than the intensive care units or the postanesthesia care units, in our institution, most intermittent bolus dosing of opioids are administered as an infusion over 20 minutes rather than "intravenous push." Although a slow administration is thought of as a somewhat safer method of intermittent dosing, careful monitoring and repeated patient assessments remain important during and after the opioid infusion. Intermittent systemic boluses cause wide fluctuations in plasma opioids concentrations. Patients therefore experience probably few side effects but increased pain just prior to their next bolus opioid dose. After the dose is administered, patients experience pain relief, but often with excessive side effects, as the plasma opioid concentration reaches supratherapeutic levels. Regular, intermittent dosing of opioids can result in dose stacking, especially if the opioids are ordered around the clock. As each next dose is administered, the prior dose has not fully cleared the plasma and the remaining plasma concentration can ramp up with each successive dose. At some point, the next bolus results in a toxic peak level, which in the frail opioid-naive patient can result in significant cardiorespiratory compromise. To avoid wide variations in plasma concentrations with resultant fluctuations in analgesia and side effects, continuous infusions and PCA are commonly used.

CONTINUOUS OPIOID INFUSIONS

Continuous opioid infusions offer the advantage of providing steady-state plasma levels and result in good analgesia in infants and children who experience relatively constant levels of pain intensity. Additional intermittent boluses are necessary for periods of increased pain, such as endotracheal tube suctioning or chest physiotherapy. Recommended starting infusion rates have been adjusted for age based on both pharmacokinetic considerations, on studies of respiratory responses, and on clinical outcome studies. Starting infusion rates for morphine have been recommended as around 0.025 to 0.030 mg/kg/hour for children and infants >6 months of age, with reductions to 0.015 mg/kg/hour from 1 to 6 months, ranging down to 0.005 mg/kg/hour for preterm neonates at 32 weeks postconception. These recommendations should be taken as population averages; individual rates should be adjusted according to clinical conditions, expected intensity of painful stimuli, and behavioral and physiologic signs.

PATIENT-, NURSE-, AND PARENT-CONTROLLED ANALGESIA

PCA is widely used among pediatric centers for variety of acute painful conditions such as cancer pain, sickle cell pain from vasooclusive crises, trauma, and acute postoperative pain. Most children 8 years of age and older have the cognitive ability to understand cause and effect relationships of pushing the PCA button and obtaining pain relief. In rare cases, experienced children younger than 6 to 8 years, who have had long-standing pain, are able to use PCA. For most children younger than 6 to 8 years, PCA has a higher failure rate in part because of the inability to understand the causal connection between button-pressing and delivery of medication to provide pain relief. However, nurse-controlled analgesia (NCA) or PNCA has been shown to provide effective analgesia with good patient, parent, and caregiver satisfaction in younger children. PNCA is also used for children with cognitive and physical limitations who are unable to use the PCA.[96–98] In our hospital, PNCA is the most common method of systemic opioid administration following major surgery in infants and in children with cognitive or physical limitations to self-administration.[99,100] At our institution, we have also adopted the use of PNCA in our neonatal population. In this population, we recommend starting your opioid dose lower at 10 μg/kg.

Commonly used opioids for PCA/NCA are morphine, hydromorphone, and fentanyl. Use of a basal infusion along with PCA boluses has been a subject of controversy and some controlled studies in adults and children. In some studies, a basal infusion improves pain scores, patient satisfaction, and the quality of nighttime sleep. In other studies, a basal infusion increased surrogate measures of hypoventilation, including brief respiratory pauses. Our view is that the recommendations regarding addition of a basal infusion depend on patient medical conditions and risk factors, on psychological factors, on expected intensity of painful stimuli, and on history of previous opioid use. For example, a basal infusion may be omitted for children who have received a regional block intraoperatively, for children with increased respiratory risks, or for those undergoing surgical procedures expected to be only moderately, but not severely, painful. Conversely, we generally include a basal infusion for patients who are opioid-tolerant or for procedures expected to cause severe pain. For those undergoing very painful operations, such as scoliosis surgery, open lateral thoracotomy, or major hip surgery, we generally maintain a basal infusion at least through the first postoperative night.

Parent-controlled analgesia is widely accepted for use among children with advanced cancer or children in palliative care. There have been several serious adverse events reported, including apnea and death with the use of parent-controlled analgesia in children with risk factors and with insufficient protocols for patient observation and education on proper use. Our view is that parent-controlled analgesia for opioid-naive children should be restricted to institutions which have formal programs for parent education, protocols for frequent assessments by nurses, and protocols for cardiorespiratory. Please see Tables 50.4 and 50.5 for PCA dosing.

TABLE 50.4 Typical Starting Doses for Patient-Controlled Analgesia (for >10 kg)

Drug	Bolus Dose (μg/kg)	Continuous Rate (μg/kg/h)	Hourly Limit (μg/kg)
Morphine	10–30	4–20	120
Hydromorphone	2–6	1–4	24
Fentanyl	0.25–1	0.25	2–4

NOTE: The usual lockout interval is 6 to 10 minutes.

TABLE 50.5 Typical Starting Doses for Patient-Controlled Analgesia (for <10 kg)

Drug	Bolus Dose (μg/kg)	Continuous Rate (μg/kg/h)	Hourly Maximum (μg/kg)
Morphine	10–30[a]	10–30	90[b]

[a]We recommend starting at 10 μg/kg per dose and no basal in infants <10 kg.
[b]Lower hourly maximum reflects differences in metabolism discussed in text in neonates.

TREATMENT OF OPIOID SIDE EFFECTS

Opioids are alike in that all produce similar side effects including nausea, vomiting, constipation, pruritus, urinary retention, respiratory depression, and sedation. In some cases, severe side effects are as distressing to children as pain. Although children may have particular side effects with individual opioids, there are few data to suggest that side effects differ greatly among the more commonly used opioids. Kehlet[101] and others have argued for multimodal approaches to postoperative analgesia that emphasize opioid-sparing, in part because of the detrimental impact of opioid side effects on the course of postoperative recovery.

There is an important role for standardized protocols for treatment of opioid side effects and for rapid institution of therapy for many patients. Nevertheless, along with prompt intervention, there is a role for clinical assessment and for consideration of a differential diagnosis. Two examples illustrate this point: (1) A patient may not only be itching due to opioids but could also have itching as part of an allergic response to a variety of other medications or physiologic processes and (2) a patient with advanced cancer, worsening back pain, and increasing opioid dosing may have urinary retention due to the opioid, but urinary retention could also be a harbinger of impending compression of the spinal cord or caudal equina. Clinicians need to balance prompt intervention with consideration of alternative diagnoses underlying these symptoms.

Opioid side effects occur by actions at both peripheral and central sites. For example, opioid-induced nausea and vomiting involves activation of receptors in the brainstem as well as in the gastrointestinal tract.[102] Similarly, some opioids may produce itching by peripheral histamine release, but the observation of profound itching with very small doses of intrathecal morphine supports the view that a predominant mechanism of opioid-induced itching is neurogenic and central, involving an imbalance of afferent signaling and neurotransmission in the spinal dorsal horn and nucleus caudalis. Local hives or itching at a site of opioid injection does not imply an allergic response.

Traditionally, treatment of opioid side effects has emphasized antagonists at nonopioid receptors; that is, use of antagonists of dopamine or serotonin receptors for treatment of nausea and vomiting or antihistamines for treatment of itching. These drugs may generate their own side effects, including extra pyramidal reactions from dopamine antagonists (phenothiazines, butyrophenones, metoclopramide); headache from serotonin antagonists (ondansetron, granisetron); and sedation, constipation, and urinary retention from antihistamines (diphenhydramine, hydroxyzine). Extrapyramidal reactions from dopamine antagonists may be treated prophylactically or as needed with antihistamines or central muscarinic anticholinergics. In our experience, extrapyramidal reactions may be misdiagnosed by some clinicians as seizures. Even among patients who do not have overt extrapyramidal signs, occasional patients report extreme dysphoria following administration of these agents. Dopamine antagonists and serotonin antagonists are partially effective in treatment of opioid-induced nausea and vomiting, but the numbers-needed-to-treat (NNTs) are higher than commonly believed by clinicians. The evidence for effectiveness of antihistamines in the treatment of opioid-induced itching is quite weak.[103]

There is a growing body of evidence supporting treating opioid side effects, especially nausea and vomiting and itching, at least in inpatients postoperatively, by ultra-low-dose infusions of opioid antagonists such as naloxone.[104] Low-dose naloxone infusions are not simply reversing opioid actions altogether, rather they are exploiting a differential dose response for reversing side effects versus reversing analgesia, in part due to differential binding to opioid receptors coupled to G-stimulatory versus G-inhibitory proteins. We could not identify studies that would guide low-dose naloxone infusions for side effect treatment in highly opioid-tolerant patients, although a preliminary report in patients with sickle cell disease suggested that a slightly higher naloxone infusion rate of 1 μg/kg/hour might be recommended.[105] At our institution, we routinely use doses between 0.5 and 2 μg/kg/hour with 1 μg/kg/hour being the most prevalent dosing. Nalbuphine is widely used for treatment of opioid-induced itching and nausea, although one pediatric study showed no benefit compared to placebo.[106]

Methylnaltrexone is a quaternized opioid antagonist that has access to the area postrema (which lacks a blood–brain barrier), but which is excluded from prominent sites of central analgesic action, such as the periaqueductal grey matter. Recent reports show methylnaltrexone to be beneficial to children and adolescents with opioid-induced constipation.[107] Alvimopan is an enterally constrained opioid antagonist that blocks opioid actions in the gastrointestinal tract, with minimal uptake in the portal vein and efficient first-pass hepatic clearance of the small quantities that do reach the liver.[108] Available evidence suggests that these two approaches hold promise for more effective treatment of opioid side effects, including nausea, vomiting, constipation, and other forms of postoperative gastrointestinal dysfunction.

Constipation is commonly seen in patients requiring opioids even for short-term use. It is such a prevalent side effect of opioids that one should employ a proactive approach of prescribing laxatives (polypropylene glycol, senna, bisacodyl, docusate) for patients expected to require more than just few doses of opioids. Please see Table 50.6 for management of common opioid side effects in children.

LOCAL ANESTHETICS AND REGIONAL ANESTHESIA IN INFANTS AND CHILDREN

Local anesthetics are widely used for a range of indications in infants and children, including topical analgesia for needle procedures, cutaneous infiltration for minor procedures, wound infiltration for surgery, peripheral and plexus blocks, and epidural and spinal anesthesia and analgesia. Work over the past 30 years has examined pharmacokinetics, safety, and clinical outcomes of local anesthesia in infants and children.

Pharmacokinetic information is available for many of the commonly used local anesthetics. Amino amides, including lidocaine, bupivacaine, and ropivacaine, have reduced clearance in neonates and younger infants due to immaturity of hepatic metabolism.[109] In the case of lidocaine, the predominant hepatic metabolite, MEGX, can accumulate in neonates, with a resultant risk of seizures. The amino ester chloroprocaine is rapidly metabolized by plasma esterases even in neonates and may be useful if prolonged infusions are required in neonates.[110]

CUTANEOUS ANALGESIA

Needle procedures are a prominent source of acute distress for infants and children. A number of local anesthetic formulations can produce good analgesia for superficial needle procedures. Several approaches can accelerate transfer across the skin, including eutectic mixtures, heating elements, iontophoresis, and jet injection. Selection among approaches may depend, in part, on local availability, cost, desired onset time, and impact of vasodilatation or vasoconstriction on the planned procedures.[111,112] A convenient jet injector device, the JTip has greatly facilitated the placement of intravenous lines, blood sampling, and skin preparation before a variety of procedures. It is easy to use, well-tolerated, and fast acting.[113,114]

WOUND INFILTRATION

Infiltration of the layers of surgical wounds is a simple approach to providing postoperative analgesia. This may be accomplished by one-time infiltration before wound closure or by placement of wound catheters for prolonged infusions of local anesthetics. Liposomal bupivacaine is now available, making it possible to have analgesia for 24 to 48 hours following infiltration. Although not approved for use in pediatrics at this time, it is available at some major pediatric centers and can be

---

TABLE 50.6	Management of Common Opioid Side Effects	
Side Effect	**Comments**	**Drug Dosage**
Nausea	Consider switching to different opioid. Use antiemetics. Exclude other processes (e.g., bowel obstruction).	Ondansetron 10–30 kg: 1–2 mg intravenously q8h >30 kg: 2–4 mg intravenously q8h Naloxone infusion 0.25–1 μg/kg/h Metoclopramide 0.1–0.2 mg/kg PO/intravenously q6h
Pruritus	Exclude other causes (e.g., drug allergy). Consider switching to different opioid. Use antipruritics.	Nalbuphine 0.1 mg/kg per dose intravenously q6h Naloxone infusion 0.25–2 μg/kg/h Diphenhydramine 0.25–0.5 mg/kg PO/intravenously q6h
Sedation	Add nonsedating analgesic (e.g., ketorolac, acetaminophen) and reduce opioid dose. Consider switching to different opioid.	Methylphenidate 0.05–0.2 mg/kg PO bid (morning and midday dosing)[a] Dextroamphetamine 5–10 mg every day[a]
Constipation	Regular use of stimulant and stool softener laxatives	Naloxone infusion 0.25–2 μg/kg/h Docusate Child: 10–40 mg PO daily Adults: 50–200 mg PO daily Dulcolax Child: 5 mg PO/PR daily Adult: 10 mg PO/PR daily Methylnaltrexone, alvimopan dosing is extrapolated from adults

[a]Generally, only for use when long-term opioids are appropriate such as in cancer pain.
bid, twice a day; PO, orally; PR, rectally.

considered for use in older children and adults. Further study is needed before recommending its use in infants and younger children.

Epidural Analgesia in Infants and Children

Epidural analgesia has widespread use in infants and children for postoperative pain management and can be considered in selected cases for children with cancer pain and for certain chronic pain conditions such as complex regional pain syndrome. Although epidural infusions can provide outstanding analgesia for children, they require specific expertise both in the techniques of placement and in management, and in our view, they should not be undertaken without a system of pediatric-specific management protocols.

A unique difference between adults and children concerns the fact that most pediatric regional anesthesia, including epidural analgesia, is performed after induction of general anesthesia or sedation because many children will not tolerate having needle procedures while awake. Although the safety track record of placement of epidural needles and catheters has been good, there remained some controversy regarding the risk–benefit ratio.[115–117] However, recent large reports from the Pediatric Regional Anesthesia Network (PRAN) have confirmed the safety and efficacy of a sleep block placement.[118]

Placing a lumbar epidural catheter in an anesthetized child is generally considered to be safe among experienced pediatric anesthesia providers. As an alternative to direct thoracic needle placement in infants, a common technique is to advance an epidural catheter from the caudal space to the desired surgical dermatome. Several studies have shown success in placing thoracic epidural catheters in infants using this technique.[119] Because neonates and infants have an increased risk of amide local anesthetic toxicity, proper placement of the epidural catheter tip is crucial in order to provide optimal analgesia while minimizing safe local anesthetic infusion rates.

For anesthetized patients who are receiving direct thoracic placement or for cephalad advancement of catheters to thoracic levels from the caudal route, our own strong personal preference is to encourage some method of objective confirmation of positioning whenever possible. Three methods can be used in different situations: (1) electrical nerve stimulation using Tsui's technique[120]; (2) radiographic confirmation, especially using fluoroscopy with radiopaque wire reinforced catheters and/or small amounts of water-soluble contrast material; and (3) ultrasound. Confirming the location of intended caudal-to-thoracic epidural catheter tip placement is strongly recommended because failure rates as high as 30% have been reported using a "blind" technique. As described by Tsui, electrical stimulation employs a saline-filled, wire-wrapped catheter, with twitches seen at the myotomal level of the catheter tip in a current range generally between 2 and 15 mA. This technique also confirms that a catheter is not subarachnoid (in which case, bilateral twitches in a broad distribution are seen at a current <0.5 to 1 mA) and not threaded out a nerve root foramen (in which case, unilateral twitches in a narrow distribution may be seen at a current <1.5 mA).

Confirming location of the epidural catheter tip in infants can be accomplished by obtaining a chest radiograph after injecting a small volume of radiocontrast dye or through the use of a radiopaque epidural catheter which can easily be seen on plain chest radiograph or fluoroscopy. An additional method of confirming epidural catheter tip location is to advance the catheter from the caudal space under direct visualization using fluoroscopy.

Ultrasound guidance can be used in guiding and confirming placement of epidural catheters in neonates and younger infants, although this technique requires two operators and significant experience in ultrasound techniques. Neuraxial structures such as ligamentum flavum, dura, and epidural space as well as depth from skin to epidural space can be clearly visualized using ultrasound in part because of incomplete ossification of the vertebrae in neonates and younger infants.[121]

DRUGS AND DRUG DOSING USED FOR EPIDURAL ANALGESIA

Continuous epidural analgesia in infants and children generally consists of dilute solutions of local anesthetics combined with fentanyl, morphine, hydromorphone, or an α_2 agonists such as clonidine.

Bupivacaine and ropivacaine are the most commonly used amide local anesthetics for epidural analgesia because they have long duration of action with slightly greater selectivity of sensory block compared to motor block. Pharmacokinetic studies of bupivacaine in children over the age of 6 months have reported good safety for infusion rates of bupivacaine of below 0.4 mg/kg/hour with plasma bupivacaine levels in a safe range of <2 to 3 μg/mL.[122] Neonates have reduced clearance of bupivacaine. Pharmacokinetic studies in neonates receiving continuous bupivacaine infusions have shown a continuous rise in plasma bupivacaine levels after the first 48 hours.

As a result of various pharmacokinetic studies, we use a maximum dose of 0.4 mg/kg/hour of bupivacaine for continuous epidural infusions in children over the age of 6 months. For children less than 4 to 6 months of age, we restrict the dose of bupivacaine to 0.2 mg/kg/hour. Because of the limitations in dosing of bupivacaine in young infants, it is reasonable to use adjuvants to epidural infusions which will have a synergistic effect with bupivacaine such as opioids and clonidine in order to maximize analgesia.

Ropivacaine is a long-acting amide local anesthetic, shown in adults, to have less central nervous system and cardiac toxicity and slightly more sensory selectivity when compared to bupivacaine. Due to this increased safety profile, ropivacaine is seeing increased use and becoming standard at many institutions such as ours. Pharmacokinetic studies in infants and children receiving single boluses of epidural ropivacaine show that, as with bupivacaine, clearances for ropivacaine are reduced in infants. In different studies, clearances for ropivacaine have ranged from around 4 to 8.5 mL/min/kg with generally lower values in younger infants. Data to support a less extensive motor block for ropivacaine have been mixed. Overall, infusion rates of 0.4 mg/kg/hour in older infants and children and 0.2 to 0.3 mg/kg/hour in neonates and younger infants appear quite safe. It is plausible that slightly higher rates than these will be shown to be safe as well.[123–125]

Chloroprocaine is used as an alternative to amide local anesthetics for continuous epidural infusions in neonates and very young infants to avoid the limitations of reduced clearance of amide local anesthetics and to safely permit sufficient epidural infusion rates for optimal analgesia. Even in neonates, chloroprocaine is rapidly metabolized with an elimination half-life of less than 6 minutes, making it an attractive choice for continuous epidural infusions in neonates. Studies of continuous epidural chloroprocaine infusions in term and preterm infants have shown good sensory blockade with no signs of neurotoxicity.[110,126]

Compared to infusions of ropivacaine or bupivacaine, higher weight-scaled infusion rates of chloroprocaine are required to achieve similar degrees of blockade. For preterm and term infants, 1.5% chloroprocaine can be infused at about 0.5 mL/kg/hour for midthoracic epidural catheters and 0.6 to 0.7 mL/kg/hour for lumbar and lower thoracic catheters. Even for neonates, additives may improve analgesia, but at roughly one-tenth the concentrations recommended earlier for infusions in older children with bupivacaine or ropivacaine. For example, fentanyl at a concentration of 0.2 µg/mL and clonidine at a concentration of 0.04 µg/mL might be considered as adjuvants.

Chloroprocaine may be used to test previously placed epidural catheters as a second loading dose. The rationale for using chloroprocaine rather than lidocaine or other amide local anesthetics for a second loading dose is based on the concern that because most patients will have had intraoperative infusions of amide local anesthetics, additional amide local anesthetics as a bolus test dose may cause serum amide local anesthetic levels to reach toxic levels. Injecting approximately 0.5 mL/kg of 3% chloroprocaine (up to a maximum total dose of around 18 mL for patients >50 kg) incrementally into the epidural catheter should result in some evidence of sensory and motor block, thereby confirming position of the catheter in the epidural space. Alternatively, lidocaine in the 0.75% to 1.5% range can also be employed. Both of these local anesthetics have relatively rapid onset to facilitate diagnosis of a working or misplaced catheter. If the patient is tachycardic or hypertensive due to pain, these parameters generally improve within 5 to 10 minutes if the catheter is in an epidural location covering the surgical field. Once proper position of the epidural catheter has been confirmed, then good analgesia should be able to be obtained through the adjustment of appropriate epidural solutions and infusion rates.

Neuraxially administered opioids have a synergistic analgesic effect when combined with local anesthetics. Due to the hydrophilic property of hydromorphone, there is a slight preference to using hydromorphone for postoperative analgesia for more extensive surgical procedures involving several dermatomes. However, due to more rostral spread of hydromorphone, the risk of respiratory depression is greater. Specific data point to no better analgesia but slightly more pruritus when morphine or hydromorphone are compared for epidural administration.[127,128] All neuraxially administered opioids can cause side effects including nausea, vomiting, urinary retention, pruritus, sedation, respiratory depression, and constipation. Nausea, vomiting, and other side effects from epidural opioids are treated similarly to those seen from parenteral opioids. Low-dose naloxone infusions significantly reduce opioid side effects without reversing opioid-induced analgesia.

Clonidine is often added to epidural local anesthetic infusions to enhance analgesia without increasing nausea, vomiting, pruritus, or respiratory depression. Studies of combinations of epidural clonidine with local anesthetics in children have shown a low side effect profile.[129,130]

Controlled trials of single-dose caudal administration of clonidine with bupivacaine have shown variable prolongation of analgesia by approximately 50% to 75% than epidural bupivacaine alone. Pharmacokinetic studies of single-dose epidural clonidine in children show wide variation in plasma concentration as well as wide variation in the time for clonidine absorption from the epidural space. Other studies have not shown significant prolongation of single-shot caudal analgesia with clonidine doses as high as 2 µg/kg.[131]

Although some clinicians perform single-shot caudal blocks routinely with clonidine doses in the range of 2 µg/kg, our view is that this dose frequently results in prolonged sedation, especially if other sedatives or systemic opioids are administered as well. Our practice for children 1 year of age and older is to use 0.5 to 1 µg/kg, to a maximum of 15 µg as a single bolus for caudal blocks and roughly 0.12 to 0.16 µg/kg/hour (0.3 to 0.4 mL/kg/hour of a solution containing 0.4 µg/mL) added to continuous epidural local anesthetic infusions (except for neonates, where lower doses and concentrations are used, as noted in the preceding text). Please see Table 50.7 for recommended doses for epidural infusions.

TABLE 50.7	Recommended Epidural Infusion Rates		
	Rate (mL/kg/hour)[a]		
Solution	<1 mo	1–4 mo	>4 mo[b]
Bupivacaine 0.1% +/– Fentanyl[c] 1–2 µg/mL +/– Clonidine 0.4 µg/mL	Rarely used	Rarely used	0.4
Ropivacaine 0.1% +/– Fentanyl 2 µg/mL +/– Clonidine 0.4 µg/mL	Rarely used	0.1–0.3	0.4–0.5
Bupivacaine 0.1% + hydromorphone 5 µg/mL	Rarely used	Rarely used	0.3–0.4
Ropivacaine 0.1% + hydromorphone 5 µg/mL	Rarely used	0.1–0.3	0.3–0.4
Chloroprocaine 1.5% + Fentanyl 0.2 µg/mL +/– Clonidine 0.04 µg/mL	0.5 (midthoracic) 0.6–0.7 (lumbar and low thoracic)	0.5 (midthoracic) 0.6–0.7 (lumbar and low thoracic)	Rarely used Rarely used

NOTE: Solutions containing hydrophilic opioids such as hydromorphone may pose a higher risk for delayed respiratory depression, so appropriate frequency of observation and continuous electronic monitoring is recommended. Higher concentrations of opioids may be considered for selected patients who are opioid-tolerant. Patient-controlled epidural anesthesia (PCEA) doses if used should be 1/4 to 1/6 the basal rate. Hourly maximums: opioid (µg/kg/h): morphine, 3–5; hydromorphone, 1.5–2.5; fentanyl, 0.1–0.5; ropivacaine, 0.4 mg/kg/h, 0.2 mg/kg/h in newborns/neonates.

[a]Infusion rates and solutions should be modified according to clinical circumstances. Little information is available on how best to adjust these rates based on degrees of prematurity.

[b]Weight scaled infusion rates should plateau at values recommended for patients weighing around 45 kg, such as maximum infusion rates for larger patients should rarely exceed 15 mL/h.

[c]In infants <6 months of age, we recommend using fentanyl at 1 µg/mL.

We recommend frequent (every 4 hour) assessment of the epidural site by the nursing staff and twice-daily inspection by the pain management team. Catheter depth should be noted with care, as the catheter can migrate either inward or outward. A small study suggests that this movement is more common in children <40 kg compared to large children and adults.[132] Assessing the site for potential signs of infection, such as tenderness, erythema, or abnormal discharge, should also be part of frequent monitoring. Care should also be taken when using adherence substances such as Mastisol to secure the epidural occlusive dressing, as there are reports of contact dermatitis with use of these agents.[133]

Peripheral Nerve Blocks in Children

Peripheral nerve blocks provide reliable and safe postoperative pain management. A report by the French-Language Society of Pediatric Anesthesiologists showed that among 24,000 regional blocks in children, the complication rate for peripheral nerve block was 0 in 1,000.[116] The PRAN database also showed the safety of peripheral nerve blocks in a cohort of 13,725 patients.[134] In 455 upper extremity blocks, the complication rate was 2%, no complications in 556 head and neck blocks, and a complication rate of 1% in 2,307 lower extremity blocks. In a retrospective review of 226 continuous peripheral nerve blocks in children over a 4-year period, no major adverse events were noted.[135] A recent study using the PRAN database also demonstrated the safety of 2,074 continuous peripheral nerve block catheters with a complication rate of 12.1% with no incidences of deep infection, persistent neurologic deficits or systemic local anesthetic toxicity.[136]

A general trend in clinical trials of peripheral nerve blockade is the observation of very good analgesia with a very low side effect profile that compares favorably to either systemic opioids or epidural infusions. In a randomized trial comparing popliteal block versus epidural analgesia for foot and ankle surgery, popliteal block results in superior analgesia with reduced incidences of nausea, vomiting, and urinary retention.[137]

A recent review shows that the use of ultrasound improves both the success rate of the block and improves the duration of the block.[138] Advantages of ultrasound guidance include direct visualization of nerves and other structures such as arteries which may reduce the likelihood of intraneural or intravascular injection and direct visualization of local anesthetic spread. Combining the use of ultrasound with peripheral nerve stimulation is sometimes used when advancing catheters for continuous use to further confirm catheter placement. The addition of clonidine to peripheral nerve blocks in children has been shown to significantly increase duration of sensory blockade by approximately 4 hours; however, the incidence of motor blockade was also significantly increased.[139]

Like epidural anesthesia, the placement of peripheral nerve block may require general anesthesia or deep sedation for most younger children. Motivated older children and adolescents will often require only minimal sedation. It is often helpful to apply a topical anesthetic, such as via a JTip, to the anticipated needle insertion site to minimize pain from needle insertion. It is our practice to perform the majority of neuraxial and peripheral nerve blocks under general sedation. Indications for using peripheral nerve blocks as the sole anesthetic technique include risk of malignant hyperthermia, risk of postoperative apnea, and patient preference.

Recommendations regarding dosing of local anesthetics for peripheral nerve block in children vary among authors. Where immediate onset is required, one group has recommended 0.5 mL/kg of a mixture of 1% lidocaine with 1:200,000 epinephrine and 0.5% ropivacaine. Several groups employ continuous perineural infusions with 0.1 to 0.15 mL/kg/hour of ropivacaine in a concentration range between 0.1% and 0.2%. As with epidural anesthesia, use of α_2 adrenergic agonists (e.g., clonidine) as adjuncts can be considered. Clonidine has been found to increase time to first use of supplemental analgesia as well as fewer doses of analgesia needed in first 24 hours following surgery at least when lower concentrations of ropivacaine or bupivacaine are used.[140] It is unclear if this remains true with higher concentrations, such as 0.2% or 0.25% of ropivacaine and bupivacaine respectively.

SUPRACLAVICULAR

A supraclavicular block is applicable to all surgeries of the upper extremity excluding shoulder surgery. Placement of a continuous catheter technique can be used in the treatment of refractory complex regional pain syndrome in children.[141] Supraclavicular block has been successfully used as the sole anesthetic for children younger than 12 years of age undergoing closed reduction of arm fractures.[142]

The trunks of the brachial plexus are located between the anterior and medial scalene muscles in the interscalene groove. Using ultrasound guidance, the first rib and subclavian artery should be located, with the pleura located just beneath the first rib. The anterior and middle scalene muscles are then located as they insert onto the first rib cephalad to the subclavian artery. The brachial plexus is located between the anterior and middle scalene muscles and superficial and lateral to the subclavian artery. Under direct ultrasound visualization, the needle is inserted from a lateral to medial direction toward the plexus, with particular attention to avoiding directing the needle medial to the anterior scalene muscles or caudally beneath the first rib to prevent pneumothorax. Only a single injection is required due to the close proximity of the trunks of the plexus in this region. If using a continuous catheter technique, we typically recommend tunneling supraclavicular catheters, particularly for patients requiring aggressive postoperative physical therapy and for catheters of longer duration such as in the treatment of complex regional pain syndrome.

INFRACLAVICULAR

Infraclavicular block is indicated for all distal upper extremity surgeries such as syndactyly repair and repairs of open forearm fractures. In the infraclavicular region, the plexus is located posterior to the pectoralis major and minor. The cords of the brachial plexus are located medial, lateral, and posterior to the axillary artery. Under direct ultrasound visualization, with the ultrasound probe medial and caudal to the coracoid process, the pectoralis muscles and the axillary artery and vein should be identified. The axillary vein is located caudal to the axillary artery. The needle is inserted under direct ultrasound visualization and advanced laterally; once the sheath surrounding the plexus is reached, spread of local anesthetic should be visualized spreading to the cords of the plexus.

SCIATIC NERVE BLOCK

The sciatic nerve block is useful in providing analgesia for a variety of surgical procedures of the lower leg or foot, for painful physical therapy following surgery, and for treatment of complex regional pain syndrome affecting the lower leg or foot. The latter study showed excellent pain relief and excellent rehabilitation with no adverse events using a continuous infusion of 0.2 % ropivacaine at 0.1 mL/kg/hour for 96 hours.[143] In the study of foot and ankle surgery by Dadure et al.,[143] the children with continuous popliteal nerve blocks received a continuous infusion of 0.2% ropivacaine at 0.1 mL/kg/hour, and a 100% satisfaction rate was reported.

Studies in adult patients comparing continuous sciatic nerve block with PCA have shown superior analgesia; reduced morphine use; and reduced frequency of nausea, vomiting, and sedation for adult patients with continuous popliteal sciatic catheters.[144] Two commonly used approaches for sciatic nerve block in children are the subgluteal approach and the popliteal approach.[145] A single-injection technique is indicated after relatively minor surgery when postoperative pain is expected to be mild and of short duration. A continuous catheter technique will provide prolonged analgesia after more extensive surgical procedures.

Sciatic-Subgluteal Approach

Because patients will need to be positioned in the prone position for a subgluteal approach to a sciatic nerve block, younger children will require general anesthesia for placement. Cooperative older children and adolescents can often tolerate the procedure in a prone procedure with sedation. The technique described in the following text uses ultrasound guidance with peripheral nerve stimulation for further confirmation. With the patient in a prone position, ultrasound is used to locate the sciatic nerve; a line marking the midpoint between the ischial tuberosity and the greater trochanter can be useful in estimating position of the sciatic nerve. Under visualization, an insulated 17G stimulating needle is advanced approximately 1 to 2 cm below the midpoint mark and is directed medially and superiorly. Initially, twitching of the gluteal muscles can be observed but will disappear as the needle advanced further. Dorsi- and plantar-flexion of foot is observed with stimulation of the sciatic nerve. A 20G stimulating catheter is advanced approximately 3 cm beyond the tip of the needle; angling the needle slightly caudally may facilitate advancing the catheter. Further nerve stimulation of the catheter confirms proper catheter placement.[146]

Popliteal Approach

Block of the sciatic nerve can also be achieved at the level of the popliteal fossa. The sciatic nerve divides into the tibial and common peroneal nerves in the popliteal fossa; proximal to the popliteal fossa crease. For this block, patients can be positioned either prone or supine with the hip and knee flexed. Our general preference is to use the prone approach when catheter placement is being considered because it makes it easier to maintain sterility and to perform tunneling of the catheter. Ultrasound is used to locate the structures in the popliteal fossa; the popliteal artery and vein are located deep and proximal to the sciatic nerve. The course of the sciatic nerve should be seen and the point at which the sciatic nerve bifurcates should be located. The tendon of the biceps femoris is located laterally, and the tendons of the semimembranosus and semitendinosus muscles are located medially. Ultrasound viewing and needle advancement can be performed using several approaches, including an in-plane approach, with the needle advancing in a lateral-to-medial direction, or an out of plane approach, with the needle advancing in a sagittal direction. Injection of local anesthetic should show local anesthetic spread around the tibial and common peroneal nerves.[146]

FEMORAL BLOCK

A femoral nerve block provides effective analgesia for knee surgery, for surgery on the anterior thigh such as a muscle biopsy, and for femur surgery or fractures. It will also provide analgesia to the medial lower extremity below the knee by blocking the saphenous nerve. Compared to PCA morphine and epidural analgesia, continuous femoral nerve block provides more effective analgesia with fewer side effects. Results indicate that using ultrasound guidance produced prolonged duration of sensory blockade with less volume of local anesthetic compared to using nerve stimulation. The typical landmarks for a femoral nerve block are the inguinal crease and the femoral arterial pulse. The femoral nerve is located lateral and deep to the femoral artery as it courses below the inguinal ligament. With the patient positioned in a supine position, ultrasound is used to locate the position of the femoral vein, artery, and nerve in the inguinal crease. Under ultrasound visualization, an insulated block needle is inserted just lateral to the arterial pulse and directed slightly cephalad. Proper placement of the needle should be seen on ultrasound, positioned alongside the femoral nerve. Nerve stimulation is an alternative method to confirm proper placement of the needle. With proper needle placement, twitching of the quadriceps and patella should be seen. Quadriceps movement alone without signs of patellar movement is due to stimulation of the sartorius muscle and does not confirm proper needle placement. If the femoral nerve is not readily located, it will be necessary to redirect the needle slightly laterally. When placing a catheter for continuous femoral block, the needle is angled slightly more cephalad and the catheter is advanced. If using nerve stimulation, twitching of the quadriceps and patella will indicate correct catheter placement. Infection rates for continuous femoral catheters appear to be low when used for short-term use. In a study examining bacterial colonization and infection rates in continuous femoral catheters, 57% of catheters had positive bacterial colonization with *Staphylococcus epidermidis* as the most common organism. However, there were no septic complications or serious infections for catheters in place for 48 hours.[147]

Recent study of femoral nerve blocks in the pediatric population found that use of ropivacaine 0.5% was superior to ropivacaine 0.2% or bupivacaine 0.25%, leading to decreased opioid use and earlier hospital discharge.[148]

TRANSVERSUS ABDOMINIS PLANE BLOCK

Transversus abdominis plane (TAP) block is a technique where local anesthetic is injected between the transversus abdominis and the internal oblique muscles. This is generally easily visualized with the use of ultrasonography. Recently, it has been gaining increasing popularity for use in pediatrics. The block may be performed as a single shot or as a continuous infusion. Applications for use include procedures such as inguinal hernia repair or other abdominal surgery.[149] A study using the PRAN database looked at the safety of 1,994 children receiving TAP blocks and found the upper incidence of overall complications was 0.3% and these complications did not require any further interventions and were considered minor.[150] Although caudal epidural blockade may provide superior pain relief, the TAP can be considered as it is less invasive and also does not cause lower extremity motor weakness.

Painful Conditions in Pediatric Hospital Care

CANCER PAIN

Infants and children with cancer experience pain from cancer treatment such as painful mucositis, postamputation pain, and peripheral neuropathies as well as from tumor spread causing bone pain, neuropathic pain, or headaches from raised intracranial pressure. Repeated painful needles procedures, such as bone marrow biopsies and lumbar punctures, are a great source of pain and distress. Several surveys have shown that as successful chemotherapeutic protocols, radiation therapy and surgical techniques have advanced, cancer treatment and painful procedures account for greater sources of cancer pain in infants and children.[151]

Frequent diagnostic and painful procedures are common for infants and children with cancer. For minor needle procedures such as intravenous line insertions and assessing implanted vascular access ports, topical analgesia should be routinely used. A number of approaches to cutaneous analgesia have been used, including local anesthetic creams or patches, with or without physical methods to accelerate transit of drug across the stratum corneum. Cognitive-behavioral interventions such as hypnosis and other relaxation techniques have also been shown to be effective for procedural pain. Children can also apply these techniques to nausea, headaches, and other symptoms. Conscious sedation or general anesthesia is typically used for more invasive needle procedures such as bone marrow biopsies and lumbar punctures. Safe sedation protocols have been developed by the American Academy of Pediatrics and are widely used by pediatric oncologists and other pediatric subspecialists for procedural sedation. Pediatric anesthesiologists are consulted for patients with risk factors that place them at increased risk for conscious sedation, for patients who fail conscious sedation, or for more invasive procedures such as central line insertions.

Mucositis is a common side effect in children receiving chemotherapy or radiation; it is especially severe and prolonged with bone marrow transplantation. Initially, pain from mucositis is often treated with topical agents, although evidence for efficacy in the prevention and treatment of mucositis has been mixed. Opioids are used for pain that persists despite topical agents. Data supports the safety and efficacy of opioid infusions and PCA for the treatment of mucositis.[80,152] Because many children with mucositis will require opioids for weeks, our practice is to eventually administer approximately 60% of the total daily opioid dose as a basal rate in order to provide sustained analgesia. NCA is used for young children.

Although a majority of children have resolution of the cancer pain after initial chemotherapy induction protocols, some children will continue to experience visceral, somatic, and neuropathic pain due to tumor invasion of solid organs, bone, nerves, and plexuses. Opioids are provided by the oral route whenever feasible. It is common practice to use a long-acting opioid, either methadone elixir or tablets or capsules of a sustained-release preparation of morphine, hydromorphone, or oxycodone, along with short-acting opioids for rescue or breakthrough pain. Currently, methadone is the most widely available long-acting opioid available as an elixir formulation. When using methadone in the cancer population, it is essential to be aware of the risk of increased QTc from other agents or due to possibility of increased serum methadone levels. Some patients with rapidly escalating pain or patients unable to tolerate oral opioids may require opioids via parenteral routes, including intravenous and subcutaneous routes. Some acute breakthrough pain can be managed with transmucosal fentanyl.[91,153] Continuous infusions and PCA or NCA allow rapid titration for escalating pain as well. In the setting of neuropathic cancer pain, we frequently prescribe anticonvulsants and antidepressants largely by extrapolation from adult practice. Opioids and other sedating medications may contribute to fatigue, somnolence, sleep disturbance, and depressed mood, but they may exist even in children not receiving opioids or sedatives. Along with treating specific or remediable causes of these symptoms, our common practice, again extrapolated from adult clinical trials, is to consider a trial of a stimulant such as methylphenidate.

A subgroup of children with cancer pain will have persistent pain despite massive dose escalation. Many of these children will have unremitting neuropathic pain associated with tumor extension to the epidural space, onto a plexus or along the course of major nerves. One approach to persistent pain in this setting is to add a low-dose ketamine infusion. At rates below 0.2 mg/kg/hour, dysphoria and dissociation are relatively uncommon.[154]

Oral ketamine has been used as well, with a provisional dose ratio of about 3:1 compared to intravenous dosing in steady state. In selected cases of refractory pain, our practice is to use regional anesthetic techniques, and most commonly in this setting, we favor implanted intrathecal ports with the catheter generally advanced to the dorsal horn level appropriate to the patient's location of greatest pain.[155] Note that for tumors predominantly in the pelvis, lumbar spine, or lower extremities, this implies having the catheter tip advanced up to around T11. The choice of drugs for these infusions must be individualized based on the nature of the patient's pain and quality of life issues, including considerations of weakness, bowel and bladder dysfunction, and sedation. In the majority of cases, we have found it necessary to include small doses of local anesthetics along with opioids, and in some cases, we have included other additives such as clonidine or ketamine. There is a small subgroup of children for whom it appears that the most feasible option for achieving relief of pain, distress, or terminal dyspnea is to provide sedation, using a range of agents, including benzodiazepines, barbiturates, or other drugs.[156]

PAIN ASSOCIATED WITH SICKLE CELL VASOOCCLUSIVE EPISODES

Pain is a common consequence of sickle cell disease due to acute vasoocclusive episodes as well as pain from compression fractures, avascular necrosis, acute cholecystitis, splenic sequestration, and stroke. Painful vasoocclusive episodes are the most common cause of pain in children with sickle cell disease and can occur in children as young as 6 months of age as fetal hemoglobin and its protection against vasoocclusive crises decreases. Children can demonstrate a range of severity and frequency of vasoocclusive episodes, from occasional episodes managed at home with oral analgesics to baseline daily pain with frequent exacerbations requiring numerous hospitalizations and systemic opioids administration. PCA is commonly used for severe pain in hospitalized patients, along with NSAIDs, hydration, red blood cell transfusion, and supplemental oxygen. Larger opioid boluses may be necessary than are typically used for postoperative pain management for patients with extreme

pain or for patients who are opioid-tolerant.[157] Often basal infusions are necessary, particularly at night to permit periods of uninterrupted sleep. Published case series indicate that even with generous PCA parameters, pain scores remain high for a high percentage of patients.[158] Recent data has shown promising results for subanesthetic dosing of ketamine in patients with sickle cell disease.

CHILDREN WITH TRAUMA

General sound principles of analgesic management should be applied to the care of children with the vast variety of traumatic injuries. Application of appropriate nerve blocks, central blocks, when possible, can facilitate recovery from the child's injuries. In addition, many injured children are fully able to take oral analgesics, avoiding the necessity of intravenous access or, even, continued stay in the hospital, once their pain is successfully managed.

CHILDREN WITH DEVELOPMENTAL DISABILITIES

Children with cognitive and developmental disabilities such as cerebral palsy and neurodegenerative disorders present unique challenges in assessing and managing pain. Many children with disabilities experience daily pain associated with muscle spasms, hip dislocation, and other musculoskeletal pains and undergo frequent painful invasive procedures such as scoliosis repair, tendon releases, and surgical treatment of gastroesophageal reflux. Children may have little or no cognitive deficits but significant motor and communication impairments, making pain assessment especially difficult. Often, parents and caretakers are able to distinguish subtle behavioral signs indicating pain. A number of pain assessment tools such as the FLACC tool and the Non-communicating Children's Pain Checklist have been used for children with cognitive and developmental disabilities. In comparing several pain assessment tools for children with cognitive limitations, physicians and nurses rated the FLACC as having higher clinical utility.[159]

Other children with severe cognitive impairment will have persistent agitation and screaming without a clear etiology and are admitted to the hospital for diagnostic evaluation and therapeutic trials. Patients should be evaluated for treatable causes of pain such as fractures, hip dislocations, esophagitis, and constipation. In some cases where no underlying cause can be eventually identified, therapeutic trials of anticonvulsants and antispasmodics may provide relief.[160]

Conclusions

Evidence is available to support safe and effective treatment of acute pain in infants, children, and adolescents in the majority of circumstances. Analgesic pharmacology has received extensive study in pediatrics over the past several decades. Individual analgesics often provide incomplete relief in standard doses, and there is a rationale for analgesic combinations and multimodal analgesia in many situations. Opioids can provide good analgesia at all ages, but with a spectrum of side effects that require active treatment, and with specific requirements for observation and monitoring according to age and patient condition–related risk factors. Techniques have been developed for neuraxial and peripheral regional anesthesia at all ages. There is a growing emphasis on ultrasound, nerve stimulation, selective use of fluoroscopy, and other approaches to provide objective confirmation of needle and/or catheter positioning. Pediatric acute pain management, whether by an acute pain service or by other delivery models, can be improved by system-wide approaches that emphasize systematic assessment of pain and other symptoms, communication, clinician education, clarification of responsibilities, and protocols for analgesic administration, side effect management, and monitoring.

References

1. Fitzgerald M, Walker SM. Infant pain management: a developmental neurobiological approach. *Nat Clin Pract Neurol* 2009;5(1):35–50.
2. Karling M, Renström M, Ljungman G. Acute and postoperative pain in children: a Swedish nationwide survey. *Acta Pædiatr* 2002;91:660–666.
3. von Baeyer CL, Chambers CT, Forsyth SJ, et al. Developmental data supporting simplification of self-report pain scales for preschool-age children. *J Pain* 2013;14(10):1116–1121.
4. Anand KJ, Hickey PR. Pain and its effects in the human neonate and fetus. *New Engl J Med* 1987;317(21):1321–1329.
5. Anand KJ, Hickey PR. Halothane-morphine compared with high-dose sufentanil for anesthesia and postoperative analgesia in neonatal cardiac surgery. *New Engl J Med* 1992;326(1):1–9.
6. Stevens BJ, Johnston CC. Physiological responses of premature infants to a painful stimulus. *Nurs Res* 1994;43(4):226–231.
7. Anand KJ. Neonatal stress responses to anesthesia and surgery. *Clin Perinatol* 1990;17(1):207–214.
8. Andrews K, Fitzgerald M. Cutaneous flexion reflex in human neonates: a quantitative study of threshold and stimulus-response characteristics after single and repeated stimuli. *Dev Med Child Neurol* 1999;41(10):696–703.
9. Franck LS. A new method to quantitatively describe pain behavior in infants. *Nurs Res* 1986;35(1):28–31.
10. Porter FL, Wolf CM, Miller JP. Procedural pain in newborn infants: the influence of intensity and development. *Pediatrics* 1999;104(1):e13.
11. Krechel S, Bildner J. CRIES: a new neonatal postoperative pain measurement score. Initial testing of validity and reliability. *Paediatr Anaesth* 1995;5(1):53–61.
12. Stevens B, Johnston C, Petryshen P, et al. Premature Infant Pain Profile: development and initial validation. *Clin J Pain* 1996;12(1):13–22.
13. Crellin DJ, Harrison D, Santamaria N, et al. Systematic review of the Face, Legs, Activity, Cry and Consolability scale for assessing pain in infants and children: is it reliable, valid, and feasible for use? *Pain* 2015;156(11):2132–2151.
14. Zhou H, Roberts P, Horgan L. Association between self-report pain ratings of child and parent, child and nurse and parent and nurse dyads: meta-analysis. *J Adv Nurs* 2008;63(4):334–342.
15. Hesselgard K, Larsson S, Romner B, et al. Validity and reliability of the Behavioural Observational Pain Scale for postoperative pain measurement in children 1–7 years of age. *Pediatr Crit Care Med* 2007;8(2):102–108.
16. McGrath PJ, Johnson G, Goodman JT. CHEOPS: a behavioral scale for rating postoperative pain in children. *Adv Pain Res Ther* 1985;9:395–402.
17. Merkel SI, Voepel-Lewis T, Shayevitz JR, et al. The FLACC: a behavioral scale for scoring postoperative pain in young children. *Pediatr Nurs* 1997;23(3):293–297.
18. Malviya S, Voepel-Lewis T, Burke C, et al. The revised FLACC observational pain tool: improved reliability and validity for pain assessment in children with cognitive impairment. *Paediatr Anaesth* 2006;16(3):258–265.
19. Voepel-Lewis T, Malviya S, Tait AR. Validity of parent ratings as proxy measures of pain in children with cognitive impairment. *Pain Manag Nurs* 2005;6(4):168–174.
20. Voepel-Lewis T, Malviya S, Tait AR, et al. A comparison of the clinical utility of pain assessment tools for children with cognitive impairment. *Anesth Analg* 2008;106(1):72–78.
21. Voepel-Lewis T, Merkel S, Tait AR, et al. The reliability and validity of the Face, Legs, Activity, Cry, Consolability observational tool as a measure of pain in children with cognitive impairment. *Anesth Analg* 2002;95(5):1224–1229.
22. Grossi E, Borghi C, Cerchiari EL, et al. Analogue Chromatic Continuous Scale (ACCS): a new method for pain assessment. *Clin Exp Rheumatol* 1983;1(4):337–340.
23. Hicks CL, von Baeyer CL, Spafford PA, et al. The Faces Pain Scale–Revised: toward a common metric in pediatric pain measurement. *Pain* 2001;93(2):173–183.
24. Stinson JN, Kavanagh T, Yamada J, et al. Systematic review of the psychometric properties, interpretability and feasibility of self-report pain intensity measures for use in clinical trials in children and adolescents. *Pain* 2006;125(1–2):143–157.
25. Alcorn J, McNamara PJ. Ontogeny of hepatic and renal systemic clearance pathways in infants: part I. *Clin Pharmacokinet* 2002;41(12):959–998.
26. Anderson BJ, Holford NH. Mechanism-based concepts of size and maturity in pharmacokinetics. *Ann Rev Pharmacol Toxicol* 2008;48:303–332.
27. Strassburg CP, Strassburg A, Kneip S, et al. Developmental aspects of human hepatic drug glucuronidation in young children and adults. *Gut* 2002;50(2):259–265.
28. Ririe DG, Prout HM, Eisenach JC. Effect of cyclooxygenase-1 inhibition in postoperative pain is developmentally regulated. *Anesthesiology* 2004;101(4):1031–1035.
29. Anderson BJ. Paracetamol (acetaminophen): mechanisms of action. *Paediatr Anaesth* 2008;18(10):915–921.
30. Miranda HF, Puig MM, Prieto JC, et al. Synergism between paracetamol and nonsteroidal anti-inflammatory drugs in experimental acute pain. *Pain* 2006;121(1):22–28.
31. Heubi JE, Barbacci MB, Zimmerman HJ. Therapeutic misadventures with acetaminophen: hepatoxicity after multiple doses in children. *J Pediatr* 1998;132(1):22–27.
32. Birmingham PK, Tobin MJ, Henthorn TK, et al. Twenty-four-hour pharmacokinetics of rectal acetaminophen in children: an old drug with new recommendations. *Anesthesiology* 1997;87(2):244–252.
33. Krenzelok EP. The FDA Acetaminophen Advisory Committee Meeting—what is the future of acetaminophen in the United States? The perspective of a committee member. *Clin Toxicology* 2009;47(8):784–789.
34. Montgomery CJ, McCormack JP, Reichert CC, et al. Plasma concentrations after high-dose (45 mg · kg^{-1}) rectal acetaminophen in children. *Can J Anaesth* 1995;42(11):982–986.
35. Yung A, Thung A, Tobias JD. Acetaminophen for analgesia following pyloromyotomy: does the route of administration make a difference? *J Pain Res* 2016;9:123–127.
36. Murat I, Baujard C, Foussat C, et al. Tolerance and analgesic efficacy of a new i.v. paracetamol solution in children after inguinal hernia repair. *Paediatr Anaesth* 2005;15(8):663–670.
37. Zuppa AF, Hammer GB, Barrett JS, et al. Safety and population pharmacokinetic analysis of intravenous acetaminophen in neonates, infants, children, and adolescents with pain or fever. *J Pediatr Pharmacol Ther* 2011;16(4):246–261.
38. Ceelie I, De Wildt SN, Van Dijk M, et al. Effect of intravenous paracetamol on postoperative morphine requirements in neonates and infants undergoing major noncardiac surgery: a randomized controlled trial. *JAMA* 2013;309(2):149–154.
39. Michelet D, Andreu-Gallien J, Bensalah T, et al. A meta-analysis of the use of nonsteroidal antiinflammatory drugs for pediatric postoperative pain. *Anesth Analg* 2012;114(2):393–406.
40. Boynton CS, Dick CF, Mayor GH. NSAIDs: an overview. *J Clin Pharmacol* 1988;28(6):512–517.
41. Kauffman RE, Lieh-Lai MW, Uy HG, et al. Enantiomer-selective pharmacokinetics and metabolism of ketorolac in children. *Clin Pharmacol Ther* 1999;65(4):382–388.
42. Zuppa AF, Mondick JT, Davis L, et al. Population pharmacokinetics of ketorolac in neonates and young infants. *Am J Therap* 2009;16(2):143–146.
43. Moffett BS, Wann TI, Carberry KE, et al. Safety of ketorolac in neonates and infants after cardiac surgery. *Paediatr Anaesth* 2006;16(4):424–428.
44. Van Overmeire B, Smets K, Lecoutere D, et al. A comparison of ibuprofen and indomethacin for closure of patent ductus arteriosus. *New Engl J Med* 2000;343(10):674–681.
45. Kokki H, Hendolin H, Maunuksela EL, et al. Ibuprofen in the treatment of postoperative pain in small children. A randomized double-blind-placebo controlled parallel group study. *Acta Anaesthesiol Scand* 1994;38(5):467–472.
46. Beukelman T, Patkar NM, Saag KG, et al. 2011 American College of Rheumatology recommendations for the treatment of juvenile idiopathic arthritis: initiation and safety monitoring of therapeutic agents for the treatment of arthritis and systemic features. *Arthritis Care Res* 2011;63(4):465–482.
47. Krishna S, Hughes LF, Lin SY. Postoperative hemorrhage with nonsteroidal anti-inflammatory drug use after tonsillectomy: a meta-analysis. *Arch Otolaryngol Head Neck Surg* 2003;129(10):1086–1089.
48. Marret E, Flahault A, Samama CM, et al. Effects of postoperative, nonsteroidal, antiinflammatory drugs on bleeding risk after tonsillectomy: meta-analysis of randomized, controlled trials. *Anesthesiology* 2003;98(6):1497–1502.
49. D'Souza JN, Schmidt RJ, Xie L, et al. Postoperative nonsteroidal anti-inflammatory drugs and risk of bleeding in pediatric intracapsular tonsillectomy. *Int J Pediatr Otorhinalaryngol* 2015;79(9):1472–1476.
50. Chan DK, Parikh SR. Perioperative ketorolac increases post-tonsillectomy hemorrhage in adults but not children. *Laryngoscope* 2014;124(8):1789–1793.
51. Vuolteenaho K, Moilanen T, Moilanen E. Non-steroidal anti-inflammatory drugs, cyclooxygenase-2 and the bone healing process. *Basic Clin Pharmacol Toxicol* 2008;102(1):10–14.
52. Sucato DJ, Lovejoy JF, Agrawal S, et al. Postoperative ketorolac does not predispose to pseudoarthrosis following posterior spinal fusion and instrumentation for adolescent idiopathic scoliosis. *Spine* 2008;33(10):1119–1124.
53. Kramer BK. Cyclo-oxygenase-2 and renal function. *Nephrol Dial Transplant* 2001;16(1):180–183.
54. Pickering AE, Bridge HS, Nolan J, et al. Double-blind, placebo-controlled analgesic study of ibuprofen or rofecoxib in combination with paracetamol for tonsillectomy in children. *Br J Anaesth* 2002;88(1):72–77.
55. Murto K, Lamontagne C, McFaul C, et al. Celecoxib pharmacogenetics and pediatric adenotonsillectomy: a double-blinded randomized controlled study. *Can J Anaesth* 2015;62(7):785–797.
56. Assouline B, Tramer MR, Kreienbuhl L, et al. Benefit and harm of adding ketamine to an opioid in a patient-controlled analgesia device for the control of postoperative pain: systematic review and meta-analyses of randomized controlled trials with trial sequential analyses. *Pain* 2016;157(12):2854–2864.
57. Michelet D, Hilly J, Skhiri A, et al. Opioid-sparing effect of ketamine in children: a meta-analysis and trial sequential analysis of published studies. *Paediatr Drugs* 2016;18(6):421–433.
58. Cha MH, Eom JH, Lee YS, et al. Beneficial effects of adding ketamine to intravenous patient-controlled analgesia with fentanyl after the Nuss procedure in pediatric patients. *Yonsei Med J* 2012;53(2):427–432.

59. Perello M, Artes D, Pascuets C, et al. Prolonged perioperative low-dose ketamine does not improve short and long-term outcomes after pediatric idiopathic scoliosis surgery. *Spine* 2017;42(5):E304–E312.

60. Rusy LM, Hainsworth KR, Nelson TJ, et al. Gabapentin use in pediatric spinal fusion patients: a randomized, double-blind, controlled trial. *Anesth Analg* 2010;110(5):1393–1398.

61. Reiter PD, Nickisch J, Merritt G. Efficacy and tolerability of intravenous valproic acid in acute adolescent migraine. *Headache* 2005;45(7):899–903.

62. Patniyot IR, Gelfand AA. Acute treatment therapies for pediatric migraine: a qualitative systematic review. *Headache* 2016;56(1):49–70.

63. Lynn AM, Nespeca MK, Bratton SL, et al. Intravenous morphine in postoperative infants: intermittent bolus dosing versus targeted continuous infusions. *Pain* 2000;88(1):89–95.

64. Lynn AM, Nespeca MK, Opheim KE, et al. Respiratory effects of intravenous morphine infusions in neonates, infants, and children after cardiac surgery. *Anesth Analg* 1993;77(4):695–701.

65. Williams DG, Hatch DJ, Howard RF. Codeine phosphate in paediatric medicine. *Br J Anaesth* 2001;86(3):413–421.

66. Sindrup SH, Brosen K. The pharmacogenetics of codeine hypoalgesia. *Pharmacogenetics* 1995;5(6):335–346.

67. Kirchheiner J, Schmidt H, Tzvetkov M, et al. Pharmacokinetics of codeine and its metabolite morphine in ultra-rapid metabolizers due to CYP2D6 duplication. *Pharmacogenetics J* 2007;7(4):257–265.

68. Kelly LE, Rieder M, van den Anker J, et al. More codeine fatalities after tonsillectomy in North American children. *Pediatrics* 2012;129(5):e1343–e1347.

69. U.S. Food and Drug Administration. FDA drug safety communication: safety review update of codeine use in children; new boxed warning and contraindication on use after tonsillectomy and/or adenoidectomy. Available at: https://www.fda.gov/downloads/Drugs/DrugSafety/UCM339116.pdf. Accessed April 3, 2018.

70. Stassinos GL, Gonzales L, Klein-Schwartz W. Characterizing the toxicity and dose-effect profile of tramadol ingestions in children [published online ahead of print February 21,1017]. *Pediatr Emerg Care.* doi:10.1097/PEC.0000000000001084.

71. Schnabel A, Reichl SU, Meyer-Friessem C, et al. Tramadol for postoperative pain treatment in children. *Cochrane Database Syst Rev* 2015;(3):CD009574.

72. U.S. Food and Drug Administration. FDA drug safety communication: FDA restricts use of prescription codeine pain and cough medicines and tramadol pain medicines in children; recommends against use in breastfeeding women. Available at: https://www.fda.gov/Drugs/DrugSafety/ucm549679.htm. Accessed April 3, 2018.

73. Valitalo P, Kokki M, Ranta VP, et al. Maturation of oxycodone pharmacokinetics in neonates and infants A population pharmacokinetic model of three clinical trials. *Pharm Res* 2017;34(5):1125–1133.

74. Kokki M, Heikkinen M, Välitalo P, et al. Maturation of oxycodone pharmacokinetics in neonates and infants: oxycodone and its metabolites in plasma and urine. *Br J Clin Pharmacol* 2017;83(4):791–800.

75. Kokki H, Rasanen I, Reinikainen M, et al. Pharmacokinetics of oxycodone after intravenous, buccal, intramuscular and gastric administration in children. *Clin Pharmacokinet* 2004;43(9):613–622.

76. Colucci RD, Swanton RE, Thomas GB, et al. Relative variability in bioavailability of oral controlled-release formulations of oxycodone and morphine. *Am J Ther* 2001;8(4):231–236.

77. Andersen G, Christrup L, Sjøgren P. Relationships among morphine metabolism, pain and side effects during long-term treatment: an update. *J Pain Symptom Manage* 2003;25(1):74–91.

78. Choonara I, Lawrence A, Michalkiewicz A, et al. Morphine metabolism in neonates and infants. *Br J Clin Pharmacol* 1992;34(5):434–437.

79. Choonara IA, McKay P, Hain R, et al. Morphine metabolism in children. *Br J Clin Pharmacol* 1989;28(5):599–604.

80. Collins JJ, Geake J, Grier HE, et al. Patient-controlled analgesia for mucositis pain in children: a three-period crossover study comparing morphine and hydromorphone. *J Pediatrics* 1996;129(5):722–728.

81. Smith HS. The metabolism of opioid agents and the clinical impact of their active metabolites. *Clin J Pain* 2011;27(9):824–838.

82. Berde CB, Beyer JE, Bournaki MC, et al. Comparison of morphine and methadone for prevention of postoperative pain in 3- to 7-year-old children. *J Pediatr* 1991;119(1)(pt 1):136–141.

83. Fredheim OM, Moksnes K, Borchgrevink PC, et al. Clinical pharmacology of methadone for pain. *Acta Anaesthesiol Scand* 2008;52(7):879–889.

84. Shaiova L, Berger A, Blinderman CD, et al. Consensus guideline on parenteral methadone use in pain and palliative care. *Palliat Support Care* 2008;6(2):165–176.

85. Chang G, Chen L, Mao J. Opioid tolerance and hyperalgesia. *Med Clin North Am* 2007;91(2):199–211.

86. Benitez-Rosario MA, Salinas-Martin A, Aguirre-Jaime A, et al. Morphine-methadone opioid rotation in cancer patients: analysis of dose ratio-predicting factors. *J Pain Symptom Manage* 2009;37(6):1061–1068.

87. Gottschalk A, Durieux ME, Nemergut EC. Intraoperative methadone improves postoperative pain control in patients undergoing complex spine surgery. *Anesth Analg* 2011;112(1):218–223.

88. Singhal NR, Jones J, Semenova J, et al. Multimodal anesthesia with the addition of methadone is superior to epidural analgesia: a retrospective comparison of intraoperative anesthetic techniques and pain management for 124 pediatric patients undergoing the Nuss procedure. *J Pediatric Surg* 2016;51(4):612–616.

89. Zernikow B, Michel E, Anderson B. Transdermal fentanyl in childhood and adolescence: a comprehensive literature review. *J Pain* 2007;8(3):187–207.

90. Koren G, Goresky G, Crean P, et al. Unexpected alterations in fentanyl pharmacokinetics in children undergoing cardiac surgery: age related or disease related? *Dev Pharmacol Ther* 1986;9:183–191.

91. Schechter NL, Weisman SJ, Rosenblum M, et al. The use of oral transmucosal fentanyl citrate for painful procedures in children. *Pediatrics* 1995;95(3):335–339.

92. Borland M, Jacobs I, King B, et al. A randomized controlled trial comparing intranasal fentanyl to intravenous morphine for managing acute pain in children in the emergency department. *Ann Emerg Med* 2007;49(3):335–340.

93. Galinkin JL, Fazi LM, Cuy RM, et al. Use of intranasal fentanyl in children undergoing myringotomy and tube placement during halothane and sevoflurane anesthesia. *Anesthesiology* 2000;93(6):1378–1383.

94. U.S. Food and Drug Administration. FDA drug safety warning: safety warnings regarding use of fentanyl transdermal (skin) patches. Available at: https://www.accessdata.fda.gov/drugsatfda_docs/label/2009/019813s044lblnew.pdf. Accessed April 3, 2018.

95. Pokela ML, Olkkola KT, Koivisto M, et al. Pharmacokinetics and pharmacodynamics of intravenous meperidine in neonates and infants. *Clin Pharmacol Ther* 1992;52(4):342–349.

96. Anghelescu DL, Burgoyne LL, Oakes LL, et al. The safety of patient-controlled analgesia by proxy in pediatric oncology patients. *Anesth Analg* 2005;101(6):1623–1627.

97. Monitto CL, Greenberg RS, Kost-Byerly S, et al. The safety and efficacy of parent-/nurse-controlled analgesia in patients less than six years of age. *Anesth Analg* 2000;91(3):573–579.

98. Voepel-Lewis T, Marinkovic A, Kostrzewa A, et al. The prevalence of and risk factors for adverse events in children receiving patient-controlled analgesia by proxy or patient-controlled analgesia after surgery. *Anesth Analg* 2008;107(1):70–75.

99. Czarnecki ML, Ferrise AS, Mano KE, et al. Parent/nurse-controlled analgesia for children with developmental delay. *Clinical J Pain* 2008;24(9):817–824.

100. Czarnecki ML, Salamon KS, Mano KE, et al. A preliminary report of parent/nurse-controlled analgesia (PNCA) in infants and preschoolers. *Clinical J Pain* 2011;27(2):102–107.

101. Kehlet H. Postoperative opioid sparing to hasten recovery: what are the issues? *Anesthesiology* 2005;102(6):1083–1085.

102. Berde C, Nurko S. Opioid side effects—mechanism-based therapy. *N Engl J Med* 2008;358(22):2400–2402.

103. Kjellberg F, Tramer MR. Pharmacological control of opioid-induced pruritus: a quantitative systematic review of randomized trials. *Eur J Anaesthesiol* 2001;18(6):346–357.

104. Maxwell LG, Kaufmann SC, Bitzer S, et al. The effects of a small-dose naloxone infusion on opioid-induced side effects and analgesia in children and adolescents treated with intravenous patient-controlled analgesia: a double-blind, prospective, randomized, controlled study. *Anesth Analg* 2005;100(4):953–958.

105. Koch J, Manworren R, Clark L, et al. Pilot study of continuous co-infusion of morphine and naloxone in children with sickle cell pain crisis. *Am J Hematol* 2008;83(9):728–731.

106. Nakatsuka N, Minogue SC, Lim J, et al. Intravenous nalbuphine 50 μg · kg⁻¹ is ineffective for opioid-induced pruritus in pediatrics. *Can J Anaesth* 2006;53(11):1103–1110.

107. Flerlage JE, Baker JN. Methylnaltrexone for opioid-induced constipation in children and adolescents and young adults with progressive incurable cancer at the end of life. *J Palliative Med* 2015;18(7):631–633.

108. Argoff CE, Brennan MJ, Camilleri M, et al. Consensus recommendations on initiating prescription therapies for opioid-induced constipation. *Pain Med* 2015;16(12):2324–2337.

109. Mazoit JX, Dalens BJ. Pharmacokinetics of local anaesthetics in infants and children. *Clin Pharmacokinet* 2004;43(1):17–32.

110. Henderson K, Sethna NF, Berde CB. Continuous caudal anesthesia for inguinal hernia repair in former preterm infants. *J Clin Anesth* 1993;5(2):129–133.

111. Schechter NL, Zempsky WT, Cohen LL, et al. Pain reduction during pediatric immunizations: evidence-based review and recommendations. *Pediatrics* 2007;119(5):e1184–e1198.

112. Zempsky WT. Pharmacologic approaches for reducing venous access pain in children. *Pediatrics* 2008;122(suppl 3):S140–S153.

113. Jimenez N, Bradford H, Seidel KD, et al. A comparison of a needle-free injection system for local anesthesia versus EMLA for intravenous catheter insertion in the pediatric patient. *Anesth Analg* 2006;102(2):411–414.

114. Lunoe MM, Drendel AL, Levas MN, et al. A randomized clinical trial of jet-injected lidocaine to reduce venipuncture pain for young children. *Ann Emerg Med* 2015;66(5):466–474.

115. Drasner K. Thoracic epidural anesthesia: asleep at the wheal? *Anesth Analg* 2004;99(2):578–579.

116. Giaufre E, Dalens B, Gombert A. Epidemiology and morbidity of regional anesthesia in children: a one-year prospective survey of the French-Language Society of Pediatric Anesthesiologists. *Anesth Analg* 1996;83(5):904–912.

117. Llewellyn N, Moriarty A. The national pediatric epidural audit. *Paediatr Anaesthesia* 2007;17(6):520–533.

118. Taenzer AH, Walker BJ, Bosenberg AT, et al. Asleep versus awake: does it matter? Pediatric regional block complications by patient state: a report from the Pediatric Regional Anesthesia Network. *Reg Anesth Pain Med* 2014;39(4):279–283.

119. Bosenberg AT, Bland BA, Schulte-Steinberg O, et al. Thoracic epidural anesthesia via caudal route in infants. *Anesthesiology* 1988;69(2):265–269.

120. Goobie SM, Montgomery CJ, Basu R, et al. Confirmation of direct epidural catheter placement using nerve stimulation in pediatric anesthesia. *Anesth Analg* 2003;97(4):984–988.

121. Rapp HJ, Folger A, Grau T. Ultrasound-guided epidural catheter insertion in children. *Anesth Analg* 2005;101(2):333–339.

122. Luz G, Wieser C, Innerhofer P, et al. Free and total bupivacaine plasma concentrations after continuous epidural anaesthesia in infants and children. *Paediatr Anaesth* 1998;8(6):473–478.

123. Bosenberg AT, Thomas J, Cronje L, et al. Pharmacokinetics and efficacy of ropivacaine for continuous epidural infusion in neonates and infants. *Paediatr Anaesth* 2005;15(9):739–749.

124. Hansen TG, Ilett KF, Lim SI, et al. Pharmacokinetics and clinical efficacy of long-term epidural ropivacaine infusion in children. *Br J Anaesth* 2000;85(3):347–353.

125. McCann ME, Sethna NF, Mazoit JX, et al. The pharmacokinetics of epidural ropivacaine in infants and young children. *Anesth Analg* 2001;93(4):893–897.

126. Bösenberg AT. Epidural analgesia for major neonatal surgery. *Paediatr Anaesth* 1998;8(6):479–483.

127. Chaplan SR, Duncan SR, Brodsky JB, et al. Morphine and hydromorphone epidural analgesia. A prospective, randomized comparison. *Anesthesiology* 1992;77(6):1090–1094.

128. Goodarzi M. Comparison of epidural morphine, hydromorphone and fentanyl for postoperative pain control in children undergoing orthopaedic surgery. *Paediatr Anaesth* 1999;9(5):419–422.

129. De Negri P, Ivani G, Visconti C, et al. The dose-response relationship for clonidine added to a postoperative continuous epidural infusion of ropivacaine in children. *Anesth Analg* 2001;93(1):71–76.

130. Constant I, Gall O, Gouyet L, et al. Addition of clonidine or fentanyl to local anaesthetics prolongs the duration of surgical analgesia after single shot caudal block in children. *Br J Anaesth* 1998;80(3):294–298.

131. Wheeler M, Patel A, Suresh S, et al. The addition of clonidine 2 μg · kg^{-1} does not enhance the postoperative analgesia of a caudal block using 0.125% bupivacaine and epinephrine 1:200,000 in children: a prospective, double-blind, randomized study. *Paediatr Anaesth* 2005;15(6):476–483.

132. Strandness T, Wiktor M, Varadarajan J, et al. Migration of pediatric epidural catheters. *Paediatr Anaesth* 2015;25(6):610–613.

133. Meikle A, Vaghadia H, Henderson C. Allergic contact dermatitis at the epidural catheter site due to Mastisol® liquid skin adhesive. *Can J Anaesth* 2012;59(8):815–816.

134. Polaner DM, Taenzer AH, Walker BJ, et al. Pediatric Regional Anesthesia Network (PRAN): a multi-institutional study of the use and incidence of complications of pediatric regional anesthesia. *Anesth Analg* 2012;115(6):1353–1364.

135. Ganesh A, Rose JB, Wells L, et al. Continuous peripheral nerve blockade for inpatient and outpatient postoperative analgesia in children. *Anesth Analg* 2007;105(5):1234–1242.

136. Walker BJ, Long JB, De Oliveira GS, et al. Peripheral nerve catheters in children: an analysis of safety and practice patterns from the pediatric regional anesthesia network (PRAN). *Br J Anaesth* 2015;115(3):457–462.

137. Dadure C, Bringuier S, Nicolas F, et al. Continuous epidural block versus continuous popliteal nerve block for postoperative pain relief after major podiatric surgery in children: a prospective, comparative randomized study. *Anesth Analg* 2006;102(3):744–749.

138. Guay J, Suresh S, Kopp S. The use of ultrasound guidance for perioperative neuraxial and peripheral nerve blocks in children: a Cochrane review. *Anesth Analg* 2017;124(3):948–958.

139. Cucchiaro G, Ganesh A. The effects of clonidine on postoperative analgesia after peripheral nerve blockade in children. *Anesth Analg* 2007;104(3):532–537.

140. Lundblad M TM, Kaabach O, Khalifa SB, et al. Alpha-2 adrenoceptor agonists as adjuncts to peripheral nerve blocks in children: a meta-analysis. *Paediatr Anaesth* 2016;26:232–238.

141. Franklin A, Austin T. The use of a continuous brachial plexus catheter to facilitate inpatient rehabilitation in a pediatric patient with refractory upper extremity complex regional pain syndrome. *Pain Pract* 2013;13(2):109–113.

142. Pande R, Pande M, Bhadani U, et al. Supraclavicular brachial plexus block as a sole anaesthetic technique in children: an analysis of 200 cases. *Anaesthesia* 2000;55(8):798–802.

143. Dadure C, Motais F, Ricard C, et al. Continuous peripheral nerve blocks at home for treatment of recurrent complex regional pain syndrome I in children. *Anesthesiology* 2005;102(2):387–391.

144. di Benedetto P, Casati A, Bertini L, et al. Postoperative analgesia with continuous sciatic nerve block after foot surgery: a prospective, randomized comparison between the popliteal and subgluteal approaches. *Anesth Analg* 2002;94(4):996–1000.

145. van Geffen GJ, Gielen M. Ultrasound-guided subgluteal sciatic nerve blocks with stimulating catheters in children: a descriptive study. *Anesth Analg* 2006;103(2):328–333.

146. Oberndorfer U, Marhofer P, Bosenberg A, et al. Ultrasonographic guidance for sciatic and femoral nerve blocks in children. *Br J Anaesth* 2007;98(6):797–801.

147. Cuvillon P, Ripart J, Lalourcey L, et al. The continuous femoral nerve block catheter for postoperative analgesia: bacterial colonization, infectious rate and adverse effects. *Anesth Analg* 2001;93(4):1045–1049.

148. Veneziano G, Tripi J, Tumin D, et al. Femoral nerve blockade using various concentrations of local anesthetic for knee arthroscopy in the pediatric population. *J Pain Res* 2016;9:1073–1079.

149. Sahin L, Sahin M, Gul R, et al. Ultrasound-guided transversus abdominis plane block in children: a randomised comparison with wound infiltration. *Eur J Anaesthesiol* 2013;30(7):409–414.

150. Long JB, Birmingham PK, De Oliveira GS Jr, et al. Transversus abdominis plane block in children: a multicenter safety analysis of 1994 cases from the PRAN (Pediatric Regional Anesthesia Network) database. *Anesth Analg* 2014;119(2):395–399.

151. Oakes LL, Anghelescu DL, Windsor KB, et al. An institutional quality improvement initiative for pain management for pediatric cancer inpatients. *J Pain Symptom Manage* 2008;35(6):656–669.

152. Ruggiero A, Barone G, Liotti L, et al. Safety and efficacy of fentanyl administered by patient controlled analgesia in children with cancer pain. *Support Care Cancer* 2007;15(5):569–573.

153. Fine PG, Marcus M, De Boer AJ, et al. An open label study of oral transmucosal fentanyl citrate (OTFC) for the treatment of breakthrough cancer pain. *Pain* 1991;45(2):149–153.

154. Finkel JC, Pestieau SR, Quezado ZM. Ketamine as an adjuvant for treatment of cancer pain in children and adolescents. *J Pain* 2007;8(6):515–521.

155. Collins JJ, Grier HE, Sethna NF, et al. Regional anesthesia for pain associated with terminal pediatric malignancy. *Pain* 1996;65(1):63–69.

156. Wolfe J, Grier HE, Klar N, et al. Symptoms and suffering at the end of life in children with cancer. *New Engl J Med* 2000;342(5):326–333.

157. Shapiro BS, Cohen DE, Howe CJ. Patient-controlled analgesia for sickle-cell-related pain. *J Pain Symptom Manage* 1993;8(1):22–28.

158. Jacob E, Miaskowski C, Savedra M, et al. Quantification of analgesic use in children with sickle cell disease. *Clin J Pain* 2007;23(1):8–14.

159. von Baeyer CL, Spagrud LJ. Systematic review of observational (behavioral) measures of pain for children and adolescents aged 3 to 18 years. *Pain* 2007;127(1–2):140–150.

160. Hauer JM, Wical BS, Charnas L. Gabapentin successfully manages chronic unexplained irritability in children with severe neurologic impairment. *Pediatrics* 2007;119(2):e519–e522.

CHAPTER 51

Acute Pain in Adults

ROBERT W. HURLEY, MICHAEL L. KENT, and **CHRISTOPHER L. WU**

Acute pain is the normal and predicable neurophysiologic response to noxious mechanical, thermal, or chemical stimuli; is generally time-limited; and resolves with the cessation of the noxious stimuli. The etiology, often, is known or understood. It is typically associated with invasive procedures, trauma, or medical diseases. The pain sensation is usually limited to the area of trauma or damage or the area that immediately surrounds it. Perhaps most importantly, the painful sensations associated with such an injury are expected to resolve over time when adequate wound healing has occurred. In contrast, chronic pain persists beyond either the course of an acute injury or illness or its expected time for healing and repair. Acute pain states can then be further divided by duration, etiology, mechanism, intensity, and/or symptoms. In this chapter, acute pain is discussed using postsurgical or postprocedural and posttraumatic pain as models.

A revolution in the management of acute pain has occurred over the past few decades. Widespread recognition of the undertreatment of acute pain by clinicians, economists, and health policy experts has led to the development of a national clinical practice guideline for acute pain management by the Agency for Healthcare Quality and Research (formerly the Agency for Health Care Policy and Research) of the U.S. Department of Health and Human Services. This landmark document includes acknowledgment of the historic inadequacies in perioperative pain management, importance of good pain control, need for accountability for adequate provision of perioperative analgesia by health care institutions, and a statement on the need for involvement of specialists in appropriate cases. In addition, several professional societies and regulatory agencies, including the American Society of Anesthesiologists[1,2] and The Joint Commission (formerly the Joint Commission on Accreditation of Healthcare Organizations [JCAHO]), have developed acute pain management standards[3] or clinical practice guidelines for acute pain management in hospitalized patients.[4] With the recent surge of opioid misuse and abuse in the United States, there has been increased focus on the influence of these pain assessment standards on opioid prescribing.[4] Although the incorrect interpretation of these standards by prescribers likely has a role in the increased use of opioids in the acute care setting, it is unlikely that it was a primary driver of the escalation in outpatient opioid prescribing. More likely causes of the increased use of opioid medications in the outpatient setting were the best intentions and overly simplistic advice of prominent physicians,[5] the incorrect interpretation of medical literature,[6] generalization from small uncontrolled studies,[7] and the intentional misuse of this same literature for financial gain by the manufacturers of the medications[8].

With their knowledge of and familiarity with pharmacology, various regional techniques, and the neurobiology of nociception, perioperative physicians such as anesthesiologists are continually on the forefront of clinical and research advances in acute pain, especially acute postoperative pain management, and have traditionally been leaders in the development of acute postoperative pain services, application of evidence-based practice to acute postoperative pain, and creation of innovative approaches to acute pain management. The effective treatment of acute pain (including postprocedural pain) needs to involve a multidisciplinary approach like that which has evolved in the treatment of chronic pain. Programs such as the enhanced recovery after surgery (ERAS) pathways that are evidence-based and multidisciplinary have demonstrated great success in the management of postoperative pain and overall patient recovery.

Acute and Chronic Effects of Acute Pain

Uncontrolled acute pain may produce a range of detrimental acute and chronic effects. Attenuation of periprocedural pathophysiology that occurs during a procedure or surgery through reduction of nociceptive input into the central nervous system (CNS) and optimization of periprocedural analgesia may decrease complications, facilitate the patient's recovery during the immediate postprocedural period,[9] reduce the length of stay,[10] and after discharge from the hospital.

The perioperative period is associated with a variety of pathophysiologic responses that may be initiated or maintained by peripheral nociceptive input. Although these responses may have had a beneficial purpose in nature, the same response to the modern-day surgery may be harmful. Uncontrolled perioperative pain may therefore be considered a major morbidity for the patient. Furthermore, attenuation of postprocedural or acute medical pain may decrease perioperative morbidity and mortality.[11]

The transmission of pain stimuli from the periphery to the spinal cord and supraspinally results in the neuroendocrine stress response. The dominant neuroendocrine response to pain involves hypothalamic–pituitary–adrenocortical and sympathoadrenal interaction, resulting in increased sympathetic tone; increased catecholamine and catabolic hormone secretion including cortisol, adrenocorticotropic hormone, antidiuretic hormone, glucagon, aldosterone, renin, and angiotensin II; and decreased secretion of anabolic hormones. The outcome of these changes includes sodium and water retention and increased levels of blood glucose, free fatty acids, ketone bodies, and lactate. A hypermetabolic, catabolic state results as metabolism and oxygen consumption are increased, and metabolic substrates are mobilized from storage depots. The negative nitrogen balance and protein catabolism may impede the patient's recovery and contribute to morbidity or mortality. Sympathetic activation may increase myocardial oxygen consumption and decrease myocardial oxygen supply, which may be important in the development of myocardial ischemia and infarction.[11,12] Sympathetic activation may also delay return of postprocedural gastrointestinal motility that may develop into an ileus.

Postprocedural acute pain may initiate several detrimental spinal reflex pathways. Respiratory function can be markedly diminished, especially with acute pain involving the upper abdomen, flank, and/or thorax. Reflex inhibition of phrenic nerve activity is an important component of this decreased pulmonary function.[11,12] However, control of acute pain is also important because patients with poor pain control may have poor inspiratory effort, have an inadequate cough, and be more likely to develop pulmonary complications.[11]

Neurobiology of Acute Pain

The neurobiology of pain is extremely complex, with redundancy and plasticity such that there is no "final common pathway" for the process of nociception. However, understanding the neurobiology of pain is crucial when contemplating which nociceptive processes to target in the treatment of acute pain. Identification of new molecular and cellular processes involved in the process of nociception has increased the number of potential targets for analgesic therapies.

PRIMARY AFFERENTS AND PERIPHERAL NERVE NEUROTRANSMITTERS

A variety of mechanical, thermal, or chemical stimuli can result in the sensation of pain. Information about these painful or noxious stimuli is carried to higher brain centers by receptors and neurons that are distinct from those that carry innocuous somatic sensory information. This topic is covered at length in Chapters 3 and 4. In brief, small-diameter Aδ and C fibers primarily transmit nociceptive information, but subsets of Aδ and C fibers are thermo receptors that transmit nonpainful cold and warm information, respectively.[13] Neurotransmission by the Aδ and C fibers is performed by numerous peptides and amino acids. Substance P (SP) was the first peptide to be defined as specific to the small diameter primary afferents and is released by noxious thermal, mechanical, and chemical stimulation of the periphery.[14–16] Exogenous application of SP into the spinal cord of rats results in dorsal horn neuronal activation[17] and behavioral responses consistent with pain.[18] Neurokinin-1 (NK-1), the receptor for SP, is found on superficial and deep neurons in the dorsal horn of the spinal cord consistent with their role in pain transmission.[19] Other peptides present in the small diameter afferents include calcitonin growth-related protein (CGRP), galanin, vasoactive intestinal polypeptide (VIP), and somatostatin (SST); however, their role in the modulation of nociceptive transmission is less well understood. In addition to these peptides, the excitatory amino acid glutamate is also present within small diameter primary afferents, released by noxious stimulation[20] and activates the second-order dorsal horn neurons.[21] The effects of glutamate are predominantly mediated by three receptor classes: alpha-amino-3-hydroxy-5-methyl-4-isoxazolepropionic acid (AMPA)/kainate, N-methyl-D-aspartate (NMDA), and metabotropic glutamate receptors (mGluR). AMPA receptors are found on postsynaptic neurons predominantly within the superficial dorsal horn.[22] NMDA receptors are found both pre- and postsynaptically (i.e., on nociceptive primary afferents and apposing second-order neurons within the superficial and deep dorsal horn).[23] mGluR are predominantly found postsynaptically on the cell body and dendrites of dorsal horns neurons.

The primary afferent's presynaptic nerve terminal in the dorsal horn of the spinal cord represents a site for a therapeutic intervention. Primary afferent fibers transmit the pain signal to the spinal cord and possess numerous receptor systems that can reduce this transmission by reducing transmitter release such as the α_2-adrenergic, glycinergic, serotoninergic, opioidergic, and GABAergic receptors[24–26] as well as ion channels sensitive to local anesthetics and anticonvulsants including voltage-gated calcium, sodium, and potassium channels.

SPINAL CORD AND SUPRASPINAL STRUCTURES

Aδ and C fiber neurons synapse primarily within laminae I, II, and V of the dorsal horn of the spinal cord. These primary afferents release neurotransmitters and neuropeptides that activate the second-order projection neurons of the spinal cord. Pain transmission through the spinal cord may be modulated by an endogenous descending pain inhibitory system and may be influenced by exogenously administered medications. The primary components of this descending pain inhibition system are the "triad" of the periaqueductal gray (PAG), the rostral ventromedial medulla (RVM), and the dorsal lateral pontine tegmentum (DLPT), which includes the locus coeruleus (LC) and the A7 nuclei. The PAG is an important site to produce analgesia following systemic administration of opioids.

The endogenous opioid [Met^5]enkephalin is present within this nucleus,[27] and opioid receptors of each subtype are present in this region.[28] The PAG provides dense projections to the RVM[29] and brainstem noradrenergic nuclei LC and A7.[30] Although each of these regions has direct projections to the spinal cord, it has been proposed that their projections to the RVM are important components in the modulation of pain by these regions.[31] The RVM can function as a relay nucleus in the production of antinociception by more rostral midbrain structures (PAG), but it also has a primary role in the suppression of nociceptive transmission at the level of the spinal cord. The suppression of nociceptive reflex behavior is thought to be mediated by the axons of RVM neurons that descend within the dorsolateral funiculus and terminate bilaterally in laminae I, II, V, VI, and VII of the spinal cord. Anatomical studies have shown these axons terminate coincident with spinothalamic tract cells and interneurons of the dorsal horn that are related to pain transmission.[32,33] Consistent with the anatomical terminations of the RVM axons, physiologic studies have shown that stimulation of the RVM results in the inhibition of a population of pain-specific neurons within the dorsal horn.[34,35] Spinally projecting neurons of the RVM possess numerous neurotransmitters including serotonin, enkephalin, γ-aminobutyric acid (GABA), glutamate, and SP.[36–38] The DLPT contains all of the noradrenergic neurons that project to the RVM and the spinal cord.[39,40] In animal models, electrical stimulation of the DLPT sites produces analgesia[41,42] and the analgesia produced by the activation of these nuclei is mediated by the α_2 adrenergic receptor.[42,43] The pain physician can pharmacologically manipulate each of these neurotransmitter systems to modulate pain transmission throughout the CNS.

Prevention

PREVENTIVE ANALGESIA

The development of central and/or peripheral sensitization after traumatic injury or surgical incision can result in the amplification of acute pain. Preventing the establishment of altered central processing by analgesic treatment may, in the short term, result in the reduction of postprocedural or traumatic pain and accelerated recovery. In the long term, the benefits may include a reduction in the development of chronic pain and an improvement in the patient's quality of recovery and satisfaction. Although experimental animal studies convincingly confirm the ability of preventive analgesia to decrease postinjury pain, the results of clinical trials are mixed.[44–46]

The precise definition of preventive analgesia is a controversy in this area of medicine and contributes to the question of whether preemptive analgesia is clinically relevant. Definitions of "preventive analgesia" include (1) any attempt to give medications prior to surgical incision, (2) administration of medications during the intraoperative or intraprocedural period, or (3) administration of medications during the intraoperative and postoperative period.[47] The first two definitions describe an exclusive preemptive approach and are relatively narrow and may contribute to the lack of a detectable effect of in clinical trials. For this text, preemptive analgesia is defined as an analgesic intervention started before the noxious stimulus arises to block peripheral and central pain transmission. This preemptive intervention is possible, primarily, in the context of surgical intervention; ideally, one in which the patient has no or minimal pain prior to the intervention. "Preventive analgesia" encompasses all three. It includes an attempt to block pain transmission prior to the injury (incision), during the noxious insult (surgery itself), and following the injury and throughout the recovery period. Unfortunately, few trials have examined the concept of preventive analgesia in a rigorous fashion. Preemptive analgesia abiding by the first one of the aforementioned three definitions has been loosely examined, although some argue that the timing of the intervention[44–46] may not be as clinically important as other aspects of preemptive analgesia including intensity and duration of the intervention. In the purest definition of preemptive analgesia, an intervention such as preoperative administration of gabapentin[48] is not necessarily preemptive if the blockade of nociceptive transmission from the periphery to central sites is incomplete or insufficient such that the development of peripheral or central sensitization would not be prevented. Incisional and inflammatory injuries are important in initiating and maintaining both peripheral and central sensitization. Confining the definition of preemptive analgesia to only the immediately preoperative or intraoperative (incisional) period may not be clinically relevant or appropriate because the inflammatory response may last well into the postoperative period and continue to maintain this sensitization. Other methodologic and study design issues also may complicate the question of whether preemptive analgesia is clinically relevant. A variety of agents and techniques[44–46] have been used to study preemptive analgesia. Using the broader definition of preventive analgesia that covers the preoperative, the intraoperative, and postoperative periods, the combination of experimental data and positive clinical trials strongly suggests that preventive analgesia is a clinically relevant phenomenon. Maximal clinical benefit is observed when there is complete blockade of noxious stimuli with extension of this blockade into the postoperative period. Recent preclinical and clinical studies provide substantial evidence that central sensitization and persistent pain after surgical incision is predominantly maintained by the incoming barrage of sensitized peripheral pain fibers throughout the perioperative period.[49] By preventing central sensitization and the peripheral input maintaining it, preventive analgesia along with intensive multimodal analgesic interventions could theoretically reduce acute postprocedure pain/hyperalgesia and chronic pain after surgery or trauma.[50] In a systematic review of clinical trials examining preemptive or preventive analgesic approaches, Katz and McCartney[51] reported an analgesic benefit of preventive analgesia but no such benefit with the strictly preemptive strategy.

Treatment Methods

Many options are available for the treatment of acute pain, including systemic (i.e., opioid and nonopioid adjuvant) analgesics and regional (i.e., neuraxial and peripheral) analgesic techniques. By considering patients' preferences and an individualized assessment of the risks and benefits of each treatment modality, the clinician can optimize the analgesic regimen for each patient. Essential aspects for postoperative monitoring for patients receiving various postoperative analgesic treatment methods are listed in Table 51.1.

SYSTEMIC ANALGESIC TECHNIQUES
Opioids

Opioid analgesics are the gold standard treatments for postprocedural, traumatic and acute medical pain. These agents generally exert their analgesic effects through μ-opioid receptors in the CNS and the periphery following an inflammatory injury, including surgical incision.[52] A theoretical advantage of full agonist opioid analgesics is that there is no analgesic ceiling. Another advantage is that opioids may be administered multiple routes including subcutaneous, transcutaneous, transmucosal, and intramuscular (IM) routes. Opioids also may be administered at specific anatomic sites such as the intrathecal (subarachnoid) or epidural space (see "Single-Dose Neuraxial Opioids" and "Continuous Epidural Analgesia" sections in the following text). Unfortunately, the effectiveness of opioids is limited by side effects including nausea, vomiting, sedation, or,

TABLE 51.1   Monitoring and Documentation of Postoperative Analgesia

Analgesic Medication[a]

- Name, concentration, and dose of drug
- Settings of PCA device: demand dose, lockout interval, continuous infusion
- Limits set (e.g., 1-h limits on dose administered)
- Supplemental or breakthrough analgesics

Routine Monitoring

- Amount of drug administered including number of unsuccessful and successful doses
- Vital signs: temperature, heart rate, blood pressure, respiratory rate, 0–10 pain score
- Analgesia
- Pain at rest and with activity, percent pain relief
- Use of breakthrough medication

Common Side Effects

- Cardiovascular: hypotension, bradycardia, or tachycardia
- Pulmonary: respiratory rate
- Gastrointestinal: nausea and vomiting, pruritus, urinary retention
- Neurologic: motor and sensory function, level of sedation

Instructions Provided

- Treatment of side effects
- Parameters for triggering notification of covering physician
- Contact information should be provided (24 h/7 d per week) if problems occur
- Emergency analgesic treatment if PCA device fails

[a]Postoperative analgesia includes systemic opioids and regional analgesic techniques. This list incorporates some of the important elements of preprinted orders, documentation, and intravenous PCA and epidural analgesia daily care described in the American Society of Anesthesiologists Practice Guidelines for Acute Pain Management.

CNS, central nervous system; PCA, patient-controlled analgesia.

the most concerning, respiratory depression. The repetitive use of opioids may induce the development of tolerance.

The most common routes of systemic opioid analgesic administration in the acute pain setting are oral, intravenous (IV), and IM. Commonly, parenteral administration of medications is necessary in the acute pain setting because the patient is unable to tolerate oral intake. Possible parenteral routes of administration include IV, IM, transdermal, and iontophoretic/transdermal (ITD). The treatment of moderate to severe acute pain often requires rapid and reliable onset of analgesia. To achieve this, the preferred medication route has traditionally been IV or IM. The development of ITD fentanyl and the validation of its efficacy in postoperative patients may expand the parenteral administration possibilities[53] but do pose a risk of misuse and diversion. Traditional transdermal fentanyl is not ideal for the use in the acute pain setting because of its slow onset of analgesia and less predictable absorption and pharmacokinetics in the postoperative recovery period. The full analgesic benefit of this medication can be up to 24 to 36 hours after application to the skin. The other important criterion for acute pain management includes reliable and predictable analgesia. Unfortunately, there is wide intersubject and intrasubject variability in serum concentration and analgesic response after systemically administered opioids in the treatment of postoperative pain.[54] The IM route of administration may result in a wider variability than the IV route and therefore may be a less ideal alternative. However, because it possesses a rapid onset time, it may be the best alternative to those who do not have immediate IV access.

The transition from parenteral to oral administration of opioids usually occurs after the patient can tolerate oral intake and his or her pain has been stabilized with parenteral opioids.

TABLE 51.2 Guidelines for Equianalgesic Dosing of Opioid Agonists in Milligrams

Medication	Parenteral (IV, SC, IM)	Oral	Transdermal
Codeine[a]	125	200	NA
Fentanyl	12.5 µg/h	NA	12.5 µg/h[b]
Hydrocodone	NA	30–60	NA
Hydromorphone	0.5–1.5	3–6	NA
Levorphanol	2	4	NA
Methadone (opioid naive)[c]	1–10	2–20	NA
Morphine	10	30	NA
Oxycodone	NA	20	NA
Oxymorphone	NA	10	NA
Tramadol	NA	300	NA

NOTE: Equianalgesic doses are approximate and are intended to serve only as an estimate of opioid requirements. Actual doses may vary, in part because of wide interpatient variability in response to opioids. Doses should be individualized and gradually titrated to effect.
[a]Not recommended due to allelic variation of CYP2D6 leading to unpredictable, slow to ultrarapid, metabolism.
[b]Not recommended for acute postoperative pain management.
[c]Methadone conversion is dependent on starting dose of morphine equivalent secondary to atypical pharmacokinetics and dynamics and is not recommended for acute pain management.
IM, intramuscular; IV, intravenous; NA, not applicable; SC, subcutaneous.

TABLE 51.4 Relative Efficacy of Single-Dose Oral Analgesics

Medication	NNT[a]	95% CI
Aspirin (650 mg)	4.4	4.0–4.9
Aspirin (1,000 mg)	4.0	3.2–5.4
Ibuprofen (400 mg)	2.7	2.5–3.0
Ibuprofen (600 mg)	2.4	1.9–3.3
Diclofenac (50 mg)	2.3	2.0–2.7
Ketorolac (10 mg)	2.6	2.3–3.1
Celecoxib (200 mg)	3.5	2.9–4.4
Celecoxib (400 mg)	2.1	1.8–2.5
Acetaminophen (650 mg)	5.3	4.1–7.2
Acetaminophen (1,000 mg)	3.8	3.4–4.4
Tramadol (50 mg)	7.1	4.6–18.0
Tramadol (100 mg)	4.8	3.4–8.2
Codeine (60 mg)	9.1	6.0–23.4
Oxycodone (15 mg)	2.4	1.5–4.9
Codeine (60 mg) + acetaminophen (650 mg)	3.6	2.9–4.5
Codeine (60 mg) + acetaminophen (1,000 mg)	2.2	1.7–2.9
Oxycodone (5 mg) + acetaminophen (325 mg)	2.5	2.0–3.2

CI, confidence interval; NNT, number needed to treat.
[a]NNT in this case refers to the number of patients who must be treated to obtain more than 50% pain relief for moderate to severe postoperative pain. NNT conveys statistical and clinical significance, is useful to compare treatment efficacy for different interventions, and summarizes treatment effects in a clinically relevant way. A lower mean NNT implies greater analgesic efficacy in this example.

The conversion from IV or IM medications can be performed by converting the parenteral opioid into the 24-hour "parenteral morphine equivalents" (PME) and converting this into the oral equivalent of the short- and long-acting opioid of choice. The division of long-acting versus short-acting medications is highly dependent on the patient, the nature of the pain, the diurnal variation of the pain, but a general rule is 50% of the daily requirement can be provided as a sustained preparation and 50% as an immediate release breakthrough preparation. Numerous "standard" tables exist for these conversions that are based on pharmacokinetic data and physician experience. Other sources of conversion tables or calculators are available including Washington State Agency Medical Directors' Group Calculator,[55] the Hopkins Opioid Program,[56] and on mobile applications from the Centers for Disease Control and Prevention[57] or in tabular form (Tables 51.2 and 51.3).

Tramadol

Tramadol is a synthetic opioid that exhibits weak µ-agonist activity and inhibits reuptake of norepinephrine and serotonin. Although tramadol exerts its analgesic effects primarily through central mechanisms, it may exhibit peripheral local anesthetic properties.[58] Tramadol is effective for treating moderate postoperative pain and comparable in analgesic efficacy to aspirin (650 mg) and acetaminophen (1,000 mg) (Table 51.4). The advantages of tramadol for mild to moderate acute pain treatment include the relative lack of respiratory depression, major organ toxicity, or depression of gastrointestinal motility, and it

TABLE 51.3 Methadone Conversion Based on Patient History of Opioid Consumption

Current Oral Morphine Equivalent (OME) (mg)	Methadone Equianalgesic Conversion (mg)
<100	OME / 4
101–300	OME / 8
301–600	OME / 10
601–800	OME / 12
801–1,000	OME / 15
>1,000	OME / 20

has a low potential for abuse.[59] Common side effects with an overall incidence ranging from 1.6% to 6.1% include dizziness, drowsiness, sweating, nausea, vomiting, dry mouth, and headache.[60] It is metabolized in the cytochrome P450 system via CYP2D6 and CYP3A4. It is, therefore, subject to the same risk of variable metabolism as codeine due to genetic differences in the CYP2D6 alleles. As a result of the CYP3A4 metabolism, it should be used with caution in patients with seizures or increased intracranial pressure and in those taking monoamine oxidase inhibitors or serotonin reuptake inhibitors, including most antidepressants.[61]

Nonsteroidal Anti-inflammatory Agents

Nonsteroidal anti-inflammatory drugs (NSAIDs) such as aspirin, ibuprofen, and naproxen exert their analgesic effect through the inhibition of the cyclooxygenase (COX) and synthesis of prostaglandins (PG). COX enzymes and PGs are important inflammatory mediators and may play an important role in the generation and maintenance of peripheral and central sensitization. Nonselective NSAIDs inhibit both COX-1 and COX-2 enzymes and thereby decrease the production of prostaglandin E_2 (PGE_2) and other PGs derived from arachidonic acid. PGs act at peripheral as well as central sites to alter nociceptive thresholds.[61] For example, administration of PGE_2 directly into the hind paw[62] or onto the spinal cord[63] of animals produces peripheral edema and hyperalgesia. Several studies have highlighted the importance of a peripheral site of action for NSAIDs. Administration in the periphery of monoclonal antibodies to PGE_2 is associated with a decrease in paw edema and hyperalgesia.[64] More recently, studies have highlighted a central component for NSAID action. In the spinal cord, PGE_2 can act presynaptically to increase the release of glutamate from primary afferent C fibers[63,65] and postsynaptically to directly excite dorsal horn neurons by activation of nonselective cation currents.[66] Both effects promote the development and maintenance of central sensitization and enhanced pain states. The systemic administration of NSAIDs reduces inflammation and the behavioral correlate of central/peripheral sensitization and hyperalgesia.[67]

NSAIDs provide effective analgesia for mild to moderate acute pain and are a useful supplement to opioids for treatment of moderate to severe pain. The NSAID may provide some opioid-sparing properties through an additive or synergistic analgesic effect. NSAIDs such as ketorolac, which can be administered either orally or parenterally, are considered an integral part of a multimodal analgesic regimen by producing analgesia through different mechanisms than opioids or local anesthetics. As with opioids, NSAIDs by themselves do not appear to have a significant impact on mortality or major morbidity when compared to other analgesic agents. However, NSAIDs may improve analgesia and patient-oriented outcomes (e.g., satisfaction and quality of life) in part by reducing opioid analgesic requirements, decreasing opioid-related side effects, and facilitating patient recovery.[68,69] When given in addition to systemic opioids, NSAIDs will improve postoperative analgesia and reduce opioid requirements by up to 50%, which may reduce some opioid-related side effects including nausea and sedation. However, not all studies note a decrease in opioid-related side effects with concurrent NSAID use.[70]

An analgesic benefit of aspirin over placebo has been shown for the 650-mg and 1,000-mg doses (see Table 51.4). The number of patients needed to treat for at least a 50% reduction in pain (number needed to treat [NNT]) was 4.4 (4.0 to 4.9) and 4.0 (3.2 to 5.4), respectively. Single-dose aspirin (650 mg) produced significantly more drowsiness and gastric irritation than placebo, with a number needed to harm (NNH) of 28 (19 to 51) and 38 (22 to 174), respectively. The authors also found that the type of pain model, pain measurement, sample size, quality of study design, and study duration had no significant impact on the results.[71] Similar NNT were obtained for naproxen 400 to 500 mg in postoperative patients.[72,73] The COX-2 selective inhibitor, celecoxib, when given at 200 mg has an NNT of 4.5 when compared to placebo in postoperative patients.[74] Neither naproxen nor celecoxib were associated with an increase in adverse events.

NSAIDs will affect osteoblastic and clastic activity in animal studies,[75] and whether NSAIDs inhibit bone healing clinically is not certain. The quality of the available literature is suboptimal, but several systematic reviews have been conducted. In one meta-analysis of case-control and cohort studies,[76] a significant association between lower quality studies and higher reported odds ratios for nonunion was observed; however, there was no increased risk of nonunion with NSAIDs when only the highest quality studies were utilized. In another meta-analysis,[77] short-time (<14 days) exposure to NSAIDs in lower/normal doses were not associated with disunion after spinal fusion but exposure to higher dose ketorolac was associated with an increased risk of nonunion.

Acetaminophen is commonly used for acute pain management as an alternative to NSAIDs, but its site of action at the molecular level is still controversial and not well defined. There are, however, some lines of evidence supporting its role in the inhibition of COX. Acetaminophen has been demonstrated to inhibit a variant of COX-2 enzymes in vivo[78] and be similar to the COX-2 selective inhibitors: It inhibits prostaglandin synthesis in intact cells at low concentrations of added arachidonic acid further suggesting that it may inhibit COX-2 function.[79] It has also been suggested that the molecular target of acetaminophen is a splice variant of COX-1, named as COX-3,[80] but its low expression level and activity suggests that this selective interaction is unlikely to be clinically relevant.[81] This suggests that acetaminophen inhibits COX-2 activity in vivo and that its analgesic effect may be a function of decreased peripheral PGE_2 synthesis in addition to centrally mediated analgesic effects of acetaminophen on descending serotoninergic pathways.[82]

Acetaminophen is very effective in the treatment of acute pain, especially that of postprocedural pain. The number of patients needed to treat for at least a 50% reduction in pain over 4 to 6 hours (NNT) for 1,000 mg of acetaminophen is 4.4, which is similar to that of 650 mg of aspirin or 100 mg of ibuprofen.[83] However, it was less effective than higher dose ibuprofen (400 mg) or diclofenac (50 mg) with NNTs of 2.3 and 2.4, respectively. Fortunately, acetaminophen is rarely associated with adverse effects in the short term; however, it is associated with hepatotoxicity after chronic use or overdose. In countries, outside of the United States, IV propacetamol, the prodrug of acetaminophen or acetaminophen itself is administered to postoperative patients who are not able to tolerate oral analgesics. In clinical trials conducted in patients with moderate to severe pain after orthopedic and gynecologic surgery, the analgesic efficacy of propacetamol was similar to that of NSAIDs.[84,85] Although providing fast and significant pain relief as well as a significant opioid-sparing effect,[84–86] it is not associated with the increased incidence of nausea, vomiting, and respiratory depression observed with opioids or the deleterious gastrointestinal, hematologic, cardiovascular, and renal effects associated with NSAIDs and selective COX-2 inhibitors. Lack of inhibition of COX-1 peripherally by acetaminophen may explain its favorable safety effect.[87] These results have been replicated with IV acetaminophen in patients recovering from major orthopedic surgery.[88] In the patient who is able to tolerate oral acetaminophen and has normal gastrointestinal absorption, there is likely minimal additional benefit of IV acetaminophen over the oral equivalent.

Excitatory Amino Acids

The excitatory amino acid neurotransmitter, glutamate, has a central role in the transmission of nociceptive signals from the periphery to the supraspinal structures and in the modulation of those signals in brainstem and spinal cord through descending bulbospinal tracts. The NMDA receptor, in particular, has been shown to have a crucial role in the development of persistent pain states including neuropathic pain.[89] Although this receptor represents an obvious target to produce analgesia, pharmacologic antagonism has met with little clinical success. IV administration of the NMDA antagonist ketamine produced a reduction in neuropathic pain; however, this came at the cost of high incidence of side effects.[90] Ketamine has had better results in the treatment of cancer pain as both a direct analgesic and by improving opioid-based analgesia.[91,92] Clinical trials of dextromethorphan and memantine have failed to show any beneficial effect when compared to placebo.[93,94] The role of NMDA antagonists in acute postprocedural or posttraumatic pain has met with less disappointing but somewhat mixed results. In one study, the addition of a single low-dose ketamine (0.25 mg/kg) administration to postoperative pain management with morphine was not found to be beneficial.[95] However, the use of low-dose (subanesthetic doses) infusions of ketamine has been successfully used to reduce morphine requirements, need for rescue analgesia and pain scores in patients recovering from abdominal surgery, spine, orthopedic surgery, and trauma.[96–100] In a recent meta-analysis, the inclusion of ketamine to a postoperative analgesic regimen improved pain relief and resulted in lower opioid requirement without adding adverse events.[101]

Anticonvulsants

Anticonvulsants, including gabapentin, carbamazepine, lamotrigine, and pregabalin, have traditionally used for the treatment of chronic neuropathic conditions. Gabapentin is an anticonvulsant that was developed as a spasmolytic and adjunct for the treatment of generalized or partial epileptic seizures resistant to conventional therapies. Although it was originally designed as a structural analog of the inhibitory neurotransmitter GABA, it does not bind to GABA receptors, and the mechanism of action of this class of drugs is not fully understood.[102] It is likely that its analgesic effects result from an action at the $\alpha_2\delta 1$ accessory unit of voltage-dependent Ca_2 channels for which it has substantial affinity[103] and which are upregulated in the dorsal root ganglia and spinal cord after peripheral nerve injury[104] as can be produced by surgical incision.[105,106] Gabapentin may produce analgesia by binding to and inhibiting presynaptic voltage-dependent Ca_2 channels, decreasing calcium influx and thereby inhibiting the release of neurotransmitters including glutamate from the primary afferent nerve fibers that synapse on and activate pain responsive neurons in the spinal cord.[107]

In clinical studies, several open-label single-center and multicenter, double-blind trials established that gabapentin was also effective for the treatment of chronic pain conditions, including postherpetic neuralgia, diabetic neuropathy, central pain, phantom pain, malignant pain, trigeminal neuralgia, and HIV-related neuropathy, which may be difficult to treat with more conventional therapies.[108–113] The role of gabapentin in the treatment of acute pain is more controversial. Although in animal and human models of acute pain the administration of gabapentin or pregabalin produces no analgesia, when it is administered prior to a variety of surgical procedures, patients report decreased pain and decreased opioid use postoperatively.[48,114,115] Gilron et al.[116] showed synergism between gabapentin and morphine in patients suffering from neuropathic pain. This synergistic effect may have played a role in the decreased pain scores of those receiving gabapentin because concomitant opioids were routinely administered in the postoperative period. Pregabalin and gabapentin have not been found to be effective in the treatment of acute chemotherapy-induced pain.[117] Pregabalin was not found to have a benefit in the treatment of acute sciatica pain.[118] Therefore, with the exception of the well-documented effectiveness of carbamazepine in the treatment of the acute exacerbation of trigeminal neuralgia, there is no evidence for the effectiveness of anticonvulsants in the treatment of acute pain not related to an operation or trauma.

α-Adrenergic Medications

α-Adrenergic receptors are widely distributed throughout the CNS and peripheral nervous system (PNS). The α_1 receptors play an essential role in the regulation of vascular tone but no significant role in nociception. Activation of α_2 receptors produces analgesia. They are linked to an inhibitory G protein on the presynaptic terminus of Aδ and C fibers and are activated by descending noradrenergic tracts from the brainstem LC and A7, which hyperpolarizes the primary afferent and reduces afferent transmitter release and pain transmission. However, depending on the α_2 receptor subtype 2a, 2b, or 2c, different physiologic consequences may occur. The α_{2b} subtype produces hemodynamic responses (hypotension), whereas the α_{2a} receptor is responsible analgesia.[119,120] Clonidine is the prototypic α_2 agonist used for analgesia, although it has substantial hemodynamic side effects because of its lack of absolute α subtype selectivity. A newer agent, dexmedetomidine, is a more selective α_2 receptor agonist that is analgesic and sedating with fewer cardiovascular effects.[121,122]

In experimental models of acute transient pain, systemically administered clonidine had no analgesic benefit.[123] In studies of postoperative patients, IV clonidine has been found to augment the local anesthetic block of the psoas compartment for hip surgery.[124] However, the benefit was short lived and provided approximately 7 hours of additional analgesia. Preoperative and perioperative administration of systemic clonidine has been found to have a very modest analgesic (and anxiolytic) effect following abdominal hysterectomy.[125,126] Perioperative use of systemic clonidine has been found to reduce overall opioid requirements following spinal surgery when given as a bolus of 3 μg/kg and followed by an infusion of 0.3 μg/kg/hour; however, modest changes in blood pressure and heart were also noted.[127]

Dexmedetomidine, although more selective for α_2 receptors and more subtype selective (α_{2a}), does not produce significant analgesia in human experimental models of acute heat or electrical pain at doses that produce modest to severe sedation.[128] In one study, dexmedetomidine infusion reduced healthy volunteer's cold pressor–induced pain by 30% at doses that produced sedation and memory loss but did not produce hemodynamic perturbations.[121] Preoperative administration of dexmedetomidine reduced postoperative opioid consumption but had no effect on postprocedure pain scores or recovery time.[129] Perioperative administration reduces opioid requirements after thoracotomy[130] and tubal ligation[131] but resulted in significant sedation and heart rate instability in some patients.

Steroids

Glucocorticoids are commonly used as prophylaxis for postoperative nausea and vomiting, but these agents may also produce an analgesic effect. Glucocorticoids may reduce acute pain in a variety of mechanisms including a reduction in inflammation and tissue damage. A recent meta-analysis examined the analgesic efficacy of a single perioperative dose of dexamethasone. Patients who received dexamethasone had lower pain scores, used less opioids, required less rescue analgesia for intolerable pain, had longer time to first dose of analgesic, and had shorter stays in the postanesthesia care unit.[132] There was no increase in infection or delayed wound healing with dexamethasone despite the finding that but blood glucose levels were higher 24 hours postoperatively. On the other hand, another meta-analysis in thyroidectomy patients[133] found that a single preoperative dose of dexamethasone did not decrease the incidence and severity of pain postoperatively. A meta-analysis of studies examining the addition of dexamethasone (4 to 10 mg) to local anesthetics for peripheral nerve blocks noted a faster onset of action and significant increase in the duration of analgesia with the addition of dexamethasone compared with local anesthetic solutions alone.[134]

Serotoninergic Medications

Serotoninergic receptors found in the spinal dorsal horn have a complex relationship to the modulation of nociceptive transmission. Three of the subtypes of serotoninergic receptors play a role in nociceptive transmission, 5-HT$_1$ and 5-HT$_2$ hyperpolarize neurons within the dorsal horn and inhibit pain transmission, whereas 5-HT$_4$ receptors depolarize dorsal horn neurons and augment the transmission of nociceptive information.[135] Presynaptic terminals of descending neurons from the RVM appear to oppose 5-HT$_1$ and 5-HT$_2$ receptors of primary afferents and interneurons in the spinal cord producing a reduction in pain like behavior in animals following activation of the RVM. Unfortunately, no subtype-specific serotoninergic agonists are available for human use for analgesia. Interestingly, a recent study found that activation of the 5-HT$_4$ receptor in the brainstem eliminates the respiratory depression associated with administration the opioid fentanyl,[136] thus having an indirect but very beneficial effect on the treatment of pain.

The only clinically available serotonergic agonists or indirect serotoninergic agonists consist of the selective serotonin reuptake inhibitors (SSRIs) that are primarily used for the treatment of depression and anxiety disorders. Unfortunately, the data regarding the use of SSRIs in acute pain are lacking or negative. The lack of clinical studies assessing the analgesic value of this class is likely due to the lack of analgesic benefit of this class of drugs in the treatment of chronic pain.[137]

NONSELECTIVE NORADRENERGIC AND SEROTONINERGIC MEDICATIONS

Although the group of nonselective noradrenergic and serotoninergic reuptake inhibitor medications, the tricyclic antidepressants (TCAs), does not carry a U.S. Food and Drug Administration indication for pain, they are a mainstay of treatment of a variety of neuropathic and nonneuropathic chronic pain states. TCAs suppress nociceptive transmission independent of their effects on depressed affect in the psychological domain. The exact mechanism of analgesic action remains unclear. As a class of agents, TCAs act to inhibit the reuptake and destruction or storage of biogenic amines including norepinephrine and serotonin. One possible mechanism is the accentuation of the descending serotoninergic and noradrenergic bulbospinal pathways on the spinal cord dorsal horn, by acting locally on $5-HT_1$, $5-HT_2$, and α_2 receptors. Interestingly, SSRIs have little if any analgesic potential[138]; yet, the TCAs with the greatest pain relieving effects have their greatest inhibition of serotonin reuptake.[139] Alternate mechanisms including histamine receptor blockade,[140] calcium channel blockade,[141] antagonism of the NMDA receptor,[142] anti-inflammatory effects,[143] and blockade of sodium channels[144] have been suggested.

The results for TCAs in experimental models of acute pain are somewhat mixed. The secondary amine, desipramine, which has the greatest norepinephrine reuptake inhibitor selectivity, has no effect on pain scores in a capsaicin-induced mechanical allodynia model.[145] In contrast, imipramine the tertiary amine precursor to desipramine produced a reduction in pain resulting from noxious stimulation of the nasal mucosa.[146] A single study found that the administration of the tertiary tricyclic amine, amitriptyline, during the acute stage of herpes zoster decreased the prevalence of postherpetic neuralgia.[147] TCAs have not been found to be effective in the treatment of postoperative pain.[148–150]

The role of the selective serotonin and norepinephrine reuptake inhibitors, duloxetine and venlafaxine, has not been fully elucidated. Like the TCAs, these drugs have been used successfully to treat chronic pain conditions. However, in the acute postoperative setting, the results are mixed. A recent randomized controlled trial (RCT) examining the perioperative administration of duloxetine found a decrease in postoperative pain and opioid consumption following spine surgery[151] and hysterectomy,[152] however was ineffective following knee arthroplasty.[153] Another selective serotonin-norepinephrine reuptake inhibitor (SSNRI), venlafaxine has similarly mixed results for postoperative pain.[154] The atypical antidepressant bupropion has not been investigated in trials of acute pain; however, it is not effective in the treatment of mechanical chronic back pain.[155]

INTRAVENOUS PATIENT-CONTROLLED ANALGESIA

Various factors, including the interpatient and intrapatient variability in analgesic needs, variability in serum drug levels (especially with IM injections), and administrative delays, may contribute to inadequate postoperative analgesia. There may be difficulty in compensating for these factors with the use of a traditional PRN analgesic regimen. By circumventing some of these issues, IV patient-controlled analgesia (IVPCA) optimizes delivery of analgesic opioids and minimizes the effects of pharmacokinetic variability among individual patients. IVPCA is based on the premise that a negative feedback loop exists, when pain is experienced, analgesic medication is self-administered, and when pain is reduced, there are no further demands. When the negative feedback loop is violated, excessive sedation or respiratory depression may occur.[156] Although some equipment-related malfunctions have been reported, the PCA device itself is relatively free of problems, and most problems related to PCA use result from user or operator errors.[156]

A PCA device can be programmed for several variables, including the demand (bolus) dose, lockout interval, and background infusion (Table 51.5). The optimal demand or bolus dose is integral to IVPCA analgesic efficacy because an insufficient demand dose may result in inadequate analgesia, whereas an excessive demand dose may result in a higher incidence of

TABLE 51.5   Intravenous Patient-Controlled Analgesia Regimens for Acute Pain

Medication	Pharmacodynamics	Bolus[a]	Lockout Interval (min)
Morphine	μ-Opioid receptor agonist	0.5–2.5 mg	5–10
Fentanyl	μ-Opioid receptor agonist	10–20 μg	5–10
Hydromorphone	μ-Opioid receptor agonist	0.5–0.25 mg	5–10
Alfentanil	μ-Opioid receptor agonist	0.1–0.2 mg	5–8
Sufentanil	μ-Opioid receptor agonist	2–5 μg	4–10
Methadone	μ-Opioid receptor agonist NMDA receptor antagonist	0.5–2.5 mg	8–20
Meperidine	μ-Opioid receptor agonist	5–25 mg	5–10
Oxymorphone	μ-Opioid receptor agonist	0.2–0.4 mg	8–10
Buprenorphine	μ-Opioid receptor partial agonist κ-Opioid receptor antagonist	0.03–0.1 mg	8–20
Nalbuphine	μ-Opioid receptor antagonist κ-Opioid receptor agonist	1–5 mg	5–15
Pentazocine	μ-Opioid receptor antagonist κ-Opioid receptor agonist	5–15 mg	5–15

[a]All doses are for adult patients. The anesthesiologist should proceed with titrated intravenous loading doses if necessary to establish initial analgesia. Individual patient's requirements vary widely, with smaller doses typically given for elderly or compromised patients. Continuous infusions are not initially recommended for opioid-naive adult patients.
NMDA, N-methyl-D-aspartate.

undesirable side effects such as respiratory depression.[157] Although the optimal demand dose is uncertain, available data suggest that the optimal demand dose for morphine is 1 mg and that for fentanyl is 40 μg for opioid-naive patients; however, the actual dose for fentanyl is often less in clinical practice.[156,157] The lockout interval may also affect the analgesic efficacy of IVPCA and is a safety feature of IVPCA. Although the optimal lockout interval is unknown, most intervals range from 5 to 10 minutes, and varying the interval within this range appears to have no effect on analgesia or side effects.[156] Most PCA devices allow the addition of a continuous or background infusion in addition to the demand dose. Initially, routine use of a background infusion was thought to confer certain advantages, including improved analgesia especially during sleep; however, subsequent trials failed to demonstrate any analgesic benefits of a background infusion in opioid-naive patients.[158] Although the routine use of continuous or background infusions in IVPCA in adult opioid-naive patients is not recommended, there may be a role for use of a background infusion for opioid-tolerant or pediatric patients. A Cochrane database meta-analysis revealed that IVPCA (compared to PRN opioids) provided significantly greater analgesia and patient satisfaction; however, patients who had IVPCA used more opioids with a higher incidence of pruritus but no difference in the incidence of other adverse events compared to PRN opioids.[159]

The incidence of opioid-related adverse events from IVPCA does not appear to differ significantly from that administered intravenously, intramuscularly, or subcutaneously. The rate of respiratory depression associated with IVPCA is low (<0.5%) and does not appear to be higher than that with systemic or neuraxial opioids.[160,161] Factors that may be associated with occurrence of respiratory depression with IVPCA include use of a background infusion, advanced age, concomitant administration of sedative or hypnotic agents, and coexisting pulmonary disease such as sleep apnea.[160,161]

REGIONAL ANALGESIC TECHNIQUES

A variety of neuraxial and peripheral regional analgesic techniques may be employed for the effective treatment of acute pain. Many these techniques were initially developed for the management of acute postoperative pain; however, their application is appropriate for the treatment of any severe acute pain. In general, epidural and peripheral techniques when local anesthetics are used can provide superior analgesia compared with systemic opioids,[162] and use of these techniques may even reduce morbidity and mortality in the postoperative population.[11,12] However, there are risks associated with the use of these techniques, and a risk versus benefit analysis of these techniques should be performed on an individual basis to determine the appropriateness of neuraxial or peripheral regional techniques for each patient, especially in light of some of the controversies about the use of these techniques in the presence of anticoagulation.

Single-Dose Neuraxial Opioids

A single dose of opioid may provide significant analgesia when administered as a sole or adjuvant analgesic agent when administered intrathecally or epidurally. One of the most important factors in determining the clinical pharmacology for an opioid is its degree of lipid solubility. Once inside the cerebrospinal fluid (CSF) through direct intrathecal injection or gradual migration from the epidural space, hydrophilic opioids (i.e., morphine and hydromorphone) tend to remain within the CSF and produce a delayed but longer duration of analgesia along with a generally higher incidence of side effects due to its cephalad spread. Neuraxial administration of lipophilic opioids, such as fentanyl and sufentanil, tends to provide rapid onset of analgesia, and the rapid clearance from the CSF may limit cephalad spread and development of certain side effects such as delayed respiratory depression but not pruritus.[163] The site of analgesic action for hydrophilic opioids is overwhelmingly spinal, but the primary site of action (spinal vs. systemic) for single-dose neuraxial lipophilic opioids is not as certain.[164]

The differences in pharmacokinetics between lipophilic and hydrophilic opioids may influence the choice of opioid to optimize analgesia and minimize side effects for a clinical situation. Single-dose intrathecal administration of a lipophilic opioid may be useful in situations (e.g., ambulatory surgical patients) in which rapid analgesic onset (minutes) combined with a moderate duration of action (<4 hours) and minimal risk of respiratory depression is needed.[165] Single-dose hydrophilic opioid administration provides effective postoperative analgesia and may be useful in patients monitored on an inpatient basis for which a longer duration of analgesia would be beneficial.

Single-dose epidural administration of lipophilic and hydrophilic opioids is used to provide analgesia, with considerations generally like those discussed with single-dose intrathecal administration of opioids. A single bolus of epidural fentanyl may be administered to provide rapid postoperative analgesia; however, diluting the epidural dose of fentanyl (typically 50 to 100 µg) in at least 10 mL of preservative-free normal saline is suggested to decrease the onset and prolong the duration of analgesia, possibly as a result of an increase in the initial spread and diffusion of the lipophilic opioid.[166] Single-dose epidural morphine is effective for postoperative analgesia and

may decrease postoperative patient morbidity in selected patients.[167,168] Use of a single-dose hydrophilic opioid may be especially helpful in providing postoperative epidural analgesia when the epidural catheter's location is not congruent with the surgical incision (e.g., lumbar epidural catheter for thoracic surgery). Lower doses of epidural morphine may be required for elderly patients and thoracic catheter sites. Commonly used dosages for intrathecal and epidural administration of neuraxial opioids are provided in Table 51.6.

An extended-release formulation of (single-dose) epidural morphine (DepoDur) encapsulated within liposomes resulting in up to 48 hours of analgesia is available.[169] The greatest benefit of liposomal morphine is its extended-release formulation and the prolonged duration of effect that may be important with the increasing use of long-acting low molecular weight heparin medications for postoperative patients for thrombosis prophylaxis. Liposomal morphine exhibits not only a dose-dependent increase in analgesia but, unfortunately, also a dose-dependent increase in adverse events including respiratory depression. This formulation is used infrequently, and therefore, no long-term data have been developed looking at patient outcomes including overall adverse event rates or any reduction in thrombosis rates as compared to traditional epidural catheter-based long-term management. As with traditional single-dose neuraxial opioids, clinicians should provide a lower dose of liposomal extended-release morphine in the elderly or those with decreased physiologic reserve or coexisting diseases, and liposomal extended-release morphine has not been approved for use in pediatric patients.

Continuous Epidural Analgesia

Analgesia delivered through an indwelling epidural catheter is a generally safe and effective method for management of acute pain.[170] Postoperative epidural analgesia can provide superior analgesia compared with systemic opioids.[171]

Epidural Medications

Epidural infusions of local anesthetic alone may be used for postoperative analgesia, but in general, they are not as effective in controlling pain as local anesthetic–opioid epidural analgesic combinations.[171] The rationale for using local anesthetic only epidural infusions has been to avoid the side effects of epidural opioids. Traditionally, this practice has resulted in inadequate analgesia and relatively high incidence of motor block and hypotension although utilizing lower concentration of local anesthetics may ameliorate some of the negative effects.

TABLE 51.6 Recommended Dosage for Neuraxial Administration of Opioids

Medication	Intrathecal Single Dose	Epidural Single Dose	Epidural Continuous Infusion
Fentanyl	5–25 µg	50–100 µg	25–100 µg/h
Morphine	0.1–0.3 mg	1–5 mg	0.1–1 mg/h
Morphine-extended release	Not recommended	5–15 mg	Not recommended
Hydromorphone	0.005–0.1 mg	0.5–1 mg	0.1–0.2 mg/h
Sufentanil	2–10 µg	1–50 µg	10–20 µg/h
Alfentanil	Not recommended	0.5–1 mg	0.2 mg/h
Methadone	Not recommended	4–8 mg	0.3–0.5 mg/h

NOTE: Doses are approximate and based on the use of the neuraxial opioid alone. No continuous intrathecal infusions are provided. Lower doses may be effective when administered to elderly patients. Units vary across medications for single dose (µg vs. mg) and continuous infusions (µg/h vs. mg/h).

Opioids may be used alone for postoperative epidural infusions in order to avoid the motor block or hypotension from local anesthetic–induced sympathetic blockade.[170] This advantage might be desirable in patients following abdominal aortic aneurysm operations as well as surgery with large fluid shifts in patients with significant cardiac or cerebrovascular disease. There are differences between continuous epidural infusions (CEIs) of lipophilic (e.g., fentanyl, sufentanil) and hydrophilic (e.g., morphine, hydromorphone) opioids. The analgesic site of action (spinal vs. systemic) for CEIs of lipophilic opioids is not clear, although several randomized clinical trials suggest that it is systemic[172] because there were no differences in plasma concentrations, side effects, or pain scores between those who received IV or epidural infusions of fentanyl. Although some data suggest a benefit from epidural of lipophilic opioids when compared to IV administration,[173] the overall advantage of administering CEIs of lipophilic opioids alone is marginal at best. Hydrophilic opioids are quite different because of their relative lack of diffusion into the systemic circulation; the primary site of their analgesic action is spinal.[172] Hydrophilic opioids can distribute throughout the CSF; therefore, the continuous infusion of these opioids may be especially useful for providing postoperative analgesia when the site of catheter insertion is not congruent with the site of surgery. CEIs of hydrophilic opioids provide superior analgesia compared with traditional PRN administration of systemic opioids.[174]

The combination of local anesthetics and opioids in a CEI may have advantages over infusions using a local anesthetic or opioid alone. Compared with a local anesthetic or opioid alone, a local anesthetic–opioid combination provides superior postoperative analgesia including improved dynamic pain relief, limits regression of sensory block, and possibly decreases the dose of local anesthetic administered,[175] although the incidence of side effects may or may not be diminished.[170] CEI of a local anesthetic–opioid combination also provides superior analgesia compared with IVPCA with opioids.[171] It is unclear whether the analgesic effect of the local anesthetic and opioid in the epidural analgesia is additive or synergistic. Experimental studies demonstrate a synergistic effect between local anesthetics and opioids[176]; however, clinical trials suggest an additive effect[177] and the lack of improvement in side effects when used in combination supports the clinical experimental data.

The choice of local anesthetic for CEIs varies. In general, bupivacaine or ropivacaine over lidocaine is chosen because of the differential and preferential clinical sensory blockade with minimal impairment of motor function.[178] The concentrations used for postoperative epidural analgesia (≤0.125% bupivacaine or ≤0.2% ropivacaine) are lower than those used for intraoperative anesthesia. The choice of opioid also varies, although many clinicians choose to use a lipophilic opioid (fentanyl, 2 to 5 μg/mL, or sufentanil, 0.5 to 1 μg/mL) to allow for rapid titration of analgesia.[170,172] However, the use of the lipophilic opioid may just provide greater analgesia than local anesthetics alone; it is not clear whether use of these highly permeable medications does not simply provide a stable systemic concentration of opioid. The use of a hydrophilic opioid (morphine, 0.05 to 0.1 mg/mL, or hydromorphone, 0.01 to 0.05 mg/mL) as part of a local anesthetic–opioid epidural analgesic regimen is more consistent with the goal of spinal delivery of opioid and also provides effective postoperative analgesia.[172]

A variety of adjuvant medications may be added to epidural infusions to enhance analgesia while minimizing side effects, but none has gained widespread acceptance. Two of the more studied adjuvants are clonidine and epinephrine. Clonidine mediates its analgesic effects primarily through its action at α_2 receptors in the spinal cord, and the epidural dose typically used ranges from 5 to 20 μg per hour.[179,180] The clinical application of clonidine is limited by its side effects: hypotension, bradycardia, and sedation.[179,180] Hypotension and bradycardia are both dose-dependent. Epinephrine may improve epidural analgesia, can increase sensory block, and is generally administered at a concentration of 2 to 5 μg/mL,[181] but it is also associated with a worsened motor block.[182] Epidural epinephrine added to local anesthetics is also associated with longer stage 2 labor and decrease Apgar scores in parturient.[182] Epidural administration of NMDA antagonists, such as ketamine, has been performed on a limited basis. Lauretti et al.[183] found no analgesic benefit when ketamine was added to the clonidine epidural infusion following orthopedic surgery. This contrasts with another trial showing a preemptive analgesic benefit of epidural ketamine prior to a thoracotomy incision.[184] The theoretical explanation for the latter result is that ketamine attenuates the development of central sensitization and might potentiate the analgesic effect of epidural opioids. The caveat to this is that the safety of neuraxial ketamine infusions is controversial and may result in neuronal apoptosis[185] and is therefore should not be used. Further safety and analgesic data are needed to justify its use.

Side Effects of Neuraxial Analgesic Drugs

Many medication-related (opioid and local anesthetic) side effects can occur with use of postoperative epidural analgesia. However, before automatically ascribing the cause to the epidural analgesic regimen, it is important to first consider other causes of the most common adverse effects of epidural analgesia; namely, hypotension, respiratory insufficiency/depression. These can include low intravascular volume, bleeding, and low cardiac output for hypotension and cerebrovascular accident, pulmonary edema, and evolving sepsis. Standing orders and nursing protocols for analgesic regimens, neurologic, hemodynamic, and respiratory monitoring; treatment of side effects; and physician notification about critical parameters should be standard for all patients receiving neuraxial and other types of postoperative analgesia.

Local anesthetics used in an epidural analgesic regimen may block sympathetic fibers and contribute to postoperative hypotension. Although the incidence of postoperative hypotension with postoperative epidural analgesia may be as high as approximately 7%, the average is closer to 0.7% to 3%.[186] Strategies to treat noncritical hypotension due to epidural analgesia include decreasing the overall dose of local anesthetic administered, or use of opioid-alone epidural because it is unlikely that neuraxial opioid alone would contribute to postoperative hypotension.[170]

Use of local anesthetics for postoperative epidural analgesia may also contribute to lower extremity motor block in approximately 2% to 3% of patients,[186] and this may contribute to development of pressure sores in the heels.[187] A lower concentration of local anesthetics and catheter-incision congruent placement of epidural catheters for abdominal or thoracic procedures may decrease the incidence of motor block.[188] Although motor block resolves in most cases after stopping the epidural infusion for approximately 2 hours, persistent or increasing motor block needs to be promptly evaluated, and spinal hematoma, spinal abscess, and intrathecal catheter migration should be considered as part of the differential diagnosis.

Nausea and vomiting associated with neuraxial administration of a single-dose opioid occurs in approximately 20% to 50% of patients,[189] and the cumulative incidence among those receiving continuous infusions of opioids may be as high as 45% to 80%.[190] Clinical and experimental data suggest that the incidence of neuraxial opioid–related nausea and vomiting is dose-dependent.[191] Nausea and vomiting from neuraxial opioids may be related to the cephalad migration of opioid within the CSF to the area postrema in the medulla.[189] Use of fentanyl alone or in combination with a local anesthetic in an epidural infusion is associated with a lower incidence of nausea and vomiting compared with infusions using morphine.[190,192] A variety of agents have been successfully used to treat neuraxial opioid–induced nausea and vomiting, including naloxone, droperidol, metoclopramide, dexamethasone, and transdermal scopolamine.[193,194]

Pruritus is one of the most common side effects of epidural or intrathecal administration of opioids, with an incidence of approximately 60% compared with about 15% to 18% for epidural local anesthetic administration or systemic opioids.[195] Although the cause of neuraxial opioid–induced pruritus is uncertain, it does not appear to be associated with peripheral histamine release but may be related to central activation of an "itch center" in the medulla or opioid receptors in the trigeminal nucleus or nerve roots with cephalad migration of the opioid[189] or through the activation of a separate population of primary afferents that mediate nonhistamine itch.[196] It is unclear whether the incidence of neuraxial opioid–related pruritus is dose-dependent because a quantitative systematic review[195] suggests no evidence of a relationship, whereas other clinical and experimental studies indicate a significant correlation.[197] Use of an epidural infusion of fentanyl alone or as part of a local anesthetic–opioid combination appears to be generally associated with a lower incidence of pruritus compared with morphine.[192] A variety of agents have been evaluated for the prevention and treatment of opioid-induced pruritus. IV naloxone, naltrexone, nalbuphine, and droperidol appear to be efficacious for the pharmacologic control of opioid-induced pruritus.[195] Although pruritus is a common side effect, it often mild, it is relatively easy to treat.[198]

Neuraxial opioids used in appropriate doses are not associated with a higher incidence of respiratory depression than that seen with systemic administration of opioids. The incidence of respiratory depression associated with neuraxial administration of opioids is dose-dependent and typically ranges from 0.1% to 0.9%.[199] The incidence of respiratory depression with continuous infusions of epidural opioids appears to be no greater than that seen after systemic opioid administration.[199] Although some institutions require patients with CEIs of hydrophilic opioids to receive monitoring in an intensive care unit setting, many large-scale trials have demonstrated the relative safety (incidence of respiratory depression <0.9%) of this technique on regular hospital wards.[200] Neuraxial lipophilic opioids are thought to cause less *delayed* respiratory depression than hydrophilic opioids, although administration of lipophilic opioids may be associated with significant, *early* respiratory depression.[201] Delayed respiratory depression is primarily associated with the cephalad spread of the hydrophilic opioids, which typically occurs within 12 hours after injection.[202] Risks factors for respiratory depression with neuraxial opioids include increasing dose, increasing age, concomitant use of systemic opioids or sedatives, and possibly prolonged or extensive surgery, presence of comorbidities, and thoracic surgery.[202] Treatment with naloxone and airway management, if necessary, is effective in 0.1- to 0.4-mg increments; however, the clinical duration of action is relatively short compared with the respiratory-depressant effect of neuraxial opioids, and a continuous infusion of naloxone (0.5 to 5 µg/kg/hour) may be needed.[203]

Urinary retention associated with neuraxial administration of opioids is the result of an interaction with the opioid receptors in the spinal cord that decreases the detrusor muscle's strength of contraction.[189] The incidence of urinary retention seems to be higher with neuraxially administered opioids than that given systemically. Urinary retention does not appear to depend on opioid dose and may be treated with the use of

low-dose naloxone, although at the risk of reversing the analgesic effects.[203] Epidural administration of local anesthetics is also associated with urinary retention, with a reported rate of approximately 10% to 30%.[204] Higher epidural infusion rates of local anesthetics (with a greater extent of sensory block and higher incidence of motor block) may be associated with a higher incidence of urinary retention.[205]

Patient-Controlled Epidural Analgesia

Epidural analgesia can be delivered as a fixed rate or continuous infusion (CEI) or through a patient-controlled device (patient-controlled epidural analgesia [PCEA]) has become more common. Like IVPCA, PCEA allows for individualization of postoperative analgesic requirements and may have several advantages over CEI, including lower drug use and greater patient satisfaction.[206] PCEA also provides superior analgesia compared with IVPCA. PCEA is a safe and effective technique for acute analgesia in hospitalized. Observational data from two series of more than 1,000 patients each reveal that more than 90% of patients with PCEA receive adequate analgesia, with a median pain score of 1 (of a possible 10) at rest and 4 with activity.[186,207] Incidences of side effects are 1.8% to 16.7% for pruritus, 3.8% to 14.8% for nausea, 13.2% for sedation, 4.3% to 6.8% for hypotension, 0.1% to 2% for motor block, and 0.2% to 0.3% for respiratory depression.[186,207] These rates are comparable to those reported with CEI, with an incidence of 10.2% to 22% for pruritus, 3.1% to 22% for nausea, 7.4% for sedation, 0.7% to 6.6% for hypotension, 3% for motor block, and 0.1% to 1.6% for respiratory depression.[200,208] The optimal PCEA analgesic solution and delivery parameters are unclear. Use of a continuous or background infusion in addition to the demand dose is more common with PCEA than with IVPCA and may provide analgesia superior to the use of a demand dose alone.[209] In general, most acute pain specialists are gravitating toward a variety of low-concentration local anesthetic–opioid combinations (Table 51.7) in an attempt to improve analgesia while minimizing side effects.

Outcome Studies of Epidural Analgesia

Use of perioperative epidural anesthesia and analgesia, especially with a local anesthetic–based analgesic solution, can attenuate the pathophysiologic response to surgery and may be associated with a reduction in mortality and morbidity compared with analgesia with systemic (opioid) agents.[11,12] A meta-analysis of randomized data (141 trials enrolling 9,559 subjects) demonstrated that perioperative use of neuraxial anesthesia and analgesia versus general anesthesia and systemic opioids reduced overall mortality (primarily in orthopedic patients) by approximately 30%.[210] In a Medicare database analysis of 68,000 surgical patients, postoperative epidural-based analgesia was associated with a decrease in overall mortality.[211] Furthermore, use of epidural analgesia can decrease the incidence of postoperative gastrointestinal, pulmonary, and possibly cardiac complications.[11,12] By inhibiting sympathetic outflow, decreasing the total opioid dose, and attenuating a spinal reflex inhibition of the gastrointestinal tract,[11] postoperative thoracic epidural analgesia can facilitate return of gastrointestinal motility without contributing to bowel dehiscence.[212] Randomized clinical trials demonstrate that use of postoperative thoracic epidural analgesia with a local anesthetic–based analgesic solution allows earlier return of gastrointestinal function and fulfillment of discharge criteria.

The benefits of perioperative epidural analgesia (compared with systemic opioid analgesia) on morbidity and mortality is best summarized in a meta-analysis in adults having surgery under general anesthesia.[213] A total of 125 trials (9,044 patients) were examined and patients who received epidural

TABLE 51.7 Neuraxial Patient-Controlled Analgesia Regimens for Acute Pain				
Location of Incision	Analgesic Solution	Continuous Rate (mL/h)	Demand Dose (mL)	Lockout Interval (min)
General regimen				
	0.05% bupivacaine + 4 µg/mL fentanyl	4–10	2–6	10
	0.0625% bupivacaine + 5 µg/mL fentanyl	4–6	3–4	10–15
	0.1% bupivacaine + 5 µg/mL fentanyl	6	2	10–15
	0.2% ropivacaine + 5 µg/mL fentanyl	5	2	20
Thoracic				
	0.0625%–0.125% bupivacaine + 5 µg/mL fentanyl	3–4	2–3	10–15
Abdominal				
	0.0625% bupivacaine + 5 µg/mL fentanyl	4–6	3–4	10–15
	0.125% bupivacaine + 0.5 µg/mL sufentanil	3–5	2–3	12
	0.1% to 0.2% ropivacaine + 2 µg/mL fentanyl	3–5	2–5	10–15
Lower extremity				
	0.0625%–0.125% bupivacaine + 5 µg/mL fentanyl	4	2	10

NOTE: Patient-controlled epidural analgesic regimens commonly used at the Johns Hopkins Hospital.

analgesia had a significantly lower risk of death (3.1% vs. 4.9%; odds ratio, 0.60; 95% confidence interval, 0.39 to 0.93) and also decreased risk of atrial fibrillation, supraventricular tachycardia, deep vein thrombosis, respiratory depression, atelectasis, pneumonia, gastrointestinal ileus, and postoperative nausea and vomiting.

The ability of postoperative epidural analgesia to attenuate postoperative pathophysiology and improve outcomes also depends on the type of drugs used (opioids vs. local anesthetics). Maximal attenuation of perioperative pathophysiology occurs with use of a local anesthetic–based epidural analgesic solution. The use of a local anesthetic–based or local anesthetic/opioid combination versus opioid-alone analgesic solution is associated with an earlier recovery of gastrointestinal motility after abdominal surgery and less frequent occurrence of pulmonary complications. Epidural analgesia is not a generic entity because different catheter locations and analgesic regimens may differentially affect perioperative morbidity.

Risks of Epidural Analgesia

The benefits of perioperative epidural anesthesia-analgesia must be weighed against the risks of this technique. Risks and benefits should be evaluated for each patient. There are complications associated with placement of an epidural catheter, with several risks associated with indwelling epidural catheters including epidural hematoma and abscess should be discussed in the context of postprocedure and/or acute pain management with epidural analgesia. The concurrent use of anticoagulants and of neuraxial anesthesia and analgesia has always been a relatively controversial issue but has been highlighted over the past decade with the increased incidence of spinal hematomas after the introduction of low molecular weight heparin in North America in 1993. Different types and classes of anticoagulants have different pharmacokinetic properties that affect the timing of neuraxial catheter or needle insertion and catheter removal. Despite several observational and retrospective studies investigating the incidence of spinal hematoma in the setting of various anticoagulants and neuraxial techniques, there is no definitive conclusion regarding the absolute safety of neuraxial anesthesia and anticoagulation. The American Society of Regional Anesthesia and Pain Medicine (ASRA) lists a series of consensus statements based on the available literature for administration (insertion and removal) of neuraxial techniques in the presence of various anticoagulants, including oral anticoagulants (warfarin), antiplatelet agents, fibrinolytics-thrombolytics, standard unfractionated heparin, and low molecular weight heparin.[214] The ASRA consensus statements include the concepts that the timing of neuraxial needle or catheter insertion or removal should reflect the pharmacokinetic properties of the specific anticoagulant, that frequent neurologic monitoring is essential, that concurrent use of multiple anticoagulants may increase the risk of bleeding, and that the analgesic regimen should be tailored to facilitate neurologic monitoring, which may be continued in some cases for 24 hours after epidural catheter removal. An updated version of the ASRA consensus statements on neuraxial anesthesia and anticoagulation can be found on their Web site,[215] and some of these statements address the newer anticoagulants. Anticoagulation risk associated with indwelling spinal cord stimulator leads, which could be considered an approximation of indwelling epidural catheters, has been addressed in a recent guideline.[216]

Infection associated with postoperative epidural analgesia may result from exogenous or endogenous sources.[170] Serious infections such as epidural abscess and meningitis associated with epidural analgesic are rare (<1 in 1,000, <1 in 50,000, respectively).[217] Epidural infections are associated with many sources of the bacteria including needle contamination, catheter contamination, epidural medication contamination, lack of the use of in-line bacterial filters, duration of catheter implantation, and patient predisposing factors for infection.[218] The use of epidural analgesia in the general surgical population with a typical duration of postoperative catheterization (approximately 2 to 4 days) is generally not associated with epidural abscess formation.[186] A trial of postoperative epidural analgesia (mean catheterization of 6.3 days) in more than 4,000 surgical cancer patients did not reveal any abscesses. Even though serious infectious complications appear to be rare after short-term (<4 days) epidural infusions, there may be a relatively higher incidence of superficial inflammation or cellulitis (4% to 14%) and even higher rate of catheter colonization (20% to 35%), with the proportion of positive cultures increasing with the duration of catheterization; however, catheter colonization rate may not be a good predictor of epidural space infection.[219]

PERIPHERAL REGIONAL ANALGESIA

The use of peripheral regional analgesic techniques as a single injection or continuous infusion can provide superior analgesia for acute pain when compared with systemic opioids and may even result in improvement in various outcomes.[220] A variety of wound infiltration and peripheral regional techniques (e.g., brachial plexus, lumbar plexus, femoral, sciatic-popliteal, and scalp nerve blocks) can be used to provide postprocedural and acute analgesia. Peripheral nerve regional analgesic techniques may have several advantages over systemic opioids including superior analgesia and decrease in opioid-related side effects and over neuraxial techniques including decreased risk of epidural hematoma formation.[221] A one-time injection of local anesthetic for peripheral regional techniques may be used primarily for intraoperative anesthesia or as an adjunct for postprocedure analgesia but can be used for acute traumatic pain management such as long bone fractures or rib fractures. Compared with placebo, peripheral nerve blocks with local anesthetics provide superior analgesia and are associated with decreased opioid use, decreased opioid-related side effects, and improvement in patient satisfaction.[220] The duration of postoperative analgesia resulting from the local anesthetic in the peripheral nerve block varies but may last up to 24 hours after injection. Continuous infusions of local anesthetics can be administered through peripheral nerve catheters. The use of continuous infusions or patient-controlled peripheral analgesia results in superior analgesia decreased opioid-related side effects, and greater patient satisfaction in comparison with systemic opioids.[221] Unfortunately, the optimal parameters including the local anesthetic, the medication concentration, the inclusion of opioid or other adjuvant medications, or continuous versus PCA versus intermittent boluses for peripheral analgesia have not been determined.

Several nonepidural regional analgesic techniques can be used for management of postoperative thoracic pain, including paravertebral and intercostal blocks, interpleural (intrapleural) analgesia, and cryoanalgesia. The most promising technique appears to be the thoracic paravertebral block, which has been used for thoracic, breast, and upper abdominal surgery and for treatment of rib fracture pain.[222] The possible sites of analgesia for the thoracic paravertebral block include direct somatic nerve, sympathetic nerve, and epidural blockade. The thoracic paravertebral block can be administered as a single injection or continuous infusion through a catheter may provide equal or superior analgesia compared with thoracic epidural analgesia and is a valuable alternative to thoracic epidural analgesia.[223] The analgesic efficacy of interpleural analgesia is controversial.[224] In a meta-analysis of RCTs examining interpleural analgesia, no difference was observed between interpleural analgesia and placebo injections. Interpleural analgesia appears to be inferior to epidural and paravertebral analgesia for postoperative pain control, preservation of lung function after thoracotomy, and reduction of postoperative pulmonary complications.[224] Intercostal blocks may provide short-term postoperative analgesia and may be repeated postoperatively; however, the incidence of pneumothorax increases with each intercostal nerve blocked (1.4% per nerve, with an overall incidence of 8.7% per patient).[225] Like interpleural analgesia, intercostal blocks do not reduce the incidence of pulmonary complications postoperatively compared to epidural analgesia. Cryoanalgesia can be used for postoperative analgesia after thoracotomy but, like interpleural analgesia and intercostal blocks, does not appear to provide any analgesic advantage over epidural analgesia and is not effective for other types of postoperative pain.[226]

Intra-articular Analgesia

Local peripheral administration of opioids including intra-articular injections after knee procedures may provide analgesia for up to 24 hours after surgery.[227] Peripheral opioid receptors are found on the peripheral terminals of primary afferent nerves and are upregulated during inflammation of peripheral tissues.[52] The results of the several randomized clinical trials investigating this topic are summarized.[227] Use of a higher dose of intra-articular morphine (5 mg vs. 1 mg) results in superior analgesia; however, there may be no advantage in the degree of analgesia provided between intra-articular and systemic opioids. The systemic absorption and action of intra-articular morphine

injection have not yet been excluded. Intra-articular injection of local anesthetics may provide a limited duration of postoperative analgesia, but the clinical benefit from intra-articular local anesthetics injections is unclear.[228] Liposomal bupivacaine, a new formulation, is now available and is approved for surgical wound infiltration. This preparation has been promoted to surgeons to reduce the need for regional anesthetic techniques, improve postoperative ambulation, and recovery. Unfortunately, the evidence from independent trials (nonmanufacturer supported trials) has not found additional benefit of this preparation over nonliposomal (standard) bupivacaine.[229] In an analysis of cost efficacy, liposomal bupivacaine was found to be equally effective and significantly more expensive.[230]

ENHANCED RECOVERY AFTER SURGERY PATHWAYS

ERAS pathways are perioperative care programs whose main goals are to improve patient recovery through research, education, and implementation of evidence-based practice. Compared to traditional care, ERAS pathways have been associated with a decrease length of stay, decreased pulmonary/cardiac complications and urinary tract infections, although there may not be any improvement in mortality or readmission rate.[231] Use of ERAS pathways have also been associated with decreases in rate of surgical site infections and even possibly cancer recurrence for oncologic surgical patients.[232] ERAS pathways have been established for many surgical procedures including colon resection, cystectomy, pancreatoduodenectomy, and liver surgery.[231,233-235]

The recent increased interest in these pathways provides many opportunities for pain management clinicians, as one of the key cornerstones of any ERAS pathway is the control of perioperative pain while minimizing analgesic-related side effects. Uncontrolled postoperative pain results in detrimental physiologic effects (e.g., delayed gastrointestinal function, decreased respiratory activity), which may delay patient recovery. The delivery of postoperative pain management in ERAS patients' needs to be tailored to facilitate patient recovery and clinicians must carefully choose from a variety of analgesic agents/techniques for the treatment of postoperative pain in ERAS patients such that the physiologic and pharmacologic benefits are maximized and side effects minimized to facilitate patient recovery and return to baseline function.

For any ERAS pathway, one of the primary pain management goals is to deliver a multimodal analgesic regimen incorporating many nonopioid analgesic agents/techniques to minimize the use of and side effects from opioids.

Multimodal analgesia commonly generally refers to use of mostly nonopioid analgesics/techniques to maximize analgesia while minimizing opioid-related side effects and may include a combination of interventional analgesic techniques (e.g., epidural catheter or peripheral nerve catheter analgesia) and systemic pharmacologic therapies (e.g., NSAID, acetaminophen, gabapentinoids). Postprocedural or posttraumatic pain is best managed through a multimodal approach.[236] The use of regional anesthesia and analgesia is an integral part of the multimodal strategy because of the superior analgesia and physiologic benefits conferred by these techniques.[9,171]

Analgesia in Special Populations

This chapter provides a general approach to the principles and practice of acute pain management, but this approach may not be applicable to certain populations that may have unique anatomic, physiologic, pharmacologic, affective, and cognitive issues. The management of acute pain should be tailored to the specific needs of a population. Although each topic by itself could merit a separate chapter in some textbooks, the general principles and essence of the issues associated with each population are outlined, and references are made to other more extensive sources.

WAR TRAUMA

The treatment of traumatic battlefield pain is largely a function of the type and acuity of injury, stability of the patient, level of treatment (Table 51.8), availability of resources, and patient diagnosis. The chain of casualty evacuation is built on levels or echelons of care, which were developed in World War II to facilitate the rapid evacuation of wounded soldiers based on their medical condition and needs. To maximize efficiency and ensure the continued availability of resources, health care providers at each level provide no more care than that which is necessary to either return the soldier to duty or safely evacuate the casualty to the next highest level. For first-level treatment, pain management consists of NSAIDs or acetaminophen, which some units dispense to individual soldiers as part of "wound packs."[237] COX-2 inhibitors possess the advantage of having minimal inhibitory effects on platelet function, which can prolong bleeding. One concern about NSAIDs is the possible increased incidence of renal failure in dehydrated and hypovolemic soldiers,[238] but this risk is mitigated by the young age, and lack of concomitant medical problems and medication usage in most deployed soldiers. Acetaminophen may be marginally safer than NSAIDs but is generally less effective as an analgesic.[239] Historically, morphine was the standard opioid analgesic used for battlefield pain control, having been first administered orally in the War of 1812 and parenterally in the US Civil War. During recent conflicts, the US military has widely incorporated Tactical Combat Casualty Care guidelines that include the suggested analgesic management of battlefield wounded service members. Patients who are injured with mild to moderate pain are administered acetaminophen and meloxicam. . However, patients with more severe injuries not suffering from hemodynamic shock or respiratory depression may additionally receive oral transmucosal fentanyl citrate (OTFC) 800 µg. The pharmacokinetics of transmucosal delivery are comparable to that of IM administration, with therapeutic blood levels being reached within 10 to 15 minutes, and peak plasma concentration occurring about 20 minutes after administration.[240]

Approximately 25% of OTFC is absorbed via the oral mucosa, with another 25% being slowly absorbed through the gastrointestinal tract.[240] The pharmacokinetics of OTFC appears to be independent of age, unaffected by multiple-dose regimens, and less prone to hemodynamic variations,[241,242] which may make it an ideal drug for battlefield analgesia. In a study by Wedmore et al.,[243] records of 286 battlefield wounded over a 7-year span who received OTFC were reviewed. Significant reductions in numerical rating scores were reported with only one soldier experiencing respiratory depression. For patients suffering from hemodynamic shock, respiratory depression, or inadequate analgesia from OTFC, ketamine 20 mg IV/intraosseous (IO) may be administered every 20 minutes with reassessment for benefit and untoward side effects. Morphine remains an alternative to OTFC in patients where IV access has been established. Other rapidly acting analgesics that may someday be used in lieu of parenteral opioids include intranasal butorphanol, intranasal ketamine, and fentanyl buccal tablets.

Second-level medical treatment facilities include mobile field surgical teams and forward surgical teams (FST), whose providers include surgeons, anesthetists, and nurses. The primary functions of FSTs are resuscitation and stabilization, with the typical duration of stay being measured in hours. Pain control at this echelon of care generally involves oral opioid and nonopioid analgesics, and IV opioids, which can be safely monitored by nurses and other personnel trained in postanesthesia recovery. PCA may be used at these facilities as resources dictate but is often unavailable. During recent conflicts, the capability to conduct regional anesthetic techniques such as single injection peripheral nerve blocks has tremendously grown with the increasing presence of ultrasound technology with FSTs.

Care at third-level military treatment facilities includes intensive care units and medical wards, which may administer continuous infusions of opioid and nonopioid (e.g., ketamine and epidural infusions of local anesthetics) analgesics for acute and subacute injuries. When pain management–trained anesthesiologists have been deployed to a combat support hospitals (CSH), more advanced interventions such as sympathetic and paravertebral blocks have been performed. Peripheral and neuraxial catheters are aggressively pursued for intermediate-term pain control directly following injury and during transport (Table 51.9).[244-246] In addition to providing safe and titratable pain relief, peripheral nerve catheters can be used for anesthesia in patients requiring repeat surgery or wound débridement. With proper maintenance and monitoring, tunneled peripheral nerve catheters can be reliably used for up to 3 weeks after placement. The limitations of peripheral nerve catheters at CSH include shortage of personnel, speed of exodus, infection risk, and concerns about compartment syndrome.

In summary, pain management in the operational setting is fraught with a unique set of challenges almost unimaginable in civilian pain treatment facilities. Because of wide variations in medical resources and personnel, there is no "optimal" pain treatment for war injuries. Instead, treatment should be

TABLE 51.8 Levels of Care in a War Zone

Level (Echelon)	Location	Type of Medical Unit	Primary Functions/ Personnel
First	Combat zone	Battalion aid station	Pain relief, stabilization, and preparation for medical evacuation; self-care/corpsmen care/buddy care
Second	Combat zone	Mobile field surgical teams or forward surgical teams	Resuscitation and surgical stabilization by surgeons, anesthetists, and nurses
Third	Controlled area of combat zone	Combat support hospital or mobile army surgical hospital	Medical and surgical care; broad array of physicians and nurses
Fourth	Communication zone	Military medical centers in United States or overseas	Medical and surgical care; may provide definitive treatment (in United States) or rehabilitation services in retained active duty personnel
Fifth	United States	VA hospitals	Definitive long-term treatment and rehabilitation in wounded or medically boarded soldiers

VA, Veteran's Affairs.

TABLE 51.9 Advantages of Peripheral Nerve Catheters for War Injuries

Can provide anesthesia for repeat surgery or wound débridement
Can provide excellent, limb-specific analgesia
Stable hemodynamics
Minimal side effects
Reduced need for opioid and other analgesics
Improved alertness
Requires only simple, easily transportable equipment

individually tailored based on a patient's injury, hemodynamic condition, available resources, and the ability to monitor treatment response. In modern warfare, the most common cause of soldier attrition is not battle-related injury but rather acute and recurrent non–battle-related injuries like those encountered in civilian pain treatment facilities and primary care offices. Recent evidence suggests that high return-to-unit rates can be obtained by the deployment of aggressive pain management capabilities in mature theaters of operation.

AMBULATORY SURGICAL PATIENTS

The percentage of surgical procedures being performed on an outpatient basis continues to increase. There is an increase in the number of outpatient surgical procedures and in the complexity of operations being performed and comorbidities of the surgical outpatients. Optimizing treatment of postoperative and postdischarge pain is especially important in patients undergoing outpatient surgery because inadequate control of postoperative pain is one of the leading causes of prolonged stays or readmission after outpatient surgery.[247] Although there has been much effort to minimize symptoms such as pain and nausea in the postanesthesia care unit and subsequent (phase II) recovery area to facilitate discharge after outpatient surgery, increasing data suggest that postdischarge pain is common and may interfere with patients' recovery and the overall health-related costs of outpatient surgery.[248,249] Despite the advances in surgical techniques that minimize surgical trauma and postoperative pain, the incidence of moderate to severe postdischarge pain is still approximately 25% to 35%[250] and can be especially troublesome for certain patients, such as those undergoing tubal ligation and orthopedic procedures.[251] After discharge, poorly controlled nausea and vomiting may interfere with the intake of oral analgesics. In light of these considerations, the traditional reliance on opioid analgesia may not be appropriate for patients undergoing ambulatory surgery because of the opioid-related side effects that may delay hospital discharge and postdischarge recovery after outpatient surgery. A multimodal or "balanced" analgesic approach using a combination of opioid and nonopioid analgesic adjuvant medications including NSAIDs or acetaminophen and local anesthetics wound infiltration or regional anesthetic techniques may be more appropriate in this surgical population. The use of local anesthetics has decreased postoperative pain, and the drugs can be administered as peripheral nerve blocks, tissue infiltration, wound instillation, or topical analgesics. Similar results have been achieved using systemic NSAIDs and acetaminophen.

Although multimodal analgesia may be especially effective in the immediate postoperative period, not all the options may be routinely available after the patient is discharged to home. For example, use of local anesthetics in peripheral nerve blocks, tissue infiltration, or wound instillation may be effective in the immediate postoperative period; however, a single dose of local anesthetic rarely provides more than 24 hours of analgesia. Realistically, most outpatients rely on a combination of short-acting analgesics including an opioid and acetaminophen or NSAID for postoperative pain control after hospital discharge.[58] Routine use of acetaminophen, especially when an NSAID is added to the regimen, is recommended to maximize postoperative analgesia,[252] although it is important to remember that when acetaminophen is used as a coanalgesic agent in combination products this limits the number of combination analgesic tablets that the patient may consume because of liver toxicity. The future of postoperative pain control in ambulatory surgical patients may include postdischarge (home) use of continuous infusion of local anesthetic solutions or even use of long-acting, "sustained-release" local anesthetics or opioids.

ELDERLY PATIENTS

The elderly population, which is expected to increase by 33% over the next two decades, accounts for approximately 12.5% of the total US population and 38% of all health care spending (approximately 5% of the US gross domestic product). There are changes in the physiology, pharmacodynamics, pharmacokinetics, and processing of nociceptive information that may influence the effectiveness of postoperative pain control in the elderly. There may be communication, affective, cognitive, social, and ideologic barriers to effective postoperative pain control in this group. The elderly generally have decreased physiologic reserves and increased comorbidities compared with younger counterparts, which may result in a higher incidence of postoperative complications such as postoperative delirium, especially in the presence of severe or uncontrolled postoperative pain.

There is a clinically significant reduction in the intensity of pain perception or symptoms with increasing age.[253,254] For instance, silent myocardial ischemia is more common in the elderly, who may instead present with other angina equivalents. Experimental studies demonstrate a decrease in Aδ and C fiber nociceptive function, delay in central sensitization, increase in pain thresholds, and decrease in sensitivity to low-intensity noxious stimuli.[255,256] However, elderly patients may have an increased response to higher intensity noxious stimuli, decreased pain tolerance, and decreased descending modulation (i.e., serotonin and noradrenergic), which may contribute to the relatively high incidence of chronic pain in elderly patients.[255,257] Despite the methodologic issues in available studies evaluating age-related differences in the perception of pain, there appears to be a clinically relevant decrease in pain perception with increasing age. However, this should not be interpreted that elderly patients experience less pain than younger patients when they do report the presence of pain.

The physiologic and pharmacokinetic effects of aging on acute pain management are complex, and the clinical implications include the slow titration of opioids that produces longer circulation times, smaller total doses because of increased sensitivity, and expectation of a longer duration of action due to reduced clearance. In general, analgesic requirements decrease with increasing age. Age has been shown to be the best predictor for postoperative requirements of intravenously and neuraxially administered morphine.[258] Similar to that seen in younger patients, there is large interpatient variability in postoperative analgesic requirements. Use of IVPCA in the elderly is appropriate to compensate for the wide interpatient variability, although postoperative titration of IV morphine can also allow successful and safe administration to elderly patients. Age per se is not an impediment to effective postprocedure or acute pain use of IVPCA or PCEA.[259] Use of postoperative epidural analgesia for elderly patients, especially in those with decreased physiologic reserves, may attenuate perioperative pathophysiology and is reported to improve postoperative outcomes such as facilitating return of gastrointestinal function after abdominal surgery, decreasing the incidence of myocardial ischemia, lowering pain scores, and decreasing pulmonary complications.

Postoperative pain management in the elderly may be especially challenging because of some of the affective, cognitive, social, and ideologic barriers. Health care providers treating geriatric patients tend to have an unfounded level of fear of complications associated with treating perioperative pain as reflected by the inadequate treatment of pain in elderly patients, even relative to younger patients.[257] Elderly patients may also contribute to inadequate pain control by their own reluctance to report pain or take opioid medications. Elderly patients have a higher incidence of affective or cognitive impairments such as depression or dementia that may interfere with effective pain management.[257] One of the most devastating complications in the elderly surgical patient is postoperative delirium, which is associated with increased mortality rates and longer hospital stays.[260] The cause of postoperative delirium is unknown, although it is believed to result from an imbalance of neurotransmitters, particularly acetylcholine and serotonin, in the presence of decreased neurophysiologic reserve and inflammatory mediators.[261,262] Although the cause of postoperative delirium is multifactorial, uncontrolled postoperative pain may be an important contributor to its development.[263] Higher pain scores predict a decline in mental status and an increased risk of delirium.[264] A multimodal analgesic approach may be useful in elderly patients but must be used with caution because adverse drug reactions in the elderly increase as the number of medications administered increases. Although the benefits of intraoperative regional anesthetic techniques on postoperative cognitive function are unclear, the postoperative or acute pain use of epidural analgesia may diminish postoperative or pain-related delirium in part through superior analgesia and a decrease in pulmonary complications.

OPIOID-TOLERANT PATIENTS

Postprocedural or acute pain may be difficult to manage in the opioid-tolerant patient because the standard approaches used for assessment and therapy in opioid-naive patients is inadequate for opioid-tolerant patients. Although opioid-tolerant patients typically require higher doses of analgesic medications in the immediate postprocedure period, many health care providers still do not provide adequate postprocedural pain relief, in part because of the fear of addiction or medication-related side effects. In dealing with patients with chronic opioid use, health care providers often mistakenly interchange several pharmacologic terms (i.e., *tolerance, physical dependence,* and *addiction*), a practice that may contribute to misunderstanding and inappropriate treatment decisions.

Tolerance refers to the pharmacologic property of an opioid in which an increasing amount is needed to maintain a given level of analgesia. Physical dependence is another pharmacologic property of opioids characterized by the occurrence of a withdrawal syndrome on abrupt discontinuation of the opioid or administration of an opioid antagonist. Tolerance and physical dependence are pharmacologic properties of opioids and not synonymous with the aberrant psychological state or behaviors associated with substance use disorder (SUD, formerly addiction), a chronic disorder characterized by the compulsive use of a substance resulting in physical, psychological, or social harm to the user and continued use despite that harm. The exaggerated fear of addiction contributes to the undertreatment of postprocedural and acute pain by health care providers; however, the data suggest that there is minimal risk of iatrogenic addiction with in-hospital or brief use of opioids for pain control in outpatients who do not have a prior history of addiction.[265,266] Several principles for pain assessment and treatment can be applied in the postprocedural or acute pain opioid-tolerant patient. The physician should expect high self-reported pain scores;[267] base treatment decisions on objective pain assessment (e.g., ability to deep breathe, cough, ambulate) in conjunction with patients' self-reported pain scores; and recognize the need to identify and treat two major problems, maintenance of a baseline (home) opioid requirement and control of incisional/procedural/acute pain. It is also appropriate to recognize that opioid detoxification is usually not an appropriate goal in this period of acute postprocedural recovery. Likewise, several general strategies can be employed for the treatment of postprocedural or acute pain in the opioid-tolerant patient. The physician can create a treatment plan early and discuss it with the patient, procedural team, and nursing staff; replace the patient's baseline opioid requirements; anticipate an increase in postprocedural analgesic

requirements; maximize the use of adjuvant drugs; consider use of regional analgesic techniques; and plan for the transition to an oral regimen.[267] Although chronic pain patients are not synonymous with opioid-tolerant patients, many of these patients are opioid-tolerant, and the same general principles and strategies may be applied to chronic pain patients who are opioid-tolerant. Recognizing and treating nonnociceptive sources of distress may be especially important for chronic pain patients. Although there is no specific threshold or time frame for when a patient becomes opioid-tolerant, after an opioid-tolerant patient is identified, a strategy for acute pain control should be created and discussed with the patient. This may include anticipation or arrangement for a longer than normal length of hospital stay, consultation with the anesthesiology or pain service, and confirmation of the patient's daily opioid intake to facilitate calculation of the patient's basal or maintenance opioid requirement in the hospitalized period. Administration of a PRN analgesic regimen alone for opioid-tolerant patients is highly discouraged because replacing the basal opioid requirement in the acute period can optimize pain relief and possibly prevent opioid withdrawal. Basal opioid requirements can be administered systemically (typically intravenously or transdermally) until the patient can tolerate an oral analgesic regimen.[156] For example, 50% to 100% of the patient's baseline opioid requirement can be administered as a continuous infusion as part of an IVPCA regimen, with a demand dose to cover the additional incisional pain. Conversion tables (see Tables 51.2 and 51.3) may facilitate equianalgesic conversion of opioids; however, these tables provide only estimations to assist health care providers in initiating opioid titration.[268] Opioid-tolerant patients generally require increased postoperative analgesic levels, including a larger demand dose.[267] Patients may require frequent adjustment (e.g., two to three times each day) of the IVPCA demand dose or continuous infusion, depending on the analgesic requirements. There is individual variability in response to different opioids, and if a decision is made to switch opioids, the choice of opioid may not as important as using an equianalgesic dose. Patients may experience different side effects with different opioids, and rotating to another opioid may be reasonable if the patient is not tolerating the first opioid.[269] Adjuvant agents such as NSAIDs should be administered on a regularly scheduled basis to optimize analgesic efficacy and possibly provide an opioid-sparing effect. Use of regional analgesic techniques with neuraxial opioids may provide excellent analgesia in opioid-tolerant patients while preventing withdrawal symptoms.[270] After the patient is tolerating oral intake, the conversion from IV opioids to a form of oral or transdermal administration that would be more suitable for discharge to home may be initiated. Opioid-tolerant patients typically can be converted to a combination of a regularly administered, controlled-release formulation of opioid such as sustained-release morphine or transdermal fentanyl and a short-acting, immediate-release opioid on a PRN basis. Although the conversion of IV opioid to an oral or transdermal form can be accomplished over a period of 1 to 2 days in opioid-tolerant patients, this process may take several days in extremely difficult cases. Converting from an IV to oral or transdermal form of opioid is not an exact science, and available conversion tables can serve only as a rough guide because of significant interpatient and intrapatient variability in the sensitivity to opioids, lack of complete cross-tolerance between opioids which may lead to greater than anticipated potency of a new opioid, and changes in the levels of pain, which may rapidly decrease in the immediate postoperative period.[268] Opioid tolerance also takes a slightly different form in those patients receiving the partial μ-opioid agonist, buprenorphine, for with medication assisted SUD therapy or chronic pain. It has broad interpatient variability in pharmacologic half-life that can range for 24 to 60 hours while having a high affinity for but low intrinsic activity at the μ-opioid receptor. Therefore, patients presenting for surgery who receive buprenorphine may not have the expected analgesic response to full agonist opioids such as morphine and the time to a usual response may be unpredictable. It has been recommended that patients on buprenorphine presenting on the day of surgery have their buprenorphine maintained throughout the perioperative period. If advance notice is given (greater than 3 days), patients can be weaned from buprenorphine prior to surgery. It is recommended that these patients be considered high-risk for difficulty in postoperative pain and recovery; therefore, all nonopioid techniques and medications should be used as appropriate. Patients with an opioid use disorder will also represent a unique challenge for the perspective of opioid tolerance, venous access, infection risk, and patient expectation of appropriate pain care. In these patients, a discussion with the surgeon should stress the importance of nonopioid management including surgical and anesthetic techniques associated with lower postoperative pain as well as a postoperative management plan. Techniques including lidocaine or ketamine infusion can be considered as a component of the postoperative pain management plan. There should also be a recognition that the postoperative period may also coincide with opioid (or polysubstance) withdrawal and may need to be addressed. An addiction medicine or addiction psychiatry consultation, if available, is likely to be beneficial for comanagement.

A more challenging, yet durable, approach to the opioid-tolerant patient will involve a presurgical prehabilitation program in which the oral morphine equivalent dosage is reduced prior to the surgical procedure. This approach would involve the coordination of multiple clinicians including anesthesiologists or pain physician/anesthesiologists in perioperative clinics, pain physicians, and the primary surgeon. Recent evidence has shown that preoperative use of moderate to high dose opioids (above the opioid-tolerant threshold of 60 mg of morphine equivalents) is associated with increased length of stay, higher readmission rates, and greater health care expenditures.[10] Therefore, this prehabilitative approach to opioids could result in improved patient outcomes and reduction in health care cost. This approach warrants future studies.

OBESITY, OBSTRUCTIVE SLEEP APNEA, AND SLEEP

Patients with obesity and obstructive sleep apnea (OSA) may be at higher risk for postoperative complications. Obesity and OSA are separate disease states, but there is some association between the two, because OSA occurs in a relatively higher percentage of obese than nonobese patients.[271] Although some data suggest that epidural analgesia may decrease postoperative complications in the obese patient,[272] the optimal postoperative analgesic and monitoring regimen for patients with OSA is not clear. Data suggest that sleep is disrupted in the immediate postoperative period and may influence postoperative morbidity and patient-oriented outcomes.

Obesity is defined as a body mass index (BMI) of more than 30 kg/m², with morbid and supermorbid obesity defined as a BMI of more than 35 kg/m² and 55 kg/m², respectively. The prevalence of obesity has increased to include approximately 22.5% of the US population.[273] Although obese patients do not necessarily have OSA, obesity is the most important physical characteristic associated with OSA. Approximately 60% to 90% of OSA patients are obese, and at least 5% of morbidly obese patients have OSA, which is defined as more than five episodes per hour of cessation of airflow for more than 10 seconds despite continued ventilatory effort.[271] It is estimated that approximately 4% of men and 2% of women (18 million Americans overall) have OSA and that up to 95% of persons with OSA are underdiagnosed.[271] Patients with OSA are generally at higher risk for chronic cognitive impairment, pulmonary

hypertension, cardiomyopathy, systemic hypertension, and possibly for myocardial infarction.[274,275] The pathophysiology of airflow obstruction is related primarily to upper airway pharyngeal collapse, including the retropalatal, retroglossal, and retroepiglottic pharynx, during sleep, especially during rapid eye movement (REM) sleep.[271] During these obstructive episodes, OSA patients may exhibit hypoxia, bradyarrhythmias or tachyarrhythmias, myocardial ischemia, abrupt decreases in left ventricular stroke volume and cardiac output, or increases in pulmonary and systemic blood pressure.[275] Based on our understanding of the pathophysiology of OSA, it is easy to see how acute pain management can be difficult in this population. Patients with OSA are at higher risk for respiratory arrest.[276] Use of sedative doses of benzodiazepines and opioids may result in frequent hypoxemia and apnea, which may be especially dangerous in the OSA patient.[276] Avoiding respiratory depressants by optimizing use of NSAIDs and epidural analgesia with a local anesthetic–based regimen may attenuate the risk for respiratory depression and arrest because the use of epidural and systemic opioids is associated with sudden postoperative respiratory arrest.[277]

The American Society of Anesthesiologists Task Force on Perioperative Management of Patients with Obstructive Sleep Apnea created guidelines that include acute pain management in patients with OSA.[278] Although the consultants acknowledged that the conclusions regarding postoperative analgesic options were based on insufficient literature evaluating the effects of various analgesic techniques, the presence of equivocal literature regarding the use of epidural opioids compared with IM or IV opioids in reducing respiratory depression, and insufficient literature regarding the addition of a basal infusion to systemic patient-controlled opioids, the consultants nevertheless recommended that regional techniques rather than systemic opioids should be used in an attempt to reduce the likelihood of adverse outcomes in patients at increased perioperative risk from OSA.[278] In addition, the consultants recommended the exclusion of opioids from neuraxial postoperative analgesia to reduce perioperative risk, and the use of NSAIDs to reduce adverse outcomes through their opioid-sparing effect. The consultants were equivocal regarding whether avoiding a basal infusion of opioids in patients with OSA reduces the likelihood of adverse outcomes.[278] Unfortunately, there is a paucity of randomized clinical trial data to provide definitive high-quality evidence-based recommendations in the provision of postoperative analgesia for OSA patients.

Gender or Sex Differences in Analgesia

A large body of data has been collected in the past 20 years concerning differences between the sexes in response to pain, including pain thresholds, and in the tolerance and response to acute pain treatment. However, the exact differences as well as their relevance are far from clear. According to the International Association for the Study of Pain (IASP), "Pain is an unpleasant sensory and emotional experience arising from actual or potential tissue damage or described in terms of such damage." This definition does not differentiate between "pain" as a woman experiences it from "pain" as a man experiences it, and thus, fundamental questions remain.

Females report more severe pain, more frequent bouts of pain, more anatomically diffuse, and longer lasting pain than males with similar disease processes, even when male- and female-specific disorders including male urologic and female gynecologic pain are excluded from the analysis. Females have a higher prevalence of pain related to musculoskeletal or to visceral origin as well as pain related to autoimmune disease (Table 51.10).[279] Substantial amounts of the accumulated data rely heavily on the subjective signs of the pain experience.

TABLE 51.10 Sex Prevalence of Clinical Pain Syndromes or Diseases

Bodily Area		Prevalence Female > Male	Prevalence Female < Male
Head	Headache	Chronic tension	Cluster
		Migraine with aura	Migraine without aura
		Postdural puncture	Posttraumatic
		Cervicogenic	War injury
		Temporal arteritis	
		Occipital neuralgia	
	Oral	Odontalgia	Paratrigeminal syndrome
		Burning mouth	Trigeminal postherpetic neuralgia
		Temporomandibular disorder	
		Trigeminal neuralgia	
Extremities	Arms	Carpal tunnel syndrome	Brachial plexus neuropathy
		Raynaud's disease	War injuries
		CRPS type I	CRPS type II
		Scleroderma	
	Legs	Chronic venous insufficiency	Meralgia paraesthetica
		Peroneal muscular atrophy	Gout
		Piriformis syndrome	Intermittent claudication
		Raynaud's disease	CRPS type II
		CRPS type I	
Viscera	Bowel	Chronic constipation	Duodenal ulcer
		Irritable bowel syndrome	
		Proctalgia fugax	
	Esophagus	Esophagitis	
	Pancreas		Pancreatic disease
	Gall bladder	Postcholecystectomy pain	
Autoimmune		Lupus erythematosus	Reiter's syndrome
		Multiple sclerosis	
		Rheumatoid arthritis	

CRPS, complex regional pain syndrome.

These are highly influenced by sociocultural variables that have little to do with a biologic difference of pain threshold or perception between women and men. An inherent reporting bias exists in the epidemiologic research related to the incidence of pain in the sexes. Females are more likely to visit a physician and are more likely to report pain as a symptom than males[280,281] reviewed in[282] which can therefore lead to an overestimation of the differences between the sexes.

In a meta-analysis of studies examining sex differences in pain response in healthy subjects less than 60 years old, the authors found women report higher pain severity at lower thresholds and have less tolerance to noxious stimulation than males.[283] In a large multicenter trial, Rolke and colleagues[254] used quantitative sensory testing (QST) to determine sensory detection thresholds and pain thresholds for thermal and mechanical noxious stimuli. Females had lower pain thresholds, with the greatest disparities for sex differences found for heat pain threshold, followed by cold pain and pain to blunt pressure.

Many other physiologic, sociocultural, and psychological variables have been identified as contributing to the differences between the two sexes about pain. One factor includes the endpoint being examined, such as pain threshold versus pain tolerance.[283–285] Pool and colleagues[286] showed that pain tolerance is highly malleable and strongly influenced by the subject's "gender" norms. Males who are highly identified with the "male" role tolerate higher levels of noxious stimuli, but those males who do not have this belief tolerate noxious stimuli at the same level as females. The age of the subject also modifies the pain threshold. Advancing age is positively associated with pain threshold.[253,254] Pickering and colleagues[285] found that the difference in score between males and females decreased with advancing age. The significant sex difference seen in thermal and mechanical threshold and in tolerance in younger volunteers became nonsignificant in volunteers greater than 40 years old.

As discussed earlier, the sex difference in humans is neither a universal nor a large effect. Furthermore, no difference between sexes is found in at least one-third of the published studies, and effect sizes are often in the small to moderate range.[283] Other investigators have sought objective measures of pain as a result of the numerous factors that have been shown to influence and in some cases abolish the pain threshold and tolerance differences between the sexes. Paulson and colleagues[284] used positron emission tomography (PET) to investigate regional brain activation after a painful somatic thermal stimulus in healthy normal volunteer male and female subjects. They reported that females had significantly greater activation of the contralateral prefrontal cortex, the contralateral insula, and the thalamus compared to males suggesting sexual dimorphism in response to pain. Unfortunately, this study reflected a difference in brain activation that was more likely the result of different pain intensities rather than a true sex difference. In a later study also using PET technology, the pain intensity was matched between the sexes and the results were the opposite of the earlier study—males had greater activation than females.[287] Finally, a study using matched pain intensity and functional magnetic resonance imaging (fMRI) showed no sex-based difference in brain activation.[288] Other PET studies have described sex differences in responses to visceral pain from rectal balloon distension, although principally with chronic visceral pain patients.[289,290] However, the differences reported were predominantly in the direction of greater activation in men. These studies were replicated using fMRI with similar results of a male predominance of neuronal activation in pain-related areas of the brain.[289]

Pain thresholds in humans vary by internal factors such as sex, gender, female menstrual phase, and psychological variables including catastrophizing, anxiety, and depression. External factors also affect the outcome including testing environment, sex, and gender of the examiner and the modality of the noxious stimuli. In the largest study assessing the role of sex on pain thresholds using multiple modalities, it was found that females had lower pain thresholds in thermal and mechanical pain testing.[254] Unfortunately, this subjective difference has not been consistently supported by other confirmatory techniques including PET or fMRI brain imaging. Awareness of the possible differences between males and females in response to pain is the only clinical application of the present data with no guidance for situations.

Unlike the abundance of literature addressing the question of drug-induced sex differences in experimental pain in rodents, the human literature is not as voluminous. Many in the literature address the response to μ-opioid receptor agonists and the remainder addresses κ-opioid receptor agonists. There has not been testing of other clinically available medications on humans in models of experimental pain. In multiple studies, either no difference[291–293] was noted between sexes or females had a significantly greater response to the medication.[294–296] Although initial studies attributed the difference to pharmacokinetic differences,[297] the metabolism of morphine to morphine-6-glucuronide (M6G), more recent work by Romberg and colleagues[292] demonstrate that no sex differences exist in M6G concentrations. To further exclude pharmacokinetic explanations for the sex differences, the same investigative group subsequently published findings using the potent synthetic μ-opioid receptor agonist alfentanil. The subject's response to alfentanil did not differ based on his or her sex.[298]

The human response to κ-opioid receptor agonists is somewhat variable. In a postsurgical model of pain, females had a greater analgesic response to κ agonist-antagonist medications including pentazocine, nalbuphine, and butorphanol.[299–301] However, in experimental models of pain, either no difference between males and females was noted[302] or males had an increased sensitivity to the medications.[303] Mogil and colleagues[303] suggest that the increased responsiveness to κ-opioid receptors agonists may be related to the absence of the MC1r gene. In an elegant study, this group studied women with fair skin and red hair who often have a functional reduction in MC1r. The women with a genetically proven loss of function polymorphisms experienced an accentuated analgesic response to pentazocine. Their analgesic response was indistinguishable from the male subjects in the study.[303] This finding has led to the proposal that the MC1r gene product acts as an antiopioid and therefore when removed unmasks the true κ-opioid effect. This enhanced effect would be inconsistent with the finding that females have an increased response to κ-opioid receptor agonists in clinical models of pain (e.g., postoperative) because fair-skinned red-headed females represent only a minority of women in general. Unfortunately, it does not explain the lack of difference or the greater analgesic response of females to μ opioids in clinical and experimental models or κ opioids in experimental models of pain.

Unfortunately, the data regarding opioid analgesics garnered from human trials is not sufficient to guide clinical practice. The studies, so far, do not justify the conclusion that males or females have a greater responsiveness to μ or κ opioid receptor agonists, and therefore, they should continue to receive similar acute pain management until more definitive studies are conducted.

Inpatient Pain Services

Although dedicated individuals can improve postoperative pain control for a few patients, more comprehensive interdisciplinary pain services developed specifically to treat this problem can address the needs for all patients within an institution. The organizational aspects of such comprehensive services are considerable. With skills in regional anesthetic techniques and knowledge of the neurobiology of nociception and the pharmacology of analgesics and local anesthetics, anesthesiologists have been leaders in postoperative pain relief and development of inpatient pain services.

Although there are several models for the development of inpatient pain services,[304,305] the key organizational aspects are similar. Development and maintenance of inpatient pain services require a commitment and financial support at the national and local level. In the United States, because there are financial burdens associated with the establishment of an acute pain service, high-volume or larger hospitals are more likely have acute pain services and have access to more high-tech analgesic techniques such as epidural analgesia.[306,307] Whether inpatient pain services improve outcomes is unclear. Two systematic reviews have examined the impact of acute pain services on patients outcomes,[308] and although systematic reviews suggest that the introduction of acute pain services is associated

with a decrease in pain scores, the effect of acute pain services on the incidence of analgesic-related side effects such as nausea and vomiting, satisfaction, and overall costs or cost reductions are uncertain.[308] Despite the direct costs (e.g., personnel, equipment, medication) associated with managing a pain service, there is no available properly conducted pharmacoeconomic study to examine the cost-effectiveness of a pain service. Use of postoperative epidural analgesia in the context of pain services may decrease the cost of patient care through shorter intensive care unit stays and a decreased rate of complications.[12]

Long-term Impact of Acute Pain

Chronic postsurgical pain (CPSP) is a largely unrecognized problem which may occur in 10% to 50% of postoperative patients (depending on type of surgery) with 2% to 10% of these patients experiencing severe CPSP.[309] Poorly controlled acute postoperative pain or acute pain in general may be an important predictive factor in the development of chronic pain.[50,310] Increasing experimental and clinical evidence suggests that the transition from acute to chronic pain occurs very quickly and that long-term behavioral and neurobiologic changes occur much earlier than previously anticipated.[311] CPSP is relatively common after procedures such as limb amputation (30% to 83%), thoracotomy (22% to 67%), sternotomy (27%), breast surgery (11% to 57%), and gallbladder surgery (up to 56%).[50] Although studies suggest that the severity of acute postoperative pain may be an important predictor in the development of CPSP, a causal relationship between severity of acute postoperative pain and subsequent CPSP has not been definitively established and other factors may be more important in predicting the development of CPSP.

Control of acute pain may improve long-term recovery or patient-oriented outcomes including quality of life or return of function. Patients whose pain is controlled in the early postoperative period (especially with use of continuous epidural or peripheral catheter techniques) may be able to actively participate in postoperative rehabilitation, which may improve short- and long-term recovery after surgery.[312] In a recent study, a multimodal approach to acute analgesia using either epidural or spinal analgesia reduced the patient's area of hyperalgesia and allodynia in the acute phase and diminished the long-term pain as well.[313] Another study examined the showed that acute postoperative pain was an important risk factor for the development of chronic pain.[314] Optimizing treatment of acute postoperative pain can improve health-related quality of life (HRQL).[315] Postsurgical chronic pain that develops as a result of poor acute pain control can interfere with patients' activities of daily living and reduce a person to a less functional status.

In addition to CPSP, long-term opioid use following surgery has emerged as a significant public health concern. One source of confusion relates to the definition of persistent opioid use after surgery as studies have commonly used time points from 90 days up to 1 year postoperatively. Although large retrospective studies have suggested a low 1-year incidence of opioid use (0.4% to 1.4%), only a certain subset of surgeries was examined.[316,317] Different surgical types such as lumbar fusion or femur fixation have been characterized by rates of 27.9% to 85% or 36% for opioid therapy 1 year following surgery, respectively.[318,319] Patient factors such as preoperative opioid use, depression, preoperative hypnotic use, and catastrophization have also been linked to persistent postsurgical opioid use.[316,320–322] Other patient risk factors (e.g., age, anxiety, pain at surgical site) have predicted persistent postsurgical opioid use is some populations but not others.[320,321] Future work must focus on surgery and population specific risk indices to account for the unique nociceptive and biopsychosocial variables that occur across surgical subtypes.

References

1. American Society of Anesthesiologists Task Force on Acute Pain Management. Practice guidelines for acute pain management in the perioperative setting. A report by the American Society of Anesthesiologists Task Force on Pain Management, Acute Pain Section. *Anesthesiology* 1995;82(4):1071–1081.
2. American Society of Anesthesiologists Task Force on Acute Pain Management. Practice guidelines for acute pain management in the perioperative setting: an updated report by the American Society of Anesthesiologists Task Force on Acute Pain Management. *Anesthesiology* 2004;100(6):1573–1581.
3. American Society of Anesthesiologists Task Force on Acute Pain Management. Practice guidelines for acute pain management in the perioperative setting: an updated report by the American Society of Anesthesiologists Task Force on Acute Pain Management. *Anesthesiology* 2012;116(2):248–273.
4. The Joint Commission. Pain management. Available at: https://www.joint commission.org/topics/pain_management.aspx. Accessed April 4, 2017.
5. Catan TP. A pain drug champion has second thoughts. *The Wall Street Journal.* December 7, 2012.
6. Porter J, Jick H. Addiction rare in patients treated with narcotics. *N Engl J Med* 1980;302(2):123.
7. Portenoy RK, Foley KM. Chronic use of opioid analgesics in non-malignant pain: report of 38 cases. *Pain* 1986;25(2):171–186.
8. Van Zee A. The promotion and marketing of OxyContin: commercial triumph, public health tragedy. *Am J Public Health* 2009;99(2):221–227.
9. Kehlet H, Holte K. Effect of postoperative analgesia on surgical outcome. *Br J Anaesth* 2001;87(1):62–72.
10. Waljee JF, Cron DC, Steiger RM, et al. Effect of preoperative opioid exposure on healthcare utilization and expenditures following elective abdominal surgery. *Ann Surg* 2017;265(4):715–721.
11. Liu S, Carpenter RL, Mulroy MF, et al. Intravenous versus epidural administration of hydromorphone. Effects on analgesia and recovery after radical retropubic prostatectomy. *Anesthesiology* 1995;82(3):682–688.
12. Wu CL, Fleisher LA. Outcomes research in regional anesthesia and analgesia. *Anesth Analg* 2000;91(5):1232–1242.
13. Darian-Smith I. Thermal sensibility. In: *Comprehensive Physiology.* Hoboken, NJ: Wiley; 2011:879–913.
14. Oh SB, Tran PB, Gillard SE, et al. Chemokines and glycoprotein120 produce pain hypersensitivity by directly exciting primary nociceptive neurons. *J Neurosci* 2001;21(14):5027–5035.
15. Oku R, Satoh M, Takagi H. Release of substance P from the spinal dorsal horn is enhanced in polyarthritic rats. *Neurosci Lett* 1987;74(3):315–319.
16. Tiseo PJ, Adler MW, Liu-Chen LY. Differential release of substance P and somatostatin in the rat spinal cord in response to noxious cold and heat; effect of dynorphin A(1-17). *J Pharmacol Exp Ther* 1990;252(2):539–545.
17. Salter MW, Henry JL. Responses of functionally identified neurones in the dorsal horn of the cat spinal cord to substance P, neurokinin A and physalaemin. *Neuroscience* 1991;43(2–3):601–610.
18. Malmberg AB, Yaksh TL. Hyperalgesia mediated by spinal glutamate or substance P receptor blocked by spinal cyclooxygenase inhibition. *Science* 1992;257(5074):1276–1279.
19. Stucky CL, Galeazza MT, Seybold VS. Time-dependent changes in Bolton-Hunter-labeled 125I-substance P binding in rat spinal cord following unilateral adjuvant-induced peripheral inflammation. *Neuroscience* 1993;57(2):397–409.
20. Jeftinija S, Jeftinija K, Liu F, et al. Excitatory amino acids are released from rat primary afferent neurons in vitro. *Neurosci Lett* 1991;125(2):191–194.
21. Aanonsen LM, Lei S, Wilcox GL. Excitatory amino acid receptors and nociceptive neurotransmission in rat spinal cord. *Pain* 1990;41(3):309–321.
22. Dougherty PM, Palecek J, Paleckova V, et al. The role of NMDA and non-NMDA excitatory amino acid receptors in the excitation of primate spinothalamic tract neurons by mechanical, chemical, thermal, and electrical stimuli. *J Neurosci* 1992;12(8):3025–3041.
23. Liu H, Wang H, Sheng M, et al. Evidence for presynaptic N-methyl-D-aspartate autoreceptors in the spinal cord dorsal horn. *Proc Natl Acad Sci USA* 1994;91(18):8383–8387.
24. Glaum SR, Miller RJ, Hammond DL. Inhibitory actions of delta 1-, delta 2-, and mu-opioid receptor agonists on excitatory transmission in lamina II neurons of adult rat spinal cord. *J Neurosci* 1994;14(8):4965–4971.
25. Hammond DL, Ruda MA. Developmental alterations in nociceptive threshold, immunoreactive calcitonin gene-related peptide and substance P, and fluoride-resistant acid phosphatase in neonatally capsaicin-treated rats. *J Comp Neurol* 1991;312(3):436–450.
26. Stone LS, Broberger C, Vulchanova L, et al. Differential distribution of α_{2A} and α_{2C} adrenergic receptor immunoreactivity in the rat spinal cord. *J Neurosci* 1998;18(15):5928–5937.
27. Beitz AJ. The organization of afferent projections to the midbrain periaqueductal gray of the rat. *Neuroscience* 1982;7(1):133–159.
28. Mansour A, Fox CA, Akil H, et al. Opioid-receptor mRNA expression in the rat CNS: anatomical and functional implications. *Trends Neurosci* 1995;18(1):22–29.
29. Beitz AJ, Mullett MA, Weiner LL. The periaqueductal gray projections to the rat spinal trigeminal, raphe magnus, gigantocellular pars alpha and paragigantocellular nuclei arise from separate neurons. *Brain Res* 1983;288(1–2):307–314.
30. Bajic D, Proudfit HK. Projections of neurons in the periaqueductal gray to pontine and medullary catecholamine cell groups involved in the modulation of nociception. *J Comp Neurol* 1999;405(3):359–379.
31. Gebhart GF. Recent developments in the neurochemical bases of pain and analgesia. *NIDA Res Monogr* 1983;45:19–35.
32. Basbaum AI, Clanton CH, Fields HL. Three bulbospinal pathways from the rostral medulla of the cat: an autoradiographic study of pain modulating systems. *J Comp Neurol* 1978;178(2):209–224.
33. Skagerberg G, Bjorklund A. Topographic principles in the spinal projections of serotonergic and non-serotonergic brainstem neurons in the rat. *Neuroscience* 1985;15(2):445–480.
34. Duggan AW, Griersmith BT. Inhibition of the spinal transmission of nociceptive information by supraspinal stimulation in the cat. *Pain* 1979;6(2):149–161.
35. Light AR, Casale EJ, Menetrey DM. The effects of focal stimulation in nucleus raphe magnus and periaqueductal gray on intracellularly recorded neurons in spinal laminae I and II. *J Neurophysiol* 1986;56(3):555–571.
36. Antal M, Petko M, Polgar E, et al. Direct evidence of an extensive GABAergic innervation of the spinal dorsal horn by fibres descending from the rostral ventromedial medulla. *Neuroscience* 1996;73(2):509–518.
37. Bowker RM, Abbott LC, Dilts RP. Peptidergic neurons in the nucleus raphe magnus and the nucleus gigantocellularis: their distributions, interrelationships, and projections to the spinal cord. *Prog Brain Res* 1988;77:95–127.
38. Menetrey D, Basbaum AI. The distribution of substance P-, enkephalin- and dynorphin-immunoreactive neurons in the medulla of the rat and their contribution to bulbospinal pathways. *Neuroscience* 1987;23(1):173–187.
39. Clark FM, Proudfit HK. The projection of noradrenergic neurons in the A7 catecholamine cell group to the spinal cord in the rat demonstrated by anterograde tracing combined with immunocytochemistry. *Brain Res* 1991;547(2):279–288.
40. Kwiat GC, Basbaum AI. The origin of brainstem noradrenergic and serotonergic projections to the spinal cord dorsal horn in the rat. *Somatosens Mot Res* 1992;9(2):157–173.
41. Proudfit HK. Pharmacologic evidence for the modulation of nociception by noradrenergic neurons. In: Fields HL, Besson JM, eds. *Progress in Brain Research.* Vol 77. New York: Elsevier; 1988:357–370.
42. Yeomans DC, Proudfit HK. Antinociception induced by microinjection of substance P into the A7 catecholamine cell group in the rat. *Neuroscience* 1992;49(3):681–691.
43. Yeomans DC, Clark FM, Paice JA, et al. Antinociception induced by electrical stimulation of spinally projecting noradrenergic neurons in the A7 catecholamine cell group of the rat. *Pain* 1992;48(3):449–461.
44. Møiniche S, Kehlet H, Dahl JB. A qualitative and quantitative systematic review of preemptive analgesia for postoperative pain relief: the role of timing of analgesia. *Anesthesiology* 2002;96(3):725–741.
45. Dahl JB, Møiniche S. Pre-emptive analgesia. *Br Med Bull* 2004;71:13–27.
46. Ong CK, Lirk P, Seymour RA, et al. The efficacy of preemptive analgesia for acute postoperative pain management: a meta-analysis. *Anesth Analg* 2005;100(3):757–773.
47. Kissin I. Preemptive analgesia. *Anesthesiology* 2000;93(4):1138–1143.
48. Hurley RW, Cohen SP, Williams KA, et al. The analgesic effects of perioperative gabapentin on postoperative pain: a meta-analysis. *Reg Anesth Pain Med* 2006;31(3):237–247.
49. Pogatzki-Zahn EM, Zahn PK. From preemptive to preventive analgesia. *Curr Opin Anaesthesiol* 2006;19(5):551–555.
50. Perkins FM, Kehlet H. Chronic pain as an outcome of surgery. A review of predictive factors. *Anesthesiology* 2000;93(4):1123–1133.
51. Katz J, McCartney CJ. Current status of preemptive analgesia. *Curr Opin Anaesthesiol* 2002;15(4):435–441.
52. Stein C. The control of pain in peripheral tissue by opioids. *N Engl J Med* 1995;332(25):1685–1690.
53. Viscusi ER, Reynolds L, Tait S, et al. An iontophoretic fentanyl patient-activated analgesic delivery system for postoperative pain: a double-blind, placebo-controlled trial. *Anesth Analg* 2006;102(1):188–194.
54. Gourlay GK. Sustained relief of chronic pain. Pharmacokinetics of sustained release morphine. *Clin Pharmacokinet* 1998;35(3):173–190.
55. Washington State Agency Medical Directors' Group. Dose opioid calculator. Available at: http://www.agencymeddirectors.wa.gov/Calculator/Dose Calculator.htm. Accessed April 4, 2017.
56. The Johns Hopkins University. Welcome to the Hopkins Opioid Program. Available at: http://www.hopweb.org/. Accessed April 4, 2017.
57. Centers for Disease Control and Prevention. Guideline resources: CDC Opioid Guideline Mobile App. Available at: https://www.cdc.gov/drugover dose/prescribing/app.html. Accessed April 4, 2017.
58. Pang WW, Huang PY, Chang DP, et al. The peripheral analgesic effect of tramadol in reducing propofol injection pain: a comparison with lidocaine. *Reg Anesth Pain Med* 1999;24(3):246–249.
59. Budd K, Langford R. Tramadol revisited. *Br J Anaesth* 1999;82(4):493–495.
60. Edwards JE, McQuay HJ, Moore RA. Combination analgesic efficacy: individual patient data meta-analysis of single-dose oral tramadol plus acetaminophen in acute postoperative pain. *J Pain Symptom Manage* 2002;23(2):121–130.
61. Svensson CI, Yaksh TL. The spinal phospholipase-cyclooxygenase-prostanoid cascade in nociceptive processing. *Annu Rev Pharmacol Toxicol* 2002;42:553–583.

62. Moncada S, Ferreira SH, Vane JR. Prostaglandins, aspirin-like drugs and the oedema of inflammation. *Nature* 1973;246(5430):217–219.

63. Ferreira SH, Lorenzetti BB. Intrathecal administration of prostaglandin E2 causes sensitization of the primary afferent neuron via the spinal release of glutamate. *Inflamm Res* 1996;45(10):499–502.

64. Portanova JP, Zhang Y, Anderson GD, et al. Selective neutralization of prostaglandin E2 blocks inflammation, hyperalgesia, and interleukin 6 production in vivo. *J Exp Med* 1996;184(3):883–891.

65. Malmberg AB, Yaksh TL. Cyclooxygenase inhibition and the spinal release of prostaglandin E2 and amino acids evoked by paw formalin injection: a microdialysis study in unanesthetized rats. *J Neurosci* 1995;15(4):2768–2776.

66. Baba H, Kohno T, Moore KA, et al. Direct activation of rat spinal dorsal horn neurons by prostaglandin E2. *J Neurosci* 2001;21(5):1750–1756.

67. Buritova J, Besson JM. Peripheral and/or central effects of racemic-, S(+)- and R(−)-flurbiprofen on inflammatory nociceptive processes: a c-Fos protein study in the rat spinal cord. *Br J Pharmacol* 1998;125(1):87–101.

68. Crews JC. Multimodal pain management strategies for office-based and ambulatory procedures. *JAMA* 2002;288(5):629–632.

69. Jin F, Chung F. Multimodal analgesia for postoperative pain control. *J Clin Anesth* 2001;13(7):524–539.

70. Grass JA, Sakima NT, Valley M, et al. Assessment of ketorolac as an adjuvant to fentanyl patient-controlled epidural analgesia after radical retropubic prostatectomy. *Anesthesiology* 1993;78(4):642–648.

71. Edwards JE, Oldman AD, Smith LA, et al. Oral aspirin in postoperative pain: a quantitative systematic review. *Pain* 1999;81(3):289–297.

72. Mason L, Edwards J, Moore RA, et al. Single dose oral indometacin for the treatment of acute postoperative pain. *Cochrane Database Syst Rev* 2004;(4):CD004308.

73. Mason L, Edwards JE, Moore RA, et al. Single dose oral naproxen and naproxen sodium for acute postoperative pain. *Cochrane Database Syst Rev* 2004;(4):CD004234.

74. Barden J, Edwards JE, McQuay HJ, et al. Single dose oral celecoxib for postoperative pain. *Cochrane Database Syst Rev* 2003;(2):CD004233.

75. Salari P, Abdollahi M. Controversial effects of non-steroidal anti-inflammatory drugs on bone: a review. *Inflamm Allergy Drug Targets* 2009;8(3):169–175.

76. Dodwell ER, Latorre JG, Parisini E, et al. NSAID exposure and risk of nonunion: a meta-analysis of case-control and cohort studies. *Calcif Tissue Int* 2010;87(3):193–202.

77. Li Q, Zhang Z, Cai Z. High-dose ketorolac affects adult spinal fusion: a meta-analysis of the effect of perioperative nonsteroidal anti-inflammatory drugs on spinal fusion. *Spine (Phila Pa 1976)* 2011;36(7):E461–E468.

78. Simmons DL, Botting RM, Robertson PM, et al. Induction of an acetaminophen-sensitive cyclooxygenase with reduced sensitivity to nonsteroid antiinflammatory drugs. *Proc Natl Acad Sci U S A* 1999;96(6):3275–3280.

79. Graham GG, Scott KF. Mechanisms of action of paracetamol and related analgesics. *Inflammopharmacology* 2003;11(4):401–413.

80. Chandrasekharan NV, Dai H, Roos KL, et al. COX-3, a cyclooxygenase-1 variant inhibited by acetaminophen and other analgesic/antipyretic drugs: cloning, structure, and expression. *Proc Natl Acad Sci USA* 2002;99(21):13926–13931.

81. Graham GG, Scott KF. Mechanism of action of paracetamol. *Am J Ther* 2005;12(1):46–55.

82. Pelissier T, Alloui A, Caussade F, et al. Paracetamol exerts a spinal antinociceptive effect involving an indirect interaction with 5-hydroxytryptamine3 receptors: in vivo and in vitro evidence. *J Pharmacol Exp Ther* 1996;278(1):8–14.

83. Moore RA, ed. *Oxford League Table of Analgesics in Acute Pain.* London: Bandolier; 2003.

84. Varrassi G, Marinangeli F, Agro F, et al. A double-blinded evaluation of propacetamol versus ketorolac in combination with patient-controlled analgesia morphine: analgesic efficacy and tolerability after gynecologic surgery. *Anesth Analg* 1999;88(3):611–616.

85. Zhou TJ, Tang J, White PF. Propacetamol versus ketorolac for treatment of acute postoperative pain after total hip or knee replacement. *Anesth Analg* 2001;92(6):1569–1575.

86. Hernandez-Palazon J, Tortosa JA, Martinez-Lage JF, et al. Intravenous administration of propacetamol reduces morphine consumption after spinal fusion surgery. *Anesth Analg* 2001;92(6):1473–1476.

87. Bonnefont J, Alloui A, Chapuy E, et al. Orally administered paracetamol does not act locally in the rat formalin test: evidence for a supraspinal, serotonin-dependent antinociceptive mechanism. *Anesthesiology* 2003;99(4):976–981.

88. Sinatra RS, Jahr JS, Reynolds LW, et al. Efficacy and safety of single and repeated administration of 1 gram intravenous acetaminophen injection (paracetamol) for pain management after major orthopedic surgery. *Anesthesiology* 2005;102(4):822–831.

89. Woolf CJ, Salter MW. Neuronal plasticity: increasing the gain in pain. *Science* 2000;288(5472):1765–1769.

90. Eide PK, Jorum E, Stubhaug A, et al. Relief of post-herpetic neuralgia with the N-methyl-D-aspartic acid receptor antagonist ketamine: a double-blind, cross-over comparison with morphine and placebo. *Pain* 1994;58(3):347–354.

91. Block BM, Hurley RW, Raja SN. Mechanism-based therapies for pain. *Drug News Perspect* 2004;17(3):172–186.

92. Cherry DA, Plummer JL, Gourlay GK, et al. Ketamine as an adjunct to morphine in the treatment of pain. *Pain* 1995;62(1):119–121.

93. Gilron I, Booher SL, Rowan MS, et al. A randomized, controlled trial of high-dose dextromethorphan in facial neuralgias. *Neurology* 2000;55(7):964–971.

94. Nikolajsen L, Gottrup H, Kristensen AG, et al. Memantine (a N-methyl-D-aspartate receptor antagonist) in the treatment of neuropathic pain after amputation or surgery: a randomized, double-blinded, cross-over study. *Anesth Analg* 2000;91(4):960–966.

95. Gillies A, Lindholm D, Angliss M, et al. The use of ketamine as rescue analgesia in the recovery room following morphine administration—a double-blind randomised controlled trial in postoperative patients. *Anaesth Intensive Care* 2007;35(2):199–203.

96. Adam F, Chauvin M, Du Manoir B, et al. Small-dose ketamine infusion improves postoperative analgesia and rehabilitation after total knee arthroplasty. *Anesth Analg* 2005;100(2):475–480.

97. Galinski M, Dolveck F, Combes X, et al. Management of severe acute pain in emergency settings: ketamine reduces morphine consumption. *Am J Emerg Med* 2007;25(4):385–390.

98. Heidari SM, Saghaei M, Hashemi SJ, et al. Effect of oral ketamine on the postoperative pain and analgesic requirement following orthopedic surgery. *Acta Anaesthesiol Taiwan* 2006;44(4):211–215.

99. Webb AR, Skinner BS, Leong S, et al. The addition of a small-dose ketamine infusion to tramadol for postoperative analgesia: a double-blinded, placebo-controlled, randomized trial after abdominal surgery. *Anesth Analg* 2007;104(4):912–917.

100. Nielsen RV, Fomsgaard JS, Siegel H, et al. Intraoperative ketamine reduces immediate postoperative opioid consumption after spinal fusion surgery in chronic pain patients with opioid dependency: a randomized, blinded trial. *Pain* 2017;158(3):463–470.

101. Wang L, Johnston B, Kaushal A, et al. Ketamine added to morphine or hydromorphone patient-controlled analgesia for acute postoperative pain in adults: a systematic review and meta-analysis of randomized trials. *Can J Anaesth* 2016;63(3):311–325.

102. Suman-Chauhan N, Webdale L, Hill DR, et al. Characterisation of [3H] gabapentin binding to a novel site in rat brain: homogenate binding studies. *Eur J Pharmacol* 1993;244(3):293–301.

103. Gee NS, Brown JP, Dissanayake VU, et al. The novel anticonvulsant drug, gabapentin (Neurontin), binds to the α2δ subunit of a calcium channel. *J Biol Chem* 1996;271(10):5768–5776.

104. Newton RA, Bingham S, Case PC, et al. Dorsal root ganglion neurons show increased expression of the calcium channel alpha2delta-1 subunit following partial sciatic nerve injury. *Brain Res Mol Brain Res* 2001;95(1–2):1–8.

105. Zahn PK, Brennan TJ. Incision-induced changes in receptive field properties of rat dorsal horn neurons. *Anesthesiology* 1999;91(3):772–785.

106. Zahn PK, Brennan TJ. Primary and secondary hyperalgesia in a rat model for human postoperative pain. *Anesthesiology* 1999;90(3):863–872.

107. Shimoyama M, Shimoyama N, Hori Y. Gabapentin affects glutamatergic excitatory neurotransmission in the rat dorsal horn. *Pain* 2000;85(3):405–414.

108. Backonja M, Beydoun A, Edwards KR, et al. Gabapentin for the symptomatic treatment of painful neuropathy in patients with diabetes mellitus: a randomized controlled trial. *JAMA* 1998;280(21):1831–1836.

109. Hahn K, Arendt G, Braun JS, et al. A placebo-controlled trial of gabapentin for painful HIV-associated sensory neuropathies. *J Neurol* 2004;251(10):1260–1266.

110. Mellick LB, Mellick GA. Successful treatment of reflex sympathetic dystrophy with gabapentin. *Am J Emerg Med* 1995;13(1):96.

111. Rosenberg JM, Harrell C, Ristic H, et al. The effect of gabapentin on neuropathic pain. *Clin J Pain* 1997;13(3):251–255.

112. Rowbotham M, Harden N, Stacey B, et al. Gabapentin for the treatment of postherpetic neuralgia: a randomized controlled trial. *JAMA* 1998;280(21):1837–1842.

113. Werner MU, Perkins FM, Holte K, et al. Effects of gabapentin in acute inflammatory pain in humans. *Reg Anesth Pain Med* 2001;26(4):322–328.

114. Clarke H, Bonin RP, Orser BA, et al. The prevention of chronic postsurgical pain using gabapentin and pregabalin: a combined systematic review and meta-analysis. *Anesth Analg* 2012;115(2):428–442.

115. Eipe N, Penning J, Yazdi F, et al. Perioperative use of pregabalin for acute pain-a systematic review and meta-analysis. *Pain* 2015;156(7):1284–1300.

116. Gilron I, Bailey JM, Tu D, et al. Morphine, gabapentin, or their combination for neuropathic pain. *N Engl J Med* 2005;352(13):1324–1334.

117. Ewertz M, Qvortrup C, Eckhoff L. Chemotherapy-induced peripheral neuropathy in patients treated with taxanes and platinum derivatives. *Acta Oncol* 2015;54(5):587–591.

118. Mathieson S, Maher CG, McLachlan AJ, et al. Trial of pregabalin for acute and chronic sciatica. *N Engl J Med* 2017;376(12):1111–1120.

119. Kamibayashi T, Maze M. Clinical uses of α₂-adrenergic agonists. *Anesthesiology* 2000;93(5):1345–1349.

120. Stone LS, MacMillan LB, Kitto KF, et al. The α₂ₐ adrenergic receptor subtype mediates spinal analgesia evoked by α₂ agonists and is necessary for spinal adrenergic-opioid synergy. *J Neurosci* 1997;17(18):7157–7165.

121. Hall JE, Uhrich TD, Barney JA, et al. Sedative, amnestic, and analgesic properties of small-dose dexmedetomidine infusions. *Anesth Analg* 2000;90(3):699–705.

122. Pandharipande PP, Pun BT, Herr DL, et al. Effect of sedation with dexmedetomidine vs lorazepam on acute brain dysfunction in mechanically ventilated patients: the MENDS randomized controlled trial. *JAMA* 2007;298(22): 2644–2653.

123. Eisenach JC, Hood DD, Curry R. Intrathecal, but not intravenous, clonidine reduces experimental thermal or capsaicin-induced pain and hyperalgesia in normal volunteers. *Anesth Analg* 1998;87(3):591–596.

124. Mannion S, Hayes I, Loughnane F, et al. Intravenous but not perineural clonidine prolongs postoperative analgesia after psoas compartment block with 0.5% levobupivacaine for hip fracture surgery. *Anesth Analg* 2005; 100(3):873–878.

125. Dimou P, Paraskeva A, Papilas K, et al. Transdermal clonidine: does it affect pain after abdominal hysterectomy? *Acta Anaesthesiol Belg* 2003; 54(3):227–232.

126. Hidalgo MP, Auzani JA, Rumpel LC, et al. The clinical effect of small oral clonidine doses on perioperative outcomes in patients undergoing abdominal hysterectomy. *Anesth Analg* 2005;100(3):795–802.

127. Marinangeli F, Ciccozzi A, Donatelli F, et al. Clonidine for treatment of postoperative pain: a dose-finding study. *Eur J Pain* 2002;6(1):35–42.

128. Angst MS, Ramaswamy B, Davies MF, et al. Comparative analgesic and mental effects of increasing plasma concentrations of dexmedetomidine and alfentanil in humans. *Anesthesiology* 2004;101(3):744–752.

129. Unlugenc H, Gunduz M, Guler T, et al. The effect of pre-anaesthetic administration of intravenous dexmedetomidine on postoperative pain in patients receiving patient-controlled morphine. *Eur J Anaesthesiol* 2005;22(5):386–391.

130. Wahlander S, Frumento RJ, Wagener G, et al. A prospective, double-blind, randomized, placebo-controlled study of dexmedetomidine as an adjunct to epidural analgesia after thoracic surgery. *J Cardiothorac Vasc Anesth* 2005;19(5):630–635.

131. Aho MS, Erkola OA, Scheinin H, et al. Effect of intravenously administered dexmedetomidine on pain after laparoscopic tubal ligation. *Anesth Analg* 1991;73(2):112–118.

132. Waldron NH, Jones CA, Gan TJ, et al. Impact of perioperative dexamethasone on postoperative analgesia and side-effects: systematic review and meta-analysis. *Br J Anaesth* 2013;110(2):191–200.

133. Li B, Wang H. Dexamethasone reduces nausea and vomiting but not pain after thyroid surgery: a meta-analysis of randomized controlled trials. *Med Sci Monit* 2014;20:2837–2845.

134. Huynh TM, Marret E, Bonnet F. Combination of dexamethasone and local anaesthetic solution in peripheral nerve blocks: a meta-analysis of randomised controlled trials. *Eur J Anaesthesiol* 2015;32(11):751–758.

135. Cardenas CG, Del Mar LP, Cooper BY, et al. 5HT₄ receptors couple positively to tetrodotoxin-insensitive sodium channels in a subpopulation of capsaicin-sensitive rat sensory neurons. *J Neurosci* 1997;17(19):7181–7189.

136. Manzke T, Guenther U, Ponimaskin EG, et al. 5-HT4(a) receptors avert opioid-induced breathing depression without loss of analgesia. *Science* 2003;301(5630):226–229.

137. Max MB, Lynch SA, Muir J, et al. Effects of desipramine, amitriptyline, and fluoxetine on pain in diabetic neuropathy. *N Engl J Med* 1992;326(19): 1250–1256.

138. Kishore-Kumar R, Schafer SC, Lawlor BA, et al. Single doses of the serotonin agonists buspirone and m-chlorophenylpiperazine do not relieve neuropathic pain. *Pain* 1989;37(2):223–227.

139. McQuay HJ, Tramer M, Nye BA, et al. A systematic review of antidepressants in neuropathic pain. *Pain* 1996;68(2–3):217–227.

140. Rumore MM, Schlichting DA. Clinical efficacy of antihistaminics as analgesics. *Pain* 1986;25(1):7–22.

141. Dickenson AH, Matthews EA, Suzuki R. Neurobiology of neuropathic pain: mode of action of anticonvulsants. *Eur J Pain* 2002;6(suppl A):51–60.

142. Eisenach JC, Gebhart GF. Intrathecal amitriptyline acts as an N-methyl-D-aspartate receptor antagonist in the presence of inflammatory hyperalgesia in rats. *Anesthesiology* 1995;83(5):1046–1054.

143. Seltzer Z, Tal M, Sharav Y. Autotomy behavior in rats following peripheral deafferentation is suppressed by daily injections of amitriptyline, diazepam and saline. *Pain* 1989;37(2):245–250.

144. Bräu ME, Dreimann M, Olschewski A, et al. Effect of drugs used for neuropathic pain management on tetrodotoxin-resistant Na⁺ currents in rat sensory neurons. *Anesthesiology* 2001;94(1):137–144.

145. Wallace MS, Barger D, Schulteis G. The effect of chronic oral desipramine on capsaicin-induced allodynia and hyperalgesia: a double-blinded, placebo-controlled, crossover study. *Anesth Analg* 2002;95(4):973–978.

146. Hummel T, Hummel C, Friedel I, et al. A comparison of the antinociceptive effects of imipramine, tramadol and anpirtoline. *Br J Clin Pharmacol* 1994;37(4):325–333.

147. Bowsher D. The effects of pre-emptive treatment of postherpetic neuralgia with amitriptyline: a randomized, double-blind, placebo-controlled trial. *J Pain Symptom Manage* 1997;13(6):327–331.

148. Levine JD, Gordon NC, Smith R, et al. Desipramine enhances opiate postoperative analgesia. *Pain* 1986;27(1):45–49.

149. Max MB, Zeigler D, Shoaf SE, et al. Effects of a single oral dose of desipramine on postoperative morphine analgesia. *J Pain Symptom Manage* 1992;7(8):454–462.

150. Wong K, Phelan R, Kalso E, et al. Antidepressant drugs for prevention of acute and chronic postsurgical pain: early evidence and recommended future directions. *Anesthesiology* 2014;121(3):591–608.

151. Bedin A, Caldart Bedin RA, et al. Duloxetine as an analgesic reduces opioid consumption after spine surgery: a randomized, double-blind, controlled study. *Clin J Pain* 2017;33(10):865–869.

152. Castro-Alves LJ, Oliveira de Medeiros AC, Neves SP, et al. Perioperative duloxetine to improve postoperative recovery after abdominal hysterectomy: a prospective, randomized, double-blinded, placebo-controlled study. *Anesth Analg* 2016;122(1):98–104.

153. YaDeau JT, Brummett CM, Mayman DJ, et al. Duloxetine and subacute pain after knee arthroplasty when added to a multimodal analgesic regimen: a randomized, placebo-controlled, triple-blinded trial. *Anesthesiology* 2016;125(3):561–572.

154. Amr YM, Yousef AA. Evaluation of efficacy of the perioperative administration of venlafaxine or gabapentin on acute and chronic postmastectomy pain. *Clin J Pain* 2010;26(5):381–385.

155. Semenchuk MR, Sherman S, Davis B. Double-blind, randomized trial of bupropion SR for the treatment of neuropathic pain. *Neurology* 2001; 57(9):1583–1588.

156. Macintyre PE. Safety and efficacy of patient-controlled analgesia. *Br J Anaesth* 2001;87(1):36–46.

157. Camu F, Van Aken H, Bovill JG. Postoperative analgesic effects of three demand-dose sizes of fentanyl administered by patient-controlled analgesia. *Anesth Analg* 1998;87(4):890–895.

158. Dawson PJ, Libreri FC, Jones DJ, et al. The efficacy of adding a continuous intravenous morphine infusion to patient-controlled analgesia (PCA) in abdominal surgery. *Anaesth Intensive Care* 1995;23(4):453–458.

159. Hudcova J, McNicol E, Quah C, et al. Patient controlled opioid analgesia versus conventional opioid analgesia for postoperative pain. *Cochrane Database Syst Rev* 2006;(4):CD003348.

160. Etches RC. Respiratory depression associated with patient-controlled analgesia: a review of eight cases. *Can J Anaesth* 1994;41(2):125–132.

161. Looi-Lyons LC, Chung FF, Chan VW, et al. Respiratory depression: an adverse outcome during patient controlled analgesia therapy. *J Clin Anesth* 1996;8(2):151–156.

162. Dolin SJ, Cashman JN, Bland JM. Effectiveness of acute postoperative pain management: I. Evidence from published data. *Br J Anaesth* 2002;89(3):409–423.

163. Hamber EA, Viscomi CM. Intrathecal lipophilic opioids as adjuncts to surgical spinal anesthesia. *Reg Anesth Pain Med* 1999;24(3):255–263.

164. Liu SS, Bernards CM. Exploring the epidural trail. *Reg Anesth Pain Med* 2002;27(2):122–124.

165. Liu SS, McDonald SB. Current issues in spinal anesthesia. *Anesthesiology* 2001;94(5):888–906.

166. Birnbach DJ, Johnson MD, Arcario T, et al. Effect of diluent volume on analgesia produced by epidural fentanyl. *Anesth Analg* 1989;68(6): 808–810.

167. Beattie WS, Buckley DN, Forrest JB. Epidural morphine reduces the risk of postoperative myocardial ischaemia in patients with cardiac risk factors. *Can J Anaesth* 1993;40(6):532–541.

168. Tsui SL, Law S, Fok M, et al. Postoperative analgesia reduces mortality and morbidity after esophagectomy. *Am J Surg* 1997;173(6):472–478.

169. Gambling D, Hughes T, Martin G, et al. A comparison of Depodur, a novel, single-dose extended-release epidural morphine, with standard epidural morphine for pain relief after lower abdominal surgery. *Anesth Analg* 2005;100(4):1065–1074.

170. Wheatley RG, Schug SA, Watson D. Safety and efficacy of postoperative epidural analgesia. *Br J Anaesth* 2001;87(1):47–61.

171. Block BM, Liu SS, Rowlingson AJ, et al. Efficacy of postoperative epidural analgesia: a meta-analysis. *JAMA* 2003;290(18):2455–2463.

172. de Leon-Casasola OA, Lema MJ. Postoperative epidural opioid analgesia: what are the choices? *Anesth Analg* 1996;83(4):867–875.

173. Salomaki TE, Laitinen JO, Nuutinen LS. A randomized double-blind comparison of epidural versus intravenous fentanyl infusion for analgesia after thoracotomy. *Anesthesiology* 1991;75(5):790–795.

174. Malviya S, Pandit UA, Merkel S, et al. A comparison of continuous epidural infusion and intermittent intravenous bolus doses of morphine in children undergoing selective dorsal rhizotomy. *Reg Anesth Pain Med* 1999;24(5):438–443.

175. Sitsen E, van Poorten F, van Alphen W, et al. Postoperative epidural analgesia after total knee arthroplasty with sufentanil 1 microg/ml combined with ropivacaine 0.2%, ropivacaine 0.125%, or levobupivacaine 0.125%: a randomized, double-blind comparison. *Reg Anesth Pain Med* 2007; 32(6):475–480.

176. Vercauteren M, Meert TF. Isobolographic analysis of the interaction between epidural sufentanil and bupivacaine in rats. *Pharmacol Biochem Behav* 1997;58(1):237–242.

177. Camann W, Abouleish A, Eisenach J, et al. Intrathecal sufentanil and epidural bupivacaine for labor analgesia: dose-response of individual agents and in combination. *Reg Anesth Pain Med* 1998;23(5):457–462.

178. Zaric D, Nydahl PA, Philipson L, et al. The effect of continuous lumbar epidural infusion of ropivacaine (0.1%, 0.2%, and 0.3%) and 0.25% bupivacaine on sensory and motor block in volunteers: a double-blind study. *Reg Anesth* 1996;21(1):14–25.

179. Curatolo M, Schnider TW, Petersen-Felix S, et al. A direct search procedure to optimize combinations of epidural bupivacaine, fentanyl, and clonidine for postoperative analgesia. *Anesthesiology* 2000;92(2):325–337.

180. Paech MJ, Pavy TJ, Orlikowski CE, et al. Postoperative epidural infusion: a randomized, double-blind, dose-finding trial of clonidine in combination with bupivacaine and fentanyl. *Anesth Analg* 1997;84(6): 1323–1328.

181. Niemi G, Breivik H. Adrenaline markedly improves thoracic epidural analgesia produced by a low-dose infusion of bupivacaine, fentanyl and adrenaline after major surgery. A randomised, double-blind, cross-over study with and without adrenaline. *Acta Anaesthesiol Scand* 1998;42(8): 897–909.

182. Soetens FM, Soetens MA, Vercauteren MP. Levobupivacaine-sufentanil with or without epinephrine during epidural labor analgesia. *Anesth Analg* 2006;103(1):182–186.

183. Lauretti GR, Rodrigues AM, Paccola CA, et al. The combination of epidural clonidine and S(+)-ketamine did not enhance analgesic efficacy beyond that for each individual drug in adult orthopedic surgery. *J Clin Anesth* 2005;17(2):79–84.

184. Ozyalcin NS, Yucel A, Camlica H, et al. Effect of pre-emptive ketamine on sensory changes and postoperative pain after thoracotomy: comparison of epidural and intramuscular routes. *Br J Anaesth* 2004;93(3):356–361.

185. Vranken JH, Troost D, de Haan P, et al. Severe toxic damage to the rabbit spinal cord after intrathecal administration of preservative-free S(+)-ketamine. *Anesthesiology* 2006;105(4):813–818.

186. Liu SS, Allen HW, Olsson GL. Patient-controlled epidural analgesia with bupivacaine and fentanyl on hospital wards: prospective experience with 1,030 surgical patients. *Anesthesiology* 1998;88(3):688–695.

187. Smet IG, Vercauteren MP, De Jongh RF, et al. Pressure sores as a complication of patient-controlled epidural analgesia after cesarean delivery. Case report. *Reg Anesth* 1996;21(4):338–341.

188. Liu SS, Moore JM, Luo AM, et al. Comparison of three solutions of ropivacaine/fentanyl for postoperative patient-controlled epidural analgesia. *Anesthesiology* 1999;90(3):727–733.

189. Chaney MA. Side effects of intrathecal and epidural opioids. *Can J Anaesth* 1995;42(10):891–903.

190. White MJ, Berghausen EJ, Dumont SW, et al. Side effects during continuous epidural infusion of morphine and fentanyl. *Can J Anaesth* 1992; 39(6):576–582.

191. Kelly MC, Carabine UA, Mirakhur RK. Intrathecal diamorphine for analgesia after caesarean section. A dose finding study and assessment of side-effects. *Anaesthesia* 1998;53(3):231–237.

192. Ozalp G, Guner F, Kuru N, et al. Postoperative patient-controlled epidural analgesia with opioid bupivacaine mixtures. *Can J Anaesth* 1998; 45(10):938–942.

193. Choi JH, Lee J, Choi JH, et al. Epidural naloxone reduces pruritus and nausea without affecting analgesia by epidural morphine in bupivacaine. *Can J Anaesth* 2000;47(1):33–37.

194. Moscovici R, Prego G, Schwartz M, et al. Epidural scopolamine administration in preventing nausea after epidural morphine. *J Clin Anesth* 1995; 7(6):474–476.

195. Kjellberg F, Tramer MR. Pharmacological control of opioid-induced pruritus: a quantitative systematic review of randomized trials. *Eur J Anaesthesiol* 2001;18(6):346–357.

196. Johanek LM, Meyer RA, Hartke T, et al. Psychophysical and physiological evidence for parallel afferent pathways mediating the sensation of itch. *J Neurosci* 2007;27(28):7490–7497.

197. Ko MC, Naughton NN. An experimental itch model in monkeys: characterization of intrathecal morphine-induced scratching and antinociception. *Anesthesiology* 2000;92(3):795–805.

198. Macario A, Scibetta WC, Navarro J, et al. Analgesia for labor pain: a cost model. *Anesthesiology* 2000;92(3):841–850.

199. de Leon-Casasola OA, Parker BM, Lema MJ, et al. Epidural analgesia versus intravenous patient-controlled analgesia. Differences in the postoperative course of cancer patients. *Reg Anesth* 1994;19(5):307–315.

200. Rygnestad T, Borchgrevink PC, Eide E. Postoperative epidural infusion of morphine and bupivacaine is safe on surgical wards. Organisation of the treatment, effects and side-effects in 2000 consecutive patients. *Acta Anaesthesiol Scand* 1997;41(7):868–876.

201. Katsiris S, Williams S, Leighton BL, et al. Respiratory arrest following intrathecal injection of sufentanil and bupivacaine in a parturient. *Can J Anaesth* 1998;45(9):880–883.

202. Mulroy MF. Monitoring opioids. *Reg Anesth* 1996;21(6 suppl):89–93.

203. Wang JJ, Ho ST, Tzeng JI. Comparison of intravenous nalbuphine infusion versus naloxone in the prevention of epidural morphine-related side effects. *Reg Anesth Pain Med* 1998;23(5):479–484.

204. Curatolo M, Petersen-Felix S, Scaramozzino P, et al. Epidural fentanyl, adrenaline and clonidine as adjuvants to local anaesthetics for surgical analgesia: meta-analyses of analgesia and side-effects. *Acta Anaesthesiol Scand* 1998;42(8):910–920.

205. Turner G, Blake D, Buckland M, et al. Continuous extradural infusion of ropivacaine for prevention of postoperative pain after major orthopaedic surgery. *Br J Anaesth* 1996;76(5):606–610.

206. Sia AT, Chong JL. Epidural 0.2% ropivacaine for labour analgesia: parturient-controlled or continuous infusion? *Anaesth Intensive Care* 1999;27(2):154–158.

207. Wigfull J, Welchew E. Survey of 1057 patients receiving postoperative patient-controlled epidural analgesia. *Anaesthesia* 2001;56(1):70–75.

208. Burstal R, Wegener F, Hayes C, et al. Epidural analgesia: prospective audit of 1062 patients. *Anaesth Intensive Care* 1998;26(2):165–172.

209. Komatsu H, Matsumoto S, Mitsuhata H. Comparison of patient-controlled epidural analgesia with and without night-time infusion following gastrectomy. *Br J Anaesth* 2001;87(4):633–635.

210. Rodgers A, Walker N, Schug S, et al. Reduction of postoperative mortality and morbidity with epidural or spinal anaesthesia: results from overview of randomised trials. *BMJ* 2000;321(7275):1493.

211. Wu CL, Hurley RW, Anderson GF, et al. Effect of postoperative epidural analgesia on morbidity and mortality following surgery in medicare patients. *Reg Anesth Pain Med* 2004;29(6):525–533.

212. Holte K, Kehlet H. Epidural analgesia and risk of anastomotic leakage. *Reg Anesth Pain Med* 2001;26(2):111–117.

213. Popping DM, Elia N, Van Aken HK, et al. Impact of epidural analgesia on mortality and morbidity after surgery: systematic review and meta-analysis of randomized controlled trials. *Ann Surg* 2014;259(6):1056–1067.

214. Horlocker TT, Wedel DJ, Rowlingson JC, et al. Regional anesthesia in the patient receiving antithrombotic or thrombolytic therapy: American Society of Regional Anesthesia and Pain Medicine Evidence-Based Guidelines (Third Edition). *Reg Anesth Pain Med* 2010;35(1):64–101.

215. American Society of Regional Anesthesia and Pain Medicine. Anticoagulation 3rd edition—interim updates. Available at: https://www.asra.com/advisory-guidelines/article/1/anticoagulation-3rd-edition. Accessed April 4, 2017.

216. Deer TR, Narouze S, Provenzano DA, et al. The Neurostimulation Appropriateness Consensus Committee (NACC): recommendations on bleeding and coagulation management in neurostimulation devices. *Neuromodulation* 2017;20(1):51–62.

217. Moen V, Dahlgren N, Irestedt L. Severe neurological complications after central neuraxial blockades in Sweden 1990-1999. *Anesthesiology* 2004;101(4):950–959.

218. Christie IW, McCabe S. Major complications of epidural analgesia after surgery: results of a six-year survey. *Anaesthesia* 2007;62(4):335–341.

219. Simpson RS, Macintyre PE, Shaw D, et al. Epidural catheter tip cultures: results of a 4-year audit and implications for clinical practice. *Reg Anesth Pain Med* 2000;25(4):360–367.

220. Wang H, Boctor B, Verner J. The effect of single-injection femoral nerve block on rehabilitation and length of hospital stay after total knee replacement. *Reg Anesth Pain Med* 2002;27(2):139–144.

221. Liu SS, Salinas FV. Continuous plexus and peripheral nerve blocks for postoperative analgesia. *Anesth Analg* 2003;96(1):263–272.

222. Karmakar MK. Thoracic paravertebral block. *Anesthesiology* 2001;95(3): 771–780.

223. Kaiser AM, Zollinger A, De Lorenzi D, et al. Prospective, randomized comparison of extrapleural versus epidural analgesia for postthoracotomy pain. *Ann Thorac Surg* 1998;66(2):367–372.

224. Pettersson N, Perbeck L, Brismar B, et al. Sensory and sympathetic block during interpleural analgesia. *Reg Anesth* 1997;22(4):313–317.

225. Shanti CM, Carlin AM, Tyburski JG. Incidence of pneumothorax from intercostal nerve block for analgesia in rib fractures. *J Trauma* 2001;51(3):536–539.

226. Miguel R, Hubbell D. Pain management and spirometry following thoracotomy: a prospective, randomized study of four techniques. *J Cardiothorac Vasc Anesth* 1993;7(5):529–534.

227. Kalso E, Smith L, McQuay HJ, et al. No pain, no gain: clinical excellence and scientific rigour—lessons learned from IA morphine. *Pain* 2002; 98(3):269–275.

228. Møiniche S, Mikkelsen S, Wetterslev J, et al. A systematic review of intra-articular local anesthesia for postoperative pain relief after arthroscopic knee surgery. *Reg Anesth Pain Med* 1999;24(5):430–437.

229. Amundson AW, Johnson RL, Abdel MP, et al. A three-arm randomized clinical trial comparing continuous femoral plus single-injection sciatic peripheral nerve blocks versus periarticular injection with ropivacaine or liposomal bupivacaine for patients undergoing total knee arthroplasty. *Anesthesiology* 2017;126:1139–1150.

230. Schroer WC, Diesfeld PG, LeMarr AR, et al. Does extended-release liposomal bupivacaine better control pain than bupivacaine after total knee arthroplasty (TKA)? A prospective, randomized clinical trial. *J Arthroplasty* 2015;30(9 suppl):64–67.

231. Lv L, Shao YF, Zhou YB. The enhanced recovery after surgery (ERAS) pathway for patients undergoing colorectal surgery: an update of meta-analysis of randomized controlled trials. *Int J Colorectal Dis* 2012;27(12): 1549–1554.

232. Gustafsson UO, Oppelstrup H, Thorell A, et al. Adherence to the ERAS protocol is associated with 5-year survival after colorectal cancer surgery: a retrospective cohort study. *World J Surg* 2016;40(7):1741–1747.

233. Tyson MD, Chang SS. Enhanced recovery pathways versus standard care after cystectomy: a meta-analysis of the effect on perioperative outcomes. *Eur Urol* 2016;70(6):995–1003.

234. Xiong J, Szatmary P, Huang W, et al. Enhanced recovery after surgery program in patients undergoing pancreaticoduodenectomy: a prisma-compliant systematic review and meta-analysis. *Medicine (Baltimore)* 2016; 95(18):e3497.

235. Song W, Wang K, Zhang RJ, et al. The enhanced recovery after surgery (ERAS) program in liver surgery: a meta-analysis of randomized controlled trials. *Springerplus* 2016;5:207.

236. Kehlet H. Multimodal approach to control postoperative pathophysiology and rehabilitation. *Br J Anaesth* 1997;78(5):606–617.

237. Wedmore IS, Johnson T, Czarnik J, et al. Pain management in the wilderness and operational setting. *Emerg Med Clin North Am* 2005;23(2):585–601, xi–xii.

238. Nakahura T, Griswold W, Lemire J, et al. Nonsteroidal anti-inflammatory drug use in adolescence. *J Adolesc Health* 1998;23(5):307–310.

239. Towheed TE, Judd MJ, Hochberg MC, et al. Acetaminophen for osteoarthritis. *Cochrane Database Syst Rev* 2003;(2):CD004257.

240. Streisand JB, Varvel JR, Stanski DR, et al. Absorption and bioavailability of oral transmucosal fentanyl citrate. *Anesthesiology* 1991;75(2):223–229.

241. Egan TD, Sharma A, Ashburn MA, et al. Multiple dose pharmacokinetics of oral transmucosal fentanyl citrate in healthy volunteers. *Anesthesiology* 2000;92(3):665–673.

242. Kharasch ED, Hoffer C, Whittington D. Influence of age on the pharmacokinetics and pharmacodynamics of oral transmucosal fentanyl citrate. *Anesthesiology* 2004;101(3):738–743.

243. Wedmore IS, Kotwal RS, McManus JG, et al. Safety and efficacy of oral transmucosal fentanyl citrate for prehospital pain control on the battlefield. *J Trauma Acute Care Surg* 2012;73(6)(suppl 5):S490–S495.

244. Buckenmaier CC III, Auton AA, Flournoy WS. Continuous peripheral nerve block catheter tip adhesion in a rat model. *Acta Anaesthesiol Scand* 2006;50(6):694–698.

245. Buckenmaier CC III, Shields CH, Auton AA, et al. Continuous peripheral nerve block in combat casualties receiving low-molecular weight heparin. *Br J Anaesth* 2006;97(6):874–877.

246. Buckenmaier C III, Mahoney PF, Anton T, et al. Impact of an acute pain service on pain outcomes with combat-injured soldiers at Camp Bastion, Afghanistan. *Pain Med* 2012;13(7):919–926.

247. Twersky R, Fishman D, Homel P. What happens after discharge? Return hospital visits after ambulatory surgery. *Anesth Analg* 1997;84(2):319–324.

248. Wu CL, Berenholtz SM, Pronovost PJ, et al. Systematic review and analysis of postdischarge symptoms after outpatient surgery. *Anesthesiology* 2002;96(4):994–1003.

249. Wu CL, Raja SN. Optimizing postoperative analgesia: the use of global outcome measures. *Anesthesiology* 2002;97(3):533–534.

250. Hendolin HI, Paakonen ME, Alhava EM, et al. Laparoscopic or open cholecystectomy: a prospective randomised trial to compare postoperative pain, pulmonary function, and stress response. *Eur J Surg* 2000;166(5):394–399.

251. Chung F, Mezei G, Tong D. Adverse events in ambulatory surgery. A comparison between elderly and younger patients. *Can J Anaesth* 1999;46(4):309–321.

252. Romsing J, Møiniche S, Dahl JB. Rectal and parenteral paracetamol, and paracetamol in combination with NSAIDs, for postoperative analgesia. *Br J Anaesth* 2002;88(2):215–226.

253. Lariviere M, Goffaux P, Marchand S, et al. Changes in pain perception and descending inhibitory controls start at middle age in healthy adults. *Clin J Pain* 2007;23(6):506–510.

254. Rolke R, Baron R, Maier C, et al. Quantitative sensory testing in the German Research Network on Neuropathic Pain (DFNS): standardized protocol and reference values. *Pain* 2006;123(3):231–243.

255. Gibson SJ, Helme RD. Age-related differences in pain perception and report. *Clin Geriatr Med* 2001;17(3):433–456, v–vi.

256. Gregoratos G. Clinical manifestations of acute myocardial infarction in older patients. *Am J Geriatr Cardiol* 2001;10(6):345–347.

257. Gloth FM III. Geriatric pain. Factors that limit pain relief and increase complications. *Geriatrics* 2000;55(10):46–48, 51–44.

258. Macintyre PE, Jarvis DA. Age is the best predictor of postoperative morphine requirements. *Pain* 1996;64(2):357–364.

259. Gagliese L, Jackson M, Ritvo P, et al. Age is not an impediment to effective use of patient-controlled analgesia by surgical patients. *Anesthesiology* 2000;93(3):601–610.

260. Marcantonio ER, Flacker JM, Michaels M, et al. Delirium is independently associated with poor functional recovery after hip fracture. *J Am Geriatr Soc* 2000;48(6):618–624.

261. Placker JM, Lipsitz LA. Neural mechanisms of delirium: current hypotheses and evolving concepts. *J Gerontol A Biol Sci Med Sci* 1999;54(6):B239–B246.

262. Flacker JM, Lipsitz LA. Serum anticholinergic activity changes with acute illness in elderly medical patients. *J Gerontol A Biol Sci Med Sci* 1999;54(1):M12–M16.

263. Schor JD, Levkoff SE, Lipsitz LA, et al. Risk factors for delirium in hospitalized elderly. *JAMA* 1992;267(6):827–831.

264. Lynch EP, Lazor MA, Gellis JE, et al. The impact of postoperative pain on the development of postoperative delirium. *Anesth Analg* 1998;86(4):781–785.

265. Aronoff GM. Medical treatment of opiate addiction. *JAMA* 2000;283(22):2931–2932.

266. Savage SR. Long-term opioid therapy: assessment of consequences and risks. *J Pain Symptom Manage* 1996;11(5):274–286.

267. Rapp SE, Ready LB, Nessly ML. Acute pain management in patients with prior opioid consumption: a case-controlled retrospective review. *Pain* 1995;61(2):195–201.

268. Anderson R, Saiers JH, Abram S, et al. Accuracy in equianalgesic dosing. conversion dilemmas. *J Pain Symptom Manage* 2001;21(5):397–406.

269. Woodhouse A, Ward ME, Mather LE. Intra-subject variability in postoperative patient-controlled analgesia (PCA): is the patient equally satisfied with morphine, pethidine and fentanyl? *Pain* 1999;80(3):545–553.

270. de Leon-Casasola OA, Myers DP, Donaparthi S, et al. A comparison of postoperative epidural analgesia between patients with chronic cancer taking high doses of oral opioids versus opioid-naive patients. *Anesth Analg* 1993;76(2):302–307.

271. Benumof JL. Obstructive sleep apnea in the adult obese patient: implications for airway management. *J Clin Anesth* 2001;13(2):144–156.

272. Rawal N, Sjostrand U, Christoffersson E, et al. Comparison of intramuscular and epidural morphine for postoperative analgesia in the grossly obese: influence on postoperative ambulation and pulmonary function. *Anesth Analg* 1984;63(6):583–592.

273. Flegal KM, Carroll MD, Kuczmarski RJ, et al. Overweight and obesity in the United States: prevalence and trends, 1960-1994. *Int J Obes Relat Metab Disord* 1998;22(1):39–47.

274. Findley LJ, Barth JT, Powers DC, et al. Cognitive impairment in patients with obstructive sleep apnea and associated hypoxemia. *Chest* 1986;90(5):686–690.

275. Roux F, D'Ambrosio C, Mohsenin V. Sleep-related breathing disorders and cardiovascular disease. *Am J Med* 2000;108(5):396–402.

276. Cullen DJ. Obstructive sleep apnea and postoperative analgesia—a potentially dangerous combination. *J Clin Anesth* 2001;13(2):83–85.

277. Garpestad E, Katayama H, Parker JA, et al. Stroke volume and cardiac output decrease at termination of obstructive apneas. *J Appl Physiol (1985)* 1992;73(5):1743–1748.

278. Gross JB, Bachenberg KL, Benumof JL, et al. Practice guidelines for the perioperative management of patients with obstructive sleep apnea: a report by the American Society of Anesthesiologists Task Force on Perioperative Management of patients with obstructive sleep apnea. *Anesthesiology* 2006;104(5):1081–1093, 1117–1118.

279. Wizemann TM, Pardue ML, eds. *Exploring the Biological Contributions to Human Health: Does Sex Matter?* Washington, DC: National Academies Press; 2001.

280. Bingefors K, Isacson D. Epidemiology, co-morbidity, and impact on health-related quality of life of self-reported headache and musculoskeletal pain—a gender perspective. *Eur J Pain* 2004;8(5):435–450.

281. Isacson D, Bingefors K. Epidemiology of analgesic use: a gender perspective. *Eur J Anaesthesiol Suppl* 2002;26:5–15.

282. Myers CD, Riley JL III, Robinson ME. Psychosocial contributions to sex-correlated differences in pain. *Clin J Pain* 2003;19(4):225–232.

283. Riley JL III, Robinson ME, Wise EA, et al. Sex differences in the perception of noxious experimental stimuli: a meta-analysis. *Pain* 1998;74(2–3):181–187.

284. Paulson PE, Minoshima S, Morrow TJ, et al. Gender differences in pain perception and patterns of cerebral activation during noxious heat stimulation in humans. *Pain* 1998;76(1–2):223–229.

285. Pickering G, Jourdan D, Eschalier A, et al. Impact of age, gender and cognitive functioning on pain perception. *Gerontology* 2002;48(2):112–118.

286. Pool GJ, Schwegler AF, Theodore BR, et al. Role of gender norms and group identification on hypothetical and experimental pain tolerance. *Pain* 2007;129(1–2):122–129.

287. Derbyshire SW, Nichols TE, Firestone L, et al. Gender differences in patterns of cerebral activation during equal experience of painful laser stimulation. *J Pain* 2002;3(5):401–411.

288. Moulton EA, Keaser ML, Gullapalli RP, et al. Sex differences in the cerebral BOLD signal response to painful heat stimuli. *Am J Physiol Regul Integr Comp Physiol* 2006;291(2):R257–R267.

289. Berman SM, Naliboff BD, Suyenobu B, et al. Sex differences in regional brain response to aversive pelvic visceral stimuli. *Am J Physiol Regul Integr Comp Physiol* 2006;291(2):R268–R276.

290. Naliboff BD, Berman S, Chang L, et al. Sex-related differences in IBS patients: central processing of visceral stimuli. *Gastroenterology* 2003;124(7):1738–1747.

291. Fillingim RB, Ness TJ, Glover TL, et al. Morphine responses and experimental pain: sex differences in side effects and cardiovascular responses but not analgesia. *J Pain* 2005;6(2):116–124.

292. Romberg R, Olofsen E, Sarton E, et al. Pharmacokinetic-pharmacodynamic modeling of morphine-6-glucuronide-induced analgesia in healthy volunteers: absence of sex differences. *Anesthesiology* 2004;100(1):120–133.

293. Wasan AD, Davar G, Jamison R. The association between negative affect and opioid analgesia in patients with discogenic low back pain. *Pain* 2005;117(3):450–461.

294. Pud D, Yarnitsky D, Sprecher E, et al. Can personality traits and gender predict the response to morphine? An experimental cold pain study. *Eur J Pain* 2006;10(2):103–112.

295. Sarton E, Olofsen E, Romberg R, et al. Sex differences in morphine analgesia: an experimental study in healthy volunteers. *Anesthesiology* 2000;93(5):1245–1254.

296. Zacny JP. Characterizing the subjective, psychomotor, and physiological effects of a hydrocodone combination product (Hycodan) in non-drug-abusing volunteers. *Psychopharmacology (Berl)* 2003;165(2):146–156.

297. Murthy BR, Pollack GM, Brouwer KL. Contribution of morphine-6-glucuronide to antinociception following intravenous administration of morphine to healthy volunteers. *J Clin Pharmacol* 2002;42(5):569–576.

298. Olofsen E, Romberg R, Bijl H, et al. Alfentanil and placebo analgesia: no sex differences detected in models of experimental pain. *Anesthesiology* 2005;103(1):130–139.

299. Gear RW, Gordon NC, Heller PH, et al. Gender difference in analgesic response to the kappa-opioid pentazocine. *Neurosci Lett* 1996;205(3):207–209.

300. Gear RW, Miaskowski C, Gordon NC, et al. Kappa-opioids produce significantly greater analgesia in women than in men. *Nat Med* 1996;2(11):1248–1250.

301. Gordon NC, Gear RW, Heller PH, et al. Enhancement of morphine analgesia by the GABAB agonist baclofen. *Neuroscience* 1995;69(2):345–349.

302. Fillingim RB, Gear RW. Sex differences in opioid analgesia: clinical and experimental findings. *Eur J Pain* 2004;8(5):413–425.

303. Mogil JS, Wilson SG, Chesler EJ, et al. The melanocortin-1 receptor gene mediates female-specific mechanisms of analgesia in mice and humans. *Proc Natl Acad Sci U S A* 2003;100(8):4867–4872.

304. Rawal N. 10 years of acute pain services—achievements and challenges. *Reg Anesth Pain Med* 1999;24(1):68–73.

305. Bardiau FM, Braeckman MM, Seidel L, et al. Effectiveness of an acute pain service inception in a general hospital. *J Clin Anesth* 1999;11(7):583–589.

306. Merry A, Judge MA, Ready B. Acute pain services in New Zealand hospitals; a survey. *N Z Med J* 1997;110(1046):233–235.

307. Carr DB, Miaskowski C, Dedrick SC, et al. Management of perioperative pain in hospitalized patients: a national survey. *J Clin Anesth* 1998;10(1):77–85.

308. Lee A, Chan S, Chen PP, et al. Economic evaluations of acute pain service programs: a systematic review. *Clin J Pain* 2007;23(8):726–733.

309. Kehlet H, Jensen TS, Woolf CJ. Persistent postsurgical pain: risk factors and prevention. *Lancet* 2006;367(9522):1618–1625.

310. Macrae WA. Chronic pain after surgery. *Br J Anaesth* 2001;87(1):88–98.

311. Carr DB, Goudas LC. Acute pain. *Lancet* 1999;353(9169):2051–2058.

312. Capdevila X, Barthelet Y, Biboulet P, et al. Effects of perioperative analgesic technique on the surgical outcome and duration of rehabilitation after major knee surgery. *Anesthesiology* 1999;91(1):8–15.

313. Lavand'homme P, De Kock M. The use of intraoperative epidural or spinal analgesia modulates postoperative hyperalgesia and reduces residual pain after major abdominal surgery. *Acta Anaesthesiol Belg* 2006;57(4):373–379.

314. Poleshuck EL, Katz J, Andrus CH, et al. Risk factors for chronic pain following breast cancer surgery: a prospective study. *J Pain* 2006;7(9):626–634.

315. Carli F, Mayo N, Klubien K, et al. Epidural analgesia enhances functional exercise capacity and health-related quality of life after colonic surgery: results of a randomized trial. *Anesthesiology* 2002;97(3):540–549.

316. Sun EC, Darnall BD, Baker LC, et al. Incidence of and risk factors for chronic opioid use among opioid-naive patients in the postoperative period. *JAMA Intern Med* 2016;176(9):1286–1293.

317. Soneji N, Clarke HA, Ko DT, et al. Risks of developing persistent opioid use after major surgery. *JAMA Surg* 2016;151(11):1083–1084.

318. Anderson JT, Haas AR, Percy R, et al. Chronic opioid therapy after lumbar fusion surgery for degenerative disc disease in a workers' compensation setting. *Spine (Phila Pa 1976)* 2015;40(22):1775–1784.

319. Al Dabbagh Z, Jansson KA, Stiller CO, et al. Long-term pattern of opioid prescriptions after femoral shaft fractures. *Acta Anaesthesiol Scand* 2016;60(5):634–641.

320. Carroll I, Barelka P, Wang CK, et al. A pilot cohort study of the determinants of longitudinal opioid use after surgery. *Anesth Analg* 2012;115(3):694–702.

321. Goesling J, Moser SE, Zaidi B, et al. Trends and predictors of opioid use after total knee and total hip arthroplasty. *Pain* 2016;157(6):1259–1265.

322. Clarke H, Soneji N, Ko DT, et al. Rates and risk factors for prolonged opioid use after major surgery: population based cohort study. *BMJ* 2014;348:g1251.

CHAPTER 52

Regional Anesthesia Techniques for Acute Pain Management

MARIE N. HANNA, JEAN-PIERRE P. OUANES, and **VICENTE GARCIA TOMAS**

Acute pain management has become a focus of the health care system and an important ethical responsibility of the medical profession. Although opioids have been the primary analgesic agents used for treating moderate and severe pain after surgery for past few decades, aggressive multimodal analgesic interventions utilizing primary a combination of nonopioid analgesic agents and techniques have become widely used during the perioperative period. Maximum benefit occurs when pain interventions are extended into the postoperative phase.[1]

Multimodal analgesia involves the administration of different agents that exert their effects via different analgesic mechanisms and act synergistically at different sites in the nervous system, thereby providing superior analgesia with fewer side effects. Multimodal analgesia can include regional analgesia with local anesthetics, acetaminophen, nonsteroidal anti-inflammatory drugs (NSAIDs), and opioids.[2]

Perioperative neuraxial and peripheral analgesia provide superior analgesia than do that from systemic opioids. Continuous analgesic techniques have the advantage of decreasing adverse perioperative pathophysiology and improving patient outcomes, including major morbidity.[3,4] This chapter focuses on regional anesthesia techniques, including central neuraxial, truncal, and peripheral perineural analgesia, for acute postoperative pain management. Indications, techniques, mechanisms of action, side effects, and complications are described.

Continuous Epidural Analgesia

THORACIC EPIDURAL ANALGESIA

Thoracic epidural analgesia (TEA) is commonly used for the treatment of pain after upper abdominal/thoracic procedures and rib fractures. TEA is often used intraoperatively as an adjunct to general anesthesia and in the postoperative period for many upper abdominal and thoracic procedures (Table 52.1). Its use in video-assisted thoracic surgery and laparoscopic procedures is less common and may be recommended only for high-risk patients. The use of TEA offers superior analgesia compared with that from systemic opioids.[5] Postoperative use of continuous epidural analgesia is associated with improved patient morbidity as it is associated with decreases in pulmonary,[6–9] cardiovascular,[6,7,9,10] and gastrointestinal[11,12] complications in high-risk patients and after high-risk procedures. It also may improve outcomes in patients with multiple rib fractures.[13]

Many factors affect the overall outcomes of continuous epidural analgesia. Among them are the congruency of epidural catheter location and surgical incision, the type of analgesic regimen used, and whether the epidural is used as part of a multimodal approach.[14,15] When compared with the systemic administration of opioids, local anesthetic-based epidural regimens provide superior analgesia and may decrease opioid-related side effects; epidural infusion of opioids alone may be used to avoid hypotension when sympathetic blockade is a concern.

The role of high TEA in cardiac surgery with cardiopulmonary bypass and in off-pump coronary artery bypass surgery remains controversial. It might improve distribution of coronary blood flow,[16] reduce the incidence of supraventricular tachycardia,[17] and decrease surgical stress response.[18] Some studies found no difference in the rates of mortality and myocardial infarction when compared with those of traditional opioids,[6] but others showed significant reduction in postoperative pulmonary and cardiac arrhythmias while improving pain scores, especially with off-pump procedures.[19]

A recent randomized control study of 600 patients undergoing elective cardiac surgery both on and off pump[20] reported no difference in 30-day mortality and morbidity, no difference in intensive care unit (ICU) stay or length of hospital stay, and no difference in quality of life at 30-day follow-up. Until there are more conclusive outcome data, the role of TEA remains controversial.

BLOCK TECHNIQUE: EPIDURAL

Epidural blockade may be performed with the patient in the sitting or lateral position through a midline or paramedian approach. With the midline approach, the epidural needle is oriented in the same plane as the spinous processes, with slight cephalad orientation toward the interlaminar space. After subcutaneous injection of local anesthetic at the needle insertion site, the epidural needle is directed through the skin wheal from the local anesthetic and slowly advanced through the supraspinous and interspinous ligaments to enter the ligamentum flavum. The practitioner inserts a syringe containing air or saline which may include a small air bubble. Upon entering the epidural space, the practitioner will feel a sudden, significant loss of resistance to plunger displacement. A 20-gauge radiopaque catheter with 1-cm graduation is passed through the epidural needle. The catheter is generally advanced 3 to 5 cm beyond the needle tip into the epidural space. The needle is then withdrawn over the catheter and the catheter secured to the patient's back. After a test dose of 3 mL of a local anesthetic

TABLE 52.1	Procedures Commonly Appropriate for Thoracic Epidural Analgesia		
Thoracic Procedures	**Upper Abdominal Procedures**	**Lower Abdominal Procedures (GI)**	**Lower Abdominal Procedures**
Thoracotomy	Gastrectomy	Bowel resection	Nephrectomy
Lobectomy	Esophagectomy	Colectomy	Cystectomy
Thymectomy	Pancreatectomy	Abdominal aortic aneurysm repair	Abdominal prostatectomy
Thoracic aortic aneurysm repair	Cholecystectomy	Exploratory laparotomy	Abdominal hysterectomy
Pectus repair	Liver resection		Pelvic exenteration
VATS			

GI, gastrointestinal; VATS, video-assisted thoracic surgery.

with 1:200,000 epinephrine is injected, the patient is observed for signs and symptoms of intrathecal (IT) or intravascular injection. The local anesthetic should be administered in 3- to 5-mL increments, ideally with intermittent aspiration to assess for accidental IT or intravascular placement, until the appropriate total dose is given.

Alternatively, a paramedian-lateral or paramedian-lateral oblique approach to the epidural space may be used. For this approach, the epidural needle insertion site is approximately one fingerbreadth lateral to the insertion site of the midline approach. The epidural needle is directed with slight cephalomedial orientation to allow the needle to bypass the supraspinous and interspinous ligaments as it is advanced to enter the triangular-shaped ligamentum flavum. Once the needle enters the ligamentum flavum, the loss-of-resistance technique is used to enter the epidural space at the midline. Although the paramedian approach may be used for both lumbar and thoracic epidurals, it is extremely advantageous in the midthoracic vertebrae (T4–T10) where the steep angle of the spinous processes limits midline access to the interlaminar foramen.

Postoperative epidural analgesia may be delivered as a fixed continuous infusion or as patient-controlled epidural analgesia (PCEA). Based on the principles of patient-controlled analgesia (PCA), PCEA allows individualization of postoperative analgesic requirements, reduces drug use, improves patient satisfaction, and provides superior analgesia.[21,22] The drug chosen for epidural analgesia is usually a local anesthetic with a long duration of action. It should exhibit preferential clinical sensory blockade and cause only minimal impairment of motor function.[23] A lipophilic opioid (e.g., fentanyl or sufentanil) or hydrophilic opioid (e.g., morphine or hydromorphone) may be added for postoperative analgesia to allow relatively rapid titration of analgesia and densening of the block.[24] Even though clonidine and epinephrine are potentially useful adjuvants, neither is widely used clinically in adults. Clonidine may enhance postoperative analgesia by activating the descending noradrenergic pathway; however, its clinical usefulness is typically limited by the presence of hypotension, bradycardia, and sedation.[25,26] Epinephrine has been shown to improve epidural analgesia and increase sensory block in the postoperative setting.[27]

Subarachnoid/Intrathecal Analgesia

Spinal analgesia may offer postoperative analgesia through additives like IT opioids for multiple procedures, including obstetric and gynecologic procedures; genitourinary procedures; orthopedic procedures of the lower extremity; and abdominal, vascular, spine, thoracic, and cardiac surgery. IT additives, including fentanyl, sufentanil, morphine, hydromorphone, and clonidine are discussed in the following text.

TECHNIQUE

Subarachnoid block may be performed with the patient in the sitting, lateral, or prone position through a midline or paramedian approach. After the patient is positioned, the appropriate interspace is identified, prepped, and draped in sterile fashion. Local anesthetic is infiltrated at the needle insertion site. The introducer needle is placed midline and advanced in the midline plane with slight cephalad angulation through the supraspinous ligament and into the interspinous ligament. The depth to the subarachnoid space must be anticipated to avoid inadvertent dural puncture with the introducer needle in thin patients. The spinal needle is then advanced through the introducer while the introducer is stabilized with the nondominant hand. As the needle passes through the ligamentum flavum, an increase in resistance is appreciated, followed by a loss of resistance, with a characteristic "pop" indicating penetration of the dura and entry into the subarachnoid space. The spinal needle stylet is

removed, and free cerebrospinal fluid (CSF) flow is confirmed through the needle. If free CSF flow is not visualized, the hub of the needle may be rotated 90 degrees, followed by slight advancement of the needle if necessary. If CSF free flow is unable to be confirmed, the needle is slowly withdrawn in slight increments, with 90-degree rotation at each increment to allow for free CSF flow. Upon obtaining free flow of CSF, the dorsal aspect of the nondominant hand is firmly placed against the patient's back with the index finger and thumb stabilizing the spinal needle hub for injection. The syringe with local anesthetic and additive is attached to the spinal needle hub and injected with the dominant hand. If redirection of the spinal needle is necessary secondary to bone contact, paresthesia, or failure to obtain CSF, the anatomy should be reevaluated and the introducer repositioned as necessary at the same or a new level. If a paresthesia is encountered at any time, needle advancement or injection should be stopped and resolution of paresthesia confirmed before and during subsequent advancement and or injection.

The paramedian-lateral and paramedian-lateral oblique approaches offer alternatives to the midline approach in patients with narrow interspinous spaces for both subarachnoid and epidural blocks. For the paramedian-lateral approach, the spinal introducer insertion site is approximately one fingerbreadth lateral to the insertion site of the midline approach. The introducer is oriented with slight medial and cephalad direction to allow the spinal needle to bypass the supraspinous and interspinous ligaments, pass through the triangular-shaped ligamentum flavum, and enter the subarachnoid space at the midline.

In the paramedian-lateral oblique approach, the caudad spinous process of the desired interspace is identified. The needle is inserted approximately one fingerbreadth lateral to this point and directed with cephalomedial orientation to bypass the supraspinous and interspinous ligaments, pass through the triangular-shaped ligamentum flavum, and enter the subarachnoid space at the midline. Alternatively, the needle is initially oriented perpendicular to the skin in all planes and advanced with the intent to contact lamina. Upon contact with lamina, the needle is walked off the superior edge of the lamina and advanced through the ligamentum flavum to enter the subarachnoid space.

CLINICAL SUBARACHNOID ANALGESIA
Opioids

Highly lipophilic, short-acting opioids, such as fentanyl, can be added to local anesthetics to improve short-term analgesia for inpatient or outpatient procedures.[28–30] The addition of 10 μg fentanyl to bupivacaine 0.5% (hyperbaric) significantly improves the quality and duration of analgesia, with no further advantage occurring if the dose is increased up to 40 μg.[31] Hydrophilic opioids, however, provide extended postoperative analgesia in the inpatient setting. Data from two meta-analyses that investigated the use of IT morphine in surgical patients suggest that use of IT morphine (0.05 to 0.2 mg) for surgical procedures will decrease pain scores and systemic opioid requirement after surgery.[32,33] Dose–response trials have shown that low doses of hydrophilic opioids maximize postoperative analgesia with a lower incidence of side effects. For example, Cole et al.[34] reported that 0.3 mg of IT morphine significantly reduces pain and PCA requirements compared to those of placebo after knee arthroplasty, with no significant difference in hypoxemia and apnea between groups. For opioid-tolerant patients, higher doses are probably acceptable, whereas doses of less than 0.3 mg may be ideal for opioid-naive individuals.[35] IT opioids have been used for cardiac surgery with improved analgesia; however, concerns with bleeding complications in patients who are receiving heparin and demonstrations of prolonged extubation times may have limited their use. Alhashemi et al.[36] showed that 250 µg is the optimal dose of IT morphine to provide significant post-operative analgesia without delaying tracheal extubation after coronary artery bypass graft surgery. IT opioid combinations provide better analgesia than systemic opioids in patients undergoing vascular and thoracic procedures. Compared to those who received intravenous (IV) PCA morphine, patients who received a mixture of either 20 µg of sufentanil with 0.2 mg of morphine, or 50 µg of sufentanil with 0.5 mg of morphine, have improved pain control with minimal side effects other than an increased frequency of urinary retention.[9,37] Although epidural analgesia with local anesthetics and opioids is likely superior to IT opioids in decreasing pulmonary complications after thoracotomy,[38] IT opioids may be a good alternative to epidural analgesia when an epidural catheter cannot be used.

Clonidine

Studies have shown that IT clonidine at doses from 15 to 150 µg improves postoperative analgesia while minimizing side effects. Adding concurrent administration of 25 to 75 µg clonidine with 250 µg morphine to a bupivacaine spinal anesthetic decreased 24-hour IV morphine consumption and improved 24-hour visual analog scale (VAS) scores as compared to adding 250 µg IT morphine alone to bupivacaine spinal anesthetic.[39–41]

Combined Spinal and Epidural

The combined spinal epidural (CSE) technique offers the advantage of both spinal and epidural techniques. CSE provides rapid-onset surgical anesthesia,[42,43] the ability to titrate to the desired sensory level and duration, and the ability to deliver postoperative analgesia through the epidural catheter.

The CSE technique is widely used in obstetric anesthesia and analgesia. In labor analgesia, CSE provides quick onset of pain relief while maintaining ambulation ability. Studies have shown great benefit of using small opioid doses (e.g., 10 to 15 µg of IT fentanyl[44]) while adding a small dose of isobaric bupivacaine,[45] ropivacaine, or levobupivacaine.[46,47] CSE may be associated with reduced duration of the first stage of labor in primiparous mothers[48] but does not shorten total labor time compared to conventional epidural analgesia.[49]

Another advantage of using this technique is that small doses of the spinal anesthetic can be used and the risk of a high spinal block and prolonged hypotension[50,51] can be avoided in patients who are already hypovolemic. Potential challenges associated with CSE are the inability to properly test the epidural catheter, increased incidence of catheter migration to the IT space, and enhanced spread of the spinal local anesthetic.[52]

TECHNIQUE OF COMBINED SPINAL EPIDURAL
Needle through Needle Technique

Neuraxial techniques in general can be performed with the patient in either a lateral or sitting position. The CSE technique is typically performed with patients sitting. It should be noted that during needle insertion, the distance from skin to epidural space is greater when patients are in the lateral position than when they are in the sitting position. After the epidural needle is inserted, a loss of resistance to plunger displacement indicates entrance into the epidural space. At that point, the plunger is carefully removed and a spinal needle is passed through the epidural needle until the characteristic "pop" is felt, indicating penetration of the dura and entry into the subarachnoid space. After free CSF flow is confirmed, the dorsal aspect of the non-dominant hand is firmly placed against the patient's back, with the index finger and thumb stabilizing the hub for injection. Local anesthetic with additive is injected, and the spinal needle is withdrawn. A 20-gauge radiopaque catheter with 1-cm graduation is passed through the epidural needle. The catheter

is advanced 4 to 5 cm beyond the needle tip into the epidural space. The needle is then withdrawn over the catheter, and the catheter secured to the patient's back. Prior to dosing, a test dose should be administered through the catheter.

Separate Needles Techniques

Two-needle, two interspace techniques: CSE could be carried out with two separate needles, one spinal and one epidural, with either the same interspace[53,54] or two different interspaces.[55–57] With the same-interspace technique, the epidural catheter will be placed first to allow proper testing before spinal anesthesia. This testing is mainly to decrease risks of IT or intravascular catheter migration. This technique carries the risk of shearing[58,59] the epidural catheter with the introduction of the spinal needle. In the different-interspaces technique, the practitioner places the spinal needle but does not inject local anesthetic. He or she then places the epidural catheter and tests it at a different interspace before administering the spinal dose. This technique allows testing of the epidural catheter while avoiding shirring of the catheter.

Regardless of which step is taken first, these techniques carry a disadvantage of taking longer to perform and requiring two separate injections. When the needle through needle (NTN) and separate needles techniques (SNT) have been compared,[60,61] some have reported better success and lower failure rate with SNT but greater patient acceptance, less discomfort, and quicker procedure time with the NTN.

COMPLICATIONS AND CHALLENGES WITH COMBINED SPINAL EPIDURAL

Spinal migration of the epidural catheter and IT administration of epidural drugs are more likely to occur with the NTN technique.[62–64] Regardless of the technique used, all epidural medications should be administered in small incremental doses while the patient's hemodynamics are closely monitored.

Failure of the spinal block is a possibility and depends on the provider's experience. Failures occur mainly as a result of the spinal needle being too short,[65] failure to puncture the dura with a small-caliber spinal needle,[66] and diverging from the midline.[67] Additionally, delay while placing the epidural catheter[68] might affect the density and level of the spinal block.

Another complication from CSE is possible nerve damage from needle or catheter trauma that occurs when the practitioner places an epidural in a patient who has received spinal anesthesia. Although this is a rare complication, the absence of sensation after spinal anesthesia may prevent identification of paresthesia that would alert anesthesiologists to needle misplacement.

Contraindications of Neuraxial Techniques

Although complications of neuraxial analgesia are extremely rare, they can be very serious. Among those complications are neuraxial hematoma, abscess, and permanent nerve injuries. Evaluation of the risks and benefits of neuraxial analgesia is always helpful and should be based on the patient's comorbidities and risk factors.

SEPSIS, FEVER, AND VIRAL INFECTIONS

Infectious complications of neuraxial techniques are extremely rare, and data are insufficient to determine whether epidural analgesia should or should not be initiated in septic patients.[69] The possibility of introducing blood-borne pathogens into the neuraxial space is a very valid concern for many practitioners. Regional anesthesia in the presence of low-grade fever should be based on an individual risk–benefit analysis. Antibiotics should be used before initiating the block, and the practitioner should use strict aseptic techniques during postprocedure monitoring to detect any signs of central nervous system (CNS) infection.

The CNS is affected early in the course of HIV infection,[70] and there is no evidence that epidural placements or an epidural blood patch for treatment of postdural puncture headache (PDPH) causes any additional spread of the virus to the CNS. It is advisable to obtain thorough documentation of any neurologic deficit before attempting a neuraxial technique in these patients. Studies have shown no reported incidence of CNS infection with neuraxial blocks in patients with recurrent herpes simplex infection.[71,72] However, a neuraxial block or catheter is contraindicated in the presence of active herpes zoster at the site of injection. Complications such as aseptic meningitis and encephalitis might develop from spread of the virus to the CNS.[73]

COAGULOPATHY, THROMBOCYTOPENIA, AND BLEEDING DISORDERS

Neuraxial techniques are contraindicated if the patient refuses it and in those with severe coagulopathy and disseminated intravascular coagulation (DIC). DIC can result from severe trauma, sepsis, amniotic fluid embolism, massive transfusion, and placental abruption, among many other diseases. Initiating an epidural in the presence of coagulopathy is an absolute contraindication, but keeping an epidural in the presence of coagulopathy is controversial. The epidural should be removed only after normal coagulation is restored. Epidural catheter removal could be as traumatic as placement, and the same precautions should be applied.[74]

Anticoagulants should be held in a timely fashion before initiation or removal of an epidural catheter. Placement of an epidural catheter is considered a relative contraindication in the presence of some bleeding disorders like hemophilia and von Willebrand disease, but it is considered safe after factor levels and partial thromboplastin time have reached normal values.

Thrombocytopenia is another relative contraindication to neuraxial anesthesia. Currently, no guidelines exist for a platelet count below which epidural placement is contraindicated. Some clinicians feel comfortable with a platelet count of 80,000, whereas others will go as low as 70,000.[75] The etiology of thrombocytopenia, the patient's bleeding status, and the trend in platelet count must be taken into consideration before placement of an epidural catheter. One can obtain a thromboelastography (TEG) to assist in determining whether to place an epidural or not. Ultimately, the decision is based on the risks and benefits for the individual patient.

CENTRAL NERVOUS SYSTEM DISORDERS

In the past, neuraxial blockade was contraindicated in patients with preexisting CNS disease, including multiple sclerosis (MS). However, a recent retrospective study[76] of 35 patients with MS showed no evidence of MS relapse after neuraxial block. It is reasonable to use low concentrations and low volumes of local anesthetics in these patients and thoroughly document any preexisting neurologic deficits before initiating a neuraxial block. A thorough informed consent should be given to the patient explaining the possibility of MS symptom aggravation.[77]

The risk of neurologic complication during a neuraxial technique is higher in anesthetized patients because they cannot respond to pain or paresthesia during needle placement.[78] The risk of neurologic complications is minimal during placement of a lumbar epidural in anesthetized patients,[79] and it is uncertain whether the risk might be higher with thoracic epidural. Previous back surgery and back pain are not considered contraindications for neuraxial techniques. In a large retrospective study of patients with a history of spinal stenosis, peripheral neuropathy, or lumbar radiculopathy, these conditions did not affect the efficacy or complications of neuraxial techniques.[80] The practitioner should discuss an informed thorough consent with the patient and explain the increased risk of technical difficulties, dural puncture, and unsuccessful block.

Analgesic Adjuvants for Central and Peripheral Analgesia

INTRODUCTION

Nociceptive pathways in the central and peripheral nervous systems are very complex and not easily blocked by one drug type or one technique. The use of agonists at inhibitory receptors and antagonists at excitatory receptors in the pain pathways allows a "multimodal" approach with optimization of pain control and reduction of adverse effects.

Neuraxial drugs such as opioids selectively decrease nociceptive afferent input from Aδ and C fibers without affecting dorsal root axons or somatosensory-evoked potentials.[81] Opioid receptors in the ventral medial medullary reticular formation may be involved in activation of noradrenergic pathways. Additionally, a descending inhibitory pathway projecting through the dorsolateral funiculus may reinforce other analgesic mechanisms.[82,83] The advantages of neuraxial opioids lay in the absence of sympathetic blockade and postural hypotension, providing for potentially easier ambulation of patients.

The last few decades have witnessed important advances in the knowledge of nociceptive transmission from the peripheral nervous system to the CNS. A number of drugs have been tested, and some have proven clinically useful when added to local anesthetics for central and peripheral nerve block (PNB). These drugs, known as analgesic adjuvants, include opioids, dexamethasone, and α_2 agonists. They may have benefit if applied in the peripheral nervous system.[84] Some adjuvants added to local anesthetics might speed their onset, prolong their effect, or reduce total required dose. Adjuncts are also used to enhance analgesia while minimizing side effects.

NEURAXIAL OPIOIDS

Opioids are classified by their lipophilic property. Lipophilic opioids (e.g., sufentanil and fentanyl) tend to provide a fast onset and short duration of analgesia as a result of rapid clearance from the CSF. Hydrophilic opioids (e.g., hydromorphone and morphine) remain within the CSF after neuraxial administration and produce a delayed but long duration of analgesia. They also tend to cause a higher incidence of side effects because of CSF spread. Hydrophilic opioids provide analgesia primarily via a spinal mechanism, whereas lipophilic opioids provide analgesia via either a spinal or systemic mechanism.[85,86] Single-shot neuraxial administration of a lipophilic opioid is appropriate for short-duration analgesia,[87] and single-shot neuraxial administration of a hydrophilic opioid is appropriate for longer duration analgesia.[88]

Neuraxial opioids are associated with side effects that could affect patients' quality of recovery. Side effects include nausea and vomiting in up to 50% of patients[89,90] and pruritus in up to 60%,[91] as opposed to 15% to 18% for PCEA with local anesthetic or systemic opioids.[92,93] Other adverse effects include urinary retention in up to 80% of patients and early or delayed respiratory depression in 0.2% to 1.9%.[90] These side effects are not limited to any specific opioid, and it is not clear whether their incidence is dose dependent. PCEA with combined local anesthetic and neuraxial opioids results in a low incidence of respiratory depression that varies from 0.07% to 0.4%,[94–96] thus making PCEA relatively safe to use in an unmonitored hospital setting. It is essential that the dose of neuraxial opioid be reduced when used in elderly patients.[97]

PERINEURAL OPIOIDS

Some systematic reviews[98,99] found little evidence for the benefit of adding opioids to local anesthetics in peripheral nerve blockade. Preliminary results suggest that buprenorphine and tramadol[98,100–102] are the two opioid agonists that have demonstrated analgesic efficacy when administered perineurally.

Buprenorphine is a partial μ-receptor agonist with a very high receptor affinity compared with that of fentanyl or morphine. In addition, it has intermediate lipid solubility, which allows it to cross the neural membrane.[103,104] Buprenorphine was found to markedly increase the duration of analgesia when added to mepivacaine and tetracaine for axillary blocks,[105] with no significant increase in adverse effects. Similar results were found when a 100-mg dose of tramadol was used as an adjuvant to mepivacaine in axillary brachial plexus block.[106,107] One study reported an increased duration of motor and sensory blockade in the axillary tramadol group that significantly ($P < .01$) outlasted both IV and placebo groups.[108]

PERINEURAL CLONIDINE AND DEXMEDETOMIDINE

Clonidine, an α_2 agonist with some α_1-stimulatory effects, is traditionally used as an antihypertensive agent but for many years has been noted to have sedative and analgesic effects. α_2 Receptors exist in the dorsal horn of the spinal cord, and their stimulation produces analgesic effects by inhibiting the presynaptic release of excitatory transmitters, including substance P and glutamate.[109–111] IT clonidine mediates analgesia by increasing acetylcholine levels. Clonidine injected close to peripheral nerves with or without local anesthetic drugs appears to mediate analgesia in a number of ways. Clonidine has local anesthetic properties[112] and has a pharmacokinetic effect on local anesthetic redistribution mediated by a vasoconstrictor effect at the α_1-receptor.[113]

Many studies have examined the effect of clonidine on local anesthetics in PNB. There is good evidence from these studies that clonidine in doses up to 1.5 μg/kg prolongs sensory block and analgesia when administered with local anesthetics for PNB.[114] Some studies have compared clonidine added to PNB to systemic clonidine. Clonidine added to the axillary brachial plexus block delayed the onset of pain twofold compared with subcutaneous clonidine injections, without producing adverse effects.[115]

A meta-analysis by Pöpping and colleagues[116] estimated that clonidine prolonged postoperative analgesia, sensory block, and motor block by 122, 74, and 141 minutes, respectively. Clonidine also increased the probability of hypotension (odds ratio [OR], 3.61), fainting (OR, 5.07), sedation (OR, 2.28), and bradycardia (OR, 3.09).

Ifield et al.[117,118] have demonstrated in two studies that the addition of clonidine to continuous PNBs is not beneficial. It failed to reduce pain scores or oral analgesic use after upper extremity surgery.

Dexmedetomidine is selective for the α_2 receptor and at present is mainly studied as a sedative agent in ICUs. Dexmedetomidine may be expected to produce not only more profound analgesia but also greater adverse effects because of the selectivity of action.[119]

PERINEURAL DEXAMETHASONE

Dexamethasone is a potent synthetic corticosteroid with approximately 7 times the anti-inflammatory potency of prednisolone.[120] The half-life is approximately 36 to 54 hours in the perioperative setting. The effectiveness of dexamethasone as a postoperative antiemetic (4 to 10 mg IV) has been confirmed by many randomized controlled trials.[121] In a recent meta-analysis that included 2,751 patients,[122] the analgesic effects of a single IV dose of dexamethasone was found to be very modest up to 24 hours postinjection.

Corticosteroids administered via perineural application are thought to exert their effect by several mechanisms, including attenuating the release of inflammatory mediators, reducing ectopic neuronal discharge, and inhibiting potassium channel–mediated discharge of nociceptive C fibers.[123–125] It is widely believed that dexamethasone improves the quality and duration of peripheral nerve blockade when administered in conjunction with local anesthetics. The U.S. Food and Drug Administration (FDA), however, has not approved dexamethasone for perineural administration.

Multiple studies have assessed the effects of using dexamethasone (4 to 10 mg) with local anesthetic for PNBs.[126–131] Dexamethasone was shown to prolong analgesia or sensory/motor block from approximately 50% to 75% beyond that of nerve blocks with local anesthetic alone. Nevertheless, some concerns have been raised over complications related to dexamethasone, such as effects on blood glucose and neurotoxicity. However, in several studies, a single dose of dexamethasone, whether administered perineurally or systemically, did not increase blood glucose to a clinically significant degree,[132–134] and IT administration did not produce neurotoxicity.[135]

Adjuvants have been added to local anesthetic for single perineural analgesia in an attempt to improve analgesia quality, spare local anesthetic consumption, and minimize motor block. To date, clinical benefits such as improving pain have been found for adding adjuncts to continuous PNBs.[117,118,136,137] No additive medications are currently approved for continuous perineural administration, and some additives that have been reported in clinical trials have undesirable side effects.[138,139]

Transversus Abdominis Plane Block, Ilioinguinal Iliohypogastric Block, Rectus Sheath Block

Innervation of the anterolateral abdominal wall arises from the anterior rami of spinal nerves T7–L1. These include the intercostal nerves (T7–T11), the subcostal nerve (T12), and the iliohypogastric and ilioinguinal nerves (L1). The anterior divisions of T7–T11 continue from the intercostal space to enter the abdominal wall between the internal oblique and transversus abdominis muscles until they reach the rectus abdominis, which they perforate and supply, ending as anterior cutaneous branches supplying the skin of the front of the abdomen. Midway in their course, they pierce the external oblique muscle giving off the lateral cutaneous branch, which divides into anterior and posterior branches that supply the external oblique muscle and latissimus dorsi respectively.

TRANSVERSUS ABDOMINIS PLANE BLOCK

It may play a role in postsurgical pain control. Transversus abdominis plane (TAP) blocks may improve analgesia in patients undergoing laparotomy for colorectal surgery, laparoscopic cholecystectomy, and open and laparoscopic appendectomy.[140–142] Blocks can be achieved by using anatomic landmarks or by ultrasound-guided techniques.[143,144]

The aim of a TAP block is to deposit local anesthetic in the plane between the internal oblique and transversus abdominis muscles, targeting the spinal nerves in this plane. The innervation to abdominal skin, muscles, and parietal peritoneum will be interrupted. If surgery traverses the peritoneal cavity, dull visceral pain (from spasm or inflammation following surgical insult) will still be experienced.

Landmark Technique

The landmark technique for performing a TAP block advocates a single entry point, the triangle of Petit, to access a number of abdominal wall nerves.[145] The lumbar triangle of Petit is situated between the lower costal margin and the iliac crest. It is bound anteriorly by the external oblique muscle and posteriorly by the latissimus dorsi. This TAP technique relies on feeling double pops as the needle traverses the external oblique and internal oblique muscles. A blunt needle will make the loss of resistance more appreciable.

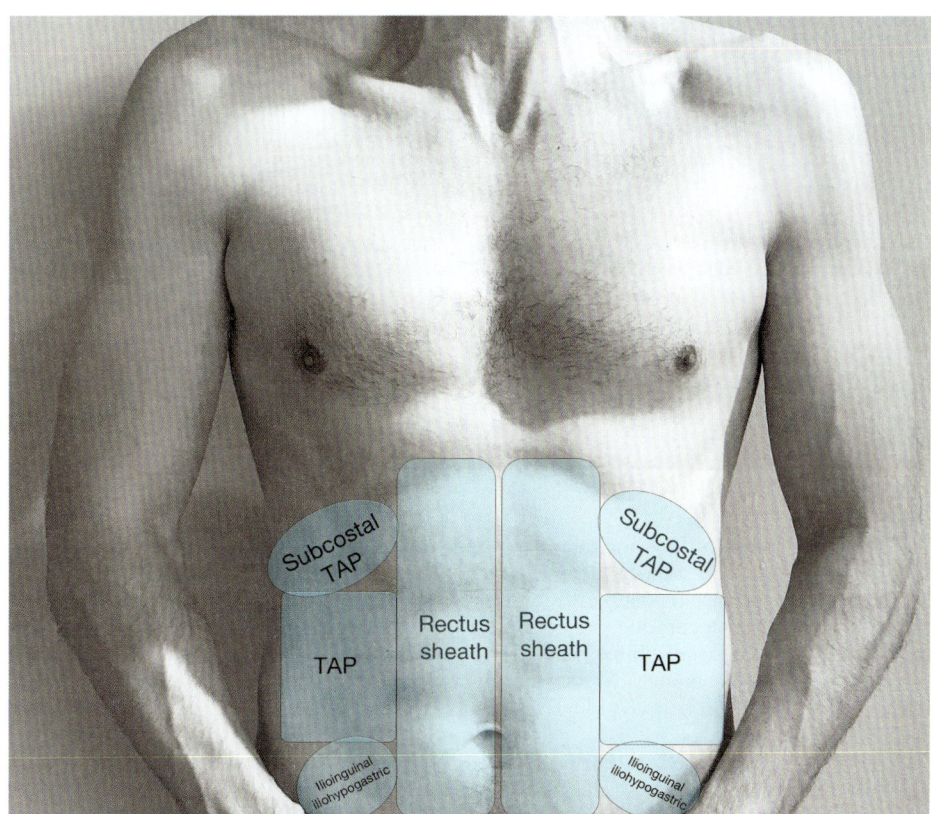

FIGURE 52.1 Surface landmarks for abdominal wall block. TAP, transversus abdominis plane. *(Reproduced with permission from Ouanes et al. http://anesthesiology.hopkins medicine.org/international-obstetric-and -regional-anesthesia/. Accessed July 18, 2018.)*

Ultrasound-Guided Transversus Abdominis Plane

Ultrasound guidance for the TAP block can help the practitioner localize and deposit the local anesthetic and thereby improve accuracy.[146] The ultrasound probe is placed in a transverse plane to the lateral abdominal wall in the midaxillary line, between the lower costal margin and the iliac crest (Figs. 52.1 and 52.2). The local anesthetic is deposited in the correct neurovascular plane between the transverse abdominis and internal oblique muscles. If prolonged analgesia is required beyond the duration of a single shot of local anesthetic, a catheter can be introduced into the TAP through a Tuohy needle. After opening up the plane with 2 mL of saline, the practitioner introduces the catheter approximately 3 cm beyond the needle tip. The position is verified by injecting a local anesthetic bolus (20 mL). An infusion of a dilute local anesthetic is started at a rate of 7 to 10 mL per hour.

There has been controversy in the literature regarding the spread and level of block achieved with a single TAP injection. Early studies showed a T7–L1 spread after a single posterior injection, making the block suitable for midline abdominal incisions.[147] Other studies, however, failed to demonstrate a spread cephalad to T10, making it more suited for lower abdominal surgery.[148] It is reasonable to expect a good analgesic effect in the region between T10 and L1 after a single posterior injection. Augmentation with a subcostal injection will help attain a higher block up to T7. The subcostal TAP is a modification of the original technique in which the ultrasound probe is placed just beneath the costal margin and parallel to it (see Fig. 52.1). The needle is then introduced from the lateral side of the rectus muscle in plane of the ultrasound beam, and 10 mL of local anesthetic is injected into the TAP to extend the analgesia provided by the posterior TAP block above the umbilicus.

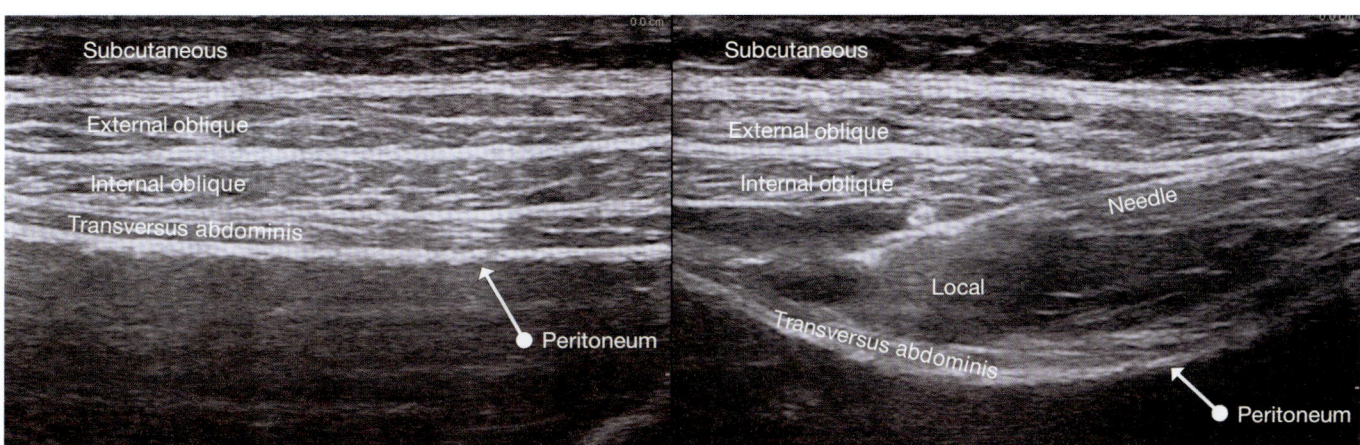

FIGURE 52.2 Ultrasound image transversus abdominis plane block. **Left:** Labeled sonoanatomy. **Right:** In-plane needle position with injection in the plane between the internal oblique and transversus abdominis. *(Reproduced with permission from Ouanes et al. http://anesthesiology.hopkinsmedicine.org /international-obstetric-and-regional-anesthesia/. Accessed July 18, 2018.)*

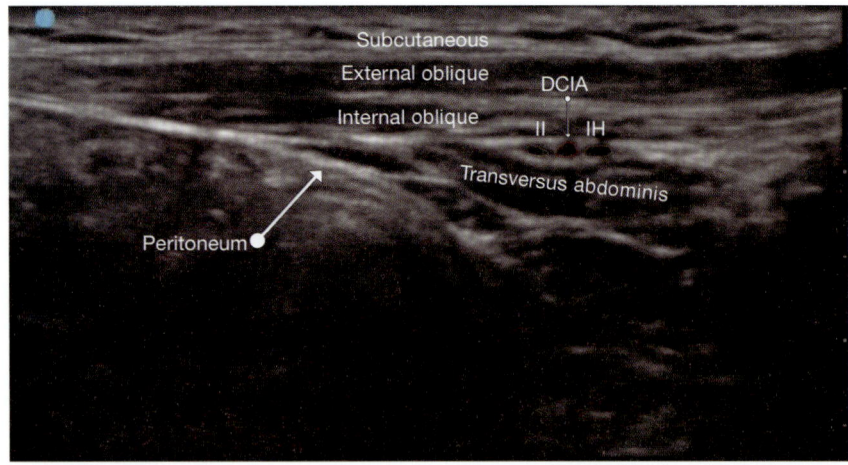

FIGURE 52.3 Ultrasound image of ilioinguinal iliohypogastric nerve block. DCIA, deep circumflex iliac artery; IH, iliohypogastric nerve; II, ilioinguinal nerve. *(Reproduced with permission from Ouanes et al. http://anesthesiology .hopkinsmedicine.org/international-obstetric-and-regional -anesthesia/. Accessed July 18, 2018.)*

Reported complications include intraperitoneal injection or hemorrhage, transient femoral nerve palsy, and local anesthetic toxicity.[149–151] One case report has been published of intrahepatic injection with blind technique.[152] Local anesthetic toxicity could also result from the large volumes required to perform this block, especially if it is done bilaterally. As with any regional technique, careful aspiration will help avoid intravascular injections.

ILIOHYPOGASTRIC AND ILIOINGUINAL BLOCK
The iliohypogastric nerve (L1) divides between the internal oblique and transversus abdominis near the iliac crest into lateral and anterior cutaneous branches, the former supplying part of the skin of the gluteal region and the latter supplying the hypogastric region. The ilioinguinal nerve (L1) communicates with the iliohypogastric nerve between the internal oblique and transversus abdominis near the anterior part of the iliac crest. It supplies the upper and medial part of the thigh and part of the skin covering the genitalia.

This block is indicated for any lower abdominal surgery, including appendectomy, hernia repair, cesarean section,[153] abdominal hysterectomy,[154] and prostatectomy.[155] Efficacy in laparoscopic surgery has also been demonstrated.[156] Bilateral blocks can be administered for midline incisions or laparoscopic surgery. The needle is introduced in plane of the ultrasound probe directly under the probe and advanced until it reaches the plane between the internal oblique and transversus abdominis muscles (see Figs. 52.1 and 52.3).

RECTUS SHEATH BLOCK
Local anesthetic deposition bilaterally within the posterior rectus sheath provides dense and predictable analgesia over the middle anterior wall from the xiphoid process to the symphysis pubis,

as shown in Figures 52.1 and 52.4. It is used for surgery with midline (or paramedian) abdominal incision. Rectus sheath block does not provide analgesia for the lateral abdomen, but it will provide somatic pain relief for abdominal wall structures superficial to the peritoneum. Patients with rectus sheath catheters typically exhibit low pain scores and low opiate requirements.[157,158]

Bilateral rectus sheath block might be helpful after emergency laparotomy. This patient group may have sepsis, coagulopathy, and hemodynamic instability. Administering an epidural postoperatively is usually not possible owing to positioning difficulty and safety concerns regarding placement of epidurals in unconscious patients.

Peripheral Nerve Blocks and Catheters

PNBs are an integral part of a postoperative multimodal analgesic regimen.[159] Use of regional anesthesia techniques have been associated with postanesthesia care unit (PACU) phase 1 bypass, fewer unplanned hospital admissions, and lower hospital costs.[160] These techniques improve analgesia and reduce the amount of IV analgesics required, thus decreasing opioid-related side effects.[161–163] Some of the benefits of single-injection nerve blocks are limited by the duration of action of the local anesthetic used.

Peripheral nerve catheters (PNCs) offer the possibility of extending the effects of the nerve block. Continuous peripheral nerve blockade (CPNB) provides postoperative analgesia equivalent to that of epidural techniques and may be associated with higher patient satisfaction, improved side-effect profile, and fewer complications than epidurals.[162,164] Strong evidence suggests that continuous perineural blockade provides superior analgesia compared to opioids for all catheter locations while

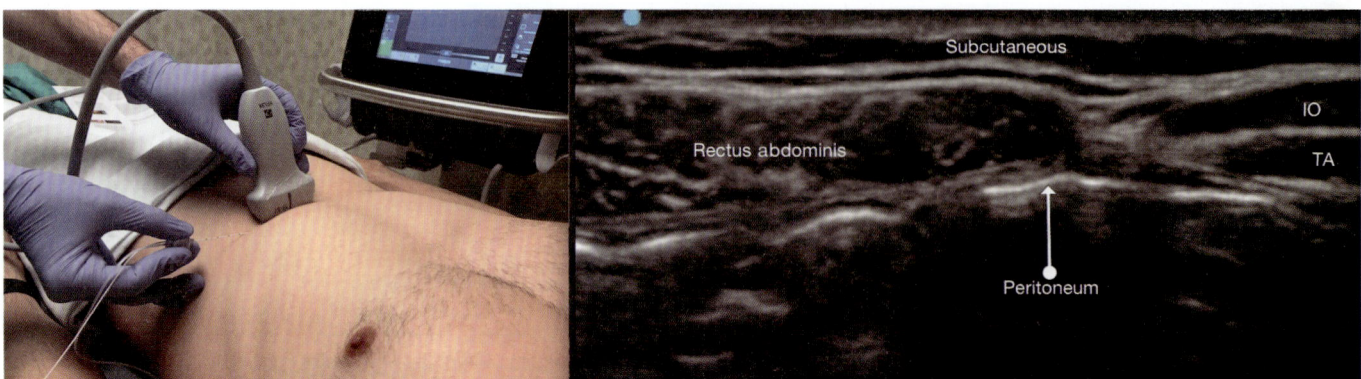

FIGURE 52.4 **Left:** Needle approach for rectus sheath block. **Right:** Labeled ultrasound image. IO, internal oblique; TA, transversus abdominis. *(Reproduced with permission from Ouanes et al. http://anesthesiology.hopkinsmedicine.org/international-obstetric-and-regional-anesthesia/. Accessed July 18, 2018.)*

reducing opioid consumption and opioid-related side effects.[4] The use of CPNB decreases the time to readiness for discharge of inpatients and allows for more aggressive rehabilitation in the postoperative period.[165] In the case of continuous interscalene nerve block for arthroscopic rotator cuff repair, its analgesic effects have been shown to extend into postoperative day 7.[166]

The use of CPNB may allow surgical procedures that traditionally required hospital admission to be performed in an outpatient setting without a significant increase in complications.[167] CPNB may be provided after discharge with a portable infusion pump, affording patients the possibility to convalesce in the comfort of their home while reducing inpatient costs.[168] Shorter inpatient stays may also have other benefits, such as lower morbidity related to nosocomial infections or medical error.[169] Complications associated with home CPNB are uncommon, the most common being block failure resulting from catheter dislodgment. Other potential complications include infection, pulmonary-related side effects as local anesthetic infusions may affect the phrenic nerve, systemic local anesthetic toxicity, and patient falls.[170] Patient selection plays a key role in the success of ambulatory CPNB, and although the optimal method and frequency of patient monitoring remains to be established, daily phone calls seem to be a widely accepted method. A retrospective review of 1,059 ambulatory supraclavicular and popliteal catheters placed over a 2-year period and infused over a mean duration of 5 days failed to reveal an increased incidence of complications.[171]

Among the different techniques for performing PNBs, ultrasound-guided regional anesthesia (UGRA) is becoming the method of choice. Compared with nerve stimulation, UGRA has been shown to provide a faster onset of blockade, better success rate, fewer needle passes with associated faster block performance, less patient discomfort, and greater patient satisfaction.[172–174] Additionally, there is level Ib evidence for a grade A recommendation that UGRA improves success of sensory block and decreases local anesthetic requirements.[175] Interscalene catheters placed under UGRA after shoulder surgery were shown to be more effective in the first 24 hours than neurostimulation.[176] Based on large prospective series, the complication rate does not seem to differ between UGRA and neurostimulation.[177,178]

Interscalene Block

INDICATIONS

The interscalene block (ISB) is usually performed for surgical procedures involving the shoulder and upper arm. The brachial plexus is targeted at the trunk level; however, it commonly results in sparing blockade of the inferior trunk (C8–T1), making

it less suitable for elbow, forearm, and hand procedures. ISB causes concomitant block of the phrenic nerve because of its close proximity, particularly at the cricoid cartilage level. At this level, the plexus and phrenic nerve are 2 to 4 mm apart. This distance increases progressively in a caudad direction.[179] Horner syndrome and recurrent laryngeal nerve block resulting in hoarseness can occur. Relative contraindications to ISB include respiratory failure, contralateral phrenic nerve lesion, and contralateral recurrent laryngeal nerve lesion. The plexus can be accessed at the interscalene groove through a lateral approach or a cervical paravertebral approach.[180,181]

LANDMARKS

The brachial plexus is formed mainly by the anterior rami of the spinal nerves C5–T1. These nerves coalesce into three trunks (superior, middle, inferior), which emerge through the interscalene groove between the anterior and middle scalene muscles.

TECHNIQUES
Nerve Stimulation

At the level of the cricoid cartilage, the interscalene groove can be palpated behind the posterior border of the sternocleidomastoid muscle (SCM). The stimulating needle is introduced in a cephalocaudal and slightly medial direction. Adequate needle placement is identified by the presence of motor response to stimulation between 0.2 and 0.5 mA in the deltoid, triceps and biceps, forearm, or hand muscles. Contraction of the diaphragm or neck musculature indicates anterior placement of the needle tip, whereas contraction of the trapezius muscle indicates posterior placement.

Ultrasound Guidance

The practitioner places the high-frequency ultrasound probe transversally at the C6 (cricoid) level and slides it laterally while observing the internal jugular, carotid artery, and SCM superficially. As the posterior border of the SCM is visualized, the anterior and middle interscalene muscles appear deep to the SCM, with the trunks of the brachial plexus emerging between them as round hypoechoic structures. Alternatively, the probe can be placed in the supraclavicular fossa, where the divisions of the brachial plexus are visualized posterior and lateral to the subclavian artery and above the first rib. The practitioner then slides the probe in a cephalad direction, observing the divisions converge into trunks at the interscalene level. The needle can be advanced in plane lateromedially, allowing for visualization of the entire needle shaft and tip (Figs. 52.5 and 52.6). Alternatively, the needle can be introduced out of plane to the

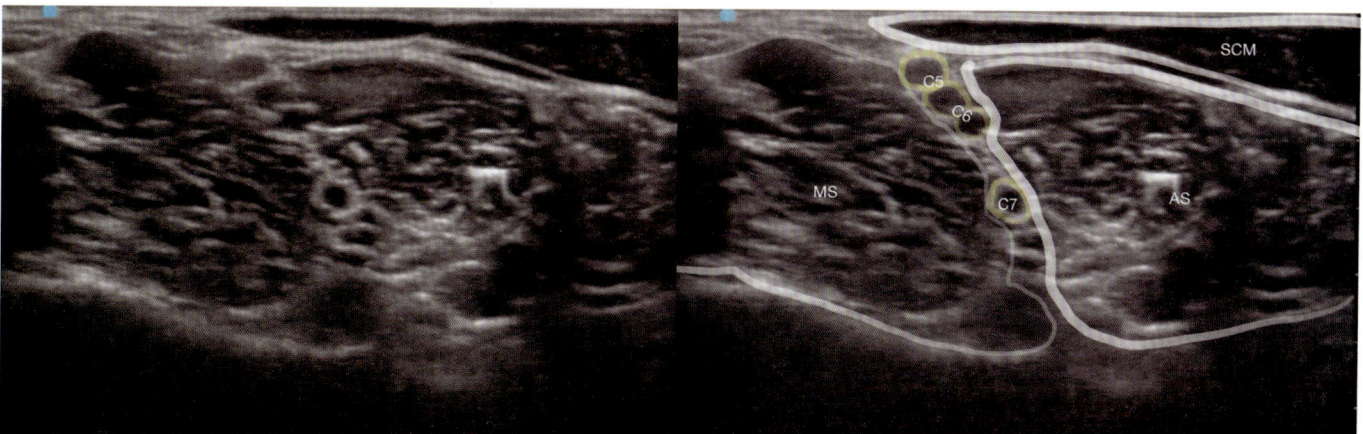

FIGURE 52.5 **Left:** Ultrasound image of interscalene anatomy. **Right:** Ultrasound image with anatomy labeled. Yellow, C5–C7 nerve roots. AS, anterior scalene; MS, middle scalene; SCM, sternocleidomastoid muscle. (*Reproduced with permission from Ouanes et al. http://anesthesiology.hopkinsmedicine.org /international-obstetric-and-regional-anesthesia/. Accessed July 18, 2018.*)

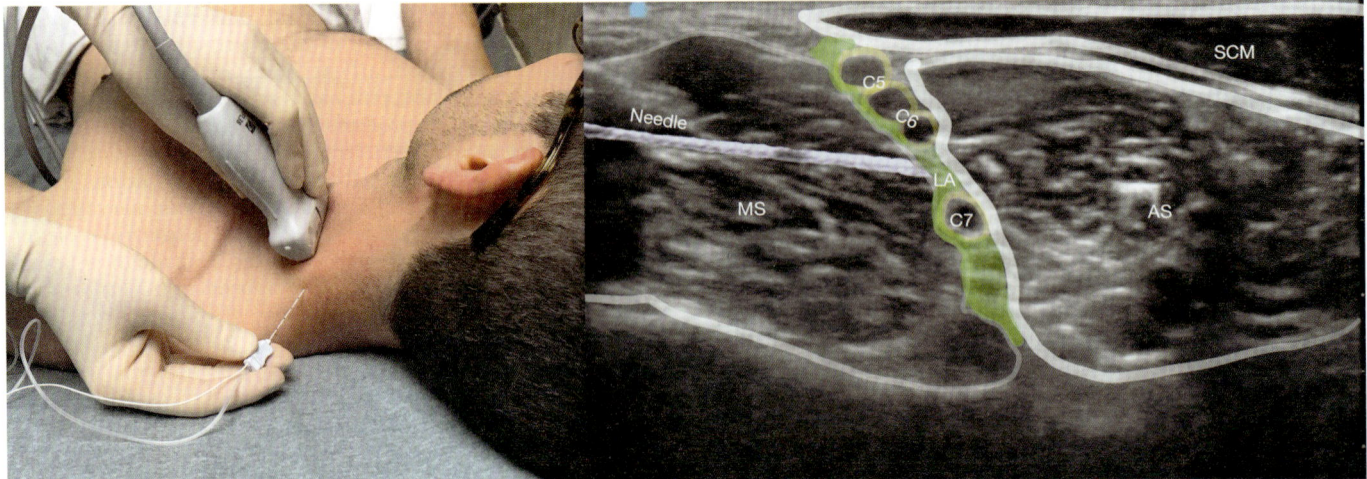

FIGURE 52.6   Left: In-plane approach of interscalene block. **Right:** Ultrasound image of in-plane approach of interscalene nerve block. *Green*, local anesthetic; *yellow*, C5–C7 nerve roots. AS, anterior scalene; MS, middle scalene; SCM, sternocleidomastoid muscle. *(Reproduced with permission from Ouanes et al. http://anesthesiology.hopkinsmedicine.org/international-obstetric-and-regional-anesthesia/. Accessed July 18, 2018.)*

ultrasound beam, resulting in a dot in the ultrasound image when the tip of the needle crosses the beam.

CLINICAL EFFECTS

Single-injection ISB for shoulder arthroscopies may be associated with fewer side effects and fewer and shorter hospital admissions than that seen with general anesthesia. In the ambulatory setting, ISB results in decreased postanesthesia unit stay and fewer unplanned hospital admissions for pain, sedation, and nausea.[182,183] ISB is effective at reducing the demand for IV PCA-delivered opioids and associated adverse effects after shoulder surgery.[163] Abdallah et al.[184] concluded in a recent meta-analysis that single-injection ISB provides effective analgesia for up to 8 hours postoperatively, whereas the opioid-sparing profile and lower adverse effects are limited to the first 12 and 24 postoperative hours respectively. In contrast to these findings, good evidence indicates that continuous ISB provides better analgesia, greater patient satisfaction, and fewer side effects than IV opioid PCA.[185–187]

In a comparison of single-injection to continuous ISB for arthroscopic rotator cuff repair, Malik et al.[188] concluded that continuous ISB for 3 days provides better analgesia than single-injection ISB and is associated with less opioid consumption and better sleep patterns. Such benefits may extend through the first postoperative week.[189] A retrospective review of continuous ISB performed for shoulder surgery revealed similar effects on analgesia and reduction of opioid requirements in the PACU, although these benefits were not associated with enhancing fast-track capability.[190] In contrast, a recent prospective randomized clinical trial comparing single-injection ISB to general anesthesia alone for shoulder arthroscopy showed significantly faster postoperative recovery time with ISB.[191] Continuous ISB with an indwelling catheter facilitates early physical therapy and enhances postoperative patient rehabilitation.[192] Better functional outcomes stemming from superior analgesia and early mobilization have also been described in patients receiving ISB for proximal humerus fracture repair.[193]

ISB should be considered with caution in patients with underlying severe pulmonary morbidity. Continuous ISB does not significantly prolong the duration of unilateral phrenic paresis compared to that with single injection ISB.[194] A clinical comparison of patients randomized to anterior and posterior approaches to ISB did not show a difference in incidence of phrenic nerve block.[195] Ghodki et al.[196] found a higher incidence of hemidiaphragmatic paresis, as assessed by ultrasonographic evaluation and pulmonary function tests, when ISB

was performed with peripheral nerve stimulation than when it was performed with ultrasound guidance. Extrafascial injection (4 mm lateral to the brachial plexus sheath) has also been reported to reduce the incidence of hemidiaphragmatic paresis compared to that with conventional intrafascial injection (between C5 and C6 within the interscalene groove) while resulting in similar analgesia.[197] Maga et al.[198] reported that faster onset was the only advantage of injection inside the brachial plexus sheath over injection outside the sheath. There was no statistically significant difference in sensory blockade after 10 minutes, but injection inside the sheath resulted in a higher incidence of transient paresthesia.

Supraclavicular Block

INDICATIONS

The supraclavicular nerve block (SCB) targets the brachial plexus at the trunks/divisions level. It has been used for surgical procedures involving the shoulder, arm, forearm, and hand. It can be performed as a single injection or with a continuous infusion through a catheter. The supraclavicular approach has a high incidence of success in blocking the ulnar and musculocutaneous nerves, which are commonly missed with interscalene and axillary blocks, respectively.[199] Therefore, the SCB has a broader spectrum of applications for both surgical anesthesia and postoperative analgesia.

LANDMARKS

At the supraclavicular level, the brachial plexus is composed of the anterior and posterior divisions of the three trunks. It is surrounded by its own fascia and located superior and lateral in relation to the subclavian artery, between the clavicle and the first rib.

ULTRASOUND TECHNIQUE

With the patient's head turned to the contralateral side of the block, the ultrasound probe is placed on the supraclavicular fossa, yielding a cross-sectional image of the brachial plexus and subclavian artery. The plexus is confirmed to lie superior and lateral to the artery. The optimal view is obtained when the first rib appears as a hyperechoic structure with its corresponding acoustic shadow just inferior to the subclavian artery and the brachial plexus. In this view, excessive advancement of the block needle should encounter the first rib, thereby reducing the risk of pneumothorax. The needle is introduced in plane from the lateral end of the ultrasound probe (Figs. 52.7 and 52.8).

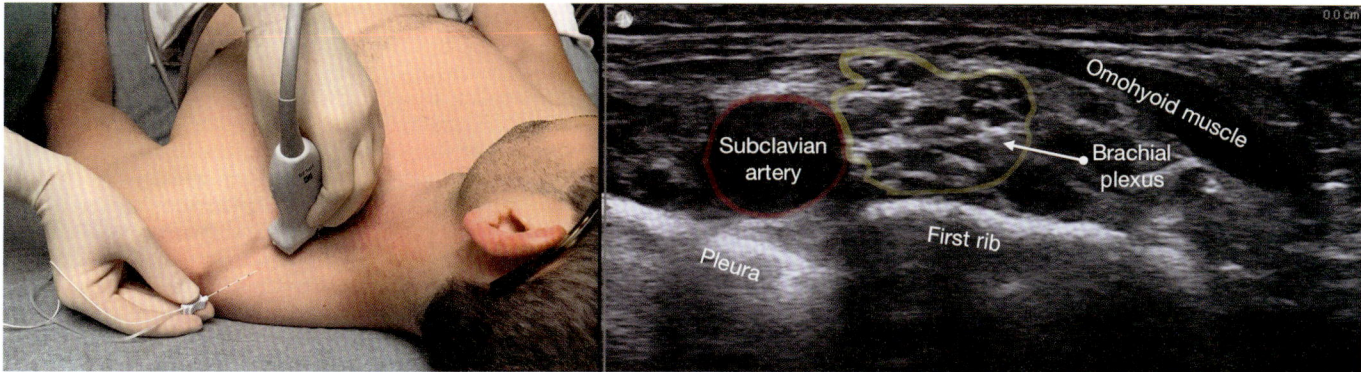

FIGURE 52.7 **Left:** Supraclavicular block. In-plane needle approach. **Right:** Ultrasound image with anatomy labeled. *(Reproduced with permission from Ouanes et al. http://anesthesiology.hopkinsmedicine.org/international-obstetric-and-regional-anesthesia/. Accessed July 18, 2018.)*

CLINICAL EFFECTS

A duration of sensory block of up to 17 hours has been described after SCB.[200] A recent randomized controlled trial of patients undergoing open rotator cuff repair found that continuous SCB provided analgesia in the 24-hour postoperative period equivalent to that of continuous ISB while reducing the incidence of hemidiaphragmatic paresis.[201] Similar results were reported when these two block modalities were compared for arthroscopic shoulder surgery.[202] SCB has been reported to cause hemidiaphragmatic paresis in approximately one-third of cases.[203] Therefore, it should be chosen carefully for patients with significant respiratory comorbidities.

Studies have shown no significant advantages of using a double-injection technique over a single-injection technique for the SCB under ultrasound guidance.[204,205] However, Arab et al.[206] found that although a triple-injection technique was associated with a longer performance time than a single-injection, it provided a more successful nerve blockade in the first 20 minutes. There was no difference in the success of surgical anesthesia between the two groups at 30 minutes. Subfascial injection of the local anesthetic (deep to the brachial plexus sheath) under ultrasound guidance resulted in a faster onset of surgical blockade and longer duration of postoperative analgesia than did an extrafascial injection (superficial to the sheath).[207]

Over the past decade, the application of ultrasound to SCB has reduced the probability of complications, including pneumothorax, Horner syndrome, phrenic nerve palsy (50% to 70% incidence), and local anesthetic systemic toxicity.[208,209] Ultrasound also allows a faster onset time of the sensory blockade, prolongs duration, and reduces the local anesthetic dose.[199,209] Because of the proximity of the pleura to the supraclavicular fossa, pneumothorax can be a significant complication of the SCB. The incidence of pneumothorax was described to be as high as 6.1% when SCB was performed without ultrasound guidance. A prospective observational study of 6,366 ultrasound-guided SCBs found a pneumothorax incidence of 0.06%, suggesting that ultrasound decreases the incidence of this complication.[210] A 5-year retrospective study confirmed the extremely low pneumothorax complication rate, including when SCB was performed by residents-in-training under direct faculty supervision. These findings suggest that ultrasound guidance has a significance in reducing pneumothorax complications.[211]

The incidence of phrenic nerve palsy after SCB is 50% to 70%. The use of ultrasonography, by virtue of reducing the volume of local anesthetic required for an effective block, has not been associated with hemidiaphragmatic paresis with volumes of 20 mL.[212] A recent prospective review of outcomes in upper limb surgery reinforced the efficacy and safety of ultrasound-guided SCB, with reported patient satisfaction in 96.7% of cases.[213]

Infraclavicular Block

INDICATIONS

The infraclavicular nerve block (ICB) targets the brachial plexus at the level of the cords and provides adequate analgesia or anesthesia of the elbow, forearm, and hand. The block can be performed as a single injection or continuously via a catheter. The infraclavicular approach is particularly well suited for continuous blockade. The pectoralis muscles aid in anchoring the catheter in place, which, in conjunction with the limited range of motion of the infraclavicular area, helps to minimize unintended catheter migration.

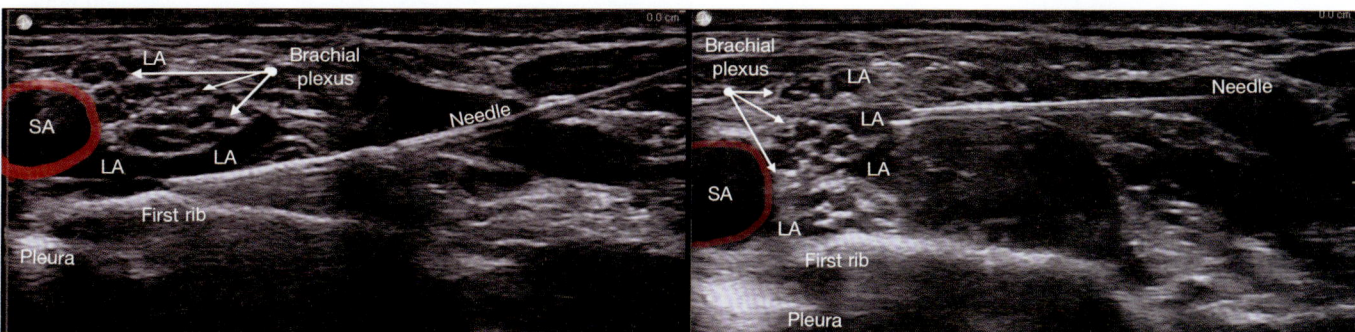

FIGURE 52.8 Supraclavicular approach to the brachial plexus block. **Left:** Initial needle approach and injection point between first rib and brachial plexus. **Right:** Additional injection point between superior and middle trunks to spread above the plexus. LA, local anesthetic; SA, subclavian artery. *(Reproduced with permission from Ouanes et al. http://anesthesiology.hopkinsmedicine.org/international-obstetric-and-regional-anesthesia/. Accessed July 18, 2018.)*

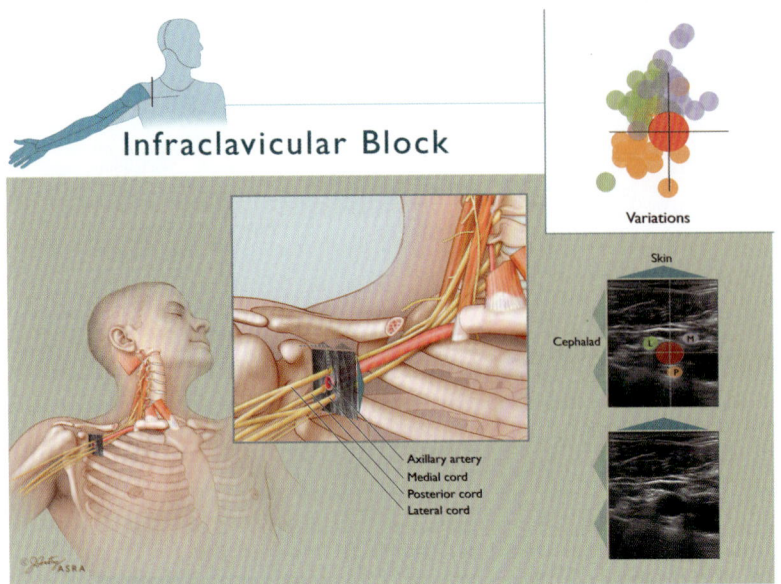

FIGURE 52.9   Infraclavicular block. Variations in cord position relative to the axillary artery. L, lateral cord; M, medial cord; P, posterior cord. *(Reprinted with permission of the American Society of Regional Anesthesia and Pain Medicine.)*

LANDMARKS

At the infraclavicular level, the brachial plexus is composed of three cords (medial, lateral, and posterior). These cords are named in accordance to their position relative to the axillary artery at the level of the pectoralis minor muscle (Pmm). However, there is significant individual variation in the position of the cords around the artery (Fig. 52.9). The level at which the block is performed is approximately 2 cm medial and 2 cm caudad to the coracoid process.

TECHNIQUE

The patient is positioned with the head turned to the contralateral side of the arm to be blocked, which is abducted and externally rotated at approximately 90 degrees. This maneuver causes the plexus to become more superficial and displaces the clavicle cephalad. The needle can then be introduced further away from the ultrasound probe at a smaller angle, thereby allowing better needle visualization (Fig. 52.10). The transducer is placed perpendicular to the clavicle in the deltopectoral groove. At this level, the pulsatile axillary artery and compressible axillary vein are visualized in cross-section deep to the Pmm (Fig. 52.11).

The needle is introduced from the superior end of the transducer and advanced in plane to the ultrasound beam. The initial injection point is deep to the axillary artery, between the artery and the posterior cord (see Fig. 52.10). Injection at this point usually results in medial spread around the artery toward the medial cord. As the needle is withdrawn, local anesthetic is injected to bathe the lateral cord. It may be necessary to redirect the needle over the artery to a point between the artery and vein to ensure proper blockade of the medial cord.

CLINICAL EFFECTS

The ICB has been shown to offer faster recovery, cause fewer adverse events, and provide better analgesia than general anesthesia with local wound infiltration.[214] A systematic review that compared ICB to other brachial plexus blocks confirmed that ICB posed a lower likelihood of tourniquet-related pain and provided more reliable blockade of the musculocutaneous nerve than did axillary block.[215] Ilfeld et al.[216] reported improved analgesia, decreased opioid use, decreased incidence of related side effects, fewer sleep disturbances, and greater patient satisfaction when continuous ICB was used for outpatients

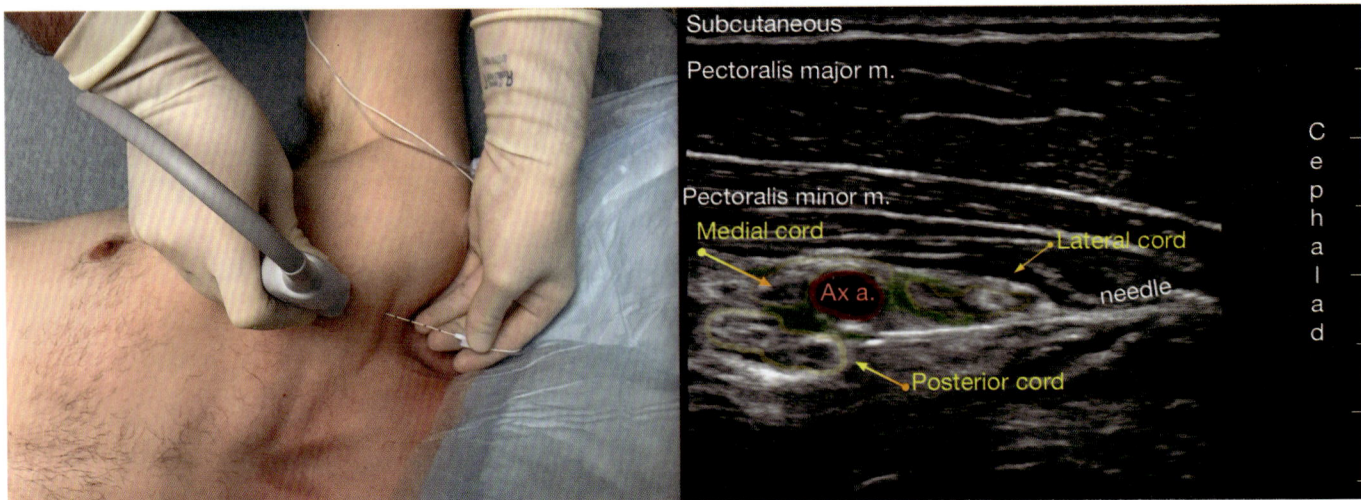

FIGURE 52.10   Infraclavicular approach to the brachial plexus block. **Left:** Infraclavicular in-plane needle insertion approach. **Right:** Corresponding ultrasound image. Ax a., axillary artery. *Green,* local anesthetic. *(Reproduced with permission from Ouanes et al. http://anesthesiology.hopkinsmedicine.org /international-obstetric-and-regional-anesthesia/. Accessed July 18, 2018.)*

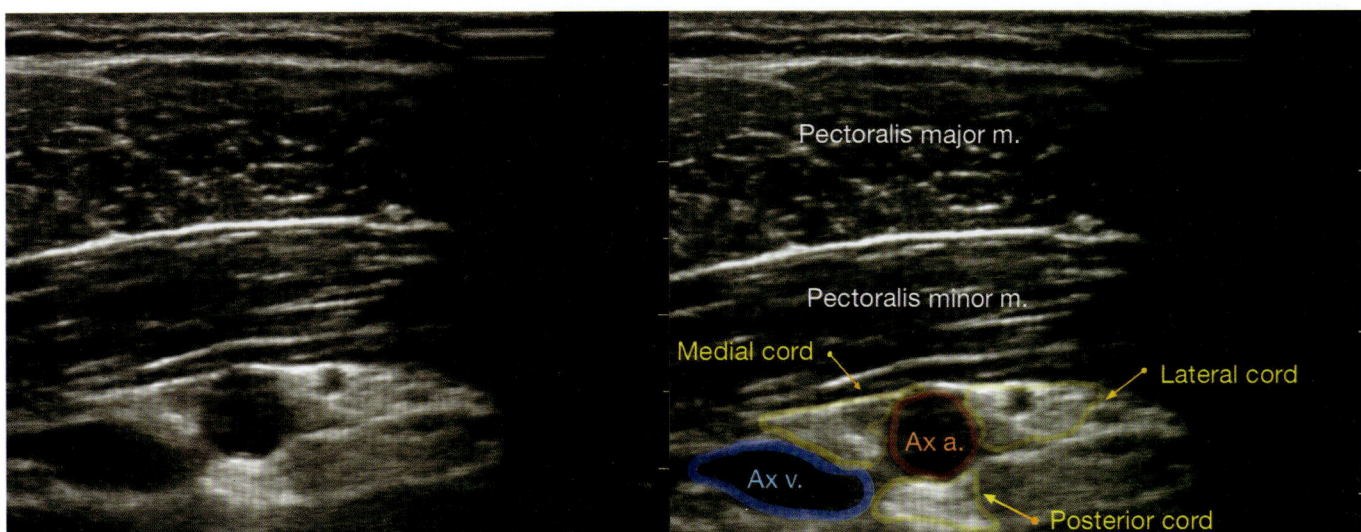

FIGURE 52.11 Infraclavicular approach to the brachial plexus block. **Left:** Ultrasound image for the infraclavicular sonoanatomy. **Right:** Ultrasound image with anatomy labeled. Ax a., axillary artery; Ax v., axillary vein; m., muscle. *(Reproduced with permission from Ouanes et al. http://anesthesiology.hopkinsmedicine .org/international-obstetric-and-regional-anesthesia/. Accessed July 18, 2018.)*

after upper extremity orthopedic surgery. An observational cohort study demonstrated a high success rate of single-injection ultrasound-guided ICB regardless of the operator's expertise.[217] In a randomized comparison study, continuous ICB provided superior analgesia to that of supraclavicular continuous block on the first postoperative day. Patients in the ICB group also required fewer oral analgesics for breakthrough pain in the first 18 to 24 postoperative hours.[218]

Axillary Block

INDICATIONS

The brachial plexus block at the axillary level targets terminal branches of the brachial plexus (ulnar, median, radial, and musculocutaneous nerves). The axillary sheath at this level is often discontinuous. At this level, the risk of pneumothorax or phrenic nerve palsy is negligible. Its low incidence of complications has made it a popular choice for elbow, forearm, wrist, and hand procedures.[219] A catheter can be placed at this level for continuous blockade. However, owing to the mobility of the axillary area and more superficial location of the plexus at this level, the catheter can be easily dislodged. This site may also be more susceptible to infection when an indwelling catheter is used.

LANDMARKS

At the axillary level, the neurovascular sheath contains the axillary artery surrounded by the radial, median, and ulnar nerves. Outside of this sheath are the intercostobrachial, axillary, and musculocutaneous nerves.

TECHNIQUES

Nerve Stimulation

The patient is positioned supine with the head turned to the contralateral side and the arm to be blocked abducted and externally rotated. The axillary artery is palpated in the axilla and stabilized with two fingers. The stimulating needle is introduced superior to it at a 30- to 45-degree angle to the skin. Finger flexion and/or thumb opposition indicate adequate needle placement. The needle should be adjusted so that muscle contraction is lost less than 0.5 mA prior to injection of local anesthetic.

At the axillary level, the musculocutaneous nerve has typically branched off the neurovascular bundle and travels within the coracobrachialis muscle. If musculocutaneous nerve block is required, a second injection is necessary. The coracobrachialis muscle is palpated underneath the biceps at the midhumeral level. The stimulating needle is introduced and its position adjusted until biceps contraction is elicited. Care must be taken not to introduce the needle into the biceps muscle itself, which could result in direct stimulation and contraction of the muscle but a failed block.

Transarterial Technique

If accidental puncture of the axillary artery occurs during the neurostimulation technique, evidenced by aspiration of blood, the needle should be advanced until blood is no longer aspirated. At this location, behind the artery, two-thirds of the local anesthetic is injected. The needle is then retracted slowly and the tip placed back inside the artery. When no blood is aspirated, the needle tip is located anterior to the axillary artery, and the remaining third of the local anesthetic is injected. Compression of the artery for a few minutes is advised to reduce the incidence of a hematoma.

Ultrasound Guidance

The patient is positioned as described earlier for the neurostimulation technique. The ultrasound probe is placed at the axillary level perpendicular to the forearm. The probe position is adjusted until a cross-sectional image of the axillary artery is obtained (Fig. 52.12). The axilla is a highly vascularized space, and releasing pressure from the probe typically exposes several axillary veins in the vicinity of the artery. The radial, median, and ulnar nerves are identified around the axillary artery as hyperechoic structures. There is significant individual variation in the position of the nerves relative to the artery. However, the radial nerve most often lies posterior to the artery, with the ulnar nerve being medial and the median nerve anterior to the axillary artery. Sequential scanning proximally and distally will reveal the trajectory of the musculocutaneous nerve and help identify it as a hypoechoic structure with a hyperechoic rim. Proximally, it lies closer to the axillary neurovascular bundle. When scanning distally, the practitioner can trace the nerve travelling toward the coracobrachialis muscle, lying between it and the biceps muscle.

The needle can be advanced from the lateral end of the probe in plane, and the needle position adjusted to allow local anesthetic spread around each nerve (Fig. 52.13).

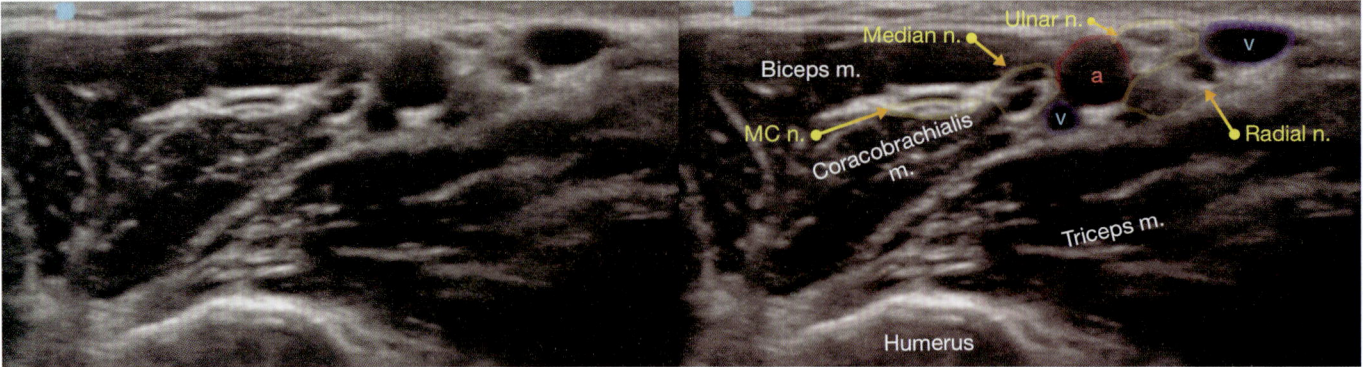

FIGURE 52.12   Axillary approach to the brachial plexus block. **Left:** Ultrasound image for the axillary anatomy. **Right:** Ultrasound image with anatomy labeled. a, axillary artery; v, axillary veins; m., muscle; MC n., musculocutaneous nerve; n., nerve. (*Reproduced with permission from Ouanes et al. http://anesthesiology.hopkinsmedicine.org/international-obstetric-and-regional-anesthesia/. Accessed July 18, 2018.*)

CLINICAL EFFECTS

Axillary brachial plexus block has been shown to provide several advantages over general anesthesia for outpatient hand surgery, including the ability to fast-track patients to phase 2, resulting in shorter PACU stays, better pain control, reduced opioid consumption prior to discharge, and lower incidence of nausea/vomiting.[220] The use of ultrasound guidance with axillary brachial plexus block has been associated with increased success rate, shorter time to onset of anesthesia, and reduced time to perform the block.[221] When studying novice practitioners, however, Barrington et al.[222] were unable to demonstrate any differences between ultrasound guidance and nerve stimulator techniques. A prospective review of axillary brachial plexus block-associated complications that included over 27,000 procedures confirmed the extremely safe profile of this block, with an overall incidence of postoperative neurologic symptoms of 0.37 per 10,000.[219]

Suprascapular and Axillary Nerve Block

INDICATIONS

Innervation to the shoulder joint from the brachial plexus is primarily carried out by the suprascapular and axillary nerves. In fact, the suprascapular nerve accounts for 70% of the sensory innervation of the shoulder.[223] Thus, the suprascapular nerve block (SSNB) has been widely used for analgesia in procedures involving the shoulder, particularly when an interscalene nerve block may be contraindicated (e.g., with severe pulmonary disease).

LANDMARKS

The suprascapular nerve emerges as a branch of the superior trunk and courses through the supraspinous groove toward the shoulder. The axillary nerve is a branch of the posterior cord.

ULTRASOUND TECHNIQUE

Positioning the ultrasound probe along the long axis of the supraspinous fossa (Fig. 52.14) enables visualization of the greater suprascapular notch. The suprascapular nerve and artery may also be visualized although not consistently. The needle is introduced in plane in a medial-to-lateral direction, and local anesthetic is deposited on the lateral aspect of the fossa, underneath the supraspinatus muscle (Fig. 52.15).

Axillary Nerve Block

The ultrasound probe is placed over the posterior surface of the humerus along its short axis, allowing visualization of the axillary artery and nerve in their short axis. Local anesthetic is deposited adjacent to the axillary artery on the posterior surface of the humerus (Fig. 52.16).

CLINICAL EFFECTS

SSNB is effective for providing analgesia in the postoperative period after shoulder surgery.[223,224] The combination of SSNB and axillary nerve block (ANB) provides superior analgesia and higher patient satisfaction after arthroscopic rotator cuff repair than SSNB alone.[225] SSNB and ANB combined with IV PCA has also proven to be a better analgesic choice than SSNB plus IV PCA, or IV PCA alone.[226] Dhir et al.[227] reported differences between the analgesic profile of SSNB combined with

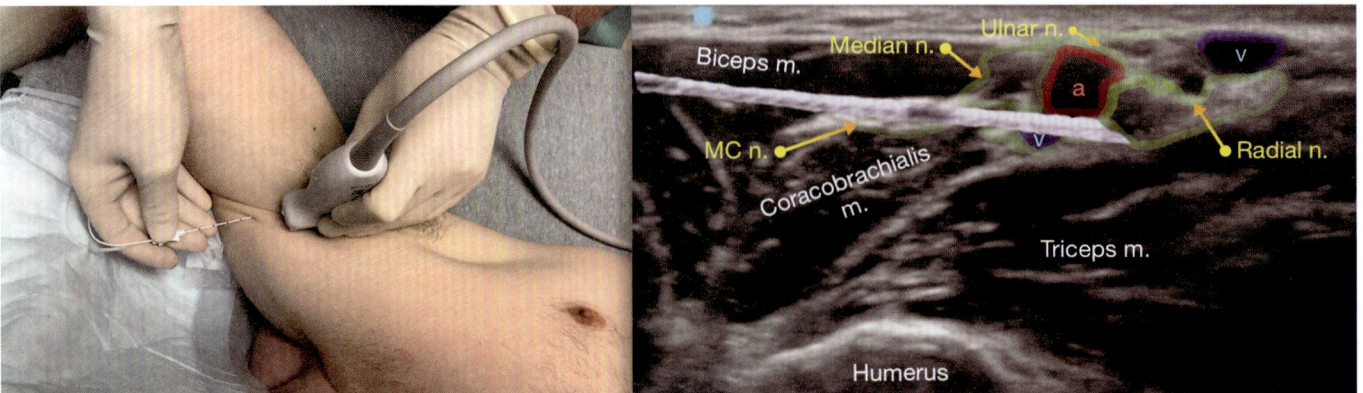

FIGURE 52.13   Axillary approach to the brachial plexus block. **Left:** In-plane needle insertion approach. **Right:** Corresponding ultrasound image. a, axillary artery; m., muscle; MC n., musculocutaneous nerve; n., nerve; v, axillary veins. (*Reproduced with permission from Ouanes et al. http://anesthesiology.hopkinsmedicine.org/international-obstetric-and-regional-anesthesia/. Accessed July 18, 2018.*)

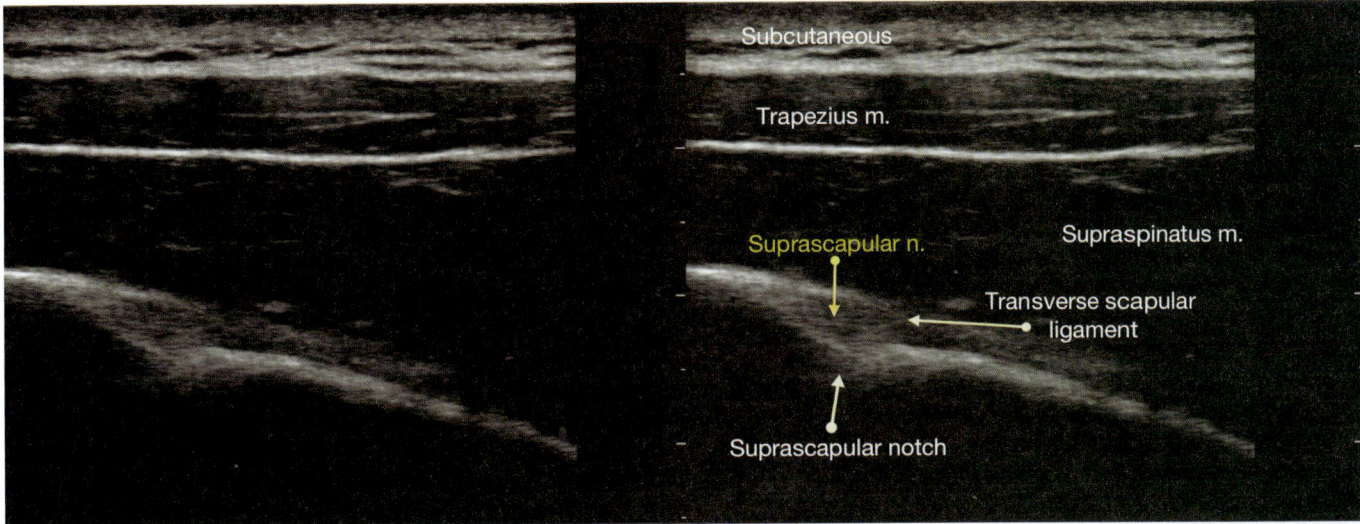

FIGURE 52.14 Suprascapular nerve block. **Left:** Ultrasound image for the suprascapular anatomy. **Right:** Ultrasound image with anatomy labeled. m., muscle; n., nerve. *(Reproduced with permission from Ouanes et al. http://anesthesiology.hopkinsmedicine.org/international-obstetric-and-regional-anesthesia/. Accessed July 18, 2018.)*

ANB and the profile of ISB. In their prospective randomized study, SSNB in combination with ANB provided better pain relief for patients at rest, with fewer side effects, whereas ISB was associated with better analgesia in the first 6 postoperative days. This difference in analgesic profile is consistent with a prior study by Pitombo et al.[228] who also described a significantly lower degree of motor blockade with the combination of SSNB and ANB. Combining ISB with SSNB provides superior analgesia to ISB alone within 48 hours after arthroscopic rotator cuff repair.[229]

Brachial Plexus Terminal Branch Blocks at the Elbow and Below

INDICATIONS
Blockade of the terminal branches of the brachial plexus at the elbow can offer certain advantages over more proximal blocks. It allows the possibility of selectively blocking a specific sensory distribution of the hand while preserving motor function of the proximal upper limb.[230] Distal blocks may cause more patient discomfort if multiple nerves are blocked, as they usually require a separate injection for each nerve. The nerve paths at this level are further restricted by surrounding muscular structures, potentially making these locations more susceptible to nerve injury associated with compression ischemia.

TECHNIQUES
Nerve Stimulation
The median nerve can be blocked by introducing the stimulating needle 2 cm above the elbow and 2 cm medial to the point at which the brachial artery is palpated. Needle position is adjusted to obtain the corresponding motor response (forearm pronation, flexion of second and third digits, thumb opposition), and then, 5 mL of local anesthetic is injected.

The ulnar nerve runs in the canal between the olecranon and the medial epicondyle. This canal is narrow and superficial, making the nerve at this point susceptible to lesion from direct needle trauma or increased pressure from the injectate. Consequently, the block is performed 1 to 2 cm proximal to this canal. The elicited motor response includes flexion of the fourth and fifth digits and wrist flexion toward the ulnar side.

To block the radial nerve at the elbow, the practitioner palpates the biceps tendon 1 to 2 cm proximal to the elbow and introduces the stimulating needle lateral to it. Radial nerve

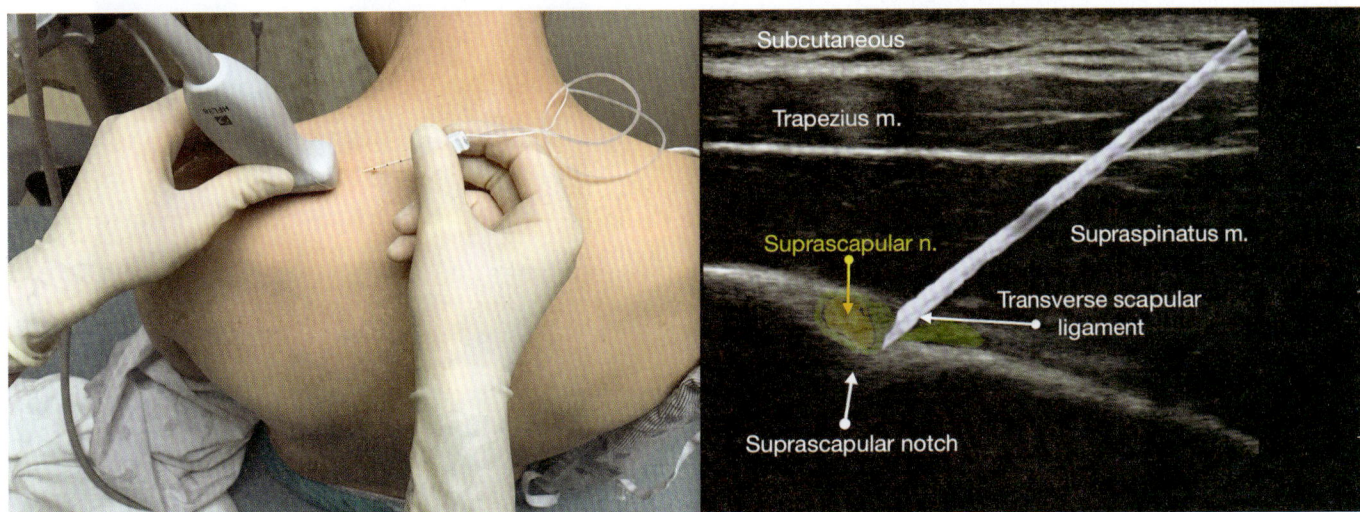

FIGURE 52.15 Needle approach and sonoanatomy for suprascapular nerve block. **Left:** In-plane needle insertion approach. **Right:** Corresponding ultrasound image. m., muscle; n., nerve. *(Reproduced with permission from Ouanes et al. http://anesthesiology.hopkinsmedicine.org/international-obstetric-and-regional-anesthesia/. Accessed July 18, 2018.)*

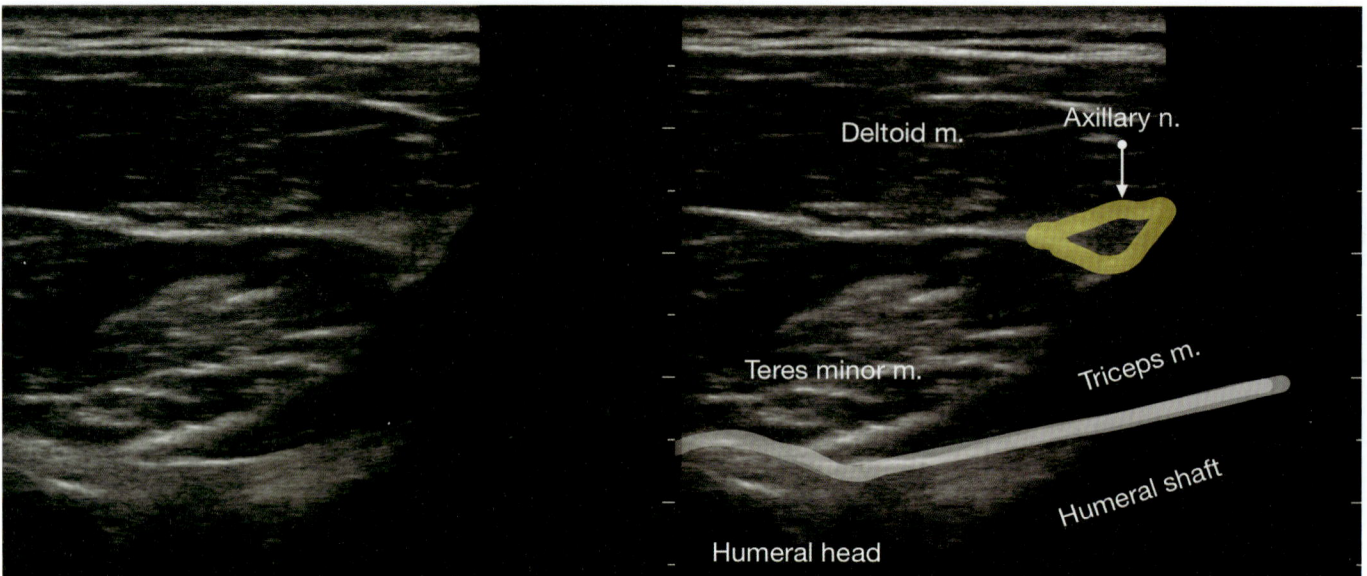

FIGURE 52.16 Axillary nerve block. **Left:** Ultrasound image for the axillary nerve anatomy. **Right:** Ultrasound image with anatomy labeled. *(Reproduced with permission from Ouanes et al. http://anesthesiology.hopkinsmedicine.org/international-obstetric-and-regional-anesthesia/. Accessed July 18, 2018.)*

stimulation should elicit extension of the hand and forearm as well as forearm supination.

Ultrasound Guidance
The individual nerves can be blocked at various locations. At the elbow, proximal forearm and midforearm are described (Fig. 52.17).

Median Nerve Block
The median nerve can be block at various locations. The patient is positioned supine with the arm abducted and forearm supinated. The nerve can be visualized in the A position medial to the brachial artery (see Figs. 52.17 and 52.18) as well as in the B and C positions of Figure 52.17 (see also Figs. 52.19 and 52.20).

Ulnar Nerve Block
With the patient supine and the arm straight and supinated, the ultrasound probe is placed over the ulnar artery at the wrist and traced proximally. The ulnar nerve can be seen medial to the artery. Eventually, the ultrasound probe is moved further away to rest in between the flexor carpi ulnaris and flexor digitorus profundus (see Figs. 52.17, 52.19, and 52.21).[230]

Radial Nerve Block
The patient is positioned supine with the arm abducted and forearm supinated. The radial nerve is visualized lying adjacent to the radius bone. It is flanked by the pronator teres muscle medially and by the brachioradialis muscle, the extensor carpi ulnaris longus muscle, and supinator muscle laterally (see Figs. 52.20 and 52.22).

CLINICAL EFFECTS
For most outpatient hand and wrist bone surgeries, an effective anesthetic and analgesic plan includes selective distal blocks with long-acting local anesthetics without vasoconstrictors like epinephrine and a concomitant axillary block with short-acting local anesthetic.[231] This combination allows for muscle function preservation in the proximal upper limb. The presence of motor block in the affected limb in the immediate postoperative period has been associated with lower patient satisfaction.[232] A prospective study that compared proximal brachial plexus blocks to terminal branch blocks performed at the level of the forearm for hand surgery found no differences in adequacy as a primary anesthetic, postoperative

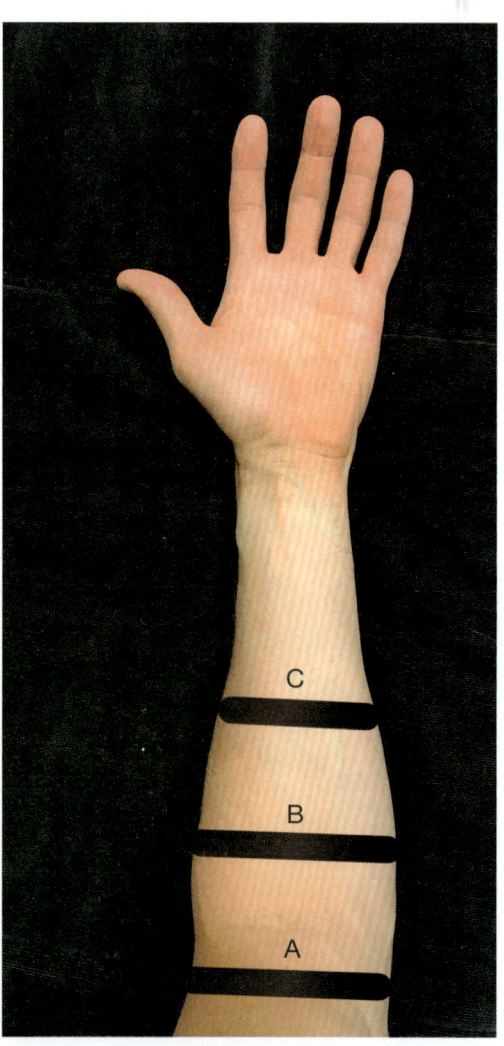

FIGURE 52.17 Terminal branch blocks: at the elbow (A), proximal forearm (B), and midforearm (C). *(Reproduced with permission from Ouanes et al. http://anesthesiology.hopkinsmedicine.org/international-obstetric-and-regional-anesthesia/. Accessed July 18. 2018.)*

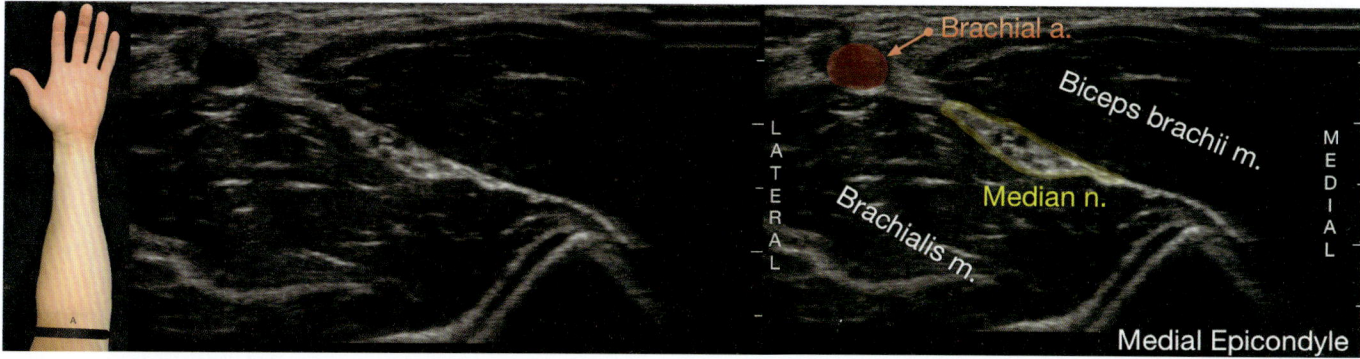

FIGURE 52.18 Median nerve at the elbow. **Left:** Location of the ultrasound cross-section. **Middle:** Ultrasound anatomy image at the elbow. **Right:** Corresponding image with anatomy labeled. a., artery; m., muscle; n., nerve. *(Reproduced with permission from Ouanes et al. http://anesthesiology.hopkinsmedicine.org /international-obstetric-and-regional-anesthesia/. Accessed July 18, 2018.)*

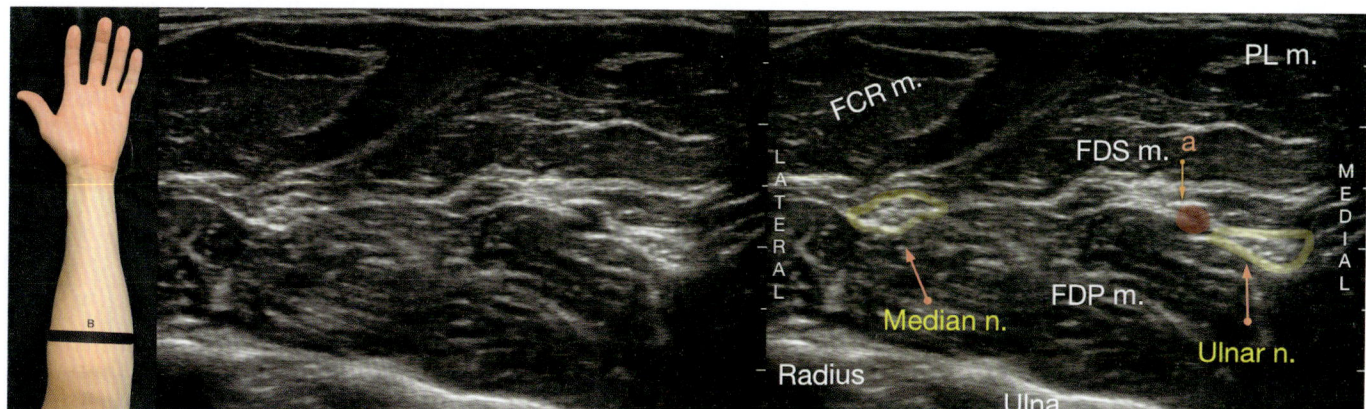

FIGURE 52.19 Median and ulnar nerves at the proximal forearm. **Left:** Location of the ultrasound cross-section. **Middle:** Ultrasound anatomy image at the proximal forearm. **Right:** Corresponding image with anatomy labeled. a, artery; FCR m., flexor carpi radialis muscle; FDP m., flexor digitorum profundus muscle; FDS m., flexor digitorum superficialis muscle; n., nerve; PL m., palmaris longus muscle. *(Reproduced with permission from Ouanes et al. http://anesthesiology.hopkinsmedicine.org/international-obstetric-and-regional-anesthesia/. Accessed July 18, 2018.)*

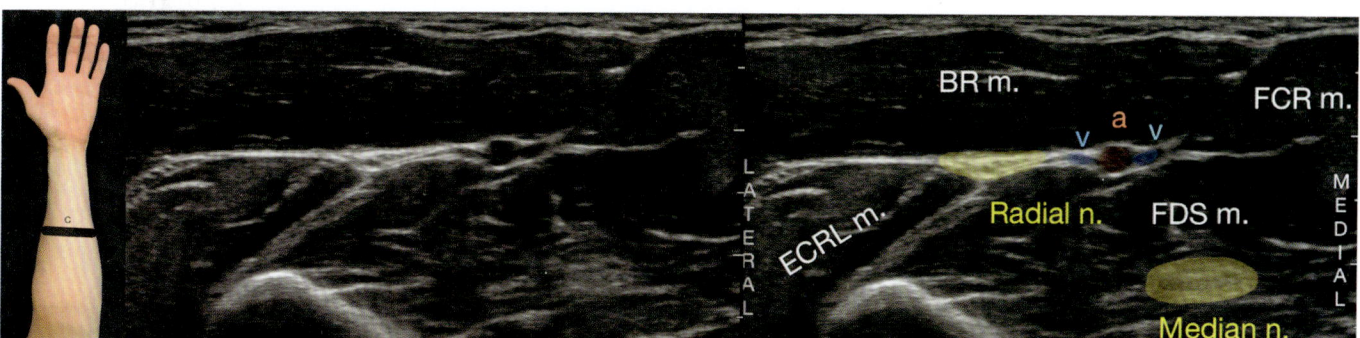

FIGURE 52.20 Median and radial nerves at the midforearm. **Left:** Location of the ultrasound cross-section. **Middle:** Ultrasound anatomy image at the midforearm. **Right:** Corresponding image with anatomy labeled. a, radial artery; BR m., brachioradialis muscle; ECRL m., extensor carpi radialis longus muscle; FCR m., flexor carpi radialis muscle; FDS m., flexor digitorum superficialis muscle; v, medial antebrachial vein. *(Reproduced with permission from Ouanes et al. http://anesthesiology.hopkinsmedicine.org/international-obstetric-and-regional-anesthesia/. Accessed July 18, 2018.)*

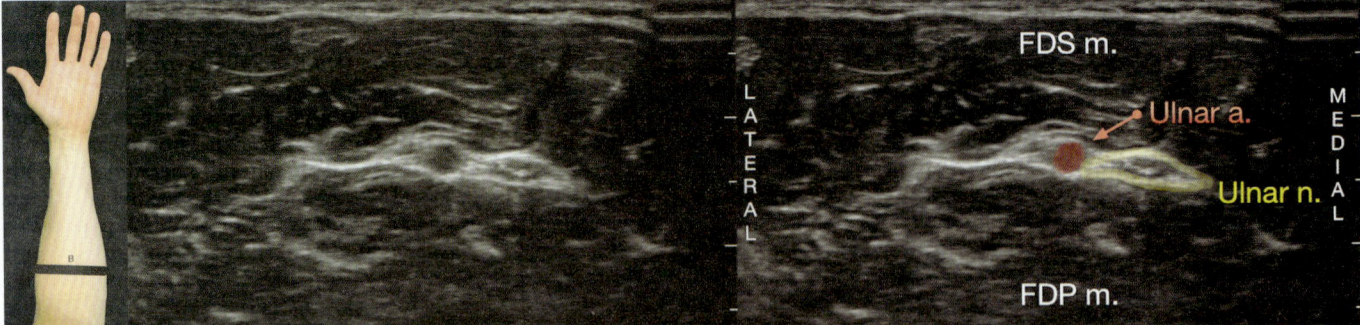

FIGURE 52.21   Ulnar nerve at the proximal forearm. **Left:** Location of the ultrasound cross-section. **Middle:** Ultrasound anatomy image at the proximal forearm. **Right:** Corresponding image with anatomy labeled. FDP m., flexor digitorum profundus muscle; FDS m., flexor digitorum superficialis muscle. (*Reproduced with permission from Ouanes et al. http://anesthesiology.hopkinsmedicine.org/international-obstetric-and-regional-anesthesia/. Accessed July 18, 2018.*)

pain scores, or opioid consumption.[233] However, terminal branch blocks at the level of the elbow will not prevent tourniquet pain in an unsedated patient because upper arm cutaneous innervation is supplied by the medial cutaneous nerve, musculocutaneous nerve, posterior cutaneous nerve, and intercostobrachial nerve.

Paravertebral Nerve Block

INDICATIONS AND LANDMARKS

Paravertebral nerve blocks (PVBs) provide anesthesia and analgesia to the thorax and abdomen. They have been successfully described for breast surgery, thoracotomy, thoracoscopy, nephrectomy, hip surgery, cardiac surgery, and lung transplant surgery.[234-238] The goal of the PVB is to deposit local anesthetic in the paravertebral space adjacent to the vertebral bodies, where spinal nerves emerge from the spinal canal and bifurcate into the ventral and dorsal rami. This space is delineated medially by the vertebral bodies and discs and the intervertebral foramina; anterolateral by the parietal pleura at the thoracic levels or iliopsoas muscle; and posterolateral by the ribs, transverse processes, and intercostal spaces. The epidural space is a continuous space in the craniocaudal dimension. Therefore, local anesthetic injected at one level will spread to adjacent levels. Contralateral spread occurs in approximately 10% of cases. PVBs can be performed with single-injection or continuous techniques.

TECHNIQUES
Landmark Technique

The patient is positioned sitting up with the neck and back flexed. The spinous processes are identified and marked. Additional marks are made 2.5 cm laterally from the spinous process on the side intended to block, which will correspond with the transverse process (Fig. 52.23). The needle is introduced at the lateral mark, perpendicular to the skin, until contact is made with the transverse process. Contact occurs at a depth of 2 to 4 cm, depending on the body habitus of the patient. If the transverse process is not encountered at 4 cm, the needle is redirected cephalad or caudad. Continuing to advance without prior contact with the transverse process carries the risk of pleural puncture. Regardless of body habitus, the paravertebral space is typically located 1 cm beyond the transverse process at the thoracic levels, or 0.5 cm at the lumbar levels because the transverse processes are thinner in this area. After contacting the transverse process, the needle is redirected caudad, walked off the transverse process, and advanced 1 cm (0.5 in the lumbar area) into the paravertebral space. It may be possible to feel a loss of resistance as the needle is advanced through the superior costotransverse ligament at the thoracic levels. However, this sensation can be very subtle and difficult to appreciate.

Ultrasound Technique
Transverse Approach

The ultrasound probe is placed transversally over the midline at the level intended to block (Figs. 52.24 and 52.25). The acoustic shadow of the spinous process is identified, along with the transverse process and costotransverse joint. The probe is then moved cephalad or caudad over the intercostal space, which allows for visualization of the pleura. The needle is introduced in plane and the local anesthetic deposited at the corner formed by the transverse process and pleura.[235,239]

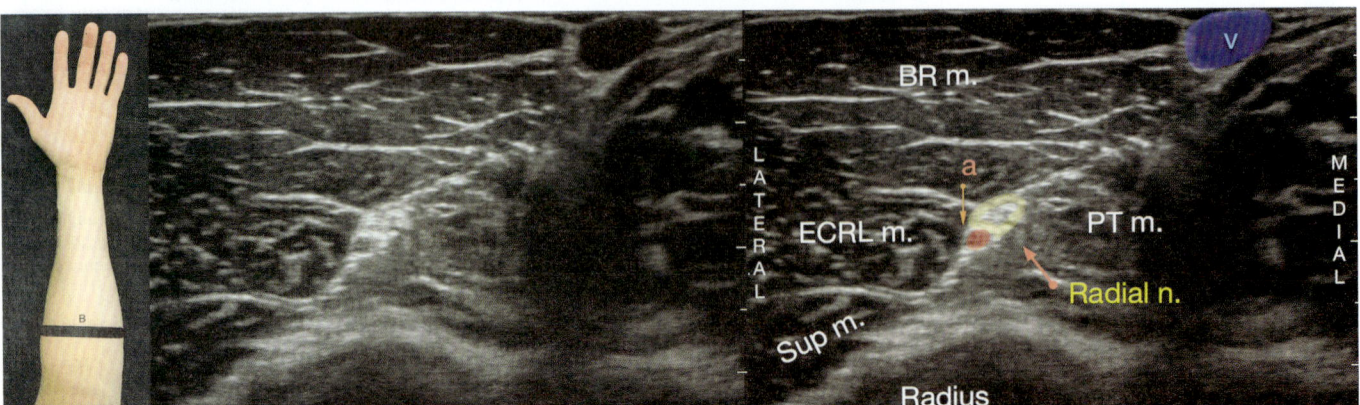

FIGURE 52.22   Radial nerve at the proximal forearm. **Left:** Location of the ultrasound cross-section. **Middle:** Ultrasound anatomy image at the proximal forearm. **Right:** Corresponding image with anatomy labeled. a, radial artery; BR m., brachioradialis muscle; ECRL m., extensor carpi radialis longus muscle; PT m., pronator teres muscle; Sup m., supinator muscle; v, medial antebrachial vein. (*Reproduced with permission from Ouanes et al. http://anesthesiology.hopkinsmedicine.org/international-obstetric-and-regional-anesthesia/. Accessed July 18, 2018.*)

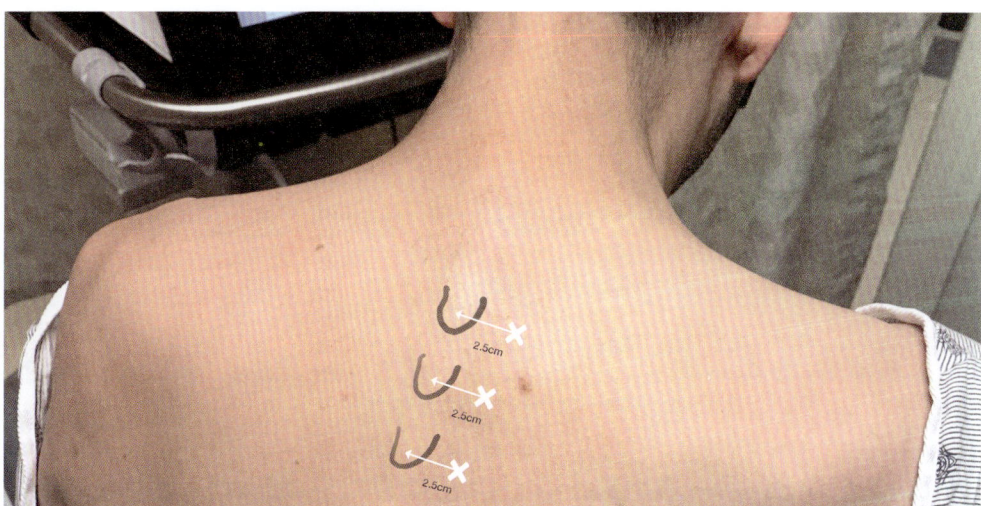

FIGURE 52.23 Thoracic paravertebral block landmarks.

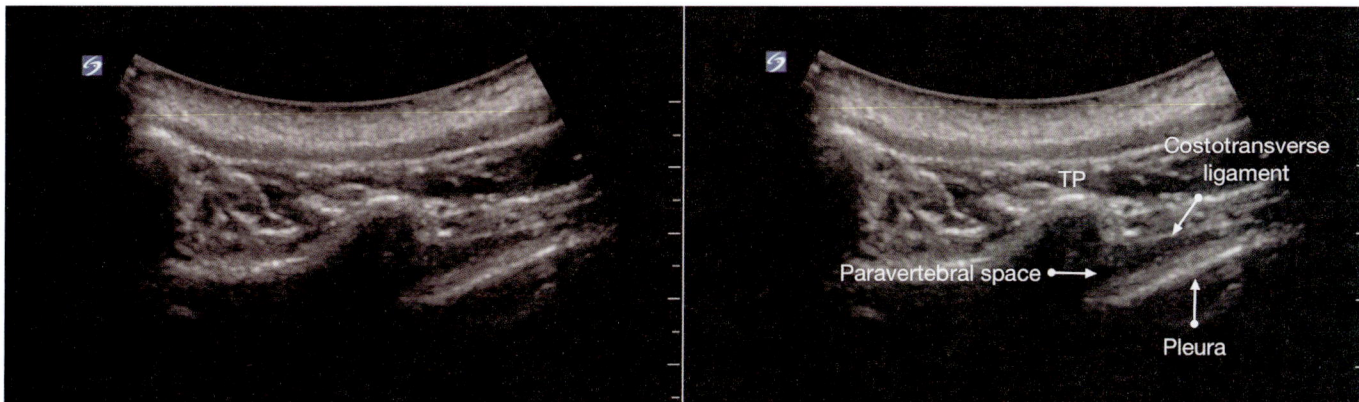

FIGURE 52.24 Thoracic paravertebral block transverse approach. **Left:** Ultrasound image for the transverse thoracic paravertebral anatomy. **Right:** Ultrasound image with anatomy labeled. TP, transversus process. *(Reproduced with permission from Ouanes et al. http://anesthesiology.hopkinsmedicine.org /international-obstetric-and-regional-anesthesia/. Accessed July 18, 2018.)*

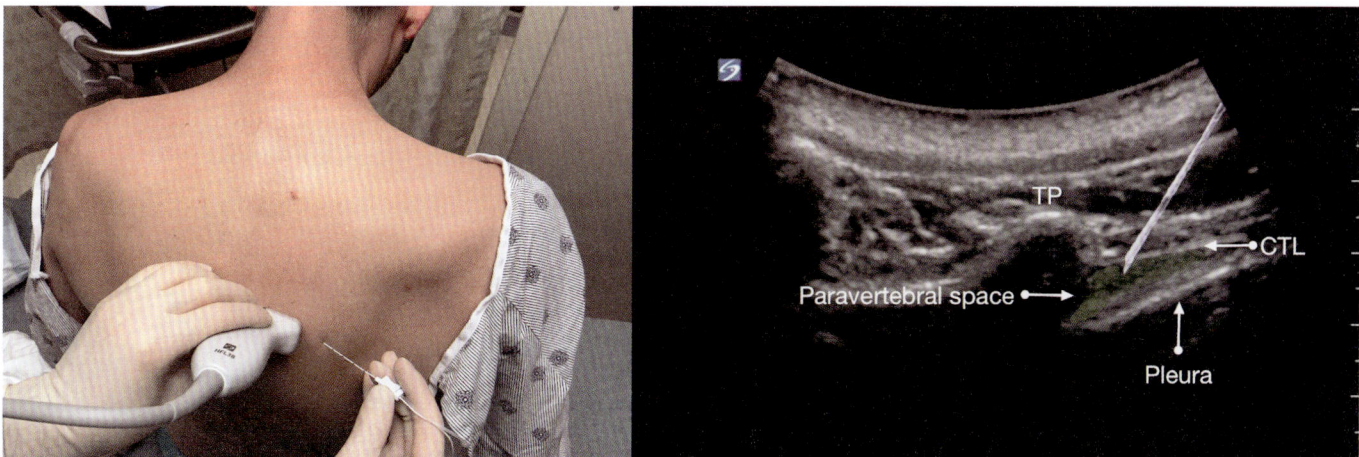

FIGURE 52.25 Needle approach and sonoanatomy for the transverse thoracic paravertebral block. **Left:** In-plane needle insertion approach. **Right:** Corresponding labeled ultrasound image. CTL, costotransverse ligament; TP, transversus process. *(Reproduced with permission from Ouanes et al. http://anesthesiology.hopkinsmedicine.org/international-obstetric-and-regional-anesthesia/. Accessed July 18, 2018.)*

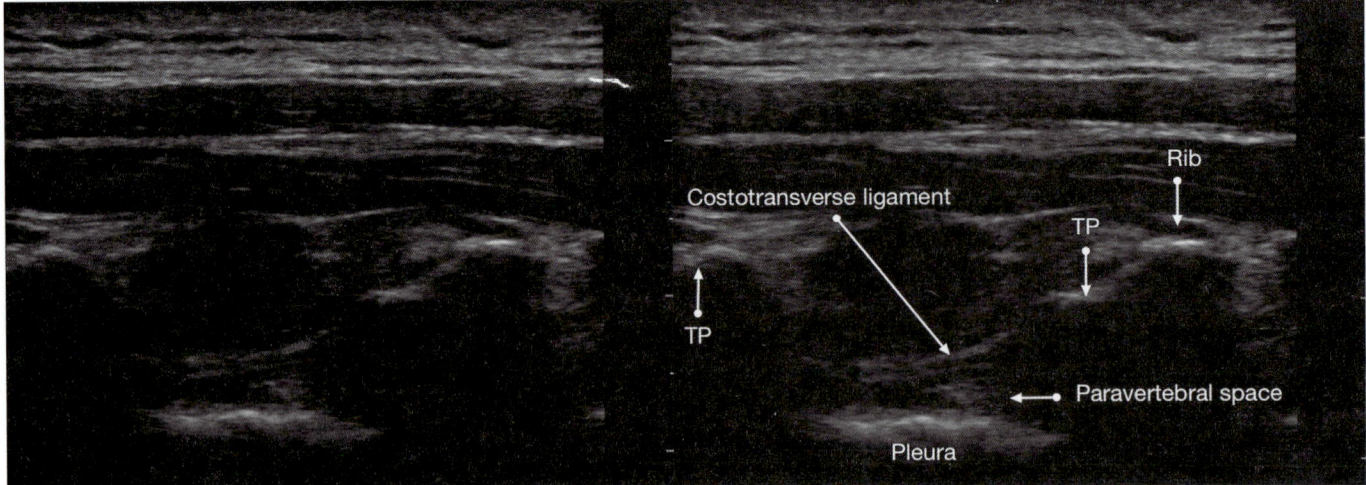

FIGURE 52.26 Thoracic paravertebral block parasagittal approach. **Left:** Ultrasound image for the parasagittal thoracic paravertebral anatomy. **Right:** Ultrasound image with anatomy labeled. TP, transversus process. *(Reproduced with permission from Ouanes et al. http://anesthesiology.hopkinsmedicine .org/international-obstetric-and-regional-anesthesia/. Accessed July 18, 2018.)*

Parasagittal Approach

The ultrasound probe is placed longitudinally 5 to 10 cm lateral to midline. At this level, the ribs are visualized in their short axis as curved structures with an acoustic shadow and the parietal pleura underneath. The probe is then slid medially and scanned over the level of the transverse processes, which appear as more square osseous structures. A slight tilt of the probe laterally will improve visualization of the pleura. The needle can be advanced in plane or out of plane into the paravertebral space (Figs. 52.26 and 52.27).[240] Injection of local anesthetic causes depression of the parietal pleura and spread to the adjacent levels.

CONTRAINDICATIONS

In addition to the general contraindications for PNBs, empyema and tumor invading the paravertebral space are specific for PVB. The same considerations for coagulopathy and neuraxial anesthesia apply to PVB.

CLINICAL EFFECTS

PVBs are effective in providing analgesia after breast cancer surgery and have been shown to decrease pain scores and mean opioid consumption up to 72% both intraoperatively and postoperatively,[235]

decrease opioid-related side effects, shorten hospitalization, and possibly decrease chronic postsurgical pain at 6 months.[239] Some of these benefits might be greatest in patients undergoing bilateral mastectomies with simultaneous breast reconstruction.[241] However, many of these benefits have been replicated in studies involving post-mastectomy breast reconstructions.[242,243] Multilevel PVB is associated with better postoperative pain control with movement as well as decreased analgesic consumption.[239,244] During infusion, continuous PVB has the additional benefit of improving analgesia and decreasing functional deficit, compared with single-injection techniques.[245] A recent study reported that PVB provided effective postoperative analgesia after thoracotomy, albeit inferior to that of epidurals.[246] However, two recent meta-analyses found no difference in pain analgesic efficacy and reported that PVB was associated with less hypotension, nausea and vomiting, and urinary retention than epidurals were.[237,238]

Nerve Blocks of the Lumbar Plexus

INDICATIONS AND LANDMARKS

The lumbar plexus (LP) is formed within the psoas muscle from the anterior rami of T12–L4. The branches of LP are

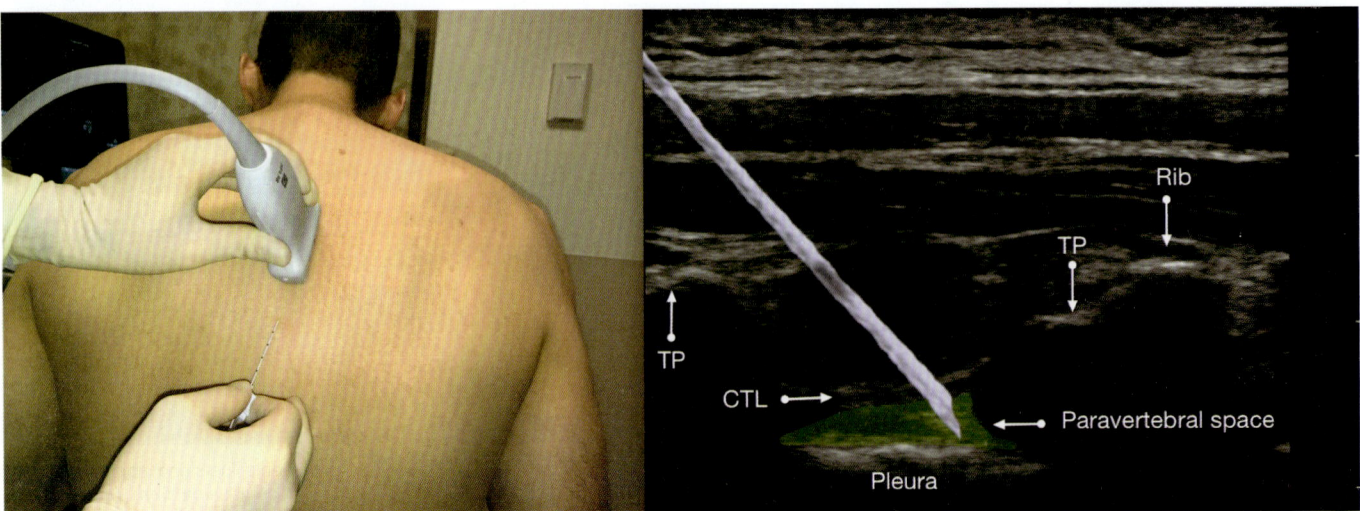

FIGURE 52.27 Needle approach and sonoanatomy for the parasagittal thoracic paravertebral block. **Left:** In-plane needle insertion approach. **Right:** Corresponding labeled ultrasound image. CTL, costotransverse ligament; TP, transversus process. *(Reproduced with permission from Ouanes et al. http://anesthesiology.hopkinsmedicine.org/international-obstetric-and-regional-anesthesia/. Accessed July 18, 2018.)*

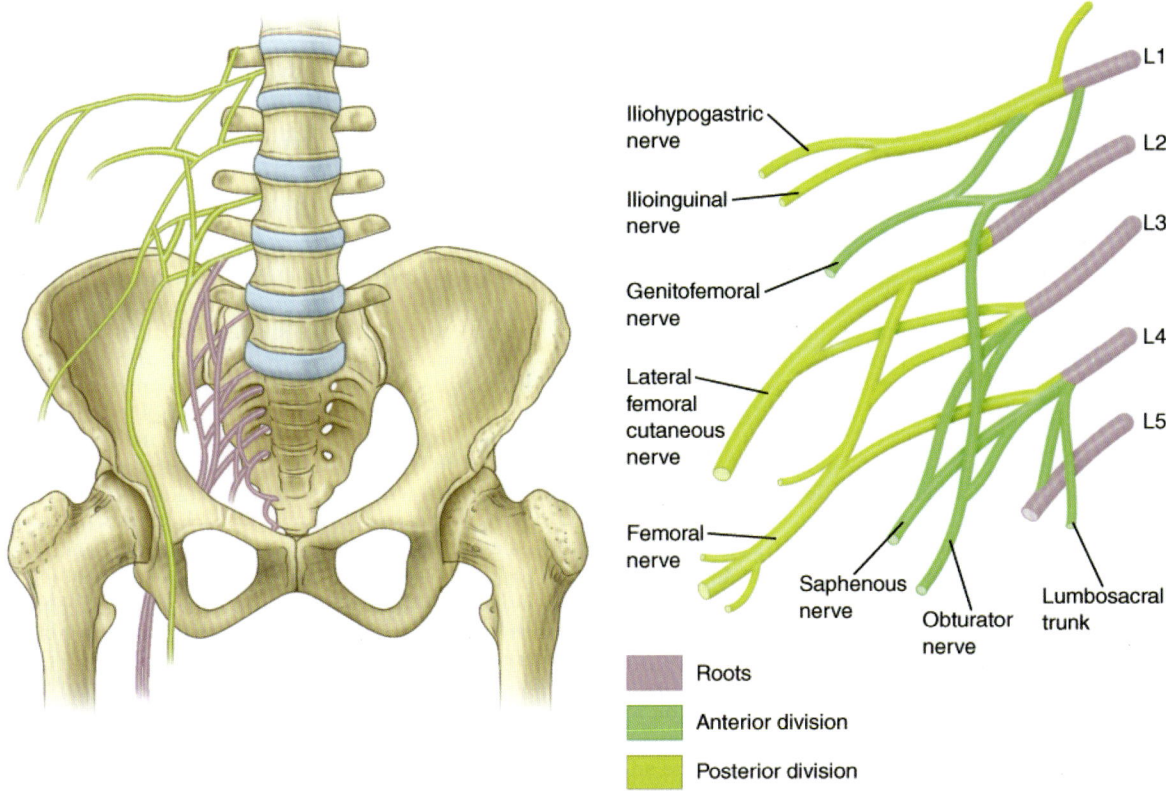

FIGURE 52.28 Lumbar plexus anatomy. *(Reprinted with permission from Anderson MK. Foundations of Athletic Training. 5th ed. Baltimore, MD: Lippincott Williams & Wilkins; 2012. Figure 12-4.)*

the iliohypogastric (T12–L1), ilioinguinal (L1), genitofemoral (L1–L2), lateral femoral cutaneous (L2–L3), femoral (L2–L4), and obturator nerves (L2–L4)[247] (Fig. 52.28). Of these, the femoral, lateral femoral cutaneous, and obturator nerves are most important for lower extremity surgery.

The LP block, also known as the psoas compartment block, was first described in 1976 by Chayen et al.[248] It is a deep block of the LP, and the local anesthetic is deposited within the body of the psoas muscle. At the L4 level, it is thought to be the most consistent approach to block the entire LP with a single injection; however, it consistently provides anesthesia or analgesia in the distributions of the femoral, lateral femoral cutaneous, and the obturator nerves.[249]

TECHNIQUES
Landmark Technique
There are two common methods of landmark-based nerve stimulation-assisted LP block.

For both techniques, the patient is placed in the lateral decubitus position with the operative side up (Fig. 52.29). Both mark palpated anatomy. In the first approach, the practitioner palpates the iliac crests and follows an imaginary line to the spinous processes of the lumbar spine to approximately the L4 spinous process. An insulated needle is inserted 4 cm lateral to the spinous process perpendicular to the skin and advanced until a quadriceps twitch is elicited or until bone is contacted. When the needle contacts bone, it is redirected off the bone either cephalad or caudad and advanced approximately 2 cm until quadriceps stimulation is obtained with current between 0.5 and 1 mA. If quadriceps stimulation is not elicited and no bony contact is made, the practitioner should reassess the landmarks.

The second commonly described landmark technique follows the same nerve stimulation principles with slightly modified landmarks (see Fig. 52.29). A line is drawn between the two iliac crests and another is drawn connecting the lumbar

spinous processes. A third line is drawn through the posterior inferior iliac spine. Finally, a line is drawn perpendicular to the other lines at the level of L4 and divided into thirds. The needle is inserted 1 cm cephalad to this line at the point of the lateral third marking.

Several descriptions of various techniques for the psoas compartment blocks have been described in the literature.[250–252]

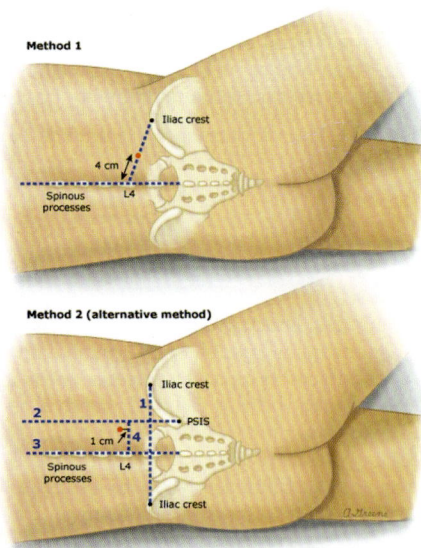

FIGURE 52.29 Landmark approaches to lumbar plexus (psoas compartment) block. PSIS, posterior superior iliac spine. *(Reproduced with permission from Jeng CL, Rosenblatt MA. Lower extremity nerve blocks: Techniques. In: UpToDate, Post TW [Ed], UpToDate, Waltham, MA. [Accessed on September 13, 2018.] Copyright © 2018 UpToDate, Inc. For more information visit www.uptodate.com.)*

All rely on bony contact with the transverse process as a guide to depth of needle placement. Chayen et al.[248] estimated the distance from the skin to the LP to be 8 cm in men (range, 6 to 10 cm) and 7 cm in women (range, 5 to 9 cm) based on CT images obtained in their patients. They found the depth of the LP from the transverse process to be consistently less than 2 cm. This relationship of transverse process to the LP was found to be independent of body mass index or gender. Thus, contact with the transverse process provides a consistent landmark to guide the user and help avoid very deep penetration.[248]

Ultrasound Guidance

Several descriptions of various techniques have been published for the use of ultrasound to guide peripheral blocks and sono-anatomy of the LP.[253,254] Using ultrasound guidance for the LP block is still challenging owing to the depth of the nerve and presence of the "acoustic shadow" formed by the transverse processes.[255,256] In clinical practice, ultrasound can be used for preprocedural scanning or for real-time guidance in combination with nerve stimulation.

With the patient in a lateral decubitus position, a curved array, low-frequency ultrasound is placed parasagittal at the lumbosacral junction. With the sacrum identified, the practitioner counts the transverse process of each vertebra cephalad until L2, L3, and L4 are identified. The longitudinal sonogram exhibits an acoustic shadow of the transverse processes produced, or what Karmakar et al.[253] call the trident sign because of its similarity to the trident (Fig. 52.30). They describe visualizing the roots of the LP within the psoas muscle in 60% of their patients. The needle is inserted from the caudal end of the probe and advanced through the space between the transverse processes of L3 and L4 into the posterior part of the psoas muscle. The needle takes a very steep angle in the plane view.[254] After negative aspiration, local anesthetic is injected, and its spread is observed within the muscle.

COMPLICATIONS

Unlike most other PNBs described, the American Society of Regional Anesthesia and Pain Medicine (ASRA) recommends that anticoagulation guidelines for neuraxial blocks be followed when performing an LP block because of its deep nature.[257]

This block has the highest incidence of complications among PNBs, although the estimated rate of complication is low overall.[249] The most common complication is neuraxial spread leading to bilateral block. Epidural spread is more common than total spinal.[247,249,258,259] Epidural spread after LP block has been reported with an incidence range from 27%[260] to 50%.[178] Cases of cardiac arrest after LP block have been reported in patients who were found to have high dermatomal block levels.[261] Other complications include injury to surrounding structures, including renal hematoma, pneumocele, total spinal anesthesia, and unintended intra-abdominal and intervertebral penetration.[247,249,258,259] Vascular injury can lead to retroperitoneal hematoma, which can go unnoticed for some time and lead to serious complications.[253,262,263] Dolan[263] pointed out in a letter to the editor that ultrasound LP allows for visualization of the

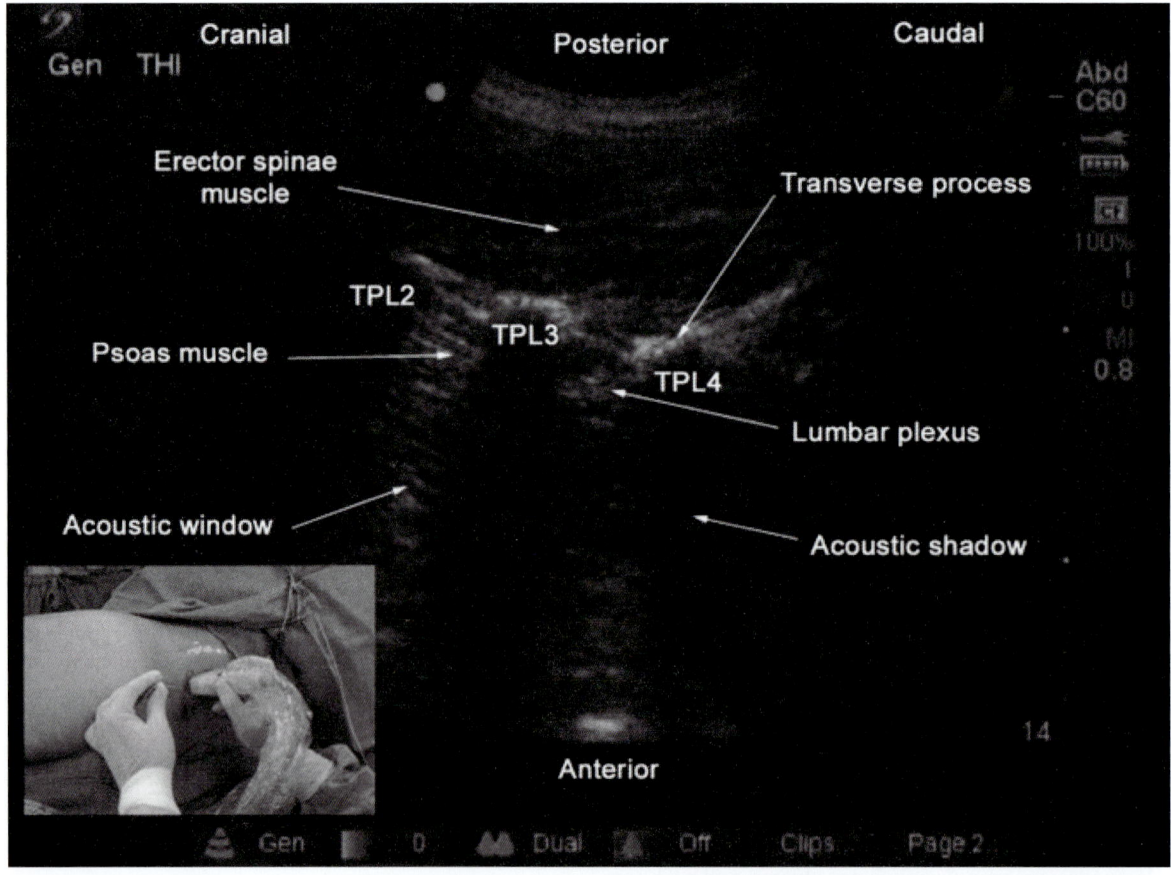

FIGURE 52.30 Longitudinal sonogram. Note the hyperechoic transverse processes with their acoustic shadow that produces the trident sign. The psoas muscle is seen in the acoustic window between the transverse processes and is recognized by its typical striated appearance. Part of the lumbar plexus is also seen as a hyperechoic shadow in the posterior part of the psoas muscle between the transverse processes of L3 (TPL3) and L4 (TPL4) vertebrae. The inset shows the orientation of the ultrasound transducer and the direction in which the needle is introduced (long axis) during an ultrasound-guided lumbar plexus block. TPL2, transverse process of L2 vertebra. (Reprinted from Karmakar MK, Ho AMH, Li X, et al. Ultrasound-guided lumbar plexus block through the acoustic window of the lumbar ultrasound trident. Br J Anaesth 2008;100[4]:533–537. Copyright © 2008 British Journal of Anaesthesia. With permission.)

distribution of local anesthetic in real time and may translate to fewer complications.[264]

To ensure the proper position of the needle during psoas compartment block and avoid excessive needle insertion, it is recommended that the transverse process be intentionally sought during the landmark approach.

CLINICAL EFFECTS

The LP block is usually used as a supplement to general anesthesia for pain control after lower extremity surgery. It may also be used as an alternative to neuraxial analgesia as a primary anesthetic to minimize the chance of sympathectomy and bilateral lower extremity block. However, if anesthesia of the lower leg or posterior thigh is required for the procedure, the sacral nerve roots must be blocked separately.[249]

LP block has been described as useful for hip and knee surgery.[265–268] The posterior approach provides analgesia to the lateral portions of the hip and knee joints.[269] In a prospective, randomized, blinded clinical trial that compared stimulating catheters and nonstimulating catheters for LP block, Cappelleri et al.[269] found that the minimum effective anesthetic volume was 12 mL with the stimulating catheter and 25 mL with the nonstimulating catheter. They reported 100% successful block in the stimulating catheter group and 69% success rate in the nonstimulating group.

Femoral Block

INDICATIONS

The femoral nerve is the main LP branch nerve (L2–L4) and responsible for sensation of the anterior medial skin of the thigh and medial leg from the tibia to the medial aspect of the foot, with articular branches innervating the hip and knee.[247] The femoral nerve block (FNB) provides adequate analgesia or anesthesia of the thigh, knee, and medial leg. It can be performed as a single injection or continuously via a catheter. The block usually requires supplementation as it does not completely cover the entire lower extremity. It usually requires supplementation with sacral plexus nerves if it is used as an anesthetic for the lower extremity.

LANDMARKS

The femoral nerve is one of the major branches of the LP. Consistently lateral to the femoral artery, it is encased by splitting of the fascia iliaca, superficial to the iliopsoas muscle. At the femoral triangle, from medial to lateral, one should locate the femoral vein (compressible), femoral artery (noncompressible/pulsating), and femoral nerve.

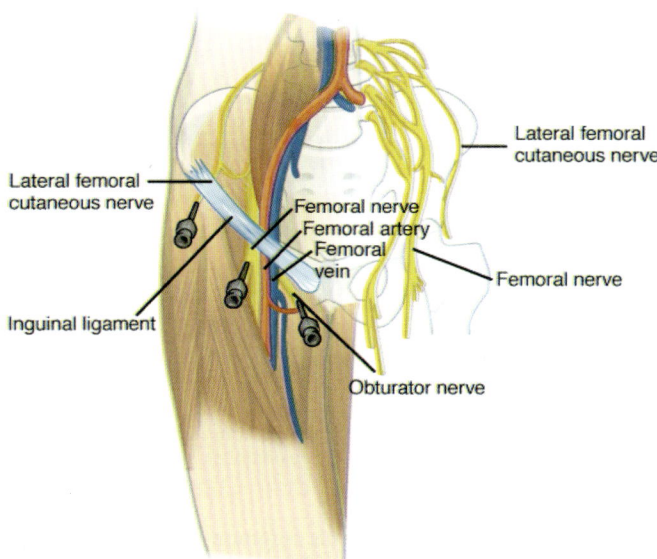

FIGURE 52.31 Anatomic landmarks for the (1) lateral femoral cutaneous, (2) femoral, and (3) obturator nerve blocks. *(Reprinted with permission from Yao FSF. Yao & Artusio's Anesthesiology. 8th ed. Baltimore, MD: Lippincott Williams & Wilkins; 2016. Figure 47.3.)*

TECHNIQUES

Nerve Stimulator-Guided Femoral Block

The common femoral artery and inguinal ligaments are palpated in the groin. The insulated needle is inserted just below the inguinal ligament and 1.5 cm lateral to the artery in an anterior-posterior direction. Stimulation of the femoral nerve produces a motor response of the quadriceps muscle. Optimal needle position is achieved when twitches are present between 0.3 and 0.5 mA. After negative aspiration, 20 to 30 mL of local anesthetic is injected in 5-mL increments, with aspiration between injections. A sartorius twitch, a band-like twitch along the medial side of the thigh, leads to unreliable analgesia because the sartorius branches run outside the femoral nerve sheath. The needle will need to be directed more posterior (Fig. 52.31).

Ultrasound Technique

With the patient supine, the practitioner places the ultrasound transducer in the inguinal crease to identify the sonoanatomy (Fig. 52.32). The hyperechoic femoral nerve can be visualized

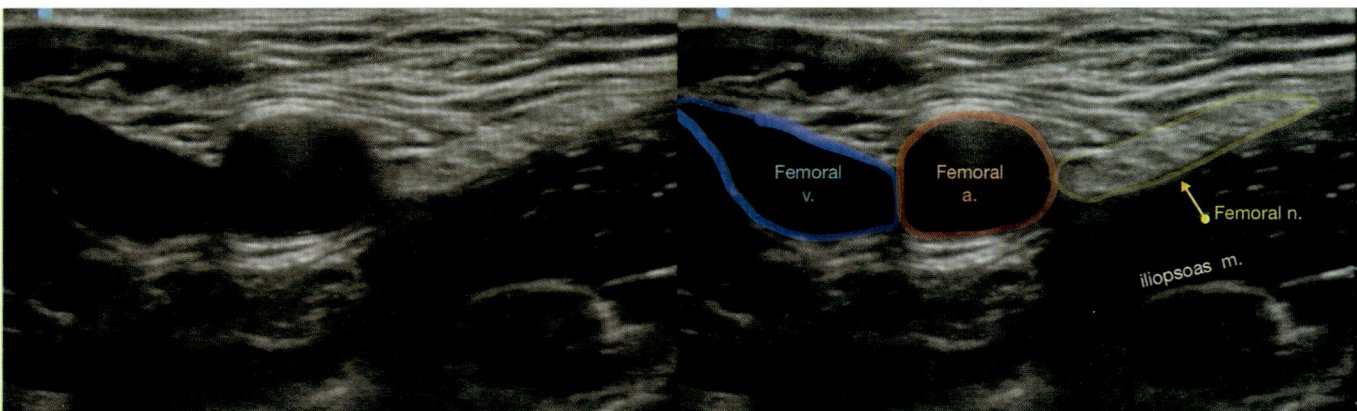

FIGURE 52.32 Femoral nerve block. **Left:** Ultrasound image for the femoral nerve sonoanatomy. **Right:** Ultrasound image with anatomy labeled. a., artery; m., muscle; n., nerve; v., vein. *(Reproduced with permission from Ouanes et al. http://anesthesiology.hopkinsmedicine.org/international-obstetric-and-regional-anesthesia/. Accessed July 18, 2018.)*

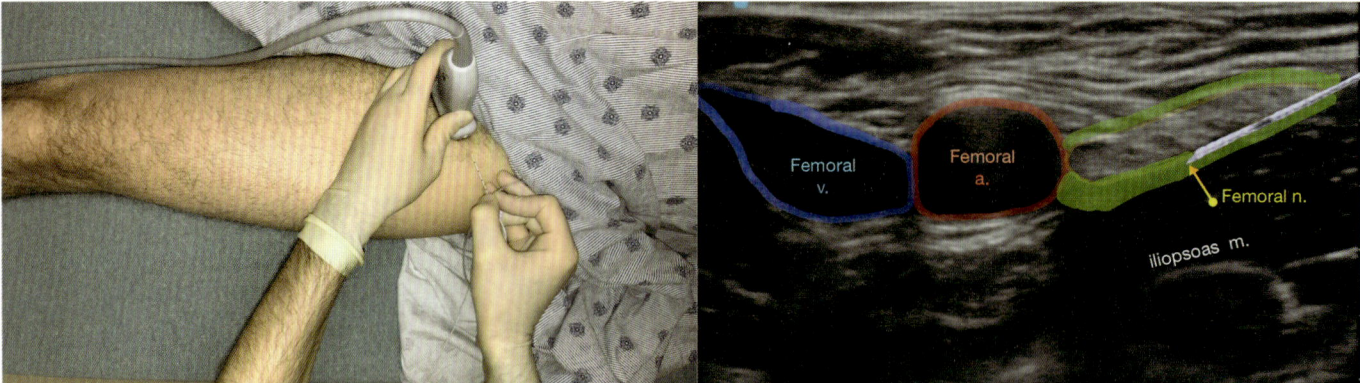

FIGURE 52.33 Patient position and transducer for in-plane femoral nerve block. **Left:** Femoral nerve block in-plane needle insertion approach. **Right:** Corresponding ultrasound image. *Green,* local anesthetic. a., artery; m., muscle; n., nerve; v., vein. *(Reproduced with permission from Ouanes et al. http://anesthesiology.hopkinsmedicine.org/international-obstetric-and-regional-anesthesia/. Accessed July 18, 2018.)*

lateral to the hypoechoic pulsatile common femoral artery and nonpulsatile femoral vein (Fig. 52.33). An in-plane or out-of-plane approach can be used. The needle is inserted and the tip placed adjacent to the nerve. The needle can be placed either above or below the femoral nerve. One should note that the nerve is enveloped in the fascia iliaca; if it is not penetrated, the block will be inadequate. Local anesthetic is injected adjacent to the nerve under ultrasound visualization (see Fig. 52.33).

COMPLICATIONS

Similar to other PNBs, complications include vascular puncture with subsequent local anesthetic toxicity, hematoma, and neurologic trauma.

Axillary and femoral PNCs pose a greater risk of infection than do other PNCs. The bacterial colonization rates have been reported to be between 13% and 57%. However, the progression to infection is between 0.05% and 3%.[270–272] Duration of catheter implant for more than 48 hours has been associated with increased risk of infection. Therefore, the block site should be examined daily for signs of inflammation.

Because of the high incidence of quadriceps weakness after FNB, adductor canal blocks (ACB) have become more popular as a postoperative analgesia choice for ambulating patients.

CLINICAL EFFECTS

When compared to IV opioids, FNBs have been shown to improve outcome after major knee and vascular surgery of the lower extremity.[273–275] Femoral nerve catheters used to be very popular for pain control after total knee arthroscopy (TKA). The perineural catheter offers an advantage over single injections as the postsurgical pain usually outlasts the duration of the longest acting single-injection PNB,[276,277] and a single-injection nerve block with a bolus of local anesthetic results in profound sensory and motor block.[278] A dense sensory and motor block provides excellent pain control, but it is undesirable because it inhibits quadriceps function mobilization.[278–280] A meta-analysis from 2013 highlights the evidence regarding FNB efficacy for postoperative pain control in patients with TKA.[281] The authors report that FNB as either a single injection or a continuous infusion provides better pain control than PCA alone.[281]

Continuous infusion of dilute ropivacaine (0.2% at 5 to 8 mL per hour) has been the recommended local anesthetic for continuous femoral nerve catheters. This dosing has been shown to provide adequate analgesia while minimizing motor block.[282] A Cochrane review showed that FNB was superior to PCA for other outcomes in addition to pain control. Chan et al.[283] reported higher patient satisfaction, less nausea and vomiting, and improved postoperative range of motion. They also reported

that continuous FNB provided equivalent analgesia for TKA with fewer side effects than epidural techniques.

Using a PNC after TKA is not without risk. A meta-analysis by Johnson et al.[284] suggested that patients who received a PNC were at greater risk for perioperative falls than were patients who received either single-injection PNB or no block. The concern for falls is legitimate as femoral nerve blockade does result in quadriceps weakness.[285] Memtsoudis et al.[286] sites the incidence of fall for patients after TKA as 1.6%. They did not attribute use of PNB to an increased risk for fall. Hence, caution should be used when mobilizing postsurgical patients with blocked lower extremities because of residual quadriceps weakness.

Adductor Canal Block

INDICATIONS

Enhanced recovery pathways and expedited early mobilization pathways after TKA have led clinicians to search for PNB sites that have minimal effect on ambulation while providing postoperative analgesia.[287] Concern has been raised over the quadriceps weakness and delayed rehabilitation caused by the FNB. These concerns have led to growing support for the ACB (Fig. 52.34).

The ACB technique was introduced in 2009 as a feasibility study.[288] In 2011, Lund et al.[289] compared quadriceps strength after ACB and FNB in a randomized controlled trial. ACB offered the potential advantage of preserving quadriceps strength[288,289] while providing pain relief comparable to that of FNB.[290] Additionally, in a placebo-controlled, double-blind, randomized controlled trial, Nader et al.[291] found that the ACB effectively reduced pain and opioid requirements in the postoperative period for TKA patients.

Three meta-analyses and systematic reviews have compared ACB and FNB.[292–294] In a meta-analysis and systematic review of randomized controlled trials, Jiang et al.[292] evaluated the efficacy and safety of the ACB for early postoperative pain management in patients undergoing TKA. The pooled results showed that the ACB resulted in less postoperative analgesic consumption than the saline group and less pain at rest and during activity. FNB and ACB had similar effects on postoperative analgesic consumption and pain, but the quadriceps strength and ability to ambulate were better in the ACB group. The two groups had similar rate of complications.

Compared with placebo groups, patients receiving ACB have demonstrated decreased perioperative opioid requirements, decreased pain during active range of motion, and early ambulation.[295,296] A noninferiority study by Abdallah et al.[297] found that when compared with FNB, the ACB preserved quadriceps

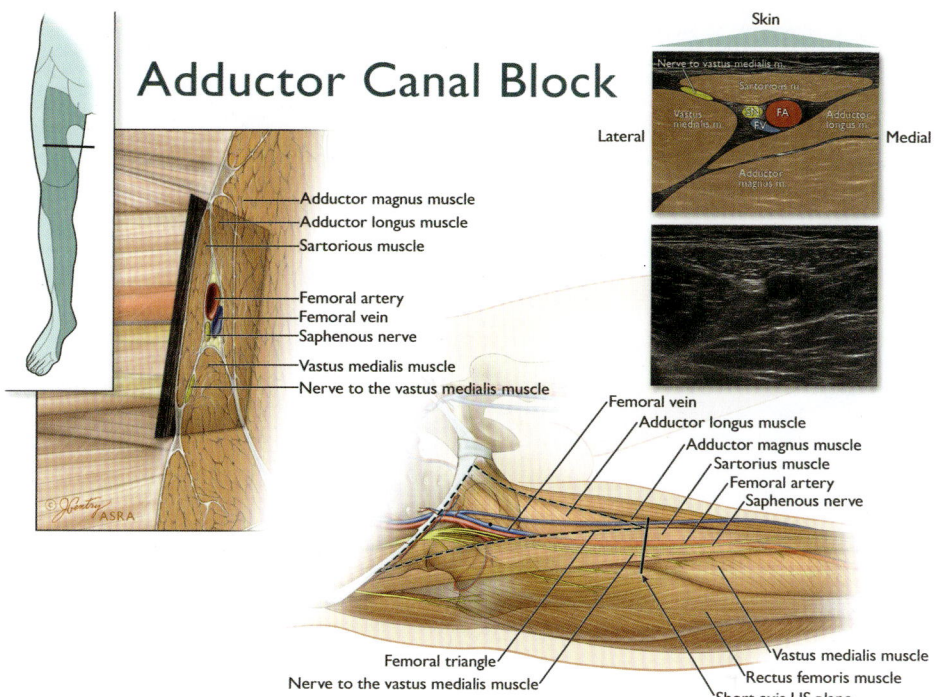

FIGURE 52.34 Adductor canal block. **Top left:** Analgesic coverage in dark blue. **Left:** Anatomic cross-section of the adductor canal. **Bottom:** Anatomic approach to the ultrasound-guided block. **Top right:** Cross-section of adductor canal with corresponding ultrasound image. *(Reprinted with permission of the American Society of Regional Anesthesia and Pain Medicine.)*

strength and provided noninferior postoperative analgesia for outpatients undergoing ACL reconstruction. However, despite evidence supporting preserved quadriceps strength, there have been case reports of quadriceps weakness after single-injection and continuous ACB.[298,299] Proximal spread of local anesthetic in the femoral triangle or anatomic variations in the motor branches to the quadriceps muscles have been suggested as possible mechanisms for quadriceps muscle weakness after ACB.[298–300]

ACBs have been described in the past to target only sensory function of the saphenous nerve.[301,302] However, in light of recent meta-analyses demonstrating noninferiority to FNBs and improved quadriceps strength over the FNBs, several studies have examined the contents of the adductor canal and spread outside the canal.[303–305] The sensory innervation of the knee is provided by branches of the femoral nerve and sciatic nerve, and some variable input from the obturator nerve. Cadaveric studies have demonstrated key nerves involved in analgesia after TKA.[306–309] The adductor canal begins at the apex of the femoral triangle and ends at the adductor hiatus.[247] The anatomic borders of the tunnel are anteriorly the aponeuroses of the surrounding muscles. The anterolateral border is the vastus medialis, the anteromedial border is the sartorius and the posterior border formed by the adductor magnus.[247] Burckett-St Laurant et al.[305] identified and traced the terminal branches of the saphenous nerve and the nerve to the vastus medialis and deep nerve plexus of the adductor canal. They found that both the vastus medialis and saphenous nerve provide innervation to the anteromedial joint capsule and subcutaneous tissues over the medial aspect of the knee.

Two studies of healthy volunteers support the claim that ACB is superior to FNB for patients undergoing TKA.[278,279] Three studies of TKA patients also demonstrated preserved quadriceps strength with ACB over FNB in both single-shot and catheter-based techniques.[280,310,311] Two cohort studies showed earlier postoperative ambulation in the continuous ACB group than in the continuous FNB group.[312,313] Mudumbai et al.[312] showed that when used in an established TKA clinical pathway, patients who received adductor canal catheters instead of femoral nerve catheters as part of a multimodal regimen were able to ambulate further on the day after surgery without any difference in pain control.[313] These findings support a functional

advantage for using ACB that does not sacrifice pain control as long as a multimodal analgesic regimen is used.

CLINICAL EFFECTS

Several authors noted motor block with the ACB.[298,299,303] Deloach and Boezaart[314] noted that the ACB spreads proximal into the femoral triangle and thus covers more nerves than just the saphenous. Gautier et al.[304] conducted a study in fresh human cadavers and demonstrated spread of the injectate outside the adductor canal and toward the popliteal fossa with some spread in the sciatic distribution. A cadaveric study by Andersen et al.[315] also noted that 15 mL of injectate into the adductor canal spread throughout the canal and beyond both proximally to the femoral triangle and distally, potentially covering some sciatic distribution.

Because the current options for local anesthetic are not very selective to motor or sensory nerve, the anesthesiologist is limited to choosing the optimal site and concentration. van der Wal et al.[316] compared the landmark transsartorial approach to the saphenous with saphenous field blocks and found that the transsartorial approach provided 94% success versus 40% success at providing complete anesthesia of the medial malleolus.

TECHNIQUE
Ultrasound Guidance

With the patient supine and leg and hip externally rotated, the practitioner places the ultrasound transducer on the midthigh, identifies the femur, and medially scans to identify the vastus medialis muscle until the sartorius muscle starts to appear superficial to the superficial femoral artery and vein. At this point, the probe is toggled to increase the echogenicity of the hyperechoic nerve lateral to the artery. The ultrasound is scanned proximally until the sartorius muscle is symmetrical above the artery (Fig. 52.35). An in-plane or out-of-plane approach can be taken to inject the local anesthetic below the sartorius muscle and adjacent to the nerve (Fig. 52.36).

Landmark Approach

The approach of van der Wal et al.[316] is to advance a 20-gauge blunt Tuohy needle through the sartorius muscle by using a loss-of-resistance technique.

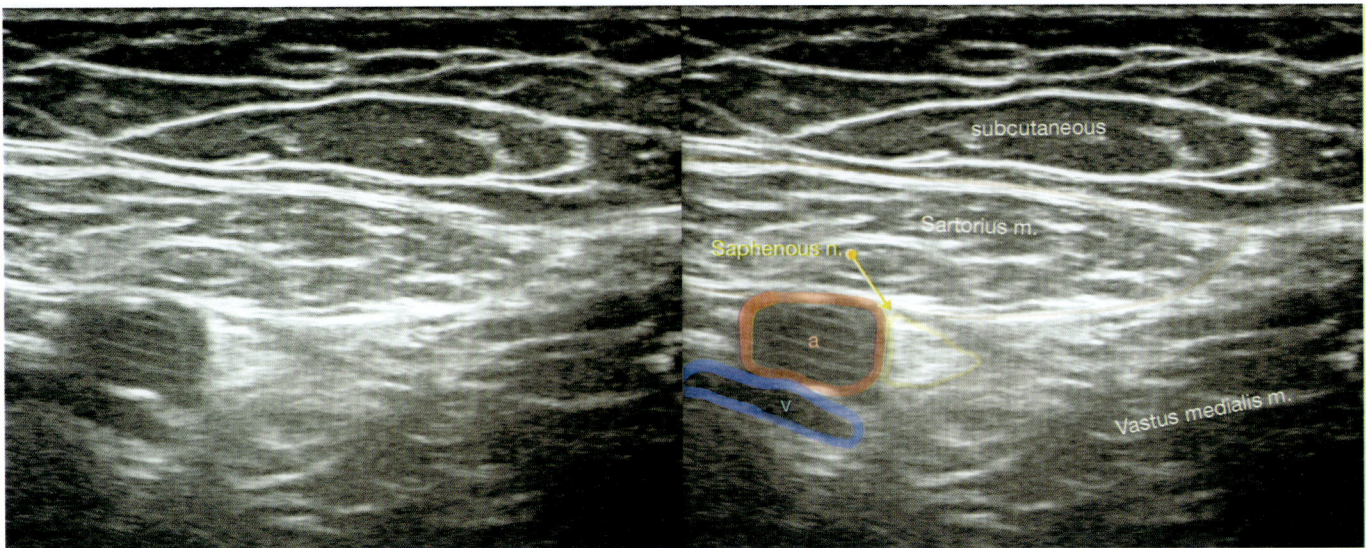

FIGURE 52.35 Adductor canal block. **Left:** Ultrasound image for the adductor canal sonoanatomy. **Right:** Ultrasound image with anatomy labeled. a, superficial femoral artery; m., muscle; n., nerve; v, superficial femoral vein. *(Reproduced with permission from Ouanes et al. http://anesthesiology .hopkinsmedicine.org/international-obstetric-and-regional-anesthesia/. Accessed July 18, 2018.)*

COMPLICATIONS

Similar to that seen in other PNBs, complications can include vascular puncture with subsequent local anesthetic toxicity, hematoma, and neurologic trauma. Neal et al.[317] reported a case series of local anesthetic-induced myotoxicity after continuous ACB that significantly impacted the patients' early rehabilitation and attributed to long-term impairment. Their institutional prevalence for this complication was 0.98/1,000. Clinical concentrations of all local anesthetics have been reported to be myotoxic in animal models, but these toxic effects are noted to be subclinical in humans.[298,299,318–321]

It was not clear[317] why clinically apparent local anesthetic-induced myotoxicity had occurred in patients who received continuous ACB but not in those with known intramuscular injection such as psoas. Continuous ACB is unique in that it occurs in a location similar to that of thigh tourniquet. The authors noted that tourniquet inflation is associated with progressive acidosis within the muscle, whereas myotoxicity is associated with alkalosis. They felt that direct tourniquet injury was unlikely; however, they introduced the idea of a "double hit" contribution of the tourniquet plus continuous ACB.

The degree to which ACB affects quadriceps function or the patient's ability to safely ambulate postoperatively is controversial. A number of studies have reported that these blocks result in little or no quadriceps weakness when compared with FNB. However, published studies have reported quadriceps weakness after ACB,

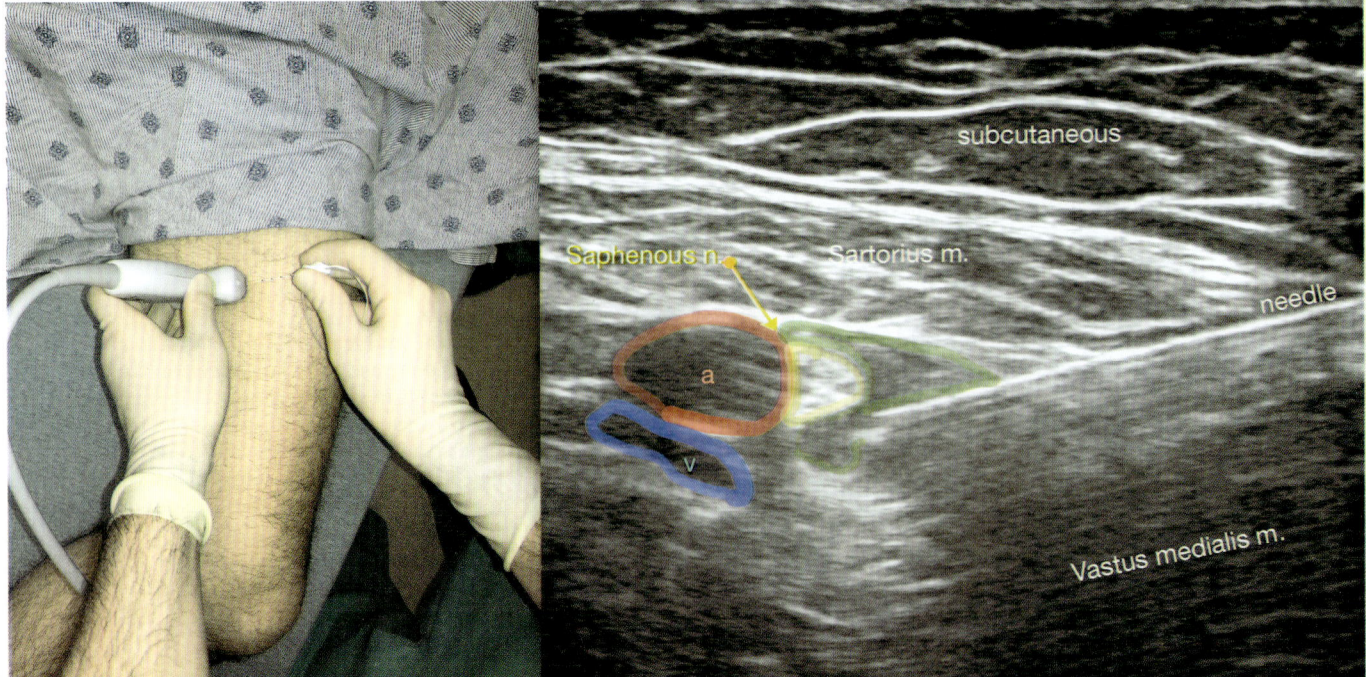

FIGURE 52.36 Left: Patient position and transducer for adductor canal block. **Right:** Needle position lateral to the nerve in the adductor canal with local anesthetic surrounding it. *Green*, local anesthetic. a, femoral artery; m., muscle; n., nerve; v, femoral vein. *(Reproduced with permission from Ouanes et al. http://anesthesiology.hopkinsmedicine.org/international-obstetric-and-regional-anesthesia/. Accessed July 18, 2018.)*

and a logical explanation would be spread of local anesthetic outside the adductor canal.[304,314] Therefore, patients should be monitored for motor strength to potentially reduce the risk of falls.

Fascia Iliaca Block

INDICATIONS

The fascia iliaca block (FIB) was originally described as the fascia iliaca compartment block in children.[322] Fascia iliaca compartment blocks are designed to be a three-in-one block. They are considered to be an anterior LP block that targets the femoral nerve, lateral femoral cutaneous nerve (LFCN), and obturator nerve.[323] The goal is to deposit local anesthetic in high volume under the fascia iliacus and allow it to spread over the three earlier mentioned nerves. As it is a fascial compartment block, the FIB is thought to cause less risk of bleeding and nerve injury than the traditional approach to the LP block. The technique has evolved from a landmark fascial click procedure with poor rate of success to an ultrasound-guided procedure with higher rates of success.

The FIB may be used in combination with other techniques to provide anesthesia and postoperative analgesia to the lower extremity. It has been used in procedures such as skin graft harvesting,[324] incisional pain,[325] postoperative analgesia after total hip or total knee arthroplasty, and prehospital analgesia in patients with femur fractures.[326,327]

TECHNIQUES

Landmark Approach

In the landmark approach, the practitioner should feel a sensation of two facial pops when the needle traverses the fascia lata and then the fascia iliaca. Penetration of both layers is essential to the success of the block. It is recommended that a short-beveled needle or pencil-point needle be used rather than a cutting needle in order to increase chances of appreciating the pops or clicks.[247]

As described by Dalens et al.,[328] a line is drawn between the pubic tubercle and the anterior superior iliac spine (ASIS). This line is divided into three equal parts and the junction of the middle and lateral thirds identified. The needle is inserted 1 cm below this point. The blunt needle is advanced until a double pop sensation is perceived. Then, the needle is presumed to have penetrated the fascia lata, and subsequently the fascia iliaca.

Ultrasound Guidance
Classic Technique

The patient is positioned supine and the ultrasound probe placed as for an FNB. The practitioner slides the ultrasound probe laterally to identify the hyperechoic lines of the fascia lata and fascia iliaca. He or she may appreciate the femoral nerve and femoral artery medially on the screen and the iliopsoas deep to the fascia layers. The block may be performed with an in-plane or out-of-plane needle approach. In the out-of-plane approach, the needle is inserted inferior to the ultrasound probe with a slight cephalad direction. Tissue displacement of the fascial planes may be appreciated. Direct visualization of local anesthetic spread below the fascia iliaca confirms correct needle placement. With the in-plane approach, the needle is advanced from the lateral edge of the ultrasound probe and visualized until it reaches below the fascia iliaca and confirmed with injection of local anesthetic.

Suprainguinal Technique

With the patient supine, the ultrasound probe is placed in the parasagittal plane on the ASIS and tilted medially. The probe is then moved medially along the inguinal ligament and kept at the same angle until the "hourglass" or "bow-tie" pattern is recognized, usually at the junction of the lateral one-third and medial two-thirds of the inguinal ligament (Fig. 52.37). The inferior part of the hourglass is formed by the sartorius muscle

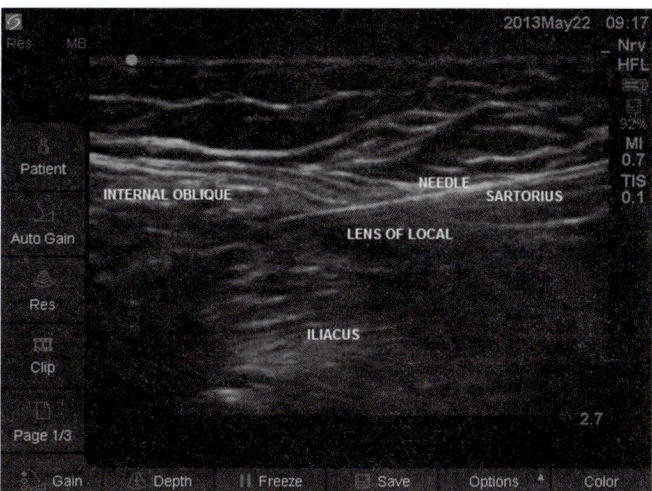

FIGURE 52.37 Suprainguinal ultrasound image of the fascia iliac block with the hourglass pattern. *(Reprinted with permission from Singh H, Jones D. Hourglass-pattern recognition simplifies fascia iliaca compartment block. Reg Anesth Pain Med 2013;38[5]:467–468.)*

and the superior part by the internal oblique. The deep circumflex iliac artery is seen just beneath the posterior part of superior hourglass (internal oblique) (see Fig. 52.1). The muscle under the hourglass is the iliacus muscle, and the fascia iliaca can be easily recognized overlying the iliacus muscle. Using an in-plane technique, the needle is introduced in an inferior-to-superior direction. It passes through the sartorius (inferior part of hourglass) and pierces the fascia iliaca. The correct placement of the needle is confirmed by the appearance of local anesthetic that pushes the iliacus down. The spread of local anesthetic is seen as a black lens sitting between the iliacus muscle and fascia. The black lens quickly disappears as the local anesthetic spreads between the fascia iliaca and the iliacus. The needle can be advanced into the hydro-dissected space for more proximal spread of local anesthetic toward the pelvic cavity.[329]

All of these blocks have been described as volume blocks and require large volumes to sufficiently spread into the fascial plane.

CLINICAL EFFECTS

When comparing the landmark approach to ultrasound-guided FIB, Dolan et al.[330] found that patients who were randomized to the ultrasound group had a greater loss of thigh sensation and greater motor blockade. They found that successful sensory loss in the anterior, medial, and lateral aspects of the thigh increased from 47% by landmark to 82% with ultrasound. The fascial pop or click landmark technique has had reported success rates of only 35% and 47%.[323,330] The success rate with ultrasound guidance has been reported as 82% and 87%.[330,331]

The evidence regarding efficacy of FIB for total hip arthroplasty is divided, as two randomized controlled trials have demonstrated no analgesic effect,[332,333] whereas two others have demonstrated efficacy at decreasing pain scores and opioid consumption.[334,335] All authors described different techniques. Shariat et al.[332] and Kearns et al.[333] each described using transverse infrainguinal techniques because they had been described as successful in previous studies.[330,334,336] Stevens et al.[334] and Bang et al.[335] used suprainguinal approaches to the FIB. Stevens et al.[334] used a double pop technique and Bang et al.[335] used a suprainguinal parasagittal ultrasound technique. Following the article by Shariat et al.,[332] several letters to the editor pointed out that the distal injection site may explain the lack of effect from the FIB in total hip arthroplasty. Hebbard et al.[337] described a novel suprainguinal parasagittal ultrasound approach that was successful in more than 150 patients. They supported their claim with a dye study in fresh cadavers, which showed consistent spread of dye in the lateral femoral cutaneous and femoral nerve distributions. Some studies have demonstrated a beneficial effect of the FIB in reducing the incidence of postoperative cognitive dysfunction and perioperative delirium in elderly patients.[336,338] Others have reported beneficial effect for treating hip fracture pain in the elderly.[339,340]

COMPLICATIONS

Transient femoral neuropathy has been reported after FIB.[341] Also a knotted fascia iliaca catheter has been reported.[342]

Lateral Femoral Cutaneous Nerve Block

INDICATIONS AND LANDMARKS

The LFCN is formed by the L2–L3 root. The nerve emerges from the lateral border of the psoas major muscle deep to the fascia iliaca. It perforates the inguinal ligament approximately 1 cm from the ASIS where it enters the thigh. The LFCN is a sensory-only nerve, and its innervation supplies an inconsistent area of skin over the lateral and anterior thigh.[247]

Small studies have reported variable success rates with landmark and nerve-stimulation techniques. Hopkins et al.[343] reported a success rate of 87.5% with the landmark nerve stimulation technique. Shannon et al.[344] reported a success rate of 100% using nerve stimulation to achieve paresthesia for confirmation of LFCN block. The same group also reported a 40% success rate when using the landmark fanning technique.

Anatomic studies have demonstrated that the distance from the LFCN at the inguinal ligament to the ASIS can range from 3 to 7.3 cm.[345–347] Ultrasound guidance is particularly suited for injection of a structure such as the LFCN because of its anatomic variability.[345–347] A study in cadavers and healthy human volunteers showed that the LFCN could be visualized consistently with ultrasound.[348]

Hurdle et al.[349] presented a technical description and case series in which they described successful and reliable blockade of the LFCN with ultrasound guidance. Others have described using the ultrasound technique as well.[349–352] Ultrasound-guided injections of the LFCN provide consistent blockade of the nerve with minimal volumes between 2 and 8 mL.[351]

TECHNIQUES

Landmark Technique

The patient position is supine. The LFCN block is performed with a modified field block technique in which a blunt needle is inserted perpendicular to the skin at a point 2 cm caudad and 2 cm medial to the ASIS (see Figs. 52.30 and 52.31). The needle is advanced until a pop is felt as it penetrates the fascia lata. Nerve stimulation can be added, and the patient should be asked if he or she feels a paresthesia or tapping in the lateral aspect of the thigh. If nerve stimulation is used, 5 to 10 mL of local anesthetic is injected whether or not the patient shows a response. If the patient shows no nerve stimulation response, the needle is withdrawn to the subcutaneous skin and redirected medially until a pop is felt and then an additional 5 mL of local anesthetic is administered. The needle is withdrawn to the subcutaneous skin and redirected laterally until a pop is felt and another 5 mL of local anesthetic administered.

Ultrasound Guidance

The ASIS is palpated and visualized with the ultrasound probe as a hyperechoic structure with posterior acoustic shadowing. The lateral end of the linear probe is placed on the ASIS, and the medial end extends medially in an anatomic transverse plane. With the probe in this position, the medial part of the probe is angled slightly in a caudal direction so the transducer is parallel with the inguinal ligament. The transducer is gently moved in

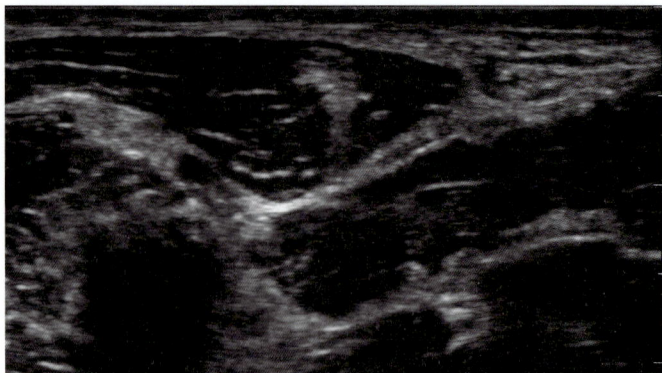

FIGURE 52.38   Ultrasound image of the lateral femoral cutaneous nerve.

a medial-caudal direction while the operator searches for the echo signature of the LFCN. With this approach, the LFCN will appear in cross-section as an oval hyperechoic structure containing several circular hypoechoic fascicles.[349] Alternately, the FNB image is obtained (see Fig. 52.32) and the probe is slid laterally identifying the sartorius muscle. Just lateral to the sartorius muscle, the LFCN can be visualized (see Fig. 52.37). This structure can be traced distally and often seen splitting into two separate structures and then retraced proximally to where it can be blocked easily (Fig. 52.38). The nerve is often found in the interfascial plane lateral to the sartorius muscle.

CLINICAL EFFECTS

Thybo et al.[353] studied the effect of ultrasound-guided LFCN in a group of patients that underwent a posterior approach to total hip arthroplasty. They reported no additional analgesic effects of the LFCN block when combined with their standard analgesic regimen of paracetamol, ibuprofen, and oxycodone. They noted that overall, the pain scores were low in all groups. A year later, Thybo et al.[354] published the effects of blocking the LFCN after total hip arthroplasty and found that movement-related pain during first hip flexion on postoperative day 1 or 2 was significantly reduced if the baseline pain was moderate or severe. They noted no effect on pain at rest.

LFCN blockade has been described for treating cases of meralgia paresthesia when patients do not respond to oral medications or conservative measures.[355,356]

COMPLICATIONS

No complications have been reported with this block.

Obturator Nerve

INDICATIONS AND LANDMARKS

The obturator nerve arises from the nerve roots of L2–L4. It exits the pelvis inferior to the superior pubic ramus. The nerve travels with the obturator artery and vein through the obturator canal and into the thigh where it branches into anterior and posterior divisions. The anterior division provides innervation to the adductor brevis, adductor longus, pectineus, and gracilis muscles. It also gives off an articular branch to the anteromedial hip capsule and cutaneous branches to the skin over the medial aspect of the thigh. The posterior branch is primarily a motor nerve for the adductors of the thigh; however, it also may provide articular branches to the medial aspect of the knee joint.

The obturator nerve block was first described by Labat[357] in his textbook in 1922. In 1973, Winnie and colleagues[358] described it as part of the 3-in-1 technique along with the LFCN and FNB. In 1993, Wassef described the interadductor approach to blocking the nerve.[359] This block provides anesthesia

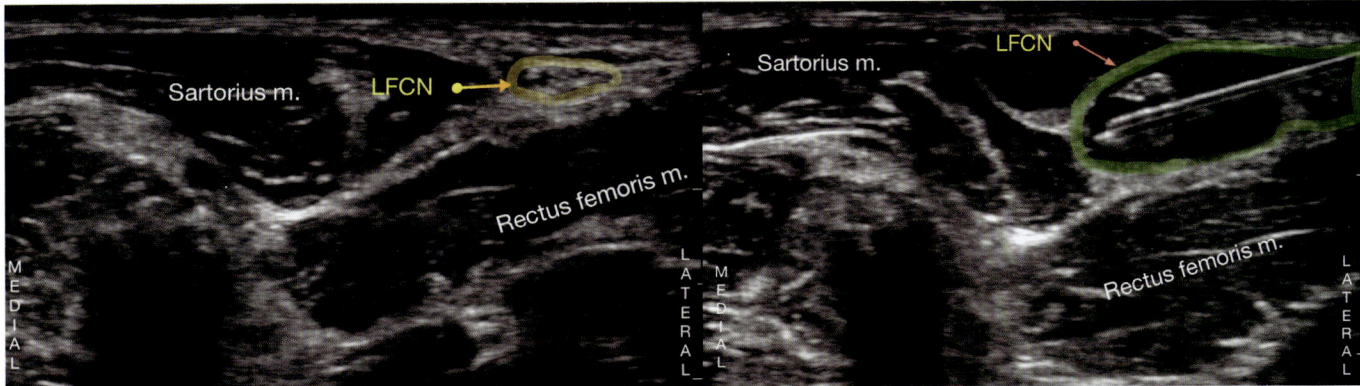

FIGURE 52.39   Lateral femoral cutaneous nerve block. **Left:** Labeled sonoanatomy. **Right:** Corresponding ultrasound image during injection. LFCN, lateral femoral cutaneous nerve; m., muscle. *Green*, local anesthetic. *(Reproduced with permission from Ouanes et al. http://anesthesiology.hopkinsmedicine .org/international-obstetric-and-regional-anesthesia/. Accessed July 18, 2018.)*

of the medial distal thigh and can be used in combination with femoral, lateral femoral cutaneous, and sciatic blocks for procedures on the distal thigh and lower leg, and prevention of tourniquet pain during lower leg surgery. The obturator nerve is occasionally blocked to prevent stimulation of the adductor muscles during transurethral resection procedures. The obturator nerve runs close to the lateral bladder wall, where direct surgical stimulation can result in adductor spasm, which causes bladder perforation and other anatomic injuries.[360] Several papers report efficacy of obturator nerve block during transurethral resection surgery.[361–364]

TECHNIQUES
Landmark Technique
With the patient positioned supine, the femoral artery is palpated and the tendon of the adductor muscle identified at the pubic tubercle. In the inguinal crease, a line is drawn from the femoral artery to the medial border of the adductor longus muscle (identified by abduction of the thigh) (Fig. 52.39). An insulated block needle is inserted at the midpoint of this line aimed cephalad and advanced until stimulation of the adductor muscle is elicited (see Figs. 52.31 to 52.33). The needle is advanced further and slightly lateral until hip adduction motor response. At that point, 10 mL of local anesthetic is injected. Then, the needle is withdrawn until the original motor response is obtained, and another 10 mL of local anesthetic is injected.

Ultrasound Guidance
With the patient supine and leg externally rotated, a linear ultrasound probe is placed in the transverse orientation in the inguinal crease, and the femoral nerve, artery, and vein are identified. The probe is moved medially to enable visualization of the pectineus, adductor longus, adductor brevis, and adductor magnus muscles. The anterior branch of the obturator nerve is a hyperechoic structure found between the adductor longus and brevis muscles. The posterior branch is a hyperechoic structure found between the adductor brevis and magnus muscles (Fig. 52.40). The needle approach may be either in plane or out of plane. The needle is directed in the fascial planes between the adductor longus and adductor brevis muscles for the anterior branch of the obturator and between the adductor brevis and adductor magnus muscles for the posterior branch.

Helayel et al.[365] described a comparison of the interductal approach in 12 cases to the traditional approach in 12 other patients of ultrasound-guided obturator nerve blocks with a success rate of 91%. Kakinohana[366] described the interductal approach to the obturator nerve block in a case series of 12 patients.

COMPLICATIONS
Intravascular injection; local anesthetic toxicity; and bladder, rectum, vagina, and spermatic cord injury have all been reported with Labat's classic approach to the block.[359]

Sacral Plexus-Sciatic Nerve Block

INDICATIONS
The sciatic nerve block is performed to achieve anesthesia and analgesia of the distal lower extremity, including the anterior and posterior lateral leg, ankle, and foot. The saphenous nerve (branch of the femoral/LP) is the only sensory nerve that innervates the medial aspect of the leg. It is required to achieve complete analgesia or anesthesia to provide sensory block to the medial aspect of the leg below the knee in addition to blockade of the sciatic nerve.

LANDMARKS
The sacral plexus is formed within the pelvis by L4–L5 and S1–S4. It provides motor and sensory innervation to portions of the entire lower extremity, including the hip, knee, and ankle. The most important nerves of the sacral plexus for surgery of the lower extremity are the sciatic nerve and its terminal branches. The sciatic nerve is a mixture of two large nerves initially bound together by connective tissue. The sciatic nerve exits the pelvis via the greater sciatic notch and beneath the piriformis muscle. In

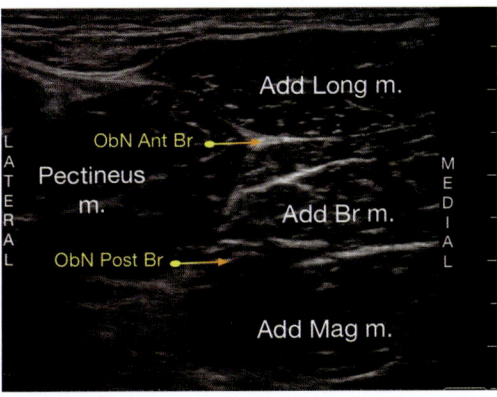

FIGURE 52.40   Ultrasound image for the obturator sonoanatomy. Anterior branch (ObN Ant Br) of the obturator nerve is located in the facial plane between the adductor longus (Add Long m.) and the adductor brevis (Add Br m.). The posterior branch (ObN Post Br) is located in the facial plane between the Add Br m. and the adductor magnus (Add Mag m.). *(Reproduced with permission from Ouanes et al. http://anesthesiology.hopkinsmedicine.org /international-obstetric-and- regional-anesthesia/. Accessed July 18, 2018.)*

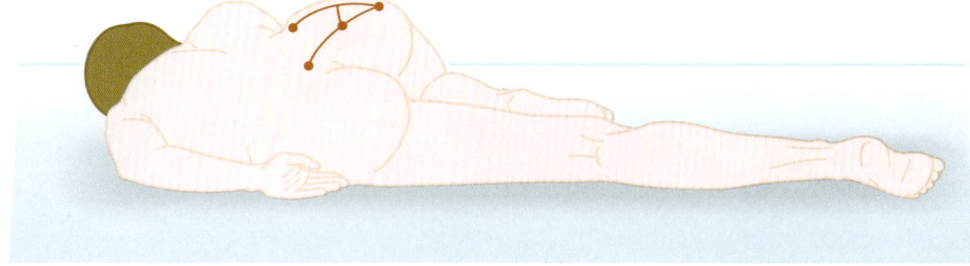

FIGURE 52.41   Patient position for the classic Labat approach to the sciatic nerve.

the upper part of the popliteal fossa, the sciatic nerve lies postero-lateral to the popliteal vesicles. The sciatic nerve usually divides into the tibial and common peroneal nerves at the upper aspect of the popliteal fossa.[247] Vloka et al.[367] reported a mean distance of 6 ± 3 cm above the popliteal crease. The tibial nerve provides motor innervation to the ankle flexors and sensory to the plantar aspect of the foot. The peroneal nerve is smaller than and lateral to the tibial nerve. It provides motor supply to the ankle extensor muscles and sensory innervation to the webspace of the first two toes. The sural nerve is purely sensory and travels with the tibial and common peroneal nerves. It supplies the posterolateral aspect of the leg and ankle and the dorsal surface of the foot.

TECHNIQUES

Several approaches can be made to this nerve. It can be targeted proximally or distally. The classic proximal approach was first described by Gaston Labat in 1922.[368] This approach has undergone several described modifications since the original description.[369–372]

Landmark Technique
Classic Labat Approach
The patient is positioned in a modified lateral Sims position with the operative side up. A line is drawn connecting the posterior superior iliac spine with the greater trochanter of the femur. A second line is drawn from the greater trochanter of the femur to the sacral hiatus. A third line is drawn from midline of line 1 to bisect line 2. At this point where the two lines cross, an insulated block needle is advanced until motor response or paresthesia is elicited. If bone is contacted, the needle is redirected laterally (Figs. 52.41 and 52.42).

Subgluteal Approach
The patient is positioned in a modified lateral Sims position with the operative side up. A line is drawn connecting the ischial

tuberosity with the greater trochanter of the femur. A second line is drawn from the center of the first line 4 to 6 cm caudad. Anywhere along line 2 is where the block can be attempted. An insulated block needle is advanced until motor response or paresthesia is elicited (Fig. 52.43). If no motor response or paresthesia is elicited, the needle is redirected medially or laterally.

Anterior Sciatic Nerve Block
With the patient supine and the surgical leg in a neutral position, the practitioner draws a line from the greater trochanter of the femur to the medial thigh parallel to the crease of the groin. At the midpoint of that line, an insulated block needle is inserted perpendicular to the skin until the femur is contacted. The needle is walked off in a cephalad medial direction until it walks off the lesser trochanter of the femur. Motor stimulation of the foot is elicited (Fig. 52.44).

Popliteal Fossa
With the patient in the prone position, the practitioner identifies the borders of the popliteal fossa by slightly bending the knee. The lateral border of this anatomical triangle is the biceps femoris, and the medial border is the semimembranosus muscle. The practitioner measures 5 to 9 cm proximal from the base of the anatomical triangle and inserts a stimulating block needle just off the medial aspect of the lateral border of the triangle until a motor response is observed with nerve stimulation or paresthesia is elicited (Fig. 52.45).

Ultrasound Technique
Classic Technique
The patient is placed in the modified lateral Sims position. Choice of an ultrasound probe depends on the patient's body habitus. Typically, a low-frequency curvilinear probe is used. The probe is placed on the posterior thigh to identify the

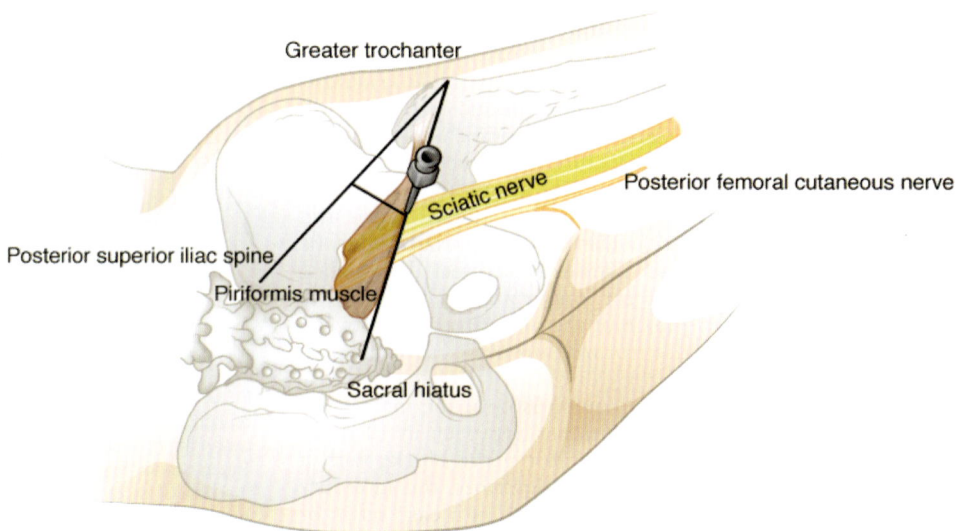

FIGURE 52.42   Illustration of the anatomic landmarks of the classic Labat approach to the sciatic nerve. *(Reprinted with permission from Yao FSF. Yao & Artusio's Anesthesiology. 8th ed. Baltimore, MD: Lippincott Williams & Wilkins; 2016: Figure 47-7.)*

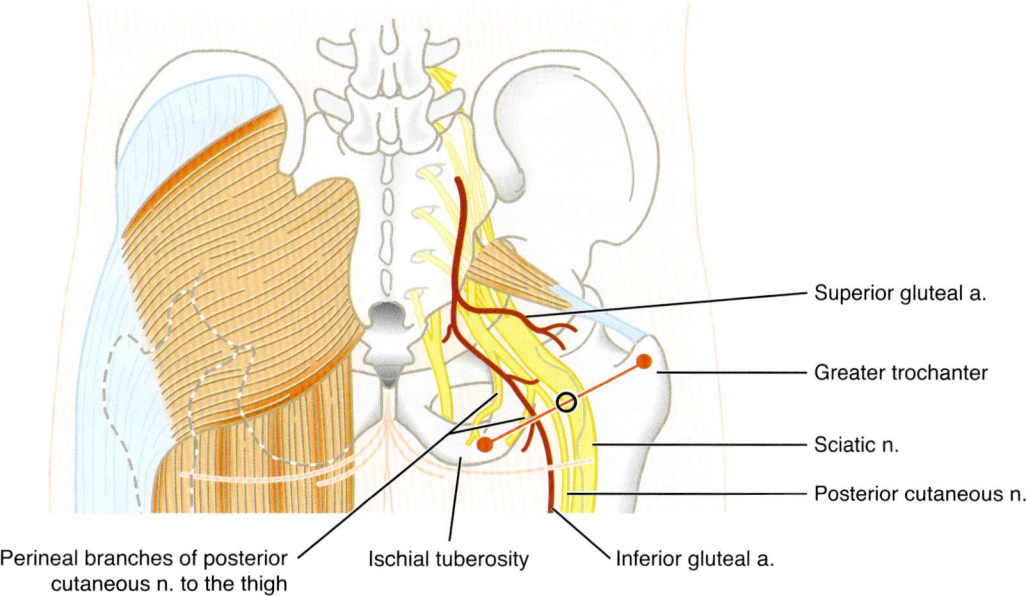

FIGURE 52.43 Illustration of the anatomic landmarks of the subgluteal approach to the sciatic nerve. *(From Horlocker TT, Kopp SL, Wedel DJ. Peripheral nerve blocks. In: Miller RD, Cohen NH, Eriksson LI, et al, eds.* Miller's Anesthesia. *8th ed. Philadelphia: Saunders; 2015:1721–1751.)*

hyperechoic femur (with dropout shadow below). The practitioner traces the femur proximally until the greater trochanter is encountered and then slides the probe medially on the gluteus maximus muscle. Deep to the gluteus maximus is the sciatic nerve, and deep to the nerve is the quadratus femoris muscle. The nerve at this level is oval or triangular. It is often visualized at the level of the bones between the ischium and the femur. An in-plane or out-of-plane technique can be employed (Figs. 52.46 and 52.47).

Alternative Technique (Anterior Approach)
The patient is positioned supine with the block leg externally rotated and knee slightly bent. The low-frequency curvilinear probe is placed in the transverse plane over the medial thigh approximately 10 cm below the femoral crease. The sciatic nerve appears as a hyperechoic nerve medial and deep to the femur. It is located between the adductor magnus muscle and the hamstrings. The nerve may be approached in an in-plane or out-of-plane technique.

Lateral Ultrasound Technique with Popliteal Approach
The patient position is usually lateral but may be prone or supine. With the patient in the lateral position, a high-frequency linear ultrasound probe is placed transversely in the popliteal crease, and the popliteal artery and popliteal vein are identified. Lateral and superficial to the vessels are the two component branches of the sciatic nerve. The tibial is usually larger and medial, and the common peroneal is usually smaller and lateral. The probe usually needs to be tilted toward the foot to increase the echogenicity of the nerves. The nerves are traced cephalad until they join to become the sciatic nerve. The needle may be inserted proximal or distal to the branch point of the nerves. Either an in-plane or out-of-plane needle technique can be used. The needle needs to be adjacent to the nerves in order to coat them with local anesthetic (Figs. 52.48 and 52.49).

CLINICAL EFFECTS
Ultrasound guidance has been shown to enhance the quality of popliteal sciatic nerve block compared to that with a single-injection, nerve stimulator-guided block that uses either a tibial or peroneal motor response.[369] According to one study, ultrasound guidance resulted in higher success rates, faster onset,

and faster progression of sensorimotor block, without increasing complications.[373] Another study reported that at the transgluteal level, ultrasounds allow a practitioner to easily identify the greater trochanter, the ischial tuberosity, and the sciatic nerve located between them.[374]

A paraneural sheath that surrounds the sciatic nerve needs to be penetrated for optimal local anesthetic spread. Two studies analyzed injections in this space.[375,376] Andersen et al.[375] showed that dye injected under the paraneurium of cadavers spread along the nerve both proximally and distally. They also noted that when the sheath was not penetrated, the dye did not spread as well. The second study compared patients who had injections of local anesthetic outside the paraneurium to those whose injections were inside the paraneurium. Using three-dimensional

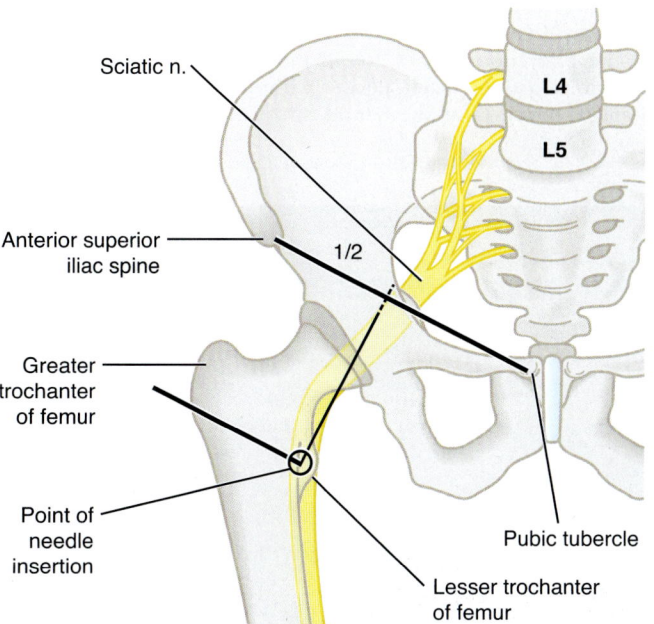

FIGURE 52.44 Landmark anterior sciatic approach.

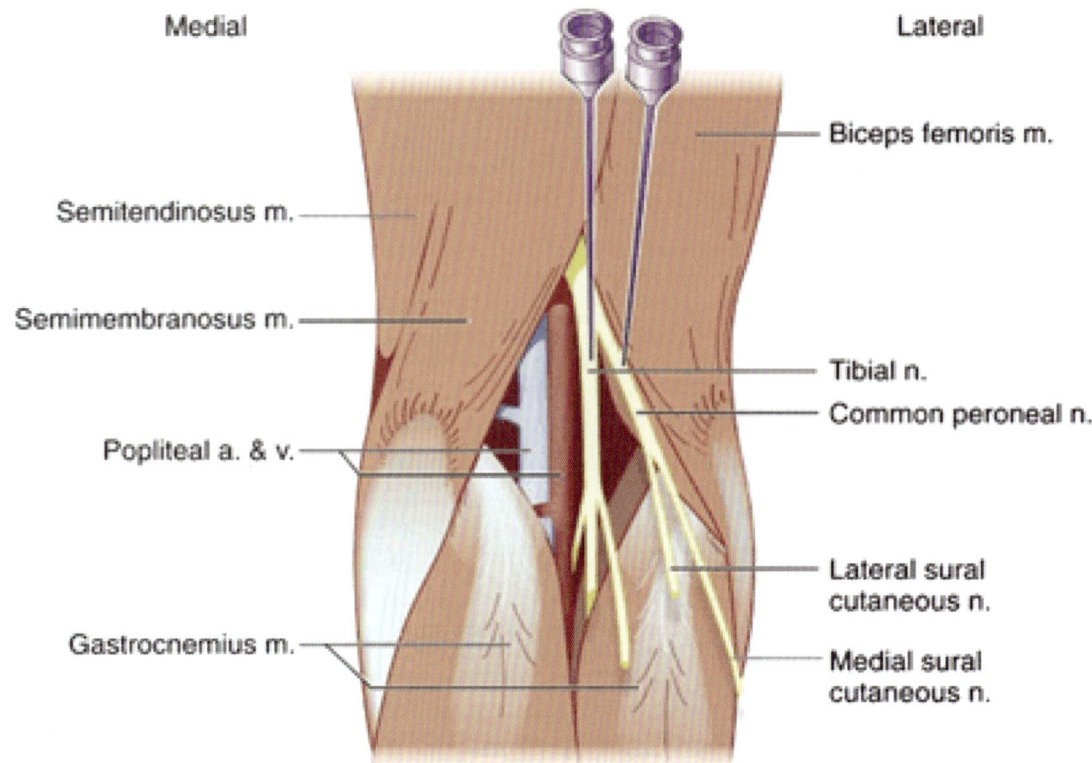

FIGURE 52.45 Landmark approach to the sciatic nerve in the popliteal fossa. a., artery; m., muscle; n., nerve; v., vein. *(Reprinted from Horlocker TT, Kopp SL, Wedel DJ. Peripheral nerve blocks. In: Miller RD, Cohen NH, Eriksson LI, et al., eds.* Miller's Anesthesia. *8th ed. Philadelphia, PA: Saunders; 2015. Fig 57-23. Copyright © 2015 Elsevier. With permission.)*

ultrasound reconstruction and clinical correlation with sensory exam, the authors concluded that block efficacy was superior when injections were made under the paraneurium.[376] A subparaneural injection hastens the onset time and also increases the duration of the sensory blockade compared to that with circumferential extraneural injection.[377] Another study supported the findings of the first study and further defined the target for local anesthetic injection as the subparaneural space.[259]

Tran et al.[378] performed a randomized comparison between ultrasound-guided subepineural popliteal sciatic nerve block proximal to the bifurcation and ultrasound-guided injection of the individual branches of the peroneal and tibial nerves distal to the bifurcation. They found that compared with separate injections around each nerve (without being subepineural), a single injection at the neural bifurcation has a faster onset time, provides higher success rates, and can be performed more quickly.[378]

Several studies have looked at minimal dosing, optimal local anesthetics, and optimal injection sites. The effective local anesthetic volume for the sciatic nerve block ranged from 0.10 to 0.15 mL/mm^2 of cross-sectional nerve area.[379,380] Other groups have identified the ED50 and ED95 for 0.5% ropivacaine in ultrasound-guided popliteal sciatic nerve block as 6 and 16 mL, respectively.[381] They had success rates of sensory blockade of 69% for the tibial nerve and 88% for the peroneal nerve.[381] Bang et al.[382] undertook a prospective study to identify the minimum effective dose of 0.75% ropivacaine in subparaneural ultrasound-guided popliteal nerve blocks. They found the ED90 to be 9 mL. Taboada et al.[383] published a prospective randomized comparison between the popliteal and

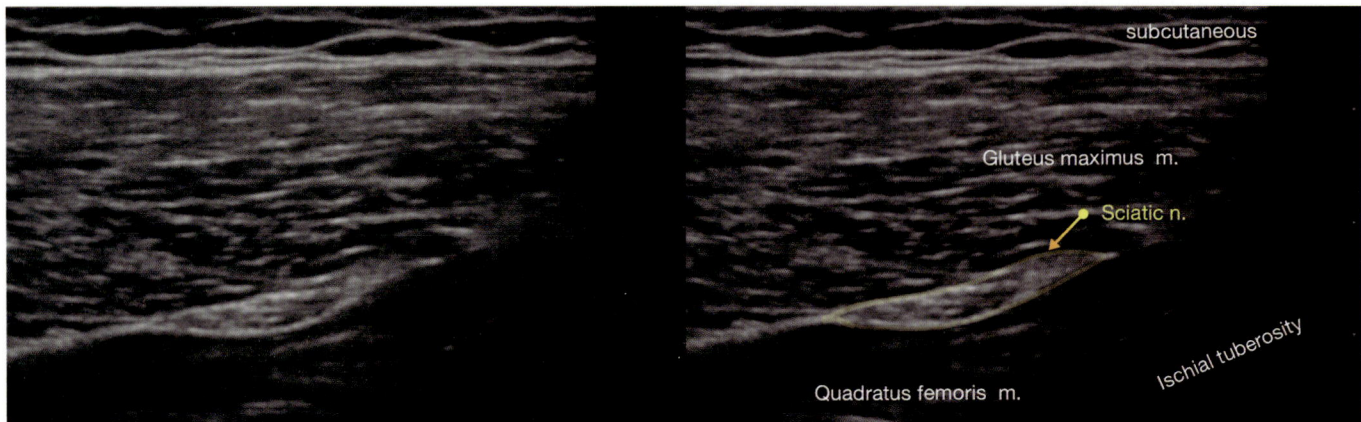

FIGURE 52.46 Subgluteal approach to the sciatic nerve block. **Left:** Ultrasound image for the subgluteal sonoanatomy. **Right:** Ultrasound image with anatomy labeled. m., muscle; n., nerve. *(Reproduced with permission from Ouanes et al. http://anesthesiology.hopkinsmedicine.org/international-obstetric -and-regional-anesthesia/. Accessed July 18, 2018.)*

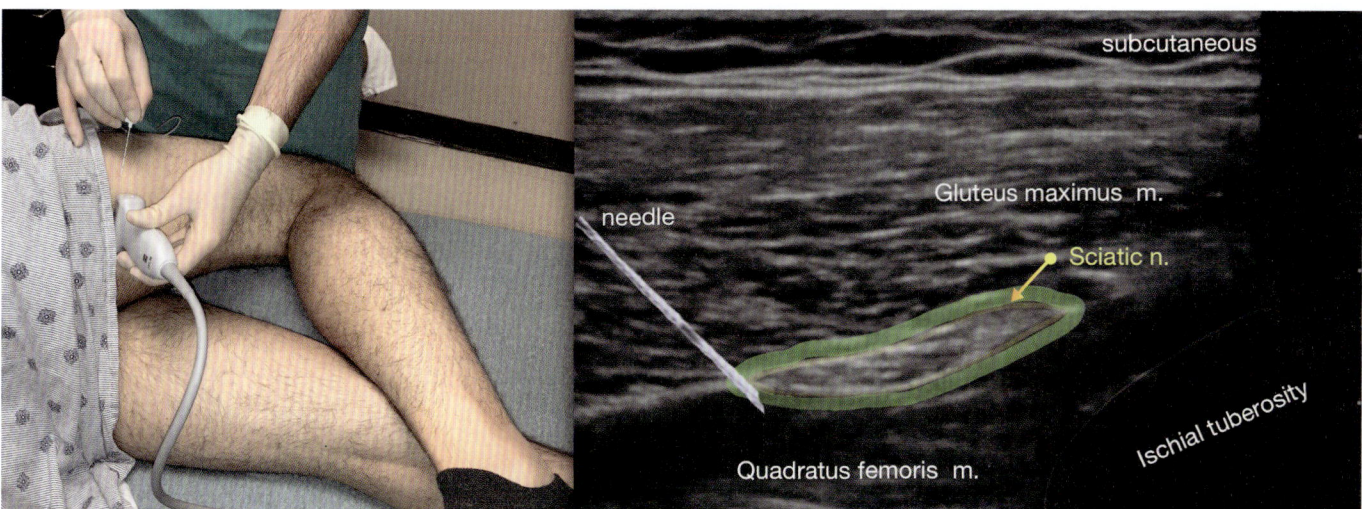

FIGURE 52.47 **Left:** Patient position and transducer for in-plane ultrasound sciatic approach. **Right:** Corresponding ultrasound image. m., muscle; n., nerve. *Green,* local anesthetic. *(Reproduced with permission from Ouanes et al. http://anesthesiology.hopkinsmedicine.org/international-obstetric-and -regional-anesthesia/. Accessed July 18, 2018.)*

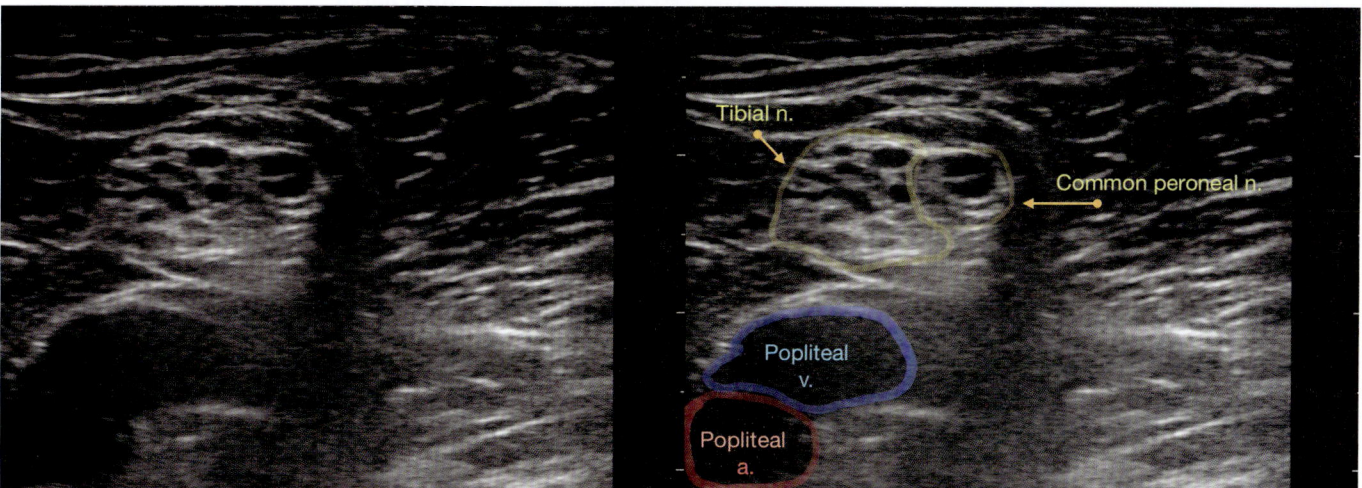

FIGURE 52.48 **Left:** Ultrasound image for the popliteal sonoanatomy. **Right:** Ultrasound image with anatomy labeled. a., artery; n., nerve; v., vein. *(Reproduced with permission from Ouanes et al. http://anesthesiology.hopkinsmedicine.org/international-obstetric-and-regional-anesthesia/. Accessed July 18, 2018.)*

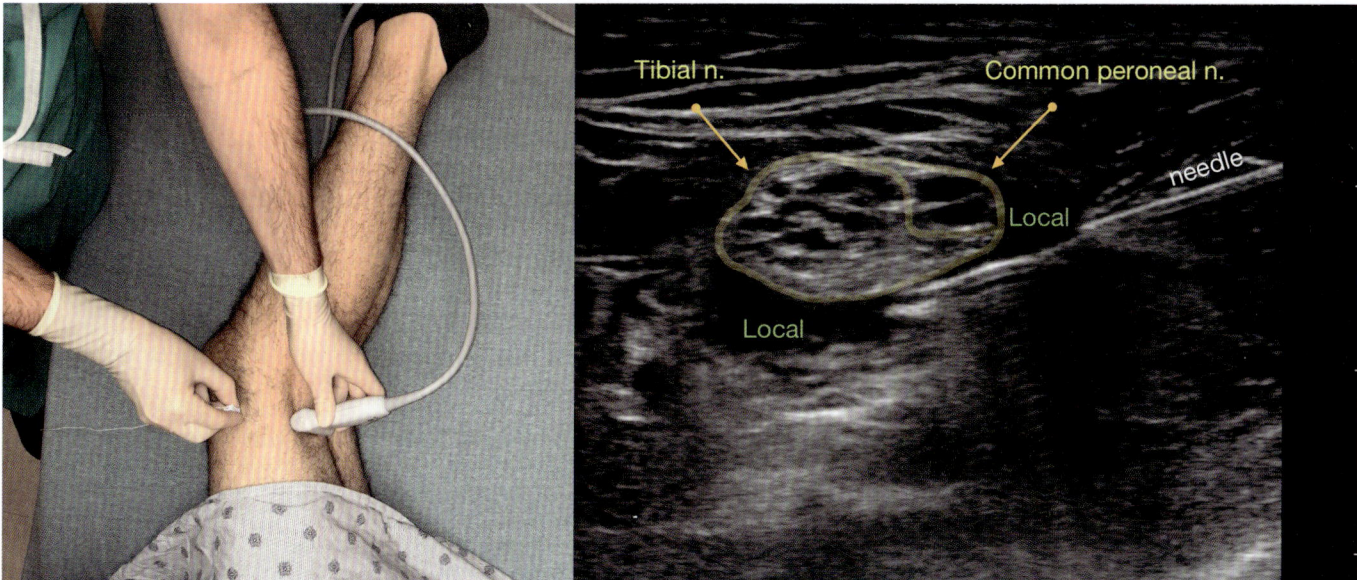

FIGURE 52.49 Patient and transducer position for ultrasound-guided lateral approach to popliteal nerve block. **Left:** Patient position in-plane needle approach. **Right:** Corresponding ultrasound image. *(Reproduced with permission from Ouanes et al. http://anesthesiology.hopkinsmedicine.org/international -obstetric-and-regional-anesthesia/. Accessed July 18, 2018.)*

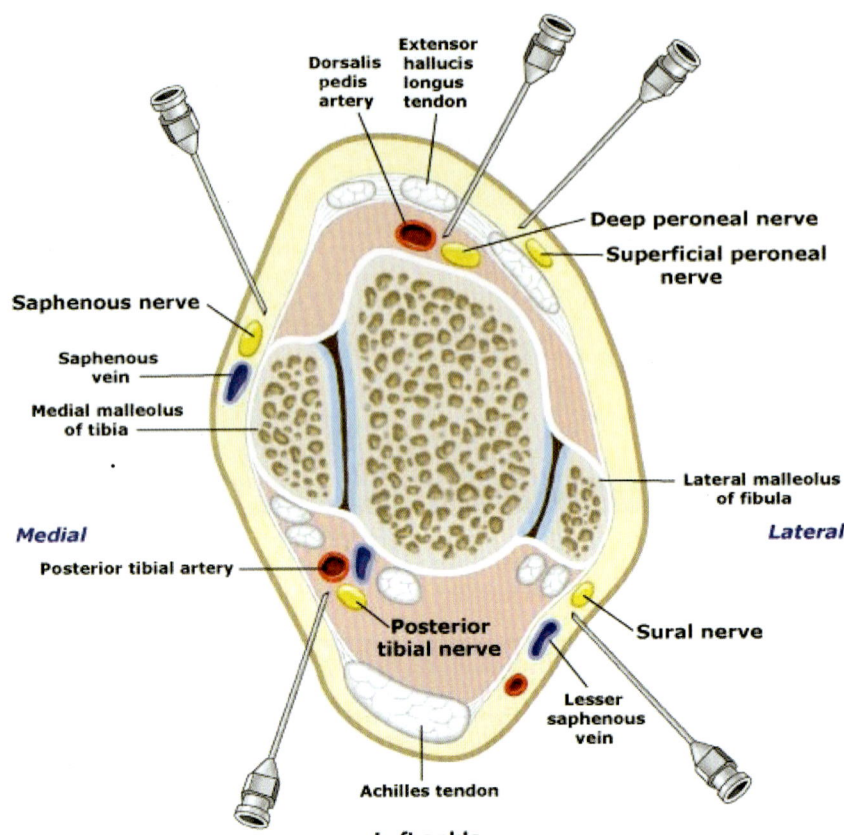

FIGURE 52.50   Illustration of the anatomic landmarks of the ankle block. *(From http://cursoenarm.net/UPTODATE/contents/mobipreview.htm?1/41 /1688. Accessed July 16, 2018.)*

subgluteal approach. They reported the ED95 for adequate block of the sciatic nerve to be 17 mL in the subgluteal group and 30 mL in the popliteal group. The authors concluded that a larger volume of local anesthetic is necessary to block the sciatic nerve at a more distal site (popliteal) than at a more proximal level (subgluteal).

COMPLICATIONS

The incidence of nerve injury associated with sciatic PNCs has ranged from 0% to 1.0%[282,384–387] and includes persistent paresthesia after a popliteal sciatic catheter in a patient population followed for an 18-month period.[282,386] Bondar et al.[388] reported a pudendal nerve injury after sciatic nerve block with the posterior approach.

Ankle Block

INDICATIONS

The ankle block was first described in 1922 by Gaston Labat in his *Textbook of Regional Anesthesia*.[389] It is carried out to achieve anesthesia and analgesia of the foot. It does not provide anesthesia or analgesia to the ankle. The ankle block targets the terminal branches of the sciatic nerve and saphenous nerve. Five nerves need to be anesthetized. Two are located beneath the deep fascia, and three are in the subcutaneous tissue. The posterior tibial nerve and deep peroneal nerve are found in the deep layer, and the superficial peroneal, saphenous, and the sural nerves are superficial.

TECHNIQUES

Landmark Technique

To anesthetize the deep fascial nerves (deep peroneal, posterior tibial), place the patient in the supine position. Start with the

deep blocks because subcutaneous infiltration can often deform the surface anatomy (Fig. 52.50).

Deep Peroneal Nerve

Palpation of the extensor hallucis longus (EHL) is often achieved by asking the patient to dorsiflex his toes. Just lateral to the EHL, the block needle is inserted until it contacts bone. Gentle pressure is released from the needle and 2 to 3 mL of local anesthetic *without* epinephrine is injected. Because this is a blind procedure, a fanning technique is used to increase the chances of successfully blocking the nerve. Fanning is redirecting the needle and repeating the block in a medial and lateral position with the same puncture site.

Posterior Tibial Nerve

The block needle is inserted posterior to the medial malleolus. Similar to the deep peroneal nerve block, the needle is advanced until bone is contacted. Then, pressure from the needle is released, and 2 to 3 mL of local anesthetic *without* epinephrine is injected. This procedure is repeated with the needle redirected in a medial and lateral position through the same puncture site.

Superficial Nerves (Sciatic Terminal Branches—Sural and Superficial Peroneal, Femoral Terminal Branch—Saphenous)

The three superficial cutaneous nerves are blocked by injecting local anesthetic *without* epinephrine into the subcutaneous tissue at the level of the medial malleolus along a line that joins both malleoli over the anterior aspect of the ankle. Usually, an injection volume of 10 to 20 mL is sufficient.[390]

Classic Ultrasound Technique

To identify the four nerves of sciatic origin, a linear high-frequency probe is used (Fig. 52.51). The tibial nerve is usually located

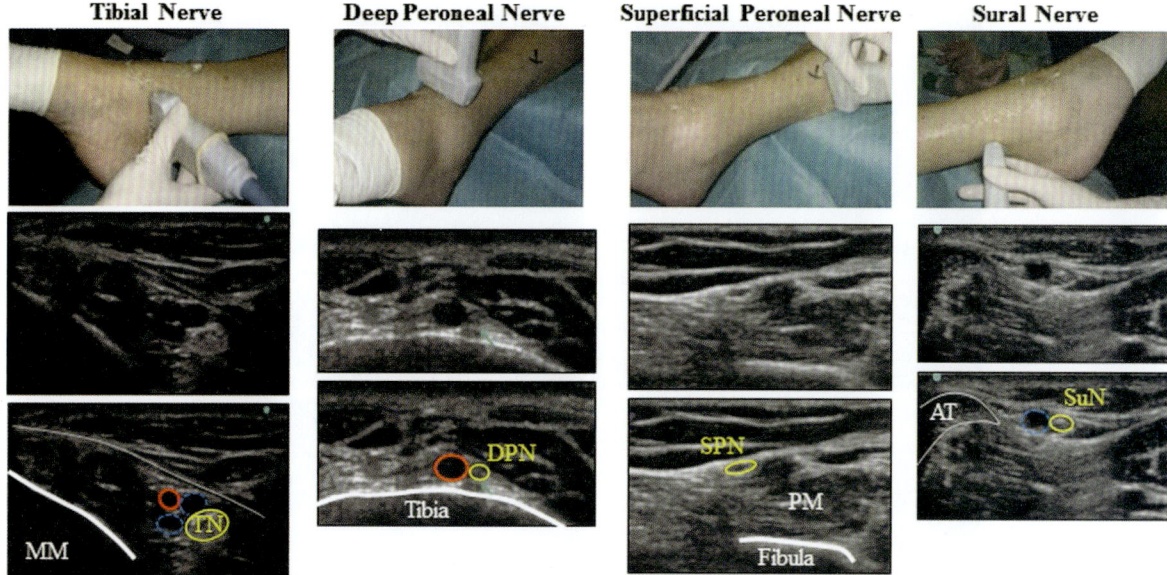

FIGURE 52.51 Probe position and ultrasound images of the nerves at the level of lower leg and ankle. AT, Achilles tendon; DPN, deep peroneal nerve; MM, medial malleolus; PM, peroneal muscles; SPN, superficial peroneal nerve; SuN, sural nerve; TN, tibial nerve. *(From López AM, Sala-Blanch X, Magaldi M, et al. Ultrasound-guided ankle block for forefoot surgery: the contribution of the saphenous nerve. Reg Anesth Pain Med 2012;37[5]:554–557.)*

between the medial malleolus and the Achilles tendon posterior to the posterior tibial artery and veins. On the anterolateral aspect of the ankle next to the anterior tibial artery, the deep peroneal nerve can be identified. The superficial peroneal nerve is scanned before it becomes subcutaneous 10 to 15 cm proximal to the lateral malleolus. The sural nerve is located between the lateral malleolus and the Achilles tendon, close to the saphenous vein.[391] Injection of 3 to 8 mL of local anesthetic per nerve has been described.[391] The goal is to surround the nerve in anesthetic.

CLINICAL EFFECTS

Compared with the conventional approach, the application of ultrasound increases the success rate and reduces the onset time of the ankle block.[392–394] Rudkin et al.[390] conducted a prospective study on 1,000 landmark ankle blocks. They found a success rate of 94.7% and attributed the short time frame between block and incision as a risk factor for block failure. Meyerson et al.[395] published their landmark ankle block experience on 1,295 patients and reported a success rate of 95%.

Redborg et al.[392] randomized 18 volunteers to ultrasound-guided or landmark sural nerve block at the ankle. They found that ultrasound use led to a more complete and longer lasting sural nerve block than did the traditional landmark technique. Although multiple techniques have been described, little evidence-based medicine is available to evaluate different techniques for blocking the tibial nerve at the ankle. Therefore, the same researchers also compared the effectiveness of ultrasound-guided and landmark-guided blocks of the tibial nerve at the ankle. The tibial nerve is arguably the most important nerve to anesthetize during an ankle block because it provides the majority of sensation to the foot. They noted a 72% success rate (defined as complete block at 30 minutes) with the ultrasound-guided technique but only a 22% success rate in the landmark group.[394] Lopez et al.[391] found that the ultrasound-guided ankle block was highly effective for bunion surgery and that every nerve in the ankle was successfully blocked within 10 minutes of injection.

COMPLICATIONS

Noorpuri et al.[396] raised concern for the possibly of masking acute compartment syndrome after forefoot revision arthroplasty in a patient with ankle block. Myerson et al.[395] published

a complication rate of 0.3% and described it as local anesthetic toxicity.

Quadratus Lumborum Block

INDICATIONS

The quadratus lumborum block (QLB) is a more posterior extension of the TAP block. It was first described by Blanco in 2007 at a scientific meeting as a technique for postoperative abdominal analgesia. He later wrote that the analgesic efficacy obtained from the TAP was superior when it spread beyond the TAP plane and into the thoracic paravertebral space.[397] Several variations of optimal injection points have been described. Blanco originally described deposition of local anesthetic at the anterolateral border of the QL, a technique he named the QL1 block. He noted that the spread pattern of local anesthetic obtained by the QL1 was similar to that of the landmark TAP with thoracic paravertebral spread.[397,398] In a randomized controlled trial for postoperative pain control, Sauter et al.[399] published a modified version of the block that used a transmuscular QL injection and clearly identifiable landmarks, which they coined the "shamrock" method. The shamrock sign is made up of the following four components: the erector spinae, the QL, the psoas major muscle, and the transverse process of the L4 vertebra (Fig. 52.52). Borglum's group[400] demonstrated that the original QLB is characterized by a 30-minute block onset time and that a single 30-mL injection of ropivacaine 0.375% will anesthetize both the lateral and anterior cutaneous branches from T7 to L1–L4. The transmuscular approach involves injection of local anesthetic in the plane between the QL and psoas major muscles. This technique has mostly been described as a single-shot procedure. Chakraborty et al.[401] reported success when they left the catheter between the QL and transversalis fascia. Blanco also offered the possibility of depositing the local anesthetic posterior to the QL muscle between the QL and transversalis fascia and coined this the QL2 block[397] (Fig. 52.53).

The QLB is indicated for abdominal surgeries because it provides analgesia to visceral and somatic nerves. Some say that it produces better analgesia than a TAP block because it not only provides analgesia to the anterior abdominal wall but also blocks visceral pain.

A landmark approach has not been described.

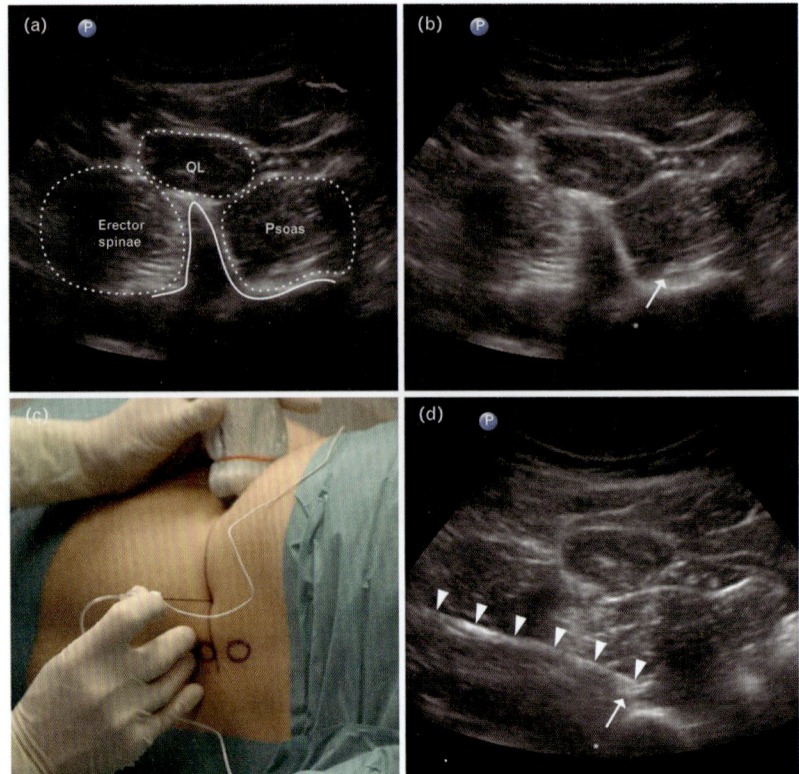

FIGURE 52.52 Shamrock lumbar plexus block. **A:** The psoas muscle, erector spinae muscle, quadratus lumborum (QL) muscle, and the L4 transverse process represent the pattern of a shamrock. **B:** The *star* and *arrow* indicates the L3 spinal nerve root. **C:** The point of needle insertion is situated on a line representing the intersection of the ultrasound beam with the skin. **D:** The cannula (marked with *arrowheads*) is advanced in a posterior-anterior direction. *(From Sauter AR, Ullensvang K, Niemi G, et al. The Shamrock lumbar plexus block: a dose-finding study. Eur J Anaesthesiol 2015;32:764–770.)*

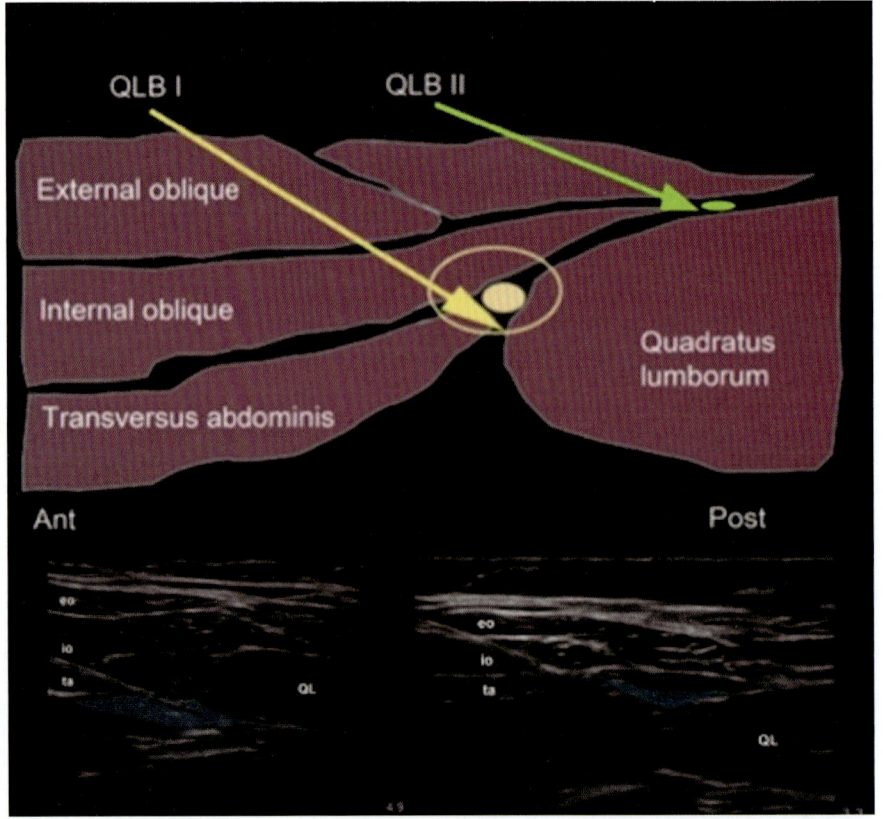

FIGURE 52.53 **Top:** Illustration of Blanco's optimal point of injection in both QLB I and II. **Bottom:** Corresponding ultrasound images, with *blue* color representing QLB I injection **(left)** and the QLB II **(right)**. eo, external oblique; io, internal oblique; QLB, quadratus lumborum block; ta, transversus abdominus.

ULTRASOUND TECHNIQUE
Quadratus Lumborum 1

With the patient in a lateral or prone position, a curvilinear probe in the transverse orientation is placed superior to the iliac crest. The transducer is then moved dorsally until the QL muscle is identified with its attachment to the lateral edge of the transverse process of the L4 vertebra. The shamrock landmarks are identified as the psoas major muscles anteriorly, the erector spinae muscle posteriorly, and the QL muscle adjacent to the transverse process[399] (Fig. 52.52A).

CLINICAL EFFECTS

The literature available for the QLB includes several case reports describing the successful use of the QLB[402] and continuous QLB catheters.[401–403] A review of the evidence by Abrahams et al.[404] in 2016 gave the evidence a grade of B based on one level Ib study, one level IIb study, and five level III studies that all supported the use of ultrasound for QLBs.

COMPLICATIONS

No complications have been reported as of the writing of this chapter. However, because possible damage to intraperitoneal structures have been reported in the TAP literature and this block was developed as an extension of the TAP, it is not unreasonable to be concerned by the potential for similar complications to that seen with TAP blocks.[152,405,406]

PECS/Serratus Anterior Plane Block

INDICATIONS

Thoracic wall blocks, which include PECS I, PECS II, and the serratus anterior plane (SAP) block, are novel, ultrasound-guided fascial plane blocks that are thought to provide anesthesia or analgesia to the chest wall without the neuraxial risk associated with epidural and paravertebral blocks. The PECS I was originally described by Blanco[407] in 2011. The report described depositing local anesthetic adjacent to the thoracoacromial artery in the fascial plane between the pectoralis major (PMm) and Pmm to target the lateral pectoral nerve and medial pectoral nerve. The original block was subsequently modified by Perez et al.[408] and further refined to include more analgesic coverage by Blanco et al.,[409] which the group called PECS II. The PECS II is performed more laterally with the local anesthetic deposited in the fascial plane between the Pmm and the serratus anterior muscle at the level of the third and fourth ribs (see Figs. 52.55 and 52.56). The broader coverage of the PECS II includes the long thoracic nerve and thoracic intercostal nerves. Sensory testing showed analgesia of T2–T4 dermatomes. Blanco et al.[409] described good results with single injections and catheters in over 100 patients. Chakraborty et al.[410] even further modified the block to a single insertion site (Fig. 52.54). Two years after the PECS I was introduced, Blanco's group[411] went on to describe a variation of the PECS II block known as the SAP block, with improved analgesia. Blanco et al.[411] described the SAP block in four healthy volunteers and reported that it provided sensory dermatomal analgesia of T2–T7. The local anesthetic could be injected either superficially or deep to the serratus anterior muscle with the superficial one providing double the analgesia (see Figs. 52.55 and 52.56).

The indications for PECS blocks include superficial anterior chest wall procedures such as pacemaker insertions[412]; postoperative analgesia for breast surgeries such as lumpectomies, mastectomies, and breast tissue expanders; and even arteriovenous fistulas revision to cover the intercostobrachial nerve.[413–415]

A landmark approach has not been described.

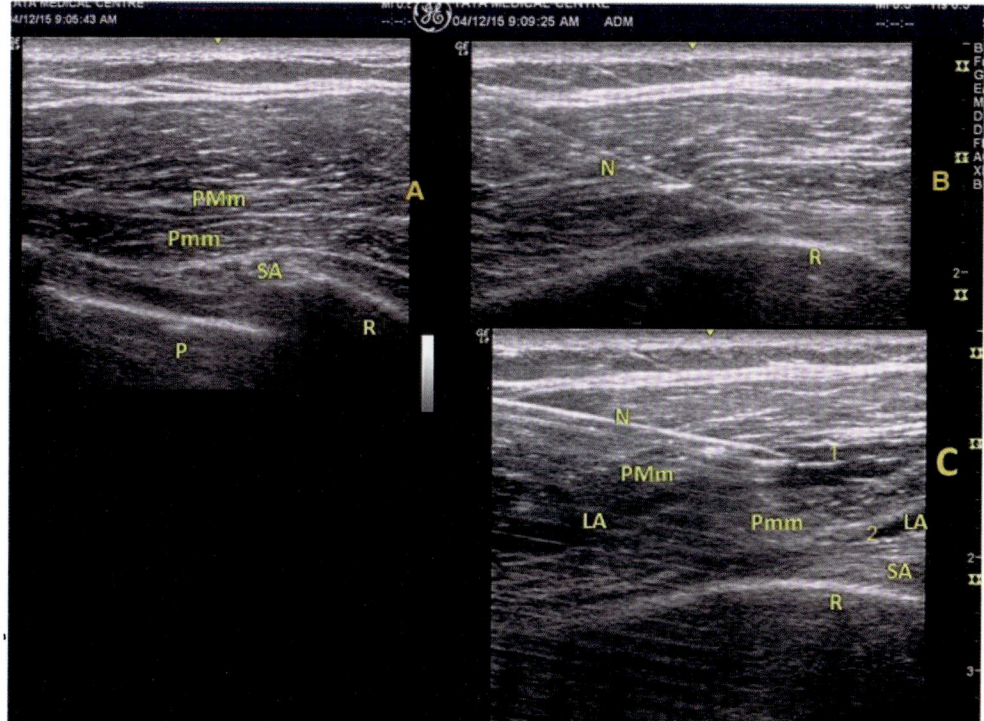

FIGURE 52.54 Modified single-injection technique for PECS I and PECS II. **A:** Scanning ultrasonogram showing the third rib (R), pleura (P), serratus anterior (SA), pectoralis minor muscle (Pmm), and pectoralis major muscle (PMm). **B:** Needle (N) enters in plane, strikes the rib, and withdraws a little to lie above SA. **C:** Needle is withdrawn to give the PECS I injection (1) between PMm and Pmm, after injecting the PECS II injection (2) between SA and Pmm. The local anesthetic (LA) is seen spreading between the muscles as a hypoechoic layer. *(From Chakraborty A, Khemka R, Datta T, et al. COMBIPECS, the single-injection technique of pectoral nerve blocks 1 and 2: a case series. J Clin Anesth 2016;35:365–368.)*

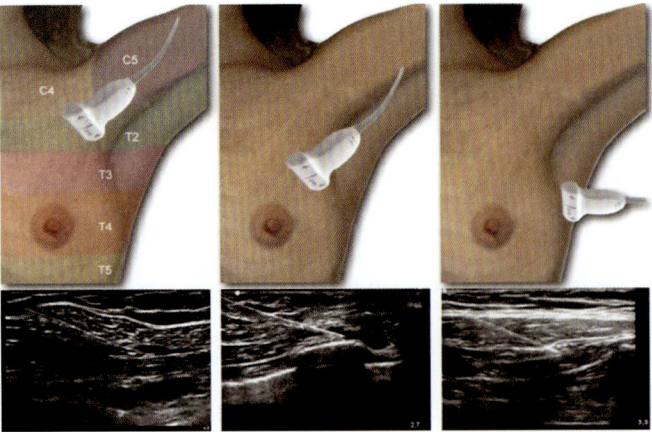

FIGURE 52.55 Graphic representing probe position and corresponding ultrasound image obtained during a PECS I block **(left)**, PECS II block **(middle)**, and serratus plane block **(right)**. *(From Blanco R, Parras T, McDonnell JG, et al. Serratus plane block: a novel ultrasound-guided thoracic wall nerve block. Anaesthesia 2013;68[11]:1107–1113.)*

ULTRASOUND TECHNIQUE
PECS I and PECS II

The patient is placed supine, and a linear array ultrasound probe is held in the parasagittal plane. The clavicle is identified cranially, and the pertinent sonoanatomy is identified from superficial to deep: the PMm and the Pmm deep to it. Between the PMm and Pmm, the thoracoacromial artery is identified. Deep to the pectoral muscles are the axillary artery, vein, and cords of the brachial plexus. With a medial tilt of the ultrasound probe, the serratus anterior muscle, intercostal muscles, ribs, and pleura are identified. The second rib is usually encountered first if the probe is traveling from a cephalad to a caudad path, with the clavicle identified first on screen. The probe is rotated toward the axilla. The needle is introduced from a cephalomedial orientation to caudolateral position. The practitioner should pass the needle through PMm, avoiding the thoracoacromial artery, and deposit 10 to 20 mL of local anesthetic between the Pmm and serratus muscle at the level of the third rib. The targeted nerves here are the lateral rami of the intercostal nerves and the long thoracic nerve. The practitioner then withdraws the needle and injects 10 mL of local anesthetic into the interfacial plane between the PMm and Pmm lateral to the thoracoacromial artery (Figs. 52.55 and 52.56).

Serratus Anterior Plane Block

With the patient lateral, the ultrasound probe is moved caudally and laterally from the PECS II position toward the midaxillary line. At the level of the fifth rib, 20 mL of local anesthetic is deposited either superficial or deep to the serratus anterior muscle. Directing the needle trajectory toward the fifth rib decreases the chance of pneumothorax by providing a bony stop for the needle if it is inadvertently advanced too deep. The described difference of analgesic duration was double if local anesthetic was injected superficial to the serratus anterior muscle (see Figs. 52.55 and 52.56).

CLINICAL EFFECTS

The advantage of the PECS blocks over paravertebral or thoracic epidural is that they are theoretically less risky and simple to perform for those facile with the ultrasound and are not contraindicated when a patient is on anticoagulation.

Because it is a relatively new block that that has undergone refinement and evolution, not many clinical studies have evaluated the efficacy of this technique. Wahba and Kamal[416] compared ultrasound-guided PECS I and PECS II blocks with landmark-guided thoracic paravertebral block at the T4 level in patients undergoing a modified radical mastectomy. They found that the PECS group required less opioid intraoperatively and reported better postoperative pain control. The study compared an ultrasound technique to landmark-guided, single-level paravertebral block with half the local anesthetic volume as the PECS group. Additional studies are warranted to compare multiple-level paravertebral blocks.

The literature available for the SAP block is limited to case reports describing successful single-shot and catheter techniques for breast surgeries and thoracotomies.[410,417–420] A review of the evidence by Abrahams et al.[404] in 2016 gave the evidence a grade of A based on one level Ib study, one level IIb study, and two level II studies that all supported the use of ultrasound for PECS blocks.

COMPLICATIONS

No complications have been reported as of the writing of this chapter. However, pneumothorax and vascular injury to the thoracoacromial vessel are possible with this technique.

Complications of Peripheral Nerve Blocks

Complications associated with PNBs are rare. In addition to the complications specific to certain blocks that were discussed earlier, some complications are relevant to all PNBs. They can be divided into two groups: neurologic complications resulting in sensory deficits, paresthesia, motor deficits, and pain; and nonneurologic complications, including those related to local anesthetic systemic toxicity, infection, and bleeding.

NEUROLOGIC COMPLICATIONS

The reported incidence of neurologic complications associated with regional anesthesia can vary because of multiple factors such as inadequate sample size, the different definitions of complications and their duration, the accuracy of patient follow-up

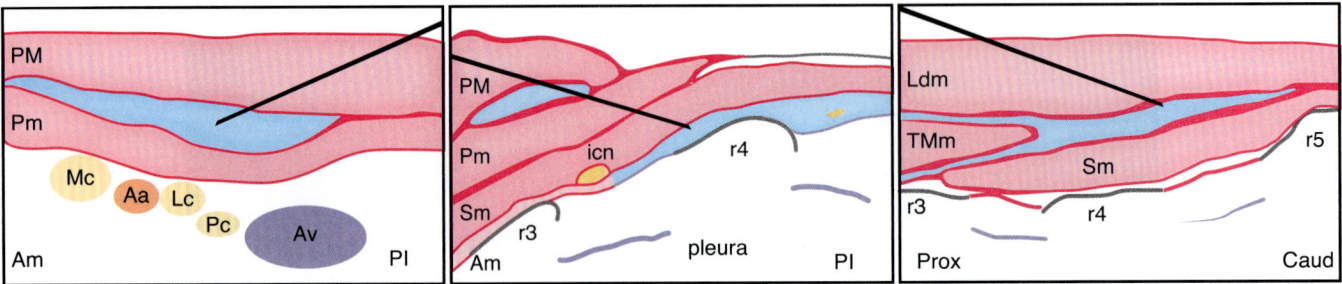

FIGURE 52.56 Graphic representing the distribution of local anesthetic *(light blue)* during a PECS I block **(left)**, PECS II block **(middle)**, and serratus plane block **(right)**. Aa, axillary artery; Am, orientation anteromedial; Av, axillary vein; Caud, caudal; icn, intercostal nerve; Lc, lateral cord; Ldm, latissimus dorsi; Mc, medial cord of the brachial plexus; Pc, posterior cord; Pl, posterolateral; PM, pectoralis major; Pm, pectoralis minor; Prox, proximal; r3, rib 3; r4, rib 4; r5, rib 5; Sm, serratus muscle; TMm, teres major. *(From Blanco R, Parras T, McDonnell JG, et al. Serratus plane block: a novel ultrasound-guided thoracic wall nerve block. Anaesthesia 2013;68[11]:1107–1113.)*

TABLE 52.2	Incidence of Neurological Complication after Peripheral Nerve Blocks					
Author	**Year**	**PNB Type**	**Technique**	**N**	**Neurologic Outcome**	**Incidence (%)**
Auroy et al.[178]	2002	All	NS, L	20,223	Neurologic complication	0.014
Barrington et al.[177]	2009	All	US, NS, L	8,189	Neurologic complication	0.02
Sites et al.[423]	2012	All	US	12,668	Postoperative neurologic symptom	0.09
Allegri et al.[424]	2016	All	US, NS, L	29,545	Postoperative neurologic symptom	0.01

L, landmark; NS, nerve stimulation; PNB, peripheral nerve block; US, ultrasound.

to identify potential complications, and the limited ability of postoperative testing to discern among different causes for postoperative neurologic injury.[421] Horlocker et al.[422] reported that 89% of postoperative neurologic injuries after ANB were the result of the surgical procedure, whereas 11% were related to the anesthetic technique. Although early postoperative neurologic symptoms are relatively frequent during the first month, their incidence reduces progressively with time. According to the largest studies performed since 2002, the incidence is 1.49/10,000 for deficits lasting up to 6 months (Table 52.2).

The mechanisms associated with peripheral nerve injury (PNI) may be mechanical, ischemic, or neurotoxic. Mechanical trauma related to the block needle may distort the nerve anatomy and cause histologic derangement, particularly when the needle tip disrupts the perineurium, resulting in an intrafascicular injection.[425,426] Intraneural injections can increase intraneural pressure, potentially causing neural ischemia. Additionally, intrafascicular injections elevate the neurotoxic effect of local anesthetics by direct exposure to the axons, while simultaneously prolonging the duration of this exposure.[425] Current ultrasound technology does not allow for differentiation between intrafascicular and interfascicular (also referred to as subepineurial) injections. The introduction of ultrasound for regional anesthesia in the last few decades has not been associated with a decrease in PNI.[208,427] Although some small studies have reported intrafascicular injections not resulting in PNI,[428,429] the American Society of Regional Anesthesia and Pain Medicine advises against intentional intraneural injections.[422] In addition to anesthetic factors, surgical-related risk factors may also result in mechanical and/or ischemic PNI from traction, stretch, transection, or compression injuries related to tourniquet, casts, dressings, hematoma formation, or compartment syndrome.[421]

Additionally, certain risk factors may also predispose patients to anesthesia-related PNI. Such factors involve preexisting neuropathies, whether clinical or subclinical, related diabetes, prior exposure to chemotherapy, entrapment neuropathies, or other metabolic diseases. A recent retrospective review of 380,680 anesthetic cases found diabetes, tobacco use, and hypertension to be independent risk factors for postoperative PNI.[430]

POSTSURGICAL INFLAMMATORY NEUROPATHY
Awareness has increased in recent years of the role of autoimmune or inflammatory pathways leading to neurologic deficits in postoperative patients. This condition has been termed *postsurgical inflammatory neuropathy* and is believed to result from an immune-mediated response to a physiologic stress such as surgery, vaccination, or infection.[431] The distinctive features that set it apart from other postsurgical neuropathies are as follows: delayed appearance (within 30 days, although immediate symptoms have also been described) with a return of neurologic function to postoperative baseline before the onset of symptoms, deficits in a distribution unrelated to anesthetic or surgical procedures, and symptoms originating with pain that subsequently subside and give rise to weakness. Radiographic imaging is negative, and the diagnosis is confirmed with a peripheral nerve biopsy, which demonstrates microvasculitis and axonal loss.[432] Current treatment of choice is immune suppression with high-dose corticosteroids or immunoglobulin.[421] It is important to consider the possibility of

postsurgical inflammatory neuropathy when confronted with patients exhibiting typical symptoms because most will improve if diagnosed and treated early. This approach is in contrast to the common management of conservative observation for other postoperative neuropathies.[431]

NONNEUROLOGIC COMPLICATIONS
Most case reports of hematomas associated with PNBs involve patients on anticoagulants despite observance of the ASRA guidelines. At highest risk are PNBs near vascular structures in expandable or noncompressible sites. Many of the cases of hematoma after PNB in patients with anticoagulation involve lumbar paravertebral blocks.[258,262,433] Consequently, these blocks traditionally have been managed according to ASRA's guidelines for neuraxial anesthesia, whereas evidence to support recommendations with most other PNBs in patients taking anticoagulation or antiplatelet therapy is lacking. In the guidelines for pain procedures in patients on anticoagulant or antiplatelet therapy, ASRA included PVBs and epidurals in the same intermediate-risk procedure category.[434] Symptoms associated with PNB hematoma include pain, drop in hemoglobin concentration, hypotension, and sensory or motor deficits. Diagnosis involves ultrasound or CT, and treatment may be conservative or require surgical evacuation.

Infectious complications related to PNBs are rare.[178,435] Capdevila et al.[384] reported the incidence of bacterial colonization of PNB catheters to be 28%, with 3% of patients exhibiting local signs of inflammation. There were no cases of bacteremia. Independent risk factors for local infection were postoperative monitoring in intensive care, catheter duration greater than 48 hours, male sex, and absence of antibiotic prophylaxis.

Local anesthetic systemic toxicity also has a very low incidence that ranges from 0.08 to 0.98/1,000 PNBs according to different studies.[423] Patients may show signs of CNS toxicity (agitation, confusion, seizure, somnolence, and apnea) and/or cardiovascular toxicity (hypertension, tachycardia, arrhythmias, hypotension, bradycardia, asystole). Cardiac toxicity occurs from binding of local anesthetic to sodium channels. Especially susceptible are patients in the extremes of age and those with heart failure or ischemic heart disease. The treatment is supportive, managing the patient's airway to prevent hypoxia and acidosis (both of which increase local anesthetic toxicity), treatment of seizures with a benzodiazepine or propofol, and lipid emulsion therapy. If cardiac arrest ensues, advanced cardiac life support (ACLS) algorithm should be initiated, with slight modifications: Epinephrine should be used with smaller initial doses because it is arrhythmogenic, and vasopressin is not recommended.[436,437]

SUMMARY OF TREATMENT OF LOCAL ANESTHETIC SYSTEMIC TOXICITY
- Get help.
- Initial focus
  - Airway management: Ventilate with 100% oxygen.
  - Seizure suppression: Benzodiazepines are preferred; avoid propofol in patients with signs of cardiovascular instability.
  - Alert the nearest facility having cardiopulmonary bypass capability.

TABLE 52.3 Upper Extremity Peripheral Nerve Block Dosing

Local Anesthetic (20–30 mL)	Anesthesia (h)	Analgesia (h)
3% 2-Chloroprocaine (+ epinephrine)	1.5	2.0
1.5% Mepivacaine	2–3	2–4
1.5% Mepivacaine (+ epinephrine)	2.5–4	3–6
2% Lidocaine (+ epinephrine)	3–6	5–8
0.5% Ropivacaine (+ epinephrine)	6–8	8–12
0.75% Ropivacaine (+ epinephrine)	8–10	12–18
0.5% Bupivacaine (+ epinephrine)	8–10	16–18

Continuous infusion ropivacaine 0.2% or dilute concentration of bupivacaine or levobupivacaine; 6–8 mL/h with a 2–4 mL hourly bolus.

TABLE 52.5 Lower Thoracic/Lumbar Paravertebral Block Dosing

Local Anesthetic (3–5 mL at Each Space for Multiple-Injection Technique or 15–20 mL for Single-Injection Technique)	Anesthesia (h)	Analgesia (h)
1.5% Mepivacaine (+ epinephrine)	2–3	3–4
2% Lidocaine (+ epinephrine)	2–3	3–4
0.5% Ropivacaine	3–5	8–12
0.75% Ropivacaine	4–6	12–18
0.5% Bupivacaine (+ epinephrine)	4–6	12–18
0.5% L-Bupivacaine (+ epinephrine)	4–6	12–18

Continuous infusion ropivacaine 0.2% or dilute concentration of bupivacaine or levobupivacaine; 10 mL/h or 5–6 mL/h with 4–5 every 30 min boluses.

- Management of cardiac arrhythmias
  - Basic and ACLS with medication adjustments
  - Avoid vasopressin, calcium channel blockers, β-blockers, or local anesthetic.
  - Reduce individual epinephrine doses to <1 μg/kg.
- Lipid emulsion (20%) therapy
  - Bolus 1.5 mL/kg (lean body mass) intravenously over 1 minute
  - Continuous infusion 0.25 mL/kg/min
  - Repeat bolus once or twice for persistent cardiovascular collapse.
  - Double the infusion rate to 0.5 mL/kg per minute if blood pressure remains low.
  - Continue infusion for at least 10 minutes after attaining circulatory stability
  - Recommended upper limit: approximately 10 mL/kg lipid emulsion over the first 30 minutes

For local anesthetics dosing recommendations, see Tables 52.3, 52.4, and 52.5.

Summary

Regional anesthesia techniques are one of the analgesic strategies available when implementing a multimodal approach to postoperative analgesia. Such techniques include neuraxial as well as PNBs and involve depositing local anesthetics perineurally. The blocks may be performed as continuous techniques for prolonged duration of action, and adjuvants can be added to the local anesthetic in order to improve analgesia, prolong the effect of the block, or reduce adverse effects. The choice of block is largely dependent on the location of the target area, and the majority of the blocks can successfully be performed via landmark techniques, nerve stimulation, ultrasound guidance, or a combination thereof.

TABLE 52.4 Lower Extremity Peripheral Nerve Block Dosing

Local Anesthetic (20–30 mL)	Anesthesia (h)	Analgesia (h)
3% 2-Chloroprocaine (+ epinephrine)	1.5	2.0
1.5% Mepivacaine	2–3	2–4
1.5% Mepivacaine (+ epinephrine)	2.5–4	3–6
2% Lidocaine (+ epinephrine)	3–6	5–8
0.5% Ropivacaine (+ epinephrine)	6–8	8–12
0.75% Ropivacaine (+ epinephrine)	8–10	12–18
0.5% Bupivacaine (+ epinephrine)	8–10	16–18

Continuous infusion ropivacaine 0.2% or dilute concentration of bupivacaine or levobupivacaine; 8–10 mL/h or 5 mL/h with 5 mL hourly bolus or 8 mL/h with 4 mL every 30 min bolus.

References

1. Kissin I, Lee SS, Bradley EL Jr. Effect of prolonged nerve block on inflammatory hyperalgesia in rats: prevention of late hyperalgesia. *Anesthesiology* 1998;88:224–232.
2. Elvir-Lazo OL, White PF. The role of multimodal analgesia in pain management after ambulatory surgery. *Curr Opin Anaesthesiol* 2010;23:697–703.
3. Wu CL, Cohen SR, Richman JM, et al. Efficacy of postoperative patient-controlled and continuous infusion epidural analgesia versus intravenous patient-controlled analgesia with opioids: a meta-analysis. *Anesthesiology* 2005;103:1079–1088.
4. Richman JM, Liu SS, Courpas G, et al. Does continuous peripheral nerve block provide superior pain control to opioids? A meta-analysis. *Anesth Analg* 2006;102:248–257.
5. Block BM, Liu SS, Rowlingson AJ, et al. Efficacy of postoperative epidural analgesia: a meta-analysis. *JAMA* 2003;290:2455–2463.
6. Liu SS, Block BM, Wu CL. Effects of perioperative central neuraxial analgesia on outcome after coronary artery bypass surgery: a meta-analysis. *Anesthesiology* 2004;101:153–161.
7. Nishimori M, Ballantyne JC, Low JH. Epidural pain relief versus systemic opioid-based pain relief for abdominal aortic surgery. *Cochrane Database Syst Rev* 2006;(3):CD005059.
8. Pöpping DM, Elia N, Marret E, et al. Protective effects of epidural analgesia on pulmonary complications after abdominal and thoracic surgery: a meta-analysis. *Arch Surg* 2008;143:990–999.
9. Svircevic V, van DD, Nierich AP, et al. Meta-analysis of thoracic epidural anesthesia versus general anesthesia for cardiac surgery. *Anesthesiology* 2011;114:271–282.
10. Beattie WS, Badner NH, Choi P. Epidural analgesia reduces postoperative myocardial infarction: a meta-analysis. *Anesth Analg* 2001;93:853–858.
11. Jørgensen H, Wetterslev J, Møiniche S, et al. Epidural local anaesthetics versus opioid-based analgesic regimens on postoperative gastrointestinal paralysis, PONV and pain after abdominal surgery. *Cochrane Database Syst Rev* 2000;(4):CD001893.
12. Marret E, Remy C, Bonnet F. Meta-analysis of epidural analgesia versus parenteral opioid analgesia after colorectal surgery. *Br J Surg* 2007;94:665–673.
13. Manion SC, Brennan TJ. Thoracic epidural analgesia and acute pain management. *Anesthesiology* 2011;115:181–188.
14. Kopacz DJ, Sharrock NE, Allen HW. A comparison of levobupivacaine 0.125%, fentanyl 4 microg/mL, or their combination for patient-controlled epidural analgesia after major orthopedic surgery. *Anesth Analg* 1999;89:1497–1503.
15. Wheatley RG, Schug SA, Watson D. Safety and efficacy of postoperative epidural analgesia. *Br J Anaesth* 2001;87:47–61.
16. Nygård E, Kofoed KF, Freiberg J, et al. Effects of high thoracic epidural analgesia on myocardial blood flow in patients with ischemic heart disease. *Circulation* 2005;111:2165–2170.
17. Scott NB, Turfrey DJ, Ray DA, et al. A prospective randomized study of the potential benefits of thoracic epidural anesthesia and analgesia in patients undergoing coronary artery bypass grafting. *Anesth Analg* 2001;93:528–535.
18. Loick HM, Schmidt C, Van AH, et al. High thoracic epidural anesthesia, but not clonidine, attenuates the perioperative stress response via sympatholysis and reduces the release of troponin T in patients undergoing coronary artery bypass grafting. *Anesth Analg* 1999;88:701–709.
19. Caputo M, Alwair H, Rogers CA, et al. Thoracic epidural anesthesia improves early outcomes in patients undergoing off-pump coronary artery bypass surgery: a prospective, randomized, controlled trial. *Anesthesiology* 2011;114:380–390.
20. Svircevic V, Nierich AP, Moons KG, et al. Thoracic epidural anesthesia for cardiac surgery: a randomized trial. *Anesthesiology* 2011;114:262–270.
21. Ferrante FM, Lu L, Jamison SB, et al. Patient-controlled epidural analgesia: demand dosing. *Anesth Analg* 1991;73:547–552.

22. Lubenow TR, Tanck EN, Hopkins EM, et al. Comparison of patient-assisted epidural analgesia with continuous-infusion epidural analgesia for postoperative patients. *Reg Anesth* 1994;19:206–211.

23. Zaric D, Nydahl PA, Philipson L, et al. The effect of continuous lumbar epidural infusion of ropivacaine (0.1%, 0.2%, and 0.3%) and 0.25% bupivacaine on sensory and motor block in volunteers: a double-blind study. *Reg Anesth* 1996;21:14–25.

24. de Leon-Casasola OA, Lema MJ. Postoperative epidural opioid analgesia: what are the choices? *Anesth Analg* 1996;83:867–875.

25. Curatolo M, Schnider TW, Petersen-Felix S, et al. A direct search procedure to optimize combinations of epidural bupivacaine, fentanyl, and clonidine for postoperative analgesia. *Anesthesiology* 2000;92:325–337.

26. Paech MJ, Pavy TJ, Orlikowski CE, et al. Postoperative epidural infusion: a randomized, double-blind, dose-finding trial of clonidine in combination with bupivacaine and fentanyl. *Anesth Analg* 1997;84:1323–1328.

27. Sakaguchi Y, Sakura S, Shinzawa M, et al. Does adrenaline improve epidural bupivacaine and fentanyl analgesia after abdominal surgery? *Anaesth Intensive Care* 2000;28:522–526.

28. Ben-David B, Solomon E, Levin H, et al. Intrathecal fentanyl with small-dose dilute bupivacaine: better anesthesia without prolonging recovery. *Anesth Analg* 1997;85:560–565.

29. Roussel JR, Heindel L. Effects of intrathecal fentanyl on duration of bupivacaine spinal blockade for outpatient knee arthroscopy. *AANA J* 1999;67: 337–343.

30. Kuusniemi KS, Pihlajamäki KK, Pitkänen MT, et al. The use of bupivacaine and fentanyl for spinal anesthesia for urologic surgery. *Anesth Analg* 2000;91:1452–1456.

31. Seewal R, Shende D, Kashyap L, et al. Effect of addition of various doses of fentanyl intrathecally to 0.5% hyperbaric bupivacaine on perioperative analgesia and subarachnoid-block characteristics in lower abdominal surgery: a dose-response study. *Reg Anesth Pain Med* 2007;32:20–26.

32. Pöpping DM, Elia N, Marret E, et al. Opioids added to local anesthetics for single-shot intrathecal anesthesia in patients undergoing minor surgery: a meta-analysis of randomized trials. *Pain* 2012;153:784–793.

33. Meylan N, Elia N, Lysakowski C, et al. Benefit and risk of intrathecal morphine without local anaesthetic in patients undergoing major surgery: meta-analysis of randomized trials. *Br J Anaesth* 2009;102:156–167.

34. Cole PJ, Craske DA, Wheatley RG. Efficacy and respiratory effects of low-dose spinal morphine for postoperative analgesia following knee arthroplasty. *Br J Anaesth* 2000;85:233–237.

35. Urban MK, Jules-Elysee K, Urquhart B, et al. Reduction in postoperative pain after spinal fusion with instrumentation using intrathecal morphine. *Spine (Phila Pa 1976)* 2002;27:535–537.

36. Alhashemi JA, Sharpe MD, Harris CL, et al. Effect of subarachnoid morphine administration on extubation time after coronary artery bypass graft surgery. *J Cardiothorac Vasc Anesth* 2000;14:639–644.

37. Mason N, Gondret R, Junca A, et al. Intrathecal sufentanil and morphine for post-thoracotomy pain relief. *Br J Anaesth* 2001;86:236–240.

38. Ballantyne JC, Carr DB, deFerranti S, et al. The comparative effects of postoperative analgesic therapies on pulmonary outcome: cumulative meta-analyses of randomized, controlled trials. *Anesth Analg* 1998;86: 598–612.

39. Strebel S, Gurzeler JA, Schneider MC, et al. Small-dose intrathecal clonidine and isobaric bupivacaine for orthopedic surgery: a dose-response study. *Anesth Analg* 2004;99:1231–1238.

40. Sites BD, Beach M, Biggs R, et al. Intrathecal clonidine added to a bupivacaine-morphine spinal anesthetic improves postoperative analgesia for total knee arthroplasty. *Anesth Analg* 2003;96:1083–1088.

41. Bernards CM. Understanding the physiology and pharmacology of epidural and intrathecal opioids. *Best Pract Res Clin Anaesthesiol* 2002;16:489–505.

42. Holmström B, Laugaland K, Rawal N, et al. Combined spinal epidural block versus spinal and epidural block for orthopaedic surgery. *Can J Anaesth* 1993;40:601–606.

43. Cherng YG, Wang YP, Liu CC, et al. Combined spinal and epidural anesthesia for abdominal hysterectomy in a patient with myotonic dystrophy. Case report. *Reg Anesth* 1994;19:69–72.

44. Sia AT, Chong JL, Chiu JW. Combination of intrathecal sufentanil 10 mug plus bupivacaine 2.5 mg for labor analgesia: is half the dose enough? *Anesth Analg* 1999;88:362–366.

45. Campbell DC, Camann WR, Datta S. The addition of bupivacaine to intrathecal sufentanil for labor analgesia. *Anesth Analg* 1995;81:305–309.

46. Hughes D, Hill D, Fee JP. Intrathecal ropivacaine or bupivacaine with fentanyl for labour. *Br J Anaesth* 2001;87:733–737.

47. Van de Velde M, Dreelinck R, Dubois J, et al. Determination of the full dose-response relation of intrathecal bupivacaine, levobupivacaine, and ropivacaine, combined with sufentanil, for labor analgesia. *Anesthesiology* 2007;106:149–156.

48. Tsen LC, Thue B, Datta S, et al. Is combined spinal-epidural analgesia associated with more rapid cervical dilation in nulliparous patients when compared with conventional epidural analgesia? *Anesthesiology* 1999;91: 920–925.

49. Pascual-Ramirez J, Haya J, Perez-Lopez FR, et al. Effect of combined spinal-epidural analgesia versus epidural analgesia on labor and delivery duration. *Int J Gynaecol Obstet* 2011;114:246–250.

50. Reyes M, Pan PH. Very low-dose spinal anesthesia for cesarean section in a morbidly obese preeclamptic patient and its potential implications. *Int J Obstet Anesth* 2004;13:99–102.

51. Ranasinghe JS, Steadman J, Toyama T, et al. Combined spinal epidural anaesthesia is better than spinal or epidural alone for Caesarean delivery. *Br J Anaesth* 2003;91:299–300.

52. Blumgart CH, Ryall D, Dennison B, et al. Mechanism of extension of spinal anaesthesia by extradural injection of local anaesthetic. *Br J Anaesth* 1992; 69:457–460.

53. Turner MA, Reifenberg NA. Combined spinal epidural anaesthesia: the single space double-barrel technique. *Int J Obstet Anesth* 1995;4:158–160.

54. Cook TM. Combined spinal epidural anaesthesia: a new technique. *Int J Obstet Anesth* 1999;8:3–6.

55. Brownridge P. Epidural and subarachnoid analgesia for elective caesarean section. *Anaesthesia* 1981;36:70.

56. Carrie LE. Epidural versus combined spinal epidural block for caesarean section. *Acta Anaesthesiol Scand* 1988;32:595–596.

57. Morris GN, Kinsella M, Thomas TA. Pencil-point needles and combined spinal epidural block. Why needle through needle? *Anaesthesia* 1998;53:1132.

58. Kestin IG. Spinal anaesthesia in obstetrics. *Br J Anaesth* 1991;66:596–607.

59. Soni AK, Sarna MC. Combined spinal epidural analgesia—single space double barrel technique. *Int J Obstet Anesth* 1996;5:206–207.

60. McAndrew CR, Harms P. Paraesthesiae during needle-through-needle combined spinal epidural versus single-shot spinal for elective caesarean section. *Anaesth Intensive Care* 2003;31:514–517.

61. Rawal N, van Zundert A, Holmström B, et al. Combined spinal-epidural technique. *Reg Anesth* 1997;22:406–423.

62. Robbins PM, Fernando R, Lim GH. Accidental intrathecal insertion of an extradural catheter during combined spinal-extradural anaesthesia for caesarean section. *Br J Anaesth* 1995;75:355–357.

63. Muranaka K, Tsutsui T. Comparison of the clinical usefulness of the two types of combined spinal epidural needles [in Japanese]. *Masui* 1994; 43:1714–1717.

64. Leighton BL, Arkoosh VA, Huffnagle S, et al. The dermatomal spread of epidural bupivacaine with and without prior intrathecal sufentanil. *Anesth Analg* 1996;83:526–529.

65. Joshi GP, McCarroll SM. Evaluation of combined spinal-epidural anesthesia using two different techniques. *Reg Anesth* 1994;19:169–174.

66. Hollway TE, Telford RJ. Observations on deliberate dural puncture with a Tuohy needle: depth measurements. *Anaesthesia* 1991;46:722–724.

67. Grau T, Leipold RW, Fatehi S, et al. Real-time ultrasonic observation of combined spinal-epidural anaesthesia. *Eur J Anaesthesiol* 2004;21:25–31.

68. Dennison B. Combined subarachnoid and epidural block for caesarean section. *Can J Anaesth* 1987;34:105–106.

69. Mutz C, Vagts DA. Thoracic epidural anesthesia in sepsis—is it harmful or protective? *Crit Care* 2009;13:182.

70. Toledano RD, Pian-Smith MC. Human immunodeficiency virus: maternal and fetal considerations and management. In: Suresh MS, Segal BS, Preston R, et al, eds. *Shnider and Levinson's Anesthesia for Obstetrics.* Philadelphia: Lippincott Williams & Wilkins; 2013:595–605.

71. Crosby ET, Halpern SH, Rolbin SH. Epidural anaesthesia for caesarean section in patients with active recurrent genital herpes simplex infections: a retrospective review. *Can J Anaesth* 1989;36:701–704.

72. Bader AM, Camann WR, Datta S. Anesthesia for cesarean delivery in patients with herpes simplex virus type-2 infections. *Reg Anesth* 1990;15:261–263.

73. Brown NW, Parsons AP, Kam PC. Anaesthetic considerations in a parturient with varicella presenting for caesarean section. *Anaesthesia* 2003;58: 1092–1095.

74. Vandermeulen EP, Van Aken H, Vermylen J. Anticoagulants and spinal-epidural anesthesia. *Anesth Analg* 1994;79:1165–1177.

75. O'Rourke N, Khan K, Hepner DL. Contraindications to neuraxial anesthesia. In: Wong CA, ed. *Spinal and Epidural Anesthesia.* New York: McGraw-Hill; 2007:127–149.

76. Hebl JR, Horlocker TT, Schroeder DR. Neuraxial anesthesia and analgesia in patients with preexisting central nervous system disorders. *Anesth Analg* 2006;103:223–228.

77. Lirk P, Birmingham B, Hogan Q. Regional anesthesia in patients with preexisting neuropathy. *Int Anesthesiol Clin* 2011;49:144–165.

78. Hebl JR, Horlocker TT, Kopp SL, et al. Neuraxial blockade in patients with preexisting spinal stenosis, lumbar disk disease, or prior spine surgery: efficacy and neurologic complications. *Anesth Analg* 2010;111:1511–1519.

79. Rosenquist RW, Birnbach DJ. Epidural insertion in anesthetized adults: will your patients thank you? *Anesth Analg* 2003;96:1545–1546.

80. Horlocker TT, Abel MD, Messick JM Jr, et al. Small risk of serious neurologic complications related to lumbar epidural catheter placement in anesthetized patients. *Anesth Analg* 2003;96:1547–1552.

81. Hamber EA, Viscomi CM. Intrathecal lipophilic opioids as adjuncts to surgical spinal anesthesia. *Reg Anesth Pain Med* 1999;24:255–263.

82. Kovelowski CJ, Ossipov MH, Hruby VJ, et al. Lesions of the dorsolateral funiculus block supraspinal opioid delta receptor mediated antinociception in the rat. *Pain* 1999;83:115–122.

83. Grabow TS, Hurley RW, Banfor PN, et al. Supraspinal and spinal delta(2) opioid receptor-mediated antinociceptive synergy is mediated by spinal alpha(2) adrenoceptors. *Pain* 1999;83:47–55.

84. Williams BA, Hough KA, Tsui BY, et al. Neurotoxicity of adjuvants used in perineural anesthesia and analgesia in comparison with ropivacaine. *Reg Anesth Pain Med* 2011;36:225–230.

85. Bernards CM. Rostral spread of epidural morphine: the expected and the unexpected. *Anesthesiology* 2000;92:299–301.

86. Cooper DW. Can epidural fentanyl induce selective spinal hyperalgesia? *Anesthesiology* 2000;93:1153–1154.

87. Liu SS, McDonald SB. Current issues in spinal anesthesia. *Anesthesiology* 2001;94:888–906.

88. Gwirtz KH, Young JV, Byers RS, et al. The safety and efficacy of intrathecal opioid analgesia for acute postoperative pain: seven years' experience with 5969 surgical patients at Indiana University Hospital. *Anesth Analg* 1999;88:599–604.

89. Chaney MA. Side effects of intrathecal and epidural opioids. *Can J Anaesth* 1995;42:891–903.

90. Gedney JA, Liu EH. Side-effects of epidural infusions of opioid bupivacaine mixtures. *Anaesthesia* 1998;53:1148–1155.

91. Walder B, Schafer M, Henzi I, et al. Efficacy and safety of patient-controlled opioid analgesia for acute postoperative pain. A quantitative systematic review. *Acta Anaesthesiol Scand* 2001;45:795–804.

92. Bucklin BA, Chestnut DH, Hawkins JL. Intrathecal opioids versus epidural local anesthetics for labor analgesia: a meta-analysis. *Reg Anesth Pain Med* 2002;27:23–30.

93. Kjellberg F, Tramer MR. Pharmacological control of opioid-induced pruritus: a quantitative systematic review of randomized trials. *Eur J Anaesthesiol* 2001;18:346–357.

94. Broekema AA, Gielen MJ, Hennis PJ. Postoperative analgesia with continuous epidural sufentanil and bupivacaine: a prospective study in 614 patients. *Anesth Analg* 1996;82:754–759.

95. de Leon-Casasola OA, Parker B, Lema MJ, et al. Postoperative epidural bupivacaine-morphine therapy. Experience with 4,227 surgical cancer patients. *Anesthesiology* 1994;81:368–375.

96. Scott DA, Beilby DS, McClymont C. Postoperative analgesia using epidural infusions of fentanyl with bupivacaine. A prospective analysis of 1,014 patients. *Anesthesiology* 1995;83:727–737.

97. Ready LB, Chadwick HS, Ross B. Age predicts effective epidural morphine dose after abdominal hysterectomy. *Anesth Analg* 1987;66:1215–1218.

98. Murphy DB, McCartney CJ, Chan VW. Novel analgesic adjuncts for brachial plexus block: a systematic review. *Anesth Analg* 2000;90:1122–1128.

99. Picard PR, Tramer MR, McQuay HJ, et al. Analgesic efficacy of peripheral opioids (all except intra-articular): a qualitative systematic review of randomised controlled trials. *Pain* 1997;72:309–318.

100. Karakaya D, Buyukgoz F, Baris S, et al. Addition of fentanyl to bupivacaine prolongs anesthesia and analgesia in axillary brachial plexus block. *Reg Anesth Pain Med* 2001;26:434–438.

101. Fanelli G, Casati A, Magistris L, et al. Fentanyl does not improve the nerve block characteristics of axillary brachial plexus anaesthesia performed with ropivacaine. *Acta Anaesthesiol Scand* 2001;45:590–594.

102. Likar R, Koppert W, Blatnig H, et al. Efficacy of peripheral morphine analgesia in inflamed, non-inflamed and perineural tissue of dental surgery patients. *J Pain Symptom Manage* 2001;21:330–337.

103. Lanz E, Simko G, Theiss D, et al. Epidural buprenorphine—a double-blind study of postoperative analgesia and side effects. *Anesth Analg* 1984;63:593–598.

104. Gutstein H, Akil H. Opioid analgesics. In: Hardman J, Limbird L, eds. *Goodman and Gilman's The Pharmacologic Basis of Therapeutics*. New York: McGraw-Hill; 2001:601.

105. Candido KD, Winnie AP, Ghaleb AH, et al. Buprenorphine added to the local anesthetic for axillary brachial plexus block prolongs postoperative analgesia. *Reg Anesth Pain Med* 2002;27:162–167.

106. Alhashemi JA, Kaki AM. Effect of intrathecal tramadol administration on postoperative pain after transurethral resection of prostate. *Br J Anaesth* 2003;91:536–540.

107. Bazin JE, Massoni C, Bruelle P, et al. The addition of opioids to local anaesthetics in brachial plexus block: the comparative effects of morphine, buprenorphine and sufentanil. *Anaesthesia* 1997;52:858–862.

108. Kapral S, Gollmann G, Waltl B, et al. Tramadol added to mepivacaine prolongs the duration of an axillary brachial plexus blockade. *Anesth Analg* 1999;88:853–856.

109. Kuraishi Y, Hirota N, Sato Y, et al. Noradrenergic inhibition of the release of substance P from the primary afferents in the rabbit spinal dorsal horn. *Brain Res* 1985;359:177–182.

110. Unnerstall JR, Kopajtic TA, Kuhar MJ. Distribution of alpha 2 agonist binding sites in the rat and human central nervous system: analysis of some functional, anatomic correlates of the pharmacologic effects of clonidine and related adrenergic agents. *Brain Res* 1984;319:69–101.

111. Fleetwood-Walker SM, Mitchell R, Hope PJ, et al. An alpha 2 receptor mediates the selective inhibition by noradrenaline of nociceptive responses of identified dorsal horn neurones. *Brain Res* 1985;334:243–254.

112. Butterworth JF, Strichartz GR. The alpha 2-adrenergic agonists clonidine and guanfacine produce tonic and phasic block of conduction in rat sciatic nerve fibers. *Anesth Analg* 1993;76:295–301.

113. Eisenach JC, Gebhart GF. Intrathecal amitriptyline. Antinociceptive interactions with intravenous morphine and intrathecal clonidine, neostigmine, and carbamylcholine in rats. *Anesthesiology* 1995;83:1036–1045.

114. Kroin JS, Buvanendran A, Beck DR, et al. Clonidine prolongation of lidocaine analgesia after sciatic nerve block in rats is mediated via the hyperpolarization-activated cation current, not by alpha-adrenoreceptors. *Anesthesiology* 2004;101:488–494.

115. Singelyn FJ, Dangoisse M, Bartholomee S, et al. Adding clonidine to mepivacaine prolongs the duration of anesthesia and analgesia after axillary brachial plexus block. *Reg Anesth* 1992;17:148–150.

116. Pöpping DM, Elia N, Marret E, et al. Clonidine as an adjuvant to local anesthetics for peripheral nerve and plexus blocks: a meta-analysis of randomized trials. *Anesthesiology* 2009;111:406–415.

117. Ilfeld BM, Morey TE, Enneking FK. Continuous infraclavicular perineural infusion with clonidine and ropivacaine compared with ropivacaine alone: a randomized, double-blinded, controlled study. *Anesth Analg* 2003;97:706–712.

118. Ilfeld BM, Morey TE, Thannikary LJ, et al. Clonidine added to a continuous interscalene ropivacaine perineural infusion to improve postoperative analgesia: a randomized, double-blind, controlled study. *Anesth Analg* 2005;100:1172–1178.

119. Abdallah FW, Brull R. Facilitatory effects of perineural dexmedetomidine on neuraxial and peripheral nerve block: a systematic review and meta-analysis. *Br J Anaesth* 2013;110:915–925.

120. Adrenal cortical steroids. In: Hebel SK, ed. *Drug Facts and Comparisons*. St. Louis, MO: Facts and Comparisons; 1997:122–128.

121. De Oliveira GSJ, Castro-Alves LJ, Ahmad S, et al. Dexamethasone to prevent postoperative nausea and vomiting: an updated meta-analysis of randomized controlled trials. *Anesth Analg* 2013;116:58–74.

122. De Oliveira GSJ, Almeida MD, Benzon HT, et al. Perioperative single dose systemic dexamethasone for postoperative pain: a meta-analysis of randomized controlled trials. *Anesthesiology* 2011;115:575–588.

123. Attardi B, Takimoto K, Gealy R, et al. Glucocorticoid induced up-regulation of a pituitary K+ channel mRNA in vitro and in vivo. *Receptors Channels* 1993;1:287–293.

124. Johansson A, Hao J, Sjolund B. Local corticosteroid application blocks transmission in normal nociceptive C-fibres. *Acta Anaesthesiol Scand* 1990;34:335–338.

125. Eker HE, Cok OY, Aribogan A, et al. Management of neuropathic pain with methylprednisolone at the site of nerve injury. *Pain Med* 2012;13:443–451.

126. Cummings KC III, Napierkowski DE, Parra-Sanchez I, et al. Effect of dexamethasone on the duration of interscalene nerve blocks with ropivacaine or bupivacaine. *Br J Anaesth* 2011;107:446–453.

127. Parrington SJ, O'Donnell D, Chan VW, et al. Dexamethasone added to mepivacaine prolongs the duration of analgesia after supraclavicular brachial plexus blockade. *Reg Anesth Pain Med* 2010;35:422–426.

128. Vieira PA, Pulai I, Tsao GC, et al. Dexamethasone with bupivacaine increases duration of analgesia in ultrasound-guided interscalene brachial plexus blockade. *Eur J Anaesthesiol* 2010;27:285–288.

129. Fredrickson MJ, Danesh-Clough TK, White R. Adjuvant dexamethasone for bupivacaine sciatic and ankle blocks: results from 2 randomized placebo-controlled trials. *Reg Anesth Pain Med* 2013;38:300–307.

130. Tandoc MN, Fan L, Kolesnikov S, et al. Adjuvant dexamethasone with bupivacaine prolongs the duration of interscalene block: a prospective randomized trial. *J Anesth* 2011;25:704–709.

131. Movafegh A, Razazian M, Hajimaohamadi F, et al. Dexamethasone added to lidocaine prolongs axillary brachial plexus blockade. *Anesth Analg* 2006;102:263–267.

132. Desmet M, Braems H, Reynvoet M, et al. I.V. and perineural dexamethasone are equivalent in increasing the analgesic duration of a single-shot interscalene block with ropivacaine for shoulder surgery: a prospective, randomized, placebo-controlled study. *Br J Anaesth* 2013;111:445–452.

133. Worni M, Schudel HH, Seifert E, et al. Randomized controlled trial on single dose steroid before thyroidectomy for benign disease to improve postoperative nausea, pain, and vocal function. *Ann Surg* 2008;248:1060–1066.

134. Thangaswamy CR, Rewari V, Trikha A, et al. Dexamethasone before total laparoscopic hysterectomy: a randomized controlled dose-response study. *J Anesth* 2010;24:24–30.

135. Taniguchi M, Bollen AW, Drasner K. Sodium bisulfite: scapegoat for chloroprocaine neurotoxicity? *Anesthesiology* 2004;100:85–91.

136. Casati A, Vinciguerra F, Cappelleri G, et al. Adding clonidine to the induction bolus and postoperative infusion during continuous femoral nerve block delays recovery of motor function after total knee arthroplasty. *Anesth Analg* 2005;100:866–872.

137. Weber A, Fournier R, Van GE, et al. Epinephrine does not prolong the analgesia of 20 mL ropivacaine 0.5% or 0.2% in a femoral three-in-one block. *Anesth Analg* 2001;93:1327–1331.

138. Brummett CM, Norat MA, Palmisano JM, et al. Perineural administration of dexmedetomidine in combination with bupivacaine enhances sensory and motor blockade in sciatic nerve block without inducing neurotoxicity in rat. *Anesthesiology* 2008;109:502–511.

139. Esmaoglu A, Yegenoglu F, Akin A, et al. Dexmedetomidine added to levobupivacaine prolongs axillary brachial plexus block. *Anesth Analg* 2010;111:1548–1551.

140. McDonnell JG, O'Donnell B, Curley G, et al. The analgesic efficacy of transversus abdominis plane block after abdominal surgery: a prospective randomized controlled trial. *Anesth Analg* 2007;104:193–197.

141. Carney J, Finnerty O, Rauf J, et al. Ipsilateral transversus abdominis plane block provides effective analgesia after appendectomy in children: a randomized controlled trial. *Anesth Analg* 2010;111:998–1003.

142. El-Dawlatly AA, Turkistani A, Kettner SC, et al. Ultrasound-guided transversus abdominis plane block: description of a new technique and comparison with conventional systemic analgesia during laparoscopic cholecystectomy. *Br J Anaesth* 2009;102:763–767.

143. Niraj G, Searle A, Mathews M, et al. Analgesic efficacy of ultrasound-guided transversus abdominis plane block in patients undergoing open appendicectomy. *Br J Anaesth* 2009;103:601–605.

144. Bharti N, Kumar P, Bala I, et al. The efficacy of a novel approach to transversus abdominis plane block for postoperative analgesia after colorectal surgery. *Anesth Analg* 2011;112:1504–1508.

145. Rafi AN. Abdominal field block: a new approach via the lumbar triangle. *Anaesthesia* 2001;56:1024–1026.

146. Hebbard P, Fujiwara Y, Shibata Y, et al. Ultrasound-guided transversus abdominis plane (TAP) block. *Anaesth Intensive Care* 2007;35:616–617.

147. McDonnell JG, Laffey JG. Transversus abdominis plane block. *Anesth Analg* 2007;105:883.

148. Shibata Y, Sato Y, Fujiwara Y, et al. Transversus abdominis plane block. *Anesth Analg* 2007;105:883.

149. Finnerty O, Carney J, McDonnell JG. Trunk blocks for abdominal surgery. *Anaesthesia* 2010;65(suppl 1):76–83.

150. Rosario DJ, Jacob S, Luntley J, et al. Mechanism of femoral nerve palsy complicating percutaneous ilioinguinal field block. *Br J Anaesth* 1997;78:314–316.

151. Kato N, Fujiwara Y, Harato M, et al. Serum concentration of lidocaine after transversus abdominis plane block. *J Anesth* 2009;23:298–300.

152. Farooq M, Carey M. A case of liver trauma with a blunt regional anesthesia needle while performing transversus abdominis plane block. *Reg Anesth Pain Med* 2008;33:274–275.

153. McDonnell JG, Curley G, Carney J, et al. The analgesic efficacy of transversus abdominis plane block after cesarean delivery: a randomized controlled trial. *Anesth Analg* 2008;106:186–191.

154. Carney J, McDonnell JG, Ochana A, et al. The transversus abdominis plane block provides effective postoperative analgesia in patients undergoing total abdominal hysterectomy. *Anesth Analg* 2008;107:2056–2060.

155. O'Donnell BD, McDonnell JG, McShane AJ. The transversus abdominis plane (TAP) block in open retropubic prostatectomy. *Reg Anesth Pain Med* 2006;31:91.

156. Mukhtar K, Singh S. Transversus abdominis plane block for laparoscopic surgery. *Br J Anaesth* 2009;102:143–144.

157. Webster K, Hubble S. Rectus sheath analgesia in intensive care patients: technique description and case series [abstract]. *Anaesth Intensive Care* 2009;37:855.

158. Cornish P, Deacon A. Rectus sheath catheters for continuous analgesia after upper abdominal surgery. *ANZ J Surg* 2007;77:84.

159. Dahl V, Raeder JC. Non-opioid postoperative analgesia. *Acta Anaesthesiol Scand* 2000;44:1191–1203.

160. Williams BA, Kentor ML, Vogt MT, et al. Economics of nerve block pain management after anterior cruciate ligament reconstruction: potential hospital cost savings via associated postanesthesia care unit bypass and same-day discharge. *Anesthesiology* 2004;100:697–706.

161. Allen HW, Liu SS, Ware PD, et al. Peripheral nerve blocks improve analgesia after total knee replacement surgery. *Anesth Analg* 1998;87:93–97.

162. Fowler SJ, Symons J, Sabato S, et al. Epidural analgesia compared with peripheral nerve blockade after major knee surgery: a systematic review and meta-analysis of randomized trials. *Br J Anaesth* 2008;100:154–164.

163. Chen HP, Shen SJ, Tsai HI, et al. Effects of interscalene nerve block for postoperative pain management in patients after shoulder surgery. *Biomed Res Int* 2015;2015:902745.

164. Gerrard AD, Brooks B, Asaad P, et al. Meta-analysis of epidural analgesia versus peripheral nerve blockade after total knee joint replacement. *Eur J Orthop Surg Traumatol* 2017;27(1):61–72.

165. Ilfeld BM, Vandenborne K, Duncan PW, et al. Ambulatory continuous interscalene nerve blocks decrease the time to discharge readiness after total shoulder arthroplasty: a randomized, triple-masked, placebo-controlled study. *Anesthesiology* 2006;105:999–1007.

166. Salviz EA, Xu D, Frulla A, et al. Continuous interscalene block in patients having outpatient rotator cuff repair surgery: a prospective randomized trial. *Anesth Analg* 2013;117:1485–1492.

167. Saporito A, Sturini E, Borgeat A, et al. The effect of continuous popliteal sciatic nerve block on unplanned postoperative visits and readmissions after foot surgery—a randomised, controlled study comparing day-care and inpatient management. *Anaesthesia* 2014;69:1197–1205.

168. Ilfeld BM. Continuous peripheral nerve blocks in the hospital and at home. *Anesthesiol Clin* 2011;29:193–211.

169. Ilfeld BM, Meunier MJ, Macario A. Ambulatory continuous peripheral nerve blocks and the perioperative surgical home. *Anesthesiology* 2015;123: 1224–1226.

170. McGraw RP III, Ilfeld BM. Toward outpatient arthroplasty: accelerating discharge with ambulatory continuous peripheral nerve blocks. *Int Anesthesiol Clin* 2012;50:111–125.

171. Gharabawy R, Abd-Elsayed A, Elsharkawy H, et al. The Cleveland Clinic experience with supraclavicular and popliteal ambulatory nerve catheters. *ScientificWorldJournal* 2014;2014:572507.

172. Bendtsen TF, Nielsen TD, Rohde CV, et al. Ultrasound guidance improves a continuous popliteal sciatic nerve block when compared with nerve stimulation. *Reg Anesth Pain Med* 2011;36:181–184.

173. Mariano ER, Loland VJ, Sandhu NS, et al. Comparative efficacy of ultrasound-guided and stimulating popliteal-sciatic perineural catheters for postoperative analgesia. *Can J Anaesth* 2010;57:919–926.

174. Lam NC, Petersen TR, Gerstein NS, et al. A randomized clinical trial comparing the effectiveness of ultrasound guidance versus nerve stimulation for lateral popliteal-sciatic nerve blocks in obese patients. *J Ultrasound Med* 2014;33:1057–1063.

175. Salinas FV. Ultrasound and review of evidence for lower extremity peripheral nerve blocks. *Reg Anesth Pain Med* 2010;35:S16–S25.

176. Fredrickson MJ, Ball CM, Dalgleish AJ. A prospective randomized comparison of ultrasound guidance versus neurostimulation for interscalene catheter placement. *Reg Anesth Pain Med* 2009;34:590–594.

177. Barrington MJ, Watts SA, Gledhill SR, et al. Preliminary results of the Australasian Regional Anaesthesia Collaboration: a prospective audit of more than 7000 peripheral nerve and plexus blocks for neurologic and other complications. *Reg Anesth Pain Med* 2009;34:534–541.

178. Auroy Y, Benhamou D, Bargues L, et al. Major complications of regional anesthesia in France: the SOS Regional Anesthesia Hotline Service. *Anesthesiology* 2002;97:1274–1280.

179. Kessler J, Schafhalter-Zoppoth I, Gray AT. An ultrasound study of the phrenic nerve in the posterior cervical triangle: implications for the interscalene brachial plexus block. *Reg Anesth Pain Med* 2008;33: 545–550.

180. Sandefo I, Iohom G, Van EA, et al. Clinical efficacy of the brachial plexus block via the posterior approach. *Reg Anesth Pain Med* 2005;30:238–242.

181. Boezaart AP, De Beer JF, Nell ML. Early experience with continuous cervical paravertebral block using a stimulating catheter. *Reg Anesth Pain Med* 2003;28:406–413.

182. D'Alessio JG, Rosenblum M, Shea KP, et al. A retrospective comparison of interscalene block and general anesthesia for ambulatory surgery shoulder arthroscopy. *Reg Anesth* 1995;20:62–68.

183. Brown AR, Weiss R, Greenberg C, et al. Interscalene block for shoulder arthroscopy: comparison with general anesthesia. *Arthroscopy* 1993;9: 295–300.

184. Abdallah FW, Halpern SH, Aoyama K, et al. Will the real benefits of single-shot interscalene block please stand up? A systematic review and meta-analysis. *Anesth Analg* 2015;120:1114–1129.

185. Al-Kaisy A, McGuire G, Chan VW, et al. Analgesic effect of interscalene block using low-dose bupivacaine for outpatient arthroscopic shoulder surgery. *Reg Anesth Pain Med* 1998;23:469–473.

186. Borgeat A, Tewes E, Biasca N, et al. Patient-controlled interscalene analgesia with ropivacaine after major shoulder surgery: PCIA vs PCA. *Br J Anaesth* 1998;81:603–605.

187. Borgeat A, Schappi B, Biasca N, et al. Patient-controlled analgesia after major shoulder surgery: patient-controlled interscalene analgesia versus patient-controlled analgesia. *Anesthesiology* 1997;87:1343–1347.

188. Malik T, Mass D, Cohn S. Postoperative analgesia in a prolonged continuous interscalene block versus single-shot block in outpatient arthroscopic rotator cuff repair: a prospective randomized study. *Arthroscopy* 2016;32: 1544–1550.

189. Brockmeier S. Continuous interscalene block provided superior analgesic control through the first postoperative week after rotator cuff repair. *J Bone Joint Surg Am* 2014;96:1924.

190. Zoremba M, Kratz T, Dette F, et al. Supplemental interscalene blockade to general anesthesia for shoulder arthroscopy: effects on fast track capability, analgesic quality, and lung function. *Biomed Res Int* 2015;2015:325012.

191. Lehmann LJ, Loosen G, Weiss C, et al. Interscalene plexus block versus general anaesthesia for shoulder surgery: a randomized controlled study. *Eur J Orthop Surg Traumatol* 2015;25:255–261.

192. Cohen NP, Levine WN, Marra G, et al. Indwelling interscalene catheter anesthesia in the surgical management of stiff shoulder: a report of 100 consecutive cases. *J Shoulder Elbow Surg* 2000;9:268–274.

193. Egol KA, Forman J, Ong C, et al. Regional anesthesia improves outcome in patients undergoing proximal humerus fracture repair. *Bull Hosp Jt Dis (2013)* 2014;72:231–236.

194. Cuvillon P, Le Sache F, Demattei C, et al. Continuous interscalene brachial plexus nerve block prolongs unilateral diaphragmatic dysfunction. *Anaesth Crit Care Pain Med* 2016;35(6):383–390.

195. Bergmann L, Martini S, Kesselmeier M, et al. Phrenic nerve block caused by interscalene brachial plexus block: breathing effects of different sites of injection. *BMC Anesthesiol* 2016;16:45.

196. Ghodki PS, Singh ND. Incidence of hemidiaphragmatic paresis after peripheral nerve stimulator versus ultrasound guided interscalene brachial plexus block. *J Anaesthesiol Clin Pharmacol* 2016;32:177–181.

197. Palhais N, Brull R, Kern C, et al. Extrafascial injection for interscalene brachial plexus block reduces respiratory complications compared with a conventional intrafascial injection: a randomized, controlled, double-blind trial. *Br J Anaesth* 2016;116:531–537.

198. Maga J, Missair A, Visan A, et al. Comparison of outside versus inside brachial plexus sheath injection for ultrasound-guided interscalene nerve blocks. *J Ultrasound Med* 2016;35:279–285.

199. Vermeylen K, Engelen S, Sermeus L, et al. Supraclavicular brachial plexus blocks: review and current practice. *Acta Anaesthesiol Belg* 2012;63:15–21.

200. Cox CR, Checketts MR, Mackenzie N, et al. Comparison of S(-)-bupivacaine with racemic (RS)-bupivacaine in supraclavicular brachial plexus block. *Br J Anaesth* 1998;80:594–598.

201. Koh WU, Kim HJ, Park HS, et al. A randomised controlled trial comparing continuous supraclavicular and interscalene brachial plexus blockade for open rotator cuff surgery. *Anaesthesia* 2016;71:692–699.

202. Wiesmann T, Feldmann C, Muller HH, et al. Phrenic palsy and analgesic quality of continuous supraclavicular vs. interscalene plexus blocks after shoulder surgery. *Acta Anaesthesiol Scand* 2016;60:1142–1151.

203. Petrar SD, Seltenrich ME, Head SJ, et al. Hemidiaphragmatic paralysis following ultrasound-guided supraclavicular versus infraclavicular brachial plexus blockade: a randomized clinical trial. *Reg Anesth Pain Med* 2015;40: 133–138.

204. Roy M, Nadeau MJ, Cote D, et al. Comparison of a single- or double-injection technique for ultrasound-guided supraclavicular block: a prospective, randomized, blinded controlled study. *Reg Anesth Pain Med* 2012;37: 55–59.

205. Tran DQ, Muñoz L, Zaouter C, et al. A prospective, randomized comparison between single- and double-injection, ultrasound-guided supraclavicular brachial plexus block. *Reg Anesth Pain Med* 2009;34:420–424.

206. Arab SA, Alharbi MK, Nada EM, et al. Ultrasound-guided supraclavicular brachial plexus block: single versus triple injection technique for upper limb arteriovenous access surgery. *Anesth Analg* 2014;118:1120–1125.

207. Sivashanmugam T, Ray S, Ravishankar M, et al. Randomized comparison of extrafascial versus subfascial injection of local anesthetic during ultrasound-guided supraclavicular brachial plexus block. *Reg Anesth Pain Med* 2015;40:337–343.

208. Neal JM. Ultrasound-guided regional anesthesia and patient safety: update of an evidence-based analysis. *Reg Anesth Pain Med* 2016;41:195–204.

209. Singh S, Goyal R, Upadhyay KK, et al. An evaluation of brachial plexus block using a nerve stimulator versus ultrasound guidance: a randomized controlled trial. *J Anaesthesiol Clin Pharmacol* 2015;31:370–374.

210. Gauss A, Tugtekin I, Georgieff M, et al. Incidence of clinically symptomatic pneumothorax in ultrasound-guided infraclavicular and supraclavicular brachial plexus block. *Anaesthesia* 2014;69:327–336.

211. Kakazu C, Tokhner V, Li J, et al. In the new era of ultrasound guidance: is pneumothorax from supraclavicular block a rare complication of the past? *Br J Anaesth* 2014;113:190–191.

212. Renes SH, Spoormans HH, Gielen MJ, et al. Hemidiaphragmatic paresis can be avoided in ultrasound-guided supraclavicular brachial plexus block. *Reg Anesth Pain Med* 2009;34:595–599.

213. Gamo K, Kuriyama K, Higuchi H, et al. Ultrasound-guided supraclavicular brachial plexus block in upper limb surgery: outcomes and patient satisfaction. *Bone Joint J* 2014;96-B:795–799.

214. Hadzic A, Arliss J, Kerimoglu B, et al. A comparison of infraclavicular nerve block versus general anesthesia for hand and wrist day-case surgeries. *Anesthesiology* 2004;101:127–132.

215. Chin KJ, Alakkad H, Adhikary SD, et al. Infraclavicular brachial plexus block for regional anaesthesia of the lower arm. *Cochrane Database Syst Rev* 2013;(8):CD005487.

216. Ilfeld BM, Morey TE, Enneking FK. Continuous infraclavicular brachial plexus block for postoperative pain control at home: a randomized, double-blinded, placebo-controlled study. *Anesthesiology* 2002;96:1297–1304.

217. Lecours M, Levesque S, Dion N, et al. Complications of single-injection ultrasound-guided infraclavicular block: a cohort study. *Can J Anaesth* 2013;60:244–252.

218. Mariano ER, Sandhu NS, Loland VJ, et al. A randomized comparison of infraclavicular and supraclavicular continuous peripheral nerve blocks for postoperative analgesia. *Reg Anesth Pain Med* 2011;36:26–31.

219. Ecoffey C, Oger E, Marchand-Maillet F, et al. Complications associated with 27 031 ultrasound-guided axillary brachial plexus blocks: a web-based survey of 36 French centres. *Eur J Anaesthesiol* 2014;31:606–610.

220. McCartney CJ, Brull R, Chan VW, et al. Early but no long-term benefit of regional compared with general anesthesia for ambulatory hand surgery. *Anesthesiology* 2004;101:461–467.

221. Qin Q, Yang D, Xie H, et al. Ultrasound guidance improves the success rate of axillary plexus block: a meta-analysis. *Braz J Anesthesiol* 2016;66: 115–119.

222. Barrington MJ, Gledhill SR, Kluger R, et al. A randomized controlled trial of ultrasound versus nerve stimulator guidance for axillary brachial plexus block. *Reg Anesth Pain Med* 2016;41:671–677.

223. Chang KV, Wu WT, Hung CY, et al. Comparative effectiveness of suprascapular nerve block in the relief of acute post-operative shoulder pain: a systematic review and meta-analysis. *Pain Physician* 2016;19:445–456.

224. Kumara AB, Gogia AR, Bajaj JK, et al. Clinical evaluation of post-operative analgesia comparing suprascapular nerve block and interscalene brachial plexus block in patients undergoing shoulder arthroscopic surgery. *J Clin Orthop Trauma* 2016;7:34–39.

225. Lee JJ, Kim DY, Hwang JT, et al. Effect of ultrasonographically guided axillary nerve block combined with suprascapular nerve block in arthroscopic rotator cuff repair: a randomized controlled trial. *Arthroscopy* 2014;30:906–914.

226. Park JY, Bang JY, Oh KS. Blind suprascapular and axillary nerve block for post-operative pain in arthroscopic rotator cuff surgery. *Knee Surg Sports Traumatol Arthrosc* 2016;24:3877–3883.

227. Dhir S, Sondekoppam RV, Sharma R, et al. A comparison of combined suprascapular and axillary nerve blocks to interscalene nerve block for analgesia in arthroscopic shoulder surgery: an equivalence study. *Reg Anesth Pain Med* 2016;41:564–571.

228. Pitombo PF, Barros RM, Matos MA, et al. Selective suprascapular and axillary nerve block provides adequate analgesia and minimal motor block. Comparison with interscalene block. *Braz J Anesthesiol.* 2013;63:45–51.

229. Lee JJ, Hwang JT, Kim DY, et al. Effects of arthroscopy-guided suprascapular nerve block combined with ultrasound-guided interscalene brachial plexus block for arthroscopic rotator cuff repair: a randomized controlled trial. *Knee Surg Sports Traumatol Arthrosc* 2017;25(7):2121–2128.

230. Sehmbi H, Madjdpour C, Shah UJ, et al. Ultrasound guided distal peripheral nerve block of the upper limb: a technical review. *J Anaesthesiol Clin Pharmacol* 2015;31:296–307.

231. Dufeu N, Marchand-Maillet F, Atchabahian A, et al. Efficacy and safety of ultrasound-guided distal blocks for analgesia without motor blockade after ambulatory hand surgery. *J Hand Surg Am* 2014;39:737–743.

232. Fredrickson MJ, Price DJ. Analgesic effectiveness of ropivacaine 0.2% vs 0.4% via an ultrasound-guided C5-6 root/superior trunk perineural ambulatory catheter. *Br J Anaesth* 2009;103:434–439.

233. Soberon JR Jr, Crookshank JW III, Nossaman BD, et al. Distal peripheral nerve blocks in the forearm as an alternative to proximal brachial plexus blockade in patients undergoing hand surgery: a prospective and randomized pilot study. *J Hand Surg Am* 2016;41:969–977.

234. Baik JS, Oh AY, Cho CW, et al. Thoracic paravertebral block for nephrectomy: a randomized, controlled, observer-blinded study. *Pain Med* 2014;15:850–856.

235. Wu J, Buggy D, Fleischmann E, et al. Thoracic paravertebral regional anesthesia improves analgesia after breast cancer surgery: a randomized controlled multicentre clinical trial. *Can J Anaesth* 2015;62:241–251.

236. Hutchins J, Apostolidou I, Shumway S, et al. Paravertebral catheter use for postoperative pain control in patients after lung transplant surgery: a prospective observational study. *J Cardiothorac Vasc Anesth* 2017;31(1): 142–146.

237. Scarfe AJ, Schuhmann-Hingel S, Duncan JK, et al. Continuous paravertebral block for post-cardiothoracic surgery analgesia: a systematic review and meta-analysis. *Eur J Cardiothorac Surg* 2016;50(6):1010–1018.

238. Yeung JH, Gates S, Naidu BV, et al. Paravertebral block versus thoracic epidural for patients undergoing thoracotomy. *Cochrane Database Syst Rev* 2016;(2):CD009121.

239. Terkawi AS, Tsang S, Sessler DI, et al. Improving analgesic efficacy and safety of thoracic paravertebral block for breast surgery: a mixed-effects meta-analysis. *Pain Physician* 2015;18:E757–E780.

240. Tighe S. The safety of paravertebral nerve block. *Anaesthesia* 2013;68:783.

241. Fahy AS, Jakub JW, Dy BM, et al. Paravertebral blocks in patients undergoing mastectomy with or without immediate reconstruction provides improved pain control and decreased postoperative nausea and vomiting. *Ann Surg Oncol* 2014;21:3284–3289.

242. Parikh RP, Sharma K, Guffey R, et al. Preoperative paravertebral block improves postoperative pain control and reduces hospital length of stay in patients undergoing autologous breast reconstruction after mastectomy for breast cancer. *Ann Surg Oncol* 2016;23:4262–4269.

243. Wolf O, Clemens MW, Purugganan RV, et al. A prospective, randomized, controlled trial of paravertebral block versus general anesthesia alone for prosthetic breast reconstruction. *Plast Reconstr Surg* 2016;137:660e–666e.

244. Kasimahanti R, Arora S, Bhatia N, et al. Ultrasound-guided single- vs double-level thoracic paravertebral block for postoperative analgesia in total mastectomy with axillary clearance. *J Clin Anesth* 2016;33:414–421.

245. Ilfeld BM, Madison SJ, Suresh PJ, et al. Treatment of postmastectomy pain with ambulatory continuous paravertebral nerve blocks: a randomized, triple-masked, placebo-controlled study. *Reg Anesth Pain Med* 2014; 39:89–96.

246. Biswas S, Verma R, Bhatia VK, et al. Comparison between thoracic epidural block and thoracic paravertebral block for post thoracotomy pain relief. *J Clin Diagn Res* 2016;10:UC08–UC12.

247. Enneking FK, Chan V, Greger J, et al. Lower-extremity peripheral nerve blockade: essentials of our current understanding. *Reg Anesth Pain Med* 2005;30:4–35.

248. Chayen D, Nathan H, Chayen M. The psoas compartment block. *Anesthesiology* 1976;45:95–99.

249. Danelli G, Fanelli A, Ghisi D, et al. Ultrasound vs nerve stimulation multiple injection technique for posterior popliteal sciatic nerve block. *Anaesthesia* 2009;64:638–642.

250. Farny J, Girard M, Drolet P. Posterior approach to the lumbar plexus combined with a sciatic nerve block using lidocaine. *Can J Anaesth* 1994; 41:486–491.

251. Brown DL. Psoas compartment block. In: Brown DL, ed. *Atlas of Regional Anesthesia.* Philadelphia: Saunders; 1999:88–91.

252. Solanski D. Posterior lumbar plexus (psoas) block. In: Chelly JE, ed. *Peripheral Nerve Blocks: A Color Atlas.* Philadelphia: Lippincott Williams & Wilkins; 1999:90–92.

253. Karmakar MK, Ho AM, Li X, et al. Ultrasound-guided lumbar plexus block through the acoustic window of the lumbar ultrasound trident. *Br J Anaesth* 2008;100:533–537.

254. Touray ST, de Leeuw MA, Zuurmond WW, et al. Psoas compartment block for lower extremity surgery: a meta-analysis. *Br J Anaesth* 2008;101:750–760.

255. Kirchmair L, Entner T, Kapral S, et al. Ultrasound guidance for the psoas compartment block: an imaging study. *Anesth Analg* 2002;94:706–710.

256. Mannion S, O'Callaghan S, Walsh M, et al. In with the new, out with the old? Comparison of two approaches for psoas compartment block. *Anesth Analg* 2005;101:259–264.

257. Kirchmair L, Entner T, Wissel J, et al. A study of the paravertebral anatomy for ultrasound-guided posterior lumbar plexus block. *Anesth Analg* 2001;93:477–481.

258. Weller RS, Gerancher JC, Crews JC, et al. Extensive retroperitoneal hematoma without neurologic deficit in two patients who underwent lumbar plexus block and were later anticoagulated. *Anesthesiology* 2003;98:581–585.

259. Karmakar MK, Shariat AN, Pangthipampai P, et al. High-definition ultrasound imaging defines the paraneural sheath and the fascial compartments surrounding the sciatic nerve at the popliteal fossa. *Reg Anesth Pain Med* 2013;38:447–451.

260. Gadsden JC, Lindenmuth DM, Hadzic A, et al. Lumbar plexus block using high-pressure injection leads to contralateral and epidural spread. *Anesthesiology* 2008;109:683–688.

261. Aida S, Takahashi H, Shimoji K. Renal subcapsular hematoma after lumbar plexus block. *Anesthesiology* 1996;84:452–455.

262. Klein SM, D'Ercole F, Greengrass RA, et al. Enoxaparin associated with psoas hematoma and lumbar plexopathy after lumbar plexus block. *Anesthesiology* 1997;87:1576–1579.

263. Dolan J. Ultrasonography or nerve stimulation for lumbar plexus blockade. *Anaesthesia* 2015;70:1329.

264. Dixon WJ. Staircase bioassay: the up-and-down method. *Neurosci Biobehav Rev* 1991;15:47–50.

265. Lang SA, Yip RW, Chang PC, et al. The femoral 3-in-1 block revisited. *J Clin Anesth* 1993;5:292–296.

266. Choi SC. Interval estimation of the LD50 based on an up-and-down experiment. *Biometrics* 1990;46:485–492.

267. Divine G, Norton HJ, Hunt R, et al. Statistical grand rounds: a review of analysis and sample size calculation considerations for Wilcoxon tests. *Anesth Analg* 2013;117:699–710.

268. Cappelleri G, Aldegheri G, Ruggieri F, et al. Effects of using the posterior or anterior approaches to the lumbar plexus on the minimum effective anesthetic concentration (MEAC) of mepivacaine required to block the femoral nerve: a prospective, randomized, up-and-down study. *Reg Anesth Pain Med* 2008;33:10–16.

269. Cappelleri G, Ghisi D, Ceravola E, et al. A randomised controlled comparison between stimulating and standard catheters for lumbar plexus block. *Anaesthesia* 2015;70:948–955.

270. Aveline C, Le HH, Le RA, et al. Perineural ultrasound-guided catheter bacterial colonization: a prospective evaluation in 747 cases. *Reg Anesth Pain Med* 2011;36:579–584.

271. Cuvillon P, Ripart J, Lalourcey L, et al. The continuous femoral nerve block catheter for postoperative analgesia: bacterial colonization, infectious rate and adverse effects. *Anesth Analg* 2001;93:1045–1049.

272. Capdevila X, Bringuier S, Borgeat A. Infectious risk of continuous peripheral nerve blocks. *Anesthesiology* 2009;110:182–188.

273. Singelyn FJ, Vanderelst PE, Gouverneur JM. Extended femoral nerve sheath block after total hip arthroplasty: continuous versus patient-controlled techniques. *Anesth Analg* 2001;92:455–459.

274. Singelyn FJ, Gouverneur JM. Extended "three-in-one" block after total knee arthroplasty: continuous versus patient-controlled techniques. *Anesth Analg* 2000;91:176–180.

275. Chelly JE, Greger J, Gebhard R, et al. Continuous femoral blocks improve recovery and outcome of patients undergoing total knee arthroplasty. *J Arthroplasty* 2001;16:436–445.

276. Ilfeld BM, Mariano ER, Girard PJ, et al. A multicenter, randomized, triple-masked, placebo-controlled trial of the effect of ambulatory continuous femoral nerve blocks on discharge-readiness following total knee arthroplasty in patients on general orthopaedic wards. *Pain* 2010;150:477–484.

277. Ilfeld BM, Le LT, Meyer RS, et al. Ambulatory continuous femoral nerve blocks decrease time to discharge readiness after tricompartment total knee arthroplasty: a randomized, triple-masked, placebo-controlled study. *Anesthesiology* 2008;108:703–713.

278. Jaeger P, Nielsen ZJ, Henningsen MH, et al. Adductor canal block versus femoral nerve block and quadriceps strength: a randomized, double-blind, placebo-controlled, crossover study in healthy volunteers. *Anesthesiology* 2013;118:409–415.

279. Kwofie MK, Shastri UD, Gadsden JC, et al. The effects of ultrasound-guided adductor canal block versus femoral nerve block on quadriceps strength and fall risk: a blinded, randomized trial of volunteers. *Reg Anesth Pain Med* 2013;38:321–325.

280. Kim DH, Lin Y, Goytizolo EA, et al. Adductor canal block versus femoral nerve block for total knee arthroplasty: a prospective, randomized, controlled trial. *Anesthesiology* 2014;120:540–550.

281. Paul JE, Arya A, Hurlburt L, et al. Femoral nerve block improves analgesia outcomes after total knee arthroplasty: a meta-analysis of randomized controlled trials. *Anesthesiology* 2010;113:1144–1162.

282. Ilfeld BM. Continuous peripheral nerve blocks: a review of the published evidence. *Anesth Analg* 2011;113:904–925.

283. Chan EY, Fransen M, Parker DA, et al. Femoral nerve blocks for acute postoperative pain after knee replacement surgery. *Cochrane Database Syst Rev* 2014;(5):CD009941.

284. Johnson RL, Kopp SL, Hebl JR, et al. Falls and major orthopaedic surgery with peripheral nerve blockade: a systematic review and meta-analysis. *Br J Anaesth* 2013;110:518–528.

285. Charous MT, Madison SJ, Suresh PJ, et al. Continuous femoral nerve blocks: varying local anesthetic delivery method (bolus versus basal) to minimize quadriceps motor block while maintaining sensory block. *Anesthesiology* 2011;115:774–781.

286. Memtsoudis SG, Danninger T, Rasul R, et al. Inpatient falls after total knee arthroplasty: the role of anesthesia type and peripheral nerve blocks. *Anesthesiology* 2014;120:551–563.

287. Webb CA, Mariano ER. Best multimodal analgesic protocol for total knee arthroplasty. *Pain Manag* 2015;5:185–196.

288. Manickam B, Perlas A, Duggan E, et al. Feasibility and efficacy of ultrasound-guided block of the saphenous nerve in the adductor canal. *Reg Anesth Pain Med* 2009;34:578–580.

289. Lund J, Jenstrup MT, Jaeger P, et al. Continuous adductor-canal-blockade for adjuvant post-operative analgesia after major knee surgery: preliminary results. *Acta Anaesthesiol Scand* 2011;55:14–19.

290. Grevstad U, Mathiesen O, Valentiner LS, et al. Effect of adductor canal block versus femoral nerve block on quadriceps strength, mobilization, and pain after total knee arthroplasty: a randomized, blinded study. *Reg Anesth Pain Med* 2015;40:3–10.

291. Nader A, Kendall MC, Manning DW, et al. Single-dose adductor canal block with local infiltrative analgesia compared with local infiltrate analgesia after total knee arthroplasty: a randomized, double-blind, placebo-controlled trial. *Reg Anesth Pain Med* 2016;41:678–684.

292. Jiang X, Wang QQ, Wu CA, et al. Analgesic efficacy of adductor canal block in total knee arthroplasty: a meta-analysis and systematic review. *Orthop Surg* 2016;8:294–300.

293. Gao F, Ma J, Sun W, et al. Adductor canal block versus femoral nerve block for analgesia after total knee arthroplasty: a systematic review and meta-analysis. *Clin J Pain* 2017;33(4):356–368.

294. Zhao XQ, Jiang N, Yuan FF, et al. The comparison of adductor canal block with femoral nerve block following total knee arthroplasty: a systematic review with meta-analysis. *J Anesth* 2016;30:745–754.

295. Jenstrup MT, Jaeger P, Lund J, et al. Effects of adductor-canal-blockade on pain and ambulation after total knee arthroplasty: a randomized study. *Acta Anaesthesiol Scand* 2012;56:357–364.

296. Hanson NA, Allen CJ, Hostetter LS, et al. Continuous ultrasound-guided adductor canal block for total knee arthroplasty: a randomized, double-blind trial. *Anesth Analg* 2014;118:1370–1377.

297. Abdallah FW, Whelan DB, Chan VW, et al. Adductor canal block provides noninferior analgesia and superior quadriceps strength compared with femoral nerve block in anterior cruciate ligament reconstruction. *Anesthesiology* 2016;124:1053–1064.

298. Veal C, Auyong DB, Hanson NA, et al. Delayed quadriceps weakness after continuous adductor canal block for total knee arthroplasty: a case report. *Acta Anaesthesiol Scand* 2014;58:362–364.

299. Chen J, Lesser JB, Hadzic A, et al. Adductor canal block can result in motor block of the quadriceps muscle. *Reg Anesth Pain Med* 2014;39:170–171.

300. Mariano ER, Kim TE, Wagner MJ, et al. A randomized comparison of proximal and distal ultrasound-guided adductor canal catheter insertion sites for knee arthroplasty. *J Ultrasound Med* 2014;33:1653–1662.

301. Andersen HL, Gyrn J, Moller L, et al. Continuous saphenous nerve block as supplement to single-dose local infiltration analgesia for postoperative pain management after total knee arthroplasty. *Reg Anesth Pain Med* 2013;38:106–111.

302. Kapoor R, Adhikary SD, Siefring C, et al. The saphenous nerve and its relationship to the nerve to the vastus medialis in and around the adductor canal: an anatomical study. *Acta Anaesthesiol Scand* 2012;56:365–367.

303. Davis JJ, Bond TS, Swenson JD. Adductor canal block: more than just the saphenous nerve? *Reg Anesth Pain Med* 2009;34:618–619.

304. Gautier PE, Hadzic A, Lecoq JP, et al. Distribution of injectate and sensory-motor blockade after adductor canal block. *Anesth Analg* 2016;122:279–282.

305. Burckett-St Laurent D, Peng P, Girón Arango L, et al. The nerves of the adductor canal and the innervation of the knee: an anatomic study. *Reg Anesth Pain Med* 2016;41:321–327.

306. Kennedy JC, Alexander IJ, Hayes KC. Nerve supply of the human knee and its functional importance. *Am J Sports Med* 1982;10:329–335.

307. Horner G, Dellon AL. Innervation of the human knee joint and implications for surgery. *Clin Orthop Relat Res* 1994;221–226.

308. Hirasawa Y, Okajima S, Ohta M, et al. Nerve distribution to the human knee joint: anatomical and immunohistochemical study. *Int Orthop* 2000;24:1–4.

309. Gardner E. The innervation of the knee joint. *Anat Rec* 1948;101:109–130.

310. Jaeger P, Zaric D, Fomsgaard JS, et al. Adductor canal block versus femoral nerve block for analgesia after total knee arthroplasty: a randomized, double-blind study. *Reg Anesth Pain Med* 2013;38:526–532.

311. Shah NA, Jain NP. Is continuous adductor canal block better than continuous femoral nerve block after total knee arthroplasty? Effect on ambulation ability, early functional recovery and pain control: a randomized controlled trial. *J Arthroplasty* 2014;29:2224–2229.

312. Mudumbai SC, Kim TE, Howard SK, et al. Continuous adductor canal blocks are superior to continuous femoral nerve blocks in promoting early ambulation after TKA. *Clin Orthop Relat Res* 2014;472:1377–1383.

313. Mariano ER, Perlas A. Adductor canal block for total knee arthroplasty: the perfect recipe or just one ingredient? *Anesthesiology* 2014;120:530–532.

314. Deloach JK, Boezaart AP. Is an adductor canal block simply an indirect femoral nerve block? *Anesthesiology* 2014;121:1349–1350.

315. Andersen HL, Andersen SL, Tranum-Jensen J. The spread of injectate during saphenous nerve block at the adductor canal: a cadaver study. *Acta Anaesthesiol Scand* 2015;59:238–245.

316. van der Wal M, Lang SA, Yip RW. Transsartorial approach for saphenous nerve block. *Can J Anaesth* 1993;40:542–546.

317. Neal JM, Salinas FV, Choi DS. Local anesthetic-induced myotoxicity after continuous adductor canal block. *Reg Anesth Pain Med* 2016;41:723–727.

318. Zink W, Graf BM. Local anesthetic myotoxicity. *Reg Anesth Pain Med* 2004;29:333–340.

319. Basson MD, Carlson BM. Myotoxicity of single and repeated injections of mepivacaine (Carbocaine) in the rat. *Anesth Analg* 1980;59:275–282.

320. Foster AH, Carlson BM. Myotoxicity of local anesthetics and regeneration of the damaged muscle fibers. *Anesth Analg* 1980;59:727–736.

321. Zink W, Bohl JR, Hacke N, et al. The long term myotoxic effects of bupivacaine and ropivacaine after continuous peripheral nerve blocks. *Anesth Analg* 2005;101:548–554.

322. Lopez S, Gros T, Bernard N, et al. Fascia iliaca compartment block for femoral bone fractures in prehospital care. *Reg Anesth Pain Med* 2003;28:203–207.

323. Capdevila X, Biboulet P, Bouregba M, et al. Comparison of the three-in-one and fascia iliaca compartment blocks in adults: clinical and radiographic analysis. *Anesth Analg* 1998;86:1039–1044.

324. Cuignet O, Pirson J, Boughrouph J, et al. The efficacy of continuous fascia iliaca compartment block for pain management in burn patients undergoing skin grafting procedures. *Anesth Analg* 2004;98:1077–1081.

325. Lako SJ, Steegers MA, van EJ, et al. Incisional continuous fascia iliaca block provides more effective pain relief and fewer side effects than opioids after pelvic osteotomy in children. *Anesth Analg* 2009;109:1799–1803.

326. Candal-Couto JJ, McVie JL, Haslam N, et al. Pre-operative analgesia for patients with femoral neck fractures using a modified fascia iliaca block technique. *Injury* 2005;36:505–510.

327. Foss NB, Kristensen BB, Bundgaard M, et al. Fascia iliaca compartment blockade for acute pain control in hip fracture patients: a randomized, placebo-controlled trial. *Anesthesiology* 2007;106:773–778.

328. Dalens B, Vanneuville G, Tanguy A. Comparison of the fascia iliaca compartment block with the 3-in-1 block in children. *Anesth Analg* 1989;69:705–713.

329. Singh H, Jones D. Hourglass-pattern recognition simplifies fascia iliaca compartment block. *Reg Anesth Pain Med* 2013;38:467–468.

330. Dolan J, Williams A, Murney E, et al. Ultrasound guided fascia iliaca block: a comparison with the loss of resistance technique. *Reg Anesth Pain Med* 2008;33:526–531.

331. Deniz S, Atim A, Kurklu M, et al. Comparison of the postoperative analgesic efficacy of an ultrasound-guided fascia iliaca compartment block versus 3 in 1 block in hip prosthesis surgery. *Agri* 2014;26:151–157.

332. Shariat AN, Hadzic A, Xu D, et al. Fascia iliaca block for analgesia after hip arthroplasty: a randomized double-blind, placebo-controlled trial. *Reg Anesth Pain Med* 2013;38:201–205.

333. Kearns R, Macfarlane A, Grant A, et al. A randomised, controlled, double blind, non-inferiority trial of ultrasound-guided fascia iliaca block vs. spinal morphine for analgesia after primary hip arthroplasty. *Anaesthesia* 2016;71:1431–1440.

334. Stevens M, Harrison G, McGrail M. A modified fascia iliaca compartment block has significant morphine-sparing effect after total hip arthroplasty. *Anaesth Intensive Care* 2007;35:949–952.

335. Bang S, Chung J, Jeong J, et al. Efficacy of ultrasound-guided fascia iliaca compartment block after hip hemiarthroplasty: a prospective, randomized trial. *Medicine (Baltimore)* 2016;95:e5018.

336. Perrier V, Julliac B, Lelias A, et al. Influence of the fascia iliaca compartment block on postoperative cognitive status in the elderly [in French]. *Ann Fr Anesth Reanim* 2010;29:283–288.

337. Hebbard P, Ivanusic J, Sha S. Ultrasound-guided supra-inguinal fascia iliaca block: a cadaveric evaluation of a novel approach. *Anaesthesia* 2011;66:300–305.

338. Mouzopoulos G, Vasiliadis G, Lasanianos N, et al. Fascia iliaca block prophylaxis for hip fracture patients at risk for delirium: a randomized placebo-controlled study. *J Orthop Traumatol* 2009;10:127–133.

339. Haines L, Dickman E, Ayvazyan S, et al. Ultrasound-guided fascia iliaca compartment block for hip fractures in the emergency department. *J Emerg Med* 2012;43:692–697.

340. Godoy MD, Vazquez J, Jauregui JR, et al. Pain treatment in post-traumatic hip fracture in the elderly: regional block vs. systemic non-steroidal analgesics. *Int J Emerg Med* 2010;3:321–325.

341. Atchabahian A, Brown AR. Postoperative neuropathy following fascia iliaca compartment blockade. *Anesthesiology* 2001;94:534–536.

342. Offerdahl MR, Lennon RL, Horlocker TT. Successful removal of a knotted fascia iliaca catheter: principles of patient positioning for peripheral nerve catheter extraction. *Anesth Analg* 2004;99:1550–1552.

343. Hopkins PM, Ellis FR, Halsall PJ. Evaluation of local anaesthetic blockade of the lateral femoral cutaneous nerve. *Anaesthesia* 1991;46:95–96.

344. Shannon J, Lang SA, Yip RW, et al. Lateral femoral cutaneous nerve block revisited. A nerve stimulator technique. *Reg Anesth* 1995;20:100–104.

345. Hospodar PP, Ashman ES, Traub JA. Anatomic study of the lateral femoral cutaneous nerve with respect to the ilioinguinal surgical dissection. *J Orthop Trauma* 1999;13:17–19.

346. de Ridder VA, de LS, Popta JV. Anatomical variations of the lateral femoral cutaneous nerve and the consequences for surgery. *J Orthop Trauma* 1999;13:207–211.

347. Grothaus MC, Holt M, Mekhail AO, et al. Lateral femoral cutaneous nerve: an anatomic study. *Clin Orthop Relat Res* 2005:164–168.

348. Damarey B, Demondion X, Boutry N, et al. Sonographic assessment of the lateral femoral cutaneous nerve. *J Clin Ultrasound* 2009;37:89–95.

349. Hurdle MF, Weingarten TN, Crisostomo RA, et al. Ultrasound-guided blockade of the lateral femoral cutaneous nerve: technical description and review of 10 cases. *Arch Phys Med Rehabil* 2007;88:1362–1364.

350. Shteynberg A, Riina LH, Glickman LT, et al. Ultrasound guided lateral femoral cutaneous nerve (LFCN) block: safe and simple anesthesia for harvesting skin grafts. *Burns* 2013;39:146–149.

351. Hara K, Sakura S, Shido A. Ultrasound-guided lateral femoral cutaneous nerve block: comparison of two techniques. *Anaesth Intensive Care* 2011;39:69–72.

352. Ng I, Vaghadia H, Choi PT, et al. Ultrasound imaging accurately identifies the lateral femoral cutaneous nerve. *Anesth Analg* 2008;107:1070–1074.

353. Thybo KH, Mathiesen O, Dahl JB, et al. Lateral femoral cutaneous nerve block after total hip arthroplasty: a randomised trial. *Acta Anaesthesiol Scand* 2016;60:1297–1305.

354. Thybo KH, Schmidt H, Hagi-Pedersen D. Effect of lateral femoral cutaneous nerve-block on pain after total hip arthroplasty: a randomised, blinded, placebo-controlled trial. *BMC Anesthesiol* 2016;16:21.

355. Grossman MG, Ducey SA, Nadler SS, et al. Meralgia paresthetica: diagnosis and treatment. *J Am Acad Orthop Surg* 2001;9:336–344.

356. Tumber PS, Bhatia A, Chan VW. Ultrasound-guided lateral femoral cutaneous nerve block for meralgia paresthetica. *Anesth Analg* 2008;106:1021–1022.

357. Labat G. *Regional Anesthesia: Its Technique and Clinical Application.* Philadelphia: Saunders; 1922.

358. Winnie AP, Ramamurthy S, Durrani Z. The inguinal paravascular technic of lumbar plexus anaesthesia: the "3-in-1 block." *Anesth Analg* 1973;52:989–996.

359. Wassef MR. Interadductor approach to obturator nerve blockade for spastic conditions of adductor thigh muscles. *Reg Anesth* 1993;18:13–17.

360. Kitamura T, Mori Y, Ohno N, et al. Case of bladder perforation due to the obturator nerve reflex during transurethral resection (TUR) of bladder tumor using the TUR in saline (Turis) system under spinal anesthesia [in Japanese]. *Masui* 2010;59:386–389.

361. Fujiwara Y, Sato Y, Kitayama M, et al. Obturator nerve block using ultrasound guidance. *Anesth Analg* 2007;105:888–889.

362. Augspurger RR, Donohue RE. Prevention of obturator nerve stimulation during transurethral surgery. *J Urol* 1980;123:170–172.

363. Deliveliotis C, Alexopoulou K, Picramenos D, et al. The contribution of the obturator nerve block in the transurethral resection of bladder tumors. *Acta Urol Belg* 1995;63:51–54.

364. Tatlisen A, Sofikerim M. Obturator nerve block and transurethral surgery for bladder cancer. *Minerva Urol Nefrol* 2007;59:137–141.

365. Helayel PE, da Conceição DB, Pavei P, et al. Ultrasound-guided obturator nerve block: a preliminary report of a case series. *Reg Anesth Pain Med* 2007;32:221–226.

366. Kakinohana M, Taira Y, Saitoh T, et al. Interadductor approach to obturator nerve block for transurethral resection procedure: comparison with traditional approach. *J Anesth* 2002;16:123–126.

367. Vloka JD, Hadzic A, April E, et al. The division of the sciatic nerve in the popliteal fossa: anatomical implications for popliteal nerve blockade. *Anesth Analg* 2001;92:215–217.

368. Jacob AK. Sciatic nerve blockade. In: Hebl JR, Lennon RL, eds. *Mayo Clinic Atlas of Regional Anesthesia and Ultrasound-Guided Nerve Blockade.* New York: Oxford University Press; 2010:405–421.

369. Raj PP, Parks RI, Watson TD, et al. A new single-position supine approach to sciatic-femoral nerve block. *Anesth Analg* 1975;54:489–493.

370. Mansour NY, Bennetts FE. An observational study of combined continuous lumbar plexus and single-shot sciatic nerve blocks for post-knee surgery analgesia. *Reg Anesth* 1996;21:287–291.

371. Di BP, Bertini L, Casati A, et al. A new posterior approach to the sciatic nerve block: a prospective, randomized comparison with the classic posterior approach. *Anesth Analg* 2001;93:1040–1044.

372. Karmakar MK, Kwok WH, Ho AM, et al. Ultrasound-guided sciatic nerve block: description of a new approach at the subgluteal space. *Br J Anaesth* 2007;98:390–395.

373. Perlas A, Brull R, Chan VW, et al. Ultrasound guidance improves the success of sciatic nerve block at the popliteal fossa. *Reg Anesth Pain Med* 2008;33:259–265.

374. Chan VW, Nova H, Abbas S, et al. Ultrasound examination and localization of the sciatic nerve: a volunteer study. *Anesthesiology* 2006;104:309–314.

375. Andersen HL, Andersen SL, Tranum-Jensen J. Injection inside the paraneural sheath of the sciatic nerve: direct comparison among ultrasound imaging, macroscopic anatomy, and histologic analysis. *Reg Anesth Pain Med* 2012;37:410–414.

376. Missair A, Weisman RS, Suarez MR, et al. A 3-dimensional ultrasound study of local anesthetic spread during lateral popliteal nerve block: what is the ideal end point for needle tip position? *Reg Anesth Pain Med* 2012;37:627–632.

377. Choquet O, Noble GB, Abbal B, et al. Subparaneural versus circumferential extraneural injection at the bifurcation level in ultrasound-guided popliteal sciatic nerve blocks: a prospective, randomized, double-blind study. *Reg Anesth Pain Med* 2014;39:306–311.

378. Tran DQ, Dugani S, Pham K, et al. A randomized comparison between subepineural and conventional ultrasound-guided popliteal sciatic nerve block. *Reg Anesth Pain Med* 2011;36:548–552.

379. Latzke D, Marhofer P, Zeitlinger M, et al. Minimal local anaesthetic volumes for sciatic nerve block: evaluation of ED 99 in volunteers. *Br J Anaesth* 2010;104:239–244.

380. Keplinger M, Marhofer P, Marhofer D, et al. Effective local anaesthetic volumes for sciatic nerve blockade: a clinical evaluation of the ED99. *Anaesthesia* 2015;70:585–590.

381. Jeong JS, Shim JC, Jeong MA, et al. Minimum effective anaesthetic volume of 0.5% ropivacaine for ultrasound-guided popliteal sciatic nerve block in patients undergoing foot and ankle surgery: determination of ED50 and ED95. *Anaesth Intensive Care* 2015;43:92–97.

382. Bang SU, Kim DJ, Bae JH, et al. Minimum effective local anesthetic volume for surgical anesthesia by subparaneural, ultrasound-guided popliteal sciatic nerve block: a prospective dose-finding study. *Medicine (Baltimore)* 2016;95:e4652.

383. Taboada M, Rodriguez J, Valino C, et al. What is the minimum effective volume of local anesthetic required for sciatic nerve blockade? A prospective, randomized comparison between a popliteal and a subgluteal approach. *Anesth Analg* 2006;102:593–597.

384. Capdevila X, Pirat P, Bringuier S, et al. Continuous peripheral nerve blocks in hospital wards after orthopedic surgery: a multicenter prospective analysis of the quality of postoperative analgesia and complications in 1,416 patients. *Anesthesiology* 2005;103:1035–1045.

385. Neuburger M, Breitbarth J, Reisig F, et al. Complications and adverse events in continuous peripheral regional anesthesia. Results of investigations on 3,491 catheters [in German]. *Anaesthesist* 2006;55:33–40.

386. Compere V, Rey N, Baert O, et al. Major complications after 400 continuous popliteal sciatic nerve blocks for post-operative analgesia. *Acta Anaesthesiol Scand* 2009;53:339–345.

387. Wiegel M, Gottschaldt U, Hennebach R, et al. Complications and adverse effects associated with continuous peripheral nerve blocks in orthopedic patients. *Anesth Analg* 2007;104:1578–1582.

388. Bondar A, Egan M, Jochum D, et al. Case report: pudendal nerve injury after a sciatic nerve block by the posterior approach. *Anesth Analg* 2010;111:573–575.

389. Labat G. *Regional Anesthesia: Its Technic and Clinical Application.* Philadelphia: W. B. Saunders; 1922.

390. Rudkin GE, Rudkin AK, Dracopoulos GC. Ankle block success rate: a prospective analysis of 1,000 patients. *Can J Anaesth* 2005;52:209–210.

391. Lopez AM, Sala-Blanch X, Magaldi M, et al. Ultrasound-guided ankle block for forefoot surgery: the contribution of the saphenous nerve. *Reg Anesth Pain Med* 2012;37:554–557.

392. Redborg KE, Antonakakis JG, Beach ML, et al. Ultrasound improves the success rate of a tibial nerve block at the ankle. *Reg Anesth Pain Med* 2009;34:256–260.

393. Chin KJ, Wong NW, Macfarlane AJ, et al. Ultrasound-guided versus anatomic landmark-guided ankle blocks: a 6-year retrospective review. *Reg Anesth Pain Med* 2011;36:611–618.

394. Redborg KE, Sites BD, Chinn CD, et al. Ultrasound improves the success rate of a sural nerve block at the ankle. *Reg Anesth Pain Med* 2009;34:24–28.

395. Myerson MS, Ruland CM, Allon SM. Regional anesthesia for foot and ankle surgery. *Foot Ankle* 1992;13:282–288.

396. Noorpuri BS, Shahane SA, Getty CJ. Acute compartment syndrome following revisional arthroplasty of the forefoot: the dangers of ankle-block. *Foot Ankle Int* 2000;21:680–682.

397. Blanco R, McDonnell JG. Optimal point of injection: the quadratus lumborum type I and II blocks. 2014. Available at: http://www.respond2articles.com/ANA/forums/post/1550.aspx. Accessed July 16, 2018.

398. Blanco R, Ansari T, Girgis E. Quadratus lumborum block for postoperative pain after caesarean section: a randomised controlled trial. *Eur J Anaesthesiol* 2015;32:812–818.

399. Sauter AR, Ullensvang K, Niemi G, et al. The Shamrock lumbar plexus block: a dose-finding study. *Eur J Anaesthesiol* 2015;32:764–770.

400. Borglum J, Christensen AF, Hoegberg LCG, et al. Bilateral-dual transversus abdominis plane (BD-TAP) block or thoracic paravertebral block (TPVB)? Distribution patterns, dermatomal anaesthesia and LA pharmacokinetics [abstract]. *Reg Anesth Pain Med* 2012;37:E137–E139.

401. Chakraborty A, Goswami J, Patro V. Ultrasound-guided continuous quadratus lumborum block for postoperative analgesia in a pediatric patient. *A A Case Rep* 2015;4:34–36.

402. Kadam VR. Ultrasound guided quadratus lumborum block or posterior transversus abdominis plane block catheter infusion as a postoperative analgesic technique for abdominal surgery. *J Anaesthesiol Clin Pharmacol* 2015;31:130–131.

403. Visoiu M, Yang C. Ultrasound-guided bilateral paravertebral continuous nerve blocks for a mildly coagulopathic patient undergoing exploratory laparotomy for bowel resection. *Paediatr Anaesth* 2011;21:459–462.

404. Abrahams M, Derby R, Horn JL. Update on ultrasound for truncal blocks: a review of the evidence. *Reg Anesth Pain Med* 2016;41:275–288.

405. Lancaster P, Chadwick M. Liver trauma secondary to ultrasound-guided transversus abdominis plane block. *Br J Anaesth* 2010;104:509–510.

406. Jankovic Z, Ahmad N, Ravishankar N, et al. Transversus abdominis plane block: how safe is it? *Anesth Analg* 2008;107:1758–1759.

407. Blanco R. The "pecs block": a novel technique for providing analgesia after breast surgery. *Anaesthesia* 2011;66:847–848.

408. Perez MF, Miguel JG, de la Torre PA. A new approach to pectoralis block. *Anaesthesia* 2013;68:430.

409. Blanco R, Fajardo M, Parras MT. Ultrasound description of Pecs II (modified Pecs I): a novel approach to breast surgery. *Rev Esp Anestesiol Reanim* 2012;59:470–475.

410. Chakraborty A, Khemka R, Datta T, et al. COMBIPECS, the single-injection technique of pectoral nerve blocks 1 and 2: a case series. *J Clin Anesth* 2016;35:365–368.

411. Blanco R, Parras T, McDonnell JG, et al. Serratus plane block: a novel ultrasound-guided thoracic wall nerve block. *Anaesthesia* 2013;68:1107–1113.

412. Fujiwara A, Komasawa N, Minami T. Pectoral nerves (PECS) and intercostal nerve block for cardiac resynchronization therapy device implantation. *Springerplus* 2014;3:409.

413. Perez MF, Duany O, de la Torre PA. Redefining PECS blocks for postmastectomy analgesia. *Reg Anesth Pain Med* 2015;40:729–730.

414. Bashandy GMN, Abbas DN. Pectoral nerves I and II blocks in multimodal analgesia for breast cancer surgery: a randomized clinical trial. *Reg Anesth Pain Med* 2015;40:68–74.

415. Chakraborty A, Khemka R, Datta T. Ultrasound-guided truncal blocks: a new frontier in regional anaesthesia. *Indian J Anaesth* 2016;60:703–711.

416. Wahba SS, Kamal SM. Thoracic paravertebral block versus pectoral nerve block for analgesia after breast surgery. *Egyptian Journal of Anaesthesia* 2014;30:129–135.

417. Madabushi R, Tewari S, Gautam SK, et al. Serratus anterior plane block: a new analgesic technique for post-thoracotomy pain. *Pain Physician* 2015;18:E421–E424.

418. Purcell N, Wu D. Novel use of the PECS II block for upper limb fistula surgery. *Anaesthesia* 2014;69:1294.

419. Khemka R, Chakraborty A, Ahmed R, et al. Ultrasound-guided serratus anterior plane block in breast reconstruction surgery. *A A Case Rep* 2016;6:280–282.

420. Bhoi D, Pushparajan HK, Talawar P, et al. Serratus anterior plane block for breast surgery in a morbidly obese patient. *J Clin Anesth* 2016;33:500–501.

421. Neal JM, Barrington MJ, Brull R, et al. The second ASRA practice advisory on neurologic complications associated with regional anesthesia and pain medicine: executive summary 2015. *Reg Anesth Pain Med* 2015;40:401–430.

422. Horlocker TT, Kufner RP, Bishop AT, et al. The risk of persistent paresthesia is not increased with repeated axillary block. *Anesth Analg* 1999;88:382–387.

423. Sites BD, Taenzer AH, Herrick MD, et al. Incidence of local anesthetic systemic toxicity and postoperative neurologic symptoms associated with 12,668 ultrasound-guided nerve blocks: an analysis from a prospective clinical registry. *Reg Anesth Pain Med* 2012;37:478–482.

424. Allegri M, Bugada D, Grossi P, et al. Italian Registry of Complications associated with Regional Anesthesia (RICALOR). An incidence analysis from a prospective clinical survey. *Minerva Anestesiol* 2016;82:392–402.

425. Farber SJ, Saheb-Al-Zamani M, Zieske L, et al. Peripheral nerve injury after local anesthetic injection. *Anesth Analg* 2013;117:731–739.

426. Hadzic A, Dilberovic F, Shah S, et al. Combination of intraneural injection and high injection pressure leads to fascicular injury and neurologic deficits in dogs. *Reg Anesth Pain Med* 2004;29:417–423.

427. Orebaugh SL, Williams BA, Vallejo M, et al. Adverse outcomes associated with stimulator-based peripheral nerve blocks with versus without ultrasound visualization. *Reg Anesth Pain Med* 2009;34:251–255.

428. Bigeleisen PE. Nerve puncture and apparent intraneural injection during ultrasound-guided axillary block does not invariably result in neurologic injury. *Anesthesiology* 2006;105:779–783.

429. Bigeleisen PE, Moayeri N, Groen GJ. Extraneural versus intraneural stimulation thresholds during ultrasound-guided supraclavicular block. *Anesthesiology* 2009;110:1235–1243.

430. Welch MB, Brummett CM, Welch TD, et al. Perioperative peripheral nerve injuries: a retrospective study of 380,680 cases during a 10-year period at a single institution. *Anesthesiology* 2009;111:490–497.

431. Kopp SL, Jacob AK, Hebl JR. Regional anesthesia in patients with preexisting neurologic disease. *Reg Anesth Pain Med* 2015;40:467–478.

432. Watson JC, Huntoon MA. Neurologic evaluation and management of perioperative nerve injury. *Reg Anesth Pain Med* 2015;40:491–501.

433. Horlocker TT, Wedel DJ, Rowlingson JC, et al. Regional anesthesia in the patient receiving antithrombotic or thrombolytic therapy: American Society of Regional Anesthesia and Pain Medicine Evidence-Based Guidelines (Third Edition). *Reg Anesth Pain Med* 2010;35:64–101.

434. Narouze S, Benzon HT, Provenzano DA, et al. Interventional spine and pain procedures in patients on antiplatelet and anticoagulant medications: guidelines from the American Society of Regional Anesthesia and Pain Medicine, the European Society of Regional Anaesthesia and Pain Therapy, the American Academy of Pain Medicine, the International Neuromodulation Society, the North American Neuromodulation Society, and the World Institute of Pain. *Reg Anesth Pain Med* 2015;40:182–212.

435. Bergman BD, Hebl JR, Kent J, et al. Neurologic complications of 405 consecutive continuous axillary catheters. *Anesth Analg* 2003;96:247–252.

436. Weinberg GL, Di GG, Ripper R, et al. Resuscitation with lipid versus epinephrine in a rat model of bupivacaine overdose. *Anesthesiology* 2008;108:907–913.

437. Di GG, Schwartz D, Ripper R, et al. Lipid emulsion is superior to vasopressin in a rodent model of resuscitation from toxin-induced cardiac arrest. *Crit Care Med* 2009;37:993–999.

CHAPTER 53

Burn Pain

SHELLEY A. WIECHMAN and **SAM R. SHARAR**

If burn injuries in themselves are not the most painful type of trauma a person can sustain, then they likely reach this status once the nature of their treatment is considered. Contemporary treatment of burn injuries involves a multitude of invasive and rehabilitative procedures that continue—often on a daily basis—for days, weeks, or months. Each intervention is critical to achieving optimal wound healing and long-term physical/occupational function yet has the potential for inflicting more pain, on a repeated basis, than that of the initial trauma. Burn injuries are pervasive in both industrial nations and developing countries around the world and affect individuals across a wide demographic span. In the United States, it is estimated that burn injuries account for 40,000 hospitalizations annually (about half of these hospitalizations are children or adolescents) and 3,275 deaths.[1] This is down from 5,500 deaths just 15 years ago. As death rates for burn injuries decline, due primarily to burn prevention strategies and improved surgical care, more patients with large burns are surviving and pose unique physical and psychological rehabilitation challenges such as scarring, contractures, amputations, psychological adjustment, and pain.[2]

Despite this increased challenge to provide effective pain relief, there has long been substantial evidence that pain from burn injuries is undertreated, particularly in children and the elderly.[3,4] Furthermore, the magnitude of pain reported after burn injury and during burn care correlates strongly with long-term adverse psychological outcome in this patient population.[5,6] Thus, there are humane, medical, and economic reasons to better control burn pain in a practical and cost-effective fashion. Pain management is closely tied to a patient's satisfaction with care, and uncontrolled pain is associated with poorer long-term outcomes in both adults and children.[7-11] Evidence-based pain management protocols have been shown to reduce pain.[12] Both the United States and New Zealand have developed clinical guidelines for the management of burn pain that were based on rigorous standards for evaluation and treatment,[13,14] and the American Burn Association has identified priority topics for research and additional clinical guidance.[15]

The Nature of Burn Pain

Treating the human suffering from burn pain is challenging from the perspectives of both the patient and clinician. It is well known that a burn injury results in one of the most intense types of sensory nociception imaginable, attributable to the unique tissue injury that results from a thermal insult to the dermal sensory organs and acute inflammatory response that, at least in the early postburn period, is related to the depth of tissue injury (Figs. 53.1 and 53.2).

First-degree burns (e.g., sunburn) are characterized by tissue injury that is limited to the epidermal skin layer and an inflammatory response in the superficial dermal layers and results in hyperemia (manifest as erythema), an intact epidermis (no skin blistering), and sensitization of dermal sensory organelles producing hyperalgesia and mild to moderate pain. Second-degree or *partial-thickness* burns involve tissue injury that extends to variable depths into the dermis; *superficial second-degree* burns involve only the upper, papillary dermis and are more likely to heal spontaneously, whereas

deep second-degree burns involve the deeper, collagen-dense reticular dermis and are more likely to require surgical treatment. Because second-degree burns consistently injure and/or inflame sensory receptors in the dermis, these burns are associated with marked hyperalgesia and produce moderate to severe pain. Third-degree burns are characterized by complete destruction of the dermis, including its sensory and vascular structures, such that although pain may still be a presenting symptom, hypalgesia to cutaneous stimulation, a leathery skin texture, and lack of capillary refill are common. Complaints of acute pain with third-degree burns are typically minimal but can be variable and are universally present with respect to the transition zone between burned and unburned skin. All burn injuries involving the dermis (i.e., second- and third-degree) result in sensitized and reorganized states of both peripheral mechanoheat receptors and dorsal horn neurons. Models of these cellular alterations provide a conceptual framework for understanding how such peripheral neuronal injuries that are present after a burn can cause acute and subacute pain, hyperalgesia, and chronic pain and are described in detail elsewhere.[16,17]

In addition to the significant pain caused by the burn injury itself, the major clinical analgesic challenge results from procedural and postoperative pain associated with contemporary burn care, which incorporates a series of aggressive procedures that stimulate nociceptive peripheral afferent fibers on a daily basis for days, weeks, or months after the initial injury. In the typical treatment paradigm, a burn injury will first be assessed as to its depth and then treated accordingly. Shallow burns will be left to heal on their own, and full-thickness thermal injuries will typically be excised and covered with a skin graft. Burns of indeterminate depth in many burn centers will

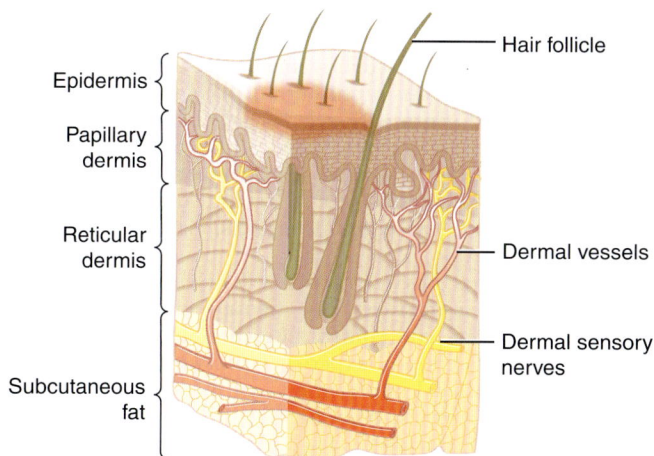

FIGURE 53.1 Anatomic layers of skin. Graphic representation of skin layers including the outer epidermis, the thin papillary dermis, the collagen-dense reticular dermis, and the deep subcutaneous fat. The dermal sensory neurons of mechanoheat receptors and dermal capillaries are shown, relative to a first-degree burn injury (confined to the outer epidermal skin layer). *(Reprinted from Sharar SR, Patterson DR, Wiechman-Askay S. Burn pain. In: Waldman SD, ed.* Pain Management. *1st ed. Philadelphia: Saunders-Elsevier; 2007:240–256. Copyright © 2007 Elsevier. With permission.)*

First Degree

Example: sunburn
Physical exam: erythema, painful,
    + capillary refill
Injury: damaged epidermis,
    inflamed papillary dermis
Treatment: spontaneous healing in
    3–4 days

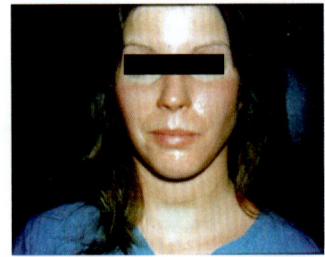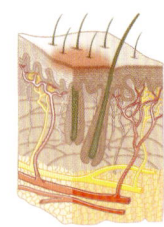

**Superficial
Second Degree
(partial thickness)**

Example: scald burn
Physical exam: pink, painful, +
    capillary refill, blisters, moist
Injury: damaged epidermis and
    papillary dermis
Treatment: spontaneous healing in
    7–10 days

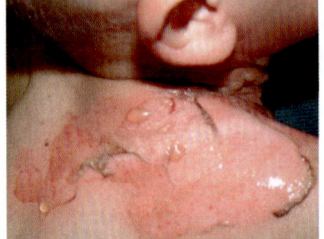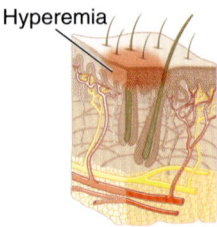

Hyperemia

**Deep
Second Degree
(partial thickness)**

Example: scald, grease burn
Physical exam: mottled red/white,
    ± painful, – capillary refill
Injury: damaged epidermis and
    papillary/reticular dermis
Treatment: spontaneous healing or
    excision/grafting

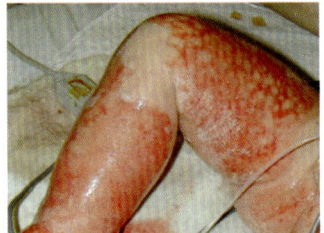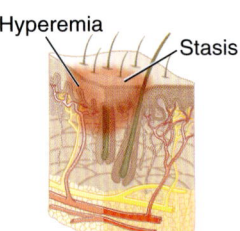

Hyperemia   Stasis

**Third Degree
(full thickness)**

Example: flame, contact burn
Physical exam: white/black,
    painless, dry, charred, leathery,
    – capillary refill
Injury: damaged epidermis,
    dermis, ± subcutaneous fat
Treatment: excision/grafting

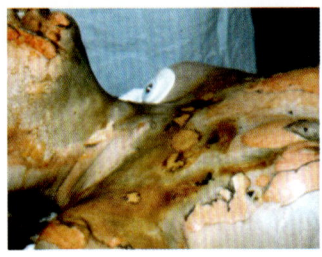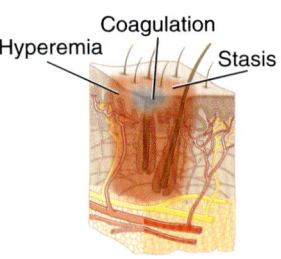

Coagulation
Hyperemia   Stasis

FIGURE 53.2   Definitions and examples of partial- and full-thickness burn injuries. Superficial and deep skin burns are defined, including clinical characteristics (etiology, physical exam findings, tissue injury, and usual treatment), photographic examples, and graphic representations of tissue injury (including zones of hyperemia, stasis, and coagulation). *(Reprinted from Sharar SR, Patterson DR, Wiechman-Askay S. Burn pain. In: Waldman SD, ed.* Pain Management. *1st ed. Philadelphia: Saunders-Elsevier; 2007:240–256. Copyright © 2007 Elsevier. With permission.)*

undergo a series of wound débridements and dressing changes, typically on a daily basis, until burn depth can be more accurately determined. Burn care–related pain can be anticipated and treated, to a large degree, based on the clinical setting in which the pain occurs. Wound débridement, limb/joint mobility exercises, therapeutic skin stretching, and other medical procedures result in *procedural pain*, which is of high intensity but limited duration. Patients who are between procedures and have minimal physical activity continue to experience *resting pain* that is relatively less intense but almost constant in duration. When pain control interventions fail to control resting pain, patients will experience *breakthrough pain*. Finally, because surgical interventions are a frequent treatment for severe burn injuries, *postoperative pain* is an additional type of pain to be considered. Each of these four types of burn pain has specific treatment strategies, as described later in this chapter.

In addition to these four distinct yet overlapping clinical settings, burn pain varies somewhat temporally with the phase of treatment, most often divided into the resuscitative, healing, and remodeling phases.[17] In the *resuscitative phase* immediately after the injury, the patient is stabilized hemodynamically and initial wound treatments are performed. This phase is

usually of short duration (e.g., hours), but depending on the size of injury can last up to 72 hours, as in the case of large surface area burns. Initial wound care in this phase is often intensely painful and, in the rush of treating life-threatening events, analgesia may be unintentionally de-emphasized. Pain in the *healing phase* is characterized by repeated episodes of burn wound care and dressing changes, wound examinations, needle sticks for intravenous (IV) access or blood sampling, and surgical procedures including débridement and grafting. The healing phase can last from days to several weeks depending on the severity of the burn and progress of the systemic response to the injury. It has been reported that hyperalgesia is more severe during this phase, independent of the size and degree of the burn. In the *remodeling phase*, the systemic and local inflammatory responses decrease, wound healing is nearing completion, and rehabilitative activities gain emphasis. Depending on the characteristics of the wound scar, this phase is characterized by not only reductions in resting pain but also ongoing episodic procedural pain associated with physical and occupational therapy sessions. It is important to note that the duration and sequence of these phases can vary depending on the clinical progress of wound treatment. For example, a patient who has progressed to the remodeling phase can return to the healing phase after a surgical procedure recreates an open wound (e.g., burn site or skin graft donor site).

Although the clinical and temporal settings of burn care can provide some prediction as to the pain a patient might experience, the magnitude and quality of a given individual's pain experience have proven extremely difficult to anticipate. The sensory and affective qualities of burn pain have received scant attention in the literature, and few studies have addressed pain patterns over the course of hospitalization. For example, Choinière and colleagues[18] observed the evolution of burn pain experienced over the course of hospitalization and found that it varied substantially both within and across patients over time. They also reported that burn pain was not accurately predicted by sociodemographic factors or burn size (the latter finding is contrary to the inaccurate assumptions of many clinicians inexperienced in treating burns). Similarly, patient pain reports do not correlate with the quantity of opioid analgesics received, a finding first published in 1981 and still reported over two decades later.[3,19] This unpredictable and often opioid-resistant nature of burn pain has been hypothetically linked to underlying sensory nerve damage[20,21] and contributes to the difficulty of effectively treating burn pain.

Although capturing the pain experience of an individual patient will likely continue to prove elusive for the reasons listed, it remains important to continue to treat burn pain aggressively. Not only can burn recovery (like that from any trauma) be hindered by the presence of acute pain,[22–24] burn pain has also been reported to influence posthospitalization emotional recovery more than the size of the burn, the duration of hospitalization, or even the patient's preinjury mental health. Ptacek and colleagues[5] reported that inpatient pain scores in adults correlated more strongly with distress and quality of life scores at 1 month after discharge than did any other independent variable studied, a finding that persisted at 1- and 2-year follow-up periods.[6] Similarly, Saxe et al.[25] reported that the amount of morphine received by burn-injured children may impact their subsequent development of posttraumatic stress disorder (PTSD). Future studies will likely further substantiate the practical utility of adequately treating burn pain.

Psychological Factors

It is well known that pain processing may be largely subjective and that the degree to which pain is interpreted as a threat will influence how much patients will suffer. A burn injury is a form of trauma that has dire emotional consequences for many survivors, and the threat value of the injury will likely have an impact on the amount of pain they perceive. Moreover, the nature of a patient's preinjury psychological makeup also has a great deal to do with how much pain he or she will perceive. In considering psychological factors, it is then important to consider the preinjury status of patients as well as their emotional adjustment during and after hospitalization.

Burn injuries often occur when people are at risk because of low social resources or because of personality and/or psychiatric factors. The estimates of preinjury psychological problems in some studies of burn patients are so high that injuries of this type should be considered to be, in part, a symptom of social ills.[26] Estimated rates of psychiatric diagnoses in patients admitted for burn care have ranged from 25% to 75%, with the most prevalent diagnoses including depression, personality disorders, and substance abuse.[26] Psychopathology and psychological problems are common in patients with burn scars that impact body function and image.[27] In addition, the nature in which the burn injury occurred is often cause for concern: suicide attempts, child and elder abuse (or neglect), domestic violence, illicit drug manufacturing (methamphetamine production, hash oil production), and juvenile fire setting are all common sources

of the injury. Psychological disturbances that predate the burn injury have the potential to increase complications, lengthen hospital stays, and lead to more serious long-term adjustment problems.[28,29] A number of these preinjury complications have direct relevance to pain control. Patients with drug and alcohol histories may show lower pain tolerance, more delirium, and higher drug-seeking behaviors. Particularly, those with a prior opioid addiction will be more sensitive to pain and greater have a greater tolerance to opioids. *Diagnostic and Statistical Manual of Mental Disorders, 5th edition* (DSM-5) Axis II character disorders can present a particular challenge to clinicians. Patients with such personality predispositions may show not only drug-seeking but also dramatic acting out behaviors, manipulation, staff splitting, and low frustration tolerance. Patients with borderline personality disorders, in particular, engage in parasuicide behavior and self-mutilation. All of these factors might complicate pain control, in addition to making the patient's overall management a challenge.

Both the burn care environment and psychological reactions to burn injuries contribute to pain and complications in its management. Patients with large unhealed burn areas or other significant medical complications are usually placed in intensive care units (ICUs). In the critical care setting, delirium and other psychotic reactions are common.[30,31] There has been recent emphasis on managing delirium more aggressively in the ICU as it leads to complications such as more infections, respiratory problems, and longer lengths of hospitalization. Unfortunately, there is a dilemma in achieving optimal management as opioids and anxiolytics are needed for pain control but are the primary contributors to delirium. Furthermore, uncontrolled pain can also increase delirium. Finding appropriate doses requires constant vigilance and adjustment. Poor communication from altered mental status or endotracheal intubation may further impede pain assessment. Anxiety is commonly reported by burn-injured patients, both at greater levels than reported to be tolerable and for prolonged periods throughout hospitalization.[32] As a result, anxiety assessment tools specific for burn-injured patients have been reported and validated and may predict burn pain and postdischarge functional capacity better than other anxiety assessment tools.[33] As hospitalization persists and patients show greater mental capacity, depression becomes increasingly common and is well known to interact with pain.[34] Depressive symptoms have a prevalence as high as 54% during postburn hospitalization[35] and are a significant predictor of physical health at 2 months postdischarge.[36] PTSD is another complication that can negatively impact pain control as PTSD can cause agitation and hypervigilance.[27,37]

The manner in which the burn environment and patients' personality factors can amplify pain is particularly notable in children, for whom the burn unit environment can be extremely strange and frightening. There is little opportunity for the burn staff to prepare children psychologically for the repeated medical procedures they must endure, and conditioned anxiety to the stimuli associated with burn care can be expected. Children will also often demonstrate regression and behavioral acting out in response to hospitalization, making pain control during procedures a particular challenge. It should be noted that although many burn centers have pediatric-specific pain protocols, their emphasis is appropriately on safety; hence, they are often not aggressive enough to adequately address pain or prevent procedural anxiety in every child. As previously mentioned, aggressive treatment of pain may serve to reduce the subsequent development of PTSD in children.[25] A comprehensive review of issues specific to pediatric burn pain can be found elsewhere.[38,39]

There is growing evidence that although pain was once thought to be a problem only during the early phases (e.g., resuscitative and healing phases) of burn care, a significant number of patients experience ongoing pain long after hospital discharge. For example, a long-term, neuropathic pain syndrome has been recently described in burned patients, presenting approximately 4 months after the initial injury[40] and persisting for an average of 13 months. Similarly, in a survey of 358 respondents of a burn survivor support group,[41] 52% reported ongoing pain, 66% said that it interfered with their rehabilitation, and 55% said the pain interfered with their daily lives. Respondents in this study also reported that thoughts of the accident and depression made their pain worse. Although much research has been done to address acute pain control after a burn injury, little is known about ongoing opioid needs once patients are discharged. Wibbenmeyer et al.[42] tracked opioid use from discharge to the outpatient setting and found that 85% of patients were on opioids at discharge with a morphine equivalent (ME) of 114. Although 90% had weaned off by 14 days postdischarge, these high doses are within the range (50 to 100 ME) associated with harmful drug effects reported in nonburn populations.[43] Furthermore, patients may show persistent depression, anxiety, or PTSD that can interfere with pain control, with both depression and anxiety predicting worse outcomes in pain, fatigue, and physical functioning assessments up to 2 years postdischarge.[44] Sleep problems are prevalent, yet frequently overlooked in postdischarge phase, and may reflect inadequate pain treatment.[45] When psychological or pain problems persist long after hospital discharge, the possibility of social or financial disincentives should be entertained. Although some patients will certainly have internally generated psychological problems, for others, the issues will persist because of such factors as litigation or the desire to avoid returning to an undesirable job.

Generalized Treatment Paradigm for Burn Pain

Because burn pain is highly variable and cannot be reliably predicted by either clinical assessment of the patient or his or her burn wound, we recommend a structured approach to burn analgesia that incorporates both pharmacologic and nonpharmacologic therapies, targets specific pain issues unique to the burn patient, and can be tailored to anticipated variations in patient need and institutional capability. One clear goal of such a paradigm is to avoid the undertreatment of burn pain.

In the generalized burn pain management paradigm, selection of an analgesic regimen is individualized and based on two broad categories: (1) the clinical need for analgesia (i.e., treatment of background vs. procedural vs. postoperative pain) and (2) limitations imposed by the patient (e.g., presence of IV access, endotracheal tube, or opioid tolerance) or by clinical facilities (available monitoring capabilities and personnel).

The presence or absence of IV access directly influences analgesic drug choice, particularly in children in whom IV access may be problematic. Patients who are endotracheally intubated and ventilated are "protected" from the risk of opioid-induced respiratory depression; thus, opioids may be more generously administered in these individuals, as is often indicated for complex burn débridement procedures in patients with more extensive or severe burn injuries. Individual differences in opioid efficacy should be considered in all patients, including opioid tolerance in patients requiring prolonged opioid analgesic therapy or in those with preexisting substance abuse histories. Due to the development of drug tolerance with prolonged medical use or recreational abuse of opioids (both commonly seen in burn patients), opioid analgesic doses needed for burn analgesia may significantly exceed those recommended in standard dosing guidelines. One clinically relevant consequence of drug tolerance is the potential for opioid withdrawal to occur during inpatient burn treatment. Thus, the period of inpatient burn care is not an appropriate time to institute deliberate opioid withdrawal or detoxification measures in the substance-abusing patient because such treatment ignores the very real analgesic needs of these patients. Similarly, when reductions in analgesic therapy are considered as burn wounds heal, reductions should occur by careful taper, in order to prevent acute opioid withdrawal syndrome.

Institutional capability to provide adequate monitoring as required for "moderate sedation" (as defined by the American Society of Anesthesiologists; Table 53.1)[46] may also dictate which agents are used for procedural analgesia, as some of the more potent opioids (e.g., fentanyl) and anesthetic agents (e.g., ketamine, propofol) may unpredictably result in potentially dangerous levels of sedation ("deep sedation" or "general anesthesia"). The use of potent opioids and anxiolytics should only occur in settings with adequate monitoring, personnel, and resuscitation equipment appropriate for the degree of sedation anticipated. For many burn wound débridement procedures and most rehabilitative therapy sessions in the hospital ward or outpatient clinic setting, opioid analgesia with "minimal sedation" is sufficient and no special monitoring is required. Larger or more potent doses of opioids, or the concurrent use of anxiolytic sedatives (e.g., benzodiazepines), may not only produce more pronounced sedation ("moderate sedation") but could also progress to "deep sedation" where patient–staff communication and/or patient consciousness are lost. Current guidelines of The Joint Commission,[47] as well as adult[46] and pediatric[48] physician specialty professional organizations, dictate both general and specific levels of monitoring (e.g., continuous pulse oximetry, presence of an independent observer specifically responsible for monitoring ventilation and vital signs) for patients requiring each of these levels of procedural analgesia and sedation.

TABLE 53.1   American Society of Anesthesiologists Continuum of Depth of Sedation

	Minimal Sedation (Anxiolysis)	Moderate Sedation/Analgesia (Conscious Sedation)	Deep Sedation/Analgesia	General Anesthesia
Responsiveness	Normal response to verbal stimulation	Purposeful* response to verbal or tactile stimulation	Purposeful* response following repeated or painful stimulation	Unrousable even with painful stimulus
Airway	Unaffected	No intervention required	Intervention may be required	Intervention often required
Spontaneous ventilation	Unaffected	Adequate	May be inadequate	Frequently inadequate
Cardiovascular function	Unaffected	Usually maintained	Usually maintained	May be impaired

*Reflex painful withdrawal from a painful stimulus is NOT considered a purposeful response.
Approved by the American Society of Anesthesiologists House of Delegates on October 13, 1999, and amended on October 27, 2004.
Reprinted with permission from American Society of Anesthesiologists Task Force on Sedation and Analgesia by Non-Anesthesiologists. Practice guidelines for sedation and analgesia by non-anesthesiologists. *Anesthesiology* 2002;96(4):1004–1017.

TABLE 53.2 Harborview Medical Center/University of Washington Burn Center Burn Analgesia and Sedation Guidelines for Adults

	ICU No PO Intake	ICU Taking PO	Ward Large Open Areas	Ward Small Open Areas/Predischarge
Background pain	Continuous morphine sulfate (IV) drip	Scheduled methadone or MS Contin	Scheduled methadone or MS Contin	Scheduled NSAIDs/acetaminophen or scheduled oxycodone or none
Procedural pain	Morphine sulfate (IV) or fentanyl (IV)	Oxycodone, fentanyl IV, or fentanyl ACTIQ	Oxycodone, fentanyl IV, Nitrox (IH) or fentanyl ACTIQ	Oxycodone
Breakthrough pain (PRN dosing)	Morphine sulfate (IV) or fentanyl (IV)	Oxycodone	Oxycodone	NSAIDs/acetaminophen or oxycodone
Background anxiolysis	Scheduled lorazepam (IV) or continuous lorazepam (IV)	Scheduled lorazepam	None or scheduled lorazepam	None
Procedural anxiolysis	Lorazepam or midazolam	Lorazepam	None or lorazepam	None
Discharge or transfer pain medications	NA	For transfer to ward: wean drips, establish PO pain meds early, anticipate dose tapering as needs decrease	Oxycodone for procedural pain; methadone taper or MS Contin taper if applicable	Oxycodone or NSAIDs for procedural pain

NOTE: Medications are to be given orally unless otherwise specified. Exception: fentanyl ACTIQ is given transmucosal. Analgesic and anxiolytic choices are simplified to a minimum number of agents to encourage staff familiarity and are targeted to specific pain and anxiety needs. Therapy can be individualized to include agents not in this guideline when clinically indicated. This chart is laminated and prominently displayed in all patient care areas.
ICU, intensive care unit; IH, inhalation; NA, not applicable; Nitrox, 50% nitrous oxide/50% oxygen inhaled; NSAIDs, nonsteroidal anti-inflammatory drugs; PRN, as needed.

Because nociception at the burn site is the predominant mechanism of pain and suffering in these patients during the resuscitative and healing phases, pharmacologic treatment with potent opioids, anxiolytics, and other agents (e.g., ketamine) is the first line of therapy. However, nonpharmacologic methods of treating burn pain are also extremely useful. Some pain control techniques should be second nature to the staff and integrated into standard care (e.g., minimizing the number and intrusiveness of dressing changes, limb elevation, brief educational approaches). Other, more novel nonpharmacologic analgesic techniques are more practically implemented after a stable pharmacologic regimen is established or may require special expertise (e.g., hypnosis). To reinforce a consistent approach to analgesic management, particularly in centers where house staff physicians or nursing staff may rotate or change frequently, the establishment of succinct yet detailed institutional guidelines may help physicians and nurses with choosing and administering analgesics that target specific analgesic needs,[12,49,50] as shown in Table 53.2. To maximize simplicity and utility, it is recommended that such guidelines be safe and effective over a broad range of ages, be explicit in their dosing recommendations, have a limited formulary to maximize staff familiarity, and allow the bedside nurse to continuously evaluate efficacy and safety.[50] In addition, the regular use of a weight-based pediatric medication worksheet (placed at the bedside and in the patient record), containing all analgesic and resuscitation drugs likely to be administered, provides a supplemental safeguard against accidental overdose, particularly in the young pediatric age group.[51]

In recent years, a number of comprehensive reviews of burn pain management that emphasize such a systematic and multidisciplinary approach to burn pain management have been published,[17,52–55] including practice guidelines from the American Burn Association.[14] The reader is referred to these sources for additional perspective and detail.

Pharmacologic Approaches

In describing pharmacologic approaches for burn analgesia, three consistent observations can be made. First, for patients with injuries extensive enough to require hospitalization, pain from the burn itself is severe. Thus, potent opioids form the cornerstones of pharmacologic pain control in these patients,

leaving few indications for the sole use of nonsteroidal anti-inflammatory drugs (NSAIDs) or acetaminophen, with notable exceptions of minor burns and outpatient treatment. Second, because burn pain has well-defined components described previously—notably background, procedural, breakthrough, and postoperative pain—pharmacologic choices for analgesia should target each pain pattern individually. Final, because burn pain will vary somewhat unpredictably throughout hospitalization due to surgical intervention and activity levels, analgesic regimens should be continuously evaluated and reassessed to avoid problems of under- or overmedication.[6] Pain assessment is facilitated by the regular use of standardized, self-report scales for adults and older children and observational scoring systems for the very young, as described in Chapter 20. A reliance on nurse assessment of patients' burn pain can be problematic, however, as it is well documented that nurses' and patients' assessment of burn pain and analgesia are not always comparable[18,56,57] with nursing staff typically underestimating the need for analgesic therapy.

OPIOIDS

Opioid agonists are the most commonly used analgesics in the treatment of burn pain, in part because (1) they are effective, (2) the benefits and risks of their use are familiar to the majority of care providers, and (3) they provide some dose-dependent degree of sedation that can be advantageous to both burn patients and staff, particularly during burn wound care procedures. The wide spectrum of opioids available for clinical use (see Chapter 79) provides dosing flexibility (i.e., variable routes of administration, variable duration of action) that is ideal for the targeted treatment of burn pain. The pharmacokinetics of opioids in burn patients are not consistently different from nonburn patients,[58,59] although decreased volume of distribution and clearance and increased elimination half-life have been reported for morphine.[60] Similarly, pharmacodynamic potency of opioids has inconsistently been reported as increased[61] and decreased[60] in burn patients.

The route of opioid administration is an important consideration in burn patients, with the principal choice between IV, oral, or transmucosal administration dictated by the severity of burn (critically ill patients require IV access and may have abnormal gut function) and high risk of burn patients for developing IV catheter–related sepsis (hence, physician reluctance to maintain long-term IV access).[62] Intramuscular opioid administration is avoided because of the need for repeated, painful injections and because of variable vascular absorption due to unpredictable compartmental fluid shifts and muscle perfusion in burn patients, particularly in the resuscitative phase. Patient-controlled analgesia (PCA) with IV opioids offers the burn patient a safe and efficient method of achieving more flexible analgesia for both background and procedural analgesia. PCA also offers the patient some degree of control over his or her medical care, this being a major issue for burn patients whose waking hours are often completely scheduled with care activities ranging from wound care to physical and rehabilitation therapy. Some studies comparing PCA opioid use to other routes of administration in the burn population have shown potential benefits of PCA.[63–65] The PCA administration of potent, short-acting opioids (e.g., fentanyl,[66] alfentanil,[67] remifentanil) for procedural analgesia may also have a useful role in burn analgesic management, but this has not been extensively investigated.

Because IV access is infrequently present in hospitalized burn patients outside of the critical care setting (for reasons noted previously), oral and transmucosal opioid delivery are frequently employed. For background pain, long-acting oral opioids (e.g., methadone) or sustained-release opioids are often utilized. However, the latter agents are not available in appropriate dose ranges for pediatric patients, so a reliance on shorter acting oral opioids is often necessary. For background pain control in this population, the use of regularly scheduled oral opioids is recommended over as needed (PRN) dosing so that more stable plasma opioid concentrations and analgesic effects may be obtained.[68] Similarly, the use of short-acting oral opioids is common for anticipated procedural pain, emphasizing early administration of the drug so that adequate plasma levels and associated analgesia are present prior to beginning the procedure. Alternatively, oral transmucosal administration of opioids is reported in burn patients to be particularly advantageous in those patients without IV access and in children, in both the inpatient[69] and outpatient[70] clinic settings.

NONOPIOIDS

The list of nonopioid analgesics in widespread use for the treatment of burn pain is relatively extensive, although clinical evidence to support such use is variably found in the published literature. Oral NSAIDs and acetaminophen, as outlined previously, are only mild analgesics and exhibit a ceiling effect in their dose–response relationship, rendering them unsuitable as sole agents for the treatment of typical, severe burn pain. However, they are of benefit in treating minor burns, particularly in the outpatient setting and in combination with more potent analgesics for their "opioid-sparing" effects. Topical application of NSAIDs on burn wounds can theoretically inhibit nociception at the injury site with minimal systemic uptake[71] yet does not result in significant analgesia.[72] The opioid agonist-antagonist drugs (e.g., nalbuphine, butorphanol) not only produce "mixed" actions at the opiate receptor level, theoretically providing analgesia (agonist property) with lesser side effects (antagonist properties) but also exhibit ceiling effects. Although studies have shown this class of drugs to be effective in treating burn pain,[73] experience with them is both limited and suggestive of efficacy in patients with only relatively mild burn pain.

Antidepressants, anticonvulsants, antipsychotics, α_2 agonists, and systemic administration of local anesthetics have been proposed as potential analgesic agents for burn pain[74] based on their known mechanisms of action in other pain states yet have not been studied extensively in the setting of burns. As neuropathic pain can occur in patients with healed burns,[21,40,41] these agents may have specific application in this setting, as suggested by a preliminary reports with a variety of nonopioid agents including gabapentin,[75,76] dexmedetomidine,[77] clonidine,[78] IV lidocaine,[79] and haloperidol.[80]

ANXIOLYTICS

Current, aggressive therapies for cutaneous burn wounds, together with the persistent and repetitive qualities of background and procedural pain, make burn care an experience that is likely to engender anxiety in both adult and pediatric patients. It is also recognized that anxiety can exacerbate acute pain.[22] This has led to the common practice of using anxiolytic drugs in combination with opioid analgesics, a practice that has persisted since the 1980s.[81] A recent survey of North American burn centers reported that up to 39% of hospitalized pediatric burn victims regularly receive anxiolytics as part of their pain and sedation management regimen.[82] Intuitively, this practice is particularly useful in premedicating patients for daily wound care procedures, due to the anticipatory anxiety experienced by these patients prior to and during débridement. Although previously shown that benzodiazepine therapy improves postoperative pain scores in nonburn settings,[83] it is also reported that low-dose benzodiazepine administration significantly reduces burn wound care pain reports.[84] It appears that the patients most likely to benefit from this therapy are not those with high trait (premorbid) anxiety but rather those with high state (at the time of the procedure) anxiety or those with high baseline pain scores.

ANESTHETICS

Inhaled nitrous oxide is an analgesic agent safe for administration by nonanesthesiology personnel to achieve moderate sedation. It provides safe and effective analgesia without loss of consciousness for moderately painful procedures in other health care settings (e.g., dentistry) and is also a commonly used, although less well-studied, agent for the treatment of burn pain.[85,86] It is typically used as a 50% mixture in 50% oxygen and is self-administered by an awake, cooperative, spontaneously breathing patient via a mouthpiece or mask. A secondary benefit of nitrous oxide use, like that of PCA opioid administration, is the element of control given to the patient for his or her care. Nitrous oxide is less useful with critically ill or uncooperative patients. It has also been implicated in a very small but measurable incidence of toxicity issues (e.g., spontaneous abortion, bone marrow suppression) to patients or staff exposed for prolonged periods,[87,88] although not in the setting of burn pain treatment.

Although it is obvious that general anesthesia is required for the surgical excision and grafting of deep burn wounds, it is not uncommon to encounter specific wound care procedures that are on a scale below that of surgical burn care yet are nevertheless difficult to perform on a conscious patient, particularly a child. These procedures are ideally suited for deep sedation or general anesthesia and include (1) the removal of hundreds of skin staples from recently grafted wounds, (2) meticulous wound care of recently grafted and often tenuous skin on the face or neck, and (3) wound care procedures in variably cooperative children. Historically, IV, intramuscular, or oral ketamine have been used for these procedures,[89,90] and there is limited evidence that ketamine administration acutely after experimental skin burns may prevent hyperalgesia and "wind-up."[91] More recently, some high-volume burn centers have developed specific training and skill retention programs in ketamine administration by nonanesthesiologists and report that satisfactory sedation for bedside procedures can be achieved in children with a low incidence of side effects.[92] However, ketamine is a dose-dependent anesthetic that can produce deep sedation and general anesthesia in an unpredictable manner; thus, appropriate patient monitoring is requisite, and nonanesthesiologists administering the drug must have specialized training and airway management skills as well as anesthesiologist backup. In addition, its use is limited by the potential risk of associated emergence delirium reactions (5% to 30% incidence), particularly in the elderly.

The extension of full anesthetic care capabilities with anesthesiology staffing outside of the operating room and into the burn unit has been successfully implemented in some specialized burn centers.[93,94] This has been facilitated by the recent introduction into clinical anesthetic practice of a variety of drugs with a rapid onset and short duration of action, a more rapid awakening/recovery, and fewer associated side effects—ideal qualities for agents to be used for procedural burn wound care. These agents include IV propofol and remifentanil and inhaled sevoflurane and desflurane. Propofol is particularly advantageous and can be titrated to effect both in terms of level of consciousness and duration of action using continuous IV infusion techniques.[95] The provision of brief, dense analgesia/anesthesia in a comprehensively monitored setting by individuals specifically trained to provide the service appears safe and efficient, both in terms of allowing wound care to proceed rapidly under ideal conditions for patient and nursing staff and in terms of cost-effective use of the operating room only for true surgical burn care procedures.

Local anesthetics are of obvious use in regional blockade for wound care procedures but have also been used for burn pain analgesia as a topical gel or IV infusion. Topical local anesthetic use on the burn wound is controversial. Prilocaine-lidocaine cream (EMLA) has no effect on burn pain in volunteers[96]; however, topical 5% lidocaine applied at 1 mg/cm² offers analgesic benefit without associated side effects.[97] Topical lidocaine use is significantly tempered by reports of local anesthetic-induced seizures due to enhanced systemic absorption at the open wound site.[98] The analgesic benefit of an IV lidocaine bolus (1 mg/kg) and 3-day continuous infusion (40 mg/kg/min) has also been reported acute burn injuries,[99] although whether its mechanism is due to anti-inflammatory or analgesic actions is unclear. Subcutaneous tumescent infiltration of local anesthetics for cutaneous surgery may provide adequate surgical anesthesia, with less blood loss from the graft donor sites.[100–102] In one feasibility study (n = 8 patients), postoperative pain was decreased by continuous infusion of subcutaneous bupivacaine into the donor sites.[103] Neuraxial administration of local anesthetics (and/or opioids) via epidural catheter would seem to be of benefit in patients with lower extremity burns, resulting in both analgesia (particularly during procedural burn care) and sympathectomy (of theoretical benefit to wound healing). However, such use has only been reported anecdotally.[104] A major drawback of this technique is the use of an indwelling catheter in patients densely colonized with infectious organisms at the wound site, thus increasing the risk for epidural abscess formation.[105] Nonneuraxial regional blocks have recently been reported to be of benefit for the pain associated with surgical skin donor site preparation on the anterolateral thigh, both a single injections[106] and as continuous infusions.[107]

PHARMACOLOGIC OPTIONS FOR BACKGROUND PAIN MANAGEMENT

Because background pain is relatively constant, it is best treated with mild to moderately potent analgesics administered so that plasma drug concentrations remain relatively constant throughout the day. Examples include the continuous IV infusion of fentanyl or morphine (± PCA), the oral administration of long-acting opioids with prolonged elimination (e.g., methadone) or prolonged enteral absorption (e.g., sustained-release morphine, sustained-release oxycodone), or oral administration on a regular schedule of short-acting oral analgesics (e.g., oxycodone, hydromorphone, codeine, acetaminophen). Background pain generally decreases with time

as the burn wounds (and associated donor sites) heal so that analgesics can be slowly tapered in the absence of significant analgesic tolerance.

PHARMACOLOGIC OPTIONS FOR PROCEDURAL PAIN MANAGEMENT

In contrast to background pain, procedural pain is significantly more intense but shorter in duration; therefore, analgesic regimens for procedural pain are best composed of moderately to highly potent opioids that have a short duration of action, with a sedation target level of moderate sedation. IV access is helpful in this setting, with ketamine and short-acting opioids (e.g., fentanyl, alfentanil) offering a potential advantage over more longer acting agents (e.g., morphine, hydromorphone). In the absence of IV access, orally administered opioids (e.g., morphine, hydromorphone, oxycodone, codeine) are commonly used, although their relatively long durations of action (2 to 6 hours) may potentially limit postprocedure recovery for other rehabilitative or nutritional activities. Oral ketamine, oral transmucosal fentanyl, and nitrous oxide are agents of particular use when IV access is not present, due to their rapid onsets and short durations of action. Finally, when a particularly painful dressing change or one that requires extreme cooperation in a noncompliant patient (e.g., face débridement in a young child) is anticipated, the provision of brief deep sedation or general anesthesia with appropriate patient monitoring, administered by anesthesiologists or appropriately trained nonanesthesiologists may be helpful. A variety of approaches to managing procedural pain associated with burn wound care have been recently summarized.[108]

PHARMACOLOGIC OPTIONS FOR POSTOPERATIVE PAIN MANAGEMENT

Postoperative pain deserves special mention because of the increased analgesic needs that should be anticipated following burn excision and grafting. This is particularly true when donor sites have been harvested, as these are often the principal source of increased postoperative pain complaints, rather than the grafted burn. Typically, this increased analgesic need is limited to 1 to 4 days following surgery before returning to preoperative levels.

Nonpharmacologic Approaches

COGNITIVE INTERVENTIONS AND COPING STYLES

In terms of pain control, cognitions can be thought of as behaviors that can be modified and that may influence the amount of pain that patients experience. Although such approaches are common in chronic pain control, there are few studies of cognitive-behavioral interventions in patients with burn injuries.[109,110] In understanding such interventions, it is important to emphasize that burn injuries are unexpected and have far-reaching consequences for patients. Furthermore, as noted previously, the aggressive procedural medical care typically associated with burn injuries adds further stress and uncertainty through the daily demands of surgery, rehabilitation, dependency on caregivers, and pain. Such uncertainty often leads to feelings of helplessness in both adult and pediatric burn patients. It is almost impossible to predict the style with which an individual patient reacts and responds to such stress; however, if one is able to determine some characteristics of the patient's cognitive style, this insight can be useful in choosing the most appropriate psychologically based interventions.

Burn patients bring different cognitive styles in the manner in which they respond to stressful medical procedures. One critical distinction lies in how much information patients desire regarding their injury and care. Whereas some patients will seek out as much information as possible, others would just as soon leave their care to health care professionals.[111–113]

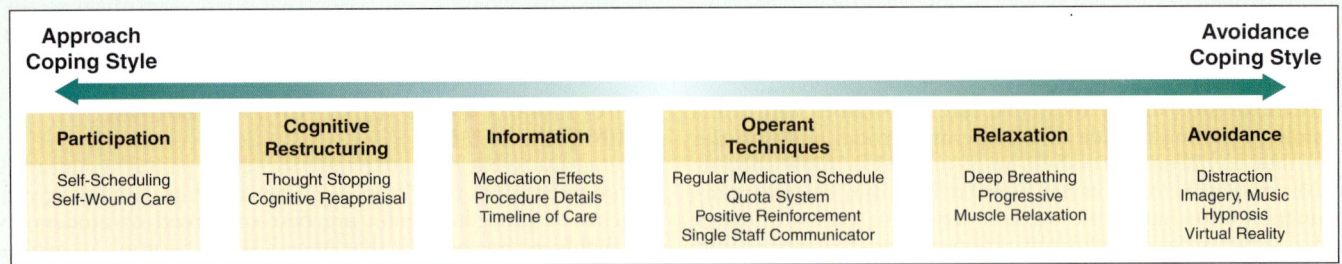

FIGURE 53.3 Control coping continuum and associated nonpharmacologic techniques. The spectrum of coping styles from approach to avoidance is depicted, including specific clinical interventions for patients whose coping styles fall on different positions along the continuum (see text for details).

In applying cognitive interventions to burn patients, it will be useful for the clinician to be aware of how they cope with stressful medical procedures. Paramount to such thinking is whether the patient will approach procedures with a tendency toward cognitive avoidance, in which case they will distract or dissociate themselves from painful stimuli. This is in contrast to patients who tend to respond to acute pain by focusing on the procedures. Such patients may take a hypervigilant stance toward pain and may find distractions difficult. Patients often fall into position along a continuum of coping styles, from an approach coping style to an avoidance coping style. If one can determine where they fall along this continuum, it is easier to determine what type of psychological intervention will be most useful (Fig. 53.3).[53,111]

If patients fall on the avoidance end of the continuum, too much information and focus on the details of care procedures will likely make them more anxious. In contrast, distraction will likely be useful for patients who possess this coping style. In the burn unit, simple distraction is more likely to be of benefit with brief procedures such as blood draws or line placements, and studies have reported that music can be effective for such simple distraction with burn pain.[114,115] Children at certain development levels may benefit from not seeing their wounds or by being more engaged by the clinicians. Such distraction will be less effective with older children or adults during the more extensive wound care procedures. In such instances, engaging patients in deep relaxation with distracting imagery will likely be more useful, although imagery often requires substantially more training time for both patients and staff. A particularly elaborate form of distraction involves the use of computer-generated immersive virtual reality (see the following text). For both children and adults, deep breathing has been found to be a simple and effective means of reducing pain during procedures.[116] In contrast, when patients cope with painful procedures by carefully focusing on them and even participating in their own care (i.e., approach coping style), they are usually less viable candidates for distraction techniques. Such patients may benefit from reappraisal techniques. Rather than focusing away from pain, reappraisal techniques might encourage patients to attend to their nociception. They can then be encouraged to differentiate sensory from affective components of pain as well as evaluate the meaning of the sensation. As is the case with chronic pain, patients may benefit from being taught to differentiate "hurt from harm" with respect to their pain sensations.[117] It is also useful to teach such patients that increased pain sensation is usually a positive sign with respect to burn wound healing. Specifically, full-thickness burns often destroy nerve endings and the capacity for nociception, but as these burn wounds heal, skin buds emerge which are highly enervated and sensitive to pain and temperature. Teaching patients the latter two principles will likely be useful to them independent of their cognitive styles in response to acute pain. Furthermore, with enough focus on

pain sensations, some patients are able to gain the sense that they are able to modify them and thus be in more control of their perceptions.

PREPARATORY INFORMATION
Providing patients with information about impending procedures can provide a powerful means of mitigating pain and anxiety. Such interventions have been found to enhance pain control with acute pain from a variety of different procedures.[118] Patients may be provided with preparatory information (what steps will be taken during a procedure) or sensory information (what they will likely feel). The use of preparatory information has not been studied with burn patients, but there is evidence that it can be useful with a variety of medical procedures such as cardiac catheterization, endoscopies, cast removal, and surgery.[119–121] Unfortunately, burn injuries often do not easily lend themselves to such interventions. Certainly, it is not possible to anticipate that a burn injury will occur and medical procedures are often performed quickly and in an invasive matter. There is little time to prepare patients, and this can be particularly difficult for children. In addition, with some medical procedures in nonburn settings, understanding what will occur may reduce anxiety and pain associated with those procedures. Unfortunately, the frequent challenge with burn care is that the procedures are very painful, invasive, and truly threatening, unlike many other types of medical procedures that simply have the appearance of being threatening.

Preparation is particularly relevant to two phenomena associated with burn care. First of all, nociceptive input may often increase as a burn wound heals. As mentioned earlier, full-thickness burn injuries may not be that painful, whereas healing injuries with new skin buds may be particularly sensitive. Care providers should take care to communicate to such patients that increased pain is actually a sign that the wound is healing, information that may help allay patient anxiety. The second beneficial instance of preparatory information involves informing patients' family members of important medical issues. For example, burn patients often show periods of delirium when in the ICU, a clinical phenomenon that can be frightening to both patients and their family members. Letting them know in advance that such confusion is a common and usually benign occurrence can mitigate subsequent anxiety.

BEHAVIORAL INTERVENTIONS
Behavioral interventions might seem more applicable to chronic pain conditions yet have surprising relevance to burn pain treatment. The application of such principles to burn can be divided into classical (stimulus) and operant (respondent) strategies. Stimulus conditioning applications have to do with the patient's state prior to wound care. Certainly, decreasing the patient's level of arousal through relaxation training, or any other means available, can minimize the ensuing cycle between anxiety and nociception. With children, the stimulus context of

painful procedures can be particularly relevant. Children and many adults will often show heightened anxiety and fear just by being exposed to the stimuli associated with painful procedures (e.g., nursing scrubs, procedures rooms). If the threatening nature of the wound care environment can be reduced, pain control can be enhanced by virtue of stimulus–response principles. As a nonburn example, some children's hospitals have instituted the creative approach of having a magnetic resonance imaging (MRI) scan tunnel appear as a cave in a jungle environment (rather than the morgue-like drawer such equipment more typically seems to resemble). What follows from this logic is that the burn-injured child's room should be considered a safe environment in which painful procedures do not occur.

Operant (reinforcement) principles are also highly applicable to burn pain management. One application has to do with medication scheduling. The tendency in many acute care settings is to simply medicate patients on a PRN schedule, an approach that is nonsensical for several reasons in burn care. Certainly, the notion of waiting until the patient hurts does not make sense from a pharmacologic perspective.[2,68,122] However, operant principles would also suggest that PRN medication schedules reinforce patients' pain complaints, both in terms of the euphoria-producing properties of opioid analgesics and the attention received from caregivers. Providing opioid analgesics on a regular schedule that reflects their pharmacokinetic properties will minimize the potential for operant factors to exacerbate the pain problem. For emotionally dependent or anxious patients, as-needed pain scheduling can actually create a paradigm for creating more pain behaviors and pain perception.[117]

A regular analgesic drug administration schedule is particularly important with patients who have substance abuse histories. Such patients may demonstrate frequent pain complaints and/or drug-seeking behaviors on the burn unit. The tendency of such patients to approach multiple caregivers for analgesics has the potential to create "staff splitting" and resentment (i.e., counter-transference) toward the patients. Accordingly, the burn unit staff may hold punitive attitudes about the patient's substance abuse history and/or the excessive nature of his or her pain complaints. Regularly scheduled medications will often minimize such conflict, as well as provide more transparent management of the patient's pain. In addition, channeling communications and negotiations about changing doses or types of medication through a single caregiver can be very useful in decreasing conflict between the patient and staff members.

In rare instances, the patient's pain behavior might be so exaggerated in the face of apparently adequate analgesia that burn staff must consider an operant-based model of pain management. Effective burn team members are trained to be highly attentive to the pain complaints of their patients. However, occasional patients may show excessive complaints based on such factors as strong dependency needs or somatic tendencies. As in any case, it is important that such patients receive adequate doses of analgesics. However, operant approaches, in which discussions of pain are minimized and patients are distracted from their complaints,[117] may become the prominent intervention. In other words, there would be discussions with the patient that medications changes will be limited to circumscribed periods and, in between such times, the patient will be encouraged to focus away from the issue of pain.

Burn rehabilitation involves continuously increasing activity levels, and patients may become simply overwhelmed with the pain associated with such movements. The quota system[123] represents a useful application of operant principles to burn care in such instances. The repeated, invasive nature of burn care has the potential to create a state of learned helplessness in patients.[124] The quota system uses rest as a reinforcement for activity and keeps activity levels well within the patient's level of physical endurance. Ehde and colleagues[123] have reported that

with overwhelmed, seemingly unmotivated patients, it is useful to encourage the burn team to reduce their overall demands, take baseline behaviors, and gradually increase demands on what the patient's baseline behavior suggests is within their range of tolerance. Such interventions can create steady increases in activity in patients who have been overwhelmed by care, and also a sense of mastery, as they are able to see steady improvement in their activities.

Avoiding the rewarding of escape behavior during procedures is a final application of operant principles. With children, it is particularly essential to do all the interventions possible to enhance pain control during procedures such as adequate analgesics and anxiolytics, sufficient emotional preparation, optimizing the wound care environment, and including parents when appropriate. Children also do better if allowed to have control of their wound care procedures, perhaps by doing their own dressing removal.[124] However, there are times when it is important to set firm limits during wound care by following through with procedures; otherwise, pain behaviors can exacerbate. Establishing this balance can certainly be a challenge for caregivers because it is not appropriate to force treatment when children are inadequately medicated. The point here is that once all that can be done that is possible in terms of analgesia, the timing of when a child can refuse or rest during wound care becomes an important issue in operant management.

HYPNOSIS

In terms of randomized controlled studies, hypnosis is one of the areas where the most evidence exists for psychologically based interventions in burn care.[125] A recent review by Patterson and Jensen[126] indicates that burn pain constitutes some of the best evidence in the literature that hypnosis can be effective. Furthermore, a number of additional reports have focused on the use of hypnosis to treat complications from burns other than pain, although with few exceptions; these reports have been anecdotal.[127,128]

There are a number of reasons why burn patients appear to be such good candidates for hypnotic-based pain control interventions.[129] First, because burn patients are in high levels of pain, they are motivated to engage in hypnosis, a technique that they might ordinarily resist. In support of this, patients with high levels of initial pain seem to show a better analgesic response to hypnosis.[130,131] Second, patients with unanticipated traumatic injuries, such as burns, may be more cooperative because of the dependency that might often be a normal reaction to trauma care (i.e., a willingness to allow others to take care of one). Third, the dissociation that may accompany a burn injury may also be a factor that moderates hypnotizability. Certainly, dissociative tendencies have been related to hypnosis,[132] as well as the acute stress disorder is a typical early reaction to burn injuries. Finally, and on a more simplistic level, hypnosis is most effective when it can be applied to a predictable, discrete event—a description that characterizes most burn wound care procedures, as painful as they are.

There have been two recent publications describing the delivery of hypnosis through immersive virtual reality technology (see the following text) in order to treat burn pain.[133,134] The advantage of this approach is that the clinician can rely on technology to achieve hypnotic induction and suggestion; thus, extensive training for hypnosis is not required. Although these reports are anecdotal, their preliminary results with this technology demonstrate analgesic effects that are equivalent to those obtained when a "live" clinician is used.

VIRTUAL REALITY

Immersive virtual reality is a particularly attention-grabbing distraction technique and is designed to give users the illusion of going inside a computer-generated virtual environment (Fig. 53.4). Virtual reality appears to provide significant cognitive

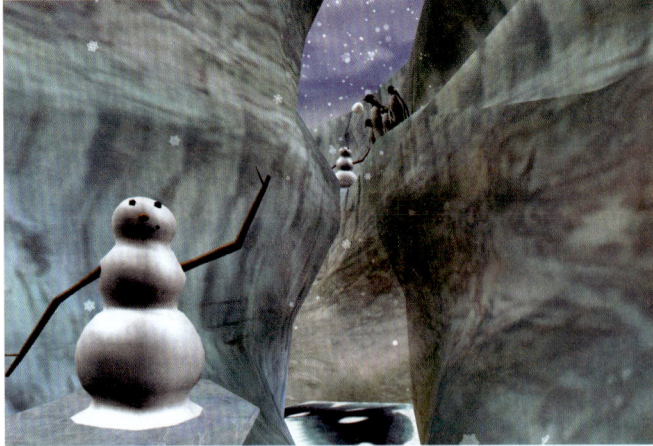

FIGURE 53.4 Virtual reality environment "SnowWorld" as seen by the patient/user. Snow/ice motif and blue/white/lavender colors suggest a cool temperature setting in direct contrast to the hot setting in which most burn injuries occur. Virtual igloos, penguins, and snowmen on canyon walls facilitate user interaction with the virtual world through user-targeted shooting of virtual snowballs at these virtual objects.

distraction to users because it is interactive and places significant cognitive demand on patients through the provision of multisensory input (visual, aural, and sometimes tactile). In addition, it utilizes a head-mounted display that blocks visual and aural input to the user from the immediate and often frightening, real-world burn care environment. Thus, virtual reality may exert its analgesic effect by diverting conscious attention away from concurrent nociceptive stimulation, resulting in an attenuated subjective pain experience. Functional brain imaging studies have shown the virtual reality results in pain reduction that is similar to that of systemic opioid administration, both in terms of magnitude of analgesia and brain activity changes, and is also additive to opioid analgesia when administered concurrently.[135] The use of adjunctive, immersive virtual reality was first reported to provide

clinically meaningful pain relief in the setting of burn wound débridement,[136] with findings subsequently replicated in larger populations of burn patients.[137,138] Virtual reality analgesia is also advantageous for the less severe pain associated with certain types of postburn rehabilitation activities[139–141] (Fig. 53.5) and has been combined with hypnotic suggestion (as noted previously) to provide nonpharmacologic analgesia for burn wound care.[133,134]

Conclusion

Effective treatment of burn injuries requires an appreciation of the unique patterns of nociception caused by this trauma and their interaction with psychological factors. Aggressive use of opioid analgesics tailored to the nature of the pain (e.g., procedural, background, postoperative) serves as the cornerstone of a multifaceted approach to burn pain. Procedural pain often involves consideration of a variety of supplemental pharmacologic approaches, ranging from mild sedation to general anesthesia. Nonpharmacologic approaches should be woven into the structure of burn care as adjuncts to pharmacologic analgesia (i.e., multimodal analgesia). The undertreatment of burn pain remains an unfortunate reality, particularly because adequate analgesia may facilitate recovery and posthospital adjustment as well as represent a more humane course of treatment.

ACKNOWLEDGMENT

The authors' work was supported in part by funding from the National Institutes of Health (RO1 GM042725 and RO1 DA 026438).

References

1. Esselman PC, Thombs BD, Magyar-Russell G, et al. Burn rehabilitation: state of the science. *Am J Phys Med Rehab* 2006;85(4):383–413.
2. Melzack R. The tragedy of needless pain. *Sci Am* 1990;262(2):27–33.
3. Carrougher GJ, Ptacek JT, Sharar SR, et al. Comparison of patient satisfaction and self-reports of pain in adult burn-injured patients. *J Burn Care Rehabil* 2003;24(1):1–8.
4. Honari S, Patterson DR, Gibbons J, et al. Comparison of pain control medication in three age groups of elderly patients. *J Burn Care Rehabil* 1997;18(6):500–504.
5. Ptacek JT, Patterson DR, Montgomery BK, et al. Pain, coping, and adjustment in patients with burns: preliminary findings from a prospective study. *J Pain Symptom Manage* 1995;10(6):446–455.
6. Patterson DR, Tininenko J, Ptacek JT. Pain during burn hospitalization predicts long-term outcome. *J Burn Care Res* 2006;27(5):719–726.
7. Sareen J, Erickson J, Medved MI, et al. Risk factors for post-injury mental health problems. *Depress Anxiety* 2013;30(4):321–327.
8. Yuxiang L, Lingjun Z, Lu T, et al. Burn patients' experience of pain management: a qualitative study. *Burns* 2012;38(2):180–186.
9. Andrews RM, Browne AL, Wood F, et al. Predictors of patient satisfaction with pain management and improvement 3 months after burn injury. *J Burn Care Res* 2012;33(3):442–452.
10. Sheridan RL, Stoddard FJ, Kazis LE, et al. Long-term posttraumatic stress symptoms vary inversely with early opiate dosing in children recovering from serious burns: effects durable at 4 years. *J Trauma Acute Care Surg* 2014;76(3):828–832.
11. Wollgarten-Hadamek I, Hohmeister J, Zohsel K, et al. Do school-aged children with burn injuries during infancy show stress-induced activation of pain inhibitory mechanisms? *Eur J Pain* 2011;15(4):423.e1–423.e10.
12. Yang HT, Hur G, Kwak IS, et al. Improvement of burn pain management through routine pain monitoring and pain management protocol. *Burns* 2013;39(4):619–624.
13. Gamst-Jensen H, Vedel PN, Lindberg-Larsen VO, et al. Acute pain management in burn patients: appraisal and thematic analysis of four clinical guidelines. *Burns* 2014;40(8):1463–1469.
14. Faucher L, Furukawa K. Practice guidelines for the management of pain. *J Burn Care Res* 2006;27(5):659–668.
15. Nedelec B, Carrougher GJ. Pain and pruritus postburn injury. *J Burn Care Res* 2017;38(3):142–145.
16. Silbert BS, Osgood PF, Carr DB. Burn pain. In: Yaksh TL, Lynch C II, Zapol WM. *Anesthesia: Biologic Foundations*. Philadelphia: Lippincott-Raven; 1997:759–773.
17. Summer GJ, Puntillo KA, Miaskowski C, et al. Burn injury pain: the continuing challenge. *J Pain* 2007;8(7):533–548.
18. Choinière M, Melzack R, Rondeau J, et al. The pain of burns: characteristics and correlates. *J Trauma* 1989;29(11):1531–1539.

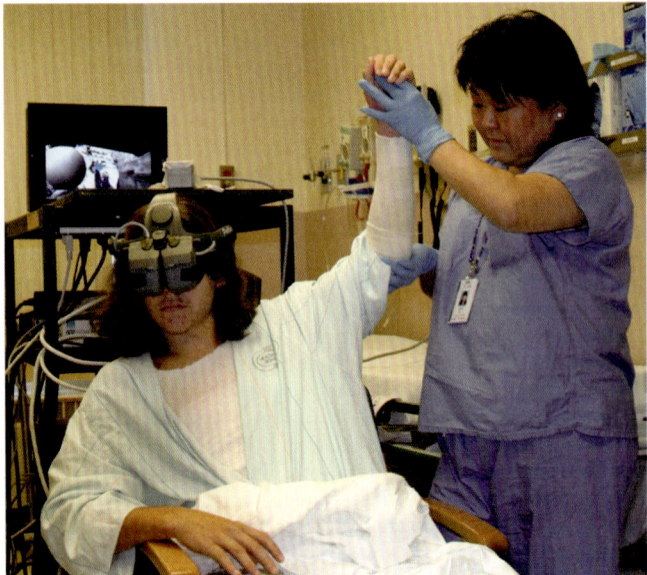

FIGURE 53.5 Clinical use of virtual reality distraction during burn wound care. A burn patient undergoes postburn skin stretching and passive joint range of motion while experiencing immersive virtual reality analgesia. Both auditory and visual stimulation are provided through a lightweight head-mounted display that can track the user's position in the virtual environment by assessment of head position, and user interaction with objects in the virtual environment is controlled by manual trackball.

19. Perry S, Heidrich G, Ramos E. Assessment of pain by burn victim patients. *J Burn Care Rehabil* 1981;2:322–326.

20. Atchison NE, Osgood PF, Carr DB, et al. Pain during burn dressing change in children: relationship to burn area, depth and analgesic regimens. *Pain* 1991;47(1):41–45.

21. Choinière M, Melzack R, Papillon J. Pain and paresthesia in patients with healed burns: an exploratory study. *J Pain Symptom Manage* 1991;6(7):437–444.

22. Chapman CR. Psychological factors in postoperative pain and their treatment. In: Smith G, Covino BG, eds. *Acute Pain*. London: Butterworths; 1985:22–41.

23. Chien S. Role of the sympathetic nervous system in hemorrhage. *Physiol Rev* 1967;47:214–288.

24. Mackersie RC, Karagianes TG. Pain management following trauma and burns. *Crit Care Clin* 1990;7:433–449.

25. Saxe G, Stoddard F, Courtney D, et al. Relationship between acute morphine and the course of PTSD in children with burns. *J Am Acad Child Adolesc Psychiatry* 2001;40(8):915–921.

26. Patterson DR, Everett JJ, Bombardier CH, et al. Psychological effects of severe burn injuries. *Psychol Bull* 1993;113(2):362–378.

27. Van Loey NE, Van Son MJ. Psychopathology and psychological problems in patients with burn scars: epidemiology and management. *Am J Clin Dermatol* 2003;4(4):245–272.

28. Berry CC, Wachtel TL, Frank HA. An analysis of factors which predict mortality in hospitalized burn patients. *Burns Incl Therm Inj* 1982;9(1):38–45.

29. Patterson DR, Finch CP, Wiechman SA, et al. Premorbid mental health status of adult burn patients: comparison with a normative sample. *J Burn Care Rehabil* 2003;24(5):347–350.

30. Agarwal V, O'Neill PJ, Cotton BA, et al. Prevalence and risk factors for development of delirium in burn intensive care unit patients. *J Burn Care Res* 2010;31(5):706–715.

31. Blank K, Perry S. Relationship of psychological processes during delirium to outcome. *Am J Psychiatry* 1984;141(7):843–847.

32. Carrougher GJ, Ptacek JT, Honari S, et al. Self-reports of anxiety in burn-injured hospitalized adults during routine wound care. *J Burn Care Res* 2006;27(5):676–681.

33. Aaron LA, Patterson DR, Finch CP, et al. The utility of a burn specific measure of pain anxiety to prospectively predict pain and function: a comparative analysis. *Burns* 2001;27(4):329–334.

34. Romano JM, Turner JA. Chronic pain and depression: does the evidence support a relationship? *Psychol Bull* 1985;97(1):18–34.

35. Thombs BD, Bresnick MG, Magyar-Russell G. Depression in survivors of burn injury: a systematic review. *Gen Hosp Psychiatry* 2006;28(6):494–502.

36. Thombs BD, Bresnick MG, Magyar-Russell G, et al. Symptoms of depression predict change in physical health after burn injury. *Burns* 2007;33(3):292–298.

37. Van Loey NE, van Son MJ, van der Heijden PG, et al. PTSD in persons with burns: an explorative study examining relationships with attributed responsibility, negative and positive emotional states. *Burns* 2008;34(8):1082–1089.

38. Stoddard FJ, Sheridan RL, Saxe GN, et al. Treatment of pain in acutely burned children. *J Burn Care Rehabil* 2002;23(2):135–156.

39. de Jong AE, Bremer M, van Komen R, et al. Pain in young children with burns: extent, course and influencing factors. *Burns* 2014;40(1):38–47.

40. Schneider JC, Harris NL, El Shami A, et al. A descriptive review of neuropathic-like pain after burn injury. *J Burn Care Res* 2006;27(4):524–528.

41. Dauber A, Osgood PF, Breslau AJ, et al. Chronic persistent pain after severe burns: a survey of 358 burn survivors. *Pain Med* 2002;3(1):6–17.

42. Wibbenmeyer L, Oltrogge K, Kluesner K, et al. An evaluation of discharge opioid prescribing practices in a burn population. *J Burn Care Res* 2015;36(2):329–335.

43. Gomes T, Mamdani MM, Dhalla IA, et al. Opioid dose and drug-related mortality in patients with nonmalignant pain. *Arch Intern Med* 2011;171(7):686–691.

44. Edwards RR, Smith MT, Klick B, et al. Symptoms of depression and anxiety as unique predictors of pain-related outcomes following burn injury. *Ann Behav Med* 2007;34(3):313–322.

45. Jaffe SE, Patterson DR. Treating sleep problems in patients with burn injuries: practical considerations. *J Burn Care Rehabil* 2004;25(3):294–305.

46. Gross JB, Bailey PL, Connis RT, et al; for American Society of Anesthesiologists Task Force on Sedation and Analgesia by Non-Anesthesiologists. Practice guidelines for sedation and analgesia by non-anesthesiologists. An updated report by the American Society of Anesthesiologists Task Force on Sedation and Analgesia by Non-Anesthesiologists. *Anesthesiology* 2002;96:1004–1017.

47. Joint Commission Resources. *Pain Management: A Systems Approach to Improving Quality and Safety*. Oak Brook, IL: Joint Commission Resources; 2012.

48. Cote CJ, Wilson S. Guidelines for monitoring and management of pediatric patients during and after sedation for diagnostic and therapeutic procedures: an update. *Pediatrics* 2006;118(6):2587–2602.

49. Cortiella J, Marvin JA. Management of the pediatric burn patient. *Nurs Clin North Am* 1997;32(2):311–329.

50. Sheridan RL, Hinson M, Nackel A, et al. Development of a pediatric burn pain and anxiety management program. *J Burn Care Res* 1997;18(5):453–459.

51. Gibbons J, Honari SR, Sharar SR, et al. Opiate-induced respiratory depression in young pediatric burn patients. *J Burn Care Rehabil* 1998;19(3):225–229.

52. Patterson DR, Hoffman HG, Weichman SA, et al. Optimizing control of pain from severe burns: a literature review. *Am J Clin Hypn* 2004;47(1):43–54.

53. Waldman SD, ed. *Pain Management*. Vol 1. Philadelphia: Saunders-Elsevier; 2006.

54. Richardson P, Mustard L. The management of pain in the burns unit. *Burns* 2009;35(7):921–936.

55. Retrouvey H, Shahrokhi S. Pain and the thermally injured patient-a review of current therapies. *J Burn Care Res* 2015;36(2):315–323.

56. Iafrati NS. Pain on the burn unit: patient vs nurse perceptions. *J Burn Care Rehabil* 1986;7(5):413–416.

57. Marvin JA. Pain assessment versus measurement. *J Burn Care Rehabil* 1995;16(3)(pt 2):348–357.

58. Perry S, Inturrisi C. Analgesia and morphine disposition in burn patients. *J Burn Care Rehabil* 1983;4(4):276–279.

59. Herman RA, Veng-Pedersen P, Miotto J, et al. Pharmacokinetics of morphine sulfate in patients with burns. *J Burn Care Rehabil* 1994;15(2):95–103.

60. Furman WR, Munster AM, Cone EJ. Morphine pharmacokinetics during anesthesia and surgery in patients with burns. *J Burn Care Rehabil* 1990;11(5):391–394.

61. Silbert BS, Lipkowski AW, Cepeda MS, et al. Enhanced potency of receptor-selective opioids after acute burn injury. *Anesth Analg* 1991;73(4):427–433.

62. Franceschi D, Gerding RL, Phillips G, et al. Risk factors associated with intravascular catheter infections in burned patients: a prospective, randomized study. *J Trauma* 1989;29(6):811–816.

63. Choinière M, Grenier R, Paquette C. Patient-controlled analgesia: a double-blind study in burn patients. *Anaesthesia* 1992;47(6):467–472.

64. Rovers J, Knighton J, Neligan P, et al. Patient-controlled analgesia in burn patients: a critical review of the literature and case report. *Hosp Pharm* 1994;29(2):106, 108–111.

65. Nilsson A, Kalman S, Sonesson LK, et al. Difficulties in controlling mobilization pain using a standardized patient-controlled analgesia protocol in burns. *J Burn Care Res* 2011;32(1):166–171.

66. Prakash S, Fatima T, Pawar M. Patient-controlled analgesia with fentanyl for burn dressing changes. *Anesth Analg* 2004;99(2):552–555.

67. Sim KM, Hwang NC, Chan YW, et al. Use of patient-controlled analgesia with alfentanil for burns dressing procedures: a preliminary report of five patients. *Burns* 1996;22(3):238–241.

68. Patterson DR, Ptacek JT, Carrougher G, et al. The 2002 Lindberg Award. PRN vs regularly scheduled opioid analgesics in pediatric burn patients. *J Burn Care Rehabil* 2002;23(6):424–430.

69. Sharar SR, Bratton SL, Carrougher GJ, et al. A comparison of oral transmucosal fentanyl citrate and oral hydromorphone for inpatient pediatric burn wound care analgesia. *J Burn Care Rehabil* 1998;19(6):516–521.

70. Sharar SR, Carrougher GJ, Selzer K, et al. A comparison of oral transmucosal fentanyl citrate and oral oxycodone for pediatric outpatient wound care. *J Burn Care Rehabil* 2002;23:27–31.

71. Alvi R, Jones S, Burrows D, et al. The safety of topical anaesthetic and analgesic agents in a gel when used to provide pain relief at split skin donor sites. *Burns* 1998;24:54–57.

72. Møiniche S, Pedersen JL, Kehlet H. Topical ketorolac has no antinociceptive or anti-inflammatory effect at thermal injury. *Burns* 1994;20:483–496.

73. Lee JJ, Marvin JA, Heimbach DM. Effectiveness of nalbuphine for relief of burn debridement pain. *J Burn Care Rehabil* 1989;10:241–246.

74. Pal SK, Cortiella J, Herndon J. Adjunctive methods of pain control in burns. *Burns* 1997;23:404–412.

75. Cuignet O, Pirson J, Soudon O, et al. Effects of gabapentin on morphine consumption and pain in severely burned patients. *Burns* 2007;33:81–86.

76. Gray P, Williams B, Cramond T. Successful use of gabapentin in acute pain management following burn injury: a case series. *Pain Med* 2008;9:371–376.

77. Walker J, Maccallum M, Fischer C, et al. Sedation using dexmedetomidine in pediatric burn patients. *J Burn Care Res* 2006;27:206–210.

78. Kariya N, Shindoh M, Nishi S, et al. Oral clonidine for sedation and analgesia in a burn patient. *J Clin Anesth* 1998;10:514–517.

79. Wasiak J, Mahar P, McGuinness SK, et al. Intravenous lidocaine for the treatment of background or procedural burn pain. *Cochrane Database Syst Rev* 2012;(6):CD005622.

80. Ratcliff SL, Meyer WJ, Cuervo LJ, et al. The use of haloperidol and associated complications in the agitated, acutely ill pediatric burn patient. *J Burn Care Res* 2004;25:472–478.

81. Perry S, Heidrich G. Management of pain during debridement: a survey of U.S. burn units. *Pain* 1982;13:267–280.

82. Martin-Herz SP, Patterson DR, Honari S, et al. Pediatric pain control practices of North American Burn Centers. *J Burn Care Rehabil* 2003;24:26–36.

83. Egan KJ, Ready LB, Nessly M, et al. Self-administration of midazolam for postoperative anxiety: a double blinded study. *Pain* 1992;49:3–8.

84. Patterson DR, Ptacek JT, Carrougher GJ, et al. Lorazepam as an adjunct to opioid analgesics in the treatment of burn pain. *Pain* 1997;72:367–374.

85. Baskett PJ, Hyland J, Deane M, et al. Analgesia for burns dressing in children: a dose-finding study for phenoperidine and droperidol with and without 50 percent nitrous oxide and oxygen. *Br J Anaesth* 1969;41:684–688.

86. Filkins SA, Cosgrav P, Marvin JA. Self-administered anesthesia: a method of pain control. *J Burn Care Rehabil* 1981;2:33–34.

87. American Society of Anesthesiologists. Report of an ad hoc committee on the effect of trace anesthetics on the health of operating room personnel. Occupational disease among operating room personnel: a national study. *Anesthesiology* 1974;41:321–340.

88. Nunn JF, Chanarin I, Tanner AG, et al. Megaloblastic bone marrow changes after repeated nitrous oxide anaesthesia. *Br J Anaesth* 1986;58:1469–1470.

89. Demling RH, Ellerbe S, Jarrett F. Ketamine anesthesia for tangential excision of burn eschar: a burn unit procedure. *The Journal of Trauma* 1978;18:269–270.

90. Humphries Y, Melson M, Gore D. Superiority of oral ketamine as an analgesic and sedative for wound care procedures in the pediatric patient with burns. *J Burn Care Rehab* 1997;18:34–36.

91. Warncke T, Stubhaug A, Jørum E. Ketamine, an NMDA receptor antagonist, suppresses spatial and temporal properties of burn-induced secondary hyperalgesia in man: a double-blind crossover comparison with morphine and placebo. *Pain* 1997;72:99–106.

92. Owens VF, Palmieri TL, Comroe CM, et al. Ketamine: a safe and effective agent for painful procedures in the pediatric burn patient. *J Burn Care Res* 2006;27:211–216.

93. Dimick P, Helvig E, Heimbach D, et al. Anesthesia-assisted procedures in a burn intensive care unit procedure room: benefits and complications. *J Burn Care Rehabil* 1993;14:446–449.

94. Powers PS, Cruse CW, Daniels S, et al. Safety and efficacy of debridement under anesthesia in patients with burns. *J Burn Care Rehabil* 1993;14:176–180.

95. Tosun Z, Esmaoglu A, Coruh A. Propofol-ketamine vs propofol-fentanyl combinations for deep sedation and analgesia in pediatric patients undergoing burn dressing changes. *Paediatr Anaesth* 2008;18:43–47.

96. Pedersen JL, Callesen T, Møiniche S, et al. Analgesic and anti-inflammatory effects of lignocaine-prilocaine (EMLA) cream in human burn injury. *Br J Anaesth* 1996;76:806–810.

97. Brofeldt BT, Cornwell P, Doherty D, et al. Topical lidocaine in the treatment of partial-thickness burns. *J Burn Care Rehabil* 1989;10:63–68.

98. Wehner D, Hamilton GC. Seizures following topical application of local anesthetics to burn patients. *Ann Emerg Med* 1984;13:456–458.

99. Jönsson A, Cassuto J, Hanson B. Inhibition of burn pain by intravenous lignocaine infusion. *Lancet* 1991;338:151–152.

100. Bussolin L, Busoni P, Giorgi L, et al. Tumescent local anesthesia for the surgical treatment of burns and postburn sequelae in pediatric patients. *Anesthesiology* 2003;99:1371–1375.

101. Fujita K, Mishima Y, Iwasawa M, et al. The practical procedure of tumescent technique in burn surgery for excision of burn eschar. *J Burn Care Res* 2008;29:924–926.

102. Gümü N. Tumescent infiltration of lidocaine and adrenaline for burn surgery. *Ann Burns Fire Disasters* 2011;24:144–148.

103. Hernandez JL, Savetamal A, Crombie RE, et al. Use of continuous local anesthetic infusion in the management of postoperative split-thickness skin graft donor site pain. *J Burn Care Res* 2013;34:e257–e262.

104. Punja K, Graham M, Cartotto R. Continuous infusion of epidural morphine in frostbite. *J Burn Care Rehabil* 1988;19:142–145.

105. Still JM, Abramson R, Law EJ. Development of an epidural abscess following staphylococcal septicemia in an acutely burned patient: case report. *J Trauma* 1995;38:958–959.

106. Cuignet O, Mbuyamba J, Pirson J. The long-term analgesic efficacy of a single-shot fascia iliaca compartment block in burn patients undergoing skin grafting procedures. *J Burn Care Rehabil* 2005;26:409–415.

107. Cuignet O, Pirson J, Boughrouph J, et al. The efficacy of continuous fascia iliaca compartment block for pain management in burn patients undergoing skin grafting procedures. *Anesth Analg* 2004;98:1077–1081.

108. Myers R, Lozenski J, Wyatt M, et al. Sedation and analgesia for dressing change: a survey of American Burn Association burn centers. *J Burn Care Res* 2017;38:e48–e54.

109. Everett JJ, Patterson DR, Chen ACN. Cognitive and behavioral treatments for burn pain. *Pain Clin* 1990;3:133–145.

110. Fauerbach JA, Lawrence JW, Haythornthwaite JA, et al. Coping with the stress of a painful medical procedure. *Behav Res Ther* 2002;40:1003–1015.

111. Martin-Herz SP, Thurber CA, Patterson DR. Psychological principles of burn wound pain in children. II: treatment applications. *J Burn Care Rehabil* 2000;21(5):458–472.

112. Thompson SC. Will it hurt less if I can control it? a complex answer to a simple question. *Psychol Bull* 1981;90:89–101.

113. Strickland BR. Internal-external expectancies and health-related behaviors. *Journal of consulting and clinical psychology*. 1978;46:1192–1211.

114. Prensner JD, Yowler CJ, Smith LF, et al. Music therapy for assistance with pain and anxiety management in burn treatment. *J Burn Care Rehabil* 2001;22:82–88.

115. Tan XMM, Yowler CJ, Super DM, et al. The effect of music therapy protocols for decreasing pain, anxiety and muscle tension levels during burn dressing changes. *J Burn Care Res* 2010;31(4):590–597.

116. Park E, Oh H, Kim T. The effects of relaxation breathing on procedural pain and anxiety during burn care. *Burns* 2013;39(6):1101–1106.

117. Fordyce WE. *Behavioral methods for chronic pain and illness*. St. Louis, MO: Mosby Year Book; 1976.

118. Tan S. Cognitive and cognitive-behavioural methods for pain control: a selective review. *Pain* 1982;12:201–228.

119. Kendall PC, Williams L, Pechacek TF, et al. Cognitive-behavioural and patient education interventions in cardiac catheterization procedures: the Palo Alto Medical Psychology Project. *J Consult Clin Psychol* 1979;47:49–58.

120. Johnson JE, Morrisey JF, Leventhal H. Psychological preparation for an endoscopic examination. *Gastrointest Endosc* 1973;19:180–182.

121. Johnson JE, Kirchhoff KT, Endress MP. Altering children's distress behaviour during orthopedic cast removal. *Nursing Res* 1975;24:404–410.

122. Paice JA, Noskin GA, Vanagunas A, et al. Efficacy and safety of scheduled dosing of opioid analgesics: a quality improvement study. *J Pain* 2005;6:639–643.

123. Ehde DM, Patterson DR, Fordyce WE. The quota system in burn rehabilitation. *J Burn Care Rehabil* 1998;19:436–439.

124. Kavanagh CK, Lasoff E, Eide Y, et al. Learned helplessness and the pediatric burn patient: dressing change behavior and serum cortisol and beta-endorphin. *Adv Pediatr* 1991;38:335–363.

125. Frenay MC, Faymonville ME, Devlieger S, et al. Psychological approaches during dressing changes of burned patients: a prospective randomised study comparing hypnosis against stress reducing strategy. *Burns* 2001;27:793–799.

126. Patterson DR, Jensen MP. Hypnosis and clinical pain. *Psychol Bull* 2003;129:495–521.

127. Chester SJ, Stockton K, De Young A, et al. Effectiveness of medical hypnosis for pain reduction and faster wound healing in pediatric acute burn injury: study protocol for a randomized controlled trial. *Trials* 2016;17:223.

128. Berger MM, Davadant M, Marin C, et al. Impact of a pain protocol including hypnosis in major burns. *Burns* 2010;36:639–646.

129. Patterson DR, Adcock RJ, Bombardier CH. Factors predicting hypnotic analgesia in clinical burn pain. *Int J Clin Exp Hypn* 1997;45:377–395.

130. Patterson DR, Everett JJ, Burns GL, et al. Hypnosis for the treatment of burn pain. *J Consult Clin Psychol* 1992;60:713–717.

131. Patterson DR, Ptacek JT. Baseline pain as a moderator of hypnotic analgesia for burn injury treatment. *J Consult Clin Psychol* 1997;65:60–67.

132. Spiegel H, Spiegel D. *Trance and Treatment*. Washington, DC: American Psychiatric Press; 1978.

133. Patterson DR, Tininenko JR, Schmidt AE, et al. Virtual reality hypnosis: a case report. *Int J Clin Exp Hypn* 2004;52:27–38.

134. Patterson DR, Wiechman SA, Jensen M, et al. Hypnosis delivered through immersive virtual reality for burn pain: a clinical case series. *Int J Clin Exp Hypn* 2006;54:130–142.

135. Hoffman HG, Richards TL, Van Oostrom T, et al. The analgesic effects of opioids and immersive virtual reality distraction: evidence from subjective and functional brain imaging assessments. *Anesth Analgesia* 2007;105:1776–1783.

136. Hoffman HG, Doctor JN, Patterson DR, et al. Use of virtual reality for adjunctive treatment of adolescent burn pain during wound care: a case report. *Pain* 2000;85:305–309.

137. Das DA, Grimmer KA, Sparnon AL, et al. The efficacy of playing a virtual reality game in modulating pain for children with acute burn injuries: a randomized controlled trial [ISRCTN87413556]. *BMC Pediatr* 2005;5:1.

138. van Twillert B, Bremer M, Faber AW. Computer-generated virtual reality to control pain and anxiety in pediatric and adult burn patients during wound dressing changes. *J Burn Care Res* 2007;28:694–702.

139. Sharar SR, Carrougher GJ, Nakamura D, et al. Factors influencing the efficacy of virtual reality distraction analgesia during postburn physical therapy: preliminary results from 3 ongoing studies. *Arch Phys Med Rehabil* 2007;88:S43–S49.

140. Faber AW, Patterson DR, Bremer M. Repeated use of immersive virtual reality therapy to control pain during wound dressing changes in pediatric and adult burn patients. *J Burn Care Res* 2013;34(5):563–568.

141. Jeffs D, Dorman D, Brown S, et al. Effect of virtual reality on adolescent pain during burn wound care. *J Burn Care Res* 2014;p35:395–408.

CHAPTER 54

Persistent Pain in Children

BOBBIE L. RILEY, TONYA M. PALERMO, GARY A. WALCO, CHARLES BERDE, and **NEIL L. SCHECHTER**

Persistent pain problems in children, as in adults, may stem from a wide variety of causes. They may be associated with ongoing illnesses such as cancer or sickle cell disease (SCD), may be the residua of pathologic processes that have resolved but have sensitized the peripheral or central nervous system such as postinfectious myalgias, or may represent a nonprogressive disorder whose main manifestation is pain such as headaches, widespread musculoskeletal pain, or functional abdominal pain. Regardless of the etiology of the pain, its assessment, its impact, and, often, the modalities used to treat are remarkably similar and often distinct from approaches used to address acute pain. For example, although the broader context of pain, including an array of genetic, developmental, environmental, and individual factors, is rarely a major focus of assessment in acute pain, these factors are essential to consider when pain is recurrent or persistent. Likewise, treatment goals may shift from pain eradication in acute pain to pain reduction, rehabilitation, and improved coping in chronic pain.

In this chapter, we describe the epidemiology of chronic pain, define its impact on children and families, and offer general approaches to its evaluation and treatment. Discussion of cancer pain is contained elsewhere in this book, as are more detailed descriptions of specific pain problems.

Epidemiology of Chronic Pain in Children

The epidemiology of the various chronic pain problems in children is often hard to ascertain primarily due to variability in the methodologies in the available research. Although this fact is an issue for adults as well, the relative limitations of the pediatric literature in the area of chronic pain, the added dimension of development when applying diagnostic criteria, child variants of adult disorders, the potential association between various pain syndromes, and the limitations in the young child's ability to report symptoms give us pause as we sift through data on the prevalence of persistent pain syndromes in children.

Recent efforts have been made to refine the taxonomy of chronic pain conditions,[1] and the need to maintain a life span developmental approach was highlighted.[2] This implies that rather than parse out pediatric conditions as separate entities, it is imperative to view the emergence of chronic pain as a developmental phenomenon from birth, through adulthood, and into the elderly years. Included is a focus on continuities and discontinuities in pain problems, highlighting longitudinal data to understand the specific genetic, epigenetic, and environmental roots of pain problems. Simply stated, children are not little adults, but adults are big children! With this as background, a sample of the epidemiology of selected persistent pain problems in children follows.

MUSCULOSKELETAL PAIN

One of the most common sites for pain in children and adolescents is the musculoskeletal system, including joint pain, bone pain, and muscle pain. Discomfort may arise from disease processes (e.g., inflammation associated with arthritis), may be related to central pain processing difficulties (e.g., juvenile fibromyalgia syndrome), or may be related to trauma or injury, typically focusing on a specific area of the body (e.g., back pain or neck pain). A recent study sought to better identify the etiology of musculoskeletal pain, which is a major first step in better grasping its epidemiology.[3] Demographic, clinical, and laboratory data were gathered on over 400 pediatric patients presenting with musculoskeletal pain, swelling, or limitation of movement. The etiology of these difficulties was identified in over 97% of cases, with by far the most common being noninflammatory and mechanical conditions (42.2%), followed by rheumatic diseases (31%), infection-related disorders (21.6%), and malignancy (2.4%). Age differences were noted, such that the prevalence of rheumatic disease was higher in those over 12 years, whereas younger age was associated with higher prevalence of infectious issues.

Arthritis

Estimates of the prevalence of juvenile arthritis have shifted a good deal over the years due to a number of factors, including diagnostic difficulties, changes in the classification schemas used, differences in research methodology, cohort effects, and factors occurring with the passage of time. Estimates of prevalence range from 10 to 220 cases per 100,000. Recent estimates suggest that 294,000 children between 0 and 17 years of age are being affected by "arthritis or other rheumatic conditions."[4]

Regarding pain in this population, Schanberg et al.[5] found that children with polyarticular juvenile arthritis had pain an average of 73% of the days. Although for most children this pain was in the mild to moderate range, 31% reported pain in the severe range. Baseline and up to 5-year follow-up data from the Childhood Arthritis Prospective Study helped identify pain trajectories over time in children with arthritis.[6] Patients between the ages of 1 and 16 years with new-onset juvenile idiopathic arthritis were followed, and three basic trajectories were identified: consistently low pain (53%), improved pain (30%), and consistently high pain (17%). A study in Canada showed similar results, with five pain severity trajectories: mild-decreasing pain (56%), moderate-decreasing pain (29%), chronically moderate pain (7%), minimal pain (4%), and mild-increasing pain (4%).[7]

Nonrheumatologic Musculoskeletal Pain

A number of studies have tried to identify the prevalence of musculoskeletal pain in children and adolescents not associated with arthritis or other rheumatologic conditions. De Inocencio[8] reported on a review of 6,500 office visits of children 3 to 14 years of age and found that 6.1% were for musculoskeletal complaints, the majority of which were for arthralgias and soft tissue pain. Common etiologies included trauma as well as mechanical or overuse pathology.

More generally, many children and adolescents report significant episodes of chronic nonspecific pain at least once in their lifetime, including limb pain (4.2% to 33.6%), knee pain (up to 18.5%), and back pain (7.6% to 34%).[9] Mikkelsson et al.[10] followed third and fifth graders over 1 year and found that pain occurring at least once per week persisted in 52.4%, with neck pain having the highest persistence.

Recognizing the risk of contiguity between chronic pain problems in children and adolescents with challenges later in life, a group of Danish researchers conducted a prospective 3-year school-based cohort study of children 8 to 14 years of age at baseline to gather information about musculoskeletal pain.[11] Through weekly mobile phone contacts, parents reported on the presence or absence of musculoskeletal pain in their children; a subset of children also underwent a more thorough clinical assessment. It was found that approximately half of the children had lower extremity pain every study year. This was hardly trivial—children experienced an average of 2.5 episodes, lasting for a total of 8 weeks each study year. Upper extremity pain was also present, but less substantial, as it occurred in approximately one quarter of the sample, lasting on average 3 weeks during a study year (about 1.5 episodes). Upper extremity pain tended to be more related to trauma than lower extremity pain. The most common sites of pain included knees and the ankle and foot area. Of note, this same research group went on to conduct a systematic review of other population based studies, with similar results.[12]

Fibromyalgia Syndrome

The prevalence of fibromyalgia syndrome in children and adolescents is difficult to determine. Mikkelsson et al.[13] used a structured pain questionnaire in a large sample of Finnish third- and fifth-grade children and found that 22 of them (1.25% overall) met criteria for fibromyalgia syndrome. In a retrospective review of patients referred to a pediatric rheumatology clinic between 1989 and 1995, 7% were diagnosed with fibromyalgia syndrome.[14] Data from the UK General Practice Research Database for the years 1990 to 2001 showed that the annual incidence of fibromyalgia increased from less than 1 per 100,000 to 35 per 100,000.[15] Female gender predominance is a well-replicated finding.[16] Although various studies have shown correlates to the presence of the syndrome, such as chronic fatigue,[17] joint hypermobility,[18] temperament,[19] familial aggregation,[20] and psychiatric symptoms,[13] causal relationships have not been shown.

Complex Regional Pain Syndrome

There are few studies reporting on the prevalence of complex regional pain syndrome (CRPS) in children and adolescents. A 2017 review found only 10 studies (only 1 population-based) with relevant data, which showed a mean age at onset of 12.5 years, with 85% of patients being female. The majority of patients (71%) had a history of trauma. Contrary to adults, lower limbs were affected in 75% of patients, with secondary site involvement in 15% of cases.[21]

Back Pain

Back pain represents a somewhat distinct form of musculoskeletal pain. A recent comprehensive review indicated that low back pain is rarely seen in children younger than school age and prevalence rates rise until age 18 years, at which time rates parallel those of adults.[22] Contrary to prior beliefs, sinister diagnoses are rare, as pain tends to be nonspecific and is self-limiting.

Beyond the incidence of chronic musculoskeletal pain, a critical issue is also the transition from the acute phase to more persistent pain problems. A recent study followed 88 10- to 17-year-olds who had presented to the emergency department or orthopedic clinic with new musculoskeletal pain complaints,

approximately 35% of whom continued to have persistent pain 4 months later. Regression analyses showed that depressive symptoms and poorer pain modulation were key risk factors related to this transition.[23]

An earlier systematic review identified 65 potential risk factors for the onset of and 43 potential prognostic factors for the persistence of musculoskeletal pain. Results showed that low socioeconomic status (strong evidence) as well negative emotional symptoms and regularly smoking in childhood or adolescence (moderate evidence) may be associated with persistence of pain. Interestingly, high body mass index, taller height, and joint hypermobility were not found to be risk factors for the onset of pain.[24]

Temporomandibular Disorders

Temporomandibular disorder (TMD) pain is often underrecognized in children and adolescents. A systematic review and meta-analysis conducted to assess the prevalence of clinical signs of temporomandibular joint (TMJ) disorders in children and adolescents captured 17,051 participants.[25] The overall prevalence of clinical signs of intra-articular joint disorders was 16%, the prevalence of TMJ sounds was 14%, clicking (10.0%), and jaw locking (2.3%). Significant correlates include bruxism and tooth-grinding as well as bite and tooth positioning.[26]

HEADACHE

Determining the incidence of headache in the pediatric population is difficult due to changing diagnostic criteria and attempts to apply adult diagnostic criteria to children. In a review by Hershey et al.,[27] it was concluded that up to 75% of children have had significant headaches by the age of 15 years, with up to 28% of adolescents describing symptoms consistent with migraine headaches. Previous meta-analytic reviews suggested a gradual increase in headache incidence over childhood with 37% to 51% of children reporting a significant headache by 7 years and up to 82% by 15 years.[28] A more recent meta-analysis of 64 cross-sectional studies (including a total of 227,249 subjects) yielded an estimated overall mean prevalence of headache was 54.4%, with an overall mean prevalence of migraine at 9.1%.[29]

The distinction between migraine and tension-type headache is often complex, particularly in pediatric headache. For example, when applying International Classification of Headache Disorders-II criteria to a large sample of German children age 7 to 14 years, Kröner-Herwig and colleagues[30] found that 7.5% of the headaches could be classified as migraine, 18.5% as tension-type, and the majority were unclassifiable. Virtanen et al.[31] found that among children who were classified as having migraines at age 6 years, half were unchanged at age 13 years, whereas for 32%, there was a shift toward tension-type headaches. Other authors found a similar lack of stability in headache type over time with headache types shifting or disappearing entirely. For example, a 10-year longitudinal study of principally preadolescent children diagnosed with migraine, only 46% continued to have migraine and the frequency of attacks had diminished.[32]

Therefore, the precise relationship between various types of headaches in children remains unclear. In addition, various authors report close relationships between headache pain and other difficulties, including neck pain,[33] back pain,[34] abdominal pain,[35] sleep disturbances,[36] fatigue,[37] epilepsy,[38,39] epistaxis,[40] psychiatric difficulties, and risk of suicide.[41–43]

Nonetheless, headaches in children appear to be quite common; however, precisely what differentiates migraine headache from tension-type headaches is difficult to discern at times. Headaches increase in frequency and severity with age with a clear shift around the time of puberty and are more common and problematic in females, and health-related quality of life (HRQOL) may be significantly impacted.[44]

CHRONIC ABDOMINAL PAIN

Chronic abdominal pain accounts for 2% to 4% of pediatric visits. Hyams et al.[45] found that 75% of middle school and high school students reported abdominal pain, whereas 21% reported it was severe enough to affect activities, and 8% visited a physician for it. Like other pain problems, various definitions and correlates of persistent abdominal pain (recurrent abdominal pain, chronic abdominal pain, functional abdominal pain, functional gastrointestinal disorder [FGID] nonorganic abdominal pain, and psychogenic abdominal pain) have led to varying perspectives in its prevalence.

A recent study of parental reports of 4- to 18-year-olds in a representative community sample of the United States indicated that 23.1% had at least one FGID, with functional constipation and abdominal migraine being the most common (Rome III criteria). The Rome III criteria for abdominal pain–related FGIDs in children and adolescents include functional dyspepsia, irritable bowel syndrome (IBS), abdominal migraine, childhood functional abdominal pain, and childhood functional abdominal pain syndrome.[46] A revision of these criteria, Rome IV, will include additional categories that include motility disturbance, visceral hypersensitivity, altered mucosal and immune functioning, altered gut microbiota, and altered central nervous system processing, all of which reflect recent advances in the field and will likely lead to more insight into incidence and etiologies.[47]

It appears that the roots of nonspecific abdominal pain may be identified quite early in development based on chart reviews of a cohort of children followed from birth to 5 years. Chitkara et al.[48] found an incidence of abdominal pain of unknown origin of 4.5/1,000 person years leading to repeated visits to the pediatrician. Finally, as was the case with prior pain problems, there is growing evidence the difficulties with chronic abdominal pain early in life are associated with the risk of future abdominal pain, other pain problems (e.g., headache), and broader somatic concerns later in childhood and beyond.[49,50]

DISEASE- OR TREATMENT-RELATED PAIN
Sickle Cell Disease

For many years, the focus of pain management in children and adolescents with SCD were episodes of vasoocclusion. Dampier and colleagues[51] gathered pain diary data in children and adolescents with SCD. They found that vasoocclusive pain is experienced on 2% of days in preschool-age children and on 5% to 10% of days in school-age children and young adolescents. School-age children tended to have less intense pain than adolescents, and girls tended to report a higher number of painful sites than boys. Subsequent data[52] showed that 40% to 50% of school-age children experience one pain episode a month, whereas about 10% experience more than two episodes a month. Although the majority of these episodes lasted 1 day or less, about 5% of episodes in older children last longer than 2 weeks.

More recently, however, it is clear that children with SCD are affected by a number of recurrent chronic pain concerns beyond those related to vasoocclusion. Although Niebanck et al.[53] found that overall the prevalence of tension-type and migraine headaches in children with SCD approximates that of healthy peers, they found that headache was more common in younger children with SCD and that there were relationships noted between frequency of headache and frequency of vasoocclusion. This suggests that factors related to SCD may increase the risk of headache pain. In addition, sequelae of splenic sequestration may lead to ongoing visceral pain in the left upper quadrant and irreversible joint damage, such as related to aseptic necrosis, may cause ongoing discomfort.

Cystic Fibrosis

Koh et al.[54] evaluated 46 children with cystic fibrosis (CF) and found that nearly half of the sample described pain occurring at least weekly with primary locations of the abdominal and pelvic region, chest, head, and neck. Although most children reported mild pain intensity and relatively short duration, a small subgroup reported moderately intense pain in the chest that was of longer duration. Pain in this group was thought to be musculoskeletal in nature, related to pulled or torn intercostal muscles, costochondritis, pleuritis, pneumothorax, or rib fracture. A Web-based study of adolescents and young adults with CF found that about half experienced moderate daily pain of 2 hours duration or less, with disability highest in areas of recreation, occupation, and social activities.[55]

Phantom Limb

Phantom pain occurs when a limb has been amputated and the individual continues to feel pain in a part of the body that is no longer there. In an early attempt to ascertain the prevalence of such conditions in children, Krane and Heller[56] conducted a retrospective survey of 5- to 19-year-olds who had undergone limb amputation in the preceding 10 years. Amputations were secondary to congenital deformity, trauma/infection, or cancer. Phantom sensations were experienced in all patients, and the overwhelming majority stated they experienced phantom pain as well. Melzack et al.[57] reported that phantom limbs are experienced by 20% of those with congenital limb deficiencies and 50% of those who underwent amputation before age 6 years. Phantom pain was reported in 20% and 42% of these groups, respectively. Using diary data, Wilkins et al.[58] found recurrent episodes of phantom pain due to congenital limb deficiencies, surgery, and trauma, with an average intensity of 6.43 out of 10.

ADDITIONAL CONSIDERATIONS

The earlier review should make it clear that there is an array of chronic and recurrent pain problems that affect children and adolescents. It is unwise, therefore, to focus on "chronic" or "recurrent" pain as a unified entity but rather as diverse syndromes, perhaps with certain common factors. As is discussed in the following text, a broad biopsychosocial perspective is deemed optimal, which embraces genetic, developmental, and environmental influences.

In the remainder of this chapter, we discuss the impact of persistent pain on children and offer a general approach to evaluating and managing it. A more detailed review on a number of more common entities is offered as well. Additional information on many of these problems is available in other sections of this book, such as Chapters 25, 49, 57, and 61.

Impact of Persistent Pain on Children and Families

Recurrent and chronic pain can have a major impact on the daily lives of children, adolescents, and their families. Whereas some children experiencing pain symptoms have minimal day-to-day impairment, other children exhibit psychological distress and have significant activity limitations due to pain. The children who seek treatment for their chronic pain symptoms likely represent the group who is experiencing the most impairment.[59] For many children, chronic pain has been associated with poorer HRQOL, psychosocial difficulties, academic problems, and disruptions in peer and family relationships.[60,61]

Disability or activity limitations that results from chronic pain is a separate concept from pain itself, and it is equally important to consider in assessment and management of pediatric pain patients.[62] Disability refers to those areas in an individual's life that are limited due to pain.[63] The domains of functioning that seem to be particularly impacted by chronic pediatric pain are participation in physical and social activities, school and academics, sleep, and family functioning. Specifically, chronic pain has been associated with more frequent school absences and academic difficulties.[64,65] Missed schooling can have direct effects on academic performance and school success as well as important effects on socialization and maintenance of peer relationships. Difficulties with peer relationships have been found in children with chronic pain, with one study of children with juvenile fibromyalgia reporting that children were more isolated, less well liked, and less socially accepted than their healthy peers.[66,67]

Activities limited due to pain vary depending on the level of pain children experience. Higher levels of pain intensity, greater pain extent, and longer pain duration have been associated with greater activity limitations and impairment.[68–71] Specific domains of activity restriction have also been associated with pain level. In one study of children with SCD, although children decreased participation in all activities (school, play, sports, social) when pain was high, they were able to maintain school attendance and social activities when pain levels were low.[69] Future research is needed to better understand the relationship between pain and activity restriction among different populations.

Sleep disturbances are highly comorbid with chronic pain, affecting over half of youth.[72,73] The most commonly experienced sleep disturbance is insomnia (i.e., difficulties falling asleep or staying asleep), which is reported by over 50% of youth with chronic pain.[73] It is associated with diminished physical function, poor quality of life, and increased depressive symptoms.[74] Untreated, insomnia symptoms persist over a 1-year period for youth with chronic pain.[67]

Psychological factors, including anxiety, depression, and coping, have been identified as important in the development and maintenance of chronic pain and disability in children (e.g., Simons and Kaczynski,[75] Nodari et al.[76]). Children with chronic pain report increased general anxiety, pain-specific anxiety, posttraumatic stress symptoms, and depressive symptoms than youth without pain conditions, which is associated with greater pain-related disability.[60,77,78] In large-scale epidemiologic studies, individuals with a history of chronic pain in adolescence subsequently report higher rates of lifetime anxiety and depressive disorders, as compared with individuals without a history of adolescent chronic pain.[79] Moreover, children's coping style (particularly maladaptive coping) and catastrophizing behaviors are associated with increased psychological distress and physical limitations.[80]

HRQOL refers to an individual's perception of the impact a disease or condition has on his or her physical health status, psychological functioning, and emotional well-being. Chronic pain may impair school attendance, mobility, self-care, interpersonal interactions, life activities, and community activities as well emotional functioning.[62] Several examinations of HRQOL in children and adolescents with pain conditions (e.g., headache, SCD, mixed pain conditions) have found that they report significantly poorer HRQOL in comparison to healthy children.[76,81] Moreover, unexplained chronic pain in adolescents has been associated with poor quality of life for the adolescent and his or her family.[59] Predictors of poor HRQOL within pain populations include the presence of sleep problems,[82] fatigue,[83] pain-related hospitalizations,[81] low socioeconomic conditions,[84] and increasing child age.

Pediatric chronic pain is embedded in a broader family context that influences the child's adjustment to chronic pain, so caregivers are a unique and integral part of pediatric chronic pain treatment.[85] Studies show that caring for a child with chronic pain has a negative impact on parent caregivers, expressed in higher anxiety, depression, and increased parental role stress.[80] Although it is unknown whether these symptoms precede the pain condition, or develop in response to parenting a child with chronic pain, high levels of parental distress have been linked to increased pain and disability in children.[85,86] Furthermore, parents may respond with increased attention, sympathy, or discouragement of activity if they perceive their child's pain as a potential sign of harm or damage. Such protective or solicitous responses can provide positive reinforcement and increase illness behavior, which may exacerbate or maintain children's pain and disability.[87,88] This bidirectional influence is illustrated in the integrative model of family and parent factors for children with chronic pain, developed by Palermo and Chambers,[89] that outlines parent and family influences on child experience of pain. Consequently, caregivers have become important targets in psychological interventions for children with chronic pain.

Parents may experience significant financial burden due to the evaluation and management of their child's recurrent and chronic pain. Pediatric chronic pain is costly to society, with estimates of $19.5 billion per year spent on pain treatment in the United States.[90] Costs to parents and caregivers include lost employment time, transportation expenses, childcare, and incidental costs. The stress of chronic pain on families is also associated with increased levels of family conflict and poorer family functioning.[91] Previous studies have shown more family problems in children with chronic pain compared to healthy children[92] and that poorer family environments are associated with increased disability.[86,93]

Clinical Evaluation of the Child with Chronic Pain

BACKGROUND

In the position statement published by the American Pain Society, chronic pain in children was defined as the result of a dynamic integration of biologic processes, psychological factors, and sociocultural factors considered within a developmental trajectory.[94] Therefore, evaluating a child with chronic pain can be time-consuming and complicated as a multitude of factors contribute to its development and maintenance. Children who present with persistent pain often receive extensive evaluations by both primary care providers and specialists in different disciplines due to the complexity of the pain presentation and the associated symptoms. If the pain appears to result from a previously or newly identified organic disease (e.g., ulcerative colitis, SCD, cancer), the treatment focus is on addressing the underlying illness while simultaneously treating the associated pain symptoms. In other situations, the source of the pain may be known and often time-limited but may not be amenable to direct treatment, and therefore, the focus is typically solely on addressing the pain (e.g., persistent postoperative, posttraumatic, or postviral pain). For both of these groups of children, there is no need for an extensive search for an explanation for their pain and the clinician can focus on its treatment.

The more challenging situations and the emphasis of the majority of this chapter occur when no obvious pathophysiologic source of the pain has been identified. The child is suffering, the parents are frustrated, extensive evaluation is often undertaken, and no treatable disease process emerges to explain the pain. In these situations, the clinician must attempt to identify those children who may have an as yet undiagnosed underlying progressive disease process and separate them from those who have chronic pain syndromes, which although uncomfortable, do not represent life-threatening illness. This is not an easy task, given the inherent vagueness and subjectivity of the symptoms, the inadequacies of children as historians, the strong desire of most children and their families for an "organic treatable diagnosis," and the vast differential diagnosis. In these situations when source of pain does not have a clear or treatable organic etiology despite adequate evaluation, the treatment focus changes and is ultimately on educating the family and patient on the pathophysiology of chronic pain including the process of central sensitization and on the value of a biopsychosocial rehabilitative approach.

Initially, however, a delicate balance must be struck between adequate evaluation and overinvestigation. The physician must be comfortable that he or she has enough information to rule out potentially serious or life-threatening causes of pain on the one hand while avoiding an endless search for the underlying etiology of the discomfort on the other. Continued laboratory investigation often convinces the child and family that there must be a biologic explanation for the problem and suggests to them that the "answer" may be found in the next laboratory test. Clinicians may report that they are ordering additional tests "for the sake of completeness" and both clinicians and families often find it difficult to draw a diagnostic line in the sand where all are content with extent of the investigation. Furthermore, pediatricians do not always agree on the diagnostic approach. Konijnenberg and colleagues[95] highlighted this problem in a series of papers in which 17 different pediatricians reviewed the medical records of 134 children with unexplained chronic pain. Consensus of the group was defined as an agreement among 80% of the pediatricians on the panel. Yet, there was disagreement on diagnostic approach in over a third of the patients and on the primary cause of the pain in over one-half.[95] Unfortunately, this diagnostic uncertainty often leads to further excessive and expensive laboratory and imaging studies. It is particularly unfortunate if, after completing an extensive battery of tests, which are negative, the doctor implies that the problem must be solely psychological and refers the child to a mental health professional.

Therefore, one of the most critical aspects of the evaluation of the child with unexplained chronic pain is the development of a trusting relationship with the child and family[96] and their acceptance that the medical investigation has been sufficient to allow the primary focus of the encounter to be on the management of the pain regardless of its etiology.

Etiologically, chronic pain is thought to stem from an interplay between biologic vulnerability, psychological variables, and environmental variables which allow for abnormalities of sensory processing, enhanced responsiveness, and excitability in the central nervous system known as *central sensitization* and *amplification. Central sensitization* is discussed in numerous other chapters throughout this book in detail, but it is the term used to describe the dysfunction or pathology of the nervous system that results in an amplified responsiveness of the central nervous system to painful and nonpainful stimuli. This increased responsiveness of the nervous system is thought to be a key element in the development and maintenance of chronic pain.[97–100]

These factors must be considered in the evaluation and treatment of all children with chronic pain. As outlined in the American Pain Society consensus statement,[94] a comprehensive clinical assessment of a child with chronic pain should include a complete medical and pain history including onset, intensity, quality, location, duration, variability, predictability, exacerbating, and alleviating factors with ongoing management and reassessment emphasizing functional improvements. The physical exam should include a complete neurologic exam, with observation of the child's general appearance, posture, and gait. Although laboratory and radiologic studies may be useful if a specific disease is suspected, the diagnosis of a chronic pain condition is predominately made by history and physical exam and best assessed by a pediatric interdisciplinary pain management team typically including pain medicine clinicians, mental health providers, and physical and occupational therapists.[94]

HISTORY

Traditional elements of the pain history for adults are applicable to evaluating chronic pain in children. Although younger children are developmentally less capable of presenting a coherent narrative, they are capable of reporting on specific aspects of their pain. Using developmentally appropriate tools, children are able to define pain intensity as well as radiation, exacerbating and relieving factors of the pain, and quality of the pain. Chronic pain in children has a significant impact on daily function which can be seen in school attendance and work quality, social relationships, and mood.[78] The history of impact on daily function should be integral in ongoing reassessment of pain management as improvement in function may occur well before a decrease in pain intensity. Roth-Isigkeit and colleagues[61] studied 750 German school children and found that 30% to 40% reported restrictions in daily living secondary to pain. Chalkiadis's[101] study of chronic pain in Australian youth revealed that 71% of children had difficulty sleeping and over 90% were unable to be involved in sports.

Because evidence supports that early exposure to painful stimuli and other adverse events potentially predisposes the child to changes in nociception, it is important to be aware of the child's medical history. Fitzgerald and colleagues'[102–105] study of rat pups has demonstrated long-lasting hypersensitivity to pain from early tissue injury. Grunau and coworkers,[106–109] in a series of papers, compared toddlers who were born prematurely to babies of normal gestation and birth weight and found differences in pain sensitivity and somatization. Measurable differences between the groups were found even when the children had reached 8 to 10 years. Anand and Scalzo[110] has even suggested that there are increased rates of attention-deficit/hyperactivity disorder (ADHD), substance abuse, and anxiety in children who have been exposed to repeated neonatal pain and stress.

Another essential element to query is the history of pain problems in the family. Although some authors, such as Borge and Nordhagen,[111] question whether chronic pain symptoms run in families, on the whole, the majority of studies have suggested that parent and family history of pain are predictors of child pain. This pattern has been identified in children with rheumatologic disease,[112] recurrent abdominal pain, migraine, and fibromyalgia.[113] The mediators of this phenomenon are unclear. They may be physiologic (such as altered pain thresholds) or psychological (e.g., social modeling of catastrophizing behavior) or most likely a combination of both. Regardless of the mediators for this phenomenon, it is essential that family history of pain be examined. The child's pain cannot be adequately addressed if the parent's pain is not recognized.

Psychological and social factors should be explored in children with chronic pain and their families regardless of the pain's etiology. Such an exploration does not imply causation, but there is clearly a transactional relationship between chronic pain and anxiety and depression.[114,115] As is evident throughout this chapter, anxiety, depression, and other mental health concerns frequently co-occur with chronic pain and need to be assessed. Questions regarding anxiety, depression, and excessive irritability should be posed to both the child and his or her family. The use of existing standardized questionnaires has been described earlier in this chapter and should be encouraged. In addition to mental health concerns in the child, Eccleston and colleagues[116] report that parents who have chronically ill children are often anxious and depressed (60% and 40%), and these symptoms may be a response to parenting a sick child or may predate the child's illness.[113] Chronic pain is likely to bring severe disruption to the social and family structure,[62,117] which should be examined as part of gathering the history of the pain and its impact.

The child's school experience should also be explored in an effort to identify further impact on daily function.[118] Increased school absenteeism is commonly reported in most chronic pain syndromes,[119] widespread musculoskeletal pain,[10] and abdominal pain.[120] This may be a result of underlying stress from learning disabilities, attentional problems, or social difficulties such as bullying. Frequent absences may also become a source of extreme stress for the child when faced with the need to reintegrate making a frank discussion about the child's grades, competencies, social skills, friendships, and existing school accommodations a necessary part of the history gathering. The Pediatric Pain Screening Tool (PPST) is a 9-item screening tool available to identify factors associated with adverse outcomes among youth who present with pain complaints, providing risk stratification and potential guidance for effective pain treatment recommendation in the clinic setting.[96]

Finally, red flags or alarm signs specific to the common functional pain syndromes that help delineate a need for additional investigation is discussed in specific sections pertaining to each syndrome (headache, abdominal pain, and musculoskeletal pain).

MEASUREMENT OF PAIN AND FUNCTIONING

A thorough biopsychosocial assessment of the child with chronic pain is critical for individualizing pain treatment strategies. The clinician aims to gather detailed information about the child's current pain and pain history and assess areas of child daily functioning that are disrupted by pain while considering the child's developmental stage. Many evidence-based self-report questionnaires have been developed and validated across the pediatric age range, which complement a semi-structured interview. Assessment is considered an iterative process, with follow-up assessment conducted throughout treatment to track progress toward treatment goals.

Measurement of aspects of recurrent and chronic pain requires tools that measure the frequency, intensity, duration, time course, and activity interference due to pain. Validated measures have been developed to capture most of these domains (e.g., Eccleston et al.,[121] Stinson et al.[122]). Developmental considerations will guide selection of the most valid and reliable tool. In children ages 4 through 12 years, Faces Pain Scales have demonstrated good validity and reliability.[123] In youth 8 years of age and older, Visual Analogue Scales, using anchors such as "no pain" and "worst pain ever," are considered most valid and reliable. The verbal Numerical Rating Scale (NRS) is often used clinically, on which participants rate their pain on an 11-point scale representing increasing pain intensity (e.g., 0 to 10). Data indicate that the NRS is a valid and reliable measure for ages 8 years and older.[124]

In addition to assessment of pain intensity, there are other characteristics of pain (e.g., duration, frequency, pain quality, spatial distribution) that are important to evaluate in children with chronic pain. Daily monitoring of pain and using a diary or log provides information about pain patterns as well as variations in children's behaviors (e.g., activities participated in) and emotions (e.g., positive or negative affect).[125] A body map identifies the spatial distribution of pain, including the number of pain locations, and indicates how widespread the pain is. It is also helpful to obtain information from parents and children about the history and course of the pain problem, including past and present treatments for pain, perceived efficacy of treatments, and beliefs about the cause of pain and expectancies for pain relief. Electronic pain diaries (e.g., smartphones and Web sites) have become increasingly used in children and adolescents to document chronic pain symptoms. For example, Stinson and colleagues[125] developed a multidimensional electronic diary to collect data on pain intensity, duration, location, and impact in adolescents with arthritis.

A critical area to assess is function. Measures such as the Functional Disability Inventory[63] and the Child Activity Limitations Interview[126] provide information about interference of pain in normal daily activities. These measures are brief and can be administered easily to document children's functional disability at baseline and treatment progress. Many children with chronic pain conditions experience significant school impairment including a high number of absences from school and difficulties making academic progress.[127,128] Role functioning can be assessed on broadband measures, such as HRQOL and pain impact measures. To supplement interview and survey assessment, objective measures of school attendance and performance (e.g., report cards, attendance records) are useful to obtain.

There are several multidomain measures that can be used for efficient assessment of multiple domains of functioning. The *Patient-Reported Outcomes Measurement Information System* (PROMIS) is a National Institutes of Health initiative. The PROMIS Pediatric Cooperative Group developed self-report item banks to assess general health domains, including depressive symptoms, anxiety, mobility, pain interference, fatigue, peer relationships, and pain intensity in children.[129] When used as a comprehensive battery, 25-, 37- and 49-item versions are available to assess multiple domains. These measures are appropriate for children ages 8 to 17 years[130] and can be supplemented by a parent proxy report. The Bath Adolescent Pain Questionnaire[131] assesses seven domains of functioning affected by pain (social functioning, physical functioning, depression, general anxiety, pain-specific anxiety, family functioning, and development), and a parent report is also available.[132] The Pediatric Quality of Life Inventory[133] is a well-validated HRQOL measure for children (age 5 to 18 years) to self-report functioning in four broad domains (physical, emotional, social, school) and has a parent proxy instrument for younger children.

Psychosocial assessment is an important component in the assessment of a child with chronic pain in order to evaluate psychological, social, and family functioning which may contribute to pain or pain-related disability. Psychosocial assessment may consist of clinical interviews, administration of standardized psychological measures, and observation of child and family members. A detailed clinical interview should cover developmental, behavioral, and psychiatric concerns in the patient's and family's history. Potential stressors and areas of maladaptive coping should be inquired about as well as a comprehensive school history and history of peer and social relationships. Ideally, a separate psychosocial assessment is conducted with child and parent alone in order to obtain their individual perspectives. Many outpatient pediatric pain clinics use intake questionnaire packets that cover demographics, developmental history, and other aspects of psychological functioning in order to consistently obtain this information in the evaluation of new patients. Review of intake packets may then provide details that serve as a springboard for more focused clinical interviews or additional psychological assessments during the intake visit.

Depending on the particular presenting concerns, standardized psychological measures may be administered to screen for mental health diagnoses, in particular, anxiety and depressive symptoms, to assess coping behaviors and family functioning. A variety of standardized instruments can be used in the clinical setting with the advantage of obtaining a quick assessment of children's psychological functioning given the limited time available for in-depth psychological evaluation in the medical setting. Many valid and reliable measures are available to assess anxiety and depression in youth such as the *Revised Child Anxiety and Depression Scale*,[134,135] and PROMIS Emotional Distress anxiety and depressive symptoms.[136] Posttraumatic stress disorder (PTSD) symptoms can be measured using standardized tools like the 24-item *Child PTSD Symptoms Scale*.[137]

When psychological measures are used to screen for psychological distress, it is important to consider the limitations of self-report and, in particular, that children may want to present themselves in a favorable light (social desirability response bias), which has been described in children and adolescents with chronic pain.[138]

Beyond general internalizing symptoms, it is also useful to assess pain-specific dimensions of anxiety (e.g., catastrophizing, pain-related fear). There are developmentally adapted versions of the Pain Catastrophizing Scale available to assess child catastrophic thoughts about pain[139] as well as parent catastrophic thinking about their child's pain.[140] Other measures are available to assess pain-related anxiety, such as the *Child Pain Anxiety Symptoms Scale*[141] and the *Fear of Pain Questionnaire*,[142] which also has a parent report.[143]

Parental and family functioning has also been a major area of focus in pediatric chronic pain assessment.[89] There are measures available to assess parent behaviors (e.g., frequently attending to pain symptoms or allowing avoidance of regular activities) that may contribute to pain-related disability (e.g., *Adult Responses to Children's Pain Questionnaire*).[144] In addition, overall family functioning can be assessed with several measures including the *Family Assessment Device*.[145] In some cases, it may be important to screen parents for their own psychological distress, given the risk for high levels of caregiver stress in this population (e.g., *Brief Symptom Inventory*). For a comprehensive review of measures available to assess parental impact of chronic pain, see Eccleston et al.[121]

There are also measures of child coping that have been validated on pediatric chronic pain samples including the Pain Response Inventory[146] and the Pain Coping Questionnaire.[147] Measures of specific areas of coping, including catastrophizing, are available such as the Pain Catastrophizing Scale, Child Version (PCS-C).[139]

Well-established measures of sleep in pediatric chronic pain include the *Children's Sleep Habits Questionnaire* (CSHQ),[148] the *Adolescent Sleep–Wake Scale* (ASWS),[149] and the *Adolescent Sleep Habits Scale* (ASHS).[149] The CSHQ is a parent-report measure used to assess multiple aspects of sleep in school-age children (ages 4 to 10 years), including bedtime behavioral issues and symptoms of sleep disordered breathing.[148] The ASWS and ASHS are complementary measures of sleep quality and sleep habits, respectively. Although reliable and relevant to pediatric pain, all three questionnaires are lengthy and potentially burdensome to complete. A short form (10-item) of the ASWS was recently developed that may be useful to integrate into quick-paced tertiary care settings.[90] For a comprehensive review of available sleep measurement tools in pediatric pain, see de la Vega and Miró.[150]

PHYSICAL EVALUATION

Information gathered from the physical examination in conjunction with the history can help differentiate a primary/functional pain disorder from pain secondary to an underlying disease. General appearance (sickly or well appearing) may be helpful, although individuals who are in pain for a prolonged period of time may look pale and wan. Growth parameters should be examined as chronic illness may well impede growth. Because of the association between chronic pain and postural orthostatic tachycardia syndrome, heart rate should be obtained both supine and standing.

The child should be asked to localize his or her pain. The differential diagnosis and intervention strategies are very different for generalized discomfort versus highly localized pain. Specific discussion of the examination of the back, abdomen, and joints is beyond the scope of this review, but regardless of the origin of the pain, the clinician should obtain general impressions of the child's mood, cooperativeness, irritability,

and eye contact along with a comprehensive neurologic exam and more focused musculoskeletal exam, noting the child's gait and posture.

Although hypermobility does not predict future musculoskeletal pain in the preteen and adolescent population, literature currently supports the association of chronic musculoskeletal pain with hypermobility.[151] The Beighton score is a valid measurement of generalized joint hypermobility in children. A score of 6/9 indicates hypermobility.[152] When positive, discussion regarding hypermobility can be helpful both in its suggestion of biologic vulnerability to pain as well as providing guidance in the development of additional goals for physical therapy such as joint protection, postural control, and improved proprioception as a part of the multidisciplinary plan.[152-154] Regardless of the origin, a Beighton score should be calculated on all children with chronic pain.[155]

CLINICAL FORMULATION

The task for the clinician is to examine the data that emerged from the history and physical and determine whether or not there are sufficient red flags to warrant further investigation for progressive disease. If there are, the child and family should be informed that the investigation is ongoing. If there are not, the clinician should report to the child and family that the child most likely has a chronic pain syndrome. In either situation, the pain should be treated appropriately, although the approach, both philosophically and practically, will vary between the two. If the pain is thought to be a manifestation of a time-limited disease process, although the approach will be multifactorial, there will often be an emphasis on more aggressive pharmacologic intervention while the disease process runs its course. If the pain is associated with a chronic condition or represents a chronic pain syndrome, the emphasis is more typically on a rehabilitative approach.

FEEDBACK WITH THE FAMILY

During initial evaluation, history and physical may warrant further investigation for progressive disease, in which case, further evaluation should be discussed with the child and family. However, if the need for additional investigation is not indicated, the clinician should review with the child and family that the more likely cause is a primary/functional pain disorder.[96] This initial feedback is, in effect, the first treatment intervention and will set the tone for the subsequent relationship with the child and family.[114,115]

Regardless of the etiology of the pain, feedback should include a number of elements. Ensuring the family at this time that the pain is "real" is critical as many families of children with chronic pain report that they have felt dismissed and feel that their child has not been believed. It is imperative that the clinician informs the family that he or she is familiar with the pain symptom complex. Even if the exact problem is not clearly defined, chronic pain problems share numerous overlapping features which need to be addressed such as sleep disturbances, school reintegration, and return to physical and social activities. Another key element is that of optimism. It is clear that expectations can influence the outcomes of chronic pain treatment.[156]

Providing an understandable explanation of the pain is a critical element of the initial feedback. The current conceptualization of chronic pain is that it results from the interplay between biologic vulnerability and psychological and environmental variables which ultimately lead to abnormalities of sensory processing, enhanced responsiveness, and excitability in the central nervous system known as *central sensitization*. Central sensitization is discussed in numerous other chapters throughout this book in detail, but it is the term used to describe the dysfunction of the nervous system that results in an amplified responsiveness to painful and nonpainful stimuli. This increased responsiveness of the nervous system is thought to be a key element in the development and maintenance of chronic pain.[97–100] Because chronic pain typically represents nerve "hypersensitivity" and not progressive disease and damage, the traditional dichotomization of pain into organic or psychological causation is inaccurate and often harmful.[98–100] It is also essential therefore that the child and family be aware that pain persistence does not serve a warning protective function as it does in acute pain and that although pain may "hurt," it is not causing "harm." This all must be explained to the child and family in an understandable way as Moseley and others have documented the importance of "neuroeducation" in promoting recovery and compliance with recommendations.[157,158] The use of metaphors ("pain is a false alarm"; "the pain is a software glitch, not a hardware problem") may be quite helpful in conveying this message.[159,160]

As previously stated, due to the complex relationship between biologic, psychological, individual, social, and environmental factors which result in chronic pain, treatment recommendations should be multidimensional. The massive stress of school, the loss of normal opportunities to socialize with friends, and the impact of the immobilization and sleep deprivation often accompanying chronic pain further contribute to its maintenance and persistence and therefore should be a part of the treatment plan elucidated during the feedback.[114] Evidence of the positive impact of a multidisciplinary approach was demonstrated in 5 out of 8 outcome domains recommended by PedIMMPACT including pain intensity, disability, school functioning, anxiety, and depressive symptoms[114] as well as by numerous other investigators.[161] Lack of acceptance of the multifactorial nature of pain and its treatment has been identified as one of the causes of treatment failure.[162]

The final element that the feedback should convey is that although the ultimate goal is reduction of pain, initially, it is the return of the child to functioning. Pain reduction or elimination will often follow.

Treatment

GENERAL PRINCIPLES OF TREATMENT

Interventions offered by multidisciplinary teams for the management of chronic pain are centered on three main components: pharmacotherapy, physical therapy, and psychological therapy for a multimodal approach focusing on improving daily function. Dimensions of daily function include "the 4 S's"[96]: sports, social, sleep, and school, with a primary goal to improve physical function and facilitate reengagement in age typical activity.[96,114,154] As mentioned previously, educating the child and family that chronic pain does not offer the warning protective function of acute nociceptive pain and stating that although the pain is unpleasant, it is not causing "harm" is essential to alleviate familial anxiety and promote participation in the main components shown to allow for improved function.

Initially, frequent scheduled follow-up appointments help the child and family build confidence through careful monitoring as the child engages in these therapies. Symptom diaries may provide interim data between appointments. This approach has been labeled "watchful waiting"[163] and can reassure parents that if new symptoms develop, a potentially unrecognized disease process will not be missed.

Interventions typically employed to address chronic pain must allow the child to return to a "normal" life. As a result, medications which significantly alter the child's sensorium are inadvisable, along with prolonged hospital or home stays. Pharmacotherapy to reduce central sensitization such as antidepressants and anticonvulsants are often the mainstay of

pharmacologic treatment regardless of the etiology of the chronic pain; however, utilized as a sole therapy for primary pain disorders, they tend to be ineffective. Although there are limited clinical trials to support their use, antidepressants and anticonvulsants are used in children for primary pain disorders. Two of the most common, amitriptyline and gabapentin, are approved for use in children; however, few other antidepressants and anticonvulsants have been.[164,165] Analgesic agents for mild acute pain, such as acetaminophen and nonsteroidal anti-inflammatory drugs (NSAIDs), may be helpful, but there is the risk of rebound headache or abdominal pain secondary to excessive nonsteroidal usage.[166,167] Guidelines for opioid use for chronic pain have not been applied to children and adolescents.[168] When used for primary pain disorders, opioids are generally associated with worse clinical outcomes.[169] That said, appropriate use may be indicated in conditions such as osteogenesis imperfecta, congenital degenerative spine conditions, other neurodegenerative conditions, and erythromelalgia.[168–170]

Physical therapy is of particular value in musculoskeletal pain syndromes such as fibromyalgia but is also valuable in any pain syndrome in which the child's activity level has been diminished and he or she has become deconditioned.[171–174] Graded exercise increases the child's feelings of well-being and provides reassurance and confidence as the child regains lost abilities.[174] Other physical and occupational therapy modalities such as desensitization, transcutaneous electrical nerve stimulation, and stretching or strengthening particular muscle groups are also helpful.[173–177] Physical therapy is also of particular benefit in individuals who are hypermobile where the focus is on joint protection and proprioception. Active mind–body techniques, such as biofeedback and guided imagery, integrate cognitive and emotional processes with physiologic function and have also demonstrated efficacy in modulating the pain pathway in chronic pain conditions.[178,179]

Evidence supports psychological interventions as effective treatment of chronic pain in children. Multiple reviews and meta-analyses confirm the strong impact of these approaches which include cognitive-behavioral as well as psychotherapeutic strategies.[180–183] Although many of the cognitive-behavioral strategies were developed to help cope during acute, painful procedures, many of these strategies, such as meditation, hypnosis, and mindfulness, are also effective for chronic pain.[178,184] Acceptance and commitment therapy (ACT) was developed to help individuals function in the context of ongoing pain.[185] Guidance of the child and the family toward resuming daily function is the overall goal of treatment. Educating parents on the best way to support their child with ongoing pain symptoms is an integral step in this process. The natural protectiveness of parents for their child with pain can hinder progress and become detrimental in primary pain syndromes. Parents often need help ushering crying, complaining children off to school when the path of least resistance is to allow them to remain in bed. Specific criteria for school attendance with modifications can help the child regain a rhythm of daily school attendance. In general, school should be mandatory except for those times when the child has a fever. When efforts to incorporate these dimensions in an outpatient setting fail to enable a child to normalize daily function, more intensive daily rehabilitation centers with an interdisciplinary team approach are shown effective in regaining daily activity and should be considered.[114]

In summary, the treatment of chronic pain in children needs to address the pain itself as well as the life context in which that pain is occurring. As a result, a multimodal approach incorporating pharmacotherapy, physical therapy, and cognitive therapy with the goal of regaining normal daily function are important dimensions of the treatment of chronic pain.

SPECIFIC INTERVENTIONS FOR CHRONIC/PERSISTENT PAIN

Children who receive care in a multidisciplinary pediatric pain clinic are typically offered a multicomponent treatment plan, which often involves psychological therapy, physical therapy, and medication management. Philosophically, most programs incorporate a rehabilitation approach in which pain is accepted as a symptom that will be diminished but might not be entirely eradicated. Therefore, the focus is typically on improving function and quality of life. The specific structure of each program differs depending on local factors with some providing inpatient rehabilitation, whereas others are solely outpatient. Many new programs are developing in the United States and abroad. Zeltzer and Schlank[186] list many pediatric pain programs in the United States, Canada, and internationally.

Pharmacologic Interventions

Pediatric analgesic pharmacology is summarized in greater detail elsewhere in this book (see Chapter 50). The current discussion emphasizes specific uses of analgesics in the setting of chronic persistent pain, as opposed to acute pain. Pharmacotherapy of chronic pain in children and adolescents requires patience and balance of risks, benefits, and side effects. For most patients coming to a chronic pain clinic, pharmacotherapy should not be used in isolation but only as a component of a multimodal treatment program. In considering a medication trial, clinicians' discussions with patients and parents strike a difficult balance. The aims of drug therapy and expected benefits should be outlined. Side effects and risks should be discussed in a manner that is honest but is tailored to the style of the individual patient and family. There is a growing literature on how patients hear risk discussions.[187]

Discussions of side effects do have the potential to generate nocebo (negative placebo) effects.

For some conditions, treatments can be specific and mechanism-driven. For example, for children with rheumatoid arthritis, pharmacotherapy is largely directed at underlying inflammatory processes, and for most patients, treatment of inflammation serves to treat the pain. Similarly, pharmacotherapy for migraine and for specific subtypes of chronic abdominal pain may be directed at underlying mechanisms in some cases.

Acetaminophen and NSAIDs are widely used for pediatric acute pain management, and NSAIDs are an integral component of management of chronic inflammatory disorders. Daily use of either of these classes of medications can produce rebound headaches. There is comparatively little studies on chronic daily administration of acetaminophen in children. Chronic administration of NSAIDs in children with rheumatoid arthritis has been associated with gastropathy and nephropathy but overall with a lower risk than has been reported in adults.

A majority of trials of cyclooxygenase (COX)-2 inhibitors in children have involved short-term use. A recent 3-month trial comparing celecoxib to naproxen showed equal efficacy and no statistically significant difference in adverse events.[188]

Opioids have been extensively studied for pediatric acute pain management and for pain in children with cancer. As with adults, there is little consensus regarding which children with chronic noncancer pain have a favorable risk–benefit ratio for long-term opioid analgesia. Overall, prospective studies on adults in pain clinic populations with non–life-shortening conditions have not shown good effect of long-term use of opioids on either pain scores or measures of quality of life or functioning. Those who defend chronic opioid therapy in adults may argue that these studies did not address ideal patient subgroups. With children and adolescents, there are additional concerns. First, opioid tolerance and opioid-induced hyperalgesia are likely to proceed more rapidly for children compared to adults.[189,190] Second, long-term opioid administration may

have detrimental effects on endocrine function. Third, with many chronic medical conditions in childhood, longevity is difficult to predict, and advances in treatment have changed prognosis for many chronic illnesses of childhood and young adult life. For these reasons, we do use opioids on a long-term basis for a small subset of children with chronic pain not due to life-limiting illnesses, but we do so with some caution and with consideration of alternatives. There is a theoretical argument in favor of selection of either methadone or buprenorphine for long-term opioid therapy in younger patients based on a hypothesis that relates the development of tolerance and hyperalgesia to differential activation of receptor-mediated activation of second messenger systems versus receptor-mediated endocytosis.[191]

For adults with many forms of chronic pain, especially neuropathic pain disorders, there is evidence for efficacy of several anticonvulsant and antidepressant medications. We cite some limited pediatric information in the following text, but at present, most information regarding efficacy must be extrapolated from clinical trials in adults. In adults, these medications are side effect–prone and inconsistently effective; they generally produce partial, rather than complete, pain relief. In adults, there are very few randomized controlled trials (RCTs) that compare one antidepressant to another[192] or that compare an antidepressant to an anticonvulsant. There is remarkably sparse evidence for selecting one medication over another in general for adults with chronic pain except for specific conditions that are uncommon in pediatrics, such as trigeminal neuralgia.

One publication is cited here mainly to recommend caution in its interpretation. The authors use an "indirect meta-analysis" to compare duloxetine to the anticonvulsants gabapentin and pregabalin for treatment of neuropathic pain in adults. What is actually done is to use outcomes from active treatment groups in studies comparing duloxetine to placebo to the active treatment groups in studies comparing gabapentin or pregabalin to placebo.[193]

For antidepressants in trials for neuropathic pain in adults, numbers needed to treat (NNTs) range from 2 to 4 for trials involving tricyclics (mostly with "global improvement" as an endpoint) to as high as 5 for trials involving duloxetine with 50% pain relief as a primary endpoint. Overall, tricyclics appear to be more effective than selective serotonin reuptake inhibitors (SSRIs) for neuropathic pain in adults.

For children and adolescents, we commonly choose nortriptyline as a first-line tricyclic. We encourage starting at a very low dose (e.g., 10 mg every night for adolescents and older children and 5 mg every night for younger children). The rate of dose escalation is determined by clinical circumstances and side effects. For an outpatient who experiences no adverse symptoms, dosing might be increased every 3 days until there is good analgesia or he or she reaches a dose around 40 or 50 mg daily. Dosing is occasionally even more rapid for inpatients with severe neuropathic cancer pain. Conversely, if the child does experience side effects, dose escalation proceeds more slowly. If there is no indication of analgesia or side effects by the time dosing is escalated to 50 mg/daily (and if we are convinced that the child is taking the medication), we will often obtain a blood level prior to further dose escalation. Clearance of tricyclics in children is enormously variable. An electrocardiogram is widely recommended either prior to initiating treatment or after dose escalation. We adhere to this recommendation while recognizing that there is little evidence that electrocardiography can identify patients at risk for sudden cardiac events.

There are a number of clinical trials and case series on antidepressants for migraine prophylaxis in pediatrics, including amitriptyline, nortriptyline, and trazodone, although many have involved open-label designs or crossover comparisons to other drugs.[194,195]

There is a widely quoted case series on the SSRI citalopram for treatment of recurrent abdominal pain in children. Although there is apparent improvement in a large percentage of patients, this should be interpreted with great caution because of the open-label and uncontrolled design of the study.[196]

There has been extensive controversy regarding potential risks of antidepressants in triggering suicidal ideation and completed suicide among adolescents. What is clear to us is that these medications require close monitoring for changes in a child's mood and behavior. Prescribing should begin in low doses, doses should be escalated in a gradual and stepwise manner, and there should be a system for frequent reassessments, ideally including regular phone calls in between clinic visits. For guidance of families, there is a well-written statement on the National Institute of Mental Health Web site.[197]

Anticonvulsants are also widely used for treatment of neuropathic pain in adults. As with antidepressants, side effects are common, treatment responses tend to be partial rather than full, and NNTs generally range from as low as 3 to over 5.

Gabapentin emerged as a widely prescribed medication for neuropathic pain in the 1990s in part because of the widespread belief that it was safer or easier to prescribe compared to other anticonvulsants. There is a remarkable dearth of trials comparing anticonvulsants to each other for neuropathic pain in adults.

As with tricyclics, our recommendation for gabapentin dosing is to start with small doses and escalate slowly, particularly in ambulatory patients. Different clinicians begin adolescents in a dose range from 100 mg daily to 300 mg daily. Our preference is to start for a few days with nighttime-only dosing, to begin morning and then afternoon dosing after about 3 days, and to escalate every few days as tolerated until there is pain relief, significant side effects, or dosing reaches a range around 1,800 mg daily over a period of about 3 weeks. Again, some patients tolerate escalation with no side effects, and others may tolerate daily doses as low as 300 mg. We commonly recommend giving half the daily dose at night, with one quarter in the morning and one quarter in the afternoon. As with tricyclics, dose escalation of gabapentin may be considerably more rapid for children with advanced cancer and refractory neuropathic pain.[198]

In our view, if trials of gabapentin or pregabalin produce minimal benefit or problematic side effects, there is reason to consider trials of anticonvulsants with different mechanisms. In particular, for peripheral neuropathic pain, we often try anticonvulsants with actions on sodium channels, such as oxcarbazepine.[199,200]

In our practice, topiramate is used primarily for migraine prophylaxis. Among the anticonvulsants, topiramate has a relatively high risk for neurocognitive side effects, especially effects on memory, word finding, and mental clarity.[201]

Some of our colleagues have tended to select anticonvulsants rather than antidepressants as first-line agents because of the aforementioned controversy regarding suicidal ideation and suicide attempts with antidepressants in pediatrics. Unfortunately, anticonvulsants may increase these risks as well. An analysis of placebo-controlled trials of anticonvulsants for a range of indications found increased frequencies of suicidal ideation and attempts in the active drug groups compared to control groups, and this increased risk was apparently not limited to a particular drug class or a particular patient group.[202]

Psychological Interventions

A range of psychological therapies has been delivered to youth with chronic pain conditions, either as single modalities or in combination with other types of interdisciplinary pain care. The evidence base for psychological therapies for children with chronic pain is moderate and growing, with 41 RCTs published across three Cochrane reviews.[203–205] Systematic reviews investigating psychological therapies for pain management including cognitive-behavioral therapy (CBT), behavioral interventions,

hypnotherapy, intensive rehabilitation, and ACT have found significant declines in children's pain intensity and disability at posttreatment, and these were small to moderate size effects. However, these treatment effects were not maintained at long-term follow-up. Psychological treatments did not have any effect on depression or anxiety outcomes at posttreatment or follow-up compared to controls. Although promising, further work is needed to enhance duration of treatment effects.

CBT is the most frequently delivered psychotherapy to youth with chronic pain conditions and typically includes a combination of education, cognitive, and behavioral skills. Cognitive skills involve teaching patients to identify and alter maladaptive cognitions related to pain. This may include working with children to recognize negative thoughts and beliefs about pain and activity engagement. Behavioral skills are intended to modify what a patient does to manage pain. Thus, these skills focus on improving patient function by increasing patient activity levels and involvement in pleasant and valued activities, such as activity pacing and pleasant activity scheduling. Relaxation is one of the most common behavioral skills used with children with chronic pain. For example, Van Der Veek et al.[206] taught deep breathing to children with functional abdominal pain by asking them to breath calmly through the abdomen (rather than the chest). Cottrell et al.[207] instructed progressive and cued muscle relaxation to youth with migraine over the phone.

Teaching parents appropriate strategies for managing their child's pain-related behaviors (e.g., reinforcing adaptive coping, discouraging maladaptive pain behaviors) is beneficial in treatment, and these strategies are increasingly being incorporated into psychological therapies.

For example, Levy et al.[208] worked with parents to recognize when their attention was directed to sickness behaviors and to redirect attention toward wellness behaviors, and this led to a reduction in maladaptive parent behaviors.

Problem-solving skills training (PSST) is based on the social problem-solving model[209,210] and focuses on teaching parents a positive orientation and rational skills for solving problems in order to reduce emotional distress. In a pilot RCT, Palermo et al.[211] delivered PSST to parents of youth with chronic pain using this model to teach five problem-solving steps (identify a problem, generate alternative solutions, decide and implement a solution, and then determine whether it worked), finding promise effects for reducing parent distress. Findings demonstrated that PSST reduced emotional distress in parents of children with chronic pain compared to a usual care condition.[211]

Although effective psychological treatments have been developed, major barriers exist for children and adolescents to access care due to the geographical distance from treatment centers with behavioral health providers, scheduling constraints, and long wait–lists, leaving a significant unmet clinical need. Availability of information and communication technology has expanded opportunities for intervening with individuals remotely. An emerging evidence base now exists for remotely delivered psychological interventions in both adult and pediatric populations; a recent systematic review of the pediatric literature identified eight RCTs, which all delivered CBT, and patients showed improvements in pain and disability.[205] As one recent example, in a large multicenter RCT with 273 adolescents with chronic abdominal, headache, or musculoskeletal pain, Palermo et al.[212] found improvements in daily physical functioning, depressive symptoms, and parent-perceived impact of pain in families receiving an 8-week Internet pain self-management program compared to an Internet pain education control group.

Pilot studies are emerging in the application of ACT to children with chronic pain.[213] ACT is an increasingly popular form of CBT that emphasizes the importance of accepting pain symptoms and working toward valued goals, using interventions such as exposure, cognitive defusion, and mindfulness.

Parents are also integrated into treatment using similar interventions emphasizing exposure to previously avoided private experiences, acceptance, and defusion exercises. In the only RCT to evaluate ACT in children with chronic pain, Wicksell et al.[214] delivered exposure treatment within an ACT framework, which emphasized acceptance of pain and negative thoughts and setting goals with youth consistent with their values to a small group of youth with chronic pain, compared to a group receiving standard multidisciplinary and pharmacologic treatment with amitriptyline. The ACT group reported reduced symptoms across all outcomes and had significantly lower pain intensity, pain-related discomfort, and fear of reinjury as well as improved perceived functional ability at posttreatment and follow-up, relative to the control group. Given the clinical interest in ACT, it is anticipated that larger scale studies will be forthcoming using this approach to treat children and adolescents with chronic pain.

Complementary and alternative medicine (CAM) interventions are becoming increasingly popular in the treatment of chronic pain and have been successful in helping children and adults manage pain symptoms.[215] CAM refers to therapies (e.g., hypnosis, acupuncture, yoga, and biofeedback) commonly used in conjunction with conventional medical treatment. Biofeedback is one type of CAM therapy effective in the treatment of persistent pediatric pain. Biofeedback involves connecting a patient to a machine that monitors physiologic responses (e.g., muscle tension, heart rate). One form of feedback, thermal biofeedback, involves using electronic instruments (e.g., a temperature probe on the finger) to measure temperature and a computer monitor to display reinforcing information back to the patient. Using relaxation approaches, patients can use the objective biofeedback information to learn to increase peripheral temperature.

Biofeedback, especially thermal biofeedback, has undergone empirical evaluation in children with migraine and tension headache, and there is evidence to recommend biofeedback and/or relaxation to any child who suffers from headaches.[216] Recently, biofeedback has been evaluated in children with chronic abdominal pain.[217,218] Although results from these studies suggest that biofeedback is effective in reducing pain, RCTs using larger sample sizes are needed. Like CBT, research shows that incorporating parenting strategies into biofeedback treatment may increase the effectiveness of treatment. Children whose parents received behavior management strategies in combination with the child's standard biofeedback treatment demonstrated more clinically significant improvement in headache pain and showed greater reductions in headache frequency than those who received biofeedback alone.[219,220]

School and Social Reintegration

School and social functioning are impaired in many children with chronic pain. In industrialized societies, school is the work of children. Numerous studies have documented that children with chronic pain have difficulties with consistent school attendance and making progress with academic work, although there may also be specific impairments in peer and social relationships that are amplified in the school setting. On average, children with chronic pain miss more school days than do children with other chronic health conditions, and they often identify school as the most problematic stressor.[62] For example, Stang and Osterhaus[119] estimated that several hundred thousand school days are missed each month as a result of pediatric headache alone. In a sample of children with SCD-related pain, Shapiro and colleagues[221] reported that on average, children missed 21% of school days, which is the equivalent of 6 to 8 weeks of the school year.

There is also evidence that children with chronic pain may experience problems with social competence and peer relationships in the school setting. In one study, adolescents with juvenile fibromyalgia syndrome were perceived as being less popular, more isolated, and withdrawn compared to matched classroom comparison peers.[66] Moreover, these adolescents were less well liked, were selected less often as a best friend, and had fewer reciprocated friendships. Negative peer interactions were explored in one study,[222] finding that children with chronic abdominal pain had higher levels of relational victimization in comparison to pain-free peers.

The school setting may also be perceived as stressful due to problematic interactions with teachers and perceptions that adults are not supportive of children with chronic pain. In a study using vignettes, teachers' attributions about the causes of chronic pain revealed a lack of knowledge of the biopsychosocial framework and a primary perception that pain was either physical or psychological.[223] Teachers responded more positively to students when medical evidence supporting the pain problem was available, and responses were associated with parental attitudes toward the school. Teachers were more likely to report children were entitled to accommodations if parents approached the school in a collaborative manner rather than using a confrontational approach.[224]

There is variability in how children and families respond to impairments that may arise in the school setting. Some children and adolescents have worked out accommodations that allow them to have reduced class time, in home tutoring, or online courses. Several mechanisms in public education laws can be used in this regard, including individualized education plans and Section 504 plans for other health impairments. Some families opt to remove their child from the school setting and engage in home schooling.

Regardless of the exact setting where school is to occur, addressing the impairments in school and social functioning are a primary focus of treatment for the child with persistent pain. Some children and adolescents have spent extensive time outside of their usual school and social settings, and therefore, graded plans for reintegration into these settings are needed. In the context of CBT, parent management guidelines have been implemented in clinical settings and in treatment studies focused on operant techniques. In general, parents are encouraged to establish a reduction of attention paid to pain symptoms in favor of increased attention paid to functional improvement. Such guidelines often include recommendations to reduce status checks, that is, allowing the child to communicate directly about pain symptoms rather than having the parent repeatedly check in with the child about his or her pain level. Most parents experience tremendous relief in being released from the role of documenting the child's pain level. Often, the focus on pain intensity and a specific numerical value (e.g., 8 out of 10) provides little in the way of adaptive coping behaviors and may lead to difficulties making decisions to reintegrate in school and social settings because of lack of change in pain levels.

Formal operant systems can be devised with families where children earn points or rewards for school attendance and participation in other social activities. The goal is to shift the pattern of contingencies so that the child experiences reinforcement for their efforts in school or social activities. An example of a point system would include specifying a target activity such as attendance at school for 4 hours each day and then developing rewards for reaching the goal (such as full computer and television privileges) and consequences for failure to achieve the goal (such as removal of access from computer and television). Psychologists and other members of the pain team can work in treatment with children and parents to develop clear, graded plans for increasing activity. Typically, an explanation to children and parents is provided that functional improvement often precedes rather than follows pain relief. It is important to start where the child is at in terms of their perceived ability to sit in a chair and focus on school work for an operant system to be successful. Sometimes, very short time periods of school attendance (e.g., 1 hour) will need to be built on gradually, and the child will need to have some control over his or her schedule. For example, it can be helpful to have the child choose what time of the day (and what classes) he or she would like to begin with upon the reintegration to school.

Carrying out a graded plan for increasing school and social functioning requires considerable effort from the parents who must arrange transportation and other logistics with getting the child to the school setting at specific times. Clinicians need to communicate sensitively to parents about their role and make clear the logical sequence of the plan to ensure its success. Additional interventions may be needed to assist children with problems related to peer relationships, interactions with teachers, or specific problems related to the school setting. There are not yet any published treatment studies evaluating school-related interventions for children with chronic pain.

Sleep

Sleep difficulties are commonly reported by children and adolescents with chronic pain in the community[61] as well as in clinical samples (e.g., juvenile rheumatoid arthritis,[225] headache,[36] SCD,[226,227] abdominal and musculoskeletal pain, and CRPS[228]). For example, a recent systematic review found that children with juvenile idiopathic arthritis experience greater difficulties with night awakenings, sleep anxiety, and excessive daytime sleepiness compared to otherwise healthy children.[229] Most commonly, across types of chronic pain conditions, children and adolescents with chronic pain describe difficulties falling asleep, frequent night and early morning awakening, and excessive daytime sleepiness.[230]

Important consequences of sleep problems have also been identified including decrements in children's HRQOL, mood, and physical functioning.[72,82] Day-to-day variability in pain, mood, and sleep has been examined in children with SCD,[227] finding that negative mood partially explained the relationship between more intense pain and poor-quality sleep on the same and subsequent days. Other studies in youth with mixed pain conditions have found temporal relationships between pain and sleep, where nighttime sleep predicted next-day pain.[231]

Early models described a bidirectional relationship between pain and sleep,[232] where uncontrolled pain can cause sleep disruptions, and in turn, disturbed sleep can enhance pain sensitivity.[233] Recent research has demonstrated that more studies now support the direction of sleep impacting pain than vice versa. That is, sleep deficiency has now been shown to *lead to* subsequent increased pain. Findings are from studies using experimental and self-report designs in multiple samples across childhood and adulthood,[234] highlighting its relevance in chronic pain treatment.

However, there has been very limited attention to either the assessment or management of sleep problems in children with chronic pain. In clinical practice, it can be very informative to assess sleep problems in all pediatric patients with chronic pain and to offer specific sleep interventions to those patients with significant sleep disturbances. In particular, a detailed history of sleep patterns should be obtained to identify problems related to insufficient sleep duration, poor sleep habits, phase delays, or difficulties falling asleep or staying asleep. Insufficient sleep duration is common during adolescence with reported sleep in healthy samples of about 7 hours per night,[235] although optimal developmental sleep requirements for adolescents have been estimated at 9 hours per night.[236] In chronic pain samples, similar restricted sleep of about 7 hours per night has been reported.[237,238] Poor sleep habits including use of caffeine in the evening, lack of consistent bedtime routines, and the presence of electronics in the bedroom can also be clear barriers to children receiving adequate sleep duration. Children with chronic pain may also develop a high level of vigilance and arousal at bedtime

and a high focus on pain when the distractions of the day are not present. These children may describe negative thoughts, worries, and somatic tension that interfere with falling asleep.

Interventions may be needed to help children increase their duration of sleep, to modify problematic sleep habits, and to teach behavioral strategies to reduce insomnia symptoms. Sleep interventions can be included as a component of CBT for chronic pain[212,239] or as a stand-alone treatment. Typically, interventions include modifying sleep hygiene (e.g., no phones or screens in bed, regular and relaxing bedtime routine), keeping a regular bedtime and wake time which allows for adequate duration of sleep, limiting naps, and reducing negative thoughts about sleep as well as teaching specific strategies to decrease insomnia symptoms. For review, see Wu et al.[240] Cognitive-behavioral therapy for insomnia (CBT-I) is recommended by the American Academy of Sleep Medicine as first-line treatment for adult insomnia.

Meta-analyses conclude that CBT-I produces reliable and durable improvement in sleep in adults with co-occurring pain conditions including arthritis and fibromyalgia.[241] There is emerging evidence suggesting that changes in sleep as a result of behavioral treatment lead to changes in pain symptoms. For example, in a recent trial of CBT-I in patients with knee osteoarthritis and insomnia, patients who received CBT-I had greater improvements in sleep and the baseline-to-posttreatment change predicted subsequent decreases in pain.[242] Moreover, CBT-I is a flexible treatment with evidence emerging that it can be delivered in group settings and remotely through the internet with similar positive benefits.

Although the treatment literature for child and adolescent insomnia interventions is more limited, there has been a recent uncontrolled trial in an adolescent pain population. In this study, adolescents with a range of physical and psychiatric comorbidities (e.g., depression, chronic pain, anxiety, GI problems) received a brief four-session CBT-I intervention.[243] CBT-I was associated with treatment improvements in insomnia symptoms, sleep quality, sleep hygiene, presleep arousal, and sleep patterns as well as improvements in psychological symptoms and HRQOL. Sleep interventions appear promising and further research is needed to understand the impact of sleep interventions on chronic pain and when these interventions should ideally be delivered to children.

Intensive Rehabilitation Therapy

Intensive rehabilitation for children with chronic pain occurs in either a day treatment or inpatient setting, during which an interdisciplinary team of three or more health care professionals works together to increase patient function. These programs have developed over the past decade in response to limitations in effectively treating children, especially those extremely disabled by pain, in the outpatient setting. Psychological treatment is typically delivered in individual or group-based treatment. A systematic review evaluating the effectiveness of intensive rehabilitation programs identified one RCT and nine nonrandomized trials.[115] At posttreatment, the meta-analysis of all included studies showed large effects for reducing disability and small to moderate effects for programs at reducing pain and depression. These benefits were maintained for 3 months after treatment and a recent study demonstrated cost-effectiveness, saving families a projected $27,000 the year following admission.[244]

Specific Entities

MUSCULOSKELETAL PAIN

Musculoskeletal pain accounts for more than 50% of all the recurrent pains reported in the pediatric population.[245] Differential diagnosis of musculoskeletal pain is vast. Two questions can help differentiate primary pain syndromes from progressive disease. Is the pain localized or widespread? Does the child appear well or unwell? If the pain is localized and the child is well, the differential diagnosis includes "growing pains," CRPS, mechanical pain, pauciarticular juvenile rheumatoid arthritis, and spondyloarthropathy. If the pain is localized and the child is unwell, the infectious arthritides should be considered. If the pain is diffuse and the child is well, hypermobility and diffuse idiopathic pain syndrome (juvenile fibromyalgia) should be considered. If the pain is diffuse and the child is unwell, malignancies or autoimmune diseases top the list. Red flags in the history to guide us in determining the differential include pain in the morning, swelling, nocturnal pain not relieved by analgesics, poor growth, or bony tenderness.[246]

Diffuse or widespread musculoskeletal pain is the term typically used for generalized musculoskeletal pain which in adults may be termed *fibromyalgia*. Diagnostic criteria for "fibromyalgia" in children and adolescents are not validated. The onset of diffuse idiopathic pain can be gradual. The pain may have an identified initial insult such as infection, but often, there is no identified trigger. A number of studies have identified an increased association between widespread muscular pain and hypermobility.[151] As more evidence is collected, hypermobility-related disorders also appear to have a strong interrelationship with many primary pain disorders.[153] This may be secondary to central sensitization, induced by constant subluxation and slippage or may have other etiologies that cause repeated microtrauma in joints and ligamentous structures with associated pain leading to disordered sensory processing.[151,153,247,248] It is also important to address syndromes that are associated with hypermobility such as Ehlers-Danlos or Marfan syndromes which may have additional problems associated with them.

Treatment for widespread musculoskeletal pain incorporates a multimodal approach and typically has physical therapy at its cornerstone.[249,250] There is the attempt to restore the normal range of movement, even if the joint is hypermobile, strengthen the surrounding musculature to add joint stability, and improve the general level of fitness in the individual. Premedicating with an analgesic prior to therapy may be warranted as pain may promote noncompliance with the prescribed regimen. Improving the child's level of fitness may help with sleep promotion and improve his or her general sense of well-being. Bulbena and others have reported an association between hypermobility and anxiety disorder in adults and believe that the tissue disorder is a predisposing factor for trait anxiety.[251-253] Even in children without hypermobility who have chronic musculoskeletal pain, cognitive-behavioral and, if necessary, pharmacologic interventions which reduce catastrophizing and panic and promote coping are often appropriate. Disordered sensory processing has been identified in many individuals with widespread musculoskeletal pain. Regardless of its origin, anticonvulsants and/or antidepressants may have a role in dampening central sensitization and therefore in the management of chronic musculoskeletal pain. Eccleston and colleagues[254] report on the success of their multidisciplinary program emphasizes family oriented CBT, physical activity, goal setting, pacing, relaxation, and communication.[255,256] As with other chronic pain problems, a holistic rehabilitation approach to musculoskeletal pain appears to have better outcomes than a unidimensional one.

COMPLEX REGIONAL PAIN SYNDROMES

CRPS1, also known as *reflex sympathetic dystrophy* (RSD), involves limb pain with neuropathic descriptors (allodynia, paresthesias, dysesthesias) and variable combinations of neurovascular disturbances (coldness, mottling, nonarticular swelling, cyanosis or rubor, delayed capillary refill), sudomotor disturbances, motor abnormalities (spasms, dystonia, "jumping movements"), and trophic changes, including

atrophy, abnormal hair growth, or joint contractures. Where these findings occur with clinical signs of injury to a nameable nerve trunk, the terms *CRPS2* or *causalgia* are used. For purposes of the current discussion, we use the term *RSD/CRPS* to refer to these disorders inclusively.

CRPS in children and adolescents has distinct epidemiologic features. It is much more common in girls than boys, it is uncommon before age 6 years, the apparent onset is most common from around ages 10 to 12 years, and the lower extremities are affected much more commonly than the upper extremities.[257]

For a majority of children with CRPS, an effective treatment program emphasizes patient and parent education about the nonprotective character of the pain, intensive rehabilitation that involves active exercise, resumption of weight-bearing, desensitization, and psychological interventions based primarily on individual and family-based CBT. For some children, this can be accomplished on an outpatient basis.[177] For others who fail to improve with outpatient treatment, a next step is to do this type of multidisciplinary rehabilitation program in an inpatient or intensive day-hospital program.[176]

In adult pain medicine practice, at least in the United States, there is a considerable emphasis on early use of nerve blocks and other invasive approaches, especially sympathetic nerve blocks; spinal cord stimulation; operative, chemical, or radiofrequency sympathectomies; and, more recently, intravenous ketamine infusions in the treatment of RSD/CRPS. In our view, these approaches are not evidence-based in adults, and they are even less supported by evidence for children and adolescents. In a previous case series, even though some of the patients did receive regional anesthetic interventions and even though some reported benefit, there was no clear association between the duration of symptoms prior to blockade and the eventual benefit.[258]

Some pediatric case series report marked improvement in function and pain scores with no use of nerve blocks.[176] Overall, most case series suggest a good long-term prognosis for the majority of children and adolescents with CRPS. Hence, in our view, the initial therapeutic approach should be to emphasize intensive rehabilitation whenever possible.

We do make selective use of regional anesthetic approaches for patients who fail to progress despite a very good rehabilitation program and for selected patients with very severe limb swelling, dystonia, or very limited limb movement. In general, our preference is to use combined somatic–sympathetic blockade using continuous catheter approaches rather than selective sympathetic blockade or other repeated single-shot blocks. For lower extremity CRPS confined to a stocking distribution in the lower leg, our practice is to place continuous popliteal fossa sciatic perineural catheters under combined ultrasound–nerve stimulation guidance.[259]

For lower extremity involvement in a wider distribution, we place an epidural catheter using fluoroscopy and/or nerve stimulation guidance to ensure proper dermatomal level and sidedness. For upper extremity CRPS, brachial plexus catheters are placed in either supraclavicular or infraclavicular sites using combined ultrasound and nerve stimulation guidance. For all forms of continuous regional anesthesia, catheters are placed with meticulous attention to sterile technique in the operating room, and they are tunneled to facilitate skin care and to reduce the chances for dislodgment. Prophylactic antibiotics are used. Patients are typically admitted to the hospital for infusions and intensive rehabilitation for periods of 5 to 8 days. Although outpatient rehabilitation assisted by peripheral blockade has been described, in our view, there is merit to inpatient admission to optimize intensive rehabilitation during the course of the infusions. In addition, our preference is to run higher infusion rates at nighttime and lower rates during the day to facilitate "cycle-breaking" at night and active mobilization during the day.

Evidence is lacking for efficacy of many types of analgesic medications commonly prescribed for adults with CRPS. Pediatric data are limited to case reports and uncontrolled case series. We do try tricyclic antidepressants and anticonvulsants for many of these patients. Responses are inconsistent.

BACK PAIN

Back pain is very common in adults and a major contributor to absence from the workplace. Persistent back pain is relatively common in adolescents but uncommon in younger children, and in younger children, its occurrence mandates earlier consideration of a range of diagnostic possibilities, including infections (osteomyelitis, pyelonephritis, intervertebral discitis), tumors, and congenital anomalies of the spine and central nervous system (tethered spinal cord, diastematomyelia).[260,261]

In specialist referral practice, back pain in adolescents is commonly seen in athletes, dancers, gymnasts, and cheerleaders and in children who are significantly overweight. For many patients with features suggestive of muscular pain and a normal neurologic exam, initial treatment should emphasize resumption of daily activities, a moderate exercise program including core stabilization and postural exercises, and avoidance of high-impact, high-velocity, or repetitive stresses on the spine. For patients with significant obesity, dietary counseling may be appropriate. Axial low back pain that worsens with back extension is commonly seen with spondylolysis and spondylolisthesis.[262,263] There is some support for bracing in the treatment of these conditions.[264]

Symptomatic lumbar disk disease is uncommon in children and relatively less common in adolescents. In our referral practice, lumbar disk disease is most commonly seen in adolescent athletes. There is an extensive literature on the advantages and disadvantages of operative treatment for lumbar radiculopathy in adults; pediatric literature is mostly limited to relatively small case series and, with few exceptions, to relatively short-term follow-up. We recently reviewed experience with fluoroscopically guided epidural steroid injections for lumbar radiculopathy in children and adolescents. A majority of patients reported reductions in pain and improvements in straight-leg raising, and the safety profile was excellent. In 2- to 5-year follow-up, less than 40% of patients in this case series came to discectomy.[265]

HEADACHE

Systematic review of pediatric headache burden found that 58% of children experience a headache at some time in childhood.[245,266] Differentiating whether the pediatric headache is primary or secondary is critical in its evaluation.[267] Primary headaches include migraine, tension-type headache, and cluster headaches. They are classified by their features as compared to secondary headaches which are classified by the underlying disorder responsible for them. Secondary headaches are those attributed to head and neck trauma; intracranial vascular and nonvascular disorders; substance administration or withdrawal; infection; or pain associated with disorders of the eyes, cranium, ears, sinuses, or teeth. Red flags in the history which suggest secondary headache are sudden onset of a severe headache, neurologic symptoms such as ataxia, lethargy, seizures, visual impairments, associated symptoms such as depressed mood or aura, headache associated with systemic illness such as hypertension and sinusitis, new headache type in a patient with cancer or human immunodeficiency virus, sudden onset of the "worst headache in your life," headaches associated with straining, change in a headache pattern, or headache in a child under 3 years old. Positive answers to these questions clearly demand additional investigation as well as imaging studies.[268–270]

Primary headaches in children are more often a continuum that may change with age rather than a discrete entity.[271–276]

Zebenholzer and colleagues[274] found that in a 1.5-year period, 30% of children were headache-free, 20% had swapped headache type, and 50% continued having the same type of headache. Such fluidity makes diagnosis and treatment complex. Criteria for the diagnosis of migraine in children require five or more headaches that last between 1 and 48 hours (shorter duration than in adults), are bilateral or unilateral, have a throbbing or pounding quality, and are aggravated by physical activities. They are typically accompanied decreased appetite, nausea, vomiting, and photophobia and phonophobia.[277] Tension headaches are typically categorized by their frequency: episodic (< once monthly), frequent (greater than once per month but <15 days per month), and chronic daily headache (>15 days per month). These headaches are typically mild to moderate pain, "band-like" pressure around the head, bilateral, not pulsating, not aggravated by physical activity, without nausea, vomiting, photophobia, or phonophobia. Precipitating factors may include illness, stress, and muscular tension.

Once the secondary causes of headache have been excluded, the general approach to primary headache treatment is similar to other primary chronic pains—a multidisciplinary approach, consisting of cognitive-behavioral approaches, physical therapy modalities with thoughtful use of medications in an overall attempt to regain function and improve pain coping abilities. Maintaining a regular routine and regular exercise is helpful.[278] Limited evidence supports a specific diet or dietary exclusion, although there may well be individuals for whom food is an important trigger.[272] Overall, SMART (Sleep, Meals, Activity, Relaxation, Trigger avoidance) lifestyles changes are recommended.[279]

Behavioral interventions are effective at reducing headache burden regardless of the headache type. These include biofeedback, progressive muscle relaxation, distraction, and hypnosis. In a systematic review of the RCTs of psychological interventions for chronic pain (12 headache and 1 recurrent abdominal pain trial), Eccleston and colleagues[182] reported the odds ratio for a 50% reduction in pain was 9.62, indicating the success of psychological interventions.

Pharmacologic treatment of pediatric headache is divided into abortive and preventative treatment. Early intervention is an essential feature of successful abortive treatment of migraine or tension headache. Early hydration, ibuprofen, naproxen, and acetaminophen are often effective. For more severe headache, NSAIDs combined with acetaminophen and/or caffeine should be tried. Triptans (5-HT-1 receptor inhibitor) such as sumatriptan nasal spray in the appropriate circumstances can be considered for severe headache. Oral triptans have also been studied in children. Rizatriptan can be used in children >6 years old and almotriptan, a combination of sumatriptan and naproxen in adolescents greater than 12 years old is approved.[280,281]

Regarding preventive therapy, it is recommended that patients with disabling headache greater than 4 days a month be considered for daily preventative therapy. Initiation of these medications should be done with the guidance that they will take 6 to 12 weeks to become effective. With this said, few medications have been studied in randomized controlled studies in pediatric populations. Of them, topiramate, tricyclic antidepressants such as amitriptyline, nortriptyline, and β-blocker, propranolol, are used.[281] More recent evaluation by the Childhood and Adolescent Migraine Prevention (CHAMP) study did not detect a difference between topiramate, amitriptyline, or placebo.[282]

There is emerging literature on the use of specific vitamins and minerals for headache prevention. High-dose riboflavin, B2 (400 mg per day), has been found to reduce migraine frequency and appears safe.[282,283] Magnesium has been shown to reduce headache frequency.[282,284] Melatonin may be beneficial in the ability to initiate sleep and promote improved lifestyle.

In summary, there is convincing evidence that cognitive-behavioral approaches are beneficial in primary pediatric headaches, regardless of etiology. The evidence on abortive and preventative medications is not limited, but a number of analgesics, 5-HT receptor agonists, anticonvulsants, antidepressants, and β-blockers have been shown to be somewhat effective in children.

FUNCTIONAL GASTROINTESTINAL PAIN

Chronic abdominal pain is defined as long-lasting intermittent or constant abdominal pain with either functional or organic etiology. Chronic abdominal pain accounts for 2% to 4% of all pediatric office visits and is one of the most common complaints in children.[285] Red flags for organic disease include pain that awakens the child from sleep, nocturnal diarrhea, persistent vomiting, weight loss, persistent right upper or lower quadrant pain, or dysphagia and should prompt a referral to a gastroenterologist. Adolescent females presenting with chronic abdominopelvic pain should be evaluated for gynecologic causes, such as endometriosis particularly those with GI symptoms and dysmenorrhea or irregular uterine bleeding. Evaluation and management of endometriosis includes hormonal and surgical intervention while incorporating a multidisciplinary approach for chronic symptoms, including neuropathic agents, physical therapy, and cognitive-behavioral strategies.[286–289]

If the history and physical examination do not suggest underlying pathology, more than likely, the patient has one of the pain predominant FGIDs. FGIDs refer to a group of disorders that are diagnosed according to the Rome IV criteria when symptoms cannot be explained by inflammatory, anatomic, metabolic, or neoplastic processes.[290] FGIDs are the most common cause of abdominal pain in children and adolescents worldwide.[285] The associated term *functional abdominal pain* has been replaced by *central mediated abdominal pain syndrome* (CAPS) central sensitization with disinhibition of pain signals as opposed to increased peripheral afferent excitability.[291] Children with chronic abdominal pain have lower quality-of-life measures compared with healthy peers and at risk for school absences, social isolation, depressive disorders, and increased somatic complaints.[292,293] Williams and colleagues[294] demonstrated this in preadolescent females with IBS when compared to healthy peers by showing an impaired endogenous inhibition of somatic pain. As previously stated, CAPS in childhood and adolescence increased the risk for a chronic primary pain disorder in adulthood.[295,296]

In addition to the general strategies for addressing chronic pain, evidence supports the efficacy of famotidine, pizotifen, CBT, biofeedback, and peppermint oil enteric-coated capsules.[218] For functional dyspepsia, they suggested treatment with antisecretory agents such as H$_2$ blockers or proton pump inhibitors is appropriate for pain predominant symptoms, whereas prokinetics seem appropriate for symptoms dominated by discomfort such as bloating. For IBS, peppermint oil is suggested, and when IBS is diarrhea-predominant, the use of antibiotics to treat bacterial overgrowth is recommended. Antidepressants and serotonergic agents had limited support in pediatrics despite their efficacy in adults. For abdominal migraine, avoidance of potential triggers such as caffeine was advised. Treatment with the preventative agents used for migraine (cyproheptadine, sumatriptan) are appropriate when paroxysms are frequent. Functional GI pain syndrome, reduction of psychosocial stressors, and behavioral treatment are effective for management.[267,275,297–300] Dietary interventions low in fermentable carbohydrates and polyols (FODMAP) and high in fiber incorporated treatment are effective in subgroups of patients reducing bloating and improving stool pattern.[275,301]

Barriers to Care

Most health care systems are stymied by the complicated care necessary to address the issues raised by children with chronic pain. The family's search for a satisfying answer may cause them to solicit multiple opinions for the pain problem. Additionally, children with chronic pain often report pain in more than one site and, as a result, multiple specialists are often involved in their care, each one focusing on one particular pain complaint. For example, headache and abdominal pain are frequent fellow travelers. The family may seek the opinion of a neurologist for the headache and a gastroenterologist for the abdominal pain. They may seek out alternative providers such as chiropractors, acupuncturists, or naturopaths as well. Laboratory and imaging studies are frequently performed in multiple settings. The primary care provider who typically provides care coordination must collate the records, reconcile often disparate opinions, be alert to the possibility of interactions among the drugs prescribed by the myriad of involved physicians, and be on the front line to address each new symptom and concern without overmedicalizing it. Care coordination is, therefore, a critical time-consuming and often unreimbursed aspect of the care for children with chronic pain, and its absence is a barrier to adequate treatment.

Another problem is the lack of facilities and practitioners capable of addressing both the biologic and psychological dimensions of chronic pain. In the outpatient arena, few individuals are comfortable addressing both realms, and multidisciplinary teams, an alternative, are often not viable economically. Inpatient facilities are rarely geared to individuals who may have both psychological and physical problems. A busy inpatient unit with desperately ill children is not the appropriate setting for a child with chronic pain, as it tends to overmedicalize the problem. Likewise, the typical psychiatric ward is often unprepared to deal with the patient who is moaning in pain and may have an as yet undiagnosed medical illness.

Finally, the inherent vagueness and poignancy of the symptom of persistent pain often leads families to seek out additional opinions and to feel that their search is never quite completed. This can create uneasiness between provider and patient which may interfere with the therapeutic alliance.

Conclusion

Persistent pain is a relatively common experience for children and may stem from a variety of causes: ongoing organic disease, persistence of pain which resulted from organic disease, as well as disorders whose primary manifestation is pain. Regardless of its origin, however, it has significant impact on the child and his or her family. In general, the goal of the clinician is to identify red flags for organic disease and, if not present, focus on symptom reduction and increasing function. Specific attention should be given to sleep, mood, school, activity, and family functioning. Typical interventions include analgesia, physical therapy, cognitive-behavioral strategies, and other medications targeted to specific symptoms. Success in the management of chronic pain should be monitored by improvement in function and not specifically through immediate reduction in pain intensity.

References

1. Fillingim RB, Bruehl S, Dworkin RH, et al. The ACTTION-American Pain Society Pain Taxonomy (AAPT): an evidence-based and multidimensional approach to classifying chronic pain conditions. *J Pain* 2014;15:241–249.
2. Walco GA, Krane EJ, Schmader KE, et al. Applying a lifespan developmental perspective to chronic pain: pediatrics to geriatrics. *J Pain* 2016;17(suppl 2): T108–T117.
3. Cavkaytar O, Düzova A, Tekşam O, et al. Final diagnosis of children and adolescents with musculoskeletal complaints. *Minerva Pediatr* 2017;69:50–58.

4. Helmick CG, Felson DT, Lawrence RC, et al. Estimates of the prevalence of arthritis and other rheumatic conditions in the United States. Part I. *Arthritis Rheum* 2008;58:15–25.

5. Schanberg LE, Anthony KK, Gil KM, et al. Daily pain and symptoms in children with polyarticular arthritis. *Arthritis Rheum* 2003;48:1390–1397.

6. Rashid A, Cordingley L, Carrasco R, et al. Patterns of pain over time among children with juvenile idiopathic arthritis [published online ahead of print November 2, 2017]. *Arch Dis Child*. doi:10.1136/archdischild-2017-313337.

7. Shiff NJ, Tupper S, Oen K, et al. Trajectories of pain severity in juvenile idiopathic arthritis: results from the Research in Arthritis in Canadian Children Emphasizing Outcomes cohort [published online ahead of print September 18, 2017]. *Pain*. doi:10.1097/j.pain.0000000000001064.

8. De Inocencio J. Epidemiology of musculoskeletal pain in primary care. *Arch Dis Child* 2004;89:431–434.

9. McGrath PA. Chronic pain in children. In: Crombie IK, Croft PR, Linton SJ, et al, eds. *Epidemiology of Pain*. Seattle, WA: IASP Press; 1999:81–101.

10. Mikkelsson M, Salminen JJ, Kautiainen H. Non-specific musculoskeletal pain in preadolescents. Prevalence and 1-year persistence. *Pain* 1997;73:29–35.

11. Fuglkjær S, Hartvigsen J, Wedderkopp N, et al. Musculoskeletal extremity pain in Danish school children—how often and for how long? The CHAMPS study-DK. *BMC Musculoskelet Disord* 2017;18:492.

12. Fuglkjær S, Dissing KB, Hestbæk L. Prevalence and incidence of musculoskeletal extremity complaints in children and adolescents. A systematic review. *BMC Musculoskelet Disord* 2017;18:418.

13. Mikkelsson M, Sourander A, Piha J, et al. Psychiatric symptoms in preadolescents with musculoskeletal pain and fibromyalgia. *Pediatrics* 1997;100:220–227.

14. Siegel DM, Janeway D, Baum J. Fibromyalgia syndrome in children and adolescents: clinical features at presentation and status at follow-up. *Pediatrics* 1998;101:377–382.

15. Gallagher AM, Thomas JM, Hamilton WT, et al. Incidence of fatigue symptoms and diagnoses presenting in UK primary care from 1990 to 2001. *J R Soc Med* 2004;97:571–575.

16. Eraso RM, Bradford NJ, Fontenot CN, et al. Fibromyalgia syndrome in young children: onset at age 10 years and younger. *Clin Exp Rheumatol* 2007;25:639–644.

17. Breau LM, McGrath PJ, Ju LH. Review of juvenile primary fibromyalgia and chronic fatigue syndrome. *J Dev Behav Pediatr* 1999;20:278–288.

18. Gedalia A, Press J, Klein M, et al. Joint hypermobility and fibromyalgia in schoolchildren. *Ann Rheum Dis* 1993;52:494–496.

19. Conte PM, Walco GA, Kimura Y. Temperament and stress response in children with juvenile primary fibromyalgia syndrome. *Arthritis Rheum* 2003;48:2923–2930.

20. Buskila D, Neumann L, Hazanov I, et al. Familial aggregation in the fibromyalgia syndrome. *Semin Arthritis Rheum* 1996;26:605–611.

21. Abu-Arafeh H, Abu-Arafeh I. Complex regional pain syndrome in children: a systematic review of clinical features and movement disorders. *Pain Manag* 2017;7:133–140.

22. MacDonald J, Stuart E, Rodenberg R. Musculoskeletal low back pain in school-aged children: a review. *JAMA Pediatr* 2017;171:280–287.

23. Holley AL, Wilson AC, Palermo TM. Predictors of the transition from acute to persistent musculoskeletal pain in children and adolescents: a prospective study. *Pain* 2017;158:794–801.

24. Huguet A, Tougas ME, Hayden J, et al. Systematic review with meta-analysis of childhood and adolescent risk and prognostic factors for musculoskeletal pain. *Pain* 2016;157:2640–2656.

25. da Silva CG, Pachêco-Pereira C, Porporatti AL, et al. Prevalence of clinical signs of intra-articular temporomandibular disorders in children and adolescents: a systematic review and meta-analysis. *J Am Dent Assoc* 2016;147:10–18.

26. Magnusson T, Egermarki I, Carlsson GE. A prospective investigation over two decades on signs and symptoms of temporomandibular disorders and associated variables. A final summary. *Acta Odontol Scand* 2005;63:99–109.

27. Hershey AD, Winner P, Kabbouche MA, et al. Headaches. *Curr Opin Pediatr* 2007;19:663–669.

28. Lewis DW, Ashwal S, Dahl G, et al. Practice parameter: evaluation of children and adolescents with recurrent headaches: report of the Quality Standards Subcommittee of the American Academy of Neurology and the Practice Committee of the Child Neurology Society. *Neurology* 2002;59:490–498.

29. Wöber-Bingöl C. Epidemiology of migraine and headache in children and adolescents. *Curr Pain Headache Rep* 2013;17:341.

30. Kröner-Herwig B, Heinrich M, Morris L. Headache in German children and adolescents: a population-based epidemiological study. *Cephalalgia* 2007;27:519–527.

31. Virtanen R, Aromaa M, Rautava P, et al. Changing headache from preschool age to puberty. A controlled study. *Cephalalgia* 2007;27:294–303.

32. Galinski M, Sidhoum S, Cimerman P, et al. Early diagnosis of migraine necessary in children: 10-year follow-up. *Pediatr Neurol* 2015;53:319–323.

33. Laimi K, Salminen JJ, Metsähonkala L, et al. Characteristics of neck pain associated with adolescent headache. *Cephalalgia* 2007;27:1244–1254.

34. Grimmer K, Nyland L, Milanese S. Repeated measures of recent headache, neck and upper back pain in Australian adolescents. *Cephalalgia* 2006;26:843–851.

35. Galli F, D'Antuono G, Tarantino S, et al. Headache and recurrent abdominal pain: a controlled study by means of the Child Behaviour Checklist (CBCL). *Cephalalgia* 2007;27:211–219.

36. Gilman DK, Palermo TM, Kabbouche MA, et al. Primary headache and sleep disturbances in adolescents. *Headache* 2007;47:1189–1194.

37. Ghandour RM, Overpeck MD, Huang ZJ, et al. Headache, stomachache, backache, and morning fatigue among adolescent girls in the United States: associations with behavioral, sociodemographic, and environmental factors. *Arch Pediatr Adolesc Med* 2004;158:797–803.

38. Stevenson SB. Epilepsy and migraine headache: is there a connection? *J Pediatr Health Care* 2006;20:167–171.

39. Wirrell EC, Hamiwka LD. Do children with benign rolandic epilepsy have a higher prevalence of migraine than those with partial epilepsies or nonepilepsy controls? *Epilepsia* 2006;47:1674–1681.

40. Jarjour IT, Jarjour LK. Migraine and recurrent epistaxis in children. *Pediatr Neurol* 2005;33:94–97.

41. Egger HL, Angold A, Costello EJ. Headaches and psychopathology in children and adolescents. *J Am Acad Child Adolesc Psychiatry* 1998;37:951–958.

42. Pakalnis A, Gibson J, Colvin A. Comorbidity of psychiatric and behavioral disorders in pediatric migraine. *Headache* 2005;45:590–596.

43. Wang SJ, Juang KD, Fuh JL, et al. Psychiatric comorbidity and suicide risk in adolescents with chronic daily headache. *Neurology* 2007;68:1468–1473.

44. Brna P, Gordon K, Dooley J. Canadian adolescents with migraine: impaired health-related quality of life. *J Child Neurol* 2008;23:39–43.

45. Hyams JS, Burke G, Davis PM, et al. Abdominal pain and irritable bowel syndrome in adolescents: a community-based sample. *J Pediatr* 1996;129:220–226.

46. Rasquin-Weber A, Hyman PE, Cucchiara S, et al. Childhood functional gastrointestinal disorders. *Gut* 1999;45(suppl 2):II60–II68.

47. Rome Foundation. What's new for Rome IV. Available at: https://theromefoundation.org/rome-iv/whats-new-for-rome-iv/. Accessed April 18, 2018.

48. Chitkara DK, Talley NJ, Weaver AL, et al. Incidence and presentation of common functional gastrointestinal disorders in children from birth to 5 years: a cohort study. *Clin Gastroenterol Hepatol* 2007;5:186–191.

49. Ramchandani PG, Hotopf M, Sandhu B, et al. The epidemiology of recurrent abdominal pain from 2 to 6 years of age: results of a large, population-based study. *Pediatrics* 2005;116:46–50.

50. Størdal K, Nygaard EA, Bentsen BS. Recurrent abdominal pain: a five-year follow-up study. *Acta Paediatr* 2005;94:234–236.

51. Dampier C, Ely E, Brodecki D, et al. Characteristics of pain managed at home in children and adolescents with sickle cell disease by using diary self-reports. *J Pain* 2002;3:461–470.

52. Dampier C, Setty BN, Eggleston B, et al. Vaso-occlusion in children with sickle cell disease: clinical characteristics and biologic correlates. *J Pediatr Hematol Oncol* 2004;26:785–790.

53. Niebanck AE, Pollock AN, Smith-Whitley K, et al. Headache in children with sickle cell disease: prevalence and associated factors. *J Pediatr* 2007;151:67–72.

54. Koh JL, Harrison D, Palermo TM, et al. Assessment of acute and chronic pain symptoms in children with cystic fibrosis. *Pediatr Pulmonol* 2005;40:330–335.

55. Hubbard PA, Broome ME, Antia LA. Pain, coping, and disability in adolescents and young adults with cystic fibrosis: a Web-based study. *Pediatr Nurs* 2005;31:82–86.

56. Krane EJ, Heller LB. The prevalence of phantom sensation and pain in pediatric amputees. *J Pain Symptom Manage* 1995;10:21–29.

57. Melzack R, Israel R, Lacroix R, et al. Phantom limbs in people with congenital limb deficiency or amputation in early childhood. *Brain* 1997;120:1603–1620.

58. Wilkins KL, McGrath PJ, Finely GA, et al. Prospective diary study of nonpainful and painful phantom sensations in a preselected sample of child and adolescent amputees reporting phantom limbs. *Clin J Pain* 2004;20:293–301.

59. Hunfeld JA, Perquin CW, Duivenvoorden HJ, et al. Chronic pain and its impact on quality of life in adolescents and their families. *J Pediatr Psychol* 2001;26(3):145–153.

60. Kashikar-Zuck S, Goldschneider KR, Powers SW, et al. Depression and functional disability in chronic pediatric pain. *Clin J Pain* 2001;17(4):341–349.

61. Roth-Isigkeit A, Thyen U, Stoven H, et al. Pain among children and adolescents: restrictions in daily living and triggering factors. *Pediatrics* 2005;115(2):e152–e162.

62. Palermo TM. Impact of recurrent and chronic pain on child and family daily functioning: a critical review of the literature. *J Dev Behav Pediatr* 2000;21(1):58–69.

63. Walker LS, Greene JW. The Functional Disability Inventory: measuring a neglected dimension of child health status. *J Pediatr Psychol* 1991;16(1):39–58.

64. Breuner CC, Smith MS, Womack WM. Factors related to school absenteeism in adolescents with recurrent headache. *Headache* 2004;44(3):217–222.

65. Lynch AM, Kashikar-Zuck S, Goldschneider KR, et al. Psychosocial risks for disability in children with chronic back pain. *J Pain* 2006;7(4):244–251.

66. Kashikar-Zuck S, Lynch AM, Graham TB, et al. Social functioning and peer relationships of adolescents with juvenile fibromyalgia syndrome. *Arthritis Rheum* 2007;57(3):474–480.

67. Palermo TM, Law E, Churchill SS, et al. Longitudinal course and impact of insomnia symptoms in adolescents with and without chronic pain. *J Pain* 2012;13(11):1099–1106. doi:10.1016/j.jpain.2012.08.003.

68. Langeveld JH, Koot HM, Passchier J. Headache intensity and quality of life in adolescents. How are changes in headache intensity in adolescents related to changes in experienced quality of life? *Headache* 1997;37(1):37–42.

69. Maikler VE, Broome ME, Bailey P, et al. Children's and adolescents' use of pain diaries for sickle cell pain. *J Soc Ped Nurs* 2001;6:161–169.

70. Tkachuk GA, Cottrell CK, Gibson JS, et al. Factors associated with migraine-related quality of life and disability in adolescents: a preliminary investigation. *Headache* 2003;43(9):950–955.

71. Rabbitts JA, Holley AL, Groenewald CB, et al. Association between widespread pain scores and functional impairment and health-related quality of life in clinical samples of children. *J Pain* 2016;17(6):678–684. doi:10.1016/j.jpain.2016.02.005.

72. Long AC, Krishnamurthy V, Palermo TM. Sleep disturbances in school-age children with chronic pain. *J Pediatr Psychol* 2008;33(3):258–268.

73. Palermo TM, Wilson AC, Lewandowski AS, et al. Behavioral and psychosocial factors associated with insomnia in adolescents with chronic pain. *Pain* 2011;152(1):89–94. doi:10.1016/j.pain.2010.09.035.

74. Kanstrup M, Holmström L, Ringström R, et al. Insomnia in paediatric chronic pain and its impact on depression and functional disability. *Eur J Pain* 2014;18(8):1094–1102.

75. Simons LE, Kaczynski KJ. The fear avoidance model of chronic pain: examination for pediatric application. *J Pain* 2012;13(9):827–835.

76. Nodari E, Battistella PA, Naccarella C, et al. Quality of life in young Italian patients with primary headache. *Headache* 2002;42(4):268–274.

77. Noel M, Wilson AC, Holley AL, et al. Posttraumatic stress disorder symptoms in youth with vs without chronic pain. *Pain* 2016;157(10):227–2284.

78. Simons LE, Sieberg CB, Claar RL. Anxiety and impairment in a large sample of children and adolescents with chronic pain. *Pain Res Manag* 2012;17(2):93–97.

79. Noel M, Groenewald CB, Beals-Erickson SE, et al. Chronic pain in adolescence and internalizing mental health disorders: a nationally representative study. *Pain* 2016;157(6):1333–1338.

80. Eccleston C, Crombez G, Scotford A, et al. Adolescent chronic pain: patterns and predictors of emotional distress in adolescents with chronic pain and their parents. *Pain* 2004;108(3):221–229.

81. Palermo TM, Schwartz L, Drotar D, et al. Parental report of health-related quality of life in children with sickle cell disease. *J Behav Med* 2002;25(3):269–283.

82. Palermo TM, Kiska R. Subjective sleep disturbances in adolescents with chronic pain: relationship to daily functioning and quality of life. *J Pain* 2005;6(3):201–207.

83. Berrin SJ, Malcarne VL, Varni JW, et al. Pain, fatigue, and school functioning in children with cerebral palsy: a path-analytic model. *J Pediatr Psychol* 2007;32(3):330–337.

84. Palermo TM, Riley CA, Mitchell BA. Daily functioning and quality of life in children with sickle cell disease pain: relationship with family and neighborhood socioeconomic distress. *J Pain* 2008;9(9):833–840.

85. Palermo TM, Valrie CR, Karlson CW. Family and parent influences on pediatric chronic pain: a developmental perspective. *Am Psychol* 2014;69(2):142–152. doi:10.1037/a0035216.

86. Logan DE, Scharff L. Relationships between family and parent characteristics and functional abilities in children with recurrent pain syndromes: an investigation of moderating effects on the pathway from pain to disability. *J Pediatr Psychol* 2005;30(8):698–707.

87. Flor H, Kerns RD, Turk DC. The role of spouse reinforcement, perceived pain, and activity levels of chronic pain patients. *J Psychosom Res* 1987;31(2):251–259.

88. Romano JM, Jensen MP, Schmaling KB, et al. Illness behaviors in patients with unexplained chronic fatigue are associated with significant other responses. *J Behav Med* 2009;32(6):558–569. doi:10.1007/s10865 -009-9234-3.

89. Palermo TM, Chambers CT. Parent and family factors in pediatric chronic pain and disability: an integrative approach. *Pain* 2005;119(1–3): 1–4.

90. Groenewald CB, Essner BS, Wright D, et al. The economic costs of chronic pain among a cohort of treatment-seeking adolescents in the United States. *J Pain* 2014;15(9):925–933. doi:10.1016/j.jpain.2014.06.002.

91. Lewandowski AS, Palermo TM, Stinson J, et al. Systematic review of family functioning in families of children and adolescents with chronic pain. *J Pain* 2010;11(11):1027–1038. doi:10.1016/j.jpain.2010.04.005.

92. Anttila P, Sourander A, Metsahonkala L, et al. Psychiatric symptoms in children with primary headache. *J Am Acad Child Adolesc Psychiatry* 2004; 43(4):412–419.

93. Larsson B, Sund AM. Emotional/behavioural, social correlates and one-year predictors of frequent pains among early adolescents: influences of pain characteristics. *Eur J Pain* 2007;11:57–65.

94. Palermo T, Eccleston C, Goldschneider K, et al. *Assessment and Management of Children with Chronic Pain. A Position Statement from the American Pain Society.* Glenview, IL: American Pain Society; 2012.

95. Konijnenberg AY, DeGraeff-Meeder ER, Kimpen JL, et al. Children with unexplained chronic pain: do pediatricians agree regarding the diagnostic approach and presumed primary cause? *Pediatrics* 2004;114:1220–1226.

96. Simons LE, Smith A, Ibagon C, et al. Pediatric Pain Screening Tool (PPST): rapid identification of risk in youth with pain complaints. *Pain* 2015; 156(8):1511–1518.

97. Woolf CJ. Central sensitization: implicatons for the diagnosis and treatment of pain. *Pain* 2011;152:S2–S15.

98. Moshiree B, Zhou Q, Price DD, et al. Central sensitization in visceral pain disorders. *Gut* 2006;55:905–908.

99. Verne GN, Price DD. Irritable bowel syndrome as a common precipitant of central sensitization. *Curr Rheumatol Rep* 2002;4:322–328.

100. Ji RR, Kohno T, Moore KA, et al. Central sensitization and LTP: do pain and memory share similar mechanisms. *Trends Neurosci* 2003;26:696–705.

101. Chalkiadis GA. Management of chronic pain in children. *Med J Aust* 2001;175:476–479.

102. Torsney C, Fitzgerald M. Age-dependent effects of peripheral inflammation upon the electrophysiological properties of neonatal rat dorsal horn neurons: development of hyperalgesia and allodynia. *J Neurophysiol* 2002; 87:1311–1317.

103. Fitzgerald M, Howard R. The neurobiological basis of pediatric pain. In: Schechter N, Berde C, Yaster M, eds. *Pain in Children and Adolescents.* 2nd ed. Philadelphia: Lippincott Williams & Wilkins; 2003:19–42.

104. Fitzgerald M, Millard C, McIntosh N. Cutaneous hypersensitivity following peripheral tissue damage in newborn infants and its reversal with topical analgesia. *Pain* 1989;39:31–36.

105. Pattinson D, Fitzgerald M. The neurobiology of infant pain: development of excitatory and inhibitory neurotransmission in the spinal dorsal horn. *Reg Anesth Pain Med* 2004;29:36–44.

106. Grunau RV, Whitfield MF, Petrie JH. Pain sensitivity and temperament in extremely low-birth-weight premature toddlers and preterm and full-term controls. *Pain* 1994;58:341–346.

107. Grunau RE, Whitfield MF, Petrie JH, et al. Early pain experience, child and family factors, as precursors of somatization: a prospective study of extremely premature and fullterm children. *Pain* 1994;56:353–359.

108. Grunau RE. Early pain in preterm infants. A model of long-term effects. *Clin Perinatol* 2002;29:373–394.

109. Grunau RE, Whitfield MF, Petrie J. Children's judgements about pain at age 8–10 years: do extremely low birthweight (< or = 1000 g) children differ from full birthweight peers? *J Child Psychol Psychiatry* 1998;39:587–594.

110. Anand KJ, Scalzo FM. Can adverse neonatal experiences alter brain development and subsequent behavior? *Biol Neonate* 2000;77:69–82.

111. Borge AI, Nordhagen R. Recurrent pain symptoms in children and parents. *Acta Paediatr* 2000;89:1479–1483.

112. Schanberg LE, Anthony KK, Gil KM. Family pain history predicts child health status in children with chronic rheumatic disease. *Pediatrics* 2001; 108:E47.

113. Burri A, Ogata S, Vehof J, et al. Chronic widespread pain: clinical comorbidities and psychological correlates. *Pain* 2015;156:1458–1464.

114. Odell S, Logan DE. Pediatric pain management: the multidisciplinary approach. *J Pain Res* 2013;6:785–760.

115. Hechler T, Kanstrup M, Holley AL, et al. Systematic review on intensive interdisciplinary pain treatment of children with chronic pain. *Pediatrics* 2015;136(1):115–127.

116. Eccleston C, Crombez G, Scotford A, et al. Adolescent chronic pain: patterns and predictors of emotional distress in adolescents with chronic pain and their parents. *Pain* 2004;108:221–229.

117. Welkom JS, Hwang W-T, Guite JW. Adolescent pain catastrophizing mediates the relationship between protective parental responses to pain and disability over time. *J Pediatr Psychol* 2013;38(5):541–550.

118. Chan ECC, Piira T, Betts G. The school functioning of children with chronic and recurrent pain. *Pediatr Pain Lett* 2005;7:11–16.

119. Stang PE, Osterhaus JT. Impact of migraine in the United States: data from the National Health Interview Survey. *Headache* 1993;33:29–35.

120. Walker LS, Guite JW, Duke M, et al. Recurrent abdominal pain: a potential precursor or irritable bowel syndrome in adolescents and young adults. *J Pediatr* 1998;132:1010–1015.

121. Eccleston C, Jordan AL, Crombez G. The impact of chronic pain on adolescents: a review of previously used measures. *J Pediatr Psychol* 2006;31(7):684–697.

122. Stinson JN, Kavanagh T, Yamada J, et al. Systematic review of the psychometric properties, interpretability and feasibility of self-report pain intensity measures for use in clinical trials in children and adolescents. *Pain* 2006;125(1–2):143–157.

123. von Baeyer CL. Children's self-reports of pain intensity: scale selection, limitations and interpretation. *Pain Res Manag* 2006;11(3):157–162.

124. Castarlenas E, Jensen MP, von Baeyer CL, et al. Psychometric properties of the Numerical Rating Scale to assess self-reported pain intensity in children and adolescents: a systematic review. *Clin J Pain* 2016;33:376–383.

125. Stinson JN, Stevens BJ, Feldman BM, et al. Construct validity of a multidimensional electronic pain diary for adolescents with arthritis. *Pain* 2008;136(3):281–292.

126. Palermo TM, Witherspoon D, Valenzuela D, et al. Development and validation of the Child Activity Limitations Interview: a measure of pain-related functional impairment in school-age children and adolescents. *Pain* 2004;109(3):461–470.

127. Logan DE, Simons LE, Stein MJ, et al. School impairment in adolescents with chronic pain. *J Pain* 2008;9(5):407–416.

128. Vervoort T, Logan DE, Goubert L, et al. Severity of pediatric pain in relation to school-related functioning and teacher support: an epidemiological study

among school-aged children and adolescents. *Pain* 2014;155(6):1118–1127. doi:10.1016/j.pain.2014.02.021.

129. Irwin DE, Stucky B, Thissen D, et al. Sampling plan and patient characteristics of the PROMIS pediatrics large-scale survey. *Qual Life Res* 2010;19(4):585–594.

130. Varni JW, Magnus B, Stucky BD, et al. Psychometric properties of the PROMIS® pediatric scales: precision, stability, and comparison of different scoring and administration options. *Qual Life Res* 2014;23(4):1233–1243.

131. Eccleston C, Jordan AL, McCracken LM, et al. The Bath Adolescent Pain Questionnaire (BAPQ): development and preliminary psychometric evaluation of an instrument to assess the impact of chronic pain on adolescents. *Pain* 2005;118(1–2):263.

132. Eccleston C, McCracken LM, Jordan A, et al. Development and preliminary psychometric evaluation of the parent report version of the Bath Adolescent Pain Questionnaire (BAPQ-P): a multidimensional parent report instrument to assess the impact of chronic pain on adolescents. *Pain* 2007;131(1–2):48–56.

133. Varni JW, Seid M, Kurtin PS. PedsQL 4.0: reliability and validity of the Pediatric Quality of Life Inventory version 4.0 generic core scales in healthy and patient populations. *Med Care* 2001;39(8):800–812.

134. Chorpita BF, Moffitt CE, Gray J. Psychometric properties of the revised child anxiety and depression scale in a clinical sample. *Behav Res Ther* 2005;43(3):309–322.

135. Chorpita BF, Yim L, Moffitt C, et al. Assessment of symptoms of DSM-IV anxiety and depression in children: a revised child anxiety and depression scale. *Behav Res Ther* 2000;38(8):835–855.

136. Irwin DE, Stucky B, Langer MM, et al. An item response analysis of the pediatric PROMIS anxiety and depressive symptoms scales. *Qual Life Res* 2010;19(4):595–607.

137. Foa EB, Johnson KM, Feeny NC, et al. The Child PTSD Symptom Scale: a preliminary examination of its psychometric properties. *J Clin Child Psychol* 2001;30(3):376–384.

138. Logan DE, Claar RL, Scharff L. Social desirability response bias and self-report of psychological distress in pediatric chronic pain patients. *Pain* 2008;36:366–372.

139. Crombez G, Bijttebier P, Eccleston C, et al. The child version of the Pain Catastrophizing Scale (PCS-C): a preliminary validation. *Pain* 2003;104(3):639–646.

140. Goubert L, Eccleston C, Vervoort T, et al. Parental catastrophizing about their child's pain. The parent version of the Pain Catastrophizing Scale (PCS-P): a preliminary validation. *Pain* 2006;123(3):254–263.

141. Pagé MG, Fuss S, Martin AL, et al. Development and preliminary validation of the Child Pain Anxiety Symptoms Scale in a community sample. *J Pediatr Psychol* 2010;35(10):1071–1082.

142. Simons LE, Sieberg CB, Carpino E, et al. The Fear of Pain Questionnaire (FOPQ): assessment of pain-related fear among children and adolescents with chronic pain. *J Pain* 2011;12(6):677–686. doi:10.1016/j.jpain.2010.12.008.

143. Simons LE, Smith AM, Kaczynski K, et al. Living in fear of your child's pain: the Parent Fear of Pain Questionnaire. *Pain* 2015;156(4):694–702.

144. Van Slyke DA, Walker LS. Mothers' responses to children's pain. *Clin J Pain* 2006;22(4):387–391.

145. Epstein NB, Baldwin LM, Bishop DS. The McMaster family assessment device. *J Marital Fam Ther* 1983;9(2):171–180.

146. Van Slyke DA, Smith CA, Walker LS, et al. Development and validation of the children's pain beliefs questionnaire. Paper presented at: the 6th Florida Conference on Child Health Psychology; April 1997; Gainesville, FL.

147. Reid GJ, Gilbert CA, McGrath PJ. The pain coping questionnaire: preliminary validation. *Pain* 1998;76(1–2):83–96.

148. Owens JA, Spirito A, McGuinn M. The Children's Sleep Habits Questionnaire (CSHQ): psychometric properties of a survey instrument for school-aged children. *Sleep* 2000;23(8):1043–1051.

149. LeBourgeois MK, Giannotti F, Cortesi F, et al. The relationship between reported sleep quality and sleep hygiene in Italian and American adolescents. *Pediatrics* 2005;115(1 suppl):257–265.

150. de la Vega R, Miró J. The assessment of sleep in pediatric chronic pain sufferers. *Sleep Med Rev* 2013;17(3):185–192.

151. Morris S, O'Sullivan PB, Murray KJ, et al. Hypermobility and musculoskeletal pain in adolescents. *J Pediatr* 2017;181:213–181.

152. Smits-Engelsman B, Klerks M, Kirby A. Beighton score: a valid measure for generalized hypermobility in children. *J Pediatr* 2011;158(1):119–123.e4.

153. Grahame R. Joint hypermobility: emerging disease or illness behavior? *Clin Med (Lond)* 2013;13(6):s50–s52.

154. Adib N, Davies K, Grahame R, et al. Joint hypermobility syndrome in childhood. A not so benign multisystem disorder? *Rheumatology* 2005;44:744–750.

155. Grahame R. The revised (Brighton 1998) criteria for the diagnosis of benign joint hypermobility syndrome (BJHS). *J Rheumatol* 2000;27:1777–1779.

156. Cormier S, Lavigne GL, Choiniere M, et al. Expectations predict chronic pain treatment outcomes. *Pain* 2016;157:329–338.

157. Moseley GL, Nicholas MK, Hodges PW. A randomized controlled trial of intensive neurophysiology education in chronic low back pain. *Clin J Pain* 2004;20:324–330.

158. Moseley L. Combined physiotherapy and education is efficacious for chronic low back pain. *Aust J Physiother* 2002;48:297–302.

159. Gallagher L, McAuley J, Moseley GL. A randomized-controlled trial of using a book of metaphors to reconceptualize pain and decrease catastrophizing in people with chronic pain. *Clin J Pain* 2013;29:20–25.

160. Coakley R, Schechter N. Chronic pain is like . . . . The clinical use of analogy and metaphor in the treatment of chronic pain in children. *Pediatric Pain Letter* 2013;15(1):1–8.

161. Flor H, Fydrich, Turk DC. Efficacy of multidisciplinary pain treatment centers: a meta-analytic review. *Pain* 1992;49:221–230.

162. Lindley KJ, Glaser D, Milla PJ. Consumerism in healthcare can be detrimental to child health: lessons from children with functional abdominal pain. *Arch Dis Child* 2005;90:335–337.

163. Herzog DB, Harper G. Unexplained disability: diagnostic dilemmas and principles of management. *Clin Pediatr* 1981;20:761–768.

164. Cooper TE, Heathcote LC, Clinch J, et al. Antidepressants for chronic non-cancer pain in children and adolescents. *Cochrane Database Syst Rev* 2017;(8):CD012535.

165. Cooper TE, Wiffen PJ, Heathcote LC, Clinch J, et al. Antiepileptic drugs for chronic non-cancer pain in children and adolescents. *Cochrane Database Syst Rev* 2017;(8):CD012536.

166. Cooper TE, Fischer E, Anderson B, et al. Paracetamol (acetaminophen) for chronic non-cancer pain in children and adolescents. *Cochrane Database Syst Rev* 2017;(8):CD012539.

167. Eccleston C, Cooper TE, Fisher E, et al. Non-steroidal anti-inflammatory drugs (NSAIDs) for chronic non-cancer pain in children and adolescents. *Cochrane Database Syst Rev* 2017;(8):CD012537.

168. Cooper TE, Fisher E, Gray AL, et al. Opioids for chronic non-cancer pain in children and adolescents. *Cochrane Database Syst Rev* 2017;(8):CD012538.

169. Schechter N, Walco GA. The potential impact on children of the CDC guideline for prescribing opioids for chronic pain: above all, do no harm. *JAMA Pediatr* 2016;170:425–426.

170. Friedrichsdorf SJ. Nugent AP. Management of neuropathic pain in children with cancer. *Curr Opin Support Palliat* 2013;7:131–138.

171. Logan DE, Carpino EA, Chiang G, et al. A day-hospital approach to treatment of pediatric complex regional pain syndrome: initial functional outcomes. *Clin J Pain* 2012;28:766–774.

172. Maynard CS, Amari A, Wieczorek B, et al. Interdisciplinary behavioral rehabilitation of pediatric pain-associated disability: retrospective review of an inpatient treatment protocol. *J Pediatr Psychol* 2010;35:128–137.

173. Wilson AC, Palermo TM. Physical activity and function in adolescents with chronic pain: a controlled study using actigraphy. *J Pain* 2012;13:121–130.

174. Verkamp EK, Flowers SR, Lynch-Jordan AM, et al. A survey of conventional and complementary therapies used by youth with juvenile-onset fibromyalgia. *Pain Manag Nurs* 2013;14:e244–e250.

175. Lynch-Jordan AM, Sil S, Peugh J, et al. Differential changes in functional disability and pain intensity over the course of psychological treatment for children with chronic pain. *Pain* 2014;155:1955–1961.

176. Sherry DD, Wallace CA, Kelley C, et al. Short- and long-term outcomes of children with complex regional pain syndrome type I treated with exercise therapy. *Clin J Pain* 1999;15:218–223.

177. Lee BH, Scharff L, Sethna NF, et al. Physical therapy and cognitive-behavioral treatment for complex regional pain syndromes. *J Pediatr* 2002;141:135–140.

178. Hunt K, Ernst E. The evidence-base for complementary medicine in children: a critical overview of systematic reviews. *Arch Dis Child* 2011;96:769–776.

179. Hemington KS, Coulombe MA. The periaqueductal gray and descending pain modulation: why should we study them and what role do they play in chronic pain? *J Neurophysiol* 2015;114:2080–2088.

180. Von Baeyer CL, Champion GD. Commentary: multiple pains as functional pain syndromes. *J Pediatr Psychol* 2011;36:433–437.

181. Schechter NL. Functional pain: time for a new name. *JAMA Pediatr* 2014;168:693–694.

182. Eccleston C, Morley S, Williams A, et al. Systematic review of randomized controlled trials of psychological therapy for chronic pain in children and adolescents with a subset meta-analysis of pain relief. *Pain* 2002;22:157–165.

183. Walco GA, Sterling CM, Conte PM, et al. Empirically supported treatments in pediatric psychology: disease related pain. *J Pediatr Psychol* 1999;24:155–167.

184. Kashikar-Zuck S, Sil S, Lynch-Jordan AM, et al. Changes in pain coping, catastrophizing, and coping efficacy after cognitive-behavioral therapy in children and adolescents with juvenile fibromyalgia. *J Pain* 2013;14:492–501.

185. Hayes SC. Acceptance and commitment therapy, relational frame theory, and the third wave of behavior therapy. *Behav Ther* 2004;35:639–665.

186. Zeltzer L, Schlank C. *Conquering Your Child's Chronic Pain.* New York: HarperCollins; 2005.

187. Moore RA, Derry S, McQuay HJ, et al. What do we know about communicating risk? A brief review and suggestion for contextualising serious, but rare, risk, and the example of cox-2 selective and non-selective NSAIDs. *Arthritis Res Ther* 2008;10(1):R20.

188. Foeldvari I, Szer IS, Zemel LS, et al. A prospective study comparing celecoxib with naproxen in children with juvenile rheumatoid arthritis. *J Rheumatol* 2009;36(1):174–182.

189. Buntin-Mushock C, Phillip L, Moriyama K, et al. Age-dependent opioid escalation in chronic pain patients. *Anesth Analg* 2005;100:1740–1745.
190. Wang Y, Mitchell J, Moriyama K, et al. Age-dependent morphine tolerance development in the rat. *Anesth Analg* 2005;100:1733–1739.
191. Williams JT, Ingram SL, Henderson G, et al. Regulation of μ-opioid receptors: desensitization, phosphorylation, internalization, and tolerance. *Pharmacol Rev* 2013;65(1):223–254
192. Sindrup SH, Bach FW, Madsen C, et al. Venlafaxine versus imipramine in painful polyneuropathy: a randomized, controlled trial. *Neurology* 2003;60:1284–1289.
193. Quilici S, Chancellor J, Löthgren M, et al. Meta-analysis of duloxetine vs. pregabalin and gabapentin in the treatment of diabetic peripheral neuropathic pain. *BMC Neurol* 2009;9:6.
194. Levinstein B. A comparative study of cyproheptadine, amitriptyline, and propranolol in the treatment of adolescent migraine. *Cephalalgia* 1991;11:122–123.
195. Hershey AD, Powers SW, Bentti A-L, et al. Effectiveness of amitriptyline in the prophylactic management of childhood headaches. *Headache* 2000;40:539–549.
196. Campo JV, Perel J, Lucas A, et al. Citalopram treatment of pediatric recurrent abdominal pain and comorbid internalizing disorders: an exploratory study. *J Am Acad Child Adolesc Psychiatry* 2004;43(10):1234–1242.
197. National Institute of Mental Health. Antidepressant medications for children and adolescents: information for parents and caregivers. Available at: http://www.nimh.nih.gov/health/topics/child-and-adolescent-mental-health/antidepressant-medications-for-children-and-adolescents-information-for-parents-and-caregivers.shtml. Accessed March 15, 2009.
198. Straube S, Derry S, McQuay HJ, et al. Enriched enrollment: definition and effects of enrichment and dose in trials of pregabalin and gabapentin in neuropathic pain. A systematic review. *Br J Clin Pharmacol* 2008;66(2):266–275.
199. Lalwani K, Shoham A, Koh JL, et al. Use of oxcarbazepine to treat a pediatric patient with resistant complex regional pain syndrome. *J Pain* 2005;6(10):704–706.
200. Sindrup SH, Jensen TS. Pharmacologic treatment of pain in polyneuropathy. *Neurology* 2000;55(7):915–920.
201. Shapiro RE. Topiramate for migraine prevention: a randomized controlled trial. *J Pediatr* 2004;145(3):419–420.
202. Mula M, Bell GS, Sander JW. Assessing suicidal risk with antiepileptic drugs. *Neuropsychiatr Dis Treat* 2010;6:613–618.
203. Eccleston C, Palermo TM, Williams AC, et al. Psychological therapies for the management of chronic and recurrent pain in children and adolescents. *Cochrane Database Syst Rev* 2014;(5):CD003968.
204. Fisher E, Heathcote L, Palermo TM, et al. Systematic review and meta-analysis of psychological therapies for children with chronic pain. *J Pediatr Psychol* 2014;39(8):763–782. doi:10.1093/jpepsy/jsu008.
205. Fisher E, Law E, Palermo TM, et al. Psychological therapies (remotely delivered) for the management of chronic and recurrent pain in children and adolescents. *Cochrane Database Syst Rev* 2015;(3):CD011118.
206. Van Der Veek SMC, Derkx BHF, Benninga MA, et al. Cognitive behavioural therapy for pediatric functional abdominal pain: a randomized controlled trial. *Pediatrics* 2013;132(5):e1163–e1172. doi:10.1542/peds.2013-0242.
207. Cottrell C, Drew J, Gibson J, et al. Feasibility assessment of telephone-administered behavioral treatment for adolescent migraine. *Headache* 2007;47(9):1293–1302. doi:10.1111/j.1526-4610.2007.00804.x.
208. Levy RL, Langer SL, Walker LS, et al. Cognitive-behavioral therapy for children with functional abdominal pain and their parents decreases pain and other symptoms. *Am J Gastroent* 201;105(4):946–956.
209. D'Zurilla TJ, Nezu AM. *Problem Solving Therapy: A Social Competence Approach to Clinical Intervention.* 2nd ed. New York: Springer; 1999.
210. D'Zurilla TJ, Nezu AM. *Problem Solving Therapy: A Positive Approach to Clinical Intervention.* 3rd ed. New York: Springer; 2007.
211. Palermo TM, Law EF, Bromberg M, et al. Problem-solving skills training for parents of children with chronic pain: a pilot randomized controlled trial. *Pain* 2016;157(6):1213–1223.
212. Palermo TM, Law EF, Fales J, et al. Internet-delivered cognitive-behavioral treatment for adolescents with chronic pain and their parents: a randomized controlled multicenter trial. *Pain* 2016;157:174–185.
213. Wicksell RK, Melin L, Olsson GL. Exposure and acceptance in the rehabilitation of adolescents with idiopathic chronic pain—a pilot study. *Eur J Pain* 2007;11(3):267.
214. Wicksell RK, Melin L, Lekander M, et al. Evaluating the effectiveness of exposure and acceptance strategies to improve functioning and quality of life in longstanding pediatric pain—a randomized controlled trial. *Pain* 2009;141(3):248–257.
215. Davis MP, Darden PM. Use of complementary and alternative medicine by children in the united states. *Arch Pediatr Adolesc Med* 2003;157(4):393–396.
216. Tsao JCI, Zeltzer LK. Complementary and alternative medicine approaches for pediatric pain: a review of the state-of-the-science. *Evid Based Complement Alternat Med* 2005;2(2):149–159.
217. Humphreys PA, Gevirtz RN. Treatment of recurrent abdominal pain: components analysis of four treatment protocols. *J Pediatr Gastroent Nutr* 2000;31(1):47–51.
218. Weydert JA, Ball TM, Davis MF. Systematic review of treatments for recurrent abdominal pain. *Pediatrics* 2003;111(1):e1–e11.
219. Allen KD, Shriver MD. Role of parent-mediated pain behavior management strategies in biofeedback treatment of childhood migraines. *Behav Ther* 1998;29:477–490.
220. Kroner-Herwig B, Mohn U, Pothmann R. Comparison of biofeedback and relaxation in the treatment of pediatric headache and the influence of parent involvement on outcome. *Appl Psychophysiol Biofeedback* 1998;23(3):143–157.
221. Shapiro BS, Dinges DF, Orne EC, et al. Home management of sickle cell-related pain in children and adolescents: natural history and impact on school attendance. *Pain* 1995;61(1):139–144.
222. Greco LA, Freeman KE, Dufton L. Overt and relational victimization among children with frequent abdominal pain: links to social skills, academic functioning, and health service use. *J Pediatr Psychol* 2007;32(3):319–329.
223. Logan DE, Catanese SP, Coakley RM, et al. Chronic pain in the classroom: teachers' attributions about the causes of chronic pain. *J Sch Health* 2007;77(5):248–256.
224. Logan DE, Coakley RM, Scharff L. Teachers' perceptions of and responses to adolescents with chronic pain syndromes. *J Pediatr Psychol* 2007;32(2):139–149.
225. Bloom BJ, Owens JA, McGuinn M, et al. Sleep and its relationship to pain, dysfunction, and disease activity in juvenile rheumatoid arthritis. *J Rheumatol* 2002;29:169–173.
226. Valrie CR, Gil KM, Redding-Lallinger R. Brief report: sleep in children with sickle cell disease: an analysis of daily diaries utilizing multilevel models. *J Pediatr Psychol* 2007;32:857–861.
227. Valrie CR, Gil KM, Redding-Lallinger R, et al. Brief report: daily mood as a mediator or moderator of the pain-sleep relationship in children with sickle cell disease. *J Pediatr Psychol* 2008;33:317–322.
228. Meltzer LJ, Logan DE, Mindell JA. Sleep patterns in female adolescents with chronic musculoskeletal pain. *Behav Sleep Med* 2005;3:193–208.
229. Stinson JN, Hayden JA, Ahola Kohut S, et al. Sleep problems and associated factors in children with juvenile idiopathic arthritis: a systematic review. *Pediatr Rheumatol Online J* 2014;12:19.
230. Valrie CR, Bromberg MH, Palermo T, et al. A systematic review of sleep in pediatric pain populations. *J Dev Behav Pediatr* 2013;34(2):120–128.
231. Lewandowski AS, Palermo TM, Motte SD, et al. Temporal daily associations between pain and sleep in adolescents with chronic pain versus healthy adolescents. *Pain* 2010;151(1):220–225.
232. Lewin DS, Dahl RE. Importance of sleep in the management of pediatric pain. *J Dev Behav Pediatr* 1999;20(4):244–252.
233. Smith MT, Edwards RR, McCann UD, et al. The effects of sleep deprivation on pain inhibition and spontaneous pain in women. *Sleep* 2007;30(4):494–505.
234. Finan PH, Goodin BR, Smith MT. The association of sleep and pain: an update and a path forward. *J Pain* 2013;14(12):1539–1552. doi:10.1016/j.jpain.2013.08.007.
235. Wolfson AR, Carskadon MA. Sleep schedules and daytime functioning in adolescents. *Child Dev* 1998;69(4):875–887.
236. Carskadon MA, Wolfson AR, Acebo C, et al. Adolescent sleep patterns, circadian timing, and sleepiness at a transition to early school days. *Sleep* 1998;21(8):871–881.
237. Palermo TM, Putnam J, Armstrong G, et al. Adolescent autonomy and family functioning are associated with headache-related disability. *Clin J Pain* 2007;23(5):458–465.
238. Tsai SY, Labyak SE, Richardson LP, et al. Brief report: actigraphic sleep and daytime naps in adolescent girls with chronic musculoskeletal pain. *J Pediatr Psychol* 2008;33:307–311.
239. Kashikar-Zuck S, Swain NF, Jones BA, et al. Efficacy of cognitive-behavioral intervention for juvenile primary fibromyalgia syndrome. *J Rheumatol* 2005;32(8):1594–1602.
240. Wu JQ, Appleman ER, Salazar RD, et al. Cognitive behavioral therapy for insomnia comorbid with psychiatric and medical conditions: a meta-analysis. *JAMA Intern Med* 2015;175(9):1461–1472. doi:10.1001/jamainternmed.2015.3006.
241. Finan PH, Buenaver LF, Coryell VT, et al. Cognitive-behavioral therapy for comorbid insomnia and chronic pain. *Sleep Med Clin* 2014;9(2):261–274.
242. Smith MT, Finan PH, Buenaver LF, et al. Cognitive-behavioral therapy for insomnia in knee osteoarthritis: a randomized, double-blind, active placebo-controlled clinical trial. *Arthritis Rheumatol* 2015;67(5):1221–1233.
243. Palermo TM, Beals-Erickson S, Bromberg M, et al. A single arm pilot trial of brief cognitive behavioral therapy for insomnia in adolescents with physical and psychiatric comorbidities. *J Clin Sleep Med* 2017;13(3):401–410.
244. Evans JR, Benore E, Banez GA. The cost-effectiveness of intensive interdisciplinary pediatric chronic pain rehabilitation. *J Pediatr Psychol* 2016;41(8):849–856.
245. King S, Chambers CT, Huguet A, et al. The epidemiology of chronic pain in children and adolescents revisited: a systematic review. *Pain* 2011;152:2729–2738.
246. Malleson PN, Beauchamp RD. Rheumatology: 16. Diagnosing musculoskeletal pain in children. *CMAJ* 2001;165:183–188.
247. Karaaslan Y, Haznedaroglu S, Oztürk M. Joint hypermobility and primary fibromyalgia: a clinical enigma. *J Rheumatol* 2000;27:1774–1776.

248. Fitzcharles MA. Is hypermobility a factor in fibromyalgia. *J Rheumatol* 2000;27:1587–1589.

249. Keer R, Grahame R. *Hypermobility Syndrome: Recognition and Management for Physiotherapists.* Edinburgh: Butterworth Heineman; 2003.

250. Clinch J, Eccleston C. Chronic musculoskeletal pain in children: assessment and management. *Rheumatology* 2009;48:466–474.

251. Bulbena A, Duro JC, Porta M, et al. Anxiety disorders in the joint hypermobility syndrome. *Psychiatry Res* 1993;46:59–68.

252. Bulbena A, Agulló A, Pailhez G, et al. Is joint hypermobility related to anxiety in a nonclinical population also? *Psychosomatics* 2004;45:432–437.

253. Martín-Santos R, Bulbena A, Porta M, et al. Association between joint hypermobility syndrome and panic disorder. *Am J Psychiatry* 1998;155:1578–1583.

254. Eccleston C, Malleson PN, Clinch J, et al. Chronic pain in adolescents: evaluation of a programme of interdisciplinary cognitive behaviour therapy. *Arch Dis Child* 2003;88:881–885.

255. Sherry DD, Brake L, Tress JL, et al. The treatment of juvenile fibromyalgia with an intensive physical and psychosocial program. *J Pediatr* 2015;167:731–737.

256. Kashikar-Zuck S, Flowers SR, Strotman D, et al. Physical activity monitoring in adolescents with juvenile fibromyalgia: findings from a clinical trial of cognitive-behavioral therapy. *Arthritis Car Res* 2013;65:398–405.

257. Wilder RT. Management of pediatric patients with complex regional pain syndrome. *Clin J Pain* 2006;22:443–448.

258. Wilder RT, Berde CB, Wolohan M, et al. Reflex sympathetic dystrophy in children. Clinical characteristics and follow-up of seventy patients. *J Bone Joint Surg Am* 1992;74:910–919.

259. Dadure C, Motais F, Ricard C, et al. Continuous peripheral nerve blocks at home in the treatment of recurrent complex regional pain syndrome I in children. *Anesthesiology* 2005;102:387–391.

260. Jones GT, Watson KD, Silman AJ, et al. Predictors of low back pain in British schoolchildren: a population-based prospective cohort study. *Pediatrics* 2003;111(4 pt 1):822–828.

261. Pellisé F, Balagué F, Rajmil L, et al. Prevalence of low back pain and its effect on health-related quality of life in adolescents. *Arch Pediatr Adolesc Med* 2009;163(1):65–71.

262. Micheli LJ, Wood R. Back pain in young athletes. Significant differences from adults in causes and patterns. *Arch Pediatr Adolesc Med* 1995;149(1):15–18.

263. Purcell L, Micheli L. Low back pain in young athletes. *Sports Health* 2009;1(3):212–222.

264. Kurd MF, Patel D, Norton R, et al. Nonoperative treatment of symptomatic spondylolysis. *J Spinal Disord Tech* 2007;20(8):560–564.

265. Berde CB, Stein JM, Moody PA, et al. Epidural steroid injections for radiculopathy +/− back pain in children and adolescents. Paper presented at: Society for Pediatric Anesthesia Annual Meeting; March 2007; Phoenix, AZ.

266. Abu-Arafeh I, Razak S, Sivaraman B, et al. Prevalence of headache and migraine in children and adolescents: a systematic review of population based studies. *Dev Med Child Neurol* 2010;52(12):1088–1097.

267. Headache Classification Subcommittee of the International Headache Society. The International Classification of Headache Disorders: 2nd ed. *Cephalalgia* 2004;24(suppl 1):9–160.

268. Lipton RB, Bigal ME, Steiner TJ, et al. Classification of primary headaches. *Neurology* 2004;63:428–435.

269. Sun H, Bastings E, Temeck J, et al. Migraine therapeutics in adolescents: a systematic analysis and historic perspectives of triptan trials in adolescents. *JAMA Pediatr* 2013;167:243–249.

270. Carville S, Padhi S, Reason T, et al. Diagnosis and management of headaches in young people and adults: summary of NICE guidance. *BMJ* 2012;345:e5765.

271. Guidetti V, Galli V. Recent development in paediatric headache. *Curr Opinion Neurol* 2001;14:335–340.

272. Lewis DW. Headaches in children and adolescents. *Am Fam Physician* 2002;65:625–632.

273. Viswanathan V, Bridges SJ, Whitehouse W, et al. Childhood headaches: discrete entities or continuum? *Dev Med Child Neurol* 1998;40:544–550.

274. Zebenholzer K, Wober C, Kienbacher C, et al. Migrainous disorder and headache of the tension-type not fulfilling the criteria: a follow-up study in children and adolescents. *Cephalalgia* 2000;20:611–616.

275. Vanuytsel T, Tack JF, Boeckxstaens GE. Treatment of abdominal pain in irritable bowel syndrome. *J Gastroent* 2014;49(8):1193–1205.

276. Turner DP, Smitherman TA, Black AK, et al. Are migraine and tension-type headache diagnostic types or points on a severity continuum? An exploration of the latent taxometric structure of headache. *Pain* 2015;156:1200–1207.

277. Winner P, Wasiewski W, Gladstein J, et al. Multicenter prospective evaluation of proposed pediatric migraine revision to the HIS criteria. Pediatric Headache Committee of the American Association for the Study of Headache. *Headache* 1998;37:545–548.

278. Marcus DA. Reducing headache disability in children and adolescents. *Am Fam Physician* 2002;554:557.

279. Youssef NN, Murphy TG, Langseder AL, et al. Quality of life for children with functional abdominal pain: a comparison study of patients' and parents' perceptions. *Pediatrics* 2006;117:54–59.

280. Saki F. Oral triptans in children and adolescents : an update. *Curr Pain Headache Rep* 2015;19(3):8.

281. Patnyiot IR, Gelfand AA. Acute treatment therapies for pediatric migraine: a qualitative systematic review. *Headache* 2016;56(1):49–70.

282. Powers SW, Coffey CS, Chamberlin LA, et al; for the CHAMP Investigators. Trial of amitriptyline, topiramate, and placebo for pediatric migraine. *N Engl J Med* 2017;376(2):115–124.

283. Schoenen J, Jacquy J, Lenaerts M. Effectiveness of high dose riboflavin in migraine prophylaxis. A randomized controlled trial. *Neurology* 1998;50:466–470.

284. Peikert A, Wilimzig C, Köhne-Volland R. Prophylaxis of migraine with oral magnesium: results of prospective, multi-center, placebo-controlled and double-blind randomized study. *Cephalalgia* 1996;16:257–263.

285. Korterink JJ, Diederen K, Benninga MA, et al. Epidemiology of pediatric functional abdominal pain disorders: a meta-analysis. *PLoS One* 2015;10(5):e0126982.

286. Powell J. The approach to chronic pelvic pain in the adolescent. *Obstet Gynecol Clinics North Am* 2014;41(3):343–355.

287. Siristatidis C, Nissotakis C, Chrelias C, et al. Immunological factors and their role in the genesis and development of endometriosis. *J Obstet Gynaecol Res* 2006;32(2):162–170.

288. Stratton P, Berkley K. Chronic pelvic pain and endometriosis: translational evidence of the relationship and implications. *Hum Reprod Update* 2011;17(3):327–346.

289. Jarrell J. Endometriosis and abdominal myofascial pain in adults and adolescents. *Curr Pain Headache Rep* 2011;15(5):368–376.

290. Palsson OS, Whitehead WE, van Tilburg MA, et al. Rome IV Diagnostic Questionnaires and tables for investigators and clinicians [published online ahead of print February 13, 2016]. *Gastroenterology.* #doi:10.1053/j.gastro.2016.02.014.

291. Keefer L, Drossman DA, Guthrie E, et al. Centrally mediated disorders of gastrointestinal pain [published online ahead of print February 19, 2016]. *Gastroenterology.* #doi:10.1053/j.gastro.2016.02.034.

292. Dengler-Crish CM, Horst SN, Walker LS. Somatic complaints in childhood functional abdominal pain are associated with functional gastrointestinal disorders in adolescence and adulthood. *J Pediatr Gastroenterol Nutr* 2011;52:162–165.

293. Dengler-Crish CM, Bruehl S, Walker LS. Increased wind-up to heat pain in women with a childhood history of functional abdominal pain. *Pain* 2011;152:802–808.

294. Williams AE, Heitkemper M, Self MM, et al. Endogenous inhibition of somatic pain is impaired in girls with irritable bowel syndrome compared with healthy girls. *J Pain* 2013;14:921–930.

295. Stabell N, Stubhaug A, Flaegstad T, et al. Widespread hyperalgesia in adolescents with symptoms of irritable bowel syndrome: results from a large population-based study. *J Pain* 2014;15:898–906.

296. Walker LS, Dengler-Crish CM, Rippel S, et al. Functional abdominal pain in childhood and adolescence increases risk for chronic pain in adulthood. *Pain* 2010;150:568–572.

297. Rasquin A, Di Lorenzo C, Forbes D, et al. Childhood functional gastrointestinal disorders: child/adolescent. *Gastroenterology* 2006;130(5):1527–1537.

298. Di Lorenzo C, Colletti RB, Lehmann HP, et al; and American Academy of Pediatrics Subcommittee on Chronic Abdominal Pain, North American Society for Pediatric Gastroenterology, Hepatology and Nutrition Committee on Abdominal Pain. Chronic abdominal pain in children: a technical report of the American Academy of Pediatrics and the North American Society for Pediatric Gastroenterology, Hepatology and Nutrition. *J Pediatr Gastroenterol Nutr* 2005;40:245–261.

299. Hoekman DR, Zeevenhooven Z, van Etten-Jamaludin FS, et al. The placebo response in pediatric abdominal pain-related functional gastrointestinal disorders: a systematic review and meta-analysis. *J Pediatr* 2017(182):155–163.

300. Teitelbaum JE, Arora R. Long-term efficacy of low-dose tricyclic antidepressants for children with functional gastrointestinal disorders. *J Pediatr Gastroenterol Nutr* 2011;53(3):260–264.

301. Horvath A, Dziechciarz P, Szajewska H. Systematic review of randomized controlled trials: fiber supplements for abdominal pain-related functional gastrointestinal disorders in childhood. *Ann Nutr Metab* 2012;61(2):95–101.

CHAPTER 55

Pain in the Older Person

PAUL M. ARNSTEIN and **KEELA HERR**

Overview

Medical science continues to expand its capacity to forestall death. As a result, people are living longer but increasingly spend their final years with daily, unrelenting pain.[1-3] Pain is emerging as a more formidable foe than death, whose conquest will demand stretching the limits of our technology and ability to provide compassionate care. Because of its increasing incidence, high economic costs, and negative impact on quality of life of patients and their families, uncontrolled pain has become a public health priority.[2,4]

Dramatic increases in people over age 65 years globally suggest that older adults will challenge the capacity of health systems with the complexity of multiple conditions contributing to pain and its sequelae. Estimates indicate that by 2050, older adults will comprise a third of the population in developed countries.[5] Although not all older adults have severe or ongoing pain, a majority do when they seek health care services. Chronic back and neck pain are the leading cause of disability worldwide, and the prevalence of chronic pain–producing diseases like arthritis, diabetes, and cancer continues to increase.[6] Older adults have the highest rates of surgery, hospitalization, injury, and disease, which increases their risk of pain.[7] The problem of pain in older adults has not diminished even though evidence to guide pain assessment and management has grown over the past decade.

THE PREVALENCE OF PAIN IN OLDER ADULTS

Although pain is not an inevitable aspect of aging, older persons are at greater risk for many disorders associated with pain. Delineating the prevalence of pain with advancing age is a challenge because epidemiologic studies differ in the age cut points, methods of data collection and measurement of pain, and the types of pain studied. However, data across settings and samples suggest that pain is prevalent and a significant factor impacting quality of life. Approximately 65% of older persons living in the community have persistent pain* conditions[8,9] with more frequent pain (up to 85%) noted in those living in institutions, particularly nursing homes,[10,11] and those in the final months of life (over 80%).[12,13] Prevalence of pain in hospitalized older adults is also high with 67% on geriatric units reporting pain present.[14]

A nationally representative sample of American adults showed back, knee, and shoulder as the most prevalent pain sites in those 65 to 69 years old, with little change in this pattern in cohorts of those 90 years old or older.[8] Over 60% of older adults report pain in multiple locations with women reporting more pain sites and a greater intensity of pain than male counterparts,[15,16] which impacts physical and psychosocial function. Older women and those with obesity, musculoskeletal conditions, and depressive symptoms are at higher risk for pain.[8]

Other common conditions associated with pain in older persons include atherosclerotic peripheral vascular disease, herpes zoster, trigeminal neuralgia, diabetic neuropathy, temporal arteritis, polymyalgia rheumatica, osteoporosis with vertebral compression fractures, lumbar spinal stenosis, and fibromyalgia.[17] Also, injuries, such as hip fractures resulting from falls, are more common in this population and may result in both acute and chronic pain.

Pain in the Older Person

IMPACT OF PAIN ON FUNCTIONING AND QUALITY OF LIFE

Pain in the older adult interferes with the ability to manage and recover from health challenges given its important and often unrecognized impact on impaired function and quality of life.[18] Acute and persistent pain have adverse health outcomes in older people.[19] Poorly managed acute pain contributes to delayed ambulation, increased incidence of delirium and cognitive dysfunction, respiratory complications, longer hospitalization, and mood disorders.[20] Additionally, long-term consequences include impaired ability to complete activities of daily living (ADL), impaired mobility development of persistent pain, and cardiovascular disease.[19,21,22]

More widely studied, persistent pain is known to negatively impact older adult physical and psychosocial function, including impaired nutrition and sleep, functional abilities, mood and cognitive function, and social interactions.[23-25] Pain from osteoporosis, osteoarthritis, and chronic back pain has been shown to significantly affect ADL, placing the older adult at risk for declining health and potentially institutionalization.[26,27] According to Hunt et al.,[9] 43% of those with dementia are able to acknowledge and self-report significant functional limitations, including the ability to perform ADL.

Combined with impaired physical health, the decline in social and recreational activities produces emotional distress, contributing to depression,[8,28] which is capable of worsening both pain and disability.[29] Pain-related factors that worsen health-related quality of life include pain presence, pain severity, and number of pain sites.[6,10,25,30-32] Persistent pain also is associated with frailty, a syndrome of physiologic decline, and should be a component assessed when determining frailty phenotype to improve the prediction of adverse outcomes.[33]

UNDERTREATMENT OF PAIN IN OLDER PERSONS

Given these potentially serious pain-related consequences, evidence that pain is commonly undertreated or untreated in older adults is disturbing. Among those with pain, a significant portion of those over age 65 years do not receive analgesics or receive inadequate treatment, including 53% of elders transitioned from acute to skilled nursing care,[34] 17% to 65% of institutionalized elders,[10,11,35] 51% of elders admitted to emergency departments with pain complaints,[20,36] and 20% of elders living with pain in the community.[37] Older patients in emergency departments are more likely to experience delays in analgesic treatment and have acute pain undertreated compared to younger patients.[38] Pain, depression, and functional limitations due to pain are particularly undertreated in low-income and minority older populations.[39]

The diagnosis and treatment of pain in older persons is more difficult in those who present with multiple medical problems and a history that reveals many potential sources of pain.

---

*The terms *chronic pain* and *persistent pain* are often used interchangeably to denote pain that lasts for more than 3 months. *Persistent pain* is used in this text to avoid negative connotation often associated with the label *chronic pain*, as is recommended by the American Geriatrics Society.

Although there is an undeniable need to prevent harm from pain-relieving treatments, this focus must be balanced with a concerted effort to avoid pain-induced harm. Guidelines for the assessment, treatment, and monitoring of older patients with pain have been widely distributed advocating for individualized approaches to pain and balancing concerns for the safety and efficacy of treatments.[40–42]

It is time to replace unrealistic fears and mistaken beliefs with guidelines that delineate prudent, safe, effective use of available treatments. Approaches to managing pain in older adults should incorporate noninvasive treatments, along with tailored pharmacologic management, based on a careful risk/benefit analysis of treatment options and the older person's unique characteristics and goals.[43]

CHANGE IN PAIN PROCESSING AND MODULATION

Mounting evidence suggests that strong unrelenting pain changes the structure and function of nerves that create widespread degenerative alterations in brain functioning,[44,45] which may explain the learning, memory, and emotional difficulties experienced by older adults with persistent pain.[46] Physiologically, aging alters functions, including a degeneration of peripheral neuronal structures, which slow transduction and transmission involved in signaling pain.[47] These changes may result in a slowed pain response, but aging does not decrease sensitivity to pain, which may actually increase with age.[48] Once pain is established, the lower density of descending inhibitory circuits and an impaired ability to recover from hyperalgesic states are attributed to aging.[49] Although some of these changes are partially reversible with effective treatment,[50,51] changes in endogenous pain modulation increase older adults' risk for developing persistent pain following an illness, surgery, or trauma.[52]

Concerns arise regarding how pain processes, including judgment of its presence and severity, is experienced in those with dementia. Although research is mixed, recent studies suggest persons with Alzheimer disease are less sensitive to the detection of thermal pain but do not differ in affective response to unpleasant stimuli, contributing to greater pain and potential damage before identifying and reporting pain.[53] Thus, cognitively impaired older adults are able to feel painful stimuli[54] and may have heightened pain sensitivity.[55] Assuming that older adults, particularly those with cognitive impairment, experience less pain makes them vulnerable to undertreatment of pain and its consequences.[56,57] Although there are instances of atypical presentations of clinical pain in older adults (e.g., silent myocardial infarctions and the absence of abdominal pain with peptic ulcer disease), these exceptions should not be used to suggest that older adults, particularly those with cognitive impairment, feel less pain.

Assessment of Pain in the Older Person

CLINICAL EVALUATION OF PAIN

A comprehensive approach to assessment is necessary when evaluating pain in older adults and developing an effective treatment approach, including identification of the underlying cause of pain, pain characteristics, and impact on physical and psychosocial function and quality of life.[58] The scope and nature of the pain assessment will depend on a number of factors such as the physiologic stability of the patient, whether the situation is an emergency or planned event, and the severity of the presenting pain complaint. If the older adult presents in moderate to severe acute pain (e.g., greater than 4 on a 0-to-10 numeric rating scale), the first priority is to complete an initial, rapid pain assessment and treat the pain.[40,59] Once the older person's pain is alleviated, a comprehensive pain assessment should be completed.

As with younger patients, self-report of pain is the criterion standard for determining pain presence and severity. The numeric rating scale, verbal descriptor scale, and faces pain scale are the most established tools for the alert, cognitively intact older adults.[60] The Iowa Pain Thermometer demonstrated comparable results to these scales and is most preferred by many older adults.[61,62] Cultural differences in tool understanding and preference also inform the need to solicit individual tool preferences.[63,64] These scales can be used more effectively in older persons by addressing sensory deficits (uses eyeglasses, hearing aids, large font/bold print written tools, etc.). Cognitive impairment can result in underreporting of pain; however, recent studies document that standard assessment techniques can be used effectively in older adults with mild to moderate cognitive impairment.[65,66] It is useful to adopt more than one validated tool for use in clinical settings to accommodate needs and preferences of different older patients. All team members (including caregivers) need to use the tool that patient prefers consistently for all pain assessments.

As a multidimensional experience, pain evaluation includes intensity, affect (how bothersome, distressing and effect on mood), sensory qualities (such as aching, stabbing, burning), spatial quality (e.g., location), temporal quality (including pattern and duration), and impact on or interference with daily activities (including physical and psychosocial functioning).[17] Multiple biopsychosocial factors (e.g., anxiety, depression, beliefs, insomnia, fear avoidance, biomechanical issues) contribute to the experience of pain and should be evaluated for their contribution to impairment or dysfunction.[67] Evidence of pain impact includes disrupted social and family relationships, changes in eating and sleeping patterns, and altered mood and ability to continue previous activities. Determining the impact of pain on the older adult's life requires gathering information on key quality of life variables from different sources, including the older adult, significant others, other health care workers, roommates, and activity therapists. The Brief Pain Inventory (BPI) is useful in many settings because it records dimensions of pain in addition to intensity (e.g., interference with functionality).[68] Other tools are available that gather data on pain and its impact in a clinically useful manner, including one called the PEG, that examines three BPI items of Pain intensity, Enjoyment in life, and General activity.[68]

Expanded assessments including the underlying conditions known to be painful and comorbid diseases, the desired and undesired effects of prior and current pain treatments, and current medications (including over-the-counter drugs) provide important information to guide treatment planning. A complete physical examination of the pain source, including potential pain contributors such as leg length discrepancy and myofascial pain, focuses on the most common sources of pain: the musculoskeletal, peripheral vascular, and neurologic systems. Laboratory tests to determine renal and hepatic functioning may be indicated, but diagnostic tests should be used sparingly given that more than half of older patients with radiographic evidence of degenerative joint disease are pain-free and imaging studies are often not necessary or useful.[69]

For a comprehensive review of pain assessment, the reader is referred to the clinical practice guidelines on acute and persistent pain available through the University of Iowa Csomay Center for Gerontological Excellence (http://www.iowanursngguidelines.com).[41,70]

NONVERBAL, COGNITIVELY IMPAIRED OLDER ADULTS

When the patient is unable to reliably self-report the presence or nature of pain due to severe cognitive impairment or critical illness, clinicians rely on a combination of assessment strategies to fill this void. An approach for recognizing pain in nonverbal older adults includes a process of data gathering that includes (1) attempting self-report, (2) identifying pathologic conditions or procedures that usually cause pain, (3) identifying behaviors associated with pain, (4) obtaining input from a family member or others knowledgeable of the older adult, and (5) attempting an analgesic trial to verify that suspected behaviors are pain-related.[58]

Even if the patient is unconscious, intubated, or chemically paralyzed, the clinician's understanding of the pain typically associated with the medical conditions/procedures allows them to make assumptions about the presence of pain and guide pain prevention and treatment interventions regardless of cognitive/verbal abilities. A good history and physical examination provides information on pain-related diagnoses and conditions that support a judgment of pain present.

Directly observable behaviors, such as grimacing, moaning, guarding, bracing, and posturing as well as those less common such as agitation, aggression, restlessness, resisting care, and changes in usual behavior patterns, are recognized as important indicators of pain in those who cannot communicate their pain verbally.[71,72] Among the behaviors displayed by people unable to communicate their pain, facial expression is being recognized as a common and essential element of the behavioral assessment.[71,73] A large number of behavioral pain assessment tools have been developed for use in this population. Systematic reviews have evaluated the strengths and limitations of existing behavioral tools reaching similar conclusions that there is no single tool appropriate for all patients and settings.[74] Updates on existing tools and psychometric properties, as well as recommendations for use, are available.[54,75] Research is ongoing to refine pain behavior indicators and tools to advance clinically useful methods of pain evaluation in this challenging population.[76]

Evidence from any of the aforementioned steps can inform clinician judgment and decision making about pain presence in the older person with advanced dementia. Use of an analgesic trial has shown positive effects in improving disturbing and distressing behaviors,[77] confirming underlying pain etiologies. Pain treatment planning is often oversimplified, expecting patients to respond similarly to the same noxious stimuli and therapeutic intervention. This may work with mild, fleeting pain, but when pain is severe and/or persistent, developing a safe, effective plan needs to be tailored to the patient's unique perceptions, capabilities, comorbid conditions, and responses. The initial goal of any pain treatment plan is to find and eliminate its source if possible and then balance concerns for pain reduction, functional improvement, and avoidance of treatment-related harm. Frequent, ongoing reassessments enhance understanding of the patient's unique pain and response to therapy and refinements need to ensure optimal safety and effectiveness.

Pharmacologic Treatment of Pain in Older Persons

PHARMACOKINETICS AND PHARMACODYNAMICS ASSOCIATED WITH AGING

With the exception of the rectal route, the rate of medication absorption is not typically affected by aging. The pattern of drug distribution does change because of less total body water and more body fat seen in many older adults. This favors the distribution and accumulation of lipophilic (fentanyl) agents while decreasing that of hydrophilic (morphine) drugs. The decline in serum protein concentrations with age can increase the bioavailability of drugs, like nonsteroidal anti-inflammatory drugs (NSAIDs), that are highly protein-bound.[78] This effect is magnified in frail, protein-depleted older adults[79] and patients taking multiple medications that displace NSAIDs from protein-binding sites.

The metabolism and excretion of NSAIDs is often compromised due to the smaller size, lower blood flow, and reduced function of the liver with age. These hepatic changes combined with fewer drug-metabolizing enzymes, increase drug elimination time, and slow the metabolism required to produce active metabolites. Reductions in renal size, glomerular filtration rate, and renal blood flow raise the risk of side effects and toxicity from slowed elimination of the drug and active and toxic metabolites.[80] NSAIDs can further contribute to this slowed clearance by lowering renal blood flow and glomerular filtration rate through its antiprostaglandin effect.

Pharmacodynamic changes with aging increase sensitivity to both the desired and undesired effects of opioids.[81] Combined with other age-related changes in the neurologic and pulmonary systems, there is a greater risk of sedation, sleep apnea, and respiratory depression with opioid analgesics.[82] Combined, these pharmacokinetic and pharmacodynamic changes warrant using lower doses and longer dosing intervals with advanced age, especially with known hepatic or renal impairment, and frailty, with or without cognitive impairment.[79]

SAFE, EFFECTIVE USE OF NONOPIOIDS IN THE OLDER PERSON
Acetaminophen

Acetaminophen is considered the safest nonopioid analgesic and is the first-line analgesic of choice for older patients when pain is mild or moderate.[17,83] Compared to other nonopioids, it has similar or lower analgesic potency but lacks undesirable gastroduodenopathy and platelet dysfunction.[40,84] Limited effectiveness compared to placebos or other analgesics call into questions its inclusion as a first-line, first-choice analgesic for older adults for all types of pain.[85] When combined with warfarin, over-anticoagulation can result.[86] Persistent excessive use of acetaminophen may impair renal function and cause hepatotoxicity, especially in frail elders and those with chronic alcohol consumption and/or liver disease. A systematic review of observational studies showed a consistent dose–response association between acetaminophen and the same serious gastrointestinal (GI), renal, and cardiovascular adverse drug events that are often observed with NSAIDs.[87] Dosage limits in the range of 2,400 to 3,250 mg daily have been suggested to minimize the risk of renal or hepatic toxicity in these populations with the caveat that most harm results from inadvertent use of multiple acetaminophen-containing drugs.[85,86]

Nonsteroidal Anti-inflammatory Drugs

NSAIDs are effective at alleviating pain, especially types that result from inflammation. When combined with acetaminophen for acute pain, NSAIDs have a similar potency to weak opioids (e.g., codeine or tramadol).[86,88] NSAIDs have both analgesic and anti-inflammatory properties; however, there is little evidence they are useful for neuropathic pain, and they have little effect on back pain.[89,90] The use of long-term NSAIDs needs careful monitoring in older people because of increased risk of GI ulceration and bleeding and renal and cardiovascular morbidity. Cautious use of NSAIDs is advised because a quarter of hospitalizations resulting from adverse drug effects are linked to NSAIDs in older patients. Thus, use of NSAIDs for more than a several days should be avoided unless alternatives are ineffective and the patient can take gastroprotective misoprostol or a proton pump inhibitor (PPI).[40,91,92] The PPI option tends to be better tolerated but exposes older adults to the risk of bone loss, fractures, *Clostridium difficile* infections, and subacute cutaneous lupus erythematosus with long-term use.[92,93]

Concerned that medication-related problems are a leading cause of hospitalization and death among older adults, the American Geriatrics Society updates the Beers Criteria, a list of medications and drug classes that are inappropriate to prescribe older adults, regardless of frailty. As a class, the chronic use of any NSAID should be avoided without gastroprotection. Any use should be avoided in those with a history of gastroduodenal ulcers, stage IV kidney disease, or congestive heart failure. Use for more than 8 days, certain products (indomethacin or ketorolac) are particularly concerning when used in older adults, as is the combination with other NSAIDs, corticosteroids, antidepressants, anticoagulants, or antiplatelet agents.[94,95] Despite these warnings, NSAIDs are prescribed to 40% of older adults with chronic pain, which may contribute to 3,300 NSAID-linked deaths and 41,000 hospitalizations observed in the United States per year.[85,92,96]

The COX-2 selective NSAIDs appear to have less risk of GI ulcerations and bleeding in the elderly than do nonselective NSAIDs.[95] However, the GI safety advantages of COX-2 selective NSAIDs are significantly reduced if high doses are used or when used in combination with aspirin or other NSAIDs. Although celecoxib has been suspected of placing patients at higher risk of cardiovascular death, a recent 3-year prospective randomized control trial using 200 mg of celecoxib per day showed a similar or better cardiovascular, GI, and renal safety profile when compared with ibuprofen or naproxen.[95] When the risks specific to rofecoxib were examined in a meta-analysis, it was that drug, rather than COX-2 selectivity, that contributed to elevated risks of cardiovascular deaths observed with long-term use of these medications.[97]

Safe Nonsteroidal Anti-inflammatory Drug Product Selection and Monitoring Use

The decision to use an NSAID in the management of persistent pain for an older adult requires individualization considering the (pain reduction and functional improvement) effectiveness balanced against potential harms considering comorbidities, concomitant medications, and associated risk factors. If short-term NSAID therapy is considered and GI risk is considered low, it may be reasonable to select celecoxib, ibuprofen, or naproxen. Continuing NSAID therapy beyond a few weeks should be done cautiously with baseline and periodic monitoring of vital signs, renal functioning, and occult GI bleeding.[98] Given an analgesic ceiling, patients are started at a low dose and asked to record the analgesic effect for 1 to 2 weeks before increasing the dose. If, after titrating to a higher dose, there is no analgesic advantage, return to the lower dose. To lessen the risk of GI and renal toxicity, urge the patient to drink a full glass of water with the NSAID to maintain adequate hydration throughout therapy.

In general, after acetaminophen is deemed inadequate or contraindicated, NSAIDs with the highest safety margin should be used in the lowest effective dose for the shortest duration.[92] For patients at highest GI risk (history of ulcers), celecoxib 100 to 200 mg per day plus a PPI is considered.[85] Because traditional NSAIDs (except naproxen) inhibit the effects of cardioprotective aspirin and increase GI risk, this combination is avoided.[99] Other options for high-risk patients include nonacetylated salicylates or topical NSAIDs and may have better safety margins than more traditional options. Salsalate (Disalcid) has advantages of minimal GI toxicity, no effects on platelets, and a twice-daily dosing regimen.[85]

Topical NSAIDs are a viable therapeutic option with a more desirable tolerability profile, less end-organ dysfunction, and GI bleed compared with their oral counterparts.[100] Topical agents are particularly beneficial when pain is localized, acute, and superficial, as it places a higher concentration at the target tissue for appropriately selected inflammatory conditions. Additional advantages include fewer systemic side effects (dry skin is the primary side effect), a lower pill burden, and avoidance of drug interactions.[85,101]

SAFE, EFFECTIVE USE OF OPIOIDS IN THE OLDER PERSON POTENTIAL RISKS OF OPIOID ANALGESICS

Declines in NSAID use by older adults have paralleled increased utilization of opioids. An estimated 9% of those older adults living in the community and 70% of those with persistent pain in nursing homes have been prescribed opioids. The American Geriatric Society guidelines identified opioids as the cornerstone for treating moderate and severe pain unresponsive to other therapy.[80,91] The place of opioid therapy is now being scrutinized given renewed concerns about potential harms, especially for older adults who are sensitive to their effects and those with renal or hepatic dysfunction.[86,102] Although older adults are generally less likely to receive opioids than their younger counterparts, they ironically are more likely to receive opioids when they sustain a fracture.[103] Despite literature continuing to support the undertreatment of older adults with pain, more opioid therapy does not guarantee better pain control.[104]

Although far from a panacea for all types of pain, a meta-analysis showed opioids to be as effective for older adults as younger patients in yielding pain reduction, functional improvement, better sleep, and quality of life.[105] As many as two-thirds of older adults who start an opioid for chronic musculoskeletal conditions achieve pain relief, but it remains unclear how long those benefits are sustained, especially because nearly half of older adults discontinue therapy because of poorly tolerated constipation, mental status changes, and nausea.[17] It isn't clear what percentage of patients would continue therapy if the GI side effects were effectively treated prophylactically, but every effort should be made to do so.[84,100] It also is unclear about the effect opioids have on mental status changes in older adults because higher pain, more intravenous fluids, and baseline antidepressant medication contribute to these changes.[106] A study examining rates of delirium after hip fracture surgery found that severe pain and the use of low doses of opioids were correlated significantly with progression to delirium. In contrast, those using higher doses of opioids did not develop or worsen delirium regardless of their baseline level of cognitive functioning.[107] What is clear is that given known risks associated with opioid use, the potential negative effects must be weighed against the consequences of untreated or partially treated pain.

Potential Safety Concerns with Opioids

Opioids increase the risk of falls, particularly during the first 2 weeks of use.[108] This risk is compounded when used in combination with other medications (e.g., benzodiazepines, antipsychotics, antidepressants) that affect the central nervous system.[80] Patients prescribed with opioids should be told to abstain from driving or other potentially dangerous activities until they have been free of visual or cognitive impairment for several days on a steady dose. As a drug class, opioids can be appropriate for older adults without a history of falls or fractures with the exception of propoxyphene, meperidine, and pentazocine which do carry additional risks for older adults.[92] Tramadol, meperidine, and fentanyl can also increase the risk of serotonin syndrome in older adults when given with other serotonergic drugs.[80]

The established risks associated with opioid use must be weighed against the consequences of poorly controlled pain. Systematic reviews express concern that effectiveness may wane over time, but the risks for serious harm remain, especially at higher doses.[102,109] Apart from estimates that tramadol is no stronger than NSAIDs, there is no evidence to support the superiority of opioid over another.[105] Reluctance to prescribe opioid drugs has probably been overly influenced by political and social pressures to control illicit drug use.[110–112]

Among adults 65 years and older, 736 fatalities were reported among the 33,091 opioid overdose deaths in 2015.[113] That represents 2% of opioid overdose deaths for the year and the lowest rate for any adult age group. Conversely, adults 45 to 54 years old had the highest death rate (8/100,000) of any age group. Aside from prescription opioids, overdoses from heroin and illicit synthetic opioids rose at an overall rate of 21% and 72%, respectively, in 2014 and 2015 accounting for 22,569 deaths compared to 12,727 deaths attributed to prescription natural and semisynthetic opioids.[113] Many prescription opioid deaths are caused by abuse or misuse of prescription opioids and being combined with benzodiazepines, which increases the overdose risk 10-fold.[114] In contrast to young adults who misuse opioids seeking euphoria, older adults may take additional medication as a result of forgetfulness, being desperate to achieve pain control, or as part of a suicidal intent.[84,102,115] The estimated prevalence of opioid misuse in older adults is 1% to 3%, which remains lower and may account for significantly less prevalent opioid overdoses than their younger counterparts.[80] Although substance abuse, diversion, and addiction disorders do occur in older adults, many are deprived prescriptions or refuse them because of overstated risks that fail to discriminate legitimate use from illicit nonmedical opioid use.[112]

Prudent Product Selection and Use

The decision to initiate opioids is made cautiously including screening patients for biopsychosocial risk factors, starting with weak, short-acting, low-dose opioids after discussing risks and the need for vigilant monitoring with the patient and caregiver.[17] Weak, atypical opioids may also be effective and have reduced likelihood of side effects such as constipation, a predictable side effect that should be treated prophylactically in older adults.[100] Tapentadol or transdermal buprenorphine are weak/mixed opioids with less risk for the toxicities associated with conventional opioids.[100,116] For adults over age 75 years with chronic arthritis or low back pain, tapentadol was shown to be as effective as oxycodone with fewer side effects over a 2-year trial period.[117,118] Transdermal buprenorphine is simple to administer (improves adherence) and avoids the first-pass metabolism which results in fewer drug–drug interactions, with less respiratory, hormonal, and immune system effects than oral opioids.[119] The absorption, distribution, metabolism, and excretion of buprenorphine, as well as the ceiling to its respiratory depressant effects, make it a good choice for older adults.[119] Given the limits of existing data, however, more familiar and less expensive opioids are generally preferred.[120]

Oxycodone and morphine are probably the best first-line opioids agents for an opioid-naive patient with acute pain. The adage, start low–go slow, would have the prudent clinician starting as low as 2.5 mg oxycodone, 5 mg oral morphine, or 1 to 2 mg parenteral morphine and then basing adjustments on the individual response. Tramadol is commonly chosen, but it has low potency and an association with seizures that requires cautious patient selection and attention to potential drug–drug interactions.[17,79]

For opioid-tolerant patients, methadone is an effective, relatively low-cost choice for carefully selected and monitored patients with refractory pain. Its use is limited by pharmacokinetic, cardiac, and drug-interaction pitfalls that require methadone to be used by highly informed experienced prescribers.[100,121] Levorphanol offers several therapeutic advantages similar to methadone but without its pharmacokinetic and drug-interaction pitfalls.[100] Drug selection decisions should ultimately depend on severity of pain, functional status, expected pain duration, and prescriber and patient preference. Regardless of selection, the lowest tolerated dose that leads to acceptable relief of pain is used, with frequent, vigilant evaluation of desired and undesired effects.[17,80]

Chronic opioid therapy requires additional safeguards be in place.[122] This is particularly true for older adults with preexisting respiratory dysfunction, including chronic obstructive pulmonary disease, emphysema, kyphoscoliosis, severe obesity, or cor pulmonale. Patients with persistent pain taking opioids often develop sleep disordered breathing, with older age and higher doses associated with both central and obstructive forms of sleep apnea that must be evaluated and treated.[82] Opioids can also cause peripheral vasodilatation which may produce orthostatic hypotension and a corresponding risk of falling. The impact of endocrine effects, immune system suppression, and opioid-induced hyperalgesia on older adults is currently being investigated,[123–127] as is the emergence of novel opioids to offset known risks that limit their use.

SAFE, EFFECTIVE USE OF ADJUVANTS IN THE OLDER PERSON

Adjuvant analgesics include a variety of agents with analgesic activity whose primary approved indication is for conditions other than pain. Many of these adjuvants are used "off-label" and have been found clinically useful for specific pain types.[128] These drugs may be used alone, or in combination with analgesics to treat persistent pain conditions, including neuropathic pain. A systematic analysis of 52 Cochrane reviews on anticonvulsants, antidepressants, behavioral, and analgesics found no treatment for chronic pain met the Centers for Disease Control and Prevention (CDC) criteria for "adequate long-term trials." Those reviews also failed to show any published evidence of a chronic pain treatment that has stronger evidence of effectiveness than opioids.[129] Thus, adjuvant therapy may need to be used in addition to, rather than instead of, opioid therapy to achieve optimal benefits.

Among antidepressants with analgesics properties, amitriptyline has the longest track record of positive trials but should be avoided in older adults due to its cardiac, anticholinergic, and sedative effects.[85] There are fewer anticholinergic adverse effects with a second-generation tricyclic antidepressants (nortriptyline or desipramine), suggesting these are better choices for older adults.[84] In hospitalized patients, however, their use is an independent predictor of postoperative delirium, increased costs, and prolonged length of stay.[106] Serotonin and norepinephrine reuptake inhibitors (SNRIs) like duloxetine and venlafaxine have fewer of these undesired effects but a greater risk of drug interactions and elevation of liver enzymes.[130] This class of drugs should be used cautiously as antidepressant-related deaths rose nearly 40% in the past 15 years, half of which were suicides.[131]

Antiepileptic drugs are first-line agents to treat neuropathic pain in older persons.[89] Gabapentin and pregabalin have labeled indications for specific neuropathic pain disorders and are frequently used for postherpetic neuralgia, painful diabetic neuropathy, and fibromyalgia. For these conditions, they provide similar analgesia to antidepressants, with improvements in mood, sleep, and quality of life.[85] Although pregabalin is regarded as the most effective in the class, a recent study found it no better than placebo for sciatica over an 8-week treatment course.[132] Thus, it cannot be assumed to be effective for all neuropathic pain types. The side effects of sedation, mental clouding, and dizziness are dose-limiting initially, and some patients are unable to tolerate these medications at the required therapeutic doses. Older antiepileptic drugs like carbamazepine may also be useful, but drug interactions, renal, liver, and hematologic toxicity make them less than ideal in older adults.[85] This class of medications carries a similar warning as opioids regarding avoiding their use in patients with a history of falls and fractures.[92]

Topical capsaicin is available over the counter at very low concentrations (0.025% to 0.075%) for the treatment of neuropathic and musculoskeletal conditions.[86] This medication is very safe except for a redness and burning sensation with thermal hyperalgesia on treated skin. Residual medication must be removed from the fingers that applied it to avoid exposing and irritating sensitive mucous membranes. The higher concentration (8%) synthetic capsaicin adhesive patch is a selective agonist of transient receptor potential vanilloid 1 channel, approved for treating peripheral neuropathic pain. A single 30-minute application of the capsaicin 8% patch significantly improves postherpetic neuralgia pain.[86] Additional studies examining a single 60-minute application or several 30-minute applications 2 months apart have provided good pain relief for different painful neuropathies.[133] Although widely used with reports of clinical success, topical lidocaine has failed to demonstrate efficacy from large, good-quality randomized controlled studies treating neuropathic pain.[134]

Other adjuvant drugs can be used in the older adult for their coanalgesic effect or to offset side effects of pain relievers. They are often selected for their general ability target mechanisms believed to cause or amplify the patient's pain, such as α_2-adrenergic or γ-aminobutyric acid ($GABA_B$) agonists, N-methyl-D-aspartate (NMDA) receptor antagonists, or cannabinoids. Effects vary considerably based on a variety of factors; therefore, it is prudent to start one agent at a time at a low dose, titrate carefully, and have frequent monitoring to establish the safety and efficacy before adding, subtracting, or adjusting other medications.[135]

Additional Treatments for Pain of Older Person

Pharmacologic management is the foundation of pain treatment in most settings; however, medications often fall short of providing optimal pain reduction and functional improvement. Guidelines are now recommending a trial of nondrug techniques before starting medications.[136] When ineffective alone, nondrug therapies should continue when analgesics are added for their medication-sparing benefits.[136] In conventional medicine, physical or psychosocial (cognitive/behavioral) modalities are often provided by a physical therapist, physiatrist, and/or psychologist. A variety of nonmainstream approaches to relieving pain when combined with conventional therapy are called complementary and integrative health (CIH) approaches. Alternative medical systems (e.g., Ayurvedic medicine, traditional Chinese medicine, homeopathy, and naturopathy) are not included as CIH approaches when they exclude conventional medical approaches.

Multidisciplinary pain treatment programs integrate physical, cognitive-behavioral, and some complementary approaches to optimize the treatment for patients with complex pain that has not responded to sequential treatment attempts.[137] Many nondrug approaches are underused in older patients, and professionals are urged to integrate these modalities, especially cognitive-behavioral therapy (CBT) and exercise into treatment plans.[17]

INTERVENTIONAL APPROACHES
Interventional approaches can provide significant benefit to older adults whose severe, disabling pain is not responsive to less invasive measures. Proper patient selection and highly trained professionals are needed to perform specific procedures with precision, followed by ongoing vigilant monitoring.[138] Many specialists use fluoroscopic verification of needle placement for many nerve blocks procedures to avoid the life-threatening risk of intravascular injections.[139,140] Older adults are particularly at higher risk in the setting of anticoagulation, uncontrolled diabetes, or cardiovascular or progressive neurologic disorders. Guidelines for interventions like facet joint and epidural spinal injections (ESIs) were developed by a Multisociety Pain Workgroup out of a concern that the number of these procedures more than doubled between 1994 and 2001 among Medicare patients. Their 17 recommendations provide strict guidance for patient selection and safety, which have been widely adopted by payers.[141] Recommendations include that cervical and lumbar interlaminar ESIs be performed with image guidance and transforaminal ESIs be conducted under real-time fluoroscopy or digital subtraction angiography. Cervical interlaminar ESIs above C6–C7 are not advised, and cervical transforaminal ESIs should only be done using nonparticulate steroids. Safety guidelines include limiting sedation levels and using precautions to prevent infections.[142] Despite these safeguards, the evidence of effectiveness is still not well established for older adults.[84]

Implanted spinal cord stimulator technology has rapidly advanced for back, leg, and phantom pain, holding promise to control pain with few if any drugs needed.[143,144] Innovative less invasive approaches are being developed that may benefit older adults who are not candidates for existing surgical procedures or dorsal column stimulation used to treat pain.[134,145] Exciting developments in noninvasive interventions, such as pulsed electromagnetic field (PEMF) therapy, hold promise for common ailments with advancing age, such as arthritis. This PEMF therapy can be administered three times a week for several weeks, or patients can self-apply bands around their affected joint (e.g., knee) every day to reduce pain, stiffness, and medication use while improving their functioning.[146,147]

PHYSICAL MODALITIES
Physical modalities to pain control range from simple applications of heat/cold, orthotics, or electrical stimulating devices patients can self-manage to more technical interventions requiring professional expertise like low-level laser treatments. Active techniques, like therapeutic exercise and aquatic therapy, work better for able-bodied older adults than passive approaches like superficial heat, transcutaneous electrical nerve stimulation (TENS), and acupuncture.[148] Physical therapists have developed graded activity programs to tailor treatments best aligned with the physical capacity of older adults with pain.[149] There are a variety of therapeutic exercises, salves, nutritional supplements and self-management techniques commonly used to reduce pain and medication use while improving well-being.[150,151]

Promoting active involvement in pain management, like home exercise programs, pacing activities, or the application of salves, are increasingly being used to provide relief while reducing medication-related problems.[150,151] Simple advice to remain physically active despite pain, in the absence of a specific exercise routine, is ineffective.[17] More structured exercise interventions for older adults with chronic pain are evidenced-based and underutilized and should be a core component of any long-term treatment plan, even for nursing home residents.[151] Moderate pressure massage and Iyengar yoga (focusing on poses) is increasingly being used to reduce pain and improve balance and mobility, even for hospitalized older patients with pain.[152,153] Physiotherapist often integrate exercises that promote balance, flexibility, body mechanics, pacing, endurance, and strengthening to not only lower pain but also reduce catastrophic thinking and avoidance behaviors known to make back pain worse.[149]

Although generally safe, some precautions are advised. Protect the skin of older adults when topical heat or cold compresses are applied and use extra lotion or gel when applying TENS pads or giving a massage.[154,155] Although commercially available natural products and supplements are safe when they do not interact with drugs, some herbal remedies have been tainted with drugs or heavy metals.[156,157] Safety precautions are needed for older adults receiving physical manipulation and body-based therapies (e.g., chiropractors, osteopaths, physical and massage therapists) because of the high risk for falls observed among individuals who use these therapies.[158]

PSYCHOSOCIAL MODALITIES

A variety of psychosocial modalities strive to change the perception of pain or alter the unhelpful thoughts, feelings, or behavioral responses that worsen pain and suffering. Specific techniques include education and counseling, distraction, coping skills training, relaxation, imagery, hypnotherapy, and facilitating emotional disclosure that help older adults with pain.[153,159,160] Structured programs like CBT, acceptance and commitment therapy (ACT), and peer-led self-management programs help older adults despite barriers to accessing them.[17,84] New models of bringing these programs to older adults are proving feasible and effective.[161–164] Although these and other psychosocial modalities help many older persons, some lack the physical or mental capacity to participate, and interventions need to be tailored to their specific (e.g., visual or auditory impairment, limited mobility) circumstance.[154,165]

When psychological attributions for pain, emotional awareness, emotional approach coping, and alexithymia are directly addressed, large effects were seen with sustained improvements in pain, functioning, and mood.[160] Pain self-management group programs suggest a smaller but significant sustained benefits can be achieved through that approach.[166] Perhaps a common thread in some of these approaches is moving away from a traditional style of trying to persuade patients to change behavior and toward asking thought-provoking questions that prompt desire, ability, reasons, and need to change, so the patient can take action based on their individual values and motivators.[167]

Older adults do benefit from structured CBT or ACT programs and may be more likely to respond than younger adults.[168] It is unclear if "booster sessions" would help because the effects of pain reduction do persist, but measures of functional improvement are not sustained.[169] Even if physical functioning is not improved, psychological flexibility, social functioning, and mental health is improved.[170]

COMPLEMENTARY AND INTEGRATIVE HEALTH

Pain is the most common health problem driving people to use CIH approaches. American spend 3 times more in out-of-pocket expenses ($15 billion per year) for complementary therapies than they do for conventional medicine.[171,172] Three-quarters of adults over age 50 years who use CIH methods reportedly did so to treat a painful condition.[173] Arthritis and low back pain are commonly treated with mind–body therapies, acupuncture, yoga, massage, spinal manipulation, thermotherapy, and tai chi.[172,174] In fact, slightly more older adults use CIH measures than conventional therapies for low back pain (96% and 95%, respectively),[150] which is aligned with recommendations of recent guidelines.[90,136] For older adults, yoga, massage, and natural products are especially appealing and are demonstrating their cost-effectiveness.[159,175] Despite a lack of strong evidence that yoga or qigong decreases low back pain, the physical postures, breathing techniques, and focused intention do improve functioning, balance, mood, self-efficacy, and quality of life.[152,176,177] Yoga may also improve memory and cognitive functioning and reverse some of the atrophic changes in the brain brought on by chronic pain and aging.[178,179]

There is evidence spinal manipulation, mind–body therapies, and natural products CIH modalities are cost-effective for older adults with pain.[175,180] Access to CIH, however, may be limited by cost, ease of access, facility policies, or physician concern. Even when they are used, patients do not disclose CIH use to health professionals.[181,182] Even though CIH is reluctantly used in frail older adults, many methods have demonstrated safety, with the added safety of reducing exposure to potentially dangerous drugs, or the need for physical or chemical restraints.[183,184] Some potential danger exists with some CIH methods, as acupuncture-related infections, nerve injuries, organ perforation, serious bleeds, and pneumothorax have been reported in older adults.[185,186] To offset these concerns, some are using the less invasive acupressure to alleviate chronic pain, but a high dropout rate suggests it is not for everyone.[187] Aromatherapy has provided transient relief of pain, improved mood, and reduced stress levels among older adults, but additional studies are needed.[188,189]

MULTIDISCIPLINARY PAIN TREATMENTS

Multidisciplinary pain treatment programs are underutilized for older adults who respond similarly as younger adults with persistent pain.[84,190,191] Multidisciplinary pain clinics have better outcomes in terms of pain reduction, functional improvement, and lower health care utilization than those who receive only single-modality interventions. About a third of patients with chronic low back pain that has not responded to other treatments gain significant control of their pain as a result of a multidisciplinary pain treatment program.[192] Even patients who do not achieve significant pain control in this type of a program are satisfied with the treatment and feel better able to self-manage their symptoms,[193] which may be why some emergency departments now provide multidisciplinary education improved pain outcomes.[194]

Although the cost–benefit ratio has not clearly been delineated for older adults, there is no compelling evidence to suggest that they should be denied such treatment. In fact, the potential adverse effects of untreated pain and/or polypharmacy suggest that multidisciplinary treatment should be considered for all geriatric patients with significant pain complaints.

Summary

Certainly, there are risks when treating older adults with severe or persistent pain. In fact, the undertreatment of pain is an important risk that can contribute to physical harm, mental despair, and social isolation during what has been dubbed "the golden years." Although much remains to be learned, we currently have sufficient knowledge to improve the way pain is assessed and treated while refining methods to further improve the safety and efficacy of pain relief efforts. Clear consistent assessment methods are needed by choosing and using tools validated for older adults. The patient's understanding of the tool should be confirmed so that meaningful information is gathered and recorded. When planning interventions, a shared decision-making approach is appropriate, where patients and their loved ones are informed of the risks, benefits, and variable responses typical for particular treatment options. This shared decision making engages the patients as active participants in the treatment process and educates them about desired and undesired effects that may be encountered and need to be recorded. Cautious drug and dose selection is needed for the older adult. Lower starting doses and longer dosing intervals are justified until the patient's response to analgesics is known. Monitoring the patient's response early in therapy for side effects, drug (or herbal) interactions, and toxicity is important, especially for those with comorbid conditions that add risks. Continued monitoring for older adults on sustained treatment is important as several late-onset toxicities (e.g., GI bleed, hypertension, liver/renal impairment, opioid-induced hyperalgesia) may not emerge until months or years of therapy have passed. The prudent use of nonoperative interventions (e.g., nerve blocks) and nondrug or complementary, integrative therapies should be considered for older adults with persistent pain. Given the breadth of options available to treat pain, allowing it to go untreated in older adults is a mistake. Whereas not all treatments are good options for older adults, failing to treat pain is unacceptable, especially for those who are so vulnerable to the harmful effects of unrelieved pain.

References

1. Shega JW, Dale W, Andrew M, et al. Persistent pain and frailty: a case for homeostenosis. *J Am Geriatr Soc* 2012;60(1):113–117.
2. Simon LS. Relieving pain in America: A blueprint for transforming prevention, care, education, and research [book review]. *J Pain Palliat Care Pharmacother* 2012;26(2):197–198.
3. Kennedy J, Roll JM, Schraudner T, et al. Prevalence of persistent pain in the U.S. adult population: new data from the 2010 national health interview survey. *J Pain* 2014;15(10):979–984.
4. Dieleman JL, Baral R, Birger M, et al. US spending on personal health care and public health, 1996-2013. *JAMA* 2016;316(24):2627–2646.
5. United Nations, Department of Economic and Social Affairs, Population Division. *World Population Ageing 2015*. New York: United Nations; 2015.
6. Stewart Williams J, Ng N, Peltzer K, et al. Risk factors and disability associated with low back pain in older adults in low- and middle-income countries. Results from the WHO Study on Global AGEing and Adult Health (SAGE). *PLoS One* 2015;10(6):e0127880.
7. Gibson SJ, Lussier D. Prevalence and relevance of pain in older persons. *Pain Med* 2012;13(suppl 2):S23–S26.
8. Patel KV, Guralnik JM, Dansie EJ, et al. Prevalence and impact of pain among older adults in the United States: findings from the 2011 National Health and Aging Trends Study. *Pain* 2013;154(12):2649–2657.
9. Hunt LJ, Covinsky KE, Yaffe K, et al. Pain in community-dwelling older adults with dementia. *J Am Geriatr Soc* 2015;63:1503.
10. Lapane KL, Quilliam BJ, Chow W, et al. The association between pain and measures of well-being among nursing home residents. *J Am Med Dir Assoc* 2012;13(4):344–349.
11. Pimentel CB, Briesacher BA, Gurwitz JH, et al. Pain management in nursing home residents with cancer. *J Am Geriatr Soc* 2015;63(4):633–641.
12. Herr K, Titler M, Fine P, et al. Assessing and treating pain in hospices: current state of evidence-based practices. *J Pain Symptom Manage* 2010;39(5):803–819.
13. Thompson GN, Doupe M, Reid RC, et al. Pain trajectories of nursing home residents nearing death. *J Am Med Dir Assoc* 2017;18(8):700–706.
14. Gianni W, Madaio RA, Di Cioccio L, et al. Prevalence of pain in elderly hospitalized patients. *Arch Gerontol Geriatr* 2010;51(3):273–276.
15. Shega JW, Tiedt AD, Grant K, et al. Pain measurement in the National Social Life, Health, and Aging Project: presence, intensity, and location. *J Gerontol B Psychol Sci Soc Sci* 2014;69(suppl 2):S191–S197.
16. Raja R, Dube B, Hensor EM, et al. The clinical characteristics of older people with chronic multiple-site joint pains and their utilisation of therapeutic interventions: data from a prospective cohort study. *BMC Musculoskelet Disord* 2016;17(1):194.
17. Reid MC, Eccleston C, Pillemer K. Management of chronic pain in older adults. *BMJ* 2015;350:h532.
18. Molton IR, Terrill AL. Overview of persistent pain in older adults. *Am Psychol* 2014;69(2):197.
19. McKeown JL. Pain management issues for the geriatric surgical patient. *Anesthesiol Clin* 2015;33(3):563–576.
20. Hwang U, Platts-Mills TF. Acute pain management in older adults in the emergency department. *Clin Geriatr Med* 2013;29(1):151–164.
21. Fayaza A, Watt HC, Langford RM, et al. The association between chronic pain and cardiac disease: a cross-sectional population study. *Clin J Pain* 2016;32(12):1062–1068.
22. Singer AE, Meeker D, Teno JM, et al. Factors associated with family reports of pain, dyspnea, and depression in the last year of life. *J Palliat Med* 2016;19(10):1066–1073.
23. Parmelee PA, Harralson TL, McPherron JA, et al. The structure of affective symptomatology in older adults with osteoarthritis. *Int J Geriatr Psychiatry* 2013;28(4):393–401.
24. Conaghan PG, Peloso PM, Everett SV, et al. Inadequate pain relief and large functional loss among patients with knee osteoarthritis: evidence from a prospective multinational longitudinal study of osteoarthritis real-world therapies. *Rheumatology (Oxford)* 2015;54(2):270–277.
25. Hermsen LA, Leone SS, Smalbrugge M, et al. Frequency, severity and determinants of functional limitations in older adults with joint pain and comorbidity: results of a cross-sectional study. *Arch Gerontol Geriatr* 2014;59(1):98–106.
26. Makris UE, Higashi RT, Marks EG, et al. Physical, emotional, and social impacts of restricting back pain in older adults: a qualitative study. *Pain Med* 2017;18(7):1225–1235.
27. Stamm TA, Pieber K, Crevenna R, et al. Impairment in the activities of daily living in older adults with and without osteoporosis, osteoarthritis and chronic back pain: a secondary analysis of population-based health survey data. *BMC Musculoskelet Disord* 2016;17(1):139.
28. Eggermont LH, Leveille SG, Shi L, et al. Pain characteristics associated with the onset of disability in older adults: the maintenance of balance, independent living, intellect, and zest in the elderly Boston study. *J Am Geriatr Soc* 2014;62(6):1007–1016.
29. Rundell SD, Sherman KJ, Heagerty PJ, et al. Predictors of persistent disability and back pain in older adults with a new episode of care for back pain. *Pain Med* 2017;18(6):1049–1062.
30. Hanssen DJ, Naarding P, Collard RM, et al. Physical, lifestyle, psychological, and social determinants of pain intensity, pain disability, and the number of pain locations in depressed older adults. *Pain* 2014;155(10):2088–2096.
31. Lacey RJ, Belcher J, Rathod T, et al. Pain at multiple body sites and health-related quality of life in older adults: results from the North Staffordshire Osteoarthritis Project. *Rheumatology (Oxford)* 2014;53(11):2071–2079. doi:10.1093/rheumatology/keu240.
32. Inoue S, Kobayashi F, Nishihara M, et al. Chronic pain in the japanese community—prevalence, characteristics and impact on quality of life. *PLoS One* 2015;10(6):e0129262.
33. Lohman MC, Whiteman KL, Greenberg RL, et al. Incorporating persistent pain in phenotypic frailty measurement and prediction of adverse health outcomes. *J Gerontol A Biol Sci Med Sci* 2017;72(2):216–222.
34. Simmons SF, Schnelle JF, Saraf AA, et al. Pain and satisfaction with pain management among older patients during the transition from acute to skilled nursing care. *Gerontologist* 2016;56(6):1138–1145.
35. Fain KM, Alexander GC, Dore DD, et al. Frequency and predictors of analgesic prescribing in U.S. nursing home residents with persistent pain. *J Am Geriatr Soc* 2017;65(2):286–293.
36. Platts-Mills TF, Esserman DA, Brown DL, et al. Older US emergency department patients are less likely to receive pain medication than younger patients: results from a national survey. *Ann Emerg Med* 2012;60(2):199–206.
37. Marcum ZA, Perera S, Donohue JM, et al. Analgesic use for knee and hip osteoarthritis in community-dwelling elders. *Pain Med* 2011;12(11):1628–1636.
38. Boccio E, Wie B, Pasternak S, et al. The relationship between patient age and pain management of acute long-bone fracture in the ED. *Am J Emerg Med* 2014;32(12):1516–1519.
39. Smith PD, Becker K, Roberts L, et al. Associations among pain, depression, and functional limitation in low-income, home-dwelling older adults: an analysis of baseline data from CAPABLE. *Geriatr Nurs* 2016;37(5):348–352.
40. Abdulla A, Adams N, Bone M, et al. Guidance on the management of pain in older people. *Age Ageing* 2013;42(suppl 1):i1–i57.
41. Arnstein P, Herr K, Butcher HK. Evidence-based practice guideline: persistent pain management in older adults. *J Gerontol Nurs* 2017;43(7):20–31.
42. Qaseem A, Wilt TJ, McLean RM, et al. Noninvasive treatments for acute, subacute, and chronic low back pain: a clinical practice guideline from the American College of Physicians. *Ann Intern Med* 2017;166(7):514–530.
43. Herr K, Arnstein P. The opioid epidemic and persistent pain management in older adults. *J Gerontol Nurs* 2016;42(12):3–4.
44. Seminowicz DA, Labus JS, Bueller JA, et al. Regional gray matter density changes in brains of patients with irritable bowel syndrome. *Gastroenterology* 2010;139(1):48.e2–57.e2.
45. Berliocchi L, Russo R, Tassorelli C, et al. Death in pain: peripheral nerve injury and spinal neurodegenerative mechanisms. *Curr Opin Pharmacol* 2012;12(1):49–54.
46. Mutso AA, Radzicki D, Baliki MN, et al. Abnormalities in hippocampal functioning with persistent pain. *J Neurosci* 2012;32(17):5747–5756.
47. Riley JL III, Cruz-Almeida Y, Glover TL, et al. Age and race effects on pain sensitivity and modulation among middle-aged and older adults. *J Pain* 2014;15(3):272–282.
48. Cole LJ, Farrell MJ, Gibson SJ, et al. Age-related differences in pain sensitivity and regional brain activity evoked by noxious pressure. *Neurobiol Aging* 2010;31(3):494–503.
49. Smith M, Davis MA, Stano M, et al. Aging baby boomers and the rising cost of chronic back pain: secular trend analysis of longitudinal Medical Expenditures Panel Survey data for years 2000 to 2007. *J Manipulative Physiol Ther* 2013;36(1):2–11.
50. Seminowicz DA, Wideman TH, Naso L, et al. Effective treatment of chronic low back pain in humans reverses abnormal brain anatomy and function. *J Neurosci* 2011;31(20):7540–7550.
51. Davis KD, Moayedi M. Central mechanisms of pain revealed through functional and structural MRI. *J Neuroimmune Pharmacol* 2013;8(3):518–534.
52. Naugle KM, Ohlman T, Naugle KE, et al. Physical activity behavior predicts endogenous pain modulation in older adults. *Pain* 2017;158(3):383–390.
53. Monroe TB, Gibson SJ, Bruehl SP, et al. Contact heat sensitivity and reports of unpleasantness in communicative people with mild to moderate cognitive impairment in Alzheimer's disease: a cross-sectional study. *BMC Med* 2016;14(1):74.
54. Hadjistavropoulos T, Herr K, Prkachin KM, et al. Pain assessment in elderly adults with dementia. *Lancet Neurol* 2014;13(12):1216–1227.
55. Defrin R, Amanzio M, de Tommaso M, et al. Experimental pain processing in individuals with cognitive impairment: current state of the science. *Pain* 2015;156(8):1396–1408.
56. Corbett A, Husebo BS, Achterberg WP, et al. The importance of pain management in older people with dementia. *Br Med Bull* 2014;111(1):139–148.
57. Gibson S, Lautenbacher S. Pain perception and report in persons with dementia. In: Lautenbacher S, Gibson SJ, eds. *Pain in Dementia*. Philadelphia: Wolters Kluwer; 2017:chap 3.
58. Booker SQ, Herr KA. Assessment and measurement of pain in adults in later life. *Clin Geriatr Med* 2016;32(4):677–692.

59. Schofield P. The assessment and management of peri-operative pain in older adults. *Anaesthesia* 2014;69(suppl 1):54–60.

60. Lukas A, Barber JB, Johnson P, et al. Observer-rated pain assessment instruments improve both the detection of pain and the evaluation of pain intensity in people with dementia. *Eur J Pain* 2013;17(10):1558–1568.

61. Herr K, Spratt KF, Garand L, et al. Evaluation of the Iowa pain thermometer and other selected pain intensity scales in younger and older adult cohorts using controlled clinical pain: a preliminary study. *Pain Med* 2007;8(7):585–600.

62. Ware LJ, Herr KA, Booker SS, et al. Psychometric evaluation of the revised Iowa Pain Thermometer (IPT-R) in a sample of diverse cognitively intact and impaired older adults: a pilot study. *Pain Manag Nurs* 2015;16(4):475–482.

63. Cruz-Almeida Y, Sibille KT, Goodin BR, et al. Racial and ethnic differences in older adults with knee osteoarthritis. *Arthritis Rheumatol* 2014;66(7):1800–1810.

64. Booker SS, Herr K. The state-of-"cultural validity" of self-report pain assessment tools in diverse older adults. *Pain Med* 2015;16(2):232–239.

65. Lukas A, Niederecker T, Günther I, et al. Self-and proxy report for the assessment of pain in patients with and without cognitive impairment: experiences gained in a geriatric hospital. *Z Gerontol Geriatr* 2013;46(3):214–221.

66. Orgeta V, Orrell M, Edwards RT, et al. Self-and carer-rated pain in people with dementia: influences of pain in carers. *J Pain Symptom Manage* 2015;49(6):1042–1049.

67. de Waal MW, Hegeman JM, Gussekloo J, et al. The effect of pain on presence and severity of depressive disorders in older persons: the role of perceived control as mediator. *J Affect Disord* 2016;197:239–244.

68. Kroenke K, Theobald D, Wu J, et al. Comparative responsiveness of pain measures in cancer patients. *J Pain* 2012;13(8):764–772.

69. Peat G, Thomas E, Duncan R, et al. Is a "false-positive" clinical diagnosis of knee osteoarthritis just the early diagnosis of pre-radiographic disease? *Arthritis Care Res (Hoboken)* 2010;62(10):1502–1506.

70. Cornelius R, Herr KA, Gordon DB, et al. Evidence-based practice guideline: acute pain management in older adults. *J Gerontol Nurs* 2017;43(2):18–27.

71. Sheu E, Versloot J, Nader R, et al. Pain in the elderly: validity of facial expression components of observational measures. *Clin J Pain* 2011;27(7):593–601.

72. Ahn H, Horgas A. The relationship between pain and disruptive behaviors in nursing home resident with dementia. *BMC Geriatr* 2013;13(1):14.

73. Beach PA, Huck JT, Miranda MM, et al. Effects of Alzheimer disease on the facial expression of pain. *Clin J Pain* 2016;32(6):478–487.

74. Lichtner V, Dowding D, Esterhuizen P, et al. Pain assessment for people with dementia: a systematic review of systematic reviews of pain assessment tools. *BMC Geriatr* 2014;14(1):138.

75. Herr K, Zwakhalen S, Swafford K. Observation of pain in dementia. *Curr Alzheimer Res* 2017;14(5):486–500.

76. Oosterman JM, Zwakhalen S, Sampson EL, et al. The use of facial expressions for pain assessment purposes in dementia: a narrative review. *Neurodegener Dis Manag* 2016;6(2):119–131.

77. Husebo BS, Ballard C, Cohen-Mansfield J, et al. The response of agitated behavior to pain management in persons with dementia. *Am J Geriatr Psychiatry* 2014;22(7):708–717.

78. Paladini A, Fusco M, Coaccioli S, et al. Chronic pain in the elderly: the case for new therapeutic strategies. *Pain Physician* 2015;18(5):E863–E876.

79. McLachlan AJ, Bath S, Naganathan V, et al. Clinical pharmacology of analgesic medicines in older people: impact of frailty and cognitive impairment. *Br J Clin Pharmacol* 2011;71(3):351–364.

80. Naples JG, Gellad WF, Hanlon JT. The role of opioid analgesics in geriatric pain management. *Clin Geriatr Med* 2016;32(4):725–735.

81. Prostran M, Vujovi KS, Vu kovi S, et al. Pharmacotherapy of pain in the older population: the place of opioids. *Front Aging Neurosci* 2016;8:144. doi:10.3389/fnagi.2016.00144.

82. Hassamal S, Miotto K, Wang T, et al. A narrative review: the effects of opioids on sleep disordered breathing in chronic pain patients and methadone maintained patients. *Am J Addict* 2016;25(6):452–465.

83. American Geriatrics Society Panel on Persistent Pain in Older Persons. The management of persistent pain in older persons. *J Am Geriatr Soc* 2002;50:S205–S224.

84. Savvas SM, Gibson SJ. Overview of pain management in older adults. *Clin Geriatr Med* 2016;32(4):635–650.

85. Marcum ZA, Duncan NA, Makris UE. Pharmacotherapies in geriatric chronic pain management. *Clin Geriatr Med* 2016;32(4):705–724.

86. Herndon CM, Arnstein P, Darnall B, et al, eds. *Principles of Analgesic Use.* 7th ed. Chicago, IL: American Pain Society Press; 2016.

87. Roberts E, Delgado Nunes V, Buckner S, et al. Paracetamol: not as safe as we thought? A systematic literature review of observational studies. *Ann Rheum Dis* 2016;75(3):552–559. doi:10.1136/annrheumdis-2014-206914.

88. McQuay HJ, Derry S, Eccleston C, et al. Evidence for analgesic effect in acute pain—50 years on. *Pain* 2012;153(7):1364–1367.

89. Finnerup NB, Attal N, Haroutounian S, et al. Pharmacotherapy for neuropathic pain in adults: a systematic review and meta-analysis. *Lancet Neurol* 2015;14(2):162–173. doi:10.1016/S1474-4422(14)70251-0.

90. Chou R, Deyo R, Friedly J, et al. Systemic pharmacologic therapies for low back pain: a systematic review for an American College of Physicians Clinical Practice Guideline. *Ann Intern Med* 2017;166(7):480–492.

91. American Geriatrics Society Panel on Pharmacological Management of Persistent Pain in Older Persons. Pharmacological management of persistent pain in older persons. *J Am Geriatr Soc* 2009;57(8):1331–1346.

92. American Geriatrics Society. American Geriatrics Society 2015 updated Beers criteria for potentially inappropriate medication use in older adults. *J Am Geriatr Soc* 2015;63(11):2227–2246.

93. Aggarwal N. Drug-induced subacute cutaneous lupus erythematosus associated with proton pump inhibitors. *Drugs Real World Outcomes* 2016;3(2):145–154.

94. Bally M, Dendukuri N, Rich B, et al. Risk of acute myocardial infarction with NSAIDs in real world use: bayesian meta-analysis of individual patient data. *BMJ* 2017;357:j1909.

95. Nissen SE, Yeomans ND, Solomon DH, et al. Cardiovascular safety of celecoxib, naproxen, or ibuprofen for arthritis. *N Engl J Med* 2016;375(26):2519–2529.

96. Ong CK, Lirk P, Tan CH, et al. An evidence-based update on nonsteroidal anti-inflammatory drugs. *Clin Med Res* 2007;5(1):19–34.

97. Gunter BR, Butler KA, Wallace RL, et al. Non-steroidal anti-inflammatory drug-induced cardiovascular adverse events: a meta-analysis. *J Clin Pharm Ther* 2017;42(1):27–38.

98. Arnstein P, Herr K. Risk evaluation and mitigation strategies for older adults with persistent pain. *J Gerontol Nurs* 2013;39(4):56–66.

99. Ruoff G. Nonsteroidal anti-inflammatory drugs and cardiovascular risk: where are we today? *J Fam Pract* 2015;64(12 suppl):S67–S70.

100. Atkinson TJ, Fudin J, Pandula A, et al. Medication pain management in the elderly: unique and underutilized analgesic treatment options. *Clin Ther* 2013;35:1669–1689.

101. Derry S, Wiffen PJ, Kalso EA, et al. Topical analgesics for acute and chronic pain in adults—an overview of Cochrane Reviews. *Cochrane Database Syst Rev* 2017;(5):CD008609. doi:10.1002/14651858.CD008609.pub2.

102. Manchikanti L, Kaye AM, Knezevic NN, et al. Responsible, safe, and effective prescription of opioids for chronic non-cancer pain: American Society of Interventional Pain Physicians (ASIPP) Guidelines. *Pain Physician* 2017;20(2S):S3–S92.

103. Hwang U, Belland LK, Handel DA, et al. Is all pain is treated equally? A multicenter evaluation of acute pain care by age. *Pain* 2014;155:2568–2574.

104. Vuong S, Pulenzas N, DeAngelis C, et al. Inadequate pain management in cancer patients attending an outpatient palliative radiotherapy clinic. *Support Care Cancer* 2016;24(2):887–892.

105. Papaleontiou M, Henderson CR Jr, Turner BJ, et al. Outcomes associated with opioid use in the treatment of chronic noncancer pain in older adults: a systematic review and meta-analysis. *J Am Geriatr Soc* 2010;58:1353–1369.

106. Brown CH IV, LaFlam A, Max L, et al. Delirium after spine surgery in older adults: incidence, risk factors, and outcomes. *J Am Geriatr Soc* 2016;64(10):2101–2108.

107. Morrison RS, Magaziner J, McLaughlin MA, et al. The impact of postoperative pain on outcomes following hip fracture. *Pain* 2003;103(3):303–311.

108. Stubbs B, Schofield P, Binnekade T, et al. Pain is associated with recurrent falls in community-dwelling older adults: evidence from a systematic review and meta-analysis. *Pain Med* 2014;15(7):1115–1128.

109. Chou R, Turner JA, Devine EB, et al. The effectiveness and risks of long-term opioid therapy for chronic pain: a systematic review for a National Institutes of Health Pathways to Prevention Workshop. *Ann Intern Med* 2015;162(4):276–286.

110. Chambers J, Gleason RM, Kirsh KL, et al. An online survey of patients' experiences since the rescheduling of hydrocodone: the first 100 days. *Pain Med* 2016;17(9):1686–1693.

111. Baker DW. History of The Joint Commission's pain standards: lessons for today's prescription opioid epidemic. *JAMA* 2017;317(11):1117–1118.

112. Scholten W, Henningfield JE. Negative outcomes of unbalanced opioid policy supported by clinicians, politicians, and the media. *J Pain Palliat Care Pharmacother* 2016;30(1):4–12.

113. Rudd RA, Seth P, David F, et al. Increases in drug and opioid-involved overdose deaths—United States, 2010–2015. *MMWR Morb Mortal Wkly Rep* 2016;65(5051):1445–1452. doi:10.15585/mmwr.mm655051e1.

114. Dasgupta N, Funk M, Proescholdbell S, et al. Cohort study of the impact of high-dose opioid analgesics on overdose mortality. *Pain Med* 2016;17:85–98.

115. Alford DP, German JS, Samet JH, et al. Primary care patients with drug use report chronic pain and self-medicate with alcohol and other drugs. *J Gen Intern Med* 2016;31(5):486–491. doi:10.1007/s11606-016-3586-5.

116. Vadivelu N, Hines RL. Management of chronic pain in the elderly: focus on transdermal buprenorphine. *Clin Interv Aging* 2008;3(3):421–430.

117. Biondi DM, Xiang J, Etropolski M, et al. Tolerability and efficacy of tapentadol extended release in elderly patients ≥75 years of age with chronic osteoarthritis knee or low back pain. *J Opioid Manag* 2015;11(5):393–403. doi:10.5055/jom.2015.0289.

118. Buynak R, Rappaport SA, Rod K, et al. Long-term safety and efficacy of tapentadol extended release following up to 2 years of treatment in patients with moderate to severe, chronic pain: results of an open-label extension trial. *Clin Ther* 2015;37(11):2420–2438.

119. Pergolizzi JV, Raffa RB, Marcum Z, et al. Safety of buprenorphine transdermal system in the management of pain in older adults. *Postgrad Med* 2017;129(1):92–101.

120. Veal FC, Peterson GM. Pain in the frail or elderly patient: does tapentadol have a role? *Drugs Aging* 2015;32(6):419–426.

121. Chou R, Cruciani RA, Fiellin DA, et al. Methadone safety: a clinical practice guideline. *J Pain* 2014;15(4):321–337.

122. Dowell D, Haegerich TM, Chou R. CDC Guideline for prescribing opioids for chronic pain—United States, 2016. *MMWR Recomm Rep* 2016;18;65(1):1–49.

123. Plein LM, Rittner HL. Opioids and the immune system—friend or foe [published online ahead of print February 18, 2017]. *Br J Pharmacol*. doi:10.1111/bph.13750.

124. Brennan MJ. The effect of opioid therapy on endocrine function. *Am J Med* 2013;126(3 suppl 1):S12–S18.

125. Hooten WM, Lamer TJ, Twyner C. Opioid-induced hyperalgesia in community-dwelling adults with chronic pain. *Pain* 2015;156(6):1145–1152.

126. Reece AS, Hulse GK. Elevation of the ACTH/cortisol ratio in female opioid dependent patients: a biomarker of aging and correlate of metabolic and immune activation. *Neuro Endocrinol Lett* 2016;37(4):325–336.

127. Ray JA, Kushnir MM, Meikle AW, et al. An exploratory study evaluating the impact of opioid and non-opioid pain medications on serum/plasma free testosterone and free estradiol concentrations. *Drug Test Anal* 2017;9:1555–1560. doi:10.1002/dta.2174.

128. Lussier D, Portenoy RK. Adjuvant analgesics. In: Doyle D, Hanks G, Cherny NI, et al, eds. *Oxford Textbook of Palliative Medicine*. 3rd ed. Oxford, United Kingdom: Oxford University Press; 2004:349–377.

129. Tayeb BO, Barreiro AE, Bradshaw YS, et al. Durations of opioid, non-opioid drug, and behavioral clinical trials for chronic pain: adequate or inadequate? *Pain Med* 2016;17(11):2036–2046.

130. Friedrich ME, Akimova E, Huf W, et al. Drug-induced liver injury during antidepressant treatment: results of AMSP, a drug surveillance program. *Int J Neuropsychopharmacol* 2016;19(4). pii:pyv126. doi:10.1093/ijnp/pyv126.

131. Nelson JC, Spyker DA. Morbidity and mortality associated with medications used in the treatment of depression: an analysis of cases reported to U.S. Poison Control Centers, 2000-2014. *Am J Psychiatry* 2017;174(5):438–450. doi:10.1176/appi.ajp.2016.16050523.

132. Mathieson S, Maher CG, McLachlan AJ, et al. Trial of pregabalin for acute and chronic sciatica. *N Engl J Med* 2017;376(12):1111–1120.

133. Burness CB, McCormack PL. Capsaicin 8% patch: a review in peripheral neuropathic pain. *Drugs* 2016;76(1):123–134.

134. Deer TR, Levy RM, Kramer J, et al. Topical lidocaine for neuropathic pain in adults. *Cochrane Database Syst Rev* 2014;(7):CD010958. doi:10.1002/14651858.CD010958.pub2.

135. Guerriero F, Bolier R, Van Cleave JH, et al. Pharmacological approaches for the management of persistent pain in older adults: what nurses need to know. *J Gerontol Nurs* 2016;42(12):49–57. doi:10.3928/00989134-20161110-09.

136. Chou R, Deyo R, Friedly J, et al. Nonpharmacologic therapies for low back pain: a systematic review for an American College of Physicians Clinical Practice Guideline. *Ann Intern Med* 2017;166(7):493–505.

137. U.S. Department of Health and Human Services. National pain strategy: a comprehensive population health-level strategy for pain. Available at: http://iprcc.nih.gov/docs/HHSNational_Pain_Strategy.pdf. Accessed November 16, 2016.

138. Rathmell JP, Benzon HT, Dreyfuss P, et al. Safeguards to prevent neurologic complications after epidural steroid injections: consensus opinions from a multidisciplinary working group and national organizations. *Anesthesiology* 2015;122(5):974–984.

139. Bernstein C, Lateef B, Fine P. Interventional pain management procedures in older patients. In: Gibson SJ, Weiner DK, eds. *Pain in Older Persons*. Seattle, WA: IASP Press; 2005:263–281.

140. Brooks AK, Udoji MA. Interventional techniques for management of pain in older adults. *Clin Geriatr Med* 2016;32(4):773–785.

141. Manchikanti L, Falco FJ. Safeguards to prevent neurologic complications after epidural steroid injections: analysis of evidence and lack of applicability of controversial policies. *Pain Physician* 2015;18(2):E129–E138.

142. Singh V. Multisociety Pain Work Group (MPW): how societies work together to make a difference. Presented at: American Academy of Pain Medicine 33rd Annual Meeting; March 16–19, 2017; Orlando, FL.

143. Verrills P, Sinclair C, Barnard A. A review of spinal cord stimulation systems for chronic pain. *J Pain Res* 2016;9:481–492.

144. Geurts JW, Joosten EA, van Kleef M. Current status and future perspectives of spinal cord stimulation in treatment of chronic pain. *Pain* 2017;158(5):771–774.

145. Radcliff K, Coric D, Albert T. Five-year clinical results of cervical total disc replacement compared with anterior discectomy and fusion for treatment of 2-level symptomatic degenerative disc disease: a prospective, randomized, controlled, multicenter investigational device exemption clinical trial. *J Neurosurg Spine* 2016;25(2):213–224. doi:10.3171/2015.12.SPINE15824.

146. Iannitti T, Fistetto G, Esposito A, et al. Pulsed electromagnetic field therapy for management of osteoarthritis-related pain, stiffness and physical function: clinical experience in the elderly. *Clin Interv Aging* 2013;8:1289–1293.

147. Bagnato GL, Miceli G, Marino N, et al. Pulsed electromagnetic fields in knee osteoarthritis: a double blind, placebo-controlled, randomized clinical trial. *Rheumatology (Oxford)* 2016;55(4):755–762.

148. Scudds RJ, Scudds RA. Physical therapy approaches to the management of pain in older adults. In: Gibson SJ, Weiner DK, eds. *Pain in Older Persons*. Seattle, WA: IASP Press; 2005:223–237.

149. Leonhardt C, Kuss K, Becker A, et al. Graded activity for older adults with chronic low back pain: program development and mixed methods feasibility cohort study. *J Geriatr Phys Ther* 2017;40(1):51–59.

150. O'Gara T, Kemper KJ, Birkedal J, et al. Survey of conventional and complementary and alternative therapy in patients with low back pain. *J Surg Orthop Adv* 2016;25(1):27–33.

151. Tse MM, Tang SK, Wan VT, et al. The effectiveness of physical exercise training in pain, mobility, and psychological well-being of older persons living in nursing homes. *Pain Manag Nurs* 2014;15(4):778–788.

152. Field T. Knee osteoarthritis pain in the elderly can be reduced by massage therapy, yoga and tai chi: a review. *Complement Ther Clin Pract* 2016;22:87–92.

153. Ardigo S, Herrmann FR, Moret V, et al. Hypnosis can reduce pain in hospitalized older patients: a randomized controlled study. *BMC Geriatr* 2016;16:14.

154. Rakel B, Herr K. Assessment and treatment of postoperative pain in older adults. *J Perianesth Nurs* 2004;19(3):194–208.

155. Pivec R, Minshall ME, Mistry JB, et al. Decreased opioid utilization and cost at one year in chronic low back pain patients treated with transcutaneous electric nerve stimulation (TENS). *Surg Technol Int* 2015;27:268–274.

156. Saper RB, Phillips RS, Sehgal A, et al. Lead, mercury, and arsenic in US- and Indian-manufactured Ayurvedic medicines sold via the Internet. *JAMA* 2008;300(8):915–923.

157. Prestwood K. Complementary and alternative medicine for the treatment of pain in older adults. In: Gibson SJ, Weiner DK, eds. *Pain in Older Persons*. Seattle, WA: IASP Press; 2005:285–307.

158. Caron A, Gallo WT, Durbin LL, et al. Relationship between falls and complementary and alternative medicine use among community-dwelling older adults. *J Altern Complement Med* 2017;23(1):41–44.

159. Bruckenthal P, Marino MA, Snelling L. Complementary and integrative therapies for persistent pain management in older adults: a review. *J Gerontol Nurs* 2016;42(12):40–48.

160. Burger AJ, Lumley MA, Carty JN, et al. The effects of a novel psychological attribution and emotional awareness and expression therapy for chronic musculoskeletal pain: a preliminary, uncontrolled trial. *J Psychosom Res* 2016;81:1–8.

161. Rini C, Porter LS, Somers TJ, et al. Automated Internet-based pain coping skills training to manage osteoarthritis pain: a randomized controlled trial. *Pain* 2015;156(5):837–848.

162. Rini C, Williams DA, Broderick JE, et al. Meeting them where they are: using the Internet to deliver behavioral medicine interventions for pain. *Transl Behav Med* 2012;2(1):82–92.

163. Riva S, Camerini AL, Allam A, et al. Interactive sections of an Internet-based intervention increase empowerment of chronic back pain patients: randomized controlled trial. *J Med Internet Res* 2014;16(8):e180.

164. Tse MM, Yeung SS, Lee PH, et al. Effects of a peer led pain management program for nursing home residents with chronic pain: a pilot study. *Pain Med* 2016;17(9):1648–1657.

165. Eccleston C, Tabor A, Edwards RT, et al. Psychological approaches to coping with pain in later life. *Clin Geriatr Med* 2016;32(4):763–771.

166. Nicholas MK, Asghari A, Blyth FM, et al. Long-term outcomes from training in self-management of chronic pain in an elderly population: a randomized controlled trial. *Pain* 2017;158(1):86–95.

167. Miller WR, Rose GS. Motivational interviewing and decisional balance: contrasting responses to client ambivalence. *Behav Cogn Psychother* 2015;43(2):129–141.

168. Wetherell JL, Petkus AJ, Alonso-Fernandez M, et al. Age moderates response to acceptance and commitment therapy vs. cognitive behavioral therapy for chronic pain. *Int J Geriatr Psychiatry* 2016;31(3):302–308.

169. Morone NE, Greco CM, Moore CG, et al. A mind-body program for older adults with chronic low back pain: a randomized clinical trial. *JAMA Intern Med* 2016;176(3):329–337.

170. Scott W, Daly A, Yu L, et al. Treatment of chronic pain for adults 65 and over: analyses of outcomes and changes in psychological flexibility following interdisciplinary acceptance and commitment therapy (ACT). *Pain Med* 2017;18(2):252–264. doi:10.1093/pm/pnw073.

171. Nahin RL, Stussman BJ, Herman PM. Out-of-pocket expenditures on complementary health approaches associated with painful health conditions in a nationally representative adult sample. *J Pain* 2015;16(11):1147–1162.

172. Nahin RL, Boineau R, Khalsa PS, et al. Evidence-based evaluation of complementary health approaches for pain management in the United States. *Mayo Clin Proc* 2016;91(9):1292–1306.

173. AARP, National Center for Complementary and Integrative Health. Complementary and alternative medicine: what people aged 50 and older discuss with their health care providers. Available at: https://nccih.nih.gov/research/statistics/2010. Accessed March 31, 2018.

174. Gong G, Li J, Li X, et al. Pain experiences and self-management strategies among middle-aged and older adults with arthritis. *J Clin Nurs* 2013;22(13–14):1857–1869. doi:10.1111/jocn.12134.

175. Herman PM, Poindexter BL, Witt CM, et al. Are complementary therapies and integrative care cost-effective? A systematic review of economic evaluations. *BMJ Open* 2012;2(5):e001046.

176. Holmberg C, Rappenecker J, Karner JJ, et al. The perspectives of older women with chronic neck pain on perceived effects of qigong and exercise therapy on aging: a qualitative interview study. *Clin Interv Aging* 2014;9:403–410.

177. Teut M, Knilli J, Daus D, et al. Qigong or yoga versus no intervention in older adults with chronic low back pain-a randomized controlled trial. *J Pain* 2016;17(7):796–805.

178. Hariprasad VR, Varambally S, Shivakumar V, et al. Yoga increases the volume of the hippocampus in elderly subjects. *Indian J Psychiatry* 2013; 55(suppl 3):S394–S396.

179. Villemure C, Čeko M, Cotton VA, et al. Neuroprotective effects of yoga practice: age-, experience-, and frequency-dependent plasticity. *Front Hum Neurosci* 2015;9:281.

180. Leininger B, McDonough C, Evans R, et al. Cost-effectiveness of spinal manipulative therapy, supervised exercise, and home exercise for older adults with chronic neck pain. *Spine J* 2016;16(11):1292–1304.

181. Rayner JA, Bauer M. "I wouldn't mind trying it. I'm in pain the whole time": barriers to the use of complementary medicines by older Australians in residential aged-care facilities. *J Appl Gerontol* 2017;36: 1070–1090.

182. Geisler CC, Cheung CK. Complementary/alternative therapies use in older women with arthritis: Information sources and factors influencing dialog with health care providers. *Geriatr Nurs* 2015;36(1):15–20.

183. McFeeters S, Pront L, Cuthbertson L, et al. Massage, a complementary therapy effectively promoting the health and well-being of older people in residential care settings: a review of the literature. *Int J Older People Nurs* 2016;11(4):266–283.

184. Leong M, Smith TJ, Rowland-Seymour A. Complementary and integrative medicine for older adults in palliative care. *Clin Geriatr Med* 2015;31(2):177–191.

185. Robinson A, Lind CR, Smith RJ, et al. Atlanto-axial infection after acupuncture. *Acupunct Med* 2016;34(2):149–151.

186. Huisma F, Konrad G, Thomas S. Pneumothorax after acupuncture. *Can Fam Physician* 2015;61(12):1071–1073.

187. Yeh CH, Morone NE, Chien LC, et al. Auricular point acupressure to manage chronic low back pain in older adults: a randomized controlled pilot study. *Evid Based Complement Alternat Med* 2014;2014:375173.

188. Tang SK, Tse MY. Aromatherapy: does it help to relieve pain, depression, anxiety, and stress in community-dwelling older persons? *Biomed Res Int* 2014;2014:430195.

189. Nasiri A, Mahmodi MA, Nobakht Z. Effect of aromatherapy massage with lavender essential oil on pain in patients with osteoarthritis of the knee: a randomized controlled clinical trial. *Complement Ther Clin Pract* 2016;25:75–80.

190. Katz B, Scherer S, Gibson SJ. Multidisciplinary pain management clinics for older adults. In: Gibson SJ, Weiner DK, eds. *Pain in Older Persons.* Seattle, WA: IASP Press; 2005:309–326.

191. Kee WG, Middaugh SJ, Redpath S, et al. Age as a factor in admission to chronic pain rehabilitation. *Clin J Pain* 1998;14(2):121–128.

192. Fishbain DA, Gao J, Lewis JE, et al. At completion of a multidisciplinary treatment program, are psychophysical variables associated with a VAS improvement of 30% or more, a minimal clinically important difference, or an absolute VAS score improvement of 1.5 cm or more? *Pain Med* 2016;17(4):781–789. doi:10.1093/pm/pnv006.

193. Moe RH, Grotle M, Kjeken I, et al. Effectiveness of an integrated multidisciplinary osteoarthritis outpatient program versus outpatient clinic as usual: a randomized controlled trial. *J Rheumatol* 2016;43(2):411–418. doi:10.3899/jrheum.150157.

194. Hogan TM, Howell MD, Cursio JF, et al. Improving Pain Relief in Elder Patients (I-PREP): an emergency department education and quality intervention. *J Am Geriatr Soc* 2016;64(12):2566–2571. doi:10.1111/jgs.14377.

CHAPTER 56

Obstetric Pain

Historical Notes

Childbirth pain is arguably the most severe pain most women will endure in their lifetimes. The modern era of childbirth analgesia began in 1847 when Dr. James Young Simpson administered ether to a woman in childbirth and later, in the same year, chloroform. The use of analgesia for childbirth aroused violent opposition from some physicians, the public, and the clergy.[1] Simpson was labeled a heretic, blasphemer, and an agent of the devil. The furor died down somewhat in 1853, when John Snow successfully administered chloroform to Queen Victoria for the birth of her eighth child.

In the ensuing years, public opinion regarding obstetric analgesia began to change, thus forcing the medical community to offer analgesia. Women enthusiastically embraced labor analgesia. Fanny Longfellow, the wife of poet Henry Wadsworth Longfellow and the first woman in the United States to receive labor analgesia in the modern era, wrote that "this is certainly the greatest blessing of this age."[2] Pain began to lose its theologic connections.[3] It was no longer considered punishment for sin or divine retribution. Instead, disease and pain were considered biologic processes that could be studied and treated.

Following this auspicious beginning in the 19th century, however, childbirth analgesia was largely neglected by the medical community. The next major step occurred in the early 20th century when *Dämmerschlaf*, or "twilight sleep," was introduced in Europe.[4] The combination of scopolamine and morphine was enthusiastically accepted by women but not by the medical profession. Medical professionals expressed concern about the effect of childbirth analgesia on the progress of labor. In addition, with the advent of twilight sleep, physicians began to appreciate that anesthetics cross the placenta and had potentially adverse effects on the newborn. This was the stimulus for Virginia Apgar, an anesthesiologist, to develop an evaluation tool to assess neonatal well-being in 1953.[5] A salutary effect of the Apgar score was that scientific studies comparing the effects of different anesthetic techniques on neonatal outcome were now possible.

Regional anesthesia was first introduced in 1884, when Carl Koller described the use of cocaine to anesthetize the eye.[6] Descriptions of regional anesthesia, including spinal, lumbar epidural, caudal, paravertebral, and pudendal nerve blocks, were published in the obstetric literature between 1900 and 1930.[3] In the 1930s and 1940s, Cleland[7] contributed to our understanding of the innervation of the uterus and applied this knowledge to regional anesthesia in the care of the obstetric patient. Continuous neuraxial analgesia, as it is practiced today, had its birth in 1943, when Hingson and Edwards[8] published the first report of continuous caudal analgesia for childbirth. Flexible, disposable catheters replaced the original malleable needles, and refinements were made, and continue to be made, in technique, drugs, doses, and delivery techniques.

Although other regional nerve block and systemic analgesic techniques are often used for analgesia, women continue to request neuraxial labor analgesia for childbirth at ever-increasing rates. In the most recent survey performed in 2012, over 85% of women in large maternity hospitals in the United States received neuraxial analgesia during labor.[9] Spinal and epidural anesthesia accounts for over 95% of the anesthetics for elective cesarean deliveries. Multimodal analgesic therapy, which often includes a regional technique component, is the norm for postcesarean analgesia. This chapter summarizes the physiology of childbirth pain, physiologic changes of pregnancy that influence the provision of analgesic and anesthetic care, specific labor analgesic techniques, the effects of analgesia on the mother and infant, and the treatment of nonobstetric pain during pregnancy and lactation.

Pain of Childbirth

Although it is a common observation that parturients vary in the amount of pain and suffering associated with labor and vaginal delivery, few well-designed studies on the prevalence, intensity, and quality of labor pain have been performed. Melzack et al.[10] used the McGill Pain Questionnaire to assess childbirth pain. The mean total pain rating index (PRI) was 34 for nulliparous and 30 for parous women. Significant differences were also found between nulliparas and parous women in the sensory qualities of pain. Labor pain scores were 8 to 10 points higher than those associated with cancer pain, phantom limb pain, and postherpetic neuralgia (Fig. 56.1A), although there was a wide range of scores ranging from mild to excruciating (Fig. 56.1B).

CHILDBIRTH PAIN MECHANISMS AND PATHWAYS

Most data support the concept that the pain of the first stage of labor originates predominantly in the cervix and the lower uterine segment rather than the body of the uterus. Dilation of the cervix and lower uterine segment results in distension, stretching, and tearing of tissues. During the late first stage and second stage of labor, the descent of the fetus and intense stretching and tearing of the tissues of the vagina and perineum become additional sources of pain.

Based on animal and human studies, Cleland[7] concluded that the sensory afferents from the uterus and cervix that transmit pain during the first stage of labor enter the spinal cord at T11 and T12 (Fig. 56.2). He demonstrated that these visceral sensory afferents are intermingled with sympathetic efferents by demonstrating that bilateral paravertebral lumbar sympathetic blockade abolished the pain of the first stage of labor. Second-stage pain from descent of the fetus in the birth canal is primarily somatic in nature and is transmitted through sacral nerves to the S2–S4 segments of the spinal cord.

Bonica[11] used a series of discrete nerve blocks of various nociceptive pathways, including paracervical, segmental epidural, caudal, and transsacral blocks, to further refine our knowledge of the nerve pathways that transmit labor pain to the central nervous system. He demonstrated that the upper part of the cervix and lower uterine segment are supplied by afferents that accompany the sympathetic nerves through the uterine and cervical plexus; the inferior, middle, and superior hypogastric plexuses; and the aortic plexuses. The nociceptive afferents then pass to the lumbar sympathetic chain and course cephalad through the lower thoracic sympathetic chain via the rami communicantes of the T10, T11, T12, and L1 spinal segments. Finally, they pass through the dorsal roots of these nerves to make synaptic contact with the interneurons of the dorsal horn.

Typical of pain arising from viscera, the pain of the first stage of labor is often referred to the T10–L1 dermatomes. Additionally, during the late first stage and second stage of labor,

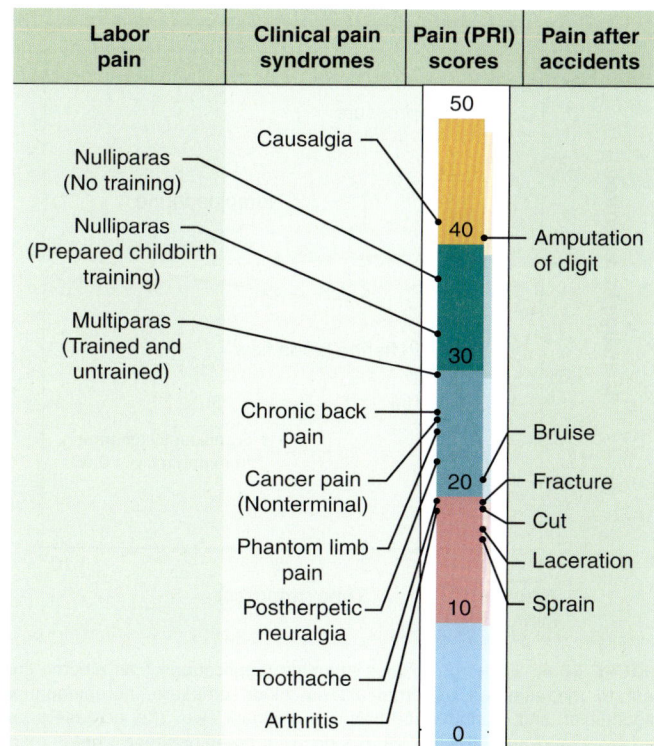

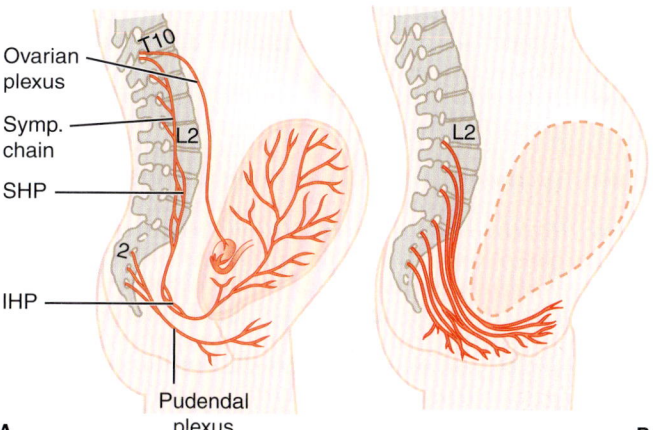

FIGURE 56.2 Schematic depiction of the peripheral nociceptive pathways involved in the pain of childbirth. **A:** The uterus, including the lower uterine segment and cervix, is supplied by afferents that pass from the uterus to the spinal cord by accompanying sympathetic nerves through the cervical plexus; the superior and inferior hypogastric plexuses (SHP, IHP); the lumbar and lower thoracic sympathetic chain; and to the T11, T12, and L1 nerve roots. The vagina and perineum are supplied by afferents that travel to the spinal cord via the pudendal nerve to the S2–S4 nerve roots. **B:** The nerves involved in the transmission of nociceptive impulses are provoked by noxious stimulation of pelvic structures.

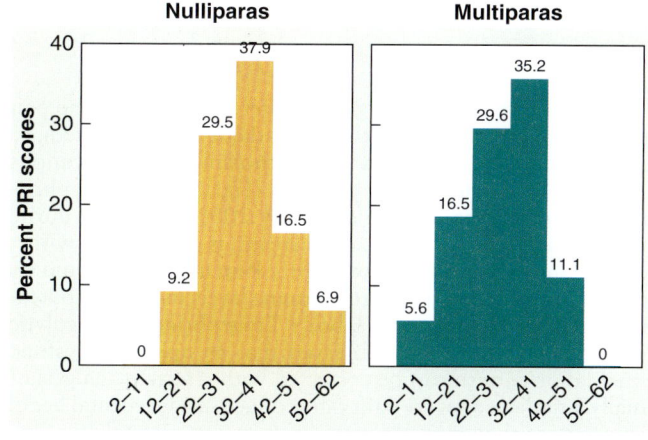

FIGURE 56.1 **A:** Comparison of pain scores using the McGill Pain Questionnaire obtained from women during labor and from patients in general hospital clinics and an emergency department. The pain rating index (PRI) represents the sum of the rank values for all words chosen from 20 sets of pain descriptions. **B:** Distribution of PRI scores from nulliparous and parous women in six intervals of the total PRI range. (*Redrawn after Melzack R. The myth of painless childbirth [the John J. Bonica lecture]. Pain 1984;19[4]:321–337, with permission.*)

superficial laminae of the dorsal horn with minimal rostrocaudal fiber extension. This explains the diffuse localization of visceral first-stage labor pain compared to somatic second-stage labor pain. It may also explain why the neuraxial administration of lipid-soluble opioids in early labor provides complete analgesia, as these drugs penetrate deeply into the spinal cord.

Understanding the anatomic basis of the transmission of labor pain underlies the current treatment of labor pain using regional anesthesia techniques. The visceral pain of the first stage of labor can be blocked with bilateral cervical plexus, lumbar sympathetic blocks, or central neuraxial blockade. The somatic pain caused by descent of the fetus in the birth canal can be blocked with bilateral pudendal nerve blocks or neuraxial blockade.

Our current understanding of the neurophysiologic basis of labor pain is superficial at best. Better understanding of the pain pathways, neurotransmitters, and receptors involved in labor pain will open up new avenues for the treatment of labor pain in the future.

FACTORS THAT AFFECT THE PAIN OF CHILDBIRTH

In addition to physiologic factors such as intensity, duration, pattern of contractions, and descent of the fetus, the amount or degree of pain and suffering associated with childbirth is influenced by physical, psychological, emotional, and motivational factors.

Physical factors that are associated with the severity and duration of childbirth pain include age, parity,[13] history of previous pain or dysmenorrhea, fatigue, the condition of the cervix at the onset of labor, and the relationship between the size and position of the fetus to the size of the birth canal. Generally, an older nullipara experiences longer and more painful labor than a younger nullipara.[10] The cervix of parous women begins to soften even before the onset of labor and is less sensitive than that of the nullipara. The intensity of uterine contractions in early labor tends to be higher in nulliparous compared to parous women, whereas the reverse is true as labor advances. Pain is greater in the presence of dystocia caused by a contracted pelvis, a large baby, or abnormal presentation or position. Women who go on to require cesarean delivery following

some parturients experience referred pain to the lower lumbar and sacral dermatomes as a result of stimulation of pain-sensitive structures within the pelvic cavity and pressure on one or more roots of the lumbosacral plexus. The pain may be severe if the fetus is in an abnormal position.

Visceral C fibers transmitting pain during the first stage of labor terminate in the spinal cord in a loose network of synapses in the ipsilateral, superficial, and deep dorsal horn and the ventral horn as well as cross the midline to the contralateral dorsal horn with extensive rostrocaudal extension.[12] In contrast, somatic afferent fibers tend to terminate in the ipsilateral a period of labor have more breakthrough pain[14] and require more epidural[14] and systemic[15] analgesia during labor than women who deliver vaginally.

Psychological factors, such as fear, apprehension, and anxiety, also influence the degree of pain and suffering during childbirth.[16] The presence of family members[17] or birthing companions[18] during labor and delivery may decrease anxiety and positively affect the progress of labor. Education, intense motivation, and cultural influences can influence the affective and behavioral dimensions of pain, although they probably minimally affect actual pain sensation. Bonica[19] observed women who had had predelivery training in psychoprophylaxis manifested little or no pain behavior during childbirth, although when questioned the next day, most of them indicated the process had been quite painful. Jewish health providers rated the labor pain of Jewish women higher than that of Bedouin women who were delivering in the same institution,[20] whereas the level of pain assessed by the women themselves was not different.

EFFECTS OF PAIN ON THE MOTHER AND FETUS

Labor and vaginal delivery produce tissue damage and, similar to tissue injury from other causes, result in pain and local segmental, suprasegmental, and cortical responses. These responses include marked stimulation of respiration and circulation as well as the hypothalamic, autonomic centers of neuroendocrine function, limbic structures, and psychodynamic mechanisms of anxiety and apprehension. These may have a deleterious impact on the mother, fetus, and newborn. Many of these responses are mitigated by effective pain relief.

The pain of childbirth is a powerful respiratory stimulus, resulting in a marked increase in minute ventilation and oxygen consumption during contractions.[21] Compensatory periods of hypoventilation between contractions cause transient maternal hypoxemia and, potentially, fetal hypoxemia (Fig. 56.3). Maternal hyperventilation causes severe respiratory alkalosis and a left shift of the maternal oxyhemoglobin dissociation

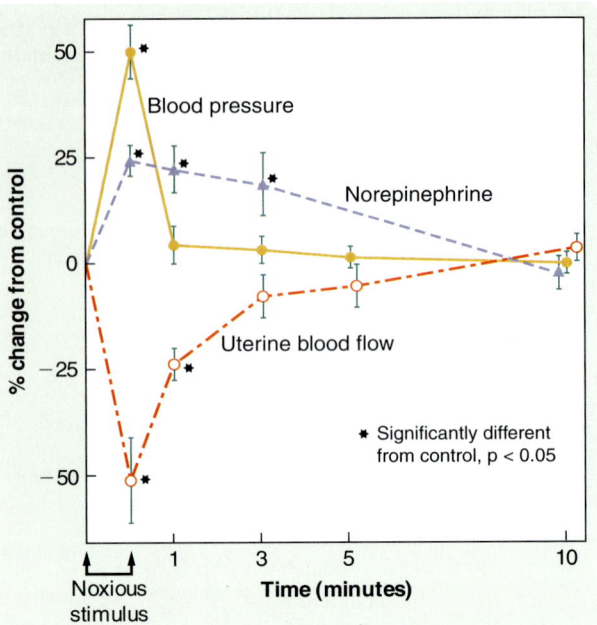

FIGURE 56.4 Effect of noxious stimulus (application of an electric current to the skin) on maternal arterial blood pressure, norepinephrine blood level, and uterine blood flow in a pregnant ewe. The increase in arterial pressure is transient, and the decay in norepinephrine level is more protracted and is reflected by a mirror image decrease in uterine blood flow. *(Redrawn after Shnider SM, Wright RG, Levinson G, et al. Uterine blood flow and plasma norepinephrine changes during maternal stress in the pregnant ewe. Anesthesiology 1979;50[6]:524–527, with permission.)*

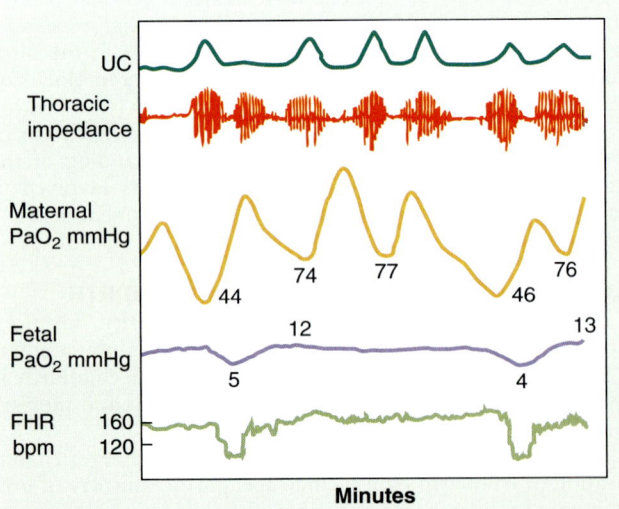

FIGURE 56.3 Continuous recording of uterine contractions (UC), maternal thoracic impedance, maternal transcutaneous oxygen tension (partial pressure of oxygen [Pao₂]), fetal oxygen tension, and fetal heart rate (FHR) in a nullipara breathing room air 120 minutes before spontaneous delivery. Marked hyperventilations during UC were followed by hypoventilation or apnea between contractions. After the first and fourth contractions, the maternal Pao₂ fell to 44 and 46 mm Hg, with a consequent decrease in fetal Pao₂, and variable decelerations, which reflect fetal hypoxemia. *(Redrawn after Huch A, Huch R, Schneider H, et al. Continuous transcutaneous monitoring of fetal oxygen tension during labour. Br J Obstet Gynaecol 1977;84[suppl 1]:1–39. Reprinted by permission of John Wiley & Sons, Inc.)*

curve, thus diminishing oxygen transfer to the fetus. The pain and stress of labor activates the sympathetic nervous system, resulting in an increase in plasma catecholamine concentrations, cardiac output, and blood pressure (Fig. 56.4). Epinephrine and norepinephrine levels increase by 200% to 600% during unmedicated labor,[22] and this increase is associated with a decrease in uterine blood flow (UBF). Pain and anxiety and the accompanying increased catecholamine levels may contribute to prolonged or dysfunctional labor.[23] Epinephrine is a tocolytic, and physicians have long observed that an apparent dysfunctional labor pattern can be corrected with effective analgesia.[24] Finally, unrelieved severe pain can produce serious mental health disturbances that may interfere with maternal–fetal bonding, future sexual relationships, and contribute to postpartum depression[10] and, rarely, posttraumatic stress disorder.

The healthy parturient easily tolerates the large increase in cardiac work, but parturients with heart disease, severe preeclampsia, or pulmonary hypertension may not tolerate these changes without adverse outcome. Similarly, the healthy fetus tolerates the changes in UBF; however, these changes may be deleterious in the setting of uteroplacental insufficiency (e.g., preeclampsia, intrauterine growth restriction).

In summary, there is large individual variation in how women experience childbirth pain and suffering. Pain associated responses to noxious stimuli during childbirth are net effects of highly complex interactions of various neural systems, modulating influences, and psychological factors. These interactions are responsible for the complex physiologic, behavioral, and affective responses that characterize the pain of childbirth.

Physiologic Changes of Pregnancy

Pregnancy is associated with significant anatomic and physiologic changes. Many of these changes impact the treatment of pain during pregnancy, parturition, and the puerperium.

TABLE 56.1	Physiologic Changes of Pregnancy and Anesthetic Implications	
Physiologic Change	**Anesthetic Implication**
Respiratory	
Increase in O_2 requirement and CO_2 production	Greater risk of desaturation after induction of general anesthesia
Decrease in FRC	Greater risk of desaturation after induction of general anesthesia
Cardiovascular	
Hyperdynamic: increased reliance on sympathetic nervous system	Increase in incidence and severity of hypotension after neuraxial analgesia/anesthesia
Decreased responsiveness to vasoactive agents	Require higher doses of vasopressors to correct hypotension
Aortocaval compression	More profound hypotension with parturient in the supine position
Aortocaval compression and engorgement of azygous veins	Less epidural space and decreased egress of drugs from the epidural space result in lower requirement for epidural drugs
Central Nervous System	
Increased lumbar lordosis and decreased thoracic kyphosis	Decreased size of lumbar interspinous space and altered movement of anesthetic agents within CSF
Rotation of pelvis	Tuffier's line more cephalad
Widening of the pelvis	Spine more "head-down" in lateral position
Decrease in CSF volume	Decrease in local anesthetic dose requirements
Decrease in CSF specific gravity	Altered baricity of spinal anesthetic solutions
Increase in CSF pH	Change in proportion of un-ionized drug
Increased susceptibility to all anesthetics	Decrease in anesthetic dose requirements
Increased progesterone levels	Increased pain threshold
Pharmacokinetics	
Altered volume of distribution	Change in drug pharmacokinetics
Altered protein binding of drugs	Change in drug pharmacokinetics
Increased renal blood flow	Change in drug elimination
Altered hepatic microsomal enzyme activity	Change in drug metabolism

CSF, cerebrospinal fluid; FRC; functional residual capacity.

Safe care of these women requires a thorough understanding of these changes and their impact on the treatment of pain. In addition, a thorough understanding of the fetal–placental complex is necessary for the safe care of the fetus and neonate. These changes and their anesthetic implications are summarized in Table 56.1 and discussed in the following text.

RESPIRATORY CHANGES

Pregnancy is associated with anatomic and physiologic changes involving the airway, lung volumes, ventilation, and the dynamics of breathing. Capillary engorgement, an increase in upper airway soft tissue mass, and enlargement of the breasts contribute to making endotracheal intubation more difficult in pregnant compared to nonpregnant women.[25] Failed intubation and pulmonary aspiration (often associated with difficult airway management) are the most common causes of anesthesia-related maternal mortality.[26] Therefore, in addition to the ability to provide complete analgesia, continuous neuraxial labor analgesia has the added benefit of avoiding the need for general anesthesia and endotracheal intubation should emergency cesarean delivery be required.

Oxygen consumption, carbon dioxide production, and minute ventilation increase during pregnancy.[27] Functional residual capacity (FRC) decreases[28] and closing capacity may exceed FRC in supine pregnant women at term. Obesity, recumbency, and anesthesia (neuraxial or general) further decrease FRC.

During parturition, minute ventilation and oxygen consumption increase markedly, and hyperventilation results in partial pressure of carbon dioxide (Pa_{CO_2}) values as low as 10 to 15 mm Hg.[29] Maternal aerobic oxygen requirements exceed oxygen consumption resulting in a progressive maternal lactic acidemia.[30]

CARDIOVASCULAR CHANGES

The cardiovascular system is hyperdynamic during pregnancy. Total blood volume increases by approximately 50% during pregnancy,[31] as does cardiac output (Fig. 56.5).[27] Plasma volume increases more than red cell mass, resulting in the physiologic anemia of pregnancy.[31] Organ perfusion is markedly increased, particularly perfusion of the uterus. Systolic blood pressure falls minimally, whereas diastolic pressure decreases by approximately 20%.[27] Both return to prepregnant levels at term. Hemodynamic stability is more highly dependent on sympathetic nervous system activity,[32] and arterial responsiveness to vasopressors is reduced.[33]

Aortocaval Compression

At term, compression of the aorta and vena cava by the gravid uterus in the supine position results in decreased right ventricular preload and a 10% to 20% decrease in cardiac output

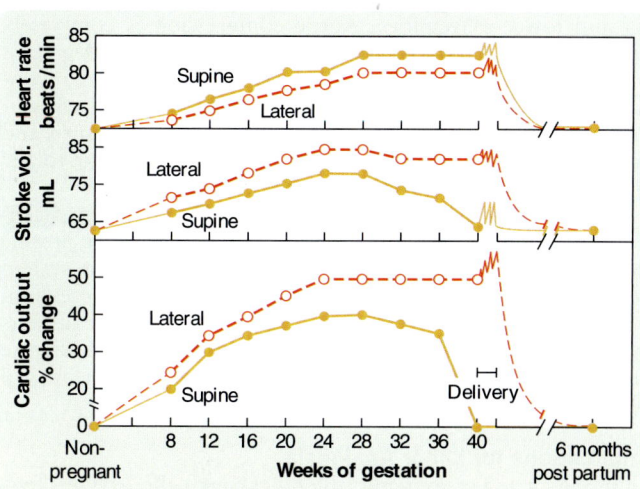

FIGURE 56.5 Changes in heart rate, stroke volume, and cardiac output during pregnancy and in the puerperium. *(Redrawn after Bonica JJ. Obstetric Analgesia and Anesthesia. 2nd ed. Seattle, WA: University of Washington Press; 1980:5. Reprinted by permission of World Federation of Societies of Anaesthesiologists.)*

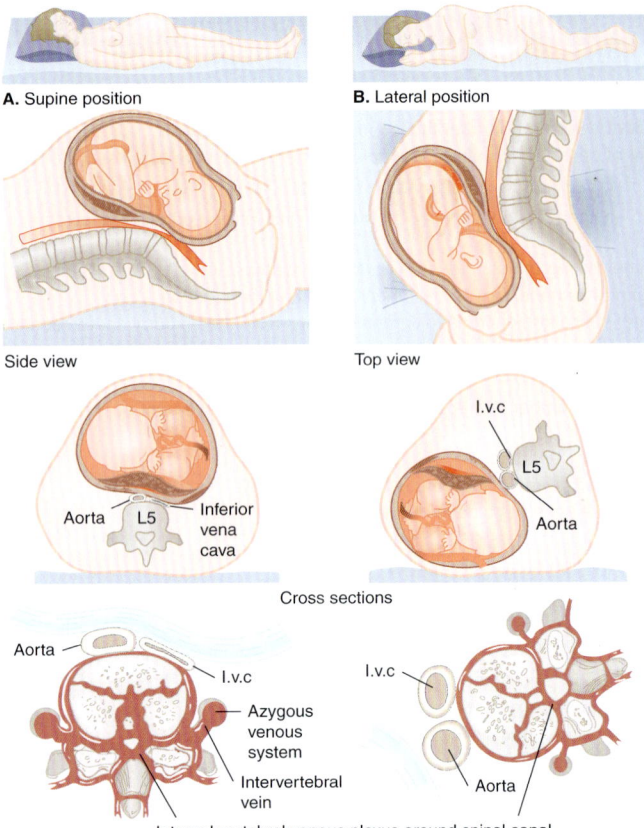

A. Supine position

B. Lateral position

Side view

Top view

I.v.c

L5

Aorta

Aorta   L5   Inferior
vena
cava

Cross sections

Aorta

I.v.c

I.v.c

Azygous
venous
system

Aorta

Intervertebral
vein

Internal vertebral venous plexus around spinal canal

FIGURE 56.6   Effect of the pregnant uterus on the inferior vena cava (I.r.c.) and the aorta in the supine position **(left)** and the lateral position **(right)**. The marked aortocaval compression in the supine position causes venous blood to be diverted to and through the vertebral venous plexus, which becomes engorged and reduces the size of the epidural and subarachnoid spaces. *(Redrawn after Bonica JJ.* Obstetric Analgesia and Anesthesia. *2nd ed. Seattle, WA: University of Washington Press; 1980:8. Reprinted by permission of World Federation of Societies of Anaesthesiologists.)*

compared to the standing position.[34] Vena cava compression begins as early as 13 to 16 weeks' gestation and may be nearly complete at term (Fig. 56.6).[35] Partial aortic compression in the supine position results in decreased blood flow to the pelvis and lower extremities. Aortic compression is completely relieved by the lateral position.[36] Data regarding the degree of compression of the vena cava in the lateral position are inconsistent[35,37]; however, in the lateral position, collateral circulation through the azygous system maintains venous return and cardiac output.[37,38] The left lateral position is superior to the right lateral position for maintenance of venous return.[39]

During labor, cardiac output increases due to increased central blood volume secondary to autotransfusion during uterine systole and because of increased sympathetic nervous system activity. Due to the adverse effects of aortocaval compression, parameters of fetal well-being deteriorate when parturients labor in the supine compared to lateral position.[40] Adverse effects may be more profound in the parturient with neuraxial blockade induced sympathetic blockade.

Implications for Labor Analgesia
Shunting of lower extremity blood through the azygous system results in venous engorgement in the epidural space. This functionally reduces the size of the epidural and subarachnoid spaces, thus reducing the amount of anesthetic necessary to produce neuroblockade. Sympathetic blockade in the term parturient (e.g., as a consequence of neuraxial analgesia/anesthesia)

results in a marked decrease in blood pressure compared to nonpregnant control subjects.[41] Pregnant women may require higher doses of vasopressors compared to nonpregnant individuals to treat hypotension.[33]

CENTRAL NERVOUS SYSTEM CHANGES
Anatomy of the Spinal Column and Analgesic Implications
Anatomic and physiologic changes in the nervous system alter responses to pain and susceptibility to both general and regional anesthesia. Specifically, anatomic changes in the spinal canal may affect neuraxial anesthesia techniques. The epidural and vertebral foraminal veins are enlarged, resulting in an increased risk of intravascular injection. Additionally, there is decreased nonvascular space in the spinal canal and decreased egress of epidural anesthetic agents from the epidural space. Engorged epidural veins[42] and increases in abdominal pressure[43] are associated with a decrease cerebral lumbosacral cerebral spinal fluid (CSF) volume.

Anatomic changes also occur to the ligamentous and bony structures of the vertebral column. The hormonal changes of pregnancy may cause the ligamentum flavum to feel less dense and "softer" in pregnant women compared to nonpregnant patients; thus, it may be more difficult to feel the passage of the epidural needle through the ligamentum flavum. Progressive accentuation of lumbar lordosis during pregnancy alters the relationship of surface anatomy to the vertebral column. The line joining the iliac crests (Tuffier's line) assumes a more cephalad relationship to the vertebral column, and accentuated lumbar lordosis results in less space between adjacent lumbar spinous processes. The apex of the lumbar lordosis is shifted caudad during pregnancy, and the typical thoracic kyphosis in women is reduced in pregnant women.[44] This may influence the spread of hypo- or hyperbaric intrathecal anesthetic solutions in supine patients.

Subarachnoid dose requirements may also be affected by the lower specific gravity of CSF in pregnant compared with nonpregnant women[45] and the higher CSF pH.[46] Widening of the pelvis may lead to a relative head-down position in women in the lateral position, thus affecting movement of hypo- or hyperbaric anesthetic solutions in the CSF. Because of the gravid uterus, it may be more difficult for a pregnant woman to achieve flexion of the lumbar spine. Finally, labor pain may make it difficult for women to assume and maintain an ideal position while the anesthesiologist initiates neuraxial anesthesia.

Neurohormonal Changes and Analgesic Implications
Pregnancy-induced neurohumoral changes may alter responses to pain. Lower plasma substance P concentrations[47] and higher CSF progesterone levels[48] are found in pregnancy. In a rat model, the pregnancy-associated increased concentration of plasma β-endorphin was associated with an increased tolerance to visceral stimulation, and this effect was reversed by naloxone.[49] Pain thresholds are increased during pregnancy[50] and labor.[51] Both peripheral and central nervous tissue from pregnant animals (including human) appears to be more susceptible to many different analgesic and anesthetic agents, including local anesthetics, volatile anesthetic agents, and thiopental. Possible mechanisms of enhanced neural blockade during pregnancy include potentiation of the analgesic effect of endogenous analgesic systems, hormone-related changes in the actions of spinal cord neurotransmitters, increased permeability of the neural sheath, or other pharmacodynamic or pharmacokinetic differences between pregnant and nonpregnant women.

Together, these anatomic and physiologic changes result in a 25% reduction in the segmental dose requirement for spinal anesthesia[48] and a similar segmental dose reduction for epidural anesthesia.[52]

PHARMACOKINETIC CHANGES

Pregnancy alters disposition of drugs by several mechanisms.[53] Volume of distribution may be altered. For example, the plasma concentration of antibiotics and, therefore, antimicrobial efficacy are decreased in pregnancy secondary to a large increase in the volume of distribution.[53] Plasma protein concentration decreases, leading to altered drug binding.[54] For example, lidocaine is less protein-bound during pregnancy, resulting in a higher free fraction in the blood.[55] Increased renal blood flow and glomerular filtration and altered hepatic microsomal activity change renal and hepatic drug clearance.

UTEROPLACENTAL UNIT

Blood flow to the uterus increases markedly during pregnancy, from 50 to 100 mL per minute before pregnancy, to 700 to 900 mL per minute at term. UBF is directly related to uterine perfusion pressure and indirectly related to uterine vascular resistance.

$$UBF = \frac{uterine\ arterial - uterine\ venous\ pressure}{uterine\ vascular\ resistance}$$

UBF is not autoregulated; therefore, decreases in uterine arterial pressure (systemic hypotension), increases in venous pressure (caval compression, uterine contraction or increase in uterine tone, Valsalva maneuver), or increases in uterine vascular resistance (increase in uterine vasoconstriction relative to systemic vasoconstriction) result in decreased UBF.

The net effect on UBF of any therapeutic intervention depends on relative changes in systemic and uterine vessels and effect on uterine tone. Labor analgesia may directly and indirectly affect UBF, both positively and negatively. For example, neuraxial analgesia may increase UBF because of decreased sympathetic outflow (secondary to both pain relief and direct sympathetic blockade), and decreased maternal hyperventilation. Conversely, neuraxial analgesia-induced maternal hypotension may decrease UBF. Additionally, neuraxial analgesia may be associated with transient uterine tachysystole secondary to an acute decrease in circulating epinephrine levels[56] and loss of its tocolytic (β₂-adrenergic agonism) effects.[57] Uterine tachysystole may also result from high concentrations of local anesthetic in uterine tissue, for example, after a paracervical block.[58]

Transfer of Drugs across the Placenta

Most drugs administrated to the mother cross the placenta to the fetus to some degree. Placental transfer depends on several factors, including plasma drug concentration and electrochemical gradients across the placenta, molecular weight, lipid solubility, degree of ionization, membrane surface area and thickness (changes during pregnancy), maternal and fetal blood flow, placental binding and metabolism, and degree of maternal and fetal protein binding. Direct drug teratogenicity may manifest as death, structural abnormalities, growth restriction, and functional deficiencies. Teratogenic potential is influenced by the timing of exposure, drug dose, duration of exposure, and genetic predisposition.[59] The risk of structural teratogenicity is greatest during the period of organogenesis (day 31 to 71 after the first day of the last menstrual period). Functional or behavioral teratogenicity may result from drug exposure during pregnancy, and even after birth, as the central nervous system continues to develop during this period.[60] Nondrug teratogens include hypoxia, hypercarbia, hyperthermia, hypoglycemia, and ionizing radiation.

Nonpharmacologic Methods of Labor Analgesia

Nonpharmacologic methods to relieve the pain and suffering of childbirth include childbirth education, emotional support, massage, aromatherapy, audiotherapy, and therapeutic use of hot and cold. More specialized techniques that require specialized training or equipment include hydrotherapy, intradermal water injections, biofeedback, transcutaneous electrical nerve stimulation (TENS), acupuncture or acupressure, and hypnosis. Many of these techniques are inadequately studied in that study quality is poor and sample size is small,[61,62] and therefore, conclusions about efficacy are not possible.

ANTENATAL CHILDBIRTH EDUCATION

Childbirth education is widely practiced. Unfortunately, studies of childbirth education lack scientific rigor. Study results are inconsistent as to whether participation in childbirth education classes influences outcomes, such as use of analgesia, duration of labor, mode of delivery, and incidence of nonreassuring fetal status.

LABOR SUPPORT

Emotional support is commonly provided by the parturient's husband or a friend. "Continuous labor support" refers to the nonmedical support of the parturient by a trained person. Prospective, controlled trials and several systematic analyses have concluded that women who receive continuous labor support have shorter labors, fewer operative deliveries, fewer analgesic interventions, and greater satisfaction.[63]

HYDROTHERAPY

Hydrotherapy is the immersion of the parturient in warm water (deep enough to cover the abdomen) during labor (not birth). Systematic reviews of randomized controlled trials have concluded that women experience less pain and use less analgesia without change in the duration of labor, rate of operative delivery, or neonatal outcome.[64]

INTRADERMAL WATER INJECTIONS

Intradermal water injection consists of the injection of 0.05 to 0.1 mL of sterile water, using an insulin or tuberculin syringe, at four sites on the lower back: over each posterior superior iliac crest, and 1 cm medial/3 cm caudad to these injections (Fig. 56.7). The technique is used to treat back pain during labor. The injections themselves are acutely painful for about 20 to 30 seconds, but as the injection pain fades, so does lower back pain. A 2012 systematic review that included seven studies and 766 study subjects reported a greater reduction in

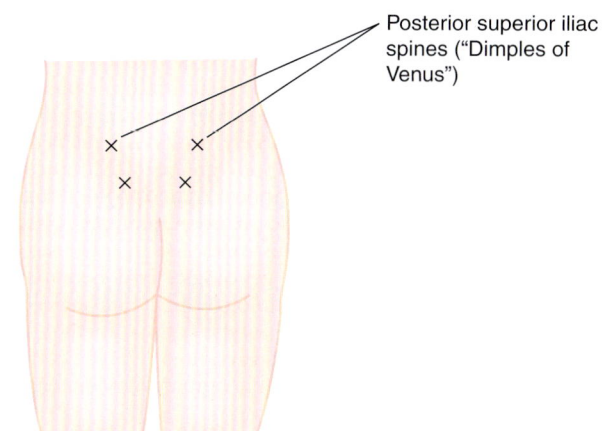

Posterior superior iliac spines ("Dimples of Venus")

FIGURE 56.7 Placement of intradermal water blocks: four intradermal injections of 0.05 to 0.1 mL of sterile water to form four small blebs over each posterior superior iliac spine and 3 cm below and 1 cm medial to each spine. The exact locations of the injections do not appear to be critical to the block success. *(Redrawn after Simkin P, Bolding A. Update on nonpharmacologic approaches to relieve labor pain and prevent suffering.* J Midwifery Womens Health *2004;49[6]:489–504. Copyright © 2004 American College of Nurse Midwives. Reprinted by permission of John Wiley & Sons, Inc.)*

pain scores in women who received sterile water injections compared with women in the control group.[65] However, the authors determined that a meta-analysis of the data was not appropriate and four studies were at high risk of bias. Further study is warranted.

HYPNOSIS

Self-hypnosis for treatment of childbirth pain has been practiced for several centuries. Hypnosis requires prenatal training of the mother, and sometimes her partner, by a trained hypnotherapist. A meta-analysis of nine randomized controlled trials that included 2,954 women found the overall use of pharmacologic analgesia methods was decreased in the hypnosis compared to control groups, but neuraxial analgesia use was not.[66] Data were inconclusive or limited regarding progress of labor and neonatal outcomes.

TRANSCUTANEOUS ELECTRICAL STIMULATION

TENS involves the application of low-intensity, high-frequency electrical impulses to the skin of the lower back. The buzzing, electrical current sensation caused by the TENS unit may reduce the mother's awareness of contraction pain. Studies of TENS are inconsistent, but in general, labor pain does not appear to be lessened or is the use of other analgesic modalities.[67]

ACUPUNCTURE AND ACUPRESSURE

Acupuncture is a component of traditional Chinese medicine that has gained popularity in Western cultures in recent years. A 2011 systematic review concluded that the use of acupuncture and acupressure during labor may have a role in reducing pain and the need for pharmacologic analgesia.[68] However, authors of a 2014 review of systematic reviews of acupuncture therapy during labor concluded that the trials included in this and other systematic reviews differ in terms of study design and outcome measures, and therefore, it may be inappropriate to include the studies in a pooled analysis.[62] Further study is warranted.

Systemic Analgesia

INHALATIONAL ANALGESIA

Inhalation analgesia for labor and vaginal delivery, common in other countries, is gaining popularity in the United States. The only inhaled anesthetic agent currently in common use is nitrous oxide. It is commercially available as a mixture of 50% nitrous oxide and 50% oxygen. Special equipment is required to ensure the safe administration of the drug without contamination of the labor room. The mother must be taught to breathe the mixture correctly, so that peak brain nitrous oxide concentrations coincide with peak contraction pain. Studies are conflicting as to whether nitrous oxide provides benefit to the parturient; most studies are of a poor quality.[69] Although the intermittent use of nitrous oxide appears safe for the fetus and neonate, neonatal studies are also of poor quality.[69] There is accumulating evidence that nitrous oxide use in other settings may not be benign; neurologic, genologic, and hematologic toxicity as well as adverse immunologic effects have been described.[70] Risk may depend on genotype[71]; thus, further study of its use for childbirth analgesia is warranted.[71,72] The concomitant use of nitrous oxide and systemic opioids may increase the risk of maternal hypoxemia.

PARENTERAL OPIOID ANALGESIA

Systemic opioid analgesia, administered by the subcutaneous, intramuscular, or intravenous route, is widely used around the world either as the sole analgesic modality or prior to the administration of regional labor analgesia.[73] The use of systemic opioids for labor analgesia lacks rigorous scientific study. There is a high incidence of side effects (e.g., sedation,

nausea, and vomiting), and analgesia is incomplete, at best, during active labor.[74,75] Historically, meperidine has been the most commonly used systemic opioid; however, its use in the United States has declined in the past decade as practitioners have come to better appreciate its long maternal and neonatal half-life and that of its active metabolite, normeperidine. There is little scientific evidence that any one opioid is better than another. All have dose-related, maternal, fetal, and neonatal side effects. Maternal side effects include nausea, vomiting, delayed gastric emptying, dysphoria, and respiratory depression. All opioids cross the placenta. In utero, opioids may result in a slower fetal heart rate and decreased beat-to-beat variability.[76] The likelihood of neonatal respiratory depression depends on the dose and timing of administration.

Patient-Controlled Intravenous Analgesia

Patient-controlled intravenous analgesia (PCIA) has theoretical advantages to nurse-administered opioid analgesia, including superior analgesia with smaller drug doses, resulting in a lower incidence of side effects. PCIA studies have been reported using meperidine, nalbuphine, fentanyl, and, more recently, remifentanil with and without a background infusion. Remifentanil has the theoretical advantage of rapid onset and offset compared to the other opioids, although its peak effect still occurs after the contraction if the parturient self-administers a bolus dose at the beginning of a contraction. Multiple studies have used different bolus doses, rates of bolus-dose administration, lockout intervals, and background infusion rates. In a 2016 review, Van de Velde and Carvalho[77] suggested a fixed bolus dose of 20 to 50 μg with a lockout interval of 1 to 3 minutes and no background infusion. The bolus dose may require upward adjustment as labor progresses. However, as with other systemic opioid techniques, it is unclear whether remifentanil PCIA can provide satisfactory analgesia without an unacceptably high incidence of side effects.[78] In a randomized trial comparing epidural to remifentanil PCIA, apnea episodes were recorded in 53% of women in the remifentanil group.[79] Monitoring oxygen saturation (SpO$_2$) was insufficient to identify most of the apnea episodes.[79] Experts agree that remifentanil PCIA should only be used when the parturient is under continuous observation by a midwife or labor nurse.[78]

Neuraxial Analgesia

Neuraxial labor analgesia is the most effective method of pain relief during childbirth and the only method that provides complete analgesia without maternal or fetal sedation. The use of neuraxial analgesia for childbirth has increased dramatically in the United States over the past 40 years.[9] The most common techniques are continuous lumbar epidural analgesia and combined spinal-epidural (CSE) analgesia. Single-shot spinal, continuous spinal, and caudal analgesia are occasionally used.

Contraindications to neuraxial analgesia and anesthesia include patient refusal, infection at the puncture site, preexisting coagulopathy, and lack of experienced anesthesia providers. Relative contraindications include hemorrhage or other causes of hypovolemia, untreated systemic infection, preload-dependent disease states, and lumbar spine pathology. The anesthesiologist should weigh the risk and benefits of a neuraxial procedure for each patient, and the specific neuraxial analgesic technique should be tailored to individual patient needs. The risks and benefits of the procedure should be discussed with each parturient, preferably early in labor. The advantages and disadvantages of specific neuraxial techniques are listed in Table 56.2.

EPIDURAL ANALGESIA

Lumbar epidural analgesia has been the mainstay of regional labor analgesia. Placement of an epidural catheter allows analgesia to be maintained until after delivery. Additionally,

TABLE 56.2 Advantages and Disadvantages of Specific Neuraxial Techniques for Labor Analgesia

	Analgesia Technique				
	Continuous Epidural	**Combined Spinal-Epidural**	**Single-Shot Spinal**	**Continuous Spinal**	**Caudal**
Advantages	• Continuous technique • No dural puncture • Ability to convert to epidural anesthesia	• Rapid onset • Early sacral block • Low dose of anesthetic • Complete early labor analgesia with opioid only[a]	• Rapid onset • Technically easier • Early sacral block	• Rapid onset • Early sacral block • Low dose of anesthetic • Continuous technique • Ability to convert to spinal anesthesia	• Ability to access epidural space in patient with lumbar epidural pathology
Disadvantages	• Slow onset • Requires greater mass of anesthetic[b] • Delayed sacral blockade/sacral sparing	• Requires dural puncture	• Requires dural puncture • Limited duration of analgesia	• Requires dural puncture with large gauge needle[c] • Potential for accidental intrathecal injection of epidural dose of anesthetic agents	• Requires large volume/mass of anesthetic to block T10 dermatome[b,d]

[a]Large doses of epidural opioid may provide near-complete analgesia for early labor but at the expense of significant systemic absorption and with accompanying side effects.
[b]Greater vascular absorption of anesthetic agents and greater likelihood for accidental intravascular injection of a toxic amount of local anesthetic.
[c]Increased risk of postdural puncture headache.
[d]May not be able to achieve T4 sensory blockade necessary for cesarean delivery.

it allows conversion to epidural anesthesia should cesarean delivery be necessary. No dural puncture is required. Randomized studies consistently demonstrate that pain scores are lower and patients are more satisfied with epidural analgesia compared to nonneuraxial analgesia.[80] Injection of anesthetics in the lumbar epidural space allows spread of the anesthetic solution both cephalad and caudad. Neural blockade to the T10 dermatome is necessary to relieve uterine and cervical pain, whereas blockade of the sacral dermatomes is necessary to block the pain of vaginal and perineal distention.

Compared to spinal analgesic techniques, the onset of epidural analgesia is significantly slower (15 to 20 minutes compared to 2 to 5 minutes), particularly the onset of sacral analgesia. It may take several hours of lumbar epidural infusion, or several bolus injections of local anesthetic into the lumbar epidural space, to achieve sacral analgesia. This is particularly disadvantageous in a rapidly laboring parturient who requires rapid onset of sacral analgesia for the late first and second stages of labor. In addition, epidural compared to spinal analgesia requires significantly more drug(s) to attain comparable analgesia, thus increasing the risk of systemic toxicity. Finally, there is significantly more systemic absorption of anesthetic agents, and therefore, maternal and fetal plasma drug concentrations are higher with epidural compared to spinal analgesia.

Lumbar epidural analgesia is initiated in either the sitting or lateral position. The epidural space is identified with a 17 or 18G epidural needle, usually using a loss-of-resistance to air of saline technique. A flexible catheter is passed through the needle approximately 4 to 5 cm into the epidural space, the epidural needle is removed, and the catheter is secured. A test dose is frequently administered to rule out intrathecal or intravascular catheter placement. The most common test dose is lidocaine 15 mg/mL with epinephrine 5 μg/mL, 3 mL. No matter whether a test dose is injected, drugs should be injected incrementally into the epidural space, as no test is 100% sensitive and catheters may migrate during use. Pregnant women are very difficult to resuscitate from local anesthetic systemic toxicity.

Analgesia is initiated by bolus injection of anesthetic(s) through the epidural needle, catheter, or both. Analgesia is maintained with intermittent bolus injections or a continuous infusion. The catheter is removed after delivery when there is no further need for analgesia/anesthesia.

Drugs for Initiation of Epidural Analgesia

Drugs commonly used for epidural labor analgesia are listed in Table 56.3. Local anesthetics, primarily bupivacaine, have been the mainstay of epidural analgesia for many years. The amount of epidural local anesthetic required for satisfactory analgesia increases as labor progresses.[81] Low bupivacaine concentrations (≤ 1.25 mg/mL) provide excellent analgesia with minimal motor block. The ED_{50} of bupivacaine 1.25 mg/mL was lower than the ED_{50} of bupivacaine 2.5 mg/mL, suggesting that the use of low concentrations is associated with less overall drug requirement.[82] Bupivacaine is highly protein-bound with minimal placental transfer,[83] and duration of analgesia is approximately 2 hours. Onset to peak effect is approximately 20 minutes. Lidocaine and 2-chloroprocaine have shorter latency, but their duration of analgesia is shorter, limiting their usefulness for routine labor analgesia. In addition, lidocaine is less protein-bound than bupivacaine and therefore has a higher umbilical vein/maternal vein ratio.[84] 2-Chloroprocaine is most useful for rapidly converting epidural *analgesia* to epidural *anesthesia* for urgent operative delivery.

TABLE 56.3 Typical Drugs for Initiation of Epidural Labor Analgesia

Drug	Concentration	
Local Anesthetics[a]		**Dose (Volume)**
Bupivacaine	1.00–1.25 mg/mL	10–15 mL
Ropivacaine	1.0–2.0 mg/mL	10–15 mL
Opioids[a]		**Dose (Mass)**
Fentanyl	—	50–100 μg
Sufentanil	—	5–10 μg
Adjuvants		
Epinephrine	1.25–5.00 μg/mL	—
Clonidine[b]	—	60–75 μg[c]

NOTE: The actual drug dose will depend on the stage of labor (women in advanced labor require higher doses), the progress of labor (women with rapid progress of labor will require higher doses), and whether or not an anesthetic containing test dose has been administered.
[a]Local anesthetics and opioids are commonly administered together, in which case a lower dose of each is required.
[b]Clonidine is not approved for use in obstetric patients in the United States.
[c]This dose should be combined with local anesthetics, as higher doses used alone cause sedation and hypotension.

Ropivacaine is a homologue of bupivacaine, formulated as a single levorotatory enantiomer. Its onset and duration of action are similar to bupivacaine,[85] but it has less potential for cardiac toxicity. Although potency studies suggest that ropivacaine is approximately 40% less potent than bupivacaine,[86] clinical studies comparing low concentrations of ropivacaine and bupivacaine for labor analgesia suggest that they are equipotent in terms of sensory blockade for labor analgesia.[87,88] However, ropivacaine may be associated with less motor blockade than equipotent doses of bupivacaine.[89] Levobupivacaine, the S-enantiomer of bupivacaine, is not available in the United States. Similar to ropivacaine and bupivacaine in its onset and duration of action, it is less cardiotoxic than bupivacaine and is associated with less motor blockade compared to bupivacaine.[87,89]

Opioids, particularly the lipid-soluble opioids, fentanyl and sufentanil, are commonly added to local anesthetics for epidural analgesia. Epidural opioids and local anesthetics interact synergistically to provide analgesia.[90,91] The addition of opioids shortens latency; allows for decreased concentration of local anesthetic, thus decreasing motor block; and prolongs analgesia. Although epidural opioids alone can provide moderate analgesia for early labor, analgesia is incomplete, and the necessary dose is accompanied by bothersome side effects (e.g., pruritus, nausea, vomiting, maternal sedation, neonatal respiratory depression). Combining local anesthetics with opioids allows for effective analgesia while minimizing the side effects of both drugs.

Fentanyl and sufentanil are ideal for labor analgesia because of their rapid onset (5 to 10 minutes). Their short duration of action (60 to 90 minutes) is overcome by maintaining analgesia with a continuous epidural infusion. Doses commonly used for epidural analgesia initiation and maintenance have been shown to be safe for both the mother and neonate.[92,93] Morphine has a much slower onset (30 to 60 minutes) and longer duration of action (12 to 24 hours) than fentanyl or sufentanil. The long duration of action is not beneficial, as the bothersome side effects of morphine (pruritus, nausea, and vomiting) continue to be present after delivery.

Adjuvants for epidural labor analgesia include epinephrine and clonidine. Epidural epinephrine may contribute to analgesia by decreasing the uptake of local anesthetics and opioids from the epidural space secondary to vasoconstriction and by binding to spinal cord α_2-adrenergic receptors.[94] Clonidine also binds to α_2-adrenergic receptors and has been shown to supplement epidural labor analgesia. The U.S. Food and Drug Administration (FDA) has not approved neuraxial clonidine for use in obstetric patients because of the risks of sedation and hypotension. However, it is useful for the treatment of breakthrough pain (75 to 100 µg) when the administration of additional local anesthetic is likely to contribute to worsening motor block; any resulting hypotension is usually readily treated.[95]

COMBINED SPINAL-EPIDURAL ANALGESIA

CSE analgesia has become increasingly popular for labor analgesia. There are advantages and disadvantages to CSE compared to traditional epidural analgesia (see Table 56.2). Onset of analgesia is significantly faster compared to epidural analgesia.[96] Complete analgesia for early labor can be accomplished with the intrathecal injection of lipid-soluble opioids without the addition of local anesthetics, thus avoiding motor blockade and decreasing the risk of hypotension. This is ideal for patients who wish to ambulate, or for those with preload-dependent conditions such as stenotic heart lesions. The effective opioid dose is significantly less than for systemic or epidural administration. Therefore, systemic drug absorption is minimal, as are direct fetal effects. The addition of local anesthetic to a lipid-soluble opioid results in sacral analgesia within several minutes. This is a decided advantage compared

to lumbar epidural analgesia, as sacral analgesia is difficult to accomplish after a single lumbar epidural dose of local anesthetic. Therefore, CSE analgesia provides more complete analgesia for women in advanced stages of labor or women whose labor is progressing rapidly. Finally, use of the CSE technique may decrease the incidence of failed epidural analgesia (e.g., a nonfunctioning epidural catheter).[97]

There are several undesirable side effects of CSE analgesia. The incidence of pruritus is higher with intrathecal versus epidural opioids.[96] Dural puncture is required to initiate CSE analgesia. The risk of postdural puncture headache (PDPH) may be minimally higher with the CSE compared to pure epidural technique (estimated excess rate of 3 in 1,000).[98] However, a more serious concern is that dural puncture in the obstetric patient may be a risk factor for postpartum neuraxial infection, a rare but potentially life-threatening complication.[99]

Several techniques for CSE analgesia/anesthesia have been described, including using two skin punctures in two interspaces, two punctures in one interspace, and the needle-through-needle technique.[98] The most common CSE technique for labor analgesia is the needle-through-needle technique in a midlumbar interspinous space. The epidural space is identified with an epidural needle in the standard fashion. The epidural needle then functions as an introducer needle as a long spinal needle is passed through it until the dura is punctured. The intrathecal drug(s) is injected through the spinal needle, the spinal needle is withdrawn, and an epidural catheter is threaded through the epidural needle. Analgesia is maintained via the epidural catheter, as with traditional epidural analgesia.

Drugs for Initiation of Combined Spinal-Epidural Analgesia

CSE labor analgesia is usually initiated with a lipid-soluble opioid (fentanyl or sufentanil) or a combination of opioid and local anesthetic (Table 56.4). Morphine is not commonly used because of its long latency and long duration of action (a disadvantage, as women usually deliver before regression of side effects). However, morphine has been successfully combined with intrathecal bupivacaine and fentanyl in order to shorten latency and increase duration of analgesia.[100] This combination of drugs may be particularly useful in settings where continuous epidural infusion techniques are impractical.[100] Meperidine is unique among the opioids in that it has weak local anesthetic properties. However, meperidine was associated with a significantly higher incidence of nausea and vomiting compared to combined fentanyl and bupivacaine.[101]

Intrathecal opioids can provide complete analgesia early in labor when the pain stimuli are primarily visceral. Onset of analgesia occurs within 5 minutes and lasts 70 to 100 minutes.[102] The reported ED_{95} of intrathecal fentanyl varies from 14 to 23 µg.[103,104] The relative potency ratio of intrathecal sufentanil

TABLE 56.4 Drugs for the Initiation of Intrathecal Labor Analgesia

Drug(s)[a]	Opioid Dose (µg)	Bupivacaine Dose (mg)
Fentanyl	15–25	—
Sufentanil	5–7.5	—
Bupivacaine-fentanyl	10–15	1.25–2.5
Bupivacaine-sufentanil	1–2.5	1.25–2.5
Bupivacaine-fentanyl-morphine[b]	Fentanyl 12.5–25	2.0–2.5
	Morphine 200–250	2.0–2.5

[a]Opioids alone provide complete analgesia for early labor, but the addition of local anesthetics is required for late first-stage and second-stage analgesia.
[b]The combination of bupivacaine-fentanyl-morphine may be advantageous in the settings where continuous epidural infusions for maintenance of analgesia are impractical and single-shot techniques are an alternative.

to fentanyl for labor analgesia is 4.4:1.[102] When administered at twice the ED_{50}, the duration of sufentanil analgesia was 25 minutes longer than fentanyl, although the incidence of side effects was not different.[102] The duration of action of intrathecal opioids is dose-related, although fentanyl doses greater than 25 μg do not increase duration of analgesia and are associated with a higher incidence of side effects.[103]

In the late first stage and second stage of labor, local anesthetic must be added to the opioid to block somatic stimuli from the vagina and perineum. The local anesthetic works synergistically with the opioid; thus, lower doses of both drugs can be used.[105] Bupivacaine is most commonly combined with fentanyl or sufentanil. The ED_{95} of bupivacaine combined with sufentanil 1.5 μg was 3.3 mg[106] and was 1.66 mg when combined with fentanyl 15 μg.[107] Bupivacaine doses between 1.25 to 2.5 mg are commonly used. Levobupivacaine and ropivacaine are not approved for intrathecal use in the United States. They are less potent than bupivacaine for intrathecal labor analgesia.[106]

Bupivacaine without opioid is not commonly used for labor analgesia. Doses high enough to provide analgesia are associated with significant motor blockade, and lower doses either do not provide satisfactory analgesia or are associated with an unacceptably short duration of action.[108]

MAINTENANCE OF EPIDURAL ANALGESIA

Epidural analgesia may be maintained with intermittent bolus injection, continuous epidural infusion, patient-controlled epidural analgesia (PCEA), with or without a background infusion or programmed intermittent epidural bolus injections. Continuous epidural infusions result in less need for bolus injections[109,110] and increased patient satisfaction[111] but higher total drug dose[109,111] compared to intermittent injections. However, the infusion of lower concentration bupivacaine at a higher rate may result in similar analgesia with less motor block and no increase in total dose.[111,112] Common infusion solutions and protocols are listed in Table 56.5.

PCEA allows for both a continuous epidural infusion and patient-titrated bolus injections. PCEA results in greater patient satisfaction and a lower average hourly dose of bupivacaine (and therefore less motor block) and less need for physician intervention.[113,114] The protocols for PCEA vary widely, and it is unclear whether this affects analgesia and outcome. At one extreme, most of the hourly dose is administered via a background infusion which the parturient may supplement with self-administered boluses. At the other extreme, there is no background infusion and the entire dose is self-administered via intermittent boluses. Bupivacaine consumption is higher with background infusions compared to a pure PCEA technique without a background infusion.[115] Although data are conflicting as to whether a background infusion improves analgesia,[114,116] it may be helpful in selected parturients (e.g., nulliparas with long labors).[114] Solutions for PCEA generally mimic those used for continuous infusions (see Table 56.5). The parturient

administered bolus dose is 5 to 10 mL, the lockout interval is 10 to 20 minutes, and the background infusion varies from 0 to 15 mL. Commonly, 30% to 50% of the hourly dose is administered as a background infusion.

The bolus administration of epidural anesthetic solution appears to result in improved analgesia with a lower total drug dose compared with continuous infusion administration. Historically, the anesthesia provider or the patient (PCEA) administered a bolus dose, whereas an infusion pump delivered a continuous infusion. In a new mode for maintaining epidural analgesia, the infusion pump is programmed to intermittently administer a bolus dose rather than a continuous infusion. Compared with continuous infusion analgesia or PCEA, programmed intermittent epidural bolus analgesia results in improved parturient satisfaction, less drug use, longer duration of analgesia, and less breakthrough pain compared to a continuous infusion of the same mass of drug per unit time.[117,118] There may be better distribution of anesthetic solution within the epidural space when large volumes are injected as a bolus compared to a slow infusion. The optimal bolus volume, interval, and administration rate have yet to be determined. Most clinicians are currently using programmed bolus volumes between 5 and 10 mL, administered every 30 to 60 minutes.[117]

OTHER CENTRAL NEURAXIAL TECHNIQUES

Single-Shot and Continuous Spinal Analgesia

In general, single-shot spinal analgesia is not useful for most laboring patients because of its limited duration of action. It may be indicated in parturients who require analgesia or anesthesia shortly before anticipated delivery or in settings where continuous epidural analgesia is not possible. Drugs for single-shot spinal analgesia mimic those used for the initiation of CSE analgesia (see Table 56.4).

Continuous spinal analgesia is currently not practical for most parturients. The 23G spinal catheter that is available in the United States is inserted using a "catheter-over-needle" technique. An initial observational trial reported that the catheter may have clinical utility[119]; however, further study is required to characterize ease of use and complications, particularly the rate of PDPH. The placement of a continuous spinal catheter is a management option in patients with unintentional dural puncture with an epidural needle or when rapid analgesia is necessary in an obese patient. In this case, the "epidural" catheter is threaded into the subarachnoid space. Care must be taken not to confuse a catheter sited in the subarachnoid space with one sited in the epidural space, given the much larger anesthetic dose required for epidural analgesia. Continuous spinal labor analgesia is commonly maintained with the same solution used for epidural analgesia but at a rate of 1 to 2 mL per hour.

Dural Puncture Epidural Analgesia

Dural puncture epidural (DPE) analgesia is a modification of CSE analgesia that aims to exploit the advantages of the CSE analgesia without its attendant disadvantages. The technique mimics that of CSE analgesia, except that no drug is injected into the subarachnoid space after puncturing the dura with a spinal needle. It is hypothesized that the dural puncture made by the spinal needle augments transdural migration of the local anesthetic/opioid solution injected into the epidural space, resulting in faster onset and improved sacral analgesia compared with epidural analgesia. Studies are conflicting as to whether DPE offers an advantage compared to epidural or CSE analgesia[120–123]; further investigation is warranted.

Caudal Analgesia

Continuous caudal epidural analgesia is used infrequently in the practice of modern obstetric anesthesia. Large volumes of local anesthetic are required for first-stage analgesia and result

TABLE 56.5	Drug Solutions for Maintenance of Epidural Labor Analgesia		
Drug Solution	Local Anesthetic Concentration (mg/mL)	Opioid Concentration (μg/mL)
Bupivacaine-fentanyl	0.625–1.25	2–4
Bupivacaine-sufentanil	0.625–1.25	0.20–0.33
Ropivacaine-fentanyl	0.8–1.5	2–4
Ropivacaine	2.0	—

NOTE: Continuous infusions rate: 10 to 15 mL/hour. Patient-controlled epidural analgesia (PCEA) parameters: PCEA bolus 5 to 10 mL, lockout interval 10 to 20 minutes, background infusion 0 to 15 mL/hour (commonly 30% to 50% of hourly dose requirement).

in higher maternal plasma concentrations of drug. There is a risk of needle/catheter misplacement and direct injection into the fetus. However, this technique is an option in patients in whom access to the lumbar neuraxial canal is not possible (e.g., fused lumbar spine).

SIDE EFFECTS OF NEURAXIAL ANALGESIA

Common side effects of neuraxial labor analgesia include hypotension and pruritus. Other side effects include urinary retention, delayed gastric emptying (after opioid techniques but not pure local anesthetic techniques), oral herpes simplex virus recrudescence, shivering, maternal hyperthermia, and fetal bradycardia.

Hypotension

Blockade of the sympathetic nervous system by local anesthetics causes vasodilation, increased venous capacitance, and decreased afterload. Hypotension may result in decreased uteroplacental perfusion and fetal heart rate decelerations or bradycardia. Therefore, maternal blood pressure and fetal heart rate should be monitored for 15 to 30 minutes after the induction of neuroblockade. Although intravenous volume expansion prior to initiating neuraxial analgesia has traditionally been used to reduce the incidence and degree of hypotension, it is not clear that this has any real benefit with modern low-dose neuraxial labor analgesia techniques.[124] The mother should be positioned in the full lateral position after initiation of neuraxial blockade, and hypotension should be treated with small bolus doses of intravenous vasopressor.

Pruritus

Pruritus is common side effect of neuraxial opioid administration. It is more common after intrathecal (as high as 100%) than epidural administration, and the incidence and severity are dose-related.[104,108] The cause is unknown, but it is not thought to be histamine-related. Pruritus may be generalized or localized to the nose, face, or chest and is typically self-limited. Concomitant local anesthetic administration decreased the incidence and severity of pruritus compared to fentanyl alone,[125] whereas the addition of epinephrine worsened the pruritus.[126] The one-time administration of naloxone (40 to 80 μg) or nalbuphine (2.5 to 5 mg) is usually effective for the treatment of pruritus induced by fentanyl or sufentanil. A naloxone infusion may be required for the treatment of morphine-induced pruritus.

Fetal Bradycardia

Fetal bradycardia, not associated with maternal hypotension, occurs after initiation of both epidural and CSE analgesia, although the incidence is likely higher after CSE analgesia.[127] Clarke and colleagues[128] hypothesized that fetal bradycardia may be due to the acute decrease in plasma epinephrine levels following the initiation of neuraxial analgesia.[56] Epinephrine is a tocolytic, and the acute decrease in maternal plasma concentration may result in temporary imbalance of uterine tocolytic/tocodynamic forces, resulting in uterine tachysystole, decreased uterine perfusion, and, ultimately, fetal bradycardia. Nitroglycerin has been used successfully to treat uterine tachysystole associated with the initiation of neuraxial analgesia.[129]

Maternal Hyperthermia

Epidural labor analgesia is associated with maternal fever (temperature ≥38° C) in some women.[130] In randomized controlled trials, the incidence ranges between 20% and 30%.[130] The mechanism is unclear; current evidence supports a noninfectious inflammatory mechanism. It is also not understood why some women become febrile and others do not.

COMPLICATIONS OF NEURAXIAL ANALGESIA

Complications of neuraxial labor analgesia include inadequate or failed analgesia, unintentional dural puncture, subdural injection, respiratory depression, high- or total-spinal anesthesia, systemic local anesthetic toxicity, needle or catheter trauma to central nervous system tissue (spinal cord and nerve roots), direct tissue local anesthetic toxicity (cauda equina syndrome, arachnoiditis), pneumocephalus, spinal or epidural hematoma, spinal or epidural abscess, and meningitis.

Unintentional Dural Puncture

Unintentional dural puncture with an epidural needle occurs in 1.5% of obstetric patients receiving epidural analgesia or anesthesia, and 52% will develop a PDPH.[131] This is a particularly troublesome complication of epidural analgesia because women are usually quickly mobile after childbirth with the need to care for their newborn infants. A therapeutic epidural blood patch with autologous blood remains the gold standard treatment. Approximately 60% to 75% of women get partial or complete relief.[132] In a multicenter randomized controlled trial comparing an epidural blood patch with 15-, 20-, or 30-mL autologous blood, there was no difference in the rate of permanent or partial headache relief among the groups, but the 20- and 30-mL groups had a higher rate of permanent relief.[132]

Other treatment modalities for the prevention and treatment of PDPH have not proven effective (e.g., epidural saline infusion, caffeine, prophylactic blood patch) or are inadequately studied (e.g., placement of an intrathecal catheter, prophylactic neuraxial morphine administration, prophylactic intravenous cosyntropin administration).

Respiratory Depression

Severe respiratory depression or arrest has been reported after the intrathecal injection of sufentanil in laboring women.[133] The risk appears to be increased when intrathecal opioids are administered before or after systemic opioids. Respiratory depression is opioid dose-dependent.[104] It generally occurs within 2 hours after the intrathecal administration of fentanyl and sufentanil. In contrast, respiratory depression after epidural and intrathecal morphine usually presents 6 to 12 hours after administration of drug.

Other Regional Analgesic Techniques

Neuraxial analgesia is the most effective and flexible analgesic technique for labor and delivery. However, some parturients may not be candidates for neuraxial analgesia or may not want it. Other nerve blocks may provide acceptable, albeit less flexible, analgesia.

PARACERVICAL BLOCK

A paracervical block blocks transmission of visceral afferent nerve impulses from the uterus and cervix through the paracervical (Frankenhäuser's) ganglion. Advantages include excellent analgesia for the first stage of labor, before fetal descent, without somatic sensory or motor block. However, the block is not continuous, and it does not relieve somatic pain caused by distension of the pelvic floor, vagina, or perineum.

Serious maternal complications are unusual; however, serious fetal complications are not uncommon. Fetal bradycardia is the most common fetal complication. Recommendations to reduce complications include (1) perform the block only in parturients with no evidence of uteroplacental insufficiency; (2) perform the block when the cervix is dilated <8 cm to avoid unintentional injection of the fetal scalp; (3) monitor uterine activity and fetal heart rate continuously; (4) after injecting local anesthetic on one side, wait 5 to 10 minutes before injecting anesthetic on the second side; and (5) consider using 2-chloroprocaine.[134]

LUMBAR SYMPATHETIC BLOCK

Paravertebral lumbar sympathetic blockade interferes with transmission of visceral afferent nerve impulses from the uterus and cervix at the level of the L2–L3 sympathetic chain. Similar to a paracervical block, it provides analgesia for the first stage but not the second stage of labor. Disadvantages include a technique that is not continuous and that it is technically difficult to learn and perform and requires bilateral injections. Advantages include that it is associated with less fetal bradycardia than a paracervical block, it provides first-stage analgesia without any motor block, it is useful for patients with previous back surgery, and the progress of labor is accelerated compared to epidural analgesia.[135]

PUDENDAL BLOCK

A pudendal nerve block interrupts pain signals from vaginal, vulvar, and perineal distension. It provides satisfactory analgesia for spontaneous vaginal and low- or outlet-forceps delivery but not midforceps delivery or exploration of the upper vagina, cervix, or uterine cavities.[136] The pudendal nerve can be blocked via the transperineal or transvaginal route. Most obstetricians in the United States employ the transvaginal route immediately before delivery.[134] Maternal and fetal complications of pudendal nerve block are rare. Fetal complications include fetal trauma and/or direct fetal injection of local anesthetic.[134]

PERINEAL INFILTRATION

Perineal infiltration is often used immediately before delivery to provide anesthesia for an episiotomy or repair. It provides no motor relaxation. Five to 10 mL of local anesthetic are injected into the posterior fourchette. Perineal infiltration may be complicated by direct injection of local anesthetic into the fetal scalp resulting in neonatal local anesthetic toxicity.[137]

Effects of Analgesia on the Progress of Labor

There has been much controversy concerning the effect of neuraxial labor analgesia on the progress of labor and mode of delivery. Early investigators noted that regional analgesia appeared to be an effective treatment for dysfunctional labor.[24,138] Observational studies, however, have uniformly found an association between neuraxial analgesia, prolonged labor, and operative delivery. A number of randomized controlled trials have compared neuraxial labor analgesia to systemic opioid analgesia, and most found no difference in the rate of cesarean delivery between groups.[80] The probable explanation for observed association between epidural analgesia and cesarean delivery is that women who have more pain during labor (and thus more likely to request analgesia) have a higher risk of cesarean delivery.[14,15] Fetal macrosomia, malposition, and dysfunctional labor are associated with more painful labor and a higher rate of cesarean delivery.

Another concern is whether neuraxial analgesia adversely affects the first stage of labor, particularly when administered in the latent phase. Again, observational studies suggest that early labor initiation of neuraxial analgesia is associated with an increased rate of cesarean delivery. Randomized controlled trials, however, uniformly demonstrated that early labor initiation of neuraxial compared to systemic opioid analgesia does not adversely affect the outcome of labor,[139] and in fact, may result in faster labor.[140,141]

Randomized controlled trials comparing neuraxial to systemic opioid analgesia have assessed the risk of instrumental vaginal delivery and duration of labor as secondary outcomes. Systematic review of these trials have found that the duration of the second stage of labor is prolonged by approximately 15 minutes and the rate of instrumental forceps delivery is increased.[80] Initiation and maintenance of epidural labor analgesia with high concentration local anesthetic solutions (defined as ≥0.1% bupivacaine, ≥0.17% ropivacaine) is associated with a higher instrumental vaginal delivery rate compared to low-concentration solutions, mostly likely secondary to the increased incidence of motor blockade with higher concentration solutions.[142] Thus, it is the responsibility of the anesthesiologist to use a neuraxial technique that minimizes motor block in order to decrease the risk of instrumental vaginal delivery.

Nonobstetric Drug Therapy during Pregnancy and Lactation

The management of pain during pregnancy is complicated by the need to limit the transfer of drugs across the placenta, particularly during the first trimester, as well as the necessity of limiting radiation exposure. Key management concepts (Table 56.6) include assessment of risk versus benefit. For example, withholding seizure medications at the risk of recurrent seizures is not sensible. In general, using older drugs with a longer history is advisable as well as using the minimum effective dose. Drugs with an active metabolite should be avoided if possible, and nerve blocks are preferable to systemic analgesia.

Most drugs administered to the mother cross into breast milk, although neonatal drug exposure is much lower than fetal exposure. Principles of drug administration during lactation are listed in Table 56.6. Drugs undergo first-pass metabolism in the neonatal gut, and neonatal exposure is generally 1% to 2% of the maternal dose.[143] Determinants of drug transfer to milk and neonatal exposure include maternal plasma concentration, drug pKa (breast milk is slightly acidotic compared to plasma), volume of milk, and the maturity of neonatal drug metabolism and elimination pathways.[143] Hepatic drug-metabolizing enzymes appear to mature at different rates but are generally reduced in the neonate compared to the adult. Glomerular filtration rate does not reach adult values until 2.5 to 5 months of age.

DRUG CLASSIFICATION DURING PREGNANCY AND LACTATION

The FDA previously required manufacturers to label drug risk for use during pregnancy using a five-category classification system (Categories A, B, C, D, X). This classification had some major limitations and was replaced in 2015 with a new Pregnancy and Lactation Labeling Rule (PLLR).[144] The new rule

---

TABLE 56.6 Principles of Drug Administration during Pregnancy and Lactation

Pregnancy

- Assess risk versus benefit.
- Consider gestational age of fetus.
- Use older drugs.
- Use the minimum effective dose.
- Avoid drugs with active metabolites.
- Consider nerve blocks.
- Consider nonpharmacologic therapies.
- Use ultrasound and MRI for imaging.

Lactation

- Assess risk versus benefit.
- Choose the safest drug.
- Use minimum effective dose.
- Use drugs with no active metabolite.
- If drug may present risk to neonate, measure neonatal drug concentration.
- Give maternal dose just after feeding.
- Consider age of infant (maturity of metabolic pathways).

MRI, magnetic resonance imaging.

requires three label sections: Pregnancy (including labor and delivery), Lactation, and Females and Males of Reproductive Potential. Each section includes a narrative text summary of the risks of using the drug, a discussion of the data supporting the summary, and information to help health care providers make decisions and counsel women about the risks of using the drug during pregnancy and lactation. Several Internet databases offer information on drug use during pregnancy and lactation as well as a well-known reference book.[59,145] Some drug companies maintain pregnancy registries for specific drugs.

The American Academy of Pediatrics has categorized drugs in terms of safety for the nursing infant.[143,146] Most drugs, including most analgesics, are listed as compatible with breastfeeding.

Analgesic Drugs during Pregnancy and Lactation

Acetaminophen is the first-line analgesic during pregnancy for the treatment of mild pain. Low-dose aspirin is considered safe; however, higher doses should be avoided as they may be associated with an increased risk for placental abruption and other bleeding problems and fetal gastroschisis.[147] Nonsteroidal anti-inflammatory drugs (NSAIDs) may cause constriction of the ductus arteriosus and may have adverse effects on fetal renal function, leading to oligohydramnios. Therefore, indomethacin and ibuprofen are not recommended for use for more than 2 days beyond the first trimester.[147] Opioids are considered safe during pregnancy, although there is a potential for neonatal abstinence syndrome after delivery.

Acetaminophen is also considered safe for nursing infants, as are NSAIDs. However, aspirin should be used with caution during lactation because of the slow elimination of salicylates by neonates and resultant drug accumulation.[146,147] Opioids are considered safe during lactation. However, meperidine should be avoided, as normeperidine has a markedly prolonged half-life in the newborn,[148] and accumulation may result in neurobehavioral depression and seizures.

References

1. Cohen J. Doctor James Young Simpson, Rabbi Abraham De Sola, and Genesis Chapter 3, Verse 16. *Obstet Gynecol* 1996;88(5):895–898.
2. Wagenknecht E. *Mrs. Longfellow Selected Letters and Journals of Fanny Appleton Longfellow (1817–1861)*. New York: Longmans, Green; 1956.
3. Caton D. The history of obstetric anesthesia. In: Chestnut DH, Wong CA, Tsen LC, et al, eds. *Obstetric Anesthesia Principles and Practice*. 5th ed. Philadelphia: Elsevier; 2014:3–12.
4. von Steinbüchel R. Vorläufige Mitteilung über die Anwendung des Skopolamin-Morphium-Injektionen in der Geburtshilfe. *Zentrallblatt Gyn* 1902;30:1304–1306.
5. Apgar V. A proposal for a new method of evaluation of the newborn infant. *Curr Res Anesth Analg* 1953;32:260–267.
6. Koller C. On the use of cocaine for producing anaesthesia on the eye. *Lancet* 1884;2:990–992.
7. Cleland JGP. Paravertebral anesthesia in obstetrics. *Surg Gynecol Obstet* 1933;57:51–62.
8. Hingson RA, Edwards WB. Continuous caudal analgesia: an analysis of the first ten thousand confinements thus managed with the report of the authors' first thousand cases. *JAMA* 1943;123:538–546.
9. Traynor AJ, Aragon M, Ghosh D, et al. Obstetric anesthesia workforce survey: a 30-year update. *Anesth Analg* 2016;122(6):1939–1946.
10. Melzack R. The myth of painless childbirth (the John J. Bonica lecture). *Pain* 1984;19(4):321–337.
11. Bonica JJ. The nature of pain in parturition. *Clin Obstet Gynecol* 1975;2:499–516.
12. Pan P, Eisenach JC. The pain of childbirth and its effect on the mother and the fetus. In: Chestnut DH, Wong CA, Tsen LC, et al, eds. *Obstetric Anesthesia. Principles and Practice*. 5th ed. Philadelphia: Elsevier; 2014:410–426.
13. Sheiner E, Sheiner EK, Shoham-Vardi I. The relationship between parity and labor pain. *Int J Gynaecol Obstet* 1998;63(3):287–288.
14. Hess PE, Pratt SD, Soni AK, et al. An association between severe labor pain and cesarean delivery. *Anesth Analg* 2000;90(4):881–886.
15. Alexander JM, Sharma SK, McIntire DD, et al. Intensity of labor pain and cesarean delivery. *Anesth Analg* 2001;92(6):1524–1528.
16. Lang AJ, Sorrell JT, Rodgers CS, et al. Anxiety sensitivity as a predictor of labor pain. *Eur J Pain* 2006;10(3):263–270.
17. Henneborn WJ, Cogan R. The effect of husband participation on reported pain and probability of medication during labor and birth. *J Psychosom Res* 1975;19(3):215–222.
18. Kennell J, Klaus M, McGrath S, et al. Continuous emotional support during labor in a US hospital: a randomized controlled trial. *JAMA* 1991;265(17):2197–2201.
19. Bonica JJ. *Principles and Practice of Obstetric Analgesia and Anesthesia*. Vol 2. Philadelphia: FA Davis; 1969.
20. Sheiner EK, Sheiner E, Shoham-Vardi I, et al. Ethnic differences influence care giver's estimates of pain during labour. *Pain* 1999;81(3):299–305.
21. Bonica JJ. Maternal respiratory changes during pregnancy and parturition. In: Marx GF, ed. *Parturient and Perinatology*. Vol 10. Philadelphia: FA Davis; 1973:1–19.
22. Shnider SM, Wright RG, Levinson G, et al. Uterine blood flow and plasma norepinephrine changes during maternal stress in the pregnant ewe. *Anesthesiology* 1979;50(6):524–527.
23. Lederman RP, Lederman E, Work B, et al. Anxiety and epinephrine in multiparous labor: relationship to duration of labor and fetal heart rate pattern. *Am J Obstet Gynecol* 1985;153(8):870–877.
24. Moir DD, Willocks J. Management of incoordinate uterine action under continuous epidural analgesia. *Br Med J* 1967;3(5562):396–400.
25. McDonnell NJ, Paech MJ, Clavisi OM, et al. Difficult and failed intubation in obstetric anaesthesia: an observational study of airway management and complications associated with general anaesthesia for caesarean section. *Int J Obstet Anesth* 2008;17(4):292–297.
26. Hawkins JL, Chang J, Palmer SK, et al. Anesthesia-related maternal mortality in the United States: 1979–2002. *Obstet Gynecol* 2011;117(1):69–74.
27. Spätling L, Fallenstein F, Huch A, et al. The variability of cardiopulmonary adaptation to pregnancy at rest and during exercise. *Br J Obstet Gynaecol* 1992;99(suppl 8):1–40.
28. Alaily AB, Carrol KB. Pulmonary ventilation in pregnancy. *Br J Obstet Gynaecol* 1978;85:518–524.
29. Hägerdal M, Morgan CW, Sumner AE, et al. Minute ventilation and oxygen consumption during labor with epidural analgesia. *Anesthesiology* 1983;59:425–427.
30. Jouppila R, Hollmen A. The effect of segmental epidural analgesia on maternal and foetal acid-base balance, lactate, serum potassium and creatine phosphokinase during labour. *Acta Anaesth Scand* 1976;20:259–268.
31. Lund CJ, Donovan JC. Blood volume during pregnancy. Significance of plasma and red cell volumes. *Am J Obstet Gynecol* 1967;98(3):394–403.
32. Kuo CD, Chen GY, Yang MJ, et al. Biphasic changes in autonomic nervous activity during pregnancy. *Br J Anaesth* 2000;84(3):323–329.
33. Annibale DJ, Rosenfeld CR, Kamm KE. Alterations in vascular smooth muscle contractility during ovine pregnancy. *Am J Physiol* 1989;256:H1282–H1288.
34. Clark SL, Cotton DB, Pivarnik JM, et al. Position change and central hemodynamic profile during normal third-trimester pregnancy and post partum. *Am J Obstet Gynecol* 1991;164:883–887.
35. Kerr MG, Scott DB, Samuel E. Studies of the inferior vena cava in late pregnancy. *Br Med J* 1964;1:532–533.
36. Abitbol MM. Aortic compression by pregnant uterus. *NY State J Med* 1976;76:1470–1475.
37. Hirabayashi Y, Shimizu R, Fukuda H, et al. Effects of the pregnant uterus on the extradural venous plexus in the supine and lateral positions, as determined by magnetic resonance imaging. *Br J Anaesth* 1997;78(3):317–319.
38. Clark SL, Cotton DB, Lee W, et al. Central hemodynamic assessment of normal term pregnancy. *Am J Obstet Gynecol* 1989;161:1439–1442.
39. Kuo CD, Chen GY, Yang MJ, et al. The effect of position on autonomic nervous activity in late pregnancy. *Anaesthesia* 1997;52(12):1161–1165.
40. Abitbol MM. Supine position in labor and associated fetal heart rate changes. *Obstet Gynecol* 1985;65:481–486.
41. Assali NS, Prystowsky H. Studies on autonomic blockade. I. Comparison between the effects of tetraethylammonium chloride (TEAC) and high selective spinal anesthesia on blood pressure of normal and toxemic pregnancy. *J Clin Invest* 1950;29:1354–1366.
42. Hirabayashi Y, Shimizu R, Fukada H, et al. Soft tissue anatomy within the vertebral canal in pregnant women. *Br J Anaesth* 1996;77(2):153–156.
43. Hogan QH, Prost R, Kulier A, et al. Magnetic resonance imaging of cerebrospinal fluid volume and the influence of body habitus and abdominal pressure. *Anesthesiology* 1996;84(6):1341–1349.
44. Hirabayashi Y, Shimizu R, Fukuda H, et al. Anatomical configuration of the spinal column in the supine position. II. Comparison of pregnant and non-pregnant women. *Br J Anaesth* 1995;75(1):6–8.
45. Richardson MG, Wissler RN. Density of lumbar cerebrospinal fluid in pregnant and nonpregnant humans. *Anesthesiology* 1996;85(2):326–330.
46. Hirabayashi Y, Shimizu R, Saitoh K, et al. Acid-base state of cerebrospinal fluid during pregnancy and its effect on spread of spinal anaesthesia. *Br J Anaesth* 1996;77(3):352–355.
47. Dalby PL, Ramanathan S, Rudy TE, et al. Plasma and saliva substance P levels: the effects of acute pain in pregnant and non-pregnant women. *Pain* 1997;69:263–267.
48. Datta S, Hurley RJ, Naulty JS, et al. Plasma and cerebrospinal fluid progesterone concentrations in pregnant and nonpregnant women. *Anesth Analg* 1986;65:950–954.

49. Iwasaki H, Collins JG, Saito Y, et al. Naloxone-sensitive, pregnancy-induced changes in behavioral responses to colorectal distention: pregnancy-induced analgesia to visceral stimulation. *Anesthesiology* 1991;74:927–933.

50. Gintzler AR, Liu NJ. The maternal spinal cord: biochemical and physiological correlates of steroid-activated antinociceptive processes. *Prog Brain Res* 2001;133:83–97.

51. Ohel I, Walfisch A, Shitenberg D, et al. A rise in pain threshold during labor: a prospective clinical trial. *Pain* 2007;132(suppl 1):S104–S108.

52. Bromage PR. Spread of analgesic solutions in the epidural space and their site of action: a statistical study. *Br J Anaesth* 1962;34:161–178.

53. Ansari J, Carvalho B, Shafer SL, et al. Pharmacokinetics and pharmacodynamics of drugs commonly used in pregnancy and parturition. *Anesth Analg* 2016;122(3):786–804.

54. Wood M, Wood AJJ. Changes in plasma drug binding and α_1-acid glycoprotein in mother and newborn infant. *Clin Pharmacol Ther* 1981;29:522–526.

55. Fragneto RY, Bader AM, Rosinia F, et al. Measurements of protein binding of lidocaine throughout pregnancy. *Anesth Analg* 1994;79(2):295–297.

56. Shnider SM, Abboud TK, Artal R, et al. Maternal catecholamines decrease during labor after lumbar epidural anesthesia. *Am J Obstet Gynecol* 1983;147(1):13–15.

57. Segal S, Csavoy AN, Datta S. The tocolytic effect of catecholamines in the gravid rat uterus. *Anesth Analg* 1998;87(4):864–869.

58. Fishburne JI, Greiss FC, Hopkinson R, et al. Responses of the gravid uterine vasculature to arterial levels of local anesthetic agents. *Am J Obstet Gynecol* 1979;133:753–761.

59. Briggs GG, Freeman RK, Towers CV, et al. *Drugs in Pregnancy and Lactation. A Reference Guide to Fetal and Neonatal Risk.* 11th ed. Philadelphia: Wolters Kluwer; 2015.

60. Davidson AJ, Becke K, de Graaff J, et al. Anesthesia and the developing brain: a way forward for clinical research. *Paediatr Anaesth* 2015;25(5):447–452.

61. Smith CA, Levett KM, Collins CT, et al. Relaxation techniques for pain management in labour. *Cochrane Database Syst Rev* 2011;(12):CD009514.

62. Levett KM, Smith CA, Dahlen HG, et al. Acupuncture and acupressure for pain management in labour and birth: a critical narrative review of current systematic review evidence. *Complement Ther Med* 2014;22(3):523–540.

63. Hodnett ED, Gates S, Hofmeyr GJ, et al. Continuous support for women during childbirth. *Cochrane Database Syst Rev* 2013;(7):CD003766.

64. Cluett ER, Burns E. Immersion in water in labour and birth. *Cochrane Database Syst Rev* 2009;(2):CD000111.

65. Derry S, Straube S, Moore RA, et al. Intracutaneous or subcutaneous sterile water injection compared with blinded controls for pain management in labour. *Cochrane Database Syst Rev* 2012;(1):CD009107.

66. Madden K, Middleton P, Cyna AM, et al. Hypnosis for pain management during labour and childbirth. *Cochrane Database Syst Rev* 2016;(5):CD009356.

67. Bedwell C, Dowswell T, Neilson JP, et al. The use of transcutaneous electrical nerve stimulation (TENS) for pain relief in labour: a review of the evidence. *Midwifery* 2011;27(5):e141–e148.

68. Smith CA, Collins CT, Crowther CA, et al. Acupuncture or acupressure for pain management in labour. *Cochrane Database Syst Rev* 2011;(7):CD009232.

69. Likis FE, Andrews JC, Collins MR, et al. Nitrous oxide for the management of labor pain: a systematic review. *Anesth Analg* 2014;118(1):153–167.

70. Sanders RD, Weimann J, Maze M. Biologic effects of nitrous oxide: a mechanistic and toxicologic review. *Anesthesiology* 2008;109(4):707–722.

71. Hogan K. Nitrous oxide genotoxicity. *Anesthesiology* 2013;118(6):1258–1260.

72. King TL, Wong CA. Nitrous oxide for labor pain: is it a laughing matter? *Anesth Analg* 2014;118(1):12–14.

73. Phillips SN, Fernando R, Girard T. Parenteral opioid analgesia: does it still have a role? *Best Pract Res Clin Anaesthesiol* 2017;31(1):3–14.

74. Bricker L, Lavender T. Parenteral opioids for labor pain relief: a systematic review. *Am J Obstet Gynecol* 2002;186(5 suppl):S94–S109.

75. Nelson KE, Eisenach JC. Intravenous butorphanol, meperidine, and their combination relieve pain and distress in women in labor. *Anesthesiology* 2005;102(5):1008–1013.

76. Hill JB, Alexander JM, Sharma SK, et al. A comparison of the effects of epidural and meperidine analgesia during labor on fetal heart rate. *Obstet Gynecol* 2003;102(2):333–337.

77. Van de Velde M, Carvalho B. Remifentanil for labor analgesia: an evidence-based narrative review. *Int J Obstet Anesth* 2016;25:66–74.

78. Van de Velde M. Remifentanil patient-controlled intravenous analgesia for labor pain relief: is it really an option to consider? *Anesth Analg* 2017;124(4):1029–1031.

79. Weiniger CF, Carvalho B, Stocki D, et al. Analysis of physiological respiratory variable alarm alerts among laboring women receiving remifentanil. *Anesth Analg* 2017;124(4):1211–1218.

80. Anim-Somuah M, Smyth RM, Jones L. Epidural versus non-epidural or no analgesia in labour. *Cochrane Database Syst Rev* 2011;(12):CD000331.

81. Capogna G, Celleno D, Lyons G, et al. Minimum local analgesia concentration of extradural bupivacaine increases with progression of labor. *Br J Anaesth* 1998;80:11–13.

82. Lyons GR, Kocarev MG, Wilson RC, et al. A comparison of minimum local anesthetic volumes and doses of epidural bupivacaine (0.125% w/v and 0.25% w/v) for analgesia in labor. *Anesth Analg* 2007;104(2):412–415.

83. Belfrage P, Berlin A, Raabe N, et al. Lumbar epidural analgesia with bupivacaine in labor. Drug concentration in maternal and neonatal blood at birth and during the first day of life. *Am J Obstet Gynecol* 1975;123:839–844.

84. Kennedy RL, Bell JU, Miller RP, et al. Uptake and distribution of lidocaine in fetal lambs. *Anesthesiology* 1990;72(3):483–489.

85. Katz JA, Bridenbaugh PO, Knarr DC, et al. Pharmacodynamics and pharmacokinetics of epidural ropivacaine in humans. *Anesth Analg* 1990;70(1):16–21.

86. Polley LS, Columb MO, Naughton NN, et al. Relative analgesic potencies of ropivacaine and bupivacaine for epidural analgesia in labor: implications for therapeutic indexes. *Anesthesiology* 1999;90(4):944–950.

87. Beilin Y, Guinn NR, Bernstein HH, et al. Local anesthetics and mode of delivery: bupivacaine versus ropivacaine versus levobupivacaine. *Anesth Analg* 2007;105(3):756–763.

88. Lee BB, Ngan Kee WD, Ng FF, et al. Epidural infusions of ropivacaine and bupivacaine for labor analgesia: a randomized, double-blind study of obstetric outcome. *Anesth Analg* 2004;98(4):1145–1152.

89. Lacassie HJ, Habib AS, Lacassie HP, et al. Motor blocking minimum local anesthetic concentrations of bupivacaine, levobupivacaine, and ropivacaine in labor. *Reg Anesth Pain Med* 2007;32(4):323–329.

90. Vercauteren M, Meert TF. Isobolographic analysis of the interaction between epidural sufentanil and bupivacaine in rats. *Pharmacol Biochem Behav* 1997;58(1):237–242.

91. Polley LS, Columb MO, Wagner DS, et al. Dose-dependent reduction of the minimum local analgesic concentration of bupivacaine by sufentanil for epidural analgesia in labor. *Anesthesiology* 1998;89(3):626–632.

92. Bader AM, Fragneto R, Terui K, et al. Maternal and neonatal fentanyl and bupivacaine concentrations after epidural infusion during labor. *Anesth Analg* 1995;81(4):829–832.

93. Porter JS, Bonello E, Reynolds F. The effect of epidural opioids on maternal oxygenation during labour and delivery. *Anaesthesia* 1996;51(10):899–903.

94. Curatolo M, Petersen-Felix S, Arendt-Nielsen L, et al. Epidural epinephrine and clonidine: segmental analgesia and effects on different pain modalities. *Anesthesiology* 1997;87(4):785–794.

95. Wong CA. Epidural and spinal analgesia/anesthesia for labor and vaginal delivery. In: Chestnut DH, Wong CA, Tsen LC, et al, eds. *Chestnut's Obstetric Anesthesia: Principles and Practice.* 5th ed. Philadelphia: Elsevier; 2014:457–517.

96. Simmons SW, Taghizadeh N, Dennis AT, et al. Combined spinal-epidural versus epidural analgesia in labour. *Cochrane Database Syst Rev* 2012;(10):CD003401.

97. Booth JM, Pan JC, Ross VH, et al. Combined spinal epidural technique for labor analgesia does not delay recognition of epidural catheter failures: a single-center retrospective cohort survival analysis. *Anesthesiology* 2016;125(3):516–524.

98. Cook TM. Combined spinal-epidural techniques. *Anaesthesia* 2000;55(1):42–64.

99. Reynolds F. Infection as a complication of neuraxial blockade. *Int J Obstet Anesth* 2005;14(3):183–188.

100. Minty RG, Kelly L, Minty A, et al. Single-dose intrathecal analgesia to control labour pain: is it a useful alternative to epidural analgesia? *Can Fam Physician* 2007;53(3):437–442.

101. Booth JV, Lindsay DR, Olufolabi AJ, et al. Subarachnoid meperidine (Pethidine) causes significant nausea and vomiting during labor. *Anesthesiology* 2000;93(2):418–421.

102. Nelson KE, Rauch T, Terebuh V, et al. A comparison of intrathecal fentanyl and sufentanil for labor analgesia. *Anesthesiology* 2002;96:1070–1073.

103. Palmer CM, Cork RC, Hays R, et al. The dose-response relation of intrathecal fentanyl for labor analgesia. *Anesthesiology* 1998;88(2):355–361.

104. Herman NL, Choi KC, Affleck PJ, et al. Analgesia, pruritus, and ventilation exhibit a dose-response relationship in parturients receiving intrathecal fentanyl during labor. *Anesth Analg* 1999;89(2):378–383.

105. Ngan Kee WD, Khaw KS, Ng FF, et al. Synergistic interaction between fentanyl and bupivacaine given intrathecally for labor analgesia. *Anesthesiology* 2014;120(5):1126–1136.

106. Van de Velde M, Dreelinck R, Dubois J, et al. Determination of the full dose-response relation of intrathecal bupivacaine, levobupivacaine, and ropivacaine, combined with sufentanil, for labor analgesia. *Anesthesiology* 2007;106(1):149–156.

107. Whitty R, Goldszmidt E, Parkes RK, et al. Determination of the ED95 for intrathecal plain bupivacaine combined with fentanyl in active labor. *Int J Obstet Anesth* 2007;16(4):341–345.

108. Wong CA, Scavone BM, Loffredi M, et al. The dose-response of intrathecal sufentanil added to bupivacaine for labor analgesia. *Anesthesiology* 2000;92(6):1553–1558.

109. Bogod DG, Rosen M, Rees GA. Extradural infusion of 0.125% bupivacaine at 10 mL/hr to women during labor. *Br J Anaesth* 1987;59(3):325–330.

110. Lamont RF, Pinney D, Rodgers P, et al. Continuous versus intermittent epidural analgesia. *Anaesthesia* 1989;44:893–896.

111. Hicks JA, Jenkins JG, Newton MC, et al. Continuous epidural infusion of 0.075% bupivacaine for pain relief in labour. *Anaesthesia* 1988;43(4):289–292.

112. Ewen A, McLeod DD, MacLeod DM, et al. Continuous infusion epidural analgesia in obstetrics: a comparison of 0.08% and 0.25% bupivacaine. *Anaesthesia* 1986;41:143.

113. van der Vyver M, Halpern S, Joseph G. Patient-controlled epidural analgesia versus continuous infusion for labour analgesia: a meta-analysis. *Br J Anaesth* 2002;89(3):459–465.

114. Halpern SH, Carvalho B. Patient-controlled epidural analgesia for labor. *Anesth Analg* 2009;108(3):921–928.

115. Vallejo MC, Ramesh V, Phelps AL, et al. Epidural labor analgesia: continuous infusion versus patient-controlled epidural analgesia with background infusion versus without a background infusion. *J Pain* 2007;8(12):970–975.

116. Heesen M, Bohmer J, Klohr S, et al. The effect of adding a background infusion to patient-controlled epidural labor analgesia on labor, maternal, and neonatal outcomes: a systematic review and meta-analysis. *Anesth Analg* 2015;121(1):149–158.

117. Carvalho B, George RB, Cobb B, et al. Implementation of programmed intermittent epidural bolus for the maintenance of labor analgesia. *Anesth Analg* 2016;123(4):965–971.

118. George RB, Allen TK, Habib AS. Intermittent epidural bolus compared with continuous epidural infusions for labor analgesia: a systematic review and meta-analysis. *Anesth Analg* 2013;116(1):133–144.

119. Tao W, Grant EN, Craig MG, et al. Continuous spinal analgesia for labor and delivery: an observational study with a 23-gauge spinal catheter. *Anesth Analg* 2015;121(5):1290–1294.

120. Thomas JA, Pan PH, Harris LC, et al. Dural puncture with a 27-gauge Whitacre needle as part of a combined spinal-epidural technique does not improve labor epidural catheter function. *Anesthesiology* 2005;103(5):1046–1051.

121. Cappiello E, O'Rourke N, Segal S, et al. A randomized trial of dural puncture epidural technique compared with the standard epidural technique for labor analgesia. *Anesth Analg* 2008;107(5):1646–1651.

122. Chau A, Bibbo C, Huang CC, et al. Dural puncture epidural technique improves labor analgesia quality with fewer side effects compared with epidural and combined spinal epidural techniques: a randomized clinical trial. *Anesth Analg* 2017;124(2):560–569.

123. Wilson SH, Wolf BJ, Bingham KN, et al. Labor analgesia onset with dural puncture epidural versus traditional epidural using a 26-gauge Whitacre needle and 0.125% bupivacaine bolus: a randomized clinical trial. *Anesth Analg* 2018;126:545–551.

124. Hofmeyr G, Cyna A, Middleton P. Prophylactic intravenous preloading for regional analgesia in labour. *Cochrane Database Syst Rev* 2004;(4):CD000175.

125. Asokumar B, Newman LM, McCarthy RJ, et al. Intrathecal bupivacaine reduces pruritus and prolongs duration of fentanyl analgesia during labor: a prospective, randomized controlled trial. *Anesth Analg* 1998;87(6):1309–1315.

126. Douglas MJ, Kim JH, Ross PL, et al. The effect of epinephrine in local anaesthetic on epidural morphine-induced pruritus. *Can Anaesth Soc J* 1986;33(6):737–740.

127. Abrao KC, Francisco RP, Miyadahira S, et al. Elevation of uterine basal tone and fetal heart rate abnormalities after labor analgesia: a randomized controlled trial. *Obstet Gynecol* 2009;113(1):41–47.

128. Clarke VT, Smiley RM, Finster M. Uterine hyperactivity after intrathecal injection of fentanyl for analgesia during labor: a cause of fetal bradycardia? *Anesthesiology* 1994;81(4):1083.

129. Mercier FJ, Dounas M, Bouaziz H, et al. Intravenous nitroglycerin to relieve intrapartum fetal distress related to uterine hyperactivity: a prospective observational study. *Anesth Analg* 1997;84(5):1117–1120.

130. Segal S. Labor epidural analgesia and maternal fever. *Anesth Analg* 2010;111(6):1467–1475.

131. Choi PT, Galinski SE, Takeuchi L, et al. PDPH is a common complication of neuraxial blockade in parturients: a meta-analysis of obstetrical studies. *Can J Anaesth* 2003;50(5):460–469.

132. Paech MJ, Doherty DA, Christmas T, et al. The volume of blood for epidural blood patch in obstetrics: a randomized, blinded clinical trial. *Anesth Analg* 2011;113(1):126–133.

133. Hughes SC. Respiratory depression following intraspinal narcotics: expect it! *Int J Obstet Anesth* 1997;6(3):145–146.

134. Chestnut DH. Alternative regional analgesic techniques for labor and vaginal delivery. In: Chestnut DH, Wong CA, Tsen LC, et al, eds. *Chestnut's Obstetric Anesthesia: Principles and Practice.* 5th ed. Philadelphia: Elsevier; 2014:518–529.

135. Leighton BL, Halpern SH, Wilson DB. Lumbar sympathetic blocks speed early and second stage induced labor in nulliparous women. *Anesthesiology* 1999;90(4):1039–1046.

136. Scudamore JH, Yates MJ. Pudendal block—a misnomer? *Lancet* 1966;1(7427):23–24.

137. DePraeter C, Vanhaesebrouch P, DePraeter N, et al. Episiotomy and neonatal lidocaine intoxication [letter]. *Eur J Pediatr* 1991;150:685–686.

138. Climie CR. The place of continuous lumbar epidural analgesia in the management of abnormally prolonged labour. *Med J Aust* 1964;2:447–450.

139. Sng BL, Leong WL, Zeng Y, et al. Early versus late initiation of epidural analgesia for labour. *Cochrane Database Syst Rev* 2014;(10):CD007238.

140. Wong CA, Scavone BM, Peaceman AM, et al. The risk of cesarean delivery with neuraxial analgesia given early versus late in labor. *N Engl J Med* 2005;352(7):655–665.

141. Ohel G, Gonen R, Vaida S, et al. Early versus late initiation of epidural analgesia in labor: does it increase the risk of cesarean section? A randomized trial. *Am J Obstet Gynecol* 2006;194(3):600–605.

142. Sultan P, Murphy C, Halpern S, et al. The effect of low concentrations versus high concentrations of local anesthetics for labour analgesia on obstetric and anesthetic outcomes: a meta-analysis. *Can J Anaesth* 2013;60(9):840–854.

143. Sachs HC. The transfer of drugs and therapeutics into human breast milk: an update on selected topics. *Pediatrics* 2013;132(3):e796–e809.

144. U.S. Food and Drug Administration. Pregnancy and lactation labeling (drugs) final rule. Available at: http://www.fda.gov/Drugs/Development ApprovalProcess/DevelopmentResources/Labeling/ucm093307.htm. Accessed July 22, 2017.

145. Brucker MC, King TL. The 2015 US Food and Drug Administration Pregnancy and Lactation Labeling Rule. *J Midwifery Womens Health* 2017;62(3):308–316.

146. American Academy of Pediatrics Committee on Drugs. Transfer of drugs and other chemicals into human milk. *Pediatrics* 2001;108(3):776–789.

147. Bloor M, Paech M. Nonsteroidal anti-inflammatory drugs during pregnancy and the initiation of lactation. *Anesth Analg* 2013;116(5):1063–1075.

148. Kuhnert BR, Kuhnert PM, Philipson EH, et al. Disposition of meperidine and normeperidine following multiple doses during labor. II. Fetus and neonate. *Am J Obstet Gynecol* 1985;151(3):410–415.

CHAPTER 57

Pain and Sickle Cell Disease

SAMIR K. BALLAS

Introduction

HISTORY

Sickle cell disease (SCD) was known in Africa before the 20th century. Inhabitants of West Africa realized that the disease was hereditary and gave it specific names such as *Chwechwechwe, Ahotutuo, Nwiiwii,* and *Nuidudui.*[1] These names are characterized by alliteration of letters that seemingly signified the recurrent clinical manifestations of the disease and the crying sounds by children in pain.

SCD was first reported in the United States in November 1910 by James B. Herrick who referred to "peculiar elongated and sickle-shaped red blood corpuscles in a case of severe anemia." In a sense and within the framework of annals, this event was of legendary mini-epic proportion. The heroes were a triumvirate of a patient, an intern, and an attending whose lives, by chance, intersected in 1904 in Presbyterian Hospital in Chicago, Illinois. The patient, Walter Clement Noel, was a student in the Chicago College of Dental Surgery, the intern was Dr. Ernest E. Irons, and the attending physician was Dr. Herrick.[2,3]

Noel came to the United States from Grenada on his own using his own funds, driven by the desire to acquire new knowledge and become a dentist.[2,3] In 2004, he had cough and fever and was admitted to the hospital under the care of Dr. Herrick. Dr. Irons was the intern who first examined a peripheral blood smear from Noel in 1904. He noticed the unusual shapes and sizes of blood cells in Noel's blood, placed a written description and a pictorial illustration of these cells in Noel's chart, and discussed his findings with his attending, Dr. Herrick.

Dr. Herrick, who already had an interest in blood and blood disorders, was baffled by these abnormal cells and could not associate them with any of the diseases known at that time. He and Dr. Irons followed Noel for about 2.5 more years without an explanation for their findings. In 1910, Dr. Herrick, after consulting with other prominent physicians and pathologists around the country on the case, published the details in an article in November 2010 in the *Archives of Internal Medicine*[2] with the hope that others might be able to shed light on the case or report similar cases.

Between 1910 and 1949, there was a plethora of descriptions of the various clinical factors of SCD by many physicians, most notably by Mason[4] who coined the term "sickle cell anemia" (SS) and by Diggs[5] who noted that the hallmark of SS is the recurrent and painful vascular occlusive crisis (VOC) interspersed with periods of stable state with no signs or symptoms other than those due to chronic hemolytic anemia.

Pauling and his associates[6] introduced the concept of SS as a molecular disease. They demonstrated that hemoglobin (Hb) isolated from red cells of patients with SCD differed electrophoretically from the Hb of normal persons and that the Hb of those with sickle cell trait was a mixture of normal and sickle Hb. Neel[7] showed that the inheritance of SS followed simple Mendelian genetics. Ingram[8] reported that the only difference between normal and sickle Hb was the replacement of glutamic acid by valine. The work of several groups established the subunit structure and primary sequences of the subunits (α, β, γ, δ) of human Hb and localized the sickle mutation to the sixth residue of the β-globin chain ($\beta 6^{Glu \to Val}$). The interaction of the sickle mutation with other Hb abnormalities clarified the spectrum of sickle cell syndromes. The advent of DNA technology in the 1970s and the 1980s paved the way for the molecular diagnosis of sickle cell disorders, prenatal diagnosis, and the identification of α-genotypes and β^S haplotypes and their effect on the clinical picture of SCD. By the 1980s, it had become clear that SCD is a highly heterogeneous disorder not only at the clinical level but also at the cellular and molecular levels. The Human Genome Project initiated several studies by many investigators to determine genetic modifiers that may predict sickle-related complications.[9] Advances by the end of the 20th century included preventative therapy by the induction of fetal Hb using hydroxyurea (HU),[10] blood transfusion to prevent primary and secondary strokes,[11,12] and curative therapy in some patients using bone marrow/stem cell transplantation.[13–19] By 2010, SCD was recognized as a global disease affecting an estimate of 100 million patients globally, mostly in Africa and India. Currently, progressive strides are underway including several randomized clinical trials, modified approaches to stem cell transplantations,[20] and promising progress in gene therapy.[21]

NATURE OF THE SICKLE MUTATION

Hemoglobinopathies are inherited disorders of the structure and/or function of the Hb molecule. Hemoglobinopathies are broadly divided into two major groups: structural variants and thalassemias. Structural variants are, most commonly, the result of single-base mutations in the globin genes. Thalassemias are characterized by decreased synthesis of any one or more of the globin chains.

The sickle mutation is the result of a single-base change (GAT→GTT) in the sixth codon of exon 1 of the β-globin gene responsible for the synthesis of the β-globin polypeptide of the Hb molecule ($\alpha_2\beta_2$). This change, in turn, results in replacement of the normal glutamic acid with valine at position 6 of the β-globin chain and the formation of sickle Hb.[7,8,22]

Over two million US residents are estimated to be either heterozygous or homozygous for the genetic substitution. Most of those affected are of African ancestry or self-identify as Black; a minority are of Hispanic or southern European, Middle Eastern, or Asian Indian descent.[23] It is estimated that between 70,000 and 100,000 Americans have SCD. Although SCD is associated with major morbidity, currently more than 90% of children with SCD in the United States and the United Kingdom survive into adulthood.[24–26] However, their life span remains shortened by two or three decades compared to the general population.[27,28]

CLASSIFICATION OF SICKLE CELL SYNDROMES

Sickle cell syndromes, also collectively referred to as SCD, comprise a group of clinically significant hemoglobinopathies in which the sickle gene is inherited from at least one parent. SS is the homozygous state where the sickle gene is inherited from both parents. Sickle cell syndromes also result from the co-inheritance of the sickle gene with Hb C gene giving rise to Hb SC diseases, with β-thalassemia genes (β^0 or β^+) giving rise to sickle-β^0-thalassemia or sickle-β^+-thalassemia, respectively, or with other β-globin structural variants giving rise to other combinations such as HbSO Arab, HbSD disease, and so on. The most prevalent SCD types include

TABLE 57.1	Major Types of Sickle Cell Syndrome and Their Typical Hematological Parameters							
Disease	Genotype	Hb (g/dL)	MCV (fl)	Hb A%	Hb A$_2$%	Hb S%	Hb F%	Hb C%
SS no α-gene deletion	β^S/β^S; αα/αα	7.0–8.0	85–110	0	2.5–3.5	75–96	1–20	0
SS deletion of 2 α- genes	β^S/β^S; −α/−α	9.0–10.0	70–80	0	3.0–4.4	75–94	1–20	0
Sickle-β^0-thal	β^S/β^0 thal	7.0–10.0	60–70	0	4.0–6.0	70–90	1–20	0
Sickle-β$^+$-thal	β^S/β$^+$ thal	>10.0	60–70	10–20	4.0–6.0	65–85	1–15	0
Hb SC disease	β^S/β^C	>10.0	75–85	0	45–50	50	1–6	45
Sickle cell trait	β^A/β^S	12–16	>82	55–57	2.5–3.5	40	<1.0	0

NOTE: All disorders may be associated with variable degrees of α-gene deletions. Hb A$_2$ and Hb C have the same electrophoretic mobility at alkaline pH and are not separable on routine analysis; they can be separated, however, by high pressure liquid chromatography.
Hb, hemoglobin; MCV, mean corpuscular volume; SS, sickle cell anemia; thal, thalassemia.

homozygous Hb SS and the compound heterozygous conditions HbSβ^0-thalassemia, HbSβ$^+$-thalassemia, and Hb SC disease. Hb SS and HbSβ^0-thalassemia are clinically very similar and therefore are commonly referred to as SS; these genotypes are associated with the most severe clinical manifestations. Table 57.1 lists the major types of sickle cell syndromes commonly seen in the United States. Certain complications of SCD may be more common in one category than another. Thus, frequent painful crises, severe anemia that requires blood transfusion, and acute chest syndrome (ACS) are more common in SS than other types of SCD. Sickle retinopathy, on the other hand, is more common in Hb SC disease than in SS. It must be emphasized that the order of severity in SCD is based on population statistics. Thus, if one compares the overall clinical picture of 100 patients with SS, for example, with that of 100 patients with Hb SC disease, then the latter will be milder as far as frequency of painful episodes, morbidity, and mortality are concerned. On the individual basis, however, there are exceptions. Thus, an individual patient with SS may have a mild disease, whereas an occasional patient with S-β$^+$-thalassemia may have a severe disease.

GENOTYPES

Sickle cell syndromes can also be divided into subcategories depending on the α genotypes and β haplotypes.[29–31] About 65% of patients with SS have normal α genotypes (β^{S}β^S; αα/αα), 30% have one α gene deleted (β^{S}β^S; −α/αα), and the remaining 5% have two α genes deleted (β^{S}β^S; −α/−α). The effect of α-gene deletion on the clinical picture of sickle cell syndromes is controversial. Generally speaking, α-gene deletion is associated with milder anemia[32] and less blood transfusion. The increased Hb level associated with α-gene deletion, however, increases the blood viscosity, which is often accompanied by increased frequency of painful crises[33,34] and vaso-occlusive episodes such as avascular necrosis (AVN).[35,36] The effect of α-gene deletion on the clinical picture is best illustrated in SS with two α-gene deletions (β^{S}β^S; −α/−α). Table 57.2 lists the unique features of this type of SCD.[37,38] Noteworthy is that HbA$_2$ is elevated in SS with two α-gene deletions, a finding that

confuses this diagnosis with S-β^0-thalassemia that is, typically, also associated with elevated HbA$_2$ levels. The clinical picture, family history, hematologic data, and molecular diagnostics can differentiate the two diagnoses.[38]

β-Haplotypes refer to the nucleotide sequence 5′ and 3′ to the sickle gene. Three major types have been described in Africans and African Americans.[30] These are the Senegalese (Sen), Benin (Ben), and Central African Republic (CAR) haplotypes. The significance of these haplotypes pertains to their effect on Hb F production. It has been established that the higher the Hb F level, the milder is the SS.[34,39] Again, these conclusions are based on population data and may not apply to an individual patient.

Pathophysiology

Pain is the hallmark of SCD and dominates its clinical picture throughout the life of the patients (Fig. 57.1). Pain, also, may precipitate or be itself precipitated by the other components of the disease. Moreover, management of sickle pain must be within the framework of the disease as a whole and not in isolation by itself. This is unlike other pain syndromes where the provider can make decisions on treatment based solely on the pain and its associated behavior. Sickle pain could, often, be the prodrome of a serious and potentially fatal complication of SCD.

TABLE 57.2	Unique Features of Sickle-α-Thalassemia (β^S/β^S; −α/−α) Compared with Sickle Cell Anemia Without α-Gene Deletion (β^S/β^S; αα/αα)

Milder anaemia
Increased Hb A$_2$ level
Splenomegaly in adults
Increased prevalence of avascular necrosis
Increased prevalence of retinopathy
Decreased prevalence of cerebrovascular accidents
Decreased prevalence of leg ulcers
Less tissue damage

Hb, hemoglobin.

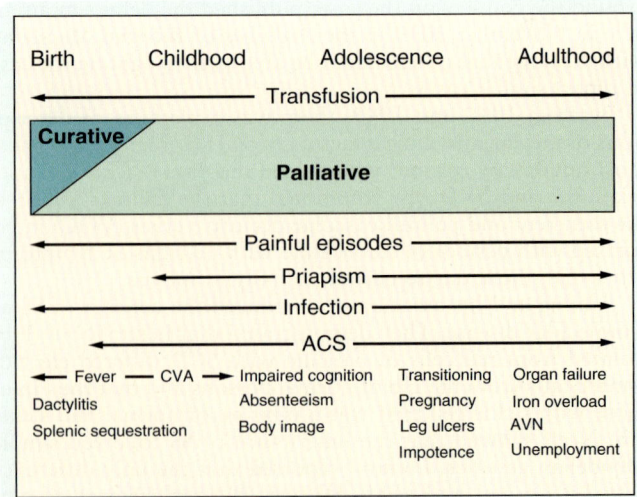

FIGURE 57.1 Sequence of complications of SS from birth through adult life. Cure is possible in selected patients. The mainstay of management in most patients is palliative, with pain management being most important. ACS, acute chest syndrome; AVN, avascular necrosis; CVA, cerebrovascular accident. *(Modified from Ballas SK. Sickle cell disease: current clinical management. Semin Hematol 2001;38[4]:308. Copyright © 2001 Elsevier. With permission.)*

TABLE 57.3 Determinants that Contribute to Vascular Occlusion in Sickle Cell Disease

Microrheology
  RBC factors
    Polymerization of deoxy Hb S
    Cellular dehydration
    Dense cells
    Fetal hemoglobin
    α-Genotype, β-haplotypes, Hb variants
    Sickling–unsickling cycles
    RBC deformability and mechanical fragility
  Factors extrinsic to RBC
    Adhesion to vascular endothelia
    Inflammatory mediators and reperfusion injury
    White blood cells
    Hemostatic factors
    Vascular factors
  Macrovascular occlusion
  Whole blood rheology
    Hematocrit
    Plasma components
    Vascular tone
  Other factors
    Epistatic genes
    The environment

Hb, hemoglobin; RBC, red blood cell.

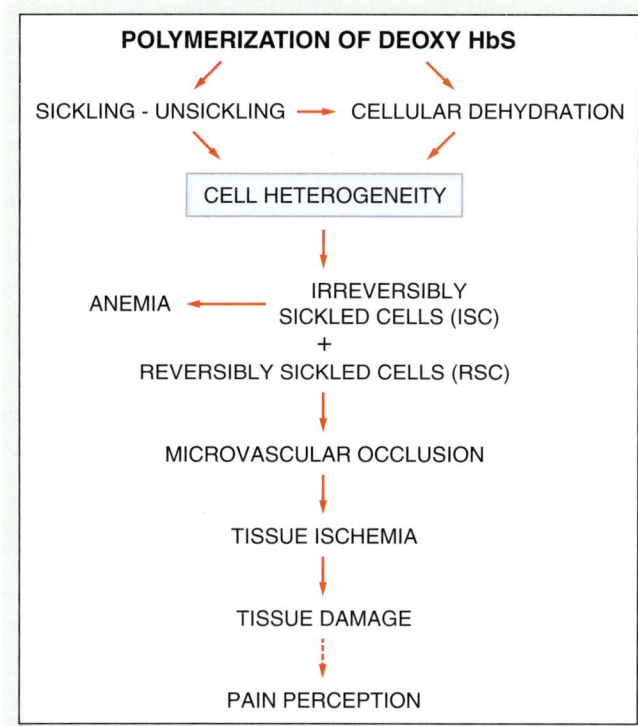

FIGURE 57.2 Sequence of pathophysiologic events that lead to vaso-occlusion and consequent pain perception. HbS, hemoglobin S. *(From Ballas SK. Sickle Cell Pain. 2nd ed. Washington DC: IASP Press; 2014. This figure has been reproduced with permission of the International Association for the Study of Pain® (IASP). The figure may not be reproduced for any other purpose without permission.)*

VASO-OCCLUSION

Vascular occlusion plays a pivotal role in explaining the clinical course of SCD.[40,41] It may involve both the microcirculation and the macrocirculation. The former underlies the VOC, and the latter is associated with organ failure including stroke and pulmonary hypertension.[42,43]

The major pathophysiologic events that lead to microvascular occlusion are (1) polymerization of deoxyhemoglobin S (deoxy Hb S); (2) generation of dense sickled cells, both reversibly and irreversibly sickled; (3) microvascular occlusion; (4) tissue ischemia; (5) tissue damage secondary to hypoxia; and (6) stimulation of peripheral nerve endings leading to pain perception (Table 57.3 and Fig. 57.2).[44,45] The precise dynamics of these events and their interrelationships are complex and poorly understood. Nevertheless, the primary process that leads to vascular occlusion is the polymerization of sickle Hb upon deoxygenation which, in turn, results in distortion of the shape of red blood

cells (RBCs), cellular dehydration, and decreased deformability and stickiness of RBC that promotes their adhesion to vascular endothelium (Fig. 57.3). Progress in the pathogenesis of vascular occlusion pertains to cellular dehydration, adhesion to endothelial cells, inflammatory state, and reperfusion injury.

CELLULAR DEHYDRATION

Cellular dehydration is secondary to loss of potassium (K⁺) and water. Two major transport mechanisms appear to play a significant role in cellular dehydration. The first mechanism is the potassium chloride (KCl) cotransport pathway activated by

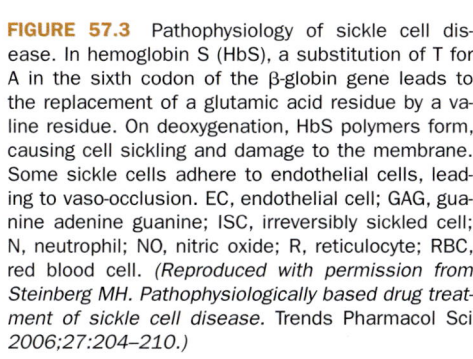
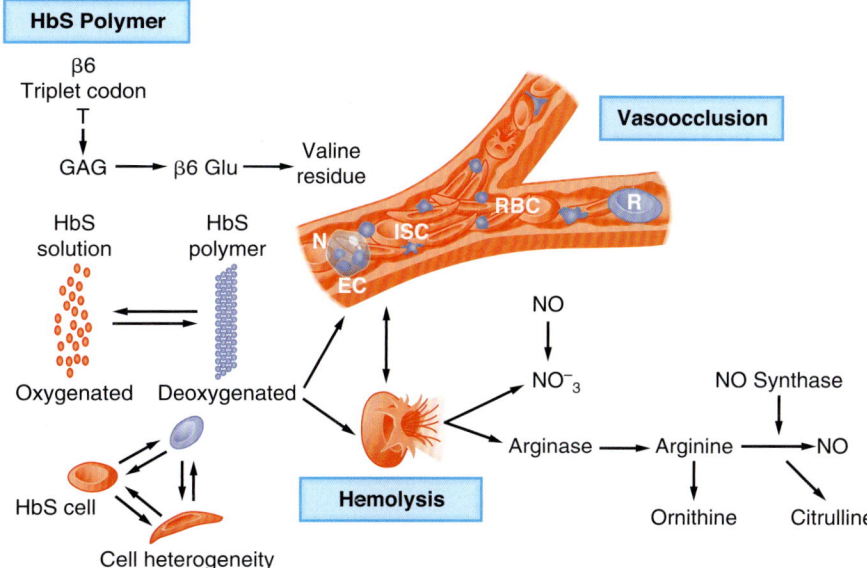

FIGURE 57.3 Pathophysiology of sickle cell disease. In hemoglobin S (HbS), a substitution of T for A in the sixth codon of the β-globin gene leads to the replacement of a glutamic acid residue by a valine residue. On deoxygenation, HbS polymers form, causing cell sickling and damage to the membrane. Some sickle cells adhere to endothelial cells, leading to vaso-occlusion. EC, endothelial cell; GAG, guanine adenine guanine; ISC, irreversibly sickled cell; N, neutrophil; NO, nitric oxide; R, reticulocyte; RBC, red blood cell. *(Reproduced with permission from Steinberg MH. Pathophysiologically based drug treatment of sickle cell disease. Trends Pharmacol Sci 2006;27:204–210.)*

acidification and cell swelling.[46-48] This pathway is most active in reticulocytes and is a feature of low-density sickle cells. Reticulocyte dehydration appears to contribute to the generation of dense sickle cells directly without going through repetitive cycles of oxygenation and deoxygenation.[49] The second transport system is the calcium (Ca^{2+})-activated K^+ channel or Gardos pathway, which is activated by Ca^{2+} reflux–induced deoxygenation.[46-48,50-52] Although much of the intracellular Ca^{2+} in sickle cells is sequestered within endocytic vesicles,[53-55] transient reflux of Ca^{2+} during deoxygenation-induced sickling appears to be responsible for stimulating the Gardos pathway. Unlike KCl cotransport, the Gardos pathway appears to be most active in the dense fraction of SS RBCs. However, in most patients, both transport systems are operative.

A phase III randomized controlled trial of senicapoc, a Gardos channel inhibitor, was terminated early because there was no difference observed between the treatment and control groups in the primary endpoint of painful crises. The reason is that rehydration of RBC increased their survival resulting in increased Hb level which, in turn, increased blood viscosity that is known to be associated with increased frequency of VOCs.[56,57]

ADHESION TO VASCULAR ENDOTHELIUM

Adhesion of sickle RBC to vascular endothelium is a pathophysiologic contributor to vaso-occlusion. Sickle RBC adhere to cultured endothelial cells in vitro under both static and dynamic conditions, whereas normal cells do not.[58-61] These findings suggest that sickle RBC have sticky surfaces that promote their attachment to monolayers of cultured endothelial cells. These in vitro observations have been documented to occur also in ex vivo perfusion studies in rats[62] and transgenic mice.[63] Both cellular and plasma factors have been reported to affect adhesion of sickle RBC to vascular endothelium. Thus, young deformable sickle RBCs appear to be more adherent to vascular endothelium than are dense, rigid, irreversibly sickled cells (ISCs).[61,64,65] Paradoxically, SS with few painful crises has been characterized by decreased red cell deformability and increased number of dense cells.[66]

Adherence of sickle RBC to vascular endothelium results in intimal hyperplasia in larger vessels that may lead to vascular occlusion and tissue infarction.[67,68] Hebbel et al.[58] reported strong correlation between the degree of adhesion of SS RBC to endothelial cells in vitro and the severity of the disease in patients with SS or other variants of SCD. Adhesive interactions of sickle erythrocytes with endothelium have been described in detail by Hebbel.[69,70]

INFLAMMATION AND REPERFUSION INJURY

In vivo studies in transgenic mice suggest that vaso-occlusion results in the creation of an inflammatory state.[71,72] The sequence of events seems to be as follows: (1) Reticulocytes carrying the $\alpha_4\beta_1$ receptor adhere to endothelial cells; (2) this is followed by logjam where there is propagation of occlusion caused by the accumulation of rigid deoxygenated mature RBC proximal to the site of adhesion; (3) the obstruction eventually clears leading to reperfusion and its associated injury; and (4) a new cycle of adhesion starts, thus creating a viscous cycle of occlusion and reperfusion. Evidence of reperfusion injury includes (1) inflammatory response in the vascular bed of the transgenic mouse with increased leucocyte rolling, adhesion, and emigration after 3 hours of mild hypoxia followed by reperfusion; (2) local production of free radicals; and (3) the complete inhibition of (1) and (2) after the infusion of monoclonal murine anti-P-selectin antibody, before reoxygenation.[71] The implication of this sequence of events is that restoration of oxygen to ischemic tissue results in the generation of free radicals associated with inflammatory endothelial and tissue damage.

Sickle RBC from patients with a high level of Hb F seem to be less adherent to vascular endothelium than those from patients with low Hb F levels. Specifically, Setty et al.[73] found that pediatric SS patients with high levels of F cells had a concomitant decrease in the number of CD36+, very late antigen (VLA) 4+, and CD71+ erythrocytes and, hence, less adherent RBC. Moreover, Hb F seems to affect the exposure of phosphatidylserine on the surface of RBC and coagulation activation. In vivo cycles of sickling/unsickling with resulting membrane changes and microvesicle formation are one factor responsible for phosphatidylserine exposure.[74] Phosphatidylserine-exposing RBC in the transgenic sickle mouse[75] were found to have shortened red cell survival. Children with SS and high Hb F levels were reported to have less phosphatidylserine-exposing RBC and, hence, milder hemolytic anemia suggesting a possibly milder clinical picture.[73]

GENETIC MARKERS

SCD is a complex genetic disorder characterized by intricate genotypic/phenotypic interactions that include correlations among multiple genetic and environmental markers and modifiers. Genetic markers may predict the severity of the disease and the possible or probable incidence of certain complications. This, in turn, allows for the implementation of certain therapeutic measures that may prevent or ameliorate the severity of some of these complications. Traditional approaches to identify genetic markers have included studies of the transgenic sickle cell mouse and natural history studies and family pedigrees.[76,77] With the advent of the Human Genome Project, novel genetic polymorphisms associated with disease have been identified, thus allowing for the performance of genetic association studies.[77-84]

The genetic markers described to date include three categories. The first includes α-thalassemia, Hb F level, and β-globin haplotypes that apply globally to SCD. These were mentioned earlier. The second category includes markers of complications associated with pain, and the third category includes complications associated with tissue damage not always associated with pain (Table 57.4 and Fig. 57.4).

Although these findings are novel and interesting, their validity and utility in predicting and treating the clinical complications of SCD should be confirmed by large controlled multi-institution studies. The studies performed to date are too small to make definite conclusions.

OTHER FACTORS

In addition to the factors mentioned earlier, there is growing evidence that psychosocial and environmental factors precipitate vaso-occlusion and affect the frequency and severity of painful episodes. Physical stress, trauma, dehydration, and infections are such known factors.

Classification of Sickle Cell Pain Syndromes

The classification of sickle cell pain syndromes entails the availability of accepted definitions of these syndromes. Such definitions would facilitate communications among providers, investigators, ancillary medical staff, administrators, insurers, the community, and patients and their families. Accepted definitions of the complications of SCD, including pain syndromes, did not exist until recently. This state of affairs made it difficult to establish cost-effective management of SCD and its complications. In an effort to fill this gap, the comprehensive sickle cell centers supported by the National Institutes of Health–published definitions of the phenotypic complications of SCD.[85,86] These were based on whatever evidence was available in the literature and the experiences of a large number of

TABLE 57.4   Association of Complications of Sickle Cell Disease with Genetic Polymorphisms

Complications	SNP	Clinical Relevance
Complications with Pain as a Major Manifestation		
• Bilirubin levels and cholelithiasis	UGT1A1	Bilirubin metabolism
• Priapism	KL, TEK, F13A1, ITGA2	Nitric oxide metabolism, angiogenesis, coagulation
• Avascular necrosis	MTHFR, ANXA2, ITGA2, KL, BMP6, TGFBR2, TGFBR3	Coagulation, cell growth, nitric oxide metabolism, TGF-β/SMAD pathway
• Leg ulcers	BMP6, BMPR1B, MAP2K1, MAP3K7, SMAD7, SMAD9, SMURF1, TGFBR2, TGFBR3, KL	TGF-β/SMAD pathway, nitric oxide metabolism
• Acute chest syndrome	NOS3, NOS1, TGFBR3, SMAD7, SMAD3, KL, ITGA2	Nitric oxide metabolism, TGF-β/SMAD pathway nitric oxide pathway, coagulation
Complications with Tissue Damage and Little or No Pain		
• Stroke	VCAM1, IL4R, TNFA, LDLR, ADRBZ, SELP, AGT, HLA, BMP6, TGFBR2, TGFBR3	Cell adhesion, inflammation, cholesterol metabolism, blood pressure, immunity, TGF-β/SMAD pathway
• Pulmonary hypertension	ACVRL1, BMP6, BMPR2, KL	TGF-β/SMAD pathway, nitric oxide metabolism
• Infection	IGF1R, CCL5, HLA, MBL2, MPO, BMP6, BMPR1A, SMAD6, TGFBR3	Cell growth, inflammation, immunity, TGF-β/SMAD pathway
• Renal impairment	BMPR1B	TGF-β/SMAD pathway

SNP, single-nucleotide polymorphism; TGF-β, transforming growth factor-β.
From Thein SL. Genetic modifiers of sickle cell disease. *Hemoglobin* 2011;35(5–6):589–606. Adapted by permission of Taylor & Francis Ltd. http://www.tandfonline.com.

hematologists caring for patients with SCD for decades. Each complication in those publications included (1) a definition, (2) diagnostic criteria, (3) a severity index if applicable, (4) classification if available, and (5) references. An accepted scheme of classification of sickle cell pain would facilitate communication and transfer of information pertinent to pain research, therapy, and clinical records. Table 57.5 shows a potential classification of sickle cell pain similar to that described by Turk and Okifuji.[87] Pathophysiologically, sickle cell pain could be nociceptive or neuropathic; temporarily, it could be acute or chronic; anatomically, it could be somatic, visceral, unilateral, bilateral, localized, or diffuse; pathologically, it could be mild, moderate, or severe (Table 57.6); and etiologically, it could be due to the disease itself or secondary to therapy or to comorbid conditions. The etiologic classifications of sickle pain are listed

in Table 57.7 and include acute pain syndromes, chronic pain syndromes, neuropathic pain syndromes, pain secondary to therapy, and pain due to comorbid conditions.

Acute Sickle Cell Pain Syndromes

THE VASCULAR OCCLUSIVE CRISIS
Vaso-occlusion is the de facto prerequisite for the development of the VOC. Tissue damage consequent to vaso-occlusion initiates a horde of complex biochemical, neurologic, electrochemical, and inflammatory sequence of events collectively referred to as nociception that culminates in the perception of acute pain. The inflammatory response due to vaso-occlusion may enhance sympathetic activity via interactions with neuroendocrine pathways and trigger release of norepinephrine, which, in the

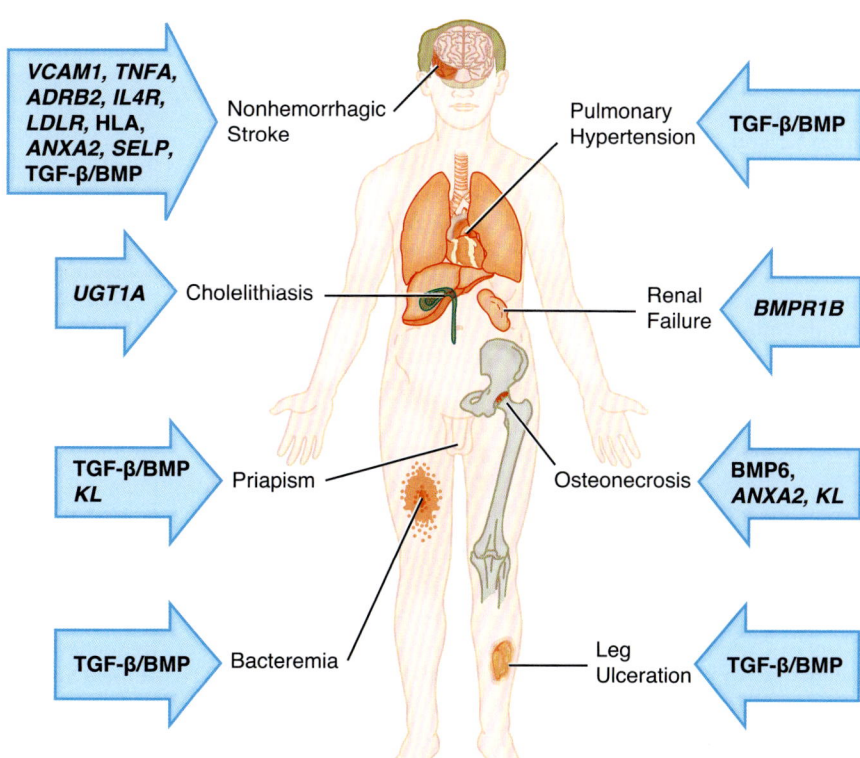

FIGURE 57.4 Genetic modifiers. Single-nucleotide polymorphisms in candidate genes suggest associations with subphenotypes of sickle cell anemia. *(From Steinberg MH. Genetic etiologies for phenotypic diversity in sickle cell anemia.* ScientificWorldJournal *2009;9: 46–67. http://dx.doi.org/10.1100/tsw.2009.10. Copyright © 2009 Martin H. Steinberg.)*

TABLE 57.5 Potential Classification of Sickle Cell Pain

Pathophysiologic

Nociceptive
Neuropathic
Psychogenic
Any combination of the above

Temporal

Acute
Chronic
Both

Anatomic

Somatic
Visceral
Deafferentation

Severity

Mild
Moderate
Severe

Etiologic

Secondary to the disease itself
Secondary to therapy
Unrelated to sickle cell disease

Regional

Head and neck pain
Chest pain
Abdominal pain
Extremities
Other regions

TABLE 57.7 Etiologic Classification of Sickle Cell Pain

Acute Pain Syndromes

Acute painful sickle cell crises
Acute chest syndrome
Acute abdominal pain syndromes
　Right upper quadrant syndrome
　Left upper quadrant syndrome
Hand–foot syndrome (dactylitis)
Priapism
Acute multiorgan failure (AMF)

Chronic Pain Syndrome

With objective signs
　Avascular (aseptic) necrosis
　Arthropathies
　Vertebral body collapse
　Leg ulcers
　Chronic osteomyelitis
Without objective signs
　Intractable chronic pain

Neuropathic Pain Syndromes

Syndromes unique/common in sickle cell disease
　Mental nerve neuropathy
　Ischemic optic neuropathy
　Spinal cord infarction
　Other neuropathies
Neuropathic pain associated with chronic intractable pain

Pain Syndromes Secondary to Therapy

Postoperative pain
Loose prosthesis (shoulders/hips)
Iatrogenic pain
　Withdrawal syndrome
　Pseudo-addiction
　Opioid-induced hyperalgesia

Pain Syndromes Due to Comorbid Conditions

Trauma
Peptic ulcer disease
Migraine headache
Arthritides (septic, rheumatoid, degenerative, collagen)
Other conditions

setting of tissue injury, causes more tissue ischemia, thus creating a vicious cycle. It is the combination of ischemic tissue damage and secondary inflammatory response that makes the pain of SCD unique in its acuteness and severity. Tissue injury generates several major pain mediators[88-91] including, but not limited to, interleukin (IL)-1, bradykinin, K+, hydrogen (H+), histamine, substance P, and calcitonin gene-related peptide (CGRP). IL-1 is an endogenous pyrogen and also upregulates the cyclooxygenase gene leading to synthesis of prostaglandins E2 and I2. Bradykinin, K+, H+, and histamine activate nociceptive afferent nerve fibers and evoke a pain response. Prostaglandins sensitize peripheral nerve endings and facilitate the transmission of painful stimuli along Aδ and C fibers that reach the cerebral cortex via the spinal cord and the thalamus. Moreover, activated nociceptors release stored substance P, which itself facilitates the transmission of painful stimuli. Bradykinin, substance P, and CGRP also cause vasodilatation and extravasations of fluids that can lead to local swelling and tenderness. The pathway for pain stimuli is subject not

only to activators, sensitizers, and facilitators but also to inhibitors. Serotonin, enkephalin, β-endorphin, and dynorphin are endogenous central pain inhibitors. Thus, in a given patient, the net outcome of tissue ischemia may be severe or mild pain, depending on the extent of tissue damage and the net balance of pain stimulators versus pain inhibitors. This may explain, in part, the considerable variation in the frequency and severity of painful sickle crises among patients and longitudinally in the same patient.

Predisposing Factors

The clinical manifestations of sickle cell syndromes vary widely from one patient to another and in the same patient over time. Some patients with SS have mild disease, whereas others suffer from a severe form and die at a relatively young age. Some patients, mostly adults, may have a clinical picture characterized by waxing and waning of the frequency and severity of VOCs.[92] Darbari et al.[93] determined markers of severe VOC frequency in children and adolescents with SS. They compared clinical and laboratory characteristics of children with SS who had three or more VOCs requiring health care in the preceding year with patients who had less than three VOCs.

Seventy-five children (20%) had severe VOCs, and 232 (61%) had none. Increasing age, α-thalassemia, iron overload,

TABLE 57.6 Classification of Painful Crisis by Severity of Pain, Duration, and Usual Place of Analgesic Therapy

Severity	Pain Score	Duration and Usual Place of Treatment	
		<4 h	>4 h
Mild	<4	Home/outpatient facility	Home/outpatient facility
Moderate	4–6	Home/outpatient facility	Home/outpatient facility/emergency department
Severe	>6	Home/emergency department	Emergency department/hospital

milder anemia, lower lactate dehydrogenase (LDH) level, and higher tricuspid regurgitation velocity were associated with a greater frequency of severe VOCs. Details of the factors proposed as indicators of severity and frequency of VOCs are as follows.

There are at least three sets of predisposing factors that predict the frequency and severity of the VOC. These are genetic, cellular, and environmental (or epigenetic) factors. Genetic factors include Hb F level, the coexistence of α-gene deletion, β-thalassemia, β-haplotypes, and epistatic gene modifiers as was mentioned earlier. They also include gender because males constitute about 60% to 66% of admissions to the hospital.[94,95] Females, however, have longer hospital stay per admission than males.[94] Cellular factors with decreased RBC deformability and increased number of dense cells in the steady state have a salutary effect, most likely because these are associated with more severe anemia and hence relatively decreased whole blood viscosity.[32,96] Patients with SS and relatively high Hb level are more likely to experience more frequent crises than those patients with SS and lower Hb level. Decreased level of vitamin A (less than 30 µg/dL) and nocturnal hypoxia are environmental factors amenable to preventative therapy.[97,98]

Precipitating Factors

Like other acute episodes of illness, the acute VOC has precipitating features. Major reported factors that seem to precipitate VOCs include dehydration, stress of any kind (physical, traumatic, physiologic, emotional), infection, acidosis, sleep apnea, and pregnancy.[99,100] Nevertheless, most painful episodes are not preceded by an obvious precipitating factor. Gil et al.[101] reported that daily mood and stress predict painful events, utilization of healthcare facilities, and work activity in adults with SCD.

In a retrospective study, Smith et al.[102] found a complex relationship between temperature changes, temperature extremes, and their relationship to emergency department (ED) visits and hospital admissions for VOCs in adults. The most relevant finding of this study was an inconsistent confirmation of a relationship between daily ambient temperature and ED visits or hospital admissions for VOCs. Jones et al.[103] studied retrospectively the number of admissions with acute pain and SCD to King's College Hospital, London, together with daily meteorologic records collected locally. Data from 1,400 days and 1,047 separate admissions were analyzed. Increased admissions were significantly associated with increased wind speed and low humidity but showed no relationship to temperature, rainfall, or barometric pressure. The strongest effect was for maximum wind speed/humidity ratio with 464 admissions on days in the lowest two quartiles of this parameter and 582 in the highest quartiles. The effect of high wind and low humidity is likely to be related to skin cooling. Anecdotally, many patients report that sudden changes in temperature seem to precipitate VOCs. The effects of windy weather were later confirmed by Nolan et al.[104] and Rogovik et al.[105]

Phases of the Acute Vaso-occlusive Crisis

The literature strongly suggests that the uncomplicated VOC requiring hospitalization has four distinct phases: prodromal, initial, established, and resolving. Figure 57.5 and Table 57.8 show the temporal relation of these phases to the severity of pain, their synonyms, and their typical estimated duration. Plotting all of the observations reported in the literature on a specific day of the VOC, whenever applicable, shows that objective clinical and laboratory signs emerge along a certain pattern (see Fig. 57.5 and Table 57.9).

The Prodromal Phase

A premonition of VOC (prodromal or pre-VOC phase) was first mentioned by Diggs,[5] who noted that one mother could predict that her child would develop a VOC by noting that the fingernails were pale. This observation was not pursued further until Murray and May[106] used a structured questionnaire with 102 patients and reported that 58% experienced a prodromal phase of an impending VOC up to 24 hours before developing features typical of their usual VOCs (see Fig. 57.5).

FIGURE 57.5 A typical profile of the events that develop during the evolution of a severe sickle cell painful crisis in an adult in the absence of overt infection or other complications. Such events are usually treated in the hospital with an average stay of 9 to 11 days. Pain becomes most severe by day 3 of the crisis and starts decreasing by day 6 or 7. The *roman numerals* refer to the phase of the crisis: I, prodromal phase; II, initial phase; III, established phase; and IV, resolving phase. *Dots* on the X axis indicate the time when changes became apparent, and *dots* on the Y axis indicate the relative value of change in comparison to the steady state indicated by the horizontal dashed line. *Arrows* indicate the time when certain clinical signs and symptoms may become apparent. *Values* shown are those reported at least twice by different investigators; *values* that were anecdotal, unconfirmed, or that were not reported to occur on a specific day of the crisis are not shown. CPK, creatinine phosphokinase; CRP, C-reactive protein; ER, emergency room; ESR, erythrocyte sedimentation rate; Hb, hemoglobin; HDW, hemoglobin distribution width; ISCs, irreversibly sickled cells; LDH, lactate dehydrogenase; RBC, red blood cells; RBC DI, red cell deformability index; RDW, red cell distribution width; SAA, serum amyloid A; WBC, white blood cell. (From Ballas SK. The sickle cell painful crisis in adults: phases and objective signs. Hemoglobin 1995;19[6]:323–333. Modified by permission of Taylor & Francis Ltd. http://www.tandfonline.com.)

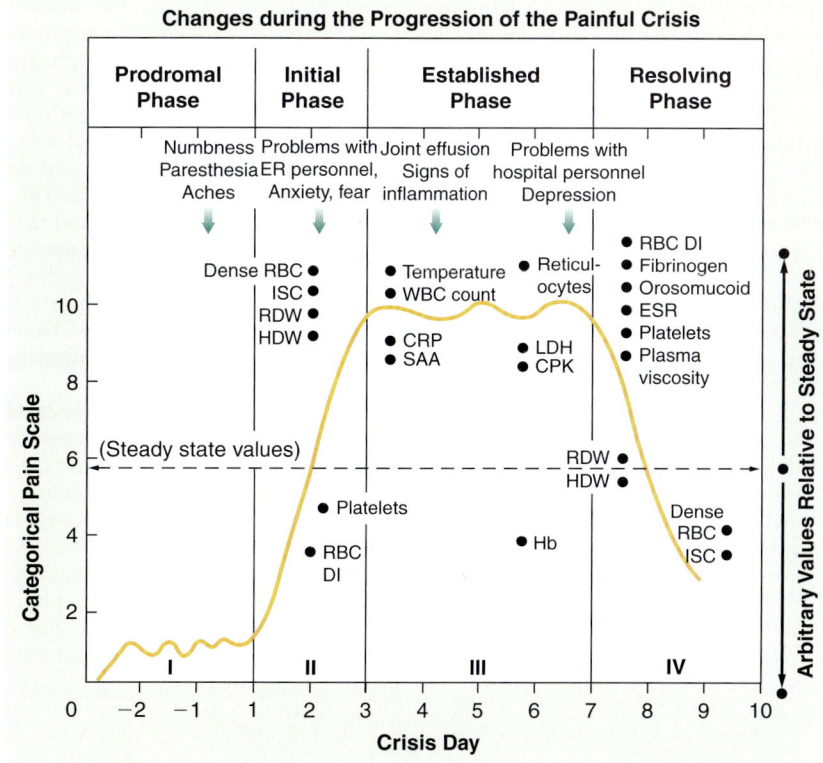

Changes during the Progression of the Painful Crisis

| Prodromal Phase | Initial Phase | Established Phase | Resolving Phase |

TABLE 57.8 Phases of the Acute Sickle Cell Painful Crisis

Phase	Possible Synonym(s)	Duration
Prodromal	Precrisis	Up to 2 d before crisis
Initial	First	Days 1 and 2 of the crisis
	Escalation	
	Evolving	
	Infarctive	
Established	Second	Days 3–7 of crisis
	Postinfarctive	
	Inflammatory	
Resolving	Last	Post day 7 of crisis
	Healing	
	Recovery	
	Postcrisis	

TABLE 57.9 Major Changes in Objective Signs during the Evolution of the Sickle Cell Painful Crisis

Prodromal Phase	Initial Phase	Established Phase	Resolving Phase
Decreasing	*Decreasing*	*Peak*	*Peak*
RBC deformability	RBC deformability	Temperature	Fibrinogen
	Platelets	WBC count	Orosomucoid
		Dense cells	ESR
		ISC	
		RDW	
		HDW	
		Reticulocytes	
		LDH	
		CRP	
		SAA	
Increasing	*Increasing*	*Nadir*	*Decreasing*
Dense RBC	Temperature	RBC deformability	Temperature
	WBC count	Hb	WBC count
	Dense cells		Dense cells
	ISC	*Increasing*	ISC
	RDW	Fibrinogen	RDW
	HDW	Orosomucoid	HDW
	ESR	Plasma viscosity	CRP
	LDH	ESR	
	CRP		*Increasing*
	Fibrinogen		RBC deformability
	Orosomucoid		Plasma viscosity
	SAA		Platelets

NOTE: Parameters shown are those reported at least twice by different investigators. CRP, C-reactive protein; ESR, erythrocyte sedimentation rate; Hb, hemoglobin; HDW, hemoglobin distribution width; ISC, irreversibly sickled cells; LDH, lactate dehydrogenase; RBC, red blood cell; RDW, red cell distribution width; SAA, serum amyloid A; WBC, white blood cell.

Symptoms mentioned during the prodromal phase included numbness, aches, and paresthesia in the sites subsequently affected by pain. Akinola et al.[107] studied 20 patients with SS over a period of 16 months. Patients were visited regularly at home by a nurse practitioner and were taught to keep a diary of clinical events and to mark a Visual Analog Scale. Twelve of 14 premonitions were followed by a typical VOC that required either home treatment (n = 4) or hospitalization (n = 8). Objective laboratory findings during this premonitory phase included decreased RBC deformability and increased number of both dense RBCs and ISCs compared to corresponding values at steady state.[107,108]

The Initial Phase
The initial phase (also called first, evolving, escalation, or infarctive phase) is heralded by the onset of typical VOC pain that increases gradually in severity and reaches a peak by the second or third day (see Fig. 57.5). Given the paucity of objective signs during this initial phase, patients experience problems with care providers in the ED.[109] Routine laboratory data may not be atypical, which often discourages the treating physician from repeating tests. Fear, anorexia, and anxiety are usually present in this initial phase.[5,109] Major RBC changes during this phase include decreased RBC deformability, increased dense cells, increased ISCs, increased red cell distribution width (RDW), and increased Hb distribution width (HDW) compared to steady state.[107,108,110–112] The increase in dense RBCs and ISCs may be (1) relative and secondary to preferential trapping of deformable discoid cells in the microvasculature, (2) absolute due to de novo formation of ISCs, or (3) a combination of both.[108] Other cellular changes in this phase include a decrease in platelet (PLT) count compared to steady state.[113–115]

The Established Phase
The established phase (also called second, postinfarctive, or inflammatory phase) is characterized by the persistence of severe steady pain and typically lasts 4 to 5 days in adults (see Fig. 57.5). Signs and symptoms of inflammation become predominant during this phase. Fever,[5,32,116] leukocytosis,[5,107,117,118] swelling, tenderness, and joint effusions[32,42,119] are common. In addition, serum levels of acute-phase reactants such as serum C-reactive protein (CRP) and serum amyloid A (SAA)[107,120,121] reach their peak values during this phase. Signs of hyperhemolysis, including decreased Hb, increased reticulocyte count, and LDH, may be seen. Tissue damage, especially bone marrow infarction, may be another source of increased LDH. An increase in creatinine phosphokinase (CPK) and aldolase usually indicates skeletal muscle injury. Billett et al.[117] reported dramatic increases in CPK values on days 5 to 8 of VOC compared to values on days 1 to 3. Depression and problems with hospital care providers,[109] who may become suspicious of patients because

of the heavy use of opioid analgesics for several days, occur toward the end of this phase and the start of the resolving phase.

The Resolving Phase
The resolving phase (also called last, healing, recovery, or post-VOC phase) is signaled by a gradual decrease in pain severity and may last 1 to 2 days (see Fig. 57.5). Significant erythrocyte changes during this phase include a decrease in the abnormalities of the initial phase, with increased RBC deformability, decreased dense cells, and decreased ISCs, below steady state. Both RDW and HDW return toward steady state. However, rebound thrombocytosis occurs, and another set of acute-phase reactants (fibrinogen and orosomucoid) reach peak values during this phase. Plasma viscosity and erythrocyte sedimentation rate (ESR) increase above baseline during this recovery phase. The significance of these changes will be addressed in the following discussion.

The Relapsing or Postdromal Phase
The resolution of the VOC is associated with rebound thrombocytosis, elevated levels of fibrinogen, orosomucoid, RBC deformability, and plasma viscosity, indicating the presence of a hypercoagulable state that may cause recurrence of the VOC (see Fig. 57.5 and Table 57.9). Ballas and Smith[108] found that approximately 20% of patients who were discharged from the hospital after the resolution of a VOC had recurrent VOC that required treatment with parenteral opioids in the ED or hospital within 1 week after discharge. A VOC appears to be a risk factor for the precipitation of another VOC. However, some patients, especially children, do well after the resolution of a VOC, with a pain-free period of variable duration before the onset of another VOC (Fig. 57.6). Others continue to have

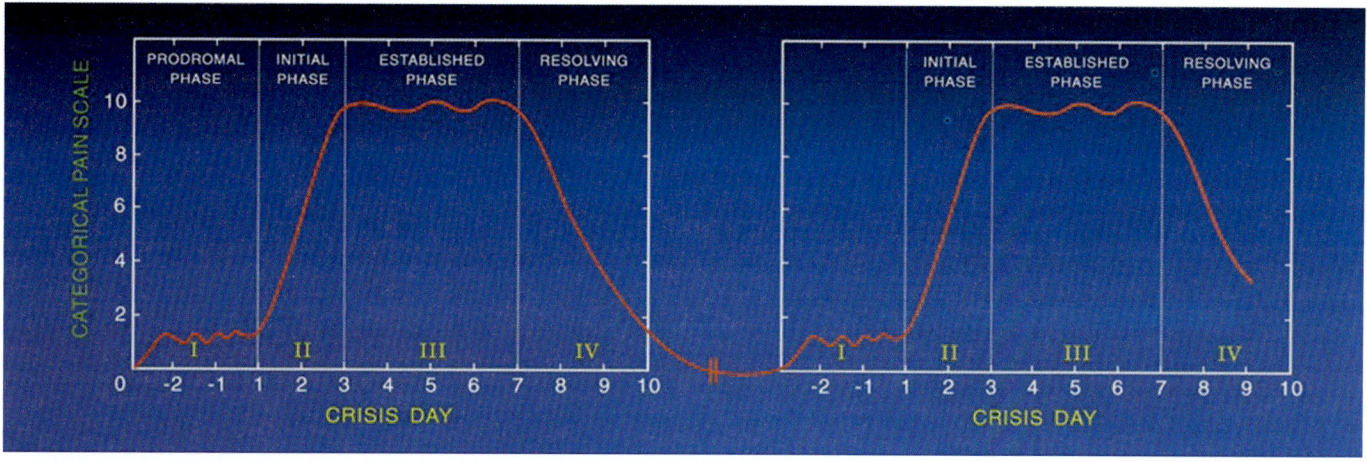

FIGURE 57.6 Two sequential painful crises with no pain during the time in between them. *(Republished with permission of American Society of Hematology from Ballas SK, Gupta K, Adams-Graves P. Sickle cell pain: a critical reappraisal. Blood 2012;120[18]:3647–3656; permission conveyed through Copyright Clearance Center, Inc.)*

pain. According to the Pain in Sickle Cell Epidemiologic Study (PiSCES), adult patients reported SCD pain at home for approximately 55% of the 31,017 days surveyed.[122] Similarly, children reported SCD pain at home for approximately 9% of the 1,515 days surveyed.[123,124] In the Multicenter Study of Hydroxyurea (MSH) study, at-home analgesics were used for SCD pain on 40% of diary days and 80% of 2-week follow-up periods, with short-acting oxycodone and acetaminophen being the most frequently used analgesics.[125,126] Descriptors and location of the pain at home were similar to those during hospitalization but milder. Patients prefer to treat pain at home with short-acting opioids rather than controlled-release opioids. In addition, those who take controlled-release opioids with short-acting opioids for breakthrough pain experience frequent attacks of breakthrough pain, resulting in the consumption of relatively large amounts of short-acting opioids. Moreover, patients prefer to be treated at a day unit rather than the ED whenever possible to avoid long hours of waiting before they are treated. Treatment of patients in day units with parenteral short-acting opioids decreased the frequency of hospital admissions and ED visits.[127]

In a prospective, longitudinal, and observational cohort study of all adult patients with SS admitted to a single institution between January 1998 and December 2002, Ballas and Lusardi[94] found the following: (1) Approximately 95% of all

of the 1,540 admissions of 136 patients were for VOCs; (2) the intensity of pain score decreased significantly during the first 4 days of hospitalization from an average of 8.7 ± 1.17 to 7.5 ± 1.00 (*P* < .001) and then reached a plateau of 7.4 until discharge (Fig. 57.7); (3) the mean score of pain intensity was >7 throughout the hospital stay; and (4) approximately 50% of hospital admissions for VOCs were associated with readmission within 1 month after discharge, and approximately 16% of all admissions were associated with readmission within 1 week after discharge (Table 57.10). The major cause of hospital readmission was the same VOC that was not controlled with analgesics at home or in the ED. Withdrawal syndrome was the cause of readmission for only five patients who were readmitted collectively 46 times (~7% of all readmissions) within 1 week after discharge. Readmission within 1 week after discharge was associated with greater mortality than otherwise.

Jacob et al.[128] showed a similar pattern of pain scores that plateaued ~5 days after hospital admission for VOCs in children. The high frequency of hospital readmission was confirmed in other studies.[129–131] In a retrospective cohort of SCD-related ED visits and hospitalizations from eight states (Arizona, California, Florida, Massachusetts, Missouri, New York, South Carolina, and Tennessee) in the 2005 and 2006 Healthcare Cost and Utilization Project State Inpatient Databases and State Emergency Department Databases, Brousseau et al.[129] found that the 30-day

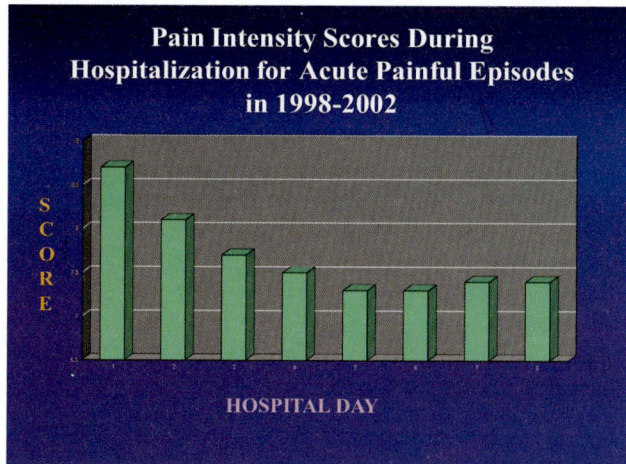

FIGURE 57.7 Pain intensity scores during hospitalization for acute painful episodes in 1998–2002. *(Republished with permission of American Society of Hematology from Ballas SK, Gupta K, Adams-Graves P. Sickle cell pain: a critical reappraisal. Blood 2012;120[18]:3647–3656; permission conveyed through Copyright Clearance Center, Inc.)*

TABLE 57.10 Incidence of Hospital Readmissions for Acute Painful Episodes in 1998–2002

	Hospital Readmissions after Discharge	
	Within 1 wk	Within 1 mo
Patients		
Males, n (%)	27/55 (49)	36/55 (66)
Females, n (%)	28/62 (45)	37/62 (60)
Total, n (%)	55/117 (47)	73/117 (62)
Readmissions		
Males, n (%)	148/871 (17)	516/871 (59)
Females, n (%)	80/586 (14)	210/586 (36)
Total, n (%)	228/1457 (16)	726/1457 (50)

NOTE: The numerator of each fraction represents the number of readmissions and the denominator represents the total number of hospital admissions before discharge. About 16% of readmissions occur 1 week after discharge, and 50% of readmissions occur 1 month after discharge.
From Ballas SK, Lusardi M. Hospital readmission for adult acute sickle cell painful episodes: frequency, etiology, and prognostic significance. *Am J Hematol* 2005;79(1):17–25. Copyright © 2005 Wiley-Liss, Inc., A Wiley Company. Reprinted by permission of John Wiley & Sons, Inc.

and 14-day readmission rates were 33.4% and 22.1%, respectively. Readmissions were highest for 18- to 30-year-old patients and for publicly insured patients. In another retrospective study in children with SCD, the most common admission and readmission (within 30 days) diagnosis was acute pain (78% and 70%, respectively).[130] The major risk factor for readmission was lack of outpatient hematology follow-up within 30 days after discharge; asthma was another risk factor for readmission within 30 days. Sobota et al.[131] performed a retrospective examination of 12,104 hospitalizations for VOC from July 1, 2006, through December 31, 2008, at 33 freestanding children's hospitals in the Pediatric Health Information System database. They identified 4,762 patients with 12,104 qualifying hospitalizations, of which 2,074 hospitalizations (17%) were readmissions for VOC within 30 days after discharge. Risk factors for readmission included older children, pain, and treatment with steroids.

ACUTE CHEST SYNDROME

Charache et al.[132] introduced the term *ACS* to define acute episodes of fever, chest pain, increased leukocytosis, and pulmonary infiltrates (Fig. 57.8) in adult patients with SS, most of whom probably had pulmonary infarction. With time, the definition of ACS has expanded to include hypoxemia, cough, shortness of breath, wheezing, chills, and worsening anemia.[133] The current definition of ACS complicating SCD includes chest pain, fever, hypoxia, dyspnea, cough, leukocytosis, decreasing Hb level, and new infiltrates on chest radiograph.[132–134] Pain is pleuritic in most patients. Abdominal pain may indicate involvement of adjacent diaphragmatic pleura. These signs and symptoms vary from mild to severe or even life-threatening. Not all of these signs and symptoms occur in all cases of ACS, with the exception of the new pulmonary infiltrates, which are considered sine qua non for the diagnosis. The presence of new infiltrates with some of the other signs and symptoms is usually enough to make the diagnosis. An infiltrate is new when compared to a previous radiograph with no infiltrate. If a previous radiograph is not available, the infiltrate in question is considered to be new. It is obvious from this description that there are gaps in making an accurate diagnosis. For example, there is no agreement on the number and nature of the accompanying signs and symptoms to make the diagnosis. Moreover, an occasional patient may have all of the signs and symptoms mentioned earlier with no new infiltrate on chest radiograph, thus generating a dilemma for the provider. Suffice it to say that ACS, like other syndromes, is a spectrum of clinical manifestations that vary from mild to very severe. Some patients may develop rapid respiratory failure and/or involvement of other organs such as the brain, kidneys, or liver, a condition referred to as multisystem organ failure.[135] Observation and careful monitoring on a daily basis, or more often if needed, are most important in ruling the diagnosis in or out.

Risk factors for developing ACS are listed in Table 57.11.[136,137] The incidence of ACS is age- and genotype-dependent, with no difference between sexes. It is approximately 3 times more common in young children than in adults but more severe in adults.[133,134] ACS is most common in SS, sickle β[0]-thalassemia, Hb SC disease, and sickle β[+]-thalassemia in decreasing order of frequency. Coexistent α-gene deletion, PLT count, and mean corpuscular volume (MCV) of RBCs do not appear to affect the incidence of ACS.[134] The incidence of ACS decreases in the presence of high Hb F level and severe anemia but is directly proportional to the steady-state white blood cell count.[134] ACS is closely associated with VOCs, especially in adults.[137,138] It occurs in approximately 50% of hospitalized patients with SS for VOC.[137,139–142] These episodes account for 15% of acute admissions and are potentially fatal.[42,142–144] Moreover, ACS appears to be the most common cause of death among patients and second to VOC as the most common cause of hospitalization of patients with SCD.[145–148] Although ACS is usually self-limited and resolves with treatment, it can be associated with respiratory failure, with a mortality rate of 1.8% in children and 4.8% in adults.[136,137]

Causes of ACS include pneumonia, bone marrow fat embolism, pulmonary infarct due to in situ sickling, rib/sternal infarction, infection, and pulmonary embolism (PE).[149–151] Approximately 50% of patients with ACS have no identifiable etiology.[137] Pulmonary bone marrow fat embolism in patients with SS appears to be more common than previously thought.[136,137] The characteristic clinical picture is that of severe bone pain, usually in long bones, followed by dyspnea, hypoxia, and fever. Tissue infarction of the bone marrow within long bones appears to generate a source of fat and necrotic tissue that has been demonstrated in the lung on autopsy (Figs. 57.9 and 57.10). "Retrograde embolization," described in the following

TABLE 57.11	Risk Factors of Acute Chest Syndrome
• High WBC count	• Rib infarction
• High Hb	• Pregnancy
• High pain rate	• Aseptic necrosis of hips
• Sickle cell anemia (SS)	• Analgesics
• S-β[0]-thalassemia	• Acute anemic events
• Fever	• Cold weather
• Age	

Hb, hemoglobin; WBC, white blood cell.

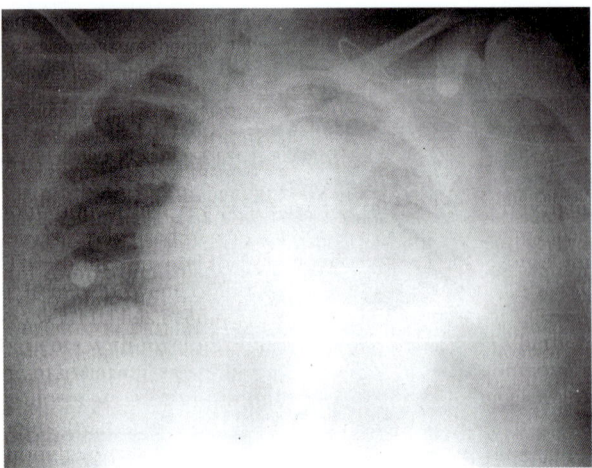

FIGURE 57.8 Chest radiograph showing diffuse pulmonary infiltrates of a patient with acute chest syndrome.

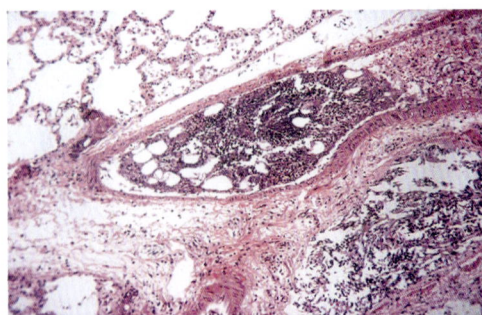

FIGURE 57.9 Autopsy specimen of lung from a patient with sickle cell anemia and fatal acute chest syndrome showing intravascular emboli composed of necrotic bone marrow elements. (*Reprinted by permission from Springer: Ballas SK. Sickle cell anaemia: progress in pathogenesis and treatment.* Drugs *2002;62[8]:1143–1172. Copyright © 2002 Adis International Limited.*)

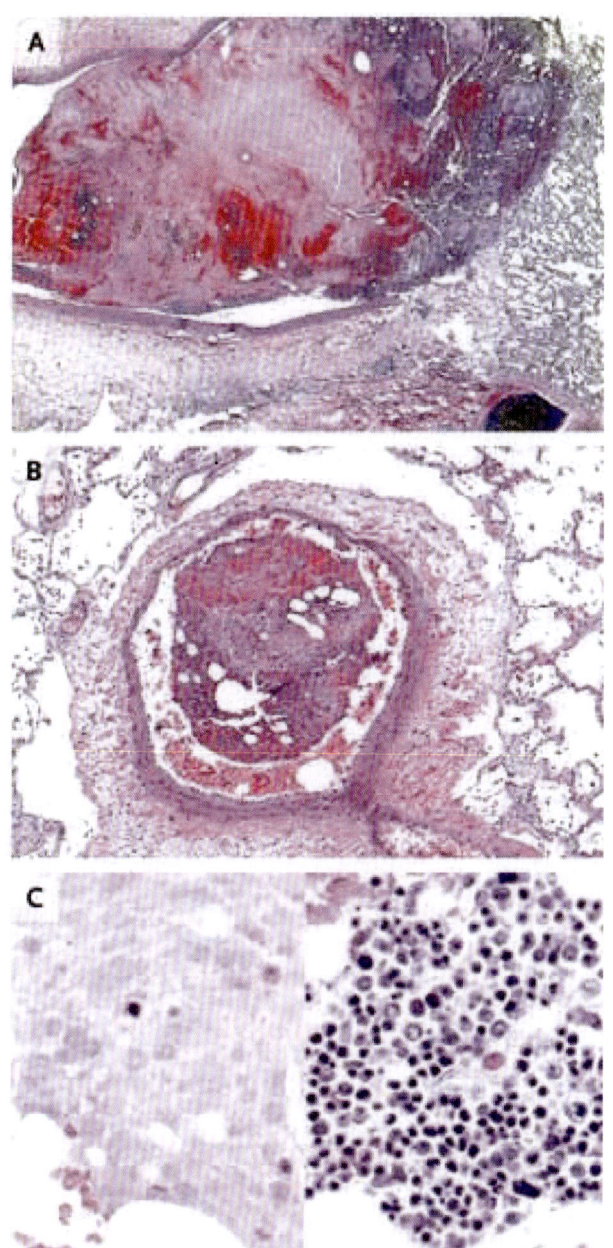

FIGURE 57.10 Photomicrographs of lung and bone marrow (hematoxylin and eosin). Bone marrow emboli, consisting of particles of bone marrow surrounded by fibrin, are present in small pulmonary arteries **(panels A and B)**. In **panel C**, a section of bone marrow shows the absence of cellular detail, indicating infarction **(left)**, as compared with a section of normal bone marrow from the same patient **(right)**. *(Medoff BD, Shepard JA, Smith RN, et al. Case records of the Massachusetts General Hospital. Case 17-2005. A 22-year-old woman with back and leg pain and respiratory failure. New Engl J Med 2005;352:2425–2434, with permission.)*

discussion, is the probable mechanism by which fat and necrotic tissue reach the lungs and other organs. At the same time, the serum level of secretary phospholipase A2 (sPLA2), an inflammatory mediator, increases in patients with ACS,[138,152] liberating free fatty acids from membrane phospholipids of the damaged tissue, which are believed to cause damage to the pulmonary endothelium, culminating in a leak syndrome, which if severe may be similar to adult respiratory distress syndrome. An elevated level of sPLA2 is both a marker and probably a predictor of ACS.

Diagnostic workup should include serial chest radiographs, cultures of sputum and blood, monitoring of arterial blood gases and Hb level, ventilation and perfusion (V/Q) scans, analysis of induced sputum, bronchial washings, analysis of urine for fat globules, and ruling out thrombophlebitis in the pelvis or lower extremities. The diagnosis of fat embolism entails the identification of fat-laden macrophages in induced deep sputum or better by bronchoalveolar lavage fluid obtained by bronchoscopy.[137,153]

The management of ACS involves multiple modalities to prevent possible catastrophic outcomes. The most important aspect of management is to maintain adequate ventilation. In mild cases, incentive spirometry may be sufficient to achieve this. However, in severe cases, mechanical ventilation in the intensive care unit is essential. Once adequate ventilation is maintained, specific treatment includes oxygen, antibiotics, simple blood transfusion or exchange transfusion, judicious use of analgesics, bronchodilators, careful hydration, and possible vasodilators. Incentive spirometry prevents splinting and atelectasis and may actually prevent ACS in patients with rib infarction.[151] Intravenous antibiotics are indicated because it is difficult to rule out pneumonia or infected lung infarcts. A combination of a third-generation cephalosporin and a macrolide or a quinolone antibiotic should be used to cover typical and atypical pathogens. Simple transfusion or exchange transfusion is indicated in patients with worsening respiratory function.[154] The beneficial effects of blood transfusion may not be due simply to decreasing the proportion of sickled RBCs; other mechanisms may be involved. These include (1) an immunomodulatory mechanism by which inflammatory cytokines (IL-8 in particular) bind to the Duffy antigen present on transfused RBCs but often absent on RBCs of Africans and African Americans[155] and (2) the albumin that is present in transfused units or used in blood exchange may bind free fatty acids, thus neutralizing their damaging effect on the pulmonary endothelium.

Although intravenous steroids may be beneficial for children with ACS,[156,157] their use in adults with ACS is controversial. Steroids appear to have two paradoxical effects in SCD. They may shorten the duration of the VOC and ACS in children, but they may increase the risk of rebound VOCs and stroke.[156–158] Huang et al.[159] reported two adult patients with SCD whose clinical picture deteriorated and was complicated by worsening pain, fat embolism, and coma after steroid therapy. Other investigators have reported similar experiences with steroids.[160,161] The mechanism by which steroids cause these undesirable complications is not well known and includes two possible mechanisms. The first mechanism pertains to their anti-inflammatory effects. Steroids stabilize cellular membranes and prevent or decrease the cleavage of membrane phospholipids by the enzyme sPLA2 to form inflammatory mediators, including free fatty acids.[138] The latter are known to cause damage to pulmonary endothelium, culminating in respiratory failure. However, once steroids are discontinued, their protective anti-inflammatory effect vanishes, with a rebound surge of inflammatory mediators that cause rebound phenomena.

The second mechanism refers to the retrograde embolization hypothesis described by Simkin and Downey.[162] Although this hypothesis was first introduced to explain the mechanisms by which steroids cause osteoporosis, it applies very well to SCD. According to this hypothesis, obstruction of the vascular channels within the bone marrow by conglomerates of sickled RBCs leads to bone marrow infarction and necrosis of hematopoietic elements and fat. The increased intramedullary pressure disrupts the endothelium of the engorged sinusoids, thus allowing the retrograde movement of necrotic bone marrow and fat into adjacent intramedullary sinusoids, which communicate directly with arteries and veins, which in turn spread necrotic material systemically, resulting in fat embolism and other VOCs. Unlike children, adults have more adipose tissue that may hypertrophy with steroids, increasing the chances of retrograde embolization. Moreover, steroids may induce or worsen AVN, which is more common in adults than in children. Together, these aspects of the VOC, the bone marrow fat, and the effects of steroids appear to explain the severe VOCs associated with systemic steroids, especially in adults.

The excessive use of opioid analgesics may precipitate ACS due to their depressive effect on respiration. Recommendations to use nonsteroidal anti-inflammatory drugs (NSAIDs) should be considered carefully.[136] Opioids have a few systemic side effects, and careful monitoring of their use ensures their safety. They should be discontinued if the respiratory rate is 10 breaths per minute, and their adverse effects can be quickly reversed with opioid antagonists. On the other hand, NSAIDs have considerable systemic side effects that may not be readily obvious. For example, NSAIDs decrease the levels of prostaglandins and prostacyclin, prostanoids that are essential in modulating the vascular tone of smooth muscle and renal blood flow. Thus, NSAIDs may worsen the clinical picture of ACS due to their vasoconstrictive effects and bronchospasm; NSAIDs are contraindicated in asthma for the same reasons.

The role of vasodilators, including nitric oxide (NO), in the management of SCD in general and ACS in particular is not finalized.[163] It has been reported than NO had a beneficial effect on VOCs in children[164] and in adults[165,166] in the ED setting. Its use in hospitalized patients with VOC had no beneficial effect.[167] An open trial using purified poloxamer 188 (Flocor), a nonionic surfactant, in patients with ACS showed no benefit.[168,169] It is hypothesized that this agent reduces blood viscosity, prevents adhesion of RBCs to vascular endothelium, and improves microvascular blood flow. Other vasodilators, such as prostacyclin and calcium channel blockers, have not been reported in the management of ACS.

Given the relative frequency of ACS in SS, and the need to monitor arterial blood gases, it is important to establish steady-state blood gases and perform oximetry and pulmonary function tests for all patients. These determinations will be of value in evaluating patients with acute onset of pulmonary signs and symptoms.[170]

ACUTE ABDOMINAL PAIN SYNDROMES

The abdomen is the second most common site of pain in SCD after musculoskeletal pain (including chest wall). The cause may be intra-abdominal pathology or pain referred from the lungs with pneumonia or from the lower ribs and the femoral heads with AVN. Specific abdominal pain syndromes due to SCD include right upper quadrant syndromes, left upper quadrant pain syndromes, and other acute abdominal episodes.

Right Upper Quadrant Pain Syndromes

Acute pain in the right upper quadrant is common in SCD.[171–173] Differential diagnosis of this entity includes VOC, acute cholecystitis, hepatic sequestration, hepatic crisis, and intrahepatic cholestasis.[174] Hemolysis of any etiology results in increased secretion of unconjugated bilirubin that precipitates in the gallbladder, causing cholelithiasis and sludge. Some reports implicate third-generation cephalosporins as causing crystallization in the gallbladder.[175]

It should be noted that liver involvement in SCD (sickle hepatopathy) is a spectrum that extends from mild (hepatic sequestration) to severe (intrahepatic cholestasis), with hepatic crisis in between. It is not unusual for the disease to progress from a mild form such as sequestration to severe intrahepatic cholestasis.[176] Detailed history; physical examination; and monitoring of the clinical picture, liver size, and laboratory data will differentiate the components of the spectrum.

Cholelithiasis, Biliary Sludge, Choledocholithiasis, and Cholecystitis

The prevalence of pigmented gallstones is approximately 30% in patients older than 10 years of age and approaches 70% to 75% in adults.[139,177] Cholelithiasis occurs as early as 2 years of age,[178] and approximately 30% of patients with SCD have gallstones by the age of 18 years.[179,180] Approximately 90% of adult patients with SS and cholelithiasis have been reported to undergo cholecystectomy either prophylactically or after an acute episode of calculous cholecystitis.[177] Acute cholecystitis may occur at any age, and the stones are often multiple and pigmented. Less than 10% of patients with cholelithiasis develop cholecystitis.[139]

The incidence of cholelithiasis appears to be affected by diet and possible genetic factors.[180] The coinheritance of α-thalassemia may reduce the incidence of stones because it may ameliorate hemolysis, which is thought to drive stone formation as mentioned earlier.[181] The same applies to any condition with a mild hemolytic component. A genetic basis for the hyperbilirubinemia pertains to mutation of UDP-glucuronosyltransferase 1 (UGT1A), the enzyme that catalyzes bilirubin glucuronidation. It appears that genetic polymorphism of the UGT1A enzyme affects the metabolism of bilirubin. The bilirubin level, as well as gallstone formation, appear to be significantly greater in patients with the 7/7 genotype compared to those with the 6/6 genotype.[182] Similar findings were reported in patients with Hb E-thalassemia.[183]

Acute cholecystitis should be treated conservatively with appropriate antibiotics and hydration until defervescence of the acute attack. Elective cholecystectomy may then be performed.[178] Treatment of asymptomatic cholelithiasis remains controversial.[179,184,185] Conservative measures, such as restriction of fatty diet, may be helpful. When gallstones are associated with chronic abdominal pain, elective cholecystectomy may be warranted. Unfortunately, only 50% of patients obtain pain relief after surgery.[139] Advocates of elective surgery for asymptomatic stones argue that surgical morbidity in a properly prepared patient with SCD is minimal, whereas morbidity in an emergency cholecystectomy is high.[139] Laparoscopic cholecystectomy is the procedure of choice for this indication. This also causes less abdominal muscle disruption and decreases postsurgical complications including ACS.[186,187]

Biliary sludge is a common finding in patients with SCD.[188,189] It is an echogenic, intraluminal sediment composed of calcium bilirubinate, cholesterol crystal, viscous bile, mucus, and protein. The natural history of biliary sludge in children with SCD shows that after a mean of 2.1 years of follow-up, approximately 65% of patients eventually develop gallstones, although not necessarily symptomatic. Approximately 40% of patients with biliary sludge do not develop gallstones despite the continued presence of sludge in most. Annual ultrasound to assess stone formation is recommended by most authors and reserve cholecystectomy only for patients with signs and symptoms of acute cholecystitis.[190]

Choledocholithiasis is the presence of gallstones in the common bile duct.[191] The prevalence of choledocholithiasis in patients with SCD appears to be <5% in patients with asymptomatic gallstones according to a survey of patients in steady state.[189,192] The rate of choledocholithiasis is higher in symptomatic patients, affecting 20% to 60% of individuals with SCD compared to 15% of those without.[193,194] Signs and symptoms are similar to those of cholelithiasis/cholecystitis. Duct obstruction is rare because pigmented stones are usually smaller than nonpigmented stones. If the common duct is obstructed, symptomatic and/or chemical pancreatitis may be present.[195] Endoscopic retrograde cholangiopancreatography and sphincterotomy are the best approach to remove the offending stones.[196]

Hepatic Sequestration

Acute hepatic sequestration is sequestration of RBCs in hepatic sinusoids, leading to liver enlargement and decreased Hb concentration. It is characterized by a decrease of ≥2 g/dL in Hb concentration from baseline with reticulocytosis, without other explanation, and liver enlargement of ≥3 cm for children and ≥5 cm for adults (from previous physical examination), without other explanation and no appreciable disturbance in liver function tests.[85] Hatton et al.[197] first described the problem in two adult patients with SS and associated infection. Davies and Brozovic[198] documented hepatic sequestration with associated infection in two young children (18 months and 4 years of age), which suggests that the syndrome may be present once autosplenectomy has occurred. Its most likely mechanism appears to be sequestration of sickled RBCs in the liver. The clinical progression is generally less acute than in splenic sequestration and develops over a few hours to days. The liver becomes progressively enlarged and palpable and may be painful as the liver capsule stretches. Other signs are falling Hb level and bone pain. Therapy is symptomatic, and blood transfusion may be indicated if the Hb level falls below 5 g/dL. Hepatic sequestration may be easily overlooked unless the size of the liver is regularly monitored in patients with VOC involving the right upper quadrant. Acute hemolysis and other causes of Hb decline should be ruled out. Recurrent episodes may occur.[199–202]

Hepatic Crisis

Hepatic crisis is the most common liver complication in SCD.[139,203] It may occur in 10% of patients admitted for VOC.[5,203] An attack is characterized by right upper quadrant abdominal pain, jaundice, hepatomegaly, fever, leukocytosis, dark urine, and often bone or joint pain. Serum transaminases and serum bilirubin are elevated to variable degrees.[204] According to some reports, the serum bilirubin level rarely goes above 15 mg/dL.[205,206] However, others reported a relatively mild course of hepatic crisis, referred to as benign extreme hyperbilirubinemia,[207] in children with serum bilirubin level as high as 57 mg/dL.[208] Most of the elevated serum bilirubin (>50%) is usually unconjugated. The clinical picture may simulate acute cholecystitis, choledocholithiasis, or viral hepatitis. Liver biopsy helps to distinguish hepatic crisis from viral hepatitis by showing sinusoidal obstruction by sickle cells, hypertrophy of Kupffer cells, and engorgement with RBCs (Fig. 57.11). Additional findings may include hemosiderosis, occasional bile stasis, and mild centrolobular necrosis. The condition is usually transient but may last 2 to 3 weeks before complete resolution.

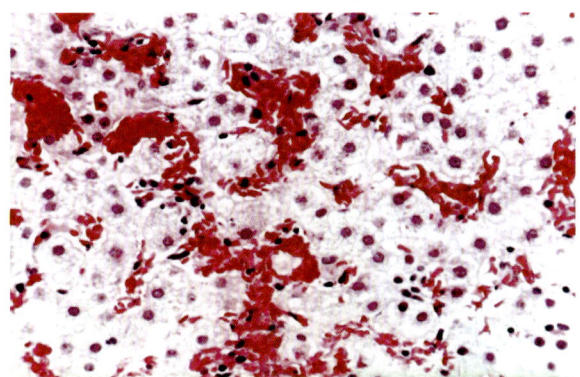

FIGURE 57.11 Liver biopsy from a patient with sickle cell anemia and hepatic crisis showing engorgement of hepatic sinusoids with sickled erythrocytes. *(From Ballas SK. Sickle cell pain. In:* Progress in Pain Research and Management. *Vol. 11. Seattle, WA: IASP Press; 1998. This figure has been reproduced with permission of the International Association for the Study of Pain® (IASP). The figure may not be reproduced for any other purpose without permission.)*

Some authors recommended treatment with intravenous fluids and antibiotics and elective cholecystectomy for gallstones.[139] Simple or exchange blood transfusion may be indicated.

Intrahepatic Cholestasis

Intrahepatic cholestasis is intrahepatic obstruction of bile formation or flow, leading to hyperbilirubinemia. It is characterized by a marked increase in direct bilirubin (>50% of total) compared to baseline, absence of extrahepatic biliary system obstruction, and absence of evidence of marked accelerated hemolysis. It may be benign, without hepatic protein synthesis failure/coagulopathy, or severe and regressive, with hepatic protein synthesis failure, thrombocytopenia, and prolongation of coagulation tests.[85,201,203,208] This severe form of hepatic crisis may, in rare cases, be complicated by fulminant cholestasis, leading to hepatic coma and death. An attack of intrahepatic cholestasis is characterized by a sudden onset of abdominal or right upper quadrant pain, increasing jaundice (with conjugated bilirubin as high as unconjugated bilirubin), a progressively enlarging liver, light-colored stools, and hyperbilirubinemia without urobilinogenuria. The clinical picture suggests cholestatic jaundice or choledocholithiasis but with no evidence of common duct obstruction or cholangitis. The prothrombin time, partial thromboplastin time, LDH, and liver enzymes are all elevated. Total serum bilirubin level may be >100 mg/dL. Liver biopsy shows similar changes to those described in hepatic crisis but in a more severe form associated with lymphocytic infiltration, paracentral necrosis, cholestasis, and dilated canaliculi containing bile plugs. Intrahepatic cholestasis is a potentially fatal complication of SCD if not treated promptly. In early reports,[206,209] only one of eight patients survived. The advent of exchange transfusion as a therapeutic modality[206] reversed this prognosis. In the author's opinion, patients who are suspected of having hepatic crisis should be watched carefully by monitoring their clinical status, hematologic parameters, serum bilirubin, liver function, and coagulation profile. If the total serum bilirubin level increases to >50 mg/dL or the prothrombin time increases to greater than 20 seconds, total blood exchange should be performed by replacing the removed blood with washed sickle-negative RBCs and fresh frozen plasma.[210] The procedure should be repeated until Hb S decreases to <30% and the serum bilirubin and prothrombin time decrease to acceptable values.[176,202,211]

Left Upper Quadrant Syndrome
Acute Splenic Sequestration Crisis

The spleen is the first organ to suffer from the destructive effects of sickle microvasculopathy that eventually lead to functional asplenia and autosplenectomy. During infancy, the spleen is enlarged in about 75% of patients with sickle anemia. Children between the ages of 5 months and 2 years are most vulnerable to splenic sequestration that varies in severity from mild to life-threatening episodes. In its full-blown picture, acute splenic sequestration is characterized by a pentad of (1) rapid fall in Hb level, (2) rise in reticulocyte count, (3) fall in PLT count, (4) sudden increase in spleen size associated with acute pain and tenderness in the left upper quadrant, and (5) signs and symptoms of hypovolemia.[212,213] Minor episodes may resolve spontaneously, but severe ones can be fatal and may be mistaken for the sudden infant death syndrome. Fibrosis occurs by the age of 8 years, and the risk for splenic sequestration decreases.[214,215] Nevertheless, older children and adults with persistent splenomegaly in certain sickle cell syndromes (SS with two α-gene deletions, Hb SC disease, and sickle-β-thalassemia) continue to be vulnerable for relatively milder episodes of splenic sequestration and for splenic infarction or splenic hemorrhage.[216] Severe splenic sequestration that could be life-threatening, however, has been described in adults with SS.[217–220]

The pathophysiologic mechanisms that lead to acute splenic sequestration are not well understood. One possible mechanism is acute obstruction of the venous flow from the spleen with a resultant damming effect associated with sudden enlargement of the spleen due to pooling of red cells and PLTs.[221,222] The acidotic environment of the spleen, due to its sluggish circulation, stimulates sickling, increases viscosity, and contributes to further obstruction of blood flow. Infection can cause more vascular engorgement in addition to the rapid acceleration of sickling. Obstruction of the venous flow may be related to abnormal rheologic properties of sickle erythrocytes.[223] Moreover, scanning electron microscopy has demonstrated trapping rigid sickle cells in the splenic cords of patients with SS.[224]

Treatment of acute splenic sequestration consists of rapid restoration of intravascular volume and oxygen-carrying capacity. This goal is achieved by the transfusion of sickle-negative RBC at a rate of 15 to 20 mL/kg with careful monitoring to avoid sudden overexpansion of blood volume that may precipitate pulmonary edema. After successful treatment, the spleen usually shrinks within a few days and gradually regains its baseline size.

Acute episodes of splenic sequestration tend to recur within a few months to a year after the initial sequestration crisis. Thus, splenectomy has been recommended for those patients who survive the initial severe episode.[225] The onset of splenic sequestration correlates with the increased risk for septicemia from *Streptococcus pneumoniae* and *Haemophilus influenza* type b, and it is recommended that all patients with sickle cell syndromes receive pneumococcal and *H. influenza* vaccines. It is important to educate the family about acute splenic sequestration so the parents can be alert for early symptoms and seek immediate medical intervention. The spleen is the major organ that produces immunoglobulin M (IgM). Patients with autosplenectomy typically have low levels of IgM, a finding that is similar to those patients with anatomic splenectomy.[226]

Other Acute Abdominal Painful Episodes

An abdominal VOC is characterized by severe, usually generalized, abdominal pain and signs of peritoneal irritation. It may also be accompanied by fever, leukocytosis, and markedly elevated LDH level. Clinically, a severe abdominal VOC may closely mimic acute abdomen and may lead to exploratory laparotomy in search of surgically correctable pathology. Patients with SCD who arrive at the ED with an acute abdominal VOC may be misdiagnosed with acute appendicitis or acute cholecystitis and undergo laparotomy and often prophylactic appendectomy and/or cholecystectomy.[227] In the author's experience, one-third of adult patients with SCD give a history of appendectomy. Whether the procedure was performed for true acute appendicitis or misdiagnosis of abdominal VOC is unknown. Nevertheless, a 30% incidence of acute appendicitis is much higher than in the general population and raises questions about the authenticity of the diagnosis. Thus, acute abdominal pain in SCD should be considered a VOC until proven otherwise.

The abdominal pain has been attributed to enlarged mesenteric and retroperitoneal lymph nodes; bone marrow hyperplasia; and infarction of the vertebral bodies, hepatobiliary disease, splenic disease, or mesenteric arterial thrombosis.[228] The abdominal pain seen in VOC may persist for several days, although protracted VOCs lasting longer than 5 days are not unusual.[229] Differentiation from other causes of acute abdominal pain may be difficult.[199,230]

Pain in the trunk in association with abdominal distention has been referred to as girdle syndrome by Davies and Brozovic.[198] It is thought to result from sickling in the mesenteric blood supply. Fluid levels may be visible on radiographs of the abdomen. Mild cases are self-limiting over a

2- to 5-day period and are treated symptomatically with intravenous fluids because gut absorption is impaired. More severe cases have associated involvement of the liver and lungs, and in very severe cases, multiorgan failure (MOF), including ACS, should be considered. Such patients may have markedly distended loops of bowel and require nasogastric suction and exchange transfusion. Infarction of segments of gut can occur, so it is important to involve surgeons in the evaluation of these patients.

HAND–FOOT SYNDROME (DACTYLITIS)

This acute pain syndrome occurs most commonly in infants and young children between the ages of 6 months and 2 years with a few case reports up to 7 years. The clinical picture is characterized by acute painful swelling of one or more extremities. It is caused by inflammation due to ischemic infarction of the bone of the affected extremity resulting in swelling, redness, and pain in affected areas. Fever and leukocytosis may be present. The episode is usually self-limited and resolves within 1 week, but recurrent attacks are common. Treatment is symptomatic, and if the attack persists, acute osteomyelitis should be ruled out.[99,100]

PRIAPISM

Priapism is a sustained, unwanted, and recurrent painful penile erection. It is one of the most debilitating complications of SCD. The word *priapism* is derived from Priapus, the Greek god of fertility and the protector of horticulture. He was also recognized as the protector of all garden produce including goats, sheep, bees, and the vine; he is depicted in sculpture with a huge tumescent penis, symbolizing fertility.

Priapism is a common complication of SCD, affecting 35% of boys and men.[231] It is most common in patients with SS, who account for approximately 80% to 90% of reported cases.[232–235] However, it does occur in males with all forms of SCD including Hb SC disease, all types of sickle thalassemia, and in those with sickle trait.[232,236] In one survey, a single episode of priapism was reported by 31% to 64% of patients, mostly children; approximately 50% of all patients had recurrent episodes, from 2 to 50 times or more, and the estimated mean duration of an episode was 125 minutes (range 50 to 480 minutes).[234,235,237,238] Priapism is not unique to SCD; it could be secondary to trauma, infection, neoplasm, hemoglobinopathies other than SCD, polycythemia, other hemolytic disorders, or hematologic malignancies.[239–243]

Clinically, priapism may be stuttering, minor, or major. Stuttering priapism is the occurrence of short, repetitive, and reversible painful episodes with detumescence occurring within a few hours after the onset of erection. This pattern has a good prognosis and is associated with normal sexual function and rarely requires medical intervention. The prevalence of stuttering priapism varies from approximately 2% of men with SCD according to some investigators[235] to 40% to 60% of men and boys with SCD according to others.[237,244]

Minor priapism is isolated and infrequent episodes of painful erection that last less than 4 hours and do not require medical intervention. By contrast, major priapism is a prolonged episode of painful erection lasting longer than 12 hours and that often requires hospitalization, with medical and/or surgical intervention, as described in the following discussion. Partial or total impotence is often associated with major episodes of priapism. Anatomically, priapism may be bicorporal or tricorporal. Magnetic resonance imaging (MRI) of the penis can differentiate these two patterns. Bicorporal priapism involves both corpora cavernosa and is common in children with stuttering pattern and with detumescence occurring within a few hours after the onset of erection. This pattern has a good prognosis and is associated with normal sexual function.

Tricorporal priapism involves both corpora cavernosa and the corpus spongiosum and is more common in older patients. It is a painful erection that may last several days or weeks and may be followed by complete or partial impotence. Its prevalence varies between 6.5%[235] and 38%[237] of men with SCD. Stroke, chronic lung disease, chronic renal failure, and chronic leg ulcers were observed more frequently in men with tricorporal priapism, and death occurred in nine adults (25% of men with priapism) within 5 years of the first episode of priapism.[235] Priapism in adult males with SCD appears to be a marker of severe disease and identifies patients who are at risk for other sickle cell-related organ failure syndromes.[241,245]

Most episodes of priapism begin during sleep.[234,238,246] Approximately 75% of priapism episodes occur between midnight and 6 AM or after sexual intercourse.[237,247,248]

Acidosis resulting from dehydration and hypoventilation during sleep may be precipitating factors. Sexual intercourse,[249] masturbation,[250] alcohol intake,[251] infection of the prostate or bladder, recent trauma, and medications with autonomic side effects are reported precipitating factors.[252] In a Jamaican study, 16% of patients reported attacks after intercourse.[244,253] However, most episodes of priapism have no obvious etiology.[254] Thrombocytosis, low Hb F level, and severity of hemolysis are reported risk factors for priapism.[237,241,245] Recent studies have linked the severity of hemolysis to priapism, leg ulcers, and pulmonary hypertension.[245] However, these associations are controversial and have been challenged by other investigators.[255]

Management of priapism is highly controversial. Controlled studies are lacking, therapeutic approaches are controversial and often conflicting, and medical and surgical therapies fail in most patients. Minor episodes of priapism and stuttering priapism usually last less than 4 hours and are often treated at home with analgesics, benzodiazepines, or pseudoephedrine and do not require treatment at the ED or hospital. Patients are advised to report to the ED if an episode lasts longer than 4 hours. Initial treatment in the ED should include hydration and opioid analgesics. Catheterization of the urinary bladder may be indicated to promote emptying. If these measures fail to cause detumescence, penile aspiration and epinephrine irrigation should be performed. Mantadakis et al.[256] recommend that aspiration of blood from the corpora cavernosa, followed by irrigation with dilute epinephrine, should be the initial therapy used for patients with SS and prolonged priapism.

Simple transfusion or exchange transfusion may be performed for patients whose priapism does not respond to aspiration and irrigation procedures and persists for 24 hours or longer.[210,247,248] Siegel et al.[257] and Rackoff et al.[258] reported significant neurologic complications (the so called Association of Sickle cell disease, Priapism, Exchange transfusion, and Neurologic events [ASPEN] syndrome) in patients with priapism who underwent exchange transfusion or partial exchange transfusion. However, analysis of their data shows that the Hb level after blood exchange was much greater than the patient's baseline level. Thus, the neurologic complications were most likely due to transfusion-induced hyperviscosity. A larger study of blood exchange transfusion in patients with priapism, which maintained the post-exchange Hb level similar to baseline values, showed no neurologic complication in any of the patients.[259] Patients responding to transfusion therapy usually experience detumescence within 24 to 48 hours after the procedure. If detumescence does not occur within 24 hours after the completion of blood exchange transfusion, surgical intervention should be considered. Surgical intervention includes various shunt procedures between the cavernosa and the spongiosum.[260,261] Without intervention, severe priapism results in impotence in >80% of patients. The combination of transfusions and surgery can decrease this to 25% to 50%. Patients who become impotent may benefit from psychological counseling and the insertion of a prosthetic penile implant.

The pharmacologic management of priapism includes approaches for acute episodes of priapism and preventative measures. The acute pain of the priapism is treated like other VOCs, with opioid analgesics and adjuvants. The adjuvants commonly used include diphenhydramine, antihistaminics, or benzodiazepines. Care should be exercised in choosing any combinations of drugs. For example, benzodiazepines should not be used with methadone because both cause prolongation of the QTc interval. A recent case report described successful management of priapism in a child with SS using neuraxial analgesia via epidural catheter.[262] There are no evidence-based recommendations for the use of preventative therapies. However, potentially beneficial anecdotes and observations were reviewed by Rogers.[234] These include HU,[263,264] pseudoephedrine, leuprolide,[265] diethylstilbestrol,[244] etilefrine (not available in the United States), flutamide, and pentoxifylline. Leuprolide, a gonadotropin-releasing hormone antagonist, is associated with hypogonadism after extended use, and diethylstilbestrol has feminizing side effects.

However, the treatments for priapism in boys and men with SCD were reviewed in a Cochrane review to assess the benefits and risks of different treatments for stuttering and fulminant priapism in SCD. The review found only one study of 11 participants who met the criteria for inclusion in the study. The study compared diethylstilbestrol to placebo. The only outcome specified in this review was reduction in frequency of stuttering priapism, and there was no significant difference between groups.[266] Three small series reported prophylactic benefit of sildenafil in sickle cell and thalassemia priapism.[267-269] However, it appears unlikely at the present that randomized trials of sildenafil versus placebo will be conducted, due to the fact that sildenafil increased the frequency of VOCs in the Treatment of Pulmonary Hypertension and Sickle Cell Disease with Sildenafil Treatment (Walk-PHaSST) trial.[270] Certain medications, such as selective serotonin reuptake inhibitors (SSRIs), tricyclic antidepressants, trazodone, and other antipsychotic drugs, are associated with priapism and hence should not be prescribed to patients with a history of priapism.[271-273]

ACUTE MULTIORGAN FAILURE

This is a catastrophic life-threatening complication of SCD in the context of VOC that may even occur in patients with otherwise mild SCD.[142,274] Fever, rapid decrease in Hb level and PLT count, nonfocal encephalopathy, and rhabdomyolysis are associated with MOF. Prompt and aggressive simple blood transfusion or blood exchange transfusion could be lifesaving with rapid recovery of organ failure in most cases. MOF may occur in patients with history of relatively mild disease with little or no evidence of chronic organ damage and may be recurrent. High Hb levels in the steady state may be a predisposing factor.

Differential diagnosis of MOF includes ACS and drug overdose. MOF is initially heralded by a rapid fall in Hb and PLT counts from baseline. Aspartate aminotransferase (AST), alanine aminotransferase (ALT), total and direct bilirubin, serum creatinine, and CPK are elevated by the third or fourth day of a VOC.

Chronic Sickle Cell Pain

AVASCULAR NECROSIS

AVN (also called ischemic necrosis or osteonecrosis) is the most commonly observed complication of SCD after the number of VOCs in adults. Although it tends to be most severe and disabling in the hip area, it is a generalized bone disorder in that the femoral and humeral heads as well as the vertebral bodies may be equally affected. Figure 57.12 shows a "fish mouth" or step-like depression seen in some patients with SCD and is probably caused by AVN or infarction of the central portion of the vertebral body and may lead to vertebral collapse.[99] The limited

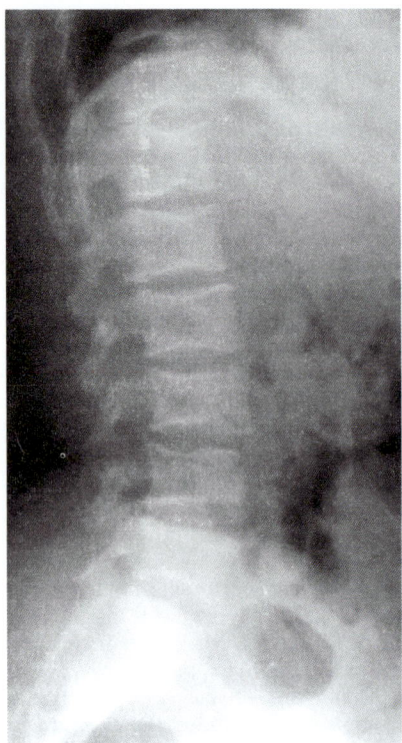

TABLE 57.12 A Combined Staging of Avascular Necrosis of the Hip by Integrating the Ficat and Steinberg Systems

Stage	Radiographic Signs
Early	
0 Preclinical	None; marrow necrosis may be present histologically
I Preradiographic	None; abnormal MRI with marrow and bone necrosis
II Before flattening of head or sequestrum formation	Diffuse porosis, sclerosis, or cysts
Transition	Femoral head flattening
	Crescent sign
Late	
III Collapse	Broken contour of head
	Sequestrum
	Joint space normal
IV Osteoarthritis	Flattened contour
	Decreased joint space
	Collapse of head

radiographic classification of AVN of the hip based on plain radiography. MRI was not available at the time. Steinberg et al.[276] expanded the Ficat staging system into six stages using MRI data.[276,277] A report from the Comprehensive Sickle Cell Centers (CSCC) investigators defined an adaptation[85] from the Ficat and Steinberg systems that combines radiography, MRI, and bone scans as shown in Table 57.12. At the time of diagnosis of AVN, 47.4% of the patients showed stage II disease, 29.6% showed stage III, and 23% showed stage IV.[36]

Medical treatment of AVN is symptomatic and includes providing nonopioid and/or opioid analgesics for pain relief as well as physical therapy. Advanced forms of the disease (stage III or IV) require total bone replacement. Core decompression (Fig. 57.14) in the management of AVN appears to be effective if done in the early stages of AVN.[278] This, however, was not supported by a prospective randomized multicenter comparing physical therapy alone with core decompression and physical therapy for femoral head AVN in 46 patients with SCD.[279] Physical therapy alone appeared to be as effective as hip core decompression followed by physical therapy in improving hip function and postponing the need for additional surgical intervention at a mean of 3 years treatment. Results of hip arthroplasty in patients with SS are not

terminal arterial blood supply and the paucity of collateral circulation make these three areas especially vulnerable to sickling and subsequent bone damage. Patients with SS and α-gene deletion have a higher incidence of AVN because the relatively high hematocrit increases blood viscosity and thus enhances microvasculopathy in the aforementioned anatomic sites.[35,36] The MCV and AST levels are negatively correlated with vascular necrosis.[36]

Figure 57.13 shows an example of the radiologic picture of AVN of the hips in SCD. The therapeutic approach to AVN depends on the stage of the disease. Ficat[275] proposed a four-stage

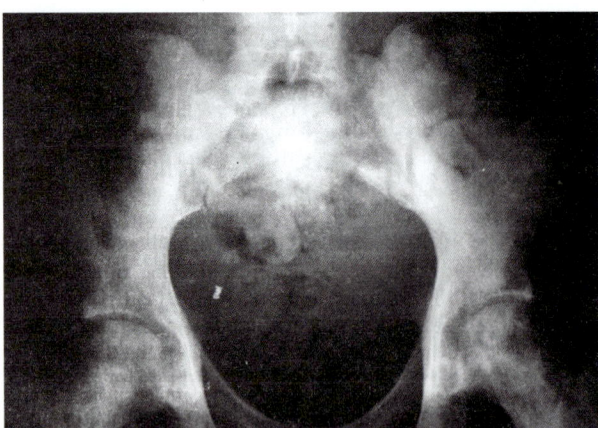

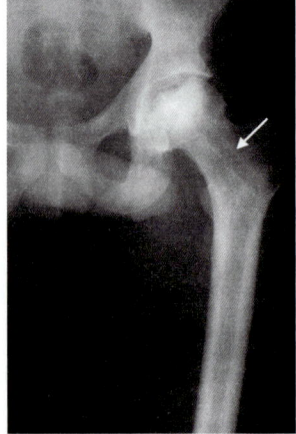

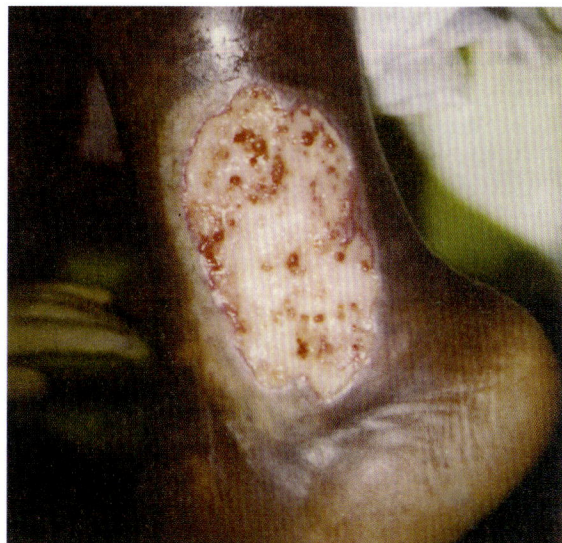
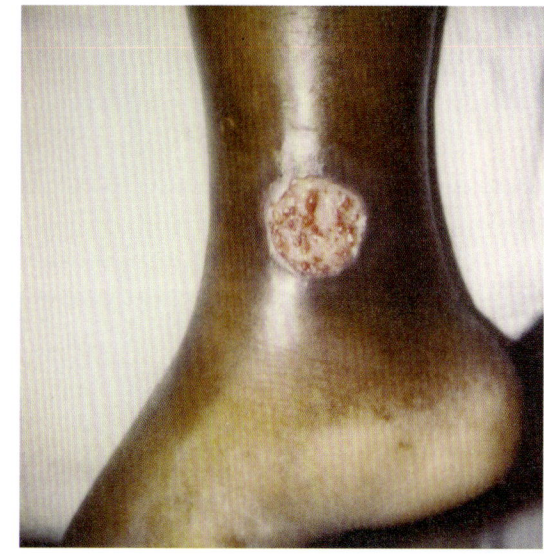

FIGURE 57.15 Leg ulcers in a patient with sickle cell anemia. *(From Ballas SK. Sickle cell pain. In: Progress in Pain Research and Management. Vol. 11. Seattle, WA: IASP Press; 1998. This figure has been reproduced with permission of the International Association for the Study of Pain® (IASP). The figure may not be reproduced for any other purpose without permission.)*

as encouraging as results of arthroplasty performed for arthritic hip.[280] Placement of an internal prosthesis may be difficult owing to the presence of hard sclerotic bone in patients with SCD. Other problems associated with hip arthroplasty in these patients include an increased incidence of infection,[281,282] a failure rate of about 50%, and a high morbidity due to loosening of both cemented and uncemented prosthesis. Recent techniques of arthroplasty may improve the life expectancy of hip prostheses.[283]

LEG ULCERS

Leg ulceration is a painful and sometimes disabling complication of SS that occurs 5% to 10% of adult patients. The most common site for the appearance of leg ulcers is the distal third of the leg, especially on the inner area, just above the ankle and over the medial malleoli (Fig. 57.15). Ulceration involves the skin and underlying tissues of the involved areas. The deeper the ulcer, the more severe. Leg ulcers are classified into stages depending on their depth and not surface area (Table 57.13). Severe pain may necessitate the use of opioid analgesics. The use of topical analgesics seems to be effective in relieving pain and decreasing the use of oral analgesics, especially opioids.[284]

Leg ulcers are more common in males and older patients and less common in patients with α-gene deletion, high total Hb level, or high levels of Hb F.[37] Leg ulcers seem to be more common in patients who are also carriers of the CAR β-gene cluster haplotype.[285] As was mentioned earlier, leg ulceration seems to be associated with priapism, pulmonary hypertension,

and death in a subtype of SCD characterized by high levels of LDH as a marker of hyperhemolysis.

Treatment of leg ulcers includes wound care using wet to dry dressings soaked in saline or Burow's solution. With good localized treatment, many ulcers heal within a few months. Oral zinc sulfate therapy (660 mg per day) may be beneficial for some patients.[42] However, a Cochrane review[286] showed that oral zinc for arterial or venous leg ulcers due to causes other than SCD had no significant difference compared to placebo. Leg ulcers that persist more than 6 months present a challenge to the treating physician and the patient. In addition, survival of patients with chronic leg ulcers seems to be decrease compared to patients without leg ulcers.[287]

Failure to respond to the measures mentioned earlier may justify the other modalities listed in Table 57.14. However, most of these modalities have been included in uncontrolled trials (controlled trials are highlighted in bold). These trials reported healing of leg ulcers in patients with SCD in response to transfusion,[210,288] erythropoietin in combination with HU,[289] arginine butyrate,[290,291] hyperbaric oxygen,[292–294] arginine-glycine-aspartic acid synthetic peptide matrix,[295] recombinant human granulocyte macrophage colony-stimulating factor,[296] collagen matrix dressing,[297] lyophilized type I collagen,[298] antithrombin III,[299] and electrical stimulation.[227] A Cochrane review[300] of the controlled trials listed in Table 57.14 showed evidence that topical application of arginine-glycine-aspartic acid peptide matrix reduced ulcer size in treated patients compared to control subjects. However, the evidence of efficacy was limited by the high risk of bias associated with the report. Moreover, heterogeneity among the controlled trials prevented performance of meta-analysis.

If all else fails, skin grafting may be considered. Some studies report a degree of success,[301–303] and others a high rate of failure.[37] To be successful, skin grafting should be performed on clean, débrided ulcers and should be preceded and followed by transfusion or exchange transfusion to keep the percentage of Hb S low (<30%) to break the cycle of sickling, vaso-occlusion, and tissue necrosis and to promote healing.

Recent modalities for the management of leg ulcers that are not commonly used in SCD include topical application of PLT-derived growth factor prepared either autologously (Procuren)[304] or by recombinant technology (Regranex)[305] and the use of cultured skin grafts.[306] In addition, mānuka honey from New Zealand has been reported to heal diabetic foot ulcers.[307,308]

TABLE 57.13	Stages of the Severity of Leg Ulceration

Stage 1: Nonblanchable erythema of intact skin, the heralding lesion of skin ulceration. In individuals with darker skin, discoloration of the skin, warmth, edema, induration, or hardness may also be indicators.

Stage 2: Partial-thickness skin loss involving epidermis, dermis, or both. The ulcer is superficial and presents clinically as an abrasion, blister, or shallow crater.

Stage 3: Full-thickness skin loss involving damage to or necrosis of subcutaneous tissue that may extend down to, but not through, underlying fascia. The ulcer presents clinically as a deep crater with or without undermining of adjacent tissue.

Stage 4: Full-thickness skin loss with extensive destruction, tissue necrosis, or damage to muscle, bone, or supporting structures (e.g., tendon, joint capsule). Undermining and sinus tracts may also be present.

TABLE 57.14 Summary of Methods Used to Treat Leg Ulcers
Local Measures
Bed rest, elevation of legs
Wet to dry dressings
Hydrotherapy (whirlpool therapy)
Disinfecting Agents
Soaps
Acetic acid (1.01%)
Hexachlorophene (pHisohex)
Hydrogen peroxide
Povidone-iodine (Betadine)
Silver sulfadiazine (Silvadene)
Sodium hypochlorite (Dakin's Solution)
Aluminum acetate (Burow's solution)
Topical antibiotics
Débridement
Surgical
Medical (enzymes)
Collagenase (Santyl, Biozyme C)
Fibrinolysin and desoxyribonuclease (Elase)
Trypsin (Granul-Derm)
Sutilains (Travase)
Solcoseryl
Hydrocolloid dressings (DuoDERM)
Agents that Promote Tissue Granulation
Benzoyl peroxide
Dextranomer (Debrisan)
Gelatin sponge (Gelfoam)
Other Modalities
Unna boots
Blood transfusion/exchange transfusion
Topical hyperbaric oxygen
Oral zinc sulfate
Erythropoietin
Arginine butyrate
Isoxsuprine hydrochloride
Propionyl-L-carnitine
RGD peptide matrix
Recombinant human granulocyte-macrophage colony stimulating factor (rh GM-CSF)
Collagen matrix dressings
Lyophilized type-1 collagen
Antithrombin III
Electrical stimulation
Skin grafting
Negative pressure therapy
Low-level laser therapy

NOTE: Controlled trials are highlighted in bold.
RGD, arginine-glycine-aspartic acid.

Amputation, a last resort for recalcitrant and severely painful ulcers, is rarely used.[309,310]

The induction of Hb F production by HU[10] would imply that it may prevent or heal leg ulcers in patients with SCD. However, HU has been reported to be associated with leg ulcers in patients with myeloproliferative disorders.[311,312] Whether the same association exists in patients with SCD is controversial. Leg ulcers were a common complication among 123 adult patients treated with HU in a retrospective French study.[313] Although controlled studies have not been reported to support the role of Hb F induction in the management of leg ulcers, future randomized, multicenter trials of HU may provide further information on this subject.

INTRACTABLE PAINFUL EPISODES

Some patients with SCD have intractable painful episodes and take opioid with or without nonopioid analgesics on a chronic basis. They have no evidence of precipitating cause such as infection, dehydration, or ischemia. Many of these patients are often referred to as "problem" patients or "difficult" patients, and their management is a challenge to the treating physician.

NEUROPATHIC PAIN

Neuropathic pain is characterized by sensations of burning, tingling, shooting, lancinating, and numbness. These symptoms may occur in the presence or absence of obvious central or peripheral nerve injury. Neuropathic pain in SCD seems to manifest itself in two forms. A number of reported neuropathic pain syndromes seem to be possibly associated with and due to the disease itself. These include mental nerve neuropathy,[314,315] trigeminal neuralgia,[316] acute proximal median mononeuropathy,[317] entrapment neuropathy,[318] acute demyelinating polyneuropathy,[318] ischemic optic neuropathy,[319] orbital infarction,[320] orbital apex syndrome,[321] and spinal cord infarction.[322]

The complications mentioned earlier are essentially neuropathies and not typical neuropathic pain as described in type 2 diabetes. Neuropathy and neuropathic pain are not synonymous. Diabetic neuropathy, for example, is not always associated with pain. The prevalence of neuropathy among diabetics is 40% to 60%, whereas neuropathic pain occurs in 10% to 16% of diabetics.[323] The prevalence of neuropathy and neuropathic pain in SCD is not well known. The nociceptive type of pain in SCD may overshadow and/or mask the neuropathic component.[324]

Management of Sickle Cell Pain

Effective management of sickle cell pain is complex and entails thorough understanding of the issues that are associated with the treatment of pain of an incurable disease on a chronic basis.[99,100,325,326] Major prerequisites for an effective and rational management of sickle cell pain pertain to the patient, the pathophysiology of the disease, the pharmacology of analgesics, and the attitude of the health care providers. A patient is as a unique human entity. The more a provider knows the patient, the more effective pain management becomes.

Knowledge of the patients should not be limited to age, sex, precise diagnosis, complications, and previous pain management methods. It should also take into consideration the biopsychosocial fabric of the patients' lives, including their level of education, employment status, occupation, family structure, source of income, ethnicity, housing conditions, fears, religion, beliefs, habits, hobbies, and perception of the severity and prognosis of their disease. This approach allows the physician to individualize pain management and avoid unfounded generalizations about patients and their consumption of opioid analgesics. Such generalizations, for instance, may result in oversedation of a patient naive to opioids or in undertreatment of a patient too tolerant of them.

Sickle cell pain is unique and, like other types of pain, is a complex human experience that is strongly affected not only by pathophysiologic factors but also by psychological, social, cultural, and spiritual ones. It is, however, consequent to tissue damage generated by the sickling process and occlusion of the microvasculature, as was described in the pathophysiology reaction. An important aspect of effective management of sickle cell pain is the intent of the care provider. Do the providers in question endeavor to treat patients in an empathetic manner by listening to, respecting, and believing them? Or do they stigmatize them as drug addicts demonstrating drug-seeking behavior and thereby justify the expulsion of some patients from their system? Do the providers actively seek management of sickle cell pain, or are they passively forced by the system to which they belong to treat patients in a cursory manner? Do some providers retain patients with mild disease and get rid of the complicated ones so that their records of hospital stay look good? As Lee et al.[189] succinctly noted that "no one knows how often physicians and hospitals try to improve measured results by declining high risk cases." These are difficult questions to answer and research. The outcome of management of sickle cell pain relies heavily on the ethical principles to which the providers in question subscribe.

Perhaps the difficulty of treating sickle cell pain can best be addressed with reference to a clinical anecdote. The patient is a young African American male who makes frequent visits to the ED for painful episodes and is labeled as an addict. The connection of the disease with race results in many ramifications that impact on care. Disparities in care arise because of the wide cultural gulf between health care providers who are predominantly white and the predominantly black patient group.[327–330] Communication and stereotyping complicate pain assessment and treatment. Frequent flyers in the ED often become labeled as drug seekers regardless of their diagnosis or the chronicity of their disease. Concerns about addiction are justified in the SCD population because these patients carry many associated risks, including disease chronicity and dismal prognosis, comorbid psychiatric disease including depression and anxiety, young age, and unremitting pain. Yet the approach needs to be one not of avoiding opioids but rather recognizing the risk while providing adequate pain management (with opioids if necessary) under controlled conditions that aim to minimize risk.

NONPHARMACOLOGIC MANAGEMENT OF PAIN

Nonpharmacologic management of pain includes cutaneous stimulation (transcutaneous electrical nerve stimulation), heat, cold and vibration, distraction, relaxation, massage, music, guided imagery, self-hypnosis, self-motivation, acupuncture, and biofeedback. Although there are no well-controlled clinical trials of the efficacy of these methods in the management of sickle cell pain, there are many anecdotal reports of their efficacy in pain management both by patients and providers.

PHARMACOLOGIC MANAGEMENT OF PAIN

Pharmacologic management of pain includes three major classes of compounds: nonopioids, opioids, and adjuvants.[99,100,326] A major difference between nonopioids and opioids is that the former have a *ceiling effect*, a term that refers to a dose above which there is no addictive analgesic effect.[328] Nonopioids include acetaminophen, NSAIDs, topical agents, tramadol, and corticosteroids. Opioids include agonists, mixed agonists-antagonists, partial agonists, and antagonists. Adjuvants commonly used in the management of sickle cell pain include antihistamines, benzodiazepines, antidepressants, anticonvulsants, and phenothiazines. Aspects of these pharmacologic agents that pertain to SCD will be discussed here.

Nonopioids and Sickle Cell Disease

Acetaminophen: This drug has been implicated in papillary necrosis of the kidney and in hepatoxicity with a dose that exceeds 4 g per day or with the recommended dose in patients with liver disease.[331–333] Because patients with SCD are at risk for renal and hepatic complications, the dosage given to them and their renal and hepatic functions have to be monitored carefully.

Nonsteroidal anti-inflammatory drugs: These drugs are well tolerated by most patients. Care has to be taken if the patients are sensitive to them, if the renal function is impaired, and if the patient has pulmonary complication especially ACS. NSAIDs should not be given to patients with impaired renal function. NSAIDs cause bronchospasm that may worsen or precipitate ACS.[333]

Opioids and Sickle Cell Disease

Depending on point of view, opioids may be considered first-line treatment for severe acute sickle cell pain. There is certainly no alternative to opioids for the treatment of severe pain, although nonopioid and nonmedical treatments should be added whenever possible as opioid-sparing adjuncts. Specific considerations for choice of opioid in SCD patients are outlined here.

Meperidine: This should be avoided whenever possible. If it has to be given, the dose has to be adjusted in the presence of abnormal renal function, and the patient has to be monitored for early signs of neurotoxicity such as myoclonus, tremors, and hyperexcitability.[99,100]

Morphine: The major metabolite of morphine (morphine-6-glucuronide) is excreted in the kidney. Accordingly, the dose of morphine has to be monitored in the presence of renal failure. Other recently reported side effects of morphine include increased risk of ACS in patients with SCD,[334,335] acceleration of renal injury,[336] and retinopathy[337] in transgenic sickle mice. In a retrospective study of hospitalized children with SCD, Buchanan et al.[335] reported that patients on morphine were more likely to develop ACS and had longer hospital stays than patients receiving nalbuphine hydrochloride (Nubain).

Methadone: Methadone is associated with several potential toxicities, including cardiotoxicity due to prolongation of the QTc interval with arrhythmia that could be fatal. In treating sickle cell pain with methadone, the provider should follow the adage "start low and go slow." Most reported fatalities due to methadone are due to overaggressive introduction of methadone to patients who have never before received the drug. This is a reflection of the drug's unusual and unpredictable pharmacokinetics. Another important point in using methadone is to be aware of the side effects of other drugs used in combination with methadone. Patients with SCD often receive antibiotics or antidepressants which also prolong the QTc interval. The electrocardiogram of such patients should be carefully monitored.[91,338]

Adjuvants and Sickle Cell Disease

Antidepressants that are known to cause priapism should not be used in patients with history of priapism. These include trazodone, SSRIs, and tricyclic antidepressants in decreasing order of risk to cure priapism.[91,338]

Management of Pain at Home

Treatment of acute VOCs at home is empiric and depends on the severity of pain and the presence or absence of complications of the disease. Ideally, painful episodes of mild severity are treated at home with nonpharmacologic measures including bed rest, hydration, massage, relaxation, diversion, heating pads, tub baths, self-hypnosis, and motivation. Patients often sense an impeding VOC, and early treatment with analgesics may abort or ameliorate an evolving VOC.[92,106,339] Home treatment of pain should follow the three-step analgesic ladder (Table 57.15) proposed by the World Health Organization.[340] This approach involves the use of analgesics in escalating potency. These medications are given alone or in combination, initially on an as-needed followed by an around-the-clock

TABLE 57.15 **Pharmacologic Home Management According to World Health Organization's Three-Step Analgesic Ladder**
Step I: mild pain
Nonopioid ± adjuvant
Step II: moderate pain
Weak opioid ± nonopioid ± adjuvant
Step III: severe pain
Strong opioid ± nonopioid ± adjuvant

administration for moderate to severe pain. This model controls pain in 90% of cancer patients.[327,341]

Chronic pain associated with SCD includes arthropathies, aseptic necrosis, vertebral body collapse, and leg ulcers.[326] In addition, some patients almost always experience persistent VOC pain.[92] These chronic pain syndromes may be treated with one of the weak or strong opioids, depending on the severity of pain. A long-acting opioid, such as methadone or oral controlled-release morphine (MS Contin, Avinza, Kadian, Oramorph) or oxycodone (OxyContin), is ideal for chronic pain.[342,343] The use of transcutaneous electrical nerve stimulation may be of value in reducing the pain intensity of these syndromes, especially if associated with leg ulcers. The use of fentanyl transdermal patches is also of potential value.[344,345] It should be noted that the presence of fever or the application of heating pads over these patches increases the absorption of fentanyl by the skin and may lead to an accumulation of a toxic plasma level,[346,347] which can be fatal.[348]

Outpatient Management of Sickle Cell Pain
Management of patients with SCD in the outpatient clinic or office is the fulcrum on which the success of comprehensive care is balanced. Because they are not in severe acute pain, patients in the clinic are receptive to counseling, education, and reinforcement of good habits by nurses, technologists, social workers, and physicians. Ideally, patients should be followed by the same personnel to maintain continuity of care. The clinic or office is where the steady state of disease is defined[339,349] clinically, hematologically, and biochemically and where a multidisciplinary approach to care is maintained by regular checkups and appropriate consultations.

Management of patients with SCD as outpatients in the clinic or office is also the basis on which future treatments and interventions are based. The most important aspect of outpatient management is the collection of baseline data including detailed medical history, physical examination, known complications, medications, and comprehensive laboratory data. The future care of patients in the ED or in the hospital depends heavily on knowing the steady state parameters of the patient. Moreover, should patients enroll in clinical trials, comparison to the steady-state status is invaluable. It is highly desirable that patients be seen and evaluated in the office or clinic by a social worker and a psychologist or psychiatrist. It is in the outpatient setting that details of care, in general, and in the ED, day unit, and hospital, in particular, are explained and discussed. The pros and cons of all medications the patient is taking will be reviewed. Prescriptions will be given as needed. Vaccines will be administered when required.[109]

Management and follow-up of outpatients in the office or clinic should culminate in an individualized treatment plan for each patient. Such a plan should summarize pertinent aspects of the medical history, physical examination, laboratory data, complications, and treatment plans for patients as outpatients, in the day unit, ED, and hospital. In some cases, the treatment plan may be transformed into an identification card to be carried by the patient and presented to the care provider as needed.[109]

Pain Management in the Day Unit
The major advantage of treating sickle cell VOCs in the day unit (or day hospital) is that patients do not have to wait for a long time before receiving treatment.[127,339,350] In the day unit, analgesic therapy is usually initiated within 15 to 20 minutes after arrival. Adult patients are admitted to the day unit if they have an uncomplicated VOC based on inclusion and exclusion criteria protocols. After a thorough assessment, treatment is initiated with intravenous hydration and a loading dose of opioid analgesic followed by assessment within 30 minutes. After the initial assessment, the patient may be medicated with 25% to 75% of the loading dose of opioid analgesic depending on the

level of pain relief and sedation. The patient's vital signs are assessed every 30 minutes for the first 2 hours of treatment and hourly thereafter. If the respiratory rate falls below 10 breaths per minute, systolic blood pressure falls below 90 mm Hg, and/or sedation occurs, the opioid is withheld and the patient is monitored closely. The duration of treatment usually lasts approximately 6 hours. Most patients (>95%) are discharged, and a few may require hospital admission.[127]

Pain Management in the Emergency Department
Treatment of VOCs in the ED follows similar principles of thorough assessment, treatment with analgesics/adjuvants, coordination of cure, monitoring, outcome, and disposition.[99,100,326,339] The major problem in the ED is the length of waiting time to initial analgesia, which could be up to several hours. Needless to say, waiting while in pain constitutes a stressful situation that could worsen the painful crises and render it no longer amenable to resolution and discharge from the ED but to hospital admission. Many EDs are in the process of determining and implementing strategies that could shorten the time to initial treatment. Specific treatment in the ED should be based on the history or the computerized version of the treatment plan, if available. Usually, analgesics are given individually every 2 hours for a total of three doses. Adjuvants may also be given intravenously or orally as needed. If the pain is resolved or reduced to a level with which the patient is comfortable, the patient is discharged with instructions for follow-up by the primary care physician and/or hematologist. Otherwise, the patient will be admitted to the hospital.

Management of Sickle Cell Pain in the Hospital
Failure to break the VOC in the ED is an indication for hospital admission. Management of pain in the hospitalized patient is essentially a continuation of the process initiated in the ED.[99,100,326,339] However, prerequisites for the rational management of acute VOCs in the hospital include knowledge of the patient, knowledge of the nature of sickle cell pain, and knowledge of the pharmacology of analgesics in general and opioids in particular. To that end, it is desirable to have patients with VOC admitted to the care of providers (preferably hematologists) who are familiar with these prerequisites and with the principles of pain management. Patient-controlled analgesia (PCA) is a useful method of delivering opioid analgesics in hospitalized patients.[351] Successful management of the acute VOC in the hospital should include the following steps:

- Multidimensional assessment to determine the location of pain, its intensity, its quality, precipitating factors, modifying factors, and triggers and to determine mood, relief, and sedation. A major component of assessment is to listen to, believe, and respect the patient with a nonjudgmental attitude.
- Choice of analgesics (opioids/nonopioids), adjuvants, and hydration, if needed. Such choices are individualized based on the patient's medical history and assessment. If the VOC is superimposed on chronic pain for which the patient is taking long-acting/controlled-release opioids with short-acting opioids for breakthrough pain, keep the long-acting/controlled-release opioids the same and discontinue the oral short-acting ones.
- Determination of the route and method of administration of short-acting analgesics. These, again, should be individualized; parenteral analgesics are usually administered either on a fixed schedule or via a PCA pump as discussed in the following discussion.
- Titration of the dose of analgesics to achieve a level of relief with which the patient is comfortable
- Maintenance of the dose that achieves adequate relief. Consider opioid rotation; that is, change the opioid selected initially to an equianalgesic opioid if its use does not achieve or maintain relief.

- Plan to treat breakthrough pain, neuropathic pain if present, and side effects of the VOC or the analgesics, if present.
- Taper the dose of analgesics once the patient uses the PCA pump less frequently or the intensity of pain decreases by two or more points.
- Gradually switch to oral analgesics using equianalgesic dose tables as an initial guide. One example would be to decrease the parenteral dose by 25% and replace it with an equianalgesic oral dose. The latter should be adjusted according to its effect of achieving a level of pain relief with which the patient is comfortable.
- Prevention of withdrawal by continued gradual reduction of the oral opioid dose after discharge or by using either a clonidine patch or methadone, if needed.
- Plan for discharge and follow-up.

Details of these steps may vary among patients, providers, and institutions. It should be emphasized that desirable outcome of management of VOCs in the hospital depends on early and aggressive treatment of pain without delay, avoidance of hasty or premature discharge from the hospital, and having a plan for follow-up after discharge, preferably within 1 week or less.

Specific Approaches to Treatment

Despite impressive "quantum leaps" in our understanding of the pathophysiology of SCD in general and SS in particular, a specific, safe, and nontoxic curative therapy has not yet been identified, with the possible exception of gradually increasing examples of bone marrow/stem cell transplant. Nevertheless, the overall medical care of patients with SCD in developed countries has improved such that their life expectancy has almost doubled since 1951.[27] Currently, there are at least five major approaches for the general management of SCD and its complications.[352] These include (1) symptomatic management, (2) supportive management, (3) preventive management, (4) abortive management, and (5) curative therapy (Table 57.16). Additional approaches pertain to the management of the patient with SCD and comorbidities[339] that complicate SCD but are not themselves complications of SCD. Examples of this new and expanding category, due to decreased morbidity and mortality of patients with SCD, include such things as the management of the patient with SCD and diabetes, obesity, cancer, etc. Most important among these measures include the preventative and curative therapies which are discussed here.

Preventive Therapies

The goal of preventive therapy is to ameliorate the clinical picture of SCD in general and to decrease the frequency and severity of VOCs in particular. For many years, the major goal of primary therapy for SCD was to identify an antisickling agent that would prevent or reverse the polymerization of sickle Hb in RBCs. Sodium cyanate inhibits polymerization of Hb S in vitro but is not beneficial in vivo at levels that provide acceptable toxicity.[353] The use of sodium cyanate was associated with peripheral neuropathy and subcapsular cataracts, which prevented its use as an antisickling agent. Although the search for beneficial antisickling compounds continues, the most promising approaches to prevent the frequency and severity of VOCs include the prevention of infection, induction of Hb F production, blood transfusion, anti-adhesion therapy and myriad agents that await confirmation of benefit in clinical trials.

Induction of Fetal Hemoglobin

High levels of Hb F have a beneficial effect in patients with SS. Platt et al.[34] demonstrated a significant inverse correlation between the frequency of VOCs and Hb F levels greater than 4%; the higher Hb F level, the milder the disease. Hb F interferes with the polymerization of Hb S; the higher (and the more pancellular) the Hb F level, the lower the intracellular concentration

TABLE 57.16	Approaches to the Management of Sickle Cell Disease and Its Complications
Approach	**Definition**
1. Supportive management	Management intended to maintain the essential requirements for good health such as balanced diet, sleep, hydration, folic acid, etc.
2. Symptomatic management	Management targeted to alleviate the symptoms of the disease as they occur. These include blood transfusion for symptomatic anemia, analgesics for pain, antibiotics for infections, etc.
3. Preventative management	Approaches to prevent the occurrence of complications of the disease. These include things like vaccination, avoidance of stressful situations, Hb F induction with hydroxyurea or other agents, transfusion to prevent the recurrence of stroke, etc.
4. Abortive management	Major purpose of this approach is to abort painful crisis, thus preventing them from getting worse or precipitating other complications. The only promising abortive approach has been nitric oxide so far.
5. Curative therapy	This is the ultimate goal of all inherited disorders. This has already been achieved in SCD by stem cell transplantation. Gene therapy is another challenging goal.

Republished with permission of American Society of Hematology from Ballas SK, Gupta K, Adams-Graves P. Sickle cell pain: a critical reappraisal. *Blood* 2012;120(18): 3647–3656; permission conveyed through Copyright Clearance Center, Inc.

of Hb S. Exceptions to this rule include some patients with high Hb F level and severe disease and vice versa.

Agents that increase the level of Hb F in humans are listed in Table 57.17. Among these, HU as monotherapy seems to be the least toxic and most effective.[10,354,355] Moreover, HU is the only drug studied for efficacy in a relatively large-scale, placebo-controlled, randomized clinical trial. All the other agents listed in Table 57.17 have been reported anecdotally to increase Hb F levels. None of the others was used in a controlled phase III clinical trial to date.

Hydroxyurea

HU is a cell-cycle specific cytotoxic agent that inhibits ribonucleotide reductase. The molecular mechanism(s) by which HU increases the production of Hb F is (are) unknown. Possible mechanisms include perturbations in cellular kinetics

TABLE 57.17	Agents that Augment Fetal Hemoglobin Production

Cell-cycle specific agents
  Azacytidine
  Cytosine arabinoside
  Myleran
  Hydroxyurea
  Decitabine
Short-chain fatty acids
  Arginine butyrate—IV
  Isobutyramide—PO
  Phenylacetate—PO
  Phenylbutyrate—PO
  Valproic acid—PO
Recombinant human erythropoietin (rHuEPO)
Combination therapy
  Hydroxyurea + rHuEPO
  Other combinations

IV, intravenous; PO, oral.
Reprinted by permission from Springer: Ballas SK. Sickle cell anaemia: Progress in pathogenesis and treatment. *Drugs* 2002;62(8):1143–1172. Copyright © 2002 Adis International Limited.

and/or recovery from cytotoxicity, recruitment of early erythroid progenitors, and recruitment of primitive erythroid progenitors (BFU-E) that lead to production of Hb F-containing reticulocytes (F-reticulocytes). Long-term HU therapy with the maximum tolerated dose (mean dose 21.3 mg/kg) with respect to myelosuppression raises Hb F by as much as 15% to 20% (mean 14.9%, range 1.9% to 26.3%).

In the randomized, placebo-controlled, double-blind MSH study, among 299 adult patients with SS with three or more VOCs per year, HU resulted in a significant ($P < .001$) reduction in the incidence of VOCs, ACS, and transfusion requirement.[10,354] HU improved the quality of life of the patients taking it.[356] There was no difference between the placebo and HU arms in the incidence of death, stroke, or hepatic sequestration. Maximum tolerated doses of HU were not required to reduce the incidence of VOCs. Although an increase in Hb F seems to be the obvious and logical explanation for the salutary effects of HU, other reasons for its beneficial effects include changes in RBC volume, cellular hydration, the cell membrane, and a direct effect on endothelial cells.

Hydroxyurea and the HUG Trials

The success of MSH prompted pediatricians to follow suit and determine the efficacy of HU in children. A multicenter phase I/II trial of HU in children with SS (HUG-KIDS) showed that HU therapy is safe for children with SS when treatment is directed by a pediatric hematologist. Treatment of children with HU induced similar laboratory changes as in adults, and children could tolerate doses of HU as high as 30 mg/kg/day.[357] Another 2-year, prospective, multicenter, open-label, single-arm, pilot study (Hydroxyurea Safety and Organ Toxicity [HUSOFT]) of HU in very young children with SS showed that HU treatment for infants with SS is feasible and well tolerated, has hematologic efficacy, and may delay functional asplenia.[358] An extension study of the HUSOFT trial, in which the dose of HU was increased to up to 30 mg/kg/day, showed that infants with SS tolerated prolonged HU therapy, with sustained hematologic benefits, fewer ACS events, and possibly preserved organ function.[359] These early studies in infants and children led to the Pediatric Hydroxyurea Phase III Clinical Trial (BABY HUG). The main objective of BABY HUG was to determine if HU can prevent the onset of chronic end-organ damage in young children with SS.[360] The primary endpoints of the study were splenic function (determined by qualitative uptake on 99Tc spleen scan) and renal function (determined by glomerular filtration rate by 99mTc-diethylene triamine pentaacetic acid [DTPA] clearance). Other endpoints included blood counts, Hb F, chemistry profiles, spleen function biomarkers, urine osmolality, neurodevelopment, transcranial Doppler ultrasonography, growth, and mutagenicity.[360] A total of 96 patients received HU, and 97 patients received placebo. The study confirmed the safety and efficacy of HU therapy for infants with SS. However, treatment with HU showed no significant differences for the primary endpoints: splenic function or glomerular filtration rate.[361] A different prospective HU study of long-term effects (HUSTLE) showed that HU at maximum tolerated dose is associated with a decrease in hyperfiltration in young children with SS.[362] In the BABY HUG trial, treatment with HU was associated with decreased pain (177 events in 62 patients on HU vs. 375 events in 75 patients in the placebo group; $P = .002$); decreased dactylitis (24 events in 14 patients on HU vs. 123 events in 42 patients in the placebo group; $P < .0001$); and decreased incidence of ACS, hospitalizations, and blood transfusions.[360] Treatment with HU increased Hb and Hb F and improved hematologic values, decreased white blood cell count, and perhaps increased preservation of organ function.[360,363] Toxicity was limited to mild to moderate neutropenia.

TABLE 57.18   Benefits of Long-Term Use of Hydroxyurea

- Decreased frequency of acute painful vaso-occlusive crises in children and adults
- Decreased frequency of acute chest syndrome in children and adults
- Decreased need for blood transfusion in children and adults
- Decreased mortality in adults; data in children not available
- Improved quality of life in adults
- Cost-effectiveness of hydroxyurea in adults
- Decreased hospital length of stay in children and adults
- Decreased utilization of analgesics in general and opioids in particular during hospitalization, outpatient acute care, and at home in adults
- A trend for more consistent employment in adults
- Decreased frequency of dactylitis in children
- Decreased glomerular hyperfiltration in young children
- Improved hematologic parameters in children and adults
- Increased Hb F levels in children and adults
- Improved RBC survival
- Improved RBC deformability
- No evidence of leukemogenicity/genotoxicity of hydroxyurea in children and adults

Benefits and Side Effects of Hydroxyurea

Benefits of the long-term use of HU (listed in Table 57.18) are numerous. Some of the parameters mentioned for adults are not available for children. These may become available later when follow-up data from the BABY HUG study are complete. The most important is decreased mortality among patients who take HU for years.[364,365] Other benefits include improved quality of life in adults,[356] cost-effectiveness,[366] decreased hospital length of stay in children and adults,[125,360] decreased use of analgesics in general and opioids in particular during hospitalization, outpatient acute care and at-home care in adults,[125,126,367] a trend for more consistent employment in adults,[368] improved RBC survival in adults,[369] and improved RBC deformability in adults.[370]

Side effects of HU are listed in Table 57.19. Toxic effects are dose- and time-dependent but can be prevented by careful monitoring of blood counts every 2 weeks after initiation of treatment. The frequency of monitoring of blood counts and blood chemistries can be decreased to once every 1 to 2 months once the patient is in a stable condition and receiving an acceptable maintenance dose. Excretion of HU is likely a linear,

---

TABLE 57.19   Side Effects of Hydroxyurea

Toxic Side Effects

Myelosuppression
Leukopenia
Thrombocytopenia
Anemia

Idiosyncratic Adverse Effects

Nausea
Vomiting
Pruritus
Skin rash
Hair loss
Leg ulcers

Effects Reported in Animals

Carcinogenesis
Teratogenesis

Long-Term Effects

Unknown

Adapted by permission from Springer: Ballas SK. Sickle cell anaemia: Progress in pathogenesis and treatment. *Drugs* 2002;62(8):1143-1172. Copyright © 2002 Adis International Limited.

first-order, renal process.[371] Accordingly, renal failure is a contraindication for the use of HU, or the dose should be adjusted according to the degree of renal impairment. Anemia is a rare toxic effect of HU; in most patients, Hb level increases.[10] Some patients experience idiosyncratic effects of HU, but the reported incidence was similar between placebo and HU.[372] Surprisingly, during the BABY HUG, a 2-year-old girl ingested an entire 35-day supply of HU at one time (612 mg/kg). Although the serum level of HU was 7,756 μM 4 hours postingestion, the only toxicity noted was transient mild myelosuppression at days 3 and 5, with complete remission by day 7; she had no hepatic or renal dysfunction, remained asymptomatic, and resumed study treatment 13 days after ingestion. No HU was detected in the serum 84 hours after ingestion.[373,374] The short half-life of HU and the presence of glomerular hyperfiltration a 2-year-old child may have been the reason why HU was cleared rapidly. In addition, HU sequesters in RBCs and leukocytes.[371] Had the patient been an adult with compromised renal function, the clinical picture might not have been so benign.

The following limitations should be considered when using HU to prevent painful crises in patients with SCD. First, HU was approved in the United States by the U.S. Food and Drug Administration for the prevention of VOCs in patients with SS and not in other types of SCD. Second, the long-term effects of HU in patients with SCD are not known, and finally, some patients do not respond to HU. Methods to identify these non-responders are being studied in order to improve the selection process for HU therapy. In some patients, combining HU with other agents that augment Hb F production may be indicated.

Other Novel Approaches to Therapy

A large number of novel preventive therapeutic modalities may have promising roles in the management of SCD in general and sickle cell pain in particular. These include, among other things, antiadhesion molecules,[375] surfactants,[168] levocarnitine, zileuton (a 5-lipoxygenase inhibitor), green tea,[376] aged garlic,[376] and herbal extracts.[377] Some of these agents are being used on an investigational basis. There are anecdotal reports of success in a few patients using some of these agents. However, the efficacy of any of these agents awaits proof in phase III, randomized, double-blind, placebo-controlled trials. Such trials will determine if a certain drug is safe, efficacious, and capable of improving the quality of life of treated patients. Recently, Singh and Ballas[378] reviewed about 38 drugs that were tried or about to be tried in several clinical trials for the prevention of VOCs and related complications. As mentioned earlier, the phase III trial of senicapoc was terminated because patients who took senicapoc had more VOCs than control subjects. A phase III trial of sildenafil to treat patients with elevated tricuspid regurgitant velocity and low exercise capacity was terminated for the same reason.[270]

CURATIVE THERAPIES
Allogeneic Hematopoietic Stem Cell Transplant

The only curative therapy available at present for SCD in general, and SS in particular, is stem cell transplant. The first two patients with SS treated by bone marrow transplant underwent this treatment not for SS but for comorbid conditions.[379–381] The first patient was an 8-year-old girl with SS who had both acute myeloid leukemia and frequent VOCs. Her clinical course after transplant was complicated by transient acute and chronic graft-versus-host disease (GVHD) involving mainly the skin and gastrointestinal tract. She also had AVN of the right hip. Further follow-up showed that she was in excellent general health and had no evidence of recurrence of SCD or leukemia.[379,380] The second patient had SS and Morquio disease, a metabolic storage disease for which bone marrow transplant was performed.[380,381] This patient failed to engraft but underwent a successful retransplant from the same donor.

In 1998, 70 patients with SS had undergone bone marrow transplant worldwide. By the end of the 20th century, at least 100 patients with SS had undergone transplant worldwide.[19,380,382,383] At that time, most patients were children who received bone marrow allografts from siblings with identical human leukocyte antigen (HLA) match and who underwent myeloablative conditioning. Although the estimated risk of mortality from HLA-identical bone marrow transplant was relatively low (~5%), there was some concern regarding short-term and long-term toxicity, lack of availability of suitable donors, and barriers to wider application.[384] Nevertheless, an interim report on the impact of bone marrow transplant for symptomatic SCD found that allogeneic bone marrow transplant establishes normal erythropoiesis and is associated with increased growth and stable central nervous system imaging results and pulmonary function in most patients.[19] Things have changed for the better since 2000; some of the barriers have been overcome, and more patients are awaiting appropriate donors for transplant. The advent of high-resolution HLA typing, the choice of stem cell sources (bone marrow, peripheral blood or cord blood), less toxic conditioning regimens, new immunosuppressive agents, facilitated immune reconstitution, and improved supportive care have made transplant a more viable option for patients with SCD.[385–389] By 2010, less than 500 patients with SCD who have undergone transplant have been reported in the Center for International Blood and Marrow Transplant Research database.[385]

Allogeneic hematopoietic stem cell transplant is the only curative treatment for SCD at present. It is successful in approximately 90% of patients. Unfortunately, conventional approaches to transplant are associated with comorbidities including, among other complications, infertility, gonadal failure, and chronic GVHD. The use of umbilical cord blood has been shown to be as effective as, and possibly safer than, traditional bone marrow transplant in children with SCD. The use of non-myeloablative conditioning regimens induce mixed chimerism in transplant recipients, resulting in decreased complications of allogeneic hematopoietic stem cell transplant in adults.[390–392]

Gene Therapy

Although allogeneic bone marrow transplant can cure SCD, its widespread use is limited by the availability of suitable donors and by the complication of GVHD. Gene therapy is an alternative approach to achieve a cure of SCD. In simple terms, gene therapy is the introduction of normal genes into abnormal cells, either in vitro or in vivo. One potential approach to cure SS is to introduce a functional β^A-globin gene into hematopoietic stem cells of the affected individual to replace the abnormal β^S-globin gene.[393] Methods to achieve this goal include the following:

- Targeted insertion of the transferred gene into the endogenous globin locus by homologous recombination such that the transferred β^A-globin gene is located in the proper chromosomal environment and expressed at the same level as endogenous β-globin. This would be the ideal approach, but it is not yet feasible in hematopoietic stem cells.
- Chimeraplasty or gene repair, which introduces chimeric oligonucleotides composed of DNA and modified RNA residues into stem cells to direct correction of the mutation in the β^S gene[394]
- Transfer of normal β^A-globin gene into hematopoietic cells via retroviral vectors that have been modified such that they do not become infective

Recent years have witnessed significant progress in the third method mentioned earlier. Basically, this is stem cell gene transfer or autologous transplant, in which the patient's own stem cells are harvested from the bone marrow or peripheral blood, genetically modified, and transplanted back into the patient.

Genetic modification involves the use of vectors carrying γ-globin genes for SCD or β-globin genes for β-thalassemia. This approach has already been established in mice and was successful in a phase I/II study, with anticipated benefit for Hb disorders. Successful conversion of a patient with β-thalassemia major to transfusion independence has been reported.[391,395–398]

Another novel gene therapy approach involves the use of somatic cells rather than stem cells to achieve a genetic cure. In this method, adult somatic cells are reprogrammed into induced pluripotent stem cells. Specifically, Hanna et al. produced pluripotent stem cells from skin fibroblasts of patients with SCD, corrected the mutation, and converted the cells in culture to hematopoietic stem cells that could be used for gene transfer as described earlier.[391,399] Research on gene therapy methods applicable to SCD and to determine the most effective and safe method of altering genetic information in hematopoietic stem cells has advanced at a faster rate than expected, and gene therapy may soon be available for clinical trials in selected patients with SS.

Conclusion

SCD is an inherited disorder of Hb structure that has no established cure in adults at the present. Cure has been achieved in selected patients with bone marrow/stem cell/cord blood transplantation from HLA-matched donors in the majority of cases after myeloablative conditioning regimen.

SCD is almost synonymous with pain, and the VOC is the insignia and the number one cause of hospitalization. Advances in the pathophysiology of SCD focused on the sequence of events that occur between polymerization of deoxy of Hb S and vaso-occlusion. Adhesion of sickle RBCs to endothelial cells, cellular dehydration, inflammatory response, reperfusion injury, and tissue damage appear to be important pathophysiologic events that culminate in the perception of pain.

The VOC evolves along four phases: prodromal, initial, established, and resolving phases. Several clinical and laboratory changes occur during the VOC provided the findings are compared to well-established baseline data. The resolving VOC may culminate in a hypercoagulable state that could precipitate another VOC in some patients. Hospital readmission seems to occur within 1 week in about 16% of patients after discharge from the hospital. Serious and potentially fatal complications of SCD such as ACS and MOF occur within 3 or 4 days after the onset of a VOC. Other types of acute sickle pain include priapism, dactylitis, hepatic crisis, and splenic sequestration.

Although management of SS continues to be primarily palliative in nature, there have been promising preventative and curative approaches to therapy. Pain management should be individualized and coupled with the proper utilization of opioid and nonopioid analgesics in order to achieve adequate pain relief. Early recognition and treatment of organ failure minimizes morbidity and improves outcome. The use of HU decreases the morbidity and mortality of SCD. Cure is possible in selected children and young adults with bone marrow or cord blood transplantation. Future research seems to focus on refining the molecular and cellular approaches to therapy including gene therapy and mechanisms that prevent the adhesion of sickle RBC to vascular endothelium.

References

1. Konotey-Ahulu FI. *The Sickle Cell Disease Patient.* London: Macmillan; 1991.
2. Herrick J. Peculiar elongated and sickle-shaped red blood corpuscles in a case of severe anemia. *Arch Intern Med* 1910;6:517–521.
3. Savitt T, Goldberg M. Herrick's 1910 case report of sickle cell anemia. *JAMA* 1989;261:266–271.
4. Mason V. Sickle cell anemia. *JAMA* 1922;79:1318–1320.
5. Diggs L. Sickle cell crises. *Am J Clin Pathol* 1965;44:1–19.
6. Pauling L, Itano H, Singer SJ, et al. Sickle cell anemia: a molecular disease. *Science* 1949;110:543–548.
7. Neel J. The inheritance of the sickling phenomenon with particular reference to sickle cell disease. *Blood* 1951;6:389–412.
8. Ingram V. A specific chemical difference between the globins of normal human and sickle-cell anemia haemoglobin. *Nature* 1956;178:792–794.
9. Steinberg MH. Predicting clinical severity in sickle cell anaemia. *Br J Haematol* 2005;129(4):465–481.
10. Charache S, Terrin ML, Moore RD, et al. Effect of hydroxyurea on the frequency of painful crises in sickle cell anemia. Investigators of the Multicenter Study of Hydroxyurea in Sickle Cell Anemia. *N Engl J Med* 1995;332(20):1317–1322.
11. Wang WC, Dwan K. Blood transfusion for preventing primary and secondary stroke in people with sickle cell disease. *Cochrane Database Syst Rev* 2013;(11):CD003146.
12. Venkataraman A, Adams RJ. Neurologic complications of sickle cell disease. *Handb Clin Neurol* 2014;120:1015–1025.
13. Walters MC, Patience M, Leisenring W, et al. Bone marrow transplantation for sickle cell disease. *N Engl J Med* 1996;335(6):369–376.
14. Gore L, Lane PA, Quinones RR, et al. Successful cord blood transplantation for sickle cell anemia from a sibling who is human leukocyte antigen-identical: implications for comprehensive care. *J Pediatr Hematol Oncol* 2000;22(5):437–440.
15. Adamkiewicz TV, Mehta PS, Boyer MW, et al. Transplantation of unrelated placental blood cells in children with high-risk sickle cell disease. *Bone Marrow Transplant* 2004;34(5):405–411.
16. Mazur M, Kurtzberg J, Halperin E, et al. Transplantation of a child with sickle cell anemia with an unrelated cord blood unit after reduced intensity conditioning. *J Pediatr Hematol Oncol* 2006;28(12):840–844.
17. Panepinto JA, Walters MC, Carreras J, et al. Matched-related donor transplantation for sickle cell disease: report from the Center for International Blood and Transplant Research. *Br J Haematol* 2007;137(5):479–485.
18. Bernaudin F, Socie G, Kuentz M, et al. Long-term results of related myeloablative stem-cell transplantation to cure sickle cell disease. *Blood* 2007;110(7):2749–2756.
19. Walters MC, Storb R, Patience M, et al. Impact of bone marrow transplantation for symptomatic sickle cell disease: an interim report. Multicenter investigation of bone marrow transplantation for sickle cell disease. *Blood* 2000;95(6):1918–1924.
20. Gluckman E, Cappelli B, Bernaudin F, et al. Sickle cell disease: an international survey of results of HLA-identical sibling hematopoietic stem cell transplantation. *Blood* 2017;129(11):1548–1556.
21. Ribeil JA, Hacein-Bey-Abina S, Payen E, et al. Gene therapy in a patient with sickle cell disease. *N Engl J Med* 2017;376(9):848–855.
22. Ingram VM. Gene mutations in human haemoglobin: the chemical difference between normal and sickle cell haemoglobin. *Nature* 1957;180(4581):326–328.
23. Farrell K, Dent L, Nguyen ML, et al. The relationship of oxygen transport and cardiac index for the prevention of sickle cell crises. *J Natl Med Assoc* 2010;102(11):1000–1007.
24. Telfer P, Coen P, Chakravorty S, et al. Clinical outcomes in children with sickle cell disease living in England: a neonatal cohort in East London. *Haematologica* 2007;92(7):905–912.
25. Quinn CT, Rogers ZR, McCavit TL, et al. Improved survival of children and adolescents with sickle cell disease. *Blood* 2010;115(17):3447–3452.
26. Artz N, Whelan C, Feehan S. Caring for the adult with sickle cell disease: results of a multidisciplinary pilot program. *J Natl Med Assoc* 2010;102(11):1009–1016.
27. Platt OS, Brambilla DJ, Rosse WF, et al. Mortality in sickle cell disease. Life expectancy and risk factors for early death. *N Engl J Med* 1994;330(23):1639–1644.
28. Powars DR, Chan LS, Hiti A, et al. Outcome of sickle cell anemia: a 4-decade observational study of 1056 patients. *Medicine (Baltimore)* 2005;84(6):363–376.
29. Steinberg MH, Embury SH. Alpha-thalassemia in blacks: genetic and clinical aspects and interactions with the sickle hemoglobin gene. *Blood* 1986;68(5):985–990.
30. Pagnier J, Mears JG, Dunda-Beklhodja O. Evidence for the multicenter origin of the sickle cell hemoglobin gene in Africa. *Proc Natl Acad Sci U S A* 1984;81:1771–1773.
31. Powars DR. Sickle cell anemia: beta s-gene-cluster haplotypes as prognostic indicators of vital organ failure. *Semin Hematol* 1991;28(3):202–208.
32. Ballas SK, Larner J, Smith ED, et al. Rheologic predictors of the severity of the painful sickle cell crisis. *Blood* 1988;72(4):1216–1223.
33. Baum KF, Dunn DT, Maude GH, et al. The painful crisis of homozygous sickle cell disease. A study of the risk factors. *Arch Intern Med* 1987;147(7):1231–1234.
34. Platt OS, Thorington BD, Brambilla DJ, et al. Pain in sickle cell disease. Rates and risk factors. *N Engl J Med* 1991;325(1):11–16.
35. Ballas SK, Talacki CA, Rao VM, et al. The prevalence of avascular necrosis in sickle cell anemia: correlation with alpha-thalassemia. *Hemoglobin* 1989;13(7–8):649–655.
36. Milner PF, Kraus AP, Sebes JI, et al. Sickle cell disease as a cause of osteonecrosis of the femoral head. *N Engl J Med* 1991;325(21):1476–1481.

37. Koshy M, Enstuah R, Koranda A. Leg ulcers in patients in sickle cell disease. *Blood* 1989;74:1403–1408.
38. Ballas SK, Gay RN, Chehab FF. Is Hb A2 elevated in adults with sickle-alpha-thalassemia (beta(S)/beta(S); -alpha/-alpha)? *Hemoglobin* 1997;21(5):405–450.
39. Steinberg MH, Hsu H, Nagel RL, et al. Gender and haplotype effects upon hematological manifestations of adult sickle cell anemia. *Am J Hematol* 1995;48(3):175–181.
40. Bouvier CA, Gaynor E, Clintron JR, et al. Circulating endothelium as an indication of vascular injury. *Thromb Diath Haemorrh* 1970;40:163–168.
41. Kaul DK, Fabry ME, Nagel RL. The pathophysiology of vascular obstruction in the sickle syndromes. *Blood Rev* 1996;10:29–44.
42. Serjeant G. *Sickle Cell Disease*. 2nd ed. Oxford, United Kingdom: Oxford University Press; 1992.
43. Expert Panel Report. *Evidence-Based Management of Sickle Cell Disease*. Bethesda, MD: National Heart, Lung, and Blood Institute; 2014. Available at: http://www.nhlbi.nih.gov/health-topics/guidelines/sickle-cell-disease-guidelines/. Accessed August 27, 2017.
44. Francis RB, Johnson CS. Vascular occlusion in sickle cell disease: current concepts and unanswered questions. *Blood* 1991;77(7):1405–1414.
45. Hebbel RP. Beyond hemoglobin polymerization. The red blood cell membrane and sickle disease pathophysiology. *Blood* 1991;77:214–237.
46. Brugnara C, Bunn HF, Tosteson DC. Regulation of erythrocyte cation and water content in sickle cell anemia. *Science* 1986;232(4748):388–390.
47. Joiner CH. Cation transport and volume regulation in sickle red blood cells. *Am J Physiol* 1993;264(2 pt 1):C251–C270.
48. Mueller BU, Brugnara C. Prevention of red cell dehydration: a possible new treatment for sickle cell disease. *Pediatr Pathol Mol Med* 2001;20(1):15–25.
49. Lew VL, Freeman CJ, Ortiz OE, et al. A mathematical model of the volume, pH, and ion content regulation in reticulocytes. Application to the pathophysiology of sickle cell dehydration. *J Clin Invest* 1991;87(1):100–112.
50. Brugnara C, Gee B, Armsby CC, et al. Therapy with oral clotrimazole induces inhibition of the Gardos channel and reduction of erythrocyte dehydration in patients with sickle cell disease. *J Clin Invest* 1996;97(5):1227–1234.
51. Brugnara C, Kopin AS, Bunn HF, et al. Regulation of cation content and cell volume in hemoglobin erythrocytes from patients with homozygous hemoglobin C disease. *J Clin Invest* 1985;75(5):1608–1617.
52. Brugnara C, Tosteson DC. Inhibition of K transport by divalent cations in sickle erythrocytes. *Blood* 1987;70(6):1810–1815.
53. Lew VL, Hockaday A, Sepulveda MI, et al. Compartmentalization of sickle-cell calcium in endocytic inside-out vesicles. *Nature* 1985;315(6020):586–589.
54. Rhoda MD, Giraud F, Craescu CT, et al. Compartmentalization of Ca2+ in sickle cells. *Cell Calcium* 1985;6(5):397–411.
55. Rubin E, Schlegel RA, Williamson P. Endocytosis in sickle erythrocytes: a mechanism for elevated intracellular Ca2+ levels. *J Cell Physiol* 1986;126(1):53–59.
56. Ataga KI, Reid M, Ballas SK, et al. Improvements in haemolysis and indicators of erythrocyte survival do not correlate with acute vaso-occlusive crises in patients with sickle cell disease: a phase III randomized, placebo-controlled, double-blind study of the Gardos channel blocker senicapoc (ICA-17043). *Br J Haematol* 2011;153(1):92–104.
57. Nagalla S, Ballas SK. Drugs for preventing red blood cell dehydration in people with sickle cell disease. *Cochrane Database Syst Rev* 2016;(3):CD003426.
58. Hebbel RP, Boogaerts MA, Eaton JW, et al. Erythrocyte adherence to endothelium in sickle-cell anemia. *N Engl J Med* 1980;302:992–995.
59. Hebbel RP, Yamada O, Moldow CF. Abnormal adherence of sickle erythrocytes to cultured vascular endothelium: possible mechanism for microvascular occlusion in sickle cell disease. *J Clin Invest* 1980;65:154–160.
60. Hoover R, Rubin R, Wise G, et al. Adhesion of normal and sickle erythrocytes to endothelial monolayer cultures. *Blood* 1979;54(4):872–876.
61. Barabino GA, McIntire LV, Eskin SG, et al. Rheological studies of erythrocyte-endothelial cell interactions in sickle cell disease. *Prog Clin Biol Res* 1987;240:113–127.
62. Fabry ME, Kaul DK. Sickle cell vaso-occlusion. *Hematol Oncol Clin North Am* 1991;5(3):375–398.
63. Kaul DK, Fabry ME, Costantini F, et al. In vivo demonstration of red cell-endothelial interaction, sickling and altered microvascular response to oxygen in the sickle transgenic mouse. *J Clin Invest* 1995;96(6):2845–2853.
64. Kaul DK, Fabry ME, Nagel RL. Microvascular sites and characteristics of sickle cell adhesion to vascular endothelium in shear flow conditions: pathophysiological implications. *Proc Natl Acad Sci U S A* 1989;86(9):3356–3360.
65. Mohandas N, Evans E. Adherence of sickle erythrocytes to vascular endothelial cells: requirement for both cell membrane changes and plasma factors. *Blood* 1984;64(1):282–287.
66. Ballas SK. Sickle cell anemia with few painful crises is characterized by decreased red cell deformability and increased number of dense cells. *Am J Hematol* 1991;36(2):122–130.
67. Stockman JA, Nigro MA, Mishkin MM, et al. Occlusion of large cerebral vessels in sickle-cell anemia. *N Engl J Med* 1972;287(17):846–849.
68. Rothman SM, Fulling KH, Nelson JS. Sickle cell anemia and central nervous system infarction: a neuropathological study. *Ann Neurol* 1986;20(6):684–690.
69. Hebbel RP. Perspectives series: cell adhesion in vascular biology. Adhesive interactions of sickle erythrocytes with endothelium. *J Clin Invest* 1997;99(11):2561–2564.
70. Hebbel RP. Adhesive interactions of sickle erythrocytes with endothelium. *J Clin Invest* 1997;100(11 suppl):S83–S86.
71. Kaul DK, Hebbel RP. Hypoxia/reoxygenation causes inflammatory response in transgenic sickle mice but not in normal mice. *J Clin Invest* 2000;106(3):411–420.
72. Platt OS. Sickle cell anemia as an inflammatory disease. *J Clin Invest* 2000;106(3):337–338.
73. Setty BN, Kulkarni S, Dampier CD, et al. Fetal hemoglobin in sickle cell anemia: relationship to erythrocyte adhesion markers and adhesion. *Blood* 2001;97(9):2568–2573.
74. Zwaal RF, Schroit AJ. Pathophysiologic implications of membrane phospholipid asymmetry in blood cells. *Blood* 1997;89(4):1121–1132.
75. de Jong K, Emerson RK, Butler J, et al. Short survival of phosphatidylserine-exposing red blood cells in murine sickle cell anemia. *Blood* 2001;98(5):1577–1584.
76. Fabry ME. Molecular genetics of the human globin genes. In: Steinberg MH, Forget BG, Higgs DR, et al, eds. *Disorders of Hemoglobin: Genetics, Pathophysiology and Clinical Management*. Cambridge, United Kingdom: Cambridge University Press; 2001:910–940.
77. Thein SL. Genetic modifiers of the beta-haemoglobinopathies. *Br J Haematol* 2008;141(3):357–366.
78. Ashley-Koch AE, Elliott L, Kail ME, et al. Identification of genetic polymorphisms associated with risk for pulmonary hypertension in sickle cell disease. *Blood* 2008;111(12):5721–5726.
79. Sebastiani P, Solovieff N, Hartley SW, et al. Genetic modifiers of the severity of sickle cell anemia identified through a genome-wide association study. *Am J Hematol* 2010;85(1):29–35.
80. Steinberg MH. SNPing away at sickle cell pathophysiology. *Blood* 2008;111(12):5420–5421.
81. Steinberg MH. Genetic etiologies for phenotypic diversity in sickle cell anemia. *Scientific WorldJournal* 2009;9:46–67.
82. Steinberg MH, Adewoye AH. Modifier genes and sickle cell anemia. *Curr Opin Hematol* 2006;13(3):131–136.
83. Steinberg MH, Sebastiani P. Genetic modifiers of sickle cell disease. *Am J Hematol* 2012;87(8):795–803.
84. Thein SL. Genetic modifiers of sickle cell disease. *Hemoglobin* 2011;35(5–6):589–606.
85. Ballas SK, Lieff S, Benjamin LJ, et al. Definitions of the phenotypic manifestations of sickle cell disease. *Am J Hematol* 2010;85(1):6–13.
86. DeBaun MR. Finally, a consensus statement on sickle cell disease manifestations: a critical step in improving the medical care and research agenda for individuals with sickle cell disease. *Am J Hematol* 2010;85(1):1–3.
87. Turk DC, Okifuji A. Pain terms and taxonomies. In: Fishman SM, Ballantyne JC, Rathmell JP, eds. *Bonica's Management of Pain*. 4th ed. Philadelphia: Lippincott Williams & Wilkins; 2010:13–23.
88. Fields HL. *Pain*. New York: McGraw-Hill; 1987.
89. Cousins MJ. Acute post operative pain. In: Wall PD, Melzack R, eds. *Textbook of Pain*. 3rd ed. New York: Churchill Livingstone; 1994:357–385.
90. Katz N, Ferrante F. Nociception. In: Ferrante FM, VadeBoncoeur TR, eds. *Postoperative Pain Management*. New York: Churchill Livingstone; 1993:17–67.
91. McMahon SB, Koltzenburg M. *Wall and Melzack's Textbook of Pain*. 5th ed. Philadelphia: Elsevier Churchill Livingstone; 2006.
92. Ballas SK, Gupta K, Adams-Graves P. Sickle cell pain: a critical reappraisal. *Blood* 2012;120(18):3647–3656.
93. Darbari DS, Onyekwere O, Nouraie M, et al. Markers of severe vaso-occlusive painful episode frequency in children and adolescents with sickle cell anemia. *J Pediatr* 2012;160(2):286–290.
94. Ballas SK, Lusardi M. Hospital readmission for adult acute sickle cell painful episodes: frequency, etiology, and prognostic significance. *Am J Hematol* 2005;79(1):17–25.
95. Udezue E, Girshab AM. Differences between males and females in adult sickle cell pain crisis in eastern Saudi Arabia. *Ann Saudi Med* 2004;24(3):179–182.
96. Lande WM, Andrews DL, Clark MR, et al. The incidence of painful crisis in homozygous sickle cell disease: correlation with red cell deformability. *Blood* 1988;72(6):2056–2059.
97. Schall JI, Zemel BS, Kawchak DA, et al. Vitamin A status, hospitalizations, and other outcomes in young children with sickle cell disease. *J Pediatr* 2004;145(1):99–106.
98. Hargrave DR, Wade A, Evans JP, et al. Nocturnal oxygen saturation and painful sickle cell crises in children. *Blood* 2003;101(3):846–848.
99. Ballas SK. *Sickle Cell Pain*. Vol 11. Seattle, WA: IASP Press; 1998.
100. Benjamin LJ. Nature and treatment of the acute painful episode in sickle cell disease. In: Steinberg MH, Forget BG, Higgs DR, et al, eds. *Disorders of Hemoglobin: Genetics, Pathophysiology, and Clinical Management*. Cambridge, United Kingdom: Cambridge University Press; 2001:671–710.
101. Gil KM, Carson JW, Porter LS, et al. Daily mood and stress predict pain, health care use, and work activity in African American adults with sickle-cell disease. *Health Psychol* 2004;23(3):267–274.
102. Smith WR, Coyne P, Smith VS, et al. Temperature changes, temperature extremes, and their relationship to emergency department visits and hospitalizations for sickle cell crisis. *Pain Manag Nurs* 2003;4(3):106–111.

103. Jones S, Duncan ER, Thomas N, et al. Windy weather and low humidity are associated with an increased number of hospital admissions for acute pain and sickle cell disease in an urban environment with a maritime temperate climate. *Br J Haematol* 2005;131(4):530–533.

104. Nolan VG, Zhang Y, Lash T, et al. Association between wind speed and the occurrence of sickle cell acute painful episodes: results of a case-crossover study. *Br J Haematol* 2008;143(3):433–438.

105. Rogovik AL, Persaud J, Friedman JN, et al. Pediatric vasoocclusive crisis and weather conditions. *J Emerg Med* 2011;41(5):559–565.

106. Murray N, May A. Painful crises in sickle cell disease—patients' perspectives. *BMJ* 1988;297(6646):452–454.

107. Akinola NO, Stevens SM, Franklin IM, et al. Rheological changes in the prodromal and established phases of sickle cell vaso-occlusive crisis. *Br J Haematol* 1992;81(4):598–602.

108. Ballas SK, Smith ED. Red blood cell changes during the evolution of the sickle cell painful crisis. *Blood* 1992;79(8):2154–2163.

109. Ballas SK. Treatment of pain in adults with sickle cell disease. *Am J Hematol* 1990;34(1):49–54.

110. Billett HH, Fabry ME, Nagel RL. Hemoglobin distribution width: a rapid assessment of dense red cells in the steady state and during painful crisis in sickle cell anemia. *J Lab Clin Med* 1988;112(3):339–344.

111. Fabry ME, Mears JG, Patel P, et al. Dense cells in sickle cell anemia: the effects of gene interaction. *Blood* 1984;64(5):1042–1046.

112. Lawrence C, Fabry ME, Nagel RL. Red cell distribution width parallels dense red cell disappearance during painful crises in sickle cell anemia. *J Lab Clin Med* 1985;105(6):706–710.

113. Alkjaersig N, Fletcher A, Joist H, et al. Hemostatic alterations accompanying sickle cell pain crises. *J Lab Clin Med* 1976;88(3):440–449.

114. Haut MJ, Cowan DH, Harris JW. Platelet function and survival in sickle cell disease. *J Lab Clin Med* 1973;82(1):44–53.

115. van der Sar A. The sudden rise in platelets and reticulocytes in sickle cell crises. *Trop Geogr Med* 1970;22(1):30–40.

116. Samuels-Reid J, Scott RB. Painful crises and menstruation in sickle cell disease. *South Med J* 1985;78(4):384–385.

117. Billett HH, Nagel RL, Fabry ME. Evolution of laboratory parameters during sickle cell painful crisis: evidence compatible with dense red cell sequestration without thrombosis. *Am J Med Sci* 1988;296(5):293–298.

118. Buchanan GR, Glader BE. Leukocyte counts in children with sickle cell disease. Comparative values in the steady state, vaso-occlusive crisis, and bacterial infection. *Am J Dis Child* 1978;132(4):396–398.

119. Schumacher HR. Rheumatological manifestations of sickle cell disease and other haemoglobinopathies. *Clin Rheum Dis* 1975;1:37–52.

120. Becton DL, Raymond L, Thompson C, et al. Acute-phase reactants in sickle cell disease. *J Pediatr* 1989;115(1):99–102.

121. Lawrence C, Fabry ME. Erythrocyte sedimentation rate during steady state and painful crisis in sickle cell anemia. *Am J Med* 1986;81(5):801–808.

122. McClish DK, Smith WR, Dahman BA, et al. Pain site frequency and location in sickle cell disease: the PiSCES project. *Pain* 2009;145(1–2):246–251.

123. Dampier C, Ely B, Brodecki D, et al. Characteristics of pain managed at home in children and adolescents with sickle cell disease by using diary self-reports. *J Pain* 2002;3(6):461–470.

124. Dampier C, Ely E, Brodecki D, O'Neal P. Home management of pain in sickle cell disease: a daily diary study in children and adolescents. *J Pediatr Hematol Oncol* 2002;24(8):643–647.

125. Ballas SK, Bauserman RL, McCarthy WF, et al. Hydroxyurea and acute painful crises in sickle cell anemia: effects on hospital length of stay and opioid utilization during hospitalization, outpatient acute care contacts, and at home. *J Pain Symptom Manage* 2010;40(6):870–882.

126. Ballas SK, Bauserman RL, McCarthy WF, et al. Utilization of analgesics in the multicenter study of hydroxyurea in sickle cell anemia: effect of sex, age, and geographical location. *Am J Hematol* 2010;85(8):613–616.

127. Benjamin LJ, Swinson GI, Nagel RL. Sickle cell anemia day hospital: an approach for the management of uncomplicated painful crises. *Blood* 2000;95(4):1130–1136.

128. Jacob E, Miaskowski C, Savedra M, et al. Changes in intensity, location, and quality of vaso-occlusive pain in children with sickle cell disease. *Pain* 2003;102(1–2):187–193.

129. Brousseau DC, Owens PL, Mosso AL, et al. Acute care utilization and rehospitalizations for sickle cell disease. *JAMA* 2010;303(13):1288–1294.

130. Frei-Jones M, Field JJ, DeBaun MR. Risk factors for hospital readmission within 30 days: a new quality measure for children with sickle cell disease. *Pediatr Blood Cancer* 2009;52(4):481–485.

131. Sobota A, Graham DA, Neufeld EJ, et al. Thirty-day readmission rates following hospitalization for pediatric sickle cell crisis at freestanding children's hospitals: risk factors and hospital variation. *Pediatr Blood Cancer* 2012;58(1):61–65.

132. Charache S, Scott JC, Charache P. "Acute chest syndrome" in adults with sickle cell anemia. Microbiology, treatment, and prevention. *Arch Intern Med* 1979;139(1):67–69.

133. Vichinsky EP, Styles LA, Colangelo LH, et al. Acute chest syndrome in sickle cell disease: clinical presentation and course. Cooperative Study of Sickle Cell Disease. *Blood* 1997;89(5):1787–1792.

134. Castro O, Brambilla DJ, Thorington B, et al. The acute chest syndrome in sickle cell disease: incidence and risk factors. The Cooperative Study of Sickle Cell Disease. *Blood* 1994;84(2):643–649.

135. Miller ST. How I treat acute chest syndrome in children with sickle cell disease. *Blood* 2011;117(20):5297–5305.

136. Claster S, Vichinsky E. Acute chest syndrome in sickle cell disease: pathophysiology and management. *J Intensive Care Med* 2000;15:59–66.

137. Vichinsky EP, Neumayr LD, Earles AN, et al. Causes and outcomes of the acute chest syndrome in sickle cell disease. National Acute Chest Syndrome Study Group. *N Engl J Med* 2000;342(25):1855–1865.

138. Styles LA, Schalkwijk CG, Aarsman AJ, et al. Phospholipase A2 levels in acute chest syndrome of sickle cell disease. *Blood* 1996;87(6):2573–2578.

139. Vichinsky EP, Lubin BH. Sickle cell anemia and related hemoglobinopathies. *Pediatr Clin North Am* 1980;27(2):429–447.

140. Sprinkle RH, Cole T, Smith S, et al. Acute chest syndrome in children with sickle cell disease. A retrospective analysis of 100 hospitalized cases. *Am J Pediatr Hematol Oncol* 1986;8(2):105–110.

141. Ashcroft MT, Serjant GR. Growth, morbidity, and mortality in a cohort of Jamaican adolescents with homozygous sickle cell disease. *West Indian Med J* 1981;30(4):197–201.

142. Athanasou NA, Hatton C, McGee JO, et al. Vascular occlusion and infarction in sickle cell crisis and the sickle chest syndrome. *J Clin Pathol* 1985;38(6):659–664.

143. Barrett-Connor E. Acute pulmonary disease and sickle cell anemia. *Am Rev Respir Dis* 1971;104(2):159–165.

144. Davies SC, Luce PJ, Win AA, et al. Acute chest syndrome in sickle-cell disease. *Lancet* 1984;1(8367):36–38.

145. Gill FM, Sleeper LA, Weiner SJ, et al. Clinical events in the first decade in a cohort of infants with sickle cell disease. Cooperative Study of Sickle Cell Disease. *Blood* 1995;86(2):776–783.

146. Thomas AN, Pattison C. Causes of death in sickle-cell disease in Jamaica. *Br Med J* 1982;285(6342):633–635.

147. van Agtmael MA, Cheng JD, Nossent HC. Acute chest syndrome in adult Afro-Caribbean patients with sickle cell disease. Analysis of 81 episodes among 53 patients. *Arch Intern Med* 1994;154(5):557–561.

148. Vichinsky EP. Comprehensive care in sickle cell disease: its impact on morbidity and mortality. *Semin Hematol* 1991;28(3):220–226.

149. Ballas SK, Park CH. Severe hypoxemia secondary to acute sternal infarction in sickle cell anemia. *J Nucl Med* 1991;32(8):1617–1618.

150. Bellet PS, Kalinyak K. Incentive spirometry to prevent acute pulmonary complications in sickle cell diseases. *N Engl J Med* 1995;333(11):699–703.

151. Rucknagel DL, Kalinyak KA, Gelfand MJ. Rib infarcts and acute chest syndrome in sickle cell diseases. *Lancet* 1991;337(8753):831–833.

152. Styles LA, Aarsman AJ, Vichinsky EP, et al. Secretory phospholipase A(2) predicts impending acute chest syndrome in sickle cell disease. *Blood* 2000;96(9):3276–3278.

153. Vichinsky E, Williams R, Das M, et al. Pulmonary fat embolism: a distinct cause of severe acute chest syndrome in sickle cell anemia. *Blood* 1994;83(11):3107–3112.

154. Alhashimi D, Fedorowicz Z, Alhashimi F, et al. Blood transfusions for treating acute chest syndrome in people with sickle cell disease. *Cochrane Database Syst Rev* 2010;(1):CD007843.

155. Abboud MR, Taylor EC, Habib D, et al. Elevated serum and bronchoalveolar lavage fluid levels of interleukin 8 and granulocyte colony-stimulating factor associated with the acute chest syndrome in patients with sickle cell disease. *Br J Haematol* 2000;111(2):482–490.

156. Bernini JC, Rogers ZR, Sandler ES, et al. Beneficial effect of intravenous dexamethasone in children with mild to moderately severe acute chest syndrome complicating sickle cell disease. *Blood* 1998;92(9):3082–3089.

157. Couillard S, Benkerrou M, Girot R, et al. Steroid treatment in children with sickle-cell disease. *Haematologica* 2007;92(3):425–426.

158. Strouse JJ, Hulbert ML, DeBaun MR, et al. Primary hemorrhagic stroke in children with sickle cell disease is associated with recent transfusion and use of corticosteroids. *Pediatrics* 2006;118(5):1916–1924.

159. Huang JC, Gay R, Khella SL. Sickling crisis, fat embolism, and coma after steroids. *Lancet* 1994;344(8927):951–952.

160. Ballas SK. Corticosteroids and sickle cell disease. *JAMA* 2009;101(3):283.

161. Darbari DS, Fasano RS, Minniti CP, et al. Severe vaso-occlusive episodes associated with use of systemic corticosteroids in patients with sickle cell disease. *J Natl Med Assoc* 2008;100(8):948–951.

162. Simkin PA, Downey DJ. Hypothesis: retrograde embolization of marrow fat may cause osteonecrosis. *J Rheumatol* 1987;14(5):870–872.

163. Atz AM, Wessel DL. Inhaled nitric oxide in sickle cell disease with acute chest syndrome. *Anesthesiology* 1997;87(4):988–990.

164. Weiner DL, Hibberd PL, Betit P, et al. Preliminary assessment of inhaled nitric oxide for acute vaso-occlusive crisis in pediatric patients with sickle cell disease. *JAMA* 2003;289(9):1136–1142.

165. Head CA, Swerdlow P, McDade WA, et al. Beneficial effects of nitric oxide breathing in adult patients with sickle cell crisis. *Am J Hematol* 2010;85(10):800–802.

166. Ikuta T, Thatte HS, Tang JX, et al. Nitric oxide reduces sickle hemoglobin polymerization: potential role of nitric oxide-induced charge alteration in depolymerization. *Arch Biochem Biophys* 2011;510(1):53–61.

167. Gladwin MT, Kato GJ, Weiner D, et al. Nitric oxide for inhalation in the acute treatment of sickle cell pain crisis: a randomized controlled trial. *JAMA* 2011;305(9):893–902.

168. Adams-Graves P, Kedar A, Koshy M, et al. RheothRx (poloxamer 188) injection for the acute painful episode of sickle cell disease: a pilot study. *Blood* 1997;90(5):2041–2046.

169. Ballas SK, Files B, Luchtman-Jones L, et al. Safety of purified poloxamer 188 in sickle cell disease: phase I study of a non-ionic surfactant in the management of acute chest syndrome. *Hemoglobin* 2004;28(2):85–102.

170. Walker BK, Ballas SK, Burka ER. The diagnosis of pulmonary thromboembolism in sickle cell disease. *Am J Hematol* 1979;7(3):219–232.

171. Karayalcin G, Rosner F, Kim KY, et al. Sickle cell anemia—clinical manifestations in 100 patients and review of the literature. *Am J Med Sci* 1975;269(1):51–68.

172. Linklater DR, Pemberton L, Taylor S, et al. Painful dilemmas: an evidence-based look at challenging clinical scenarios. *Emerg Med Clin North Am* 2005;23(2):367–392.

173. Magid D, Fishman EK, Charache S, et al. Abdominal pain in sickle cell disease: the role of CT. *Radiology* 1987;163(2):325–328.

174. Al-Mulhim AS, Al-Mulhim FM, Al-Suwaiygh AA. The role of laparoscopic cholecystectomy in the management of acute cholecystitis in patients with sickle cell disease. *Am J Surg* 2002;183(6):668–672.

175. Lopez AJ, O'Keefe P, Morrissey M, et al. Ceftriaxone-induced cholelithiasis. *Ann Intern Med* 1991;115(9):712–714.

176. Singh NK, el-Mangoush M. Hepatic sequestration crisis presenting with severe intrahepatic cholestatic jaundice. *J Assoc Physicians India* 1996;44(4):283–284.

177. Ballas SK, Lewis CN, Noone AM, et al. Clinical, hematological, and biochemical features of Hb SC disease. *Am J Hematol* 1982;13(1):37–51.

178. Walker TM, Hambleton IR, Serjeant GR. Gallstones in sickle cell disease: observations from The Jamaican Cohort study. *J Pediatr* 2000;136(1):80–85.

179. Curro G, Meo A, Ippolito D, et al. Asymptomatic cholelithiasis in children with sickle cell disease: early or delayed cholecystectomy? *Ann Surg* 2007;245(1):126–129.

180. Nzeh DA, Adedoyin MA. Sonographic pattern of gallbladder disease in children with sickle cell anaemia. *Pediatr Radiol* 1989;19(5):290–292.

181. Haider MZ, Ashebu S, Aduh P, et al. Influence of alpha-thalassemia on cholelithiasis in SS patients with elevated Hb F. *Acta Haematol* 1998;100(3):147–150.

182. Passon RG, Howard TA, Zimmerman SA, et al. Influence of bilirubin uridine diphosphate-glucuronosyltransferase 1A promoter polymorphisms on serum bilirubin levels and cholelithiasis in children with sickle cell anemia. *J Pediatr Hematol Oncol* 2001;23(7):448–451.

183. Premawardhena A, Fisher CA, Fathiu F, et al. Genetic determinants of jaundice and gallstones in haemoglobin E beta thalassaemia. *Lancet* 2001;357(9272):1945–1946.

184. Bond LR, Hatty SR, Horn ME, et al. Gall stones in sickle cell disease in the United Kingdom. *Br Med J (Clin Res Ed)* 1987;295(6592):234–236.

185. Papadaki MG, Kattamis AC, Papadaki IG, et al. Abdominal ultrasonographic findings in patients with sickle-cell anaemia and thalassaemia intermedia. *Pediatr Radiol* 2003;33(8):515–521.

186. Jawad AJ, Kurban K, el-Bakry A, et al. Laparoscopic cholecystectomy for cholelithiasis during infancy and childhood: cost analysis and review of current indications. *World J Surg* 1998;22(1):69–74.

187. St. Peter SD, Keckler SJ, Nair A, et al. Laparoscopic cholecystectomy in the pediatric population. *J Laparoendosc Adv Surg Tech A* 2008;18(1):127–130.

188. Al-Salem AH, Qaisruddin S. The significance of biliary sludge in children with sickle cell disease. *Pediatr Surg Int* 1998;13(1):14–16.

189. Lee SP, Maher K, Nicholls JF. Origin and fate of biliary sludge. *Gastroenterology* 1988;94(1):170–176.

190. Werlin SL, Scott JP. Is biliary sludge a stone-in-waiting? *J Pediatr* 1996;129(3):321–322.

191. Vicari P, Gil MV, Cavalheiro Rde C, et al. Multiple primary choledocholithiasis in sickle cell disease. *Intern Med* 2008;47(24):2169–2170.

192. McCall IW, Desai P, Serjeant BE, et al. Cholelithiasis in Jamaican patients with homozygous sickle cell disease. *Am J Hematol* 1977;3:15–21.

193. Cameron JL, Maddrey WC, Zuidema GD. Biliary tract disease in sickle cell anemia: surgical considerations. *Ann Surg* 1971;174(4):702–710.

194. Lee SP, Nicholls JF, Park HZ. Biliary sludge as a cause of acute pancreatitis. *N Engl J Med* 1992;326(9):589–593.

195. Ahmed S, Siddiqui AK, Siddiqui RK, et al. Acute pancreatitis during sickle cell vaso-occlusive painful crisis. *Am J Hematol* 2003;73(3):190–193.

196. Issa H, Al-Salem AH. Role of ERCP in the era of laparoscopic cholecystectomy for the evaluation of choledocholithiasis in sickle cell anemia. *World J Gastroenterol* 2011;17(14):1844–1847.

197. Hatton CS, Bunch C, Weatherall DJ. Hepatic sequestration in sickle cell anaemia. *Br Med J (Clin Res Ed)* 1985;290(6470):744–745.

198. Davies SC, Brozovic M. The presentation, management and prophylaxis of sickle cell disease. *Blood Rev* 1989;3(1):29–44.

199. Ahmed N, Chizhevsky V. Acute hepatic sequestration associated with pneumococcal infection in a 5-year-old boy with sickle beta degrees-thalassemia: a case report and review of the literature. *J Pediatr Hematol Oncol* 2007;29(10):720–724.

200. Ahn H, Li CS, Wang W. Sickle cell hepatopathy: clinical presentation, treatment, and outcome in pediatric and adult patients. *Pediatr Blood Cancer* 2005;45(2):184–190.

201. Banerjee S, Owen C, Chopra S. Sickle cell hepatopathy. *Hepatology* 2001;33(5):1021–1028.

202. Norris WE. Acute hepatic sequestration in sickle cell disease. *J Natl Med Assoc* 2004;96(9):1235–1239.

203. Johnson CS, Omata M, Tong MJ, et al. Liver involvement in sickle cell disease. *Medicine (Baltimore)* 1985;64(5):349–356.

204. Lacaille F, Lesage F, de Montalembert M. Acute hepatic crisis in children with sickle cell disease. *J Pediatr Gastroenterol Nutr* 2004;39(2):200–202.

205. Sheehy TW. Sickle cell hepatopathy. *South Med J* 1977;70(5):533–538.

206. Sheehy TW, Law DE, Wade BH. Exchange transfusion for sickle cell intrahepatic cholestasis. *Arch Intern Med* 1980;140(10):1364–1366.

207. Kaine WN, Udeozo IO. Sickle cell hepatic crisis in Nigerian children. *J Trop Pediatr* 1988;34(2):59–64.

208. Buchanan GR, Glader BE. Benign course of extreme hyperbilirubinemia in sickle cell anemia: analysis of six cases. *J Pediatr* 1977;91(1):21–24.

209. Wade FA. Sickle cell crisis resembling obstructive (cholangiolar type) jaundice. Report of a case and review of the literature. *Va Med Mon (1918)* 1960;87:474–478.

210. Talacki CA, Ballas SK. Modified method of exchange transfusion in sickle cell disease. *J Clin Apher* 1990;5(4):183–187.

211. Hernandez P, Dorticos E, Espinosa E, et al. Clinical features of hepatic sequestration in sickle cell anaemia. *Haematologia (Budap)* 1989;22(3):169–174.

212. Emond AM, Collis R, Darvill D, et al. Acute splenic sequestration in homozygous sickle cell disease: natural history and management. *J Pediatr* 1985;107(2):201–206.

213. Solanki DL, Kletter GG, Castro O. Acute splenic sequestration crises in adults with sickle cell disease. *Am J Med* 1986;80(5):985–990.

214. Powars DR. Natural history of sickle cell disease—the first ten years. *Semin Hematol* 1975;12(3):267–285.

215. Topley JM, Rogers DW, Stevens MC, et al. Acute splenic sequestration and hypersplenism in the first five years in homozygous sickle cell disease. *Arch Dis Child* 1981;56(10):765–769.

216. Moll S, Orringer EP. Case report: splenomegaly and splenic sequestration in an adult with sickle cell anemia. *Am J Med Sci* 1996;312(6):299–302.

217. De Ceulaer K, Serjeant GR. Acute splenic sequestration in Jamaican adults with homozygous sickle cell disease: a role of alpha thalassaemia. *Br J Haematol* 1991;77(4):563–564.

218. Bowcock SJ, Nwabueze ED, Cook AE, et al. Fatal splenic sequestration in adult sickle cell disease. *Clin Lab Haematol* 1988;10(1):95–99.

219. Sarma PS. Acute splenic sequestration crisis in a young woman with homozygous sickle cell anaemia. *Postgrad Med J* 1989;65(760):105–107.

220. Koduri PR. Acute splenic sequestration crisis in adults with sickle cell anemia. *Am J Hematol* 2007;82(2):174–175.

221. Altman KI, Watman RN, Salomon K. Surgically induced splenogenic anaemia in the rabbit. *Nature* 1951;168(4280):827.

222. Itzchak Y, Glickman MG, Gottschalk A, et al. Hemodynamic and morphologic evaluation of the spleen after splenic vein ligation in the dog. *Invest Radiol* 1978;13(2):155–160.

223. Jensen WN, Lessin LS. Membrane alterations associated with hemoglobinopathies. *Semin Hematol* 1970;7(4):409–426.

224. Barnhart MI, Henry RL, Lusher JM. *Sickle Cell*. 2nd ed. Kalamazoo, MI: The Upjohn Company; 1976:15–35.

225. Serjeant GR, Serjeant BE. *Sickle Cell Disease*. 3rd ed. Oxford, United Kingdom: Oxford University Press; 2001.

226. Ballas SK, Burka ER, Lewis CN, et al. Serum immunoglobulin levels in patients having sickle cell syndromes. *Am J Clin Pathol* 1980;73(3):394–396.

227. Ballas SK. The sickle cell painful crisis in adults: phases and objective signs. *Hemoglobin* 1995;19(6):323–333.

228. Gage TP, Gagnier JM. Ischemic colitis complicating sickle cell crisis. *Gastroenterology* 1983;84(1):171–174.

229. Lukens JN. Sickle cell disease. *Dis Mon* 1981;27(5):1–56.

230. Nault JC, Amathieu R, Luis D, et al. Acute hepatic failure in sickle cell vaso-occlusive crisis. *Ann Fr Anesth Reanim* 2009;28(4):393–395.

231. Olujohungbe AB, Adeyoju A, Yardumian A, et al. A prospective diary study of stuttering priapism in adolescents and young men with sickle cell anemia: report of an international randomized control trial—the priapism in sickle cell study. *J Androl* 2011;32(4):375–382.

232. Adeyoju AB, Olujohungbe AB, Morris J, et al. Priapism in sickle-cell disease; incidence, risk factors and complications—an international multicentre study. *BJU Int* 2002;90(9):898–902.

233. Powars DR, Johnson CS. Priapism. *Hematol Oncol Clin North Am* 1996;10(6):1363–1372.

234. Rogers ZR. Priapism in sickle cell disease. *Hematol Oncol Clin North Am* 2005;19(5):917–928, viii.

235. Sharpsteen JR Jr, Powars D, Johnson C, et al. Multisystem damage associated with tricorporal priapism in sickle cell disease. *Am J Med* 1993;94(3):289–295.

236. Okpala I, Westerdale N, Jegede T, et al. Etilefrine for the prevention of priapism in adult sickle cell disease. *Br J Haematol* 2002;118(3):918–921.

237. Emond AM, Holman R, Hayes RJ, et al. Priapism and impotence in homozygous sickle cell disease. *Arch Intern Med* 1980;140(11):1434–1437.

238. Mantadakis E, Cavender JD, Rogers ZR, et al. Prevalence of priapism in children and adolescents with sickle cell anemia. *J Pediatr Hematol Oncol* 1999;21(6):518–522.

239. Allue Lopez M, Garcia de Jalon Martinez A, Pascual Regueiro D, et al. Priapism as an initial presentation of chronic myeloid leukaemia. *Actas Urol Esp* 2004;28(5):387–389.

240. Gregory AB, Ates K, Trinity JB, et al. Priapism: pathogenesis, epidemiology, and management. *J Sex Med* 2010;7:476–500.

241. Kato GJ. Priapism in sickle-cell disease: a hematologist's perspective. *J Sex Med* 2011;1:70–78.

242. Morano SG, Latagliata R, Carmosino I, et al. Treatment of long-lasting priapism in chronic myeloid leukemia at onset. *Ann Hematol* 2000;79(11):644–645.

243. Rodgers R, Latif Z, Copland M. How I manage priapism in chronic myeloid leukaemia patients. *Br J Haematol* 2012;158(2):155–164.

244. Serjeant GR, de Ceulaer K, Maude GH. Stilboestrol and stuttering priapism in homozygous sickle-cell disease. *Lancet* 1985;2(8467):1274–1276.

245. Kato GJ, Gladwin MT, Steinberg MH. Deconstructing sickle cell disease: reappraisal of the role of hemolysis in the development of clinical subphenotypes. *Blood Rev* 2007;21(1):37–47.

246. Hamre MR, Harmon EP, Kirkpatrick DV, et al. Priapism as a complication of sickle cell disease. *J Urol* 1991;145(1):1–5.

247. Baron M, Leiter E. The management of priapism in sickle cell anemia. *J Urol* 1978;119(5):610–611.

248. Seeler RA. Intensive transfusion therapy for priapism in boys with sickle cell anemia. *J Urol* 1973;110(3):360–363.

249. Krauss L, Fitzpatrick T. The treatment of priapism by penile aspiration under controlled hypotension. *J Urol* 1961;85:595–598.

250. Karayalcin G, Imran M, Rosner F. Priapism in sickle cell disease: report of five cases. *Am J Med Sci* 1972;264(4):289–293.

251. Conrad ME, Perrine GM, Barton JC, et al. Provoked priapism in sickle cell anemia. *Am J Hematol* 1980;9(1):121–122.

252. Galloway SJ, Harwood-Nuss AL. Sickle-cell anemia—a review. *J Emerg Med* 1988;6(3):213–226.

253. Serjeant GR. The emerging understanding of sickle cell disease. *Br J Haematol* 2001;112(1):3–18.

254. Pohl J, Pott B, Kleinhans G. Priapism: a three-phase concept of management according to aetiology and prognosis. *Br J Urol* 1986;58(2):113–118.

255. Bunn HF, Nathan DG, Dover GJ, et al. Pulmonary hypertension and nitric oxide depletion in sickle cell disease. *Blood* 2010;116(5):687–692.

256. Mantadakis E, Ewalt DH, Cavender JD, et al. Outpatient penile aspiration and epinephrine irrigation for young patients with sickle cell anemia and prolonged priapism. *Blood* 2000;95(1):78–82.

257. Siegel JF, Rich MA, Brock WA. Association of sickle cell disease, priapism, exchange transfusion and neurological events: ASPEN syndrome. *J Urol* 1993;150(5 pt 1):1480–1482.

258. Rackoff WR, Ohene-Frempong K, Month S, et al. Neurologic events after partial exchange transfusion for priapism in sickle cell disease. *J Pediatr* 1992;120(6):882–885.

259. Ballas SK, Lyon D. Safety and efficacy of blood exchange transfusion for priapism complicating sickle cell disease. *J Clin Apher* 2016;31(1):5–10.

260. Dawson C, Whitfield H. ABC of urology. Urological emergencies in general practice. *BMJ* 1996;312(7034):838–840.

261. Gradisek RE. Priapism in sickle cell disease. *Ann Emerg Med* 1983;12(8):510–512.

262. McHardy P, McDonnell C, Lorenzo AJ, et al. Management of priapism in a child with sickle cell anemia; successful outcome using epidural analgesia. *Can J Anaesth* 2007;54(8):642–645.

263. Al Jam'a AH, Al Dabbous IA. Hydroxyurea in the treatment of sickle cell associated priapism. *J Urol* 1998;159(5):1642.

264. Saad ST, Lajolo C, Gilli S, et al. Follow-up of sickle cell disease patients with priapism treated by hydroxyurea. *Am J Hematol* 2004;77(1):45–49.

265. Levine LA, Guss SP. Gonadotropin-releasing hormone analogues in the treatment of sickle cell anemia-associated priapism. *J Urol* 1993;150(2 pt 1):475–477.

266. Chinegwundoh F, Anie KA. Treatments for priapism in boys and men with sickle cell disease. *Cochrane Database Syst Rev* 2004;(4):CD004198.

267. Bialecki ES, Bridges KR. Sildenafil relieves priapism in patients with sickle cell disease. *Am J Med* 2002;113(3):252.

268. Burnett AL, Bivalacqua TJ, Champion HC, et al. Feasibility of the use of phosphodiesterase type 5 inhibitors in a pharmacologic prevention program for recurrent priapism. *J Sex Med* 2006;3(6):1077–1084.

269. Tzortzis V, Mitrakas L, Gravas S, et al. Oral phosphodiesterase type 5 inhibitors alleviate recurrent priapism complicating thalassemia intermedia: a case report. *J Sex Med* 2009;6(7):2068–2071.

270. Machado RF, Barst RJ, Yovetich NA, et al. Hospitalization for pain in patients with sickle cell disease treated with sildenafil for elevated TRV and low exercise capacity. *Blood* 2011;118(4):855–864.

271. Compton MT, Miller AH. Priapism associated with conventional and atypical antipsychotic medications: a review. *J Clin Psychiatry* 2001;62(5):362–366.

272. Hosseini SH, Polonowita AK. Priapism associated with olanzapine. *Pak J Biol Sci* 2009;12(2):198–200.

273. Songer DA, Barclay JC. Olanzapine-induced priapism. *Am J Psychiatry* 2001;158(12):2087–2088.

274. Hassell KL, Eckman JR, Lane PA. Acute multiorgan failure syndrome: a potentially catastrophic complication of severe sickle cell pain episodes. *Am J Med* 1994;96(2):155–162.

275. Ficat RP. Treatment of avascular necrosis of the femoral head. In: Hungerford DS, ed. *The Hip.* St. Louis, MO: CV Mosby; 1983:279–295.

276. Steinberg ME, Hayken GD, Steinberg DR. A quantitative system for staging avascular necrosis. *J Bone Joint Surg Br* 1995;77(1):34–41.

277. Steinberg ME, Steinberg DR. Classification systems for osteonecrosis: an overview. *Orthop Clin North Am* 2004;35(3):273–283, vii–viii.

278. Styles LA, Vichinsky EP. Core decompression in avascular necrosis of the hip in sickle-cell disease. *Am J Hematol* 1996;52(2):103–107.

279. Neumayr LD, Aguilar C, Earles AN, et al. Physical therapy alone compared with core decompression and physical therapy for femoral head osteonecrosis in sickle cell disease. Results of a multicenter study at a mean of three years after treatment. *J Bone Joint Surg Am* 2006;88(12):2573–2582.

280. Saito S, Saito M, Nishina T, et al. Long-term results of total hip arthroplasty for osteonecrosis of the femoral head. A comparison with osteoarthritis. *Clin Orthop Relat Res* 1989(244):198–207.

281. Hanker GJ, Amstutz HC. Osteonecrosis of the hip in the sickle-cell diseases. Treatment and complications. *J Bone Joint Surg Am* 1988;70(4):499–506.

282. Clarke HJ, Jinnah RH, Brooker AF, et al. Total replacement of the hip for avascular necrosis in sickle cell disease. *J Bone Joint Surg Br* 1989;71(3):465–470.

283. Learmonth ID, Young C, Rorabeck C. The operation of the century: total hip replacement. *Lancet* 2007;370(9597):1508–1519.

284. Ballas SK. Treatment of painful sickle cell leg ulcers with topical opioids. *Blood* 2002;99(3):1096.

285. Powars D, Chan LS, Schroeder WA. The variable expression of sickle cell disease is genetically determined. *Semin Hematol* 1990;27(4):360–376.

286. Wilkinson EA. Oral zinc for arterial and venous leg ulcers. *Cochrane Database Syst Rev* 2012;(8):CD001273.

287. Minniti CP, Eckman J, Sebastiani P, et al. Leg ulcers in sickle cell disease. *Am J Hematol* 2010;85(10):831–833.

288. Chernoff AI, Shapleigh JB, Moore CV. Therapy of chronic ulceration of the legs associated with sickle cell anemia. *JAMA* 1954;155:1487–1491.

289. al-Momen AK. Recombinant human erythropoietin induced rapid healing of a chronic leg ulcer in a patient with sickle cell disease. *Acta Haematol* 1991;86(1):46–48.

290. McMahon L, Tamary H, Askin M, et al. A randomized phase II trial of arginine butyrate with standard local therapy in refractory sickle cell leg ulcers. *Br J Haematol* 2010;151(5):516–524.

291. Sher GD, Olivieri NF. Rapid healing of chronic leg ulcers during arginine butyrate therapy in patients with sickle cell disease and thalassemia. *Blood* 1994;84(7):2378–2380.

292. Heng MC. Local hyperbaric oxygen administration for leg ulcers. *Br J Dermatol* 1983;109(2):232–234.

293. Heng MC, Pilgrim JP, Beck FW. A simplified hyperbaric oxygen technique for leg ulcers. *Arch Dermatol* 1984;120(5):640–645.

294. Ravina A, Minuchin O, Kehrmann H. A simple, disposable, hyperbaric oxygen device for the treatment of wounds. *Isr J Med Sci* 1983;19(9):845–847.

295. Wethers DL, Ramirez GM, Koshy M. The RGD study group. *Blood* 1994;84:1775–1779.

296. Pieters RC, Rojer RA, Saleh AW, et al. Molgramostim to treat SS-sickle cell leg ulcers. *Lancet* 1995;345(8948):528.

297. Reindorf CA, Walker-Jones D, Adekile AD, et al. Rapid healing of sickle cell leg ulcers treated with collagen dressing. *J Natl Med Assoc* 1989;81(8):866–868.

298. Mian E, Mian M, Beghe F. Lyophilized type-I collagen and chronic leg ulcers. *Int J Tissue React* 1991;13(5):257–269.

299. Cacciola E, Giustolisi R, Musso R, et al. Antithrombin III concentrate for treatment of chronic leg ulcers in sickle cell-beta thalassemia: a pilot study. *Ann Intern Med* 1989;111(6):534–536.

300. Marti-Carvajal AJ, Knight-Madden JM, Martinez-Zapata MJ. Interventions for treating leg ulcers in people with sickle cell disease. *Cochrane Database Syst Rev* 2012;(11):CD008394.

301. Heckler FR, Dibbell DG, McCraw JB. Successful use of muscle flaps or myocutaneous flaps in patients with sickle cell disease. *Plast Reconstr Surg* 1977;60(6):902–908.

302. Khouri RK, Upton J. Bilateral lower limb salvage with free flaps in a patient with sickle cell ulcers. *Ann Plast Surg* 1991;27(6):574–576.

303. Spence RJ. The use of a free flap in homozygous sickle cell disease. *Plast Reconstr Surg* 1985;76(4):616–619.

304. Gilsanz F, Escalante F, Auray C, et al. Treatment of leg ulcers in beta-thalassaemia intermedia: use of platelet-derived wound healing factors from the patient's own platelets. *Br J Haematol* 2001;115(3):710.

305. Papanas N, Maltezos E. Benefit-risk assessment of becaplermin in the treatment of diabetic foot ulcers. *Drug Saf* 2010;33(6):455–461.

306. Marcelo D, Beatriz PM, Jussara R, et al. Tissue therapy with autologous dermal and epidermal culture cells for diabetic foot ulcers. *Cell Tissue Bank* 2012;13(2):241–249.

307. Casey G, van Rij A. Manuka honey and leg ulcers. *N Z Med J* 1997;110(1045):216.

308. Gethin G, Cowman S. Case series of use of manuka honey in leg ulceration. *Int Wound J* 2005;2(1):10–15.

309. Queiroz AM, Campos J, Lobo C, et al. Leg amputation for an extensive, severe and intractable sickle cell anemia ulcer in a Brazilian patient. *Hemoglobin* 2014;38(2):95–98.

310. Maximo C, Olalla Saad ST, Thome E, et al. Amputations in sickle cell disease: case series and literature review. *Hemoglobin* 2016;40(3):150–155.

311. Dissemond J. Medications. A rare cause for leg ulcers. *Hautarzt* 2011;62(7): 516–523.

312. Kikuchi K, Arita K, Tateishi Y, et al. Recurrence of hydroxyurea-induced leg ulcer after discontinuation of treatment. *Acta Derm Venereol* 2011;91(3):373–374.

313. Nzoukakou R, Bachir D, Lavaud A, et al. Clinical follow-up of hydroxyurea-treated adults with sickle cell disease. *Acta Haematol* 2011;125(3): 145–152.

314. Konotey-Ahulu FI. Mental-nerve neuropathy: a complication of sickle-cell crisis. *Lancet* 1972;2(7773):388.

315. Kirson LE, Tomaro AJ. Mental nerve paresthesia secondary to sickle-cell crisis. *Oral Surg Oral Med Oral Pathol* 1979;48(6):509–512.

316. Asher SW. Multiple cranial neuropathies, trigeminal neuralgia, and vascular headaches in sickle cell disease, a possible common mechanism. *Neurology* 1980;30(2):210–211.

317. Shields RW Jr, Harris JW, Clark M. Mononeuropathy in sickle cell anemia: anatomical and pathophysiological basis for its rarity. *Muscle Nerve* 1991;14(4):370–374.

318. Ballas SK, Reyes PE. Peripheral neuropathy in adults with sickle cell disease. *Am J Pain Med* 1997;71:53–58.

319. Salvin ML, Barondes MJ. Ischemic optic neuropathy in sickle cell disease. *Am J Ophthalmology* 1988;105:221–223.

320. Blank JP, Gill FM. Orbital infarction in sickle cell disease. *Pediatrics* 1981;67(6):879–881.

321. Al-Rashid RA. Orbital apex syndrome secondary to sickle cell anemia. *J Pediatr* 1979;95(3):426–427.

322. Rothman SM, Nelson JS. Spinal cord infarction in a patient with sickle cell anemia. *Neurology* 1980;30(10):1072–1076.

323. Erbas T, Ertas M, Yucel A, et al. Prevalence of peripheral neuropathy and painful peripheral neuropathy in Turkish diabetic patients. *J Clin Neurophysiol* 2011;28(1):51–55.

324. Ballas SK, Darbari DS. Neuropathy, neuropathic pain, and sickle cell disease. *Am J Hematol* 2013;88(11):927–929.

325. Benjamin LJ, Payne R. Pain in sickle cell disease: a multidimensional construct. In: Pace B, ed. *Renaissance of Sickle Cell Disease Research in the Genomic Era*. London: Imperial College Press; 2007:99–118.

326. Benjamin LJ, Dampier CD, Jacox AK. *Guideline for the Management of Acute and Chronic Pain in Sickle Cell Disease*. Glenview, IL: American Pain Society; 1999.

327. Dunlop RJ, Bennett KC. Pain management for sickle cell disease. *Cochrane Database Syst Rev* 2006;(2):CD003350.

328. Todd KH, Green C, Bonham VL Jr, et al. Sickle cell disease related pain: crisis and conflict. *J Pain* 2006;7(7):453–458.

329. Green CR, Anderson KO, Baker TA, et al. The unequal burden of pain: confronting racial and ethnic disparities in pain. *Pain Med* 2003;4(3):277–294.

330. Labbe E, Herbert D, Haynes J. Physicians' attitude and practices in sickle cell disease pain management. *J Palliat Care* 2005;21(4):246–251.

331. Lipton RB, Stewart WF, Ryan RE Jr, et al. Efficacy and safety of acetaminophen, aspirin, and caffeine in alleviating migraine headache pain: three double-blind, randomized, placebo-controlled trials. *Arch Neurol* 1998;55(2):210–217.

332. Sunshine A, Olzon NZ. Non-narcotic analgesics. In: Wall PD, Melzack R, eds. *Textbook of Pain*. 2nd ed. New York: Churchill Livingstone; 1989:670–685.

333. Ferrante M. Non-steroidal anti-inflammatory drugs. In: Ferrante M, VadeBoncouer TR, eds. *Postoperative Pain Management*. New York: Churchill Livingstone; 1993:133–143.

334. Kopecky EA, Jacobson S, Joshi P, et al. Systemic exposure to morphine and the risk of acute chest syndrome in sickle cell disease. *Clin Pharmacol Ther* 2004;75(3):140–146.

335. Buchanan ID, Woodward M, Reed GW. Opioid selection during sickle cell pain crisis and its impact on the development of acute chest syndrome. *Pediatr Blood Cancer* 2005;45(5):716–724.

336. Weber ML, Hebbel RP, Gupta K. Morphine induces kidney injuryin transgenic sickle cell mice. *Blood* 2005;106(suppl 1):884a–885a.

337. Gupta K, Chen C, Lutty GA, et al. Morphine exaggerates retinopathy in transgenic sickle mice [abstract no. 209]. *Blood* 2005;106(suppl 1):64a–65a.

338. Loeser JD, Butler SH, Chapman CR, et al. *Bonica's Management of Pain*. 3rd ed. Philadelphia: Lippincott Williams & Wilkins; 2001.

339. Ballas SK. *Sickle Cell Pain*. 2nd ed. Washington DC: International Association for the Study of Pain; 2014.

340. World Health Organization. *Cancer Pain Relief*. Geneva, Switzerland: World Health Organization; 1986.

341. Jacox A, Carr DB, Payne R. New clinical-practice guidelines for the management of pain in patients with cancer. *N Engl J Med* 1994;330(9):651–655.

342. Jaffe JH, Martin WR. Opioid analgesics and antagonists. In: Goodman LS, Gilman A, Rall TW, et al, eds. *Goodman and Gilman's the Pharmacological Basis of Therapeutics*. 8th ed. New York: Pergamon Press; 1990:485–521.

343. Khojasteh A, Evans W, Reynolds RD, et al. Controlled release morphine in the treatment of cancer pain with pharmacokinetic correlation. *J Clin Oncol* 1987;5:956–961.

344. Payne R. Pain management in sickle cell disease. Rationale and techniques. *Ann N Y Acad Sci* 1989;565:189–206.

345. Rowbotham DJ, Wyld R, Peacock JE, et al. Transdermal fentanyl for the relief of pain after upper abdominal surgery. *Br J Anaesth* 1989;63(1):56–59.

346. Elander J, Lusher J, Bevan D, et al. Understanding the causes of problematic pain management in sickle cell disease: evidence that pseudoaddiction plays a more important role than genuine analgesic dependence. *J Pain Symptom Manage* 2004;27(2):156–169.

347. Elander J, Marczewska M, Amos R, et al. Factors affecting hospital staff judgments about sickle cell disease pain. *J Behav Med* 2006;29(2):203–214.

348. Biedrzycki OJ, Bevan D, Lucas S. Fatal overdose due to prescription fentanyl patches in a patient with sickle cell/beta-thalassemia and acute chest syndrome: a case report and review of the literature. *Am J Forensic Med Pathol* 2009;30(2):188–190.

349. Ballas SK. More definitions in sickle cell disease: steady state v base line data. *Am J Hematol* 2012;87(3):338.

350. Adewoye AH, Nolan V, McMahon L, et al. Effectiveness of a dedicated day hospital for management of acute sickle cell pain. *Haematologica* 2007;92(6):854–855.

351. van Beers EJ, van Tuijn CF, Nieuwkerk PT, et al. Patient-controlled analgesia versus continuous infusion of morphine during vaso-occlusive crisis in sickle cell disease, a randomized controlled trial. *Am J Hematol* 2007;82(11): 955–960.

352. Ballas SK, Kesen MR, Goldberg MF, et al. Beyond the definitions of the phenotypic complications of sickle cell disease: an update on management. *ScientificWorldJournal* 2012;2012:949535.

353. Stevens MC, Padwick M, Serjeant GR. Observations on the natural history of dactylitis in homozygous sickle cell disease. *Clin Pediatr (Phila)* 1981;20(5):311–317.

354. Charache S, Barton FB, Moore RD, et al. Hydroxyurea and sickle cell anemia. Clinical utility of a myelosuppressive "switching" agent. The Multicenter Study of Hydroxyurea in Sickle Cell Anemia. *Medicine* 1996;75(6):300–326.

355. Shaiova L, Wallenstein D. Outpatient management of sickle cell pain with chronic opioid pharmacotherapy. *J Natl Med Assoc* 2004;96(7):984–986.

356. Ballas SK, Barton FB, Waclawiw MA, et al. Hydroxyurea and sickle cell anemia: effect on quality of life. *Health Qual Life Outcomes* 2006;4:59.

357. Kinney TR, Helms RW, O'Branski EE, et al. Safety of hydroxyurea in children with sickle cell anemia: results of the HUG-KIDS study, a phase I/II trial. Pediatric Hydroxyurea Group. *Blood* 1999;94(5):1550–1554.

358. Wang WC, Wynn LW, Rogers ZR, et al. A two-year pilot trial of hydroxyurea in very young children with sickle-cell anemia. *J Pediatr* 2001;139(6): 790–796.

359. Hankins JS, Ware RE, Rogers ZR, et al. Long-term hydroxyurea therapy for infants with sickle cell anemia: the HUSOFT extension study. *Blood* 2005;106(7):2269–2275.

360. Wang WC, Ware RE, Miller ST, et al. Hydroxycarbamide in very young children with sickle-cell anaemia: a multicentre, randomised, controlled trial (BABY HUG). *Lancet* 2011;377(9778):1663–1672.

361. Alvarez O, Miller ST, Wang WC, et al. Effect of hydroxyurea treatment on renal function parameters: results from the multi-center placebo-controlled BABY HUG clinical trial for infants with sickle cell anemia. *Pediatr Blood Cancer* 2012;59(4):668–674.

362. Aygun B, Mortier NA, Smeltzer MP, et al. Hydroxyurea treatment decreases glomerular hyperfiltration in children with sickle cell anemia. *Am J Hematol* 2013;88(2):116–119.

363. Lebensburger JD, Miller ST, Howard TH, et al. Influence of severity of anemia on clinical findings in infants with sickle cell anemia: analyses from the BABY HUG study. *Pediatr Blood Cancer* 2012;59(4):675–678.

364. Steinberg MH, Barton F, Castro O, et al. Effect of hydroxyurea on mortality and morbidity in adult sickle cell anemia: risks and benefits up to 9 years of treatment. *JAMA* 2003;289(13):1645–1651.

365. Steinberg MH, McCarthy WF, Castro O, et al. The risks and benefits of long-term use of hydroxyurea in sickle cell anemia: a 17.5 year follow-up. *Am J Hematol* 2010;85(6):403–408.

366. Moore RD, Charache S, Terrin ML, et al. Cost-effectiveness of hydroxyurea in sickle cell anemia. Investigators of the Multicenter Study of Hydroxyurea in Sickle Cell Anemia. *Am J Hematol* 2000;64(1):26–31.

367. Smith WR, Ballas SK, McCarthy WF, et al. The association between hydroxyurea treatment and pain intensity, analgesic use, and utilization in ambulatory sickle cell anemia patients. *Pain Med* 2011;12(5):697–705.

368. Ballas SK, Bauserman RL, McCarthy WF, et al. The impact of hydroxyurea on career and employment of patients with sickle cell anemia. *J Natl Med Assoc* 2010;102(11):993–999.

369. Ballas SK, Marcolina MJ, Dover GJ, et al. Erythropoietic activity in patients with sickle cell anaemia before and after treatment with hydroxyurea. *Br J Haematol* 1999;105(2):491–496.

370. Ballas SK, Dover GJ, Charache S. Effect of hydroxyurea on the rheological properties of sickle erythrocytes in vivo. *Am J Hematol* 1989;32(2):104–111.

371. Drugs contributor. Hydroxyurea. *Drugs.com*. Available at: http://www.drugs.com/ppa/hydroxyurea.html. Accessed August 28, 2017.

372. Charache S, Terrin ML, Moore RD, et al. Design of the multicenter study of hydroxyurea in sickle cell anemia. Investigators of the Multicenter Study of Hydroxyurea. *Control Clin Trials* 1995;16(6):432–446.

373. Miller ST, Rey K, He J, et al. Massive accidental overdose of hydroxyurea in a young child with sickle cell anemia. *Pediatr Blood Cancer* 2012;59(1):170–172.

374. Ware RE, Rees RC, Sarnaik SA, et al. Renal function in infants with sickle cell anemia: baseline data from the BABY HUG trial. *J Pediatr* 2010;156(1):66–70.

375. Kaul DK, Tsai HM, Liu XD, et al. Monoclonal antibodies to alphaVbeta3 (7E3 and LM609) inhibit sickle red blood cell-endothelium interactions induced by platelet-activating factor. *Blood* 2000;95(2):368–374.

376. Ohnishi ST, Ohnishi T, Ogunmola GB. Green tea extract and aged garlic extract inhibit anion transport and sickle cell dehydration in vitro. *Blood Cells Mol Dis* 2001;27(1):148–157.

377. Ballas SK. Hydration of sickle erythrocytes using a herbal extract (Pfaffia paniculata) in vitro. *Br J Haematol* 2000;111(1):359–362.

378. Singh PC, Ballas SK. Emerging drugs for sickle cell anemia. *Expert Opin Emerg Drugs* 2015;20(1):47–61.

379. Johnson FL, Look AT, Gockerman J, et al. Bone-marrow transplantation in a patient with sickle-cell anemia. *N Engl J Med* 1984;311(12):780–783.

380. Johnson FL, Mentzer WC, Kalinyak KA, et al. Bone marrow transplantation for sickle cell disease. The United States experience. *Am J Pediatr Hematol Oncol* 1994;16(1):22–26.

381. Mentzer WC, Packman S, Wara W. Successful bone marrow transplant in a child with sickle cell anemia and Morquio's disease [abstract]. *Blood* 1990;76:69a.

382. Vermylen C, Cornu G. Bone marrow transplantation for sickle cell disease. The European experience. *Am J Pediatr Hematol Oncol* 1994;16(1):18–21.

383. Vermylen C, Cornu G, Ferster A, et al. Haematopoietic stem cell transplantation for sickle cell anaemia: the first 50 patients transplanted in Belgium. *Bone Marrow Transplant* 1998;22(1):1–6.

384. Walters MC. Bone marrow transplantation for sickle cell disease: where do we go from here? *J Pediatr Hematol Oncol* 1999;21(6):467–474.

385. Buchanan G, Vichinsky E, Krishnamurti L, et al. Severe sickle cell disease—pathophysiology and therapy. *Biol Blood Marrow Transplant* 2010;16 (1 suppl):S64–S67.

386. Krishnamurti L, Kharbanda S, Biernacki MA, et al. Stable long-term donor engraftment following reduced-intensity hematopoietic cell transplantation for sickle cell disease. *Biol Blood Marrow Transplant* 2008;14(11):1270–1278.

387. Shenoy S, Grossman WJ, DiPersio J, et al. A novel reduced-intensity stem cell transplant regimen for nonmalignant disorders. *Bone Marrow Transplant* 2005;35(4):345–352.

388. Walters MC, Patience M, Leisenring W, et al. Barriers to bone marrow transplantation for sickle cell anemia. *Biol Blood Marrow Transplant* 1996;2(2):100–104.

389. Walters MC, Quirolo L, Trachtenberg ET, et al. Sibling donor cord blood transplantation for thalassemia major: Experience of the Sibling Donor Cord Blood Program. *Ann N Y Acad Sci* 2005;1054:206–213.

390. Al Jefri AH. Advances in allogeneic stem cell transplantation for hemoglobinopathies. *Hemoglobin* 2011;35(5–6):469–475.

391. Friedrich MJ. Advances reshaping sickle cell therapy. *JAMA* 2011;305(3):239–240.

392. Locatelli F, Pagliara D. Allogeneic hematopoietic stem cell transplantation in children with sickle cell disease. *Pediatr Blood Cancer* 2012;59(2):372–376.

393. Forget B, G. Gene therapy. In: Embury SH, Hebble RP, Mohandas N, et al, eds. *Sickle Cell Disease: Basic Principles and Clinical Practice*. New York: Raven Press; 1994:853–860.

394. Cole-Strauss A, Yoon K, Xiang Y, et al. Correction of the mutation responsible for sickle cell anemia by an RNA-DNA oligonucleotide. *Science* 1996;273(5280):1386–1389.

395. Cavazzana-Calvo M, Payen E, Negre O, et al. Transfusion independence and HMGA2 activation after gene therapy of human beta-thalassaemia. *Nature* 2010;467(7313):318–322.

396. Dong A, Rivella S, Breda L. Gene therapy for hemoglobinopathies: progress and challenges. *Transl Res* 2013;161(4):293–306.

397. Payen E, Leboulch P. Advances in stem cell transplantation and gene therapy in the β-hemoglobinopathies. *Hematology Am Soc Hematol Educ Program* 2012;2012:276–283.

398. Persons DA. Hematopoietic stem cell gene transfer for the treatment of hemoglobin disorders. *Hematology Am Soc Hematol Educ Program* 2009:690–697.

399. Hanna J, Wernig M, Markoulaki S, et al. Treatment of sickle cell anemia mouse model with iPS cells generated from autologous skin. *Science* 2007;318(5858):1920–1923.

CHAPTER 58

Pain in HIV

SVETLANA FAKTOROVICH and **DAVID M. SIMPSON**

On June 5, 1981, the Centers for Disease Control and Prevention (CDC) described five cases of a rare lung infection, *Pneumocystis carinii* along with other unusual opportunistic infection in previously healthy, young homosexual men, two of whom died by the time of publication. This was the first report of a disease that has become known as HIV/AIDS, tremendously impacting the health and economy of many countries around the world.

There are currently around 36.9 million people living with HIV around the world.[1] With the development of antiretroviral combination therapy (ART), life expectancy has improved and the rates of opportunistic infections and malignancies have dramatically declined. However, despite medical advancements, this disease remains one of the most complex entities in the realm of human illness, with the potential of affecting any system of the human body.

Pain remains a common and difficult to manage symptom in HIV-infected patients, both early in the course of the disease as well as in the later stages. Resulting in psychological distress, decreased quality of life, and decreased functional ability, pain is one of the most significant causes of disability in HIV/AIDS.[2–4] It can vary dramatically in presentation, with one individual sometimes experiencing multiple types of pain simultaneously. Furthermore, management is especially complicated in the setting of comorbid mental illness and substance abuse, both of which are more prevalent in the HIV population.[5] Pain management therefore must be an essential part in the care of an HIV/AIDS patient.

This chapter focuses on pain syndromes afflicting the HIV/AIDS population with special focus on neurologic pain in these patients, along with regimens for pain management. Particular attention is also placed on higher risk populations.

Prevalence of Pain in HIV/AIDS

Pain has long been recognized as an important and disabling feature of HIV/AIDS. The development of combination therapy in the late 1990s has in many ways revolutionized the treatment of HIV, allowing patients to live long, relatively healthy lives. However, pain, estimated to affect 20% to 90% of those infected depending on the stage of the disease, remains a significant problem.[6–8]

Among HIV-positive individuals, studies suggest that 20% to 30% experience moderate- to severe-intensity pain.[7,9] However, the etiology can be variable, including unrelated comorbid conditions, HIV infection and its associated illnesses as well as side effects of ART. Not surprisingly, poorly controlled pain is a risk factor for comorbid depression and poor compliance on ART.

One study conducted in the United Kingdom by Lawson et al.[8] looked at more than 800 HIV-positive subjects in an outpatient setting, of whom 62.8% reported pain over the prior month. Of those subjects, 58% were otherwise asymptomatic (CDC category A) and 76% were on ART. Most experienced pain that day, with a median of two areas affected. However, up to 24% reported whole-body pain. Another multicenter study reported more than 300 individuals with HIV in an ambulatory setting and demonstrated prevalence of pain in 55% of subjects, 82% of whom rated the intensity at "severe–very severe."[10] Those reporting pain were more likely to have a lower

CD4 count as well as comorbid medical problems. Notably, these findings are similar to those of several studies conducted in the pre-ART era, when AIDS was the inevitable outcome of HIV infection.[11–12]

The majority of the literature available focuses mainly on acute/subacute pain in HIV. However, as this population ages, chronic pain, defined as greater than 3 months duration, has become an important, although poorly studied, problem. Lawson et al.[8] found the mean duration of pain in their subjects to be 3 years. Another prospective study conducted in Denmark in the pre-ART era found that lower extremities were the most common site of pain, followed by head, gastrointestinal (GI) tract, and muscles/bones. Of those who suffered from pain for longer than 1 year, neuropathic pain was the predominant cause.

Pain in Women with HIV/AIDS

Multiple studies on the treatment of pain in HIV/AIDS have noted greater reported pain intensity among seropositive women than their male counterparts.[11,13] Disproportionate undertreatment of pain is at least in part to blame. Breitbart et al.[14] estimated that women were twice as likely to be undertreated as men. However, the cause for this difference is unknown. Physicians' view of women as well as patient-specific factors, such as unwillingness to report pain, fear of addiction to pain medication, and wanting to be a "good patient" have all been considered.

In addition, several pain syndromes exist that are unique to women. Opportunistic infections and malignancies of the pelvic and genitourinary tract can be a significant cause of pain. HIV-infected women have a higher rate of gynecologic surgeries such hysterectomy for cervical neoplasia and resection of tuboovarian abscesses from pelvic inflammatory disease.[15] Disorders of the menstrual cycle also occur. Heavy menses, or menorrhagia, seen in the setting of thrombocytopenia associated directly with HIV or secondary to ART such as indinavir, can be a significant cause of pain.[16]

Certain disorders of aging, such as osteoporosis with secondary bone fractures, are also being seen with higher frequency in the HIV population, both from HIV-induced bone loss and long-term effects of ART.[15,17] Although not restricted to the female gender, this risk becomes especially high in HIV-infected peri- and postmenopausal women.

Pain in Children with HIV/AIDS

Children infected with HIV also suffer from pain, with an estimated prevalence of 20% to 60%.[18,19] Similar to adults, pain in children can be complex and related to the disease process itself, opportunistic infections or secondary to treatment. One large prospective cohort study of HIV-infected children found higher incidence of pain with female gender and lower CD4 count.[18] The most common, pain-specific diagnoses included candidiasis, varicella zoster infection, and sinusitis. Furthermore, several studies suggest that pain in children with HIV is associated with increased mortality.[18] However, treating children is often complicated by reluctance by both physicians and parents to use strong analgesics as well as the challenges in quantitating pain in the younger ages.

Specific Pain Syndromes in HIV/AIDS

GASTROINTESTINAL PAIN

The GI tract is a common site of complications for the HIV/AIDS population. Opportunistic infections and HIV-related neoplasms are especially seen in patients that are either non-compliant or fail ART. When evaluating a patient with GI symptoms, the first step is to identify the level of immunodeficiency, including whether the patient is on ART or is treatment-naive. CD4 count is the best serologic marker for immune status. Those with CD4 less than 200 cells/mm³ are at greatest risk for an opportunistic infection, with a further exponential increase at CD4 less than 100 cells/mm³.[20] Treating the underlying problem is the primary treatment goal, although analgesia is often required especially in the acute setting.

OROPHARYNGEAL PAIN

Oral and throat pain is a very commonly seen symptom in HIV. Candidiasis of the oral cavity, which often presents as white lesions or red patches, has been estimated to affect 50% to 95% of HIV-infected patients at some point in their disease course.[21] It is one of the most common causes of oral pain, although can be asymptomatic. Oral candidiasis can also be one of the first signs of HIV infection and therefore warrants testing in a patient without a known immunodeficiency. Although most commonly caused by *Candida albicans*, other *Candida* species have been identified.[22] Necrotizing periodontal diseases, such as necrotizing gingivitis and ulcerative periodontitis, are also strongly associated with HIV infection.[23] Multiple viruses including Herpes simplex (HSV), cytomegalovirus (CMV), Epstein-Barr virus (EBV), invasive fungal species, and bacteria have been implicated in some of these cases.

ESOPHAGEAL PAIN

Although esophageal symptoms are often unrelated to HIV disease, opportunistic disease can be seen including in patients on ART. One study evaluated seropositive patients undergoing endoscopy and found an opportunistic infection in 26% of subjects on highly active antiretroviral therapy (HAART), 48% of subjects on non-ART mono- or polytherapy (no protease inhibitor), and 80% of those not on any ART.[24] In patients with upper GI symptoms (e.g., odynophagia, nausea, vomiting, hematemesis) with AIDS, an upper endoscopy results in a diagnosis in approximately 75% of patients.[25] *C. albicans* is the most common infectious agent affecting the esophageal tract in HIV, followed by viruses (e.g., CMV esophagitis and duodenitis, HSV esophagitis).[20]

Candida esophagitis is typically seen in the setting of a CD4 count less than 200 cells/mm³, whereas *Mycobacterium avium* complex (MAC) is typically seen at when CD4 falls below 50 cells/mm³. CMV, the most common agent causing viral esophagitis, occurs with CD4 below 100 cells/mm³.[26] Upper endoscopy is the standard of care for upper GI symptoms, and in patients where an opportunistic infection is suspected, aggressive tissue sampling and biopsy should be done. In CMV disease, for example, multiple biopsies may increase the likelihood of diagnosis.[27] Kaposi sarcoma and lymphoma can also cause invasive disease of the esophagus, resulting in dysphagia, pain, and ulceration.[28]

ABDOMINAL PAIN

Abdominal pain is another common site of pain in the HIV/AIDS population and in many cases may be associated with diarrhea. Prevalence among AIDS patients has been estimated to be 12% to 20%.[29–31] In addition to the common causes of abdominal pain in non-HIV patients, inflammation and direct mucosal invasion by HIV, opportunistic infections, and neoplasms are all potential causes to consider when evaluating an HIV patient.[32] The risk of opportunistic infections and neoplasms is related to the level of immunosuppression. For patients with CD4 count less than 100 cells/mm³, for example, pathogens to consider include CMV, *Cryptosporidium*, and *Microsporidium*.[20] Colitis secondary to MAC infection, seen with CD4 less than 100 cells/mm³, is increasingly rare in the ART era. This entity is mostly seen in patients that first present with late-stage HIV.[33]

CMV is the most common opportunistic pathogen of the bowel, with abdominal pain often being the primary presenting symptom. In addition, small and large bowel perforation has been described with CMV ileitis.[34] Furthermore, with patients being on ART and various prophylactic antimicrobial agents, drug-induced side effects and *Clostridium difficile* colitis must also be considered. Lymphoma of the GI tract can also present with abdominal pain potentially leading to intestinal obstruction or perforation. Diffuse large B-cell lymphoma (DLBCL) and mucosa-associated lymphoid tissue (MALT) lymphoma are the most common subtypes of GI lymphomas.[35]

Pancreatitis is another potential cause of abdominal pain. Acute pancreatitis, often presenting with severe epigastric pain, nausea, vomiting, and fever, has an estimated yearly incidence of 0.6% to 15% in HIV-infected individuals.[36,37] Medication-induced pancreatic toxicity is considered the most common cause and has been well described with various agents including but not limited to nucleoside analogues, pentamidine, nonnucleoside reverse transcriptase inhibitors (NNRTIs) and protease inhibitors (PIs).[38] Furthermore, hypertriglyceridemia secondary to ART is associated with pancreatitis. Identification and discontinuation of the offending agent is critical. Treatment is otherwise supportive. Multiple opportunistic infections have also been implicated, usually in the setting of disseminated infection. These agents include CMV, MAC, *Cryptococcus*, *Mycobacterium tuberculosis*, and toxoplasmosis.[39] However, their incidence in causing pancreatitis is unclear given that many of these patients have also had exposure to pancreotoxic agents. In addition, pancreatitis has also been described as part of primary HIV infection with multisystem involvement.[40] Comorbid conditions such as alcohol abuse should also be considered.

Hepatobiliary symptoms, including right upper quadrant pain, are other common sites of pain. Opportunistic infections can be responsible for these cases, typically with CD4 count less than 50 cells/mm³, suggesting this is part of a systemic disseminated disease process, with MAC being the mostly frequently seen pathogen.[33] One study reporting liver biopsies and autopsies in AIDS patients with liver disease found 38% of specimens testing positive for MAC.[41] Hepatic tuberculosis can occur earlier in the disease course. CMV and cryptosporidial infections have also been described as causes of cholecystitis and secondary sclerosing cholangitis.[42] Drug-induced liver injury (DILI) is also a common adverse effect of ART and antituberculous drugs, including but not limited to efavirenz, pyrazinamide, and isoniazid.[43] It is estimated that 8% to 23% of patients on HAART will develop DILI.[44,45]

ANORECTAL

It is estimated that up to 30% of HIV-infected patients experience anorectal symptoms during the course of their illness.[46] Pain is the most common presenting symptom, affecting more than 50% of individuals.[47,48] Other common symptoms include rectal bleeding, discharge, and pruritus. Anorectal ulcers are a common cause of pain. Although most commonly idiopathic, malignancy and infectious causes including HSV, CMV, mycobacteria, and syphilis must be ruled out. It is also important to note that other sexually transmitted diseases can present in the anorectal region especially in homosexual individuals, including gonorrhea, chlamydia, and *M. tuberculosis* especially in cases of nonhealing ulcers. Perirectal abscesses are also common, typically presenting with fever and pain, and generally require surgical drainage.

Anorectal malignancy is also a major concern in HIV patients. Anal squamous intraepithelial lesions have a very high rate of occurrence in HIV-infected men that practice anal intercourse and can progress into anal cancer, although rate of progression is unknown. Risk factors include HPV subtypes 16 and 18, perirectal HSV, low CD4 count, and cigarette smoking.[46] Lymphoma and disseminated Kaposi sarcoma can also present as perianal lesions.

Chest Pain Syndromes

Chest pain is another complaint seen among HIV-infected patients, with estimated occurrence of 13% in one outpatient based study.[31] Multiple potential etiologies include but are not limited to cardiac, pulmonary, mediastinal, and esophageal. The latter is discussed in the section entitled "Gastrointestinal Pain."

CARDIAC PAIN

Multiple studies have suggested that HIV-infected patients are at risk of early coronary artery disease (CAD), although the exact relationship is not fully understood. Hyperlipidemia and insulin resistance secondary to PIs are significant contributors, although necropsy studies prior to use of these agents also showed high rates of early CAD.[49–52] Presentation of CAD may potentially differ in HIV-infected patients compared to noninfected individuals, with one study suggesting pain being a less prominent symptom in HIV patients.[53]

PULMONARY/PLEURITIC PAIN

Pulmonary infections are another important entity, typically presenting with fever, chills, cough, and occasionally pleuritic chest pain. Bacterial pneumonia is up to 25 times more common in HIV-infected patients, with the median CD4 count in affected patients being 200 cells/ mm³.[54] Recurrent bacterial pneumonias is considered an AIDS-defining illness. *Streptococcus pneumoniae* is the most common pathogen in both HIV-positive and HIV-negative individuals in the community, followed by *Haemophilus influenzae* and *Staphylococcus aureus*. Other, less common infectious agents include *Nocardia asteroides* and *Legionella*. *Pneumocystis pneumonia*, another AIDS-defining illness, can be associated with pneumothorax.

Malignancies can also be a source of pleuritic pain. Primary lung cancer is a leading cause of cancer death in HIV-positive patients. Although there is a higher rate of cigarette use among this population, HIV is considered an independent risk factor for lung cancer for unclear mechanisms.[55] In addition, opportunistic malignancies such as Kaposi sarcoma and lymphoma can involve pain. Furthermore, HIV is considered a prothrombotic state especially in advanced disease states, with a higher rate of pulmonary embolism than the general population.[56]

CHEST WALL PAIN

Osteomyelitis of the chest wall is a rare entity, with *S. aureus* and *Pseudomonas aeruginosa* being the most common infectious agents.[57] Tuberculosis can also cause abscesses within the chest wall, constituting up to 5% of musculoskeletal cases of tuberculosis.[58] Lymphoma, especially non-Hodgkin type, has also been known to present within the chest wall.

Musculoskeletal Pain

ARTHROPATHY

Arthralgia, including pain and stiffness of the joints, is a common symptom reported by HIV patients. It most commonly affects the knee, elbow, and shoulder and occurs intermittently. Studies have shown variable prevalence, and it remains unclear whether its presentation differs from that in the general population.[59,60]

HIV-associated arthritis is a controversial disease entity that has been described in advanced HIV since 1988, with a reported prevalence between 0.4% and 13.8%.[60] According to one study, it manifests as an acute-onset, large-joint arthritis, lasting less than 6 weeks, without radiologic changes, in individuals that are HLA-B27–negative and do not fit any other known rheumatologic or infectious arthritis.[61] Assuming its existence, this condition is self-limiting and responds to oral anti-inflammatory agents and intra-articular steroid injection.

Reactive arthritis triggered by multiple infectious agents, most commonly sexually transmitted diseases, is also seen among HIV patients. Reiter's syndrome, involving the triad of arthritis, urethritis, and conjunctivitis, has been described in association with the HIV itself, although studies have not clearly demonstrated an increased prevalence of this condition compared to the general population.[62–64] A wide range of inflammatory arthropathies such as psoriatic arthritis and rheumatoid arthritis (RA) can also be seen in HIV patients. Pre-ART studies suggest that remission or improvement of RA may occur in the setting of HIV, presumably secondary to CD4+ helper lymphocyte depletion.[65,66] However, more recent research has demonstrated that both conditions can exist simultaneously.[67]

Management of autoimmune arthritis in this population depends on the disease severity and level of immunosuppression. Most mild cases do well with oral, nonsteroidal anti-inflammatory medications (NSAIDs). Moderate-severity arthritis often responds better to intra-articular steroid injection. In severe cases, oral steroids and disease-modifying therapies such as hydroxychloroquine and methotrexate have been used safely in patients on ART, with close monitoring of their CD4 count and viral load.[59,68,69]

Septic arthritis is uncommon in the HIV population, with an estimated prevalence of 1% in one study, although appears to be more frequent in developing countries and among IV drug users.[59,67] *Staphylococcus aureus* and *Streptococcus pneumoniae* are the two most common infectious agents, most often involving the knees.[70,71] There is a poor correlation between CD4 count and septic joints secondary to these typical bacterial infections.[70] However, opportunistic infections of the joints, such as atypical mycobacteria and fungal infections including *Candida* and *Nocardia*, typically occur in individuals with CD4 count less than 100/mm³.

OSTEOPOROSIS

Osteoporosis and osteopenia also have an increased prevalence in the HIV population, making these individuals at higher risk of bone fractures. ART, specifically PIs are largely responsible for this.[72] Furthermore, HIV itself may play a role as well as comorbidities commonly seen with HIV including hypogonadism, liver disease, kidney disease, and malnutrition.[72,73]

Neurologic Manifestations

PERIPHERAL NEUROPATHY

Peripheral neuropathy (PN) is the most common neurologic complaint in HIV patients. Although studies have shown significant variability, PN is thought to affect between 30% to 60% of infected individuals.[74,75] Although most frequently seen in older patients with later stages of illness, this condition is known to affect all stages of HIV. Furthermore, with the development of ART, patients are living longer lives, and as a result, the prevalence of this condition is increasing.[76] PN is thought to be influenced by several factors, including the HIV itself, the neurotoxic effect of the ART, as well as other comorbidities. Multiple types of neuropathy can occur, and here, we address the ones that have pain as a major symptom. Table 58.1 outlines many of these conditions.

TABLE 58.1   Neuropathy in HIV

Immune-Mediated Neuropathy

1. Distal symmetric polyneuropathy
2. Inflammatory demyelinating polyneuropathy
   a. Acute inflammatory demyelinating polyneuropathy (AIDP or Guillain-Barré syndrome)
   b. Chronic inflammatory demyelinating polyneuropathy (CIDP)
3. Mononeuritis multiplex

Infectious Neuropathy

1. Progressive polyradiculopathy (PP)—typically cytomegalovirus (CMV) related, however can be due to other infectious agents or lymphoma
2. CMV-related mononeuritis multiplex—presentation similar to inflammatory presentation
3. HIV, herpes simplex virus (HSV), or herpes zoster virus (varicella zoster virus [VZV])-related mononeuropathy
4. Hepatitis C–related peripheral neuropathy with or without cryoglobulinemia
5. Other less common infectious neuropathies
   a. HSV radiculomyelitis
   b. VZV radiculitis

Toxic Neuropathy

1. Antiretroviral therapy
   a. Nucleoside reverse transcriptase inhibitors (NRTIs)
   b. Protease inhibitors (PIs)
2. Antibacterial agents
   a. Isoniazid
   b. Rifampin
   c. Ethambutol
   d. Nitrofurantoin
   e. Metronidazole
3. Antiviral
   a. Foscarnet
4. Vitamin deficiencies
   a. Vitamin B_{12}
   b. Vitamin B_6
   c. Vitamin D
5. Alcohol
6. Heavy metals

Other Medical Conditions

1. Diabetes
2. Hypo- or hyperthyroidism
3. Postherpetic neuralgia
4. Multiple myeloma
5. Autoimmune diseases
   a. Rheumatoid arthritis
   b. Sjögren's syndrome
   c. Systemic lupus erythematosus

DISTAL SYMMETRIC POLYNEUROPATHY

Distal symmetric polyneuropathy (DSP) is the most common type of polyneuropathy afflicting the HIV population. It is a predominantly sensory axonopathy that typically presents with symptoms including numbness, paresthesia, and burning-type pain. It progresses in a "stocking-glove" distribution, first in the soles of the feet and ascending up the body to later involve the hands. These individuals often also experience allodynia, sensation of pain to ordinarily nonpainful stimuli and hyperesthesia, and increased skin sensitivity. It is estimated to affect up to 35% of patients with HIV, many of whom are asymptomatic.[77] Studies have suggested that almost all HIV-infected patients at autopsy have pathologic evidence of peripheral neuropathy.

Neurologic testing usually reveals diminished or absent ankle reflexes, increased vibratory threshold, and decreased sensation to pain and temperature. Proprioception is typically preserved until later in the disease course. Muscle weakness

can also manifest in advanced stages. Electrodiagnostic studies may be useful in diagnosing this condition. Findings typically demonstrate symmetrical sensory and motor axonal damage despite predominantly sensory symptoms. Skin biopsy can also be helpful, demonstrating loss of epidermal nerve fibers that may correlate with clinical and electrodiagnostic severity of DSP as demonstrated by Zhou and colleagues.[78]

The risk and severity of DSP is associated with high HIV viral load, although it can be found in the setting of undetectable viral load.[79] The underlying pathogenesis of DSP from HIV infection is not fully understood. However, it is felt to be an indirect, immune-mediated process. Neuronal damage in DSP occurs from the production of neurotoxic, proinflammatory agents including free radicals and cytokines such as tumor necrosis factor alpha (TNF-α), interleukin (IL) 1, and IL-6.[80,81] Macrophage and lymphocyte infiltration along with presence of these cytokines has been found in dorsal root ganglia of AIDS patients. Plasma levels of TNF-α and IL-6 are higher in HIV-1–infected individuals.[82]

ART may help to prevent this neurotoxic process, likely via indirect immune-mediated mechanisms. However, several of the commonly used agents, including nucleoside reverse transcriptase inhibitors (NRTI) and PI are felt to have neurotoxic effects that also increase the risk of neuropathy. Two studies estimated the prevalence of ART-induced neuropathy in 8% and 16% of patients, although there is significant variability.[83,84] It can often be difficult to differentiate drug-induced from HIV-associated neuropathy. However, the primary feature that appears to distinguish the drug-induced form is the rapidly progressive course, with onset often within a few weeks of starting the medication and improvement after its discontinuation. It has been suggested that the greatest risk of developed ART-induced PN is within the first few months of starting the medication.[75]

TREATMENT OF HIV-ASSOCIATED SENSORY NEUROPATHY

Current guidelines on treating neuropathic pain, such as those by American Academy of Neurology, focus on other forms of PN, such as diabetic and postherpetic neuropathy, and therefore may not be equally applicable to HIV. Many classes of drugs, including antidepressants, antiepileptics, oral analgesics, and topical agents, have been used and studied in treating this disabling condition, while only targeting positive symptoms such as paresthesias and pain. Research has also mostly focused on symptomatic relief, not disease modification. One meta-analysis conducted by Phillips and colleagues[85] looked at 14 prospective, double-blind, randomized controlled trials studying 10 different pharmacologic therapies in HIV-related sensory neuropathy. Only 3 showed superiority over placebo, including high-dose topical capsaicin, smoked cannabis, and recombinant human nerve growth factor (rhNGF). The other agents such as amitriptyline, mexiletine, gabapentin, pregabalin, lamotrigine, and low-dose capsaicin cream did not show any significant benefit over placebo. Please refer to the treatment section for additional information on these agents.

INFLAMMATORY DEMYELINATING POLYNEUROPATHY

Since the 1980s, an association between HIV and inflammatory demyelinating polyneuropathy (IDP) has been recognized. It can occur at any point in the HIV disease course and can take on the form of acute inflammatory demyelinating polyneuropathy (AIDP), also known as Guillain-Barré syndrome, or the chronic form (chronic inflammatory demyelinating polyneuropathy [CIDP]). Presentation is often similar to those not infected by HIV. AIDP is typically monophasic with recovery occurring around 3 to 4 weeks and has been more commonly described during seroconversion, often with CD4 >200.[86,87] CIDP has a course of greater than 8 weeks. Clinical features include progressive, ascending weakness of the extremities with areflexia on exam and relative sparing of sensation. In addition, more than 80% of patients complain of moderate to severe pain, most commonly describing a deep, aching pain of the back or legs and dysesthesias of the extremities.[88]

The pathophysiology of IDP in early HIV cases is likely immune-mediated, as opposed to AIDS patients in whom opportunistic viral infections (such as CMV) may be the cause.[83]

Electrodiagnostic studies typically show a primary demyelinating neuropathy, with evidence of axonal loss in cases of CIDP. Cerebrospinal fluid (CSF) analysis is not as reliable in diagnosing IDP in HIV patients with high CD4 count as it is in the non-HIV population. CSF studies in HIV-negative patients with IDP typically show albuminocytologic dissociation including high protein without pleocytosis. High protein and mild lymphocytic pleocytosis can also be found in asymptomatic HIV-positive patients with high CD4 count.[89]

Treatment in early HIV is similar to non-HIV patients, including immunomodulating therapy such as intravenous immunoglobulin (IVIG), plasmapheresis, and corticosteroids but with caution due to their associated immunosuppressant effects. Antiviral therapy targeting CMV is used in AIDS patients with advanced immune compromise, especially when virologic studies or nerve biopsy indicate evidence of CMV infection.

MONONEURITIS MULTIPLEX

Mononeuritis multiplex (MM) typically manifests as asymmetric and multifocal peripheral neuropathies that can involve motor and sensory disturbances. Pain is also a common symptom, often described as a deep, aching pain; however, burning pain and allodynia in affected regions can also be seen.

Similar to IDP, MM can also occur anywhere in the HIV disease process. Cases early on are also likely immune-mediated, with a milder and often self-limiting course.[86] In late-stage HIV, an opportunistic infectious process is the likely cause, often with a worse prognosis. CMV infection of nerve fibers has been well established as a potential cause of MM in AIDS. HIV or coinfected hepatitis C–related vasculitis is also a potential cause of MM. Electrodiagnostic studies typically show multifocal axonal neuropathy.

PROGRESSIVE POLYRADICULOPATHY

Progressive polyradiculopathy (PP) typically occurs in advanced stages of HIV/AIDS and has a severe and rapidly progressive course. Presentation can resemble cauda equina syndrome, involving radicular pain, flaccid paraplegia, sensory changes, sphincter dysfunction, and areflexia.[76,77] Magnetic resonance imaging (MRI) with contrast is a helpful diagnostic study, both to rule out a compressive lesion as well as looking for signal changes/contrast enhancement of the lumbosacral roots.[90] CSF testing typically reveals a pleocytosis and positive CMV polymerase chain reaction (PCR) confirming the infection. Electrodiagnostic studies are also useful in supporting a polyradicular process. Due to risk of irreversible damage from root necrosis, early antiviral therapy for CMV is crucial, including agents such as ganciclovir and foscarnet.

INFLAMMATORY MYOPATHIES

HIV-associated polymyositis is the most common myopathy associated with HIV infection. Presentation is similar to that in noninfected patients, including a slowly progressive course affecting predominantly proximal muscles in a symmetrical distribution. Muscle pain in affected muscles is common. Diagnostic criteria include muscle weakness, elevated creatine kinase (CK), and evidence of myopathy on electrodiagnostic studies and muscle biopsy. Although no treatment guidelines have been established, immunomodulatory therapy including corticosteroids and IVIG has been successfully used.[90] Mechanisms

by which HIV leads to inflammatory myopathy are unclear. However, a T cell–mediated process has been proposed. A similar myopathy has also been described with immune reconstitution inflammatory syndrome (IRIS) as well as a potential side effect of zidovudine (ZDV).[91]

There have been various other myopathies seen in the setting of HIV, including pyomyositis secondary to opportunistic infections in AIDS patients, such as *S. aureus*. Dermatomyositis and inclusion body myositis have also been described.[90]

Headache

Headache is a very common symptom in the HIV population, affecting potentially up to 38% to 61% of individuals, especially in advanced stages of illness.[92] Etiology can vary widely. From benign migraine or tension headache to a life-threatening intracranial infection or malignancy, headaches can be a diagnostic dilemma for the treating physician.

PRIMARY HEADACHES

Migraine and tension-type headaches are the most common primary headaches seen in the HIV population.[93–95] Few studies have looked into the rates of primary headache phenotypes in this population and whether ART plays a role. Kirkland et al.[92] conducted one of the few large, post-ART studies characterizing headaches in the HIV/AIDS population, the majority of whom were on combination therapy. The overwhelming majority had primary headaches, most commonly migraines, with only 2.8% secondary to opportunistic encephalic infection. A significant inverse relationship was found between CD4 count and headache frequency, severity, and associated level of disability. Notably, there was no relationship with duration of HIV infection.

Commonly used migraine therapies are summarized in Table 58.2, including both preventative and abortive regimens. Opiates are not recommended for the use of aborting primary headaches due to poor efficacy and risk of medication overuse headache (MOH), especially in those with comorbid substance abuse problems. When choosing a regimen, comorbidities and other medications (including ART) must be considered. For example, ergotamines (such as dihydroergotamine) are contraindicated in patients taking PIs and NNRTIs due to risk of psychosis, seizures, and gangrene and are therefore are not typically used in the HIV population.

SECONDARY HEADACHES

HIV is able to easily cross the blood–brain barrier, allowing central nervous system (CNS) manifestation to occur at all stages of illness. Headache may be part of the prodromal illness of the primary infection of HIV-1, usually occurring 2 to 4 weeks after exposure, often described as a dull, bilateral ache.[92,96] Aseptic meningitis, characterized by fever, meningismus, and cranial neuropathies, can also occur with primary infection, usually self-limited but with the potential to recur at a later time.

The onset of headaches in a known HIV-infected patient warrants workup to rule out a wide range of secondary, opportunistic causes, especially with more advanced stages of illness even in the absence of focal neurologic deficits.

In the United States and other developed countries, the most common, focal infectious lesions in advanced disease include toxoplasmosis and progressive multifocal leukoencephalopathy (PML), caused by the John Cunningham (JC) virus.[97] The former often presents as focal granulomas or abscesses within the parenchyma, although leptomeningeal processes can also occur. The latter presents as focal, at times confluent lesions within the white matter. Focal neurologic deficits are common; however, presentations can be vague,

TABLE 58.2 Migraine Therapy

Prophylactic Agents

	Starting dose:	Optimal daily dose:	Additional conditions that may benefit:	Side effects include:	Caution:
Antidepressants					
Tricyclic antidepressants (TCAs)					
• Amitriptyline	10–25 mg at bedtime	25–150 mg daily (Tepper[171])	Depression, neuropathic pain, anxiety, sleep disturbance	Sedation, cardiac arrhythmia, anticholinergic side effects (constipation, blurred vision, urinary retention), cognitive dysfunction, extrapyramidal symptoms, narrow-angle glaucoma	Elderly, mood disorders as may increase suicidality, cardiovascular disease, seizure disorders, renal impairment; FDA box warning—risk of suicidality with antidepressants
• Nortriptyline	25 mg at bedtime	25–100 mg daily (Tepper[171])			
Serotonin norepinephrine reuptake inhibitors (SNRIs)					
• Venlafaxine	37.5 mg daily	150 mg daily (Tepper[171])	Depression, neuropathic pain, anxiety	Insomnia, drowsiness, anxiety, dizziness, nausea, sexual dysfunction, anorexia, hypertension, tachycardia, SIADH	Elderly, with other serotonergic drugs, seizure disorders, renal impairment; FDA box warning—risk of suicidality with antidepressants
• Duloxetine	30 mg daily	60–120 mg daily			
Antiepileptics					
• Valproic acid	250 mg BID	500–1,500 mg daily (Tepper[171])	Epilepsy, difficulty gaining weight, mood stabilization	Drowsiness, dizziness, alopecia, thrombocytopenia, tremor, pancreatitis, transaminitis, fetal neural tube defects, hyperammonemia	Women of childbearing age, hematologic disorders, mitochondrial disease; Contraindicated in severe hepatic disease and pregnancy
• Topiramate	15–25 mg daily	100 mg daily (Tepper[171])	Epilepsy, obesity, cluster headaches	Paresthesias, drowsiness, memory impairment, nephrolithiasis, secondary angle-closure glaucoma, hyperammonemia	Elderly, renal impairment, nephrolithiasis, glaucoma; Extended-release contraindicated on recent alcohol use
• Gabapentin	300 mg every 8 h	900–2,400 mg daily (Tepper[171])	Neuropathic pain, epilepsy, difficulty gaining weight	Dizziness, drowsiness, weight gain, leukopenia	Renal dysfunction
• Levetiracetam	250–500 mg BID	500–1,000 mg daily (Linde et al.[172])	Epilepsy	Agitation, suicidality, personality changes, sedation	Depression, behavioral disorders
β-Blockers					
• Propranolol	20 mg every 8–12 h	120–240 mg daily (Tepper[171])	Essential tremor, hypertension, cardiac arrhythmias	Bradycardia, hypotension, dizziness, disorientation, dyspnea, bronchospasm	Cardiac conduction abnormalities, compensated heart failure, peripheral vascular disease; Contraindicated in bronchial asthma, heart block greater than first degree
• Nadolol	20–40 mg daily	80–240 mg daily (Tepper[171])	Hypertension, cardiac arrhythmias		
• Atenolol	25 mg daily	100 mg daily (Tepper[171])	Hypertension, cardiac arrhythmias		
• Metoprolol	50 mg every 12 h	20 mg daily (Tepper[171])	Hypertension, cardiac arrhythmias		
• Timolol	10 mg every 12 h	20–30 mg daily (Tepper[171])	Hypertension, cardiac arrhythmias		
Angiotensin receptor blocker					
• Candesartan	4 mg daily	16 mg daily (Tepper[171])	Hypertension, heart failure	Hypotension, palpitations, tachycardia, dizziness, hyperkalemia, increase serum creatinine, angioedema	Heart failure, renal impairment, hepatic impairment; Contraindicated in pregnancy for migraine prevention
Triptan[a]					
• Frovatriptan	2.5 mg every 12–24 h	2.5–7.5 mg daily (Maasumi et al.[173])		Flushing, chest pain, dizziness, paresthesias, palpitations	Contraindicated in ischemic coronary artery disease, coronary artery vasospasm, history of stroke or TIA, basilar or hemiplegic migraine, severe hepatic impairment
• Naratriptan	1 mg every 12 h	1–5 mg daily (Maasumi et al.[173])			
• Zolmitriptan	2.5 mg every 8–12 h	5–7.5 mg daily (Maasumi et al.[173])			
Additional agents					
• Magnesium		400–600 mg chelated magnesium (Tepper[171])	Hypomagnesemia	Diarrhea with excessive intake	
• Botulinum toxin injection	Varies with formulation		Cosmetic	Brow ptosis, eyelid ptosis, diplopia, excessive tearing, eye closure weakness, injection site reaction, distant toxin spread	Myasthenia gravis, pregnancy, renal impairment; Pregnancy, pediatric use; FDA box warning—distant spread causing dysphagia, respiratory failure and death has been reported

Abortive Agents[b]

	Usual dose:	Side effects:	Caution:
Nonsteroidal anti-inflammatory agents (NSAIDS)			
• Ibuprofen	400 mg; maximum 2,400 mg/d (Becker[174])	Dizziness, pruritus, rash, GI upset, GI ulceration	Cardiovascular disease, renal disease, history of GI ulcers
• Naproxen	500 mg; maximum 1,375 mg/d (Becker[174])		
Acetaminophen	1,000 mg; maximum 4,000 mg/d (Becker[174])	GI upset, dose-related hepatic injury	Regular alcohol use, hepatic impairment, renal impairment, known G6PD deficiency
Triptans			
• Sumatriptan	50–100 mg; maximum 200 mg/d (Becker[174])	Paresthesias, flushing, chest discomfort, nausea, dizziness	Contraindicated in ischemic coronary artery disease, coronary artery vasospasm, history of stroke or TIA, basilar or hemiplegic migraine
• Naratriptan	2.5 mg; maximum 5 mg/d (Becker[174])		
• Rizatriptan	10 mg; maximum 20 mg/d (Becker[174])		
• Zolmitriptan	2.5–5 mg; maximum 10 mg/d (Becker[174])		
Antiemetics			
• Metoclopramide	10 mg; up to 4 times daily (Becker[174])	Drowsiness, dystonic reaction, restlessness, akathisia, tardive dyskinesia, seizure, bradycardia, hematologic abnormalities, drug-induced parkinsonism (rare), neuroleptic malignant syndrome (rare)	Cardiac disease, Parkinson disease, with other agents with extrapyramidal side effects
Muscle relaxants			
• Tizanidine	4–8 mg; maximum 36 mg daily	Hypotension, drowsiness, dizziness, weakness, bradycardia	Elderly, renal impairment, hepatic impairment Contraindicated with CYP1A2 inhibitors such as ciprofloxacin
Ergotamines[c]			
• Oral ergotamine		Bradycardia, cold extremities, hypertension, vasospasm, pleuropulmonary fibrosis, cardiac valvular sclerosis	Triptan use, pregnancy, lactation, elderly Contraindicated in coronary artery disease, in patients on protease inhibitors
• Dihydroergotamine (DHE)			

BID, twice a day; FDA, U.S. Food and Drug Administration; GI, gastrointestinal; G6PD, glucose-6-phosphate dehydrogenase; SIADH, syndrome of inappropriate antidiuretic hormone secretion; TIA, transient ischemic attack.
[a]Short-term prophylaxis preceding known migraine triggers (such as menstrual migraine).
[b]Should be taken within 2 hours of migraine onset, and all abortive therapy should be limited to 3 days per week to avoid medication overuse headache.
[c]Avoid with protease inhibitors and nonnucleoside reverse-transcriptase inhibitors.

with indolent headache as the primary feature. CMV, another opportunistic agent affecting those with advanced AIDS, typically causes diffuse encephalitis. Cryptococcus is the most common agent causing meningitis, often presenting with headache and confusion without overt meningismus.[98] Neurosyphillis can be variable in presentation, including meningeal spread, focal lesions in the parenchyma, or extracranial causing cranial neuropathies.

Opportunistic malignancies can also occur, most commonly primary CNS lymphoma. However, metastatic, systemic lymphoma, and intracranial Kaposi sarcoma can present as focal parenchymal lesions, often causing constitutional symptoms as well as symptoms of increased intracranial pressure including headache, nausea, and vomiting.

Any HIV patient with new onset headaches, independent of age or CD4 count, warrants radiologic imaging, preferably MRI over computed topography due to higher sensitivity and better visualization of the posterior fossa. Additional workup often includes lumbar puncture. Brain biopsy may be necessary in certain cases for a definitive diagnosis.

Treatment of pain in secondary headaches focuses on treating the underlying condition. However, in cases of refractory or prolonged pain despite treatment of the underlying condition, many of the abortive therapies used for primary headaches may be used (see Table 58.2). Opiates can also be considered in the acute setting for severe, refractory pain due to a secondary headache. Preventative agents used for migraines may also be used for chronic pain. Steroids should also be used with caution due to potential of worsening immunosuppression.

Management of Pain

EVALUATION GUIDELINES

When evaluating an HIV patient for pain, a clinician must have a working knowledge of the various etiologies and treatment options of pain in this population, including those discussed in this chapter. A comprehensive assessment includes a detailed history and physical examination, as well as a clinical measurement tools to quantify and describe the pain being experienced.

A standard pain history should include intensity, quality, location, temporal pattern, and response to any previously used analgesics. The pain history as well as the ability to categorize the pain experienced based on its pathophysiology can provide significant clues regarding the underlying etiology and assist in

choosing an appropriate treatment regimen. Pain assessment should be repeated at every clinical encounter. In addition, a complete medical and psychosocial assessment, including any psychiatric and substance abuse comorbidities, must be completed and readdressed during the course of treatment. It may be appropriate to involve family members and significant others in treatment planning.

PAIN MEASUREMENT/ASSESSMENT TOOLS

Given that pain is a subjective symptom, self-reporting is the standard of care.[99] Many assessment tools, based on the patient's own perception of the pain, have been developed that allow a practitioner to monitor pain over time using a validated scale. Two commonly used tools are the Numerical Rating Scale, where pain is rated from 0 to 10, and the Visual Analog Scale (VAS), both of which address pain intensity. Wong-Baker FACES pain scale is an alternative intensity scale that can be used in children. The Brief Pain Inventory (BPI)[100] is a commonly used tool in cancer and AIDS-associated pain, addressing both pain intensity and interference, including the effect of pain on seven domains of functioning. It has also been validated in many languages. The Short-Form McGill Pain Questionnaire[101] is another validated questionnaire, which addresses 15 sensory and affective pain descriptors and may be useful in determining medication effect on various pain qualities. For patients that are unable to communicate verbally, the Behavioral Pain Scale[102] can be useful.

MULTIMODAL TREATMENT APPROACH

Although medication is the primary approach in treating chronic pain, the optimal treatment in this complicated population is multimodal, incorporating psychotherapy, cognitive-behavioral therapy, rehabilitation, and other non-pharmacologic therapies.

PHARMACOLOGIC TREATMENT

When choosing a pharmacologic approach, it is important to classify pain as being either nociceptive or neuropathic (Fig. 58.1). Nociceptors are receptors that respond to potentially tissue damaging stimuli by signaling to the CNS, resulting in the perception of pain. Nociception can be augmented by various substances, including proinflammatory cytokines and prostanoids; however, a stimulus is needed to produce the sensation of pain, whether it be thermal, mechanical, or chemical.[103] Neuropathic pain results from damage of the peripheral

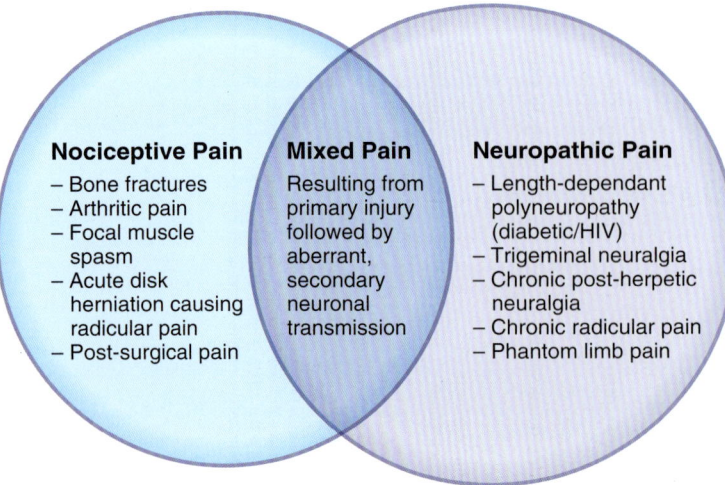

Nociceptive Pain
– Bone fractures
– Arthritic pain
– Focal muscle spasm
– Acute disk herniation causing radicular pain
– Post-surgical pain

Mixed Pain
Resulting from primary injury followed by aberrant, secondary neuronal transmission

Neuropathic Pain
– Length-dependant polyneuropathy (diabetic/HIV)
– Trigeminal neuralgia
– Chronic post-herpetic neuralgia
– Chronic radicular pain
– Phantom limb pain

FIGURE 58.1 Nociceptive versus neuropathic pain.

or CNS, resulting in transmission abnormalities even in the absence of additional damaging stimuli. Chronic neuropathic pain is felt to be secondary to aberrant signaling after the nervous system is reorganized after an injury.[103] Pharmacotherapy works to reduce the noxious stimulus and/or dampen pain transmission through the nervous system.

Few pain management guidelines have been developed to specifically target the HIV population. Treatment approaches have been adapted primarily based on published guidelines for cancer pain and nonmalignant chronic pain. Newshan and Staats[99] conducted a literature review with a proposed set of guidelines on the use of various pharmacologic and nonpharmacologic interventions in HIV pain. Among agents likely to be effective include acetaminophen, NSAIDs, and short-term opioids. Chronic opioid use is not recommended both due to poor evidence for long-term efficacy as well as safety concerns.

World Health Organization (WHO) guidelines on treating cancer pain at the end of life have also been widely used, especially for individuals in the terminal stages of HIV infection. Initially developed in 1986 and updated a decade later, these guidelines provide a comprehensive, stepwise approach with a three-step ladder based on pain intensity (Fig. 58.2). Step 1, in the setting of mild pain, suggests the use of acetaminophen or NSAIDs. Step 2, consisting of persistent and moderate-intensity pain, recommends a weak opioid agent, such as codeine or tramadol, to be added to the step 1 regimen. Step 3, in the setting of persistent, severe pain, involves treatment with a strong opioid such as morphine or hydromorphone in combination with nonopioid therapy. The guideline suggests administering the medication at regular intervals as opposed to on an as-needed basis. Adjuvant agents such as stimulants and laxatives may be used to prevent and treat side effects of opioid analgesics. In addition, antidepressants and anticonvulsants are recommended as adjuvant agents especially in cases of neuropathic pain. For long-term pain control in nonterminal patients, this approach is not recommended due to potential long-term risks of opiate use. Other guidelines such as those published by the American Pain Society have also been applied in the setting of pain in HIV.[104] Table 58.3 lists many of these agents, including dosing approach and side effects/risks.

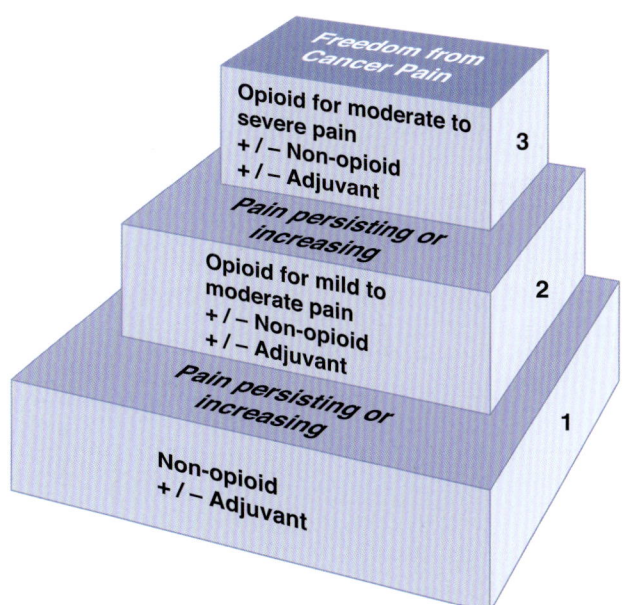

FIGURE 58.2 World Health Organization pain ladder. *(From World Health Organization. WHO's cancer pain ladder for adults. Available at: http://www.who.int/cancer/palliative/painladder/en/. Accessed February 15, 2017.)*

Acetaminophen

Acetaminophen is often considered a first-line agent for pain and is the most commonly used analgesic in the world.[105] WHO guidelines recommend it as a first-line agent in a wide variety of mild to moderate pain conditions. In addition to having a favorable side effect profile, its efficacy is comparable to that of NSAIDs.[106] U.S. Food and Drug Administration (FDA) recommends a maximum daily dose of 4 g per day. However, according to the American Geriatrics Society, the maximum daily dosing recommended for chronic acetaminophen use is 3 g per day due to concern of liver toxicity. Caution should be taken in patients with severe renal disease, liver disease, and/or regular alcohol use. Although FDA guidelines list severe hepatic impairment as a contraindication to its use, one review by Chandok and Watt[107] suggests that 2 g per day or less is a safe option in patients with cirrhosis. Long-term data is unfortunately not available.

Nonsteroidal Anti-inflammatory Drugs

NSAIDs are another commonly used group of agents in the treatment of mild to moderate pain, providing analgesia, anti-inflammation, and antipyresis. Their primary mechanism is the inhibition of prostaglandin formation through the blockade of cyclooxygenase in the periphery. Concerning side effects include GI ulceration, cardiovascular toxicity, renal and hepatic dysfunction, and bleeding. Much of the data available on their efficacy have been focused on their use in musculoskeletal conditions. A Cochrane review found that NSAIDs were superior to acetaminophen for pain relief and improving function in osteoarthritis.[108] Another review reported that NSAIDs were effective in the short-term treatment of acute and chronic low back pain without sciatica.[109] Topical NSAIDs such as ibuprofen and diclofenac were also found to provide pain relief with less concern of systemic adverse events in patients with acute musculoskeletal pain. Caution should be taken when used in patients with bleeding diathesis as well as those with cardiac, renal, and GI comorbidities.

Opioid Analgesics

The use of opioids for the treatment of chronic pain among noncancer populations is controversial. The undertreatment of pain has been well documented in the medical literature, primarily due to fear of overdose and addiction, especially in a population with high rates of drug abuse. However, in patients with severe, disabling pain that is not responsive to other forms of therapy, opioids may be an effective treatment. Multiple, randomized controlled trials have shown good short-term efficacy (most <6 weeks) in decreasing pain and improving function in nociceptive and neuropathic chronic pain (defined as lasting greater than 3 months).[110] However, little data exists for long-term effects of opioid use in individuals with chronic pain.[111]

According to the 2016 CDC guidelines, nonopioid therapies are preferred. However, when used, opioids should be used in combined with nonpharmacologic and nonopioid therapy. When starting treatment, immediate-release formulations should be prescribed instead of extended release agents, at the lowest effective dose. Extra caution should be taken when prescribing total opioid doses of greater than or equal to 50 morphine milligram equivalent (MME) per day, and doses greater than 90 MME per day should be avoided. MME calculation method for various opiates in listed in Table 58.4. According to CDC guidelines, patients have at least 2 times greater risk of overdose at or above 50 MME per day compared to 20 MME per day. Benefits and risks should be assessed regularly, initially within 1 to 4 weeks of starting therapy followed by every 3 months or more frequently. Opioid regimens should be tapered or discontinued once benefits no longer outweigh the risks. Furthermore, urine drug testing is recommended prior

TABLE 58.3   Nonopiate Analgesics

	Dose	Side Effects Include	Caution
Acetaminophen	650 mg every 4–6 h	Increased liver function tests, renal toxicity	Liver disease, renal disease, G6PD deficiency
Nonsteroidal anti-inflammatory drugs (NSAIDs) • Ibuprofen • Naprosyn • Meloxicam • Etodolac • Nabumetone	600 mg TID-QID or 800 mg TID 250 mg BID, 375 mg BID, or 500 mg BID 7.5–15 mg daily 200–400 mg TID-QID (max dose 1,000 mg daily) 500–1,000 mg daily or BID	Abdominal discomfort, gastritis, gastrointestinal (GI) bleeding, prolonged bleeding time	Caution in elderly, patients on anticoagulants and patients with history of GI bleeding FDA box warning—NSAIDs increase risk of cardiovascular and cerebrovascular events

Adjuvant Agents

	Dose	Side Effects Include	Caution
Antidepressants Tricyclic antidepressants (TCAs) • Amitriptyline • Nortriptyline	 Starting dose: 25 mg QHS (10 mg daily if >65 y old); titrate up by 25 mg Maximum dose: 100 mg daily Starting dose: 25 mg QHS (10 mg daily if >65 y old); titrate up by 25 mg Maximum dose: 75–100 mg daily	Sedation, cardiac arrhythmia, anticholinergic side effects (constipation, blurred vision, urinary retention), cognitive dysfunction, extrapyramidal symptoms, narrow-angle glaucoma	Elderly, mood disorders as may increase suicidality, cardiovascular disease, seizure disorders, renal impairment FDA box warning—risk of suicidality with antidepressants
Serotonin norepinephrine reuptake inhibitors (SNRIs) • Venlafaxine • Duloxetine	Starting dose: 37.5 mg daily; may be titrated weekly by 37.5 mg/d Maintenance dose: 75–225 mg daily Starting dose: 30–60 mg daily Maintenance dose: 60 mg daily	Insomnia, drowsiness, anxiety, dizziness, nausea, sexual dysfunction, anorexia, hypertension, tachycardia, SIADH	Elderly, with other serotonergic drugs, seizure disorders, renal impairment FDA box warning—risk of suicidality with antidepressants
Antiepileptics • Gabapentin • Pregabalin • Lamotrigine	 Starting dose: 300 mg daily (often divided into TID dosing); may be slowly titrated up Maximum dose: 3,600 mg daily Starting dose: 150 mg daily (often divided into BID dosing); may be titrated up weekly Maximum dose: 300 mg (150 mg BID) Starting dose: 50 mg daily; may increase dose weekly by 50 mg/d (for BID dosing) Maintenance dose: 200–400 mg daily (100–200 mg BID)	Dizziness, drowsiness, weight gain, leukopenia Agitation, suicidality, personality changes, sedation Drowsiness, dizziness, ataxia, Stevens-Johnson syndrome	Renal dysfunction Depression, behavioral disorders Liver dysfunction

Opioids (Manchikanti et al.[175])

Agent	Starting Dose for Opioid-Naive Patients	Starting Dose for Opioid-Exposed Patients	Titrate as Needed to Daily Maintenance Dose	Side Effects	Caution
Tramadol	50 mg every 8–12 h	50 mg every 6–8 h	150–300 mg daily	Nausea, vomiting, constipation, drowsiness, somnolence, dizziness, pruritus, sexual dysfunction, difficulty urinating, neuroendocrine dysfunction with long-term use, respiratory depression	Caution in elderly and cachectic patients. FDA box warning—respiratory depression Patients with respiratory conditions such as asthma and sleep apnea are at higher risk for respiratory depression Caution when in combination with other sedating and respiratory depressing agents such as benzodiazepines, diphenhydramine, alcohol, etc.
Codeine	15 mg every 8–12 h	30 mg every 6–12 h	120–160 mg daily		
Fentanyl transdermal patch	Not recommended in opioid naive patients	Dose calculated by MME per day based on opioid requirements; 12.5–25 µg every 72 h	12.5–50 µg every 72 h		
Hydrocodone	5–10 mg every 8–12 h	5–10 mg every 6–8 h	30–40 mg daily		
Hydromorphone	2 mg every 8–12 h	2–4 mg every 8–12 h	8–16 mg daily		
Morphine immediate-release	Not recommended	10 mg every 8–12 h	30–60 mg daily		
Oxycodone immediate-release	5–10 mg every 8–12 h	5–10 mg every 6–8 h	30–40 mg daily		
Oxymorphone	5 mg every 8–12 h	5–10 mg every 8–12 h	30–40 mg daily		

BID, twice a day; FDA, U.S. Food and Drug Administration; G6PD, glucose-6-phosphate dehydrogenase; QHS, every bedtime; QID, four times a day; SIADH, syndrome of inappropriate antidiuretic hormone secretion; TID, three times a day.

TABLE 58.4	Morphine Milligram Equivalents per Day (MME per day)

Instructions for calculating total opioid MME per day
1. Take total daily dosage of each opioid agent used.
2. Multiple daily dosage of each opioid by conversion factor listed.
3. Add them together.

Opioid (Doses in mg/day Except Where Noted)	Conversion Factor
Codeine	0.15
Fentanyl transdermal patch (in µg/h)	2.4
Hydrocodone	1
Hydromorphone	4
Methadone	
1–20 mg/d	4
21–40 mg/d	8
41–60 mg/d	10
≥61–80 mg/d	12
Morphine	1
Oxycodone	1.5
Oxymorphone	3

NOTE: These dose conversions are estimated and cannot account for all individual differences in genetics and pharmacokinetics.
From Centers for Disease Control and Prevention. Calculating total daily dose of opioids for safer dosage. Available at: https://www.cdc.gov/drugoverdose/pdf/calculating_total_daily_dose-a.pdf. Accessed February 15, 2017.

TABLE 58.5	Interactions between Opiates and Antiretroviral Therapy (ART)	
Opiate	Effect on Blood Level of Opiate	Effect on Blood Level of ART
Tramadol	Level increases and efficacy decreases in presence of ritonavir (CYP2D6 inhibition) which metabolizes tramadol to active form.	
Morphine	Level decreases with ritonavir, indinavir through stimulation of glucuronidation; risk of opiate withdrawal	
Oxycodone	Level increases with ritonavir (CYP2D6 inhibition); may cause opiate toxicity	
Methadone	Level decreases with nevirapine and efavirenz; may cause withdrawal. Level decreases after 2- to 3-week period with lopinavir/ritonavir and darunavir/ritonavir.	Decreases level of stavudine and didanosine Increases level of zidovudine, with risk of toxicity
Buprenorphine	Level increases with atazanavir, with risk of toxicity. Level may increase with efavirenz, with unclear clinical significance.	

From Krashin DL, Merrill JO, Trescot AM. Opioids in the management of HIV-related pain. *Pain Physician* 2012;15(3)(suppl):ES157–ES168.

to starting therapy followed by periodic testing. Informed consent should be obtained. "Pain agreement," a written document given to the patient detailing the circumstances under which opioids will be prescribed as well as discontinued, have been proposed to help educate patients and minimize harm.[112] However, there are insufficient data that this approach minimizes abuse. The most consistent risk factor for potential opioid abuse is a prior history of alcohol or drug abuse. Male sex, younger age, comorbid psychiatric illness, and history of sexual abuse have also been associated with higher levels of abuse.[113–115]

Another concern for opioid use in the HIV population is the potential for drug–drug interactions with ART. Table 58.5 summarizes many of these interactions. By stimulating glucuronidation, ritonavir can increase morphine metabolism and provoke withdrawal.[116] Ritonavir can also inhibit CYP2D6, which metabolizes oxycodone/long-acting OxyContin, resulting in higher blood levels. Therefore, patients may warrant lower oxycodone dosing to avoid toxicity in the setting of this ART.[117] Methadone, which is used to treat opioid addiction as well as severe, chronic pain, has been found to interact with multiple ART agents. When combined with ZDV, methadone may increase ZDV levels, increasing the risk of toxicity.[118] Methadone has also been found to decrease didanosine (ddI) and stavudine (d4T) levels. Although the exact mechanism of the latter effect is unclear, methadone-induced slowing of GI motility may be responsible. Enteric-coated ddI was found to have higher bioavailability than the tablet form in the presence of methadone and is therefore the preferred formulation.[118] Nevirapine and efavirenz may also decrease methadone levels and precipitate withdrawal symptoms.

Antidepressant Agents

Antidepressants are another class of medications that have long been used to treat numerous chronic pain syndromes. These include serotonin norepinephrine reuptake inhibitors (SNRIs), tricyclic antidepressants (TCAs), and selective serotonin reuptake inhibitors (SSRIs), among others, which are felt to affect pain pathways by multiple mechanisms. In addition to regulating serotonin and norepinephrine, both of which are

critical in pathophysiology of chronic pain, they alter nociceptive pathways by potentiating monoaminergic activity and targeting various receptors in pain production such as adrenergic, histaminergic, and N-methyl-D-aspartate receptors.[119,120] In addition, the onset of pain relief occurs both faster and at lower doses than what is often required for the treatment of depression, usually within a few days of initiating therapy.[121] When used to treat neuropathic pain, the rationale is derived from evidence in diabetic and postherpetic neuralgia because few studies have looked directly at the use of these agents in HIV-related neuropathy.

Although not FDA-approved for the treatment of chronic pain, TCAs such as amitriptyline and nortriptyline have been widely used as first-line agents in the treatment of chronic pain. Amitriptyline is effective in treating a variety of neuropathic pain syndromes such as diabetic neuropathy and postherpetic neuralgia.[122,123] However, in HIV-related neuropathic pain, it failed to show analgesic benefit.[124,125] Similar evidence exists for the use of nortriptyline, which has a more favorable side effect profile, especially in the elderly, due to less anticholinergic and sedative effects.[126] In addition, TCAs have some benefit in other chronic pain syndromes including headache of both tension and migraine origin, low back pain, chronic pelvic pain, and fibromyalgia.[126] Other TCAs such as imipramine and desipramine have also been used. Of note, PIs such as ritonavir can increase TCA blood levels and increase side effects and risk of toxicity.[116]

Duloxetine, an SNRI, is FDA-approved for chronic musculoskeletal pain, fibromyalgia, and neuropathic pain due to diabetic polyneuropathy. Studies to date have not looked at duloxetine for its use in HIV-related neuropathy; however, data exist for its use in other forms of painful peripheral neuropathy.[121] Although few studies have compared it head to head with other antidepressants, one study found equal if not greater efficacy than amitriptyline in neuropathic pain.[127] Venlafaxine, another SNRI, has demonstrated analgesic benefit in the treatment of painful peripheral neuropathy when used in higher doses (at least 150 mg per day) with a better side effects profile compared to TCAs.[128] In addition, these agents have also been used successfully in migraine prevention.[129] However, in prevention of tension-like headaches, benefit has not been demonstrated.[130]

SSRIs have also been used in the treatment of pain, although evidence is conflicting.[131] One randomized study found fluoxetine to be inferior in its ability to control neuropathic pain compared to TCAs but better tolerated.[132] No analgesic benefit has been shown in other etiologies of chronic pain, such as low back pain or arthritis.[133] Furthermore, one meta-analysis showed no benefit of SSRIs over placebo at 2 months of treatment.[134] Other antidepressants that have been studied for the treatment of chronic pain but failed to show efficacy include mirtazapine and trazodone.

Although antidepressants can be used alone, they are often used in combination with other analgesic agents such as opioids, in patients with moderate to severe pain. As adjuvant agents, they can increase the therapeutic value of opiates by decreasing the required dose and reducing side effects.[135]

Anticonvulsants

Gabapentin has long been used as a first-line agent in treating neuropathic pain in a wide variety of conditions, with several studies in HIV-related distal sensory polyneuropathy (HIV-DSP). The mechanism of action of gabapentinoids in neuropathic pain is not entirely clear. Although a structural analogue of γ-aminobutyric acid (GABA), it is felt to exert its analgesic affect by interacting with α_2 voltage-gated calcium channel as well as inhibition of nociceptive transmission from damaged, peripheral nerves.[136] One small study of 26 patients showed significant pain reduction and improved sleep with gabapentin in HIV-DSP.[136]

Pregabalin, another gabapentinoid that exerts its effect on the voltage-gated α_2-channel, is also commonly prescribed for neuropathic pain. Although efficacious in multiple other etiologies of neuropathic pain, little data support its use in HIV. Two large, multicenter randomized controlled trials looking at pregabalin in HIV-DSP, were conducted by the same group and failed to show a benefit in pain reduction over placebo, although in one study patients on pregabalin demonstrated less hyperalgesia.[137,138] Furthermore, there was no significant improvement in sleep quality, an effect that has previously been demonstrated with pregabalin in other neuropathic pain states.

There are several studies of lamotrigine in neuropathic pain likely due to its sodium channel blocking effect. Efficacy has been demonstrated in multiple forms of neuropathic pain including trigeminal neuralgia, diabetic neuropathy, complex regional pain syndrome, and poststroke pain.[139] Pain relief has also been shown to be correlated with plasma concentration of lamotrigine in patients with trigeminal neuralgia. Two randomized studies, one small and one larger performed by the same group, studied lamotrigine in HIV-related neuropathy.[140,141] Both showed a significant improvement in pain with lamotrigine compared to placebo. However, when the larger study sample was stratified based on exposure to neurotoxic ART, only the group receiving neurotoxic ARTs showed a benefit over placebo.[141] However, lamotrigine has relatively little use in neuropathic pain, due in part to a complex titration schedule and concern of potentially serious allergic reaction including rash and Stevens-Johnson syndrome. Lamotrigine blood levels may also decrease in the setting of ritonavir/atazanavir and therefore require increased dosing.[142]

Topical Capsaicin

Capsaicin, an active ingredient derived from chili peppers, has been studied as a topical therapeutic agent for various types of painful neuropathy. It acts as an agonist for the vanilloid receptor (TRPV1), a ligand-gated cation channel selectively expressed on small, nociceptive nerve fibers.[143] Initial application results in immediate channel excitation, release of substance P and increase in pain perception, followed by the depletion of nociceptive neuropeptides and decrease in nociceptive fiber density leading to prolonged analgesia.[144] One study successfully demonstrated a transient epidermal denervation using biopsy following the use of capsaicin in a human model.[145]

Multiple studies have been conducted looking at low-dose (up to 0.075%) topical capsaicin for a wide range of painful conditions such as postherpetic neuralgia and diabetic neuropathy, which have shown significant pain relief.[146,147] Three large, randomized studies have been conducted using high-dose (8%, 640 μg/cm²) capsaicin patch in patients with HIV-DSP. Two of the studies found successful pain reduction 12 weeks posttreatment and good tolerability of the drug.[143,148] The third study, however, did not find significant pain improvement compared to controls.[149] Treatment-related pain was managed with topical lidocaine preceding patch application, along with local cooling and short-acting opioids as needed.

Cannabinoids

Due to the need for additional therapeutic options, exogenous cannabinoids have also emerged as a potential therapy for chronic neuropathic pain. Currently, 29 states, as well as the District of Colombia, Guam, and Puerto Rico, have medical marijuana and cannabis programs. Multiple studies in animal models have demonstrated efficacy of systemic cannabinoids in treating various types of pain such as thermal and mechanical pain.[150,151] A study by Abrams et al.[152] randomized patients with painful HIV-DSP to smoking cannabis versus placebo for 5 days in an inpatient setting and found significant pain reduction in the cannabis group and specifically an antihyperalgesic effect. Another study looking at subjects with HIV-DSP refractory to two analgesics, similarly found improvement in pain intensity among subjects given cannabis versus placebo.[153] Although controversial and with significant legal hurdles, the evidence supporting the use of cannabinoids is promising. Furthermore, the high rate of comorbid substance abuse in the HIV population creates an additional level of complexity in considering these agents in affected patients.

Recombinant Human Nerve Growth Factor

NGF is a neurotrophic agent typically produced by damaged nerve fibers in the process in regeneration and is therefore a potential target in the treatment of neuropathic pain. McArthur and colleagues[154] studied rhNGF in the treatment of HIV-DSP and found an improvement in pain but no change in epidermal nerve fiber density to suggest nerve regeneration at 18 weeks. Hypothesizing that nerve regeneration may take longer than 18 weeks, the same group published results of the trial at 48 weeks. Once again, dose-dependent improvement in pain was demonstrated; however, no change in nerve fiber density was seen.[155]

Combination Pharmacotherapy

Combination therapy has become an increasingly common treatment strategy in treating neuropathic pain due to concerns of limited efficacy and dose-related side effects of individual agents. The rationale behind this approach includes additive or synergistic analgesia, using agents with different mechanisms of action to create better pain control, lower dose requirements, and greater tolerability.[156] No studies to date have looked specifically at combination therapy in HIV-related neuropathy. In other forms of neuropathic pain, combination therapy has been demonstrated to provide better pain control, although no improvement in side effects was seen. Gabapentin and opiates, including prolonged-release oxycodone and sustained-release morphine, have been shown to be superior to individual therapy.[157,158] Another study found that combination nortriptyline and gabapentin was more effective in controlling pain than either agent alone in patients with diabetic polyneuropathy and postherpetic neuralgia.[156]

NONPHARMACOLOGIC THERAPIES

Self-management strategies such as physical activity, spending time with loved ones, and medication compliance as well as cognitive methods such as positive thinking and relaxation are all important techniques by which patients with chronic pain can work to improve their overall quality of life.[159]

Alternative, nonpharmacologic therapies have also been investigated in the treatment of HIV-related pain, including cognitive-behavioral therapy, acupuncture, and hypnosis. Two studies looked at 12 weeks of cognitive-behavioral therapy among HIV patients with various chronic pain syndromes of moderate to severe intensity.[160,161] Although limited by poor attendance to treatment groups, these studies found small improvements in pain at 12 and 24 weeks.

Two studies have looked at acupuncture for the treatment of HIV-DSP. One randomized placebo-controlled study looking at 250 patients found no benefit of acupuncture over placebo in pain control.[124] However, a smaller, more recent study of 50 HIV patients treated with acupuncture and moxibustion (burning of mugwort leaf) versus placebo did demonstrate symptomatic improvement in neuropathic pain among the treatment group.[162]

Hypnosis is useful in a variety of different pain syndromes.[163] In addition to being safe, patients can be taught self-hypnosis to help manage pain on a day-to-day basis.[164] One small study in patients with HIV-DSP looking at three weekly sessions of hypnosis found improvement in pain levels, quality of life, and decreased depressive symptoms 7 weeks posttreatment.[164] Although the available evidence is limited, these therapies may be a useful addition to the pharmacologic therapies offered to patients.

UNDERTREATMENT OF PAIN

Pain has long been recognized as an important cause of disability in patients living with HIV/AIDS, leading to psychological and physical stress as well as decreased quality of life. Unfortunately, undertreatment of pain has been a long-standing issue in this population, with multiple studies showing greater than 60% of HIV-positive individuals living with pain affecting their daily living.[3,14] Individuals with higher levels of pain have higher levels of health care utilization, with one study showing a near linear relationship between pain and outpatient visits.[165]

Individuals with HIV/AIDS have a higher rate of psychiatric illness, with higher rates of depressive symptoms such as hopelessness, anhedonia, difficulty with sleep, and poor appetite as well as anxiety.[2] Pain often exacerbates these psychiatric conditions and overall suffering. Individuals with comorbid major depression and chronic pain, when compared to those with major depression without chronic pain, have longer duration and more severe depressive symptoms as well as higher risk of suicidal ideation.[166]

Multiple sociodemographic factors, including female gender, intravenous drug use, unemployment, and lower education, have also been associated with higher reported levels of pain.[2] This raises concern regarding societal factors that may be barriers for receiving appropriate pain relief. Certain minority groups, such as Alaskan Natives, Native Americans, and Asian Americans, were found to also have lower health care utilization related to pain, possibly due to language and cultural barriers to pain treatment.[165]

BARRIERS TO PAIN MANAGEMENT

Many barriers to effective pain treatment exist on the part of both physicians and patients. Illicit drug use occurs at a higher rate among individuals with HIV/AIDS than the general population, which can affect a clinician's perception and treatment of a patient's pain syndrome. The fear of opioid addiction can be a barrier for both the clinician and the patient as well. Although estimates of opioid abuse among chronic pain patients have been variable depending on the definition, one systematic review suggested up to 20% to 30% rate of misuse and 8% to 12% rate of addiction.[167] In individuals with a history of substance use, increased monitoring is warranted; however, pain relief should remain an important treatment priority.

One study surveyed close to 500 providers on the most important barriers in pain management in AIDS.[168] Lack of knowledge about pain management, lack of access to pain specialists, and concern regarding abuse and addiction were the most commonly perceived barriers. Additional barriers include fear of medication side effects and limited access to drug treatment services. Another study looking at patient-specific barriers in a group of ambulatory AIDS patients found that the most commonly reported barriers included fear of side effects and physical discomfort of opiates as well as misconceptions about the concept of tolerance.[169] Other common patient-specific barriers include wanting to minimize number of pills taken, preference for nonpharmacologic methods of pain management, not being able to afford to fill a prescription, and fear of family/friends thinking they are abusing opiates.[170]

Summary

The development of ART has revolutionized the treatment of HIV, allowing individuals to live much longer, healthier lives. However, pain remains a significant issue, affecting the quality and daily functioning of the lives of these patients. Although many therapies are available for the treatment of pain in HIV-positive patients, efficacy is limited and additional HIV-specific research is necessary to determine the best treatment approaches. Furthermore, awareness and education about pain management for both patients and clinicians is crucial to overcome the many barriers that exist in treatment.

References

1. Centers for Disease Control and Prevention. HIV/AIDS, statistics overview. Available at: https://www.cdc.gov/hiv/statistics/overview/index.html. Accessed February 15, 2017.
2. Douaihy AB, Stowell KR, Kohnen S, et al. Psychiatric aspects of comorbid HIV/AIDS and pain, part 1. *AIDS Read* 2007;17(6):310–314.
3. Frich LM, Borgbjerg FM. Pain and pain treatment in AIDS patients: a longitudinal study. *J Pain Symptom Manage* 2000;19(5):339–347.
4. Kirsh KL, Whitcomb LA, Donaghy K, et al. Abuse and addiction issues in medically ill patients with pain: attempts at clarification of terms and empirical study. *Clin J Pain* 2002;18(4)(suppl):S52–S60.
5. Bing EG, Burnam MA, Longshore D, et al. Psychiatric disorders and drug use among human immunodeficiency virus-infected adults in the United States. *Arch Gen Psychiatry* 2001;58(8):721–728.
6. Merlin JS, Cen L, Praestgaard A, et al. Pain and physical and psychological symptoms in ambulatory HIV patients in the current treatment era. *J Pain Symptom Manage* 2012;43(3):638–645.
7. Glare PA. Pain in patients with HIV infection: issues for the new millennium. *Eur J Pain* 2001;5(suppl A):43–48.
8. Lawson E, Sabin C, Perry N, et al. Is HIV painful? An epidemiologic study of the prevalence and risk factors for pain in HIV-infected patients. *Clin J Pain* 2015;31:813–819.
9. Singer EJ, Zorilla C, Fahy-Chandon B, et al. Painful symptoms reported by ambulatory HIV-infected men in a longitudinal study. *Pain* 1993;54(1):15–19.
10. Aouizerat BE, Miaskowski CA, Gay C, et al. Risk factors and symptoms associated with pain in HIV-infected adults. *J Assoc Nurses AIDS Care* 2010;21(2):125–133.
11. Breitbart W, McDonald MV, Rosenfeld B, et al. Pain in ambulatory AIDS patients. I: pain characteristics and medical correlates. *Pain* 1996;68(2–3):315–321.
12. McCormack JP, Li R, Zarowny D, et al. Inadequate treatment of pain in ambulatory HIV patients. *Clin J Pain* 1993;9(4):279–283.
13. Miaskowski C, Penko JM, Guzman D, et al. Occurrence and characteristics of chronic pain in a community-based cohort of indigent adults living with HIV infection. *J Pain* 2011;12(9):1004–1016.

14. Breitbart W, Rosenfeld BD, Passik SD, et al. The undertreatment of pain in ambulatory AIDS patients. *Pain* 1996;65(2–3):243–249.

15. Cejtin HE. Gynecologic issues in the HIV-infected woman. *Infect Dis Clin North Am* 2008;22(4):709–739.

16. Stricker RB. Hemostatic abnormalities in HIV disease. *Hematol Oncol Clin North Am* 1991;5(2):249–265.

17. Weitzmann MN, Ofotokun I, Titanji K, et al. Bone loss among women living with HIV. *Curr HIV/AIDS Rep* 2016;13(6):367–373.

18. Gaughan DM, Hughes MD, Seage GR, et al. The prevalence of pain in pediatric human immunodeficiency virus/acquired immunodeficiency syndrome as reported by participants in the Pediatric Late Outcomes Study (PACTG 219). *Pediatrics* 2002;109(6):1144–1152.

19. Hirschfeld S, Moss H, Dragisic K, et al. Pain in pediatric human immunodeficiency virus infection: incidence and characteristics in a single-institution pilot study. *Pediatrics* 1996;98(3 pt 1):449–452.

20. Wilcox CM, Saag MS. Gastrointestinal complications of HIV infection: changing priorities in the HAART era. *Gut* 2008;57(6):861–870.

21. Rabeneck L, Crane MM, Risser JM, et al. A simple clinical staging system that predicts progression to AIDS using CD4 count, oral thrush, and night sweats. *J Gen Intern Med* 1993;8(1):5–9.

22. Clark-Ordóñez I, Callejas-Negrete OA, Aréchiga-Carvajal ET, et al. Candida species diversity and antifungal susceptibility patterns in oral samples of HIV/AIDS patients in Baja California, Mexico. *Med Mycol* 2016;55:285–294.

23. Ryder MI, Nittayananta W, Coogan M, et al. Periodontal disease in HIV/AIDS. *Periodontol 2000* 2012;60(1):78–97.

24. Mönkemüller KE, Lazenby AJ, Lee DH, et al. Occurrence of gastrointestinal opportunistic disorders in AIDS despite the use of highly active antiretroviral therapy. *Dig Dis Sci* 2005;50(2):230–234.

25. Bashir RM, Wilcox CM. Symptom-specific use of upper gastrointestinal endoscopy in human immunodeficiency virus-infected patients yields high dividends. *J Clin Gastroenterol* 1996;23(4):292–298.

26. Mönkemüller KE, Wilcox CM. Esophageal ulcer caused by cytomegalovirus: resolution during combination antiretroviral therapy for acquired immunodeficiency syndrome. *South Med J* 2000;93(8):818–820.

27. Wilcox CM, Straub RF, Schwartz DA. Prospective evaluation of biopsy number for the diagnosis of viral esophagitis in patients with HIV infection and esophageal ulcer. *Gastrointest Endosc* 1996;44(5):587–593.

28. O'Neill WM, Sherrard JS. Pain in human immunodeficiency virus disease: a review. *Pain* 1993;54(1):3–14.

29. Barone JE, Gingold BS, Arvanitis ML, et al. Abdominal pain in patients with acquired immune deficiency syndrome. *Ann Surg* 1986;204(6):619–623.

30. Lebovits AH, Lefkowitz M, McCarthy D, et al. The prevalence and management of pain in patients with AIDS: a review of 134 cases. *Clin J Pain* 1989;5(3):245–248.

31. Hewitt DJ, McDonald M, Portenoy RK, et al. Pain syndromes and etiologies in ambulatory AIDS patients. *Pain* 1997;70(2–3):117–123.

32. Dworkin B, Wormser GP, Rosenthal WS, et al. Gastrointestinal manifestations of the acquired immunodeficiency syndrome: a review of 22 cases. *Am J Gastroenterol* 1985;80(10):774–778.

33. Al Anazi AR. Gastrointestinal opportunistic infections in human immunodeficiency virus disease. *Saudi J Gastroenterol* 2009;15(2):95–99.

34. Michalopoulos N, Triantafillopoulou K, Beretouli E, et al. Small bowel perforation due to CMV enteritis infection in an HIV-positive patient. *BMC Res Notes* 2013;6:45.

35. Peng JC, Zhong L, Ran ZH. Primary lymphomas in the gastrointestinal tract. *J Dig Dis* 2015;16(4):169–176.

36. Cappell MS, Marks M. Acute pancreatitis in HIV-seropositive patients: a case control study of 44 patients. *Am J Med* 1995;98(3):243–248.

37. Dutta SK, Ting CD, Lai LL. Study of prevalence, severity, and etiological factors associated with acute pancreatitis in patients infected with human immunodeficiency virus. *Am J Gastroenterol* 1997;92(11):2044–2048.

38. Manfredi R, Calza L. HIV infection and the pancreas: risk factors and potential management guidelines. *Int J STD AIDS* 2008;19(2):99–105.

39. Dassopoulos T, Ehrenpreis ED. Acute pancreatitis in human immunodeficiency virus-infected patients: a review. *Am J Med* 1999;107(1):78–84.

40. Paño-Pardo JR, Alcaide ML, Abbo L, et al. Primary HIV infection with multisystemic presentation. *Int J Infect Dis* 2009;13(4):e177–e180.

41. Schneiderman DJ, Arenson DM, Cello JP, et al. Hepatic disease in patients with the acquired immune deficiency syndrome (AIDS). *Hepatology* 1987;7(5):925–930.

42. Goldin RD, Hunt J. Biliary tract pathology in patients with AIDS. *J Clin Pathol* 1993;46(8):691–693.

43. Yimer G, Gry M, Amogne W, et al. Evaluation of patterns of liver toxicity in patients on antiretroviral and anti-tuberculosis drugs: a prospective four arm observational study in Ethiopian patients. *PLoS One* 2014;9(4):e94271.

44. Núñez M. Clinical syndromes and consequences of antiretroviral-related hepatotoxicity. *Hepatology* 2010;52(3):1143–1155.

45. Jones M, Núñez M. Liver toxicity of antiretroviral drugs. *Semin Liver Dis* 2012;32(2):167–176.

46. Wallace MR, Brann OS. Gastrointestinal manifestations of HIV infection. *Curr Gastroenterol Rep* 2000;2(4):283–293.

47. Barrett WL, Callahan TD, Orkin BA. Perianal manifestations of human immunodeficiency virus infection: experience with 260 patients. *Dis Colon Rectum* 1998;41(5):606–612.

48. Yuhan R, Orsay C, DelPino A, et al. Anorectal disease in HIV-infected patients. *Dis Colon Rectum* 1998;41(11):1367–1370.

49. Sullivan AK, Nelson MR, Moyle GJ, et al. Coronary artery disease occurring with protease inhibitor therapy. *Int J STD AIDS* 1998;9(11):711–712.

50. Henry K, Melroe H, Huebsch J, et al. Severe premature coronary artery disease with protease inhibitors. *Lancet* 1998;351(9112):1328.

51. Behrens G, Schmidt H, Meyer D, et al. Vascular complications associated with use of HIV protease inhibitors. *Lancet* 1998;351(9120):1958.

52. Tabib A, Greenland T, Mercier I, et al. Coronary lesions in young HIV-positive subjects at necropsy. *Lancet* 1992;340(8821):730.

53. Perelló R, Calvo M, Miró O, et al. Clinical presentation of acute coronary syndrome in HIV infected adults: a retrospective analysis of a prospectively collected cohort. *Eur J Intern Med* 2011;22(5):485–488.

54. Chou SH, Prabhu SJ, Crothers K, et al. Thoracic diseases associated with HIV infection in the era of antiretroviral therapy: clinical and imaging findings. *Radiographics* 2014;34(4):895–911.

55. Sigel K, Makinson A, Thaler J. Lung cancer in persons with HIV. *Curr Opin HIV AIDS* 2017;12(1):31–38.

56. Patra S, Nagesh CM, Reddy B, et al. Acute pulmonary embolism being the first presentation of undetected HIV infection: report of two cases. *Int J STD AIDS* 2013;24(6):497–499.

57. Chen YL, Tsai SH, Hsu KC, et al. Primary sternal osteomyelitis due to Peptostreptococcus anaerobius. *Infection* 2012;40(2):195–197.

58. Papavramidis TS, Papadopoulos VN, Michalopoulos A, et al. Anterior chest wall tuberculous abscess: a case report. *J Med Case Rep* 2007;1:152.

59. Mody GM, Parke FA, Reveille JD. Articular manifestations of human immunodeficiency virus infection. *Best Pract Res Clin Rheumatol* 2003;17(2):265–287.

60. Fox C, Walker-Bone K. Evolving spectrum of HIV-associated rheumatic syndromes. *Best Pract Res Clin Rheumatol* 2015;29(2):244–258.

61. Reveille JD, Conant MA, Duvic M. Human immunodeficiency virus-associated psoriasis, psoriatic arthritis, and Reiter's syndrome: a disease continuum? *Arthritis Rheum* 1990;33(10):1574–1578.

62. Clark MR, Solinger AM, Hochberg MC. Human immunodeficiency virus infection is not associated with Reiter's syndrome. Data from three large cohort studies. *Rheum Dis Clin North Am* 1992;18(1):267–276.

63. Hochberg MC, Fox R, Nelson KE, et al. HIV infection is not associated with Reiter's syndrome: data from the Johns Hopkins Multicenter AIDS Cohort Study. *AIDS* 1990;4(11):1149–1151.

64. Altman EM, Centeno LV, Mahal M, et al. AIDS-associated Reiter's syndrome. *Ann Allergy* 1994;72(4):307–316.

65. Bijlsma JW, Derksen RW, Huber-Bruning O, et al. Does AIDS 'cure' rheumatoid arthritis? *Ann Rheum Dis* 1988;47(4):350–351.

66. Calabrese LH, Wilke WS, Perkins AD, et al. Rheumatoid arthritis complicated by infection with the human immunodeficiency virus and the development of Sjögren's syndrome. *Arthritis Rheum* 1989;32(11):1453–1457.

67. Yao Q, Frank M, Glynn M, et al. Rheumatic manifestations in HIV-1 infected in-patients and literature review. *Clin Exp Rheumatol* 2008;26(5):799–806.

68. Ornstein MH, Sperber K. The antiinflammatory and antiviral effects of hydroxychloroquine in two patients with acquired immunodeficiency syndrome and active inflammatory arthritis. *Arthritis Rheum* 1996;39(1):157–161.

69. Maurer TA, Zackheim HS, Tuffanelli L, et al. The use of methotrexate for treatment of psoriasis in patients with HIV infection. *J Am Acad Dermatol* 1994;31(2 pt 2):372–375.

70. Vassilopoulos D, Chalasani P, Jurado RL, et al. Musculoskeletal infections in patients with human immunodeficiency virus infection. *Medicine (Baltimore)* 1997;76(4):284–294.

71. Hughes RA, Rowe IF, Shanson D, et al. Septic bone, joint and muscle lesions associated with human immunodeficiency virus infection. *Br J Rheumatol* 1992;31(6):381–388.

72. Brown TT, Qaqish RB. Antiretroviral therapy and the prevalence of osteopenia and osteoporosis: a meta-analytic review. *AIDS* 2006;20(17):2165–2174.

73. Walker-Bone K, Doherty E, Sanyal K, et al. Assessment and management of musculoskeletal disorders among patients living with HIV. *Rheumatology (Oxford)* 2016;56:1648–1661.

74. Bhatia NS, Chow FC. Neurologic complications in treated HIV-1 infection. *Curr Neurol Neurosci Rep* 2016;16(7):62.

75. Ghosh S, Chandran A, Jansen JP. Epidemiology of HIV-related neuropathy: a systematic literature review. *AIDS Res Hum Retroviruses* 2012;28(1):36–48.

76. Verma S, Estanislao L, Mintz L, et al. Controlling neuropathic pain in HIV. *Curr HIV/AIDS Rep* 2004;1(3):136–141.

77. Estanislao LB, Morgello S, Simpson DM. Peripheral neuropathies associated with HIV and hepatitis C co-infection: a review. *AIDS* 2005;19(suppl 3):S135–S139.

78. Zhou L, Kitch DW, Evans SR, et al. Correlates of epidermal nerve fiber densities in HIV-associated distal sensory polyneuropathy. *Neurology* 2007;68(24):2113–2119.

79. Simpson DM, Haidich AB, Schifitto G, et al. Severity of HIV-associated neuropathy is associated with plasma HIV-1 RNA levels. *AIDS* 2002;16(3):407–412.

80. Schifitto G, McDermott MP, McArthur JC, et al. Markers of immune activation and viral load in HIV-associated sensory neuropathy. *Neurology* 2005;64(5):842–848.

81. Kolson DL, Gonzalez-Scarano F. HIV-associated neuropathies: role of HIV-1, CMV, and other viruses. *J Peripher Nerv Syst* 2001;6(1):2–7.
82. de Larrañaga GF, Petroni A, Deluchi G, et al. Viral load and disease progression as responsible for endothelial activation and/or injury in human immunodeficiency virus-1-infected patients. *Blood Coagul Fibrinolysis* 2003;14(1):15–18.
83. Morgello S, Estanislao L, Simpson D, et al. HIV-associated distal sensory polyneuropathy in the era of highly active antiretroviral therapy: the Manhattan HIV Brain Bank. *Arch Neurol* 2004;61(4):546–551.
84. Pettersen JA, Jones G, Worthington C, et al. Sensory neuropathy in human immunodeficiency virus/acquired immunodeficiency syndrome patients: protease inhibitor-mediated neurotoxicity. *Ann Neurol* 2006;59(5):816–824.
85. Phillips TJ, Cherry CL, Cox S, et al. Pharmacological treatment of painful HIV-associated sensory neuropathy: a systematic review and meta-analysis of randomised controlled trials. *PLoS One* 2010;5(12):e14433.
86. Lyons J, Venna N, Cho TA. Atypical nervous system manifestations of HIV. *Semin Neurol* 2011;31(3):254–265.
87. Brannagan TH, Zhou Y. HIV-associated Guillain-Barré syndrome. *J Neurol Sci* 2003;208(1–2):39–42.
88. Moulin DE, Hagen N, Feasby TE, et al. Pain in Guillain-Barré syndrome. *Neurology* 1997;48(2):328–331.
89. Marshall DW, Brey RL, Cahill WT, et al. Spectrum of cerebrospinal fluid findings in various stages of human immunodeficiency virus infection. *Arch Neurol* 1988;45(9):954–958.
90. Robinson-Papp J, Simpson DM. Neuromuscular diseases associated with HIV-1 infection. *Muscle Nerve* 2009;40(6):1043–1053.
91. Illa I, Nath A, Dalakas M. Immunocytochemical and virological characteristics of HIV-associated inflammatory myopathies: similarities with seronegative polymyositis. *Ann Neurol* 1991;29(5):474–481.
92. Kirkland KE, Kirkland K, Many WJ, et al. Headache among patients with HIV disease: prevalence, characteristics, and associations. *Headache* 2012;52(3):455–466.
93. Mirsattari SM, Power C, Nath A. Primary headaches in HIV-infected patients. *Headache* 1999;39(1):3–10.
94. Evers S, Wibbeke B, Reichelt D, et al. The impact of HIV infection on primary headache. Unexpected findings from retrospective, cross-sectional, and prospective analyses. *Pain* 2000;85(1–2):191–200.
95. Berger JR, Stein N, Pall L. Headache and human immunodeficiency virus infection: a case control study. *Eur Neurol* 1996;36(4):229–233.
96. Holloway RG, Kieburtz KD. Headache and the human immunodeficiency virus type 1 infection. *Headache* 1995;35(5):245–255.
97. Brew BJ, Miller J. Human immunodeficiency virus-related headache. *Neurology* 1993;43(6):1098–1100.
98. Sheikh HU, Cho TA. Clinical aspects of headache in HIV. *Headache* 2014;54(5):939–945.
99. Newshan G, Staats JA. Evidence-based pain guidelines in HIV care. *J Assoc Nurses AIDS Care* 2013;24(1 suppl):S112–S126.
100. Daut RL, Cleeland CS, Flanery RC. Development of the Wisconsin Brief Pain Questionnaire to assess pain in cancer and other diseases. *Pain* 1983;17:197–210.
101. Melzack R. The Short-Form McGill Pain Questionnaire. *Pain* 1987;30(2):191–197.
102. Payen JF, Bru O, Bosson JL, et al. Assessing pain in critically ill sedated patients by using a behavioral pain scale. *Crit Care Med* 2001;29(12):2258–2263.
103. Argoff CE. Pharmacologic management of chronic pain. *J Am Osteopath Assoc* 2002;102(9)(suppl 3):S21–S27.
104. Chou R. 2009 Clinical guidelines from the American Pain Society and the American Academy of Pain Medicine on the use of chronic opioid therapy in chronic noncancer pain: what are the key messages for clinical practice? *Pol Arch Med Wewn* 2009;119(7–8):469–477.
105. Ennis ZN, Dideriksen D, Vaegter HB, et al. Acetaminophen for chronic pain: a systematic review on efficacy. *Basic Clin Pharmacol Toxicol* 2016;118(3):184–189.
106. Bradley JD, Brandt KD, Katz BP, et al. Comparison of an antiinflammatory dose of ibuprofen, an analgesic dose of ibuprofen, and acetaminophen in the treatment of patients with osteoarthritis of the knee. *N Engl J Med* 1991;325(2):87–91.
107. Chandok N, Watt KD. Pain management in the cirrhotic patient: the clinical challenge. *Mayo Clin Proc* 2000;85(5):451–458.
108. Towheed TE, Maxwell L, Judd MG, et al. Acetaminophen for osteoarthritis. *Cochrane Database Syst Rev* 2006;(1):CD004257.
109. Roelofs PD, Deyo RA, Koes BW, et al. Non-steroidal anti-inflammatory drugs for low back pain. *Cochrane Database Syst Rev* 2008;(1):CD000396.
110. Furlan A, Chaparro LE, Irvin E, et al. A comparison between enriched and nonenriched enrollment randomized withdrawal trials of opioids for chronic noncancer pain. *Pain Res Manag* 2011;16(5):337–351.
111. Chou R, Turner JA, Devine EB, et al. The effectiveness and risks of long-term opioid therapy for chronic pain: a systematic review for a National Institutes of Health Pathways to Prevention Workshop. *Ann Intern Med* 2015;162(4):276–286.
112. Payne R, Anderson E, Arnold R, et al. A rose by any other name: pain contracts/agreements. *Am J Bioeth* 2010;10(11):5–12.
113. Robinson-Papp J, Elliott K, Simpson DM, et al. Problematic prescription opioid use in an HIV-infected cohort: the importance of universal toxicology testing. *J Acquir Immune Defic Syndr* 2012;61(2):187–193.
114. Ives TJ, Chelminski PR, Hammett-Stabler CA, et al. Predictors of opioid misuse in patients with chronic pain: a prospective cohort study. *BMC Health Serv Res* 2006;6:46.
115. Wasan AD, Butler SF, Budman SH, et al. Psychiatric history and psychologic adjustment as risk factors for aberrant drug-related behavior among patients with chronic pain. *Clin J Pain* 2007;23(4):307–315.
116. Krashin DL, Merrill JO, Trescot AM. Opioids in the management of HIV-related pain. *Pain Physician* 2012;15(3)(suppl):ES157–ES168.
117. Nieminen TH, Hagelberg NM, Saari TI, et al. Oxycodone concentrations are greatly increased by the concomitant use of ritonavir or lopinavir/ritonavir. *Eur J Clin Pharmacol* 2010;66(10):977–985.
118. Bruce RD, Altice FL, Gourevitch MN, et al. Pharmacokinetic drug interactions between opioid agonist therapy and antiretroviral medications: implications and management for clinical practice. *J Acquir Immune Defic Syndr* 2006;41(5):563–572.
119. Bair MJ, Robinson RL, Katon W, et al. Depression and pain comorbidity: a literature review. *Arch Intern Med* 2003;(20):2433–2445.
120. Jann MW, Slade JH. Antidepressant agents for the treatment of chronic pain and depression. *Pharmacotherapy* 2007;27(11):1571–1587.
121. Lunn MP, Hughes RA, Wiffen PJ. Duloxetine for treating painful neuropathy, chronic pain or fibromyalgia. *Cochrane Database Syst Rev* 2014;(1):CD007115.
122. Moore RA, Derry S, Aldington D, et al. Amitriptyline for neuropathic pain in adults. *Cochrane Database Syst Rev* 2015;(7):CD008242.
123. Bryson HM, Wilde MI. Amitriptyline. A review of its pharmacological properties and therapeutic use in chronic pain states. *Drugs Aging* 1996;8(6):459–476.
124. Shlay JC, Chaloner K, Max MB, et al. Acupuncture and amitriptyline for pain due to HIV-related peripheral neuropathy: a randomized controlled trial. Terry Beirn Community Programs for Clinical Research on AIDS. *JAMA* 1998;280(18):1590–1595.
125. Kieburtz K, Simpson D, Yiannoutsos C, et al. A randomized trial of amitriptyline and mexiletine for painful neuropathy in HIV infection. AIDS Clinical Trial Group 242 Protocol Team. *Neurology* 1998;51(6):1682–1688.
126. Khouzam HR. Psychopharmacology of chronic pain: a focus on antidepressants and atypical antipsychotics. *Postgrad Med* 2016;128(3):323–330.
127. Kaur H, Hota D, Bhansali A, et al. A comparative evaluation of amitriptyline and duloxetine in painful diabetic neuropathy: a randomized, double-blind, cross-over clinical trial. *Diabetes Care* 2011;34(4):818–822.
128. Aiyer R, Barkin RI, Bhatia A. Treatment of neuropathic pain with venlafaxine: a systematic review. *Pain Med* 2017;18(10):1999–2012.
129. Ozyalcin SN, Talu GK, Kiziltan E, et al. The efficacy and safety of venlafaxine in the prophylaxis of migraine. *Headache* 2005;45(2):144–152.
130. Banzi R, Cusi C, Randazzo C, et al. Selective serotonin reuptake inhibitors (SSRIs) and serotonin-norepinephrine reuptake inhibitors (SNRIs) for the prevention of tension-type headache in adults. *Cochrane Database Syst Rev* 2015;(5):CD011681.
131. Saarto T, Wiffen PJ. Antidepressants for neuropathic pain: a Cochrane review. *J Neurol Neurosurg Psychiatry* 2010;81(12):1372–1373.
132. Max MB, Lynch SA, Muir J, et al. Effects of desipramine, amitriptyline, and fluoxetine on pain in diabetic neuropathy. *N Engl J Med* 1992;326(19):1250–1256.
133. Dharmshaktu P, Tayal V, Kalra BS. Efficacy of antidepressants as analgesics: a review. *J Clin Pharmacol* 2012;52(1):6–17.
134. Moja PL, Cusi C, Sterzi RR, et al. Selective serotonin re-uptake inhibitors (SSRIs) for preventing migraine and tension-type headaches. *Cochrane Database Syst Rev* 2005;(3):CD002919.
135. Khan MI, Walsh D, Brito-Dellan N. Opioid and adjuvant analgesics: compared and contrasted. *Am J Hosp Palliat Care* 2011;28(5):378–383.
136. Hahn K, Arendt G, Braun JS, et al. A placebo-controlled trial of gabapentin for painful HIV-associated sensory neuropathies. *J Neurol* 2004;251(10):1260–1266.
137. Simpson DM, Schifitto G, Clifford DB, et al. Pregabalin for painful HIV neuropathy: a randomized, double-blind, placebo-controlled trial. *Neurology* 2010;74(5):413–420.
138. Simpson DM, Rice AS, Emir B, et al. A randomized, double-blind, placebo-controlled trial and open-label extension study to evaluate the efficacy and safety of pregabalin in the treatment of neuropathic pain associated with human immunodeficiency virus neuropathy. *Pain* 2014;155(10):1943–1954.
139. McCleane GJ. Lamotrigine in the management of neuropathic pain: a review of the literature. *Clin J Pain* 2000;16(4):321–326.
140. Simpson DM, Olney R, McArthur JC, et al. A placebo-controlled trial of lamotrigine for painful HIV-associated neuropathy. *Neurology* 2000;54(11):2115–2119.
141. Simpson DM, McArthur JC, Olney R, et al. Lamotrigine for HIV-associated painful sensory neuropathies: a placebo-controlled trial. *Neurology* 2003;60(9):1508–1514.
142. Birbeck GL, French JA, Perucca E, et al. Antiepileptic drug selection for people with HIV/AIDS: evidence-based guidelines from the ILAE and AAN. *Epilepsia* 2012;53(1):207–214.
143. Simpson DM, Brown S, Tobias J, Group NS. Controlled trial of high-concentration capsaicin patch for treatment of painful HIV neuropathy. *Neurology* 2008;70(24):2305–2313.

144. Holzer P. Local effector functions of capsaicin-sensitive sensory nerve endings: involvement of tachykinins, calcitonin gene-related peptide and other neuropeptides. *Neuroscience* 1988;24(3):739–768.

145. Polydefkis M, Hauer P, Sheth S, et al. The time course of epidermal nerve fibre regeneration: studies in normal controls and in people with diabetes, with and without neuropathy. *Brain* 2004;127(pt 7):1606–1615.

146. Zhang WY, Li Wan Po A. The effectiveness of topically applied capsaicin. A meta-analysis. *Eur J Clin Pharmacol* 1994;46(6):517–522.

147. Kingery WS. A critical review of controlled clinical trials for peripheral neuropathic pain and complex regional pain syndromes. *Pain* 1997;73(2):123–139.

148. Brown S, Simpson DM, Moyle G, et al. NGX-4010, a capsaicin 8% patch, for the treatment of painful HIV-associated distal sensory polyneuropathy: integrated analysis of two phase III, randomized, controlled trials. *AIDS Res Ther* 2013;10(1):5.

149. Clifford DB, Simpson DM, Brown S, et al. A randomized, double-blind, controlled study of NGX-4010, a capsaicin 8% dermal patch, for the treatment of painful HIV-associated distal sensory polyneuropathy. *J Acquir Immune Defic Syndr* 2012;59(2):126–133.

150. Buxbaum DM. Analgesic activity of 9-tetrahydrocannabinol in the rat and mouse. *Psychopharmacologia* 1972;25(3):275–280.

151. Moss DE, Johnson RL. Tonic analgesic effects of delta 9-tetrahydrocannabinol as measured with the formalin test. *Eur J Pharmacol* 1980;61(3):313–315.

152. Abrams DI, Jay CA, Shade SB, et al. Cannabis in painful HIV-associated sensory neuropathy: a randomized placebo-controlled trial. *Neurology* 2007;68(7):515–521.

153. Ellis RJ, Toperoff W, Vaida F, et al. Smoked medicinal cannabis for neuropathic pain in HIV: a randomized, crossover clinical trial. *Neuropsychopharmacology* 2009;34(3):672–680.

154. McArthur JC, Yiannoutsos C, Simpson DM, et al. A phase II trial of nerve growth factor for sensory neuropathy associated with HIV infection. AIDS Clinical Trials Group Team 291. *Neurology* 2000;54(5):1080–1088.

155. Schifitto G, Yiannoutsos C, Simpson DM, et al. Long-term treatment with recombinant nerve growth factor for HIV-associated sensory neuropathy. *Neurology* 2001;57(7):1313–1316.

156. Gilron I, Bailey JM, Tu D, et al. Nortriptyline and gabapentin, alone and in combination for neuropathic pain: a double-blind, randomised controlled crossover trial. *Lancet* 2009;374(9697):1252–1261.

157. Gilron I, Bailey JM, Tu D, et al. Morphine, gabapentin, or their combination for neuropathic pain. *N Engl J Med* 2005;352(13):1324–1334.

158. Hanna M, O'Brien C, Wilson MC. Prolonged-release oxycodone enhances the effects of existing gabapentin therapy in painful diabetic neuropathy patients. *Eur J Pain* 2008;12(6):804–813.

159. Merlin JS, Walcott M, Kerns R, et al. Pain self-management in HIV-infected individuals with chronic pain: a qualitative study. *Pain Med* 2015;16(4):706–714.

160. Cucciare MA, Sorrell JT, Trafton JA. Predicting response to cognitive-behavioral therapy in a sample of HIV-positive patients with chronic pain. *J Behav Med* 32(4):340–348.

161. Trafton JA, Sorrell JT, Holodniy M, et al. Outcomes associated with a cognitive-behavioral chronic pain management program implemented in three public HIV primary care clinics. *J Behav Health Serv Res* 2012;39(2):158–173.

162. Anastasi JK, Capili B, McMahon DJ, et al. Acu/Moxa for distal sensory peripheral neuropathy in HIV: a randomized control pilot study. *J Assoc Nurses AIDS Care* 2013;24(3):268–275.

163. Montgomery GH, DuHamel KN, Redd WH. A meta-analysis of hypnotically induced analgesia: how effective is hypnosis? *Int J Clin Exp Hypn* 200;48(2):138–153.

164. Dorfman D, George MC, Schnur J, et al. Hypnosis for treatment of HIV neuropathic pain: a preliminary report. *Pain Med* 2003;14(7):1048–1056.

165. Dobalian A, Tsao JC, Duncan RP. Pain and the use of outpatient services among persons with HIV: results from a nationally representative survey. *Med Care* 2004;42(2):129–138.

166. Uebelacker LA, Weisberg RB, Herman DS, et al. Chronic pain in HIV-infected patients: relationship to depression, substance use, and mental health and pain treatment. *Pain Med* 2015;16(10):1870–1881.

167. Vowles KE, McEntee ML, Julnes PS, et al. Rates of opioid misuse, abuse, and addiction in chronic pain: a systematic review and data synthesis. *Pain* 2015;156:569–576

168. Breitbart W, Kaim M, Rosenfeld B. Clinicians' perceptions of barriers to pain management in AIDS. *J Pain Symptom Manage* 1999;18(3):203–212.

169. Breitbart W, Passik S, McDonald MV, et al. Patient-related barriers to pain management in ambulatory AIDS patients. *Pain* 1998;76(1–2):9–16.

170. Breitbart W, Dibiase L. Current perspectives on pain in AIDS. *Oncology (Williston Park)* 2002;16(6):818–829, 834–835.

171. Tepper SJ. The role of prevention. *Handb Clin Neurol* 2002;97:195–205.

172. Linde M, Mulleners WM, Chronicle EP, et al. Antiepileptics other than gabapentin, pregabalin, topiramate, and valproate for the prophylaxis of episodic migraine in adults. *Cochrane Database Syst Rev* 2013;(6):CD010608.

173. Maasumi K, Tepper SJ, Kriegler JS. Menstrual migraine and treatment options: review. *Headache* 2017;57(2):194–208.

174. Becker WJ. Acute migraine treatment. *Continuum (Minneap Minn)* 2015;21(4):953–972.

175. Manchikanti L, Abdi S, Atluri S, et al. American Society of Interventional Pain Physicians (ASIPP) guidelines for responsible opioid prescribing in chronic non-cancer pain: part 2—guidance. *Pain Physician* 2012;15(3 suppl):S67–S116.

CHAPTER 59

The Treatment of Chronic Pain in Patients with History of Substance Abuse

HOWARD A. HEIT and **DOUGLAS L. GOURLAY**

Chronic pain has no positive physiologic value, whereas acute pain is an adaptive, beneficial response necessary for the preservation of tissue integrity.[1] Recurrent migraine headache, painful peripheral neuropathy, or metastatic bone cancer serves no useful physiologic purpose. In addition, pain remains the most common complaint presenting to the primary health care professional and should be treated in all populations.[2,3] This is no less true in those persons suffering from an active or remote history of substance misuse disorder. A substance use disorder does not decrease the likelihood of a treatable pain condition, it simply complicates it.

The U.S. Census Bureau reported in 2016 that the nation's population had reached ~323 million.[4] Approximately 16% to 23% (~52 to 74 million) of the population suffers pain which is undertreated or not treated at all.[2,5] In the third world, the statistics are even grimmer. Three percent to 16% of the American population may have the disease of addiction.[6] Substance use disorders alone pose a heavy societal burden, endangering individual and family health and well-being and sapping resources from the health care system.[7] In fact, the current data on prevalence of addiction is extremely difficult to interpret. Part of the reason for this is the continued interchangeable use of the terms *addiction* and *dependence*.[8] For example, in a recent article in *The New England Journal of Medicine*, the authors cite Centers for Disease Control and Prevention (CDC) Guideline data which states that the prevalence of opioid dependence may be as high as 26% among patients in primary care receiving opioids for chronic noncancer-related pain.[9] Because we know that there is some degree of physical dependency associated with the chronic use of opioid agonist class of drugs in all patients, the term *opioid dependency* seems to be used to denote opioid addiction. This uncertainty in terminology makes data collection, interpretation, and comparisons between studies extremely difficult. This also makes the determination of incidence and percentage of chronic pain and addiction in other developed countries equally difficult. Furthermore, in certain subsets of the general population, we expect the incidence of pain to be considerably greater as has been reported, for example, in methadone maintenance treatment (MMT) programs.[10] Opioids may be indicated in a small percentage of these MMT patients with moderate to severe pain. However, this population is at increased risk for relapse even in the context of a comprehensive treatment plan that includes "rational pharmacotherapy." In addition, regulatory scrutiny often leaves the health care professional in a position of real or perceived vulnerability when prescribing a controlled substance. This may put both health care professionals and their patients at risk of a suboptimal outcome for an often-treatable medical condition.

The use of controlled substances including opioids in persons who may suffer from concurrent substance use disorders presents additional challenges to the health care professional. Success in the treatment of either condition requires an approach that encompasses the entire biopsychosocial needs of the patient. Pain management necessitates the need for careful boundary setting within the therapeutic relationship. Unfortunately, it is impossible to determine beforehand, with any degree of certainty, who will become problematic users of prescription medications.[11] Despite our best efforts, no risk assessment tool has been developed which can reliably define risk of aberrant drug-taking behavior in patients prescribed opioids for the treatment of chronic pain.[12,13] Risk is a part of the human condition: "If you have a pulse, you have a risk." What is more important is to make a credible attempt at assessing these risks in all patients and to manage these risks to the best of our abilities. By recognizing the need to carefully assess all patients, in a biopsychosocial model, stigma can be reduced, patient care improved, and overall risk contained.[14] The fact is that no matter how carefully we try to limit the use of opioids to the "lowest class of risk," there will *always* be a need to assess treatment goals and outcomes and modify them according to specific patient needs.

The goals of this chapter are to address the complex issues associated with the treatment of pain in persons with problematic behavior and to offer the health care professional an approach that may reduce risk and, hopefully, improve outcome.

Principle of Balance

Health care professionals who treat patients at the interface of pain and addiction and officials who formulate and enforce regulations must understand the central principle of "balance" as it relates to the use of any controlled substance including opioids.

That principle provides for a system of controls to reduce the risk of diversion, abuse, or trafficking of opioids, balanced against the assurance of the availability of opioids for legitimate medical and scientific purposes and accessibility of opioids to all who need them for the relief of pain.[15] Health care professionals must embrace this principle as should our patients, dispensing pharmacists, and our communities.

By applying the principle of balance, it stands to reason that health care professionals should be able to treat pain in patients with the disease of addiction who are willing to simultaneously address both conditions. One can successfully treat acute pain in the face of an active addiction, but one will not achieve the stated goals in chronic pain management with an untreated substance use disorder.[11] Mutual support programs such as Alcoholics Anonymous and Narcotics Anonymous are quite clear in terms of their position on the management of any medical condition: These are side issues and should not interfere with the 12 steps and traditions of their respective programs.[16] Inappropriate use of prescription medications, even when legitimately prescribed by a licensed professional, can interfere in the recovery process. A legitimate indication for a given drug does not necessarily imply an "appropriate" indicate for that drug. For this reason, patients "in recovery" from drug or alcohol misuse need to ensure that their physicians are knowledgeable in the recovery process or have guidance from someone with such knowledge involved in their care.

THE IMPORTANCE OF THE DEFINITIONS

Using precise definitions at the interface of pain and addiction medicine will allow health care providers to improve their clinical practice of pain management (Table 59.1).[17-19]

Confusion between physical dependence and addiction may contribute to the undertreatment of chronic pain. Ballantyne and LaForge[20] have expressed concern over the apparent lack of distinction between physical and psychological dependence in the diagnosis of addiction, preferring to consider these as entirely separable phenomena. Although the following definitions share many elements in common, "continued use despite harm" remains the behavioral marker in the chronic pain patient that will define, over time, an addictive disorder, if present.[21] Physical dependence does not mean addiction, nor is it necessarily devoid of psychological components. Physical dependence and addiction can coincide, but physical dependence is neither necessary nor sufficient to make a diagnosis of addiction. Physical dependence is an expected, neuropharmacologic adaptation that occurs because of chronic exposure to an agonist class of drug. Addiction is a much more complex biobehavioral phenomenon.[17-19]

TABLE 59.1 Definitions

1. **Addiction** is a primary, chronic, neurobiologic disease, with genetic, psychosocial, and environmental factors influencing its development and manifestations. It is characterized by behaviors that include one or more of the following: impaired control over drug use, compulsive use, continued use despite harm, and craving.

2. **Physical dependence** is a state of adaptation that is manifested by a drug class–specific withdrawal syndrome that can be produced by abrupt cessation, rapid dose reduction, decreasing blood level of the drug, and/or administration of an antagonist.

3. **Tolerance** is a state of adaptation in which exposure to a drug induces changes that result in a diminution of one or more of the drug's effects over time.

4. **Pseudoaddiction** is a syndrome that causes patients to seek additional medications due to inadequate pharmacotherapy being prescribed. Typically when the pain is treated appropriately, the inappropriate behavior ceases.

5. **Pseudotolerance** is the need to increase medication such as opioids for pain when other factor(s) are present such as disease progression, new disease, increased physical activity, lack of compliance, change in medication, drug interaction, addiction, and/or deviant behavior.

6. **Iatrogenic addiction** occurs when a patient, with a negative personal or family history for alcohol or drug addiction or abuse, is appropriately prescribed a controlled substance and subsequently in the therapeutic course meets the diagnostic criteria for addiction to that substance.

7. **Misuse** is use of a medication (for a medical purpose) other than as directed or as indicated, whether willful or unintentional, and whether harm results or not.

8. **Abuse** is any use of an illicit drug with the intentional self-administration of a medication for nonmedical purpose such as altering one's state of consciousness (e.g., getting high). A licit substance such as alcohol can be abused.

9. **Diversion** is the intentional removal of a medication from legitimate distribution and dispensing channels for illicit sale or distribution.

10. **Aberrant behavior** is when the patient steps outside the boundaries of the agreed-on treatment plan which is established as early as possible in the doctor–patient relationship.

From Passik SD, Weinreb HJ. Managing chronic nonmalignant pain: overcoming obstacles to the use of opioids. *Adv Ther* 2000;17(2):70–83; Weissman DE, Haddox JD. Opioid pseudoaddiction—an iatrogenic syndrome. *Pain* 1989;36(3): 363–366; Pappagallo M. The concept of pseudotolerance to opioids. *J Pharm Care Pain Symptom Control* 1998;6:95–98. Katz NP, Adams EH, Chilcoat H, et al. Challenges in the development of prescription opioid abuse-deterrent formulations. *Clin J Pain* 2007;23(8):648–660; and Gourlay DL, Heit H. Pain and addiction: managing risk through comprehensive care. *J Addict Dis* 2008;27(3):23–30.

Physical dependence is a natural expected neuroadaptive response that can occur with opioids, alcohol, benzodiazepines, corticosteroids, antidepressants, diabetic agents, cardiac medications, and many other medications used in clinical medicine. Abrupt cessation of these medications can produce a withdrawal syndrome that can include, but is not limited to, nausea, vomiting, diaphoresis, diarrhea, abdominal cramps, seizures, anhedonia, dysphoria, and, in some cases, even death.[17-19] For example, a heroin addict may be both physically dependent and addicted to the narcotic, whereas the pain patient taking opioids is physically dependent but not necessarily addicted. Both will experience some degree of withdrawal if the drug is abruptly stopped. In the pain patient, physical dependence with withdrawal may also be associated with withdrawal-mediated hyperalgesia.[22]

In fact, one of the greatest challenges in the interpretation of adverse outcomes in the context of opioid medication management is that related to equivalency of dose, given the wide range of medications we have within the opioid class of drugs.

The concept of morphine milligram equivalence (MME) has come under significant fire in recent years due to the perceived shortcomings of trying to equate molecules of different therapeutic potencies and intrinsic activities. The concept, however flawed, is in our opinion a worthwhile one.

Although the debate rages on as to what effect chronic versus acute exposure, medication tolerance, and individual pharmacogenetics variabilities to mention only a few of the relevant variables have on equivalent doses, there are several immutable points to consider.

The first is that there is, without a doubt, a significant prescription drug abuse problem in America.[23] Although many drug classes are abused, the opioid class of medication has come under direct fire in terms of increased morbidity and mortality as drugs of abuse.

The second point is that regardless of where the line is drawn, be it 90-mg morphine equivalence or 200-mg morphine equivalences per day, risk clearly rises as daily dose increases.[24,25]

The final point, and perhaps one that might be open to the greatest expert debate, is that as dose of drug continues to increase, despite inadequate therapeutic response, the probability of achieving a successful therapeutic outcome diminishes.[9] What impact the comorbid conditions of substance abuse and/or addiction might contribute toward adverse outcomes in this context remains to be seen.

Iatrogenic addiction is not clearly defined in the literature.[3,26] The true incidence of iatrogenic addiction to opioids is not known.[26] It is therefore important to set limits and boundaries for all patients before writing the first prescription.[14]

It is only by careful evaluation and rational pharmacotherapeutic management of the pain that concurrent diagnoses such as addiction or pseudoaddiction[27] can be confirmed. Although a diagnosis of addiction is made prospectively over time, a diagnosis of pseudoaddiction is usually made retrospectively.[11] When reasonable limits and boundaries are placed on a patient, and yet they continue to step out of bounds, addiction or drug abuse should be considered.

Health care professionals with improved understanding of the definitions on basic scientific and clinical levels will be better able to more effectively evaluate and treat chronic pain patients with or without the disease of addiction.

Basic Science of the Disease of Addiction

Drugs of misuse act at local cellular and membrane sites that are within a neurochemical system that is called the reward and withdrawal pathway (Fig. 59.1).[28] This pathway is in the mesolimbic dopamine system, and it involves, among other structures, the ventral tegmental area, nucleus accumbens,

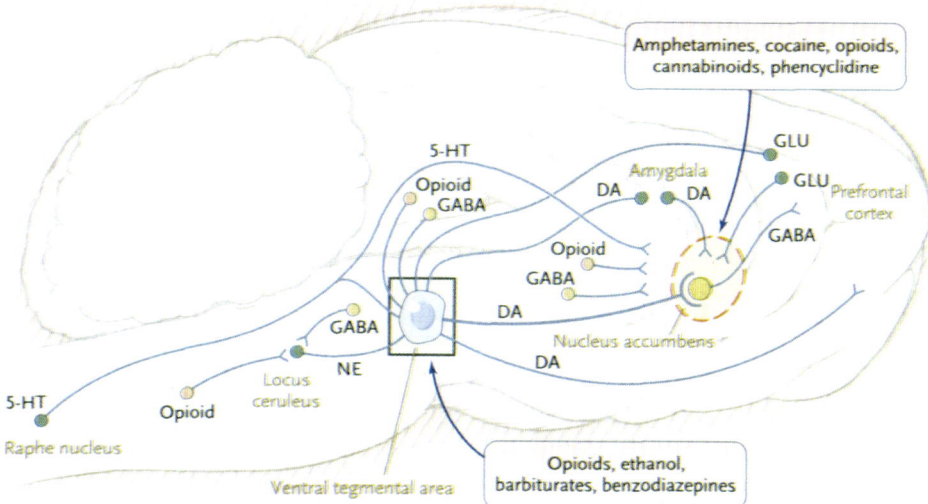

FIGURE 59.1 Common reward pathway: mesocorticolimbic dopamine system. 5-HT, 5-hydroxytrypophan; DA, dopamine; GABA, gamma aminiobutyric acid; GLU, glutamate; NE, norephinephrine. *(Reproduced from Cami J, Farre M. Drug addiction.* N Engl J Med *2003;349[10]:975–986. Copyright © 2003 Massachusetts Medical Society. Reprinted with permission from Massachusetts Medical Society.)*

amygdala, and prefrontal cortex of the primitive brain. Addiction is a neurobiologic disease that causes disruption of these pathways. This disruption is mediated via receptor sites and neurotransmitters. Central to this reward and withdrawal pathway is the neurotransmitter dopamine, which has been shown to be relevant not only to drug reward but also to food, drink, sex, and social reward.[29,30] Disruption of this neurochemical pathway by drugs of abuse may lead to addiction. Drug withdrawal can intensify with repeated drug use and can persist during prolonged periods of drug abstinence, a symptom complex known as the protracted abstinence syndrome.[31] This sensitization of a neural process related to drug cravings or to environmental stimuli such as sights, smells, and sounds associated with drugs (referred to as cues) leads to the progressive increase in drug-seeking behavior that characterizes addiction. Such sensitization appears to increase the attractiveness of the drug taking and that of the drug-associated stimuli.[32]

One of the most common reasons for relapse is stress.[28] It stands to reason that if a chronic pain patient is in recovery from drug or alcohol use and his or her pain is inadequately treated, he or she may turn to the street for licit or illicit drugs and/or alcohol to cope with the pain.

The health care professional must recognize addiction as a treatable brain disease[33,34]; that is, a distinct medical condition that may or may not be associated with the patient's pain syndrome. However, when these do coexist, the successful treatment of either will require addressing both problems. In fact, as a general principle, all pain doctors should be talented amateurs in the context of identifying and treating substance use disorders (D. L. Gourlay, personal communication, verbal, July 2017).

Opioids can cause physical dependence and, upon abrupt discontinuation, withdrawal as a result of upregulation of the cyclic adenosine monophosphate (cAMP) pathway at the locus coeruleus.[31] This is a normal physiologic response to this class of medications. It should be noted that most of the medications capable of producing physical dependence are not associated with the disease of addiction.

Tolerance is also a natural, expected physiologic response that can occur with exposure to certain classes of drugs, especially alcohol and opioids. The *key* to this definition is that all other factors remain stable so that just the physiologic response to the drug can be evaluated.[17] In fact, tolerance is neither good

nor bad. It occurs at different rates, to different effects in different people, over time. So, although there is relatively rapid tolerance development to the cognitive blunting effects of the opioid class of drug, tolerance to the constipating effects of opioids rarely occurs. Unappreciated disease progress that is associated with dose escalation is termed *pseudotolerance*,[35] a term that was coined to describe the apparent loss of analgesic effect in cancer patients with unrecognized increases in tumor burden.[35] Pharmacodynamic tolerance involves adaptations that occur at both the site of the drug action (e.g., receptor, ion channel, as well as in related systems more distal to it). For example, pharmacodynamic tolerance to opioids is evident at both the level of the opioid receptor in the locus coeruleus (primary) and in the dopaminergic reward pathways afferent to the site of this discrete drug action (secondary).[32] Persons addicted to heroin and chronic pain patients taking opioids can both exhibit tolerance to the drug.

BINARY CONCEPT OF PAIN AND ADDICTION

In the past, the literature has suggested that pain conditions and addictive disorders might be dichotomous phenomena.[11,14,36] It has been said that in the context of a "legitimate" pain diagnosis, which usually meant a condition that made sense to the assessing health care professional, the likelihood of there being an addictive disorder was so small as to not even merit investigation. Unfortunately, if the patient had an obvious substance use disorder, very real and treatable pain conditions were often ignored. With time, this thinking was tempered somewhat to suggest that in the absence of a current or past personal or family history of a substance use disorder, the risk of addiction was very low indeed.[14] This dichotomous approach to pain and addiction has not served patients, health care professionals, or society well.

In reality, there is nothing about a genuine pain condition that is protective against having a concurrent substance use disorder[3]; however, untreated pain, as a stressor, should always be considered in the assessment of relapse risk.[28] Although there are some data in the animal literature to suggest that acute pain may blunt the euphoric reward of some drugs including opioids,[37,38] this concept has largely been discounted. Patients with a substance use disorder are often disproportionate consumers of health care resources, especially in the context of trauma.[39,40] The presence of a preexisting substance use disorder is not mitigated by a concurrent pain problem; it is complicated by it.

Although there is no evidence in the literature to suggest that those patients without past histories or apparent increased risk of substance use disorders become addicted as a result of rational pharmacotherapy for the treatment of any medical condition, including chronic pain, there is little credible evidence to the contrary either. Perhaps more relevant questions to ask are whether rational pharmacotherapeutic management of acute or chronic pain can reactivate a previously dormant substance use disorder or express an as yet unidentified genetic predisposition[3] toward substance misuse or addiction. In the authors' opinion, the answer to both questions very likely is "Yes."[11]

Risk, of course, varies with circumstance. For example, the prevalence of alcoholism in the hospitalized general medical population is estimated at 19% to 26%,[41] whereas in the trauma subset, the prevalence rises to 40% to 62%.[40] Regardless of what the actual risk is, it is clear that no one specific marker can reliably identify the at-risk pain patient, so careful boundary setting for all patients is strongly recommended.[14] However, boundary setting is not without potential risk. It is interesting to note that in some cases, aberrant behavior on the part of the patients may be driven, if not created by overly proscriptive rules and demands placed on them by their treatment provider/team.

Take, for example, the patient that is forced to provide urine drug samples on a twice-weekly basis. It might be considered "aberrant" if the patient appears unwilling to comply. In fact, many would consider even weekly urine drug testing (UDT) onerous and so the disruption in the patients' life might well be considered unacceptable. If boundaries and limits are set excessively tight, even "normal" patients will be forced to step out of bounds. Not only is this excessive, but there is no evidence in the literature to suggest this pattern of testing is either clinically useful or medically necessary.[42]

Not all aberrant behavior reflects drug misuse or addiction. Some individuals who do not meet the diagnostic criteria for addiction may also use medications and other drugs problematically. This group is sometimes referred to as "chemical copers."[43] These individuals lack the skills commonly acquired during childhood and adolescence and tend to turn to external sources for support in dealing with life's problems. Often, however, these patients suffer from complex, multidimensional problems that may only be partially responsive to even optimum pharmacotherapy in the absence of a biopsychosocial treatment plan. Unidimensional problems may respond to unidimensional pharmacologic solutions. Multidimensional problems however may transiently respond to pharmacologic interventions but rarely in a sustainable fashion.[11]

It is only by aggressive investigation and rational pharmacotherapeutic management of the pain that this diagnosis can be made. *The diagnosis of addiction is often made prospectively over time.*[11] When the patient's behavior remains aberrant despite the appropriate management of the underlying painful condition with reasonably set limits, substance misuse or addiction should be considered. In contrast, *the diagnosis of pseudoaddiction is made retrospectively,*[11] meaning that with appropriate management of pain, aberrant behavior is reduced or eliminated.[11,14] Boundary setting may include interval dispensing and contingency prescribing. Interval dispensing requires the patient to see other members of the health care team, such as a staff member of the prescriber or the pharmacist, on a more frequent basis than the actual prescriber. Thus, interval dispensing can be a simple and effective means to help patients keep from "borrowing (medications) from tomorrow to pay for today," thereby reducing the risk of running out of medications early. With contingency prescribing, receiving the

next prescription is contingent on something such as bringing bottles in for "pill counts" or mandatory attendance at all appointments.

It might be worth expanding on the point of "pill counts." For many practitioners, the frequency of appointments and quantity of medication prescribed are such that the "correct" answer to any pill count is "zero." The problem with this approach is the physician has no idea exactly when the bottle became empty. A more useful approach is to calculate the number of pills required to reach the next appointment and add 3 days' worth of pills to that prescription. In the authors' experience, it is far more difficult for a patient who tends to overuse the medications to bring back the correct number of tablets for the count if her or she are, in fact, struggling with control. The extra medication fulfills the added purpose of adding a buffer between the patient and practitioner in case one or the other is unable to attend the next appointment precisely as scheduled. It is always useful to clarify this practice, in advance with the patient's pharmacist, so that the prescription will make sense in the context that it was written in.

PAIN AND OPIOID ADDICTION—A CONTINUUM APPROACH

Although pain and addiction can and sometimes do exist as comorbid conditions, they may also be present as part of a dynamic continuum with pain at one end of the spectrum and addiction at the other (Fig. 59.2).[11,36] In cases where the identified substance of misuse is one in which there can be no doubt about the medical appropriateness of its use, such as with alcohol or cocaine, a comorbid pain *and* substance use disorder should be considered. However, when the drug in question can arguably be both the *problem* and the *solution*, depending on the health care professionals' training and perspective, a continuum model may better apply.[11,36] With chronic pain, appropriateness of ongoing opioid use should be periodically evaluated, especially when there is little or no objective evidence of improvement in pain relief or function.

In cases in which pain and addiction coexist either as a continuum or comorbid condition, it is important to identify which aspect of the illness is dominant. Failure to treat both conditions, when present, will undoubtedly lead to frustration and poor outcomes in both domains. It is equally important to realize that this continuum is dynamic, with substance use disorder symptoms becoming dominant during periods of stress even after years of stable recovery.[11,36]

SEPARATING THE "MOTIVE" FROM "BEHAVIOR" WHEN DEALING WITH PAIN AND ADDICTION

One of the greatest challenges facing practitioners treating complex pain patients is dealing with the patient who explains his or her aberrant behavior in terms of his or her chronic pain. Not infrequently, the health care professional will hear the

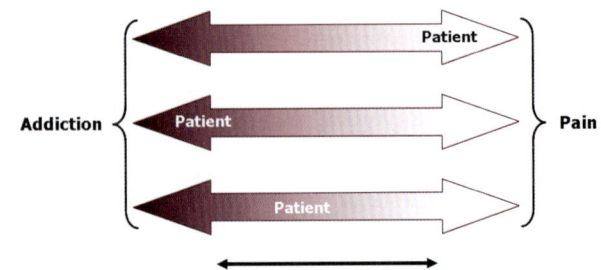

FIGURE 59.2 Pain and addiction continuum. (*From Heit HA, Gourlay D. Chronic pain and addiction. In: Pasricha PJ, Willis WD, Gebhart GF, eds.* Chronic Abdominal and Visceral Pain: Theory and Practice. *1st ed. New York: Taylor & Francis; 2006:231–244. Copyright © 2007 by Taylor & Francis Group, LLC. Reproduced by permission of Taylor and Francis Group, LLC, a division of Informa plc.*)

patient say "But I'm not an addict, I'm a pain patient" when challenged with explaining why he or she has run out of medication early, yet again. Of course, interpreting such behavior can be challenging.[44] The differential diagnosis is long and includes dependence, pseudoaddiction, true addiction, comorbid psychopathology, "chemical coping,"[43] and even criminal behavior such as diversion.[11] More often than not, the patient and/or patient's family can identify and are willing to discuss the aberrant behavior in the context of a "problem" rather than as evidence of a definitive substance use disorder.

Take for example the patient who has unilaterally escalated his daily dose of medication, necessitating an early return for prescription renewal. Although this may occur occasionally for quite legitimate reasons especially during the induction phase of treatment, repeated unilateral dose increases reflect behavior that must be carefully evaluated. In such a case, it may be more useful to focus on the problematic behavior (running out early) rather than the motive behind the behavior (i.e., addiction/abuse, chemical coping, etc.) when exploring this with the patient. Once the problematic behavior is identified and a remedial course of action selected, the ease with which the patient adheres to this "solution" will help to identify which aspect of the aberrant behavior differential is likely at work. Patients whose problematic behavior remains unchanged despite conservative efforts likely suffer from more complex problems that would best be referred on to a substance use disorder professional or other clinician with greater experience and resources to assess and manage these more challenging cases.[45] Nonforensic, patient-centered UDT, which is discussed in Chapter 60, can be a very useful tool in these cases.[14,46,47]

In the case of criminal behavior such as diversion of the prescribed medications, this behavior and the motive behind it are clearly unacceptable. In the authors' opinion, this may be cause to sever the doctor–patient relationship and dismiss the patient from the practice. Dismissing patients for such criminal behavior is unlikely to be construed as abandonment in most jurisdictions. On the other hand, where possible, simply abandoning the molecule may be a more effective and patient-centered approach to take in cases where questionable behavior leaves the prescriber with concerns about the safety of ongoing prescription of controlled substances. In some cases, the patient will simply abandon the practitioner who no longer supplies the controlled substances; in such cases, careful documentation of the process will ensure that any adverse consequences that might befall the patient reflect the severity of the underlying illness, not a result of any action that the prescriber might have taken. In fact, when addressing aberrant behavior, there are many "correct answers" that might be considered in addressing these issues, but in the authors' opinion, there is only one, wrong answer, and that is to simply do nothing.

In fact, one of the sometimes unrealized opportunities that come with addressing aberrant behavior is the chance to simply "do things differently" from this point onward. In many respects, this is an opportunity for the patient and the practitioner to implement therapeutic change in the hopes of improving treatment outcome. This is particularly true when addressing the new patient in your practice, who is already on considerable doses of controlled substances.[48]

OPIOIDS FOR ANALGESIA OR OPIOID-STABILIZING EFFECT?

Not all pain syndromes are equally responsive to opioids.[49] Neuropathic pain may be less opioid responsive, often requiring higher doses.[50] In cases in which a patient is physically dependent on opioids, as one would expect with prolonged use of this class of drug, it can sometimes be useful to consider the appropriateness of continuation of opioid therapy, especially when treatment goals of improved function and decreased pain remain unmet.

Most pain is, to some degree, opioid-responsive. Yet despite years of experience with opioid therapy, it remains unclear who in advance will achieve a *sustained* response. In fact, the vast majority of efficacy data for the use of opioids involving randomized controlled trials are of 6 weeks or less duration.[9,51,52] Further, chronic opioid therapy has been shown to worsen pain levels and function. This makes the evaluation of any "trial of opioid therapy" even more important because it is becoming clear that if the continued prescription of opioids is not leading to a clear benefit, it must be a problem. Of course, the challenges associated with opioid tapering are considerable.

When the patient and clinician define the need to remain on opioid therapy not by how well the patient is doing but rather by how poorly things go when they try to reduce or discontinue the drug, it is time to reexamine the therapeutic role of opioids. When opioid levels in a physically dependent pain patient become inadequate, early withdrawal may occur. In the context of opioid-abstinence-induced hyperalgesia, it would be expected that the pain complaint might worsen.[22] It is something of a myth that patients who no longer need opioids always come off them easily. *In any trial of therapy, including opioid pharmacotherapy, there must be a clear exit strategy in addition to an entrance, stabilization, and maintenance strategy before writing the first prescription.*[11,48] This is not to say that those patients who are clearly benefiting from opioid pharmacotherapy should be weaned from these medications on the assumption that they "may no longer need them" but rather that not all persons who have inadequate pain relief or function while on opioids should remain on this class of drugs. In fact, some persons with poorly controlled pain while on opioid therapy may improve with a carefully executed opioid taper. The term *taper* is used here rather than *detoxification*, which is a term more commonly associated with the disease of addiction. Pain patients are "tapered," and addiction patients are "detoxed." In some jurisdictions, this can be a critical distinction in medicolegal terminology. Again, to restate a critical point: "Words matter."

Recommendations for Terminating Opioid Therapy

A trial of opioid therapy is just that: a trial. In some cases, a decision to discontinue opioids must be made. Although the optimum case is one in which both the clinician and the patient feel this is the appropriate course to take, not infrequently, it is the clinician alone who has made this decision. Discontinuation of the opioid class of drugs should, when possible, be done respecting that the patient may have become physically dependent. Although no one taper schedule should be considered the "gold standard," it is important to bear the following in mind. The speed with which the dose can be reduced at the beginning of the taper does not necessarily predict the speed with which the patient will be able to finish.

In any taper, there is a tension between neuroadaptation and time. The taper should be as fast as possible, so as to minimize lingering withdrawal symptoms while being slow enough to allow for neuroadaptation. Never forget that for some patients, regardless of slowness of taper, withdrawal symptoms cannot be eliminated, only prolonged until the goal of opioid discontinuation is obtained. Even then, post-acute withdrawal symptoms may further frustrate the goal.

As a rule, dropping 10% every 1 to 2 weeks until the patient reaches the bottom third, after which the dose is reduced by 5% every 2 to 4 weeks until completed is a gentle taper that most patients will tolerate well. During the taper, worsening pain scores, especially in the morning, may indicate too rapid a dose reduction, frustrating the efforts at tapering the drug. Although there certainly is merit in adjusting the rate of taper in a symptom-responsive fashion, there is a significant risk of even the best of intended tapers turning into an unintended maintenance program of ongoing medication management. In some cases, the correct approach is to simply "push through" the difficult times and remember the original goal, which is to get off the opioid medication. It is important to remember that opioid termination should not be synonymous with termination of care. Although for some patients, the net effect is that they will seek care elsewhere if opioids are not being prescribed.

A very real challenge in the treatment of chronic pain in the context of aberrant behavior is the determination of which aspect of the patient's pathology dominates. Some clinicians have argued that as long as their medical record clearly records that the primary intent behind the prescription of controlled substances is for the treatment of chronic pain, any substance use–related disorder should be seen as a secondary issue. In fact, it is more complicated than that. For example, if a patient being treated for chronic pain is, by any reasonable peer assessment, a dominant substance use disorder, it will, in most cases, be the assessment of peers which will be taken as correct. In some cases, it may appear to be clear, for example, the pain patient who acknowledges the parenteral use of the oral medications. This would seem to most as incontrovertible evidence of an addictive disorder. However, some practitioners, especially those who have arbitrarily restricted their care to those patients without apparent addictive disorders, will continue to see any aberrant behavior as evidence of inadequate treatment of pain. In the authors' opinion, the safest course of action to take in such cases is to refer the patient on for further assessment and, if necessary, treatment of a concurrent substance use disorder. Failure to do so puts the patient at significant risk of harm due to inadequate treatment of a potentially lethal, substance use disorder. It also may expose the treating clinician to adverse regulatory scrutiny.

It is tempting to think that finding the correct molecule (i.e., the "right" drug) will achieve the desired outcomes in terms of achieving patient stability. For example, buprenorphine is a drug with considerable utility in terms of pain management and maintenance treatment of an opioid substance use disorder. Unfortunately, it is not simply the buprenorphine that leads to a good outcome in the maintenance treatment of opioid dependency. It is also the structure and support that is integral to the use of this drug in achieving satisfactory treatment outcomes. Interested readers are encouraged to read information regarding Drug Addiction Treatment Act of 2000 (DATA 2000) or to attend a DATA 2000 buprenorphine course for further insights into this potentially lifesaving treatment option.[53-55]

The purpose of effective pain management in any patient population, including those suffering from substance use disorders, is to reduce pain while improving function. When a drug appears to do more harm than good and yet continues to be used, an active addictive disorder must be considered. Although risk can never be eliminated, it can usually be managed. Failure to identify pain and addiction, where they exist, can render even the most ardent efforts at pain management ineffective and frustrating.

Assessment Tools

There are multiple assessment tools that are available for health care professionals to stratify the risk of drug/alcohol abuse or addiction. These tools may be used in pain management if one is considering prescribing a controlled substance, especially an opioid. There are a variety of tools that have been proposed to help the clinician identify the "at-risk" patient for aberrant behavior including but not exclusively the Alcohol Use Disorders Identification Test (AUDIT),[56] the Screener and Opioid Assessment for Patients with Pain (SOAPP),[57,58] the CAGE-AID (Alcohol Including Drugs) (Table 59.2),[59,60] and the Opioid Risk Tool (ORT).[61]

TABLE 59.2 CAGE-AID (Alcohol Including Drugs) Questionnaire

- Have you tried to **C**ut down or **C**hange your pattern of drinking or drug use?
- Have others been **A**nnoyed or **A**ngry by others' concern about your drinking or drug use?
- Have you felt **G**uilty about the consequences of your drinking or drug use?
- Have you had a drink or used a drug in the morning (**E**ye-opener) to decrease hangover or withdrawal symptoms?

ORT is a five-question clinical interview or patient questionnaire to assess patients at risk for aberrant behavior with prescription opioids prior to treatment initiation. It quantifies the level of risk for patients in an easy-to-use format. Its scoring is based on gender, family history of substance abuse, personal history of substance abuse, age, history of sexual abuse, and psychological disease (Table 59.3).[61]

Of course, an increased risk does not mean that any given patient will behave aberrantly, and for those who do, not all behavior is equally significant in terms of meaning. In this respect, it is important to remember that "predisposed" does not mean "predestined" in terms of expression of risk. In fact, all assessment tools only offer a "statistical" probability of aberrant behavior in any single patient. Ultimately, individual risk is evaluated over time. The importance of clinical judgment supported by object evaluations of stability (e.g., UDT, pill counts) in the ongoing evaluation of risk cannot be overstated. However, for those patients clearly at increased risk, the need for closer monitoring should be evident. It is also important to note that on initial evaluation of all patients, the health care professional should always ask respectfully and in a nonjudgmental manner about a history of drug or alcohol abuse/addiction, physical or sexual abuse, or any current or history of mental disorders. This information allows the treating health care professional to formulate the appropriate treatment plan with boundary settings that are tailored to individual risk. It also offers the opportunity to bring another

---

TABLE 59.3 Stratifying Risk: Opioid Risk Tool

		Female	Male
• Five-question clinical interview to assess patients			
• Specifically developed to screen patients with chronic pain who will be using opioids	**Family history of substance abuse**		
	Alcohol	[ ] 1	[ ] 3
	Illegal drugs	[ ] 2	[ ] 3
	Prescription drugs	[ ] 4	[ ] 4
	Personal history of substance abuse		
	Alcohol	[ ] 3	[ ] 3
	Illegal drugs	[ ] 4	[ ] 4
• Quantifies the level of risk for patient	Prescription drugs	[ ] 5	[ ] 5
• Three risk categories	**Age** (if between 16 and 45)	[ ] 1	[ ] 1
• Low: 0–3 points	**History of preadolescent sexual abuse**	[ ] 3	[ ] 0
• Moderate: 4–7 points	**Psychological disease**		
• High: 8 points and above	Attention deficit disorder, obsessive-compulsive disorder, bipolar, schizophrenia	[ ] 2	[ ] 2
	Depression	[ ] 1	[ ] 1
	Scoring Total: _____		

Adapted from Webster LR, Webster RM. Predicting aberrant behaviors in opioid-treated patients: preliminary validation of the Opioid Risk Tool. *Pain Med* 2005;6(6):432–442. Reproduced by permission of American Academy of Pain Medicine.

member(s) into the treatment team to begin to address the bio-psychosocial issues of the patient. This increases the chances of the patient reaching his or her therapeutic goals of pain management.

Universal Precautions in Pain Medicine

The heightened interest in pain management is making the need for appropriate boundary setting within the clinician–patient relationship even more apparent. Unfortunately, it is impossible to determine beforehand, with any degree of certainty, who will become problematic users of prescription medications. A parallel can be drawn between the chronic pain management paradigm and our experience with problems identifying the "at-risk" individuals from an infectious disease model.

The term *universal precautions* as it applies to infectious disease came out of the realization that it was impossible for a health care professional to reliably assess risk of infectivity during an initial assessment of a patient.[62] Lifestyle, past history, and even aberrant behavior such as tattoos and injection drug use were unreliable indicators that led to patient stigmatization and increased health care professional risk. It was only after research into the prevalence of such diseases as hepatitis B, hepatitis C, and HIV that we realized the safest and most reasonable approach to take was to apply an appropriate minimum level of precaution to *all* patients to reduce the risk of transmission of potentially life-threatening infectious disease to health care professionals. Fear was replaced by knowledge, and with knowledge came the practice we know as universal precautions in infectious disease.

Universal precautions (UP) in pain medicine is a risk management concept introduced in 2005 which proposes adopting a minimum level of inquiry and care applicable to *all* patients presenting with chronic pain. UP offers an assessment and ongoing management scheme for all chronic pain patients.[14] It recognizes the need to carefully assess all patients within a multidimensional biopsychosocial model, including past history of and present aberrant behaviors that might be associated with drug or alcohol use. By applying careful and reasonably set limits in the clinician–patient relationship, it is possible to triage chronic pain patients into three categories according to risk as presented later in this chapter.[11]

UP were introduced to open a dialogue between the pain management and addiction communities around the assessment and management of risk. They were not proposed as complete but rather as a good starting point for those treating chronic pain. It is important to note that UP are not simply about opioid therapy but rather stress the importance of assessing and, where necessary, managing treatable comorbid conditions including substance use disorders.[63] As with UP in infectious disease, by applying the following recommendations, patient care may be improved, stigma reduced, and overall risk contained.[14]

THE 10 PRINCIPLES OF UNIVERSAL PRECAUTIONS IN PAIN MEDICINE

The 10 principles of UP are listed in Table 59.4. Treatable causes for pain should be identified where they exist and therapy directed toward the pain generator. Even in the absence of specific objective findings, pain can and should be treated. Any comorbid conditions, including substance use disorders and other psychiatric illness, must also be identified and addressed. A complete inquiry into past personal and family history of substance misuse is essential to adequately assess and treat any patient. It is a common misconception that people with alcohol and drug use disorders will always lie about their use: In fact, it is more often the case that the practitioner simply did not bother to ask the patient, when this information

TABLE 59.4 The 10 Principles of Universal Precautions
1. Diagnosis with appropriate differential
2. Psychological assessment including risk of addictive disorders
3. Informed consent (verbal or written/signed)
4. Treatment agreement (verbal or written/signed)
5. Preintervention/postintervention assessment of pain level and function.
6. Appropriate trial of opioid therapy +/− adjunctive medication
7. Reassessment of pain score and level of function
8. Regularly assess the "four A's" of pain medicine: Analgesia, Activity, Adverse reactions, and Aberrant behavior.[a]
9. Periodically review pain and comorbidity diagnoses, including addictive disorders.
10. Documentation

[a]From Frieden TR, Houry D. Reducing the risks of relief—the CDC Opioid-Prescribing Guideline. *N Engl J Med* 2016;374(16):1501–1504.
Adapted from Gourlay DL, Heit HA, Almarhezi A. Universal precautions in pain medicine: a rational approach to the management of chronic pain. *Pain Med* 2005;6(2):107–112. Reproduced by permission of American Academy of Pain Medicine.

is not obtained. People tend not to lie about that which they think is normal. A sensitive and respectful assessment of risk should not be seen in any way as diminishing a patient's complaint of pain. Patient-centered UDT should be discussed with all patients regardless of what medications they are currently taking. In the authors' opinion, the prescription of controlled substances to patients who are "philosophically opposed" to UDT is relatively contraindicated.

Informed consent is part of an initial evaluation. Health care professionals must discuss with and answer any questions about the proposed treatment plan including anticipated benefits and foreseeable risks. The specific issues of addiction, physical dependence, and tolerance should be explored at a level appropriate to the patient's understanding.

Written opioid agreements facilitate the documentation of informed consent, patient education, and compliance in the management of chronic pain.[64] A well-written agreement establishes the responsibilities of clinician to patient and vice versa. It outlines the treatment plan and documents informed consent. The opioid agreement helps to establish boundaries and consequences for drug misuse or diversion. Noncompliance with the agreement can aid in the diagnosis of the disease of addiction or substance misuse, which would often require a change in the treatment plan.

Opioid agreements have the potential to improve the therapeutic relationship.[64–66] The agreement, whether written and signed or informal and simply documented in the medical record, must be part of an environment of care that emphasizes honest and open communication. A practice policy for all patients prescribed with opioids to sign a medication management agreement is often a simple and effective way to approach this sometimes uncomfortable issue. In the authors' opinion, the agreement should be *reasonable*, *readable*, and *flexible*. Sometimes, such agreements are erroneously called *opioid contracts*. However, these rarely reach the level of legally binding contracts and, as such, are better referred to as medication management agreements. Where written agreements are used, both the patient and clinicians should sign two copies. The patient should be offered a copy to share with whomever he or she thinks appropriate. Effective agreements clearly define both the clinician's and patient's responsibilities (Table 59.5).[64–66]

Preintervention or postintervention assessment of pain level and function must emphasize that any treatment plan begins with a "trial of therapy." This is particularly true when controlled substances are contemplated or used. Without a documented assessment of preintervention pain scores and level

TABLE 59.5 Treatment Agreement for Opioid Maintenance Therapy for Noncancer or Cancer Pain
• Goals of therapy
• Single prescriber if possible
• Informed consent on all opioid risks
• Definition of addiction, tolerance, and physical dependence
• Need for patient disclosure of substance abuse history; psychiatric history including history of sexual, physical, or verbal abuse; and medications currently prescribed
• Need for complete, honest self-report of pain relief, side effects, and function at each medical visit
• Establishment of regular medical visits
• Requirement for prescription renewal only during regular office hours
• Conditions of noncompliance (e.g., evidence of drug hoarding or use of any illegal drug *may* cause termination of the clinician–patient relationship)
• Use of the word *may* instead of *will* in the agreement, so clinical judgment can be used in each situation
• Patient consent to random urine drug tests and pill counts
• Permission for the practice to contact appropriate sources to obtain or provide information about the patient's care or actions
• Recovery program for substance misuse or addiction (patients must agree to concurrent assessment and treatment of their substance use disorder)

Adapted from Heit HA. Creating and implementing opioid agreements. *Dis Manag Digest* 2003;7(1):2–3.

TABLE 59.6 Triage of the Chronic Pain Patient
Group I—Primary Care Patients
This group has no past or current history of substance use disorders. They have a noncontributory family history with respect to substance use disorders and lack major or untreated psychopathology. This group clearly represents the majority of patients who will present to the primary care practitioner.
Group II—Primary Care Patient with Specialist Support
In this group, there may be a past history of a treated substance use disorder or a significant family history of problematic drug use. They may also have a past or concurrent psychiatric disorder. These patients, however, are not actively addicted but do represent increased risk which may be managed in consultation with appropriate specialist support. This consultation may be formal and ongoing (co-managed) or simply with the option for referral back for reassessment should the need arise.
Group III—Specialty Pain Management
This group of patients represents the most complex cases to manage due to an active substance use disorder or major, untreated psychopathology. These patients are actively addicted and pose significant risk to both themselves and to the practitioners who often lack the resources or experience to manage them. The prescription of controlled substances should generally be left to those persons with the experience and resources to manage the active addict.

Adapted from Gourlay DL, Heit HA, Almarhezi A. Universal precautions in pain medicine: a rational approach to the management of chronic pain. *Pain Med* 2005;6(2):107–112. Reproduced by permission of American Academy of Pain Medicine.

of function, it may be difficult to demonstrate success in any medication trial. The ongoing assessment and documentation of goals met will help support the continuation of any mode of therapy. Failure to meet these goals should necessitate reevaluation and possible change in the treatment plan.

An appropriate trial of opioid therapy, generally with adjunctive medication, may be warranted in moderate to severe pain. Although opioids should not routinely be thought of as treatment of first choice, they must also not be considered as agents of last resort. Recently, the CDC has published a set of guidelines for the use of opioids in the treatment of chronic noncancer pain.[9,67] Pharmacologic regimens must be individualized based on subjective as well as objective clinical findings. The appropriate combination of agents, including opioids and adjunctive medications, may be "rational pharmacotherapy" and provide a stable therapeutic platform from which to base treatment changes. In an ideal world, rational pharmacotherapy should be coupled with an integrated structure of biopsychosocial support. Unfortunately, the financial resources to support such integrated approaches is often lacking.

Regular reassessment of the patient's pain score and level of function, combined with corroborative support from family or other knowledgeable third parties, will help document the rationale to continue or modify the current therapeutic trial. The routine assessment of the "four *A*'s" of pain medicine: Analgesia, Activity, Adverse effects, and Aberrant behavior will help to direct therapy and support pharmacologic options taken.[68] It may also be useful to document a fifth A: Affect (E. Covington, personal communication, verbal, July 2005). The prescriber should periodically review pain diagnosis and comorbid conditions, including substance use disorders. Underlying illnesses evolve. Diagnostic tests change with time. In the pain and addiction continuum, it is not uncommon for a patient to move from a dominance of one disorder to the other. As a result, treatment focus may need to change over the course of time. If an addictive disorder predominates, aggressive treatment of an underlying pain problem will likely fail if not coordinated with treatment for the concurrent addictive disorder.

Careful and complete documentation of the initial evaluation and at each follow-up is both medicolegally indicated and in the best interest of all parties. Thorough documentation, combined with an appropriate doctor–patient relationship, will reduce medicolegal exposure and risk of regulatory sanction. If you do not document it, it did not happen.

PATIENT TRIAGE

One of the goals in the initial assessment of a pain patient is to obtain a reasonable assessment of risk of a concurrent substance use disorder or major psychopathology. In this context, patients can be stratified into three basic groups. The UP's triage scheme offers a practical framework to help determine which patients they may safely manage in the primary care setting, those who should be co-managed with specialist support, and those who should be referred on for definitive management of their chronic pain condition in a specialist setting (Table 59.6).[14]

It is important to remember that Groups II and III can be dynamic; Group II becoming Group III with relapse to active addiction, whereas Group III patients can move to Group II with appropriate treatment. In some cases, as more information becomes available to the practitioner, the patient who was originally thought to be low risk (Group I) may become Group II or even Group III. It is important to continually reassess risk over time.

Treating the Pain Patient on Opioid Agonist Treatment

The treatment of pain in a patient on opioid agonist treatment (OAT) with methadone or sublingual (S/L) buprenorphine for the disease of opioid addiction can be particularly challenging. Here is an example when the controlled substance prescribed for pain can be the solution, the problem, or both.[11]

Methadone and S/L buprenorphine (with or without naloxone) can be used for the dual purpose of treating the disease of addiction and pain, but they pose an interesting challenge for the prescriber. For appropriate prescribing of these medications, their unique pharmacokinetic and pharmacodynamic properties must be understood. This allows for proper patient selection and evaluation to optimize outcomes in the treatment of pain, addiction, or the comorbid conditions of pain and addiction.

In the disease of addiction, the dose of methadone or S/L buprenorphine is usually given once a day. In the clinical experience of the authors, methadone and buprenorphine are best dosed every 6 to 8 hours for the most effective treatment of opioid responsive pain.[69] However, it should be noted that this dosing schedule for S/L buprenorphine for analgesia is not documented in the peer-reviewed literature.[69]

Buprenorphine's high receptor affinity may theoretically interfere with effectiveness of other full μ analgesics, although this concept has come under review in recent publications.[70,71] As with other partial μ agonists, buprenorphine is typically contraindicated in opioid-dependent patients because it may precipitate severe withdrawal.[72,73]

Pain management for patients who are using S/L buprenorphine for the disease of addiction requires an individualized approach. The literature has suggested that to treat pain in a patient on OAT with S/L buprenorphine, one must discontinue the S/L buprenorphine and do a re-induction of the drug after the acute pain syndrome resolves.[74] This may not be necessary in some instances. In certain circumstances, the patient may be spared the discomfort of having to go into withdrawal as the full μ agonist is discontinued and he or she is rotated back to S/L buprenorphine. In most cases, the pain can simply be managed by titrating the S/L dose upward to effect with a 6- to 8-hour dosing regimen up to maximum dose of 32 mg per day.[69] If breakthrough medication is needed, consider using one with high potency such as transmucosal fentanyl lozenges, fentanyl buccal tablets, or hydromorphone because of their high affinity to the opioid receptor.[69] It is important to remember that even at maximal maintenance agonist doses of buprenorphine, μ receptor occupancy is less than 100%.[75] In the authors' opinion, rapid-onset opioid formulations should be used with caution in this population, primarily for acute pain, with tightly set boundaries as per UP with limited "pill load" prescribed between evaluations of the acute pain (see Chapter 60). It is important to remember that it is always possible to add a full μ agonist to a patient who is maintained on buprenorphine without fear of precipitating withdrawal. The reverse is, however, not always true. The risk of precipitated withdrawal may in fact be as much a function of the molecule chosen as the route of administration (e.g., the rapid onset of a large S/L preparation vs. the slow onset of a transdermal delivery system.)

The patient who is on OAT and requires chronic pain management must agree to the principles of UP or some similarly integrated approach to risk management. It may also be useful to place this patient in an appropriate group for risk stratification (Group II or Group III) and monitor accordingly.

The Treatment of Pain and Suffering in Our Society

There is a debate over whether opioids are "good" or "bad" and whether they should be available for widespread use. Of course, opioids are "good" when used appropriately and "bad" when they are misused. In fact, the debate has become even more granular: Is there any justification for chronic opioid therapy in the context of noncancer-related pain when we carefully consider an honest risk/benefit assessment? We believe that in a selected patient population, there are some patients who, at least in the short run, seem to benefit from the chronic use of opioids. It is likely fair to say that some patients, especially those who were initiated on opioid therapy in the past, might

well do better off these medications than on them. However, this should not alter the fact that for those patients who need them, they must be made available, even if availability requires appropriate monitoring and oversight individualized to each case.[76] The chronic pain population is incredibly heterogeneous and varies tremendously in terms of vulnerability to addiction and misuse. The best way to accomplish the goal of keeping opioids available to those who need them and may truly benefit from them is for all stakeholders involved in legitimate opioid therapy to openly address the complexity of the issue and to do so in a collaborative fashion.[76]

Major stakeholders in achieving an appropriate balance in the treatment of pain and the prevention of drug abuse and diversion are health care professionals, patients, third-party payers, regulatory bodies, law enforcement, pharmaceutical industry, the public at large, and the media. If these groups reconcile themselves to the need for thoughtful and unemotional dialogue, opioid treatment can remain a viable option while efforts are made to stem the tide of prescription drug misuse and addiction. Everyone has a stake in this complex issue. We are all aging, and many of us will have pain. Societal solutions are needed now so that we can all enjoy the comfort of knowing that safe and effective pain treatment will be there for us if we need it. It is the responsibility of all to make this a reality.[76] Unfortunately, the very issue of chronic opioid therapy being "safe and effective pain treatment" is clearly open to debate.[77]

This brings us to the issue of compliance with medication management in the context of the treatment of chronic pain.

One wonders if pain patients are being held to an unrealistically high standard regarding compliance with their treatment plan. For example, in the treatment of any chronic illness such as diabetes mellitus, 100% adherence to the treatment plan, although desirable, is obviously not achieved in most patients. In fact, a recent review indicates that approximately 20% to 50% of patients are not adherent to recommended medical therapy.[78] The failure to comply is a complex interplay of a multitude of biopsychosocial factors including but not limited to patient motivation. To expect 100% compliance with any pharmacotherapeutic agent, including controlled substances is to ignore this fact. Again, the moral imperative of elimination of prescription drug misuse in America has significantly altered our understanding of the core components of treatment adherence.

In fact, there is ample evidence that the whole field of pain medicine may be being held to an unrealistic standard. Clearly, in the practice of the art of medicine, clinicians are expected to know certain things. Take for example, the execution of a trial of opioid therapy. In the prescription of these potent medications, clinicians are expected to thoroughly discuss with their patients the risks and potential benefits of this course of treatment. Initial prescriptions of potentially dangerous medications must be sufficiently detailed as to reasonably guide the patient to their safe use. Similarly, the prescriber is expected to ensure, through the course of the clinical encounter, how exactly the patient is using this medication and where necessary adjust the treatment strategy. These two aspects of the clinical encounter are clearly within the reasonably prudent prescribers' mandate of best practices. There is, however, a third piece of information that is only known to the patient; that is, how they are "actually" using the medication.

In some circumstances, it may be helpful to treat the clinical encounter as a "worst case scenario." For example, a patient who repeatedly runs out of medication *could* simply be a victim of incredibly bad luck—but it is much more likely that they are over using their medications and running out early as a result. Under more dire circumstances, the prescriber might be becoming an unwitting accomplice to the criminal act of drug diversion. It often is very difficult to tell, in advance which explanation is the correct one. Unfortunately, in recent department of justice prosecutions, it often seems that the physician is expected to approach the patient (in the prescription of controlled substances) *as if he or she were lying*, until there is unequivocal evidence to prove that he or she *is not lying* about the use of prescription medications. Sadly, there is rarely ever absolute proof of these things—yet judicial assessment after the fact often takes the position of "doctor knew, or ought to have known" about the patient's misbehavior. Clearly, such an approach would very much undermine the therapeutic relationship to the detriment of many patient's care.

Worse still is the fact that many patients and more than a few prescribers view opioid therapy as the "gold standard" in pain management.[79,80] This has at least been in part due to a growing use of the opioid class drugs in the management of chronic pain. Although this may be true in the context of acute pain, there is mounting evidence that long-term efficacy of the opioid class of drugs in the treatment of chronic pain is lacking.[3] What role chronic opioid therapy will play in any patient population, especially those with the added risk of a preexisting substance use disorder, remains to be seen.

Conclusion

The purpose of effective pain management in any patient population, including those suffering from substance use disorders, is to reduce pain while improving function. Although achieving this goal may be more difficult in patients with substance use disorders, it is not impossible. Risk can never be eliminated, but it can usually be managed. By approaching these patients within a biopsychosocial model using the information presented in this chapter, the health care professional can give the patient the best quality of life possible given the reality of his or her clinical situation.

References

1. Oaklander A. The pathology of pain. *Neuroscientist* 1999;5(5):302–310.
2. Krames ES, Olson K. Clinical realities and economic considerations: patient selection in intrathecal therapy. *J Pain Symptom Manage* 1997;14(3 suppl):S3–S13.
3. Volkow ND, McLellan AT. Opioid abuse in chronic pain—misconceptions and mitigation strategies. *N Engl J Med* 2016;374(13):1253–1263.
4. U.S. and world population clock. Available at: https://www.census.gov/popclock/. Accessed April 22, 2016.
5. Center for Behavioral Health Statistics and Quality. *Behavioral Health Trends in the United States: Results for the 2014 National Survey on Drug Use and Health.* Rockville, MD: Substance Abuse and Mental Health Services Administration; 2015.
6. Savage SR. Long-term opioid therapy: assessment of consequences and risks. *J Pain Symptom Manage* 1996;11(5):274–286.
7. Crowley R, Kirschner N, Dunn AS, et al. Health and public policy to facilitate effective prevention and treatment of substance use disorders involving illicit and prescription drugs: an American College of Physicians position paper. *Ann Intern Med* 2017;166(10):733–736.
8. Heit HA, Gourlay DL. *DSM-V* and the definitions: time to get it right. *Pain Med* 2009;10(5):784–786.
9. Frieden TR, Houry D. Reducing the risks of relief—the CDC Opioid-Prescribing Guideline. *N Engl J Med* 2016;374(16):1501–1504.
10. Rosenblum A, Joseph H, Fong C, et al. Prevalence and characteristics of chronic pain among chemically dependent patients in methadone maintenance and residential treatment facilities. *JAMA* 2003;289(18):2370–2378.
11. Gourlay DL, Heit H. Pain and addiction: managing risk through comprehensive care. *J Addict Dis* 2008;27(3):23–30.
12. Jones T, Moore T, Levy JL, et al. A comparison of various risk screening methods in predicting discharge from opioid treatment. *Clin J Pain* 2012;28(2):93–100.
13. Passik SD, Lowery A. Psychological variables potentially implicated in opioid-related mortality as observed in clinical practice. *Pain Med* 2011;12(suppl 2):S36–S42.
14. Gourlay DL, Heit HA, Almahrezi A. Universal precautions in pain medicine: a rational approach to the management of chronic pain. *Pain Med* 2005;6(2):107–112.
15. Joranson DE, Gilson AM, Ryan KM, et al. *Achieving Balance in Federal and State Pain Policy: A Guide to Evaluation.* 2nd ed. Madison, WI: University of Wisconsin Comprehensive Cancer Center; 2003. Available at: http://www.medsch.wisc.edu/painpolicy. Accessed December 19, 2004.
16. Shoemaker S, Wilson B. *The Big Book of Alcoholics Anonymous.* New York: Works Publishing; 1939.
17. Heit HA. Addiction, physical dependence, and tolerance: precise definitions to help clinicians evaluate and treat chronic pain patients. *J Pain Palliat Care Pharmacother* 2003;17(1):15–29.
18. American Academy of Pain Medicine, American Pain Society, American Society of Addiction Medicine. *Definitions Related to the Use of Opioids for the Treatment of Pain.* Glenview, IL: American Academy of Pain Medicine; 2001.
19. Savage SR, Joranson DE, Covington EC, et al. Definitions related to the medical use of opioids: evolution towards universal agreement. *J Pain Symptom Manage* 2003;26(1):655–667.
20. Ballantyne JC, LaForge KS. Opioid dependence and addiction during opioid treatment of chronic pain. *Pain* 2007;129(3):235–255.
21. Inturrisi CE. Clinical pharmacology of opioids for pain. *Clin J Pain* 2002;18(4 suppl):S3–S13.
22. Li X, Clark JD. Hyperalgesia during opioid abstinence: mediation by glutamate and substance p. *Anesth Analg* 2002;95(4):979–984.
23. Califf RM, Woodcock J, Ostroff S. A proactive response to prescription opioid abuse. *N Engl J Med* 2016;374(15):1480–1485.
24. Von Korff M, Dublin S, Walker RL, et al. The impact of opioid risk reduction initiatives on high-dose opioid prescribing for patients on chronic opioid therapy. *J Pain* 2016;17(1):101–110.
25. Washington State Agency Medical Directors' Group. *Interagency Guideline on Opioid Dosing for Chronic Non-Cancer Pain: An Educational Aid to Improve Care and Safety with Opioid Therapy.* Washington State Agency Medical Directors' Group; 2010.
26. Wasan AD, Correll DJ, Kissin I, et al. Iatrogenic addiction in patients treated for acute or subacute pain: a systematic review. *J Opioid Manag* 2006;2(1):16–22.
27. Weissman DE, Haddox JD. Opioid pseudoaddiction—an iatrogenic syndrome. *Pain* 1989;36(3):363–366.
28. Koob GF, Le Moal M. Drug addiction, dysregulation of reward, and allostasis. *Neuropsychopharmacology* 2001;24(2):97–129.
29. Nestler EJ, Landsman D. Learning about addiction from the genome. *Nature* 2001;409(6822):834–835.
30. Nestler EJ. Molecular basis of long-term plasticity underlying addiction. *Nat Rev Neurosci* 2001;2(2):119–128.
31. Kasser CL, Geller A, Howell EH, et al. Principles of detoxification. In: Graham AW, Schultz TK, eds. *Principles of Addiction Medicine.* 2nd ed. Chevy Chase, MD: American Society of Addiction Medicine; 1998.
32. Nestler EJ, Hyman SE, Malenka RC. Reinforcement and addictive disorders. In: *Molecular Neuropharmacology: A Foundation for Clinical Neuroscience.* New York: McGraw-Hill; 2001.
33. Leshner AI. Addiction is a brain disease, and it matters. *Science* 1997;278(5335):45–47.
34. Wise RA. Addiction becomes a brain disease. *Neuron* 2000;26(1):27–33.
35. Pappagallo M. The concept of pseudotolerance to opioids. *J Pharm Care Pain Symptom Control* 1998;6:95–98.
36. Heit H, Gourlay D. Chronic pain and addiction. In: Pasricha P, Willis W, Gebhart G, eds. *Chronic Abdominal and Visceral Pain: Theory and Practice.* New York: Taylor & Francis; 2006:231–244.
37. Ozaki S, Narita M, Narita M, et al. Suppression of the morphine-induced rewarding effect and G-protein activation in the lower midbrain following nerve injury in the mouse: involvement of G-protein-coupled receptor kinase 2. *Neuroscience* 2003;116(1):89–97.
38. Ozaki S, Narita M, Narita M, et al. Suppression of the morphine-induced rewarding effect in the rat with neuropathic pain: implication of the reduction in mu-opioid receptor functions in the ventral tegmental area. *J Neurochem* 2002;82(5):1192–1198.
39. Graham AW. Screening for alcoholism by life-style risk assessment in a community hospital. *Arch Intern Med* 1991;151(5):958–964.
40. Reyna TM, Hollis HW Jr, Hulsebus RC. Alcohol-related trauma. The surgeon's responsibility. *Ann Surg* 1985;201(2):194–197.
41. Moore RD, Bone LR, Geller G, et al. Prevalence, detection, and treatment of alcoholism in hospitalized patients. *JAMA* 1989;261(3):403–407.
42. Gourlay D, Heit H, Caplan YH. *Urine Drug Testing in Clinical Practice: The Art and Science of Patient Care.* 5th ed. Baltimore, MD: Johns Hopkins University School of Medicine; 2012.
43. Bruera E, Moyano J, Seifert L, et al. The frequency of alcoholism among patients with pain due to terminal cancer. *J Pain Symptom Manage* 1995;10(8):599–603.
44. Passik SD, Kirsh KL, Whitcomb L, et al. Pain clinicians' rankings of aberrant drug-taking behaviors. *J Pain Palliat Care Pharmacother* 2002;16(4):39–49.
45. Houry D, Baldwin G. Announcing the CDC guideline for prescribing opioids for chronic pain. *J Safety Res* 2016;57:83–84.
46. Gourlay D, Heit H, Caplan Y. *Urine Drug Testing in Primary Care: Dispelling the Myths & Designing Strategies.* 3rd ed. Available at: http://www.familydocs.org/assets/Professional_Development/CME/UDT.pdf. Accessed March 7, 2006.
47. Heit HA, Gourlay DL. Urine drug testing in pain medicine. *J Pain Symptom Manage* 2004;27(3):260–267.
48. Gourlay DL, Heit HA. Universal precautions revisited: managing the inherited pain patient. *Pain Med* 2009;10(suppl 2):S115–S123.

49. Dellemijn P. Are opioids effective in relieving neuropathic pain? *Pain* 1999;80(3):453–462.

50. Scadding JW. Treatment of neuropathic pain: historical aspects. *Pain Med* 2004;5(suppl 1):S3–S8.

51. Chou R, Turner JA, Devine EB, et al. The effectiveness and risks of long-term opioid therapy for chronic pain: a systematic review for a National Institutes of Health Pathways to Prevention Workshop. *Ann Intern Med* 2015;162(4):276–286.

52. Kalso E, Edwards JE, Moore RA, et al. Opioids in chronic non-cancer pain: systematic

53. Resnick RB. Food and Drug Administration approval of buprenorphine-naloxone for office treatment of addiction. *Ann Intern Med* 2003;138(4):360.

54. Resnick RB, Galanter M, Resnick E, et al. Buprenorphine treatment of heroin dependence (detoxification and maintenance) in a private practice setting. *J Addict Dis* 2001;20(2):75–83.

55. *The Drug Addiction Treatment Act of 2000*. Available at https://www.samhsa.gov/programs-campaigns/medication-assisted-treatment/training-materials-resources/buprenorphine-waiver. Accessed April 20, 2018.

56. Saunders JB, Aasland OG, Babor TF, et al. Development of the Alcohol Use Disorders Identification Test (AUDIT): WHO Collaborative Project on Early Detection of Persons with Harmful Alcohol Consumption—II. *Addiction* 1993;88(6):791–804.

57. Butler SF, Budman SH, Fernandez K, et al. Validation of a screener and opioid assessment measure for patients with chronic pain. *Pain* 2004;112 (1–2):65–75.

58. Akbik H, Butler SF, Budman SH, et al. Validation and clinical application of the Screener and Opioid Assessment for Patients with Pain (SOAPP). *J Pain Symptom Manage* 2006;32(3):287–293.

59. Brown RL, Rounds LA. Conjoint screening questionnaires for alcohol and other drug abuse: criterion validity in a primary care practice. *Wis Med J* 1995;94(3):135–140.

60. Fiellin DA, Reid MC, O'Connor PG. Outpatient management of patients with alcohol problems. *Ann Intern Med* 2000;133(10):815–827.

61. Webster LR, Webster RM. Predicting aberrant behaviors in opioid-treated patients: preliminary validation of the Opioid Risk Tool. *Pain Med* 2005;6(6):432–442.

62. Centers for Disease Control and Prevention. Recommendations for prevention of HIV transmission in health-care settings. *MMWR* 1987;36(suppl 2S):1–16.

63. Gourlay D, Heit H. Universal precautions: a matter of mutual trust and responsibility. *Pain Med* 2006;7(2):210–212.

64. Fishman SM, Bandman TB, Edwards A, et al. The opioid contract in the management of chronic pain. *J Pain Symptom Manage* 1999;18(1):27–37.

65. Fishman SM, Kreis PG. The opioid contract. *Clin J Pain* 2002;18(suppl 4): S70–S75.

66. Heit HA. Creating and implementing opioid agreements. *Dis Manag Digest* 2003;7(1):2–3.

67. Olsen Y. The CDC Guideline on Opioid Prescribing: rising to the challenge. *JAMA* 2016;315(15):1577–1579.

68. Passik SD, Weinreb HJ. Managing chronic nonmalignant pain: overcoming obstacles to the use of opioids. *Adv Ther* 2000;17(2):70–83.

69. Heit HA, Gourlay DL. Buprenorphine: new tricks with an old molecule for pain management. *Clin J Pain* 2008;24(2):93–97.

70. Pergolizzi JV Jr, Scholten W, Smith KJ, et al. The unique role of transdermal buprenorphine in the global chronic pain epidemic. *Acta Anaesthesiol Taiwan* 2015;53(2):71–76.

71. Pergolizzi J, Aloisi AM, Dahan A, et al. Current knowledge of buprenorphine and its unique pharmacological profile. *Pain Pract* 2010;10(5):428–450.

72. Clark NC, Lintzeris N, Muhleisen PJ. Severe opiate withdrawal in a heroin user precipitated by a massive buprenorphine dose. *Med J Aust* 2002;176(4):166–167.

73. Sporer KA. Buprenorphine: a primer for emergency physicians. *Ann Emerg Med* 2004;43(5):580–584.

74. Center for Substance Abuse Treatment. *Clinical Guidelines for the Use of Buprenorphine in the Treatment of Opioid Addiction*. A Treatment Improvement Protocol (TIP) Series 40. Rockville, MD: Substance Abuse and Mental Health Services Administration; 2004.

75. Zubieta J, Greenwald MK, Lombardi U, et al. Buprenorphine-induced changes in mu-opioid receptor availability in male heroin-dependent volunteers: a preliminary study. *Neuropsychopharmacology* 2000;23(3):326–334.

76. Passik SD, Heit H, Kirsh KL. Reality and responsibility: a commentary on the treatment of pain and suffering in a drug-using society. *J Opioid Manag* 2006;2(3):123–127.

77. Ballantyne JC. Opioid therapy in chronic pain. *Phys Med Rehabil Clin N Am* 2015;26(2):201–218.

78. Kripalani S, Yao X, Haynes RB. Interventions to enhance medication adherence in chronic medical conditions: a systematic review. *Arch Intern Med* 2007;167(6):540–550.

79. Alford DP. Opioid prescribing for chronic pain—achieving the right balance through education. *N Engl J Med* 2016;374(4):301–303.

80. Thielke SM, Turner JA, Shortreed SM, et al. Do patient-perceived pros and cons of opioids predict sustained higher-dose use? *Clin J Pain* 2014;30(2):93–101.

CHAPTER 60

Compliance Monitoring in Chronic Pain Management

DOUGLAS L. GOURLAY and **HOWARD A. HEIT**

The pain management practitioner faces several challenges in the safe and effective management of chronic pain. One of these relates to the important issue of monitoring compliance with a previously agreed-on course of therapy. Unfortunately, in today's medicolegal climate, the need for clinicians to take steps to reduce the risk of diversion and misuse of controlled substances has become apparent. Although the debate continues as to what degree prescribers contribute to the overall source of controlled substance that reaches the street,[1-4] there should be no debate about the prescriber's responsibility to ensure a decreased need for these drugs by addressing demand reduction strategies in all susceptible individuals. All pain patients are not potential diverters: All aberrant behavior does not represent drug addiction or misuse.[5] However, we tend to adopt a more casual attitude toward prescription drugs, including opioids, despite the fact that there is a disturbing trend toward prescription drug abuse by adolescents and others who have found their family medicine chests a ready supply of abusable drugs.[4,6] Whether this is because of an implicit sense of safety associated with prescription products or due to a simple comparison with typical illicit drugs of abuse found on the street is unclear. In fact, there has been a marked increase in counterfeit drugs on the street, typically adulterated with potent opioids such as fentanyl and carfentanil. In many cases, the first exposure to these drugs results in a fatal outcome. The emergence of naloxone rescue protocols in so many cities in North America is a testament to this growing problem.[7,8]

How Communication Influences Compliance Assessment

Clinicians have less control over how our prescriptions are used than we would like to believe. In fact, there are three dimensions to consider when examining the prescription of any controlled substance.

The first is "what the patient is told to do." Obviously, a prescriber must inform and document the instructions around the prescription of any medication, especially controlled substances. To this end, a physician might reasonably be held to account for a bad outcome in the context of medication use if the only documented instructions to the patient were "Use as directed." Treatment compliance assumes that the clinician is clear about how the patient was instructed and that the patient clearly understood these instructions. In the author's opinion, this is rarely the case.

The second is "what the patient is telling the prescriber he is doing." Communication between patient and prescriber is key not only to ensuring the best possible treatment outcomes but also in identifying possible miscommunications between prescriber and patient around treatment plans, especially with opioids. So, the patient who is advised to take medications in a "three-times-daily fashion" might remain clinically unstable—until the prescriber finds out that the patient is actually taking medications at 0900h, 1000h, and 1100h, respectively. Clearly, the prescriber and the patient are not on the same page around the dosing interval of this medication. Again, assessment of treatment requires careful communication.

But the final possibility is "what the patient *might* be doing with the medication, in a worst-case scenario." Take for example the patient who is becoming obviously impaired during the first week of a recent prescription refill. Although the patient never run out of medications early (over the course of a 1-month prescription), he may be overusing his medications during the initial phase of the prescription, only to struggle on toward the end of the month because he has literally "borrowed from tomorrow to pay for today" in his dosing schedule.[9] Simply asking what is the most medication he has had to use in 24 hours will help to get a better understanding of how the medication is actually being used.

In the aforementioned examples, the clinician is clearly responsible for the instructions given to the patient and to some extent is responsible for clarifying those instructions if necessary based on what the patient tells the clinician he or she is doing. In the third case, however, the patient alone must be held responsible for any adverse outcomes based on what he is *actually* doing if this information is withheld from the prescriber.

A considerable effort has been expended in teaching clinicians how to initiate pharmacotherapy ("entrance strategy"), but unfortunately, there has not been an equal effort expended in teaching the technique of terminating these medications ("exit strategy"),[10,11] some of which may have considerable withdrawal syndromes associated with their rapid taper or abrupt discontinuation. No matter how selective we appear to be in offering opioid trials to "low-risk" patient populations, prescribers will always need to (1) assess the opioid trial as either successful/failed and (2) have a defensible, rational, and compassionate exit strategy.[12]

For the purposes of this chapter, compliance monitoring may be defined as those steps taken by a prescriber to ensure that treatment plans are adhered to and prescribed medications are appropriately used. Many factors contribute to a patient's failure to adhere to an agreed-on treatment plan.[13] To expect 100% adherence, even when controlled substances are involved, is to ignore this fact.[13]

Compliance monitoring should begin with an individual assessment of risk. As outlined in Chapter 59, it is unwise to assume that you can assess risk, with any degree of certainty, at the first visit. Risk assessment and management is best performed over time. Treatment agreements, interval and contingency prescribing, pill counts, prescription monitoring programs (PMP), and urine drug testing (UDT) can all play important parts in helping to manage risk and so improve outcomes.[14-17]

The fact is we have little evidence to support this practice.[18] Beyond this, there is little evidence to support the notion that risk evaluation and mitigation strategies (REMS) accomplish any of their stated goals. In fact, the recent push toward abuse-deterrent/abuse-resistant has also been without scientific or clinical support of efficacy.[19] Only time will tell if these approaches have a meaningful and positive impact on the problem of prescription drug abuse in America. In the authors' opinion, placing too much confidence in the ability of clever delivery systems to prevent aberrant drug-taking behavior in the high-risk patient population may cause us to revisit many of the same problems we have had to deal with over the past 25 years. As with the diabetic patient who self-reports optimum glycemic control at a follow-up visit, the clinician still performs a glycated hemoglobin (HgBA$_1$C) test (which is a measure of glycemic control over time) as an objective measure of treatment success.[9,20] Because hyperglycemia is not illegal, there is little prejudice created in the clinician's mind when the objective test is at odds with the patient's self-report. Just as with HgBA$_1$C, the clinician can use a discordant UDT result to motivate change on the part of the patient and to monitor healthy changes already made.

For the most part, monitoring efforts should be based on the initial then subsequent assessments of risk over time. In this regard, frequency of drug testing might reasonably be expected to be greater in an identified "high-risk" patient population compared to a "low-risk" population. In fact, even in high-risk populations, UDT can be overused. Medically necessary testing must be tailored to the patient.

A variety of tools have been developed to aid the clinician with this important task.[21-26] Regardless of the tool used, the result is only an estimate of the risk of the patient engaging in aberrant behavior. High risk is not an absolute contraindication for the prescribing of controlled substances but might cause a prudent clinician to seek formal consultation with or referral to other appropriate health care professionals who have sufficient experience and resources to manage these often challenging cases.[14] It is important to remember that having a legitimate reason for prescribing a controlled substance does not in itself make it appropriate to do so.

Interpreting Aberrant Behavior

Even with the most reasonable treatment plan, a patient's ability to comply is based on a multitude of potentially conflicting factors. When a patient fails to comply, the treating clinician needs to have an approach that allows the patient and prescriber to adequately address these issues. Not all aberrant behavior represents abuse, addiction, or criminal intent.[9] Similarly, what may seem like reasonable treatment goals for any given patient may be more difficult for some patients to comply with than others, even in the context of a previously signed treatment agreement. When a patient steps out of previously defined limits and boundaries, the clinician should examine the context of this behavior.

It is often surprising for clinicians to realize that some aberrant behavior can be iatrogenic in nature. Unreasonably set limits or demands on a patient can cause even the lowest risk patients to "step out of bounds." However, in some cases, this behavior can be framed in the context of a "Golden Moment" where the patient may begin to see things for the way they are rather than the way he or she wished they were. In this way, both clinician and patient can improve their level of communication that is inherent in all positive therapeutic relationships. Rather than simply dismissing the patient for breaking the treatment agreement, which can perpetuate the patient's revolving-door approach to health care, both parties become better educated to move forward in a strengthened therapeutic relationship based on mutual trust and honesty. This approach best serves the mutual interests of patient, practitioner, and the community in which they live.

Some patients, however, are not ready to make these changes; they may need to seek care elsewhere. It is important to remember that it is generally better for a patient to abandon a reasonable and prudent course of therapy offered by a knowledgeable practitioner than it is for that patient to be dismissed from the practice. Although it may be necessary and appropriate to discontinue the prescription of controlled substances such as the opioid class of medication, this should rarely be equivalent to dismissal from care, although a drug-seeking patient may

interpret the two as being the same. From a medical legal perspective, it is usually better to "abandon the molecule" rather than be perceived as having abandoned the patient.

POTENTIAL TREATMENT TRAPS IN COMPLIANCE MONITORING
Borrowing from Tomorrow to Pay for Today

For most patients, problematic prescription drug use does not involve misuse or diversion. For those patients who do exhibit aberrant behavior such as running out of medications early, the most common problem relates to simply taking more than prescribed. The concept of *borrowing from tomorrow to pay for today* is something that many patients can relate to.[5] In these circumstances, prescribing multiple prescriptions for smaller quantities of medications, to be dispensed by the pharmacist on an interval basis, can assist the patient with treatment adherence. In many states, regulations now allow for appropriately dated prescriptions to be written and filled sequentially by a pharmacist ("Do not fill until").[17] Patients who need more oversight than weekly medication pickup should likely be referred on for more formal assessment of potential comorbid conditions such as substance use disorders or other significant psychopathology.

Avoiding Excessive Pill Loads

In the management of chronic pain, medications must be carefully titrated to their optimum dose. Traditional teaching for a trial of opioid therapy suggests using immediate-release medications to establish drug responsiveness followed by conversion to sustained-release medication, typically in a two- or three-times-daily dosing schedule with a suitable amount of immediate-release medication for breakthrough pain management. More recent guidelines from the Centers for Disease Control and Prevention have suggested that, where possible, immediate-release medications are to be used over their sustained-release counterparts.[27] Although the addiction literature continues to suggest that from the perspective of abuse/addiction risk, patients are likely to do better on sustained-release or truly long-acting (e.g., methadone/buprenorphine) opioids for the long-term treatment of chronic pain, there are no recent long-term perspective studies in the literature to confirm this important clinical point.[28-31]

By definition, a successful trial is one in which the patient is clearly improved either in terms of pain relief, functional restoration, or ideally both. Properly chosen patients may do well with this approach. Some, however, improve initially but lack the sustainable relief seen with truly opioid-responsive pain. In these cases, there is often seen a gradual dose escalation with diminishing returns as the side effect profile begins to overtake the therapeutic effect. For some patients, efficacy is measured by the subtle cognitive effects transiently seen with a new drug or drug dose rather than the marked reduction in pain scores and improved function typically seen with treatment-responsive pain. Unfortunately, tolerance to these effects can develop quickly, leading to significant dose escalation. Sometimes, to reduce drug use, the prescriber provides the patient with smaller dose tablets in the hopes the patient will be able to titrate the dose down, reducing the overall dose taken and so the adverse effects often seen with higher medication levels.

For example, a patient who is using 80 mg of controlled-release oxycodone in an every-8-hours dosing schedule may request 20-mg tablets rather than the 80-mg tablets, indicating that the patient often feels he or she does not need to take the entire dose to keep the pain under control. To reduce the total daily dose, the 80-mg tablets are changed to 20-mg tablets. In this case now, instead of receiving 3 tablets per day, 21 tablets per week, the patient receives 12 tablets per day (to be used "as directed" in a three-times-daily divided dose). This is a total of

84 tablets per week. In a monthly prescription, this amounts to 336 tablets. Although some patients may achieve the desired goal of dose reduction, others will ultimately begin to redistribute the controlled-release drug, often taking the medication more frequently during the day than the agreed-on 8-hour interval. With such large quantities of tablets available, *borrowing from tomorrow to pay for today* can become a problem.[5] In such cases when patients have asked for smaller unit doses as described earlier, it can be revealing to ask the patient to bring in extra medications at the next visit. It is a minority of patients who can comply with this request, indicating that they use the medication up eventually. In these cases, closer inquiry may show that the duration of action for the modified-release drug is only 3 or 4 hours, necessitating six or more dosing intervals per day to achieve "stability." Clearly, the use of a modified-release medication in the same fashion as an immediate-release preparation is inappropriate. In a sense, the patient can be legitimately advised that the "clever delivery system" has failed them. In these cases, the answer is not to dose more frequently with the controlled-release preparation but rather to consider rotating to another modified-release system or to a truly long-acting medication such as methadone or buprenorphine.

Using Pill Load Limits to Modify Behavior

Many practitioners use the time between visits as a guide to how many unit doses any given prescription will need. So, if a prescription is written for 3 tablets daily and the follow-up appointment is in 30 days, many clinicians would write the script for 90 tablets (possibly adding 2 or 3 days' worth to cover for exigent circumstances). For most, writing a prescription for less than 100 tablets is quite reasonable. In some cases, that same 30-day interval will require many more than 100 tablets. As an example, a person might use 10 hydrocodone/acetaminophen tablets per day. In this case, a 1-month supply would require you to write for 300 tablets. Practically, this would mean the patient would have to fill prescriptions on a 10-day interval (to allow for unit dose limits of 100 or fewer tablets per prescription). This is both inconvenient for the patient as well as costlier due to co-pays for filling multiple scripts.

This may also present an opportunity for the patient to consider tapering the daily dose of medication used and so allowing for more time between prescriptions filled. At least one recent guideline has indicated that individual prescriptions for excessive numbers of tablets or milligrams of drug will trigger an investigation by the appropriate regulatory body.[32]

Compliance Monitoring Tips and Traps

There is some literature examining compliance failures and aberrant behaviors, but most seem to examine this from a patient perspective. Physicians have rarely been taught to consider their own role in the patient behaviors that they are struggling with.

Take for example the patient who is demonstrating aberrant behavior including symptom magnification and drug-seeking behaviors. Many clinicians can identify this as abnormal, either at the conscious or gut levels, and act accordingly. Few have ever considered the possibility that this may be iatrogenic in etiology.

If a patient believes that the ongoing prescription of medications is "contingent" on the doctor believing that he or she "still needs" these drugs, the patient is likely to behave in a way that he or she believes will result in continuation of the status quo. However, if the prescriber has caused the patient to believe (either consciously or unconsciously) that he or she is uncomfortable with these prescriptions and at some point will ultimately stop writing prescriptions for them, the behavior can be seen in a totally different light. It should not be a surprise that when the patient sees that today is not the day to begin the feared taper or worse simple discontinuation of the drugs on which the patient has at least become physically dependent that the demeanor changes almost magically. Yes, it is clearly abnormal behavior, but it is not entirely clear what this behavior means. As a general rule, it is easier to identify abnormal behavior than it is to accurately interpret what it means. In the context of abnormal behavior, there can be a variety of "correct" responses: The one absolutely incorrect thing to do is to simply ignore it.[17]

Urine Drug Testing in Pain Medicine

UDT is a useful tool in pain management that provides valuable objective information to assist in diagnostic and therapeutic decision making.[16] Results of UDT can assist in assessing compliance with a previously agreed-on treatment plan (adherence/compliance); they may also identify relapse or drug misuse as early as possible, and finally, the results can be used to advocate for the patient with third-party interests.[17] Of course, any diagnostic test used in the context of patient care must meet the basic test of medical necessity. The topic of medical necessity will be examined in greater detail later in the chapter.

To assess compliance, the clinician may look for the presence of prescribed medications and/or metabolites as evidence of their recent use. Not finding the prescribed drug or finding unprescribed or illicit drugs in the urine merits further discussion with the patient while recognizing that laboratory error and test insensitivity can result in misleading data. Bingeing by the patient can result in unexpected negative urine reports if the patient runs out of medication prior to sample collection. Therefore, these results by themselves cannot be relied on to prove drug diversion and may be consistent with addiction, pseudoaddiction, or the use of an opioid for nonpain purposes—so-called chemical coping.[33] The purpose of UDT should be explained to the patient at the initial evaluation. UDT should be used, like all other diagnostic tests, to improve patient care. UDT can also enhance the relationship between clinicians and patients by providing documentation of adherence to mutually agreed-on treatment plans.[16,34]

Reports of unprescribed or illicit substances in the urine aid in the assessment and diagnosis of drug misuse or addiction. UDT results can be used to encourage change to more functional behaviors while supporting the positive changes previously made. Thus, the appropriate use of a UDT result requires documentation in the medical record and an understanding on the part of both the patient and the clinician of how these results are to be used.[35]

In the pain management setting, the presence of an illicit or unprescribed drug does not necessarily negate the legitimacy of the patient's pain complaints, but it may suggest a concurrent disorder such as drug abuse or addiction. Although acute pain can be treated in a patient with an active addictive disorder, it is unlikely that one can successfully treat chronic pain in a patient with untreated addiction. The patient must be willing to accept assessment and treatment of both disorders to receive adequate outcomes in either.[11] Thus, the diagnosis of a concurrent addictive disorder, when it exists, does nothing to negate a legitimate pain disorder, but rather, it complicates it. In some cases, the very nature of the patients' diagnosis may change because of information gained through drug testing.

SPECIMEN CHOICE

Urine has been the preferred biologic specimen for determining the presence or absence of most drugs since the 1970s.[36] This is in part due to the increased window of detection of 1 to 3 days for most drugs and/or their metabolites.[37] When compared to serum samples, the relatively noninvasive nature of sample collection, ease of storage, and low cost of testing favor urine as the specimen of choice. Although there are currently other matrix options, including saliva, hair, and even breath (tetrahydrocannabinol [THC]), urine remains the most commonly used specimen.[17,38]

WHOM TO TEST

The question of whom to test is made easier by having a uniform practice policy that helps reduce individual stigma. Beyond this, any risk of patient profiling based on racial, cultural, or other physical appearances is reduced. Careful explanation of the purpose of testing normally allays patient concerns.[16]

FREQUENCY OF TESTING

Testing frequency is a function of many factors, some of which are patient-based and others are a function of the practice. For example, in a pain practice where the patient referral base is typically more complex, a policy of testing all patients on admission and thereafter to be determined by clinical assessment of risk is recommended. On the other hand, in the average primary care setting, where the prevalence of individuals with substance use disorder should be no greater than the population, it may be sufficient to discuss UDT with all patients and reserve actual testing to a behaviorally triggered paradigm. Unfortunately, this latter approach does subject the patient and practitioner to the risk of missing a potentially treatable comorbid disorder (substance misuse/addiction).[2,39,40]

In those practices with a disproportionate percentage of high-risk patients, determining how frequently to use UDT can be a real challenge. Contrary to popular belief, even high-risk patients can be tested too frequently. In a perfect world, we would *not* be testing everyone "all the time." It is not simply cost that requires us to use appropriate clinical judgment in the rational use of laboratory resources, including UDT. It is important to remember that drug testing is not a therapeutic measure. It is only through the judicial use of UDT with careful integration of clinical and behavioral components that optimum clinical care can be delivered.

Regardless, as time moves forward, the use of UDT is fast becoming a standard of care. What is becoming clear is that the risk to the patient and practitioner alike is a function of what is done with the data thus obtained and not fundamentally in the data itself.[40]

TESTING STRATEGIES

The literature is clear that there is often a disconnect between the reason a UDT was ordered, the results obtained, and, most importantly, the clinical consequences to the patient because of these tests. The fundamental problem is a lack of testing strategy or plan for the clinician to use in response to results obtained. So, for the cocaine-misusing, chronic noncancer pain patient who refuses to give up the use of this drug, the clinical course correction necessary may, for the sake of safety, simply involve the termination of the use of controlled substances such as the opioid class of drug. On the other hand, in the palliative care case where there may be a moral imperative to the continued use of controlled substances for pain management, the decision to move this person into a more supervised setting for medication management might be made based on this new information.

The clinician must know the drugs for which to test, appropriate methods to use, and the expected use of the results obtained. If the purpose of testing is to find unprescribed or illicit drug use, a combined chromatographic and spectroscopic method such as gas chromatography/mass spectroscopy or liquid chromatography/tandem mass spectroscopy (GC/MS or LC/MS-MS) or similar technologies are the most specific for identifying individual drugs or their metabolites.[41] Caution must be exercised when interpreting UDT results in a pain practice. True-negative urine results for prescribed medication may indicate a pattern of bingeing rather than drug diversion.

TABLE 60.1 Retention Times and Detection Windows of Common Analytes

Drug	Approximate Retention Time
Amphetamines	48 h
Barbiturates	Short-acting (e.g., secobarbital) 24 h
	Long-acting (e.g., phenobarbital) 2–3 wk
Benzodiazepines	3 d if therapeutic dose ingested
	Up to 4–6 wk after extended dosage (i.e., 1 or more years)
Cocaine	
Metabolite	2–4 d
Ethanol	2–4 h
Methadone	Approximately 3 d
Opioids	2 d
Cannabinoids	Moderate smoker (four times a week) 5 d
	Heavy smoker (smoking daily) 10 d
	Retention time for chronic smokers may be 20–28 d
Phencyclidine	Approximately 8 d
	Up to 30 d in chronic users
	(mean value = 14 d)

NOTE: Interpretation of retention time must consider variability of urine specimens, drug metabolism and half-life, patient's physical condition, fluid intake, and method and frequency of ingestion. These are general guidelines only.

Time of last use of the drug(s) can be helpful in the interpretation of negative UDT results. Table 60.1 lists retention times/detection windows of common analytes.

PRESUMPTIVE VERSUS DEFINITIVE TESTING

For many years, the terms using in clinical drug testing were borrowed from the forensic world of UDT. The concept of preliminary or "screen testing" by various immunoassay techniques followed by more specific "confirmatory testing" by what is often termed a *second, scientific method* is one more suited to criminal justice rather than clinical care. More recently, the terms have begun to change in clinical care: Preliminary testing is now "presumptive testing," and confirmatory testing has been replaced with "definitive testing." In the former case, presumptive testing often provides indirect evidence of specific drug or drug classes, whereas the latter case uses sophisticated methodologies that definitively identify the drug and/or drug metabolite in any given sample. The specifics of these methods are beyond the scope of this chapter, but readers are invited to review *Urine Drug Testing in Clinical Practice*, 6th edition, for specifics.[17]

A routine UDT presumptive panel* might include the following drugs/drug classes:
- Cocaine
- Amphetamines / methamphetamine
- Opioids
- Methadone
- Marijuana
- Benzodiazepines

To reduce the risk of an undetected substituted or adulterated test sample, random urinary creatinine, pH, and temperature should be included in the test panel to assist with interpretation and to increase specimen reliability. The temperature of a urine sample within 4 minutes of voiding should be between 90° and 100° F.[42] Urinary pH undergoes physiologic fluctuations throughout the day but should remain within the range of 4.5 to 8.0.[42]

---

*Any test panel element should include consideration of the population of donor's being tested as well as the local drugs of abuse common to their setting.

Urinary creatinine varies with daily water intake and hydration; normal human urine has a creatinine concentration greater than 20 mg/dL. Values lower than 20 mg/dL indicate dilution, and findings lower than 5 mg/dL are inconsistent with human urine.[42,43] Test results outside of these ranges should be discussed with the patient and/or the laboratory, as necessary.[16]

The detection time of most drugs or their metabolites in urine is usually 1 to 3 days, which is influenced by several factors including but not limited to dose, route of administration, metabolism, urine concentration, and pH.[41,44] Chronic use of a lipid-soluble drug such as marijuana may extend the window of detection to a week or more.[42,45] Benzodiazepines and their metabolites differ widely in their elimination half-lives, which affect their clinical effect, excretion, and detection (see Table 60.1).[46]

There has been much debate about the role of "passive marijuana smoke" and the possibilities of a "contact high" through passive inhalation of smoke from cannabis users.[47–52] The literature is at best contradictory about whether a low-level THC UDT specimen can be accounted for based on "secondhand smoke." Much of this literature is based on cannabis strains that are an order of magnitude less potent than that which is available today. In the author's opinion, further research into this area is necessary to come to a meaningful conclusion in terms of passive THC exposure as a cause for a positive presumptive or definitive test with the availability today's high potency cannabis.

The method chosen to detect a drug will depend on the reason for undertaking the test. Immunoassay drug tests (i.e., presumptive tests) are, at the current time, most commonly used. They are designed to classify substances as either present or absent and are generally highly sensitive. They are not, however, able to definitively identify the agent leading to the positive result and so are referred to as "presumptive tests." In pain management, specific drug identification using more sophisticated identification tests is often needed. Combined techniques such as GC/MS make accurate identification of a specific drug and/or its metabolites possible and so are commonly referred to as "definitive tests." When the patient is being prescribed with drugs from several different classes of compounds, such as is often the case with many pain patients, specific drug identification may be necessary, especially in cases of contested results.

Immunoassay drug tests for natural opioids are very responsive to morphine and codeine but do not distinguish between the two. UDT by immunoassay also shows a low sensitivity for semisynthetic/synthetic opioids such as oxycodone and fentanyl.[46,53] A negative result does not exclude their use. Even though an immunoassay may be negative for consumed oxycodone, it should be positive by more definitive testing such as GC/MS if the drug was used within the window of detection. The clinical importance of this fact with UDT cannot be overstated because compliant patients have been dismissed from pain management practices in response to a false-negative immunoassay test when looking specifically for prescribed oxycodone. More recently, drug-specific immunoassay tests have been developed for such drugs as oxycodone or methadone, which are semisynthetic and synthetic drugs, respectively. The previous detection of an analyte, especially semisynthetic drugs, does not ensure future detection, even when dose and dosing interval have not changed.[16] This is especially true when the drug concentration is "peri threshold" as would be the case when the concentration is 302 ng/mL and the cutoff is 300 ng/mL. Small changes in the state of hydration could easily make the sample "negative" one day and positive another.

LIMITATIONS OF TEST INTERPRETATION

The legitimate presence of a prescribed drug in the urine sample may make monitoring of that class of drugs impossible by immunoassay technique alone. Specific drug identification by

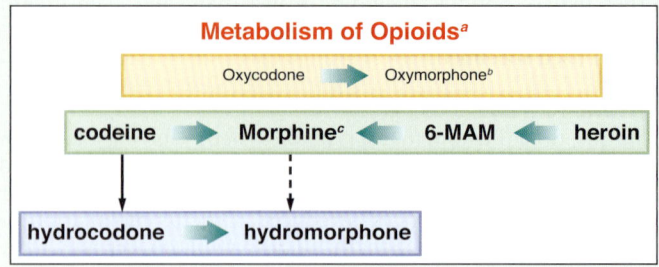

FIGURE 60.1 Basic opioid metabolic pathways. Not comprehensive pathways but may explain the presence of apparently unprescribed drugs. [a]From Gourlay D, Heit H, Caplan Y. Urine Drug Testing in Primary Care: Dispelling the Myths & Designing Strategies. 3rd ed. Available at: http://www.familydocs .org/assets/Professional_Development/CME/UDT.pdf. Accessed March 7, 2006. [b]From Sloan PA, Barkin RL. Oxymorphone, and oxymorphone extended release: a pharmacotherapeutic review. J Opioid Manag 2008;4(3):131–144. [c]From Cone EJ, Heit HA, Caplan YH, et al. Evidence of morphine metabolism to hydromorphone in pain patients chronically treated with morphine. J Anal Toxicol 2006;30(1):1–5. 6-MAM, 6-monoacetylmorphine (an intermediate metabolite).

chromatographic testing (i.e., GC/MS, LC/MS-MS) may also be necessary to identify which member of the detected class is responsible for the positive screen.[16]

The clinician also must understand the basic metabolism of commonly prescribed drugs, especially opioids, so he or she will be able to explain a UDT result that is positive for the prescribed medication and/or its metabolite(s). For example, codeine is a prodrug that has no intrinsic analgesic activity but is metabolized to morphine and other compounds for its analgesic properties. See Figure 60.1 for basic opioid metabolic pathways.

The amount of drug and/or metabolite(s) (i.e., nanogram per milliliter) within a urine sample should not be used to extrapolate backward and make specific determinations regarding compliance with prescribed medication. Software and laboratory products have not been scientifically validated and reported in the peer-reviewed literature to give this information at this time. Interpreting UDT beyond the current scientific knowledge may put clinicians and patients at medical and/or legal risk.[54] In addition, UDT cannot diagnose addiction, physical dependence, or diversion and should always be verified and correlated with the clinical picture. Health care professionals should use UDT results in conjunction with other clinical information when deciding to continue with or adjust the established boundaries of the treatment plan.

Dealing with Unexpected Urine Toxicology Results

Unlike drug testing that is forensically based, such as workplace testing, drug testing in clinical practice must have relevance to patient care. Unfortunately, these test results may come back unexpectedly negative for a prescribed drug or positive for an unprescribed one. The first step in interpreting these results is to contact the lab to ensure that no clerical errors have been made. Occasionally, a negative urine is falsely reported as positive either due to a simple clerical error (i.e., lab wrote positive when they meant negative) or the patient has taken some other product or medication that is causing an unexpected result. In some cases, more definitive testing as recommended by the lab will give answers to these questions, but they should never be ignored. There must be a process to follow that ultimately should include discussing the unexpected result with the patient.[16,34]

Unfortunately, drug tests may yield results that appear to be at odds with the patient's apparent level of clinical stability. Once confirmed as accurate, it is important to speak with the patient, carefully documenting the results and ensuing discussion in the medical record. When the patient acknowledges recreational use of prohibited substances, he or she should be advised of the clinical consequences of continued use including referral on to a specialist in substance use disorders or, if the patient indicates an unwillingness to stop using, discontinuation of the prescription of any controlled substances. When the patient indicates that he or she will no longer use, the patient should be tested more frequently—and, when possible, randomly—to ensure that this drug use has indeed stopped.[16,34] There are far more illicit/unprescribed drug users who *think* they are recreational users than are recreational users.

Decision to Terminate Opioid Therapy

The decision to change therapeutic direction should ideally be one made through mutual consultation and agreement between the patient and the physician. Unfortunately, occasions arise when the decision to discontinue a therapeutic agent or class of drugs must be made unilaterally. When mutually agreed-on therapeutic goals have not been met, the trial of therapy should be considered a failure and an exit strategy implemented. One commonly held myth is that those patients who no longer need opioid therapy come off these agents easily. This is often untrue. In fact, many articles have been written about pharmacologic efforts at attenuating the withdrawal symptoms associated with opioid withdrawal.[55-58] Unfortunately, most of these articles are contained in the addiction medicine literature: The pain management literature has been surprisingly quiet on this issue. Interestingly, many medications other than the opioid class of drugs can pose significant challenges to the prescriber and patient alike when the decision is made to discontinue a course of therapy.[59-64]

Generally, it is better to taper a drug than to abruptly discontinue it. Furthermore, the ease with which a patient can reduce a large dose to a smaller one may not predict the ease with which the patient ultimately discontinues the drug altogether. For this reason, a reasonable taper schedule for drugs with a known discontinuation syndrome is to reduce the agent by ~10% to 20% every 1 to 2 weeks until the last one-third of the dose is reached, at which point the agent should be reduced by ~5% to 10% every 2 to 4 weeks until the agent is stopped. When withdrawal symptoms present themselves, it may be helpful to suspend the taper until these symptoms resolve.

The speed with which a drug is discontinued is a function of many different variables. For example, a taper that is initiated following resolution of a chronic pain generator might be expected to be slower than one that is initiated in response to use of a prohibited substance such as cocaine. Of course, there are situations where it may not be advisable to taper the drug at all. In these cases, the drug will be abruptly discontinued. It should be noted that although abrupt cessation of the opioid class of drug is often distressing, it is unlikely to result in direct harm to the patient. This is not the case with the sedative class of drugs which usually require some form of pharmacologic assistance to safely terminate these agents.

In some cases, certain therapeutic agents can be used to blunt the withdrawal process, especially toward the end of the taper. In the case of opioid withdrawal, the α agonist clonidine can be useful to offset the hyperadrenergic symptoms associated with opioid withdrawal.[65] For the sedative class of drugs, gabapentinoids have been used with some success to both reduce the risk of withdrawal seizures as well as the significant distress associated with this class of drug. For the most part, the stimulant class of drugs does not have physical withdrawal syndromes associated with discontinuation; however, psychological support is often needed to successfully discontinue this class of drugs.

When the decision is made to discontinue a certain class of medication, it is important to remember that this should not be misinterpreted as discontinuation of treatment. Unfortunately for some patients, discontinuation of a certain drug may result in their abandoning the practitioner who has made the decision to no longer provide this medication. From a medicolegal perspective, it is much easier to defend against a patient who abandons a practitioner who makes a patient-centered decision to alter treatment based on sound medical judgment than it is to defend against an assertion of abandonment by a practitioner who becomes aware that his or her patient may have a problem with drugs.

FUTURE CONSIDERATIONS

An unfortunate reality of the massive expansion of drug testing in clinical care has been an excessive burden on the limited health care dollar.[66] The sale of desktop analyzers has seen an explosion of costs, often with very little evidence of clinical necessity or value added in terms of improved patient care. Clearly, the future of rational drug testing will have to rely on more reasonable compensation models that reflect the actual costs of performing these tests.

In fact, the science of drug testing is in evolution. One of the challenges in clinical care is finding a reliable and cost-effective method to identify specific drugs and their metabolites. The "two-step" approach of presumptive testing by an indirect, immunologic method followed by definitive testing using a combination chromatographic/spectroscopic method is both labor- and time-intensive. The necessary delays which result between sample collection and being able to act on a result are costly. More recently, other methods and approaches to drug testing have appeared.

One approach is to skip presumptive testing altogether and go directly to more definitive methodologies such as LC/MS-MS. To keep costs down and to reduce reporting delays, preliminary testing can be done using a "dilute and shoot" approach which requires very little sample preparation.[67,68] Now, our current "per analyte" method of laboratory compensation is lagging behind the fact that this method generates a vast amount of reliable data with very little sample preparation.

Even more exciting is the application of techniques such as substrate-enhanced Raman spectroscopy, which can identify specific compounds in a urine sample in both a timely and cost-effective manner. Sample preparation is minimal and relies on a nondestructive testing method to accurately test samples for clinical care.[69]

In conclusion, it is important to remember that a patient's failure to adhere rigorously to a treatment protocol should not be interpreted as definitive evidence of a substance use disorder or, worse, criminal intent. Patients fail to comply for a complex variety of reasons that must be assessed on an individual basis. Remember, aberrant behavior is much easier to identify than it is to interpret. By separating the motive from the behavior in assessing and interpreting departures from an agreed-on treatment plan, a patient-centered approach to problem solving can be implemented.[5]

References

1. Joranson DE, Gilson AM. Drug crime is a source of abused pain medications in the United States. *J Pain Symptom Manage* 2005;30(4):299–301.
2. Katz NP, Adams EH, Benneyan JC, et al. Foundations of opioid risk management. *Clin J Pain* 2007;23(2):103–118.
3. Joranson DE, Gilson AM. A much-needed window on opioid diversion. *Pain Med* 2007;8(2):128–129.
4. Center for Disease Control and Prevention. *Injury Prevention & Control: Opioid Overdose*. Atlanta, GA: U.S. Department of Health and Human Services; 2016.
5. Gourlay D, Heit H. Pain and addiction: managing risk through comprehensive care. *J Addict Dis* 2008;27(3):8.
6. Stopping drug use before it starts. In: *National Drug Control Strategy Annual Report*. Rockville, MD: Office of National Drug Control Policy; 2008:17–19.

7. Park TW, Lin LA, Hosanagar A, et al. Understanding risk factors for opioid overdose in clinical populations to inform treatment and policy. *J Addict Med* 2016;10(6):369–381.

8. Frank RG, Pollack HA. Addressing the fentanyl threat to public health. *N Engl J Med* 2017;376(7):605–607.

9. Gourlay DL, Heit H. The use of drug testing in promoting treatment adherence in pain medicine. In: Cheatle MD, Fine PG, eds. *Facilitating Treatment Adherence in Pain Medicine.* New York: Oxford University Press; 2017:57–82.

10. Gourlay DL, Heit HA. Universal precautions revisited: managing the inherited pain patient. *Pain Med* 2009;10(suppl 2):S115–S123.

11. Gourlay D, Heit H, Almarhezi A. Universal precautions in pain medicine: a rational approach to the management of chronic pain. *Pain Med* 2005;6(2):107–112.

12. Gourlay DL, Heit HA. Pain and addiction: managing risk through comprehensive care. *J Addict Dis* 2008;27(3):23–30.

13. Kripalani S, Yao X, Haynes RB. Interventions to enhance medication adherence in chronic medical conditions: a systematic review. *Arch Intern Med* 2007;167(6):540–550.

14. Gourlay D, Heit H. Universal precautions: a matter of mutual trust and responsibility. *Pain Med* 2006;7(2):210–212.

15. Fishman SM, Kreis PG. The opioid contract. *Clin J Pain* 2002;18(4 suppl):S70–S75.

16. Heit HA, Gourlay DL. Urine drug testing in pain medicine. *J Pain Symptom Manage* 2004;27(3):260–267.

17. Gourlay DL, Heit H, Caplan YH. *Urine Drug Testing in Clinical Practice: The Art and Science of Patient Care.* 6th ed. Stamford, CT: PharmaCom Group; 2015.

18. Starrels JL, Becker WC, Alford DP, et al. Systematic review: treatment agreements and urine drug testing to reduce opioid misuse in patients with chronic pain. *Ann Intern Med* 2010;152(11):712–720.

19. Becker WC, Fiellin DA. Abuse-deterrent opioid formulations—putting the potential benefits into perspective. *N Engl J Med* 2017;376(22):2103–2105.

20. Heit HA, Gourlay DL. Using urine drug testing to support healthy boundaries in clinical care. *J Opioid Manag* 2015;11(1):7–12.

21. Saunders JB, Aasland OG, Babor TF, et al. Development of the Alcohol Use Disorders Identification Test (AUDIT): WHO Collaborative Project on Early Detection of Persons with Harmful Alcohol Consumption—II. *Addiction* 1993;88(6):791–804.

22. Butler SF, Budman SH, Fernandez K, et al. Validation of a screener and opioid assessment measure for patients with chronic pain. *Pain* 2004;112(1–2):65–75.

23. Akbik H, Butler SF, Budman SH, et al. Validation and clinical application of the Screener and Opioid Assessment for Patients with Pain (SOAPP). *J Pain Symptom Manage* 2006;32(3):287–293.

24. Brown RL, Rounds LA. Conjoint screening questionnaires for alcohol and other drug abuse: criterion validity in a primary care practice. *Wis Med J* 1995;94(3):135–140.

25. Fiellin DA, Reid MC, O'Connor PG. Outpatient management of patients with alcohol problems. *Ann Intern Med* 2000;133(10):815–827.

26. Webster LR, Webster RM. Predicting aberrant behaviors in opioid-treated patients: preliminary validation of the Opioid Risk Tool. *Pain Med* 2005;6(6):432–442.

27. Houry D, Baldwin G. Announcing the CDC guideline for prescribing opioids for chronic pain. *J Safety Res* 2016;57:83–84.

28. Dole VP. Implications of methadone maintenance for theories of narcotic addiction. *JAMA* 1988;260(20):3025–3029.

29. Brookoff D. Abuse potential of various opioid medications. *J Gen Intern Med* 1993;8(12):688–690.

30. Zacny JP. Should people taking opioids for medical reasons be allowed to work and drive? *Addiction* 1996;91(11):1581–1584.

31. Haythornthwaite JA, Menefee LA, Quatrano-Piacentini AL, et al. Outcome of chronic opioid therapy for non-cancer pain. *J Pain Symptom Manage* 1998;15(3):185–194.

32. Busse JW, Guyatt GH, Carrasco A, et al. *The 2017 Canadian Guideline for Opioids for Chronic Non-Cancer Pain.* Ontario, Canada: National Pain Centre; 2017. Available at: http://nationalpaincentre.mcmaster.ca/. Accessed April 20, 2018.

33. Bruera E, Moyano J, Seifert L, et al. The frequency of alcoholism among patients with pain due to terminal cancer. *J Pain Symptom Manage* 1995;10(8):599–603.

34. Gourlay D, Heit H, Caplan Y. *Urine Drug Testing in Primary Care: Dispelling the Myths & Designing Strategies.* 3rd ed. Available at: http://www.familydocs.org/assets/Professional_Development/CME/UDT.pdf. Accessed March 7, 2006.

35. Passik SD, Schreiber J, Kirsh KL, et al. A chart review of the ordering and documentation of urine toxicology screens in a cancer center: do they influence patient management? *J Pain Symptom Manage* 2000;19(1):40–44.

36. Caplan YH, Goldberger BA. Alternative specimens for workplace drug testing. *J Anal Toxicol* 2001;25(5):396–399.

37. Conigliaro C, Reyes C, Schultz J. Principles of screening and early intervention. In: Graham AW, Schultz TK, Mayo-Smith MF, et al, eds. *Principles of Addiction Medicine.* 3rd ed. Chevy Chase, MD: American Society of Addiction Medicine; 2003:323–336.

38. Hammett-Stabler CA, Pesce AJ, Cannon DJ. Urine drug screening in the medical setting. *Clin Chim Acta* 2002;315(1–2):125–135.

39. Katz NP, Sherburne S, Beach M, et al. Behavioral monitoring and urine toxicology testing in patients receiving long-term opioid therapy. *Anesth Analg* 2003;97(4):1097–1102.

40. Katz N, Fanciullo GJ. Role of urine toxicology testing in the management of chronic opioid therapy. *Clin J Pain* 2002;18(suppl 4):S76–S82.

41. Vandevenne M, Vandenbussche H, Verstraete A. Detection time of drugs of abuse in urine. *Acta Clin Belg* 2000;55(6):323–333.

42. Cook JD, Caplan YH, LoDico CP, et al. The characterization of human urine for specimen validity determination in workplace drug testing: a review. *J Anal Toxicol* 2000;24(7):579–588.

43. Lipman A, Jackson K. Opioid pharmacotherapy. In: Warfield C, Bajwa Z, eds. *Principles and Practice of Pain Management.* New York: McGraw Hill; 2003:583–600.

44. Casavant MJ. Urine drug screening in adolescents. *Pediatr Clin North Am* 2002;49(2):317–327.

45. Huestis MA, Mitchell JM, Cone EJ. Detection times of marijuana metabolites in urine by immunoassay and GC-MS. *J Anal Toxicol* 1995;19(6):443–449.

46. Simpson D, Braithwaite RA, Jarvie DR, et al. Screening for drugs of abuse (II): Cannabinoids, lysergic acid diethylamide, buprenorphine, methadone, barbiturates, benzodiazepines and other drugs. *Ann Clin Biochem* 1997;34(pt 5):460–510.

47. Zeidenberg P, Bourdon R, Nahas GG. Marijuana intoxication by passive inhalation: documentation by detection of urinary metabolites. *Am J Psychiatry* 1977;134(1):76–77.

48. Falck R. Passive inhalation of marijuana smoke. *JAMA* 1983;250(7):898.

49. Mason AP, Perez-Reyes M, McBay AJ, et al. Cannabinoid concentrations in plasma after passive inhalation of marijuana smoke. *J Anal Toxicol* 1983;7(4):172–174.

50. Cone EJ, Johnson RE. Contact highs and urinary cannabinoid excretion after passive exposure to marijuana smoke. *Clin Pharmacol Ther* 1986;40(3):247–256.

51. Cone EJ, Johnson RE, Darwin WD, et al. Passive inhalation of marijuana smoke: urinalysis and room air levels of delta-9-tetrahydrocannabinol. *J Anal Toxicol* 1987;11(3):89–96.

52. Cone EJ, Roache JD, Johnson RE. Effects of passive exposure to marijuana smoke. *NIDA Res Monogr* 1987;76:150–156.

53. Shults T, St. Clair S. *The Medical Review Officer Handbook.* Triangle Park, NC: Quadrangle Research; 1999.

54. Shults T. *MRO Alert.* Triangle Park, NC: Quadrangle Research;1–4.

55. Stock C, Shum JH. Buprenorphine: a new pharmacotherapy for opioid addictions treatment. *J Pain Palliat Care Pharmacother* 2004;18(3):35–54.

56. Bisaga A, Comer SD, Ward AS, et al. The NMDA antagonist memantine attenuates the expression of opioid physical dependence in humans. *Psychopharmacology (Berl)* 2001;157(1):1–10.

57. Bickel WK, Stitzer ML, Liebson IA, et al. Acute physical dependence in man: effects of naloxone after brief morphine exposure. *J Pharmacol Exp Ther* 1988;244(1):126–132.

58. Fishman SM, Wilsey B, Mahajan G, et al. Methadone reincarnated: novel clinical applications with related concerns. *Pain Med* 2002;3(4):339–348.

59. Tran KT, Hranicky D, Lark T, et al. Gabapentin withdrawal syndrome in the presence of a taper. *Bipolar Disord* 2005;7(3):302–304.

60. Hirose S. Restlessness related to SSRI withdrawal. *Psychiatry Clin Neurosci* 2001;55(1):79–80.

61. Mareth TR, Brown TM. SSRI withdrawal. *J Clin Psychiatry* 1996;57(7):310.

62. Kotzalidis G, de Pisa E, Patrizi B, et al. Similar discontinuation symptoms for withdrawal from medium-dose paroxetine and venlafaxine after nine years in the same patient. *J Psychopharmacol* 2008;22(5):581–584.

63. Campagne DM. Venlafaxine and serious withdrawal symptoms: warning to drivers. *MedGenMed* 2005;7(3):22.

64. Johnson H, Bouman WP, Lawton J. Withdrawal reaction associated with venlafaxine. *BMJ* 1998;317(7161):787.

65. Lowenson J, ed. *Substance Abuse.* 4th ed. Philadelphia: Lippincott Williams & Wilkins; 2005.

66. Zhang Y, Kwong TC. Utilization management in toxicology. *Clin Chim Acta* 2014;427:158–166.

67. Kong TY, Kim JH, Kim JY, et al. Rapid analysis of drugs of abuse and their metabolites in human urine using dilute and shoot liquid chromatography-tandem mass spectrometry. *Arch Pharm Res* 2017;40(2):180–196.

68. Eichhorst JC, Etter ML, Hall PL, et al. LC-MS/MS techniques for high-volume screening of drugs of abuse and target drug quantitation in urine/blood matrices. *Methods Mol Biol* 2012;902:29–41.

69. Inscore F, Shende C, Sengupta A, et al. Detection of drugs of abuse in saliva by surface-enhanced Raman spectroscopy (SERS). *Appl Spectrosc* 2011;65(9):1004–1008.

CHAPTER 61

Headache

PETER J. GOADSBY

Headache is a remarkably common problem in neurology and even in general medicine and, by definition, has a substantial pain component. Books are devoted to the topic, and interested readers are directed to recent editions for more detail on the subjects covered here.[1-5] The headache disorders are classified by the International Classification of Headache Disorders,[6] now in its third edition, as being either primary, where the headache syndrome is itself the problem, or secondary, where the headache syndrome is driven by other pathologic processes. This chapter is designed to cover the primary headaches with a broad view. Facial neuralgias and facial pain syndromes are covered elsewhere in this book. Where a primary headache causes face pain, and most primary headaches can do this, it will be included here for completeness. This chapter covers the broad principles, the generic anatomy, and physiology of head pain and then discusses in turn the currently defined primary headache syndromes. There is much opportunity in headache to make patients significantly better and much research advancement in this very exciting area of medicine.[7,8]

General Principles

A general system for headache nosology is outlined in Table 61.1 The clinical challenge remains that although life-threatening headache is relatively uncommon in most societies, it occurs and its detection requires suitable awareness by the doctors of its clinical markers (Table 61.2). Primary headache often confers considerable disability over time and, although not life-threatening, certainly robs patients of a good quality of life.[9]

PRIMARY HEADACHE SYNDROMES

The primary headaches are a group of remarkable disorders in which headache and associated features are seen in the absence of any exogenous cause. First, the general anatomy and physiology will be described as it applies to most of the syndromes. Then, the primary headache syndromes will be addressed in turn.

ANATOMY AND PHYSIOLOGY

The most common *disabling* primary headaches, migraine and cluster headache, have been studied extensively in recent times, and they are now relatively well understood insofar as neurologic disorders that involve the brain are concerned. The word *disabling* is emphasized as the writer takes the view that there are not sufficient clear data that tension-type headache provides a substantial and disabling community problem.[10] In experimental animals, the detailed anatomy of the connections of the pain-producing dura mater and intracranial extracerebral vessels has built on the classical human observations of Wolff[11] and Feindel et al.[12,13] It is these structures, and not the brain itself, that primarily generate, or are perceived to generate, head pain.

The key structures involved are[7]

- The large intracranial vessels and dura mater
- The peripheral terminals of the trigeminal nerve that innervate these structures
- The central terminals and second-order neurons of the caudal trigeminal nucleus and dorsal horns of C_1 and C_2 (trigeminocervical complex)
- Higher center processing in the thalamus, ventroposteromedial and posterior thalamus, and cortex
- Modulatory centers in the diencephalon and brainstem, such as periaqueductal gray matter, locus coeruleus, and parts of the hypothalamus

The innervation of the large intracranial vessels and dura mater by the trigeminal nerve is known as the *trigeminovascular system*. The cranial parasympathetic autonomic innervation provides the basis for symptoms such as lacrimation and nasal stuffiness, which are prominent in the trigeminal autonomic cephalalgias,[14,15] although they may also be seen in migraine.[16] It is clear from human functional imaging studies that vascular changes in migraine and cluster headache are driven by these neural vasodilator systems so that these headaches should be regarded as *neurovascular*.[17] The concept of a primary *vascular* headache should be abandoned because it neither explains the pathogenesis of what are complex central nervous system disorders, nor does it necessarily predict treatment outcomes.[18] The term *vascular headache* has no place in modern medical practice when referring to primary headache.

Migraine is an episodic syndrome of headache with sensory sensitivity, such as to light, sound, and head movement, probably due to dysfunction of aminergic brainstem/diencephalic sensory control systems (Fig. 61.1). The first of the migraine genes has been identified for familial hemiplegic migraine and includes mutations in the *CACNA1A* gene for the $Ca_V 2.1$ (α_{1A})

TABLE 61.1	Common Causes of Headache		
Primary Headache		**Secondary Headache**	
Type	**Prevalence (%)**	**Type**	**Prevalence (%)**
Migraine	16	Systemic infection	63
Tension-type	69	Head injury	4
Cluster headache	0.1	Subarachnoid hemorrhage	<1
Idiopathic stabbing	2	Vascular disorders	1
Exertional	1	Brain tumor	0.1

Data from Olesen J, Tfelt-Hansen P, Ramadan N, et al. *The Headaches*. Philadelphia: Lippincott Williams & Wilkins; 2005.

TABLE 61.2	Warning Signs in Head Pain

- Sudden-onset pain
- Fever
- Marked change in pain character or timing of attacks
- Neck stiffness
- Pain associated with higher center complaints
- Pain associated with neurologic disturbance, such as clumsiness or weakness
- Pain associated with local tenderness, such as of the temporal artery

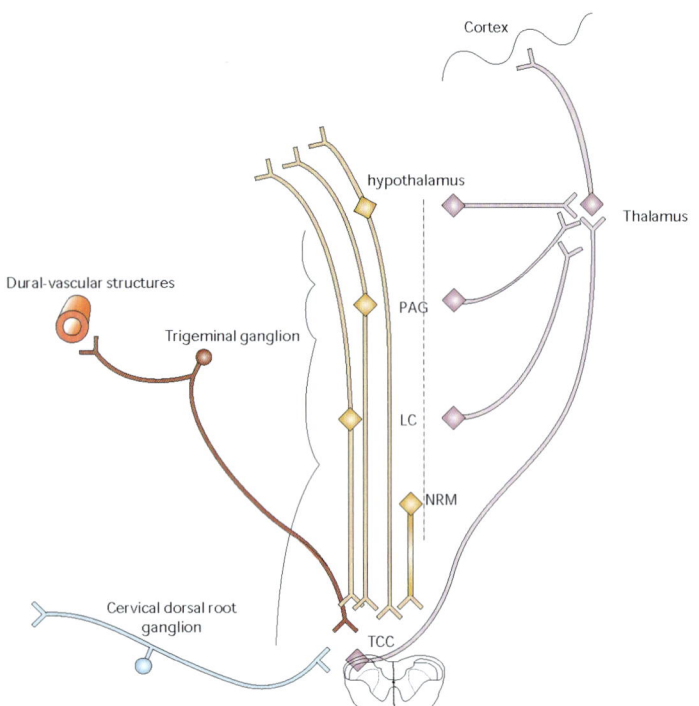

FIGURE 61.1   Pathophysiology of migraine. Diagram of some structures involved in the transmission of trigeminovascular nociceptive input and the modulation of that input that form the basis of a model of the pathophysiology of migraine.[7] Afferents from dural-vascular structures innervated predominantly by branches of the first (ophthalmic division) of the trigeminal nerve whose cell bodies are found in the trigeminal ganglion (Vg) project to second-order neurons in the trigeminocervical complex (TCC). The TCC extends from trigeminal nucleus caudalis to the caudal portion of the dorsal horn of the C_2 spinal cord. Input from cervical structures, such as joints or muscle, project through cell bodies in the upper cervical dorsal root ganglia (DRG) to the TCC. TCC neurons project to ventrobasal thalamus (thalamus) and then to cortex. Sensory modulation can occur by descending influences onto the TCC that largely respect the midline (*dashed line*), such as those from hypothalamus, midbrain periaqueductal gray (PAG), pontine locus coeruleus (LC), and nucleus raphe magnus (NRM). These influences are cartooned as being direct, but both direct and indirect projections are recognized. In addition, sensory modulation can occur from at least LC, PAG, and hypothalamic projects to thalamus nuclei as ascending systems again that largely respect the midline.

subunit of the neuronal P/Q voltage-gated calcium channel,[19] the Na/K ATP pump α_2 subunit gene *ATP1A2*[20] and the voltage-gated sodium channel *SCN1A*.[21] These findings and the clinical features of migraine suggest it might be part of the spectrum of diseases known as channelopathies, or now ionopathies: disorders involving dysfunction of ion channel fluxes.[22] Functional neuroimaging has suggested that brainstem regions,

in migraine (Fig. 61.2), and the posterior hypothalamic region, in cluster headache (Fig. 61.3), are good candidates for specific involvement in primary headache.[17]

SECONDARY HEADACHE

It is imperative to establish in the patient presenting with any form of head pain whether there is an important secondary

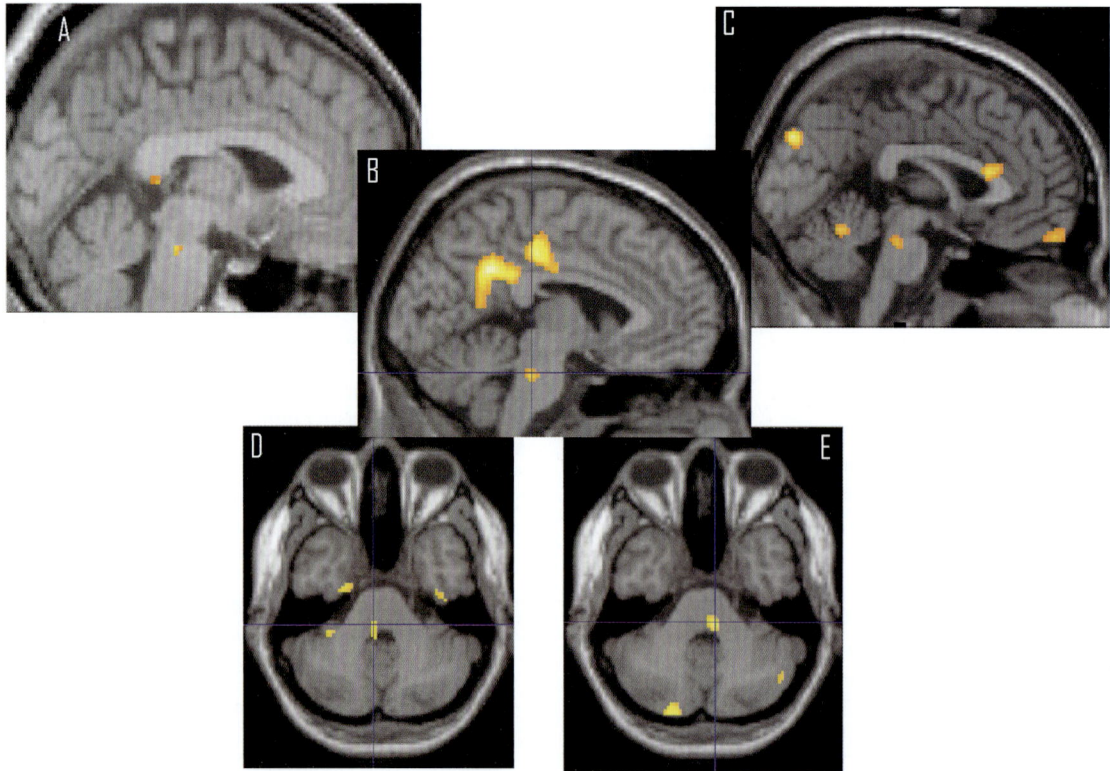

FIGURE 61.2   Activations identified on positron emission tomography in migraine. Consistently, there is dorsolateral pons activation in episodic migraine without aura, triggered by nitroglycerin[144] **(A)** or spontaneously studied[145] **(B)**, and in chronic migraine[146] **(C)**. Moreover, there is lateralization to the right **(D)** and left **(E)** in this structure that parallels the unilateral presentation of the pain.[147]

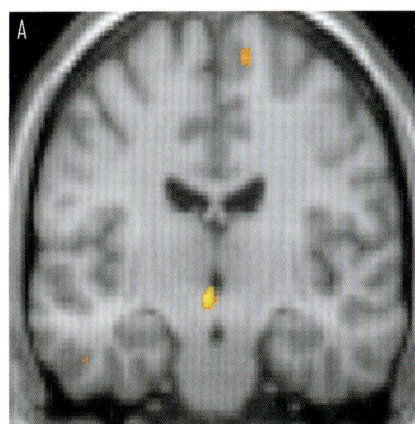
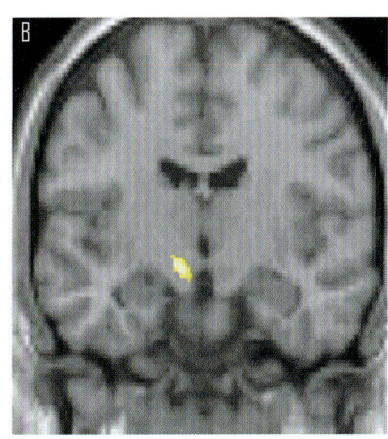

FIGURE 61.3 Activations on positron emission tomography in the posterior hypothalamic gray matter in patients with acute cluster headache **(A)**. The activation demonstrated is lateralized to the side of the pain.[23] When comparing the brains of patients with cluster headache with a control population using an automatic anatomical technique known as *voxel-based morphometry* (VBM) that employs high-resolution T1 weighted magnetic resonance imaging, a similar region is demonstrated **(B)** and has increased gray matter.[24]

headache. Perhaps, the most crucial clinical feature to elicit is the length of the history. Patients with a short history require prompt attention and may require prompt investigation and management. Patients with a longer history generally require time and patience rather than alacrity. There are some important general features, including associated fever or sudden onset of pain (see Table 61.2). Patients with a history of recent-onset headache or neurologic signs need a positive diagnosis of a benign disorder or require brain imaging with computed tomography (CT) or magnetic resonance imaging (MRI). Patients with a history of recurrent headache over a period of 1 year or more, fulfilling International Headache Society (IHS) criteria for migraine (Table 61.3) and with a normal physical examination, have positive brain imaging findings in only about 1/1,000 images.[25] In general, it should be noted that brain tumor is a rare cause of headache and rarely a cause of isolated long-term histories of headache. A notable exception to the general rules about secondary headache is pituitary tumor, which can trigger underlying primary headache biologies and should always be considered, especially in the differential diagnosis of trigeminal autonomic cephalalgias (see the following text; Levy et al.[26]). The management of secondary headache is generally self-evident: treatment of the underlying condition, such as an infection or mass lesion. One notable exception is the condition of persistent posttraumatic headache. This is an important problem that may be seen after central nervous system infection; trauma, both blunt and surgical; intracranial bleeds; and other precipitants, using the term *trauma* in its broader context to mean a biologic insult. The prevalence of the problem in returning service personnel has served to draw attention to the condition.[27,28] It can certainly often be both prolonged and disabling.

MIGRAINE
Clinical Features
Migraine is an episodic brain disorder that affects about 12% to 15% of the population[29] and can be highly disabling.[9] It has

been estimated to be the most costly neurologic disorder in the European Community at more than €27 billion per year,[30] and its cost to the US economy was a staggering $19.6 billion per year more than a decade ago.[31] Migraine presents with headache generally accompanied by features, such as sensitivity to light, sound, or movement, and often with nausea, or less often vomiting (see Table 61.3). None of the features is compulsory and indeed, given that the migraine aura, visual disturbances with flashing lights or zigzag lines moving across the fields or other neurologic symptoms, is reported in only about 25% of patients, a high index of suspicion is required to diagnose migraine. In a controlled study of patients presenting to primary care physicians with a main complaint of headache over the previous 3 months, migraine was the diagnosis on more than 90% of occasions[10]; thus, a high index of suspicion is important. A headache diary can often be helpful in making the diagnosis, although in reality, usually the diary helps more in assessing disability or recording how often patients use acute attack treatments. Phenotyping remains an essentially clinical art mixing experience and an understanding of the problems likely to present: *Good headache histories are taken not given.* In differentiating the two main primary headache syndromes seen in clinical practice, *migraine at its simplest is headache with associated features, and tension-type headache is headache that is featureless*; furthermore, *most disabling headache presentations in primary care are probably migrainous in biology.* By features, here is meant throbbing pain; sensitivity to sensory stimuli: visual, auditory, olfactory; or to head movement itself.

Frequent Migraine
If headache with associated features describes migraine attacks, then *headachy* describes the migraine sufferer over his or her lifetime. It is important to realize that the word migraine can both describe the attacks using standard criteria (see Table 61.3) and describe the disorder itself, which is more than just the attacks. The migraine sufferer inherits a tendency to have headache that is amplified at various times by their interaction with their environment, the much-discussed triggers. The brain of the migraineur seems more sensitive to sensory stimuli and to change, and this tendency is notably amplified in females during their menstrual cycle. Migraine sufferers may have headache when they oversleep, when tired, when they skip meals, when they overexert, when stressed, or when they relax from a stressor. They are less tolerant to change, and part of successful management is to advise them to maintain regularity in their lives in the knowledge of this fluctuating biology. It is this biology that marks migraine and in clinical practice must override the phenotype of individual headaches. Chronic migraine is the largest part of the group of headaches known collectively as *chronic daily headache*, a term best not often employed because almost invariably, a more specific diagnosis can be made.

TABLE 61.3	Simplified Diagnostic Criteria for Migraine

Repeated attacks of headache lasting 4–72 h that have these features, normal physical examination and no other reasonable cause for the headache

At Least Two of	At Least One of
• Unilateral pain	• Nausea/vomiting
• Throbbing pain	• Photophobia and phonophobia
• Aggravation by movement	
• Moderate or severe intensity	

Adapted from Headache Classification Committee of the International Headache Society. The International Classification of Headache Disorders, 3rd Edition. *Cephalalgia* 2018;38:1–211.

INSTRUCTIONS: Please answer the following questions about ALL your headaches you have had over the last 3 months. Write your answer in the box next to each question. Write zero if you did not do the activity in the last 3 months (Please refer to the calendar below, if necessary)

1. On how many days in the last 3 months did you miss work or school because of your headaches? .... |__|__| days

2. How many days in the last 3 months was your productivity at work or school reduced by half or more because of your headaches *(Do not include days you counted in question 1 where you missed work or school)*? .... |__|__| days

3. On how many days in the last 3 months did you **not** do household work because of your headaches? .... |__|__| days

4. How many days in the last 3 months was your productivity in household work reduced by half or more because of your headaches *(Do not include days you counted in question 3 where you did not do household work)*? .... |__|__| days

5. On how many days in the last 3 months did you miss family, social, or leisure activities because of your headaches? .... |__|__| days

A. On how many days in the last 3 months did you have a headache? (If a headache lasted more than one day, count each day) .... |__|__| days

B. On a scale of 0 - 10, on average how painful were these headaches?

(where 0 = no pain at all, and 10 = pain as bad as it can be) .... |__|__|

FIGURE 61.4 Migraine Disability Assessment Score Questionnaire. This survey was developed by Richard B. Lipton, MD, Professor of Neurology, Albert Einstein College of Medicine, New York, NY, and Walter F. Stewart, MPH, PhD, Associate Professor of Epidemiology, Johns Hopkins University, Baltimore, MD. Reprinted from Stewart, WF, Lipton RB, Downson, AJ et al. Development and testing of the Migraine Disability Assessment (MIDAS) Questionnaire to assess headache-related disability. *Neurology* 2001;56(S1) with permission.

Chronic migraine currently requires some 15 days a month of headache of which 8 are clearly migrainous and with a predating history of migraine.[6] After making a diagnosis, the second step in the clinical process is to be sure that the disease burden has been captured, how much headache does the patient have and more important, what can the patient not do; what is his or her degree of disability? One can ask the patient directly to get a flavor for this, keep a diary or get a quick but accurate estimate using the Migraine Disability Assessment Scale (MIDAS), which is well validated and very easy to use in practice (Fig. 61.4).

Principles of Management of Migraine
After diagnosis, the management of migraine begins with an explanation of some aspects of the disorder to the patient.
- Migraine is an inherited tendency to have headache; this is caused by the patient's genes; therefore, it cannot be cured, *but*
- Migraine can be modified and controlled by lifestyle adjustment and the use of medicines;
- Migraine is not life-threatening nor associated with serious illness with the exception of females who smoke and use estrogenic oral contraceptives but migraine can make life a misery; and
- Migraine management takes time and cooperation when, for example, a headache diary has to be collected or inquiry made concerning the disability.

Nonpharmacologic Management of Migraine
This approach aims to help the migrainous patient identify things making the problem worse and encouraging them to modify these. Patients need to know that the brain sensitivity to triggers in migraine varies. Patient associations are often very helpful in supporting migraineurs to identify triggers. The knowledge that there is variability will remove considerable frustration on the patient's part and will ring true to most as they have had the experience. The crucial lifestyle advice is to explain to the patient that migraine is a state of brain sensitivity to change. This implies that the migraine sufferer needs to regulate their lives: healthy diet, regular exercise, regular sleep patterns, avoiding excess caffeine and alcohol, and, as far as practical, modifying or minimizing changes in stress. The balanced life with less highs and lows will benefit most migraine sufferers.

Preventive Treatments of Migraine
The patient needs to understand they have an inherited, noncurable but manageable problem. To start a preventive, they need to have sufficient disability to wish to take a medicine to reduce the effects of the disease on their life. The basis of considering preventive treatment from a medical viewpoint is a combination of acute attack frequency and attack tractability that is conferring an unacceptable degree of disability. Patients with attacks unresponsive to abortive medications are easily considered for prevention, whereas patients with simply treated

TABLE 61.4 Preventive Treatments in Migraine[a]

Drug	Dose	Selected Side Effects
Pizotifen	0.5–2 mg daily	Weight gain Drowsiness
β-Blocker		
Propranolol	40–120 mg bid	Reduced energy Tiredness Postural symptoms *Contraindicated in asthma*
Tricyclics		
• Amitriptyline • Dosulepin (dothiepin) • Nortriptyline	25–75 mg every night	Drowsiness *Note:* Some patients are very sensitive and may only need a total dose of 10 mg, although generally 1–1.5 mg/kg body weight is required.
Anticonvulsants		
• Valproate • Topiramate	400–600 mg twice daily 50–200 mg/d	Drowsiness Weight gain Tremor Hair loss Foetal abnormalities Hematologic or liver abnormalities Paraesthesia Cognitive dysfunction Weight loss Care with a family history of glaucoma Nephrolithiasis Dizziness Sedation
Candesartan	4–24 mg daily	Postural dizziness
Flunarizine	5–15 mg daily	Drowsiness Weight gain Depression Parkinsonism
Chronic migraine only		
• Onabotulinum toxin type A	155 units	Injection site pain
Single studies[b]		
• Lisinopril	20 mg daily	Cough
• Single-pulse transcranial magnetic stimulation	2–24 pulses daily	Neck discomfort (5%)
Nutraceuticals[c]		
• Riboflavin	400 mg daily	GI upset
• Coenzyme Q10	100 mg three times daily	
• Butterbur	75 mg twice daily	
• Feverfew	6.25 mg three times daily	
No convincing controlled evidence		
• Verapamil		
Controlled trials to demonstrate *no effect*		
• Nimodipine		
• Clonidine		
• SSRIs: fluoxetine		

GI, gastrointestinal. SSRI, selective serotonin reuptake inhibitor.
[a]Commonly used preventives are listed with reasonable doses and common side effects. The local national formulary should be consulted for detailed information.
[b]Compounds not widely considered mainstream but with a positive randomized control trial against placebo.
[c]Nonpharmaceuticals with at least one positive randomized controlled trial against placebo.

attacks may be less obvious candidates. Another important consideration is disease progress. If a patient diary shows a clear trend of an increasing frequency of attacks, it is better to initiate a preventive than wait for the problem to worsen.

A simple rule for frequency might be that for one to two headaches a month, there is usually no need to start a preventive; for three to four, it may be needed but not necessarily; and for five or more per month, prevention should definitely be considered. Options available for treatment are covered in detail in Table 61.4 and vary by country. One problem with preventives is that they have fallen into use for migraine from other indications and often bring unwanted or intolerable side effects. It is not clear how preventives work, although it seems likely that they modify the brain sensitivity that underlies migraine. Another key clinical point is that generally, each drug should be started at a low dose and gradually increased to a reasonable maximum if there is going to be a clinical effect.

New advances: The development of migraine-specific preventives is on us as monoclonal antibodies to the calcitonin gene-related peptide (CGRP) pathway are nearing the clinic; effective and well tolerated, a new era is beginning.[32] There are four monoclonal antibodies effective in both episodic and chronic migraine: three to CGRP, eptinezumab,[33,34] fremanezumab,[35,36] and galcanezumab,[37,38] and one to the receptor, erenumab.[39,40] Neuromodulation or neurostimulation approaches are promising as patients and physicians seek nonpharmaceutical approaches to treatment[41]; the best established of these being single-pulse transcranial magnetic stimulation (sTMS).[42,43]

Acute Attack Therapies of Migraine
Acute attack treatments for migraine can be usefully divided into disease-nonspecific treatments, analgesics and nonsteroidal anti-inflammatory drugs (NSAIDs), disease-specific treatments, ergot-related compounds, and triptans (Table 61.5). It is important to be aware that most acute attack medications seem to have

TABLE 61.5	Acute Migraine Treatments
Nonspecific Treatments	**Specific Treatments**
Often used with antiemetic/prokinetics, such as domperidone (10 mg) or metoclopramide (10 mg)	
Aspirin (900 mg) Paracetamol (acetaminophen— 1,000 mg) NSAIDs • Naproxen (500–1,000 mg) • Ibuprofen (400–800 mg) • Tolfenamic acid (200 mg)	Ergot derivatives • Ergotamine (1–2 mg) Triptans • Sumatriptan (50 or 100 mg) • Naratriptan (2.5 mg) • Rizatriptan (10 mg) • Zolmitriptan (2.5 or 5 mg) • Eletriptan (40 or 80 mg) • Almotriptan (12.5 mg) • Frovatriptan (2.5 mg) Neuromodulation • Single-pulse transcranial magnetic stimulation (sTMS) • Noninvasive vagus nerve stimulation (nVNS)

NSAIDs, nonsteroidal anti-inflammatory drugs.

a propensity to aggravate headache frequency and can induce a state of refractory daily, near-daily, or medication overuse headache. As evidence is gathered, this seems to occur in patients with migraine, either a previous clear history or a family or personal history of *headacheyness*.[44] Codeine-containing analgesics are particularly troublesome when available in over-the-counter (OTC) preparations. One should advise patients with migraine to avoid taking acute attack medicines on more than 2 days a week. A proportion of patients who stop taking regular analgesics will have substantial improvement in their headache with a reduction in frequency; however, for some, it will not make any difference. It is crucial to emphasize to the patient that standard preventive medications often simply do not work in the presence of regular analgesic use.

Treatment strategies: Given the array of options to control an acute attack of migraine, how does one start? The simplest approach to treatment has been described as *stepped care*. In this model, all patients are treated, assuming no contraindications, with the simplest treatment, such as aspirin 900 mg or paracetamol (acetaminophen) 1,000 mg with an antiemetic. Aspirin is an effective strategy, has been proven so in double-blind controlled clinical trials, and is best used in its most soluble formulations. The alternative would be a strategy known as *stratified care*, by which the physician determines, or stratifies, treatment at the start based on likelihood of response to levels of care. An intermediate option may be described as stratified care by attack. The latter is what many headache authorities suggest and what patients often do when they have the options.[45] Patients use simpler options for their less severe attacks relying on more potent options when their attacks or circumstances demand them.

Nonspecific acute migraine attack treatments: Simple drugs, such as aspirin and paracetamol (acetaminophen), are cheap and can be effective. Dosages should be adequate and the addition of domperidone (10 mg orally) or ondansetron (4 mg) or aprepitant (80 mg) can be very helpful. NSAIDs can very useful when tolerated. Their success is often limited by inappropriate dosing, and adequate doses of naproxen (500 to 1,000 mg orally or rectally, with an antiemetic), ibuprofen (400 to 800 mg orally),[46] or tolfenamic acid (200 mg orally)[47] can be extremely effective.

Specific acute migraine attack treatments: When simple analgesic measures fail or more aggressive treatment is required, the specific antimigraine treatments are required (Table 61.6). Although ergotamine remains a useful treatment, it can no longer be considered the treatment of choice in acute migraine.[48] There are particular situations in which ergotamine is very helpful, but its use must be carefully controlled as ergotamine overuse produces dreadful headache in addition to a host of

TABLE 61.6	Stratification of Acute Specific Migraine Treatments
Clinical Situation	**Treatment Options**
Failed analgesics/ NSAIDs	First tier Sumatriptan 50 mg or 100 mg po Almotriptan 12.5 mg po Rizatriptan 10 mg po Eletriptan 40 mg po Zolmitriptan 2.5 mg po Slower effect/better tolerability Naratriptan 2.5 mg po Frovatriptan 2.5 mg po Infrequent headache Ergotamine 1–2 mg po Dihydroergotamine nasal spray 2 mg
Early nausea or difficulties taking tablets	Zolmitriptan 5 mg nasal spray Sumatriptan 20 mg nasal spray Rizatriptan 10 mg MLT wafer
Headache recurrence	Ergotamine 2 mg (most effective pr/usually with caffeine) Naratriptan 2.5 mg po Almotriptan 12.5 mg po Eletriptan 40 mg
Tolerating acute treatments poorly	Naratriptan 2.5 mg Almotriptan 12.5 mg Single-pulse transcranial magnetic stimulation (sTMS) Noninvasive vagus nerve stimulation (nVNS)
Early vomiting	Zolmitriptan 5 mg nasal spray Sumatriptan 25 mg pr Sumatriptan 6 mg sc
Menstrually related headache	Prevention Ergotamine po every night Oestrogen patches Treatment Triptans Dihydroergotamine nasal spray
Very rapidly developing symptoms	Zolmitriptan 5 mg nasal spray Sumatriptan 6 mg sc Dihydroergotamine 1 mg IMI

IMI, intramuscular injection; MLT, Maxalt-MLT.

vascular problems. The triptans, serotonin 5-HT$_{1B/1D}$ receptor agonists, have revolutionized the life of many patients with migraine and are clearly the most powerful option available to stop a migraine attack. They can be rationally applied by considering their pharmacologic, physicochemical, and pharmacokinetic features[49] as well as the formulations that are available.[45] Recent data suggests that combining a triptan with an NSAID can improve efficacy and reduce headache recurrence.[50]

New advances: There are exciting new developments in acute therapy of migraine that are on the horizon. Neuromodulation approaches with supraorbital stimulation,[51] noninvasive vagus nerve stimulation (nVNS),[52] and transcranial magnetic stimulation[53] each have controlled trials and an interesting physiologic basis.[54,55] They offer patients a nonpharmaceutical option. What has been sought almost since the launch of the triptans is effective acute antimigraine treatments without vasoconstrictor effects.[8] The development of lasmiditan, a serotonin 5-HT$_{1F}$ receptor agonist, or *ditan*, that is without vasoconstrictor effects,[56] yet works in clinic in phase II[57] and now in two phase III studies,[58] is an important development. Similarly, the development of small molecule CGRP receptor antagonists, or *gepants*, notably now rimegepant[59] and ubrogepant,[60] which are both effective in treating acute migraine, and come from a clearly safe class of treatments,[61] again offers the real promise of an important advance for patients.

Medication Overuse

An important clinical issue, which is probably a consequence of the interplay between migrainous biology and acute attack treatment, is what is described as medication overuse.

Medication overuse is defined as consuming an acute attack therapy on 10 days or more per month. This issue can be conflated with "medication overuse headache" as if every patient using analgesics at that frequency has a headache driven by acute attack medicines. The issue has been recently questioned.[62] It can certainly be helpful clinically to encourage analgesic overuse be reduced and eliminated if one is to see the underlying headache phenotype and commence to manage the problem.[63] Patients can reduce their use either by, as an example, 10% every week or two, depending on their circumstances, or if they wish, and there is no contraindication, by immediate cessation of use. Either approach can be facilitated by first keeping a careful diary over a month or two to be sure of the size of the problem. A small dose of an NSAID, such as naproxen 500 mg two to three times daily if tolerated, will take the edge off the pain as the analgesic use is reduced, as does a greater occipital nerve injection. It is useful aside that NSAID overuse does not seem to be a common issue in practice.[64] When the patient has reduced their analgesic use substantially, a preventive should be introduced. It is widely considered that medication overuse is a common cause of intractability to preventive treatments. This seems true in practice, although it is not invariable and not well studied.

Some patients with medication overuse will require admission for treatment. Broadly, this consists of two groups, those who fail outpatient withdrawal or those who have a significant complicating medical indication, such as brittle diabetes mellitus, or complicating medicines, such as opioids, where withdrawal may be problematic as an outpatient. When such patients are admitted, acute medications are withdrawn completely on the first day, unless there is some contraindication. Antiemetics, such as domperidone,[65] ondansetron, or aprepitant,[66] and fluids are administered as required as well as clonidine for opioid withdrawal symptoms. For acute intolerable pain during the waking hours, aspirin (1 g intravenously) is useful,[67] and at night, chlorpromazine by injection, after ensuring adequate hydration. If the patient does not settle over 3 to 5 days, a course of intravenous dihydroergotamine (DHE) can be employed.[68,69]

TENSION-TYPE HEADACHE
Clinical Features
As its name suggests, tension-type headache (TTH) is the headache form most seeking of understanding. TTH is diagnosed often, and although the phenotype is common, much of the disabling headache that goes under the name TTH is likely to be chronic migraine in terms of its biology. TTH has two forms, episodic TTH, where attacks occur on less than 15 days a month, and chronic TTH, where attacks, on average over time, are seen on 15 days or more a month. The IHS seeks to subdivide episodic TTH into an infrequent variety, arguably of little practical impact on the patient's life, and a more frequent but nonchronic version. Patients with the chronic form are part of the broader clinical syndrome of chronic daily headache, but chronic TTH and chronic daily headache are not equal concepts.

TTH has been defined by the IHS both for its episodic and chronic forms, although the admixture of symptoms allowed has consistency problems. A useful clinical approach is to diagnose TTH using the appendix criteria,[6] when the headache is completely featureless: no nausea, no vomiting, no photophobia, no phonophobia, no osmophobia, no throbbing, and no aggravation with movement. Such an approach neatly divides migraine, which has one of more of these features and is the main differential diagnosis, from TTH.

Pathophysiology
The pathophysiology of TTH is poorly understood. This results from the fact that the name implies to most that it is a product of *nervous tension*, for which there is no clear evidence, and

the definitions employed have undoubtedly admitted patients with migraine to the studies. Moreover, the concept that TTH in some way involves muscle contraction is incorrect because the evidence is that muscle contraction is no more likely that it is in migraine.[70] It seems likely that TTH will be due to a primary disorder of central nervous system pain modulation alone in contrast with migraine, which is a more generalized disturbance of sensory modulation.

Management
Adopting the clinical approach to TTH outlined in the preceding text results in diagnosing a headache form that is usually less disabling, more often described by patients as irritating.[71] Its episodic form is generally amenable to simple analgesics, paracetamol (acetaminophen), aspirin, or other NSAIDs, which can be purchased OTC. There are clear clinical studies to demonstrate that triptans in TTH alone are not helpful, although, germane to the earlier discussion, triptans are effective in TTH where the patient also has migraine.[72] For chronic TTH, amitriptyline is the only treatment with clear evidence of efficacy[73–75]; the other tricyclics, selective serotonin reuptake inhibitors, or the benzodiazepines have not been shown in controlled trials to be effective. Similarly, there is no controlled evidence for the use of electromyography (EMG) biofeedback, relaxation therapy, or acupuncture. Botulinum toxin has been shown reasonably clearly to be ineffective.[76] Stress management has been shown to be an effective approach in a controlled trial.[75]

TRIGEMINAL-AUTONOMIC CEPHALALGIAS
Cluster Headache
Cluster headache is a rare form of primary headache with a population frequency of approximately 0.1%.[77] As a clinical anchor, it is about as common as multiple sclerosis in the United Kingdom[78] and must be regarded as a disorder best managed by neurologists or headache specialists. It is perhaps the most painful condition of humans; in the cohort of more than 1,000 patients seen by the author, and in patient-based assessments,[79] not a single one has had a more painful experience, including childbirth, multiple fractures of the limbs, or renal stones. It is one of a group of conditions known now as trigeminal-autonomic cephalalgias (TACs) and thus needs to be differentiated from other TACs[14,80] and the short-lasting headaches without cranial autonomic symptoms, such as lacrimation or conjunctival injection (Table 61.7).

The core feature of cluster headache is periodicity, be it circadian or in terms of active and inactive bouts over weeks and months (Table 61.8). The typical cluster headache patient is male, with a 3:1 predominance, with bouts of one to two attacks of relatively short duration unilateral pain every day for 8 to 10 weeks a year. They are generally perfectly well between times. Patients with cluster headache tend to move about during attacks, pacing, rocking, or even rubbing their head for relief.

TABLE 61.7 Cluster Headache, Other Trigeminal Autonomic Cephalalgias, and Short-Lasting Headaches	
Trigeminal Autonomic Cephalalgias[a]	**Other Short-Lasting Headaches**
• Cluster headache	• Primary stabbing headache
• Paroxysmal hemicrania	• Trigeminal neuralgia
• SUNCT/SUNA syndrome	• Primary cough headache
	• Primary exertional headache
	• Primary sex headache
	• Hypnic headache

SUNA, short-lasting unilateral neuralgiform headache attacks with cranial autonomic features; SUNCT, short-lasting unilateral neuralgiform headache attacks with conjunctival injection and tearing.
[a]Beware of pituitary tumor-related headache in the differential diagnosis of these trigeminal autonomic cephalalgias.

TABLE 61.8 Diagnostic Criteria for Cluster Headache

Diagnostic Criteria

A. At least five attacks fulfilling B–D
B. Severe or very severe unilateral orbital, supraorbital, and/or temporal pain lasting 15–180 min if untreated
C. Headache is accompanied by at least one of the following:
  1. Ipsilateral conjunctival injection and/or lacrimation
  2. Ipsilateral nasal congestion and/or rhinorrhea
  3. Forehead and facial sweating
  4. Ipsilateral eyelid edema
  5. Ipsilateral forehead and facial sweating
  6. Ipsilateral miosis and/or ptosis
  7. A sense of restlessness or agitation
D. Attacks have a frequency from one every other day to eight per day.
E. Not attributed to another disorder

Episodic Cluster Headache

Description: occurs in periods lasting 7 d to 1 y separated by pain-free periods lasting 3 mo or more
Diagnostic criteria:
A. All fulfilling criteria A–E of 3.1
B. At least two cluster periods lasting from 7 to 365 d and separated by pain-free remissions of ≥3 mo.

Chronic Cluster Headache

Description: Attacks occur for more than 1 y without remission or with remissions lasting less than 3 mo.
Diagnostic criteria:
A. All alphabetical headings of 3.1
B. Attacks recur over >1 y without remission periods or with remission periods <3 mo

After Headache Classification Committee of the International Headache Society (IHS). The International Classification of Headache Disorders, 3rd Edition. *Cephalalgia* 2018;38(1):1–211. Copyright © International Headache Society 2013–2018.

The pain is usually retroorbital, boring, and very severe. It is associated with ipsilateral symptoms of cranial (parasympathetic) autonomic activation: a red or watering eye, the nose running or blocking, or cranial sympathetic dysfunction (eyelid droop). Cluster headache is likely to be a disorder involving central pacemaker regions of the posterior hypothalamus and perhaps other neurons of this region (see Fig. 61.2).[23,24]

The TACs (cluster headache, paroxysmal hemicrania [PH], and short-lasting unilateral neuralgiform headache attacks with conjunctival injection and tearing [SUNCT] syndrome) present a distinct group to be differentiated from short-lasting headaches that do not have prominent cranial autonomic syndromes, notably trigeminal neuralgia, idiopathic (primary)

stabbing headache, and hypnic headache.[81] By determining the cycling pattern, length of attack, frequency of attack, and timing of the attacks, most patients can be usefully classified. The importance of clinical classification of this group is threefold. First, the clinical phenotype determines the likely secondary causes that must be considered and appropriate investigations ordered. Second, the appropriate classification gives clarity to the patient with a clear diagnosis and allows the physician to draw on available literature to comment on natural history. Third, the correct diagnosis determines therapy that can be very different in these conditions, being very good if the diagnosis is correct but largely ineffective if it is not (Table 61.9).

Managing Cluster Headache

Cluster headache is managed using acute attack treatments and preventive agents. Acute attack treatments are usually required by all cluster headache patients at some time, whereas preventives can seem almost lifesaving for the patients with chronic cluster headache and are often needed to shorten the active periods in patients with the episodic form of the disorder. Episodic cluster headache is diagnosed if patients have a treatment-free period of 3 consecutive months in a year and chronic when that is not the case.[6]

Preventive treatments: The options for preventive treatment in cluster headache depend on the bout length (Table 61.10). Patients with short bouts require medicines that act quickly but will not necessarily be taken for long periods, whereas those with long bouts or indeed those with chronic cluster headache require safe, effective medicines that can be taken for long periods. Verapamil is now widely considered as the first-line preventive treatment when the bout is prolonged or in chronic cluster headache. By contrast, limited courses of oral corticosteroids can be very useful strategies when the bout is relatively short.[82]

Verapamil has been suggested as a useful option for the last decade and compares favorably with lithium. What has clearly emerged from clinical practice is the need to use higher doses than had initially been considered and certainly higher than those used in cardiologic indications. Although most patients will start on doses as low as 40 to 80 mg twice daily, doses up to 960 mg daily are often required. Side effects, such as gingival hyperplasia, constipation, and leg swelling, are recognized as are cardiac dysrhythmias. Verapamil can cause heart block by slowing conduction in the atrioventricular (AV) node, monitored clinically by the PR interval on the electrocardiogram (ECG). Given that the effects on the AV node take up to 10 days to manifest, 2-week intervals are recommended between dose changes on the first exposure, with ECGs prior

TABLE 61.9 Differential Diagnosis of Short-Lasting Headaches

Feature	Cluster Headache	Paroxysmal Hemicrania	SUNCT/SUNA[a]	Primary Stabbing Headache	Trigeminal Neuralgia[a]	Hypnic Headache
Gender	M > F 3:1	F = M	M > F	F > M	F > M	M = F
Pain						
Type	Boring/throbbing	Boring/throbbing	Stabbing/throbbing	Stabbing	Stabbing	Throbbing
Severity	Very severe	Very severe	Very severe	Severe	Very severe	Moderate
Cranial location	Any	Any	Any	Any	V2/V3 > V1	Generalized
Duration	15–180 min	1–45 min	15–600 s	Seconds to 3 min	<5 s	15–30 min
Frequency	1–8/d	1–40/d	1/d–30/hr	Any	Any	1–3 per night
Autonomic	+	+	+	−	−	−
Alcohol	+	One-third	−	−	−	−
Cutaneous trigger to attacks	−	−	+	−	+	−
Indomethacin	−	+	−	+	−	−

[a]SUNCT/SUNA generally has no refractory period to trigger additional attacks, although this is a very common feature of trigeminal neuralgia.
F, female; M, male; SUNA, short-lasting unilateral neuralgiform headache attacks with cranial autonomic symptoms; SUNCT, short-lasting unilateral neuralgiform headache attacks with conjunctival injection and tearing; +, present; −, absent.

TABLE 61.10	Preventive Management of Cluster Headache
Short-term Prevention	**Long-term Prevention**
Episodic cluster headache	*Episodic cluster headache and prolonged chronic cluster headache*
• Prednisolone	• Verapamil
• Verapamil	• Lithium
• Greater occipital nerve injection	• Melatonin
• (Daily nocturnal ergotamine)	• ?Topiramate
	• ?Noninvasive vagus nerve stimulation
	• Sphenopalatine ganglion stimulation

?, unproven but promising.

the next escalation, and routine six monthly ECGs after the dose is established.[83]

The development of nVNS for the preventive treatment of cluster headache is a promising way forward.[84] It compares with standard of care[85] and is particularly useful when patients have contraindications or intolerability to standard therapies.

Acute attack treatment: Cluster headache attacks often peak rapidly and thus require a treatment with quick onset. Many patients with acute cluster headache respond very well to treatment with oxygen inhalation. This should be given as 100% oxygen at 10 to 12 L per minute for 15 to 20 minutes.[86] It is important to have a high-flow and high oxygen content. Injectable sumatriptan 6 mg is effective, rapid in onset,[87] and has no evidence of tachyphylaxis.[88] Sumatriptan 20 mg[89] and zolmitriptan 5 mg[90,91] nasal sprays are effective in acute cluster headache in controlled trials and offer a useful option. Sumatriptan is not effective when given preemptively as 100 mg orally three times daily,[92] and there is no evidence that it is useful when used orally in the acute treatment of cluster headache; indeed, it can be associated with medication overuse headache problems.[61] The most recent development in the treatment of acute cluster headache has been the completion of two randomized sham-controlled studies of nVNS. The two studies worked for acute attacks in patients with episodic cluster headache but not in chronic cluster headache.[93,94]

Surgical treatment: The surgical treatment of cluster headache has been completely transformed by the introduction of neurostimulation therapies. Surgical treatment of cluster headache is reserved for the most refractory patients, typically with chronic cluster headache. Destructive procedures, such as sphenopalatinectomy or radiofrequency lesions of the trigeminal ganglion, have been used. The former is without clear effects, with the latter being helpful but often at significant cost, including ocular complications or anesthesia dolorosa. Trigeminal rhizotomy has also been employed, with all the complications of radiofrequency lesions and the occasional death.[95] Set against this, the functional imaging work describing activations in the posterior hypothalamic region[23] directly lead to deep brain stimulation approaches in the same region that seem highly effective,[96] although not without morbidity and mortality. Occipital nerve stimulation is a less invasive approach to the management of intractable chronic cluster headache,[97,98] although with time its limitations have become clearer. The most promising surgical option at this time is sphenopalatine ganglion stimulation, which is reported in a controlled trial to be effective for both acute attack treatment and prevention,[99] with good long-term outcomes.[100]

PAROXYSMAL HEMICRANIA

Sjaastad and Dale[101] first reported eight cases of a frequent unilateral severe but short-lasting headache without remission coining the term *chronic paroxysmal hemicrania* (CPH). The mean daily frequency of attacks varied from 7 to 22 with the pain persisting from 5 to 45 minutes on each occasion. The site and associated autonomic phenomena were similar to cluster headache, but the attacks of CPH were suppressed completely by indomethacin.

The essential features of PH that we have seen from a substantial cohort of patients are[102]:

- Unilateral very severe pain
- Short-lasting attacks typically 20 minutes in length
- Very frequent attacks (usually more than 5 times a day)
- Marked autonomic features ipsilateral to the pain
- Robust, quick (less than 72 hour), excellent response to indomethacin

The pathophysiology of PH is marked by activations on positron emission tomography (PET) in the contralateral posterior hypothalamus and contralateral ventral midbrain.[103] The posterior hypothalamic activity is shared with cluster headache, SUNCT, and hemicrania continua, whereas the ventral midbrain activity is only seen in hemicrania continua, which remarkably is also an indomethacin-sensitive primary headache.[104]

The therapy of PH may be complicated by gastrointestinal side effects seen with indomethacin, in which topiramate may be helpful.[105] When indomethacin is poorly tolerated, nVNS may be very useful and is well tolerated in patients with PH.[106] Secondary PH is more likely if the patient requires high doses (>200 mg per day) of indomethacin and raised cerebrospinal fluid (CSF) pressure should be suspected in apparent bilateral PH. It is worth noting that indomethacin reduces CSF pressure by an unknown mechanism.[107] It is appropriate to image patients, with MRI if practical, when a diagnosis of PH is being considered.

SHORT-LASTING UNILATERAL NEURALGIFORM HEADACHE ATTACKS WITH CONJUNCTIVAL INJECTION AND TEARING OR CRANIAL AUTONOMIC ACTIVATION

Sjaastad and colleagues[108] reported three male patients whose brief attacks of pain in and around one eye were associated with sudden conjunctival injection and other autonomic features of cluster headache. The attacks lasted only 15 to 60 seconds and recurred 5 to 30 times per hour and could be precipitated by chewing or eating certain foods, such as citrus fruits. They were not abolished by indomethacin. Brain imaging has suggested that they share with cluster headache and PH the feature on activation studies of involvement of the posterior hypothalamic region.[109] Of the patients recognized with this problem, males dominate slightly and the paroxysms of pain may last between 5 and 300 seconds, although longer duller interictal pains are recognized, as are longer attacks with a sawtooth pattern.[104] The conjunctival injection seen with SUNCT is often the most prominent autonomic feature, and tearing may be very obvious. If one of either conjunctival injection or tearing is absent, or neither is present but another cranial autonomic symptom is seen, the term *short-lasting unilateral neuralgiform headache attacks with cranial autonomic symptoms* (SUNA) is used.[6] The two key clinical features of SUNCT/SUNA are the attacks being triggerable with no refractory period to triggering. The latter serves as a very useful distinction between SUNCT/SUNA and trigeminal neuralgia. SUNCT/SUNA can be treated very often with lamotrigine and if that is unhelpful topiramate or gabapentin.[110] Carbamazepine often has a useful but incomplete effect. Given what has been reported, cranial MRI with pituitary and posterior fossa views is highly recommended when SUNCT/SUNA is considered as a diagnosis.[110]

OTHER PRIMARY HEADACHES
Primary Stabbing Headache

Short-lived jabs of pain, defined by the Headache Classification Committee of the IHS as primary stabbing headache,[6] are well documented in association with most types of primary headache.

The essential clinical features are:
- Pain confined to the head, although rarely is it facial
- Stabbing pain lasting from 1 to many seconds and occurring as a single stab or a series of stabs
- Recurring at irregular intervals (hours to days)

These pains have been called ice-pick pains or jabs and jolts. They generally respond to indomethacin (25 to 50 mg twice to three times daily). The symptoms tend to wax and wane, and after a period of control on indomethacin, it is appropriate to withdraw treatment and observe the outcome. Most patients will not want treatment when the nature of the problem is explained, and they are reassured that the attacks are not sinister in any way.

Primary Cough Headache

Sharp pain in the head on coughing, sneezing, straining, laughing, or stooping has long been regarded as a symptom of organic intracranial disease, commonly associated with obstruction of the CSF pathways. The presence of an Arnold-Chiari malformation or any lesion causing obstruction of CSF pathways or displacing cerebral structures must be excluded before cough headache is assumed to be benign. Cerebral aneurysm, carotid stenosis, and vertebrobasilar disease may also present with cough or exertional headache as the initial symptom. The term *benign Valsalva's maneuver–related headache* covers the headaches provoked by coughing, straining, or stooping, but *cough headache* is more succinct and so widely used it is unlikely to be displaced.[6]

The essential clinical features of primary cough headache are:
- Bilateral headache of sudden onset, lasting minutes, precipitated by coughing
- May be prevented by avoiding coughing
- Diagnosed only after structural lesions, such as posterior fossa tumor, have been excluded by neuroimaging

Indomethacin is the medical treatment of choice in cough headache. Raskin[111] followed up an observation of Sir Charles Symonds reporting that some patients with cough headache are relieved by lumbar puncture.[112] This is a simple option when compared to prolonged use of indomethacin. The mechanism of this response remains unclear.

Primary Exertional Headache

The relationship of this form of headache to cough headache is unclear and certainly much is shared. Indeed, the relationship to migraine also requires delineation.

The clinical features are[6]:
- Pain specifically brought on by physical exercise
- Bilateral and throbbing in nature at onset and may develop migrainous features in those patients susceptible to migraine
- Lasts from 5 minutes to 24 hours
- Prevented by avoiding excessive exertion, particularly in hot weather or at high altitude

The acute onset of headache with straining and breath holding as in weightlifter's headache may be explained by acute venous distension. The development of headache after sustained exertion, particularly on a hot day, is more difficult to understand. Anginal pain may be referred to the head, probably by central connections of vagal afferents and may present as exertional headache, so called cardiac cephalgia.[113] The link to exercise is the important clinical clue. Pheochromocytoma may occasionally be responsible for exertional headache. Intracranial lesions or stenosis of the carotid arteries may have to be excluded as discussed for benign cough headache. Headache may be precipitated by any form of exercise and often has the pulsatile quality of migraine. The most obvious form of treatment is to take exercise gradually and progressively whenever possible.

Indomethacin at daily doses varying from 25 to 150 mg is generally very effective in benign exertional headache. Indomethacin 50 mg or frovatriptan 2.5 mg po are useful short-term preventive measures.

Primary Sex Headache

Sex headache may be precipitated by masturbation or coitus and usually starts as a dull bilateral ache while sexual excitement increases, suddenly becoming intense at orgasm. The term *orgasmic cephalgia* is not accurate because not all sex headaches require orgasm. Two types of primary sex headache are recognized: a dull ache in the head and neck that intensifies as sexual excitement increases and a sudden severe ("explosive") headache occurring at orgasm.[6] Low CSF volume headache may also be precipitated by a sexual activity and is considered as a form of new daily persistent headache (NDPH) (see the following text).

The essential clinical features of sex headache are:
- Precipitation by sexual excitement
- Bilateral at onset
- Prevented or eased by ceasing sexual activity before orgasm

Headaches developing at the time of orgasm are not always benign, and consideration of a diagnosis of subarachnoid headache is essential. Sex headache affects men more often than women and may occur at any time during the years of sexual activity. It may develop on several occasions in succession and then not trouble the patient again, despite no obvious change in sexual technique. In patients who stop sexual activity when headache is first noticed, it may subside within a period of 5 minutes to 2 hours, and it is recognized that more frequent orgasm can aggravate established sex headache. About one-third of the patients with sex headache have a history of exertional headaches, but there is no excess of cough headache in patients with sex headache. In about 50% of patients, sex headache will settle in 6 months. Migraine is reported in about 25% of patients with sex headache.

Primary sex headaches are usually irregular and infrequent in occurrence, so management can often be limited to reassurance and advice about ceasing sexual activity if a milder, warning headache develops. When the condition recurs regularly or frequently, it can be prevented by the administration of propranolol; the dosage required varies from 40 to 200 mg daily. An alternative is the calcium channel blocking agent diltiazem 60 mg three times daily, which this author finds particularly useful in such patients. Indomethacin (25 to 50 mg) or frovatriptan (2.5 mg) taken about 30 to 45 minutes prior to sexual activity can also be helpful.

Hypnic Headache

This syndrome was first described by Raskin[114] in patients aged from 67 to 84 years who had headache of a moderately severe nature that typically came on a few hours after going to sleep.[114] These headaches last from 15 to 30 minutes, are typically generalized, although may be unilateral, and can be throbbing. Patients may report falling back to sleep only to be awoken by a further attack a few hours later with up to three repetitions of this pattern over the night. In a series of 19 patients, 16 (84%) were female, and the mean age at onset was 61 ± 9 years.[115] Headaches were bilateral in two-thirds and unilateral in one-third and in 80% of cases mild or moderate. Three patients reported similar headaches when falling asleep during the day. None had photophobia or phonophobia, and nausea is unusual.

Patients with this form of headache generally respond to a bedtime dose of lithium carbonate (200 to 600 mg) and in those that do not tolerate this, verapamil at bedtime may be alternative strategies).[116] Dodick and colleagues[115] reported that one to two cups of coffee or caffeine 60 mg orally at bedtime was helpful. This is a simple approach that is effective in about one-third of patients. An important secondary cause of hypnic headache is hypertension which should be carefully pursued and appropriately investigated as treatment of the blood pressure will arrest the headache problem.[117]

Primary Thunderclap Headache

Sudden-onset severe headache may occur in the absence of sexual activity, and the differential diagnosis includes the sentinel bleed of an intracranial aneurysm, cervicocephalic arterial dissection, and cerebral venous thrombosis. Headaches of explosive onset may also be caused by the ingestion of sympathomimetic drugs or tyramine-containing foods in a patient who is taking monoamine oxidase inhibitors and can also be a symptom of pheochromocytoma. Whether thunderclap headache can be the presentation of an unruptured cerebral aneurysm is unclear. Day and Raskin[118] reported a woman with three episodes of sudden-onset very severe headache who was found to have an unruptured aneurysm of the internal carotid artery, with adjacent areas of segmental vasospasm. In the absence of CT scan or CSF evidence of subarachnoid hemorrhage, studies indicate that such patients do very well, and there indeed seems a form of benign or primary thunderclap headache.

Wijdicks and colleagues[119] followed up 71 patients for an average of 3.3 years whose CT scans and CSF findings were negative. Twelve patients had further such headache, and 31 (44%) later had regular episodes of migraine or TTH. Factors identified as precipitating the headache were sexual intercourse in 3 cases, coughing in 4, and exertion in 12, whereas the remainder had no obvious cause. A history of hypertension was found in 11 and of previous headache in 22. Markus[120] compared the presentation of 37 patients with subarachnoid hemorrhage and 189 with a similar thunderclap headache and normal CSF examination and could not discern any characteristic to distinguish the two conditions.

Investigation of any sudden-onset severe headache, be it in the context of sexual excitement or isolated thunderclap headache, should be driven by the clinical context. The first presentation should be vigorously investigated with x-ray CT and CSF examination and, where possible, MRI/magnetic resonance venography (MRV)/magnetic resonance angiography (MRA). Formal cerebral angiography should be reserved for when no primary diagnosis is forthcoming, and the clinical situation is particularly suggestive of intracranial aneurysm. Bearing in mind the entity of diffuse multifocal reversible cerebral vasospasm,[121] which may be seen in apparent primary thunderclap headache without there being an intracranial aneurysm, caution in interpretation of findings is crucial.

Hemicrania Continua

Two patients were initially reported with this syndrome, a woman aged 63 years and a man of 53 years, who developed unilateral headache without obvious cause. Both patients were relieved completely by indomethacin, whereas other NSAIDs were of little or no benefit. Newman and colleagues[122] reviewed the 24 previously reported cases and added 10 of their own, including some with pronounced autonomic features resembling cluster headache. They divided their case histories into remitting and unremitting forms. Of the 34 patients reviewed, 22 were women and 12 men with the age of onset ranging from 11 to 58 years. The symptoms were controlled by indomethacin 75 to 150 mg daily. The essential features of hemicrania continua are[6]:

- Unilateral pain
- Pain is continuous but with exacerbations that may be severe
- Complete resolution of pain with indomethacin
- Exacerbations may be associated with autonomic features

Apart from analgesic overuse as an aggravating factor, and a report in an HIV-infected patient, the status of secondary hemicrania continua is unclear. Antonaci and colleagues[123] proposed the "indotest" by which the intramuscular injection of indomethacin 50 mg could be used as a diagnostic tool. In hemicrania continua, pain was relieved in 73 ± 66 minutes and the pain-free period was 13 ± 8 hours. A placebo-controlled modification of this test is preferred where possible to the open-label version. Using the latter method in conjunction with PET, it has been shown that there is activation of the contralateral posterior hypothalamus and ipsilateral dorsal rostral pons in association with the headache of hemicrania continua as well as activation of the ipsilateral ventrolateral midbrain.[124] The alternative is a trial of oral indomethacin, initially 25 mg 3 times daily, then 50 mg 3 times daily, and then 75 mg 3 times daily. One should allow up to 2 weeks for any dose to have a useful effect. Acute treatment with sumatriptan has been employed and reported to be of no benefit. Cyclooxygenase 2 (COX-2) antagonists seem effective, although undesirable now, and topiramate is helpful in some patients as is greater occipital nerve injection. nVNS is helpful in these patients and well tolerated.[106]

New Daily Persistent Headache

NDPH is a clinically useful concept with a range of important possible causes because some are very treatable (Table 61.11). From a nosologic point of view, all that are mentioned here could be placed within various categories of the IHS classification,[6] and indeed, the IHS refers to primary NDPH. However, the term as employed here serves both patients and clinicians by highlighting a group of conditions, some of which are curable and encompasses the IHS term under as the primary featureless form of NDPH.[125]

The patient with NDPH presents with a history of headache on most if not all days that began from one day to the next. The onset of headache is abrupt, often moment-to-moment but at least in less than a few days where three is suggested as an upper limit. The typical history is for the patient to recall the exact day and circumstances, so from one moment to the next, a headache develops that never leaves them. This presentation triggers certain key questions about the onset and behavior of the pain. The pressing issues arise from considering the secondary headache possibilities. Although subarachnoid hemorrhage is listed for some logical consistency, as the headache may certainly come on from one moment to the next, it is not likely to produce diagnostic confusion in this group of patients. Suffice to say that subarachnoid hemorrhage is so important that it must always be considered if only to be excluded, either by history or appropriate investigation.

Primary new daily persistent headache: Case series of primary NDPH showed it to occur in both males and females.[126] Migrainous features are common, with unilateral headache in about one-third and throbbing pain in about one-third. Nausea was reported in about half the patients, as was photophobia and phonophobia observed again in about half. A number of

TABLE 61.11   Differential Diagnosis of New Daily Persistent Headache

Primary	Secondary
• Migrainous-type	• Subarachnoid hemorrhage
• Featureless (tension-type)	• Low CSF volume headache
	• Raised CSF pressure headache
	• Posttraumatic headache[a]
	• Chronic meningitis

[a]Includes postinfective forms.
CSF, cerebrospinal fluid.

these patients have a previous history of migraine but not more than one might expect given the population prevalence of migraine.[126,127] It is remarkable that the initial report noted that 86% of patients were headache free at 24 months. It is general experience among those interested in headache management that primary NDPH is perhaps the most intractable and least therapeutically rewarding form of headache. In general, one can classify the dominant phenotype, migraine or TTH, and treat with preventives according to that subclassification.

Secondary new daily persistent headache: The secondary causes of the syndrome of NDPH are worthy of consideration, as they have distinctive clinical pictures that can guide investigation (see Table 61.11).

Low Cerebrospinal Fluid Volume Headache

The syndrome of persistent low CSF volume headache is an important diagnosis not to miss. The more immediately obvious version of this problem is encountered commonly after lumbar puncture. In that situation, the headache usually settles rapidly with bed rest. In the chronic situation, the patient typically presents with a history of headache from one day to the next. The pain is generally not present on waking, worsens during the day, and is relieved by lying down. Recumbency usually improves the headache in minutes, and it takes only minutes to an hour for the pain to return when the patient is again upright. The patient may give a history of an index event: lumbar puncture or epidural injection or a vigorous Valsalva, such as with lifting, straining, coughing, clearing the Eustachian tubes in an aeroplane, or multiple orgasms. Patients may volunteer, or a history may be obtained, that soft drinks with caffeine provide temporary respite. Spontaneous leaks are recognized, and the clinician should not be put off the diagnosis if the headache history is typical when there is no obvious index event. As time passes from the index event, the postural nature may be less obvious; certainly, cases whose index event was several years prior to the eventual diagnosis are recognized. The term *low volume* rather than *low pressure* is used because there is no clear evidence at which point the pressure can be called low. Although low pressures, such as 0 to 5 are often identified, a pressure of 16 cm CSF has been recorded with a documented leak. One should be aware of the possibility of the development of subdural collections in patients with low CSF volume headaches, which makes imaging before any invasive studies all the more important.

The investigation of choice is MRI with gadolinium (Fig. 61.5), which produces a striking pattern of diffuse pachymeningeal enhancement,[128] although in about 10% of cases a leak can be documented without enhancement.[129] The finding of diffuse meningeal enhancement is so typical that in clinical context immediate treatment is appropriate. It is also common to see Chiari malformations on MRI with some degree of descent of the cerebellar tonsils. This is important because surgery in such settings simply worsens the headache problem. It seems appropriate that any patient being considered for such surgery for a headache indication should be reviewed by a neurologist first. To investigate further, CSF pressure may be determined or preferably a leak sought with ^{111}In-DPTA CSF studies that can demonstrate the site, early emptying of tracer into the bladder, or lack of progression of tracer over the cerebral convexities, although with MR-myelography, this method is becoming redundant.[130]

Treatment is bed rest in the first instance. False-positive transient improvement in persistent low CSF volume headache with chiropractic and other similar therapies is recognized where the treatment necessitates the patient lying down for a prolonged period for the therapy. Intravenous caffeine (500 mg in 500-mL saline administered over 2 hours) is the standard and often very efficacious treatment. The ECG should be checked for any

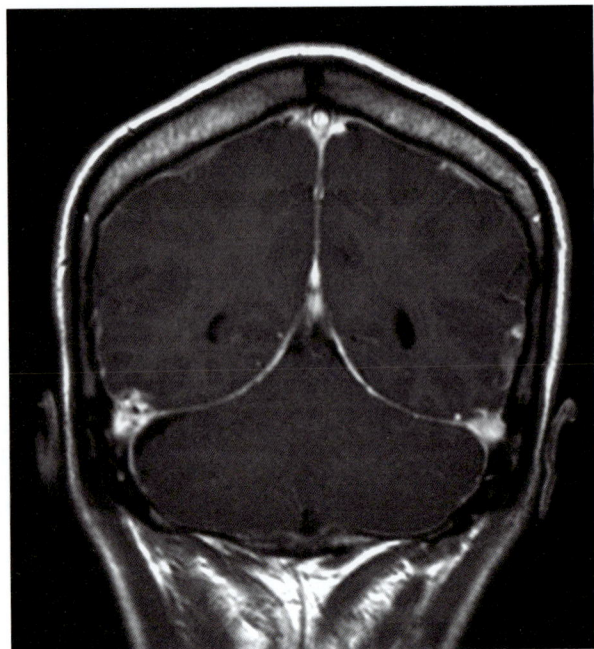

FIGURE 61.5 Magnetic resonance image showing diffuse meningeal enhancement after gadolinium administration in a patient with low cerebrospinal fluid volume (pressure) headache.

arrhythmia prior to administration. A reasonable practice is to carry out at least two infusions separated by 4 weeks after obtaining the suggestive clinical history and MRI with enhancement. Because intravenous caffeine is safe, and can be curative, by an unknown mechanism, it spares many patients the need for further tests. If that is unsuccessful, an abdominal binder may be helpful. If a leak can be identified, either by the radioisotope study, or by CT myelogram, or spinal T2-weighted MRI, an autologous blood patch is usually curative. In more intractable situations, theophylline is a useful alternative that offers outpatient management, although its onset of action is rather slow. An important phenotypically identical headache can be seen in the postural orthostatic tachycardia syndrome (POTS)[131] and should be considered when investigating this group of patients.

Raised Cerebrospinal Fluid Pressure Headache

As is the case for low CSF pressure states, raised CSF pressure as a cause of headache is well recognized by neurologists. Brain imaging can often reveal the cause, such as raised pressure due to a space-occupying lesion. The particular setting in which patients enter the spectrum of NDPH are those with idiopathic intracranial hypertension who present with headache without visual problems, particularly with normal fundi. It is recognized that intractable chronic migraine can be triggered by persistently raised intracranial pressure.[132] These patients typically give a history of generalized headache that is present on waking and gets better as the day goes on. It is generally worse with recumbency. Visual obscurations are frequently reported. Fundal changes on raised intracranial pressure would make the diagnosis relatively straightforward, but it is in those without such changes that the history must drive investigation. Patients often report a curious whooshing sensation in the occipital region.

Brain imaging is mandatory if raised pressure is suspected, and it is most simple in the long run to obtain an MRI and include MRV. The CSF pressure should be measured by lumbar puncture taking care to do so when the patient is symptomatic so that both the pressure and response to removal of CSF can be determined. A raised pressure and improvement in headache with removal of CSF is diagnostic of the problem. The fields should be formally documented even in the absence of overt ophthalmic involvement. Initial treatment can be with acetazolamide (250 to 500 mg twice daily). The patient may respond in weeks with improvement in headache. If this is not effective, topiramate has many actions that may be useful in this setting: carbonic anhydrase inhibition, weight loss, and neuronal membrane stabilization, probably through actions on phosphorylation pathways. A small number of severely disabled patients who do not respond to medical treatment will come to intracranial pressure monitoring and even shunting. This is exceptional and not undertaken without careful work up.

Posttraumatic Headache

NDPH may be seen after a blow to the head but more commonly after an infective episode, typically viral, or even malarial meningitis. A recent series identified one-third of all patients with NDPH reported the headache starting after a flu-like illness. The patient may note a period in which they had a significant infection: fever, neck stiffness, photophobia, and marked malaise. The headache starts during that period and never stops. Investigation reveals no current cause for the headache. It has been suggested that some patients with this syndrome have a persistent Epstein-Barr infection,[133] but this syndrome is anything but clearly delineated. A complicating factor will often be that the patient had a lumbar puncture during that illness, so a persistent low CSF volume headache needs to be considered first. Posttraumatic headache may be seen after carotid artery dissection, subarachnoid hemorrhage, and following intracranial surgery for a benign mass. The underlying theme seems to be that a traumatic event involving the dura mater can trigger a headache process that lasts for many years after that event.

The treatment of this form of NDPH is substantially empirical. Tricyclics, notably amitriptyline, and anticonvulsants, valproate, topiramate, and gabapentin, have been used with good effects.

OTHER IMPORTANT FORMS OF SECONDARY HEADACHE

Giant Cell Arteritis

This is an important cause of headache because delay in steroid treatment may result in blindness due to retinal artery ischaemia (Table 61.12). It is also known as temporal arteritis or cranial arteritis. Patients are usually elderly with focal tenderness of the scalp which may be provoked markedly by resting the head on the pillow. Jaw claudication provoked by chewing is a characteristic but relatively uncommon feature. Constitutional symptoms are common, particularly weight loss, malaise, or polymyalgia rheumatica. An elevated erythrocyte sedimentation rate (ESR) is a strong pointer to the diagnosis. The temporal artery may be tenderly inflamed, swollen, or pulseless. On suspicion of this diagnosis, steroid treatment should be started pending the result of temporal artery biopsy. Treatment is very often long term and requires careful monitoring for reactivation and the side effects of corticosteroids.

TABLE 61.12   Other Secondary Headaches

- Giant cell arteritis
- Cervicogenic headache
- Reader's paratrigeminal neuralgia[139]
- Tolosa-Hunt syndrome[140,141]
- Headache as a presentation of cervical dystonia[5]
- Headache in temporomandibular dysfunction
- Cardiac cephalalgia[113]
- Headache with endocrine disturbance, particularly pituitary tumor[26]
- Neck-tongue syndrome[142]
- Red-ear syndrome[143]

Cervicogenic Headache

It is a time-honored concept that the neck is responsible for much headache. Unfortunately, as with much of history, the good story is often ruined by the facts. Although there is little doubt that there is a rich overlap between the innervation of intracranial pain-producing structures by the ophthalmic division of the trigeminal nerve, and the posterior fossa and high cervical innervation by branches especially of the C_2 dorsal root,[134] causality is another issue. The Headache Classification Committee of the IHS recognizes that head pain can arise from the neck and labels this cervicogenic headache.[6] The term has been used by others to define a syndrome[135] that is so poorly described as to be useless in practice.[136] Most patients with neck discomfort and headache referred to specialty practice have migraine. They will have neck stiffness or discomfort as a premonitory symptom that can clearly persist in all stages of the attack.[137] They may respond to local therapies, such as greater occipital nerve injection[138]; however, this implies no more than triggering and is to be expected. The pursuit of neck pathology and the treatment of patients who have migraine by manipulative or physical means has no support in the controlled literature and is rarely of long-lasting value.

ACKNOWLEDGMENT

PJG is funded by the NIHR-Maudsley Biomedical Research Centre.

References

1. Lance JW, Goadsby PJ. *Mechanism and Management of Headache*. 7th ed. New York: Elsevier; 2005.
2. Silberstein SD, Lipton RB, Goadsby PJ. *Headache in Clinical Practice*. 2nd ed. London: Martin Dunitz; 2002.
3. Olesen J, Tfelt-Hansen P, Ramadan N, et al. *The Headaches*. Philadelphia: Lippincott Williams & Wilkins; 2005.
4. Lipton RB, Bigal M. *Migraine and Other Headache Disorders*. New York: Marcel Dekker; 2006.
5. Goadsby PJ, Dodick D, Silberstein SD. *Chronic Daily Headache for Clinicians*. Hamilton, Canada: BC Decker Inc; 2005.
6. Headache Classification Committee of the International Headache Society. The International Classification of Headache Disorders, 3rd Edition. *Cephalalgia* 2018;38:1–211.
7. Goadsby PJ, Holland PR, Martins-Oliveira M, et al. Pathophysiology of Migraine—a disorder of sensory processing. *Psychol Rev* 2017;97:553–622.
8. Oakes T, Zhang Q, Ferguson M, et al. Efficacy and safety of LY2951742 in a randomized, double-blind, placebo-controlled, dose-ranging study in patients with migraine. *Headache* 2016;56(suppl 1):68.
9. Vos T, Abajobir AA, Abate KH, et al. Global, regional, and national incidence, prevalence, and years lived with disability for 328 diseases and injuries for 195 countries, 1990-2016: a systematic analysis for the Global Burden of Disease Study 2016. *Lancet* 2017;390(10100):1211–1259.
10. Tepper SJ, Dahlof CG, Dowson A, et al. Prevalence and diagnosis of migraine in patients consulting their physician with a complaint of headache: data from the landmark study. *Headache* 2004;44:856–864.
11. Wolff HG. *Headache and Other Head Pain*. New York: Oxford University Press; 1948.
12. Feindel W, Penfield W, McNaughton F. The tentorial nerves and localization of intracranial pain in man. *Neurology* 1960;10:555–563.
13. McNaughton FL, Feindel WH. Innervation of intracranial structures: a reappraisal. In: Rose FC, editor. *Physiological Aspects of Clinical Neurology*. Oxford: Blackwell Scientific Publications; 1977:279–293.
14. Goadsby PJ, Lipton RB. A review of paroxysmal hemicranias, SUNCT syndrome and other short-lasting headaches with autonomic features, including new cases. *Brain* 1997;120:193–209.
15. May A, Goadsby PJ. The trigeminovascular system in humans: pathophysiological implications for primary headache syndromes of the neural influences on the cerebral circulation. *J Cereb Blood Flow Metab* 1999;19:115–127.
16. Obermann M, Yoon M-S, Dommes P, et al. Prevalence of trigeminal autonomic symptoms in migraine: a population-based study. *Cephalalgia* 2007;27:504–509.
17. Sprenger T, Goadsby PJ. What has functional neuroimaging done for primary headache . . . and for the clinical neurologist? *J Clin Neurosci* 2010;17: 547–553.
18. Charles A. Vasodilation out of the picture as a cause of migraine headache. *Lancet Neurol* 2013;12:419–420.
19. Ophoff RA, Terwindt GM, Vergouwe MN, et al. Familial hemiplegic migraine and episodic ataxia type-2 are caused by mutations in the Ca^{2+} channel gene CACNL1A4. *Cell* 1996;87:543–552.

20. De Fusco M, Marconi R, Silvestri L, et al. Haploinsufficiency of ATP1A2 encoding the Na$^+$/K$^+$ pump a2 subunit associated with familial hemiplegic migraine type 2. *Nature Gen* 2003;33:192–196.

21. Dichgans M, Freilinger T, Eckstein G, et al. Mutation in the neuronal voltage-gated sodium channel *SCN1A* causes familial hemiplegic migraine. *Lancet* 2005;366:371–377.

22. Goadsby PJ. Advances in the understanding of headache. *Br Med Bull* 2005;73:83–92.

23. May A, Bahra A, Buchel C, et al. Hypothalamic activation in cluster headache attacks. *Lancet* 1998;352:275–278.

24. May A, Ashburner J, Buchel C, et al. Correlation between structural and functional changes in brain in an idiopathic headache syndrome. *Nat Med* 1999;5:836–838.

25. Quality Standards Subcommittee of the American Academy of Neurology. The utility of neuroimaging in the evaluation of headache patients with normal neurologic examinations. *Neurology* 1994;44:1353–1354.

26. Levy M, Matharu MS, Meeran K, et al. The clinical characteristics of headache in patients with pituitary tumours. *Brain* 2005;128:1921–1930.

27. Theeler BJ, Erickson JC. Posttraumatic headache in military personnel and veterans of the Iraq and Afghanistan conflicts. *Curr Treat Options Neurol* 2012;14(1):36–49.

28. Neely ET, Midgette LA, Scher AI. Clinical review and epidemiology of headache disorders in US service members: with emphasis on post-traumatic headache. *Headache* 2009;49(7):1089–1096.

29. Lipton RB, Stewart WF, Diamond S, et al. Prevalence and burden of migraine in the United States: data from the American Migraine Study II. *Headache* 2001;41:646–657.

30. Andlin-Sobocki P, Jonsson B, Wittchen HU, et al. Cost of disorders of the brain in Europe. *Eur J Neurol* 2005;12(suppl 1):1–27.

31. Stewart WF, Ricci JA, Chee E, et al. Lost productive time and cost due to common pain conditions in the US workforce. *JAMA* 2003;290:2443–2454.

32. Tso AR, Goadsby PJ. Anti-CGRP monoclonal antibodies: the next era of migraine prevention? *Curr Treat Options Neurol* 2017;19:27.

33. Dodick DW, Goadsby PJ, Silberstein SD, et al. Randomized, double-blind, placebo-controlled, phase II trial of ALD403, an anti-CGRP peptide antibody in the prevention of frequent episodic migraine. *Lancet Neurol* 2014;13:1100–1107.

34. Smith J, Dodick DW, Goadsby PJ, et al. Randomized, double-blind, placebo-controlled trial of ALD403 (eptinezumab), an anti-CGRP monoclonal antibody for the prevention of chronic migraine. *Headache* 2017;57(suppl 3):130.

35. Bigal ME, Dodick DW, Rapoport AM, et al. Safety, tolerability, and efficacy of TEV-48125 for preventive treatment of high-frequency episodic migraine: a multicentre, randomised, double-blind, placebo-controlled, phase 2B study. *Lancet Neurol* 2015;14:1081–1090.

36. Dodick D, Goadsby P, Silberstein S, et al. Randomized, double-blind, placebo-controlled trial of ALD403, an anti-CGRP peptide antibody in the prevention of chronic migraine. *Neurology* 2017;88(16 suppl):S52.003.

37. Skljarevski V, Oakes TM, Zhang Q, et al. Galcanezumab for episodic migraine prevention: a randomized phase 2B placebo-controlled dose-ranging clinical trial. *JAMA Neurol* 2017;75:187–193.

38. Detke HC, Wang S, Skljarevski V, et al. A phase 3 placebo-controlled study of galcanezumab in patients with chronic migraine: results from the 3-month double-blind treatment phase of the REGAIN study. *Headache* 2017;57:1336–1337.

39. Goadsby PJ, Reuter U, Hallstrom Y, et al. A controlled trial of erenumab for episodic migraine. *N Engl J Med* 2017;377:2123–2132.

40. Tepper SJ, Ashina M, Reuter U, et al. A phase 2, randomised, double-blind, placebo-controlled study to evaluate the efficacy and safety of erenumab in chronic migraine prevention. *Lancet Neurol* 2017;16:425–434.

41. Puledda F, Goadsby PJ. An update on non-pharmacological neuromodulation for the acute and preventive treatment of migraine. *Headache* 2017;57:685–691.

42. Bhola R, Kinsella E, Giffin N, et al. Single-pulse transcranial magnetic stimulation (sTMS) for the acute treatment of migraine: evaluation of outcome data for the UK post market pilot program. *J Headache Pain* 2015;16:51.

43. Starling AJ, Tepper SJ, Marmura MJ, et al. A multicenter, prospective, single arm, open label, observational study of sTMS for migraine prevention (ESPOUSE Study). *Cephalalgia* 2018;38:1038–1048.

44. Goadsby PJ. Pathophysiology of migraine. *Continuum* 2006;12:52–66.

45. Goadsby PJ, Lipton RB, Ferrari MD. Migraine—current understanding and treatment. *N Engl J Med* 2002;346:257–270.

46. Kellstein DE, Lipton RB, Geetha R, et al. Evaluation of a novel solubilized formulation of ibuprofen in the treatment of migraine headache: a randomized, double-blind, placebo-controlled, dose-ranging study. *Cephalalgia* 2000;20:233–243.

47. Myllyla VV, Havanka H, Herrala L, et al. Tolfenamic acid rapid release versus sumatriptan in the acute treatment of migraine: comparable effect in a double-blind, randomized, controlled, parallel-group study. *Headache* 1998;38:201–207.

48. Tfelt-Hansen P, Saxena PR, Dahlof C, et al. Ergotamine in the acute treatment of migraine—a review and European consensus. *Brain* 2000;123:9–18.

49. Goadsby PJ. The pharmacology of headache. *Prog Neurobiol* 2000;62:509–525.

50. Brandes JL, Kudrow D, Stark SR, et al. Sumatriptan-naproxen for acute treatment of migraine: a randomized trial. *JAMA* 2007;297:1443–1454.

51. Chou DE, Gross GJ, Casadei CH, et al. External trigeminal nerve stimulation for the acute treatment of migraine: open-label trial on safety and efficacy. *Neuromodulation* 2017;20(7):678–683.

52. Tassorelli C, Grazzi L, de Tommaso M, et al. Non-invasive vagus nerve stimulation (nVNS) for the acute treatment of migraine: a randomised controlled trial. *Cephalalgia* 2017;37(1 suppl):319–320.

53. Lipton RB, Dodick DW, Silberstein SD, et al. Single-pulse transcranial magnetic stimulation for acute treatment of migraine with aura: a randomised, double-blind, parallel-group, sham-controlled trial. *Lancet Neurol* 2010;9:373–380.

54. Andreou AP, Holland PR, Akerman S, et al. Transcranial magnetic stimulation and potential cortical and trigeminothalamic mechanisms in migraine. *Brain* 2016;139:2002–2014.

55. Akerman S, Simon B, Romero-Reyes M. Vagus nerve stimulation suppresses acute noxious activation of trigeminocervical neurons in animal models of primary headache. *Neurobiol Dis* 2017;102:96–104.

56. Nelson DL, Phebus LA, Johnson KW, et al. Preclinical pharmacological profile of the selective 5-HT1F receptor agonist lasmiditan. *Cephalalgia* 2010;30:1159–1169.

57. Farkkila M, Diener HC, Geraud G, et al. Efficacy and tolerability of lasmiditan, an oral 5-HT(1F) receptor agonist, for the acute treatment of migraine: a phase 2 randomised, placebo-controlled, parallel-group, dose-ranging study. *Lancet Neurol* 2012;11:405–413.

58. Kuca B, Wietecha L, Berg P, et al. Lasmiditan (100 mg and 100 mg) compared to placebo for acute treatment of migraine. *Headache* 2017;57:1311.

59. Marcus R, Goadsby PJ, Dodick D, et al. BMS-927711 for the acute treatment of migraine: a double-blind, randomized, placebo controlled, dose-ranging trial. *Cephalalgia* 2014;34:114–125.

60. Voss T, Lipton RB, Dodick DW, et al. A phase IIb randomized, double-blind, placebo-controlled trial of ubrogepant for the acute treatment of migraine. *Cephalalgia* 2016;36:887–898.

61. Ho TW, Edvinsson L, Goadsby PJ. CGRP and its receptors provide new insights into migraine pathophysiology. *Nat Rev Neurol* 2010;6:573–582.

62. Scher AI, Rizzoli PB, Loder EW. Medication overuse headache: an entrenched idea in need of scrutiny. *Neurology* 2017;89(12):1296–1304.

63. Paemeleire K, Bahra A, Evers S, et al. Medication-overuse headache in cluster headache patients. *Neurology* 2006;67:109–113.

64. Bahra A, Walsh M, Menon S, et al. Does chronic daily headache arise *de novo* in association with regular analgesic use? *Headache* 2003;43:179–190.

65. Robbins N, Ito H, Scheinman M, et al. Safety of domperidone in treating nausea associated with dihydroergotamine infusion and headache. *Neurology (Minneap)* 2016;87:2522–2526.

66. Chou DC, Tso AR, Goadsby PJ. Aprepitant for the management of nausea with inpatient intravenous dihydroergotamine (DHE). *Neurology (Minneap)* 2016;87:1613–1616.

67. Weatherall MW, Telzerow AJ, Cittadini E, et al. Intravenous aspirin (lysine acetylsalicylate) in the in-patient management of headache. *Neurology* 2010;75:1098–1103.

68. Nagy AJ, Gandhi S, Bhola R, et al. Intravenous dihydroergotamine (DHE) for inpatient management of refractory primary headaches. *Neurology* 2011;77:1827–1832.

69. Eller M, Gelfand AA, Riggins NY, et al. Exacerbation of headache during dihydroergotamine for chronic migraine does not alter outcome. *Neurology (Minneap)* 2016;86(9):856–859.

70. Schoenen J, Wang W. Tension-type headache. In: Goadsby PJ, Silberstein SD, eds. *Headache*. Oxford: Butterworth-Heinemann; 1997:177–200.

71. Goadsby PJ. Chronic tension-type headache. *AM Fam Phys* 2003;89:36–40.

72. Lipton RB, Stewart WF, Cady R, et al. Sumatriptan for the range of headaches in migraine sufferers: results of the Spectrum Study. *Headache* 2000;40:783–791.

73. Diamond S, Baltes BJ. Chronic tension headache treated with amitriptyline: a double-blind study. *Headache* 1971;11:110–116.

74. Gobel H, Hamouz V, Hansen C, et al. Chronic tension-type headache: amitriptyline reduces clinical headache-duration and experimental pain sensitivity but does not alter pericranial muscle activity readings. *Pain* 1994;59:241–249.

75. Holroyd KA, O'Donnell FJ, Lipchik GL, et al. Management of chronic tension-type headache with (tricyclic) antidepressant medication, stress-management therapy and their combination: a randomized controlled trial. *JAMA* 2001;285:2208–2215.

76. Silberstein SD, Göbel H, Jensen R, et al. Botulinum toxin type A in the prophylactic treatment of chronic tension-type headache: a multicentre, double-blind, randomized, placebo-controlled, parallel-group study. *Cephalalgia* 2006;26:790–800.

77. Sjaastad O, Bakketeig LS. Cluster headache prevalence. Vågå study of headache epidemiology. *Cephalalgia* 2003;23:528–533.

78. Ford HL, Gerry E, Johnson M, et al. A prospective study of the incidence, prevalence and mortality of multiple sclerosis in Leeds. *J Neurol* 2002;249:260–265.

79. Schor LI. Cluster headache: investigating severity of pain, suicidality, personal burden, access to effective treatment, and demographics among a large international survey sample. *Cephalalgia* 2017;37(1 suppl):172.

80. May A, Goadsby PJ. The enigma of the interconnection of trigeminal pain and cranial autonomic symptoms. *Cephalalgia* 2016;36:727–729.

81. Goadsby PJ. Trigeminal autonomic cephalalgias. *Continuum* 2012;18:883–895.

82. Nesbitt AD, Goadsby PJ. Cluster headache. *BMJ* 2012;344:e2407.
83. Cohen AS, Matharu MS, Goadsby PJ. Electrocardiographic abnormalities in patients with cluster headache on verapamil therapy. *Neurology* 2007;69:668–675.
84. Nesbitt AD, Marin JCA, Tompkins E, et al. Initial experience with a novel non-invasive vagus nerve stimulation device for the treatment of cluster headache. *Neurology (Minneap)* 2015;84:1–5.
85. Gaul C, Diener HC, Silver N, et al. Non-invasive vagus nerve stimulation for PREVention and Acute treatment of chronic cluster headache (PREVA): a randomised controlled study. *Cephalalgia* 2016;36:534–546.
86. Cohen AS, Matharu MS, Burns B, et al. Randomized double-blind, placebo-controlled trial of high-flow inhaled oxygen in acute cluster headache. *Cephalalgia* 2007;27:1188.
87. The Sumatriptan Cluster Headache Study Group. Treatment of acute cluster headache with sumatriptan. *N Engl J Med* 1991;325:322–326.
88. Ekbom K, Waldenlind E, Cole JA, et al. Sumatriptan in chronic cluster headache: results of continuous treatment for eleven months. *Cephalalgia* 1992;12:254–256.
89. van Vliet JA, Bahra A, Martin V, et al. Intranasal sumatriptan in cluster headache—randomized placebo-controlled double-blind study. *Neurology* 2003;60:630–633.
90. Cittadini E, May A, Straube A, et al. Effectiveness of intranasal zolmitriptan in acute cluster headache. A randomized, placebo-controlled, double-blind crossover study. *Arch Neurol* 2006;63:1537–1542.
91. Rapoport AM, Mathew NT, Silberstein SD, et al. Zolmitriptan nasal spray in the acute treatment of cluster headache: a double-blind study. *Neurology* 2007;69:821–826.
92. Monstad I, Krabbe A, Micieli G, et al. Preemptive oral treatment with sumatriptan during a cluster period. *Headache* 1995;35:607–613.
93. Silberstein SD, Mechtler LL, Kudrow DB, et al. Non-invasive vagus nerve stimulation for the ACute Treatment of cluster headache: findings from the randomized, double-blind, sham-controlled ACT1 study. *Headache* 2016;56(8):1317–1332.
94. Goadsby PJ, de Coo IF, Silver N, et al. Non-invasive vagus nerve stimulation for the acute treatment of episodic and chronic cluster headache: a randomized, double-blind, sham-controlled ACT2 study [published online ahead of print January 1, 2017]. *Cephalalgia*. doi:10.1177/0333102417744362.
95. Jarrar RG, Black DF, Dodick DW, et al. Outcome of trigeminal nerve section in the treatment of chronic cluster headache. *Neurology* 2003;60:1360–1362.
96. Leone M, Franzini A, D'Amico D, et al. Hypothalamic deep brain stimulation to relieve intractable chronic SUNCT: the first case. *Neurology* 2004;62(suppl 5):A356.
97. Burns B, Watkins L, Goadsby PJ. Successful treatment of medically intractable cluster headache using occipital nerve stimulation (ONS). *Lancet* 2007;369:1099–1106.
98. Magis D, Allena M, Bolla M, et al. Occipital nerve stimulation for drug-resistant chronic cluster headache: a prospective pilot study. *Lancet Neurol* 2007;6:314–321.
99. Schoenen J, Jensen RH, Lanteri-Minet M, et al. Stimulation of the sphenopalatine ganglion (SPG) for cluster headache treatment—pathway CH-1: a randomized, sham-controlled study. *Cephalalgia* 2013;33:816–830.
100. Jurgens TP, Barloese M, May A, et al. Long-term effectiveness of sphenopalatine ganglion stimulation for cluster headache. *Cephalalgia* 2017;37:423–434.
101. Sjaastad O, Dale I. A new (?) clinical headache entity "chronic paroxysmal hemicrania". *Acta Neurol Scand* 1976;54:140–159.
102. Cittadini E, Matharu MS, Goadsby PJ. Paroxysmal hemicrania: a prospective clinical study of thirty-one cases. *Brain* 2008;131:1142–1155.
103. Matharu MS, Cohen AS, Frackowiak RSJ, et al. Posterior hypothalamic activation in paroxysmal hemicrania. *Ann Neurobiol* 2006;59:535–545.
104. Cohen AS, Matharu MS, Goadsby PJ. Short-lasting unilateral neuralgiform headache attacks with conjunctival injection and tearing (SUNCT) or cranial autonomic features (SUNA). A prospective clinical study of SUNCT and SUNA. *Brain* 2006;129:2746–2760.
105. Cohen AS, Goadsby PJ. Paroxysmal hemicrania responding to topiramate. *J Neurol Neurosurg Psychiatry* 2007;78:96–97.
106. Tso AR, Marin JCA, Goadsby PJ. Non-invasive vagus nerve stimulation for treatment of indomethacin-sensitive headaches. *JAMA Neurol* 2017;74:e1–e2.
107. Jensen K, Ohrstrom J, Cold GE, et al. The effects of indomethacin on intracranial pressure, cerebral blood flow and cerebral metabolism in patients with severe head injury and intracranial hypertension. *Acta Neurochir (Wien)* 1991;108:116–121.
108. Sjaastad O, Saunte C, Salvesen R, et al. Shortlasting unilateral neuralgiform headache attacks with conjunctival injection, tearing, sweating, and rhinorrhea. *Cephalalgia* 1989;9:147–156.
109. May A, Bahra A, Buchel C, et al. Functional MRI in spontaneous attacks of SUNCT: short-lasting neuralgiform headache with conjunctival injection and tearing. *Ann Neurol* 1999;46:791–793.
110. Weng H, Cohen AS, Schankin C, et al. Phenotypic and treatment outcome data on SUNCT and SUNA, including a randomised placebo-controlled trial [published online ahead of print January 1, 2017]. *Cephalalgia*. doi:10.1177/0333102417739304.
111. Raskin NH. The cough headache syndrome: treatment. *Neurology* 1995;45:1784.
112. Symonds C. Cough headache. *Brain* 1956;79:557–568.
113. Lance JW, Lambros J. Headache associated with cardiac ischemia. *Headache* 1998;38:315–316.
114. Raskin NH. The hypnic headache syndrome. *Headache* 1988;28:534–536.
115. Dodick DW, Mosek AC, Campbell JK. The hypnic ("alarm clock") headache syndrome. *Cephalalgia* 1998;18:152–156.
116. Holle D, Naegel S, Krebs S, et al. Clinical characteristics and therapeutic options in hypnic headache. *Cephalalgia* 2010;30(12):1435–1442.
117. Gil-Gouveia R, Goadsby PJ. Secondary "hypnic headache." *J Neurol* 2007;254:646–654.
118. Day JW, Raskin NH. Thunderclap headache: symptom of unruptured cerebral aneurysm. *Lancet* 1986;2(8518):1247–1248.
119. Wijdicks EF, Kerkhoff H, van Gijn J. Long-term follow up of 71 patients with thunderclap headache mimicking subarachnoid hemorrhage. *Lancet* 1988;2:68–70.
120. Markus HS. A prospective follow-up of thunderclap headache mimicking subarachnoid hemorrhage. *J Neurol Neurosurg Psychiatry* 1991;54:1117–1125.
121. Dodick DW, Brown RD, Britton JW, et al. Nonaneurysmal thunderclap headache with diffuse, multifocal, segmental, and reversible vasospasm. *Cephalalgia* 1999;19:118–123.
122. Newman LC, Lipton RB, Russell M, et al. Hemicrania continua: attacks may alternate sides. *Headache* 1992;32:237–238.
123. Antonaci F, Pareja JA, Caminero AB, et al. Chronic paroxysmal hemicrania and hemicrania continua. Parenteral indomethacin: the 'Indotest.' *Headache* 1998;38:122–128.
124. Matharu MS, Cohen AS, McGonigle DJ, et al. Posterior hypothalamic and brainstem activation in hemicrania continua. *Headache* 2004;44:747–761.
125. Goadsby PJ, Boes CJ. New daily persistent headache. *J Neurol Neurosurg Psychiatry* 2002;72(suppl 6):ii6–ii9.
126. Vanast WJ. New daily persistent headaches: definition of a benign syndrome. *Headache* 1986;26:317.
127. Li D, Rozen TD. The clinical characteristics of new daily persistent headache. *Cephalalgia* 2002;22:66–69.
128. Mokri B, Piepgras DG, Miller GM. Syndrome of orthostatic headaches and diffuse pachymeningeal gadolinium enhancement. *Mayo Clin Proc* 1997;72(5):400–413.
129. Mokri B, Atkinson JL, Dodick DW, et al. Absent pachymeningeal gadolinium enhancement on cranial MRI despite symptomatic CSF leak. *Neurology* 1999;53:402–404.
130. Monteith TS, Kralik SF, Dillon WP, et al. The utility of radioisotope cisternography in low csf/volume syndromes compared to myelography. *Cephalalgia* 2016;36:1291–1295.
131. Mokri B, Low PA. Orthostatic headaches without CSF leak in postural tachycardia syndrome. *Neurology* 2003;61:980–982.
132. Mathew NT, Ravishankar K, Sanin LC. Coexistence of migraine and idiopathic intracranial hypertension without papilledema. *Neurology* 1996;46:1226–1230.
133. Diaz-Mitoma F, Vanast WJ, Tyrrell DLJ. Increased frequency of Epstein-Barr virus excretion in patients with new daily persistent headaches. *Lancet* 1987;1:411–415.
134. Bartsch T, Goadsby PJ. Anatomy and physiology of pain referral patterns in primary and cervicogenic headache disorders. *Headache Curr* 2005;2:42–48.
135. Antonaci F, Fredriksen T, Sjaastad O. Cervicogenic headache: clinical presentation, diagnostic criteria, and differential diagnosis. *Curr Pain Headache Rep* 2001;5:387–392.
136. Goadsby PJ. A critical view of cervicogenic headache. In: Sjaastad O, Fredriksen TA, Bono G, et al, eds. *Cervicogenic Headache.* London: Smith-Gordon; 2004:131–136.
137. Giffin NJ, Ruggiero L, Lipton RB, et al. Premonitory symptoms in migraine: an electronic diary study. *Neurology* 2003;60:935–940.
138. Afridi SK, Shields KG, Bhola R, et al. Greater occipital nerve injection in primary headache syndromes- prolonged effects from a single injection. *Pain* 2006;122:126–129.
139. Goadsby PJ. Raeder's syndrome: "paratrigeminal" paralysis of oculopupillary sympathetic system. *J Neurol Neurosurg Psychiatry* 2002;72:297–299.
140. Tolosa E. Periarteritic lesions of the carotid siphon with the clinical features of a carotid infraclinoidal aneurysm. *J Neurol Neurosurg Psychiatry* 1954;17:300–302.
141. Hunt WE, Meagher JN, LeFever HE, et al. Painful ophthalmoplegia. Its relation to indolent inflammation of the cavernous sinus. *Neurolgy (Minneap)* 1961;11:56–62.
142. Bogduk N. An anatomical basis for the neck-tongue syndrome. *J Neurol Neurosurg Psychiatry* 1981;44:202–208.
143. Lance JW. The red ear syndrome. *Neurology* 1996;47:617–620.
144. Bahra A, Matharu MS, Buchel C, et al. Brainstem activation specific to migraine headache. *Lancet* 2001;357:1016–1017.
145. Afridi S, Giffin NJ, Kaube H, et al. A positron emission tomographic study in spontaneous migraine. *Arch Neurol* 2005;62:1270–1275.
146. Matharu MS, Bartsch T, Ward N, et al. Central neuromodulation in chronic migraine patients with suboccipital stimulators: a PET study. *Brain* 2004;127:220–230.
147. Afridi S, Matharu MS, Lee L, et al. A PET study exploring the laterality of brainstem activation in migraine using glyceryl trinitrate. *Brain* 2005;128:932–939.

CHAPTER 62

Noncardiac Chest Pain

RONNIE FASS and **TAKAHISA YAMASAKI**

Noncardiac chest pain (NCCP) is defined as recurring angina-like retrosternal chest pain of noncardiac origin. A patient's history and characteristics do not reliably distinguish between cardiac and esophageal causes of chest pain.[1] This is compounded by the fact that patients with a history of coronary artery disease (CAD) may also experience chest pain of noncardiac origin. The heightened awareness about the potentially devastating ramifications of chest pain may drive patients to seek medical attention despite a negative cardiac workup.[2] Furthermore, almost half of NCCP patients are not convinced by their negative cardiac diagnosis, and reassurance alone has proved to be an ungratifying therapeutic strategy.[3] There are many causes for NCCP, and they are not limited to the esophagus (Table 62.1).[4] Compared to patients with cardiac angina, those with NCCP are usually younger, less likely to have typical symptoms, and more likely to have a normal resting electrocardiogram.[5] Additionally, levels of anxiety of NCCP patients seen in a rapid access chest pain clinic significantly exceeded those of patients with cardiac angina and remained above community norms for at least 2 months after clinic visit.[6] NCCP patients view their condition as significantly less controllable and less understandable than those whose pain is of cardiac origin.[6]

NCCP may be the manifestation of non-gastrointestinal (GI) or GI-related disorders (Fig. 62.1). An important step toward understanding of the underlying mechanisms of NCCP was the recognition that gastroesophageal reflux disease (GERD) is the most common contributing factor for chest pain. Although chest pain has been considered an atypical manifestation of GERD, it is an integral part of the limited repertoire of esophageal symptoms. In patients with non–GERD-related NCCP, esophageal motility disorders and functional chest pain (FCP) are the main underlying mechanism for symptoms. The Rome IV Committee uses the term *functional chest pain* to describe recurrent episodes of substernal chest pain of visceral quality with no apparent explanation (Table 62.2). As with all other functional esophageal disorders, GERD, major esophageal motor disorders, and eosinophilic esophagitis should also be ruled out before the diagnosis is established.[7]

Up to 20% of the patients with FCP exhibit other functional disorders, primarily irritable bowel syndrome (IBS) (27%) and abdominal bloating (22%).[8] The mechanisms responsible for FCP include abnormal mechanophysical properties of the esophagus, central and peripheral hypersensitivity, altered central processing of visceral stimuli, and psychological comorbidity (Table 62.3). The latter may include depression, anxiety, panic attack, and somatization.[9]

Epidemiology

Information about the epidemiology of NCCP in the United States and around the world is relatively limited. Presently, chest pain is the second most common presentation to hospital emergency departments; however, only 25% of individuals who experience chest pain actually present to a hospital.[10]

The mean annual prevalence of NCCP in six population-based studies was approximately 25%. However, these studies differ in many aspects such as NCCP definition, geography, sample size, sampling order, and ethnic disparities.[11] A population-based survey in the United States assessed the prevalence of GERD in Olmsted County, Minnesota, and reported an overall NCCP prevalence of 23%.[12] Gender distribution among NCCP patients was similar (24% among males and 22% among females). Using the Rome criteria for functional GI disorders, Drossman et al.[13] reported a prevalence of 13.6% in 8,250 households in the United States. In this study, FCP was diagnosed rather than NCCP. Eslick[14] and Eslick et al.[15] recently evaluated the prevalence of NCCP in Australia by using a mailing of a validated Chest Pain Questionnaire to 1,000 randomly selected individuals. The study demonstrated a prevalence rate of 33% with almost equal gender distribution (32% in males vs. 33% in females). This study also showed that the population prevalence of NCCP decreases with increasing age.[14,15]

A nationwide population-based study from South America found that the annual prevalence of NCCP was 23.5% and that NCCP has been equally reported by both sexes.[16] In this study, frequent typical GERD symptoms (at least once a week) were significantly and independently associated with NCCP. Another recently published epidemiologic study demonstrated that the annual prevalence of NCCP in a Chinese population was 19%.[17] Although females with NCCP tend to consult health care providers more often than men, the disorder affects both sexes equally.[12,14,16] Additionally, females are more likely to present to hospital emergency departments with NCCP than males, but there are no sex differences regarding chest pain intensity.[18] Overall, women tend to use terms like *burning* and *frightening* more often than men.[19]

Epidemiologic studies report a decrease in the prevalence of NCCP with increasing age. Women under 25 years of age and those between 45 and 55 years of age have the highest prevalence rates.[15] Patients with NCCP are younger, consume greater amounts of alcohol and tobacco, and are more likely to suffer from anxiety than their counterparts with ischemic heart disease. Patients with NCCP continue to seek treatment on a regular basis after the diagnosis was established for both chest pain and other unrelated symptoms, but few are in contact with hospital services.[20] A meta-analysis of the epidemiology of NCCP in the community revealed pooled prevalence of 13%, lack of age and gender predilection, and increased prevalence in subjects with GERD (odds ratio [OR], 4.71).[21]

In one study, almost a fourth of individuals with NCCP had sought health care for chest pain within the previous 12 months. None of the GI (heartburn, dysphagia, and acid regurgitation) or psychological (anxiety, depression, and neuroticism) risk factors was significantly associated with pursuing consultation for NCCP.[15] A recent US-based survey revealed that cardiologists manage by themselves about half of the patients who are diagnosed with NCCP.[22] Of those NCCP patients who were referred, 45.9% were sent back to the primary care physician (PCP) and only 29.3% to a gastroenterologist (Fig. 62.2).

In a survey of PCPs, Wong et al.[23] demonstrated that most NCCP patients were diagnosed and treated by PCPs (79.5%) without being referred to a gastroenterologist. The most preferred subspecialty for the initial diagnostic evaluation of a patient presenting with chest pain was cardiology (62%), followed by gastroenterology (17%). The mean percentage of such referrals was only 22%. The most preferred subspecialty for further management of NCCP was gastroenterology (76%),

TABLE 62.1 Noncardiac, Nonesophageal Etiologies for Chest Pain

Musculoskeletal
  Tietze syndrome
  Costochondritis
  Fibromyalgia
  Precordial catch syndrome
  Slipping rib syndrome

Gastrointestinal
  Eosinophilic esophagitis
  Gastric
  Biliary tree
  Pancreatic
  Intra-abdominal masses (benign and malignant)

Pulmonary
  Pneumonia
  Pulmonary embolus
  Lung cancer
  Sarcoidosis
  Pneumothorax and pneumomediastinum
  Pleural effusions
  Intrathoracic masses (benign and malignant)

Miscellaneous
  Aortic disorders
  Pericarditis and myocarditis
  Pulmonary hypertension
  Herpes zoster
  Drug-induced pain
  Sickle cell crisis
  Psychological disorders

Reprinted from Fass R, Achem SR. Noncardiac chest pain: epidemiology, natural course and pathogenesis. *J Neurogastroenterol Motil* 2011;17:110–123, with permission.

TABLE 62.2 Rome IV Diagnostic Criteria for Functional Chest Pain of Presumed Esophageal Origin

Must include all of the following:
• Retrosternal chest pain or discomfort
• Absence of associated esophageal symptoms, such as heartburn and dysphagia
• Absence of evidence that major esophageal motility disorders, gastroesophageal reflux, or eosinophilic esophagitis are the cause of the symptom
Criteria must be fulfilled for the last 3 months with symptoms onset at least 6 months prior to diagnosis with a frequency of at least once a week.

followed by cardiology (8%). The mean percentage of the actual referral rate was 29.8% for gastroenterologists and 14% for cardiologists.[23]

A study by Eslick and Talley[24] reported that 78% of patients who presented to a hospital emergency department with acute chest pain had seen a health care provider in the last 12 months. The most common health care provider seen was a general practitioner (85%), followed by cardiologist (74%), gastroenterologist (30%), pulmonologist (14%), alternative therapist (8%), and psychologist (10%).[24] A multiple logistic regression analysis revealed that patients with chest pain who are also suffering from heartburn were 16 times more likely to see a general practitioner (OR, 16.40; 95% confidence interval [CI], 1.98 to 135.99) and 3 times more likely to consult a gastroenterologist (OR, 3.10; 95% CI, 1.26 to 7.62). Additionally, work

absenteeism rates (29%) and interruptions to daily activities (63%) were high because of NCCP.

Many patients with NCCP report poor quality of life and admit taking cardiac medications despite lack of evidence for a cardiac cause. Only a small fraction of patients feels reassured. Consequently, the economic burden of the disease has been proposed to be very high, although studies evaluating the cost impact of NCCP on the health care system are very scarce. In one study, the health care cost for NCCP was estimated to be more than $315 million annually primarily because of multiple clinic visits, emergency room visits, hospitalizations, and prescription medications.[25] This cost estimate does not include indirect costs such as lost days of work or the impact of symptoms on patients' quality of life, which have been demonstrated to be more significant when evaluating the economic burden of patients with functional bowel disorders. In Australia, the annual cost associated with NCCP presentations to the Nepean Hospital amounts to approximately $1.4 million.[26] The researchers extrapolated these costs to the Australian health care system and conservatively estimated that NCCP accounts for at least a $30 million of the health care budget annually.

Natural History

Thus far, very few studies have prospectively evaluated the natural course of NCCP. Obviously, the main concern is the likelihood of these patients developing true ischemic heart disease if followed long term. One of the early studies by Wielgosz et al.[27] followed 821 patients with chest pain and normal coronary arteries for a period of 1 year. The authors demonstrated that only three (0.3%) patients died, and all were due to non-ischemic reasons.[27] However, most of the patients (67%) continued to experience chest pain to some degree (39% less pain, 26% the same pain, and 2% more severe pain). In a study

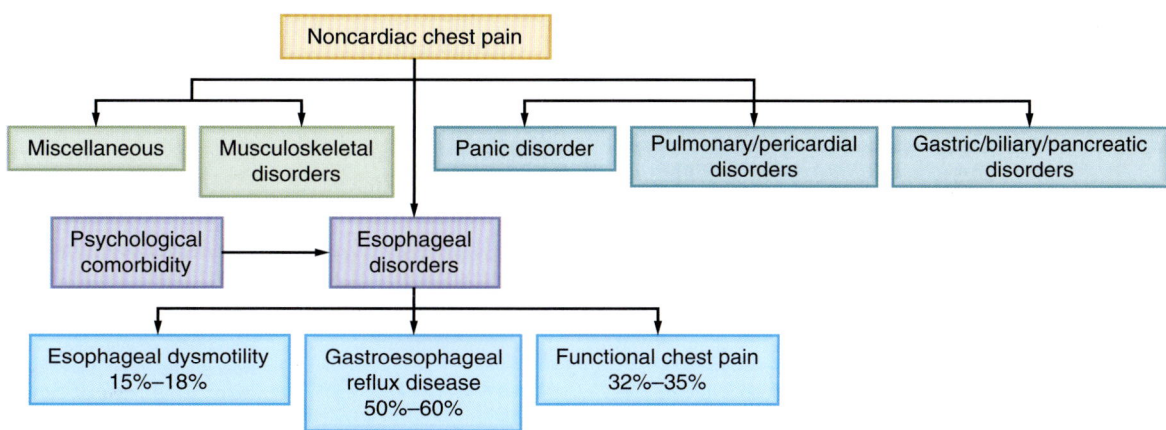

FIGURE 62.1 The different underlying mechanisms of noncardiac chest pain.

TABLE 62.3 The Main Proposed Underlying Mechanisms of Functional Chest Pain

- Abnormal mechanophysical properties
  - Hyperactive esophagus
  - ↓ Compliance
- Visceral hypersensitivity
  - Peripheral and central sensitization
  - Altered central processing of visceral stimuli (altered autonomic activity)
- Psychological abnormalities
  - Panic attack
  - Anxiety
  - Depression

that followed 46 NCCP patients over a period of 11 years, only 2 (4.3%) of the subjects died from a cardiovascular-related event (stroke and ischemic heart disease). Again, as in the previous study, 74% of the surviving NCCP patients continued to report chest pain 11 years later, and of those, 34% reported chest pain symptoms weekly.[28] Other studies also documented a very limited long-term mortality in NCCP patients but with continuous debilitating symptoms, impaired functional status, chronic use of drugs (GI, cardiac, and psychiatric), repeated admissions to the hospital, and repeated cardiac and noncardiac procedures.[20,29–33] In a survey study, 119 NCCP patients, of which 63 were diagnosed as having pain from the esophagus, were followed for a period of 21.8 months.[34] Patients with esophageal-related chest pain usually continued to have recurrent pain. Interestingly, a specific diagnosis did not significantly increase the likelihood of pain resolution. However, patients who understood that the esophagus was the source of their pain were significantly less likely to feel disabled by their pain and therefore were less likely to require continued physician evaluation. This study was published prior to the proton pump inhibitor (PPI) era. It is unlikely that patients with NCCP

due to GERD will continue to have symptoms long term if they are compliant with their antireflux treatment. In another study that compared long-term natural history between NCCP and GERD patients, the authors found no significant difference in survival between the two groups (hazard ratio, 1.1; 95% CI, 0.8 to 1.5). Interestingly, the diagnosis of NCCP disappeared from the electronic hospital record in 96% of the patients within 2 years of follow-up.[35]

In a recent study that followed 355 NCCP patients, the authors demonstrated that 49% sought care in the emergency department, 42% underwent repeated cardiac workup, and only 15% were seen by a gastroenterologist.[36] Survival free of cardiac death in the subset with NCCP and a GI disorder was 90.2% at 10 years and 84.8% at 20 years compared to 93.7% at 10 years and 88.1% at 20 years for those with NCCP of unknown origin. Less than a handful of studies reported similar mortality between patients with NCCP and those with CAD.[33,37] A more recent study by Eslick and Talley[38] followed 126 NCCP and 71 cardiac patients who were seen in the emergency room for a period of 4 years. The majority of the NCCP (71%) and the CAD patients (81%) continued to have symptoms 4 years later. The authors found no difference in the mortality rate between the two groups (CAD, 11.0%, vs. NCCP, 5.5%; $P = .16$). However, the study may suffer from type II error, and the results need to be confirmed in a larger cohort of patients.

Overall, the aforementioned data support the overall conclusion that increased mortality is uncommon in NCCP patients. However, patients with NCCP demonstrate poor quality of life primarily due to continuation of symptoms many years after diagnosis.

Pathophysiology

GASTROESOPHAGEAL REFLUX DISEASE

Many studies have shown an association between GERD and NCCP. However, association does not confer causality. Resolution or improvement of chest pain symptoms in response

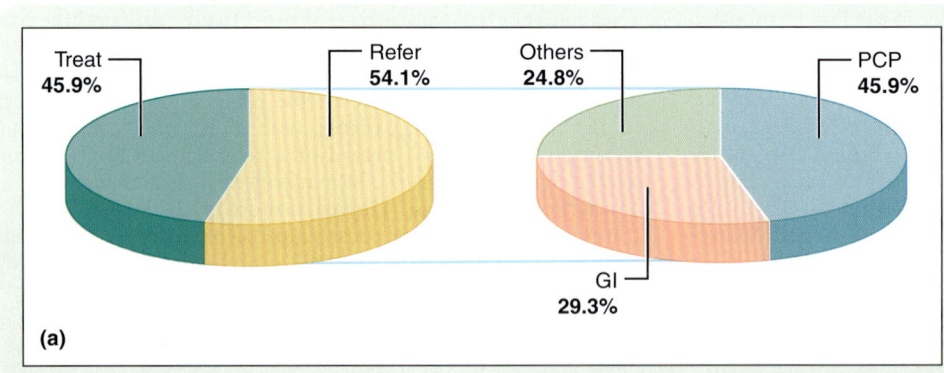

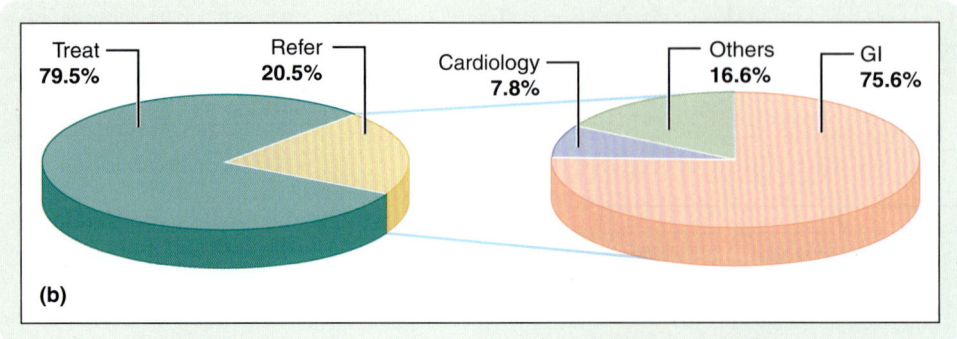

FIGURE 62.2 A: A survey of 246 cardiologists determined that approximately half self-managed noncardiac chest pain patients. (Reprinted with permission from Wong WM, Risner-Adler S, Beeler J, et al. Noncardiac chest pain: the role of the cardiologist—a national survey. J Clin Gastroenterol 2005;39[10]:858–862, with permission.) **B:** A similar survey of 205 primary care physicians demonstrated that the majority self-managed noncardiac chest pain patients. (Redrawn after Wong WM, Risner-Adler S, Beeler J, et al. Noncardiac chest pain: the role of the cardiologist—a national survey. J Clin Gastroenterol 2005;39[10]:858–862, with permission.)

to treatment with antireflux medications provides the missing causal link.

Locke et al.[12] have demonstrated that NCCP is more commonly reported by patients (37%) who experience heartburn symptoms at least weekly, as compared with 30.7% of those who have infrequent heartburn (less than once a week) and 7.9% of those without any GERD symptoms. In another community-based study, the authors found that 53% of all patients with NCCP experienced heartburn and 58% acid regurgitation.[15] Stahl et al.[39] found in a small sample of NCCP patients that 61.5% had GERD-related symptoms. In three different studies evaluating the role of the PPI test in patients with NCCP, the authors found GERD-related symptoms in 68% to 90% of the patients.[40–42]

Ambulatory 24-hour esophageal pH testing studies have demonstrated that about half of NCCP patients have an abnormal esophageal acid exposure. Stahl et al.[39] evaluated 13 consecutive NCCP patients and found that 69.2% had an abnormal pH test. Beedassy et al.[43] evaluated 104 patients with NCCP and documented that 48% of them had an abnormal pH test. It should be noted that only 21% of the 52 patients who reported chest pain during the study had a concomitant acid reflux event. Interestingly, only 10 of the 52 subjects had a positive symptom index (>50%). Similarly, DeMeester et al.[44] demonstrated that 46% of patients with chest pain had symptoms associated with an acid reflux event as documented during pH testing. Pandak et al.[45] found an abnormal pH test in 42% of NCCP patients. In three different studies evaluating the role of the PPI test, the authors found abnormal pH test in 37.5% to 67% of the NCCP patients.[40–42] In a study from Asia, 34.3% of the NCCP patients had at least one abnormal pH parameter.[46] Even in patients with CAD who continued to have atypical chest pain symptoms, 49% to 67% had some of their painful episodes associated with acid reflux.[47,48]

The presence of esophageal mucosal abnormalities consistent with GERD appears to be less common in NCCP patients than GERD symptoms or excess esophageal acid exposure. From different studies, the range has been between 2.5% and 75%.[46,49–52] In three different studies evaluating the role of the PPI test in patients with NCCP, the authors found GERD-related endoscopic findings in 44% to 75% of the NCCP patients.[40–42] In all of these studies, low-grade erosive esophagitis was the main GERD-related endoscopic finding. A recent study by Dickman et al.[53] evaluated upper GI findings in patients with NCCP as compared with those having only GERD-related symptoms using a large multicenter consortium. Of the NCCP group, 28.6% had hiatal hernia, 19.6% erosive esophagitis, 4.4% Barrett esophagus (BE), and 3.6% esophageal stricture/stenosis. The prevalence of these findings was significantly lower in the NCCP group when compared with the GERD group. From this study, it appears that GERD-related mucosal abnormalities are not uncommon in the esophagus of NCCP patients. However, the prevalence of these anatomical findings is lower than what has been observed in GERD patients. Importantly, NCCP patients may also demonstrate BE, albeit uncommonly.

The mechanism by which gastroesophageal reflux causes NCCP remains poorly understood. It is still unclear why esophageal exposure to gastric content in some patients causes heartburn, and in others, chest pain. This is compounded by the fact that some patients may experience chest pain at one time and heartburn at other times. Characteristics of the individual reflux episodes (duration and pH) have been proposed to influence patients' symptoms. Smith et al.[54] studied 25 individuals with NCCP to determine the relation between the sensation of pain in GERD and pH of the refluxate. They found that all 25 patients had reproduction of their pain during intra-esophageal infusion of solutions with pH 1 and 1.5. Reflux events resulting in pain were significantly longer than

those without pain and were more often associated with a recently preceding painful episode.

Esophageal hypersensitivity has been suggested to be another important mechanism for chest pain in patients with GERD. In one study,[55] healthy subjects underwent perfusion of the distal esophagus with normal saline or 0.1 N hydrochloric acid. Perceptual responses to intraluminal esophageal balloon distension were evaluated using an electronic barostat. As compared with saline, acid perfusion reduced the perception threshold (innocuous sensation) and tended to reduce the pain threshold (aversive sensation). This study demonstrated short-term sensitization of mechanosensitive afferent pathways by transient exposure to acid. The authors suggested that in patients with NCCP, acid reflux induces sensitization of the esophagus, which may subsequently alter the way the esophagus perceives otherwise normal esophageal distention. Sarkar et al.[56] recruited 19 healthy volunteers and 7 patients with NCCP. Hydrochloric acid was infused into the distal esophagus over 30 minutes. Sensory responses to electrical stimulation were monitored within the acid-exposed distal esophagus and the nonexposed proximal esophagus before and after infusion. In the healthy subjects, acid infusion into the distal esophagus lowered the pain threshold in the upper esophagus. Patients with NCCP already had a lower resting esophageal pain threshold than healthy subjects. After acid perfusion, their pain threshold in the proximal esophagus fell further and for a longer duration than was the case for the healthy subjects (Fig. 62.3). Additionally, there was a decrease in pain threshold after acid infusion in the anterior chest wall. This study demonstrated the development of secondary allodynia (visceral hypersensitivity to an innocuous stimulus in normal tissue that is in proximity to the site of tissue injury) in the proximal esophagus by repeated acid exposure of the distal esophagus. The concurrent visceral and somatic pain hypersensitivity is most likely caused by central sensitization (an increase in excitability of spinal cord neurons induced by activation of nociceptive C fibers in the area of tissue injury). The patients with NCCP demonstrated visceral hypersensitivity and amplified secondary allodynia in the esophagus.

Another explanation how GERD may cause chest pain was provided by studies using high-frequency, intraluminal ultrasonography. Balaban et al.[57] demonstrated a temporal

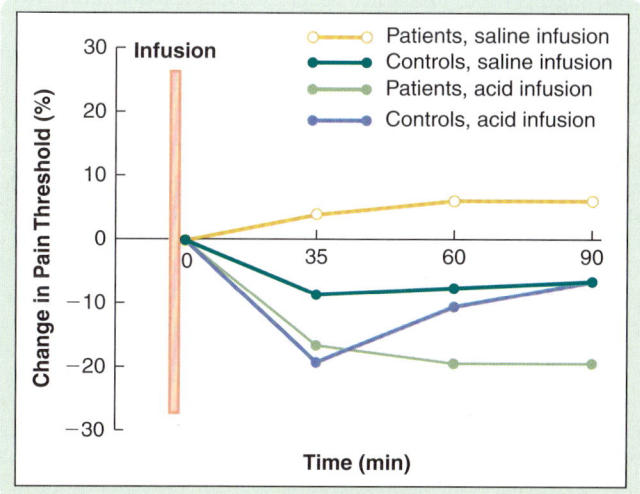

FIGURE 62.3   Mean change in pain threshold in the upper esophagus after 5 minutes infusion of acid or saline into the lower esophagus (noncardiac chest pain vs. control). *(Redrawn after Sarkar S, Aziz Q, Woolf CJ, et al. Contribution of central sensitization to the development of non-cardiac chest pain. Lancet 2000;356[9236]:1154–1159. Copyright © 2000 Elsevier. With permission.)*

correlation between sustained contractions of the esophageal longitudinal muscle and spontaneous as well as provoked esophageal chest pain. In a follow-up study, the authors suggested that the duration of sustained esophageal contraction determines the type of symptom perceived by patients.[58] Heartburn was associated with shorter duration contractions, whereas chest pain was associated with contractions of longer duration. In a recent study, the authors suggested that esophageal muscle thickness per se, in the absence of esophageal motility abnormality, can lead to chest pain symptoms.[59] Utilization of pH impedance in patients with GERD-related NCCP suggested that the presence of gas in the refluxate may drive the chest pain symptom.[60]

Studies have demonstrated that NCCP patients with evidence of GERD (endoscopic findings and/or abnormal pH test) commonly respond to antireflux treatment. Between 78% and 92% of NCCP patients with objective evidence of GERD demonstrated symptoms improvement on antireflux treatment.[40,42,45,46] In contrast, response to PPI treatment in NCCP patients without objective evidence of GERD ranged between 10% and 14%.[40–42] Kushnir et al.[61] have demonstrated that a positive symptom association probability and elevated acid exposure time predicted response to PPI treatment in patients with NCCP. When used hierarchically, response to antireflux treatment was best predicted when GERD parameters (acid exposure time, symptom association probability, and symptom index) were all abnormal and poorest when all normal. These data suggest a causal relationship between patients' GERD and chest pain symptoms.

In patients with CAD and atypical chest pain, a higher incidence and longer duration of ischemic events were more commonly observed in those with GERD.[48]

LINKED ANGINA

It is well known that the esophagus and the heart share similar sensory innervation, and several studies have demonstrated that acidification of the distal esophagus may influence the flow of the coronary circulation.[62–64] Chauhan et al.[65] have shown a reduction in coronary artery blood flow in response to acid perfusion into the distal esophagus in patients with syndrome X. Syndrome X is defined as typical chest pain and electrocardiographic changes suggestive of myocardial ischemia on stress test but patent coronary arteries on angiogram.[64] The reduction in coronary blood flow was also associated with typical anginal pain, suggesting the presence of an esophagocardiac inhibitory reflex.[65] These findings were later confirmed by Rosztoczy et al.[66] who showed a decrease in coronary artery blood flow in 19 out of 42 (45%) patients undergoing acid perfusion of the esophagus.

ESOPHAGEAL DYSMOTILITY

Several large studies demonstrated that approximately 30% of NCCP patients had abnormal esophageal manometry.[67–69] In one study that included 910 NCCP patients, the authors found that 70% had normal esophageal motility (Fig. 62.4).[67] Nutcracker esophagus (14.4%) was the most commonly documented esophageal motility abnormality, followed by nonspecific esophageal motor disorder (10.8%). Diffuse esophageal spasm (DES), achalasia, and hypertensive lower esophageal sphincter (LES) were very uncommon in this NCCP group. In another study, Dekel et al.[68] evaluated 140 NCCP patients using the Clinical Outcomes Research Initiative database. Unlike the previous study that included patients from one major center with interest in esophageal motility, the study by Dekel et al.[68] included patients from more than 60 academic, veteran affairs, and private centers from around the United States. The authors also found that 70% of the subjects had a normal esophageal motility test. Hypotensive LES (61%) was the most common motility abnormality diagnosed, followed by hypertensive LES,

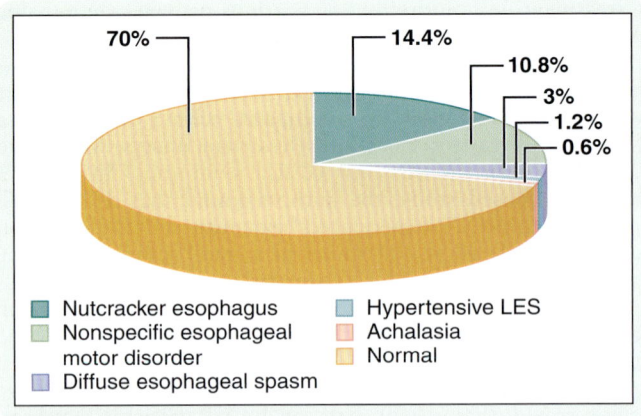

FIGURE 62.4 Distribution of esophageal motility abnormalities in noncardiac chest pain patient without gastroesophageal reflux disease (N = 910). (Redrawn after Katz PO, Dalton CB, Richter JE, et al. Esophageal testing of patients with noncardiac chest pain or dysphagia. Results of three years' experience with 1161 patients. Ann Intern Med 1987;106[4]:593–597. Copyright © 1987 American College of Physicians. All Rights Reserved. Reprinted with the permission of American College of Physicians, Inc.)

nonspecific esophageal motor disorder, and nutcracker esophagus (10% each). In this study, achalasia and DES were also very uncommon. The difference in the distribution of motility abnormalities between the two studies reflects the different study designs. In the first study, only non–GERD-related NCCP patients were included, whereas all newcomers were enrolled into the second study. A recent study from Chile evaluated 100 newly diagnosed NCCP patients and found that 8% of them had an abnormal esophageal manometry.[70] In this study, 36% of patients had nutcracker esophagus, 28% hypotensive LES, and 16% nonspecific esophageal motor disorder. The reason for the discrepancy between the results of this study and the other two is unclear. It appears, however, that the high rate of esophageal motility abnormalities recorded in NCCP patients in this study may reflect a local referral bias.

There are very few studies assessing NCCP patients with high-resolution esophageal manometry (HREM). One study demonstrated impaired peristalsis in 60% of NCCP patients, including ineffective esophageal motility, fragmented peristalsis, and absent contractility.[60]

The relationship between NCCP and esophageal dysmotility remains an area of intense controversy because documentation of esophageal dysmotility during manometry is rarely associated with reports of chest pain symptoms.[71] In addition, unlike GERD, we are still devoid of highly effective pharmacologic compounds that can eliminate esophageal dysmotility and thus can be used to demonstrate a causal relationship.[72] Furthermore, in NCCP patients who underwent simultaneous esophageal manometry and pH testing, chest pain was more commonly associated with acid reflux events than motility abnormalities.[69,73] Even the past usage of ambulatory 24-hour esophageal manometry was unable to improve the sensitivity of the test in NCCP. In fact, studies have demonstrated that 27% and 43% of patients did not report any chest pain symptoms during the test.[69,74] Moreover, the investigators were able to relate pain episodes to recorded esophageal dysmotility in only 13% to 24% of patients. Consequently, the routine usage of ambulatory 24-hour esophageal manometry has been questioned, and the technique is rarely performed in clinical practice. In one study, the authors were able to demonstrate improvement of NCCP symptoms in patients with nutcracker esophagus receiving antireflux treatment but with no effect on esophageal motility.[75]

Some authorities have proposed using esophageal motility abnormalities in NCCP patients as a marker for an underlying motor disorder that may be responsible for patients' symptoms.[76] However, it is plausible that our current evaluative techniques of the esophagus provide only crude information about esophageal motor function. Future tests will require providing a more comprehensive evaluation of anatomical structure and biomechanics of the esophagus and their relationship to pain.

SUSTAINED ESOPHAGEAL CONTRACTIONS

High-frequency intraluminal ultrasonography, a technique useful for the evaluation of smooth muscle contraction, has been employed to assess the esophageal motor corollary of chest pain in NCCP patients.[57] By using high-frequency intraluminal ultrasonography, Balaban et al.[57] have shown a close correlation between longitudinal muscle contractions and reports of chest pain. When evaluating the 10 participating subjects, the authors demonstrated esophageal longitudinal muscle contractions preceding 18 of 24 spontaneous chest pain events. These muscle contractions cannot be detected by conventional esophageal pressure recordings that solely evaluate the esophageal circular muscle. Balaban et al.[57] further showed that edrophonium-induced chest pain was also preceded by sustained esophageal muscle contractions.[57] The authors also demonstrated that swallow-associated contractions of the longitudinal muscles lasted an average of 6.4 seconds, whereas contractions associated with chest pain lasted a mean of 68.0 seconds. Pehlivanov et al.[58] demonstrated that the duration of the sustained esophageal muscle contractions might be correlated with the type of symptom perceived by patients. Shorter durations of these contractions were associated more with heartburn, whereas longer durations were linked more with chest pain.[58] Furthermore, sustained esophageal muscle contractions were observed in patients who reported heartburn that was unrelated to an acid reflux event giving further credence to the hypothesis that sustained esophageal contractions are responsible for the generation of esophageal-related symptoms such as chest pain. Unfortunately, high-frequency intraluminal ultrasonography is highly operator-dependent and consequently may not always be an objective evaluative tool. None of the initial studies have been replicated by other investigators. Although sustained esophageal muscle contractions appear to be predictable markers for chest pain, it is still unclear if they are the direct underlying mechanism or just an epiphenomenon.

ESOPHAGEAL HYPERSENSITIVITY

Studies have consistently documented alteration in pain perception regardless of whether dysmotility was present or absent in patients with NCCP.

Visceral hypersensitivity is a phenomenon in which conscious perception of visceral stimulus is enhanced independently of the intensity of the stimulus.[77] Peripheral and central mechanisms have been proposed to be responsible for visceral hypersensitivity in patients with NCCP. It has been hypothesized that peripheral sensitization of esophageal sensory afferents leads to subsequently heightened responses to physiologic or pathologic stimuli of the esophageal mucosa.[78] Additionally, central sensitization at the brain level or the dorsal horn of the spinal cord may modulate afferent neural function and thus enhance perception of intraluminal stimuli.[79] What causes peripheral or central sensitization remains to be determined. Studies have shown that acute tissue irritation results in subsequent peripheral and central sensitization, which is manifested as increased background activity of sensory neurons, lowering of nociceptive thresholds, changes in stimulus response curves, and enlargement of receptive fields.[80] Peripheral sensitization involves the reduction of esophageal pain threshold and increase in the transduction processes of primary afferent neurons.[81] Esophageal tissue injury, inflammation, spasm, or repetitive mechanical stimuli can all sensitize peripheral afferent nerves. There is immune dysfunction, for example, stimulated lymphocyte expression of interleukin (IL)-5 and IL-13.[82] There is also increased mucosal mast cells in patients with esophageal hypersensitivity and specifically those with FCP.[83] The presence of esophageal hypersensitivity can be subsequently demonstrated long after the original stimulus is no longer present and the esophageal mucosa has healed. However, it is still unclear what factors are pivotal for the persistence of esophageal hypersensitivity.

Studies have demonstrated that patients with non–GERD-related NCCP have lower perception thresholds for pain. Richter et al.[84] used balloon distension protocol in the distal esophagus and found that 50% of patients with NCCP developed pain at volumes of 8 mL or less in comparison with 9 mL or more in healthy subjects who developed pain (Fig. 62.5). The authors found no difference in the pressure–volume curve of the two groups as well as no difference in esophageal motility. When the balloon was inflated to 10 mL, patients with a history of NCCP were more likely to experience pain (18/30) than the control subjects (6/30). Barish et al.[81] evaluated 50 patients with NCCP and 30 healthy volunteers using graded balloon distension protocol. Of the patients with NCCP, 56% (28/50) experienced their "typical" chest pain during balloon distension as compared with 20% (6/30) of the normal controls. Of those with NCCP who experienced pain, 85% reported pain at values below the usual sensory threshold (20 cm H_2O). There was no difference in esophageal tone between the two groups.

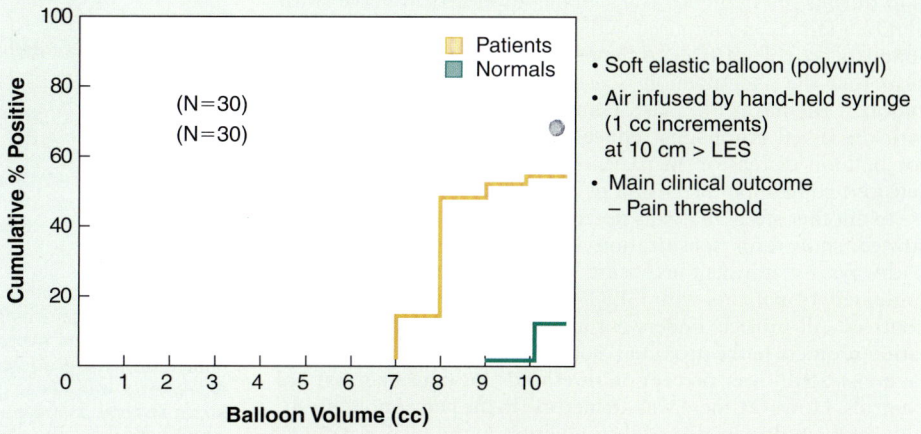

FIGURE 62.5 Pain thresholds in noncardiac chest pain patients versus normal controls using a balloon distension protocol. *(Redrawn after Richter JE, Barish CF, Castell DO. Abnormal sensory perception in patients with esophageal chest pain. Gastroenterology 1986;91[4]:845–852. Copyright © 1986 Elsevier. With permission.)*

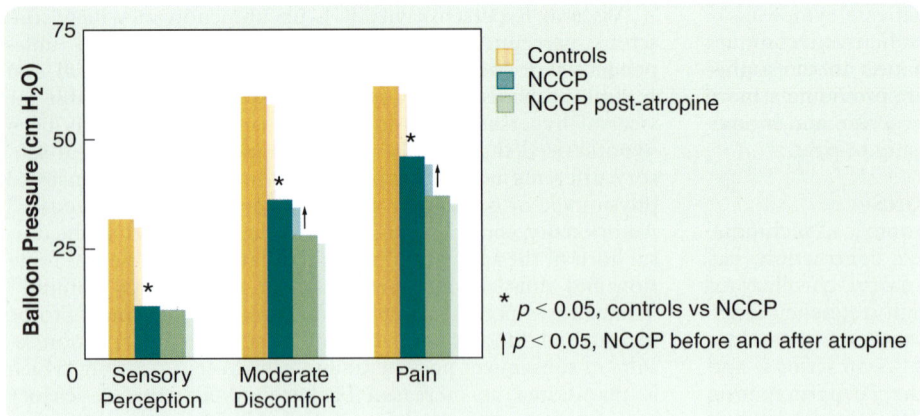

FIGURE 62.6 Mean pressure thresholds in controls and in patients with noncardiac chest pain (NCCP) before and after atropine was given. *(Reprinted by permission from Nature: Rao S, Hayek B, Summers RW. Functional chest pain of esophageal origin: hyperalgesia or motor dysfunction. Am J Gastroenterol 2001;96[9]:2584–2589. Copyright © 2001 Springer Nature.)*

Rao et al.[85] used impedance planimetry to evaluate 24 patients with NCCP and 12 healthy controls. Using balloon distention, they demonstrated that those with NCCP had lower perception thresholds for first sensation and moderate discomfort and pain in comparison to the healthy controls. Typical chest pain was reproduced in 83% of the NCCP patients. In addition, the reactivity of the esophagus to balloon distension was increased in those with NCCP, as was the pressure elastic modulus. Rao et al.[86] also performed graded balloon distensions of the esophagus using impedance planimetry in 16 consecutive patients with NCCP (normal esophageal evaluation) and 13 healthy control subjects. Patients who experienced chest pain during balloon distension were subsequently restudied after receiving intravenous atropine (Fig. 62.6). Balloon distensions reproduced chest pain at lower sensory thresholds in most NCCP patients as compared with controls. Similar findings were documented after atropine administration despite relaxed and more deformable esophageal wall. Thus, the investigators concluded that esophageal hypersensitivity, rather than motor dysfunction, is the predominant mechanism for FCP.

As noted earlier, it was demonstrated the development of secondary allodynia in the proximal esophagus by repeated acid exposure of the distal esophagus.[56] The patients with NCCP demonstrated both visceral hypersensitivity and amplified secondary allodynia in the esophagus. However, it is unclear from the study what mechanism is responsible for the exaggerated secondary allodynia and what initiates central sensitization in patients with NCCP. It is interesting to note that other studies in NCCP, using a similar human model of acute tissue irritation by acid infusion, showed no significant effect on pain thresholds.[87]

Börjesson et al.[87] also demonstrated that patients with NCCP have reduced sensitivity to esophageal balloon distension during simultaneous transcutaneous electrical nerve stimulation (TENS) as compared with healthy controls. This further supports the role of visceral hypersensitivity in NCCP and suggests that the phenomenon is probably due to central sensitization.[88] Mehta et al.[88] also demonstrated that acid infusion into the distal esophagus reduces esophageal pain thresholds for balloon distension in patients with NCCP not previously sensitive to balloon distension or acid infusion.

In another study that was noted earlier,[55] the authors demonstrated short-term sensitization of mechanosensitive afferent pathways by transient exposure to acid. Sarkar et al.[89] also evaluated 14 patients with GERD-related NCCP and 8 healthy controls. All subjects underwent an esophageal electrical stimulation protocol in the proximal esophagus, and those with NCCP demonstrated lower perception thresholds for pain than normal controls. However, there was an increase in the perception thresholds for pain during electrical stimulation in the NCCP patients after a 6-week course of high-dose PPI (omeprazole 20 mg twice daily) (Fig. 62.7).[89] This study demonstrated that patients with NCCP and evidence of GERD have a component of esophageal hypersensitivity that is responsive to high-dose PPI therapy.

In another small study that enrolled 22 NCCP patients with documented nutcracker esophagus, the authors demonstrated that stepwise balloon distensions reproduced pain symptoms at a lower threshold in 90% of NCCP patients as compared with 20% of healthy controls.[90] It was concluded that patients with NCCP and nutcracker esophagus also exhibit visceral hypersensitivity. Additionally, visceral hypersensitivity is the likely main underlying mechanism for patients' symptoms rather than the presence of the high amplitude contractions (nutcracker esophagus). Unfortunately, the presence of GERD in these patients was not determined in this study.

In a recent study, 75% of patients with FCP who underwent impedance planimetry demonstrated esophageal hypersensitivity.[91] These patients had larger cross-sectional areas, decreased esophageal wall strain, distensibility, and lower thresholds for perception, discomfort, and pain as compared with FCP patients without esophageal hypersensitivity or healthy controls. Another recent study showed that pain evoked by bag distention in FCP patients is dependent primarily on stress and to a lesser degree on strain.[92] The pain does not appear to be related to mucosal perfusion.

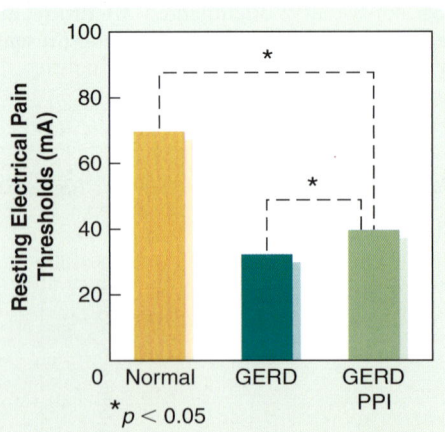

FIGURE 62.7 Patients with chest pain and occult gastroesophageal reflux disease (GERD) demonstrate visceral hypersensitivity that may be partially responsive to acid suppression with a proton pump inhibitor (PPI). *(Reprinted by permission from Nature: Sarkar S, Thompson DG, Woolf CJ, et al. Patients with chest pain and occult gastroesophageal reflux demonstrate visceral pain hypersensitivity which may be partially responsive to acid suppression. Am J Gastroenterol 2004;99[10]:1998–2006. Copyright © 2004 Springer Nature.)*

ALTERED AUTONOMIC ACTIVITY

Tougas et al.[93] have performed several studies exploring autonomic nervous system function and its role in the pathogenesis of NCCP. In one study, the investigators assessed autonomic activity, using spectral analysis of heart rate variability, before and during distal esophageal acidification of patients with NCCP and matched healthy controls.[93] Of those with NCCP, 68% developed angina-like symptoms during the esophageal acidification. These patients had a higher baseline heart rate and a lower baseline vagal activity than patients without acid sensitivity. During acid infusion, vagal cardiac outflow increased in acid-sensitive patients as compared with patients without acid sensitivity. Additionally, Tougas[94] have also documented increased vagal activity in patients with NCCP during other intra-esophageal stimuli, both mechanical and electrical. These studies indicate that autonomic dysregulation may be present in at least a subset of patients with NCCP. The authors further hypothesized that increased perception of esophageal stimulation may also reflect an exaggerated brainstem response. However, Tougas[94] has hypothesized that in most cases in which both central and autonomic factors are involved, central factors will likely lead to autonomic dysregulation.

PSYCHOLOGICAL COMORBIDITY

Psychological comorbidity has been shown to be common in NCCP and affects up to 75% of patients. It has yet to be determined if the high level of psychological comorbidity may be related to referral bias to tertiary referral centers or if it is the result of long-term experience of pain. Regardless, studies reported a high prevalence (>50%) of panic disorder, anxiety, and major depression in NCCP patients.[15,95–108] Other psychological abnormalities have also been reported including neuroticism, hypochondriac behavior, obsessive-compulsive disorder, phobic disorder, and somatization.[15,100–103,109–113] In a small study of 36 subjects with NCCP, the authors found that 58% had some type of psychological abnormality.[114] Of those, anxiety, depression, and panic disorder were the most common. In a large population-based study in Australia, the authors surveyed a random sample of 1,000 residents in the Sydney area.[15] Among those with NCCP, the prevalence of anxiety was 23% and depression 7%. In a telephone survey from Hong Kong that included 2,209 subjects, the authors demonstrated that depression and anxiety were significantly more common in NCCP patients than those without NCCP.[104]

Among all esophageal symptoms, chest pain was shown to closely correlate with psychometric abnormalities. In some patients, chest pain is part of a host of symptoms that characterize panic attack. Panic attack is a common cause for emergency room visits due to chest pain. In a large study that encompassed 441 consecutive ambulatory patients presenting with chest pain to the emergency department of a heart center, 25% were diagnosed as suffering from a panic attack.[110] Although the reason for the observed association between NCCP and panic disorder remains to be fully elucidated, hyperventilation was demonstrated to precipitate chest pain in 15% of patients with NCCP.[115] Additionally, it was demonstrated that hyperventilation could provoke reversible esophageal manometric abnormalities such as esophageal spasm (4%) and a nonspecific esophageal motor disorder (22%).[116] Furthermore, studies have demonstrated that hyperventilation may precipitate a panic attack.

Anxiety and depression influence reports of pain and thus contribute to the pathophysiology of NCCP. Lantinga et al.[117] found that patients with NCCP had higher levels of neuroticism and psychiatric comorbidity before and after cardiac catheterization than did patients with CAD. This finding appears to have prognostic significance because

these patients display less improvement in pain, more frequent pain episodes, greater social maladjustment, and more anxiety at 1-year follow-up than individuals with relatively low initial levels of psychosocial disturbances. In a large epidemiologic study from England, a significant relationship between NCCP and psychiatric disorders was demonstrated in young adults.[118] Two independent variables were associated with chest pain: parental illness and fatigue during childhood.

Studies have been inconsistent when the frequency of panic disorder, anxiety, and depression were compared between NCCP patients and those with CAD. Some studies reported increased panic disorder, anxiety, and depression in NCCP patients, whereas others found no significant difference in the prevalence of psychological disorders between the two groups.[9,111,119–122] In one study of 199 participants, panic disorder was more common in NCCP as compared with those with CAD (41% vs. 22%).[119] However, other psychiatric disorders were highly prevalent (72%) but without any difference between the two groups. In contrast, Cormier et al.[123] demonstrated that 98 NCCP patients scored higher on measures of anxiety and negative life events and had a significantly greater prevalence of *Diagnostic and Statistical Manual of Mental Disorders* (3rd ed.; DSM-III) panic disorder (47% vs. 6%), major depression (39% vs. 8%), and two or more simple phobias (43% vs. 12%) than did patients with CAD. In a recent multivariate analysis, the authors were able to develop a predictive model for distinguishing between NCCP and CAD that includes alexithymia (a condition in which patients are unable to express their feelings with words), quality of life, and coping based on religion and seeking medical help (85.4% sensitivity and 80.0% specificity).[124]

NCCP patients with psychological disorders show diminished quality of life, more frequent chest pain, and less treatment satisfaction than NCCP patients without psychological comorbidity.[108] One study suggested that NCCP patients with more than one psychological disorder are more difficult to treat than those with a single psychological disorder.[125]

Cheng et al.[126] demonstrated that patients with NCCP, when compared to patients with rheumatism and healthy controls, tended to monitor more, use more problem-focused coping, display a coping pattern with a poorer strategy–situation fit, and receive less emotional support in times of stress. Additionally, monitoring perceptual style and problem-focused coping were associated with higher levels of anxiety and depression. Jerlock et al.[127] evaluated 231 NCCP patients and compared their psychosocial profile with 1,069 healthy subjects without NCCP. The authors found that NCCP patients had more sleep problems, mental strain at work, stress at home, and negative life events as compared with the healthy group.

Gender differences related to psychological factors have also been observed in NCCP patients. Men reported less depression and trait anxiety than women.[128]

Diagnosis of Noncardiac Chest Pain

CARDIOLOGY EVALUATION

A cardiology evaluation is required in patients with angina-like pain. This recommendation is primarily driven by the recognition that the morbidity and mortality of CAD far exceeds that of esophageal-related causes of NCCP. Furthermore, a patient's history and characteristics do not reliably distinguish between cardiac and esophageal causes of chest pain.[1] NCCP patients may report squeezing or burning substernal chest pain, which may radiate to the back, neck, arms, and jaw and is indistinguishable from cardiac-related chest pain.[129–131]

The description of chest pain obtained during a careful history is categorized as typical angina (80% to 90% likelihood of obstructive CAD), atypical angina (40% to 80% likelihood), or as noncardiac (20% to 70% likelihood). Typical angina is characterized by the following three characteristics:

- Retrosternal chest discomfort experienced as pressure or heaviness
- Duration of 5 to 15 minutes
- Induced by stress or exertion, a large meal, or exposure to cold and relieved by rest or nitroglycerin

Atypical angina is diagnosed when two of these are present, and NCCP is likely if none or only one of these cardinal features exists.[132] Therefore, a patient who describes the spontaneous onset of "an elephant sitting on my chest" for 1 minute, with left arm involvement, diaphoresis, and nausea, actually has NCCP.[132] Although some of the patients may have a high probability of CAD for their chest pain and others low probability, the majority of the patients with chest pain fall into the intermediate range and thus require further testing to determine the presence of significant CAD. Diagnosis of NCCP is more likely in younger patients with chest pain, particularly females, and those without personal or strong family history of CAD.

A unique relationship between the esophagus and the heart has been proposed because the two organs share similar sensory innervation, and several studies have demonstrated that acidification of the distal esophagus may influence the flow of the coronary circulation.[62–64] Chauhan et al.[65] have shown a reduction in coronary artery blood flow in response to acid perfusion into the distal esophagus in patients with syndrome X. Syndrome X is defined as typical chest pain and electrocardiographic changes suggestive of myocardial ischemia on stress test but patent coronary arteries on angiogram.[65] The reduction in coronary blood flow was also associated with typical angina pain, suggesting the presence of an esophagocardiac inhibitory reflex. These findings were later confirmed by Rosztoczy et al.[66] who showed a decrease in coronary artery blood flow in 19 out of 42 (45%) patients undergoing acid perfusion of the esophagus.

In a subset of patients, ischemic heart disease and GERD or esophageal dysmotility may coincide.[133] It is the role of the cardiologist to determine if the chest pain is related to the underlying heart disease. Only after the cardiologist confirmed that symptoms are unrelated to the underlying ischemic heart disease, then further esophageal workup is warranted.

In conclusion, patients presenting for the first time with chest pain should initially undergo an evaluation by a cardiologist to exclude a cardiac cause.

GERD-RELATED NCCP

There is no gold standard for diagnosing GERD-related NCCP. The currently available diagnostic tests to detect GERD in patients with NCCP include barium swallow, upper endoscopy, the acid perfusion test, ambulatory 24-hour esophageal pH monitoring, and the PPI test.

BARIUM ESOPHAGRAM

Barium esophagram has very little use in the diagnosis of GERD. Barium esophagram has a low sensitivity (20%) for diagnosing GERD in general due to lack of anatomical and mucosal abnormalities in most of the GERD patients.[134] Furthermore, the significance of barium reflux during the procedure as a diagnostic for GERD is questionable. Johnston et al.[134] found that the proportion of patients with an abnormal 24-hour esophageal pH study was similar to the proportion of patients with a normal 24-hour esophageal pH study who had spontaneous barium reflux during the test. Additionally, spontaneous barium reflux has been demonstrated in up to 20% of healthy subjects.[135]

The role of barium esophagram is unclear in patients with GERD-related NCCP primarily due to the rare presence of esophageal mucosal abnormalities. However, one may consider performing a barium esophagram as the initial diagnostic test in patients who report dysphagia in addition to chest pain.

UPPER ENDOSCOPY

Upper endoscopy is frequently used as a diagnostic tool in the evaluation of unexplained upper digestive complaints and specifically in patients with NCCP. In 1990, the American Gastroenterological Association guidelines for chest pain of esophageal origin recommended the routine use of endoscopy in the evaluation of NCCP.[136] Since then, several studies have reported a variable rate of diagnostic yield in NCCP. In one of the earlier endoscopic studies, Hsia et al.[50] evaluated 100 consecutive patients with NCCP (mean age 50 years). In this single-center study, the authors found that 38% of the patients had a normal test, 24% erosive esophagitis (grades II to IV), 18% gastritis and/or duodenitis, 14% a sliding hiatal hernia without evidence of erosive esophagitis, and 6% gastric or duodenal ulcer.[50]

Several studies from different countries have also evaluated the value of upper endoscopy in NCCP. In a study of a northern Mexican population, only 10% of the NCCP patients demonstrated mucosal abnormalities during endoscopy. The vast majority of those were acid peptic–related.[137] A study from Denmark evaluated 49 patients with NCCP (28 women, mean age 51.6 years) who were referred to a tertiary cardiology center. The authors detected grade I erosive esophagitis in 15 patients (31%), grade II erosive esophagitis in 1 patient, and peptic ulcer in 3 patients (6%).[51] A study from China reported that in 70 consecutive patients with NCCP (mean age 58.5 ± 10), only 11% had endoscopic abnormalities (three with duodenal ulcer, three with gastric ulcer, and two with erosive esophagitis).[138] In a study from Italy, 61 consecutive patients with NCCP underwent endoscopy, and only 10% demonstrated mucosal findings (most erosive esophagitis).[133] In the largest study thus far addressing the role of upper endoscopy in NCCP, Dickman et al.[53] reported mucosal findings in 3,688 consecutive patients undergoing endoscopic evaluation for NCCP (mean age 55.1 years, range 18 to 99.6 years). Patients were seen in 76 community, university, and Veteran Health Administration Care Centers. The authors found that 44% of the NCCP patients had a normal upper endoscopy. Endoscopic findings in those with abnormal tests included hiatal hernia (28.6%), erosive esophagitis (19.4%), BE (4.4%), esophageal stricture or stenosis (3.6%), and peptic ulcer (2%) (Table 62.4).[53] The authors

TABLE 62.4   **The Value of Upper Endoscopy in Chest Pain Patients as Compared to Those with Reflux-Related Symptoms Using a Large Multicenter Consortium**

Findings	Chest Pain Group N = 3,688 (%)	Reflux Group N = 32,981 (%)	P Value
Barrett esophagus	163 (4.4%)	3,016 (9.1%)	<.0001
Esophageal inflammation	715 (19.4%)	9,153 (27.8%)	<.0001
Hiatal hernia	1,053 (28.6%)	14,775 (44.8%)	<.0001
Normal	1,627 (44.1%)	12,801 (38.8%)	<.0001
Stricture/stenosis	132 (3.6%)	1,223 (3.7%)	0.69

Reprinted by permission from Nature: Dickman R, Mattek N, Holub J, et al. Prevalence of upper gastrointestinal tract findings in patients with noncardiac chest pain versus those with gastroesophageal reflux disease (GERD)-related symptoms: results from a national endoscopic database. *Am J Gastroenterol* 2007;102(6):1173–1179. Copyright © 2007 Springer Nature.

concluded that the mucosal findings in NCCP patients were primarily GERD-related. An important finding of this study is that 4.4% of the patients with NCCP also had BE. This was significantly lower than the BE rate (9.1%) observed in GERD patients in the same study. Two other small studies have also reported the presence of BE in 5.2% and in 6.7% of NCCP patients undergoing endoscopy.[137,139]

Presently, there is no evidence that upper GI tract neoplasia presents solely with chest pain, possibly explaining the absence of these lesions in the aforementioned endoscopic studies. In one recent series of 307 patients who presented between 1991 and 1996 with esophageal adenocarcinoma or squamous cell carcinoma, 21 (7%) reported chest pain but usually in addition to dysphagia. Only two (<1%) had chest pain as the sole presenting symptom.[140]

It appears that upper endoscopy has a variable diagnostic yield (10% to 44%) in NCCP patients. Almost all of the mucosal findings are acid peptic–related and likely responsive to antireflux treatment. Consequently, upper endoscopy should be reserved for patients with NCCP and alarm symptoms such as dysphagia, odynophagia, weight loss, or anemia. Because BE can be identified in GERD-related NCCP patients, albeit in lower frequency than in heartburn patients, screening endoscopy in this particular subset population of NCCP patients is appropriate.

In conclusion, upper endoscopy reveals potential explanations for NCCP in a minority of patients and should be reserved for subjects with alarm features or in whom endoscopic evaluation is indicated.

AMBULATORY 24-HOUR ESOPHAGEAL pH MONITORING

The introduction of the PPI test and the growing utilization of PPI empirical therapy in NCCP have diminished the value of the traditional 24-hour pH test. This was further supported by a study demonstrating that the PPI test was at least as sensitive as ambulatory 24-hour esophageal pH monitoring.[141] As a result, the use of pH testing appears to have value in patients with NCCP in whom objective evidence is required (off therapy). For example, in patients with NCCP who are candidates for antireflux surgery, objective evidence of abnormal 24-hour esophageal pH monitoring off PPI treatment is needed. The pH test could also be helpful in patients with equivocal or negative PPI therapeutic trial. In patients with NCCP undergoing the PPI test, 24-hour esophageal pH monitoring has a therapeutic predictive value in addition to its diagnostic merit.[142] Patients with greater esophageal acid exposure appear to have a greater response to antireflux treatment. Consequently, in nonresponders to a therapeutic trial of PPI, pH monitoring on therapy may disclose patients who still have an abnormal pH test or positive symptom association with acid reflux events (symptom index or symptoms association probability). The value of the pH test in patients with NCCP nonresponsive to PPI treatment has yet to be elucidated. Although impedance + pH sensor has been proposed to be more sensitive in evaluating patients with typical or atypical manifestations of GERD who failed double-dose daily PPIs therapy, studies addressing specifically NCCP patients are still lacking.[143,144] This is compounded by the fact that the role of nonacid reflux in causing NCCP remains insufficiently studied. However, future studies are needed to compare the value of impedance + pH sensor versus pH testing alone in evaluating NCCP patients, either on or off PPI treatment.

In conclusion, ambulatory 24-hour esophageal pH monitoring should be reserved for NCCP patients in whom objective evidence of GERD is required (off therapy) or in whom response to a therapeutic PPI trial is equivocal or negative (on therapy).

THE WIRELESS pH SYSTEM

Ambulatory 24-hour esophageal pH testing of the esophagus was developed nearly 40 years ago. This technique allows detection of acid reflux for prolonged periods of time.[145] Until recently, all pH studies involved the use of catheter-based equipment. By using this catheter-based system, it has been shown that abnormal esophageal acid exposure occurred in 21% to 53% of patients with NCCP. A correlation between chest pain and acid reflux event was found in 12% to 50% of the cases. However, traditional pH testing using a pH probe has been shown to impact patient's lifestyle and consequently reflux-provoking activities.[27]

Recent developments led to the introduction and successful use of catheter-free pH system to diagnose GERD.[146] This pH system offers the additional advantage of recording esophageal pH monitoring for an extended period of time (i.e., 48 to 96 hours) while improving patient tolerance for the test. The wireless pH monitoring system (Bravo pH System, Given Imaging, Yoqneam, Israel) consists of a small radiotelemetry capsule that is attached to the esophageal mucosa (located at 6 cm above the squamocolumnar junction). Although it does not require a transnasal wire, it can be placed transnasally.[147]

Presently, there is only a single study that evaluated the value of extended pH testing (48 hours) in patients with NCCP.[148] In this study, Prakash and Clouse[148] evaluated 63 patients with NCCP suspected of having GERD. The authors found that extended pH testing provided a 10% gain in detecting abnormal acid exposure time and 7.3% in the number of subjects reporting symptoms. The number of chest pain episodes available for association with reflux events doubled regardless of whether subjects were on or off antireflux therapy. Extended testing also improved the ability to detect more episodes of chest pain in 21% of the subjects. Overall, extending pH testing to 48 hours provided meaningful information in 19.4% of the NCCP patients.[148]

Potential disadvantages of the wireless pH system include the need to perform endoscopy prior to placement of the capsule to ensure proper position inside the esophagus. Premature detachment of the capsule has been reported in up to 12% of early studies, but rates have improved with additional modifications by the manufacturer.[149] Chest discomfort has been described by a number of patients, some even requiring removal of the capsule.[147] This could be of concern, particularly in patients who are already complaining of chest pain. However, in a study of 452 patients undergoing wireless pH testing, fewer than 2% required removal of the capsule because of discomfort.[150] Of the eight patients requiring removal of the capsule, the majority (62.5%) had chest pain as the indication for the study. Thus, patients with NCCP may be more susceptible to develop chest discomfort after capsule placement than other patients who undergo wireless pH testing.

Overall, the aforementioned studies suggest that extended wireless pH testing provides a modest but meaningful advantage over traditional 24-hour pH probe in the evaluation of patients with NCCP suspected to be GERD-related. It increases the window of opportunity for detecting more symptoms associated with gastroesophageal reflux events.

In conclusion, extending pH monitoring (48 hours) using wireless pH capsule improves detection of reflux-associated chest pain symptoms.

THE PROTON PUMP INHIBITOR TEST

A therapeutic trial in the form of empirical therapy (vide infra) or the PPI test is recommended prior to any invasive or noninvasive testing to diagnose GERD-related NCCP. There are two therapeutic trial approaches in NCCP that are markedly different from each other. Empirical therapy with PPIs, usually lasting 2 to 3 months, is often used by physicians as the initial treatment of patients with atypical manifestations of GERD including NCCP.[79] In contrast, the PPI test or short therapeutic trial is defined as a short course of high-dose PPI for diagnosing GERD-related NCCP.[79] The latter test is considered a simple and noninvasive diagnostic tool. It is readily available and at the disposal of PCPs as well as specialists. Additionally, it increases the role of PCPs in evaluating and treating patients with atypical manifestations of GERD. Studies have also shown that it offers significant cost savings when compared with the other diagnostic tests for GERD.

The doses used in the PPI test have ranged from 40 to 80 mg daily for omeprazole, 30 to 90 mg daily for lansoprazole, and 40 mg daily for rabeprazole, over duration of treatment of 1 to 28 days, in patients with symptoms suggestive of GERD or NCCP.[41,42,45,46,151-158] In patients with laryngeal manifestations of GERD, the doses ranged from 40 to 80 mg omeprazole daily and the duration of treatment from 1 to 4 weeks.[159-162] By far, the most commonly used PPI in most of the PPI test trials was omeprazole, which has led to the term the *omeprazole test*.[40,45,151-157] However, studies using other PPIs demonstrated that they are equally efficacious as short therapeutic trials.[41,42,46]

An important factor in determining the sensitivity of a PPI test is the definition of a positive test. In most studies, a symptom score cutoff was used: If the symptom assessment scores for heartburn, chest pain, or other symptoms improved by more than 50% to 75% (depending on the study) relative to baseline, the test was considered positive. As with any diagnostic test, the optimal cutoff is critical in defining test accuracy.[158] The symptom score cutoff values that were used among studies that evaluated PPI tests for GERD were chosen arbitrarily. Rarely, studies calculated the receiver operator curve by varying the percentage reduction in the symptom tested to ascertain the optimal value for detecting patients with GERD.[153,158] This cutoff point provides the greatest sensitivity, specificity, positive predictive value, and accuracy of the short therapeutic trial tested.

The diagnostic accuracy of the PPI test is limited by the lack of gold standard for the diagnosis of GERD. In the absence of a gold standard, studies evaluating the PPI test have used a combination of upper endoscopy and ambulatory 24-hour esophageal pH monitoring as the closest one can get to a gold standard. Factors that may determine the sensitivity of the PPI test include type of antireflux medication used, dosage, treatment duration, definition of a positive test (symptom score cutoff, change in symptom grading, receiver operating characteristics curve analysis), and the GERD-related symptom evaluated.

Only one study attempted to compare the accuracy of the PPI test (omeprazole) to 24-hour esophageal pH monitoring in diagnosing GERD.[141] The study used the presence of erosive esophagitis as indicative of GERD in patients who are not on aspirin or nonsteroidal anti-inflammatory drugs. Thirty-five patients were included, and they underwent both pH testing and the PPI test (omeprazole 40 mg before breakfast and 20 mg before dinner). The PPI test was significantly more sensitive than total acid contact time during pH testing (83% vs. 60%, $P < .03$). The sensitivity of the pH test increased to 80%, only after adding patients with positive symptom index and patients with abnormal acid contact time, in the supine and/or erect positions despite normal total acid contact time. The authors concluded that the PPI test was at least as sensitive as ambulatory 24-hour esophageal pH monitoring in diagnosing GERD in patients with documented erosive esophagitis. In different studies, the sensitivity of the PPI test for GERD-related NCCP ranged from 69% to 95% and the specificity from 67% to 86%.[40,45,46,156,157,163-165]

In a double-blind, placebo-controlled trial, 37 patients with NCCP were randomized to either placebo or high-dose omeprazole (40 mg before breakfast and 20 mg before dinner) for 7 days.[40] After a washout period and repeated baseline symptom assessment, patients crossed over to the opposite arm. The PPI test was considered positive if the chest pain improved by at least 50% after treatment. The combination of upper endoscopy and 24-hour esophageal pH monitoring was used as the gold standard. Sixty-two percent (23/37) of the patients had evidence of GERD: Seven had abnormal esophageal acid exposure by pH testing only, eight had erosive esophagitis only, and eight had both. Of the GERD-positive group, 78.3% had a positive PPI test, and 22.7% had a positive placebo response. In contrast, of the GERD-negative group, 14.2% had a positive PPI test, and 7.1% had a positive placebo response. Thus, the calculated sensitivity was 78.3%, specificity 85.7%, and the positive predictive value was 90%.[40] When different reductions in chest pain were evaluated as previously mentioned, the greater accuracy of predicting GERD-related NCCP was obtained with 65% symptom reduction, producing a sensitivity of 85.7% and specificity of 90.9%.[40] Using similar design, other investigators confirmed the usefulness of the PPI test for diagnosing GERD-related NCCP.[45,46] Furthermore, subsequent studies demonstrated that short therapeutic trials with PPIs other than omeprazole achieved similar efficacy for the diagnosis of GERD-related NCCP.[164,165] A study in the Chinese population showed that the PPI test, using lansoprazole 30 mg daily for a period of 4 weeks, was useful in diagnosing endoscopy-negative GERD-related NCCP.[46]

As with the PPI test in patients with classic GERD symptoms, the value of the PPI test in NCCP has been assessed by several meta-analyses.[166-168] One meta-analysis of randomized, controlled trials (parallel group and crossover design), the authors evaluated the pooled risk ratio for continued chest pain after PPI therapy, overall number needed to treat, pooled sensitivity, specificity, and diagnostic OR for the PPI test versus reference standards.[166] Eight studies were included in the PPI efficacy analysis. The pooled risk ratio for continued chest pain after PPI therapy was 0.54 (95% CI, 0.41 to 0.71). The overall number needed to treat was 3 (95% CI, 2 to 4). The pooled sensitivity, specificity, and diagnostic OR for the PPI test versus 24-hour pH monitoring and upper endoscopy were 80, 73, and 13.83 (95% CI, 5.48 to 34.91), respectively. All studies were small, and there was evidence for publication bias or other small study effects. The authors concluded that PPI therapy reduces symptoms in NCCP and may be useful as a diagnostic test in identifying abnormal esophageal acid reflux.

Wang et al.[167] have also performed a meta-analysis of the PPI test in patients with NCCP. Unlike the previous meta-analysis, the authors found only six studies that met inclusion criteria. The overall sensitivity and specificity of a PPI test were 80% (95% CI, 71% to 87%) and 74% (95% CI, 64% to 83%), respectively, compared with 19% (95% CI, 12% to 29%) and 77% (95% CI, 62% to 87%), respectively, in the placebo group. The PPI test showed significant higher discriminative power, with a summary diagnostic OR of 19.35 (95% CI, 8.54 to 43.84) compared with 0.61 (95% CI, 0.20 to 1.86) in the placebo group. Thus, the authors concluded that the use of PPI treatment as a diagnostic test for detecting GERD in patients with NCCP has an acceptable sensitivity and specificity that could be used as an initial approach by PCPs to detect GERD in selected patients with NCCP.

When using the PPI test, there is a significant correlation between the extent of esophageal acid exposure in the distal esophagus as determined by ambulatory 24-hour esophageal pH monitoring and the change in symptom intensity score after treatment. This suggests that the higher the esophageal acid exposure, the greater the response to the PPI test in patients with GERD-related NCCP.[142] Economic analysis has also shown that the PPI test for GERD-related NCCP is a cost-saving approach primarily because of the significant reduction in the usage of various costly, invasive diagnostic tests.[40]

In patients with NCCP, the PPI test was evaluated using a cost minimization analysis.[40] The PPI test was found to save $573 per average patient with NCCP undergoing diagnostic evaluation. The test was associated with an 81% reduction in the number of upper endoscopies and 79% reduction in the number of ambulatory 24-hour esophageal pH tests. This significant reduction is because of the high positive predictive value of the PPI test for patients with GERD-related NCCP.

When a decision-analytic model utilizing Bayesian analysis was developed to compare the costs and outcomes of alternative diagnostic strategies for NCCP, noninvasive strategies utilizing the PPI test as the initial step resulted in significant cost savings compared with invasive strategies. These cost savings were a direct result of a significant reduction in the utilization of invasive diagnostic tests that are of unproven utility in the diagnosis and subsequent management of patients with NCCP.[169]

In conclusion, a therapeutic trial with a PPI should precede any other testing for GERD unless objective evidence of GERD is required. The PPI test is a cost-effective diagnostic strategy for GERD-related NCCP.

MULTICHANNEL INTRALUMINAL IMPEDANCE

The combination of an impedance catheter and a pH probe provides a unique opportunity to study physiologic and pathologic events within the esophagus and their relationship to symptoms. In addition, the recording assembly can disclose the characteristics of the gastric refluxate (acidic, weakly acidic, alkaline, gas, liquid, and mixed gas and liquid). The specific value of the multichannel intraluminal impedance plus pH sensor and the documentation of weakly acidic reflux in patients with NCCP remains to be elucidated. The combined multichannel intraluminal impedance and manometry testing has also been useful in determining bolus transport patterns, bolus transit parameters, and bolus clearance in patients with esophageal motor disorders and a variety of symptoms including chest pain.[170]

A recent study evaluated 120 NCCP patients with 24-hour multichannel intraluminal impedance. The authors demonstrated that 40% of the NCCP patients were having reflux as the underlying cause of their chest pain.[171] Reflux episodes that were associated with chest pain had a higher proximal extent, a higher volume clearance time, a higher 15-minute acid burden, more often acidic, a lower nadir pH, and a longer acid duration time than reflux episodes which were not followed by chest pain.

ESOPHAGEAL DYSMOTILITY

In approximately a third of the patients with non–GERD-related NCCP, various esophageal motility abnormalities have been described.[67,68,172] Thus, in NCCP, esophageal manometry is commonly performed if GERD has been excluded as the underlying cause.[16] The role of esophageal manometry in NCCP has evolved over the last few years primarily due to lack of effective treatment for the various esophageal motility abnormalities. This was compounded by clinical evidence that patients with non–GERD-related NCCP reported symptom improvement on pain modulators regardless if esophageal dysmotility was present or absent (except for achalasia).[173] Consequently, the role of esophageal manometry in non–GERD-related NCCP appears to be limited to identifying the small number of patients with achalasia.[174]

ESOPHAGEAL MANOMETRY

Esophageal manometry remains the best tool to detect esophageal motility disorders. However, studies have demonstrated that 70% of NCCP patients have normal esophageal motility during manometry testing.[67,68] The esophageal motor disorders commonly diagnosed in NCCP patients include nutcracker esophagus, hypotensive LES, DES (recently renamed distal esophageal spasm), hypertensive LES, nonspecific esophageal motility disorders, ineffective motility, and achalasia. Although esophageal motility disorders are noted in up to 30% of patients with NCCP, the relationship between these motor abnormalities and chest pain remains unclear. Patients rarely have chest pain at the time these motility abnormalities are recorded. Therapeutic trials aimed at improving abnormal motility in NCCP patients have not consistently resulted in symptomatic improvement.[75,175,176] This has led investigators to speculate that the motility abnormalities represent either a marker of sensory motor deficiency in NCCP patients or just an epiphenomenon rather than the direct cause of pain. Hitherto, the precise cause of esophageal pain in NCCP remains unknown.

It is possible that the abnormal motor response observed in NCCP patients originates from "activated" esophageal sensory afferents that trigger a secondary motor contraction in response to some type of intraluminal stimulus. Another theory speculates that chest pain may arise from intramural ischemia that is induced by increased esophageal motor activity.[177] However, studies that evaluated the blood supply of the esophagus suggested that the presence of vast arterial perfusion for this organ argues against the validity of this theory.[178] Recent studies have suggested that esophageal pain may originate from other muscle layers of the esophagus that escape detection during conventional esophageal manometry. Investigators have proposed that sustained longitudinal muscle contractions may be the cause of esophageal induced chest pain.[57] In contrast, Rao et al.[85] have suggested that the chest pain in NCCP patients is caused by hyperactive and stiffer esophageal wall as compared with controls. Thus, all of the aforementioned observations suggest that the source of chest pain in NCCP patients is the result of pathophysiologic mechanisms other than abnormal esophageal motility per se.

Achalasia is uncommon in NCCP, occurring in only 2% of patients presenting for manometric evaluation.[67,68] Achalasia typically presents with dysphagia and weight loss. Nevertheless, a number of series have shown that chest pain occurs in 48% to 64% of patients with achalasia.[179,180] It is unclear why some patients have dysphagia alone, whereas others also experience chest pain. In a recent study that included 211 patients with achalasia, chest pain occurred in 117 (55%), dysphagia in 173 (81%), regurgitation in 147 (69%), and heartburn in 121 patients (57%).[181] Thus, in patients with recurrent NCCP, diagnosis of achalasia is important because treatment of this entity differs substantially from the treatment of patients with other esophageal motility disorders. Frequently, patients with achalasia will require either esophageal balloon dilation or Heller myotomy.

The value of high-resolution esophageal manometry in NCCP awaits more research in the future.[182] Several studies evaluated the distribution of esophageal motor disorders in NCCP patients using HREM. Akinsiku et al.[183] compared the value of HREM with conventional manometry in 300 NCCP patients. The HREM also established that normal esophageal motility was the most common finding (46.67%). In addition, ineffective esophageal motility was the most commonly documented esophageal motor disorder (25.33%), followed by achalasia (7.33%), hypotensive LES (4.67%), absent contractibility (4%), and jackhammer/nutcracker esophagus (3.33%). Another study, using 24-hour ambulatory pressure-pH-impedance monitoring and HREM, revealed esophageal dysmotility (distal esophageal spasm) only in 4 out of 59 NCCP patients (6.8%).[184]

Overall, esophageal manometry can identify an esophageal motility disorder in approximately one-third of NCCP patients.

However, the relationship between these motility disorders and chest pain is unclear and remains to be elucidated. Although only a small number of patients with non–GERD-related NCCP have achalasia, identifying this disorder is necessary because therapeutic modalities such as Heller myotomy or esophageal balloon dilation have been shown to be efficacious.

In conclusion, esophageal manometry is indicated in patients with non–GERD-related NCCP primarily to exclude achalasia.

PROVOCATIVE TESTING

In order to enhance the value of esophageal manometry in providing a definitive diagnosis, pharmacologic provocative agents have been used to elicit chest pain while monitoring changes in esophageal amplitude contractions.

EDROPHONIUM (TENSILON) TEST

The edrophonium (Tensilon) test has been used pharmacologically to induce esophageal dysmotility and chest pain in patients with NCCP. Edrophonium is an anticholinesterase that increases cholinergic activity at muscarinic receptors.[185] The pharmacologic action of this short-acting drug is manifested within 30 to 60 seconds after injection and lasts an average of 10 minutes. The aim of the edrophonium test is to induce greater esophageal body amplitude contractions in the hope of provoking the patient's typical chest pain.[186] The test is performed by injection of either 80 mg/kg or 10 mg edrophonium intravenously, immediately followed by 5 to 10 swallows of 5 to 10 mL of water over a period of 5 to 10 minutes. The pain occurs during swallowing within 5 minutes after the administration of the drug and disappears as the drug is quickly metabolized.[187] Overall, the side effects are minimal, and the antidote atropine is rarely required. Side effects include increased salivation, nausea, vomiting, and abdominal cramps.

The sensitivity of the edrophonium test is relatively low. Studies have shown that the edrophonium test is positive in approximately 30% of patients with normal baseline esophageal manometry.[188,189] Consequently, the usage of the edrophonium test has declined in the last decade.

ERGONOVINE STIMULATION TEST

The ergonovine stimulation test has been demonstrated to induce augmentation of esophageal contractions and chest pain in patients with NCCP. Ergonovine is a sympathomimetic agent of the ergot alkaloid group. The drug is reportedly as effective as edrophonium in the provocation of chest pain in NCCP patients, but the side effects are more common and could potentially be fatal (coronary artery spasm). Thus, ergonovine is rarely used today in clinical practice in the evaluation of NCCP.[187]

PENTAGASTRIN STIMULATION TEST

Pentagastrin directly stimulates esophageal smooth muscle, especially in patients with primary esophageal dysmotility. Its sensitivity to inducing pain in patients with NCCP is low, and presently, the drug is no longer used for NCCP provocative testing.[187]

Sensory Testing of the Esophagus

The esophagus, like the rest of the viscera, receives dual sensory innervation, traditionally referred to as parasympathetic and sympathetic because the sensory nerves are anatomically associated with the autonomic nervous system but more properly based on the actual nerves, vagal, and spinal (Fig. 62.8).[190] The vagal afferent neurons compose 80% of the vagal trunk and have cell bodies in the nodose ganglia.[191] Vagal afferents whose receptive fields are located in the esophageal smooth muscle layer are sensitive to mechanical distension, whereas polymodal (responding to multiple modalities of stimuli) vagal afferents with receptive fields in the mucosa are sensitive to various chemical or mechanical intraluminal stimuli, which, under normal circumstances, are not associated with conscious perception.[192] In general, vagal afferents do not play a direct role in visceral pain transmission at the level of the gut, except for certain types of vagal afferents that appear to have a pain modulatory effect.[193] Recent reports suggest that vagal afferents may also play a role in perception of esophageal distension.[193,194] In contrast, spinal afferents, which have their cell bodies in the dorsal root ganglia, are primarily acting as nociceptors and are central to the perception of discomfort and pain.[195] Spinal afferents with receptive fields in the muscle layer and serosa are primarily mechanosensitive. The intraepithelial nerve endings of spinal afferent are likely to be involved in mediating acid-induced pain during topical exposure to intraluminal acid.[196,197] Many of the afferents contain calcitonin gene-related peptide and substance P, which are neurotransmitters that are important in mediating visceral nociception.[191]

Data regarding cortical loci involved in processing of esophageal sensation in humans are relatively scarce.[198] Nonpainful esophageal balloon distensions elicit bilateral activation along the central sulcus, the insular cortex, and the frontal and parietal operculum.[199] In contrast, painful esophageal balloon distensions result in intense activation of the same areas

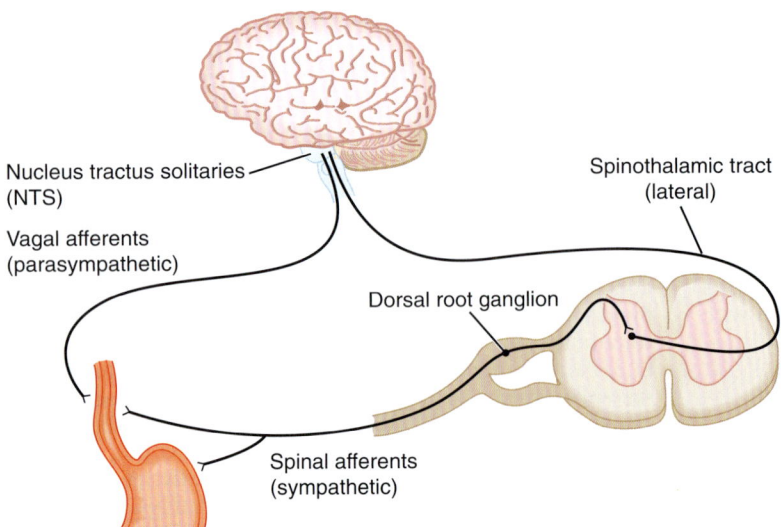

FIGURE 62.8 Esophageal sensory afferent pathways. *(Redrawn after Fass R. Sensory testing of the esophagus. J Clin Gastroenterol 2004;38[8]:628–641, with permission.)*

Nucleus tractus solitaries (NTS)

Vagal afferents (parasympathetic)

Spinothalamic tract (lateral)

Dorsal root ganglion

Spinal afferents (sympathetic)

and additional activation of the right anterior insular cortex (important in affective processing) and anterior cingulate gyrus (important in pain processing and generating an affective and cognitive response to pain).[200–202] Nonpainful infusion of 0.1 N hydrochloric acid resulted in cerebral cortical activity that was concentrated in the posterior cingulate and the parietal and anteromesial frontal lobes.[203] The superior frontal lobe regions activated corresponded to Brodmann area 32, the insula, the operculum, and the anterior cingulate.

Chest pain symptoms may represent an activation of a common pathway in response to different intraesophageal stimuli. Different intraesophageal stimuli (e.g., acid and balloon distension) may elicit similar symptoms in different patients or different symptoms in the same patient.[196,204] Thus, esophageal symptoms such as heartburn or chest pain are not stimulus-specific.

A recent study demonstrated that chest pain and heartburn may be provoked in normal subjects during esophageal balloon distension either in the proximal or distal portion of the esophagus.[196] Volume thresholds for heartburn and chest pain in both esophageal locations were similar, suggesting that, for a specific volume, some patients develop chest pain, and others, heartburn. Furthermore, volume thresholds for both chest pain and heartburn did not differ significantly at each esophageal location and between locations. In this study, esophageal balloon distension reproduced typical heartburn symptoms in some patients with documented GERD and chest pain in others. This study clearly demonstrates that balloon distension may result in different types of esophageal symptoms.

The mechanism by which an esophageal stimulus causes heartburn in some patients and chest pain in others remains poorly understood. Balaban and colleagues[57] have demonstrated a temporal correlation between sustained contractions of the esophageal longitudinal muscle and both spontaneous and provoked esophageal chest pain. In a subsequent study that assessed the temporal relationship between sustained esophageal longitudinal muscle contractions and heartburn, the investigators suggested that shorter duration of the sustained esophageal contraction was associated with heartburn and longer duration with chest pain.[58]

Perception of intraesophageal events, either physiologic or pathologic, is a complicated process that involves central and peripheral mechanisms. Several studies have shown that most intraesophageal stimuli are not perceived by subjects. For example, less than 20% of all acid reflux events result in GERD symptoms regardless of whether mucosal injury is present.[205] It is yet to be elucidated what factors determine perception of an intraesophageal event, leading to symptom generation. In GERD, it has been demonstrated that the actual hydrogen ion concentration (H+) of the refluxate, the summation of several short reflux events, the distribution of acid along the esophagus (proximal migration), or the nadir or duration of acid reflux events.[198] Several studies have demonstrated that fat and other nutrients can modulate perception of intraluminal events that are mediated by gut neurotransmitters, hormones, or enzymes. Meyer and colleagues[206] have shown that intraduodenal fat significantly shortened latency to onset of heartburn and intensified the perception of acid-induced heartburn in subjects with GERD who underwent intraesophageal acid perfusion.

Central neural mechanisms seem to have an important role in modulating esophageal perception also.[207] Psychological comorbidity (e.g., anxiety and depression) can modulate esophageal perception and cause subjects to perceive low-intensity esophageal stimuli (pathologic or physiologic) as being painful.[208] Another important factor is stress that seems to enhance perception of intraesophageal stimuli by reducing perception thresholds for pain.[200] Stress has recently emerged as an important factor in symptom generation and exacerbation of both functional and organic GI disorders.[201] Traditionally, stress is considered a domain of psychology and, thus, commonly lumped together with the role of psychiatric comorbidity.[209] However, recent developments in the understanding of brain–gut interactions in functional bowel disorders resulted in reassessment of the role of chronic stress in the pathophysiology and management of GI disorders such as NCCP. Certain stressful life events have been associated with the onset or symptom exacerbation of functional bowel disorders. In addition, daily experiences of stress seem to have an important modulating effect on perception of intraluminal events.

Other central factors, such as sleep quality, may also alter perception of intraesophageal events. Further research is needed to better define the brain–gut (or gut–brain) relationship as it relates to symptom generation in esophageal disorders.

ACID PERFUSION TEST (BERNSTEIN TEST)

The acid perfusion test was introduced as an objective method to identify esophageal chemosensitivity to acid.[202] A nasogastric tube was passed through the nares of a fasting, sitting subject and into the stomach.[202,210] After the gastric content was aspirated, the tube was withdrawn until it measured 30 cm from the nares to the tip.[210] This maneuver assumed that the solution would be delivered at a level near the junction of the upper and middle thirds of the esophagus. The tube was connected to an intravenous bottle. A control administration of 0.9% NaCl was perfused for 10 to 15 minutes at a rate of 6 to 7.5 mL per minute. This was followed by administration of 0.1 N hydrochloric acid, at a similar rate, for 30 minutes or until discomfort was induced.[210] If symptoms appeared, the test was discontinued and saline solution was given.

The acid perfusion test was originally devised to distinguish between chest pain of cardiac and esophageal origin. However, since the initial description, many modifications have been made to the original Bernstein test. Although the basic principle of the test remained similar, many investigators have tried different acid perfusion rates, concentrations, and durations in the hope of increasing the sensitivity of the test.[211–218] Furthermore, some have even suggested the addition of bile salts to the acid solution.[219]

Many attempts were made to change the test from a qualitative to a quantitative tool. Time to onset of symptoms during acid perfusion was used to compare the extent of chemosensitivity to acid between GERD and Barrett patients.[220] Fass and colleagues[196] placed a manometry catheter 10 cm above the upper border of the LES to ensure sufficient exposure of the esophageal mucosa to acid. Saline was infused initially for 2 minutes, and then without the patient's knowledge, 0.1 N hydrochloric acid was infused for 10 minutes at a rate of 10 mL per minute. Patients were instructed to report whenever their typical symptoms were reproduced. Esophageal chemosensitivity was assessed by both the latency until typical symptom perception was induced (expressed in seconds) and the total sensory intensity rating reported by the subject at the end of acid perfusion by using a verbal descriptor scale. The scale consisted of a 20-cm vertical bar flanked by descriptors of increasing intensity (no sensation, faint, very weak, weak, very mild, mild, moderate, barely strong, slightly intense, strong, intense, very intense, and extremely intense). Placement of words along the side of the scale was determined from their relative log intensity rating in a normative study.[221] The validity of these scales for assessing the perceived intensity of visceral sensations has been confirmed.[222]

An acid perfusion test intensity score (cm × seconds) was then calculated as follows: $I \times T/100$, where I is the total intensity rating at the end of acid perfusion and T is the duration of report of typical symptom perception during the test. For convenience, the score was divided by 100. The test is highly specific, but the sensitivity ranges from 6% to 60%.[73,129,222–230] A negative test has no clinical relevance and does not exclude esophageal origin.

Presently, the acid perfusion test is rarely performed in clinical practice because of its limited diagnostic value in NCCP and other esophageal disorders. Because of the low sensitivity and the emergence of noninvasive and highly sensitive modalities, such as the PPI test and empirical therapy with a PPI, many authors have considered the acid perfusion test to be obsolete.[135,211,228]

ELECTRICAL STIMULATION

Electrical stimulation of the esophagus has been used by several research groups to study visceral perception and cortical responses to different intensities of intraesophageal stimuli. The technique has yet to be standardized, and published protocols are difficult to compare.

Electrical stimulation of the esophageal mucosa is performed by using a 5-mm stainless steel electrode attached to a standard manometric catheter assembly.[229] The electrode is made from fine stainless-steel wire wrapped around the end of the catheter and fixed with surgical silk.[230] The electrodes are connected to an electrical stimulator. The catheter assembly is then passed through the nostril, and the electrode is placed in the esophagus. Electrical stimuli are applied repeatedly in a series of 24 stimuli (duration 200 μs at 0.2 Hz). A reference electrode is placed on the abdominal wall, 5 cm below the xiphoid process. Electrical stimulation of the upper and lower esophagus can be achieved by two pairs of silver/silver chloride bipolar ring electrodes located at 5 and 20 cm proximal to the tip of the catheter.[56]

The ascending stimulus paradigm includes stimuli that are delivered at a frequency of 0.2 Hz at intensities between 0 and 100 mA.[56] Severity and qualitative perceptual responses are usually assessed by a verbal descriptor.[231] Descriptors are used in ascending order of severity. Sensory threshold is the intensity (measured in milliampere [mA]) at which the participant reports faint sensation, and pain threshold is the intensity at which the participant reports an intense sensation.[56] A somewhat different stimulus paradigm is used in patients who undergo recording of cerebral evoked responses to esophageal electrical stimulation.[78]

INTRALUMINAL ULTRASONOGRAPHY

High-frequency intraluminal ultrasonography has been introduced as a novel modality to study the relationship between esophageal motor events and symptoms. The technique has been a useful tool for evaluating smooth muscle contractions.[232] Esophageal ultrasonography can be performed continuously using a catheter-based probe, which allows direct visualization of changes in smooth muscle conformation.[57] The capability of intraluminal ultrasonography to evaluate changes in the thickness of the longitudinal muscle of the esophagus has been used to determine the relationship between esophageal symptoms and motor changes of the esophageal wall. Although the technique has yet to be standardized, investigators have used an esophageal catheter assembly that included a 12.5-MHz ultrasound transducer, solid-state pressure catheter, and monopolar antimony pH catheter.[57] The ultrasound transducer was placed 5 cm above the LES. The 24-hour recordings were analyzed every 2 seconds for a period of 2 minutes before and 30 seconds after the onset of the studied symptom. Rules for image analysis remain at the discretion of the investigator. Because of the limited number of centers that are proficient with this technique, image analysis is primarily operator-dependent, and interobserver and intraobserver agreements have yet to be determined.

Using intraluminal ultrasonography, Balaban and colleagues[57] demonstrated that most chest pain episodes in patients with NCCP were preceded by sustained thickening of the esophageal smooth muscle wall due to longitudinal muscle contraction that was not detected by esophageal manometry catheter. The same muscular changes were noted after edrophonium-induced chest pain. The authors suggested that the duration rather than the magnitude of the longitudinal muscle contraction is the determining factor for generating esophageal pain. In this study, swallow-associated longitudinal muscle contractions lasted an average of 6.4 seconds, whereas contractions associated with chest pain persisted for a mean

of 68.0 seconds. Similar studies in patients with GERD revealed that the mean duration of sustained longitudinal muscle contractions during heartburn was 44.9 seconds.[58] The motor changes were also observed in patients who reported heartburn that was unrelated to acid reflux events, further supporting the investigator's hypothesis that this sustained esophageal muscle contraction is responsible for generation of esophageal symptoms, such as chest pain and heartburn.

Even though high-frequency intraluminal ultrasonography has been a valuable research tool to assess the biomechanics of the human esophagus, its exact role in evaluating esophageal-related symptoms has not been fully elucidated.[233] Initial studies provided intriguing data, but other investigators have yet to replicate these findings. Additionally, sustained contractions of the esophageal longitudinal muscle may represent an epiphenomenon that occurs with symptoms rather than being the trigger for symptoms.

BALLOON DISTENSION

Balloon distension has been used primarily for research purposes to determine perception thresholds for pain. This modality has been used extensively in studies of various functional bowel disorders, most notably IBS, functional dyspepsia, and NCCP.[84,234,235]

More than 40 years ago, intraesophageal balloon distension in humans was reported to produce pain referred to the chest.[236] Early data indicated that, in patients with documented ischemic heart disease, balloon distension of the esophagus produced pain indistinguishable from anginal pain but without ECG changes.[237] This may be explained by convergence of sensory pathways at the level of spinal cord or in the midbrain. Despite this similarity in pain, it seems that esophageal balloon distension itself has no effect on coronary function or blood flow.[238]

Balloon distension was reintroduced during the mid-1980s in a seminal study that evaluated perception thresholds for pain in patients with NCCP.[84] The latex balloon was attached to a manometric catheter and filled with air. The balloon was positioned 10 cm above the LES and distended in a stepwise fashion using a handheld syringe.

A further development in the balloon distension technique was the introduction of a pump that was powered by compressed air.[81] The pump ensured inflations at a predetermined rate, which was difficult to achieve with a handheld syringe. However, neither system was able to provide concomitant pressure measurements that could have been helpful to determine whether the balloon remained within the esophageal lumen during each inflation. This was particularly critical in protocols that inflated balloons within the distal portion of the esophagus. Fass and colleagues[196] demonstrated that balloon distension in the esophagus resulted in phasic esophageal contractions that increased with increase in balloon volume. These powerful contractions, in association with shortening of the esophagus, may propel the balloon into the stomach without being recognized by the subject or the investigator. Concomitant pressure measurements would have been helpful to detect the migration of the balloon into the gastric fundus by demonstrating a sudden decrease in intraluminal pressure despite continued increase in the balloon's volume.

The introduction of the electronic barostat, a computer-driven volume-displacement device, has helped to ensure proper location of the balloon regardless of inflation paradigm that was used.[239] The basic principle of the barostat is to maintain a constant pressure within the balloon/bag in the lumen despite muscular contractions and relaxations.[172,239] To maintain a constant pressure, the barostat aspirates air with contractions and injects air with relaxations. Presently, many prefer the use of a polyethylene bag to that of a latex balloon. Bags are infinitely compliant and show no increase in intra-bag pressure until about 90% of the maximum bag volume has been achieved.[239,240] In contrast, latex balloons resist inflation and thus show a rapid increase in intra-balloon pressure with small volumes of distension.[196,239,241] When the pressure increases above the elastance threshold, the balloon becomes plastic and accommodates large volumes of air with very little change in pressure.[239,240] For tubular organs in the GI tract, such as the esophagus, experts recommend the use of a cylindrical bag (rather than the spherical) with a fixed length.[196,239]

Barostats have been used extensively in studies evaluating rectosigmoid and gastric perception thresholds for pain. However, this technique has been rarely used to assess esophageal mechanosensitivity in humans. Unlike the rectum and the stomach, the esophagus does not serve as a storage organ but rather as a conduit. Consequently, intraesophageal distensions do not mimic a normal, physiologic stimulus, and thus, perceptual responses to such a stimulus may have no scientific merit. This factor, in addition to the patient's difficulties in tolerating balloon distension, which commonly results in poor recruitment rates as well as the potential for esophageal perforation, has made esophageal balloon distensions by a barostat a less attractive research tool.

Various distension protocols have been used in different studies. Like any other technique that assesses esophageal sensation, balloon distension has yet to be standardized. Slow ramp distension is an ascending method that involves slow (rate varies from one study to another) increase in volume or pressure of the balloon usually until the desired perceptual response has been reported by the subject.[55,196,242] In contrast, phasic distensions are rapid inflations of the balloon that can be delivered in random sequence or double random staircase.[55,196] The latter includes two series of distension stimuli (staircases), and the computer alternates between the two staircases on a random basis.[196,239,242] With the tracking method, the barostat is programmed to deliver a series of intermittent phasic stimuli separated by interpulse rest period within an interactive stimulus tracking procedure.[196,243,244] If the subject indicates a sensation below the tracked intensity, then the following stimulus will increase in pressure. If the subject reports the desired sensation, then the following pressure step is randomized to stay the same or decrease. The random element is placed to mask the relationship between ratings and subsequent stimulus change and, therefore, decrease potential scaling bias.[81]

Quantification of perceptual responses depends on the characteristics of the mechanoreceptors in a specific region of the GI tract. Volume or pressure distension can be considered the most physiologic stimuli.[245] The most reliable reports of esophageal sensory thresholds are obtained during volume distension. Although the overall pressure–volume curve is linear, the pressure at any given volume may vary because of the presence or absence of a superimposed esophageal phasic contractions.[196] Despite this physiologic phenomenon, other investigators rely primarily on pressure when performing balloon studies in the esophagus.

Commonly, qualitative and quantitative perceptual responses are evaluated during balloon distension studies. Qualitative perceptual responses include symptom reports in response to balloon distension, such as chest pain, heartburn, bloating, and fullness, among others.[196,246] Heartburn is a common sensation that occurs during balloon distension and may mimic the patient's typical heartburn symptom.[246] Quantitative perceptual responses are commonly obtained during slow-ramp distension and include the minimal distension volume or pressure at which the individual first reports moderate sensation (innocuous sensation), discomfort, and pain (aversive sensation).[196] Discomfort threshold is commonly defined as the first unpleasant esophageal sensation, and pain threshold is defined as the first sensation of pain.[196]

Pitfalls that may modify perceptual responses to balloon distension include the following: Increased rate of balloon distension results in reported perception at lower volumes or pressures,[247] longer durations of balloon distension are more likely to elicit sensation than shorter durations,[247] elderly subjects demonstrate diminished visceral pain perception and female patients seem to have lower perception thresholds for pain compared with male patients,[248–250] and the proximal esophagus has been suggested to be more sensitive to chemical and mechanical stimuli than the distal esophagus.[196,251] Additionally, reduced sensitivity to intraluminal stimuli has been demonstrated in specific patient populations, such as those with Barrett mucosa or esophageal stricture.[220,252,253] A recent study demonstrated the development of secondary hypersensitivity in the adjacent portion of the esophagus that was not sensitized by a chemical stimulus (acid).[56]

Balloon studies are primarily designed to assess the presence of visceral hypersensitivity in various esophageal disorders. Early studies demonstrated that pain develops with balloon distension more frequently in NCCP patients than in normal control subjects and that their pain occurs at smaller volumes.[81,84,254] Short-term sensitization of mechanosensitive afferent pathways by transient exposure to irritants has been shown in both humans and animal models of visceral hypersensitivity.[88,255] Human studies that evaluated the effect of esophageal acid perfusion on perception of esophageal distension in healthy control subjects and patients with GERD had varying results.[88,134,256,257]

Mehta and colleagues[88] reported that perfusion of the esophagus with 0.1 N hydrochloric acid for 30 minutes resulted in enhanced sensitivity to esophageal balloon distension. Similarly, Sarkar and colleagues[258] reported that acid perfusion into the distal esophagus was associated with the development of mechanical hypersensitivity in the proximal esophagus, which had not been exposed to acid, suggesting the development of secondary visceral hypersensitivity. Peghini and coworkers[259] found a lowering of the pain threshold to distension only in those individuals who were symptomatic during acid perfusion. In contrast, DeVault[257] reported that a 15-minute acid perfusion had no significant effect on pain perception during esophageal distension. The mechanisms underlying the sensitizing effect of acute tissue irritation on visceral afferent pathways have been well characterized in the form of peripheral and central sensitization.[195] Such sensitization manifests as increased background activity of sensory neurons, the lowering of nociceptive thresholds, changes in stimulus response curves, and enlargement of receptive fields. During a noxious event, a series of counterregulatory mechanisms are activated that are aimed at containing the development of both the acute and any long-lasting sensitization.[195]

Studies evaluating balloon distensions in patients with chronic acid exposure or esophageal mucosal injury are scarce. Fass and colleagues[196] demonstrated that mild to moderate chronic tissue injury in GERD differentially affects mechanosensitive and chemosensitive afferent pathways. GERD patients showed enhanced perception of acid perfusion but not of esophageal distension. Chemosensitivity but not mechanosensitivity was correlated with reflux symptoms and with the degree of endoscopically shown tissue injury at baseline. Trimble and coworkers[208] evaluated patients with heartburn and excess reflux defined by abnormal upper endoscopy or 24-hour esophageal pH monitoring and compared them with patients with heartburn and a normal 24-hour pH test. The results demonstrated that the latter group had lower volume thresholds for perception of esophageal balloon distension and discomfort. This study suggests that patients with typical heartburn who lack any evidence of excess acid are highly sensitive to mechanical stimuli.

Balloon distension has been commonly used to assess the effect of various drugs on esophageal sensory perception. Imipramine, octreotide, and nifedipine have all been shown to increase perception thresholds for pain in normal controls or patients with NCCP.[258–262] Balloon distention is rarely used in clinical practice primarily because of the complexity of the procedure and lack of standardization despite a recent study demonstrating its diagnostic utility in third of the NCCP subjects.[263]

ESOPHAGEAL EVOKED POTENTIALS

Cerebral evoked potentials reflect electrical activity of the brain in response to visual, auditory, somatosensory, and visceral stimuli. There is a clear relationship between stimulus frequency, using esophageal electrical stimulation, and amplitude of cerebral evoked potentials.[264] Studies have demonstrated that a significant and progressive decrease of evoked potential amplitudes is associated with increasing stimulus frequency. This suggests a rapid attenuation of the cerebral autonomic responses with increased frequency of electrical stimulation.[264] Furthermore, a stimulus intensity–response relationship has been shown in brain response to increasing stimulus intensity, which is probably explained by increased recruitment of afferent fibers.[264,265]

Balloon distension and electrical stimulation protocols have been used in studies assessing cerebral evoked potentials in response to esophageal stimulation. It is unclear if one of the sensory testing methods is better than the other.

Esophageal balloon distension triggers a characteristic triphasic evoked potential.[266] Two negative peaks (N1 and N2) and one positive peak (P1) can be demonstrated. Latency is the time in milliseconds from the stimulus to the peak. There is a considerable intersubject variability but almost no intrasubject variability when recording cerebral evoked potentials. Studies in normal subjects have shown significantly shorter latencies during balloon distension in the proximal esophagus as compared with the distal esophagus.[267]

Assessment of patients with NCCP, using the esophageal balloon distension paradigm, revealed that amplitude and quality of cerebral evoked potentials increased with increasing sensation, whereas the latencies remained stable.[266] Additionally, the amplitude and quality of evoked potentials were lower in NCCP patients as compared with controls. Similar levels of sensation were produced by lower balloon volumes in NCCP patients.[264]

Esophageal stimulation and cerebral evoked potentials may provide clues to the pathway and type of neurons involved in nociception.[268] Additionally, cerebral evoked potentials were used to identify brain areas that are responsible for esophageal pain sensation.[269,270]

BRAIN IMAGING

In addition to cortical evoked potentials, other techniques have been increasingly used to evaluate the brain–gut relationship in patients with esophageal disorders. These techniques include positron emission tomography (PET) and functional magnetic resonance imaging (fMRI). The GI is intricately connected to the central nervous system by pathways that are continuously sampling and modulating gut function.[271]

PET scanning is an established method to study the functional neuroanatomy of the human brain.[272,273] Radio-labeled compounds allow the study of biochemical and physiologic processes involved in cerebral metabolism.[271] Tomographic images represent spatial distribution of radioisotopes in the brain. Regional cerebral blood flow is studied with labeled water ($H_2^{15}O$) and glucose metabolism with 18Fl-labeled fluorodeoxyglucose. Unlike PET, fMRI does not require radioisotopes and, hence, is considered a safer imaging technique. fMRI detects increases in oxygen concentration in areas of heightened neuronal activity.[266,272,274] This imaging technique is best suited for locating the site but not the sequence or duration of neuronal activity. Overall, fMRI provides both anatomic and functional information.

Thus far, only a few studies have attempted to assess the cortical process of esophageal sensation in humans. Aziz and colleagues[199] examined the human brain loci involved in the process of esophageal sensation using PET and distal esophageal balloon distension in eight healthy volunteers. Nonpainful stimuli elicited bilateral activation along the central sulcus, insular cortex, and the frontal and parietal operculum. Painful stimuli resulted in intense activation of the same

areas and additional activation of right anterior insular cortex and anterior cingulate gyrus. The former is important in affective processing, whereas the latter is important in pain processing and generating an affective and cognitive response to pain.[275–277] In another study, Kern and colleagues[203] evaluated activation of cerebral cortical responses to esophageal mucosal acid exposure using fMRI. Ten healthy subjects underwent intraesophageal perfusion of 0.1 N hydrochloric acid over 10 minutes. None of the study subjects reported GERD symptoms during acid perfusion. Cerebral cortical activity was concentrated in the posterior cingulate, parietal, and anteromesial frontal lobes. The superior frontal lobe regions activated in this study corresponded to Brodmann area 32, the insula, the operculum, and the anterior cingulate.

Further studies are needed to assess cerebral activation in patients with different esophageal disorders. In addition, it would be of great interest to determine whether there are differences in central processing of an intraesophageal stimulus in patients with NCCP, nonerosive reflux disease, or functional heartburn. It is also important to begin to examine the role of psychophysiologic states such as stress, anxiety, and depression and their effects on central nuclei involved with perception of esophageal stimuli.

SENSORY TESTING—PITFALLS IN STUDY DESIGN

Surprisingly, many studies using esophageal sensory testing to evaluate sensory perception thresholds are afflicted with design flaws that make interpretation of the results very difficult. Studies using balloon distension paradigms in the distal esophagus, without simultaneously measuring intraesophageal pressure, are inherently flawed because of the tendency of the balloon to migrate into the stomach due to esophageal contraction and shortening in response to distension of the balloon. Other common pitfalls include using different rates of balloon distension or acid perfusion, different balloon distension paradigms, or more commonly using an inappropriate control group. For example, a study that compares esophageal sensory testing of patients with BE versus normal controls, and uses a younger control group, is likely to bias the study results. Patients with BE are commonly older, and age per se (being older) increases perception thresholds for pain.[252] Thus, it will be difficult to discern if the Barrett epithelium or the difference in age is responsible for patients' alteration in pain perception.

Studies that evaluate esophageal sensory testing in IBS patients, as compared with normal controls and use a more gender-diverse control group, are also hard to interpret. IBS patients are commonly women, and a control group that is composed of a significant number of men may bias the results toward the IBS group unrelated to the underlying disorder (IBS). Men, as compared with women, demonstrate an increase of perception thresholds for pain in response to esophageal stimuli.

Ensuring a similar study protocol and age- as well as gender-matched control group will reduce the potential bias in esophageal sensory testing studies. However, because of lack of standardization in study design, comparison between studies remains a difficult task.

PSYCHOLOGICAL EVALUATION

Between 17% and 43% of the patients with NCCP are estimated to suffer from some type of psychological abnormality.[177] Psychological comorbidity can modulate esophageal pain perception and cause subjects to perceive low-intensity esophageal stimuli as being painful.[57,85,178,179] Anxiety, depression, neuroticism, and hypochondriac behavior have all been described in NCCP patients.[180–182,210] Consequently, patients, especially those who are unresponsive to medical intervention and those suspected to have psychological comorbidity, should be referred to a psychologist or psychiatrist for further evaluation.[131]

TABLE 62.5	Treatment Plan for NCCP
GERD-related NCCP	PPIs, endoscopic and surgical therapy
Dysmotility-related NCCP	• Achalasia: medical, endoscopic, and surgical therapy
	• Jackhammer esophagus: Treat for GERD first. If no response, pain modulator.
	• Spastic motility disorder: pain modulator or smooth muscle relaxants
Functional chest pain	Pain modulators, low dose, and at bedtime (long term)

GERD, gastroesophageal reflux disease; NCCP, noncardiac chest pain; PPI, proton pump inhibitor.

Treatment

Treatment for NCCP should be targeted toward the specific underlying mechanism responsible for the patient's symptoms. Table 62.5 provides a general treatment plan for NCCP.

GERD-RELATED NCCP

Lifestyle modifications include elevation of the head of the bed; weight loss; smoking cessation; and avoidance of alcohol, coffee, fresh citrus juice, and other food products as well as medications that can exacerbate reflux such as opioids, benzodiazepines, and calcium-channel blockers.[278,279] Although these lifestyle modifications are commonly advocated as first-line treatment in GERD patients, there is no evidence to support their efficacy in GERD-related NCCP. Regardless, enthusiasm about lifestyle modifications is very high among physicians, and thus, it is highly likely that GERD-related NCCP subjects will be instructed to follow them.

The efficacy of histamine (H_2) receptor antagonists in controlling symptoms in patients with GERD-related NCCP has been shown to range from 42% to 52%.[280] In one study, cimetidine (unknown dose) and antacids were shown to be effective in only 42% of the patients with GERD-related NCCP who were followed for a period of 2 to 3 years.[281] Stepping down GERD therapy from a PPI to an H_2 receptor antagonist has been disappointing in GERD-related NCCP patients.

Omeprazole (Prilosec) 20 mg twice daily or placebo was administered over a period of 8 weeks to GERD-related NCCP patients in the only double-blind, placebo-controlled trial that has been performed.[44] Patients who received omeprazole had a significant reduction in both the number of days with chest pain and in their chest pain severity scores compared to the patients who received placebo. Thus far, most of the studies assessing the efficacy of PPIs in NCCP primarily utilized omeprazole. However, it is likely that all other PPIs would demonstrate similar efficacy. In fact, a recent open-label study with esomeprazole (Nexium) administered 40 mg once daily over a period of 1 month demonstrated complete resolution of symptoms in 57.1% of subjects with either NCCP or laryngeal manifestations of GERD.[282] In another open-label study, 85% of NCCP patients reported symptom relief or improvement after receiving PPI twice daily (different brands) for a period of 3 months.[283]

A retrospective review of patients' files revealed that PPIs reduce the number of chest pain episodes, emergency department visits, and hospitalizations due to chest pain in subjects with documented CAD.[284] It is likely that GERD-related symptoms contribute to the medical-seeking behavior of this patient population.

Patients with GERD-related NCCP should be treated with at least double the standard dose of PPI until symptoms remit, followed by dose tapering to determine the lowest PPI dose that can control symptoms. As with other extraesophageal manifestations of GERD, NCCP patients may require more than 2 months of therapy for optimal symptom control. A single randomized placebo-controlled study evaluated symptom scores in 599 NCCP patients treated with esomeprazole 40 mg twice daily for 2 weeks.[285] Several questionnaires, including the Reflux Disease Questionnaire (RDQ), Short Form-36 (SF-36), Hospital Anxiety and Depression Questionnaire (HAD), McGill Pain Questionnaire (MPQ), Chest pain visual analogue scale (VAS), Brief Pain Inventory (BPI), and Quality of Life in Reflux and Dyspepsia (QOLRAD), were used for symptom assessment in this study. Chest pain symptom relief was defined as being less than or equal to 1 day of minimal symptoms during the last 7 days of treatment. Patients were stratified into two groups based on clinical judgment of the presence or absence of GERD-related symptoms. Importantly, pH testing was not done to demonstrate pathologic acid reflux. Patients without GERD symptoms demonstrated significant improvement in chest pain symptoms on esomeprazole as compared to placebo (38.7% vs. 25.5% respectively; $P = .018$). Post-hoc analysis of the combined populations (patients with and without GERD symptoms) indicated positive treatment response to esomeprazole for chest pain in patients with acid reflux–related symptoms as compared with placebo (33.1% vs. 24.9% respectively; $P = .035$).[285] Long-term maintenance PPI treatment has been shown to be highly effective.[286] Borzecki and colleagues[287] developed a decision tree to compare empiric treatments for NCCP patients with H_2 receptor antagonists or standard-dose PPI for 8 weeks with initial investigations (upper endoscopy or upper GI series). Empiric treatment was more cost-effective in the initial investigation strategy, with a cost of $849 per patient versus $2,187 per patient.

Only one trial has been published using the EndoCinch endoluminal gastroplication (ELGP) as a treatment modality for atypical GERD symptoms, including NCCP. ELGP is an endoscopic suture technique that places sutures, using the EndoCinch device, 1 cm below the esophagogastric junction (OGJ).[288] In an open-label trial evaluating ELGP in patients with atypical GERD symptoms (n = 39), including NCCP (18/39), the authors demonstrate that 72% (n = 13/18) of patients reported improvement in symptoms of chest pain at 6 months postprocedure as compared to baseline symptoms ($P = .0003$).[289]

The value of antireflux surgery in GERD-related NCCP is unclear. Several studies have demonstrated a significant improvement in symptoms following laparoscopic fundoplication in patients with GERD-related NCCP. For instance, Patti and associates[290] reported improvement in chest pain symptoms following laparoscopic fundoplication in 85% of patients with GERD-related NCCP. In addition, Farrell and coworkers[291] reported that 90% of NCCP patients who underwent antireflux surgery experienced improvement in chest pain and 50% reported complete symptom resolution. In contrast, So and colleagues[292] reported that after laparoscopic fundoplication, relief of atypical GERD symptoms (e.g., chest pain) was less satisfactory than relief of typical GERD symptoms (e.g., heartburn). In their study, the authors evaluated symptom improvement with a questionnaire given 3 months and 12 months after antireflux surgery. Overall, heartburn was relieved in 93% of patients, whereas only 48% of patients reported relief of chest pain symptoms.

NON–GERD-RELATED NCCP

The treatment of non–GERD-related NCCP is primarily based on esophageal pain modulation (Table 62.6). An important development in this field was the recognition that NCCP patients with spastic esophageal motor disorders (except achalasia), as documented by esophageal manometry, are more likely to respond to pain modulators than to muscle relaxants. Unfortunately, no large, well-designed studies to assess pain modulators in patients with non–GERD-related NCCP have been performed thus far.

Several recent studies have shown that most NCCP patients are managed by cardiologists and PCPs who appear to know little about the role and treatment of esophageal hypersensitivity in

TABLE 62.6 Therapeutic Modalities of Non–GERD-Related NCCP

- Smooth muscle relaxants (nitrates, calcium channel blockers, sildenafil)
- Botulinum toxin injection
- Pain modulators (trazodone, TCAs, SSRIs, theophylline)
- Surgery for motility disorders
- Cognitive-behavioral therapy, hypnotherapy, and others

GERD, gastroesophageal reflux disease; NCCP, noncardiac chest pain; SSRIs, selective serotonin reuptake inhibitors; TCAs, tricyclic antidepressants.

NCCP.[22,23,293] Even gastroenterologists appeared somewhat uninformed about the role of visceral hypersensitivity in NCCP.[294]

Nitroglycerin and long-acting nitrates cause relaxation of GI smooth muscles by stimulating cyclic guanosine monophosphate (GMP)-dependent pathways. Several open-label studies have reported that nitrates improve symptoms and esophageal motility patterns in patients with chest pain and esophageal dysmotility. Several investigators reported symptomatic improvement in patients with DES, accompanied by normalization of esophageal motility during treatment with nitrates.[295,296] In one small study, five patients with DES experienced a 4-year clinical and manometric remission.[297] However, other studies have failed to demonstrate similar efficacy.[298,299] Long-acting nitrates in doses of 10 to 20 mg two to three times daily, as well as short-acting, sublingual nitrates for acute episodes of chest pain in NCCP patients, were used in these studies.

Overall, studies that evaluated the value of nitrates in NCCP have been limited by small numbers of patients and inconsistent results in regard to drug efficacy. A placebo-controlled trial that excludes patients with GERD has yet to be performed.

Because calcium plays an important role in esophageal muscle contraction, the role of calcium channel blocking agents in patients with NCCP and esophageal spastic motility disorders has been the focus of investigation. Nifedipine (10 to 30 mg, by mouth, three times a day) decreases the amplitude and duration of esophageal contractions in patients with nutcracker esophagus after only 2 weeks.[189] Unfortunately, the effect of the drug disappeared after 6 weeks of treatment with the complete recurrence of symptoms. Davies and associates[300] used a placebo-controlled trial to assess the efficacy of nifedipine in the prevention of symptomatic episodes of esophageal spasm in eight NCCP patients over a 6-week period. The authors were unable to find statistically significant differences in symptom improvement between the two therapeutic arms. In contrast, symptom improvement was noted in 20 NCCP patients with various esophageal motility disorders, including hypertensive LES, nutcracker esophagus, DES, and vigorous achalasia, treated with nifedipine (10 mg, by mouth, three times a day).[301] Nifedipine was also found to significantly decrease LES resting pressure, with a direct correlation to the plasma levels of drug.[302]

Diltiazem (60 to 90 mg, by mouth, four times a day) for 8 weeks significantly improved mean chest pain scores and esophageal motility studies in patients with nutcracker esophagus when compared to placebo.[303,304] However, in a study evaluating eight patients with DES, the effect of diltiazem in relieving chest pain was not different from the effect of placebo, probably due to the small number of patients who participated in the study.[305]

Other calcium channel blockers have been evaluated in patients with primary esophageal motor disorders including verapamil, fendiline, nimodipine, and nisoldipine, with various effects on LES resting pressure and esophageal amplitude contractions. Regardless, calcium channel blockers appear to have a transient esophageal motor effect that translates to a short-lived improvement in symptoms, compounded by a variety of side effects such as hypotension, bradycardia, and pedal edema.

Sildenafil is a potent selective inhibitor of cyclic GMP-specific phosphodiesterase 5 (PDE5), which inactivates nitric oxide–stimulated GMP. Intracellular accumulation of the latter induces smooth muscle relaxation. The drug has been shown to improve esophageal motility in patients with nutcracker esophagus or hypertensive LES by lowering LES resting pressure, reducing distal esophageal amplitude contractions, and prolonging the duration of LES relaxation.[306,307] However, thus far, there have been no studies that specifically addressed NCCP patients, so the value of this compound in NCCP remains unknown. Additionally, the usage of this compound in NCCP will likely be limited by its cost and side effects.

The antispasmodic cimetropium bromide has been shown to be efficacious in eight NCCP patients with nutcracker esophagus when taken intravenously,[308] but clinical data regarding the efficacy of an oral formulation are still lacking. Hydralazine, an antihypertensive compound that directly dilates peripheral vessels, was shown to improve chest pain and dysphagia by decreasing the amplitude and duration of esophageal contractions in a small study of only five patients.[299] Overall, evidence to support the therapeutic benefit of anticholinergic agents for the treatment of NCCP remains very limited.

Multiple case series evaluating peroral endoscopic myotomy (POEM) for the treatment of spastic oesophageal motility disorders (diffuse oesophageal spasm, jackhammer esophagus, nutcracker esophagus, and hypertensive LES) have shown symptomatic improvement in chest pain symptoms reaching 91%.[308] Some controversy exists on whether a longer myotomy extending into the full length of the spastic oesophageal muscle or short-segment myotomy should be pursued in patients with spastic oesophageal motor disorders.[309] It appears that patients with achalasia demonstrate better symptom response to POEM compared to patients with spastic oesophageal motor disorders. However, larger trials are needed to further determine the value of POEM in NCCP patients with esophageal hypercontractility.

PAIN MODULATORS

Visceral hypersensitivity is thought to be the primary underlying mechanism of patients with non–GERD-related NCCP regardless of the presence or absence of esophageal motor disorder. Consequently, drugs that can alter esophageal pain perception have become the mainstay of therapy in these patients.

Several drugs have been shown to have a pain modulatory or a visceral analgesic effect, thus alleviating chest pain symptoms. These drugs include tricyclic antidepressants (TCAs), selective serotonin reuptake inhibitors (SSRIs), theophylline, and trazodone. Table 62.7 provides a hierarchy of antidepressants of choice for chest pain reduction and global health improvement.[310]

The only TCA that has been studied in a randomized double-blind, placebo-controlled trial is imipramine. In one study, 60 NCCP patients were divided into three groups and treated with either imipramine 50 mg, clonidine 0.1 mg, or placebo daily. Treatment with imipramine, clonidine, and placebo showed a mean reduction in chest pain frequency (± standard

TABLE 62.7 Hierarchy of Antidepressants of Choice for Chest Pain Reduction and Global Health Improvement

Pain Reduction	Global Health Improvement
1. Venlafaxine	1. Venlafaxine
2. Sertraline	2. Sertraline
3. Imipramine	3. Trazodone
4. Trazodone	4. Imipramine
5. Paroxetine	5. Paroxetine

From Nguyen TM, Eslick GD. Systematic review: the treatment of noncardiac chest pain with antidepressants. *Aliment Pharmacol Ther* 2012;35(5):493–500. Copyright © 2012 Blackwell Publishing Ltd. Reprinted by permission of John Wiley & Sons, Inc.

deviation [SD]) compared to the placebo phase of 52% (±25%), 39% (±51%), and 1% (±86%), respectively. Only imipramine treatment showed significant reduction in chest pain frequency (approximately 50%) compared to the placebo phase ($P = .03$) as well as decreased right ventricular sensitivity to pain. Both imipramine and clonidine had improved symptoms of chest pain intensity compared to placebo ($P = .001$ and .002, respectively). There was no difference in treatment effect when patients with normal and those with abnormal esophageal motility studies were compared. There was no change in esophageal sensitivity to balloon distension during treatment as compared to baseline. Fifteen patients treated with imipramine had a slight but significant prolongation of the corrected QT interval ($P = .02$). No patients reported symptoms suggestive of a proarrhythmic effect.[260] Cox et al.[311] performed a randomized, double-blind, crossover trial of imipramine versus placebo in 18 women with chest pain and normal coronary angiograms who were suffering anginal episodes despite conventional anti-anginal medication. All patients were randomized to treatment with either imipramine 50 mg or placebo daily for a period of 5 weeks, followed by a 2-week washout period. Patients were then crossed over to the other arm for an additional 5 weeks. The total number of chest pain episodes was significantly less with imipramine compared to placebo (11 vs. 21, respectively; $P = .01$). However, no significant improvement was detected in any of the six quality of life domains when imipramine was compared to placebo. This was most likely due to the high incidence of side effects with imipramine compared to placebo (83% vs. 44% respectively; $P = .01$). Furthermore, three patients were withdrawn from the study due to side effects. The most common side effects reported were dry mouth and dizziness.

Park et al.[312] conducted a randomized, open-label trial in FCP patients refractory to standard-dose PPI. The study compared treatment outcomes between standard-dose PPI (rabeprazole 20 mg daily) plus low-dose amitriptyline (10 mg at bedtime) ($n = 17$) versus double-dose PPI therapy alone (rabeprazole 20 mg twice a day) ($n = 19$). Patients who had both negative pH testing for GERD and less than 50% improvement in global symptoms scores after treatment with standard-dose rabeprazole for 1 month were enrolled into the study. Daily symptom diaries were used to evaluate global symptom scores each week. Mean global symptom scores were not statistically significant between the two treatment groups (3.75 ± 0.31 vs. 4.35 ± 0.29; $P = .172$); however, within the groups, differences in global symptom scores were significant at week 8 ($P < .001$). After 8 weeks, 71% of patients treated with both amitriptyline and standard-dose rabeprazole had greater than 50% global symptom improvement, whereas only 26% of patients treated with double-dose rabeprazole had a similar degree of symptom improvement ($P = .008$). In addition, those patients who received both amitriptyline and standard-dose rabeprazole were noted to have significant improvement in scores of body pain and general health perception compared with those receiving double-dose rabeprazole ($P = .031$ and .01, respectively).[312] Other new TCAs known to have fewer anticholinergic side effects, such as nortriptyline, are attractive treatment options due to more favorable side effect profiles but have not been formally studied in NCCP.

Trazodone

Trazodone, dosed between 100 and 150 mg, was evaluated in 29 patients with contraction abnormalities and NCCP using a double-blind, placebo-controlled trial for 6 weeks. Questionnaires that were used to evaluate symptom improvement with treatment included the Oesophageal Distress Symptom Score, Symptom Checklist 90-Revised (SCL-90-R), Global Symptom Index, positive symptom index, and the Montgomery-Åsberg Depression Rating Scale (MADRS). All patients underwent the Bernstein test with acid perfusion into the esophagus at the time of esophageal manometry. Those patients with positive acid perfusion testing, findings of esophagitis on upper endoscopy or barium studies, were excluded. Trazodone-treated patients reported a significantly greater global improvement (per VAS) compared to placebo at 6 weeks posttreatment (trazodone: 48% vs. placebo: 11%; $P = .02$) despite no effect on esophageal motility. In addition, patients treated with trazodone had a statistically significant reduction in esophageal distress symptom scores (including NCCP) compared to placebo ($P = .03$). However, there was no significant difference in chest pain intensity or frequency in patients treated with trazodone versus placebo. Side effects were generally mild and consisted of dry mouth in two patients and dizziness, drowsiness, and fatigue in five patients receiving trazodone.[173]

Serotonin Norepinephrine Reuptake Inhibitors

Venlafaxine 75 mg per day was compared with placebo for the treatment of 43 patients with FCP. Symptom diaries documented scores of frequency and severity of chest pain. Symptom intensity scores were calculated by adding daily severity for the week multiplied by daily frequency. Additional questionnaires included SF-36 and the Beck Depression Inventory (BDI). Symptom score improvement of greater than 50% was considered to be treatment success. On the intention-to-treat analysis, more than 50% improvement in symptoms was seen in 52% of patients treated with venlafaxine versus 4% treated with placebo (OR 26.0; 95% CI, 5.7 to 118.8; $P < .001$). Furthermore, patients in the venlafaxine group had a significantly greater improvement in body pain and emotional state compared with the placebo group ($P = .002$ and .002, respectively).[313] Overall, the side effects were minimal and primarily consisted of sleep disturbances.

Selective Serotonin Reuptake Inhibitors

A double-blind, randomized placebo-controlled trial evaluating paroxetine in dosages ranging from 5 to 50 mg was performed in 43 NCCP patients. Patients were evaluated by the physician-rated scales (Clinical Global Impression of Illness Severity and Clinical Global Impression of Improvements), BDI, Short Form MPQ, Medical Outcomes Study SF-36, and a patient-rated scale of symptom severity (VAS) to assess symptoms throughout the study period. No GI evaluation had been performed before or during enrolment into the study. Only on Clinical Global Impression of Improvements questionnaire did paroxetine treatment show superiority to placebo ($P < .05$).[314]

Sertraline was evaluated as a treatment for NCCP in a single-site, double-blind, placebo-controlled study consisting of 30 patients.[315] The sertraline group received 50 mg at the beginning of the study, with titration of the dose to 200 mg based on clinical response. Patients were evaluated with daily pain diaries (VASs), SF-36 Health Survey Manual, and the BDI at enrollment. Patients treated with sertraline had greater reduction in chest pain scores (week 0: 3.94, week 9: 1.49) compared to those treated with placebo (week 0: 3.50, week 9: 2.96; 95% CI, -3.49, -0.36; $P = .02$), with pain scores decreasing by approximately 0.2 units for each week of the study. The SF-36 subscore for general health had significantly improved at the end of treatment compared to placebo. Side effects were generally mild and reported as restlessness, nausea, decreased libido, and delayed ejaculation.[315]

Adenosine Antagonists

A few studies have evaluated the role of theophylline in the treatment of esophageal chest pain. Rao et al.[316] first conducted a 3-month open-label trial of theophylline infusion in 21 patients with FCP. Patients underwent impedance planimetry as well as balloon distension of the esophagus, with esophageal hypersensitivity being defined as reproduction of chest pain symptoms with balloon distension ≤ 55 cm H_2O pressure. Chest pain intensity and improvement in chest pain symptoms were measured by VASs. Sensory responses to balloon distension were graded on a scale of 0 to 3 (0 = no pain, 1 = fullness/distension, 2 = discomfort, 3 = pain). Of those who demonstrated reproducible chest pain with graded balloon distension (16/21), 12 (75%) had increased chest pain thresholds ($P < .05$). The median threshold for discomfort increased to 45 cm H_2O (vs. pretreatment: 20 cm H_2O; $P < .05$) and for chest pain to greater than 65 cm H_2O (vs. pretreatment: 40 cm H_2O; $P < .05$). Eight of the 12 patients who received oral theophylline (6 mg/kg/day) completed the second portion of the study. Six of eight patients (75%) had greater than 50% reduction in chest pain frequency and intensity ($P < .05$) with intravenous theophylline compared to baseline scores ($P < .05$). These six patients were subsequently transitioned to the oral theophylline phase of the trial.

Adverse effects were noted in four patients including transient insomnia, nausea, palpitations, and tremor. Two patients who were transitioned to oral theophylline discontinued treatment due to symptoms of nausea, transient insomnia, and palpitations.[316]

Rao et al.[317] also performed two randomized placebo-controlled trials in a single cohort of NCCP patients several years later involving intravenous and oral theophylline. The first trial with intravenous administration of theophylline treatment in 16 NCCP patients demonstrated increased chest pain thresholds ($P = .027$), increased esophageal cross-sectional area ($P = .03$), and a more distensible esophageal wall ($P = .04$) after treatment, as compared with placebo, suggesting a more relaxed esophagus after theophylline infusion. The second trial evaluated oral theophylline treatment response in 19 NCCP patients compared to placebo. Patients treated with oral theophylline (200 mg capsules twice daily for 4 weeks) had a 58% reduction in symptoms, compared to 6% on placebo ($P < .02$). Patients were noted to have less chest pain episodes ($P = .025$) as well as decreased duration ($P = .002$) and severity ($P = .031$) of symptoms (Fig. 62.9). Theophylline was reasonably tolerated, with reported side effects of nausea, insomnia, tremor, and light-headedness.[317]

Octreotide

Octreotide, a synthetic analog of somatostatin, has been shown to increase rectal and sigmoid perception thresholds for pain in IBS subjects as well as healthy subjects.[318,319] It has been postulated that the effect of octreotide is mediated by the activation of somatostatin receptors at the spinal cord and/or the supraspinal level. Octreotide, administered 100 mg subcutaneously, was found to significantly increase perception thresholds for pain as compared to placebo in healthy subjects undergoing intraesophageal balloon distension.[320] Unfortunately, due to cost and the lack of an oral formulation, octreotide is rarely utilized for NCCP in clinical practice.

Benzodiazepines

Alprazolam has been shown in a study to ameliorate chest pain at a mean dose of 4.3 mg daily in patients with NCCP and panic disorder.[321] In this study, 15 out of 20 patients reported at least a 50% reduction in panic attack episodes and a corresponding decline in the frequency of chest pain episodes. Clonazepam, given 1 to 4 mg daily, was also shown to be effective in the treatment of patients with NCCP and panic disorder.[322] The treatment of a functional disorder such as NCCP with benzodiazepines has been greatly discouraged primarily due to the likelihood of becoming addicted to this class of drugs.

ENDOSCOPIC TREATMENT AND SURGERY FOR NCCP

Botulinum toxin (BOTOX; Allergan, Irvine, CA) interacts selectively with cholinergic neurons to inhibit the release of acetylcholine at the presynaptic terminals. Botulinum toxin injection into the LES has been used in several uncontrolled trials that included patients with NCCP and documented esophageal spastic motility disorder. Injecting botulinum toxin into the LES in a small, uncontrolled study resulted in 50% reduction of chest pain episodes in 72% of the subjects for a mean duration of 7.3 months (Fig. 62.10).[323]

Laparoscopic fundoplication relieves heartburn and acid regurgitation in most patients with GERD, but its effect on chest pain is less clear. DeMeester and associates[44] identified a temporal correlation between chest pain and acid reflux events in 12 of 23 patients with NCCP. Chest pain resolved in all 12 patients treated either by surgery (eight patients) or acid-reducing agents (four patients). Patti and coworkers[290] reviewed patients who complained of chest pain in addition to heartburn and acid regurgitation. Overall, chest pain improved in 85% of these patients after undergoing laparoscopic fundoplication for GERD. Improvement in chest pain increased to 96% in patients whose chest pain correlated with GERD most of the time. Farrell and colleagues[291] evaluated the effectiveness of antireflux surgery for patients with atypical manifestations of GERD. Chest pain improved in 90% of patients after laparoscopic fundoplication, with symptom

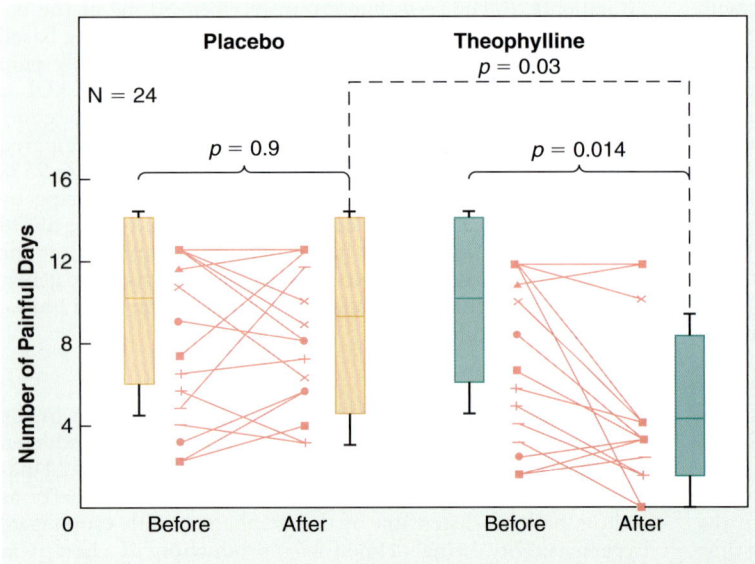

FIGURE 62.9 The effect of oral theophylline versus placebo on the number of painful days in each individual with non–gastroesophageal reflux disease-related noncardiac chest pain at baseline and after drug administration (200 mg twice daily for 4 weeks). (Reprinted by permission from Nature: Rao SS, Mudipalli RS, Remes-Troche JM, et al. Theophylline improves esophageal chest pain—a randomized, placebo-controlled study. Am J Gastroenterol 2007;102[5]:930–938. Copyright © 2007 Springer Nature.)

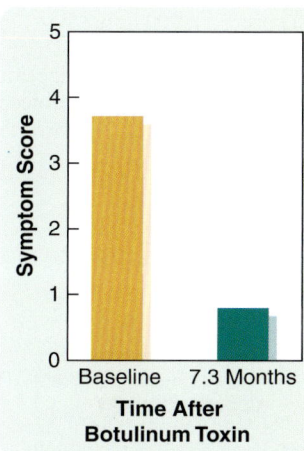

FIGURE 62.10 The effect of botulinum toxin injection in 29 non–gastroesophageal reflux disease-related noncardiac chest pain patients with spastic esophageal motility disorder. *(Reprinted by permission from Nature: Miller LS, Pullela SV, Parkman HP, et al. Treatment of chest pain in patients with noncardiac, nonreflux, nonachalasia spastic esophageal motor disorders using botulinum toxin injection into the gastroesophageal junction. Am J Gastroenterol 2002;97[7]:1640–1646. Copyright © 2002 Springer Nature.)*

resolution in 50% of patients. Although surgical studies demonstrated a high success rate of antireflux surgery in GERD-related NCCP patients, the patients included were carefully selected.

Very few studies to date have specifically evaluated the value of endoscopic treatment for GERD in patients with GERD-related NCCP. Liu et al.,[289] who treated 18 NCCP patients with ELGP, demonstrated short-term symptomatic response (6 months) in 72% of them. During long-term follow-up (1 to 3 years) 75% of nonresponders became symptom-free, and 40% of responders became symptomatic.

JOHREI THERAPY

Johrei therapy is a technique by which a healer transmits healing energy to the patient. Gasiorowska et al.[324] conducted a randomized controlled pilot study evaluating the effect of Johrei versus wait-list (no intervention) in controlling symptoms of 39 patients with FCP. All patients enrolled had normal ambulatory esophageal pH testing, upper endoscopy, and esophageal manometry. Patients were evaluated by the SF-36, SCL-90-R, Perceived Stress Scale (PSS), and HAD scale. Symptom intensity scores were calculated by adding the reported daily symptom severity multiplied by frequency. Eighteen Johrei sessions delivered by the same certified practitioner were conducted over a 6-week period. The study demonstrated a significant posttreatment reduction in symptom intensity scores (7.0) in the Johrei group as compared to baseline (20.28; $P = .0023$). In contrast, the wait-list group demonstrated no difference in symptom intensity scores compared to baseline (23.06) and posttreatment (20.69; P = not significant) scores.[324] Johrei was well tolerated with no side effects reported.

PSYCHOLOGICAL TREATMENT

Psychological comorbidity, mainly depression and anxiety, is common in patients with NCCP. Psychotherapy may be helpful in the treatment of patients with NCCP, particularly those who also have hypochondriasis, anxiety, or panic disorder.

Several studies have demonstrated that patients with NCCP who are treated with cognitive-behavioral therapy report significant improvement in quality of life and reduction in chest pain symptoms. Additionally, cognitive-behavioral therapy has been successfully used for the treatment of NCCP patients without an existing panic disorder.[325] A study evaluating patients who were treated with cognitive-behavioral therapy reported that 48% of these patients remained pain-free at 12-month

follow-up, as compared to only 13% of the patients in the nonintervention group. Other psychological interventions that have been suggested to be effective in patients with NCCP include reassurance, education, relaxation techniques, breathing training, and biofeedback. Biofeedback was assessed in a study that compared it to primary care visits only in patients with NCCP.[326] Patients in the biofeedback group demonstrated a significantly lower symptom frequency and severity. However, a large group of patients assigned to the biofeedback arm (52%) did not complete the study.

Keefe et al.[327] randomized 116 NCCP patients to a combination of coping skills plus sertraline, sertraline alone, coping skills plus placebo, or placebo. Patients recorded chest pain intensity and unpleasantness scores using VASs (0 to 100) and completed the State-Trait Anxiety Inventory (STAI), Pain Catastrophizing Scale (PCS), BDI, Sickness Impact Profile (SIP), Stone and Neale's Coping Inventory, and Coping Strategies Questionnaire. The rate of change in chest pain intensity and unpleasantness with coping skills and sertraline, either alone or in combination, was statistically significant compared to those treated with placebo alone. Of note, patients treated with coping skills plus sertraline also had a significant improvement in catastrophizing of pain symptoms and anxiety compared to the other groups ($P = .02$).[327]

Hypnotherapy has been recently evaluated in the treatment of NCCP patients. Jones and colleagues[328] reported an 80% improvement in symptoms, with a significant reduction in pain intensity, among patients who were receiving 12 sessions of hypnotherapy, compared to only a 23% symptom improvement in the control group (Fig. 62.11). The study concluded that hypnotherapy appears to have a role in treating NCCP and that further studies are needed.

FUTURE THERAPY

Future research in NCCP will continue to focus on mechanisms for pain and will attempt to identify new therapeutic modalities aimed to reduce visceral pain. Research will likely concentrate primarily on the role of central and peripheral sensitization in enhancing perception of intra-esophageal stimuli. Furthermore, currently available treatments for other functional GI disorders, such as IBS and non-ulcer dyspepsia, may be tested in NCCP as well.

The serotonin-related drugs, such as 5-HT3 receptor antagonists and 5-HT4 receptor agonists, appear to have a pain-modulatory effect, probably by altering the initiation, transmission, or processing of extrinsic sensory information

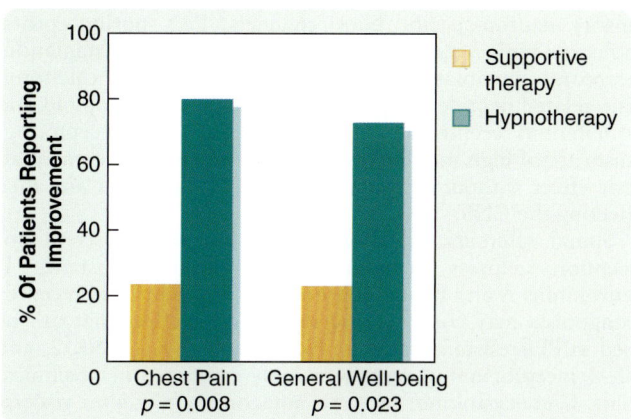

FIGURE 62.11 Percentage of patients reporting a global improvement in chest pain or general well-being with either hypnotherapy (N = 15) or supportive therapy (N = 13). *(Redrawn after Jones H, Cooper P, Miller V, et al. Treatment of non cardiac chest pain: a controlled trial of hypnotherapy. Gut 2006;55[10]:1403–1408, with permission from BMJ Publishing Group Ltd.)*

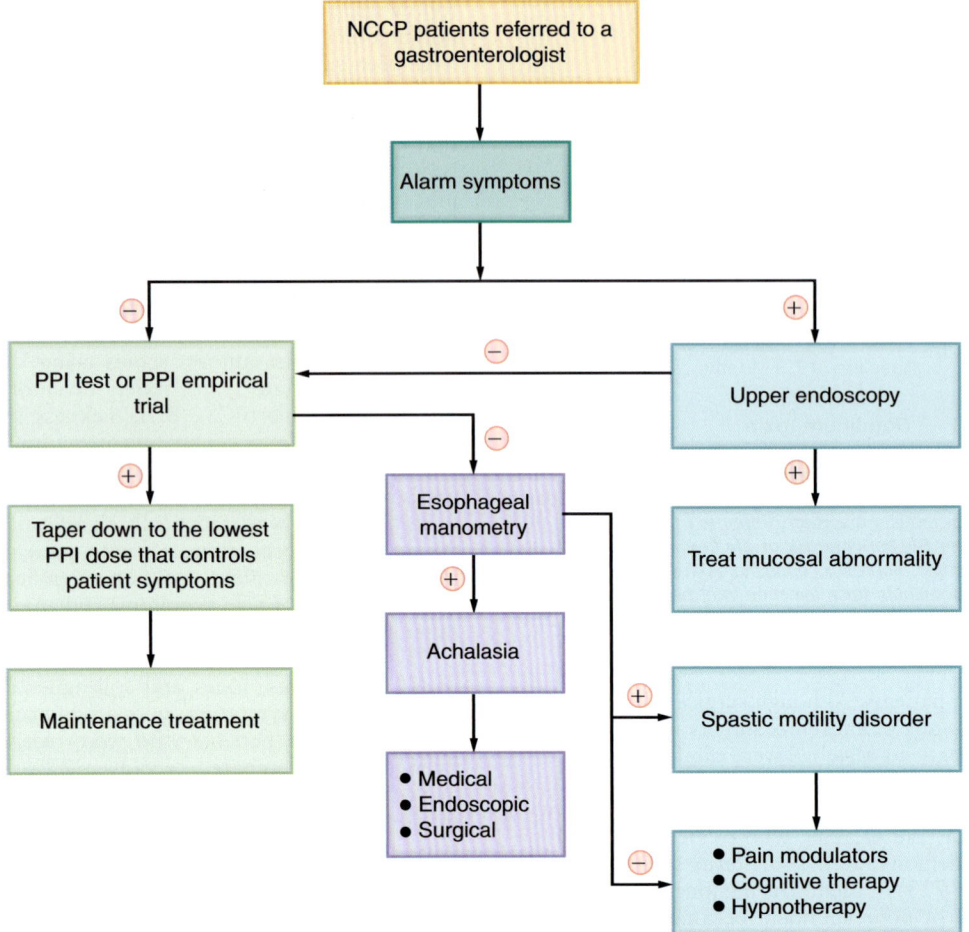

FIGURE 62.12 Proposed management algorithm for noncardiac chest pain. NCCP, noncardiac chest pain; PPI, proton pump inhibitor. *(Redrawn after George N, Abdallah J, Maradey-Romero C, et al. Review article: the current treatment of non-cardiac chest pain.* Aliment Pharmacol Ther *2016;43[2]:213–239. Copyright © 2015 John Wiley & Sons Ltd. Reprinted by permission of John Wiley & Sons, Inc.)*

from the GI tract. Phosphorylation of *N*-methyl-D-aspartate (NMDA) receptors expressed by dorsal horn neurons leads to central sensitization via an increase in their excitability and subsequent increase in receptive field size.[56] Potentially, this central sensitization may be prevented or even reversed by antagonism of NMDA receptors within the spinal cord.

Potential targets that are currently under consideration include vanilloid receptor ion channels, acid-sensing ion channels, sensory neuron-specific Na+ channels, P2X purinoceptors, cholecystokinin receptors, bradykinin and prostaglandin receptors, glutamate receptors, tachykinin, and calcitonin gene-related peptide receptors as well as peripheral opioid and cannabinoid receptors.[329,330] The peripheral opioid receptor agonists are of high interest because they may offer visceral analgesic effect without crossing the blood–brain barrier and thus affecting the CNS.

Spinal afferents, which may play a role in visceral nociception, express tachykinins that include substance P, neurokinins A and B, and neuropeptide K. Tachykinin receptor antagonists may confer a visceral analgesic effect that can be used in PPI-resistant patients. Neurokinin (NK)-1, NK-2, and NK-3 receptor antagonists were only evaluated in preclinical trials. Cholecystokinin receptor antagonists may alter visceral pain perception.[331]

Another important area that is likely to attract future attention when treating patients with NCCP is complementary and alternative therapeutic modalities that can interfere with the mind and body axis. Figure 62.12 provides a proposed management algorithm for NCCP.

References

1. Jerlock M, Welin C, Rosengren A, et al. Pain characteristics in patients with unexplained chest pain and patients with ischemic heart disease. *Eur J Cardiovasc Nurs* 2007;6:130–136.
2. Ockene IS, Shay MJ, Alpert JS, et al. Unexplained chest pain in patients with normal arteriograms. *N Engl J Med* 1980;303:1249–1252.
3. Dumville JC, MacPherson H, Griffith K, et al. Non-cardiac chest pain: a retrospective cohort study of patients who attended a Rapid Access Chest Pain Clinic. *Fam Pract* 2007;24:152–157.
4. Fass R, Achem SR. Noncardiac chest pain: epidemiology, natural course and pathogenesis. *J Neurogastroenterol Motil* 2011;17:110–123.
5. Sekhri N, Feder GS, Junghans C, et al. How effective are rapid access chest pain clinics? Prognosis of incident angina and non-cardiac chest pain in 8762 consecutive patients. *Heart* 2007;93:458–463.
6. Robertson N, Javed N, Samani N, et al. Psychological morbidity and illness appraisals of patients with cardiac and non-cardiac chest pain attending a Rapid Access Chest Pain Clinic: a longitudinal cohort study. *Heart* 2008;94:e12.
7. Aziz Q, Fass R, Gyawali CP, et al. Functional esophageal disorders. *Gastroenterology* 2016;150:1368–1379.
8. Mudipalli RS, Remes-Troche JM, Andersen L, et al. Functional chest pain: esophageal or overlapping functional disorder. *J Clin Gastroenterol* 2007;41:264–269.
9. Mourad G, Jaarsma T, Hallert C, et al. Depressive symptoms and healthcare utilization in patients with noncardiac chest pain compared to patients with ischemic heart disease. *Heart Lung* 2012;41:446–455.
10. Potokar JP, Nutt DJ. Chest pain: panic attack or heart attack? *Int J Clin Pract* 2000;54:110–114.
11. Katerndahl DA, Trammell C. Prevalence and recognition of panic states in STARNET patients presenting with chest pain. *J Fam Pract* 1997;45:54–63.
12. Locke GR III, Talley NJ, Fett SL, et al. Prevalence and clinical spectrum of gastroesophageal reflux: a population-based study in Olmstead County, Minnesota. *Gastroenterology* 1997;112:1448–1456.
13. Drossman DA, Li Z, Andruzzi E, et al. U.S. householder survey of functional gastrointestinal disorders. Prevalence, sociodemography, and health impact. *Dig Dis Sci* 1993;38:1569–1580.

14. Eslick GD. Noncardiac chest pain: epidemiology, natural history, health care seeking, and quality of life. *Gastroenterol Clin North Am* 2004;33:1–23.

15. Eslick GD, Jones MP, Talley NJ. Non-cardiac chest pain: prevalence, risk factors, impact and consulting—a population-based study. *Aliment Pharmacol Ther* 2003;17:1115–1124.

16. Chiocca JC, Olmos JA, Salis GB, et al. Prevalence, clinical spectrum and atypical symptoms of gastro-oesophageal reflux in Argentina: a nationwide population-based study. *Aliment Pharmacol Ther* 2005;22:331–342.

17. Wong WM, Lai KC, Lam KF, et al. Prevalence, clinical spectrum and health care utilization of gastro-oesophageal reflux disease in a Chinese population: a population-based study. *Aliment Pharmacol Ther* 2003;18:595–604.

18. Kennedy JW, Killip T, Fisher LD, et al. The clinical spectrum of coronary artery disease and its surgical and medical management, 1974-1979. The Coronary Artery Surgery study. *Circulation* 1982;66(5 pt 2):III16–III23.

19. Mousavi S, Tosi J, Eskandarian R, et al. Role of clinical presentation in diagnosing reflux-related non-cardiac chest pain. *J Gastroenterol Hepatol* 2007;22:218–221.

20. Tew R, Guthrie E, Creed F, et al. A long-term follow-up study of patients with ischemic heart disease versus patients with nonspecific chest pain. *J Psychosom Res* 1995;39:977–985.

21. Ford AC, Suares NC, Talley NJ. Meta-analysis: the epidemiology of noncardiac chest pain in the community. *Aliment Pharmacol Ther* 2011;34:172–180.

22. Wong WM, Risner-Adler S, Beeler J, et al. Noncardiac chest pain: the role of the cardiologist—a national survey. *J Clin Gastroenterol* 2005;39:858–862.

23. Wong WM, Beeler J, Risner-Adler S, et al. Attitudes and referral patterns of primary care physicians when evaluating subjects with noncardiac chest pain—a national survey. *Dig Dis Sci* 2005;50:656–661.

24. Eslick GD, Talley NJ. Non-cardiac chest pain: predictors of health care seeking, the types of health care professional consulted, work absenteeism and interruption of daily activities. *Aliment Pharmacol Ther* 2004;20:909–915.

25. Richter JE, Bradley LA, Castell DO. Esophageal chest pain: current controversies in pathogenesis, diagnosis, and therapy. *Ann Intern Med* 1989;110:66–78.

26. Eslick GD, Talley NJ. Non-cardiac chest pain: squeezing the life out of the Australian healthcare system? *Med J Aust* 2000;173:233–234.

27. Wielgosz AT, Fletcher RH, McCants CB, et al. Unimproved chest pain in patients with minimal or no coronary disease: a behavioral phenomenon. *Am Heart J* 1984;108:67–72.

28. Potts S, Bass CM. Psychological morbidity in patients with chest pain and normal or near-normal coronary arteries: a long-term follow-up study. *Psychol Med* 1995;25:339–347.

29. Gurevitz O, Jonas M, Boyko V, et al. Clinical profile and long-term prognosis of women < or = 50 years of age referred for coronary angiography for evaluation of chest pain. *Am J Cardiol* 2000;85:806–809.

30. Launbjerg J, Fruergaard P, Hesse B, et al. The long-term prognosis of patients with acute chest pain of various origins. *Ugeskr Laeger* 1997;159:175–179.

31. Kisely S, Guthrie E, Creed F, et al. Predictors of mortality and morbidity following admission with chest pain. *J R Coll Physicians Lond* 1997;31:177–183.

32. Karlson BW, Wiklund I, Bengtson A, et al. Prognosis, severity of symptoms, and aspects of well-being among patients in whom myocardial infarction was ruled out. *Clin Cardiol* 1994;17:427–431.

33. Hallani H, Eslick GD, Cox M, et al. Chest pain? Cause. *Lancet* 2004;363:452.

34. Ward BW, Wu WC, Richter JE, et al. Long-term follow-up of symptomatic status of patients with noncardiac chest pain: is diagnosis of esophageal etiology helpful? *Am J Gastroenterol* 1987;82:215–218.

35. Williams JF, Sontag SJ, Schnell T, et al. Non-cardiac chest pain: the long-term natural history and comparison with gastroesophageal reflux disease. *Am J Gastroenterol* 2009;104:2145–2152.

36. Leise MD, Locke GR III, Dierkhising RA, et al. Patients dismissed from the hospital with a diagnosis of noncardiac chest pain: cardiac outcomes and health care utilization. *Mayo Clin Proc* 2010;85:323–330.

37. Wilhelmsen L, Rosengren A, Hagman M, et al. "Nonspecific" chest pain associated with high long-term mortality: results from the primary prevention study in Göteborg, Sweden. *Clin Cardiol* 1998;21:477–482.

38. Eslick GD, Talley NJ. Natural history and predictors of outcome for non-cardiac chest pain: a prospective 4-year cohort study. *Neurogastroenterol Motil* 2008;20:989–997.

39. Stahl WG, Beton RR, Johnson CS, et al. Diagnosis and treatment of patients with gastroesophageal reflux and noncardiac chest pain. *South Med J* 1994;87:739–742.

40. Fass R, Fennerty MB, Ofman JJ, et al. The clinical and economic value of a short course of omeprazole in patients with noncardiac chest pain. *Gastroenterology* 1998;115:42–49.

41. Dickman R, Emmons S, Cui H, et al. The effect of a therapeutic trial of high-dose rabeprazole on symptom response of patients with non-cardiac chest pain: a randomized, double-blind, placebo-controlled, crossover trial. *Aliment Pharmacol Ther* 2005;22:547–555.

42. Bautista J, Fullerton H, Briseno M, et al. The effect of an empirical trial of high-dose lansoprazole on symptom response of patients with non-cardiac chest pain—a randomized, double-blind, placebo-controlled, crossover trial. *Aliment Pharmacol Ther* 2004;19:1123–1130.

43. Beedassy A, Katz PO, Gruber A, et al. Prior sensitization of esophageal mucosa by acid reflux predisposes to a reflux-induced chest pain. *J Clin Gastroenterol* 2000;31:121–124.

44. DeMeester TR, O'Sullivan GC, Bermudez G, et al. Esophageal function in patients with angina-type chest pain and normal coronary angiograms. *Ann Surg* 1982;196:488–498.

45. Pandak WM, Arezo S, Everett S, et al. Short course of omeprazole: a better first diagnostic approach to noncardiac chest pain than endoscopy, manometry, or 24-hour esophageal pH monitoring. *J Clin Gastroenterol* 2002;35:307–314.

46. Xia HH, Lai KC, Lam SK, et al. Symptomatic response to lansoprazole predicts abnormal acid reflux in endoscopy-negative patients with non-cardiac chest pain. *Aliment Pharmacol Ther* 2003;17:369–377.

47. Singh S, Richter JE, Hewson EG, et al. The contribution of gastroesophageal reflux to chest pain in patients with coronary artery disease. *Ann Intern Med* 1992;117:824–830.

48. Liu Y, He S, Chen Y, et al. Acid reflux in patients with coronary artery disease and refractory chest pain. *Intern Med* 2013;52:1165–1171.

49. Faybush EM, Fass R. Gastroesophageal reflux disease in noncardiac chest pain. *Gastroenterol Clin North Am* 2004;33:41–54.

50. Hsia PC, Maher KA, Lewis JH, et al. Utility of upper endoscopy in the evaluation of noncardiac chest pain. *Gastrointest Endosc* 1991;37:22–26.

51. Frøbert O, Funch-Jensen P, Jacobsen NO, et al. Upper endoscopy in patients with angina and normal coronary angiograms. *Endoscopy* 1995;27:365–370.

52. Park SH, Choi JY, Park EJ, et al. Prevalence of gastrointestinal diseases and treatment status in noncardiac chest pain patients. *Korean Circ J* 2015;45:469–472.

53. Dickman R, Mattek N, Holub J, et al. Prevalence of upper gastrointestinal tract findings in patients with noncardiac chest pain versus those with gastroesophageal reflux disease (GERD)-related symptoms: results from a national endoscopic database. *Am J Gastroenterol* 2007;102:1173–1179.

54. Smith JL, Opekun AR, Larkai E, et al. Sensitivity of the esophageal mucosa to pH in gastroesophageal reflux disease. *Gastroenterology* 1989;96:683–689.

55. Hu WH, Martin CJ, Talley NJ. Intraesophageal acid perfusion sensitizes the esophagus to mechanical distension: a Barostat study. *Am J Gastroenterol* 2000;95:2189–2194.

56. Sarkar S, Aziz Q, Woolf CJ, et al. Contribution of central sensitisation to the development of non-cardiac chest pain. *Lancet* 2000;356:1154–1159.

57. Balaban DH, Yamamoto Y, Liu J, et al. Sustained esophageal contraction: a marker of esophageal chest pain identified by intraluminal ultrasonography. *Gastroenterology* 1999;116:29–37.

58. Pehlivanov N, Liu J, Mittal RK. Sustained esophageal contraction: a motor correlate of heartburn symptom. *Am J Physiol Gastrointest Liver Physiol* 2001;281:G743–G751.

59. Dogan I, Puckett JL, Padda BS, et al. Prevalence of increased esophageal muscle thickness in patients with esophageal symptoms. *Am J Gastroenterol* 2007;102:137–145.

60. Ribolsi M, Balestrieri P, Biasutto D, et al. Role of mixed reflux and hypomotility with delayed reflux clearance in patients with non-cardiac chest pain. *J Neurogastroenterol Motil* 2016;22:606–612.

61. Kushnir VM, Sayuk GS, Gyawali CP. Abnormal GERD parameters on ambulatory pH monitoring predict therapeutic success in noncardiac chest pain. *Am J Gastroenterol* 2010;105:1032–1038.

62. Kaski JC. Cardiac syndrome X and microvascular angina. In: Kaski JC, ed. *Chest Pain with Normal Coronary Angiograms: Pathogenesis, Diagnosis and Management*. London: Kluwer Academic Publishers; 1999:1–12.

63. Kaski JC, Rosano GM, Collins P, et al. Cardiac syndrome X: clinical characteristics and left ventricular function. Long-term follow-up study. *J Am Coll Cardiol* 1995;25:807–814.

64. Kaski JC. Pathophysiology and management of patients with chest pain and normal coronary arteriograms (cardiac syndrome X). *Circulation* 2004;109:568–572.

65. Chauhan A, Petch MC, Schofield PM. Cardio-oesophageal reflex in humans as a mechanism for "linked angina." *Eur Heart J* 1996;17:407–413.

66. Rosztoczy AI, Vass A, Wittmann T, et al. Esophageal acid stimulation combined with transesophageal echocardiography shows high clinical impact in the establishment of esophago-cardiac reflex. *Gastroenterology* 2003;124(suppl 4):A534, #T1618.

67. Katz PO, Dalton CB, Richter JE, et al. Esophageal testing of patients with noncardiac chest pain or dysphagia. Results of three years' experience with 1161 patients. *Ann Intern Med* 1987;106:593–597.

68. Dekel R, Pearson T, Wendel C, et al. Assessment of oesophageal motor function in patients with dyspepsia or chest pain—the Clinical Outcomes Research Initiative experience. *Aliment Pharmacol Ther* 2003;18:1083–1089.

69. Lam HG, Dekker W, Kan G, et al. Acute noncardiac chest pain in a coronary care unit. Evaluation by 24-hour pressure and pH recording of the esophagus. *Gastroenterology* 1992;102:453–460.

70. Rencoret G, Csendes A, Henríquez A. Esophageal manometry in patients with non cardiac chest pain [in Spanish]. *Rev Med Chil* 2006;134:291–298.

71. Fass R, Navarro-Rodriguez T. Noncardiac chest pain. *J Clin Gastroenterol* 2008;42:636–646.

72. Fass R. Chest pain of esophageal origin. *Curr Opin Gastroenterol* 2002;18:464–470.

73. Peters L, Maas L, Petty D, et al. Spontaneous noncardiac chest pain. Evaluation by 24-hour ambulatory esophageal motility and pH monitoring. *Gastroenterology* 1988;94:878–886.

74. Breumelhof R, Nadorp JH, Akkermans LM, et al. Analysis of 24-hour esophageal pressure and pH data in unselected patients with noncardiac chest pain. *Gastroenterology* 1990;99:1257–1264.

75. Achem SR, Kolts BE, Wears R, et al. Chest pain associated with nutcracker esophagus: a preliminary study of the role of gastroesophageal reflux. *Am J Gastroenterol* 1993;88:187–192.

76. DiMarino AJ Jr, Allen ML, Lynn RB, et al. Clinical value of esophageal motility testing. *Dig Dis* 1998;16:198–204.

77. Lembo AJ. Visceral hypersensitivity in noncardiac chest pain. *Gastroenterol Clin North Am* 2004;33:55–60.

78. Hollerbach S, Bulat R, May A, et al. Abnormal cerebral processing of oesophageal stimuli in patients with noncardiac chest pain (NCCP). *Neurogastroenterol Motil* 2000;12:555–565.

79. Fass R, Naliboff B, Higa L, et al. Differential effect of long-term esophageal acid exposure on mechanosensitivity and chemosensitivity in humans. *Gastroenterology* 1998;115:1363–1373.

80. Handwerker HO, Reeh PW. Nociceptors: chemosensitivity and sensitization by chemical agents. In: Willis WD Jr, ed. *Hyperalgesia and Allodynia.* New York: Raven Press; 1992:107.

81. Barish CF, Castell DO, Richter JE. Graded esophageal balloon distention. A new provocative test for noncardiac chest pain. *Dig Dis Sci* 1986;31:1292–1298.

82. Kindt S, Van Oudenhove L, Broekaert D, et al. Immune dysfunction in patients with functional gastrointestinal disorders. *Neurogastroenterol Motil* 2009;21:389–398.

83. Lee H, Chung H, Park JC, et al. Heterogeneity of mucosal mast cell infiltration in subgroups of patients with esophageal chest pain. *Neurogastroenterol Motil* 2014;26:786–793.

84. Richter JE, Barish CF, Castell DO. Abnormal sensory perception in patients with esophageal chest pain. *Gastroenterology* 1986;91:845–852.

85. Rao SS, Gregersen H, Hayek B, et al. Unexplained chest pain: the hypersensitive, hyperreactive, and poorly compliant esophagus. *Ann Intern Med* 1996;124:950–958.

86. Rao SS, Hayek B, Summers RW. Functional chest pain of esophageal origin: hyperalgesia or motor dysfunction. *Am J Gastroenterol* 2001;96:2584–2589.

87. Börjesson M, Pilhall M, Eliasson T, et al. Esophageal visceral pain sensitivity: effects of TENS and correlation with manometric findings. *Dig Dis Sci* 1998;43:1621–1628.

88. Mehta AJ, De Caestecker JS, Camm AJ, et al. Sensitization to painful distension and abnormal sensory perception in the esophagus. *Gastroenterology* 1995;108:311–319.

89. Sarkar S, Thompson DG, Woolf CJ, et al. Patients with chest pain and occult gastroesophageal reflux demonstrate visceral pain hypersensitivity which may be partially responsive to acid suppression. *Am J Gastroenterol* 2004;99:1998–2006.

90. Mujica VR, Mudipalli RS, Rao SS. Pathophysiology of chest pain in patients with nutcracker esophagus. *Am J Gastroenterol* 2001;96:1371–1377.

91. Nasr I, Attaluri A, Hashmi S, et al. Investigation of esophageal sensation and biomechanical properties in functional chest pain. *Neurogastroenterol Motil* 2010;22:520–526.

92. Hoff DA, Gregersen H, Ødegaard S, et al. Sensation evoked by esophageal distension in functional chest pain patients depends on mechanical stress rather than on ischemia. *Neurogastroenterol Motil* 2010;22:1170–1176.

93. Tougas G, Spaziani R, Hollerbach S, et al. Cardiac autonomic function and oesophageal acid sensitivity in patients with non-cardiac chest pain. *Gut* 2001;49:706–712.

94. Tougas G. The autonomic nervous system in functional bowel disorders. *Gut* 2000;47:iv78–iv80.

95. Bass C, Wade C, Hand D, et al. Patients with angina with normal and near normal coronary arteries: clinical and psychosocial state 12 months after angiography. *Br Med J (Clin Res Ed)* 1983;287:1505–1508.

96. Bass C, Wade C. Chest pain with normal coronary arteries: a comparative study of psychiatric and social morbidity. *Psychol Med* 1984;14:51–61.

97. Channer KS, Papouchado M, James MA, et al. Anxiety and depression in patients with chest pain referred for exercise testing. *Lancet* 1985;2:820–823.

98. Costa PT Jr. Influence of the normal personality dimension of neuroticism on chest pain symptoms and coronary artery disease. *Am J Cardiol* 1987;60:20J–26J.

99. McCroskery JH, Schell RE, Sprafkin RP, et al. Differentiating anginal patients with coronary artery disease from those with normal coronary arteries using psychological measures. *Am J Cardiol* 1991;67:645–646.

100. Flugelman MY, Weisstub E, Galun E, et al. Clinical, psychological and thallium stress studies in patients with chest pain and normal coronary arteries. *Int J Cardiol* 1991;33:401–408.

101. Mayou R, Bryant B, Forfar C, et al. Non-cardiac chest pain and benign palpitations in the cardiac clinic. *Br Heart J* 1994;72:548–553.

102. Chignon JM, Lepine JP, Ades J. Panic disorder in cardiac outpatients. *Am J Psychiatry* 1993;150:780–785.

103. Tennant C, Mihailidou A, Scott A, et al. Psychological symptom profiles in patients with chest pain. *J Psychosom Res* 1994;38:365–371.

104. Wong WM, Lam KF, Cheng C, et al. Population based study of noncardiac chest pain in southern Chinese: prevalence, psychosocial factors and health care utilization. *World J Gastroenterol* 2004;10:707–712.

105. Clouse RE, Lustman PJ. Psychiatric illness and contraction abnormalities of the esophagus. *N Engl J Med* 1983;309:1337–1432.

106. Cannon RO III, Benjamin SB. Chest pain as a consequence of abnormal visceral nociception. *Dig Dis Sci* 1993;38:193–196.

107. Fleet RP, Dupuis G, Marchand A, et al. Panic disorder in emergency department chest pain patients: prevalence, comorbidity, suicidal ideation, and physician recognition. *Am J Med* 1996;101:371–380.

108. Demiryoguran NS, Karcioglu O, Topacoglu H, et al. Anxiety disorder in patients with non-specific chest pain in the emergency setting. *Emerg Med J* 2006;23:99–102.

109. Jones M, Lewis A. Effort syndrome. *Lancet* 1941;237:813–818.

110. Huffman JC, Pollack MH. Predicting panic disorder among patients with chest pain: an analysis of the literature. *Psychosomatics* 2003;44:222–236.

111. Alexander PJ, Prabhu SG, Krishnamoorthy ES, et al. Mental disorders in patients with noncardiac chest pain. *Acta Psychiatr Scand* 1994;89:291–293.

112. Carter CS, Maddock RJ. Chest pain in generalized anxiety disorder. *Int J Psychiatry Med* 1992;22:291–298.

113. Dammen T, Ekeberg O, Arnesen H, et al. Personality profiles in patients referred for chest pain. Investigation with emphasis on panic disorder patients. *Psychosomatics* 2000;41:269–276.

114. Husser D, Bollmann A, Kühne C, et al. Evaluation of noncardiac chest pain: diagnostic approach, coping strategies and quality of life. *Eur J Pain* 2006;10:51–55.

115. Stollman NH, Bierman PS, Ribeiro A, et al. CO2 provocation of panic: symptomatic and manometric evaluation in patients with noncardiac chest pain. *Am J Gastroenterol* 1997;92:839–842.

116. Cooke RA, Anggiansah A, Wang J, et al. Hyperventilation and esophageal dysmotility in patients with noncardiac chest pain. *Am J Gastroenterol* 1996;91:480–484.

117. Lantinga LJ, Sprafkin RP, McCroskery JH, et al. One-year psychosocial follow-up of patients with chest pain and angiographically normal coronary arteries. *Am J Cardiol* 1988;62:209–213.

118. Hotopf M, Mayou R, Wadsworth M, et al. Psychosocial and development antecedents of chest pain in young adults. *Psychosom Med* 1999;61:861–867.

119. Dammen T, Arnesen H, Ekeberg O, et al. Psychological factors, pain attribution and medical morbidity in chest-pain patients with and without coronary artery disease. *Gen Hosp Psychiatry* 2004;26:463–469.

120. Katon W, Hall ML, Russo J, et al. Chest pain: relationship to psychiatric illness to coronary arteriographic results. *Am J Med* 1988;84:1–9.

121. Eken C, Oktay C, Bacanli A, et al. Anxiety and depressive disorders in patients presenting with chest pain to the emergency department: a comparison between cardiac and non-cardiac origin. *J Emerg Med* 2010;39:144–150.

122. Cheung TK, Hou X, Lam KF, et al. Quality of life and psychological impact in patients with noncardiac chest pain. *J Clin Gastroenterol* 2009;43:13–18.

123. Cormier LE, Katon W, Russo J, et al. Chest pain with negative cardiac diagnostic studies. Relationship to psychiatric illness. *J Nerv Ment Dis* 1988;176:351–358.

124. García-Campayo J, Rosel F, Serrano P, et al. Different psychological profiles in non-cardiac chest pain and coronary artery disease: a controlled study. *Rev Esp Cardiol* 2010;63:357–361.

125. Beitman BD, Basha I, Flaker G, et al. Atypical or nonanginal chest pain. Panic disorder or coronary artery disease? *Arch Intern Med* 1987;147:1548–1552.

126. Cheng C, Wong WM, Lai KC, et al. Psychosocial factors in patients with noncardiac chest pain. *Psychosom Med* 2003;65:443–449.

127. Jerlock M, Kjellgren KI, Gaston-Johansson F, et al. Psychosocial profile in men and women with unexplained chest pain. *J Intern Med* 2008;264:265–274.

128. Fagring AJ, Gaston-Johannson F, Kjellgren KI, et al. Unexplained chest pain in relation to psychosocial factors and health-related quality of life in men and women. *Eur J Cardiovasc Nurs* 2007;6:329–336.

129. Nevens F, Janssens J, Piessens J, et al. Prospective study on prevalence of esophageal chest pain in patients referred on an elective basis to a cardiac unit for suspected myocardial ischemia. *Dig Dis Sci* 1991;36:229–235.

130. Richter JE. Chest pain and gastroesophageal reflux disease. *J Clin Gastroenterol* 2000;30:S39–S41.

131. Eslick GD. Usefulness of chest pain character and location as diagnostic indicators of an acute coronary syndrome. *Am J Cardiol* 2005;95:1228–1231.

132. Fenster PE. Evaluation of chest pain: a cardiology perspective for gastroenterologists. *Gastroenterol Clin North Am* 2004;33:35–40.

133. Battaglia E, Bassotti G, Buonafede G, et al. Noncardiac chest pain of esophageal origin in patients with and without coronary artery disease. *Hepatogastroenterology* 2005;52:792–795.

134. Johnston BT, Troshinsky MB, Castell JA, et al. Comparison of barium radiology with esophageal pH monitoring in the diagnosis of gastroesophageal reflux disease. *Am J Gastroenterol* 1996;91:1181–1185.

135. Eslick GD, Fass R. Noncardiac chest pain: evaluation and treatment. *Gastroenterol Clin North Am* 2003;32:531–552.

136. Browning TH. Diagnosis of chest pain of esophageal origin. A guideline of the Patient Care Committee of the American Gastroenterological Association. *Dig Dis Sci* 1990;35:289–293.

137. García-Compeán D, González MV, Galindo G, et al. Prevalence of gastroesophageal reflux disease in patients with extraesophageal symptoms referred from otolaryngology, allergy, and cardiology practices: a prospective study. *Dig Dis Sci* 2000;18:178–182.

138. Wong WM, Lai KC, Lau CP, et al. Upper gastrointestinal evaluation of Chinese patients with non-cardiac chest pain. *Aliment Pharmacol Ther* 2002;16:465–471.

139. Canavan JB, Grainger RJ, Murray FE, et al. The diagnostic value of endoscopy in evaluating non-cardiac chest pain. *Gastrointest Endosc* 2005;61:AB128.

140. Gibbs JF, Rajput A, Chadha KS, et al. The changing profile of esophageal cancer presentation and its implication for diagnosis. *JAMA* 2007;99:620–626.

141. Fass R, Ofman JJ, Sampliner RE, et al. The omeprazole test is as sensitive as 24-h oesophageal pH monitoring in diagnosing gastro-oesophageal reflux disease in symptomatic patients with erosive oesophagitis. *Aliment Pharmacol Ther* 2000;14:389–396.

142. Fass R, Fennerty MB, Johnson C, et al. Correlation of ambulatory 24-hour esophageal pH monitoring results with symptom improvement in patients with noncardiac chest pain due to gastroesophageal reflux disease. *J Clin Gastroenterol* 1999;28:36–39.

143. Zerbib F, Roman S, Ropert A, et al. Esophageal pH impedance monitoring and symptom analysis in GERD: a study in patients off and on therapy. *Am J Gastroenterol* 2006;101:1956–1963.

144. Fass R, Sifrim D. Management of heartburn not responding to proton pump inhibitors. *Gut* 2009;58:295–309.

145. Spencer J. Prolonged pH recording in the study of gastroesophageal reflux. *Br J Surg* 1969;56:912–914.

146. Pandolfino JE, Richter JE, Ourts T, et al. Ambulatory esophageal pH monitoring using a wireless system. *Am J Gastroenterol* 2003;98:740–749.

147. Wong WM, Bautista J, Dekel R, et al. Feasibility and tolerability of transnasal/per-oral placement of the wireless pH capsule vs. traditional 24-h oesophageal pH monitoring—a randomized trial. *Aliment Pharmacol Ther* 2005;21:155–163.

148. Prakash C, Clouse RE. Wireless pH monitoring in patients with non-cardiac chest pain. *Am J Gastroenterol* 2006;101:446–452.

149. Hirano I, Richter JE. Practice Parameters Committee of the American College of Gastroenterology. ACG practice guidelines: esophageal reflux testing. *Am J Gastroenterol* 2007;102:668–685.

150. Prakash C, Jonnalagadda S, Azar R, et al. Endoscopic removal of the wireless pH monitoring capsule in patients with severe discomfort. *Gastrointest Endosc* 2006;64:828–832.

151. Schindlbeck NE, Klauser AG, Voderholzer WA, et al. Empiric therapy for gastroesophageal reflux disease. *Arch Intern Med* 1995;155:1808–1812.

152. Johnsson F, Weywadt L, Solhaug J, et al. One-week omeprazole treatment in the diagnosis of gastrooesophageal reflux disease. *Scand J Gastroenterol* 1998;33:15–20.

153. Fass R, Ofman JJ, Gralnek IM, et al. Clinical and economic assessment of the omeprazole test in patients with symptoms suggestive of gastroesophageal reflux disease. *Arch Intern Med* 1999;150:2161–2168.

154. Bate C, Riley S, Chapman R, et al. Evaluation of omeprazole as a cost-effective diagnostic test for gastro-oesophageal reflux disease. *Aliment Pharmacol Ther* 1999;13:59–66.

155. Juul-Hansen P, Rydning A, Jacobsen C, et al. High-dose proton-pump inhibitors as a diagnostic test of gastroesophageal reflux disease in endoscopy-negative patients. *Scand J Gastroenterol* 2001;36:806–810.

156. Squillace SJ, Young MF, Sanowski RA. Abstract: single dose omeprazole as a test for noncardiac chest pain. *Gastroenterology* 1993;107:A197.

157. Young MF, Sanowski RA, Talbert GA, et al. Omeprazole administration as a test for gastroesophageal reflux [abstract]. *Gastroenterology* 1992;102:192.

158. Fass R. Empirical trials in treatment of gastroesophageal reflux disease. *Dig Dis* 2000;18:20–26.

159. Metz D, Childs M, Ruiz C, et al. Pilot study of the oral omeprazole test of reflux laryngitis. *Otolaryngol Head Neck Surg* 1997;116:41–46.

160. Ours T, Kavuru M, Schilz R, et al. A prospective evaluation of esophageal testing and a double-blind, randomized study of omeprazole in a diagnostic and therapeutic algorithm for chronic cough. *Am J Gastroenterol* 1999;94:3131–3138.

161. Jaspersen D, Diehl K, Geyer P, et al. Diagnostic omeprazole test in suspected reflux-associated chronic cough. *Pneumologie* 1999;53:438–441.

162. Kiljander T, Salomaa E, Heitanen E, et al. Chronic cough and gastro-oesophageal reflux: a double-blind placebo-controlled study with omeprazole. *Eur Respir J* 2000;16:633–638.

163. Maev IV, Iurenev GL, Burkov SG, et al. Rabeprazole test and comparison of the effectiveness of course treatment with rabeprazole in patients with gastroesophageal reflux disease and non-coronary chest pain [in Russian]. *Klin Med (Mosk)* 2007;85:45–51.

164. Fass R, Pulliam G, Hayden CW. Patients with noncardiac chest pain (NCCP) receiving an empirical trial of high dose rabeprazole, demonstrate early symptom response—a double blind, placebo-controlled trial [abstract]. *Gastroenterology* 2001;129:1162.

165. Fass R, Fullerton H, Hayden CW, et al. Patients with noncardiac chest pain (NCCP) receiving an empirical trial of high dose rabeprazole, demonstrate early symptom response—a double blind, placebo-controlled trial [abstract]. *Gastroenterology* 2002;122:(A-221):11620.

166. Cremonini F, Wise J, Moayyedi P, et al. Diagnostic and therapeutic use of proton pump inhibitors in noncardiac chest pain: a meta-analysis. *Am J Gastroenterol* 2005;100:1226–1232.

167. Wang W, Huang J, Zheng G, et al. Is proton pump inhibitor testing an effective approach to diagnose gastroesophageal reflux disease in patients with noncardiac chest pain? *Arch Intern Med* 2005;165:1222–1228.

168. Wertli MM, Ruchti KB, Steurer J, et al. Diagnostic indicators of non-cardiovascular chest pain: a systematic review and meta-analysis. *BMC Med* 2013;11:239.

169. Ofman JJ, Gralnek IM, Udani J, et al. The cost-effectiveness of the omeprazole test in patients with noncardiac chest pain. *Am J Med* 1999;107:219–227.

170. Savarino E, Tutuian R. Combined multichannel intraluminal impedance and manometry testing. *Dig Liver Dis* 2008;40:167–173.

171. Herregods MC, Bredenoord AH, Oors JM, et al. Determinants of the association between non-cardiac chest pain and reflux. *Am J Gastroenterol* 2017;112:1671–1677.

172. Azpiroz F, Malagelada JR. Physiological variations in canine gastric tone measured by electronic barostat. *Am J Physiol* 1985;248:G229–G237.

173. Clouse RE, Lustman PJ, Eckert TC, et al. Low-dose trazodone for symptomatic patients with esophageal contraction abnormalities. A double-blind, placebo-controlled trial. *Gastroenterology* 1987;92:1027–1036.

174. Fass R, Winters GF. Evaluation of the patient with noncardiac chest pain: is gastroesophageal reflux disease or an esophageal motility disorder the cause? *Medscape Gastroenterol* 2001;3:1–10.

175. Richter JE, Dalton CB, Bradley LA, et al. Oral nifedipine in the treatment of noncardiac chest pain in patients with the nutcracker esophagus. *Gastroenterology* 1987;93:21–28.

176. Kahrilas PJ. Nutcracker esophagus: an idea whose time has gone? *Am J Gastroenterol* 1993;88:167–169.

177. MacKenzie J, Belch J, Land D, et al. Oesophageal ischaemia in motility disorders associated with chest pain. *Lancet* 1988;2:592–595.

178. Liebermann-Meffert DM, Luescher U, Neff U, et al. Esophagectomy without thoracotomy: is there a risk of intramediastinal bleeding? A study on blood supply of the esophagus. *Ann Surg* 1987;206:184–192.

179. Eckardt VF, Stauf B, Bernhard G. Chest pain in achalasia: patient characteristics and clinical course. *Gastroenterology* 1999;116:1300–1304.

180. Camacho-Lobato L, Katz PO, Eveland J, et al. Vigorous achalasia: original description requires minor change. *J Clin Gastroenterol* 2001;33:375–377.

181. Perretta S, Fisichella PM, Galvani C, et al. Achalasia and chest pain: effect of laparoscopic Heller myotomy. *J Gastrointest Surg* 2003;7:595–598.

182. Kahrilas PJ, Ghosh SK, Pandolfino JE. Challenging the limits of esophageal manometry. *Gastroenterology* 2008;134:16–18.

183. Akinsiku O, Yamasaki T, Brunner S, et al. High resolution vs conventional esophageal manometry in the assessment of esophageal motor disorders in patients with noncardiac chest pain [published online ahead of print December 29, 2017]. *Neurogastroenterol Motil.* doi:10.1111/nmo.13282.

184. Barret M, Herregods TV, Smout AJ, et al. Diagnostic yield of 24-hour esophageal manometry in non-cardiac chest pain. *Neurogastroenterol Motil* 2016;28:1186–1193.

185. London RL, Ouyang A, Snape WJ Jr, et al. Provocation of esophageal pain by ergonovine or edrophonium. *Gastroenterology* w1981;81:10–14.

186. Nostrant TT. Provocation testing in noncardiac chest pain. *Am J Med* 1992;92:56S–64S.

187. Dekel R, Martinez-Hawthorne SD, Guillen RJ, et al. Evaluation of symptom index in identifying gastroesophageal reflux disease-related noncardiac chest pain. *J Clin Gastroenterol* 2004;38:24–29.

188. Lee CA, Reynolds JC, Ouyang A, et al. Esophageal chest pain. Value of high-dose provocative testing with edrophonium chloride in patients with normal esophageal manometries. *Dig Dis Sci* 1987;32:682–688.

189. Richter J, Dalton C, Buice R, et al. Nifedipine: a potent inhibitor of contractions in the body of the human esophagus. Studies in healthy volunteers and patients with the nutcracker esophagus. *Gastroenterology* 1985;89:549–554.

190. Gebhart GF, Bielefeldt K. Visceral pain. In: Bushnell MC, Basbaum AI, eds. *Pain*. San Diego, CA: Academic Press; 2008:543–570. *The Senses: A Comprehensive Reference*; vol 5.

191. Goyal RK, Hirano I. The enteric nervous system. *N Engl J Med* 1996;334:1106–1115.

192. Grundy D, Scratcherd T. Sensory afferents from the gastrointestinal tract. In: Schultz SG, Wood JD, Rauner BB, eds. *Handbook of Physiology*. New York: Oxford University; 1989:593–620.

193. Randich A. Visceral nerve stimulation and pain modulation. In: Johsn LR, ed. *Physiology of the Gastrointestinal Tract*. 3rd ed. Amsterdam, The Netherlands: Elsevier; 1993:126–139.

194. Tougas G, Fitzpatrick D, Upton ARM, et al. The cortical evoked responses produced by balloon distention and electrical stimulation of the esophagus involve different vagal fibers [abstract]. *Gastroenterology* 1993;104.

195. Mayer EA, Gebhart GF. Basic and clinical aspects of visceral hyperalgesia. *Gastroenterology* 1994;107:271–293.

196. Fass R, Malagon I, Schmulson M. Chest pain of esophageal origin. *Curr Opin Gastroenterol* 2001;17:376–380.

197. Rodrigo J, Hernandez CJ, Vidal MA, et al. Vegetative innervation of the esophagus. III. Intraepithelial endings. *Acta Anat (Basel)* 1975;92:242–285.

198. Fass R, Tougas G. Functional heartburn—the stimulus, the pain and the brain. *Gut* 2002;51:885–892.

199. Aziz Q, Andersson JL, Valind S, et al. Identification of human brain loci processing esophageal sensation using positron emission tomography. *Gastroenterology* 1997;113:50–59.

200. Fass R, Naliboff BD, Fass SS, et al. The effect of auditory stress on perception of intraesophageal acid in patients with GERD. *Gastroenterology* 2008;134:696–705.

201. Schey R, Dickman R, Parthasarathy S, et al. Sleep deprivation is hyperalgesic in patients with gastroesophageal reflux disease. *Gastroenterology* 2007;133:1787–1795.

202. Fass R, Malagon I, Pulliam G, et al. Gender differences in perceptual and emotional ratings of intra-esophageal stimuli in GERD patients undergoing auditory-induced stress [abstract]. *Gastroenterology* 2002;122:A187.

203. Kern MK, Birn RM, Jaradeh S, et al. Identification and characterization of cerebral cortical response to esophageal mucosal acid exposure and distention. *Gastroenterology* 1998;115:1353–1362.

204. Takeda T, Liu J, Gui A, et al. Heartburn not chest pain, is the most common symptoms in response to esophageal distension in normal subjects [abstract]. *Gastroenterology* 2001;120(suppl 5):A-222, #1167.

205. Baldi F, Ferrarini F, Longanesi A, et al. Acid gastroesophageal reflux and symptom occurrence. Analysis of some factors influencing their association. *Dig Dis Sci* 1989;34:1890–1893.

206. Meyer JH, Lembo AJ, Elashoff JD, et al. Duodenal fat intensifies the perception of heartburn. *Gut* 2001;49:624–628.

207. Fass R. Focused clinical review—nonerosive reflux disease. *Medscape Gastroenterol* 2001;3:1–13.

208. Trimble KC, Pryde A, Heading RC. Lowered oesophageal sensory thresholds in patients with symptomatic but not excess gastro-oesophageal reflux: evidence for a spectrum of visceral sensitivity in GORD. *Gut* 1995;37:7–12.

209. Mayer EA. The neurobiology of stress and gastrointestinal disease. *Gut* 2000;47:861–869.

210. Bernstein LM, Baker LA. A clinical test for esophagitis. *Gastroenterology* 1958;34:760–781.

211. Hewson EG, Sinclair JW, Dalton CB, et al. Twenty-four-hour esophageal pH monitoring: the most useful test for evaluation of noncardiac chest pain. *Am J Med* 1991;90:576–583.

212. Bernot R, Norton RA. The esophageal acid perfusion test. *Lahey Clin Found Bull* 1965;14:58–63.

213. Fisher RS, Cohen S. Gastroesophageal reflux. *Med Clin North Am* 1978; 62:3–20.

214. Breen KJ, Whelan G. The diagnosis of reflux oesophagitis: an evaluation of five investigative procedures. *Aust N Z J Surg* 1978;48:156–161.

215. Behar J, Biancani P, Sheahan DG. Evaluation of esophageal tests in the diagnosis of reflux esophagitis. *Gastroenterology* 1976;71:9–15.

216. Battle WS, Nyhus LM, Bombeck CT. Gastroesophageal reflux: diagnosis and treatment. *Ann Surg* 1973;177:560–565.

217. Howard PJ, Maher L, Pryde A, et al. Symptomatic gastro-oesophageal reflux, abnormal oesophageal acid exposure, and mucosal acid sensitivity are three separate, though related, aspects of gastro-oesophageal reflux disease. *Gut* 1991;32:128–132.

218. Kaul B, Petersen H, Grette K, et al. The acid perfusion test in gastroesophageal reflux disease. *Scand J Gastroenterol* 1986;21:93–96.

219. Price SF, Smithson KW, Castell DO. Food sensitivity in reflux esophagitis. *Gastroenterology* 1986;75:240–243.

220. Bachir GS, Leigh-Collis J, Wilson P, et al. Diagnosis of incipient reflux esophagitis: a new test. *South Med J* 1981;74:1072–1074.

221. Johnson DA, Winters C, Spurling TJ, et al. Esophageal acid sensitivity in Barrett's esophagus. *J Clin Gastroenterol* 1987;9:23–27.

222. Gracely RH, McGrath F, Dubner R. Ratio scales of sensory and affective verbal pain descriptors. *Pain* 1978;5:5–18.

223. Silverman DH, Munakata JA, Ennes H, et al. Regional cerebral activity in normal and pathological perception of visceral pain. *Gastroenterology* 1997;112:64–72.

224. Vantrappen G, Janssens J, Ghillebert G. The irritable oesophagus—a frequent cause of angina-like pain. *Lancet* 1987;1:1232–1234.

225. Hewson EG, Dalton CB, Richter JE. Comparison of esophageal manometry, provocative testing, and ambulatory monitoring in patients with unexplained chest pain. *Dig Dis Sci* 1990;35:302–309.

226. Ghillebert G, Janssens J, Vantrappen G, et al. Ambulatory 24 hour intraesophageal pH and pressure recordings versus provocation tests in the diagnosis of chest pain of oesophageal origin. *Gut* 1990;31:738–744.

227. De Caestecker JS, Pryde A, Heading RC. Comparison of intravenous edrophonium and oesophageal acid perfusion during oesophageal manometry in patients with non-cardiac chest pain. *Gut* 1988;29:1029–1034.

228. Richter JE. Provocative tests in esophageal diseases. In: Scarpignato C, Galmiche JP, eds. *Functional Evaluation in Esophageal Diseases*. Basel, Switzerland: Karger; 1994.

229. Hewson EG, Sinclair JW, Dalton CB, et al. Acid perfusion test: does it have a role in the assessment of non cardiac chest pain? *Gut* 1989;30:305–310.

230. Hollerbach S, Klamath MV, Fitzpatrick D, et al. The cerebral response to electrical stimuli in the oesophagus is altered by increasing stimulus frequencies. *Neurogastroenterol Motil* 1997;9:129–139.

231. Tougas G, Hudoba P, Fitzpatrick D, et al. Cerebral-invoked potential responses following direct vagal and esophageal electrical stimulation in humans. *Am J Physiol* 1993;294:G486–G491.

232. Nguyen HN, Silny J, Matern S. Multiple intraluminal electrical impedancometry for recording of upper gastrointestinal motility: current results and further implications. *Am J Gastroenterol* 1999;94:306–317.

233. Heft MW, Parker SR. An experimental basis for revising the graphic rating scale for pain. *Pain* 1984;19:153–161.

234. Takeda T, Kssab G, Liu J, et al. A novel ultrasound technique to study the biomechanics of the human esophagus in vivo. *Am J Physiol Gastrointest Liver Physiol* 2002;282:G785–G793.

235. Ritchie J. Pain from distention of the pelvic colon by inflating a balloon in the irritable colon syndrome. *Gut* 1973;14:125–132.

236. Mertz H, Walsh JH, Sytnik B, et al. The effect of octreotide on human gastric compliance and sensory perception. *Neurogastroenterol Motil* 1995;7:175–185.

237. Kramer P, Hollander W. Comparison of experimental esophageal pain with clinical pain of angina pectoris and esophageal disease. *Gastroenterology* 1955;29:719–743.

238. Lipkin M, Sleisenger MH. Studies of visceral pain: measurements of stimulus intensity and duration associated with the onset of pain in esophagus, ileum, and colon. *J Clin Invest* 1958;37:28–34.

239. Yakshe PN, Tong LJ, Andreini SJ, et al. Does provocative esophageal testing influence coronary blood flow or coronary flow reserve? Preliminary results of concurrent esophageal and cardiac testing [abstract]. *Gastroenterology* 1993;104:A227.

240. Whitehead WE, Delvaux M, Team TW. Standardization of barostat procedures for testing smooth muscle tone and sensory thresholds in the gastrointestinal tract. *Dig Dis Sci* 1997;42:223–241.

241. Toma TD, Zighelboim J, Phillips SF, et al. Methods for studying intestinal sensitivity and compliance: in vitro studies of balloons and a barostat. *Neurogastroenterol Motil* 1996;8:19–28.

242. Khan MI, Feinle C, Read DW. Investigating gastric and sensory response to distention: comparative studies using flaccid bags and latex balloons. *2nd United European Gastroenterology Meeting* 1992:13:175.

243. Sun WM, Read NW, Prior A, et al. Sensory and motor responses to rectal distention vary according to rate and pattern of balloon inflation. *Gastroenterology* 1990;99:1008–1015.

244. Munakata J, Naliboff B, Harraf F, et al. Repetitive sigmoid stimulation induces rectal hyperalgesia in patients with irritable bowel syndrome. *Gastroenterology* 1997;112:55–63.

245. Whitehead WE, Crowell MD, Shone D, et al. Sensitivity to rectal distention: validation of a measurement system [abstract]. *Gastroenterology* 1993;104:A600.

246. Lembo T, Niazi M, Mayer EA. Do mucosal mechanoreceptors contribute to rectal hyperalgesia in IBS patients? [abstract]. *Gastroenterology* 1993; 104:A540.

247. Pehlivanov M, Liu J, Mittal R. Sustained esophageal contraction: a motor correlate of heartburn symptom [abstract]. *Gastroenterology* 1999;116:A1062.

248. Nguyen P, Castell DO. Stimulation of esophageal mechanoreceptors is dependent on rate and duration of distention. *Am J Physiol* 1994;267:G115–G118.

249. Lasch H, Castell DO, Castell JA. Evidence of diminished visceral pain with aging: studies using graded intraesophageal balloon distention. *Am J Physiol* 1997;272:G1–G3.

250. Fass R, Pulliam G, Johnson C, et al. Symptom severity and oesophageal chemosensitivity to acid in older and young patients with gastro-oesophageal reflux. *Age Aging* 2000;29:125–130.

251. Nguyen P, Lee SD, Castell DO. Evidence of gender differences in esophageal pain threshold. *Am J Gastroenterol* 1995;90:901–905.

252. Niemantsverdriet EC, Timmer R, Breumelhof R, et al. Regional differences in esophageal acid sensitivity studied with pH-controlled segmental acid perfusion [abstract]. *Gastroenterology* 1997;112:A237.

253. Grade A, Pulliam G, Johnson C, et al. Reduced chemoreceptor sensitivity in patients with Barrett's esophagus may be related to age and not to the presence of Barrett's epithelium. *Am J Gastroenterol* 1997;92:2040–2043.

254. Winwood PJ, Mavrogiannis CC, Smith CL. Reduced sensitivity to intra-oesophageal acid in patients with reflux-induced strictures. *Scand J Gastroenterol* 1993;28:109–112.

255. Clouse RE, McCord GS, Lustman PJ, et al. Clinical correlates of abnormal sensitivity to intraesophageal balloon distention. *Dig Dis Sci* 1991;36: 1040–1045.

256. Garrison DW, Chandler MJ, Foreman RD. Viscerosomatic convergence onto feline spinal neurons from esophagus, heart and somatic fields: effects of inflammation. *Pain* 1992;49:373–382.

257. DeVault KR. Acid infusion does not affect intraesophageal balloon distention-induced sensory and pain thresholds. *Am J Gastroenterol* 1997;92:947–949.

258. Sarkar S, Woolf CJ, Aziz Q, et al. Secondary hyperalgesia is induced by acid in the healthy human oesophagus [abstract]. *Gut* 1997;41:A26.

259. Peghini PL, Katz PO, Castell DO. Imipramine decreases oesophageal pain perception in human male volunteers. *Gut* 1998;42:807–813.

260. Cannon RO III, Quyyumi AA, Mincemoyer R, et al. Imipramine in patients with chest pain despite normal coronary angiograms. *N Engl J Med* 1994;330:1411–1417.

261. Castell DO, Wood JD, Frieling T, et al. Cerebral electrical potentials evoked by balloon distension of the human esophagus. *Gastroenterology* 1990;98:662–666.

262. DeVault KR. Nifedipine does not alter barostat determined esophageal smooth muscle tone [abstract]. *Gastroenterology* 1995;108:A591.

263. Nasr I, Attaluri A, Coss-Adame E, et al. Diagnostic utility of the oesophageal balloon distension test in the evaluation of oesophageal chest pain. *Aliment Pharmacol Ther* 2012;35:1474–1481.

264. Smout AJ, DeVore MS, Dalton CB, et al. Effects of nifedipine on esophageal tone and perception of esophageal distension. *Dig Dis Sci* 1992;37:598–602.

265. DeVault KR. Provocative tests for pain of esophageal origin. In: Castell DO, Richter JE, eds. *The Esophagus*. 3rd ed. Philadelphia: Lippincott Williams & Wilkins; 1999:135–143.

266. Hollerbach S, Kamath MV, Chen Y, et al. The magnitude of the central response to esophageal electrical stimulation is intensity dependent. *Gastroenterology* 1997;112:1137–1146.

267. Smout AJ, DeVore MS, Castell DO. Cerebral potentials evoked by esophageal distension in human. *Am J Physiol* 1990;259:G955–G959.

268. Frieling T, Enck P, Wienbeck M. Cerebral responses evoked by electrical stimulation of rectosigmoid in normal subjects. *Dig Dis Sci* 1989;34:202–205.

269. DeVault KR, Beacham S, Castell DO, et al. Esophageal sensation in spinal cord-injured patients: balloon distension and cerebral evoked potential recording. *Am J Physiol* 1996;271:G937–G941.

270. Franssen H, Weusten BL, Wieneke GH, et al. Source modeling of esophageal evoked potentials. *Electroencephalogr Clin Neurophysiol* 1996;100:85–95.

271. Aziz Q, Furlong PL, Barlow J, et al. Topographic mapping of cortical potentials evoked by distension of the human proximal and distal oesophagus. *Electroencephalogr Clin Neurophysiol* 1995;96:219–228.

272. Aziz Q, Thompson DG. Brain-gut axis in health and disease. *Gastroenterology* 1998;114:559–578.

273. Hartshorne MF. Positron emission tomography. In: Orrison WW, Lewine JD, Sanders JA, et al, eds. *Functional Brain Imaging*. St. Louis, MO: Mosby-Year Book; 1995:187–212.

274. Aine CJ. A conceptual overview and critique of functional neuroimaging techniques in humans: I. MRI/FMRI and PET. *Crit Rev Neurobiol* 1995;9:229–309.

275. Sanders JA, Orrison WW. Functional magnetic resonance imaging. In: Orrison WW, Lewine JD, Sanders JA, et al, eds. *Functional Brain Imaging*. St. Louis, MO: Mosby-Year Book; 1995:239–326.

276. Vogt BA, Sikes RW, Vogt LJ. Anterior cingulate cortex and the medial pain system. In: Vogt BA, Gabriel M, eds. *Neurobiology of Cingulate Cortex and Limbic Thalamus*. Boston, MA: Birkhauser; 1994:313–344.

277. Talbot JD, Marrett S, Evans AC, et al. Multiple representations of pain in human cerebral cortex. *Science* 1991;251:1355–1358.

278. Minshohima S, Maorrow TJ, Koeppe RA. Involvement of insular cortex in central autonomic regulation during painful thermal stimulation. *J Cereb Blood Flow Metab* 1995;15:1355–1358.

279. Fass R, Bautista J, Janarthanan S. Treatment of gastroesophageal reflux disease. *Clin Cornerstone* 2003;5:18–29.

280. Kitchin L, Castell D. Rationale and efficacy of conservative therapy for gastroesophageal reflux disease. *Arch Intern Med* 1991;151:448–454.

281. Fang J, Bjorkman D. A critical approach to noncardiac chest pain: pathophysiology, diagnosis, and treatment. *Am J Gastroenterol* 2001;96:958–968.

282. Achem S, Kolts B, MacMath T, et al. Effects of omeprazole versus placebo in treatment of noncardiac chest pain and gastroesophageal reflux. *Dig Dis Sci* 1997;42:2138–2145.

283. Louis E, Jorissen L, Bastens B, et al. Atypical symptoms of GORD in Belgium: epidemiological features, current management and open label treatment with 40 mg esomeprazole for one month. *Acta Gastroenterol Belg* 2006;69:203–208.

284. Dore MP, Pedroni A, Pes GM, et al. Effect of antisecretory therapy on atypical symptoms in gastroesophageal reflux disease. *Dig Dis Sci* 2007;52:463–468.

285. Flook NW, Moayyedi P, Dent J, et al. Acid-suppressive therapy with esomeprazole for relief of unexplained chest pain in primary care: a randomized, double-blind, placebo-controlled trial. *Am J Gastroenterol* 2013;108:56–64.

286. Liuzzo JP, Ambrose JA, Diggs P. Proton-pump inhibitor use by coronary artery disease patients is associated with fewer chest pain episodes, emergency department visits and hospitalizations. *Aliment Pharmacol Ther* 2005;22:95–100.

287. Borzecki A, Pedrosa M, Prashker M. Should noncardiac chest pain be treated empirically? A cost-effectiveness analysis. *Arch Intern Med* 2000;160:844–852.

288. Ozawa S, Kumai K, Higuchi K, et al. Short-term and long-term outcome of endoluminal gastroplication for the treatment of GERD: the first multicenter trial in Japan. *J Gastroenterol* 2009;44:675–684.

289. Liu JJ, Carr-Locke DL, Osterman MT, et al. Endoscopic treatment for atypical manifestations of gastroesophageal reflux disease. *Am J Gastroenterol* 2006;101:440–445.

290. Patti M, Molena D, Fisichella P, et al. Gastroesophageal reflux disease (GERD) and chest pain. Results of laparoscopic antireflux surgery. *Surg Endosc* 2002;16:563–566.

291. Farrell T, Richardson W, Trus T, et al. Response of atypical symptoms of gastro-oesophageal reflux to antireflux surgery. *Br J Surg* 2001;88:1649–1652.

292. So J, Zeitels S, Rattner D. Outcomes of atypical symptoms attributed to gastroesophageal reflux treated by laparoscopic fundoplication. *Surgery* 1998;124:28–32.

293. Cheung TK, Lim PW, Wong BC. Noncardiac chest pain—an Asia-Pacific survey on the views of primary care physicians. *Dig Dis Sci* 2007;52:3043–3048.

294. Cheung TK, Lim PW, Wong BC. The view of gastroenterologists on noncardiac chest pain in Asia. *Aliment Pharmacol Ther* 2007;26:597–603.

295. Orlando R, Bozymski E. Clinical and manometric effects of nitroglycerin in diffuse esophageal spasm. *N Engl J Med* 1989;289:23–25.

296. Millaire A, Ducloux G, Marquand A, et al. Clinical effects and effects on esophageal motility. *Arch Mal Coeur Vaiss* 1989;82:63–68.

297. Swamy N. Esophageal spasm: clinical and manometric response to nitroglycerine and long acting nitrites. *Gastroenterology* 1977;72:23–27.

298. Kikendall J, Mellow M. Effect of sublingual nitroglycerin and long-acting nitrate preparations on esophageal motility. *Gastroenterology* 1980;79:703–706.

299. Mellow M. Effect of isosorbide and hydralazine in painful primary esophageal motility disorders. *Gastroenterology* 1982;83:364–370.

300. Davies H, Lewis M, Rhodes J, et al. Trial of nifedipine for prevention of oesophageal spasm. *Digestion* 1987;36:81–83.

301. Nasrallah S, Tommaso C, Singleton R, et al. Primary esophageal motor disorders: clinical response to nifedipine. *South Med J* 1985;78:312–315.

302. Konrad-Danlhoff I, Baunack A, Ramsch K, et al. Effect of the calcium antagonists nifedipine, nitrendipine, nimodipine and nisoldipine on oesophageal motility in man. *Eur J Pharmacol* 1991;41:313–316.

303. Richter J, Spurling T, Cordova C, et al. Effects of oral calcium blocker, diltiazem, on esophageal contractions. Studies in volunteers and patients with nutcracker esophagus. *Dig Dis Sci* 1984;29:649–656.

304. Cattau E Jr, Castell D, Johnson D, et al. Diltiazem therapy for symptoms associated with nutcracker esophagus. *Am J Gastroenterol* 1991;86:272–276.

305. Drenth J, Bos L, Engels L. Efficacy of diltiazem in the treatment of diffuse oesophageal spasm. *Aliment Pharmacol Ther* 1990;4:411–416.

306. Lee LI, Park H, Kim TH, et al. The effect of sildenafil on esophageal motor function in healthy subjects and patients with nutcracker esophagus. *Neurogastroenterol Motil* 2003;15:617–623.

307. Bortolotti M, Pandolfo N, Giovannini M, et al. Effect of sildenafil on hypertensive lower esophageal sphincter. *Eur J Clin Invest* 2002;32:682–685.

308. Sharata AM, Dunst CM, Pescarus R, et al. Peroral endoscopic myotomy (POEM) for esophageal primary motility disorders: analysis of 100 consecutive patients. *J Gastrointest Surg* 2015;19:161–170.

309. Minami H, Isomoto H, Yamaguchi N, et al. Peroral endoscopic myotomy: emerging indications and evolving techniques. *Dig Endosc* 2015;27:175–181.

310. Nguyen TM, Eslick GD. Systematic review: the treatment of noncardiac chest pain with antidepressants. *Aliment Pharmacol Ther* 2012;35:493–500.

311. Cox ID, Hann CM, Kaski JC. Low dose imipramine improves chest pain but not quality of life in patients with angina and normal coronary angiograms. *Eur Heart J* 1998;19:250–254.

312. Park SW, Lee H, Lee HJ, et al. Low-dose amitriptyline combined with proton pump inhibitor for functional chest pain. *World J Gastroenterol* 2013;19:4958–4965.

313. Lee H, Kim JH, Min BH, et al. Efficacy of venlafaxine for symptomatic relief in young adult patients with functional chest pain: a randomized, double-blind, placebo-controlled, crossover trial. *Am J Gastroenterol* 2010;105:1504–1512.

314. Doraiswamy PM, Varia I, Hellegers C, et al. A randomized controlled trial of paroxetine for noncardiac chest pain. *Psychopharmacol Bull* 2006;39:15–24.

315. Varia I, Logue E, O'Connor C, et al. Randomized trial of sertraline in patients with unexplained chest pain of noncardiac origin. *Am Heart J* 2000;140:367–372.

316. Rao SS, Mudipalli RS, Mujica V, et al. An open-label trial of theophylline for functional chest pain. *Dig Dis Sci* 2002;47:2763–2768.

317. Rao SS, Mudipalli RS, Remes-Troche JM, et al. Theophylline improves esophageal chest pain—a randomized, placebo-controlled study. *Am J Gastroenterol* 2007;102:930–938.

318. Bradette M, Delvaux M, Staumont G, et al. Octreotide increases thresholds of colonic visceral perception in IBS patients without modifying muscle tone. *Dig Dis Sci* 1994;39:1171–1178.

319. Schwetz I, Naliboff B, Munakata J, et al. Anti-hyperalgesic effect of octreotide in patients with irritable bowel syndrome. *Aliment Pharmacol Ther* 2004;19:123–131.

320. Johnston B, Shils J, Leite L, et al. Effects of octreotide on esophageal visceral perception and cerebral evoked potentials induced by balloon distension. *Am J Gastroenterol* 1994;94:65–70.

321. Crea F, Pupita G, Galassi A, et al. Role of adenosine in pathogenesis of anginal pain. *Circulation* 1990;81:164–172.

322. Wulsin L, Maddock R, Beitman B, et al. Clonazepam treatment of panic disorder in patients with recurrent chest pain and normal coronary arteries. *Int J Psychiatry Med* 1999;29:97–105.

323. Miller L, Pullela S, Parkman H, et al. Treatment of chest pain in patients with noncardiac, nonreflux, nonachalasia spastic esophageal motor disorders using botulinum toxin injection into the gastroesophageal junction. *Am J Gastroenterol* 2002;97:1640–1646.

324. Gasiorowska A, Navarro-Rodriguez T, Dickman R, et al. Clinical trial: the effect of Johrei on symptoms of patients with functional chest pain. *Aliment Pharmacol Ther* 2009;29:126–34.

325. van Peski-Oosterbaan A, Spinhoven P, van Rood Y, et al. Cognitive-behavioral therapy for noncardiac chest pain: a randomized trial. *Am J Med* 1999;106:424–429.

326. Ryan M, Gervirtz R. Biofeedback-based psychophysiological treatment in a primary care setting: an initial feasibility study. *Appl Psychophysiol Biofeedback* 2004;29:79–93.

327. Keefe FJ, Shelby RA, Somers TJ, et al. Effects of coping skills training and sertraline in patients with noncardiac chest pain: a randomized controlled study. *Pain* 2011;152:730–741.

328. Jones H, Cooper P, Miller V, et al. Treatment of non-cardiac chest pain: a controlled trial of hypnotherapy. *Gut* 2006;55:1403–1408.

329. Holzer P. Gastrointestinal afferents as targets of novel drugs for the treatment of functional bowel disorders and visceral pain. *Eur J Pharmacol* 2001;429:177–193.

330. Zheng Y, Medda BK, Banerjee B, et al. Prevention of gastroesophageal reflux-induced ulceration by selective TPRV1 receptor antagonist in rats [abstract]. *Gastroenterology* 2007;132:A275.

331. Scarpignato C, Pelosini I. Management of irritable bowel syndrome: novel approaches to the pharmacology of gut motility. *Can J Gastroenterol* 1999;13:50A–65A.

CHAPTER 63

Abdominal, Peritoneal, and Retroperitoneal Pain

DAVID JUSTIN LEVINTHAL and **KLAUS BIELEFELDT**

Abdominal pain is one of the leading causes for patients to seek consultation with a physician (Fig. 63.1). Determining the precise mechanisms that underlie such abdominal pain symptoms and providing effective therapies both remain major clinical challenges. The experience of visceral pain is shaped by multiple factors including peripheral mechanisms, such as acute injury or active inflammation, and central processes, such as visceral hypersensitivity and somatization. Ultimately, the pain experience is neurally encoded and perceived at the level of the brain. Thus, a complex interplay of factors that are capable of influencing the activity of neurons located throughout the neuraxis should be considered as drivers or modulators of visceral perception in general and particularly in the experience of visceral pain.

What separates visceral pain, and thus many of the abdominal pain syndromes, from somatic pain is an often vague or diffuse localization, a different quality of pain, radiation to somatic referral sites, and a disproportionate degree of unpleasantness. Some of these distinguishing features are related to neuroanatomic differences in the peripheral and central pathways that process visceral and somatic pain information. For example, the sensory nerve innervation density of internal organs is much lower than that of many somatic structures, particularly when compared to the skin. In addition, individual visceral afferent neurons may project to more than one receptive field within an organ or between different organs and may respond to more than one sensory modality.[1,2] Lastly, information from more the one anatomical site or organ converges within higher centers of the central nervous system,[3] which further adds to the vague nature of visceral sensation. The aim of this chapter is to discuss the clinical features of abdominal pain and diagnostic strategies designed to identify its causes, to explore the general mechanisms that account for visceral pain, and to evaluate the efficacy of current treatment paradigms for alleviating abdominal pain.

Clinical Approach to Abdominal Pain

The abdominopelvic area contains many different organs that include most of the gastrointestinal tract, parenchymal organs such as the liver and pancreas, the urogenital tract, large vessels, and the various somatic structures that comprise the abdominal wall. Several characteristics of pain serve to identify underlying mechanisms that help clinicians in the decision making related to diagnostic or therapeutic approaches. *Acute pain* is more likely driven by peripheral mechanisms. Archetypical examples include the acute colicky pain of ureteral obstruction due to kidney stones or the severe pain of acute pancreatitis. *Chronic pain conditions* more often involve central sensitizing processes. Common chronic conditions characterized by persistent abdominal pain include irritable bowel syndrome (IBS), functional dyspepsia, and interstitial cystitis. Patients with these disorders may still experience acute fluctuations in pain that correlate with peripheral sensory input, but the magnitude of pain responses is often more closely linked to anxiety, stress, or other psychological variables that impact the processing of pain information at the level of the brain.

Somatic and *visceral* components of abdominal pain classically have distinct clinical features. Somatic pain is more clearly localized and often sharper in character, whereas typical visceral pain is more often perceived as dull, diffuse, and perhaps deeper in location. These differences in clinical features reflect anatomical differences in somatic and visceral nerves, as somatic nociception originates from the parietal peritoneum, abdominal body wall, or skin, whereas sensors for visceral pain are located within the walls of hollow structures or within the parenchyma of abdominal organs. A classic example showing the distinct manifestation of these pain types is the evolution of acute appendicitis: Early in the course of the disease, the pain is often vague and referred to mid-abdominal regions but then shifts to McBurney's point (a focal position within the right lower quadrant), where it is becomes highly localized and sharper in quality as the parietal peritoneum becomes inflamed later on in the disease course.

PAIN LOCALIZATION AND CHARACTER

As is true for all disorders associated with pain and discomfort, pain localization provides key information about the source of possible underlying problems. Peripheral visceral neural pathways reflect the embryologic origin or anatomical position of visceral structures, whereas the mapping of somatic pain is clearly organized along spinal segmental afferent pathways throughout the neuraxis. For example, pain from the proximal gastrointestinal tract tends to project to the upper abdomen (e.g., stomach), from the midgut (e.g., jejunum) to the periumbilical region, and from the hindgut (e.g., colon) to the lower abdomen. Processes involving the pelvic organs tend to trigger pain felt in the groin, suprapubic, or perineal area and often radiate toward the sacrum or genitals. Due to the retroperitoneal location of the pancreas, kidneys, and ureters, pain that arises from these structures projects more toward the flank, back, or groin. Yet, many patients experience the localization and quality of visceral pain in "atypical" ways. Experiments using a distension stimulus within the esophagus, stomach, small bowel, or colon triggered pain responses that fell within

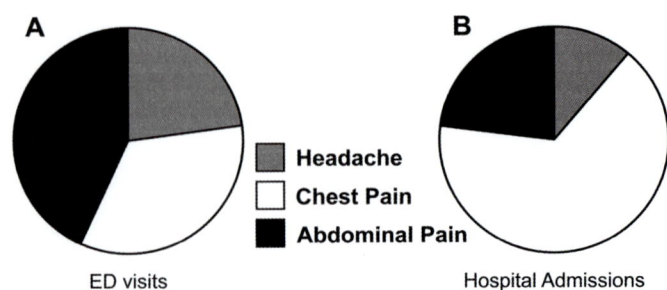

FIGURE 63.1 Relative contribution of abdominal pain, compared to headache and chest pain, as the primary chief complaint in emergency department (ED) visits **(A)** and in ED visits ultimately leading to hospital admission **(B)**. Data is derived from the National Emergency Department Sample (NEDS) in 2016. Abdominal pain accounted for 43.1% of 1.38 million ED encounters **(A)**, whereas complaints of chest pain accounted for a majority of ED visits that led hospital admission.

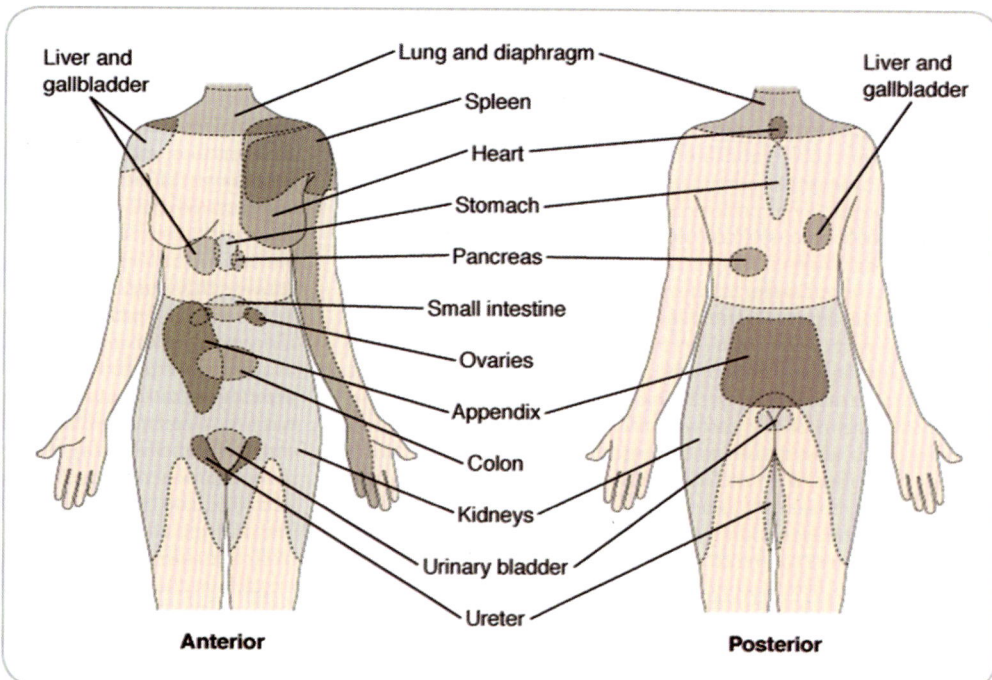

FIGURE 63.2 Classic patterns of cutaneous sites of pain referred from visceral structures. *(Reprinted with permission from Anderson MK. Foundations of Athletic Training. 6th ed. Philadelphia, PA: Lippincott Williams & Wilkins; 2016. Figure 6-1.)*

predicted somatic areas in just more than half of participants.[4–7] In addition, the terms used to describe a perceived stimulus poorly correlated with the modality of the administered stimulus. For example, about one-third of subjects experienced a feeling of heartburn during esophageal luminal distension.[8] Conversely, direct jejunal stimulation with capsaicin often was reported as a pressure sensation rather than an expected burning sensation.[4] These observations could be explained by the fact that many visceral afferents are polymodal, meaning they can be activated by more than a single stimulus type.[9]

Sensory input from the viscera often is *referred* to distant sites within somatic structures, a phenomenon attributed to the convergence of primary visceral and somatic sensory input onto the same second-order neurons within the spinal cord.[10] Although radiating pain is not always present or follows a consistent pattern, the pattern of radiating pain can provide important clinical clues to the true anatomical source of pain. For example, retrosternal pain radiating to the left shoulder or arm occurs during myocardial ischemia, right upper abdominal pain radiating to the right scapula in cases of cholecystitis, or flank pain radiating to the groin or genitals is a hallmark of a migrating kidney stone (Fig. 63.2).

TIME COURSE

The time course of more acute pain can provide important diagnostic clues about the source of the problem. For example, very sudden onset and intense pain suggests perforation, acute ischemia, or acute pancreatitis. In contrast, most inflammatory processes and obstructions tend to present with a more gradual and escalating intensity, may fluctuate in intensity over minutes, and, as already described earlier for appendicitis, change in character and location. Distension of the capsule of a parenchymal organ can trigger more constant discomfort, as can inflammation or infiltrative processes, such as pancreatic cancer. Constant pain also predicts a more significant impact on quality of life and is associated with increased health care resource utilization.[11] Recurring, intermittent pain is more common and characterized by a regular pattern of waxing and waning, often referred to as "colicky" in nature, and is frequently related to the obstruction of luminal structures.

CONTEXTUAL INFORMATION

Additional information about *triggering* or *alleviating factors*, associated symptoms, prior medical problems and surgeries, and current medical therapies can provide other important clues about the source of abdominal pain. Food intake most commonly influences abdominal pain of gastrointestinal origin, typically functioning as an exacerbating factor. The lag time between the ingestion of food and the onset or exacerbation of pain can help identify the potential source. For example, close to immediate onset of pain with swallowing (i.e., odynophagia) points at the esophagus as a pain generator. Discomfort due to gastric disorders typically manifests within 30 minutes of ingesting a meal, while underlying small bowel abnormalities may have more significant delays of onset. However, gastric filling or lipid nutrient exposure of the duodenum stimulates colonic contractions (gastrocolonic response), which may secondarily trigger discomfort.[12] Ingesting acidic or spicy material often triggers symptoms in patients with gastroesophageal reflux or functional dyspepsia, and bland food or drink may dilute or neutralize these exposures. Thus, food may have a range of effects on pain of gastrointestinal origin.

As gastroduodenal filling may increase pain symptoms, emptying may ease pain. The rate of emptying of an ingested meal is typically relatively slow (hours), which explains a gradual and delayed improvement of postprandial discomfort. However, vomiting, although obviously unpleasant to experience, may more rapidly alleviate pain by quickly decompressing the proximal small bowel and stomach. If the physiologic processes of urination or defecation alter abdominal pain, then this implicates a bladder, distal colon, or rectal source of pain.

Body position and activity may also influence pain intensity. During many acute pain episodes or significant pain exacerbations, increased activity or stretching out in the supine position tends to worsen pain, whereas crouching in the fetal position eases pain. This common phenomenon may be related to decreased tension in the abdominal wall muscles but lacks specificity in discriminating somatic from visceral pain. Abdominal wall sources of abdominal pain by definition are of somatic rather than visceral origin, yet when not recognized as such, abdominal wall pain frequently triggers recurrent physician visits and extensive testing in search of a visceral source.[13] Somatic abdominal pain typically has some positional component and is clearly exacerbated by physical activity, such as lifting, or tensing the abdominal muscles (Carnett's sign). In contrast, levator ani syndrome involves somatic pain from the pelvic floor muscles experienced as perineal pressure and pain that typically worsens when sitting or standing and improves with laying down.[14]

Learning about *associated symptoms and signs* often narrows down the list of possible underlying problems. Dysphagia in patients with chest pain implicates an esophageal source. Nausea and vomiting are common symptoms that may suggest an upper gastrointestinal problem, such as peptic ulcer disease or an obstruction of the gastrointestinal tract. Yet, nausea and vomiting may also result as an autonomic response to acute pain, as described with the intense and colicky pain of passing kidney stones. Similarly, concurrent changes in bowel patterns can provide important diagnostic information pointing to the colon as a source of pain. Tenesmus, an intense cramp-like pain felt in the lower abdominal or pelvic area with associated urgency to defecate and frequent evacuations of only small volumes of often loose and/or bloody feces, suggests a rectal source of pain. This symptom is analogous to the clinical manifestations of bladder infection, which more commonly are felt as pain in the suprapubic region and similarly are accompanied by a high frequency of low volume and often painful urination that may also be bloody (hematuria). Cramps felt within the pelvis that may be associated with vaginal bleeding or discharge, but that are not associated with changed bowel patterns or micturition, may indicate a uterine or ovarian disorder.

Information about *prior illnesses or operations and coexisting diseases* is essential when approaching patients with abdominal pain. Late complications from abdominal surgeries due to adhesive disease may result in partial or complete bowel obstruction that are among the most common reasons for hospitalization in surgical units.[15] An underlying inflammatory bowel disease may manifest with pain due to a flare or disease-related complications, such as abscess formation or strictures. Patients with medical illnesses such as cardiovascular disease and hypertension have higher risks of aortic aneurysm and mesenteric ischemia. Those with hyperuricemia or hypercalcemia risk the formation of kidney stones. Functional syndromes, such as IBS, functional dyspepsia, or bladder pain syndrome, are often associated with other chronic pain disorders, such as fibromyalgia or migraines.[16] Psychiatric disorders similarly correlate with such functional diseases, partially mediated through hypervigilance, catastrophizing, or somatization.[17-21]

Medication and drug use, including over-the-counter agents and illicit drugs, may either cause or exacerbate problems that manifest with abdominal pain. For example, nonsteroidal anti-inflammatory drugs (NSAIDs) increase ulcer risk through well-described mechanisms.[22] Less common but more serious complications of medical therapy include acute pancreatitis, as seen with azathioprine, eluxadoline, and diuretics, or ischemic colitis with alosetron.[23,24] More commonly, medications (including opioids, antidepressants, anticholinergics, and antibiotics) may influence the motility of the stomach or bowel to generate dyspeptic symptoms and changes in bowel movement patterns. Opioid withdrawal, an increasing problem in the context of the current opioid use epidemic, is characterized by a number of intense physical symptoms. Acute opiate withdrawal may not only lead to psychomotor activation but also to intense abdominal pain that is associated with repeated vomiting and diarrhea. Similarly, the clinical presentation of cyclic vomiting syndrome (CVS) in adults overlaps with such withdrawal symptoms. Although refractory CVS appears to more common

in those chronically using opioids, CVS is more commonly associated with long-term cannabinoid use and in such cases is referred to as cannabinoid hyperemesis syndrome.[25]

PHYSICAL EXAMINATION

The physical examination provides critical information in the evaluation of new and sudden onset pain. Simple inspection may immediately reveal signs of distress; show pallor, jaundice, or diaphoresis; or implicate more chronic processes, such as malignancy, if cachexia is present. Vital signs add important details and guide decisions about the potential need for immediate interventions, such as fluid resuscitation or antibiotics for sepsis. A distended abdomen indicates either the presence of ascites or potential intestinal obstruction. Scars or hernias provide additional important information. A vesicular rash with dermatomal distribution suggests shingles, which can cause significant pain. The direct examination of the abdomen should proceed in a stepwise manner to minimize undue stress and limit the impact of anticipated pain and voluntary abdominal muscle contractions. A light touch or stroking movement over the skin may reveal significant cutaneous allodynia. This allodynia could be indicative of a peripheral somatic neuropathy, such as is seen in postherpetic neuralgia, or that may additionally represent a central sensitization process, such as is typically seen in patients presenting with chronic abdominal discomfort and functional pain syndromes. Intense pain with rigid abdominal musculature and transiently intensified discomfort when the pressure is released (rebound tenderness) suggests involvement of the parietal peritoneum. More detailed palpation can reveal masses or an enlarged liver or identify possible hernias and assess whether they can be reduced. Highly localized pain without involuntary guarding or rebound tenderness should prompt an additional assessment by asking the patient to tense their abdominal wall muscles (Carnett's sign), which can identify a possible role of the abdominal wall as a source of pain.[13,26] Listening for a bruit or abnormal bowel sounds should complete the abdominal examination. Other findings ranging from cutaneous changes of scleroderma to joint hypermobility, an irregular pulse, or a perirectal fistula may provide additional clues that will lead to the diagnosis or guide decisions about further testing.

DIAGNOSTIC TESTING IN ABDOMINAL PAIN

The goal of diagnostic evaluations in patients with abdominal pain is to identify the anatomical site of pain generation and, ideally, to determine the mechanism of illness (i.e., gallstone pancreatitis, nephrolithiasis, endometriosis, etc.). The choices of diagnostic modalities range from blood or stool tests to endoscopic evaluations or radiographic studies. Yet, the most common disorders presenting with abdominal pain are "functional disorders" defined by chronic pain and a variety of other symptoms in the absence of distinct structural or other findings on standard diagnostic testing. A better understanding of mechanisms that contribute to such functional disorders has driven the search for biomarkers that may support, perhaps even establish their diagnosis, or at least act as prognostic indicators that can predict treatment outcomes. Isolated tests largely have fallen short of expectations. Composite scores derived from survey data and fecal or serologic biomarkers may hold more promise but have yet to be established as clinically useful tools.

Mechanisms of Visceral Pain

The principles underlying visceral sensation and pain share key mechanisms with somatic sensory pathways (see Chapters 3 and 9). Yet, there are several important differences between somatic and visceral sensation that aid in understanding the clinical presentation and treatment of patients with visceral pain.

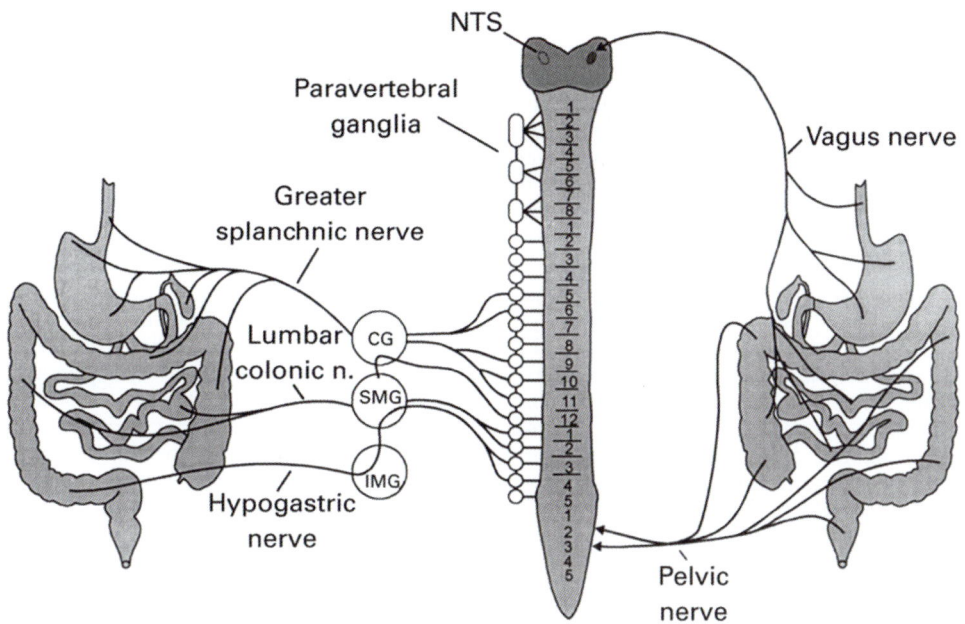

FIGURE 63.3 Schematic diagram that demonstrates the pattern of afferent pathways from abdominal and pelvic organs to the central nervous system. Visceral spinal afferents **(left side)** travel in parallel along sympathetic pathways but have cell bodies contained in dorsal root ganglia and central projections that innervate the spinal cord. Vagal afferents **(right side)** travel along vagal pathways and have cell bodies within the nucleus of the solitary tract of the brainstem, whereas pelvic visceral nerves travel along the pelvic nerve and target sacral segments of the spinal cord. CG, celiac ganglion; IMG, inferior mesenteric ganglion; NTS, nucleus tractus solitarii; SMG, superior mesenteric ganglion. *(Reprinted from Gebhart GF. Visceral pain—peripheral sensitization. Gut 2000;47(suppl 4):iv54–iv55, with permission from BMJ Publishing Group Ltd.)*

Abdominal viscera largely emerge as midline structures and receive bilateral sensory input from both spinal and vagal sensory afferents (Fig. 63.3). These two complementary sensory systems both convey information to the brain and contribute to the perception of visceral stimuli from organs. The cell bodies of spinal afferents are located in the dorsal root ganglia and send central terminals into the dorsal spinal cord. Vagal afferents, which innervate most abdominal and some pelvic structures, have their cell bodies in the nodose ganglion and send central terminals to the nucleus of the solitary tract in the brainstem. Traditionally, only spinal afferent pathways were believed to relay information about painful stimuli, whereas vagal fibers presumably contributed only to homeostatic regulation. However, recent findings suggest some overlapping roles of these anatomically distinct pathways, as vagal afferents may encode chemo-nociceptive or higher intensity mechanosensitive signals that trigger unpleasant feelings such as nausea and shape the complex human experience of pain.

VISCERAL NOCICEPTION

Detailed physiologic investigations of visceral spinal afferents have identified distinct response patterns to low- or high-intensity stimuli.[27] These foundational data suggested that painful stimuli can specifically engage specialized nociceptive pathways that are activated only by high-threshold stimulation (*specificity coding*). However, many visceral afferents that are activated by low-intensity stimuli encode a range of stimulus intensities that extends well into the noxious range. These visceral afferents appear to sensitize after exposure to heat, acid, or inflammatory mediators.[28] These findings argue against an exclusive role of specialized, high-threshold nociceptors in mediating painful sensations and instead suggest that the summation of sensory inputs ultimately shapes the perception of discomfort and pain (*intensity coding*). Furthermore, several neurophysiologic properties that presumably characterize nociceptive neurons are also commonly found in most visceral afferents, including an ability to respond to more than a single

stimulus modality, the expression of ion channels and other neurochemical markers classically associated with nociceptors, and axonal conduction velocities in the C-fiber range.[29–31]

Due to their relatively low innervation density, smaller axonal size, and the difficulty in gaining access to their target organs for precise experimental manipulation, investigators have only recently started to gain insight into the structure–function relationship of afferent nerve endings within the viscera. Detailed anatomic and physiologic studies have identified branching patterns with linear arrays of nerves that run parallel to muscle fibers of the muscular layer of the gut and encode changes in length or stretch.[32] Actively generated muscle tension activates fibers with sensory terminals that spread through ganglia of the enteric nervous system.[33,34] Less distinct branching patterns are found along other structures, such as the epithelium or vasculature, and the role of these possible transduction sites in generating visceral sensations and/or pain is only partially understood.[35,36]

Most visceral spinal afferents terminate in the superficial layers (lamina I and II) of the dorsal horn. The central terminals branch within the spinal cord and may extend several spinal segments rostral or caudal to their original entry point within these laminae. This anatomical feature contributes to the vague localization of visceral inputs, including pain.[37] The second-order neurons within the spinal cord typically also receive convergent input from somatic, often cutaneous sites, explaining the pattern of referred pain described earlier (see Fig. 63.2). Second-order neurons project rostrally primarily through the spinothalamic tract. However, some visceral nociceptive afferents terminate in second-order neurons located within lamina X, surrounding the spinal canal. These second-order neurons send their ascending axons through the dorsal columns, creating a recently recognized pain pathway that may account for descriptions of visceral pain that persists despite bilateral injury or transection of the spinothalamic tract.[38]

The neural activity of second-order neurons acts as a "gate" that can diminish or enhance pain signals from being relayed to higher brain centers. Importantly, descending projections from the midbrain and brainstem directly influence the critical synaptic connection between primary afferents and these second-order neurons. Thus, there is a neural substrate for the brain to effectively inhibit or augment visceral and somatic pain signaling at the level of the spinal cord (for more information, see Chapters 5 and 6), and such descending pathways may well provide some of the neuroanatomical basis for the influence of stress, cognitive, and emotional factors on pain perception (see Chapter 7).

CENTRAL PROCESSING OF SOMATIC AND VISCERAL PAIN

The precise cerebral cortical mapping of spinothalamic inputs from the viscera is poorly understood. Classical neurophysiologic experiments in nonhuman primates found that visceral spinal afferents can ultimately project to the trunk representation within primary and secondary somatosensory cortical regions.[39] Yet, neuroanatomical tracing experiments in nonhuman primates that mapped spinothalamocortical projections from purely somatic spinal afferents found that only a minority of neurons project directly to the primary somatosensory cortex. Rather, the majority of direct spinothalamic input was received in the dorsal insular cortex, secondary somatosensory cortex, and within the midcingulate motor areas.[40] Functional brain imaging studies of humans obtained during painful cutaneous and visceral stimulation have led to a wider understanding of central mechanisms that contribute to pain. These studies have largely corroborated the neuroanatomical and neurophysiologic observations from studies in nonhuman primates. Both cutaneous and visceral pain were associated with an overlapping pattern of activation within some subcortical and cortical structures, preferentially including the ventromedial thalamus, anterior cingulate cortex, secondary sensory cortex, and regions of the insula. However, some important differences emerged, such as a greater activation of the primary sensory cortex during visceral pain compared to cutaneous pain. Many of the areas involved in visceral pain processing are also involved in emotional processing, an association that may well account for the disproportionate unpleasantness of visceral pain.[41] Interestingly, the pattern of brain activation triggered by visceral pain is qualitatively similar to patterns observed during less intense or even unperceived visceral stimulation. This observation argues against specific "labeled lines" for visceral nociception and raises the possibility that visceral stimulation in general influences the visceral pain experience (for a more detailed discussion on central pain processing, see Chapter 6).[42,43]

SENSITIZATION AND VISCERAL HYPERSENSITIVITY

Detailed in vitro and in vivo physiologic studies, including investigations in human volunteers, have clearly demonstrated that both peripheral and central visceral sensory mechanisms exhibit significant functional plasticity. Sensitization is defined as an increase in the response magnitude to the same stimulus intensity, and it is the primary form of plasticity that drives the development of *visceral hypersensitivity*. Visceral hypersensitivity is the key to the clinical manifestations of many functional visceral pain disorders, ranging from functional dyspepsia to chronic pancreatitis and interstitial cystitis.[44–48] Peripheral and central sensitization can be experimentally dissociated (for detailed discussions on mechanisms of sensitization, see Chapters 3, 4, and 6). Although they are mechanistically distinct, published investigations typically have shown a close interaction between peripheral and central sensitization processes. For example, acid perfusion sensitized the esophagus to subsequent mechanical stimulation and, at the same time, increased its somatic referral area.[6] Similarly, repeated rectal stimulation led to increased pain ratings and an increase in the

somatic territory of referred pain.[5] Two examples of chronic disorders illustrate the clinical relevance of the complex, reciprocal interaction between peripheral and central mechanisms, which ultimately lead to heightened and long-lasting pain. First, chronic pancreatitis is a disease with ongoing inflammation and significant changes in the structure of peripheral nerves.[49–51] The disease typically manifests with pain as the predominant symptom. Despite the often striking abnormalities in pancreatic structure and abnormalities in peripheral nerves, a small but important cohort study demonstrated that a complete neuroaxial block, which abolished all but the vagal sensory input from the pancreas, completely relieved pain in only less than a quarter of the patients.[52] This observation reflects the ability of increases in peripheral input to drive central sensitization as a secondary process that may ultimately even become more relevant in the clinical manifestation of a disease. Second, several cohort studies have demonstrated that there is a higher incidence of IBS after acute bacterial or viral infections.[53–56] Although the severity of the initiating infection (i.e., a peripheral factor) functioned as one important independent predictor of lasting symptoms, preexisting anxiety and depression (i.e., central factors) were also independently associated with a higher risk of developing IBS.[57] The presence of these affective spectrum disorders may play a role in different aspects that characterize this disorder, ranging from influences on descending modulatory pathways to altered vigilance and the cortical processing of pain to increased symptom reporting or health care–seeking behavior.[58] The impact of psychiatric diseases has been demonstrated in other common pain syndromes, implying that these factors drive more generalized increases in pain sensitivity.[59,60]

Detailed neuroimaging studies have revealed changes in cortical thickness within areas activated during pain processing in both chronic pancreatitis and IBS, providing a structural correlate and potential biomarker for the observations described earlier.[61,62] Interestingly, such apparent differences in brain structure may not only be a consequence of ongoing painful input but could also reflect the impact of other factors, such as early adverse life events,[63] or correlate with behavioral patterns, such as enhanced stress responses or catastrophizing.[64] Recognizing these complex interactions between peripheral and central sensitization in individuals with chronic pain conditions may not only improve our mechanistic understanding of visceral pain but could also personalize treatment choices and improve treatment outcomes.[65,66]

Susceptibility Factors

GENETIC FACTORS

Genetic studies of patients with pain syndromes do not only have to contend with the interactions between genes and environmental factors but also the fact that different pain disorders may result from a variety of underlying mechanisms (see Chapter 8). Most investigations of genetic influences on abdominal pain have focused on the IBS population primarily because this disorder is highly prevalent throughout the world. However, the theoretical advantage of studying this common disorder is unfortunately confounded its phenotypic variability, as IBS can manifest with diarrhea, constipation, or mixed bowel patterns and varying degrees of pain. Perhaps not surprisingly, studies have identified multiple mechanisms that contribute to IBS, such as differences in nutritional intake, microbial flora, and subtle changes in peripheral inflammation, and to psychological traits that affect health care–seeking behavior. Despite these caveats, a large genetic study in IBS patients showed higher symptom concordance between first-degree rather than second-degree relatives, which is consistent with some contribution of genetic traits to the development of IBS. However, partners had nearly similar rates of symptom overlap, which points to the role of shared environmental factors.[67] These results are in line with a large twin study in IBS that failed to show differences between mono- and dizygotic twins.[68] Thus, there is mixed evidence for a clear genetic underpinning to IBS.

Serotonin (5-HT) plays an important role in gastrointestinal signaling,[69] and thus, many genetic investigations in IBS have used a candidate gene approach focused on polymorphisms of the gene for the 5-HT transporter. These studies showed variable results. Independent of the inconclusive findings, these same genetic markers are associated with psychiatric comorbidity, making it difficult to attribute the associations to IBS itself rather than to risk factors or cofactors that may influence its clinical manifestations, such as symptom severity.[70–72] Genes encoding other components of the 5-HT signaling system have not been as closely examined but may also be associated with altered emotional responses,[73] bowel patterns,[74] or responses to drugs that target 5-HT receptors.[75] The catechol-O-methyltransferase (COMT) gene has been inconsistently linked to functional pain disorders.[76] As was true for 5-HT signaling, COMT variants also correlate with psychological traits that influence symptom severity and reporting in IBS.[77–79] Similar links between emotional responses and genetic markers have been reported for allelic variants of signaling molecules in the hypothalamic-pituitary-adrenal (HPA) axis, which plays an important role in mediating stress reactions.[80,81]

Genes involved in mucosal permeability, innate immunity,[82] or absorptive pathways[83,84] may sensitize individuals to develop IBS after apparently banal enteric infections. A possible link between innate or adaptive immunity and IBS supports a concept in which interactions between environmental factors, in this context microbial colonization or infection, and host responses contribute to IBS development.[85–88] Although these studies do not allow us to determine which aspect of the clinical manifestations of IBS are associated with the various genetic traits, the available data point at differences between constipation and diarrhea-predominant IBS, suggesting that these genetic markers may correlate more with bowel patterns rather than the pain of IBS per se.[74,89,90]

ADVERSE LIFE EVENTS AND STRESS

Nearly three decades ago, studies first linked the exposure to physical and sexual abuse to an increased risk of developing IBS.[91] Subsequent controlled animal experiments have explored the impact of exposure to adverse life events and have shown changes in bowel function and responses to noxious stimuli,[92,93] presumably due to the increased plasticity of the nervous system during this critical phase of development. More detailed assessments argue against specific links between IBS or other abdominal pain syndromes and such traumatic events early on in life[94–97] and instead suggest that such exposures may alter the activation of the HPA axis and enhance stress responses.[98] Although the association between abuse or other adverse life events and diseases manifesting with pain may well be more indirect, mediated by heightened vigilance or catastrophizing, it remains clinically relevant as it affects perceived symptom severity and health care–seeking behavior.[99–101]

Chronic stress also affects the manifestation of IBS and other abdominal pain syndromes. Mechanistic studies described a link between stress experiences, enhanced activation of the HPA axis, and altered attention to and processing of visceral stimuli.[102] As is true for the impact of adverse life events, increased stress exposures negatively influence health outcomes.[103]

PSYCHIATRIC DISEASES

Several cohort studies examined the incidence of IBS after large outbreaks of waterborne illnesses and demonstrated that preexisting anxiety and depression independently predict the development of IBS after the infection.[104–106] Complex modeling studies indicate that depression may increase somatization,[107–109] whereas anxiety may drive vigilance, catastrophizing, and avoidance.[110] A simple "common sense model" (Fig. 63.4) highlights the interaction of various psychological factors that contribute to generating increases in perceived symptom intensity.[111] More comprehensive conceptual models incorporate additional factors such as social and environmental interactions that shape these various psychological factors. In addition, a more comprehensive model needs to consider the impact of autonomic responses, which may alter visceral function and thereby indirectly influence visceral sensory inputs. Consistent with such explanatory models, psychiatric comorbidity plays a central role in illness perception, health care–seeking behavior, and resource utilization.[112]

MICROBIAL COLONIZATION

Within the last decade, an increasing number of studies suggest that the microbial colonization of the gastrointestinal tract contributes to symptoms, presumably via effects on epithelial function, permeability, and immune activation.[113] Animal studies and some small human investigations raise questions about an impact on pain experiences, endocrine function, and even emotional responses.[114–117] Several studies have demonstrated changes in the microbiome, with secondary changes in fermentation of luminal contents, short-chain fatty acid concentrations, and bile acid metabolism, in IBS.[118,119] Although most of these investigations focused on bacteria, potential differences also involve fungal organisms[120] and may even include parasites and viruses. Defining dysbiosis as a disrupted pattern of microbial colonization, 70% of IBS patients had abnormal findings, as opposed to 17% of healthy controls; yet, results did not differentiate IBS from inflammatory bowel disease, and patterns

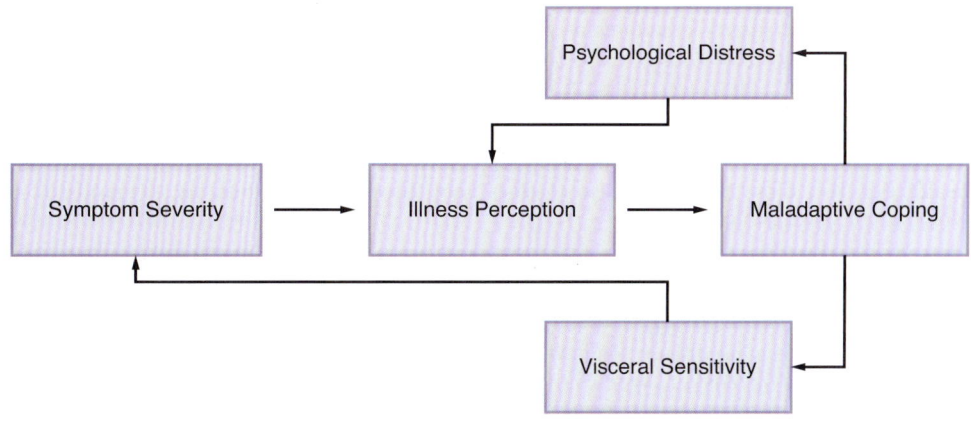

FIGURE 63.4 Schematic model that highlights the interactions and influences between psychological factors and symptom severity in those with functional pain disorders. *(From Knowles SR, Austin DW, Sivanesan S, et al. Relations between symptom severity, illness perceptions, visceral sensitivity, coping strategies and well-being in irritable bowel syndrome guided by the common sense model of illness.* Psychol Health Med *2017;22[5]:524–534. Reprinted by permission of Taylor & Francis Ltd. http://www.tandfonline.com.)*

did not seem to reflect whether the inflammatory bowel disease was active or in apparent remission.[121] The impact of microbial colonization of the gut on gastrointestinal function becomes even more complex when we examine the influence of dietary factors. Prospective studies clearly demonstrated that the composition of luminal contents changes the microbial colonization, which, in turn, is associated with changes in gastrointestinal symptoms, raising the question whether the dysbiosis observed in IBS patients is the true cause for symptoms or if it is an epiphenomenon, largely reflecting dietary habits.[122,123]

Biomarkers of Abdominal Pain

As already mentioned earlier, chronic visceral pain is frequently caused by functional illnesses, which are largely defined by characteristic symptom patterns and the absence of obvious objective abnormalities on standard medical tests. Consensus diagnostic criteria for a variety of functional pain syndromes were formulated not only to standardize research populations but also to allow a positive diagnosis. Yet, common clinical practice still follows a path in which exhaustive testing is used to repeatedly exclude alternative etiologies, often including rare diseases. This practice is costly, inefficient, and in some cases leads to iatrogenic injury. Investigators have therefore continued to search for biomarkers that could aid in the diagnosis or treatment of functional abdominal pain syndromes.

Nearly half a century ago, Ritchie[124] first reported a heightened sensitivity of IBS patients to rectal distension. Those findings fit a conceptual model that revolves around visceral hypersensitivity as a primary mechanism in IBS and related pain disorders. The paradigm of provoking defined peripheral sensory inputs has since been refined and applied to many different disorders with mostly similar results.[125–127] About 50% to 70% of patients with functional abdominal pain syndromes experience pain with lower intensity stimuli than normal people, suggesting visceral hypersensitivity is indeed a key mechanism. Yet, such enhanced pain responses are not consistently limited to the bodily regions presumably directly involved in the underlying disorder.[59,60,128] Furthermore, even the anticipation of a stimulus often triggered discomfort in patients.[129–131] Situational anxiety and enhanced vigilance are important factors that drive the apparent hypersensitivity to anticipated rather than actual stimulation,[132] highlighting the importance of central factors in chronic visceral pain. More importantly, a longitudinal study showed a dissociation between time-dependent changes in symptom severity ratings related to the underlying disorder and the pain levels experienced during acute visceral stimulation. Thus, responses to acute painful stimulation may correlate with mechanisms that contribute to chronic visceral pain syndromes, but these responses lack utility as diagnostic or prognostic markers and are also not appropriate surrogate targets to determine treatment effects. Several other biomarkers or diagnostic algorithms have been developed and range from enhanced sensitivity in cutaneous pain referral sites[133] to grey matter changes determined with morphometric analyses of brain scans[134] or composite measures of multiple biomarkers and psychological variables.[135] Although some of these data appear conceptually appealing, confirmatory studies are required to determine if such markers not only differentiate disease from health but also differentiate between distinct pain disorders, which often share clinical features.

Treatment of Abdominal Pain

As is true for all pain disorders, it is paramount to identify and treat the underlying disease to alleviate the driver of pain. However, pain may persist in chronic illnesses, or, in the case of functional pain disorders, pain may be a key symptom that is not linked to clearly understood and/or easily correctable mechanisms. In such cases, pain itself becomes the target for symptomatic management strategies. Therapeutic options range from localized interventions, psychological therapies, systemic medications that directly or indirectly influence pain, and surgery. Commonly used analgesic medications have side effects that need to be considered along with the potential benefits of the medications. Opioids, NSAIDs, and many antidepressant medications adversely affect gastrointestinal function or structure, drive nausea, dyspeptic symptoms, constipation, or diarrhea and may thus negatively affect quality of life despite their possibly beneficial effects on pain. Concerns about such side effects are even more relevant in patients who already suffer from abdominal problems, which may further limit the utility of these medications.

LIFESTYLE MODIFICATIONS

Stress and other environmental or lifestyle factors may influence disease development and manifestations. In functional gastrointestinal disorders, food intake is an important treatment target, as it has complex impacts on the gut, either directly from filling and distension of stomach, or indirectly by altering the gut's microbiome, resulting in differences in fermentation of luminal contents. More than 80% of IBS patients experience symptom exacerbations in response to foods, with poorly absorbed carbohydrates, dairy, and legumes being the most commonly reported culprits.[136] As is true for many factors that influence symptom severity, dietary patterns also correlate with resource utilization.[137] Thus, assessing such habits and considering modifications of meal size, frequency, consistency, or nutrient composition should be a routine part of any treatment plan in gastrointestinal disorders. Consuming foods low in poorly absorbed, poorly fermented foods (i.e., a low-fermentable oligo-di-monosaccharides and polyols [FODMAP] diet) appears to be a viable strategy to treat IBS, particularly in patients that have associated diarrhea, bloating, and increased flatulence.[138,139] A low-FODMAP diet may not only alter food-derived luminal contents but also secondarily changes the microbial colonization of the gut, which could further benefit epithelial and immune function.[122]

As already described earlier, adverse life events and stress heighten vigilance, influence autonomic output, and alter gut function, thereby contributing to symptom severity.[111,140] Experimentally, acute stress clearly worsens symptoms in IBS patients.[102,141] The close correlation between perceived stress and symptom severity ratings suggests potential feed-forward interactions in which symptoms contribute to increasing levels of stress, increased anxiety, and heightened vigilance, creating an amplifying effect on pain.[142] Social and interpersonal strains may also influence the clinical picture. Shared life experiences and exposures as well as reinforcing responses with learned illness behavior contribute to illness development.[143] Negative experiences, such as conflict or social stressors,[144,145] affect symptom severity but will have less negative an impact in a more supportive environment.[146] Consistent with such results, treatments that strengthen social support decrease perceived stress levels and improve stress tolerance, thereby indirectly alleviating pain symptoms.[147]

The restorative effect of sleep is yet another important consideration, as disruptions of normal sleep patterns or sleep deprivation increase the likelihood of developing IBS.[148,149] Thus, the demands of modern life, such as travel across time zones or shift work, may contribute to the high prevalence of visceral pain syndromes[150] and affect symptom severity, mood, and overall quality of life.[151] Although not always easily addressed and implemented, assessing lifestyle factors as cause, modulator, and/or treatment target may allow patients to better understand and hopefully also better control their disease, without encountering risks of adverse events that may come with the more conventional pharmacologic interventions.

PATIENT–PROVIDER RELATIONSHIP

Close listening is required to identify the many psychosocial factors that contribute to symptoms and may thus be appropriate treatment targets. Yet, the act of listening is inherently therapeutic. When asked to define their expectations from a provider, patients seek education and look for empathy and good listening skills.[152] A well-designed study compared two different sham interventions, differing only in the formalized communication strategy. Displays of active listening behavior and empathy were shown to be clearly superior to more transactional communications focused solely on treatment options, the therapist's experience, and expected beneficial treatment response.[153] These results are consistent with detailed analyses of placebo responses in a large study, which suggest that effective communication provides patients with an improved sense of control, an increased feeling of being understood, and promotes trust in the provider.[154] Based on such findings, experts advocate a patient-centered approach that may offer repeated opportunities to describe important illness experiences.[155] Although these data and recommendations may seem intuitively obvious and in line with a long-standing tradition that emphasizes the therapeutic relationship between "healer" and patient, only about half of the patients with visceral pain syndromes report that health care providers meet their expectations.[156]

PLACEBO RESPONSE

Placebo responses are not unique to visceral pain or functional abdominal disorders, but the magnitude and prevalence of placebo responses in this population are generally high, ranging between 30% and 40%. Such high placebo response rates complicate the interpretation of smaller case series or uncontrolled trials. Interestingly, even when informed that they will be receiving a placebo, IBS patients still improved in a recent trial when compared to a control group.[157] Systematic analyses highlight the importance of supportive patient–provider relationship,[153] which may be especially important in reclusive patients and individuals with prior negative treatment experiences.[155] For investigators, the placebo response constitutes a challenge that requires larger sample sizes and a study design that controls for important confounders contributing to these nonspecific effects. Yet, these very confounders also present an opportunity for clinicians, whose listening skills, empathy, and educational efforts may significantly influence treatment effects independently of the modality chosen.

OPIOIDS

The more widespread use of opioids for benign disorders has influenced approaches to noncancer pain involving the abdomen. Depending on the underlying problem, chronic opioid use varies between 15% and 50% as shown in large cohort studies of diseases characterized by inflammation, structural changes, or functional abnormalities only.[158–161] Yet, opioid therapy is associated with increased health care resource utilization and even functions as a predictor for poor treatment outcomes.[162–164] In inflammatory bowel disease, the negative prognostic impact of opioid management may even be associated with higher mortality.[165] Such findings add to more general concerns about the opioid epidemic, which was in part driven by shifts in medical practice patterns to rely on opiate medications to treat pain. Chronic opioid exposure often comes with adverse effects on gastrointestinal function and may even negatively impact pain sensitivity, prompting some investigators to define the *narcotic bowel syndrome* as a distinct illness. This syndrome is characterized by ongoing and worsening pain despite high and often escalating opioid doses, which is presumably driven by opioid-induced hyperalgesia (see also Chapter 79) and changes in gut motility.[166,167]

Opioid receptors are expressed peripherally and alter many gastrointestinal functions, and several peripherally acting opioid agonists or antagonists have been developed that impact gastrointestinal function. The role of peripheral opiate receptors in visceral pain is less clear. Despite promising preclinical data, local administration of μ-opioid receptor agonists did not blunt acute pain during rectal distension in human volunteers.[168] The peripherally restricted μ-opioid agonist loperamide decreases diarrhea but has inconsistent effects on pain in IBS. Loperamide caused constipation and subsequent discomfort in healthy volunteers, again arguing against a clinically relevant role of peripheral μ-opioid receptors in mediating visceral pain per se.[169,170] Peripherally acting κ-opioid receptor agonists decreased esophageal pain in humans[171] but had no or at best marginal effects on satiety or pain in response to gastric distension.[172,173] Clinical trials using such a κ-opioid agonist did not demonstrate benefit in spontaneous pain exacerbations in IBS or chronic symptoms in dyspepsia.[174,175] Only a post-hoc analysis suggested some improvement in diarrhea predominant IBS, which was confounded by the expected changes in bowel patterns associated with opioid use.[176] Agents with penetration into the central nervous system seemed more promising, as they lowered pain ratings in IBS during rectal distension[177] and were superior compared to placebo when used in patients with functional dyspepsia or IBS.[178,179] However, the utility of these κ-opioid drugs was limited due to their central side effects.[180]

NONOPIOID ANALGESICS

Case-control studies show that patients with abdominal pain syndromes are more likely to use NSAIDs.[181] These results may simply be a surrogate marker for pain but may be confounded by the known NSAID-induced adverse effects that often involve the gastrointestinal tract, causing dyspeptic symptoms, ulcers, and intestinal or colonic inflammation.[182–185] Prostaglandins play an essential role in uterine contractions. Consistent with this role, NSAID therapy is more effective than placebo or acetaminophen in dysmenorrhea and chronic pelvic pain but is associated with more side effects, mostly due to the already mentioned impact on the gastrointestinal tract.[186,187] Parenteral administration of an NSAID is also beneficial in biliary[188] and renal colic,[189] with data suggesting superiority not only over spasmolytics but also over morphine.[190] Although intravenous acetaminophen was inferior to parenteral NSAIDs, pain reduction in renal colic equaled that of morphine.[191] These data indicate that parenteral NSAID therapy should be preferred over opioids in the management of acute abdominal pain. However, the common adverse effects from the gut limit its utility in chronic abdominal pain treatment. Studies examining acetaminophen focused on acute pain management with intravenous infusion, therefore not allowing conclusions about the potential impact of prolonged use. The one exception is primary dysmenorrhea, in which acetaminophen apparently alleviated pain but was inferior to an NSAID.[192,193]

NEUROMODULATORS

Gabapentin and pregabalin as well as other anticonvulsive agents alter neuronal excitability and have found widespread acceptance as mood stabilizing, neuromodulating agents. After early reports suggested benefit in neuropathic pain, these drugs and other anticonvulsive agents have become commonly used adjuncts in analgesic therapy. Yet, there is only limited evidence supporting the use of gabapentin or pregabalin in disorders associated with chronic visceral pain. Pregabalin improved pain ratings in a randomized controlled trial of chronic pancreatitis, but this effect was not associated with a benefit in perceived quality of life or in overall functional status.[194] Interestingly, pain ratings remained lower over several months in a subsequent trial that combined pregabalin with antioxidants.[195] The only published trial in a small cohort with IBS did not show significant symptom relief when compared to placebo, with similar results having been reported in chronic pelvic pain.[196–198]

Although confounded by the unclear benefit of tricyclic antidepressants (see following discussion), gabapentin was superior when compared to such agents in patients with pelvic pain.[199] Data on other anticonvulsive drugs are too limited to allow conclusions. The published information, largely based on relatively small trials, fits with the results of meta-analyses, which indicate that gabapentin is effective in postherpetic and diabetic neuropathy but not in other conditions with neuropathic pain,[200] in fibromyalgia, or in phantom limb pain.[201,202]

ANTIDEPRESSANTS

Antidepressants are commonly used as adjunct in chronic pain syndromes. Several mechanisms have been invoked to explain a possible analgesic effect of tricyclic antidepressants, which affect a variety ion channels and thus decrease neuron excitability. Serotonin norepinephrine reuptake inhibitors (SNRIs) influence central targets to increase the impact of descending modulation on nociceptive pathways. It is also possible that these medications improve pain indirectly by improving mood, which may be especially relevant in depressed individuals who show parallel changes in mood and pain independent of the type of medication used.[203]

Most studies addressing the possible benefit of antidepressants in visceral pain focus on IBS. Drugs, dosages, study designs, and endpoints differ among studies and complicate cross-study comparisons. The largest study did not show a significant decrease in pain ratings when compared to placebo.[204] Meta-analyses point at a potential benefit, yet results are not consistent and raise questions about the utility of selective serotonin reuptake inhibitors (SSRIs).[205,206] The apparent discrepancies similarly surface in trials targeting other disorders manifesting with chronic visceral pain. In functional dyspepsia, only a small study suggests a benefit during treatment with a tricyclic agent, while the SSRI escitalopram was not superior to placebo.[207] In contrast, the largest trial examining tricyclic antidepressants in functional foregut disorders did not show a benefit of nortriptyline in gastroparesis.[208] Only one appropriately designed study addressed the effects of SNRI with negative results in functional dyspepsia.[209] When used as part of multidrug intervention, the duloxetine-containing treatment arm improved urinary symptoms, mood, and quality of life in patients with chronic prostatitis but was associated with a high dropout rate due to side effects.[210] Overall, the contradictory results provide only limited empiric support for the commonly held view that antidepressants function as neuromodulators and have analgesic properties in visceral pain syndromes.[211–217] The primary role for these agents lies in their true role as antidepressants that can improve coexisting psychiatric illness burden. Considering the role of psychiatric disorders and psychological mechanisms in the development and clinical presentation of functional visceral pain, antidepressants may exert their influence more indirectly in these disorders through their effect on mood.

PSYCHOLOGICAL THERAPIES

As may well be true for antidepressants, psychological treatment strategies target key mechanisms, such somatization, hypervigilance, and catastrophizing that are important in the development and maintenance of functional pain syndromes.[20,218,219] A meta-analysis clearly showed beneficial effects of treatments that range from cognitive-behavioral therapy to mindfulness.[220] Although true comparative studies are still lacking, an analysis of published data suggests that cognitive-behavioral therapy may be more effective than other strategies.[221] The initial investment in time and resources to deliver these interventions may constitute a significant burden. In addition, the specialized therapists needed to provide the care are not universally available. Thus, several alternative models have emerged to deliver psychological therapies. Shorter treatments courses may indeed work equally as well as longer interventions but obviously come

with a lower cost.[222] Educational group sessions can improve central processing and fear of visceral symptoms with an overall benefit in quality of life.[223] The widespread use of social media and the Internet has driven the development of virtual programs, which seem promising based on pilot studies.[224,225] Overall, cognitive-behavioral therapy and hypnotherapy have an established role in the management of functional and possibly also other chronic visceral pain syndromes. The remaining question is if group or virtual therapy can improve access, lower treatment costs, and still have long-term outcomes comparable to the conventional one-on-one treatment model.

BLOCKING AFFERENT PATHWAYS

Based on the importance of sensory input and peripheral sensitization, blocking visceral nerve activity should theoretically improve visceral pain. The need for more invasive steps to reach inner organs and the complex innervation complicates the practical and widespread use of approaches that directly target this afferent input. Data are thus limited and often inconclusive. Using sensory thresholds during rectal distension as a surrogate endpoint, intrarectal lidocaine blunted experimentally induced and, in a follow-up study, also spontaneous pain in IBS.[226,227] The short response duration and need for repeated enemas limit the utility of this approach. Other studies demonstrated changes in the structure and function of presumed nociceptive fibers after exposure to capsaicin or resiniferatoxin. These small and uncontrolled studies do not allow clear conclusions but suggest some potential improvement of pain ratings, with more consistent changes in bladder symptoms in patients with interstitial cystitis.[228–230] An alternative approach exploits the renal excretion of pentosan polysulfate to deliver a locally active agent believed to reduce urothelial injury in cystitis. Although not superior to wait-listing only in interstitial cystitis, pentosan polysulfate improved symptoms in men in chronic prostatitis.[231,232] The recent introduction of uroguanylin analogues as treatment for constipation triggered interest in a signaling cascade that involves cyclic guanosine monophosphate (cGMP). Mechanistic studies demonstrate that the secondary messenger is also released at the basolateral side of intestinal epithelial cells and has inhibitory effects of afferent nerve firing and behavioral responses to acute rectal distension, apparently restricted to experimental conditions with hypersensitivity.[233,234] However, agents approved for the management of constipation, in general, were found in a meta-analysis to be associated with decreases in abdominal discomfort in proportion to the improvement in bowel patterns, thus arguing against a specific antinociceptive action of uroguanylin analogues.[235]

Local anesthetic agents also play a potential therapeutic role in myofascial pain affecting abdominal wall muscles, labeled by some anterior cutaneous nerve entrapment syndrome based on the presumed mechanisms. A controlled trial clearly demonstrated a benefit of local infiltration with lidocaine.[236] The effect is only transient in most of the affected persons, but up to one-third of the patients reported longer lasting benefit.[237,238] Given the transient benefit of blocking afferent input, some clinicians advocate neurectomy as a more definitive approach. Controlled trials are difficult as the associated cutaneous anesthesia with neurectomy would, by definition, exclude effective blinding of participants and investigators. Keeping this caveat in mind, a small controlled trial showed superiority of neurectomy over sham surgery when patients were followed for a 6-week period[239] with long-term data from the same group suggesting a lasting benefit.[240]

As already mentioned earlier, the complex anatomy and difficulty in accessing the neural innervation of abdominal and pelvic viscera have been obstacles in developing and routinely using peripheral nerve blocks in the management of chronic visceral pain. The increased availability of cross-sectional imaging or endoscopic ultrasound allows the direct identification of targets, with cohort studies showing good short-term results.[241–243] The longer lasting impact is less clear as retrospective case series suggest transient benefits with ongoing pain and opioid use in more than 50% even after neurolytic interventions.[244,245] The largest controlled trial in pancreatic cancer demonstrated decreased pain levels but failed to show a lasting decrease in opioid use or an impact on quality of life.[246] Clinical practice seems to reflect these findings, as a survey of physicians with a professional focus on pancreatic disease suggested that celiac plexus block is not commonly used and is generally considered to be ineffective.[247] Data on chronic pelvic pain are more positive. Although controlled studies are limited, studies suggest pelvic pain improvement after block or neurectomy,[248] with response rates between 30% and 70%.[249,250]

The contradictory results of studies examining transient nerve blocks or more definitive approaches (neurolysis and neurectomy) point at the importance of central sensitization and fit with limited data on the clinical impact of spinal blockade. During a differential neuroaxial block with complete anesthesia up to the lower chest area, less than 30% of patients with chronic pancreatitis experienced complete resolution of their pain.[52] A similar investigation targeted patients with unexplained chronic abdominal pain and reported comparable results.[251] In the aggregate, treatments that limit or even eliminate peripheral input can decrease pain but often do not lead to a complete resolution of pain, again likely a consequence of central processes that may still be affected by the activity of sensory nerves but can become the primary mechanism driving chronic pain.

SMOOTH MUSCLE RELAXANTS

Many of the hollow visceral structures undergo rhythmic contractions, which can be temporally linked to the experience of abdominal pain. Indeed, detailed physiologic examination showed a correlation between changes in visceral contractile phenomena and the perception of pain in human volunteers and in patients with functional gastrointestinal diseases.[252,253] Thus, weakening such contractions can be an important therapeutic mechanism in patients with patterns or descriptors of pain suggesting an enhanced perception of such contractile activity.[254,255] Anticholinergic agents, typically referred to as "spasmolytics," have become a routine component of the medical management of IBS. The clinical practice is backed by data that show benefit in pain and global symptom ratings in IBS patients.[256] The L-type calcium channel blocker otilonium bromide also functions as smooth muscle relaxant and was shown to be superior to placebo in IBS.[257–259] Other commonly used calcium channel blockers, such as nifedipine, amlodipine, or diltiazem, have not been systematically examined in IBS but have been studied in spastic esophageal disorders. Consistent with their mechanism of action, there were significant effects of these agents on esophageal contractions, which were not matched by symptomatic improvement.[260,261] Anticholinergic or other spasmolytic agents have also been investigated in other abdominal pain disorders. Acute administration alleviated bladder cramps after catheterization.[262] On demand, therapy alleviated abdominal cramps independent of the presumed underlying cause but was not superior to acetaminophen.[263,264] In renal colic, spasmolytics were not superior to placebo when used alone[265] and did not improve pain control when added to NSAID therapy.[266] Although not necessarily mediated by changes in smooth muscle function, NSAIDs show a significant benefit in dysmenorrhea, which could be partly due to the role of prostaglandins in uterine smooth *muscle contractions.*[186]

ACID SUPPRESSANTS

Ever since William Beaumont's foundational observations of gastric function, changes in gastric acid production have been invoked a driver of illness and dyspeptic symptoms.[267] Current clinical guidelines for the management of functional dyspepsia promote the initial use of acid-suppressive medications.[268] Although heartburn and other manifestations of gastroesophageal reflux clearly respond to such a strategy, studies of acid suppression in functional dyspepsia show at best marginal improvements over placebo, with the benefit being largely restricted to patients with coexisting reflux symptoms.[269–271]

ALTERING THE MICROBIOME

The highest density of microbial colonization of the human body is found within the colon. As already discussed earlier, there is mounting interest in the effect of changes in the microbiome on gastrointestinal function and symptoms. Probiotics have become an accepted option in the management of gastrointestinal disorders, particularly in IBS, even though their beneficial effects are only marginal. Many questions remain regarding the most effective type or mixture of organisms to target for therapy.[272] Conversely, antibiotic therapy is used to treat other symptoms of IBS, with the underlying assumption that small intestinal bacterial overgrowth or dysbiosis is relevant mechanism.[273,274] Although the subjective benefit of gut targeted antibiotics outlasts the immediate treatment effects, the presumably abnormal bacterial flora generally recovers within few weeks after treatment cessation, and symptoms often recur. Repeat treatment cycles may well be helpful but raise concerns about the more frequent use of antibiotics in a chronic but benign and noninfectious condition such as IBS, concerns that are especially relevant in an era of characterized by increasingly widespread antibiotic resistance.

SEROTONIN

More than 90% of the body's 5-HT is found in the gastrointestinal tract, where it plays an important role in regulating motility and secretion.[69] 5-HT signaling is complex, with many different receptor subtypes expressed in cells that range from neurons in the central and enteric nervous system to lymphocytes and platelets. Clinically exploited 5-HT effect on visceral sensation largely revolve around pathways mediating nausea and vomiting, with 5-HT$_3$ receptor antagonists having become the most commonly used antiemetics in clinical medicine. The same 5-HT$_3$ receptors reside in the enteric neurons and impact gut motility and secretion. Several 5-HT$_3$ receptor antagonists have been studied in diarrhea-predominant IBS, and results show decreases in bowel frequency, increased stool consistency, and, in most studies, improved pain ratings.[275–277] Detailed mechanistic studies have failed to demonstrate a true effect on sensory mechanisms, suggesting an indirect impact of the reported changes in bowel patterns.[278–281] Several partial 5-HT$_4$ agonists have been developed, which enhance motility and transit in the gut to alleviate constipation and related symptoms including pain.[282,283] Although one study showed a shift in the pain threshold to mechanical but not chemical stimulation of the esophagus,[284] other investigators have not identified consistent changes in gastrointestinal sensation.[285–289] Thus, as was true for the 5-HT$_3$ antagonists, these results highlight the indirect benefit on pain that is likely derived from changes in underlying gut motor function, transit, and luminal filling rather than direct action on nociceptive pathways. Documented adverse events with cardiac arrhythmias, myocardial, or bowel ischemia have led to the withdrawal of several agents targeting 5-HT signaling, leaving us largely with the antiemetics mentioned earlier. Antidepressants also affect 5-HT signals, primarily by interfering with its uptake. Although some agents, such as buspirone or mirtazapine, also interact with 5-HT receptors, they currently have no established role in pain management.

SUBSTANCE P

Substance P acts on neurokinin 1 (NK1) receptors that play a key role in visceral and somatic nociception (see Chapters 3 and 4). Despite a strong evidence basis from anatomical studies and physiologic experiments in normal and genetic knockout rodent models, NK1 antagonists do not appear to have notable analgesic properties in humans.[290] The NK1 receptor antagonist aprepitant functions as a potent antiemetic,[291] but it does not affect perception of gastric distension in human volunteers[292] and had only minor effects on overall symptom severity in patients with gastroparesis.[293] Therefore, NK1 receptor inhibitors do not appear to have good use for treating disorders primarily characterized by pain.

COMPLEMENTARY AND ALTERNATIVE MEDICINE THERAPY

Given the significant impact of chronic visceral discomfort on quality of life and the at times limited benefit of conventional therapies, many patients turn to complementary and alternative medicine (CAM) therapies, ranging from physical movement interventions to the use of herbal remedies, various devices, and acupuncture.[294-297] Systematic studies are limited, and thus, it is difficult to assess the efficacy of many CAM approaches. Physical approaches, such as reflexology, massage therapy, or manipulations based on osteopathic principles, do not seem to be more effective than placebo interventions.[298,299] One exception is the application of local heat patches, which are comparable to NSAID therapy in dysmenorrhea.[300,301] Although acupuncture has gained popularity, well-designed controlled trials failed to show benefit beyond the placebo effect. However, high response rates in both active and sham acupuncture demonstrate the power of placebo interventions in modulating chronic pain.[302-305]

It is also difficult to assess the true utility of herbal preparations, which often contain mixtures of different plant extracts, some of which may have laxative effects that obviously change gut function and thus indirectly affect symptoms. Trials of peppermint oil on visceral pain in IBS show the most convincing evidence of efficacy. Detailed physiologic studies in human volunteers demonstrate a spasmolytic effect with a decrease in the amplitude of colonic contractions but also possible effects on visceral sensory function.[306,307] When used to treat IBS, peppermint oil was superior to placebo.[308,309]

Ginger may have weak inhibitory effects on muscarinic and 5-HT receptors.[310] Although ginger extracts showed some benefit in dyspepsia and dysmenorrhea, randomized trials did not demonstrate efficacy in IBS.[311-313] Iberogast, a mixture containing peppermint among other herbal extracts, alleviated dyspeptic symptoms.[314,315] Small studies in IBS patients suggest a potential benefit of curcumin with fennel oil or anise extract.[316,317] In contrast, another commonly used agent, St. John's Wort, was ineffective in IBS.[318]

Many supplements include digestive enzymes based on the underlying assumption that gastrointestinal discomfort is a sign of impaired digestion. Systematic studies in patients with chronic pancreatitis did not support an independent impact on pain[319] but confirmed the expected benefit in patients with coexisting exocrine insufficiency.[320] As oxidative damage may contribute to tissue injury in inflammatory processes, antioxidants could play a role in reducing injury and blunting symptoms, a concept that has some empiric backing in chronic pancreatitis.[321,322] The aggregate data demonstrate that the widespread use of herbal remedies and supplements continues despite limited supportive evidence of efficacy beyond placebo responses.

Conclusion

Visceral pain is a common problem made more impactful due to disproportionate unpleasantness compared to similarly intense somatic pain. There has been increasing understanding of the neurobiologic underpinnings that account for key differences in the clinical features of visceral and somatic abdominal pain.

For example, visceral pain is often poorly localized, in part due to the low innervation density of viscera, and patterns of visceral pain referral to distant, mostly cutaneous sites are the result of convergence of visceral and somatic sensory pathways within the central nervous system. These clinical features of abdominal pain can help in the identification of underlying medical problems. Many of the abdominal viscera are hollow organs that accommodate, propel, and ultimately expel their contents. Therefore, the filling state and degree of muscle tension or contractile activity are peripheral factors that influence visceral pain intensity, and as such present clues to not only diagnosis but also treatment options using dietary interventions, altering bowel patterns, or inhibiting muscle activity. Changes in the complex interactions between the microbial flora, luminal contents, the gut epithelium, and the enteric nervous system may also influence visceral pain in syndromes such as IBS. Pharmacologic management of abdominal pain relies primarily on strategies that are used in other conditions characterized by acute or chronic pain. However, the deeper location and typically bilateral innervation of viscera complicates the use of local therapies, such as nerve blocks or topical agents. Frequently used analgesic medications such as opiates and NSAIDs have some limited utility when used chronically due to direct effects on the gut mucosa and motility that lead to commonly experienced side effects. On the other hand, agents that interfere with cholinergic and serotoninergic signaling can alter visceral function, often with secondary improvement of pain or discomfort and without significant impact on somatic function or sensation. Future research into the neurobiologic mechanisms of visceral and somatic abdominal pain pathways will hopefully identify specific targets that can translate into novel therapies for a host of common, chronic pain syndromes.

References

1. Zhong F, Christianson JA, Davis BM, et al. Dichotomizing axons in spinal and vagal afferents of the mouse stomach. *Dig Dis Sci* 2008;53:194–203.
2. Christianson JA, Liang R, Ustinova EE, et al. Convergence of bladder and colon sensory innervation occurs at the primary afferent level. *Pain* 2007;128:235–243.
3. Bruggemann J, Shi T, Apkarian AV. Squirrel monkey lateral thalamus. II. Viscerosomatic convergent representation of urinary bladder, colon, and esophagus. *J Neurosci* 1994;14:6796–6814.
4. Schmidt B, Hammer J, Holzer P, et al. Chemical nociception in the jejunum induced by capsaicin. *Gut* 2004;53:1109–1106.
5. Munakata J, Naliboff B, Harraf F, et al. Repetitive sigmoid stimulation induces rectal hyperalgesia in patients with irritable bowel syndrome. *Gastroenterology* 1997;112:55–63.
6. Drewes AM, Reddy H, Staahl C, et al. Sensory-motor responses to mechanical stimulation of the esophagus after sensitization with acid. *World J Gastroenterol* 2005;11:4367–4374.
7. Mertz H, Fullerton S, Naliboff B, et al. Symptoms and visceral perception in severe functional and organic dyspepsia. *Gut* 1998;42:814–822.
8. Takeda T, Nabae T, Kassab G, et al. Oesophageal wall stretch: the stimulus for distension induced oesophageal sensation. *Neurogastroenterol Motil* 2004;16:721–728.
9. Bielefeldt K, Zhong F, Koerber HR, et al. Phenotypic characterization of gastric sensory neurons in mice. *Am J Physiol Gastrointest Liver Physiol* 2006;291:G987–G997.
10. Garrison DW, Chandler MJ, Foreman RD. Viscerosomatic convergence onto feline spinal neurons from esophagus, heart and somatic fields: effects of inflammation. *Pain* 1992;49:373–382.
11. Mullady DK, Yadav D, Amann ST, et al. Type of pain, pain-associated complications, quality of life, disability and resource utilisation in chronic pancreatitis: a prospective cohort study. *Gut* 2011;60:77–84.
12. Simrén M, Abrahamsson H, Björnsson ES. An exaggerated sensory component of the gastrocolonic response in patients with irritable bowel syndrome. *Gut* 2001;48:20–27.
13. Glissen Brown JR, Bernstein GR, Friedenberg FK, et al. Chronic abdominal wall pain: an under-recognized diagnosis leading to unnecessary testing. *J Clin Gastroenterol* 2016;50:828–835.
14. Rao SS, Bharucha AE, Chiarioni G, et al. Functional anorectal disorders [published online ahead of print March 25, 2016]. *Gastroenterology*. doi:10.1053/j.gastro.2016.02.009.
15. Kossi J, Salminen P, Rantala A, et al. Population-based study of the surgical workload and economic impact of bowel obstruction caused by postoperative adhesions. *Br J Surg* 2003;90:1441–1444.

16. Whitehead W, Palsson O, Jones K. Systematic review of the comorbidity of irritable bowel syndrome with other disorders: what are the causes and implications? *Gastroenterology* 2002;122:1140–1156.

17. Lifford KL, Barbieri RL. Diagnosis and management of chronic pelvic pain. *Urol Clin North Am* 2002;29:637–647.

18. Henningsen P, Zimmermann T, Sattel H. Medically unexplained physical symptoms, anxiety, and depression: a meta-analytic review. *Psychosom Med* 2003;65:528–533.

19. North CS, Downs D, Clouse RE, et al. The presentation of irritable bowel syndrome in the context of somatization disorder. *Clin Gastroenterol Hepatol* 2004;2:787–795.

20. Lackner JM, Quigley BM. Pain catastrophizing mediates the relationship between worry and pain suffering in patients with irritable bowel syndrome. *Behav Res Ther* 2005;43:943–957.

21. Spiegel BM, Kanwal F, Naliboff B, et al. The impact of somatization on the use of gastrointestinal health-care resources in patients with irritable bowel syndrome. *Am J Gastroenterol* 2005;100:2262–2273.

22. Musumba C, Jorgensen A, Sutton L, et al. The relative contribution of NSAIDs and *Helicobacter pylori* to the aetiology of endoscopically-diagnosed peptic ulcer disease: observations from a tertiary referral hospital in the UK between 2005 and 2010. *Aliment Pharmacol Ther* 2012;36:48–56.

23. U.S. Food and Drug Administration. FDA Drug Safety Communication: FDA warns about increased risk of serious pancreatitis with irritable bowel drug Viberzi (eluxadoline) in patients without a gallbladder. Available at: https://www.fda.gov/Drugs/DrugSafety/ucm546154.htm.

24. Friedel D, Thomas R, Fisher RS. Ischemic colitis during treatment with alosetron. *Gastroenterology* 2001;120:557–560.

25. Levinthal DJ, Bielefeldt K. Adult cyclical vomiting syndrome: a disorder of allostatic regulation. *Exp Brain Res* 2014;232:1–7.

26. Suleiman S, Johnston DE. The abdominal wall: an overlooked source of pain. *Am Fam Physician* 2001;64:431–438.

27. Sengupta JN, Gebhart GF. Characterization of mechanosensitive pelvic nerve afferent fibers innervating the colon of the rat. *J Neurophysiol* 1994;71:2046–2060.

28. Kang Y-M, Bielefeldt K, Gebhart GF. Sensitization of mechanosensitive gastric vagal afferent fibers in the rat by thermal and chemical stimuli and gastric ulcers. *J Neurophysiol* 2004;91:1981–1989.

29. Akopian AN, Souslova V, England S, et al. The tetrodotoxin-resistant sodium channel SNS has a specialized function in pain pathways. *Nature Neuroscience* 1999;2:541–548.

30. McCleskey EW, Gold MS. Ion channels of nociception. *Annu Rev Physiol* 1999;61:835–856.

31. Stucky CL, Lewin GR. Isolectin B4-positive and -negative nociceptors are functionally distinct. *J Neurosci* 1999;19:6497–6505.

32. Phillips RJ, Powley TL. Tension and stretch receptors in gastrointestinal smooth muscle: re-evaluating vagal mechanoreceptor electrophysiology. *Brain Res Brain Res Rev* 2000;34:1–26.

33. Zheng H, Lauve A, Patterson LM, et al. Limited excitatory local effector function of gastric vagal afferent intraganglionic terminals in rats. *Am J Physiol* 1997;273:G661–G669.

34. Lynn P, Olsson C, Zagorodnyuk V, et al. Rectal intraganglionic laminar endings are transduction sites of extrinsic mechanoreceptors in the guinea pig rectum. *Gastroenterology* 2003;125:786–794.

35. Song X, Chen BN, Zagorodnyuk VP, et al. Identification of medium/high-threshold extrinsic mechanosensitive afferent nerves to the gastrointestinal tract. *Gastroenterology* 2009;137:274.e1–284.e1.

36. Spencer NJ, Zagorodnyuk V, Brookes SJ, et al. Spinal afferent nerve endings in visceral organs: recent advances. *Am J Physiol Gastrointest Liver Physiol* 2016;311:G1056–G1063.

37. Sugiura Y, Tonosaki Y. Spinal organization of unmyelinated visceral afferent fibers in comparison with somatic afferent fibers. In: Gebhart GF, ed. *Progress in Pain Research and Management.* Vol 5. Seattle, WA: IASP Press; 1995:41–59.

38. Willis WD, Al-Chaer ED, Quast MJ, et al. A visceral pain pathway in the dorsal column of the spinal cord. *Proc Natl Acad Sci U S A* 1999;96:7675–7679.

39. Amassian VE. Cortical representation of visceral afferents. *J Neurophysiol* 1951;14:433–444.

40. Dum RP, Levinthal DJ, Strick PL. The spinothalamic system targets motor and sensory areas in the cerebral cortex of monkeys. *J Neurosci* 2009;29:14223–14235.

41. Strigo IA, Bushnell MC, Boivin M, et al. Psychophysical analysis of visceral and cutaneous pain in human subjects. *Pain* 2002;97:235–246.

42. Lu CL, Wu YT, Chen LF, et al. Neuronal correlates of gastric pain induced by fundus distension: a 3T-fMRI study. *Neurogastroenterol Motil* 2004;16:575–587.

43. Kern M, Hofmann C, Hyde J, et al. Characterization of the cerebral cortical representation of heartburn in GERD patients. *Am J Physiol Gastrointest Liver Physiol* 2004;286:G174–G181.

44. Twiss C, Kilpatrick L, Craske M, et al. Increased startle responses in interstitial cystitis: evidence for central hyperresponsiveness to visceral related threat. *J Urol* 2009;181:2127–2133.

45. Tack J, Caenepeel P, Fischler B, et al. Symptoms associated with hypersensitivity to gastric distention in functional dyspepsia. *Gastroenterology* 2001;121:526–535.

46. Dizdar V, Gilja OH, Hausken T. Increased visceral sensitivity in Giardia-induced postinfectious irritable bowel syndrome and functional dyspepsia. Effect of the 5HT3-antagonist ondansetron. *Neurogastroenterol Motil* 2007;19:977–982.

47. Buscher HC, Wilder-Smith OH, van Goor H. Chronic pancreatitis patients show hyperalgesia of central origin: a pilot study. *Eur J Pain* 2006;10:363–370.

48. Olesen SS, Brock C, Krapup AL, et al. Descending inhibitory pain modulation is impaired in patients with chronic pancreatitis. *Clin Gastroenterol Hepatol* 2010;8:724–730.

49. Friess H, Zhu ZW, di Mola FF, et al. Nerve growth factor and its high-affinity receptor in chronic pancreatitis. *Ann Surg* 1999;230:615–624.

50. Shrikhande SV, Friess H, di Mola FF, et al. NK-1 receptor gene expression is related to pain in chronic pancreatitis. *Pain* 2001;91:209–217.

51. Shrikhande SV, Martignoni ME, Shrikhande M, et al. Comparison of histological features and inflammatory cell reaction in alcoholic, idiopathic and tropical chronic pancreatitis. *Br J Surg* 2003;90:1565–1572.

52. Conwell DL, Vargo JJ, Zuccaro G, et al. Role of differential neuroaxial blockade in the evaluation and management of pain in chronic pancreatitis. *Am J Gastroenterol* 2001;96:431–436.

53. Marshall J, Thabane M, Garg AX, et al. Incidence and epidemiology of irritable bowel syndrome after a large waterborne outbreak of bacterial dysentery. *Gastroenterology* 2006;131:445–450.

54. Borgaonkar MR, Ford DC, Marshall JK, et al. The incidence of irritable bowel syndrome among community subjects with previous acute enteric infection. *Dig Dis Sci* 2006;51:1026–1032.

55. Zanini B, Ricci C, Bandera F, et al. Incidence of post-infectious irritable bowel syndrome and functional intestinal disorders following a water-borne viral gastroenteritis outbreak. *Am J Gastroenterol* 2012;107:891–899.

56. Wensaas K-A, Langeland N, Hanevik K, et al. Irritable bowel syndrome and chronic fatigue 3 years after acute giardiasis: historic cohort study. *Gut* 2012;61:214–219.

57. Marshall JK, Thabane M, Garg AX, et al. Eight year prognosis of postinfectious irritable bowel syndrome following waterborne bacterial dysentery. *Gut* 2010;59:605–611.

58. Naliboff BD, Derbyshire SW, Munakata J, et al. Cerebral activation in patients with irritable bowel syndrome and control subjects during rectosigmoid stimulation. *Psychosom Med* 2001;63:365–375.

59. Stabell N, Stubhaug A, Flægstad T, et al. Widespread hyperalgesia in adolescents with symptoms of irritable bowel syndrome: results from a large population-based study. *J Pain* 2014;15:898–906.

60. Stabell N, Stubhaug A, Flægstad T, et al. Increased pain sensitivity among adults reporting irritable bowel syndrome symptoms in a large population-based study. *Pain* 2013;154:385–392.

61. Frøkjær JB, Bouwense SA, Olesen SS, et al. Reduced cortical thickness of brain areas involved in pain processing in patients with chronic pancreatitis. *Clin Gastroenterol Hepatol* 2012;10:434.e1–438.e1.

62. Blankstein U, Chen J, Diamant NE, et al. Altered brain structure in irritable bowel syndrome: potential contributions of pre-existing and disease-driven factors. *Gastroenterology* 2010;138:1783–1789.

63. Labus JS, Dinov ID, Jiang Z, et al. Irritable bowel syndrome in female patients is associated with alterations in structural brain networks. *Pain* 2014;155:137–149.

64. Piche M, Chen JI, Roy M, et al. Thicker posterior insula is associated with disease duration in women with irritable bowel syndrome (IBS) whereas thicker orbitofrontal cortex predicts reduced pain inhibition in both IBS patients and controls. *J Pain* 2013;14:1217–1226.

65. Bouwense SA, Ahmed Ali U, ten Broek RP, et al. Altered central pain processing after pancreatic surgery for chronic pancreatitis. *Br J Surg* 2013;100:1797–1804.

66. Lelic D, Olesen SS, Hansen TM, et al. Functional reorganization of brain networks in patients with painful chronic pancreatitis. *Eur J Pain* 2014;18:968–977.

67. Waehrens R, Ohlsson H, Sundquist J, et al. Risk of irritable bowel syndrome in first-degree, second-degree and third-degree relatives of affected individuals: a nationwide family study in Sweden. *Gut* 2015;64:215–221.

68. Mohammed I, Cherkas LF, Riley SA, et al. Genetic influences in irritable bowel syndrome: a twin study. *Am J Gastroenterol* 2005;100:1340–1344.

69. Gershon MD, Tack J. The serotonin signaling system: from basic understanding to drug development for functional GI disorders. *Gastroenterology* 2007;132:397–414.

70. Kohen R, Tracy JH, Haugen E, et al. Rare variants of the serotonin transporter are associated with psychiatric comorbidity in irritable bowel syndrome. *Biol Res Nurs* 2016;18:394–400.

71. Colucci R, Gambaccini D, Ghisu N, et al. Influence of the serotonin transporter 5HTTLPR polymorphism on symptom severity in irritable bowel syndrome. *PLoS One* 2013;8:e54831.

72. Mujakovic S, ter Linde JJ, de Wit NJ, et al. Serotonin receptor 3A polymorphism c.-42C> T is associated with severe dyspepsia. *BMC Med Genet* 2011;12:140.

73. Kilpatrick LA, Labus JS, Coveleskie K, et al. The HTR3A polymorphism c.-42C>T is associated with amygdala responsiveness in patients with irritable bowel syndrome. *Gastroenterology* 2011;140:1943–1951.

74. Grasberger H, Chang L, Shih W, et al. Identification of a functional TPH1 polymorphism associated with irritable bowel syndrome bowel habit subtypes. *Am J Gastroenterol* 2013;108:1766–1774.

75. Shiotani A, Kusunoki H, Ishii M, et al. Pilot study of biomarkers for predicting effectiveness of ramosetron in diarrhea-predominant irritable bowel syndrome: expression of S100A10 and polymorphisms of TPH1. *Neurogastroenterol Motil* 2015;27:82–91.

76. Karling P, Danielsson A, Wikgren M, et al. The relationship between the val158met catechol-O-methyltransferase (COMT) polymorphism and irritable bowel syndrome. *PLoS One* 2011;6:e18035.

77. Hall KT, Tolkin BR, Chinn GM, et al. Conscientiousness is modified by genetic variation in catechol-O-methyltransferase to reduce symptom complaints in IBS patients. *Brain Behav* 2015;5:39–44.

78. Hall K, Lembo A, Kirsch I, et al. Catechol-O-methyltransferase val158met polymorphism predicts placebo effect in irritable bowel syndrome. *PLoS One* 2012;7:e48135.

79. Orand A, Gupta A, Shih W, et al. Catecholaminergic gene polymorphisms are associated with GI symptoms and morphological brain changes in irritable bowel syndrome. *PLoS One* 2015;10:e0135910.

80. Orand A, Naliboff B, Gadd M, et al. Corticotropin-releasing hormone receptor 1 (CRH-R1) polymorphisms are associated with irritable bowel syndrome and acoustic startle response. *Psychoneuroendocrinology* 2016;73:133–141.

81. Komuro H, Sato N, Sasaki A, et al. Corticotropin-releasing hormone receptor 2 gene variants in irritable bowel syndrome. *PLoS One* 2016;11:e0147817.

82. Villani A-C, Lemire M, Thabane M, et al. Genetic risk factors for post-infectious irritable bowel syndrome following a waterborne outbreak of gastroenteritis. *Gastroenterology* 2010;138:1502–1513.

83. Camilleri M, Carlson P, Acosta A, et al. Colonic mucosal gene expression and genotype in irritable bowel syndrome patients with normal or elevated fecal bile acid excretion. *Am J Physiol Gastrointest Liver Physiol* 2015;309:G10–G20.

84. Henström M, Diekmann L, Bonfiglio F, et al. Functional variants in the sucrase-isomaltase gene associate with increased risk of irritable bowel syndrome. *Gut* 2018;67:263–270.

85. Saito YA, Locke GR, Zimmerman JM, et al. A genetic association study of 5-HTT LPR and GNbeta3 C825T polymorphisms with irritable bowel syndrome. *Neurogastroenterol Motil* 2007;19:465–470.

86. Swan C, Duroudier NP, Campbell E, et al. Identifying and testing candidate genetic polymorphisms in the irritable bowel syndrome (IBS): association with TNFSF15 and TNF. *Gut* 2013;62:985–994.

87. Zucchelli M, Camilleri M, Nixon Andreasson A, et al. Association of TNFSF15 polymorphism with irritable bowel syndrome. *Gut* 2011;60:1671–1677.

88. Srivastava D, Ghoshal U, Mittal RD, et al. Associations between IL-1RA polymorphisms and small intestinal bacterial overgrowth among patients with irritable bowel syndrome from India. *Neurogastroenterol Motil* 2014;26:1408–1416.

89. Wouters MM, Lambrechts D, Knapp M, et al. Genetic variants in CDC42 and NXPH1 as susceptibility factors for constipation and diarrhoea predominant irritable bowel syndrome. *Gut* 2014;63:1103–1111.

90. van der Veek PP, van den Berg M, de Kroon YE, et al. Role of tumor necrosis factor-alpha and interleukin-10 gene polymorphisms in irritable bowel syndrome. *Am J Gastroenterol* 2005;100:2510–2516.

91. Drossman DA, Leserman J, Nachman G, et al. Sexual and physical abuse in women with functional or organic gastrointestinal disorders. *Ann Intern Med* 1990;113:828–833.

92. Al-Chaer ED, Kawasaki M, Pasricha PJ. A new model of chronic visceral hypersensitivity in adult rats induced by colon irritation during postnatal development. *Gastroenterology* 2000;119:1276–1285.

93. Coutinho SV, Plotsky PM, Sablad M, et al. Neonatal maternal separation alters stress-induced responses to viscerosomatic nociceptive stimuli in rat. *Am J Physiol Gastrointest Liver Physiol* 2002;282:G307–G316.

94. Blanchard EB, Keefer L, Lackner JM, et al. The role of childhood abuse in Axis I and Axis II psychiatric disorders and medical disorders of unknown origin among irritable bowel syndrome patients. *J Psychosom Res* 2004;56:431–436.

95. Latthe P, Mignini L, Gray R, et al. Factors predisposing women to chronic pelvic pain: systematic review. *BMJ* 2006;332:749–755.

96. Ringel Y, Drossman DA, Leserman JL, et al. Effect of abuse history on pain reports and brain responses to aversive visceral stimulation: an fMRI study. *Gastroenterology* 2008;134:396–404.

97. Geeraerts B, van Oudenhove I, Fischler B, et al. Influence of abuse history on gastric sensorimotor function in functional dyspepsia. *Neurogastroenterol Motil* 2009;21:33–41.

98. Videlock EJ, Adeyemo M, Licudine A, et al. Childhood trauma is associated with hypothalamic-pituitary-adrenal axis responsiveness in irritable bowel syndrome. *Gastroenterology* 2009;137:1954–1962.

99. Talley NJ, Boyce PM, Jones M. Predictors of health care seeking for irritable bowel syndrome: a population based study. *Gut* 1997;41:394–398.

100. Guthrie E, Creed F, Fernandes L, et al. Cluster analysis of symptoms and health seeking behaviour differentiates subgroups of patients with severe irritable bowel syndrome. *Gut* 2003;52:1616–1622.

101. Kanuri N, Cassell B, Bruce SE, et al. The impact of abuse and mood on bowel symptoms and health-related quality of life in irritable bowel syndrome (IBS). *Neurogastroenterol Motil* 2016;28:1508–1517.

102. Posserud I, Agerforz P, Ekman R, et al. Altered visceral perceptual and neuroendocrine response in patients with irritable bowel syndrome during mental stress. *Gut* 2004;53:1102–1108.

103. Bennett EJ, Tennant CC, Piesse C, et al. Level of chronic life stress predicts clinical outcome in irritable bowel syndrome. *Gut* 1998;43:256–261.

104. Gwee KA, Read NW, Graham JC, et al. Psychometric scores and persistence of irritable bowel after infectious diarrhoea. *Lancet* 1996;347:150–153.

105. Gwee K-A, Leong Y-L, Graham C, et al. The role of psychological and biological factors in postinfective gut dysfunction. *Gut* 1999;44:400–406.

106. Lowe B, Lohse A, Andresen V, et al. The development of irritable bowel syndrome: a prospective community-based cohort study. *Am J Gastroenterol* 2016;111:1320–1329.

107. Van Oudenhove L, Vandenberghe J, Geeraerts B, et al. Determinants of symptoms in functional dyspepsia: gastric sensorimotor function, psychosocial factors or somatisation? *Gut* 2008;57:1666–1673.

108. Nicholl B, Halder S, Macfarlane G, et al. Psychosocial risk markers for new onset irritable bowel syndrome—results of a large prospective population-based study. *Pain* 2008;137:147–155.

109. Choung RS, Locke GR, Zinsmeister AR, et al. Psychosocial distress and somatic symptoms in community subjects with irritable bowel syndrome: a psychological component is the rule. *Am J Gastroenterology* 2009;104:1772–1779.

110. Wolitzky-Taylor K, Craske MG, Labus JS, et al. Visceral sensitivity as a mediator of outcome in the treatment of irritable bowel syndrome. *Behav Res Ther* 2012;50:647–650.

111. Knowles SR, Austin DW, Sivanesan S, et al. Relations between symptom severity, illness perceptions, visceral sensitivity, coping strategies and well-being in irritable bowel syndrome guided by the common sense model of illness. *Psychol Health Med* 2017;22:524–534.

112. Lackner JM, Ma CX, Keefer L, et al. Type, rather than number, of mental and physical comorbidities increases the severity of symptoms in patients with irritable bowel syndrome. *Clin Gastroenterol Hepatol* 2013;11:1147–1157.

113. Jalanka-Tuovinen J, Salojärvi J, Salonen A, et al. Faecal microbiota composition and host–microbe cross-talk following gastroenteritis and in postinfectious irritable bowel syndrome. *Gut* 2014;63:1737–1745.

114. Goebel A, Buhner S, Schedel R, et al. Altered intestinal permeability in patients with primary fibromyalgia and in patients with complex regional pain syndrome. *Rheumatology (Oxford)* 2008;47:1223–1227.

115. Mayer EA, Tillisch K, Gupta A. Gut/brain axis and the microbiota. *J Clin Invest* 2015;125:926–938.

116. Dinan TG, Cryan JF. Melancholic microbes: a link between gut microbiota and depression? *Neurogastroenterol Motil* 2013;25:713–719.

117. Moloney RD, Johnson AC, O'Mahony SM, et al. Stress and the microbiota-gut-brain axis in visceral pain: relevance to irritable bowel syndrome. *CNS Neurosci Ther* 2016;22:102–117.

118. Dior M, Delagreverie H, Duboc H, et al. Interplay between bile acid metabolism and microbiota in irritable bowel syndrome. *Neurogastroenterol Motil* 2016;28:1330–1340.

119. Ringel-Kulka T, Choi CH, Temas D, et al. Altered colonic bacterial fermentation as a potential pathophysiological factor in irritable bowel syndrome. *Am J Gastroenterol* 2015;110:1339–1346.

120. Botschuijver S, Roeselers G, Levin E, et al. Intestinal fungal dysbiosis associates with visceral hypersensitivity in patients with irritable bowel syndrome and rats. *Gastroenterology* 2017;153:1026–1039.

121. Casén C, Vebo HC, Sekelja M, et al. Deviations in human gut microbiota: a novel diagnostic test for determining dysbiosis in patients with IBS or IBD. *Aliment Pharmacol Ther* 2015;42:71–83.

122. Bennet SMP, Böhn L, Störsrud S, et al. Multivariate modelling of faecal bacterial profiles of patients with IBS predicts responsiveness to a diet low in FODMAPs [published online ahead of print April 17, 2017]. *Gut*. doi:10.1136/gutjnl-2016-313128.

123. McIntosh K, Reed DE, Schneider T, et al. FODMAPs alter symptoms and the metabolome of patients with IBS: a randomised controlled trial. *Gut* 2017;66:1241–1251.

124. Ritchie J. Pain from distension of the pelvic colon by inflating a balloon in the irritable colon syndrome. *Gut* 1973;14:125–132.

125. Trimble KC, Pryde A, Heading RC. Lowered oesophageal sensory thresholds in patients with symptomatic but not excess gastro-oesophageal reflux: evidence for a spectrum of visceral sensitivity in GORD. *Gut* 1995;37:7–12.

126. Vandenberghe J, Vos R, Persoons P, et al. Dyspeptic patients with visceral hypersensitivity: sensitisation of pain specific or multimodal pathways? *Gut* 2005;54:914–919.

127. Cremonini F, Houghton LA, Camilleri M, et al. Barostat testing of rectal sensation and compliance in humans: comparison of results across two centres and overall reproducibility. *Neurogastroenterol Motil* 2005;17:810–820.

128. Zhou Q, Fillingim RB, Riley III JL, et al. Central and peripheral hypersensitivity in the irritable bowel syndrome. *Pain* 2010;148:454–461.

129. Song GH, Venkatraman V, Ho KY, et al. Cortical effects of anticipation and endogenous modulation of visceral pain assessed by functional brain MRI in irritable bowel syndrome patients and healthy controls. *Pain* 2006;126:79–90.

130. Berman SM, Naliboff BD, Suyenobu B, et al. Reduced brainstem inhibition during anticipated pelvic visceral pain correlates with enhanced brain response to the visceral stimulus in women with irritable bowel syndrome. *J Neurosci* 2008;28:349–359.

131. Yáguez L, Coen S, Gregory LJ, et al. Brain response to visceral aversive conditioning: a functional magnetic resonance imaging study. *Gastroenterology* 2005;128:1819–1829.

132. Naliboff BD, Berman S, Suyenobu B, et al. Longitudinal change in perceptual and brain activation response to visceral stimuli in irritable bowel syndrome patients. *Gastroenterology* 2006;131:352–365.

133. Olesen SS, Graversen C, Bouwense SA, et al. Quantitative sensory testing predicts pregabalin efficacy in painful chronic pancreatitis. *PLoS One* 2013;8:e57963.

134. Labus JS, Van Horn JD, Gupta A, et al. Multivariate morphological brain signatures predict patients with chronic abdominal pain from healthy control subjects. *Pain* 2015;156:1545–1554.

135. Jones MP, Chey WD, Singh S, et al. A biomarker panel and psychological morbidity differentiates the irritable bowel syndrome from health and provides novel pathophysiological leads. *Aliment Pharmacol Ther* 2014;39: 426–437.

136. Bohn L, Storsrud S, Tornblom H, et al. Self-reported food-related gastrointestinal symptoms in IBS are common and associated with more severe symptoms and reduced quality of life. *Am J Gastroenterol* 2013;108:634–641.

137. Gudleski GD, Satchidanand N, Dunlap LJ, et al. Predictors of medical and mental health care use in patients with irritable bowel syndrome in the United States. *Behav Res Ther* 2017;88:65–75.

138. de Roest RH, Dobbs BR, Chapman BA, et al. The low FODMAP diet improves gastrointestinal symptoms in patients with irritable bowel syndrome: a prospective study. *Int J Clin Pract* 2013;67:895–903.

139. Halmos EP, Power VA, Shepherd SJ, et al. A diet low in FODMAPs reduces symptoms of irritable bowel syndrome. *Gastroenterology* 2014;146:67. e5–75.e5.

140. Salvioli B, Pellegatta G, Malacarne M, et al. Autonomic nervous system dysregulation in irritable bowel syndrome. *Neurogastroenterol Motil* 2015; 27:423–430.

141. Murray CD, Flynn J, Ratcliffe L, et al. Effect of acute physical and psychological stress on gut autonomic innervation in irritable bowel syndrome. *Gastroenterology* 2004;127:1695–1703.

142. Blanchard EB, Lackner JM, Jaccard J, et al. The role of stress in symptom exacerbation among IBS patients. *J Psychosom Res* 2008;64:119–128.

143. van Tilburg MA, Levy RL, Walker LS, et al. Psychosocial mechanisms for the transmission of somatic symptoms from parents to children. *World J Gastroenterol* 2015;21:5532–5541.

144. Thakur ER, Gurtman MB, Keefer L, et al. Gender differences in irritable bowel syndrome: the interpersonal connection. *Neurogastroenterol Motil* 2015;27:1478–1486.

145. Drossman DA, Chang L, Schneck S, et al. A focus group assessment of patient perspectives on irritable bowel syndrome and illness severity. *Dig Dis Sci* 2009;54:1532–1541.

146. Lackner JM, Gudleski GD, Firth R, et al. Negative aspects of close relationships are more strongly associated than supportive personal relationships with illness burden of irritable bowel syndrome. *J Psychosom Res* 2013;74:493–500.

147. Lackner JM, Brasel AM, Quigley BM, et al. The ties that bind: perceived social support, stress, and IBS in severely affected patients. *Neurogastroenterol Motil* 2010;22:893–900.

148. Lee SK, Yoon DW, Lee S, et al. The association between irritable bowel syndrome and the coexistence of depression and insomnia. *J Psychosom Res* 2017;93:1–5.

149. Nicholl BI, Halder SL, Macfarlane GJ, et al. Psychosocial risk markers for new onset irritable bowel syndrome—results of a large prospective population-based study. *Pain* 2008;137:147–155.

150. Nojkov B, Rubenstein JH, Chey WD, et al. The impact of rotating shift work on the prevalence of irritable bowel syndrome in nurses. *Am J Gastroenterol* 2010;105:842–847.

151. Patel A, Hasak S, Cassell B, et al. Effects of disturbed sleep on gastrointestinal and somatic pain symptoms in irritable bowel syndrome. *Aliment Pharmacol Ther* 2016;44:246–258.

152. Halpert A, Dalton CB, Palsson O, et al. What patients know about irritable bowel syndrome (IBS) and what they would like to know. National Survey on Patient Educational Needs in IBS and development and validation of the Patient Educational Needs Questionnaire (PEQ). *Am J Gastroenterol* 2007;102:1972–1982.

153. Kaptchuk TJ, Kelley JM, Conboy LA, et al. Components of placebo effect: randomised controlled trial in patients with irritable bowel syndrome. *BMJ* 2008;333:999–1003.

154. Weinland S, Morris C, Dalton C, et al. Cognitive factors affect treatment response to medical and psychological treatments in functional bowel disorders. *Am J Gastroenterol* 2010;105:1397–1406.

155. Conboy LA, Macklin E, Kelley J, et al. Which patients improve: characteristics increasing sensitivity to a supportive patient-practitioner relationship. *Soc Sci Med* 2010;70:479–484.

156. Halpert A, Dalton CB, Palsson O, et al. Irritable bowel syndrome patients' ideal expectations and recent experiences with healthcare providers: a national survey. *Dig Dis Sci* 2010;55:375–383.

157. Kaptchuk T, Friedlander E, Kelley J, et al. Placebos without deception: a randomized controlled trial in irritable bowel syndrome. *PLoS One* 2010;12:e15591.

158. Niemann T, Madsen L, Larsen S, et al. Opioid treatment of painful chronic pancreatitis. *Int J Pancreatol* 2000;27:235–240.

159. Nusrat S, Yadav D, Bielefeldt K. Pain and opioid use in chronic pancreatitis. *Pancreas* 2012;41:264–270.

160. Cross RK, Wilson KT, Binion DG. Narcotic use in patients with Crohn's disease. *Am J Gastroenterol* 2005;100:2225–2229.

161. Parkman HP, Yates K, Hasler WL, et al. Similarities and differences between diabetic and idiopathic gastroparesis. *Clin Gastroenterol Hepatol* 2011;9:1056–1064.

162. Olesen SS, Poulsen JL, Broberg MC, et al. Opioid treatment and hypoalbuminemia are associated with increased hospitalisation rates in chronic pancreatitis outpatients. *Pancreatology* 2016;16:807–813.

163. Stefaniak T, Vingerhoets A, Makarewicz W, et al. Opioid use determines success of videothoracoscopic splanchnicectomy in chronic pancreatic pain patients. *Langenbecks Arch Surg* 2008;393:213–218.

164. Maranki JL, Lytes V, Meilahn JE, et al. Predictive factors for clinical improvement with Enterra gastric electric stimulation treatment for refractory gastroparesis. *Dig Dis Sci* 2008;53:2072–2078.

165. Lichtenstein GR, Feagan BG, Cohen RD, et al. Serious infections and mortality in association with therapies for Crohn's disease: TREAT registry. *Clin Gastroenterol Hepatol* 2006;4:621–630.

166. Grunkemeier D, Cassara J, Dalton C, et al. The narcotic bowel syndrome: clinical features, pathophysiology, and management. *Clin Gastroenterol Hepatol* 2007;5:1126–1139.

167. Farmer AD, Gallagher J, Bruckner-Holt C, et al. Narcotic bowel syndrome. *Lancet Gastroenterol Hepatol* 2017;2:361–368.

168. Brokjaer A, Olesen AE, Christrup LL, et al. The effects of morphine and methylnaltrexone on gastrointestinal pain in healthy male participants. *Neurogastroenterol Motil* 2015;27:693–704.

169. Marcus SN, Heaton KW. Irritable bowel-type symptoms in spontaneous and induced constipation. *Gut* 1987;28:156–159.

170. Efskind PS, Bernklev T, Vatn MH. A double-blind placebo-controlled trial with loperamide in irritable bowel syndrome. *Scand J Gastroenterol* 1996;31:463–468.

171. Arendt-Nielsen L, Olesen A, Staahl C, et al. Analgesic efficacy of peripheral kappa-opioid receptor agonist CR665 compared to oxycodone in a multi-modal, multi-tissue experimental human pain model: selective effect on visceral pain. *Anesthesiology* 2009;111:616–624.

172. Floyd BN, Camilleri M, Busciglio I, et al. Effect of a kappa-opioid agonist, i.v. JNJ-38488502, on sensation of colonic distensions in healthy male volunteers. *Neurogastroenterol Motil* 2009;21:281–290.

173. Delgado-Aros S, Chial HJ, Camilleri M, et al. Effects of a kappa-opioid agonist, asimadoline, on satiation and GI motor and sensory functions in humans. *Am J Physiol Gastrointest Liver Physiol* 2003;284:G558–G566.

174. Talley NJ, Choung RS, Camilleri M, et al. Asimadoline, a kappa-opioid agonist, and satiation in functional dyspepsia. *Aliment Pharmacol Ther* 2008;27:1122–1131.

175. Szarka LA, Camilleri M, Burton D, et al. Efficacy of on-demand asimadoline, a peripheral kappa-opioid agonist, in females with irritable bowel syndrome. *Clin Gastroenterol Hepatol* 2007;5:1268–1275.

176. Mangel AW, Bornstein JD, Hamm LR, et al. Clinical trial: asimadoline in the treatment of patients with irritable bowel syndrome. *Aliment Pharmacol Ther* 2008;28:239–249.

177. Delvaux M, Louvel D, Lagier E, et al. The agonist fedotozine relieves hypersensitivity to colonic distention in patients with irritable bowel syndrome. *Gastroenterology* 1999;116:38–45.

178. Dapoigny M, Abitbol JL, Fraitag B. Efficacy of peripheral kappa agonist fedotozine versus placebo in treatment of irritable bowel syndrome. A multicenter dose-response study. *Dig Dis Sci* 1995;40:2244–2249.

179. Read NW, Abitbol JL, Bardhan KD, et al. Efficacy and safety of the peripheral kappa agonist fedotozine versus placebo in the treatment of functional dyspepsia. *Gut* 1997;41:664–668.

180. Rivière PJ-M. Peripheral kappa-opioid agonists for visceral pain. *Br J Pharmacol* 2004;141:1331–1334.

181. Keszthelyi D, Dackus GH, Masclee GM, et al. Increased proton pump inhibitor and NSAID exposure in irritable bowel syndrome: results from a case-control study. *BMC Gastroenterol* 2012;12:121.

182. Verhaegh BP, de Vries F, Masclee AA, et al. High risk of drug-induced microscopic colitis with concomitant use of NSAIDs and proton pump inhibitors. *Aliment Pharmacol Ther* 2016;43:1004–1013.

183. Ananthakrishnan AN, Higuchi LM, Huang ES, et al. Aspirin, nonsteroidal anti-inflammatory drug use, and risk for Crohn disease and ulcerative colitis: a cohort study. *Ann Intern Med* 2012;156:350–359.

184. Talley N, Weaver A, Zinsmeister A. Smoking, alcohol, and nonsteroidal anti-inflammatory drugs in outpatients with functional dyspepsia and among dyspepsia subgroups. *Am J Gastroenterol* 1994;89:524–528.

185. Shaib Y, El-Serag HB. The prevalence and risk factors of functional dyspepsia in a multiethnic population in the United States. *Am J Gastroenterol* 2004;99:2210–2216.

186. Marjoribanks J, Ayeleke RO, Farquhar C, et al. Nonsteroidal anti-inflammatory drugs for dysmenorrhoea. *Cochrane Database Syst Rev* 2015;(7): CD001751.

187. Moore RA, Derry S, Wiffen PJ, et al. Overview review: comparative efficacy of oral ibuprofen and paracetamol (acetaminophen) across acute and chronic pain conditions. *Eur J Pain* 2015;19:1213–1223.

188. Fraquelli M, Casazza G, Conte D, et al. Non-steroid anti-inflammatory drugs for biliary colic. *Cochrane Database Syst Rev* 2016;(9):CD006390.

189. Pathan SA, Mitra B, Straney LD, et al. Delivering safe and effective analgesia for management of renal colic in the emergency department: a double-blind, multigroup, randomised controlled trial. *Lancet* 2016;387: 1999–2007.

190. Afshar K, Jafari S, Marks AJ, et al. Nonsteroidal anti-inflammatory drugs (NSAIDs) and non-opioids for acute renal colic. *Cochrane Database Syst Rev* 2015;(6):CD006027.

191. Serinken M, Eken C, Turkcuer I, et al. Intravenous paracetamol versus morphine for renal colic in the emergency department: a randomised double-blind controlled trial. *Emerg Med J* 2012;29:902–905.

192. Milsom I, Minic M, Dawood MY, et al. Comparison of the efficacy and safety of nonprescription doses of naproxen and naproxen sodium with ibuprofen, acetaminophen, and placebo in the treatment of primary dysmenorrhea: a pooled analysis of five studies. *Clin Ther* 2002;24: 1384–1400.

193. Dawood MY, Khan-Dawood FS. Clinical efficacy and differential inhibition of menstrual fluid prostaglandin F2alpha in a randomized, double-blind, crossover treatment with placebo, acetaminophen, and ibuprofen in primary dysmenorrhea. *Am J Obstet Gynecol* 2007;196: 35.e1–35.e5.

194. Olesen SS, Bouwense SA, Wilder-Smith OH, et al. Pregabalin reduces pain in patients with chronic pancreatitis in a randomized, controlled trial. *Gastroenterology* 2011;141:536–543.

195. Talukdar R, Lakhtakia S, Nageshwar Reddy D, et al. Ameliorating effect of antioxidants and pregabalin combination in pain recurrence after ductal clearance in chronic pancreatitis: results of a randomized, double blind, placebo-controlled study. *J Gastroenterol Hepatol* 2016;31:1654–1662.

196. Houghton LA, Fell C, Whorwell PJ, et al. Effect of a second-generation $\alpha_2\delta$ ligand (pregabalin) on visceral sensation in hypersensitive patients with irritable bowel syndrome. *Gut* 2007;56:1218–1225.

197. Pontari MA, Krieger JN, Litwin MS, et al. Pregabalin for the treatment of men with chronic prostatitis/chronic pelvic pain syndrome: a randomized controlled trial. *Arch Intern Med* 2010;170:1586–1593.

198. Lewis SC, Bhattacharya S, Wu O, et al. Gabapentin for the management of chronic pelvic pain in women (GaPP1): a pilot randomised controlled trial. *PLoS One* 2016;11:e0153037.

199. Sator-Katzenschlager SM, Scharbert G, Kress HG, et al. Chronic pelvic pain treated with gabapentin and amitriptyline: a randomized controlled pilot study. *Wien Klin Wochenschr* 2005;117:761–768.

200. Wiffen PJ, Derry S, Bell RF, et al. Gabapentin for chronic neuropathic pain in adults. *Cochrane Database Syst Rev* 2017;(6):CD007938.

201. Cooper TE, Derry S, Wiffen PJ, et al. Gabapentin for fibromyalgia pain in adults. *Cochrane Database Syst Rev* 2017;(1):CD012188.

202. Alviar MJ, Hale T, Dungca M. Pharmacologic interventions for treating phantom limb pain. *Cochrane Database Syst Rev* 2016;(10):CD006380.

203. Gebhardt S, Heinzel-Gutenbrunner M, Konig U. Pain relief in depressive disorders: a meta-analysis of the effects of antidepressants. *J Clin Psychopharmacol* 2016;36:658–668.

204. Drossman DA, Toner BB, Whitehead WE, et al. Cognitive-behavioral therapy versus education and desipramine versus placebo for moderate to severe functional bowel disorders. *Gastroenterology* 2003;125:19–31.

205. Xie C, Tang Y, Wang Y, et al. Efficacy and safety of antidepressants for the treatment of irritable bowel syndrome: a meta-analysis. *PLoS One* 2015;10:e0127815.

206. Ford AC, Talley NJ, Schoenfeld PS, et al. Efficacy of antidepressants and psychological therapies in irritable bowel syndrome: systematic review and meta-analysis. *Gut* 2009;58:367–378.

207. Talley NJ, Locke GR, Saito YA, et al. Effect of amitriptyline and escitalopram on functional dyspepsia: a multicenter, randomized controlled study. *Gastroenterology* 2015;149:340.e2–349.e2.

208. Parkman HP, Van Natta ML, Abell TL, et al. Effect of nortriptyline on symptoms of idiopathic gastroparesis: the norig randomized clinical trial. *JAMA* 2013;310:2640–2649.

209. van Kerkhoven LA, Laheij RJ, Aparicio N, et al. Effect of the antidepressant venlafaxine in functional dyspepsia: a randomized, double-blind, placebo-controlled trial. *Clin Gastroenterol Hepatol* 2008;6:746–752.

210. Giannantoni A, Porena M, Gubbiotti M, et al. The efficacy and safety of duloxetine in a multidrug regimen for chronic prostatitis/chronic pelvic pain syndrome. *Urology* 2014;83:400–405.

211. Cheong YC, Smotra G, Williams AC. Non-surgical interventions for the management of chronic pelvic pain. *Cochrane Database Syst Rev* 2014;(3):CD008797.

212. Papandreou C, Skapinakis P, Giannakis D, et al. Antidepressant drugs for chronic urological pelvic pain: an evidence-based review. *Adv Urol* 2009;2009:797031.

213. Lunn M, Hughes R, Wiffen P. Duloxetine for treating painful neuropathy, chronic pain or fibromyalgia. *Cochrane Database Syst Rev* 2014;(1): CD007115.

214. Lunn MP, Hughes RA, Wiffen PJ. Duloxetine for treating painful neuropathy, chronic pain or fibromyalgia. *Cochrane Database Syst Rev* 2014;(1): CD007115.

215. Moore RA, Derry S, Aldington D, et al. Amitriptyline for fibromyalgia in adults. *Cochrane Database Syst Rev* 2015;(7):CD011824.

216. Moore RA, Derry S, Aldington D, et al. Amitriptyline for neuropathic pain in adults. *Cochrane Database Syst Rev* 2015;(7):CD008242.

217. Derry S, Wiffen PJ, Aldington D, et al. Nortriptyline for neuropathic pain in adults. *Cochrane Database Syst Rev* 2015;(1):CD011209.

218. Garland EL, Gaylord SA, Palsson O, et al. Therapeutic mechanisms of a mindfulness-based treatment for IBS: effects on visceral sensitivity, catastrophizing, and affective processing of pain sensations. *J Behav Med* 2012;35: 591–602.

219. van Tilburg MA, Palsson OS, Whitehead WE. Which psychological factors exacerbate irritable bowel syndrome? Development of a comprehensive model. *J Psychosom Res* 2013;74:486–492.

220. Ford AC, Quigley EM, Lacy BE, et al. Effect of antidepressants and psychological therapies, including hypnotherapy, in irritable bowel syndrome: systematic review and meta-analysis. *Am J Gastroenterol* 2014;109:1350–1366.

221. Laird KT, Tanner-Smith EE, Russell AC, et al. Comparative efficacy of psychological therapies for improving mental health and daily functioning in irritable bowel syndrome: a systematic review and meta-analysis. *Clin Psychol Rev* 2017;51:142–152.

222. Lackner JM, Gudleski GD, Keefer L, et al. Rapid response to cognitive behavior therapy predicts treatment outcome in patients with irritable bowel syndrome. *Clin Gastroenterol Hepatol* 2010;8:426–432.

223. Labus J, Gupta A, Gill HK, et al. Randomised clinical trial: symptoms of the irritable bowel syndrome are improved by a psycho-education group intervention. *Aliment Pharmacol Ther* 2013;37:304–315.

224. Hunt MG, Moshier S, Milonova M. Brief cognitive-behavioral internet therapy for irritable bowel syndrome. *Behav Res Ther* 2009;47:797–802.

225. Ljótsson B, Falk L, Vesterlund AW, et al. Internet-delivered exposure and mindfulness based therapy for irritable bowel syndrome—a randomized controlled trial. *Behav Res Ther* 2010;48:531–539.

226. Verne GN, Sen A, Price DD. Intrarectal lidocaine is an effective treatment for abdominal pain associated with diarrhea-predominant irritable bowel syndrome. *J Pain* 2005;6:493–496.

227. Lembo T, Munakata J, Mertz H, et al. Evidence for the hypersensitivity of lumbar splanchnic afferents in irritable bowel syndrome. *Gastroenterology* 1994;107:1686–1696.

228. Fagerli J, Fraser MO, deGroat WC, et al. Intravesical capsaicin for the treatment of interstitial cystitis: a pilot study. *Can J Urol* 1999;6:737–744.

229. Peng CH, Kuo HC. Multiple intravesical instillations of low-dose resiniferatoxin in the treatment of refractory interstitial cystitis. *Urol Int* 2007;78:78–81.

230. Apostolidis A, Gonzales GE, Fowler CJ. Effect of intravesical resiniferatoxin (RTX) on lower urinary tract symptoms, urodynamic parameters, and quality of life of patients with urodynamic increased bladder sensation. *Eur Urol* 2006;50:1299–1305.

231. Sands BE, Sandborn WJ, Creed TJ, et al. Basiliximab does not increase efficacy of corticosteroids in patients with steroid-refractory ulcerative colitis. *Gastroenterology* 2012;143:356.e1–364.e1.

232. Nickel JC, Forrest JB, Tomera K, et al. Pentosan polysulfate sodium therapy for men with chronic pelvic pain syndrome: a multicenter, randomized, placebo controlled study. *J Urol* 2005;173:1252–1255.

233. Eutamene H, Bradesi S, Larauche M, et al. Guanylate cyclase C-mediated antinociceptive effects of linaclotide in rodent models of visceral pain. *Neurogastroenterol Motil* 2010;22:312–e84.

234. Castro J, Harrington A, Hughes P, et al. Linaclotide inhibits colonic nociceptors and relieves abdominal pain via guanylate cyclase-C and extracellular cyclic guanosine 3′,5′-monophosphate. *Gastroenterology* 2013;145:1334–1346.

235. Bielefeldt K, Levinthal DJ, Nusrat S. Effective constipation treatment changes more than bowel frequency: a systematic review and meta-analysis. *J Neurogastroenterol Motil* 2016;22:31–45.

236. Boelens OB, Scheltinga MR, Houterman S, et al. Randomized clinical trial of trigger point infiltration with lidocaine to diagnose anterior cutaneous nerve entrapment syndrome. *Br J Surg* 2013;100:217–221.

237. Boelens OB, Scheltinga MR, Houterman S, et al. Management of anterior cutaneous nerve entrapment syndrome in a cohort of 139 patients. *Ann Surg* 2011;254:1054–1058.

238. Siawash M, Mol F, Tjon ATW, et al. Anterior rectus sheath blocks in children with abdominal wall pain due to anterior cutaneous nerve entrapment syndrome: a prospective case series of 85 children. *Paediatr Anaesth* 2017;27:545–550.

239. Boelens OB, van Assen T, Houterman S, et al. A double-blind, randomized, controlled trial on surgery for chronic abdominal pain due to anterior cutaneous nerve entrapment syndrome. *Ann Surg* 2013;257:845–849.

240. van Assen T, Boelens OB, van Eerten PV, et al. Long-term success rates after an anterior neurectomy in patients with an abdominal cutaneous nerve entrapment syndrome. *Surgery* 2015;157:137–143.

241. Santosh D, Lakhtakia S, Gupta R, et al. Clinical trial: a randomized trial comparing fluoroscopy guided percutaneous technique vs. endoscopic ultrasound guided technique of coeliac plexus block for treatment of pain in chronic pancreatitis. *Aliment Pharmacol Ther* 2009;29:979–984.

242. Sahai A, Lemelin V, Lam E, et al. Central vs. bilateral endoscopic ultrasound-guided celiac plexus block or neurolysis: a comparative study of short-term effectiveness. *Am J Gastroenterol* 2009;104:326–329.

243. Puli SR, Reddy JB, Bechtold ML, et al. EUS-guided celiac plexus neurolysis for pain due to chronic pancreatitis or pancreatic cancer pain: a meta-analysis and systematic review. *Dig Dis Sci* 2009;54:2330–2337.

244. Johnson C, Berry D, Harris S, et al. An open randomized comparison of clinical effectiveness of protocol-driven opioid analgesia, celiac plexus block or thoracoscopic splanchnicectomy for pain management in patients with pancreatic and other abdominal malignancies. *Pancreatology* 2009;9:755–763.

245. Edelstein MR, Gabriel RT, Elbich JD, et al. Pain outcomes in patients undergoing CT- guided celiac plexus neurolysis for intractable abdominal visceral pain. *Am J Hosp Palliat Care* 2017;34:111–114.

246. Wong GY, Schroeder DR, Carns PE, et al. Effect of neurolytic celiac plexus block on pain relief, quality of life, and survival in patients with unresectable pancreatic cancer: a randomized controlled trial. *JAMA* 2004;291:1092–1099.

247. Burton F, Alkaade S, Collins D, et al. Use and perceived effectiveness of non-analgesic medical therapies for chronic pancreatitis in the United States. *Aliment Pharmacol Ther* 2011;33:149–159.

248. Latthe PM, Proctor ML, Farquhar CM, et al. Surgical interruption of pelvic nerve pathways in dysmenorrhea: a systematic review of effectiveness. *Acta Obstet Gynecol Scand* 2007;86:4–15.

249. Nezhat CH, Seidman DS, Nezhat FR, et al. Long-term outcome of laparoscopic presacral neurectomy for the treatment of central pelvic pain attributed to endometriosis. *Obstet Gynecol* 1998;91:701–704.

250. Zullo F, Palomba S, Zupi E, et al. Long-term effectiveness of presacral neurectomy for the treatment of severe dysmenorrhea due to endometriosis. *J Am Assoc Gynecol Laparosc* 2004;11:23–28.

251. Rizk MK, Tolba R, Kapural L, et al. Differential epidural block predicts the success of visceral block in patients with chronic visceral abdominal pain. *Pain Pract* 2012;12:595–601.

252. Cuomo R, Vandaele P, Coulie B, et al. Influence of motilin on gastric fundus tone and on meal-induced satiety in man: role of cholinergic pathways. *Am J Gastroenterol* 2006;101:804–811.

253. Steens J, Van Der Schaar PJ, Penning C, et al. Compliance, tone and sensitivity of the rectum in different subtypes of irritable bowel syndrome. *Neurogastroenterol Motil* 2002;14:241–247.

254. Gilbert QO. The spastic colon. *Cal West Med* 1929;30:330–334.

255. Hare DC. Therapeutic observations on non-specific colitis: (section of therapeutics and pharmacology). *Proc R Soc Med* 1935;29:19–30.

256. Ruepert L, Quartero A, de Wit N, et al. Bulking agents, antispasmodics and antidepressants for the treatment of irritable bowel syndrome. *Cochrane Database Syst Rev* 2011;(8):CD003460.

257. Clavé P, Acalovschi M, Triantafillidis JK, et al. Randomised clinical trial: otilonium bromide improves frequency of abdominal pain, severity of distention and time to relapse in patients with irritable bowel syndrome. *Aliment Pharmacol Ther* 2011;34:432–442.

258. Battaglia G, Morselli-Labate AM, Camarri E, et al. Otilonium bromide in irritable bowel syndrome: a double-blind, placebo-controlled, 15-week study. *Aliment Pharmacol Ther* 1998;12:1003–1010.

259. Glende M, Morselli-Labate A, Battaglia G, et al. Extended analysis of a double-blind, placebo-controlled, 15-week study with otilonium bromide in irritable bowel syndrome. *Eur J Gastroenterol Hepatol* 2002;14:1331–1338.

260. Richter JE, Dalton CB, Bradley LA, et al. Oral nifedipine in the treatment of noncardiac chest pain in patients with the nutcracker esophagus. *Gastroenterology* 1987;93:21–28.

261. Drenth JP, Bos LP, Engels LG. Efficacy of diltiazem in the treatment of diffuse oesophageal spasm. *Aliment Pharmacol Ther* 1990;4:411–416.

262. Nam K, Seo JH, Ryu JH, et al. Randomized, clinical trial on the preventive effects of butylscopolamine on early postoperative catheter-related bladder discomfort. *Surgery* 2015;157:396–401.

263. Lacy BE, Wang F, Bhowal S, et al. On-demand hyoscine butylbromide for the treatment of self-reported functional cramping abdominal pain. *Scand J Gastroenterol* 2013;48:926–935.

264. Mueller-Lissner S, Tytgat GN, Paulo LG, et al. Placebo- and paracetamol-controlled study on the efficacy and tolerability of hyoscine butylbromide in the treatment of patients with recurrent crampy abdominal pain. *Aliment Pharmacol Ther* 2006;23:1741–1748.

265. Holdgate A, Oh CM. Is there a role for antimuscarinics in renal colic? A randomized controlled trial. *J Urol* 2005;174:572–575.

266. Jones JB, Giles BK, Brizendine EJ, et al. Sublingual hyoscyamine sulfate in combination with ketorolac tromethamine for ureteral colic: a randomized, double-blind, controlled trial. *Ann Emerg Med* 2001;37:141–146.

267. Bielefeldt K. From ischochymia to gastroparesis: proposed mechanisms and preferred management of dyspepsia over the centuries. *Dig Dis Sci* 2014;59:1088–1098.

268. Talley NJ, Vakil N. Guidelines for the management of dyspepsia. *Am J Gastroenterol* 2005;100:2324–2337.

269. Peura D, Kovacs T, Metz D, et al. Lansoprazole in the treatment of functional dyspepsia: two double-blind, randomized, placebo-controlled trials. *Am J Med* 2004;116:740–748.

270. Talley NJ, Meineche-Schmidt V, Paré P, et al. Efficacy of omeprazole in functional dyspepsia: double-blind, placebo-controlled trials (the Bond and Opera studies). *Aliment Pharmacol Ther* 1998;12:1055–1065.

271. Rabeneck L, Souchek J, Wristers K, et al. A double blind, randomized, placebo-controlled trial of proton pump inhibitor therapy in patients with uninvestigated dyspepsia. *Am J Gastroenterol* 2002;97:3045–3051.

272. Ford AC, Quigley EM, Lacy BE, et al. Efficacy of prebiotics, probiotics, and synbiotics in irritable bowel syndrome and chronic idiopathic constipation: systematic review and meta-analysis. *Am J Gastroenterol* 2014;109:1547–1561.

273. Sharara AI, Aoun E, Abdul-Baki H, et al. A randomized double-blind placebo-controlled trial of rifaximin in patients with abdominal bloating and flatulence. *Am J Gastroenterol* 2006;101:326–333.

274. Pimentel M, Lembo A, Chey WD, et al. Rifaximin therapy for patients with irritable bowel syndrome without constipation. *N Engl J Med* 2011;364:22–32.

275. Fukudo S, Kinoshita Y, Okumura T, et al. Ramosetron reduces symptoms of irritable bowel syndrome with diarrhea and improves quality of life in women. *Gastroenterology* 2016;150:358.e8–366.e8.

276. Camilleri M, Mayer EA, Drossman DA, et al. Improvement in pain and bowel function in female irritable bowel patients with alosetron, a 5-HT3 receptor antagonist. *Aliment Pharmacol Ther* 1999;13:1149–1159.

277. Garsed K, Chernova J, Hastings M, et al. A randomised trial of ondansetron for the treatment of irritable bowel syndrome with diarrhoea. *Gut* 2014;63:1617–1625.

278. Delvaux M, Louvel D, Mamet J-P, et al. Effect of alosetron on responses to colonic distension in patients with irritable bowel syndrome. *Aliment Pharmacol Ther* 1998;12:849–855.

279. Thumshirn M, Coulie B, Camilleri M, et al. Effects of alosetron on gastrointestinal transit time and rectal sensation in patients with irritable bowel syndrome. *Aliment Pharmacol Ther* 2000;14:869–878.

280. Janssen P, Vos R, Van Oudenhove L, et al. Influence of the 5-HT3 receptor antagonist ondansetron on gastric sensorimotor function and nutrient tolerance in healthy volunteers. *Neurogastroenterol Motil* 2011;23:444–449, e175.

281. Hammer J, Phillips SF, Talley NJ, et al. Effect of a 5HT3-antagonist (ondansetron) on rectal sensitivity and compliance in health and the irritable bowel syndrome. *Aliment Pharmacol Ther* 1993;7:543–551.

282. Müller-Lissner SA, Fumagalli I, Bardhan KD, et al. Tegaserod, a 5-HT4 receptor partial agonist, relieves symptoms in irritable bowel syndrome patients with abdominal pain, bloating and constipation. *Aliment Pharmacol Ther* 2001;15:1655–1666.

283. Novick J, Miner P, Krause R, et al. A randomized, double-blind, placebo-controlled trial of tegaserod in female patients suffering from irritable bowel syndrome with constipation. *Aliment Pharmacol Ther* 2002;16:1877–1888.

284. Rodriguez-Stanley S, Zubaidi S, Proskin HM, et al. Effect of tegaserod on esophageal pain threshold, regurgitation, and symptom relief in patients with functional heartburn and mechanical sensitivity. *Clin Gastroenterol Hepatol* 2006;4:442–450.

285. Coffin B, Farmachidi JP, Rueegg P, et al. Tegaserod, a 5-HT4 receptor partial agonist, decreases sensitivity to rectal distension in healthy subjects. *Aliment Pharmacol Ther* 2003;17:577–585.

286. Tack J, Janssen P, Bisschops R, et al. Influence of tegaserod on proximal gastric tone and on the perception of gastric distention in functional dyspepsia. *Neurogastroenterol Motil* 2011;23:e32–e39.

287. Corsetti M, Tack J. Tegaserod: a new 5-HT(4) agonist in the treatment of irritable bowel syndrome. *Expert Opin Pharmacother* 2002;3:1211–1218.

288. Manes G, Domínguez-Muñoz JE, Leodolter A, et al. Effect of cisapride on gastric sensitivity to distension, gastric compliance and duodeno-gastric reflexes in healthy humans. *Dig Liver Dis* 2001;33:407–413.

289. Tack J, Broeckaert D, Coulie B, et al. The influence of cisapride on gastric tone and the perception of gastric distension. *Aliment Pharmacol Ther* 1998;12:761–766.

290. Hill R. NK1 (substance P) receptor antagonists—why are they not analgesic in human? *Trends Pharmacol Sci* 2000;21:244–246.

291. Curran M, Robinson D. Aprepitant: a review of its use in the prevention of nausea and vomiting. *Drugs* 2009;69:1853–1878.

292. Ang D, Pauwels A, Akyuz F, et al. Influence of a neurokinin-1 receptor antagonist (aprepitant) on gastric sensorimotor function in healthy volunteers. *Neurogastroenterol Motil* 2013;25:e830–e838.

293. Pasricha PJ, Yates KP, Sarosiek I, et al. Aprepitant has mixed effects on nausea and reduces other symptoms in patients with gastroparesis and related disorders. *Gastroenterology* 2018;65.e11–76.e11.

294. Donker GA, Foets M, Spreeuwenberg P. Patients with irritable bowel syndrome: health status and use of health care services. *Br J Gen Pract* 1999;49:787–792.

295. Kong SC, Hurlstone DP, Pocock CY, et al. The incidence of self-prescribed oral complementary and alternative medicine use by patients with gastrointestinal diseases. *J Clin Gastroenterol* 2005;39:138–141.

296. Tillisch K. Complementary and alternative medicine for functional gastrointestinal disorders. *Gut* 2006;55:593–596.

297. Drossman DA, Morris CB, Schneck S, et al. International survey of patients with IBS: symptom features and their severity, health status, treatments, and risk taking to achieve clinical benefit. *J Clin Gastroenterol* 2009;43:541–550.

298. Florance BM, Frin G, Dainese R, et al. Osteopathy improves the severity of irritable bowel syndrome: a pilot randomized sham-controlled study. *Eur J Gastroenterol Hepatol* 2012;24:944–949.

299. Tovey P. A single-blind trial of reflexology for irritable bowel syndrome. *Br J Gen Pract* 2002;52:19–23.

300. Akin MD, Weingand KW, Hengehold DA, et al. Continuous low-level topical heat in the treatment of dysmenorrhea. *Obstet Gynecol* 2001;97:343–349.

301. Navvabi Rigi S, Kermansaravi F, Navidian A, et al. Comparing the analgesic effect of heat patch containing iron chip and ibuprofen for primary dysmenorrhea: a randomized controlled trial. *BMC Womens Health* 2012;12:25.

302. Lowe C, Aiken A, Day AG, et al. Sham acupuncture is as efficacious as true acupuncture for the treatment of IBS: a randomized placebo controlled trial [published online ahead of print March 2, 2017]. *Neurogastroenterol Motil*. doi:10.1111/nmo.13040.

303. Proctor ML, Smith CA, Farquhar CM, et al. Transcutaneous electrical nerve stimulation and acupuncture for primary dysmenorrhoea. *Cochrane Database Syst Rev* 2002;(1):CD002123.

304. Lembo AJ, Conboy L, Kelley JM, et al. A treatment trial of acupuncture in IBS patients. *Am J Gastroenterol* 2009;104:1489–1497.
305. Schneider A, Enck P, Streitberger K, et al. Acupuncture treatment in irritable bowel syndrome. *Gut* 2006;55:649–654.
306. Micklefield G, Jung O, Greving I, et al. Effects of intraduodenal application of peppermint oil (WS(R) 1340) and caraway oil (WS(R) 1520) on gastroduodenal motility in healthy volunteers. *Phytother Res* 2003;17:135–140.
307. Papathanasopoulos A, Rotondo A, Janssen P, et al. Effect of acute peppermint oil administration on gastric sensorimotor function and nutrient tolerance in health. *Neurogastroenterol Motil* 2013;25:e263–e271.
308. Cash BD, Epstein MS, Shah SM. A novel delivery system of peppermint oil is an effective therapy for irritable bowel syndrome symptoms. *Dig Dis Sci* 2016;61:560–571.
309. Khanna R, MacDonald JK, Levesque BG. Peppermint oil for the treatment of irritable bowel syndrome: a systematic review and meta-analysis. *J Clin Gastroenterol* 2014;48:505–512.
310. Pertz HH, Lehmann J, Roth-Ehrang R, et al. Effects of ginger constituents on the gastrointestinal tract: role of cholinergic M3 and serotonergic 5-HT3 and 5-HT4 receptors. *Planta Med* 2011;77:973–978.
311. Giacosa A, Guido D, Grassi M, et al. The effect of ginger (*Zingiber officinalis*) and artichoke (*Cynara cardunculus*) extract supplementation on functional dyspepsia: a randomised, double-blind, and placebo-controlled clinical trial. *Evid Based Complement Alternat Med* 2015;2015:915087.
312. van Tilburg MA, Palsson OS, Ringel Y, et al. Is ginger effective for the treatment of irritable bowel syndrome? A double blind randomized controlled pilot trial. *Complement Ther Med* 2014;22:17–20.
313. Chen CX, Barrett B, Kwekkeboom KL. Efficacy of oral ginger (*Zingiber officinale*) for dysmenorrhea: a systematic review and meta-analysis. *Evid Based Complement Alternat Med* 2016;2016:6295737.
314. Braden B, Caspary W, Börner N, et al. Clinical effects of STW 5 (Iberogast®) are not based on acceleration of gastric emptying in patients with functional dyspepsia and gastroparesis. *Neurogastroenterol Motil* 2009;21:632–638.
315. von Arnim U, Peitz U, Vinson B, et al. STW 5, a phytopharmacon for patients with functional dyspepsia: results of a multicenter, placebo-controlled double-blind study. *Am J Gastroenterol* 2007;102:1268–1275.
316. Mosaffa-Jahromi M, Lankarani KB, Pasalar M, et al. Efficacy and safety of enteric coated capsules of anise oil to treat irritable bowel syndrome. *J Ethnopharmacol* 2016;194:937–946.
317. Portincasa P, Bonfrate L, Scribano ML, et al. Curcumin and fennel essential oil improve symptoms and quality of life in patients with irritable bowel syndrome. *J Gastrointestin Liver Dis* 2016;25:151–157.
318. Saito YA, Rey E, Almazar-Elder AE, et al. A randomized, double-blind, placebo-controlled trial of St John's wort for treating irritable bowel syndrome. *Am J Gastroenterolog* 2009;105:170–177.
319. Yaghoobi M, McNabb-Baltar J, Bijarchi R, et al. Pancreatic enzyme supplements are not effective for relieving abdominal pain in patients with chronic pancreatitis: meta-analysis and systematic review of randomized controlled trials. *Can J Gastroenterol Hepatol* 2016;2016:8541839.
320. D'Haese JG, Ceyhan GO, Demir IE, et al. Pancreatic enzyme replacement therapy in patients with exocrine pancreatic insufficiency due to chronic pancreatitis: a 1-year disease management study on symptom control and quality of life. *Pancreas* 2014;43(6):834–841.
321. Rustagi T, Njei B. Antioxidant therapy for pain reduction in patients with chronic pancreatitis: a systematic review and meta-analysis. *Pancreas* 2015;44:812–818.
322. Ahmed Ali U, Jens S, Busch OR, et al. Antioxidants for pain in chronic pancreatitis. *Cochrane Database Syst Rev* 2014;(8):CD008945.

CHAPTER 64

Pelvic Pain in Females

KATY VINCENT and **JANE MOORE**

Pelvic pain is common in women, frequently leading to disability, social disruption, and loss of economic productivity. Many women do not seek help, often having lived with the pain since adolescence and accepting it as normal. In New Zealand, only 34% of a community sample of women aged between 18 and 50 years reported no pelvic pain, with 55.2% reporting dysmenorrhea, 25.4% chronic pelvic pain (CPP), and 19.7% dyspareunia.[1] In the United States, 14.7% of women of the same age range reported CPP with estimated outpatient medical costs of $881.5 million per year, 15% reporting work absenteeism, and 45% reduced productivity.[2] Similarly in the United Kingdom, 24% of 18- to 49-year-olds reported CPP[3] and 37 of every 1,000 women consulting their general practitioner presented with CPP[4]; this was comparable to asthma (37/1,000) and back pain (41/1,000) and higher than migraine (21/1,000).

Pelvic pain is a frustrating symptom for both the patient and the doctor. Presentation can be variable, involving many organ systems, and severity can fluctuate over time. The frequent lack of an obvious initial diagnosis in both acute and CPP means that women frequently undergo large numbers of investigations and often unnecessary surgical procedures with associated morbidity and mortality. There is often a long interval between presentation and diagnosis with 25% remaining without a diagnosis after 3 to 4 years and more than 30% of women having had their pain for more than 5 years.[4]

The aim of this chapter is to provide an overview of the common causes of pelvic pain as well as to detail some of the less well known but easily treated causes with up-to-date evidence and a clear rationale for investigation and treatment. Because of the complexity of the innervation of the pelvis and the anatomical proximity of pelvic viscera, there is frequently overlap between what has traditionally been considered the domain of gynecology, urology, or gastroenterology. Therefore, some conditions will only be briefly discussed here when they are considered in more detail in other chapters of this book.

We discuss acute pelvic pain and CPP separately as, although there are overlaps, presentation and management are often very different. In addition, we also consider pelvic pain in pregnancy, dysmenorrhea, and mittelschmerz and pain associated with the complications of assisted conception. Finally, we discuss dyspareunia and the vulval pain syndromes which frequently coexist with other pelvic pain and whose etiology and management may be similar.

TABLE 64.1 Nongynecologic Causes of Acute Pelvic Pain

- Appendicitis
- IBS
- Constipation
- Inflammatory bowel disease
- Mesenteric adenitis
- Diverticulitis
- Strangulation of a hernia
- Urinary tract infection
- Renal/bladder calculi
- Acute muscle spasm

IBS, irritable bowel syndrome.

Acute Pelvic Pain

INTRODUCTION

The maxim that "acute pelvic pain in a woman of reproductive age is an ectopic pregnancy until proven otherwise" needs always to be borne in mind as ruptured ectopic pregnancies are associated with high morbidity and mortality and the consequences of a missed diagnosis are severe.[5] However, there are many other causes of acute pain in the lower abdominal/pelvic area that also need to be considered in the differential diagnosis. Many of these are not gynecologic (Table 64.1), although the symptom frequently presents, or is referred, to the gynecologist. Unless the patient is extremely unwell, assessment should begin as always with a detailed history followed by examination and appropriate investigations.

OVERVIEW OF ASSESSMENT

Where at all possible, the history should be taken in private, allowing the woman (whatever her age) to have with her only those people she requests to be present. A detailed history of the pain should be taken and associated bowel and urinary symptoms and vaginal discharge/bleeding should be enquired about directly. It is also important to ascertain with accuracy the date of her last menstrual period (LMP) and whether this was normal as well as a contraceptive history and any recent episodes of unprotected sexual intercourse (UPSI). In all cases, but particularly with adolescents, these areas need to be approached sensitively. The presence of any risk factors for ectopic pregnancy (Table 64.2) should be established and the woman's obstetric history ascertained. With an acute exacerbation of a chronic pain, it is important to inquire whether any precipitating factors (either physical or psychological) are present. At all times, clinicians should consider safeguarding issues and be alert to the possibility of assault, knowing where to access appropriate help locally if required.

Initial examination should ascertain that she is hemodynamically stable before examining the abdomen. The exact site of the pain should be established and evidence of an acute abdomen or abdominal/pelvic masses looked for. Pelvic pain in a sexually active woman (especially with a positive pregnancy test) should prompt a gentle digital internal examination, looking specifically for adnexal tenderness/masses and cervical excitation. Any discharge should be noted and appropriate swabs taken. If vaginal bleeding is present, a speculum examination should also be performed. Rectal examination may be indicated depending on the history. Again, privacy should be ensured, although a chaperone is recommended.

TABLE 64.2 Risk Factors for an Ectopic Pregnancy

- Past history of PID
- Progesterone-only contraceptive pill
- Previous ectopic pregnancy
- Previous tubal surgery
- IVF
- Endometriosis
- Uterotubal anomalies
- Fetal exposure to diethylstilbestrol

IVF, in vitro fertilization; PID, pelvic inflammatory disease.

TABLE 64.3 Investigation of Acute Pelvic Pain

- Urinary/serum hCG
- MSU
- Vaginal swabs (including appropriate culture to detect *Chlamydia*)
- Urethral swab
- FBC, G&S (cross-match if ectopic suspected)
- CRP
- Pelvic US–TA or TV as appropriate
- Abdominal radiograph (+/− contrast)
- Pelvic MRI
- Diagnostic laparoscopy

CRP, C-reactive protein; FBC, full blood count; G&S, group and save; hCG, human chorionic gonadotrophin; MRI, magnetic resonance imaging; MSU, midstream urine; TA, transabdominal; TV, transvaginal; US, ultrasound.

All women should have a urinary pregnancy test, but otherwise, investigations should be prompted by the history and examination findings rather than routinely ordered. Initially, investigations should be kept to a minimum in the case of an acute exacerbation of CPP. Investigations that might be considered are listed in Table 64.3.

GYNECOLOGIC FACTORS
Pelvic Inflammatory Disease
Pelvic inflammatory disease (PID) is a common cause of acute pelvic pain, and the incidence is increasing. It is an upper genital tract infection and can include one or more of the following: endometritis, salpingitis, tubo-ovarian abscess, and pelvic peritonitis. Prompt treatment and effective contact tracing are important as long-term sequelae include CPP, subfertility, and ectopic pregnancy. Although infection usually ascends from the cervix, cervical swabs can be negative even when pathogenic organisms are isolated from the fallopian tubes. The pain is thought to be due to inflammation, tissue destruction, irritation of peritoneal surfaces, and distortion of anatomy. Right upper quadrant pain and perihepatic adhesions occur in the Fitz-Hugh-Curtis syndrome, which is seen in 10% to 20% of women with PID.[6,7] Clinical features of PID lack sensitivity and specificity but include lower abdominal pain and tenderness, deep dyspareunia, abnormal vaginal/cervical discharge, cervical excitation and adnexal tenderness, and fever.[8] Evidence of acute infection will not always be seen on diagnostic laparoscopy, and therefore, this investigation should be reserved for cases where alternative pathology needs to be excluded or if a pelvic mass is seen on ultrasound (US).[9] Where there is a high index of suspicion, it is recommended that empirical antibiotic treatment should be commenced once swabs have been taken without waiting for culture results or performing further investigations.[9] This is particularly important if other features of sepsis are present, in which instance admission and adherence to local sepsis guidelines is recommended. A number of different organisms are associated with PID, including *Chlamydia trachomatis*, *Neisseria gonorrhoea*, *Mycoplasma genitalium*, and anaerobes.[8] The most commonly implicated organisms vary geographically, and therefore, local guidelines for appropriate antibiotic treatment regimens should always be consulted. There are now high rates of quinolone-resistant gonorrhoea in the Unites States, and, since April 2007, fluoroquinolone antibiotics have no longer been recommended for the treatment of PID in the United States[10]; this is increasingly also the case in the United Kingdom. Antibiotic treatment is usually continued for 14 days (with intravenous doses converted to oral once apyrexial), and therefore, patient compliance can be an issue. The presence of an intrauterine contraceptive device (IUCD) only increases the risk of developing PID in the first few weeks after insertion. Leaving the device in situ while mild PID is being treated does not appear to affect the outcome. In severe cases, however, it is recommended that the IUCD be removed.[9]

When there is definite evidence of a pelvic abscess or severe disease, surgery is recommended (either laparoscopy or laparotomy), to drain the abscess and divide pelvic adhesions, there is no good evidence to recommend division of perihepatic adhesions, however.[9] Depending on location, it may also be possible to drain pelvic collections under US guidance. This has been shown to be effective with fewer complications than surgery.[11]

To prevent reinfection, contact tracing and treatment of all sexual partners from 6 months prior to presentation is recommended.[9] This may be best done through a local genitourinary medicine (GUM) clinic, which will have experience of contact tracing and counseling about the long-term consequences of sexually transmitted infections. If admission is not required and appropriate facilities exist, it may be more effective to refer the woman to a GUM clinic immediately, to be seen the same day, before treatment is started. Sexual intercourse should be avoided until both the patient and her partner have completed a full course of treatment.

Adnexal Pathology
The adnexa comprise the fallopian tubes and the ovaries, the overlying peritoneum, and accompanying blood vessels. Common adnexal problems causing pain are discussed here.

Adnexal Torsion
Unlike the testes, it is rare for normal adnexa to undergo torsion. However, the ovaries and the distal ends of the fallopian tubes hang free and, if enlarged by an ovarian cyst or hydrosalpinx for example, are able to twist and cause ischemia and thus pain, with necrosis ensuing if the torsion is not resolved. Initially, the pain may be a dull ache that comes and goes; however, once necrosis occurs, the pain becomes constant and severe and may be accompanied by pyrexia, nausea, leucocytosis, and raised inflammatory markers. Clinically, a tender pelvic mass will be found on internal examination, and this can be confirmed with US. Management is surgical, ideally by urgent laparoscopy. If the adnexa appear healthy, then the torsion can be untwisted and the cyst/hydrosalpinx dealt with appropriately. Traditionally, removal of the mass was performed if the tissues appeared gangrenous. However, there is increasing evidence that the appearance of the tissues does not correlate well with residual ovarian function and recovery, and follow-up studies where de-torsion was performed suggest that ovarian function recovers in the majority of cases. It is therefore now recommended that de-torsion be performed and the clinical condition observed with an interval salpingo-oophorectomy performed only if clinically indicated.[12]

Other Ovarian Cyst Accident
As well as undergoing torsion, an ovarian cyst (either functional or pathologic) can also cause pain by rupturing or by hemorrhaging into itself. Ruptured cysts usually cause acute pain followed by a generalized dull ache; however, if enough fluid/blood is released into the pelvis to irritate the diaphragm, then shoulder pain may also be present. Diagnosis is usually clinical, although, a US may show fluid in the pelvis and the absence of a previously noted ovarian cyst. Pregnancy must always be excluded (usually with a urinary pregnancy test), but if the pain is resolving and the woman is hemodynamically stable, then management is conservative, providing symptom relief. However, if she is unstable or a significant amount of fluid is present in the pelvis, laparoscopy may be required. In this instance, it is obviously important to be sure the diagnosis is correct and that an ectopic pregnancy, for example, has not been missed.

Hemorrhage into a cyst may be self-limiting or require surgery. Again, this decision should be based on the clinical picture.

In all these cases, if there is any doubt as to the nature of the cyst, then surgery should be performed so that tissue for histology can be obtained.

Hematometra/Hematocolpos

A relatively rare cause of acute, or acute-on-chronic, pelvic pain is a hematometra or hematocolpos (literally blood in the uterus or blood in the cervix). This can be primarily from a congenital anomaly or secondary to procedures such as transcervical resection of the endometrium if cervical stenosis occurs. With congenital anomalies where a bifid uterus exists with one blind ending horn, it is possible to have normal menstrual flow from one horn and a gradually increasing hematometra in the other.

Diagnosis is by US or magnetic resonance imaging (MRI), and management is surgical, which may be as simple as cervical dilatation or incising an imperforate hymen. The discovery of a congenital müllerian anomaly should prompt a thorough investigation of the renal and urogenital system as many of these anomalies coexist.[13]

Acute Exacerbation of Chronic Pelvic Pain

An emergency presentation with acute pelvic pain can be an exacerbation of a much more chronic problem. Often, the patient is known to the department, but for others, the sudden worsening of chronic pain can be the final straw that causes the woman to present for the first time. As well as organizing appropriate analgesia (remaining alert to the possibility of an opioid addiction) and treating any associated symptoms, a careful search for the factor(s) precipitating the exacerbation should be made. This may be disease-related, such as an ovarian cyst accident; treatment-related, such as reactivation of endometriosis by add-back hormone replacement therapy (HRT) or constipation secondary to increased analgesia use; or lifestyle-related, such as increased activity worsening musculoskeletal pain or a bereavement worsening psychological status. If such precipitating factors can be identified, they should be discussed with the patient. Coping strategies can be taught to prevent future emergency presentations, which may also be reduced by easy access to a health care professional who knows the woman well.

If a women presents for the first time to a department but is managed elsewhere for their CPP, it is always advisable to contact the team responsible for her care to ensure that management of the acute exacerbation/presentation does not interfere with the long-term plan. Although certainly not the case for the majority of women, there is a small group of patients who attend a variety of different hospitals with the aim of procuring the treatment (be it surgery, opioids, or other options) they desire. Although these women clearly have the right to seek a second or third opinion, it can be helpful to be fully informed of this behavior and the results of previous investigations/surgeries when forming a management plan and deciding which other clinicians may need to be involved.

COMPLICATIONS SPECIFIC TO PREGNANCY

A number of complications specific to pregnancy can present with pelvic pain and need always to be borne in mind in a woman of reproductive age. It is also worth noting, however, that the physiologic and anatomical adaptations of pregnancy can alter the presenting features of many non–pregnancy-related conditions such as appendicitis. When treating pain in a possibly ongoing pregnancy, nonsteroidal anti-inflammatory drugs (NSAIDs) are contraindicated because of effects on implantation, fetal renal function, and premature closure of the ductus arteriosus. Acetaminophen (paracetamol) and opioids, however, are safe. Reassurance and explanation are perhaps more important than ever in these cases to avoid anxiety about the pregnancy further clouding the clinical picture.

Ectopic Pregnancy

An ectopic pregnancy is one in which the conceptus implants outside the uterine cavity. Most commonly, this is within the fallopian tube (98.3%) but more rarely can be in the abdominal cavity,

on the ovary, or on the cervix. The incidence is approximately 1 in 100 pregnancies[14]; however, this is likely to increase with the increasing incidence of pelvic infection and assisted conception. Rarely, a heterotopic pregnancy can occur, which is effectively a twin pregnancy in two different sites (e.g., one intrauterine and one ectopic pregnancy). These cases can be easily missed with false reassurance given once the intrauterine pregnancy is seen on US. With the rising prevalence of assisted conception techniques, the incidence of heterotopic pregnancies is increasing.[15]

Classically, presentation is with a period of amenorrhoea followed by brown vaginal loss and then onset of pelvic pain. Realistically, however, presentation is varied, ranging from asymptomatic (an incidental finding at routine scan), through any combination of pain and/or old or fresh vaginal bleeding, to collapse secondary to hypovolemia. Initial pain is thought to be secondary to stretching of the peritoneum covering the distended fallopian tube; however, with rupture of the tube, peritonitis occurs and tracking of the blood up to the diaphragm can cause shoulder tip pain.

In the collapsed patient with a positive pregnancy test, diagnosis is assumed and resuscitation commenced with surgery performed immediately when she is stable. At the opposite extreme, in a hemodynamically stable woman with minimal symptoms, diagnosis can be difficult. In early pregnancy, an intrauterine gestation may not be visible even with transvaginal ultrasound (TVUS). A combination of serial human chorionic gonadotrophin (hCG) levels and repeated US may be required to determine the location and viability of the pregnancy. If a high index of suspicion is present or the woman is isolated socially, this observation may best be done as an inpatient; however, in the majority of cases, early pregnancy clinics facilitate safe outpatient management.

Appropriate management depends on the severity of presentation. With an unstable patient, urgent laparotomy or laparoscopy should be performed depending on the skills of the available surgeon. With a stable patient, the majority of cases should be able to be managed laparoscopically, reducing postoperative pain, recovery time, and hospital stay. Some units now manage appropriate cases medically using methotrexate; however, this is not without risks and requires careful surveillance and a motivated patient.[16]

However, the pregnancy is managed, the risks of an ectopic pregnancy in the future are considerably higher than in the background population, and the woman should be counseled about this prior to discharge and advised to get an early scan in her next pregnancy. It should not be forgotten that a pregnancy has been lost, and many women/couples value the opportunity to talk this through either at the time or at a later date.

Miscarriage

Miscarriage is defined as pregnancy loss prior to viability (currently considered to be 24 weeks) and occurs in 10% to 20% of clinical pregnancies.[17] Because of connotations of blame, the medical term *abortion* should no longer be used when pregnancy loss is spontaneous. The different types of miscarriage are shown in Table 64.4. Bleeding is not always the presenting feature. Classically, bleeding precedes pain in a miscarriage as opposed to an ectopic pregnancy where the pain occurs first. As this is not reliable, all pain or bleeding in early pregnancy should be referred to an early pregnancy unit for further assessment and management. Management may be expectant, medical (using prostaglandin analogues ± antiprogesterone) or surgical (traditionally known as *evacuation of retained products of conception* [ERPC] but now more frequently called a *surgical management of miscarriage* [SMoM] as this terminology is more acceptable to women and their partners). If the woman is hemodynamically unstable or the bleeding is very heavy, then surgery is recommended; otherwise, the choice of

TABLE 64.4	Types of Miscarriage[17,157]
Threatened	May be continuing to bleed
	Viable pregnancy
Inevitable	Bleeding
	Cervical os open
Complete	Bleeding settled
	All products of conception passed
Incomplete	May be continuing to bleed
	Products still present
Delayed	No/minimal bleeding
	Fetal demise, all products still present
Anembryonic pregnancy	May have bleeding
	Gestational sac present but no yolk sac or embryo

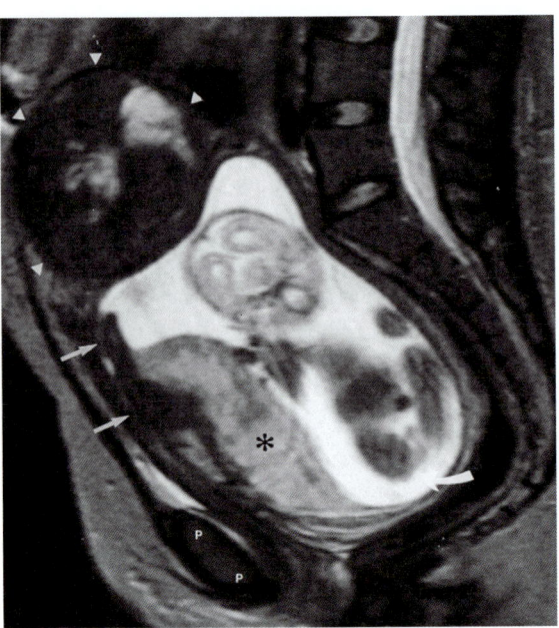

FIGURE 64.1 Magnetic resonance imaging of persistent retroversion of the uterus at 20 weeks' gestation. The uterine fundus containing the breech (*curved arrow*) can be seen in the pouch of Douglas. The placenta (*asterisk*) is attached to the posterior uterine wall with a large intramural fibroid (*arrowheads*) superiorly on the lower portion of the anterior wall, and the cervix (*arrows*) just below, above the level of the symphysis pubis (*P*). (*From Hamoda H, Chamberlain PF, Moore NR, et al. Conservative treatment of an incarcerated gravid uterus. BJOG 2002;109:1074–1075, with permission.*)

management should be made by the woman. Nonsurgical options are associated with longer periods of bleeding but avoid the risks of a general anesthetic and may allow the woman to feel more in control. Contrary to previous beliefs, there is no increase in infection rate with expectant management.[18] All nonimmunized, Rhesus-negative women who miscarry after 12 weeks' gestation should be given prophylaxis with anti-D immunoglobulin. Prior to 12 weeks, anti-D immunoglobulin should be given for medical or surgical evacuation or if the bleeding is very heavy and associated with pain.[17] The negative psychological impact of early pregnancy loss can be enormous, both for the woman and her family, and therefore, counseling and support should be offered. Ideally, this should be at a local level, although national support groups also exist.

Fibroid Degeneration

Uterine fibroids (leiomyomas) are benign tumors of the uterus, which are found in approximately 20% of women of reproductive age. They are usually asymptomatic and are more common in older women and women of African origin. They possess estrogen receptors and are thus stimulated to grow during pregnancy. As their blood supply is mainly peripheral, central areas can suffer from ischemia if enlargement is rapid, causing pain. This is known as red degeneration. The pain is generally well localized with tenderness over the area of the fibroid only (as opposed to placental abruption where the whole uterus is tender and woody hard) and may be accompanied by a mild pyrexia and leukocytosis. Opioid analgesia is often required and admission may be necessary, if only for observation and fetal monitoring if there is any doubt about the diagnosis.

Ovarian Cyst Accident

As in the nonpregnant state, hemorrhage into or rupture or torsion of an ovarian cyst can occur during pregnancy. In general, presentation and management are as for the nonpregnant woman; however, symptoms can be masked and nonspecific during pregnancy. Rupture of a cyst can present with severe pain and shock, and in early pregnancy, laparoscopy may be necessary to exclude ectopic pregnancy. However, if pain is resolving and no other symptoms are present, conservative management is recommended. If surgical management is required beyond early pregnancy, laparotomy may have to be considered because of the risks and technical difficulties of a laparoscopy with an enlarged uterus.

Ligamentous Stretch

As the uterus enlarges, it moves out of the pelvis and becomes an abdominal organ. During this process, the supporting round ligaments are stretched and cause pain in the late first/early second trimester in 10% to 30% of pregnancies. Management is by simple analgesia and reassurance; however, it is important to ensure that other causes of pain are not missed, such as rupture of a heterotopic pregnancy or acute appendicitis.

Urinary Retention and Uterine Incarceration

Uterine retroversion occurs in up to 15% of pregnancies in the first trimester, but by 15 weeks' gestation, spontaneous anteversion almost always occurs. It is reported that retroversion persists into the second trimester in 1 in 3,000 pregnancies.[19] Rarely, it may not be noticed until a cesarean section is performed at term; however, it can become impacted and present with urinary frequency, urgency, abdominal pain, and urinary retention. Pelvic adhesions secondary to infection or endometriosis and posterior wall fibroids can predispose to incarceration. Diagnosis can be aided by US or MRI (Fig. 64.1); however, fetal parts may be palpable vaginally and an enlarged bladder abdominally. Gentle manual decompression is usually possible after emptying the bladder with a Foley catheter. Intermittent catheterization is occasionally necessary for a few days subsequently, but an indwelling catheter is not recommended because of the risk of infection.[20] If asymptomatic retroversion persists until term, delivery should be by cesarean section and a classical incision is often required.[19]

COMPLICATIONS OF ASSISTED CONCEPTION
Ovarian Hyperstimulation Syndrome

Ovarian hyperstimulation syndrome (OHSS) is a serious and sometimes fatal complication of assisted conception techniques. It is a systemic disease secondary to the release of proinflammatory mediators, including vasoactive products, from the hyperstimulated ovaries. It can be subdivided into early, within 9 days of the ovulatory hCG dose, or late and is classified according to severity (Table 64.5). Mild disease has been reported to complicate up to 33% of in vitro fertilization (IVF) cycles, whereas the severe form occurs in around 1%. OHSS is more likely in women with polycystic ovaries, young women, and in cycles where conception occurs, especially if multiple pregnancies.[21] Presentation is variable depending on severity (see Table 64.5) but should always be borne in mind in a woman with abdominal/pelvic pain who has recently

TABLE 64.5	Symptoms and Signs of Ovarian Hyperstimulation Syndrome
Mild OHSS	Abdominal bloating
	Mild abdominal pain
	Ovarian size usually <8 cm
Moderate OHSS	Moderate abdominal pain
	Nausea ± vomiting
	US evidence of ascites
	Ovarian size usually 8–12 cm
Severe OHSS	Clinical ascites (occasionally hydrothorax)
	Oliguria (<300 mL/d)
	Hematocrit >45%
	Hyponatremia (sodium <135 mmol/L)
	Hypo-osmolality (osmolality <282 mOsm/kg)
	Hyperkalemia (potassium >5 mmol/L)
	Hypoproteinemia
	Ovarian size usually >12 cm
Critical OHSS	Tense ascites or large hydrothorax
	Hematocrit >55%
	White cell count >25,000/mL
	Oligo/anuria
	Thromboembolism
	Acute respiratory distress syndrome

OHSS, ovarian hyperstimulation syndrome; US, ultrasound.
Adapted from Mathur RS, Drakeley AJ, Raine-Fenning NJ, et al. *The Management of Ovarian Hyperstimulation Syndrome.* London: Royal College of Obstetricians and Gynaecologists; 2016.

TABLE 64.6	Causes of Dysmenorrhea

- Endometriosis
- Adenomyosis
- Müllerian anomalies
- PID
- Fibroids
- Cervical stenosis
- Pelvic venous congestion
- Intrauterine device

PID, pelvic inflammatory disease.

undergone assisted conception. Mild and moderate disease can be managed on an outpatient basis, but more severe forms or concerns about a worsening condition require admission. In general, management involves symptom control: analgesia with either acetaminophen (paracetamol) or codeine but avoiding NSAIDs and antiemetics suitable for early pregnancy (e.g., prochlorperazine, metoclopramide), continuing progesterone luteal support but stopping hCG support and avoiding strenuous exercise and sexual intercourse because of the risk of ovarian torsion. In severe cases, multidisciplinary management is advised to deal with issues of fluid balance and thromboembolic risk (0.7% to 10%).[22] Paracentesis may be necessary but should always be done under US guidance because of the risk of injury to enlarged, vascular ovaries. Importantly, women should be reassured that pregnancy may continue normally despite OHSS.[21]

Pelvic Infection

Pelvic infection can occur after investigation of tubal patency with a hysterosalpingogram (HSG) or laparoscopy and dye test or after oocyte retrieval. Prior to such investigations being arranged, all women should have cervical swabs performed, and any infection should be treated with an appropriate antibiotic regimen. Oocyte retrieval is usually performed transvaginally under US guidance. Rates of pelvic infection secondary to this procedure vary between units and published series but are generally low, between 0% and 1%.[23] Initial management is with antibiotics and US to exclude a pelvic abscess. Progressive worsening of symptoms or failure to improve should prompt a further search for a pelvic collection and consideration of the possibility of bowel damage, for which laparoscopy or laparotomy would be required.

Dysmenorrhea

Dysmenorrhea is defined as pain with menstruation and was excluded from older definitions of CPP.[24] However, there is increasing evidence of psychological distress, reduced quality of life, and long-term alterations in central nervous system structure and function in women with dysmenorrhea[25–28] such that the most recent International Association for the Study of Pain (IASP) Taxonomy does include it as a subcategory of CPP.[29] Estimates of prevalence range from 20% to 90%, and it has a major social and economic impact, being the leading cause of school and work absenteeism in young women.[30] Traditionally, dysmenorrhea has been subdivided into primary and secondary. Primary (functional) dysmenorrhea is not associated with other pathology; is thought to be due to overproduction of prostaglandins and leukotrienes in the myometrium causing strong, painful contractions of the uterus; and is common in adolescents.[31] It is frequently considered to be a "normal" part of development and assumed to improve with age or after pregnancy, although this has not been shown to be true in longitudinal studies. Secondary dysmenorrhea is associated with other pathology (Table 64.6) and therefore often occurs with other symptoms such as dyspareunia and menorrhagia. It is traditionally considered to affect women in their 30s and over, but it is worth remembering that children as young as 8 years old have been shown to have biopsy-proven endometriosis,[32] and congenital uterine anomalies probably occur in around 4% of the population, increasing to 10% in adolescents with pelvic pain.[31] Clinically, therefore, we find this distinction to be unhelpful and consider dysmenorrhea as a symptom which deserves to be treated and investigated as appropriate, no matter what age the patient.

Initial assessment should include a detailed history, including risk factors for pathology associated with dysmenorrhea and other symptoms. In young girls who are not sexually active and without associated symptoms, a pelvic examination is not necessary before commencing empirical treatment. If there are concerns about structural anomalies, an abdominal US can offer reassurance but cannot diagnose or exclude endometriosis.

NONSTEROIDAL ANTI-INFLAMMATORY DRUGS

Many women, especially teenagers, self-medicate for their dysmenorrhea, and NSAIDs are often the drugs of choice. NSAIDs act by inhibiting cyclooxygenase and therefore reduce prostaglandin production and associated uterine contractions. Mefenamic acid has been shown to also inhibit the lipoxygenase pathway.[33] Systematic reviews have concluded that NSAIDs are an effective treatment for dysmenorrhea but that there is insufficient evidence to determine which, if any, is the most effective.[34] A greater improvement of symptoms can be obtained if treatment is started 24 hours prior to the onset of bleeding and, if a loading dose of twice the regular dose is used initially, followed by regular doses as needed.[35]

HORMONAL TREATMENTS

The combined oral contraceptive pill (COCP) has been used as a treatment for dysmenorrhea for many years. It acts to inhibit ovulation and limit endometrial growth, reducing progesterone and subsequent prostaglandin and leukotriene production.[31] A number of trials have shown a significant improvement in dysmenorrhea with COCP use, both high and lower dose formulations.[36] Many clinicians would suggest running the pill packets back-to-back without having a withdrawal bleed in between packets, as if the pain is only associated with bleeding inducing amenorrhea will effectively treat the problem. If this is not acceptable for cultural or other reasons, tricycling the COCP (i.e., taking three packets of pills back-to-back) has also been shown to reduce symptoms as well as decreasing the frequency of menstruation[37] and thus may be a good alternative.

Depot medroxyprogesterone acetate (DMPA), a long-acting injectable contraceptive, also reliably inhibits ovulation in both its intramuscular and subcutaneous formulations,[38] and amenorrhea is common. In one study, 64% of adolescents reported an improvement in dysmenorrhea symptoms with DMPA[39]; however, concerns about loss of bone mineral density (BMD) limit its prolonged use in adolescence. For women also requiring long-term contraception, a levonorgestrel-releasing intrauterine system (LNG-IUS) is another alternative. The majority of women are amenorrheic with the system in place, and even for those who continue to bleed, menses tend to be lighter and less painful, although bleeding can be erratic for the first 6 months. In some instances, this may be the most appropriate option for nulliparous young adults, in which case a brief general anesthetic may be necessary for insertion. For severe symptoms, a therapeutic trial of a gonadotrophin-releasing hormone (GnRH) agonist (see the following text) could also be considered.

SURGICAL TREATMENTS

Surgery for dysmenorrhea should only be considered as an investigation for other pathologies if there is no response to medical treatment (e.g., diagnostic laparoscopy) or as a last resort. Systematic reviews suggest that there is insufficient evidence to support the use of surgical nerve interruption[40] (either laparoscopic uterine nerve ablation [LUNA] or presacral neurectomy [PSN]) in dysmenorrhea, and the rates of complications are high.

NONPHARMACOLOGIC INTERVENTIONS

A number of other interventions have been studied to improve dysmenorrhea with varying success. Both high-frequency transcutaneous electrical nerve stimulation (TENS) and acupuncture have shown benefit in some studies[41,42] as has topical heat therapy[43]; however, neither psychological interventions nor dietary supplements have been shown to be beneficial in pure dysmenorrhea.[44,45] As always, the role of education and validation of symptoms cannot be emphasized strongly enough, and this is particularly true for adolescents.

Mittelschmerz

Mittelschmerz (literally "middle pain" in German) is one-sided, lower abdominal pain that occurs at or around ovulation. It can last from minutes to 48 hours and requires no treatment other than simple analgesics. It is thought to occur in approximately 50% of women at some point. What causes the pain is not known, but possible suggestions include tubal, uterine, or cecal spasm; increased tension in the ovary or Graafian follicle; or peritoneal irritation due to leak of blood or fluid from the follicle. However, the latter is probably unlikely as in one study, 33 out of 34 women experienced the pain prior to follicular rupture (as confirmed with US),[46] and pain is on the same side as follicular rupture in only 86% of women.[47] Mittelschmerz probably causes most concern when a woman recommences ovulation after a long period of treatment with an ovulation inhibitor. Because it is not expected, the sudden, acute pain can then lead to investigation for other conditions such as appendicitis or an ovarian cyst accident. Similar, but more severe, pain can occur with trapped ovary syndrome and endometriosis, as discussed in the following text.

Chronic Pelvic Pain

INTRODUCTION

CPP is a symptom, not a diagnosis. As is seen, the causes are diverse, often multifactorial, and not always evident on routine examinations or even laparoscopy. As well as the economic impact already alluded to, CPP has major psychological, social, and cultural consequences not only for the woman but also for her partner, family, and society as a whole. It is acknowledged that it is frequently poorly managed; yet, it is as common as migraine and back pain and affects all races and social classes.

FACTORS ASSOCIATED WITH CHRONIC PELVIC PAIN

A number of factors are thought to be associated with CPP and should be explored during the consultation at an appropriate point.

Social

CPP is seen in women of all social classes with no variation in prevalence depending on marital or employment status.[48] However, social support can be an important factor in how a woman deals with her pain and social isolation can make the situation very difficult. It is easy to see how a vicious circle is set up with pain leading to the loss of the woman's social role and thus her self-esteem, causing isolation and contributing to further pain.

Abuse

Although frequently alluded to, the relationship between physical or sexual abuse and CPP is still not clear. The majority of studies is retrospective and only target women who have already developed the symptom. It appears that women in secondary care with any chronic pain condition are more likely to report a history of childhood abuse than pain-free women. When CPP is considered, sexual abuse is more commonly reported than in other pain conditions. It could be, however, that childhood sexual abuse is a predisposing factor for the development of depression, anxiety, and somatization which may then lead to the development of CPP.[24] In a rare prospective study,[49] children who had been abused were followed until their 20s and were not found to have an increase in medically unexplained symptoms when compared to a population who were not known to have been abused. However, those with unexplained symptoms were more likely to report their abuse. Thus, a revealed abuse history should not be assumed to be the cause of the pain, but failure to respond to treatments should perhaps prompt an exploration of these areas if a good therapeutic relationship already exists.

A recent study assessed whether a history of abuse is associated with the development of gynecologic disorders associated with CPP. In a cohort of 473 women undergoing laparoscopy, they found no increased risk of endometriosis, fibroids, or ovarian cysts in those with an abuse history but did find that a history of physical abuse was associated with a higher likelihood of pelvic adhesions.[50]

Psychological

Women with CPP display an increased incidence of "negative" psychological features, such as depression, anxiety, and catastrophization.[51] This is common with other chronic pain conditions, such as fibromyalgia and irritable bowel syndrome (IBS). However, it is not possible to know whether these factors predispose a woman to develop CPP, contribute to a perpetuation of the pain, or are a consequence of years of living with pain and attempts to justify its severity or even existence to friends, family, and health care professionals. What is known is that psychological state can alter the experience of pain, and this is the area that should be emphasized to the woman when a referral to a psychologist is suggested. Improving sleep patterns alone can both improve mood and have a significant effect on ability to function.

Personality

Similarly, whether personality types predispose to the development of chronic pain conditions or merely alter the way in which they are dealt with is not known. Some personality traits can make recovery more difficult. "Driven types," for example, are unable to pace themselves and do too much on a "good day" so that on the following day, symptoms are worse again. On the other hand, those who take easily to the "sick role" can be hard to persuade to engage in therapeutic options and may also fail to respond. Women with diagnosed personality disorders should be managed in conjunction with a psychiatrist.

OVERVIEW OF ASSESSMENT

The initial assessment of a woman with CPP is very important. Complete recovery at follow-up is associated with a favorable patient rating of the quality of the initial consultation.[52] The woman needs to be given time to tell her story, without interruptions, but with the support of whomever she would like to be present (which may be no one but the doctor). The extra time taken to listen to the history in the patient's own words may well give valuable information about the context of the pain, its effects on her life, and her beliefs about its cause and prognosis. In fact, an explanation for the pain has been shown to be one of things women with CPP most want out of their consultation (Table 64.7).[53] The process of telling her story and of the examination can, in itself, be therapeutic. Once a cycle of chronic pain has been set up, it is unlikely that a single cause for the pain will be identified, and the clinician should be alert for any contributing factors that may be revealed.

History

A detailed history of the pain should be taken including when and how it began; its associations, such as bowel, bladder, and psychological symptoms; and the effects of posture and movement. The circumstances surrounding the start of the pain and whether they recently changed should be discussed, as should the reasons why she has presented now. Cyclicity of symptoms or exacerbation with intercourse need to be established as does her current and future fertility aspirations. Relevant information may well be gleaned from her obstetric history, and a contraceptive and smear history should also be taken. It should be ascertained that no "red flag" symptoms, such as rectal bleeding or weight loss, exist. Although a history of past or present abuse (verbal, physical, or sexual) may also be present, it may not be appropriate to discuss this at the first consultation. If abuse is revealed, these experiences need to be accepted as stated, and it is important to know where to access specialist help locally should this be required.[24]

Examination

Examination requires more time than is routine in gynecology, and as it is the time when the patient is most vulnerable, new information is often revealed at this point.[54] The decision as to whether to have a chaperone present is a personal one that will depend on both the doctor's and patient's wishes. However,

the presence of a third person may alter the dynamic and prevent certain information being revealed. Examination should begin, as always, with observation. This includes evidence of not only skin alterations or damage and posture but also of both the patient's attitude to the examination and the doctor's response to this. Evidence of altered sensation (hypersensitivity or allodynia[55]) should be sought before abdominal palpation is performed. The effect of movement should be assessed, which might suggest musculoskeletal pain. The extent to which an internal examination is performed will depend on the history. With marked vaginismus, anything more than a gentle, one-finger examination may be inappropriate. Altered sensation on the vulva and perineum should be looked for and pelvic floor muscle tone assessed if possible. Rectal examination should only be performed if there is a clear indication in the history.

Investigations

Investigations should be guided by the history, but care should be taken to avoid overinvestigation initially. Many women will have already seen a number of doctors, often of many specialities, and had a variety of frequently invasive investigations. One particularly useful strategy is to ask the woman to keep a detailed pain diary over 1 to 2 months. This can reveal information about the timing of the pain and its associations to the doctor and to the patient.[24]

Therapeutic Trial

Very cyclical symptoms are usually gynecologic in origin, although pain perception itself may vary with the menstrual cycle as can symptoms of both interstitial cystitis (IC)/bladder pain syndrome (BPS) and IBS. Where symptoms are markedly cyclical, a therapeutic trial of a GnRH analogue could be considered before a laparoscopy is performed.[24] This group of drugs, given initially as monthly subcutaneous injections, cause a prolonged activation of the GnRH receptor leading to an initial worsening of symptoms (the "initial flare"). This is followed by a reduction in luteinizing hormone (LH) and follicle-stimulating hormone (FSH), such that serum estradiol levels are suppressed by 21 days and remain at levels equivalent to postmenopausal women with continued dosing. Common adverse effects are shown in Table 64.8. The most common complaints of hot flushes and emotional symptoms are often well tolerated if pain is relieved. The biggest concern, however, is the loss of BMD which can be up to 6% after 6 months of treatment.[57] If the trial is successful, then treatment can continue with the addition of low-dose combined HRT, and this combination has been shown to be safe and effective for up to 2 years. After this time, many women are not prepared to continue with monthly injections (although three monthly preparations exist and can be effective in some women) and seek alternative management options. However, in those who would like to continue with treatment, there is now evidence from small studies that the combination is safe for up to 10 years, with one of these women having stopped treatment to conceive and then recommenced treatment after delivery.[58]

Diagnostic Laparoscopy

If no relief is gained from a therapeutic trial of GnRH analogue or if there are other indications such as subfertility or a pelvic mass, diagnostic laparoscopy should be performed. However, laparoscopy is not without risks with large series quoting approximately 3% risk of minor complications and 0.6 to 1.8/1,000 risk of major complications such as bowel perforation and vascular damage.[59] Furthermore, although it was initially thought that a negative laparoscopy would reassure a woman, more recent studies have shown this not to be the case[60] and it may reaffirm her beliefs that the doctors do not believe her and think the pain is of psychological origin.

TABLE 64.7 What Women Would Like from the Chronic Pelvic Pain Consultation[53]

- Personal care
- To be understood and taken seriously
- Explanation
- Reassurance

TABLE 64.8 Hormonal Treatments for Endometriosis-Related Pain[158]

Treatment	Main Adverse Effects
COCP[36,159] (continuous or tricycling)	Thromboembolic disorders, altered serum lipid profile, hypertension, skin reactions, migraine, intermenstrual bleeding, depression, altered libido
Danazol[160]	Deepening of voice, acne, hirsutism, clitoral hypertrophy, vaginal dryness, hematologic disturbances, altered serum lipid profile, thromboembolic disorders, depression, weight gain, altered libido, muscle cramps
Gestrinone[161]	Headache, depression, weight gain, voice changes, acne, hirsutism, intermenstrual spotting, gastrointestinal disturbances, muscle cramps
Progestogens (e.g., medroxyprogesterone acetate)[161]	Depression, weight gain, altered libido, acne, vaginal bleeding, breast tenderness, thromboembolic disorders, gallbladder disease, worsening of ovarian cysts
LNG-IUS[56,162]	Irregular vaginal bleeding, depression, weight gain, reduced libido, breast tenderness, vaginal discharge, uterine perforation, ovarian cysts
GnRH agonists[57]	Initial flare in symptoms, bruising/pain at injection site, depression, emotional lability, reduced libido, vaginal dryness, hot flushes, headache, pituitary apoplexy
GnRH antagonists[163]	Same as for GnRH agonists except that no initial flare occurs

COCP, combined oral contraceptive pill; GnRH, gonadotrophin-releasing hormone; LNG-IUS, levonorgestrel-releasing intrauterine system.

Empirical Treatment

Even if no clear cause of the pain can be found on investigation, the pain should still be treated empirically. Analgesia or hormonal treatments may be appropriate, but it is often worth considering drugs such as amitriptyline, gabapentin, pregabalin, and duloxetine in addition. Although there is very limited evidence of efficacy for these drugs in CPP specifically,[61,62] there is increasing evidence of both somatic and visceral sensory disturbance in women with CPP.[63–65] Thus, a trial of these drugs which are effective in neuropathic pain and may have a role in reducing visceral hypersensitivity[66] may be worthwhile. Topical capsaicin cream on the skin of the abdomen (not the vulva) may be useful for hyperalgesia and allodynia. Nonpharmacologic treatments such as acupuncture, TENS, chiropractic, and osteopathic manipulations may be beneficial, and pain management techniques and support groups can also be of value.[67]

THE IMPORTANCE OF VISCERAL HYPERSENSITIVITY IN CHRONIC PELVIC PAIN

Visceral hypersensitivity (and subsequent viscerovisceral/ viscerosomatic referral) is thought to have an important role in CPP.[65] It can be the primary pain generator, perpetuating factor, or cause of secondary symptoms. Visceral hypersensitivity should therefore always be borne in mind, especially when symptoms from multiple organs are present or where there is no clear demonstrable cause. This area is covered in more detail in Chapters 3, 4, and 65. Sex steroid hormones are known to act at multiple sites throughout the peripheral and central nervous system, and it is thus not surprising that these symptoms often show cyclicity and can respond to hormonal manipulation.

GYNECOLOGIC FACTORS IN CHRONIC PELVIC PAIN
Endometriosis

Endometriosis is defined as "an inflammatory disease process, characterized by lesions of endometrial-like tissue outside the uterus that is associated with pelvic pain and/or infertility."[68] Although it is a common cause of CPP and dysmenorrhea, it is also a common incidental finding in asymptomatic women. Therefore, it is imperative that a detailed history and examination are undertaken even in a woman who has previously been diagnosed with endometriosis, as it may not be the sole cause of, or even related to, her pain.

Endometriosis is a complex condition, with much still unknown about its etiology, natural history, and incidence. In 1927, Sampson[69] suggested it was due to retrograde menstruation. However, this process can be demonstrated in more than 90% of women; therefore, a combination of retrograde menstruation and an altered immune environment,[70] allowing implantation and the development of a nerve and blood supply, is currently considered to be the most likely etiology. In order to make a definitive diagnosis of endometriosis, direct visualization of ectopic endometrial implants must occur,[71] preferably with biopsy and histologic confirmation.

The prevalence of endometriosis is difficult to establish, as the vast majority of implants are in the pelvic cavity (although extrapelvic disease does occur) and not every woman will have a laparoscopy or laparotomy. Clinical presentation can be variable (Table 64.9), and to confuse matters further, the extent of disease seen at laparoscopy correlates poorly with the severity of symptoms.[72] There remains considerable debate as to how endometriosis causes pain. However, increasing evidence is appearing for peripheral and central nervous system involvement and musculoskeletal factors in addition to the more traditionally considered roles of inflammation and fibrosis from the lesions themselves.[64,73–75]

Although laparoscopy and lesion histology is the criterion standard diagnostic test, current guidelines recommend that if the history and clinical examination are suggestive of endometriosis, a definitive diagnosis is not required before commencing empirical treatment.[71] There are a large variety of treatment options currently available for endometriosis, and the appropriate treatment(s) should be decided in discussion with the woman depending on her specific constellation of symptoms and current and future fertility wishes. A full discussion of these options is beyond the scope of this chapter; however, an overview of the management of endometriosis-related pain (but not infertility) is given in the following text. More detailed reviews can be found elsewhere.[71,76]

Medical Management of Endometriosis

As with dysmenorrhea, traditionally, NSAIDs have been used to treat pain secondary to endometriosis. However, there is no evidence to suggest that they have any greater effect than placebo.[77] Women need to also be informed of the inhibitory effect of NSAIDs on ovulation when taken midcycle. The enzyme

TABLE 64.9 Symptoms and Signs of Endometriosis

Symptoms	Signs
Dysmenorrhea	Fixed, retroverted uterus
Dyspareunia	Enlarged ovary
Dyschezia	Uterosacral nodules
CPP	Rectovaginal nodules
Infertility	
Hematuria	
Hematochezia	
Chronic fatigue	

CPP, chronic pelvic pain.

cyclooxygenase-2 (COX-2) is involved in both pain and inflammation, and specific COX-2 inhibitors have shown promising results in human studies of endometriosis-related pain.[78] However, because of concerns over the safety of this class of drugs,[79] they cannot currently be recommended.

The majority of endometriotic tissue is hormonally sensitive, and hormonal suppression has been shown to reduce endometriosis-associated pain.[71] The available hormonal treatments are shown in Table 64.8. They all appear to be equally effective at controlling endometriosis-related pain but have differing adverse effect profiles. In general, however, symptoms return over time after stopping the treatment. For example, in one study, the median time to recurrence of pain was 6.1 months after stopping danazol and 5.2 months after a GnRH analogue.[80]

Over recent years, it has become apparent that endometriotic deposits express aromatase and are thus able to synthesize estradiol,[81] possibly explaining why some women continue to have symptoms while in a hypoestrogenic state. Recent small trials of nonsteroidal aromatase inhibitors (AIs) in combination with hormonal treatments have shown promising results, especially as the women concerned were refractory to other treatments.[82] AI, such as anastrazole and letrozole, are used in the treatment of postmenopausal women with estrogen-sensitive breast cancers and are known to have a mild adverse effect profile, although, as with GnRH analogues, there are concerns about loss of BMD.[83]

Surgical Management of Endometriosis

As is apparent from the discussion of medical treatments, these options only keep the disease suppressed but do not affect a cure; once treatment is stopped, symptoms may recur. Complete surgical excision of disease can be performed and has been shown to significantly reduce pain scores, improve sexual function, and improve quality of life. In one series, for example, 67% of women reported an improvement following surgery, 8% felt their symptoms to be unchanged, 25% were worse, but only 33% required further surgery during the 5-year follow-up period.[84] However, particularly with deeply infiltrating endometriosis (DIE), there are significant risks associated with surgery (including bowel perforation, fistula formation, and ureteric damage), and this should therefore only be undertaken at specialist centers by a multidisciplinary team with the necessary expertise.[71] Despite these risks, recent cohort studies do suggest significant improvements in quality of life and pain scores at 1-year follow-up after resection of severe disease at specialized centers.[85] If a diagnostic laparoscopy is being undertaken and mild disease is seen, then current recommendations are that this should be excised or ablated at the time[71]; however, there is no convincing evidence that this offers long-term benefit for those with only mild peritoneal disease. Neither pre- nor postoperative hormonal treatment has been shown to improve outcome measures, including pain scores.[86] However, if retrograde menstruation is an etiologic factor, it makes sense to induce an amenorrheic state in women not currently wishing to conceive. The LNG-IUS has been shown to significantly reduce the risk of recurrence of moderate-severe dysmenorrhea at 1 year[56] and is therefore worth considering.

Novel Concepts in Endometriosis-Associated Pain

Traditionally, endometriosis has been considered to cause pain either due to inflammation, fibrosis or direct infiltration of pelvic nerves. This view is being increasingly challenged as evidence emerges of alterations in both the peripheral and central nervous system and musculoskeletal factors, too.[73,74,87,88] There is also now an awareness that patients want management of their pain and are interested in nonsurgical, nonhormonal treatments.[89] There are no published studies on the use of neuropathic adjuncts in endometriosis-associated pain and only very limited data on either physical or psychological therapies.[90–93]

However, the similarities increasingly being demonstrated between women with endometriosis-associated pain and those with other chronic pain conditions[64] suggest that for those patients refractive to standard treatments or who only show a partial response, it may well be beneficial to consider a more holistic approach, potentially including the use of neuropathic adjuncts and psychological and physical therapies. We would argue that review by a clinician skilled in identifying such factors should be considered before undertaking repeated surgical treatments if pain is the sole indication for surgery.

Adenomyosis

Adenomyosis is defined as the presence of endometrial glands and stroma within the myometrium.[94] Typically, the surrounding myometrium is hypertrophic and hyperplastic. Very little research has been undertaken on adenomyosis specifically, with much of the management being extrapolated from that of endometriosis—a condition with which it has not only many similarities but also a number of differences. Previously, the diagnosis was made histologically after hysterectomy, and it was a common finding in women undergoing hysterectomy for menorrhagia. It is now possible to make the diagnosis radiologically with MRI or TVUS.[95] In experienced units, these two methods are equally accurate, but MRI is less user-dependent and usually considered to be the investigation of choice. However, a relatively high rate of false positives will be seen, with, for example, uterine contractions being falsely diagnosed as adenomyosis. Without reliable diagnostic criteria, clinical trials of treatments are difficult and a true prevalence is unknown.

There appear to be two distinct forms of the condition: diffuse, where endometrial cells are widely distributed throughout the myometrium, and focal, where a discrete collection of cells are seen, also known as an adenomyoma.[96] Surgical excision of the former is not possible; thus, treatment options are limited to either medical management or hysterectomy. Although some cases of focal disease may be amenable to surgical management, it is possibly not as responsive to hormonal treatment. As many women undergoing conservative surgery (as opposed to hysterectomy) for this condition will be doing so to maintain their fertility, it is important that they are fully counseled about complications such as the risk of future uterine rupture before embarking such a procedure.[97] In a similar manner to fibroids, it has been suggested that it might be possible to embolize or use focused US to ablate adenomyotic tissue. Preliminary results from these therapies are promising,[98,99] but substantially more research still needs to be undertaken in this area.

Adenomyosis causes menorrhagia, metrorrhagia, dysmenorrhea, and infertility and is thought to occur secondary to a breach in the integrity of the myometrial–endometrial junction, such as occurs in pregnancy, especially those complicated by abnormal placentation and surgery (including ERPC/SMoM and cesarean section), or after blunt trauma to the abdomen. As with endometriosis, the ectopic endometrial tissue is hormone-sensitive and has been shown to express aromatase.[100] GnRH agonists, danazol, AIs, and the LNG-IUS have all been shown to be successful in the treatment of adenomyosis, although all have side effects.[101] Perhaps, the most promising of these is the LNG-IUS because of its mild adverse effect profile and apparent tolerability by patients.

Adhesions

Adhesions are a common finding in women with and without pelvic pain. They are formed after trauma to the visceral or parietal peritoneum and so can be secondary to surgery, infection, and endometriosis. Between 70% and 85% are thought to occur after surgery[102] and are thus iatrogenic. The relationship between adhesions and pain is still unclear, with only limited data relating their presence causally to pain.[103,104] Traditionally, surgery has been performed to divide adhesions (adhesiolysis); however, this is associated with a high rate of complications (~4%) including bowel injury, and meta-analyses suggest little long-term benefit.[105] Therefore, although adhesiolysis cannot be recommended in general as a treatment for CPP, in those women who have severe adhesions involving the bowel, it may be successful but associated with significant risk.[104,106]

There are, however, two other distinct cases where adhesions are known to cause pain: trapped ovary syndrome and ovarian remnant syndrome. In the former, a retained ovary becomes trapped in dense adhesions after hysterectomy, whereas in the latter, a small piece of ovary is unintentionally left behind at oophorectomy and again becomes trapped in adhesions. In both cases, the pain is cyclical and can be suppressed with a GnRH analogue. It may be possible to surgically remove the ovary/remnant; however, with distorted anatomy, this is not without risk, and some women may prefer to remain on the combination of GnRH analogue and low-dose HRT instead.[24]

Chronic Pelvic Inflammatory Disease

Chronic inflammation with scar tissue and distortion of pelvic structures can be seen in women who have had repeated episodes of acute PID or those in whom infection has been asymptomatic initially (as is frequently the case with *Chlamydia*). US may demonstrate features of chronic salpingitis, such as dilated fallopian tubes and poor mobility,[107] and severe adhesions may be seen at laparoscopy. These can be divided surgically, especially if they are causing anatomical distortion. However, although this may improve fertility as has been discussed, it may not have any effect on the pain. Chronic inflammation can cause sensitization of peripheral nerves, and therefore, a trial of a neuropathic adjunct may be indicated, especially if there are other symptoms suggesting a generalized visceral hypersensitivity syndrome. An exploration of the woman's attitudes to and beliefs about her pain may be beneficial. Guilt about earlier sexual behavior or concerns about current or future fertility may be revealed.

Pelvic Venous Congestion

Pelvic venous congestion syndrome is described as CPP arising from dilated and refluxing pelvic veins and is often proposed as a cause of pelvic pain with menstrual exacerbation. However, there is little convincing data supporting a causative relationship. Research in this area is hampered by the lack of consistent diagnostic criteria for the condition and the failure of the majority of studies to exclude other causes of CPP.[108] Although dilated pelvic veins are found in ~30% of women with CPP,[109,110] they are also found in at least 10% of the general population with increasing incidence in multiparous women. Proposed treatments for the syndrome would in many cases be effective for other pathologies associated with CPP (including continuous medroxyprogesterone acetate[111] and hysterectomy and bilateral oophorectomy[112]). However, a more specific treatment, embolization of incompetent pelvic veins, does appear to provide symptomatic relief, although the authors of a recent systematic review note that the quality of the evidence is low.[113] This is therefore an area where more research is needed.

GASTROINTESTINAL FACTORS IN CHRONIC PELVIC PAIN

As with acute pelvic pain, CPP secondary to a nongynecologic cause can present to gynecologists because of the site of the pain and its presumed etiology. It is therefore important that a detailed history of bowel function and its relation to and/or effect on the pain is taken. The gastrointestinal (GI) tract can be both the initial pain generator and the cause of secondary symptoms in a visceral hypersensitivity syndrome. IBS and constipation are very common and may be provoked by other conditions or medication and thus need to always be

borne in mind. Deep endometriosis frequently presents with bowel symptoms; however, it is important to remember that similar symptoms can be the presenting features of GI tract malignancies and inflammatory bowel disease and to fully investigate any "red flag" symptoms, such as rectal bleeding or unexplained weight loss.

Irritable Bowel Syndrome

IBS is a functional disorder of the GI tract and is discussed in detail in Chapter 63. We have mentioned it here, however, to draw attention to the fact that cyclical changes in the severity of symptoms are seen. Healthy, pain-free women frequently show alterations in their bowel habit around menstruation, possibly secondary to prostaglandin release, and this is often amplified in women with IBS.[114] It has been shown that rectal sensitivity to balloon distension varies with the menstrual cycle in women with IBS but not in those without.[115] Interestingly, in women whose IBS is clearly cyclical even without evidence of other gynecologic symptoms, the use of GnRH analogue treatment to suppress endogenous hormone production has been shown to be successful.[116]

Constipation

Constipation is a common cause of pelvic pain and can be easily avoided. It may be due to poor diet, lack of exercise, or reduced fluid intake; however, it is frequently iatrogenic, secondary to opioid use. It is therefore important to emphasize the need for fluid intake and dietary fiber as well as prescribing laxatives whenever such analgesics are required.

UROLOGIC FACTORS IN CHRONIC PELVIC PAIN

Pain originating in the urinary tract will also often be pelvic and therefore present to gynecologists. Again, symptoms may be cyclical or associated with symptoms in other organs. This coexistence of symptoms and the common embryologic origin of the structures involved have led to the suggestion of a "urogenital pain syndrome," including some or all of IC/BPS, vulvodynia, urethral syndrome, coccyodynia, and perineal pain.[117]

Interstitial Cystitis/Bladder Pain Syndrome

Pelvic pain experienced as arising from the bladder and associated with urinary symptoms, including urgency and frequency, was known as *interstitial cystitis* (IC).[118] However, there is ongoing debate as to the appropriateness of this terminology given the lack of evidence for bladder inflammation (cystitis) in many patients and the clear similarities with other chronic pain conditions. Alternative terminology has been proposed including *bladder pain syndrome* (BPS) and *painful bladder syndrome* (PBS).[29,119–121] A full description of these discussions and the advantages/disadvantages of each name are beyond the scope of this chapter. Here, we use IC/BPS in line with the American Urological Society[121]; however, we acknowledge that this is not the standard throughout the world and that there is a current push from some areas, including patient groups, to change back to IC due to issues with coding, funding, and recognition of the condition.

Until relatively recently, urologic pelvic pain had received little research funding, and progress toward both our understanding of the problem and potential novel treatments was very slow. However, there is now a large program of research in this area (Multidisciplinary Approach to the Study of Chronic Pelvic Pain [MAPP]; http://www.mappnetwork.org) that will potentially completely change the field, hopefully with significant patient benefit. One arm of this program addresses phenotyping with the aim of being better able to subtype patients with IC/BPS. However, until this program completes, current practice tends toward subdividing based on the presence or absence of Hunner lesions.[118]

Both the presentation and the impact of the condition on women's lives are very variable, and thus, treatment needs to be individualized. In general, however, multidisciplinary treatment regimens are likely to be most successful, including a combination of dietary modification, pharmacologic agents such as pentosan polysulfate sodium, and physical therapy. A key feature of the condition is the variation over time with both predictable and unpredictable flares in pain and associated urologic symptoms.[122] With the exception of sexual activity, triggers for flares appear to be relatively individual,[123] suggesting that it may be worth the woman keeping a detailed diary for a number of months with the aim of identifying her triggers and then aiming to either avoid these or learn strategies to manage the associated flare.

Urethral Syndrome

Urethral syndrome is also characterized by urinary urgency, frequency, dysuria, and suprapubic/lower back pain without any obvious cause. Dysfunction of the pelvic floor may be involved as success is often achieved with skeletal muscle relaxants or electrostimulation and biofeedback. Because of similarities in presentation to prostatitis in men, a chronic low-grade infection of the paraurethral glands has been suggested to be a possible cause. If tenderness can be elicited just lateral to the urethra through the anterior vaginal wall, this may be a possibility, and a prolonged course of antibiotics may be justified.[124]

MUSCULOSKELETAL FACTORS IN CHRONIC PELVIC PAIN

Dysfunction in the musculoskeletal system can be both the primary cause of CPP or secondary to pathology elsewhere. Although it may not be the first thought in a gynecologic consultation, it is surprisingly common, with one retrospective study suggesting that 75% of 132 nonconsecutive patients with CPP had musculoskeletal abnormalities.[125] Importantly, we are increasingly realizing that musculoskeletal factors coexist with other pathologies (e.g., endometriosis)[74,88] and a failure to identify them may contribute to the poor response often seen to treatment of the peripheral pathology. It is therefore important that the musculoskeletal system is appropriately assessed in all women with CPP and any issues dealt with in order that a good response to treatment occurs. A detailed description of appropriate assessment is not possible here but can be found elsewhere.[126] Some of the important musculoskeletal factors to be borne in mind are discussed briefly in the following text and in more detail in Chapters 35 and 36.

Fibromyalgia

Many women with fibromyalgia complain of pain in their lower back and pelvis with two of the tender points that were previously used to diagnose the condition being in the gluteal muscles in the upper outer quadrants of the buttocks. Pain here can easily be confused with the lower back pain often described by women with CPP. Furthermore, fibromyalgia may have cyclical exacerbations,[127] and therefore, symptoms are often assigned to a gynecologic cause.

Trigger Points

Trigger points are frequently found in abdominal and pelvic floor muscles causing or exacerbating both CPP and dyspareunia. These can be the primary pain generator or can be secondary, either to other musculoskeletal abnormalities such as sacroiliac joint (SIJ) dysfunction or to repeated episodes of visceral pain as occurs in adenomyosis. The continued presence of a trigger point can explain a partial response to treatment of the underlying pathology and is an indication for a careful reexamination of the patient at her follow-up visit.

Pelvic Floor Abnormalities

In women, pelvic floor abnormalities can be secondary to postural alterations caused by pain or other musculoskeletal conditions, visceromuscular referral patterns, or trauma as occurs during childbirth or certain surgical procedures. Unilateral or bilateral pelvic floor abnormalities can cause CPP, dyspareunia (with secondary vaginismus), perineal pain, and dyschezia and yet are frequently overlooked. In a woman with dyspareunia, demonstrating that pressure on a tender, tense pelvic floor muscle recreates her pain during intercourse can help toward relieving concerns about her reproductive organs. Good response to treatment is frequently obtained from physiotherapy. Recent studies on the injection of botulinum toxin into the pelvic floor muscles have shown some promise.[128] However, it would be prudent to combine any such treatment with a physiotherapy assessment and exercise program to ensure the underlying cause of the spasm is addressed and that the dysfunction does not recur.

Hernia

Acute obstruction of a hernia will cause acute pain; however, a number of different types of hernias can also be responsible for CPP, although the exact mechanism by which they cause pain is debated. Most commonly, these include inguinal, femoral, and obturator hernias. Imaging modalities such as computed tomography or MRI may be useful in making the diagnosis if a clear examination finding is not present. Surgical repair is usually the recommended treatment, and this can either be open or laparoscopic with both having their own advantages and disadvantages.[129]

Sacroiliac Joint Pain

The SIJ is the largest axial joint in the body. A network of muscles support the joint and deliver regional muscular forces to the pelvic bones. The associated ligaments are weaker in women to allow mobility and facilitate parturition. The innervation of the joint is complex and still debated but probably includes fibers from L4 to S4.[130] It is widely accepted that SIJ dysfunction causes lower back pain, and pelvic pain appears to occur in a significant percent of patients. In general, the pain is unilateral (unless both joints are affected) and below the L5 spinous process, sometimes radiating down as far as the foot. SIJ dysfunction and pain can occur for a number of reasons, including pregnancy, trauma, and prolonged bending and lifting. A number of possible treatments exist with varying degrees of success. Conservative options include physiotherapy and joint stabilization which have been shown to be successful in some series.[131] Intra-articular joint injections under radiologic guidance have been shown to produce good to excellent pain relief in most studies. Surgical fusion of the joint may be required in some cases, although adequately powered, prospective studies are lacking.

NEUROLOGIC FACTORS IN CHRONIC PELVIC PAIN

It has already been mentioned that in many conditions causing pelvic pain, secondary sensitization of the peripheral or central nervous system can occur, perpetuating or increasing pain and extending referral areas and involving other organ systems.[63,64,132] There are also situations where damage to a nerve or nerve roots can be the primary cause of the pain. The specific nerve(s) involved will determine the precise distribution of pain and associated symptoms; however, a number of general features are usually associated with a neuropathy. Classically, the pain is shooting, burning, or stabbing in nature. Initially at least, the pain will be in a clearly defined area, although secondary changes may blur this. Trophic skin changes may also be present. Symptoms may be exacerbated or relieved by movements which stretch/relax the nerve or increase/decrease

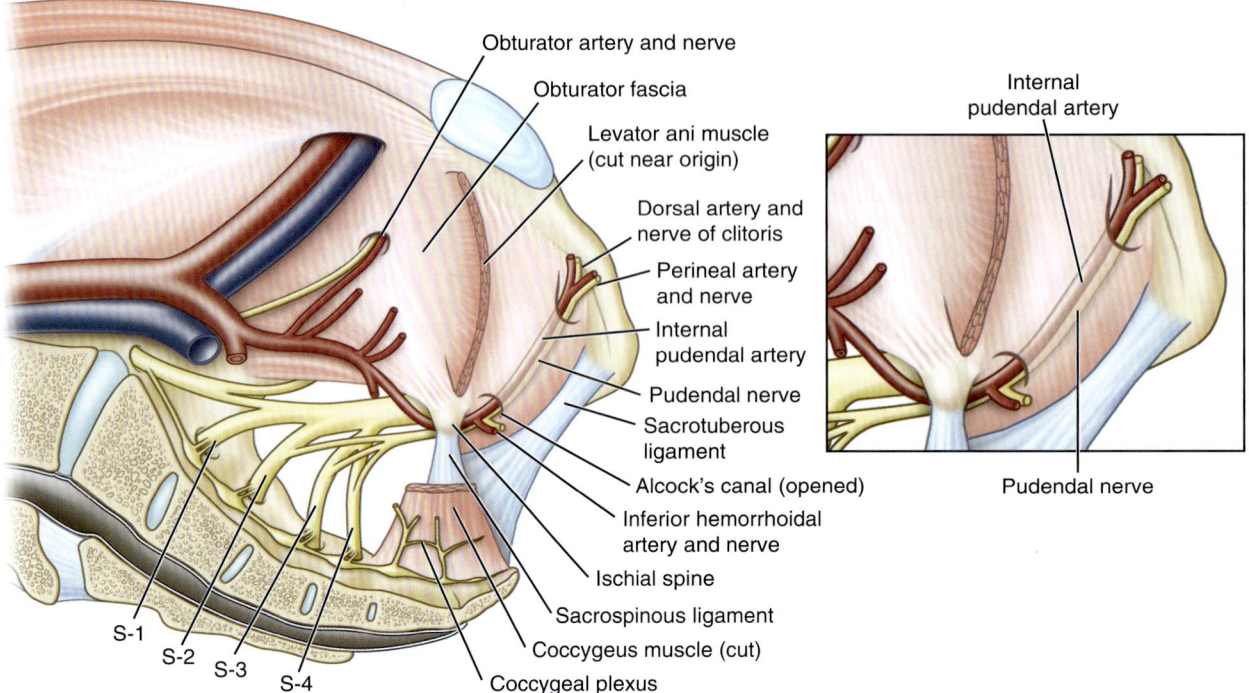

FIGURE 64.2 Course of the pudendal nerve.

compression by surrounding structures. Local anesthetic block-ade of the specific nerve may relieve the pain entirely; however, it is also possible that pain can be worsened by this procedure perhaps because the injected fluid volume worsens compres-sion. Because of the complex innervation of the pelvis, there are many different neuropathies that can occur. We discuss in detail here only the most common, pudendal neuropathy; however, a careful consideration of innervation patterns may point to an unusual neuropathy in a woman whose symptoms cannot otherwise be explained. We also consider neuropathies second-ary to a Pfannenstiel incision because of the prevalence of this procedure in obstetrics and gynecology. More information on other pelvic neuropathies can be found elsewhere.[133]

Pudendal Neuropathy

The pudendal nerve arises from the sacral plexus in the ventral rami of sacral nerves 2, 3, and 4 (S2–S4) and exits the pelvis through the greater sciatic foramen between the piriformis and coccygeus muscles. It then winds around the sacrospinous lig-ament and passes through Alcock's canal to enter the pelvis again through the lesser sciatic foramen before branching into clitoral, superficial perineal, deep perineal, and posterior rec-tal branches (Fig. 64.2).[134] It can be seen that there are many points where nerve entrapment could occur and many situa-tions in which this nerve could be damaged including surgery and childbirth.[135]

Pain is felt in the distribution of the nerve and is exacerbated by sitting and relieved to a variable extent by standing or lying on the unaffected side. Perineal sensation is usually preserved as is muscle tone, although pain may be recreated during rectal examination. Local anesthetic nerve blocks may be successful and can also aid with diagnosis; however, they may have to be repeated regularly. Although surgical decompression may be an option, damage to the nerve may not be reversible.[136]

Neuropathy Secondary to a Pfannenstiel Incision

A Pfannenstiel incision is a low transverse abdominal incision which was first described in 1900. It is commonly used for ce-sarean sections and many benign gynecologic procedures but more rarely in general surgery. Aesthetically, it is more pleas-ing to the woman, being below the "bikini" line. It also has a number of advantages over other abdominal incisions, in-cluding lower incisional hernia rates, fewer wound infections, less hematoma formation, and less direct postoperative pain. However, the ilioinguinal and iliohypogastric nerves have a superficial course and are relatively easily injured by a Pfan-nenstiel incision.[137] In the literature, the reported incidence of nerve damage after a Pfannenstiel incision is 3.7%[138]; however, the true incidence may well be higher as many cases are not reported or diagnosed. Typically, the pain is burning or lanci-nating near the incision and radiates to the area supplied by the nerve with associated sensory impairment. The nerves can be damaged in a number of ways: direct nerve trauma with neuroma formation, suture incorporation of the nerve during fascial closure, and constriction of the nerve during scar or wound healing.[138] Optimal treatment is still unclear. In many cases, the symptoms resolve over time without treatment. The nerve can be blocked with local anesthetic, which will at least confirm the diagnosis even if the pain is not entirely removed. In some cases, surgery is required; even in these cases, however, long-term recovery is good.[138] Education is clearly required, about both careful surgical techniques to reduce the incidence of nerve entrapment and the presentation, such that diagnosis and treatment occur more rapidly.

Dyspareunia

OVERVIEW

Dyspareunia is defined as genital pain just before, during, or after sexual intercourse. It can be subdivided into primary, having always occurred in association with intercourse, and secondary, having developed after a period of pain-free sex-ual activity. Additionally, it can also be divided into superficial, with pain only on entry, and deep, thought to be associated with organic pathology. As with so many pain conditions, these subdivisions are overly simplistic and frequently clinically un-helpful. Whatever the initial trigger for an episode of painful intercourse, fear of further pain can set up a cycle of muscular

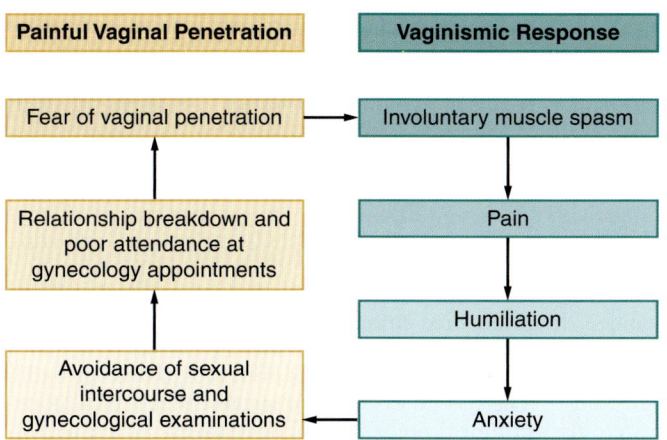

FIGURE 64.3 Cycle of vaginismus. *(Adapted from Butcher J. Female sexual problems II: sexual pain and sexual fears.* BMJ *1999;318[7176]:110–112, with permission from BMJ Publishing Group Ltd.)*

tension and vaginismus (Fig. 64.3), ensuring that future episodes will be painful, reinforcing that fear. Furthermore, the psychological consequences of an inability to have pain-free intercourse on both the woman and her partner should not be underestimated. Psychological morbidity can worsen the experience. However, dyspareunia should not be assumed to be psychological in origin just because no pathology is evident at initial examination.

Possible causes of dyspareunia are listed in Table 64.10. Superficial vulval pain is a common cause of dyspareunia and is discussed in detail in the following section. If superficial dyspareunia occurs after childbirth, time should be taken to explore the woman's beliefs and to reassure her. Occasionally, hypoestrogenism may be the cause, but it is very rare for surgery to be required in these cases. Deep dyspareunia can be secondary to many abdominopelvic pathologies but is also often positional. If a woman complains of pain on contact with the cervix, this may be due to inadequate arousal and failure of the upper vagina to balloon and therefore move the cervix out of reach.[139] Whatever the initial cause of pain, vaginismus is a frequent sequela and is therefore discussed here in more detail.

Vaginismus

The term *vaginismus* was first used in 1862 and is now thought to be one of the commonest female sexual problems. The true prevalence is unknown; however, it is identified in 10% to 20% of women requesting help for sexual dysfunction.[140] Definitions vary as to whether spasm of the muscles surrounding the lower third of the vagina is included or whether it is difficulty in allowing vaginal entry, often associated with involuntary pelvic muscle contraction.[141] Although pain with intercourse is usually the presenting feature, there is often fear of any object being placed in the vagina; thus, tampons are not used and gynecologic examinations not well tolerated. Some women are so fearful that they avoid smear tests and other essential health checks.

Vaginismus is thought to occur as a conditioned response secondary to adverse physical or psychological stimuli. Early traumatic experiences are thought to predispose to the condition, including traumatic sexual experiences, unsympathetic gynecologic examinations, and assault, although a history of abuse (physical or sexual) is not usually associated with vaginismus.[141] A background of religious orthodoxy has, however, been shown to be associated. Psychosexual fantasies often coexist such as that the vagina is too small to accommodate a penis or that it is a delicate, fragile organ which will be damaged during intercourse. These can arise secondary to comments made inadvertently, for example, at the time of episiotomy repair, and clinicians should therefore think carefully about what is said at vulnerable times. Male sexual dysfunction can develop as a consequence of vaginismus, although the reverse can also occur with vaginismus arising secondary to a male partner's impotence.

Treatment should be individualized to the specific woman or couple and her or their desires. For most women, successful vaginal penetrative intercourse and an improved sexual experience for both partners is the aim. However, in some instances, the woman may not feel comfortable with intercourse even after the vaginismus has resolved. Current guidelines suggest that the basis of treatment should be to enable the woman to become more comfortable with her genitals, followed by graded exposure to different types of vaginal penetration in order to overcome her fear of penetration.[142] At all times during treatment, the woman should feel that she is in control and the extent to which her partner is involved should be her decision, although involvement should be encouraged. For some couples, fertility is the ultimate aim and an appropriate referral may need to be made.

A number of different approaches are described, one of which is a combination of behavioral and desensitization exercises using relaxation and graded vaginal trainers. Education is also important, and there may be a need for exploration of fantasies before they can be dispelled. Hypnotherapy, physiotherapy using biofeedback, amitriptyline, and local injections with botulinum toxin have all been reported to have good results. If physical causes have been excluded, treatment is usually highly successful with some authors reporting up to 100% success.[142]

Vulval Pain Syndromes

Although not truly pelvic pain, the vulval pain syndromes (vulvodynia and vestibulodynia) exhibit many features which are similar to CPP, and the two can coexist in a urogenital pain syndrome. Much of what has already been discussed in relation to the assessment and multidisciplinary management of CPP is just as relevant for vulval pain. It is therefore appropriate to include a brief overview of these conditions in a chapter devoted to pelvic pain in females.

As with CPP, there is frequently a delay between presentation and diagnosis, and many unsuccessful, often inappropriate, and sometimes damaging treatments may have already been tried.[143] It is therefore not surprising that many of these women report anger and frustration and that psychological morbidity

TABLE 64.10	Causes of Dyspareunia			
Vulval	**Vaginal**	**Pelvic**	**Musculoskeletal**	**Systemic**
Vulval pain syndrome	Vaginismus	Endometriosis	Pelvic floor tension	Hypoestrogenism
Vestibular pain syndrome	Congenital abnormality	IBS	Pelvic floor trigger point	Inadequate arousal
Herpes simplex	Inadequate lubrication	IC/BPS/urethral syndrome		Psychological
Postepisiotomy	Radiation vaginitis	Chronic PID		Abuse history
		Adnexal pathology		

BPS, bladder pain syndrome; IBS, irritable bowel syndrome; IC, interstitial cystitis; PID, pelvic inflammatory disease.

is more prevalent than in asymptomatic women.[144] There is no evidence to suggest that these psychological features are a cause rather than a consequence of the conditions. Because vulval pain syndromes are almost invariably associated with dyspareunia in sexually active women, sexual dysfunction is also common, with secondary problems such as vaginismus and anorgasmia developing. However, there is no evidence of higher rates of previous sexual or physical abuse in these women as compared to healthy controls.[145]

The vulval pain syndromes were first described in the late 1800s; however, there has been confusion surrounding their nomenclature, etiology, and management ever since. Further difficulties occur as vulval pain can present to gynecologists, dermatologists, or GUM specialists, each of whom historically had different preferred treatments. The International Society for the Study of Vulvovaginal Disease (ISSVD), a multispecialty society, is working to redress this and has recently reclassified these syndromes as either vulvodynia (which can be localized or generalized, and provoked or unprovoked) or vestibulodynia.[146] These terms replace dysesthetic vulvodynia and vestibulitis. Many women will, however, present with symptoms of both vulvar and vestibular pain. The ISSVD defines vulvodynia as "vulvar discomfort, most often described as burning pain, occurring in the absence of relevant visible findings or a specific, clinically identifiable, neurologic disorder."[146] The term *vestibulodynia* has replaced vestibulitis as there is no evidence of inflammation and is defined by the ISSVD as "provoked vulval dysesthesia localized to the vestibule."[146] Pain can also occur on urination and defecation. It should be noted, however, that the IASP use different terminologies, aiming to bring the conditions in line with other pain syndromes (e.g., vulval pain syndrome).[29]

By definition, a thorough history and examination with appropriate investigations should be undertaken to exclude other causes of vulval pain, such as those listed in Table 64.11, before a label of a vulval pain syndrome is given. To date, the true prevalence remains unknown, with the large reported variation in numbers of women attending clinics likely due to variation in the type of clinic and known interests of the clinicians. However, as more specialized vulval clinics become established, the number of referrals for vulval pain syndromes continues to increase. The etiology remains unknown but is likely to be multifactorial.[143] Although it is unlikely that irritation from topical

agents (e.g., antifungal agents, bubble bath) is the precipitating factor, their use may well exacerbate symptoms and should be discouraged. Examination will reveal either focal or generalized pain in response to light touch with a cotton-tipped swab but is otherwise unremarkable.

A number of treatments have been shown to be successful; however, treatment needs to be carefully tailored to the individual patient, and a multidisciplinary approach is usually of benefit. Basic advice on vulval care should be given, recommending careful hygiene but with avoidance of perfumed products and overdrying. Although topical products in general should be avoided, fragrance-free emollient creams can be soothing and local anesthetic gel such as topical lidocaine can be particularly useful prior to intercourse acting as both a pain reliever and a lubricant.[143] There is no evidence to suggest that topical corticosteroids, antifungal preparations, or testosterone are helpful and only minimal evidence to support the use of topical estrogens.[146] Recent work has suggested a central component to vulvodynia,[147,148] which may explain the success of drugs such as amitriptyline, gabapentin, pregabalin, and lamotrigine in the condition.[149-151] There is also recent evidence suggesting topical gabapentin may be helpful.[152]

Whether tension in the pelvic floor muscles (a common finding in women with vulvodynia) is involved in perpetuating the pain remains unknown; however, physiotherapists can be very successful in treating vulval pain syndromes. In one series, 71% of women had a greater than 50% improvement in symptoms, 62% experienced improvement in sexual functioning, and 50% had an increase in quality of life.[153]

Surgery should be considered as a last resort. However, it can be successful in a subgroup of women and should not be dismissed entirely. In general, it appears to be less successful in women with coexisting vaginismus and more successful in women who had a good response to lidocaine gel preoperatively. Postoperative psychosexual counseling and the use of dilators and physical therapy have been shown to improve outcome.[146]

As with other chronic pain syndromes, the value of patient support groups, such as the Vulval Pain Society, should not be underestimated as the vulval pain syndromes are a particularly isolating group of disorders. The effect of the conditions on relationships can be devastating and, unlike conditions such as endometriosis which are coming more and more into the public's awareness, vulval pain is still seen as a taboo subject and not discussed.

Conclusion

Research in many fields over recent years has led to an improved understanding of both the basic science of visceral pain and of many of the conditions causing pelvic pain. However, time to listen to and explore a woman's story as well as to perform a careful examination must be invested in order to make the best use of this knowledge. Sociologic research has identified the recurrent theme of the social meaninglessness of pain without a medical diagnosis[154] and encouraged us to consider chronic pain in a biopsychosociocultural context.[155] The more recent move toward multidisciplinary CPP clinics is a positive step forward in these respects and acknowledges that the secondary consequences of the pain (be they musculoskeletal, psychological, gastrointestinal, sexual, etc.) must also be managed in order to facilitate a full recovery.[156]

TABLE 64.11	Causes of Secondary Vulval Pain

- Infection
  - *Candida albicans*
  - Herpes simplex
- Inflammation
  - Lichen sclerosus
  - Eczema
  - Contact dermatitis
  - Psoriasis
  - Crohn's disease
- Iatrogenic
  - Postepisiotomy
  - Postsurgical scar
- Musculoskeletal
  - Pelvic floor tension
- Hormonal
  - Hypoestrogenism
- Trauma
- Rare
  - Symptomatic dermographism
  - Aphthous ulceration
  - Bullous disorders
  - Sacral meningeal cysts
  - Pudendal nerve entrapment

References

1. Grace VM, Zondervan KT. Chronic pelvic pain in New Zealand: prevalence, pain severity, diagnoses and use of the health services. *Aust N Z J Public Health* 2004;28(4):369–375.
2. Mathias SD, Kuppermann M, Liberman RF, et al. Chronic pelvic pain: prevalence, health-related quality of life, and economic correlates. *Obstet Gynecol* 1996;87(3):321–327.

3. Zondervan KT, Yudkin PL, Vessey MP, et al. The community prevalence of chronic pelvic pain in women and associated illness behaviour. *Br J Gen Pract* 2001;51(468):541–547.

4. Zondervan KT, Yudkin PL, Vessey MP, et al. Prevalence and incidence of chronic pelvic pain in primary care: evidence from a national general practice database. *Br J Obstet Gynaecol* 1999;106(11):1149–1155.

5. Knight M, Nair M, Tuffnell D, et al. *Saving Lives, Improving Mothers' Care—Lessons Learned to Inform Maternity Care from the UK and Ireland Confidential Enquiries into Maternal Deaths and Morbidity 2013–15.* Oxford, United Kingdom: National Perinatal Epidemiology Unit, Oxford University; 2017.

6. Curtis AH. A cause of adhesion in the right upper quadrant. *JAMA* 1930;94:1221–1222.

7. Fitz-Hugh T Jr. Acute gonococcic peritonitis of the right upper quadrant in women. *JAMA* 1934;102:2094–2096.

8. Bevan CD, Johal BJ, Mumtaz G, et al. Clinical, laparoscopic and microbiological findings in acute salpingitis: report on a United Kingdom cohort. *Br J Obstet Gynaecol* 1995;102:407–414.

9. Ross J, McCarthy G. *UK National Guideline for the Management of Pelvic Inflammatory Disease, 2011.* London: British Association for Sexual Health and HIV; 2011.

10. Rio CD, Hall G, Hook EW III, et al. Update to CDC's Sexually Transmitted Diseases Treatment Guidelines, 2006: fluoroquinolones no longer recommended for treatment of gonococcal infections. *MMWR Morb Mortal Wkly Rep* 2007;56(14):332–336.

11. Aboulghar MA, Mansour RT, Serour GI. Ultrasonographically guided transvaginal aspiration of tuboovarian abscesses and pyosalpinges: an optional treatment for acute pelvic inflammatory disease. *Am J Obstet Gynecol* 1995;172:1501–1503.

12. Damigos E, Johns J, Ross J. An update on the diagnosis and management of ovarian torsion. *Obstet Gynecol* 2012;14:229–236.

13. Creighton SM. Common congenital anomalies of the female genital tract. *Rev Gynaecol Prac* 2005;5(4):221–226.

14. Bakken IJ, Skjeldestad FE. Time trends in ectopic pregnancies in a Norwegian county 1970-2004—a population-based study. *Hum Reprod* 2006;21(12):3132–3136.

15. Braude P, Rowell P. Assisted conception. III—problems with assisted conception. *BMJ* 2003;327(7420):920–923.

16. Elson CJ, Salim R, Potdar N, et al. *Diagnosis and Management of Ectopic Pregnancy.* London: Royal College of Obstetricians and Gynaecologists; 2016. Green-top guideline no. 21.

17. National Institute for Health and Care Excellence. *Ectopic Pregnancy and Miscarriage: Diagnosis and Initial Management in Early Pregnancy of Ectopic Pregnancy and Miscarriage.* London: Royal College of Obstetricians and Gynaecologists; 2012.

18. Jurkovic D. Modern management of miscarriage: is there a place for non-surgical treatment? *Ultrasound Obstet Gynecol* 1998;11:161–163.

19. Hamoda H, Chamberlain PF, Moore NR, et al. Conservative treatment of an incarcerated gravid uterus. *BJOG* 2002;109(9):1074–1075.

20. Yohannes P, Schaefer J. Urinary retention during the second trimester of pregnancy: a rare cause. *Urology* 2002;59(6):946.

21. Mathur RS, Drakeley AJ, Raine-Fenning NJ, et al. *The Management of Ovarian Hyperstimulation Syndrome.* London: Royal College of Obstetricians and Gynaecologists; 2016.

22. Stewart JA, Hamilton PJ, Murdoch AP. Thromboembolic disease associated with ovarian stimulation and assisted conception techniques. *Hum Reprod* 1997;12:2167–2173.

23. Ludwig AK, Glawatz M, Griesinger G, et al. Perioperative and post-operative complications of transvaginal ultrasound-guided oocyte retrieval: prospective study of >1000 oocyte retrievals. *Hum Reprod* 2006;21(12):3235–3240.

24. Kennedy SH, Moore J. *The Initial Management of Chronic Pelvic Pain.* London: Royal College of Obstetricians and Gynaecologists; 2012. Green-top guideline no. 41.

25. Vincent K, Warnaby C, Stagg CJ, et al. Dysmenorrhoea is associated with central changes in otherwise healthy women. *Pain* 2011;152(9):1966–1975.

26. Iacovides S, Avidon I, Baker FC. Women with dysmenorrhoea are hypersensitive to experimentally induced forearm ischaemia during painful menstruation and during the pain-free follicular phase. *Eur J Pain* 2015;19(6):797–804.

27. Tu C-H, Niddam DM, Chao H-T, et al. Abnormal cerebral metabolism during menstrual pain in primary dysmenorrhea. *Neuroimage* 2009;47(1):28–35.

28. Tu C-H, Niddam DM, Chao H-T, et al. Brain morphological changes associated with cyclic menstrual pain. *Pain* 2010;150(3):462–468.

29. Baranowski A, Abrams P, Berger RE, et al. *Taxonomy of Pelvic Pain. Classification of Chronic Pain.* 2nd ed. Seattle, WA: IASP Press; 2012.

30. French L. Dysmenorrhea. *Am Fam Phys* 2005;71(2):285–291.

31. Harel Z. Dysmenorrhea in adolescents and young adults: etiology and management. *J Pediatr Adolesc Gynecol* 2006;19(6):363–371.

32. Laufer MR, Sanfilippo J, Rose G. Adolescent endometriosis: diagnosis and treatment approaches. *J Pediatr Adolesc Gynecol* 2003;16(3 suppl):S3–S11.

33. Boctor AM, Eickholt M, Pugsley TA. Meclofenamate sodium is an inhibitor of both the 5-lipoxygenase and cyclooxygenase pathways of the arachidonic acid cascade in vitro. *Prostaglandins Leukot Med* 1986;23(2–3):229–238.

34. Marjoribanks J, Ayeleke RO, Farquhar C, et al. Nonsteroidal anti-inflammatory drugs for dysmenorrhoea. *Cochrane Database Syst Rev* 2015;(7):CD001751.

35. DuRant RH, Jay MS, Shoffitt T, et al. Factors influencing adolescents' responses to regimens of naproxen for dysmenorrhea. *Am J Dis Child* 1985;139(5):489–493.

36. Wong CL, Farquhar C, Roberts H, et al. Oral contraceptive pill for primary dysmenorrhoea. *Cochrane Database Syst Rev* 2009;(4):CD002120.

37. Sulak PJ, Cressman BE, Waldrop E, et al. Extending the duration of active oral contraceptive pills to manage hormone withdrawal symptoms. *Obstet Gynecol* 1997;89(2):179–183.

38. Jain J, Dutton C, Nicosia A, et al. Pharmacokinetics, ovulation suppression and return to ovulation following a lower dose subcutaneous formulation of Depo-Provera. *Contraception* 2004;70(1):11–18.

39. Harel Z, Biro FM, Kollar LM. Depo-Provera in adolescents: effects of early second injection or prior oral contraception. *J Adolesc Health* 1995;16(5):379–384.

40. Proctor M, Latthe P, Farquhar C, et al. Surgical interruption of pelvic nerve pathways for primary and secondary dysmenorrhoea. *Cochrane Database Syst Rev* 2005;(4):CD001896.

41. Proctor ML, Smith CA, Farquhar CM, et al. Transcutaneous electrical nerve stimulation and acupuncture for primary dysmenorrhoea. *Cochrane Database Syst Rev* 2002;(1):CD002123.

42. Smith CA, Armour M, Zhu X, et al. Acupuncture for dysmenorrhoea. *Cochrane Database Syst Rev* 2016;(4):CD007854.

43. Akin MD, Weingand KW, Hengehold DA, et al. Continuous low-level topical heat in the treatment of dysmenorrhoea. *Obstet Gynecol* 2001;97(3):343–349.

44. Proctor ML, Murphy PA, Pattison HM, et al. Behavioural interventions for primary and secondary dysmenorrhoea. *Cochrane Database Syst Rev* 2007;(3):CD002248.

45. Pattanittum P, Kunyanone N, Brown J, et al. Dietary supplements for dysmenorrhoea. *Cochrane Database Syst Rev* 2016;(3):CD002124.

46. O'Herlihy C, Robinson HP, Ch de Crespigny LJ. Mittelschmerz is a preovulatory symptom. *BMJ* 1980;280:986.

47. Marinho AO, Sallam HN, Goessens L, et al. Ovulation side and occurrence of mittelschmerz in spontaneous and induced ovarian cycles. *BMJ* 1982;284(6316):632.

48. Zondervan K, Barlow DH. Epidemiology of chronic pelvic pain. *Baillieres Best Pract Res Clin Obstet Gynaecol* 2000;14(3):403–414.

49. Raphael KG, Widom CS, Lange G. Childhood victimization and pain in adulthood: a prospective investigation. *Pain* 2001;92:283–293.

50. Schliep KC, Mumford SL, Johnstone EB, et al. Sexual and physical abuse and gynecologic disorders. *Hum Reprod* 2016;31(8):1904–1912.

51. Newton-John T. The psychology of pain. In: MacLean A, Stones RW, Thornton S, eds. *Pain in Obstetrics and Gynaecology.* London: Royal College of Obstetricians and Gynaecologists; 2001:59–69.

52. Selfe SA, Matthews Z, Stones RW. Factors influencing outcome in consultations for chronic pelvic pain. *J Womens Health* 1998;7(8):1041–1048.

53. Price J, Farmer G, Harris J, et al. Attitudes of women with chronic pelvic pain to the gynaecological consultation: a qualitative study. *BJOG* 2006;113(4):446–452.

54. Skrine R, Mountford H, eds. *Psychosexual Medicine: An Introduction.* London: Arnold; 2001.

55. Jarrell J. Demonstration of cutaneous allodynia in association with chronic pelvic pain. *J Vis Exp* 2009;28:e1232.

56. Vercellini P, Frontino G, De Giorgi O, et al. Comparison of a levonorgestrel-releasing intrauterine device versus expectant management after conservative surgery for symptomatic endometriosis: a pilot study. *Fertil Steril* 2003;80(2):305–309.

57. Brown J, Pan A, Hart RJ. Gonadotrophin-releasing hormone analogues for pain associated with endometriosis. *Cochrane Database Syst Rev* 2010;(12):CD008475.

58. Bedaiwy MA, Casper RF. Treatment with leuprolide acetate and hormonal add-back for up to 10 years in stage IV endometriosis patients with chronic pelvic pain. *Fertil Steril* 2006;85(1):220–222.

59. Chapron C, Querleu D, Bruhat MA, et al. Surgical complications of diagnostic and operative gynaecological laparoscopy: a series of 29,956 cases. *Hum Reprod* 1998;13(4):867–872.

60. Onwude JL, Thornton JG, Morley S, et al. A randomised trial of photographic reinforcement during postoperative counselling after diagnostic laparoscopy for pelvic pain. *Eur J Obstet Gynecol Reprod Biol* 2004;112:89–94.

61. Sator-Katzenschlager SM, Scharbert G, Kress HG, et al. Chronic pelvic pain treated with gabapentin and amitriptyline: a randomized controlled pilot study. *Wie Klin Wochenschr* 2005;117(21–22):761–768.

62. Lewis SC, Bhattacharya S, Wu O, et al. Gabapentin for the management of chronic pelvic pain in women (GaPP1): a pilot randomised controlled trial. *PLoS One* 2016;11(4):e0153037.

63. Whitaker LH, Reid J, Choa A, et al. An exploratory study into objective and reported characteristics of neuropathic pain in women with chronic pelvic pain. *PLoS One* 2016;11(4):e0151950.

64. Brawn J, Morotti M, Zondervan KT, et al. Central changes associated with chronic pelvic pain and endometriosis. *Hum Reprod Update* 2014;20(5):737–747.

65. Berkley K. Multiple mechanisms of pelvic pain: lessons from basic research. In: MacLean A, Stones RW, Thornton S , eds. *Pain in Obstetrics and Gynaecology*. London: Royal College of Obstetricians and Gynaecologists; 2001:26–39.

66. Kuiken SD, Tytgat GN, Boeckxstaens GE. Review article: drugs interfering with visceral sensitivity for the treatment of functional gastrointestinal disorders—the clinical evidence. *Aliment Pharmacol Ther* 2005;21(6):633–651.

67. Cheong YC, Smotra G, Williams AC. Non-surgical interventions for the management of chronic pelvic pain. *Cochrane Database Syst Rev* 2014;(3):CD008797.

68. Johnson NP, Hummelshoj L, Adamson GD, et al. World Endometriosis Society consensus on the classification of endometriosis. *Hum Reprod* 2017;32(2):315–324.

69. Sampson JA. Peritoneal endometriosis due to the menstrual dissemination of endometrial tissue into the peritoneal cavity. *Am J Obstet Gynecol* 1927;14:422–469.

70. Kyama C, Debrock S, Mwenda J, et al. Potential involvement of the immune system in the development of endometriosis. *Reprod Biol Endocrinol* 2003;1(1):123.

71. Dunselman GA, Vermeulen N, Becker C, et al. ESHRE guideline: management of women with endometriosis. *Hum Reprod* 2014;29:400–412.

72. Vercellini P, Fedele L, Aimi G, et al. Association between endometriosis stage, lesion type, patient characteristics and severity of pelvic pain symptoms: a multivariate analysis of over 1000 patients. *Hum Reprod* 2007;22(1):266–271.

73. Stratton P, Berkley KJ. Chronic pelvic pain and endometriosis: translational evidence of the relationship and implications. *Hum Reprod Update* 2011;17(3):327–346.

74. Stratton P, Khachikyan I, Sinaii N, et al. Association of chronic pelvic pain and endometriosis with signs of sensitization and myofascial pain. *Obstet Gynecol* 2015;125(3):719–728.

75. Morotti M, Vincent K, Brawn J, et al. Peripheral changes in endometriosis-associated pain. *Hum Reprod Update* 2014;20(5):717–736.

76. Vercellini P, Somigliana E, Vigano P, et al. Endometriosis: current therapies and new pharmacological developments. *Drugs* 2009;69(6):649–675.

77. Brown J, Crawford TJ, Allen C, et al. Nonsteroidal anti-inflammatory drugs for pain in women with endometriosis. *Cochrane Database Syst Rev* 2017;(1):CD004753.

78. Cobellis L, Razzi S, De Simone S, et al. The treatment with a COX-2 specific inhibitor is effective in the management of pain related to endometriosis. *Eur J Obstet Gynaecol Reprod Biol* 2004;116(1):100–102.

79. Juni P, Nartey L, Reichenbach S, et al. Risk of cardiovascular events and rofecoxib: cumulative meta-analysis. *Lancet* 2004;364:2021–2029.

80. Miller JD, Shaw RW, Casper RF, et al. Historical prospective cohort study of the recurrence of pain after discontinuation of treatment with danazol or a gonadotropin-releasing hormone agonist. *Fertil Steril* 1998;70(2):293–296.

81. Kitawaki J, Kusuki I, Koshiba H, et al. Detection of aromatase cytochrome P-450 in endometrial biopsy specimens as a diagnostic test for endometriosis. *Fertil Steril* 1999;72:1100–1106.

82. Attar E, Bulun SE. Aromatase inhibitors: the next generation of therapeutics for endometriosis? *Fertil Steril* 2006;85(5):1307–1318.

83. Howell A, Cuzick J, Baum M, et al. Results of the ATAC (Arimidex, Tamoxifen, Alone or in Combination) trial after completion of 5 years' adjuvant treatment for breast cancer. *Lancet* 2005;365(9453):60–62.

84. Abbott JA, Hawe J, Clayton RD, et al. The effects and effectiveness of laparoscopic excision of endometriosis: a prospective study with 2-5 year follow-up. *Hum Reprod* 2003;18(9):1922–1927.

85. Kent A, Shakir F, Rockall T, et al. Laparoscopic surgery for severe rectovaginal endometriosis compromising the bowel: a prospective cohort study. *J Minim Invasive Gynecol* 2016;23(4):526–534.

86. Yap C, Furness S, Farquhar C. Pre and post operative medical therapy for endometriosis surgery. *Cochrane Database Syst Rev* 2004;(3):CD003678.

87. Morotti M, Vincent K, Becker CM. Mechanisms of pain in endometriosis. *Eur J Obstet Gynecol Reprod Biol* 2017;209:8–13.

88. Raimondo D, Youssef A, Mabrouk M, et al. Pelvic floor muscle dysfunction on 3D/4D transperineal ultrasound in patients with deep infiltrating endometriosis: a pilot study. *Ultrasound Obstet Gynecol* 2017;50:527–532.

89. Horne AW, Saunders PTK, Abokhrais IM, et al. Top ten endometriosis research priorities in the UK and Ireland. *Lancet* 2017;389(10085):2191–2192.

90. Petrelluzzi KFS, Garcia MC, Petta CA, et al. Physical therapy and psychological intervention normalize cortisol levels and improve vitality in women with endometriosis. *J Psychosom Obst Gyn* 2012;33(4):191–198.

91. Meissner K, Schweizer-Arau A, Limmer A, et al. Psychotherapy with somatosensory stimulation for endometriosis-associated pain: a randomized controlled trial. *Obstet Gynecol* 2016;128(5):1134–1142.

92. Darai C, Deboute O, Zacharopoulou C, et al. Impact of osteopathic manipulative therapy on quality of life of patients with deep infiltrating endometriosis with colorectal involvement: results of a pilot study. *Eur J Obstet Gynecol Reprod Biol* 2015;188:70–73.

93. Zhao LP, Wu HS, Zhou XH, et al. Effects of progressive muscular relaxation training on anxiety, depression and quality of life of endometriosis patients under gonadotrophin-releasing hormone agonist therapy. *Eur J Obstet Gyn Reprod Biol* 2012;162(2):211–215.

94. Ferenczy A. Pathophysiology of adenomyosis. *Hum Reprod Update* 1998;4:312–322.

95. Dueholm M, Lundorf E. Transvaginal ultrasound or MRI for diagnosis of adenomyosis. *Curr Opin Obstet Gynecol* 2007;19(6):505–512.

96. Bergeron C, Amant F, Ferenczy A. Pathology and pathophysiology of adenomyosis. *Best Prac Res Clin Obstet Gynaecol* 2006;20:511–521.

97. Oliveira MAP, Crispi CP Jr, Brollo LC, et al. Surgery in adenomyosis. *Arch Gynecol Obstet* 2018;297:581–589.

98. de Bruijn AM, Smink M, Lohle PNM, et al. Uterine artery embolization for the treatment of adenomyosis: a systematic review and meta-analysis. *J Vasc Interven Radiol* 2017;28(12):1629–1642.e1.

99. Zhang L, Rao F, Setzen R. High intensity focused ultrasound for the treatment of adenomyosis: selection criteria, efficacy, safety and fertility. *Acta Obstet Gynecol Scand* 2017;96(6):707–714.

100. Urabe M, Yamamoto T, Kitawaki J, et al. Estrogen biosynthesis in human uterine adenomyosis. *Acta Endocrinol* 1989;121(2):259–264.

101. Pontis A, D'Alterio MN, Pirarba S, et al. Adenomyosis: a systematic review of medical treatment. *Gynecol Endocrinol* 2016;32(9):696–700.

102. Peters AAW, Bakkum EA, Hellebrekers BWJ. Clinical significance of adhesions in patients with chronic pelvic pain. In: MacLean A, Stones RW, Thornton S, eds. *Pain in Obstetrics and Gynaecology*. London: Royal College of Obstetricians and Gynaecologists; 2001:214–223.

103. Cheong Y, Saran M, Hounslow JW, et al. Are pelvic adhesions associated with pain, physical, emotional and functional characteristics of women presenting with chronic pelvic pain? A cluster analysis. *BMC Womens Health* 2018;18(1):11.

104. Peters AA, Trimbos-Kemper GC, Admiraal C, et al. A randomized clinical trial on the benefit of adhesiolysis in patients with intraperitoneal adhesions and chronic pelvic pain. *Br J Obstet Gynaecol* 1992;99(1):59–62.

105. van den Beukel BA, de Ree R, van Leuven S, et al. Surgical treatment of adhesion-related chronic abdominal and pelvic pain after gynaecological and general surgery: a systematic review and meta-analysis. *Hum Reprod Update* 2017;23(3):276–288.

106. Swank DJ, Swank-Bordewijk SCG, Hop WCJ, et al. Laparoscopic adhesiolysis in patients with chronic abdominal pain: a blinded randomised controlled multi-centre trial. *Lancet* 2003;361:1247–1251.

107. Timor-Tritsch IE, Lerner JP, Monteagudo A, et al. Transvaginal sonographic markers of tubal inflammatory disease. *Ultrasound Obstet Gynecol* 1998;12(1):56–66.

108. Champaneria R, Shah L, Moss J, et al. The relationship between pelvic vein incompetence and chronic pelvic pain in women: systematic reviews of diagnosis and treatment effectiveness. *Health Technol Assess* 2016;20(5):1–108.

109. Beard RW, Reginald PW, Wadsworth J. Clinical features of women with chronic lower abdominal pain and pelvic congestion. *Br J Obstet Gynaecol* 1988;95:153–161.

110. Gültaþlý NZ, Kurt A, Ýpek A, et al. The relation between pelvic varicose veins, chronic pelvic pain and lower extremity venous insufficiency in women. *Diagn Interv Radiol* 2006;12(1):34–38.

111. Farquhar CM, Rogers V, Franks S, et al. A randomized controlled trial of medroxyprogesterone acetate and psychotherapy for the treatment of pelvic congestion. *Br J Obstet Gynaecol* 1989;96(10):1153–1162.

112. Beard RW, Kennedy RG, Gangar KF, et al. Bilateral oophorectomy and hysterectomy in the treatment of intractable pelvic pain associated with pelvic congestion. *Br J Obstet Gynaecol* 1991;98(10):988–992.

113. Daniels JP, Champaneria R, Shah L, et al. Effectiveness of embolization or sclerotherapy of pelvic veins for reducing chronic pelvic pain: a systematic review. *J Vasc Interven Radiol* 2016;27(10):1478.e8–1486.e8.

114. Whorwell PJ. Abdominal pain. In: MacLean A, Stones RW, Thornton S, eds. *Pain in Obstetrics and Gynaecology*. London: Royal College of Obstetricians and Gynaecologists; 2001:209–213.

115. Houghton LA, Lea R, Jackson N, et al. The menstrual cycle affects rectal sensitivity in patients with irritable bowel syndrome but not healthy volunteers. *Gut* 2002;50:471–474.

116. Palomba S, Orio F, Manguso F, et al. Leuprolide acetate treatment with and without coadministration of tibolone in pre-menopausal women with menstrual cycle-related irritable bowel syndrome. *Fertil Steril* 2005;83(4):1012–1020.

117. Wesselmann U. Pain of urogenital origin. *Pain Clin Updates* 2000;8(5):1–4.

118. Dell JR. Interstitial cystitis/painful bladder syndrome: appropriate diagnosis and management. *J Womens Health* 2007;16(8):1181–1187.

119. Fall M, Baranowski AP, Elneil S, et al. EAU guidelines on chronic pelvic pain. *Eur Urol* 2010;57(1):35–48.

120. Doggweiler R, Whitmore KE, Meijlink JM, et al. A standard for terminology in chronic pelvic pain syndromes: a report from the Chronic Pelvic Pain Working Group of the International Continence Society. *Neurourol Urodyn* 2016;36:984–1008.

121. Hanno P, Burks DA, Clemens JQ, et al. *Diagnosis and Treatment of Interstitial Cystitis/Bladder Pain Syndrome*. Linthicum, MD: American Urological Association; 2014.

122. Sutcliffe S, Colditz GA, Goodman MS, et al. Urological chronic pelvic pain syndrome symptom flares: characterisation of the full range of flares at two sites in the Multidisciplinary Approach to the Study of Chronic Pelvic Pain (MAPP) Research Network. *Brit J Urol* 2014;114(6):916–925.

123. Sutcliffe S, Jemielita T, Lai HH, et al. A case-crossover study of urologic chronic pelvic pain syndrome flare triggers in the MAPP research network [published online ahead of print December 27, 2017]. *J Urol.* doi:10.1016/j.juro.2017.12.050.
124. Gittes RF, Nakamura RM. Female urethral syndrome: a female prostatitis? *West J Med* 1996;164:435–438.
125. King PM, Myers CA, Ling FW, et al. Musculoskeletal factors in chronic pelvic pain. *J Psychosom Obstet Gynaecol* 1991;12:87–98.
126. Prendergast SA, Weiss J. Screening for musculoskeletal causes of pelvic pain. *Clin Obstet Gynecol* 2003;46(4):773–782.
127. Macfarlane TV, Blinkhorn A, Worthington HV, et al. Sex hormonal factors and chronic widespread pain: a population study among women. *Rheumatol* 2002;41(4):454–447.
128. Abbott JA, Jarvis SK, Lyons SD, et al. Botulinum toxin type A for chronic pain and pelvic floor spasm in women—a randomized controlled trial. *Obstet Gynecol* 2006;108(4):915–923.
129. Perry CP, Echeverri JDV. Hernias as a cause of chronic pelvic pain in women. *J Soc Lap Surg* 2006;10:212–215.
130. Cox M, Ng G, Mashriqi F, et al. Innervation of the anterior sacroiliac joint. *World Neurosurg* 2017;107:750–752.
131. Cohen SP. Sacroiliac joint pain: a comprehensive review of anatomy, diagnosis, and treatment. *Anesth Analg* 2005;101(5):1440–1453.
132. Kaya S, Hermans L, Willems T, et al. Central sensitization in urogynecological chronic pelvic pain: a systematic literature review. *Pain Physician* 2013;16(4):291–308.
133. Perry CP. Peripheral neuropathies and pelvic pain: diagnosis and management. *Clin Obstet Gynecol* 2003;46(4):789–796.
134. Moore KL. *Clinically Oriented Anatomy.* 3rd ed. Baltimore, MD: Williams & Wilkins; 1992.
135. Robert R, Prat-Pradal D, Labat JJ, et al. Pudendal nerve entrapment. *Surg Radiol Anat* 1998;20:93–98.
136. Robert R, Labat JJ, Bensignor M, et al. Decompression and transposition of the pudendal nerve in pudendal neuralgia: a randomized controlled trial and long-term evaluation. *Eur Urol* 2005;47(3):403–408.
137. Luijendijk RW, Jeekel J, Storm RK, et al. The low transverse Pfannenstiel incision and the prevalence of incisional hernia and nerve entrapment. *Ann Surg* 1997;225(4):365–369.
138. Whiteside JL, Barber MD, Walters MD, et al. Anatomy of ilioinguinal and iliohypogastric nerves in relation to trocar placement and low transverse incisions. *Am J Obstet Gynecol* 2003;189(6):1574–1578.
139. Butcher J. Female sexual problems II: sexual pain and sexual fears. *BMJ* 1999;318:110–112.
140. Schnyder U, Schnyder-Luthi C, Balinari P, et al. Therapy for vaginismus: In vivo versus in vitro desensitization. *Can J Psych* 1998;43:941–944.
141. Lahaie MA, Boyer SC, Amsel R, et al. Vaginismus: a review of the literature on the classification/diagnosis, etiology and treatment. *Womens Health* 2010;6(5):705–719.
142. Crowley T, Richardson D, Goldmeier D. Recommendations for the management of vaginismus: BASHH Special Interest Group for Sexual Dysfunction. *Int J STD AIDS* 2006;17:14–18.
143. Nunns D. Vulval pain syndromes. *BJOG* 2000;107:1185–1193.
144. Nunns D, Mandal D. Psychological and psychosexual aspects of vulval vestibulitis. *Genitourin Med* 1997;73:541–544.
145. Edwards L, Mason M, Phillips M, et al. Childhood sexual and physical abuse: incidence in patients with vulvodynia. *J Reprod Med* 1997;42:135–139.
146. Haefner HK, Collins ME, Davis GD, et al. The vulvodynia guideline. *J Low Genit Tract Dis* 2005;9(1):40–51.
147. Pukall CF, Strigo IA, Binik YM, et al. Neural correlates of painful genital touch in women with vulvar vestibulitis syndrome. *Pain* 2005;115(1–2):118–127.
148. Hampson JP, Reed BD, Clauw DJ, et al. Augmented central pain processing in vulvodynia. *J Pain* 2013;14(6):579–589.
149. van Beekhuizen HJ, Oost J, van der Meijden WI. Generalized unprovoked vulvodynia: a retrospective study on the efficacy of treatment with amitriptyline, gabapentin or pregabalin. *Eur J Obstet Gynecol Reprod Biol* 2018;220:118–121.
150. Munday PE. Response to treatment in dysaesthetic vulvodynia. *J Obstet Gynaecol* 2001;6:610–613.
151. Meltzer-Brody SE, Zolnoun D, Steege JF, et al. Open-label trial of lamotrigine focusing on efficacy in vulvodynia. *J Reprod Med* 2009;54(3): 171–178.
152. Boardman LA, Cooper AS, Blais LR, et al. Topical gabapentin in the treatment of localized and generalized vulvodynia. *Obstet Gynecol* 2008;112(3): 579–585.
153. Hartmann EH, Nelson C. The perceived effectiveness of physical therapy treatment on women complaining of chronic vulvar pain and diagnosed with either vulvar vestibulitis syndrome or dysesthetic vulvodynia. *J Womens Health* 2001;25:13–18.
154. Grace VM. Mind/body dualism in medicine: The case of chronic pelvic pain without organic pathology: a critical review of the literature. *Int J Health Serv* 1998;28(1):127–151.
155. Grace VM. Chronic pelvic pain: sociocultural perspectives. In: MacLean A, Stones RW, Thornton S, eds. *Pain in Obstetrics and Gynaecology.* London: Royal College of Obstetricians and Gynaecologists; 2001:12–25.
156. Chen I, Money D, Yong P, et al. An evaluation model for a multidisciplinary chronic pelvic pain clinic: application of the re-aim framework. *J Obstet Gynaecol Can* 2015;37(9):804–809.
157. Kolte AM, Bernardi LA, Christiansen OB, et al. Terminology for pregnancy loss prior to viability: a consensus statement from the ESHRE early pregnancy special interest group. *Hum Reprod* 2015;30(3):495–498.
158. Joint Formulary Committee. *British National Formulary 74.* London: BMJ Publishing Group, Royal Pharmaceutical Society; 2017.
159. Davis L, Kennedy SS, Moore J, et al. Modern combined oral contraceptives for pain associated with endometriosis. *Cochrane Database Syst Rev* 2007;(3):CD001019.
160. Selak V, Farquhar C, Prentice A, et al. Danazol for pelvic pain associated with endometriosis. *Cochrane Database Syst Rev* 2007;(4):CD00068.
161. Prentice A, Deary AJ, Bland E. Progestagens and anti-progestagens for pain associated with endometriosis. *Cochrane Database Syst Rev* 2000; (2):CD002122.
162. Lockhat FB, Emembolu JO, Konje JC. The efficacy, side-effects and continuation rates in women with symptomatic endometriosis undergoing treatment with an intra-uterine administered progestogen (levonorgestrel): a 3 year follow-up. *Hum Reprod* 2005;20(3):789–793.
163. Taylor HS, Giudice LC, Lessey BA, et al. Treatment of endometriosis-associated pain with elagolix, an oral GnRH antagonist. *N Engl J Med* 2017;377:28–40.

CHAPTER 65

Pelvic Pain in Males

ANDREW BARANOWSKI

This chapter is about pain *perceived* to be in the male pelvis—the pelvic pain syndromes. For the purpose of this chapter, the pelvis is considered as the anatomical bony pelvis and the structures both within and adjacent to it, including the male external genitalia, nervous system structures, and soft tissue/muscular structures, that is, the pelvis in its broadest sense. Although this chapter focuses primarily on the male urogenital pelvic pain syndromes, the importance of other systems, particularly the musculoskeletal, nervous, and other viscera, is emphasized when appropriate.

There are many well-recognized, well-defined pathologies that may result in pain perceived within the male urogenital system, such as infections of the organs; infiltration of somatic, visceral, and nervous tissue by cancer; and referred sensations from the musculoskeletal system. However, for less defined pathologies, the mechanisms underlying the pains have been less widely appreciated outside of pain medicine. The mechanisms for this second group, which is probably the majority of male pelvic pain patients, involve neurologic mechanisms—in particular, central sensitization that may involve the whole neuraxis. These are the primary chronic pain syndromes.

The latest classification approaches have taken this dichotomy of mechanisms into account. To emphasize the differences, those conditions where the main mechanisms are related to central sensitization are known as the pelvic pain syndromes, and they are considered separately from those conditions with ongoing nociceptive, acute pain mechanisms, such as those due to chronic infection. Pelvic pain syndromes are defined by their symptoms and signs and typically by the presence of sensitization, including visceral hypersensitivity, viscerovisceral hypersensitivity (i.e., cross-organ sensitization), and viscerosomatic hypersensitivity (e.g., expanded area of referred sensation and/or increased sensitivity to palpation). Often, an important part of the process of diagnosing the pelvic pain syndromes is excluding other pathologies.

Classification of the pelvic pain syndromes involves terminology, phenotyping, and taxonomy. The phenotype describes the condition in terms of symptoms, signs, and, where possible, mechanisms. Incorporating the phenotype into a hierarchy of phenotypes produces a taxonomy that allows comparisons between phenotypes. This approach enables appropriate prognosis and treatment. The terminology used can be very emotive, and careful description of the meaning of the terms is often required. The classification of pelvic urogenital pain has been rapidly evolving over the past 15 years and is likely to continue to do so.[1-9] This ongoing change in classification not only reflects our increasing knowledge but also has caused problems for research and evidence-based treatment. The classification will be covered in depth as it is the key to understanding male pelvic pain syndromes.

The central nervous system mechanisms of central sensitization and the psychological responses that result in the chronic pain syndrome are covered in other chapters within this book; those processes that are specific to urogenital pain are expanded on in this chapter. There are some obvious differences between the male and female urogenital systems that will result in specific pain syndromes; however, it is important to recognize that there is much overlap as well. Those differences due to gender and sex are covered in Chapter 7.

This chapter supports that in most men with chronic pain perceived in the pelvic organs, the cause of the pain is not often due to classical pathologies of infection or infiltration but more commonly due to chronic pain mechanisms involving a number of systems with referred pain, sensory and functional consequences (e.g., urinary and fecal incontinence, urge and urgency, urinary hesitance, impotence), and chronic pain psychological responses.[8]

Taxonomy and Phenotyping Chronic Pelvic Pain

A realization has occurred that pain *perceived* within the pelvis may be associated with classical pathology of the pelvic structures *or* that it may result secondary to central nervous system pain mechanisms. It is the latter conditions that this chapter primarily concentrates on.

CLASSICAL PATHOLOGIES

Classical pathologies include infection, inflammation, degeneration, neoplastic, and autoimmune mechanisms of any of the pelvic or adjacent pelvic structures (referred pain). In the case of classical pathology, chronic persistent pain is the result of ongoing local pathology, persistent nociceptor activation with peripheral sensitization, and possibly a central sensitization process. Treatment will primarily be focused on managing the underlying pathology and the use of analgesics where required. Removing the peripheral cause should resolve the pain.

PELVIC PAIN SYNDROMES AND NONPELVIC PAIN SYNDROMES

Most of the recent attempts at classification, taxonomy, and phenotyping have tried to separate out the classical pathologies from those conditions without classical pathology that have become known as the pelvic pain syndromes.[3,7,10] The pelvic pain syndromes are the conditions where there is no peripheral pathology maintaining the pain experience (peripheral stimuli may however maintain the central sensitization). In its attempt to separate out the pelvic pain syndromes from those with a nociceptive cause, the European Association of Urology (EAU) in their 2004 classification system called those conditions associated with classical pathology as "well-defined" conditions and the European Society for the Study of Interstitial Cystitis (ESSIC) called them "confusable diseases."[3,10] Both of those terms have a disadvantage. The term *well-defined* suggests that the pain syndromes are poorly defined; however, as an understanding of chronic pain mechanisms (including visceral pain mechanisms) and central sensitization develops, this is clearly not the case. ESSIC used the term *confusable* to separate out the pain syndromes from those conditions that they might be confused with, a very difficult concept. In future classifications, one way forward is that chronic pelvic urogenital pain syndromes will become a differential diagnosis with the classical pathologies, and the taxonomy will be divided into pelvic pain syndromes and nonpelvic pain syndromes.[11] The World Health Authority working with the International Association for Pain in ICD11 is using the term primary chronic pain. The emphasis is thus on the pelvic pain syndromes, which is probably correct as in most individuals classical disease processes are not present. Table 65.1 illustrates the division of

TABLE 65.1 The Division of Chronic Pelvic Pain into Pelvic Pain Syndromes and Nonpelvic Pain Syndromes

Axis I Region	Axis II System	Axis III End Organ as Pain Syndrome as Identified from Hx, Ex, and Ix	Axis IV Referral Characteristics	Axis V Temporal Characteristics	Axis VI Character	Axis VII Associated Symptoms	Axis VIII Psychological Symptoms
Chronic pelvic pain	Urologic	Pelvic pain syndrome Bladder pain syndrome Urethral pain syndrome Prostate pain syndrome Scrotal pain syndrome Penile pain syndrome (See Table 65.2 on ESSIC classification) Type A inflammatory Type B noninflammatory Testicular pain syndrome Epididymal pain syndrome Postvasectomy pain syndrome	Suprapubic Inguinal Urethral Penile/clitoral Perineal Rectal Back Buttocks	ONSET Acute Chronic ONGOING Sporadic Cyclical Continuous TIME Filling Emptying Immediate post Late post PROVOKED	Aching Burning Stabbing Electric Other	URINARY Frequency Nocturia Hesitance Poor flow Pis en deux Urge Urgency Incontinence Other GYNECOLOGIC, for example, menstrual SEXUAL, for example, female dyspareunia impotence, anorectal, incontinence, constipation MUSCULAR, for example, hyperalgesia, dysfunction CUTANEOUS, for example, allodynia	Cognitive Behavioral Emotional
	Gynecologic	Vaginal pain syndrome Vulvar pain syndrome Generalized vulvar pain syndrome Localized vulvar pain syndrome Vestibular pain syndrome Clitoral pain syndrome					
		Other	Endometriosis associated pain syndrome				
	Anorectal Neurologic Muscular	Anorectal pain syndrome Pudendal pain syndrome Pelvic floor muscle pain syndrome					
Nonpelvic pain syndromes	Neurologic Urologic	Pudendal neuralgia					

From Fall M, Baranowski AP, Elneil S, et al. Guidelines on chronic pelvic pain. Paper presented at: 23rd European Association of Urology Annual Congress; March 2008; Milan, Italy.

TABLE 65.2 Definitions of Pelvic Pain
• *Chronic pelvic pain* is nonmalignant pain perceived in structures related to the pelvis of either men or women. In the case of documented nociceptive pain that becomes chronic, the pain must have been continuous or recurrent for at least 6 months. If nonacute pain mechanisms and central sensitization mechanisms are well documented, then the pain may be regarded as chronic, irrespective of the time period. In all cases, there often are associated negative cognitive, behavioral, sexual, and emotional consequences.[3,11] • *Pelvic pain syndrome* is the occurrence of persistent or recurrent episodic pelvic pain associated with symptoms suggestive of lower urinary tract, sexual, bowel, or gynecologic dysfunction. There is no proven infection or other obvious pathology.[3,11]

TABLE 65.3 Phenotype Classification of the Male Pelvic Urogenital Pain Syndromes
• *Penile pain syndrome* is the occurrence of pain within the penis that is not primarily in the urethra, with the absence of proven infection or other obvious pathology.[3,11] • *Prostate pain syndrome* is the occurrence of persistent or recurrent episodic prostate pain, which is associated with symptoms suggestive of urinary tract and/or sexual dysfunction. There is no proven infection or other obvious pathology.[3,11] (This definition of prostate pain syndrome was adapted from the National Institutes of Health [NIH] consensus definition and classification of prostatitis[4] and includes those conditions that they term *chronic pelvic pain syndrome*. Using their classification system, prostate pain syndrome may be further subdivided into type A, inflammatory, and type B, noninflammatory.) • *Scrotal pain syndrome* is the occurrence of persistent or recurrent episodic scrotal pain that is associated with symptoms suggestive of urinary tract or sexual dysfunction. There is no proven epididymo-orchitis or other obvious pathology.[3,11] • *Testicular pain syndrome* is the occurrence of persistent or recurrent episodic pain localized to the testis on examination that is associated with symptoms suggestive of urinary tract or sexual dysfunction. There is no proven epididymoorchitis or other obvious pathology. (This is a more specific definition than scrotal pain syndrome.)[3,11] • *Postvasectomy pain syndrome* is a scrotal pain syndrome that follows vasectomy.[3,11] • *Epididymal pain syndrome* is the occurrence of persistent or recurrent episodic pain localized to the epididymis on examination that is associated with symptoms suggestive of urinary tract or sexual dysfunction. There is no proven epididymoorchitis or other obvious pathology (more specific definition than scrotal pain syndrome).[3,11]

chronic pelvic pain into pain syndromes and nonpelvic pain syndromes. Table 65.2 provides the definitions for chronic pelvic pain and the pelvic pain syndromes. The latest World Health Organization *International Classification of Diseases*, 11th Revision, recognizes pain as a condition in its own right, although uses some outdated terminology. The International Continence Society has tried by working with other published guidelines to achieve international consensus. However, their "Standard for Terminology" did not have any pain medicine representation and reverted to older terminology in places.[12] It will take a lot more time for consensus to be reached.

This chapter uses the EAU and International Association for the Study of Pain (IASP) accepted classifications, which the author was involved in.

Male Urogenital Pain Syndromes

Traditionally, pelvic pain conditions would be classified into those of the male, female, or both. This approach is currently being reconsidered, as the mechanisms discussed earlier may be common to both sexes with the only difference being the sex organ that the pain is perceived in. However, as there has been a lot of research looking at the end-organ pain syndromes and their treatment, this is summarized in the following text as relevant for the male.

MALE-SPECIFIC PELVIC PAIN SYNDROMES

The unique male pelvic pain syndromes are those where the pain is *perceived* in the male sex organs. Table 65.3 summarizes these conditions. The definitions serve to emphasize that classical pathologies are absent.

SUBCLASSIFICATION OF THE PELVIC PAIN SYNDROMES BY ORGAN

Much discussion has been had about whether it is appropriate to divide the pelvic pain syndromes by the end organ that the pain is perceived in. Many would rather maintain a more generic approach and keep to the term *pelvic pain syndrome* to cover all pains perceived within the pelvis and not associated with a classical pathology. The EAU approach (see Table 65.1) uses a progressive step-by-step approach to classification.[3,11] That is, classification starts at the left end of the table if pain is perceived within the pelvis or the external sex organs. Further subclassification only occurs if there are distinct localizing factors within an end organ. Such an approach to taxonomy is very similar to that used to classify life and the animal and plant kingdoms. For instance, we would progress from animal to mammal to elephant only as the evidence allowed. The primary localizing factor for pelvic pain is pain produced by local physical stimulation, such as palpation. If an end organ is clearly associated with the area of perceived pain, then the pain may be labeled with that end organ name as in Table 65.1.

If more than one organ is deemed to be involved, then either two names may be given to the condition, or it may be more appropriate to consider the pain in more generic terms as a pelvic pain syndrome.

THE IMPORTANCE OF TAXONOMY AND PHENOTYPING

The mentioned taxonomy (hierarchical classification of conditions) and phenotyping (identifying of the physical characteristics—symptoms and signs—and mechanisms of the diseases within the taxonomy) is important.

Appropriate taxonomy and phenotyping is a prerequisite for epidemiology, diagnosis, management, and prognosis. With traditional management of pelvic pain, there has been a tendency to use inappropriate treatments with inappropriate expectations; the result is increased distress and a worse prognosis.[8]

Currently, it is not unusual for inappropriate treatments to be instigated due to a failure to understand the pain syndromes.[1] For example, classic mismanagement would be the recurrent use of antibiotics or the use of surgery for the complaint of pain. Whereas surgery may have a role for functional reasons (e.g., incontinence), there is a serious debate about its use for pain management. Appropriate taxonomy and phenotyping allows appropriate expectation of both the patient and those providing medical care. Unfortunately, many patients and doctors have inappropriate expectations for treatments aimed at cure. This produces distress, and the increased distress is associated with a worse prognosis.[13,14]

An appropriate taxonomy and phenotyping encourages interdisciplinary and multidisciplinary management. In the case of most pelvic pain syndromes, where there may be a reduction in symptoms with appropriate treatment, cure is often not possible. The best outcomes in terms of reduced disability and improved quality of life will come from a symptom management approach involving multiple interdisciplinary teams (e.g., urology, pain medicine, neurology) and multiple members of the team (e.g., nurses, doctors, psychologists, physiotherapists). This is a standard approach for other pain syndromes and should be the standard approach for the urogenital/pelvic pain syndromes.

Epidemiology

Epidemiology requires a clear understanding of the disease that is being studied. Unfortunately, as the phenotyping and taxonomy of male pelvic pain is ongoing, clear-cut epidemiologic data for specific pelvic urogenital pain syndromes are not available.

INCIDENCE/PREVALENCE
Prostate Pain Syndrome
Male pain perceived deep within the pelvis is usually labeled as prostatitis despite the absence of infection and, frequently, the absence of inflammation within fluids extracted from the prostate. The National Institutes of Health (NIH) classification[4] of "prostatitis" includes pain perceived in the prostate without evidence of inflammation or infection and has reinforced this misnomer. Therefore, most of the data relating to pain perceived within the prostate stems from the "prostatitis" literature. As well as pain, these patients often have urinary urge (constant need to void as a result of a sensory disturbance), frequency (secondary to the urge), hesitancy, and poor flow, but they do not have urgency (need to void because of a fear of incontinence).

Several studies have looked at the demographic distribution of the disease. Prostatitis appears to be more common in men younger than 50 years of age, although there may be a second cohort aged greater than 74 years.[15-17] The Nickel et al.[16] study identified 9.7% of men as having "chronic prostatitis-like" symptoms as defined by the NIH-Chronic Prostatitis Symptom Index. This index includes urinary "irritative" and "obstructive" symptoms as well as measures of quality of life as these are frequently disrupted.[18]

Scrotal Pain Syndrome
Testicular pain in isolation and without obvious cause is well defined as an example of chronic visceral pain. It is essential to rule out pain referred to the testis, such as from an adductor enthesitis or from the spine. Thoracic pathology with or without involvement of the nerve roots may also produce pain perceived in the testis.

Despite being well defined, the testicular pain syndrome is poorly researched and information about its incidence is scanty. The majority of the information stems from postvasectomy surgery,[19] where the incidence may be as high as 19% following this operation. Once more, the problem appears to be more frequent in younger men.[20-23] In a large cohort study of 625 postvasectomy men, the likelihood of scrotal pain after 6 months was 14.7%. The mean pain severity on a VAS score was 3.4/10. In the pain group, 0.9% had quite severe pain, noticeably affecting their daily life. In this cohort, different techniques were used to perform the vasectomy. The risk of postvasectomy pain was significantly lower in the no-scalpel vasectomy group (11.7% vs. the scalpel group 18.8%).[24]

Penile Pain Syndrome
There are very few data on this condition, which also appears to be unusual in the pain clinic. The condition must not be confused with the penile pain of pudendal neuralgia or pain sensation referred from the bladder or urethra. This condition is also quite different from the psychiatric obsession associated with the sex organs that can occur in certain patients. A painful penis without obvious cause has been seen to follow circumcision and may represent a central sensitization process.

PRECIPITATING FACTORS
Very little is known about the factors that predispose men to urogenital pain syndromes.[25,26] In certain, but probably only a small proportion of, cases, some form of trauma or infection may be the precipitating factor.[27] Surgical trauma in the form of vasectomy may result in testicular pain.[28] Recurrent minor injury may be a predisposing factor, as for any pain syndrome.

The role of the pudendal nerve is disputed by different experts in the field. There is no doubt that pudendal neuralgia (pain associated with pudendal nerve damage) exists.[29] The mechanism(s) presumably will be the same as for all nerves, and the pain would be perceived in the appropriate dermatome. Depending on the site of damage, the pain may be perceived in the anus, perineum, deeper within the pelvis, the bladder base, or the penis.[30] Whether the sexual function and the central sensitization of the sexual process imparts any specific properties on the damaged pudendal nerve is not known. As may be expected, the nerve damage may be associated with a range of sensory abnormalities such as dysesthesia, allodynia, or numbness. The pudendal nerve is suggested to be at risk from recurrent injuries (such as cycling or long hours of sitting) and from acute trauma, including surgical interventions, such as for cancer or orthopedics.[31-34] Sitting while working at a computer appears to be a predisposing factor among young men (personal observation).

The role of the musculature is also highly debated.[28,35-41] In general, it is now well accepted that the pelvic muscles (including the core muscles of the abdomen and spine) may be involved in the pelvic pain syndromes and that these muscles are subject to the same causes as any other muscle. Trauma, as during sports injury, birth injury for women, and accidents, may produce a muscle-based pain. A report from the Chronic "Prostatitis Cohort Study" showed that 51% of patients with "prostatitis" and only 7% of controls had any muscle tenderness. Tenderness in the pelvic floor muscles was only found in the chronic pelvic pain group.[42]

Stress is said to be responsible for pelvic muscle tension and hence pain in certain cases, although it must be appreciated that chronic pain will also be associated with psychological responses and even psychiatric disorders.[43-45]

The role of negative sexual encounters (NSE) continues to be disputed.[46,47] The prevalence of childhood male sexual abuse may be as high as 16% in some countries; in the United Kingdom, it has been estimated as 5%. Three percent of male adults may also have had an NSE. Victims of torture are frequently subjected to sexual abuse. What is not clear is the relationship of this abuse to male urogenital pain syndromes. In our editorial,[8] it was suggested that there is little sound evidence to support NSEs as a cause of chronic urogenital pain in patients. However, there is no doubt that in a patient who has suffered an NSE, that incident may require management in its own right.

There are now several articles that indicate that the psychological status of the patient is relevant to the pelvic pain experience. Patients exhibiting high distress associated with catastrophizing and poor coping strategies do less well.[48-51]

Mechanisms

DIFFERENCES BETWEEN VISCERAL AND NONVISCERAL SOMATIC PAINS
In a proportion of patients with pain perceived to be in the pelvis, ongoing classical visceral pain mechanisms may be involved. A number of these mechanisms are listed in Table 65.4 and compared to somatic pain mechanisms. In certain patients with persistent pelvic pain, chronic central sensitization mechanisms are predominant.

TABLE 65.4	Differences between Visceral and Nonvisceral Somatic Pains	
	Visceral Pain Mechanism	**Nonvisceral Somatic Pain Mechanisms**
Effective painful stimuli	Stretching, distension, ischemia, inflammation, producing poorly localized pain	Mechanical, thermal, chemical, and electrical stimuli, producing well localized pain
Summation	Widespread stimulation produces a significantly magnified pain	Widespread stimulation produces a modest increase in pain
Autonomic involvement	Autonomic features (e.g., nausea and sweating) frequently present	Autonomic features less frequent
Referred pain	Pain perceived at a site distant to the cause of the pain is common.	Pain is well localized.
Referred hypersensitivity	Referred cutaneous and muscle hypersensitivity is common as is involvement of other viscera. **This is very important.**	Hypersensitivity tends to be localized.
Innervation	Low-density, unmyelinated C fibers, and thinly myelinated Aδ	Dense innervation with a wide range of nerve fibers
Primary afferent physiology	Intensity coding. As stimulation increases, afferent firing increases with an increase in sensation and ultimately pain.	Two fiber coding; there are separate well-defined peripheral nerves for nociceptive pain and normal sensation. For pain to be perceived, under normal circumstances without central sensitization, the smaller C and Aδ-associated nociceptors have to be activated.
Silent afferents[a,b]	Approximately 20% of visceral afferents are silent until the time they are switched on. These fibers are very important in the central sensitization process.	Similar to viscera with around 20% of afferents being silent
Central mechanisms	Play an important part in the viscerovisceral, visceromuscular, and musculovisceral hypersensitivities. Sensations not normally perceived become perceived and nonnoxious sensations become painful.	Responsible for the allodynia and hyperalgesia of chronic somatic pain
Abnormalities of function	Central mechanisms associated with visceral pain may be responsible for organ dysfunction.	Somatic pain associated with somatic dysfunction
Central pathways and representation	As well as classical pathways, there is evidence for a separate dorsal horn pathway and central representation.	Classical pain pathways

[a]From Feng B, Gebhart GF. Characterization of silent afferents in the pelvic and splanchnic innervations of the mouse colorectum. *Am J Physiol* 2011;300:G170–G180.
[b]From Gebhart GF, Bielefeldt K. Physiology of visceral pain. *Comprehensive Physiol* 2016;6:1609–1633.

PERIPHERAL MECHANISMS[52–55]

Sensitization of visceral afferents and activation of silent afferents by endogenous mediators, including nerve growth factor (NGF), is considered pivotal for the development of visceral pain. NGF is able to both directly activate primary afferents and indirectly activate them (such as through the regulation of the expression of bradykinin).[56] Multiple tachykinins are implicated in both the normal control of bladder contraction and in the heightened stimulation and sensitization of the afferent loop of the micturition reflex after inflammation. Similar mechanisms are known for the other organs. Adenosine triphosphate released from hollow organs, such as when the bladder is distended, acts on purinergic P2X3 receptors found on visceral afferents and on small-diameter dorsal root ganglion (DRG) neurons. Once more, these mechanisms may be involved in normal function as well as pain. Voltage-gated ion channels (tetrodotoxin resistant sodium channel, NaV1.8) are also implicated in the visceral pain states.

CENTRAL MECHANISMS[57–61]

In visceral pain, excitatory amino-acid receptors such as N-methyl-D-aspartate (NMDA) and α-amino-3-hydroxy-5-methyl-4-isoxazolepropionic acid (AMPA) play a vital role in the production of viscerovisceral, musculovisceral, and visceromuscular hypersensitivity. Both clinical studies and basic science support that central mechanisms activated as a result of an insult in one organ can result in nonnoxious sensations being perceived and noxious sensations becoming more painful both in the same organ and in different organs and the muscles. Such mechanisms explain why many patients have multiple end organ sensitivities. For example, patients with the bladder pain syndrome may also have muscle trigger points and anorectal sensitivity (e.g., irritable bowel syndrome). Once triggered, the changes in the central nervous system can persist for great lengths of time.

MUSCLES AND PELVIC PAIN

As with any pain syndrome, muscle tenderness and trigger points may be implicated as a source of pain in the urogenital pain syndromes. Central mechanisms are of great importance in the pathogenesis of these muscle hypersensitivities. The muscles involved may form a part of the spinal, abdominal, or pelvic complex of muscles. It is not unknown for adjacent muscles of the lower limbs and the thorax to become involved. Pain may be well localized to the trigger points but is more often associated with classical referral patterns. As well as trigger points, inflammation of the attachments to the bones (enthesitis) and of the bursa (bursitis) may be found.[41,62–64]

Numerous events have been suggested as causative factors. A local infection, such as a bladder infection, may produce local muscle spasm and subsequent muscle-associated pain. Renal stones are clearly associated with spinal muscle hyperalgesia.[65] The onset of pain may be due to some form of minor strain or may be associated with a more obvious injury, such as those associated with sports.[66] Certain postures will affect the different muscles in different ways and, consequently, may either exacerbate the pain or reduce it. Stress has been implicated as being both an initiator of pelvic myalgia and as a maintenance factor; as a consequence, NSE may also have a precipitating effect.[47]

Pelvic Muscle Pain Syndromes[67,68]

The following are some examples of pelvic muscle pain syndromes.

Piriformis[69,70]

This muscle originates from the anterior part of the sacrum and inserts onto the greater trochanter. The muscle produces external rotation of the leg. It starts within the pelvis, leaving it by the greater sciatic foramen. It is the relationship of the piriformis at this level to the nerves that allows the possibility of nerve irritation by the piriformis (see the following text). Pain associated with this muscle refers to the buttock and is worse on passive internal rotation or active external rotation against resistance. Trigger points are usually identified at the level of the greater sciatic foramen.

Obturator Internus[71,72]

This muscle arises from the inner surface of the anterolateral wall of the pelvis, where it covers the majority of the foramen ovale and is attached to the obturator membrane, the inferior rami of the pubis, and the ischium. It leaves the pelvis via the lesser sciatic notch to attach to the greater trochanter. It may develop trigger points deep in its body (detected by internal pelvic examination) or in its external part. Pain may refer anteriorly, deep within the pelvis, and to the genitalia and/or posteriorly to the rectum and buttocks. Bursitis may occur as the muscle passes out of the pelvis and around the ischium. This muscle may be associated with pudendal nerve irritation (see following text).

Levator Ani[73]

The levator ani is inserted into the inner surface of the anatomical lesser pelvis and is composed of three parts—iliococcygeus, puborectalis, and pubococcygeus. The muscles form a sling with fibers uniting in the midline and blending with the sphincters of the pelvic organs (Fig. 65.1). Trigger points produce a range of referral patterns from the anus to the penis and into the testis. It has been suggested that levator plate hypersensitivity, trigger points, and referred pain are responsible for the prostate pain syndrome.[38,74]

The relationship of these muscles to the pelvic organs results in a wide range of other symptoms, such as urinary urge with associated frequency. Pain may be exacerbated by use of the muscles, such as during intercourse, ejaculation, voiding of urine, and defecation.

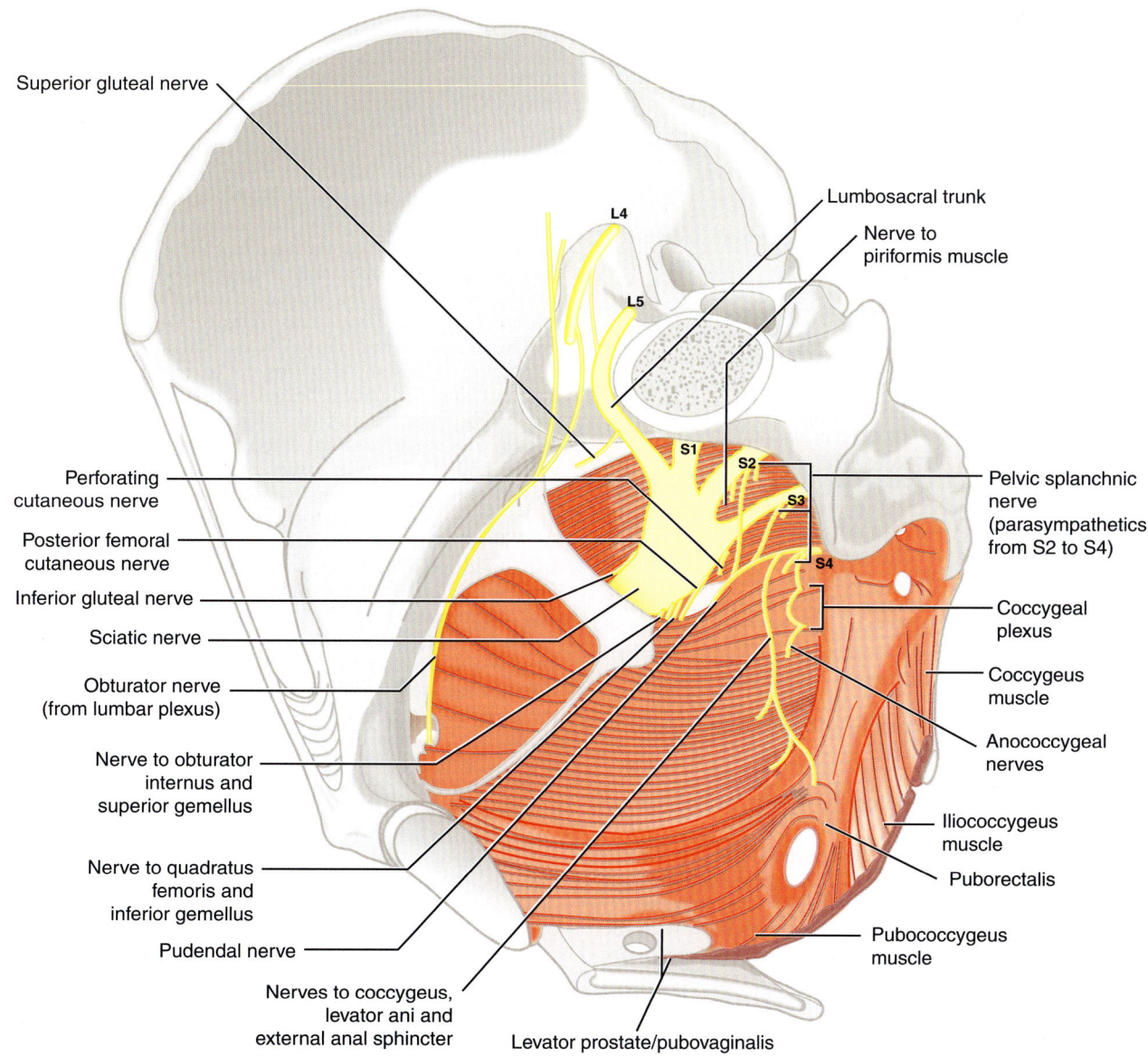

FIGURE 65.1 Male pelvic anatomy.

Coccygeus[38]

The coccygeus originates from the spine of the ischium and inserts into the coccyx.

Psoas[75]

The psoas originates from the transverse process of the lumbar vertebrae; leaving the pelvis below the inguinal ligament, it inserts into the lesser trochanter of the femur. Pain can refer to the back, pelvis, and groin.

Spinal and Abdominal Muscle Pain Syndromes

The spinal and abdominal muscle pain syndromes often have a close relationship with the pelvic muscle pain syndromes. Muscle pains may be seen to spread from the site of the original pain (either the pelvis or the spinal/abdominal muscles) to involve adjacent muscles. Sometimes, this progression may be picked up from the history; in other patients, it may be impossible to separate out the history around what appears to be total body pain. Kinesophobia and subsequent immobility are predisposing factors to the spread of muscle pain.[76,77] Stress and tension are also negative prognostic factors. The thoracolumbar junction is an important source of referred pain to the buttocks, hips, groin, and testicles.[78]

As in the pelvic muscle pain syndromes, spasm of the abdominal and spinal musculature may be associated with local nerve irritation, such as the genitofemoral nerve with psoas spasm and the anterior cutaneous branches of the intercostals nerves as they transgress the rectus abdominis. Disease at the thoracolumbar junction may result in L1 and/or T12 root irritation and, consequently, pain perceived in the groin and testicles.

PELVIC NERVES AND PAIN

It is well established that nerve injury may be associated with a range of symptoms that include dysesthesia, allodynia, hyperalgesia, and constant or intermittent pain. The mechanisms are well established (see other chapters in this book). In some cases, the onset of pain is clearly associated with the nerve damage. However, in many cases, arriving at the diagnosis of peripheral nerve injury generated pain can be difficult. This is particularly so for the urogenital pains:

1. Due to the difficulty in identifying the nerves and examining their relevant dermatomes
2. Pelvic dermatomes overlap widely, and consequently, signs of nerve injury are difficult to identify.
3. Many pelvic nerves are primarily sensory or autonomic, and as a result, there is little somatic motor data available to aid the diagnosis of nerve damage.
4. Even when there are motor fibers present, significant nerve damage has to be present for there to be abnormal neurophysiology, and the muscles are difficult to access.
5. Referred sensations (including cutaneous dysesthesia, allodynia, and hyperalgesias) from the muscle hypersensitivities, tendonitis, and enthesitis are common and frequently confuse the picture.

Peripheral Nerve Pain Syndromes

Nerves and the Male Genitalia

The afferents from the skin of the male genitals pass via a complex of multiple sensory nerves, and this makes the diagnosis of nerve injury as a cause of pain difficult. The anterolateral part of the scrotum has afferents primarily associated with the genitofemoral nerve; there is some possible involvement of the ilioinguinal and iliohypogastric nerves. The posterior scrotal branches of the pudendal nerve transmit sensation from the posterior scrotum. The penis shaft is innervated on its dorsal surface by the genitofemoral, ilioinguinal, and iliohypogastric nerves and the ventral surface by the perineal branches of the posterior femoral cutaneous nerve and cutaneous branches of the pudendal nerve. The glans penis is associated with the dorsal nerve of the penis, the terminal branch of the pudendal nerve. All the nerves that are associated with the scrotum may also receive afferents from the testis, although classically, the nerves from the testis are usually associated with the genito-femoral nerve. The superficial branches of the pudendal superficial perineal nerve and the perineal branch of the posterior femoral cutaneous nerve receive afferents from the perineal skin. Deeper afferents from the perineum and from some of the pelvic organs pass to the pudendal nerve via its deep perineal branch.

The course of the afferents from the pelvic organs is well described in most anatomy books, as are the sources of innervation. For the aims of this chapter, the involvement of the pudendal nerve must be emphasized. It must also be recognized that the pelvic plexus is both associated with the parasympathetic and sympathetic nerves and that, as well as efferents associated with these pathways, afferents may travel back to both the sacral roots and the thoracolumbar roots with these autonomic nerves. Sites for injury and for possible intervention may thus include the ganglion impar, superior hypogastric plexus, inferior hypogastric plexus, and lumbar sympathetic trunk as well as more central spinal root areas.

Pain Arising from Damage to the Anterior Groin Nerves

The iliohypogastric nerve arises from L1, and its anterior branch supplies the skin above the pubis where its lateral cutaneous branch is distributed to the anterolateral part of the buttock. Nerve damage may be associated with surgical trauma during operations on the groin or loin. More proximal lesions are rare but should be considered as they may represent sepsis or neoplastic infiltration.

The ilioinguinal nerve is smaller than the iliohypogastric nerve; arising from L1, it is distributed to the skin of the groin and mons pubis. Nerve damage may be associated with surgical trauma during operations on the groin or loin. More proximal lesions are rare but should be considered as they may also represent sepsis or neoplastic infiltration.

The genitofemoral nerve arises from L1 and L2. It passes through the psoas and then down it to emerge through the deep inguinal ring. Its genital branch supplies the cremaster and a part of the anterior and lateral scrotum. The femoral branch passes close to the external iliac artery, the deep circumflex iliac artery, and the femoral artery to be distributed to the upper part of the femoral triangle. As the two branches of the genitofemoral nerve may separate at any level, sensory phenomena associated with nerve damage will depend on the level of the lesion and individual variability. Genitofemoral neuralgia may suggest a vascular aneurysm, local sepsis, or be associated with loin or groin surgery.

The lateral cutaneous nerve of the thigh arises from L2 and L3 and passes to eventually leave the abdomen behind or through the inguinal ligament at a variable distance medial to the anterior superior iliac spine. In the thigh, it divides into an anterior branch that supplies the anterolateral skin of the thigh, approximately 10 cm down from the inguinal ligament to the knee. The posterior branch supplies the skin more laterally from the greater trochanter, down to midthigh.

Obturator nerves L2, L3, and L4 descend through the psoas, around the pelvis closely approximated to the obturator internus muscle and obturator vessels to leave the pelvis via the obturator foramen. This nerve has significant motor innervation; its cutaneous branch is distributed primarily to the inner thigh.

Pain Arising from Damage to the Posterior Triangle Nerves

The posterior triangle area is the area defined by the upper border of the piriformis superiorly; the lower border of quadratus femoris inferiorly; the greater trochanter laterally; and the lateral border of the sacrum, lateral border of the sacrotuberal ligament, and lateral border of the ischial tuberosity medially. It is in this region that the sciatic nerve, the posterior femoral cutaneous nerve (which branches into the posterior cutaneous perineal branch as well as the cluneal nerves), the nerve to obturator internus muscle, and the pudendal nerve can be found; they pass deep to the piriformis and superficial to the superior gemellus and obturator internus muscles.

The pudendal nerve has its roots at the S2, S3, and S4 levels. It has three main branches: the inferior anal/rectal nerve; the superficial perineal nerve (which terminates as cutaneous branches in the perineum and posterior aspect of the scrotum); and the deep perineal nerve, which is distributed to the pelvic structures (possibly innervating parts of the bladder, prostate, and urethra) and terminates as the dorsal nerve of the penis, innervating the glans penis. It has been suggested that the pudendal nerve may be damaged at the level of the piriformis muscle, the sacrospinal ligament, or within Alcock's canal, medial to the obturator internus muscle. The site of injury will determine the site of perceived pain and the nature of associated symptoms (e.g., the more distal the damage, the less likely the anal region will be involved). There is also a school of thought that suggests that the fine nerve endings of the pudendal may become trapped in the muscle planes producing neuropathic pain, possibly with mechanisms similar to complex regional pain syndrome.[30,79] Magnetic resonance neurography may have a diagnostic role.[80]

Functional Problems and Male Pelvic Pain

In addition to pain, many patients with urogenital pain syndromes suffer with abnormalities of organ function. The exact mechanisms involved may not be clear. It is well described that certain drugs (Table 65.5) and surgical interventions can produce organ dysfunction.

The mechanisms, both central and peripheral, involved in the production of the pain may also be the cause of some of the functional disorders. Certainly, those functions that are reliant on voluntary control may be affected by changes in sensory perception. The sensation of urge perceived with a more or less empty bladder may be associated with urinary frequency, and similarly, the sensation of rectal fullness may be associated with frequent attempts to defecate. Because of convergence of visceral afferent input within the central nervous system, abnormalities of sensation perceived primarily in one organ may result in functional abnormalities further afield[60,81,82] and widespread muscle spasm.[82,83] Abnormal visceral motor function may also occur.[84] The role of the neuroendocrine and neuroimmune systems is poorly understood. The effect of these conditions on fertility is also poorly understood. In males, most frequent effects on sexual function are erectile dysfunction and

TABLE 65.5 Drugs Prescribed in Pain Clinics and Some of Their Effect on Organ Function

Drugs	Effects
Opioids, including tramadol	Constipation Urinary hesitance Reduced sexual desire and erectile ability
Antidepressants	Constipation Urinary hesitance and retention Reduce orgasmic sensation Delay or inhibit ejaculation
Anticonvulsants	Carbamazepine may block testosterone production with subsequent testicular atrophy, gynecomastia, galactorrhea. May inhibit ejaculation

premature ejaculation. These can be evaluated by proper questionnaires, namely, International Index of Erectile Function (IIEF) and Premature Ejaculation Diagnostic Tool (PEDT).

Psychological Consequences of Male Pelvic Pain

The effect of gender on illness and illness behavior is clearly established; however, there is little research on the effect of illness on gender identity and sexual psychology. One may assume that disorders of the male urogenital system will be prone to produce problems within both of these areas with a risk that the male either fails to achieve meaningful relationships or that established relationships have an increased chance of breaking down. All chronic pain is associated with depression and cognitive-behavioral problems. The severity of the pain appears to be the main determinant. Depression and catastrophizing are poor prognostic factors. Tripp et al.'s paper and more recent work by the same group[51] are key studies. Problems with work, relationships, sex, and loss of meaning of life appeared to be as equally important as the pain itself. For the successful management of a patient with chronic pelvic pain, a multidisciplinary team approach is essential (see the following text).

Male Urogenital Pelvic Pain Syndromes— Treatment

SEX DIFFERENCES AND THERAPIES

There are some fundamental differences between males and females that may affect drug pharmacokinetics and pharmacodynamics. In contrast to women, men usually have greater muscle mass, lower percentage body fat, and less fluctuations in hormones. Other genetic-related factors may be at play. Men appear to require significantly more morphine than women per kg body weight,[85] and women seem to achieve statistically significantly more analgesia with κ-opioid agonists (e.g., nalbuphine, buprenorphine, and pentazocine) than do men. The effect of sex differences on other therapies is poorly researched.

SPECIFIC PAIN SYNDROME TREATMENTS

A more complex review can be obtained in the current EAU guidelines for chronic pelvic pain.[11]

Prostate Pain Syndrome

Because the exact nature of this condition is poorly understood, specific drug treatment options do not exist.

Most patients will receive one or more courses of antibiotics. The current EAU guidelines[3] indicate that because some patients have been observed to improve with antimicrobial therapy a trial treatment with antibiotics is recommended. They go on to say that "patients responding to antibiotics should be maintained on the medication for 4 to 6 weeks or even longer." If antibiotics are used, other therapeutic options should be offered after one unsuccessful course of a quinolone or tetracycline antibiotic over 6 weeks. The only randomized placebo-controlled trials that have been done for oral antibiotic treatment are for ciprofloxacin (6 weeks),[86] levofloxacin (6 weeks),[87] and tetracycline hydrochloride (12 weeks). Network meta-analysis has suggested significant effects in decreasing total symptoms: pain, voiding, and quality of life scores compared with placebo.

Recently, there have been many studies that demonstrate an improvement of symptoms in patients with NIH III a/b prostatitis when α-adrenoceptor blockers are used. α-Adrenoceptors are found in the bladder neck and prostate, and α-adrenoceptor blockers are conventionally used to improve flow in the presence of lower urinary tract obstructive symptoms.[88–91] These studies demonstrate an improvement in pain as well as voiding and quality of life.[92-101] Combined α blockers with antibiotics may be superior to monotherapy.

Analgesics are often considered the mainstay of symptomatic management. Simple analgesics containing paracetamol (acetaminophen) are often first line but unfortunately, in many cases, with little benefit. Nonsteroidal anti-inflammatory medications can be considered but should only be used long term if there is evidence of inflammation. Opioids should only be used if one or the other of the national guidelines has been followed (e.g., The British Pain Society/Faculty of Pain Medicine guidelines).

Symptom control is primarily aimed at reducing spasm in the bladder outflow system (smooth and/or striated muscles) or the use of simple analgesics.[102,103] Striated muscle relaxants may help if there is pelvic floor muscle spasm or in the presence of pelvic floor muscle trigger points.[87]

Studies have looked at the role of hormone manipulation with the 5-α-reductase inhibitor finasteride. In a small percentage of patients, finasteride has been found efficacious with an improvement in voiding and a reduction in pain.[87,104,105] The EAU does not recommend 5-α-reductase inhibitors for use in pelvic pain syndrome in general, but symptom scores may be reduced in a restricted group of older men with an elevated prostate-specific antigen (PSA).[3]

The role for anticholinergics is debatable. Meares[106] has suggested they may be beneficial in reducing urinary urgency.

In a systematic review and meta-analysis, patients treated with phytotherapy were found to have significantly lower pain scores than those treated with placebo. In addition, overall response rate in network meta-analysis was in favor of phytotherapy (risk ratio [RR], 1.6; 95% confidence interval [CI], 1.1 to 1.6).[101]

There is little evidence for immune modulation using cytokine inhibitors.[107,108]

There are advocates for therapies, such as biofeedback, relaxation exercises, lifestyle changes (e.g., diet, discontinuing bike riding, changing a work station), acupuncture, massage therapy, chiropractic therapy, and meditation.[87,102] Pelvic floor exercises and biofeedback pelvic floor training, independent of other influences, may benefit this group of patients.[109] The debate about exercise versus trigger point therapy continues with very little research.[109] It appears that managing the associated muscle hypersensitivity is important, whether it is the primary problem or secondary. If we draw comparisons with other musculoskeletal-related pain syndromes, managing the patient as a whole appears appropriate. The physical treatment options should probably consist of exercises, postural/core work, trigger point release, and pacing. Maintaining the locus of control with the patient is important.

Heat therapy, such as transrectal hyperthermia[110-112] and transurethral thermotherapy,[113-115] has been reported to produce favorable results in some patients. Generally, the evidence is weak and the treatments rarely used.

In summary, the mainstay of treatment appears to be antibiotics, α-adrenoceptor blockers, various simple analgesics, hands-on physiotherapy, and pain management psychology and behavioral physiotherapy. There does not appear to be a role for surgery.

Scrotal/Testicular/Epididymal Pain Syndromes

There is very limited research on this condition, and as a result, the evidence for efficacy is limited.[8] Some groups have advocated the use of antibiotics, but, as with the prostate pain syndrome, there appears to be limited supporting evidence in the absence of an identified infection.

If urinary symptoms are present, then those symptoms may be managed as in the prostate pain syndrome. Similarly, the use of nonsteroidal anti-inflammatory drugs (NSAIDs) may have a role if inflammation is present. Analgesics, including opioids and neuropathic analgesics, may be tried; the effect must be monitored and appropriate guidelines adhered to.

There is still debate as to what scrotal contents may be associated with pain. However, there is a suggestion that in the presence of a hydrocele, spermatocele, or varicocele, on average, 50% of patients may see benefit from surgery.[116-118] In the absence of such a lesion, the role of surgery is debatable and may even be detrimental.[8]

In the scrotal pain syndrome, microsurgical testicular denervation has been advocated; however, the number of studies are limited and not double blind for technical reasons.[117,119] The results of epididymectomy and orchidectomy are considered even worse (although 20% and 60% success rates, respectively, have been suggested).[120,121] It should be of concern that these procedures are still undertaken despite the fact that pain may be increased by the procedure.

Nerve blocks (L1 dorsal root renal/sympathectomy, groin blocks, and pudendal/perineal [posterior triangle] blocks) are regularly used in the treatment of scrotal pain syndrome. As well as a possible therapeutic role (for which there are no supporting studies), they are also important for the differential diagnosis process. Although the evidence for therapeutic benefit is limited, the risks are either small or extremely rare.

GENERIC TREATMENT APPROACH

Urogenital pain syndromes should be managed with the same general approach that is used for any of the pain syndromes. Where possible, the consultation and therapeutic procedure environment should be purpose-built, allowing privacy and comfort (many of these patients would prefer to stand or lie for the consultation). Anatomical models and diagrams, including drawings or photographs of genitalia, that will facilitate the consultation should be available. As well as doctors, nurses skilled in the management of this group of patients should be at hand to reinforce the discussion from the consultation.

Psychology and Sexual Counseling

In view of the psychological consequences of urogenital pain, experienced pain management psychologists should be at hand. The full range of their skills utilized for chronic pain management will be required, but psychosexual counseling and relationship work is often required as well. For the sexual problems, we operate a system where the medical and nursing staff not only undertake the medical management of the sexual problems but also provide medical information on normality and variants to enable the patient to place their sexual problems in context. Psychological interventions are instigated early and often while physical treatments are ongoing—the aim is to support and prevent psychological and sexual problem deterioration. Under such circumstances, both the patient and the psychologist have to be able to work with this model of early psychology and ongoing physical treatment.

Trigger Point Therapy

As discussed earlier, trigger points and hypersensitive muscles should be managed as appropriate with treatment options that include drugs, stretching, exercise, relaxation, and injections. Injections into pelvic trigger points are no different than injections into muscles elsewhere but require the expertise of a specialist with skills using imaging such as computed tomography (CT), ultrasound, or possible procedural magnetic resonance imaging (MRI). The agent injected is not agreed on but usually is a local anesthetic and steroid mixture. Botulinum toxin injections into some of the deeper pelvic muscles has been advocated.[122,123]

Nerve Blocks

Nerve blocks may not only have a role in the management of specific nerve injuries but also serve to relax muscles. Nerve blocks may be therapeutic or diagnostic.

Surgery

Surgery was discussed earlier and, in view of the risks with minimal proven benefit, should not be undertaken without a good surgical reason. If the surgery is significant, psychological evaluation and intervention should be considered first.[124,125] Surgery has a role in proven pudendal neuralgia with the site of entrapment being situated at the ischial spine between the sacrospinous ligament (or ischial spine) and the sacrotuberous ligament in 74% of patients.[126]

Drugs
Centrally Acting Analgesics

Chong and Hester[125] summarized the current knowledge in relation to the role of targeting neuropathic pain in urogenital pain syndromes. There is a debate as to when and whether such drugs have a role in the management of the pelvic pain syndromes. Tricyclic and tetracyclic antidepressant drugs may have a role if there are neuropathic qualities to the pain. The best evidence is for amitriptyline. Selective serotonin reuptake inhibitors (SSRIs) and serotonin and norepinephrine inhibitors (SNRIs) are also considered to have a role. Venlafaxine has the strongest evidence but is troubled with cardiac side effects. Duloxetine may have an advantage where stress incontinence is a problem.

Gabapentin and pregabalin have become very popular in the management of chronic pelvic pain, and several studies have suggested they may have a role (still to be published). Other antiepileptics could be considered, as for the management of any neuropathic pain.

Opioids should be considered providing appropriate precautions are undertaken and guidelines adhered to.

Neuromodulation

The evidence base for neuromodulation in chronic pelvic/urogenital pain is limited. However, some very good guidelines do exist for the use of neuromodulation in peripheral nerve injury and complex regional pain syndrome.[127] Hence, one would expect neuromodulation to help certain urogenital pain conditions. Case history reports support this. The main problem is achieving stimulation in the appropriate area, and although some specialists do claim to gain benefit by stimulating the lower thoracic region, it appears that most specialist implanters would now stimulate the sacral roots either by a lumbar retrograde or transsacral approach. The stimulation is thus preganglionic/ganglionic and not dorsal horn or true peripheral sensory nerve only. The transsacral approach is easy to trial and also has the benefit of some excellent guidelines for bowel and bladder dysfunction neuromodulation.[128,129] It is our policy to try transforaminal/transsacral neuromodulation first, and if that fails to reduce the pain, but the patient wishes to try other approaches, we then try lumbar retrograde or lumbar anterograde approaches. The EAU[3] says, "The role of neuromodulation in the management of pelvic pain should only be considered by specialists in pelvic pain management." Neuromodulation appears to have the strongest benefit in those with bladder pain syndrome.[130]

Overview and Conclusion

Male urogenital pain may arise from the specific male urogenital organs. However, there is a strong literature pointing out that in many men, the pain may arise from other sources but is perceived in the male sex organs. It is now well established that when a man presents with urogenital pelvic pain, the nervous system, musculoskeletal system, and other organs should be looked at as potential sources of the pain. The role of the central nervous system in altering afferent perception and producing efferent dysfunction is now well understood. The central nervous system is also key as a cause for the widespread distribution of the pain syndrome. Often, multiple organs and systems are involved. The nervous system may also be key in the association between the pelvic pain syndromes and systemic disorders such as fibromyalgia and chronic fatigue syndrome. In view of this complex of interacting mechanisms, a single therapeutic option is rarely rewarding. Antibiotics and surgery for pain are also rarely rewarding. Multimodal approaches to pain management appear to provide the best results. Management should be aimed at not only the pain but also the other sensory symptoms and functional disorders. The more distressed the patient, the worse the prognosis; hence, early pain management and early psychological, sexual, and relationship support is crucial to a good outcome.

References

1. Abrams P, Baranowski AP, Berger RE, et al. A new classification is needed for pelvic pain syndromes—are existing terminologies of spurious diagnostic authority bad for patients? *J Urol* 2006;175(6):1989–1990.
2. Abrams P, Cardozo L, Fall M, et al. The standardisation of terminology of lower urinary tract function: report from the Standardisation Sub-committee of the International Continence Society. *Neurourol Urodyn* 2002;21(2):167–178.
3. Engeler D, Baranowski AP, Borovicka J, et al. *EAU Guidelines on Chronic Pelvic Pain*. Arnhem, The Netherlands: European Association of Urology; 2017.
4. Gillenwater JY, Wein AJ. Summary of the National Institute of Arthritis, Diabetes, Digestive and Kidney Diseases Workshop on Interstitial Cystitis, National Institutes of Health, Bethesda, Maryland, August 28–29, 1987. *J Urol* 1988;140(1):203–206.
5. Kreiger JN, Nyberg L, Nickel JC. NIH consensus definition and classification of prostatitis. *JAMA* 1999;82:236–237.
6. Hanno P, Baranowski AP, Rosamilia A, et al. International Continence Society guidelines on chronic pelvic pain. Paper presented at: Changing paradigms for chronic pelvic pain: a report from the Chronic Pelvic Pain/Chronic Prostatitis Scientific Workshop; October 2005; Baltimore, MD.
7. van de Merwe JP, Nordling J, Bouchelouche P, et al. Diagnostic criteria, classification, and nomenclature for painful bladder syndrome/interstitial cystitis: an ESSIC proposal. *Eur Urol* 2008;53:60–67.
8. Baranowski AP, Abrams P, Berger RE, et al. Urogenital pain—time to accept a new approach to phenotyping and, as a consequence, management. *Eur Urol* 2008;53:33–36.
9. Engeler DS, Baranowski AP, Dinis-Oliveira P, et al. The 2013 EAU guidelines on chronic pelvic pain: is management of chronic pelvic pain a habit, a philosophy, or a science? 10 years of development. *Eur Urol* 2013;64: 431–439. Available at: https://www.ncbi.nlm.nih.gov/pubmed/23684447. Accessed April 19, 2018.
10. Van de Merwe JP, Nordling J. Interstitial cystitis: definitions and confusable diseases. Paper presented at: Third ESSIC Meeting; June 2005; Baden, Austria.
11. Fall M, Baranowski AP, Elneil S, et al. Guidelines on chronic pelvic pain. Paper presented at: 23rd European Association of Urology Annual Congress; March 2008; Milan, Italy.
12. Doggweiler R, Whitmore KE, Meijlink JM, et al. A standard for terminology in chronic pelvic pain syndromes: a report from the Chronic Pelvic Pain Working Group of the International Continence Society. *Neurourol Urodyn* 2017;36(4):984–1008.
13. Tripp D, Nickel CJ, Wang Y, et al. Catastrophizing and pain-contingent rest predict patient adjustment in men with chronic prostatitis/chronic pelvic pain syndrome. *J Pain* 2006;7(10):697–708.
14. Rothrock NE, Lutgendorf S, Kreder KJ. Coping strategies in patients with interstitial cystitis: relationships with quality of life and depression. *J Urol* 2003;169:233–236.
15. Roberts RO, Lieber MM, Rhodes T, et al. Prevalence of a physician-assigned diagnosis of prostatitis: the Olmsted County study of urinary symptoms and health status among men. *Urology* 1998;51(4):578–584.
16. Nickel JC, Downey J, Hunter D, et al. Prevalence of prostatitis-like symptoms in a population based study using the National Institutes of Health Chronic Prostatitis Symptom Index. *J Urol* 2001;165,842–845.
17. Krieger JN, Lee SW, Jeon J, et al. Epidemiology of prostatitis. *Int J Antimicrob Agents* 2008;31(suppl 1):S85–S90.
18. Litwin MS, McNaughton-Collins M, Fowler FJ Jr, et al. The National Institutes of Health Chronic Prostatitis Symptom Index: development and validation of a new outcome measure. Chronic Prostatitis Collaborative Research Network. *J Urol* 1999;162(2):369–375.
19. Nariculam J, Minhas S, Adeniyi A, et al. A review of the efficacy of surgical treatment for and pathological changes in patients with chronic scrotal pain. *BJU Int* 2007;99(5):1091–1093.
20. Granitsiotis P, Kirk D. Chronic testicular pain: an overview. *Eur Urol* 2004;45(4):430–436.
21. Ahmed I, Rasheed S, White C, et al. The incidence of post-vasectomy chronic testicular pain and the role of nerve stripping (denervation) of the spermatic cord in its management. *Br J Urol* 1997;79(2):269–270.

22. McMahon AJ, Buckley J, Taylor A, et al. Chronic testicular pain following vasectomy. *Br J Urol* 1992;69(2):188–191.
23. Eklund A, Montgomery A, Bergkvist L, et al. Chronic pain 5 years after randomized comparison of laparoscopic and Lichtenstein inguinal hernia repair. *Br J Surg* 2010;97(4):600–608.
24. Leslie TA, Illing RO, Cranston DW, et al. The incidence of chronic scrotal pain after vasectomy: a prospective audit. *BJU Int* 2007;100(6):1330–1333.
25. Wesselmann U, Burnett AL, Heinberg LJ. The urogenital and rectal pain syndromes. *Pain* 1997;73(3):269–294.
26. Nickel JC, Siemens DR, Nickel KR, et al. The patient with chronic epididymitis: characterization of an enigmatic syndrome. *J Urol* 2002;167(4):1701–1704.
27. Hahn L. Treatment of ilioinguinal nerve entrapment—a randomized controlled trial. *Acta Obstet Gynecol Scand* 2011;90(9):955–960.
28. Davis BE, Noble MJ, Weigel JW, et al. Analysis and management of chronic testicular pain. *J Urol* 1990;143(5):936–939.
29. Labat JJ, Riant T, Robert R, et al. Diagnostic criteria for pudendal neuralgia by pudendal nerve entrapment (Nantes criteria). *Neurourol Urodyn* 2008;27(4):306–310.
30. Robert R, Prat-Pradal D, Labat JJ, et al. Anatomic basis of chronic perineal pain: role of the pudendal nerve. *Surg Radiol Anat* 1998;20:93–98.
31. Kao JT, Burton D, Comstock C, et al. Pudendal nerve palsy after femoral intramedullary nailing. *J Orthop Trauma* 1993;7:58–63.
32. Lyon T, Koval KJ, Kummer F, et al. Pudendal nerve palsy induced by fracture table. *Orthop Rev* 1993;22:521–525.
33. Alevizon SJ, Finan MA. Sacrospinous colpopexy: management of postoperative pudendal nerve entrapment. *Obstet Gynecol* 1996;88:713–715.
34. Ricchiuti VS, Haas CA, Seftel AD, et al. Pudendal nerve injury associated with avid bicycling. *J Urol* 1999;162:2099–2100.
35. Glazer HI. Dysesthetic vulvodynia. Long-term follow-up after treatment with surface electromyography-assisted pelvic floor muscle rehabilitation. *J Reprod Med* 2000;45:798–802.
36. Wise D. *A Headache in the Pelvis: A New Understanding and Treatment for Prostatitis and Chronic Pelvic Pain Syndromes*. 3rd ed. San Francisco, CA: National Center for Pelvic Pain Research; 2005.
37. Fon LJ, Spence RA. Sportsman's hernia. *Br J Surg* 2000;87(5):545–552.
38. Hetrick DC, Ciol MA, Rothman I, et al. Musculoskeletal dysfunction in men with chronic pelvic pain syndrome type III: a case-control study. *J Urol* 2003;170(3):828–831.
39. Clemens JQ, Nadler RB, Schaeffer AJ, et al. Biofeedback, pelvic floor re-education, and bladder training for male chronic pelvic pain syndrome. *Urology* 2000;56(6):951–955.
40. Carter JE. Abdominal wall and pelvic myofascial trigger points. In: Howard FM, ed. *Pelvic Pain, Diagnosis and Management*. Philadelphia: Lippincott Williams & Wilkins; 2000:314–358.
41. Slocumb JC. Neurological factors in chronic pelvic pain: trigger points and the abdominal pelvic pain syndrome. *Am J Obstet Gynecol* 1984;149:536–543.
42. Shoskes DA, Berger R, Elmi A, et al. Muscle tenderness in men with chronic prostatitis/chronic pelvic pain syndrome: the chronic prostatitis cohort study. *J Urol* 2008;179(2):556–560.
43. Egan KJ, Krieger JN. Psychological problems in chronic prostatitis patients with pain. *Clin J Pain* 1994;10:218–226.
44. Berghuis JP, Heiman JR, Rothman I, et al. Psychological and physical factors involved in chronic idiopathic prostatitis. *J Psychosom Res* 1996;41(4):313–325.
45. Wenninger K, Heiman JR, Rothman I, et al. Sickness impact of chronic nonbacterial prostatitis and its correlates. *J Urol* 1996;155(3):965–968.
46. Royal College of Obstetricians and Gynaecologists. *The Initial Management of Chronic Pelvic Pain*. London: Royal College of Obstetricians and Gynaecologists; 2005. Green-top guideline no. 41.
47. Savidge CJ, Slade P. Psychological aspects of chronic pelvic pain. *J Psychosom Res* 1997;42(5):433–444.
48. Vlaeyen JW, Linton SJ. Fear-avoidance and its consequences in chronic musculoskeletal pain: a state of the art. *Pain* 2000;85:317–332.
49. Newton-John T, Brooke S. Treating sexual dysfunction in chronic pain patients. In: Gifford L, ed. *Topical Issues in Pain 2: Biopsychosocial Assessment and Management Relationships and Pain*. Cornwall, United Kingdom: CNS Press; 2000:177–186.
50. Tripp DA, Nickel JC, Wang Y, et al. Catastrophizing and pain-contingent rest predict patient adjustment in men with chronic prostatitis/chronic pelvic pain syndrome. *J Pain* 2006;7(10):697–708.
51. Tripp DA, Nickel JC, Wang Y, et al. Biopsychosocial factors in quality of life in CP/CPPS. *BJU Int* 2008;101:59–64.
52. Nazif O, Teichman JM, Gebhart GF. Neural upregulation in interstitial cystitis. *Urology* 2007;69(4 suppl):24–33.
53. Pezet S, McMahon SB. Neurotrophins: mediators and modulators of pain. *Annu Rev Neurosci* 2006;29:507–538.
54. McMahon SB, Jones NG. Plasticity of pain signaling: role of neurotrophic factors exemplified by acid-induced pain. *J Neurobiol* 2004;61(1):72–87.
55. Pontari MA, Ruggieri MR. Mechanisms in prostatitis/chronic pelvic pain syndrome. *J Urology* 2004;172(3):839–845.
56. Petersen M, Segond von Banchet G, Heppelmann B, et al. Nerve growth factor regulates the expression of bradykinin binding sites on adult sensory neurons via the neurotrophin receptor p75. *Neuroscience* 1998;83(1):161–168.
57. Giamberardino MA. Visceral pain. *Pain* 2005;13(6):1–6.
58. Roza C, Laird JM, Cervero F. Spinal mechanisms underlying persistent pain and referred hyperalgesia in rats with an experimental ureteric stone. *J Neurophysiol* 1998;79(4):1603–1612.
59. Vecchiet L, Giamberardino MA, de Bigontina P. Referred pain from viscera: when the symptom persists despite the extinction of the visceral focus. *Adv Pain Res Ther* 1992;20:101–110.
60. Melzack R, Coderre TJ, Katz J, et al. Central neuroplasticity and pathological pain. *Ann N Y Acad Sci* 2001;933:157–174.
61. McMahon SB, Dmitrieva N, Koltzenburg M. Visceral pain. *Br J Anaesth* 1995;75(2):132–144.
62. Akermark C, Johansson C. Tenotomy of the adductor longus tendon in the treatment of chronic groin pain in athletes. *Am J Sports Med* 1992;20:640–643.
63. Taylor DC, Meyers WC, Moylan JA, et al. Abdominal musculature abnormalities as a cause of groin pain in athletes. *Am J Sports Med* 1991;3:239–242.
64. Gajraj NM. Botulinum toxin A injection of the obturator internus muscle for chronic pelvic pain. *J Pain* 2005;6(5):333–337.
65. Giamberardino MA, de Bigontina P, Martegiani C, et al. Effects of extracorporeal shock-wave lithotripsy on referred hyperalgesia from renal/ureteral calculosis. *Pain* 1994;56:77–83.
66. Lloyd-Smith R, Bernard AM, Herry JY, et al. Survey of overuse and traumatic hip and pelvic injuries in athletes. *Phys Sports Med* 1985;10:131–141.
67. Weiss JM. Pelvic floor myofascial trigger points: manual therapy for interstitial cystitis and the urgency-frequency syndrome. *J Urol* 2001;166:2226–2231.
68. Prendergast SA, Weiss JM. Screening for musculoskeletal causes of pelvic pain. *Clin Obstet Gynecol* 2003;46:773–782.
69. Fishman LM, Schaefer MP. The piriformis syndrome is underdiagnosed. *Muscle Nerve* 2003;28:646–649.
70. McCrory P. The "piriformis syndrome"—myth or reality? *Br J Sports Med* 2001;35:209–210.
71. Cox JM, Bakkum BW. Possible generators of retrotrochanteric gluteal and thigh pain: the gemelli-obturator internus complex. *J Manipulative Physiol Ther* 2005;28(7):534–538.
72. Meknas K, Christensen A, Johansen O. The internal obturator muscle may cause sciatic pain. *Pain* 2003;104:375–380.
73. Salvati EP. The levator syndrome and its variant. *Gastroenterol Clin North Am* 1987;16:71–78.
74. Segura JW, Opitz JL, Greene LF. Prostatosis, prostatitis or pelvic floor tension myalgia? *J Urol* 1979;122:168–169.
75. Ingber RS. Iliopsoas myofascial dysfunction: a treatable cause of "failed" low back syndrome. *Arch Phys Med Rehabil* 1989;70(5):382–386.
76. Nederhand MJ, Hermens HJ, Ijzerman MJ, et al. The effect of fear of movement on muscle activation in posttraumatic neck pain disability. *Clin J Pain* 2006;22(6):519–525.
77. Klaber Moffett JA, Jackson DA, Richmond S, et al. Randomised trial of a brief physiotherapy intervention compared with usual physiotherapy for neck pain patients: outcomes and patients' preference. *BMJ* 2005;330(7482):75.
78. Maigne R. Le syndrome de la jonction dorso-lombaire. Douleur lombaire basse, douleur pseudo-viscérale, pseudo douleur de hanche et pseudo douleur pubienne. *Sem Hop (Paris)* 1981;57:545–554.
79. Ramsden CE, McDaniel MC, Harmon RL, et al. Pudendal nerve entrapment as source of intractable perineal pain. *Am J Phys Med Rehabil* 2003;82:479–484.
80. Wadhwa V, Hamid AS, Kumar Y, et al. Pudendal nerve and branch neuropathy: magnetic resonance neurography evaluation. *Acta Radiol* 2017;58(6):726–733.
81. Cervero F, Laird JM. Understanding the signalling and transmission of visceral nociceptive events. *J Neurobiol* 2004;61(1):45–54.
82. Procacci P, Maresca M. Clinical approach to visceral sensation. In: Cervero F, Morrison JFB, eds. *Visceral Sensation. Progress in Brain Research*. Amsterdam, The Netherlands: Elsevier; 1986;67:21–28.
83. Vecchiet L, Giamberardino MA, Dragani L et al. Pain from renal/ureteral calculosis: evaluation of sensory thresholds in the lumbar area. *Pain* 1989;36:289–295.
84. Laird JM, Roza C, Cervero F. Effects of artificial calculosis on rat ureter motility: peripheral contribution to the pain of ureteric colic. *Am J Physiol* 1997;272:R1409–R1416.
85. Chia YY, Chow LH, Hung CC, et al. Gender and pain upon movement are associated with the requirements for postoperative patient-controlled *iv* analgesia: a prospective survey of 2,298 Chinese patients. *Can J Anaesth* 2002;49:249–255.
86. Curtis Nickel J, Baranowski AP, Pontari M, et al. Management of men diagnosed with chronic prostatitis/chronic pelvic pain syndrome who have failed traditional management. *Rev Urol* 2007;9(2):63–72.
87. Nickel JC, Downey J, Clark J, et al. Levofloxacin for chronic prostatitis/chronic pelvic pain syndrome in men: a randomized placebo-controlled multicenter trial. *Urology* 2003;62(4):614–617.
88. Barbalias GA, Meares EM Jr, Sant GR. Prostatodynia: clinical and urodynamic characteristics. *J Urol* 1983;130:514–517.
89. Osborn DE, George NJ, Rao PN, et al. Prostatodynia—physiological characteristics and rational management with muscle relaxants. *Br J Urol* 1981;53:621–623.

90. de la Rosette JJ, Karthaus HF, van Kerrebroeck PE, et al. Research in 'prostatitis syndromes': the use of alfuzosin (a new alpha 1-receptor-blocking agent) in patients mainly presenting with micturition complaints of an irritative nature and confirmed urodynamic abnormalities. *Eur Urol* 1992;22:222–227.

91. Neal DE Jr, Moon TD. Use of terazosin in prostatodynia and validation of a symptom score questionnaire. *Urology* 1994;43:460–465.

92. Cheah PY, Liong ML, Yuen KH, et al. Terazosin therapy for chronic prostatitis/chronic pelvic pain syndrome: a randomized, placebo controlled trial. *J Urol* 2003;169(2):592–596.

93. Gül O, Eroğlu M, Ozok U. Use of terazosine in patients with chronic pelvic pain syndrome and evaluation by prostatitis symptom score index. *Int Urol Nephrol* 2001;32(3):433–436.

94. Mehik A, Alas P, Nickel JC, et al. Alfuzosin treatment for chronic prostatitis/chronic pelvic pain syndrome: a prospective, randomized, double-blind, placebo-controlled, pilot study. *Urology* 2003;62(3):425–429.

95. Evliyaoğlu Y, Burgut R. Lower urinary tract symptoms, pain and quality of life assessment in chronic non-bacterial prostatitis patients treated with alpha-blocking agent doxazosin; versus placebo. *Int Urol Nephrol* 2002;34(3):351–356.

96. Tuğcu V, Tağçi AI, Fazlioğlu A, et al. A placebo-controlled comparison of the efficiency of triple- and monotherapy in category III B chronic pelvic pain syndrome (CPPS). *Eur Urol* 2007;51(4):1113–1117.

97. Chen Y, Wu X, Liu J, et al. Effects of a 6-month course of tamsulosin for chronic prostatitis/chronic pelvic pain syndrome: a multicenter, randomized trial. *World J Urol* 2011;29(3):381–385.

98. Nickel JC, Downey J, Pontari MA, et al. A randomized placebo-controlled multicentre study to evaluate the safety and efficacy of finasteride for male chronic pelvic pain syndrome (category IIIA chronic nonbacterial prostatitis). *BJU Int* 2004;93(7):991–995.

99. Nickel JC, O'Leary MP, Lepor H, et al. Silodosin for men with chronic prostatitis/chronic pelvic pain syndrome: results of a phase II multicenter, double-blind, placebo controlled study. *J Urol* 2011;186(1):125–131.

100. Cohen JM, Fagin AP, Hariton E, et al. Therapeutic intervention for chronic prostatitis/chronic pelvic pain syndrome (CP/CPPS): a systematic review and meta-analysis. *PLoS One* 2012;7(8):e41941.

101. Anothaisintawee T, Attia J, Nickel JC, et al. Management of chronic prostatitis/chronic pelvic pain syndrome: a systematic review and network meta-analysis. *JAMA* 2011;305(1):78–86.

102. Nickel JC, Weidner W. Chronic prostatitis: current concepts and antimicrobial therapy. *Infect Urol* 2000;13:22.

103. Nickel JC. Prostatitis: evolving management strategies. *Urol Clin North Am* 1999;26:737–751.

104. Golio G. The use of finasteride in the treatment to chronic nonbacterial prostatitis. In: Abstracts of the 49th Annual Meeting of the Northeastern Section of the American Urological Association. Phoenix, AZ: Northeastern Section of the American Urological Association; 1997. Abstract 128.

105. Holm M, Meyhoff HH. Chronic prostatic pain. A new treatment option with finasteride? *Scand J Urol Nephrol* 1997;31:213–215.

106. Meares EJ. Prostatitis and related disorders. In: Walsh PC, Retik AB, Stamey TA, et al, eds. *Campbell's Urology*. Philadelphia: WB Saunders; 1992: 807–822.

107. Canale D, Scaricabarozzi I, Giorgi P, et al. Use of a novel non-steroidal anti-inflammatory drug, nimesulide, in the treatment of abacterial prostatovesiculitis. *Andrologia* 1993;25:163–166.

108. Canale D, Turchi P, Giorgi PM, et al. Treatment of abacterial prostatovesiculitis with nimesulide. *Drugs* 1993;46(suppl 1):147–150.

109. Kamihira O, Sahashi M, Yamada S, et al. Transrectal hyperthermia for chronic prostatitis. *Nippon Hinyokika Gakkai Zasshi* 1993;84:1095–1098.

110. Kumon H, Ono N, Uno S, et al. Transrectal hyperthermia for the treatment of chronic prostatitis. *Nippon Hinyokika Gakkai Zasshi* 1993;84:265–271.

111. Montorsi F, Guazzoni G, Bergamaschi F, et al. Is there a role for transrectal microwave hyperthermia of the prostate in the treatment of abacterial prostatitis and prostatodynia? *Prostate* 1993;22:139–146.

112. Shaw TK, Watson GM, Barnes DG. Microwave hyperthermia in the treatment of chronic abacterial prostatitis and prostatodynia: results of a double-blind placebo controlled trial. *J Urol* 1993;149:405A.

113. Nickel JC, Sorenson R. Transurethral microwave thermotherapy of nonbacterial prostatitis and prostatodynia: initial experience. *Urology* 1994; 44:458–460.

114. Nickel JC, Sorensen R. Transurethral microwave thermotherapy for nonbacterial prostatitis: a randomized double-blind sham controlled study using new prostatitis specific assessment questionnaires. *J Urol* 1996;155: 1950–1955.

115. Gray CL, Powell CR, Amling CL. Outcomes for surgical management of orchalgia in patients with identifiable intrascrotal lesions. *Eur Urol* 2001;39:455–459.

116. Yaman O, Ozdiler E, Anafarta K, et al. Effect of microsurgical subinguinal varicocele ligation to treat pain. *Urology* 2000;55:107–108.

117. Padmore DE, Norman RW, Millard OH. Analyses of indications for and outcomes of epididymectomy. *J Urol* 1996;156:95–96.

118. Heidenreich A, Olbert P, Engelmann UH. Management of chronic testalgia by microsurgical testicular denervation. *Eur Urol* 2002;41:392–397.

119. Choa RG, Swami KS. Testicular denervation. A new surgical procedure for intractable testicular pain. *Br J Urol* 1992;70:417–419.

120. Sweeney P, Tan J, Butler MR, et al. Epididymectomy in the management of intrascrotal disease: a critical reappraisal. *Br J Urol* 1998;81:753–755.

121. Thomson AJ, Jarvis SK, Lenart M, et al. The use of botulinum toxin type A (BOTOX) as treatment for intractable chronic pelvic pain associated with spasm of the levator ani muscles. *BJOG* 2005;112(2):247–249.

122. Bennett JD, Miller TA, Richards RS. The use of Botox in interventional radiology. *Tech Vasc Interv Radiol* 2006;9(1):36–39.

123. Naja MZ, Al-Tannir MA, Maaliki H, et al. Nerve-stimulator-guided repeated pudendal nerve block for treatment of pudendal neuralgia. *Eur J Anaesthesiol* 2006;23(5):442–444.

124. Robert R, Labat JJ, Bensignor M et al. Decompression and transposition of the pudendal nerve in pudendal neuralgia: a randomized controlled trial and long-term evaluation. *Eur Urol* 2005;47(3):403–408.

125. Chong MS, Hester J. Pharmacotherapy for neuropathic pain with special reference to urogenital pain. In: Baranowski AP, Abrams P, Fall M, eds. *Urogenital Pain in Clinical Practice*. New York: Informa Healthcare USA; 2007:427–440.

126. Ploteau S, Perrouin-Verbe MA, Labat JJ, et al. Anatomical variants of the pudendal nerve observed during a transgluteal surgical approach in a population of patients with pudendal neuralgia. *Pain Physician* 2017;20(1): E137–E143.

127. British Pain Society. Spinal cord stimulation for the management of pain. Available at: http://www.britishpainsociety.org/pub_professional.htm#spinalcord. Accessed April 19, 2018.

128. National Institute for Health and Care Excellence. Urge incontinence and urinary frequency. Available at: http://www.nice.org.uk/guidance/index.jsp?action=download&o=30827. Accessed April 19, 2018.

129. National Institute for Health and Care Excellence. Faecal incontinence in adults: management. Available at: http://www.nice.org.uk/guidance/index.jsp?action=download&o=30919. Accessed April 19, 2018.

130. Peters KM, Feber KM, Bennett RC. A prospective, single-blind, randomized crossover trial of sacral vs pudendal nerve stimulation for interstitial cystitis. *BJU Int* 2007;100(4):835–839.

CHAPTER 66

Cranial Neuralgias

MUHAMMAD HASSAN MAJEED and **ZAHID H. BAJWA**

Since the last edition of this book was written, advances in diagnostic modalities have improved our understanding of the etiology and pathogenesis of the neuralgias of the face, head, and neck. Recent modifications in the nomenclature have also occurred which reflect a more accurate organization and classification of the cranial neuralgias and facial pain. Although the nomenclature of these severe and often incapacitating pain syndromes remains controversial, immense efforts have been made to scientifically categorize these syndromes based on causal factors, when known, or strict diagnostic criteria, when causal factors are not known.[1–3] Although imperfect, the International Classification of Headache Disorders, 3rd edition (ICHD-III) (beta version), classification system continues to be refined and to serve as a valuable instrument to further advance the scientific understanding and treatment of these disorders.[4] The importance of accurate diagnosis and classification of these conditions is particularly critical as it pertains to treatment of many of the neuralgias for which successful medical and surgical treatments have been developed.

Cranial neuralgias refer to paroxysmal pain in the distribution of a specific cranial nerve. Previous classifications separated facial pain into *typical*, *atypical*, and *symptomatic* neuralgias. Because a great portion of the current literature continues to utilize these terms, it is important to understand the meaning of both the previously used nomenclature and the revised nomenclature.[3] Other features ascribed to the previous classification system are described in Table 66.1.

The revised classification system utilizes the terms *classical* and *painful trigeminal neuropathy*. The term *classical* refers to trigeminal neuralgia (TN) including both idiopathic cases and those related to vascular compression of trigeminal nerve. The term *classical* rather than *primary* has been applied to those patients with a typical history even though a vascular or other source of compression or demyelination may be discovered during its course. The term *painful trigeminal neuropathy* (PTN) can then be reserved for those patients in whom a neuroma, tumor, multiple sclerosis (MS), or other cause has been demonstrated. In the past, the term *symptomatic trigeminal neuralgia* represented these cases.

The term *persistent idiopathic facial pain* has replaced *atypical facial pain* in the taxonomy. This change reflects a lack of known mechanisms, continued recognition of the potential contribution of multiple etiologic factors to this syndrome, and an emerging knowledge of the pathophysiology of diffuse pain syndromes previously not well understood.[5–8]

This chapter is organized around the current classification of neuralgias of the cranial nerves and associated disorders. We cover most of these with particular emphasis on TN as this single disorder is best studied among cranial neuralgias and offers the most reports of diverse clinical experiences. Emphasis is made on updates in classification, diagnosis, and treatment of cranial neuralgias. A narrative bridge from past literature and understanding is included to enhance the reader's understanding of more recent research, insights, and therapeutic approaches.

TABLE 66.1 Characteristics of Facial Pain Syndromes

Feature	Typical Neuralgia	Atypical Neuralgia Unilateral Facial Pain	Persistent Idiopathic Facial Pain (Formerly Atypical Facial Pain)
Frequency	Intermittent: every few moments to once a day or less	Constant, can fluctuate	Constant, not much variation
Pain-free intervals	Always	Rarely	Never
Description	Electric shock, stabbing, shooting	Burning, aching, can have superimposed shocks	Burning, aching
Location	Unilateral; usually trigeminal, rarely nervus intermedius, glossopharyngeal, vagus, upper cervical	Trigeminal or upper cervical; unilateral, rarely bilateral	Not restricted to specific cranial nerve distribution Poorly localized Intraoral or facial Can extend to neck or nasolabial fold Starts unilateral May progress to bilateral
Sensory changes	None or mild hypesthesia	Often hypesthesia	Common hypesthesia Dysesthesia, paresthesias
Precipitating factors	Triggered by nonnoxious stimulation, often in anterior face and remote from face	Rarely triggered; trigger usually in area of pain	Not triggered
Autonomic changes	None	Rarely present	None
Local tenderness	None	Rare	Rare
Causative factors	Vascular compression of nerve in subarachnoid space; rarely MS	Tumor, infection, trauma, or mechanical impingement on nerve; MS, often no cause found	None known
Common age at onset (years)	>50	30	Variable
Gender	60% female	75% female	90% female

Classical Trigeminal Neuralgia

HISTORY

TN was described as early as the first century AD in the writings of Aretaeus (Fig. 66.1). Treatments at that time included bloodletting and the application of bandages containing arsenic, mercury, hemlock, cobra, and bee venom as well as other poisons. Eleventh-century Arab physician Jurjani advanced the vascular compression theory as the causative factor of the severe pain and spasm of this syndrome.[9] The first clinical descriptions of TN in the European literature have been ascribed to Johannes Bausch in 1672 and John Locke in 1677. French physician Nicolas André, who in 1756 described five cases of "unbearably painful twitch," is credited with first recognizing this condition as a unique medical entity. It was André who coined the term *tic douloureux* ("painful spasm"). English physician John Fothergill similarly published a full account of the syndrome and presented the paper to the Medical Society of London in 1773 and thus the disorder has sometimes been referred to him.[9–11] Other historical names for TN include *prosopalgia* and *neuralgia* of the fifth.

In a treatise on neuralgia published by Massachusetts physician E. P. Hurd[12] in 1890, the following description of the clinical presentation of TN is found: "Probably no more atrocious suffering is known . . . During the attack, the patients utter loud outcries, toss about on their beds and smite their heads. The muscles of the affected side of the face are often the seat of rapid contractions, convulsive shocks, which have given to this disease one of the names by which it is known, [tic douloureux]. These contractions may be limited to single groups of muscles, as the zygomaticus, or the frontal part of the occipito-frontales . . . then the paroxysmal shocks diminish in frequency and intensity, and all becomes calm; the storm has passed, to be renewed again under the same form in a time not far distant."

In the 19th century, susceptibility to this condition was thought to be secondary to hereditary factors (with "the ancestors of the neuralgic subject being either neuralgic or sufferers from hysteria, epilepsy, or other neurosis"), in combination with other factors such as disease, intemperance, or insufficient diet. Medical treatment was ineffective until the introduction of trichloroethylene inhalation in the 1920s. Prior to this, treatment in the late 1800s focused on advocating a nutritious diet, adequate sleep, hydrotherapy, vigorous exercise, and moderation in all things. Patients were advised to avoid strain, reading, and brainwork, which were felt to be instrumental in initiating an attack, as well as alcohol, tobacco, and other stimulants. Successful nonsurgical treatment for TN was reported by such notable 19th-century physicians as Wilhelm Erb and Duchenne de Boulogne. These included the use of electrotherapy in the form of interrupted current and galvanism.[11,12]

Although early attempts at surgical treatment of TN by Mareschal, surgeon to King Louis XIV of France, around 1750 and Veillard and Dussans in 1768 were unsuccessful, Bell and Magendie's clarification of the anatomy and function of the trigeminal and facial nerves in the early 19th century is thought to have contributed to subsequent effective surgical treatments for facial pain. Successful neurectomy of the inferior maxillary nerve was reported by Dr. Joseph Pancoast of Philadelphia in 1840 and in 1851. Dr. J. M. Carnochan described successful resection of the maxillary nerve and removal

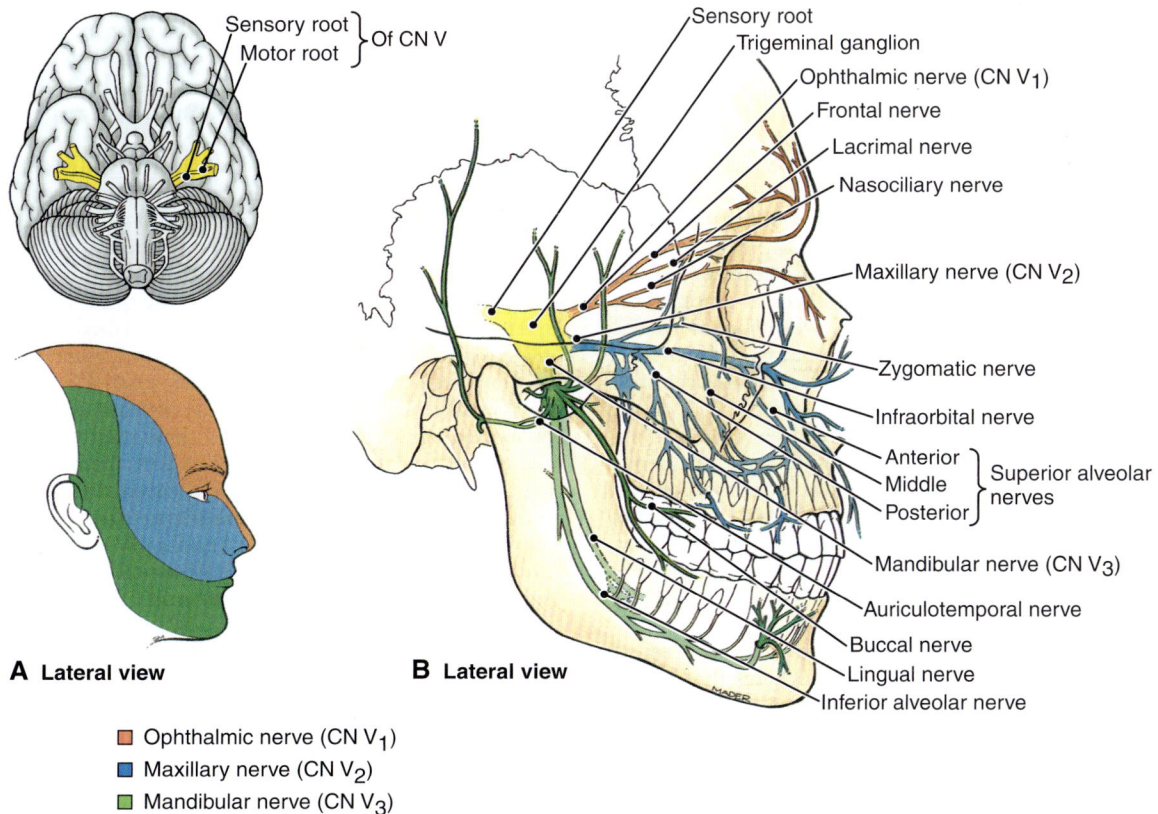

A Lateral view **B** Lateral view

■ Ophthalmic nerve (CN V1)
■ Maxillary nerve (CN V2)
■ Mandibular nerve (CN V3)

FIGURE 66.1 Distribution of the trigeminal nerve (cranial nerve V). The trigeminal nerve gives rise to three divisions: V1, the ophthalmic nerve; V2, the maxillary nerve; and V3, the mandibular nerve. Each division provides sensory innervations to the skin, subcutaneous tissue, and dura mater. The sensory fibers from each division pass through an autonomic ganglion and project the postsynaptic parasympathetic fibers from that ganglion (V1 for the ciliary ganglion, V2 for the pterygopalatine ganglion, and V3 for the submandibular and otic ganglia). V3 additionally supplies motor innervations to four pairs of muscles: temporal, masseter, lateral, and medial pterygoid muscles. *(Reprinted with permission from Moore KL, Dalley AF. Clinically Oriented Anatomy. 6th ed. Baltimore, MD: Lippincott Williams & Wilkins; 2009. Figure 9-9.)*

of Meckel's ganglion from the foramen rotundum to the infraorbital foramen. Subsequent surgical advances in technique were made by Horsley, Taylor, and Coleman in 1891 (middle fossa approach) and Hartley and Krause in 1892 (subtemporal approach). Cushing's modification to this approach, reported in 1900, involved approaching the trigeminal ganglion from below the middle meningeal artery. His contribution was credited with decreasing the mortality rate of the surgery to 5%. In 1921, Frazier suggested electrical stimulation to clearly define and spare the motor root, and in 1928, Stookey recommended differential sectioning of the sensory fibers of only the affected divisions of the trigeminal nerve. In 1925, Dandy reported a novel lateral suboccipital or cerebellar approach that preserved the motor root and was associated with little blood loss. Because of his posterior fossa approach, he was able to observe vascular loops impinging on the root entry zone (REZ) in many patients and inferred that this was the cause of TN.[11,12]

In 1967, Peter Jannetta reported use of the posterior fossa approach with the aid of an operating microscope.[13,14] He was able to confirm Dandy's observations of vascular loops compressing the REZ and subsequently performed a large series of successful surgical treatment of patients with TN using a technique that became known as microvascular decompression (MVD). MVD involves decompression of the nerve by moving the offending vascular loop(s), which are then restrained with nonabsorbent Teflon felt. Due to its low complication and high success rates, MVD has become the surgical procedure of choice for the treatment of intractable TN. The history of the medical and surgical treatments for TN has been thoroughly reviewed by Cole et al.[1,11,12]

EPIDEMIOLOGY

Several epidemiologic studies have collected data on the incidence of TN. Although there is some variation in the reported incidence, in all cases, it continues to be reported as a rare neurologic disorder. A UK study by Brewis et al.[15] published in 1966 reported an incidence of 2 per 100,000. This number was thought to be low due to lack of inclusion of patients seen by otolaryngologists. US studies by Kurtzke[16] in 1982 and Katusic et al.[17] in 1990 reported an incidence of 4 and 4.8, respectively (age and sex adjusted per 100,000 per year). A prospective UK study by MacDonald et al.[18] reported an incidence of 8 per 100,000 per year. An epidemiologic study that was also performed in the United Kingdom reported an incidence of 26 per 100,000 per year between January 1992 and April 2002.[19] This study reviewed patients diagnosed with TN by general practitioners rather than those referred to specialists.

The incidence of TN has consistently been found to be higher in females with a 1.74:1 female/male ratio. Incidence increased with age, usually after age 40 years with peak occurrence between ages 50 and 80 years. Occurrence in patients younger than age 40 years should raise suspicion of secondary causes such as tumor or MS. TN occurs rarely in children.[20,21]

ETIOLOGY AND PATHOPHYSIOLOGY

The various pathologic findings reported and complex theories advanced in the TN literature attempt to explain the combination of unique clinical features of TN such as the following:

- Stereotyped paroxysms of lancinating pain which occur in a limited part of the trigeminal territory
- Separation of the trigger area from the painful region
- Nonnoxious triggers
- Absence of sensory or motor deficit
- Characteristic response of TN to antiepileptic medications

New diagnostic techniques are now challenging theories that were previously advanced to resolve the many questions which remain regarding the etiology and pathophysiology of TN.

Observation of surgical findings led to the 20th-century vascular compression theory of TN. This theory was proposed when Dandy, Gardner, and Miklos recognized the presence of a groove or distortion of the trigeminal nerve root by vessels, or rarely tumors. Jannetta produced convincing evidence that this was the cause of TN by his large series of effective MVD surgeries using the operating microscope. He also demonstrated the absence of trigeminal nerve compression in patients undergoing suboccipital craniotomy for other reasons and in a series of fresh cadaver studies.[11,13,14] Jannetta's review of 4,400 operative procedures from 1969 to 1999 revealed a rostroventral superior cerebellar artery loop compressing the trigeminal nerve either at the brainstem or distally to be the most common cause of vascular compression.[22] Compression by the posterior inferior cerebellar, vertebral, and anterior inferior cerebellar arteries has been also been found. Other reported causes of compression of the trigeminal nerve have included meningiomas, epidermoid cysts, arachnoid cysts, and schwannomas arising from the nerve root itself.[23] Malis[24] proposed petrous ridge and fibrous dural band compression as a cause of TN and demonstrated successful alleviation of TN in a case series of 43 patients undergoing decompression of these fibrous bands.

Kerr[25] and King further argued a peripheral versus a central mechanism for TN. Kerr's[25] peripheral hypothesis, based on epidemiology, surgical resections, and cadaver and animal studies, suggested that the paroxysmal neuralgic pain of TN with associated trigger zones is consistent with minor mechanical or pulsatile compression superimposed on predisposing axonal degenerative changes due to hypertension, atherosclerosis, or disease such as MS. He also noted that with aging, replacement of the bony roof of the carotid canal with connective tissue is known to occur. He argued that these degenerative bony changes would permit pulsatile contact with areas of the ventral ganglion which correlate with the anatomic area in which most trigger zones are known to occur.[14,25]

King argued a central etiology for TN based on injections of alumina gel into the spinal nucleus of the fifth nerve in cats which resulted in a syndrome of dysesthesia of the face with overreaction to tactile stimulation.[21,25] Calvin et al.[26] proposed electrophysiologic mechanisms which required both peripheral and central events to produce the symptoms of TN. Fromm and colleagues[27] published studies which implicated an initial peripheral injury followed by failure of central inhibitory mechanisms as causative factors leading to the onset of TN.

The compression theory of TN, described by the findings of Dandy, Gardner, Miklos, Jannetta, and others, postulates a mechanism for production of the complex of TN symptoms that involves degenerative changes to the central peripheral myelin transitional zone of the trigeminal nerve due to either direct or indirect effects of compression along the course of the nerve from the pons to its entry into Meckel's cave.[28] Ultrastructure analysis of trigeminal root biopsy specimens of patients with TN obtained during surgery for MVD support this theory. They reveal axonopathy, axonal loss, demyelination, and axon apposition without intervening glial processes consistent with the "ignition hypothesis" of TN. This model correlates the mentioned pathophysiologic changes with the paroxysmal symptoms of TN based on similar foci of nerve root demyelination and juxtaposition of axons which have been demonstrated in patients with MS and TN together with experimental studies which indicate that this anatomic arrangement favors the ectopic generation of spontaneous nerve impulses and their ephaptic conduction to adjacent fibers. These studies also demonstrate that spontaneous nerve activity is likely to be increased by deformity of the nerve and frequently associated pulsatile vasculature.[29–32]

More conclusive evidence supporting both peripheral and central etiologies of TN can be found in electrophysiologic studies. One such study has revealed evidence of peripheral damage to small Aδ fibers of the trigeminal nerve near the REZ in the brainstem. Findings revealed demyelination and axonal degeneration or isolated advanced axonal damage on the symptomatic side in patients with classic TN (CTN). In patients with TN and concomitant chronic facial pain, facilitation of central trigeminal processing at the supraspinal level was found. This is consistent with divergent results of MVD in these two groups of patients. Outcome data from MVD in patients with TN shows excellent or good pain relief in 97% immediately postoperatively and in 80% of those with 5-year follow-up. In patients with TN and concomitant persistent facial pain, previously defined as "atypical," only 51% show good or excellent pain relief at 5 years.[33,34] Pre- and postoperative electrophysiologic recording sessions revealed that relief of pain correlates with normalization of previously prolonged trigeminal reflex responses. Electrophysiologic testing has also been able to differentiate TN from symptomatic TN with a high degree of sensitivity and specificity (94% and 98%).[35] Although not practical for routine patient diagnostic purposes, this research is helpful in understanding the decreased response rates in these distinct groups of patients.

SYMPTOMS AND SIGNS

Clear and concise criteria are essential in establishing a diagnosis and conducting research for TN. This is particularly true for a condition such as TN where there is no objective laboratory test to confirm the clinical diagnosis. White and Sweet[36,37] helped to achieve these goals by publishing precise and succinct criteria which facilitated early and accurate clinical recognition of TN and facilitated subsequent research (Table 66.2). The International Headache Society recently established new clinical diagnostic criteria for TN as part of the ICHD-III, which have gained wide acceptance and reflect a significant advance that should further promote communication and stimulate research regarding TN.

TN has well-described pathognomonic features which differentiate it from other types of facial pain. It is characterized by intense paroxysmal, electrical pain which may be accompanied by muscular spasms on the affected side of the face. The attacks generally last from fractions of a second to 2 minutes and are followed by a refractory period during which no pain can be triggered. Pain is abrupt in onset and termination. Between paroxysms, "The patient is in dreaded fear of the next flash of pain."[38] Occurrence of spontaneous remission of pain for weeks, months, or years is another feature of TN which may complicate accurate assessment of therapies.[39]

The pain of TN is limited to the distribution of one or more divisions of the trigeminal nerve and occurs most frequently in V2, V3, or a combination of V2 and V3. First division pain is rare in TN.[40] The pain of TN occurs on the right side of the face more often than the left with predominance ranging from 59% to 66%. Reviews have reported a 3% to 5% occurrence of bilateral pain. Pain rarely occurs on both sides simultaneously. Rather, the painful spasms occur on one side for weeks or months and then, following a period of remission, occur on the opposite side.[38,41-43] Pain occurring on both sides simultaneously or the presence of an abnormal neurologic exam should raise concerns of a secondary etiology such as tumor or MS.[44,45]

Trigger zones, or areas of the face or head that upon nonnoxious stimulation elicit a TN episode, are also a characteristic

---

TABLE 66.2 The International Classification of Headache Disorders, 3rd Edition (ICHD-III) (Beta Version), Diagnostic Criteria for Classical Trigeminal Neuralgia

ICHD-III Beta Diagnostic Criteria for Classical Trigeminal Neuralgia

Description:
Trigeminal neuralgia developing without apparent cause other than neurovascular compression
Diagnostic criteria:
A. At least three attacks of unilateral facial pain fulfilling criteria B and C
B. Occurring in one or more divisions of the trigeminal nerve, with no radiation beyond the trigeminal distribution
C. Pain has at least three of the following four characteristics:
    1. Recurring in paroxysmal attacks lasting from a fraction of a second to 2 min
    2. Severe intensity
    3. Electric shock-like, shooting, stabbing, or sharp in quality
    4. Precipitated by innocuous stimuli to the affected side of the face
D. No clinically evident neurologic deficit
E. Not better accounted for by another ICHD-III diagnosis

Classical Trigeminal Neuralgia, Purely Paroxysmal

Description:
Trigeminal neuralgia without persistent background facial pain
Diagnostic criteria:
A. Recurrent attacks of unilateral facial pain fulfilling criteria for classical trigeminal neuralgia
B. No persistent facial pain between attacks
C. Not better accounted for by another ICHD-III diagnosis
Comment:
Classical trigeminal neuralgia, purely paroxysmal, is usually responsive, at least initially, to pharmacotherapy (especially carbamazepine or oxcarbazepine).

Classical Trigeminal Neuralgia with Concomitant Persistent Facial Pain

Previously used terms:
Atypical trigeminal neuralgia; trigeminal neuralgia type 2
Description:
Trigeminal neuralgia with persistent background facial pain
Diagnostic criteria:
A. Recurrent attacks of unilateral facial pain fulfilling criteria for classical trigeminal neuralgia
B. Persistent facial pain of moderate intensity in the affected area
C. Not better accounted for by another ICHD-III diagnosis

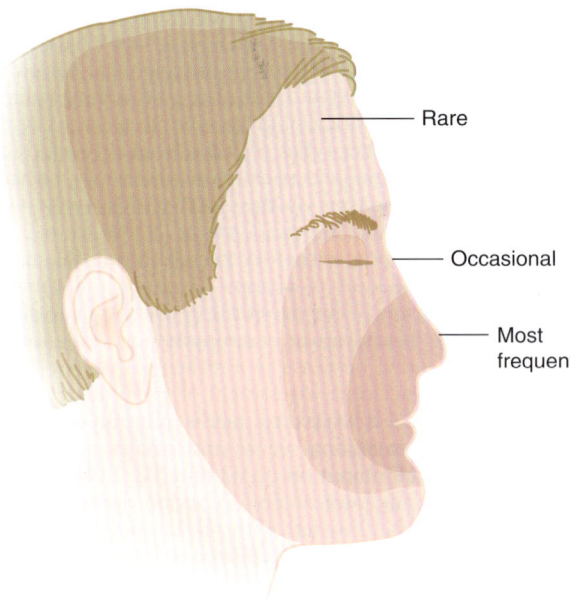

FIGURE 66.2 The most likely sites of triggering for tic douloureux are in the anterior face.

feature of TN. In two large series of patients with TN, trigger zones were reported to be present in 91%.[36,46] Trigger zones may be found in more than one division of the trigeminal nerve. The pain can also be triggered in a different zone from the trigger. The central part of the face near the nose and lips is the area in which triggers most often occur (Fig. 66.2). Touch and vibration have been found to be the most effective stimuli.[47] Attacks are reported to be set off by washing the face, shaving, talking, chewing, brushing of the hair and scalp, or a light breeze on the face of a patient. This can lead to poor hygiene, weight loss, dehydration, and social withdrawal. The ICHD-III criteria also list precipitation of pain paroxysms by "trigger areas" or "trigger factors." These triggers may include stimuli outside of the trigeminal distribution, such as a limb movement, and may include other sensory stimulation such as bright lights, loud noises, or tastes.[2]

Pre-TN is an additional syndrome reported initially in 1949 by Symonds.[48] In these patients, a dull aching or burning pain involving a part of the upper or lower jaw develops for hours, days, or weeks and may be triggered by jaw movements or liquids. They may have several bouts of this pain with remissions for weeks, months, or years followed by sudden onset of the paroxysmal pain of TN. Carbamazepine (CBZ) and/or baclofen have been effective in most cases. Unfortunately, some patients undergo multiple dental procedures before the syndrome is recognized as an early sign of TN.[48–50]

DIFFERENTIAL DIAGNOSIS

The diagnosis of TN is made essentially on clinical information. Differentiating TN from PTN and other causes of facial pain is of great relevance in treating underlying disease or lesions and for instituting effective medical or surgical therapy. This requires a thorough history to obtain the patient's detailed description of defining characteristics, frequency and duration of pain, exacerbating factors, presence or absence of triggers, and associated symptoms. A complete physical exam is necessary to confirm the presence or absence of neurologic deficits. Appropriate tests, such as magnetic resonance imaging/angiography (MRI/MRA) with fast imaging

employing steady-state acquisition (FIESTA) is often indicated to confirm the suspected diagnosis and exclude secondary causes. Development of time-of-flight (TOF) MRA, 3T MRI and 3D T2-weighted driven equilibrium (DRIVE) MRI provide excellent multidimensional images of brain structures, neighboring blood vessels, nerves, and cerebrospinal fluid. These technologic advancements help to locate exactly the site of neurovascular conflict (NVC) loop or any other secondary cause such as plaque and/or space occupying lesions.

Because TN is itself a rare disease, rare presentations of other disease processes fulfilling the diagnostic criteria of TN may require close examination. Rare cases of sinusitis presenting as TN involving first and second division of the trigeminal nerve have been reported with one report of fatal progression in a diabetic patient.[51,52] Because involvement of the ophthalmic branch occurs in less than 5% of TN patients, a high degree of suspicion is indicated in such cases.

As the example earlier illustrates, it is important to differentiate TN and PTN because PTN may be secondary to a progressive lesion or disease process. Expedient treatment of the underlying disease process or lesion in these cases may limit patient morbidity and mortality and improve overall patient outcome. Although most patients with malignant and benign tumors present with sensory deficit or persistent idiopathic facial pain, the literature does contain reports of patients with tumors initially presenting with TN and no neurologic deficits.[53,54]

MS is a common cause of secondary TN which should be considered in any person under 50 years who presents with TN. Brainstem auditory evoked potential and blink reflex testing are sensitive methods for examining patients with TN. When the patient's neurologic exam is abnormal or if the patient does not respond to standard medical therapy, increasingly sensitive methods of CT or MRI/MRA result in accurate diagnosis in almost all cases.[34,55–58]

The cranial neuralgias covered in greater depth later in this chapter must also be differentiated from TN. Glossopharyngeal neuralgia presents with paroxysmal, electrical pain, spontaneous remissions, and triggers associated with swallowing, chewing, coughing, and talking in some patients. Pain occurs most frequently in the ear, tonsils, larynx, and tongue and may radiate to the neck, shoulder, or face. In less than 10% of cases, there is an association with TN. Glossopharyngeal neuralgia is also rarely found in patients with MS.[59]

Intense and stabbing pain localized in the depth of the ear canal is also described in by patients with geniculate ganglion or nervus intermedius neuralgia, a rare disorder affecting the sensory branch of the facial nerve. Other cranial neuralgias which may be confused with TN include "tic convulsif" and hemifacial spasm.

Patients with tic convulsif present with severe otalgia combined with unilateral facial spasm. This rare neuralgic disease is thought to be due to vascular compression of the sensory and motor components of the facial nerve at their junction with the brainstem. Hemifacial spasm is a neuralgia involving the facial nerve which is characterized by intermittent, involuntary, irregular, unilateral contractions of muscles supplied by the ipsilateral facial nerve.[60–62]

Cluster headache pain is unilateral and usually occurs in the ocular, frontal, and temporal areas (although it may occur in the infraorbital and maxillary regions). It usually presents initially in men who are between 18 and 40 years old. Pain is severe, constant, stabbing, burning, and throbbing with associated ipsilateral ptosis, miosis, tearing, and rhinorrhea. Bouts often occur for several weeks to months with one to three attacks in a 24-hour period. Patients will not infrequently be woken from sleep with an attack. Pain-free intervals of several months may occur between bouts of attacks. These headaches tend to respond to ergot preparations, prednisone, and methysergide.[63]

Pain arising from a group of disorders known as trigeminal autonomic cephalgias may also be confused with TN. These include cluster headaches, chronic paroxysmal hemicranias, and short-lasting unilateral neuralgiform headaches with conjunctival injection and tearing (SUNCT). Knowledge of their epidemiology and a careful history will assist with accurate diagnosis.[64]

Chronic paroxysmal hemicrania usually occurs in women. It generally involves the ocular, frontal, and temporal areas. Occasionally, it may involve the occipital, infraorbital, aural, mastoid, and nuchal areas on the same side. Attacks vary in frequency in duration but may last 5 to 45 minutes. Pain is excruciating and is associated with ipsilateral conjunctival injection, lacrimation, nasal stuffiness, and rhinorrhea. These headaches respond well to indomethacin.[65]

SUNCT is a rare syndrome which typically affects males between age 23 and 77 years of age. It is characterized by unilateral burning, stabbing, or electric pain which is usually near the eye. Episodes generally last from 15 to 120 seconds, and multiple episodes can occur daily. Patients present with cutaneously triggered attacks in up to 75% of cases. These attacks are differentiated from TN by lack of a refractory period and presence of associated conjunctival injection, tearing, rhinorrhea, and facial sweating or flushing. As in TN, primary and secondary forms occur. Secondary forms may be due to cerebellopontine angle arteriovenous malformation, infection, and pituitary tumors.[64,66,67]

Painful ophthalmoplegia such as seen in Tolosa-Hunt syndrome, ocular diabetic neuropathy, ophthalmic herpes zoster (HZ), and ophthalmoplegic migraine must also be differentiated from TN.

Tolosa-Hunt syndrome is a painful ophthalmoplegia caused by granulomatous inflammation in the cavernous sinus. It is characterized by episodic unilateral or bilateral orbital pain associated with paralysis of one or more of the third, fourth, or sixth cranial nerves. Involvement of the V2 and V3 divisions of the trigeminal nerve, the optic nerve, and the facial nerve has been reported. The pain is typically described as steady gnawing or boring. Spontaneous resolution may be followed by remissions and relapses of symptoms. Involvement of the optic, facial, acoustic, or trigeminal nerves has been reported. Treatment with corticosteroids results in resolution of pain and paresis in most cases within 72 hours. Failure of response to steroids or recurrence of symptoms should prompt further workup.[2]

Ocular diabetic neuropathy may present as eye and forehead pain associated with ocular cranial nerve paresis (usually cranial nerve III). As in other diabetic neuropathies, pain improves with glucose control, treatment with tricyclics, and anticonvulsant medications.[2]

HZ involving the trigeminal ganglion affects the ophthalmic division in the majority of cases. Ophthalmic herpes may be accompanied by palsies of the third, fourth, and/or sixth cranial nerves or with facial palsy. Burning pain, sometimes accompanied by neuralgic pain, is typically followed by vesicular eruption within 7 days. Pain may resolve or persist as postherpetic neuralgia.[2]

Ophthalmoplegic migraine is a rare clinical entity presenting as recurrent migraine-like headaches accompanied by paresis of one or more of the ocular cranial nerves in the absence or other intracranial lesion. There may be a latent period of up to 4 days from onset of headache to onset of ocular cranial nerve paresis. Demonstration on MRI of thickening and enhancement of the cisternal part of the occulomotor nerve in these patients suggests the etiology of recurrent demyelinating neuropathy.[2]

Other common causes of facial pain include pain caused by sinusitis or other inflammatory conditions involving the eyes, tumors of the nose or sinuses, disorders of the teeth, jaws, or related structures such as temporomandibular joint (TMJ) pain and posttraumatic pain of the peripheral branches of the trigeminal nerve.

Sinusitis presents with pain involving the periocular, frontal, nasal, and maxillary areas. It is generally described as deep and constant and is associated with purulent discharge, fever, and fullness of the nose and ears. CT reveals opacification of the sinuses. In older patients or immunocompromised individuals, tumors or mycoses should be ruled out.[68]

Pain related to the teeth is often triggered by chewing or by hot, cold, sweet, and sour substances. It may have occasional sharp and shooting characteristics but usually will also have a diffuse, continuous aching, throbbing, or burning component which is difficult to localize. This type of pain is also differentiated from TN by lack of trigger zones or periods of spontaneous remissions. TMJ pain and myofascial pain related to the jaw is described as aching, burning, or cramping pain associated with use of the jaw or muscles of mastication. Clicking and other signs of joint dysfunction are associated features.[69,70] These topics are discussed in further detail in Chapter 67 on facial pain within this text.

Trauma to peripheral branches of the trigeminal nerve after surgery, blunt or penetrating trauma, or dental procedures generally presents as constant pain with burning, tingling, or stabbing components as well as a dull background pain. One study comparing patients with facial pain after nerve injury to patients with pain of spontaneous origin found decreased temperature and tactile thresholds and abnormal temporal summation of pain in patients with nerve injury but not in patients with spontaneous pain.[71]

Persistent idiopathic facial pain is typically described as a continuous, dull ache that is poorly localized. It fluctuates in intensity and is generally unresponsive to analgesics. It occurs most frequently in women with a mean age of 44.6 years and range of 17 to 87 years. Most of these patients have multiple diagnoses including depression, headache, neck and back pain, and irritable bowel disease. Neurologic and radiologic exams are normal by definition. These patients often have undergone multiple dental procedures.[72]

TREATMENT

Treatment—Medical Management

The use of the antiepileptic medications for the treatment of TN was first suggested by Bergougan[73] in 1942. His trial of phenytoin in these patients was based on Trousseau's theory that the paroxysmal pain of TN was similar to the paroxysmal brain activity occurring in patients with epilepsy.[74]

Medical therapy of TN is largely based on the efficacy of drugs that have undergone double-blind evaluation. This is particularly important in light of the need to obtain expedient relief of the excruciating pain of the paroxysms suffered by these patients with proven therapies. The occurrence of unpredictable periods of prolonged spontaneous remission in patients with TN creates a greater likelihood of attributing successful treatment of this disease to ineffective agents. Surgical consultation should be sought early for patients with structural lesions and in patients refractory to medical treatment. For patients unresponsive to medical therapy who are not surgical candidates due to coexisting medical conditions, treatment with radiation or percutaneous therapies, as described in the following paragraphs, may be effective.

Of the medications studied in the treatment of TN, CBZ is considered the drug of choice according to the European Federation of Neurological Societies and the Quality Standards Subcommittee of the American Academy of Neurology.[75] Current evidence suggests that oxcarbazepine (OXC) should be the first-line agent in patients with intolerable side effects or inadequate pain control with CBZ.[76] The combination of CBZ with baclofen or lamotrigine has been shown to be effective in cases where patients do not respond to CBZ alone or in whom it loses efficacy.[76]

CBZ is an anticonvulsant, structurally similar to a tricyclic antidepressant, imipramine. It is metabolized primarily by cytochrome P450 isoenzyme CYP3A4. It slows the recovery rate of voltage-gated sodium channels, modulates activated calcium channel activity, and activates the descending inhibitory modulation system. Although it is one of the oldest antiepileptic drugs and many new drugs in this class exist with fewer side effects and fewer drug–drug interactions, four placebo-controlled studies and a systematic review have established its effectiveness in reducing the intensity and frequency of attacks and the number of triggers with a combined number needed to treat of 1.7.[77-81] In a cumulative analysis, CBZ showed a 58% to 100% success in achieving pain control, whereas in comparison, a placebo showed a mere 0% to 40% response.[35]

CBZ is the only U.S. Food and Drug Administration (FDA)-approved drug for TN. Although CBZ has been shown to have an initial response rate of over 70% in TN patients, one long-term study which evaluated its efficacy over a 16-year period reported that by 5 to 16 years, only 22% of participants continued to have effective relief with 44% requiring additional or alternative treatment.[82] The recommended starting dose is 100 to 200 mg twice daily with gradual increase by 200 mg until pain relief or intolerable side effects occur. The typical maintenance dose of CBZ is 600 to 1,200 mg daily in divided doses. Therapeutic level is 4 to 12 μg/mL. Side effects occur in up to 40% of patients initially but generally subside in most patients after a few weeks. The HLA-B*15:02 allele is a genetic susceptibility marker in Asians that is associated with an increased risk of developing Stevens-Johnson syndrome and/or toxic epidermal necrolysis. Screening for this allele in patients with Asian ancestry is recommended before to starting CBZ. If genetic testing results are positive for the presence of at least one copy of the HLA-B*15:02 allele, CBZ should be avoided. The biologic half-life of CBZ is 30 to 35 hours when first administered. This decreases to 12 hours with autoinduction of liver enzymes which occurs after a few weeks. Because pain relief appears to be closely related to serum level, slow-release formulations may be effective in maintaining serum drug concentration.[83]

The efficacy of CBZ is limited by side effects that include drowsiness, dizziness, constipation, nausea, and ataxia. More severe adverse effects include rashes, leukopenia, abnormal liver function, and, rarely, aplastic anemia and hyponatremia due to inappropriate secretion of antidiuretic hormone. Compared with placebo, it has a number needed to harm of 3 for minor side effects and 24 for major side effects. Monitoring of complete blood count, liver function, and sodium is recommended.[84-86]

OXC is the 10-keto analogue of CBZ. Due to its better tolerability, fewer drug–drug interaction, and proven efficacy, OXC is often considered as an initial medication for the treatment of TN. In three head-to-head randomized controlled trials (RCTs), CBZ and OXC both proved to be equally effective in 88% of patients who experienced greater than a 50% reduction in pain attacks.[76] Tolerability was reported as "good" to "excellent" by 62% of patients receiving OXC compared with 48% of patients receiving CBZ. In comparison to CBZ, OXC only needs the monitoring of serum sodium levels.

Lamotrigine also decreases repetitive firing of sodium channels by slowing the recovery rate of voltage-gated channels. In a small, double-blind, crossover, RCT evaluating patients on CBZ or phenytoin who were refractory to treatment with these medications, lamotrigine (400 mg) versus placebo increased the number of patients who improved after 4 weeks of treatment.[87] A case series also suggests its efficacy as monotherapy for TN. Side effects include dizziness, constipation, nausea, and drowsiness. Stevens-Johnson syndrome has been reported to occur in 1 in 10,000 patients taking lamotrigine. Its utility as a single agent may be limited by its long titration schedule.[88,89]

Phenytoin is one of our oldest anticonvulsants with a molecular structure similar to the barbiturates. It acts by blocking sodium channels in rapidly discharging neurons and by inhibiting presynaptic glutamate release. Although it is has been used longer than any other antiepileptic drug in the treatment of TN, there are no controlled trials supporting its efficacy. Uncontrolled observations report that it is effective in relieving symptoms in 23 of 30 patients when 3 to 5 mg/kg was given intravenously for acute therapy.[90-92] Phenytoin interacts with many drugs including digoxin and warfarin. Severe rashes can occur in 1 of 10 to 20 patients. There is also a possibility of hyperglycemia, hepatotoxicity, gingival hyperplasia, and megaloblastic anemia. Fosphenytoin, a prodrug of phenytoin that is better tolerated intravenously, also appears to be effective in acutely ill patients.[93]

Baclofen is an analog of the neurotransmitter γ-aminobutyric acid. Its effectiveness in the treatment of TN may be due to depression of excitatory synaptic transmission in the spinal trigeminal nucleus.[94] In three small RCTs, baclofen was shown to be effective as both monotherapy and add-on therapy to CBZ in the treatment of patients with TN. The starting dose is 5 to 10 mg three times a day, with gradual titration to a maintenance dose of 50 to 60 mg per day. Sedation, dizziness, and dyspepsia can occur with treatment. The dose should be adjusted in patients with decreased renal function because baclofen is excreted primarily by the kidneys. Baclofen has central nervous system and cardiovascular depressant effects, and thus, careful titration should occur in patients on other sedating medications and on antihypertensive agents. Antidiabetic medications may need to be adjusted secondary to increases in blood glucose. Baclofen should be discontinued slowly because seizures and hallucinations have been reported upon withdrawal.[95-97]

Intranasal lidocaine has shown some efficacy in trials. Intranasal 8% lidocaine spray was examined in 25 patients with V2 division TN in an RCT crossover study resulting in moderate or better pain relief in 23 of 25 subjects receiving lidocaine spray and 1 subject receiving placebo. Relief lasted from 0.5 to 24 hours.[98]

In a small open-label perspective study, 53 patients with TN received pregabalin 150 to 600 mg daily and were followed for 1 year. After 8 weeks of treatment, a quarter of the patients were pain-free and almost half of them had significant pain reduction with an overall response rate of 74%.[99] In a small open-label pilot study, 4 out of 10 subjects taking levetiracetam for TN responded with 50% to 90% improvement in pain intensity.[100] In another small open-label study, 23 patients who took levetiracetam for TN reported a 62% decrease in daily episodes of pain.[101]

Uncontrolled observations and case studies have shown efficacy in the treatment of TN with valproic acid, clonazepam, and pimozide.[102-105] The efficacy of pimozide is severely limited by its significant side effects which include Parkinsonism, mental retardation, and memory impairment. The anticonvulsant drugs gabapentin and topiramate have been shown to be effective in the treatment of neuropathic pain; however, there are no controlled studies of their effectiveness in the treatment of TN. Small case series report their effectiveness in the treatment of symptomatic TN secondary to MS.[106-108] In a meta-analysis of effectiveness in TN, overall topiramate results did not differ from CBZ after 2 months of treatment.[109] A small prospective randomized study and a case report demonstrated relief of TN symptoms with injection of botulinum toxin (16 to 100 units).[110,111] A six-patient retrospective analysis and an eight-patient prospective trial of intravenous lidocaine, in doses ranging from 2 to 5 mg/kg/hour, resulted in partial or complete relief of TN pain paroxysms provoked by vibratory symptoms.[47,112]

In summary, the current literature supports CBZ as first-line therapy for TN, although data also supports use of OXC as first-line therapy, particularly in patients refractory to CBZ monotherapy or who have intolerable side effects. Those patients who do not respond to monotherapy of CBZ or OXC may benefit from combination therapy with gabapentin, lamotrigine, levetiracetam, pregabalin, topiramate, or baclofen. Intravenous phenytoin, fosphenytoin, or lidocaine or botulinum toxin injections may be effective in refractory cases of TN for treatment of severe, frequent attacks which may affect the patient's ability to eat or drink. Infusions should be conducted in a carefully monitored setting with appropriate medical attention and emergency equipment available. Due to reports of spontaneous intermittent or permanent remissions of TN, periodic withdrawal of medications is warranted in patients who have prolonged pain-free periods on oral medications.

Treatment—Nerve and Neurolytic Blockade
Local anesthetic injection or infusion has been used for diagnostic purposes and for temporizing treatment in patients with unbearable pain refractory to medical therapy and/or awaiting MVD.[113] No controlled studies of nerve blockade for relief of TN have been reported, and controlled studies are needed to validate this approach. Small case series include significant reduction of pain and triggers in five elderly patients for a median of 2 months subsequent to injection of the infraorbital nerve in patients with second division TN using a combination of 4% tetracaine dissolved in 0.5% bupivacaine. Another study looking at relief of pain following injection of the infraorbital nerve reported greater than 3 months of relief with 4% tetracaine and 0.5% bupivacaine (compared to 3 days or less with 0.5% bupivacaine or 1% mepivacaine alone).[114,115] A combination of ketamine, morphine, and bupivacaine produced similar pain relief and duration as reported following a series of injections of symptomatic peripheral trigeminal nerve branches in patients with TN.[116]

A case report of stimulator-guided mandibular and maxillary division nerve blockade using a combination of lidocaine, bupivacaine, clonidine, and fentanyl at monthly intervals for 1 year in two patients describes prolongation of relief after 3 months and pain-free status with no recurrence at 9-month follow-up. No sensory or motor disturbances were reported.[117] Peripheral injections are of value in elderly patients who have not responded to medical or other surgical therapies. Standard precautions to avoid intravascular injection of drugs should be taken, and care should be taken when performing V2 and V3 blockade as total brainstem anesthesia with respiratory arrest following extraoral trigeminal V2 to V3 blocks has been reported.[118]

Careful aspiration, fluoroscopic guidance when available, utilizing contrast (when no contraindication exists), and digital subtraction can decrease the risk of intravascular or intrathecal injection. As with intravenous infusions, injections should be performed in a monitored setting with appropriate medical attention and readily available emergency equipment.

Alcohol, phenol, or glycerol injection has long been reported in the treatment of TN. Percutaneous gangliolysis using glycerol is discussed under surgical techniques. A retrospective case audit of patients who received peripheral alcohol injections for TN from 1994 to 1999 found a mean duration of effect of 11 months.[119] In a retrospective review of 100 patients with TN who were treated with 1 to 1.5 mL of absolute alcohol injection, 86% reported pain control. The duration of analgesia varied widely from a period of 2 to 56 months.[120] In a prospective study from South Korea, 98 patients who received mandibular nerve blocks with alcohol had pain relief. At 1 year, 90.4%, at 2 years 69%, at 3 years 53.5%, and at 7 years 33% remained pain-free.[121] Glycerol injections provided a mean of 7 months of pain relief.[122] A retrospective analysis of 157 cases of intractable idiopathic TN treated with

peripheral glycerol injections reported an initial 98% success rate with 60 patients having recurrent pain between 25 and 36 months. The study reports complete or near-complete pain relief in 154 patients at 4 years (with inclusion of patients with recurrent pain who were reinjected).[123] Postinjection facial swelling, discomfort, and numbness are reported complications of alcohol injections. More serious complications occurred in 3 of 413 injections over a 20-year period.[124] A small case series of 60 peripheral injections in 18 patients of the infraorbital, supraorbital, and mandibular nerves using 10% phenol in glycerol reported 87% initial marked or total pain relief and a median of 9 months of continued relief. Most patients with recurrent pain requested a repeated procedure rather than surgery or a ganglion nerve block. No serious complications or dysesthetic pain were reported. In patients with facial sensory loss, sensation was recovered within 6 months and was well tolerated.[125] In a randomized control trial of 42 patients with TN, 68% of the subjects who received botulinum toxin type A (BTX-A) in comparison to only 15% of the placebo group subjects, showed significant improvement in pain intensity and frequency after 2 weeks.[126] In an RCT, both 25 and 75 units of BTX-A were better (70.4% and 86.2%) than placebo (32.1%) in the treatment of TN at 8 weeks follow-up. There was no significant difference between two doses of BTX-A.[127]

Treatment—Surgical
Surgical therapies are aimed at either damaging or destroying pain transmitting nerve fibers or relieving pressure on the nerve from vascular loops, fibrous bands, or mass lesions. Radiation therapy may relieve pain in patients who are not surgical candidates and who are refractory to medical management of TN.

Microvascular Decompression
MVD is performed under general anesthesia using a microscope to visualize the trigeminal nerve as it leaves the pons via a suboccipital craniectomy. Compression of the nerve by a vein or artery is relieved by repositioning the artery or coagulating the vein. Although MVD is invasive, it is associated with the best long-term outcome and overall mortality and complication rates are low. An analysis of long-term follow-up data of 1,324 patients with TN who underwent MVD between 1976 and 2000 revealed an increase in the postoperative cure rate from 92.9% to 96.7% in patients operated on after 1986. Recurrence rate decreased from 10.2% to 6.5% in the patients operated on between 1986 and 2000 compared to the patients who underwent MVD between 1976 and 1986.[128] Barker et al.[129] reported results of 1,185 patients who underwent MVD over a 20-year period. It was noted that the rate of complications was significantly reduced, and no deaths occurred after 1980 when intraoperative monitoring of brainstem evoked response was used. Female gender, symptoms lasting more than 8 years, venous compression of the terminal REZ, and the lack of immediate postoperative cessation of pain were significant predictors of eventual recurrence.[129] Endoscopic microvascular decompression (E-MVD) was used in 47 patients with TN. In the follow-up period of 15 ± 8 months after the surgery, patients reported overall excellent pain control. One patient had permanent hearing loss as a complication of the surgery. E-MVD was deemed to be safe and effective in the treatment of TN.[130] In a comparative study of endoscopic versus traditional microscopic microvascular decompression (M-MVD) for TN, 167 subjects were followed up from 2006 to 2013. Out of 167 patients, 93 patients underwent M-MVD and 74 underwent E-MVD. Overall outcome and complications rates were comparable.[131] In a retrospective comparative analysis of 225 patients who underwent MVD and 206 having undergone percutaneous trigeminal radiofrequency rhizotomy, 64% of patients who underwent MVD remained

completely pain-free 20 years postoperatively versus 50% risk of recurrence of pain 2 years after radiofrequency rhizotomy.[132] Hospital and surgeon volume was found to be a significant factor affecting morbidity in a study conducted from 1996 to 2000 by Kalkanis and associates.[133] The overall mortality rate was 0.3% with volume and mortality not statistically related. The rate of discharge other than to home was 3.8%, with hospitals and/or surgeons who performed the surgeries at low volumes being 5.1% as compared to 1.6% for high volume.[133] Percutaneous rhizotomy or gangliolysis is useful in treating the elderly or debilitated patient who is refractory or intolerant to medical therapy and for whom surgery is not warranted due to risk factors. Gangliolysis is performed under fluoroscopic guidance by placing a needle percutaneously through the foramen ovale and advancing it to the trigeminal cistern.

The three techniques currently used for gangliolysis include percutaneous radiofrequency ablation/thermocoagulation, trigeminal ganglion compression, and retrogasserian glycerol rhizolysis. Percutaneous radiofrequency trigeminal gangliolysis involves the use of radiofrequency to create anatomically distinct lesions in cycles of 45 to 90 seconds at 60° to 90° C. Percutaneous trigeminal ganglion compression is performed under general anesthesia utilizing a Fogarty catheter that is inserted via a 14G catheter into the trigeminal cistern and inflated with radiocontrast to compress the gasserian ganglion. Careful observation of heart rate and blood pressure is required due to the possibility of severe bradycardia and hypotension which may require treatment with atropine and vasopressors. Percutaneous glycerol rhizolysis is performed in a sitting position. After confirmation of needle location with radiocontrast, 0.1 to 0.4 mL of anhydrous glycerol is injected into the cistern of Meckel's cave.

In a prospective longitudinal study of 48 patients with TN, 31 had pure TN and the remainder presented with atypical facial pain and mixed TN. They were treated with radiofrequency thermocoagulation of the gasserian ganglion with overall favorable outcomes after the treatment. The mean time for reoccurrence of pain was 40 months for the CTN cohort and 36 months for TN patients with atypical facial pain.[134] An analysis of 100 subjects who underwent percutaneous balloon compression (PBC) of the trigeminal rootlets showed initial pain relief in 90% of patients. Twenty months was the median time to be symptom-free without the help of any medications.[135] A systematic review of radiofrequency ablation/thermocoagulation techniques for the treatment of TN demonstrated complete pain relief without medication in a median of 88% in patients undergoing radiofrequency thermocoagulation at 6-month follow-up.[136] This dropped to 61% at the 3-year follow-up. Retrospective analysis of patients undergoing percutaneous glycerol rhizolysis showed complete pain relief in 84% of patients with or without medication at 6 months following treatment. This dropped to a median of 54% at 3-year follow-up.

Complications with any of the ablative techniques described earlier have been noted to include dysesthetic disturbances in 4% to 10% of patients treated. Up to 30% of patients treated with radiofrequency thermocoagulation experienced significant permanent sensory loss. Other complications included corneal numbness and keratitis, anesthesia dolorosa, transient masseter weakness, cranial nerve deficits, and vascular injuries. The complication rate was highest in patients undergoing radiofrequency thermocoagulation, although most complications were transient.[136]

Ablative procedures are less invasive than MVD and are generally associated with a high initial response rate. Recurrence is common, however, and the incidence of facial numbness is higher than with MVD. Patients who have a recurrence of TN after an ablative procedure can successfully undergo MVD.[129]

Stereotactic Radiosurgery

The first radiosurgical device was developed in the 1950s by Professor Lars Leksell at the Karolinska Institute in Stockholm. This work resulted in the development of the gamma knife which is able to precisely irradiate small intracranial targets with gamma ray photons.

Of 149 patients who received gamma knife stereotactic radiosurgery (GKS) for TN, 76%, 69%, and 60% reported pain control at 1, 2, and 3-year follow-up, respectively. Twenty-seven patients were treated with repeat GKS; 70% and 62% reported freedom from pain at 1 and 2 years.[137] Pain relief with GKS occurs after a lag time of about 1 month.[3,138] A systematic review of these data found that approximately 75% of patients report complete relief within 3 months, and 50% of patients can permanently stop drug therapy after surgery. Sensory disturbances (e.g., numbness, paresthesias, and dysesthesias) are the most frequent complications.[138]

CyberKnife radiosurgery is a more recently developed system to incorporate a miniature linear accelerator mounted on a flexible, robotic arm. This system offers targeting accuracy without the need for the invasive head frame and is able to treat tumors anywhere in the body. Although GKS has the advantage of over 30 years of clinical use, observational studies using the CyberKnife system for the treatment of TN report a 92.7% initial success for pain relief at a median latency to pain relief of 7 days. Long-term response rate at 11 months was 78%.[139] Larger study groups and longer follow-up is needed to further evaluate long-term pain relief and complications. In an analysis of outcomes in 27 patients who had refractory TN who received CyberKnife radiosurgery, 42.9% were pain-free within 1 month after the procedure. The time for reoccurrence of pain widely varied.[140] Although radiosurgery is less effective than MVD, it is an effective, minimally invasive treatment option for patient's refractory to medical therapy who are not surgical candidates or in whom the risks of surgery are not acceptable. Patients who fail to respond to radiosurgery or who have recurrence of symptoms may respond to repeat treatment.[141,142]

In a retrospective analysis, 870 patients who received stereotactic radiosurgery for TN (95% CTN), based on treatment dose, were divided into three groups: 352 patients received the dose of ≤82 Gy, 85 patients received 83 to 86 Gy, and 433 patients ≥90 Gy. In a 4-year follow-up, pain control was 79%, 82%, and 92%, respectively.[143] In a recent analysis, the stereotactic radiosurgery outcome of 112 patients who had type 1 (TN1) or 2 (TN2) TN (old classification) and treated between 1994 and 2016 was reviewed. At 5, 10, and 15 months, symptom relief was 75%, 90%, and 90% for TN1 and 47%, 77%, and 87% for TN2. In a long-term follow-up at 24 and 36 months, 67% and 52% for TN1 and 32% and 32% for TN2 reported symptom relief.[144]

Peripheral Neurectomy

Surgical destruction of the peripheral branches of the trigeminal nerve is indicated for patients who have failed medical therapy, who have failed gangliolysis, or who have severe cardiopulmonary disease and are unable to tolerate a suboccipital craniectomy and MVD. Duration of good to excellent relief varies from less than 1 year to a range of 2 to 5 years in reported series. In one series, the median pain-free period among 88 patients was 41 months with a mean of 52.5 months. Analysis of 40 patients found excellent to good results in all patients for a period of time ranging from 2 to 5 years.[145,146] The procedure can be repeated; however, the risk of neuroma is increased as is diminished success. Following neurectomy, dense numbness in the distribution of the eradicated nerve can occur.

Cryoablation of the peripheral branches of the trigeminal nerve can be performed using a 1.4- to 2-mm probe which incorporates a nerve stimulator to test both sensory and motor function as well as a thermistor to identify temperature at the tip of the probe. A 3.5- to 5.5-mm ice ball is produced which results in disruption of the nerve structure with wallerian degeneration while leaving the myelin sheath and endoneurium intact (axonotmesis).[147] The use of cryotherapy to successfully treat patients with TN has been reported by several authors to provide analgesia for periods ranging from 6 to 13 months. No permanent sensory loss was reported; however, in one review, up to one-third of patients developed atypical facial pain following the procedure.[148–150]

Painful Trigeminal Neuropathy

PTN is differentiated from TN through demonstration of a causative lesion other than vascular compression. Sensory impairment and bilaterality may be present as well as lack of a refractory period after a paroxysm.[2] MS and benign or malignant neoplasms are the most common cause of PTN, although fungal infection and bacterial sinusitis with intracranial extension, scrub typhus, hardened felt from previous MVD surgery, and TN as the first manifestations of mixed connective tissue disorder have also been reported.[139,151–155]

MULTIPLE SCLEROSIS

MS is an inflammatory autoimmune systemic disease which is characterized by demyelinating lesions and plaques within the central nervous system. Widespread neuronal loss with periods of remyelination may be associated with periods of remission.

MS affects women more than men with a cumulative ratio of females to males of 1.77 to 1.0. Median and mean age of onset of MS is 23.5 and 30 years of age, respectively.[156] TN occurs in up to 2% of patients with MS, although this represents only about 0.5% of patients presenting with TN.[157,158] These patients can present with symptoms which mimic CTN but often present with bilateral symptoms and persistent background facial pain.[158]

The pathophysiology of TN in MS continues to be debated. Although demyelinating lesions affecting the trigeminal REZ have been found on autopsy and on MRI, 24 MS patients out of a series of 851 studied at one institution were found to have entry zone lesions which were clinically silent.[159,160]

Although MVD was once thought to be contraindicated in MS patients with PTN, a report of MVD performed in 35 MS patients with severe neurovascular compression at the REZ resulted in a 39% excellent and 22% fair to good long-term pain relief. Seventy-four percent of these patients had demyelinating lesions affecting the brainstem trigeminal pathway on the painful side in addition to neurovascular compression.[161] In a series of five patients with TN and MS who were refractory to medical treatment and had undergone multiple unsuccessful percutaneous procedures, those patients undergoing MVD combined with partial sectioning of the nerve did better than those undergoing MVD alone.[162] A study reported 43 patients with MS related TN who were treated with GKS, 91% reported initial symptom relief. The actuarial probability to live pain-free was 87.2%, 71.8%, 43.1%, 38.3%, and 20.5%, at 6 months, 1, 3, 5, and 10 years, respectively.[163]

In general, patients with PTN secondary to MS respond less favorably to medical and interventional therapies and may require significantly more treatment than their cohorts with CTN.[164]

NEOPLASM

The presentation of TN does not rule out the presence of a tumor. Some authors advocate advanced imaging of all patients presenting with TN due to delayed neurologic symptoms in patients with space-occupying lesions.[154] Among 2,972 patients diagnosed with TN at the Mayo Clinic between 1976 and 1990, tumors were the cause of facial pain in approximately

10% (296 patients). Sex and pain distributions paralleled those in TN; however, patients presenting with tumors were younger than those with TN. Delay in tumor diagnosis averaged 6.3 years. The development of neurologic deficits prompted further imaging and diagnosis of tumor in 47% of these patients. These patients were often successfully treated medically for many years prior to onset of neurologic symptoms.[53,165]

Meningioma and epidermoid and acoustic neuroma are the most frequent posterior fossa tumors associated with PTN. In a review of 161 and 80 consecutive posterior fossa tumors from 1993 to 1999 and 1979 to 2003 at separate institutions, cranial nerve dysfunction was the most common neurologic sign on admission. Intracranial hypertension and disturbance of gait also presented in up to 44% of these patients.[166,167] Twenty cases of TN caused by contralateral tumors of the posterior fossa have been reported. Only 4 of these cases symptomatically conformed to CTN. The mechanism of contralateral tumor causing TN is thought to be distortion and displacement of the brainstem and compression of the contralateral Meckel's cave.[168,169]

Pain in all three divisions of the trigeminal nerve is the first symptom of a tumor in Meckel's cave in over 65% of cases. The most common cavernous sinus tumors are trigeminal schwannomas and meningiomas. Tumors in this location make up only 0.5% of all intracranial tumors.[170] Case reports of metastatic disease to Meckel's cave presenting as TN include colorectal cancer, esophageal cancer, breast cancer, renal cell carcinoma, and lymphoma.[170–174] Primary melanoma, adenocarcinoma, and lymphoma involving Meckel's cave and associated with TN have also been reported.[175–178] TN with subacute onset of numbness in one or more divisions of the trigeminal nerve is thought to be associated with rapidly expanding tumor in this region.[174]

Other reported causes of symptomatic TN include platybasia (a skull base deformity),[179] sarcoid granuloma of the trigeminal nerve, and infarction of the REZ of the trigeminal nerve in the pons.[180,181] TN has also been seen in adults and children as the only manifestation of Chiari type I malformations.[182–184] Patients with hydrocephalus from remote causes such as a lumbar myxopapillary ependymoma and a quadrigeminal arachnoid cyst have also presented with TN.[185,186] Shunting and relief of hydrocephalus resulted in resolution of symptoms in these cases.

Five percent to 10% of TN has been reported to be PTN secondary to brain tumors.[187] Although persistent pain, numbness, palsies, and gait disturbances along with other neurologic signs often differentiate these patients from those with TN, delay in the presentation of neurologic deficits is not infrequent. Expedient workup including advanced imaging is indicated in cases of TN with new onset of neurologic signs such as numbness or palsies.

HERPES ZOSTER AND POSTHERPETIC NEURALGIA

HZ and postherpetic neuralgia is classified by ICHD-III as a subgroup of TN under subclassification of PTN caused by HZ infection, whereas the International Association for the Study of Pain (IASP) categorizes it as postherpetic neuralgia.

Etiology

Acute HZ results from the reactivation of the varicella zoster virus which is referred to as "chickenpox" in children or "shingles" in adults. The virus remains dormant in the dorsal root ganglia of cranial or spinal nerves after resolution of the original infection. As cellular immunity wanes with disease, chemotherapy, or age, the virus is reactivated and is transported along peripheral nerves producing an acute neuritis. Viral replication results in direct nerve sheath and neuronal injury. Destruction of tissue and inflammation result in excitation of nociceptors and dorsal horn sensitization. The dorsal horns of patients who do not develop postherpetic neuralgia show less tissue damage and more rapid resolution of inflammatory changes.[188]

Epidemiology

The rate of HZ and the rate of HZ-associated complications increase with age, with 68% of cases occurring in those aged 50 years and older. Postherpetic neuralgia occurs in 18% of adult patients with HZ and in 33% of those aged 79 years and older.[189]

In HZ involving the trigeminal nerve, neuronal spread of the virus occurs along the ophthalmic (first) and less frequently the maxillary (second) division of the fifth cranial nerve. Vesicular eruptions usually occur at the terminal points of sensory innervation, causing extreme pain. HZ involving the ophthalmic ganglion of the trigeminal nerve, or zoster ophthalmicus, accounts for as many as 10% to 25% of HZ cases. Nasociliary involvement will most likely cause ocular inflammation. Inflammation of the eye can lead to impairment of vision and in some cases temporary blindness. Such cases are considered emergent, and prompt treatment is required to prevent chronic inflammation or long-term vision loss.

Contiguous spread of the virus may lead to the involvement of other cranial nerves, resulting in optic neuropathy (cranial nerve II) or isolated cranial nerve palsies (cranial nerve III, IV, or VI).

Symptoms and Signs

Acute HZ typically presents with a prodrome consisting of hyperesthesia, paresthesias, burning dysesthesias, or pruritus along the affected dermatome(s). This prodrome is usually accompanied by fever and general malaise. It generally lasts 1 to 2 days but may precede the appearance of skin lesions by up to 3 weeks. Manifestation of prodromal symptoms without development of the characteristic rash may occur in some patients. This presentation is known as "zoster sine herpete" and may delay correct diagnosis and treatment.

Following the prodromal period, a vesicular skin rash appears along the affected nerve. Involvement of the trigeminal nerves characteristically respects the vertical midline. The vesicles will discharge fluid and begin to scab over after about 1 week. The pain is extreme during the inflammatory stage. Vesicles at the tip of the nose are known as Hutchinson sign and signal a 75% likelihood of ocular sequelae which may include follicular conjunctivitis; epithelial and/or interstitial keratitis; dendritic keratitis; uveitis; scleritis chorioretinitis; optic neuropathy; and palsies of the third, fourth, or sixth cranial nerves.

Pain that persists beyond healing of the rash but which resolves within 4 months of onset is referred to as subacute herpetic neuralgia. Postherpetic neuralgia refers to pain persisting longer than 4 months from initial onset of rash.[190] Affected patients usually report constant, severe, burning, lancinating pain in the distribution of the affected nerve(s). Patients may also complain of pain in response to nonnoxious stimuli (allodynia). Even the slightest pressure from clothing, bedsheets, or a slight breeze may elicit severe pain.

Diagnosis

The diagnosis of acute HZ is essentially clinical, based on the characteristic unilateral appearance of a vesicular rash limited to the distribution of a specific nerve or nerve root. As discussed in the "Symptoms and Signs" section earlier, this is preceded most commonly by a painful prodrome characterized by burning dysesthesias or paresthesias along the affected dermatome. The criterion standard of laboratory diagnosis is polymerase chain reaction testing together with direct identification of varicella zoster virus in culture. Immunocompromised patients may benefit from immunoglobulin (Ig) G- and IgA anti-varicella zoster virus antibodies.[191,192]

Treatment

The goals of treatment of acute HZ include treatment of the acute viral infection, treatment of the severe acute pain associated with HZ infection, and prevention of postherpetic neuralgia.

Acute HZ infection should be treated with antiviral medication within 72 hours of vesicular eruption to reduce the duration and severity of pain associated with the infection. The use of antivirals may produce a moderate reduction in the risk of development of postherpetic neuralgia. Oral steroids may also be beneficial in reducing the severe pain of acute HZ.[193]

Acute treatment of acute HZ with neuropathic analgesics (i.e., anticonvulsants or tricyclic antidepressants) starting within 48 hours of onset of rash may also reduce acute pain and incidence of postherpetic neuralgia.[194-197] Patients with ocular involvement should have immediate evaluation and treatment of ophthalmic complications by a specialist.

The varicella zoster vaccine was approved by the FDA in May 2006 and was found to reduce the incidence of shingles by 51% in a randomized double-blind study. Pain was reduced by 61% in those who received the vaccine but still developed the infection, and postherpetic neuralgia was reduced by two-thirds compared with placebo.[198] The FDA recently approved a new shingles vaccine called Shingrix for adults age 50 years and older.[199]

Nutritional counseling may also be indicated in populations at risk for HZ. In a review of 243 HZ cases, it was determined that individuals, particularly those over age 60 years, who ate less than one serving of fruit or vegetables weekly had a threefold greater risk of HZ compared to those who ate more than three servings daily independent of vitamin supplement intake.[200] An association between deficiency of vitamin A (a key immune modulator involved in the synthesis of lymphocytes, neutrophils, cytokines, and immunoglobulins) and increased risk of HZ has also been observed.[201]

Systematic reviews of the literature have concluded that pharmacologic therapies shown to be more effective than placebo for postherpetic neuralgia include tricyclic antidepressants, opioids, gabapentin, pregabalin, tramadol, capsaicin, and lidocaine 5% patch. Intrathecal methylprednisolone was shown to be of benefit in patients refractory to pharmacologic therapies.[202,203] Safety and tolerability should be considered when selecting pharmacologic treatments. Older patients may have more intolerable side effects at standard doses and thus may require smaller doses and more gradual titration. They may also be on multiple medications for coexisting medical conditions with potential for drug–drug reactions. In a 13-week RCT for the treatment of 370 patients with postherpetic neuralgia, pregabalin showed efficacy from week 1 and continued for 13 weeks. Most common side effects were dizziness (5.8%), somnolence (2.9%), and ataxia (2.5%).[204]

Sympathetic blockade, including stellate ganglion block, has commonly been used to provide pain relief of variable duration in both acute HZ and in postherpetic neuralgia. Although a review of sympathetic blocks in the treatment of acute HZ and postherpetic neuralgia found the evidence to be inconclusive due to lack of properly controlled studies, it found available data to suggest that sympathetic blocks may provide considerable pain relief during acute HZ but appear to provide only short-term relief in postherpetic neuralgia.[188]

Nervus Intermedius Neuralgia

Nervus intermedius neuralgia is an uncommon disorder affecting the sensory branch of the facial nerve (cranial nerve VII) (Fig. 66.3). It is located between the motor component of the facial nerve and the vestibulocochlear nerve (cranial nerve VIII). Sensory fibers contained in the nervus intermedius nerve carry afferent sensory input from the skin of the external auditory meatus; mucous membranes of the nasopharynx and nose; and taste from the anterior two-thirds of the tongue, floor of the mouth, and the palate. The geniculate ganglion contains the cell bodies of the sensory fibers of the nervus intermedius. Compression of the geniculate ganglion therefore can also result in nervus intermedius neuralgia.

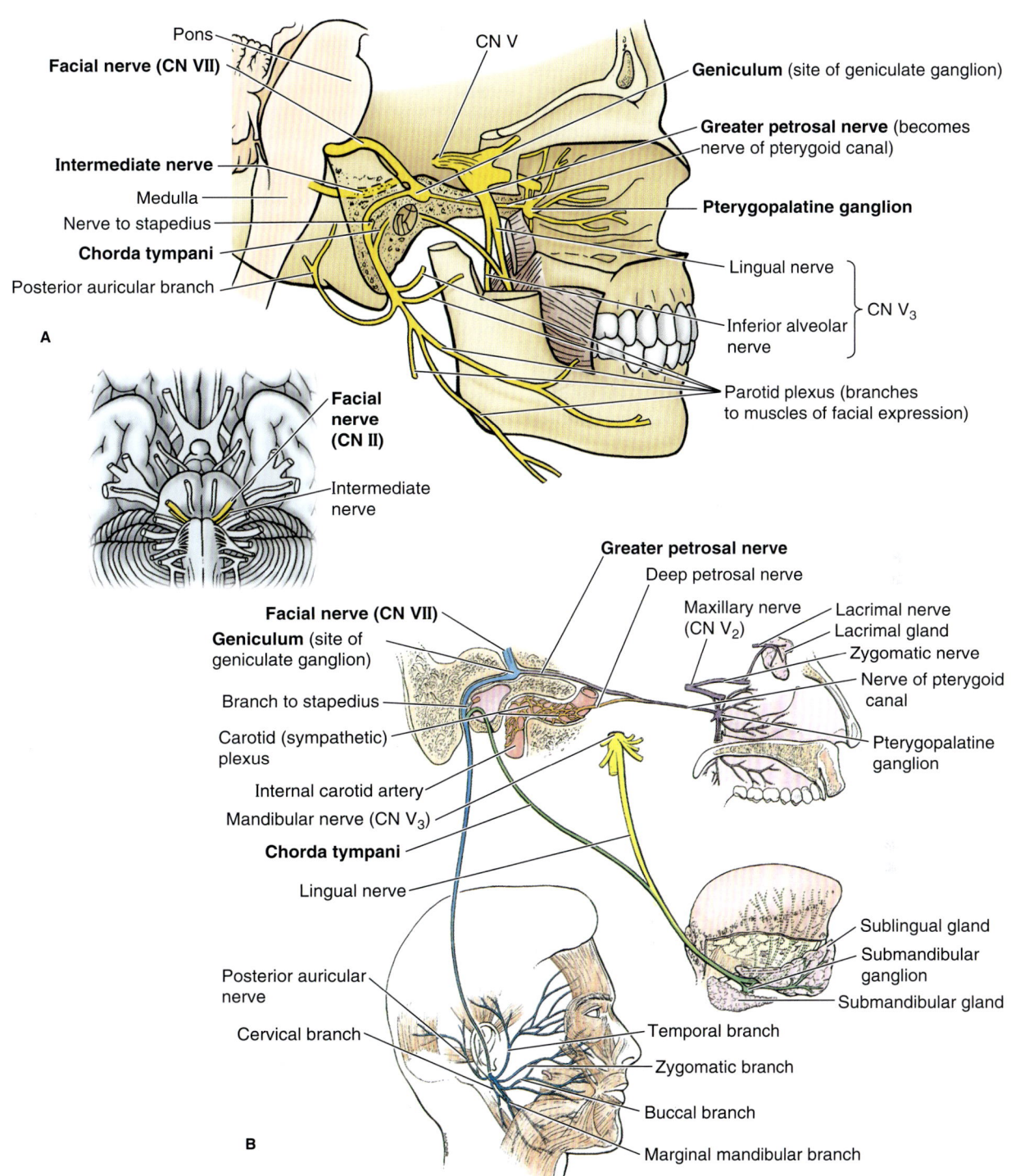

FIGURE 66.3 A,B: Distribution of the facial nerve (cranial nerve VII). The facial nerve emanates from the brainstem between the pons and the medulla. The motor part of the facial nerve arises from the facial nerve nucleus in the pons and divides into five branches after coursing through the petrous temporal bone, the internal auditory meatus, the facial canal, the stylomastoid foramen, and the parotid gland. It is responsible for muscles of facial expression and supplies preganglionic parasympathetic fibers to ganglia of the head and neck. It also supplies taste sensation to the anterior two-thirds of the tongue, partial afferent innervations of the oropharynx, as well as some cutaneous sensation around the auricle. *(Reprinted with permission from Moore KL, Dalley AF. Clinically Oriented Anatomy. 6th ed. Baltimore, MD: Lippincott Williams & Wilkins; 2009. Figure 9-10.)*

The cell bodies of parasympathetic axons within the nervus intermedius are contained within the superior salivatory nucleus. These axons synapse with neurons which supply parasympathetic innervations to the lachrymal gland as well as the submandibular and sublingual glands.

Nervus intermedius neuralgia involves severe pain deep in the ear which may radiate to the outer ear, mastoid, or eye region. The syndrome was reported as "tic douloureux of the sensory filaments of the facial nerve" by Clark and Taylor in 1909.[205] Rare cases continue to be reported.

ETIOLOGY

Vascular compression is suggested as the cause of many cases of nervus intermedius neuralgia. Jannetta[206] described relief of nervus intermedius and other cranial neuralgias following MVD in 1976. He reviewed 14 cases of nervus intermedius neuralgia, which, after failed conservative treatment, went on to MVD. Over 71% experienced an excellent outcome, over 21% experienced partial relief, and 7% had no relief following MVD. Good long-term results were seen in 90% of patients.

In a 1991 review of 18 cases of "primary otalgia" seen over a 15-year period, vascular loops, adhesions, thickened arachnoid, and benign osteoma were among abnormalities involving the nervus intermedius. The authors reported decompression of cranial nerves V, IX, X, the tympanic nerve and the chorda tympani in addition to the nervus intermedius in many of these cases.[207,208] Nonetheless, the existence of nervus intermedius as a unique entity has been questioned due to the similarity of its presentation to that of glossopharyngeal neuralgia.

SYMPTOMS AND SIGNS

The pain of nervus intermedius neuralgia is sharp, lancinating, and paroxysmal. Painful attacks are unilateral and can be triggered by cold, noise, swallowing, or touch. Patients may also experience symptoms such as increased salivation, bitter taste, tinnitus, and vertigo during paroxysms. Patients with nervus intermedius neuralgia may also rarely have pain in the trigeminal distribution. This may be due to cross compression of cranial nerve V in addition to the nervus intermedius (as has been seen on surgical exploration).[209]

DIAGNOSIS

Sensation is supplied to the area of the ear by the cranial nerves V, VII, VIII, IX, and X and the second and third cervical nerves. A thorough history should be taken to ascertain the exact distribution and character of the pain as well as any triggers or precipitating factors. A comprehensive examination should rule out other causes of otalgia before the diagnosis of geniculate ganglion neuralgia can be made. This should include examinations of the nose, paranasal sinuses, mouth, teeth, nasopharynx, pharynx, and larynx to rule out other causes of pain, audiogram, auditory evoked response potentials, and vestibular tests. MRI with gadolinium enhancement of the brain, cerebellopontine angle, and facial nerve and MRA should be performed. As described earlier, vascular compression or other pathology may involve more than one of the cranial nerves in the middle fossa.

As described in the previous section, nervus intermedius neuralgia can be caused by HZ infection. The pain from acute HZ involving the geniculate ganglion is usually constant and burning as opposed to the lancinating paroxysmal pain of nervus intermedius neuralgia. Onset of the pain from acute HZ is generally followed by a vesicular eruption involving the eardrum and external auditory canal.

TREATMENT

Pharmacologic treatment of nervus intermedius neuralgia is similar to that of TN. When conservative management fails, a thorough workup to exclude other causes of pain should be investigated. The nervus intermedius or geniculate ganglion cannot be injected with local anesthetic or other solution; however, blockade of other nerves supplying the area of the ear can be anesthetized to exclude them as causes of the otalgia. Surgical management consists of MVD or section of the nervus intermedius. Excision of the nervus intermedius and geniculate ganglion has also been advocated along with selective retrolabyrinthine V nerve section in extreme cases.[208]

Glossopharyngeal Neuralgia

Glossopharyngeal neuralgia is a rare neuralgia with a reported relative frequency of 0.75% to 1% compared to TN.[210,211] It is defined as paroxysmal pain in the areas supplied by cranial nerves IX and X. The glossopharyngeal or ninth cranial nerve exits the upper medulla just rostral to the vagus nerve.

Sensory fibers carried in the glossopharyngeal nerve supply the posterior one-third of the tongue, the tonsils, pharynx, the middle ear, and the carotid body. The glossopharyngeal nerve also supplies parasympathetic fibers to the parotid gland via the otic ganglion, motor fibers to the stylopharyngeus muscle, and contributes to the pharyngeal plexus. The symptoms associated with glossopharyngeal neuralgia can be better understood upon review of its branches, which include the tympanic nerve, stylopharyngeal nerve, tonsillar nerve, nerve to the carotid sinus, branches to the posterior third of the tongue, lingual branches, and a communicating branch to the vagus nerve (Fig. 66.4).

ETIOLOGY

Similar to TN nomenclature, classical or idiopathic and secondary or symptomatic forms of glossopharyngeal neuralgia exist. Idiopathic glossopharyngeal neuralgia occurs most commonly from vascular compression of cranial nerve IX (often in association with cranial nerve X). Symptomatic causes include tumors, peritonsillar abscess, carotid aneurysm, Chiari type I malformations, and Eagle syndrome (in which cranial nerve IX is compressed against an ossified stylohyoid ligament).[212-214] The vertebral artery or posterior inferior cerebellar arteries are most often implicated on surgical exploration.

SYMPTOMS AND SIGNS

The character of pain in the patient with glossopharyngeal neuralgia is similar to that of TN. The unbearable, electrical, lancinating pain is located unilaterally in the ear, larynx, tonsillar fossa, or base of the tongue. It is rarely bilateral. It may radiate toward the ear, the angle of the jaw, or the upper and lateral aspect of the neck. Paroxysms of pain are often triggered by swallowing, yawning, coughing, or talking.

DIAGNOSIS

A careful history and physical exam is essential in the evaluation of a patient suspected of suffering from glossopharyngeal neuralgia. MRI/MRA should be performed to rule out a mass lesion or vascular pathology. An ossified stylohyoid ligament (consistent with Eagle syndrome) may be identified on roentgenogram. As in TN, the paroxysms of glossopharyngeal neuralgia may last from seconds to minutes. Dozens of attacks may occur daily with episodes lasting from weeks to months followed by periods of remission. The patient is generally free from pain between attacks, although dull background pain may persist. Investigation should also exclude MS in younger patients with bilateral symptoms or neurologic deficits. The branch of the glossopharyngeal nerve to the carotid sinus is involved in maintenance of blood pressure and is thought to play a role in some profound cardiac arrhythmias or even asystole which occur in some patients in association with pain paroxysms. The differential diagnosis includes geniculate or nervus intermedius neuralgia. Rare glossopharyngeal zoster has been reported.[215]

TREATMENT

The pharmacologic treatment of glossopharyngeal neuralgia is similar to TN. When conservative therapy has failed, surgical exploration and vascular decompression has been shown to be highly effective on long-term follow-up with a low complication rate.[216,217] When a source of neurovascular compression is not found, successful relief of symptoms has been obtained with section of the glossopharyngeal nerve together with the upper fibers of the vagus nerve.[218,219]

Vagal Neuralgia

The two sensory branches of the vagus nerve, the auricular branch and the superior laryngeal nerve, are involved in this rare neuralgia (Fig. 66.5). The auricular branch of the vagus nerve, or Alderman's nerve, divides into two branches: the posterior

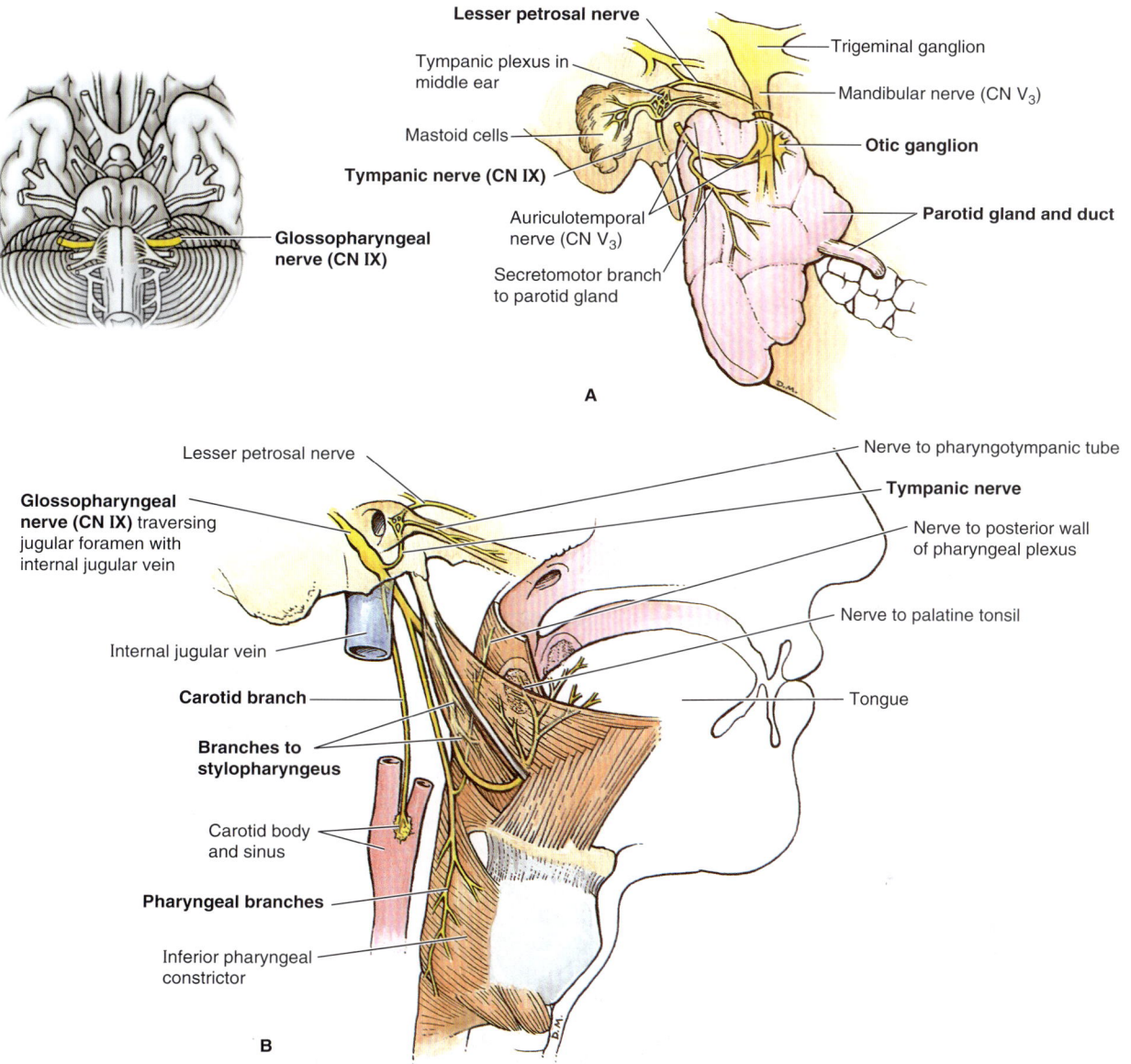

FIGURE 66.4 Distribution of the glossopharyngeal nerve. **A:** The glossopharyngeal nerve exits the skull via the jugular foramen between the internal jugular vein and internal carotid artery, lateral and ventral to the vagus and accessory nerves. It receives general sensory fibers via the tympanic nerve, the nerve to the palatine tonsils, and pharyngeal nerve branches. It receives special sensory fibers (taste) from the posterior one-third of the tongue and visceral sensory fibers from the carotid bodies and carotid sinus. **B:** The parasympathetic component of the glossopharyngeal nerve supplies the postsynaptic innervations to the parotid gland via the otic ganglion. The glossopharyngeal nerve is responsible for the afferent limb of the gag reflex, and thus, the gag reflex is absent in patients with damage to the glossopharyngeal nerve. The efferent limb of the gag reflex is supplied by the vagus nerve. *(Reprinted with permission from Moore KL, Dalley AF. Clinically Oriented Anatomy. 6th ed. Baltimore, MD: Lippincott Williams & Wilkins; 2009. Figure 9-13.)*

auricular nerve and the nerve supplying the auricula and posterior part of the external acoustic meatus. The superior laryngeal nerve descends behind the internal carotid artery and divides into the internal and external laryngeal nerves. The internal laryngeal nerve supplies sensation to the base of the tongue, epiglottis, and the larynx to above the vocal cords. The external laryngeal nerve supplies the cricothyroid muscle and the inferior pharyngeal constrictor and communicates with the superior cardiac nerve behind the common carotid artery.

ETIOLOGY

Idiopathic or classic vagal neuralgia is characterized by lack of a known precipitating lesion or by vascular compression of the upper fibers of the vagus nerve as they leave the brainstem. Secondary or symptomatic vagal neuralgia involving the superior laryngeal branch has been reported to be secondary to multiple causes including deviation of the hyoid bone, lateral

pharyngeal diverticulum, and as a complication following carotid endarterectomy.[220–222]

SYMPTOMS AND SIGNS

Vagal neuralgia is characterized by severe pain paroxysms in the submandibular region, throat, and/or under the ear. Attacks are triggered by swallowing, talking, yawning, coughing, or straining and turning the head. A trigger zone is generally present in the larynx or lateral aspect of the throat overlying the hyoid bone. Compression of the vagus nerve has also been reported to be associated with intractable hiccups, coughing, spontaneous gagging, and dysphagia.[223,224]

DIAGNOSIS

The diagnosis of vagal neuralgia is based on a thorough history to define the distinct characteristics and precipitating factors of the patient's pain. A careful exam of the head and neck

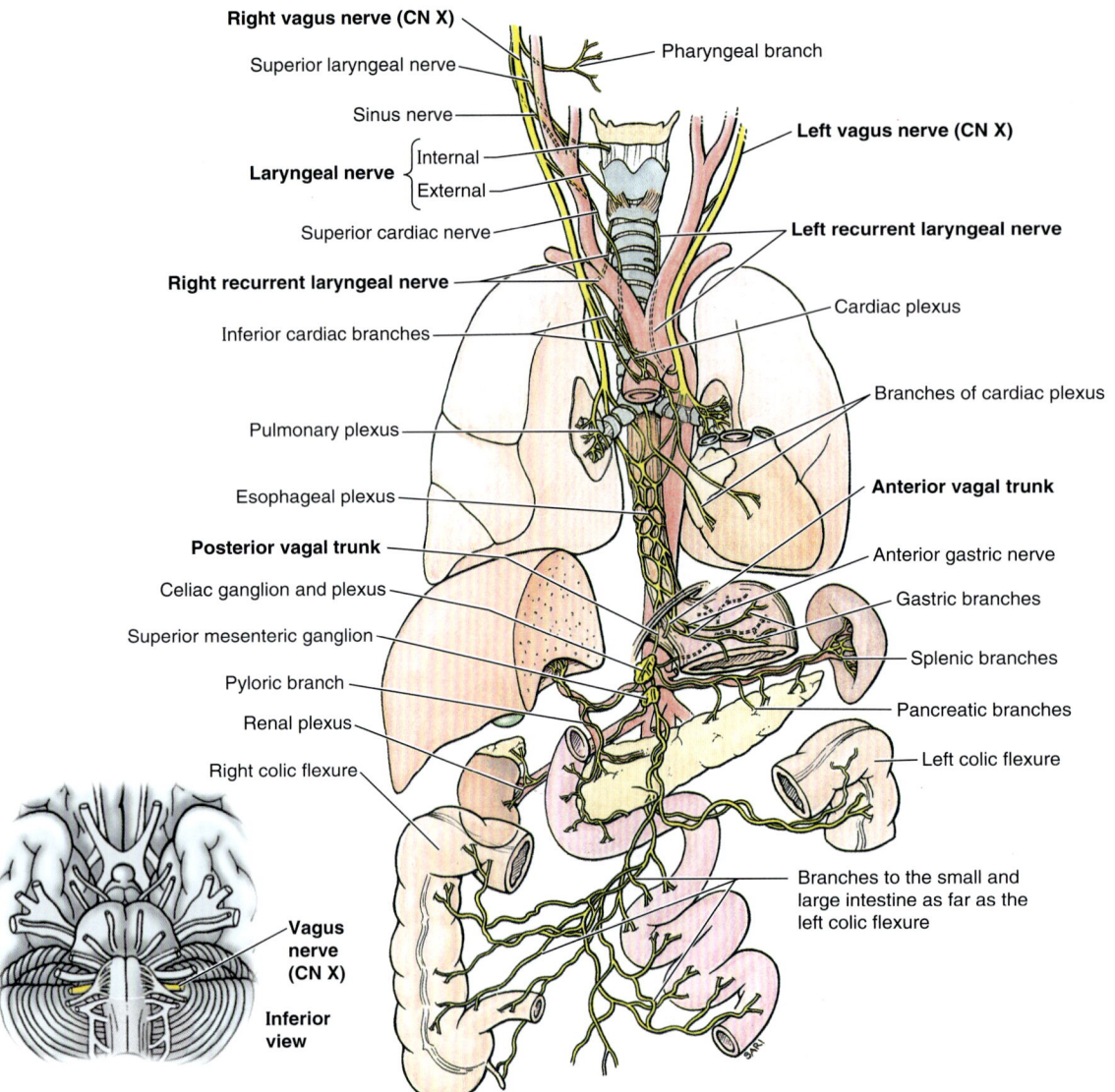

FIGURE 66.5 Distribution of the vagus nerve (cranial nerve X). The vagus nerve originates in the brainstem and courses through the jugular foramen to extend into the head, neck, thorax, and abdomen where it provides efferent motor parasympathetic innervation to viscera as well as afferent innervation that delivers information about the state of organs to the brain. (*Reprinted with permission from Moore KL, Dalley AF. Clinically Oriented Anatomy. 6th ed. Baltimore, MD: Lippincott Williams & Wilkins; 2009. Figure 10-16.*)

should be performed to rule out other pathology. MRI/MRA should be performed to rule out compressive mass lesions or neurovascular compression. Hoarseness of speech and a trigger point superolateral to the thyroid cartilage may be noted on exam of the patient. Differential diagnosis includes glossopharyngeal neuralgia, geniculate neuralgia, and carotidynia.

TREATMENT
Pharmacologic therapy of vagal neuralgia is identical to that of TN. Successful treatment of superior laryngeal neuralgia with high concentration lidocaine injections after CBZ treatment failure has been reported.[225] Surgical treatment following pharmacologic therapy failure warrants consideration. MVD has been successful when neurovascular compression of the vagus is identified. When no compressive lesion is identified, relief of pain can be obtained following section of the glossopharyngeal nerve and the upper rootlets of the vagus nerves. The medial aspect of the descending trigeminal tract has also been sectioned in refractory cases to produce loss of pain and temperature sensation in the pharynx.[226] Kandan et al.[227] reported that

21 patients with glossopharyngeal and vagus nerves neuralgias underwent surgery over 19 years, with MVD being the most common procedure. Treatment outcomes were reported as similar to surgical treatments of TN.

Other Terminal Branch Neuralgias

Rare neuralgias involving branches of the trigeminal nerve have been reported. These include supraorbital neuralgia, nasociliary neuralgia, infraorbital neuralgia, and nummular headache. Injury or entrapment of other peripheral branches of the trigeminal nerve such as the lingual, alveolar, or mental nerves may result in pain in the area supplied by that branch.

Supraorbital neuralgia is characterized by paroxysmal or constant pain in the region of the supraorbital notch. It is unilateral and radiates to the medial aspect of the forehead in the area supplied by the supraorbital nerve. It can be caused by injury or entrapment of the supraorbital nerve at its outlet. The pain is transiently relieved by injection of a small volume of local anesthetic at the supraorbital notch. Medical treatment is often unsuccessful when entrapment of the nerve is present. Successful treatment with cryoablation and surgical release of the nerve at its outlet has been reported.[228,229]

Nasociliary neuralgia, or Charlin's neuralgia, is a rare condition characterized by stabbing pain lasting seconds to hours in one side of the nose. The pain radiates to the medial frontal region and is triggered by touching the lateral aspect of the ipsilateral nostril. Temporary relief from pain following local anesthetic blockade of the nasociliary nerve is diagnostic. Inflammatory cutaneous lesions and chronic sinusitis have been implicated as secondary causes of nasociliary neuralgia.[230,231] Relief following surgical section of the nasociliary nerve, turbinectomy, and septoplasty has been described.[232]

Infraorbital neuralgia has been reported most frequently in association with posttraumatic entrapment syndromes.[233] If pain is not successfully alleviated by reduction of zygomatic fracture and mobilization of surrounding soft tissue and bone, pharmacologic therapy with antiepileptic agents alone or combined with antidepressants such as the tricyclics or serotonin norepinephrine reuptake inhibitors may be effective.

Nummular headache is thought to be neuralgia related to a terminal cutaneous branch of the trigeminal nerve. It has been described as a primary disorder characterized by head pain felt exclusively in a small round area generally 2 to 6 cm in diameter. The pain is not attributed to another disorder, and neurologic and neuroimaging exams are normal by definition. A constant background pain may be described as well as exacerbations which are spontaneous or triggered by combing the hair or touch in the affected area. A 2013 review found that gabapentin was effective in 60% of subjects, TCAs in about 45% and peripheral nerve block in 42% of the cases.[234] In patients refractory to pharmacologic therapy, nerve blocks are also effective. Despite small sample size, onabotulinum toxin A was reported to reduce pain for an average of 14 weeks after initial and repeat injections.[235]

In all cases of idiopathic neuralgia of the terminal branches of the trigeminal nerve, a careful history and physical exam to rule out other causes of facial pain the is imperative. Age less than 40 years and presence of neurologic deficit should prompt further diagnostic radiologic exams to rule out compressive lesions.

Other Cranial Neuralgia–Related Causes of Pain: Anesthesia Dolorosa

Anesthesia dolorosa is also known as painful posttraumatic trigeminal neuropathy.

ETIOLOGY

Anesthesia dolorosa is defined as perception of pain in an area that is anesthetic. It is a dreaded complication of trigeminal nerve surgery, including partial nerve sections, MVD, percutaneous gangliolysis, neurolytic injections, and stereotactic radiosurgery. It has also been reported after penetrating cranial injury.[236] The area of persistent and painful anesthesia is in the distribution of the injured nerve.

SYMPTOMS AND SIGNS

The patient with anesthesia dolorosa complains of burning, pulling, or stabbing pain which can also include a sharp, stinging, shooting, or electrical component. The pain often increases with cold or with rapid temperature changes.

DIAGNOSIS

As it pertains to the head and face, anesthesia dolorosa typically involves the territory of a specific branch or branches of the trigeminal nerve or the occipital nerve. Quantitative sensory testing may be used to confirm lack of sensation.

TREATMENT

There are no controlled trials evaluating pharmacologic therapy for anesthesia dolorosa. Empiric treatment of pain by clinical characteristics has led to use of anticonvulsants in patients with lancinating and electrical pain; tricyclic antidepressants, and serotonin norepinephrine reuptake inhibitors in patients with burning pain; and intravenous lidocaine and ketamine infusions in patients unresponsive to other pharmacologic therapy.[237,238] Motor cortex stimulation was the recommended surgical treatment of choice for facial anesthesia dolorosa according to authors of a review of the literature on central and neuropathic pain over the last 15 years. Motor cortex stimulation may act by replacing nociceptive with nonnociceptive sensory input at the cortical, thalamic, brainstem, and spinal level. It may also interfere with the emotional component of nociceptive perception.[239] In a prospective study of 10 patients undergoing trial and treatment with motor cortex stimulation, patients with facial weakness and sensory loss regained both strength and discriminative sensation during stimulation.[240] Raslan et al.[241] reported positive results of motor cortex stimulation for trigeminal neuropathic or deafferentation pain. Anesthesia dolorosa did not appear to respond to deep brain stimulation according to one 15-year series of 141 patients.[242]

Conclusion

Diagnosis of trigeminal or other cranial neuralgias requires knowledge of the features of neuralgic pain, a thorough understanding of the unique characteristics and specific anatomic distribution of each cranial nerve, and familiarity with the distinctive features of other pain syndromes involving the structures of the head and neck is essential to establishing. Although the cranial neuralgias are rare when compared with other neuropathic pain syndromes, the extreme suffering encountered in patients who present with these syndromes, together with the need to distinguish between classical and symptomatic presentations, mandates advanced neuroimaging in all cases to rule out progressive processes such as intracranial tumors, infection, or MS. Pharmacologic, surgical, and percutaneous therapies for the cranial neuralgias have continued to advance with development of new agents and techniques which are associated with fewer side effects and complications. Improved monitoring in the case of surgical and percutaneous therapies have also been instrumental in reducing patient morbidity and mortality.

References

1. Burchiel KJ. A new classification for facial pain. *Neurosurgery* 2003;53: 1164–1166.
2. Headache Classification Committee of the International Headache Society. The International Classification of Headache Disorders, 3rd edition (beta version). *Cephalalgia* 2013;33(9):629–808.
3. Nurmikko TJ, Eldridge PR. Trigeminal neuralgia—pathophysiology, diagnosis and current treatment. *Br J Anaesth* 2001;87(1):117–132.
4. Zebenholzer K, Wöber C, Vigl M, et al. Facial pain and the second edition of the International Classification of Headache Disorders. *Headache* 2006;46(2):259–263.
5. Jääskeläinen SK, Forssell H, Tenovuo O. Electrophysiological testing of the trigeminofacial system: aid in the diagnosis of atypical facial pain. *Pain* 1999;80:191–200.
6. Nielsen LA, Henriksson KG. Mechanisms in chronic musculoskeletal pain (fibromyalgia): the role of central and peripheral sensitization and pain disinhibition. *Best Pract Res Clin Rhematol* 2007;21(3):465–480.
7. Burchiel KJ. Trigeminal neuropathic pain. *Acta Neurochir Suppl (Wien)* 1993;58:145–149.
8. Merskey H, Bogduk N. *Classification of Chronic Pain. Descriptions of Chronic Pain Syndromes and Definitions of Pain Terms.* Seattle, WA: IASP Press; 1994:59–71.
9. Cowan JA, Brahma B, Sagher O. Surgical treatment of trigeminal neuralgia: comparison of microvascular decompression, percutaneous ablation, and stereotactic radiosurgery. Surgical management of chronic pain. *Tech Neurosurg* 2003;8(3):157–167.

10. Block A, Kremer EF, Fernandez E. *Handbook of Pain Syndromes: Biopsychosocial Perspectives.* Mahwah, NJ: Lawrence Erlbaum Associates; 1999;435–436.

11. Cole CD, Liu JK, Apfelbaum RI. Historical perspectives on the diagnosis and treatment of trigeminal neuralgia. *Neurosurg Focus* 2005;18(5):1–10.

12. Hurd EP. *A Treatise on Neuralgia.* Detroit, MI: George S. Davis; 1890.

13. Jannetta P. Neurovascular compression in cranial nerve and systemic disease. *Ann Surg* 1980;192:518–525.

14. Jannetta PJ. Arterial compression of the trigeminal nerve at the pons in patients with trigeminal neuralgia. *J Neurosurg* 1967;17:159–180.

15. Brewis M, Poskanzer DC, Rolland C, et al. Neurological disease in an English city. *Acta Neurol Scand* 1966;42(suppl 24):1–89.

16. Kurtzke JF. The current neurologic burden of illness and injury in the United States. *Neurology* 1982;32:1207–1214.

17. Katusic S, Beard CM, Bergstralh E, et al. Incidence and clinical features of trigeminal neuralgia, Rochester, Minnesota, 1945–1984. *Ann Neurol* 1990;27(1):89–95.

18. MacDonald BK, Cockerell OC, Sander JW, et al. The incidence and lifetime prevalence of neurological disorders in a prospective community based study in the UK. *Brain* 2000;123:664–676.

19. Hall GC, Carroll D, Parry D, et al. Epidemiology and treatment of neuropathic pain: the UK primary care perspective. *Pain* 2006;122(1–2):156–162.

20. Lopes PG, Castro ES Jr, Lopes LH. Trigeminal neuralgia in children: two case reports. *Pediatr Neurol* 2002;26(4):309–310.

21. Ramanathan M, Parameshwarman AA, Jayakumar N, et al. Reactivation of trigeminal neuralgia following distraction osteogenesis in an 8-year-old child: report of a unique case. *J Indian Soc Pedod Prev Dent* 2007;25(1):49–51.

22. Love S, Coakham HB. Trigeminal neuralgia: pathology and pathogenesis. *Brain* 2001;124(12):2347–2360.

23. McLaughln MR, Jannetta PJ, Clyde BL, et al. Microvascular decompression of cranial nerves: lessons learned after 4400 operations. *J Neurosurg* 1999;90:1–8.

24. Malis LI. Petrous ridge compression and its surgical correction. *J Neurosurg* 2007;107:220–224.

25. Kerr FW. Evidence for a peripheral etiology of trigeminal neuralgia. *J Neurosurg* 2007;107:225–231.

26. Calvin WH, Loeser JD, Howe JF. A neurophysiological theory for the pain mechanism of tic douloureux. *Pain* 1977;3:147–154.

27. Fromm GH, Chattha AS, Terrence CF, et al. Role of inhibitory mechanisms in trigeminal neuralgia. *Neurology* 1981;31:683–687.

28. Selçuk P, Kurtkaya O, Uzün I, et al. Microanatomy of the central myelin-peripheral myelin transition zone of the trigeminal nerve. *Neurosurgery* 2006;59:354–359.

29. Devor M, Govrin-Lippmann R, Rappaport ZH. Mechanism of trigeminal neuralgia: an ultrastructural analysis of trigeminal root specimens obtained during microvascular decompression surgery. *J Neurosurg* 2002;96(3):532–543.

30. Rappaport ZH. An electron-microscopic analysis of biopsy samples of the trigeminal root taken during microvascular decompressive surgery. *Stereotact Funct Neurosurg* 1997;68(1–4 pt 1):182–186.

31. Love S, Gradidge T, Coakham HB. Trigeminal neuralgia due to multiple sclerosis: ultrastructural findings in trigeminal rhizotomy specimens. *Neuropathol Appl Neurobiol* 2001;27(3):238–244.

32. Obermann M, Yoon MS, Ese D, et al. Impaired trigeminal nociceptive processing in patients with trigeminal neuralgia. *Neurology* 2007;69:835–841.

33. Watson JC. From paroxysmal to chronic pain in trigeminal neuralgia implications of central sensitization. *Neurology* 2007;69:817–818.

34. Cruccu G, Biasiotta A, Galeotti F, et al. Diagnostic accuracy of trigeminal reflex testing in trigeminal neuralgia. *Neurology* 2006;66:139–141.

35. Gronseth G, Cruccu G, Alksne J, et al. Practice parameter: the diagnostic evaluation and treatment of trigeminal neuralgia (an evidence-based review): report of the Quality Standards Subcommittee of the American Academy of Neurology and the European Federation of Neurological Societies. *Neurology* 2008;71(15):1183–1190.

36. White JC, Sweet WH. *Pain and the Neurosurgeon.* Springfield, IL: Charles C. Thomas; 1969.

37. White JC, Sweet WH. *Pain, Its Mechanisms and Neurosurgical Control.* Springfield, IL: Charles C. Thomas; 1969.

38. Davies EW, Naffziger HC. Major trigeminal neuralgia. An analysis of two hundred and forty-five cases. *Calif Med* 1948;68:130–134.

39. Rushton JG, MacDonald HN. Trigeminal neuralgia: special considerations of nonsurgical treatment. *JAMA* 1957;165:437.

40. Wilkins R. Trigeminal neuralgia: introduction. In: Wilkins R, Rengachary S, eds. *Neurosurgery.* New York: McGraw-Hill; 1985:2337–2344.

41. Peet MM, Schneider RC. Trigeminal neuralgia: a review of six hundred and eighty-nine cases with a follow-up study on sixty-five percent of the group. *J Neurosurg* 1957;9:367–377.

42. Harris W. An analysis of 1,433 cases of paroxysmal trigeminal neuralgia (trigeminal-tic) and the en-results of gasserian alcohol injection. *Brain* 1940;63:209–224.

43. Ruge D, Brochner R, Davis L. A study of the treatment of 637 patients with trigeminal neuralgia. *J Neurosurg* 1958;15:528–536.

44. Jackson EM, Bussard GM, Hoard MA, et al. Trigeminal neuralgia: a diagnostic challenge. *Am J Emerg Med* 1999;17:597–600.

45. Gass A, Kitchen N, MacManus DG, et al. Trigeminal neuralgia in patients with multiple sclerosis: lesion localization with magnetic resonance imaging. *Neurology* 1997;49:1142–1144.

46. Albrecht K, Krump J. Diagnosis, differential diagnosis and possibilities for treatment of trigeminal neuralgia: with special reference to the conservative treatment with hydantoin drugs and vitamin B12 [in German]. *Munch Med Wochenschr* 1954;96:985.

47. Kugelberg E, Lindblom U. The mechanism of the pain in trigeminal neuralgia. *J Neurol Neurosurg Psychiatry* 1959;22:36–43.

48. Symonds C. Facial pain. *Ann R Coll Surg Engl* 1949;4:206.

49. Mitchell RG. Pre-trigeminal neuralgia. *Br Dent J* 1980;149:167.

50. Fromm GH, Graff-Radford SB, Terrence CF, et al. Pre-trigeminal neuralgia. *Neurology* 1990;40:1493–1495.

51. Sawaya RA. Trigeminal neuralgia associated with sinusitis. *ORL J Otorhinolaryngol Relat Space* 2000;62:160–163.

52. Lin YW, Lin SK, Weng IH. Fatal paranasal sinusitis presenting as trigeminal neuralgia. *Headache* 2006;46(1):174–178.

53. Cheng TM, Cascino TL, Onofrio BM. Comprehensive study of diagnosis and treatment of trigeminal neuralgia secondary to tumors. *Neurology* 1993;43:2298–2302.

54. Mathews ES, Scrivani SJ. Percutaneous stereotactic radiofrequency thermal rhizotomy for the treatment of trigeminal neuralgia. *Mt Sinai J Med* 2000;67:288–299.

55. Metzer SW. Trigeminal neuralgia secondary to tumor with normal exam, responsive to carbamazepine. *Headache* 1991;31(3):164–166.

56. Jamjoom AB, Jamjoom ZA, al-Fehaily M, et al. Trigeminal neuralgia related to cerebellopontine angle tumors. *Neurosurg Rev* 1996;19(4):237–241.

57. Meng L, Yuguang L, Feng L, et al. Cerebellopontine angle epidermoids presenting with trigeminal neuralgia. *J Clin Neurosci* 2005;12(7):784–786.

58. Tanaka T, Morimoto Y, Shiiba S, et al. Utility of magnetic resonance cisternography using three-dimensional fast asymmetric spin-echo sequences with multiplanar reconstruction: the evaluation of sites of neurovascular compression of the trigeminal nerve. *Oral Surg Oral Med Oral Pathol Oral Radiol Endod* 2005;100(2):215–225.

59. Laha RK, Jannetta PJ. Glossopharyngeal neuralgia. *J Neurosurg* 1977;47:316–320.

60. Yentür EA, Yegül I. Nervus intermedius neuralgia: an uncommon pain syndrome with an uncommon etiology. *J Pain Symptom Manage* 2000;19(6):407–408.

61. Yeh HS, Tew JM Jr. Tic convulsif, the combination of geniculate neuralgia and hemifacial spasm relieved by vascular decompression. *Neurology* 1984;34(5):682–683.

62. Samii M, Günther T, Iaconetta G, et al. Microvascular decompression to treat hemifacial spasm: long-term results for a consecutive series of 143 patients. *Neurosurgery* 2002;50(4):712–718.

63. Goadsby PJ. Pathophysiology of cluster headache: a trigeminal autonomic cephalgia. *Lancet Neurol* 2002;1(4):251–257.

64. Bussone G, Usai S. Trigeminal autonomic cephalgias: from pathophysiology to clinical aspects. *Neurol Sci* 2004;25(suppl 3):S74–S76.

65. Boes CJ, Swanson JW. Paroxysmal hemicrania, SUNCT and hemicrania continua. *Semin Neurol* 2006;26(2):260–270.

66. Cohen AS, Matharu MS, Goadsby PJ. Short-lasting unilateral neuralgiform headache attacks with conjunctival injection and tearing (SUNCT) or cranial autonomic features (SUNA)—a prospective clinical study of SUNCT and SUNA. *Brain* 2006;129(10):2746–2760.

67. Bigal ME, Lipton RB. The differential diagnosis of chronic daily headaches: an algorithm-based approach. *J Headache Pain* 2007;8(5):263–272.

68. Rosenfeld RM. Clinical practice guideline on adult sinusitis. *Otolaryngol Head Neck Surg* 2007;137(3):365–377.

69. Zakrzewska JM. *Trigeminal Neuralgia. Major Problems in Neurology: 28.* London: WB Saunders; 1995:63–72.

70. Israel HA, Scivani SJ. The interdisciplinary approach to oral, facial and head pain. *J Am Dent Assoc* 2000;131(7):919–926.

71. Eide PK, Rabben T. Trigeminal neuropathic pain: pathophysiological mechanisms examined by quantitative assessment of abnormal pain and sensory perception. *Neurosurgery* 1998;43(5):1103–1110.

72. Lang E, Kaltenhäuser M, Seidler S, et al. Persistent idiopathic facial pain exists independent from somatosensory input from the painful region: findings from quantitative sensory functions and somatotopy of the primary somatosensory cortex. *Pain* 2005;118(1–2):80–91.

73. Bergougan M. Cures hereuses de nevralgies faciales essentielles par le diphenyl-hydantoinate de soude. *Rev Laryng Otol Rhino* 1942;63:34.

74. Trousseau A. De la nevralgie epileptiforme. *Arch Gen Med* 1853;1:33.

75. Jorns TP, Zakrzewska JM. Evidence-based approach to the medical management of trigeminal neuralgia. *Br J Neurosurg* 2007;21(3):253–261.

76. Cruccu G, Gronseth G, Alksne J, et al. AAN-EFNS guidelines on trigeminal neuralgia management. *Eur J Neurol* 2008;15(10):1013–1028.

77. Campbell FG, Graham JG, Zilkha KJ. Clinical trial of carbamazepine (Tegretol) in trigeminal neuralgia. *J Neurol Neurosurg Psychiatry* 1966;29:265–267.

78. Rockliff BW, Davis EH. Controlled sequential trials of carbamazepine in trigeminal neuralgia. *Arch Neurol* 1966;15:129–136.

79. Killian JM, Fromm GH. Carbamazepine in the treatment of neuralgia. *Arch Neurol* 1968;19:129–136.

80. Nichol CF. A four year double-blind study of Tegretol in facial pain. *Headache* 1969;9:54–57.
81. Wiffen P, Collins S, McQuay H, et al. Anticonvulsant drugs for acute and chronic pain. *Cochrane Database Syst Rev* 2005;(3):CD001133.
82. Taylor JC, Brauer S, Espir ML. Long-term treatment of trigeminal neuralgia. *Postgrad Med J* 1981;57:16–18.
83. Tomson T, Ekbom K. Trigeminal neuralgia: time course of pain in relation to carbamazepine dosing. *Cephalalgia* 1981;1:91–97.
84. Hart RG, Easton DJ. Carbamazepine and hematologic monitoring. *Ann Neurol* 1982;11:309–312.
85. Liebel JT, Menger N, Langohn H. Oxcarbaepine in der Behandlung der Trigeminusneuralgie. *Nervenheikunde* 2001;20:461–465.
86. Gronseth G, Gruccu G, Alksne J, et al. The diagnostic evaluation and treatment of trigeminal neuralgia. (An evidence based review: Report of the Quality Standards Subcommittee of the American Academy of Neurology and the European Federation of Neurological Societies). *Neurology* 2008;71(15):1183–1190.
87. Zakrezewsk JM, Chaudhry Z, Nurmikko TJ, et al. Lamotrigine (Lamictal) in refractory trigeminal neuralgia: results from a double-blind placebo controlled crossover trial. *Pain* 1997;73:223–230.
88. Leandri M, Lundardi G, Inglese M, et al. Lamotrigine in trigeminal neuralgia secondary to multiple sclerosis. *J Neurol* 2000;247:556–558.
89. Canavero S, Bonicalzi V, Ferroli P, et al. Lamotrigine control of idiopathic trigeminal neuralgia [letter]. *J Neurol Neurosurg Psychiatry* 1995;59:646.
90. Iannone A, Baker AB, Morrell F. Dilantin in the treatment of trigeminal neuralgia. *Neurology* 1958;8:126–128.
91. Braham J, Saia A. Phenytoin in the treatment of trigeminal and other neuralgias. *Lancet* 1960;2:892–893.
92. McCleane GJ. Intravenous infusion of phenytoin relieves neuropathic pain: a randomized, double-blinded, placebo-controlled, crossover study. *Anesth Analg* 1999;89:985–988.
93. Cheshire WP. Fosphenytoin: an intravenous option for the management of acute trigeminal neuralgia crisis. *J Pain Symptom Manage* 2001;21:506–510.
94. Fromm GH, Terrence CF, Chattha AS, et al. Baclofen in trigeminal neuralgia: its effect on the spinal trigeminal nucleus: a pilot study. *Arch Neurol* 1980;37:768–771.
95. Fromm GH, Terrence CF, Chattha AS. Baclofen in the treatment of trigeminal neuralgia: double-blind study and long-term follow-up. *Ann Neurol* 1984;15:240–244.
96. Fromm GH, Terrence CF. Comparison of L-baclofen and racemic baclofen in trigeminal neuralgia. *Neurology* 1987;37:1725–1728.
97. Parekh S, Shah K, Kotdawalla H, et al. Baclofen in carbamazepine resistant trigeminal neuralgia-a double blind clinical trial. *Cephalalgia* 1989;9:392–393.
98. Kanai A, Suzuki A, Kobayashi M, et al. Intranasal lidocaine 8% spray for second division trigeminal neuralgia. *Br J Anaesth* 2007;98(2):275.
99. Obermann M, Yoon M, Sensen K, et al. Efficacy of pregabalin in the treatment of trigeminal neuralgia. *Cephalalgia* 2008;28(2):174–181.
100. Jorns TP, Johnston A, Zakrzewska JM. Pilot study to evaluate the efficacy and tolerability of levetiracetam (Keppra) in treatment of patients with trigeminal neuralgia. *Eur J Neurol* 2009;16(6):740–744.
101. Mitsikostas DD, Pantes GV, Avramidis TG, et al. An observational trial to investigate the efficacy and tolerability of levetiracetam in trigeminal neuralgia. *Headache* 2010;50(8):1371–1377.
102. Peiris JB, Perera GL, Devendra SV, et al. Sodium valproate in trigeminal neuralgia. *Med J Aust* 1980;2:278.
103. Karlov VA, Savitskaia ON. Comparative effectiveness of antiepileptic preparations in the treatment of patients with trigeminal neuralgia. *Zh Nevropatol Psikhiatr Im S S Korsakova* 1980;80:530–535.
104. Court JE, Kase CS. Treatment of tic douloureux with a new anticonvulsant (clonazepam). *J Neurol Neurosurg Psychiatry* 1976;39:297–299.
105. Lechin F, vad der Dijs B, Lechin ME, et al. Pimozide therapy for trigeminal neuralgia. *Arch Neurol* 1989;46:960–963.
106. Wiffen PJ, McQuay HJ, Edwards JE, et al. Gabapentin for acute and chronic pain. *Cochrane Database Syst Rev* 2005;(3):CD005452.
107. Gilron I, Booher SL, Rowan JS, et al. Topiramate in trigeminal neuralgia: a randomized, placebo-controlled multiple cross-over pilot study. *Clin Neuropharmacol* 2001;24:109–112.
108. Zvartau-Hind M, Din MU, Gilani A, et al. Topiramate relieves refractory trigeminal neuralgia in MS patients. *Neurology* 2000;55:1587–1588.
109. Wang Q, Bai M. Topiramate versus carbamazepine for the treatment of classical trigeminal neuralgia. *CNS Drugs* 2011;25(10):847–857.
110. Türk U, Ihan S, Alp R, et al. Botulinum toxin and intractable trigeminal neuralgia. *Clin Neuropharmacol* 2005;28(4):161–162.
111. Allam N, Brasis-Neto JP, Brown G, et al. Injections of botulinum toxin type a produce pain alleviation in intractable trigeminal neuralgia. *Clin J Pain* 2005;21(2):182–184.
112. Galer BS, Miller KV, Rowbotham MC. Response to intravenous lidocaine infusion differs based on clinical diagnosis and site of nervous system injury. *Neurology* 1993;43:1233–1235.
113. Umino M, Kohase H, Ideguchi S, et al. Long-term pain control in trigeminal neuralgia with local anesthetics using and indwelling catheter in the mandibular nerve. *Clin J Pain* 2002;18(3):196–199.
114. Radwan IA, Saito S, Goto F. High-concentration tetracaine for the management of trigeminal neuralgia: quantitative assessment of sensory function after peripheral nerve block. *Clin J Pain* 2001;17(4):323–326.
115. Goto F, Ishizaki K, Yoshikawa D, et al. The long lasting effects of peripheral nerve blocks for trigeminal neuralgia using high concentration of tetracaine dissolved in bupivacaine. *Pain* 1999;79(1):101–103.
116. Chang FS, Huang GS, Cherng CH, et al. Repeated peripheral nerve blocks by the co-administration of ketamine, morphine, and bupivacaine attenuate trigeminal neuralgia. *Can J Anesh* 2003;50(2):201–202.
117. Naja MZ, Al-Tannir M, Ziade MF, et al. Repeated nerve blocks with clonidine, fentanyl and bupivacaine for trigeminal neuralgia. *Anaesthesia* 2006;61:70–71.
118. Nique TA, Bennett CR. Inadvertent brainstem anesthesia following extraoral trigeminal V2-V3 blocks. *Oral Surg Oral Med Oral Pathol* 1981;51(5):468–470.
119. McLeod NM, Patton DW. Peripheral alcohol injections in the management of trigeminal neuralgia. *Oral Surg Oral Med Oral Pathol Oral Radiol Endod* 2007;104(1):12–17.
120. Shah SA, Khan MN, Shah SF, et al. Is peripheral alcohol injection of value in the treatment of trigeminal neuralgia? An analysis of 100 cases. *Int J Oral Maxillofac Surg* 2011;40(4):388–392.
121. Han KR, Kim C. Brief report: the long-term outcome of mandibular nerve block with alcohol for the treatment of trigeminal neuralgia. *Anesth Analg* 2010;111(2):550–553.
122. Fardy MJ, Zakrzewska JM, Patton DW. Peripheral surgical techniques for the management of trigeminal neuralgia-alcohol and glycerol injections. *Acta Neurochir (Wien)* 1994;129(3–4):181–184.
123. Erdem E, Alkan A. Peripheral glycerol injections in the treatment of idiopathic trigeminal neuralgia: retrospective analysis of 157 cases. *J Oral Maxillofac Surg* 2001;59(10):1176–1180.
124. Fardy MJ, Patton DW. Complications associated with peripheral alcohol injections in the management of trigeminal neuralgia. *Br J Oral Maxillofac Surg* 1994;32(6):387–391.
125. Wilkenson HA. Trigeminal nerve peripheral branch phenol/glycerol injections for tic douloureux. *J Neurosurg* 1999;90(5):828–832.
126. Wu C-J, Lian Y-J, Zheng Y-K, et al. Botulinum toxin type A for the treatment of trigeminal neuralgia: results from a randomized, double-blind, placebo-controlled trial. *Cephalalgia* 2012;32(6):443–450.
127. Zhang H, Lian Y, Ma Y, et al. Two doses of botulinum toxin type A for the treatment of trigeminal neuralgia: observation of therapeutic effect from a randomized, double-blind, placebo-controlled trial. *J Headache Pain* 2014;15(1):65.
128. Kondo A. Microvascular decompression surgery for trigeminal neuralgia. *Stereotact Funct Neurosurg* 2001;77(1–4):187–189.
129. Barker FG, Jannetta PJ, Bissonette PAC, et al. The long-term outcome of microvascular decompression for trigeminal neuralgia. *N Engl J Med* 1996;334(17):1077–1083.
130. Bohman L-E, Pierce J, Stephen JH, et al. Fully endoscopic microvascular decompression for trigeminal neuralgia: technique review and early outcomes. *Neurosurg Focus* 2014;37(4):E18. doi:10.3171/2014.7.FOCUS14318.
131. Lee JYK, Pierce JT, Sandhu SK, et al. Endoscopic versus microscopic microvascular decompression for trigeminal neuralgia: equivalent pain outcomes with possibly decreased postoperative headache after endoscopic surgery. *J Neurosurg* 2017;126(5):1676–1684.
132. Tronnier VM, Rasche D, Hamer J, et al. Treatment of idiopathic trigeminal neuralgia: comparison of long-term outcome after radiofrequency rhizotomy and microvascular decompression. *Neurosurgery* 2001;48(6):1261–1267.
133. Kalkanis SN, Eskandar EN, Carter BS, et al. Microvascular decompression surgery in the United States, 1996–2000: mortality rates, morbidity rates, and the effects of hospital and surgeon volumes. *Neurosurgery* 2003;52:1251–1261.
134. Zakrzewska JM, Jassim S, Bulman JS. A prospective, longitudinal study on patients with trigeminal neuralgia who underwent radiofrequency thermocoagulation of the Gasserian ganglion. *Pain* 1999;79(1):51–58.
135. Bergenheim AT, Asplund P, Linderoth B. Percutaneous retrogasserian balloon compression for trigeminal neuralgia: review of critical technical details and outcomes. *World Neurosurg* 2013;79(2):359–368. doi:10.1016/j.wneu.2012.03.014.
136. Lopez BC, Jamlyn PJ, Zakrzewska JM. Systematic review of ablative neurosurgical techniques for the treatment of trigeminal neuralgia. *Neurosurgery* 2004;54:973–983.
137. Baschnagel AM, Cartier JL, Dreyer J, et al. Trigeminal neuralgia pain relief after gamma knife stereotactic radiosurgery. *Clin Neurol Neurosurg* 2014;117:107–111.
138. Sheehan J, Pan HC, Stroila M, et al. Gamma knife surgery for trigeminal neuralgia: outcomes and prognostic factors. *J Neurosurg* 2005;102:434–441.
139. Lim M, Villavicencio AT, Burneikiene S, et al. CyberKnife for idiopathic trigeminal neuralgia. *Neurosurg Focus* 2005;18(5):E9.
140. Karam SD, Tai A, Snider JW, et al. Refractory trigeminal neuralgia treatment outcomes following CyberKnife radiosurgery. *Radiat Oncol* 2014;9(1):257. doi:10.1186/s13014-014-0257-8.

141. Shetter AG, Rogers CL, Ponce R, et al. Gamma knife radiosurgery for recurrent trigeminal neuralgia. *J Neurosurg* 2002;97:536–538.

142. Pollock BE, Foote RL, Link MJ, et al. Repeat radiosurgery for idiopathic trigeminal neuralgia. *Int J Radiat Oncol Biol Phys* 2005;61:192–195.

143. Kotecha R, Kotecha R, Modugula S, et al. Trigeminal neuralgia treated with stereotactic radiosurgery: the effect of dose escalation on pain control and treatment outcomes. *Int J Radiat Oncol Biol Phys* 2016;96(1):142–148. doi:10.1016/j.ijrobp.2016.04.013.

144. Chen C-J, Paisan G, Buell TJ, et al. Stereotactic radiosurgery for type 1 versus type 2 trigeminal neuralgias. *World Neurosurg* 2017;108:581–588. doi:10.1016/j.wneu.2017.09.055.

145. Quinn JH, Weil T. Trigeminal neuralgia: treatment by repetitive neurectomy. Supplemental report. *J Oral Surg* 1975;33(8):591–595.

146. Murali R, Rovit RL. Are peripheral neurectomies of value in the treatment of trigeminal neuralgia? An analysis of new cases and cases involving previous radiofrequency gasserian thermocoagulation. *J Neurosurg* 1996;85(3):435–437.

147. Trescott AM. Cryoanalgesia in interventional pain management. *Pain Physician* 2003;6:345–360.

148. Jakrewska JM. Cryotherapy in the management of paroxysmal trigeminal neuralgia. *J Neurol Neurosurg Psychiatry* 1987;50(4):485–487.

149. Pradel W. Cryosurgical treatment of genuine trigeminal neuralgia. *Br J Oral Maxillofac Surg* 2002;40(3):244–247.

150. Zakrzewska JM, Nally FF. The role of cryotherapy (cryoanalgesia) in the management of paroxysmal neuralgia: a six year experience. *Br J Oral Maxillofac Surg* 1988;26(1):18–25.

151. Kiya K, Sacoda K, Gen M, et al. A case of aspergillotic meningoencephalitis associated with trigeminal neuralgia. *No Shinkei Geka* 1982;10(8):861–866.

152. Suzuki K, Iwabucchi N, Kuramochi S, et al. Aspergillus aneurysm of the middle cerebral artery causing a fatal subarachnoid hemorrhage. *Intern Med* 1995;34(6):550–553.

153. Arai M, Nakamura A, Shichi D. Case of tsutsugamushi disease (scub typhus) presenting with fever and pain indistinguishable from trigeminal neuralgia. *Rinsho Shinkeigaku* 2007;47(6):362–364.

154. Vitali AM, Sayer FT, Honey CR. Recurrent trigeminal neuralgia secondary to Teflon felt. *Acta Neuochir (Wien)* 2007;149(7):719–722.

155. Hojaili B, Barland P. Trigeminal neuralgia as the first manifestation of mixed connective tissue disorder. *J Clin Rheumatol* 2006;12(3):145–147.

156. Irizarry MC. Multiple sclerosis. In: Cudkowicz ME, Irizarry MC, eds. *Neurologic Disorders in Women.* Boston, MA: Butterworth-Heinemann; 1997:85.

157. Solaro C, Brichetto G, Amato MP, et al. The prevalence of pain in multiple sclerosis: a multicenter cross sectional study. *Neurology* 2004;16(5):919–921.

158. Rovitt RL. *Trigeminal Neuralgia.* Baltimore, MD: Williams & Wilkins; 1990.

159. da Silva CJ, da Roch AJ, Mendes MF, et al. Trigeminal involvement in multiple sclerosis: magnetic resonance imaging findings with clinical correlation in a series of patients. *Mult Scler* 2005;11(3):282–285.

160. van der Meijs AH, Tan IL, Barkhof F. Incidence of enhancement of the trigeminal nerve on MRI in patients with multiple sclerosis. *Mult Scler* 2002;8(1):64–67.

161. Broggi G, Ferroli P, Franzini A, et al. Operative findings and outcomes of microvascular decompression for trigeminal neuralgia in 35 patients affected by multiple sclerosis. *Neurosurgery* 2004;55(4):830–838.

162. Resnick DK, Jannetta PJ, Lunsford LD, et al. Microvascular decompression for trigeminal neuralgia in patients with multiple sclerosis. *Surg Neurol* 1996;46(4):358–361.

163. Tuleasca C, Carron R, Resseguier N, et al. Multiple sclerosis-related trigeminal neuralgia: a prospective series of 43 patients treated with gamma knife surgery with more than one year of follow-up. *Stereotact Funct Neurosurg* 2014;92(4):203–210. doi:10.1159/000362173.

164. Cheng JS, Sanchez-Mejia RO, Limbo M, et al. Management of medically refractory trigeminal neuralgia in patients with multiple sclerosis. *Neurosurg Focus* 2005;18(5):e13.

165. Puca A, Meglio M. Typical trigeminal neuralgia associated with posterior cranial fossa tumors. *Ital J Neurol Sci* 1993;14(7):549–452.

166. Roberti F, Sekhar LN, Kalavakonda C, et al. Posterior fossa meningiomas: surgical experience in 161 cases. *Surg Neurol* 2001;56(1):8–20.

167. Lobato RD, Gonzaáez P, Alday R, et al. Meningiomas of the basal posterior fossa. Surgical experience in 80 cases. *Neurocirugia (Astur)* 2004;15(6):525–542.

168. Haddad FS, Taha JM. An unusual cause for trigeminal neuralgia: contralateral meningioma of the posterior fossa. *Neurosurgery* 1990;26(6):1033–1038.

169. Florensa R, Llovet J, Pou S, et al. Contralateral trigeminal neuralgia as a false localizing sign in intracranial tumors. *Neurosurgery* 1987;20(1):1–3.

170. Mewes H, Schroth I, Deinsberger W, et al. Pain of the trigeminal nerve as the first symptom of metastasis from an oesohaguscarcinoma in Meckel's cave—case report [in German]. *Zentralbl Neurochir* 2001;62(2):65–68.

171. Mastronardi L, Lunardi P, Osman FJ, et al. Metastatic involvement of the Meckel's cave and trigeminal nerve. A case report. *J Neurooncol* 1997;32(1):87–90.

172. Nakano I, Iwwsuki K, Kondo A. Solitary metastatic breast carcinoma in a trigeminal nerve mimicking a trigeminal neuroma. Case report. *J Neurosurg* 1996;85(4):677–680.

173. Hirota N, Fujimoto T, Takahashi M, et al. Isolated trigeminal nerve metastases from breast cancer: an unusual cause of trigeminal mononeuropathy. *Surg Neurol* 1998;49(5):558–561.

174. Kuntzer T, Bogousslavsky J, Rilliet B, et al. Herald facial numbness. *Eur Neurol* 1992;32(5):297–301.

175. Inatomi Y, Inoue T, Nagata S, et al. Trigeminal neuralgia caused by the metastasis of malignant lymphoma to the trigeminal nerve: a case report. *No Shinkei Geka* 1998;26(5):401–405.

176. Falavigna A, Borba LA, Ferraz FA, et al. Primary melanoma of Meckel's cave: case report. *Arq Neuropsiquatr* 2004;62(2A):353–356.

177. Tacconi L, Arulampalam T, Johnston F, et al. Adenocarcinoma of Meckel's cave: case report. *Surg Neurol* 1995;44(6):553–555.

178. Abdel Aziz KM, van Loveren HR. Primary lymphoma of Meckel's cave mimicking trigeminal schwannoma: case report. *Neurosurgery* 1999;44(4):859–862.

179. Kanpolat Y, Tatli M, Ugur HC, et al. Evaluation of platybasia in patients with idiopathic trigeminal neuralgia. *Surg Neurol* 2007;67(1):78–81.

180. Quinones-Hinojosa A, Chang EF, Khan SA, et al. Isolated trigeminal nerve sarcoid granuloma mimicking trigeminal schwannoma: case report. *Neurosurgery* 2003;52(3):700–705.

181. Golby AJ, Norbash A, Silverberg GD. Trigeminal neuralgia resulting from infarction of the root entry zone of the trigeminal nerve: case report. *Neurosurgery* 1998;43(3):620–622.

182. Ivánez V, Moreno M. Trigeminal neuralgia in children as the only manifestation of Chiari I malformation. *Rev Neuro* 1999;28(5):485–487.

183. Rosetti P, Ben Taib NO, Brotchi J, et al. Arnold Chiari Type I malformation presenting as a trigeminal neuralgia: case report. *Neurosurgery* 1999;44(5):1122–1123.

184. Teo C, Nakaji P, Serisier D, et al. Resolution of trigeminal neuralgia following third ventriculostomy for hydrocephalus associated with Chiari I malformation: case report. *Minim Invasive Neurosurg* 2005;48(5):302–305.

185. Schwartz NE, Rosenberg S, So YT. Action at a distance: a lumbar spine tumor presenting as trigeminal neuralgia. *Clin Neurol Neurosurg* 2006;108(8):806–808.

186. Ohnishi YI, Fujimoto Y, Taniguchi M, et al. Neuroendoscopically assisted cyst-cisternal shunting for a quadrigeminal arachnoid cyst causing typical trigeminal neuralgia. *Minim Invasive Neurosurg* 2007;50(2):124–127.

187. Uzumi N, Hasegawa J, Kaoru K, et al. Pain relief by stellate ganglion block in a case with trigeminal neuralgia caused by a cerebellopontine angle tumor. *Anesth Prog* 2002;49:88–91.

188. Wu CL, March A, Dworkin RH. The role of sympathetic nerve blocks in acute herpes zoster and postherpetic neuralgia. *Pain* 2007;87:121–129.

189. Wollan PC, St Sauver JL, Kurland MJ, et al. A population-based study of the incidence and complication rates of herpes zoster before zoster vaccine introduction. *Mayo Clin Proc* 2007;82(11):1341–1349.

190. Dworkin RH, Portenoy RK. Pain and its persistence in herpes zoster. *Pain* 1996;67:241.

191. Sampathkumar P, Drage LA, Martin DP. Herpes zoster(shingles) and post herpetic neuralgia. *Mayo Clin Proc* 2009;84(3):274–280.

192. Gross G, Schöfer H, Wassilew S, et al. Herpes zoster guideline of the German Dermatology Society (DDG). *J Clin Virol* 2003;26(3):277–289.

193. Schmader K. Management of herpes zoster in elderly patients. *Infect Dis Clin Pract* 1995;4:293–299.

194. Crooks RJ, Jones DA, Fiddian AP. Zoster associated chronic pain: an overview of clinical trials with acyclovir. *Scand J Infect Dis Suppl* 1991;80:62–68.

195. Whitley RJ, Weiss H, Gnann J, et al. Acyclovir with and without prednisone for treatment of herpes zoster. A randomized, placebo-controlled trial. *Ann Intern Med* 1996;125:376–383.

196. Bowsher D. The effects of pre-emptive treatment of postherpetic neuralgia with amitriptyline: a randomized, double-blind, placebo controlled trial. *J Pain Symptom Manage* 1997;13:327–331.

197. Kuraishi Y, Takasaki I, Nojima H, et al. Effects of the suppression of acute herpetic pain by gabapentin and amitriptyline on the incidence of delayed postherpetic pain in mice. *Life Sci* 2004;74:2619–2626.

198. Oxman MN, Levin MJ, Johnson GR, et al. A vaccine to prevent herpes zoster and postherpetic neuralgia in older adults. *N Engl J Med* 2005;352(22):2271–2284.

199. Bharucha T, Ming D, Breuer J. A critical appraisal of "Shingrix," a novel herpes zoster subunit vaccine (HZ/Su or GSK1437173A) for varicella zoster virus. *Hum Vaccin Immunother* 2017;13(8):1789–1797. doi:10.1080/21645515.2017.1317410.

200. Thomas SL, Wheeler JG, Hall AJ. Micronutrient intake and the risk of herpes zoster: a case-control study. *Int J Edidemiol* 2006;35:307–314.

201. High KP, Legault C, Sinclair JA, et al. Low plasma concentrations of retinol and alpha-tocopherol in hematopoietic stem cell transplant recipients: the effect of mucositis and the risk of infection. *Am J Clin Nutr* 2002;76:1358–1366.

202. Alper BS, Lewis PR. Treatment of postherpetic neuralgia: a systematic review of the literature. *J Fam Pract* 2002;51:121–128.

203. Hempenstal K, Nurmikko TJ, Johnson RW, et al. Analgesic therapy in postherpetic neuralgia: a quantitative systematic review. *PLoS Med* 2005;2:e164.

204. van Seventer R, Feister HA, Young JP, et al. Efficacy and tolerability of twice-daily pregabalin for treating pain and related sleep interference in postherpetic neuralgia: a 13-week, randomized trial. *Curr Med Res Opin* 2006;22(2):375–384.

205. Clark LP, Taylor AS. True tic douloureux of the fibers of the sensory filaments of the facial nerve. *JAMA* 1909;53:2144–2146.

206. Jannetta PJ. Microsurgical approach to the trigeminal nerve for tic douloureux. *Prog Neurosurg* 1976;7:180–200.

207. Lovely TJ, Jannetta PJ. Surgical management of geniculate neuralgia. *Am J Otol* 1997;18(4):512–517.

208. Rupa V, Sauders RL, Weider DJ. Geniculate neuralgia: the surgical management of primary otalgia. *J Neurosurg* 1991;75(4):505–511.

209. Pulek JL. Geniculate neuralgia: long-term results of surgical treatment. *Ear Nose Throat J* 2002;81(1):30–33.

210. Bohm E, Strann RR. Glossopharyngeal neuralgia. *Brain* 1962;85:371–388.

211. Chawla JC, Falconer MA. Glossopharyngeal and vagal neuralgia. *BMJ* 1967;3:529–531.

212. Bryun GW. Glossopharyngeal neuralgia. In: Vinkin PJ, Gruyn GW, Klawans HL, eds. *Handbook of Clinical Neurology*. Amsterdam, The Netherlands: Elsevier; 1985:459–473.

213. Fini G, Gasparini G, Filippini F, et al. The long styloid process syndrome or Eagle's syndrome. *J Craniomaxillofac Surg* 2000;28:123–127.

214. Soh KB. The glossopharyngeal nerve, glossopharyngeal neuralgia and the Eagle's syndrome-current concepts and management. *Singapore Med J* 1999;40:659–665.

215. Nakagawa H, Nagasao M, Kusuyama T, et al. A case of glossopharyngeal zoster diagnosed by detecting viral antigen in the pharyngeal mucous membrane. *J Laryngol Otol* 2007;121(2):163–165.

216. Sampson JH, Grossi PM, Asaoka K, et al. Microvascular decompression for glossopharyngeal neuralgia: long-term effectiveness and complication avoidance. *Neurosurgery* 2004;54(4):884–889.

217. Zhao K, Zuo H, Zhang L, et al. Long-term follow-up results of microsurgical treatment for glossopharyngeal neuralgia. *Zhonghua Wai Ke Za Zhi* 2000;38(8):598–600.

218. Resnick DK, Jannetta PJ, Bissonnette D, et al. Microvascular decompression for glossopharyngeal neuralgia. *Neurosurgery* 1995;36:64–68.

219. Patel A, Kassam A, Horowitz M, et al. Microvascular decompression in the management of glossopharyngeal neuralgia: analysis of 217 cases. *Neurosurgery* 2002;50:705–710.

220. Kodama S, Oribe K, Suzuki M. Superior laryngeal neuralgia associated with deviation of the hyoid bone. *Auris Nasus Larynx* 2007;35(3):429–431.

221. Bagatzounis A, Geyer G. Lateral pharyngeal diverticulum as a cause of superior laryngeal nerve neuralgia. *Laryngorhinootologie* 1994;73(4):219–221.

222. O'Neill BP, Aronson AE, Pearson BW, et al. Superior laryngeal neuralgia: carotidynia or just another pain in the neck? *Headache* 1982;22(1):6–9.

223. Johnson DL. Intractable hiccups: treatment by microvascular decompression of the vagus nerve. Case report. *J Neurosurg* 1993;78(5):813–816.

224. Resnick DK, Jannetta PJ. Hyperactive rhizopathy of the vagus nerve and microvascular decompression. Case report. *J Neurosurg* 1999;90(3):580–582.

225. Takahashi SK, Suzuki M, Izuha A, et al. Two cases of idiopathic superior laryngeal neuralgia treated by superior laryngeal nerve block with a high concentration of lidocaine. *J Clin Anesth* 2007;19(3):237–238.

226. Kunc Z. Treatment of essential neuralgia of the ninth nerve with selective tractotomy. *J Neurosurg* 1965;23:494–500.

227. Kandan SR, Khan S, Jeyaretna DS, et al. Neuralgia of the glossopharyngeal and vagal nerves: long-term outcome following surgical treatment and literature review. *Br J Neurosurg* 2010;24(4):441–446. doi:10.3109/02688697.2010.487131.

228. Trescott AM. Headache management in an interventional pain practice. *Pain Physician* 2000;3(2):197–200.

229. Sjaastad O, Stolt-Nielsen A, Pareja JA, et al. Supraorbital neuralgia. On the clinical manifestation and a possible therapeutic approach. *Headache* 1999;39(3):204–212.

230. Lambert WC, Okorodudu AO, Schwartz RA. Cutaneous nasociliary neuralgia. *Acta Derm Venereol* 1985;65(3):257–258.

231. Spokoinaia VA. Neuralgia of the trigeminal nerve and pterygopalatine ganglion as a complication of paranasal sinusitis [in Russian]. *Vestn Otorinolaringol* 1989;4:49–53.

232. Zhao Y, Li H, Cai Q, et al. Partial middle turbinectomy and folded for nasociliary neuralgia by transnasal endoscopic surgery [in Chinese]. *Lin Chuang Er Bi yan Hou Ke Za Zhi* 2004;18(2):91–92.

233. Rath EM. Surgical treatment of maxillary nerve injuries. The infraorbital nerve. *Atlas Oral Maxillofac Surg Clin North Am* 2001;9(2):31–41.

234. Schwartz DP, Robbins MS, Grosberg BM. Nummular headache update. *Curr Pain Headache Rep* 2013;17(6):340. doi:10.1007/s11916-013-0340-0.

235. Mathew NT, Kailasam J, Meadors L. Botulinum toxin type A for the treatment of nummular headache: four case studies. *Headache* 2007;48(3):442–447.

236. Tatli M, Keklikci U, Aluclu U, et al. Anesthesia dolorosa caused by penetrating cranial injury. *Eur Neurol* 2006;56(3):162–165.

237. Stillman M. Clinical approach to patients with neuropathic pain. *Cleve Clin J Med* 2006;73(8):726–739.

238. Wallace MS. Pharmacologic treatment of neuropathic pain. *Curr Pain Headache Rep* 2001;5:138–150.

239. Lazorthes Y, Sol JC, Fowo S, et al. Motor cortex stimulation for neuropathic pain. *Acta Neurochir Suppl* 2007;97(pt 2):37–44.

240. Brown JA, Pilitsis JG. Motor cortex stimulation for central and neuropathic facial pain: a prospective study of 10 patients and observations of enhanced sensory and motor function during stimulation. *Neurosurgery* 2005;56(2):290–297.

241. Raslan AM, Nasseri M, Bahgat D, et al. Motor cortex stimulation for trigeminal neuropathic or deafferentation pain: an institutional case series experience. *Stereotact Funct Neurosurg* 2011;89(2):83–88.

242. Levy RM, Lamb S, Adams JE. Treatment of chronic pain by deep brain stimulation: long term follow-up and review of the literature. *Neurosurgery* 1987;21(6):885–893.

CHAPTER 67

Facial Pain

ALAA ABD-ELSAYED, PAMELA J. HUGHES, and **AHMED M.T. RASLAN**

Facial pain syndromes are common in clinical practice. Many of these syndromes are also unique, given the complex anatomy and specialized sensory innervation of the head, face, and neck. The complexity of the anatomy can pose diagnostic challenges when endeavoring to treat facial pain syndromes.

The common descriptive terms for facial pain complaints are frequently misleading. To avoid confusion, clinicians should be familiar with the International Headache Society's Diagnostic Classification for Head, Face, and Neck Pain Disorders (Table 67.1).

The aforementioned grouping of diagnose(s) is a rather exhaustive differential diagnosis of facial pain. This includes acute and subacute conditions that affect a vast majority of the structures of the human head. This would include ocular, nasal, sinus, dental, oral, muscular, mucosal, and any other causes specific to the region of the head and face.

Although such a list is good for an all-encompassing reference, it is not necessarily helpful for pain practitioners who deal mostly with chronic pain conditions. In this chapter, the focus is on chronic pain conditions that would present as facial pain. Because the primary differential diagnosis of facial pain is trigeminal neuralgia and the nociceptive pain pathway responsible for facial pain, conditions that present in a similar fashion to trigeminal neuralgia or could be misdiagnosed as such are discussed in detail here.

Trigeminal and Other Cranial Nerve Neuropathic Conditions

TRIGEMINAL NEUROPATHY

Trigeminal neuropathy is a spectrum, the earliest of which is classically called trigeminal neuralgia. Because the most classic description of trigeminal neuralgia is episodic, sharp shooting pain without any detectable sensory or motor deficit, there are also other forms of trigeminal neuropathic pain that signify a higher degree of neuropathy. The best description of the spectral nature of trigeminal facial pain is found in the classification offered by Burchiel et al.[2,3] in 2003 and 2005.

In that classification, pain is classified based on the understanding of the pathophysiology of neuralgia (Table 67.2).

Trigeminal Neuralgia Type 1

This represents the classic description of trigeminal neuralgia in its purest form; it is idiopathic, sharp, shooting, electrical shock-like, episodic pain lasting several seconds, with pain-free intervals between attacks. This diagnosis is fairly straightforward, and most neurosurgeons are familiar with this clinical entity. The condition is caused usually by a vascular compression near the root entry zone because it is the junction of the central and peripheral myelin that renders that zone susceptible to the pathology. Vascular compression leads to demyelination, which in turn leads to ectopic action potential generation that is suspected to allegedly drive the sharp lancinating episodes of facial pain. A full description of the pathophysiology of pain triggering is best described by Devor in 2002 as the ignition hypothesis.[4,5]

Trigeminal Neuralgia Type 2

This is still a variant of the classic idiopathic trigeminal neuralgia; however, the crucial feature of this condition is the presence of dull aching or background pain for more than 50% of time. This represents a form of trigeminal neuralgia with more evidence of sensory neuropathy compared to type 1. Some of these patients do progress from type 1, and some present as such on initial presentation. Several studies suggest that surgical treatment for trigeminal neuralgia is more successful and durable in patients with trigeminal neuralgia type 1 compared to type 2.[6] It is fairly common to have a normal bedside sensory examination testing in cases of idiopathic trigeminal neuralgia regardless of the type.

Symptomatic Trigeminal Neuralgia

In contrast to idiopathic forms of trigeminal neuralgia, this is not an idiopathic form, it is caused by either a diagnosed demyelinating disorder such as multiple sclerosis, a tumor, a vascular malformation, or other structural pathology leading to compression of the trigeminal root entry zone, other than the

TABLE 67.1	International Headache Society International Classification of Headache Disorders[1]	
Primary headaches	• Migraine without aura, with aura • Tension-type headache • Cluster headache and other trigeminal autonomic cephalalgias • Other primary headaches
Secondary headaches	• Attributed to head and/or neck trauma • Attributed to cranial or cervical vascular disorder • Attributed to nonvascular intracranial disorder • Attributed to a substance or its withdrawal • Attributed to infection • Attributed to disorder of homeostasis • Headache or facial pain attributed to disorder of cranium, neck, eyes, ears, nose, sinuses, teeth, mouth, or other facial or cranial structures • Attributed to psychiatric disorder
Headache or facial pain attributed to disorders of cranium, neck, eyes, ears, nose, sinuses, teeth, mouth, or other facial or cranial structures	• Cranial bones • Neck • Eyes • Ears • Rhinosinusitis (sinus disorders) • Teeth, jaws, or related structures • TMJ disorders (TMD) • Other
Cranial neuralgias, central and primary facial pain, and other headaches	• Trigeminal neuralgia • Glossopharyngeal neuralgia • Occipital neuralgia • Constant pain caused by compression, irritation, or distortion of cranial nerves or upper cervical roots by structural lesions • Head or facial pain attributed to herpes zoster • *Postherpetic neuralgia* • Central causes of facial pain • Anesthesia dolorosa • Central poststroke pain • *Facial pain attributed to multiple sclerosis* • *Persistent idiopathic facial pain* • *Burning mouth syndrome*

TMD, temporomandibular disorder; TMJ, temporomandibular joint.

TABLE 67.2 Classifications and Pathophysiology of Neuralgia

Type 1 Neuralgia	Type 2 Neuralgia	Symptomatic	Neuropathic	Postherpetic	Deafferentation	Atypical
Sharp stabbing episodic pain for >50% of the time Constitute the typical TN	Sharp stabbing pain <50% with predominant component of dull aching or burning pain Advanced from of TN	Due to: 1. MS 2. Tumor 3. AVM 4. Aneurysm etc.	Unintentional injury 1. Surgical ENT, ophthalmic, plastic 2. Traumatic idiopathic	Herpes zoster outbreak Severe neuropathy	Intentional neurosurgical injury for treatment of TN	Somatoform Pain disorder Cannot be diagnosed by history only

AVM, arteriovenous malformation; ENT, eyes, nose, and throat; MS, multiple sclerosis; TN, trigeminal neuralgia.

vascular compression described in idiopathic forms. It is noteworthy that clinically patients may present in either a type 1– or type 2–like presentation; however, constant dull aching pain (type 2 like) is more common in patients with symptomatic trigeminal neuralgia.

Neuropathic Trigeminal Neuralgia

In this entity, the degree of trigeminal neuropathy is more advanced compared to idiopathic trigeminal neuralgia; there is an objective sensory loss in the distribution of the trigeminal nerve and it is associated with classic manifestations of neuropathic pain including but not limited to allodynia, hyperalgesia, and burning pain. Neuropathic trigeminal neuralgia is usually caused by either intentional or unintentional injury to the trigeminal nerve. Examples of unintentional injuries would include trauma; postdental injection; postprocedural in maxillofacial surgeries; skull bases surgery; ear, nose, and, throat (ENT) surgery; or poststroke. Examples of intentional injuries include trigeminal neuropathy following neurosurgical ablation of the one or more branches of the trigeminal nerve for the purpose of alleviation of pain. Spontaneous neuropathic trigeminal neuralgia had been also described, albeit, a rare condition.[7]

Postherpetic Trigeminal Neuralgia

Postherpetic trigeminal neuralgia is the condition that follows herpes zoster viral infection to the trigeminal ganglion. It is a more severe form of neuropathy manifested by significant allodynia, hyperalgesia, and burning dysesthesia. It commonly affects the first division of the trigeminal nerve.

Deafferentation Trigeminal Neuralgia

Deafferentation trigeminal neuralgia, otherwise known as anesthesia dolorosa, is the most severe form of neuropathy and trigeminal neuralgia. The features of this pathology suggest a marked sensory loss or even corneal anesthesia in severe cases. Unfortunately, this is an iatrogenic condition that is induced by surgical interventions to denervate the trigeminal distribution. It is common with techniques such as rhizotomy or alcohol denervation and less common (or require repeated exposure) after techniques with rather smaller quantifiable ablation such as radiofrequency rhizotomy, glycerol rhizotomy, balloon compression, or radiosurgery.

Atypical Facial Pain

In this particular classification, atypical facial pain refers to somatoform disorder, in which a psychological disorder can be unequivocally diagnosed. Obviously, this is a difficult condition to treat and would be a contraindication to interventional therapies.

Treatment of various forms of trigeminal neuralgia is mentioned elsewhere in this textbook, but the degree of neuropathy determines the possible reversibility and therefore dictates the treatment options. Medical treatments for most of cranial

nerve neuropathy–related pain is medical at first with medications such as carbamazepine, gabapentin, and topiramate. Should medical treatment fail, interventional therapies are introduced, and these are introduced based on the degree of neuropathy. As such, early neuropathy such as trigeminal neuralgia type 1 would benefit from a potentially curative option such as microvascular decompression, whereas postherpetic neuralgia requires advanced interventions such as neuromodulation of the central nervous system.

GLOSSOPHARYNGEAL NEURALGIA

Glossopharyngeal neuralgia (GN) is a rare condition in which patients experience paroxysmal episodes of pain along the auricular and pharyngeal branches of both the glossopharyngeal and vagus nerves. Patients will often complain of severe, lancinating pain "attacks" along one side of the throat, with occasional radiation to the ear, that are often precipitated by swallowing, chewing, coughing, or yawning.[8] It can be particularly debilitating when the vagus nerve is involved as patients may experience loss of sympathetic tone that can lead to syncope and seizures in up to 10% of the cases.[9]

GN is most often caused by neurovascular compression at the root entry zone of the brainstem—most often, it is the posterior inferior cerebellar artery that is responsible for the compression, although the anterior inferior cerebellar artery (AICA) has been documented as well.[10] With an incidence of just 1% when compared to its better known counterpart, trigeminal neuralgia, GN is notoriously hard to diagnose.[11] Given this diagnostic dilemma, high-sensitivity, high-specificity magnetic resonance imaging (MRI) is recommended to rule out any other potential causes such as neoplasm or an elongated styloid process.[10]

Treatment is initially medical, as with most cranial neuralgias, and if this fails, surgical decompression or sectioning may be very effective in alleviating pain.[12] Ruling out mimicking conditions such as Eagle syndrome is critical prior to administering an interventional therapy.

NERVUS INTERMEDIUS NEURALGIA

Nervus intermedius neuralgia (NIN), also known as geniculate neuralgia, is a rare pain condition characterized by paroxysmal, deep ear pain. Patients commonly describe the pain as "being stabbed in the ear with an icepick." These attacks can be debilitating and socially isolating. The posterior wall of the auditory canal as well as the superficial ear drum are common trigger zones for the paroxysms, for example, by loud noises or cold wind.[13] Sensory innervation to the skin of the external ear and auditory canal is complex, including contributions from cranial nerves (CN) V, IX, and X; the nervus intermedius (NI); and upper cervical dorsal roots.[14] This complicated innervation leads to confusion about the culprit nerve in primary otalgia and contributes ultimately to confusion in diagnosis. Medical treatment is the first-line therapy for this condition, and, as with other cranial neuralgia, surgical decompression or section can be effective.[15]

Odontogenic and Temporomandibular Joint Disorders

ODONTOGENIC PAIN

Facial pain emanating from an odontogenic source can be a challenge to distinguish from other causes of facial pain. This section guides the clinician to identify potential sources of odontogenic pain, understand the different characteristics of those sources of pain, and ultimately provide for a differential diagnosis. To fully understand the mechanisms to which odontogenic pain arises, a review of dental anatomy and the process of how dental pathology progresses is required.

The normal anatomy of a tooth is characterized by three layers (from the surface to the middle of the tooth): enamel, dentin and dental pulp on the crown of the tooth and cementum, and dentin and dental pulp on the roots of the teeth (Fig. 67.1).

The dental pulp is the generative part of the tooth and is made up of connective tissue and generative cells called odontoblasts. This part of the tooth is also innervated and when insulted causes tooth pain. Dental caries is the typical etiology of dental pain and begins by invading the enamel, progressing to the dentin, and then, if unrestored by a dentist, will progress to invade the pulp, seeding the pulp tissue with harmful bacteria that causes infection and inflammation. This leads to an acute episode of pain and then can lead to abscess formation. As the dental caries progresses through the layers of the tooth, the characteristics of dental pain change, as does the dental or pulpal diagnosis. Once the dental pulp becomes necrotic, the pain may subside, but the necrotic tissue will act as a substrate for pathogenic bacteria that then can cause spread of infection to surrounding tissues.

A second source of odontogenic pain stems from the tissues surrounding the dentition. Periodontitis is a chronic, periradicular disease characterized by inflammation of the gingiva causing soft tissue attachment loss and bone loss surrounding the tooth. In its early stages, the process may be painless but, if untreated, culminates in mobility of teeth and ultimately tooth loss. The degree of pain associated with periodontal disease in the absence of abscess formation is typically mild and not limited to one particular area of the mouth. It is also important to note that periodontal disease is an inflammatory process that is associated with other systemic, chronic disease such as diabetes.

Pericoronitis is a type of gingival inflammation that typically occurs around an erupting or partially erupted third molar (wisdom tooth). The inflammatory response in acute pericoronitis can be significant causing severe pain and trismus and may lead to severe cellulitis and abscess spreading to the deep spaces of the neck and posterior oropharynx.

Steps for Diagnosis

A good clinical exam begins with a thorough history. The timing, location, and characteristics of the patient's pain must be investigated. A head and neck exam should include palpation of the neck, facial bones, muscles, and soft tissues. The temporomandibular joint (TMJ) should also be included in the head and neck exam and is discussed in another section in this text. Any asymmetries or swellings should be noted, and in the presence of pain, cellulitis or abscess should be suspected. Tenderness to the muscles of mastication without swelling or dental findings should lead the clinician down the path of myofascial origins. The oral examination should include inspection of the dentition, oral mucosa, tongue, floor of the mouth, and the oropharynx.

Dental Findings

The clinician should look for presence of dental disease including dental caries, fractured teeth, or mobile teeth. Dental caries is characterized by the presence of dark areas of the tooth that have invaded or cavitated the enamel (Fig. 67.2).

Stains may sometimes mimic dental caries but will not exhibit loss of tooth structure. In general, the more tooth structure that is involved, the more invasive the decay and the closer to invasion of the pulp causing pain. The decay may start on

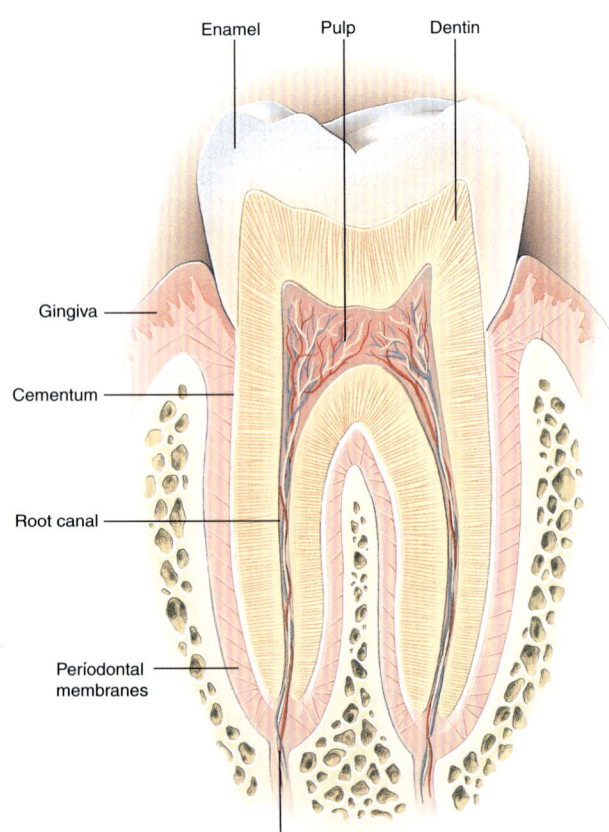

Longitudinal Section of a Tooth

Enamel · Pulp · Dentin

Gingiva

Cementum

Root canal

Periodontal membranes

Apical foramina with artery, vein, and nerve

FIGURE 67.1 Normal tooth anatomy.

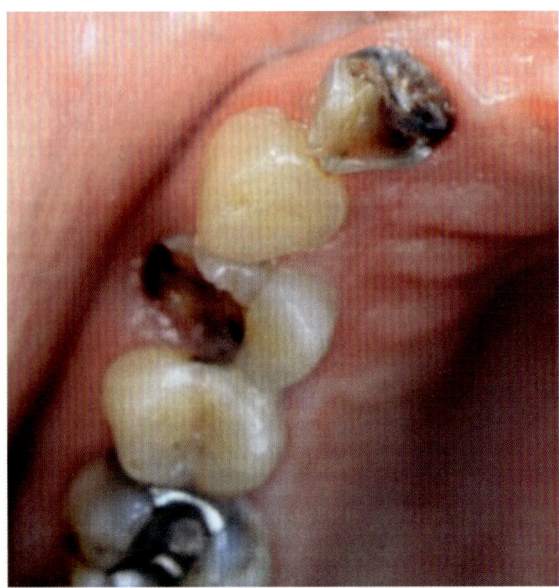

FIGURE 67.2 Dental caries. *(Source: Anatomical Chart Company. Disorders of the Teeth and Jaw Anatomical Chart, 2004.)*

TABLE 67.3	Characteristics of Facial Odontogenic Pain by Dental Diagnosis				
Dental Diagnosis	Pain Characteristics	Localization of Pain	Factors that Aggravate	Examination Findings	Radiographic Findings
Dentin sensitivity	Mild to moderate; ceases when aggravant is removed	The affected teeth	Cold	Gingival recession	None
Reversible pulpitis	Sharp, throbbing, moderate to severe, intermittent	Affected tooth	Cold/heat, sweets, chewing/percussion	Dental caries or dental trauma (fractured tooth)	Caries or fracture approaching the pulp
Irreversible pulpitis	Sharp, throbbing, moderate to severe, can be constant	Generalized to ipsilateral side of face or jaw	Cold/heat, sweets, chewing/percussion	Caries, may exhibit gingival or facial swelling	Caries approaching or invading pulp, widened periodontal ligament or periapical radiolucency
Pericoronitis	Constant aching or throbbing; moderate to severe pain	Depending on severity, can be localized to the posterior mandible or can be diffuse to include the entire side of the face extending to the neck	Chewing/functioning	Erythematous, edematous mucosa overlying the third molar area. Purulence may be present. Patient may exhibit trismus. In more severe cases, the patient may exhibit malaise, fever, and abscess formation extending into the neck.	Submerged or impacted wisdom tooth

Adapted from Zakrzewska JM. Differential diagnosis of facial pain and guidelines for management. *Br J Anaesth* 2013;111(1):95–104.

the occlusal surface of the tooth, between the teeth, or at the gingival cervical margins. If the decay begins between the teeth, the caries may not be easily identified clinically and may require radiographic evaluation. Teeth with periapical or pulpal inflammation many times will be tender to percussion and will elicit a more painful response then percussion of the surrounding, unaffected teeth. Additionally, the same teeth may elicit painful response to thermal stimulation compared to the surrounding dentition. The degree to which these findings are positive leads to a diagnosis of reversible or irreversible pulpitis (Table 67.3). Mobility of a tooth in the presence of pain may indicate a periapical abscess, or chronic periodontitis. An abscess typically will be limited to one tooth or one area of the mouth, where in chronic periodontitis, multiple teeth usually are affected in several areas of the mouth.

Oral Soft Tissue Findings

The oral mucosa, gingiva, tongue, floor of mouth, and oropharynx should be inspected and palpated for any masses, ulcerations, bleeding, suppuration, or swelling. Areas of acute inflammation will typically be painful and characterized by erythema. If the inflammation and pain is in the area of a carious tooth, an acute inflammatory process should be suspected (pulpitis or acute abscess). Any fistulas present on the gingiva indicate chronic periapical abscess and a necrotic tooth. These are not necessarily painful, but at some point, prior to the fistula formation, may have been a source of pain to the patient. Any suppuration emanating from the gingival crevice of a tooth or multiple teeth in the presence of mobility suggests severe, chronic periodontitis. The gingiva, in this instance, may bleed easily when manipulated.

Most dental pain is limited to the general area of the offending tooth. Pericoronitis and pain secondary to third molars may be more precarious and generalized to the face, jaw, and ear on the affected side. When severe, the patient will exhibit trismus and may have signs of cellulitis.

Radiographic Examination

Dental radiographs in conjunction with clinical findings are needed for definitive diagnosis in most cases. Dental caries are characterized by radiolucencies within the tooth structure. The depth of invasion of the decay will most likely correlate with the level of reported pain.

Periapical pathology indicating pulpal invasion and necrosis may reveal a widened periodontal ligament (PDL) and possible radiolucency at the apex of the tooth. Bone levels below the cementoenamel junction (CEJ) of the tooth indicate periodontal disease (Fig. 67.3).

Evaluating for odontogenic causes of pain should be ruled out when the patient presents with facial pain. Performing a thorough history and clinical exam should lead the clinician to a reasonable suspicion and differential diagnosis; however, a basic understanding of the pathologic process and clinical signs and symptoms of dental disease is helpful in identifying the causes of the odontogenic origin and progression of disease (see Table 67.3).

TEMPOROMANDIBULAR DISORDERS

TMJ disorders are considered the most common musculoskeletal disorders that cause orofacial pain.[16] These disorders can typically be separated into two entities: myofascial pain disorders and interarticular disorders (internal derangements). Although these two entities can, and many times do coexist, they have very specific pain patterns that characterize each process. It is important for the clinician to understand the differences, as treatment of these two groups may vary widely. Israel[17] defines internal derangement as a condition in which there are damaged intra-articular tissues leading to disturbances in the biomechanical functioning of the TMJ. Fricton[18] describes myofascial pain as a regional muscle pain disorder

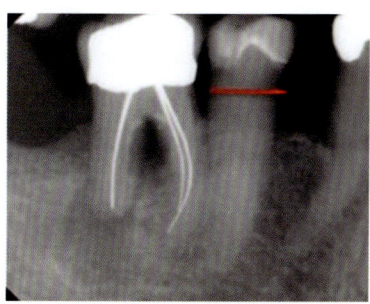

FIGURE 67.3 Bone levels (*red line*) below the cementoenamel junction of the tooth, indicate periodontal disease.

characterized by localized muscle tenderness, limited range of motion, and regional pain.

As with any pain disorder, recognition and diagnosis starts with taking a thorough history. Elements specific to temporomandibular disorder (TMD) include the following: severity and character of pain, time of onset, factors that exacerbate the pain or factors that decrease pain, history of trauma or other temporal event, progression of the pain over time, history of joint noises, functional impairment, or range of motion issues. Additionally, quality-of-life questions such as work or life stressors, habits such as bruxism, history of depression, chronic pain, anxiety, or other mental health issues should be addressed as these may contribute to the development of myofascial pain/TMD, or may develop as a result of these disorders.[19]

Clinical exam should begin with inspection of the face to look for jaw relationship discrepancies including asymmetry, retrognathia, or prognathism. Palpation of the facial, cervical, and occipital musculature should be performed, noting any discomfort to palpation and radiation of that pain within a referral zone of the muscle. Additionally, palpation of muscle bands and firm, localized nodules, or "trigger points" should be noted.[3] Palpation of the lateral poles of the mandibular condyle, just anterior to the tragus of the ear, should be performed. Any pain on palpation should be noted. The clinician should also palpate the condyles while the patient performs mandibular movements (opening and closing, lateral excursive movements, and protrusion of the jaw). During this, the clinician should note any clicking, popping, or grinding sensations. Some would advocate for listening with a stethoscope over the joint as the patient performs the aforementioned movements and documenting any joint noises. Range of motion measurements should be obtained. Normal mandibular opening is typically 40 to 45 mm, measured between the incisal edges of the upper and lower incisor teeth. The clinician should also observe for any deviations upon opening. Deviations on opening and the inability to move the jaw laterally either to the right or left should be noted.

Myofascial pain is typically characterized by pain in the muscles of mastication and may exhibit bands and/or trigger points and typically have a zone of referred pain surrounding the tender point.[18] The characteristics are summarized in Table 67.4.

The aim of treatment of this disorder is to decrease muscle activity and increase range of motion. This can be accomplished with pharmacotherapy, occlusal splint therapy, and physical therapy.[17]

Internal derangements can be complex with respect to the pathology and etiology of the disorder. The characteristics of internal derangements are summarized in Table 67.5 but vary widely depending on the type of internal derangement. Common findings include joint capsule tenderness, decreased range of motion, and joint noises.

The American Association of Orofacial Pain introduced a taxonomic classification of TMD (Table 67.6).

TABLE 67.5 Clinical Characteristics of Internal Derangement

- Localized pain in the preauricular area to palpation
- Localized pain on opening and closing
- Deviation of mandible to affected side on opening
- Minimal lateral excursive movement opposite of the affected side
- Appreciation of joint noises on opening or closing
- Decreased mouth opening (hypomobility of the mandible)

Internal derangements can also be classified according to severity of disease. The Wilkes Staging System (Table 67.7) is commonly used by TMJ surgeons to help provide a guide for treatment based on the severity of the damage to the joint. Depending on the physical findings in the clinical exam, imaging may be beneficial for finalizing a diagnosis.

MRI is typically used when an internal derangement is thought to involve disk displacement, disk perforation, or other soft tissue abnormalities. Computed tomography (CT) imaging can be beneficial to identify degenerative processes, neoplasms, or bony ankylosis of the joint. The treatment of internal derangement is typically aimed at decreasing inflammation and increasing range of motion.[17] Treatment modalities vary widely but most often begin with nonsurgical interventions if possible including pharmacotherapy, occlusal splint therapy, and physical therapy. If symptoms persist, surgical options may then be considered.

TABLE 67.6 Taxonomic Classification for Temporomandibular Disorders

I. Temporomandibular joint disorders
  1. Joint pain
     A. Arthralgia
     B. Arthritis
  2. Joint disorders
     A. Disk disorders
        1. Disk displacement with reduction
        2. Disk displacement with reduction with intermittent locking
        3. Disk displacement without reduction with limited opening
        4. Disk displacement without reduction without limited opening
     B. Hypomobility disorders other than disk disorders
        1. Adhesions/adherence
        2. Ankylosis
           a. Fibrous
           b. Osseous
     C. Hypermobility disorders
        1. Subluxation
        2. Luxation
  3. Joint diseases
     A. Degenerative joint disease
        1. Osteoarthrosis
        2. Osteoarthritis
     B. Systemic arthritides
     C. Condylysis/idiopathic condylar resorption
     D. Osteochondritis dissecans
     E. Osteonecrosis
     F. Neoplasm
     G. Synovial chondromatosis
  4. Fractures
  5. Congenital/developmental disorders
     A. Aplasia
     B. Hypoplasia
     C. Hyperplasia

Republished with permission of Quintessence Publishing Company Inc. from Schiffman E, Ohrbach R, Truelove E, et al. Diagnostic Criteria for Temporomandibular Disorders (DC/TMD) for Clinical and Research Applications: Recommendations of the International RDC/TMD Consortium Network and Orofacial Pain Special Interest Group. *J Oral Facial Pain Headache.* 2014;28(1):6–27; permission conveyed through Copyright Clearance Center, Inc.

TABLE 67.4 Clinical Characteristics of Myofascial Pain

- Trigger points in muscle bands
- Tenderness to muscles on palpation
- Consistent points of tenderness
- Pain in zone of referral/reference
- Constant pain
- Dull ache
- Pain fluctuates in intensity.
- Consistent patterns of referral
- Alleviation with extinction of trigger point

Adapted from Fricton J. Myofascial pain: mechanisms to management. *Oral Maxillofac Surg Clin North Am* 2016;28:289–311.

TABLE 67.7 Wilkes Classification of Internal Derangement of the Temporomandibular Joint

Stage		Clinical	Radiographic
I.	Early	Painless clicking, no limitation on opening	Mild displacement of disk with reduction; normal disk morphology
II.	Early/ intermediate	Occasional painful clicking, intermittent locking	Anterior disk displacement with reduction
III.	Intermediate	Joint tenderness, frequent prolonged locking, restricted motion	Anterior disk displacement with or without reduction; no degenerative changes
IV.	Intermediate/ late	Chronic pain, no clicking, restricted motion	Anterior disk displacement without reduction; degenerative changes; adhesions
V.	Late	Variable pain, painful/reduced function, crepitus	Anterior disk displacement without reduction; advanced degenerative changes; advanced adhesions; gross disk deformity and/or perforation

Chronic Headache Disorders Causing Facial Pain

PRIMARY HEADACHE CONDITIONS
Migraine Headache

The International Classification of Headache (ICHD) prescribed migraine headache as frequent headaches with a migrainous nature.

The ICHD determined the following criteria for diagnosing migraine headache.

At least five attacks fulfilling the following criteria (1 to 3)[1]:
1. Attacks lasting 4 to 72 hours whether untreated or unsuccessfully treated
2. The headache has at least two of the following four characteristics:
   a. Unilateral
   b. Pulsating in nature
   c. Moderate to severe in intensity
   d. Aggravation by or causing avoidance of routine physical activity
3. Headache is associated with at least one of the following:
   a. Nausea and/or vomiting
   b. Photophobia and phonophobia

Not better accounted for by another ICHD-3 diagnosis

History taking is the most important step in diagnosing migraine headaches. Investigations may be performed to exclude other causes of headache as brain tumors, intracranial hemorrhage, and other physical lesions.

Patients may report certain triggers that initiate their headache. Migraine headache may occur in the following phases[20]:

Prodrome: Patients may experience vague affective symptoms as long as 24 hours before the onset of the headache attack.

Aura: Some patients will have neurologic symptoms that may last up to 1 hour. Symptoms may be visual, sensory, or brainstem related.

Resolution: occurs after the headache resolves and usually characterized by deep sleep

Migraine hangover: Some patients may experience malaise, fatigue, and head pain after sudden movement or coughing.

The pathophysiology of migraine is a complex neurobiologic process; several theories have been proposed to explain its pathophysiology including neuronal hyperexcitability, hypersensitivity to stimuli, recurrent activation and sensitization of the trigeminovascular pathway, reduced activation of descending inhibitory pathways, and structural/functional changes in the pain pathways.[21-23]

Treatment includes the following approaches:

Lifestyle modifications: It is very important to recognize if there are any triggers that initiate the headache and work on avoiding those triggers.[24]

Treatment of acute headache: Patients may use abortive medication early when headaches start and mild. Some of the medications that can be used include paracetamol, aspirin, ibuprofen, naproxen, and triptans. A combination of triptans and naproxen can also be used. It has been recently suggested that noninvasive stimulation techniques as transcranial magnetic stimulation and vagal stimulation can be used for same purpose.[25,26]

Preventive treatment: Preventive treatment is usually considered when headache frequency and severity increase in a way that interferes with patient's work and social life. First-line treatment includes β-blockers and tricyclics. Second-line medications include anticonvulsants, onabotulinum toxin A, flunarizine, and supplements as riboflavin and magnesium.[27,28]

Interventions can be utilized for patients who do not respond to medications. Some of the procedures performed are botulinum toxin type A injection, occipital nerve blocks, occipital nerve stimulator, and deep brain stimulation.[29]

Tension Headache

Tension-type headaches (TTHs) are recurrent episodes of headache that can persist for minutes to weeks. Pain is typically bilateral, described as tightening in nature, and of variable intensity. It may be associated with photophobia and phonophobia, but nausea and vomiting are usually absent.[30]

It has been proposed that TTH is related to some component of specified stress-related disorders or muscular tension, but large number of clinical trials proposed neurobiologic basis decreasing the belief in psychological diseases as a cause.[31-33]

Patient history is the main tool of diagnosis. As mentioned earlier, tension headaches are bilateral, tightening in nature, usually not associated with nausea and vomiting but might be associated with photophobia and phonophobia. Patients may report triggering factors as stress, lack of sleep, not eating, alcohol, and menstruation.[34]

On physical examination, a focus on palpating head and neck muscles is important to identify any tender points.

Although the main pathophysiology remains a matter of debate, some mechanisms have been proposed. Pericranial myofascial mechanisms may explain episodic TTH. Sensitization of central pain pathways due to prolonged nociceptive stimuli from the pericranial myofascial tissues may explain the change from episodic to chronic TTH.[32]

Nonsteroidal anti-inflammatory drugs (NSAIDs) are the mainstays in the treatment of acute headache. Other medications that can be added in combination with NSAIDs include acetaminophen, caffeine, codeine, sedatives, and tranquilizers.[35,36] Preventing an attack can be achieved by avoiding triggers and by using amitriptyline. In addition, nonpharmacologic treatment as relaxation therapy and biofeedback can be equally effective but require skilled personnel to administer.[37]

For chronic TTH, amitriptyline has been an effective medication. Some studies found modest efficacy of the following medications: citalopram, sertraline, mianserin, fluvoxamine, paroxetine, venlafaxine, sulpiride, and mirtazapine.[38-43] Muscle relaxants may play a role in the treatment. There is some evidence that tizanidine may be beneficial in treating chronic TTH.[44] There has been conflicting data on its use in TTH and botulinum toxin type A, and therefore, it is not recommended.

Nonpharmacologic therapy may be used in patients who fail pharmacologic therapy or in conjunction with it; examples include physical therapy, psychological therapy, and nerve blocks.[45]

Cluster Headache

Cluster headache is typically unilateral associated with ipsilateral autonomic symptoms.

It is important to note that cluster headache is more common in men.

Diagnostic criteria requires that patients should have at least 5 attacks fulfilling criteria 1 to 4.
1. Severe unilateral orbital, supraorbital, and/or temporal pain lasting 15 to 180 minutes if not treated
2. Headache accompanied by at least one of the following:
   a. Ipsilateral conjunctival injection and/or lacrimation
   b. Ipsilateral nasal congestion and/or rhinorrhea
   c. Ipsilateral eyelid edema
   d. Ipsilateral forehead and facial sweating
   e. Ipsilateral miosis and/or ptosis
3. A sense of restlessness or agitation
4. Attacks have a frequency of 1 every other day to 8 per week.
No other disorder that can explain those symptoms.[30]

The pathophysiology of cluster headache is still unknown. The hypothalamus as the supraordinate center may be responsible for initiating attacks. The pain in the cranial autonomic nervous system is introduced and maintained by activation of the parasympathetic and trigeminal nuclei.[46]

Treatment of acute attack includes inhaling oxygen 8 to 12 L per minute, which is effective in resolving the headache in the majority of patients within 15 minutes.[47] Serotonin receptor agonists, triptans, have been also shown to be effective and of rapid effect.

Should a patient develop frequent, severe, acute attacks, preventive therapy should be initiated. Calcium channel blockers such as verapamil have been identified as an effective preventive medication. Lithium is an alternative therapy to verapamil but requires closer monitoring for blood levels and side effects. In addition, corticosteroids have been found to be effective and can be used on a temporary basis until verapamil or lithium is started.[48,49]

Oral ergotamines are alkaloids that have been found to be an effective treatment strategy. However, their serious side effects have limited their use. The sodium channel blocker, topiramate, can be effective if used in high-dosage limits or in combination with other medications.

Interventions can be performed for patients resistant to pharmacotherapy. Some of these interventions include occipital nerve blocks, sphenopalatine ganglion blocks, specified neuromodulation, and rhizotomy.[50–52]

Exertional Headache

Exertional headache is an uncommon, self-limited, and short-lasting headache condition that is precipitated by exertion. The diagnosis of exertional headache can be difficult as it shares symptoms and signs with other headache conditions. Diagnosis is usually made based on clinical grounds, but imaging can be used to exclude other serious conditions such as brain tumors or intracranial hemorrhage.

Exertional headache can be diagnosed based on the following diagnostic criteria[53–55]:
Headache is associated with physical activities.
Bilateral, throbbing, and may develop migrainous features
Can last 5 minutes to 24 hours
Avoiding physical exercise prevents the headache.
No other disorders to explain those symptoms.

There are several theories proposed to explain the mechanism of exertional headache. Most believe it is vascular in origin. According to one theory, exertion increases cerebral arterial pressure causing pain sensitive venous sinuses at the base of the brain to dilate.[54,56] The treatment of exertional headache is not well studied. Although several medications have been proposed, indomethacin is the most frequently suggested.

Hypnic Headache

It is a primary headache condition occurring exclusively during sleep and mainly in the elderly.[30]

Based on ICHD-3 beta version, hypnic headache can be diagnosed based on following criteria[57,58]:
Recurrent headache fulfilling criteria 1 to 4
1. Develops only during sleep
2. Occurs >10 times per month for >3 months
3. Lasts 15 minutes and up to 4 hours after waking
4. No cranial autonomic symptoms or restlessness
Not accounted for by any other condition

Although pathophysiology remains unclear, several mechanisms have been proposed as posterior hypothalamic condition and central sensitization of trigeminal processing but with conflicting results.[59]

Several medications were studied for treatment of acute attacks, but results have been controversial. Caffeine-containing analgesics seem to be the most effective.[60]

Preventive medications including lithium, caffeine, indomethacin, and topiramate have been proposed for treatment of chronic hypnic headaches.

Secondary Headache Conditions

MEDICATION OVERUSE HEADACHE

Medication-overuse headache (MOH) is a headache condition that occurs in patients with previously existing primary headache that occurs on more than or equal to 15 days per month for more than 3 months. It is a headache condition that is caused by overuse of medications used for treating headache. MOH is diagnosed by fulfilling the following criteria[1]: headache on ≥15 days per month, preexisting headache disorder, overuse of acute and/or symptomatic headache drugs for >3months, and no other condition can explain those symptoms.

The pathophysiology of MOH is not fully understood, and several theories have been proposed including angiotensin-converting enzyme polymorphism, brain-derived neurotrophic factor polymorphism, catechol-O-methyltransferase polymorphism, and serotonin transporter polymorphism. Additionally, it has been postulated that headache may result from interactions with various neurotransmitter systems, neuronal hyperexcitability, and drug dependence.[61–66]

Treatment of MOH can be challenging, as medication used for treating the primary headache condition is the cause of the headache. It is important to start the treatment with educating the patient on MOH. Reducing the doses of medications used for treating the primary headache condition should follow dedicated education. Sometimes, detoxification with abrupt withdrawal may be necessary with reinstating the preventive therapy later at lower doses.[67,68]

Prevention is the best option to avoid MOH. Patients and providers need to work on avoiding very high doses of medications for treating primary headache with close follow-up and monitoring for early detection and treatment.

SINUS HEADACHES

Sinus headache, although commonly used, specialists consider it an inaccurate term. It refers to headache or facial pain associated with sinus disease. A more accurate term proposed by specialists is *rhinogenic headache*.[69]

The HIS diagnostic criteria for headache attributed to rhinosinusitis include the following[70]:
Frontal headache associated with pain in one or more regions of the face and fulfilling criteria 2 and 3
1. Presence of clinical, nasal endoscopic, CT and/or MRI, and/or laboratory evidence of acute or acute on top of chronic rhinosinusitis

2. Headache and facial pain that develops simultaneously with onset of rhinosinusitis
3. Headache and/or facial pain that resolves within 7 days after remission or treatment of acute rhinosinusitis

Management includes treatment of sinusitis, which is essential, migraine-directed therapy,[71] and nasal surgery for mucosal contact point.[72]

HEAD INJURY HEADACHES

Posttraumatic headache (PTHA) is a form of secondary headache that develops within 7 days after a head trauma.[73]

There is no specific pattern for PTHA, as it can share criteria of migraine and tension headaches, but the most important factor is its association with a trauma or traumatic brain injury (TBI). The pathophysiology has been proposed to possibly be related to peripheral or central sensitization mechanisms. Treatment strategies should match the type of headache associated with the trauma. A multidisciplinary approach is highly recommended.[74]

SHORT-LASTING, UNILATERAL, NEURALGIFORM HEADACHE ATTACKS WITH CONJUNCTIVAL INJECTION AND TEARING

Short-lasting, unilateral, neuralgiform headache attacks with conjunctival injection and tearing (SUNCT) syndrome is a unilateral headache/facial pain characterized by brief paroxysmal attacks accompanied by ipsilateral local autonomic signs, usually conjunctival injection and lacrimation.[75]

Diagnostic features include the following[76–78]:

Unilateral, mostly described as ocular-related pain but can involve larger area of the head

Typically does not change sides or cross midline

Moderate to severe

Usually stabbing or pulsating in nature

Pain lasts from 5 to 240 seconds

Three patterns of attacks are described as follows:

Classical single attacks

Groups of a number of attacks

"Sawtooth" pattern with numerous attacks lasting minutes

The frequency of attacks is from 3 to 200 daily.

Additional features include the following: It is accompanied by marked ipsilateral conjunctival injection and lacrimation that appear rapidly with onset of an attack. Whereas nasal stuffiness and rhinorrhea are common, sweating is rare to accompany the attack.

Pathophysiology: The mechanism of SUNCT is still unclear, but studies suggested the presence of a relationship between the hypothalamus and the condition. MRI has allowed for recognition of activation within the hypothalamus during an attack. There is a direct connection between the trigeminal nucleus caudalis within the brainstem and the posterior hypothalamus. It is possible that stimulation of the peripheral trigeminal nerve activates the hypothalamus, and the hypothalamus in turn communicates with the trigeminal nucleus caudalis via the release of neurotransmitters. In support of this possible hypothalamic mechanism, elevated levels of prolactin has been associated with SUNCT.[79–81]

SUNCT is refractory to most treatment modalities except for the antiepileptic drug group. Lamotrigine is proposed to be the first-line medication.[82,83] However, intravenously delivered lidocaine and phenytoin have shown some efficacy.

SHORT-LASTING, UNILATERAL, NEURALGIFORM HEADACHE ATTACKS WITH CRANIAL AUTONOMIC FEATURES

Short-lasting, unilateral, neuralgiform headache attack with cranial autonomic features (SUNA) is a novel type of headache. It can be difficult to differentiate from SUNCT. One of the main differences is that the attack duration can be extended to 10 minutes with a similar treatment paradigm as SUNCT.

PAROXYSMAL HEMICRANIAS

This type of chronic headache is usually continuous with a small percentage of patients who suffer with episodic paroxysmal hemicrania.[84] Clinically, it is usually unilateral; severe orbital or periorbital pain; rarely becomes bilateral; may extend to a larger area in the head; can refer to the shoulder, neck, and arm; lasts 2 to 30 minutes; and sharp in nature. Additionally, it is accompanied by at least one of these ipsilateral autonomic phenomena/signs: conjunctival injection/lacrimation, nasal congestion, eyelid edema, facial sweating, and miosis/ptosis. Attacks may occur more than five times daily, might be seasonal temporal, periauricular, maxillary, and rarely the occipital region. Referral to the shoulder, neck, and arm is also quite common, and strong pain may cross the midline; the vast majority of attacks do not change sides.

The response to indomethacin is absolute, but the mechanism is not well understood. Other alternatives include calcium channel blockers, naproxen, and carbamazepine.[84–87]

CONTACT POINT HEADACHE

Another headache responsible for facial pain features is the contact point headache. The contact point headache is also called anterior ethmoidal neuralgia, Sluder's neuralgia, sphenopalatine ganglion neuralgia, and pterygopalatine ganglion neuralgia.

It presents as a persistent stabbing or sharp pain in a single localized area/spot on the face.[88] It is thought to develop due to nerve compression related to a structural abnormality usually inside the nose, such as a septal spur or a deviated septum.

The nerve affected is usually the anterior ethmoid nerve, a nerve that branches off sphenopalatine ganglion (pterygopalatine ganglion).

Clinically, it presents with a pain syndrome that usually starts after the patient has had an upper respiratory infection and presents as localized pain on one spot and one side of the face; it can be localized to the roof of the mouth and upper teeth. Pain is commonly localized to an area between the eye and cheek but can radiate to other parts of the face.

The only single medication that had shown effectiveness in providing relief of contact point headache is an over-the-counter decongestant. Surgery is the main treatment to cure the condition and relieve the pressure on the nerve.[89]

References

1. Headache Classification Committee of the International Headache Society. The International Classification of Headache Disorders, 3rd edition (Beta version). *Cephalalgia* 2013;33:629–808.
2. Burchiel KJ. A new classification for facial pain. *Neurosurgery* 2003;53:1164–1167.
3. Eller JL, Raslan AM, Burchiel KJ. Trigeminal neuralgia: definition and classification. *Neurosurg Focus* 2005;18(5):E3.
4. Devor M, Amir R, Rappaport H. Pathophysiology of trigeminal neuralgia: the ignition hypothesis. *Clin J Pain* 2002;18:4–13.
5. Devor M, Govrin-Lippmann R, Rappaport ZH. Mechanism of trigeminal neuralgia: an ultrastructural analysis of trigeminal root specimens obtained during microvascular decompression surgery. *J Neurosurg* 2002;96:532–543.
6. Burchiel KJ, Slavin KV. On the natural history of trigeminal neuralgia. *Neurosurgery* 2000;46:152–154.
7. Peñarrocha M, Alfaro A, Bagán JV, et al. Idiopathic trigeminal sensory neuropathy. *J Oral Maxillofac Surg* 1992;50:472–476.
8. Reddy GD, Viswanathan A. Trigeminal and glossopharyngeal neuralgia. *Neurol Clin* 2014;32(2):539–552.
9. Rey-Dios R, Cohen-Gadol AA. Current neurosurgical management of glossopharyngeal neuralgia and technical nuances for microvascular decompression surgery. *Neurosurg Focus* 2013;34(3):E8.
10. Haller S, Etienne L, Kövari E, et al. Imaging of neurovascular compression syndromes: trigeminal neuralgia, hemifacial spasm, vestibular paroxysmia, and glossopharyngeal neuralgia. *AJNR Am J Neuroradiol* 2016;37(8):1384–1392.
11. Chen J, Sindou M. Vago-glossopharyngeal neuralgia: a literature review of neurosurgical experience. *Acta Neurochir (Wien)* 2015;157(2):311–321.

12. Ma Y, Li YF, Wang QC, et al. Neurosurgical treatment of glossopharyngeal neuralgia: analysis of 103 cases. *J Neurosurg* 2016;124(4):1088–1092.

13. Rupta V, Saunders RL, Wieder DJ. Geniculate neuralgia: the surgical management of primary otalgia. *J Neurosurg* 1991;75:505–511.

14. Tubbs RS, Steck DT, Mortazavi MM, et al. The nervus intermedius: a review of its anatomy, function, pathology and role in neurosurgery. *World Neurosurg* 2013;79(5):763–767.

15. Tang IP, Freeman SR, Kontorinis G, et al. Geniculate neuralgia: a systemic review. *J Laryngol Otol* 2014;128:394–399.

16. Dym H, Israel H. Diagnosis and treatment of temporomandibular disorders. *Dent Clin North Am* 2012;56:149–161.

17. Israel H. Internal derangement of the temporomandibular joint: new perspectives on an old problem. *Oral Maxillofac Surg Clin North Am* 2016;28:313–333.

18. Fricton J. Myofascial pain: mechanisms to management. *Oral Maxillofac Surg Clin North Am* 2016;28:289–311.

19. Scrivani S, Spierings E. Classification and differential diagnosis of oral and maxillofacial pain. *Oral Maxillofac Surg Clin North Am* 2016;28:233–246.

20. Blau JN. Migraine: theories of pathogenesis. *Lancet* 1992;339:1202–1207.

21. Lance JW, Goadsby PJ. *Mechanism and Management of Headache*. London: Butterworth-Heinemann; 1998.

22. Silberstein SD, Lipton RB, Goadsby PJ. *Headache in Clinical Practice*. 2nd ed. London: Martin Dunitz; 2002.

23. Olesen J, Tfelt-Hansen P, Welch KMA. *The Headaches*. 2nd ed. Philadelphia: Lippincott Williams & Wilkins; 2000.

24. Lipton RB, Silberstein SD, Saper JR, et al. Why headache treatment fails. *Neurology* 2003;60(7):1064–1070.

25. Lipton R, Dodick D, Silberstein S, et al. Single-pulse transcranial magnetic stimulation for acute treatment of migraine with aura: a randomised, double-blind, parallel-group, sham-controlled trial. *Lancet Neurol* 2010;9:373–380.

26. Goadsby P, Grosberg B, Mauskop A, et al. Effect of noninvasive vagus nerve stimulation on acute migraine: an open-label pilot study. *Cephalalgia* 2014;34:986–993.

27. Dodick D, Freitag F, Banks J, et al. Topiramate versus amitriptyline in migraine prevention: a 26-week, multicentre, randomized, double-blind, double-dummy, parallel-group noninferiority trial in adult migraineurs. *Clin Ther* 2009;31:542–559.

28. Linde K, Rossnagel K. Propranolol for migraine prophylaxis. *Cochrane Database Syst Rev* 2004;(2):CD003225.

29. Magis D, Schoenen J. Advances and challenges in neurostimulation for headaches. *Lancet Neurol* 2012;11:708–719.

30. Headache Classification Subcommittee of the International Headache Society. The International Classification of Headache Disorders: 2nd edition. *Cephalalgia* 2004;24(suppl 1):9–160.

31. Ashina M. Neurobiology of chronic tension-type headache. *Cephalalgia* 2004;24:161–172.

32. Bendtsen L. Central sensitization in tension-type headache—possible pathophysiological mechanisms. *Cephalalgia* 2000;20:486–508.

33. Jensen R. Pathophysiological mechanisms of tension-type headache: A review of epidemiological and experimental studies. *Cephalalgia* 1999;19:602–621.

34. Ulrich V, Russell MB, Jensen R, et al. A comparison of tension-type headache in migraineurs and non-migraineurs: a population-based study. *Pain* 1996;67:501–506.

35. Steiner TJ, Lange R, Voelker M. Aspirin in episodic tension-type headache: placebo-controlled dose-ranging comparison with paracetamol. *Cephalalgia* 2003;23:59–66.

36. Ashina S, Ashina M. Current and potential future drug therapies for tension-type headache. *Curr Pain Headache Rep* 2003;7:466–474.

37. Bendtsen L, Mathew NT. Prophylactic pharmacotherapy of tension-type headache. In: Olesen J, Goadsby PJ, Ramadan N, et al. *The Headaches*. 3rd ed. Philadelphia: Lippincott Williams & Wilkins; 2005:735–741.

38. Bendtsen L, Jensen R, Olesen J. A non-selective (amitriptyline), but not a selective (citalopram), serotonin reuptake inhibitor is effective in the prophylactic treatment of chronic tension-type headache. *J Neurol Neurosurg Psychiatry* 1996;61:285–290.

39. Singh NN, Mishra S. Sertaline in chronic tension-type headache. *J Assoc Physicians India* 2002;50:873–878.

40. Manna V, Bolino F, Di Cicco L. Chronic tension-type headache, mood depression and serotonin: therapeutic effects of fluvoxamine and mianserine. *Headache* 1994;34:44–49.

41. Langemark M, Olesen J. Sulpiride and paroxetine in the treatment of chronic tension-type headache. An explanatory double-blind trial. *Headache* 1994;34:20–24.

42. Zissis N, Harmoussi S, Vlaikidis N, et al. A randomized, double-blind, placebo-controlled study of venlafaxine XR in out-patients with tension-type headache. *Cephalalgia* 2007;27:315–324.

43. Bendtsen L, Jensen R. Mirtazapine is effective in the prophylactic treatment of chronic tension-type headache. *Neurology* 2004;62:1706–1711.

44. Shimmomura T, Awaki E, Kowa H, et al. Treatment of tension type headache with tizanidine hydrochloride, its efficacy and relationship with plasma MHPG concentration. *Headache* 1991;31:601–604.

45. Holroyd KA, Martin PR, Nash JM. Psychological treatments of tension-type headache. In: Olesen J, Goadsby PJ, Ramadan N, et al, eds. *The Headaches*. 3rd ed. Philadelphia: Lippincott Williams & Wilkins; 2005:711–719.

46. May A, Bahra A, Büchel C, et al. Hypothalamic activation in cluster headache attacks. *Lancet* 1998;352:275–278.

47. Cohen AS, Burns B, Goadsby PJ. High-flow oxygen for treatment of cluster headache: a randomized trial. *JAMA* 2009;302:2451–2457.

48. May A, Leone M, Afra J, et al. EFNS guidelines on the treatment of cluster headache and other trigeminal-autonomic cephalalgias. *Eur J Neurol* 2006;13:1066–1077.

49. Rasche D, Klase D, Tronnier VM. Neuromodulation in cluster headache. Clinical follow-up after deep brain stimulation in the posterior hypothalamus for chronic cluster headache, case report—part II [in German]. *Schmerz* 2008;22(suppl 1):37–40.

50. Ansarinia M, Rezai A, Tepper SJ, et al. Sphenopalatine ganglion (SPG) stimulation during acute migraine and cluster headaches. *Headache* 2010;50:1164–1174.

51. May A, Leone M, Boecker H, et al. Hypothalamic deep brain stimulation in positron emission tomography. *J Neurosci* 2006;26:3589–3593.

52. Broggi G, Messina G, Franzini A. Cluster headache and TACs: rationale for central and peripheral neuromodulation. *Neurol Sci* 2009;30(suppl 1):S75–S79.

53. Rooke D. Benign exertional headache. *Med Clin North Am* 1968;52:801–808.

54. McCrory P. Recognizing exercise-related headache. *Phys Sports Med* 1997;25:33–43.

55. Paulson GW. Weightlifters headache. *Headache* 1983;23:193–194.

56. MacDougall JD, Tuxen D, Sale DG, et al. Arterial blood pressure response to heavy resistance exercise. *J Appl Physiol* 1985;58:785–790.

57. Liang JF, Wang SJ. Hypnic headache: a review of clinical features, therapeutic options and outcomes. *Cephalalgia* 2014;34(10):795–805.

58. Dodick D. Patient perceptions and treatment preferences in migraine management. *CNS Drugs* 2002;16 (suppl 1):19–24.

59. de Tommaso M, Valeriani M, Guido M, et al. Abnormal brain processing of cutaneous pain in patients with chronic migraine. *Pain* 2003;101:25–32.

60. Holle D, Naegel S, Krebs S, et al. Clinical characteristics and therapeutic options in hypnic headache. *Cephalalgia* 2010;30:1435–1442.

61. Phillips MI. Functions of angiotensin in the central nervous system. *Annu Rev Physiol* 1987;49:413–435.

62. Binder DK, Scharfman HE. Brain-derived neurotrophic factor. *Growth Factors* 2004;22:123–131.

63. Cargnin S, Viana M, Ghiotto N, et al. Functional polymorphisms in COMT and SLC6A4 genes influence the prognosis of patients with medication overuse headache after withdrawal therapy. *Eur J Neurol* 2014;21:989–995.

64. Srikiatkhachorn A, Tarasub N, Govitrapong P. Effect of chronic analgesic exposure on the central serotonin system: a possible mechanism of analgesic abuse headache. *Headache* 2000;40:343–350.

65. Ayzenberg I, Obermann M, Nyuis P, et al. Central sensitization of the trigeminal and somatic nociceptive systems in medication overuse headache mainly involves cerebral supraspinal structures. *Cephalalgia* 2006;26:1106–1114.

66. Fuh JL, Wang SJ, Lu SR, et al. Does medication overuse headache represent a behavior of dependence? *Pain* 2005;119:49–55.

67. Rossi P, Di Lorenzo C, Faroni J, et al. Advice alone vs. structured detoxification programmes for medication overuse headache: a prospective, randomized, open-label trial in transformed migraine patients with low medical needs. *Cephalalgia* 2006;26:1097–1105.

68. Rossi P, Faroni JV, Tassorelli C, et al. Advice alone versus structured detoxification programmes for complicated medication overuse headache (MOH): a prospective, randomized, open-label trial. *J Headache Pain* 2013;14:10.

69. Cady RK, Dodick DW, Levine HL, et al. Sinus headache: a neurology, otolaryngology, allergy, and primary care consensus on diagnosis and treatment. *Mayo Clin Proc* 2005;80(7):908–916.

70. Levine HL, Setzen M, Cady RK, et al. An otolaryngology, neurology, allergy, and primary care consensus on diagnosis and treatment of sinus headache. *Otolaryngol Head Neck Surg* 2006;134:516–523.

71. Ishkanian G, Blumenthal H, Webster CJ, et al. Efficacy of sumatriptan tablets in migraineurs self-described or physician-diagnosed as having sinus headache: a randomized, double-blind, placebo-controlled study. *Clin Ther* 2007;29:99–109.

72. Welge-Luessen A, Hauser R, Schmid N, et al. Endonasal surgery for contact point headaches: a 10-year longitudinal study. *Laryngoscope* 2003;113:2151–2156.

73. Walker WC, Seel RT, Curtiss G, et al. Headache after moderate and severe traumatic brain injury: a longitudinal analysis. *Arch Phys Med Rehabil* 2005;86(9):1793–1800.

74. Ivanhoe CB, Hartman ET. Clinical caveats on medical assessment and treatment of pain after TBI. *J Head Trauma Rehabil* 2004;19:29–39.

75. Sjaastad O, Saunte C, Salvesen R, et al. Shortlasting unilateral neuralgiform headache attacks with conjunctival injection, tearing, sweating, and rhinorrhea. *Cephalalgia* 1989;9(2):147–156.

76. Cohen AS, Matharu MS, Goadsby PJ. Short-lasting unilateral neuralgiform headache attacks with conjunctival injection and tearing (SUNCT) or cranial autonomic features (SUNA): a prospective clinical study of SUNCT and SUNA. *Brain* 2006;129(pt 10):2746–2760.

77. Sjaastad O, Kruszewski P. Trigeminal neuralgia and "SUNCT" syndrome: similarities and differences in the clinical pictures. An overview. *Funct Neurol* 1992;7(2):103–107.

78. Pareja JA, Cuadrado ML. SUNCT syndrome: an update. *Expert Opin Pharmacother* 2005;6(4):591–599.

79. Auer T, Janszky J, Schwarcz A, et al. Attack-related brainstem activation in a patient with SUNCT syndrome: an ictal fMRI study. *Headache* 2009;49(6):909–912.

80. Goadsby PJ, Lipton RB. A review of paroxysmal hemicranias, SUNCT syndrome and other short-lasting headaches with autonomic feature, including new cases. *Brain* 1997;120(pt 1):193–209.

81. Bosco D, Labate A, Mungari P, et al. SUNCT and high nocturnal prolactin levels: some new unusual characteristics. *J Headache Pain* 2007;8(2):114–118.

82. Cohen AS. Short-lasting unilateral neuralgiform headache attacks with conjunctival injection and tearing. *Cephalalgia* 2007;27:824–832.

83. Cohen AS, Matharu MS, Goadsby PJ. Trigeminal autonomic cephalalgias: current and future treatments. *Headache* 2007;47:969–980.

84. Boes CJ, Dodick DW. Refining the clinical spectrum of chronic paroxysmal hemicrania: a review of 74 patients. *Headache* 2002;42(8):699–708.

85. Antonaci F, Sjaastad O. Chronic paroxysmal hemicrania (CPH): a review of the clinical manifestations. *Headache* 1989;29(10):648–656.

86. Matharu MS, Goadsby PJ. Bilateral paroxysmal hemicrania or bilateral paroxysmal cephalalgia, another novel indomethacin-responsive primary headache syndrome? *Cephalalgia* 2005;25(2):79–81.

87. Boes CJ, Vincent M, Russell D. Chronic paroxysmal hemicrania. In: Olesen J, Goadsby PJ, Ramadan NM, et al, eds. *The Headaches.* 3rd ed. Philadelphia: Lippincott Williams & Wilkins; 2006:815–822.

88. Ahamed SH, Jones NS. What is Sluder's neuralgia? *J Laryngol Otol* 2003;117(6):437–443.

89. Karlov VA, Tebloev IK, Savitskaia ON, et al. Facial autonomic and trophic disorders [in Russian]. *Zh Nevropatol Psikhiatr Im S S Korsakova* 1979;79(4):416–420.

CHAPTER 68

Neck and Arm Pain

ANITA H. HICKEY and **ZAHID H. BAJWA**

The unique anatomy of the cervical spine and upper extremity balances the attributes of strength and stability with those of flexibility and range of motion. The biomechanical properties associated with these combined properties allow for a high incidence of degenerative changes. These increase with aging and are often associated with episodic or chronic pain. Although the origin of pain in the neck is often categorized as axial pain versus radicular pain and musculoskeletal pain versus neuropathic pain, the patient presenting for treatment in the clinical setting may not always be representative of these categorical descriptions.

An understanding of the normal anatomy of the neck and upper extremity, pathophysiology of common disorders of the cervical spine, diversity of clinical presentations of neck and arm pain, and the potential contribution of systemic and psychological factors is critical in forming a differential diagnosis, referring the patient for appropriate diagnostic tests and evaluations and instituting timely and appropriate treatment. This chapter focuses on the anatomy of the cervical spine and upper extremity; recent data regarding the epidemiology of neck and arm pain; the critical role of the clinician in performing a thorough and targeted history and physical examination; and finally, a discussion of the etiology and treatment of neck and arm pain.

The common causes of mechanical neck and arm pain, including cervical spondylosis and myelopathy, cervical radiculopathy, cervicogenic headache (CEH), brachial plexopathy, peripheral nerve entrapment syndromes of the upper extremity, and thoracic outlet syndrome (TOS), are discussed in this chapter. Myofascial pain syndromes, fibromyalgia, and acute musculoskeletal disorders can involve the neck and upper extremities and are covered in detail elsewhere in this text. Neck and arm pain may also be secondary to primary or metastatic disease. Cancer pain is discussed more thoroughly elsewhere as well. Therapeutic modalities are covered more extensively in Part V: Methods for Symptomatic Control.

Anatomy of the Neck and Arm

CERVICAL SPINE

The anatomy of the cervical spine is complex in order to allow for support of the weight of the cranium, to provide protection and support of the neurovascular elements of the cervical spine, and to simultaneously permit functional mobility in relation to the surrounding structures. It is composed of 7 vertebrae, 5 intervertebral disks, 12 joints of Luschka, and 14 zygapophyseal joints, uniquely bound and connected to numerous ligaments and muscles which both limit and permit varying degrees of motion of the cervical spine.[1]

With the exception of the first two cervical vertebrae, which have unique characteristics, each of the seven cervical vertebrae is composed of a segmental unit, which includes a vertebral body, an intervertebral disk, four uncovertebral joints of Luschka, two pedicles, two lamina, two inferior, and two superior zygapophyseal (articular facet) joints. Between each vertebral segment, a spinal nerve, radicular blood vessels, and the sinuvertebral (recurrent meningeal) nerves pass through neural openings or foramina on each side of the cervical spine (Fig. 68.1).[1]

The upper two segments of the cervical spine have unique anatomic and biomechanical characteristics when compared with the lower five segments of the cervical spine. The atlas, or C1 vertebra, is a ring-shaped vertebra with paired lateral pillars, which function as articulating joints or facets. The upper ellipsoid facets articulate superiorly with the occipital condyles to form the atlantooccipital joints, whereas the round and concave inferior facets articulate inferiorly with the axis to form the atlantoaxial joints. The anterior arch of the atlas incorporates an articular surface which contacts the anterior surface of the dens or odontoid process of the axis. The atlas is the widest of the cervical vertebrae, allowing for the spinal cord, dens, and a surrounding cushion of spinal fluid. It has a mean internal, anteroposterior dimension of approximately 31.7 mm and an internal width of 32.2 mm. The atlas is the only cervical vertebra not associated with an intervertebral disk. Its transverse process is longer than the other cervical vertebrae to support the attachments of the muscles that rotate the head, and its transverse foramen contains the vertebral artery, veins, and sympathetic nerves (Fig. 68.2).

The axis, or C2 vertebra, has a small body anteriorly from which the odontoid process arises and projects upward. Its oval-shaped anterior face articulates with that on the anterior arch of the atlas. The posterior surface of the odontoid process articulates with the transverse ligament. The facets on the upper and lower surfaces of the lateral masses of the axis articulate with the atlas above and the C3 facet joints below. The atlas also has a large palpable bifid spinous process and small transverse processes with transverse openings or foramina through which the vertebral artery, veins, and the vertebral sympathetic plexuses pass. Because both the atlas and the axis lack pedicles and intervertebral foramen, the nerve roots of the first and second spinal nerves pass above and posterior to the articulating lateral masses of each vertebrae. The hypoglossal nerves traverse the occipital condyles anterolaterally through the hypoglossal foramen a mean of 12.2 mm from the posterior margin of the occipital condyle (see Fig. 68.2).[1]

The five lower cervical vertebrae share common characteristics in that they are composed of a vertebral body, an intervening intervertebral disk, two pedicles, two laminae, two vertebral arches, and a spinous process. The upper and lower surfaces of the pedicles form the articulating facets of the cervical zygapophyseal joints. The transverse processes are situated anterolaterally to the facet joints. Their trough-shaped surfaces contain the roots of the cervical spinal nerves and a foramen through which the vertebral artery, veins, and vertebral sympathetic nerve pass.[1]

The anterior portions of the C2 through C7 vertebral bodies, like those of the thoracic and lumbar spine, are connected at their upper and lower surfaces by intervertebral disks, which make up the main joints of the spinal column. Each disk is made up of a central nucleus pulposus surrounded by a thick ring of fibrous cartilage called the annulus fibrosis. The disk is connected to the vertebral body above and below by a hyaline cartilage endplate whose fibers interface with the disk and the vertebral body.[1]

The nucleus pulposus contains collagen and elastin fibers embedded in a colloidal proteoglycan gel which is osmotically active

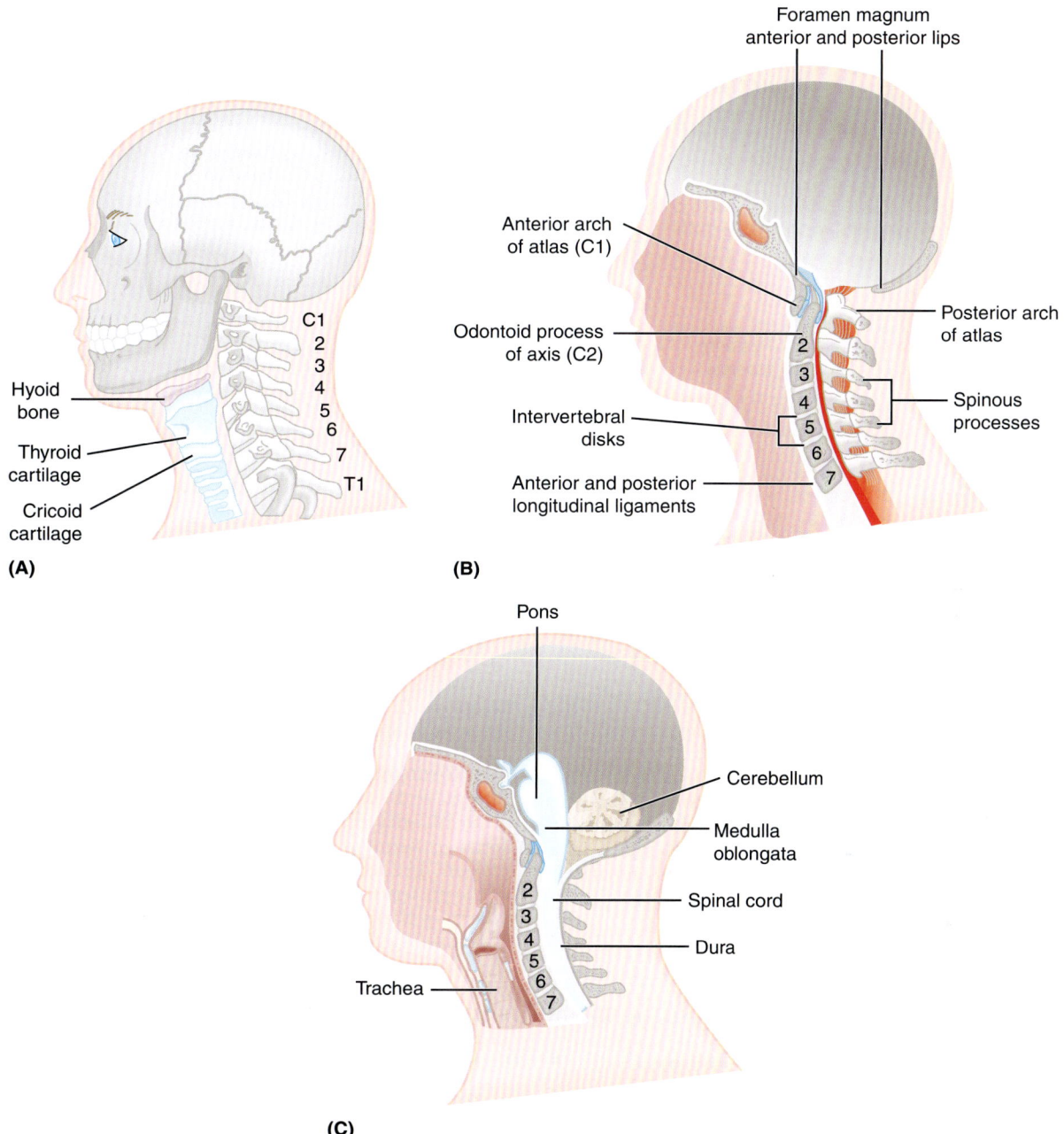

FIGURE 68.1 Anatomy of the cervical spine. **A:** Lateral view, showing landmarks of the spine, including the hyoid bone, thyroid and cricoid cartilages, and transverse and spinous processes. **B:** View of the skeletal portion of the lower skull and cervical spine. The skull and spinous processes are shown in sagittal section, whereas the vertebral bodies are shown as normal. **C:** Sagittal view of the cervical spine showing the relationship of the brainstem, medulla oblongata, foramen magnum, and spinal canal, containing the spinal cord. Normally, the lower portion of the medulla is outside and below the foramen magnum so that subluxation of the atlas on the axis and compression of the lower brainstem can occur by compression from the odontoid process, which moves posteriorly against the neuraxis. *(Modified from Bland JH*. Disorders of the Cervical Spine: Diagnosis and Medical Management. *Philadelphia, PA: Saunders; 1987. Copyright © 1987 Elsevier. With permission.)*

in healthy disks with an approximately 80% water content. The annulus is made up of 15 to 25 concentric rings or lamellae made up of collagen fibers oriented in an alternating criss-cross oblique fashion with elastin fibers layered between the lamellae. The annulus attaches around the entire circumference of the upper and lower endplates and, together with the nucleus pulposus, forms a fluid elastic system. These properties allow the disk to absorb and more evenly distribute the mechanical stress of high-impact activity. By the third decade of life, the disk has become avascular and must rely on diffusion of nutrients and water through the endplates and lymph. The properties of the healthy disk permit disk hydration by way of compression and relaxation of the viscoelastic system, similar to the action of squeezing a sponge. With aging, atherosclerosis, and trauma, degenerative changes occur within the disk. A decrease in protein polysaccharide content and thus its water composition leads to loss of its viscoelastic properties. Degeneration of the disk increases the axial load and shear on the zygapophyseal joints and contributes to simultaneous degenerative changes of these posterior spinal elements (Fig. 68.3).[1]

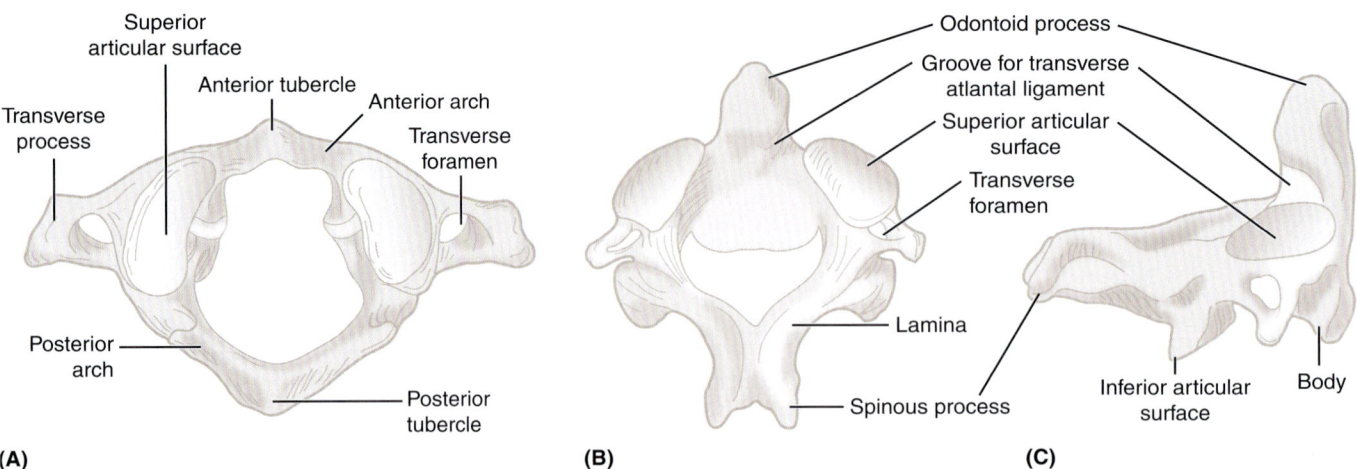

FIGURE 68.2   Anatomy of the atlas and axis. **A:** Superior view of the atlas. **B:** The axis viewed from a superior and posteroanterior aspect. **C:** Lateral view of the axis.

The posterior elements of the lower segments of the cervical spine consist of two vertebral arches, a central posterior spinous process, two transverse processes, and a paired articulation. The transverse processes and posterior spinous processes serve as sites for attachment of supporting ligaments and neck muscles. The zygapophyseal facet joints are true joints with cartilaginous surfaces lined with synovium, containing synovial fluid and surrounded with a ligamentous joint capsule. As such, they are subject to the same inflammatory and degenerative diseases found in other synovial joints. The cervical zygapophyseal joints provide a guiding and gliding movement between the adjacent cervical vertebrae. The movements allowed at the atlantooccipital and atlantoaxial joint are much different from those allowed at the C2–C3 through C7–T1 joints. Differences between the cervical and lumbar spine are summarized in Table 68.1 and Figure 68.4.[1]

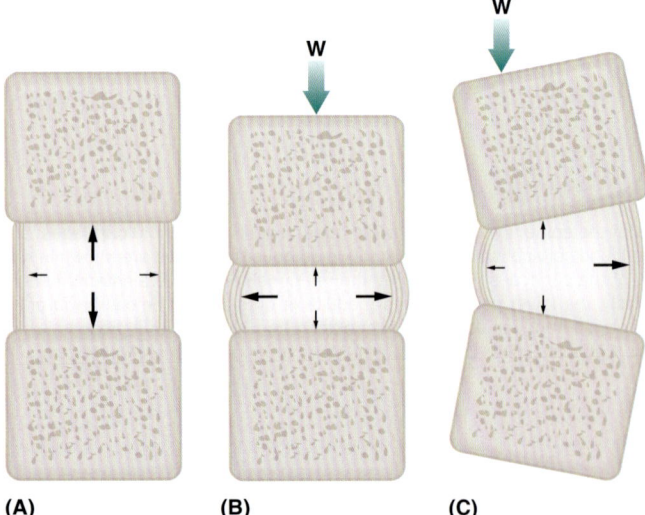

FIGURE 68.3   Schematic depiction of the hydraulic mechanism of the intervertebral disk. **A:** Normal disk at rest. The internal pressure is exerted in all directions, and the fibers of the annulus are taut. **B:** When the disk is compressed, the fluid within the nucleus pulposus cannot compress, so the annulus must bulge. **C:** With flexion of the spine, the fluid shifts within the intervertebral disk; the cubic contents remain the same, but the fluid shift causes fibers of the anterior annulus to shorten and those of the posterior annulus to elongate. W, weight. *(From Cailliet R. Neck and Arm Pain. 2nd ed. Philadelphia: FA Davis; 1981. Reproduced with permission of F.A. Davis Co., in the format Republish in a book via Copyright Clearance Center.)*

Ligaments of the Cervical Spine

The ligaments of the cervical spine provide essential protection to the spinal cord and nerves during various stresses which occur owing to a top-heavy and eccentrically balanced head atop a relatively narrow elastic cervical spine. The greatest range and amplitude of movement in the cervical spine occurs between the occiput and the C3 vertebra, whereas nodding in an up and down movement in the sagittal plane occurs between the atlas and the axis.[1]

Atlantooccipital Unit

Flexion and extension at the occiput to C1 level is limited to 23 to 24.5 degrees by impingement of the tip of the dens on the foramen magnum in flexion and the tectorial membrane in extension. The tectorial membrane is a fan-shaped continuation of the posterior longitudinal ligament to the base of the occiput where its fibers connect with the dura mater. Lateral bending is resisted by the anatomy of the occipital-C1 articulation and the alar ligaments and averages 3.4 to 5.5 degrees per side. The alar ligaments are enclosed in a synovial membrane and extend to the margin of the foramen magnum from each side of the odontoid process. Axial rotation is also limited by the

TABLE 68.1   Differences between the Cervical and Lumbar Spine

Characteristic	Cervical	Lumbar
Disk to vertebral body height ratio	1:2	1:3
Vertical height of disk	Anterior height 2× that of posterior height/ wedge shaped	Anterior height slightly greater anterior
Vertebral end-plates	Convex and concave, nucleus in anterior portion of disk	Flat and parallel, nucleus centrally located
Joints of von Luschka	False joints or pseudo-arthrosis, appear at 10–20 years of age	Not present in lumbar or thoracic spine
Posterior longitudinal ligament	Double layered between vertebrae Broad, thick, and complete across post-vertebra	Incomplete posteriorly from L3 to S1
Movement between vertebrae	Forward and backward gliding motion	Rocking movement

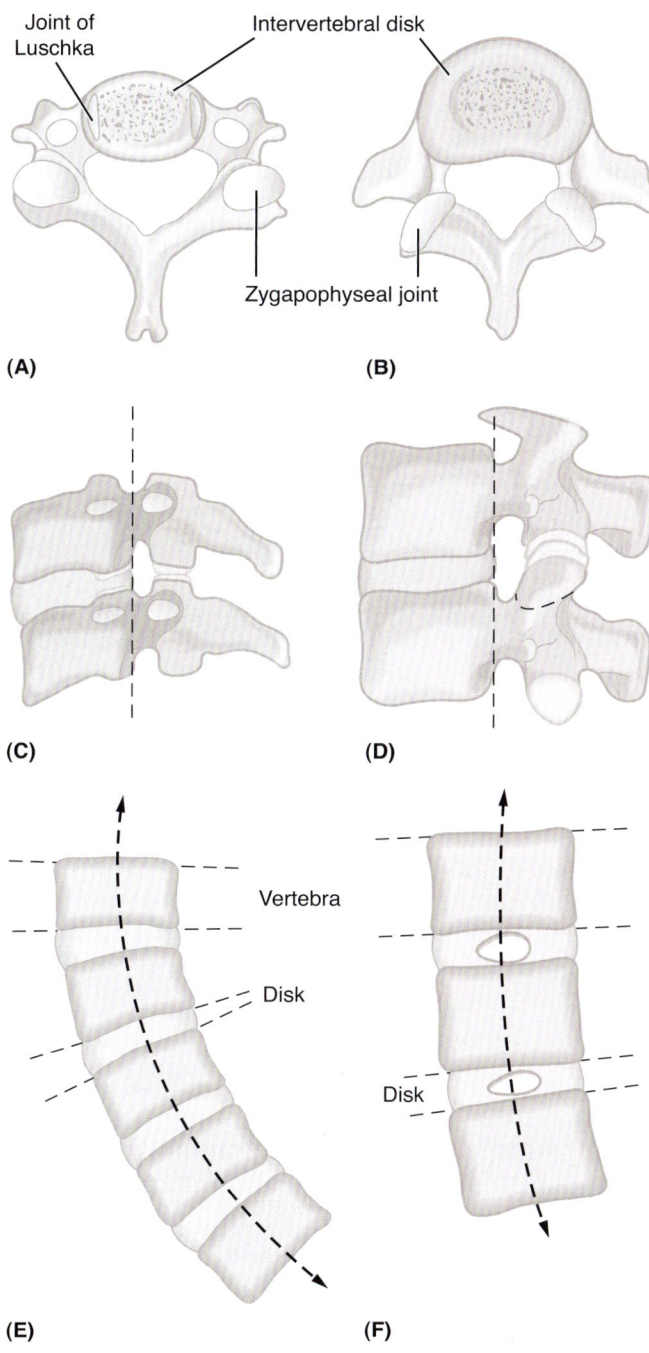

(A)

(B)

Joint of Luschka

Intervertebral disk

Zygapophyseal joint

(C)

(D)

(E) **(F)**

Cervical **Lumbar**

Vertebra

Disk

Disk

FIGURE 68.4 Comparative views of the cervical and lumbar functional units. **A:** Cross-section of the five joints of the cervical spine, which include an intervertebral disk, the paired uncovertebral (Luschka) joints, and the paired posterior articulations. **B:** Cross-section of the three joints of the lumbar spine, which include an intervertebral disk and the paired posterior articulations. **C,D:** Lateral views of the same vertebrae shown in **A** and **B.** The *dashed lines* divide the anterior supporting portion from the posterior gliding portion of each functional unit. **E,F:** Lateral views of the bodies of the vertebrae of the cervical and lumbar spines, depicting particularly the shapes of the intervertebral disks. Note that in the cervical region, the anterior portion of the disk is larger (higher) than the posterior portion, whereas in the lumbar region, the difference between the anterior and posterior portions is much less. *(Modified from Cailliet R. Neck and Arm Pain. 2nd ed. Philadelphia: FA Davis; 1981. Reproduced with permission of F.A. Davis Co., in the format Republish in a book via Copyright Clearance Center.)*

atlantooccipital joint and the alar ligament, 2.4 to 7.2 degrees per side. Lateral translation, stretch and compression, and sagittal plane translation are restricted by the tectorial membrane, the alar, and the apical ligaments as well as the occipital-C1 articulation. The apical ligament is a vestigial remnant of the notochord and attaches from the peak of the odontoid process to the anterior foramen magnum. Other ligaments at this level include the posterior atlantooccipital membrane, which forms the connection between the anterior margin of the foramen magnum and the anterior arch of the atlas, and the posterior atlantooccipital membrane, which extends posteriorly over the vertebral artery.[1]

Atlantoaxial Unit

Axial rotation is the primary movement of the C1–C2 segment. The average 23.3 to 38.9 degree per side rotation is limited by the atlantoaxial joints, the transverse ligament of the ipsilateral side, the alar ligaments of the contralateral side, and capsular ligaments. Flexion rotation is 10.1 to 22.4 degrees and is resisted by the transverse ligament during flexion, the tectorial membrane and joint anatomy. Lateral bending is limited to 6.7 degrees mostly by the alar ligament. Posterior movement or translation at this level is resisted by abutment of the dens on the arch of C1. The transverse ligament extends posteriorly to the odontoid process between the lateral pillars of the atlas. The destabilizing effect of a tear of the transverse ligament is equal to that of a fracture of the odontoid process.[1,2]

Other Cervical Ligaments

The posterior longitudinal ligament and the anterior longitudinal ligaments limit the degree of flexion, extension, and transverse sliding of the C2 to C7 vertebrae. The anterior longitudinal ligament blends with the annulus as it crosses the disk spaces and adheres to the front of the vertebral bodies. The posterior longitudinal ligament is a double-layered structure which is firmly bound to the posterior surface of the cervical disks and loosely bound to the posterior cervical vertebrae. It reinforces the capsular ligaments and the anterior border of the cervical spinal canal.[1]

The ligamentum flavum is a paired structure forming the posterior border of the epidural space. Collectively referred to as ligament flava, they extend between the anterior-inferior surface of the lamina above and to the posterior-superior surface of the lamina below. Posterior to the ligamentum flavum, the interspinous ligaments extend between and connect each spinous process. The ligamentum nuchae is the superior continuation of the supraspinous ligaments of the thoracic and lumbar vertebrae. It is a strong fibrous posterior ligament which extends from the base of the skull to the tips of the posterior cervical spinous process and vertebra (Fig. 68.5).[1]

MUSCULATURE OF THE NECK

The capital movers are the muscles of the neck that flex and extend the head. The capital extensors include the posterior rectus capitis minor and major and the obliquus capitis superior and inferior. The groups of longer muscles that act as capital extensors while working together bilaterally include the longissimus capitis, semispinalis capitis, and splenius capitis. The capital flexors are the short recti and the longus capitis muscles. The most extension and extensor musculature is at the atlantoaxial and C6 through T1 joints. The cervical extensors include the splenius cervicis, longissimus cervicis, and semispinalis cervicis. Maximum flexion of the cervical spine and maximum cervical lordosis occur at C4–C5. The flexors of the cervical spine consist of the scalenus anterior, medius, and posterior. Unilateral rotators of the head include the splenius cervicis, splenius capitis, longissimus capitis, and sternocleidomastoid. The erector muscles of the vertebral column are also involved in movement of the neck (Fig. 68.6).[1]

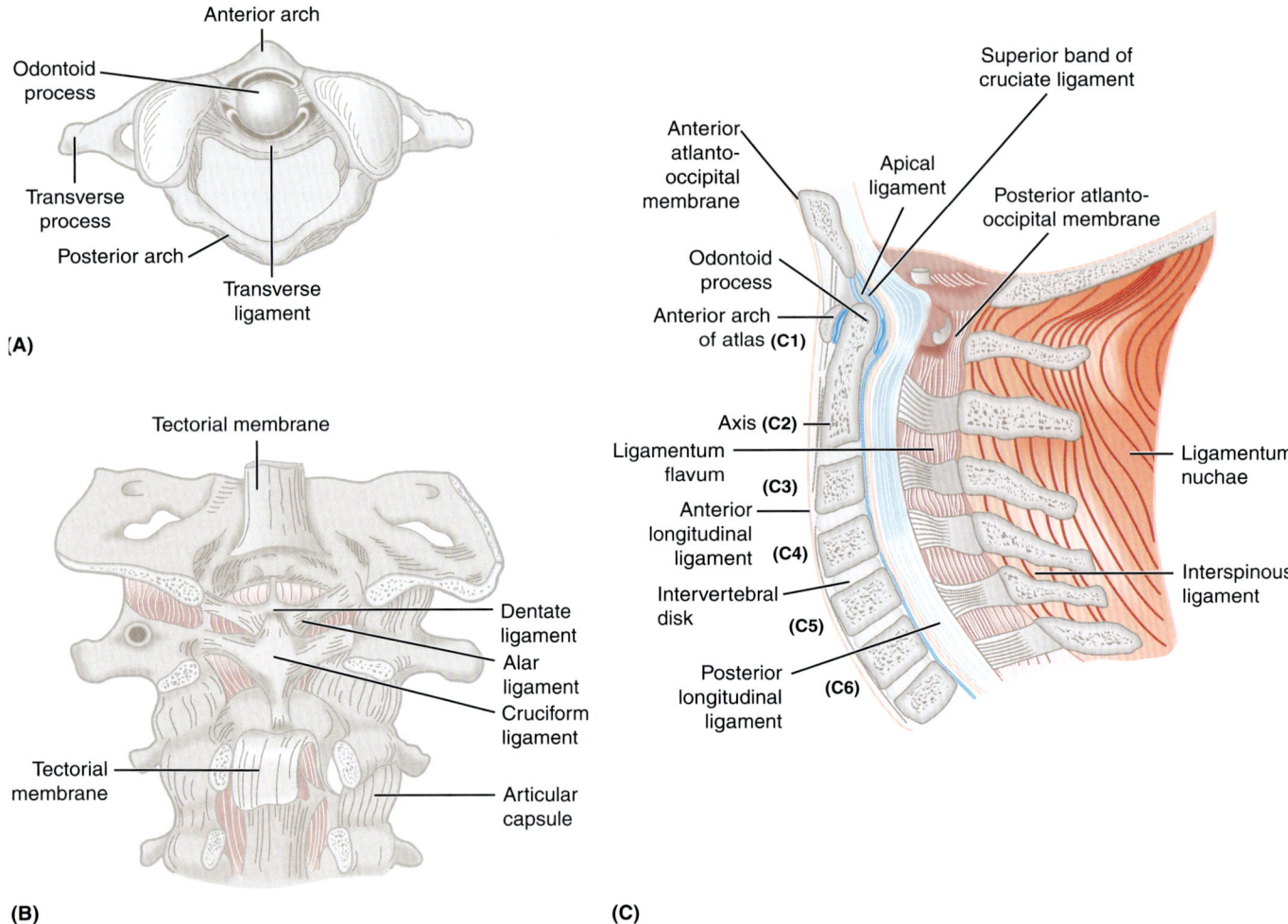

(A)

(B)

(C)

FIGURE 68.5 **A–C:** Ligaments of various parts of the cervical spine (see text for details).

THE VERTEBRAL CANAL

A transverse cut through the cervical vertebral canal reveals its triangular shape with the base or anterior wall made of the vertebra, disk, posterior longitudinal ligament, pedicle, and neural foramina. The lateral and dorsolateral aspects of the other two sides of the triangle include the zygapophyseal joints, laminae, and ligament flava. The canal has its largest sagittal diameter, a range of 16 to 30 mm, at the C1–C2 level and its smallest sagittal diameter, a range of 14 to 23 mm, at the C5–C6 level. The cervical canal lengthens and the intervertebral foramina enlarge during flexion, whereas shortening of the cord and a decrease in the size of the foramen occurs with extension. Lateral flexion or rotation causes the ipsilateral foramina to decrease in size and the contralateral foramina to enlarge. These changes in size of the foramen become significant in the degenerative spine (Fig. 68.7).[1]

The spinal cord is covered by meninges which consist of the delicate pia matter attached to the cord, the web-like arachnoid membrane, and the strong outer dura mater. The dura mater is attached to the foramen magnum and the dorsal surfaces of the C2 and C3 vertebra. The spinal cord is suspended in and protected by surrounding cerebrospinal fluid and is attached laterally to the dural sheath by the dentate ligaments, which are thickenings of the pia mater between and anterior and posterior roots. The anterior and posterior rootlets join the anterior and posterior roots, respectively, at the inner aspect of the intervertebral foramina (Fig. 68.8). An enlargement of the cervical cord occurs from the C3–T1 levels. It is larger than the lumbar enlargement as it contains the ascending and descending long tracts for the trunk as well as the upper and lower limbs. The transverse diameter of the cervical spinal cord is greater than its sagittal diameter, and the cervical cord occupies approximately 40% of the canal. With neck extension, the dura relaxes to form a corrugated appearance and the vertebra above approximates the arch of the vertebra below causing encroachment into the cervical canal. These factors, together with shortening of the cord during extension, increase the risk of impingement of the cord during neck extension.[1]

VERTEBRAL ARTERIES

The vertebral arteries are the first branches from the subclavian trunk and pass cephalad as they course through the transverse foramina of C6–C2 anterior to the cervical nerves. They are accompanied by the vertebral venous plexus and the vertebral nerve and sympathetic plexus, whose fibers originate from neurons in the stellate and intermediate cervical sympathetic ganglia. Branches from the vertebral artery pass through the intervertebral foramina where they supply ligaments, dura, and bone and communicate with the posterior and anterior spinal arteries, which are also branches of the vertebral arteries. The vertebral arteries are supplied by fibers from the

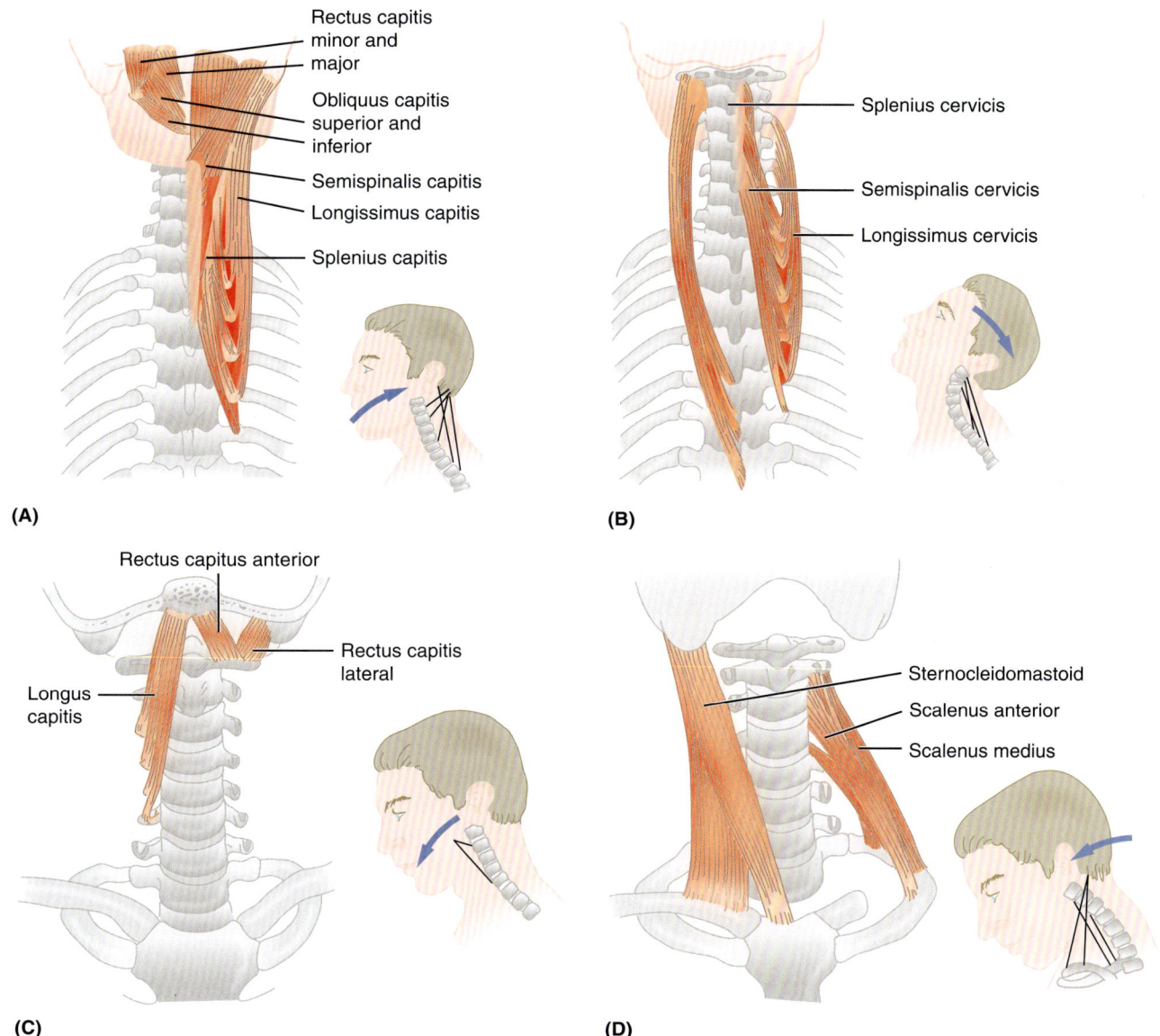

FIGURE 68.6 Musculature of the head and neck. **A:** The capital extensors attach on the skull and move the head on the neck. **B:** The cervical extensors originate from and attach on the cervical spine and alter the curvature of the spine. **C:** The capital flexors flex the head on the neck. **D:** The cervical flexors attach occlusively on the cervical vertebrae and have no significant functional attachment to the skull. *(Modified from Clemente CD, ed. Gray's Anatomy of the Human Body. 30th ed. Philadelphia: Lea & Febiger; 1985; and from Cailliet R. Neck and Arm Pain. 2nd ed. Philadelphia: FA Davis; 1981. Reproduced with permission of F.A. Davis Co., in the format Republish in a book via Copyright Clearance Center.)*

vertebral sympathetic plexus as are the basilar artery, circle of Willis, superior cerebellar, and posterior cerebellar artery (Fig. 68.9).[1]

CERVICAL NERVES

A more detailed discussion of peripheral and spinal pain mechanisms and applied anatomy relevant to pain can be found in earlier chapters of this text. The spinal nerve roots are composed of a dorsal sensory root and a ventral motor root. The posterior root breaks into 12 or more rootlets which attach in series to the dorsolateral sulcus of the cord near Lissauer's tract and then project into the dorsal and ventral horns. Peripherally, the sensory rootlets converge into the fascicule radiculae which unite to form the dorsal root ganglion. A smaller number of rootlets make up the anterior root which arises from the ventrolateral sulcus of the cord. Each rootlet is covered by pia mater, and as they coalesce to form

dorsal and ventral roots, they become separately covered in arachnoid-dural sleeves which are attached to the bony margin of the intervertebral foramen. The anterior roots are in contact with Luschka's joint, and the disk annulus and the dorsal root approximates the articular process and zygapophyseal joint capsule as they pass through the cervical intervertebral foramen. The dorsal and anterior roots join slightly beyond the dorsal root ganglion to form the composite spinal nerve.[1]

The figure eight-shaped intervertebral foramina are largest at the C2–C3 level and progressively narrow and shorten to the C6–C7 level with an average vertical diameter of 10 mm and transverse diameter of 5 mm. The first and second cervical nerves are unique in that they do not pass through an intervertebral foramen. The first cervical nerve passes between the occiput and C1 lateral to the occipital condyle and the second between C1 and C2 posterior to the lateral pillars.[1]

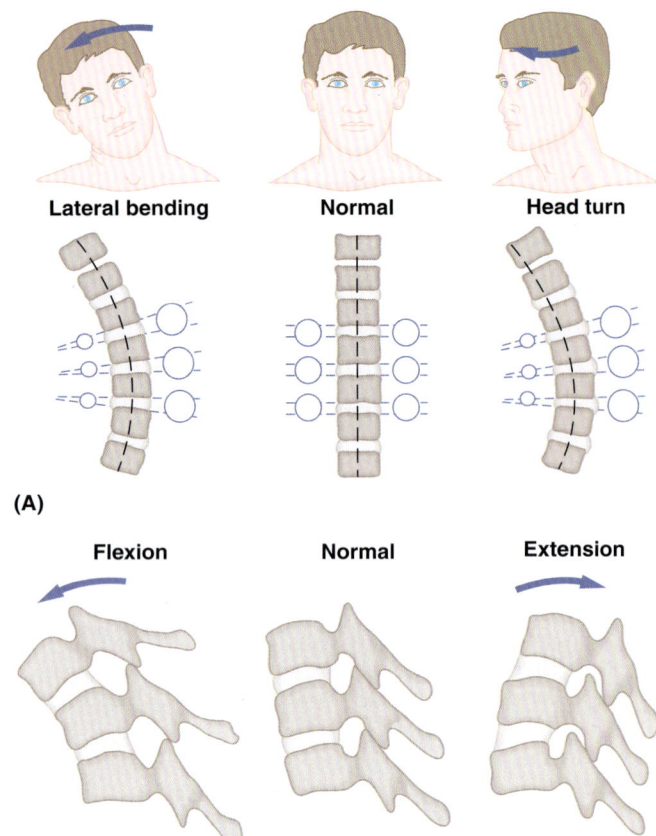

(A)

Lateral bending   Normal   Head turn

Flexion   Normal   Extension

(B)

FIGURE 68.7 Changes in the size of the intervertebral foramina with movement of the neck. **A:** With lateral flexion and rotation of the head, the foramina become smaller on the side of the head to which the head flexes laterally or rotates, and they are open on the opposite side. **B:** With forward flexion, the intervertebral foramina become larger, whereas with extension they become smaller. *(Modified from Cailliet R. Neck and Arm Pain. 2nd ed. Philadelphia: FA Davis; 1981. Reproduced with permission of F.A. Davis Co., in the format Republish in a book via Copyright Clearance Center.)*

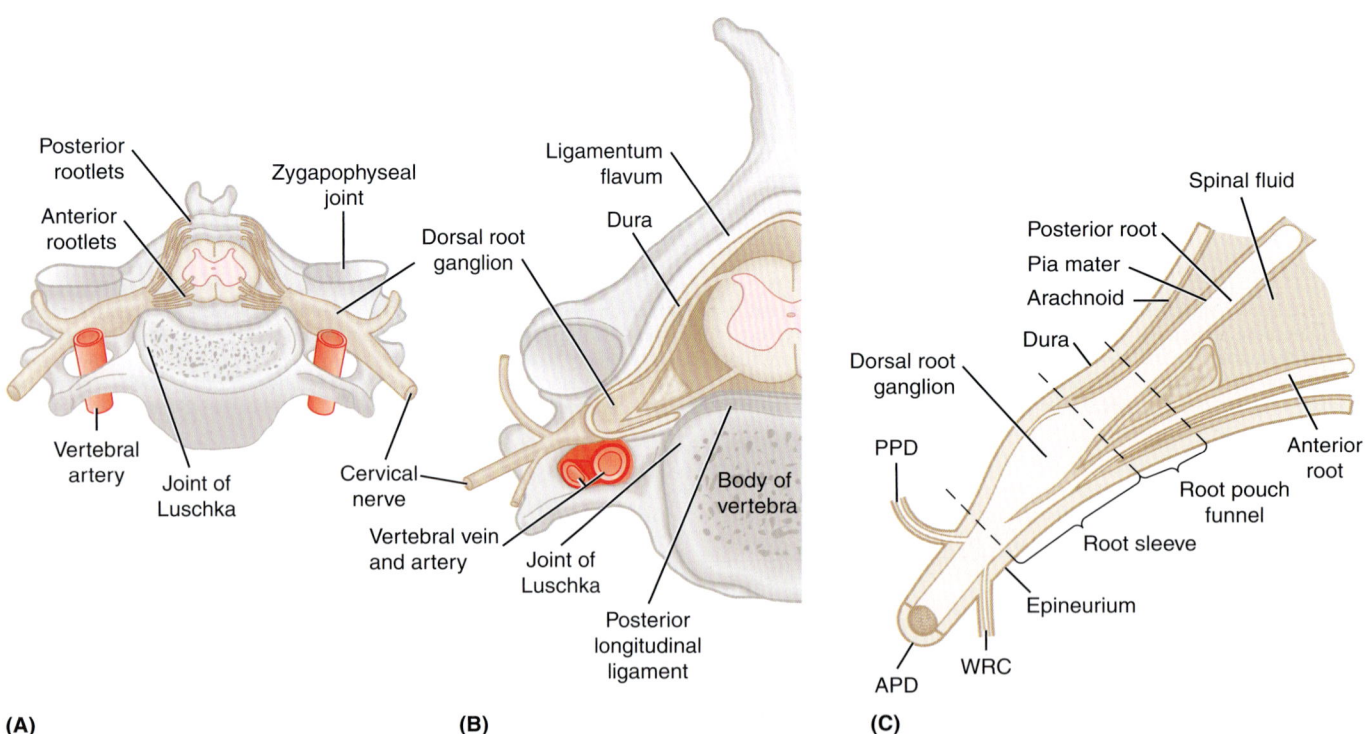

(A)   **(B)**   **(C)**

FIGURE 68.8 Transverse sections of the cervical spine. **A:** The spinal cord and anterior and posterior rootlets join to form the spinal nerve. Note the relationship of the nerves to the Luschka and zygapophyseal joints and the two vertebral arteries, which pass through the transverse foramina and are located just anterior to the nerve. **B:** Cross-section of a cervical vertebra showing some details of the relationship of the posterior root to the lateral aspect of the ligamentum flavum, which covers the zygapophyseal joint just posterior to it. The anterior root and its dural covering are close to the lateral part of the posterior longitudinal ligaments and to the capsules of the joint of Luschka. The proximal portion of the dorsal root ganglion is in the outer portion of the intervertebral foramen, whereas the remainder is in the gutter of the transverse process. **C:** Detailed anatomy of a nerve root and its meningeal covering. Note the extent of the root pouch and root sleeve. Just distal to the joining of the anterior and posterior roots is the short spinal nerve covered by epineurium (the continuation of the dura), which promptly divides into the anterior primary division (APD) and posterior primary division (PPD) and gives off a white ramus communicantes (WRC). *(A, Modified from Bland JH. Disorders of the Cervical Spine: Diagnosis and Medical Management. 2nd ed. Philadelphia, PA: Saunders; 1987. Copyright © 1987 Elsevier. With permission.; B and C, Modified from Cailliet R. Neck and Arm Pain. 2nd ed. Philadelphia: FA Davis; 1981. Reproduced with permission of F.A. Davis Co., in the format Republish in a book via Copyright Clearance Center.)*

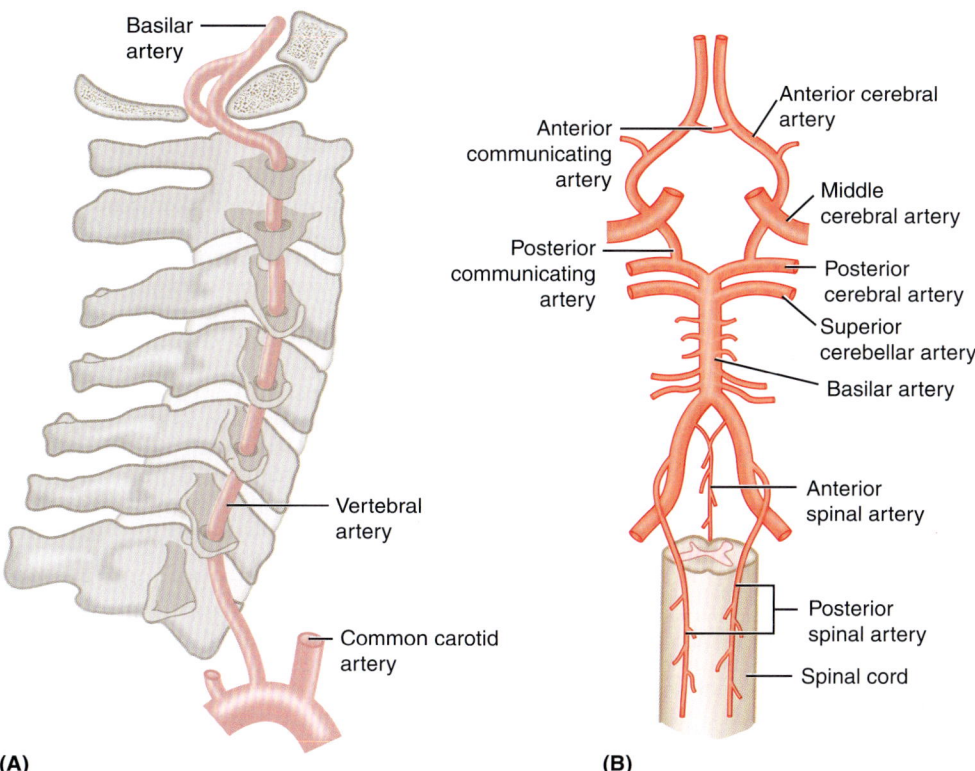

(A)   **(B)**

FIGURE 68.9 A: Lateral view of the cervical vertebrae depicting the course of the vertebral artery from C6 to C1 through bony ridges of the foramina transversaria. Note the double U turn the artery makes from C2 to C1 in its posterior course around the lateral mass of the atlas. **B:** The two vertebral arteries join to form the basal arteries. Also shown is the circle of Willis. Note the origin of the anterior spinal artery and the two posterior spinal arteries from the two vertebral arteries.

In addition to the nerve roots, the foramina contain the spinal radicular arteries, intervertebral veins, and venous plexuses together with loose areolar tissue and fat from the adjoining extension of the epidural space. These provide a protective cushion in the healthy spine. Each spinal nerve receives one or more gray rami communicantes from the cervical sympathetic ganglia after exiting the spinal canal. Spinal nerves 1 through 4 receive fibers from the superior cervical sympathetic ganglion, spinal nerves 5 and 6 from the intermediate ganglia, spinal nerves 7 and 8 from the inferior cervical ganglion, and spinal cervical nerve 8 and thoracic 1 from the first thoracic ganglion. The meninges are supplied from a branch of the cervical spinal nerve at each level (Figs. 68.8 and 68.10).[1]

Lateral to the intervertebral foramen, posterior to the vertebral artery, the spinal nerves separate into posterior and anterior primary divisions with the anterior motor divisions being much larger than the posterior divisions, with the exception of C1. Each spinal nerve supplies muscles (myotomes) and skin (dermatomes) as well as ligamentous and bony structures (sclerotomes). The posterior primary division passes over the posterior portion of the transverse process around the articular pillar and divides into the medial sensory and lateral muscular branches, with the exception of the C1 nerve.[1]

The first cervical nerve or suboccipital nerve remains as one trunk and supplies the muscles of the suboccipital triangle. Sensory fibers from the C1 nerve supply the periosteum and body of the atlas and occiput, the atlantooccipital and atlantoaxial joints, and ligaments around these joints. It may occasionally supply skin of the scalp and communicate with the greater and lesser occipital nerves. The posterior primary divisions of the other cervical spinal nerves supply the muscles

of the posterior neck (lateral branches) and skin of the neck (medial branches).[1]

The greater occipital nerve is the medial or sensory branch of the posterior division of the second cervical nerve. It communicates with the third cervical nerve to supply the scalp over the vertex and top of the head and gives muscular branches to

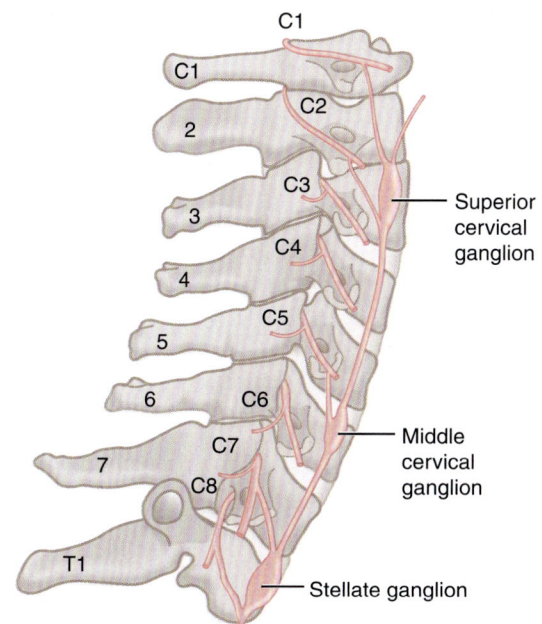

FIGURE 68.10 Lateral view showing the course and relation of the cervical nerves and the cervical sympathetic chain.

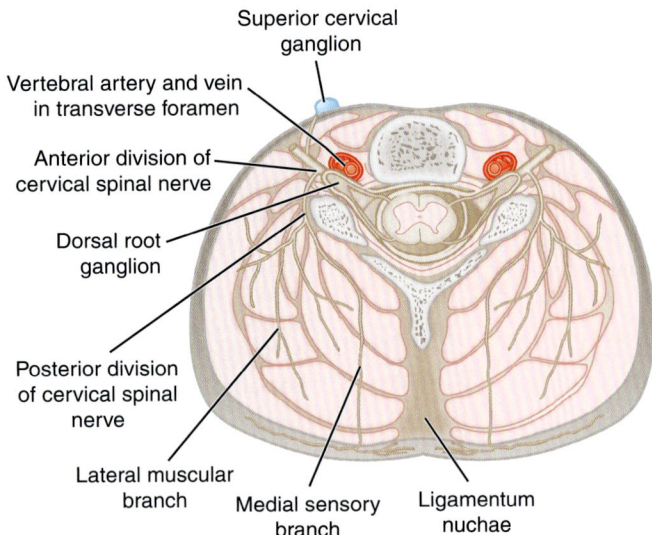

FIGURE 68.11 Cross-section of the third cervical segment showing the course and distribution of the posterior primary division, with its medial branch passing posteriorly to supply the skin and subcutaneous structures and the lateral branch supplying the muscles. Also shown is a cross-section of the superior cervical ganglion and its connection to the nerve by the white ramus communicantes. Note the vertebral vessels just anterior to the nerve.

the semispinalis capitis. The third or least occipital nerve arises from the medial sensory branch of the posterior division of the third cervical nerve (Figs. 68.11 and 68.12).[1]

THE CERVICAL AND BRACHIAL PLEXUS

The cervical plexus is made up of the anterior primary divisions of the upper four cervical nerves. The brachial plexus is formed from the lower four cervical nerves, C5 through C8, together with T1 (Fig. 68.13).[1]

The anterior trunks from cervical nerves two through four divide into ascending and descending branches which form a series of three loops. These are located lateral to the vertebrae, anterior to the levator scapulae and scalenus medius muscles, and beneath the sternocleidomastoid muscle. The deep branches of the cervical plexus lie beneath the sternocleidomastoid muscle and are divided into the lateral or external group and the medial or internal group. The lateral group of branches supplies muscular branches to the scalenus medius, sternocleidomastoid, trapezius, and levator scapulae. It also sends communicating branches to the spinal accessory nerve. The medial or internal branches send off communicating fibers which join the vagus, hypoglossal and descendens hypoglossi nerves, the superior cervical sympathetic ganglion, and, by means of the ansa hypoglossi, supply the thyrohyoid, geniohyoid, omohyoid, sternothyroid, and sternohyoid muscles. The medial branches also supply the rectus capitis, lateralis, and anticus, the longus capitis and longus colli muscles, as well as the diaphragm by way of the phrenic nerve.[1]

The superficial or cutaneous branches of the cervical plexus are often referred to as the superficial cervical plexus and include the lesser occipital nerve, the great auricular nerve, the anterior cutaneous nerve, and the supraclavicular nerve. The lesser occipital nerve joins with the greater occipital and greater auricular nerves to supply the posterior scalp. Its auricular branch supplies the upper and posterior auricula and communicates with the mastoid branch of the great auricular nerve. The great auricular nerve supplies the skin of the face over the parotid gland and communicates with the facial nerve via its anterior or facial branch. Another branch supplies the lobule and lower part of the concha of the ear and communicates with the lesser occipital nerve, the auricular branch of the vagus, and the posterior auricular branch of the facial nerve. The anterior cutaneous nerve supplies the cranial, ventral, and lateral aspects of the neck as far as the sternum.[1]

Finally, the supraclavicular nerve supplies the skin and superficial fascia of the clavicular region as well as the periosteum and bone of the clavicle. Via its medial or supraclavicular branches known also as the suprasternal nerves, it supplies the skin of the infraclavicular region medially as far as the midline and laterally to the junction of the medial and middle third of the clavicle. The intermediate supraclavicular nerve supplies the skin over the pectoralis major as far as the second or third rib and communicates with the cutaneous branches of the second and third intercostals nerves. The lateral supraclavicular nerves or supraacromial nerves supply the skin of the top and dorsal parts of the shoulder (Figs. 68.14 and 68.15).[1]

The brachial plexus is formed from the primary anterior divisions of the fifth through eighth cervical nerves and the first

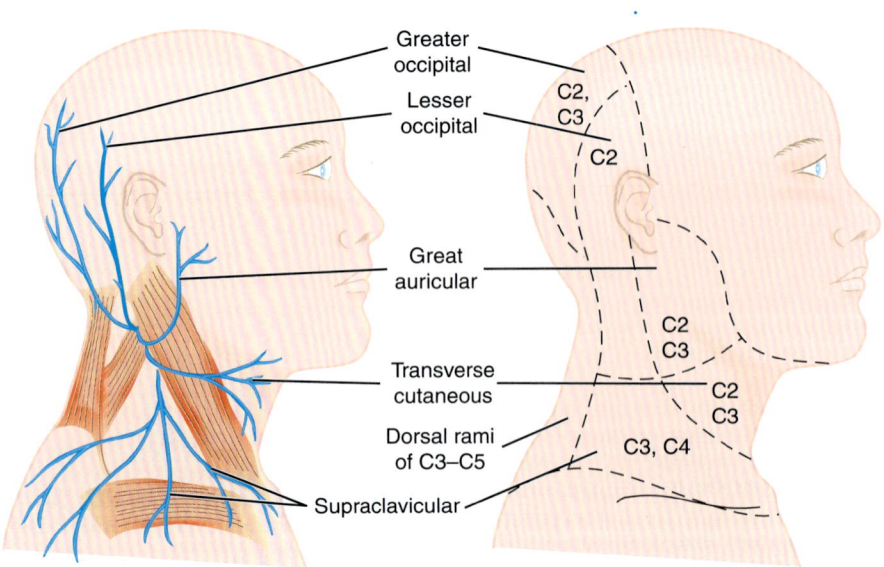

FIGURE 68.12 Cutaneous nerves derived from the cervical plexus (see text for details).

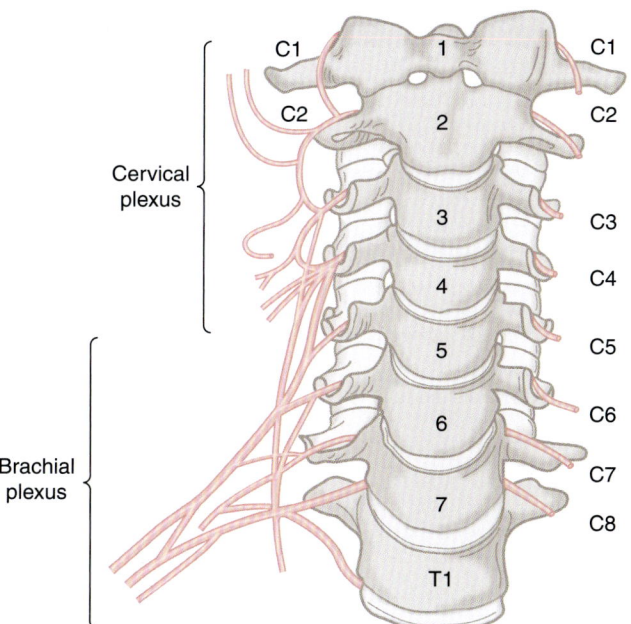

FIGURE 68.13   Anterior view showing the formation of the cervical and brachial plexuses.

These further divide into anterior and posterior divisions which pass beneath the midclavicular region to enter the apex of the axilla. Within the axilla, the anterior and posterior divisions form the lateral, medial, and posterior cords. The anterior divisions of the upper and middle trunks, containing fibers from the fifth, sixth, and seventh cervical nerves, form the lateral cord. The anterior division of the lower trunk continues as the medial cord and contains fibers from the eighth cervical and first thoracic nerves. The union of all the posterior divisions makes up the posterior cord, which thus contains fibers from all nerves of the brachial plexus. The three cords divide to give rise to the peripheral nerves of the upper extremity at the lateral border of the pectoralis minor. The lateral aspect of the median nerve and the musculocutaneous nerves derive from the lateral cord. The medial cord divides into the medial head of the median nerve, the ulnar nerve, and the medial antebrachial and brachial cutaneous nerves as well as a branch to the intercostobrachial nerve. The axillary and radial nerves are terminating branches from the posterior cord.[1]

In addition to supplying terminal branches to the upper extremity, the brachial plexus carries postganglionic sympathetic

thoracic nerve with occasional contributing branches from the anterior primary divisions of the fourth cervical and second thoracic nerves. These combine to form three trunks which include (1) the upper trunk, formed from the primary divisions of the fifth and sixth cervical nerves; (2) the middle trunk, formed from the seventh primary division; and (3) the lower trunk, formed from the eighth cervical and first thoracic primary divisions.[1] The upper trunk gives off the suprascapular nerve which supplies the shoulder joint, the supraspinatus and infraspinatus muscles, and the subclavius nerve, which supplies the subclavius muscle.

The three trunks continue from the interscalenus space in an anterolateral and inferior direction toward the first rib.

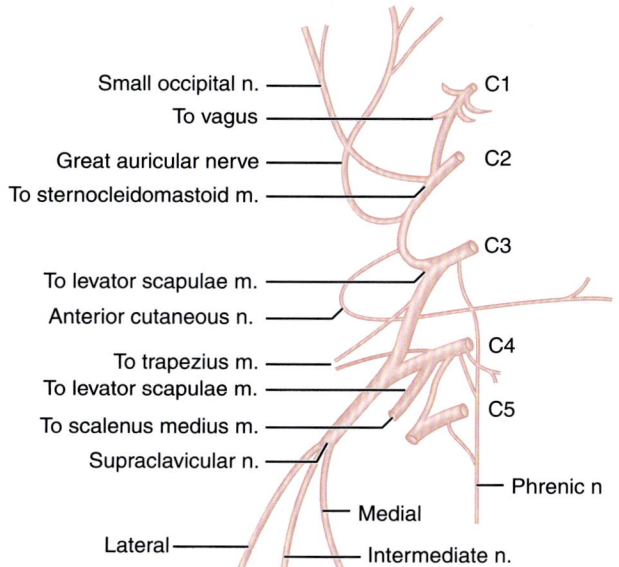

FIGURE 68.14   Origin and composition of the cervical plexus. m., muscle; n., nerve.

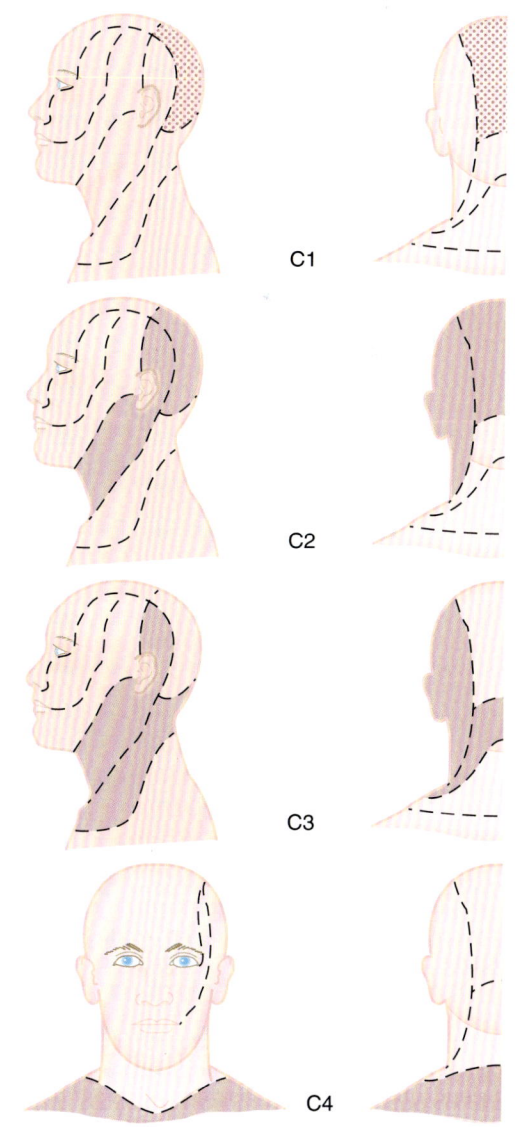

FIGURE 68.15   Dermatomes of the neck and head derived from the upper four cervical nerves.

TABLE 68.2	**Organization and Branches of the Brachial Plexus**			
Structure	Neurotome		Structure	Neurotome
Branches of Cervical Nerves			**Branches**	
To phrenic nerve	C5		Anterior pectoral	C5–C7
To longus colli and scaleni muscles	C5–C7		**Terminal Branches**	
Branches from Roots			Musculocutaneous nerve	C5–C7
Dorsal scapular nerve	C4, C5		Median nerve, lateral portion	C6, C7
Long thoracic nerve	C5–C7		Medial cord origin (inferior trunk)	C8–T1
Branches from Trunks (Superior Trunk)			**Branches**	
Nerve to subclavius	C5, C6		Medial brachial cutaneous nerve	C8–T1
Suprascapular nerve	C5, C6		Medial antebrachial cutaneous nerve	C8–T1
Posterior cord origin (from all trunks)	C5–C8, T1		**Terminal Branches**	
Branches			Median nerve (medial portion)	C8–T1
Superior subscapular nerve	C5, C6		Ulnar nerve	C8–T1
Inferior subscapular nerve	C5, C6			
Thoracodorsal nerve	C6–C8			
Terminal Branches				
Axillary	C5, C6			
Radial	C5–C8, T1			
Lateral cord origin (superior and middle trunk)	C5–C7			

fibers from the cervical and thoracic sympathetic chain to the upper limbs. The brachial plexus also supplies branches to the longus colli muscle and the scalene muscles. The fifth cervical nerve sends fibers to the phrenic nerve, the rhomboid muscles, and the levator scapulae muscles via the dorsal scapular nerve. Fibers from the anterior divisions of the fifth, sixth, and sev-

enth cervical nerves supply the serratus anterior muscle via the long thoracic nerve (Table 68.2 and Figs. 68.16 and 68.17). The segmental and peripheral nerve supply of the neck and arm is summarized in Figures 68.18 and 68.19 as well as Tables 68.3, 68.4, and 68.5. Sympathetic nervous system contributions to the upper extremity from the cervical and thoracic preganglionic

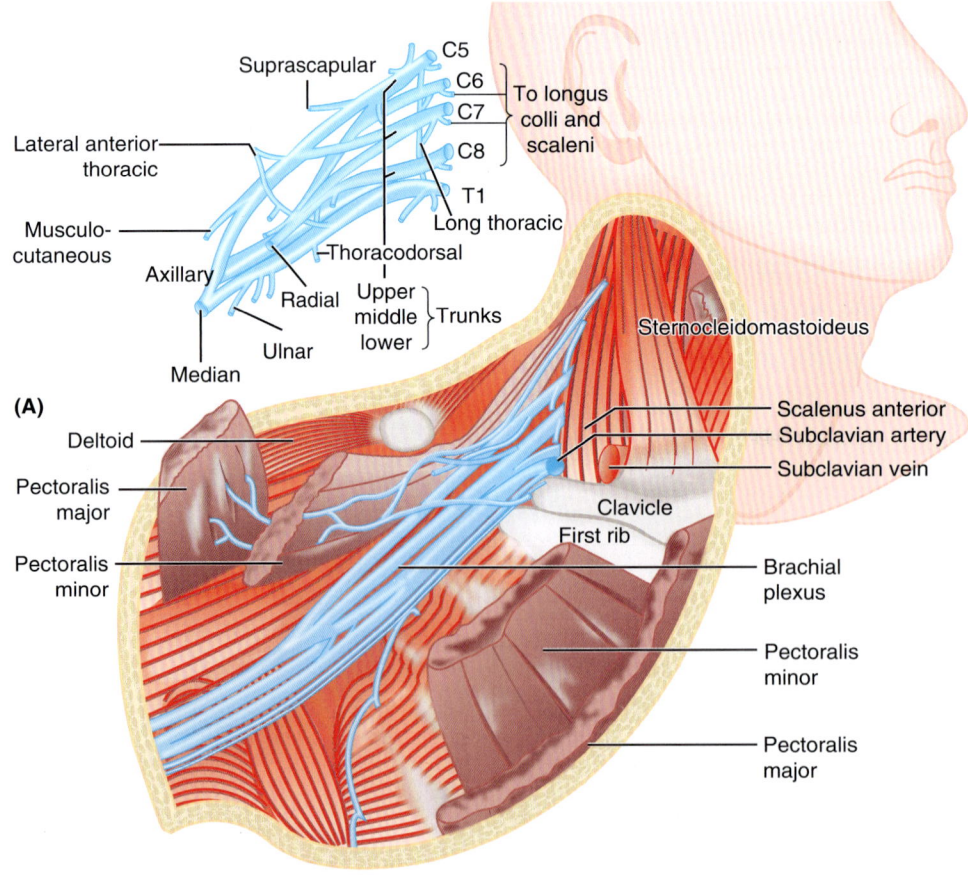

FIGURE 68.16   Anatomy of the brachial plexus. **A:** Schematic depiction of the brachial plexus. **B:** Relation of the roots of the brachial plexus to the scalene muscles showing the position of the plexus over the first rib and its course into the axilla.

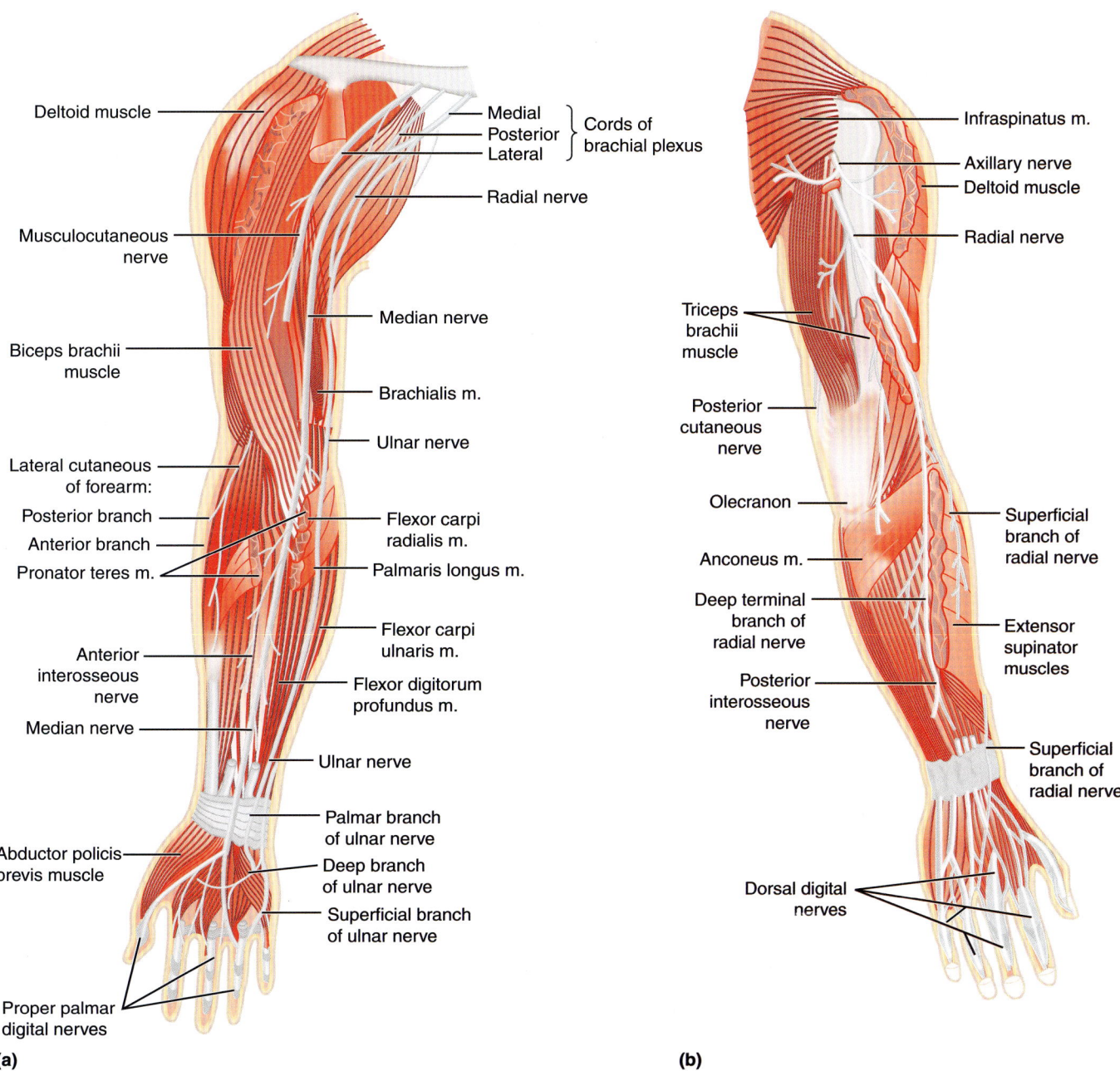

FIGURE 68.17 Anatomy of the median, ulnar, and radial nerves. Anterior view **(A)** and posterior view **(B)** of the upper limb showing the course of the three nerves and some of the muscles (m.) they supply.

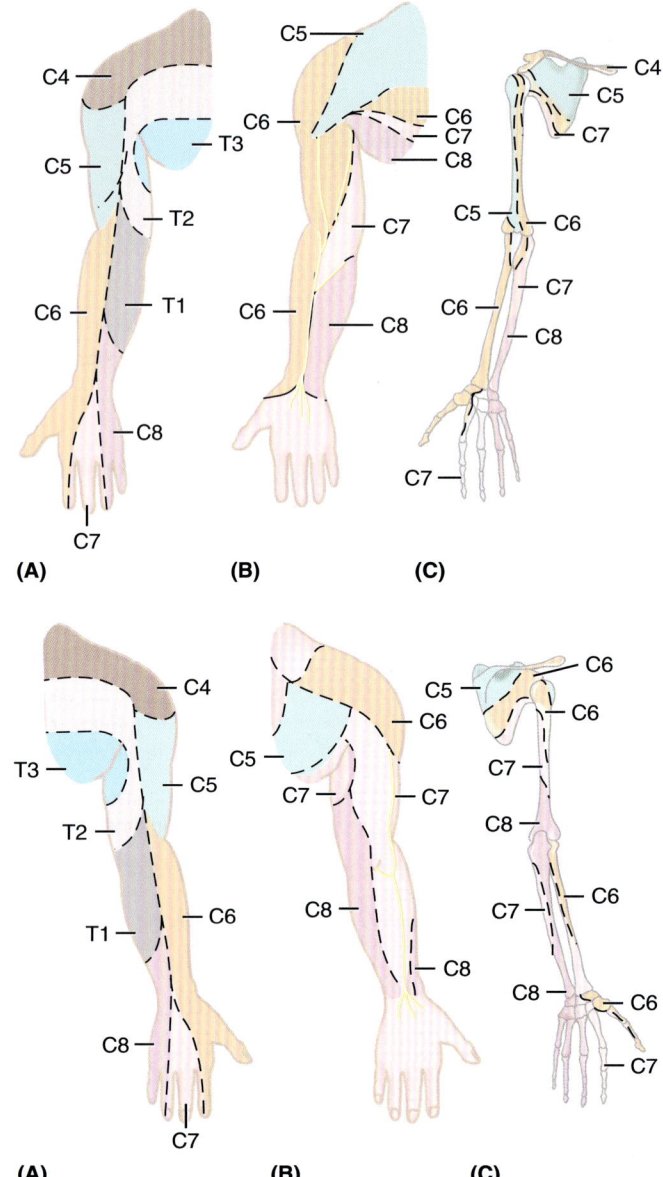

FIGURE 68.18   Segmental nerve supply to the upper limb showing the anterior view (**above**) and posterior view (**below**). **A:** Dermatomes. **B:** Myotomes. **C:** Sclerotomes.

neurons are illustrated and described in Figure 68.20. Contributions from the anterolateral and posterolateral subclavian sympathetic nerves, which supply the subclavian artery and its branches distal to the scalene muscles, contain both sympathetic and sensory fibers.[1]

PECTORAL GIRDLE AND SHOULDER ANATOMY

The differential diagnosis of neck and arm pain includes many disorders of the pectoral girdle and shoulder which can result not only in shoulder pain but also in radiation of pain to the neck and/or arm. Common disorders involving the shoulder and pectoral girdle include rotator cuff tears, tendonitis, impingement syndromes, and arthritis (Figs. 68.21 and 68.22). An understanding of the complex anatomy and biomechanics of pectoral girdle and shoulder is thus essential for the diagnosis and treatment of pain in this region.[1]

The pectoral girdle is made up of the scapula and clavicle, the sternoclavicular and acromioclavicular joints, and the scapulothoracic and humeroacromial interfaces. Unlike the lower

limb, which is built for weight bearing as well as locomotion, the upper limb function is primarily to allow mobility and a wide range of motion for the arm and hand. The girdle does not articulate with the vertebral column, as does the pelvic girdle, but with the thoracic cage at the saddle-shaped sternoclavicular joint. The sternoclavicular joint is divided into two spaces by an articular disk and is surrounded by a strong, lax capsule. In addition to the capsule, the joint is stabilized by the interclavicular ligament superiorly, inferiorly by the costoclavicular ligament (which limits elevation and rotation of the clavicle and serves as the fulcrum of movements at the sternoclavicular joint), and the posterior sternoclavicular ligament. Dislocation of the costoclavicular joint is rare but tends to occur anteriorly where the joint is weakest when it does occur (Fig. 68.23).

The acromioclavicular joint of the pectoral girdle is surrounded by a weak and lax capsule. It is stabilized by the acromioclavicular ligament superiorly; the fan-shaped coracoclavicular ligament, which serves as a vertical axis for scapular rotation; and the trapezoid ligament, which serves as a hinge

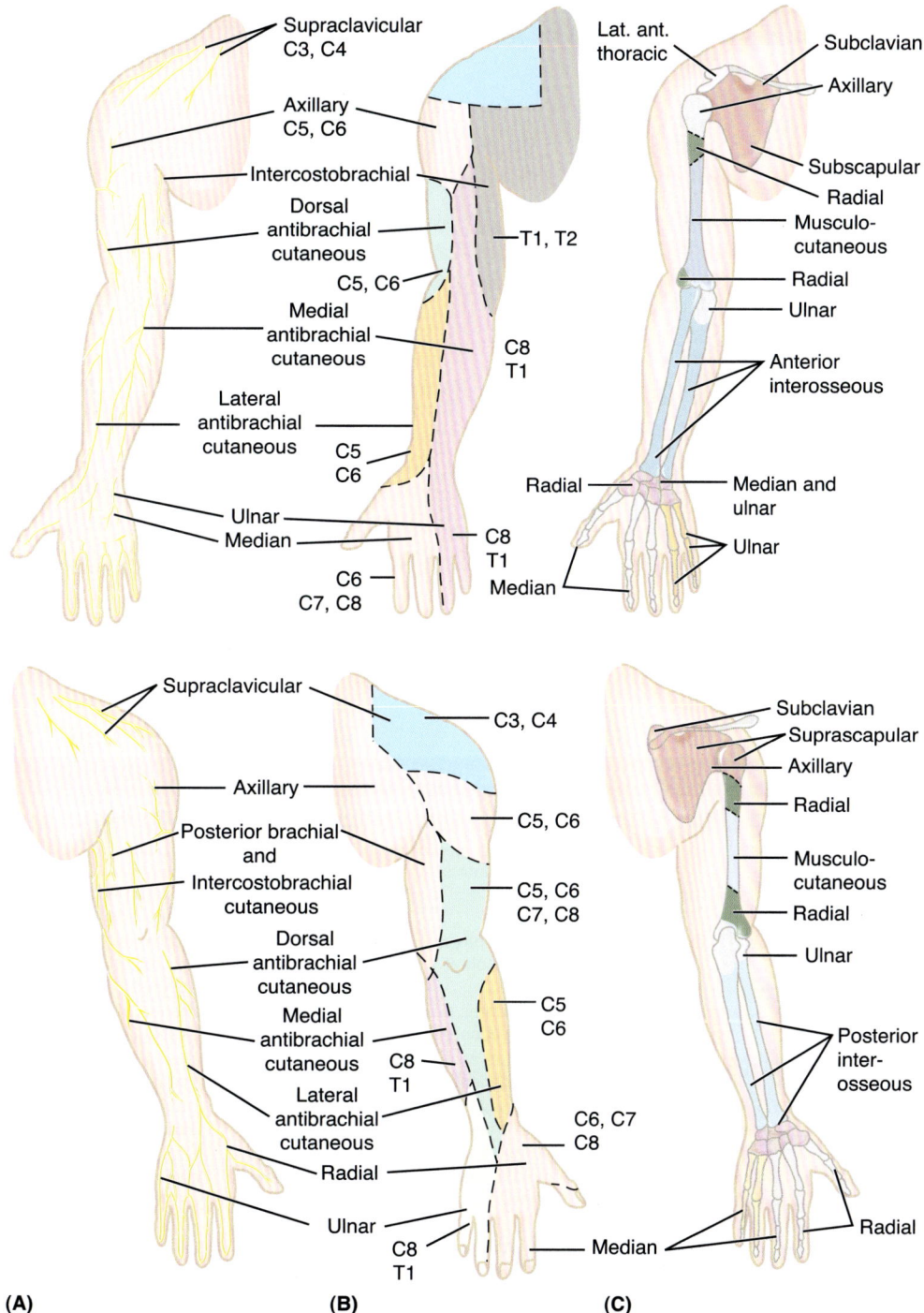

(A) (B) (C)

FIGURE 68.19 Peripheral nerve supply to the upper limb showing the anterior view **(above)** and posterior view **(below)**. **A:** Various cutaneous nerves and their territories **(B)**. **C:** Nerve supply to the bones and joints.

TABLE 68.3	Nerve Supply of Muscles of the Neck		
Muscle	**Nerve Supply**	**Muscle**	**Nerve Supply**
Capital Flexors		*Cervical Spine Extensors*	
Rectus capitis anterior	C1, C2	Splenius cervicis	C2–C7
Rectus capitis lateralis	C1, C2	Longissimus cervicis	C1–C8[a]
Longus capitis	C1–C4	Semispinalis cervicis	C1–C8[a]
Capital Extensors		Multifidus	C3–T1
Rectus capitis posterior major	C1	*Head Rotators[a]*	
Rectus capitis posterior minor	C1	Sternocleidomastoid	See above
Oblique capitis superior	C1	Splenius cervicis	
Oblique capitis inferior	C1	Semispinalis cervicis	
Longus capitis	C1–C4	Longissimus cervicis	
Splenius capitis	C3–C5	*Other Neck Muscles*	
Semispinalis capitis	C3–C5	Geniohyoid	C1
Cervical Spine Flexors		Thyrohyoid	C1
Scalenus anterior	C4–C7	Sternohyoid	C1–C3
Scalenus medius	C3–C8	Sternothyroid	C1–C3
Scalenus posterior	C5–C8	Omohyoid	C1–C3
Longus colli	C2–C8		
Sternocleidomastoid	Cranial nerve XI; C2, C3[b]		

[a]When the muscle of one side contracts.
[b]When muscles of both sides contract.

TABLE 68.4	Sclerotomal Distribution Pattern of the Cervical and First Thoracic Nerves		
Segment	**Sclerotome**	**Joints**	**Ligaments**
C1	Periosteum and body of atlas	Atlantoaxial, medial, atlantoaxial, lateral, atlantoaxial	Alar, cruciform, apical dental, accessory atlantoaxial, articular capsules, nuchal, anterior atlantooccipital membrane, posterior atlantooccipital membrane
C2	Periosteum and body of axis	Medial atlantoaxial, lateral atlantoaxial, intervertebral	Anterior longitudinal, atlantoaxial membrane, atlantoaxial, capsular, cruciform, nuchal
C3	Periosteum and body of C3 vertebra and clavicle	Intervertebral, Luschka, sternoclavicular, zygapophyseal	Anterior longitudinal, posterior longitudinal, capsular, nuchal
C4	Periosteum and body of C4 vertebra and clavicle	Intervertebral, Luschka, sternoclavicular, zygapophyseal	Anterior longitudinal, posterior longitudinal, capsular, ligamentum flavum, nuchal
C5	Periosteum and body of C5 vertebra and portions of humerus, scapula, and proximal ulna	Acromioclavicular, glenohumeral Luschka, intervertebral, elbow, zygapophyseal, sternoclavicular	Anterior longitudinal, posterior longitudinal, capsular, nuchal, ligamentum flavum
C6	Periosteum and body of C6 vertebra and portions of humerus, radius, scapula, and first metacarpal bone	Glenohumeral, intervertebral, Luschka, elbow, zygapophyseal	Anterior longitudinal, posterior longitudinal, capsular, nuchal, ligamentum flavum
C7	Periosteum and body of C7 vertebra and portions of humerus, scapula, radius, and ulna	Elbow, Luschka, intervertebral, zygapophyseal	Anterior longitudinal, posterior longitudinal, nuchal, ligamentum flavum
C8	Periosteum and body of C8 vertebra and portions of humerus, ulna, carpal bones, and bones of fourth and fifth fingers	Intervertebral, Luschka, zygapophyseal, elbow, wrist, hand	Supraspinous, interspinous, anterior longitudinal, posterior longitudinal
T1	Periosteum and body of T1 vertebra	Intervertebral, zygapophyseal, costovertebral, elbows, wrist, hand	Anterior longitudinal, posterior longitudinal, supraspinous, interspinous, ligamentum flavum

TABLE 68.5   Nerve Supply of the Muscles of the Upper Limbs

Region/Muscle Group/Function[a]	Peripheral Nerve Supply	Segmental Nerve Supply[b]
Shoulder rotator cuff		
Supraspinatus	Suprascapular	C5, C6
Infraspinatus	Suprascapular	C5, C6
Subscapularis	Nerve to subscapularis	C5, C6
Teres minor	Axillary	C5, C6
Scapular motion		
Elevation		
Levator scapulae	Dorsal scapular	C4, C5
Rhomboideus	Dorsal scapular	C4, C5
Trapezius (superior fibers)	Spinal accessory	CN XI
Depression		
Trapezius (inferior fibers)	Spinal accessory	CN XI
Pectoralis major	Medial/lateral pectorals	C5, C6, C7, C8, T1
Subclavius	Nerve to subclavius	C5, C6
Upward rotation		
Serratus anterior	Long thoracic	C5, C6, C7
Trapezius (upper/lower fibers)	Spinal accessory	CN XI
Downward rotation		
Levator scapulae	Dorsal scapular	C4, C5
Rhomboideus	Dorsal scapular	C4, C5
Pectoralis major and minor	Lateral/medial pectorals	C5, C6, C7, C8, T1
Latissimus dorsi	Thoracodorsal	C6, C7, C8
Abduction (protraction)		
Serratus anterior	Long thoracic	C5, C6, C7
Pectoralis major	Medial/lateral pectorals	C5, C6, C7, C8, T1
Adduction (retraction)		
Trapezius (middle fibers)	Spinal accessory	CN XI
Rhomboideus	Dorsal scapular	C4, C5
Latissimus dorsi	Thoracodorsal	C6, C7, C8
Arm motion		
Flexion		
Pectoralis major (clavicular head)	Medial/lateral pectorals	C5, C6, C7, C8, T1u
Deltoid (anterior fibers)	Axillary	C5, C6
Coracobrachialis	Musculocutaneous	C6, C7
Biceps brachii	Musculocutaneous	C5, C6
Extension		
Latissimus dorsi	Thoracodorsal	C6, C7, C8
Teres major	Subscapular	C5, C6
Deltoid (posterior fibers)	Axillary	C5, C6
Triceps brachii	Radical	C7, C8
Abduction		
Deltoid (middle fibers)	Axillary	C5, C6
Supraspinatus	Suprascapular	C5, C6
Infraspinatus	Suprascapular	C5, C6
Teres minor	Axillary	C5, C6
Adduction		
Pectoralis major and minor	Medial/lateral pectorals	C5, C6, C7, C8, T1
Latissimus dorsi	Thoracodorsal	C6, C7, C8
Teres major	Subscapular	C5, C6
Medial rotation		
Subscapularis	Nerve to subscapularis	C5, C6
Latissimus dorsi	Thoracodorsal	C6, C7, C8
Pectoralis major and minor	Medial/lateral pectorals	C5, C6, C7, C8, T1
Lateral rotation		
Infraspinatus	Suprascapular	C5, C6
Teres minor	Axillary	C5, C6

(continued)

TABLE 68.5 (Continued)

Region/Muscle Group/Function[a]	Peripheral Nerve Supply	Segmental Nerve Supply[b]
Elbow/forearm motion		
Extension		
Triceps brachii	Radial	C6, <u>C7</u>, C8
Anconeus	Radial	<u>C7</u>, C8
Flexion		
Biceps brachii	Musculocutaneous	<u>C5</u>, C6
Brachialis	Musculocutaneous	<u>C5</u>, C6
Brachioradialis	Radial	<u>C5</u>, C6
Wrist motion		
Flexion		
Flexor carpi radialis	Median	C6, <u>C7</u>
Flexor carpi ulnaris	Ulnar	C7, <u>C8</u>
Palmaris longus	Median	<u>C7</u>, C8
Extension		
Extensor carpi radialis longus/brevis	Radial	<u>C6</u>, C7
Extensor carpi ulnaris	Radial (posterior interosseus)	<u>C7</u>, C8
Radial deviation		
Flexor carpi radialis	Median	<u>C6</u>, C7
Extensor carpi radialis longus/brevis	Radial	<u>C6</u>, C7
Ulnar deviation		
Flexor carpi ulnaris	Ulnar	C7, <u>C8</u>
Extensor carpi ulnaris	Radial (posterior interosseus)	<u>C7</u>, C8
Digits (2–5)		
Flexion		
Flexor digit superficialis	Median	C7, <u>C8</u>, T1
Flexor digit profundus	Median (anterior interosseus)	C7, <u>C8</u>, T1
Extension		
Extensor digit communis	Radial (posterior interosseus)	<u>C7</u>, C8
Extensor digit minimi	Radial (posterior interosseus)	<u>C7</u>, C8
Extensor indicis	Radial (posterior interosseus)	<u>C7</u>, C8
Abduction		
Dorsal interossei	Ulnar	C8, <u>T1</u>
Adduction		
Palmar interossei	Ulnar	C8, <u>T1</u>
Motion of thumb		
Flexion		
Flexor pollicis longus	Median (anterior interosseus)	C7, <u>C8</u>
Extension		
Extensor pollicis longus	Radial (posterior interosseus)	C7, <u>C8</u>
Extensor pollicis brevis	Radial (posterior interosseus)	C7, <u>C8</u>
Abductor pollicis longus	Radial (posterior interosseus)	C7, <u>C8</u>
Adduction		
Adductor pollicis	Ulnar	C8, <u>T1</u>
Abduction		
Abduction pollicis brevis	Median	C8, <u>T1</u>
Opponens pollicis	Median	C8, <u>T1</u>
Opposition		
Opponens pollicis	Median	C8, <u>T1</u>
Hypothenar group (motion of fifth finger)		
Abduction digiti minimi	Ulnar	C8, <u>T1</u>
Flexor digiti brevis	Ulnar	C8, <u>T1</u>
Opponens digiti minimi	Ulnar	C8, <u>T1</u>

CN, cranial nerve.
[a]Only the primary muscle nerves are included.
[b]Main root is underlined.

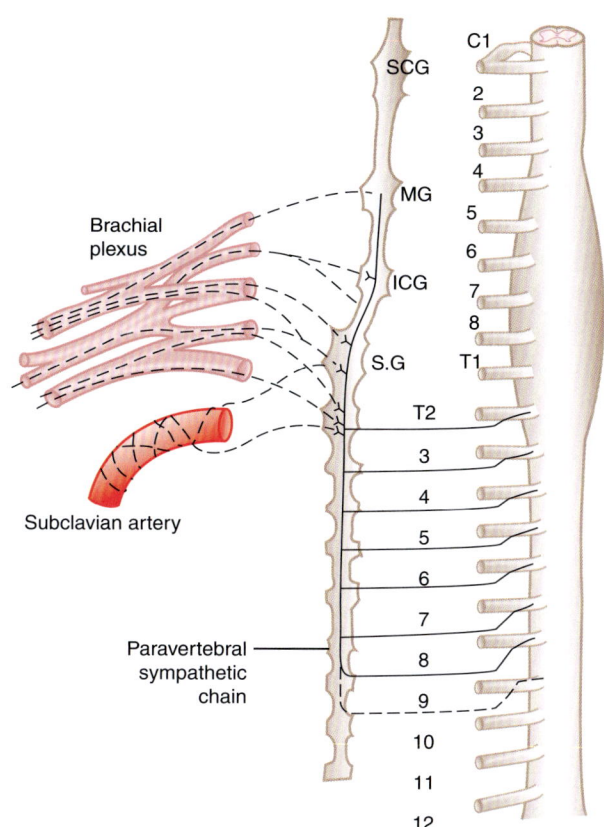

FIGURE 68.20 Schematic depiction of the origins and courses of preganglionic sympathetic neurons destined to supply the upper limbs. Note that the axons of the preganglionic neurons, which are located in spinal segments T2–T8 (and occasionally T9), pass through the anterior root as white rami communicantes and from there to the paravertebral sympathetic chain, where they ascend and synapse with postganglionic fibers primarily in the second thoracic, stellate, and intermediate and middle cervical ganglia, and occasionally in the third cervical ganglion (not shown). Some of the postganglionic fibers pass directly to the subclavian artery, but most pass as gray rami communicantes to the roots of the brachial plexus. ICG, inferior cervical ganglion; MG, middle cervical ganglion; SCG, superior cervical ganglion; SG, stellate ganglion.

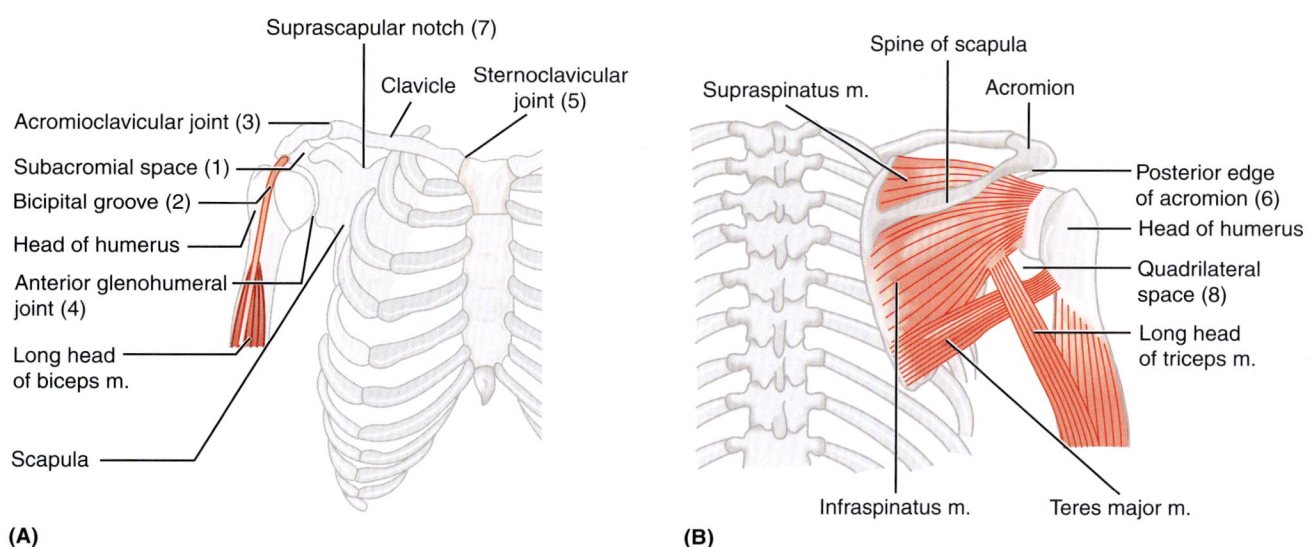

(A)   **(B)**

FIGURE 68.21 Anterior **(A)** and posterior **(B)** views of the shoulder identifying the various bones and joints and also the sites of pathologic processes that produce pain and tenderness. (*1*) Subacromial space, which can be involved with calcific tendinitis, rotator cuff tendinitis and impingement syndrome, and rotator cuff tear; (*2*) bicipital groove, which can be involved in bicipital tendinitis and biceps tendon subluxation and tear; (*3*) acromioclavicular joint, which can be involved with degenerative and infectious processes; (*4*) anterior glenohumeral joint, which can be the site of glenohumeral arthritis, osteonecrosis, glenoid labial tears, and adhesive capsulitis; (*5*) sternoclavicular joint, which can be the site of pain caused by infection, degenerative changes, or trauma; (*6*) posterior edge of the acromion, which can contribute to rotator cuff tendinitis, calcific tendinitis, and rotator cuff tear; (*7*) suprascapular notch, which can be the site of suprascapular nerve entrapment; and (*8*) quadrilateral space, which can be the site of axillary nerve entrapment. m., muscle.

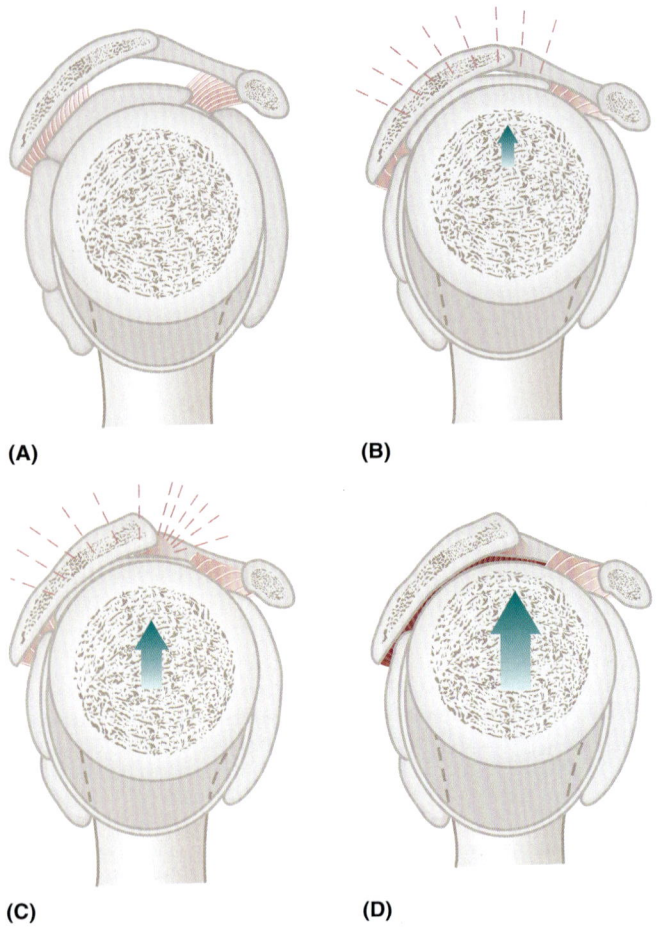

(A) (B)

(C) (D)

FIGURE 68.22 With progressive cuff fiber failure, the head moves upward against the coracoacromial arch. **A:** Normal relationships of the cuff and the coracoacromial arch. **B:** Upward displacement of the head, squeezing the cuff against the acromion and the coracoacromial ligament. **C:** Greater contact and abrasion, giving rise to a traction spur in the coracoacromial ligament. **D:** Still greater upward displacement, resulting in abrasion of the humeral articular cartilage and cuff tear arthropathy. *(Reprinted from Matsen FA. Practical Evaluation and Management of the Shoulder. 1st ed. Philadelphia, PA: Saunders; 1994:123. Copyright © 1994 Elsevier. With permission.)*

for scapular motion about the horizontal axis. A partial or complete disruption of the coracoclavicular ligament, resulting in separation of the acromioclavicular joint, may occur with a fall on the shoulder.

The scapulothoracic interface allows a gliding movement between the ventral surface of the scapula and the thorax overlying the second through the seventh ribs. The scapula is held in close approximation to the thorax by the serratus anterior, the trapezius, and the rhomboid muscles. For full abduction and forward flexion of the shoulder to occur, the scapula must undergo upward rotation. Movements of the pectoral girdle consist of upward-downward rotation, protraction-retraction, and elevation-depression (Table 68.6 and Figs. 68.24 and 68.25).

The glenohumeral joint is a synovial joint that consists of the interface of the head of the humerus with the pear-shaped glenoid cavity and ring of fibrocartilage known as the glenoid labrum. These deepen the socket of the scapula and assist with stability of the glenohumeral joint. The supraglenoid

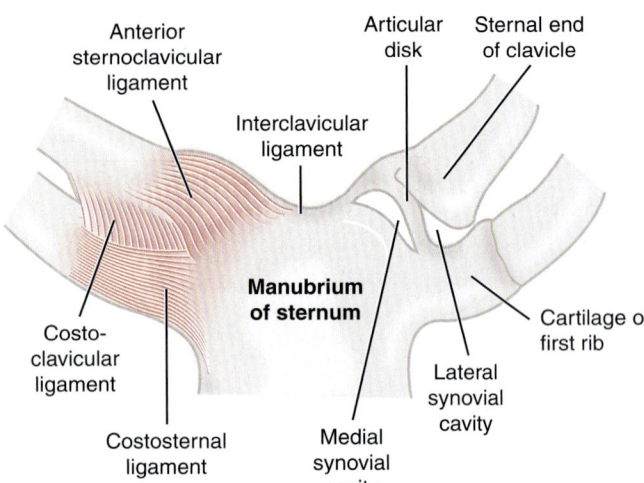

FIGURE 68.23 Anatomy of the sternoclavicular joints viewed from the front. *(Adapted with permission from Clement CD. Gray's Anatomy of the Human Body. 30th ed. Philadelphia, PA: Lea & Febiger; 1985:366–367.)*

TABLE 68.6	Prime Movers of the Pectoral Girdle
Movement	**Muscles**
Elevation	Trapezius (upper fibers)
	Rhomboids
	Levator scapulae
Depression	Latissimus dorsi
	Pectoralis major (costal fibers)
	Trapezius (lower fibers)
Protraction	Serratus anterior
	Pectoralis minor
	Pectoralis major
Retraction	Trapezius
	Rhomboids
Upward rotation	Trapezius
	Serratus anterior
Downward rotation	Rhomboids

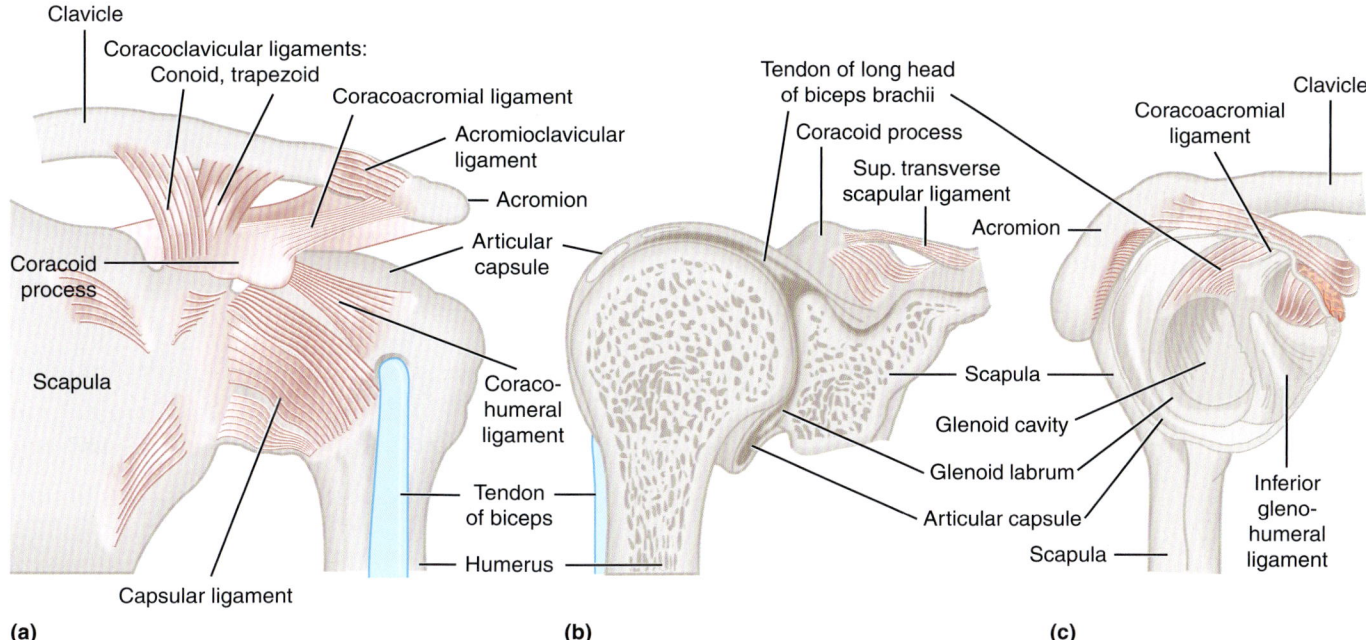

(a)

(b)

(c)

FIGURE 68.24 Anatomy of the shoulder joint. **A:** Anterior view of ligaments of the left shoulder. **B:** Coronal section through the head of the left humerus and shoulder joint, anterior half viewed from behind. **C:** Interior of the right shoulder viewed from its lateral aspect. *(Adapted with permission from Clement CD.* Gray's Anatomy of the Human Body. *30th ed. Philadelphia, PA: Lea & Febiger; 1985368–372.)*

and infraglenoid tubercles above and below the glenoid cavity are attachment sites for the long head of the biceps and triceps, respectively. The joint capsule is strong but lax, to allow for mobility, and attaches to the scapula proximally and distally to the articular margins of the head of the humerus superiorly and the surgical neck of the humerus inferiorly. The ligaments of the glenohumeral joint consist of the superior, middle, and inferior glenohumeral ligaments (thickenings of the anterior capsule); the coracohumeral ligament (which attaches to the greater and lesser tuberosities and limits flexion and extension); and the coracoacromial ligament (which extends from the undersurface of the acromion to the coracoid process and acts as an articulating surface for the head of the humerus). The subacromial and subdeltoid bursae lie between the coracoacromial arch and the rotator cuff tendons and have been implicated in shoulder impingement (see Fig. 68.24).

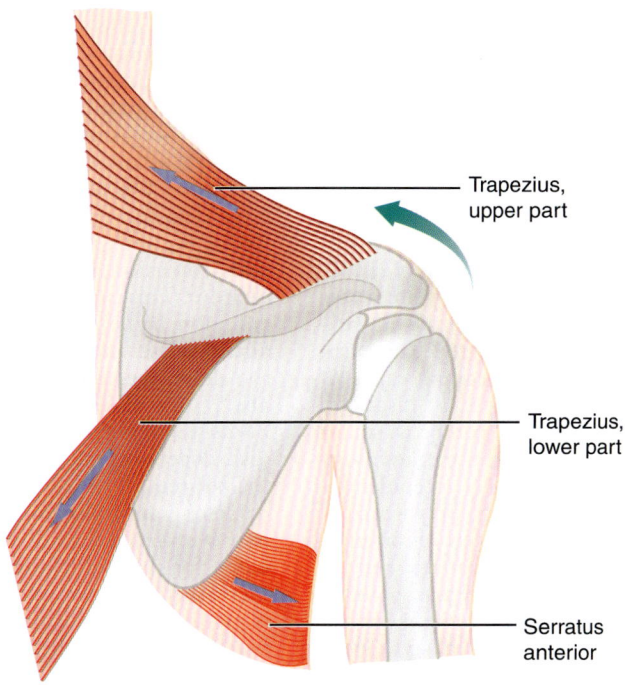

FIGURE 68.25 The muscles that rotate the scapula upward during abduction of the arm. Note that the upper part of the trapezius, which is attached to the outer part of the scapular spine, pulls upward and that the lower part of the serratus anterior, attached to the lower part of the scapula, pulls the inferior angle laterally, whereas the lower portion of the trapezius, attached to the medial part of the scapular spine, pulls downward. *(Reprinted with permission from Rosse C, Gaddum-Rosse P.* Hollinshead's Textbook of Anatomy. *5th ed. Philadelphia, PA: Lippincott–Raven; 1997:235.)*

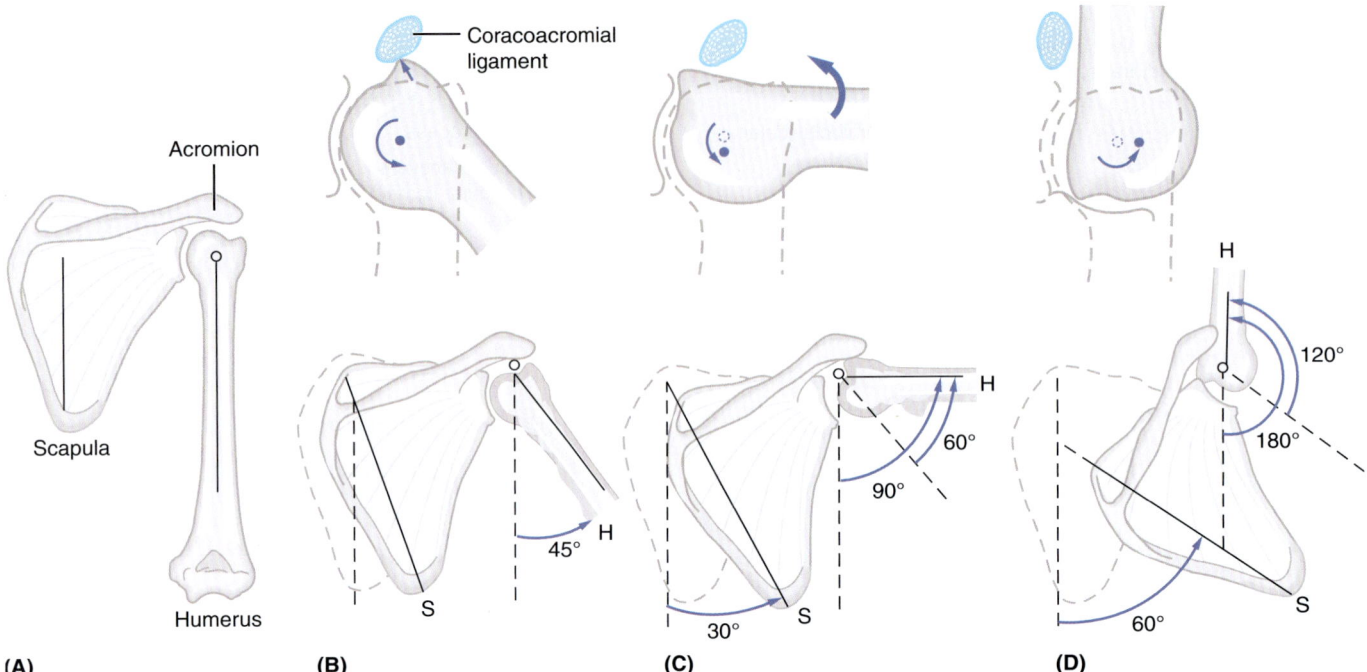

FIGURE 68.26 Biomechanics of the glenohumeral movements of arm abduction. **A:** Normal position of the head and shaft of the humerus. The circle in the head of the humerus indicates the center of rotation. **B:** Humerus (H) abducted 45 degrees and the scapula (S) beginning upward rotation. The upper panel shows that the incongruity of the articulating surface of the head of the humerus and the surface of the glenoid cavity causes the greater tuberosity of the humerus to impinge on the coracoacromial ligament. The upper panel in **C** shows that to allow the greater tuberosity to pass under the coracoacromial hood during arm abduction, the humeral head is depressed (depicted by downward movement of the center of rotation) and the humeral head rotated (*thin arrow*). The abduction movement of the arm is accomplished in a smooth coordinated movement during which for each 15 degrees of arm abduction, 10 degrees of motion occurs at the glenohumeral joint, and 5 degrees occurs because of scapular rotation on the thorax. Thus, as noted in **C**, abduction of the arm to 90 degrees is accomplished by 60 degrees rotation of the humerus and 30 degrees rotation of the scapula. Full abduction of the arm, as shown in **D**, is accomplished by 120 degrees of rotation at the glenohumeral joint and 60 degrees rotation of the scapula. *(Modified from Cailliet R. Shoulder Pain. 2nd ed. Philadelphia: FA Davis; 1981. Reproduced with permission of F.A. Davis Co., in the format Republish in a book via Copyright Clearance Center.)*

Movement at the shoulder requires the combined motion of the glenohumeral joint and the pectoral girdle for flexion or abduction greater than 90 degrees. For example, the abduction or elevation of the arm to 180 degrees requires 60 degrees of scapular rotation to alter the angle of the glenoid fossa during its articulation with the head of the humerus (Figs. 68.26 and 68.27). Prime movers of the pectoral girdle and glenohumeral joint are listed in Tables 68.6 and 68.7.[1]

Epidemiology of Neck and Arm Pain

According to The Global Burden of Disease Study 2013, which evaluated the national disability-adjusted life years (DALYs) for 306 diseases and injuries and healthy life expectancy (HALE) for 188 countries from 1990 to 2013, back and neck pain have risen from the seventh leading cause of disability in 1990 to the fourth leading cause of disability in 2013, following ischemic heart disease, cerebrovascular disease, and lower respiratory infections.[3] The methodology and definition of neck pain varies significantly in epidemiologic studies of neck and arm pain. An average prevalence of 15% to 50% with a mean of 37.2% have been reported in most epidemiologic studies and a recent systematic review. Associated conditions identified with neck and arm pain include psychosocial factors such as anxiety, depression, kinesiophobia, poor coping skills as well as sedentary lifestyle, sleep disorders, smoking, and genetic risk factors. Associated poor health, as well as musculoskeletal and psychological health complaints, were prognostic for poor outcome. Prevalence was found to be overall higher in females with prevalence peaking in middle age.[4]

Controversy exists regarding the relationship between radiologic evidence of cervical spine degeneration and neck pain, with some finding no significant difference in the degree of neck pain in patients with or without radiographic evidence of cervical spine degenerative changes, with others correlating neck pain with increasing grade of disk degeneration.[5] Zapletal et al.[6] showed increasing evidence of neck pain with increasing prevalence of atlantoodontoid degenerative changes.

Up to 78% of asymptomatic subjects have been found to have degenerative changes on magnetic resonance imaging (MRI) accompanied by positive findings such as disk bulging and protrusion, foraminal stenosis, and abnormal spinal cord contour. This evidence suggests that degenerative findings are common in both asymptomatic and symptomatic individuals, increase linearly with age, and cannot be assumed to be the definitive cause of neck pain in symptomatic individuals.[7-9] One study comparing cervical spine MRIs of fighter pilots to age-matched controls showed premature cervical disk degeneration among pilots exposed frequently to high +Gz forces.[10]

Neck pain following whiplash-associated disorders is common with more than 300 persons per 100,000 population evaluated for this complaint each year according to recent data.[11] Increased symptom severity and presence of neurologic signs is predictive of poor prognosis. Postinjury feelings of helplessness in controlling the consequences of pain, fear of movement, catastrophizing, and postinjury anxiety have also been found to be associated with higher risk of long-term disability,[12] as has changing the insurance system from a no-fault to a tort system of compensation.[13] Studies from hospital populations report that at an average follow-up of 2 years, 20% to 45%

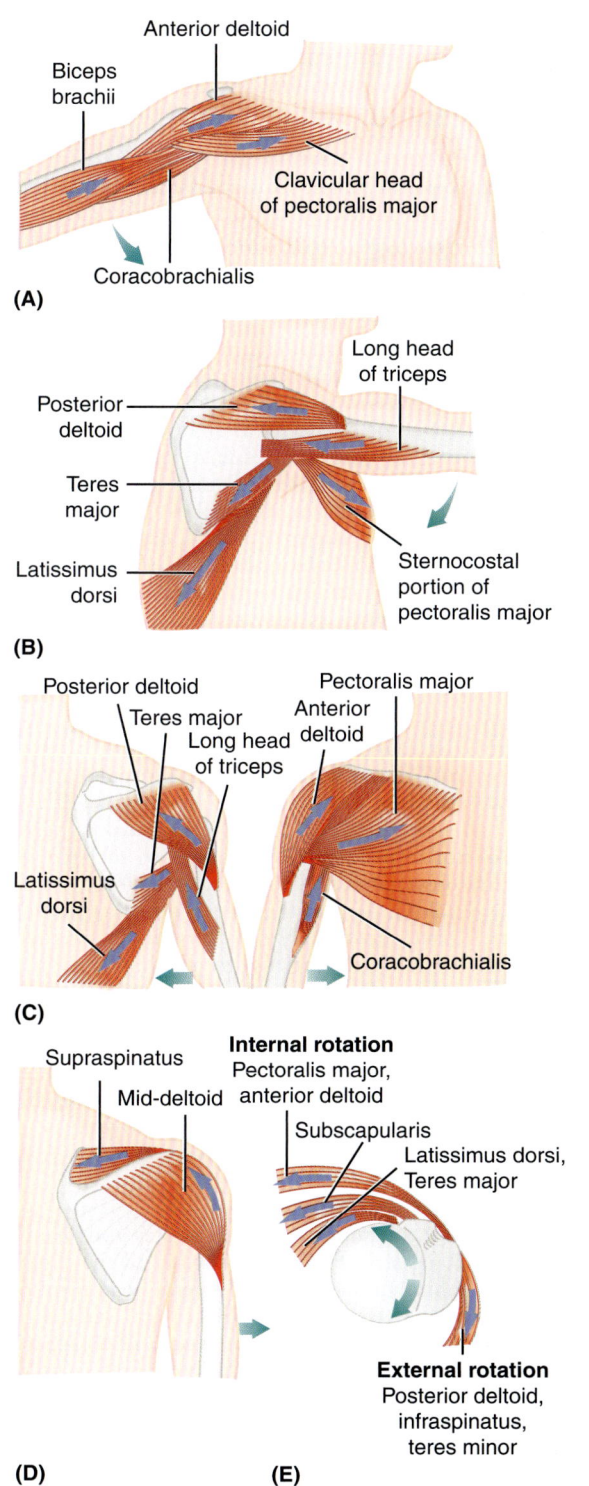

FIGURE 68.27   Muscles that move the shoulder and arm: flexors **(A)**, extensors **(B)**, adductors **(C)**, abductors **(D)**, and rotators **(E)**. *(Adapted with permission from Hollinshead WH. Anatomy for Surgeons. Vol 3: The Back and Limbs. 3rd ed. New York: Harper & Row; 1982:325–330.)*

TABLE 68.7	Prime Movers of the Glenohumeral Joint
Flexion	Pectoralis major (clavicular head)
	Deltoid (anterior fibers)
Extension	Latissimus dorsi
	Deltoid (posterior fibers)
Internal rotation	Pectoralis major
	Latissimus dorsi
	Teres major
	Subscapularis
External rotation	Infraspinatus
	Teres minor
	Deltoid (posterior fibers)
Abduction	Deltoid
	Supraspinatus
Adduction	Pectoralis major
	Latissimus dorsi
	Teres major
	Subscapularis

Neck, shoulder, and arm pain associated with generalized pain or pain at other anatomical sites has been associated with greater persistence and disability than more localized neck, shoulder, and arm pain. Neck and arm pain associated with more generalized pain is also more likely to be associated with somatization, poor psychological health, older age, and less correlation with occupation or activity. More localized neck and shoulder pain is more strongly associated with use of keyboards at work and less frequent at older age.[18]

Evaluation of the Patient

HISTORY AND PHYSICAL EXAMINATION

The patient in pain is prompted to seek help not only to alleviate the suffering which accompanies their condition but also to address the accompanying condition of impairment or disability. The psychological, physical, or functional handicap which coexists with pain results in loss of ability to perform normal activities and fulfill roles that are fundamental to personal identity. Ultimately, the goal of a successful evaluation should be the ability to answer the patient's three fundamental questions: (1) "What's happening to me?" (2) "What's going to happen to me?" and (3) "What can be done to improve what happens to me?"[19]

The differential diagnosis of neck and arm pain is broad and encompasses acute pain from work-related injury, motor vehicle trauma and infection, emerging symptoms from enlarging tumors, vascular abnormalities or infections, manifestations of complex systemic disease processes, and exacerbation of chronic degenerative or inflammatory processes. The initial evaluation should be comprehensive in order to ascertain not only the etiology of physical symptomology but also the impact the patient's disability has on their psychosocial environment.

History

A thorough history of the patient with neck and arm pain is essential to separate acute from chronic, emergent from urgent and routine complaints, and focal and regional injuries and degenerative changes from systemic disorders. Pain in the neck and arm may also be referred from the thorax or abdomen requiring a thorough review of systems. The differential diagnosis is frequently based on the history, which then guides further focus during the physical exam and diagnostic testing.

Immediate consideration must be made regarding the severity and urgency of the complaint. Emergent conditions can often be discerned at the time of phone request for urgent evaluation or by nurses when the patient is screened at check-in. Severe neck

of patients with soft tissue neck injuries following whiplash reported discomfort sufficient enough to interfere with their capacity to work.[14]

Onset of neck and arm pain in the workplace varies widely across various occupations. Highly repetitive work, low job satisfaction, and a high level of fear avoidance are associated with development of neck and arm pain as are jobs which require prolonged bending or flexion of the neck such as computer work.[15–17] pain accompanied by progressive disturbance of gait, progressive motor or sensory deficits, or urinary and fecal incontinence requires prompt physician evaluation. Enlarging tumor, acute infection, and unstable inflammatory spondyloarthropathy can progress to respiratory failure and death if not treated promptly and requires immediate surgical and medical intervention. Acute progressive neurologic and cognitive deficits accompanied by hemodynamic instability may also present with dissecting vertebral and extracranial carotid artery aneurysms.[20,21] Other red flags include significant head trauma in the presence of a neurologic deficit. Night pain or unrelenting pain with associated weight loss is suggestive of a neoplastic or infectious process.

Location/Radiation
Pain in the neck and arm may be skeletal, myofascial, or neuropathic. Neuropathic pain can be further divided into peripheral or segmental nerve pathology versus autonomic and central nervous system pathology or sensitization. Cohen[22] suggests the diagnostic construct of mechanical versus nonmechanical pain. Mechanical pain is exacerbated by movement and occurs in the essentially well patient. Nonmechanical pain is often related to a medical source such as infection, neoplasm, or an inflammatory process generally seen in patients with systemic manifestations of their disease process.

The purpose of a thorough history with determination of the location, pattern, and distribution of the patient's pain is to establish an initial differential diagnosis which can subsequently be confirmed or ruled out by physical examination, diagnostic laboratory, radiologic, and electrophysiologic testing. Localized pain is usually caused by disorders of joints and muscles. Segmental pain conforming to dermatomal distributions may implicate lesions of nerve roots. Pain conforming to a peripheral dermatomal and/or myotomal distribution suggests lesions of the cervical or brachial plexus or their branches. Knowledge of dermatomal, myotomal, sclerotomal, and zygapophyseal referral patterns as well as distribution of peripheral nerves of the cervical and brachial plexus are essential for determining a rational differential diagnosis (see Figs. 68.11 through 68.19 and Tables 68.3 through 68.5).

In addition to cervical nerve root inflammation or impingement, cervical and brachial referral patterns may be secondary to myofascial trigger points or referred pain from cervical zygapophyseal joints. Widespread pain may implicate fibromyalgia syndrome, rheumatologic disease such as mild systemic lupus erythematosus, polyarticular osteoarthritis, rheumatoid arthritis, polymyalgia rheumatica, hypermobility syndromes, and even osteomalacia. Nonrheumatologic syndromes must also be considered in patients presenting with widespread pain. These include neoplastic and neurologic diseases, hypothyroidism, and other endocrine disorders, chronic infections, and a variety of psychiatric conditions.[23]

Location of the patient's pain cannot in isolation lead to a correct diagnosis. All aspects of the history of present illness; past medical and surgical history; family history of hereditary illness; and social, occupational, behavioral, psychological, and demographic information are necessary to identify predisposing factors or mechanisms of injury. A review of systems and detailed physical exam are essential to rule out manifestations of systemic disease and presence or absence of significant neurologic deficits. Even then, further diagnostic tests as well as pharmacologic and interventional trials may be required in complex cases to confirm or rule out etiologic hypothesis.

Onset
Acute onset of pain may occur after trauma, injury, or following an unaccustomed increase in activity in a deconditioned patient; however, an acute exacerbation of a chronic condition cannot be excluded. More gradual or insidious onset is common in progressive degenerative, inflammatory, or malignant process. It is important to elicit the time at which the pain first occurred, characteristics of the pain during the interval between onset, and evaluation of precipitating events or factors.

Intensity and Pattern of Severity with Time
A cardinal principle of diagnosis is assessment of the intensity of pain both at baseline and in response to time, activities, and treatment. Although the visual analogue or numerical rating pain score system is subjective and may be influenced by psychological, social, and occupational factors, it is essential to evaluate the trend of each patient's pain over time in order to assess the effects of pharmacologic, psychological, behavioral, physical, and interventional therapies. Patterns of pain severity over time are often associated with certain diseases. Chronic unrelenting pain may be due to inflammatory disease or a more centralized pain syndrome. Pain due to cervical spondylosis and stenosis may be severe with activities requiring neck flexion and rotation and absent or significantly reduced when the patient's neck is held in a neutral position. Patient complaint of night pain or pain of spontaneous onset which is constant and not relieved by rest or modified by movement may raise suspicion for an infectious or neoplastic process.

Quality
Electrical, shooting, stabbing, lancinating, burning, tingling, and pins and needles are common terms used to describe neuropathic pain. Dull, aching, cramping, or throbbing pain is more often associated with pain of a musculoskeletal nature. Stiffness is often described in association with degenerative arthritis or diffuse idiopathic skeletal hyperostosis (DISH). It is not unusual for the patient to include sensory changes (numbness, pins and needles, or burning) as well as cramping and aching pain in their description of cervical radiculopathy. This is most likely due to both the cutaneous or dermatomal and muscular or myotomal distribution of the cervical nerve roots. Burning pain associated with allodynia and thermohyperesthesia suggests complex regional pain syndrome (CRPS). The more chronic the pain condition, the more likely the patient will report a poorly localized, widespread, nondermatomal pain pattern due to changes in central pain processing known to occur following persistent painful peripheral input.[24]

Modifying Factors and Drug History
Asking the patient the question "What makes your pain better or worse?" will assist in further narrowing of the differential diagnosis. Coughing or sneezing and lateral head rotation and extension may cause exacerbation of cervical radicular pain. Chronic inflammatory pain is often worse after a period of inactivity and improves with exercise. Degenerative arthritis is often exacerbated by exercise and improves with rest. In patients with multiple pain complaints, response to medication may help guide diagnosis. In patients who have failed multiple medication trials, it is important to elicit specific reactions to medications, duration of use, dosages reached, and titration schedules implemented. An elderly patient, for example, who gives a history of intolerable sedation with an antiepileptic medication, may have been started at a standard adult dose and subsequently titrated upward using an aggressive titration schedule. This patient may be able to benefit from this same medication if it is titrated more gradually from a low dose.

Associated Symptoms
A history of neck and arm pain associated with frequently dropping objects, difficulty with writing, or other fine motor skills is useful in separating motor weakness from guarding secondary to pain. Associated symptoms may help to broaden or further refine the differential diagnosis. A patient with neck

and arm pain which occurs with increased activity and is associated with diaphoresis and shortness of breath may broaden the differential diagnosis to include coronary artery disease. Indeed, the first clinical description of cervical radiculopathy by Semmes and Murphy[25] in 1943 was entitled "The Syndrome of Unilateral Rupture of the Sixth Cervical Vertebral Disc with Compression of the Seventh Cervical Root: A Report of Four Cases with Symptoms Simulating Coronary Disease." Association of neck and radicular arm pain with positional headaches accompanied with nausea, photophobia, and blurred vision may lead the physician to rule out low-pressure headache.[26]

Family History

In addition to more common hereditary arthritides such as rheumatoid arthritis (more common in females), ankylosing spondylitis (predominantly seen in males), psoriatic arthritis, and Reiter's syndrome, there are also more uncommon hereditary diseases which can involve the cervical spine. Compression of the cervical cord from cervical root neurofibromas in patients with neurofibromatosis type 1 has been reported to present with progressive neurologic deficit.[27] Tophaceous gout of the odontoid process and larynx, epidural, mediastinal, and subcutaneous emphysema in a patient with Marfan's disease following forceful coughing, and cervical dystonia in spinocerebellar ataxia type 2 are other inherited disorders manifesting with neck pain.[28-31]

Age and Psychosocial History

The patient's age, sex, occupational, and social history is important in determining risk factors known to be associated with the development of persistent neck and upper limb pain. Whereas sports or trauma injury and congenital defects such as Chiari I malformations are common causes of neck pain in pediatric or adolescent patients, degenerative changes are common in older patients. Jobs or activities which require repeated lifting of heavy objects, prolonged bending of the neck, working with arms at/above shoulder height, and which involve little job control and little social support are associated with the development of neck pain. Specific jobs and activities associated with the development of neck pain include prolonged computer work and bicycling.[16,17,32] Extensive neck and upper extremity pain is independently associated with psychological ill health, female sex, unemployed status, and smoking.[18]

Questions regarding use of pillows at night and bifocals as well as any other activities which put the patient's neck under prolonged flexion strain should be included in the social and occupational history. In some cases, simple correction of repetitive strain with postural reeducation may result in relief of symptoms.

Depression and anxiety may occur as a reaction to persistent pain and are also independent risk factors for the development of chronic pain. The depressed individual may lack the psychological and social capabilities to cope with the complex physical, emotional, cognitive, and behavioral components of the pain experience.[33] Patients with coexisting histories of depression and anxiety may benefit from referral to a psychopharmachologist and from psychological consultation for cognitive and behavioral therapies to assist the patient with coping strategies.

Past Medical History and Review of Systems

The past medical history, past surgical history, and review of systems may provide essential clues tying the patient's symptoms to an associated disease process. Table 68.8 lists a few coexisting diseases which may present with neck pain and radiculopathy, whereas Table 68.9 lists a review of systems checklist which may identify systemic involvement or an urgent, rapidly progressing process.

TABLE 68.8	Noncompressive Infectious, Inflammatory, and Neoplastic Causes of Neck Pain and Radiculopathy

- Infection (most common in immunosuppressed patients)
  - Herpes zoster, human immunodeficiency virus, cytomegalovirus, tuberculosis, *Borrelia burgdorferi* (Lyme disease)
- Inflammatory
  - Systemic lupus erythematosus, sarcoidosis, Bruns-Garland syndrome (diabetic radiculopathy), Parsonage-Turner syndrome (neuralgic amyotrophy), multiple sclerosis, "pseudopolyneuropathy," gout

Surgical History

A past surgical history of neck fusion may signal risk of pseudoarthrosis or increased risk of recurrent disk disease above or below the level of fusion. Poststernotomy lesions following cardiac surgery with the clinical appearance of a C8 radiculopathy have been described. The causal mechanism is thought to be related to an occult fracture of the first thoracic rib. These are often mistaken for ulnar neuropathy at the elbow thought to be associated with surgical positioning.[34]

TABLE 68.9	A Comprehensive Checklist of Associated Features of Neck Pain that Might Indicate a Red Flag Condition

System	Past History	Symptoms Of	Feature or Condition
Nervous	Yes/No	Yes/No	Weakness
	Yes/No	Yes/No	Numbness
	Yes/No	Yes/No	Bladder dysfunction
	Yes/No	Yes/No	Impaired balance
	Yes/No	Yes/No	Impaired vision
	Yes/No	Yes/No	Altered speech
	Yes/No	Yes/No	Disorientation
	Yes/No	Yes/No	Altered consciousness
Cardiovascular	Yes/No	Yes/No	Risk factors
	Yes/No	Yes/No	Chest pain
	Yes/No	Yes/No	Anticoagulants
	Yes/No	Yes/No	Transient ischemic attacks
Respiratory	Yes/No	Yes/No	Carcinoma
	Yes/No	Yes/No	Tuberculosis
	Yes/No	Yes/No	Cough
	Yes/No	Yes/No	Weight loss
Alimentary	Yes/No	Yes/No	Carcinoma
	Yes/No	Yes/No	Weight loss
	Yes/No	Yes/No	Loss of appetite
	Yes/No	Yes/No	Dysphagia
	Yes/No	Yes/No	Diarrhea
	Yes/No	Yes/No	Altered bowel habits
Urinary	Yes/No	Yes/No	Incontinence
	Yes/No	Yes/No	Obstruction
Reproductive	Yes/No	Yes/No	Breast lump
	Yes/No	Yes/No	Uterine dysfunction
Endocrine	Yes/No	Yes/No	Thyroid cancer
	Yes/No	Yes/No	Hyperparathyroidism
Reticulo-endothelial	Yes/No	Yes/No	Lymph nodes
Skin	Yes/No	Yes/No	Rash
Musculoskeletal	Yes/No	Yes/No	Other joint pain
	Yes/No	Yes/No	Other muscle pain
	Yes/No	Yes/No	Risk of Paget's disease
	Yes/No	Yes/No	Risk of myeloma

Reprinted from Bogduk N. The neck. *Baillieres Best Pract Res Clin Rheumatol* 1999;13(2):261–285. Copyright © 1999 Harcourt Publishers Ltd. With permission.

Physical Examination

General Observations

Many important observations can be made during the initial interview and even as the patient travels from the waiting area to the exam room. The general health and independence of the patient can be surmised from skin and muscle tone, posture, gait, and use of assistive devices. Cachexia may be a sign of debilitation due to cancer or long-standing depression. Mood, affect, and cognitive state can be ascertained during questioning as well as during the physical exam. Other important general observations include symmetry of the shoulders; abnormal head positions including lateral flexion, rotation, or protrusion; and evidence of muscle wasting or deformity of the neck, shoulders, or upper limbs.

A complete physical exam is paramount in the patient with neck, shoulder, and arm pain. Inspection of the skin for lesions may reveal psoriasis which may be associated with psoriatic arthritis. Vesicles typifying herpes zoster may be found in a patient complaining of radicular symptoms. Lesions typical of erythema nodosum may be indicative of inflammatory disease or cancer, and needle marks (intravenous drug abuse) may raise suspicion for vertebral column infections. Acute pain from viscera sharing the same embryologic segmental derivation as the cervical spine can present as neck, shoulder, or arm pain. These include the submandibular glands, lymph nodes, thyroid, esophagus, heart, lungs, stomach, gallbladder, pancreas, and diaphragm, necessitating a general inspection and palpation of these areas.[35] In general, a systematic approach which includes a neurologic exam, inspection and palpation of bony and soft tissue structures followed by range of motion and special tests used in the diagnosis of neck pain should supplement but not replace the full physical examination.

Exam of the Neck

Neurologic Exam. Examination of the neck must include a neurologic exam. Tumors, infections, and carotid dissections which present as neck pain are also associated with cranial nerve palsies and sensory deficits. Delay in recognition of neurologic deficits in these cases can lead to progression of tumor or infection with poor surgical or medical outcome and prognosis.[36–38] A summary of the motor, sensory, and autonomic functions of the cranial nerves is found in Table 68.10.

In addition to examination of the cranial nerves, general head, neck, and upper extremity sensory; motor and deep tendon exam; sensory, motor, and deep tendon exam of the lower extremities are essential. Exam findings signaling a possible cervical myelopathy include unilateral or bilateral spastic,

TABLE 68.10 Summary of the Motor, Sensory, and Autonomic Functions of the Cranial Nerves

Cranial Nerve (CN)	Cranial Point Exit	Peripheral Innervation of Head	Function	Symptom/Sign of Damage
Olfactory (CN I)	Cribriform plate	Mucosa of nasal cavity	Smell	Anosmia
Optic (CN II)	Optic foramen	Retina of eye	Vision	Blindness
Occulomotor (CN III)	Superior orbital fissure	All extraocular eye muscles except superior oblique and lateral rectus	Eye movement (elevation, adduction)	Eye deviates down and out. Loss of papillary accommodation reflexes
Trochlear (CN VI)	Superior orbital fissure	Superior oblique (extraocular eye muscle)	Eye movement (depression of adducted eye)	Diplopia, lateral deviation of eye
Trigeminal (CN V)	V1—superior orbital fissure V2—foramen rotundum V3—foramen ovale	V1—cutaneous sensation of nose, eyes, and scalp V2—sensation of face: maxilla, nasal mucosa, upper lip, and teeth V3—cutaneous sensation of lower face: mouth mucosa, lower jaw teeth, TMJ, anterior two-thirds of tongue Motor supply to muscles of mastication	Facial sensation, mastication	Facial anesthesia Loss of pain sensation Weakness/loss of mastication
Abducent (CN VI)	Superior orbital fissure	Lateral rectus (extraocular eye muscle)	Eye movement (abduction)	Medial eye deviation
Facial (CN VII)	Entry: internal acoustic meatus Exit: stylomastoid foramen	Motor: muscles of facial expression and scalp	Facial expression, taste, salivation, lacrimation	Paralysis of facial muscles Loss of taste (anterior two-thirds of tongue) Dry mouth, loss of lacrimation
Vestibulocochlear (CN VIII)	Internal acoustic meatus	Inner ear labyrinth structures (semicircular canal and cochlear apparatus)	Balance hearing	Vertigo, disequilibrium, nystagmus, hearing loss
Glossopharyngeal (CN IX)	Jugular foramen	Posterior one-third of tongue Parotid gland Mucosa and elevator muscles of pharynx	Taste salivation Innervation of pharynx	Loss of taste (posterior one-third of tongue) Loss of gag reflex
Vagus (CN X)	Jugular foramen	Palatal muscles, pharyngeal constrictors, vocal cords Taste and sensation to epiglottis	Swallowing and talking Cardiac, gastrointestinal tract Respiration Taste	Dysphagia and hoarseness Loss of cough reflex, loss of taste
Cranial accessory Spinal accessory (CN XI)	Jugular foramen —	Motor supply to larynx and pharynx Head rotation and shoulder shrugging	Pharynx/larynx muscles Trapezius, sternocleidomastoid	Head turning Shoulder shrug weakness
Hypoglossal (CN XII)	Hypoglossal canal	Intrinsic and some extrinsic tongue muscles	Tongue movement	Atrophy of tongue muscles, deviation on protrusion, fasciculations

TMJ, temporomandibular joint.

TABLE 68.11 Muscle Strength Grading

- Grade 0: total paralysis
- Grade 1: palpable or visible contraction
- Grade 2: full range of motion with gravity eliminated
- Grade 3: full range of motion against gravity
- Grade 4: full range of motion with decreased strength
- Grade 5: normal strength
- NT: not testable

ataxic, spastic-ataxic or Trendelenburg gait, hyperreflexia of lower extremity deep tendon reflexes and Babinski sign, and decreased sphincter tone or loss of the anal "wink."

Sensory Exam. The sensory exam is particularly useful in the patient with neuropathic pain. Sensory testing should include brush touch for allodynia; light pressure for tenderness and hyperalgesia; and palpation for painful areas as well as vibration, hot, cold, and sharp versus dull discrimination. Positive sensations, stimulus-evoked hypersensitivities such as allodynia to innocuous stimulation including light touch and cold, and hyperalgesia to noxious stimulation such as pinprick occur focally in mononeuropathies and distally and symmetrically in polyneuropathies. In neuropathic pain syndromes such as CRPS, allodynia, and hyperalgesia may spread outside the area of the original injury or to homologous sites in the opposite limb. These sensory findings are often associated with focal autonomic abnormalities such as sweating, skin temperature and color changes, and edema are also present in CRPS. In central pain and anesthesia dolorosa, allodynia, hyperalgesia, and aftersensation (persistence of pain after the stimulus has ceased) can occur in areas demonstrated to have loss of sensation. In small-fiber neuropathies, loss of thermal, pain, and sometimes touch perception with sparing of large-fiber functions such as muscle strength, deep tendon reflexes, and vibratory and proprioceptive perception is seen. These functions are all compromised in combined large- and small-fiber polyneuropathies.[39] The sensory exam should include evaluation for dermatomal patterns of sensory abnormality and for altered sensation in peripheral nerve distributions in patients with suspected peripheral nerve injury or entrapment syndromes. A "cord" level of sensory disturbance may be confined to the upper extremities due to "central cord syndrome" with involvement of decussating anterior sensory fibers.[40]

Motor Exam. Motor exam is tested using the standard muscle strength scale from 0 to 5 (Table 68.11).

In addition to testing of motor function of the cranial nerves, myotomal or segmental nerve root motor supply should be systematically evaluated (Table 68.12).

Deficits consistent with peripheral nerve lesions or injury should also be ruled out (Table 68.13).

TABLE 68.12 Segmental Motor Function Evaluation

- C2: breathing
- C3–C4: spontaneous breathing, trapezius function
- C4–C6: shoulder flexion, extension
- Upper extremity strength
- C5: deltoid abduction at shoulder
- C6: biceps flexion at forearm
- C6: wrist extension (extensor carpi radialis)
- C7: wrist flexion
- C7: elbow extension (triceps)
- C7: finger extension
- C8: fingers flexion middle finger (flex dig profundus)
- T1: small finger abductors (abductor digiti minimi)
- T1: interossei (spread fingers)

Reflex testing should include upper and lower extremities because lesions of the cervical spine may manifest with hypoactive reflexes at the level of the lesion, hyperactive reflexes below the lesion, and pathologic reflexes. Cutaneous reflexes will also be lost below the lesion. Reflexes are tested using the following standard scale:

- 0: absent reflex
- 1+: trace or seen only with reinforcement
- 2+: normal
- 3+: brisk
- 4+: nonsustained clonus (i.e., repetitive vibratory movements)
- 5+: sustained clonus

Using this scale, 1+, 2+, or 3+ reflex is considered normal unless there is a significant difference between sides. In contrast, 0, 4+, and 5+ are considered abnormal.

Upper extremity normal and pathologic reflexes are outlined in Table 68.14.

Inspection and Palpation. After observation for abnormal posture such as abnormal loss of cervical lordosis, torticollis, and obvious atrophic musculature of the neck or upper extremity, the patient should be asked to lay supine to relax the musculature of the neck. This allows optimal examination of the bony structures of the neck.[35] While standing at the patient's side, one hand supports the neck from behind while the other is used to palpate the anterior neck structures.

The most superior bony structure of the anterior neck is the hyoid bone. It is the only bone in the skeletal structure not articulated to any other bone. It supports the root of the tongue and in turn is supported by the muscles of the neck and suspended by the stylohyoid ligaments from the styloid processes of the temporal bones. The body of the hyoid bone is palpated in the midline, whereas the lesser and greater cornu are palpated laterally to each side of the body forming a horseshoe-like structure. The hyoid bone lies at the lower level of C3 or at the intervertebral disk between C3 and C4. Although injuries of the hyoid bone are rare outside of strangulation, fractures of the hyoid due to trauma, cardiopulmonary resuscitation, and sports injuries have been reported with complications including carotid pseudoaneurysm, pharyngeal laceration, and airway compromise.[41–44] Insertion tendonitis of the hyoid bone has also been reported as an unrecognized source of neck pain with recognizable radiologic features.[45] Below the hyoid bone, at the level of C4 to C5, is the thyroid cartilage. The first cricoid ring forms the upper border of the trachea. It lies at the level of C6. The carotid tubercle, also known as Chassaignac's tubercle, is the anterior tubercle of the C6 transverse process and can be palpated approximately 3 cm lateral to the first cricoid ring. The carotid arteries overlie the tubercles. Caution should be taken to examine the carotid pulses individually to prevent bradycardia and/or syncope.

Soft tissues of the anterior neck include the H-shaped thyroid gland which extends from the thyroid cartilage cranially to the fourth to sixth tracheal rings inferiorly. This area should be inspected to preclude generalized enlargement of the gland and palpated to exclude thyroid masses. The exam should include inspection for palpable lymph nodes which may be due to infection or metastatic disease. Unknown primary carcinoma presents as painless enlarged cervical lymph nodes and

TABLE 68.13 Manifestations of Peripheral Nerve Injuries of Upper Extremities

- Ulnar nerve: claw hand
- Radial nerve: wrist drop
- Median nerve: cannot make "OK" sign

TABLE 68.14   Upper Extremity Deep Tendon Reflexes and Pathologic Reflexes

Reflex	Nerve Root or Function Tested	Location	Response
Scapulohumeral reflex	Tests integrity of cord segments from C4 to C6	Lower aspect of medial border of scapula	Adduction and lateral rotation of the arm
Biceps reflex	C5, C6	Tap thumb placed over biceps tendon in antecubital fossa	Flexion of forearm
Brachioradialis reflex	C6	Proximal to radial aspect of wrist	Radial and dorsiflexion at wrist
Triceps reflex	C7	Tendon of triceps muscle as it crosses olecranon fossa	Extension at elbow
Hoffmann sign (pathologic if positive; upper extremity equivalent of Babinski sign)	Test for upper motor neuron lesion	Patient's long finger in slight extension	Involuntary flexion of thumb and little finger to make "OK" sign
		DIP flicked downward by examiner's thumb	
Jaw reflex	Upper motor neuron lesions	Tap finger placed over mental area of chin	Jaw closing (abnormal if hyperactive)
Chvostek sign (pathologic if positive)	Hypocalcemia or other metabolic abnormality	Tap over facial nerve anterior to ear	Hyperactive response

DIP, distal interphalangeal joint.

accounts for approximately 5% of all head and neck malignancies. If malignancy is suspected, the patient should be referred for more advanced imaging and diagnostic testing.[46] By having the patient turn his or her head to the opposite side, the sternocleidomastoid muscle may be examined from the origins on the sternum and clavicle to its insertion on the mastoid process of the temporal bone. The anterior border of this muscle from origin to insertion defines the lateral limit of the anterior triangle of the neck and the posterior border, the anterior limit of the posterior triangle of the neck. The exam should include palpation for painful or painless masses, trigger points with associated referral patterns, and pain associated with swallowing.

Palpation of the bony landmarks of the posterior cervical spine includes the inion or external occipital protuberance in the midline, which makes the midpoint of the superior nuchal line extending laterally from the inion bilaterally. The occipital nerves run medial to the occipital arteries over the occiput approximately 3 cm from the midline. Tenderness or pain with examination of this area may be seen with occipital neuralgia. Palpation of the cervical spine is performed in a systematic way, starting with the spinous processes, and followed by the zygapophyseal joints. Pain over the midline structures

may indicate a structural problem of the cervical spine. The zygapophyseal joints are located 2 to 3 cm from the midline. Palpation of the lateral atlantoaxial joint of C1–C2 is undertaken by rotating the patient's head to the ipsilateral side. C2, C3, C4, and C5 are usually difficult to palpate because of the normal cervical lordosis but can be easily identified if it is remembered that the C3–C4 joint is at the level of the hyoid bone and the C4–C5 joint is at the superior aspect of the thyroid cartilage. The C6 spinous process can be easily identified as it is usually easily palpable and disappears under the examining finger on extension of the neck. The level of the C6–C7 joint can also be confirmed by its location at the level of the cricoid ring. The largest "fixed" prominence is the spinous process of C7. Referral patterns from the zygapophyseal joints have recently been studied in patients with neck, head, and shoulder pain with the most common referral patterns based on areas in which patients are relieved of pain by controlled blocks are depicted in Figures 68.28 through 68.33.[47]

Examination of the soft tissues of the posterior neck includes palpation of the suboccipital muscles and trapezius which, like the sternocleidomastoid, may be a source of CEH. The trapezius extends from the external occipital protuberance, the

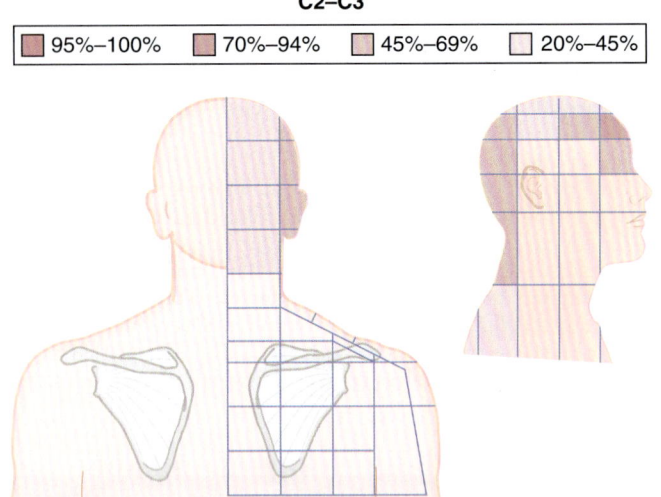

FIGURE 68.28 Distribution of pain and pain frequency in each grid area as reported by patients with pain originating from C2 to C3. *(From Cooper G, Bailey B, Bogduk N. Cervical zygapophysial joint pain maps. Pain Medicine 2007;8[4]:344–853. Reproduced by permission of American Academy of Pain Medicine.)*

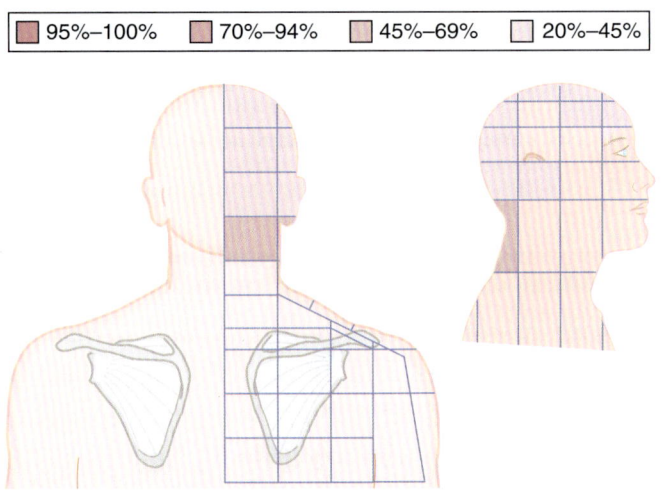

FIGURE 68.29 Distribution of pain and pain frequency in each grid area as reported by patients with pain originating from C3 to C4. *(From Cooper G, Bailey B, Bogduk N. Cervical zygapophysial joint pain maps. Pain Medicine 2007;8[4]:344–853. Reproduced by permission of American Academy of Pain Medicine.)*

C4–C5

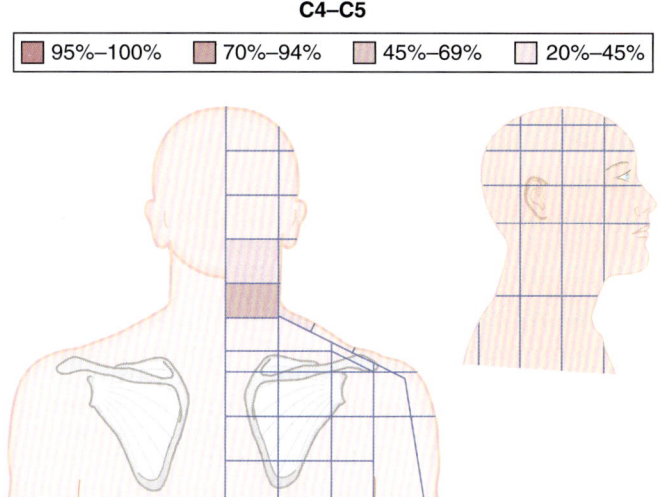

FIGURE 68.30 Distribution of pain and pain frequency in each grid area as reported by patients with pain originating from C4 to C5. (*From Cooper G, Bailey B, Bogduk N. Cervical zygapophysial joint pain maps. Pain Medicine 2007;8[4]:344–353. Reproduced by permission of American Academy of Pain Medicine.*)

C6–C7

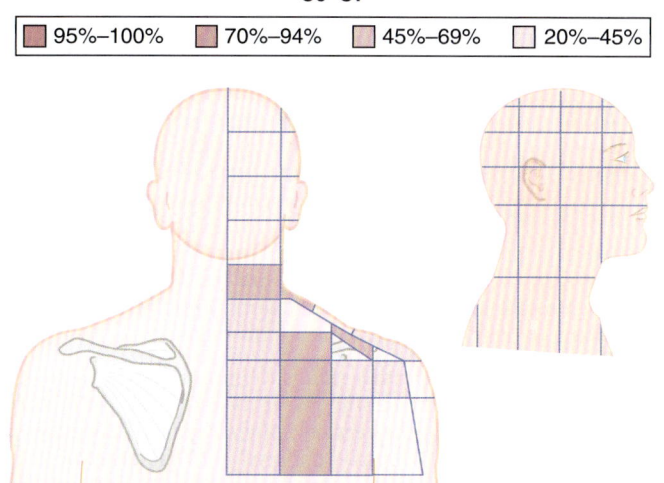

FIGURE 68.32 Distribution of pain and pain frequency in each grid area as reported by patients with pain originating from C6 to C7. (*From Cooper G, Bailey B, Bogduk N. Cervical zygapophysial joint pain maps. Pain Medicine 2007;8[4]:344–353. Reproduced by permission of American Academy of Pain Medicine.*)

medial third of the superior nuchal line of the occipital bone, the ligamentum nuchae, spinous processes of the seventh cervical, and all thoracic vertebrae to the posterior border of the lateral third of the clavicle, the medial margin of the acromion, and the posterior border of the scapular spine. The scalene muscles should not be neglected in patients with neck ache, arm ache, and headache. Neck pain, occipital headache, extremity paresthesia, pain, and weakness may occur from scarring of the scalene muscles secondary to neck trauma such as whiplash injuries.[48] As with examination of the anterior neck, a chain of lymph nodes lies along the anterolateral border of the trapezius. Enlargement or tenderness of these may indicate infection or metastatic disease.

Special Tests for Neck and Upper Extremity

Spurling's Maneuver. This maneuver is used to confirm the presence of a cervical radiculopathy. It is performed by extending and rotating the head to the right or left. This narrows the

intervertebral foramen by 20% to 30%. It has been shown to have a sensitivity of 30% and a specificity of 93% on 235 individuals referred for electrodiagnosis of upper extremity nerve pain.[49] It also increases pressure on the cervical facet joints and may intensify facet mediated pain.

Valsalva Test. This test is performed by having the patients place their thumb in their mouth and blow, as if to push the thumb out of their mouth. This maneuver increases the intraspinal pressure and may reveal the presence of space-occupying lesions of the cervical spine such as large intervertebral disk herniations, tumors, and stenosis due to spondylosis or osteophytes. If the mass involves the area of the spine adjacent to nerve roots, radicular pain may be reproduced.

Distraction Test. This test reduces pressure on the intervertebral disk and exiting nerve roots and simulates the effect that traction may have on treatment of neck and radicular symptoms.

C5–C6

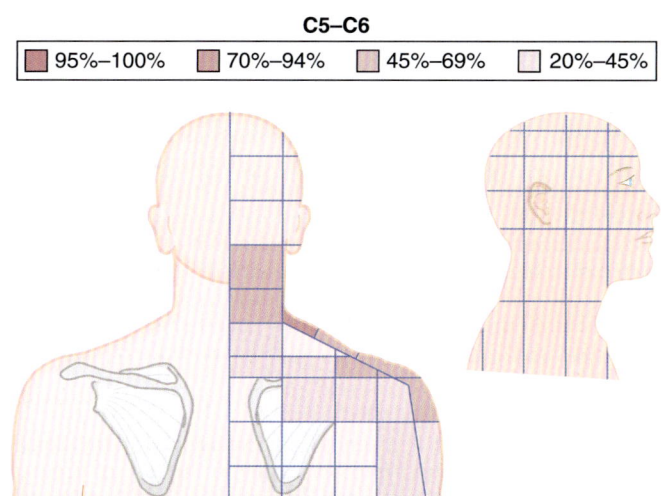

FIGURE 68.31 Distribution of pain and pain frequency in each grid area as reported by patients with pain originating from C5 to C6. (*From Cooper G, Bailey B, Bogduk N. Cervical zygapophysial joint pain maps. Pain Medicine 2007;8[4]:344–353. Reproduced by permission of American Academy of Pain Medicine.*)

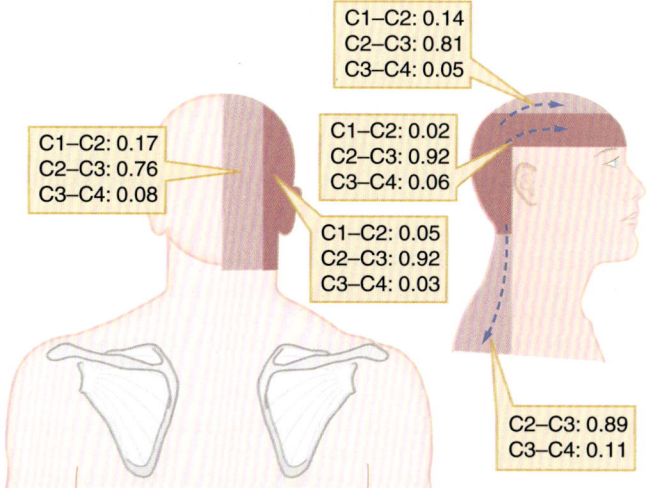

FIGURE 68.33 The probability of neck and head pain in areas depicted being secondary to C1–C2, C2–C3, and C3–C4 segments. (*From Cooper G, Bailey B, Bogduk N. Cervical zygapophysial joint pain maps. Pain Medicine 2007;8[4]:344–353. Reproduced by permission of American Academy of Pain Medicine.*)

It is performed by placing one hand underneath the jaws, the other beneath the occiput, and applying gentle upward pressure over 30 to 60 seconds. Increased pain with this maneuver may be due to inflammatory or degenerative disease or muscle or ligamentous pathology.

Jackson's Compression Test. As with Spurling's maneuver, this test places increased pressure on the cervical facet joints and causes narrowing of the neural foramen. It may reproduce neck pain due to facet arthropathy and/or upper extremity radicular pain due to nerve root compression. To perform this test, the patient is instructed to rotate his or her head first to the right and then to the left. The examiner exerts gentle pressure to the top of the patient's head after each movement.

Lhermitte's Sign. Lhermitte's sign is the production of a sensation of lightening-like paresthesias or dysesthesias in the arms or legs upon flexion of the cervical spine. It may be caused by a large disk herniation or bony compression of the anterior cord in patients with a narrowed central canal. It may also occur in patients with rheumatoid arthritis with associated instability or in patients with multiple sclerosis affecting the cervical spinal cord, tumors, and syringomyelia.[50]

Shoulder Depression and Abduction Tests. The shoulder depression and abduction tests are useful for evaluation of radicular pain. The shoulder depression test is performed by having the patient laterally flex his or her neck while placing downward pressure on the shoulder opposite the direction of flexion. This produces stretch on irritated nerve roots and may accentuate or reproduce radicular symptoms. The shoulder abduction test relieves pressure on the cervical nerve roots and may relieve or reduce cervical radicular symptoms. It is performed by having the patient place the hand from the painful side on the top of their head. This maneuver shortens the distance between the cervical spine and the coracoid process, thus relieving tension on the nerve root.

In vivo studies using kinematic MRI of 21 patients with cervical spine disk herniations or cervical spondylosis demonstrated an increase of foraminal size with flexion, axial rotation to the opposite side of pain, and flexion combined with axial rotation to the opposite side of the pain. Foraminal size decreased at extension combined with axial rotation to the side of the pain. A decrease or no change of foraminal size was observed at either extension or axial rotation to the side of the pain alone. Cervical cord rotation or displacement was noted with axial rotation in 24% of these patients.[51] Active versus passive range-of-motion testing is advised in patients with neurologic symptoms or those at risk of instability of the cervical spine (i.e., patients with progressive rheumatoid arthritis involving the cervical spine). In these patients, limitation of active range of motion due to pain may be protective.

Adson Maneuver. This test is used to rule out compression of the subclavian artery by an extra cervical rib or scalene muscle bands, which may result in TOS. It was first described by Alfred Washington Adson in 1927. It is performed by having the patient sit with his or her arms resting on the knees with his or her head extended and rotated toward the affected side. The patient is then instructed to breathe deeply and hold his or her breath while the radial pulse is monitored. The test is considered positive if the radial pulse disappears. More recently, the positioning often includes abduction and external rotation of the arm. Current testing methods include use of Doppler ultrasound to record significant changes in subclavian artery flow characteristics during the earlier mentioned maneuvers.[52] Although the clinical validity of the Adson test has been questioned, a 2006 study showed complete relief of symptoms following surgery in 87% of patients with a positive Adson test using Doppler ultrasound compared to significant relief of pain in only 50% of patients with a negative Doppler-assisted Adson test.[53]

Halsted Maneuver (Exaggerated Military Position). The Halsted maneuver is a test of neurovascular compression at the costoclavicular space. The patient assumes a military posture with the shoulders rolled backward and downward so to narrow the costoclavicular space. The radial pulse is monitored. The maneuver is considered positive if the radial pulse disappears.

Roos Test or Elevated Arm Stress Test. The Roos or elevated arm stress test (EAST) is a test for TOS during which the patient abducts both arms to 90 degrees with elbows flexed to 90 degrees thus narrowing the scalene triangle. The patient then opens and closes his or her hands for a period of 3 minutes. Patients without TOS will have pain, fatigue, or distress in the forearms only. Patients with TOS will have significant symptomology which replicates their normal TOS symptoms and may not be able to complete the test.

Further diagnostic tests for shoulder pathology are outlined in Table 68.15.

Examination of the Shoulder and Arm

Detailed anatomy of the neck, shoulder, and upper extremities, including normal range of motion, is covered in the initial part of this chapter and is essential to understanding the anatomic and functional correlates of this portion of the physical exam. Physical examination of the shoulder, arm, elbow, forearm, wrist, and hand should include the following:
- Blood pressure
- Inspection of position, shape, muscle atrophy, swelling
- Inspection of skin for allodynia, changes in color, temperature, or trophic changes
- Palpation of muscles and tendon for tenderness, pain, trigger points, dysesthesias, and radiation patterns
- Palpation over joints during range of motion testing for crepitus, popping, or locking
- Active and passive range of motion at shoulder: abduction, adduction, internal and external rotation, flexion, and extension at shoulder
- Other tests for shoulder, see Table 68.15
- Range of motion at forearm: flexion, extension, pronation, and supination
- Range of motion at wrist: dorsal flexion, palmar flexion, ulnar flexion, and radial flexion
- Range of motion of fingers: flexion, extension, adduction, abduction, opponens, and grip
- Observation of effect on pain of each movement

Waddell Signs. In their study of illness behavior, Waddell et al.[54] described five categories of nonanatomic signs (Table 68.16) and reported that the presence of at least three signs was indicative of significant psychosocial stress. Although the presence of three or more signs is often interpreted as a sign of malingering, no association with malingering or secondary gain has been demonstrated in controlled studies.[55] Fishbain et al.[56] reported that Waddell signs decreased following comprehensive pain management. Pain behaviors are known to be a means for patients to communicate pain and distress. They can be positively reinforced by attention from family members or by being excused from undesirable obligations. Pain behaviors may also be "unlearned" using cognitive and behavioral therapies.[57,58]

LABORATORY EVALUATION

Pain must be seen as a diagnosis of exclusion, for the consequences of treating pain symptomatically in the face of progressive systemic disease can result in a tragic delay of diagnosis and treatment. In general, laboratory testing is guided by the patient's history of present illness, past medical history, and physical exam. A patient who is systemically ill requires more extensive testing guided by affected organs and systems. For example, patients who are febrile or those with weight loss, anorexia, and other signs suggesting infection or neoplasm would benefit from complete blood

TABLE 68.15 Tests Used in Shoulder Pain Diagnosis and Significance of Positive Findings

Test	Maneuver/Description	Diagnosis Suggested by Positive Result
Apley scratch test	Patient touches superior and inferior aspects of opposite scapula.	Loss of range of motion of the shoulder: rotator cuff problem
Neer test	The examiner should stabilize the patient's scapula with one hand while passively flexing the arm while it is internally rotated. If the patient reports pain in this position, then the result of the test is considered to be positive.	Subacromial impingement syndrome
Hawkins-Kennedy test	Patient is examined while sitting with shoulder flexed to 90 degrees and their elbow flexed to 90 degrees. Examiner grasps and supports proximal to the wrist and elbow; the examiner and the patient then quickly rotate the arm internally. Pain located below the acromioclavicular joint with internal rotation is considered a positive test result.	Subacromial impingement syndrome
Drop arm test	Examiner will passively abduct the patient's shoulder (humerus) to 90 degrees. The patient is then asked to slowly lower or adduct the shoulder to their side. If the patient is unable to perform this motion, the examiner can hold the humerus at 90 degrees of abduction and apply slight pressure to the distal forearm.	Inability to controllably lower the arm can indicate a rotator cuff dysfunction.
Empty can test	The patient's arm should be elevated to 90 degrees in the scapular plane, with the elbow extended, full internal rotation, and pronation of the forearm. This results in a thumbs-down position, as if the patient were pouring liquid out of a can. Examiner stabilizes the shoulder while applying a downwardly directed force to the arm; the patient tries to resist this motion. This test is considered positive if the patient experiences pain or weakness with resistance.	Supraspinatus muscle/tendon tear or suprascapular nerve dysfunction
Lift-off test	Patient stands and places the dorsum of the hand against mid-lumbar spine. The patient then lifts his hand away from the back.	An inability to perform this action indicates a lesion of the subscapularis muscle. Abnormal motion of the scapula during the test may indicate scapular instability.
Cross-arm test (scarf test)	With the arm to be tested in 90 degrees of elbow flexion and 90 degrees of shoulder flexion (forward elevation), the patient then cross adducts/horizontally adducts, resting the hand on top of the opposite shoulder. The examiner pushes the arm into further cross/horizontal adduction. The position and movement mimics throwing a "scarf" over the shoulder, hence the name of the test. A positive test is indicated by localized pain over the acromioclavicular joint.	A positive test commonly indicates acromioclavicular joint osteoarthritis or acromioclavicular joint ligament injury.
O'Brien test (active compression test)	The upper extremity to be tested is placed in 90 degrees of shoulder flexion and 10–15 degrees of horizontal adduction. The patient then fully internally rotates the shoulder and pronates the elbow. The examiner provides a distal stabilizing force as the patient is instructed to apply an upward force. The procedure is then repeated in a neutral shoulder and forearm position. A positive test occurs with pain reproduction or clicking in the shoulder with the first position and reduced/absent with the second position.	Labral (superior labral tear from anterior to posterior or SLAP) lesion or acromioclavicular lesions as cause for shoulder pain
Apprehension test	Examiner stands either behind or at the involved side, grasps the wrist with one hand, and passively externally rotates the humerus to end range with the shoulder in 90 degrees of abduction. Forward pressure is then applied to the posterior aspect of the humeral head by the examiner or the table (if the patient is in supine). A positive test for anterior instability is if apprehension is presented by the patient or if the patient reports pain.	A positive test indicates a possible torn labrum or anterior instability problem.
Relocation test	With the patient supine, the examiner pre-positions the shoulder at 90 degrees of abduction and maximal external rotation. The examiner grasps the subject's wrist and hand with his or her distal hand while applying a posterior force to the humeral head while externally rotating the shoulder. The test is considered positive if the patient is able to be moved into a greater range of external rotation before apprehension is expressed as compared to when there is no posterior pressure exerted by the examiner.	Checks for glenohumeral instability, dislocation, and subluxation. This test should be done following the apprehension test especially if anterior instability is suspected.
Sulcus sign	With the arm straight and relaxed to the side of the patient, the elbow is grasped, and traction is applied in an inferior direction. With excessive inferior translation, a depression occurs just below the acromion. The appearance of this sulcus is a positive sign.	A positive test indicates glenohumeral instability.
Yergason test	The patient should be seated or standing, with the humerus in neutral position and the elbow in 90 degrees of flexion. The patient is asked to externally rotate and supinate their arm against the manual resistance of the therapist. Yergason test is considered positive if pain is reproduced in the bicipital groove during the test.	A positive test indicates biceps tendon pathology, such as bicipital tendonitis.
Speed maneuver	The examiner places the patient's arm in shoulder flexion, external rotation, full elbow extension, and forearm supination; manual resistance is then applied by the examiner in a downward direction. The test is considered to be positive if pain in the bicipital tendon or bicipital groove is reproduced.	A positive test indicates a superior labral tear or bicipital tendonitis.
Clunk test	Have the patient lie supine. The examiner places one hand on the posterior aspect of the shoulder over the humeral head and places the other hand on the humerus above the elbow. Fully abduct the arm over the patient's head and then push anteriorly with the hand over the humeral head while the other hand rotates the humerus into external rotation. A clunk or grinding sound is a positive test.	A positive test indicates a tear of the labrum.
Crank test	With the subject standing, the examiner places the distal hand on the subject's elbow and the proximal hand on the subject's proximal humerus and then passively elevates the subjects shoulder to 160 degrees in the scapular plane. With the distal hand, the examiner applies a load along the long axis of the humerus while the proximal hand externally and internally rotates the humerus. A positive test is when there is reproduction of symptoms with or without a click during the maneuver (usually during external rotation).	A positive test indicates a glenohumeral ligament lesion and may also be used to assess anterior shoulder instability or a labral tear.

SLAP, superior labrum anterior and posterior.

TABLE 68.16 Waddell Signs

1. Superficial and widespread tenderness or nonanatomic tenderness (it is "one" sign)
2. Stimulation tests: axial loading and pain on simulated rotation (it's another "one" sign)
3. Distracted straight leg raise
4. Nonanatomic sensory changes: regional sensory changes and regional weakness (it's another "one" sign)
5. Overreaction

TABLE 68.17 NEXUS Criteria for Radiologic Evaluation of the Neck in Patients after Trauma

- No midline cervical tenderness
- No focal neurologic deficit
- Normal alertness
- No intoxication
- No painful, distracting injury

NEXUS, National Emergency X-Radiography Utilization Study.

count and differential analysis. Those with a history of hepatitis or other risk factors for liver disease would benefit from a liver enzyme panel. Patients with cold intolerance, weight gain, and lethargy should undergo thyroid function test analysis.

Morning stiffness, polyarticular involvement, rigidity, or cutaneous manifestations suggest an inflammatory arthritic component requiring a more extensive rheumatologic evaluation. Patients with a diagnosis of fibromyalgia should undergo testing of both thyroid function and vitamin D levels because hypothyroidism and vitamin D deficiency can both result in diffuse pain syndromes which mimic fibromyalgia.

Laboratory analysis of the erythrocyte sedimentation rate and C-reactive protein may also assist in evaluating inflammatory phenomena such as an autoimmune disease, infection, or neoplasm. These may be significantly elevated with an upward trend in patients who are afebrile, who have a normal white blood cell count, and who culture negative (even in the face of sepsis).[59,60]

Other laboratory tests which may be useful in ruling out systemic disease in select patients include serum calcium, which among other diagnoses may be elevated in patients with malignancy, and serum alkaline phosphatase, which is elevated in metastatic spine tumors and Paget disease.[1]

RADIOGRAPHIC STUDIES

Diagnostic and functional imaging is covered in detail in Chapters 18 and 19. In general, imaging of the neck and arm should be performed in patients with a history of trauma, persistent or progressive pain, and in patients with neurologic deficits involving the neck and/or upper extremities in order to confirm or rule out treatable organic causes of pain or neurologic deficits and to guide therapeutic decision making.

Although the clinical usefulness of cervical spine radiographs for evaluation of neck pain has been questioned,[61,62] cervical spine fractures occur frequently following relatively minor trauma in the elderly patient[63] with a relative risk of up to three times more fractures in elderly versus younger adults evaluated in the emergency room.[64] Although significant cervical spine injury is infrequent in younger patients, diagnosis is often delayed following motor vehicle and sports trauma. In published series, missed cervical spine injuries following trauma have been reported to occur in 4.6% to 33% of patients.[65,66] C2 and C5–C6 level fractures are the most commonly seen injuries.[65,67,68] In a recent report of 100 consecutive patients who underwent operative fixation or halo stabilization for cervical spine injuries, 10% of injuries were missed due to failure to perform plain cervical films versus failure of interpretation or failure to utilize more advanced imaging techniques.[67] A recent prospective, multicenter US study designed to validate clinical criteria developed to evaluate patients with neck pain following blunt trauma[69–71] confirmed sensitivity of the set of five criteria (Table 68.17) approaching 100% for clinically important injuries.[72]

Even fewer injuries were missed in a more recent multicenter study, when the Canadian C-spine rule was applied (Fig. 68.34).[73] Anteroposterior, neutral lateral, and odontoid plain film views are recommended. A patient with persistent neck pain or tenderness despite normal plain film radiology or suspected ligamentous injury may benefit from flexion-extension views to evaluate for listhesis or instability. These views may also be helpful in determining the amount of motion occurring with flexion and extension in patients with degenerative spondylolisthesis. Prior to flexion-extension imaging, the patient should perform active range of motion in the presence of a physician to confirm that no significant neurologic deficit occurs during these maneuvers.

In patients with chronic neck pain, plain film views can reveal degenerative changes such as loss of disk height, bone spurs, endplate irregularity, and endplate sclerosis. In patients with prior cervical spine fusion, instability secondary to pseudoarthrosis can be appreciated.

Computerized tomography (CT) is recommended for patients with acute or chronic neck pain who have normal plain films and clinically suspected cervical spine pathology or to further define abnormalities seen on plain films.[74] It is also useful for evaluating the size and shape of the spinal canal, facet and uncovertebral joints, and transverse foramina.[75,76] When possible, patients with neurologic deficits or pain due to suspected neurologic or soft tissue injury or pathology should undergo MRI. According to a systematic analysis and multicenter study comparing CT to MRI for assessment of cervical spine injuries following trauma to the cervical spine, midsagittal T1- and T2-weighted MRI provides an objective, quantifiable, and reliable assessment of spinal cord compression that cannot be adequately assessed by CT alone.[77] MRI and magnetic resonance myelography are comparable to CT myelography in assessing spinal stenosis and spinal nerve roots. Although CT is superior in imaging canal foraminal osteophytes, MRI is superior to CT in assessment of spinal cord gray matter and nerve root signal changes and well as ligamentous and intervertebral disk changes.[78] Use of gadolinium-enhanced MRI in symptomatic patients who have undergone surgery of the cervical spine is valuable in identifying changes consistent with postoperative infection in the acute postoperative period and in defining the extent of epidural scar formation versus reherniation of intervertebral disks in patients with recurrent neck and radicular pain.[79]

If MRI is contraindicated (i.e., due to a pacemaker or spinal cord stimulator), CT using 45-degree oblique reconstruction is superior to sagittal reconstructions oriented at 90 degrees for evaluation of the foramen for bony spurs.[80]

In regard to imaging of the shoulder, a standard series of shoulder radiographs excludes or confirms arthritis, bursitis, tendonitis, calcification, dislocation, tumor, and old or new fractures.[81] CT is useful for diagnosing bony lesions, subtle dislocation, labral tears, and full rotator cuff tears. MRI is more

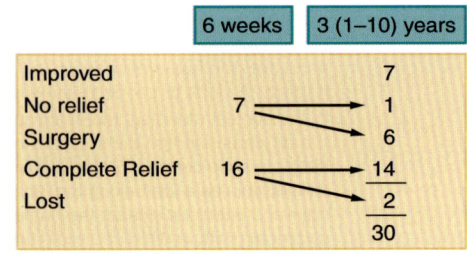

FIGURE 68.34 Canadian C-Spine rule.

expensive, time-consuming, and less readily available in some areas, and certain pathologies such as the glenoid labrum and the surrounding ligaments may be difficult to evaluate with MRI. MRI is able to evaluate partial or full rotator cuff tears and has the advantages of noninvasive nature, lack of contrast exposure, nonionizing radiation, high degree of resolution, and ability to evaluate multiple pathologies.

Ultrasound is used to diagnose rotator cuff tears, is noninvasive, rapid, and relatively inexpensive; however, it has been shown to have more interoperator variability in performance and interpretation of imaging.[81–85]

Advanced imaging as well as electromyography and nerve conduction velocity testing should be performed as needed for the purpose of guiding treatment decision making. Electrodiagnostic evaluation of acute and chronic pain is discussed in Chapter 16.

Multiple plain radiographic views are often needed to visualize the elbow, forearm, wrist, and hand and can also be used to confirm or rule out fractures, tendonitis, and dislocations. Minimal evaluation of the elbow should include anteroposterior views for the distal humerus and proximal forearm as well as lateral views in maximal flexion and extension. Additional views such as radiocapitellar, cubital tunnel, oblique, and stress views may be utilized based on history or mechanism of injury and physical exam findings.[1]

Common Causes of Neck and Arm Pain

MECHANICAL NECK PAIN AND CERVICOGENIC HEADACHE

Neck pain from similar mechanisms may be axial, associated with radicular pain, headache, and/or symptoms suggesting spinal cord compression. The complex and highly interdependent structures of the neck may preclude identification of a single pain generator in patients with advanced disease. Muscle and ligamentous injury or pain may result from factors related to posture, poor ergonomics, stress, injury, and/or chronic muscle fatigue. Pain may also result from degenerative changes of the cervical facet joints and disks and atlantooccipital and atlantoaxial joints and irritation, inflammation, and mechanical distortion of the cervical nerve roots and spinal cord. These processes may occur independently or concurrently and require a careful history and physical examination together with the judicial use of diagnostic tests to rule out systemic disease and rapidly progressive processes. Recent data reports a 12-month prevalence of 30% to 50% for neck pain and associated disorders in adults.[3] A knowledge and application of recent prospective studies, systemic reviews, and meta-analysis proposing guidelines for evaluation and treatment of these patients may assist with assessing the risk versus benefit for effective conservative versus interventional and surgical therapies in this large and heterogeneous population.

Cervical Spondylosis and Radiculopathy

Degenerative changes of the cervical spine reach a prevalence of nearly 95% by age 65 years. These changes are associated with positive changes such as disk protrusion, neural foraminal narrowing, and spinal cord contour changes in up to 78% of asymptomatic individuals.[7–9,86] In symptomatic individuals, the risk versus benefit of surgery and other interventional therapy[87] mandates an understanding of the natural course of symptomatic patients with cervical spondylosis and radiculopathy. Although the outcome of these patients when treated conservatively versus surgically is controversial,[88,89] recent investigations reveal clinical and radiographic correlates with outcome in this population, which may be of assistance in timely surgical referral when symptoms continue to progress following conservative treatment.[90–92]

Cervical spondylosis was first distinguished from acute cervical disk protrusion by Brain et al.[93] in 1948. The latter occurs more commonly in individuals younger than age 55 years, is often traumatic in origin, and most frequently compresses the nerve roots versus the spinal cord. The former is a chronic degenerative condition of the cervical spine associated with formation of osteophytes. It is a universal finding associated with aging and is associated with compression of the spinal cord in most symptomatic cases. Patients older than age 55 years are more likely to have central canal or neural foraminal stenosis due to spondylosis.[94] In a population-based study conducted from 1976 to 1990 in Rochester, Minnesota, a confirmed disk herniation was found to account for approximately 20% of all cervical radiculopathies and approximately 70% of all spondylosis. The average age-adjusted incidence rate per 100,000 population was 107.3 for males, 63.5 for females, and reached a peak of 202.9 for the age group between ages 50 to 54 years.[95,96]

Spondylosis refers to degenerative changes of the spine involving the intervertebral disks, uncovertebral joints of Lushcka, zygapophyseal joints, ligaments, and connective tissue of the cervical vertebrae. Degenerative changes of the cervical spine are seen in approximately 10% of individuals by age 25 years and in 95% by age 65 years. The process is believed to begin with fibrosis and loss of elasticity of the disk which occurs with loss of water, protein, and mucopolysaccharides from the nucleus pulposus. Loss of disk space height initially occurs ventrally and leads to loss of cervical lordosis. This shift of biomechanical forces results in ventral vertebral body compression with resultant pathologic cervical spine kyphosis, dissection of the annulus fibrosus, posterior longitudinal ligament, and Sharpey's fibers away from the edges of the posterior vertebral body, formation of reactive bone on the edges of exposed dorsal vertebral bodies, and increased axial load bearing by the uncovertebral and zygapophyseal joints, with resultant hypertrophy and osteophytic formation ventral and posterior to the neural foramen.

Spondylotic spurs may eventually span the width of the vertebral canal in some patients. Because the osteophytes form in response to increased motion or segmental instability, the levels most commonly affected, both by disk herniation and chronic spondylosis are C6–C7 followed by C5–C6 because these are the cervical segments at which the most extension and flexion occur.

The reduction in sagittal spinal canal diameter in cervical spondylosis results from a combination of static and dynamic factors. Static reduction of the sagittal diameter of the spinal canal occurs from disk herniation or bulging; vertebral body osteophyte growth into the anterior spinal canal; and degenerative hypertrophy of the uncovertebral joints, facet joints, and ligamentum flavum combined with calcification of the posterior longitudinal ligament. The addition of dynamic factors such as flexion, extension, or subluxation can further increase the risk for compression and injury to the contents of the spinal canal and neural foramen including the spinal cord, nerve roots, arteries, and veins. These combined pathologic features are thought to be responsible for the production of the wide spectrum of clinical symptoms associated with cervical spondylosis including neck and shoulder pain, occipital pain and headaches, radicular symptoms, and cervical radiculopathies and cervical spondylotic myelopathy (CSM). Compression of the spinal cord may occur from spondylotic bars and calcified posterior longitudinal ligament ventrally or from the hypertrophic ligamentum flavum dorsally. Cumulative repetitive injury to the spinal cord is thought to occur with flexion, due to a "bowstring effect" over the ventral spondylotic bars and kyphotic spine, and compression dorsally by buckling of the ligamentum flavum. MRI flexion and extension studies observed increased cervical stenosis in twice as many patients during extension versus flexion. Risk for compression of the spinal cord is increased in individuals with congenital narrowing of the spinal canal.

CSM refers to clinically evident spinal cord dysfunction with the presence of long-tract signs due to compression of the spinal cord. Weakness or stiffness in the legs with unsteady gait together with weakness or clumsiness of the hands is pathognomonic of CSM. Progression of weakness may be gradual in some patients or sudden in others following minor trauma. In a prospective study at a UK regional neuroscience center, 23.6% of 585 patients admitted with tetraparesis or paraparesis were found to have CSM. Some patients may complain of hesitancy on urination; however, loss of sphincter control or urinary incontinence is rare and considered a late sign of myelopathy.

Patients with CSM generally present with neck and shoulder pain and stiffness. The patient may also present with pain in the arm, elbow, wrist, or fingers described as combined or isolated sensations of stabbing, dull, or aching pain. Arm pain may be nondermatomal in distribution and accompanied by numbness or tingling in the hands. Pain which conforms to a dermatomal distribution with associated motor and sensory deficits is referred to a radiculopathy rather than myelopathy. Some patients may present with both myelopathy and radiculopathy.

Signs of CSM on physical exam include an electrical sensation radiating down the back to the legs with flexion of the neck (Lhermitte's sign); atrophy of the intrinsic musculature of the hands; and variable sensory, vibratory, or proprioceptive loss in the extremities. Deep tendon reflexes may be reduced or absent at the level of compression with hyperreflexia below the level of the lesion together with upper motor signs such as clonus, Hoffmann, and Babinski sign.[76,93,97,98]

There are two commonly used classification systems for CSM. The classification of Crandall and Batzdorf[99] divides CSM patients into five groups of spinal cord dysfunction. These include the transverse lesion syndrome, the motor system syndrome, the central cord syndrome, the Brown-Séquard syndrome, and the brachialgia cord syndrome. These are summarized in Table 68.18. Ferguson and Caplan[100] categorize CSM into four overlapping syndromes, which are summarized in Table 68.19.

The differential diagnosis of CSM includes amyotrophic lateral sclerosis, multiple sclerosis, hereditary spastic paraplegia, spinal cord tumors, and subacute combined degeneration of the spinal cord associated with vitamin B_{12} deficiency.

MRI is the imaging technique of choice for evaluating the patient with CSM. T2- and T1-weighted signals on MRI have been found to correlate with various degrees of injury

TABLE 68.18 Crandall and Batzdorf[99] Classification of Clinical Syndromes in Cervical Spondylotic Myelopathy

Transverse lesion syndrome	Most common lesion. Involves posterior column, spinothalamic and corticospinal tracts, and often anterior horn cells. Posterior column involvement uncommon and late.
Motor system syndrome	Involves anterior horn cells and corticospinal tracts primarily. Little sensory involvement. Upper and lower extremity weakness, gait disturbance, and spasticity.
Central cord syndrome	Upper extremities weaker than lower extremities. Profound hand weakness. Posterior column involved often presenting as painful paresthesias of hands.
Brown-Séquard syndrome	Unilateral spinal cord dysfunction. Involvement of corticospinal tract. Posterior column sensory loss (position, vibration) and long tract motor signs (hemiplegia) are found ipsilateral to the lesion, whereas pain and temperature are lost contralaterally. One or two levels below highest level of motor involvement.
Brachialgia cord syndrome	Upper extremity nerve root compression combined with long tract signs (analogous to Ferguson and Caplan's[100] combined medial and lateral syndrome).

TABLE 68.19 Ferguson and Caplan[100] Classification of Clinical Syndromes in Cervical Spondylotic Myelopathy

Lateral syndrome	Represents a spondylotic radiculopathy. Absence of long tract signs.
Medial syndrome	Upper motor neuron symptoms. Variable weakness of all extremities, gait abnormalities, spasticity below level of compression.
Combined medial and lateral syndrome	Most common clinical presentation.
Vascular syndrome	Acute onset and rapid progression of myelopathy. Thought to represent insufficiency or compression of anterior spinal artery and its branches to the spinal cord.

to the spinal cord on histologic studies. Edema is seen as a high-intensity T2-weighted image. Necrotic changes in the gray matter correspond to low signals on T1-weighted studies but high signals on T2-weighted studies. T1-weighted hypointensity is an expression of irreversible damage and, therefore, the worst prognosis.[92,101] A less favorable surgical outcome is predicted by the presence of a T1-weighted hypointense signal and the presence of clonus or spasticity. A high intramedullary T2-weighted signal without clonus or spasticity is associated with a more favorable surgical outcome with a greater likelihood of reversal of MRI signal changes.[102] A recent investigation reported multiple regression analysis of various risk factors associated with surgical outcome. According to this analysis, the most significant prognostic factor was the transverse area of the spinal cord, followed by the duration of symptoms and the presence of multisegmental areas of high-signal intensity on T2-weighted MRI. The latter was associated with upper extremity muscle atrophy and less favorable surgical recovery of neurologic function.[91]

Controversy exists regarding optimal treatment for patients with CSM, and many authors recommend conservative treatment due to significant risks associated with surgery and lack of data supporting long-term improved outcome in patients undergoing surgery versus conservative care.[103–106] A recent prospective 3-year follow-up study did not show, on average, that the effects of surgery in the treatment of mild and moderate forms of CSM were better than the conservative approach. Nevertheless, there was a slight but statistically significant increase in the number of patients with a negative trend in the score for daily activities in the conservatively treated group. The authors of this study recommend conservative treatment for patients with mild SCM along with careful follow-up evaluation and reassessment 3 months after the start of conservative treatment. Decompression surgery is recommended for patients who experience neurologic deterioration during this period.[88] A prospective, multicenter study with independent clinical review evaluating conservative versus surgical treatment for patients with moderate to severe CSM found that although surgical treatment was not found to improve neurologic outcome, overall pain and functional status improved significantly. When medical and surgical treatments were compared, surgically treated patients appeared to have better outcomes, despite exhibiting a greater number of neurologic and nonneurologic symptoms and greater functional disability before treatment.[89]

Conservative treatment for CSM consists of intermittent cervical immobilization with a soft collar, the use of anti-inflammatory medications, active discouragement of high-risk activities, and avoidance of risky environments involving physical overloading, excess cold, movement on slippery surfaces, manipulation therapies, or vigorous or prolonged flexion of the head. Additional conservative measures include a rehabilitation program with physiotherapy and referral to a multidisciplinary pain team. Patients with moderate to severe symptoms on presentation and progressive neurologic symptoms should be referred for surgical evaluation. The aim of the surgery in these patients is to stop the progression of neurologic deterioration and prevent sudden deterioration after minor injury or in particular situations such as swimming, cycling, and physical overloading.[88,89]

Cervicogenic Headache

The term *cervicogenic headache* (CEH) was coined by Sjaastad et al.[107] in 1983. He later organized the Cervicogenic Headache International Study Group (CHISG), and diagnostic criteria for CEH were published by the CHISG in 1990.[108] A revision of criteria for CEH was published by the CHISG in 1998.[109]

CEH was recognized as a unique category of headaches by the International Association for the Study of Pain in 1994, using criteria similar to that published by Sjaastad et al.[110] Revised criteria for CEH were published by the International Headache Society (IHS) in 2004.[111]

Although controversy exists regarding the defining characteristics and prevalence of CEH, there is emerging evidence of valid clinical, diagnostic, and therapeutic criteria which differentiates this syndrome from migraine headache, tension-type headache, hemicrania continua, and chronic paroxysmal hemicrania.[112,113]

CEH is defined as unilateral head or face pain which starts in the neck and is triggered by neck movement or sustained awkward neck posture. Although pain begins in the neck or occipital region, it may spread to the retroorbital, temporal, and frontal areas of the head and face where maximum pain may be perceived. Pain may occur to a lesser degree on the contralateral side; however, profound unilateral dominance should exist. CEH is typically described as deep and nonthrobbing with intermittent attacks lasting hours to days. In time, headaches may become constant with superimposed attacks of more intense pain. Pain in CEH should be reproducible upon palpation or stimulation of cervical spine or neck structures. It is accompanied by reduced range of motion of the neck and ipsilateral nonradicular neck, shoulder, or arm pain. Nausea, vomiting, photophobia, dizziness, blurred vision, lacrimation, and conjunctival injection may occur.

The new IHS criteria requires clinical, laboratory, or imaging evidence of a lesion or disorder within the neck or cervical spine known to be associated with the causation of headache. This should be validated by reproducible clinical signs or by controlled diagnostic blockade (Tables 68.20 and 68.21 show comparison of IHS and CHISG criteria for CEH).

The prevalence of CEH in the literature varies widely from 0% to 80%, depending on the population of patients studied, diagnostic criteria, and methodology.[112] A recent Norwegian study reported that 75% of tractor drivers suffered from moderate to severe generalized headache only when working on their tractor because of consecutively turning or twisting their

TABLE 68.20   International Headache Society Diagnostic Criteria for Cervicogenic Headache

A. Pain referred from a source in the neck and perceived in one or more regions of the head and/or face fulfilling criteria C and D

B. Clinical, laboratory, and/or imaging evidence of a disorder or lesion within the cervical spine or soft tissues of the neck known to be, or generally accepted as, a valid cause of headache

C. Evidence that the pain can be attributed to the neck disorder or lesion based on at least one of the following:
   1. Demonstration of clinical signs that implicate a source of pain in the neck
   2. Abolition of headache following diagnostic blockade of a cervical structure or its nerve supply using placebo or other adequate controls

D. Pain resolves within 3 months after successful treatment of the causative disorder or lesion.

TABLE 68.21   Cervicogenic Headache International Study Group Cervicogenic Headache Diagnostic Criteria[109]

Major Criteria

A. Symptoms and signs of neck involvement; it is obligatory that one or more of the phenomena 1 to 3 are present.
   1. Precipitation of head pain, similar to the usually occurring one:
      a. By neck movement and/or sustained, awkward head positioning, and/or
      b. By external pressure over the upper cervical or occipital region on the symptomatic side
   2. Restriction of the range of motion in the neck
   3. Ipsilateral neck, shoulder, or arm pain of a rather vague, nonradicular nature, or, occasionally, arm pain of a radicular nature

B. Confirmatory evidence by diagnostic anesthetic blockages

C. Unilaterality of the head pain, without side shift

Head Pain Characteristics

D. Moderate to severe, nonthrobbing pain, usually starting in the neck

   Episodes of varying duration, or

   Fluctuating, continuous pain

Other Characteristics of Some Importance

E. Only marginal effect or lack of effect of indomethacin

   Only marginal effect or lack of effect of ergotamine and sumatriptan

   Female sex

   Not infrequent occurrence of head or indirect neck trauma by history, usually of more than only medium severity

Other Features of Lesser Importance

F. Various attack-related phenomena, only occasionally present and/or moderately expressed when present
   1. Nausea
   2. Phonophobia and photophobia
   3. Dizziness
   4. Ipsilateral "blurred vision"
   5. Difficulties on swallowing
   6. Ipsilateral edema, mostly in the periocular area

neck for many hours daily.[114] In a series of 100 consecutive patients with neck pain following whiplash, Lord et al.[115] reported a prevalence of associated headache in 88%. Of those patients with headache as the dominant symptom, 54% were found to have neck pain originating from a C2–C3 cervical zygapophyseal joint following diagnostic blocks. This was associated with tenderness over the affected joint on physical examination.[115] In a study of 34 patients with the complaint of headache emanating from the occipital region, tenderness to exam over the tip of the transverse process of C1 and worsening of their usual headache with passive rotation of the C1 vertebra, 60% were found to have complete relief of their pain following diagnostic blockade of the atlantoaxial joint.[116] Pain maps based on regions of the head and neck in which patients were relieved of pain following controlled blocks revealed radiation of pain from the C1–C2 through the C3–C4 facet joints to the suboccipital and occipital regions as well as the vertex, frontal, orbital, and temporoparietal region of the head.[47]

The anatomic basis by which pain from the cervical spine and neck can be perceived in the face and head derives from the convergence of afferents from the trigeminal nerve with those of the first three spinal nerves in the caudal aspect of the trigeminal nucleus in the brainstem.[117,118] Musculoskeletal structures innervated by the first three cervical nerves are outlined in Table 68.22. Convergence with the spinal trigeminal nucleus and the extradural convergence of the first three cervical nerves may account for the difficulty encountered in localizing the pain in patients with CEH.

TABLE 68.22 Musculoskeletal Structures of the Neck Innervated by C1 through C3

- Muscles: capital flexors and extensors, cervical spine flexors including the scalenus medius, scalenus posterior, longus colli and sternocleidomastoid, cervical spine extensors, head rotators, and other neck muscles including the hyoid muscles, the sternothyroid, and diaphragm
- Periosteum and body of the atlas, axis and C3 vertebra and clavicle, atlantooccipital, atlantoaxial, intervertebral, Luschka, sternoclavicular and zygapophyseal joints associated with the C1–C3 spinal segments, associated ligaments

The anatomy of the sinuvertebral nerve may also contribute to the variation of pain patterns among patients and the presence of diffuse neck and head pain in the presence of discrete injuries. The sinuvertebral nerves supply structures within the spinal canal. They arise from the rami communicantes and enter the spinal canal by way of the intervertebral foramina. Branches ascend and descend one or more levels, interconnecting with the sinuvertebral nerves from other levels and innervating the anterior and posterior longitudinal ligaments dura mater and blood vessels as well as sending nociceptive fibers to degenerative intervertebral disks.[119,120] Neurogenic inflammation from compression ischemia of the cervical nerve and inflammatory response following exposure of spinal tissues to proinflammatory mediators such as phospholipase A2 from extruded nucleus pulposus may also contribute to neck pain and CEH.

In addition to the evidence of atlantoaxial and zygapophyseal joint evidence discussed earlier, there is evidence that CEH may arise from a discogenic origin. Reproduction of patient's usual headache by cervical provocation discography has been reported, as has relief of headache following decompressive surgery of the upper and lower cervical spine.[121,122] The mechanisms by which headaches are provoked by levels below C3 have caused speculation regarding the possibility of convergence of afferents from lower spinal nerves with trigeminal afferents in the spinal trigeminal nucleus. An alternate explanation could lie in the anatomy of the sinuvertebral nerves, which descend from higher levels in the cervical spine to communicate with those at lower levels. An inflammatory response could also be causative with proinflammatory mediators resulting from disk degeneration at lower cervical spinal segments precipitating a nociceptive response at adjacent spinal segments.[119]

Greater and lesser occipital nerve injections using local anesthetic and/or steroid have been reported as useful for diagnosis and short-term relief of CEH. Many authors consider entrapment of the greater occipital nerve to be one of the major underlying causes of CEH.[123–125] A recent controlled trial of nerve stimulator-guided greater and lesser occipital nerve blocks with adjuvant agents provided greater than 50% relief versus placebo with significant reduction of associated headache features and medication use in the treatment group.[126] A case report of pulsed radiofrequency for the treatment of intractable occipital headache reported 70% relief for 4 months followed by an additional 5 months of 70% relief with repeat pulsed radiofrequency.[127]

Percutaneous radiofrequency cervical medial branch neurotomy has been shown, in a rigorous double-blind controlled trial, to provide relief in 70% of patients diagnosed with cervical zygapophyseal joint pain following whiplash injuries. Other therapies found to have efficacy in the treatment of CEH include the physical therapy modalities of manipulation and/or mobilization in conjunction with exercise and intramuscular lidocaine injections. In chronic neck disorders associated with a radicular component, epidural injection of methylprednisolone and lidocaine improved pain greater than cervical intramuscular injections with the same solution at 1-year follow-up.[128–130]

DIFFUSE IDIOPATHIC SKELETAL HYPEROSTOSIS

DISH is a form of osteoarthritis that is characterized by the calcification and ossification of soft tissues including ligaments and tendons. It may involve both the peripheral joints and the axial skeletal structures in 25% and 15% of men and women, respectively, who are older than 50 years of age. Its prevalence increases to 35% and 26%, respectively, in individuals older than 70 years. Classical axial involvement results in calcification of the ligamentum flavum in the lumbar spine, the anterior longitudinal ligament in the thoracic spine, and the posterior longitudinal ligament in the cervical spine. It is distinguished from degenerative spondylosis of the spine by earlier onset; sparing of the intervertebral disk; and its association with a number of risk factors including diabetes mellitus, obesity, hyperuricemia, dyslipidemia, hypertension, coronary artery disease, and prolonged use of isoretinal (vitamin A supplementation).

The patient with DISH typically presents with stiffness and decreased range of motion. Older patients with cervical spine involvement may complain of dysphagia due to pharyngeal encroachment from large anterior osteophytes. Other potential sequelae include cervical myelopathy and cervical spine fractures following relatively trivial trauma. The diagnosis of cervical spine fractures is often delayed due to the presence of baseline neck and spine pain.

The diagnosis of DISH is radiographic and is based on the criteria established by Resnick and Niwayama.[131] These include the presence of "flowing" ossification along anterolateral margins of at least four contiguous vertebrae and the absence of changes associated with degenerative spondylosis. Treatment consists of conservative measures similar to cervical degenerative spondylosis. Operative treatment is reserved for those patients who fail to respond to conservative measures.[132,133]

CERVICAL RADICULOPATHIES

The classical definition and clinical manifestation of cervical radiculopathies is pain, sensory loss, and motor weakness in the distribution of the affected nerve root. Although the cause of radicular symptoms has been presumed to be secondary to compression of the nerve root because of adjacent soft disk herniation or progressive degenerative changes of the cervical spine, the poor correlation between radiologic evidence of degenerative change and incidence of painful symptoms in the cervical spine has been well documented.[134–138] Other factors thought to contribute to the pathogenesis of radiculopathic symptoms include vascular insufficiency, venous engorgement, nerve root fibrosis, and inflammation. Type-C cell distortion in dorsal root ganglion of cervical nerve roots has been proposed as a mechanism of accentuated neuropeptide production and increased hypersensitivity in patients with acute and chronic neural foraminal compression or edema.[139]

The patient with cervical radiculopathy typically complains of burning, aching, cramping, electrical, or sharp pain which radiates to the neck and head, shoulder, arm, or chest depending on the involved nerve root(s). In acute radiculopathy, pain classically presents in a myotomal distribution versus a distal dermatomal distribution. The pain is generally accompanied by numbness and paresthesias. Motor weakness and diminution or loss of deep tendon reflexes may also be seen. Spurling's maneuver, Valsalva, coughing, and sneezing will often provoke or aggravate the patient's symptoms, whereas the shoulder abduction sign (having the patient abduct the shoulder and place their hand on top of their head) will generally relieve their pain.

The C1 nerve passes between the occiput and C1. It is also known as the suboccipital nerve and supplies sensory fibers to the periosteum and body of the atlas, occiput, atlantooccipital joint, and atlantoaxial joint. It is also distributed to the muscles of the suboccipital triangle. The C2 nerve passes between C1 and C2. The medial or sensory branch of C2 is also known as the greater occipital nerve. It supplies the scalp over the vertex and top of the head and supplies muscular branches to the semispinalis.

C3 arises between C2 and C3. The medial sensory branch of the posterior division of the third cervical nerve forms the third or least occipital nerve. The anterior rami of the upper four cervical nerves communicate to form the cervical plexus. Pathologic processes which affect the C1 through C3 nerves cause pain radiating to the head and neck. Pain of the upper cervical spine was covered in more detail in the section on CEHs.[140,141] The greater auricular nerve and the anterior cutaneous nerve are also derived from the second and third cervical nerves. Processes affecting these nerves can also result in pain involving the mastoid process, the lobule and concha of the ear, the skin of the face over the parotid gland, and the skin of the anterolateral aspect of the neck as far as the sternum. Via the deep cervical plexus, the second and third cervical nerves also communicate with the vagus, the hypoglossal nerve, the superior cervical sympathetic ganglion, and the diaphragm by way of the phrenic nerve (see Table 68.3).

Radiculopathy of the fourth cervical nerve root results from pathologic changes between the C3 and C4 vertebrae and is more common than a C3 radiculopathy. The supraclavicular nerve arises mainly from the fourth cervical nerve and supplies the skin and superficial fascia of the clavicular region, the periosteum, and bony structure of the clavicle as far as the midline and the skin over the pectoralis major as far as the second or third rib. It additionally communicates with the cutaneous branches of the second and third rib. The lateral supraclavicular nerve supplies the skin of the top and dorsal parts of the shoulder. Involvement of the C3 nerve may be a cause of unexplained pain along the base of the neck that radiates to the superior aspect of the shoulder and posteriorly to the scapula. Pain in the distribution of the supraclavicular nerve may also be a cause of chronic breast pain in women.

The rhomboid, trapezius, and levator scapulae muscles are supplied in part by the fourth cervical nerve root, but a motor deficit may be difficult to detect. A sensory deficit may be present over the anterolateral aspect of the neck, along the distribution of the transverse cervical and supraclavicular nerves. Because the C3, C4, and C5 nerve roots innervate the diaphragm, involvement of these three nerve roots may lead to diaphragmatic weakness.

The brachial plexus is formed by the fifth, sixth, seventh, and eighth cervical nerves together with the first thoracic nerve and frequently contributing branches from the anterior division of the fourth cervical and second thoracic nerve. The variation of brachial plexus and extradural cervical nerve connections may contribute to variations in radicular patters among patients.

Pathologic changes at the C4–C5 level result in a C5 radiculopathy. The principal motor deficit seen in classical C5 radiculopathy is supraspinatus and deltoid muscle weakness with impaired shoulder abduction. Weakness of the clavicular head of the pectoralis major, biceps, and infraspinatus muscles can also occur. The pectoralis reflex and the biceps reflex, which are innervated by the fifth and sixth cervical nerve roots, may be decreased or absent. The numbness follows the C5 sensory distribution, which is located over the top of the shoulder along its midportion, and extends laterally to the midportion of the arm. The component fibers of the suprascapular nerve are derived primarily from the fifth and sixth cervical nerves. It supplies sensory, motor, and sympathetic fibers which supply the supraspinatus and infraspinatus muscles, the shoulder joint, and periarticular structures as well as an area of skin at the apex of the shoulder. Patients often present with numbness and localized shoulder pain that can be confused with a pathologic shoulder condition. The absence of pain with a range of motion of the shoulder and the absence of impingement signs at the shoulder help to differentiate radiculopathy of the fifth cervical nerve root from a pathologic shoulder condition.

The sixth cervical nerve root is the second most commonly involved in cervical radiculopathy. Patients with pathology at this level typically present with pain radiating from the neck to the lateral aspect of the biceps, lateral aspect of the forearm, dorsal aspect of the web space between the thumb and index finger, and into the tips of those digits. Numbness occurs in the same distribution. Motor deficits are best elicited in the wrist extensors, but weakness of the biceps, supinator, pronator, teres, and triceps muscles may be present. The brachioradialis and biceps reflexes may be decreased or absent. The pain and paresthesias of C6 radiculopathy may mimic carpal tunnel syndrome (CTS), which is caused by median nerve entrapment at the transverse carpal ligament.

The seventh cervical nerve root is most frequently involved by cervical radiculopathy according to many clinical studies. The patient with C7 radiculopathy complains of pain radiating along the back of the shoulder, often extending into the scapular region, down along the triceps, along the dorsum of the forearm and into the dorsum of the long finger. Motor weakness is most often appreciated in the latissimus dorsi muscle, the triceps, wrist flexors, and finger extensors. The triceps reflex may be lost or diminished. Entrapment of the posterior interosseus nerve may be mistaken for the motor component of seventh cervical radiculopathy and presents with weakness in the extensor digitorum communis, extensor pollicis longus, and extensor carpi ulnaris. With entrapment of the interosseus nerve, sensory changes are absent and the triceps and wrist flexors show normal strength.

Pathology at the C7–T1 level results in radiculopathy of the eighth cervical nerve root. Patients with a C8 radiculopathy generally present with sensory changes extending over the medial aspect of the arm and forearm and into the medial hand and the fourth and fifth digits. Numbness usually involves both the dorsal and volar aspects of the digits and hand and may extend proximal to the wrist over the medial aspect of the forearm. Weakness may involve the small muscles of the hand, particularly the interossei, and the flexors and extensors of the wrist and fingers (with the exception of the flexor carpi radialis and extensor carpi radialis muscles). This may cause patients to complain of difficulty using their hands for routine tasks such as buttoning shirts and grasping objects. Compression of the C8 nerve root may initially be difficult to differentiate from ulnar entrapment at the elbow. C8 nerve root compression may affect the function of the flexor digitorum profundus in the index and long fingers, the flexor pollicis longus in the thumb, and the pronator quadratus, but these muscles are not affected by entrapment of the ulnar nerve. Also, the short thenar muscles, except for the adductor pollicis, may be involved with C8 or T1 compression but are spared with ulnar nerve involvement. Furthermore, sensory changes seen with ulnar neuropathies include numbness, tingling, and/or pain in the fourth and fifth fingers and the hand just below these fingers but not proximal to the wrist (medial antebrachial cutaneous nerve distribution), as may be seen with C8 radiculopathy. Anterior interosseus nerve entrapment may also mimic C8 or T1 radiculopathy but lacks sensory changes, and thenar muscle involvement is absent.

Although uncommon, occurrence of T1–T2 disk herniations or other pathology at this level may result in a T1 radiculopathy. The T1 nerve is the main contributor to the adductor pollicis, the thenar muscles, the interossei, and the first two lumbricals. Classic T1 radiculopathy results in intrinsic hand weakness. Numbness occurs in the axilla, and Horner syndrome can occur ipsilaterally.[1,98,142]

Epidemiologic data suggest that up to 90% of patients with cervical radiculopathy improve with conservative medical treatment alone.[95,96,143–145] However, due to lack of standardized diagnostic criteria and comparative randomized controlled trials comparing conservative with surgical treatment, evidence-based guidelines have been difficult to establish.

Conservative therapy in patients with cervical radiculopathy includes activity modification, education, and physical therapy with progressive passive and active modalities. Pharmacologic therapy requires a large armamentarium of medications due to the heterogeneity in this patient population and the various mechanisms involved in the production of neuropathic pain. Options include over-the-counter analgesics, anticonvulsants, tricyclic antidepressants, and selective serotonin norepinephrine reuptake inhibitors, topical anesthetic agents, nonsteroidal anti-inflammatory drugs, antiarrhythmics, muscle relaxants, nonnarcotic analgesics, and opioids.[146,147] Multiple studies including a recent systematic review support the efficacy of interlaminar cervical epidural steroid injections for the management of cervical radiculitis, discogenic pain without facet joint pain, and postsurgery syndrome.[130,148] Use of fluoroscopic guidance in interlaminar epidural steroid injections and use of nonparticulate steroid in transforaminal injections may significantly reduce the risk of complications.[149–151]

Outcome in patients with cervical radiculopathy following medical versus operative treatment was recently reported following a prospective, multicenter study with independent clinical review. Comparison of results of patients undergoing medical versus surgical treatments showed that, although both medically and surgically treated patients reported statistically significant improvement in their overall pain, more improvement was observed in the surgery group. Improvement in worst pain and average pain was also statistically significant in both groups. Surgically treated patients had more neurologic and nonneurologic symptoms and more functional disability before treatment. However, despite high satisfaction in surgically treated patients, a significant number of patients continued to report horrible or excruciating pain, multiple neurologic symptoms, and minimal or no work activity. These results are similar to those in patients with CSM in that the majority of patients improve with conservative therapy, whereas those with persistent severe pain and progressive neurologic symptoms are generally referred for operative management, which attempts to improve pain and arrest the progression of neurologic symptoms.[89,145]

UPPER EXTREMITY PERIPHERAL NERVE ENTRAPMENT SYNDROMES AND BRACHIAL PLEXUS NEUROPATHY

Acute trauma with resultant fibrosis and scar tissue, chronic trauma from overuse injuries, or space-occupying lesions can result in entrapment of peripheral nerves. An understanding of peripheral nerve distribution and common entrapment sites is essential for the diagnosis and treatment of peripheral nerve entrapment syndromes. Entrapment typically occurs at sites where a segment of nerve passes through a fibro-osseous tunnel or through an opening in fibrous, tendinous, or muscular bands of tissue. Sustained mechanical compression and ischemia may result in neurapraxia. Peripheral nerve entrapment syndromes typically present with pain at the site of entrapment. Pain can radiate both distally and proximally to this point. Sensory, motor, or sympathetic changes can occur in the nerve distribution distal to the site of entrapment.

The diagnosis of nerve compression or nerve entrapment is based on a careful history of the mechanism of injury or repetitive use and a thorough physical exam together with neurologic and electrodiagnostic examinations. MRI is helpful in identifying the cause of the neuropathy, identifying the site of entrapment based on muscle denervation patterns, and detecting unsuspected space-occupying lesions.[152,153] Nerve entrapment and radiculopathies may infrequently exist simultaneously. In a retrospective analysis of 12,736 cases of CTS and ulnar neuropathy at the elbow, 435 (3.4%) of these cases were found to have a coexisting cervical root lesion. However, lesions were on the same nerve in only 98 (0.8%) of these cases.[154] Upper extremity nerve entrapment syndromes are characterized in Table 68.23. Two most common nerve entrapment syndromes of the upper extremity, CTS and cubital tunnel syndrome (CuTS), are discussed in the following text in greater detail.

Carpal Tunnel Syndrome

CTS is the most common upper extremity entrapment syndrome estimated to affect 3% to 6% of adults in the United States. Risk factors for the development of CTS include age, smoking, obesity, rheumatoid arthritis, diabetes, lupus, hypothyroidism, acromegaly, flexor tenosynovitis, ganglion, pregnancy, multiple sclerosis, work with vibrating tools, and repetitive hand and wrist tasks. CTS is more common in women, with higher risk in those taking birth control pills and those going through menopause.

TABLE 68.23	Upper Extremity Entrapment Syndromes			
Nerve	**Usual Cause**	**Location of Pain**	**Sensory Changes**	**Weakness**
Dorsal scapular	Scalenus medius hypertrophy	Medial scapula, lateral arm	None	Rhomboids, levator scapulae Weak with pressing elbow backward against resistance with hands on hip or pushing palm backward against resistance with arm folded behind back
Suprascapular	Band in supraspinatus notch	Posterolateral, shoulder, lateral arm; tender at suprascapular notch	None	Supraspinatus, infraspinatus Weakness in abduction and external rotation of arm
Long thoracic	Downward pressure on shoulder	Not usually painful; can have diffuse ache in shoulder or scapula	None	Serratus anterior Weak with raising arms above head
Musculocutaneous	Entrapment by coracobrachialis	Anterior arm, proximal lateral forearm	Anterolateral forearm	Biceps, brachialis Elbow flexor and forearm supination weakness
Posterior interosseous	Entrapment at proximal forearm	Proximal radial forearm	None	Wrist and finger extensors and abductors
Ulnar (at elbow)	Entrapment at cubital tunnel	Elbow, ulnar forearm, and hand	Ulnar hand, fourth and fifth digits	Flexor carpi ulnaris and intrinsics
Ulnar (at wrist)	Entrapment at Guyon's canal	Ulnar side of hand, fourth and fifth digits	Ulnar hand, fourth and fifth digits	Adductor pollicis, interossei, hypothenar muscles
Median (at elbow)	Entrapment at ligament of Struthers or pronator teres	Elbow, volar forearm	Radial hand; first, second, and third digits	Pronator teres, flexor carpi radialis, flexor digitorum superior
Median (at wrist)	Entrapment at carpal tunnel	Wrist; radial hand; first, second, and third digits	Radial hand; first, second, and third digits	Thenar muscles, first and second lumbricals
Anterior interosseous	Entrapment at pronator teres or flexor digitorum superior	Elbow, volar forearm	None	Pronator quadratus, flexor pollicis longus, first and second flexor digitorum profundus
Digital nerve	Entrapment at intermetacarpal tunnel	Finger	Half of finger	None

The incidence of CTS is also high in wheel chair athletes, cyclists, wrestlers, and football athletes (from blocking technique).

It is useful to review the anatomy of the carpal tunnel, the fibro-osseous outlet which lies between the flexor retinaculum, and the carpal bones. Its contents include the tightly packed median nerve and nine extrinsic flexor tendons of the thumb and fingers. Pressure within the carpal tunnel averages 2 to 31 mm Hg in healthy individuals and as high as 32 to 110 mm Hg in patients with CTS. Carpal tunnel pressure increases up to 8-fold with wrist flexion and 10-fold with wrist extension.

The clinical diagnosis of CTS includes a history of paresthesia affecting the median nerve distribution (generally the thumb and first two and a half fingers although some patients complain of paresthesias radiating up the arm to the shoulder), often bilaterally but initially in the dominant hand in most patients. Other signs and symptoms may include brachialgia paraesthetica nocturna, thenar atrophy, loss of two-point sensory discrimination, and reduced manual dexterity. Clinical diagnosis includes a positive Phalen test (sustained wrist flexion for 60 seconds [78% to 80% sensitivity and 73% to 83% specificity]), Tinel sign (reproduction of paresthesias in median nerve distribution with percussion over the carpal tunnel at the wrist [20% to 50% sensitivity and 76% to 77% specificity]), and Durkan or carpal compression test (87% sensitivity and 90% specificity). Electrodiagnostic studies (EDS) have a 49% to 84% sensitivity and a 95% to 99% specificity. Although EDS are often used to confirm clinical diagnosis, other more expensive imaging modalities may be indicated in complex cases to rule out additional suspected etiologies of patient symptomology.

In regard to treatment of CTS, although patients with mild to moderate symptoms may respond to conservative treatment, with splinting and steroid injections having the best evidence of nonoperative treatments, several high-quality studies have demonstrated superior outcome with operative versus nonoperative treatment of CTS.[155,156]

Cubital Tunnel Syndrome

Second only to CTS, CuTS is the second most common nerve entrapment syndrome in both the general population and due to sports. CuTS occurs slightly more in males versus females, increases with age and is seen more frequently in occupations with frequent elbow flexion such as carpenters, musicians, and painters. It is seen in athletes from sports such as baseball, wrestling, and football. Risk factors also include prolonged pressure over the forearm with the elbows in a flexed position such as when resting forearms on a hard surface.

The cubital tunnel consists of the medial epicondyle medially, the olecranon laterally, the elbow capsule at the posterior aspect of the ulnar collateral ligament which forms the floor of the cubital tunnel, and the deep forearm fascia of the flexor carpi ulnaris and the arcuate ligament of Osborne or cubital tunnel retinaculum which forms the roof. The ulnar nerve is most commonly compressed beneath Osborne's ligament, although it may also be compressed proximately at the arcade of Struthers and distally by the deep pronator aponeurosis. Intraneural pressure sharply increases with elbow flexion greater than 90 degrees.

Clinical signs and symptoms in patients with CuTS include pain localized to the elbow or radiating to medial forearm and wrist, atrophy of intrinsic hand muscles, flexion weakness of the fourth and fifth fingers, and sensory deficit in fourth and fifth fingers. Weakness of the interossei may result in Wartenberg sign (inability to fully adduct the small finger with finger held abducted and extended). Weakness of the adductor pollicis may result in Froment sign (positive Froment sign consists of flexion of interphalangeal [IP] joint of the thumb as compensation for weakness of adductor pollicis by using the flexor pollicis longus when asked to perform a pinch). Weakness of the ulnar lumbrical muscles may result in claw hand deformity. Routine provocative testing also includes ulnar nerve percussion at the retrocondylar groove and the elbow flexion test. In more severe CuTS, severe weakness, atrophy of intrinsic

hand musculature, and loss of two-point sensory discrimination may also be seen. Electrodiagnostic and nerve conduction studies may be helpful in localizing the site of compression.[153]

Conservative or nonoperative treatment is recommended in patients with mild CuTS as up to 88% of patients with mild symptoms reported relief of paresthesia with nonsurgical management. A 2012 Cochrane review of treatment for ulnar neuropathy at the elbow found that giving information on avoiding prolonged movements or positions causing traction and compression on the cubital tunnel (avoid full flexion and direct pressure) was effective for mild to moderate symptoms. Nonoperative therapies which are commonly prescribed include discontinuing triceps strengthening exercises, avoidance of direct pressure to the medial aspect of the elbow on firm surfaces, maintaining a resting elbow position of 45 to 50 degree of flexion, and using a nighttime elbow towel orthosis to prevent elbow flexion beyond 50 degrees. In regard to surgical treatment, the 2012 Cochrane review found no difference between simple decompression and transposition of the ulnar nerve but higher rates of infections in the transposition cases.[153]

Early recognition is essential for timely diagnosis and treatment of nerve entrapment syndromes involving the upper extremity as they are thought to affect the function of many individuals, including musicians, athletes, and as many as one in four office workers.[155] Most patients respond to conservative treatment including rest splints, rehabilitative exercises, passive physical therapy modalities, relative rest, and correction of training and equipment use errors. Other measures may include anti-inflammatory medications, protective padding or bracing, and injections with local anesthetic and steroids. In patients with severe or progressive neurologic deficit or intractable pain, surgical decompression may be necessary.[156]

LESIONS OF THE BRACHIAL PLEXUS

Injury to the brachial plexus resulting in functional impairment of the upper extremity can occur secondary to penetrating or blunt trauma, severe traction, or acceleration-deceleration injuries. Other etiologies include congenital, developmental or exogenous compression, vascular or infectious disease, and neoplastic disease. The relative incidence of these lesions of the brachial plexus is presented in Table 68.24.

Brachial plexus injury (BPI) can be classified into preganglionic lesions, postganglionic lesions, and a combination of preganglionic and postganglionic lesions. In a preganglionic lesion, the nerve root is avulsed. A postganglionic lesion involves the nerve distal to the sensory ganglion and is further divided into nerve ruptures or lesions in continuity.

TABLE 68.24	Causes of Brachial Plexus Lesions	
Cause	**Example(s)**	**Incidence (% of cases)**
Trauma	Penetrating injuries (e.g., gunshot, knife); closed injuries: obstetric (newborn), mechanical distortion	70
Compression	Exogenous (knapsack paralysis); congenital abnormality; developmental abnormality	10
Vascular	Local disease of major vessels; generalized vasculopathy (lupus erythematosus, arteritis); secondary to radiation therapy	5
Infectious	Viral; bacterial (local sepsis, abscess, or cellulitis)	3
Neoplastic	Primary tumors of brachial plexus; secondary involvement of plexus by tumors of surrounding tissues (Pancoast's tumor)	10
Miscellaneous causes	Electric shock; parainfectious; following serum therapy; unknown	2

Clinical exam and electrodiagnostic and imaging studies may help in determining the location and severity of injury, which is essential in therapeutic decisions regarding these injuries. CT myelography is considered most reliable in detecting avulsion injuries. MRI, as well as new techniques such as MR myelography, diffusion-weighted neurography, and Bezier surface reformation, provides additional useful data in the evaluation and management of BPI.[157,158]

Treatment of traumatic BPI is conservative versus surgical and is based on various factors such as the degree of damage, the site and type of injury, the time interval between injury and surgery, and the patient's age and occupation. Surgical treatment includes neurolysis, nerve grafting, nerve transfer, and other reconstructive procedures.[159–161] Physical therapy and pain control is essential for recovery of function following operative cases and for optimization of function and palliation of pain in nonoperative cases. In addition to pharmacologic treatment options, successful treatment of pain related to brachial plexus lesions has been reported following implantation of spinal cord and deep brain stimulator systems.[162,163]

Acute Brachial Plexus Neuritis

Acute brachial plexus neuritis is an uncommon disorder of unknown etiology that is commonly misdiagnosed as cervical spondylosis or cervical radiculopathy. It was first described by Spillane[164] in 1943 and is also known as Parsonage-Turner syndrome or neuralgic amyotrophy due to the case series of this condition by Parsonage and Turner[165] in 1948. Other names by which it is referred include brachial plexus neuropathy, paralytic neuritis, and acute shoulder neuritis.

The classical presentation of the patient with acute brachial plexus neuritis is the acute onset of severe burning pain in the neck, shoulder, and upper arm not associated with a precipitating injury or trauma. The pain may or may not be associated with sensory deficit and generally subsides over the following days to weeks. It is followed by a profound weakness, sometimes to the extent of flaccidity, involving the supraspinatus, infraspinatus, and deltoid and/or biceps muscles. Involvement of the sternomastoid or diaphragm has also been described, as has isolated or single nerve involvement. Bilateral brachial plexus involvement is not uncommon. Gradual recovery of muscle strength over 3 to 4 months is the usual course of brachial neuritis; however, some patients may experience several years of permanent muscle weakness. Chronic scapulocostal pain syndromes may occur due to dysfunctional mechanics following profound weakness.

Although a viral etiology has been proposed, various infections have been reported as preceding the onset of this disorder in up to 25% of cases. Onset following influenza, hepatitis B, or other vaccinations in up to 15% of cases suggests an immunologic etiology. Familial and recurrent cases are encountered. Other reported precipitating factors include childbirth, trauma, and surgery. Pathologic studies favor an immune-mediated demyelinating pathogenesis over an axon-loss mechanism.[166,167]

The annual incidence of acute brachial plexus neuritis is reported to be 1.64 cases per 100,000, although this figure is presumed to be low because of misdiagnosis. It occurs most often between age 20 and 60 years with a reported male predominance of 2:1 to 11.5:1.[166]

Diagnosis of brachial neuritis requires a high level of suspicion. A case series report of electrodiagnostic results reports no evidence of prolongation of F latencies and no reduction of conduction velocity or conduction block in conventional peripheral ulnar and median nerve motor studies. Proximal nerve stimulation of the cervical roots and brachial plexus revealed axonal degeneration in most cases as well as evidence of proximal conduction block consistent with demyelination. MRI is useful in evaluating muscle denervation, muscle signal intensity changes, and muscle volume loss.[168]

Treatment of brachial neuritis is primarily supportive with use of analgesic medications followed by range-of-motion exercises. An arm sling may be helpful in preventing injury and strain from the weight of the arm distracting the humeral head from the glenoid fossa.[59] Full functional recovery is expected in 80% to 90% of patients, although the course may be protracted. Ten percent to 20% of patients may continue to have significant residual muscle weakness. In cases of profound and early weakness, intravenous immunoglobulin treatment has been proposed due to its usefulness in treating other focal demyelinating peripheral nerve diseases.[169,170] Acupuncture may also be effective in treating pain and improving function.[171,172]

Thoracic Outlet Syndrome

The definition, diagnosis, and treatment of TOS are among the most disputed of any clinical entity. The syndrome generally refers to a variety of symptoms in the upper extremity due to compression of the brachial plexus, subclavian artery, and subclavian vein. Compression of the neurovascular bundle can occur as it passes through the interscalene triangle, the costoclavicular triangle, and subcoracoid space during its passage from the base of the neck to the proximal aspect of the arm. Structural compressive etiologies include fibrous bands, scar tissue, hypertrophied or fibrous muscles, anomalous soft tissue, and cervical ribs. Previous to the coining of the term *TOS* in 1956 by Peet,[173] the name of this syndrome was assigned according to the etiologies of compression including scalenus anticus syndrome, costoclavicular syndrome, hyperabduction, cervical rib syndrome, or first rib syndrome. The lower trunk of the brachial plexus (C8 and T1) is most often affected. Other factors associated with the development of TOS include repetitive trauma to the brachial plexus, median sternotomy, or traumatic events such as motor vehicle accidents.[174]

TOS is variably divided into arterial, venous, or neurogenic. Alternatively, it has been classified as vascular, neurogenic, and nonspecific. The latter classification system reflects both diagnostic criteria and therapeutic recommendations and outcome.

Vascular TOS occurs in only 2% to 5% of thoracic outlet cases and is described most frequently in young individuals following vigorous arm activity or strenuous work. Patients with subclavian artery compression frequently present with pallor, pulselessness, and coolness of the affected upper extremity; transient ischemic attack; or infarcts of the hand and fingers. Decreased blood pressure in the affected arm when compared with the opposite arm of more than 20 mm Hg may also be present. Claudication may occur only with arm hyperabduction in some patients. Injury may include thrombosis, aneurysm, and/or stenosis.

Subclavian vein compression typically presents with edema and cyanosis of the upper limb with hyperabduction of the upper extremity. Thrombosis of the axillary-subclavian vein (also known as Paget-von Schröetter syndrome), occurs in association with vigorous shoulder activity.

Doppler and duplex ultrasonography, magnetic resonance arteriography, CT angiography, and arteriography are used to confirm the diagnosis of vascular TOS. Decompression procedures or vessel reconstruction may be indicated in urgent cases and in cases not responsive to conservative therapy.[174–177]

Neurogenic and nonspecific categories of TOS comprise 95% to 98% of cases. A syndrome of painless atrophy of the hand primarily involving the abductor pollicis brevis with lesser atrophy of the interossei and hypothenar muscles known as Gilliatt-Sumner hand is the classic presentation of the true neurogenic type of TOS. This is associated with positive neurologic and electrodiagnostic findings. Sensory loss typically involves the ulnar aspect of the forearm and hand consistent with lower trunk compression, although upper trunk compression has also been reported. Pain is not the primary symptom of true neurogenic TOS; however, the patient may complain of diffuse, dull pain in the neck, shoulder, axillary region, and arm which may worsen with overhead activities and repetitive use of the arm.

The most common form of TOS is the nonspecific type. Patients generally present with the primary complaint of pain, often following a motor vehicle– or work-related injury. EAST, upper limb tension test, and Adson tests may be positive, but specificity is limited as they have been shown to be positive in many asymptomatic individuals. The specificity of Adson test and EAST tests was 76% and 30%, respectively, and 82% when combined. Physical examination findings are often inconclusive and nonspecific, although physical exam may guide further diagnostic electrophysiologic and imaging studies and subsequent treatment decisions.[177–179] The differential diagnosis of TOS includes cervical radiculopathy or myelopathy, acute brachial neuritis, Reynaud's disease, multiple sclerosis, ulnar or median nerve entrapment syndromes, acute coronary syndrome, and CRPS.

The diagnosis of nonspecific TOS requires a detailed history and physical exam to rule out other causes of neck and upper extremity pain. Electrodiagnostic testing may help localize and quantify a brachial plexus lesion in true neurogenic TOS and rule out other segmental or systemic neuropathies.[180,181] Radiographic studies used in evaluation with the patient with suspected TOS include cervical spine and chest radiographs to rule out bony abnormalities and MRI and CT to evaluate the cervical spine for soft tissue anomalies, tumors, or degenerative disease of the cervical spine.[182]

Conservative treatment of TOS is indicated in the majority of cases and consists of activity modification education with instructions to avoid provocative positions and activities. Physical therapy programs to restore normal posture and strengthen the muscles of the pectoral girdle have also been successful in alleviating symptoms in greater than 50% of cases.[183] Surgical approaches to treatment are undertaken in intractable or urgent cases. Surgery in the nonspecific type of TOS is associated with the least favorable outcome and is generally discouraged due to the significant risks associated with surgeries in this region. New minimally invasive techniques are now being investigated and may offer reduced risk of complications.[184,185]

References

1. Loeser JD. *Bonica's Management of Pain.* 3rd ed. Philadelphia: Lippincott Williams & Wilkins; 2001:1008.
2. Wolfla CE. Anatomical, biomechanical, and practical considerations in posterior occipitocervical instrumentation. *Spine J* 2006;6(6 suppl):225S–232S.
3. Murray CJ, Barber RM, Foreman KJ, et al; for GBD 2013 DALYs and HALE Collaborators. Global, regional, and national disability-adjusted life years (DALYs) for 306 diseases and injuries and healthy life expectancy (HALE) for 188 countries, 1990–2013: quantifying the epidemiological transition. *Lancet* 2015;386(10009):2145–2191.
4. Cohen SP. Epidemiology, diagnosis, and treatment of neck pain. *Mayo Clin Proc* 2015;90(2):284–299.
5. Peterson C, Bolton J, Wood AR, et al. A cross-sectional study correlating degeneration of the cervical spine with disability and pain in United Kingdom patients. *Spine (Phila Pa 1976)* 2003;28(2):129–133.
6. Zapletal J, Hekster RE, Straver JS, et al. Relationship between atlanto-odontoid osteoarthritis and idiopathic suboccipital neck pain. *Neuroradiology* 1996;38(1):62–65.
7. Matsumoto M, Fujimura Y, Suzuki N, et al. MRI of cervical intervertebral discs in asymptomatic subjects. *J Bone Joint Surg Br* 1998;80(1):19–24.
8. Okada E, Matsumoto M, Fujiwara H. Disc degeneration of cervical spine on MRI in patients with lumbar disc herniation: comparison study with asymptomatic volunteers. *Eur Spine J* 2011;20(4):585–591.
9. Siivloa SM, Levoska S, Tervonen O, et al. MRI changes of cervical spine in asymptomatic and symptomatic young adults. *Eur Spine J* 2002;11(4):358–363.
10. Hämäläinen O, Vanharanta H, Kuusela T. Degeneration of cervical intervertebral disks in fighter pilots frequently exposed to high +Gz forces. *Aviat Space Environ Med* 1993;64(8):692–696.
11. Holm LW, Carroll LJ, Cassidy D, et al. The burden and determinants of neck pain in whiplash-associated disorders after traffic collisions: results of the bone and joint decade 2000–2010 task force on neck pain and its associated disorders. *Eur Spine J* 2008;17(suppl 1):S52–S59.
12. Carroll LJ, Holm LW, Hogg-Johnson S, et al. Course and prognostic factors for neck pain in whiplash-associated disorders (WAD): results of the Bone and Joint Decade 2000–2010 Task Force on Neck Pain and Its Associated Disorders. *J Manipulative Physiol Ther* 2009;32(2 suppl):S97–S107.
13. Berglund A, Alfredsson L, Jensen I, et al. Occupant- and crash-related factors associated with risk of whiplash injury. *Ann Epidemiol* 2003;13(1):66–72.
14. Merskey H, Teasell RW. Problems with insurance-based research on chronic pain. *Med Clin North Am* 2007;91(1):31–43.
15. Andersen JH, Haahr JP, Frost P. Risk factors for more severe regional musculoskeletal symptoms: a two-year prospective study of a general working population. *Arthritis Rheum* 2007;56(4):1355–1364.
16. Ostegren PO, Hanson BS, Balogh I, et al. Incidence of shoulder and neck pain in a working population: effect modification between mechanical and psychosocial exposures at work? Results from a one year follow-up of the Malmö shoulder and neck study cohort. *J Epidemiol Community Health* 2005;59(9):721–728.
17. Hannan LM, Monteilh CP, Gerr F, et al. Job strain and risk of musculoskeletal symptoms among a prospective cohort of occupational computer users. *Scand J Work Environ Health* 2005;31(5):375–386.
18. Sarquis LMM, Coggon D, Ntani G, et al. Classification of neck/shoulder pain in epidemiological research: a comparison of personal and occupational characteristics, disability and prognosis among 12,195 workers from 18 countries. *Pain* 2016;157(5):1028–1036.
19. Cohen JJ. Remembering the real questions. *Ann Intern Med* 1998;128(7):563–566.
20. Arnold M, Cumurciuc R, Stapf C, et al. Pain as the only symptom of cervical artery dissection. *J Neurol Neurosurg Psychiatry* 2006;77(9):1021–1024.
21. Bassi P, Lattuada P, Gomitoni A. Cervical cerebral artery dissection: a multicenter prospective study (preliminary report). *Neurol Sci* 2003;24(suppl 1):S4–S7.
22. Cohen ML. Cervical and lumbar pain. *Med J Aust* 1996;165(9):504–508.
23. McBeth J, Macfarlane GJ, Benjamin S, et al. Features of somatization predict the onset of chronic widespread pain: results of a large population-based study. *Arthritis Rheum* 2001;44(4):940–946.
24. Navarro X, Vivó M, Valero-Cabré A. Neural plasticity after peripheral nerve injury and regeneration. *Prog Neurobiol* 2007;82(4):163–201.
25. Semmes RE, Murphy F. The syndrome of unilateral rupture of the sixth cervical vertebral disc with compression of the seventh cervical root: a report of four cases with symptoms simulating coronary disease. *JAMA* 1943;121(15):1209–1214.
26. Albayram S, Wasserman BA, Yousem DM, et al. Intracranial hypotension as a cause of radiculopathy from cervical epidural venous engorgement: case report. *AJNR Am J Neuroradiol* 2002;23(4):618–621.
27. Leonard JR, Ferner RE, Thomas N, et al. Cervical cord compression from plexiform neurofibromas in neurofibromatosis 1. *J Neurol Neurosurg Psychiatry* 2007;78(12):1404–1406.
28. Fraser JF, Anand VK, Schwartz TH. Endoscopic biopsy sampling of tophaceous gout of the odontoid process. Case report and review of the literature. *J Neurosurg Spine* 2007;7(1):61–64.
29. Tsikoudas A, Coateswortth AP, Martin-Hirsch DP. Laryngeal gout. *J Laryngol Otol* 2002;116(2):140–142.
30. Fujimoto K, Matsunaga R, Yamamoto F, et al. Epidural, mediastinal and subcutaneous emphysema in a patient with suspected forme fruste of Marfan syndrome [in Japanese]. *Nihon Kokyuki Gakkai Zasshi* 2004;42(10):909–913.
31. Boesch SM, Müller J, Wenning GK, et al. Cervical dystonia in spinocerebellar ataxia type 2: clinical and polymyographic findings. *J Neurol Neurosurg Psychiatry* 2007;78(5):520–522.
32. Asplund S, Webb C, Barkdull T. Neck and back pain in bicycling. *Curr Sports Med Rep* 2005;4(5):271–274.
33. Leino P, Magni G. Depressive and distress symptoms as predictors of low back pain, neck shoulder pain, and other musculoskeletal morbidity: a 10-year follow-up of metal industry employees. *Pain* 1993;53(1):89–94.
34. Wilbourn AJ. Brachial plexus lesions. In: Dyck PJ, Thomas PK, eds. *Peripheral Neuropathy.* 4th ed. Philadelphia: Elsevier Saunders; 2005:1339–1373.
35. Bland JH. *Disorders of the Cervical Spine: Diagnosis and Medical Management.* 2nd ed. Philadelphia: Saunders; 1994.
36. Blum CA, Yaghi S. Cervical artery dissection: a review of the epidemiology, pathophysiology, treatment, and outcome. *Arch Neurosci* 2015;2(4):e26670.
37. Chennupati SK, Norris R, Dunham B, et al. Osteosarcoma of the skull base: case report and review of literature. *Int J Pediatr Otorhinolaryngol* 2008;72(1):115–119.
38. Kumanda S, Per H, Gumu H, et al. Torticollis secondary to posterior fossa and cervical spine tumors: report of five cases and literature review. *Neurosurg Rev* 2006;29(4):333–338.
39. Horowitz SH. The diagnostic workup of patients with neuropathic pain. *Med Clin North Am* 2007;91(1):21–30.
40. Voskuhl RR, Hinton RC. Sensory impairment in the hands secondary to spondolytic compression of the cervical spinal cord. *Arch Neurol* 1990;47(3):309–311.
41. Levine E, Taub PJ. Hyoid bone fractures. *Mt Sinai J Med* 2006;73(7):1015–1018.
42. Wang W, Kong L, Dong R, et al. Fracture of the hyoid bone associated with atlantoaxial subluxation: a case report and review of the literature. *Am J Forensic Med Pathol* 2007;28(4):345–347.
43. Hashimoto Y, Moriya F, Furumiya J. Forensic aspects of complications resulting from cardiopulmonary resuscitation. *Leg Med (Tokyo)* 2007;9(2):94–99.
44. Sethi A, Sareen D, Chopra S, et al. Pharyngeal perforation with deep neck abscess secondary to isolated hyoid bone fracture. *J Laryngol Otol* 2005;119(12):1007–1009.
45. Aydil U, Ekinci O, Köybaşioğlu A, et al. Hyoid bone insertion tendinitis: clinicopathologic correlation. *Eur Arch Otorhinolaryngol* 2007;264(5):557–560.
46. Schmalbach CE, Miller FR. Occult primary head and neck carcinoma. *Curr Oncol Rep* 2007;9(2):139–146.
47. Cooper G, Bailey B, Bogduk N. Cervical zygapophysial joint pain maps. *Pain Medicine* 2007;8(4):344–853.

48. Sanders RJ, Hammond SL, Rao NM. Diagnosis of thoracic outlet syndrome. *J Vasc Surg* 2007;46(3):601–604.

49. Tong HC, Haig AJ, Yamakawa K. The Spurling test and cervical radiculopathy. *Spine (Phila Pa 1976)* 2002;27(2):156–159.

50. Ventafridda V, Caraceni A, Martini C, et al. On the significance of Lhermitte's sign in oncology. *J Neurooncol* 1991;10(2):133–137.

51. Muhle C, Bischoff L, Weinert D, et al. Exacerbated pain in cervical radiculopathy at axial rotation, flexion, extension, and coupled motions of the cervical spine: evaluation by kinematic magnetic resonance imaging. *Invest Radiol* 1998;33(5):279–288.

52. Kuwayama DP, Lund JR, Brantigan CO, et al. Choosing surgery for neurogenic tos: the roles of physical exam, physical therapy, and imaging. *Diagnostics (Basel)* 2017;7(2):E37.

53. Ledd AD, Agarwal S, Sadhu D. Doppler Adson's test: predictor of outcome of surgery in non-specific thoracic outlet syndrome. *World J Surg* 2006;30(3):291–292.

54. Waddell G, McCulloch HA, Kummel E, et al. Non-organic physical signs in low-back pain. *Spine* 1980;5:117–125.

55. Fishbain DA, Rosomoff HL, Cutler RB, et al. Secondary gain concept: a review of the scientific evidence. *Clin J Pain* 1995;11(1):6–21.

56. Fishbain DA, Cutler RB, Rosomoff HL, et al. Is there a relationship between nonorganic physical findings (Waddell signs) and secondary gain/malingering? *Clin J Pain* 2004;20(6):399–408.

57. Turk DC, Wack JT, Kerns RD. An empirical examination of the "pain-behavior" construct. *J Behav Med* 1985;8(2):119–130.

58. McCahon S, Strong J, Sharry R, et al. Self-report and pain behavior among patients with chronic pain. *Clin J Pain* 2005;21(3):223–231.

59. Lossos IS, Yossepowitch O, Kandel L, et al. Septic arthritis of the glenohumeral joint. A report of 11 cases and review of the literature. *Medicine (Baltimore)* 1998;77(3):177–187.

60. Unkila-Kallio L, Kallio MJ, Peltola H. The usefulness of C-reactive protein levels in the identification of concurrent septic arthritis in children who have acute hematogenous osteomyelitis. A comparison with the usefulness of the erythrocyte sedimentation rate and the white blood-cell count. *J Bone Joint Surg Am* 1994;76(6):848–853.

61. Heller CA, Stanley P, Lewis-Jones B, et al. Value of x ray examinations of the cervical spine. *Br Med J (Ciln Res Ed)* 1983;287(6401):1276–1278.

62. Johnson MJ, Lucas GL. Value of cervical spine radiographs as a screening tool. *Clin Orthop Relat Res* 1997;340:102–108.

63. Malik SA, Murphy M, Connolly P, et al. Evaluation of morbidity, mortality and outcome following cervical spine injuries in elderly patients. *Eur Spine J* 2008;17(4):585–591.

64. Touger M, Gennis P, Nathanson N, et al. Validity of a decision rule to reduce cervical spine radiography in elderly patients with blunt trauma. *Ann Emerg Med* 2002;40(3):287–293.

65. Davis JW, Phreaner DL, Hoyt DB, et al. The etiology of missed cervical spine injuries. *J Trauma* 1993;34(3):342–346.

66. Bohlman HH. Acute fractures and dislocations of the cervical spine. An analysis of three hundred hospitalized patients and review of the literature. *J Bone Joint Surg Am* 1979;61(8):1119–1140.

67. MacDonald RL, Schwartz MD, Mirich MD, et al. Diagnosis of cervical spine injury in motor vehicle crash victims: how many x-rays are enough. *J Trauma* 1990;30(4):392–397.

68. Brohi K, Wilson-Macdonald J. Evaluation of unstable cervical spine injury: a 6-year experience. *J Trauma* 2000;49(1):76–80.

69. Hoffman JR, Schriger DL, Mower WR, et al. Low-risk criteria for cervical-spine radiography in blunt trauma: a prospective study. *Ann Emerg Med* 1992;21(12):1454–1460.

70. Hoffman JR, Wolfson AB, Todd KH, et al. Selective cervical spine radiography in blunt trauma: methodology of the National Emergency X-Radiography Utilization Study (NEXUS). *Ann Emerg Med* 1998;32(4):461–469.

71. Mahadevan S, Mower WR, Hoffman JR, et al. Interrater reliability of cervical spine injury criteria in patients with blunt trauma. *Ann Emerg Med* 1998;31(2):197–201.

72. Hoffman JR, Mower WR, Wolfson B, et al. Validity of a set of clinical criteria to rule out injury to the cervical spine in patients with blunt trauma. *N Engl J Med* 2000;343(2):94–99.

73. Stiell IG, Clement CM, McKnight RD, et al. The Canadian C-spine rule versus the NEXUS low-risk criteria in patients with trauma. *N Engl J Med* 2003;349(26):2510–2518.

74. Klein GR, Vaccaro AR, Albert TJ, et al. Efficacy of magnetic resonance imaging in the evaluation of posterior cervical spine fractures. *Spine (Phila Pa 1976)* 1999;24(8):771–774.

75. Sanchez B, Waxman K, Jones T, et al. Cervical spine clearance in blunt trauma: evaluation of a computed tomography-based protocol. *J Trauma* 2005;59(1):179–183.

76. Shedid D, Benzel EC. Cervical spondylosis anatomy: pathophysiology and biomechanics. *Neurosurgery* 2007;60(1 suppl 1):S7–S13.

77. Fehlings MG, Rao SC, Tator CH, et al. The optimal radiologic method for assessing spinal canal compromise and cord compression in patients with cervical spinal cord injury. Part II: results of a multicenter study. *Spine (Phila Pa 1976)* 1999;24(6):605–613.

78. Maus TP. Imaging of the spine and nerve roots. *Phys Med Rehabil Clin N Am* 2002;13(3):487–544.

79. Babar S, Saifuddin A. MRI of the post-discectomy lumbar spine. *Clin Radiol* 2002;57(11):969–981.

80. Dorenbeck U, Schreyer AG, Schlaier J, et al. Degenerative diseases of the cervical spine: comparison of a multiecho data image combination sequence with a magnetization transfer saturation pulse and cervical myelotraphy and CT. *Neuroradiology* 2004;46(4):306–309.

81. Stevenson JH, Trojian T. Evaluation of shoulder pain. *J Fam Pract* 2002;51(7):605–611.

82. Woodward TW, Best TM. The painful shoulder: part II. Acute and chronic disorders. *Am Fam Physician* 2000;61(11):3291–3300.

83. Uri DS. MR imaging of shoulder impingement and rotator cuff disease. *Radiol Clin North Am* 1997;35(1):77–96.

84. Ertl JP, Kovacs G, Burger RS. Magnetic resonance imaging of the shoulder in the primary care setting. *Med Sci Sports Exerc* 1998;30(4 suppl):S7–S11.

85. Stiles RG, Otte MT. Imaging of the shoulder. *Radiology* 1993;188(3):603–613.

86. Garfin SR. Cervical degenerative disorders: etiology, presentation, and imaging studies. *Instru Course Lect* 2000;49:335–338.

87. Carragee EJ, Hurwitz EL, Cheng I, et al. Treatment of neck pain: injections and surgical interventions: results of the Bone and Joint Decade 2000–2010 Task Force on Neck Pain and Its Associated Disorders. *Spine (Phila Pa 1976)* 2008;33(4 suppl):S153–S169.

88. Kadanka Z, Mares M, Bednarik J, et al. Approaches to spondylotic cervical myelopathy: conservative versus surgical results in a 3 year follow-up study. *Spine (Phila Pa 1976)* 2002;27(20):2205–2211.

89. Sampath P, Bendebba M, Davis JD, et al. Outcome of patients treated for cervical myelopathy. A prospective, multicenter study with independent clinical review. *Spine (Phila Pa 1976)* 2000;25(6):670–676.

90. Alafifi T, Kern R, Fehlings M. Clinical and MRI predictors of outcome after surgical intervention for cervical spondylotic myelopathy. *J Neuroimaging* 2007;17(4):315–322.

91. Wada E, Yonenobu K, Suzuki S, et al. Can intramedullary signal change on magnetic resonance imaging predict surgical outcome in cervical spondolytic myelopathy? *Spine (Phila Pa 1976)* 1999;24(5):455–461.

92. Mastronardi L, Elsawaf A, Roperto R, et al. Prognostic relevance of the postoperative evolution of intramedullary spinal cord changes in signal intensity on magnetic resonance imaging after anterior decompression for cervical spondylotic myelopathy. *J Neurosurg Spine* 2007;7(6):615–622.

93. Brain WR, Northfield D, Wilkinson M. The neurological manifestations of cervical spondylosis. *Brain* 1952;75(2):187–225.

94. Truumees E, Herkowitz HN. Cervical spondylotic myelopathy and radiculopathy. *Instr Course Lect* 2000;49:339–360.

95. Malanga GA. The diagnosis and treatment of cervical radiculopathy. *Med Sci Sports Exerc* 1997;29(7 suppl):S236–S245.

96. Radhakrishnan K, Litchy WJ, O'Fallon WM, et al. Epidemiology of cervical radiculopathy. A population-based study from Rochester, Minnesota, 1976 through 1990. *Brain* 1994;117(pt 2):325–335.

97. Malcolm GP. Surgical disorders of the cervical spine: presentation and management of common disorders. *J Neurol Neurosurg Psychiatry* 2002;73(suppl 1);i33–i41.

98. Polston DW. Cervical radiculopathy. *Neurol Clin* 2007;25(2):373–385.

99. Crandall PH, Batzdorf U. Cervical spondylotic myelopathy. *J Neurosurg* 1966;25(1):57–66.

100. Ferguson RJL, Caplan LR. Cervical spondylotic myelopathy. *Neurol Clin* 1985;3(2):373–382.

101. Ito T, Oyanagi K, Takahashi H, et al. Cervical spondylotic myelopathy: clinicopathologic study on the progression pattern and thin myelinated fibers of the lesions of seven patients examined during complete autopsy. *Spine (Phila Pa 1976)* 1996;21(9):827–833.

102. Fujii H, Yone K, Sakou T. Magnetic resonance imaging study of experimental acute spinal cord injury. *Spine (Phila Pa 1976)* 1993;18(14):2030–2034.

103. Hunt WE. Cervical spondylosis: natural history and rare indications for surgical decompression. *Clin Neurosurg* 1980;27:466–480.

104. Long DM. Lumbar and cervical spondylosis and spondylotic myelopathy. *Curr Opin Neurol Neurosurg* 1993;6(4):576–580.

105. Lunsford LD, Bissonette DJ, Zorub DS. Anterior surgery for cervical disc disease. Part 2: treatment of cervical spondylotic myelopathy in 32 cases. *J Neurosurg* 1980;53(1):1–11.

106. Rowland LP. Surgical treatment of cervical spondylotic myelopathy: time for a controlled trial. *Neurology* 1992;42(1):5–13.

107. Sjaastad O, Saunte C, Hovdal H, et al. "Cervicogenic" headache. An hypothesis. *Cephalalgia* 1983;3(4):249–256.

108. Sjaastad O, Fredriksen TA, Pfaffenrath V. Cervicogenic headache: diagnostic criteria. *Headache* 1990;30:725–726.

109. Sjaastad O, Fredriksen TA, Pfaffenrath V. Cervicogenic headache: diagnostic criteria. The Cervicogenic Headache International Study Group. *Headache* 1998;38(6):442–445.

110. Merskey H, Bogduk N. *Classification of Chronic Pain: Description of Chronic Pain Syndromes and Definition of Pain Terms.* Seattle, WA: IASP Press; 1994.

111. Headache Classification Subcommittee of the International Headache Society. The international classification of headache disorders: second edition. *Cephalalgia* 2004;24(suppl 1):1–155.

112. Haldeman S, Dagenais S. Cervicogenic headaches: a critical review. *Spine J* 2001;1(1):31–46.

113. Antonaci F, Bono G, Chimento P. Diagnosing cervicogenic headache. *J Headache Pain* 2006;7(3):145–148.

114. Sjaastad O, Bakketeig LS. Tractor drivers' head and neckache: Vågå study of headache epidemiology. *Cephalalgia* 2002;22(6):462–467.

115. Lord SM, Barnsley L, Wallis BJ, et al. Third occipital nerve headache: a prevalence study. *J Neurol Neurosurg Psychiatry* 1994;57(10):1187–1190.

116. Aprill C, Axinn MJ, Bogduk N. Occipital headaches stemming from the lateral atlanto-axial (C1-2) joint. *Cephalalgia* 2002;22(1):15–22.

117. Kerr FWL. Central relationships of trigeminal and cervical primary afferents in the spinal cord and medulla. *Brain Res* 1972;43(2):561–572.

118. Busch V, Jakob W, Juergens T, et al. Functional connectivity between trigeminal and occipital nerves revealed by occipital nerve blockade and nociceptive blink reflexes. *Cephalalgia* 2006;26(1):50–55.

119. Groen GJ, Baljet B, Drukker J. Nerves and nerve plexuses of the juman vertebral column. *Am J Anat* 1990;188(3):282–296.

120. Schellhas KP, Garvey TA, Johnson BA, et al. Cervical diskography: analysis of provoked responses at C2-C3, C3-C4, and C4-C5. *AJNR Am J Neuroradiol* 2000;21(2):269–275.

121. Ahn Y, Lee SH, Chung SE, et al. Percutaneous endoscopic cervical discectomy for discogenic cervical headache due to soft disc herniation. *Neuroradiology* 2005;47(12):924–930.

122. Diener HC, Kaminski M, Stappert G, et al. Lower cervical disc prolapse may cause cervicogenic headache: prospective study in patients undergoing surgery. *Cephalalgia* 2007;27(9):1050–1054.

123. Biondi DM. Cervicogenic headache: a review of diagnostic and treatment strategies. *J Am Osteopath Assoc* 2005;105(4 suppl 2):16S–22S.

124. Leone M, D'Amico D, Grazzi L, et al. Cervicogenic headache: a critical review of the current diagnostic criteria. *Pain* 1998;78(1):1–5.

125. Bovim G, Sand T. Cervicogenic headache, migraine without aura and tension-type headache. Diagnostic blockade of the greater occipital and supra-orbital nerves. *Pain* 1992;51(1):43–48.

126. Naja ZM, El-Rajab M, Al-Tannir MA, et al. Occipital nerve blockade for cervicogenic headache: a double-blind randomized controlled clinical trial. *Pain Pract* 2006;6(2):89–95.

127. Navani A, Mahajan G, Kreis P, et al. A case of pulsed radiofrequency lesioning for occipital neuralgia. *Pain Med* 2006;7(5):453–456.

128. Lord SM, Barnsley L, Wallis BJ, et al. Percutaneous radio-frequency neurotomy for chronic cervical zygapophyseal-joint pain. *New Engl J Med* 1996;335(23):1721–1726.

129. Gross AR, Hoving JL, Haines TA, et al. Manipulation and mobilisation for mechanical neck disorders. Cochrane Database Syst Rev 2004;(1):CD004249.

130. Peloso P, Gross A, Haines T, et al. Medicinal and injection therapies for mechanical neck disorders. *Cochrane Database Syst Rev* 2007;(3):CD000319.

131. Resnick D, Niwayama G. Radiographic and pathologic features of spinal involvement in diffuse idiopathic skeletal hyperostosis (DISH). *Radiology* 1976;119(3):559–568.

132. Sarzi-Puttine P, Atzeni F. New developments in our understanding of DISH (diffuse idiopathic skeletal hyperostosis). *Curr Opin Rheum* 2004;16(3):287–292.

133. Childs SG. Diffuse idiopathic skeletal hyperostosis: Forestier's disease. *Orthop Nurs* 2004;23(6):375–382.

134. Marshall LL, Trethewie ER, Curtain CC. Chemical radiculitis. A clinical, physiological and immunological study. *Clin Orthop Relat Res* 1977;129:61–67.

135. Hoyland JA, Freemont AJ, Jayson MI. Intervertebral foramen venous obstruction. A cause of periradicular fibrosis? *Spine (Phila Pa 1976)* 1989;14(6):558–568.

136. Jayson MI. The role of vascular damage and fibrosis in the pathogenesis of nerve root damage. *Clin Orthop Relat Res* 1992;279:40–48.

137. Hasue M. Pain and the nerve root. An interdisciplinary approach. *Spine (Phila Pa 1976)* 1993;18(14):2053–2058.

138. Garfin SR, Rydevik B, Lind B, et al. Spinal nerve root compression. *Spine (Phila Pa 1976)* 1995;20(16):1810–1820.

139. Boyd-Clark LC, Briggs CA, Galea MP. Segmental degeneration in the cervical spine and associated changes in dorsal root ganglia. *Clin Anat* 2004;17(6):468–477.

140. Kouwenhoven JW, Wuisman PI, Ploegmakers JF. Headache due to an osteochondroma of the axis. *Eur Spine J* 2004;13(8):746–749.

141. Bogduk N. Cervicogenic headache: anatomic basis and pathophysiologic mechanisms. *Curr Pain Headache Rep* 2001;5(4):382–386.

142. Harrop JS, Hanna A, Silva MT, et al. Neurological manifestations of cervical spondylosis: an overview of signs, symptoms, and pathophysiology. *Neurosurgery* 2007;60(1 suppl 1):S14–S20.

143. Wainner RS, Gill H. Diagnosis and nonoperative management of cervical radiculopathy. *J Orthop Sports Phys Ther* 2000;30(12):728–744.

144. Wolff MW, Levine LA. Cervical radiculopathies: conservative approaches to management. *Phys Med Rehabil Clin N Am* 2002;13(3):589–608.

145. Sampath P, Bendebba M, Davis JD, et al. Outcome in patients with cervical radiculopathy: prospective, multicenter study with independent clinical review. *Spine (Phila Pa 1976)* 1999;24(6):591–597.

146. Galluzze KE. Managing neuropathic pain. *J Am Osteopath Assoc* 2007;107(10 suppl 6):ES39–ES48.

147. Chen H, Lamer TJ, Rho RH, et al. Contemporary management of neuropathic pain for the primary care physician. *Mayo Clin Proc* 2004;79(12):1533–1545.

148. Manchikanti L, Nampiaparampil DE, Candido KD, et al. Do cervical epidural injections provide long-term relief in neck and upper extremity pain? A systematic review. *Pain Physician* 2015;18:39–60.

149. Scanlan GC, Moeller-Bertram T, Romanowsky SM, et al. Cervical transforaminal epidural steroid injections more dangerous than we think? *Spine (Phila Pa 1976)* 2007;32(11):1249–1256.

150. Manchikanti L, Bakhit CE, Pakanati RR, et al. Fluoroscopy is medically necessary for the performance of epidural steroids. *Anesth Analg* 1999;89(5):1330–1331.

151. Hessiion WG, Stanczak JD, Davis KW, et al. Epidural steroid injections. *Semin Roentgenol* 2004;39(1):7–23.

152. Wahab KW, Sanya EO, Adebayo PB, et al. Carpal tunnel syndrome and other entrapment neuropathies. *Oman Med J.* 2017;32(6):449–454.

153. Cass S. Upper extremity nerve entrapment syndromes in sports: an update. *Curr Sports Med Rep* 2014;13(1):16–21.

154. Morgan G, Wilbourn A. Cervical radiculopathy and coexisting distal entrapment neuropathies: double-crush syndromes? *Neurology* 1998;50(1):78–83.

155. Wellik GM. Nerve entrapments of the wrist: early treatment preserves function. JAAPA 2005;18(4):18–23.

156. Callandruccio JH, Thompson NB. Carpal tunnel syndrome: making evidence-based treatment decisions. *Orthop Clin North Am* 2018;49(2):223–229.

157. Yoshikawa T, Hayashi N, Yamamoto S, et al. Brachial plexus injury: clinical manifestations, conventional imaging findings, and the latest imaging techniques. *Radiographics* 2006;26(suppl 1):S133–S143.

158. Bertelli JA, Ghizoni MF. Use of clinical signs and computed tomography myelography findings in detecting and excluding nerve root avulsion in complete brachial plexus palsy. *J Neurosurg* 2006;105(6):835–842.

159. Kawabata H, Shibata T, Matsui Y, et al. Use of intercostals nerves for neurotization of the musculocutaneous nerve in infants with birth-related brachial plexus palsy. *J Neurosurg* 2001;94(3):386–391.

160. Samii A, Carvalho GA, Samii M. Brachial plexus injury: factors affecting functional outcome in spinal accessory nerve transfer for the restoration of elbow flexion. *J Neurosurg* 2003;98(2):307–312.

161. Norkus T, Norkus M, Pranckevicius S, et al. Early and late reconstruction in brachial plexus palsy: a preliminary report. *Medicina (Kaunas)* 2006;42(6):484–491.

162. Owen SL, Green AL, Nandi DD, et al. Deep brain stimulation for neuropathic pain. *Acta Neurochir Suppl* 2007;97(pt 2):111–116.

163. Verdolin MH, Stedje-Larsen ET, Hickey AH. Ten consecutive cases of complex regional pain syndrome of less than 12 months duration in active duty United States military personnel treated with spinal cord stimulation. *Anesth Analg* 2007;104(6):1557–1560.

164. Spillane JD. Localized neuritis of the shoulder girdle. A report of 46 patients in the MEF. *Lancet* 1943;2:532–535.

165. Parsonage M, Turner J. Neuralgic amyotrophy: the shoulder-girdle syndrome. *Lancet* 1948;1:973–978.

166. Miller JD, Pruitt S, Mcdonald TJ. Acute brachial plexus neuritis: an uncommon cause of shoulder pain. *Am Fam Phys* 2000;62(9):2067–2072.

167. Sierra A, Prat J, Bas J, et al. Blood lymphocytes are sensitized to brachial plexus nerves in patients with neuralgic amyotrophy. *Acta Neurol Scand* 1991;83(3):183–186.

168. Lo YL, Mills KR. Motor root conduction in neuralgic amyotrophy: evidence of proximal conduction block. *J Neurol Neurosurg Psychiatry* 1999;66(5):586–590.

169. Tsairis P, Dyck PJ, Mulder DW. Natural history of brachial neuritis. *Arch Neurol* 1972;27:109–117.

170. Jaspert A, Claus D, Grehl H, et al. Multifocal motor neuropathy: clinical and electrophysiologic findings. *J Neurol* 1996;243(10):684–692.

171. Inoue M, Hojo T, Yano T, et al. The effects of electroacupuncture on peripheral nerve regeneration in rats. *Acupunct Med* 2003;21(1–2):9–17.

172. Patel G, Euler D, Audette JF. Complementary and alternative medicine for noncancer pain. *Med Clin North Am* 2007;91(1):141–167.

173. Peet RM, Henriksen JD, Anderson TP, et al. Thoracic-outlet syndrome: evaluation of a therapeutic exercise program. *Proc Staff Meet Mayo Clin* 1956;31(9):281–287.

174. Urschel HC Jr, Kourlis H Jr. Thoracic outlet syndrome: a 50-year experience at Baylor University Medical Center. *Proc (Bay Univ Med Cent)* 2007;20(2):125–135.

175. Durham JR, Yao JS, Pearce WH, et al. Arterial injuries in the thoracic outlet syndrome. *J Vasc Surg* 1995;21(1):57–70.

176. Huang JH, Zager EL. Thoracic outlet syndrome. *Neurosurg* 2004;55(4):897–902.

177. Davidovic LB, Kostic DM, Jakovljevic NS, et al. Vascular thoracic outlet syndrome. *World J Surg* 2003;27(5):545–550.

178. Kuhn JE, Lebus GF, Bible JE. Thoracic outlet syndrome. *J Am Acad Orthop Surg* 2015;23(4):222–232.

179. Gergoudis R, Barnes RW. Thoracic outlet arterial compression: prevalence in normal persons. *Angiology* 1980;31(8):538–541.

180. Povlsen S, Povlsen B. Diagnosing thoracic outlet syndrome: current approaches and future directions. *Diagnostics (Basel)* 2018;8(1):21.

181. Rousseff R, Tzvetanov P, Valkov I. Utility (or futility?) of electrodiagnosis in thoracic outlet syndrome. *Electromyogr Clin Neurophysiol* 2005;45(3):131–133.

182. Demondion X, Herbinet P, Van Sint Jan S, et al. Imaging assessment of thoracic outlet syndrome. *Radiographics* 2006;26(6):1735–1750.

183. Mackinnon SE, Patterson GA, Navak CB. Thoracic outlet syndrome: a current overview. *Semin Thorac Cardiovasc Surg* 1996;8(2):176–182.

184. Degeorges R, Reynaud C, Becquemin JP. Thoracic outlet syndrome surgery: long-term functional results. *Ann Vasc Surg* 2004;18(5):558–565.

185. Rochkind S, Shemesh M, Patish H, et al. Thoracic outlet syndrome: a multidisciplinary problem with a perspective for microsurgical management without rib resection. *Acta Neurochir Suppl* 2007;100:145–147.

CHAPTER 69

Chest Wall Pain

NARASIMHA R. GUNDAMRAJ and **STEVEN H. RICHEIMER**

General Considerations

The chest wall is a common site of pain encountered in clinical practice. The origin of pain can be from various structures of the chest wall. These include pain from skeletal components including the spine, muscles, and nerves or pain that is referred from outside the chest wall (Table 69.1). For instance, visceral pain from the chest can be perceived as chest wall pain. It is important to distinguish the origin of pain as arising from the chest wall or from the viscera inside. Focusing on some key points in the history and physical examination can assist in diagnosing the origin of pain. A thorough knowledge of the anatomy and physiology of the chest wall and its relationship to the vital organs enclosed inside is essential for any clinician involved in treatment of chest wall pain.

Anatomy of the Chest Wall

The chest wall is made up of skeletal structures, muscular elements, and neurovascular components. The skeletal structures of the chest wall include the ribs, vertebrae, and the sternum. From a functional standpoint, the skeletal components of the chest wall provide protection for the specialized organs that support the vital functions of the human body.

SKELETAL STRUCTURES OF THE CHEST WALL

The chest wall is made up of the vertebrae posteriorly, ribs and costal cartilages laterally, and the sternum anteriorly. The superior boundary of the thorax includes the T1 vertebra posteriorly, 1st rib laterally, and superior margin of the sternum (Fig. 69.1). Inferiorly, the thorax is bounded by the T12 vertebra and the 12th rib posteriorly, 7th to 10th ribs and their cartilages laterally joining anteriorly to the xiphisternum.[1,2] The anteroposterior and lateral diameter of the thorax is smaller at the top compared to the inferior portion. A compromise in the space at the thoracic inlet due to pathology of the skeletal structures or thoracic viscera can compromise the neurovascular structures and also result in chest wall pain.[3,4]

Thoracic Spine

The thoracic spine is made up of 12 thoracic vertebrae (Fig. 69.2). Each thoracic vertebra is heart-shaped with long and inclined spinous processes (Fig. 69.3). Costal facets are present laterally on either side of the body for articulation with the ribs. Costal facets are also present on the transverse processes (except T11 and T12) for articulation with the tubercles of the ribs.

Ribs

There are 12 pairs of ribs attached posteriorly to the spine. The upper 7 pairs of ribs are attached anteriorly to the sternum by costal cartilages and are called true ribs (Fig. 69.4). The 8th, 9th, and 10th ribs are attached to each other, and the 7th rib by their costal cartilages forming small synovial joints. These ribs are called false ribs. The 11th and 12th ribs have no anterior attachments and are called floating ribs. A typical rib is a long, curved, flat bone. The superior border is smooth and rounded. The inferior border is sharp and thin, and it overhangs the costal groove, which encloses the intercostals vessels and the nerves. The head of the rib has two facets for articulation with

the corresponding vertebral body and the one above it. The neck is a constricted portion of the rib after the head. A prominence on the outer surface of the rib at the junction of the shaft and the neck is called the tubercle. It also has a facet for articulation with the transverse process of the corresponding vertebra. A cervical rib arising from the transverse process of the 7th cervical vertebra is seen in 0.5% of humans. It can cause pressure on the adjacent neurovascular structures—the brachial plexus and the subclavian artery.

TABLE 69.1 Chest Pain Caused by Neuropathic, Musculoskeletal, and Other Disorders
I. Pain primarily of neuropathic origin
A. Disease of the spinal cord (myelopathy)
B. Lesions of the rootlets or roots of thoracic spinal nerves (radiculopathy)
C. Lesions of the formed spinal nerves (neuropathy)
D. Lesions of the intercostal nerves (intercostal neuropathy)
E. Disorders of the peripheral branches of spinal nerves (peripheral neuropathy)
II. Pain primarily of musculoskeletal origin
A. Lesions or disease of bones
1. Disease or lesions of the thoracic vertebrae
2. Disease or lesions of the ribs
3. Diseases or disorders of the costal cartilages
4. Disease or disorders of the sternum
5. Disease of the sternoclavicular joint
B. Disorders of muscles
1. Myofascial pain syndromes
2. Chest pain caused by other disorders of muscles
III. Diseases of the skin
A. Burns and other trauma
B. Cicatrices
C. Postoperative pain syndromes
D. Mastodynia
E. Deep axillary abscess
F. Adiposis dolorosa
G. Phlebitis of the anterolateral chest
H. Other dermatologic painful disorders
IV. Chest pain caused by extrathoracic diseases
A. Disorders of the cervical spine and shoulder
1. Intervertebral disk disease
2. Thoracic outlet syndromes
B. Abdominal diseases
1. Gas entrapment syndromes
2. Disorders of the gastrointestinal tract
3. Disease of the biliary tract
4. Disease of the pancreas
5. Other abdominal visceral disease
C. Diseases of the diaphragm
1. Acute primary diaphragmatitis
2. Subphrenic abscess
3. Diaphragmatic flutter
V. Chest pain primarily of psychological origin
A. Abnormal emotional reactions to visceral disease
B. Anxiety syndrome
C. Depression syndrome
D. Conversion reaction
E. Hypochondriasis
F. Psychiatric syndromes

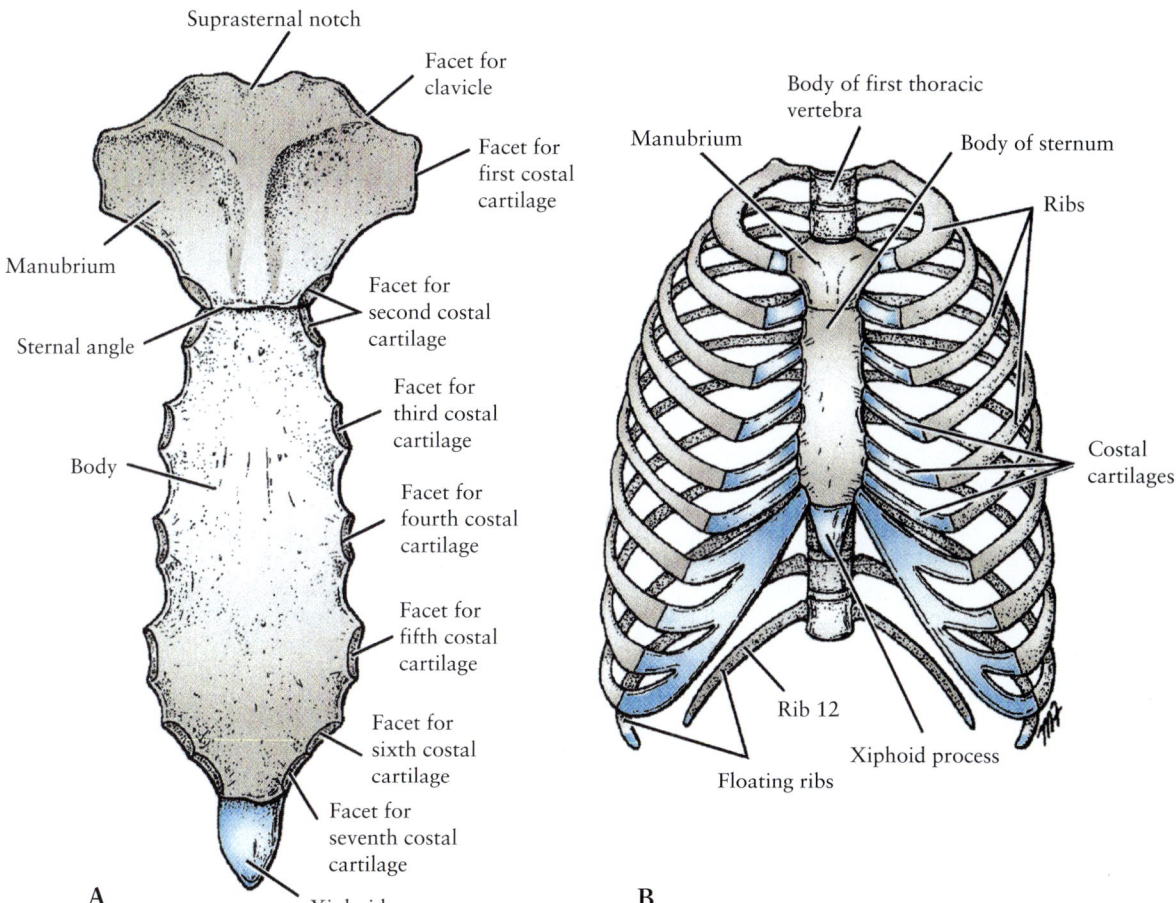

FIGURE 69.1 **A:** Anterior view of the sternum. **B:** Sternum, ribs and costal cartilages forming the thoracic skeleton. *(Reprinted with permission from Snell RS. Clinical Anatomy by Regions. 9th ed. Philadelphia, PA: Lippincott Williams & Wilkins; 2011. Figure 2-1.)*

Sternum

The sternum is a flat bone in the middle of the anterior chest wall. It is divided into three parts: manubrium, body, and xiphoid process. The manubrium is the upper portion of the sternum that articulates with the body of the sternum at the manubriosternal joint. It also articulates at the clavicles, the first costal cartilage, and the upper portion of the second costal cartilage. The body of the sternum on each side articulates with the second to seventh costal cartilages. The xiphoid process is a roughly triangular cartilaginous structure that becomes ossified in adulthood. The angle of Louis or sternal angle is the junction between the manubrium and the body of the sternum. This useful anatomic landmark is palpated by feeling for a transverse ridge on the anterior aspect of the sternum. It correlates to the second costal cartilage anteriorly and the intervertebral disk between the fourth and fifth thoracic vertebrae posteriorly.

JOINTS OF THE CHEST WALL

The chest wall includes many joints. The manubriosternal joint and xiphisternal joints are fixed joints. The costochondral connections of ribs with costal cartilages are also nonsynovial joints. These costochondral joints can become the source of painful irritation. The costal cartilages often calcify with age, reducing the flexibility of the chest wall. The joints of the heads of the ribs with the vertebral bodies, and the joints of the tubercles with the transverse processes of the ribs, are synovial joints that allow for the expansion movements of the chest wall. The joints of the costal cartilages with the sternum are synovial (with the exception of the first rib), but these joints allow for only slight motion and they tend to disappear with age.

INTERCOSTAL SPACES

The intercostal space between the ribs is covered with three muscles: the external intercostals, internal intercostals, and the innermost intercostals muscle (Fig. 69.5). The innermost intercostal muscle is lined by the endothoracic fascia, which in turn covers the parietal pleura. The intercostal nerves and blood vessels run between the internal and the innermost intercostals muscles in the intercostals groove. The intercostal muscles play an important role in the mechanics of respiration. They are supplied by the corresponding intercostal nerves. The neurovascular structures in the intercostal groove are arranged from above downward as vein, artery, and nerve.

INTERCOSTAL NERVES

The anterior rami of the first 11 thoracic spinal nerves form the intercostals nerves. The anterior ramus of the 12th nerve lies in the abdominal wall as the subcostal nerve. The rami communicantes connect the intercostals nerve to the sympathetic trunk. The collateral branch runs forward inferiorly to the intercostal nerve on the upper border of the rib below. The lateral cutaneous branch runs in the skin on the side of the chest and divides in to the anterior and posterior branches. The anterior cutaneous branch is the terminal portion of the intercostal nerves and reaches the skin near the midline anteriorly (Fig. 69.6). Muscular branches are given out to the intercostals muscles. Pleural sensory branches go to the pleura. Peritoneal sensory branches from the 7th to 11th intercostal nerves run to the parietal peritoneum. The 1st intercostal nerve has a branch joining the brachial plexus. The second intercostal nerve joins the medial

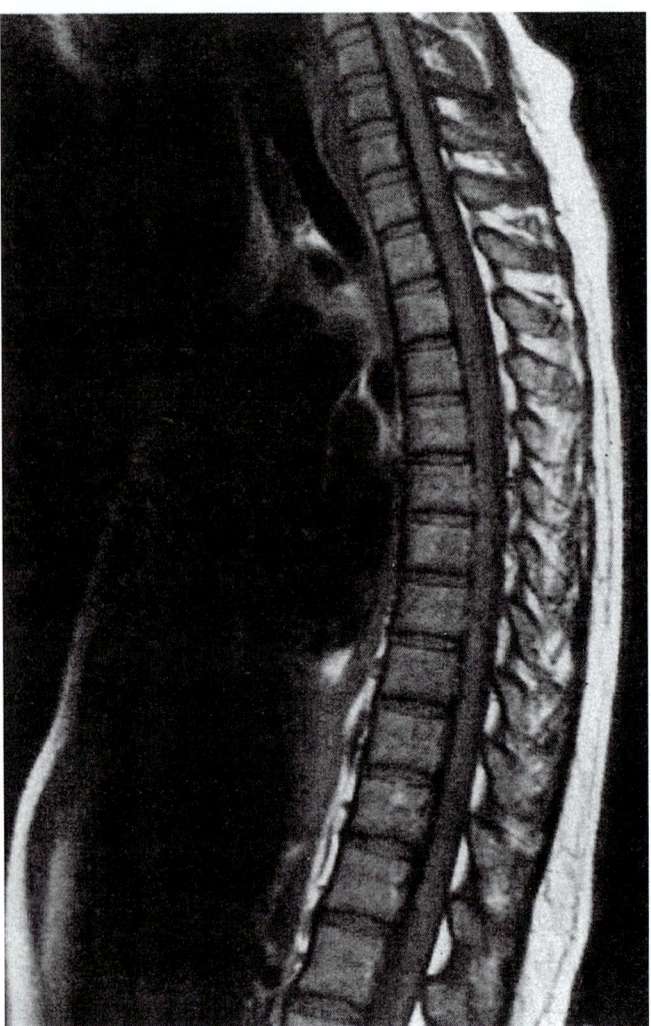

FIGURE 69.2 Magnetic resonance imaging normal thoracic spine, midsagittal T1-weighted image. *(Reprinted with permission from Lee JKT, Sagel SS, Stanley RJ, et al. Computerized Body Tomography with MRI Correlation. 4th ed. Philadelphia, PA: Lippincott Williams & Wilkins; 2006. Figure 23.3A.)*

cutaneous nerve of the arm by the intercostobrachial nerve. In coronary artery disease, referred pain to the arm might be through this nerve.[5]

Neoplastic Chest Wall Pain

A thorough history and physical examination is necessary to rule out pain caused by neoplasms of the thorax. Associated symptoms of cough, dyspnea, brachial plexopathy, and hoarseness due to recurrent laryngeal nerve involvement or Horner syndrome should arouse the suspicion of possible neoplastic disease. Diagnostic radiologic tests can confirm the diagnosis and the extent of involvement. If there is a high level of suspicion for neoplastic disease in a patient presenting with chest wall pain, diagnosis of the condition should be undertaken prior to any interventional procedures. Pain due to neoplastic disease is treated with a comprehensive or multimodal approach with opioid and nonopioid analgesics, physical therapy, interventional treatment with intercostal nerve blocks or epidural injections, and psychotherapy. In patients with refractory cancer pain, neuraxial delivery of opioid and local anesthetics by continuous infusion pumps or neurolytic ablation may be necessary for pain control.

Lung and breast cancers account for the majority of the thoracic neoplasms. Other neoplasms include metastatic lesions of the lung and the skeletal structures. Neoplasms of the lung present with symptoms of cough, dyspnea, hemoptysis, or obstructive symptoms due to compression of the neurovascular structures. Pain is not a common symptom with lung cancers except when there is pleural involvement. Nociceptive pain is usually localized, constant, or associated with chest wall movement and is caused by the invasion of the pleura, vertebrae, or other soft tissues of the chest wall. Deafferentation or neuropathic pain is caused by compression, infiltration, or damage to the involved spinal nerves and produces allodynia, hyperalgesia, dysesthesia, or hyperesthesia in a segmental fashion.[6] Involvement of the superior pulmonary sulcus produces Pancoast syndrome. It is characterized by pain in the shoulder and arm, motor weakness and wasting of muscles of the hand, as well as Horner syndrome.[7] A mass in the superior sulcus of the lung can cause compression of the lower trunk of the brachial plexus. Pain and motor symptoms are most commonly seen in the distribution of the ulnar nerve. Brachial plexopathy can also result from other causes such as metastatic tumors, radiation, or thoracic surgery.[6,8]

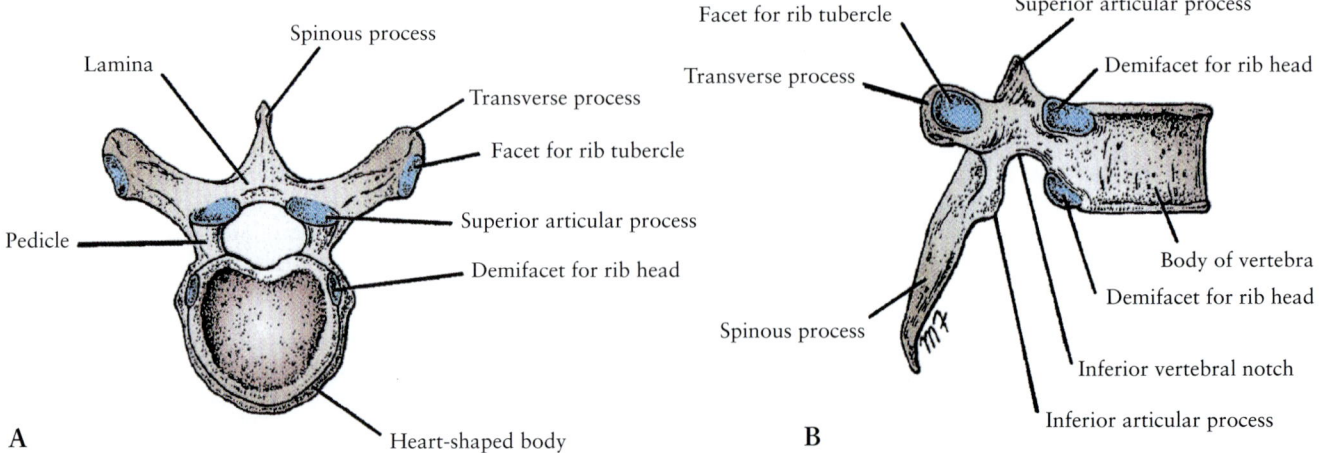

FIGURE 69.3 Thoracic vertebra. **A:** Superior surface. **B:** Lateral surface. *(Reprinted with permission from Snell RS. Clinical Anatomy by Regions. 9th ed. Philadelphia, PA: Lippincott Williams & Wilkins; 2011. Figure 2-3.)*

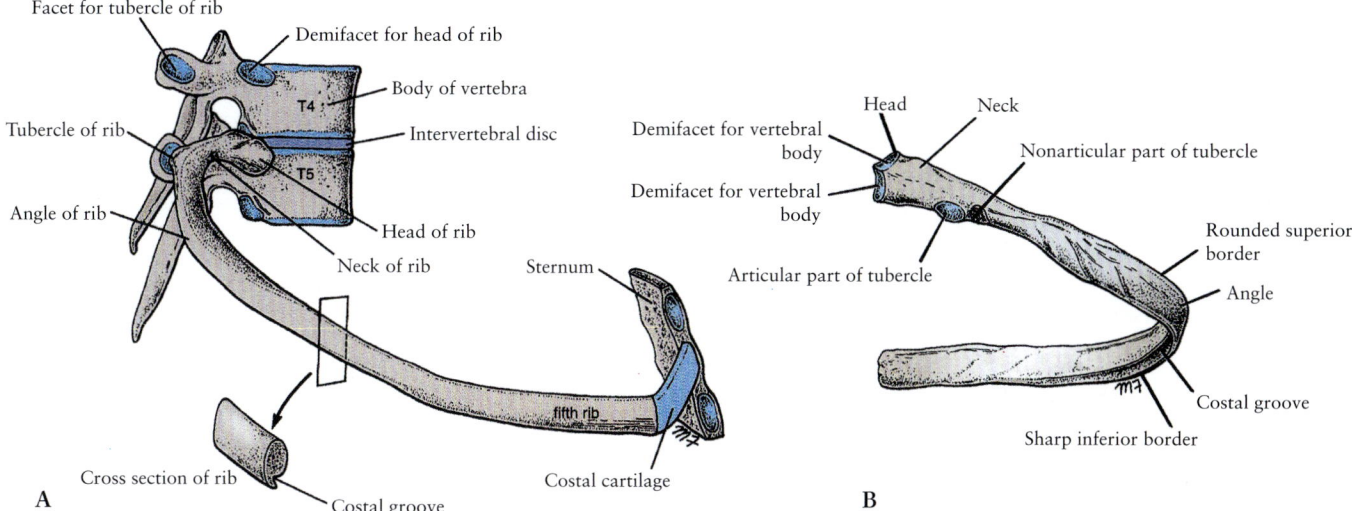

FIGURE 69.4 Fifth rib as it articulates with the vertebral column posteriorly and the sternum anteriorly. *(Reprinted with permission from Snell RS. Clinical Anatomy by Regions. 9th ed. Philadelphia, PA: Lippincott Williams & Wilkins; 2011. Figures 2-4 and 2-5.)*

EPIDURAL SPINAL CORD COMPRESSION

Epidural spinal cord compression is the second most common central neurologic complication of systemic cancer. Pain is the initial symptom before the development of other neurologic signs and symptoms. The pain can be misdiagnosed as musculoskeletal in origin. Appropriate imaging studies can aid in the diagnosis. Treatment includes corticosteroids and radiation. Surgical decompression with laminectomy or vertebral body resection is recommended in patients who are relatively healthy.[9,10]

SUPERIOR VENA CAVA SYNDROME

Obstruction of the blood flow through the superior vena cava results in superior vena cava syndrome. The obstruction can be due to external compression from pathology of the lung, lymph nodes, or mediastinum. It can also result from internal obstruction due to thrombus formation. Chest wall pain, cough, dyspnea along with collateral venous engorgement of the chest wall and neck, and facial edema are the common signs and symptoms. Dyspnea is the most common symptom. Lung cancer is the most common cause followed by lymphoma.

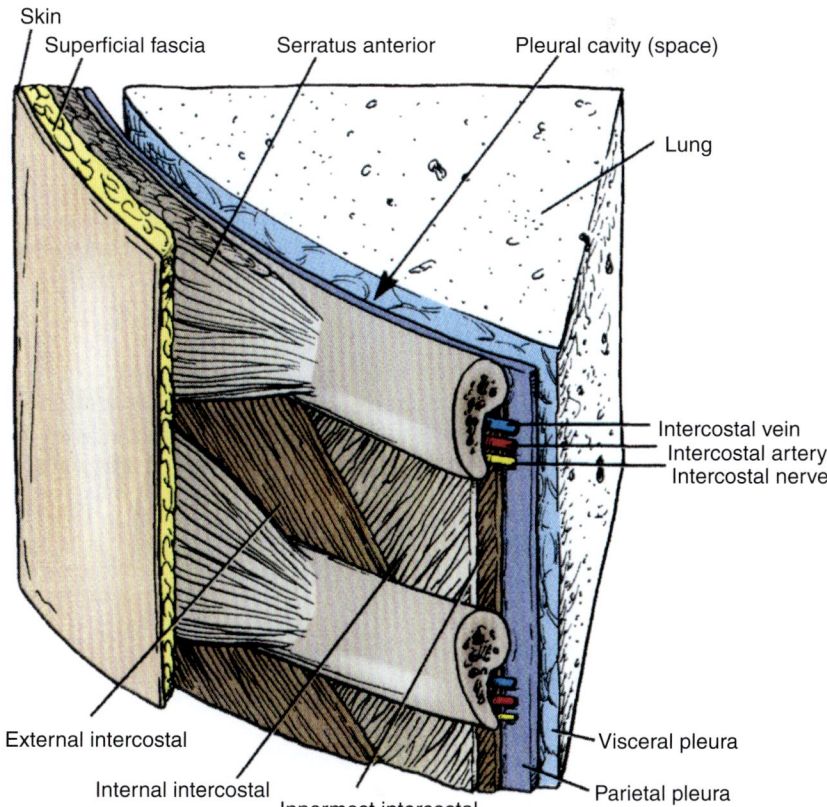

FIGURE 69.5 Intercostal space, its boundaries, and contents. *(Reprinted with permission from Snell RS. Clinical Anatomy by Regions. 9th ed. Philadelphia, PA: Lippincott Williams & Wilkins; 2011. Figure 2-3.)*

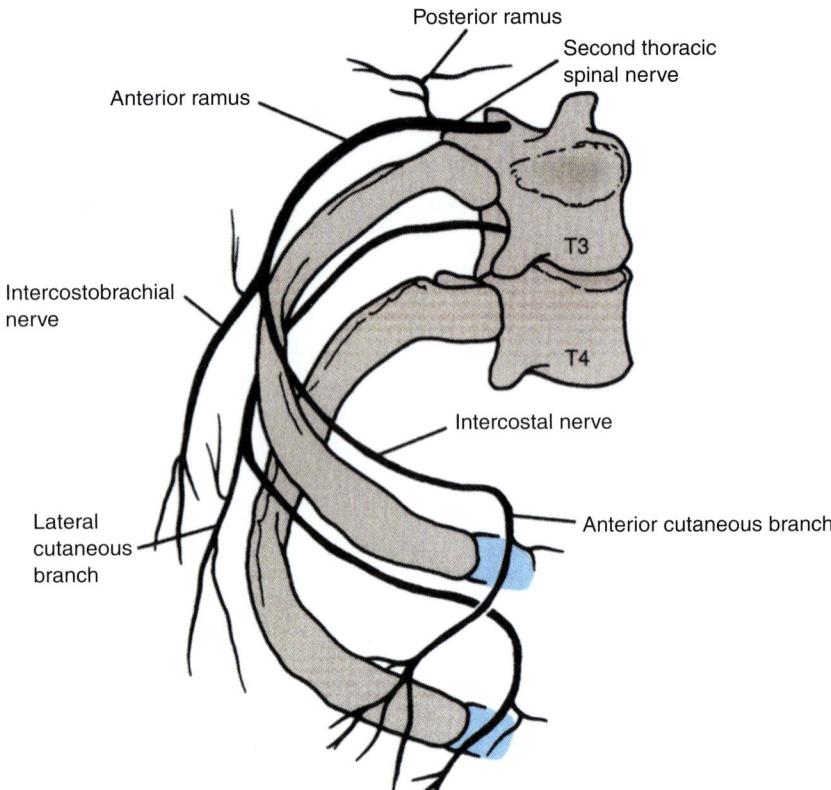

FIGURE 69.6   The distribution of two intercostals nerves to the rib cage. *(Reprinted with permission from Snell RS. Clinical Anatomy by Regions. 9th ed. Philadelphia, PA: Lippincott Williams & Wilkins; 2007. Figure 2-12.)*

Malignancy accounts for 60% to 85% of all cases of superior vena cava syndrome with small-cell lung cancer serving as the most common type of lung malignancy causing this syndrome.[11] Non-Hodgkin lymphoma is the most common type of lymphoma resulting in obstruction of the superior vena cava. The widespread use of central venous catheters, ports, pacemakers, and defibrillators has increased the incidence of benign superior vena cava syndrome (SVCS) due to endovascular obstruction.[12] Diagnosis is made based on clinical symptoms and the findings of abnormal lesions in the chest radiograph. Confirmatory studies include contrast-enhanced computed tomography (CT) scan and venous angiography. Current treatment strategies include chemotherapy, radiation, or endovascular stenting.[13] Surgical treatment is performed with spiral saphenous interposition graft or other grafts. Radiation treatment is indicated for emergency relief of airway obstruction.

COSTOPLEURAL SYNDROME
Tumor invasion of the pleura, ribs, and soft tissues of the chest wall with or without involvement of the intercostals nerves can result in sharp, aching, or burning pain (Fig. 69.7). Pain is exacerbated by movements of the chest wall, deep breathing, and coughing. Lesions of the pleura closer to the diaphragm can cause localized pain in the shoulder region or referred dull aching pain in the back or upper abdomen. Mediastinal pleural involvement causes pain deep in the central portion of the chest or the shoulder region. This type of pain is often potently responsive to steroidal or nonsteroidal anti-inflammatory analgesics.

Nonneoplastic Chest Wall Pain

Chest wall pain from other than neoplasms and visceral pain is discussed in this section. This section includes a discussion of chest wall pain due to neuropathy including neuraxial pain, myofascial, skeletal, and joint pain.

NEUROPATHIC PAIN
Pain due to neuropathy can arise anywhere along the nervous system supplying the chest wall. The pain can be neuraxial involving the spinal cord and nerve roots or related to peripheral nerves (Table 69.2).

Neuropathic Pain of Central Origin
Thoracic myelopathy can cause chest wall pain, back pain, or abdominal pain. Lesions can be present within the spinal cord or extramedullary or epidural spaces. Thoracic disk herniation can also result in chest wall pain (Fig. 69.8). Pain is usually the initial symptom before other neurologic symptoms. Pain is

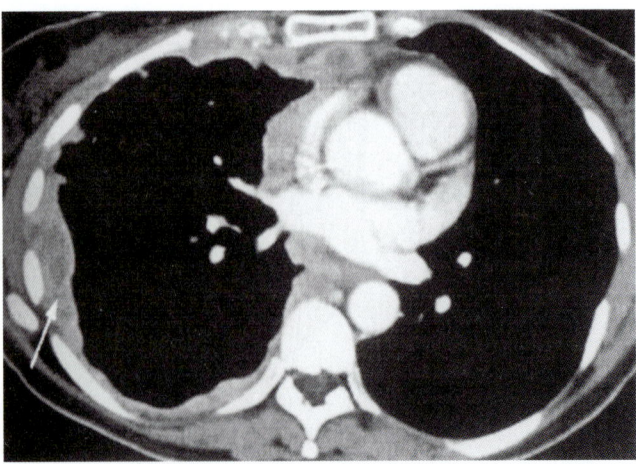

FIGURE 69.7   Computed tomography image showing right pleural thickening due to mesothelioma. *(Reprinted with permission from Lee JKT, Sagel SS, Stanley RJ, et al. Computerized Body Tomography with MRI Correlation. 4th ed. Philadelphia, PA: Lippincott Williams & Wilkins; 2006. Figure 8-71A.)*

TABLE 69.2 Chest Pain Primarily of Neuropathic Origin

I. Diseases of the spinal cord (myelopathy)
   A. Intrinsic spinal cord diseases: primary tumors, metastatic tumors, syringomyelia, trauma, multiple sclerosis, infarction, abscess
   B. Extramedullary intrathecal disorders
      1. Primary tumors: meningioma, neurofibroma
      2. Metastatic tumors
   C. Epidural spinal cord compression
      1. Primarily caused by vertebral pathology
      2. Metastatic neoplasm from breast, lung, prostate
      3. Epidural abscess
      4. Hematoma
      5. Adhesive arachnoiditis
II. Diseases of the rootlets and roots of spinal nerves (radiculopathy)
   A. Infection and inflammation
      1. Herpes zoster
      2. Syphilis (tabes dorsalis)
      3. Meningitis
      4. Systemic infection
      5. Tuberculosis
      6. Other infectious diseases
   B. Mechanical compression or injury
      1. Osteoarthritis
      2. Other arthritides
      3. Ruptured intervertebral disk
      4. Fracture of vertebra
      5. Abscess or tumor of the vertebra
      6. Paget disease of the spine
III. Diseases of the formed thoracic spinal nerves (neuropathy)
   A. Vertebral compression (same as IIB)
   B. Paravertebral compression
      1. Paravertebral adenopathy
      2. Mediastinal tumors
      3. Paravertebral abscess
      4. Aortic aneurysm
   C. Primary nerve tumors
      1. Neurofibroma
      2. Schwannoma
   D. Systemic infection, neuropathy
   E. Other neuritides
      1. Alcoholism
      2. Avitaminosis
      3. Intoxication by heavy metals, food, amoebae
      4. Vitamin metabolic disorders and others
IV. Disorders of the intercostal nerves (intercostal neuralgia)
   A. Compression or injury secondary to fracture or tumors of ribs
   B. External trauma (e.g., stab wounds)
   C. Postinfectious intercostal neuropathy
   D. Postoperative neuropathy
      1. Postmastectomy syndrome
      2. Postthoracotomy syndrome

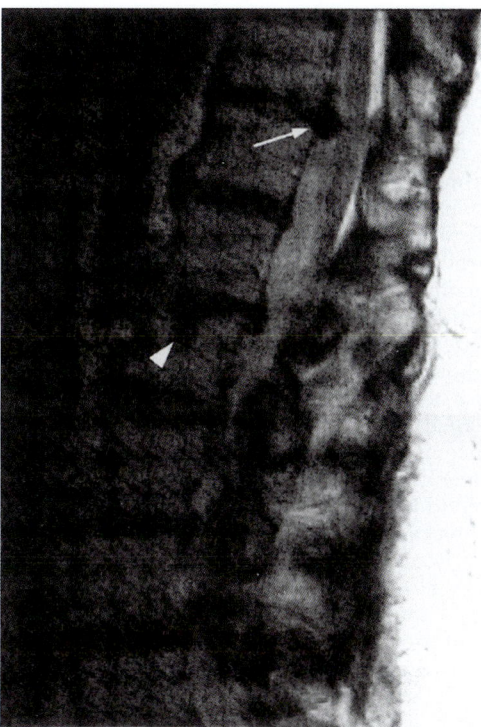

FIGURE 69.8 Sagittal T2-weighted magnetic resonance imaging showing a central thoracic disk herniation at T11–T12 (*arrow*). The cord is displaced posteriorly. The *arrowhead* shows a Schmorl nodule. (*Reprinted with permission from Lee JKT, Sagel SS, Stanley RJ, et al. Computerized Body Tomography with MRI Correlation. 4th ed. Philadelphia, PA: Lippincott Williams & Wilkins; 2006. Figure 23-37B.*)

(MRI) can help make the diagnosis. Stopping the infusion may decrease the size of the mass. Consensus guidelines to improve safety and mitigate risk of granulomas are available and updated every few years. Surgical removal of the symptomatic granuloma is rarely necessary.[17]

Peripheral Neuropathic Chest Wall Pain
Herpes Zoster and Postherpetic Neuralgia
Acute herpes zoster, also called shingles, is caused by the DNA virus, varicella zoster virus (VZV). The incidence of herpes zoster is higher in older and immunocompromised patients. Factors that decrease immune function such as chronic corticosteroid use, human immunodeficiency virus infection, cancer, and chemotherapy can increase the risk of developing herpes zoster.[18] Following a primary VZV infection, the virus remains dormant in the dorsal root ganglia. Acute herpes zoster is characterized by the reactivation of the latent virus in the dorsal root ganglion. It typically presents as a mononeuropathy involving the intercostal nerves. Clinically, the presentation begins with burning pain, hyperesthesia, or tingling followed by the characteristic vesicular rash. The prodromal sensory symptoms may be present for 1 to 2 weeks prior to the appearance of the rash.[19] The characteristic rash is initially maculopapular and progresses into vesicles with erythematous bases. The rash of herpes zoster is commonly seen involving one or two contiguous thoracic dermatomes, almost always unilateral. T5 and T6 dermatomes are most commonly affected.[20] Pain is sharp, burning, and superficial in nature. Pain can be worsened with ulceration and secondary infection of the vesicles. Associated muscle spasms can worsen the pain.

Diagnosis of the condition is made by the clinical presentation of the characteristic rash.

worsened in the recumbent position. If pain is the only symptom, it is often confused as myofascial or skeletal pain. Prompt diagnosis is important in light of potentially evolving cord compression. Pain that is progressive and not relieved by conventional therapy for musculoskeletal pain requires prompt attention to rule out neoplasm. Acute neurologic symptoms are initially treated with corticosteroids and radiation therapy.[14] Surgical decompression with laminectomy may be necessary if the symptoms are not relieved by nonsurgical methods. Lower cervical disk herniation can also present as neuropathic chest wall pain.[15,16] A relatively rare cause of thoracic neuropathic pain is seen in the form of an extramedullary granuloma in patients with neuraxial infusion pumps. Stopping the implanted infusion pump and radiographic exam with contrast through the catheter, CT myelography, or magnetic resonance imaging

The main goal of treatment of acute herpes zoster infection is not only to treat the acute condition but also to prevent central sensitization and postherpetic neuralgia. Treatment of the acute condition is initially pharmacologic. Elderly patients are more susceptible to developing postherpetic neuralgia; therefore, more aggressive treatment with additional interventional modalities is recommended. Pharmacologic therapy involves initiating treatment with oral antiviral agents as soon as the diagnosis has been made. Studies have shown efficacy of antiviral agents if started within 72 hours.[21,22] Interventional treatments include segmental epidural blockade with dilute local anesthetic solutions, intercostal nerve blocks, and sympathetic blockade of the cervicothoracic chain with stellate ganglion blocks are recommended. For an elderly patient suffering with a very painful bout of acute zoster, aggressive interventional treatment can reduce the severity of pain and may reduce the risk of severe pain of postherpetic neuralgia. The number of interventional treatments can range anywhere from three to four in a 2-week period. Continuous segmental epidural blockade with thoracic epidural catheter is also recommended; however, it may require hospitalization of the patient. Continuous blockade of the intercostal nerves can be achieved by placing a catheter in the intercostal space connected to an isomeric infusion pump. Such therapy can be used effectively on an outpatient basis. Use of dilute local anesthetics with less toxicity can reduce complications due to local anesthetic toxicity in older patients.

Postherpetic neuralgia presents with persistence of severe sharp, burning pain in the affected dermatomes after the disappearance of the acute rash. About 20% of elderly patients with herpes zoster develop postherpetic neuralgia. The pain may persist for months to years without treatment. Hyperalgesia and allodynia of the effected dermatome is seen. The chronicity of the pain can result in behavioral changes affecting sleep and mood. Psychosocial symptoms and depression can worsen the pain. Treatment of postherpetic neuralgia includes symptomatic treatment of pain with medications and interventions. Medical management involves the use of neuropathic analgesics which are discussed extensively elsewhere in this text. These may include tricyclic antidepressants, duloxetine, and anticonvulsants.[23-25] Systemic corticosteroids are ineffective in preventing postherpetic neuralgia. However, their use during the acute phase has not been associated to worsening of the disease.[26,27] Topical treatment with local anesthetic patches, local anesthetic ointments, preparations with capsaicin, and compounded creams can be used to achieve symptomatic treatment of the condition.[28-30] Transcutaneous electrical nerve stimulation (TENS) can also be helpful.[31] Interventional treatment with intercostal nerve blocks or epidural injections may be required. Permanent implants like dorsal column spinal cord

stimulators and peripheral intercostal nerve stimulators offer a novel approach to pain control in patients who require repeated interventional treatments. A trial of such a stimulator is recommended before permanent implantation. Along with the interventional treatments, aggressive behavioral therapy is highly recommended. Chronic opioid therapy may be needed. A comprehensive approach using pharmacologic, interventional, rehabilitative, and behavioral treatments will help achieve pain relief and improve functional capacity of the patient.

Intercostal and Peripheral Neuropathy

Chronic intercostal neuralgia can result from trauma or compression of the intercostals nerves. Due to the proximity of the nerves to the inferior aspect of the ribs, any abnormalities of the ribs such as fractures and metastatic lesions can result in intercostal neuralgia. Prior thoracic or breast surgery and surgical lesion of the nerves can result in chronic intercostal neuralgia. Other causes include trauma or infection. Pain is characterized as sharp, superficial, burning, or lancinating in the distribution of the affected nerve. Pain is worsened by respirations and movements of the chest wall similar to the clinical presentation of pleuritic lesions. Localized tenderness to palpation may be appreciated in the intercostal space. A thorough history looking for previous trauma or surgeries can assist in the diagnosis.

Medical management of intercostal neuralgia consists of treatment with nonsteroidal anti-inflammatory agents, tricyclic antidepressants, and anticonvulsants. Intercostal nerve blocks with long-acting local anesthetics and corticosteroids can be effective (Fig. 69.9). Cryoablation or radiofrequency neurolysis of the intercostal nerves can provide longer pain relief.[32] Ultrasound guidance can provide accuracy in identification of the nerves for radiofrequency neurolysis.[33] We avoid chemolysis of the intercostals nerves because of concerns of postlysis neuralgia and neuritis. Dorsal root ganglion radiofrequency ablation has been described for treatment of intercostal neuralgia.[34-36] Long-term relief can also be achieved by implantable dorsal column or peripheral nerve stimulators.[37]

CHEST WALL PAIN OF SKELETAL ORIGIN

Skeletal chest wall pain can originate from the thoracic spine, ribs, costal cartilages, or sternum.

Abnormalities of the Thoracic Spine

Localized pain in the back can result from abnormalities of the thoracic spine. Pain is caused by stimulation of nociceptive fibers in the periosteum, joints, and ligaments. Reflex muscle spasms of the paraspinal muscles are also associated with pain. Deep palpation of the thoracic spinous processes, the paravertebral region, and movement of the spine can elicit pain.

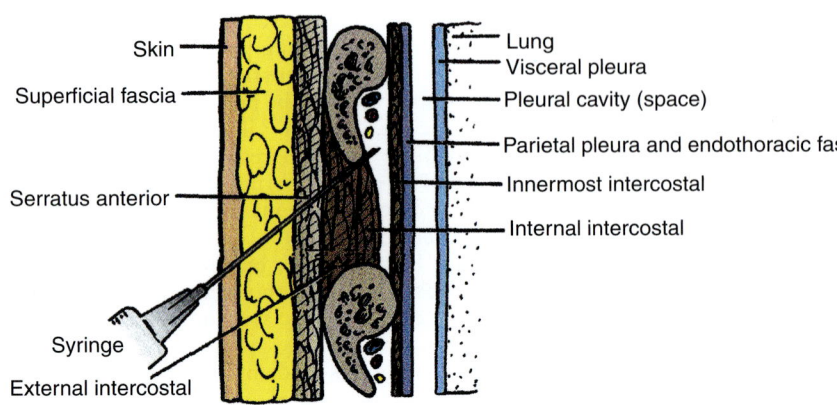

Skin — Superficial fascia — Serratus anterior — Syringe — External intercostal — Lung — Visceral pleura — Pleural cavity (space) — Parietal pleura and endothoracic fascia — Innermost intercostal — Internal intercostal

FIGURE 69.9 Intercostal nerve block. *(Modified with permission from Snell RS. Clinical Anatomy by Regions. 7th ed. Philadelphia, PA: Lippincott Williams & Wilkins; 2003. Figure 2-8B.)*

Congenital abnormalities of the spinal curvature resulting in scoliosis can cause chest wall pain as the patient ages. Structural changes in the thoracic spine due to postural kyphosis, trauma, or disease can result in pain. Correction of lateral scoliosis with surgical or nonsurgical interventions can help alleviate the pain. Posture training with strengthening exercises and relief of muscle spasms is helpful.

Vertebral Fractures

Fractures of the vertebral body can be very painful. The pain can be particularly severe and may radiate into the chest wall. Vertebral fractures are the result of trauma, metastatic disease, or osteoporosis. Compression fractures in younger patients are mostly due to trauma. However, corticosteroid use can also result in compression fractures in younger patients. Osteoporosis is a major public health concern in the modern world. It is estimated that by the eighth decade, 50% of all women will develop vertebral fractures.[38] There is significant impact on the patient with an osteoporotic vertebral fracture resulting in pain, deformity, dependence, and fear of falling. More than 200,000 people per year with osteoporotic fractures require opioid pain medications.[39,40] Radiologic diagnosis with plain films, CT scan, or MRI can assist in the diagnosis of a patient who presents with acute onset posterior axial pain with or without radicular symptoms (Fig. 69.10).

Physical examination may reveal deformity of the spine. A prominent spinous process can sometimes be palpated above or below the level of the compression fracture. Pain may not be present initially, and about 50% of the patients present at a later time with the onset of pain. Most of the fractures are due to a combination of flexion with axial compression resulting in collapse of the anterior portions of the vertebral body. With osteoporosis, as the load-bearing capacity of the vertebral bodies decreases, minor movements such as bending or lifting can result in a fracture in older patients. Crushed fracture of the anterior and middle columns of the vertebral body, the so-called burst fractures, can result in neurologic compromise. The main goal of therapy is prevention. Treatment options for pain due to vertebral compression fractures include analgesics, bracing, and interventional treatments. Surgical treatment is indicated if there is neurologic compromise. However, surgery can be invasive and result in failure of fixation in the osteoporotic spine.

Vertebral body augmentations with vertebroplasty or balloon kyphoplasty have had promising results. It involves mechanical augmentation of the compressed vertebral body by injecting acrylic bone cement material. Use of polymethylmethacrylate for vertebral compression fractures was reported in France in 1991 with good results of pain relief. Polymethylmethacrylate is injected into the vertebral body via a posterolateral approach. The posterior cortex of the vertebral body must be intact prior to injection. Studies have recognized the best timing of interventional procedures to be within 6 weeks of the fracture.[41,42] No differences in pain were reported when vertebroplasty is compared to balloon kyphoplasty.[43] Both techniques have their own advantages and disadvantages.[44] Medial branch nerve blockade and radiofrequency ablation is an emerging option with lower risk than other interventional approaches described earlier, albeit without an extensive evidentiary basis.[45]

Ankylosing Spondylitis

Ankylosing spondylitis results in a stiff spine due to arthritic changes in the intervertebral joints including the costovertebral,

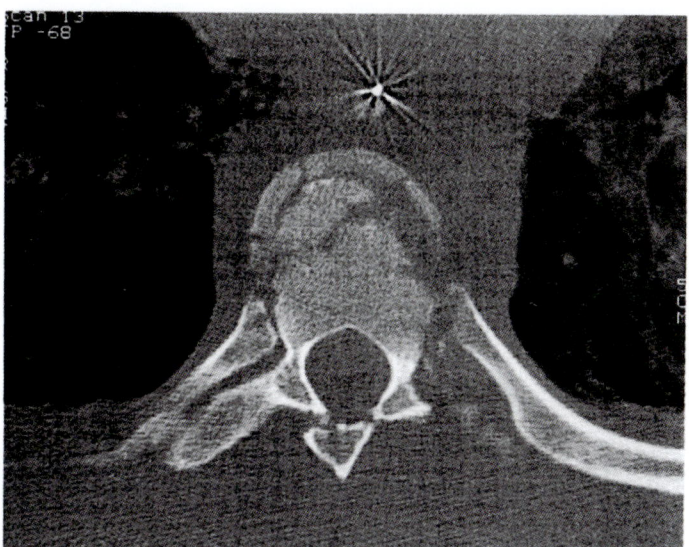
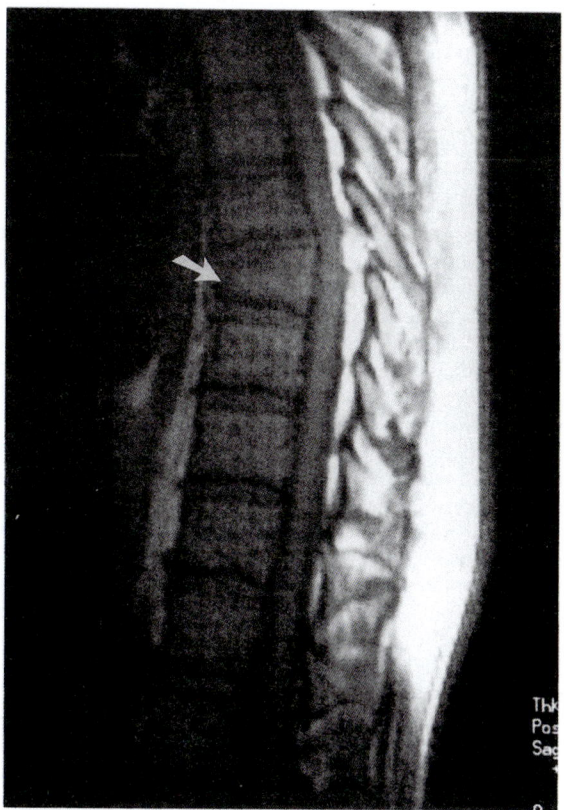

FIGURE 69.10 Thoracic spine compression fracture. **A:** Axial computed tomography shows compression fracture involving mainly the anterior aspect of T7 vertebral body. **B:** Midsagittal T1-weighted image shows the wedged T7 vertebral body (*arrow*). The posterior margin is displaced into the spinal canal, producing spinal cord compression. (*Reprinted with permission from Lee JKT, Sagel SS, Stanley RJ, et al. Computerized Body Tomography with MRI Correlation. 4th ed. Philadelphia, PA: Lippincott Williams & Wilkins; 2006. Figure 23-14B.*)

costotransverse, and apophyseal joints. The sternoclavicular joints can also be involved.[46] Patients can typically present with mild to moderate pain in the posterior chest wall. Anterior chest wall pain has also been reported in patients with ankylosing spondylitis.[47] Physical examination demonstrates limited movements of the spine with contracted tender paraspinal muscles. Diagnosis is made by plain films that show characteristic fused spine or "bamboo spine." Occasionally, involvement of the nerve roots due to arthritic changes in the joints can result in radicular pain. Secondary contracture of the paraspinal muscles can worsen the pain. Effective treatment involves physical therapy, trigger point muscle injections, and muscle relaxants. Progression of the arthropathy should be addressed with the expertise of a rheumatologist. Paravertebral blocks can provide relief from radicular pain. Thoracic facet joint injections with corticosteroid and local anesthetics can provide significant relief of pain. If good results are encountered with facet joint injections, longer term relief of pain can be obtained with radiofrequency ablation of the nerve supply of the facet joint. The radiofrequency technique is generally considered to be safer than chemical ablation because there are additional risks associated with the potential unwanted spread of the chemolysis agent.

Costovertebral Arthritis

Arthritis of the costovertebral and costotransverse joints can cause posterior chest wall pain. Pain is localized, aching, and deep in character. Pain can be increased with deep breathing, coughing, or lateral compression of the chest. Physical examination may reveal localized deep tenderness that may be hard to distinguish from thoracic facet syndrome. Characteristics of pain and radiologic examination can delineate the pathology.[48,49] Treatment is provided with nonsteroidal anti-inflammatory agents and physical therapy. Interventional treatment with injection of the joints with local anesthetic, corticosteroid mixture with fluoroscopic confirmation can alleviate the pain. It can also be diagnostic. Low-dose opioid medications may be needed for treatment of chronic pain from the arthritis.[50] Rarely, resection of the joints is considered for refractory pain from isolated costovertebral joint arthritis.[51]

Diffuse Idiopathic Skeletal Hyperostosis

Another cause of posterior chest wall pain in elderly patients can be due to diffuse idiopathic skeletal hyperostosis (DISH), also called Forestier disease. Patients present with dull aching thoracic back pain, posterior chest wall pain, dysphagia, myelopathy due to involvement of the posterior longitudinal ligaments, fractures, subluxation, and, rarely, intercostal neuralgia. Physical findings include slight increase in dorsal kyphosis, minimal reduction in motion, and localized tenderness. Diagnosis is confirmed with radiologic exams with plain films and CT scans showing spinal hyperostosis resulting in linear ossification and bridging osteophytosis along the anterior and anterolateral aspects of the vertebral bodies. DISH most commonly affects the thoracic spine. Absence of sacroiliitis, true syndesmophytes, and ankylosing apophyseal joints distinguishes this syndrome from ankylosing spondylitis.[52,53] The syndrome of synovitis, acne, pustulosis, hyperostosis, and osteitis (SAPHO syndrome) can also be a cause of anterior chest wall hyperostosis.[54] Treatment is symptomatic with nonsteroidal anti-inflammatory drugs (NSAIDs) and physical therapy.

Thoracic Facet Syndrome

Thoracic facet syndrome results from abnormal locking or binding of the facet joints. Sudden or rapid turning movements of the trunk, working with hands over the head, or lifting with the trunk in a twisted position can result in this syndrome.

Symptoms include moderate to severe pain on the side of the spine or anterolateral chest wall.[55,56] The pain is worsened with extension of the spine and relieved with flexion. Localized deep tenderness can be elicited to deep palpation over the facet joint. Tenderness and spasms of the erector spinae muscles can exacerbate the pain. It can mimic the pain from costovertebral arthropathy. Injection of the joint can assist in making the correct diagnosis. Treatment includes NSAIDs, physical therapy, and injection of the facet joints and medial branches with corticosteroid and local anesthetics. Radiofrequency denervation offers long-term pain relief but for unknown reasons may be associated with higher rates of postlytic neuritis than comparable radiofrequency denervation of medial branch nerves in the lumbar or cervical regions.[57–59]

Chest Wall Pain Arising from the Ribs

Rib fractures account for one of the most common causes of acute chest wall pain of skeletal origin. Blunt trauma to the ribs is the usual cause of fractures. Other causes include severe paroxysmal coughing (tussive fracture), metastatic disease, osteoporosis, osteomalacia, and Paget disease of the bone (Fig. 69.11). Elder or child abuse should be sought in unexplained rib fractures after all other etiologies are eliminated.

Fractures may involve several ribs or multiple fractures of the same rib. Acute pain from rib fractures is usually aching, sharp, and worsened with respirations. Pain from multiple fractures can restrict breathing leading to additional pulmonary complications. Acute pain from rib fractures is treated with NSAIDs, low-dose opioids, or continuous intercostal nerve blocks. Chest wall pain from multiple rib fractures in trauma patients, in which serious consequences might occur from hypoventilation due to pain-related splinting, are candidates for a thoracic epidural catheter with a continuous epidural infusion.[60,61] Multiple studies in selected trauma patients have shown better outcomes of

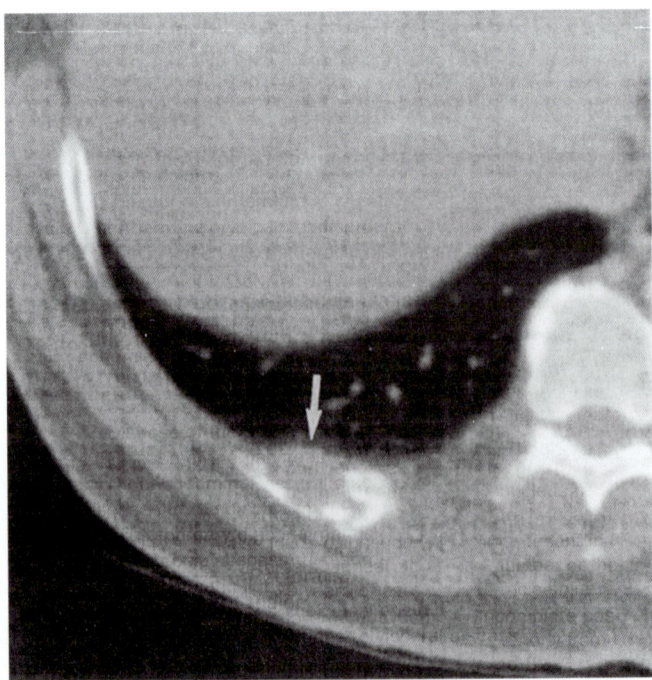

FIGURE 69.11 Computed tomography showing rib destruction from multiple myeloma (*arrow*). (*Reprinted with permission from Lee JKT, Sagel SS, Stanley RJ, et al. Computerized Body Tomography with MRI Correlation. 4th ed. Philadelphia, PA: Lippincott Williams & Wilkins; 2006. Figure 8-82.*)

pain relief and reduction in pulmonary complications with thoracic epidural infusion compared to systemic opioids or intrapleural catheters.[62–66]

Ultrasound-guided serratus plane blocks have been used recently for pain control after multiple rib fractures.[67,68]

Occasionally, rib trauma without radiographically apparent fracture can cause localized pain and swelling with point tenderness in the area. If these are related to hypoventilation due to splinting from pain, they may be considered the same as rib fractures potentially requiring neuroaxial analgesia. Local injections with local anesthetics, intercostals nerve blocks, and NSAIDs can help relieve the pain. Topical local anesthetic patches with 5% lidocaine may be helpful for some with pain from single rib fractures or rib injuries without a fracture. Metastatic disease from the breast, lungs, and prostate can cause isolated rib tenderness. Plain radiographs and nuclear medicine bone scans can aid in the diagnosis.

Slipping Rib Syndrome

Slipping rib syndrome was described first in 1922 by Davies-Colley.[69] It is characterized by chest wall or abdominal pain due to irritation of the intercostal nerves. The etiology is thought to be due to trauma. There is increased mobility of the costal cartilages of 8th to 10th ribs near the sternum. The syndrome is also referred to as clicking rib, gliding rib, or displaced ribs.[70] It is also seen in children.[71,72] The cause for pain is due to anatomic variation of the 8th to 10th ribs, which, instead of articulating directly with the sternum, articulate with the costal cartilages of the upper rib. As such, the sternal ends of these ribs are more prone to trauma. Injury can cause separation of the cartilages causing slipping movements of the ribs with respiration. A characteristic click can be felt with the movement of the ribs over the border of the upper cartilage. Diagnosis of the condition can be accomplished by the "hooking maneuver." The examiner's curled fingers are placed over the inferior border of the rib and the rib is pulled up anteriorly. A positive test produces a clicking noise and increases the pain.[73] Slipping rib syndrome is treated conservatively with reassurance and nonopioid analgesics. Injection of the painful site (between the detached cartilage and the rib) with local anesthetic steroid combination medications may relieve pain for a longer period. Surgical excision of the involved rib and costal cartilages has also been suggested for refractory cases.

Tietze Syndrome

Tietze syndrome is characterized by a benign, nonsuppurative, painful swelling of the second or third costal cartilages.[74] It was first described in 1921 by Tietze. Straining, severe cough, heavy manual work, nutritional deficiencies, and arthritic conditions have all been implicated as the possible causes. In 80% of the patients, the condition is unilateral.[75] Pain is usually localized but occasionally can radiate over the anterior chest wall to the shoulder or neck. Pain is characterized as heaviness, tightness, or soreness. Pain is exacerbated by coughing and deep breathing. There is localized tenderness and swelling over the involved cartilage.[76] The overlying skin is normal. Radiologic diagnosis by bone scans is nonspecific.[77] Treatment includes use of nonopioid anti-inflammatory medications. The condition usually is self-limited with occasional exacerbations and remissions.

Costochondritis

Costochondritis is one of the most common causes of anterior chest wall pain often confusing or coexisting with the pain due to coronary artery disease.[78–80] Pain is characterized as aching, sharp, or tightness in the anterior chest wall. Unlike Tietze syndrome, it involves multiple sites. No swelling is palpated. There is localized tenderness involving multiple costochondral regions of the anterior chest wall. Second to fifth costal cartilages are frequently involved. Pain is aggravated with movement of the chest. Pain can radiate anteriorly or to the back. In adolescents, it can cause chest wall or abdominal pain. Firm steady pressure applied over the sternum, intercostal spaces, costochondral junctions, and the ribs can reproduce the pain. The horizontal flexion test consists of having the arm flexed across the anterior chest wall and applying steady traction in a horizontal direction while the patient's head is rotated toward the ipsilateral shoulder. The crowing rooster maneuver involves having the patient extend the neck as much as possible by looking toward the ceiling while the clinician, standing behind the patient, exerts traction on the posteriorly extended arms.

It is important to distinguish pain due to costochondritis (especially left-sided) from that of coronary artery disease or abdominal pathology.[78] Pain due to costochondritis is usually located to the lateral side of the sternum unlike substernal cardiac pain.[81,82] Pain can radiate to the left arm or shoulder. The patient gives a history of pain with movement and postural changes. Localized concordant tenderness can be palpated. Pain usually lasts for a few minutes to hours, distinguishing it from pain of acute cardiac origin. Intercostal nerve blocks and injection of the tender costochondral areas with local anesthetic have been used for diagnostic purposes. Rarely, emergency room physicians experience a patient with both costochondritis and coronary artery disease. Careful history and physical exam along with treatment with sublingual nitroglycerin can aid in prompt diagnosis of the cardiac pain, which is relieved with nitroglycerin.

Treatment of costochondritis is initiated with NSAIDs, physical therapy, heat application, and less commonly with low-dose opioids. Once the diagnosis has been made, reassuring the patent about the benign nature of the condition can prevent patient anxiety and avoid unnecessary expensive diagnostic workup. Localized injection of the costochondral junction with local anesthetics and corticosteroids can help relieve the pain.

Costochondral Dislocation

Costochondral dislocation is commonly seen after trauma in young patients.[83] It is also encountered after thoracic surgery with rib retraction. The pain is typically dull, aching, or burning and is usually continuous. Localized tenderness is present. Sometimes, a mass is felt due to cartilaginous excess from the injury. Treatment is similar to other conditions as described earlier with oral analgesics and intercostals nerve blocks. Manipulation and reduction of the dislocation after adequate analgesia can correct the condition.

Chest Wall Pain of Sternal Origin

Sternoclavicular joint arthritis can be caused due to various arthritic conditions (osteoarthritis, rheumatoid arthritis, psoriatic) and rarely infections due to central venous catheters.[84–86] Infections are also seen in intravenous drug users. Traumatic subluxation and dislocation can also cause pain.[87] Apart from trauma, such conditions are also seen after cardiac surgery when the sternum is retracted. Pain is localized to the affected joint. Localized tenderness of the joint is seen with palpation along with pain from shrugging the shoulders. Treatment consists of oral NSAIDs and injection of the joints with local anesthetic and corticosteroid. Such intervention must be avoided in infectious joints which are treated with antibiotics and analgesics.

Blunt injuries to the sternum can cause subluxation of the manubriosternal joint.[87] Manubriosternal arthritis can occur due to various arthritic conditions.[88–90] Septic arthritis of the joint is also seen.[91,92] Pain is localized to the anterior sternum or angle of Louis with occasional radiation parasternally. Pain is characterized as sharp aggravated with deep breathing, coughing, or yawning. Pain may mimic anginal pain. Diagnosis is made by physical examination. Bone scans can be positive.[93] Treatment consists of systemic analgesics, topical lidocaine patches, heat, infiltration of the joint with local anesthetics, and corticosteroids. Rarely, surgical intervention to correct the manubriosternal displacement is necessary.

Xiphoidalgia (Painful Xiphoid Syndrome, Xiphoid Cartilage Syndrome, Hypersensitive Xiphoid)

Intermittent, inferior substernal, or epigastric pain associated with tenderness of the xiphoid to palpation is characteristic of xiphoidalgia.[94,95] Pain is spontaneous without any obvious precipitating cause. It is sometimes seen along with coronary artery disease, intestinal disease, and metabolic disorders. Movements of the xiphoid with bending, stooping, or turning precipitates or exacerbates the pain more commonly after a full meal. Along with NSAIDs, local injection of the xiphisternal joint with local anesthetic and corticosteroid can alleviate the pain.

Chest Wall Pain of Myofascial Origin

Myofascial strain can be caused by excessive muscular activity. Repeated stress due to exercise, coughing, straining, or repetitive movements (chopping wood, painting a ceiling) can result in generalized tenderness over the anterior chest wall. Pain in the intercostals or accessory thoracic muscles is usually due to trauma. Pain from the pectoralis muscles can be exacerbated with adduction movements of the shoulder. Pain between the scapula and spine from an injured rhomboid is increased with bracing of the shoulders backward. Treatment consists of reassurance, local heat or cold, NSAIDs, topical lidocaine patches, physical therapy, and avoiding precipitating activities. Infiltration of the muscle with local anesthetic can be undertaken if there is localized tenderness. Caution regarding the risk of pneumothorax is necessary for all chest wall injections.

Precordial Catch Syndrome (Chest Wall Twinge Syndrome)

This is characterized by episodes of sudden, brief, sharp precordial or periapical pain. This is a benign, self-limited condition.[96,97] Sharp pains, stitches, or catches are felt in the chest wall in the left parasternal on or near the cardiac apex. Some patients report pain from assuming a slouching or bent position. Pain may last for a few seconds to up to 3 minutes. Deep breathing exacerbates the pain, whereas shallow breathing relieves it. There is no localized tenderness. The cause is unknown. Intercostal muscle spasms and pain from the pleura have been postulated as possible causes. Treatment consists of reassurance and correction of posture. Due to the unpredictability and the benign short duration of pain, analgesics are not necessary.

Epidemic Myalgia (Bornholm Disease, Epidemic Pleurodynia, Devil's Grip)

This condition is characterized by paroxysms of intense sharp chest wall and upper abdominal pain due to viral infection with coxsackie or echoviruses.[98] The paroxysms of pain are separated by pain-free intervals. Frequently, there is associated fever, headache, and pharyngitis. The condition is self-limited.

Breast Pain

Pain arising from the breast is a common and nonspecific symptom in women.[99,100] Usual causes include benign cysts, fibrocystic change, or cyclical pain due to hormonal cycle changes of the menstrual cycle. Other causes of breast pain include malignancy, mastitis, ductal ectasia, breast abscess, hormone replacement therapy, or large breasts. Careful clinical evaluation and mammography to rule out malignancy should be undertaken. Pain due to malignant breast lesions does not usually present until the tumor is large (greater than 2 cm in diameter).

Axillary lymph node involvement can present as either localized or sharp pain in the arm with involvement of the intercostobrachial nerves. Extramammary sources of breast pain should be evaluated if no other etiology is suggestive. Causes include skeletal and myofascial pain from the chest wall, radicular pain, or pain from peripheral nerves.

Chronic severe breast pain that persists for years without any obvious cause characterizes idiopathic mastalgia. Pain can be unilateral or bilateral, cyclical or noncyclical, which is usually seen in the third or early fourth decades of life. Without any organic diagnosis, the etiology is often misdiagnosed as psychologic.[100] Cyclical mastalgia responds to danazol, bromocriptine, or tamoxifen. Hormonal events such as pregnancy, menopause, or use of oral contraceptives may lead to relief.[101–103]

Breast pain is often treated with NSAIDs and acetaminophen. Warm compresses, ice packs, or gentle massage can also help relieve pain. Pain arising from the cervical or thoracic spine requires appropriate treatment of the cause as discussed elsewhere in this book. Peripheral myofascial and skeletal pain, also discussed elsewhere in this book, can be treated with injection of local anesthetic and corticosteroid.[104,105]

Adiposis Dolorosa (Dercum Disease)

This syndrome is characterized by painful subcutaneous fatty tumors in various parts of the body, including the breast.[106] This can result in chronic pain in the breast. Treatment with intravenous lidocaine and resection of the fatty lesions is helpful.

Mondor Disease

Thrombosis of the superficial veins of the thoracic wall can cause pain in the anterolateral chest wall.[107] This is seen occasionally in patients who abuse intravenous drugs.[108] The disease is mostly seen in middle-aged women with pendulous breasts and can cause pain in the breast.[109] Presence of a palpable tender cord is characteristic. The disease can cause anxiety in the patient. Mondor disease is self-limited. Treatment involves management of pain with NSAIDs.

Postsurgical Chest Wall Pain

Pain can persist for several months to years after surgery. It is often additively perplexing for the patient to live with pain after the original pathology has been corrected with surgery. Chronic postsurgical pain is most commonly seen after thoracotomy, mastectomy, and cardiac surgery. Other rare causes of chronic postsurgical chest wall pain include video-assisted thoracoscopy, mediastinoscopy, breast reconstruction, and surgery of the cervical or thoracic spine.

Postsurgical Breast Pain and Postmastectomy Pain Syndrome

Persistent pain in the anterior chest wall, axilla, and the arm can be seen in a few patients after mastectomy.[110–112] It can also occur after minor breast surgeries, such as lumpectomy. Breast reconstruction or other cosmetic breast surgeries can be also associated with such pain. Submuscular implants and capsule formation around the implant can cause injury or impinge on the thoracodorsal, long thoracic, lateral, or medial pectoral nerves. Postsurgical complications such as wound infection, fluid or hematoma retention, and reexploration can frequently result in pain. Although previous studies describe pain in less than 10% of patients, more recent studies report pain, paresthesias, and phantom sensations in about half of the patients.[113,114] In about half of the cases pain resolves with time. Pain is described as burning, sharp, or tight constriction of the axilla. Pain can be associated with surgical scar sensitivity. There can be associated dysesthesia or hyperesthesia of the anterior chest wall. It is presumed that injury to the intercostobrachial nerves and, rarely, the intercostal nerves is the cause. However, pain management interventions have included intercostal nerve blocks and not blockade of the intercostobrachial nerves,[115] but it should be noted that the intercostobrachial nerves are branches of the second and third intercostal nerves, so blocks of the second and third intercostal nerves will also block the intercostobrachial nerves. Patients are at risk for developing upper extremity problems due to restricted movement of the arm secondary to pain. Treatment consists of analgesic and neuropathic medications, physical therapy, reassurance, intercostal or paravertebral nerve blocks, or epidural analgesia.[116,117] Intraoperative infiltration of botulinum toxin into the chest wall musculature has also been suggested.[118] Ultrasound-guided pectoral blocks have demonstrated pain control similar to thoracic paravertebral blocks.[119] Persistent pain should arouse suspicion for recurrent breast disease.

Phantom breast syndrome has been a common occurrence after a mastectomy in the past.[120–122] The incidence has decreased with adequate psychosocial supportive therapy.[123,124] It can present as painful or nonpainful sensations in the region of the missing breast as if it is still present. It can develop within 3 months after the surgery. Risk factors for development of the syndrome include psychosocial factors, damaged body image, and impaired sexual function. Affected women are usually younger, premenopausal with children. Predisposing factors for phantom breast pain are similar to phantom limb syndrome and include pain in the involved breast prior to surgery.[125] Preoperative analgesia may be effective in preventing this syndrome; however, it has not been significantly studied.

Postthoracotomy Pain

Chronic chest wall pain after thoracotomy can be disabling to the patient.[126,127] Characteristics of postthoracotomy pain can be burning, aching, hyperesthesia, or allodynia along the surgical incision and the involved dermatome. Women experience more pain than men after major thoracotomy.[128] No difference has been seen in the incidence of acute or chronic pain with different types of thoracotomy incisions.[129] Prospective studies have predicted that adequate management of acute postsurgical pain can prevent the chronicity of pain.[130,131] Preoperative psychosocial factors were not associated with development of chronic pain after thoracic surgery. There was no difference in the incidence and severity of chronic pain after thoracotomy versus thoracoscopy.[132]

Management of acute pain with thoracic epidural placed prior to surgery has been shown to decrease the severity of perioperative pain and decrease the incidence of chronic pain. Other causes of radicular chest wall pain and recurrent cancer have to be excluded, especially in postthoracotomy patients who experience onset of severe pain several months after the thoracotomy. Management is similar to treatment for intercostal neuralgia.[133,134] Thoracic paravertebral blocks are also helpful to control acute and chronic pain.[135,136] Pulsed radio frequency of dorsal root ganglia or intercostal nerves is recommended for refractory pain.[137] Prior to any injections of the surgical scar site, a careful examination is necessary to avoid injury to herniated lung tissue in rare cases.[138,139] A multimodal approach to pain management provides higher success in controlling chronic postthoracotomy pain.

Postcardiac Surgery Pain

Persistent anterior chest wall pain has been reported in about 28% of patients after cardiac surgery.[140,141] Myocardial ischemia, infection, sternal or costosternal instability, sternal wires, and intercostal neuralgia (especially after dissection of the internal mammary artery from the chest wall) can be possible causes.[142] Pain can persist up to 2 years postoperatively. Initial attempts at treatment should be focused on eliminating obvious serious causes. Treatment consists of analgesic and neuropathic medications, costosternal joint injections, and surgical removal of sternal wires.[143]

CHEST PAIN AND PSYCHOLOGICAL FACTORS

Patients with sudden acute chest pain, regardless of the cause, experience varying degrees of anxiety, apprehension, and fear, depending on their interpretation of the cause of pain. Those who believe they are experiencing a heart attack become extremely frightened of possible impending death. Patients with persistent angina develop reactive depression, which, if untreated, produces progressive physical and psychological deterioration.[144] Musculoskeletal chest pain can cause a great deal of anxiety and apprehension until the patients are reassured about the benign nature of the condition.[145,146] Adolescents can often present with chest pain that is mostly myofascial or psychogenic in origin.

Chest pain can also result from psychological mechanisms. Because of the potential seriousness of a physical cause of chest pain, thorough history, physical examination, and diagnostic workup is essential. Some of the features of psychological chest pain include pain at the apex of the heart, patients describing the character of pain dramatically, development of pain unrelated to physiologic events, and possible presence of an emotional precipitating event prior to the pain. Once the diagnosis of psychological chest pain has been made, reassurance, relaxation techniques, anxiolytic drugs, sedatives, tranquilizers, and time can reduce the anxiety.

Patients with chronic anxiety can present with chest pain and other symptoms. This syndrome has been called Da Costa syndrome, neurocirculatory asthenia, vasoregulatory asthenia, effort syndrome, and soldier's heart.[147,148] Patients can present with symptoms of apical chest pain, shortness of breath, nervousness, anxiety, fatigue, generalized weakness, and low energy level. Treatment consists of reassurance, behavioral therapy, and treatment of underlying psychiatric disorders, if any. Other psychiatric disorders, such as depression, conversion reactions, hypochondriasis, and learned behavior, can manifest as chest pain.

CHEST WALL PAIN OF CARDIAC ORIGIN

In any patient who presents with chest pain, the differential diagnosis must include chest pain of cardiac origin. Angina presents as substernal chest pain or tightness. However, atypical presentations of chest pain or gastric symptoms can be seen from cardiac disease. Evaluation of risk factors may help assist in making the diagnosis in atypical presentations. Chronic refractory angina pectoris is a condition where patients present with chronic and disabling chest pain despite optimal medical treatment. In such patients who are not candidates for invasive cardiac procedures, spinal cord stimulation (SCS) offers adequate pain control and improvement in the quality of life.[149,150] SCS is also mentioned as an available adjunct by the task force on the management of stable angina pectoris of the European Society of Cardiology.[151] Angina due to acute myocardial infarction is not masked by SCS.[152]

Conclusion

Chest wall pain can result from lesions within the chest wall or referred pain from the thoracic viscera (Figs. 69.12 and 69.13). A comprehensive assessment and examination is needed to differentiate these and to further determine if the lesion involves skeletal, muscular, or neurologic components of the chest wall or thoracic and abdominal viscera (Table 69.3).

Our growing treatment armamentarium includes analgesic and neuropathic medications, nerve blocks and ablations, joint injections, implanted pumps, and transcutaneous or implanted peripheral or dorsal column stimulators as well as behavioral medicine approaches. In recent years, portable ultrasound has become an easily accessible, user-friendly tool in diagnosis and interventional treatment of chest wall pain. In most cases of chest wall pain, conservative, multidisciplinary approaches are initially preferred, saving invasive treatments for the more refractory cases.

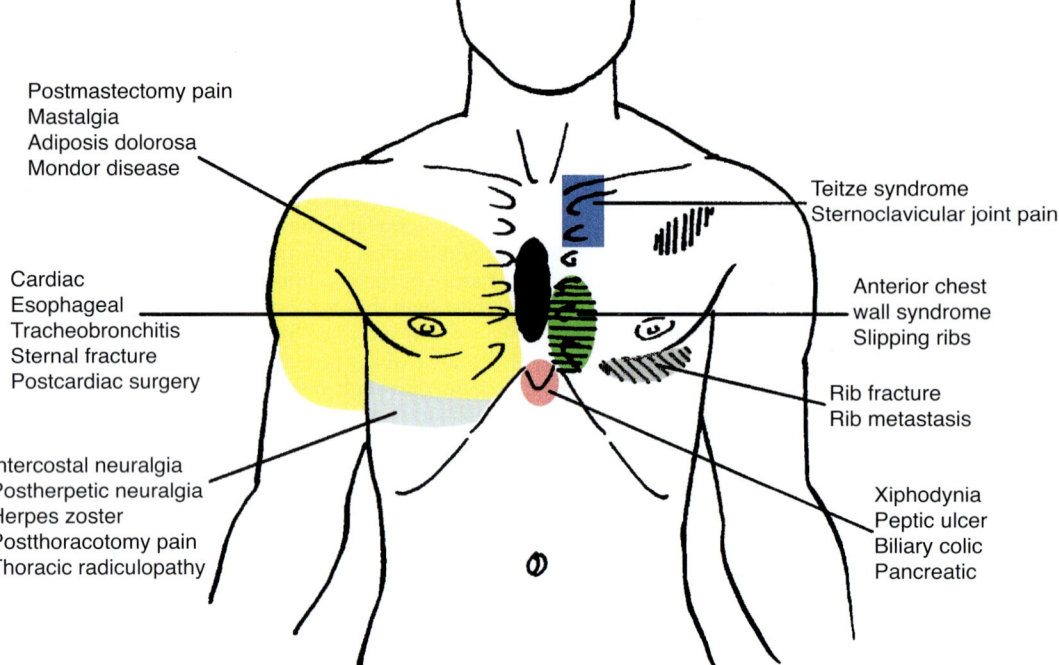

FIGURE 69.12 Common sites of anterior chest wall pain due to chest wall structures or referred pain.

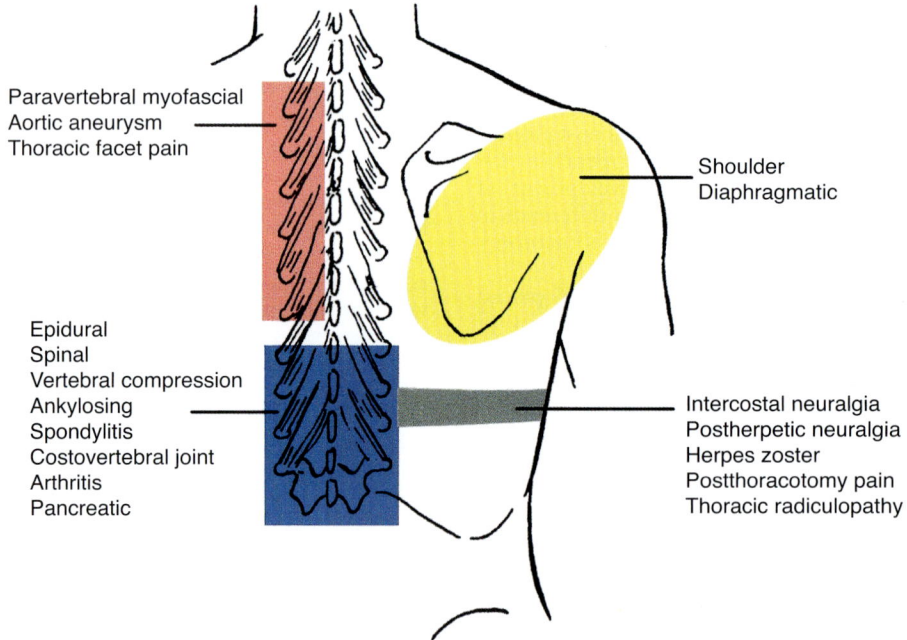

FIGURE 69.13 Common sites of posterior chest wall pain due to chest wall structures or referred pain.

TABLE 69.3 **Pain in the Chest: Summary of Differential Diagnosis**

Etiology (Disease)	International Association for the Study of Pain Code Reference[a]	Important Diagnostic Features	
		Characteristics of the Pain	Associated Symptoms and Signs
I. Pain caused by disease of the heart and aorta			
A. Angina pectoris (stable angina, unstable angina, variant angina)	XVII-4	Mild, moderate, severe, or excruciating anterior chest pain felt predominantly retrosternally with radiation to parasternal region, left arm or right arm or both, epigastrium, and, less frequently, to the interscapular region, neck, and lower jaw; discomfort felt as severe oppression or heaviness on the chest, a sense of constriction or bandlike pressure, or a feeling of choking, strangling, or tight pressure on the neck; pain provoked by physical effort, severe emotional stress, or a large meal (except unstable angina, which occurs at rest or with little or no provocation); lasts 2–5 min with stable angina, 15–30 min or longer with unstable angina and variant angina; promptly relieved with nitroglycerin or discontinuation of effort	History of previous anginal attacks; can have normal ECG at rest, but ST depression and other ECG changes during stress test; positive evidence with radionuclide stress testing and coronary arteriography; demonstration of coronary artery spasm in variant angina
B. Acute myocardial infarction	XVII-5	Pain of same character, location, and reference as angina but of sudden onset, much more severe, and of longer duration (1–8 h or more); little or no relief with nitroglycerin; intense pain often accompanied by strong alarm reaction and feeling of impending death	Frequent nausea, vomiting, and profuse sweating; many patients develop tenderness in pectoral muscle and deep muscle of interscapular region; some develop bradycardia and hypotension and others tachycardia and hypertension; ECG changes include Q-wave and ST-segment elevation and increased creatine kinase and other serum enzyme levels
C. Aortic stenosis	—	Dyspnea first symptom but angina occurs with severe aortic stenosis; chest pain occurs during physical exertion as a result of increased oxygen demand from increased myocardial mass and high ventricular systolic pressure	With severe disease, exertional syncope is caused by decline in arterial pressure; left ventricular failure, palpitation, fatigue, weakness, peripheral cyanosis, narrow pulse pressure, and palpable systolic murmur; increased QRS complex and ST- and T-wave alterations
D. Aortic regurgitation	—	Asymptomatic early in disease; dyspnea on exertion; pain late symptom of severe disease that can occur at rest as well as with exertion and persists longer than angina of coronary artery disease; some patients have neck and abdominal pain	Dyspnea on exertion, flushing, sweating, palpitation; increased fatigue progresses to orthopnea and eventually to paroxysmal nocturnal dyspnea; high-pitched crescendo diastolic murmur along left sternal border
E. Mitral valve prolapse	—	Sharp, stabbing chest pain not provoked by exertion and unresponsive to nitroglycerin; more frequent in female subjects	Cardiac arrhythmia produces palpitation and rarely dizziness, syncope, or even sudden death; midsystolic click and late systolic murmur
F. Hypertrophic cardiomyopathy	—	Most patients asymptomatic; symptomatic patients have dyspnea on exertion because of increased stiffness of left ventricular walls; typical angina pectoris with exertion	Atrial and ventricular arrhythmias produce palpitation, dizziness, and syncope; ECG shows QRS changes of left ventricular hypertrophy and abnormal Q wave
G. Acute pericarditis	XVII-6	Severe, sharp chest pain; worse in supine position, partially relieved by sitting; markedly aggravated by deep breathing; pain usually retrosternal (central), radiates to the neck and trapezius ridge but not to the arms	Dyspnea occurs because of marked increase in pain with normal respiration; triphasic pericardial friction rub occurs with atrial systole, ventricular systole, and ventricular diastole, occasionally only biphasic; ECG initially shows ST-segment elevation and later T-wave flattening
H. Diseases of the thoracic aorta			
1. Dissecting aneurysm	—	Sudden, severe excruciating pain with maximal intensity at its onset; location of pain helps to localize dissection: ascending aortic dissection produces anterior chest pain in 65% of patients and posterior chest pain in 50%; dissection in descending thoracic aorta produces back pain in nearly all patients; radiation to the neck, throat, jaw, and abdomen in a small percentage of patients	Nausea, vomiting, diaphoresis, bradycardia, and hypotension or tachycardia and hypertension; loss of one or more arterial pulses; sense of impending death, apprehension

(continued)

TABLE 69.3   (Continued)

Etiology (Disease)	International Association for the Study of Pain Code Reference[a]	Important Diagnostic Features	
		Characteristics of the Pain	**Associated Symptoms and Signs**
2. Nondissecting aneurysm	XVII-7	Mild to severe continuous burning, aching pain with bouts of lancinating pain; radiation to the chest, shoulder, and back caused by mechanical compression or injury of thoracic spinal nerves; erosion of bone causes boring, agonizing, intractable back pain	Dyspnea, cough, dysphagia, hoarseness; Horner syndrome; pulsating mass; radiographic evidence
II. Diseases of the respiratory system			
A. Diseases of the tracheobronchial tree			
1. Acute tracheobronchitis (infectious, irritative, thermal injury)	—	Mild to moderate burning, aching pain in the retrosternal and parasternal regions; pain severe with thermal injury; associated with sore throat	Preceded by upper respiratory infection: coryza, malaise, chilliness, slight fever, back and muscle pain; with bronchitis, initially dry and nonproductive cough but later mucoid or mucopurulent, dyspnea might be present
2. Bronchiectasis	—	Mild to moderate aching pain in retrosternal and parasternal regions	Chronic cough and sputum production; with progression, cough becomes more productive, hemoptysis common, recurrent pneumonia frequent; wheezing, dyspnea in severe cases
B. Diseases of the pulmonary circulation			
1. Acute pulmonary hypertension	—	Severe crushing, gripping pain in the center of the chest simulating that of acute myocardial infarction, but does not radiate to arms or jaw and seldom to back	Usually decrease in arterial PO_2 can have dyspnea, cyanosis, sweating
2. Chronic pulmonary hypertension (primary, secondary)	—	Pain in anterior chest, primarily retrosternal; radiation to neck; some patients have typical angina pectoris complicated by myocardial ischemia	Primary hypertension usually in female subjects; dyspnea, easy fatigue, less frequently syncope; right ventricular hypertrophy can progress to failure
3. Pulmonary embolism	—	With large embolus pain is sudden, severe, crushing, and of a visceral central type; simulates pain of myocardial infarction but does not radiate to the jaw or arms; lasts for minutes to several hours; small embolus produces localized severe pleuritic pain that is persistent and lasts a week or longer; aggravated by deep breathing or coughing	Feeling of impending death (angor animi), pressure on throat, desire to defecate; history of thrombi in leg, pelvis, occasionally in upper extremity; rarely, embolic fluid or fat emboli; initially the large embolus usually produces pulmonary hypertension from increased pulmonary vascular resistance, leading to decreased cardiac output, hypotension that can progress to shock, with sweating, tachypnea, dyspnea, arterial hypoxemia; hemoptysis, pleural friction rub with small embolus; radiography reveals wedge-shaped shadow
C. Diseases of the lungs			
1. Pneumonia	—	With lobar pneumonia, patient develops pleuritis with moderate to severe pain in lateral chest or shoulder aggravated by deep breathing and coughing (because of involvement of central diaphragmatic pleura); little or no pain with bronchopneumonia	Systemic symptoms and signs of infection: fever, cough, occasionally nausea, vomiting, malaise, and muscle pain; blood-streaked sputum, occasionally hemoptysis; rhonchi; percussion reveals dullness; radiographic evidence
2. Lung abscess	—	Typical pleuritic chest pain if abscess produces pleuritis; characteristics similar to those of lobar pneumonia (see earlier)	Malaise, anorexia, sputum-producing cough, sweats, severe prostration, and fever; putrid odor (anaerobic infection); fine moist rales
3. Atelectasis	—	Rapid occlusion with massive lung collapse causes moderate to severe pain on the affected side	Rapid collapse causes dyspnea, cyanosis, hypotension, tachycardia, fever, and shock; percussion, dullness, or flatness; diminished or absent breath sounds; decreased chest excursion of affected side
D. Disorders of the pleura			
1. Pneumothorax (spontaneous)	—	Sudden moderate to severe stabbing, sharp pain felt across the chest or over abdomen or corresponding shoulder, can simulate pain of acute myocardial infarction or acute abdomen	Dyspnea, absent breath sounds; with large or tension pneumothorax tympany on percussion; decreased excursion of affected side; cardiac dullness and apex felt away from affected side; radiographic evidence

TABLE 69.3 (Continued)

Etiology (Disease)	International Association for the Study of Pain Code Reference[a]	Important Diagnostic Features	
		Characteristics of the Pain	**Associated Symptoms and Signs**
2. Pleuritis (pneumonitis, pulmonary infarct, pleural tumors, lung abscess, actinomycosis, coccidiomycosis, other infectious processes)	—	Localized, sharp, knifelike stabbing, piercing pain in various regions of the chest depending on the site of pathology (side, shoulder, epigastrium); markedly aggravated by deep breathing, coughing, laughing, movement of the chest; pain can be continuous with pleural carcinoma	Diagnostic pleural friction rub; history and systemic symptoms and signs of infection; chest signs (rales, rhonchi); radiographic evidence
3. Epidemic pleurodynia (Bornholm disease)	—	Severe paroxysmal sharp pain in side of chest wall, epigastrium, costovertebral region, and abdomen	Fever, headache; occasionally orchitis, encephalitis, and pericarditis occur during epidemic pleurodynia
E. Bronchogenic and metastatic carcinoma of the lung, bronchial pleura (squamous cell carcinoma, undifferentiated small or large cell adenocarcinoma, bronchoalveolar carcinoma)	—	Location, quality, and severity of pain depend on location and type of spread: a. Endobronchial carcinoma: sternal and parasternal pain b. Intrapulmonary carcinoma: vague central (visceral) pain c. Pleural spread: sharp, stabbing, chest wall pain markedly aggravated by breathing, coughing, movement d. Mediastinal spread: neuropathy with segmental pain e. Pancoast syndrome (brachial plexopathy): pain in shoulder, scapula, medial arm	Weight loss; paraneoplastic syndromes; other signs and symptoms: a. Cough, hemoptysis b. Hypoxia, dyspnea, atelectasis c. Signs and symptoms of pleuritis (see earlier) d. Compression of superior vena cava ∅ superior vena cava syndrome e. Horner syndrome, hoarseness, weakness of all muscles supplied by the ulnar nerve
III. Diseases of the esophagus A. Esophagitis 1. Gastroesophageal reflux disease	XIX-4	Retrosternal pain extends from suprasternal notch to xiphoid process; radiation to epigastrium, neck and back, and, rarely, arms; simulates pain of myocardial ischemia; lasts seconds to many hours; aggravated by stooping or lifting, recumbency, citrus juices, exercise, heavy meal, coffee, alcohol, aspirin, tobacco, and obesity; relieved by antacids	Dysphagia, odynophagia, regurgitation, and occasionally aspiration; diagnosis helped by pH monitoring, acid perfusion test, and esophagoscopy
2. Acute and chronic esophagitis caused by infection or chemical agents	XIX-4	Corrosive agents: immediate, severe, burning pain in throat and behind the whole length of the sternum down to epigastrium, pain is constant with periodic increases in intensity produced by esophageal spasm; infection: pain appears gradually over a period of hours or days and is constant, mild to moderate, and burning in character; both are markedly aggravated by swallowing (odynophagia) and by citrus juices and other factors listed previously for gastroesophageal reflux disease	Infection: signs and symptoms of inflammation (e.g., fever, chills); chemical esophagitis: pharyngeal erythema; moniliasis; typical soft white patches in tongue, tonsil, and buccal mucosa; other associated symptoms as earlier (e.g., dysphagia, odynophagia)
B. Esophageal motor disorders (achalasia; diffuse spasm unclassified motor disorders)	XIX-3	Moderate to severe retrosternal pain; radiation to epigastrium and back, neck, jaw, teeth, left arm, or both arms; aggravated by cold liquids, solids, and emotional stress; partially relieved by nitroglycerin; lasts seconds to many hours and can awaken patient from sleep; simulates pain of myocardial infarction	Dysphagia, odynophagia; diagnosis aided by manometry, scintigraphy, provocative tests (e.g., edrophonium- or methacholine-induced esophageal spasm)
C. Esophageal laceration and rupture (Mallory-Weiss syndrome, Boerhaave syndrome)	—	Mallory-Weiss syndrome: laceration of distal esophagus and proximal stomach during retching, vomiting, or hiccup causes pain in lower sternum and epigastrium; Boerhaave syndrome: spontaneous rupture occurs during intense vomiting following a large meal and causes sudden, severe, excruciating crushing or tearing pain in lower retrosternal region and epigastrium, with radiation to the back	Dysphagia, odynophagia; rupture ∅ mediastinitis ∅ acute illness, epigastric tenderness, and later subcutaneous emphysema and left pleural effusion

(continued)

TABLE 69.3 (Continued)			
	International Association for the Study of Pain Code Reference[a]	**Important Diagnostic Features**	
Etiology (Disease)		**Characteristics of the Pain**	**Associated Symptoms and Signs**
D. Carcinoma	—	Moderate to severe retrosternal pain; radiation to epigastrium with lower lesions and to upper sternum with upper lesions; radiation to neck, interscapular region; pain continuous and aggravated by food ingestion	Dysphagia, odynophagia, weight loss; esophageal obstruction; radiographic, CT, and esophagoscopic evidence
E. Paraesophageal hiatal hernia	XIX-2	Generally asymptomatic; might be feeling of epigastric fullness and lower retrosternal discomfort; with incarceration and strangulation severe, excruciating epigastric and retrosternal pain	Possible massive gastrointestinal hemorrhage; radiographic and esophagoscopic evidence
IV. Diseases of the mediastinum and diaphragm			
A. Mediastinal disorders			
1. Spontaneous mediastinal emphysema	—	Sudden intense, violent, agonizing retrosternal or precordial pain; radiation to nape of neck and shoulder associated with pleural pain; persists for hours	Signs of emphysema: crunching sound in area of pain, decreased or obliterated cardiac dullness, pneumothorax, subcutaneous emphysema (crepitus); radiographic evidence
2. Acute or chronic mediastinitis	—	Continuous; mild to moderate; retrosternal, central; oppressive or burning, aching sensation; can be severe	Systemic signs of infection; history of esophageal rupture or other trauma
3. Neoplasms (anterior compartment, superior compartment, middle compartment, posterior compartment)	—	One-third of patients asymptomatic: remainder have chest pain, cough, dyspnea, and symptoms caused by compression or invasion of structures in mediastinum	Middle compartment: dysphagia, hoarseness; anterior compartment, superior compartment: retrosternal and suprasternal discomfort, local chest pain from pressure on sternum; posterior compartment: neurogenic tumors, vague chest pain, cough, radicular pain from neuropathy, superior vena cava syndrome
B. Diseases of the diaphragm			
1. Diaphragmatic pleuritis	—	Sharp, stabbing *pleuritic* pain along the nape and shoulder or in the posterior and lateral parts of the lower chest and upper abdomen, or both; aggravated by diaphragmatic motion	Signs and symptoms of pneumonitis or infectious processes with inflammation of diaphragmatic pleura
2. Acute primary diaphragmatitis (Hedblom syndrome)	—	Moderate to severe pain in lower chest, upper abdomen, and shoulder	Chills and fever; muscle spasm of abdomen; decreased lung expansion on inspiration; radiographic evidence of flattened diaphragm
3. Diaphragmatic spasm	—	Precordial pain; radiation to shoulder	Dyspnea during sustained spasm of the diaphragm can cause occlusion of esophagus; some patients develop progressive dyspnea, pallor, sweating, hypotension, and angor animi simulating that of acute myocardial infarction; occlusion of the esophagus causes dysphagia and odynophagia
4. Diaphragmatic flutter	—	Lower chest pain felt along the diaphragmatic attachment in the epigastrium, precordium; radiation to the shoulder and occasionally to the neck and arm	Dyspnea, palpitation; symptoms and signs of various causative factors (e.g., encephalitis, intoxication)
V. Pain of neuropathic origin			
A. Lesions or diseases of the spinal cord (myelopathy)			
1. Intramedullary lesion (tumor, syringomyelia, trauma, multiple sclerosis, abscess, hemorrhage)	I-6	Spontaneous, burning, diffuse, poorly localized pain; bouts of explosive pain; later radicular pain involving several segments, depending on the size of the lesion	Dissociation of sensation, loss of pain and temperature sensation but little effect on proprioception; sensory changes often "spotty"; lower motor neuron signs; with multiple sclerosis spotty paresthesia, pain, symptoms and signs of other involved parts of CNS
2. Extramedullary lesion (primary or metastatic tumor; abscess; hemorrhage)	I-6	Initially localized back pain but subsequently pain is radicular; aggravated by increase in CSF pressure, such as that caused by straining, sneezing, coughing	Paravertebral tenderness, paresthesia, followed by sensory loss, muscular weakness; lower motor neuron signs at level of lesion; increased deep reflexes; CSF changes early and marked; spinal cord compression with large lesion

TABLE 69.3 (Continued)

Etiology (Disease)	International Association for the Study of Pain Code Reference[a]	Important Diagnostic Features	
		Characteristics of the Pain	**Associated Symptoms and Signs**
3. Epidural spinal cord compression (primary or metastatic tumor, hemorrhage, posterior disk protrusion, abscess, hemorrhage)	—	Localized back pain at level of site of lesion in 95% of patients; bilateral radicular pain in segments affected by lesion in 55%; aggravated by neck flexion, straight leg raising, coughing, sneezing, Valsalva maneuver	Back tenderness on deep palpation, fist pounding; no other early signs, but later muscle weakness ranging from mild degree to paraplegia; numbness and paresthesia in 50%; bladder and bowel dysfunction with low thoracic epidural spinal cord compression
B. Lesions of rootlets or roots of T1–T12 (radiculopathy)			
1. Herpes zoster	I-1	Continuous aching, itching, or burning pain, often with superimposed bouts of severe lancinating pain; hyperalgesia; aggravated by trunk motion, palpation of vesicles; persists until healing of rash (1–4 wk)	Appearance of rash, later vesicles form and then crust; hyperalgesia and hyperesthesia of skin in affected segments; occasionally systemic symptoms of infection; mood and behavioral changes with unrelieved pain
2. Postherpetic neuralgia	I-1	Severe, continuous, unrelenting burning pain, itching; accompanied by severe paroxysms of stabbing, lancinating pain that persist long after acute phase	Hyperalgesia, hypesthesia, hyperpathia; scar in area of vesicles; reactive depression, sleep disturbances, anorexia, lassitude, constipation, decreased libido; high suicide rate among those with unrelieved postherpetic neuralgia
3. Tabes dorsalis	I-6	Severe, sharp, lancinating, girdle-like (segmental) pain of brief duration with intervals of remission	History of syphilis; CSF evidence; other symptoms of CNS syphilis
4. Mechanical compression (tumor, disk protrusion, vertebral fracture, osteophyte, adhesive arachnoiditis)	—	Segmental sharp, burning pain; aggravated by cough, sneezing, straining, and movement of trunk	Hyperalgesia, hyperesthesia, hypesthesia, dysesthesia; radiographic evidence of pathology
C. Diseases of formed thoracic spinal nerves (neuropathy)			
1. Vertebral compression (arthritis, metastatic or traumatic fracture, tumor of vertebrae, osteomyelitis)	—	Segmental neuralgia usually present: continuous burning or sharp pain affecting part or entire segment of nerve, associated with paroxysms of stabbing pain; compression of anterior root produces dull, aching, occasionally stabbing pain in part of affected segment; both aggravated by movement of thoracic spine; often worse at night	Paravertebral tenderness and segmental hyperalgesia, hyperesthesia, hypesthesia; radiographic evidence (CT scan)
2. Paravertebral compression (mediastinal tumors, aortic aneurysm, paravertebral abscess, or adenopathy)	—	Continuous moderate to severe burning, aching segmental pain; aggravated by movement of spine; occasional bouts of lancinating pain	Paravertebral tenderness; segmental hyperalgesia, hypesthesia; radiographic evidence
3. Primary neurogenic tumors (neurofibroma, schwannoma, ganglioneuroma, neuroblastoma)	—	Possibly localized back pain and tenderness but usually continuous burning, aching pain; associated with lancinating pain in distribution of affected nerve	Sensory deficit (hypesthesia), paresthesia, dysesthesia; CT scan and radiographic evidence
4. Other neuropathies (systemic infection, alcoholism, avitaminosis, diabetes, metals)	—	Continuous or intermittent mild to moderate burning pain; associated with paroxysms of stabbing pain in one or more dermatomes	History of infection, alcoholism, nutrition deficiency, exposure to ingestion of metals; hyperesthesia, hyperalgesia, hypesthesia, paresthesia, dysesthesia; other signs and symptoms of primary disorder
D. Lesion or disease of the intercostal nerves—intercostal neuropathy (compression or irritation secondary to rib fracture; trauma; primary or metastatic tumor of ribs; pleuritis)	—	Superficial continuous burning pain in distribution of affected intercostal nerve; also, local pain with rib fracture or tumor, pleuritic pain with pleuritis	History of trauma or infection; paresthesia, hyperesthesia, dysesthesia, hypesthesia; superficial and deep tenderness; radiographic evidence; palpable tumor or fracture
VI. Pain of musculoskeletal origin			
A. Lesions of the thoracic spine			
1. Fracture (trauma, neoplasm, osteoporosis, subluxation, dislocation)	—	Initially localized dull, aching pain, often referred to anterior part of chest; aggravated by motion, worse and throbbing at night; segmental pain with root compression	History of trauma; radiographic evidence; localized tenderness paravertebrally and over spinous processes; possibly segmental hyperalgesia, paresthesia

(continued)

TABLE 69.3   (Continued)

Etiology (Disease)	International Association for the Study of Pain Code Reference[a]	Important Diagnostic Features	
		Characteristics of the Pain	**Associated Symptoms and Signs**
2. Metastatic or primary tumors	—	Intense aching, boring circumscribed pain; aggravated by motion and local pressure	Local tenderness or segmental hyperalgesia and hyperesthesia; CT scan and radiographic evidence
3. Arthritis or deformity of spine	—	Usually circumscribed aching pain in back and side; segmental pain with neuropathy	Signs of arthritis in other areas; deformity of spine evident; local tenderness; reflex muscle spasm; radiographic evidence
4. Ankylosing spondylitis	—	Usually circumscribed dull aching pain in back; later paraspinal contractures develop with compression of nerve root, which causes segmental pain	Tenderness on deep palpation; radiographic evidence
5. Diffuse idiopathic skeletal hyperostosis	—	Mild to moderate localized, dull, aching pain; aggravated by inactivity and cold	Tenderness and stiffness in thoracic spine; dorsal kyphosis; reduction of range of movement and in chest expansion; characteristic radiographic evidence
6. Inflammatory disease of vertebrae (osteomyelitis, actinomycosis, tuberculosis, syphilis, subperiosteal hematoma)	—	Circumscribed, continuous, aching pain; moderate to severe; aggravated by pressure, often worse at night	Local and systemic symptoms and signs of inflammation; localized tenderness paravertebrally and over spinous process
7. Costovertebral joint arthritis	—	Localized deep aching pain similar to that arising from vertebral pathology; aggravated by movement; relieved by local infiltration of joint	Tenderness on deep palpation; radiographic evidence
8. Apophyseal facet syndrome	—	Moderate to severe, dull, aching, localized pain and tenderness; aggravated by hyperextension; relieved by flexion of the spine	Tenderness; limitation of motion, flattening of normal kyphotic thoracic curve; paraspinal muscle spasm
B. Rib lesions			
1. Fracture or trauma (severe cough, osteoporosis, metastatic tumor)	—	Localized sharp pain at site of lesion; widespread chest pain with multiple rib fractures; pain aggravated by deep breathing, coughing, movement of thorax	History of accidental trauma or severe coughing; evidence of osteoporosis; exquisite tenderness on palpation of fracture site; radiographic evidence; with compound fracture can have pneumothorax and damage to lung, with respiratory symptoms and signs
2. Primary metastatic rib tumor (myeloma, chondrosarcoma, granuloma)	—	Mild to moderate or severe continuous unilateral dull, aching, chest pain; relatively localized but can also produce intercostal neuralgia	Palpable mass and tenderness to pressure; radiographic evidence
3. Other bone diseases (osteitis deformans, acromegaly, Paget disease, osteoporosis, hyperostosis)	—	Localized continuous aching pain; intercostal neuralgia if lesion irritates nerve	Evidence of disease elsewhere; tenderness on palpation; radiographic evidence
C. Disorders of the costal cartilages			
1. Costochondritis (anterior chest wall syndrome)	—	Unilateral or bilateral aching pain in lower anterior chest wall usually in region of cartilages of third, sixth, and seventh ribs; aggravated by deep breathing, coughing, palpation	No swelling of costochondral region; more frequent in younger than older people; development of anxiety and concern about heart disease if pain is on left side
2. Tietze syndrome	—	Localized moderate dull, aching pain in upper anterior chest in region of second and perhaps third costochondral junction; aggravated by palpation, movement of chest wall, coughing, respiratory infection; worse when lying down; recurs between intervals of remission	Palpable tender tumorlike swelling at site of costochondral joint; occurs mostly in people older than 50 y; radiography not diagnostic; development of anxiety, fatigue, concern about heart disease
3. Slipping rib syndrome (rib tip syndrome, slipped cartilage)	XVII-10	Unilateral lower chest and upper abdominal localized aching or sharp pain; aggravated by hyperextension and raising of arms; relieved by forward bending to the affected side	Palpation produces tenderness and reveals upward curling of loosened end of cartilages of 8th, 9th, and 10th ribs; hooking flexed finger under costal cartilage and exerting pressure anteriorly produces clicking noise
4. Fracture of cartilage or dislocation of costochondral joint	—	Sudden sharp pain from fracture or dislocation followed by continuous dull aching, burning discomfort in area of costal margin; reference to back	History of injury; tenderness on palpation; displaced cartilage is palpable and feels like lump

TABLE 69.3 (Continued)

Etiology (Disease)	International Association for the Study of Pain Code Reference[a]	Important Diagnostic Features	
		Characteristics of the Pain	Associated Symptoms and Signs
D. Lesions or disorders of the sternum			
1. Fracture of sternum	—	Localized pain in region of sternum, usually sharp initially but then continuous and aching; aggravated by deep breathing or palpation	History of blunt trauma to anterior chest; tenderness to palpation; leads to manubriosternal arthralgia
2. Rheumatoid arthritis or osteoarthritis	—	Continuous or intermittent pain localized to the angle of Louis; aggravated by deep breathing, coughing, sneezing, and yawning	Mild swelling of joint; exquisite tenderness to palpation; systemic arthritis present; radiographic evidence of arthropathy
3. Xiphoidalgia (hypersensitive xiphoid syndrome, xiphodynia)	—	Spontaneous deep aching or sharp pain varying in intensity from a slight to agonizing discomfort that simulates pain of myocardial infarction; aggravated by movements that act on xiphoid process (e.g., bending, stooping, turning) and by increase in intragastric pressure caused by a large meal; can be constant or recurs several times a day; lasts for minutes to several hours	Pressure on xiphoid process produces spontaneous pain that can radiate deep retrosternally and to the precordium, epigastrium, and across shoulder and back; persists for weeks or months but usually disappears spontaneously
4. Arthritis of sternoclavicular joint	—	Localized sharp or aching pain in region of joint; radiation to shoulder and upper chest	Joint swollen, tender on palpation; radiographic evidence
E. Muscle disorders			
1. Myofascial pain syndromes with trigger points			
a. Anterior chest (major and minor, pectoralis; scaleni; sternalis; intercostals)	—	Frequent cause of pain in anterior chest; pain is deep and aching; aggravated by activity; sternalis and pectoralis pain can simulate pain of angina pectoris; pain relieved by injection of trigger points with local anesthetic	History of severe strain by heavy lifting; local tenderness, trigger points present; unaffected body activity
b. Lateral chest (serratus anterior; intercostals)	—	Deep aching pain on the lateral aspect of the chest extending from the lower axilla to about the seventh to the sixth ribs; pain also in area near the inferior angle of the scapula; with intercostal syndrome site of pain varies with site of trigger points; relief with trigger point injection	Localized tenderness and trigger point about the level of the sixth rib; pressure on trigger points produces spontaneous pain
c. Posterior chest (rhomboidei, latissimus dorsi multifidi, serratus posterior superior, iliocostalis thoracis)	—	Deep aching pain in different parts of the back depending on the site of the trigger point and the muscles involved; aggravated by activity of muscles, unaffected by bodily activity	Localized tenderness and trigger points
2. Acute muscle spasm	—	Sharp localized pain in area of the spastic muscle; some radiation to anterior and posterior chest; complete relief with infiltration of muscle	Palpation of spastic muscle; generalized tenderness
3. Muscle contractures	—	Constant deep aching pain, often associated with early spondylosis	Possible localized tenderness of affected muscle or in an area of reference
4. Dermatomyositis and polymyositis	—	Rarely a cause of chest pain; when present, pain aching and aggravated by palpation	Generalized weakness; elevated serum levels of skeletal muscle enzyme
VII. Pain of tegumentary origin (including the breast)			
A. Acute disorders			
1. Burns and other trauma	—	Sharp burning pain following burns, aching pain with trauma	History of injury or burn; emotional reactions
2. Postoperative pain	—	Fairly localized sharp, burning, aching pain primarily at the site of incision; can radiate to involve adjacent segments	Reflex muscle spasm, tenderness; hyperalgesia; tachycardia response; signs of neuroendocrine stress
3. Acute mastodynia (inflammatory)	—	Sharp, aching, burning pain in chest; radiation to axilla and inner arm; aggravated by movement of the breast	Extreme tenderness, tumefaction; evidence of infection
4. Deep axillary abscess	—	Sharp localized, diffuse dull, aching pain in axilla; radiation to anterior chest and medial arm	Tenderness, fluctuating mass; signs of infection

(continued)

TABLE 69.3   (Continued)

Etiology (Disease)	International Association for the Study of Pain Code Reference[a]	Important Diagnostic Features	
		Characteristics of the Pain	**Associated Symptoms and Signs**
5. Acute dermatologic disorders (vesicles, furuncles, bullae, pustules, ulcers, erythema, cellulitis)	—	Aching, burning, itching pain localized to lesion	Possible evidence of local or systemic disease
B. Chronic disorders			
1. Postmastectomy syndrome		Sharp, burning, aching pain and tingling in the chest wall, armpit or arm sometimes associated with numbness or unbearable itching.	Hyperesthesia, hyperalgesia, hypesthesia, paresthesia; neuroma often palpable; evidence of recurrent cancer by use of CT scan or other diagnostic procedures
2. Postthoracotomy syndrome		Sharp, burning, aching pain; accompanied by bouts of lancinating pain in distribution of the dermatomes supplied by the injured nerve or in part of the segment; aggravated by light touch of skin, palpation of neuroma, and emotional stress	Hyperesthesia, hyperalgesia, hypesthesia, paresthesia; neuroma often palpable; evidence of recurrent cancer by use of CT scan or other diagnostic procedures
3. Adiposis dolorosa (Dercum disease)	—	Enlarged painful fatty subcutaneous nodule most commonly in the chest and arms but can affect any part except the face; usually darting, shooting, or stabbing pain; occurs spontaneously or provoked by palpation	Usually occurs in obese women; weakness, fatigue, emotional instability, occasional dementia
4. Chronic mastalgia	—	Chronic persistent pain; cyclic in two-thirds of patients and continuous in the other third; deep, aching, diffuse pain over entire breast without palpable evidence of pathology; about 20% have spontaneous intermittent relief, whereas others have relief at menopause or pregnancy or with use of oral contraceptives; those with noncyclic pain have pain that can persist for 2–3 y or for as long as 30 y	Psychological tests usually reveal no abnormality; positive response to hormonal manipulation suggests a hormonal basis to the condition
5. Scleroderma (dermatomyositis, disseminating lupus erythematosus, polyarteritis nodosa)	—	Dull, aching, occasionally burning pain in the chest wall, usually in the area of the lesion; with scleroderma, chest pain can arise from skin, thoracic wall, or myocardial or esophageal lesions	Symptoms and signs of systemic disease; many types produce widespread visceral involvement
6. Other chronic dermatologic diseases	—	(See Chapter 31 for detailed discussion)	
7. Mondor disease (phlebitis of anterolateral chest)	—	Rare condition manifested by thrombosis of superficial vein of thoracic wall that produces palpable painful cord within the skin; usually sharp and persistent; intensified by deep inspiration or flexion of the trunk	Presence of painful, tender, subcutaneous cord running obliquely across thorax in distribution of one or more superficial veins; lesion indolent after several weeks
C. Cancer of the breast	—	Early breast cancer not painful; in far advanced disease, skin nodule eventually breaks down and formation also causes localized breast pain; metastasis to the pleura produces pleuritic pain; metastasis to the ribs causes localized pain and can be associated with segmental neuralgia; metastasis to the spine produces back pain and later can cause epidural spinal cord compression or plexopathy	Early: retracted nipple, bleeding, distorted areola or breast contour, skin dimpling (*peau d'orange*); later: axillary supraclavicular adenopathy; metastatic lesion demonstrated by radiography and CT scan
VIII. Chest pain referred from extrathoracic disorders			
A. Disorders of the cervical spine that cause neuropathy			
1. Posterolateral protrusion of intervertebral disk (C7, C8)		Pain in the neck, shoulder, medial aspect of the arm, and pectoral region of the chest; with left-sided lesion, pain can simulate that of myocardial ischemia but is differentiated by aggravation by lateral flexion and the Spurling test (see Chapter 54); unaffected by activity if neck and arms not moved	Paravertebral and pectoral muscle tenderness; hyperalgesia, hyperesthesia, and paresthesia of the arm; decrease in reflexes and some muscle weakness in the upper limbs
2. Arthritis, osteophyte, fracture or other lesion that compresses root or nerve			

TABLE 69.3 (Continued)

Etiology (Disease)	International Association for the Study of Pain Code Reference[a]	Important Diagnostic Features	
		Characteristics of the Pain	**Associated Symptoms and Signs**
3. Thoracic inlet syndromes (scalenus anticus syndrome; cervical rib or abnormal first rib; costoclavicular compression)	—	Pain most prominent in the shoulder and upper limbs; radiation to the upper pectoral region; aggravated by severe arm abduction and walking with swinging arms; unaffected by activity if arms not moved	Supraclavicular (scaleni) tenderness and fullness; neurovascular signs and symptoms in the upper extremities; radiographic evidence of abnormal cervical rib
4. Pancoast syndrome	—	Pain in shoulder, scapula, medial aspect of arm, and superior anterior chest; aggravated by extreme abduction of the arm and paravertebral pressure; unaffected by activity if neck and limbs are not moved	Signs and symptoms of plexopathy with paresthesia, dysesthesia, numbness in the medial aspects of the forearm and fourth and fifth fingers, also medial aspect of arm; marked weakness of muscles supplied by ulnar nerve; radiographic and CT scan evidence of lesion
B. Diseases of the abdominal viscera			
1. Gas entrapment syndromes (e.g., caused by aerophagia, excess production of gas in bowel)	—	Bloated sensation associated with pain in the epigastrium and central lower chest; if diaphragm irritated, pain also in shoulder; dull, aching pain worsens as day progresses; transiently relieved by belching; gas entrapment in hepatic flexure of colon produces discomfort in right upper quadrant and lower part of right chest, gas in splenic flexure causes pain in left upper quadrant and left lower chest	History of aerophagia, abdominal tympany; radiographic evidence
2. Peptic ulcer disease	—	Ulcer in cardia of stomach produces pain in the epigastrium and central lower anterior chest, ulcer in other locations not associated with chest pain; duodenal ulcer causes pain that radiates to xiphoid process but not higher	Peptic ulcer confirmed by radiography and endoscopy
3. Perforated ulcer	—	Sudden severe epigastric pain that can radiate to lower chest with severe hypotension; myocardial ischemia; anginal pain	History, physical signs (e.g., muscle spasm, shock, diaphoresis, hematemesis)
4. Biliary colic	—	Sudden moderate to severe epigastric pain; radiation to back; right subcostal region and low central portion of right chest; rarely, pain confined only to chest mimicking that of myocardial infarction, but no radiation to arm or jaw	Patient can have nausea but no vomiting; in distress but no fever; subcostal tenderness
5. Acute cholecystitis	—	Pain usually localized to right upper quadrant; lasts few days rather than a few hours; chest pain rare except in patients with coexisting coronary artery disease: in these patients, biliary pain provokes angina pectoris and ECG changes (low amplitude and inversion of T wave)	Nausea, vomiting, fever, jaundice, and tender right upper quadrant mass; abdominal muscle spasm
6. Acute pancreatitis	—	Sudden severe epigastric pain associated with retrosternal oppression; radiation to lower part of left side of chest; unaffected by effort; often provokes ECG changes similar to those of myocardial ischemia and infarction	Severe abdominal muscle spasm; often hypotension, hypoventilation, elevated blood amylase level
7. Subphrenic abscess	—	Pus from perforated viscus produces subdiaphragmatic abscess with inflammation of the diaphragm; pleuritic pain in the lower chest and often the shoulder; intrapleural rupture of amebic liver abscess; sudden severe chest pain	Dyspnea, fever, pleural effusion and, occasionally, hepatomegaly
IX. Chest pain primarily of psychological origin			
A. Acute anxiety state	—	Sudden acute diffuse pain in chest in the precordial region near cardiac apex (not retrosternal); severe, sharp, stabbing pain or dull, heavy pressure experienced after effort, not during	Dyspnea (air hunger) leading to hyperventilation, tachycardia, dizziness, palpitations, perspiration, tremor, weakness, chest tightness; psychological evaluation and testing reveal evidence of anxiety

(continued)

TABLE 69.3 (Continued)

Etiology (Disease)	International Association for the Study of Pain Code Reference[a]	Important Diagnostic Features	
		Characteristics of the Pain	Associated Symptoms and Signs
B. Chronic anxiety (cardiac neurosis, soldier's heart, neurocirculatory asthenia, irritable heart, effort syndrome)	—	Pain usually at apex of the heart; felt as dull ache with or without attacks of sharp pain over same area; either of brief duration or continuous for hours and days; associated with fatigue rather than effort; responds poorly to all medication	Chronic anxiety and apprehension; severe dyspnea; respiratory distress both at rest and with exertion, sighing respirations; possible ECG changes; low energy level; psychological evaluation and testing reveal psychopathology
C. Depression	—	Endogenous depression can cause atypical chest pain described as a heavy feeling or deep ache or tightness; possible radiation to left arm; usually worse in the morning, lessens as the day goes on	Feeling of overconcern with the heart; in primary affective disorder, patient complains of feelings of depression, guilt, worthlessness, withdrawal, disinterest; occasional suicidal preoccupation, anorexia, weight loss, fatigue, low energy level, malaise, insomnia; psychological evaluation and testing reveal psychopathology
D. Hypochondriasis	—	Precordial or apical pain; pain described by patient in minute detail regarding location, quality, and duration but does not fit pattern of any organic disease, and description of the pain changes from one visit to another	Feeling of overconcern with the heart; many other complaints (e.g., dysfunction of gastrointestinal tract); may present different complaints at different visits; psychological evaluation and testing produces evidence of psychopathology
E. Operant pain (learned pain)	—	Initially, patient has chest pain from disease of the heart or lungs that persists after healing because of reinforcing environmental factors; develops chronic pain behavior and abnormal illness behavior	Progressive physical deterioration over time because of inactivity, muscle weakness, and other factors that cause pain and reinforce the behavior; psychological evaluation and testing reveal psychopathology

CNS, central nervous system; CSF, cerebrospinal fluid; CT, computed tomography; ECG, electrocardiogram; PO_2, partial pressure of oxygen;
[a]See Table 2.2.

References

1. Snell RS, ed. The thorax: part I—the thoracic wall. In: *Clinical Anatomy by Regions*. 8th ed. Philadelphia: Lippincott Williams & Wilkins; 2007:45–73.
2. Standring S, ed. *Gray's Anatomy: The Anatomical Basis of Clinical Practice*. 39th ed. London: Churchill Livingstone; 2005:951–968.
3. Sanders RJ. *Thoracic Outlet Syndrome*. Philadelphia: Lippincott; 1991.
4. Schaumburg HH, Berger AR, Thomas PK. *Disorders of Peripheral Nerves*. 2nd ed. Philadelphia: FA Davis; 1992.
5. White JC. Cardiac pain: anatomic pathways and physiologic mechanisms. *Circulation* 1957;16:644–655.
6. Watson PN, Evans RJ. Intractable pain with lung cancer. *Pain* 1987;29:163–173.
7. Pancoast HK. Superior pulmonary sulcus tumor. *JAMA* 1932;99:1391–1394.
8. Hepper NGG. Thoracic inlet tumors. *Ann Int Med* 1966;64:979–989.
9. Kori S, Foley KM, Posner JB. Brachial plexus lesions in patients with cancer: clinical findings in 100 cases. *Neurology* 1981;31:45–50.
10. Gilbert RW, Kim JH, Posner JB. Epidural spinal cord compression from metastatic tumor. *Ann Neurol* 1978;3:40–51.
11. Posner JB. Back pain and epidural spinal cord compression. *Med Clin North Am* 1987;71:185–205.
12. Sfyroeras GS, Antonopoulos CN, Mantas G. A review of open and endovascular treatment of superior vena cava syndrome of benign etiology. *Eur J Vasc Endovasc Surg* 2017;53:238–254.
13. Rusch V, Ginsberg RJ. Chest wall, pleura, lung, and mediastinum. In: Schwartz SI, Shires GT, eds. *Principles of Surgery*. New York: McGraw-Hill; 1999:667–790.
14. Gucalp R, Dutcher J. Oncologic emergencies. In: Fauci AS, Harrison TR, eds. *Harrisons Principles of Internal Medicine*. New York: McGraw-Hill; 1998:627–634.
15. Yeung MC, Hagen NA. Cervical disc herniation presenting with chest wall pain. *Can J Neurol Sci* 1993;20:59–61.
16. O'Connor RC, Andary MT, Russo RB, et al. Thoracic radiculopathy. *Phys Med Rehabil Clin N Am* 2002;13:623.
17. Deer TR, Pope JE, Hayek SM, et al. The Polyanalgesic Consensus Conference: recommendations for intrathecal drug delivery: guidance for improving safety and mitigating risks. *Neuromodulation* 2017;20:155–176.
18. Donahue JG, Choo PW, Manson JE, et al. The incidence of herpes zoster. *Arch Intern Med* 1995;155:1605–1609.
19. Choo PW, Galil K, Donahue JG, et al. Risk factors for postherpetic neuralgia. *Arch Intern Med* 1997;157:1217–1224.
20. Bowsher D. Pathophysiology of postherpetic neuralgia. *Neurology* 1995;45:S58–S60.
21. Wu JJ, Huang DB, Tyring SK. Dermatologic virology. In: Hall JC, ed. *Sauer's Manual of Skin Diseases*. 9th ed. Philadelphia: Lippincott Williams & Wilkins; 2006:228–229.
22. Schmader K. Management of herpes zoster in elderly patients. *Infect Dis Clin Pract* 1995;4:293–299.
23. Dworkin RH, Perkins FM, Nagasako E. Prospects for the prevention of post herpetic neuralgia in herpes zoster patient. *Clin J Pain* 2000;16:S90–S100.
24. Rowbotham M, Harden N, Stacey B, et al. Gabapentin for the treatment of postherpetic neuralgia. *JAMA* 1998;280:1837–1842.
25. Dworkin RH, Corbin AE, Young JP Jr, et al. Pregabalin for the treatment of post herpetic neuralgia. *Neurology* 2003;60:1274–1283.
26. Chen N, Yang M, He L, et al. Corticosteroids for preventing postherpetic neuralgia. *Cochrane Database Syst Rev* 2010;(12):CD005582.
27. Chen N, Li Q, Zhang Y, et al. Vaccination for preventing postherpetic neuralgia. *Cochrane Database Syst Rev* 2011;(3):CD007795.
28. Argoff C, Katz N, Backonja M. Treatment of postherpetic neuralgia: a review of therapeutic options. *J Pain Symptom Manage* 2004;28:396–411.
29. Rowbotham M, Davies PS, Verkempinck C, et al. Lidocaine patch: double-blind controlled study of a new treatment method for postherpetic neuralgia. *Pain* 1996;65:39–44.
30. Watson CP, Tyler KL, Bickers DR, et al. A randomized vehicle controlled trial of topical capsaicin in the treatment of post herpetic neuralgia. *Clin Ther* 1993;15:510–526.
31. Nathan PW, Wall PD. Treatment of post-herpetic neuralgia by prolonged electrical stimulation. *BMJ* 1974;3:645–647.
32. Trescot AM. Cryoanalgesia in interventional pain management. *Pain Physician* 2003;6:345–360.
33. Akkaya T, Ozkan D. Ultrasound-guided pulsed radiofrequency treatment of the intercostal nerve: three cases. *J Anesth* 2013;27:968–969.
34. Best C. Use of radiofrequency ablation of dorsal root ganglion technique for precision diagnosis and treatment of intercostal neuralgia. *J Pain* 2016;17:S92–S93.
35. Bogduk NB. Assessing a new procedure: thoracic radiofrequency dorsal root ganglion lesions. *Clin J Pain* 1996;12:76–77.

36. Stolker RJ, Vervest AC, Groen GJ. The treatment of chronic thoracic segmental pain by radiofrequency percutaneous partial rhizotomy. *J Neurosurg* 1994;80:986–992.

37. Kang S, Singh J, Vidal Melo M, et al. Spinal cord stimulation for intercostal neuralgia in a patient with implantable cardiac defibrillator and biventricular pacing. *Neuromodulation* 2014;17:386–388.

38. Kostuik JP. Osteoporotic fractures of the spine. In: Vaccaro AR, ed. *Fractures of the Cervical, Thoracic and Lumbar Spine*. New York: Marcel Dekker; 2003:635–653.

39. Cohen MS, Blair B, Garfin SR. Thoracolumbar compression fractures. In: Levine AM, Eismont FJ, Garfin SR, et al, ed. *Spine Trauma*. Philadelphia: WB Saunders; 1998:388–401.

40. Schwartz ED, Flanders AE. *Spinal Trauma*. Philadelphia: Lippincott Williams & Wilkins; 2007.

41. Barr J, Barr M, Lemley T, et al. Percutaneous vertebroplasty for pain relief and spinal stabilization. *Spine* 2000;25:923–928.

42. Mathis JM, Barr JD, Belkoff M. Percutaneous vertebroplasty: a developing standard of care for vertebral compression fractures. *Am J Neuroradiol* 2001;22:373–381.

43. Rodriguez AJ, Fink HA, Mirigian L, et al. Pain, quality of life and safety outcomes of kyphoplasty for vertebral compression fractures: report of a task force of the American Society for Bone and Mineral Research. *J Bone Miner Res* 2017;32(9):1935–1944.

44. Goz V, Errico TJ, Weinreb JH, et al. Vertebroplasty and kyphoplasty: national outcomes and trends in utilization from 2005 through 2010. *Spine J* 2015;15:959–965.

45. Solberg J, Copenhaver D, Fishman SM. Medial branch nerve block and ablation as a novel approach to pain related to vertebral compression fracture. *Curr Opin Anaesthesiol* 2016;29(5):596–599.

46. Reuler JB, Girard DE, Nardone DA. Sternoclavicular joint involvement in ankylosing spondylitis. *South Med J* 1978;71:1480–1481.

47. Wendling D, Prati C, Demattei C, et al. Anterior chest wall pain in recent inflammatory back pain suggestive of spondyloarthritis. Data from DESIR cohort. *J Rheumatol* 2013;40:1148–1152.

48. Nathan H, Weinberg H, Robin GC. The costovertebral joints: anatomical-clinical observations in arthritis. *Arthritis Rheum* 1964;7:228–240.

49. Sanzhang C, Rothschild BM. Zygapophyseal and costovertebral/costotransverse joints: an anatomic assessment of arthritis impact. *Br J Rheumatol* 1993;32:1066–1071.

50. Roth SH. A new role for opioids in the treatment of arthritis. *Drugs* 2002;62:255–263.

51. Sales JR, Beals RK, Hart RA. Osteoarthritis of the costovertebral joints: the results of resection arthroplasty. *J Bone Joint Surg Br* 2007;89(10):1336–1339.

52. Resnick D, Niwayama G. Radiographic and pathologic feature of spinal involvement in diffuse skeletal hyperostosis. *Radiology* 1976;119:559–568.

53. Forestier J, Rotes-Querol J. Senile ankylosing hyperostosis of the spine. *Ann Rheum Dis* 1950;9:321–330.

54. Amital H, Applbaum YH, Aamar DS, et al. SAPHO syndrome treated with pamidronate: an open-label study of 10 patients. *Rheumatology* 2005;44:137–138.

55. Fukui S, Ohseto K, Shiotani M. Patterns of pain induced by distending the thoracic zygapophyseal joints. *Reg Anesth* 1997;22:332–336.

56. Dreyfuss P, Tibiletti C, Dreyer S. Thoracic zygapophyseal joint pain patterns. A study in normal volunteers. *Spine* 1994;19:807–811.

57. Manchikanti L, Kaye AD, Boswell MV, et al. A systematic review and best evidence synthesis of the effectiveness of therapeutic facet joint interventions in managing chronic spinal pain. *Pain Physician* 2015;18:535–582.

58. Manchikanti KN, Atluri S, Singh V, et al. An update of evaluation of therapeutic thoracic facet joint interventions. *Pain Physician* 2012;15:463–481.

59. Chua WH, Bogduk N. The surgical anatomy of thoracic facet denervation. *Acta Neurochir* 1995;136:140–144.

60. Cicala RS, Voeller GR, Fox T, et al. Epidural analgesia in thoracic trauma: effects of lumbar morphine and thoracic bupivacaine on pulmonary function. *Crit Care Med* 1990;18:229–231.

61. Ullman DA, Fortune JB, Greenhouse BB, et al. The treatment of patients with multiple rib fractures using continuous thoracic epidural narcotic infusion. *Reg Anesth* 1989;14:43–47.

62. Mackersie RC, Karagianes TG, Hoyt DB, et al. Prospective evaluation of epidural and intravenous administration of fentanyl for pain control and restoration of ventilatory function following multiple rib fractures. *J Trauma* 1991;31:443–449.

63. Haenel JB, Moore FA, Moore EE, et al. Extrapleural bupivacaine for amelioration of multiple rib fracture pain. *J Trauma* 1995;38:22–27.

64. Luchette FA, Radafshar SM, Kaiser R, et al. Prospective evaluation of epidural versus intrapleural catheters for analgesia in chest wall trauma. *J Trauma* 1994;36:865–870.

65. Moon MR, Luchette FA, Gibson SW, et al. Prospective randomized comparison of epidural vs parenteral opioid analgesia in thoracic trauma. *Ann Surg* 1999;229:684.

66. Shinora K, Iwama H, Akama Y, et al. Interpleural block for patients with multiple rib fractures: comparison with epidural block. *J Emerg Med* 1994;12:441–446.

67. Kunhabdulla NP, Agarwal A, Gaur A, et al. Serratus anterior plane block for multiple rib fractures. *Pain Physician* 2014;17:E651–E653.

68. Bossolasco M, Bernardi E, Fenoglio LM. Continuous serratus plane block in a patient with multiple rib fractures. *J Clin Anesth* 2017;38:85–86.

69. Davies-Colley R. Slipping rib. *BMJ* 1922;1:432.

70. Wright JT. Slipping rib syndrome. *Lancet* 1980;2:632–634.

71. Mooney DP, Shortner NA. Slipping rib syndrome in childhood. *J Pediatr Surg* 1997;32:1081–1082.

72. Porter GE. Slipping rib syndrome: an infrequently recognized entity in children: a report of three cases and review of literature. *Pediatrics* 1985;76:810–813.

73. Heinz GJ, Zavala DC. Slipping rib syndrome. *JAMA* 1977;237:794–795.

74. Motulsky A, Rohn RJ. Teitze's syndrome: cause of chest pain and chest wall swelling. *JAMA* 1953;152:504–506.

75. Gill GV. Epidemic of Teitze's syndrome. *BMJ* 1977;2:499.

76. Kayser HL. Teitze's syndrome: a review of literature. *Am J Med* 1956;21:982–989.

77. Sain AK. Bone scan in Teitze's syndrome. *Clin Nucl Med* 1978;3:470–471.

78. Fossgreen O, Fossgreen J, Sondergaard-Petersen J, et al. Musculo-skeletal pathology in patients with angina pectoris and normal coronary angiograms. *J Int Med* 1999;245:237–246.

79. Scobie BA. Costochondral pain in gastroenterologic practice [letter]. *N Engl J Med* 1976;295:1261.

80. Peyton FW. Unexpected frequency of idiopathic costochondral pain. *Obstet Gynecol* 1983;62:605–608.

81. Wolf E, Stern S. Costosternal syndrome: its frequency and importance in differential diagnosis of coronary heart disease. *Arch Intern Med* 1976;136:189–191.

82. Epstein SE, Gerber LH, Borer JS. Chest wall syndrome: a common cause of unexplained cardiac pain. *JAMA* 1979;241:2793–2797.

83. Brown RT. Costochondritis in adolescents. *J Adolesc Health Care* 1981;1:198–201.

84. Aglas F, Gretler J, Rainer F, et al. Sternoclavicular septic arthritis: a rare but serious complication of subclavian venous catheterization. *Clin Rheumatol* 1994;13:507–512.

85. Prevo RL, Rasker JJ, Kruijsen MW. Sternocostoclavicular hyperostosis or pustulotic arthrosteitis? *J Rheumatol* 1989;16:1602–1605.

86. Resnick CS, Ammann AM. Cervical spine involvement in sternoclavicular hyperostosis. *Spine* 1985;10:846–848.

87. Dastgeer GM, Mikolich DJ. Fracture-dislocation of manubriosternal joint: an unusual complication of seizures. *J Trauma* 1987;27:91–93.

88. Doube A, Clarke AK. Symptomatic manubriosternal joint involvement in rheumatoid arthritis. *Ann Rheum Dis* 1989;48:516–517.

89. Kernodle GW Jr, Allen NB. Acute gout presenting in the manubriosternal joint. *Arthritis Rheum* 1986;29:570–572.

90. Sebes JI, Salazar JE. The manubriosternal joint in rheumatoid disease. *Am J Roentgenol* 1983;140:117–121.

91. Gruber BL, Kaufman LD, Gorevic PD. Septic arthritis involving manubriosternal joint. *J Rheumatol* 1985;12:803–804.

92. Van Linthoudt D, De Torrente A, Humair L, et al. Septic manubriosternal arthritis in a patient with Reiter's disease. *Clin Rheumatol* 1987;6:293–295.

93. Parker VS, Malhotra CM, Ho G Jr, et al. Radiographic appearance of the sternomanubrial joint in arthritis and related conditions. *Radiology* 1984;153:343–347.

94. Lipkin M, Fulton LA, Wolfson EA. Xiphoidalgia syndrome. *N Engl J Med* 1955;253:591–597.

95. Howell JM. Xiphodynia. *J Emerg Med* 1992;10:435–438.

96. Miller AJ, Texidor TA. Precordial catch: a neglected syndrome of precordial pain. *JAMA* 1955;159:1364–1365.

97. Reynolds JL. Precordial catch syndrome in children. *South Med J* 1989;82:1228–1230.

98. Hopkins JH. Bornholm disease. *BMJ* 1950;27:1230–1232.

99. Preece PE, Mansel RE, Bolton PM et al. Clinical syndromes of mastalgia. *Lancet* 1976;2:670–673.

100. Wisbey JR, Kumar S, Mansel RE, et al. Natural history of breast pain. *Lancet* 1983;2:672–674.

101. Preece PE, Mansel RE, Hughes LE. Mastalgia: psychoneurosis or organic disease? *BMJ* 1978;1:29–30.

102. Mansel RE, Preece PE, Hughes LE. A double blind trial of prolactin inhibitor bromocriptine in painful benign breast disease. *Br J Surg* 1978;65:724–727.

103. Mansel RE, Wisbey JR, Hughes LE. Controlled trial of the antigonadotropin danazol in painful nodular benign breast disease. *Lancet* 1982;1:928–930.

104. Gately CA, Maddox PR, Mansel RE, et al. Mastalgia refractory to drug treatment. *Br J Surg* 1990;77:1110–1112.

105. Khan HN, Rampaul R, Blamey RW. Local anesthetic and steroid combined injection therapy in the management of non-cyclical mastalgia. *Breast* 2004;13:129–132.

106. Petersen P, Kastrup J. Dercum's disease (adiposis dolorosa). Treatment of severe pain with intravenous lidocaine. *Pain* 1987;28:77–80.

107. Lunn GM, Potter JM. Mondor's disease. *BMJ* 1954;1:1074–1076.

108. Cooper RA. Mondor's disease secondary to intravenous drug abuse. *Arch Surg* 1990;125:807–808.

109. Camiel MR. Mondor's disease in the breast. *Am J Obstet Gynecol* 1985;152:879–881.

110. Stevens PE, Dibble SL, Miaskowski C. Prevalence, characteristics and impact of postmastectomy pain syndrome: an investigation of women's experiences. *Pain* 1995;61:61–68.

111. Carpenter JS, Andrykowski MA, Sloan P, et al. Post mastectomy and post lumpectomy pain in breast cancer survivors. *J Clin Epedemiol* 1998;51:1285.

112. Vecht CJ, Vande Brand HJ, Wajer OJ. Post-axillary dissection pain in breast cancer due to a lesion of the intercostobrachial nerve. *Pain* 1989;38:171–176.

113. Wallace SW, Wallace AM, Lee J, et al. Pain after breast surgery: a survey of 282 women. *Pain* 1996;66:195–205.

114. Smith WC, Bourne D, Squair J, et al. A retrospective cohort study of post mastectomy pain syndrome. *Pain* 1999;83:91–95.

115. Wijayasinghe N, Anderson KG, Kehlet H. Neural blockade for persistent pain after breast cancer surgery. *Reg Anesth Pain Med* 2014;39:272–278.

116. Reuben SS, Makari-Judson G, Lurie SD. Evaluation of efficacy of the perioperative administration of venlafaxine XR in the prevention of postmastectomy pain syndrome. *J Pain Symptom Manage* 2004;27:133–139.

117. Crawford JS, Simpson J, Crawford P. Myofascial release provides symptomatic relief from chest wall tenderness occasionally seen following lumpectomy and radiation in breast cancer patients. *Int J Radiat Oncol Biol Phys* 1996;15:1188–1199.

118. Layeeque R, Hochberg J, Siegel E, et al. Botulinum toxin infiltration for pain control after mastectomy and expander reconstruction. *Ann Surg* 2004;240:608–614.

119. Kulhari S, Bharti N, Bala I, et al. Efficacy of pectoral nerve block versus thoracic paravertebral block for postoperative analgesia after radical mastectomy: a randomized controlled trial. *Br J Anaesth* 2016;117:382–386.

120. Jamison K, Wellisch DK, Katz RL, et al. Phantom breast syndrome. *Arch Surg* 1979;114:93–95.

121. Krøner K, Knudsen UB, Lundby L, et al. Long-term phantom breast syndrome after mastectomy. *Clin J Pain* 1992;8:346–350.

122. Staps T, Hoogenhout J, Wobbes T. Phantom breast sensations following mastectomy. *Cancer* 1985;56:2898–2901.

123. Gottrup H, Andersen J, Arendt-Nielsen L, et al. Psychophysical examination in patients with post mastectomy pain. *Pain* 2000;87:275–284.

124. Tasmuth T, Von Smitten K, Kalso E. Effect of present pain and mood on the memory of past postoperative pain in women treated surgically for breast cancer. *Pain* 1996;68:343–345.

125. Kroner K, Krebs B, Skov J, et al. Immediate and long-term phantom breast syndrome after mastectomy: incidence, clinical characteristics and relationship to pre-mastectomy breast pain. *Pain* 1989;36:327–334.

126. Keller SM, Carp NZ, Levy MN, et al. Chronic post thoracotomy pain. *J Cardiovasc Surg* 1994;35:161–164.

127. Daczman E, Gordon A, Kreisman H, et al. Long-term postthoracotomy pain. *Chest* 1991;99:270–274.

128. Ochroch EA, Gottschalk A, Troxel AB, et al. Women suffer more short and long term pain than men after major thoracotomy. *Clin J Pain* 2006;22:491–498.

129. Athanassiadi K, Kakaris S, Theakos N, et al. Muscle-sparing versus posterolateral thoracotomy: a prospective study. *Eur J Cardiothorac Surg* 2007;31:496–500.

130. Katz J, Jackson M, Kavanaugh BP, et al. Acute pain after thoracic surgery predicts long term postthoracotomy pain. *Clin J Pain* 1996;12:50–55.

131. Bayman EO, Parekh KR, Keech J, et al. A prospective study of chronic pain after thoracic surgery. *Anesthesiology* 2017;126:938–951.

132. Springer JS, Karlsson P, Madsen CS, et al. Functional and structural assessment of patients with and without persistent pain after thoracotomy. *Eur J Pain* 2017;21:238–249.

133. Sihoe ADL, Lee TW, Wan IYP, et al. The use of gabapentin for postoperative and posttraumatic pain in thoracic surgery patients. *Eur J Cardiothorac Surg* 2006;26:795–799.

134. Senturk M, Ozcan PE, Talu GK, et al. The effects of three different analgesia techniques on long term postthoracotomy pain. *Anesth Analg* 2002;94:11.

135. Kirvela O, Antila H. Thoracic paravertebral block in chronic postoperative pain. *Reg Anesth* 1992;17:348–350.

136. Kamakar MK. Thoracic paravertebral block. *Anesthesiology* 2001;95: 771–780.

137. Cohen SP, Sireci A, Wu CL, et al. Pulsed radiofrequency of the dorsal root ganglia is superior to pharmacotherapy or pulsed radiofrequency of the intercostal nerves in the treatment of chronic postsurgical thoracic pain. *Pain Physician* 2006;9:227–236.

138. Meek JC, Bollen E, Koudstaal J, et al. Pain in scar as an early symptom of acquired thoracic lung hernia. *Eur Respir J* 1991;4:505–507.

139. Fitzpatrick C, Coppola CP, Eichelberger MR. Intercostal hernia and spontaneous pneumothorax in a liver transplant recipient: a case report. *J Pediatr Surg* 2007;42:E5–E8.

140. Eisenberg E, Pultorak Y, Pud D, et al. Prevalence and characteristics of post coronary artery bypass graft surgery pain (PCP). *Pain* 2001;92:11–17.

141. Bruce J, Drury N, Poobalan AS, et al. The prevalence of chronic chest and leg pain following cardiac surgery: a historical cohort study. *Pain* 2003;104:265–273.

142. Mailis A, Umana M, Feindel CM. Anterior intercostal nerve damage after coronary artery bypass graft surgery with use of internal thoracic artery graft. *Ann Thorac Surg* 2000;69:1455–1488.

143. Norgaard MA, Andersen TC, Lavrsen MJ, et al. The outcome of sternal wire removal on persistent anterior chest wall pain after median sternotomy. *Eur J Cardiothorac Surg* 2006;29:920–924.

144. Billings RF. Chest pain related to emotional disorders. In: Levine DL, Billings RF, eds. *Chest Pain: An Integrated Diagnostic Approach*. Philadelphia: Lea & Febiger; 1977:133–150.

145. Mukerji B, Mukerji V, Alpert MA, et al. The prevalence of rheumatologic disorders in patients with chest pain and angiographically normal coronary arteries. *Angiology* 1995;46:425–430.

146. Wise CM, Semble EL, Dalton CB. Musculoskeletal chest wall syndromes in patients with noncardiac chest pain: a study of 100 patients. *Arch Phys Med Rehabil* 1992;73:147–149.

147. Vaisrub S. Da costa syndrome revisited [editorial]. *JAMA* 1975;232:164.

148. Wheeler EO, White PD, Reed EW, et al. Neurocirculatory asthenia (anxiety, neurosis, effort syndrome, neurasthenia): a 20-year follow-up study of 173 patients. *JAMA* 1950;142:878–889.

149. Borjesson M, Andrell P, Lundberg D, et al. Spinal cord stimulation in severe angina pectoris—a systematic review based on the Swedish Council on Technology assessment in health care report on long-standing pain. *Pain* 2008;140:501–508.

150. Di Pede F, Lanza GA, Zuin G, et al. Immediate and long-term clinical outcome after spinal cord stimulation for refractory stable angina pectoris. *Am J Cardiol* 2003;91:951–955.

151. Fox K, Garcia MAA, Ardissino D, et al. Guidelines on the management of stable angina pectoris: the Task Force on the Management of Stable Angina Pectoris of the European Society of Cardiology. *Eur Heart J* 2006;27(11):1341–1381.

152. Anderson C, Hole P, OXhoj H. Does pain relief with spinal cord stimulation for angina conceal myocardial infarction. *Br Heart J* 1994;71:419–421.

CHAPTER 70

Lower Extremity Pain

GAGAN MAHAJAN and **DAVE LOOMBA**

The information in this chapter is presented in three major sections detailing (1) specific causes of lumbosacral plexopathy, (2) specific lower extremity peripheral nerve lesions, and (3) specific causes of foot pain.

Lumbosacral Plexopathy

Although the lumbar and sacral plexuses are separate structures, they are often referred to as a single structure—the lumbosacral plexus—that provides motor and sensory innervation to the pelvis and leg (Fig. 70.1). The lumbar plexus, which is made up of the ventral rami of the T12–L3 and a portion of the L4 nerve roots, is contained within the psoas muscle and lies anterior to the L2–L5 vertebral bodies.[1–3] The anterior and posterior divisions of the ventral rami form the terminal branches of the lumbar plexus and include the iliohypogastric (T12, L1), ilioinguinal (L1), genitofemoral (L1, L2), lateral femoral cutaneous (L2, L3), obturator nerves (L2, L3, L4), and femoral (L2, L3, L4) nerves.[3] The saphenous nerve is a branch of the femoral nerve.

The sacral plexus (Fig. 70.2), which is made up of the ventral rami of the S1–S5 nerve roots, connects with the lumbar plexus via the lumbosacral trunk. It is made up of the ventral rami of the L4–L5 nerve roots and lies just anterior to the piriformis muscle, posterior to the internal iliac vessels, and in close proximity to the hypogastric arteries and veins, lateral rectum, pelvic colon, and ureters.[2,3] Similar to the lumbar plexus, terminal branches arise from the anterior and posterior divisions of the ventral rami of the sacral plexus. The tibial nerve (made up of the anterior divisions of the ventral rami) and the common fibular (peroneal) nerve (made up of the posterior divisions) form the terminal branches of the sciatic nerve on bifurcating from their common epineural sheath.[3] Additional terminal branches of the sacral plexus include the superior gluteal (L4, L5, S1), inferior gluteal (L5, S1, S2), posterior femoral cutaneous (S1, S2, S3), and pudendal (S2, S3, S4) nerves.[3]

There are multiple causes of lumbosacral plexopathy. These include space-occupying masses (invasive neoplasm, compression by retroperitoneal or pelvic mass), vascular/metabolic diseases (diabetes, chronic idiopathic peripheral polyneuropathy, vasculitis, aneurysmal dilation), trauma (pelvic fractures, complications from surgery or radiation therapy), and idiopathic causes.[4] Nontraumatic lesions are the most common, as evidenced by one report of 86 cases revealing a neoplastic etiology in more than 50% and trauma in only 6%.[3] Patellar reflex impairment along with hip flexion, knee extension, and/or dorsiflexion weakness suggests lumbar plexopathy, whereas ankle reflex impairment along with hip extension, knee flexion, and/or plantarflexion weakness suggests sacral plexopathy.

Depending on the cause, diagnostic workup for plexopathy can include plain film x-ray imaging, detailed neuroimaging (computed tomography [CT] and magnetic resonance imaging [MRI]), angiography, ultrasonography, electrodiagnostic studies (electromyography [EMG] and nerve conduction study [NCS]), and laboratory studies. Diagnostic studies in isolation of the patient's medical history and physical exam findings, however, have limitations. For example, neuroimaging may not be able to differentiate between benign tumor versus malignant tumor versus radiation-induced plexopathy. Likewise, electrodiagnostic studies may not be able to differentiate between

peripheral neuropathy versus plexopathy.[3] Electrodiagnostic studies, however, may be able to provide information on the extent of motor axon loss or on the presence of muscle denervation when clinical assessment is limited by the cause of injury.

Treatment options depend on the cause, location, symptom severity, physical exam findings, and duration of the plexopathy.[3] In certain situations, surgery may be the initial treatment of choice, whereas in other circumstances, observation and symptom management may be the preferred approach. Conservative therapy for symptomatic relief includes medications (corticosteroids, acetaminophen, nonsteroidal anti-inflammatory drugs [NSAIDs], anticonvulsants, tricyclic antidepressants, opioids, topical analgesics, and lidocaine patch) and injections. Spinal cord stimulation or intrathecal therapies may be considered for those who have a suboptimal response to the aforementioned and/or those who are not surgical candidates. Physical therapy is important for those with evidence of motor weakness in order to minimize muscle atrophy, prevent muscle contractures, and maintain ambulatory status. Assessment for orthotic devices (e.g., ankle-foot orthosis [AFO]) and gait assistive devices (e.g., crutches, cane, walker) also may be necessary in order to prevent falls.

NEOPLASMS

In comparison to neoplastic involvement of the lumbosacral spinal nerves, cauda equina, or conus medullaris, lumbosacral plexus involvement is relatively uncommon and has a reported incidence of 0.71%.[5,6] Neoplastic plexopathies can involve the sacral plexus (50%), lumbar plexus (33%), or lumbosacral plexus (17%).[3,7] Most are of malignant origin, with 75% occurring by direct extension (most commonly from gastrointestinal tumors, genitourinary tumors lymphomas, sarcomas), or metastasis.[3,5] Breast cancer is the most common primary source, and rarely is the diagnosis of neoplastic plexopathy made before discovery of the primary neoplasm.

Neoplastic plexus involvement portends a poor prognosis, with death often occurring within 6 months of diagnosis.[5] Insidious onset of low back pain (lumbar plexus) and/or leg pain (sacral plexus) are often the primary heralding features and can precede other neurologic symptoms.[1,3,5,7] At initial onset, unilateral leg pain is present in 90% of patients and tends to be more prominent than low back pain.[8] The pain can have both nociceptive and neuropathic features and is worse with recumbency, movement, and Valsalva maneuvers.[1] Lumbar plexus involvement, also known as malignant psoas syndrome, is suggested by localization of pain over the costovertebral angle, anterior abdominal wall, groin, or thigh and by painful fixed flexion of the hip worsened by passive or active hip.[1,9,10] Within 13 months of pain onset, many patients develop additional neurologic symptoms: weakness (86%), gait dysfunction, sensory loss (73%), reflex impairment (64%), and paroxysmal or continuous paresthesias or dysesthesias.[1,3,5,6,8] Additional physical exam findings may include (1) lower extremity edema (seen in 50%), (2) warm and dry foot (seen with sympathetic nerve involvement), (3) palpable rectal mass and perineal pain (seen in more than one-third with sacral involvement), (4) incontinence and impotence (seen in 10%, usually implying extensive sacral involvement with bilateral sacral plexopathy), and (5) abdominal and pelvic pain.[1,3,6,11] The differential diagnosis, however, must also include radiation-induced plexopathy, peripheral neuropathy,

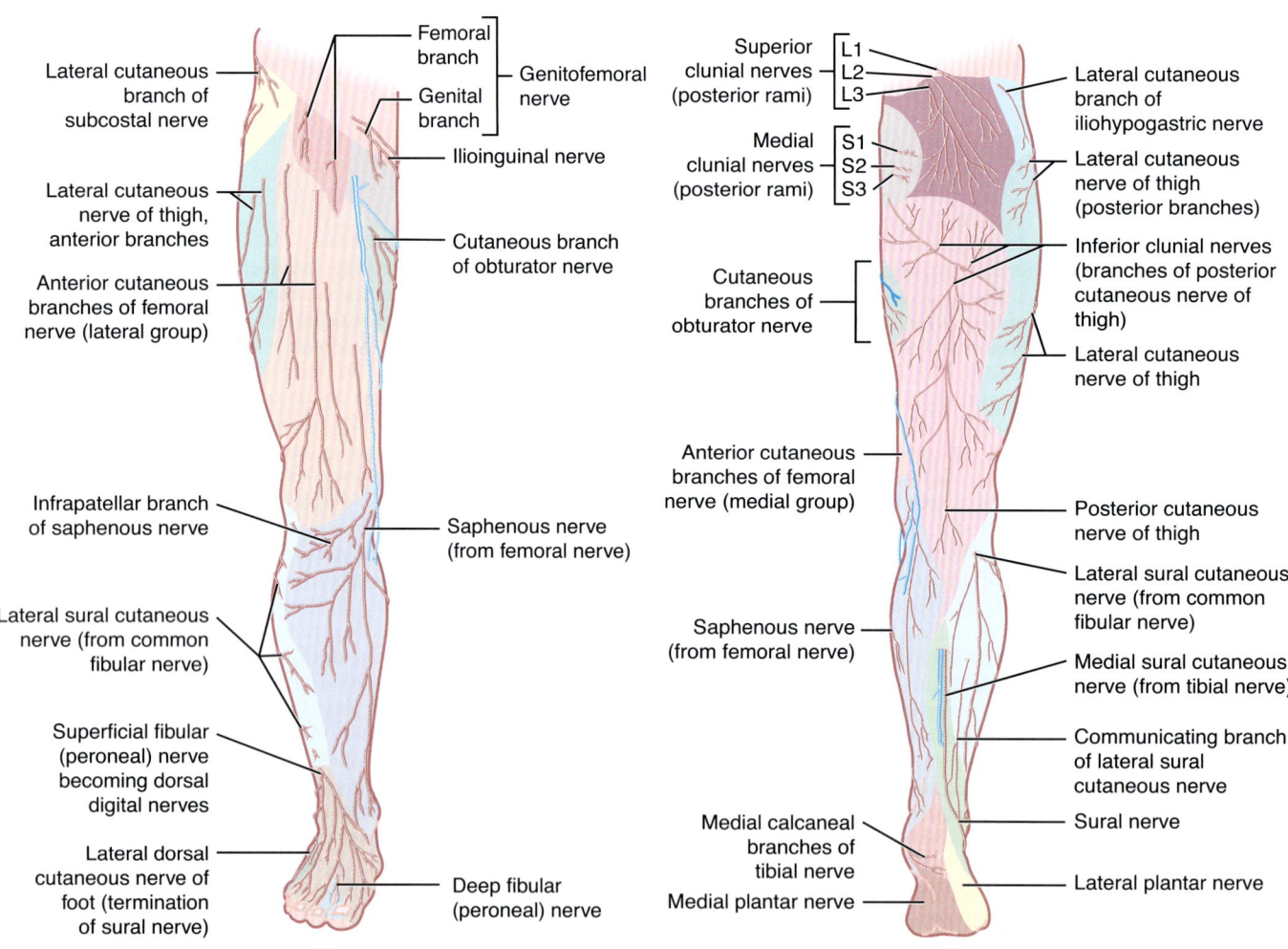

FIGURE 70.1   A: Anatomy of the lumbosacral plexus. Anterior **(B)** and posterior **(C)** views of cutaneous innervation of the lumbosacral plexus.

radiculopathy, cauda equina syndrome, retroperitoneal hematoma, and vertebral compression fracture.[1]

Tumors can be broadly classified as intrinsic or extrinsic. Intrinsic tumors can be benign (e.g., neurofibromas and plexiform lesions) or malignant (e.g., schwannomas or neurogenic sarcomas).[1] Neurofibromas, which are common in patients with neurofibromatosis type 1, are commonly seen in the paraspinal,

sacral plexus, sciatic notch, and perirectal regions.[12] Patients may or may not have symptoms with benign or malignant tumors, and an MRI alone may be insufficient to differentiate one from the other. Symptomatic relief with analgesic medications may be necessary until the tumor can be excised.

Extrinsic tumors are malignant. Lymphoma can cause a plexopathy due to enlarged lymph nodes (most common),

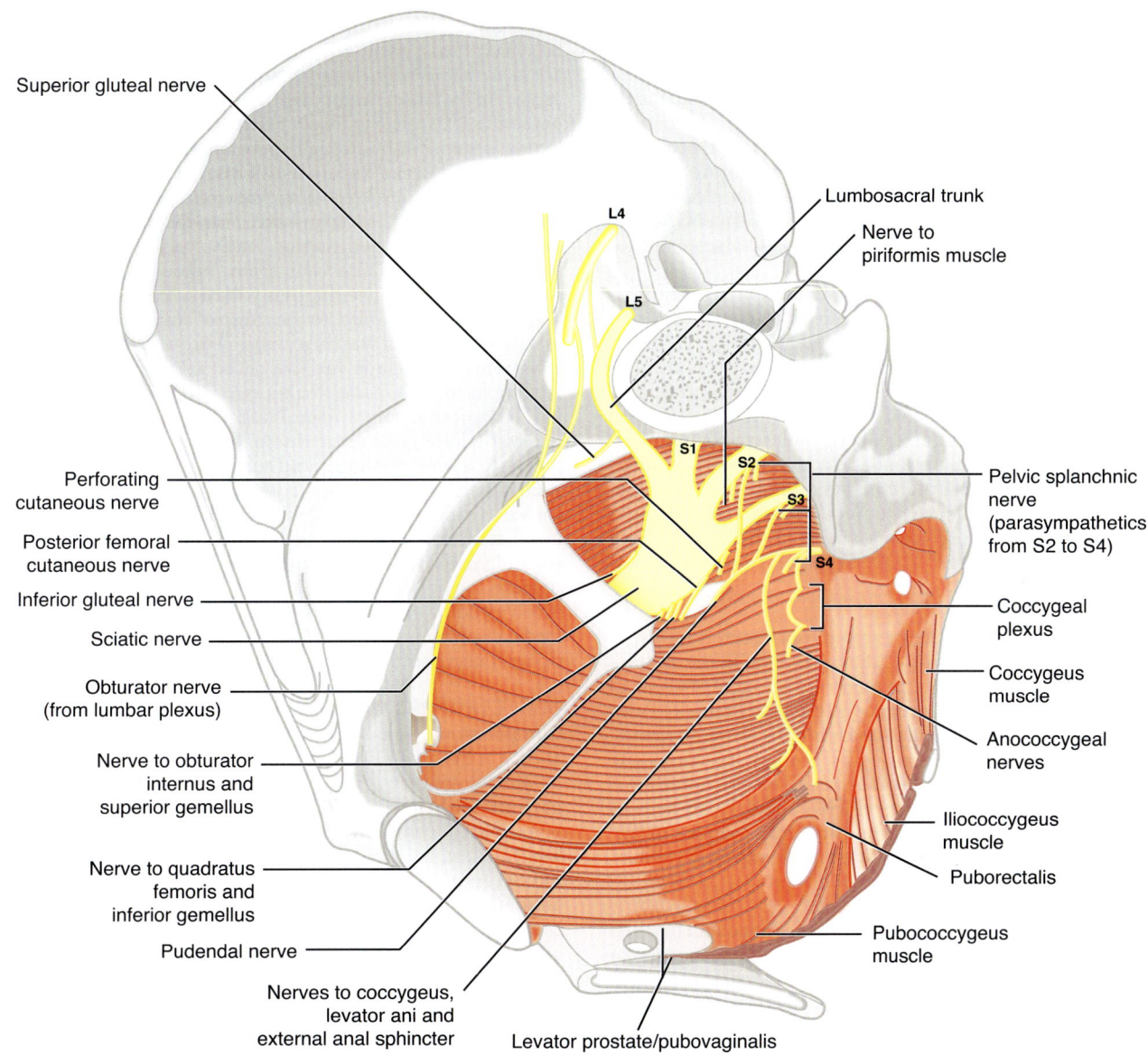

FIGURE 70.2 Oblique sagittal view of the sacral plexus.

extranodal disease in the muscle (e.g., psoas, iliacus, piriformis, and gluteal muscles) or subcutaneous fat, or direct sciatic nerve involvement (rare).[2] Carcinomas (colorectal, genitourinary, breast, lung, and prostate) and retroperitoneal sarcomas can cause a plexopathy by encasement of the plexus by the primary tumor itself, metastasis into the surrounding soft and bony tissue, or metastasis into the plexus itself.[1,2] Sacral chordomas, which can cause constipation, urinary frequency, and sciatica, are the most common primary malignant sacral tumors.[2] Imaging with MRI, CT, or positron emission tomography computed tomography (PET-CT) may help with the workup of these extrinsic tumors. Chemotherapy, radiation therapy, and/or surgical resection of the tumor is usually indicated.

RADIATION-INDUCED PLEXOPATHY
Pelvic radiation therapy to treat urologic cancers, gynecologic cancers, and lymphomas can result in radiation-induced lumbar, sacral, or lumbosacral plexopathy. Unlike neoplastic plexopathy, which is often associated with significant pain and weakness, radiation plexopathy is primarily associated with weakness, with significant pain being present in fewer than 25% of patients.[8] Weakness is noted predominantly in the

distal L5–S1 innervated muscles and may be accompanied by reflex and sensory impairment, skin changes, and lymphedema; bowel or bladder disturbance is rare.[8,11] The mean duration of symptom onset is 5 years but can vary from a few months to more than three decades.[3,11] Skin changes and lymphedema are commonly seen.[8] Because of obvious therapeutic implications, neuroimaging studies are critically important in order to discriminate between tumor recurrence, radiation fibrosis, and surgical scar tissue. Electrodiagnostic studies should be included to help establish the diagnosis when neuroimaging findings are nonspecific. Characteristic electrodiagnostic findings include demyelinating conduction block and myokymia.[3] If electrodiagnostic findings are also nonspecific, the diagnosis usually needs to be confirmed by biopsy or surgical exploration. For those with only radiation-induced plexopathy, treatment is nonsurgical and involves symptom management.[3]

DIABETIC AND NONDIABETIC LUMBOSACRAL RADICULOPLEXUS
Diabetic lumbosacral radiculoplexus (diabetic amyotrophy) involves microvasculitic ischemic nerve injury. It most commonly occurs in elderly patients with chronic type 2 diabetes mellitus

and does not occur in isolation of diabetic peripheral polyneuropathy.[3] Patients usually report weight loss and low back and/or leg pain that is worse at night. These symptoms are often followed by signs of weakness, atrophy, and sensory deficits involving the anterior thigh along with an absent patellar reflex. Electrodiagnostic findings include axonal loss, demyelination, and denervation changes in muscles innervated by the obturator and femoral nerves.[3] Neuroimaging is necessary to rule out other potential causes of lumbosacral plexopathy. Because the plexopathy is due to ischemic nerve injury, treatment focuses on symptom management, physical therapy, and assessment for a gait assistive device.

Nondiabetic lumbosacral radiculoplexus is an underappreciated cause of lumbosacral plexopathy. Similar to diabetic lumbosacral radiculoplexus, nondiabetic lumbosacral radiculoplexus involves microvasculitic (motor, sensory, and autonomic) nerve injury; initially involves the legs; and is associated with pain, weight loss, prolonged morbidity and mortality, and incomplete recovery.[13] Both nondiabetic and diabetic lumbosacral radiculoplexus also share similar electrodiagnostic findings and treatment strategies. Unlike diabetic lumbosacral radiculoplexus, however, nondiabetic lumbosacral radiculoplexus is not associated with hyperglycemia and is probably due to an autoimmune phenomenon.[13]

ABSCESS

Psoas, gluteal, and pelvic abscesses can present acutely or insidiously with painful fixed flexion of the hip or pain in the abdominal, pelvic, or gluteal regions. In their retrospective analysis of 23 retroperitoneal collections related to the psoas muscle, Paley et al.[14] confirmed 5 were hematomas and 18 were abscesses, and of the abscesses, 3 were caused by primary infections and the remainder by infections of spinal, renal, or gastrointestinal origin. Because their appearance on MRI and CT can be confused with lymphoma or tumor deposits, image-guided percutaneous drainage can be of diagnostic and therapeutic value.[2]

RETROPERITONEAL HEMATOMA

Retroperitoneal hematomas can occur from anticoagulant therapy, hemophilia, ruptured aortic aneurysms, idiopathically, or iatrogenically (e.g., cardiac catheterization).[15] The degree of neurologic deficit depends on the size of the hematoma: (1) A small hematoma compresses the intrapelvic portion of the femoral nerve within the iliacus muscle; (2) a large hematoma compresses the lumbar plexus within the psoas muscle, affecting both the obturator and femoral nerves; and (3) a widespread hematoma affects the lumbosacral plexus.[2] Signs and symptoms may include ecchymosis (flank, low back, and/or thigh) and acute or subacute onset of lower abdominal or groin pain radiating to the anterior thigh. Neuroimaging facilitates the diagnosis. EMG and NCS findings include abnormalities in the adductor muscle and axonal loss in the distribution of the femoral nerve or lumbar plexus (although involvement of the lumbosacral plexus can also occur).[3] Even though retroperitoneal hematomas are considered compartment syndromes, treatment is nonsurgical.[3]

ANEURYSMS

Aneurysms of the distal aorta, iliac arteries, intrapelvic arteries, and hypogastric arteries and arteriovenous malformations can injure the lumbosacral plexus via direct compression or ischemia from embolism of feeding vessels.[2,3] Symptoms may include low back pain with or without radicular symptoms, sensory loss, and weakness. The initial diagnostic workup includes an abdominal and pelvic ultrasound, followed by neuroimaging and angiography. The electrodiagnostic finding includes axonal loss, but pinpointing the location is often challenging.[3] Treatment involves surgical repair of the aneurysm.

TRAUMA

Traumatic injuries to the lumbosacral plexus, in comparison to the brachial plexus, occur infrequently because the neural structures are (1) relatively distant to highly mobile structures and (2) well protected by muscle and bone.[3] Therefore, trauma-induced lumbosacral plexopathy typically results from penetrating or violent injuries—gunshot blast, high-speed motor vehicle or motorcycle accident, pedestrian versus motor vehicle accident, or fall from a tall height—and is often associated with pelvic bony fractures. Isolated fractures involving the non–weight-bearing anterior one-third of the pelvic ring are often stable and do not result in neurovascular injury. Conversely, because the posterolateral two-thirds of the pelvic ring is involved with weight bearing and lays in close proximity to neurovascular structures, fractures in this area lead to instability and neurovascular compromise.[3] Symptoms can include variable degrees of pain, sensory and reflex impairment, muscle weakness, atrophy, and gait abnormality. Treatment involves identifying the extent of neurovascular injury. Because most nerve traumatic injuries spontaneously improve (to a certain degree) and surgical repair can be technically challenging, surgery is not recommend as the initial treatment of choice.[3] Of those who do require surgery, outcomes are relatively better with repair of the lumbar instead of sacral plexus.[3] Neuropathic pain persisting beyond the anticipated healing process suggests the presence of a neuroma or scar tissue. Treatment may involve additional surgery to remove the neuroma or scar tissue, medication management, or implantation of a spinal cord or peripheral nerve stimulator.

OBSTETRIC-RELATED PLEXOPATHY

Compression of the lumbosacral plexus between the pelvic rim and fetal head can occur during the latter stages of pregnancy or during delivery (Fig. 70.3).[3] Katirji et al.[16] described seven patients with intrapartum maternal lumbosacral plexopathy who shared common features: short maternal stature, prolonged labor, pain and demyelination in an L5 nerve root distribution, foot drop, and complete resolution of symptoms within 5 months. A large fetal head or the use of forceps can also cause compression of the lumbosacral plexus. Neuroimaging may be of limited benefit when the fetus is present. EMG and NCS abnormalities include abnormalities in muscles innervated by the L5 nerve root and a demyelinating conduction block of nerves supplying the muscles of the anterolateral leg.[3] Aside from delivery of the fetus, treatment is nonsurgical.[3]

Specific Nerve Entrapment Syndromes

LATERAL FEMORAL CUTANEOUS NERVE ENTRAPMENT

The lateral femoral cutaneous nerve (LFCN), a purely sensory nerve, originates from the lumbar plexus and conveys fibers from posterior divisions of the ventral rami of the L2 and L3 nerve roots (Fig. 70.4). Near the anterior superior iliac spine (ASIS), the LFCN divides into anterior and posterior branches and conveys sensory information from the anterolateral and lateral surfaces of the thigh, respectively. Compression of the LFCN most commonly occurs as the nerve exits the pelvis and pierces or crosses the inguinal ligament and attaches to the ASIS.[17] Entrapment of the LFCN, also known as lateral femoral cutaneous neuralgia, was first characterized by Bernhard in 1878. In 1895, Roth coined the name meralgia paresthetica (MP), which is derived from the Greek words *meros* (meaning thigh) and *algos* (meaning pain).[18,19]

Although MP is not rare, its exact prevalence remains unknown. It can occur at any age but is most commonly seen in patients 30 to 60 years of age.[19,20] After looking at the relationship between comorbidity (e.g., carpal tunnel syndrome, pregnancy, hip osteoarthritis, obesity, symptoms of the pubic

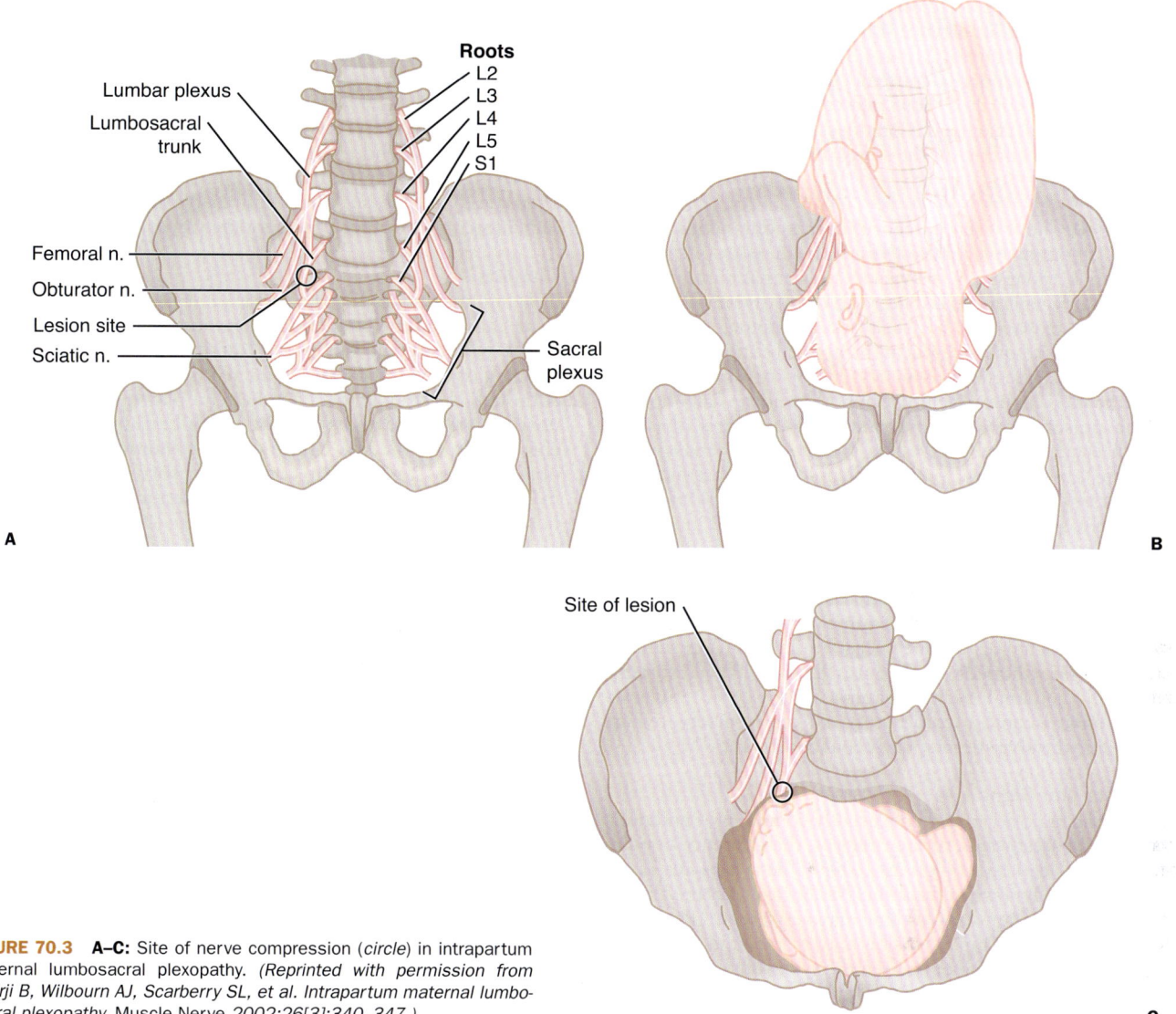

Roots
L2
L3
L4
L5
S1

Lumbar plexus
Lumbosacral trunk
Femoral n.
Obturator n.
Lesion site
Sciatic n.
Sacral plexus

A

B

Site of lesion

C

FIGURE 70.3   A–C: Site of nerve compression (*circle*) in intrapartum maternal lumbosacral plexopathy. *(Reprinted with permission from Katirji B, Wilbourn AJ, Scarberry SL, et al. Intrapartum maternal lumbosacral plexopathy. Muscle Nerve 2002;26[3]:340–347.)*

Lateral cutaneous nerve of thigh (anterior branches)

Lateral cutaneous nerve of thigh (posterior branches)

A

B

FIGURE 70.4   Cutaneous branches of the lateral femoral cutaneous nerve. Anterior **(A)** view and posterior **(B)** view.

bone, thrombosis of the leg, diabetes mellitus, and the use of corticosteroids) and the occurrence of MP, van Slobbe et al.[20] concluded the incidence rate of MP is 4.3 per 10,000 person-years. Although probably underdiagnosed in children, it has been seen in as many as one-third of those treated for osteoid osteoma.[19] Whether there is a true gender predilection remains unknown, as results vary depending on the study referenced.[17,20–23]

Etiology

Causes of MP have been categorized as spontaneous or iatrogenic.[21] Spontaneous causes result from entrapment due to intrapelvic (pregnancy, pelvic or abdominal tumors, uterine fibroids, degenerative pubic symphysis, diverticulitis, and appendicitis), extrapelvic (seatbelt trauma, tight garments or belts, and obesity), or mechanical (prolonged sitting, prolonged standing, and leg length discrepancy) factors or from metabolic derangements (diabetes mellitus, hypothyroidism, alcoholism, and lead poisoning).[19,24] The greatest risk factor is obesity.[24] Mondelli et al.[23] noted that obese patients (body mass index ≥ 30 kg/m^2), but not overweight patients (body mass index 25 to 29.9 kg/m^2), showed twofold greater risk for developing MP. Interestingly, some have even reported cases of MP in patients who have lost weight.[25,26] Postulated mechanisms may include the presence of other compressive factors, lack of nutritional factors, or underlying systemic disease.[23] Iatrogenic causes of MP result from orthopedic procedures (pelvic osteotomy, iliac crest bone graft harvest, spine surgery, and total hip replacement) and nonorthopedic procedures (gastric bypass surgery, laparoscopic inguinal herniorrhaphy, laparoscopic cholecystectomy, laparoscopic myomectomy, coronary artery bypass grafting, aortic valve surgery, and renal transplant).[19,26]

Symptoms and Signs

Although the majority of patients usually complain of unilateral sensory loss, paresthesias, or dysesthesias, the incidence of bilateral symptoms can be as high as 20%.[17] The symptoms rarely radiate proximally toward the spine.[19] Hair loss over the anterolateral thigh due to constant rubbing may be present.[19] Prolonged standing, walking, or hip extension may worsen the symptoms. Hip flexion may alleviate or worsen the symptoms. A Tinel sign (paresthesias radiating to the anterolateral thigh) sometimes can be elicited by percussing medial to the ASIS.[23] For those patients in whom inguinal ligament LFCN entrapment is suspected, the pelvic compression test should be performed (Fig. 70.5).

With the patient lying in a lateral decubitus position on the unaffected limb, the examiner maintains downward pressure on the pelvis for 45 seconds. Transient improvement of symptoms is considered a positive result.[27] Nouraei et al.[27] showed this test had a sensitivity of 95% and a specificity of 93.3% in those with electrodiagnostically proven MP.

Symptoms extending beyond the territory of the nerve, reflex changes, muscle weakness, or muscle atrophy suggest an alternate diagnosis, such as a lumbar plexopathy, high lumbar radiculopathy, or other peripheral neuropathy.

Diagnosis

Imaging and laboratory studies should be considered when a clear cause cannot be identified: radiograph or neuroimaging of the pelvis to rule out pelvic tumor or fracture and neuroimaging of the lumbosacral spine to rule out disk herniation.[19] Although electrodiagnostic studies can play a role in the diagnosis of MP, some argue its utility may be hampered by inherent technical difficulty, challenges in obtaining a response in obese patients, and small recordable sensory responses (absent in 71% and prolonged in 24%).[24] Furthermore, in order to obtain the best recordings one must use needle electrodes instead of surface electrodes. Others, however, claim that electrodiagnostics should play a central role in diagnosing MP. Instead of strictly looking at the absolute value of the sensory nerve action potential (SNAP) amplitude, Seror and Seror[22] demonstrated a specificity of 98.75% in their study of 120 patients when the side-to-side amplitude ratio was greater than 2.3 and the amplitude was less than 3 microvolts. Because the nerve is purely sensory, EMG testing of muscles should be normal. The value of somatosensory-evoked potentials (SSEPs) in making the diagnosis is debatable.[19] Ultimately, the greatest benefit of performing an electrodiagnostic is to rule out other entities—high lumbar radiculopathy, lumbar plexopathy, or other peripheral neuropathy—that can cause similar symptoms.

Treatment

Nonsurgical treatment for MP is typically successful, as symptoms are often mild and self-limited. In their study of 277 patients, Williams and Trzil[28] reported conservative management was successful in 91% of patients. Initial recommendations include advising patients to avoid wearing tight-fitting garments or belts, advising obese patients to lose weight, and correcting leg-length discrepancies. If symptoms persist, other treatment

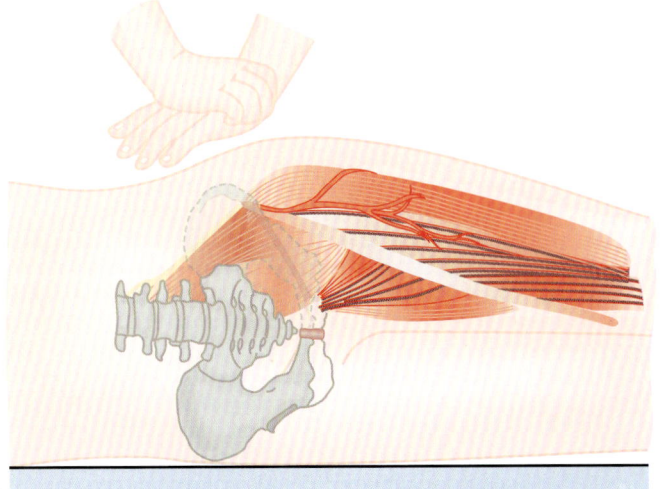
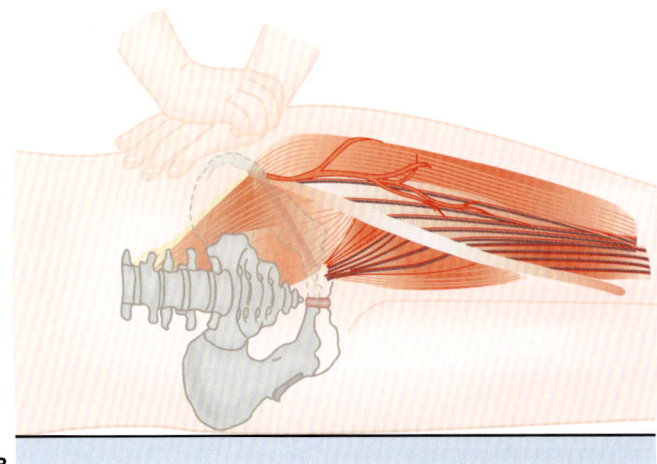

A   **B**

FIGURE 70.5 Pelvic compression test. Place the patient in a lateral decubitus position **(A)** and apply downward pressure on the pelvis for 45 seconds **(B)**. Transient improvement of symptoms is a positive test.

options include ice, transcutaneous electrical nerve stimulation (TENS) unit, and analgesic medications and injections. Because no controlled studies have been performed, the long-term efficacy of a local anesthetic LFCN block (with or without corticosteroids) is unclear. Furthermore, whether temporary relief of symptoms alters the long-term prognosis is unknown. Using a standard treatment algorithm in 79 patients, Haim et al.[17] showed symptomatic improvement in 21 patients requiring conservative therapy and medical management, 48 patients requiring LFCN blocks using corticosteroid and local anesthetic, and 10 patients requiring surgery. At 1-year follow-up, the authors reported none of the patients had recurrence of MP symptoms.

Traditionally, the target site of injection is identified based on anatomic landmarks (1 cm medial and 1 cm inferior to the ASIS), with a large volume of medication being injected using a fanning technique. Although large volumes may increase the success rate of blocking the LFCN to obtain useful diagnostic information, it can also come at the risk of inadvertently blocking the femoral and/or obturator nerves. However, absence of immediate analgesia does not necessarily rule out the diagnosis of MP given the LCFN's anatomic variability and given failure rate of this technique being as high as 60%.[29] In a prospective, randomized, crossover study involving 20 patients, the same authors demonstrated a 100% versus 40% success rate with blocking the LFCN using a stimulating needle versus a fanning technique, respectively.[29] Ultrasound guidance can also improve the success rate of identifying the correct nerve. In their study of 20 patients, Tagliafico et al.[30] described a technically successful LFCN block in 100% of the patients and no short-term or long-term complications. Similarly, Hurdle et al.[31] reported a technically successful LFCN block in their study of 10 patients, 5 of whom were obese. The advantages to using ultrasound-guidance include real-time visualization of the needle position and the adjacent structures, use of lower volumes of injectate, and avoidance of blockage of the femoral and/or obturator nerves.[30,31]

For those who do not obtain long-term benefit from corticosteroid injections, other treatments that have been tried include cryoanalgesia, pulsed or continuous radiofrequency (RF), alcohol neurolysis, peripheral nerve stimulation, and spinal cord stimulation. The successful outcomes reported in some of these studies need to be interpreted with caution, though, as they tend to be case reports, case series, or retrospective studies.[32–35] For those patients whose symptoms are refractory to analgesic medications, LFCN blocks, and neurostimulation, operative interventions may include transecting the LFCN at the level of the inguinal ligament (neurectomy) or incising the inguinal ligament to decompress the LFCN (neurolysis).[28] Based on their systematic review of the literature, Payne et al.[36] could not identify one treatment as being superior to the other due to the lack of high-quality studies. As with any neurodestructive procedure, there is a risk of nerve injury or neuroma formation.

FEMORAL NERVE ENTRAPMENT

The femoral nerve is a sensory (Fig. 70.6) and motor nerve and is the largest nerve of the lumbar plexus. It originates within the psoas muscle and arises from the posterior divisions

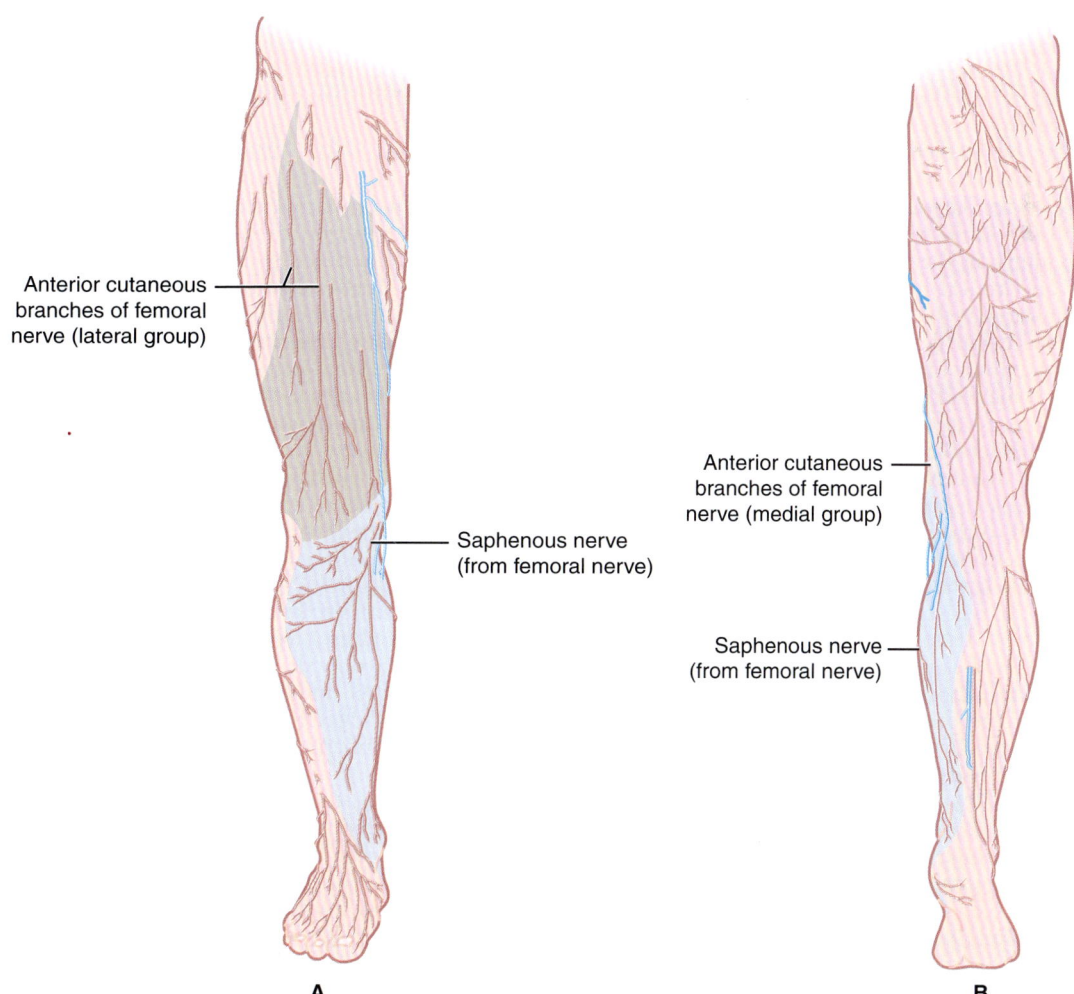

Anterior cutaneous branches of femoral nerve (lateral group)

Saphenous nerve (from femoral nerve)

Anterior cutaneous branches of femoral nerve (medial group)

Saphenous nerve (from femoral nerve)

A **B**

FIGURE 70.6 Cutaneous branches of the femoral nerve. Anterior **(A)** view and posterior **(B)** view.

of the ventral rami of the L2, L3, and L4 nerve roots (see Fig. 70.1A).[37] (The anterior divisions of the same nerve roots form the obturator nerve.) In the abdomen, the femoral nerve gives off branches to the iliacus and psoas muscles, and as it passes under the inguinal ligament, it gives off a branch to the pectineus muscle. The nerve then enters the femoral triangle lateral to the femoral artery, and upon exiting the triangle, it splits into an anterior and posterior division. The anterior division provides motor innervation to the sartorius muscle and sensory innervation (via the medial and intermediate femoral cutaneous nerves) to the anterior thigh as far distally as the knee. The posterior division provides motor innervation to the quadriceps muscles (rectus femoris, vastus lateralis, vastus intermedius, and vastus medialis) and sensory innervation (via the saphenous nerve) to the anteromedial aspect of the knee, medial calf, medial malleolus, and part of the medial arch of the foot and great toe.[37,38]

Isolated femoral neuropathy, originally known as anterior crural neuritis, was first reported in 1822 in a thesis by Descot. Although most lesions are unilateral, bilateral involvement has been observed.[26] Because an isolated unilateral femoral neuropathy is uncommon, its true incidence remains unknown. Kuntzer et al.[39] reported that of 7,252 electrodiagnostic examinations performed at their institution between 1988 and 1994, femoral neuropathy accounted for the diagnosis is only 32 patients (0.5%). Femoral neuropathies can cause either motor and sensory disturbances or sensory disturbances only. The latter occurs when the saphenous nerve, which is the distal sensory continuation of the femoral nerve, is involved.

Etiology

The causes of femoral neuropathy may be divided into the following categories: (1) direct nerve trauma (gunshot or knife wound, hip or pelvic fracture, hip replacement, hip prosthesis displacement, thermal energy from methyl methacrylate, inguinal herniorrhaphy, or femoral nerve block), (2) nerve ischemia due to interrupted vascularization at the intrapelvic level (common iliac artery occlusion, vascular or aortic surgery, or renal transplant with graft in the iliac fossa), (3) nerve compression (femoral artery injury in the femoral triangle, retroperitoneal hematoma, retroperitoneal mass, lithotomy positioning, prolonged hyperextension of the hip, or entrapment under the inguinal ligament with hip flexion), (4) metabolic (diabetes or pelvic radiation therapy), and (5) idiopathic.[37,39–41]

Because of a somewhat differential blood supply, the left femoral nerve is more susceptible to ischemic injury than the right.[42] The most vulnerable site of injury is located 4 to 6 cm above the inguinal ligament, which is where the nerve exits from the psoas muscle.[26] Because most pelvic surgical maneuvers occur proximal to the psoas muscle and out of the direct path of the nerve, neuropathy due to a compressive injury from retractors is more likely than that due to nerve transection and is independent of the type of incision (horizontal, midline, or lateral).

Most surgery-related causes of femoral neuropathy are preventable as long as retractors are used with care and positional factors are taken into account.[41] In their analysis of 32 patients with electrodiagnostically confirmed femoral neuropathy, Kuntzer et al.[39] identified an iatrogenic cause in 65% of the cases, and of these, 87% were related the hip surgeries. The incidence of femoral neuropathy after total hip arthroplasty is estimated to be as high as 3%.[42] A significant number of cases of femoral neuropathy occur with gynecologic, urologic, orthopedic, and vascular surgeries.[26,39,42] The incidence of neuropathy after abdominal hysterectomy, for example, ranges from 7% to 12%.[42] Based on their prospective study looking at femoral neuropathy subsequent to abdominal hysterectomy, Goldman et al.[43] reported the incidence of femoral neuropathy

decreased from 7.45% to 0.7% when self-retaining retractors were eliminated. The compression is often indirect, as the nerve becomes entrapped between the pelvic wall and the psoas muscle on which the retractor rests.[26] In those instances where a compressive neuropathy has occurred, direct ischemia of vasa nervorum due to deficient vascularization is the most likely mechanism of action. Urologic procedures (renal transplant, radical cystectomy, transurethral resection of the bladder with exploration and biopsy of a tumor mass, percutaneous nephrolithotomy of a pelvic kidney, radical cystoprostatectomy and continent urinary diversion, and psoas hitch vesicopexy) can also be a cause of femoral nerve injury.[37] For patients undergoing renal transplant with graft in the iliac fossa, the occurrence of femoral neuropathy ranges from 0.5% to 2.2%.[26,42] Possible explanations for the cause include nerve compression combined with potential hematoma in the iliac space and prolonged vascular anastomosis or arterial clamping time.

Symptoms and Signs

Unilateral sensory loss, paresthesias, or dysesthesias in the distribution of the femoral nerve and its branches, an impaired patellar reflex, and/or hip flexion and knee extension weakness may be present. Quadriceps atrophy may be noted in chronic and severe cases. Patients with hip flexion and knee extension weakness describe frequent buckling of the knee and/or falls while ambulating.[37] Navigating stairs is often difficult, requiring patients to ascend by leading with the unaffected leg and to descend by leading with the affected leg. Kuntzer et al.[39] reported weakness and dysesthesias in 88% and 44%, respectively. Pain, if present, can be at the site of the causative lesion (iliac fossa and inguinal region) or in the distribution of the nerve itself (anterior thigh or medial calf). Inguinal pain suggests a retroperitoneal mass.[37] Pain may be exacerbated by hip extension and partially relieved with hip flexion and external rotation.[24]

Diagnosis

If femoral neuropathy is noted in the immediate postoperative period, appropriate neuroimaging and radiographic studies should be ordered to determine the cause. Because motor weakness and reflex changes can also be seen with lumbar plexopathies or radiculopathies, these diagnoses must be included in the differential. Electrodiagnostic testing can help isolate the location and extent of nerve injury. Although the presence of EMG abnormalities in the vastus medialis muscle was not predictive of prognosis, the presence of NCS abnormalities, especially percentage of axonal loss, was predictive of prognosis.[44] Axonal loss, which is indicative of axonotmesis, portends a slower and possibly incomplete recovery. Kuntzer et al.[39] concluded that all patients with less than 50% axonal loss showed improvement within 1 year, whereas less than half the patients with greater than 50% axonal loss improved with conservative management alone. Irrespective of cause of injury, no improvement occurs after 2 years. Prognosis of recovery is greater if testing reveals only demyelinating abnormalities.[41] However, if abnormal EMG findings are found in the lumbar paraspinal muscles, this suggests a lumbar radiculopathy or plexopathy and not a peripheral neuropathy.

Treatment

If imaging studies identify a treatable cause, then the appropriate surgery should be performed as soon as possible to minimize the extent of neurologic deficit. Based on their retrospective series (1967 to 2000) of 119 surgically treated patients with intrapelvic or thigh-level femoral nerve lesions (89 traumatic injuries and 30 tumors), Kim et al.[45] recommended surgery in the absence of improvement at 3 to 4 months: neurolysis if intraoperative nerve action potentials across the nerve lesion are present and resection with grafting if intraoperative nerve action potentials are absent.[45] Although fewer patients underwent neurolysis compared to resection with grafting, the extent of recovery was greater in the former group, consistent with the severity of nerve injury. If there is no evidence of clinical or electrodiagnostic improvement after 3 to 6 months in those with iatrogenic or idiopathic femoral neuropathy, then surgical exploration with neurolysis should be considered.[41]

Assuming the femoral neuropathy is not due to traumatic injury or mass effect that necessitates surgery, recovery is typically the rule, and conservative treatment is usually sufficient. In their retrospective analysis of 2,175 patients undergoing a combined sciatic-femoral nerve block, Fanelli et al.[46] found 45 patients (2%) experienced transient neurologic dysfunction and all, but 1, improved within 4 to 12 weeks.[46] Extent of recovery (none, partial, or complete) and time to recovery after abdominal surgery is much more variable, the latter ranging from 2 weeks to 1 year.[41] Nonoperative treatment options include rest, analgesic medications, injections, and physical therapy. Whether temporary relief of symptoms with medications or injections alters the long-term prognosis is unknown, as the extent of recovery depends on the causative factor, extent of nerve damage, and location of injury. Longer recovery times should be anticipated when nerve damage is extensive and/or more proximal. Recovery is excellent if the etiology is due to lithotomy positioning, but it is less than satisfactory when due to hip surgery or inguinal procedures.[44,47] Kuntzer et al.,[39] however, reported no association between etiology and outcome. Physical therapy is important for those with evidence of motor weakness in order to prevent muscle contractures, minimize muscle atrophy, and maintain ambulatory status. For those with significant quadriceps weakness and knee instability, orthotic and/or gait assistive devices should be considered.

SAPHENOUS NERVE ENTRAPMENT

The saphenous nerve is the terminal sensory branch of the posterior division of the femoral nerve and is the longest cutaneous branch of the femoral nerve (Fig. 70.7). It originates near the inguinal ligament and descends within the quadriceps muscles in the subsartorial (Hunter's) canal and emerges from the canal to become subcutaneous approximately 10 cm proximal to the medial femoral condyle. The canal, which is located in the middle third of the medial thigh, also contains the femoral artery and vein. The saphenous nerve along with its two main divisions, the sartorial and infrapatellar nerves, supplies cutaneous sensation from the anteromedial aspect of the knee, medial calf, medial malleolus, and part of the medial arch of the foot.[37,38]

Etiology

Saphenous nerve injury can occur anywhere along the course of the nerve. Most saphenous neuropathies are iatrogenic or related to surgical procedures, although spontaneous neuropathies with unidentified causes can also occur.[37,48] Saphenous nerve trauma during femoral vascular surgeries and from saphenous vein harvesting for coronary artery bypass graft surgery can result in saphenous neuropathy.[49–55] After undergoing vascular reconstructions below the inguinal ligament, Adar et al.[49] reported variable degrees of saphenous neuropathy in 27 of 55 (49%) of patients, which were unrelated to surgical technical flaws. Inadvertent transection of the infrapatellar or sartorial nerves, such as during knee surgery (medial arthrotomy, medial meniscectomy, patellar realignment, total knee arthroplasty, and secondary repair for medial instability with pes transfer) can occur.[38,48,56,57] Schwabegger et al.[58] reported how a retained hemostatic clip on the infrapatellar nerve after a gracilis muscle flap resulted in neuralgia due to neuroma formation and moderate fibrosis within the subsartorial (Hunter's) canal. Resection of the neuroma resolved the pain, but sensory impairment remained. Another case report describes nerve damage resulting following a medial knee joint injection.[59]

Saphenous nerve entrapment can occur as it travels through the subsartorial (Hunter's) canal.[37,48] One case report documents distal tibial pain mimicking a tibial stress fracture from entrapment of the saphenous nerve caused by pes anserine bursitis.[60] Compression or thrombosis of the superficial femoral artery within the adductor canal can cause claudication pain in the lower leg.[53] Neural compression from the femoral vessels and adductor magnus tendons, which is more proximal to the subsartorial (Hunter's) canal, has also been reported.[61] Other case reports describe compression of the nerve due to an osteochondroma and from sitting astride and gripping a surfboard between the knees.[62,63]

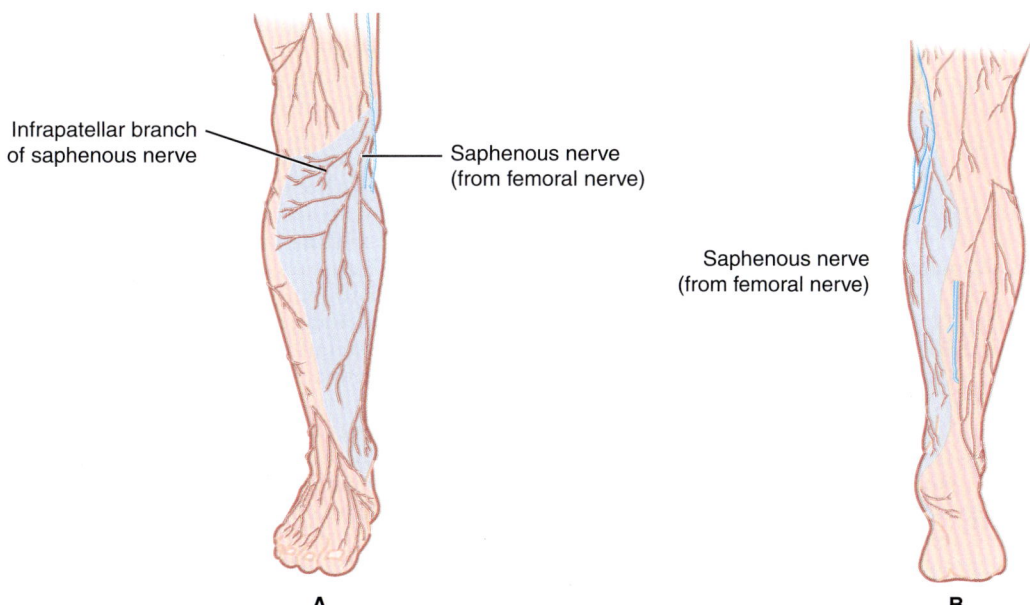

Infrapatellar branch of saphenous nerve

Saphenous nerve (from femoral nerve)

Saphenous nerve (from femoral nerve)

A

B

FIGURE 70.7   Cutaneous branches of the saphenous nerve. Anterior **(A)** view and posterior **(B)** view.

Symptoms and Signs

Knee pain is the main complaint, occurring in 90% of patients in one study, and tends to be worst with walking or any exercise involving active knee extension.[49,53,63] In another study involving 15 cases of saphenous nerve entrapment, patients most commonly reported medial knee and leg pain after prolonged walking (87%) and standing (47%).[48] Additional symptoms reported by these same patients included hypoesthesia (47%), no change in sensation (47%), and hyperesthesia (6%). Point tenderness over the subsartorial canal may be elicited in some of those with a suspected entrapment neuropathy but it is unlikely to be present in those with a traumatic nerve injury.[48,49,63] Because it is a purely sensory nerve, motor strength is unaffected. Therefore, sensory abnormalities or pain beyond the territory of the nerve, reflex changes, muscle atrophy, or muscle weakness suggests a lumbar plexopathy, lumbar radiculopathy, or other peripheral neuropathy.

Diagnosis

Electrodiagnostic studies can be helpful, but performing a saphenous NCS can be challenging. Instead of strictly looking at the absolute value of the SNAP amplitude or latency in the affected limb, it is more important to compare the side-to-side SNAP amplitudes.[37] A SNAP amplitude of less than 50% of the unaffected limb suggests the lesion is at or distal to the dorsal root ganglion.[37] Because the nerve is purely sensory, the EMG result should be normal. The clinical utility of saphenous nerve SSEPs is low. A pelvic MRI or CT should be considered if one suspects a mass lesion in the subsartorial canal.

Treatment

Nonsurgical treatment options include rest, analgesic medications, and injections. For those with a suspected entrapment neuropathy, a saphenous nerve block (with or without corticosteroid) over the subsartorial or transsartorial canal can be tried. Both of these approaches have been described as part of the anesthetic plan for lower extremity surgery.[64,65] Although the long-term efficacy of doing a saphenous nerve block in the setting of saphenous neuralgia remains unclear, the nerve block might yield a diagnostic answer. A local anesthetic saphenous nerve block provided relief in 12 of 32 (38%) cases described by Mozes et al.,[66] but they did not provide lasting relief in any of the 15 cases described by Worth et al.[48] With corticosteroid added to the local anesthetic in 30 patients undergoing a series of saphenous nerve blocks, Romanoff et al.[53] reported favorable outcomes (80%), no change (13%), and increased pain (7%). Whether temporary relief of symptoms alters the long-term prognosis is unknown. An ultrasound-guided saphenous nerve block can improve chances of obtaining a successful block.[67] Of 39 patients undergoing an ultrasound-guided subsartorial saphenous nerve block, Tsai et al.[64] reported a 77% success rate. For those with unremitting symptoms, neurolysis or neurectomy may be indicated, although which surgical approach offers the best outcome with the fewest complications is debatable.[48,66]

OBTURATOR NERVE ENTRAPMENT

The obturator nerve, which is a sensory and motor nerve, originates from the anterior divisions of the ventral rami of the L2, L3, and L4 nerve roots (Fig. 70.8; see Fig. 70.1A). (The posterior divisions of the same nerve roots form the femoral nerve.) The obturator nerve emerges from the medial surface of the psoas major muscle at the pelvic brim and descends along the lateral pelvic wall where it passes through the fibroosseous obturator foramen. Within the foramen, the obturator nerve splits into an anterior and posterior branch, finally emerging through the obturator foramen and entering the thigh. At the point of origin, the anterior branch supplies an articular branch to the hip joint

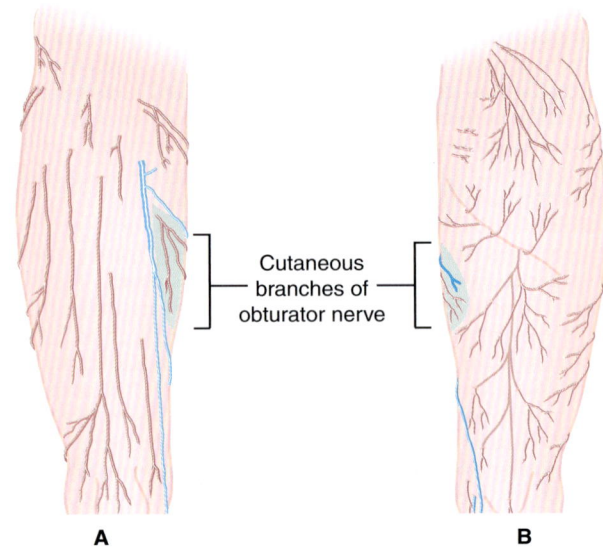

FIGURE 70.8 Cutaneous branches of the obturator nerve. Anterior (**A**) view and posterior (**B**) view.

followed by motor branches to the adductor longus and brevis, gracilis, and pectineus muscles. The sensory fibers of the anterior branch convey cutaneous information from the distal two-thirds of the medial thigh. The posterior branch supplies motor branches to the obturator externus and adductor magnus muscles and sensory branches to the articular capsule, cruciate ligaments, and synovial membrane of the knee joint. A normal variant in approximately 8% to 13% of the population, the accessory obturator nerve supplies the pectineal muscles and hip joint.[68]

Etiology

An isolated obturator neuropathy is uncommon because the nerve is well protected within the pelvis and medial thigh.[69,70] Causes of obturator neuropathy include entrapment (obturator hernia or local infection), compression (pelvic trauma, pelvic hematoma, pelvic tumor, retroperitoneal mass, fetal head or forceps in the pelvic canal during delivery, trauma or hematoma caused by cesarean section, acetabular labral cyst, extrapelvic synovial cyst, prolonged tourniquet use, or myositis ossificans), surgery (orthopedic, gynecologic, or pelvic laparoscopy), lithotomy positioning, and diabetes.[37,68–76] Of 22 patients with electrodiagnostic evidence of obturator neuropathy, Sorenson et al.[69] found perioperative complications or pelvic trauma were the most common causes. Because laparoscopic pelvic procedures could result in inadvertent electrocautery of the wrong nerve, careful visualization of the adjacent neurovascular structures should be undertaken.[37,70] The mechanism of entrapment is unclear, but Bradshaw et al.[68] concluded from their study of 32 athletes that electrodiagnostic and surgical findings (nerve entrapment by fascia and vessels over the obturator externus and adductor brevis muscles) suggest entrapment occurs at the level of the obturator foramen and proximal thigh, instead of within the obturator tunnel. Gender differences in the bony pelvic anatomy also play a role. Higher iliac bones, a smaller transverse pelvic inlet diameter, and a narrower subpubic angle, which all contribute to a greater bend in the obturator nerve within the obturator canal, probably accounts for the higher incidence of obturator neuropathy in men.[68]

Symptoms and Signs

Symptoms of obturator neuropathy include weakness, paresthesias, sensory loss, and/or pain along the medial thigh with extension as far distally as the knee. Sorenson et al.[69] reported that patients most commonly complained of medial thigh or groin pain (73%) followed by muscle weakness (27%) and sensory impairment (27%). Unfortunately, the complaints of pain can make it challenging to differentiate whether it is due to obturator neuropathy versus a traumatic or surgical procedure. Similar to Sorenson et al.,[69] Bradshaw et al.[68] found that self-reports of numbness or paresthesia among their 32 athletes were uncommon except in those with chronic obturator neuropathy. Additional symptoms included referred pain to the ASIS, exercise-induced exacerbation of pain with radiation from the medial thigh to knee, resolution of pain with rest, exercise-induced adductor muscle weakness and spasm, and wide-based gait. Because the femoral and sciatic nerves provide partial innervation to the adductor longus and magnus, respectively, muscle weakness may be difficult to appreciate on physical exam. With chronic and severe obturator neuropathy, though, medial thigh atrophy may occur. The adductor tendon reflex may even be diminished, but because this reflex can be absent in those without neuropathy, it must be obtainable in the unaffected limb.[37] A positive Howship-Romberg's sign—pain provocation along the medial thigh to the knee with passive abduction and extension of the affected hip or passive internal rotation of the hip—suggests the diagnosis.[77] This neural tension maneuver is felt to be pathognomonic of an obturator hernia, occurring in 15% to 50% of cases.[77,78]

Diagnosis

Because motor weakness and reflex changes can also be seen with lumbar plexopathies or radiculopathies, these diagnoses must be included in the differential. When the physical exam is nonspecific, sensory and motor findings can be confirmed with electrodiagnostic testing. Sorenson et al.[69] were able to diagnose a different disorder in 15 of 38 (39%) of patients who carried a presumptive diagnosis of obturator neuropathy. Radiographs of the pelvis are typically normal, unless osteitis pubis is present, and bone scans may show increased uptake in the pubic ramus on the affected side that presumably represents an inflammatory reaction that tracks along the fascia to entrap the nerve.[68] Alternatively, the periosteal changes may represent adductor insertion avulsion syndrome ("thigh splints"). If an intrapelvic or extrapelvic lesion is suspected, neuroimaging should be obtained.

Treatment

Recovery after sustaining an obturator nerve insult appears good in those with an acute neuropathy and poor in those with a chronic neuropathy. Conservative treatment measures include rest, physical therapy to stretch the groin muscles and to strengthen the adductor and pelvic muscles, soft tissue massage, and analgesic medications. Physical therapy is important for those with evidence of motor weakness in order to prevent muscle contractures, minimize muscle atrophy, and maintain ambulatory status. Among patient with an acute obturator neuropathy, Sorenson et al.[69] found that 93% of patients improved with conservative treatment or surgical exploration, indicating conservative management is the preferred course of care. Conversely, a chronic obturator neuropathy portends a poor prognosis as none of the patients with this diagnosis improved. Controversy exists as to whether severity of nerve injury affects long-term prognosis. Bradshaw et al.[68] noted failure with conservative treatment in those with electrodiagnostic evidence of denervation, instead preferring definitive surgical neurolysis. Conversely, Sorenson et al.[69] found three of four patients with electrodiagnostic evidence of a complete lesion improved without surgical exploration. For those who have limited benefit with noninjection therapies, a fluoroscopically guided obturator nerve block at the obturator foramen can be attempted.[68] Successful treatment of groin pain, medial and lateral thigh

pain, and hip joint pain with continuous RF and pulsed RF of the articular branches of the obturator and femoral nerves has also been described in various case reports.[79–81] For those with persistent symptoms or severe injuries (pelvic trauma, intraoperative nerve laceration, or tumor), surgery is recommended.[37]

SCIATIC NERVE ENTRAPMENT

The sciatic nerve arises from the lumbosacral plexus and is composed of the L4, L5, S1, S2, and S3 nerve roots (Fig. 70.9). It enters the lower extremity by exiting the pelvis through the sciatic notch. Variability exists, however, in the course the sciatic nerve takes as it exits the pelvis through the greater sciatic notch near the piriformis muscle. Beaton and Anson[82] found that among 1,510 cadaveric extremities, in 88%, the sciatic nerve exited below the piriformis muscle; in 11%, the piriformis muscle was divided in two parts such that the fibular division of the sciatic nerve passed in between both parts of the piriformis muscle and the tibial division passed below the bottom-most part of the muscle; in 0.86%, the fibular and tibial division of the nerve either passed above and below the muscle, respectively; and in 0.13%, the entire sciatic nerve pierced an undivided piriformis muscle (Fig. 70.10). The two anatomic variations where the sciatic nerve or its divisions pass in between the nerves lead to the nontraumatic variant of piriformis syndrome. Upon leaving the gluteal region, the sciatic nerve travels posterior and medial to the hip joint.

Commonly perceived of as a single nerve, the sciatic nerve is composed of lateral (fibular division) and medial (tibial division) trunks that actually lay adjacent to each other. Around the middle to distal aspect of the posterior thigh, the divisions

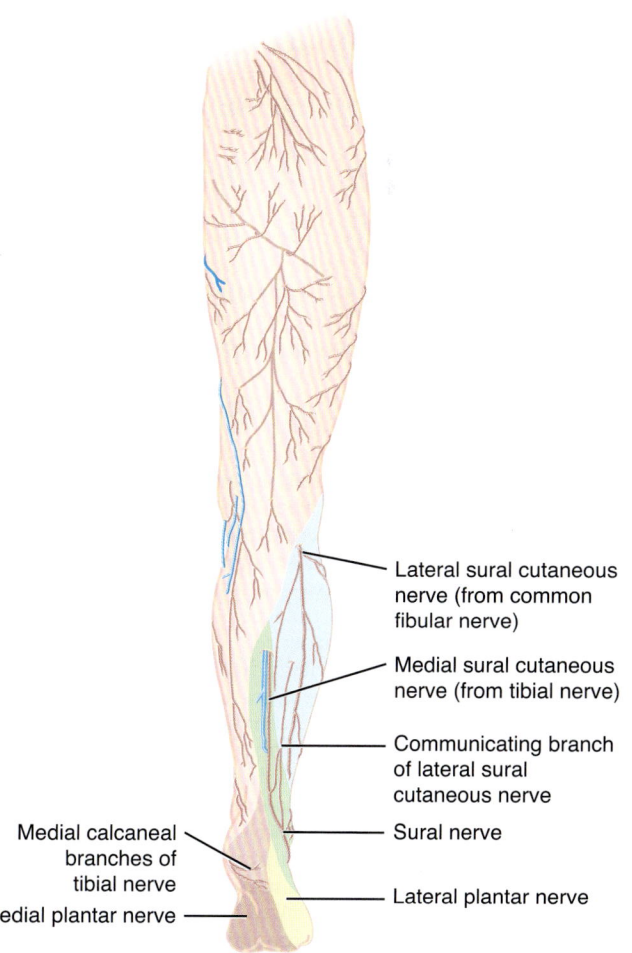

Lateral sural cutaneous nerve (from common fibular nerve)

Medial sural cutaneous nerve (from tibial nerve)

Communicating branch of lateral sural cutaneous nerve

Sural nerve

Medial calcaneal branches of tibial nerve

Lateral plantar nerve

Medial plantar nerve

FIGURE 70.9 Cutaneous branches of the sciatic nerve.

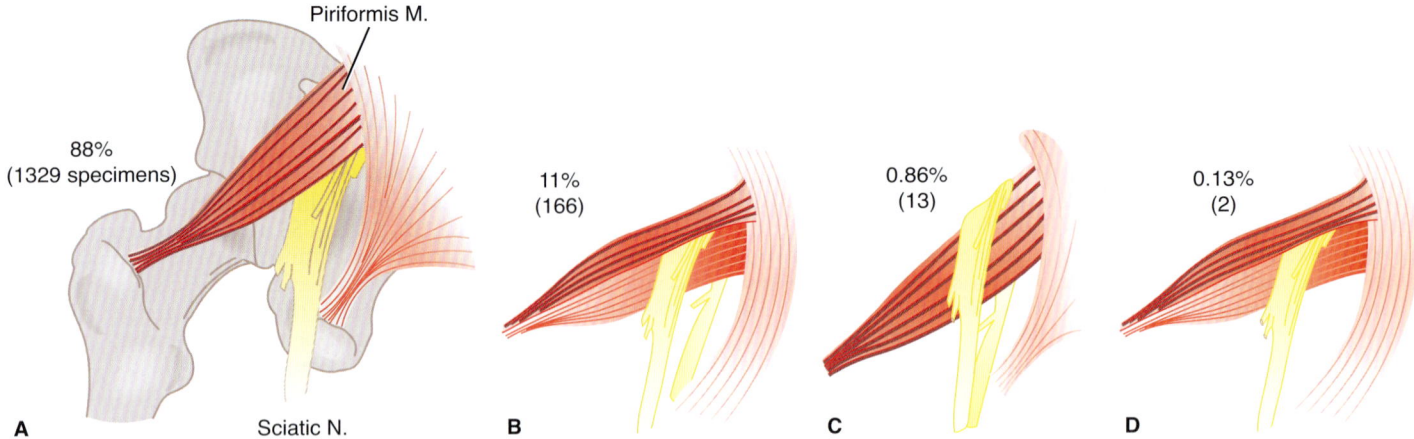

FIGURE 70.10 **A–D:** Relationship of the sciatic nerve to the piriformis muscle in 1,510 extremities studied. *(From Beaton LE, Anson BJ. The relation of the sciatic nerve and its subdivisions to the piriformis muscle. Anat Rec 1938;70:1–5.)*

diverge to form the common fibular and tibial nerves. Prior to diverging, the fibular division innervates the short head of the biceps femoris muscle, with tibial nerve branches innervating the remaining hamstring (semitendinosus, semimembranosus, and long head of the biceps femoris) muscles. With the exception of the saphenous nerve, branches of the sciatic nerve supply the sensory innervation below the knee, and branches of the sciatic nerve supply the entire motor innervation below the knee.

Etiology
After fibular neuropathy, sciatic neuropathy is the second most common lower extremity peripheral neuropathy.[83] Injury can occur anywhere along the course of the nerve from the gluteal region to the posterior thigh. Causes of sciatic neuropathy include compression (hematoma, abscess, piriformis syndrome, benign or malignant tumor, myositis ossificans, endometriosis, prolonged sitting or supine positioning without adequate pressure relief, lithotomy position, vaginal delivery due to nerve compression from the fetus's head, or pneumatic thigh tourniquet), contusion (fall from a height without fracture or dislocation), trauma (gunshot wound, laceration, femur fracture, intramuscular injection of medication into the gluteal region), stretch injury (hip arthroplasty, hip dislocation, hip or femur fracture), nerve ischemia (vasculitis, arterial thrombosis, arterial bypass surgery, diabetes mellitus, postradiation therapy), and idiopathic.[44,84–86] Based on 492 reported cases of sciatic neuropathy in the English literature from 1967 to 1997, Plewnia et al.[86] found that the five most common causes were hip arthroplasty (34%), intramuscular injection of medication into the gluteal region (28%), hip fracture or dislocation (9%), benign or malignant tumor (8%), and external compression (8%).

Sciatic nerve injury is the most common neurologic complication of total hip arthroplasty—with an estimated incidence of 0.6% to 6.7% of all arthroplasties—and can be caused by stretch injury, direct trauma from retractors or fixation screws, infarction, intraneural hemorrhage, hip dislocation, thermal injury from methyl methacrylate extravasation, or compression from the prosthesis or a bony prominence.[84] In their study of 100 patients with electrodiagnostically confirmed sciatic neuropathy, Yuen et al.[83] reported that hip arthroplasty occurred in 22% and accounted for the most common cause of sciatic nerve injury. Kline et al.,[84] however, discovered that of 380 patients seen from 1967 to 1991, hip arthroplasty only accounted for a minority (3%) of cases and that injection injury from intramuscular drug administration accounted for the majority (36%) of cases. Although most cases of hip arthroplasty–related sciatic neuropathy occur in the perioperative setting, delayed onset can also be seen.[85]

Sciatic nerve entrapment by the piriformis muscle, also known as *piriformis syndrome*, can be another cause of sciatica. Although its diagnosis remains controversial, it is reported to occur with a 6:1 female-to-male predominance.[87] It is less commonly due to sciatic nerve entrapment by the piriformis muscle and instead is more commonly associated with direct trauma to the sciatic notch and the gluteal regions; prolonged sitting; prolonged combined hip flexion, adduction, and internal rotation; and certain athletes (cyclists who ride for prolonged periods of time, tennis players who constantly internally rotate their hip with an overhead serve, and ballet dancers who constantly externally rotate their hip while dancing).[82,88–91] Although the mechanism of injury may be postulated, the etiology of the signs and symptoms remains less clear. Traumatic injury to the piriformis muscle may generate inflammatory and edematous changes to the muscle and surrounding fascia, subsequently compressing the sciatic nerve against the wall of the pelvis and leading to a compression neuropathy.[90] The trauma itself may induce focal hyperirritability in the piriformis muscle, which can be further exacerbated by muscle spasm or hypertrophy.

Symptoms and Signs
Signs and symptoms of sciatic neuropathy include weakness, impaired ankle reflex, paresthesias, sensory loss, and/or pain in the distribution of the nerve. Weakness of toe extension and flexion, ankle dorsiflexion and plantarflexion, and ankle eversion and inversion are the most prominent signs.[85] Clinically, absence of complete weakness of ankle dorsiflexion and plantarflexion predicts earlier or better recovery.[92] Of the two nerve trunks, weakness more commonly affects fibular-innervated versus tibial-innervated muscles.[85,93] This is especially true in sciatic neuropathy after hip replacement.[83] Although it is not entirely understood why the fibular division is more selectively injured compared to the tibial division, various reasons have been postulated: (1) superficial and lateral position, thereby placing the fibular division in closer proximity to the hip joint and exposing it to injury from hip joint trauma or surgery; (2) smaller blood supply; (3) fewer and larger fascicles; (4) less supportive endoneurium and perineurium between fascicles; and (5) relative tethering of the nerve at the sciatic notch and fibular head, thereby making it vulnerable to stretch injuries.[84,94] The exception to this rule appears to be femur fractures or gunshot wounds to the thigh, in which case the tibial division can be involved to an equal or greater extent.[83] Because of preferential fibular involvement, knee flexion weakness is commonly insignificant, and isolated injury to the fibular division can masquerade as a fibular neuropathy at the knee or fibular head.

The most common presenting symptoms with piriformis syndrome are a deep, aching buttock pain that is often associated with a limp and sitting intolerance on the affected side.[90] Squatting, climbing stairs, walking, and prolonged sitting (especially on hard surfaces) typically worsen the pain. In addition, the piriformis muscle's compression of the pudendal nerve and blood vessels may cause labial pain and dyspareunia in females and scrotal pain and impotence in males. Painful bowel movements have also been reported, presumably due to the close proximity of the piriformis muscle and the rectum.[95] The two most consistent physical exam findings are tenderness to palpation in the greater sciatic notch and reproduction of pain with maximum flexion, adduction, and internal rotation of the hip.[90] Various physical exam maneuvers can be tried in an attempt to reproduce these findings: Freiberg sign (buttock pain with passive, forced internal rotation of the hip), Lasègue's sign (pain and tenderness to palpation in the greater sciatic notch with the hip passively flexed to 90 degrees and the knee passively extended 180 degrees), Pace's maneuver (buttock pain with resisted abduction of the affected leg while in the seated position), and Beatty's maneuver (while lying in a lateral decubitus position on the unaffected side, buttock pain is elicited in the affected extremity when the patient actively abducts the affected hip and holds the knee several inches off the table).[87,96,97]

Diagnosis

Because the differential diagnosis can include radiculopathy, plexopathy, or fibular neuropathy, neuroimaging of the pelvis and/or lumbosacral spine may be necessary to help establish the cause of nerve damage based on the mechanism of injury. Electrodiagnostic testing can be performed to confirm the location of the lesion and to offer prognostic information based on the chronicity and severity of nerve damage. Because muscles innervated by the nerve roots are uninvolved, the lumbar paraspinal muscles are unaffected. In their retrospective analysis of 100 patients, Yuen et al.[83] noted greater severity of injury of the fibular division (64%), significant axonal loss (93%), tibialis anterior muscle EMG abnormality (92%), and low or absent extensor digitorum brevis (EDB) compound muscle action potential (CMAP) amplitude (80%). A more favorable prognosis—earlier or better recovery—was noted in those with a recordable EDB, CMAP, and presence of demyelination instead of axonal loss.[83] Because normal sural and superficial fibular SNAP amplitudes were obtained in 29% and 9% of patients, respectively, the authors concluded that sparing of the tibial division does not necessarily exclude the diagnosis of sciatic neuropathy.

To diagnose piriformis syndrome, the symptoms and clinical exam findings must be correlated with neuroimaging of the pelvis (asymmetry of the piriformis muscle, mass effect, or anatomic variation consistent with entrapment) and electrodiagnostic studies (evidence consistent with extrapelvic compression of the sciatic nerve at the level of the piriformis muscle).[95,98,99]

Treatment

Conservative therapy for symptomatic relief includes analgesic medications, injections, and physical therapy. Physical therapy is important for those with evidence of motor weakness in order to prevent muscle contractures, minimize muscle atrophy, and maintain ambulatory status. An AFO should be considered for those with significant ankle dorsiflexion and plantarflexion weakness. Spinal cord stimulation or intrathecal therapies should be considered for those who have a suboptimal response to the aforementioned and/or those who are not surgical candidates.

Surgical treatment of sciatic neuropathy is directed at identifying the cause of nerve injury. Surgery should be considered for cases of compression due to obvious mass effect or traumatic neuropathy that fails to improve with time. Surgical exploration for trauma-induced injuries, however, requires careful deliberation. Kline et al.[84] found that medical management in those patients with a partial deficit and/or improvement in function and pain resulted in an 80% and 60% chance of useful return of function in the tibial and fibular divisions, respectively. In those patients in whom surgery (neurolysis, suture repair, or nerve graft) was performed because of evidence of a nerve action potential distal to the lesion, good-to-excellent outcomes were common for the tibial division but less common for the fibular division. Kline et al.[84] suggested that the paucity of successful functional outcomes with fibular division surgeries may be related to uncoordinated muscle reinnervation (as opposed to insufficient nerve regeneration), further calling into question the practicality of fibular division surgery.

If the diagnosis of piriformis syndrome is confirmed and conservative management with physical therapy and medication fails to adequately relieve symptoms, an intramuscular piriformis injection of corticosteroid and local anesthetic can be undertaken with image guidance (fluoroscopy, CT, or ultrasound) alone or in combination with EMG guidance or nerve stimulation.[88,100–104] Comparing ultrasound guidance versus fluoroscopic guidance, Finnoff et al.[105] found the accuracy of needle placement was 95% versus 30%, respectively. Because the duration of analgesia with corticosteroid can be short-lived, some have even advocated the use of botulinum toxin for prolonged analgesia in those that at least respond diagnostically to the local anesthetic.[106–109] The use of botulinum toxin for this diagnosis, though, is an off-label use of the medication. Surgical consultation for evaluation of piriformis tendon release and sciatic neurolysis should be considered as a last resort.[90,110]

FIBULAR (PERONEAL) NERVE ENTRAPMENT

The fibular nerve is derived from the L4, L5, S1, and S2 nerve roots as a part of the sciatic nerve (Fig. 70.11). The fibular nerve, along with the tibial nerve, is a division of the sciatic nerve. Approximately 8 cm proximal to the popliteal fossa, the fibular nerve separates from the tibial nerve and forms the common fibular nerve. As it descends into the popliteal fossa, it innervates the short head of the biceps femoris muscle. Proximal to the fibular head, the common fibular nerve gives off two branches: the sural communicating branch and the lateral cutaneous branch. The sural communicating branch becomes part of the sural nerve after receiving a branch from the tibial nerve. The lateral cutaneous branch conveys sensory information from the proximal and lateral aspect of the leg. As it winds around the fibular head, covered only by skin and a thin layer of subcutaneous tissue, the common fibular nerve is most vulnerable to injury. Approximately 1 to 2 cm distal to

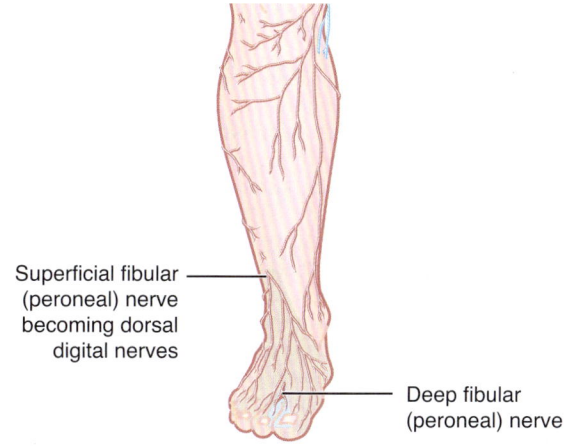

Superficial fibular (peroneal) nerve becoming dorsal digital nerves

Deep fibular (peroneal) nerve

FIGURE 70.11   Cutaneous branches of the fibular nerve.

the fibular head, the common fibular nerve dives into the fibular tunnel which is made up of the aponeurosis of the soleus muscle and a wide, thick, and inflexible fibrous arch.[111] Distal to the fibular tunnel, the common fibular nerve separates into the superficial and deep fibular nerves. The superficial fibular nerve innervates the ankle evertors and plantar flexors (peroneus longus and brevis muscles), after which it divides into the medial and intermediate dorsal cutaneous nerves to provide sensory innervation to most of the dorsal aspect of the foot, with the exception of the web space between the first and second toes. (Ankle inversion is unaffected because the tibial nerve innervates the tibialis posterior muscle.) The deep fibular nerve innervates the ankle and toe dorsiflexors (tibialis anterior, extensor hallucis longus, extensor digitorum longus, and peroneus tertius muscles). Distal to the ankle mortise, the deep fibular nerve gives off lateral and medial branches. The former innervates the EDB and extensor hallucis brevis, and the latter supplies cutaneous sensation to the web space between the first and second toes.

Etiology

Fibular neuropathy is the most common lower extremity mononeuropathy, but its exact gender or age prevalence is unknown.[112] In a retrospective analysis looking at 5,777 trauma patients, Noble et al.[113] noted 79 lower extremity peripheral nerve injuries involving the fibular (39), sciatic (28), tibial (8), and femoral (4) nerves. Although fibular nerve trauma most commonly occurs at the fibular head where it is superficially protected only by the skin and thin underlying fascia, injury to the fibular nerve and its branches can occur anywhere along the course of the nerve. Aprile et al.[112] demonstrated that most (83%) causes of fibular neuropathy are identifiable, with the majority (31%) being due to perioperative issues. Various causes of fibular nerve injury include entrapment, compression (improperly applied casts or braces, tight stockings, vascular abnormality, osteophytes, and intraneural or extraneural tumor), traction (leg-crossing, prolonged squatting or kneeling, prolonged ankle plantarflexion, surgical positioning, high-heeled shoes), trauma (fracture of the proximal fibular head, knee dislocation, ankle sprain or fracture, nerve laceration, and gunshot injury), metabolic (rapid weight-loss, hyperthyroidism, diabetes mellitus, vasculitic disorders, and leprosy), surgery (orthopedic surgery, vascular surgery, and plastic surgery), or idiopathic.[24,111,113–128] In their study of 146 fibular nerve injuries requiring surgery, Piton et al.[129] classified the causes as fibular tunnel syndrome (62), external compression (16), trauma (33), iatrogenic injury (16), tumor (9), wound injury (7), contusion (2), and burn injury (1). In a larger and more recent study involving 318 fibular nerve injuries requiring surgery, Kim et al.[130] classified the causes as stretch or contusion without fracture or dislocation (141), tumor (40), laceration (39), entrapment (30), stretch or contusion with fracture or dislocation (22), external compression (21), iatrogenic (13), and gunshot (12). Looking at 60 patients who only had entrapment, Fabre et al.[111] classified the causes as idiopathic (53), postural (5), and dynamic (2). True entrapment can be classified as postural (which is associated with kneeling, crouching, squatting, or ankle plantarflexion) or dynamic (which is associated with activities such as running).[24,131–133] For those with entrapment, it is postulated that chronic nerve irritation within the fibrous arch of the fibular tunnel causes edema, which subsequently causes scar tissue formation as the nerve glides in the narrow tunnel during knee flexion and extension.[111]

Superficial fibular nerve entrapment is relatively uncommon and usually is due to compression of the nerve as it exits the anterolateral compartment 10 cm proximal to the ankle.[134–136] Although deep fibular nerve entrapment can occur anywhere along its course, it is known as "anterior tarsal tunnel syndrome" when it becomes compressed beneath the inferior extensor retinaculum.[136–138] Postural causes of deep fibular entrapment include prolonged plantarflexion, such as with wearing high-heeled shoes.[24]

Symptoms and Signs

Symptoms of fibular neuropathy may include weakness, paresthesias, sensory loss, and/or pain in the distribution of the fibular nerve and its various branches. Patients with dynamic entrapment report activity-related leg pain with or without sensory impairment.[24] The degree and extent of neuromuscular deficit and atrophy depends on the location (common vs. superficial vs. deep fibular), severity, and chronicity of nerve injury. Common fibular injury typically causes dorsiflexion (ankle and toes) and eversion (ankle) weakness, leading to tripping due to dragging of toes, excessive hip and knee flexion in an attempt to clear the foot (steppage gait), and foot slap.[136] When the injury is proximal to the knee, knee flexion weakness also occurs because the biceps femoris muscle is affected. A positive Tinel sign at the fibular head, 10 cm proximal to the ankle, or over the dorsal aspect of the ankle suggests a common fibular, superficial fibular, or deep fibular neuropathy, respectively. Fabre et al.[111] noted a positive Tinel sign at the fibular head in 60 of the 62 (97%) cases of common fibular entrapment. Sensory abnormalities, motor weakness, or pain beyond the territory of the nerve suggest an alternate diagnosis, such as a lumbar plexopathy, a lumbar radiculopathy, or other peripheral neuropathy.

Diagnosis

Electrodiagnostic studies can be performed to confirm the diagnosis, location, and extent of fibular neuropathy. Without axonal loss, the NCS reveals slowing of the nerve conduction velocity. However, when long-standing compression or direct nerve injury results in axonal loss, a decreased SNAP amplitude, a decreased compound muscle action potential amplitude, and a conduction block can be seen on NCS. The EMG portion of the study not only helps confirm axonal loss but the extent of muscle involvement can also aid in determining whether the lesion involves the common fibular, superficial fibular, or deep fibular nerve. For those with exercise-induced (dynamic) fibular neuropathy, electrodiagnostic studies may need to be done before and after exercising.[24] Once a fibular neuropathy has been confirmed electrodiagnostically, additional imaging (radiograph, CT, and MRI) or laboratory studies may be needed to isolate the cause of nerve injury.

Treatment

Nonsurgical treatment options include rest, modification of footwear or garments, analgesic medications, injections, and physical therapy. Physical therapy is important for those with evidence of motor weakness in order to prevent muscle contractures, minimize muscle atrophy, and maintain ambulatory status. Whether temporary relief of symptoms with medications or injections alters the long-term prognosis is unknown, as the extent of recovery depends on the causative factor, extent of nerve damage, and location of injury. The degree of pain relief after doing a fibular nerve block at the fibular head can provide diagnostic information. Significant fibular nerve damage resulting in ankle and foot weakness may necessitate an AFO and customized orthopedic shoes to correct any gait disturbance.

Depending on the etiology of fibular nerve injury, surgery is advocated within 2 to 4 months if there is lack of clinical and electrophysiologic improvement.[111,129,130] In their retrospective analysis of 318 patients with preoperatively confirmed EMG evidence of knee-level common fibular nerve lesions, Kim et al.[130] reported recovery of useful function in 88% and 84% of those undergoing neurolysis and end-to-end suture repair, respectively; recovery of useful function in 75%, 38%, and 16% for those requiring nerve grafting less than 6 cm, 6 to

12 cm, and 13 to 24 cm, respectively; and preservation of preoperative clinical function in 80% of those requiring tumor resection.[130] For patients with idiopathic entrapment, surgical decompression is recommended when symptoms fail to resolve within 3 to 4 months because the time needed for recovery is shorter than that associated with conservative management.[111]

Foot Pain

PES PLANUS

Etiology

Pes planus, a condition also known as flatfoot, refers to the loss of the normal longitudinal arch of the medial foot (Fig. 70.12). The most common cause of pes planus is insufficiency or dysfunction of the posterior tibial tendon.[139] Congenital flatfoot is used to describe a flatfoot present since birth. Trauma, such as Lisfranc joint injuries and calcaneal fractures, can also lead to pes planus due to joint subluxation. Degenerative changes secondary to arthritis can also lead to pes planus. Tarsal coalition—a congenital fibrous union or fusion between the bones of the hindfoot and midfoot—has also been implicated as a cause of flatfoot.[140]

Symptoms and Signs

Symptoms of pes planus can vary among patients with different forms of anatomic pathology and biomechanics leading to the condition. Examination of the feet should begin with the patient in standing position. Typically, the longitudinal arch flattens upon standing and appears when the foot is not bearing weight. Heel eversion often accompanies pes planus. Severe pes planus may result in significant pain, particularly along the course of the posterior tibial tendon, which may be tender upon palpation.[141]

Diagnosis and Treatment

Radiographic imaging should be performed of the foot and ankle in three weight-bearing views—anteroposterior, oblique, and lateral. Loss of the longitudinal arch is best visualized on the weight-bearing lateral radiographs.[142] MRI can also be useful in assessing this condition, particularly in evaluation of the posterior tibial tendon. Treatment is often conservative through the use of arch supports and plantar inserts. Surgical treatment may involve posterior tibial advancement, subtalar fusion, or osteotomies, depending on the initial cause of the condition.

PES CAVUS

Etiology

Cavus foot deformity is an abnormal elevation of the longitudinal arch (Fig. 70.13). This results in increased stress forces on the metatarsal heads and decreased weight bearing by the plantar region of the foot.[143] Causes of pes cavus include

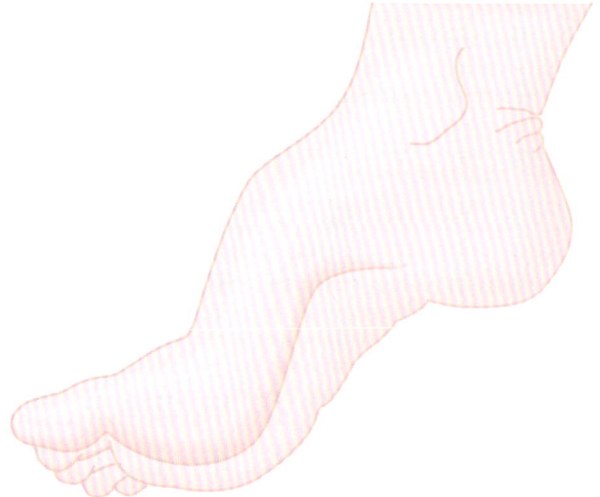

FIGURE 70.13 Pes cavus.

neuromuscular disease (such as muscular dystrophy, cerebral palsy, and spinal tumors), residual clubfoot, malunion of calcaneal or talar fractures, and burns.[143]

Symptoms and Signs

Symptomatology varies based on the extent of the deformity. Lateral foot pain can develop as a result of increased weight bearing by the lateral foot. Metatarsalgia is frequently associated with pes cavus. Intractable plantar keratosis is often seen as well. Clawing of the toes—hyperextension at the metatarsophalangeal joints and flexion of the proximal and distal interphalangeal joints—may also be present.[143] Patients may experience generalized stiffness of the joint, leading to disuse of the affected foot.

Diagnosis and Treatment

Physical examination should elucidate if the deformity is flexible or rigid. This can be determined by performance of the Coleman block test.[142] A 1-in wood block is placed beneath the heel and lateral foot while the first, second, and third metatarsals are allowed to hang freely into plantarflexion and pronation. If heel varus corrects in this stance, the deformity is flexible. If the hindfoot does not correct, the deformity is rigid. Weight-bearing radiographs of the ankle and foot aid in the diagnosis through demonstration of hindfoot varus. MRI of the spine may be necessary to evaluate for possible spinal tumor presence if the deformity is unilateral and no inciting traumatic event is noted. In addition, a neurologic consultation and an EMG/NCS can be obtained to evaluate for polio, Charcot-Marie-Tooth disease, and other neurologic causes of pes cavus. Conservative therapy for pes cavus includes the use of orthotic shoe inserts to offset increased weight-bearing forces on the metatarsal heads. Surgical intervention is warranted if the condition is severe and is aimed at construction of a plantigrade foot. This may be accomplished through tendon transfers, osteotomies, and arthrodesis.[142]

PLANTAR FASCIITIS

Etiology

Plantar fasciitis is a painful inflammatory condition involving the insertion of the plantar fascia on the medial process of the calcaneal tuberosity. Pes planus, pes cavus, leg-length discrepancy, overpronation, and running all involve increased stress forces placed on the plantar fascia and thus can lead to plantar fasciitis.[144]

Symptoms and Signs

Patients typically complain of intense sharp heel pain after the first few steps in the morning or after a period of rest. The pain

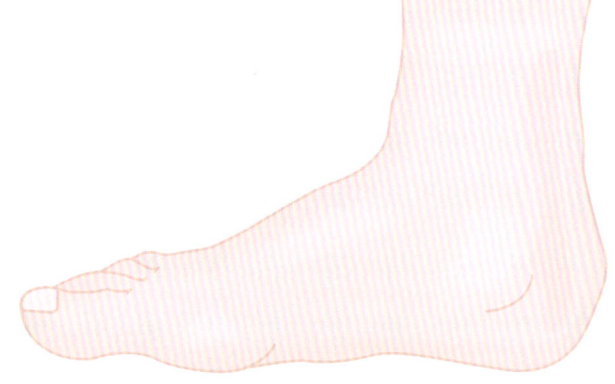

FIGURE 70.12 Pes planus.

is usually located along the anterior portion of the heel, with radiation into the sole of the foot.[145] The pain is exacerbated by weight-bearing activities and relieved by rest. Patients may also experience generalized stiffness of the foot and swelling of the heel.

Diagnosis and Treatment

Pain can be reproduced on palpation of the anteromedial aspect of the calcaneus as well as the proximal plantar fascia. Passive dorsiflexion of the toes and toe walking can also reproduce pain secondary to plantar fasciitis.[145] Radiographic imaging can reveal soft tissue calcifications in the heel and may be more useful to investigate for bony tumor or fractures as an underlying cause. Ultrasound may reveal a thicker heel aponeurosis, which can be associated with plantar fasciitis. MRI can demonstrate thickening of the plantar fascia. Because of the poor sensitivity and specificity of these imaging techniques, diagnosis of plantar fasciitis is usually made through the history and physical examination. Conservative treatment involves the use of medial arch support inserts in footwear, shoe modifications, stretching exercises focusing on the plantar fascia, ice therapy, and NSAIDs.[145,146] Night splints can be worn to allow the plantar fascia to heal in an elongated position as opposed to the natural plantarflexed position of the foot during sleep. Some studies have demonstrated that corticosteroid injections, botulinum toxin injections, and autologous platelet-rich plasma therapy can also be useful in treating plantar fasciitis.[147,148] It should be noted that injection of botulinum toxin for plantar fasciitis is considered an off-label use of the medication. The injection of either corticosteroid or botulinum toxin is performed with a medial or lateral approach into the site of maximal tenderness. Complications of corticosteroid injections include plantar fascia rupture and fat pad atrophy.[149] When these treatment modalities are unsuccessful, surgical release of the plantar fascia may be indicated. However, extracorporeal shockwave therapy (ESWT) could be an alternative to a surgical remedy that also happens to be noninvasive and safe. In their systematic review of ESWT (2005 to 2016), Roerdink et al.[146] found no complications at 1-year follow-up.

HEEL PAD DEFICIENCY
Etiology

The fat pad of the heel is made of individual fibrous septa containing fat and elastic fibrous tissue. The fat pad absorbs shock and distributes mechanical forces to the calcaneus.

The fat pad atrophies with age, multiple glucocorticoid injections, and trauma.[150]

Symptoms and Signs

Patients typically experience deep, diffuse plantar heel pain that is exacerbated upon standing and walking/running on hard surfaces. Direct palpation of this area reproduces this pain. There is palpable atrophy of the heel pad, and underlying bone may be palpated. Scar tissue and calcification can be observed.

Diagnosis and Treatment

Diagnosis is usually made through history and physical examination. NSAIDs can provide significant analgesia. Long-acting local anesthetics, such as bupivacaine, can be infiltrated into the affected area for severe, painful crises. Corticosteroids are contraindicated, as they can worsen the condition.[149] Shock-absorbing footwear inserts can be helpful by providing cushion and absorbing shock.

TARSAL TUNNEL SYNDROME
Anatomy

The tarsal tunnel is bounded by the flexor retinaculum, a strong fibrous band that extends from the medial malleolus to the margin of the calcaneus, and the medial surfaces of both the calcaneus and talus.[151] The posterior tibial nerve courses beneath the flexor retinaculum through this tunnel and divides into the medial and lateral plantar nerves, which innervate the small muscles of the foot and the skin on the plantar aspect of the foot and toes (Fig. 70.14).

Etiology

Compression of the posterior tibial nerve as it passes behind the medial malleolus in the tarsal tunnel may lead to tarsal tunnel syndrome, a painful condition of the ankle and plantar aspect of the foot. The branches of the posterior tibial nerve are vulnerable to compressive injury (restrictive footwear), entrapment from space-occupying lesions (i.e., ganglion cysts, osteophytes, and tumors), direct trauma, overuse injuries, and inflammation within the tarsal tunnel.[152] Hindfoot valgus deformities can further exacerbate tarsal tunnel syndrome symptoms due to increased neural tension that is secondary to an increase in eversion and dorsiflexion foot positioning. All of these conditions can lead to edema and scar tissue formation, which further limit the vascular supply and cause increased traction of the nerve between joint movements. This ultimately can result in axonal and wallerian degeneration.

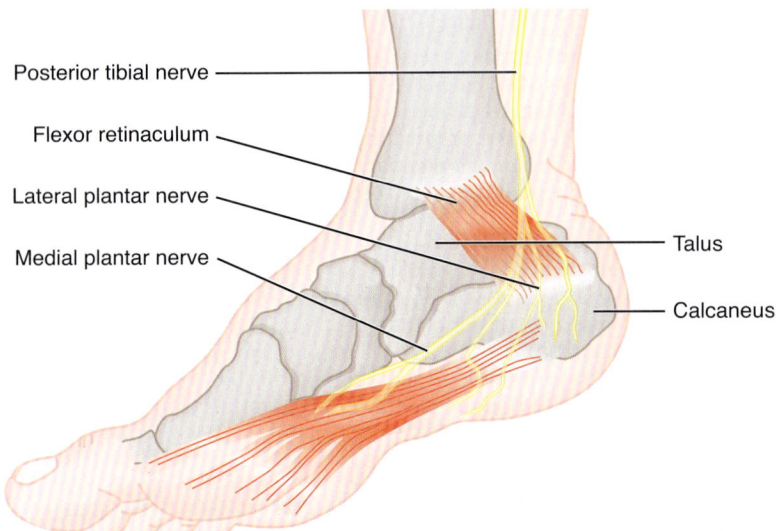

Posterior tibial nerve

Flexor retinaculum

Lateral plantar nerve

Medial plantar nerve

Talus

Calcaneus

FIGURE 70.14 Anatomy of the tarsal tunnel and posterior tibial nerve.

Symptoms and Signs

Pain or paresthesias in the heel, medial malleolus, or plantar surface of the foot may occur, depending on which nerve branch is compressed and the severity of the compression. When both plantar nerves are affected, symptoms extend from the posterior malleolus to the plantar aspect of the foot and dorsal surfaces of the distal aspect of the toes. Pain can be experienced in both the standing and reclining positions and may be worse at night.[151] Simultaneous dorsiflexion and eversion of the ankle exacerbates the pain due to increased nerve tension. Advanced disease leads to weakness of the intrinsic muscles of the foot and of the toe plantar flexor muscles. Physical examination typically reveals tenderness to palpation of the tibial nerve. Percussion at the medial malleolus (Tinel sign) causes radiation of pain and paresthesias along the path of the posterior tibial nerve and its branches.[151] In addition, symptoms may be reproduced through continuous compression of the nerve for 30 seconds (Phalen's sign).[151] Sensory deficits are uncommon but can affect the sole of the foot if present.

Diagnosis

An EMG/NCS often reveals prolonged motor terminal latency of the medial or plantar nerves to the abductor hallucis and abductor digiti quinti muscles, absent nerve potentials, or slow nerve conduction velocities.[153] Although electrodiagnostic testing can aid in the diagnosis of tibial neuropathy, neuroimaging may still be necessary to demonstrate whether a space-occupying lesion within the tarsal tunnel is the source of the symptoms.[153] An MRI demonstrates the anatomy of the tarsal tunnel and its contents and can prove useful in planning for surgical decompression.

Treatment

The initial treatment includes nonsurgical measures such as avoidance of exacerbating activities, medications (corticosteroids, acetaminophen, NSAIDs, antiseizure medications, opioids, tricyclic antidepressants, topical analgesics, lidocaine patch), TENS, physical therapy, shoe inserts, and night splints with the foot in plantarflexion. An injection of local anesthetic and corticosteroid into the tarsal tunnel may provide analgesia.[153] Surgical decompression with release of the flexor retinaculum, is employed if nonoperative measures fail. If present, space-occupying lesions of the tarsal tunnel, such as varicose veins and ganglions, are removed along with release of the flexor retinaculum. Decompression may also be accomplished through division of the proximal ridge of the abductor hallucis.[152] Surgical complications primarily involve incomplete release of the flexor retinaculum, resulting in persistent pain.[152]

LISFRANC JOINT INSTABILITY
Etiology

The Lisfranc joint (tarsometatarsal joint or metatarsal cuneiform joint) is a six-bone complex that connects the forefoot and the midfoot. It is made up of the articulation of the bases of the first three metatarsals with the cuneiforms and the fourth and fifth metatarsals with the cuboid. The joint aids in pronation and supination of the foot.[154] The great majority of Lisfranc joint injuries are associated with fractures, especially the metatarsals. Although injury to the joint is generally associated with high-energy mechanisms (e.g., falls or motor vehicle collisions), resulting in severe inversion or plantarflexion, low-impact mechanisms (e.g., direct trauma in sports-related injuries) are also known to cause injury.[155] The Lisfranc injury may be classified by the direction of the dislocation.

Symptoms and Signs

Lisfranc joint instability is characterized by severe midfoot pain and the inability to bear weight. Point tenderness over the midfoot is noted on exam. Bruising on the plantar surface of the midfoot represents an occult sign of an injury. Depending on the mechanism of injury, there may be soft tissue damage, such as edema, a wound, or vascular impairment. Pain or edema that persists after soft tissue healing is expected to have occurred should raise the index of suspicion for a Lisfranc joint injury.[155]

Diagnosis

Conventional radiography is the initial imaging modality of choice. Radiographs will reveal fractures of the joint and displacement of the metatarsals. Because sprains are more difficult to detect, weight-bearing plain radiographs and stress radiographs taken with the foot plantarflexed and inverted have been suggested to establish the diagnosis.[156] Advanced imaging, however, should be considered in the following circumstances: (1) CT for identifying occult fractures or subtle subluxations and (2) MRI for soft tissue and ligamentous injuries.[157]

Treatment

Treatment depends on the type and severity of the injury as well as the length of time between injury and diagnosis. Ligamentous injury can benefit from casting or a fitted boot. If these conservative treatments fail, surgical open reduction or joint fusion may be required.

POSTERIOR TIBIAL TENDON INSUFFICIENCY
Etiology

Posterior tibial tendon insufficiency is the most common cause of acquired adult flatfoot deformity.[158] Flatfoot deformities result from flattening of the medial longitudinal arch of the foot with failing of the supporting soft tissue structures of the ankle and hindfoot. The posterior tibial tendon is the principle supporting mechanism of this arch, although ligament involvement is extensive.[139] Dysfunction of the posterior tibial tendon leads to the collapse of the arch and the formation of a pes planovalgus deformity. Arthritis may develop secondary to the foot deformity. Insufficiency of the posterior tibial tendon may result from a variety of insults, including trauma and arthritic damage. Patients are most often middle-aged females and are often obese.[159]

Symptoms and Signs

Initially, patients report pain along the medial aspect of the foot and ankle due to stretching of medial ligaments and soft tissues. On physical exam, erythema, edema, and tenderness to palpation along the course of the posterior tibial tendon can be appreciated. Later, as the arch begins to collapse, the ankle starts to roll inward, resulting in pain along the lateral aspect of the foot.[159] There may be difficulty in performing a single leg heel rise. Persistent dull aching pain due to destruction of the midfoot may culminate in difficulty with standing and ambulation.

Diagnosis

Radiographic imaging should include weight-bearing anteroposterior and lateral radiographs of the foot to evaluate the biomechanical relationships and detect secondary arthritic changes.[159] MRI is utilized to assess the integrity of the posterior tibial tendon.

Treatment

Initial treatment is supportive and involves immobilization, analgesic medications, and orthotic devices to correct pronation. Steroid injections have not been proven to be efficacious and remain controversial. When supportive measures fail, treatment consists of surgical augmentation of the posterior tibial tendon alone or in combination with osteotomy or arthrodesis.[159]

DORSAL FOOT GANGLIA
Etiology

The etiology of dorsal foot ganglia is uncertain. However, they are the most common nodules found in the foot, with women accounting for up to 85% of the cases.[160]

Symptoms and Signs

Ganglia are generally asymptomatic. However, pain can occur as a result of inflammatory pressure points created while walking or from wearing tight-fitting footwear.[160]

Diagnosis and Treatment

Ganglia are fluid-filled nodules that typically arise from a joint or tendon sheath and are most commonly located over the dorsum of the midfoot, forefoot, and toes.[160] Upon palpation, they are firm and well-circumscribed. Nonsurgical treatment options include use of footpads, compression of the ganglion with an arch strap, or fine needle aspiration of the ganglion. Recurrence of the ganglion after aspiration is not uncommon. When conservative measures fail, surgical excision of the ganglion and stalk from its origin on the ligament or joint capsule and capsular excision should be performed.

METATARSALGIA
Etiology

Metatarsalgia refers to pain involving one or more of the metatarsal heads and distal metatarsal shafts secondary to chronically elevated stress forces as the total body weight is transferred to the forefoot during the midstance and push-off phases of walking and running.[161] Abnormal biomechanics resulting from excessive pronation, cavus deformities, foot surgeries (e.g., osteotomies), and high-heeled shoes can further increase the weight distribution on the metatarsal heads.[162] The increased prevalence of metatarsalgia among women is likely due to wearing high-heeled shoes. Other causes of metatarsalgia include intermetatarsal bursitis/neuritis, metatarsal stress fracture, metatarsophalangeal joint stress syndrome, sesamoiditis, inflammatory arthritis, interdigital neuroma, and aseptic necrosis of the second metatarsal head (Freiberg disease).[162]

Symptoms and Signs

Pain severity is gradual in nature and is aggravated with walking and running activities. Over time, calluses can form over the second and third metatarsal heads and can further increase weight bearing on the metatarsal heads. On physical examination, palpable point tenderness is elicited at the distal end of the plantar metatarsal fat pad and also can be reproduced by squeezing the metatarsal head between the thumb and index finger.[162] Interdigital neuromas can lead to metatarsalgia and should be considered when pain is present in the interdigital web spaces. Over time, the pain may progress to diffuse forefoot and midfoot pain.

Diagnosis

Laboratory and imaging studies are not performed to confirm the diagnosis of metatarsalgia but instead are performed to rule out other diagnoses that may have a similar presentation. Radiographic imaging (weight-bearing anteroposterior, lateral, and oblique views) of the affected foot should be obtained to exclude metatarsal stress fractures, which may also lead to forefoot pain. Ultrasound and MRI may be necessary if a neuroma, cyst, bursitis, or other soft tissue anomaly is suspected. A serum C-reactive protein, uric acid level, and erythrocyte sedimentation rate should be obtained to exclude gout, which often presents as metatarsal pain at the base of the great toe.

Treatment

Conservative treatment includes the use of analgesic medications and semirigid orthotic inserts to reduce pressure on the metatarsal heads. Kang et al.[163] showed that the use of metatarsal pads resulted in decreased maximal peak pressures and pressure time intervals during exercise, which translated to improved function and analgesia. Athletes can achieve significant pain reduction through the use of metatarsal bar appliances that can be placed in footwear. Surgical procedures are aimed at equalizing weight-bearing forces on the metatarsal heads and may include metatarsal shaft osteotomy or metatarsal head condyle excision.[164]

HALLUX VALGUS
Etiology

Hallux valgus, also known as bunion deformity, is the most common deformity of the metatarsophalangeal joint.[165] Subluxation results in lateral deviation of the proximal phalanx of the great toe and the formation of a medial prominence by the first metatarsal head (Fig. 70.15). The deformity can be congenital or can result from biomechanical instability. Use of improper footwear, such as high-heeled shoes with tight-fitting and small toe boxes, may explain the higher prevalence hallux valgus among women.[165]

Symptoms and Signs

Pain occurs in the first metatarsophalangeal joint and can be described as deep, aching, and/or lancinating. Pain is worsened with ambulation and relieved upon shoe removal. Physical examination reveals a prominence on the medial aspect of the first metatarsal head and valgus deformity of the great toe. Adventitial bursa formation over the prominent medial metatarsal head can also be observed.[166] Bursitis and overlying skin inflammation may be present. Osteoarthritic changes that occur over time may result in significant reduction in joint range of motion associated with pain.

Diagnosis

Radiographic imaging (weight-bearing anteroposterior, lateral, and oblique views) should be obtained in order to measure the angular degree of deformity, which provides diagnostic and prognostic information.[166]

Treatment

Conservative treatment involves wearing footwear with wide toe boxes and placing pads in the first web space and over the median prominence to relieve pressure-induced pain. Oral analgesic medications and corticosteroid injections into

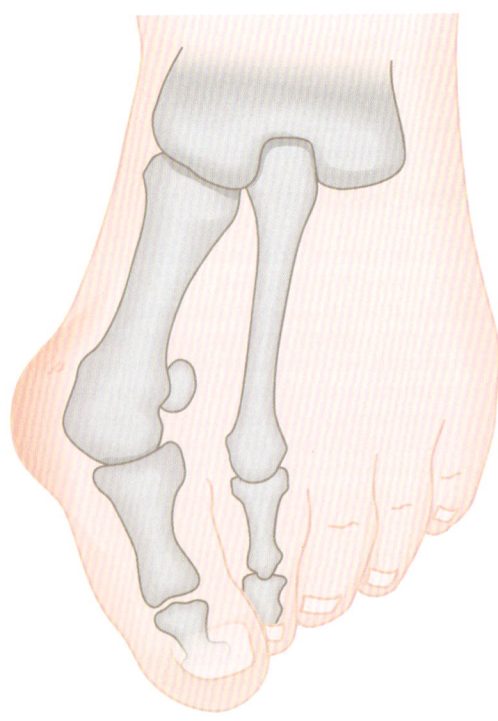

FIGURE 70.15 Hallux valgus. See text for details.

the first metatarsophalangeal joint can be used to address acute, painful inflammatory states. Surgical treatment is indicated for intractable pain associated with significant functional impairment. Surgical options include osteotomy, exostectomy, resectional arthroplasty, resectional arthroplasty with implant, capsulotendon balancing, first metatarsophalangeal joint arthrodesis, and first metatarsocuneiform joint arthrodesis.[166] A majority of these techniques involve excision of the medial prominence of the metatarsal head (bunionectomy), adductor hallucis tendon release, and occasional excision of the lateral sesamoid bone. Major surgical complications include overcorrection and recurrence.[166]

HALLUX RIGIDUS
Etiology
Hallux rigidus is osteoarthritis of the first metatarsophalangeal joint and is associated with restricted range of motion and pain (Fig. 70.16). This results from cartilage degeneration, altered joint mechanics, and osteophyte formation. Impingement of the dorsal osteophytes results in inflammation and pressure point pain.[167] Athletic activities involving running have been associated with development of hallux rigidus.

Symptoms and Signs
Patients describe a dull, aching pain on the dorsal surface of the first metatarsophalangeal joint that occurs during weight-bearing activities involving the forefoot and often results in an antalgic gait. Unlike hallux valgus, pain from hallux rigidus is associated with or without wearing shoes. Neuropathic pain can result from first dorsal digital nerve entrapment. Physical examination reveals an osteophyte formation on the dorsal surface of the first metatarsophalangeal joint and extremely limited range of motion.

Diagnosis
Radiographic imaging reveals degenerative changes of the first metatarsophalangeal joint. Early changes include dorsal and marginal osteophyte formation. Severe changes that can be visualized include joint space narrowing, sclerosis, joint irregularities, and sesamoid and cystic degeneration. Coughlin and Shurnas[168] proposed a grade 0 to 4 classification system based on range of motion, physical exam findings, and radiographic results.

Treatment
Conservative treatment includes rest, customized foot orthotics, and wearing low-heeled, rigid rocker bottom soled shoes with soft surfaces lining the dorsum of the foot. Corticosteroids can

be injected in to the first metatarsal interspace lateral to the joint, along with local anesthetic application in the region of the first dorsal digital nerve.[167] Several surgical treatments can be attempted to correct the condition. The least invasive, a cheilectomy, involves the excision of all irregular bony spurs contributing to decreased range of motion. This can provide significant pain relief and gain in function, although a successful outcome is inversely proportional to the degree of arthritic changes. A resection arthroplasty (Keller procedure), which involves excision of the base of the proximal phalanx, is usually reserved for patients with low functional demands.[167] A proximal phalanx and metatarsal osteotomy can also be performed. Complications, such as flaccidity and motor weakness of the hallux, are quite high.[167] Although a joint arthrodesis can provide analgesia, it results in loss of joint motion. Despite this, patients can continue to remain physically active.

INTRACTABLE KERATOSIS
Etiology
Intractable keratosis is characterized by hard callus formation that develops underneath the metatarsal heads due to plantar flexion.[169] Callus formation results in point pressure on the plantar fat pad.

Symptoms and Signs
Intractable keratosis presents as a painful discrete lesion that is aggravated by weight-bearing activities and causes an antalgic gait. Physical examination reveals a 1-cm focal, white-colored lesion with circumferential erythema found on the plantar aspect of the forefoot.[170]

Diagnosis
Radiographic imaging should be performed to exclude other pathology, including fractures and metatarsal avascular necrosis.

Treatment
Conservative treatment involves wearing shoes with wide toe boxes and placing a pad underneath the uninvolved metatarsal heads in order to off-load weight from the involved metatarsal head. Pumice stones and prescription creams containing lactic acid can be used to reduce the mass of the keratosis and thereby provide symptomatic relief. Analgesic medications can provide minor relief. Corticosteroid injections are controversial as they can create fat-pad atrophy and further exacerbate the condition.[171] Surgical options can include callus tissue reduction and core removal, a variety of distal metatarsal osteotomies, and segmental resection of the proximal metatarsal.[170]

SESAMOIDITIS
Etiology and Pathophysiology
Sesamoiditis refers to inflammation of the two sesamoid bones on the plantar of the first metatarsophalangeal joint. This state of inflammation can occur as a result of increased stress forces on the sesamoid bones from repetitive trauma due to increased activity, ill-fitting foot wear, anatomic variations, infection, osteoarthritis, or inflammatory arthropathies. Postural abnormalities may also contribute to this condition.

Symptoms and Signs
Pain is localized on the plantar aspect of the foot and is aggravated by weight-bearing activities. Physical examination reveals pain with direct palpation of the sesamoid bone and on dorsiflexion of the metatarsophalangeal joint.[172]

Diagnosis
Radiographic studies should be performed to exclude fractures and other anatomic abnormalities. If plain film radiographs are nondiagnostic, a bone scan, CT, or MRI can prove useful.[172]

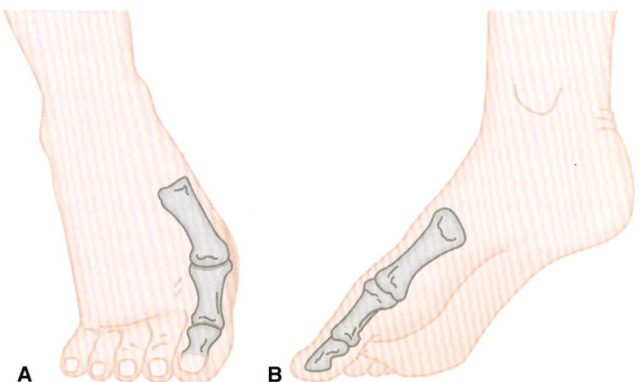

FIGURE 70.16 Hallux rigidus. **A:** Anterior view. **B:** Medial view. Arthritis of the metatarsophalangeal joint reduces motion, especially in dorsiflexion. Push-off is painful.

Treatment

The initial treatment includes reducing loading forces on the sesamoid bones, immobilization with rocker bottom shoes or orthoses, activity modification, and NSAIDs.[172] If conservative management fails, then surgical options should be considered.[172]

GOUT
Etiology

Elevated systemic uric acid levels—due to increased uric acid production, decreased renal excretion of uric acid, or both—cause gout.[173] When serum uric acid concentrations exceed 7.0 mg/dL, precipitation of uric acid crystal occurs.[174] Gout typically manifests in men with a peak age of onset in the fifth decade of life and in women in the sixth decade of life.[174]

Symptoms and Signs

The natural history of gout can be divided into three distinct stages: asymptomatic hyperuricemia, acute and intermittent gout, and chronic tophaceous gout.[173] Asymptomatic hyperuricemia can last for 10 to 30 years before an acute gouty arthritis event occurs. This event is characterized by severe pain in conjunction with edema, erythema, and rubor of the affected joint, after which resolution occurs within 1 to 2 weeks. Gout typically involves only one joint in the early course of the disease, and it is usually the first metatarsophalangeal joint. The acute and intermittent phase involves asymptomatic periods interrupted by acute attacks. These intervals can vary from months to years, but over time, the frequency and duration of attacks and number of joints involved increases. Although it remains uncertain, the attacks may be associated with rapid fluctuations of serum uric acid levels. Chronic gouty arthritis typically develops after more than 10 years of acute intermittent gout. There are no pain-free intervals in this stage.

Diagnosis

Patients report multiple painful, stiff, edematous joints, particularly in the toes, ankles, and knees. Although elevated serum uric acid levels (greater than 7.0 mg/dL) are commonly seen in gout, there may be periods of time when serum uric acid levels are normal.[173] In addition to hyperuricemia, leukocytosis, elevated erythrocyte sedimentation rates, and elevated C-reactive protein levels may be present in acute attacks. The criterion standard of diagnosis, however, remains aspiration and examination of synovial fluid from an actively affected joint. Under polarized microscopy, monosodium uric acid crystals are seen as negatively birefringent needle-like structures engulfed by polymorphonuclear neutrophils.

Treatment

Treatment of acute gouty arthritis focuses on decreasing the inflammation within the joints.[175] This is best accomplished through NSAIDs. In patients who cannot take NSAIDs, corticosteroids can be given via the oral, intravenous, or intra-articular routes. If taken within the first 12 hours of an acute gouty attack, oral colchicine can have an anti-inflammatory effect and can prevent uric acid crystal deposition. Although colchicine does not lower the uric acid levels, in low doses, it can be used to prevent or reduce the severity of future attacks. Patients, however, may not be able to tolerate the side effects of nausea, vomiting, and diarrhea. Chronic therapy to prevent recurrence of gouty arthritic attacks is aimed at normalizing serum uric acid levels. Uricosuric agents, such as probenecid, work by increasing uric acid secretion into the urine. Xanthine oxidase inhibitors, such as allopurinol, work by inhibiting uric acid synthesis. Surgical resection of large nodular deposits of uric acid crystals, also known as tophi, can offer improvement in terms of mechanical function.[176]

INTERDIGITAL (MORTON'S) NEUROMA
Etiology

An interdigital neuroma is characterized by a well-localized area of pain on the plantar aspect of the forefoot that radiates into the web space. It typically involves the third interspace of the foot. Although this condition is termed *interdigital neuroma*, it is not a true neuroma. The histopathologic changes include the degeneration of nerve fibers associated with deposition of amorphous eosinophilic material that is more congruent with neuropathy secondary to an entrapment phenomenon.[177] What causes an interdigital neuroma is unclear, although it has been hypothesized that it arises from constant traction of nerve fibers against the transverse metatarsal ligament during dorsiflexion of the toes.[178] Interdigital neuromas occur approximately 10 times more frequently in women than men. This may be explained by the state of continuous dorsiflexion of the feet when wearing high-heeled shoes.[178]

Symptoms and Signs

Patients typically complain of localized pain in the region of the metatarsal head. The third interspace is more frequently involved than the second interspace, but it rarely involves the first or fourth interspace.[179] The pain is aggravated by wearing tight-fitting shoes and walking and is alleviated by rest and removal of shoes. Upon palpation of the involved interspace, patients report a sharp pain that radiates into the toes. Often, a mass located in the interspace can be palpated. Palpating the affected interspace with one hand and squeezing the entire foot at the same time with the other hand, resulting in narrowing of the intermetatarsal space and compression of the mass can often reproduce symptoms. This can elicit an audible click, known as Mulder's sign.[170] The differential diagnosis of interdigital neuroma should include stress fracture, tendon sheath ganglion, foreign-body reaction, nerve sheath tumor, strain of the plantar capsule, and capsulitis or bursitis at the level of the plantar metatarsophalangeal joint.[179] In many of these conditions, inflammation of the adjacent nerve also may be present, causing the neuritic sensation of an interdigital neuroma, thus complicating proper diagnosis. It is also important to distinguish interdigital pain from metatarsalgia, which gives rise to a host of other possible pathologies including avascular necrosis, synovial cysts, and tarsal tunnel compression.

Diagnosis

Although interdigital neuromas are often diagnosed based solely on clinical findings, MRI, CT, and ultrasound have all been utilized for diagnostic purposes as well. MRI has emerged as the preferred imaging modality due to superior contrast resolution and precision. Interdigital neuromas are best visualized on short-axis (transverse) T1-weighted images through the metatarsal heads. Due to their highly vascular nature, intravenous contrast agents typically result in visual enhancement. They appear as bulbous masses arising between the metatarsal heads (Fig. 70.17).[180] Although radiographs may reveal pathology at the metatarsophalangeal joint, they are not useful in the diagnosis of interdigital neuromas.

Conservative management of interdigital neuromas includes wearing shoes with wider toe boxes, adequate cushioning, and heels no higher than 1 in. Neuroma pads—soft support inserts that are placed proximal to the affected metatarsal head—are designed to separate the metatarsal heads and prevent rubbing or irritating the affected neuroma when stepping down. Oral NSAIDs and corticosteroid injections into the affected interspace can be tried.[178] However, corticosteroids can result in local fat atrophy and metatarsalgia. Phenol neurolysis of the common interdigital nerve has also been reported to be effective.[181] When conservative management fails, surgical intervention may be indicated. This involves a dorsal incision in

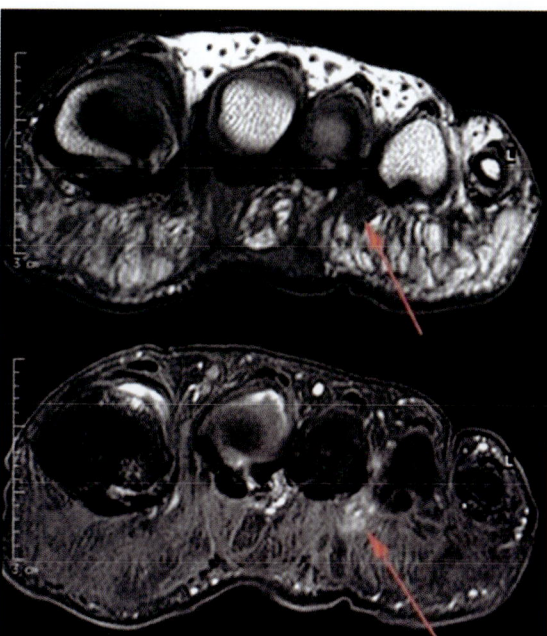

FIGURE 70.17 Interdigital neuroma. Transverse T1-weighted **(top)** and contrast-enhanced fat-suppressed T1-weighted **(bottom)**. Magnetic resonance images show the bulbous morphology of the perineural mass with plantar extension. The administration of contrast material reveals enhancement of the lesion.

the midline of the affected interdigital space in order to release the transverse metatarsal ligament, as the nerve typically lies beneath this ligament. Postoperative recovery includes a compression dressing worn for several weeks after wound closure. Ambulation is permitted in a postoperative boot.[182] It is important to note that patients may experience decreased sensation in the interdigital web space.

HAMMERTOES
Etiology
Hammertoe deformities are primarily flexible or fixed plantarflexion deformities of the proximal interphalangeal (PIP) joint, with hyperextension of the metatarsophalangeal joint and extension deformities of the distal interphalangeal joint (Fig. 70.18).[173,183] This results in a dorsal prominence on the PIP, which can cause pain secondary to compression and inflammation from footwear. Physical examination must include determining if the deformity is fixed or flexible. Other deformities may be present, such as hallux valgus or cavus foot deformities. Examination of the extensor surface of the PIP joint may reveal callus or ulcer formation. Intractable keratosis can develop underneath the metatarsal head of the involved toe.[162]

Diagnosis
Radiographic imaging should include weight-bearing anteroposterior and lateral radiographs of the involved foot.

Treatment
Conservative management involves the use of metatarsal pads and shoes with wide toe boxes. Surgical treatment involves metatarsophalangeal joint correction, but the type of surgery is influenced by whether the deformity is fixed or flexible. Fixed hammertoe deformities are corrected through resection arthroplasty of the PIP joint, with the aim of reducing soft tissue contraction forces through toe shortening. Additional procedures such as flexor/extensor tenotomies, metatarsophalangeal joint release, or arthroplasty may be necessary. Weil osteotomies, which primarily involve metatarsal shortening, have also been used to correct the deformity.[184] Flexible hammertoe deformities are surgically corrected with a Girdlestone flexor tendon transfer. This involves harvesting the long flexor tendon from the plantar aspect of the foot and surgically affixing this into the extensor hood. Thus, the tendon functions as both an extensor of the interphalangeal joints and a flexor the metatarsophalangeal joint.[179] The major complication of Girdlestone flexor tendon transfer is a failure to identify a contracture of the flexor digitorum longus tendon during surgery, resulting in inadequate correction.[183]

CLAW TOE DEFORMITY
Etiology
Claw toe deformity results from dorsiflexion of the proximal phalanx on the lesser metatarsophalangeal joint and concurrent flexion of the PIP and distal interphalangeal joints (Fig. 70.19).[183] Pain results from friction between the interphalangeal joints and the shoe. In addition, patients experience pain underneath the metatarsal heads from being in plantarflexion.[179] As with hammertoes, claw toe deformities may be flexible or fixed. They typically involve all four of the lesser toes. The clinical evaluation is similar to that of hammertoe deformities, including inspection for possible callus and ulcer formation along the extensor surface of the PIP joints.

Diagnosis
Radiographic imaging should include weight-bearing anteroposterior and lateral radiographs of the involved foot.[179]

Treatment
Conservative management includes wearing shoes that have increased depth to reduce pressure on the lesser toes and placement of arch supports underneath the metatarsal heads. Shoe inserts can be positioned proximal to the metatarsophalangeal joints in flexible deformities that are mild. The flexible deformity is corrected with a Girdlestone flexor tendon transfer. The fixed deformity requires a DuVries proximal phalangeal condylectomy in conjunction with the Girdlestone tendon transfer procedure.[179] As with hammertoe surgical correction, the major complication is inadequate correction and subsequent recurrence of the deformity.[183]

HARD CORN (CLAVUS DURUM)
Corns are painful, hyperkeratotic skin lesions located over bony prominences that result from excessive pressure on the skin.

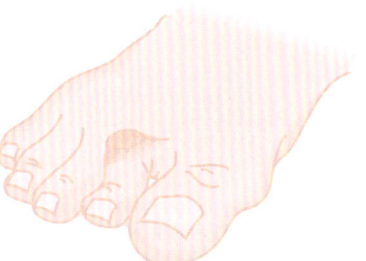

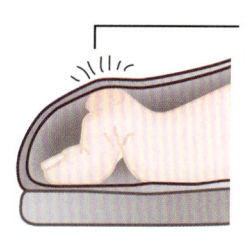

Sites of pressure

FIGURE 70.18 Hammertoe deformity, a typical small toe deformity, often causes corns and calluses with standard footwear. Extra deep shoes avoid these problems.

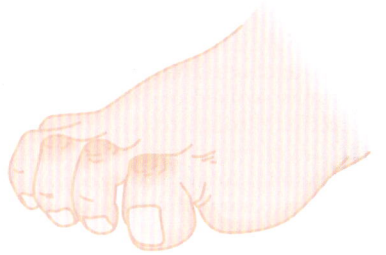

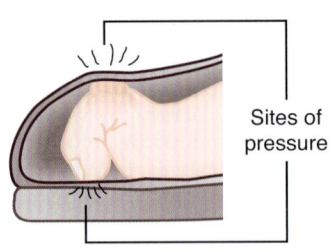

Sites of pressure

FIGURE 70.19   Claw toe deformity, a typical small toe deformity, often causes corns and calluses with standard footwear. Extra deep shoes avoid these problems.

Histologic specimens reveal hyperplasia of the epidermis, especially proliferation of the stratum corneum.[185] Hard corns are notable for their dry, horny appearance that develops over the dorsal and lateral surfaces of the fifth toe, on the lateral condyle of the proximal phalanx.

Treatment

Conservative treatment is aimed at reducing pressure on the bony prominences by wearing shoes with large toe boxes. Surgical correction involves débridement of the lesion and, occasionally, necessitates removal of the distal portion of the proximal phalanx. The most common complication of the latter surgical procedure is excessive bone removal, resulting in a flaccid fifth toe.[186]

SOFT CORN (CLAVUS MOLLUM)

Soft corns are macerated lesions that frequently occur in the fourth web space between the base of the proximal of the fourth toe and the medial condyle of the head of the proximal phalanx of the fifth toe.[179] These typically develop as a result of small bony protrusion anomalies that cause pressure points, which can then result in ulceration.[186]

Treatment

As with hard corns, management first focuses on reducing pressure on the bony prominences through utilization of footwear with large toe boxes. Other treatment modalities include the use of keratolytics such as salicylic acid.[187] Surgical treatment involves removal of the bony protrusion.

INGROWN TOENAIL (ONYCHOCRYPTOSIS)

An ingrown toenail is a painful condition resulting from nail plate penetration on the medial or lateral nail fold epithelium (Fig. 70.20). This typically involves the great toe. It is associated with trauma, tight-fitting footwear, improperly trimming the nails at the nail margins, and aberrant nail curvature.[188]

Treatment

If no infection is present, initial treatment includes elevation of the nail by placing cotton between the nail plate and the skin. This can be aided by daily foot soaks and removal of any pressure points on the nail. Additional treatment involves trimming an oblique portion of the affected nail toward the posterior nail fold under a digital block.[188] The nail groove is then débrided and dressed. If infection or granulation occurs, treatment is focused on partial removal of the nail plate. This involves performing a digital nerve block, followed by a longitudinal incision from the base to the tip of the affected region of the nail plate, including the nail beneath the cuticle. The nail is then grasped with a hemostat and removed from the nail groove using a rocking motion. The nail groove is then débrided and dressed.[188]

References

1. Ramchandren S, Dalmau J. Metastases to the peripheral nervous system. *J Neurooncol* 2005;75(1):101–110.
2. Planner AC, Donaghy M, Moore NR. Causes of lumbosacral plexopathy. *Clin Radiol* 2006;61(12):987–995.
3. Wilbourn AJ. Plexopathies. *Neurol Clin* 2007;25(1):139–171.
4. Yee T. Recurrent idiopathic lumbosacral plexopathy. *Muscle Nerve* 2000;23(9):1439–1442.
5. Taylor BV, Kimmel DW, Krecke KN, et al. Magnetic resonance imaging in cancer-related lumbosacral plexopathy. *Mayo Clinic Proc* 1997;72(9):823–829.
6. Yadav R. Neoplastic lumbosacral plexopathy. Available at: http://emedicine.medscape.com/article/316390-overview. Accessed August 26, 2009.
7. Jaeckle KA. Neurological manifestations of neoplastic and radiation-induced plexopathies. *Semin Neurol* 2004;24(4):385–393.
8. Portenoy RK. Cancer pain. Epidemiology and syndromes. *Cancer* 1989;63(11 suppl):2298–2307.
9. Agar M, Broadbent A, Chye R. The management of malignant psoas syndrome: case reports and literature review. *J Pain Symptom Manage* 2004;28(3):282–293.
10. Stevens MJ, Gonet YM. Malignant psoas syndrome: recognition of an oncologic entity. *Australasian Radiol* 1990;34(2):150–154.
11. Falah M, Schiff D, Burns TM. Neuromuscular complications of cancer diagnosis and treatment. *J Support Oncol* 2005;3(4):271–282.
12. Tonsgard JH, Kwak SM, Short MP, et al. CT imaging in adults with neurofibromatosis-1: frequent asymptomatic plexiform lesions. *Neurology* 1998;50(6):1755–1760.
13. Dyck PJ, Windebank AJ. Diabetic and nondiabetic lumbosacral radiculoplexus neuropathies: new insights into pathophysiology and treatment. *Muscle Nerve* 2002;25(4):477–491.
14. Paley M, Sidhu PS, Evans RA, et al. Retroperitoneal collections—aetiology and radiological implications. *Clin Radiol* 1997;52(4):290–294.
15. Ozcakar L, Sivri A, Aydinli M, et al. Lumbosacral plexopathy as the harbinger of a silent retroperitoneal hematoma. *Southern Med J* 2003;96(1):109–110.
16. Katirji B, Wilbourn AJ, Scarberry SL, et al. Intrapartum maternal lumbosacral plexopathy. *Muscle Nerve* 2002;26(3):340–347.
17. Haim A, Pritsch T, Ben-Galim P, et al. Meralgia paresthetica: a retrospective analysis of 79 patients evaluated and treated according to a standard algorithm. *Acta Orthop* 2006;77(3):482–486.
18. Roth V. Meralgia paresthetica. *Med Obozr* 1895;43:678.
19. Harney D, Patijn J. Meralgia paresthetica: diagnosis and management strategies. *Pain Med* 2007;8(8):669–677.
20. van Slobbe AM, Bohnen AM, Bernsen RM, et al. Incidence rates and determinants in meralgia paresthetica in general practice. *J Neurol* 2004;251(3):294–297.

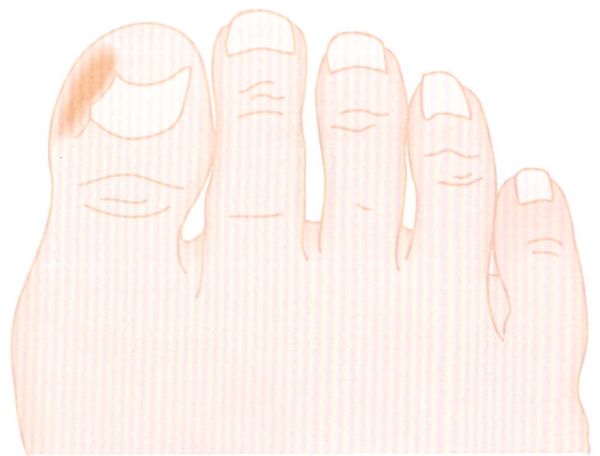

FIGURE 70.20   Ingrown toenail is often caused by improper nail cutting techniques or by wearing ill-fitting footwear that creates pressure against the lateral nail fold producing exquisite pain and tenderness.

21. Grossman MG, Ducey SA, Nadler SS, et al. Meralgia paresthetica: diagnosis and treatment. *J Am Acad Orthopc Surg* 2001;9(5):336–344.

22. Seror P, Seror R. Meralgia paresthetica: clinical and electrophysiological diagnosis in 120 cases. *Muscle Nerve* 2006;33(5):650–654.

23. Mondelli M, Rossi S, Romano C. Body mass index in meralgia paresthetica: a case-control study. *Acta Neurol Scand* 2007;116(2):118–123.

24. Hollis M, Lemay D. Nerve entrapment syndromes of the lower extremity. Available at: https://emedicine.medscape.com/article/2225774-overview. Accessed August 26, 2009.

25. Kitchen C, Simpson J. Meralgia paresthetica. A review of 67 patients. *Acta Neurol Scand* 1972;48(5):547–555.

26. Pastor Guzman JM, Pastor Navarro H, Donate Moreno MJ, et al. Femoral neuropathy in urological surgery. *Actas Urol Esp* 2007;31(8):885–894.

27. Nouraei SA, Anand B, Spink G, et al. A novel approach to the diagnosis and management of meralgia paresthetica. *Neurosurgery* 2007;60(4):696–700.

28. Williams PH, Trzil KP. Management of meralgia paresthetica. *J Neurosurg* 1991;74(1):76–80.

29. Shannon J, Lang SA, Yip RW, et al. Lateral femoral cutaneous nerve block revisited. A nerve stimulator technique. *Reg Anesth* 1995;20(2):100–104.

30. Tagliafico A, Serafini G, Lacelli F, et al. Ultrasound-guided treatment of meralgia paresthetica (lateral femoral cutaneous neuropathy): technical description and results of treatment in 20 consecutive patients. *J Ultrasound Med* 2011;30(10):1341–1346.

31. Hurdle MF, Weingarten TN, Crisostomo RA, et al. Ultrasound-guided blockade of the lateral femoral cutaneous nerve: technical description and review of 10 cases. *Arch Phys Med Rehabil* 2007;88(10):1362–1364.

32. Shah RV, Racz GB. Pulsed mode radiofrequency lesioning of the suprascapular nerve for the treatment of chronic shoulder pain. *Pain Phys* 2003;6(4):503–506.

33. Trescot AM. Cryoanalgesia in interventional pain management. *Pain Phys* 2003;6(3):345–360.

34. Barna SA, Hu MM, Buxo C, et al. Spinal cord stimulation for treatment of meralgia paresthetica. *Pain Phys* 2005;8(3):315–318.

35. Rozen D, Ahn J. Pulsed radiofrequency for the treatment of ilioinguinal neuralgia after inguinal herniorrhaphy. *Mt Sinai J Med* 2006;73(4):716–718.

36. Payne R, Seaman S, Sieg E, et al. Evaluating the evidence: is neurolysis or neurectomy a better treatment for meralgia paresthetica? *Acta Neurochir* 2017;159(5):931–936.

37. Busis NA. Femoral and obturator neuropathies. *Neurol Clin* 1999;17(3):633–653, vii.

38. Hunter LY, Louis DS, Ricciardi JR, et al. The saphenous nerve: its course and importance in medial arthrotomy. *Am J Sports Med* 1979;7(4):227–230.

39. Kuntzer T, van Melle G, Regli F. Clinical and prognostic features in unilateral femoral neuropathies. *Muscle Nerve* 1997;20(2):205–211.

40. Carter GT, McDonald CM, Chan TT, et al. Isolated femoral mononeuropathy to the vastus lateralis: EMG and MRI findings. *Muscle Nerve* 1995;18(3):341–344.

41. Ducic I, Dellon L, Larson EE. Treatment concepts for idiopathic and iatrogenic femoral nerve mononeuropathy. *Ann Plastic Surg* 2005;55(4):397–401.

42. Brasch RC, Bufo AJ, Kreienberg PF, et al. Femoral neuropathy secondary to the use of a self-retaining retractor. Report of three cases and review of the literature. *Dis Colon Rectum* 1995;38(10):1115–1118.

43. Goldman JA, Feldberg D, Dicker D, et al. Femoral neuropathy subsequent to abdominal hysterectomy. A comparative study. *Eur J Obstet Gynecol Reprod Biol* 1985;20(6):385–392.

44. Schmalzried TP, Noordin S, Amstutz HC. Update on nerve palsy associated with total hip replacement. *Clin Orthop Relat Res* 1997;344:188–206.

45. Kim DH, Murovic JA, Tiel RL, et al. Intrapelvic and thigh-level femoral nerve lesions: management and outcomes in 119 surgically treated cases. *J Neurosurg* 2004;100(6):989–996.

46. Fanelli G, Casati A, Garancini P, et al. Nerve stimulator and multiple injection technique for upper and lower limb blockade: failure rate, patient acceptance, and neurologic complications. Study Group on Regional Anesthesia. *Anesth Analg* 1999;88(4):847–852.

47. Walsh C, Walsh A. Postoperative femoral neuropathy. *Surg Gynecol Obstet* 1992;174(3):255–263.

48. Worth RM, Kettelkamp DB, Defalque RJ, et al. Saphenous nerve entrapment. A cause of medial knee pain. *Am J Sports Med* 1984;12(1):80–81.

49. Adar R, Meyer E, Zweig A. Saphenous neuralgia: a complication of vascular reconstructions below the inguinal ligament. *Ann Surg* 1979;190(5):609–613.

50. Chauhan BM, Kim DJ, Wainapel SF. Saphenous neuropathy: following coronary artery bypass surgery. *NY State J Med* 1981;81(2):222–223.

51. Lederman RJ, Breuer AC, Hanson MR, et al. Peripheral nervous system complications of coronary artery bypass graft surgery. *Ann Neurol* 1982;12(3):297–301.

52. Roder OC, Kamper A, Jorgensen SJ. Incidence of saphenous neuralgia in arterial surgery. *Acta Chir Scand* 1984;150(1):23–24.

53. Romanoff ME, Cory PC Jr, Kalenak A, et al. Saphenous nerve entrapment at the adductor canal. *Am J Sports Med* 1989;17(4):478–481.

54. Lavee J, Schneiderman J, Yorav S, et al. Complications of saphenous vein harvesting following coronary artery bypass surgery. *J Cardiovasc Surg* 1989;30(6):989–991.

55. Senegor M. Iatrogenic saphenous neuralgia: successful therapy with neuroma resection. *Neurosurgery* 1991;28(2):295–298.

56. Miller DB Jr. Arthroscopic meniscus repair. *Am J Sports Med* 1988;16(4):315–320.

57. Tennent TD, Birch NC, Holmes MJ, et al. Knee pain and the infrapatellar branch of the saphenous nerve. *J Royal Soc Med* 1998;91(11):573–575.

58. Schwabegger AH, Rhomberg M, Ninkovic MM, et al. Saphenous nerve neuralgia after gracilis muscle flap harvest. *Br J Plastic Surg* 1998;51(5):410.

59. Iizuka M, Yao R, Wainapel S. Saphenous nerve injury following medial knee joint injection: a case report. *Arch Phys Med Rehabil* 2005;86(10):2062–2065.

60. Hemler DE, Ward WK, Karstetter KW, et al. Saphenous nerve entrapment caused by pes anserine bursitis mimicking stress fracture of the tibia. *Arch Phys Med Rehabil* 1991;72(5):336–337.

61. Murayama K, Takeuchi T, Yuyama T. Entrapment of the saphenous nerve by branches of the femoral vessels. A report of two cases. *J Bone Joint Surg* 1991;73(5):770–772.

62. Fabian RH, Norcross KA, Hancock MB. Surfer's neuropathy. *N Engl J Med* 1987;316(9):555.

63. Hattori H, Asagai Y, Yamamoto K. Sudden onset of saphenous neuropathy associated with hereditary multiple exostoses. *J Orthop Sci* 2006;11(4):405–408.

64. Tsai PB, Karnwal A, Kakazu C, et al. Efficacy of an ultrasound-guided subsartorial approach to saphenous nerve block: a case series. *Can J Anaesth* 2010;57(7):683–688.

65. Benzon HT, Sharma S, Calimaran A. Comparison of the different approaches to saphenous nerve block. *Anesthesiology* 2005;102(3):633–638.

66. Mozes M, Ouaknine G, Nathan H. Saphenous nerve entrapment simulating vascular disorder. *Surgery* 1975;77(2):299–303.

67. Bianchi S. Ultrasound of the nerves of the knee region. Technique of examination and normal US appearance. *J Ultrasound* 2006;10:68–75.

68. Bradshaw C, McCrory P, Bell S, et al. Obturator nerve entrapment. A cause of groin pain in athletes. *Am J Sports Med* 1997;25(3):402–408.

69. Sorenson EJ, Chen JJ, Daube JR. Obturator neuropathy: causes and outcome. *Muscle Nerve* 2002;25(4):605–607.

70. Jirsch JD, Chalk CH. Obturator neuropathy complicating elective laparoscopic tubal occlusion. *Muscle Nerve* 2007;36(1):104–106.

71. Kleiner JB, Thorne RP. Obturator neuropathy caused by an aneurysm of the hypogastric artery. A case report. *J Bone Joint Surg* 1989;71(9):1408–1409.

72. Redwine DB, Sharpe DR. Endometriosis of the obturator nerve. A case report. *J Reprod Med* 1990;35(4):434–435.

73. Rogers LR, Borkowski GP, Albers JW, et al. Obturator mononeuropathy caused by pelvic cancer: six cases. *Neurology* 1993;43(8):1489–1492.

74. Nakayama T, Kobayashi S, Shiraishi K, et al. Diagnosis and treatment of obturator hernia. *Keio J Med* 2002;51(3):129–132.

75. Yamashita K, Hayashi J, Tsunoda T. Howship-Romberg sign caused by an obturator granuloma. *Am J Surg* 2004;187(6):775–776.

76. Stuplich M, Hottinger AF, Stoupis C, et al. Combined femoral and obturator neuropathy caused by synovial cyst of the hip. *Muscle Nerve* 2005;32(4):552–554.

77. Yokoyama Y, Yamaguchi A, Isogai M, et al. Thirty-six cases of obturator hernia: does computed tomography contribute to postoperative outcome? *World J Surg* 1999;23(2):214–217.

78. Kammori M, Mafune K, Hirashima T, et al. Forty-three cases of obturator hernia. *Am J Surg* 2004;187(4):549–552.

79. Kawaguchi M, Hashizume K, Iwata T, et al. Percutaneous radiofrequency lesioning of sensory branches of the obturator and femoral nerves for the treatment of hip joint pain. *Reg Anesth Pain Med* 2001;26(6):576–581.

80. Malik A, Simopolous T, Elkersh M, et al. Percutaneous radiofrequency lesioning of sensory branches of the obturator and femoral nerves for the treatment of non-operable hip pain. *Pain Phys* 2003;6(4):499–502.

81. Wu H, Groner J. Pulsed radiofrequency treatment of articular branches of the obturator and femoral nerves for management of hip joint pain. *Pain Pract* 2007;7(4):341–344.

82. Beaton LE, Anson BJ. The relation of the sciatic nerve and its subdivisions to the piriformis muscle. *Anat Rec* 1938;70:1–5.

83. Yuen EC, So YT, Olney RK. The electrophysiologic features of sciatic neuropathy in 100 patients. *Muscle Nerve* 1995;18(4):414–420.

84. Kline DG, Kim D, Midha R, et al. Management and results of sciatic nerve injuries: a 24-year experience. *J Neurosurg* 1998;89(1):13–23.

85. Yuen EC, So YT. Sciatic neuropathy. *Neurol Clin* 1999;17(3):617–631, viii.

86. Plewnia C, Wallace C, Zochodne D. Traumatic sciatic neuropathy: a novel cause, local experience, and a review of the literature. *J Trauma* 1999;47(5):986–991.

87. Pace JB, Nagle D. Piriform syndrome. *Western J Med* 1976;124(6):435–439.

88. Fishman SM, Caneris OA, Bandman TB, et al. Injection of the piriformis muscle by fluoroscopic and electromyographic guidance. *Reg Anesth Pain Med* 1998;23(6):554–559.

89. Thiele GH. Coccygodynia and pain in the superior gluteal region. *JAMA* 1937;109:1271–1275.

90. Benson ER, Schutzer SF. Posttraumatic piriformis syndrome: diagnosis and results of operative treatment. *J Bone Joint Surg* 1999;81(7):941–949.

91. Travell JG, Simons DG. *Myofascial Pain and Dysfunction: The Trigger Point Manual.* Baltimore, MD: Williams & Wilkins; 1992.

92. Yuen EC, Olney RK, So YT. Sciatic neuropathy: clinical and prognostic features in 73 patients. *Neurology* 1994;44(9):1669–1674.

93. Kim DH, Murovic JA, Tiel R, et al. Management and outcomes in 353 surgically treated sciatic nerve lesions. *J Neurosurg* 2004;101(1):8–17.

94. Feinberg J, Sethi S. Sciatic neuropathy: case report and discussion of the literature on postoperative sciatic neuropathy and sciatic nerve tumors. *HSS J* 2006;2(2):181–187.

95. Wallace MS, Staats P, eds. *Pain Medicine and Management: Just the Facts.* New York: McGraw-Hill; 2004.

96. Freiburg AH. Sciatic pain and it's relief by operations on muscle and fascia. *Arch Surg* 1937;34:337–350.

97. Beatty RA. The piriformis muscle syndrome: a simple diagnostic maneuver. *Neurosurgery* 1994;34(3):512–514.

98. Fishman LM, Zybert PA. Electrophysiologic evidence of piriformis syndrome. *Arch Phys Med Rehabil* 1992;73(4):359–364.

99. Filler AG, Haynes J, Jordan SE, et al. Sciatica of nondisc origin and piriformis syndrome: diagnosis by magnetic resonance neurography and interventional magnetic resonance imaging with outcome study of resulting treatment. *J Neurosurg* 2005;2(2):99–115.

100. Bevilacqua Alen E, Diz Villar A, Curt Nuno F, et al. Ultrasound-guided piriformis muscle injection. A new approach. *Rev Esp Anestesiol Reanim* 2016;63(10):594–598.

101. Jeong HS, Lee GY, Lee EG, et al. Long-term assessment of clinical outcomes of ultrasound-guided steroid injections in patients with piriformis syndrome. *Ultrasonography* 2015;34(3):206–210.

102. Fabregat G, Rosello M, Asensio-Samper JM, et al. Computer-tomographic verification of ultrasound-guided piriformis muscle injection: a feasibility study. *Pain Phys* 2014;17(6):507–513.

103. Fowler IM, Tucker AA, Weimerskirch BP, et al. A randomized comparison of the efficacy of 2 techniques for piriformis muscle injection: ultrasound-guided versus nerve stimulator with fluoroscopic guidance. *Reg Anesth Pain Med* 2014;39(2):126–132.

104. Fanucci E, Masala S, Sodani G, et al. CT-guided injection of botulinic toxin for percutaneous therapy of piriformis muscle syndrome with preliminary MRI results about denervative process. *Eur Radiol* 2001;11(12):2543–2548.

105. Finnoff JT, Hurdle MF, Smith J. Accuracy of ultrasound-guided versus fluoroscopically guided contrast-controlled piriformis injections: a cadaveric study. *J Ultrasound Med* 2008;27(8):1157–1163.

106. Childers MK, Wilson DJ, Gnatz SM, et al. Botulinum toxin type A use in piriformis muscle syndrome: a pilot study. *Am J Phys Med Rehabil* 2002;81(10):751–759.

107. Fishman LM, Anderson C, Rosner B. BOTOX and physical therapy in the treatment of piriformis syndrome. *Am J Phys Med Rehabil* 2002;81(12):936–942.

108. Yoon SJ, Ho J, Kang HY, et al. Low-dose botulinum toxin type A for the treatment of refractory piriformis syndrome. *Pharmacotherapy* 2007;27(5):657–665.

109. Rodriguez-Piñero M, Vidal Vargas V, Jimenez Sarmiento AS. Long-term efficacy of ultrasound-guided injection of incobotulinumtoxinA in piriformis syndrome. *Pain Med* 2018;19(2):408–411.

110. Diop M, Parratte B, Tatu L, et al. Anatomical bases of superior gluteal nerve entrapment syndrome in the suprapiriformis foramen. *Surg Radiol Anat* 2002;24(3–4):155–159.

111. Fabre T, Piton C, Andre D, et al. Peroneal nerve entrapment. *J Bone Joint Surg* 1998;80(1):47–53.

112. Aprile I, Padua L, Padua R, et al. Peroneal mononeuropathy: predisposing factors, and clinical and neurophysiological relationships. *Neurol Sci* 2000;21(6):367–371.

113. Noble J, Munro CA, Prasad VS, et al. Analysis of upper and lower extremity peripheral nerve injuries in a population of patients with multiple injuries. *J Trauma* 1998;45(1):116–122.

114. Takao M, Ochi M, Shu N, et al. A case of superficial peroneal nerve injury during ankle arthroscopy. *Arthroscopy* 2001;17(4):403–404.

115. Yilmaz S, Altinbas H, Senol U, et al. Common peroneal nerve palsy after retrograde popliteal artery puncture. *Eur J Vasc Endovasc Surg* 2002;23(5):467–469.

116. Yilmaz E, Karakurt L, Serin E, et al. Peroneal nerve palsy due to rare reasons: a report of three cases. *Acta Orthop Traumatol Turcica* 2004;38(1):75–78.

117. Flores JP, Koerbel A, Tatagiba M. Peroneal nerve compression resulting from fibular head osteophyte-like lesions. *Surg Neurol* 2005;64(3):249–252.

118. Hems TE, Jones BG. Peroneal nerve damage associated with the proximal locking screws of the AIM tibial nail. *Injury* 2005;36(5):651–655.

119. Niall DM, Nutton RW, Keating JF. Palsy of the common peroneal nerve after traumatic dislocation of the knee. *J Bone Joint Surg Br* 2005;87(5):664–667.

120. Giannas J, Bayat A, Watson SJ. Common peroneal nerve injury during varicose vein operation. *Eur J Vasc Endovasc Surg* 2006;31(4):443–445.

121. Atkin GK, Round T, Vattipally VR, et al. Common peroneal nerve injury as a complication of short saphenous vein surgery. *Phlebology* 2007;22(1):3–7.

122. Drosos GI, Stavropoulos NI, Kazakos KI. Peroneal nerve damage by oblique proximal locking screw in tibial fracture nailing: a new emerging complication? *Arch Orthop Trauma Surg* 2007;127(6):449–451.

123. Ersozlu S, Ozulku M, Yildirim E, et al. Common peroneal nerve palsy from an untreated popliteal pseudoaneurysm after penetrating injury. *J Vasc Surg* 2007;45(2):408–410.

124. O'Neill PJ, Parks BG, Walsh R, et al. Excursion and strain of the superficial peroneal nerve during inversion ankle sprain. *J Bone Joint Surg* 2007;89(5):979–986.

125. Prasad AR, Steck JK, Dellon AL. Zone of traction injury of the common peroneal nerve. *Ann Plast Surg* 2007;59(3):302–306.

126. Hamdan FB, Jaffar AA, Ossi RG. The propensity of common peroneal nerve in thigh-level injuries. *J Trauma* 2008;64(2):300–303.

127. Sanger JR, Kao DS, Hackbarth DA. Peroneal nerve compression by lateral gastrocnemius flap. *J Plast Reconstr Aesthet Surg* 2009;62(8):e280–e282.

128. Jowett AJ, Johnston JF, Gaillard F, et al. Lateral meniscal cyst causing common peroneal palsy. *Skeletal Radiol* 2008;37(4):351–355.

129. Piton C, Fabre T, Lasseur E, et al. Common fibular nerve lesions. Etiology and treatment. Apropos of 146 cases with surgical treatment. *Rev Chir Orthop Reparatrice Appar Mot* 1997;83(6):515–521.

130. Kim DH, Murovic JA, Tiel RL, et al. Management and outcomes in 318 operative common peroneal nerve lesions at the Louisiana State University Health Sciences Center. *Neurosurgery* 2004;54(6):1421–1429.

131. Marwah V. Compression of the lateral popliteal (common peroneal) nerve. *Lancet* 1964;2(7374):1367–1369.

132. Moller BN, Kadin S. Entrapment of the common peroneal nerve. *Am J Sports Med* 1987;15(1):90–91.

133. Leach RE, Purnell MB, Saito A. Peroneal nerve entrapment in runners. *Am J Sports Med* 1989;17(2):287–291.

134. McAuliffe TB, Fiddian NJ, Browett JP. Entrapment neuropathy of the superficial peroneal nerve. A bilateral case. *J Bone Joint Surg Br* 1985;67(1):62–63.

135. Styf J, Morberg P. The superficial peroneal tunnel syndrome. Results of treatment by decompression. *J Bone Joint Surg Br* 1997;79(5):801–803.

136. Fernandez E, Pallini R, Lauretti L, et al. Neurosurgery of the peripheral nervous system: entrapment syndromes of the lower extremity. *Surg Neurol* 1999;52(5):449–452.

137. Krause KH, Witt T, Ross A. The anterior tarsal tunnel syndrome. *J Neurol* 1977;217(1):67–74.

138. Hetherington V, ed. *Textbook of Hallux Valgus and Forefoot Surgery.* Cleveland, OH: Churchill Livingstone; 2000.

139. Deland J, de Asla R, Sung I, et al. Posterior tibial tendon insufficiency: which ligaments are involved? *Foot Ankle Int* 2005;26(6):427–435.

140. Lemley F, Berlet G, Hill K, et al. Current concepts review: tarsal coalition. *Foot Ankle Int* 2006;27(12):1163–1169.

141. Pomeroy G, Pike R, Beals T, et al. Acquired flatfoot in adults due to dysfunction of the posterior tibial tendon. *J Bone Joint Surg* 1999;81(8):1173–1182.

142. Younger A, Hansen S. Adult cavovarus foot. *J Am Acad Orthop Surg* 2005;13(5):302–315.

143. Wapner K, Myerson M, eds. *Pes Cavus.* Philadelphia: WB Saunders; 2000.

144. Buchbinder R. Clinical practice plantar fasciitis. *N Engl J Med* 2004;350(21):2159–2166.

145. Cole C, Seto C, Gazewood J. Plantar fasciitis: evidence-based review of diagnosis and therapy. *Am Fam Physician* 2005;72(11):2237–2242.

146. Roerdink RL, Dietvorst M, van der Zwaard B, et al. Complications of extracorporeal shockwave therapy in plantar fasciitis: systematic review. *Int J Surg* 2017;46:133–145.

147. Ahmad J, Ahmad SH, Jones K. Treatment of plantar fasciitis with botulinum toxin. *Foot Ankle Int* 2017;38(1):1–7.

148. Monto RR. Platelet-rich plasma efficacy versus corticosteroid injection treatment for chronic severe plantar fasciitis. *Foot Ankle Int* 2014;35(4):313–318.

149. Young C, Rutherford D, Niedfeldt M. Treatment of plantar fasciitis. *Am Fam Phys* 2001;63(3):467–474.

150. Aldridge T. Diagnosing heel pain in adults. *Am Fam Phys* 2004;70(2):332–338.

151. ÜrgÜden M, Bilbaşar H, Özdemir H, et al. Tarsal tunnel syndrome—the effect of the associated features on outcome of surgery. *Int Orthop* 2002;26(4):253–256.

152. DiDomenico L, Masternick E. Anterior tarsal tunnel syndrome. *Clin Podiatr Med Surg* 2006;23(3):611–620.

153. Franson J, Baravarian B. Tarsal tunnel syndrome: a compression neuropathy involving four distinct tunnels. *Clin Podiatr Med Surg* 2006;23(3):597–609.

154. Englanoff G, Anglin D, Hutson H. Lisfranc fracture-dislocation: a frequently missed diagnosis in the emergency department. *Ann Emerg Med* 1995;26(2):229–233.

155. Ross G, Cronin R, Hauzenblaus J, et al. Plantar ecchymosis sign: a clinical aid to diagnosis of occult Lisfranc tarsometatarsal injuries. *J Orthop Trauma* 1996;10(2):119–122.

156. Faciszewski T, Burks R, Manaster B. Subtle injuries of the Lisfranc joint. *J Bone Joint Surg* 1990;72(10):1519–1522.

157. Siddiqui NA, Galizia MS, Almusa E, et al. Evaluation of the tarsometatarsal joint using conventional radiography, CT, and MR imaging. *Radiographics* 2014;34(2):514–531.

158. Beals T, Pomeroy G, Manoli A. Posterior tendon insufficiency: diagnosis and treatment. *J Am Acad Orthop Surg* 1999;7(3):112–118.

159. Kohls-Gatzoulis J, Angel J, Singh D, et al. Tibialis posterior dysfunction: a common and treatable cause of adult acquired flatfoot. *BMJ* 2004;329(7478):1328–1333.

160. Macdonald DJ, Holt G, Vass K, et al. The differential diagnosis of foot lumps: 101 cases treated surgically in North Glasgow over 4 years. *Ann Royal Coll Surg Engl* 2007;89(3):272–275.

161. Hockenbury R. Forefoot problems in athletes. *Med Sci Sports Exerc* 1999;31(7 suppl):448–458.

162. Loeser J, ed. *Bonica's Management of Pain.* 3rd ed. Philadelphia: Lippincott Williams & Wilkins; 2001.

163. Kang J, Chen M, Chen S, et al. Correlations between subjective treatment responses and plantar pressure parameters of metatarsal pad treatment in metatarsalgia patients: a prospective study. *BMC Musculoskelet Disord* 2006;7(95):1471–2474.

164. O'Kane C, Kilmartin T. The surgical management of central metatarsalgia. *Foot Ankle Int* 2002;23(5):415–419.

165. Mann R, Coughlin M. Hallux valgus—etiology, anatomy, treatment and surgical considerations. *Clin Orthop Relat Res* 1981;157:31–41.

166. Ajis A. Tailor's bunion: a review. *J Foot Ankle Surg* 2005;44(3):236–245.

167. Beertema W, Draijer W, van Os J, et al. A retrospective analysis of surgical treatment in patients with symptomatic hallux rigidus: long-term follow-up. *J Foot Ankle Surg* 2006;45(4):244–251.

168. Coughlin M, Shurnas P. Hallux rigidus: demographics, etiology, and radiographic assessment. *Foot Ankle Int* 2003;24(10):731–743.

169. Kitaoka H, Patzer G. Chevron osteotomy of lesser metatarsals for intractable plantar callosities. *J Bone Joint Surg* 1998;80(3):516–518.

170. Coughlin M. Common causes of pain in the forefoot in adults. *J Bone Joint Surg* 2000;82(6):781–790.

171. Tsai W. Treatment of proximal plantar fasciitis with ultrasound-guided steroid injection. *Arch Phys Med Rehabil* 2000;81(10):1416–1421.

172. York PJ, Wydra FB, Hunt KJ. Injuries to the great toe. *Curr Rev Musculoskelet Med* 2017;10(1):104–112.

173. Eggebeen A. Gout: an update. *Am Fam Physician* 2007;76(6):801–808.

174. Ruddy S, Harris EJ, Harris C, et al, eds. *Kelly's Textbook of Rheumatology.* 7th ed. Philadelphia: Elsevier Saunders; 2001.

175. Shekelle PG, Newberry SJ, FitzGerald JD, et al. Management of gout: a systematic review in support of an American College of Physicians clinical practice guideline. *Ann Intern Med* 2017;166(1):37–51.

176. Lee S, Sun I, Lu Y, et al. Surgical treatment of the chronic tophaceous deformity in upper extremities—the shaving technique. *J Plast Reconstr Aesthet Surg* 2009;62:669–674.

177. Graham C, Graham D. Morton's neuroma: a microscopic evaluation. *Foot Ankle* 1984;5(150):150–153.

178. Hassouna H. Morton's metatarsalgia: pathogenesis, aetiology and current management. *Acta Orthop Belgica* 2005;71(6):646–655.

179. Skinner H, ed. *Current Diagnosis and Treatment in Orthopedics.* 4th ed. Philadelphia: McGraw-Hill; 2006.

180. George VA, Khan AM, Hutchinson CE, et al. Morton's neuroma: the role of MR scanning in diagnostic assistance. *Foot* 2005;15(1):14–16.

181. Magnan B, Marangon A, Frigo A, et al. Local phenol injection in the treatment of interdigital neuritis of the foot (Morton's neuroma). *Chir Organi Mov* 2005;90(4):371–377.

182. Klenerman L. Morton's neuroma. *Curr Orthop* 1997;11(1):15–18.

183. Kirchner J, Wagner E. Girdlestone-Taylor flexor extensor tendon transfer techniques. *Foot Ankle Surg* 2004;3(2):91–99.

184. Trnka H, Gebhard C, Muhlbauer M. The Weil osteotomy for treatment of dislocated lesser metatarsophalangeal joints: good outcome in 21 patients with 42 osteotomies. *Acta Orthop Scand* 2002;73(2):190–194.

185. Wolff K, ed. *Fitzpatrick's Dermatology in General Medicine.* 7th ed. New York: McGraw-Hill; 2008.

186. Canale T, ed. *Campbell's Operative Orthopaedics.* 10th ed. St. Louis, MO: Mosby; 2003.

187. Cordoro K, Ganz J. Training room management of medical conditions: sports dermatology. *Clin Sports Med* 2005;24(3):565–598.

188. Tintinalli J, ed. *Tintinalli's Emergency Medicine: A Comprehensive Study Guide.* 6th ed. Philadelphia: McGraw-Hill; 2004.

CHAPTER 71

Neck Pain

ANDREW J. ENGEL and **NIKOLAI BOGDUK**

Definition

In its taxonomy, the International Association for the Study of Pain (IASP)[1] construed neck pain to be pain arising from the cervical spine. It defined cervical spinal pain from a posterior perspective as pain anywhere in a region bounded superiorly by the superior nuchal line, laterally by the margins of the neck, and inferiorly by an imaginary transverse line through the T1 spinous process[1] (Fig. 71.1). The definition allowed for the identification of upper and lower cervical spinal pain, for pain located in the respective halves of this region.

Neck pain was defined in this way primarily because patients with neck pain typically indicate the location of their pain as behind the cervical spine. A supplementary reason was to distinguish neck pain of spinal origin from pain arising from the viscera of the neck, which lie anterior to the cervical spine.[1]

Referred Pain

Numerous experiments in human volunteers[2–7] have shown that pain from various somatic structures, such as the posterior neck muscles, cervical synovial joints, and cervical intervertebral disks, can be referred to various extents in various directions, depending on the segmental location of the source of pain. This type of pain is known as somatic referred pain and is different and distinct from cervical radicular pain. It does not involve irritation of nerve roots. It arises because of convergence of primary afferents on common neurones in the spinal cord.[1] Thus, pain that is mediated by a particular nerve, and relayed to a particular spinal cord segment, may be perceived in the territory subtended by other nerves that relay to that spinal cord segment. Characteristically, somatic referred pain is dull and aching in quality, in contrast to the lancinating quality of radicular pain. Furthermore, somatic referred pain tends to be sessile; it occupies a particular region and may expand slowly, in contrast to radicular pain which tends to shoot or travel in a linear pattern.[1]

From upper cervical segments (C1, C2, C3), pain can be referred into the occipital region, across the parietal region of the skull, and into the frontal region or orbit (Fig. 71.2). From lower cervical segments (C5, C6, C7), pain can be referred across the shoulder or shoulder girdle (see Fig. 71.2).

Older studies, using injections of hypertonic saline into the interspinous spaces of the neck, reported patterns of referred pain extending into the arm, forearm, and hand,[2,4] but these observations have not been corroborated using modern techniques. Although some physicians have reported anecdotally that they have encountered such distant patterns of somatic referred pain, these patterns have not been formally documented in the modern literature. That literature indicates that the common patterns of somatic referred pain from the cervical spine are more proximal in distribution.

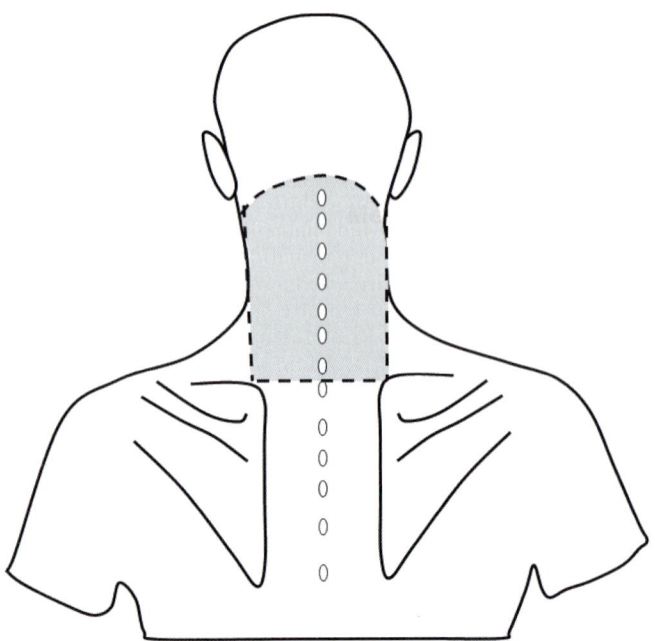

FIGURE 71.1 Neck pain is defined as pain perceived within a region bounded superiorly by the superior nuchal line, laterally by the margins of the neck, and inferiorly by an imaginary transverse line through the T1 spinous process.[1]

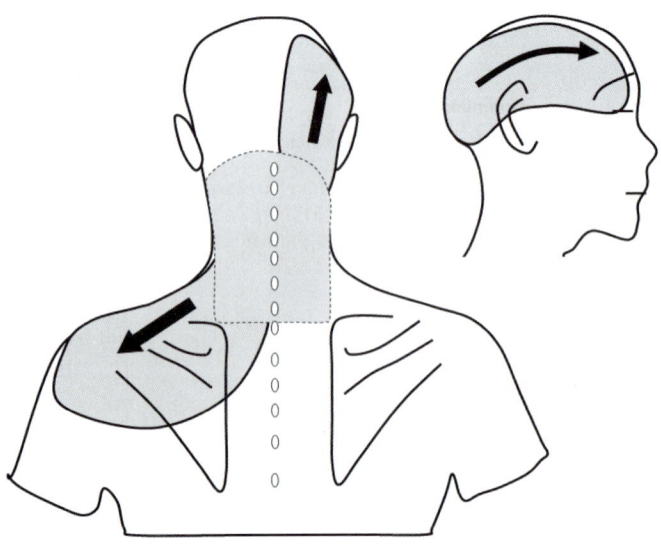

FIGURE 71.2 Referred pain from the cervical spine. From upper cervical segments, pain can be referred into the occiput and into the head (*inset*). From lower cervical segments, pain can be referred into the region of the shoulder and shoulder girdle.

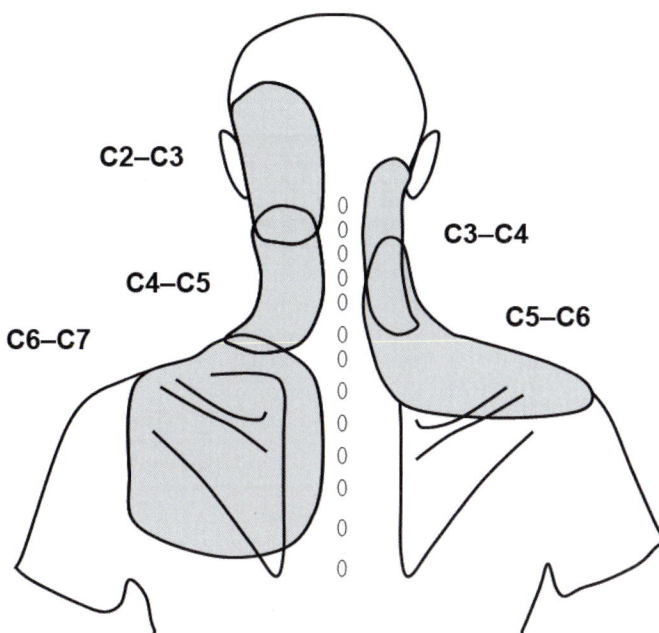

FIGURE 71.3 Patterns of referred pain from the cervical zygapophysial joints or the intervertebral disks at the segments indicated.

Patterns of referred pain are not dependent on the structure that is the source of pain. The pattern is dictated by which segmental nerves innervate the source. Consequently, for example, the cervical zygapophysial joints[5,6] and cervical intervertebral disks[7] in the same vertebral segments have similar patterns of referred pain because they share a similar segmental nerve supply (Fig. 71.3).

These patterns of referred pain, evoked by noxious stimuli in volunteers, have been corroborated and elaborated by studies of patients whose neck pain has been abolished temporarily by controlled diagnostic blocks of the cervical zygapophysial joints and lateral atlantoaxial joints.[8]

Pain from the C3–C4 segment may extend into the occipital region but largely tends to lie topographically over the levator scapulae muscle. Pain from C4–C5 tends to nestle into the angle between the neck and the top of the shoulder.

Pain from the C5–C6 segments tends to radiate over the deltoid region of the shoulder. Pain from C6–C7 segments tends to spread more posteriorly, over the shoulder girdle, but there can be considerable overlap between the distributions of referred pain from C5–C6 and C6–C7.

Pain from C1–C2 and C2–C3 structures radiates into the occipital region but can extend across or through the head into the forehead or orbit. Although there is considerable overlap between the pain patterns of C1–C2 and C2–C3, pain from C1–C2 tends to spread somewhat more rostrally across the vertex and into the forehead rather than across the parietal region and into the orbit.[8]

CERVICOGENIC HEADACHE

In some patients with neck pain referred to the head, headache is their dominant complaint. Consequently, they seek the attention of neurologists or other specialists in headache. In those circles, this type of headache is referred to as *cervicogenic headache*, if and once the cervical origin of pain is established.[9–11]

Pursuing Diagnosis

The rubric "neck pain" is not a diagnosis; it is simply a restatement of the patient's presenting complaint. A diagnosis requires a statement of the source of pain, if not also its cause.

However, because a diagnosis is not often possible, most practitioners avoid pursuing a diagnosis and manage neck pain as a symptom rather than a diagnosis.

Neck pain does not include neurologic symptoms or signs. If a patient exhibits features of radiculopathy or myelopathy, those features take precedence. The pursuit of diagnosis converts from a pursuit of neck pain to a pursuit of the neurologic disorder.

Traditional means of pursuing a diagnosis are history, examination, and imaging. To these have been added minimally invasive tests. These approaches or tools have different utility depending on the category of neck pain established by history.

Very few causes of neck pain can be diagnosed from history alone, but history does provide cues that define different categories of neck pain. The five useful categories are trauma, acute, chronic, whiplash, and cervicogenic headache. These categories differ in terms of the nature, volume, and quality of evidence that apply to each, both for diagnosis and subsequent treatment.

Although physical examination may provide an assessment of the patient's disability to move his or her neck, it does not contribute to diagnosis. Features such as range of movement, aggravation of pain, and tenderness are nonspecific; they can be affected or produced by virtually any cause of neck pain. Moreover, most signs elicited by physical examination of the neck lack either reliability or validity or both.[12] Therefore, they cannot be relied on to make a diagnosis.

Medical imaging can detect fractures, tumors, and infections, but these are rare causes of neck pain. For most patients, imaging provides no diagnostic information. Medical imaging, therefore, has no role in the routine screening of patients with acute neck pain. In order to be efficient, and not wasteful, its use should be predicated by particular features in the patient's history or presentation.

Minimally invasive tests have no established or proven role in the investigation of acute neck pain. Their role lies in the pursuit of the causes of chronic neck pain.

TRAUMA

Serious injuries to the neck can arise from motor vehicle accidents, falls, or a blow to the head. This etiology will be evident from the history.

The lesions of concern are fractures to the cervical spine, particularly fractures that threaten the integrity of the spinal cord, for these may require specialist management by immobilization or urgent surgery. However, fractures are not common, even among patients with a history of significant injury. A review of studies in departments of emergency medicine found that only $3.5\% \pm 0.5\%$ of patients suspected of possibly having a fracture proved to have a fracture on imaging.[13]

Studies looking for predictors of fractures have shown that the alerting features are loss of consciousness, neurologic signs, and immediate onset of pain.[14] These features have been captured in the Canadian C-Spine Rules,[15] which are validated guidelines for the use of imaging in the pursuit of fractures (Fig. 71.4). Given the low pretest likelihood of fractures, even in patients at risk, these rules serve to eliminate unnecessary imaging in patients in whom the likelihood of fractures is essentially zero and in whom any missed fractures are unlikely to be of practical consequence.

ACUTE NECK PAIN

Technically, the definition of acute neck pain is pain that has been present for less than 3 months.[1] However, in practice, acute neck pain would be pain of recent onset, measured in hours or days. Whereas other considerations will apply later, the prime imperative of assessment of acute neck pain is the recognition of conditions that involve a serious cause of pain, or systemic conditions in which involvement of the neck is only part of the problem (Table 71.1).

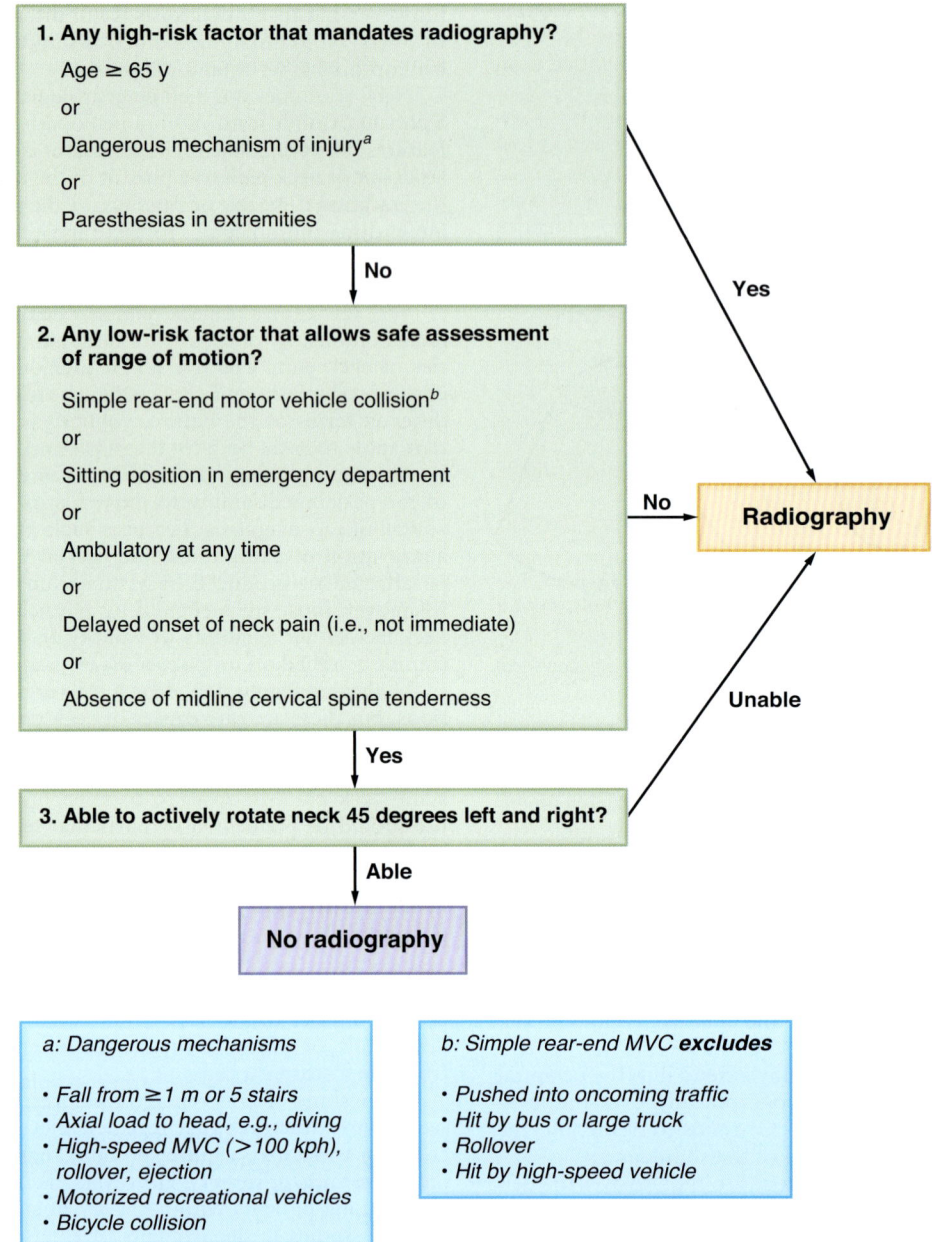

FIGURE 71.4   The Canadian C-Spine Rules.[1] MVC, motor vehicle collision.

TABLE 71.1	A Synopsis of the Causes of Acute Neck Pain	
	Uncommon or Rare	**Common**
Serious	Fractures	
	Tumors	
	Discitis	
	Septic arthritis	
	Osteomyelitis	
	Meningitis	
	Epidural abscess	
	Epidural hematoma	
	Aneurysms	
	Intracranial lesions	
Nonserious	Rheumatoid arthritis	Unknown
	Ankylosing spondylitis	
	Polymyalgia rheumatica	
	Longus colli tendonitis	
	Crystal arthropathies	
	Neuromas	

Serious Conditions

Serious causes of acute neck pain are rare. Two population studies of plain radiography of the cervical spine, each involving over 1,000 patients, both reported not detecting any serious disorder that was not otherwise suspected from the patient's history.[16,17] By inference, this zero prevalence of undiagnosed fractures, tumors, or infections has an upper 95% confidence limit of 0.4%. Thus, it can be deduced that *serious causes of neck pain have a prevalence substantially less than 0.4%.* This rarity argues against wanton application of medical imaging to screen for conditions that are extremely unlikely to be present.

Screening for suspected fractures should be governed by the Canadian C-Spine Rules (see Fig. 71.4). For tumors and infections, no guidelines have been validated for the cervical spine, but in principle, those for the lumbar spine would seem applicable.[18] For tumors, the indications for imaging would be a past history of cancer or persistence of pain and failure to improve on treatment. For infections, the indications would be a history of possible inoculation, an evident source for infection, immunosuppression, systemic features of infection, or failure to improve. Meningitis is readily suspected on clinical grounds (fever, neck stiffness, Kernig's sign).

Epidural hematoma is a serious condition because it threatens the spinal cord. Once neurologic signs appear, the window of opportunity for successful neurosurgical decompression is only a matter of hours.[19] However, the initial presenting feature may simply be neck pain,[20,21] but motor and sensory deficits develop usually within hours of the onset of pain.[20,22–24] Patients presenting with neck pain should be warned to report immediately the onset of any new clinical features, at which time the instigation of investigations can be considered.

Aneurysms most commonly present with headache, but neck pain alone can be the sentinel feature of dissections of the internal carotid artery, the vertebral artery, or the aorta.[25–29] The alerting features to these conditions are a history of cardiovascular risk factors, direct trauma to the neck, and the onset of cerebrovascular features.

A case report records two patients in whom neck pain was the presenting feature of intracranial lesions: one a subarachnoid hemorrhage and the other a glioblastoma multiforme.[30] The mechanism of pain was neither determined nor discussed but possibly involves irritation of the dura mater of the posterior cranial fossa, which is innervated by cervical nerves. The rarity of such cases, however, excuses intracranial lesions from the differential diagnosis of acute neck pain in the first instance, but physicians should remain alert to this possibility in patients with persistent, unresponsive neck pain.

Inflammatory Disorders

Neck pain can be, or can become, an additional feature for systemic inflammatory disorders such as rheumatoid arthritis, seronegative spondyloarthropathies, polymyalgia rheumatica, Reiter's syndrome, and psoriatic arthritis. In such cases, the neck pain does not warrant pursuit of diagnosis, for the diagnosis is evident from the primary features of these conditions, such as widespread distribution of arthritis, arthralgia, or muscle pain.

Longus colli tendonitis is a rare condition that involves inflammation and edema of the upper portion of the longus colli muscle. The presenting features are neck pain, limitation of neck movement, and difficulties swallowing.[31] Medical imaging reveals edema in the prevertebral space and prevertebral muscles of the neck, and calcification can occur in the longus colli. Although alarming, the condition is self-limiting within about 2 weeks.[31]

Widespread Pain

The neck can be one of several regions affected in widespread pain conditions such as fibromyalgia, but in such cases, the diagnosis is that of the widespread pain. A pursuit of the cause of the neck pain in particular is neither warranted nor required.

Rare Conditions

Because the cervical spine contains many synovial joints, in principle, these could be affected by crystal arthropathies, which need to be considered in the differential diagnosis of neck pain. However, gout has a predilection for joints of the appendicular skeleton, and although it can affect the spine, it does so rarely.[32] Other crystal arthropathies have not been reported affecting the cervical spine.

Injuries to peripheral nerves of the shoulder girdle, such as the long thoracic nerve and the spinal accessory nerve, may not be readily apparent because they do not cause sensory problems, and patients may not be immediately aware of their motor deficits. Pain occurs not because of a cervical lesion but as a result of a neuroma developing on the proximal stump of the severed nerve and affecting deep sensory afferents.[33] Because these afferents relay to cervical segments, the pain of the neuroma will be perceived as cervical pain.

Spurious Conditions

Diffuse idiopathic skeletal hyperostosis, ossification of the posterior ligament, and Paget disease are conditions that can affect the neck, but there is no evidence that they cause neck pain. Paget disease has been expressly reported as not causing pain when it has affected the cervical spine.[34]

Although commonly invoked as a diagnosis, cervical spondylosis is no more than a radiographic change with age; it is no more frequent in patients with neck pain than in patients with no pain.[35–37] Likewise, osteoarthritis of the cervical spine has no relationship to neck pain. If anything, the data show that patients with osteoarthritis of the cervical synovial joints are slightly less likely to have pain, although not significantly so statistically.[37]

A rubric commonly used for the diagnosis of neck pain is "soft tissue injury," but this term means no more than neck pain in the absence of a fracture, without the nature of the "injury" and its location being specified.

"Myofascial pain" is purportedly a diagnosis of neck pain when it affects the muscles of the neck. However, no signs for the diagnosis of this condition have been shown to be reliable,[38] and none has been shown to be valid.

Unknown

Because detectable causes of acute neck pain are rare, for most cases, the cause is unknown. For this reason, the IASP offered the rubric *cervical spinal pain of unknown origin*. However, although this term serves the strict requirements of taxonomy, it is unwieldy. No less wieldy is the term *neck pain of unknown origin*. For this reason, a term commonly used is *idiopathic neck pain*.

CHRONIC NECK PAIN

The literature provides little evidence concerning the diagnosis of chronic neck pain. In contrast, there is an abundance of evidence concerning neck pain after whiplash, but it is not clear the extent to which the latter can be translated legitimately to chronic neck pain of spontaneous origin.

Chronic neck pain amounts to neck pain that has persisted beyond 3 months.[1] Commonly in practice, chronic neck pain is attributed to cervical spondylosis or cervical osteoarthritis, but as discussed earlier, these radiographic features have no statistically significant relationship to pain. By some practitioners, chronic neck pain is attributed to myofascial pain, but for this concept, there are no reliable or validated diagnostic criteria.

To some extent, the guidelines for the pursuit of diagnosis of acute neck pain apply to chronic neck pain, but by the time neck pain has become chronic, many of the serious causes of neck pain will have declared themselves. However, some exceptions apply.

Some tumors may be slow growing. Some spinal infections may remain cryptic for a long time. For the diagnosis of cervical spondylodiscitis, delays of 12 to 15 weeks have been reported.[39] It is, therefore, appropriate to use cervical magnetic resonance imaging (MRI) to clear patients with chronic neck pain of cryptic lesions before pursuing other diagnostic tests. Other cryptic lesions include osteitis fibrosa cystica[40] and other bone lesions.

The reason for the lack of evidence on the diagnosis of chronic neck pain is that, apart from cryptic lesions, no feature on history, physical examination, or medical imaging has been shown to be diagnostic of any cause of chronic neck pain. It is for that reason that some physicians resort to minimally invasive tests for the diagnosis of chronic neck pain.

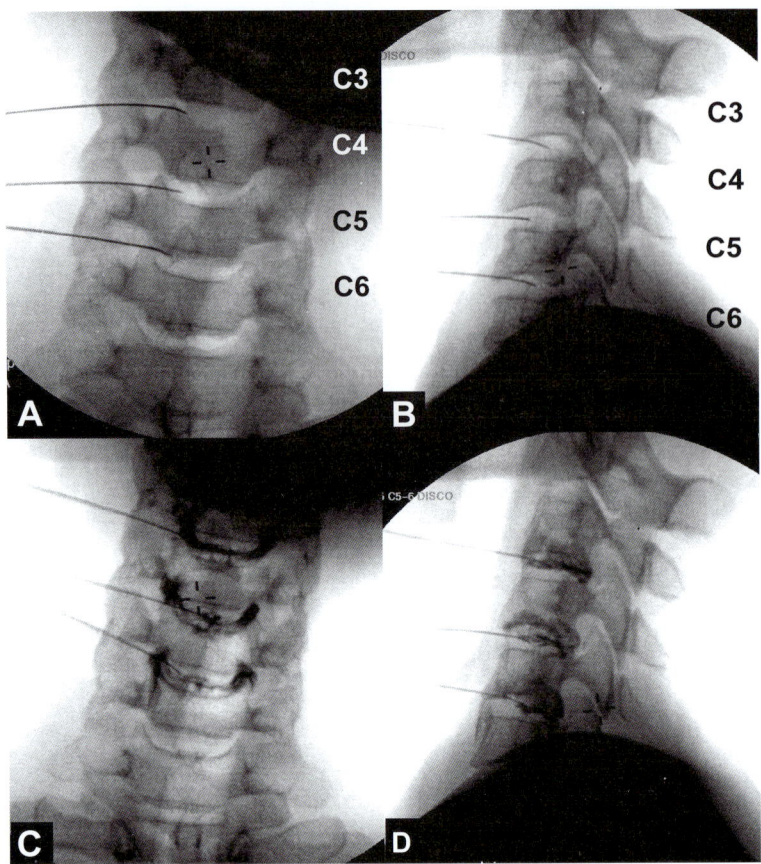

FIGURE 71.5 Fluoroscopy images of stages in cervical disk stimulation. **A:** Anterior view of needles inserted into the C4, C5, and C6 intervertebral disks. **B:** Lateral view of needles inserted. **C:** Anterior view after injection of contrast medium into each of the intervertebral disks. **D:** Lateral view after injection of contrast medium. *(Reproduced with permission from Bogduk N, ed. Practice Guidelines for Spinal Diagnostic and Treatment Procedures. 2nd ed. San Francisco, CA: International Spine Intervention Society; 2013.)*

Cervical Disk Stimulation

Cervical disk stimulation is a test for neck pain stemming from a cervical intervertebral disk. The test involves introducing spinal needles, along an anterolateral approach, into the disk suspected of being the source of pain and into adjacent disks that serve as controls[41] (Fig. 71.5). Once the tip of the needle is placed at the center of the disk, a small volume of contrast medium, or normal saline, is injected into the disk in order to stress it (see Fig. 71.5). A positive response is one in which stimulation of the suspected disk reproduces the patient's pain but stimulation of adjacent disks evokes no pain.[41] However, caveats apply to the validity of cervical disk stimulation.

In the first instance, cervical disk stimulation can be false positive in patients whose neck pain stems from the cervical zygapophysial joints at the tested segment.[42] In such patients, anesthetizing the zygapophysial joints relieves their pain completely. Because the innervation of the zygapophysial joints is topographically separate from that of the disk, local anesthetic blocks of the joints cannot anesthetize the disk. Therefore, the positive response to disk stimulation must be false either because disk stimulation also stresses the zygapophysial joints or because the tested segment is rendered hyperalgesic by the zygapophysial joint pain. Consequently, in order to be valid, cervical disk stimulation should only be performed in patients in whom cervical zygapophysial joint pain has been excluded.[42]

It has been conventional to perform cervical disk stimulation typically at segmental levels C4–C5, C5–C6, and C6–C7, on the grounds that the C5–C6 and C6–C7 disks are the most likely sources of cervical discogenic pain. However, this practice introduces another source of false-positive responses. A study showed that if all disks are tested, rather than just the usual three, there are often disks at other than accustomed levels that happen to be positive.[43] Consequently, restricting the application of disk stimulation to just the lower three cervical disks generates both false-positive and false-negative responses. If one of the three disks is positive to stimulation, the response will be false positive if there happens also to be a positive disk at a segment not tested. Conversely, testing just the lower three disks will be false negative if no disk at these levels is positive but a positive disk at higher levels remains untested. To avoid these problems, the standard of care has to be that all cervical disks must be tested.[42]

Medial Branch Blocks

Cervical medial branch blocks are a test for pain stemming from a cervical zygapophysial joint. The test involves anesthetizing the medial branches that innervate the joint suspected of being the source of pain[44] (Fig. 71.6). In order to be valid, the blocks must be controlled. Placebo-controlled blocks are the consummate standard, but an acceptable compromise is comparative local anesthetic blocks.[44–46] On the occasion of the first block, the patient is randomized to receive either a short-acting (lidocaine) or a long-acting (bupivacaine) local anesthetic. If the response is positive, the block is repeated using the same or other agent.[44–46] A positive result is defined as complete relief of the index pain on both occasions that the joint is anesthetized.[44–46]

Prevalence

No studies have provided data on the prevalence of either cervical discogenic pain or cervical zygapophysial joint pain in patients with chronic neck pain of spontaneous origin (i.e., idiopathic neck pain). The only data come from three studies conducted in pain clinics, on mixed samples of patients with neck pain with or without a history of minor trauma to the neck.[47–49]

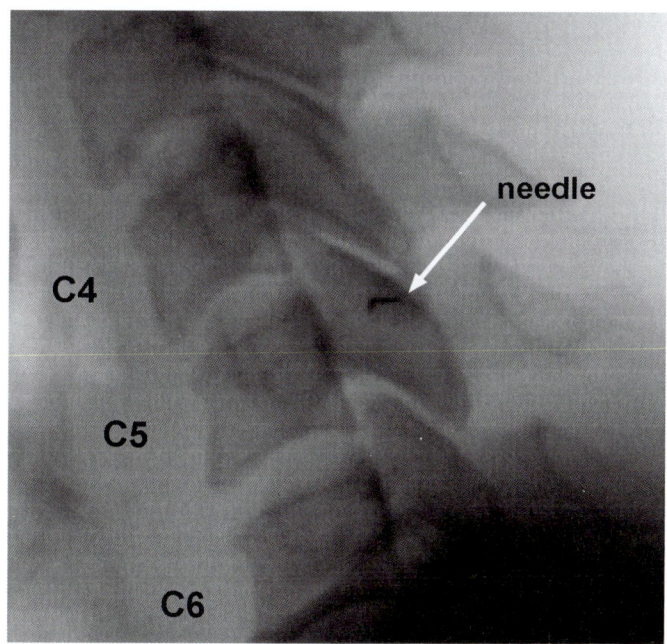

FIGURE 71.6 A lateral fluoroscopy view of a needle in position for the conduct of a C5 medial branch block. *(Reproduced with permission from Bogduk N, ed.* Practice Guidelines for Spinal Diagnostic and Treatment Procedures. *2nd ed. San Francisco, CA: International Spine Intervention Society; 2013.)*

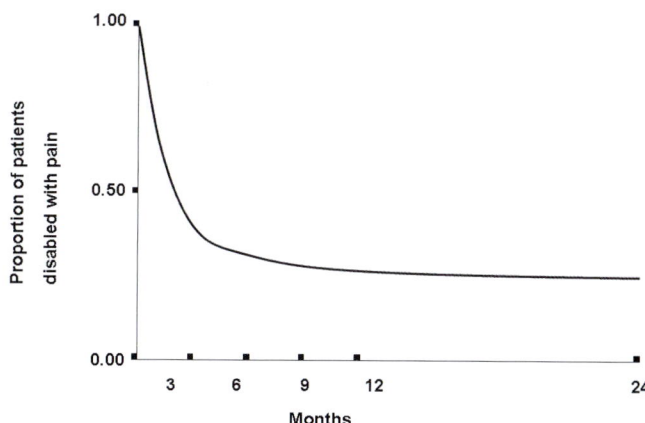

FIGURE 71.7 The recovery curve for whiplash. Most patients recover within 3 months or so, leaving a tail of about 25% with chronic neck pain. *(Based on the data of Radanov BP, Sturzenegger M, Di Stefano G. Long-term outcome after whiplash injury: a 2-year follow-up considering features of injury mechanism and somatic, radiologic, and psychosocial findings.* Medicine *1995;74:281–297.)*

Two of these studies reported only on the prevalence of cervical zygapophysial joint pain, which they found to be 36%[47] and 60%.[48] In the third study, the prevalence of zygapophysial joint pain was 45%, and the prevalence of discogenic pain was 13%.[49] These data show that the cervical zygapophysial joints are the most common, detectable source of chronic neck pain, and that discogenic pain is substantially less common.

WHIPLASH

Neck pain after whiplash can be distinguished from other categories of neck pain by the precipitating event: a read-end motor vehicle collision. This distinction is made because the motor vehicle accident constitutes circumstantial evidence that the patient possibly has an injury that could be the cause of their pain. For patients with idiopathic neck pain, no such etiology is available.

Etiology

Studies of car crash dummies[50] and of human volunteers[51] have shown that, during a whiplash event, the cervical spine is initially compressed from below by a rising thorax. This causes a sigmoid deformation of the spine, during which the entire spine does not move outside the normal physiologic range of motion, but individual segments, typically C5–C6, undergo an abnormal posterior sagittal rotation. Later, the head catapults forward, and the cervical spine is passively flexed. During this phase, stresses are applied to the capsules of the zygapophysial joints, particularly those at C2–C3. The stresses are not large enough to tear the capsules but are nevertheless large in magnitude.[52]

Clinical Features

The cardinal feature of a whiplash injury is neck pain. However, the prognosis is quite favorable. Some 60% of patients fully recover within 3 months, and 75% within a year (Fig. 71.7). Only about 25% of patients suffer disabling chronic pain, of whom a fifth are severely disabled.[53]

Mathematically, the recovery curve for whiplash (see Fig. 71.7) suggests that it is a composite of two populations, as shown in Figure 71.8. Group A are patients who recover rapidly regardless of treatment and respond well to reassurance, activation, and exercises. Group B are patients who do not recover and do not benefit even from tailored conservative care. These patients have greater pain, disability, and psychological distress at onset and exhibit cold hyperalgesia and mechanical hyperalgesia remote from the cervical spine.[54] These differences suggest that the two groups suffer different injuries or injuries of different severity.

For lack of reliability, validity, or both, no features on history or physical examination have been able to identify any source or cause of neck pain after whiplash. For patients with temporary pain, which recovers spontaneously, "muscle sprain" is the most plausible conjecture, but it has never been identified in patients in a valid manner.

In case reports or small, descriptive series, lesion such as small fractures,[55,56] aneurysms of the vertebral artery or internal carotid artery[57–59] have been reported in individual patients but not in any substantial proportion of patients with either acute or chronic neck pain after whiplash.

In clinical studies, the source of chronic neck pain after whiplash has been traced to the cervical zygapophysial joints

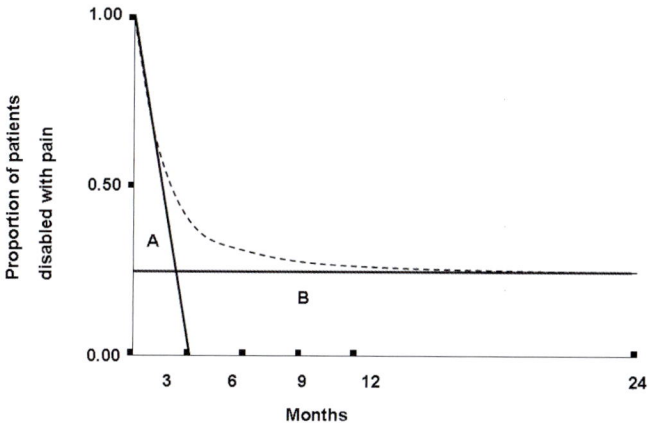

FIGURE 71.8 A graph showing how the recovery curve in Figure 71.7 can be resolved into two populations of patients: those who recover quickly (A) and those destined ab initio to have persistent disability (B).

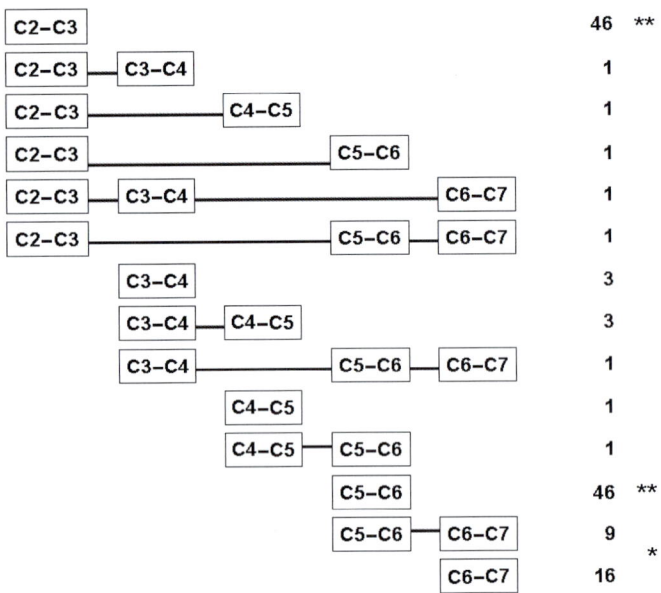

C2–C3		46	**
C2–C3 — C3–C4		1	
C2–C3 ———— C4–C5		1	
C2–C3 ————————— C5–C6		1	
C2–C3 — C3–C4 —————— C6–C7		1	
C2–C3 ———— C5–C6 — C6–C7		1	
C3–C4		3	
C3–C4 — C4–C5		3	
C3–C4 ———— C5–C6 — C6–C7		1	
C4–C5		1	
C4–C5 — C5–C6		1	
C5–C6		46	**
C5–C6 — C6–C7		9	*
C6–C7		16	

FIGURE 71.9 The segmental location of painful zygapophysial joints in patients with chronic neck pain after whiplash, as determined by controlled, diagnostic, medial branch blocks.[8] *Asterisks* indicate the segments most commonly responsible.

in 54%[60] and 60%[61] of patients. Studies in laboratory animals have shown that the lesion responsible for chronic zygapophysial joint pain is a submaximal strain of the joint capsule.[62] After such strains, the affected joint becomes a source of persistent nociceptive output which generates, in the dorsal root ganglion and central pain pathways, metabolic changes that are the hallmark of chronic pain.[63–74]

Diagnosis

For acute neck pain after whiplash, pursuit of diagnosis is not warranted. The condition is self-evident from the presenting complaint and history of injury. Imaging is not indicated according to the Canadian C-Spine Rules[15] (see Fig. 71.4). Multiple studies using MRI have not identified any lesions that might the cause of pain.[75–80]

For chronic neck pain after whiplash, the only investigation that has been shown to have utility are cervical medial branch blocks. With a prevalence of 54% to 60%, cervical zygapophysial joint pain is the single most common basis for chronic neck pain after whiplash.[52,60,61] The joints most commonly responsible are those at C2–C3 and C5–C6[8] (Fig. 71.9).

Most often, the neck pain arises from the joints at one or other of these segments. Patients with C2–C3 zygapophysial joint pain have upper cervical pain and headache. Those with C5–C6 pain have lower neck pain and referred pain into the shoulder region. In patients with unilateral pain, the ipsilateral joint is the cause. In patients with bilateral pain, both joints at the responsible segment are typically the source.

Less frequently, the C6–C7 zygapophysial joint is the source of pain, either alone or in combination with the C5–C6 joint. Other combinations can occur, although far less frequently such as C2–C3 together with adjacent or remote joints and C5–C6 together with joints above.

CERVICOGENIC HEADACHE
Differential Diagnosis

By definition, cervicogenic headache is explicitly pain referred to the head from the cervical spine. That implies a source of pain in the cervical spine. The differential diagnosis encompasses other causes of headache that do not lie in the cervical spine but are nonetheless innervated by cervical spinal nerves. These include aneurysms of the vertebral artery or internal carotid artery and lesions in the posterior cranial fossa that irritate or stretch the dura mater, such as tumors, hemorrhage, and infection. These conditions would be distinguished from cervicogenic headache by the onset of neurologic features or features of infection.

Diagnosis

A variety of causes of cervicogenic headache have been postulated and promoted,[9–11] but few have satisfied the diagnostic criteria required by the International Headache Society.[81] Those criteria allow for clinical diagnosis provided that the diagnostic tests used have proven reliability and validity (Table 71.2), but no clinical features have been shown to have these properties. Otherwise, the diagnostic criteria require relief of pain by controlled, diagnostic blocks.

Certain clinical features have been shown to be reliable for establishing a diagnosis of *probable* cervicogenic headache.[82] These are unilateral headache and pain starting in the neck, and three additional features such as pain radiating to the shoulder and arm, varying duration or fluctuating continuous pain, moderate, nonthrobbing pain, and history of neck trauma. The definitive diagnosis, however, requires establishing a source of pain in the cervical spine by minimally invasive tests.

Sources

Notionally, any of the structures innervated by the upper three cervical spinal nerves could be a source of cervicogenic headache.[9–11] However, no diagnostic tests have been developed and validated for headache stemming from the upper cervical muscles, the transverse or alar ligaments, or the dura mater. Tests are available only for the C2–C3 intervertebral disk and the upper cervical synovial joints.

TABLE 71.2   Diagnostic Criteria for Cervicogenic Headache as Proposed by the International Headache Society[81]

Diagnostic Criteria

A. Pain referred from a source in the neck and perceived in one or more regions of the head and/or face, fulfilling criteria C and D

B. Clinical, laboratory, and/or imaging evidence of a disorder or lesion within the cervical spine or soft tissues of the neck known to be, or generally accepted as, a valid cause of headache[a]

C. Evidence that the pain can be attributed to the neck disorder or lesion based on at least one of the following:
  1. Demonstration of clinical signs that implicate a source of pain in the neck[b]
  2. Abolition of headache following diagnostic blockade of a cervical structure or its nerve supply using placebo or other adequate controls[c]

D. Pain resolves within 3 mo after successful treatment of the causative disorder or lesion

[a]Tumors, fractures, infections, and rheumatoid arthritis of the upper cervical spine have not been validated formally as causes of headache but are nevertheless accepted as valid causes when demonstrated to be so in individual cases. Cervical spondylosis and osteochondritis are not accepted as valid causes fulfilling criterion B. When myofascial tender spots are, the headache should be coded under 2. Tension-type headache.
[b]Clinical signs acceptable for criterion C1 must have demonstrated reliability and validity. The future task is the identification of such reliable and valid operational tests. Clinical features such as neck pain, focal neck tenderness, history of neck trauma, mechanical exacerbation of pain, unilaterality, coexisting shoulder pain, reduced range of motion in the neck, nuchal onset, nausea, vomiting, photophobia, etc., are not unique to cervicogenic headache. These may be features of cervicogenic headache, but they do not define relationship between the disorder and the source of the headache.
[c]Abolition of headache means complete relief of headache, indicated by a score of zero on a Visual Analogue Scale (VAS). Nevertheless, acceptable as fulfilling criterion C2 is >90% reduction in pain to a level of <5 on a 100-point VAS.

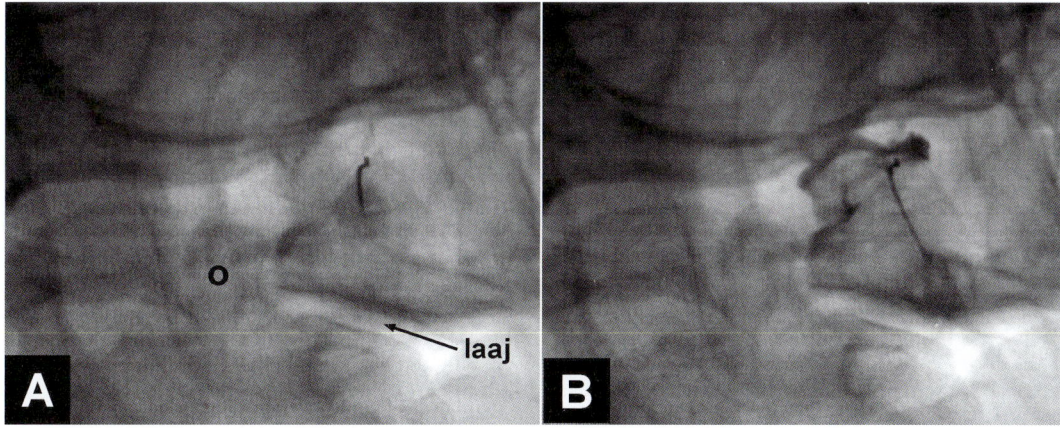

FIGURE 71.10 Fluoroscopy images of an atlantooccipital joint block. **A:** An oblique posterior view of a needle having pierced the capsule of the joint. O, odontoid process; laaj, lateral atlantoaxial joint. **B:** An oblique posterior view after injection of contrast medium into the joint. *(Images kindly provided by Dr. Paul Dreyfuss, Seattle, Washington.)*

Minimally Invasive Tests

For pain stemming from an intervertebral disk, disk stimulation is the only available diagnostic test. The test is positive if provocation of a disk reproduces the patient's headache, provided that stimulation of other disks does not reproduce pain.[41]

Pain stemming from the atlantooccipital or lateral atlantoaxial joints can be tested with intra-articular injections of local anesthetic[83] (Figs. 71.10 and 71.11). The test is positive if blocking the joint fully relieves the headache. However, to guard against false-positive responses, some form of control block is required, such as placebo block or a block of a nearby structure that is not the target joint. No equivalent test has been developed for pain stemming from the median atlantoaxial joint.

Pain from the C2–C3 zygapophysial joint can be diagnosed using comparative local anaesthetic blocks of the third occipital nerve, which is the nerve that innervates this joint. The nerve can be anesthetized where it crosses the lateral aspect of the joint[84] (Fig. 71.12).

Prevalence

No studies have provided data on the prevalence of headache stemming from the C2–C3 disk. The evidence is limited to observations that disk stimulation reproduces headache in some patients[7,43] and that discectomy and fusion can relieve the headache.[85]

Diagnostic blocks of the atlantooccipital joints have not been applied in systematic population studies to determine the prevalence of headache stemming from these joints. The literature is limited to reports of positive responses to blocks in small samples of patients, which do not provide prevalence data, but nonetheless constitute proof of principle, namely, that in some patients, the headache can be traced to an atlantooccipital joint.[86]

Responses to lateral atlantoaxial joint blocks have been reported in a few case series.[49,87,88]

In these studies, the source of pain could be traced to the lateral atlantoaxial joints in 16%,[87] 13%,[88] and 9%[49] of patients presenting with headache.

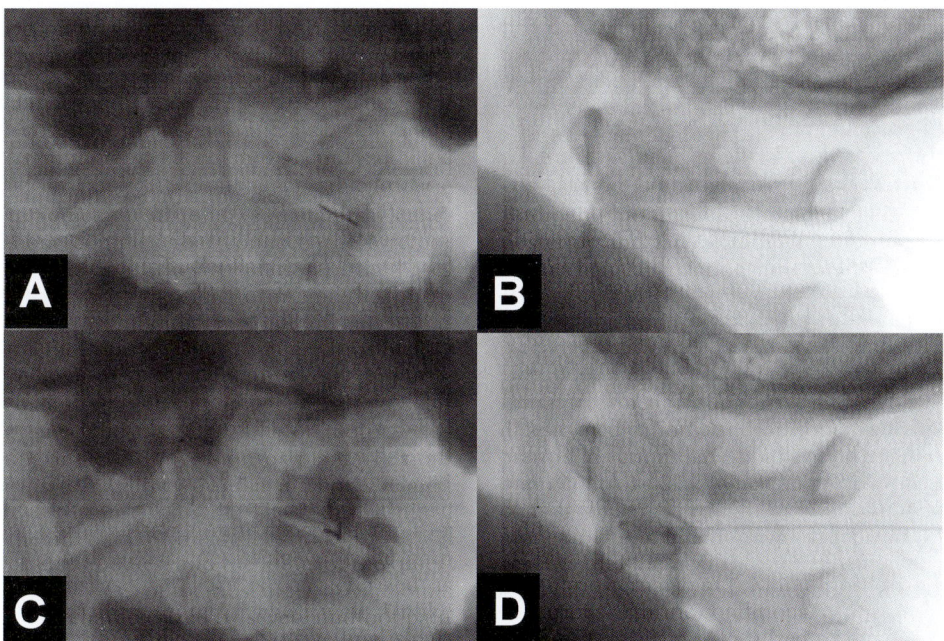

FIGURE 71.11 Fluoroscopy images of a lateral atlantoaxial joint block. **A:** Posterior view of a needle inserted into the right lateral atlantoaxial joint. **B:** Lateral view of needle in the joint. **C:** Posterior view after injection of contrast medium into the joint. **D:** Lateral view after injection of contrast medium.

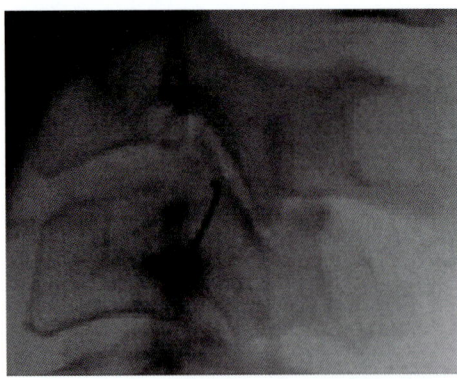

FIGURE 71.12 Lateral fluoroscopy view of a needle in one of three positions for a third occipital nerve block. *(Reproduced with permission from Bogduk N, ed.* Practice Guidelines for Spinal Diagnostic and Treatment Procedures. *2nd ed. San Francisco, CA: International Spine Intervention Society; 2013.)*

The most common, documented source of cervicogenic headache is the C2–C3 zygapophysial joint. It is the source of pain in some 56% of patients with headache after whiplash.[89]

Treatment

NECK PAIN
Conservative Therapy
Traditionally, conservative therapy for neck pain has consisted of medications and therapies, delivered alone or in combination. Despite the large number of studies that have been conducted, convincing evidence of efficacy is lacking. Variously, the literature provides no evidence of effectiveness or efficacy, evidence that certain therapies are no more effective than sham therapy or other therapies, or no evidence of any lasting benefit. In particular, no conservative therapy has been shown to eliminate neck pain, or to reduce it sufficiently to allow restoration of activities of daily living, with no further need for other health care.

There is no evidence that nonsteroidal anti-inflammatory drugs (NSAIDs), opioids, or antidepressants provide short- or long-term benefits.[90] Usual care using analgesics or NSAIDs is no more effective than placebo physical therapy,[91] and adding NSAIDs to manipulative therapy provides no greater relief of pain.[91] Muscle relaxants are no more effective than placebo or have not been studied beyond 8 days.[90]

Soft collars do not provide any greater reduction in pain than rest, exercises, usual care, or no care, and rigid collars are no more effective than usual care.[90] Traction is no more effective than sham traction.[92]

Electrotherapies, such as ultrasound, or diathermy, provide no better outcome than exercises or manual therapy, usual care, or sham therapy.[90] For lack of adequate studies, the evidence on transcutaneous electrical nerve stimulation is inconclusive.[93]

Patient education is equal to or less effective than other conservative care. Any benefits are small and short lived.[94]

There is no evidence to support relaxation therapy, cognitive-behavioral therapy, or biofeedback.[95] In the short term, cognitive-behavioral therapy is more effective than no treatment but is no more effective than other treatments.[96] Adding behavioral therapy to exercises does not improve the outcomes.[96,97]

There is no literature on the effectiveness of multidisciplinary pain management for acute neck pain. For chronic neck pain, the few studies that have been conducted show no benefit,[98,99] or minimal benefit for pain and disability,[100] but no better than that of continuing primary care.[101]

Acupuncture is either no better than sham acupuncture[102] or slightly more effective than sham treatment or no treatment but only in the short term.[103] There is no evidence of long-term benefit.

There is evidence of moderate to high quality that cervical manipulation provides outcomes similar to those of cervical mobilization, but the literature comparing these two therapies with inactive treatments is of low quality. It shows benefits immediately after treatment but not in the short or long term.[104] Spinal manipulative therapy is somewhat more effective than medications alone but not more effective than a home exercise program[105] or exercise in general.[90,102]

Dry needling of trigger points is no more effective than sham needling.[106]

Multimodal therapy involves combinations of exercises, manual therapy, and education. It may be of benefit,[107] but the evidence is inconsistent that multimodal therapy is any more effective than usual care, collars, or advice to stay active.[90]

Exercise is the most studied of the conservative therapies for neck pain, but nonetheless, conclusions are limited. There is no high-quality evidence for exercise therapy, and its effectiveness remains uncertain.[108] Any benefits are inconsistent, small in magnitude, and only short lived.[108,109] The evidence is stronger for strengthening exercises.[110]

For chronic neck pain after whiplash, the evidence on exercises is conflicting. Some have found neck-specific exercises to be more often effective than instructions to pursue physical activity,[97] whereas others found exercises to be no more effective that advice to stay active.[111,112]

Injections
A systematic review found that injections of botulinum toxin were no more effective than placebo for chronic neck pain.[91] Of studies published since, one found botulinum toxin to be more effective than placebo in a small proportion of patients with chronic neck pain,[113] but another found no superiority over placebo.[114]

Trigger point injections appear to be as effective as ultrasound treatment[115] but ultrasound is no more effective than placebo treatment.[116]

Interventional Pain Medicine
For the use of cervical epidural injection of steroids to treat chronic neck pain, in patients with no radicular features, the formal literature is limited. A brief descriptive study reported that 56% of 41 patients with idiopathic neck pain had 90% relief maintained for 6 months after treatment.[117] No other outcomes corroborating pain relief were provided. Another outcome study reported 6 of 58 patients achieving complete relief of pain, and a further 8 each achieving 51% to 75% or 75% to 95% relief at 3 weeks after treatment with up to three injections.[118] A systematic review found no other admissible evidence.[119] A controlled study found no difference in outcome if epidural injections contained steroids or only local anesthetic.[120] These data provide little support for the use of epidural steroids in the treatment of neck pain.

Intra-articular injection of steroids into the cervical zygapophysial joints was introduced as a treatment for neck pain during the 1980s. Some have advocated this treatment since then.[121] A controlled trial, however, showed limited value for this treatment. In patients proven to have neck pain stemming from a zygapophysial joint, intra-articular injection of steroids was no more effective than intra-articular injection of local anesthetic, and few patients benefited from either therapy beyond 15 days.[122]

The only treatment that has been shown to relieve neck pain completely is percutaneous radiofrequency medial branch neurotomy. The treatment involves carefully coagulating the

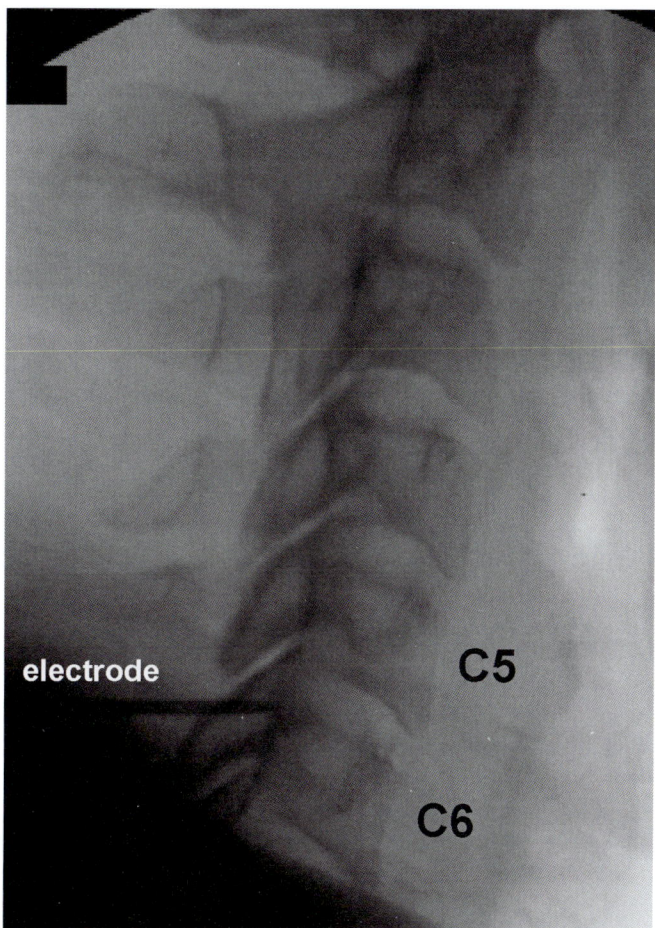

FIGURE 71.13 A lateral radiograph of the cervical spine, showing an electrode in place for radiofrequency neurotomy of a C5 medial branch, in the course of treatment of C5–C6 zygapophysial joint pain.

medial branches of the dorsal rami that are responsible for mediating the patient's pain[123] (Fig. 71.13). The singular indication is complete relief of pain following controlled diagnostic blocks of these nerves.[124]

A placebo-controlled trial showed that this is a valid procedure.[125] The results of the original investigators[125–127] have been corroborated by others.[128,129] Complete relief of pain is achieved in some 70% of patients treated.[125–127] Errors in diagnosis account for the failures. Some patients have false-positive responses to diagnostic blocks, even when these are controlled. In other patients, neurotomy unmasks latent or previously undiagnosed sources of pain (e.g., at adjacent segmental levels).

The pooled data indicate that about 60% of patients maintain complete relief of pain at 6 months and between 30% and 50% do so at 12 months.[130] Success rates are not demonstrably different between patients with legal claims and those without.[126,127,129,131] Recurrence of pain is to be expected because the treated nerves regenerate. Repeat neurotomy reinstates relief. Repetition has been reported to reinstate relief up to seven times, with the average duration of relief ranging between 8 and 18 months per repetition.[126–129,132]

Complete relief of pain is accompanied by restoration of activities of daily living and no need for other health care.[125,126,130] These outcomes occur only if the technique recommended by the International Spine Intervention Society[123] is used and only if the selection criteria are complete relief of pain following controlled diagnostic blocks of the medial branches to be targeted.[130] If lesser diagnostic criteria are used, success rates and the degree of relief are substantially lower.[133,134]

Conspicuously, radiofrequency medial branch neurotomy is the only treatment that has been shown to provide complete relief of chronic neck pain, with restoration of activities of daily living, and no other need for health care.[125,126,130] Moreover, it also resolves psychological distress immediately upon relieving pain[135,136] and reduces central sensitization and hyperalgesia.[137] No other treatment for chronic neck pain has been shown to have these properties. A Cochrane review found that the evidence for cervical radiofrequency neurotomy was limited but only in the sense that there have not been more controlled trials; there was no dispute concerning the quality of the published studies.[138] An independent review reported that radiofrequency neurotomy sets a benchmark for the treatment of chronic neck pain.[139]

CERVICOGENIC HEADACHE

For the treatment of cervicogenic headache diagnosed clinically, no drugs have been shown to be effective, injections of botulinum toxin are not effective, and most conservative therapies are either ineffective or, at best are partially effective, in some patients, for a short time.[9–11] The only consistent evidence is that exercises offer some benefit.[108,140]

The best available evidence indicates that manual therapy or exercises are equally effective but to limited extents.[141] In the short term, some 76% of patients achieve at least 50% reduction in pain, with 35% achieving complete relief. In the long term, 72% have a reduction of greater than 50% in the frequency of headache, but data on relief of pain are lacking.

Although intra-articular injections of steroids have been advocated for the treatment of headache stemming from the atlantooccipital or lateral atlantoaxial joints,[86–88] this treatment has not been evaluated in patients in whom the target joint had been proven to be the source of pain using controlled diagnostic blocks. No controlled studies have validated the use of steroids.

For patients whose headache can be relieved by lateral atlantoaxial joint blocks, an option for treatment is arthrodesis of the joint. The surgical literature attests to complete relief of pain being achieved, albeit in small numbers of patients, for over 2 years.[142–144]

In those patients in whom the source of headache can be traced to the C2–C3 intervertebral disk, disk excision and anterior cervical fusion reportedly can be effective.[85] For pain from the C2–C3 zygapophysial joint, intra-articular injection of steroids has been advocated,[145] but a controlled trial that included patients with C2–C3 zygapophysial joint pain found intra-articular steroids to be no more effective than intra-articular local anesthetic.[122]

The most abundant evidence for headache stemming from the C2–C3 zygapophysial joints applies to thermal radiofrequency neurotomy of the third occipital nerve.[123] When the third occipital nerve has been shown, using controlled diagnostic blocks,[84] to be responsible for mediating the headache (Fig. 71.14), lasting relief can be achieved by coagulating that nerve. The available evidence shows that the effectiveness of radiofrequency neurotomy is contingent on the rigor of diagnosis and the rigor of treatment.

Three controlled trials have provided salutary evidence on practices that are not effective.[146–148] Radiofrequency neurotomy is not effective: when patients are selected for treatment simply on the basis of clinical criteria; when nerves are indiscriminately targeted, without having been subjected previously to controlled diagnostic blocks; or when techniques for radiofrequency neurotomy are used that have not been validated.[9–11]

Radiofrequency neurotomy becomes effective when patients are selected whose headache has been completely relieved by controlled diagnostic blocks of the third occipital nerve[84] and

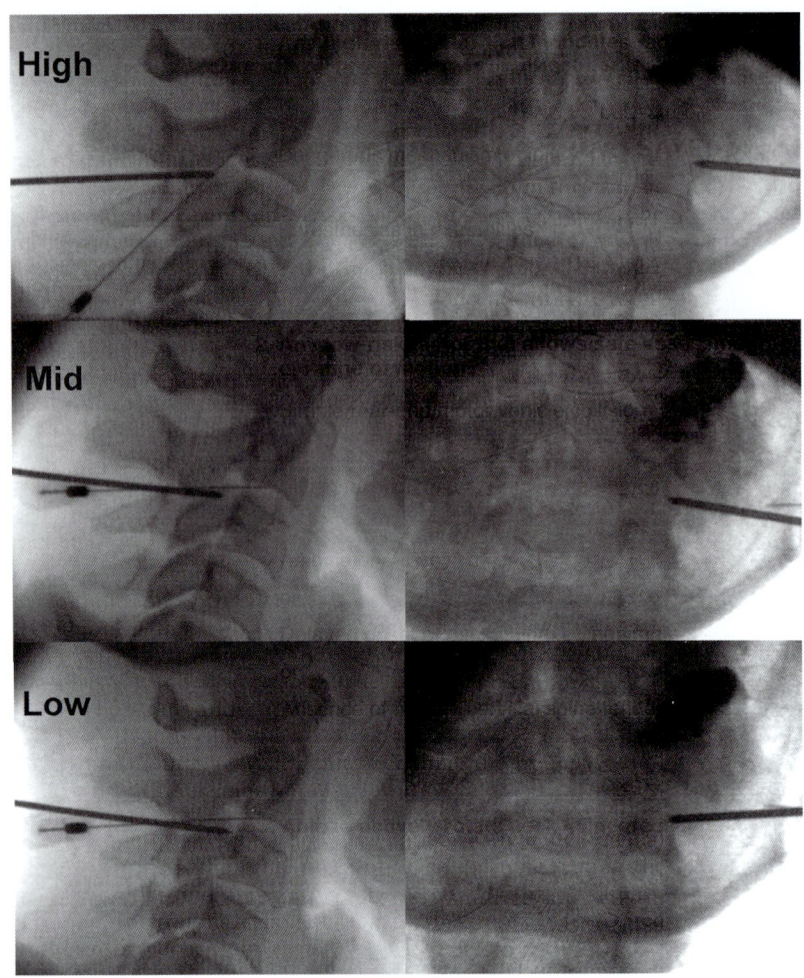

High

Mid

Low

FIGURE 71.14 Lateral and posterior fluoroscopy views of an electrode placed in high, middle, and low positions for a third occipital thermal radiofrequency neurotomy. The electrode is placed in three positions in order to encompass variations in the possible location of the third occipital nerve as it crosses the C2–C3 zygapophysial joint.

when third occipital neurotomy is performed according to prescribed standards.[123] If these diagnostic criteria are satisfied and correct technique is used, complete relief of pain can be achieved in 88% of patients, for a median duration of some 297 days,[149] that relief being associated with restoration of activities of daily living, and no need for other health care. Such results have been corroborated by other studies.[127–129] For patients in whom headaches recur, relief can be reinstated by repeating the neurotomy. By repeating neurotomy as required, some patients have been able to maintain relief of their headache for longer than 2 years,[149] for up to 5 years,[129] and beyond.[127]

A surgical alternative for cervicogenic headache has been explored.[150] Based on complete, or near-complete, relief of headache following nerve root blocks and likewise following zygapophysial joint blocks, 34 patients underwent posterior fusion of C1–C3 using Brook's triple wire fusion. Another 10 patients underwent fusion variously at C1–C2, C2–C3, or C1–C3 based on positive responses to nerve root blocks but no response to zygapophysial joint blocks. At 1 year after surgery, 3 patients had no pain, 22 had only mild pain, and 16 had moderate pain rated as less than 5/10. At 4 years, 7 patients had no pain, 22 had mild pain, and 10 had moderate pain. In only 2 patients did pain scores deteriorate to preoperative levels.

Summary

The literature provides few options for the evidence-based management of neck or cervicogenic headache. A minimalist clinical pathway captures the practices and advice for which the evidence is most consistent or for which outcomes are strongest (Fig. 71.15).

For acute neck pain, the best advice is to avoid passive therapies[102] and to provide advice to remain active, coupled with home exercises to maintain neck movements.[90,107,151–154] If physicians are tempted to prescribe analgesics, they should do so aware that the effect may be no more than that of a placebo.

Resolution may occur as a result of the treatment or because of natural recovery. Nevertheless, if resolution commences, the treatment should be reinforced in order to encourage recovery until resolution is complete.

If pain continues, the best option remains advice coupled with formal exercise therapy.[90,108,110] However, the evidence is conflicting as to whether advice alone[111,112] or exercises alone[97] are sufficient, and the effect may be small.[109]

Beyond conservative therapy, medial branch blocks should be entertained, on the grounds that the cervical zygapophysial joints are the most likely, identifiable source of pain. If controlled blocks are positive, then thermal radiofrequency neurotomy becomes an option for treatment.

If blocks are negative, or if medial branch neurotomy fails to provide relief, there are no proven options. With that understanding, physicians and their patients might explore unproven options.

For neck pain, those options include other conservative therapies or surgery. For cervicogenic headache, the options include investigation of the atlantooccipital and atlantoaxial joints or the C2–C3 disk, with treatment by intra-articular steroids or arthrodesis.[9–11]

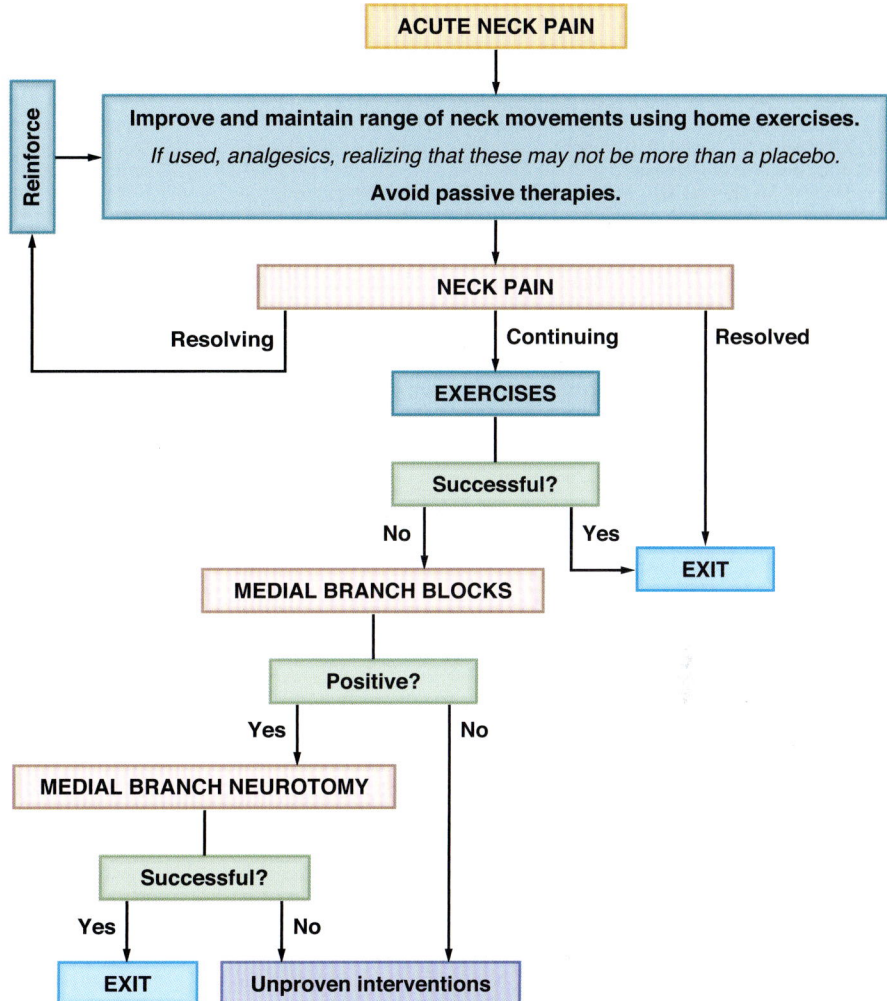

FIGURE 71.15 A clinical pathway for the management of acute and chronic neck pain.

References

1. Merskey H, Bogduk N, eds. Spinal pain, section 1: spinal and radicular pain syndromes. In: *Classification of Chronic Pain: Descriptions of Chronic Pain Syndromes and Definition of Pain Terms*. 2nd ed. Seattle, WA: IASP Press; 1994:11–16.
2. Kellgren JH. On the distribution of pain arising from deep somatic structures with charts of segmental pain areas. *Clin Sci* 1939;4:35–46.
3. Campbell DG, Parsons CM. Referred head pain and its concomitants. *J Nerv Ment Dis* 1944;99:544–551.
4. Feinstein B, Langton JN, Jameson RM, et al. Experiments on referred pain from deep somatic tissues. *J Bone Joint Surg Am* 1954;36A:981–997.
5. Dwyer A, Aprill C, Bogduk N. Cervical zygapophyseal joint pain patterns I: a study in normal volunteers. *Spine* 1990;15:453–457.
6. Fukui S, Ohseto K, Shiotani M, et al. Referred pain distribution of the cervical zygapophyseal joints and cervical dorsal rami. *Pain* 1996;68:79–83.
7. Schellhas KP, Garvey TA, Johnson BA, et al. Cervical diskography: analysis of provoked responses at C2–C3, C3–C4, and C4–C5. *Am J Neuroradiol* 2000;21:269–275.
8. Cooper G, Bailey B, Bogduk N. Cervical zygapophysial joint pain maps. *Pain Med* 2007;8:344–353.
9. Bogduk N, Bartsch T. Cervicogenic headache. In: Silberstein SD, Lipton RB, Dodick DW, eds. *Wolff's Headache*. 8th ed. New York: Oxford University Press; 2008:551–570.
10. Bogduk N, Govind J. Cervicogenic headache: an assessment of the evidence on clinical diagnosis, invasive tests, and treatment. *Lancet Neurol* 2009;8:959–968.
11. Bogduk N. The neck and headaches. *Neurol Clin* 2014;32:471–487.
12. Bogduk N, McGuirk B. Acute neck pain: physical examination. In: *Medical Management of Acute and Chronic Neck Pain. An Evidence-Based Approach*. Amsterdam, The Netherlands: Elsevier; 2006:43–49.
13. Roberge RJ, Wears RC, Kelly M, et al. Selective application of cervical spine radiography in alert victims of blunt trauma: a prospective study. *J Trauma* 1988;28:784–788.
14. McNamara RM. Post-traumatic neck pain: a prospective and follow-up study. *Ann Emerg Med* 1988;17:906–911.
15. Stiell IG, Wells GA, Vandemheen KL, et al. The Canadian C-spine rule for radiography in alert and stable trauma patients. *JAMA* 2001;286:1841–1848.
16. Heller CA, Stanley P, Lewis-Jones B, et al. Value of x ray examinations of the cervical spine. *Br Med J* 1983;287:1276–1278.
17. Johnson MJ, Lucas GL. Value of cervical spine radiographs as a screening tool. *Clin Orthop* 1997;340:102–108.
18. Deyo RA, Diehl AK. Lumbar spine films in primary care: current use and effects of selective ordering criteria. *J Gen Inter Med* 1986;1:20–25.
19. Lawton MT, Porter RW, Heiseman JE, et al. Surgical management of spinal epidural hematoma: relationship between surgical timing and neurological outcome. *J Neurosurg* 1995;83:1–7.
20. Williams JM, Allegra JR. Spontaneous cervical epidural haematoma. *Ann Emerg Med* 1994;23:1368–1370.
21. Lobitz B, Grate I. Acute epidural hematoma of the cervical spine: an unusual cause of neck pain. *South Med J* 1995;88:580–582.
22. Beatty RM, Winston KR. Spontaneous cervical epidural haematoma: a consideration of etiology. *J Neurosurg* 1984;61:143–148.
23. Matsumae M, Shimoda M, Shibuya N, et al. Spontaneous cervical epidural hematoma. *Surg Neurol* 1987;28:381–384.
24. Benyamin RM, Vallejo R, Wang V, et al. Acute epidural hematoma formation in cervical spine after interlaminar epidural steroid injection despite discontinuation of clopidogrel. *Reg Anesth Pain Med* 2016;41:398–401.
25. Silbert PL, Makri B, Schievink WI. Headache and neck pain in spontaneous internal carotid and vertebral artery dissections. *Neurology* 1995;45:1517–1522.
26. Biousse V, D'Anglejan-Chatillon J, Massiou H, et al. Head pain in non-traumatic carotid artery dissection: a series of 65 patients. *Cephalalgia* 1994;14:33–36.
27. Sturzenegger M. Headache and neck pain: the warning symptoms of vertebral artery dissection. *Headache* 1994;34:187–193.
28. Garrard P, Barnes D. Aortic dissection presenting as a neurological emergency. *J R Soc Med* 1996;89:271–272.
29. Hirst AE, Johns VJ, Kime FW. Dissecting aneurysm of the aorta: a review of 505 cases. *Medicine* 1958;37:217–275.

30. Schattner A. Pain in the neck. *Lancet* 1996;348:411–412.
31. Shawky A, Elnady B, El-Morshidy E, et al. Longus colli tendinitis. A review of literature and case series. *SICOT J* 2017;3:48.
32. Hardin JG, Halla JT. Cervical spine syndromes. In: Koopman WJ, ed. *Arthritis and Allied Conditions. A Textbook of Rheumatology*. 14th ed. Philadelphia: Lippincott Williams & Wilkins; 2001:2009–2018.
33. Cherington M, Hendee R. Accessory nerve palsy—a painful cranial neuropathy: surgical cure. *Headache* 1978;18:274–275.
34. Harinck HI, Buvoet OL, Vellenga CJ, et al. Relation between signs and symptoms in Paget's disease of bone. *Quart J Med* 1986;58:133–151.
35. Gore DR, Sepic SB, Gardner GM. Roentgenographic findings of the cervical spine in asymptomatic people. *Spine* 1986;1:521–524.
36. Elias F. Roentgen findings in the asymptomatic cervical spine. *N Y State J Med* 1958;58:3300–3303.
37. Fridenberg ZB, Miller WT. Degenerative disc disease of the cervical spine. A comparative study of asymptomatic and symptomatic patients. *J Bone Joint Surg* 1963;45A:1171–1178.
38. Lucas N, Macaskill P, Irwig L, et al. Reliability of physical examination for diagnosis of myofascial trigger points. A systematic review of the literature. *Clin J Pain* 2009;25:80–89.
39. Heyde CE, Boehm H, El Saghir H, et al. Surgical treatment of spondylodiscitis in the cervical spine: a minimum 2-year follow-up. *Eur Spine J* 2006;15:1380–1387.
40. Khalatbari MR, Moharamzad Y. Brown tumor of the spine in patients with primary hyperparathyroidism. *Spine* 2014;39:E1073–E1079.
41. International Spine Intervention Society. Cervical disc stimulation. In: Bogduk N, ed. *Practice Guidelines for Spinal Diagnostic and Treatment Procedures*. 2nd ed. San Francisco, CA: International Spine Intervention Society; 2013:283–302.
42. Bogduk N, Aprill C. On the nature of neck pain, discography and cervical zygapophysial joint pain. *Pain* 1993;54:213–217.
43. Grubb SA, Kelly CK. Cervical discography: clinical implications from 12 years of experience. *Spine* 2000;25:1382–1389.
44. International Spine Intervention Society. Cervical medial branch blocks. In: Bogduk N, ed. *Practice Guidelines for Spinal Diagnostic and Treatment Procedures*. 2nd ed. San Francisco, CA: International Spine Intervention Society; 2013:101–139.
45. Engel A, MacVicar J, Bogduk N. A philosophical foundation for diagnostic blocks, with criteria for their validation. *Pain Med* 2014;15:998–1006.
46. Engel AJ, Bogduk N. Mathematical validation and credibility of diagnostic blocks for spinal pain. *Pain Med* 2016;17:1821–1828.
47. Speldewinde GC, Bashford GM, Davidson IR. Diagnostic cervical zygapophysial joint blocks for chronic cervical pain. *Med J Aust* 2001;174:174–176.
48. Manchikanti L, Singh V, Rivera J, et al. Prevalence of cervical facet joint pain in chronic neck pain. *Pain Physician* 2002;5:243–249.
49. Yin W, Bogduk N. The nature of neck pain in a private pain clinic in the United States. *Pain Med* 2008;9:196–203.
50. McConnell WE, Howard, RP, Guzman HM, et al. Analysis of human test subject kinematic responses to low velocity rear end impacts. In: *Proceedings of the 37th Stapp Car Crash Conference*. San Antonio, TX: Society of Automotive Engineers; 1993:21–30.
51. Kaneoka K, Ono K, Inami S, et al. Motion analysis of cervical vertebrae during whiplash loading. *Spine* 1999;24:763–770.
52. Bogduk N. On cervical zygapophysial joint pain after whiplash. *Spine* 2011;36:S194–S199.
53. Radanov BP, Sturzenegger M, Di Stefano G. Long-term outcome after whiplash injury: a 2-year follow-up considering features of injury mechanism and somatic, radiologic, and psychosocial findings. *Medicine* 1995;74:281–297.
54. Jull G, Kenardy J, Hendrikz J, et al. Management of acute whiplash: a randomized controlled trial of multidisciplinary stratified treatments. *Pain* 2013;154:1798–1806.
55. Signoret F, Feron JM, Bonfait H, et al. Fractured odontoid with fractured superior articular process of the axis. *J Bone Joint Surg* 1986;68B:182–184.
56. Craig JB, Hodgson BF. Superior facet fractures of the axis vertebra. *Spine* 1991;16:875–877.
57. Hinse P, Thie A, Lachenmayer L. Dissection of the extracranial vertebral artery: report of four cases and review of the literature. *J Neurol Neurosurg Psychiat* 1991;54:863–869.
58. Janjua KJ, Goswami V, Sagar G. Whiplash injury associated with acute bilateral internal carotid arterial dissection. *J Trauma* 1996;40:456–458.
59. Tulyapronchote R, Selhorst JB, Malkoff MD, et al. Delayed sequelae of vertebral artery dissection and occult cervical fractures. *Neurology* 1994;44:1397–1399.
60. Barnsley L, Lord SM, Wallis BJ, et al. The prevalence of chronic cervical zygapophysial joint pain after whiplash. *Spine* 1995;20:20–26.
61. Lord S, Barnsley L, Wallis BJ, et al. Chronic cervical zygapophysial joint pain after whiplash: a placebo-controlled prevalence study. *Spine* 1996;21:1737–1745.
62. Winkelstein BA. How can animal models inform on the transition to chronic symptoms in whiplash? *Spine* 2011;36:S218–S225.
63. Quinn KP, Winkelstein BA. Cervical facet capsular ligament yield defines the threshold for injury and persistent joint-mediated neck pain. *J Biomech* 2007;40:2299–2306.
64. Lu Y, Chen C, Kallakuri S, et al. Neural response of cervical facet joint capsule to stretch: a study of whiplash pain mechanism. *Stapp Car Crash J* 2005;49:49–65.
65. Lu Y, Chen C, Kallakuri S, et al. Development of an in vivo method to investigate biomechanical and neurophysiological properties of spine facet joint capsules. *Eur Spine J* 2005;14:565–572.
66. Quinn KP, Dong L, Golder FJ, et al. Neuronal hyperexcitability in the dorsal horn after painful facet joint injury. *Pain* 2010;151:414–421.
67. Kallakuri S, Singh A, Lu Y, et al. Tensile stretching of cervical facet joint capsule and related axonal changes. *Eur Spine J* 2008;17:556–563.
68. Lee KE, Davis MB, Winkelstein BA. Capsular ligament involvement in the development of mechanical hyperalgesia after facet joint loading: behavioral and inflammatory outcomes in a rodent model of pain. *J Neurotrauma* 2008;25:1383–1393.
69. Lee KE, Winkelstein BA. Joint distraction magnitude is associated with different behavioral outcomes and substance P levels for cervical facet joint loading in the rat. *J Pain* 2009;10:436–445.
70. Dong L, Odeleye AO, Jordan-Sciutto KL, et al. Painful facet joint injury induces neuronal stress activation in the DRG: implications for cellular mechanisms of pain. *Neurosci Lett* 2008;443:90–94.
71. Dong L, Winkelstein BA. Simulated whiplash modulates expression of the glutamatergic system in the spinal cord suggesting spinal plasticity is associated with painful dynamic cervical facet loading. *J Neurotrauma* 2010;27:163–174.
72. Winkelstein BA, Santos DG. An intact facet capsular ligament modulates behavioral sensitivity and spinal glial activation produced by cervical facet joint tension. *Spine* 2008;33:856–862.
73. Lee KE, Davis MB, Mejilla RM, et al. In vivo cervical facet capsule distraction: mechanical implications for whiplash and neck pain. *Stapp Car Crash J* 2004;48:373–395.
74. Lee KE, Thinnes JH, Gokhin DS, et al. A novel rodent neck pain model of facet-mediated behavioral hypersensitivity: implications for persistent pain and whiplash injury. *J Neurosci Methods* 2004;137:151–159.
75. Ellertsson AB, Sigurjonsson K, Thorsteinsson T. Clinical and radiographic study of 100 cases of whiplash injury. *Acta Neurol Scand* 1978;5(suppl 67):269.
76. Pettersson K, Hildingsson C, Toolanen G, et al. MRI and neurology in acute whiplash trauma. *Acta Orthop Scand* 1994;65:525–528.
77. Fagerlund M, Bjornebrink J, Pettersson K, et al. MRI in acute phase of whiplash injury. *Eur Radiol* 1995;5:297–301.
78. Borchgrevink GE, Smevik O, Nordby A, et al. MR imaging and radiography of patients with cervical hyperextension-flexion injuries after car accidents. *Acta Radiol* 1995;36:425–428.
79. Ronnen HR, de Korte PJ, Brink PR, et al. Acute whiplash injury: is there a role for MR imaging? A prospective study of 100 patients. *Radiology* 1996;201:93–96.
80. Voyvodic F, Dolinis J, Moore VM, et al. MRI of car occupants with whiplash injury. *Neuroradiology* 1997;39:25–40.
81. International Headache Society. The International Classification of Headache Disorders, 2nd edition. *Cephalalgia* 2004;24(suppl 1).
82. Antonaci F, Ghirmai S, Bono S, et al. Cervicogenic headache: evaluation of the original diagnostic criteria. *Cephalalgia* 2001;21:573–583.
83. International Spine Intervention Society. Lateral atlanto-axial joint access. In: Bogduk N, ed. *Practice Guidelines for Spinal Diagnostic and Treatment Procedures*. 2nd ed. San Francisco, CA: International Spine Intervention Society; 2013:29–51.
84. International Spine Intervention Society. Third occipital nerve blocks. In: Bogduk N, ed. *Practice Guidelines for Spinal Diagnostic and Treatment Procedures*. 2nd ed. San Francisco, CA: International Spine Intervention Society; 2013:141–163.
85. Schofferman J, Garges K, Goldthwaite N, et al. Upper cervical anterior diskectomy and fusion improves discogenic cervical headaches. *Spine* 2002;27:2240–2244.
86. Busch E, Wilson PR. Atlanto-occipital and atlanto-axial injections in the treatment of headache and neck pain. *Reg Anesth* 1989;14(suppl 2):45.
87. Aprill C, Axinn MJ, Bogduk N. Occipital headaches stemming from the lateral atlanto-axial (C1-2) joint. *Cephalalgia* 2003;22:15–22.
88. Narouze SN, Casanova J, Maekhail N. The longitudinal effectiveness of lateral atlantoaxial intra-articular steroid injection in the treatment of cervicogenic headache. *Pain Med* 2007;8:184–188.
89. Lord S, Barnsley L, Wallis B, et al. Third occipital headache: a prevalence study. *J Neurol Neurosurg Psychiat* 1994;57:1187–1190.
90. Hurwitz EL, Carragee EJ, van der Velde G, et al. Treatment of neck pain: non-invasive interventions. Results of the Bone and Joint Decade 2000-2010 Task Force on Neck Pain and Its Associated Disorders. *Spine* 2008;33:S123–S152.
91. Peloso PM, Gross A, Haines T, et al. Medicinal and injection therapies for mechanical neck disorders. *Cochrane Database Syst Rev* 2007;(3):CD000319. doi:10.1002/14651858.CD000319.pub4.
92. Graham N, Gross A, Goldsmith CH, et al. Mechanical traction for neck pain with or without radiculopathy. *Cochrane Database Syst Rev* 2008;(3):CD006408. doi:10.1002/14651858.CD006408.pub2.
93. Kroeling P, Gross A, Goldsmith CH, et al. Electrotherapy for neck pain. *Cochrane Database Syst Rev* 2009;(4):CD004251. doi:10.1002/14651858.CD004251.pub4.

94. Yu H, Côté P, Southerst D, et al. Does structured patient education improve the recovery and clinical outcomes of patients with neck pain? A systematic review from the Ontario Protocol for Traffic Injury Management (OPTIMa) Collaboration. *Spine J* 2016;16:1524–1540.

95. Shearer HM, Carroll LJ, Wong JJ, et al. Are psychological interventions effective for the management of neck pain and whiplash-associated disorders? A systematic review by the Ontario Protocol for Traffic Injury Management (OPTIMa) Collaboration. *Spine J* 2016;16:1566–1581.

96. Monticone M, Cedraschi C, Ambrosini E, et al. Cognitive-behavioural treatment for subacute and chronic neck pain. *Cochrane Database Syst Rev* 2015;(5):CD010664. doi:10.1002/14651858.CD010664.pub2.

97. Ludvigsson ML, Peterson G, Dedering Å, et al. One- and two-year follow-up of a randomized trial of neck-specific exercise with or without a behavioural approach compared with prescription of physical activity in chronic whiplash disorder. *J Rehabil Med* 2016;48:56–64.

98. Karjalainen K, Malmivaara A, van Tulder M, et al. Multidisciplinary biopsychosocial rehabilitation for neck and shoulder pain among working age adults. A systematic review with the framework of the Cochrane collaboration back review group. *Spine* 2001;26:174–181.

99. Karjalainen K, Malmivaara A, van Tulder M, et al. Multidisciplinary biopsychosocial rehabilitation for neck and shoulder pain among working age adults. *Cochrane Database Syst Rev* 2003;(2):CD002194. doi: 10.1002/14651858.CD002194.

100. Vendrig AA, van Akkerveeken PF, McWhorter KR. Results of a multimodal treatment program for patients with chronic symptoms after a whiplash injury of the neck. *Spine* 2000;25:238–244.

101. Lindell O, Johansson SE, Strender LE. Subacute and chronic, non-specific back and neck pain: cognitive-behavioural rehabilitation versus primary care. A randomized controlled trial. *BMC Musculoskelet Disord* 2008;9:172.

102. Wong JJ, Shearer HM, Mior S, et al. Are manual therapies, passive physical modalities, or acupuncture effective for the management of patients with whiplash-associated disorders or neck pain and associated disorders? An update of the Bone and Joint Decade Task Force on Neck Pain and Its Associated Disorders by the OPTIMa collaboration. *Spine J* 2016;16:1598–1630.

103. Trinh K, Graham N, Irnich D, et al. Acupuncture for neck disorders. *Cochrane Database Syst Rev* 2016;(5):CD004870. doi:10.1002/14651858 .CD004870.pub4.

104. Gross A, Langevin P, Burnie SJ, et al. Manipulation and mobilisation for neck pain contrasted against an inactive control or another active treatment. *Cochrane Database Syst Rev* 2015;(9):CD004249. doi:10.1002/14651858 .CD004249.pub4.

105. Bronfort G, Evans R, Anderson AV, et al. Spinal manipulation, medication, or home exercise with advice for acute and subacute neck pain: a randomized trial. *Ann Intern Med* 2012;156:1–10.

106. Sterling M, Vicenzino B, Souvlis T, et al. Dry-needling and exercise for chronic whiplash-associated disorders: a randomized single-blind placebo-controlled trial. *Pain* 2015;156:635–643.

107. Sutton DA, Côté P, Wong JJ, et al. Is multimodal care effective for the management of patients with whiplash-associated disorders or neck pain and associated disorders? A systematic review by the Ontario Protocol for Traffic Injury Management (OPTIMa) Collaboration. *Spine J* 2016;16:1541–1565.

108. Gross A, Kay TM, Paquin JP, et al. Exercises for mechanical neck disorders. *Cochrane Database Syst Rev* 2015;(1):CD004250. doi:10.1002/14651858 .CD004250.pub5.

109. Southerst D, Nordin MC, Côté P, et al. Is exercise effective for the management of neck pain and associated disorders or whiplash-associated disorders? A systematic review by the Ontario Protocol for Traffic Injury Management (OPTIMa) Collaboration. *Spine J* 2016;16:1503–1523.

110. Gross AR, Paquin JP, Dupont G, et al. Exercises for mechanical neck disorders: A Cochrane review update. *Man Ther* 2016;24:25–45.

111. Stewart MJ, Maher CG, Refshauge KM, et al. Randomized controlled trial of exercise for chronic whiplash-associated disorders. *Pain* 2007;128: 59–68.

112. Michaleff ZA, Maher CG, Lin CW, et al. Comprehensive physiotherapy exercise programme or advice for chronic whiplash (PROMISE): a pragmatic randomised controlled trial. *Lancet* 2014;384:133–141.

113. Miller D, Richardson D, Aisa M, et al. Botulinum neurotoxin-A for treatment of refractory neck pain: a randomized, double-blind study. *Pain Med* 2009;10:1012–1017.

114. Padberg M, de Bruijn SF, Tavy DL. Neck pain in chronic whiplash syndrome treated with botulinum toxin. A double-blind, placebo-controlled clinical trial. *J Neurol* 2007;254:290–295.

115. Esenyel CZ, Caglar N, Aldemir T. Treatment of myofascial pain. *Am J Phys Med Rehabil* 2000;79:48–52.

116. Gam AN, Warming S, Larsen LH, et al. Treatment of myofascial trigger points with ultrasound combined with massage and exercise—a randomised controlled trial. *Pain* 1998;77:73–79.

117. Cicala RS, Thoni K, Angel JJ. Long-term results of cervical epidural steroid injections. *Clin J Pain* 1989;5:143–145.

118. Purkis IE. Cervical epidural steroids. *Pain Clinic* 1986;1:3–7.

119. Benyamin R, Singh V, Parr AT, et al. Systematic review of the effectiveness of cervical epidurals in the management of chronic neck pain. *Pain Physician* 2009;12:137–157.

120. Manchikanti L, Cash KA, Pampati V, et al. Two-year follow-up results of fluoroscopic cervical epidural injections in chronic axial or discogenic neck pain: a randomized, double-blind, controlled trial. *Int J Med Sci* 2014;11:309–320.

121. Kim KH, Choi SH, Kim TK, et al. Cervical facet joint injections in the neck and shoulder pain. *J Korean Med Sci* 2005;20:659–662.

122. Barnsley L, Lord SM, Wallis BJ, et al. Lack of effect of intraarticular corticosteroids for chronic pain in the cervical zygapophyseal joints. *N Engl J Med* 1994;330:1047–1050.

123. International Spine Intervention Society. Percutaneous radiofrequency cervical medial branch neurotomy. In: Bogduk N, ed. *Practice Guidelines for Spinal Diagnostic and Treatment Procedures*. San Francisco, CA: International Spine Intervention Society; 2004:249–284.

124. International Spine Intervention Society. Cervical medial branch blocks. In: Bogduk N, ed. *Practice Guidelines for Spinal Diagnostic and Treatment Procedures*. San Francisco, CA: International Spine Intervention Society; 2004:112–137.

125. Lord SM, Barnsley L, Wallis BJ, et al. Percutaneous radio-frequency neurotomy for chronic cervical zygapophysial-joint pain. *N Engl J Med* 1996;335:1721–1726.

126. Lord SM, McDonald GJ, Bogduk N. Percutaneous radiofrequency neurotomy of the cervical medial branches: a validated treatment for cervical zygapophysial joint pain. *Neurosurg Quart* 1998;8:288–308.

127. McDonald G, Lord SM, Bogduk N. Long-term follow-up of patients treated with cervical radiofrequency neurotomy for chronic neck pain. *Neurosurgery* 1999;45:61–68.

128. Barnsley L. Percutaneous radiofrequency neurotomy for chronic neck pain: outcomes in a series of consecutive patients. *Pain Med* 2005;6: 282–286.

129. MacVicar J, Borowczyk J, MacVicar AM, et al. Cervical medial branch radiofrequency neurotomy in New Zealand. *Pain Med* 2012;13:647–654.

130. Engel A, Rappard G, King W, et al; for the Standards Division of the International Spine Intervention Society. The effectiveness and risks of fluoroscopically-guided cervical medial branch thermal radiofrequency neurotomy: a systematic review with comprehensive analysis of the published data. *Pain Med* 2016;17:658–669.

131. Sapir DA, Gorup JM. Radiofrequency medial branch neurotomy in litigant and nonlitigant patients with cervical whiplash. *Spine* 2001;26: E268–E273.

132. Husted DS, Orton D, Schofferman J, et al. Effectiveness of repeated radiofrequency neurotomy for cervical facet joint pain. *J Spinal Disord Tech* 2008;21:406–408.

133. Royal M, Wienecke G, Movva V, et al. Retrospective study of efficacy of radiofrequency neurolysis for facet arthropathy. *Pain Med* 2001;2:249.

134. Shin WR, Kim HI, Shin DG, et al. Radiofrequency neurotomy of cervical medial branches for chronic cervicobrachialgia. *J Korean Med Sci* 2006;21:119–125.

135. Smith AD, Jull G, Schneider G, et al. Cervical radiofrequency neurotomy reduces psychological features in individuals with chronic whiplash symptoms. *Pain Physician* 2014;17:265–274.

136. Wallis BJ, Lord SM, Bogduk N. Resolution of psychological distress of whiplash patients following treatment by radiofrequency neurotomy: a randomised, double-blind, placebo-controlled trial. *Pain* 1997;73:15–22.

137. Smith AD, Jull G, Schneider G, et al. Cervical radiofrequency neurotomy reduces central hyperexcitability and improves neck movement in individuals with chronic whiplash. *Pain Med* 2014;15:128–141.

138. Niemisto L, Kalso EA, Malmivaar A, et al. Radiofrequency denervation for neck and back pain. *Cochrane Database Syst Rev* 2003;(1):CD004058. doi:10.1002/14651858.CD004058.

139. Centre for Health Services and Policy Branch. *Percutaneous Radio-Frequency Neurotomy Treatment of Chronic Cervical Pain Following Whiplash Injury*. Vancouver, Canada: University of British Columbia, British Columbia Office of Health Technology Assessment; 2001.

140. Varatharajan S, Ferguson B, Chrobak K, et al. Are non-invasive interventions effective for the management of headaches associated with neck pain? An update of the Bone and Joint Decade Task Force on Neck Pain and Its Associated Disorders by the Ontario Protocol for Traffic Injury Management (OPTIMa) Collaboration. *Eur Spine J* 2016;25:1971–1999.

141. Jull G, Trott P, Potter H, et al. A randomized controlled trial of exercise and manipulative therapy for cervicogenic headache. *Spine* 2002;27: 1835–1843.

142. Ghanayem AJ, Leventhal M, Bohlman HH. Osteoarthrosis of the atlanto-axial joints—long-term follow-up after treatment with arthrodesis. *J Bone Joint Surg* 1996;78A:1300–1307.

143. Joseph B, Kumar B. Gallie's fusion for atlantoaxial arthrosis with occipital neuralgia. *Spine* 1994;19:454–455.

144. Schaeren S, Jeanneret B. Atlantoaxial osteoarthritis: case series and review of the literature. *Eur Spine J* 2005;14:501–506.

145. Slipman CW, Lipetz JS, Plastara CT, et al. Therapeutic zygapophyseal joint injections for headache emanating from the C2-3 joint. *Am J Phys Med Rehabil* 2001;80:182–188.

146. Haspeslagh SR, van Suijlekom HA, Lame IE, et al. Randomised controlled trial of cervical radiofrequency lesions as a treatment for cervicogenic headache. *BMC Anesthesiol* 2006;6:1.

147. Stovner LJ, Kolstad F, Helde G. Radiofrequency denervation of facet joints C2–C6 in cervicogenic headache: a randomised, double-blind, sham-controlled study. *Cephalalgia* 2004;24:821–830.

148. van Suijlekom HA, van Kleef M, Barendse GAM, et al. Radiofrequency cervical zygapophyseal joint neurotomy for cervicogenic headaches: a prospective study of 15 patients. *Funct Neurol* 1998;13:297–303.

149. Govind J, King W, Bailey B, et al. Radiofrequency neurotomy for the treatment of third occipital headache. *J Neurol Neurosurg Psychiat* 2003;74: 88–93.

150. Long DM, Davis RF, Speed WG. Fusion for occult posttraumatic cervical facet injury. *Neurosurg Q* 2006;16:129–134.

151. Kjaer P, Kongsted A, Hartvigsen J, et al. National clinical guidelines for non-surgical treatment of patients with recent onset neck pain or cervical radiculopathy. *Eur Spine J* 2017;26(9):2242–2257.

152. Peeters GG, Verhagen AP, de Bie RA, et al. The efficacy of conservative treatment in patients with whiplash injury. A systematic review of clinical trials. *Spine* 2001;26: E64–E73.

153. Verhagen AP, Peeters GG, de Bie RA, et al. Conservative treatment for whiplash. *Cochrane Database Syst Rev* 2007;(2):CD003338.

154. Verhagen AP, Scholten-Peeters GG, van Wijngaarden S, et al. Conservative treatment for whiplash. *Cochrane Database Syst Rev* 2004;(1):CD003338 .pub2.

CHAPTER 72

Acute Low Back Pain

WADE KING and **NIKOLAI BOGDUK**

Introduction

There are three imperatives for the practitioner when they encounter a new patient with what seems to be acute low back pain. The first imperative is to determine whether or not the presenting complaint is, indeed, low back pain as conventionally defined and whether or not it is acute. The second imperative is to determine whether any associated referred pain is somatic referred pain or radicular pain. The third imperative is to identify if the pain is caused by serious pathologies. Once those imperatives are addressed, the management of acute low back pain becomes very straightforward.

DEFINITION

The International Association for the Study of Pain (IASP) construed low back pain as pain arising from one or other of the components of the lumbar spine and referred to it by the rubric: lumbar spinal pain.[1] It defined lumbar spinal pain as pain perceived anywhere in the region bounded by the lateral margins of the erector spinae muscles, an imaginary transverse line through the tip of the last thoracic spinous process, and an imaginary transverse line through the tip of the first sacral spinous process (Fig. 72.1).[1] This definition serves to distinguish lumbar spinal pain from thoracic spinal pain, gluteal pain, and loin pain, for pain in these latter regions invites a

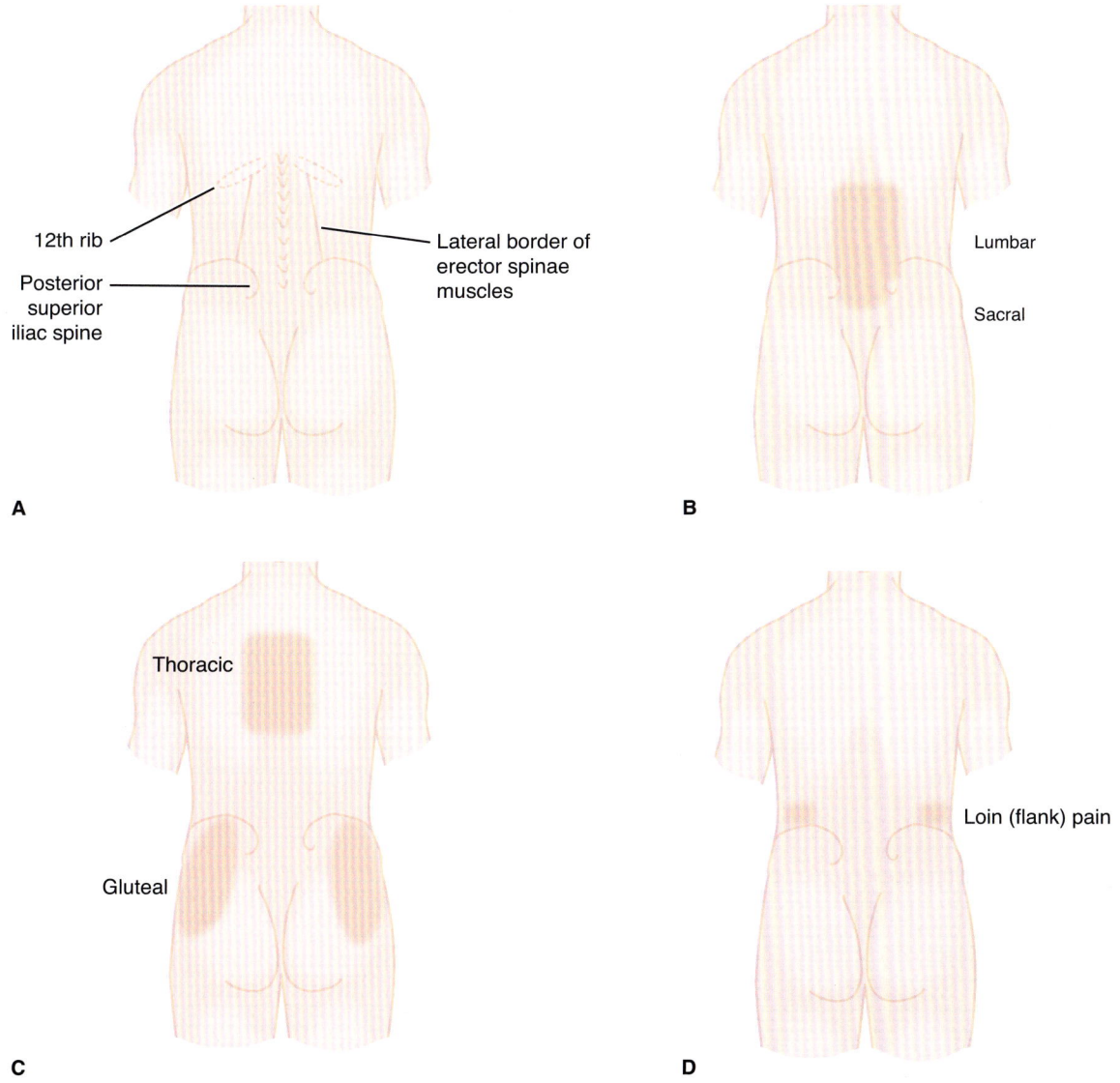

FIGURE 72.1 The definition of what is back pain and what is not. **A:** Landmarks for the definition of lumbar spinal pain. **B:** The topographical location of lumbar spinal pain and sacral spinal pain, any combination of which amounts to low back pain. **C:** Thoracic spinal pain and gluteal pain. **D:** Loin pain.

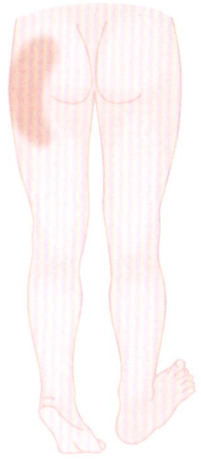 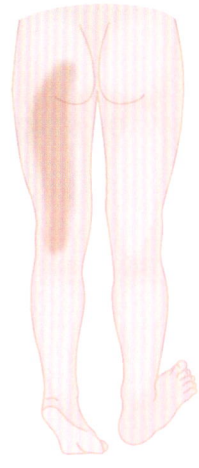 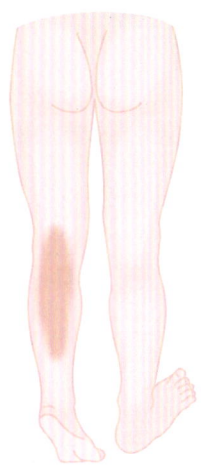

FIGURE 72.2 Various patterns of distribution of somatic referred pain from the lumbar spine.

different approach to diagnosis and management because its causes are likely to lie outside the lumbar spine. Gluteal pain invites a consideration of disorders of the hip or pelvis. Loin pain invites consideration of disorders of the urinary tract and other viscera.

The adjective *acute* serves to indicate pain of recent origin. In practice, this means pain that has started within recent hours or days. For taxonomic purposes, the IASP set an upper limit and defined acute pain as pain that has been present for no longer than 12 weeks.[1] A further refinement identifies subacute pain as pain that has been present for longer than 5 or 7 weeks but less than 12 weeks.[2] These distinctions are pertinent because the evidence on effective management differs for acute, subacute, and chronic low back pain.

REFERRED PAIN

The definition of lumbar spinal pain does not restrict the location of pain to the region of the lumbar spine. The emphasis is where the pain is primarily perceived or where it appears to start. However, lumbar spinal pain can spread to distant regions, in which case it is known as somatic referred pain.

Somatic referred pain is caused by convergence.[1,3] Second-order neurons in the spinal cord that receive afferent nerves from the lumbar spine also subtend afferent nerves from distant sites. In the absence of other, localizing information, the central nervous system cannot distinguish the exact source of input, whereupon spinal pain can be perceived as also arising from distant sites. The precise definition of somatic referred pain, therefore, becomes pain perceived in regions innervated by nerves other than those that innervate the actual source of pain (but which share the same central connections).

Experiments in human volunteers and studies in patients undergoing invasive tests or treatments have shown that somatic referred pain can be perceived in the gluteal region, groin, thigh, leg, and even as far as the foot.[4–11] The referred pain typically spreads as a continuous area extending from the back into the lower limb, but it can sometimes "skip" regions to become a remote island of pain (Fig. 72.2). The distinction between somatic referred pain and local pain in the lower limb is that referred pain is always concurrent with back pain. If the back pain ceases so does the referred pain. Conversely, when the back pain is more severe, the referred pain tends to spread further into the lower limb.[6]

Somatic referred pain is distinctly different from radicular pain, otherwise known in the lower limb as sciatica.[3] Somatic referred pain is perceived as a dull, aching sensation; it radiates slowly over relatively wide areas; it tends to be sessile, meaning that once it occupies a particular region; it tends to stay there, although perhaps waxing or waning in intensity. Patients can have difficulties identifying the boundaries of an area of somatic referred pain, but they can clearly identify its centroid or principal location. In contrast, radicular pain is lancinating in quality, like an electric shock, and travels into the lower limb along a narrow band (Fig. 72.3).[12]

CAUSES

The serious causes of back pain are those conditions that threaten the welfare of the patient if not recognized and treated. Variously, they are conditions that threaten the integrity of the spinal cord or cauda equina, can spread to become systemic, or can compromise circulatory homeostasis.

Extrinsic disorders are ones, which by way of hemorrhage or inflammation, can irritate the anterior surface of the lumbar spine, with or without actually penetrating the anterior muscles or vertebrae. Notable among them are aneurysms of the abdominal aorta[13,14] or aneurysms of retroperitoneal arteries such as the gastroduodenal artery.[15] Back pain may be a feature of visceral disorders, such as pancreatitis, that cause retroperitoneal inflammation, but in these disorders, back

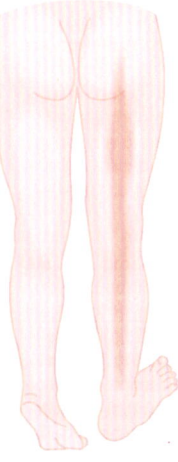

FIGURE 72.3 The pattern of radicular pain. Radicular pain is felt along a narrow band traveling into the lower limb.

pain is typically additional to abdominal pain. Aneurysms, however, can present with back pain as the sole symptom. Indeed, back pain has been the sole symptom of substantial proportions of patients who have died suddenly from ruptured aortic aneurysm.[16]

Serious intrinsic causes of back pain encompass fractures of the lumbar spine; primary tumors and metastases; and infections of the vertebrae, intervertebral disks, or paraspinal muscles. However, these causes of low back pain are rare. In primary care settings, fractures occur in between 1% and 4% of presentations, malignancy occurs in less than 0.2%, and infection in 0.01%.[17,18] Other serious causes are so rare that they have been described only in case reports, and their prevalence has not been estimated.

Although not serious in the sense of being life-threatening, nonetheless notable causes of back pain are the several seronegative spondylarthropathies, such as ankylosing spondylitis and Reiter's syndrome. These conditions need to be recognized because they require specialist rheumatology management.

For the remaining 96% to 99% of cases, the causes of acute low back pain are unknown. The principal reason for this is that conventional investigations, such as medical imaging, are not able to identify causes of back pain other than fractures, malignancy, or infection. So, when applied in mass surveys, they have not detected elusive sources of pain. However, such surveys have served to refute certain conditions as causes of back pain.

Spondylosis or degenerative changes, spondylolisthesis, and spondylolysis occur commonly in subjects without back pain, and their appearance on medical imaging is not related to low back pain to either a statistically significant or clinically significant extent. Therefore, none of these conditions is diagnostic of the cause of pain.[19]

Certain causes of back pain can be identified using invasive, diagnostic tests, but these are not indicated for acute low back pain and have not been systematically applied to samples of patients with acute low back pain in order to determine the cause of their pain. Their utility is limited to the investigation of chronic back pain (see Chapter 73). However, it should be understood that among patients with acute low back pain are ones whose pain will eventually become chronic. Therefore, the diagnosable causes of chronic back pain will be present among patients with acute low back pain. However, there is no imperative to diagnose these conditions while patients are in the acute phase. Investigations can be reserved until the patient approaches having chronic pain (see Chapter 73).

Management Algorithm

Because it will not be possible to make a diagnosis in the vast majority of patients with acute low back pain, their management cannot be based on finding and treating a particular cause of pain. Ultimately, their back pain, and any associated disabilities, will need to be treated as undiagnosed symptoms, using what is known to work. However, for that approach to be safe, the practitioner must be confident both that the patient does, indeed, have lumbar spinal pain and that he or she has not missed any serious causes of pain.

Figure 72.4 describes a suitable algorithm based on these principles. The algorithm starts with TRIAGE, which calls for consideration of extraneous and serious causes of back pain. The algorithm proceeds to MANAGEMENT but is promptly followed by CONCERN. Concern not only involves checking if the patient is responding or not to management but also introduces VIGILANCE. Vigilance means checking for the emergence of features of serious conditions that may not have been present or evident at the time of presentation. If a serious condition is not evident, management is resumed either

to REINFORCE previous interventions or to SUPPLEMENT these with additional measures if required. The algorithm continues in an anticlockwise spiral, until the patient exits the algorithm because he or she has recovered, because a serious condition has been detected, or because his or her pain has become chronic or threatens to do so, whereupon a new algorithm is followed.

An important feature of this algorithm is that it neither supposes nor expects that a practitioner will necessarily detect serious causes of acute back pain on the occasion of the first consultation. Indeed, for some conditions, it may not be biologically possible to do so. Some tumors and infections may not be detectable, clinically or on medical imaging, for several weeks after the onset of pain. For this reason, the algorithm emphasizes vigilance for the emergence of serious conditions. Conversely, the algorithm reminds practitioners to consider, and keep being alert to, serious conditions for the opposite of vigilance is negligence.

TRIAGE

Triage serves to check that the patient does indeed have back pain, that the pain is not a symptom of a vascular or visceral disorder, that the pain is likely to be of spinal origin, but that a serious cause is not responsible. Questions about these issues will not necessarily be answered in a single step. Rather, if a systematic approach to history and examination is taken, cues will emerge at various stages in the inquiry that will alert the practitioner to possibilities. These cues should be collected so that if sets of cues implicate a serious condition, the diagnosis of that condition can be pursed further. On the other hand, if cues are sought but do not arise, the practitioner can be confident that because of the absence of cues, a serious condition is unlikely. The discipline required, however, is that cues are looked for, and their absence is established by having looked for them and not by assuming that they will not be present because they are unlikely to be present.

A disciplined approach involves taking a comprehensive history thoroughly and can be assisted by reference to a "red flag" checklist (Fig. 72.5). A "red flag" is a clinical feature that alerts the practitioner to the possibility of a serious cause of pain and invites further consideration of that cause. Alone, a "red flag" is not meant to be diagnostic; it is only an alerting feature. Therefore, it is not surprising that individual "red flags" have poor positive predictive value.[22] The diagnosis of a serious cause of back pain requires other measures. A "red flag" serves only to invite consideration of applying those other measures.

The "red flag" checklist (see Fig. 72.5) is not based on the positive predictive value of "red flags." Rather, it was derived on the basis of case reports of conditions that were overlooked but could have been detected earlier if only the right questions were asked.[20,21] The "red flag" checklist therefore serves to remind practitioners not to overlook various, rare possibilities. In a large study, the checklist proved effective in detecting all serious conditions while missing none.[21]

The cardinal risk factors for fractures of the lumbar spine are trauma and the prolonged use of corticosteroids, particularly in the elderly.[17] Therefore, inquiry should be made about these factors, particularly in the elderly.

Asymptomatic stress fractures of the pars interarticularis are common in the general population, but among sportspeople, they are a likely cause of acute back pain. Therefore, participation in sport should be on the agenda in any inquiry of the patient's history.

Infections of the lumbar spine are often cryptic at onset; pain may be the only feature. Among the risk factors for infection is any reason for the patient to have an infection. This includes any history of a breach in the body's defense mechanisms, such a penetrating injury, a surgical or dental procedure,

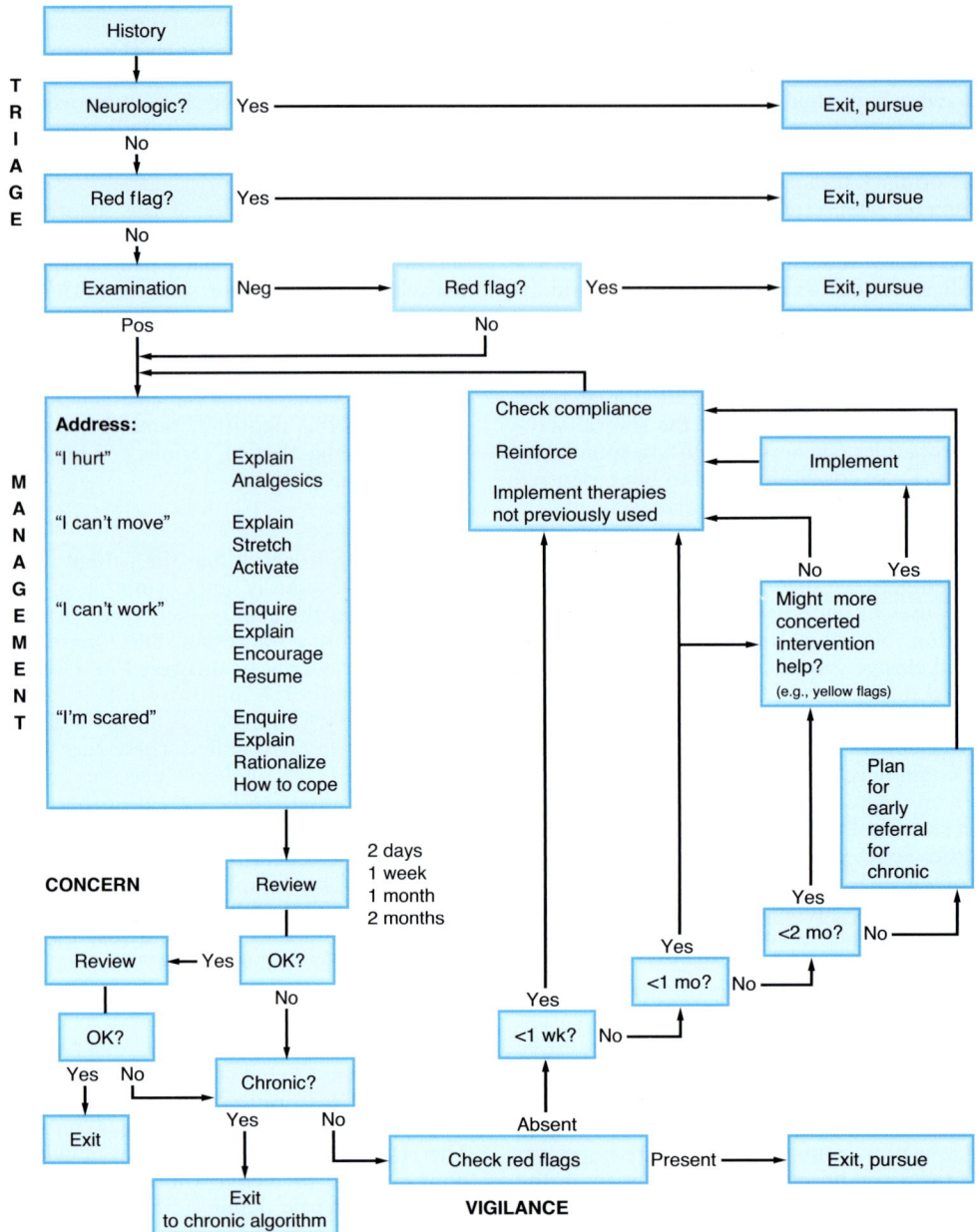

FIGURE 72.4 An algorithm for the management of acute low back pain.

tattooing, venipuncture, catheterization, skin lesions, immunosuppression, and diabetes mellitus. Otherwise, malaise and fever are strong alerting features to infection as a possible cause of back pain.

Unusual domains of inquiry pertain to hobbies, occupational exposure, and travel. These domains relate to the acquisition of unusual infections by fungi, parasites such as hydatid, and other exotic organisms. When these conditions have been missed in practice, it has not been for lack of clinical acumen but because elementary questions about exposure have not been asked. A particularly exotic example is exposure to spear grass (a plant found in Northern Australia), whose seed can burrow into tissues using an osmotically driven corkscrew action. In an unpublished case, a patient suffered unremitting pain, due to a seed buried in the patient's spine, whose diagnosis was delayed because no one asked about exotic exposures.

A past history of cancer and weight loss are the cardinal features of malignancy affecting the lumbar spine that is not yet producing other features.[17] Otherwise, the checklist (see Fig. 72.5) reminds practitioners to undertake a systems review

for associated features. These are elaborated in the following text under the "Medical History" section.

Medical History

Eliciting the medical history systematically is the cardinal tool for triage. Taking a history serves not only to check for serious conditions but also to help the practitioner understand subjective aspects of the patient's condition and helps develop the rapport to forge the doctor–patient relationship that is essential for effective medical care.[23]

A comprehensive history can be elicited systematically by pursuing an inquiry strategy in several domains that, generically, are pertinent to any pain problem (Table 72.1). For acute low back pain, some of these domains are rarely relevant, but several are pivotal.

The extent to which each domain of history is explored will depend on the practitioner's role in the patient's management. Physicians will need to elicit a more detailed history because they are expected to identify any "red flag" conditions, they will be responsible for ordering any special investigations that

Name:			LOW BACK PAIN		
Date of birth:			Medical Record No.		
History of:			**Cardiovascular**			**Endocrine**		
Trauma	Y	N	Risk factors?	Y	N	Diabetes?	Y	N
Sports injury	Y	N	**Respiratory**			Corticosteroids?	Y	N
Fever, night sweats	Y	N	Cough?	Y	N	Parathyroid	Y	N
Recent surgery	Y	N	**Urinary**			**Musculoskeletal**		
Catheterization	Y	N	Infection?	Y	N	Pain elsewhere?	Y	N
Venipuncture	Y	N	Hematuria?	Y	N	**Neurologic**		
Illicit drug use	Y	N	Retention?	Y	N	Symptoms/signs?	Y	N
Weight loss	Y	N	Stream problems?	Y	N	**Skin**		
Past history of cancer	Y	N	**Reproductive**			Infection?	Y	N
Occupational exposure	Y	N	Menstrual?	Y	N	Rashes?	Y	N
Hobby exposure	Y	N	**Hemopoietic**			**GIT**		
(Overseas) travel	Y	N	Problems?	Y	N	Diarrhea?	Y	N
Comments:				**Signature**	
				Date:	

FIGURE 72.5 A checklist for "red flag" clinical indicators, suitable for inclusion in medical records used in general practice, based on Bogduk and McGuirk[20] and McGuirk et al.[21]

might be required, and they will have responsibility for the longer term management of those patients whose pain persists. In such cases, the history elicited initially will be useful for monitoring the progress of the condition and the development of any of its features.

TABLE 72.1 Domains of Inquiry for the Systemic History of Any Pain Problem

Site
Distribution
Duration of illness
Quality
Intensity
Frequency
Periodicity
Time of onset
Mode of onset
Precipitating factors
Aggravating factors
Relieving factors
Associated features

A paramedical practitioner will not need to elicit such a detailed history if he or she is working in cooperation with, and on referral from, a physician who has assumed primary responsibility for the patient and who has already taken a comprehensive history. However, he or she should still address the basic features of history and any cues alerting to a "red flag" condition and any other aspect of the history that pertains to his or her role in the management of the acute condition. A paramedical practitioner acting as the sole health care provider inherits the responsibility for taking a comprehensive history and the responsibility for alerting the appropriate medical practitioner if a "red flag" condition is suspected.

Site

Establishing the site of pain is fundamental to assessment. Although the patient might report pain in the back, the actual location of pain may not accord with the definition of lumbar spinal pain. Pain in the loin, or pain in the buttock, are not back pain and invite a different algorithm for assessment.

Likewise, radicular pain is not back pain. Although its cause may lie in the lumbar spine, radicular pain is perceived in the lower limb, not in the back. Its assessment requires a different algorithm (see Chapter 70).

If a patient with back pain also has pain in the abdomen or pelvis, the latter takes priority. The patient should be assessed for visceral or vascular disease before back pain is the focus of attention.

Distribution

A patient with back pain may also have somatic referred pain. The distribution of referred pain does not help in the diagnosis of the source of pain for the patterns of referral are related to the segmental innervation of the source, not to the specific source itself. However, the distribution of referred pain is one factor that helps distinguish somatic referred pain from radicular pain. Of all the things that have been revealed by research over the last 70 years, this distinction still seems to have failed to permeate education on back pain.[3]

Somatic referred pain tends to spread over broad areas. The patient usually finds it difficult to identify the boundaries of where it is felt, but he or she can indicate its centroid. Once established, somatic referred pain is sessile in nature; although the area in which it is felt may fluctuate in size with the intensity of the pain, the center of its location tends to be fixed. In contrast, radicular pain is typically perceived along a narrow band that travels longitudinally into the lower limb (see Fig. 72.3). Other distinguishing features relate to the quality of pain.

Duration of Illness

It is pertinent to confirm that the patient has acute low back pain, and not recurrent or chronic pain, for the evidence pertaining to management and treatment is quite different for each of these conditions. The present algorithm pertains to acute low back pain. So, the practitioner should confirm that the pain has been present for less than 12 weeks. If the pain is subacute, its initial management will not be different from that of acute pain, but different options for treatment may later apply.

Quality

Determining the quality of pain is perhaps the most difficult domain of inquiry for patients with back pain. Patients often find it difficult to describe the quality of their pains and may default to describing their impacts using words like *severe* or *horrible*. In such a case, the practitioner should explain that intensity is a different feature that will be assessed separately (see the following text) and should steer the patient back to considering the quality. The practitioner should not prompt the patient with suggestions as that may lead to unreliable recording of the quality.

Somatic low back pain and somatic referred pain tend to be dull and aching in quality; in some instances, the pain feels like an expanding pressure. If patients can find such words to describe the quality of their pain, it serves to corroborate a somatic source of the pain.

Radicular pain is lancinating, shooting, or electric in quality. Although not diagnostic of the source or cause of pain, these features distinguish radicular pain from somatic referred pain.[3] Making this distinction is pivotal to the efficient and effective management of patients with somatic referred pain. It protects them from mistakenly undergoing investigations in the pursuit of disk herniations or other causes of neuropathy. It protects them from undergoing presumptive treatment for radicular pain, such as epidural steroids, which do not work for back pain or somatic referred pain.

Intensity

Intensity of pain means its magnitude as measured on a valid scale. A seminal article stated that if pain is not measured initially, it cannot later be said to have been relieved.[24]

A patient can provide a measure of the intensity of his or her pain by using a validated instrument such as a Visual Analog Scale[25,26] or a Numerical Pain Rating Scale.[26,27] High scores, however, are difficult to interpret in a valid manner. Although they might indicate severe pain because of serious pathology, high scores may be no more than an indication that the patients feel that they are suffering because of the pain's impact, even though the cause of their pain may not be serious. Other features help to indicate if the patient has a serious cause for severe pain (see "Associated Features" section in the following text).

The particular relevance of establishing the intensity of pain is that it is a relative risk factor for poor outcome.[28] Patients with pain of high intensity may require more concerted management regardless of whether the reason for high intensity is physiologic or psychological.

Periodicity

Periodicity is a domain of inquiry that is not relevant to back pain. It pertains more to visceral disorders and headache, in which pain can occur in bouts with regular frequency during a day or during a month. It is nevertheless mentioned here in the interests of complying with a generic, systematic approach to taking a history for any pain.

Time of Onset

Time of onset pertains to when pain that is not constant actually starts. That may be at a particular time each day or a particular day in a given week or given month. This domain of inquiry is more pertinent for certain types of headache or for visceral pain, which may be cyclical, but it is not irrelevant for back pain. Characteristic, and almost pathognomonic, of ankylosing spondylitis is early morning stiffness. In this context, regardless of whether or not patients distinguish back stiffness from back pain or conflate the two, the key feature is that the symptom is perceived in the morning.

Mode of Onset

The mode of onset means the manner in which pain commences: for example, suddenly or gradually. Pain of sudden onset invites exploration of any event (such as an accident) associated with the onset. The magnitude and directions of forces involved may provide clues to the structure(s) likely to have been injured. A sudden onset of severe pain, for no obvious reason, is not diagnostic of any cause but constitutes an alerting feature to possible serious causes. When the onset of back pain has been gradual, or otherwise unremarkable, there is little relevance to this variable.

Precipitating Factors

Precipitating factors are events, activities, or movements that brought on the original onset of pain or that trigger episodes of intermittent pain. A history of significant trauma is an alerting feature to fracture being the cause of pain, but otherwise particular precipitating factors have no bearing on the cause of pain. However, inquiry into precipitating factors becomes relevant to understanding how the patient may be disabled for undertaking work, domestic, or other physical activities.

Aggravating Factors

Aggravating factors are activities, movements, or postures that worsen the intensity of pain. These factors are of little value for diagnostic purposes because regardless of its cause, back pain is typically aggravated by movement of the spine or by sustained postures. More informative—and alerting—is low back pain that is not aggravated by particular postures or movements. That suggests a source which is not subject to compression loading in the lumbar spine or tension in its joints and ligaments. Visceral and vascular disorders have this property, as can malignancy until it starts to affect spinal joints.

Relieving Factors

Relieving factors are those that things that lessen the intensity of pain and/or that decrease the frequency of episodic pain.

They are the complement to aggravating factors. Pain that is not relieved by rest should invite a concerted consideration of possible, sinister causes.

Associated Features

The domain of associated features is the most critical and revealing domain of inquiry about low back pain. Serious causes of pain will usually be evident through the features that they produce, other than pain. Conversely, case reports that describe missed diagnoses often show that the diagnosis could have been made earlier if only a thorough inquiry about associated features had been conducted earlier. Inquiry into associated features is prompted by the second and third columns of the "red flag" checklist (see Table 72.1).

Risk factors for cardiovascular disease constitute alerting features to aortic aneurysm in the differential diagnosis of back pain. These include a family history of cardiovascular disease, high cholesterol, hypertension, older age, and smoking. The risk is amplified by a history of cerebrovascular disease, ischemic heart disease, or peripheral vascular disease.[13]

The lung is one of several sites of primary tumors that metastasize to the spine, but there are few clinical features of early lung cancer. Asking about respiratory problems, and cough in particular, as well as smoking as a risk factor, serves to remind practitioners about the possibility of lung metastases.

Inquiry about urinary function is indicated for a variety of reasons. The urinary tract may be a source of infection. Prostatic cancer may cause problems with urinary stream or voiding. Spinal tumors can affect the sacral nerves and thereby cause problems with bladder continence. Urethritis, especially if concurrent with uveitis, is pathognomonic of Reiter's syndrome.

Similar considerations apply to the reproductive system, which includes the breast in females, because the breast, ovary, and testis can be sources of metastases to the spine. However, primary tumors in the reproductive system will not be detected by history unless they happen to produce associated features.

Even more cryptic are disorders of the hematopoietic system. These may be impossible to detect clinically, but the oncology literature is replete with case reports of patients, with a history of neoplastic blood diseases, presenting with back pain.[29-33]

The endocrine system harbors several possible causes or risk factors for back pain. These include thyroid cancer as a source of spinal metastases, diabetes mellitus as a risk factor for spinal infection, and osteoporosis either primary or caused by corticosteroids as a cause of pathologic fracture. Osteitis fibrosa cystica, caused by hyperparathyroidism, can be a cause of spinal pain with no other features.

The musculoskeletal system should be assessed in order to determine if back pain is but one manifestation of a systemic disease such as rheumatoid arthritis or polymyalgia rheumatica. These conditions are declared by pain in the appendicular skeleton, and the condition is no longer one of isolated back pain.

The presence of neurologic features is a game changer. The diagnostic pursuit of numbness, weakness, or disturbed control of the bladder or bowel immediately takes precedence over the assessment of back pain. If the cause of back pain is not revealed on finding the cause of the neurologic features, the assessment of back pain can be resumed once the neurologic disorder has been diagnosed and stabilized.

Inquiry about skin lesion is relevant on two counts. Superficial infections could be the source of spinal infections. Otherwise, skin lesions are among the features of seronegative spondylarthropathies. Likewise, disturbed gastrointestinal function can be a feature of bowel cancer, which can metastasize to the spine, or be a feature of seronegative spondylarthropathies.

Psychological and Social History

To complete a comprehensive medical history, the practitioner should explore relevant aspects of the patient's affect and his or her social situation. Sensitive appraisal of these aspects can enhance rapport which is so important to the doctor–patient relationship and help the practitioner develop empathy.

One psychological feature of particular relevance in acute low back pain is fear. Patients with back pain may be scared of its possible association with serious pathology; they may be scared of making the pain worse by what they do; they may be scared of what they think may be its prognosis. Other psychological features of relevance in acute low back pain are anxiety and depression caused by what the patient thinks the implications of the pain might be. These features need to be identified because they are as much a part of the presenting complain as the back pain itself. If the back pain cannot be promptly stopped, fears will need to be managed, along with the back pain, because persistent fears or misapprehensions can impede the patient's rehabilitation.

Social features of relevance include the patient's home situation and the degree of support he or she has from family members, friends, and his or her employer. Delving gently into the effects of the pain on the patient's home relationships, on his or her work, and on his or her leisure interests helps the practitioner understand the interplay of disability and handicap in each area of the patient's life.

Physical Examination

Examination of the lumbar spine has traditionally involved inspection, palpation, and movement testing, or as described in an aphorism by Apley "look, feel, move."[34] There is very little evidence of the validity of physical signs detected by examination of the lumbar spine.[34,35] So, arguably, there is not much point in going through the process. Nevertheless, there are two reasons for conducting a physical examination. In the first instance, patients expect to be examined, and performing an examination is an indication that the physician is interested in the patient and concerned about them. The fact that nothing found on examination is diagnostic is immaterial in this context. The second reason is ironic. Of greater significance than finding positive features on examination is finding no physical features in the lumbar spine. Absence of somatic signs prompts a serious consideration of visceral and vascular causes of low back pain. A pertinent aphorism is if patients have no signs in their back, turn them over and examine their abdomen and pelvis.

Inspection

Physical signs detectable by visual inspection of the patient include general and specific features. General observations are static posture both standing and sitting (for signs of scoliosis, kyphosis and loss of lordosis), dynamic posture when walking (for antalgic gait), and bodily deformity. Specific observations include scars, puncture marks, swelling, and other local changes of shape.

Palpation

Physical signs detectable by palpation include altered sensitivity (hypoesthesia or hyperesthesia), relationships of bony landmarks, and tenderness. If tenderness is present, it may be diffuse or focal, and if focal, the practitioner may note its relationship to bony landmarks such as spinous processes.

Movement Testing

Movement testing may include assessing active, passive, and accessory ranges of movement. Active and passive ranges of thoracolumbar movement can be tested in the three basic planes of the body: flexion and extension in the sagittal plane, left and right side bending in the frontal plane, and left and right rotation in the transverse plane. If appropriate, movements can be tested in combinations of those ranges such as "quadrant extension" (extension with rotation, as in looking backward over the shoulder).

Some craft groups contend that the accessory ranges of passive intervertebral motion can and should be tested. The evidence from the available literature indicates that conventional, physical examination procedures lack reliability, validity, or both.[35] Nothing found by various maneuvers or tests of the accessory ranges of spinal movement reliably implicates any source of cause of pain with any validity.

The exception to this may be spinal assessment by the McKenzie method. Two studies have shown that careful, specialized examination can identify patients with sacroiliac joint pain[36] and patients with internal disk disruption.[37] These studies, however, were based on patients with chronic low back pain, in whom these two conditions are common. Their prevalence in patients with acute low back pain is not known, and therefore, the validity of McKenzie assessment in these patients has not been established.

Other Examination

Although classical teaching prescribes a neurologic examination for patients with low back pain, it is neither warranted nor justified. If a patient reports a history of neurologic symptoms, such as weakness or numbness, a neurologic examination becomes mandatory, but in that context, the indications for neurologic examination are the neurologic symptoms—not the back pain. Neurologic diseases do not present with back pain as the only feature. In patients with back pain as the sole feature, physicians might elect to perform a neurologic examination in order to appear thorough, but they should be under no illusion that it serves to establish a diagnosis. This guideline should not be confused with neurologic examination in a patient with radicular pain. Neurologic examination is, indeed, indicated if the patient has radiculopathy, but in that context, it is pain in the leg—not pain in the back—that is the indication for neurologic examination.

Given the possibility of vascular and visceral disorders, examination of the abdomen is pertinent in the initial assessment of a patient with acute low back pain. This includes auscultation for bruits and checking for hypotension, both of which are signs of aortic aneurysm.[13]

A component of physical examination that has not been formally studied pertains to the demeanor of the patient. This can be helpful in identifying patients with serious causes of pain. Patients with infections and cancer are typically serious, subdued, or quietly guarded in their presentation. They avoid movement and are apprehensive about being examined. Their general demeanor is grim—as if, intuitively, they know that something serious is wrong. That appearance is distinctly not histrionic. Although they may rate their pain as severe, they do not incessantly draw attention to it. Beware the quiet patient with severe pain.

Ancillary Investigations

Much evidence from research has overturned past habits of routine investigations for acute low back pain. Imaging investigations, such as plain radiography, computed tomography (CT) scanning, or magnetic resonance imaging (MRI), are not justified either "just in case" or to reveal something that is not evident on history. The same may be said for blood tests such as erythrocyte sedimentation rate (ESR), C-reactive protein (CRP), alkaline phosphatase, serum calcium, and (especially) human leukocyte antigen (HLA) B27. In the absence of specific clinical indicators, the yield of these investigations is zero or close to it.

Further investigations should be pursued only if triggered by an alerting "red flag" feature, and in that event, the investigations should be tailored to the particular entity of concern. For that purpose, Table 72.2 lists various options for first- and second-line investigations for particular suspected pathologies. In some instances, laboratory investigations precede imaging.

Plain radiography lacks sensitivity and specificity for any cause of back pain other than fractures. It is indicated only to those patients who have risk factors for fracture (see Table 72.2).

Neither CT nor MRI has ever been shown to demonstrate a cause of back pain in patients with no clinical indicators

TABLE 72.2 Clinical Indicators and Preferred Investigations for Possible Serious Causes of Spinal Pain			
Suspected Pathology	**Clinical Indicators**		**Preferred Test**
Fracture	Severe trauma	First line	X-ray
Stress fracture	Sporting activity involving spinal extension, rotation, or both	First line	Bone scan or MRI
		Second line	X-ray
Pathologic fracture	Osteoporosis	First line	X-ray
	Prolonged use of corticosteroids	Second line	MRI
	Past history of cancer		
Infection	Fever, sweating	First line	ESR, FBC, CRP
	Risk factors for infection (invasive medical procedure, injection, illicit drug use, trauma to skin or mucous membrane, immunosuppression, diabetes mellitus, alcoholism)	Second line	MRI
Tumor	Past history of malignancy	All cases	1: ESR, CRP
	Age greater than 50 years	First line	2: MRI
	Failure to improve	Second line	
	Weight loss	Prostate	PSA
	Pain not relieved by rest	Myeloma	IEPG, serum protein electrophoresis
Aortic aneurysm	Cardiovascular risk factors	First line	ultrasound
Other aneurysm	Anticoagulants	Second line	CT, MRI
	No musculoskeletal signs		
	Hypotension		
	Palpable mass		
	Bruits		

CRP, C-reactive protein; CT, computed tomography; ESR, erythrocyte sedimentation rate; FBC, full blood count; IEPG, immunoelectrophoretogram; MRI, magnetic resonance imaging; PSA, prostate specific antigen.

of fracture, infection, or cancer or in the absence of neurologic signs. In that regard, the use of CT or MRI in patients with back pain should not be confused with its use in patients with radicular pain or with neurologic signs. In those conditions, it is the neurologic features that are the indication for investigation—not the back pain.

Apart from not being diagnostic, medical imaging has the liability of needlessly alarming patients. To the uninformed patient, the vocabulary of radiology reports sounds serious and significant. Terms such as *spondylosis*, *spondylolisthesis*, and *degenerative changes* sound like the patient has a disease that both explains his or her pain and requires treatment. Yet, the evidence shows that these conditions are not related to pain.[19] Moreover, applying these false and alarming labels is associated with worse prognosis.[38]

Nor is it an argument that patients expect imaging. They do so only when they remain uninformed. A controlled study has shown that 5 minutes of explanation deters most patients from wanting unnecessary radiographs.[39] The arguments against imaging include their lack of sensitivity and specificity, the very low likelihood of finding anything, the possibility of false-positive findings and the distress that they can cause, the possible false sense of security from a negative result, and the health hazards of radiation exposure.

Studies have shown that imaging did not detect an occult cancer if patients were under 50 years, had no history of cancer, with no weight loss, and no signs of systemic illness.[40,41] In patients over the age of 50 years, or with unexplained weight loss, or with signs of systemic illness, imaging did not detect cancer if their ESR was less than 20 mm per hour. Therefore, for suspected cancer, the indications for imaging are either a past history of cancer or a raised ESR. The appropriate imaging is either bone scan or MRI. Both are equally sensitive, but MRI has greater specificity.

In sportspeople in whom a stress fracture is suspected, the imperative is to detect a stress reaction before actual fracture. Doing so allows the pars interarticularis to be protected from further stress and allowed to heal. Once fractures occur, there is no guarantee that they will unite. Bone scan has been the traditional investigation, but it lacks specificity; it cannot distinguish between a stress reaction and an actual fracture. MRI can detect and distinguish both and should be the preferred investigation.

Formulation

After taking a comprehensive history, performing an examination, and reviewing any previous investigations, a practitioner will have noted any alerting "red flags," and appropriate further investigations will have confirmed a serious cause for back pain or excluded it for the time being. Conversely, if none of the "red flags" on the "red flag" checklist are present, the practitioner can be confident that there is no serious cause of pain currently detectable. However, the practitioner must nonetheless remain vigilant for any change in symptoms or new symptoms that might herald the manifestation of a serious condition. That includes instructing the patient to report immediately any such change in symptoms.

Having excluded serious causes, for the time being, the practitioner can formulate an assessment based on the information gathered from history and examination. For purposes of forthcoming management that formulation would encompass the location and extent of pain, its intensity, any fears or beliefs that the patient may have about the pain, and the disabilities that either the pain or fears are producing. Each of these becomes a target of management. The formulation will not be an attempt at diagnosis of the specific source and cause of the pain; that is inappropriate in the acute phase.

INITIAL MANAGEMENT

All contemporary practice guidelines recommend that the first line of care for all patients with acute low back pain should be explanation, reassurance, encouragement to continue physical activity, and supporting the patient to take responsibility for his or her own rehabilitation.[42–46]

Practice guidelines hold in reserve certain second-line interventions, but their effectiveness is either questionable or small. Therefore, it is imperative that first-line interventions be as effective as possible. Fortunately, medical management based on these first-line recommendations has been found to be effective in field trials.[21,47,48]

The precepts of good medical management of a patient with acute low back pain can be encapsulated by the patient's cardinal complaints: "I hurt; I can't move; I can't work; and I'm scared."[49,50] For effective management, all these issues need to be addressed.

Pain

Modalities used in the management of acute low back pain include patient education, medication, physical therapies, and activation. Of these, the only ones well supported by evidence are patient education and activation, and they are the mainstays of caring for patients with acute low back pain.

Patient Education

Effective patient education has two elements: explanation and information. The practitioner should provide explanation of the pain and information about the good prognosis based on the favorable natural history. These elements should be delivered with a good dose of reassurance.

Explanation is the foremost tool for the management of acute low back pain. It has two aspects: what the patient does not have and what the patient does have.

The practitioner should explain to patients that the chances of a serious cause are extremely low and are even lower because of their negative responses to the "red flag" checklist. If pressed, the practitioner can explain why there is no need for any special investigations. If patients ask about x-rays, the practitioner should take the time to explain why they are not indicated and what the health risks of x-rays are.

Lumbar spine radiographs may be false-negative in up to 41% of patients with known vertebral cancer.[51] Osteomyelitis does not appear before 2 to 8 weeks of evolution of the disease; a normal radiologic picture does not exclude the diagnosis of spinal infection.[52] A lumbar spine series delivers 40 times the radiation dose received from a chest x-ray[51,53] and delivers to the gonads a radiation dose equivalent to that from having a daily chest radiographs for 6 years.[51,54–56] Explaining this to patients constitutes evidence-based practice.

Once the "red flag" issues have been covered, the practitioner should provide a calm and clear explanation of why the patient has pain. It does not matter if this explanation is not biologically valid; it simply has to indicate to the patient that the practitioner does know what is going on. In this regard, it is not so much what the practitioner says that is important but the manner in which they say it. Providing a confident explanation is the opposite of appearing uncertain, or alarmed, about what the problem might be. Providing such an explanation is the opposite of panicking and pursuing unnecessary investigations that alarm the patients and reinforce their fears that something serious is wrong.

Individual practitioners may develop their own pattern, in offering an explanation. One that has been tested[47,48] is to explain to patients, in simple terms, that they have internal disk disruption: a small injury that is presently inflamed and sore but which will settle.[47] Depending on the situation, practitioners might prefer an alternative model that does not

TABLE 72.3	The Eight C's that Define the Attributes of Good Explanation of a Patient's Acute Low Back Pain
Calm	
Clear	
Credible	
Confident	
Convincing	
Concerted	
Caring	
Concern	

nominate a specific diagnosis that may later prove wrong. They might care to explain to patients that they have strained their back muscles or that their muscles are sore because they have been undertaking activities in an inefficient manner.

Whatever the model used, the art of explanation can be encapsulated by the eight C's (Table 72.3). The explanation should be **calm** (delivered in such a way as to allay anxiety), **clear** (expressed in terms the patient can readily understand), and **credible** (fitting the patient's circumstances and intelligible to him or her). The practitioner's manner in presenting the explanation should be **confident** (precluding uncertainty which breeds doubts in the patient's mind), **convincing** (which requires monitoring the patient's response to the explanation and addressing any uncertainties), and **concerted** (which means the practitioner should show he or she is trying hard to help the patient). Throughout the explanation, the practitioner should show that he or she **cares** about the patient and his or her complaint and have **concern** (which does not mean alarm about possible, serious causes of pain; it is related to caring, taking the patient seriously). All of these attributes amount to the opposite of being fast, perfunctory, and dismissive.

Explanation is reinforced by the second tool at the disposal of the practitioner: information. This involves informing the patient of the evidence on the natural history of acute low back pain. Provided that patients are managed properly, the natural history is very favorable. Some 80% can be expected to recover fully, if managed well.[21] Explaining this fact constitutes evidence-based practice. The practitioner should explain to the patient, in terms that the patient will understand, that the odds are in his or her favor and that there is every chance of recovering (even regardless of treatment), but that it may take time. During that time, there are certain measures that both the practitioner and the patient can take to ease the situation while this recovery takes place.

The evidence for this approach is strong. A systematic review found 24 studies, of which 14 (58%) were of high quality, and showed that patient education is effective for the management of patients with acute or subacute low back pain.[57]

Some guidelines recommend issuing the patient with an educational booklet about back pain. This might serve to standardize information provided, and practitioners might consider it an aid in their endeavors, but booklets have little effect when used alone.[58,59] They are not a substitute for explanation, support, and encouragement provided personally by a practitioner following the eight C's (see Table 72.3).

Medication

Medications have no proven place in the management of acute low back pain. Paracetamol (acetaminophen), at a dose of 4 g per day, is no better than placebo for relieving acute low back pain, in either the short term or long term.[60] Nonsteroidal anti-inflammatory drugs (NSAIDs) are statistically more effective, on average, than placebo but barely so.[61,62] Their superiority over placebo is less than the minimally important clinical change for back pain.[52] Meanwhile, the risk of harm, from the side effects of NSAIDs, outweighs any trivial effect that they have on pain.

An earlier Cochrane review recommended that muscle relaxants be used with caution because of their side effects.[63] More recent reviews found that muscle relaxants were more effective than placebo but only in the short term, that is, over a matter of days,[62,64] and that they had a significantly higher risk of harm from side effects.[62] However, a recent series of controlled trials have shown that adding orphenadrine or methocarbamol,[65] or diazepam,[66] or cyclobenzaprine[67] did not improve outcomes for pain or function achieved by treatment with naproxen alone. Benzodiazepines have been shown to be no more effective than placebo.[62]

There is no published evidence that antidepressants[45,62] or antiseizure drugs[45,62] are effective for acute low back pain. Nor is there evidence that opioids are effective.[45,62] The use of these agents for acute low back pain lacks any evidence base.

Superficial Heat

Instead of drugs, an expedient and effective alternative for the short-term relief of acute low back pain is superficial heat, in the form of low-level heat wrap therapy. Applying heat to the back has been shown to be more effective than placebo, both in general patients[68–71] and in workers with back pain,[72] and is more effective than either ibuprofen or paracetamol (acetaminophen).[73] It has been rated as a cost-effective intervention.[74]

Physical Therapies

Evidence is not lacking on the effectiveness of physical therapies commonly used to treat acute low back pain. The available evidence shows either that these therapies provide relief of pain to no greater degree than does sham therapy or that any superiority over sham treatments is small in magnitude and clinically insignificant.[75]

For the relief of pain, exercises are no more effective than no exercises.[75] When exercise therapy has been compared with other therapies, the evidence is inconsistent as to which is better if at all.[75] Manipulative therapy is not more effective than either inactive treatments (such as education pamphlets) or active treatments such as exercise.[75–77] Two trials of acupuncture showed inconsistent effects, and two trials showed reduction of pain by an average of 9 points out of 100, compared with sham therapy,[75] but the minimal clinically important change for back pain is greater than 20/100. Meanwhile, five trials show no clear effects on function, which is the cardinal problem for patients with acute low back pain.[75] Massage may provide short-lasting but small benefits greater than those of sham therapy or other, active therapies.[45,75]

Other interventions, commonly used in the past, for the relief of acute low back pain, either lack formal evidence of efficacy or have been shown to be ineffective. They should be avoided not only because they are ineffective but also because they conflict with the precept of empowering the patient to become responsible for his or her own rehabilitation. In this category are application of cold,[68,78] therapeutic ultrasound,[79] low-level laser,[80] bed rest,[81] lumbar supports,[82] traction,[83] transcutaneous electrical nerve stimulation,[84] and back school.[85]

Multidisciplinary pain management has explicitly been shown to be not effective for acute low back pain,[86] so it is not indicated early in the course of management. For subacute back pain, a systematic review found low-quality evidence that multidisciplinary rehabilitation might improve pain and function more than does usual care but not more than do other interventions, such as light mobilization, graded activity, a brief clinical intervention including education and advice on exercise, and psychological counseling.[87]

Activation

Multiple studies and reviews have consistently shown that maintaining activity is a crucial component in the management of acute low back pain.[21,47,88] The emphasis lies not in treating a particular pathology but in resuming or maintaining activity, in a holistic sense, in order to prevent the patient being disabled by his or her pain. The intervention should be combined with explanation, information, reassurance, and encouragement in empowering the patient to take responsibility for his or her own management.

The practitioner should explain to the patient that the evidence shows that those who resume activities have a much more favorable prognosis: They recover more quickly and more thoroughly than patients who resort to rest and avoidance of activities.[88] A model of explanation that has successfully been used is to explain that muscle tightness is a normal reaction to pain but one that can be deleterious; allowing the back to seize up or become stiff not only interferes with movement but can also add to the pain.[47] The objective of treatment, therefore, is to prevent and overcome stiffness.

This can be achieved by teaching the patient a set of simple stretching exercises.[89] These are not exercises that require supervision or attendance at a facility, such as a physiotherapy practice or gymnasium. They are exercises that can, and should, be executed virtually anywhere that the patient needs them. In order to reduce stiffness and keep the patient mobile, the patient should perform the exercises at strategic times of the day, such as upon rising, before going to work, at coffee breaks, or lunchtime. In the sense of a "warm-up," they can be applied as a preparatory and preventive measure prior to undertaking a major activity, such as commencing chores. As a first-aid measure, they can be applied to ease exacerbations of pain, after sustained activity or after prolonged sitting. Providing a first-aid measure is one of the crucial steps in empowering the patient to be able to look after themselves. Exercises that the patient can do by themselves, and for themselves, are crucial to avoiding passive interventions and becoming dependent on them.

Work

All guidelines on occupational low back pain emphasize the benefits of returning to work or remaining at work.[90–92] Patients who do so inherit a better prognosis than those who do not.

The obstructing factor in this context lies not in the patient but in the attitude of the treating practitioner. It is easier, and faster, to write a certificate for time off work than to explain to the patient why they do not need one.[93] What is difficult is to change the attitudes of practitioners. Changing patients is far less of a problem.

The practitioner should share with the worker the evidence of the benefits of returning to work. They should inquire as to why the patient feels or believes that he or she cannot return to work.

Fears of aggravating the pain will already have been partly addressed by confidently providing a credible explanation for the pain, coupled with an explanation that activity will not do harm. That message is reinforced by helping the patient resume movements and empowering them to do so. Those movements include work.

Some patients may have pain of high intensity that temporarily impedes their ability and capacity to resume their accustomed work. For such patients, modified work duties may be required. Unfortunately, there is no evidence, in the form of controlled trials, that vindicates the prescription of modified duties. Their reputation rests on anecdotal and observational data. The strongest evidence lies in a cohort study, which found that keeping patients at work, with modified duties as required, resulted in a greater proportion of patients fully recovered, and fewer recurrences, than did usual care.[93]

Prescribing modified duties imposes a responsibility. The practitioner should not forget the patient. The objective of modified duties is to have the patients remain at work but progressively to restore their capacity for former duties. During this period, the patients and their progress need to be monitored. As soon as they are able, the patients should return to full work. A certificate and its expiry date do not magically achieve this. It is the continued involvement of the practitioner that does so.

Inquiry into the patient's beliefs about work may reveal extraneous but pertinent issues. They may resent their work environment or their supervisor. They may harbor fears about recurrences of accidents in which they were injured. Such issues raise agendas that are separate and additional to the back pain. Those agendas need to be pursued and managed parallel to the back pain itself.

In the first instance, the practitioner needs to elicit from the worker the beliefs and concerns that they have. Mistaken beliefs can be discussed and corrected. Misplaced concerns can be allayed. Otherwise, workplace intervention may be required. If the practitioner themselves cannot exercise this, the services of a skilled practitioner in occupational medicine should be recruited.

The evidence strongly supports the efficacy of workplace intervention. Whether as an isolated intervention, or adding it to medical management, workplace intervention improves outcomes.[94] It is conspicuous, however, that the contents of the workplace intervention are immaterial. The effective ingredient does not lie in the specifics of ergonomic or related changes. What counts is that the worker has an advocate who acts on his or her behalf and in his or her interests. This is done in the context of solving problems with the participation of supervisors and management. Solutions may lie in modifying the physical work environment, the social work environment, work flow, or work demands. The solution should be cast in a manner such as to benefit all parties. The worker returns to an improved environment. The employer avoids the problem of additional injuries and claims and the burden of increased insurance premiums. Advocacy is paramount in these negotiations. Workers typically do not have access to management, whom they may regard as intransigent and uncaring. The occupational physician has the appropriate "social rank" to appear before management and to explain the circumstances to them.

Workplace intervention takes time and requires a particular, skilled aptitude. General practitioners and others may not have this time or aptitude. That, however, is not a pretext for overlooking or neglecting workplace intervention. Persisting problems with return to work, in a practice or in a region, are an indication that specialist skills need to be recruited.

Fear

Fear is the most damaging characteristic that a patient with acute low back pain can harbor. Their fears might pertain to biologically, what is wrong; medically, what is going to be done; or socially, what is going to happen. Such fears inhibit the patient's recovery. It is important, therefore, that any such fears be discovered and addressed.

It is not necessary, nor expected, for a practitioner to address the fears that a patient might have at the first consultation. However, the possibility of fears should be noted and their exploration resumed at follow-up visits.

The practitioner can explore possible fears in the course of a normal consultation, either by being alert to what the patient might mention, or allude to, spontaneously, or they can check for fears through simple questions, such as what do you think is the cause of pain, what do you think needs to be done, and what do you think is going to happen.

Fears about the biology of back pain are covered by providing a credible, convincing explanation, reinforced by repetition if necessary. Fears about prognosis and consequences are covered by providing information to the patient about the favorable natural history of acute low back pain. Fears about management are covered by providing the patient with a concerted plan, which empowers them and does not leave them abandoned. Fears about work, employment, and future are encompassed by the workplace intervention.

If required, formal behavioral therapy can be of benefit. A systematic review found that for patients with acute low back pain, cognitive-behavioral therapy was effective for reducing fear-avoidance beliefs, although having no effect on pain or disability.[95]

REVIEW

An old medical myth is that if the patient does not return, he or she must be alright. This myth has been dispelled. A longitudinal study, in British primary care, followed patients after they presented to general practitioners with acute low back pain.[96] They did not return to the general practitioners, who possibly assumed that they had recovered. Research nurses found that only 25% of patients had recovered and the remainder continued to suffer, but they did not return to their general practitioner because they felt that they had not been helped.

Patients with acute low back pain should not be abandoned, and they should not feel abandoned. The risk of doing so is that patients will exaggerate and prolong their disability, if left to fend for themselves. The singular measure against this eventuality is planned concern.

The treating practitioner should schedule a follow-up of the patient. This might be a conventional consultation, or it might be no more than a telephone follow-up. If patients have recovered, and report that they do not need further care, no more need be done, but if patients have not recovered, face-to-face follow-up is indicated.

An algorithm with scheduled follow-up allows busy practitioners to divide their management into initial triage, at the first consultation, and further exploration, at subsequent consultation(s). This removes the perceived burden of having to get everything done on the first occasion.

If the patient is progressing well, further follow-up can be decreased or dispensed with. If they are not progressing, the review consultation provides the opportunity for the succeeding steps in the algorithm

VIGILANCE

Vigilance in this context means the practitioner keeping careful watch for any development in the patient's condition that may require intervention. This is most easily done in review consultations. Serious disorders may not be evident at the first consultation. Repeating the checklist for "red flags" serves to detect the emergence of any new features, which may require changes to the management plan. Relying on clinical monitoring, in this way, obviates the need for precipitous, and inappropriate, use of investigations at the first consultation.

If "red flag" features emerge, management appropriate for those features can be pursued. If "red flag" features do not emerge, the previous management can continue.

REINFORCEMENT

During the review consultation, the practitioner should assess the progress of the patient. If previous management appears to be working, no change is required. If progress to recovery seems to be slow, the practitioner should assess why this might be the case.

The practitioner should check if the patient understood the previous plan of management and if they are complying with it. The review consultation provides the opportunity to reinforce previous explanations, if they were not understood, and to check, for example, if the patient has been able to undertake an activation program correctly.

If the patient is not complying, the reasons for that need to be elicited. Misunderstandings can be corrected. If unjustified resistance is the reason, that raises an agenda in the management plan that is not back pain.

If progress is not occurring despite adequate compliance, consideration needs to be given to implementing interventions not previously used. If activation exercises were not prescribed at the first consultation, they can be introduced now. If the patient is having difficulties restoring movement, a supervised exercise program, conducted in a cognitive-behavioral milieu, can be effective.[97]

Yellow Flags

Slow progress to recovery may be due to undetected, or unrevealed, psychosocial factors, referred to as "yellow flag" indicators.[98] These pertain to the patient's beliefs and behaviors concerning physical activity and domestic, social, and vocational responsibilities.

When patients believe that physical activity might harm their back, and that they should not undertake activities that make their pain worse, they avoid activities. For most patients with acute low back pain, these beliefs are not justified. Explanation, reassurance, and encouragement to resume activities are the cardinal tools for overcoming these mistaken beliefs. If required, a graded plan of resuming activities can be developed and followed. Some patients may take longer to regain activities. The guiding principle is that increments should be pursued, even if they are small.

Patients may seek to avoid domestic activities and responsibilities, such as cooking, cleaning, maintenance, shopping, and housework, for fear of pain. Avoiding such activities amplifies their disability. Encouragement to resume these activities may be not enough to convince some patients. The accustomed manner in which they do things may not be efficient. They may need help to analyze how else they might acquit the required activity in a manner that does not aggravate their pain. The guiding principle is not to abandon the activity but to find alternative means to achieve its purpose. In this regard, the practitioner provides his or her own intellect to help solve the patient's problem.

Patients may avoid social activities, claiming that their back pain prevents them from doing so. But back pain does not directly preclude social activity. The mediating factor is fear that social activity will aggravate their pain. If the patients can regain movement at home, they can apply the same principles away from home. They should be helped to understand that becoming a recluse will not improve their prognosis; if anything, it will hinder their recovery. Encouragement should be coupled with suggestions of what to do if their pain threatens to be aggravated when they are "out." Instead of being an embarrassment, doing the stretching exercises can be turned into an asset.

If psychosocial problems prove insurmountable, they—rather than the back pain itself—become the paramount problem, and referral to a psychologist may be warranted. Trained psychologists are more likely to achieve better outcomes if they can see patients early in the development of problems.

Perhaps, the most destructive of the "yellow flags" is aversion to work. Patients may believe that work caused their pain, that work aggravates their pain, that work is too heavy for them, and that they should not work. Such beliefs require sensitive analysis and discussion. In the majority of cases, the patient's beliefs about work will not be valid. The practitioner cannot afford to be dismissive and assertive. They need to understand the patient's work and, in a compassionate manner, be able to indicate how work can be resumed in a safe manner. It may be helpful to engage the services of an occupational physician who is familiar with the patient's industry and can develop a return to work plan in the context of a workplace intervention.

Discussion

Acute low back pain is unlike other conditions encountered in primary care. A specific diagnosis is rarely possible. No treatment constitutes a quick fix. It is not a complaint that can be cured by writing a prescription, a referral, or a request for imaging.

Acute low back pain requires an unconventional approach. Because there is no specific treatment, its management relies on supporting the patient while natural history takes its course. If managed well, some 70% of patients can expect to recover, with recurrence rates as low as 16%.[21] Good outcomes can be obtained even in patients eligible for workers compensation claims.[93]

The imperative is to avoid nocebo effects. These arise if the practitioner is dismissive or trivializes the complaint, if they say "nothing is wrong" or "it's all in your head," or if they behave as if they do not know what is wrong or appear disinterested.

The opposite is achieved by being calm, clear, credible, confident, convincing, concerted, caring, and concerned. Patients recognize this and appreciate it as helpful. They rate their care as excellent, significantly more often those under usual care.[21]

Although this approach is consonant with contemporary practice guidelines, unfortunately, it has not been widely adopted. The reasons for this have not been explored. It may be that acute low back pain requires a unique aptitude and attitude. It may be that the effort required, particularly for patients with psychosocial dimensions to their complaint, requires unfamiliar or new skills. It may be that the recommended algorithm is incompatible with busy practice and the reimbursement that primary physicians attract. These, however, are ideologic, political, and socioeconomic matters. They are not scientific evidence that refutes what can be made to work in primary care.

The recommended algorithm does not provide a cure for all patients. Among patients with acute low back pain are ones destined (statistically) to develop chronic pain. If reiteration and reinforcement of simple interventions does not result in progress and resolution, patients at risk of becoming chronic should be identified before they do so. Appointments to pain clinics or spine specialists may take time to obtain, and they are easier to cancel than to obtain. Therefore, for patients with persistent pain, steps for early referral to appropriate resources become part of the closing phases of the algorithm for acute low back pain. The management of these patients follows a different algorithm, with a different evidence base (see Chapter 73).

Conclusion

The chances of a successful outcome for a patient with acute low back pain are governed largely by the natural history of the condition. Most patients with acute low back pain will recover spontaneously if simply left alone. There is no need for diagnostic interventions other than to pursue any suggestion of "red flag" conditions such as infection and neoplasm, but mercifully, they are rare. There is no need for therapeutic interventions other than those that provide symptomatic relief and even they are only required if the pain is very intense. What patients with acute low back pain need is a caring approach by practitioners who understand the relevant scientific evidence; reassurance that the pain will very likely, on the basis of the natural history, settle by spontaneous healing; and follow-up with vigilance by a practitioner keeping careful watch for any development in the patient's condition that may require intervention if the pain does not resolve.

The patient may have associated problems in other domains, the psychological and social phenomena that may coexist with low back pain, but those are secondary problems that generally will resolve when the pain settles. Caring practitioners will address, or have addressed, the psychological and social concomitants of pain if they impact on the patient sufficiently to warrant specific treatment but will never allow those issues to obscure the main aim of helping the patient cope with the pain until it goes away.

References

1. Merskey H, Bogduk N, eds. *Classification of Chronic Pain. Descriptions of Chronic Pain Syndromes and Definitions of Pain Terms.* 2nd ed. Seattle, WA: IASP Press; 1994.
2. King W. Acute, subacute and chronic pain. In: Schmidt RF, Willis WD Jr, eds. *Encyclopedic Reference of Pain.* Berlin: Springer; 2007:35–36.
3. Bogduk N. On the definitions and physiology of back pain, referred, pain and radicular pain. *Pain* 2009;147:17–19.
4. Kellgren JH. On the distribution of pain arising from deep somatic structures with charts of segmental pain areas. *Clin Sci* 1939;4:35–46.
5. Feinstein B, Langton JN, Jameson RM, et al. Experiments on pain referred from deep somatic tissues. *J Bone Joint Surg* 1954;35A:981–987.
6. Mooney V, Robertson J. The facet syndrome. *Clin Orthop* 1976;115:149–156.
7. Bogduk N. Lumbar dorsal ramus syndrome. *Med J Aust* 1980;2:537–541.
8. Fairbank JC, Park WM, McCall IW, et al. Apophyseal injections of local anaesthetic as a diagnostic aid in primary low-back pain syndromes. *Spine* 1981;6:598–605.
9. Fortin JD, Dwyer AD, West S, et al. Sacroiliac joint: pain referral maps upon applying a new injection/arthrography technique. Part I: asymptomatic volunteers. *Spine* 1994;19:1475–1482.
10. Fukui S, Ohseto K, Shiotani M, et al. Distribution of referred pain from the lumbar zygapophyseal joints and dorsal rami. *Clin J Pain* 1997;13:303–307.
11. O'Neill CW, Kurgansky ME, Derby R, et al. Disc stimulation and patterns of referred pain. *Spine* 2002;27:2776–2281.
12. Smyth MJ, Wright V. Sciatica and the intervertebral disc. An experimental study. *J Bone Joint Surg* 1959;40A:1401–1418.
13. Keisler B, Carter C. Abdominal aortic aneurysm. *Am Fam Physician* 2015;91:538–543.
14. Li Y, Li L, Zhang D, et al. A contained ruptured abdominal aortic aneurysm presenting with vertebral erosion. *Ann Vasc Surg* 2017;41:279.
15. Huang CF, Liu YT, Wu YC, et al. Spontaneous pseudoaneurysm rupture of gastroduodenal artery: a rare and life-threatening condition of back pain. *J Formos Med Assoc* 2014;113:756–757.
16. El-Farhan N, Busuttil A. Sudden unexpected deaths from ruptured abdominal aortic aneurysms. *J Clin Forensic Med* 1997;4:111–116.
17. Bardin LD, King P, Maher CG. Diagnostic triage for low back pain: a practical approach for primary care. *Med J Aust* 2017;206:268–273.
18. Downie A, Williams CM, Henschke N, et al. Red flags to screen for malignancy and fracture in patients with low back pain: systematic review. *BMJ* 2013;347:f7095.
19. Bogduk N. Degenerative joint disease of the spine. *Radiol Clin N Am* 2012;50:613–628.
20. Bogduk N, McGuirk B. History. In: *Medical Management of Acute and Chronic Low Back Pain. An Evidence-Based Approach.* Amsterdam, The Netherlands: Elsevier; 2002:27–40.
21. McGuirk B, King W, Govind J, et al. The safety, efficacy, and cost-effectiveness of evidence-based guidelines for the management of acute low back pain in primary care. *Spine* 2001;26:2615–2622.
22. Verhagen AP, Downie A, Maher CG, et al. Most red flags for malignancy in low back pain guidelines lack empirical support: a systematic review. *Pain* 2017;158:1860–1868.
23. King W. Diagnosis of pain, medical history. In: Schmidt RF, Willis WD Jr, eds. *Encyclopedic Reference of Pain.* Berlin: Springer; 2007:1112–1115.
24. Huskisson EC. Measurement of pain. *Lancet* 1974;2:1127–1131.
25. Strong J, Ashton R, Chant D. Pain intensity measurement in chronic low back pain. *Clin J Pain* 1991;7:209–218.
26. Briggs M, Closs JS. A descriptive study of the use of visual analogue scales and verbal rating scales for the assessment of postoperative pain in orthopedic patients. *J Pain Symptom Manage* 1999;18:438–446.
27. Farrar JT, Young JP, La Moreaux L, et al. Clinical importance of changes in chronic pain intensity measured on an 11-point numerical pain rating scale. *Pain* 2001;94:149–158.
28. Hill JC, Whitehurst DG, Lewis M, et al. Comparison of stratified primary care management for low back pain with current best practice (STarT Back): a randomised controlled trial. *Lancet* 2011;378:1560–1571.
29. Oliveira E, Lavrador JP, Teixeira J, et al. A purely extradural lumbar nerve root cavernoma mimicking acute myeloid leukemia recurrence: case report and literature review. *Surg Neurol Int* 2016;7(suppl 38):S908–S910.
30. Wu SC, Huang TC, Yu WY, et al. Unusual lower back pain with monocytosis: a case report. *Oncol Lett* 2016;12:4048–4050.
31. Socola F, Insuasti-Beltran G, Henrich Lobo R, et al. Chronic lymphocytic leukemia with translocation (2;14)(p16;q32): a case report and review of the literature. *Case Rep Oncol Med* 2016;2016:9037436.
32. He Z, Tao S, Deng Y, et al. Extramedullary relapse in lumbar spine of patient with acute promyelocytic leukemia after remission for 16 years: a case report and literature review. *Int J Clin Exp Med* 2015;8:22430–22434.
33. Tsunemine H, Umeda R, Nohda Y, et al. Acute myeloid leukemia complicated by giant cell arteritis. *Intern Med* 2016;55:289–293.
34. Apley AG, Solomon L, eds. The back. In: *Apley's System of Orthopaedics and Fractures.* 7th ed. Oxford, United Kingdom: Butterworth-Heinemann; 1993:367–369.

35. Bogduk N, McGuirk B. Physical examination. In: *Medical Management of Acute and Chronic Low Back Pain. An Evidence-Based Approach*. Amsterdam, The Netherlands: Elsevier; 2002:41–47.

36. Laslett M, Young SB, Aprill CN, et al. Diagnosing painful sacroiliac joints: a validity study of a McKenzie evaluation and sacroiliac provocation tests. *Aust J Physiother* 2003;49:89–97.

37. Laslett M, Oberg B, Aprill CN, et al. Centralization as a predictor of provocation discography results in chronic low back pain, and the influence of disability and distress on diagnostic power. *Spine J* 2005;5:370–380.

38. Sloan TJ, Walsh DA. Explanatory and diagnostic labels and perceived prognosis in chronic low back pain. *Spine* 2010;35:E1120–E1125.

39. Deyo RA, Diehl AK, Rosenthal M. Reducing roentgenography use: can patient expectations be altered? *Arch Int Med* 1987;147:141–145.

40. Deyo RA, Diehl AK. Cancer as a cause of back pain: frequency, clinical presentation and diagnostic strategies. *J Gen Intern Med* 1988;3:230–238.

41. Joines JD, McNuff RA, Carey TS, et al. Finding cancer in primary care outpatients with low back pain. A comparison of diagnostic strategies. *J Gen Intern Med* 2001;16:14–23.

42. National Institute for Health and Care Excellence. *Low Back Pain and Sciatica in Over 16s: Assessment and Management*. London: National Institute for Health and Care Excellence; 2001. NICE guideline NG59.

43. Stochkendahl MJ, Kjaer P, Hartvigsen J, et al. National clinical guidelines for non-surgical treatment of patients with recent onset low back pain or lumbar radiculopathy. *Eur Spine J* 2018;27:30–75.

44. Van Wambeke P, Desomer A, Ailliet L, et al. *Low Back Pain and Radicular Pain: Assessment and Management—Summary*. Brussels, Belgium: Belgian Health Care Knowledge Centre; 2017.

45. Qaseem A, Wilt TJ, McLean RM, et al. Noninvasive treatments for acute, subacute, and chronic low back pain: a clinical practice guideline from the American College of Physicians. *Ann Intern Med* 2017;166:514–530.

46. Spearing M, March L, Bellamy N, et al. Management of acute musculoskeletal pain. *APLAR J Rheumatol* 2005;8:5–15.

47. Indahl A, Velund L, Reikeraas O. Good prognosis for low back pain when left untampered: a randomized clinical trial. *Spine* 1995;20:473–477.

48. Indahl A, Haldorsen EH, Holm S, et al. Five-year follow-up study of a controlled clinical trial using light mobilization and an informative approach to low back pain. *Spine* 1998;23:2625–2630.

49. Bogduk N, McGuirk B. Algorithm for acute low back pain. In: *Medical Management of Acute and Chronic Low Back Pain. An Evidence-Based Approach*. Amsterdam, The Netherlands: Elsevier; 2002:73–81.

50. Watson P. The MSM quartet. *Aust Musculoskelet Med* 1999;4(2):8–9.

51. Frazier LM, Carey TS, Lyles MF, et al. Selective criteria may increase lumbosacral spine roentgenogram use in acute low-back pain. *Arch Int Med* 1989;149:47–50.

52. Waldvogel FA, Vasey H. Osteomyelitis: the past decade. *N Engl J Med* 1980;303:360–370.

53. Whalen JP, Balter S. Radiation risks associated with diagnostic radiology. *Dis Mon* 1982;28:73.

54. Reinus WR, Strome G, Zwemer F. Use of lumbosacral spine radiographs in a level II emergency department. *AJR Am J Roentgenol* 1998;170:443–447.

55. Hall FM. Back pain and the radiologist. *Radiology* 1980;137:861–863.

56. Ardran GM, Crooks HE. Gonad radiation dose from diagnostic procedures. *Br J Radiol* 1957;30:295–297.

57. Engers AJ, Jellema P, Wensing M, et al. Individual patient education for low back pain. *Cochrane Database Syst Rev* 2008;(1):CD004057.

58. Roland M, Dixon M. Randomized controlled trial of an educational booklet for patients presenting with back pain in general practice. *J Roy Coll Gen Pract* 1989;39:244–246.

59. Little P, Roberts L, Blowers H, et al. Should we give detailed advice and information booklets to patients with back pain? A randomized controlled factorial trial of a self-management booklet and doctor advice to take exercise for back pain. *Spine* 2001;26:2065–2072.

60. Saragiotto BT, Machado GC, Ferreira ML, et al. Paracetamol for low back pain. *Cochrane Database Syst Rev* 2016;(6):CD012230.

61. Machado GC, Maher CG, Ferreira PH, et al. Non-steroidal anti-inflammatory drugs for spinal pain: a systematic review and meta-analysis. *Ann Rheum Dis* 2017;76:1269–1278.

62. Chou R, Deyo R, Friedly J, et al. Systemic pharmacologic therapies for low back pain: a systematic review for an American College of Physicians Clinical Practice Guideline. *Ann Intern Med* 2017;166:480–492.

63. van Tulder MW, Touray T, Furlan AD, et al. Muscle relaxants for nonspecific low back pain: a systematic review within the framework of the Cochrane collaboration. *Spine* 2003;28:1978–1992.

64. Abdel Shaheed C, Maher CG, Williams KA, et al. Efficacy and tolerability of muscle relaxants for low back pain: systematic review and meta-analysis. *Eur J Pain* 2017;21:228–237.

65. Friedman BW, Cisewski D, Irizarry E, et al. A randomized, double-blind, placebo-controlled trial of naproxen with or without orphenadrine or methocarbamol for acute low back pain. *Ann Emerg Med* 2017;71:348.e5–356.e5. doi:10.1016/j.annemergmed.2017.09.031.

66. Friedman BW, Irizarry E, Solorzano C, et al. Diazepam is no better than placebo when added to naproxen for acute low back pain. *Ann Emerg Med* 2017;70:169–176.

67. Friedman BW, Dym AA, Davitt M, et al. Naproxen with cyclobenzaprine, oxycodone/acetaminophen, or placebo for treating acute low back pain: a randomized clinical trial. *JAMA* 2015;314:1572–1580.

68. French SD, Cameron M, Wlaker BF, et al. A Cochrane review of superficial heat or cold for low back pain. *Spine* 2006;31:998–1006.

69. Mayer JM, Ralph L, Look M, et al. Treating acute low back pain with continuous low-level heat wrap therapy and/or exercise: a randomized controlled trial. *Spine J* 2005;5:395–403.

70. Nadler SF, Steiner DJ, Ersala GN, et al. Continuous low-level heatwrap therapy for treating acute nonspecific low back pain. *Arch Phys Med Rehabil* 2003;84:329–334.

71. Nadler SF, Steiner DJ, Petty SR, et al. Overnight use of continuous low-level heatwrap therapy for relief of low back pain. *Arch Phys Med Rehabil* 2003;84:335–342.

72. Tao XG, Bernacki EJ. A randomized clinical trial of continuous low-level heat therapy for acute muscular low back pain in the workplace. *J Occup Environ Med* 2005;47:1298–1306.

73. Nadler SF, Steiner DJ, Ersala GN, et al. Continuous low-level heat wrap therapy provides more efficacy than ibuprofen and acetaminophen for acute low back pain. *Spine* 2002;27:1012–1017.

74. Lloyd A, Scott DA, Akehurst RL, et al. Cost-effectiveness of low-level heat wrap therapy for low back pain. *Value Health* 2004;7:413–422.

75. Chou R, Deyo R, Friedly J, et al. Nonpharmacologic therapies for low back pain: a systematic review for an American College of Physicians Clinical Practice Guideline. *Ann Intern Med* 2017;166:493–505.

76. Rubinstein SM, Terwee CB, Assendelft WJJ, et al. Spinal manipulative therapy for acute low-back pain. *Cochrane Database Syst Rev* 2012;(9):CD008880.

77. Rubinstein SM, Terwee CB, Assendelft WJ, et al. Spinal manipulative therapy for acute low back pain: an update of the Cochrane review. *Spine* 2013;38:E158–E177.

78. French SD, Cameron M, Walker BF, et al. Superficial heat or cold for low back pain. *Cochrane Database Syst Rev* 2006;(1):CD004750.

79. Seco J, Kovacs FM, Urrutia G. The efficacy, safety, effectiveness, and cost-effectiveness of ultrasound and shock wave therapies for low back pain: a systematic review. *Spine J* 2011;11:966–977.

80. Yousefi-Nooraie R, Schonstein E, Heidari K, et al. Low level laser therapy for nonspecific low-back pain. *Cochrane Database Syst Rev* 2008;(2):CD005107.

81. Dahm KT, Brurberg KG, Jamtvedt G, et al. Advice to rest in bed versus advice to stay active for acute low-back pain and sciatica. *Cochrane Database Syst Rev* 2010;(6):CD007612.

82. van Duijvenbode I, Jellema P, van Poppel M, et al. Lumbar supports for prevention and treatment of low back pain. *Cochrane Database Syst Rev* 2008;(2):CD001823.

83. Wegner I, Widyahening IS, van Tulder MW, et al. Traction for low-back pain with or without sciatica. *Cochrane Database Syst Rev* 2013;(8):CD003010.

84. Melzack R, Vetere P, Finch L. Transcutaneous electrical nerve stimulation for low back pain. A comparison of TENS and massage for pain and range of motion. *Phys Ther* 1983;63:489–493.

85. Poquet N, Lin CW, Heymans MW, et al. Back schools for acute and subacute non-specific low-back pain. *Cochrane Database Syst Rev* 2016;(4):CD008325. doi:10.1002/14651858. CD008325.pub2.

86. Sinclair SJ, Hogg-Johnson S, Mondloch MV, et al. The effectiveness of an early active intervention program for workers with soft-tissue injuries. The early claimant cohort study. *Spine* 1997;22:919–931.

87. Marin TJ, Van Eerd D, Irvin E, et al. Multidisciplinary biopsychosocial rehabilitation for subacute low back pain. *Cochrane Database Syst Rev* 2017;(6):CD002193. doi:10.1002/14651858.CD002193.pub2.

88. Waddell G, Feder G, Lewis M. Systematic reviews of bed rest and advice to stay active for acute low back pain. *Brit J Gen Pract* 1997;47:647–652.

89. Bogduk N, McGuirk B. The "Indahl" exercises for low back pain. *Aust Musculosket Med* 2008;13(1):8–14.

90. Carter JT, Birrell LN, eds. *Occupational Health Guidelines for the Management of Low Back Pain at Work—Principal Recommendations*. London: Faculty of Occupational Medicine; 2000.

91. Waddell G, Burton AK. Occupational health guidelines for the management of low back pain at work: evidence review. *Occup Med* 2001;51:124–135.

92. Staal JB, Hlobil H, van Tulder MW, et al. Occupational health guidelines for the management of low back pain: an international comparison. *Occ Environ Med* 2003;60:618–626.

93. McGuirk B, Bogduk N. Evidence-based care for low back pain in workers eligible for compensation. *Occup Med* 2007;57:36–42.

94. Loisel P, Abenhaim L, Durand P, et al. A population-based, randomized clinical trial on back pain management. *Spine* 1997;22:2911–2918.

95. Baez S, Hoch MC, Hoch JM. Evaluation of cognitive behavioral interventions and psychoeducation implemented by rehabilitation specialists to treat fear-avoidance beliefs in patients with low back pain: a systematic review [published online ahead of print December 14, 2017]. *Arch Phys Med Rehabil*. doi:10.1016/j.apmr.2017.11.003.

96. Croft PR, Macfarlane GJ, Papageorgiou AC, et al. Outcome of low back pain in general practice: a prospective study. *BMJ* 1998;316:1356–1359.

97. Klaber Moffett J, Torgerson D, Bell-Syer S, et al. Randomised controlled trial of exercise for low back pain: clinical outcomes, costs, and preferences. *BMJ* 1999;319:279–283.

98. Kendall NAS, Linton SJ, Main CJ. *Guide to Assessing Psychosocial Yellow Flags in Acute Low Back Pain: Risk Factors for Long-term Disability and Work Loss*. Wellington, New Zealand: Accident Rehabilitation and Compensation Insurance Corporation of New Zealand and the National Health Committee; 1997.

CHAPTER 73

Chronic Low Back Pain

WADE KING and **NIKOLAI BOGDUK**

Introduction

Chronic low back pain is a huge problem in terms of its prevalence and the effects it has on people who suffer it. The size of the problem is magnified by the effects it has on the family and friends of those who suffer it, on health care practitioners who seek to address it, and on funding authorities and governments that organize or provide health care for it.

Health care practitioners who encounter a new patient with what seems to be chronic low back pain face three or four imperatives.

- The first imperative is to determine the type of pain, meaning whether or not it is, in fact, low back pain as conventionally defined, and if it is chronic.
- The second imperative is to consider any associated referred pain, to determine whether it is somatic referred pain or radicular pain.
- The third imperative is to identify any "red flag" condition that may be present, meaning serious pathologies like infection and neoplasia, which are rare but important causes of low back pain.

When those issues are addressed, the practitioner can decide whether or not to pursue definitive diagnosis of the source and cause of the pain. That decision governs the options that will then become available for management of the patient's problem. Treatments for chronic low back pain fall into two categories, general and specific. General measures are those that can be applied to all patients irrespective of the source and cause of their pain. Specific measures are those that can be applied to particular sites of pain generation and so require precise identification of the source of the pain, and if possible also its cause. For those practitioners who would employ specific treatments, a fourth imperative applies.

- The fourth imperative is to diagnose at least the source of the pain, if not also its cause, for a specific diagnosis is crucial to the application of specific, targeted treatments for chronic low back pain.

Once the practitioner has decided either to pursue definitive diagnosis or not and has addressed the imperatives pertinent to that decision, management of the patient becomes a matter of considering the various therapeutic options and offering treatment(s) with the best evidence of effectiveness for the condition as the practitioner conceives it. The decision to apply any treatment must be based on a mutual agreement with the patient after he or she has been given enough information about the treatment to enable him or her to give informed consent (or informed dissent, if the patient does not want to undergo a particular treatment).

DEFINITION

The International Association for the Study of Pain (IASP) construed back pain as synonymous with lumbar spinal pain, which it defined as pain perceived anywhere in the region bounded by the lateral margins of the erector spinae muscles, an imaginary transverse line through the tip of the last thoracic spinous process, and an imaginary transverse line through the tip of the first sacral spinous process (see Fig. 72.1).[1]

This definition serves to distinguish lumbar spinal pain from thoracic spinal pain, gluteal pain, and loin pain, for pain in these latter regions invites a different approach to diagnosis and management because its causes are likely to lie outside the lumbar spine. Gluteal pain invites a consideration of disorders of the hip or pelvis. Loin pain invites consideration of disorders of the urinary tract and other viscera.

Chronic low back pain is defined, by convention, as back pain that has persisted for longer than 3 months.[1,2] Some authorities consider this rubric can be applied earlier if the pain shows no signs of improving.[3] Establishing the duration of pain is relevant because the evidence base for the causes and management of chronic low back is distinctly different from that which applies to acute or subacute low back pain.

REFERRED PAIN

The definition of low back pain does not restrict the location of pain to the region of the lumbar spine. The emphasis is where the pain is primarily perceived, or where it appears to start. Thereafter, lumbar spinal pain can spread to distant regions, in which case it is known as somatic referred pain.

When assessing a patient with chronic low back pain, a prime consideration is making the distinction between somatic referred pain and radicular pain. Identifying which of the two types the patient has is pivotal to management because the causes of somatic referred pain and radicular pain are quite different, and their mechanisms are different. So they invite different investigations and different treatments. Investigations and treatments that may be appropriate for radicular pain are totally inappropriate for a patient who only has somatic referred pain. The cardinal distinctions between somatic referred and radicular pain lie in the quality of pain and its manner of spread.[4]

Somatic referred pain is typically dull and aching in quality; patients sometimes compare it to a feeling of deep pressure. Its distribution tends to occupy a broad area with diffuse boundaries that are hard to define, and the patient may demonstrate it with an open hand rather than with a pointing finger. Although the distribution may extend further into the lower limb when severe, the center of the pain is relatively fixed in location and the patient can usually indicate it readily, whereas its boundaries may be harder to delineate.

Somatic referred pain arises because of convergence, in the central nervous system, between nociceptive afferents from the lower back and from the lower limb onto common second-order neurons.[1,4] In the absence of accurate, somatotopic information, the patient cannot identify the actual source of pain and perceives it as arising throughout the area subtended by the common neuron and, therefore, in the lower limb.

Typically, somatic referred pain spreads from the lumbar spinal region in a contiguous fashion, as if expanding from the lumbar region (see Fig. 72.2). As a rule, the more severe the back pain, the more distant is the spread of the referred pain.[5] However, in some patients, the referred pain can "skip" regions such as the thigh and be perceived only in the calf.[6]

Radicular pain, in contrast, is typically sharp and shooting ("lancinating") in quality; it is often described by patients as "stabbing" pain and sometimes as "like electric shocks." Its distribution is much more precisely defined. Typically, it travels down the length of the lower limb in a narrow strip (see Fig. 72.3)[4,7,8] that the patient can demonstrate with one finger.

Also, it more often extends all the way down the lower limb to the foot. The mechanism of radicular pain is irritation of the dorsal root ganglion of a spinal nerve.[4]

Some authors maintain that somatic referred pain does not extend below the knee and that, therefore, pain below the knee must be radicular in origin. This is not correct, for it has been shown that pain from the lumbar zygapophysial joints and intervertebral disks can be referred beyond the knee, even into the foot.[5,6,9,10]

SOURCES

Experiments in normal volunteers have shown that noxious stimulation of the muscles of the back,[11,12] the interspinous ligaments,[12–14] the zygapophysial joints,[5,9,10] the sacroiliac joints,[15] and the intervertebral disks[6,16–18] can all evoke pain in the back. Back pain can also be evoked by mechanical[18] or chemical irritation of the dura mater.[19] All these structures, therefore, become the possible sources of pain in patients who present with low back pain. Notably, of all the structures in the lumbar spine, the intervertebral disks appear to be the most sensitive to experimental, noxious stimulation.[18]

CAUSES

Although the possible sources of back pain have been demonstrated, its causes have been more elusive. Pain arising from muscles or ligaments in the back is presumed to be caused by strains of these structures, but direct evidence of the resultant pathology has not been produced. However, the structures for which the cause of pain has been well established are the lumbar intervertebral disks and the lumbar zygapophysial joints.

Lumbar Intervertebral Disks

When intervertebral disks are affected by overt pathology such as infection, there is no dispute about the source or cause of pain. The inflammation caused by infection constitutes a source of chemical irritation of the nociceptive fibers that innervate the affected disk.[20] Less obvious are the mechanisms of pain in mechanical disorders of the disk.

Lumbar disks can be affected by internal disk disruption. As described in greater detail in Chapter 101, this condition has a distinctly different epidemiology and different structural features from those of disk degeneration.[20] It is caused by fracture or fatigue failure of the vertebral endplate and is characterized by degradation of the nuclear matrix and the development of internal radial and circumferential fissures.[20] It has been produced in laboratory animals[20] and can be diagnosed in patients, if special tests are used (see "Prevalence" section in the following text). The prevailing model is that pain arises from chemical irritation of nociceptors around the internal fissures and from mechanical stimulation of nociceptors in the posterior anulus fibrosus because it is subjected to greater than normal compression loading as a result of degradation of the nuclear matrix (see Chapter 101).[20]

Lumbar Zygapophysial Joints

Laboratory studies have shown that the lumbar zygapophysial joints are susceptible to small fractures, or avulsions of the capsule, when subjected to compression or excessive torsion.[21,22] Postmortem pathoanatomic studies have shown such injuries in people who have been injured in motor vehicle accidents.[23,24] However, no studies have validated antemortem methods of diagnosing such injuries, for example, by high-resolution computerized tomography (CT) scan.

PREVALENCE

Conventional methods of assessment and investigation typically fail to identify the cause of chronic low back pain in the majority of patients. This has fostered belief in the claim that a cause cannot be found in over 80% of patients with chronic low back pain.

This figure has been used to justify not pursuing a diagnosis of chronic low back pain but moreover to regard chronic back pain as being not due to injury or disease but as a psychosocial complaint. This figure has been endorsed and enshrined by various authorities in the past in support of disdaining pursuit of diagnosis.[25–28]

The source of this figure is rarely, if at all, quoted by its advocates, but it can be found by a simple search of the literature.[29,30] The source is a study of acute low back pain, published in 1966, in which British general practitioners claimed that a diagnosis was not possible in 80% of cases.[31] For diagnosis, the study relied on history, conventional examination, and plain radiography, for these were the only methods available in 1966. Given the limitations of history, physical examination, and plain radiography, it is not surprising that a diagnosis could not be established. In the intervening 50 years, methods have been developed and applied in order to pinpoint, if not the actual cause, then at least the source of pain in large proportions of patients with chronic low back pain. These methods are not indicated for acute low back pain even today, as explained in Chapter 72, so, in that sense, what was written in 1966 would still be considered correct about acute low back pain, but it is totally inappropriate for chronic low back pain in the modern era.

Although it may not be possible to identify the actual cause of back pain, in many instances, the source of pain can be established by using diagnostic nerve blocks (see Chapter 98). The paradigm is that if a structure is the source of pain, it can be identified as such if anesthetizing the structure (or its nerve supply) abolishes the pain. However, in patients with chronic pain, diagnostic blocks are susceptible to false-positive responses. Therefore, in order to be valid, diagnostic blocks need to be controlled.[32,33] Furthermore, other variables need to be rigorously defined and measured, such as magnitude of relief and duration of relief of pain.[32,33]

Diagnostic blocks can be applied to pursue sources of pain in the ligaments or muscles of the lumbar spine or its synovial joints. Although diagnostic blocks have, from time to time, been performed as tests for pain from muscles or ligaments, no studies have performed the blocks rigorously. So, no dependable data are available as to the prevalence of low back pain stemming from muscles or ligaments. The opposite applies to synovial joints.

Using physiologic controls, multiple studies have purported to trace the source of chronic low back pain to the lumbar zygapophysial joints. Prevalence rates of 15%,[34] 40%,[35] and 45%[36–38] have been reported. What is contentious about these figures, however, is that complete relief of pain was not a diagnostic criterion. Rather, the investigators accepted 50% relief or 80% relief. They assumed that any pain not relieved stemmed from another, concurrent source, but that source was not identified. Meanwhile, other studies have shown that rarely do patients with chronic low back pain have concurrent sources of pain: from the zygapophysial joints, the sacroiliac joint, or the intervertebral disks.[39,40] Therefore, insofar as concurrent sources of pain have not been identified, partial relief of pain must be viewed as a spurious diagnostic criterion. Placebo responses have not been excluded.

When studies have looked for complete relief of pain following blocks of the lumbar zygapophysial joints, substantially lesser prevalence estimates have been encountered. In general populations, the prevalence of complete relief of pain is about 5% or less.[41–44] Therefore, lumbar zygapophysial joint pain may not be as common as has been held to date.

One study, using placebo controls, however, did find that 34% of an elderly population obtained at least 90% relief of pain.[35]

A later study found that zygapophysial joint pain was age dependent. Among patients in whom a source of pain can be established, the likelihood of a zygapophysial joint being the source of back pain is only 2% in patients aged 20 to 35 years; it rises to between 5% and 10% in patients aged 35 to 50 years and 20% in patients aged 50 to 65 years.[45,46] In patients over the age of 65 years, the likelihood rises to between 30% and 40%, and in this age group, zygapophysial joints are the most likely source of back pain.[45,46]

In elderly patients, it is tempting to attribute their pain to osteoarthrosis, but there is no correlation between the joint being painful and the radiologic features of osteoarthrosis on plain radiographs[4,47–49] or on CT scan.[50] It has been proposed that painful lumbar zygapophysial joints express inflammatory changes evident on magnetic resonance imaging (MRI) using a fat-saturation setting,[51] but this has yet to be corroborated by studies using controlled diagnostic blocks.

Earlier studies using controlled, intra-articular blocks traced the source of chronic low back pain to the sacroiliac joints in about 20% of patients.[40,52] A later study corroborated this prevalence as an average figure[45] but showed that the prevalence of sacroiliac joint pain differed with age.[46] The likelihood of the sacroiliac joint being the source of pain was low (2% to 10%) in patients under 65 years of age, but in older patients, it varied between 5% and 21% depending on body mass index.[46]

Pain stemming from the posterior sacroiliac ligaments (or "posterior sacroiliac complex"[53]) can be diagnosed using controlled blocks of the lateral branches of the sacral dorsal rami. However, although techniques for such blocks have been described and validated,[54] they have not been applied in population studies. So, the prevalence of sacroiliac ligament pain is not yet known.

The diagnosis of internal disk disruption requires disk stimulation and postdiscography CT. The disk is stimulated with an injection of contrast medium in order to determine if stimulating it mechanically reproduces the patient's pain. CT scanning is performed after disk stimulation to determine if the painful disk exhibits the radial or circumferential fissures that are characteristic of internal disk disruption.[20]

In patients with chronic low back pain, the prevalence of internal disk disruption is about 40%.[20] Of the diagnosable causes of chronic low back pain, the likelihood of internal disk disruption being the cause of pain is effectively 90% in patients under the age of 50 years, falling to 60% after the age of 50 years, and 20% after the age of 65 years.[46]

REFUTED CAUSES

Research has shown that many conditions, traditionally considered to be possible causes of chronic low back pain, are actually not causes. Multiple studies have shown that spondylolysis or spondylolisthesis cannot be held as causes of back pain in adults. These conditions occur with equal prevalence in subjects with no symptoms and in patients with back pain.[4] Similarly, so-called "degenerative changes" (better called "spondylosis") occur only slightly more frequently in patients with back pain than they do in asymptomatic individuals.[4] The difference in prevalence is so small as to render "degenerative changes" not diagnostic. They represent no more than normal age changes.

ACCEPTED CAUSES

There is no dispute that tumors and infections can cause low back pain, but these conditions are rare. Although specialist practitioners may be accustomed to greater prevalences because they are in referral practice, the prevalence of serious causes of back pain in primary care can be estimated to be no more than 5%. Given that the prevalence of tumors and infections is less than 1% in patients with acute low back pain,[55,56] if all patients

with acute low back pain progressed to chronic back pain, the prevalence of tumors and infections would remain less than 1%. If only 20% of patients progressed to chronic back pain, included all those with tumors or infections, the prevalence of those conditions would be concentrated by a factor of 5, to 5%.

UNTESTED CAUSES

In its Classification of Chronic Pain, the IASP recognizes, in principle, certain causes of chronic low back pain that are promoted by some practitioners.[1] These include muscle sprain, ligament sprain, segmental dysfunction, and trigger points. However, the IASP requires that for the diagnosis of these conditions, techniques be used that are of known reliability and validity, but no technique has been shown to be both reliable and valid for the diagnosis of these entities. Therefore, they remain as only theoretical or imaginary constructs.

Assessment

The assessment of a patient with chronic low back pain serves three objectives. Foremost, the practitioner has a duty of care not to miss any serious causes of pain. Second, information should be gathered to formulate the type of diagnosis on which the practitioner intends to base treatment. Third, information should be gathered to determine the physical and emotional state of the patients, along with their social circumstances so that any management plan takes these into consideration.

Chronic pain is often accompanied by associated psychological and social problems. The relationships between them are encapsulated in the biopsychosocial model of pain, expounded in 1977.[57] According to this model, chronic pain has three domains, the biologic, the psychological, and the social. The biologic domain includes the causative bodily impairment and the neurophysiologic mechanisms that generate the experience of pain in the patient's cerebral cortex; these biologic features of pain are essential to it: Without them, there would be no pain. The psychological domain includes affective features of distress and suffering, such as anxiety and depression; these psychological features are secondary to the experience of pain[58]: They result from the patient's response to the pain experience, and without that experience, they would not exist. The social domain includes issues such as impacts on family relationships and social activities[59]: They are largely secondary to affective changes, so their existence depends on both the biologic and psychological domains. The biologic domain of pain is the crux of the condition, the sine qua non of the patient's problems.[57] In assessing a patient with chronic low back pain, the practitioner should focus on the biologic domain as the core issue but is advised to be aware of psychological and social issues that may relate to it.

As described in greater detail in Chapter 72, the initial assessment relies heavily on eliciting a medical history,[60] undertaking physical examination,[61] and then employing, judiciously, ancillary investigations indicated by the clinical features. The processes of history taking and physical examination, if undertaken empathetically, help in developing the rapport which underlies an effective doctor–patient relationship; more than that, they yield cues that guide the rational utilization of ancillary investigations, both to pursue any suspicions of serious causes of pain and to explore the possibilities of source(s) and cause(s) of pain consistent with the clinical features.

The extent to which each domain of patient assessment is explored will depend on the practitioner's role in the patient's management. Physicians will seek information that is more or less diagnostic information depending on whether they pursue definitive diagnosis that would enable specific, targeted treatment, or intend to apply only general treatments that do not require precise identification of the pain source. All physicians will need to elicit a more detailed history than paramedical practitioners because physicians are expected to identify any "red flag" conditions, they will be responsible for ordering any special investigations that might be required, and they will have responsibility for the longer term management of those patients whose pain persists. In such cases, the history elicited initially will be useful for monitoring the progress of the condition and the development of any of its features.

Paramedical practitioners will not need to undertake a detailed assessment if they are working in cooperation with, and upon referral from, a physician who has assumed primary responsibility for the patient and who has already taken a comprehensive assessment. However, they should still address the basic features of history and any cues alerting to a "red flag" condition and any other aspect of assessment that pertains to their role in the management of the patient's condition. A paramedical practitioner acting as the sole health care provider assumes the responsibility for taking a comprehensive assessment and the responsibility for alerting the appropriate medical practitioner if a "red flag" condition is suspected.

In order for the medical history to be comprehensive, that is, not neglecting anything, it can be guided by a systematic approach that is applicable to any form of pain (see Table 72.1). Being systematic ensures that no domain of inquiry is overlooked or forgotten, but which could have yielded valuable cues toward diagnosis.

That systematic approach can be supplemented by reference to a "red flag" checklist (see Fig. 72.5). As explained in Chapter 72, a "red flag" is a feature, identified in the history, that alerts the practitioner to the possibility of a serious cause of pain. A "red flag" of itself is not diagnostic, nor is it intended to be. Serious causes of pain will be diagnosed (or excluded) by subsequent investigations. A "red flag" serves only to alert the practitioner to consider the serious cause that is prompted by the "red flag" and to decide if investigations should be pursued or not.[62] The "red flag" checklist was not developed on the basis of the predictive power of particular features. Rather, it was developed on the basis of case reports of unusual, unexpected, or cryptic causes of back pain that were overlooked during the patient's original management but which would have been identified if relevant questions had been asked at the time or if remotely possible causes of pain had been entertained.[62,63]

Triage is much more important when patients present with chronic low back pain than it is for those with acute low back pain. With acute low back pain, there is little point in trying to establish the exact source and cause of the pain because such information will not affect the approach to management (as explained in Chapter 72).[64] With chronic low back pain, diagnosis is pivotal to management: If the precise source of the pain can be identified, specific, targeted treatment can be applied.

MEDICAL HISTORY

Before commencing inquiry into the history of the patient's complaint of pain, it is convenient to establish the patient's age. This is pertinent because certain malignancies are distinctly more common in the elderly, and because certain diagnosable conditions are more likely in the elderly, or conversely in younger patients. In this regard, age alone is not an absolute determining factor, but it raises the threshold of suspicion. Other features in the history may subsequently raise or reduce that threshold.

Confirming the *site of pain* is important to establish whether the patient has lumbar spinal pain, as defined,[1] rather than loin pain or gluteal pain. Loin pain suggests a visceral source (perhaps a ureter, a kidney, or its vessels), whereas primary gluteal pain suggests a hip disorder rather than spinal pain.

Pain located in the lumbar or sacral spinal region can arise from many sources, but there is a partial rule concerning

sacroiliac pain. Pain from the sacroiliac joint, or from the posterior sacroiliac complex of ligaments and muscles, tends to be located over that sacroiliac region, and radiates distally[15,40]; rarely, if ever, has it been found to extend above the L5 level. So, pain located exclusively below L5 increases the likelihood of the sacroiliac joint or the posterior sacroiliac ligaments being the source.

Another consideration of site is to distinguish between the pain which is the focus of the assessment (the "index pain") and any other pain the patient may have. For example, a patient may have a painful knee, but subsequently, he or she may develop pain in the lower back and leg on that side. For the purpose of the assessment, the antecedent knee pain should be excluded from the description of the "index pain" (namely, that in the low back and leg), although the knee pain should also be noted as a concurrent problem.

If the patient with back pain also has abdominal pain, the presentation converts from one of back pain to one of abdominal pain. Assessment of the abdominal pain takes precedence and requires a different algorithm (see Chapter 47).

The *duration of illness* means how long the patient has been experiencing the pain, and it establishes whether the pain is chronic; if so, it is somewhat reassuring with respect to pathology. Patients are unlikely to have a serious cause if their condition has not deteriorated over several months or if new signs or associated features have not developed. However, the practitioner should not be complacent about "red flags," for there are exceptions. Tumors may grow slowly. Chronic spinal infections can remain indolent and not produce additional features for a long time; in one study, delays of 1 to 8 years were encountered in 47% of infected patients.[65]

The *distribution* of pain needs to be interpreted carefully as it is a discriminating variable between somatic referred and radicular pain. The first point to note is that pain in the buttock and/or lower limb can stem from any source of pain in the lumbar spine. The cardinal distinctions between somatic referred pain and radicular pain lie in the quality of pain and its manner of spread, as described earlier (see "Referred Pain" section in the preceding text). Making this distinction prevents mistaking somatic referred pain for radicular pain, and thereupon pursuing the diagnosis and treatment of disk herniation, which is a cause of radicular pain but not a cause of back pain.

The *quality* of pain is the other cardinal discriminating variable between somatic referred and radicular pain. Somatic referred pain is typically dull and aching in quality, whereas radicular pain is typically sharp and shooting in quality; it is often described by patients as "stabbing" pain and sometimes as "like electric shocks."

The *intensity* of pain is a very significant feature and should be assessed with care. Ideally, it should be measured by the patient themselves, using (under supervision) a valid instrument. Suitable instruments include a visual analogue scale (VAS) or a numerical pain rating scale (see Chapter 23). If the intensity tends to fluctuate, scores should be recorded for the average intensity when the patient is active and the most intense pain experience recently. The resultant score(s) should be recorded for monitoring with the progress of the condition.

The importance of pain intensity is twofold. First, it signifies the significance of the pain to the patient and is the single most important factor in the patient's decision to seek medical treatment. Few people would bother to seek medical advice about pain of very slight intensity. Consequently, regardless of the actual score recorded by the patient, that degree of pain is patently concerning enough to the patient for them to seek medical treatment. In that regard, it is worth noting that when a patient describes severe pain, he or she is usually conveying the degree of suffering that the pain induces and suffering is a function of many factors additional to noxious stimulation by the pain generator (see "Psychosocial History" section in the following text).

Second, the pain intensity recorded at the initial assessment provides an invaluable guide to the progress of the condition and the effectiveness or otherwise of treatment(s) applied; a relevant aphorism is that pain cannot be said to have been relieved unless it has been measured.[66]

Although important for the reasons outlined, measuring pain intensity is not usually helpful as a discriminating variable in the assessment of chronic low back pain. Serious causes of pain may cause intense pain but so can conditions such as internal disk disruption. Meanwhile, some patients may rate their pain as intense because of the suffering that it causes, in which case the intensity is not necessarily proportional to magnitude of nociception arising from the source of pain.

The *periodicity* means whether the pain is constant or intermittent, it is not usually helpful as a discriminating variable in the assessment of chronic low back pain because most patients will complain of constant pain. If the pain is reported as intermittent, the practitioner should distinguish between pain that is present constantly but waxes and wanes in intensity and pain that is truly intermittent and occurs in episodes. If the pain is truly intermittent, practitioner should record the frequency and duration of the episodes.

The variables *periodicity*, *time of onset*, and *mode of onset* pertain to pain that occurs in distinct episodes. They describe the frequency of episodes; when the pain starts during a particular day, week, or month; and if it comes on suddenly or gradually. These variables are relevant in the diagnosis of various forms of headache and visceral pain, which have metabolic triggers, but they are not pertinent to chronic low back, which is typically constant. If the pain is reported as intermittent, the practitioner should be careful to distinguish between pain that is present constantly but waxes and wanes in intensity and pain that is truly intermittent and occurs in episodes. If the latter, practitioner should record the frequency and duration of the episodes.

Time of onset becomes relevant in the assessment of chronic low back pain if the patient describes early morning stiffness, which later is relieved on commencing movements. This feature is highly alerting to the possibility of ankylosing spondylitis being the cause. If it has not been noted previously when the patient was in the acute phase, noting it now, when the patient has chronic pain, still serves to engage a rheumatologist in the management of the patient.

Precipitating factors are events or movements that trigger an episode of pain. *Aggravating factors* are postures or activities that make the pain worse. *Relieving factors* are actions that reduce the pain. None of these factors is diagnostic of any particular cause of pain, but they construct a picture of the patient's disabilities.

Features such as aggravation of pain by flexion, extension, or rotation are not valid determinants of pain stemming from intervertebral disks, zygapophysial joints, or sacroiliac joints.[35,40,67] Anecdotally, however, sacroiliac joint pain is strongly suggested when a patient's pain is triggered or aggravated by sitting on the ipsilateral buttock and relieved by sitting on the contralateral buttock.

Associated features, as explained in detail in Chapter 72, often provide cues to serious causes of pain. The "red flag" checklist (see Fig. 72.5) itemizes features that amount to past history and features that amount to a systems review.

Fever or night sweats raise the possibility of infection. Otherwise, the risk factors for infection encompass any manner of penetration or breach of the body's first line of defense: epithelium. These include surgical or dental procedures, catheterization or venipuncture, tattooing, illicit drug use, and skin lesions.

A history of weight loss—especially unexplained weight loss—or a past history of cancer constitutes grounds for suspecting malignancy.

Inquiring about occupation, leisure interests, and travel is relevant for what might be called exotic disorders, such as fungal infections and parasitic infections. Urban dwellers would not normally be exposed to such organisms, but individuals with unusual occupations or hobbies may be exposed, and individuals who live in or travel to rural or tropical environments may get exposed. Not inquiring about these domains can result in exotic conditions, such as hydatid cysts, being overlooked.

A systems review should address cardiovascular risk factors, for these are major alerting features for aortic and other aneurysms as a cause of back pain. Inquiring about respiratory, urinary, and reproductive functions may identify sources of malignancy in these systems. Symptoms of urinary dysfunction may alert the practitioner to urinary tract infection, and the combination of back pain, urethritis, and uveitis is pathognomonic of Reiter syndrome.

Hematopoietic neoplasms are notoriously cryptic causes of persistent back pain. They escape early diagnosis because they typically produce no other manifestations and are not regularly considered in the differential diagnosis. However, the oncology literature is replete with case reports of patients, with a history of blood diseases, who present with back pain (see Chapter 72).

The endocrine system should be assessed for possible sites of primary tumors, but more particularly, chronic use of corticosteroids is a risk factor for osteoporosis fractures of the lumbar spine, and diabetes mellitus is a risk factor for cryptic infection. Osteitis fibrosa cystica, as a manifestation of hyperparathyroidism, may present with spinal pain as the sole feature.

Assessing the musculoskeletal systems serves to identify conditions in which back pain is but one feature, the others being arthropathies in the appendicular skeleton. These include rheumatoid arthritis and the seronegative spondyloarthropathies. Likewise, inquiry should be made about the skin and gastrointestinal tract because the spondyloarthropathies are associated with rashes or vesicles and with diarrhea.

Neurologic symptoms are a game changer. If a patient reports or acknowledges numbness, weakness, or impaired continence of the bladder or bowel, the presentation converts from one of back pain to one of a neurologic disorder. Assessment of the neurologic disease takes precedence and requires a different algorithm. Once the neurologic disease has been diagnosed, if back pain continues to be unexplained, its assessment can be resumed.

The *circumstances of onset* pertain to what was happening when the complaint of pain originally started and its manner of onset at that time. Having the patient describe the first episode of pain can help determine the etiology of the pain: whether there was an apparent external cause or not or if the pain is truly idiopathic. In this regard, no particular features are diagnostic, but certain features of history constitute circumstantial evidence when matched with what is known from biomechanical studies.

Serious falls are an obvious risk factor for fractures of the lumbar spine. For the average individual, a serious fall would be one from a height. Older patients, however, who have osteoporosis, can suffer fractures after minimal trauma.

The biomechanics evidence implicates compression injuries in the etiology of internal disk disruption (see Chapter 101). These injuries can occur acutely, as in falls onto the buttocks or as a result of repetitive compressions incurred during heavy lifting or pulling over a period of time. However, internal disk disruption is a progressive disorder. Pain may not occur at the time of injury or may be not more than sense of discomfort. Overt or significant pain may be delayed until fissures develop in the anulus fibrosus, and the anulus becomes chemically irritated or mechanically stressed. The pattern of internal disk disruption, therefore, is one in which a reason for compression injury can be implicated, followed by a subsequent, progressive onset of disabling pain.

Otherwise, a knowledge of biomechanics can provide useful information from an accurate description of the circumstances in which injury may have occurred.[68,69] Assessing the magnitudes of forces (i.e., "stresses") applied, the directions in which those stresses were likely to be acting, and the patient's posture at the time can, when combined with knowledge of the anatomy and the loading capacities of the various structures of the lumbar spine, enable the practitioner to make a reasonable guess as to the structure(s) likely to have been injured. Sudden, severe rotation invites consideration of torsional injuries to the zygapophysial joints or the anulus fibrosus. Falls onto a buttock, or a longitudinal impact to an extended lower limb during a motor vehicle accident, are postulated risk factors for injuries to the sacroiliac joint. Sportspeople, whose activities involve forceful or repeated extension and rotation, are at risk of sustaining painful stress reactions in the pars interarticularis, or overt fractures of the pars.[70,71]

PSYCHOSOCIAL HISTORY

The *psychological and social history* bring to light psychological and social factors that are of greater significance when low back pain is chronic rather than acute. Persistence of pain over a long period tends to generate associated issues which if left unchecked may give rise to significant psychological comorbidities and social disruptions.

In the psychological domain, these may range from minor affective disquiets like uncertainty, mild fear, and diminished quality of life to major affective disorders such as anxiety, depression, and catastrophizing. As part of the initial assessment, the practitioner should probe gently for clues to disturbances of affect and, if any are apparent, record them to be addressed as part of the management plan.

In the social domain, issues of concern may include inability to work, loss of income, diminished contact with people outside the family, inability to perform usual tasks around the home and disturbances of family relationships. Again, the practitioner should probe sensitively for clues to such issues and plan to address any that become evident.

PHYSICAL EXAMINATION

After completing the medical history, the practitioner should proceed to perform a physical examination of the patient. There are several reasons for this. First, the examination may yield clues that clarify any suspicions raised by "red flag" features. Second, examination findings may reinforce clues from the history to the presence of injuries or impairments that are known sources and causes of chronic low back pain. Third, physical examination undertaken sensitively helps in developing the rapport which underlies an effective doctor–patient relationship. Finally, but not least importantly, many patients expect to be examined and they may feel that a practitioner who does not examine them is not very interested in their case.

Conventional physical examination will not provide a definitive diagnosis of chronic low back pain because there are no physical signs that are pathognomonic of its known sources and causes. The diagnostic purpose of physical examination is to reveal features that may be added to cues gained from the other domains of patient assessment to guide the rational application of valid ancillary investigations which can determine the source of low back pain. Some practitioners use physical features to guide treatment and/or to monitor progress, for example, in focusing on improving range of motion, or to classify patients, but these applications are not diagnostic in a pathoanatomic sense.

A systematic physical examination encompasses inspection, palpation, and movement testing.[61] The notes in the following text should be read in conjunction with the corresponding sections of Chapter 72.

Inspection may reveal general and specific features. General observations may include bodily deformity (malformations, amputations, prostheses), static posture both standing and sitting (for signs of scoliosis and kyphosis and loss of lordosis), dynamic posture when walking (for antalgic gait, other gait abnormalities), and performing gross movements (for transfers of weight such as pushing on the thighs while bending forward and straightening afterward). Specific observations include scars, puncture marks, swelling, and other local changes of shape.[72,73]

Palpation reveals features such as altered sensitivity (hypoesthesia or hyperesthesia), relationships of bony landmarks, and tenderness.[72,73] If tenderness is present, it may be diffuse or focal, and if focal, the clinician may note its relationship to bony landmarks such as spinous processes.

Movement testing addresses ranges of active thoracolumbar extension, flexion, sidebending, and rotation,[74,75] which may be restricted mechanically or by pain. Although not diagnostic, these abnormalities provide an indication of the disabilities that the patient has because of the pain. If one or more active ranges are restricted, the examiner should test the patient in the corresponding passive ranges to determine whether the restriction is due to anatomic limitation or to pain. No valid diagnostic information can be gained by testing accessory ranges of movement.

In one arena, developments have occurred. A specialized protocol of examination, based on detecting centralization of pain and other features, has been tested. The resultant data show the method has reliability for the detection of sacroiliac joint pain[76] and of internal disk disruption[77]; the data for its validity for definitive diagnosis of those entities is less convincing. It does not detect zygapophysial joint pain.[76,77] Whatever its value, this protocol requires special training.[78]

As for acute low back pain (see Chapter 72), physical examination is perhaps most informative when the patient exhibits no signs in the lumbar region. In that event, consideration needs to be given to a visceral or vascular cause of pain. Palpation for a pulsating mass and auscultation for bruits are cardinal actions for the assessment of aortic aneurysms.

Neurologic examination is neither necessary nor productive in the assessment of patients with chronic low back pain. Neurologic examination is indicated if the patient has neurologic symptoms, but in that event, the presenting feature is the neurologic disturbance and not back pain. In the absence of neurologic symptoms, neurologic examination serves only to satisfy the examiner that features which should not be present are, indeed, not present.

REVIEW OF PREVIOUS INVESTIGATIONS

Many patients with chronic low back pain will present with the films or digital images of multiple imaging studies they have undergone before. Before considering these, the practitioner should take pause and reflect on two caveats.

The first caveat is that a great deal of evidence[4] shows that imaging appearances do not correlate with pain, so the practitioner should be careful not to be misled by appearances that are irrelevant to the patient's index pain. The second caveat is that radiologic reports have been shown to have much less than perfect reliability,[79] so the practitioner should inspect the images themselves rather than rely on printed reports. With those two cautions in mind, it is suggested that before looking at any imaging, practitioners should formulate an idea, based on the clues gained from the history and examination, of what they might expect to see on the imaging. Then, they should peruse the images (not the reports) and note whether what they expected, or anything like it, is apparent; if so, that reinforces the impression gained from other clues; if not, such as when there are abnormal radiologic appearances at distant spinal levels or on the other side from the index pain, they can probably regard those appearances as irrelevant. Practitioners unfamiliar with spine imaging should consult a colleague who can help them read and interpret the images.

Patients may have undergone an invasive diagnostic or treatment procedure, but this may have not been performed in an optimal manner. The patient's response may or may not have been recorded accurately. Practitioners with appropriate knowledge can review any films to check for accuracy of the procedure, and they can check with the patient or any post-procedural pain charts to see what the response to the test was. Practitioners without pertinent knowledge should check with a colleague who does have the appropriate knowledge to confirm the validity of any procedures.

With these precautions in mind, previous investigations can serve either or both of two purposes: They can complement and enhance the assessment developed from history and examination, and they can be used to avoid requesting the same or additional investigations.

Provisional Diagnosis

To complete the patient assessment, the practitioner who wishes to pursue definitive diagnosis and specific, targeted treatment should formulate a provisional diagnosis. This is achieved by combining the symptoms and other subjective features apparent from the medical history with the physical signs elicited by clinical examination, and the relevant appearances seen on previous imaging (and the results of any other previous investigations such as blood tests, if any), to form a concept of the patient's presentation. This concept should then be developed into a hypothesis of the most likely explanation(s) for the patient's pain. Otherwise, the practitioner might raise a diagnostic hypothesis on the basis of the pretest probabilities (i.e., what is likely according to epidemiologic data). The practitioner's hypothesis should be expressed as one or a short list of the known sources of chronic low back pain as described in the *Classification of Chronic Pain*[1] published by the IASP; the putative diagnoses include discogenic pain (most commonly, internal disk disruption), zygapophysial joint pain, and sacroiliac pain (from either the sacroiliac joint or the posterior sacroiliac complex).

The evidence base shows that a definitive diagnosis can rarely, if ever, be determined after the initial assessment of a patient with chronic low back pain. So the provisional diagnosis should be appreciated as nothing more than a "best guess" of the known sources and causes of chronic low back pain. Its purpose is as a guide to further investigation, designed to test the provisional diagnosis and either confirm the pain source by the results of valid diagnostic tests or refute that "guess" and guide the practitioner to arrange other valid tests that allow definitive diagnosis of the actual pain source.

Definitive diagnosis will enable specific, targeted treatment. In the rare case in which the pain proves to be due to a "red flag" condition, it can be treated as appropriate to its nature. In the much more common situation in which the pain is proven due to one of the known spinal injuries and impairments that cause chronic low back pain, it can then be treated with a specific, targeted treatment with predictable effectiveness (see "Treatment" section in the following text).

If, after performing a comprehensive patient assessment, a practitioner who intends to apply targeted treatment is not able to formulate a provisional diagnosis of the likely source(s) of the patient's pain, he or she should make no attempt at specific treatment. The evidence base shows that specific treatment not based on valid diagnosis is unlikely to abolish the pain but is

likely to aggravate the patient's situation by subjecting them to (further) interventions that only add to the frustration of undergoing misguided treatments which prove ineffective. The moral and ethical imperatives for a practitioner who wishes to apply specific treatment but cannot formulate a provisional diagnosis of likely source(s) and cause(s) of chronic low back pain is to refer the patient to someone else who can.

If, after performing patient assessment, a practitioner intends to apply only general forms of treatment, there is no need for them to formulate a provisional diagnosis of the likely specific sources and causes of the patient's pain. If no particular cause is evident, or if the practitioner chooses not to venture a putative diagnosis, the IASP Classification of Chronic Pain[1] includes the diagnostic term *lumbar spinal pain of unknown or uncertain origin*. Although technically and literally correct, this label is unwieldy and may be somewhat unpalatable. In the past when the knowledge base was very limited, "nonspecific chronic low back pain" was an alternative preferred by some, but this is neither a default nor legitimate diagnosis. It means no more than the cause of back pain has not been pursued. Yet, it is misused to imply, in a definitive sense, that there is no cause or that no cause can be found. This rubric is particularly egregious, when it is used to convince patients that they should not pursue diagnosis. There is no term in common use that means "I chose not to look."

If a "red flag" has been identified during the initial assessment, the suspected serious cause of pain becomes the provisional diagnosis. Further investigations should be undertaken either to confirm or to rule out the suspected condition. Table 72.2 provides a guideline for the selection of appropriate investigations. If investigations prove positive, further management becomes that for the condition diagnosed. The problem is no longer one of back pain.

If no "red flags" are detected, the practitioner can be reasonably confident that a serious condition is not the cause of pain. In that event, the practitioner can formulate a provisional diagnosis of spinal causes of chronic low back pain.[1]

For confirmation, whether the provisional diagnosis is a "red flag" or a hypothesis of known spinal causes of pain, the provisional diagnosis must be tested by applying ancillary investigations.

Ancillary Investigations

Special investigations can be undertaken for either or both of two purposes. One is to "clear" the patient of serious or cryptic causes of pain that may not be evident from history and physical examination. The second is to test a putative diagnosis.

CLEARANCE

The best investigation for "clearing" the patient is MRI. MRI has sufficient sensitivity and specificity to detect unusual causes of pain, such as occult tumors, and neoplastic infiltrations that would otherwise escape detection.

There is no justification for progressing through plain radiography, bone scan, and CT before considering MRI. Each of those other investigations has little or limited ability to detect cryptic disorders. For screening purposes, MRI can detect fractures, which would be seen on plain radiographs, but MRI will also detect soft tissue lesions, which plain radiography cannot do. The increased vascular uptake that bone scan demonstrates will be evident on MRI with greater specificity. Although CT provides better resolution of bone, bony lesions will not escape detection by MRI.

NOT INDICATED

Electrophysiologic testing is one investigation not indicated for chronic low back pain. There is no lesion that causes low back pain and produces conduction block in the nerves of the lower limb, so nerve conduction studies cannot show anything useful about back pain. Some practitioners are accustomed to using conduction studies because they confuse somatic referred pain with radicular pain and explain that they are testing for radiculopathy, but even that practice is without foundation. It has been shown that even in patients with radicular pain, conduction studies are not diagnostic.[80,81] Conduction studies are indicated only if peripheral neuropathy is in the differential diagnosis of radiculopathy. Back pain is not radiculopathy, and peripheral neuropathy is not a differential diagnosis for chronic low back pain.

Likewise, CT is not an appropriate investigation for chronic low back pain. Its use is based on confusion between radicular pain and somatic referred pain. CT is useful for the detection of disk herniations in patients with radicular pain, but somatic referred pain is not caused by disk herniation. The only role for CT in back pain would be as a substitute when MRI is not available as a screening test. In that regard, CT is not an alternative to MRI, for there are conditions that MRI can detect that CT cannot detect. CT is an alternative to MRI for bureaucratic or economic reasons, not for medical ones.

Plain radiography is not indicated in patients with chronic low back pain. The lesions that it can detect are some fractures and gross lesions of bone. These are rare causes of chronic low back pain and are better detected by MRI or CT if it must be an alternative.

Establishing a definitive diagnosis has merit and purpose on either of two fronts. A definitive diagnosis might be made of a condition for which there is no proven treatment. This might appear to lack utility because establishing a diagnosis does not lead to better treatment. However, that argument assesses only the positive utility of establishing a diagnosis; investigations can also have negative utility. Establishing a diagnosis serves to protect patients from futile pursuit of other diagnoses and to protect them from trials of therapy that have no prospect of fixing the condition that has been diagnosed. It also protects patients from false accusations that their pain is only psychological, that they are imagining it, or that there is nothing wrong. Otherwise, there is positive utility to establishing a diagnosis of conditions for which there is a proven treatment.

MAGNETIC RESONANCE IMAGING

Certain features evident on MRI are fairly indicative of internal disk disruption. These are described in greater detail in Chapter 101. In summary, here, the two features are Modic lesions and high-intensity zones (HIZs).

Modic lesions occur in the spongiosa of the vertebral body above or below a disk with internal disruption (Fig. 73.1). Type 1 lesions appear dark on T1-weighted images but bright on T2-weighted images and represent bone marrow edema. Type 2 lesions appear bright both on T1-weighted images and T2-weighted images and represent fat deposition (implicitly postinflammatory). They occur in about 33% of patients with chronic back pain and correlate significantly with the affected

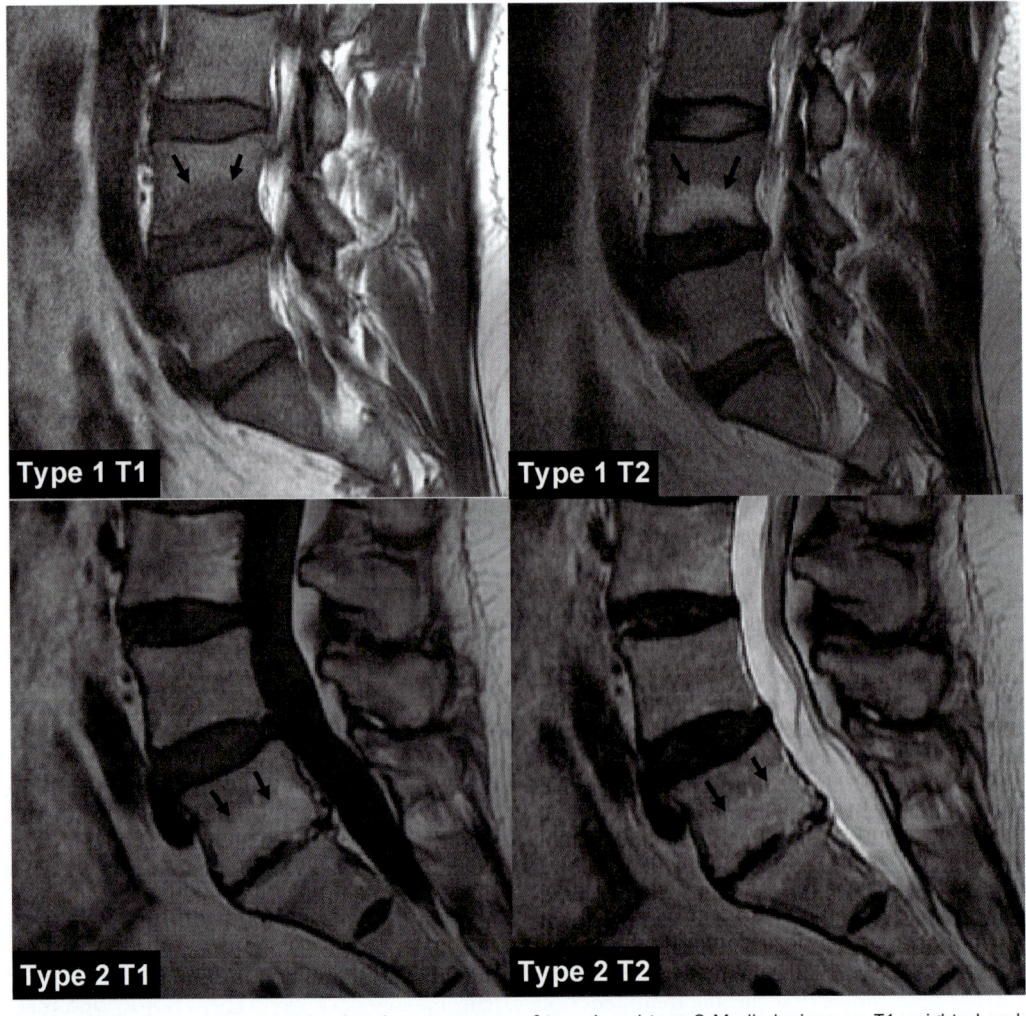

FIGURE 73.1 Sagittal magnetic resonance scans showing the appearance of type 1 and type 2 Modic lesions on T1-weighted and T2-weighted scans. *(Images kindly provided by Dr. Tim Maus, Mayo Clinic, Rochester, Minnesota.)*

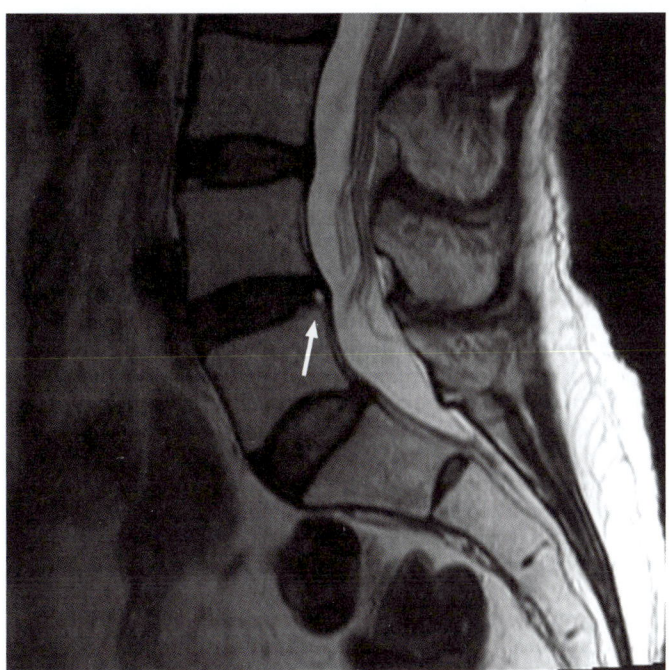

FIGURE 73.2 A T2-weighted, midline, sagittal magnetic resonance scan showing a high-intensity zone (*arrow*) in the anulus fibrosus of the L4–L5 disk. *(Image kindly provided by Dr. Milton Landers, Wichita, Kansas.)*

disk being painful, the pooled data indicating a positive likelihood ratio of about 3 (see Chapter 101).[20]

HIZs in the posterior anulus (Fig. 73.2) represent the cross-sectional appearance of a circumferential fissure. They occur in 20% to 30% of patients with chronic low back pain and correlate with the affected disk being painful. Although figures differ between studies, the pooled data show that an HIZ has a positive likelihood ratio greater than 3 for the affected disk being the source of pain (see Chapter 101).[20]

Modic lesions and HIZs each have similar positive likelihood ratios. Either sign inherits the same diagnostic power. Given that the pretest probability of internal disk disruption is 40%, a likelihood ratio of 3 increases diagnostic confidence to 67% that the affected disk is the source of pain. For most purposes, this degree of confidence may be enough. It is enough on which to base conservative therapy, if that therapy is appropriate for internal disk disruption. It is enough for medicolegal purposes because 67% exceeds the threshold for "on balance of probabilities," that is, 50%. This level of confidence, however, may not be enough if invasive therapies are contemplated.

DISK STIMULATION

The definitive, diagnostic test for internal disk disruption is disk stimulation supplemented by postdiscography CT scanning (see Chapter 101).[20] The test involves placing needles into the center of the disk to be tested and into two adjacent disks which serve as controls (Fig. 73.3). Contrast medium is injected into each of the disks with manometry to measure the

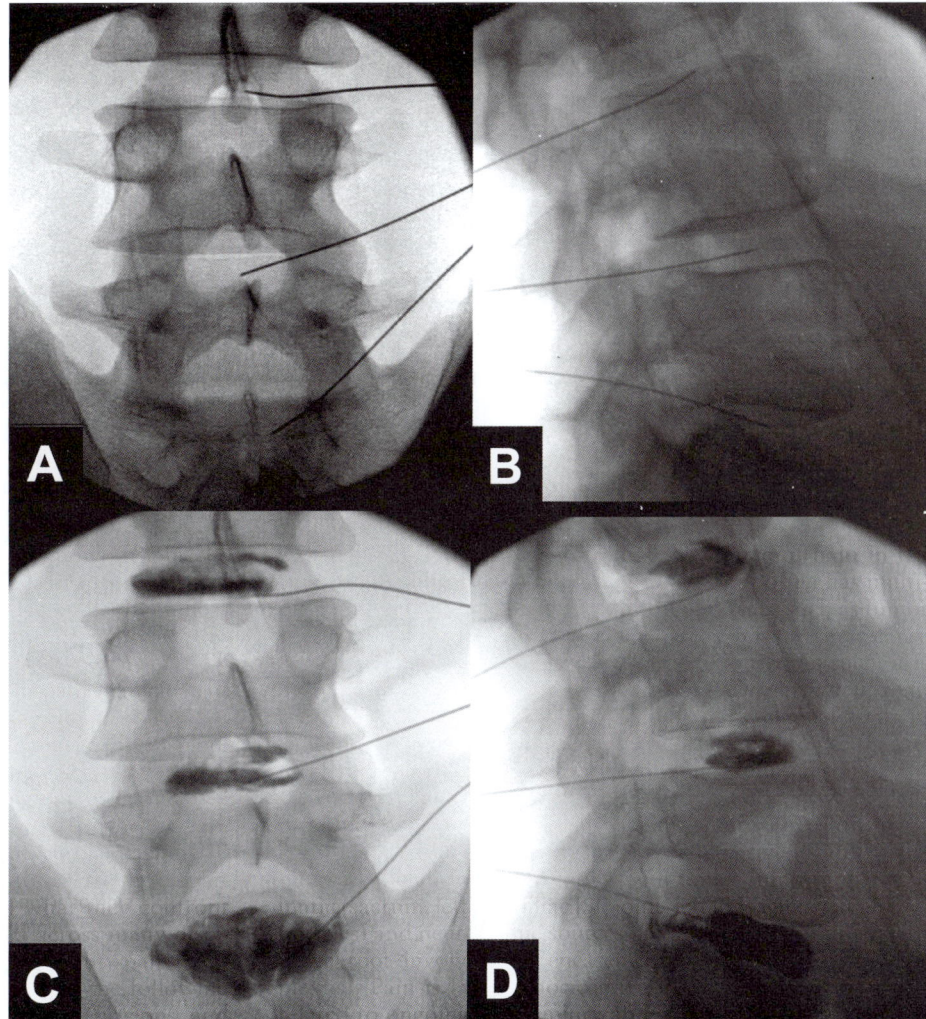

FIGURE 73.3 Fluoroscopy images of stages in the conduct of lumbar disk stimulation. **A:** Posteroanterior view of needles having been placed into the centers of the L3–L4, L4–L5, and L5–S1 disks. **B:** Lateral view of needles having been placed. **C:** Posteroanterior view after injection of contrast medium into each of the disks. **D:** Lateral view after injection of contrast medium. *(Images reproduced with permission from Bogduk N, ed.* Practice Guidelines for Spinal Diagnostic and Treatment Procedures. *2nd ed. San Francisco, CA: International Spine Intervention Society; 2013.)*

intradiscal pressure, and the patient's response to stimulation is recorded. Further details about the conduct of the test have been published elsewhere.[82] Upon completion of the disk stimulation, a CT scan of each of the disks is obtained.

The criteria for a positive test are that stimulation of the target disk, to an injection pressure less than 20 psi (0.14 kPa), reproduces the patient's pain to an intensity greater than 7/10, provided that stimulation of adjacent disks is not painful. Subsequently, the CT scan should show a grade III or IV fissure in the disk.

The validity of disk stimulation has been challenged on the alleged grounds that it has too high a false-positive rate. That challenge has been refuted by studies that collectively show that the false-positive rate is not greater than 10% and may be substantially less.[20]

The indication for disk stimulation is the need to establish a diagnosis of discogenic pain in general or internal disk disruption in particular. Depending on the circumstances, the test could be used for its negative diagnostic utility. For example, establishing a diagnosis of discogenic pain could protect patients from undergoing futile therapy for a presumed diagnosis of sacroiliac joint pain. A negative response to disk stimulation could protect patients from undergoing surgery based on a presumption of discogenic pain. The positive diagnostic utility lies in selecting patients, and disks, for treatments that target painful disks.

SINUVERTEBRAL NERVE BLOCKS

The sinuvertebral nerves (also known as recurrent meningeal nerves or recurrent nerves of Luschka) innervate the meninges, ligaments, and periosteum of the spinal canal and the anulus fibrosus of the intervertebral disk and carry sensory information, including pain, from those structures.[83]

Sinuvertebral nerve block (SVNB) is a diagnostic intervention aimed at identifying a painful disk by interrupting transduction of pain in the sinuvertebral nerve(s) that supply the target disk. The procedure is also sometimes called selective nerve root sleeve block. It involves introducing a spinal needle, under fluoroscopy, through the relevant intervertebral foramen and injecting a local anesthetic agent in such a way as to ensure the injectate flows inward and upward to reach the vicinity of the back of the disk. Somatic discogenic pain is relieved by anesthetic agent that reaches the disk, whereas associated radicular pain is relieved by agent that reaches the vicinity of the dorsal root ganglion.[84]

SVNBs have been reported as useful in numerous publications.[85-87] Although such papers suggest that SVNBs have roles in the diagnosis of discogenic pain, they do not provide data that evaluate their diagnostic validity.

An exploratory study assessed the potential utility of SVNB as an alternative to the more invasive disk stimulation test.[88] The results showed the sensitivity of SVNB was 73.3% (95% confidence interval [CI], 50.9% to 95.7%), but technical issues resulted in a target specificity of only 40% (95% CI, 15.2% to 64.8%). These results indicate that SVNB cannot yet replace disk stimulation but encourage future studies to improve its target specificity.

LUMBAR MEDIAL BRANCH BLOCKS

Lumbar medial branch blocks (LMBBs) are the diagnostic test for pain stemming from one or more of the lumbar zygapophysial joints. Intra-articular blocks are used by some practitioners, but intra-articular blocks have not been formally validated. LMBBs have been validated for face validity (target specificity) and for construct validity (the extent to which they achieve their purpose).[89] In other words, LMBBs do not anesthetize other structures that might be an alternative source of pain,[90] and they protect normal volunteers from experimentally induced pain from the joint anesthetized.[91]

LMBBs involve placing the tips of needles onto each of the two nerves that innervate the target zygapophysial joint and injecting 0.3 to 0.5 mL of local anesthetic onto each nerve (Fig. 73.4). Details for the conduct of the procedure are available elsewhere.[89]

Single, diagnostic blocks carry a high false-positive rate.[36,38,92] Therefore, for valid diagnosis, LMBBs have to be controlled. Comparative local anesthetic blocks have been used in the past, but doubts have been raised about their validity (see Chapter 98). Because of the low prevalence of lumbar zygapophysial joint pain and false-positive responses, even comparative blocks still have substantial false-positive rates. Consequently, operators who use comparative blocks need to appreciate that some of their positive responses will be doubtful. The only way to reduce this doubt is to perform placebo-controlled blocks.

With these reservations in mind, it is possible to use LMBBs to determine if a patient has back pain stemming from one or more lumbar zygapophysial joints. An algorithm for the efficient use of blocks has been described.[93] It recommends multilevel screening blocks in the first instance in order to identify patients who do not have zygapophysial joint pain, which is the most common response. Patients who report relief of the pain from screening blocks can then be subjected to repeat testing, with controlled blocks, in order to identify the joint or joints that are the source(s) of pain (see Chapter 98).

In terms of positive diagnostic utility, positive responses to medial branch blocks are the singular indication for treatment by lumbar medial branch thermal radiofrequency neurotomy (RFN) (see Chapter 102). This is the only treatment specific for lumbar zygapophysial joint pain for which there is rigorous evidence of effectiveness.

SACROILIAC JOINT BLOCKS

The definitive test for sacroiliac joint pain is controlled blocks of the joint using intra-articular injections of local anesthetic. These blocks require accurate access to the cavity of the joint, which at times, may be difficult to achieve (Fig. 73.5). Details concerning the procedure are available elsewhere.[94] Once access to the joint has been achieved, and confirmed by injection of a small volume of contrast medium to create an arthrogram, 1 to 2 mL of local anesthetic agent can be injected in order to anesthetize the joint.

The criteria for a positive response should be complete relief of pain, on each occasion, after controlled blocks are performed.[94] For reasons not fully articulated and defended, some practitioners settle for the criterion being greater than 75% relief of pain.[95] Intuitively, the greater the degree of relief, the more convincing the response would be that the joint is, indeed, the source of pain.[94]

The positive diagnostic utility of sacroiliac joint blocks (SIJBs) is that patients with a positive response can be directed to treatments specific for sacroiliac joint pain. The negative diagnostic utility is that establishing a diagnosis of sacroiliac joint pain protects patients from the futile pursuit of other diagnoses or from undertaking treatments that lack any rationale for treating sacroiliac joint pain.

SACRAL LATERAL BRANCH BLOCKS

In principle, it seems plausible that the ligaments behind the sacroiliac joint could be a source of pain. These ligaments are innervated by the lateral branches of the S1–S3 dorsal rami and are not anaesthetized by intra-articular blocks of the sacroiliac joint. A plausible diagnostic test for pain stemming from these ligaments would be blocks of the sacral lateral branches. However, no studies have yet systematically established the prevalence of this source of pain and whether it occurs in isolation or in company with sacroiliac joint pain. Furthermore, technical concerns have arisen.

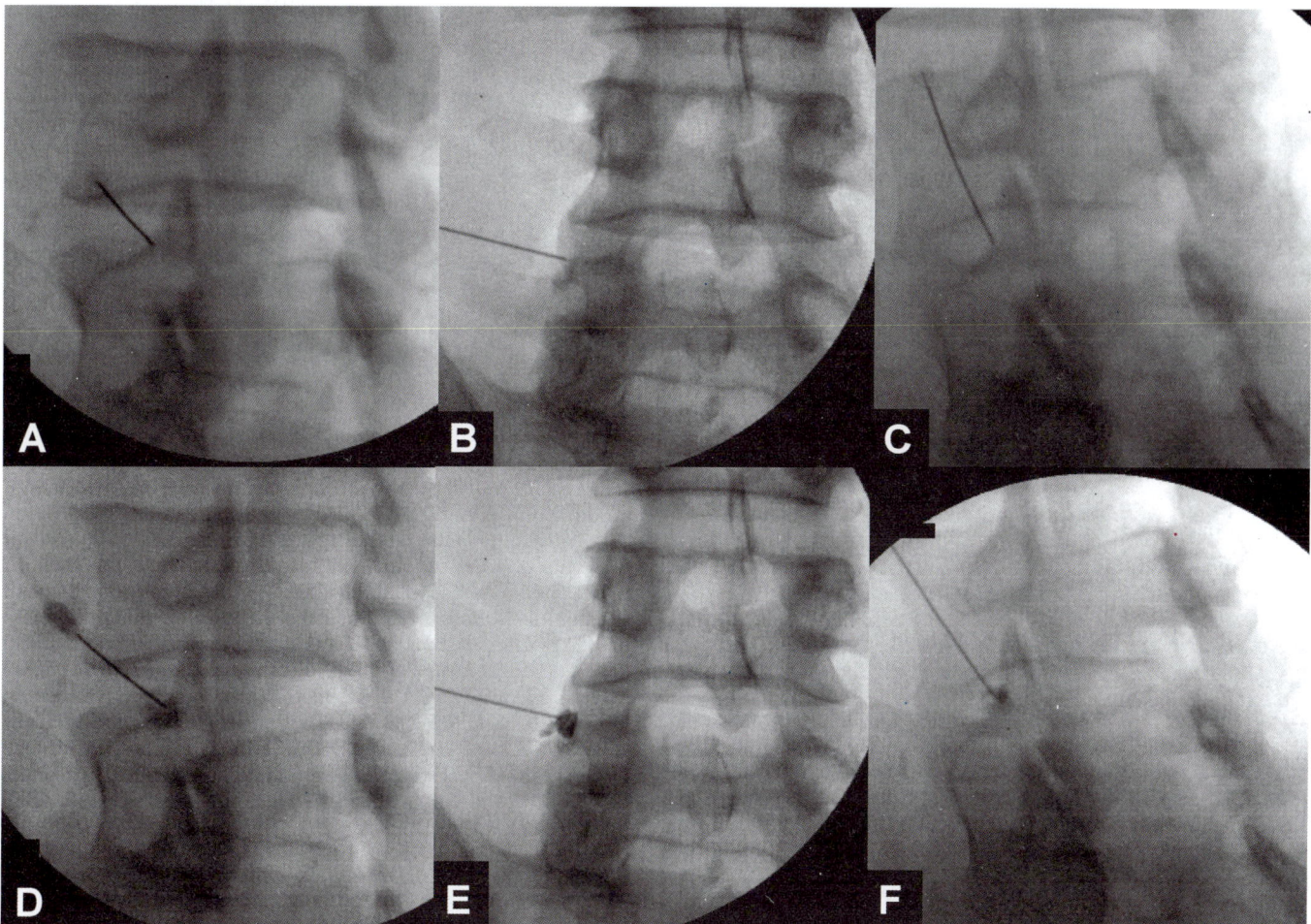

FIGURE 73.4 Fluoroscopy views of stages in the conduct of a left L4 medial branch block. **A:** Oblique view of a needle placed at the target point of the L4 medial branch on the neck of the L5 superior articular process. **B:** Posterior view of the needle resting on the target point. **C:** Declined oblique view showing the needle on the neck of the superior articular process. **D:** Oblique view after injection of a test does of contrast medium. **E:** Posterior view showing contrast medium concentrated around the target point. **F:** Declined oblique view showing contrast medium against the neck of the superior articular process. *(Reproduced with permission from Bogduk N, ed.* Practice Guidelines for Spinal Diagnostic and Treatment Procedures. *2nd ed. San Francisco, CA: International Spine Intervention Society; 2013.)*

Sacral lateral branches are elusive targets. They run at various depths within multiple layers of dense ligaments. Consequently, the original technique which involved injecting local anesthetic at a single site, lateral to each dorsal sacral foramen, fails to capture the target nerves reliably.[95] Needles need to be placed at multiple sites, at multiple depths, in order to capture the nerves, but even that technique is imperfect.[54]

Missing a nerve invalidates a block, but only in a negative sense: Patients who might have had a positive response are missed. If a technique manages to capture all the target nerves, and if the response to blocks is positive, for that response to be valid, it needs to be corroborated by controlled blocks.

No studies in the literature have reported using controlled blocks of the sacral lateral branches. One study used an approximation.[96] Blocks using bupivacaine were performed twice to corroborate responses, but different agents or placebo controls were not used. This study did not explicitly report the prevalence of positive responses, but implicitly, the yield was at least about 17% in 304 patients with pain predominantly caudal to L5, with the criterion for a positive response being at least 75% relief of pain following each of the two blocks.

The cardinal application of sacral lateral branch blocks is to select patients for sacral lateral branch neurotomy. The rationale is that if blocks of these nerves temporarily relieve the patient's pain, then coagulating the nerves should provide long-lasting relief.

Treatment

The patient whose main complaint is chronic low back pain primarily wants that pain to be treated effectively so he or she becomes pain free.[97] In the light of the literature on the treatment of chronic low back pain, such a wish by the patient may seem naive, as most publications on the effectiveness of treatments for chronic low back pain report partial relief only and then only for relatively short periods. Some publications on treatments report no relief of pain at all but instead report relief of para-phenomena such as pain-related disability or pain-related depression. Although such treatments may be of some benefit in their own ways, they cannot and should not be considered legitimate treatments for chronic low back pain. Pain relief is what patients want and it should be the primary goal of treatment. Ideally the relief should be total and enduring, so patients can return to activities and a quality of life they have not enjoyed since the pain came on.

Complete and enduring relief of chronic low back pain is not an unrealistic expectation, even when the pain has been present for a long time before treatment. Complete and enduring relief is the normal expectation when other types of pain are treated effectively and it is the usual outcome achieved when pains such as chronic angina pectoris, chronic hip pain, or chronic toothache are treated by methods that

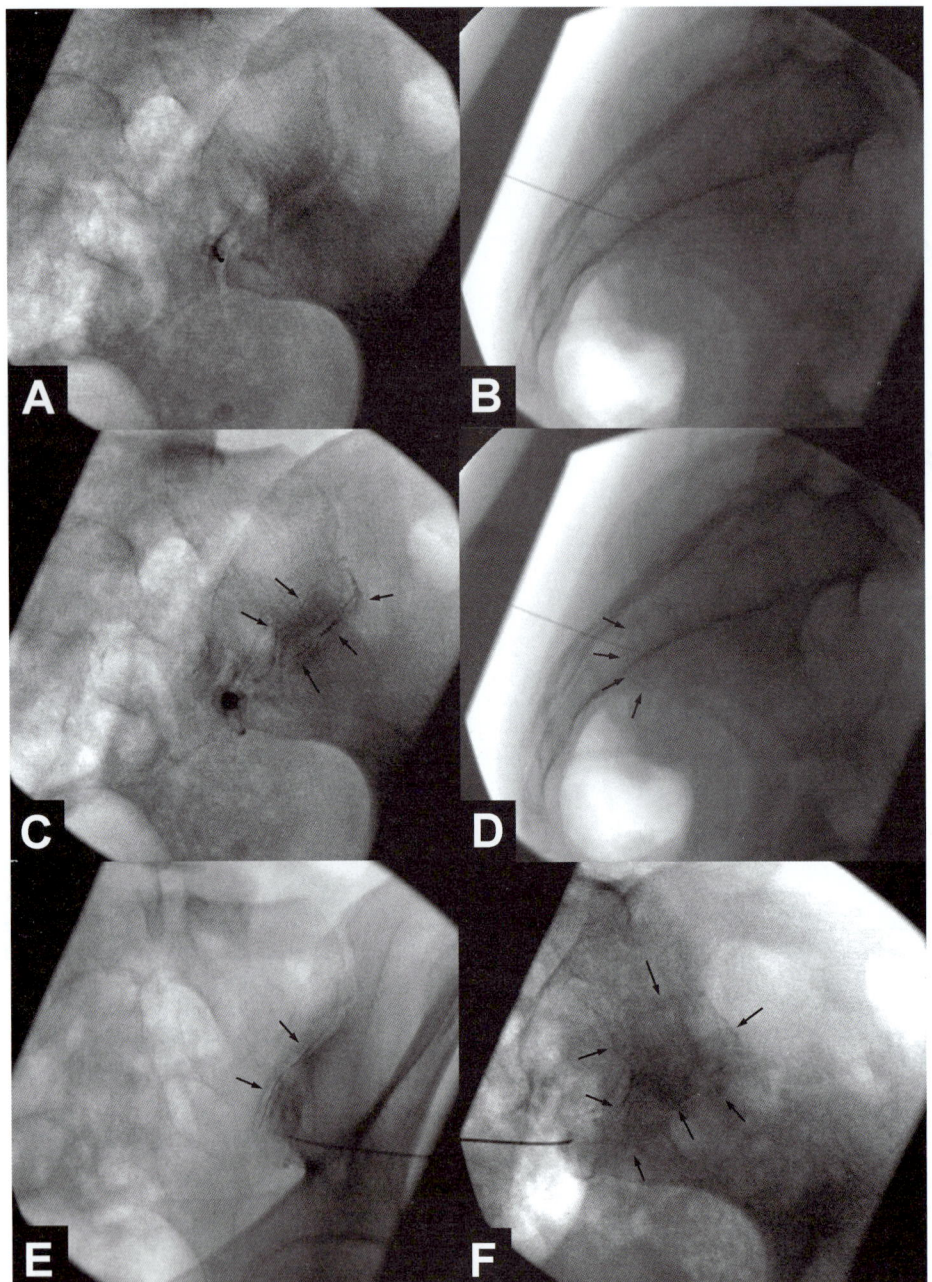

FIGURE 73.5 Fluoroscopy views of stages in the conduct of an intra-articular injection into a right sacroiliac joint. **A:** A near anteroposterior view, slightly contralateral oblique, showing a needle having entered the joint. **B:** A lateral view showing the needle having entered the joint. **C:** A near anteroposterior view after injection of a small volume of contrast medium. Linear streaks run between the various silhouettes of the joint margins (*arrows*), and the cavity of the joint blushes. **D:** A lateral view after injection of contrast medium. The image of the contrast medium is faint. It can be seen to outline the inferior perimeter of the joint cavity (*arrows*). **E:** An ipsilateral oblique view after injection of more contrast medium, showing contrast medium forming linear streaks between the joint margins. **F:** A contralateral oblique view through the right ilium showing how the contrast medium outlines the perimeter of the joint (*arrows*) and forms an auricular-shaped blush across the surface of the joint. *(Images reproduced with permission from Bogduk N, ed.* Practice Guidelines for Spinal Diagnostic and Treatment Procedures. *2nd ed. San Francisco, CA: International Spine Intervention Society; 2013.)*

address their mechanisms of pain generation effectively. The key to achieving complete and enduring relief is to identify the mechanism of the index pain and to address that mechanism with some intervention which deactivates it. The various treatments offered for chronic low back pain should be considered with the objective of complete and enduring pain relief clearly in mind.

Metaphorically, the literature on the treatment of chronic low back pain is a political and ideologic minefield. Various craft groups appear intent in proving that their therapy is effective and should be used. Some groups promote their ideology as

the preferred approach and condemn the approaches of others. Those who choose not to make a pathoanatomic diagnosis rely on nonspecific therapies, whereas those who do pursue a diagnosis are intent on having an intervention that works for the condition that they diagnose.

Common to all participants is the evolution of the literature and the standards applied to evaluating the evidence. Enthusiasm for particular therapies in the past has been tempered either by additional research or by reappraisal of previous evidence. New therapies confront higher standards of analysis and reporting than did their predecessors.

GENERAL TREATMENTS

Contemporary evidence is not flattering for conservative, general therapies for chronic low back pain. The evidence shows that various therapies either have no attributable effect or have small effects. This applies as much to physical therapies as to drug therapies.

Conspicuously, no general therapy has been shown to abolish chronic low back pain or to reduce it substantially so that the patient can resume normal activities of daily living and requires not other health care for the back pain. Yet, this is what patients want. When surveyed, patients with chronic low back pain indicate that although they consider 30% reductions in pain or disability worthwhile, they desire at least 80% reduction, if not complete relief.[97] General therapies do not meet these expectations.

DRUG THERAPY
Paracetamol (Acetaminophen)

For chronic low back pain, there is very low-quality evidence (based on a single trial that has been retracted) for no effect of paracetamol (acetaminophen).[98] No other studies have tested paracetamol for the treatment of chronic low back pain.[99] For acute low back pain, paracetamol has been shown to be no more effective than a placebo.[98,99]

Nonsteroidal Anti-inflammatory Drugs

For the relief of pain, nonsteroidal anti-inflammatory drugs (NSAIDs) have a small effect greater than that of placebo.[99,100] According to one review, the effect amounts to a mean difference in pain scores of 12/100, at 12 weeks after commencing treatment.[99] Another review calculated the difference to be on 3/100.[101] Compared with placebo, NSAIDs increase the chances of obtaining 30% relief of pain from about 30% to 50%.[99] Studies have detected no differences in effectiveness between different NSAIDs.

Muscle Relaxants

There is little evidence on which to base valid conclusions about the effectiveness of muscle relaxants for chronic low back pain.[99] A Cochrane review found muscle relaxants are effective for short-term symptomatic relief in patients with acute and chronic low back pain, but the incidence of drowsiness, dizziness, and other side effects is high, so muscle relaxants must be used with caution.[102]

Benzodiazepines

There are no long-term data on the effectiveness or otherwise of benzodiazepines.[100]

Antidepressants

In the treatment of chronic low back pain, tricyclic antidepressants and selective serotonin reuptake inhibitors are not more effective than placebo, for the relief of pain, or improving depression, or improving function.[99]

Recent studies have provided favorable results for duloxetine, a selective serotonin norepinephrine reuptake inhibitor (SSNRI) drug. It is significantly more effective than placebo for the relief of pain and for improving function, but the effect sizes are small.[99,100]

Pregabalin

Pregabalin has no effects greater than those of placebo for low back pain or associated disability.[99]

Opioids

In the short term, strong opioids achieve greater relief of pain than that from placebo. The effect is statistically significant, but its clinical significance is small, amounting to a mean difference of 1/10 for pain and for disability.[99,100] The same small superiority applies for tramadol and for buprenorphine patches.[99] No long-term data are available. Meanwhile, opioids have a higher risk than placebo for side effects such as nausea, dizziness, constipation, vomiting, and somnolence.[99]

PHYSICAL MODALITIES
Physiotherapy

Physiotherapy involves a range of physical modalities of treatment including massage; mobilization; traction; taping and provision of lumbar supports; and often heat, cold, laser, ultrasound, and various electrical therapies used singly or in combination at the individual physiotherapist's discretion. Some physiotherapists offer special forms of physiotherapy, such as McKenzie therapy, and some provide formal manual therapy, including spinal manipulation. The effectiveness of these modalities can best be considered singly.

Massage

A systematic review found very little evidence that massage is an effective treatment for chronic low back pain; patients with chronic low back pain had improvements in pain outcomes after massage but only briefly, and the relief was not sustained.[103] Massage provides small effects on disability, more than those achieved in usual care, at 12 weeks, but the magnitude of the difference reduces by 52 weeks.[104] Massage is significantly more effective than manual therapy, exercise, relaxation therapy, acupuncture, physiotherapy, or transcutaneous electrical nerve stimulation (TENS) in the short term.[104]

Traction

The latest systematic review found that "traction, either alone or in combination with other treatments, has little or no impact on pain intensity, functional status, global improvement or return to work among people with low back pain; there was no difference regarding the type of traction (manual or mechanical); side-effects reported included increased pain, aggravation of neurological signs and subsequent surgery."[105]

Manual Therapy

Manual therapy, the laying on of hands by a therapist to perform soft tissue stretching, joint mobilization, and spinal manipulation, has been one of the most frequently used modalities of treatment for many decades since it developed in the late 19th century. It is the main practice of several craft groups including osteopaths, chiropractors, and manipulative therapists (specially trained physiotherapists); it is also performed by many medical practitioners practicing musculoskeletal medicine, manual medicine, and physiatry. Over the years, manual therapy has developed an aura of mystique, and many patients with chronic low back pain view it as something they rely on for almost magical relief of their condition. By its advocates, manual therapy is promoted variously as a therapeutic skill based on special understanding of bodily functions or as an orthodox remedy for musculoskeletal dysfunction.

In fact, manual therapy achieves small but statistically nonsignificant effects on pain when compared with sham therapy.[104] It provides better short-term relief than other active therapies, but the differences between therapies are small. There is no evidence of lasting, long-term effects.[104]

A systematic review found "high quality evidence that there is no clinically relevant difference between spinal manipulative therapy and other interventions for reducing pain and improving function in patients with chronic low-back pain; spinal manipulative therapy appears to be as effective as other common therapies prescribed for chronic low-back pain, such as exercise therapy, standard medical care or physiotherapy."[106]

McKenzie Therapy

Systematic reviews have found limited evidence concerning the efficacy of McKenzie therapy for chronic low back pain.[107,108] Advocates of the treatment cite a study that showed no superiority over stabilization exercises and a study that showed slightly better outcomes than those of strengthening exercise at 2 months after treatment but not at 8 months.[109]

Transcutaneous Electrical Nerve Stimulation

TENS is often used as an adjunct in the management of low back pain. However, despite the widespread use of TENS machines, the analgesic effectiveness of TENS still remains uncertain.[110] A systematic review found "conflicting evidence regarding the benefits of TENS for chronic low back pain, which does not support the use of TENS in the routine management of chronic low back pain."[111]

Other Physical and Electrical Modalities

There is little published evidence for interferential, shortwave diathermy, ultrasound, laser, or taping.[104] Ultrasound is no more effective than sham therapy, and low-level laser therapy is only slightly better than sham laser therapy.[100] A systematic review of low-level laser found "there are insufficient data to either support or refute the effectiveness of low-level laser therapy for the treatment of non-specific low back pain."[112]

Lumbar Supports

The available evidence shows that lumbar supports provide no benefit in terms of pain relief; the authors of a systematic review reported that there was little or no difference in short-term pain reduction or overall improvement between patients with chronic low-back pain who used back supports and those who received no treatment.[113]

Exercise Therapy

The evidence on exercise therapy is mixed, depending on which studies are reviewed.[104] Some reviews have found that exercise therapy reduces pain by 10/100 more than having no exercises but offers no benefit for function. Other reviews have found that exercise therapy reduces pain by 9/100 more than does usual care and improves function by 12/100. Differences decrease to about 4/100 for pain and 3/100 for function in the long term. When compared with minimal interventions, exercise therapy provides the same differences in benefit.[104]

Proponents of high-intensity strengthening exercises have sought evidence of efficacy within the general literature on exercise for chronic low back pain but found no clear evidence of benefit over other exercises or other interventions such as physiotherapy and massage.[114] Others, likewise, found trunk-strengthening exercises to be more effective than no exercises but not more effective than aerobics or McKenzie treatment.[115]

Proponents of core stabilization exercises found moderate evidence that this form of exercise is effective in improving pain and function but strong evidence that it was not more effective than physiotherapy, manual therapy, general exercises, and minimal care.[116] Another review found that stabilization exercises were superior to usual medical care and education, but not to manipulative therapy, and no additional effect was found when stabilization exercises were added to a conventional physiotherapy program.[117]

Tai chi provides greater relief of pain than does being put on a waiting list but only by 10/100 points.[104] Low-quality evidence shows that yoga offers small effects on pain and function that are better than those achieved in usual care.[100,104]

SIMPLE NEEDLE TREATMENTS

Many practitioners offer a range of special needle treatments, including acupuncture, trigger point injection, and prolotherapy.

Some perform these as monotherapies, and others provide them in combination with other treatments within the framework of musculoskeletal medicine and physiatry.

Acupuncture

The only positive evidence of the effectiveness of acupuncture for chronic low back pain comes from trials that showed acupuncture was more effective than no acupuncture, but these benefits were evident only immediately after treatment and not beyond.[104] When compared with sham treatment, acupuncture is minimally more effective for reducing pain, but only immediately after treatment, and provides no better effect for improving function. There is no evidence of any lasting beneficial effects beyond the immediate effects of treatment.[104]

Trigger Point Injection

Trigger point injection is an intervention that has been popular with general practitioners and physiatrists because it requires no special equipment and is easy to perform in consulting rooms. Despite its popularity for the treatment of various musculoskeletal conditions, there are few studies of its efficacy, and even fewer of its efficacy specifically in patients with chronic low back pain.[118] Studies limited to immediate and short-term outcomes (7 days) report conflicting results. No studies have provided long-term data.

Prolotherapy

Prolotherapy involves the injection of sclerosing agents, such as hypertonic dextrose or phenol, into tender areas of the back muscles, ostensibly at muscle attachment sites.

Multiple reviews have found no evidence of efficacy for prolotherapy.[119–121] Studies of prolotherapy and cointerventions have found some positive results for the combination of treatments, but studies in which prolotherapy alone was tested have found only negative results.[121]

One study provided intriguing results[122]; it showed that prolotherapy was not significantly more effective than injections of normal saline; the success rates from either treatment were the same. However, at 12 months, 46% of patients had at least 50% relief from their chronic back pain, and 20% had complete relief. These outcomes—obtained in a randomized controlled trial—dwarf those of any other conservative therapy for chronic back pain. They prompted one review of drug therapy for back pain to conclude that the most powerful drug for the treatment of back pain appears to be normal saline delivered by charismatic injection.[123]

BACK SCHOOL

The evidence on back schools is low in quality and shows that back school is not more effective than no treatment.[124] It offers no benefits greater than those of usual care or physical therapy or exercises.

PSYCHOLOGICAL INTERVENTIONS

The evidence base shows that a patient with chronic low back pain has little if anything to gain from psychological therapies in terms of pain relief or even relief of psychological para-phenomena. A systematic review found that "overall there is an absence of evidence for behavior therapy, except a small improvement in mood immediately following treatment; cognitive behavioral therapy (CBT) has small positive effects on disability and catastrophizing, but not on pain or mood, when compared with active controls; CBT has small to moderate effects on pain, disability, mood and catastrophizing, immediately post-treatment when compared with waiting list, but all except a small effect on mood had disappeared at follow-up."[125]

Other reviews have not changed this summary. Psychology therapies, such as progressive relaxation, operant therapy, and CBT, are each slightly more effective than being put on a waiting list, by about 20/100 for pain, in the short term, but there are no long-term outcome data.[100,104] Adding psychology therapies to physiotherapy does not improve the outcomes achieved by physiotherapy alone.[104] Behavioral therapy is slightly more effective than usual care for the relief of pain in the short term but provides no benefit in the long term for either pain or function.[126] For pain or depression, the outcomes of behavioral therapy are not different from those of exercise, and adding behavioral therapy to an inpatient rehabilitation program provides no additional benefit.[127]

Mindfulness-based stress reduction offers improvements in pain that are greater, by 1/10, than those achieved under usual care, and similar improvements in function.[100,104] However, it is not shown to be better than CBT, which is only very slightly and temporarily more effective than being put on a waiting list.[100,104]

MULTIDISCIPLINARY PAIN MANAGEMENT

In its original form, multidisciplinary pain management involves the collaboration of practitioners of all relevant disciplines working closely as a team to manage patients with chronic pain. A pain physician elicits the patient's history and performs physical examination, radiologists assist by interpreting diagnostic imaging, nurses contribute their observations, physiotherapists and exercise physiologists assess any musculoskeletal disabilities, and a psychologist or psychiatrist assesses the patient's psychological state. Others, such as occupational therapists and social workers assess the patient's vocational, social, and financial situation. When all relevant diagnostic information is gathered, the team formulates a provisional diagnosis and applies diagnostic investigations such as nerve blocks and perhaps discography to develop a definitive diagnosis. Management is then undertaken with each team member contributing where they can help. The pain physician coordinates the management and provides pharmacologic interventions and perhaps other interventions such as specific, targeted needle treatments. Orthopedic surgeons and neurosurgeons provide surgical interventions, if indicated. Physiotherapists provide interventions in their realm and psychologists address affective issues. A rehabilitation physician supervises the patient's recovery and rehabilitation, with the help of occupational therapists and social workers, and perhaps assisted by an occupational physician to facilitate the patient's return to work. If required, additional specialists such as neurologists can also be involved in the management team.

Such an approach seems ideal as a concept, for it provides the patient with the best care available in each of the areas of need. Where such truly multidisciplinary pain clinics operate, outcomes are potentially as good as those achievable by all the disciplines involved. When first developed, this model of multidisciplinary pain management held promise as an appropriate way to handle complex problems such as chronic back pain, and multidisciplinary pain management soon became the iconic, preferred method of care.

Unfortunately, that ideal model has been subverted in many places by those who seek to assume the expertise of a large multidisciplinary team but in fact focus on only two or three disciplines, most commonly psychologists and physiotherapists with a physician as nominal leader. Such people operate what they call "pain clinics" that claim to take the biopsychosocial approach to chronic pain but actually focus mainly if not exclusively on the psychological and social domains of a patient's problem and largely or totally ignore the biologic domain. In such "multidisciplinary biopsychosocial rehabilitation," there is usually no attempt at specific diagnosis, the underlying belief being that chronic pain is essentially of psychological origin and is best treated with psychological interventions, with perhaps input from a physiotherapist to make the treatment seem holistic.

The belief that chronic pain is psychological stems from early in the second half of the 20th century, when scientific knowledge of the neuroanatomy and pathology of the lumbar spine was sparse. In the 1950s and 1960s, some authors promoted the psychoanalytic concept that intractable pain is a defense against unconscious psychic conflict.[127,128] Chronic pain was attributed to repressed hostility and aggression, guilt, resentment, loss, masked depression, and various personality disorders. Behavioral therapy was advocated as a means of managing chronic low back pain defined in that way. This model of pain was reinforced by the belief that chronic low back pain has no physical cause.

Over the 50 years since these beliefs were first espoused, research has either refuted or dispelled each of these beliefs. Multiple studies have shown that a source of pain can be established, in the majority of patients with chronic low back pain, if appropriate investigations are undertaken. Meanwhile, the concepts of chronic pain being due to psychological abnormalities, although eloquently espoused, have not found support from evidence, particularly from controlled studies.[128] Thus, "multidisciplinary" clinics that purport to manage chronic pain without pursuing biomedical diagnosis operate on a false premise, and the outcome data show they do not provide any clinically significant relief, and certainly not total and enduring relief, of chronic low back pain.

Another belief on which "multidisciplinary biopsychosocial rehabilitation" is based is the idea that once pain becomes chronic, the process of central sensitization occurs, and the pain becomes permanent and intractable, in effect a permanent disease in its own right.[129] This contention has been refuted explicitly by several studies[130–133]; it is also refuted implicitly by the many studies which show chronic low back pain can be eliminated, with restoration of function and no need for ongoing health care.

In relation to effectiveness, a systematic review of the current evidence on "multidisciplinary biopsychosocial rehabilitation" shows it is barely more effective than usual care in reducing pain and disability, with outcomes of 0.5 to 1.4 units on a 0 to 10 numerical rating scale for pain and 1.4 to 2.5 on the 0 to 24 Roland-Morris disability scale.[134]

A systematic review of the current evidence on behavioral therapy for patients with chronic low back pain shows little or no difference between behavioral treatment and group exercise either for relieving pain or for alleviating depressive symptoms.[126] A recent systematic review of the current evidence on psychological therapies for low back pain found "overall there is an absence of evidence for behavior therapy, except a small improvement in mood immediately following treatment; cognitive behavioral therapy (CBT) has small positive effects on disability and catastrophizing, but not on pain or mood, when compared with active controls; CBT has small to moderate effects on pain, disability, mood and catastrophizing, immediately post-treatment when compared with waiting list, but all except a small effect on mood had disappeared at follow-up."[125]

Referring doctors need to be aware of the skills, outcomes, and reputation of any clinic to which they may send their patients. Worthwhile clinics are not defined by using the title "multidisciplinary"; they are defined by the outcomes they achieve. A truly multidisciplinary approach to the management of patients with chronic low back pain has the potential to address all problems in the biologic, psychological, and social domains of chronic pain. However, patients and practitioners should not be hoodwinked into trying an intervention that is similar in name only. The summary of the evidence on "multidisciplinary biopsychosocial rehabilitation" is that it does little or nothing to help patients with chronic low back pain; socalled "pain clinics," which use that approach are misnamed because they do not address pain, let alone relieve it.

FUNCTIONAL RESTORATION

Functional restoration is also "multidisciplinary" in nature, but it was more prompted by the discipline of sports medicine than by psychology. It arose from the proposition that injured workers could rehabilitate by work hardening in the way that athletes are known to overcome musculoskeletal injuries by concerted training and perseverance.[135] The objective was to restore function, virtually regardless of the pain.

It has become difficult to disentangle functional restoration from "multidisciplinary biopsychosocial rehabilitation," particularly when it comes to the literature on efficacy. So-called "multidisciplinary biopsychosocial rehabilitation" has adopted some of the principles and practices of functional restoration, particularly those of intensive training, whereas functional restoration has adopted behavioral therapy from "multidisciplinary biopsychosocial rehabilitation." It is unclear the extent to which behavioral therapy is a critical component of functional restoration, but the evidence of its ineffectiveness is as quoted earlier[126]; the evidence on a group program of exercise and education using a cognitive-behavioral approach shows it is not significantly more effective than providing an educational booklet.[136]

SPECIFIC, TARGETED TREATMENTS

For certain sources of pain, minimally invasive treatments can be used to relieve that pain. These treatments are the ones that involved penetrating the body with needles electrodes, or other devices, but without actually opening the body in order to achieve access. The rationale for minimally invasive treatments is that if the source or cause of back pain can be identified, then rectifying the cause, ablating the cause, or ablating the nerves that innervate the source should relieve the patient's pain (and any disabilities caused by that pain). Minimally invasive therapies are, therefore, target specific and can be addressed according to their target.

Discogenic Pain

Discogenic low back pain is pain arising from an intervertebral disk. Ostensibly, it is caused by stimulation of nociceptors in the disk that are stimulated by internal chemical processes or mechanical loading of the anulus fibrosis. The cardinal cause is internal disk disruption (see Chapter 101).

A variety of interventions have been explored for the management of lumbar discogenic pain. Variously, they target the pathology of internal disk disruption at a macroscopic or molecular level or target the nerves that transduce the pain. They involve coagulating fissures in the anulus fibrosis or the nociceptors around them, injecting chemicals intended to antagonize degradative processes in the disk, and injecting "biologics" designed to inhibit cytokines and proteolytic enzymes and to promote healing of connective tissues. These interventions and their effectiveness are covered in detail in Chapter 101 and are only summarized briefly here. In essence, however, none has been proven to be effective, as promised by the rationale for minimally invasive treatments.

Intradiscal Therapies

Of the treatments that use coagulation, intradiscal biacuplasty has been shown to be more effective than usual care, but it is successful in only a proportion of patients and only to a small degree. Although fair to reasonable success rates have been reported for other ablative therapies for the relief of pain, none has yet been vindicated in terms of restoring function and eliminating the need for other health care.

For various chemical therapies, the literature shows that intradiscal steroids are not effective, and etanercept has only short-term effects. Open-label studies have not been able to reproduce the outcomes reported in a controlled trial of methylene blue, and good results reported for proliferants have not been reproduced by anyone else.

Studies of biologics are in their infancy. For agents such as fibrin sealant, platelet-rich plasma, and α_2-macroglobulin, pilot studies have announced modest, positive outcomes, but rigorous controlled studies have not been conducted. An open-label study reported good results from intradiscal injection of stem cells, but a controlled trial found no convincing superiority over sham therapy.

In effect, although many investigators have promoted or evaluated intradiscal treatments specifically targeting painful disks, none has yet been proven to be a useful solution to this common source of chronic low back pain.

Epidural Injection of Corticosteroid

Epidural injections of corticosteroids, by the caudal or interlaminar route, have been used extensively to treat lumbar radicular pain, for which they had a reputation of effectiveness (see Chapter 99). Because of this reputation, and because they are relatively easy to perform, they have also been used to treat presumed discogenic back pain. The evidence shows that such injections are no more effective than epidural injections of local anesthetic.[137–139] Injection of either agent may be palliative for a limited period, but neither has been shown to provide lasting relief. Notionally, chronic low back pain might be palliated by repeated caudal or interlaminar blocks, but the efficacy, safety, and cost-effectiveness of perpetual blocks have not been established.

Meanwhile, epidural injections are not without dangers. Complications and side effects of caudal injections include dural puncture, increased intracranial pressure, nerve damage, vascular injury, hematoma formation, cerebrovascular or pulmonary embolism, intravascular injection, intracranial air injection, chemical meningitis, arachnoiditis, infection, abscess formation, increased back pain, and increased leg pain, among others.[140] Unwanted effects of interlaminar epidural injections of steroid reported include epidural hematomas; spinal cord or cauda equina injuries; infectious complications such as epidural abscess, meningitis, discitis, and osteomyelitis; dural puncture; subdural air; pneumocephalus; arterial gas embolism; seizures; transient blindness; retinal necrosis; chorioretinopathy; stroke; chemical meningitis; and increased pain.[141]

Transforaminal Injection of Steroid

Transforaminal injection of steroids (TFIS) offers the prospect of delivering corticosteroids across the back of a painful disk. In that location, they putatively can combat the inflammatory effects of exudates from the disk into the retrodiscal, epidural space, and if they diffuse into the disk, they could exert the same effects within the disk. Given that steroids have a local anesthetic effect,[142] TFIS could also block the sinuvertebral nerves that innervate the posterior disk. A suitable indication for such injections would be relief of pain following bilateral diagnostic blocks of the four sinuvertebral nerves that principally supply the disk.

Evidence for the effectiveness of TFIS for discogenic low back pain is only in its infancy. A small pilot study, published only as a university thesis, showed that TFIS was moderately effective in patients with discogenic chronic low back pain but no radicular pain.[143] With success defined as complete or at least good relief on the Oxford Pain Chart scale, 81% (95% CI, 66% to 96%) of 27 patients had a successful outcome at 1 week, and 52% (95% CI, 33% to 71%) at 6 weeks, after a single TFIS treatment.

Zygapophysial Joint Pain

Intra-articular Steroids

Zygapophysial joint pain has been, and still is, treated by intra-articular injection of steroid. However, this treatment was never been evaluated in patients with back pain proven to arise from the zygapophysial joints.[144] It is not surprising, therefore, that multiple controlled trials have found it to be no more effective than sham therapy.[41,145,146]

Facet Joint Nerve Blocks

For patients with positive responses to controlled diagnostic blocks of the lumbar medial branches, some physicians advocate repeating the blocks as a treatment, whenever the pain returns.[147] This intervention amounts to converting a diagnostic procedure into a therapeutic one. The outcomes are the same regardless of whether steroids are added or not to the local anesthetic agent used.[147]

Patients can obtain at least 50% relief of pain, for several weeks after each injection, but the treatment is not curative.[147] Blocks need to be repeated in order to maintain relief. However, although pain can be reduced, the treatment makes little to no difference in terms of return to work or use of opioids for pain.[147]

Lumbar Medial Branch Thermal Radiofrequency Neurotomy

Lumbar medial branch thermal RFN is a procedure designed to treat pain stemming from one or more lumbar zygapophysial joints. It involves coagulating the nerves that innervate the painful joint, using electrodes that generate a heat lesion around their tip (Fig. 73.6).

The procedure advocated by the International Spine Intervention Society, and described in its Practice Guidelines,[148] was developed over many years on the basis of anatomical studies, laboratory studies, and pilot clinical studies. In particular, the technique described recognizes the importance of placing electrodes parallel to the target nerve, to ablate the nerve adequately and along a maximal length; using a large-gauge (16 gauge) electrode placed at multiple sites, in order to accommodate variations in the location of the nerve; and creating multiple lesions over the nerve at 80° C. Furthermore, the indication for the procedure is complete, or near complete, relief of pain following controlled diagnostic blocks of the target nerve.[148]

This procedure was validated in an early benchmark study.[149] That study showed that at 12 months after treatment, some 60% of patients had 80% relief of their pain, and 80% of patients had 60% relief. It also showed denervation in the myotomes of multifidus that were innervated by the target nerves, which meant that the procedure had adequately coagulated those nerves.

A larger benchmark study has since corroborated and extended these outcomes. The study was conducted in two neighboring practices.[150] The data from each practice differed only in that one practice performed treatments over a longer period of survey and performed more repeat treatments when pain recurred. Patients were selected on the basis of complete relief of pain following comparative local anesthetic blocks.

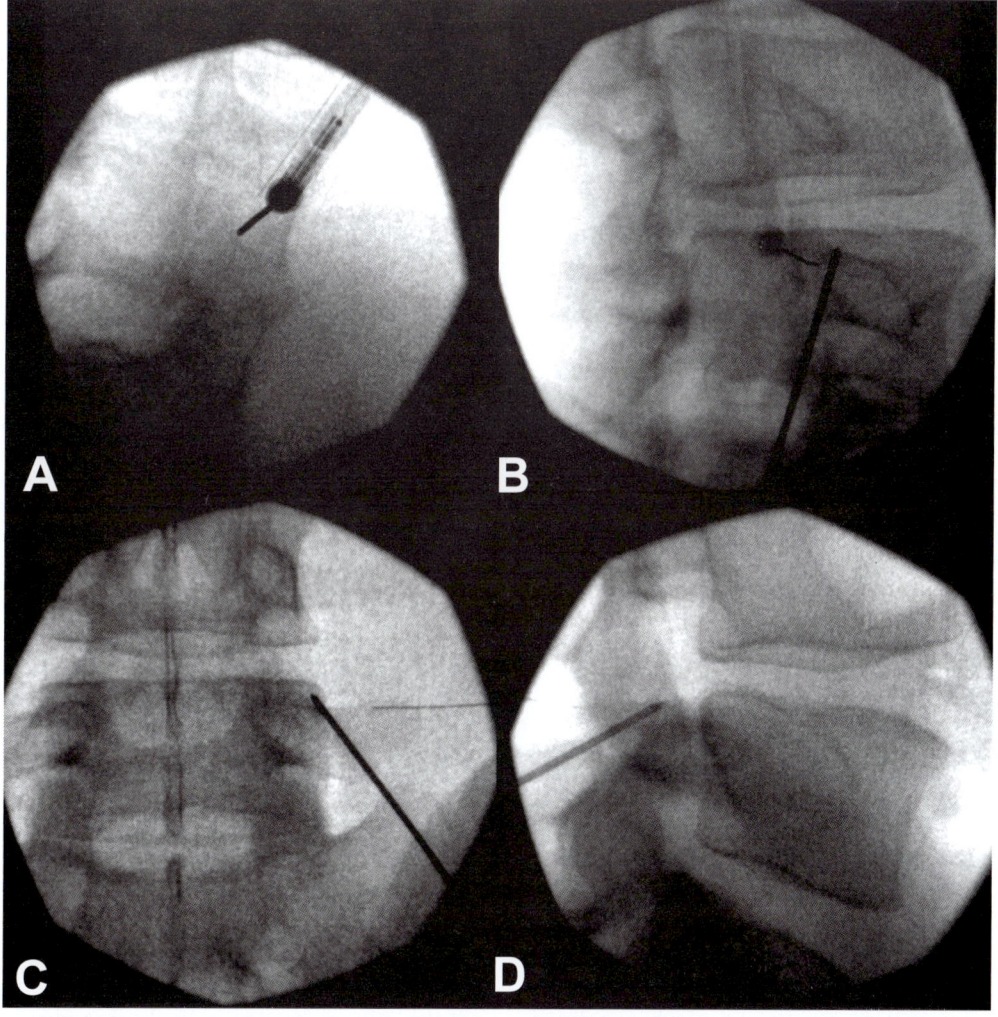

FIGURE 73.6 Fluoroscopy views of an electrode placed for radiofrequency coagulation of a right L4 medial branch. **A:** Declined view showing the electrode crossing the neck of the L5 superior articular process. **B:** Oblique view showing the electrode crossing the superior articular process as far as the rostral edge of the transverse process of L5. **C:** Posterior view showing the abducted trajectory of the electrode, which is applied against the neck of the superior articular process. **D:** Lateral view showing that the active tip of the electrode lies opposite the middle two quarters of the neck of the superior articular process. *(Images reproduced with permission from Bogduk N, ed.* Practice Guidelines for Spinal Diagnostic and Treatment Procedures. *2nd ed. San Francisco, CA: International Spine Intervention Society; 2013.)*

Successful outcome was defined as complete relief of pain, accompanied by restoration of activities of daily living, and no need for continuing care for back pain. In the two practices, the initial success rates were 58% (44% to 72%) and 53% (40% to 66%). In the first practice, the median duration of relief from the first treatment was 15 months, with an interquartile range of 10 to 28 months. In the second practice, the corresponding figures were 15 (10 to 29) months. Repeat treatments were performed to reinstate relief if pain recurred after the first treatment. A total of 35 treatments in 29 patients were performed in the first practice, and 66 treatments in 30 patients in the second practice, resulting in a median duration of relief, per treatment, of 13 months, over a 5-year period.

This study is the only one that has achieved complete relief of back pain, coupled with restoration of function, and eliminated of any other health care. It sets the benchmark for outcomes from lumbar RFN. Critically, however, it assiduously followed the guidelines for selecting patients and for technique used.[148] Patients were treated only if they reported complete relief of pain from controlled, diagnostic blocks, and meticulous surgical technique was used. These outcomes have never been matched by any other study, but no other study has followed the same rigorous guidelines for selecting patients or for surgical technique.

Other studies, including controlled trials, have selected patients on the basis of single diagnostic blocks, with the definition of a positive response being 70% relief in one study[151] and only 50% or less in others.[152–156] Single blocks incur a high false-positive rate,[36–38,92,157,158] and they do not identify the 30% or so of patients who fail to get any relief when blocks are simply repeated.[159] Therefore, studies that used single blocks to select patients for lumbar RFN must have been confounded by patients who did not have the condition for which they were treated, which would substantially decrease their success rate. This effect could only be compounded by using 50% relief for the definition of a positive block.

Three controlled trials[153,160,161] placed their electrodes at locations remote from any nerve. Therefore, by definition, they performed a sham treatment. The controlled trials that did this amount to comparing one sham with another. Other controlled trials did not disclose where they placed their electrodes.[154]

Two controlled trials[152,155] placed electrodes perpendicular to the target nerve. Doing so does not necessarily prevent coagulation of the nerve, but the coagulation would be limited in length, which reduces the duration of effect. The studies would underestimate the duration of effect and would be compromised for showing differences between treatments over time.

Mixed in with the literature on thermal RFN, which applies lesions to the target nerve at 80° C, are reports of "pulsed RFN" which uses electrodes placed well away from the target nerve and heated to only 41° C, with indifferent results.[156]

The studies with these technical and procedural flaws do not constitute valid evidence of the effectiveness or otherwise of lumbar thermal RFN, more so when a study has multiple flaws, such as suboptimal selection of patients and suboptimal surgical technique. Yet, almost all of the literature on lumbar RFN is so affected. Most egregious in this regard is the fact that authors of reviews have ignored these technical flaws and wide variations of technique, despite having been warned about them in the literature,[162,163] and despite the authors of one controlled trial having acknowledged the flaws of their own study.[164] The negative conclusions of reviews are not valid if they are based on flawed studies. Those conclusions might well apply to lumbar RFN when performed poorly, but they do not apply to lumbar thermal RFN being performed correctly in appropriately selected patients.

The latter theme has been highlighted when authors of controlled trials have responded to letters to the editor criticizing their studies. In particular, on two occasions now, studies have been criticized for inaccurate surgical technique and for poor selection of patients.[162,165–167] In both instances, the authors expressly replied that they studied how lumbar RFN was practiced in The Netherlands.[168,169] Consequently, their results cannot be generalized to how lumbar RFN is practiced elsewhere and especially not when it is practiced according to the International Spine Intervention Society guidelines.[148]

Only two controlled trials have used correct surgical technique, but both were compromised by patient selection. The study of Tekin et al.[156] selected patients on the basis of a single diagnostic block. This would have compromised the success rate of their treatment but would not have compromised the comparison with a credible sham treatment—because the study was randomized. It showed a clear superiority of success rates in favor of lumbar RFN. The study of Nath et al.[170] used comparative blocks to select patients, but those patients had concurrent, other pain problems, such as radicular pain. So, complete relief of pain and restoration of function could not be achieved in this sample. Nevertheless, insofar as the patients could distinguish their back pains from their other pains, those who underwent active treatment report greater improvements in pain, greater reduction in use of analgesics, and greater global satisfaction than those treated with sham therapy.

Sacroiliac Pain

Sacroiliac pain includes pain stemming from the sacroiliac joint and pain stemming from its posterior ligaments. The quest for effective treatments is hampered by confusion between sacroiliac joint pain and sacroiliac ligament pain. The two conditions differ with respect to the structures that are the source of pain, and the means by which the two conditions can be diagnosed. Yet, in many published trials of possible treatments, this distinction has not been made. So, it is not evident which condition was being treated or, indeed, if the patients did, in fact, have sacroiliac pain of either type.

Sacroiliac Joint Injection of Steroids

The mainstay for treating sacroiliac joint pain has been intra-articular injection of steroids. The attraction of this form of treatment is that it is relatively simple to perform, for anyone with an access to a fluoroscope (or CT scanner). Moreover, there is no proven alternative treatment for sacroiliac joint pain, although other methods have been tried.

The reputation of intra-articular steroids for sacroiliac joint pain rests on descriptive studies, of various degrees of quality, that report various degrees of success for short or longer periods.[171,172] The best quality, outcome study investigated 150 patients with presumptive sacroiliac joint pain based on clinical examination.[173] All underwent a first intra-articular injection of bupivacaine and triamcinolone, from which 88 had at least 75% pain relief. Of these 88, 58 underwent a second injection of the same agents, from which 39 had relief again. Of these 39 patients, 13 had at least 50% relief that lasted less than 6 weeks, but 26 (45%) had relief that lasted longer than 6 weeks (36.8 ± 9.9 weeks).

This study hints that intra-articular steroids might be a useful treatment for sacroiliac joint pain, but several caveats apply. For a condition for which there is no other treatment, the modest success rate (45%) is notionally tolerable. The limited duration of relief (36 weeks) is also tolerable, for the treatment could be repeated if pain recurred.[171] However, the definition of success (50% relief) is weak. No studies have produced evidence that this limited degree of relief reduces the burden of illness. No studies have shown that reducing sacroiliac joint pain by 50% is enough to restore function to reasonable levels and to reduce, if not eliminate, the need for other health care.

More rigorous data are required before intra-articular steroids can be promoted as a mainstream treatment for sacroiliac joint pain. Without such evidence, this treatment is destined to remain contentious, for pundits and those who pay for treatment will not be able to distinguish between something that physicians do and something from which patients genuinely benefit to a worthwhile degree.

Sacral Lateral Branch Neurotomy

Sacral lateral branch thermal RFN is a procedure in which the lateral branches of the S1–S3 dorsal rami are coagulated with radiofrequency electrodes. Rationale for this treatment should be to relieve pain stemming from the posterior sacroiliac ligaments, and the indication should be complete relief of pain following controlled, diagnostic blocks of the target nerves, but this has not been expressed in the literature.

The literature is both confused and confusing.[53] Sacral lateral branch RFN was portrayed, adopted, and is still applied as a treatment for sacroiliac joint pain. In nearly all studies of this procedure, the initial indication for treatment has been a positive response to injections of local anesthetic and steroid into the sacroiliac joint.[53] Indeed, a recent Appropriate Use Criteria for sacroiliac procedures[174] reinforced this attitude. It maintained that if sacroiliac joint pain was diagnosed by an intra-articular block, it would be appropriate to entertain treatment by sacral lateral branch RFN, and the next step would be to perform sacral lateral branch blocks. This recommendation portrays intra-articular blocks and lateral branch blocks as complementary, but they are not.[175]

It has been shown in normal volunteers that anesthetizing the sacral lateral branches protects subjects from posterior ligament pain, but it does not protect them from sacroiliac joint pain.[54] Consequently, sacral lateral branch RFN cannot be a logical treatment for sacroiliac joint pain. It is a logical treatment only for posterior sacroiliac ligament pain. Under those conditions, intra-articular blocks are immaterial and irrelevant.[175] They have no role in the selection of patients for sacral lateral branch RFN. The sole indication for sacral lateral branch RFN becomes relief of pain following controlled blocks of the sacral lateral branches.

Because of this confusion, most studies of sacral lateral branch RFN are ill founded. Three studies[176–178] selected patients on the basis of positive responses to a single SIJB. Four studies required two intra-articular SIJBs.[179–182] None of these blocks constitute evidence that the patients had pain that might be relieved by sacral lateral branch RFN. Therefore, the outcomes reported amount to no more than what to expect when the procedure is performed arbitrarily in patients with sacroiliac joint pain.

Two studies selected patients on the basis of an initial intra-articular SIJB and a subsequent lateral branch block.[183,184] Neither of the blocks was controlled. Under this protocol, the intra-articular block was irrelevant, but the lateral branch block at least provided prima facie evidence that the patients had pain from the posterior ligament complex. However, because the lateral branch blocks were not controlled, uncertain is the extent to which responses were contaminated by false-positive responses.

In those studies,[183,184] 56% and 52% of patients reported at least 50% relief of pain at 9 months and at 6 months, respectively. This is a modest outcome both in terms of success rate and in terms of degree of relief. The pilot study[183] reported only on relief of pain. The later study[184] reported that disability scores also improved, but only 23% of patients reduced their opioid use.

Only one study has selected patients solely on the basis of lateral branch blocks.[96] The blocks were not controlled, but patients had to report at least 75% relief on both occasions that a block using bupivacaine was performed. The patients were randomized to active or sham treatment. At 6 months after sacral lateral branch RFN, 27% of patients had greater than 50% relief of pain, and 18% reported being totally free of pain. At 9 months, these figures were 52% and 15%. The proportion of patients who achieved good outcomes at 1 month was nearly six times greater than that of patients who underwent sham therapy, but the small sample size prevented demonstrating an absolute statistically significant difference. This study constitutes the only evidence for sacroiliac joint pain RFN in appropriately selected patients.

Although the development of sacral lateral branch RFN was inspired by the success of cervical and lumbar medial branch neurotomy, the outcomes of lateral branch neurotomy have not mirrored those achieved by medial branch neurotomy. Most studies have reported only the achievement of 50% relief of pain. The one study that most closely adhered to the rationale for lateral branch neurotomy[96] achieved complete relief of pain in only 18% of patients. The reason for this low yield is not known. There may be limitations to surgical technique, or it may be that 75% relief from diagnostic blocks, and not using controls, is not a sufficiently rigorous selection criterion. For medial branch neurotomy, the best outcomes have been achieved after complete relief of pain following controlled diagnostic blocks (see "Lumbar Medial Branch Thermal Radiofrequency Neurotomy" section in the preceding text).

A systematic review rated the evidence on sacral lateral branch RFN as moderate.[53] The treatment seems effective for providing some relief of pain mediated by sacral lateral branches, but that relief is limited in extent and duration, and the indications for the procedure are unclear.

INVASIVE TREATMENTS

Invasive treatments are ones in which the body must be opened and entered. In the context of chronic low back pain, invasive treatments are those in which subcutaneous pockets are created for the implantation of devices and those in which the lumbar spine is exposed for direct access.

Implanted Devices

For the control of severe, chronic low back pain unresponsive to any other treatment, devices can be implanted to deliver drugs intrathecally or to provide spinal cord stimulation. Intrathecal drugs and spinal cord stimulators are not routine treatments for uncomplicated chronic low back pain. Typically, they have been reserved for the treatment of patients in whom surgery has failed to provide relief and whose diagnosis has become failed back surgery syndrome. The assessment and treatment of these patients is described in Chapter 75.

Spinal Surgery

In the past, surgery had a reputation as a successful treatment for chronic low back pain. However, because surgery is a major undertaking with serious hazards, it was reserved for patients in whom conservative therapy had failed, as a "last port of call."

The reputation of surgery was established by the early literature, which claimed high success rates for the treatment of low back pain. With the advent of evidence-based medicine, the tenor of that literature has changed (see Chapter 74). Randomized controlled trials showed firstly that surgery was not substantially more effective than concerted conservative care, and secondly that, although it might improve pain and function, surgery was not curative. The language in the literature changed from success rates in terms of patients free of pain and not using analgesics to success rates for achieving only a minimal clinically important change, with patients still taking opioids.

As with other interventions, the selection of patients is a critical factor in determining the outcomes of spinal surgery. Operations performed on the indications of imaging findings are doomed to failure in proportion to the extent that imaging findings do not correlate with pain. Despite this, many surgeons continue to operate on "bulging disks" as if this is a sufficient diagnostic criterion for the cause of pain, with predictable results for their unfortunate patients.

The literature on the effectiveness of surgery for chronic low back pain is explored in greater detail in Chapter 74. In essence, the contemporary evidence shows that surgery offers the prospect of some degree of relief of pain, greater on average than that offered by conservative therapies, but absent from the modern literature are any data on success rates for achieving complete relief of pain, or sufficient relief to restore function and eliminate the need for further health care. The effectiveness of surgery is contentious. Indeed, in the United Kingdom, the National Institute for Health and Care Excellence has decreed that surgery for back pain should be performed only in the context of a controlled trial.[185] Disk stimulation might be required for entry into such trials, but there is no justification for it to be a part of routine practice.

Conclusion

Patients with chronic low back pain wants their pain to be relieved completely.[97] Against this standard, the literature reflects the parlous state of medical science for the treatment of chronic low back pain. Treatments and interventions for which there was enthusiasm in the past have proved not to be real answers. However, there are some treatments that do provide satisfactory outcomes, and those options can be considered as general and specific.

General measures are available for practitioners who cannot apply specific, targeted interventions (or refer patients for them) and for those patients who for any reason will not undergo specific, targeted treatment. General treatment options vary greatly in their effectiveness. Those used more commonly include drugs, physical modalities, exercises, singular needle treatments, and "multidisciplinary biopsychosocial rehabilitation."

No drugs eliminate chronic low back pain. Analgesics are at best palliative and might be used for maintenance care. It is questionable whether NSAIDs should be used. They provide benefits only marginally greater than those of a placebo, but they carry risks of side effects and complications that cannot be ignored. Opioids also offer minimal benefits greater than those of placebo, and side effects are common. By trial and error, a practitioner might find patients who can tolerate side effects and for whom opioids provide a satisfactory level of relief. Unfortunately, care has to be taken to avoid the problem of tolerance, let alone the ever-growing problem of diversion. Duloxetine may prove to be a viable alternative.

Physical modalities offer temporary relief, especially of the muscular stiffness that often accompanies chronic low back pain. Massage is more effective than physiotherapy, manual therapy, exercise, acupuncture, or TENS for relief in the short term. Ultrasound treatment and TENS are no more effective than sham therapy, and low-level laser therapy is only slightly better than sham laser therapy. There is little published evidence for interferential, shortwave diathermy, or taping. Lumbar supports confer no benefit.

Contemporary guidelines advocate exercise as preferred management for chronic low back pain.[100,186–188] The effectiveness of exercise, however, is only palliative. Massage might be employed for respite relief. Psychological therapy might help patients for the stress that they suffer and might be used for this purpose, but in that event, the indication for referral is stress not pain.

"Multidisciplinary biopsychosocial rehabilitation" has been proven both inappropriate and ineffective for relief of chronic low back pain. It is inappropriate because the main beliefs on which it was founded have been proven false. The belief that a cause cannot be found in over 80% of patients with chronic low back pain has been shown clearly to be false. The belief that chronic pain becomes permanent and intractable, and a disease in its own right, has also been shown to be false. Otherwise, no studies have produced data that show that "multidisciplinary biopsychosocial rehabilitation" provides any clinically significant benefit.

No general treatment has been proven, on a regular basis, to abolish pain or reduce it to tolerable levels, restore function, and eliminate the need for further health care. At best, various general therapies might reduce pain by a modest or small degree and improve function slightly, but this amounts to palliative care.

The patient may well have associated problems in other domains: the psychological and social phenomena that may coexist with chronic low back pain, but those are secondary problems that may resolve or be greatly diminished if the pain is eliminated. Caring practitioners will address, or have addressed, the psychological and social concomitants of chronic pain if they impact on the patient sufficiently to warrant specific treatment, but doing so is not a surrogate for treating the pain.

Special investigations can be undertaken to determine the cause or source of pain in a large proportion of patients. Establishing a definitive diagnosis can rationalize management, by preventing an aimless and futile pursuit of a cure, and it may, but does not necessarily, lead to a successful specific treatment.

For investigations to be clinically useful, they need to be conducted rationally and in a valid manner. Even in the published literature, this has not always been the case. Unknown is the extent to which investigations in conventional practice are conducted in a valid manner. Failure to do so compromises the outcomes of subsequent treatment and tarnishes the reputation of the investigation and the associated treatment.

Although clinics might offer diagnostic blocks, they do not necessarily perform them according to established guidelines. Diagnostic blocks involve more than just placing a needle and injecting a small volume of local anesthetic. Patients need to be assessed and informed of the purpose of the procedure and the protocol to be followed. That protocol needs to be rigorous and disciplined, for which reason detailed guidelines have been published.[89,94]

MRI serves two purposes. It can provide "clearance" of serious causes of back pain, and with reasonable confidence, it can identify many cases of discogenic pain. Disk stimulation can be used to establish a diagnosis of discogenic pain but is not indicated for routine practice. It can be reserved for special instances, such as when a particular disk needs to be targeted for specific therapy.

However, no treatment for discogenic pain has yet been properly validated. Intradiscal therapies are at best experimental. Ablative treatments have not proved successful. Intradiscal injection of biologic agents is still being explored. Surgery might be entertained, but surgery carries no guarantee of success.

Lumbar zygapophysial joint pain can be diagnosed using controlled medial branch blocks. These are simple procedures and pose little or no hazard when performed competently. The problem, however, is that lumbar zygapophysial joint pain is not common, especially in younger patients. Consequently, it is appropriate to start with screening blocks, in order to identify the majority of patients who are going to have negative responses. If screening blocks are negative, no further pursuit of zygapophysial joint pain is indicated. If the blocks are positive, additional blocks will need to be performed to refine the diagnosis and confirm it. Patients who prove positive to controlled blocks can be treated with lumbar thermal RFN.

If performed meticulously, in correctly selected patients, lumbar thermal RFN is the one treatment that has been shown to be capable of providing complete relief of pain, accompanied by restoration of function, and elimination of further health care. If it is to be successful, it must be thermal RFN not "pulsed radiofrequency."[148] A useful precaution for any referral to a clinic offering radiofrequency treatment is to ask for the guidelines that the clinic follows, the information it gives to its patients, the diagnostic strategies and the assessment instruments that it uses, and the details of the RFN procedure(s) it provides. Such documents provide a prima facie appraisal of the integrity of the clinic.

Sacroiliac joint pain can be investigated using intra-articular diagnostic blocks. Posterior sacroiliac ligament pain can be investigated using sacral lateral branch blocks. In both instances, a single block will rule out the condition if the response is negative. If the block is positive, and confirmed by controls, the patient becomes a potential candidate for treatment. Sacroiliac joint pain could be treated with intra-articular steroids. Sacroiliac ligament pain could be treated with sacral lateral branch RFN. In both instances, whether or not it is worthwhile to pursue a 50% chance of getting 50% relief for 6 months or so is matter for discussion between the physician, the patient, and those who shall pay for the treatment. More rigorous studies could either refute these treatments or refine their disciplined application.

Many other "treatments" for chronic low back pain have not been addressed in this chapter because there is no evidence by which they can be evaluated. Yet, they are still practiced. In this regard, Dr. Archie Cochrane, the founder of evidence-based medicine, once posed the rhetorical question, "I wonder how many things are done in medicine because they can be, rather than because they should be?"[189]

References

1. Merskey H, Bogduk N, eds. *Classification of Chronic Pain. Descriptions of Chronic pain Syndromes and Definitions of Pain Terms.* 2nd ed. Seattle, WA: IASP Press; 1994.
2. van Tulder MW, Koes BW, Bouter LM. Conservative treatment of acute and chronic nonspecific low back pain: a systematic review of randomized controlled trials of the most common interventions. *Spine* 1997;22:2128–2156.
3. Waddell G. *The Back Pain Revolution.* Edinburgh: Churchill Livingstone; 1998.
4. Bogduk N. On the definitions and physiology of back pain, referred, pain and radicular pain. *Pain* 2009;147:17–19.
5. Mooney V, Robertson J. The facet syndrome. *Clin Orthop* 1976;115:149–156.
6. O'Neill CW, Kurgansky ME, Derby R, et al. Disc stimulation and patterns of referred pain. *Spine* 2002;27:2776–2781.
7. Smyth MJ, Wright V. Sciatica and the intervertebral disc. An experimental study. *J Bone Joint Surg* 1959;40A:1401–1418.
8. Norlen G. On the value of the neurological symptoms in sciatica for the localization of a lumbar disc herniation. *Acta Chir Scandinav* 1944;95(suppl):1–96.
9. McCall IW, Park WM, O'Brien JP. Induced pain referred from posterior lumbar elements in normal subjects. *Spine* 1979;4:441–446.
10. Fukui S, Ohseto K, Shiotani M, et al. Distribution of referred pain from the lumbar zygapophyseal joints and dorsal rami. *Clin J Pain* 1997;13:303–307.
11. Kellgren JH. Observations on referred pain arising from muscle. *Clin Sci* 1938;3:175–190.
12. Bogduk N. Lumbar dorsal ramus syndrome. *Med J Aust* 1980;2:537–541.
13. Kellgren JH. On the distribution of pain arising from deep somatic structures with charts of segmental pain areas. *Clin Sci* 1939;4:35–46.
14. Feinstein B, Langton JN, Jameson RM, et al. Experiments on pain referred from deep structures. *J Bone Joint Surg* 1954;36A:981–997.
15. Fortin JD, Dwyer AP, West S, et al. Sacroiliac joint: pain referral maps upon applying a new injection/arthrography technique: part I: asymptomatic volunteers. *Spine* 1994;19:1475–1482.
16. Wiberg G. Back pain in relation to the nerve supply of the intervertebral disc. *Acta Orthop Scandinav* 1947;19:211–221.
17. Falconer MA, McGeorge M, Begg AC. Observations on the cause and mechanism of symptom-production in sciatica and low-back pain. *J Neurol Neurosurg Psychiat* 1948;11:13–26.
18. Kuslich SD, Ulstrom CL, Michael CJ. The tissue origin of low back pain and sciatica: a report of pain response to tissue stimulation during operations on the lumbar spine using local anesthesia. *Orthop Clin North Am* 1991;22:181–187.
19. El Mahdi MA, Latif FY, Janko M. The spinal nerve root "innervation," and a new concept of the clinicopathological interrelations in back pain and sciatica. *Neurochirurgia* 1981;24:137–141.
20. Bogduk N, April C, Derby R. Lumbar discogenic pain: state-of-the-art review. *Pain Med* 2013;14:813–836.
21. Farfan HF, Cossette JW, Robertson GH, et al. The effects of torsion on the lumbar intervertebral joints: the role of torsion in the production of disc degeneration. *J Bone Joint Surg* 1970;52A:469–497.
22. Yang KH, King AI. Mechanism of facet load transmission as a hypothesis for low back pain. *Spine* 1984;9:557–565.
23. Twomey LT, Taylor JR, Taylor MM. Unsuspected damage to lumbar zygapophyseal (facet) joints after motor vehicle accidents. *Med J Aust* 1989;151:210–217.
24. Taylor JR, Twomey LT, Corker M. Bone and soft tissue injuries in post mortem lumbar spines. *Paraplegia* 1990;28:119–129.
25. Kirwan EO. Back pain. In: Wall PD, Melzack R, eds. *Textbook of Pain*, 2nd ed. Edinburgh: Churchill Livingstone; 1989:335–340.
26. White AA. The 1980 symposium and beyond. In: Frymoyer JW, Gordon SL, eds. *New Perspectives on Low Back Pain.* Park Ridge, IL: American Academy of Orthopaedic Surgeons; 1989:3–17.
27. Frymoyer W. Epidemiology. In: Frymoyer JW, Gordon SL, eds. *New Perspectives on Low Back Pain.* Park Ridge, IL: American Academy of Orthopaedic Surgeons; 1989:19–33.
28. Quebec Task Force on Spinal Disorders. Scientific approach to the assessment and management of activity-related spinal disorders: a monograph for clinicians. *Spine* 1987;12:S1–S59.
29. Bogduk N. Myths and critical reasoning. *Aust Musculoskelet Med* 2012;17:6–8.
30. DePalma MJ. Diagnostic nihilism toward low back pain: what once was accepted, should no longer be. *Pain Med* 2015;16:1453–1454.
31. Dillane JB, Fry J, Kalton G. Acute back syndrome—a study from general practice. *Brit Med J* 1966;2:82–84.
32. Engel A, MacVicar J, Bogduk N. A philosophical foundation for diagnostic blocks, with criteria for their validation. *Pain Med* 2014;15:998–1006.
33. Engel AJ, Bogduk N. Mathematical validation and credibility of diagnostic blocks for spinal pain. *Pain Med* 2016;17:1821–1828.
34. Schwarzer AC, Aprill CN, Derby R, et al. Clinical features of patients with pain stemming from the lumbar zygapophysial joints. Is the lumbar facet syndrome a clinical entity? *Spine* 1994;19:1132–1137.
35. Schwarzer AC, Wang S, Bogduk N, et al. Prevalence and clinical features of lumbar zygapophysial joint pain: a study in an Australian population with chronic low back pain. *Ann Rheum Dis* 1995;54:100–106.
36. Manchikanti L, Pampati V, Fellows B, et al. Prevalence of lumbar facet joint pain in chronic low back pain. *Pain Phys* 1999;2:59–64.
37. Manchikanti L, Pampati V, Fellows B, et al. The inability of the clinical picture to characterize pain from facet joints. *Pain Phys* 2000;3:158–166.
38. Manchikanti L, Pampati V, Fellows B, et al. The diagnostic validity and therapeutic value of lumbar facet joint nerve blocks with or without adjuvant agents. *Curr Rev Pain* 2000;4:337–344.
39. Schwarzer AC, Aprill CN, Derby R, et al. The relative contributions of the disc and zygapophyseal joint in chronic low back pain. *Spine* 1994;19:801–806.
40. Schwarzer AC, Aprill CN, Bogduk N. The sacroiliac joint in chronic low back pain. *Spine* 1995;20:31–37.
41. Carette S, Marcoux S, Truchon R, et al. A controlled trial of corticosteroid injections into facet joints for chronic low back pain. *N Engl J Med* 1991;325:1002–1007.
42. Jackson RP, Jacobs RR, Montesano PX. Facet joint injection in low back pain. A prospective study. *Spine* 1988;13:966–971.
43. Laslett M, Oberg B, Aprill CN, et al. Zygapophysial joint blocks in chronic low back pain: a test of Revel's model as a screening test. *BMC Musculoskelet Disord* 2004;5:43.
44. Laslett M, McDonald B, Aprill CN, et al. Clinical predictors of screening lumbar zygapophyseal joint blocks: development of clinical prediction rules. *Spine* J 2006;6:370–379.
45. DePalma MJ, Ketchum JM, Saullo T. What is the source of chronic low back pain and does age play a role? *Pain Med* 2011;12:224–233.
46. DePalma MJ, Ketchum JM, Saullo TR. Multivariable analyses of the relationships between age, gender, and body mass index and the source of chronic low back pain. *Pain Med* 2012;13:498–506.
47. Magora A, Schwartz A. Relation between the low back pain syndrome and x-ray findings. *Scand J Rehabil Med* 1976;8:115–126.
48. Torgerson WR, Dotter WE. Comparative roentgenographic study of the asymptomatic and symptomatic lumbar spine. *J Bone Joint Surg* 1976;8:115–126.
49. van Tulder MW, Assendelft WJJ, Koes BW, et al. Spinal radiographic findings and nonspecific low back pain. A systematic review of observational studies. *Spine* 1997;22:427–434.
50. Schwarzer AC, Wang S, O'Driscoll D, et al. The ability of computed tomography to identify a zygapophysial joint in patients with chronic low back pain. *Spine* 1995;20:907–912.
51. Czervionke LF, Fenton DS. Fat-saturated MR imaging in the detection of inflammatory facet arthropathy (facet synovitis) in the lumbar spine. *Pain Med* 2008;9:400–406.
52. Maigne JY, Aivaliklis A, Pfefer F. Results of sacroiliac joint double block and value of sacroiliac pain provocation tests in 54 patients with low-back pain. *Spine* 1996;21:1889–1892.
53. King W, Ahmed S, Baisden J, et al. Diagnosis and treatment of posterior sacroiliac complex pain: a systematic review with comprehensive analysis of the published data. *Pain Med* 2015;16:257–265.
54. Dreyfuss P, Henning T, Malladi N. et al. The ability of multi-site, multi-depth sacral lateral branch blocks to anesthetize the sacroiliac joint complex. *Pain Med* 2009;10:679–688.

55. Bardin LD, King P, Maher CG. Diagnostic triage for low back pain: a practical approach for primary care. *Med J Aust* 2017;206:268–273.

56. Downie A, Williams CM, Henschke N, et al. Red flags to screen for malignancy and fracture in patients with low back pain: systematic review. *BMJ* 2013;347:f7095.

57. Engel G. The need for a new medical model: a challenge for biomedicine. *Science* 1977;196:129–136.

58. Nicholas MK, Linton SJ, Watson PJ, et al; and "Decade of the Flags" Working Group. Early identification and management of psychological risk factors ("yellow flags") in patients with low back pain: a reappraisal. *Phys Ther* 2011;91:737–753.

59. Turk DC, Kerns RD, Rosenberg R. Effects of marital interaction on chronic pain and disability: examining the down side of social support. *Rehabil Psych* 1992;37:259–274.

60. King W. Diagnosis of pain, medical history. In: Schmidt RF, Willis WD Jr, eds. *Encyclopedic Reference of Pain*. Berlin: Springer; 2007:1112–1115.

61. King W. Diagnosis of pain, musculoskeletal examination. In: Schmidt RF, Willis WD Jr, eds. *Encyclopedic Reference of Pain*. Berlin: Springer; 2007:1230–1232.

62. Verhagen AP, Downieb A, Maher CG, et al. Most red flags for malignancy in low back pain guidelines lack empirical support: a systematic review. *Pain* 2017;158:1860–1868.

63. Bogduk N, McGuirk B. History. In: Bogduk N, McGuirk B, eds. *Medical Management of Acute and Chronic Low Back Pain. An Evidence-Based Approach*. Amsterdam, The Netherlands: Elsevier; 2002:27–40.

64. McGuirk B, King W, Govind J, et al. The safety, efficacy, and cost-effectiveness of evidence-based guidelines for the management of acute low back pain in primary care. *Spine* 2001;26:2615–2622.

65. Malawski SK, Lukawski S. Pyogenic infection of the spine. *Clin Orthop* 1991;272:58–66.

66. Huskisson EC. Measurement of pain. *Lancet* 1974;2:1127–1131.

67. Schwarzer AC, Aprill CN, Derby R, et al. The prevalence and clinical features of internal disc disruption in patients with chronic low back pain. *Spine* 1995;20:1878–1883.

68. Roaf R. A study of the mechanics of spinal injuries. *J Bone Joint Surg* 1960; 42B:810–823.

69. Adams MA, Dolan P. Recent advances in lumbar spinal mechanics and their clinical significance. *Clin Biomech* 1995;10:3–19.

70. Cyron BM, Hutton WC. The fatigue strength of the lumbar neural arch in spondylolysis. *J Bone Joint Surg* 1978;60B:234–238.

71. Farfan HF, Osteria V, Lamy C. The mechanical etiology of spondylolysis and spondylolisthesis. *Clin Orthop* 1976;117:40–55.

72. Frisch H. Examination of the LPH region in the supine position (E/II). In: Frisch H, ed. *Systematic Musculoskeletal Examination*. Berlin: Springer; 1994:155–179.

73. McRae R. *Clinical Orthopaedic Examination*. 2nd ed. Edinburgh: Churchill Livingstone; 1987:71–96.

74. Russe OA, Gerhardt JJ. *International SFTR Method of Measuring and Recording Joint Motion*. Bern, Switzerland: Hans Huber; 1975:44–47.

75. Greene WB, Hechman JD. The thoracic and lumbar spine. In: Greene WB, Hechman JD, eds. *The Clinical Measurement of Joint Motion*. Rosemont, IL: American Academy of Orthopaedic Surgeons; 1994:69–98.

76. Laslett M, Young SB, Aprill CN, et al. Diagnosing painful sacroiliac joints: a validity study of a McKenzie evaluation and sacroiliac provocation tests. *Aust J Physiother* 2003;49:89–97.

77. Laslett M, Oberg B, Aprill CN, et al. Centralization as a predictor of provocation discography results in chronic low back pain, and the influence of disability and distress on diagnostic power. *Spine J* 2005;5:370–380.

78. Aina A, May S, Clare H. The centralization phenomenon of spinal symptoms—a systematic review. *Man Ther* 2004;9:134–143.

79. Coste J, Paolaggi JB, Spira A. Reliability of interpretation of plain lumbar spine radiographs in benign, mechanical low-back pain. *Spine* 1991;16:426–428.

80. Dvorak J. Neurophysiologic tests in diagnosis of nerve root compression caused by disc herniation. *Spine* 1996;21(suppl 24S):39S–44S.

81. Andersson GBJ, Brown MD, Dvorak J, et al. Consensus summary on the diagnosis and treatment of lumbar disc herniation. *Spine* 1996;21(suppl 24S):75S–78S.

82. International Spine Intervention Society. Lumbar disc access. In: Bogduk N, ed. *Practice Guidelines for Spinal Diagnostic and Treatment Procedures*. 2nd ed. San Francisco, CA: International Spine Intervention Society; 2013:317–375.

83. Bogduk N, Tynan W, Wilson AS. The nerve supply to the lumbar intervertebral discs. *J Anat* 1981;132:39–56.

84. Tajima T, Furukawa K, Kuramochi E. Selective lumbosacral radiculography and block. *Spine* 1980;1:68–77.

85. Blankenbaker DG, Davis KW, Choi JJ. Selective nerve root blocks. *Sem Roentgenol* 2004;39:24–36.

86. Gajraj NM. Selective nerve root blocks for low back pain and radiculopathy. *Reg Anesth Pain Med* 2004;29:243–256.

87. Eckel TS, Bartynski WS. Epidural steroid injections and selective nerve root blocks. *Tech Vasc Interv Radiol* 2009;12:11–21.

88. Schliessbach J, Siegenthaler A, Heini P, et al. Blockade of the sinuvertebral nerve for the diagnosis of lumbar diskogenic pain: an exploratory study. *Anesth Analg* 2010;111:204–206.

89. International Spine Intervention Society. Lumbar medial branch blocks. In: Bogduk N, ed. *Practice Guidelines for Spinal Diagnostic and Treatment Procedures*. 2nd ed. San Francisco, CA: International Spine Intervention Society; 2013:457–488.

90. Dreyfuss P, Schwarzer AC, Lau P, et al. Specificity of lumbar medial branch and L5 dorsal ramus blocks: a computed tomographic study. *Spine* 1997;22:895–902.

91. Kaplan M, Dreyfuss P, Halbrook B, et al. The ability of lumbar medial branch blocks to anesthetize the zygapophysial joint. *Spine* 1998;23:1847–1852.

92. Schwarzer AC, Aprill CN, Derby R, et al. The false-positive rate of uncontrolled diagnostic blocks of the lumbar zygapophysial joints. *Pain* 1994;58:195–200.

93. International Spine Intervention Society. An algorithm for the investigation of low back pain. In: Bogduk N, ed. *Practice Guidelines for Spinal Diagnostic and Treatment Procedures*. 2nd ed. San Francisco, CA: International Spine Intervention Society; 2013:523–529.

94. International Spine Intervention Society. Sacroiliac joint access. In: Bogduk N, ed. *Practice Guidelines for Spinal Diagnostic and Treatment Procedures*. 2nd ed. San Francisco, CA: International Spine Intervention Society; 2013:533–555.

95. Dreyfuss P, Snyder BD, Park K, et al. The ability of single site, single depth sacral lateral branch blocks to anesthetize the sacroiliac joint complex. *Pain Med* 2008;9:844–850.

96. Patel N, Gross A, Brown L, et al. A randomized, placebo-controlled study to assess the efficacy of lateral branch neurotomy for chronic sacroiliac joint pain. *Pain Med* 2012;13:383–398.

97. Yelland MJ, Schluter PJ. Defining worthwhile and desired responses to treatment of chronic low back pain. *Pain Med* 2006;7:38–45.

98. Saragiotto BT, Machado GC, Ferreira ML, et al. Paracetamol for low back pain. *Cochrane Database Syst Rev* 2016;(6):CD012230.

99. Chou R, Deyo R, Friedly J, et al. Systemic pharmacologic therapies for low back pain: a systematic review for an American College of Physicians Clinical Practice Guideline. *Ann Intern Med* 2017;166:480–492.

100. Qaseem A, Wilt TJ, McLean RM, et al. Noninvasive treatments for acute, subacute, and chronic low back pain: a clinical practice guideline from the American College of Physicians. *Ann Intern Med* 2017;166:514–530.

101. Enthoven WT, Roelofs PD, Deyo RA, et al. Non-steroidal anti-inflammatory drugs for chronic low back pain. *Cochrane Database Syst Rev* 2016;(2):CD012087. doi:10.1002/14651858.CD012087.

102. van Tulder MW, Touray T, Furlan AD, et al. Muscle relaxants for non-specific low-back pain. *Cochrane Database Syst Rev* 2003;(2):CD004252.

103. Furlan AD, Giraldo M, Baskwill A, et al. Massage for low-back pain. *Cochrane Database Syst Rev* 2015;(9):CD001929.

104. Chou R, Deyo R, Friedly J, et al. Nonpharmacologic therapies for low back pain: a systematic review for an American College of Physicians Clinical Practice Guideline. *Ann Intern Med* 2017;166:493–505.

105. Wegner I, Widyahening IS, van Tulder MW, et al. Traction for low-back pain with or without sciatica. *Cochrane Database Syst Rev* 2013;(8):CD003010.

106. Rubinstein SM, Bronfort G, Haas M, et al. Evidence-informed management of chronic low back pain with spinal manipulation and mobilization. *Spine J* 2008;8:213–225.

107. Clare HA, Adams R, Maher CG. A systematic review of efficacy of McKenzie method for low back pain. *Aust J Physiother* 2004;50:209–216.

108. Machado LA, de Souza MS, Ferreira PH, et al. The McKenzie method for low back pain: a systematic review of the literature with a meta-analysis approach. *Spine* 2006;31:E254–E262.

109. May S, Donelson R. Evidence-informed management of chronic low back pain with the McKenzie method. *Spine J* 2008;8:134–141.

110. Nnoaham KE, Kumbang J. Transcutaneous electrical nerve stimulation (TENS) for chronic pain. *Cochrane Database Syst Rev* 2014;(7):CD003222.

111. Odebiyi DO, Henschke N, Ferreira ML, et al. Transcutaneous electrical nerve stimulation (TENS) for chronic low-back pain. *Cochrane Database Syst Rev* 2013;(4):CD010500.

112. Yousefi-Nooraie R, Schonstein E, Heidari K, et al. Low level laser therapy for nonspecific low-back pain. *Cochrane Database Syst Rev* 2008;(2):CD005107.

113. van Duijvenbode I, Jellema P, van Poppel M, et al. Lumbar supports for prevention and treatment of low back pain. *Cochrane Database Syst Rev* 2008;(2):CD001823.

114. Mayer J, Mooney V, Dagenais S. Evidence-informed management of chronic low back pain with lumbar extensor strengthening exercises. *Spine J* 2008;8:96–113.

115. Slade SC, Keating JL. Trunk-strengthening exercises for chronic low back pain: a systematic review. *J Manip Physiol Ther* 2006;29:163–173.

116. Standaert CJ, Weinstein SM, Rumpeltes J. Evidence-informed management of chronic low back pain with lumbar stabilization exercises. *Spine J* 2008;8:114–120.

117. Ferreira PH, Ferreira ML, Maher CG, et al. Specific stabilization exercise for spinal and pelvic pain: a systematic review. *Aust J Physiother* 2006;52:79–88.

118. Malanga G, Wolff E. Evidence-informed management of chronic low back pain with trigger point injections. *Spine J* 2008;8:243–252.

119. Dagenais S, Mayer J, Haldeman S, et al. Evidence-informed management of chronic low back pain with prolotherapy. *Spine J* 2008;8:203–212.

120. Yelland MJ, Del Mar C, Pirozzo S, et al. Prolotherapy injections for chronic low-back pain. *Cochrane Database Syst Rev* 2004;(2):CD004059.

121. Dagenais S, Yelland MJ, Del Mar C, et al. Prolotherapy injections for chronic low-back pain. *Cochrane Database Syst Rev* 2007;(2):CD004059.

122. Yelland MJ, Glasziou PP, Bogduk N, et al. Prolotherapy injections, saline injections, and exercises for chronic low-back pain: a randomized trial. *Spine* 2004;29:9–16.

123. Bogduk N. Pharmacological alternatives for the alleviation of back pain. *Expert Opin Phamacother* 2004;5:2091–2098.

124. Parreira P, Heymans MW, van Tulder MW, et al. Back Schools for chronic non-specific low back pain. *Cochrane Database Syst Rev* 2017;(8):CD011674. doi:10.1002/14651858.CD011674.pub2.

125. Williams AC, Eccleston C, Morley S. Psychological therapies for the management of chronic pain (excluding headache) in adults. *Cochrane Database Syst Rev* 2012;(11):CD007407.

126. Henschke N, Ostelo RW, van Tulder MW, et al. Behavioural treatment for chronic low-back pain. *Cochrane Database Syst Rev* 2010;(7): CD002014.

127. Gamsa A. The role of psychological factors in chronic pain. I. A half century of study. *Pain* 1994;57:5–15.

128. Gamsa A. The role of psychological factors in chronic pain. II. A critical appraisal. *Pain* 1994;57:17–29.

129. Siddall PJ, Cousins MJ. Persistent pain as a disease entity: implications for clinical management. *Anesth Analg* 2004;99:510–520.

130. Ruscheweyh R, Sandkühler J. Opioids and central sensitisation: II. Induction and reversal of hyperalgesia. *Eur J Pain* 2005;9:149–152.

131. Curatolo M, Arendt-Nielsen L, Petersen-Felix S. Central hypersensitivity in chronic pain: mechanisms and clinical implications. *Phys Med Rehabil Clin N Am* 2006;17:287–302.

132. Cohen M, Quintner J, Buchanan D. Is chronic pain a disease? *Pain Med* 2013;14:1284–1288.

133. Smith A, Jull G, Schneider G, et al. Cervical radiofrequency neurotomy reduces psychological features in individuals with chronic whiplash symptoms. *Pain Phys* 2014;17:265–274.

134. Kamper SJ, Apeldoorn AT, Chiarotto A, et al. Multidisciplinary biopsychosocial rehabilitation for chronic low back pain: Cochrane systematic review and meta-analysis. *BMJ* 2015;350:h444.

135. Mayer TG, Gatchel RJ, Kishino N, et al. Objective assessment of spine function following industrial injury. A prospective study with comparison group and one-year follow-up. *Spine* 1985;10:482–493.

136. Johnson RE, Jones GT, Wiles NJ, et al. Active exercise, education, and cognitive behavioral therapy for persistent disabling low back pain: a randomized controlled trial. *Spine* 2007;32:1578–1585.

137. Manchikanti L, Cash KA, McManus CD, et al. One year results of a randomized, double-blind, active controlled trial of fluoroscopic caudal epidural injections with or without steroids in managing chronic discogenic low back pain without disc herniation or radiculitis. *Pain Phys* 2011;14:25–36.

138. Manchikanti L, Cash KA, McManus CD, et al. Preliminary results of randomized, equivalence trial of fluoroscopic caudal epidural injections in managing chronic low back pain: part 1. Discogenic pain without disc herniation or radiculitis. *Pain Phys* 2008;11:785–800.

139. Manchikanti L, Cash KA, McManus CD, et al. A randomized, double-blind, active-controlled trial of fluoroscopic lumbar interlaminar epidural injections in chronic axial or discogenic low back pain: results of a 2-year follow-up. *Pain Phys* 2013;16:E491–E504.

140. Conn A, Buenaventura RM, Datta S, et al. Systematic review of caudal epidural injections in the management of chronic low back pain. *Pain Phys* 2009;12:109–135.

141. Parr AT, Diwan S, Abdi S. Lumbar interlaminar epidural injections in managing chronic low back and lower extremity pain: a systematic review. *Pain Phys* 2009;12:163–188.

142. Johansson A, Hao J, Sjolund B. Local corticosteroid application blocks transmission in normal nociceptive C-fibres. *Acta Anaesthesiol Scand* 1990;34:335–338.

143. King W. *Sinuvertebral Nerve Blocks and Transforaminal Corticosteroid Injections in the Management of Lumbar Discogenic Pain* [master's thesis]. Sydney, Australia: University of Sydney; 1999.

144. Bogduk N. A narrative review of intra-articular corticosteroid injections for low back pain. *Pain Med* 2005;6:287–296.

145. Lilius G, Laasonen EM, Myllynen P, et al. Lumbar facet joint syndrome: a randomised clinical trial. *J Bone Joint Surg* 1989;71B:681–684.

146. Lilius G, Harilainen A, Laasonen EM, et al. Chronic unilateral back pain: predictors of outcome of facet joint injections. *Spine* 1990;15:780–782.

147. Manchikanti L, Singh V, Falco FJE, et al. Evaluation of lumbar facet joint nerve blocks in managing chronic low back pain: a randomized, double-blind, controlled trial with a 2-year follow-up. *Int J Med Sci* 2010;7:124–135.

148. International Spine Intervention Society. Lumbar medial branch thermal radiofrequency neurotomy. In: Bogduk N, ed. *Practice Guidelines for Spinal Diagnostic and Treatment Procedures*. 2nd ed. San Francisco, CA: International Spine Intervention Society; 2013:489–522.

149. Dreyfuss P, Halbrook B, Pauza K, et al. Efficacy and validity of radiofrequency neurotomy for chronic lumbar zygapophysial joint pain. *Spine* 2000;25:1270–1277.

150. MacVicar J, Borowczyk JM, MacVicar AM, et al. Lumbar medial branch radiofrequency neurotomy in New Zealand. *Pain Med* 2013;14:639–645.

151. Gofeld M, Jitendra J, Faclier G. Radiofrequency denervation of the lumbar zygapophysial joints: 10-year prospective audit. *Pain Phys* 2007;10: 291–300.

152. van Kleef M, Barendse GA, Kessels A, et al. Randomized trial of radiofrequency lumbar facet denervation for chronic low back pain. *Spine* 1999;24:1937–1942.

153. van Wijk RM, Geurts JW, Wynne HJ, et al. Radiofrequency denervation of lumbar facet joints in the treatment of chronic low back pain. A randomized, double-blind sham lesion-controlled trial. *Clin J Pain* 2004;21: 335–344.

154. Juch JNS, Maas ET, Ostelo RWJG, et al. Effect of radiofrequency denervation on pain intensity among patients with chronic low back pain the Mint randomized clinical trials. *JAMA* 2017;318:68–81.

155. van Tilburg CW, Stronks DL, Groeneweg JG, et al. Randomised sham-controlled double-blind multicentre clinical trial to ascertain the effect of percutaneous radiofrequency treatment for lumbar facet joint pain. *Bone Joint J* 2016;98-B:1526–533.

156. Tekin I, Mirzai H, Ok G, et al. A comparison of conventional and pulsed radiofrequency denervation in the treatment of chronic facet joint pain. *Clin J Pain* 2007;23:524–529.

157. Manchikanti L, Boswell MV, Singh V, et al. Prevalence of facet joint pain in chronic spinal pain of cervical, thoracic, and lumbar regions. *BMC Musculoskelet Disord* 2004;5:15.

158. Manchukonda R, Manchikanti KN, Cash KA, et al. Facet joint pain in chronic spinal pain: an evaluation of prevalence and false-positive rate of diagnostic blocks. *J Spinal Disord Tech* 2007;20:539–545.

159. Lord SM, Barnsley L, Bogduk N. The utility of comparative local anaesthetic blocks versus placebo-controlled blocks for the diagnosis of cervical zygapophysial joint pain. *Clin J Pain* 1995;11:208–213.

160. Gallagher J, Petriccione di Valdo PL, Wedley Jr, et al. Radiofrequency facet joint denervation in the treatment of low back pain: a prospective controlled double-blind study to assess its efficacy. *Pain Clin* 1994;7:193–198.

161. Leclaire R, Fortin L, Lambert R, et al. Radiofrequency facet joint denervation in the treatment of low back pain: a placebo-controlled clinical trial to assess efficacy. *Spine* 2001;26:1411–1416.

162. Bogduk N. Lumbar radiofrequency neurotomy. *Clin J Pain* 2006;22:409.

163. Bogduk N, Dreyfuss P, Govind J. A narrative review of lumbar medial branch neurotomy for the treatment of back pain. *Pain Med* 2009;10:1035–1045.

164. Dreyfuss P, Baker R, Leclaire R, et al. Radiofrequency facet joint denervation in the treatment of low back pain: a placebo-controlled clinical trial to assess efficacy. *Spine* 2002;27:556–557.

165. Vorobeychik Y, Stojanovic MP, McCormick ZL. Radiofrequency denervation for chronic low back pain. *JAMA* 2017;318:2254–2255.

166. Rimmalapudi V, Buchalter J, Calodney A. Radiofrequency denervation for chronic low back pain. *JAMA* 2017;318:2255–2256.

167. Ming-Chih Kao MC, Leong MS, Mackey S. Radiofrequency denervation for chronic low back pain. *JAMA* 2017;318:2256.

168. van Wijk RM, Geurts JW, Groen GJ. Comments on efficacy of radiofrequency facet denervation procedures. *Pain Med* 2012;13:843–845.

169. Maas E, Juch J, Huygen F. Radiofrequency denervation for chronic low back pain. *JAMA* 2017;318:2256–2257.

170. Nath S, Nath CA, Pettersson K. Percutaneous lumbar zygapophysial (facet) joint neurotomy using radiofrequency current, in the management of chronic low back pain: a randomized double-blind trial. *Spine* 2008;33:1291–1297.

171. Hawkins J, Schofferman J. Serial therapeutic sacroiliac joint injections: a practice audit. *Pain Med* 2009;10:850–853.

172. Hart R, Wendshce P, Kočiš J, et al. Injection of anaesthetic-corticosteroid to relieve sacroiliac joint pain after lumbar stabilisation. *Acta Chir Orthop Traimatol Cech* 2011;78:339–342.

173. Liliang PC, Lu K, Weng HC, et al. The therapeutic efficacy of sacroiliac joint blocks with triamcinolone acetonide in the treatment of sacroiliac joint dysfunction without spondyloarthropathy. *Spine* 2009;34:896–900.

174. MacVicar J, Kreiner DS, Duszynski B, et al. Appropriate use criteria for fluoroscopically guided diagnostic and therapeutic sacroiliac interventions: results from the spine intervention society convened multispecialty collaborative. *Pain Med* 2017;18:2081–2095.

175. Bogduk N. A commentary on appropriate use criteria for sacroiliac pain. *Pain Med* 2017;18:2055–2057.

176. Buijs EJ, Kamphuis ET, Groen GJ. Radiofrequency treatment of sacroiliac joint-related pain aimed at the first three sacral dorsal rami: a minimal approach. *Pain Clin* 2004;16:139–147.

177. Speldewinde GC. Outcomes of percutaneous zygapophysial and sacroiliac joint neurotomy in a community setting. *Pain Med* 2001;12:209–218.

178. Stelzer W, Aiglesberger M, Stelzer D, et al. Use of cooled radiofrequency lateral branch neurotomy for the treatment of sacroiliac joint-mediated low back pain: a large case series. *Pain Med* 2013;14:29–35.

179. Kapural L, Nageeb F, Kapural M, et al. Cooled radiofrequency (RF) system for the treatment of chronic pain from sacroiliitis: the first case-series. *Pain Pract* 2008;8:348–354.

180. Karaman H, Kavak GO, Tüfek A, et al. Cooled radiofrequency application for treatment of sacroiliac joint pain. *Acta Neurochir* 2011;153:1461–1468.

181. Cheng J, Pope JE, Dalton JE, et al. Comparative outcomes of cooled versus traditional radiofrequency ablation of the lateral branches for sacroiliac joint pain. *Clin J Pain* 2013;29:132–137.

182. Cohen SP, Hurley RW, Buckenmaier CC, et al. Randomized placebo-controlled study evaluating lateral branch radiofrequency denervation for sacroiliac joint pain. *Anesthesiology* 2008;109:279–288.

183. Cohen SP, Abdi S. Lateral branch blocks as a treatment for sacroiliac joint pain: a pilot study. *Reg Anesth Pain Med* 2003;28:113–119.

184. Cohen SP, Strassels SA, Kurihara C, et al. Outcome predictors for sacroiliac joint (lateral branch) radiofrequency denervation. *Reg Anesth Pain Med* 2009;34:206–214.

185. Todd NV. The surgical treatment of non-specific low back pain. *Bone Joint J* 2017;99-B:1003–1005.

186. National Institute for Health and Care Excellence. *Low Back Pain and Sciatica in Over 16s: Assessment and Management*. London: National Institute for Health and Care Excellence. NICE guideline 59.

187. Stochkendahl MJ, Kjaer P, Hartvigsen J, et al. National clinical guidelines for non-surgical treatment of patients with recent onset low back pain or lumbar radiculopathy. *Eur Spine J* 2018;27:60–75.

188. Van Wambeke P, Desomer A, Ailliet L, et al. *Low Back Pain and Radicular Pain: Assessment and Management—Summary*. Brussels, Belgium: Belgian Health Care Knowledge Centre; 2017.

189. Cochrane AL. *Effectiveness and Efficiency*. Cambridge, United Kingdom: Cambridge University Press; 1972.

CHAPTER 74

Surgery for Low Back Pain

YOUSSEF GHABRIAL and **NIKOLAI BOGDUK**

Fusion of the lumbar spine was initially developed to treat tuberculosis of the spine and to stabilize spinal deformities.[1-3] Later, it was used to treat the instability of spondylolisthesis and to prevent iatrogenic instability after disk excision for disk herniation. In due course, fusion was applied to treat chronic low back pain.

The procedures commonly used in the treatment of back pain are summarized in Figure 74.1. The procedures differ according to the direction of approach: whether the spine is fused or not, whether disks are excised or not, and if a bone graft or instruments or both are used to achieve fusion. Other, more avant-garde techniques include minimally invasive approaches through the psoas muscle.[4]

Posterolateral fusions were originally performed using only a bone graft. They were later supplemented by pedicle screws and plates when it was shown that instrumentation improved fusion rates. Likewise, posterior interbody fusions are now supplemented by pedicle screws in order to enhance arthrodesis. Anterior interbody fusions are classically performed using a bone dowel, but some surgeons add screws and plates or an interbody cage to promote bone union.

Rationale

It is difficult to find in the literature an explicit, stated rationale for fusion in the treatment of low back pain. Implicitly, the earliest rationale was that because back pain was aggravated by movement of the lumbar spine, instability must be causing the pain, and, therefore, stabilizing the spine should relieve the pain. According to this rationale, a specific diagnosis was not required; persistent pain was the sole indication for surgery. Some surgeons applied nominal diagnostic rubrics, such as spondylosis or degenerative disk disease, despite these conditions being no more than normal age changes,[5] a paradox that some surgeons acknowledge.[4]

Later, some surgeons proposed that the intervertebral disk was the source of pain and adopted discography as the diagnostic test. Painful disks could be protected from aggravation

by posterolateral fusion, or the disk could be excised and replaced by a bone graft.

A contentious indication for fusion is spondylolisthesis. This condition is an attractive target for surgery because it constitutes a deformity and has been reputed to be unstable, both of which can be rectified by surgery. However, research has shown that spondylolisthesis is commonly asymptomatic, such that its presence on radiographs has no statistically significant or clinically significant association with back pain.[5,6] Furthermore, studies have shown no detectable instability in spondylolisthesis.[7-10] Other studies have found evidence of abnormal motion and paradoxical motion in patients with spondylolisthesis, but at the segment above, not at the affected segment.[11]

Spondylolisthesis remains an indication for surgery in patients with radicular pain or radiculopathy, when it can be shown that the deformity is causing nerve root compression. In that event, surgery is remarkably successful at relieving radicular pain.[12,13] In patients with concurrent back pain, surgery is less often effective and, to a lesser degree, for the relief of back pain.[12,13]

A literature review summarized the success rates of surgery for spondylolisthesis as reported in 34 original studies.[14] For posterior fusion alone, the success rates ranged between 37.5% and 98%, with an average of 74.8%. For anterior fusion, the success rates ranged between 80% and 95%. These data, however, were based on irregular and sometimes ill-defined criteria for clinical success. Some studies measured success in terms of patients achieving complete relief of symptoms, whereas others reported only the proportion of patients achieving some degree of improvement. Few studies, however, reported the degree of impairment before surgery and rarely have outcomes been corroborated by quantitative measures of pain, disability, return to work, and use of other health care.

Better data are available from randomized controlled trials. Surgery for spondylolisthesis is patently more effective than conservative therapy,[15-17] but surgery is neither universally nor completely effective. Only 56% of patients rate themselves as "much better," whereas 11% consider themselves unchanged and consider their condition to be worse.[16] Surgery is, therefore, an imperfect solution for spondylolisthesis. The implication is that fusion does not effectively target the cause of back pain in spondylolisthesis.

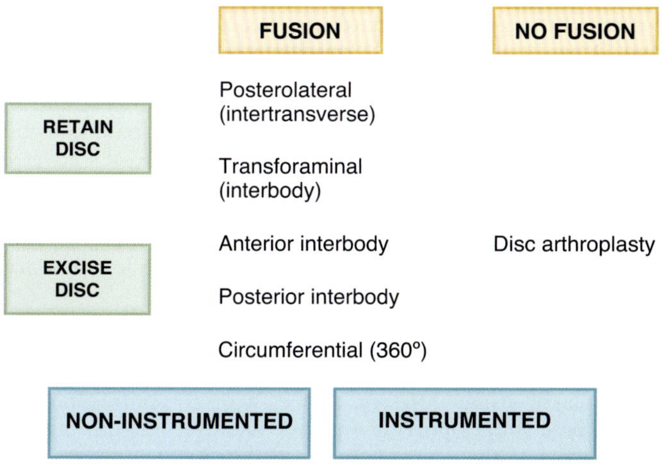

Effectiveness

Pivotal to the use of fusion for low back pain is the evidence for its effectiveness and efficacy. This evidence should be as much of interest to physicians who might refer patients for surgery as it is to surgeons who might perform the surgery. That evidence has evolved. Three epochs can be described, according to whether studies were performed before, during, or after the advent of the principles and demands of evidence-based medicine (EBM), which occurred around the turn of the 20th century.

BEFORE EVIDENCE-BASED MEDICINE

Before the advent of EBM, surgeons reported good outcomes from fusion in the treatment of chronic low back pain. These reports created the reputation of surgery of being a decisive option for patients for whom conservative therapy had failed to provide relief.

FIGURE 74.1 A classification of types of surgery used for low back pain.

FUSION / NO FUSION

RETAIN DISC — Posterolateral (intertransverse); Transforaminal (interbody)

EXCISE DISC — Anterior interbody / Disc arthroplasty; Posterior interbody; Circumferential (360°)

NON-INSTRUMENTED / INSTRUMENTED

However, studies during that epoch used methods that nowadays would not be held in high regard. These include the following:

- Surgeons evaluating their own outcomes, as opposed to having an independent, third party assessing outcomes
- Reporting qualitative outcomes, such as "excellent" or "very good" results, without supporting quantitative data
- Not providing baseline data
- Reporting outcomes without stratifying for different presenting conditions or symptoms
- Not using validated instruments for outcome measures
- Not reporting on all variables of interest, such as pain, disability or function, and use of other health care for back pain

For example, the success rates reported during this epoch were summarized in terms such as "61% excellent and 31% good outcomes," "88% excellent or good outcomes," and "100% satisfactory outcomes" for posterior interbody fusion and "89% relieved," "95% clinically favorable," and "74% satisfactory outcomes" for anterior lumbar interbody fusion.[18] For patients with persistent, disabling pain, or their treating physicians, such numbers are appealing.

Table 74.1 lists the outcomes reported by various studies for anterior lumbar interbody fusion in patients diagnosed by discography as having discogenic pain. Although the success

TABLE 74.1   Outcomes Reported by Various Studies that Used Discography to Select Segments for Treatment by Fusion

Source	Criteria	Success Rate
Blumenthal et al.[19]	Normal activities and no medications or NSAIDs only	74%
Kozak and O'Brien[20]	At least 75% relief of pain and return to work or Slight restriction of activities and no analgesics	74%
Kostuik et al.[21]	Absence of significant back or leg pain Occasional use of nonnarcotic analgesics	31%
Gill and Blumenthal[22]	At least 75% relief of pain and return to work or Return to normal activities and no opioids	66%
Lee et al.[23]	No pain	26%
	Mild pain	61%
	No medications	59%
	No opioids	30%
	No restricted activities	50%
	Mild or moderate restriction	30%
	Return to full work	81%
	Return to restricted work	11%
Wetzel et al.[24]	Minimal symptoms and no analgesics, or marked improvement, and rare use of analgesics	46%
Parker et al.[25]	Pain less than 4/10 No medications other than NSAIDs Return to at least 75% previous work capacity	39%
Penta and Fraser[26]	Complete relief or Good deal of relief	39% / 39%
Greenough et al.[27]	Complete or almost complete relief A good deal of relief	17% / 23%

NSAIDs, nonsteroidal anti-inflammatory drugs.

rates are more modest than those of the earlier literature, many are still attractive. One in five patients, or better, could expect to achieve complete relief of their back pain.

ADVENT OF EVIDENCE-BASED MEDICINE

At the turn of the 20th century, the precepts, principles, and demands of EBM were increasingly applied to studies in pain medicine and were applied to studies of surgery for back pain. This encompassed conducting randomized controlled trials and prospectively using multiple, validated outcome measures. The first target was conventional fusion for chronic low back pain.

In nearly rapid succession, three randomized controlled trials were conducted in which spinal fusion was compared with conservative care. In the first trial,[28] surgeons were allowed to perform their procedure of choice, which encompassed anterior lumbar interbody fusion, posterior lumbar interbody fusion, and posterolateral fusion with or without pedicle screws. (A companion report showed that outcomes were not significantly different between these various options.[29]) In the second study,[30] all patients were treated with posterolateral fusion with pedicle screw fixation. In the third study,[31] surgeons were allowed to use their procedure of choice, but the type of surgery used for each patient was not reported.

In the first study, conservative therapy consisted of physical therapy supplemented with other forms of treatment such as information and education, transcutaneous electrical nerves stimulation, acupuncture, injections, cognitive and functional training, and coping strategies.[28] That study found significant differences in favor of surgery (Fig. 74.2). Nonsurgical care provided no change in mean scores for back pain, whereas fusion provided a 50% decrease in pain over 6 to 12 months. By 24 months, this improvement had attenuated to a 30% reduction in pain but was still significantly greater than that achieved by nonsurgical care.

These outcomes were not corroborated by the second and third trials. In the second trial,[30] mean scores for pain and disability improved marginally, but to the same extent, in patients treated by fusion as in patients treated with behavioral therapy plus exercises (see Fig. 74.2). Similarly, in the third study,[31] scores for pain and function improved slightly, but to the same degree, in patients treated by fusion or in a rehabilitation program (see Fig. 74.2).

These studies became the standing evidence base for spinal fusion. Whereas one study showed significant superiority over conservative therapy, two others did not. Notwithstanding this dissonance, none of the three studies reproduced the high success rates claimed for surgery in the literature of the past.

The second target of EBM was total disc replacement, alias disc arthroplasty. Although there had been a few earlier studies, the introduction of disc arthroplasty into the United States was subjected to rigorous standards, particularly by the U.S. Food and Drug Administration. Consequently, all of the literature was of high quality methodologically.

Disc arthroplasty was heralded as offering the potential of restoring joint mechanics, and thereby reducing pain and improving function, and preserving motion would lessen adverse loading and changes in range of motion at adjacent segments.[32] Preliminary results from descriptive studies were good in some studies[33] and yielded outcomes comparable to those of fusion for low back pain.[32] Recovery time seemed to be less than for fusion.[33]

In the early controlled trials, Blumenthal et al.[34] compared disc arthroplasty, using a particular device, with a form of anterior lumbar interbody fusion, and Zigler et al.[35] compared arthroplasty, using different device, with circumferential fusion. These studies provide outcome data not only on disc arthroplasty but also on the conventional fusion procedures with which it was compared.

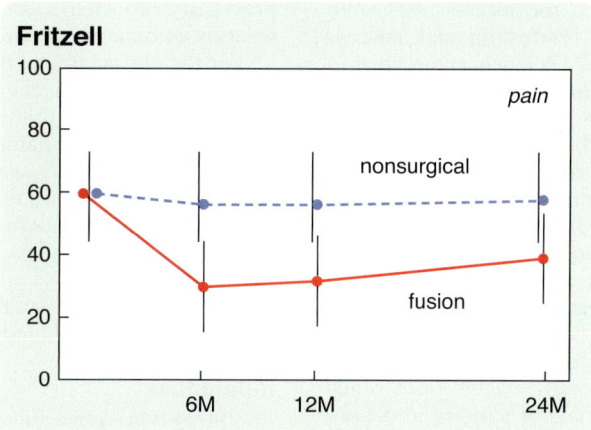

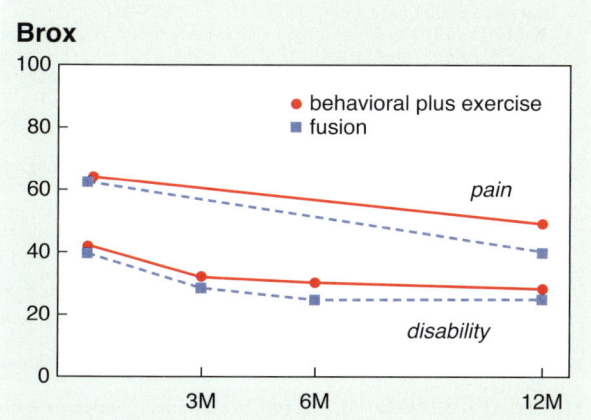

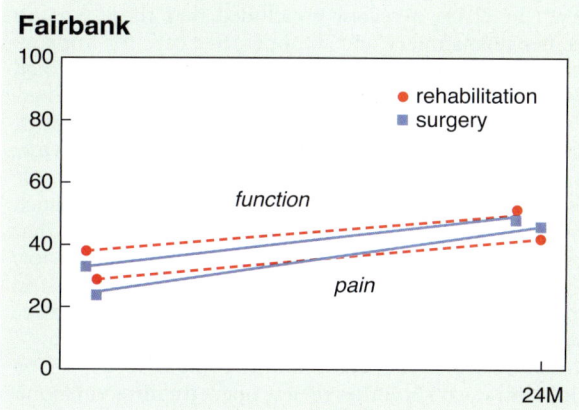

FIGURE 74.2 Graphic summaries of the outcomes of three controlled trials of fusion for low back pain. The trials used different outcome instruments. In the trials of Fritzell et al.[28] and of Brox et al.,[30] lower scores indicate improvement. In the trial of Fairbank et al.,[31] higher scores indicate improvement.

Although the Blumenthal et al.[34] study found disc arthroplasty to be noninferior to fusion, the outcomes of both arthroplasty and anterior lumbar interbody fusion were modest. Mean pain scores improved from 70 to 30, which exceeds the minimal clinically important change (MCIC) of 20 points; and Oswestry Disability Index (ODI) improved from 50 to 25, but 64% of patients treated by surgery still took opioids, and although 64% returned to work, 53% had been working before surgery. These latter figures do not attest to any substantial decrease in the burden of illness; surgery did not seem to alter the patients' use of other health care or restore their ability to work. The proportion of patients who were completely relieved of pain was not reported. One reviewer recommended that these data argue for caution by patients and surgeons.[36]

The Zigler et al.[35] study found disc arthroplasty to be slightly more effective, on average, than circumferential fusion, but it, too, reported only modest results for both surgical treatments. After arthroplasty, ODI improved from 63.4 at inception to 34.5 at 24 months but with a standard deviation of 24.8. This latter figure indicates that a large proportion of patients were still substantially disabled. Pain scores improved from just above 70 to 37 but with a standard deviation of 30.1. This study judged outcomes as a success if the ODI improved by 15 points, which is the MCIC required by the U.S. Food and Drug Administration.[37] On this basis, a 72% success rate was claimed. But this misrepresents MCIC. The MCIC does not amount to the least value at which success occurs. It is no more than the least value that patients equate with a detectable level of improvement. The study did not report the proportion of patients rendered substantially better or free of pain.

Of patients considered to have a successful outcome, 39% still took opioids, which seems contradictory. Reviewers concluded that this study lacked sufficient detail for the interested reader to perform an independent evaluation of the data to confirm or reject the authors' conclusions.[38]

These results from controlled trials of arthroplasty are starkly inferior to those of a well-reported descriptive study. In the study of Bertagnoli et al.,[39] at 2 years, 32% of patients had no back pain, and a further 59% had only occasional pain; 90% took no opioids; only 41% required nonsteroidal anti-inflammatory drugs (NSAIDs) for pain. The latter figures are the sorts of outcomes that referring physicians and their patients would like to expect from surgery for back pain. Opinion leaders, however, put more stock in data from controlled trials rather than observational studies, no matter how well reported the latter might be.

SINCE EVIDENCE-BASED MEDICINE
The epoch since the advent of EBM is characterized by fewer pivotal studies but a continuing, steady stream of reviews, systematic or otherwise. The themes that have emerged for total disc replacement have differed from those for fusion.

On total disc replacement, reviews published in 2006 concluded that total disc replacement was not inferior to fusion, but the difference in benefit was less than 15 points for disability,[40] and at 24 months, 64% of patients were still taking opioids after disc replacement, and 80% after fusion.[41] In 2012, a Cochrane review remarked that the outcomes between disc replacement and fusion differed by only 5/100 for pain, and 4/100 for disability.[42] A review in 2013 reiterated this small difference in outcomes and added that the success rates were 53% for disc replacement and 41% for fusion, with success being defined as achieving the MCIC.[43] A Cochrane review in 2013 concluded that such differences in outcome were not clinically relevant.[44]

More recent reviews have included more recent studies and newer devices, but their conclusions remain unchanged. Outcomes from disc replacement are minimally better than those of fusion.[45,46] For these reasons, in the United Kingdom, it has been recommended that, for the treatment of low back pain, disc replacement be offered only in the context of a randomized controlled trial.[47] Despite an increasing literature, the Italian review concluded that disc arthroplasty could be a reliable option in the treatment of degenerative disk disease in years to come.[47]

With respect to fusion, conventional reviews have relied essentially on the three controlled trials of surgery and non-operative therapy (see Fig. 74.2). One published in 2006 concluded that there was insufficient evidence on the effectiveness of surgery.[48] In 2015, a review concluded that there was no difference between surgery and nonoperative care for improving disability.[49] A dissenting review concluded that the pooled data showed that fusion had moderate treatment effects, better than those of nonsurgical care, at 12 months, 24 months, and longer than 48 months after treatment.[50] Another review acknowledged that the outcomes of fusion were comparable with those of intensive rehabilitation but commented that such rehabilitation programs might not always be available and that fusion constituted a valid alternative.[51] Yet, another review concluded that because outcomes were not different, fusion and nonoperative care both remain acceptable methods of care for intractable back pain.[52]

Whereas these reviews focused on the comparison of fusion with nonoperative care, another review opened a different front. It harvested data from trials not limited to those comparing fusion with nonoperative care and focused on the magnitude of outcomes from fusion. On the grounds that fusion offered an average improvement of 37/100 for pain, and 27/100 for disability, it advocated that fusion should be considered a valid treatment for back pain.[53] The implied argument seems to be that because surgery offers improvements greater than those reported for any conservative therapy, it should constitute a valid treatment. However, for a major undertaking such as surgery, these average improvements are small and do not amount to success rates. The data from controlled trials show that in terms of success rates, fusion has a success rate of 41% for achieving just an MCIC.[43] In an uncontrolled study, only 16% of patients with workers compensation achieved MCIC, and only 36% of patients without claims did so.[54]

Discussion

Over the last 40 years, the literature on surgery for low back pain has evolved. More rigorous standards have been applied both to the design of studies and to how they are reported. The language has changed. Early studies proclaimed impressive success rates. These have not been corroborated by modern controlled trials. When compared with nonoperative care or with other surgical procedures, the outcomes of surgery are modest. Success rates are no longer defined in terms of the proportions of patients rendered free of pain or no longer requiring health care. That language has been replaced by a new definition of success: the proportion achieving just an MCIC.

It is not evident from the literature whether this change is due to a decrease in the effectiveness of surgery or to an exaggeration of outcomes in earlier studies. Curious in that regard is that surgeons who earlier proclaimed impressive outcomes from anterior lumbar interbody fusion[19] became advocates for disc replacement[34] but were unable to reproduce their own

previously reported success rates. It would seem that tighter scrutiny of outcomes makes a difference to success rates.

For the physician and patient who are seeking a solution for intractable back pain, the literature and evidence on surgery is less attractive than it used to be. If there is a prospect of achieving complete relief of pain, or reducing pain to a tolerable level, only occasional studies speak of it, most do not. If surgery is to restore its former reputation, its former successes need to be re-established under modern conditions of reporting and reestablished by multiple studies. Success defined as achieving only an MCIC will not be marketable. Nor will surgery be marketable if some patients make small gains, whereas other patients suffer the consequences of failed surgery (see Chapter 75).

References

1. Hibbs RH. An operation for progressive spinal deformities. *New York Med J* 1911;93:1013–1016.
2. Albee FH. Transplantation of a portion of the tibia into the spine for Pott's disease: a preliminary report. *JAMA* 1911;57:885–886.
3. Wiltberger BR. The dowel intervertebral-body fusion as used in lumbar-disc surgery. *J Bone Joint Surg Am* 1957;39-A:284–292.
4. Lee YC, Zotti MGT, Osti OL. Operative management of lumbar degenerative disc disease. *Asian Spine J* 2016;10:801–819.
5. Bogduk N. Degenerative joint disease of the spine. *Radiol Clin N Am* 2012;50:613–628.
6. van Tulder MW, Assendelft WJJ, Koes BW, et al. Spinal radiographic findings and nonspecific low back pain. A systematic review of observational studies. *Spine* 1997;22:427–434.
7. Olsson TH, Selvik G, Willner S. Vertebral motion in spondylolisthesis. *Acta Radiol Diagn* 1976;17:861–868.
8. Penning L, Blickman JR. Instability in lumbar spondylolisthesis: a radiographic study of several concepts. *Am J Radiol* 1980;134:293–301.
9. Wood K, Popp C, Transfeldt E, et al. Radiographic evaluation of instability in spondylolisthesis. *Spine* 1994;19:1697–1703.
10. Pearcy M, Shepherd J. Is there instability in spondylolisthesis? *Spine* 1985;10:175–177.
11. Schneider G, Pearcy MJ, Bogduk N. Abnormal motion in spondylolytic spondylolisthesis. *Spine* 2005;30:1159–1164.
12. Ghahreman A, Ferch RD, Rao PJ, et al. Minimal access versus open posterior lumbar interbody fusion in the treatment of spondylolisthesis. *Neurosurgery* 2010;66:296–304.
13. Cheung NK, Ferch RD, Ghahreman A, et al. Long-term follow-up of minimal-access and open posterior lumbar interbody fusion for spondylolisthesis. *Neurosurgery* 2013;72:443–450.
14. Kwon BK, Hilibrand AS, Malloy K, et al. A critical analysis of the literature regarding surgical approach and outcome for adult low-grade isthmic spondylolisthesis. *J Spinal Disord Tech* 2005;18:S30–S40.
15. Weinstein JN, Lurie JD, Tosteson TD, et al. Surgical versus nonsurgical treatment for lumbar degenerative spondylolisthesis. *New Engl J Med* 2007;356:2257–2270.
16. Moller H, Hedlund R. Surgery versus conservative management in adult isthmic spondylolisthesis—a prospective randomized study: part 1. *Spine* 2000;25:1711–1715.
17. Moller H, Hedlund R. Instrumented and noninstrumented posterolateral fusion in adult spondylolisthesis—a prospective randomized study: part 2. *Spine* 2000;25:1716–1721.
18. Schechter NA, France MP, Lee CK. Painful internal disc derangements of the lumbosacral spine: discographic diagnosis and treatment by posterior lumbar interbody fusion. *Orthopedics* 1991;14:447–451.
19. Blumenthal SL, Baker J, Dossett A, et al. The role of anterior lumbar fusion for internal disc disruption. *Spine* 1988;13:566–569.
20. Kozak JA, O'Brien JP. Simultaneous combined anterior and posterior fusion. An independent analysis of a treatment for the disabled low-back pain patient. *Spine* 1990;15:322–328.
21. Kostuik JP, Errico TJ, Gleason TF. Luque instrumentation in degenerative conditions of the lumbar spine. *Spine* 1990;15:318–321.
22. Gill K, Blumenthal SL. Functional results after anterior lumbar fusion at L5-S1 in patients with normal and abnormal MRI scans. *Spine* 1992;17:940–942.
23. Lee CK, Vessa P, Lee JK. Chronic disabling low back pain syndrome cause by internal disc derangements. The results of disc excision and posterior lumbar interbody fusion. *Spine* 1995;20:356–361.
24. Wetzel FT, La Rocca SH, Lowery GL, et al. The treatment of lumbar spinal pain syndromes diagnosed by discography: lumbar arthrodesis. *Spine* 1994;19:792–800.
25. Parker LM, Murrell SE, Boden SD, et al. The outcome of posterolateral fusion in highly selected patients with discogenic low back pain. *Spine* 1996;21:1909–1917.
26. Penta M, Fraser RD. Anterior lumbar interbody fusion. A minimum 10-year follow-up. *Spine* 1997;22:2429–2434.

27. Greenough CG, Peterson MD, Hadlow S, et al. Instrumented posterolateral lumbar fusion. Results and comparison with anterior interbody fusion. *Spine* 1998;23:479–486.
28. Fritzell P, Hagg O, Wessberg P, et al; and the Swedish Lumbar Spine Study Group. 2001 Volvo Award Winner in clinical studies: lumbar fusion versus nonsurgical treatment for chronic low back pain. A multicenter randomized controlled trial from the Swedish Lumbar Spine Study Group. *Spine* 2001;26:2521–2532.
29. Fritzell P, Hägg O, Wessberg P, et al; and the Swedish Lumbar Spine Study Group. Chronic low back pain and fusion: a comparison of three surgical techniques. A prospective multicenter randomized study from the Swedish Lumbar Spine Study Group. *Spine* 2002;27:1131–1141.
30. Brox JI, Sorensen R, Friis A, et al. Randomized clinical trial of lumbar instrumented fusion and cognitive intervention and exercises in patients with chronic low back pain, and disc degeneration. *Spine* 2003;28:1913–1921.
31. Fairbank J, Frost H, Wilson-MacDonald J, et al; Spine Stabilisation Trial Group. Randomised controlled trial to compare surgical stabilisation of the lumbar spine with an intensive rehabilitation programme for patients with chronic low back pain: the MRC spine stabilisation trial. *BMJ* 2005;330:1233.
32. Anderson PA, Rouleau JP. Intervertebral disc arthroplasty. *Spine* 2004;29:2779–2786.
33. Gamradt SC, Wang JC. Lumbar disc arthroplasty. *Spine J* 2005;5:95–103.
34. Blumenthal S, McAfee PC, Guyer RD, et al. A prospective, randomized, multicenter Food and Drug Administration investigational device exemptions study of lumbar total disc replacement with the CHARITÉ™ artificial disc *versus* lumbar fusion. Part I: evaluation of clinical outcomes. *Spine* 2005;30:1565–1575.
35. Zigler J, Delamarter R, Spivak JM, et al. Results of the prospective, randomized, multicenter Food and Drug Administration investigational device exemption study of the ProDisc®-L total disc replacement *versus* circumferential fusion for the treatment of 1-level degenerative disc disease. *Spine* 2007;32:1155–1162.
36. Mirza SK. Point of view. Commentary on the research reports that led to Food and Drug Administration approval of an artificial disc. *Spine* 2005;30:1561–1564.
37. Mirza SK, Deyo RA. Systematic review of randomized trials comparing lumbar fusion surgery to nonoperative care for treatment of chronic back pain. *Spine* 2007;32:816–823.
38. Zindrick MR, Spratt KF. Point of view. *Spine* 2007;32:1163.
39. Bertagnoli R, Yue JJ, Shah R, et al. The treatment of disabling single-level lumbar discogenic low back pain with total disc arthroplasty utilizing the Prodisc prosthesis: a prospective study with 2-year minimum follow-up. *Spine* 2005;30:2230–2236.
40. McCrory DC, Turner DA, Patwardhan MB, et al. *Spinal Fusion for Treatment of Degenerative Disease Affecting the Lumbar Spine.* Rockville, MD: Agency for Healthcare Research and Quality; 2006.
41. Health Quality Ontario. Artificial discs for lumbar and cervical degenerative disc disease -update: an evidence-based analysis. *Ont Health Technol Assess Ser* 2006;6(10):1–98.
42. Jacobs W, Van der Gaag NA, Tuschel A, et al. Total disc replacement for chronic back pain in the presence of disc degeneration. *Cochrane Database Syst Rev* 2012;(9):CD008326. doi:10.1002/14651858.CD008326.pub2.
43. Wei J, Song Y, Sun L, et al. Comparison of artificial total disc replacement versus fusion for lumbar degenerative disc disease: a meta-analysis of randomized controlled trials. *Int Orthop* 2013;37:1315–1325.
44. Jacobs WC, van der Gaag NA, Kruyt MC, et al. Total disc replacement for chronic discogenic low back pain: a Cochrane review. *Spine* 2013;38:24–36.
45. Formica M, Divano S, Cavagnaro L, et al. Lumbar total disc arthroplasty: outdated surgery or here to stay procedure? A systematic review of current literature. *J Orthop Traumatol* 2017;18:197–215.
46. Salzmann SN, Plais N, Jennifer Shue J, et al. Lumbar disc replacement surgery—successes and obstacles to widespread adoption. *Curr Rev Musculoskelet Med* 2017;10:153–159.
47. Todd NV. The surgical treatment of non-specific low back pain. *Bone Joint J* 2017;99-B:1003–1005.
48. van Tulder MW, Koes B, Seitsalo S, et al. Outcome of invasive treatment modalities on back pain and sciatica: an evidence-based review. *Eur Spine J* 2006;15:S82–S92.
49. Wang X, Wanyan P, Tian JH, et al. Meta-analysis of randomized trials comparing fusion surgery to non-surgical treatment for discogenic chronic low back pain. *J Back Musculoskelet Rehabil* 2015;28:621–627.
50. Noshchenko A, Hoffecker L, Lindley EM, et al. Long-term treatment effects of lumbar arthrodeses in degenerative disk disease. A systematic review with meta-analysis. *J Spinal Disord Tech* 2015;28:E493–E521.
51. Eck JC, Sharan A, Ghogawala Z, et al. Guideline update for the performance of fusion procedures for degenerative disease of the lumbar spine. Part 7: lumbar fusion for intractable low-back pain without stenosis or spondylolisthesis. *J Neurosurg Spine* 2014;21:42–47.
52. Bydon M, De la Garza-Ramos R, Macki M, et al. Lumbar fusion versus nonoperative management for treatment of discogenic low back pain: a systematic review and meta-analysis of randomized controlled trials. *J Spinal Disord Tech* 2014;27:297–304.
53. Phillips FM, Slosar PJ, Youssef JA, et al. Lumbar spine fusion for chronic low back pain due to degenerative disc disease: a systematic review. *Spine* 2013;38:E409–E422.
54. Carreon LY, Glassman SD, Kantamneni NR, et al. Clinical outcomes after posterolateral lumbar fusion in workers' compensation patients: a case-control study. *Spine* 2010;35:1812–1817.

CHAPTER 75

Failed Back Surgery

Failed back surgery (FBS) is a nonspecific term that implies the outcome of spine surgery did not meet the expectations established *before* surgery of the patient and the surgeon. It does not mean that the patient failed to get total pain relief or return to full function. Such expectations are not reliably attainable. It might be argued that when the patient is not satisfied, but the surgeon feels the outcome meets expectations, it is a failure of communication rather than the surgery.

There can be wide discrepancies between patient and surgeon with regard to expectations of outcome with patients usually having higher expectations than their surgeon.[1] Factors associated with higher patient expectations of outcome include younger age, not widowed, prior chiropractic care, poorer function as measured by Oswestry Disability Index (ODI), and worse mental health score.[2]

A surgeon's expectations for outcome in a specific patient should be based on published medical evidence, the nature of the structural problem, the number and types of prior surgeries, the psychological health of the patient, and the skills and experience of the surgeon. When the surgeon communicates reasonable expectations, there is greater chance the patient will be satisfied if those expectations are met.[3]

There are almost too many options for the treatment of patients with FBS. It seems logical that the best outcome will occur when treatment is matched to each specific patient's structural, neuropathic, or psychological cause. This often requires a multidisciplinary approach. To be prepared to treat these challenging patients, physicians should know the reasons spine surgery might fail, the structural causes of FBS, and the best treatment options for each situation.

Causes of Failed Back Surgery

It has been said that the best surgical outcome occurs when the right surgeon does the right surgery for the right problem on the right patient at the right time. There is a significant risk for FBS when any of these rights goes wrong.

There are several studies that have looked at the structural and neuropathic causes of FBS.[4-7] Clinically, it is most important to determine the structural cause for the pain whenever possible. If a structural etiology is identified, it is useful to decide whether the cause is a residual, recurrent, or new problem. Residual or recurrent structural pathology may be due to inadequate evaluation before surgery or mismatch of the surgery needed versus the surgery performed, unrecognized complications, or technical failure. New structural problems are those that developed after surgery, which might or might not be a consequence of the surgery itself.

Another model is based on the time course of the residual, recurrent, or new pain after surgery. Patients who never improve or who deteriorate in the first 4 weeks or so after surgery are likely to have residual pathology, a complication, or a technical failure. Most of these patients will still be under the care of their surgeon rather than a pain medicine specialist. Patients who get somewhat better initially but then deteriorate may have developed instability, instrumentation failure, recurrent disk herniation, or delayed infection. Those who get better but then deteriorate after 6 months or so might have new pathology at the same or adjacent segment, which can include for example facet or sacroiliac joint (SIJ) pain or pseudarthrosis.

MISMATCH: SURGERY NEEDED VERSUS SURGERY PERFORMED ("WRONG SURGERY")

When a surgeon chooses an operation that is not appropriate for the structural problem, the operation is likely to fail. It might prove useful, in this model, to appreciate the distinction between surgery for leg pain as opposed to surgery for back pain. True radicular (rather than referred) leg pain is usually caused by neural compression. Surgeries aimed at improving leg pain include decompression of involved neural structures in the neural foramen, central canal, or by a disk herniation. Assuming facet and SIJ source of pain have been excluded, surgeries directed toward improving axial low back pain (LBP) include fusion for pain arising from a disk (discogenic pain) or instability, for example. It follows that if a patient had predominantly axial LBP but had a decompression or discectomy without fusion, it might not have been the "right surgery" for the clinical problem, and there is a high likelihood of poor result. In other words, there was a mismatch between the clinical problem and the surgery. The surgeon performed a "leg pain operation" for LBP.

A second type of mismatch occurs when the surgery does not address all the patient's pathology. For example, there are patients who have pathology such as disk degeneration, disk herniations, spinal stenosis, or combinations at multiple motion segments. The surgeon might have elected to operate on only the worst segment or segments, thereby leaving the patient with residual problems at the adjacent segments. This type of patient might have required multilevel surgery or, if the number of levels is excessive, perhaps no surgery at all.

Another example is the patient with both central and foraminal stenosis. The surgeon achieves decompression of the central canal but does not achieve adequate decompression of the lateral canal. The patient may be left with leg pain due to remaining foraminal stenosis, which might incorrectly be thought to be neuropathic pain. Yet, another example is the patient with severe foraminal stenosis. A surgeon may decide to perform a limited decompression for fear of causing instability that might necessitate fusion. As a result, there is inadequate decompression and the patient does not get better. The patient needed decompression and fusion but only had decompression. This is another mismatch between the surgery needed and the surgery performed.

Another example of a mismatch between the surgery needed and the surgery performed occurs when the surgeon fails to fully consider the effect of surgery on the motion segment. For example, consider a patient with spinal stenosis and very slight spondylolisthesis and spinal stenosis who has leg pain. If the surgeon chooses decompression without fusion, many times, the spondylolisthesis progresses and the patient develops progressive LBP.

Finally, and not to be minimized, some spinal pathology is not treatable by surgery. An example would be four or five levels of painful disks.

INCOMPLETE EVALUATION AND/OR DIAGNOSIS ("RESIDUAL PATHOLOGY")

If a patient has not been fully evaluated, it is more likely that the surgery will fail. Surgery performed after an incomplete evaluation might leave significant structural pathology unattended.

Incomplete evaluation is often due to over reliance on imaging studies, particularly magnetic resonance imaging (MRI), without fully appreciating the information from the history and examination. Many spine specialists use confirmatory diagnostic spinal injections to complement the other information. Plain radiographs done standing with flexion and extension views can be very valuable to disclose spondylolisthesis or deformity that was not seen on supine MRI.[8] Pain relief after transforaminal epidural injection would suggest any foraminal stenosis seen on MRI is in fact the pain generator.[9–11] Discography had been used frequently but is rarely used now due to the possibility of creating long-term degeneration of otherwise normal disks coupled with the great improvements in the quality of MRI scans.[12]

Psychological health is one of the most important variables with respect to the outcome of surgery.[13,14] Therefore, psychological evaluation is especially important for patients ("right patient") with long-standing pain and impairment or when the surgeon has any inkling that there might be a significant psychological problem. Neither surgeons nor physiatrists perform well in identifying patients with psychological illness compared to objective psychological testing and so referral is often in the best interests of all.[15]

Most psychological illness in the postoperative patient was present before surgery but not considered or was underestimated. Many patients with long-standing chronic LBP have some degree of psychological illness, some mild but some more severe, which might have altered surgery decision making.[13] The most common problems described are depression, anxiety disorder, and substance use disorder.[14] Although these disorders may not be a contraindication for surgery, treatment before surgery and psychological follow-up afterward might prove useful to increase the chances of a good result. In addition to these familiar illnesses, there is growing evidence that a patient's coping abilities, fear and fear-avoidance behavior, and history of sexual or physical abuse may play important roles in continuing pain, impairment, and disability and contributing to a poor outcome.[16–23]

COMPLICATIONS

Many of the complications of spinal surgery occur early in the postoperative period and should have been recognized by the surgeon. Infection usually occurs early but occasionally does not appear for weeks or months. Misplaced pedicle screws can cause new leg pain, usually in a single dermatome, and is often present immediately after surgery but can occur slightly later. Neural injury during surgery has similar symptoms and appears right after surgery. Complications that occur or are discovered later include facet or pedicle fractures; pedicle screw misplacement; and bone graft collapse, resorption, or dislocation (after interbody fusion). In addition, surgery might have been performed at the wrong level.

Pedicle screws can cause LBP by any of several mechanisms. There can be pain over the screws, sometimes attributed to chronic irritation of overlying soft tissues and bursa formation. This usually is seen months after surgery. Pedicle screw misplacement can cause leg pain if a screw breaches a pedicle and irritates or injures a nerve. This can be mistaken for neural injury due to surgical trauma. Therefore, if there is leg pain in a single dermatome, it is necessary to obtain computed tomography (CT) scan to see if there has been even slight breach of the pedicle.

Pseudarthrosis is a failure of fusion. Some patients with nonunions have pain, but others do not. Therefore, one cannot assume that the nonunion is the cause of the pain. Plain radiographs are not reliable to show if a fusion is solid. However, if standing films with sagittal flexion and extension views show motion, it would indicate nonunion. The most useful test is a CT scan that includes reformatted curved coronal sections that are taken out to the tips of the transverse processes in addition to the usual sagittal and axial images.[24,25] CT also allows visualization of the anterior column to look for lucency surrounding an interbody fusion device.

Some patients undergo surgery and then develop instability, defined as greater than 3 mm translation on standing flexion/extension x-rays. It is not uncommon to see patients with very slight spondylolisthesis before surgery for disk herniation or spinal stenosis in whom no fusion was done because the slip was so slight. Then some months after surgery, the back pain worsens, and plain x-rays reveal progression of the slip.

TECHNICAL FAILURE

Even though the surgery was appropriate for the symptoms and pathology, the surgeon may not have accomplished the technical goals. Technical failure is usually apparent on good-quality imaging studies. Inadequate decompression of a foramen is not uncommon. There may be incomplete removal of a disk herniation, especially if it was a far lateral herniation. There may be misplacement of screws or incorrect connection of internal fixation.

RESIDUAL PATHOLOGY
Spinal Pathology
Residual pathology implies that surgery did not correct all the structural problems that had been causing pain. Problems such as pain arising from facet or SIJ might not have been recognized. There might have been pathology at other levels in addition to the operated segment.

Extraspinal Pathology
Residual pathology also includes extraspinal disorders that can mimic spinal problems.[26–30] When an extraspinal disorder is the cause of pain, it might have been present prior to surgery and not recognized or occurred afterward. Some of the more common problems that can mimic motion segment spine pain are shown in Table 75.1 and include primary hip disorders, SIJ pain, greater trochanteric pain syndromes (GTPS), and peripheral nerve injury or entrapment.[26–30]

TABLE 75.1 Differential Diagnosis of Some of the More Common Extraspinal Causes of Failed Back Surgery by Symptoms, Signs, Radiology, and Injections				
Diagnosis	**Symptoms**	**Signs**	**Radiology**	**Injections**
Hip	Groin pain	Limp; limited hip internal rotation	Standing x-rays of pelvis + hips	Relief with intra-articular anesthetic
Trochanteric pain syndrome	Lateral thigh pain	Tenderness over GT and muscle insertions	Not helpful	Relief with injection of GT and muscle insertions
Nerve entrapment or neuroma	Pain in peripheral nerve distribution	Allodynia, + Tinel sign	MRI, EMG, and nerve conduction	Relief with anesthesia of affected nerve
Peripheral arterial insufficiency	Arterial claudication	Poor pulses	Positive arterial studies	N/A

EMG, electromyography; GT, greater trochanter; MRI, magnetic resonance imaging; N/A, not applicable.

Painful disorders of the hip region most often are independent of spinal pathology but, at times, can coexist, especially in older patients.[30] This is a challenging problem because there is considerable overlap between their respective symptoms and signs. Brown et al.[31] studied a referral population with leg pain to determine if there were signs or symptoms that might differentiate between osteoarthritis of the hip and a spinal disorder. The factors that were suggestive of primary hip pathology were the presence of a limp, groin pain, or limited internal rotation of the hip. Factors more suggestive of spinal stenosis were lateral thigh pain, buttock pain, and pain below the knee, particularly in the absence of groin pain. Weight-bearing radiographs of the hip can serve as an initial screening tool.

Disorders of the structures near the hip that can mimic spine pain include GTPS, subtle sacral fractures, gluteal tendonitis, hamstring syndrome, ischial bursitis, or tendonitis. Patients with GTPS typically complain of pain in the proximal lateral thigh, often with radiation to the distal thigh and occasionally below the knee.[26,29] Pain is usually increased by lying on the affected side, climbing stairs, and transition from sitting to standing. Pain may arise from the bursa itself or from the gluteal medius and minimus.[32] On exam, there is tenderness over the greater trochanter, but in the variants of GTPS, there may be tenderness at the local muscle insertion sites. Diagnosis is confirmed by relief of pain with the injection of local anesthetic into the bursa and nearby muscles.

Peripheral nerve trauma or entrapment can mimic radiculopathy.[27] In the patient with FBS, the most relevant problems are lateral femoral cutaneous nerve entrapment or injury (meralgia paresthetica), which presents with pain in the lateral or anterolateral thigh, peroneal nerve entrapment, and sciatic nerve entrapment.[27,28] With entrapments, pain will be in the distribution of the peripheral nerve involved, not in a true lumbar dermatome. There may be a positive Tinel sign over the area of pathology. Diagnosis can often be confirmed by nerve conduction studies, and there will be temporary relief of pain after injection with local anesthetic in the area of presumed entrapment.

RECURRENT PATHOLOGY

Recurrent pathology can recur even after perfect surgery. Disk herniations recur in up to 15% of patients after discectomy. Foraminal stenosis can recur after if there is progressive degeneration of the same motion segment.

NEW PATHOLOGY

Pain after prior spine surgery may be totally unrelated to the index surgery. The usual structural causes of LBP can occur after an index surgery.

Structural Etiologies of Failed Back Surgery

Despite the many reasons for FBS, there are a limited number of structural etiologies for the residual or recurrent pain. The studies that looked at the most common structural causes of FBS had very similar findings (Table 75.2).[4-7] The most common structural causes of pain after surgery are foraminal stenosis, recurrent or residual disk herniation, one or more painful disks, facet joints (FJs), SIJ, and neuropathic pain.

There are four studies that reported on the causes of FBS in individual series. Unfortunately, one is from 1981 and two from 2002. The most recent study was in 2010 but only looked at patients with prior fusion. It does not appear that there have been more recent descriptions despite FBS being fairly common. Because of the age of the data, some considerations are necessary. There has been much greater recognition of neuropathic pain and pain arising from the SIJ pain and FJs. Surgical techniques have improved. There is greater

TABLE 75.2 Most Common Spinal Causes of Failed Back Surgery in Three Reported Studies[5-7]

Diagnosis	Waguespack et al.[5]	Slipman et al.[6]	DePalma et al.[7a]
Number of patients	181[b]	197[b]	28
Foraminal stenosis	64 (35%)	25 (15%)	
Disk herniation	12 (7%)	12 (13%)	
Discogenic pain	45 (25%)	40 (30%)	7 (25%)
Neuropathic pain	18 (10%)	25 (13%)	
Instability	9 (5%)	4 (2%)	
Pseudarthrosis	26 (14%)	0	
Facet joint	Not evaluated	5 (3%)	5 (18%)
Sacroiliac joint	Not evaluated	3 (2%)	12 (43%)
No primary diagnosis	11 6(%)	11 (5.6%)	0
Other	7 (4%)		4[c] (14%)

[a]All postfusion.
[b]Some patients had >1 diagnosis.
[c]Irritation from hardware.

recognition of foraminal stenosis. It is too early to know all the causes in patients who have undergone total disk replacement. That said, the data we have is what we have to work with, coupled with experience.

Burton et al.[4] in 1981 reported an analysis of several hundred patients with FBS. About 58% had foraminal stenosis, 7% to 14% had central canal stenosis, 12% to 16% had recurrent (or residual) disk herniations, 6% to 16% had arachnoiditis, and 6% to 8% had epidural fibrosis. Other less common causes in their series included neuropathic pain, chronic mechanical pain, painful disk above a fusion, pseudarthrosis, foreign body, and surgery performed at the wrong level. They were unable to establish a diagnosis in less than 5% of their patients, even though their patients were evaluated early in the CT scan era and well before MRI scans. They did use discography. In 1981, surgeons were less aware of foraminal stenosis and discogenic pain.

In a retrospective review of 181 patients with FBS seen at a tertiary care spine center, Waguespack et al.[5] could make a diagnosis in 94% of patients. Slipman et al.[6] also could make a diagnosis in about 89% of patients. Some patients had more than one primary diagnosis. DePalma et al.[7] looked at the etiology of pain in patients who had lumbar fusions. The details are shown in Table 75.2

In the following section, I have used functional definitions of structural abnormalities that are a composite of those proposed by the North American Spine Society.[33] The differential diagnoses of some of the more common causes of FBS along with some helpful symptoms, signs, radiologic findings, and response to injections are shown in Table 75.3.

FORAMINAL STENOSIS

Foraminal stenosis was found in 15% and 35% of FBS patients in the studies of Waguespack et al.[5] and Slipman et al.,[6] half of what was seen 25 years ago.[4] The lower prevalence may be due to increased awareness of the problem, improved imaging studies, and/or better understanding of the need for meticulous decompression. Patients with foraminal stenosis have pain that is predominantly in the leg or buttock region, often in the distribution of a single dermatome. Pain is usually worsened by standing and walking and relieved by sitting. MRI or CT scan shows narrowing of the canal at the index level or an adjacent segment.

There are no data regarding the utility of selective nerve root blocks in FBS. There are suggestions that when performed with excellent technique, they can provide some information, especially perhaps when there is no relief, which might suggest the targeted root was not the cause of pain.[10] According to one systematic review, there is good evidence that lumbar

TABLE 75.3 Differential Diagnosis of Common Causes of Failed Back Surgery by Symptoms, Signs, Radiology, and Injections

Diagnosis	Symptoms	Signs	Radiology	Injections
Lateral canal stenosis	Leg pain > LBP; relief with sitting	Loss of lumbar lordosis	MRI: foraminal stenosis	Relief with transforaminal epidural
Painful disk	LBP; ? worse with sitting	Restricted flexion in standing	MRI: degenerated disk(s)	No sustained relief
Neuropathic pain	Leg pain burning Dysesthesia	Hypoalgesia Allodynia	No alternative diagnosis	+/− relief with sympathetic block
Facet syndrome	Left or right LBP	? Facet tenderness	Not specific	Medial branch block relieves pain
Recurrent HNP	Vary with location; leg pain > LBP	Variable	HNP on MRI	Epidural may provide temporary relief
SI joint pain	Gluteal pain with referral to leg and groin	May have + provocative testing	Not helpful	SI joint injection relieves pain

HNP, herniated nucleus pulposus; LBP, low back pain; MRI, magnetic resonance imaging; SI, sacroiliac; +/−, may be helpful.

selective nerve root blocks can aid with the identification of one or more symptomatic roots.[9] There is moderate evidence that identifying or excluding a root as cause of pain improves surgical outcome.[9] Other systematic reviews did not find the evidence convincing.[11]

PAINFUL DISK (DISCOGENIC PAIN)

Pain that arises from within a disk is often referred to as discogenic pain. One or more painful disks was found to be the cause of FBS in 25% to 30% of patients.[4–7] Painful disks can occur at the level of prior surgery, at an adjacent segment, or rarely at the index level despite prior posterolateral fusion.[34,35] When there is a residual painful disk at the index surgical level, it is likely that it was not treated adequately by performing a fusion, especially an interbody fusion. When there is a painful disk at an adjacent segment, it was either present prior to surgery and not addressed or the disk degenerated after surgery.[35] Risk factors for adjacent segment degeneration include body mass index >25 kg/m, preoperative disk degeneration, and superior FJ violation during surgery

Although there is no totally consistent symptom complex for discogenic LBP, especially after surgery, the diagnosis is more likely when there is dominant midline LBP that might radiate to the left and right of the midline, the gluteal regions, and often to the leg in a nondermatomal fashion. Pain is usually worse sitting and during transition from sitting to standing. It may improve with standing or walking. Physical examination is not specific. There may be decreased flexion in standing due to pain. There may be tenderness over the spinous processes but not over the FJs.

When the diagnosis of discogenic pain is suggested by history and examination, MRI shows a single degenerated disk, and other potential causes of chronic LBP have been excluded, it is likely that the diagnosis is correct.

DISK HERNIATION

Recurrent or residual disk herniation was seen in 7% to 12% of patients with FBS.[4–6] There are two common presentations of pain from a disk herniation: radicular and axial. The topography of the pain is primarily due to the location of the herniation. A posterolateral herniation is more likely to compress or irritate a nerve root and therefore present with predominant leg pain. A midline herniation, unless very large, does not compress neural elements and presents with predominant LBP. A disk that is degenerated and herniated can cause both leg pain and LBP. In the presence of epidural or perineural fibrosis, a disk herniation may cause more leg pain than expected than if there were no fibrosis.

Diagnosis of recurrent or residual disk herniation is inferred from the history and physical examination and confirmed by MRI.

FACET JOINT PAIN

The FJs were the cause of pain in 3% to 18% of patients with FBS.[6,7,36,37] FJ injury may occur during surgery because of progressive degeneration of the motion segment at the surgical level or degeneration due to the mechanical stresses of fusion at an adjacent segment.

There has been increased interest in the role of FJs since the introduction of total disk arthroplasty (TDR). Van Ooij et al.[38] reported that FJ arthrosis was responsible for clinical failure in 11 of 27 patients. Shim et al. reported radiologic degradation of the facets in 32% to 36% of patients after TDR.[38,39]

There are no reports of definitively correlated symptoms and signs of FJ pain in patients with FBS. Based on best evidence and clinical expertise, it is reasonable to perform medial branch blocks on most FBS patients as part of the routine evaluation when back pain (vs. leg pain) predominates unless there is another obvious cause for the problem.[36,40] Features of the history that increase the likelihood of FJ pain being present are age greater than 65 years, absence of midline pain, and improvement in pain by lying supine. Other features are pain is not worse with forward flexion including sitting, not worse when rising from sitting to standing, and not worse with coughing. Features from the examination are tenderness to palpation over the FJs or transverse processes. The diagnosis of FJ pain is made when there is excellent relief of the target pain on two occasions after medial branch block.[36]

SACROILIAC JOINT PAIN

There is consistent evidence that the SIJ can be a cause of pain in at least 2% to 3% in patients with FBS and may be as high as 42% in patients who have had fusion to the sacrum.[5–7,41–43] The SIJ can become painful due to transfer of stress after fusion or might have been present before surgery but not recognized.[44,45]

Again, there are no specific signs or symptoms specific for SIJ pain, but there are clues to the diagnosis. Virtually all patients have pain distal to the posterior iliac crest and lateral to the midline spine. Some patients will point directly over the SIJ when asked to show where the pain is centered. Pain is frequently referred to the groin, thigh, calf, and occasionally the foot—patterns that might otherwise suggest radiculopathy or even hip joint pathology. Pain may increase with single-leg weight bearing. Most often, there is tenderness directly over the SIJ. Plain radiographs, MRI, and CT are not definitive. The confirmation of SIJ pain requires relief of the target pain after fluoroscopically guided local anesthetic SIJ injection.

SPINAL STENOSIS AND AXIAL LOW BACK PAIN

The classic symptom of central spinal stenosis is leg pain with walking (neurogenic claudication) or standing. In addition, many if not most patients with spinal stenosis also report LBP.[46–48] Anecdotally and experientially, there are patients with spinal stenosis with predominant LBP, especially in the gluteal region. Pain is worse with standing or walking, and there is complete or near-complete relief of pain sitting. This symptom complex is quite the opposite of discogenic pain but similar to FJ pain. Patients usually experience at least temporary relief of pain after epidural steroid injection and no relief after medial branch block, again just the opposite of FJ pain. The patients with FBS and predominant LBP might have spinal stenosis at the index level or an adjacent segment that developed after surgery or was not addressed at surgery.

NEUROPATHIC PAIN

Neuropathic pain is pain due to injury or physiologic dysfunction of the peripheral or central nervous system (CNS). Neuropathic pain was the predominant problem in 10% to 13% of FBS patients.[4–6] It is likely that there is increased attention being paid to neuropathic pain as better treatments have become available.

There are several potential mechanisms for neuropathic pain after spine surgery. A nerve root could have been damaged prior to surgery due to either sudden injury (acute disk herniation) or prolonged compression from foraminal stenosis or disk herniation. In the latter two examples, radicular type pain continues despite technically successful surgery. Alternatively, a nerve could be damaged during the surgery itself, which is sometimes referred to as a *battered nerve*. There can be peripheral nerve injuries such as cluneal neuroma due to nerve injury at an iliac crest donor site. Meralgia paresthetica can also be seen.[28,49]

Neural injury or dysfunction can be responsible for both amplification and persistence of pain. Neuropathic pain of spinal origin usually presents with a predominance of leg pain in one or two adjacent dermatomes or along the path of a peripheral nerve. In classic presentations, the pain is described as burning, dysesthetic, or electrical, but in neuropathic disorders after spine surgery, pain is more frequently described as aching and stabbing. Pain may be constant or intermittent. It is often precipitated or aggravated by simple activities because the damaged nerves are hyperexcitable and respond abnormally to even minor mechanical changes.

In pure and uncomplicated neuropathic pain, there is no evidence of nerve root compression on imaging studies. It is important to distinguish neuropathic pain from what I call neurogenic pain. Neurogenic pain implies that a nerve is being compressed or irritated rather than its being permanently damaged. To further complicate matters, some patients have both neuropathic pain plus ongoing neural compression (neurogenic), which is referred to as a mixed pain syndrome.

Neuropathic pain can also be due to physiologic dysfunction in the peripheral nervous system or CNS without obvious structural nerve damage. Because of prolonged or repeated chemical or mechanical damage to afferent nerves, these nociceptors may become sensitized and hyperexcitable (peripheral sensitization). There is lowering of their activation thresholds and subsequent increased responsiveness to all stimuli. In this physiologically altered setting, innocuous stimuli may be perceived as painful (allodynia), minimally noxious stimuli may be perceived as very painful (hyperalgesia), and there can be stimulus-independent pain as well.

A similar sensitization can develop in the CNS because of "constant bombardment" by painful afferent stimuli (central sensitization). In patients with persistent axial LBP (rather than the more typical neuropathic extremity pain) despite perfect surgery and no other explanation for pain, it has been proposed that the back pain represents central sensitization and neuropathic pain.[50,51]

EPIDURAL FIBROSIS

Epidural fibrosis has been reported to occur in 16% of patients with FBS when assessed by MRI and 83% when assessed by epiduroscopy.[52] Some believe epidural fibrosis is a frequent cause of pain after back surgery, but others have found no relation between amount or location of scar and pain or disability.[52–54] Most spine surgeons feel that most often fibrosis is an incidental finding that does not in and of itself causes pain but perhaps has the potential to make other problems such as radiculopathy due to disk herniation or spinal stenosis worse.[53] That said, it is true that some patients with FBS and fibrosis do improve after lysis of adhesions, but this is not proof that the scar itself was the cause.[55] Most authors feel that further research is necessary before epidural lysis becomes standard practice.

DECONDITIONING

Deconditioning has been considered to be at least partially responsible for the persistent pain and pain-related impairment and disability in many patients with chronic LBP and FBS. I view three models for this so-called *deconditioning syndrome*. The pure physical deconditioning model holds that loss of muscle strength and endurance is responsible for reduced activity, impairment, and disability.[56] The cognitive-behavioral model emphasizes the fear-avoidance paradigm, which holds that some patients with chronic LBP avoid activities out of pain-related catastrophic thinking and fear.[56] They believe that attempts to increase their function will result in increased pain and progressive structural damage, and, as a result, they markedly curtail their activity. A third model is a combination of the two in which patients have both the maladaptive fear avoidance and true physical deconditioning. As a result of the fear-avoidant decreased activity, there is disuse (perhaps better termed *underuse*) with progressive loss of muscle strength and endurance.[56–60]

In patients with chronic LBP and deconditioning, the paraspinal musculature is most affected.[57] There is MRI, CT scan, and ultrasound evidence that after spine surgery, many patients have decreased cross-sectional area (CSA) of their lumbar muscles.[58] Motosuneya et al.[59] looked at the changes in muscle CSA after five different types of spine surgery and surprisingly found some loss of muscle strength even in those patients who had anterior spine surgery. They opined that rigid fixation and resultant protection of the paraspinal muscles was at least partly responsible.[59]

There is consistent evidence that posterior spine surgery (and possibly anterior as well) can cause loss of muscle density, histologic changes, and probably decreased strength. There is a trend in the evidence that suggests a correlation between greater muscle changes and LBP after surgery. Nearly all investigators agree there is good evidence that exercise is effective in reducing impairment and disability, but the mechanisms are not straightforward. Most likely, the deconditioning syndrome has both physical and psychological components. There can be loss of muscle volume and strength from the surgery itself and disuse. There might be a psychological component due to fear avoidance.

Psychological Factors in Failed Back Surgery ("Right Patient")

It has been well documented and fully accepted that many patients with chronic LBP have a psychological condition.[13,14] It is no wonder then that presurgical psychological testing can predict the outcome of spine surgery quite well.[13,61] It is also of note that spine surgeons and other spine specialists do not do well in the identification of psychological distress.[15] In patients with chronic LBP, the most common psychological illnesses are depression, anxiety disorder, and substance abuse disorder, and so, it is logical that many of these same factors are present in patients with sufficient structural abnormalities to potentially warrant surgery.[14] Most often, it appears that these psychological illnesses develop because of the injury.[62] Although rarely the only cause of pain, psychological factors can make pain and function worse.

Although preoperative depression correlates with postoperative symptoms, the literature suggests that the early psychological response is a very important predictor of longer term outcome.[21,22] This might be particularly relevant to management of FBS and warrants special attention to depressive illness and fear avoidance. For example, Adogwa et al.[63] showed that patient outcome for revision surgery for spinal stenosis, adjacent segment degeneration, and pseudoarthrosis correlated best with preoperative Zung Depression Scale score.

In a different very useful framework, the fear-avoidance model is important for patients with FBS. Preoperative fear avoidance does not appear to be a significant risk factor of FBS, but its early appearance after surgery appears to be predictive of eventual poor outcome.[22,23,64]

Fear avoidance, in the postoperative setting, is the avoidance of movements or activities due to fears of ruining the surgery, causing more pain, and/or reinjury. Fear avoidance can lead to inactivity and then disuse and deconditioning, which might worsen any disability. In turn, increased pain and depressive mood disorder might follow.

Archer and associates[22] prospectively studied fear avoidance and other psychological factors before and after spine surgery. In their series, fear avoidance 6 weeks after surgery was predictive of level of pain, physical health, and disability at 6 months. In addition, preoperative depression predicted similar poor results.

Catastrophic thinking, again in this context, is an exaggerated negative interpretation of the meaning of the pain.[65] Patients dwell on the most negative conceivable aspects and feel helpless and hopeless. Such thinking can be present in the postoperative period and appears to correlate to some degree with fear avoidance.

Yet, another model revolves around dysfunctional childhood and with what is now termed *adverse childhood events.* Such patients might be at higher risk for chronic pain, impairment, disability, and FBS.[8,66] Identified disruptions include childhood physical or sexual abuse; abandonment; or parents who had addictive disease, chronic pain syndromes, or severe psychological illness, among others.

It is also important to recognize that some of the psychological problems that can arise after surgery might be due to the psychological trauma of surgery itself (posttraumatic stress disorder [PTSD]) or the fear of making things worse afterward (fear avoidance and catastrophizing).[67,68] Hart et al.[67] reported a 22% prevalence of PTSD after spine surgery. This postoperative psychological distress was correlated with poorer outcome. The same authors also reported that preoperative psychiatric diagnosis was the strongest predictor of PTSD and seemed to be a stronger predictor of worse outcome than preoperative mental health.[68]

Establishing the Diagnosis

ROLE OF THE HISTORY

The history is the most important part of the evaluation of a patient with FBS. When possible, preoperative notes and imaging studies should be part of the history. The history provides the information necessary to order and interpret other diagnostic elements. The most important elements of the history include a thorough description of the current pain, a comparison of the pain before and after surgery, the time course of the reappearance of the pain, and the response of the pain to specific activities. It is also very valuable to analyze whether the type of surgery performed was appropriate for the preoperative symptoms and condition. The history should lead to a limited differential diagnosis, suggest the emphasis for the physical

examination, and provide guidelines for selecting appropriate imaging studies and diagnostic injections. It is important to remember there may be more than one diagnosis present.

Preoperative Versus Current Pain

Pain that is essentially the same before and after surgery in terms of severity, location, quality, and response to mechanical maneuvers suggests that the original problem was not corrected. There may have been an error in diagnosis, an error selecting the correct surgery, or an incomplete surgery. On the other hand, when symptoms have changed significantly, it is most likely that there is new pathology, either a complication of surgery, technical failure, or progression of the underlying disease.

Location of Pain (Especially Low Back Pain Versus Leg Pain)

It is useful to divide FBS patients into those with predominantly LBP and those with predominantly leg pain. In general, when LBP is greater than leg pain, the most common causes are discogenic pain at the level of the index surgery or at adjacent levels, FJ pain, SIJ pain, or instability. If fusion was attempted, there may be a pseudarthrosis, although pseudarthrosis itself can be an incidental finding rather than the cause of pain. When leg pain predominates, the more common causes include residual foraminal stenosis; recurrent or residual disk herniation; neuropathic pain; and also SIJ dysfunction, hip disease, or peripheral nerve injury or entrapment.

Response to Mechanical Changes

There are no studies that document the changes in pain in response to common activities in patients with FBS. Therefore, these correlations are extrapolated from studies in patients with chronic LBP and no prior surgery. These responses to biomechanical stresses are clues but obviously cannot be considered definitive.

Response to Sitting

LBP or leg pain that increases with sitting and with flexion in standing is more likely due to one or more painful disks or instability Leg pain that improves with sitting is usually due to spinal stenosis.

Transition from Sitting to Standing

LBP that worsens during the transition from sit to stand suggests disk pain or SIJ and speaks against FJ pain.[14] LBP that increases with standing suggests posterior element pathology such as FJ pain. Leg pain that increases with standing or walking suggests spinal stenosis.

Quality of Pain

The word the patient uses to describe the pain is occasionally helpful. Burning, electric shock-like pain, dysesthesia, or superficial (skin) tenderness to light touch (allodynia) suggests neuropathic pain. However, neuropathic pain after spine surgery may not fit these classical descriptors. Screening tests for neuropathic pain, although useful before surgery, are not as helpful after spine surgery.[51]

TIME COURSE OF APPEARANCE OF PAIN
Preoperative Low Back Pain or Leg Pain Never Improves or Early Onset of Old Symptoms

When LBP never improves or recurs within days to a month or so after surgery, it is most likely that the symptomatic structural pathology was not adequately addressed by surgery, there was a complication such as wrong level surgery or the wrong procedure for this particular patient was done. Partial pain relief implies correction of only part of the structural problem. This outcome falls in the category of residual pathology, and the differential diagnosis has already been outlined.

New Leg Pain Soon after Surgery

The early appearance of new leg pain suggests direct neural injury during surgery, misplacement of a pedicle screw, or, less commonly, deep venous thrombosis.[49]

Pain Improves but Recurs 1 to 6 Months after Surgery

Pain that improved initially but recurred in 1 to 6 months may be due to residual, recurrent, or new pathology. If pain location and description resemble preoperative symptoms, residual, or recurrent pathology is likely. Pain that has new characteristics is more likely due to new pathology. There may be recurrent disk herniation, failure (loosening of pedicle screws) of internal fixation, instability, and late infection.

Pain Improves but Recurs and Is Different

Pain that recurs late and has a different location or quality compared to the preoperative pain is more likely due to new pathology, which can occur at the index level or adjacent segment. Adjacent segment problems include painful degenerated disk, herniation, stenosis, or facet dysfunction. In addition, SIJ problems occur, especially if there is fusion to L5 or the sacrum.

ROLE OF RADIOLOGIC EVALUATION OF FAILED BACK SURGERY

The radiologic evaluation is important. The choice of the type of imaging is determined by the surgery performed and clues from the history and physical examination, which usually allow for a reasonable differential diagnosis. The best information will be obtained if the clinician consults with the radiologist regarding the suspected diagnosis, type of prior surgery, and current symptoms. The radiologist can then follow along with the testing in real time, which should yield the best information.

Radiologic examination should include plain x-rays and MRI scan.[8,25,69,70] CT is important if there is suspicion that the problem involves the bony structures, nonunion of fusion or location, or fracture of internal fixation screws, or if the patient is very claustrophobic.[8,24,69] There are only rare indications for nuclear imaging studies (infection, possible malignancy, possible rheumatologic illness), myelography (pseudomeningocele), or CT myelography.

Standard radiographs with standing flexion and extension lateral views and anteroposterior (AP) view are very important and are too frequently not performed.[8] These standard films are used to evaluate whether the desired segment(s) were addressed as an assessment of the alignment in multiple planes, extent of disk space narrowing if any, spondylolisthesis, and when fusion has been attempted, pseudarthrosis, or broken or misplaced internal fixation devices.[8,24] There are several excellent reviews of postoperative imaging that demonstrate the normal findings based on type of surgery as well as findings that indicate a structural problem.[25,69,70]

MRI is usually the optimal exam for most FBS patients. It is important that the radiologist knows this is a patient with FBS so the proper imaging sequences are obtained. MRI is excellent for the diagnosis of spinal stenosis, disk herniation, disk degeneration, and infection. It will show if decompression was adequate to decompress the nerve root. Arachnoiditis can easily be detected with MRI but is less valuable when there are certain types of instrumentation.

ROLE OF DIAGNOSTIC INJECTIONS
Anesthetic Injections

There are little data on the utility of diagnostic spinal injections in patients with FBS.[9,36] Anesthetic injections are the standard for the diagnosis of FJ and SIJ pain.[36,71,72] A transforaminal injection (TFI) is sometimes used to determine if a nerve that appears compressed on MRI or CT scan is in fact the pain generator.[73,74] A positive TFI may be defined as relief of the target pain after anesthetizing a specific spinal nerve.

Provocation Disk Injections (Discography)

Discography had been used extensively in the evaluation of patients with chronic LBP and FBS who were suspected of having discogenic pain. However, discography has fallen into disfavor because of data that suggests injection into a disk can result in long-term degeneration.[12] That said, it might play a very limited role in patients with FBS when definitive diagnosis is elusive, pain is refractory, and surgery is being considered.[7,75]

Treatments

There is a spectrum of treatments for FBS that ranges from manual therapy, exercise, and medication through interventional pain treatments and repeat surgery.[76] The treatment of each patient should be based on the cause of the pain and then the best available published evidence integrated with the physician's clinical expertise and each patient's values and circumstances. It must be recognized that just as pain management is not necessarily a failure of spine surgery, neither is corrective spine surgery a failure of pain management.

NONSPECIFIC TREATMENTS
Rehabilitation and Exercise

Rehabilitation is usually the first line of treatment for patients with FBS. The premise is that many patients are weak and deconditioned and exercise therapy will help overcome these factors.[60] In addition, there is evidence that exercise therapy helps patients overcome their fear avoidance, which leads to improvement in many domains, physical and psychological.[66]

Several studies have looked at the response to exercise and rehabilitation in patients with FBS.[77-79] Timm[77] compared five types of treatment for FBS: high-tech exercise, low-tech exercise, modalities, manipulation, and control group with no treatment. Both active forms of exercise were better than control, passive modalities and manipulation. Brox et al.[78] reported outcomes in patients treated for FBS after discectomy. The program was 25 hours per week for 3 weeks and included cognitive-behavioral therapy and lectures. At 1 year, LBP (0 to 100) improved from 65 to 51 and ODI improved from 45 to 32. Miller et al.[79] compared the outcomes of chronic LBP and FBS patients in an interdisciplinary functional restoration program. Both groups did well with significant decreases in pain and disability. The chronic LBP patients without prior surgery had greater reductions in pain and disability, but the FBS patients were significantly more improved in strength and endurance measures, activities of daily living, and fear of exercise after the program. Karahan et al.[80] compared isokinetic, lumbar stabilization, home exercises, and no treatment in a single-blind randomized trial of patients with FBS. They used both psychological and physical outcome measures. The isokinetic and lumbar stabilization groups had equivalent clinical and statistical improvement, both better than home exercise. All exercise groups did better than control.

Medications

The use of medications for patients with FBS is based on clinical experience, expert opinion, case series, and extrapolation from studies on patients with chronic LBP and other pain states rather than proof of efficacy in FBS.[81] Medications might play an adjunctive role while a patient is in rehabilitation, but in some patients, medication becomes a long-term treatment.

Acetaminophen (APAP), although commonly used, has been shown to be no more effective than placebo in acute LBP.[82,83] There are no studies of APAP in chronic LBP or FBS. Risk of liver disease is significant at doses above 3 g per day. There is little to recommend APAP in patients with FBS.

Nonsteroidal anti-inflammatory drugs (NSAIDs) are commonly prescribed for acute LBP. However, the data are mixed regarding efficacy. Newer trials report no advantage over placebo in chronic LBP.[81,84] NSAIDs have side effects that can be very serious, including myocardial infarction, gastrointestinal hemorrhage, and renal and liver toxicity, among others. Although the risk of major cardiovascular event is not high, it is important. Of note is that recent studies suggest that cardiac events can occur in the first week of use with a second peak before 30 days.[85] It is prudent to avoid NSAIDs in the elderly and patients with underlying medical problems, especially cardiac, who are at greatest risk of serious adverse events.

For most patients skeletal muscle relaxants do not provide much benefit for chronic LBP.[84] The antiseizure medications such as gabapentin, pregabalin, and topiramate might offer some benefit, although good data are lacking.

Neither tricyclic nor selective serotonin uptake inhibitors are effective for chronic LBP.[84] Duloxetine has been shown to be useful in some patients with chronic LBP but does not seem to have been studied in patients with FBS.

Opioid analgesics have become the most controversial medications for the treatment of pain not related to malignancy and are discussed in detail elsewhere. The most recent guideline of the American College of Physicians (ACP) states that pharmacologic therapies should be considered in patients who have not responded to nonpharmacologic therapies. They suggest NSAIDs and tramadol as first-line therapies, and tramadol or duloxetine as second-line therapies.[84] Paradoxically, this is the recommendation even though NSAIDs have little value and potentially serious adverse events. The guideline goes on to state,

> Clinicians should only consider opioids as an option in patients who have failed the aforementioned treatments and only if the potential benefits outweigh the risks for individual patients and after a discussion of known risks and realistic benefits with patients (grade: weak recommendation, moderate-quality evidence).

SOME OF THE SPECIFIC TREATMENTS FOR SPECIFIC DISORDERS
Discogenic Pain
Discogenic pain can occur at the index level of prior surgery or adjacent segment. In the setting of FBS, rehabilitation and fusion surgery have been compared. For patients with mild to moderate pain after discectomy, a 3-week interdisciplinary functional rehabilitation program was equal to fusion surgery.[78]

Facet Joint Pain
Klessinger[36] studied the efficacy of radiofrequency neurotomy (RFN) in 120 patients who had undergone microsurgical lumbar disk surgery and had residual axial LBP. There were 34 who had a positive response to diagnostic medial branch blocks and then were treated with RFN. Twenty patients (58.8%) achieved at least 50% reduction in pain for a minimum of 6 months. Good results have been seen in patients with chronic LBP of FJ origin as well.[86] Successful RFN relieves pain to a meaningful degree for about 9 to 12 months. When pain recurs, RFN can be repeated. Repeat RFN is usually successful unless there has been disease progression or technical failure.[87]

Sacroiliac Joint Pain
There do not appear to be studies of nonsurgical therapies for the treatment of SIJ pain after lumbar surgery.[41] The noninterventional options that have been reported in SIJ pain without fusion include medications (topical and oral), physical therapy, support belts, and manual therapy. If response is poor, SIJ corticosteroid injection can be considered the next step. The duration of relief after steroid injection varies greatly. Some patients achieve long-lasting relief after one to three injections, but others require several injections each year.[88] For patients who do not respond to these treatments, SIJ RFN can be effective in well-selected patients and sustained for 12 months in some.[89-91] Finally, for patients with severe and refractory pain, SIJ fusion has been reported to be helpful.[92]

Spinal Stenosis
As previously noted, spinal stenosis may involve the central canal or foramen or both. Foraminal stenosis is more common than central stenosis in patients with FBS. Central stenosis can be treated initially with rehabilitation and epidural corticosteroid injections. Patients who fail medical treatment and rehabilitation usually do well with surgery.[93-96] The same paradigm seems appropriate for foraminal stenosis. If stenosis is severe and extensive decompression is needed, fusion may be required. For mixed pain syndromes, if decompression is not sufficient, medications and/or spinal cord stimulation (SCS) may be useful.

Neuropathic Pain
Neuropathic pain is best treated sequentially with medication trial first and perhaps SCS if medications prove ineffective. If there is limited success, SCS is often useful.[97] SCS is discussed in detail elsewhere. Newer 10-kHz high-frequency SCS appears to improve efficacy and even provide improvement in the LBP component.

There are case series regarding the treatment of cluneal nerve injuries with injections of corticosteroids and sometimes with alcohol.[98]

Lysis of Adhesions
As noted earlier, most patients develop fibrosis after back surgery, and there is debate about its significance. In one theory, the fibrosis is responsible for the pain, and therefore, lysis of the adhesions will result in improvement. There are several studies and reviews that present evidence of effectiveness in a small number of well-selected patients.[76,99,100]

Psychological Interventions
Psychological illness, just like structural problems, is treated according to its severity and type with a detailed discussion elsewhere in this book. Depression, anxiety disorder, substance abuse disorder, and PTSD might best be treated with some combination of individual psychotherapy, group therapy, and, when necessary, medications. In addition, time-limited cognitive-behavioral therapy can be useful for reducing catastrophic thinking with its maladaptive interpretation of pain, increasing function, insomnia, and other stress-related problems.

Indirect forms of cognitive-behavioral treatments—physical rehabilitation, for example—can be useful for fear avoidance and even catastrophic thinking. Physical rehabilitation can provide both of strength and body mechanics training and at the same time help patients overcome some of the fear avoidance, catastrophic thinking, and even depression.[66,101]

Mindfulness training, also known as mindfulness-based stress reduction (MBSR), has been evaluated in a randomized controlled but short-term study in patients with FBS.[102] One group received usual care plus MBSR weekly for 8 weeks, and the other usual care alone. The MBSR group had clinically and significantly greater improvement than the control group in level of pain, pain acceptance, function, and sleep quality. Results were clinically and statistically significant. In a systematic review, Reiner et al.[103] found evidence that MBSR reduced pain intensity in patients with chronic pain. Schütze and associates[104] showed in a small study that the combination of MBSR and physical therapy produced meaningful improvements in pain catastrophizing, physical function, and depression.

Reoperation

The role of reoperation is complex and depends on the structural cause of the FBS, levels of pain, and disability and psychological status. If there is an anatomical abnormality that corresponds to the patient's pain, and the patient has failed all reasonable conservative care, surgery might be a viable option. Surgery is not likely to benefit neuropathic pain but might be beneficial for radicular pain.

Brox et al.[78] showed that reoperation after failure of discectomy was not better than aggressive conservative care consisting of an inpatient program for several weeks. Therefore, it appears reasonable to offer rehabilitation before contemplating surgery, although the magnitude of the conservative care used by Brox et al.[78] is rarely available to most patients.

Indications for surgery can include recurrent disk herniation, residual spinal stenosis, pseudarthrosis, progressive deformity, and severe adjacent segment disease.[93-96]

References

1. Lattig F, Fekete T, O'Riordan D, et al. A comparison of patient and surgeon preoperative expectations of spinal surgery. *Spine* 2013;38:1040–1048.
2. Mancuso C, Duculan R, Stal M, et al. Patients' expectations of lumbar spine surgery. *Eur Spine J* 2015;24:2362–2369.
3. Mancuso C, Duculan R, Cammisa F, et al. Fulfillment of patients' expectations of lumbar and cervical spine surgery. *Spine J* 2016;16:1167–1174.
4. Burton C, Kirkaldy-Willis W, Yong-Hing K, et al. Causes of failure of surgery on the lumbar spine. *Clin Orthop* 1981;157:191–199.
5. Waguespack A, Schofferman J, Slosar P, et al. Etiology of long-term failures of lumbar spine surgery. *Pain Med* 2002;3:18–22.
6. Slipman CW, Shin CH, Patel RK, et al. Etiologies of failed back surgery syndrome. *Pain Med* 2002;3:200–214.
7. DePalma M, Ketchum J, Saullo T. Etiology of chronic low back pain inpatients having undergone lumbar fusion. *Pain Med* 2011;12:732–739.
8. Kizilkilic O, Yalcin O, Sen O, et al. The role of standing flexion-extension radiographs for spondylolisthesis following single level disk surgery. *Neurol Res* 2007;29:540–543.
9. Cohen SP, Hurley RW. The ability of diagnostic spinal injections to predict surgical outcomes. *Anesth Analg* 2007;105:1756–1775.
10. Yeom JS, Lee JW, Park K, et al. Value of diagnostic lumbar selective nerve root block: a prospective controlled study. *AJNR Am J Neuroradiol* 2008;29:1017–1023.
11. Datta S, Manchikanti L, Falco FJ, et al. Diagnostic utility of selective nerve root blocks in the diagnosis of lumbosacral radicular pain: systematic review and update of current evidence. *Pain Physician* 2013;16:SE97–SE124.
12. Cuellar J, Stauff M, Herzog R, et al. Does provocative discography cause clinically important injury to the lumbar intervertebral disc? A 10-year matched cohort study. *Spine J* 2016;16:273–280.
13. Block AR, Ohnmeiss DD, Guyer RD, et al. The use of presurgical psychological screening to predict the outcome of spine surgery. *Spine J* 2001;1:274–282.
14. Dersh J, Gatchel R, Mayer T, et al. Prevalence of psychiatric disorders in patients with chronic disabling occupational spinal disorders. *Spine* 2006;31:56–62.
15. Daubs M, Patel A, Willick S, et al. Clinical impression versus standardized questionnaire: the spinal surgeon's ability to assess psychological distress. *J Bone Joint Surg Am* 2010;92:2878–2883.
16. Crombez G, Vlaeyen J, Heuts P, et al. Pain-related fear is more disabling than pain itself: evidence on the role of pain-related fear in chronic back pain disability. *Pain* 1999;80:329–339.
17. Mercado A, Carroll L, Cassidy J, et al. Passive coping is a risk factor for disabling neck or low back pain. *Pain* 2005;117:51–57.
18. Hasenbring M, Plaas H, Bischbein B, et al. The relationship between activity and pain in patients 6 months after lumbar disc surgery: do pain-related coping modes act as moderator variables? *Eur J Pain* 2006;10:701–709.
19. Schofferman J, Anderson D, Hines R, et al. Childhood psychological trauma correlates with unsuccessful spine surgery. *Spine* 1992;17:S138–S144.
20. Schofferman J, Hines R, Anderson D, et al. Childhood psychological trauma and chronic refractory low back pain. *Clin J Pain* 1993;9:260–265.
21. Burgstaller JM, Wertli MM, Steurer J, et al. The influence of pre- and postoperative fear avoidance beliefs on postoperative pain and disability in patients with lumbar spinal stenosis: analysis of the Lumbar Spinal Outcome Study (LSOS) data. *Spine* 2017;42:E425–E432.
22. Archer K, Seebach C, Mathis S, et al. Early postoperative fear of movement predicts pain, disability, and physical health six months after spinal surgery for degenerative conditions. *Spine J* 2014;14:759–767.
23. Archer K, Wegener S, Seebach C, et al. The effect of fear of movement beliefs on pain and disability after surgery for lumbar and cervical degenerative conditions. *Spine* 2011;36:1554–1562.
24. Herzog R, Marcotte P. Imaging corner. Assessment of spinal fusion. Critical evaluation of imaging techniques. *Spine* 1996;21:1114–1118.
25. Zampolin R, Erdfarb A, Miller T. Imaging of lumbar spine fusion. *Neuroimaging Clin N Am* 2014;24:269–286.
26. Bolt P, Wahl M, Schofferman J. The roles of the hip, spine, sacroiliac joint and other structures in patients with persistent pain after back surgery. *Semin Spine Surg* 2008;20:14–19.
27. Saal J, Dillingham M, Gamburd R, et al. The pseudoradicular syndrome. Lower extremity peripheral nerve entrapment masquerading as lumbar radiculopathy. *Spine* 1988;13:926–930.
28. Harney D, Patijn J. Meralgia paresthetica: diagnosis and management strategies. *Pain Med* 2007;8:669–677.
29. Tortolani P, Carbone J, Quartararo L. Greater trochanteric pain syndrome in patients referred to orthopedic spine specialists. *Spine J* 2002;2:251–254.
30. Sembrano J, Polly D. How often is low back pain not coming from the back? *Spine* 2009;34:E27–E32.
31. Brown MD, Gomez-Marin O, Brookfield KF, et al. Differential diagnosis of hip disease versus spine disease. *Clin Orthop Relat Res* 2004;419:280–284.
32. Fardon D. Letter to the editor. *Spine J* 2003;3:251.
33. Fardon DF, Williams AL, Dohring EJ, et al. Lumbar disc nomenclature: version 2.0: recommendations of the combined task forces of the North American Spine Society, the American Society of Spine Radiology and the American Society of Neuroradiology. *Spine J* 2014;14:2525–2545.
34. Barrick W, Schofferman J, Reynolds J, et al. Anterior fusion improves discogenic pain at levels of posterolateral fusion. *Spine* 2000;25:853–857.
35. Wang H, Ma L, Yang D, et al. Incidence and risk factors of adjacent segment disease following posterior decompression and instrumented fusion for degenerative lumbar disorders. *Medicine* 2017;96:e6032.
36. Klessinger S. Zygapophysial joint pain in post lumbar surgery syndrome. The efficacy of medial branch blocks and radiofrequency neurotomy. *Pain Med* 2013;14:374–377.
37. Steib K, Proescholdt M, Brawanski A, et al. Predictors of facet joint syndrome after lumbar disc surgery. *J Clin Neurosci* 2012;19:418–422.
38. van Ooij A, Oner F, Verbout A. Complications of artificial disc replacement. *J Spinal Dis Tech* 2003;16:369–383.
39. Shim C, Lee S, Shin H, et al. Charite versus ProDisc. A comparative study of a minimum 3-year follow-up. *Spine* 2007;32:1012–1018.
40. Manchikanti L, Manchukonda R, Pampati V, et al. Prevalence of facet joint pain in chronic low back pain in postsurgical patients by controlled comparative local anesthetic blocks. *Arch Phys Med Rehabil* 2007;88:449–455.
41. Yoshihara H. Sacroiliac joint pain after lumbar/lumbosacral fusion: current knowledge. *Eur Spine J* 2012;21:1788–1796.
42. Katz V, Schofferman J, Reynolds J. The sacroiliac joint: a potential cause of pain after lumbar fusion. *J Spinal Disord Tech* 2003;16:96–99.
43. Polly DW Jr. The sacroiliac joint. *Neurosurg Clin N Am* 2017;28:301–312.
44. Chou L, Slipman CW, Bhagia SM, et al. Inciting events initiating injection-proven sacroiliac joint syndrome. *Pain Med* 2004;5:26–32.
45. Longo UG, Loppini M, Berton A, et al. Degenerative changes of the sacroiliac joint after spinal fusion: an evidence-based systematic review. *Br Med Bull* 2014;112(1):47–56.
46. Yamashita K, Ohzono K, Hiroshima K. Five-year outcomes of surgical treatment for degenerative lumbar spinal stenosis. *Spine* 2006;31:1484–1490.
47. Simotas A, Dorey F, Hansraj K, et al. Nonoperative treatment for lumbar spinal stenosis. *Spine* 2000;25:197–204.
48. Malmivaara A, Statis P, Heliovaara M, et al. Surgical or nonoperative treatment for lumbar spinal stenosis. A randomized controlled trial. *Spine* 2007;32:1–8.
49. Antonacci M, Eismont F. Neurologic complications after lumbar spine surgery. *J Am Acad Orthop Surg* 2001;9:137–145.
50. Blond S, Mertens P, David R, et al. From "mechanical" to "neuropathic" back pain concepts in FBSS patients. A systematic review based on factors leading to the chronification of pain. *Neurochirurgie* 2015;61(suppl 1):S45–S56.
51. Markman J, Kress B, Frazer M, et al. Screening for neuropathic characteristics in failed back surgery syndromes: challenges for guiding treatment. *Pain Med* 2015;16:520–530.
52. Bosscher H, Heavner J. Incidence and severity of epidural fibrosis after back surgery: an endoscopic study. *Pain Pract* 2010;10:18–24.
53. Rönnberg K, Lind B, Zoega B, et al. Peridural scar and its relation to clinical outcome: a randomised study on surgically treated lumbar disc herniation patients. *Eur Spine J* 2008;17:1714–1720.
54. Almeida DB, Prandini MN, Awamura Y, et al. Outcome following lumbar disc surgery: the role of fibrosis. *Acta Neurochirurgica* 2008;150:1167–1176.
55. Hsu E, Atanelov L, Plunkett A, et al. Epidural lysis of adhesions for failed back surgery and spinal stenosis: factors associated with treatment outcome. *Anesth Analg* 2014;118:215–224.
56. Smeets R, Vlaeyen J, Hidding A, et al. Active rehabilitation for chronic low back pain: cognitive-behavioral, physical, or both? First direct post-treatment results from a randomized controlled trial. *BMC Musculoskeletal Disord* 2006;7:1–16.
57. Smeets R, Wade D, Hidding A, et al. The association of physical deconditioning and chronic low back pain: a hypothesis-oriented systematic review. *Disabil Rehabil* 2006;28:673–693.

58. Gille O, Jolivet E, Dousset V, et al. Erector spinae muscle changes on magnetic resonance imaging following lumbar surgery through a posterior approach. *Spine* 2007;32:1236–1241.

59. Motosuneya T, Asazuma T, Tsuji T, et al. Postoperative change of the cross-sectional area of back musculature after 5 surgical procedures as assessed by magnetic resonance imaging. *J Spinal Disord Tech* 2006;19:318–322.

60. Bousema E, Verbunt J, Seelen H, et al. Disuse and physical deconditioning in the first year after the onset of back pain. *Pain* 2007;130:279–286.

61. Marek R, Block A, Ben-Porath Y. The Minnesota Multiphasic Personality Inventory-2-Restructured Form (MMPI-2-RF): incremental validity in predicting early postoperative outcomes in spine surgery candidates. *Psychol Assess* 2015;27:114–124.

62. Dersh J, Mayer T, Theodore B, et al. Do psychiatric disorders first appear preinjury or postinjury in chronic disabling occupational spinal disorders? *Spine* 2007;32:1045–1051.

63. Adogwa O, Parker SL, Shau DN, et al. Preoperative Zung Depression Scale predicts outcome after revision lumbar surgery for adjacent segment disease, recurrent stenosis, and pseudarthrosis. *Spine J* 2012;12:179–185.

64. Havakeshian S, Mannion A. Negative beliefs and psychological disturbance in spine surgery patients: a cause or consequence of a poor treatment outcome? *Eur Spine J* 2013;22:2827–2835.

65. Smeets R, Viaeyen J, Kester A, et al. Reduction of pain catastrophizing mediates the outcome of both physical and cognitive-behavioral treatment in chronic low back pain. *J Pain* 2006;7(4):261–271.

66. Kernan T, Rainville J. Observed outcomes associated with a quota-based exercise approach on measures of kinesiophobia in patients with chronic low back pain. *J Orthop Sports Phys Ther* 2007;11:679–687.

67. Hart R, Perry E, Hiratzka S, et al. Post-traumatic stress symptoms after elective lumbar arthrodesis are associated with reduced clinical benefit. *Spine* 2013;38:1508–1515.

68. Deisseroth K, Hart R. Symptoms of post-traumatic stress following elective lumbar spinal arthrodesis. *Spine* 2012;37:1628–1633.

69. Bittane RM, de Moura AB, Lien RJ. The postoperative spine: what the spine surgeon needs to know. *Neuroimaging Clin N Am* 2014;24:295–303.

70. Willson MC, Ross JS. Postoperative spine complications. *Neuroimaging Clin N Am* 2014;24:305–326.

71. Bogduk N. Lumbar medial branch blocks. In: Bogduk N, ed. *Practice Guidelines for Spinal Diagnostic and Treatment Procedures*. San Francisco, CA: International Spine Intervention Society; 2004:47–64.

72. Bogduk N. Sacroiliac joint blocks. In: Bogduk N, ed. *Practice Guidelines for Spinal Diagnostic and Treatment Procedures*. San Francisco, CA: International Spine Intervention Society; 2004:66–86.

73. Bogduk N. Lumbar spinal nerve blocks. In: Bogduk N, ed. *Practice Guidelines for Spinal Diagnostic and Treatment Procedures*. San Francisco, CA: International Spine Intervention Society; 2004:3–19.

74. van Akkerveeken P. The diagnostic value of nerve root sheath infiltration. *Acta Orthop Scand* 1993;64:61–63.

75. Verrills P, Nowesenitz G, Barnard A. Prevalence and characteristics of discogenic pain in tertiary practice: 223 consecutive cases utilizing lumbar discography. *Pain Med* 2015;16:1490–1499.

76. Amirdelfan K, Webster L, Poree L, et al. Treatment options for failed back surgery syndrome patients with refractory chronic pain: an evidence based approach. *Spine* 2017;42(suppl 14):S41–S52.

77. Timm KE. A randomized-control study of active and passive treatments for chronic low back pain following L5 laminectomy. *J Orthop Sports Phys Ther* 1994;20:276–286.

78. Brox J, Reikeras O, Nygaard Ø, et al. Lumbar instrumented fusion compared with a cognitive intervention and exercises in patients with chronic back pain after previous surgery for disc herniation: a prospective randomized controlled study. *Pain* 2006;122:145–155.

79. Miller B, Gatchel R, Lou L, et al. Interdisciplinary treatment of failed back surgery syndrome (FBSS): a comparison of FBSS and non-FBSS patients. *Pain Pract* 2005;5:190–202.

80. Karahan AY, Sahin N, Baskent A. Comparison of effectiveness of different exercise programs in treatment of failed back surgery syndrome: a randomized controlled trial. *J Back Musculoskelet Rehabil* 2017;30(1):109–120.

81. Chou R, Deyo R, Friedly J, et al. Systemic pharmacologic therapies for low back pain: a systematic review for an American College of Physicians clinical practice guideline. *Ann Intern Med* 2017;166:480–492.

82. Williams CM, Maher CG, Latimer J, et al. Efficacy of paracetamol for acute low-back pain: a double-blind, randomised controlled trial. *Lancet* 2014;384:1586–1596.

83. Saragiotto B, Machado G, Ferreira M, et al. Paracetamol for low back pain. *Cochrane Database Syst Rev* 2016;(6):CD012230.

84. Qaseem A, Wilt TJ, McLean RM, et al; for Clinical Guidelines Committee of the American College of Physicians. Noninvasive treatments for acute, subacute, and chronic low back pain: a clinical practice guideline from the American College of Physicians. *Ann Intern Med* 2017;166:514–530.

85. Bally M, Dendukuri N, Rich B, et al. Risk of acute myocardial infarction with NSAIDs in real world use: bayesian meta-analysis of individual patient data. *BMJ* 2017;357:j1909.

86. Lee CH, Chung CK, Kim CH. The efficacy of conventional radiofrequency denervation in patients with chronic low back pain originating from the facet joints: a meta-analysis of randomized controlled trials. *Spine J* 2017;17:1770–1780.

87. Schofferman J, Kine G. The effectiveness of repeated radiofrequency neurotomy for lumbar facet pain. *Spine* 2004;29:2471–2473.

88. Hawkins J, Schofferman J. Serial therapeutic sacroiliac joint injections: a practice audit. *Pain Med* 2009;10:850–853.

89. Leggett L, Soril L, Lorenzetti D, et al. Radiofrequency ablation for chronic low back pain: a systematic review of randomized controlled trials. *Pain Res Manag* 2014;19:e146–e153.

90. Romero F, Vital R, Zanini M, et al. Long-term follow-up in sacroiliac joint pain patients treated with radiofrequency ablative therapy. *Arq Neuropsiquiatr* 2015;73:476–479.

91. Cohen SP, Hurley RW, Buckenmaier CC III, et al. Randomized placebo-controlled study evaluating lateral branch radiofrequency denervation for sacroiliac joint pain. *Anesthesiology* 2008;109:279–288.

92. Zaidi H, Montoure A, Dickman C. Surgical and clinical efficacy of sacroiliac joint fusion: a systematic review of the literature. *J Neurosurg Spine* 2015;23:59–66.

93. Adogwa O, Carr RK, Kudyba K, et al. Revision lumbar surgery in elderly patients with symptomatic pseudarthrosis, adjacent-segment disease, or same-level recurrent stenosis. Part 1. Two-year outcomes and clinical efficacy: clinical article. *J Neurosurg Spine* 2013;18:139–146.

94. Brodke DS, Annis P, Lawrence BD, et al. Reoperation and revision rates of 3 surgical treatment methods for lumbar stenosis associated with degenerative scoliosis and spondylolisthesis. *Spine* 2013;38:2287–2294.

95. Javalkar V, Cardenas R, Tawfik T, et al. Reoperations after surgery for lumbar spinal stenosis. *World Neurosurg* 2011;75:737–742.

96. Kim CH, Chung CK, Park CS, et al. Reoperation rate after surgery for lumbar spinal stenosis without spondylolisthesis: a nationwide cohort study. *Spine J* 2013;13:1230–1237.

97. Lad SP, Babu R, Bagley JH, et al. Utilization of spinal cord stimulation in patients with failed back surgery syndrome. *Spine* 2014;39:E719–E727.

98. Jeong Y, Ahn K, Kim H, et al. The effects of the local steroid injection in the patients with medial superior cluneal nerve entrapments. *J Korean Acad Rehabil Med* 2005;29:276–280.

99. Helm S II, Racz GB, Gerdesmeyer L, et al. Percutaneous and endoscopic adhesiolysis in managing low back and lower extremity pain: a systematic review and meta-analysis. *Pain Physician* 2016;19:E245–E282.

100. Jamison D, Hsu E, Cohen S. Epidural adhesiolysis: an evidence-based review. *J Neurosurg Sci* 2014;58:65–76.

101. Rainville J, Hartigan C, Jouve C, et al. The influence of intense exercise-based physical therapy program on back pain anticipated before and induced by physical activities. *Spine J* 2004;4:176–183.

102. Esmer G, Blum J, Rulf J, et al. Mindfulness-based stress reduction for failed back surgery syndrome: a randomized controlled trial. *J Am Osteopath Assoc* 2010;110:646–652.

103. Reiner K, Tibi L, Lipsitz J. Do mindfulness-based interventions reduce pain intensity? A critical review of the literature. *Pain Med* 2013;14:230–242.

104. Schütze R, Slater H, O'Sullivan P, et al. Mindfulness-based functional therapy: a preliminary open trial of an integrated model of care for people with persistent low back pain. *Front Psychol* 2014;5:839. doi:10.3389/fpsyg.2014.00839.

CHAPTER 76

Psychological Screening of Candidates for Spine Surgery or Placement of Implanted Devices

ROBERT EDWARDS and **ROBERT N. JAMISON**

Introduction

Chronic pain, generally defined as pain persisting for more than 3 months, or past the normal healing time, affects nearly 100 million adults in the United States.[1] It is estimated that 25 million adults report suffering with daily pain at any one time, and pain as a symptom accounts for 50 million primary care office visits.[2] Patients with persistent pain often report depression, anxiety, irritability, sexual dysfunction, and decreased energy.[3] Family roles are altered and worries about financial limitations and the consequences of a restricted lifestyle are common.[4] Chronic pain is one of the major reasons to seek health care and can impose a tremendous burden on the quality of life of those affected by this condition.[5] According to the Global Burden of Disease Initiative of the World Health Organization, chronic pain is ranked first in associated disability and overall burden.[6] It has been determined that chronic pain adversely affects individuals at a higher frequency than depression, substance abuse, arthritis, and Alzheimer disease.[7,8]

Despite multiple medical interventions and numerous treatment efforts, the incidence of chronic pain continues to rise and represents one of the costliest health care conditions in the United States.[9] In fact, chronic pain imposes the greatest economic burden of any health condition[10,11] and affects more people than diabetes, heart disease, and cancer combined.[9] Persistent back pain in particular is one of the principal drivers of these costs, both in the United States[12] and internationally,[13] with indirect costs (e.g., lost or reduced work productivity) accounting for more than half of this economic burden.[14]

Although there are many accepted and recommended treatments for chronic pain, the efficacy of these treatments is limited, and many individuals receiving treatments for their pain continue with disabling pain despite these therapies. The Agency for Healthcare Research and Quality (AHRQ) listed 20 common treatments for persons with chronic pain.[15] They reported that the long-term effect sizes for most medical interventions for pain, including back surgery and implanted devices, tend to be small. The AHRQ article recommended that selection of therapies that have the lowest cost and lowest chance for harm be considered first because there was no clear comparative advantage for most treatments compared to another.[16] The AHRQ also set as a priority the identification of those chronic pain patients who would most likely benefit from specific treatments for chronic pain.[15]

Studies suggest that most patients with chronic pain present with some psychiatric symptoms. Close to 50% of patients with chronic pain have a comorbid psychiatric condition, and 35% of patients with chronic back and neck pain have a comorbid depression or anxiety disorder.[17] Many chronic pain patients have a history of physical or sexual abuse, or a past history of a mood disorder.[18] In surveys of chronic pain clinic populations, between 50% and 70% of patients have significant psychopathology, making psychiatric comorbidity the most prevalent comorbidity in patients with chronic noncancer pain.[19] In addition, the presence of a long-lasting pain syndrome is a leading risk factor for suicide.[20]

Psychological assessment is designed to identify problematic emotional reactions, maladaptive thinking and behavior, and social problems that contribute to pain and disability. When psychosocial issues are identified, treatment can be tailored to address these challenges in the patient's life, thereby improving the likelihood and speed of recovery and prevention of ongoing or more severe problems. (4) When various first-line treatment options such as trials of medication and physical therapy fail or are ineffective, spinal surgery, spinal cord stimulation (SCS), or placement of an intrathecal drug delivery system (IDDS) are considered as treatment options, especially for those with severe intractable pain.

The purpose of this chapter is to review the major psychosocial variables that have been shown to be associated with poor outcome from surgery or an implanted device. We provide a brief critical review of factors that contribute to poor outcome from surgery, SCS, or an IDDS, present accepted strategies for assessing those psychological and social factors that predict outcome from surgery and implantable devices for pain and offer recommendations for future evaluation procedures in order to improve outcomes.

SPINAL SURGERY

Lumbar surgery with or without bone grafts and with or without implanted hardware can be controversial when employed for treating chronic pain alone. Radiologic studies have shown that 80% of asymptomatic individuals have evidence of degenerative disk disease or a bulging or herniated disk,[21] conditions often considered an indication for surgery. Yet, no clear indicators currently exist to determine which patients with low back pain would benefit from surgery.[22] In the United States, rates of spine surgery for back and leg pain have been steadily increasing, and there is a wide variation of the frequency of back surgery from one region of the country to the next.[23] Outcome trials of surgery for individuals with chronic low back pain have indicated success rates that range between 41% and 57%.[24] A number of controlled trials, however, have indicated that surgery is no better than physical therapy and multidisciplinary rehabilitation.[25–29] A troublesome component of back surgery is postsurgical complications and increased pain. Rates of complications and reoperations after spine surgery have ranged from 5% to 16%.[24]

Deyo and Mirza,[30] found that 2 years after surgery, there was no significant difference between back pain patients of similar diagnosis who were treated surgically or nonsurgically. Turner et al.,[31] reviewing all published research on spinal fusion, found that approximately 65% to 75% of all patients achieved satisfactory clinical outcomes. In these studies, poorer outcome was associated with a number of factors, including greater numbers of fused levels and the use of instrumentation. Similarly, Hoffman and colleagues,[32] in a literature review on laminectomy and discectomy, found that the mean success rate of these procedures for relief of spine pain was 67%. The popular media have highlighted these and similar results, which appear to provide support for declarations about treatments for back pain such as that of a recent issue of *Consumer Reports* (June 2017) that stated "conventional approaches don't always work and can cause other serious problems."

Failed spine surgery can significantly impact the patient, the physician, the employer, and the third-party payer. The patient often continues to remain disabled, with perhaps even greater pain, increased medication dependence, and more emotional difficulty than prior to the surgery. The pain may be so great, or the surgery so unsuccessful, that reoperation is required, as is the case in an estimated 10% of those who undergo laminectomy and discectomy,[32] and 23% of those who undergo spinal fusion.[31] The patient after failed surgery places many demands on the health care system, often requiring increasing medications and multiple additional treatments. Patients often feel frustrated and discouraged. The physician may become angry with the patient for not responding to treatment and the employer can be concerned about his or her obligation to pay compensation to a permanently disabled worker.

Given that spine surgery can be effective yet the implications of failed spine surgeries can be so profound, it becomes critical to determine factors that may lead to poor results from such procedures. Improper pre- and postoperative information and treatments may also worsen surgical results. A growing body of research indicates that psychosocial factors are among the most significant influences on spine surgery results. For example, DeBerard et al.[33] compared the outcomes of spinal fusion in patients who had been recommended for a preoperative psychological evaluation (based on surgeon recognition of the presence of psychosocial concerns) versus those who were not recommended for such evaluations. Those recommended for a psychological evaluation did less well after surgery, suggesting that even the surgeons' perception of psychological issues was predictive of outcome. In another study, DeBerard and colleagues[34] demonstrated that those who were identified with more negative affect (high psych) before back surgery had more repeat surgeries, had greater disability, had higher medical expenses, and had a higher incidence of disability after surgery than those with less emotional distress. Thus, presurgical evaluation and careful patient selection can be extremely important in helping to identify those individuals who might benefit the most from lumbar surgery.

SPINAL CORD STIMULATION AND INTRATHECAL DRUG DELIVERY SYSTEMS

SCS with implantable or externalized systems has been available since the 1960s.[35] The theoretical basis of the efficacy of SCS is based on Melzack and Wall's[36] gate control theory that proposes that stimulation of large nerve fibers overrides the transmission of small nerve fibers that transmit pain. SCS is expected to reduce, not eliminate pain by blocking the conduction of primary nerve pathways.[37] It seems to be most successful in relieving pain in the limbs (e.g., the leg or arm), although more recently, neurostimulation devices have been developed that target axial back pain.[38,39] Throughout the years, there have been improvements in SCS systems allowing for better coverage of painful areas with multiple channels, higher frequency stimulation, burst technology, electrode surfaces with increased number of contacts, and leads that are shaped to provide varying degrees of coverage.[40] Spinal cord stimulators have reported success rates ranging from 20% to 70%.[41] They have been found to be efficacious for neuropathic pain[42] and radiculopathy.[43] There has been a rapid increase in the number of implanted spinal cord stimulators, and some econometric analyses have indicated that SCS may be a cost-effective treatment option, particularly for patients with persistent neuropathic pain syndromes and complex regional pain syndrome.[44]

Spinal infusion of analgesics, with use of an IDDS has been utilized since the 1980s.[45] Spinally administered analgesics had

initially been used for treatment of cancer pain[46] and with the subsequent development of implantable components for continuous intrathecal infusions became an acceptable method to treat patients with intractable spasticity as well as pain.[47] This technology consists of implanting a drug delivery device designed for long-term continuous infusion of medication. The drug delivery system consists of a collapsible drug reservoir into which the drug is injected and, powered by a battery and computer chip, allows for variable infusion rates and bolus injections through a catheter anchored in the back with the tip of the catheter positioned within the thecal sac to deliver drug to the cerebrospinal fluid (CSF).[48] Such infusions for cancer pain have good success rates (defined as a reduction of pain by one-third), ranging from 60% to 90%.[49] Collectively, intrathecal infusion devices have provided pain relief in noncancer pain patients who had failed more conservative therapies[50] and patients with an IDDS have demonstrated a reduction in side effects from oral medications, decreased need for oral analgesia, and improvement in their physical assessment.[51] The data indicate variable success rates for noncancer pain ranging from 25% to 70%.[52]

Although outcome studies report that SCS and/or an IDDS are efficacious in treating chronic pain, decisions for implantation have historically been based on clinical judgment of the implanting physician.[49] Recent empirical work, though, has begun to investigate the clinical characteristics that are associated with outcomes for implantable devices. A study by Hassenbusch and colleagues[53] compared SCS with intrathecal infusions by measuring postoperative verbal numeric scores and activity levels. The findings of this study and others suggest that IDDS were useful in reducing bilateral or axial pain (e.g., pain just in the low back), whereas SCS is better for unilateral radicular symptoms (e.g., pain down one leg stemming from nerve damage in the back).[50] In general, patients considered for an implantable device often are not seen as poor candidates for spinal surgery, either due to previous failed surgery or lack of clear pathology accounting for the pain, and have failed to respond to conservative approaches and long-term use of oral opioids.

Implantation of these devices, however, is not without risks. Reports of infection or intrathecal granulomas causing neurologic injury are documented,[54] and the safety of these devices for use with chronic noncancer pain patients is an important consideration. The risks associated with SCS include possible nerve injury, spinal cord puncture, bleeding, and infection. Similar risks also exist for IDDS including discomfort at the implantation site as well as possible disconnections, kinking, catheter migration, and inflammatory masses (granulomas) that build up at the tip of the catheter. Risks also include increased depression if the device becomes ineffective in reducing pain.[48] Because of the risks associated with implantation of these devices, as well as their substantial costs, there has been a good deal of emphasis on patient selection. As noted earlier, some studies have focused on identifying pain phenotypes that are most responsive to implantable therapies[48,53]; other areas of investigation include evaluation of psychosocial factors that might predict success or failure of stimulators or IDDS. Thus, a careful evaluation of each candidate for surgery or for an implantable device is judged to be important, and in clinical practice, a psychological evaluation is often a recommended or mandatory part of the evaluation process for patients being considered for implantable pain-management devices.

AFFECTIVE DISORDERS AS PREDICTORS OF OUTCOME

Many chronic pain patients experience some level of depression. For up to 85%, the intensity of this emotional experience is sufficient to meet the diagnostic criteria for clinical depression.[17] Depressive symptoms include depressed mood, diminished interest in almost all activities, weight loss or gain, insomnia or hypersomnia, agitation or psychomotor retardation, fatigue or energy loss, feelings of worthlessness or guilt, impaired concentration, and recurrent thoughts of death unrelated to other comorbidities.[55] Several studies have assessed depression using different instruments and found that it can be predictive of greater disability and poor outcomes of spinal surgery.[56] Kjelby-Wendt et al.[57] examining discectomy results found that patient satisfaction with surgery was strongly related to elevated scores on the Beck Depression Inventory (BDI)—in fact, elevated scores were found in 55% of dissatisfied patients but in only 18% of satisfied patients. Schade et al.[58] found that depression, as assessed on a simple Likert-type scale, had strong negative correlations with return to work and overall recovery. Trief et al.[59] found that high scores on the Zung depression inventory were associated with little reduction in back pain and elevated work disability after spine surgery. Finally, DeBerard et al.[34] found that depression was strongly related to total medical costs in workers' compensation patients undergoing spinal fusion.

Patients with chronic pain and a comorbid psychiatric disorder are more likely to report greater pain intensity, more pain-related disability, and a larger affective component to their pain than those without psychiatric comorbidity.[60,61] Patients with chronic pain and psychopathology, especially those with chronic low back pain, also typically have poorer pain and disability outcomes with treatment.[62–64] There is a significantly poorer return-to-work rate 1 year after injury among patients with chronic pain and anxiety and/or depression compared with those without any psychopathology.[65] Thus, psychiatric comorbidity, primarily major depression and anxiety disorders, is associated with greater levels of chronic pain, more disability, and a worse response to treatment.

Given the significant interpatient variability in treatment outcomes, it would be of tremendous value, from both a societal and patient perspective, to identify in advance who is most and least likely to benefit from surgery or an implanted device. In general, some risk factors have been identified that correlate with greater risk for pain or poor outcomes from treatment for pain. These include variables such as pain chronicity, psychological distress, a history of abuse or trauma, poor social support, and significant cognitive deficits.[65] In particular, psychopathology and/or extreme emotionality have been seen as contraindications for certain therapies.[66] Outcome studies highlight the poor response of patients with psychiatric comorbidity to many treatments.[67,68] For example, spinal pain patients with both anxiety and depression have a 62% worse return-to-work rate than those with no psychopathology.[69] Epidemiologic research suggests a bidirectional association between back pain and emotional distress; pain increases symptoms of depression and individuals with a preexisting depressive disorder have a disproportionately high risk for developing spinal pain.[70] Similarly, cognitive processes such as maladaptive beliefs and pessimistic expectations are associated with a greater likelihood of developing chronic pain and with poorer functional outcomes among chronic low back pain patients.[71] There is also evidence of a genetic predisposition toward increased depression and anxiety among persons with low back pain based on twin studies.[72]

Numerous factors are likely to play a role in shaping outcomes following surgical interventions or placement of an implanted device in patients with chronic back pain. However, there does not seem to be a consensus on what factors are the strongest and most consistently predictive of outcomes, and there is no universally accepted standard approach for screening surgical candidates or individuals considered for an implanted device. Nonetheless, a presurgical psychological evaluation is often recommended based on research demonstrating the predictive value of spine presurgical psychological evaluations.[73]

A recent systematic review was carried out of the current literature, using critical appraisal and strategies to limit bias, to determine the strength of the evidence for the assumption that careful screening will help to predict pain-related and functional outcomes from lumbar surgery or SCS.[74] Collectively, a statistically significant relationship was found between psychological factors and treatment outcome (e.g., high preimplant levels of distress were prospectively associated with less SCS-related pain relief) in 92% of the studies reviewed. In particular, presurgical somatization, depression, anxiety, and poor coping were most useful in helping to predict poor response (i.e., less treatment-related benefit) to lumbar surgery and SCS. Older age and longer pain duration were also predictive of poorer outcome in some studies, whereas pretreatment physical findings, activity interference, and pain intensity were minimally predictive. Interestingly, several studies have confirmed that younger patients treated earlier in the course of their pain condition derive the most benefit from SCS,[75] which might suggest that using SCS as a "last resort" could be a suboptimal management strategy.

A review of psychosocial characteristics as predictors of outcomes following SCS suggests that depression is most robustly linked to poor SCS outcomes.[76] Indeed, Sparkes and colleagues[76] cite multiple well-designed studies suggesting that higher levels of preimplantation depressive symptoms impact negatively on the efficacy of SCS treatment.

Trief and colleagues[59] found that patients with elevated state anxiety scores on the State Trait Anxiety Inventory (STAI) achieved less pain relief and lower return to work rates after surgery than did patients with lower anxiety. One particularly troublesome type of anxiety centers on the belief that increasing function and activity may increase the likelihood of reinjury. This type of fear measure has been assessed by several questionnaires including the Tampa Scale for Kinesiophobia.[77] Den Boer et al.[78] found that elevated scores on the Tampa scale were associated with delayed return to work after lumbar disk surgery. One plausible explanation for this result is that patients with a heightened fear of movement might be less likely to engage in aggressive postoperative rehabilitation. Kiecolt-Glaser et al.[79] suggest that anxiety may increase postoperative pain and such increased noxious sensations could then downregulate immune function, further compromising the surgery healing process.

SOMATIZATION

Estimated rates of chronic pain patients with somatization (sometimes known as *hypochondriasis*) vary, ranging from 1% to 12%, even though unexplained symptoms are a common problem in medical settings.[80,81] The classical concept of somatization that implies that there is no pathophysiologic basis for physical complaints is quite problematic to apply to patients with chronic pain. This is because the majority of patients with chronic pain have some underlying physical condition that is at least partially responsible for their pain. The pain symptoms due to a physical or somatic cause (such as degenerative disk disease in the lumbar spine) may then be amplified by psychiatric factors, such as depression, anxiety, pain catastrophizing, fear of movement, and/or poor coping.[82] Areas in the brain which process pain and mood together (such as the prefrontal and anterior cingulate cortices, and insula, commonly termed the *medial pain system*) may be the underlying brain substrates by which pain signals coming from the spinal cord are then amplified and perceived as heightened pain sensations. Hence, it is more appropriate to think of somatization as a process of amplification of bodily signals centered in the brain. There may or may not be a physical basis in the body for the abnormal physical sensations.[83] The "somatoform pain disorders" fall within the "Somatization Disorders" classification in *Diagnostic and Statistical Manual of Mental Disorders, 5th edition* (DSM-5) and are meant to capture this concept of amplification of bodily perceptions, which is made worse by concomitant depression. The two diagnoses most commonly used with chronic pain patients are Pain disorders associated with psychological factors and a general medical condition, and Pain disorders associated with psychological factors. For patients with a strong component of heightened awareness of pain, the evidence is strong that repeated invasive procedures and implanted devices almost uniformly are unsuccessful.[61,74] Education about the nature of the problem and helping patients understand the risk associated with repeated treatments is also important.

Providers should resist a dualistic model that postulates that pain is either all physical or all mental in origin. This model alienates patients who may feel blamed for their pain and is not consistent with modern models of pain causation. Multiple lines of evidence suggest that pain is a product of efferent as well as afferent activity in the nervous system. We know that tissue damage and nociception are not necessary or sufficient for pain and the relationship between pain and nociception is highly complex. We are only beginning to understand the complexities of the relationship between pain and suffering, which appears to be a central phenomenon.[84]

PAIN SENSITIVITY

Recent studies have also suggested that quantitative sensory testing (QST) may be a useful adjunct to psychological evaluation in the assessment of patients under consideration for spinal surgery or for placement of an implantable device. QST involves the administration of standardized noxious stimuli under highly controlled conditions; often, parameters such as pain threshold and tolerance in response to a variety of stimulus modalities are measured as indices of pain sensitivity. Our group recently reported that high levels of pain sensitivity may be associated with elevated risk for pain medication misuse[85] and individual differences in QST responses may be useful as prognostic indicators in a variety of settings. For example, among neuropathic pain patients undergoing SCS, the degree of pretrial mechanical allodynia was inversely associated with the amount of pain relief reported by patients.[86] That is, the most mechanosensitive patients reported the least SCS-related analgesic benefit. Functional neuroimaging studies have revealed that SCS functions in part by activating cortical pain-modulatory circuitry,[87] and it may be that the most preoperatively pain-sensitive individuals are those whose pain-modulatory systems are the most difficult to engage. Patients with chronic low back pain exhibit generalized patterns of hypersensitivity to pain that are consistent with central sensitization-like processes,[88–90] indicating that heightened pain sensitivity in the central nervous system may represent an important pain mechanism in patients with chronic back pain.

Assessment of pain sensitivity is potentially useful in several surgical contexts. First, there is some evidence that a higher degree of preoperative pain sensitivity is associated with poorer pain and disability outcomes following spinal surgery.[91–93] Such findings are consistent with data from other surgical procedures indicating that preoperative sensory phenotyping with QST can provide valuable prognostic data.[94,95] Second, assessment of sensory responses to provocative tests such as discography, which involves injection of radiographic dye into the nucleus pulposus of a putatively disrupted disk, can be illuminating. The injection, performed under fluoroscopy and combined with postdiscogram CT, gives evidence of the presence and extent of disk disruption. Interestingly, the injection of a disrupted disk has been demonstrated to act as a stimulus that provokes pain, often with a pattern and intensity similar to the patient's normally occurring pain. For example, Vanharanta et al.[96] found that injection of moderately to severely disrupted disks provoked pain that was similar or an exact reproduction of normally occurring pain in approximately 65%

of cases. On the other hand, injection into normal-appearing disks provoked exact or similar reproduction of pain in only 18% of cases. Even stronger results along the same lines were obtained by Walsh et al.[97] Thus, discography may provide a laboratory method for administering controlled stimulation of the disk in order to assess whether certain patients with low back pain display heightened pain sensitivity.

ANGER

Anger is a common and prominent emotion in patients with chronic pain. Patients with low back pain, in particular, may experience and express anger about past medical care; about unfair treatment by employers, friends, and family; and about the physical and functional limitations that are endemic to low back pain.[98] A study by Fernandez and Milburn[99] demonstrates just how frequently patients experience this emotion. These researchers asked chronic pain patients to endorse the intensity of 10 different emotions they were experiencing and found that anger was given the highest ratings of all emotions assessed.[99] High levels of anger have also been associated with postoperative complications and elevated levels of postoperative pain for spinal surgeries as well as other procedures.[100] There are numerous reasons why anger may have a negative impact on pain-related outcomes. First, anger may lead to maladaptive lifestyle changes, such as poor health habits, lack of physical exercise, or excessive use of drugs or alcohol. Such poor health behavior profiles may impair the benefits of physical interventions and have a negative impact on the patient's commitment to postoperative rehabilitation. Second, anger can lead to the desire for vindication or revenge, and certainly, this can influence treatment results.[101,102] Similarly, DeGood and Kiernan[103] have found chronic pain patients who are angry and blame their employer for their injuries report high levels of emotional distress and have poorer response to treatment. Third, anger has been shown to have an adverse effect on many health conditions, such as cardiovascular disease, headaches, asthma, and many others, which may in turn exacerbate the negative effects of pain.[104] Final, anger appears to directly impact physiologic pain perception by increasing muscle tension near the site of the injury, activating neural circuits underlying regulation of pain, and interfering with the analgesic effects of endogenous opioids.[105,106]

Cognitive Factors

A growing body of research is examining the ways in which patients' thoughts and beliefs concerning their pain, independent of personality or emotional factors, can strongly affect treatment outcome.[95] Such cognitions and coping strategies have been demonstrated to influence the level of pain experienced by the patient, level of functional ability, and adjustment to the pain and efforts to overcome it.[95] For example, catastrophizing is a pain-specific psychosocial construct composed of negative cognitive and emotional processes such as helplessness, pessimism, rumination about pain-related symptoms, and magnification of pain reports.[70,107] Overall, higher catastrophizing has been shown to be a risk factor for the development of long-term pain and for negative sequelae of pain such as worsening physical disability, higher health care costs, and the amplification of pain sensitivity among patients with low back pain and joint pain. Retrospective survey studies in patients with musculoskeletal pain have indicated that catastrophizing often emerges as one of the most important pretreatment variables predicting surgical outcomes[108,109] and a risk factor that impairs the effectiveness of pain-relieving interventions. Fortunately, catastrophizing is a modifiable risk factor that can be ameliorated with a variety of nonpharmacologic treatments, from physical therapy to meditation.[60,70,107] As such, it should be assessed as part of any psychosocial screening.

COPING STRATEGIES

Coping strategies may be defined as specific thoughts and behaviors individuals use to manage their pain or their emotional reactions to pain.[110] For example, "active" pain coping generally includes engaging in positive thinking, making encouraging self-statements, distracting one's attention from pain, undertaking as much physical activity as possible within pacing guidelines, or using physical pain-reducing techniques such as relaxation exercises and stretching. Facilitating such coping strategies seems to be an important part of many nonpharmacologic treatments for chronic pain. One recent prospective study of multidisciplinary treatment revealed that patients who entered treatment with stronger personal beliefs in their ability to control pain, and those who increased their use of positive self-statements and cognitive reinterpretation of pain showed the most substantial decreases in pain-related interference at 6 months and 18 months posttreatment.[111] Coping strategies may affect the patient's level of attentiveness to pain, the ability to persist in the face of pain, and the extent to which the patient feels entitled to be taken care of as a result of the pain. There are a number of questionnaires available to assess pain-related coping strategies, including the Vanderbilt Pain Management Inventory (PMI).[112] However, the largest body of research on coping in chronic pain (and the only research directly applied to surgical screening) has used the Coping Strategies Questionnaire (CSQ).[113] Gross[114] administered the CSQ preoperatively to 50 lumbar laminectomy candidates. Patients who obtained good results from surgery indicated on the CSQ that they felt better able to control the pain and also indicated they were more self-reliant. Other coping strategies assessed by the CSQ, such as hoping and praying and catastrophizing, were associated with poor surgical outcomes. These results are consistent with several other studies demonstrating that more passive coping strategies and perceived lack of pain control tend to be associated with greater pain levels, higher opioid consumption, greater levels of depression, and poorer treatment outcome.[107,115] Recent research by den Boer et al.[78,116] provides further support for the strong influence of coping strategies on surgical outcome. In this study, patients undergoing spine surgery for lumbar radicular syndrome were examined. "Passive pain coping" was assessed preoperatively using the Pain-Coping Inventory. Results indicated that passive pain coping, along with negative surgical outcome expectancy, predicted more severe disability and reduced work capacity at 6 months after surgery. Taken together with the just-cited study by Gross,[114] these results demonstrate that the effectiveness of surgery may be partially mediated by the manner in which the patient thinks about the experience of pain and the strategies he or she has available to cope with the pain.

Behavioral Factors

All the psychosocial factors discussed up to this point are components of a patient's internal milieu: thoughts, feelings, and personality. Factors external to the patient can also exert profound influences upon recovery from spine surgery. Especially powerful in this regard are the responses of others to the patient's pain. Pain behavior almost always occurs in a social context, communicating to observers that the patient is in distress. Observers, in turn, may react to such behavior with attempts to relieve the patient's pain, help him or her to avoid further problems, or be supportive of limitations in activity. Employers, and even the insurance system, may also inadvertently support pain behaviors through provision of disability benefits or time off of work. Unfortunately, such solicitous responses from others, although well intentioned, may serve to reinforce or reward pain behaviors, increasing the likelihood that patients will continue to show and experience pain.[117,118]

Moreover, the patients' individual attachment style is an important predictor of outcomes; individuals with anxious or insecure attachment styles are at elevated risk for poorer mental and physical health and for less treatment-related improvement.[119] These social factors are especially important in the occupational setting. Anema and colleagues[120] compared return-to-work rates in injured workers across numerous countries and found that differences in job characteristics and social disability systems were more important than medical interventions, patient, and injury-related factors in predicting occupational outcomes. In addition, these same home- and work-related social forces contribute to shaping important outcomes after spine surgery, as patients with minimal social and occupational support have more postoperative complications, pain, and disability following a variety of operative procedures.[121-123]

EARLY-LIFE TRAUMA AND ABUSE

Strong prospective links have been observed between early traumatic experiences and the subsequent development of chronic pain.[95,124] Childhood physical, sexual, and psychological abuse are reported to be risk factors for the adult development of musculoskeletal pain conditions.[125] In adulthood, posttraumatic stress disorder (PTSD) has been identified as a risk factor for chronic pain, for the transition from acute to chronic pain, and for elevated severity of pain and disability in abuse victims.[126-128] Overall, a disproportionately high number of chronic back pain patients have been the victims of abuse or abandonment as either adults or as children. In one study, more than half of the patients with chronic refractory low back pain evaluated at a multidisciplinary pain clinic had a history of at least one form of such childhood psychological trauma.[129] These figures are substantially higher than the base rate in the US population. At present, the treatment implications for patients are unknown. Whereas some studies[130] find less positive outcomes following spine surgery among patients with a significant history of childhood abuse, others have not confirmed this finding, highlighting the need for additional research.[129]

SUBSTANCE ABUSE

Excessive use and abuse of opioid medications and alcohol appear to be red flags for poor surgical outcome.[131,132] To the extent that patients depend on such substances, their responsibility for pain relief and improvements in functional ability through participation in postoperative rehabilitation may be diminished.[133] Many chronic pain patients use excessive amounts of opioids. For example, Polatin and colleagues[134] found that 19% of spine pain patients entering a work-hardening program had a history of substance use disorder, and even higher rates were reported in other studies. Unfortunately, there is little research addressing the relationship of substance use disorder and spine surgery outcome, although the results suggest that there is a higher incidence of spine surgery failures among those who continually abuse prescription medication and alcohol.[135] The medical literature is clearer in demonstrating a relationship between poor surgical outcomes and smoking cigarettes.[136]

COMPONENTS OF PSYCHOLOGICAL EVALUATIONS

Generally speaking, a goal of lumbar surgery and an implanted device for pain is to reduce pain. There are other potential positive outcomes from surgery or placement of an implanted device for pain including (1) relying less on prescription medication, (2) improving activities of daily living, and (3) returning individuals to productive lifestyles. A psychological evaluation is designed to help identify patients at risk for poor outcome and to prepare the patient so that they can achieve maximum benefit from surgery or implanted device.[137] Regarding implanted devices, Medicare and many health insurance companies in the United States require implant candidates to have a psychological evaluation. As part of the evaluation, patients need to be informed of the risks as well as possible benefits from surgery or placement of an implanted device and to address realistic expectations. For SCS and IDDS, patients undergo a trial designed to determine the likely efficacy of a permanent implant. For SCS, the trial consists of temporary placement of a stimulator lead for 4 to 10 days and a successful trial, often required by Medicare and third-party payers, includes self-reported pain reduction by 50% and overall patient satisfaction. For IDDS patients, the trial is often conducted during a brief inpatient stay. It is important to remind patients with an IDDS that they would need to return periodically to refill their drug delivery system and for SCS patients that their time using the device directly affects battery longevity. Showing prospective implant patients a model of the device so that they can hold it and understand how it works can be important. Open discussion of any concerns about having a device implanted can also be useful. For some SCS patients, there may be some loss of normal sensation and having future magnetic resonance imaging (MRI) studies may be contradicted with some systems. For any device, future revisions or explants may be necessary in the event of infection, failed batteries, or any severe complication.

Psychological evaluations should include the assessment of sensory, affective, cognitive, and behavioral components of the pain experience, expectations of benefit of an implanted device, and identification of personality and psychosocial factors that can influence treatment outcome.[137] Table 76.1 presents the major categories that should be addressed during a psychological interview. The sensory experience is usually best understood through description of the severity, location, and temporal characteristics of chronic pain. Distressing emotional qualities of the experience of pain as well as preexisting emotional dispositions need to be understood, as fear[138] and depression[17] are powerful determinants of the response and emotional reactions to pain, related disability, and overall care. Patterns of thinking may exacerbate and maintain dysfunctional pain as well as facilitate coping that enhance adjustment during painful flare-ups. There is variability in the extent to which chronic pain interferes with activities of daily living or contributes to substantial functional impairment. Clinicians have long relied on careful appraisal of nonverbal behavior in the course of physical examinations and through observation of patients outside the examining situation, for example, when engaged in spontaneous behavior elsewhere in clinics or in everyday situations. Self-report can also be useful in assessing nonverbal behavior by focusing on overt activity rather than subjective experience, for example, functional capacity or competence and disability in different situations. Finally, family socialization and important life experiences influence both effective and ineffective patterns of attempts to cope with pain. History gathering typically is the primary source of this information.

Ethnic and cultural variation and family histories of managing pain and illness may be of importance. For example, when significant others in a patient's family have had a history of recurrent, persistent, or particularly severe pain, there is a disposition to similar patterns in the patient themselves.[139]

Of comparable importance are current social contexts. Patients experiencing social distress (e.g., with employers, family members or others) either directly related to painful episodes (reduced employment, isolation from the community) or unrelated to painful episodes (e.g., financial distress, difficult relationships) are likely to increase demands on the health care system. Furthermore, the presence of a supportive social environment is associated with lower levels of pain and less physical disability following surgical intervention.[140]

Although clinicians must be aware of the objectives of referral sources, patients similarly are typically carefully attuned to the expectations and goals of referral agencies and those engaged in the assessment. Patients frustrated with lack of success in treating pain or provision of financial and other support when unable to earn a livelihood bring different concerns to the assessment than patients who are not worried by such situations and expect the assessment will lead to effective care. Long histories of inadequate care or denial of care are more likely to lead to hostile behavior.

VALIDATED PSYCHOLOGICAL MEASURES

A psychological evaluation should include valid and reliable assessments of subjective pain intensity, mood and personality, activity interference, pain beliefs, and coping (Table 76.2). The following categories include some popular assessment tools used to measure these constructs.

TABLE 76.1 Categories to Be Addressed during a Psychological Interview

1. Pain description
2. Aggravating and minimizing factors
3. Past and current treatments, including medication use
4. Daily activities: content and level
5. Relevant medical history
6. Development, education, and employment history
7. Compensation status, engagement in litigation
8. History of drug or alcohol abuse
9. History of psychiatric disturbance
10. Current emotional status
11. Financial and social support
12. Perceived directions for treatment

TABLE 76.2 Assessment Categories and Frequently Used Psychometric Measures

1. Pain intensity
   Numerical rating scales (NRS)
   Visual analogue scales (VAS)
   Verbal rating scales (VRS)
   Pain drawings (PD)
2. Mood and personality
   Minnesota Multiphasic Personality Inventory (MMPI)
   Symptom Checklist 90 (SCL-90)
   Beck Depression Inventory (BDI)
   Hospital Anxiety and Depression Scale (HADS)
3. Functional capacity
   Short-Form Health Survey (SF-36)
   Multidimensional Pain Inventory (MPI)
   Pain Disability Index (PDI)
   Oswestry Disability Index (ODI)
   Roland-Morris Questionnaire (RMQ)
   Waddell Disability Instrument
   Functional Rating Scale
   Back Pain Function Scale
4. Pain beliefs and coping
   Coping Strategies Questionnaire (CSQ)
   Pain Management Inventory (PMI)
   Pain Self-Efficacy Questionnaire (PSEQ)
   Survey of Pain Attitudes (SOPA)
   Inventory of Negative Thoughts in Response to Pain (INTRP)
   Chronic Pain Self-Efficacy Scale (CPSS)
   Pain Catastrophizing Scale (PCS)
5. Medication monitoring and adverse effects
   Screener and Opioid Assessment for Pain Patients (SOAPP-R)
   Current Opioid Misuse Measure (COMM)
   Opioid Compliance Checklist (OCC)
   Opioid Risk Testing (ORT)
   Side Effects Checklist (SEC)

Pain Intensity Measures

Because one of the obvious primary goals of surgery or placement of an implanted device for chronic pain is to decrease the intensity of the pain, it is important to monitor pain intensity for a period before surgery or a device trial and after treatment. There are a number of ways to measure pain intensity, including numerical pain ratings, visual analogue scales, verbal rating scales, pain drawings, and a combination of standardized questionnaires. Pain intensity rating methods have evolved from designs originally developed by Budzynski[141] and Melzack.[142] Studies have shown that self-monitored pain intensity ratings are both reliable and valid.[143] The daily monitoring of multiple measures of pain intensity over a 1- to 2-week period before considering a trial of SCS or IDDS has a number of benefits. First, more information is obtained than can be gained from a single index of perceived pain intensity. More specifically, averaging multiple measures of pain intensity over time increases the reliability and validity of the assessment and is preferable to a single rating of pain intensity.[141] Second, in the case of a trial of SCS or IDDS, average pain intensity ratings can serve as a baseline to help establish whether continued treatment is needed after an appropriate trial period. Baseline measures are essential to making judgments about the overall impact of treatment for pain.

Numerical pain ratings often involve the patient's rating of his or her pain on a scale of 0 to 10 or 0 to 100. Ideally, the external validity of the measure is improved by descriptive anchors that help the patient understand the meaning of each numerical value (e.g., 1 to 2, pain can be ignored at times; 3 to 4, pain is present but does not interfere with activity; 5 to 6, the pain is very noticeable and begins to limit function; 7 to 8, pain is quite severe and performing average daily activities is impaired; 9 to 10, pain is as worse as it can be and all activity is significantly impaired). Another popular means of measuring pain intensity is the visual analog scale (VAS), which uses a straight line with extreme limits of pain at either end.[143] Some clinics employ electronic pain ratings available on a laptop computer, cell phone, or Internet Web site that can be used at home on a daily basis to get multiple time-stamped assessments of pain in the patient's natural environment.[144,145]

There are a number of verbal rating scales,[143] that consist of phrases chosen by the patients—as few as four or as many as 15, often ranked in order of severity from "no pain" to "excruciating pain"—to describe the intensity of their pain. Other verbal scales can be used to describe the quality of pain, for example, piercing, stabbing, shooting, burning, throbbing.[146] Among the self-report measures, numerical rating scales are most popular among professionals. However, there is no evidence to suggest that VAS or verbal rating scales are any less sensitive to treatment effects. All these types of measures have been shown to be acceptable in the quantification of clinical pain.[143,147]

Mood and Personality

Patients with chronic pain often report depression, anxiety, irritability, a history of physical or sexual abuse, or a past history of a mood disorder.[148,149] Patients with chronic low back pain with evidence of a personality disorder or high ratings of depression and neuroticism respond more favorably to conservative management rather than surgery or placement of an implanted device.[150–152] Mental health professionals continue to debate the best way to measure psychopathology and/or emotional distress in chronic pain patients. Although most measures are helpful in ruling out severe psychiatric disturbance, unfortunately, no measure can boast perfect validity in predicting treatment outcome.[153] The measures commonly used to evaluate personality and emotional distress include the Minnesota Multiphasic Personality Inventory-2 (MMPI-2),[154]

the Symptom Checklist 90 (SCL-90-R),[155] the BDI,[156] the Hospital Anxiety and Depression Scale (HADS),[157] and others.

The MMPI and its successor, the MMPI-2, had been the instruments traditionally used in assessing chronic pain patients and to predict outcome following spine surgery and SCS.[154,158] This measure consists of 567 true/false items and yields a distinct profile for each pain patient. Studies have shown that these profiles can predict return-to-work in males as well as response to surgical treatment.[159] Although this test was widely used to measure psychopathology, the profiles obtained for chronic pain patients could be misinterpreted because of the physical symptoms frequently reported by these patients.[160] Patients also reported disliking the test's emphasis on psychopathology that seemed to be unrelated to their pain problem.

The SCL-90 is a 90-item checklist with a 5-point scale that offers a global index score as well as nine subscale scores as a general assessment of emotional distress and has been used to evaluation outcomes from surgery[161] and SCS.[162] This self-report instrument offers easy inspection of individual items that may pertain specifically to persons with chronic pain. However, its disadvantages include the high correlation between subscales and the absence of validity scales to detect subtle inconsistencies in responses.[163]

The BDI assesses depressive symptoms in chronic pain patients. This 21-item self-report questionnaire measures the severity of depression and is commonly used to evaluate the outcome of treatment. It is easy to administer and score, although one limitation is the potential for misinterpretation of an elevated depression score as a result of the frequent endorsement of somatic items by chronic pain patients, for example, fatigue, sleep disturbances, and loss of sexual interest. The BDI has been used to predict outcome of lumbar disk surgery,[164] surgical management of spinal stenosis,[165] and benefit of peripheral nerve stimulation.[166] The Center for Epidemiologic Studies Depression (CES-D) scale is an additional tool for assessment of depressive symptoms in pain patients.[167]

The HADS is a 14-item scale designed to assess the presence and severity of anxious and depressive symptoms. Seven items assess anxiety, and seven items measure depression, each coded from 0 to 3. The HADS has been used extensively in clinics and has adequate reliability (Cronbach's $\alpha = .83$) and validity, with optimal balance between sensitivity and specificity. It has been translated into many languages and is widely used around the world in clinical and research settings.[168]

Functional Capacity and Activity Interference Measures

Some clinicians consider pain reduction meaningless unless accompanied by a noticeable change in function. Thus, some reliable measurement of functional capacity is often desirable before the onset of therapy. Research has shown that physical impairment, defined as an objective medical condition such as an amputation, is not very predictive of disability, which is an inability to work because of a medical impairment. Rather, beliefs about an injury predict disability and physical performance after surgery better than pain ratings or a physical impairment.[169,170] Measures that can be used to assess activity level and function include the Short-Form Health Survey (SF-36),[171] the West Haven–Yale Multidimensional Pain Inventory (WHYMPI, mostly known now as the MPI),[172] and the Pain Disability Index (PDI).[173] It is preferable to consider functional measures that are specific to the chronic pain condition being assessed, for example, back pain patients will have different activity limitations than someone with upper extremity pain.

The SF-36, which was initially developed from the Medical Outcomes Study to survey health status, includes eight scales that measure (1) limitations in physical activities due to health problems, (2) limitations in social activities due to physical and emotional problems, (3) limitations in usual role activities due to physical health problems, (4) bodily pain, (5) general mental health, (6) limitations in usual role activities due to emotional problems, (7) vitality (energy and fatigue), and (8) general health perceptions.[171] Although the SF-36 is a popular measure, pain patients tend to score very low (severe limitations) such that modest improvements can go undetected. An expanded measure known as the Treatment Outcomes of Pain System (TOPS),[174] that incorporates the SF-36, has been modified specifically for patients with pain to improve sensitivity and reliability of measurement of treatment outcome.

The MPI is a 56-item measure made up of 7-point rating scales. The subscales assess activity interference, perceived support, pain severity, negative mood, and perceived control. The advantage of this self-report instrument is that it was created specifically for chronic pain patients and can be useful in classifying those patients into three types: dysfunctional, interpersonally distressed, and adaptive copers.[175] Strong evidence supports the presence of these three types in the assessment of chronic pain patients.[176]

Other popular functional measures include the Oswestry Disability Questionnaire,[177] the Roland-Morris Functional Disability Scale,[177] the Waddell Disability Instrument,[178] the Functional Rating Scale,[179] and the Back Pain Functional Scale.[180]

Pain Beliefs

Pain perception, beliefs about pain, and approaches to self-managing pain are important in predicting the outcome of treatment and are particularly relevant as predictors for implantable devices. Unrealistic or negative thoughts about an ongoing pain problem may contribute to increased pain and emotional distress, decreased functioning, a greater reliance on medication, and poor outcome from surgery.[181] Certain chronic pain patients are prone to maladaptive beliefs about their condition that may not be compatible with the physical nature of their pain.[182] Patients with adequate psychological functioning exhibit a greater tendency to ignore their pain, use coping self-statements, remain active, and use less medication after joint replacement surgery.[183]

Because efficacy expectations have been shown to influence the efforts patients will make to manage their pain, measures of self-efficacy or perceived control are useful in assessing a patient's attitude after surgery.[184] Several self-report measures assess coping and pain attitudes. The most popular tests used to measure maladaptive beliefs include the CSQ,[113] the PMI,[185] the Pain Self-Efficacy Questionnaire (PSEQ),[186] the Survey of Pain Attitudes (SOPA),[187] and the Inventory of Negative Thoughts in Response to Pain (INTRP).[188] Other instruments include the Pain Beliefs and Perceptions Inventory (PBPI),[189] and the Chronic Pain Self-Efficacy Scale (CPSS).[190] Finally, the Pain Catastrophizing Scale (PCS)[191] is a well-validated, widely used, self-report measure of catastrophic thinking associated with pain. The construct of catastrophizing incorporates magnification of pain-related symptoms, rumination about pain, feelings of helplessness, and pessimism about pain-related outcomes. Assessment of catastrophizing is important when evaluating candidacy for an implanted device because it adversely affects outcome and is a strong predictor for continued disability following surgery.[192] Individuals rate the extent to which they experience the thought or feeling described by each item when they are in pain; scores on this 13-item measure can range from 0 to 52 (each item is scored 0 = not at all to 4 = all the time). The PCS has good psychometric properties in pain patients and controls.[193] In recent studies of chronic pain patients, Cronbach's α for the PCS has been reported as above 0.9, indicating very high levels of internal item consistency.[194] Distraction has been useful in reducing catastrophizing,[195] as is even a brief course of cognitive behavioral therapy.[196]

It is suspected that patients who have unrealistic beliefs and expectations about their condition are also poor candidates for pain treatment.[197] Patients who have a high catastrophizing score, who endorse passive coping on the PMI, who demonstrate low self-efficacy regarding their ability to manage their pain on the PSEQ, who describe themselves as disabled by their pain on the SOPA, and who report frequent negative thoughts about their pain on the INTRP are at greatest risk for poor treatment outcome following placement of an implanted device.

ELECTRONIC PAIN ASSESSMENT PROGRAMS

There has been recent interest in implementing electronic pain assessment programs in clinic settings to assess and monitor persons with chronic pain prior to surgery or a trial of an implanted device.[198,199] Evidence exists of the benefits of such programs in assessing risk of poor outcomes, to reduce personnel time, and to document change along the continuum of pain care.[200] Preliminary studies suggest that a Web-based secure electronic assessment program outweighs the benefits of a paper questionnaire.[201] In a study designed to determine the impact of an electronic pain evaluation program, chart reviews were conducted between pain patients who completed an electronic pain assessment program (N = 89) and controls who represented standard care (N = 120).[202] Chart review findings suggested that posted reports on the patient medical record from an electronic assessment increased the presence of key pain assessment information that were not found when incorporating notes from a traditional paper-and-pencil questionnaire. In particular, information on past treatments; adverse effects; psychological symptoms of depression, anxiety, and irritability; mental health treatment; past history of smoking; litigation; and substance abuse were documented more frequently (P < .001).[200] It is thought that a detailed evaluation would be beneficial when determining benefit from an implanted device or spinal surgery. In a second related study by Butler and colleagues,[202] two groups of chronic pain patients (treatment as usual = 75, electronic pain assessment = 72) were interviewed after completing their initial clinic visit and completed mailed questionnaires 3 months later. Results from this study showed that those subjects who had completed the electronic pain assessment program reported more discussion about legal issues, substance use history, and medication safety compared with those patients who were not given the electronic assessment program (P < .05). Satisfaction questionnaire responses supported both provider and patient perceived benefit of using the electronic pain assessment program. Overall, results indicate that use of a comprehensive electronic pain assessment program improves documentation of chart elements in clinic notes and can be associated with increased discussion of key, pain-relevant topics during the clinical visit and in assessing patients considered for surgery or an implanted device.

Conclusion

A growing body of research reviewed in this chapter indicates that psychosocial factors can strongly influence spine surgery outcome and long-term benefit from an implanted device. These results suggest that a comprehensive psychological screening should be included as a component of the diagnostic process in many spine surgery candidates and patients considered for placement of an implanted device for pain. Table 76.3 provides a set of general referral guidelines that a physician can keep in mind when considering the need for a psychological assessment.[203] When the provider judges that a patient displays four or more of these points (listed in Table 76.3), a referral for a comprehensive psychological screening should be initiated. Such a referral is especially critical if there is a planned

TABLE 76.3 Referral Guidelines for Presurgical Psychological Screening[203]

- Excessive pain behavior
- Symptoms inconsistent with identified pathology
- High levels of depression or anxiety
- Sleep disturbance: insomnia or hypersomnia
- Excessively high or low expectations about surgical outcome
- A high degree of pain-related catastrophizing
- Limited pain coping skills
- High levels of social/interpersonal conflict
- Negative attitude toward work or employer
- Emotional lability or mood swings
- Inability to work or greatly decreased functional ability (<3 mo)
- Escalating or large doses of narcotics or anxiolytics
- Litigation or continuing disability benefits resulting from spine injury
- Referral considerations

0–1 items: not necessary to refer unless desired by patient

2–3 items: consider referral for presurgical psychological screening

4+ items: strongly consider referral for presurgical psychological screening

surgery that will be exploratory and highly invasive, for example, involving multiple levels and instrumentation, or involves a reoperation, or when placement of an implanted device is being considered for a condition that is complex and particularly protracted.

The major psychosocial risk factors contributing to poor surgical outcome are listed in Table 76.4.[204] A comprehensive psychological evaluation helps to identify these risk factors. Research from several laboratories has found that using a scorecard approach to identifying risk factors has predictive value and that patients with a high level of overall risk respond poorly to spine surgery or invasive procedures.[205–207] The results reviewed in this chapter demonstrate that spine surgery or placement of an implanted device may not be effective for patients with a high level of psychosocial risk. For such patients, a more conservative intervention may be more appropriate and effective. Fortunately, a cost-effective alternative to surgery or implantation exists—the multidisciplinary chronic pain management program (CPMP). Such programs teach patients to manage and cope with pain and its impact, through a combination of physical conditioning, education, psychological treatment, relaxation training, and vocational counseling.

TABLE 76.4 Presurgical Psychological Screening Risk Factors for Poor Surgical Outcome[204]

- Personality factors (assessed by objective tests)
  - Pain sensitivity
  - Anger
  - Depression
  - Anxiety and obsessions
- Poor coping strategies (assessed by objective tests)
  - Catastrophizing
  - Low self-efficacy or pain control
- Behavioral factors
  - Spousal reinforcement of pain
  - Litigation pending
  - Workers' compensation
  - Blaming employer for injury
- Historic factors
  - Abuse and abandonment
  - Past psychological treatment
  - Multiple previous medical problems
  - Substance abuse

Several recent studies have shown that the CPMP approach can be as effective in treating patients with spinal pain as is spine surgery.[25–28] The studies comparing CPMPs to spine surgery suggest that even when medical diagnostics reveal spinal pathology potentially amenable to surgery, many patients may achieve comparable results with less long-term risk by undergoing treatment in a CPMP.

Using a comprehensive psychological screening, the surgeon or the pain physician can reduce the costs arising from procedures that have a relatively low probability of benefit and can help the high-risk patient avoid a downward slide into increasing pain and disability. Based on the results of the psychological screening, surgeons or pain physicians may decide to (1) refer the patient for treatment at a CPMP, (2) postpone elective surgery or placement of an implanted device until psychosocial factors are addressed, (3) avoid surgery and invasive procedures altogether, or (4) proceed with surgery or implantation but involve psychologists early during rehabilitation. Psychological screening offers the potential to sharpen patient selection for spine surgery and for implanted devices and tailor treatments to both the patient's physical and psychological needs.

References

1. Institute of Medicine Committee on Advancing Pain Research, Care, and Education. *Relieving Pain in America: A Blueprint for Transforming Prevention, Care, Education and Research*. Washington, DC: National Academies Press; 2011.
2. Nahin RL. Estimates of pain prevalence and severity in adults: United States, 2012. *J Pain* 2015;16:769–780.
3. Alschuler KN, Ehde DM, Jensen MP. The co-occurrence of pain and depression in adults with multiple sclerosis. *Rehabil Psychol* 2013;58:217–221.
4. Jamison RN, Edward RR. Integrating pain management into clinical practice. *J Clin Psych Med Settings* 2012;19:49–64.
5. Koes BW, Van Tulder MW, Ostelo RW, et al. Clinical guidelines for the management of low back pain in primary care: an international comparison. *Spine* 2001;26:2504–2513.
6. Murray CJ, Vos T, Lozano R, et al. Disability-adjusted life years (DALYs) for 291 diseases and injuries in 21 regions, 1990–2010: a systematic analysis for the Global Burden of Disease Study 2010. *Lancet* 2013;380:2197–2223.
7. Murray CJ, Barber RM, Foreman KJ, et al. Global, regional, and national disability-adjusted life years (DALYs) for 306 diseases and injuries and healthy life expectancy (HALE) for 188 countries, 1990-2013: quantifying the epidemiological transition. *Lancet* 2015;386(10009):2145–2191.
8. Murray CJ, Atkinson C, Bhalla K, et al. The state of US health, 1990-2010 burden of diseases, injuries, and risk factors. *JAMA* 2013;310(6):591–606.
9. Gaskin D, Richard P. The economic costs of pain in the United States. *J Pain* 2012;13:715–724.
10. Ferrari R, Russell AS. Regional musculoskeletal conditions: neck pain. *Best Pract Res Clin Rheumatol* 2003;17:57–70.
11. Stewart WF, Ricci JA, Chee E, et al. Lost productive time and cost due to common pain conditions in the US workforce. *JAMA* 2003;290:2443–2454.
12. Becker A, Held H, Redaelli M, et al. Low back pain in primary care: costs of care and prediction of future health care utilization. *Spine (Phila Pa 1976)* 2010;35(18):1714–1720.
13. Hoy D, March L, Brooks P, et al. Measuring the global burden of low back pain. *Best Pract Res Clin Rheumatol* 2010;24(2):155–165.
14. Phillips CJ, Harper C. The economics associated with persistent pain. *Curr Opin Support Palliat Care* 2011;5:127–130.
15. Chou R, Deyo R, Friedly J, et al. *Noninvasive Treatments for Low Back Pain. Comparative Effectiveness Review No. 169*. Rockville, MD: Agency for Healthcare Research and Quality; 2016.
16. Chou R, Deyo R, Friedly J, et al. Nonpharmacological therapies for low back pain: a systematic review. *Ann Intern Med* 2017;166:493–505.
17. Jamison RN, Wasan AA. Depression in the patient with chronic pain. In: Barsky AJ, Siberswieg DA, eds. *Depression in Medical Illness*. New York: McGraw-Hill; 2017:287–298.
18. Bair M, Robinson R, Katon W, et al. Depression and pain comorbidity: a literature review. *Arch Int Med* 2003;163:2433–2445.
19. Von Korff M, Deyo R. Potent opioids for chronic musculoskeletal pain: flying blind? *Pain* 2004;109:207–209.
20. Edwards RR, Smith MT, Kudel I, et al. Pain-related catastrophizing as a risk factor for suicidal ideation in chronic pain. *Pain* 2006;126:272–279.
21. Brinjikji W, Luetmer PH, Comstock B, et al. Systematic literature review of imaging features of spinal degeneration in asymptomatic populations. *AJNR Am J Neuroradiol* 2015;36:811–816.
22. Malik KM, Cohen SP, Walega DR, et al. Diagnostic criteria and treatment of discogenic pain: a systematic review of recent clinical literature. *Spine J* 2013;13(11):1675–1689.

23. Rajaee SS, Bae HW, Kanim LE, et al. Spinal fusion in the United States: analysis of trends from 1998 to 2008. *Spine* 2012;37:67–76.

24. Wei J, Song Y, Sun L, et al. Comparison of artificial total disc replacement versus fusion for lumbar degenerative disc disease: a meta-analysis of randomized controlled trials. *Int Orthop* 2013;37:1315–1325.

25. Brox JI, Sørensen R, Friis A, et al. Randomized clinical trial of lumbar instrumented fusion and cognitive intervention and exercises in patients with chronic low back pain and disc degeneration. *Spine* 2003;28:1913–1921.

26. Brox JI, Reikeras O, Nygaard O, et al. Lumbar instrumented fusion compared with cognitive intervention and exercises in patients with chronic back pain after previous surgery for disc herniation: a prospective randomized controlled study. *Pain* 2006;122:145–155.

27. Brox JI, Nygaard ØP, Holm I, et al. Four-year follow-up of surgical versus non-surgical therapy for chronic low back pain. *Ann Rheum Dis* 2010; 69(9):1643–1648.

28. Fairbank J, Frost H, Wilson-MacDonald J, et al; for Spine Stabilisation Trial Group. Randomised controlled trial to compare surgical stabilisation of the lumbar spine with an intensive rehabilitation programme for patients with chronic low back pain: the MRC Spine Stabilisation Trial. *BMJ* 2005; 330(7502):1233.

29. Fritzell P, Hagg O, Wessberg P, et al. Lumbar fusion versus nonsurgical treatment for chronic low back pain: a multicenter randomized controlled trial from the Swedish Lumbar Spine Study Group. *Spine* 2001;26(23):2521–2532.

30. Deyo RA, Mirza SK. Trends and variations in the use of spine surgery. *Clin Orthop Relat Res* 2006;443:139–146.

31. Turner JA, Ersek M, Herron L, et al. Patient outcomes after lumbar spinal fusions. *JAMA* 1992;268:907–911.

32. Hoffman RM, Wheeler KJ, Deyo RA. Surgery for herniated lumbar discs: a literature synthesis. *J Gen Intern Med* 1993;8:487–496.

33. DeBerard MS, Masters KS, Colledge AL, et al. Outcomes of posterolateral lumbar fusion in Utah patients receiving worker's compensation. *Spine* 2001;26:738–747.

34. DeBerard MS, Masters KS, Colledge AL, et al. Presurgical biopsychosocial variables predict medical and compensation costs of lumbar fusion in Utah workers' compensation patients. *Spine J* 2003;3:420–429.

35. Shealy C, Mortimer JT, Reswick JB. Electrical inhibition of pain by stimulation of dorsa columns: preliminary clinical report. *Anesth Analg* 1967;46:489–491.

36. Melzack R, Wall PD. Pain mechanisms: a new theory. *Science* 1965;150: 971–979.

37. North RB, Linderoth B. Spinal cord stimulation. In: Fishman SM, Ballantyne JC, Rathmell JP, eds. *Bonica's Management of Pain*. 4th ed. Philadelphia: Lippincott Williams & Wilkins; 2010:1379–1392.

38. Stidd Da, Rivero S, Weinand ME. Spinal cord stimulation with implanted epidural paddle lead relieves chronic axial low back pain. *J Pain Res* 2014;7:465–470.

39. Lamer TJ, Deer TR, Hayek SM. Advanced innovations for pain. *Mayo Clin Proc* 2016;91:246–258.

40. Hou S, Kemp K, Grabois M. A systematic evaluation of burst spinal cord stimulation for chronic back and limp pain. *Neuromodulation* 2016;19: 398–405.

41. Kemler MA, van Kleef M, et al. Spinal cord stimulation in patients with chronic reflex sympathetic dystrophy. *N Engl J Med* 2000;343:618–624.

42. Monhemius RS. Efficacy of spinal cord stimulation for neuropathic pain: assessment by abstinence. *Eur J Pain* 2003;7:513–519.

43. Lee N, Vasudevan S. Spinal cord stimulation use in patients with failed back surgery syndrome. *Pain Manag* 2012;2:135–140.

44. Hoelscher C, Riley J, Wu C, et al. Cost-effectiveness data regarding spinal cord stimulation for low back pain. *Spine* 2017;42:S72–S79.

45. Harbaugh RE, Reeder TM. Continuous drug delivery by an implantable drug delivery system. *Am J Hosp Care*, 1984;1:17–20.

46. Onofrio BM, Yaksh TL, Arnold PG. Continuous low-dose intrathecal morphine administration in the treatment of chronic pain of malignant origin. *Mayo Clinic Proc* 1981;56:516–520.

47. Saulino M, Ivanhoe CB, McGuire JR, et al. Best practices for intrathecal baclofen therapy: patient selection. *Neuromodulation* 2016;19:607–615.

48. Osenbach RK. Intrathecal drug delivery in the management of pain. In: Fishman SM, Ballantyne JC, Rathmell JP, eds. *Bonica's Management of Pain*. 4th ed. Philadelphia: Lippincott Williams & Wilkins; 2010:1437–1458.

49. Veizi E, Hayek S. Interventional therapies for chronic low back pain. *Neuromodulation* 2014;17:S31–S45.

50. Bagnall D. The use of spinal cord stimulations and intrathecal drug delivery in the treatment of low back-related pain. *Phys Med Rehabil Clin N Am* 2010;21:851–858.

51. Kumar K, Kelly M, Pirlot KM. Continuous intrathecal morphine treatment for chronic pain of non-malignant etiology: long-term benefits and efficacy. *Surg Neurology* 2001;55:79–86.

52. Roberts LJ, Finch PM, Goucke CR, et al. Outcome of intrathecal opioids in chronic non-cancer pain. *Eur J Pain* 2001;5:353–361.

53. Hassenbusch SJ, Stanton-Hicks M, Covington EC. Spinal cord stimulation versus spinal infusion for low back and leg pain. *Acta Neurochir Suppl* 1995;64:109–115.

54. Deer TR, Raso LJ, Garten RL. Inflammatory mass of an intrathecal catheter in patients receiving baclofen as a sole agent: a report of two cases and a review of the identification and treatment of the complication. *Pain Medicine* 2007;8:259–262.

55. Sharpe L, McDonald S, Correia H, et al. Pain severity predicts depression symptoms over and above individual illnesses and multimorbidity in older adults. *BMC Psychiatry* 2017;17:166.

56. Hung CI, Liu CY, Fu TS. Depression: an important factor associated with disability among patients with chronic low back pain. *Int J Psychiatry Med* 2015;49:187–198.

57. Kjelby-Wendt G, Styf J, Carlsson SG. The predictive value of psychometric analysis in patients treated by extirpation of lumbar intervertebral disc herniation. *J Spinal Disord* 1999;12:375–379.

58. Schade V, Semmer N, Main CJ, et al. The impact of clinical, morphological, psychosocial, and work-related factors on the outcome of lumbar discectomy. *Pain* 1999;80:239–249.

59. Trief PM, Ploutz-Snyder R, Fredrickson BE. Emotional health predicts pain and function after fusion: a prospective multicenter study. *Spine* 2006;31:823–830.

60. Lazaridou A, Franceschelli O, Buliteanu A, et al. Influence of catastrophizing on pain intensity, disability, side effects, and opioid misuse among pain patients in primary care. *J Appl Behav Res* 2017;22:e12081.

61. Campbell CM, Jamison RN, Edwards RR. Psychological screening/phenotyping as predictors for spinal cord stimulation. *Curr Pain Headache Rep* 2013;17:307–314.

62. Rakvåg TT, Klepstad P, Baar C, et al. The Val158Met polymorphism of the human catechol-O-methyltransferase (COMT) gene may influence morphine requirements in cancer pain patients. *Pain* 2005;116:73–78.

63. Rooks DS, Huang J, Bierbaum BE, et al. Effect of preoperative exercise on measures of functional status in men and women undergoing total hip and knee arthroplasty. *Arthritis Care Res* 2006;55:700–708.

64. Wasan AD, Kaptchuk TJ, Davar G, et al. The association between psychopathology and placebo analgesia in patients with discogenic low back pain. *Pain Med* 2006;7:217–228.

65. Tunks ER, Crook J, Weir R. Epidemiology of chronic pain with psychological comorbidity: prevalence, risk, course, and prognosis. *Can J Psychia* 2008;53:224–234.

66. Bruehl S, Liu X, Burns J, et al. Associations between daily chronic pain intensity, daily anger expression, and trait anger expressiveness: an ecological momentary assessment study. *Pain* 2012:153:2352–2358.

67. Wasan AD, Michna E, Edwards RR, et al. Psychiatric comorbidity is associated prospectively with diminished opioid analgesia and increased opioid misuse in patients with chronic low back pain. *Anesthesiology* 2015;123: 861–872.

68. Evers A, Kraaimaat F, van Reil P, et al. Cognitive, behavioral and physiological reactivity to pain as a predictor of long-term pain in rheumatoid arthritis patients. *Pain* 2001;93:139–146.

69. Boersma K, Linton SJ. Screening to identify patients at risk: profiles of psychological risk factors for early intervention. *Clin J Pain* 2005;21:38–43.

70. Edwards RR, Calahan C, Mensing G, et al. Pain, catastrophizing, and depression in the rheumatic diseases. *Nature Rev Rheumatol* 2011;7:216–224.

71. Harkins S, Price D, Braith J. Effects of extraversion and neuroticism on experimental pain, clinical pain, and illness behavior. *Pain* 1989;36:209–218.

72. Fernandez M, Colodro-Conde L, Hartvigsen J, et al. Chronic low back pain and the risk of depression or anxiety symptoms: insights from a longitudinal twin study. *Spine J* 2017;17:905–912.

73. Block AR, Gatchel RJ, Deardorff WW. *The Psychology of Spine Surgery*. Washington, DC: American Psychological Association, 2003.

74. Celestin J, Edwards RR, Jamison RN. Pretreatment psychosocial variables as predictors of outcomes following lumbar surgery and spinal cord stimulation: a systematic review and literature synthesis. *Pain Med* 2009;10:639–653.

75. Kumar K, Rizvi S, Bnurs SB. Spinal cord stimulation is effective in management of complex regional pain syndrome I: fact or fiction. *Neurosurgery* 2011;69:566–578.

76. Sparkes E, Raphael JH, Duarte RV, et al. A systematic literature review of psychological characteristics as determinants of outcome for spinal cord stimulation therapy. *Pain* 2010;150:284–289.

77. Roelofs J, Goubert L, Peters ML, et al. The Tampa Scale for Kinesiophobia: further examination of psychometric properties in patients with chronic low back pain and fibromyalgia. *Eur J Pain* 2004;8:495–502.

78. den Boer JJ, Oostendorp RA, Beems T, et al. Reduced work capacity after lumbar disc surgery: the role of cognitive-behavioral and work-related risk factors. *Pain* 2006;126:72–78.

79. Kiecolt-Glaser JK, Page GG, Marucha PT, et al. Psychological influences on surgical recovery. Perspectives from psychoneuroimmunology. *Am Psychol* 1998;53:1209–1218.

80. Snider KT, Johnson JC, Snider EJ, et al. Increased incidence and severity of somatic dysfunction in subjects with chronic low back pain. *J Am Osteopath Assoc* 2008;108:372–378.

81. Rosmalen JG, Tak LM, de Jonge P. Empirical foundations for the diagnosis of somatization: implications of DSM-5. *Psychol Med* 2001;41:1133–1142.

82. Dijkstra-Kersten SM, Sitnikova K, van Marwijk HW, et al. Somatisation as a risk factor for incident depression and anxiety. *J Psychosom Res* 2015;79:614–619.

83. Tomenson B, McBeth J, Chew-Graham CS, et al. Somatization and health anxiety as predictors of health care use. *Psychosom Med* 2012;74:656–664.

84. Manning JS, Jackson WC. Depression, pain, and comorbid medical conditions. *J Clin Psychiatry* 2013;74(2):e03.

85. Edwards RR, Wasan A, Michna E, et al. Elevated pain sensitivity in chronic pain patients at risk for opioid misuse. *J Pain* 2011;9:953–963.

86. van Eijs F, Smits H, Geurts JW, et al. Brusk-evoked allodynia also predicts outcome of spinal cord stimulation in complex regional pain syndrome type I. *Eur J Pain* 2010;14:164–169.

87. Stancák A, Kozák J, Vrba I, et al. Functional magnetic resonance imaging of cerebral activation during spinal cord stimulation in failed back surgery syndrome patients. *Eur J Pain* 2008;12:137–148.

88. Hübscher M, Moloney N, Rebbeck T, et al. Contributions of mood, pain catastrophizing, and cold hyperalgesia in acute and chronic low back pain: a comparison with pain-free controls. *Clin J Pain* 2014;30:886–893.

89. O'Neill S, Manniche C, Graven-Nielsen T, et al. Generalized deep-tissue hyperalgesia in patients with chronic low-back pain. *Eur J Pain* 2007;11:415–420.

90. O'Neill S, Manniche C, Graven-Nielsen T, et al. Association between a composite score of pain sensitivity and clinical parameters in low-back pain. *Clin J Pain* 2014;30:831–838.

91. Kim HJ, Lee JI, Kang KT, et al. Influence of pain sensitivity on surgical outcomes after lumbar spine surgery in patients with lumbar spinal stenosis. *Spine* 2015;40:193–200.

92. Kim HJ, Park JH, Kim JW, et al. Prediction of postoperative pain intensity after lumbar spinal surgery using pain sensitivity and preoperative back pain severity. *Pain Med* 2014;15:2037–2045.

93. Kim HJ, Suh BG, Lee DB, et al. Gender difference of symptom severity in lumbar spinal stenosis: role of pain sensitivity. *Pain Physician* 2013;16:E715–E723.

94. Grosen K, Fischer IW, Olesen AE, et al. Can quantitative sensory testing predict responses to analgesic treatment? *Eur J Pain* 2013;17:1267–1280.

95. Schreiber KL, Kehlet H, Belfer I, et al. Predicting, preventing and managing persistent pain after breast cancer surgery: the importance of psychosocial factors. *Pain Manag* 2014;4:445–459.

96. Vanharanta H, Sachs BL, Spivey MA, et al. The relationship of pain provocation to lumbar disc deterioration as seen by CT/discography. *Spine* 1987;12:295–298.

97. Walsh TR, Weinstein JN, Spratt KF, et al. Lumbar discography in normal subjects. A controlled, prospective study. *J Bone Joint Surg Am* 1990;72(7):1081–1088.

98. Burns JW, Gerhart JI, Bruehl S, et al. Anger arousal and behavioral anger regulation in everyday life among people with chronic low back pain: relationships with spouse responses and negative affect. *Health Psychol* 2016;35:29–40.

99. Fernandez E, Milburn TW. Sensory and affective predictors of overall pain and emotions associated with affective pain. *Clin J Pain* 1994;10:3–9.

100. Mavros MN, Athanasiou S, Gkegkes ID, et al. Do psychological variables affect early surgical recovery? *PLoS One* 2011;6:e20306.

101. Scott W, Trost Z, Bernier E, et al. Anger differentially mediates the relationship between perceived injustice and chronic pain outcomes. *Pain* 2013;154:1691–1698.

102. Sullivan MJ, Scott W, Trost Z. Perceived injustice: a risk factor for problematic pain outcomes. *Clin J Pain* 2012;28(6):484–488.

103. DeGood DE, Kiernan B. Perception of fault in patients with chronic pain. *Pain* 1996;64:153–159.

104. Bruehl S, Burns JW, Chung OY, et al. Pain-related effects of trait anger expression: neural substrates and the role of endogenous opioid mechanisms. *Neurosci Biobehav Rev* 2009;33:475–491.

105. Burns JW, Bruehl S, Chont M. Anger regulation style, anger arousal and acute pain sensitivity: evidence for an endogenous opioid "triggering" model. *J Behav Med* 2014;37:642–653.

106. Burns JW, Bruehl S, France CR, et al. Endogenous opioid function and responses to morphine: the moderating effects of anger expressiveness. *J Pain* 2017;18:923–932.

107. Edwards RR, Dworkin RH, Sullivan MD, et al. The role of psychosocial processes in the development and maintenance of chronic pain. *J Pain* 2016;17:S70–S92.

108. Khan RS, Ahmed K, Blakeway E, et al. Catastrophizing: a predictive factor for postoperative pain. *Am J Surg* 2011;201:122–131.

109. Rabbitts JA, Fisher E, Rosenbloom BN, et al. Prevalence and predictors of chronic postsurgical pain in children: a systematic review and meta-analysis. *J Pain* 2017;18:605–614.

110. Hassett AL, Finan PH. The role of resilience in the clinical management of chronic pain. *Curr Pain Headache Rep* 2016;20:39.

111. de Rooij A, de Boer MR, Roorda LD, et al. Cognitive mechanisms of change in multidisciplinary treatment of patients with chronic widespread pain: a prospective cohort study. *J Rehabil Med* 2014;46:173–180.

112. Snow-Turek AL, Norris MP, Tan G. Active and passive coping strategies in chronic pain patients. *Pain* 1996;64:455–462.

113. Rosenstiel AK, Keefe FJ. The use of coping strategies in chronic low back pain patients: relationship to patient characteristics and current adjustment. *Pain* 1983;17:33–44.

114. Gross AR. The effect of coping strategies on the relief of pain following surgical intervention for lower back pain. *Psychosom Med* 1986;48:229–241.

115. Edwards RR, Dolman AJ, Michna E. Changes in pain sensitivity and pain modulation during oral opioid treatment: the impact of negative affect. *Pain Med* 2016;17:1882–1891.

116. den Boer JJ, Oostendorp RA, Evers AW, et al. The development of a screening instrument to select patients at risk of residual complaints after lumbar disc surgery. *Eur J Phys Rehabil Med* 2010;46:497–503.

117. Wilson SJ, Martire LM, Sliwinski MJ. Daily spousal responsiveness predicts longer-term trajectories of patients' physical function. *Psychol Sci* 2017;28:786–797.

118. Jensen MP, Moore MR, Bockow TB, et al. Psychosocial factors and adjustment to chronic pain in persons with physical disabilities: a systematic review. *Arch Phys Med Rehabil* 2009;92:146–160.

119. Kowal J, McWilliams LA, Peloquin K, et al. Attachment insecurity predicts responses to an interdisciplinary chronic pain rehabilitation program. *J Behav Med* 2015;38:518–526.

120. Anema JR, Schellart AJ, Cassidy JD, et al. Can cross country differences in return-to-work after chronic occupational back pain be explained? An exploratory analysis on disability policies in a six country cohort study. *J Occup Rehabil* 2009;19:419–426.

121. Dorow M, Lobner M, Stein J, et al. The course of pain intensity in patients undergoing herniated disc surgery: a 5-year longitudinal observational study. *PLoS One* 2016;11:e0156647.

122. Mancuso CA, Duculan R, Craig CM, et al. Psychosocial variables contribute to length of stay and discharge destination after lumbar surgery independent of demographic and clinical variables. *Spine* 2018;43:281–286.

123. Tripp DA, Abraham E, Lambert M, et al. Biopsychosocial factors predict quality of life in thoracolumbar spine surgery. *Qual Life Res* 2017;26:3099–3110. doi:10.1007/s11136-017-1654-x.

124. Afari N, Ahumada SM, Wright LJ, et al. Psychological trauma and functional somatic syndromes: a systematic review and meta-analysis. *Psychosom Med* 2014;76:2–11.

125. Jones GT, Power C, Macfarlane GJ. Adverse events in childhood and chronic widespread pain in adult life: results from the 1958 British Birth Cohort Study. *Pain* 2009;143:92–96.

126. Kongsted A, Bendix T, Qerama E, et al. Acute stress response and recovery after whiplash injuries. A one-year prospective study. *Eur J Pain* 2008;12:455–463.

127. Lang AJ, Laffaye C, Satz LE, et al. Relationships among childhood maltreatment, PTSD, and health in female veterans in primary care. *Child Abuse Negl* 2006;30:1281–1292.

128. Wuest J, Ford-Gilboe M, Merritt-Gray M, et al. Pathways of chronic pain in survivors of intimate partner violence. *J Womens Health* 2010;19:1665–1674.

129. Nickel R, Egle UT, Hardt J. Are childhood adversities relevant in patients with chronic low back pain? *Eur J Pain* 2002;6:221–228.

130. Schofferman J, Anderson D, Hines R, et al. Childhood psychological trauma and chronic refractory low-back pain. *Clin J Pain* 1993;9:260–265.

131. Sharifzadeh Y, Kao MC, Sturgeon JA, et al. Pain catastrophizing moderates relationships between pain intensity and opioid prescription: nonlinear sex differences revealed using a learning health system. *Anesthesiology* 2017;127:136–146.

132. Jamison RN, Mao J. Opioid analgesics. *Mayo Clinic Proc* 2015;90:957–968.

133. Jurcik DC, Sundaram AH, Jamison RN. Chronic pain, negative affect, and prescription opioid abuse. *Curr Opin Psychol* 2015;5:42–49.

134. Polatin PB, Kinney RK, Gatchel RJ, et al. Psychiatric illness and chronic low-back pain. The mind and the spine—which goes first? *Spine* 1993;18:66–71.

135. Spengler DM, Freeman C, Westbrook R, et al. Low-back pain following multiple lumbar spine procedures. Failure of initial selection? *Spine* 1980;5:356–360.

136. Lee SM, Landry J, Jones PM, et al. Long-term quit rates after a perioperative smoking cessation randomized controlled trial. *Anesth Analg* 2015;120:582–587.

137. Jamison RN. Psychological evaluation and treatment of chronic pain. In: Vacanti CA, Sikka PK, Urman RD, et al, eds. *Essential Clinical Anesthesia.* New York: Cambridge University Press; 2011:901–905.

138. Vlaeyen JW, Linton SJ. Fear-avoidance and its consequences in chronic musculoskeletal pain: a state of the art. *Pain* 2000;85:317–322.

139. Hermann C, Hohmeister J, Zohsel K, et al. The assessment of pain coping and pain-related cognitions in children and adolescents: current methods and further development. *J Pain* 2007;8:802–813.

140. Hack TF, Kwan WB, Thomas-Maclean RL, et al. Predictors of arm morbidity following breast cancer surgery. *Psychooncology* 2010;19:1205–1212.

141. Budzynski TS, Stoyva JM, Adler LS, et al. EMG biofeedback and tension headache: a controlled study. *Psychosom Med* 1973;35:484–496.

142. Melzack R. The McGill Pain Questionnaire: major properties and scoring methods. *Pain* 1975;1:277–299.

143. Jensen MP, Karoly P. Self-report scales and procedures for assessing pain in adults. In: Turk DC, Melzack R, eds. *Handbook of Pain Assessment.* 2nd ed. New York: Guilford Press; 2001:15–34.

144. Jamison RN, Gracely RH, Raymond SA, et al. Comparative study of electronic vs. paper VAS ratings: a randomized, crossover trial using healthy volunteers. *Pain* 2002;99:341–347.

145. Marceau LD, Link CL, Smith LD, et al. In-clinic use of electronic pain diaries: barriers of implementation among pain physicians. *J Pain Symptom Manage* 2010;40:391–404.

146. Ferreira-Valente MA, Pais-Ribeiro JL, Jensen MP. Validity of four pain intensity rating scales. *Pain* 2011;152:2399–2404.

147. Miro J, Castarlenas E, de la Vega R, et al. Validity of three rating scales for measuring pain intensity in youths with physical disabilities. *Eur J Pain* 2016;20:130–137.

148. Von Korff M, Lane D, Miglioretti G, et al. Chronic spinal pain and physical-mental comorbidity in the United States: results from the National Comorbidity Survey Replication. *Pain* 2005;113:331–339.

149. Kalso E, Edwards JE, Moore RA, et al. Opioids in chronic non-cancer pain: systematic review of efficacy and safety. *Pain* 2004;112:372–380.

150. Daubs MD, Norvell DC, McGuire R, et al. Fusion versus nonoperative care for chronic low back pain: do to psychological factors affecting outcome? *Spine* 2011;36:S96–S109.

151. Sinikallio S, Airaksinen O, Aalto T, et al. Coexistence of pain and depression predicts a poor 2-year surgery outcome among lumbar spinal stenosis patients. *Nord J Psychiatry* 2010;64:391–396.

152. Sinikallio S, Aalto T, Airaksinen O, et al. Depression is associated with a poorer outcome of lumbar spinal stenosis surgery: a two-year perspective follow-up study. *Spine* 2011;36:677–682.

153. Dworkin RH, Turk DC, Wyrwich KW, et al. Interpreting the clinical importance of treatment outcomes in chronic pain clinical trials: IMMPACT recommendations. *J Pain* 2008;9:105–121.

154. Hathaway SR, McKinley JC, Butcher JN, et al. *Minnesota Multiphasic Personality Inventory—2: Manual for Administration.* Minneapolis, MN: University of Minnesota Press; 1989.

155. Derogatis LR, Melisaratos N. The Brief Symptom Inventory: an introductory report. *Psychol Med* 1983;13:595–605.

156. Beck AT, Ward CH, Mendelson M, et al. An inventory for measuring depression. *Archives Gen Psychia* 1961;4:561–571.

157. Zigmond AS, Snaith RP. The Hospital Anxiety and Depression Scale. *Acta Psychiatrica Scandinavica* 1983;37:361–370.

158. Block AR, Marek RJ, Ben-Porath YS, et al. Associations between pre-implant psychological factors and spinal cord stimulation outcome: evaluation using the MMPI-2-RF. *Assessment* 2017;24:60–70.

159. Tarescavage AM, Scheman J, Ben-Porath YS. Reliability and validity of the Minnesota Multiphasic Personality Inventory-2-Restructured Form (MMPI-2-RF) in evaluations of chronic low back pain patients. *Psychol Assess* 2015;27:433–446.

160. Moore JE, McFall ME, Kivlahan DR, et al. Risk of misinterpretation of MMPI Schizophrenia scale elevations in chronic pain patients. *Pain* 1988;32:207–213.

161. Stokvis A, van der Avoort DJ, van Neck JW, et al. Surgical management of neuroma pain: a prospective follow-up study. *Pain* 2010;151:862–869.

162. Spincemaille GH, Beersen N, Dekkers MA, et al. Neuropathic limb pain and spinal cord stimulation: results of the Dutch prospective study. *Neuromodulation* 2004;7:184–192.

163. Jamison RN, Rock DL, Parris WC. Empirically derived Symptom Checklist 90 subgroups of chronic pain patients: a cluster analysis. *J Behav Med* 1988;11:147–158.

164. Tschugg A, Lener S, Hartmann S, et al. Preoperative support improves the outcome of lumbar disc surgery: a perspective monocentric cohort study. *Neurosurg Rev* 2017;40:597–604.

165. Urban-Baeza A, Zarate-Kalfopulos B, Romero-Vargas S, et al. Influence of depression symptoms on patient expectations and clinical outcomes in the surgical management of spinal stenosis. *J Neurosurg Spine* 2015;22:75–79.

166. Reverberi C, Dario A, Barolat G. Spinal cord stimulation (SCS) in conjunction with peripheral nerve field stimulation (PNfS) for treatment of complex pain in failed back surgery syndrome (FBSS). *Neuromodulation* 2013;16:78–82.

167. Radloff LS. The CES-D scale: a self-report depression scale for research in the general population. *Appl Psychol Measures* 1977;1:385–401.

168. Bjelland I, Dahl AA, Huag TT, et al. The validity of the Hospital Anxiety and Depression Scale. An updated literature review. *J Psychosom Res* 2002;52:69–77.

169. Dance C, DeBerard MS, Gunday CJ. Pain acceptance potentially mediates the relationship between pain catastrophizing and post-surgery outcomes among compensated lumbar fusion patients. *J Pain Res* 2016;10:65–72.

170. Turk DC, Okifuji A, Sinclair JD, et al. Differential responses by psychosocial subgroups of fibromyalgia syndrome patients to an interdisciplinary treatment. *Arthritis Care* 1998;11:397–404.

171. Ware JE, Sherbourne CD. The MOS 36-item Short-Form Health Survey (SF-36). I. Conceptual framework and item selection. *Med Care* 1992;20:473–483.

172. Kerns RD, Turk DC, Rudy TE. The West Haven-Yale Multidimensional Pain Inventory (WHYMPI). *Pain* 1985;23:345–356.

173. Pollard CA. Preliminary validity study of the Pain Disability Index. *Percept Motor Skills* 1984;59:974.

174. Ho MJ, LaFleur J. The Treatment Outcomes of Pain Survey (TOPS): a clinical monitoring and outcomes instrument for chronic pain practice and research. *J Pain Palliative Care Pharm* 2004;18:49–59.

175. Turk DC, Rudy TE. Towards an empirically derived taxonomy of chronic pain patients: integration of psychological assessment data. *J Consult Clin Psychol* 1988;56:233–238.

176. Flor H, Turk DC. *Chronic Pain: An Integrated Biobehavioral Approach.* Seattle, WA: IASP Press; 2011.

177. Leclaire R, Blier F, Fortin L, et al. A cross-sectional study comparing the Oswestry and Roland-Morris Functional Disability scales in two populations of patients with low back pain of different levels of severity. *Spine* 1997;22:68–71.

178. Waddell G, Main CJ. Assessment of severity in low-back disorders. *Spine* 1984;9:204–208.

179. Evans JH, Kagan A. The development of a functional rating scale to measure the treatment outcome of chronic spinal patients. *Spine* 1986;11:277–281.

180. Stratford PW, Binkley JM. A comparison study of the Back Pain Functional Scale and the Roland Morris Questionnaire. *J Rheumatol* 2000;27:1928–1936.

181. Coronado RA, George SZ, Devin CJ, et al. Pain sensitivity and pain catastrophizing are associated with persistent pain and disability after lumbar spine surgery. *Arch Phys Med Rehabil* 2015;96:1763–1770.

182. Wenzel HH, Veld RH, Melman WP, et al. Psychological risk factors in back pain patients at an orthopaedic outpatient clinic. *J Back Musculoskelet Rehabil* 30(1):71–78.

183. Pinto P, Maintyre T, Araujo-Soares V, et al. The role of pain catastrophizing in the provision of rescue analgesia by healthcare providers following major joint arthroplasty. *Pain Physician* 2014;17:515–524.

184. Helmerhorst GT, Vranceanu AM, Vrahas M, et al. Risk factors for continued opioid use two to two months after surgery for musculoskeletal trauma. *J Bone Joint Surg Am* 2014;19:495–499.

185. Brown GK, Nicassion PM, Wallston KA. Pain coping strategies and depression in rheumatoid arthritis. *J Consult Clin Psychol* 1989;57:652–657.

186. Lorig K, Chastain RL, Ung E, et al. Development and evaluation of a scale to measure perceived self-efficacy in people with arthritis. *Arthritis Rheum* 1989;32:37–44.

187. Karoly P, Jensen MP. *Multimethod Assessment of Chronic Pain.* New York: Pergamon Press; 1987.

188. Gil K, Williams DA, Keefe FJ, et al. The relationship of negative thoughts to pain and psychological distress. *Behavioral Ther* 1990;21:349–362.

189. Williams DA, Robinson ME, Geiser ME. Pain beliefs: assessment and utility. *Pain* 1994;59:71–78.

190. Anderson KO, Noel-Dowds B, Pelletz RE, et al. Development and initial validation of a scale to measure self-efficacy beliefs in patients with chronic pain. *Pain* 1995;63:77–84.

191. Sullivan MJ, Pivik J. The Pain Catastrophizing Scale: development and validation. *Psychol Assess* 1995;7:524–532.

192. Kim HJ, Park JW, Chang BS, et al. The influence of catastrophizing on treatment outcomes after surgery for lumbar spinal stenosis. *Bone Joint J* 2015;97:1546–1554.

193. Van Damme S, Crombez G, Bijttebier P, et al. A confirmatory factor analysis of the Pain Catastrophizing Scale: invariant factor structure across clinical and non-clinical populations. *Pain* 2002;96:319–324.

194. Edwards RR, Giles J, Bingham CO, et al. Moderators of the negative effects of catastrophizing in arthritis. *Pain Medicine* 2010;11:591–599.

195. Schreiber KL, Campbell C, Martel MO, et al. Distraction analgesia in chronic pain patients: the impact of catastrophizing. *Anesthesiology* 2014;121:1292–1301.

196. Rolving N, Nielsen CV, Christensen FB, et al. Does a preoperative cognitive-behavioral intervention affect disability, pain behavior, pain, and return to work the first year after lumbar spinal fusion surgery? *Spine* 2015;40:593–600.

197. Jamison RN. The role of psychological testing and diagnosis in patients with pain. In: Dworkin RH, Breitbart WS, eds. *Psychosocial Aspects of Pain: A Handbook for Health Care Providers.* Seattle, WA: IASP Press; 2004:117–137.

198. Provenzano D, Fanciullo G, Jamison R, et al. Computer assessment and diagnostic classification of chronic pain patients. *Pain Med* 2007;S3:167–175.

199. Marceau LD, Smith LD, Jamison RN. Electronic pain assessment in clinical practice. *Pain Med* 2011;1:325–336.

200. Butler SF, Zacharoff K, Charity S, et al. Electronic opioid risk assessment program for chronic pain patients: barriers and benefits of implementation. *Pain Pract* 2014;14:98–105.

201. Marceau LD, Carolan S, Schuth B, et al. Pain diaries as a tool to improve pain management: is there any evidence? *Pain Med* 2007;S3:101–109.

202. Butler SF, Zacharoff KL, Charity S, et al. Impact of an electronic pain and opioid risk assessment program: are there improvements in patient encounters and clinic notes? *Pain Med* 2016;17:2047–2060.

203. Block AR. Psychological screening of spine surgery candidates. In: Fishman SM, Ballantyne JC, Rathmell JP, eds. *Bonica's Management of Pain.* 4th ed. Philadelphia: Lippincott Williams & Wilkins; 2010:1149.

204. Block AR, Ohnmeiss DD, Guyer RD, et al. The use of presurgical psychological screening to predict the outcome of spine surgery. *Spine J* 2001;1:274–282.

205. Epker J, Block AR. Presurgical psychological screening in back pain patients: a review. *Clin J Pain* 2001;17:200–205.

206. Marek RJ, Block AR, Ben-Porath YS. Validation of a psychological screening algorithm for predicting spine surgery outcomes [published online ahead of print July 1, 2017]. *Assessment.* doi:10.1177/1073191117719512.

207. Azimi P, Benzel EC, Shahzadi S, et al. Use of artificial neural networks to predict surgical satisfaction in patients with lumbar spinal canal stenosis: clinical article. *J Neurosurg Spine* 2014;20:300–305.

PART FIVE

Methods for Symptomatic Control

PHARMACOLOGIC THERAPIES

CHAPTER **77**

Rational Pharmacotherapy for Pain

ARTHUR G. LIPMAN

Pharmacology is the science that deals with the origin, nature, chemistry, effects, and uses of drugs. Commonly, pharmacology is subdivided into pharmacodynamics (how drugs work; mechanisms of action) and pharmacokinetics (how drugs are absorbed, distributed, biotransformed [metabolized], and eliminated) in the body. Pharmacology is nonclinical science done largely in animal and in vitro models in the laboratory setting. Clinical pharmacology, often termed *therapeutics* in the United Kingdom and some other countries, is the discipline intended to translate findings from the laboratory bench to the patient bedside. Despite attempts in the United States to develop clinical pharmacology as a subspecialty of internal medicine, and subsequently pediatrics and psychiatry, very few clinical pharmacologists are in practice and fewer still are in training programs today. By definition, the terms *pharmacology* and even *clinical pharmacology* are somewhat restrictive.

Pharmacotherapy is, simply put, the treatment of disease by medicines. This is now a recognized health science discipline and describes the practice of clinicians including many physicians, pharmacists, advanced practice nurses, pharmacologically oriented psychologists, and others. Pharmacotherapy encompasses what those who attempted to develop clinical pharmacology envisioned without restricting practice to subspecialty-certified physicians. It is an academic discipline and numerous respected journals, and an increasing number of health science textbooks now have pharmacotherapy in their titles. This more inclusive term includes those aspects of pharmacology and findings from clinical pharmacology that apply directly to the use of pharmacologically active substances in patient care.

Clinicians must have access to contemporary information on how drugs work to use them optimally in managing pain. Pharmacology is the science of how the drugs work, not their application in treating patients. Thus, this section of *Bonica's Management of Pain* has been renamed Pharmacotherapy.

Pharmacotherapy is a potent tool in pain management. However, we must use drugs wisely to provide optimal patient benefit. Several core concepts in rational pharmacotherapy are introduced in this chapter as a prelude to the four subsequent chapters on specific pharmacotherapy for pain management.

Drugs Are Both Underused and Overused in Pain Management

There is a broad consensus among pain clinicians that pain, especially chronic nonmalignant pain, is often undertreated.[1] One of the reasons for this is concern about medication misuse.

Increasing reports of adverse events and even fatalities associated with analgesic use indicate that some practitioners may use analgesic pharmacotherapy unwisely or excessively. It is important to view drugs as tools that can be used well or poorly. Adverse events are not due to the drugs per se; they are due to the way the drugs are used. Clinicians are encouraged not to label any class of drugs as "good" or "bad" but to recognize that they only become so designated because of the way they are used. However, there are some drugs within various classes that one should consider suboptimal, for example, meperidine,[2] as discussed in more detail in the opioids chapter (Chapter 79). This section attempts to identify medication use that is more apt to have positive outcomes than adverse outcomes.

Pharmacotherapy Alone Is Rarely Optimal Therapy for Chronic Pain

Analgesic pharmacotherapy often is appropriate alone for acute pain. However, chronic malignant and nonmalignant pain usually responds better to multimodal treatment.[3] Many adverse events due to medications might not occur if lower drug doses are used, and concurrent nonpharmacologic therapy often reduces drug dose requirements (Table 77.1). Using multiple drugs to address symptoms of other drugs, that is, polypharmacy, sometimes leads to complex regimens with adverse events.[4] Although it is usually wise to simplify drug regimens, use of more than one drug in combination may reduce the risk of adverse events when the drugs are additive or synergistic and the adverse events are commonly dose-related. A common

TABLE 77.1 Examples of Pain Intervention Alternatives to Increasing Opioid Dose

Etiology	Treatment
Bony pain	NSAID with opioid
Neuropathic pain	TCAs, anticonvulsants, local anesthetics, topical capsaicin, nerve blocks
Infectious damage	Incision and drainage, anti-infectives
GI spasm	Anticholinergic agents
Constipation	Stimulating laxatives
Lymphedema	Physical therapy, compression

GI, gastrointestinal; NSAID, nonsteroidal anti-inflammatory drug; TCA, tricyclic antidepressant.
Reprinted with permission from Lipman AG. Comments on Fitzgibbon and Galer. *Pain* 1994;58:429–431. *Pain.* 1995;63(1):135.

example is concurrent use of an opioid and a nonsteroidal anti-inflammatory drug (NSAID) because these two drug classes are mutually dose sparing. One might consider such use of multiple drugs for pharmacotherapy as "rational polypharmacy."

It is often useful to consider medications for chronic non-malignant pain as temporary interventions to facilitate the patient's adapting to self-management techniques such as physical activation, cognitive restructuring, or responding to medical procedures such as serial nerve blocks.

EVERY USE OF MEDICATION FOR PAIN IS AN EXPERIMENT

It is axiomatic that every drug has the potential to do harm. We should only use pharmacotherapy when the potential benefit outweighs the potential harm; that is, there is a favorable risk-to-benefit ratio. Clinicians should consider initial pain pharmacotherapy as a trial to determine outcome before committing to ongoing pharmacotherapy. All medication orders should expire at a predetermined time and only be continued after it is clear that the benefits outweigh the risks. It is helpful in most cases to tell patients that new medications are being ordered for a limited time to determine if they should be continued. This practice would eliminate many adverse outcomes from ongoing drug therapy. This practice might also lessen inappropriate patient expectations about their drug therapy for pain. It is usually unwise to continue any medication without a clear determination that it is more helpful than harmful.

In addition to risk-to-benefit considerations, clinicians should always consider cost–benefit issues. Frequently, new drugs and dosage forms offer incremental advantages over previously available agents, but the new agents do so at a markedly greater cost. The pharmaceutical industry often aggressively markets new and patent-protected drugs and dosage forms, although there is rarely a financial incentive for a pharmaceutical manufacturer or distributor to promote generic drugs because pharmacists can legally substitute generic equivalent drugs unless the prescriber specifies otherwise. At the extreme, entire older classes of drugs, which may still be agents of choice, have been largely replaced by newer, far more expensive agents. For example, tricyclic antidepressants are still drugs of choice for neuropathic pain, but no company promotes them. Aggressive marketing of various antiepileptic and serotonin norepinephrine reuptake-inhibiting drugs that are as effective or nearly as effective as the tricyclic antidepressants for this indication has resulted in the newer, more expensive drugs being considered by many clinicians as the only drugs for neuropathic pain.

PATIENT PREFERENCE: SYMPTOM CONTROL VERSUS SIDE EFFECTS

Patients vary both in their desire to take medications to manage their pain and in their response to the medications. Many patients are highly averse to taking medications, especially opioids, even when those medications can greatly reduce the pain. This aversion may be due to fears or misconceptions about the medications, and clinicians should inquire about their patients' beliefs and preferences when considering pharmacotherapy. When a patient with allergies indicates a preference for a particular antihistamine, we normally provide that medication. However, when a chronic pain patient expresses a preference for a particular opioid, many clinicians become suspect that there is an ulterior motive for specifying a drug of choice. The perceived preference may be due to prior experience, observation of other patients' good or bad response to opioids, or misconceptions. We should ascertain the basis for our patients' expressed preferences when feasible rather than draw our own—often inaccurate—conclusions. Obviously, we should correct wrong information on which patients express preferences.

Some chronic pain patients prefer to be more alert even though the trade-off may be more intense pain. Others prefer

as much pain relief as possible with the accompanying dulling of their senses. Neither preference is right or wrong. It is very reasonable to counsel patients about the side effects of the analgesics and adjuvants we are considering and ask them their preferences regarding comfort versus alertness. One of the most problematic misconceptions among chronic pain patients is that medication will "cure" their pain. It is important to determine if the patient harbors such beliefs and to correct them when possible.

There is great interpatient variability in response to analgesics. We see this commonly with NSAIDs but cannot explain the mechanism. With opioids, it also is common, and we know several sources of genetic polymorphism that cause interpatient variability[5] as described in more detail in Chapter 79. Clinicians should actively counsel patients about the need to adjust medications and doses to optimize response: One size does not fit all.

WHENEVER POSSIBLE TREAT THE CAUSE OF THE PAIN

A commonly espoused concept in opioid pharmacotherapy is to increase the medication dose until the patient experiences either adequate pain relief or unacceptable side effects. Although there may be some wisdom in this approach, it also has two major problems.[6] One is that opioids are not the therapy of choice for all types of pain. For example, bone pain in which there is inflammation often responds better to NSAIDs than to opioids and nearly always responds better to a combination of these two drug classes than to opioids alone. Likewise, neuropathic pain nearly always responds better to a combination of opioids and tricyclic antidepressants or anticonvulsant medications with fewer side effects than will be seen with one class alone. Again, a combination of both a neuropathic pain-specific agent with an opioid is usually synergistic. Opioids can actually blunt pain from constipation but would probably exacerbate the constipation. It is far better to identify the cause of the pain and to treat it with specific modalities than to simply use opioids and increase the dose to response. Examples of painful conditions that are indications for such alternate modalities include incision and drainage with anti-infective agents for painful infected cysts, physical therapy for myofascial pain, and massage with pressure for pain due to painful lymphatic drainage blockade.

The second limitation is that several opioid dosage forms, most notably the newer long-acting ones, are very expensive. The great interpatient variability in response to opioids supports changing drugs when a patient does not respond as expected after two or three dose increments. Such patients may well respond better to other opioids to which they are rotated. Thus, serial trials of different opioids to find the optimal drug are sometimes indicated.

SYNERGISM AND POTENTIATION

Additive effects may occur when we use two pharmacologic agents concurrently and the combined effect equals the sum of the two agents' effects. Unless doing so provides a specific benefit, for example, dose sparing with drugs that have problematic dose-related adverse effects, additive pharmacotherapy usually is not warranted. It simply complicates the regimen, reducing patient adherence (compliance) and often increasing cost. Synergism occurs when two drugs act together to produce a supra-additive action. This often is desirable. An example is using an NSAID with an opioid for their mutually synergistic effects. Synergism occurs because of the two different mechanisms and the NSAID being anti-inflammatory with the opioid acting largely centrally while NSAID provides peripheral anti-inflammatory activity. Potentiation is an effect in which one drug enhances the action of another. An example is the concurrent use of acetaminophen and morphine, which has been demonstrated in rat model.[7] Both drugs are simple analgesics, that is, they have no anti-inflammatory activity. The opioid is far more active than the acetaminophen, but the latter increases the effectiveness of the former by acting at the serotonergic system in the brain. Although the concurrent use of acetaminophen can be clinically useful, the net clinical advantage of combination therapy is less than occurs when an opioid is used with an NSAID producing the two-way advantage of synergism.

OUTCOMES ANALYSES OF PAIN PHARMACOTHERAPY

Clinical studies of analgesics have traditionally focused largely, if not exclusively, on efficacy. Efficacy is defined simply as the ability of an agent to have a desired effect. Studies of analgesic efficacy for chronic pain typically last only 3 to 6 weeks. Commonly, reduction in pain intensity is the measured outcome. Every pain clinician knows that long-term effectiveness is the outcome measure needed to determine the usefulness of a drug for chronic pain and that patients' ability to function, to carry out activities of daily living, is often more important than pain intensity per se. These should be the criteria for effectiveness.

The pharmaceutical industry is beginning to conduct true effectiveness studies in support of their products. When more clinicians insist on such evidence before adopting new drugs that are supported only by the short-term efficacy studies needed for the drugs to be approved for human use, we will see more true effectiveness studies.

Clinical outcomes studies compose only one of the three types of studies needed to assess the place of drugs in pain management. Health-related quality of life (HRQoL) research is a relatively new discipline that provides important information for a wide range of subjective complaints, including pain.[8] A commonly used measurement tool for HRQoL is the Medical Outcomes Study Short-Form 36 (MOS SF-36).[9] More recently, the National Institutes of Health (NIH) has been developing a state-of-the-art group of assessment tools for self-reported health, using modern technology with computerized testing and data collection (the Patient-Reported Outcome Measurement Information Systems, PROMIS). This is a measurement tool that is capable of measuring HRQoL in a wide range of clinical disease states, including pain.[10] It has been widely adopted since its introduction in 2004, and researchers both in the United States and internationally are using it with increasing frequency, with substantial integration into clinical settings. Although these instruments provide useful population data, they lack the specificity, sensitivity, and brevity needed for utility as a clinical monitoring tool in chronic pain management. For that purpose, several tools are in development such as the 3-item PEG Scale (measures pain intensity and pain interference with enjoyment of life and general wellbeing)[11] and PainTracker, a more extensive measurement tool that in addition measures pain location, sleep interference, activity interference, depression, anxiety, side-effects, medication utilization and satisfaction with treatment (https://www.nva.org/wp-content/uploads/2015/01/Pain-Tracker-Form.pdf). HRQoL studies provide valuable clinical information on how interventions affect patients' ability to function, not just their subjective pain intensity report.

The third type of study that is becoming increasingly important is pharmacoeconomics (PE) analyses. Pain management has become more complex, more invasive, and more expensive in recent years. Five types of PE studies that help define which interventions are apt to provide the most benefit are listed in Table 77.2.[12]

TABLE 77.2 **Types of Pharmacoeconomic Analyses**
• Cost-effectiveness
• Cost-utility
• Cost-benefit
• Cost-minimization
• Cost-consequence

From Asche CV, Seal B, Jackson KC, et al. Economic evaluations in pain management: principles and methods. *J Pain Palliat Care Pharmacother* 2006;20(3):15–23. Adapted by permission of Taylor & Francis Ltd. http://www.tandfonline.com.

APPROVED DRUGS AND DRUGS FOR NONAPPROVED USES

For a drug to be available for routine clinical use in the United States, the manufacturer or distributor (sponsor) must hold an approved new drug application (NDA) from the U.S. Food and Drug Administration (FDA). The FDA can legally approve an NDA only after the sponsor has completed three phases of clinical studies under a license for those studies called an investigational new drug exemption (IND). The IND specifies exactly how and in whom the investigators can use the drug and use outside of those restrictions can lead to criminal penalties. Only clinicians explicitly named on the IND or persons under their direct supervision can legally participate in the studies. Once the FDA licenses a new drug for human use, any licensed prescriber can legally use it for any human use. However, the sponsor cannot legally advertise or market the newly approved drug for indications outside of the labeling even when good scientific evidence supports such use. This includes any continuing professional education activities directly supported by the sponsor. Furthermore, the indications that are listed in the labeling (package insert) for the newly approved drug can, by law, only include those indications approved by the FDA based on clinical studies submitted by the sponsor in support of the NDA.

If the sponsor provides an unrestricted educational grant to a professional society, hospital, or other such uninterested party, that organization can sponsor continuing professional education in which presenters can discuss nonapproved ("off-label") uses of the drug based on scientific and professional publications and findings. Thus, for example, a sponsor cannot legally promote an antiepileptic drug that is not FDA-approved for neuropathic pain management for that indication even if there is good scientific evidence of the efficacy of the drugs for that indication. Neither can professionals paid directly by the sponsor make continuing education presentations in which they discuss off-label use in any program. That would be defined as marketing the drug for a nonapproved use. However, this in no way constrains licensed prescribers from prescribing the medication for off-label use as long as an NDA has been issued for another human use.

If a patient suffers an adverse event from a drug prescribed off label, the harmed parties can initiate civil (malpractice) litigation against the prescriber and the health care facility where this occurred. There normally are no grounds for criminal action against the practitioner for prescribing an approved drug even though it was for a nonapproved indication. Published scientific evidence supporting the use of the drug as prescribed is normally a good defense in such actions. The lack of such evidence greatly increases the prescribers' exposure to civil litigation.

Pain patients often have comorbid mood disorders, and sometimes, they are already involved in litigation relating to the cause of their pain. These factors may increase the risk of litigation against pain clinicians if the patients are dissatisfied with the care they receive. Therefore, pain clinicians should remain aware of legal issues when planning and implementing pharmacotherapy for such patients. Opioids and other such potent medications are essential in pain management, however, and clinicians should not hesitate to use such pharmacotherapy when indicated. Clinicians should always carefully document what they are doing as recommended by the Federation of State Medical Boards of the United States. In its 2017 Guidelines for the Chronic Use of Opioid Analgesics (https://www.fsmb.org/Media/Default/PDF/Advocacy/Opioid%20Guidelines%20As%20Adopted%20April%202017_FINAL.pdf), the Federation explicitly states that the diagnosis and treatment of pain is integral to the practice of medicine and clinicians must understand the relevant pharmacologic and clinical issues in the use of opioid analgesics. Criteria for evaluating the use of controlled substances and information to document in the medical record when doing so are listed in Table 77.3.

TABLE 77.3 Guidelines for the Chronic Use of Opioid Analgesics

- Patient evaluation and risk stratification
- Development of a treatment plan and goals
- Informed consent and treatment agreement
- Initiating an opioid trial
- Ongoing monitoring and adapting the treatment plan
- Periodic and unannounced drug testing
- Adapting treatment
- Accurate and complete medical records to include:
  - Copies of the signed informed consent and treatment agreement
  - The patient's medical history
  - Results of the physical examination and all laboratory tests
  - Results of the risk assessment, including results of any screening instruments used
  - A description of the treatments provided, including all medications prescribed or administered (including the date, type, dose, and quantity)
  - Instructions to the patient, including discussions of risks and benefits with the patient and any significant others
  - Results of ongoing monitoring of patient progress (or lack of progress) in terms of pain management and functional improvement
  - Notes on evaluations by and consultations with specialists
  - Results of queries to the state PDMP
  - Any other information used to support the initiation, continuation, revision, or termination of treatment and the steps taken in response to any aberrant medication use behaviors. These may include actual copies of, or references to, medical records of past hospitalizations or treatments by other providers.
  - Authorization for release of information to other treatment providers
- Compliance with controlled substance laws and regulations

PDMP, prescription drug monitoring program.
Adopted as policy by the Federation of State Medical Boards, April 2017. Available online at: https://www.fsmb.org/Media/Default/PDF/Advocacy/Opioid%20 Guidelines%20As%20Adopted%20April%202017_FINAL.pdf. Accessed January 13, 2018. Copyright © 2017 Federation of State Medical Boards, Inc.

RATIONAL PHARMACOTHERAPY

The criteria for rational pharmacotherapy are simple. The drug must be legal; that is, there must be an NDA for at least one human use. If the drug is used for a nonapproved use, the clinician should assure that there is good evidence supporting that use. The clinician must be confident that the potential benefit for use of the drug in that specific patient in the regimen prescribed presents potential benefits that outweigh the potential risks. To make that determination, the clinician must understand both the pharmacodynamics and pharmacokinetics of the drug. The recent increase in deaths due to methadone is attributable in part to the prescribers not understanding the long elimination half-life of the opioid. When any opioid dose is increased before the drug has reached steady-state serum levels, there is risk of toxicity from drug accumulation. Due to the relatively high cost of commercially available long-acting opioids, several third-party payers encouraged primary care clinicians to change their patients from the more expensive analgesics to methadone. However, methadone, a pharmacologically long-acting opioid, has a much longer half-life than pharmaceutically long-acting opioids such as sustained-acting oxycodone. That difference in half-life necessitates changes in the opioid regimen when initiating methadone. After initiation, the dose should not be increased before serum levels near steady state are reached and that may require 5 to 7 days for methadone. Practitioners unawareness of the implications of this aspect of methadone's pharmacology appears to be at least one factor in the increased number of methadone deaths observed in the last decade.[13]

Conclusion

Pharmacotherapy is essential in the management of nearly all acute pain and the majority of chronic pain patients. Safe and rational use requires attention to the risk-to-benefit ratio in each clinical situation. It is not logical to provide analgesics for every patient in pain, nor is it reasonable to deny analgesic medication when it is needed.

Pharmacotherapy is the most common modality used to treat pain. Too often, pharmacotherapy is used as a sole intervention. Most patients with moderate to severe acute pain or any chronic pain would benefit more from multimodal therapy.

Recent statements and publications emphasizing the risks of pharmacotherapy without providing a balanced discussion of the benefits of these drugs have discouraged some clinicians from using needed medications for pain. The U.S. Drug Enforcement Administration (DEA) has taken positions that discourage opioid pharmacotherapy,[14] and the American Heart Association has discouraged NSAID use due to cardiovascular risk without addressing the major improvement in quality of life that millions of patients receive from these medications.[15] The DEA posits that reducing opioid use will reduce opioid abuse. Although that may be true, it would occur at the cost of countless pain patients suffering unnecessarily. The American Heart Association position looks at the cardiovascular risks associated with NSAIDs. However, it does not consider the impact of painful inflammatory diseases such as osteoarthritis, which erode the quality of life of millions of patients.

Pain clinicians must be effective advocates for rational pharmacotherapy for their patients. To do so, we must be knowledgeable about the drugs we use. We also must assure that our patients and their families have accurate information to help them use the medications correctly. The following four chapters provide a scientific basis for that advocacy and use.

References

1. Symposium: the undertreatment of pain—legal, regulatory, and research perspectives and solutions. *J Law Med Ethics* 2001;29(1).
2. Cohen MJ, Schecter WP. Perioperative pain control: a strategy for management. *Surg Clin North Am* 2005;85(6):1243–1257.
3. White PF. Multimodal pain management—the future is now! *Curr Opin Investig Drugs* 2007;8(7):517–518.
4. Nogueras C, Miralles R, Roig A, et al. Polypharmacy as part of comprehensive geriatric assessment: disclosure of false diagnosis of atrial fibrillation by drug revision. *J Am Geriatr Soc* 2007;55(9):1476–1478.
5. Somogyi AA, Barratt DT, Coller JK. Pharmacogenetics of opioids. *Clin Pharmacol Ther* 2007;81(3):429–444.
6. Lipman AG. Efficacy of opioids in cancer pain syndromes. *Pain* 1995;63:135.
7. Sandrini M, Vitale G, Ottani A, et al. The potential of analgesic activity of paracetamol plus morphine involves the serotonergic system in rat brain. *Inflam Res* 1999;48(3):120–127.
8. Moinpour CM, Donaldson GW, Redman MW. Do general dimensions of quality of life add clinical value to symptom data? *J Natl Cancer Inst Monogr* 2007;(37):31–38.
9. Ware JE Jr, Sherbourne CD. The MOS 36-item Short-Form Health Survey (SF-36) I. Conceptual framework and item selection. *Med Care* 1992; 30(6):473–483.
10. Amtmann D, Cook KF, Jensen MP, et al. Development of a PROMIS item bank to measure pain interference. *Pain* 2010;150:173–182.
11. Kean J, Monahan PO, Kroenke K, et al. Comparative responsiveness of the PROMIS Pain Interference Short Forms, Brief Pain Inventory, PEG, and SF-36 Bodily Pain Subscale. *Med Care* 2016;54:414–421.
12. Asche CV, Seal B, Jackson KC II, et al. Economic in pain management: principles and methods. *J Pain Palliat Care Pharmacother* 2006;20(3):15–23.
13. Centers for Disease Control and Prevention. Increase in poisoning deaths due to non-illicit drugs—Utah, 1991–2003. *MMWR Morb Mortal Wkly Rep* 2005;54:33–36.
14. Lipman AG. Does the DEA truly seek balance in pain medicine? A chronology of confusion that impedes good patient care. *J Pain Palliat Care Pharmacother* 2005;19(1):7–9.
15. Antman EM, Bennett JS, Daugherty A, et al. Use of nonsteroidal anti-inflammatory drugs: an update for clinicians: a scientific statement from the American Heart Association. *Circulation* 2007;115:1634–1642.

CHAPTER 78

Nonsteroidal Anti-inflammatory Drugs and Acetaminophen

ADAM C. YOUNG and **ASOKUMAR BUVANENDRAN**

Nonsteroidal anti-inflammatory drugs (NSAIDs) are a diverse group of compounds with analgesic, antipyretic, and anti-inflammatory activity. Newer compounds, more specific for reducing pain and inflammation while promoting safety and tolerability, have largely replaced the prototypical NSAID, aspirin. NSAIDs remain the most widely prescribed drugs in the world with an estimated 30 million users worldwide and sales greater than \$12 billion globally.[1] They are valuable in the management of both acute and chronic painful and inflammatory conditions and are administered by both systemic and local (topical) routes.

The earliest agent in this class, which has been used in folk medicine for millennia, is willow bark. Hippocrates wrote about the use of powdered willow bark for pains and fever in the fifth century before the Common Era. Edward Stone formally reported salicylic acid extracted from the bark and leaves of willow, myrtle, and a number of other plants as a medication for fever in 1763. Felix Hoffmann, a chemist at Bayer Pharmaceuticals in Germany, rediscovered the acetylsalicylic acid formulation, which Bayer then named *Aspirin* and marketed as a remedy for pain, fever, and inflammation early in the 20th century. Only in the mid-20th century did aspirin become the generic name for that compound.

The next generation of NSAIDs were introduced in the 1960s, the first being indomethacin which was soon followed by ibuprofen. Numerous other NSAIDs followed, most of which claimed better efficacy and safety than earlier compounds. In the past two decades, several NSAIDs have been removed from commercial availability due to potentially lethal side effects after they were in general use. Phenylbutazone and oxyphenbutazone lost popularity and were withdrawn due to blood dyscrasias. Suprofen caused nephrotoxicity. Benoxaprofen, bromfenac, and ibufenac (which was marketed in the United Kingdom, not the United States) caused serious hepatotoxicity. Two of the three cyclooxygenase (COX)-2 selective NSAIDs approved in the United States in the 1990s were subsequently withdrawn from the market, as noted in the following discussion of the COX-2 selective agents. Today, over two dozen NSAIDs are commercially available in the United States for clinical use (Table 78.1), and several others are available in other countries as well.

Mechanism of Action

PROSTAGLANDIN SYNTHESIS AND PHARMACOLOGY

NSAIDs act by inhibiting prostaglandin synthesis in vivo. Prostaglandins (PGs) are derived from arachidonic acid and other polyunsaturated fatty acids; the 20-carbon polyunsaturated essential fatty acid (arachidonic acid) is the major source in mammalian tissues. PGs derived from arachidonic acid contain two double bonds. These are PGE_2, thromboxane and prostacyclin. Analogous compounds synthesized from icosatrienoic (linoleic) and eicosapentaenoic acids contain one fewer or one more double bond in the side chains (PGE_1, PGE_3, respectively).[2] The PGs, thromboxanes, hydroxy acids, and leukotrienes, which retain the 20-carbon unsaturated fatty acid backbone, are collectively known as eicosanoids.[3] Their release, usually as a result of trauma, is the major stimulus for eicosanoid production as PGs cannot be stored and are released as soon as they are synthesized.[4] Cell membrane disruption causes phospholipid release which is converted to arachidonic acid by the action of phospholipase A_2 (PLA_2). Arachidonic acid then acts as a substrate for the COX enzyme.

CENTRAL SITES OF ACTION

PGs also are involved in the pyretic response. After injection of pyrogens, cerebrospinal fluid (CSF) PG levels rise. That effect can be prevented by pretreatment with aspirin alluding to the central sites of action.[5] Acetaminophen (paracetamol) is analgesic and antipyretic but lacks clinically useful peripheral anti-inflammatory activity. Acetaminophen blocks PG synthetase within the blood–brain barrier; the same effect is not seen in the periphery. Therefore, it is not an NSAID per se, although it is commonly used for many of the same indications as NSAIDs. Acetaminophen is discussed in more detail later in the chapter.

PERIPHERAL SITES OF ACTION

Prostanoids do not generally activate nociceptors directly; they sensitize them to mechanical stimuli and chemical mediators of nociception such as bradykinin.[6] PGE_2 is the predominant eicosanoid released from endothelial cells of small blood vessels[7] and is a key mediator of both peripheral and central pain sensitization.[3] Because it is the prostanoid most associated with inflammatory responses, the formation of PGE_2 at inflammatory sites is often considered an indicator of local COX activity, and suppression of PGE_2 is an indicator of a reduced inflammatory process.[8] The production of PGE_2 is slow in onset and of long duration in response to inflammation.[9]

COX-1 AND COX-2 SELECTIVITY

COX is encoded by two genes.[10] Although the isomerization of PGH_2 into PGE_2 has been well characterized biochemically and pharmacologically, the enzyme responsible, PGE synthase (PGES), was only recently purified and cloned.[11,12] The existence of more than one COX isoform, and specifically one that is positively regulated by cytokines and negatively regulated by glucocorticoids, was long suspected. In the early 1990s, an inducible COX isoenzyme was cloned.[13] The recognition of two COX isoforms, then designated COX-1 and COX-2, generated intense efforts to characterize the relative contribution of each isoform to prostanoid production in specific situations (Fig. 78.1).

COX-1 and COX-2 are membrane-associated enzymes with a 60% amino acid sequence homology.[14] In spite of their structural similarity, the two COX isoforms have different gene expression profiles, distinct kinetic properties, and different interactions with PLA_2s and synthases.[15] COX-1 is expressed constitutively and produces prostanoids that fine-tune physiologic processes requiring instantaneous or continuous regulation (e.g., hemostasis).[14] COX-2 expression is usually low but

TABLE 78.1   Acetaminophen and Nonsteroidal Anti-inflammatory Drugs Available in the United States—Indications for Pain Relief

Generic Name	Trade Name(s)	Half-life (h)	Protein Bound (%)	Maximum Daily Adult (Pediatric) Dose	Adult Daily Dose	Pediatric Daily Dose
Para-aminophenol Derivative						
Acetaminophen (paracetamol)	Tylenol, Panadol, Anacin, Mapap	1–4	25	≥12 y: 1 g/4 h, 4 g/d (neonate: 60 mg/kg/d, infant/child: 75 mg/kg/d)	325–1,000 mg PO q4–6h; <50 kg: 15 mg/kg IV q6h; >50 kg: 1 g IV q6h	Neonates: 10–15 mg/kg PO q6–8h; infant/child: 10–15 mg/kg PO q4–6h; ≥12 y: 325–650 mg PO q4–6h; 2–12 y: 15 mg/kg IV q6h; 13+ y <50 kg: 15 mg/kg IV q6h; 13+ y >50 kg: 1 g IV q6h
Salicylates						
Aspirin	Bufferin, Ecotrin	2–4.5	50–80	4 g (60–80 mg/kg/d)	325–650 mg PO q4h	10–15 mg/kg PO q4–6h
Choline magnesium trisalicylate	Generic only	2–3	90–95	3 g	1,500 mg PO bid	12–37 kg: 50 mg/kg/d PO divided bid; >37 kg: 2,250 mg/d PO divided bid to tid
Diflunisal	Dolobid	8–12	98–99	1,500 mg	500–750 mg PO bid	N/A
Salsalate	Generic only	1	90–95	3 g	1,500 mg PO bid	N/A
Propionic Acid Derivatives						
Fenoprofen	Nalfon	3	99	3,200 mg	300–600 mg PO tid to qid	N/A
Flurbiprofen	Ansaid	4.7–5.7	>99	300 mg	50–100 mg PO bid to tid	N/A
Ibuprofen	Advil, Caldolor, Motrin	2–4	90–99	2,400 mg PO; 3,200 mg IV (6 mo–11 y: 40 mg/kg/d)	400 mg PO q4–6h; 400–800 mg IV q6h	6 mo–11 y: 5–10 mg/kg PO q6–8h, 10 mg/kg IV q4–6h; 12+ y: 400 mg PO/IV q4–6h
Ketoprofen	Orudis	1.1–4	99	300 mg	50 mg PO q6–8h	N/A
Naproxen	Naprosyn	15	>99	1,250 mg (1,000 mg)	250–500 mg PO q12h bid	≥2 y: 10–20 mg/kg/d PO divided q8–12h
Naproxen sodium	Aleve, Anaprox	15	>99	1,100–1,375 mg (1,100 mg)	275–550 mg PO q12h	≥2 y: 11–22 mg/kg/d PO divided q8–12h
Oxaprozin	Daypro	54.9	>99.5	1,200 mg (1,200 mg)	1,200 mg PO qd	10–20 mg/kg PO qd
Fenamates						
Meclofenamate	Meclomen	2–3	99	400 mg	50–100 mg PO q4–6h	N/A
Diclofenac sodium	Zorvolex, Dyloject	2	>99	105 mg PO; 150 mg IV	18–35 mg PO tid; 37.5 mg IV q6h	N/A
Tolmetin	Tolectin	5	99	1,800 mg (30 mg/kg/d)	200–600 mg PO tid	≥2 y: 15–30 mg/kg/d divided tid to qid
Ketorolac	Toradol	2.5–5	99	40 mg PO, 120 mg IM/IV (120 mg IM, 60 mg IV)	30 mg IM/IV q6h, 10 mg PO q4–6h	≥6 mo: 0.5 mg/kg IM/IV q6h for up to 72 h
Mefenamic acid	Ponstel	2	90	1,000 mg	250 mg PO q6h up to 7 d	≥14 y: 250 mg PO q6h for up to 7 d
Enolic Acid Derivatives (Oxicams)						
Meloxicam	Mobic	15–20	>99	15 mg (7.5 mg)	7.5–15 mg PO qd	60+ kg: 7.5 mg PO qd
Piroxicam	Feldene	30–86	99	20 mg	20 mg PO qd	N/A
Nabumetone	Relafen	23	>99	2,000 mg	1,000–2,000 mg divided qd to bid	N/A
Acetic Acid Derivatives						
Etodolac	Lodine	7.3	>99	1,000 mg (20–30 kg: 400 mg/d, 31–45 kg: 600 mg/d, 46–60 kg: 800 mg/d, >60 kg: 1,000 mg/d)	200–400 mg PO q6–8h	(≥6 y only) 20–30 kg: 400 mg PO qd; 31–45 kg: 600 mg PO qd; 46–60 kg: 800 mg PO qd; >60 kg: 1,000 mg PO qd
Indomethacin	Indocin	4.5	97	200 mg (4 mg/kg/d up to 150–200 mg/d)	25–50 mg PO tid	1–2 mg/kg/d PO divided bid to qid
Sulindac	Clinoril	7.8	93	400 mg	150–200 mg PO bid up to 7–14 d	N/A
COX-2 Selective NSAID (Coxib)						
Celecoxib	Celebrex	11	97	400 mg	100–200 mg PO qd to bid	(≥2 y only) 10–25 kg: 50 mg PO bid; >25 kg: 100 mg PO bid

bid, twice a day; COX, cyclooxygenase; IM, intramuscular; IV, intravenous; N/A, not available; NSAID, nonsteroidal anti-inflammatory drug; PO, by mouth; q12h, every 12 hours; q4–6h, every 4 to 6 hours; q4h, every 4 hours; q6–8h, every 6 to 8 hours; q6h, every 6 hours; q8–12h, every 8 to 12 hours; qd, every day; qid, four times a day; tid, three times a day.

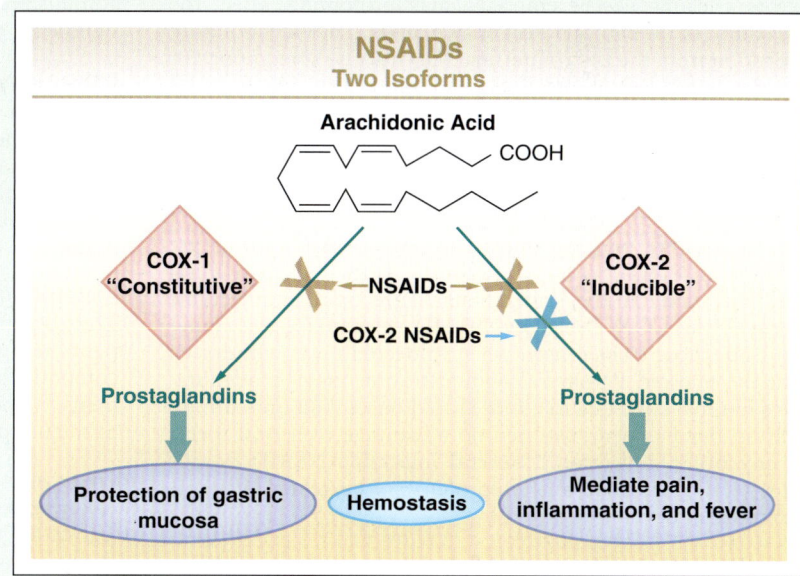

FIGURE 78.1 Simplified arachidonic acid pathway differentiating COX-1 and COX-2 effects.

can be induced by numerous factors including neurotransmitters, growth factors, pro-inflammatory cytokines, lipopolysaccharide, calcium, phorbol esters, and small peptide hormones.[16] However, there are exceptions to the original constitutive versus inducible theory of COX expression. COX-1 expression can be induced in some stress conditions, such as nerve injury, and many tissues, including the central nervous system (CNS) and the kidney, constitutively express COX-2.[16] In the spinal cord, there are detectable basal levels of both COX-1 and COX-2. That might enable immediate reactions to transmitter release that results in prostanoid production.[17] A third isoform designated COX-3 that was identified in dogs is formed as a splice variant of COX-1.[18] Because canine COX-3 can be inhibited by therapeutic concentrations of acetaminophen, initial reports postulated that COX-3 inhibition was the mechanism of action of acetaminophen, However, this does not appear to be true; more recent evidence indicates that COX-3 is not expressed in humans.[19]

Induction of COX-2

The original hypothesis formulated by John Vane in his Nobel prize–winning work on the mechanism of action of NSAIDs was that these compounds inhibited prostanoid production in the periphery preventing a sensitizing action of PGE_2 on the peripheral terminals of sensory fibers.[20] Peripheral inflammation induces an increase in COX-2[21] and PGES expression in the CNS. The pro-inflammatory cytokine interleukin 1β (IL-Iβ) is upregulated at the site of inflammation and plays a major role in inducing COX-2 in local inflammatory cells by activating the transcription factor nuclear factor kappa B (NF-κB).[22] IL-1β is also responsible for the induction of COX-2 in the CNS in response to peripheral inflammation. However, this is not the consequence either of neural activity arising from the sensory fibers innervating the inflamed tissue or of systemic IL-1β in the plasma. Rather, peripheral inflammation produces some other signal molecule that enters the circulation, crosses the blood-brain barrier, and acts to elevate IL-1β, leading to COX-2 expression in neurons and nonneuronal cells in many different areas of the spinal cord.[3,23] An elevation of COX-2 also occurs at many levels in the brain and spinal cord, mainly in the endothelial cells of the brain vasculature.[24] Thus, there appear to be two forms of input from peripheral inflamed tissue to the CNS. The first is mediated by electrical activity in sensitized nerve fibers innervating the inflamed area, which signals the location

of the inflamed tissue as well as the onset, duration, and nature of any stimuli applied to this tissue.[21] This input is sensitive to peripherally acting COX-2 inhibitors (and to neural blockade with local anesthetics, e.g., epidural anesthesia).[25] The second is a humoral signal originating from the inflamed tissue, which acts to produce a widespread induction of COX-2 in the CNS. Regional anesthesia does not affect this[23,26]; it only is blocked by centrally acting COX-2 inhibitors.[23,25] One implication of this is that patients who receive neuraxial anesthesia for surgery may require a centrally acting COX-2 inhibitor to optimally reduce postoperative pain and the postoperative stress response.[25] Therefore, the permeability of the blood–brain barrier to both nonselective and COX-2 selective NSAIDs is important.[27,28] Inhibitors of COX-2 that better penetrate the blood–brain barrier might represent more efficient analgesics and could also act to reduce many of the more diffuse aspects of inflammatory pain, such as generalized aches and pains, depression, and loss of appetite, which are key aspects in determining the "quality of life" response to treatment.[29] The main process by which a drug passes from the circulation into the CNS is passive diffusion. Lipophilicity and ionization are critical determinants of this transfer.[30] The CSF represents a convenient sampling point for drugs that enter the CNS; however, there are very few NSAIDs for which the CSF pharmacokinetics has been defined.[31] The high lipid solubility of indomethacin allows it to rapidly cross into the CSF and equilibrate with the free plasma concentration.[32] Similar results are seen with ketoprofen.[33]

Pharmacokinetics

NSAIDs are weak acids with pK_a values typically lower than 5. Because weak acids will be 99% ionized 2 pH units above their pK_a, these anti-inflammatory agents are present in the body mostly in the ionized form. Although NSAIDs differ in their individual pharmacokinetic properties, some general factors affecting NSAID pharmacokinetics can enable clinicians to select among the different agents available.

ABSORPTION
Oral

Most NSAIDs are rapidly absorbed following oral administration, with peak plasma concentrations generally reached within 2 to 3 hours, although slow-release dosage forms have been developed to maintain active plasma levels for prolonged times.

Factors affecting gastric emptying may profoundly affect the time course of the clinical effect of an NSAID. The extent of drug absorption from the gastrointestinal (GI) tract is more important than the rate.[34] Rectal and topical administration minimize GI side effects that are common with these agents. In general, the rate and extent of NSAID absorption is comparable for the rectal and oral routes.[35]

Injectables

Intravenous (IV) and intramuscular (IM) NSAIDs forms are available in several countries. Ketorolac is the only parenteral NSAID available in the United States. Parecoxib, an injectable analog of the COX-2 selective NSAID valdecoxib, was under study, but those trials ceased when valdecoxib was withdrawn from the market. Parenteral administration may be advantageous in renal colic due to a more rapid onset than oral administration but has demonstrated no advantage over oral forms for any other indication.[36] Several injectable NSAID dosage forms (e.g., diclofenac and ibuprofen) are currently available with more in development.

Topical

There is good evidence that topical NSAIDs can be safe and effective and that they produce less GI toxicity than systemic forms of the same drugs.[37,38] These topical forms can be effective for inflammation of the knee and surface tissues; they generally are not effective for deeper structures. Topical NSAIDs must be properly formulated. Although extemporaneously compounded topical NSAIDs have been used, these often are ineffective. The vehicle and formulation can profoundly influence the efficacy of the topical dosage form.[39] In the United States, a diclofenac topical patch (Flector), gel (Voltaren Gel), and liquid (PENNSAID) are commercially available. Topical NSAID dosage forms available in several countries are listed in Table 78.2.

Intranasal

As an alternative to IM administration, intranasal (IN) ketorolac has gained popularity among those treating acute pain in situations where IV access is not readily available and/or oral administration is contraindicated. Following IN administration of ketorolac, there is a short time to peak plasma concentration of about 30 minutes.[40] This is not only true for adolescents but also for adults and the elderly.[41]

DISTRIBUTION

NSAIDs other than aspirin are generally lipid-soluble, weakly acidic, and highly bound to plasma proteins, primarily albumin. In most cases, <1% of the total plasma concentration exists in the unbound form. Hypoalbuminemia increases the free fraction of NSAIDs in the plasma, thus affecting the distribution and elimination of these agents.[42] The high degree of serum protein binding increases interaction risk with other highly serum protein bound drugs. Most NSAIDs have distribution volumes between 0.1 and 0.15 L/kg.

In inflammatory joint disease, NSAID effectiveness corresponds to the affected joint synovial fluid drug levels. Those correlate closely with the drug concentration at the active site because there is simple transport of drugs across the synovial membrane.[43,44] The amount of drug in synovial fluid is dependent on the amount of albumin in the joint, which is lower than in plasma.[45]

ELIMINATION

Hepatic biotransformation is the major elimination pathways for most NSAIDs,[46] which are metabolized by cytochrome P450–mediated oxidation and/or glucuronide conjugation. Renal excretion of unmetabolized drug is a minor elimination pathway for most NSAIDs accounting for less than 10% of the

administered dose. Some NSAID metabolites are excreted to a significant extent via the bile.

PATHOPHYSIOLOGIC CONDITIONS AFFECTING THE KINETICS OF NSAIDS

Renal Failure

Renal failure influences NSAID kinetics by reducing renal excretion of the drugs and metabolites normally eliminated in the urine and by affecting the distribution and biotransformation of drugs.

Absorption and Distribution

The absorption of NSAIDs is not impaired in renal failure patients. However, the plasma protein binding of many acidic compounds such as the NSAIDs is impaired in renal failure patients.[47] The result is an increase in the volume of distribution of the unbound fraction of the drug in plasma.

Elimination

An increase in the unbound fraction of the drug in plasma may lead to an increase in total plasma clearance of the NSAID. The clearance of those NSAIDs for which formation of acyl glucuronides is a major elimination pathway is significantly reduced in patients with renal failure.[48] The acyl glucuronide forming NSAIDs (diflunisal, ketoprofen, naproxen, indoprofen, benoxaprofen, tiaprofenic acid) are usually rapidly excreted in urine but accumulate in plasma of patients with renal failure. The effect of renal failure on the oral clearance of several NSAIDs (e.g., ibuprofen, fenbufen, isoxicam and piroxicam) is small.[49] Most of these compounds are metabolized by oxidative pathways. All NSAIDs are very highly bound to plasma proteins, and hemodialysis will not likely result in increased elimination of these agents. No dosage adjustments are therefore necessary for patients receiving NSAIDs who are undergoing hemodialysis.[48]

Hepatic Disease

Absorption and Distribution

Because the majority of NSAIDs are low clearance drugs, mild to moderate liver disease should theoretically not interfere with their oral bioavailability. Because the liver is the major organ for the synthesis of albumin which is the major binding protein for NSAID in plasma, hepatic dysfunction would be expected to cause alterations in the unbound drug fraction in plasma.

Elimination

Because most NSAIDs have a small total intrinsic clearance (oral clearance) relative to blood flow, hepatic clearance is essentially independent of flow and reflects drug metabolizing capacity. The elimination of ibuprofen does not seem to be affected in patients with mild to moderate liver disease.[50]

Specific Drugs

All NSAIDs are analgesic, anti-inflammatory, and antipyretic. Differences among the drugs in their approved label indications reflect the studies submitted for approval rather than the actual indications for which the drugs are effective. Characteristics and available dosage forms of commercially available NSAIDs in the United States and much of the world are listed in Table 78.2. Initial selection of an NSAID for a specific patient should be based on several factors—including the patient's past experience, dosing frequency compatibility with the patient's lifestyle, and cost. No population studies suggest that any one NSAID is more effective than another, but interpatient variability in response does occur. Because patients respond differently to various NSAIDs for reasons that are not well understood, it is appropriate to try an NSAID at full dose for about 3 weeks and then to rotate to another NSAID if the desired effect does

TABLE 78.2 Approved Topical NSAIDs in the United States, Canada, New Zealand, Ireland, Finland, France, and Israel

Country (Database)	Diclofenac	Ketoprofen	Ibuprofen	Piroxicam
United States (U.S. Food and Drug Administration, http://www.fda.gov)	**Flector patch** (diclofenac epolamine 1.3% patch, Alphama Pharmaceuticals, Britol, TN) **Voltaren Gel** (diclofenac sodium 1% gel, Endo Pharmaceuticals, Malvern, PA)	NA	NA	NA
Canada (Health Canada Drug Product Database, http://www.hc-sc.gc.ca/dhp-mps/prodpharma/databasdon/index-eng.php)	**PENNSAID** (diclofenac sodium 1.5% topical solution, Square Pharmaceuticals, Dhaka, Bangladesh) **Voltaren Emulgel** (diclofenac 1% topical gel, Novartis, Parsippany, NJ)	NA	NA	NA
New Zealand (MEDSAFE, http://www.medsafe.govt.nz/profs/Datasheet/DSForm.asp)	NA	**Oruvail topical gel** (ketoprofen 2.5%, Sanofi Aventis, Surrey, England)	NA	NA
Ireland (Irish Medicines Board, http://www.imb.ie/EN/Medicines/HumanMedicines/HumanMedicinesListing.aspx)	**Diclac 1% gel** (diclofenac sodium 1%, Rowex, Cork, Ireland) **Difene gel** (diclofenac sodium1%, Astellas Pharma, Dublin, Ireland) **Difene spray gel** (diclofenac sodium 4%, Astellas Pharma, Dublin, Ireland) **Flector tissugel 1% medicated plaster** (diclofenac epolamine 1%, Novartis, Prispanny, NJ) **Voltarol emulgel** (diclofenac diethylamine 1%, Novartis, Prispanny, NJ)	**Fastum 2.5 gel** (ketoprofen 2.5% gel, Menarini, Florence, Italy) **Oruvail** (ketoprofen 2.5% gel, Sanofi Aventis, Surrey England)	**Ibugel 5%** (ibuprofen 5% gel, Dermal Laboratories, Herts, United Kingdom) **Nurofen gel** (ibuprofen 5% gel, Reckitt Benckiser Ireland, Dublin, Ireland), **Phorpain** (ibuprofen 5% gel, Goldshield Pharmaceuticals, Surrey, England)	**Feldene gel** (piroxicam 0.5% gel, Pfizer, New York, NY)
Finland (National Agency for Medicines, http://namweb.nam.fi/namweb/do/haku/view?locale=en)	**EEZE spray** (diclofenac 4% spray, Antula Healthcare, Stockholm, Sweden) **Flector** (diclofenac epolamine 1% plaster IBSA Farmaceutici Italia Srl, Lodi, Italy) **Voltaren Emulgel** (diclofenac diethylamine 1%, Novartis, Parsippany, NJ)	**Ketorin 2.5%** (ketoprofen 2.5% gel, Orion Oyj, Epsoo, Finland) **Orudis gel** (ketoprofen 2.5% gel, Sanofi Aventis, Surrey, England)	NA	**Feldene gel** (piroxicam 0.5% gel, Pfizer, New York, NY)
France (French Health Products Safety Agency, http://agmed.sante.gouv.fr/htm/1/amm/amm0.htm)	**Flector** (1% diclofenac epolamine plaster (Laboratoires Genevrier SA, Antibes, France) **Voltaren Emulgel** (diclofenac diethylamine 1% gel, Novartis, Prispanny, NJ) **Diclofenac 1% gel** (diclofenac diethylamine 1% gel, Merck, Whitehouse Station, NJ)	**Ketoprofen 2.5 % gel** (multiple manufacturers)	**Ibuprofen 5% gel, solution** (multiple manufacturers)	**Piroxicam gel** (piroxicam 0.5% gel, Pfizer, New York, NY)
Israel (The Israel Drug Registry, http://www.health.gov.il/units/pharmacy/trufot/index.asp?safa=e)	**Dicloplast** (diclofenac sodium patch 140 mg, CTS Chemical Industries, Tel Aviv, Israel) **Voltaren Emulgel** (diclofenac diethylamine 1% gel, Novartis, Parsippany, NJ) **Diclofenac sodium 1%** (diclofenac sodium 1% gel, Vitamed, Benyamina, Israel) **Dicloren gel** (diclofenac sodium 1%, Trima, Kibbutz Maabarot, Israel)	**Fastum gel** (ketoprofen 2.5% gel, Menarini, Florence, Italy)	**Deep relief** (ibuprofen 5% and levomenthol 3%, Mentholatum, Hertfordshire, England) **Nurofen gel** (5% ibuprofen gel, Reckitt Benckiser Healthcare, Hull, England)	**Exipan** (piroxicam 0.5% gel, Perrigo Israel Pharmaceuticals, Bnei Brak, Israel) **Feldene gel** (piroxicam 0.5% gel, Pfizer, New York, NY)

NOTE: Websites accessed in December 2008.
NA, not available.

not occur. There is no evidence that a patient who does not respond to an NSAID in one chemical subclass (e.g., propionic acid derivatives) will respond any better to an NSAID from another chemical subclass class than to a different propionic acid derivative NSAID.

SALICYLATES
Aspirin
The aspirin elimination half-life increases from 2.5 hours at low doses to 19 hours at high doses. It is well absorbed from the stomach and small intestine, with peak blood levels achieved 1 hour after an oral dose. There is then rapid conversion of aspirin to salicylates from a high first-pass effect, which occurs in the wall of the small intestine and the liver. The metabolic pathways follow first-order and zero-order kinetics.[51]

Aspirin inhibits the biosynthesis of PGs through irreversible acetylation and consequent inactivation of COX. This differs from contemporary NSAIDs, which are reversible COX inhibitors.[52] Most cells can synthesize COX; platelets cannot. Thus, the acetylation of their microsomal enzyme lasts for the life of the platelet (10 to 14 days). The ability of aspirin to acetylate proteins helps explain its anti-inflammatory superiority over most other salicylates. Aspirin is the only NSAID that has been associated with Reye syndrome, a potentially lethal disorder that produces seizures and coma. It has occurred with the use of aspirin during a viral illness in children.[53] As a consequence, aspirin is now rarely if ever used in pediatrics.

Diflunisal
Diflunisal has potentially better GI tolerability than aspirin because diflunisal is not metabolized to salicylic acid in plasma according to the results of a study comparing it at 250 mg and 500 mg twice a day to aspirin at 600 mg four times a day.[54] Diflunisal has a shorter half-life and causes less inhibition of platelet aggregation than aspirin.

ACETIC ACID DERIVATIVES
Indomethacin
Indomethacin is well absorbed following oral and rectal administration, but the extent of absorption varies widely among patients. There is also a large interpatient variability in elimination half-life caused by extensive enterohepatic recirculation of the drug. It is highly bound to serum albumin. Metabolism involves demethylation and deacetylation in the liver with subsequent excretion of inactive metabolites and unchanged drug in the bile and urine.[55] Its clinical application is somewhat limited by a relatively high incidence of gastritis and renal dysfunction. It is used in patients with acute gouty arthritis, osteoarthritis, and headaches (such as the hemicranias). Indomethacin is often used in neonatology to facilitate closure of a patent ductus arteriosus (PDA).

Sulindac
Sulindac resulted from the search for a drug similar to indomethacin but with less toxicity. Sulindac is an inactive prodrug that is converted after absorption by liver microsomal enzymes to sulindac disulfide, the active metabolite.[56] As few as 25% of the patients have GI problems, primarily constipation.[57] Sulindac was considered in early studies to be the least nephrotoxic of the NSAIDs, but subsequent studies failed to support this contention.[58]

Tolmetin and Etodolac
These two NSAIDs claim fewer side effects than others in the class. Tolmetin is excreted in the urine partly unchanged, partly conjugated and as an inactive dicarboxylic acid metabolite.[59] Tolmetin can cause edema due to sodium retention and abnormal liver function, both of which are reversible upon discontinuation of this NSAID.

Etodolac is an acidic compound with a pK_a of 4.65 and is available as tablets and capsules with a dosage of up to 1 g daily and maximum of 1.2 g. Clinical doses of 200 to 300 mg twice a day for the relief of low back or shoulder pain have been equated to analgesia with naproxen 500 mg twice a day.[60] Large clinical trials demonstrated a similar incidence of abdominal pain and dyspepsia is similar to several other NSAIDs, and GI ulceration occurs in less than 0.3% of patients.[61] Dyspepsia occurs with etodolac in 10% of patients with a somewhat lower incidence of abdominal pain.

Ketorolac
Oral ketorolac was approved for use in the United States approximately 3 years after the parenteral form and has an efficacy similar to that of naproxen and ibuprofen.[62] The oral dose is 10 to 20 mg every 4 to 6 hours for no more than 5 days continuous use because of the potential for toxicity. Ketorolac tromethamine has a pK_a of 3.5. It is formulated in a racemic mixture with the S form providing analgesia. Following oral administration, bioavailability is near 100%; however, concomitant administration with high-fat meals will result in decreased peak and time-to-peak concentrations. Time-to-peak effect is estimated at 2 to 3 hours with no difference based on dosage. However, increased dosages will provide prolonged durations of analgesia. With oral and IV administration, it is almost entirely bound to plasma proteins (>99%). This results in a small apparent volume of distribution with extensive metabolism by conjugation and renal excretion.[63] Hypoalbuminemia will result in a higher concentration of free drug. Clearance relies on hepatic conjugation, with the metabolites primarily (92%) renal excretion. The S enantiomer is preferentially metabolized, with some studies suggesting a half-life of 2.5 hours compared to 5 hours for the R enantiomer.[64]

Ketorolac was the first parenteral NSAID available for clinical analgesic use in the United States, having gained U.S. Food and Drug Administration (FDA) approval in 1989. The parenteral form of ketorolac can be administered at single doses of 15, 30, or 60 mg IV or as 30 mg IM every 6 hours, again up to 5 days use out of concerns for toxicity. The analgesic effect with IV ketorolac is more rapid and occurs within 30 minutes, peak effect between 1 and 2 hours, and duration of analgesia of 4 to 6 hours (FDA-approved labeling).[64] It has demonstrated antipyretic effects 20 times that of aspirin and thus can mask febrile response when given routinely to patients postoperatively. Some have suggested that ketorolac may act at the CNS in addition to the peripheral mode of action,[32] and dental surgery studies with ketorolac also indicate that ketorolac acts centrally.[65] However, CSF studies contradict this claim as measurements of the drug in CSF show poor penetration.[66]

The effectiveness of ketorolac has been well established as several studies have demonstrated efficacy comparable to or exceeding that of morphine for treatment of moderate postoperative pain treatment and with fewer side effects.[67] Notwithstanding are concerns for side effects such as bleeding and renal injury. Ketorolac is known to prolong bleeding time but does not alter it beyond the upper limits of normal.[68] In fact, there is evidence that indicates no clinically significant effect on surgical site bleeding when compared to placebo.[69] There were early reports of death due to GI and operative site bleeding[70] resulting in the drug being recalled in Germany and France. In a response to these adverse events, the drug's manufacturer recommended reducing the dose of ketorolac from 150 to 120 mg per day.[64] The European Committee for Proprietary Medicinal Products recommended a further reduction of the maximum daily dose to 60 mg for the elderly and to 90 mg for the non-elderly.[71] Currently, there is consensus that the dose should be as low as 7.5 to 10 mg every 6 hours.[72,73] When first used postoperatively at an initial dose of 60 mg followed by 30-mg doses every 4 hours, ketorolac was associated with acute tubular necrosis, especially in patients who had undergone procedures that required fluid restriction. Some deaths resulted. Subsequently, to minimize this risk, doses were commonly reduced by 50% to 75%, but concerns about nephrotoxicity continue. The appropriate analgesic dose of parenteral ketorolac is controversial. The IN route of administration may produce higher levels of the drug in the CNS and CSF[74] with minimal GI side effects. Studies are underway to determine the efficacy of this drug when administered intranasally.[75]

Ketorolac is the only IN NSAID commercially available. It has been praised for its rapid onset of action with its unique route of administration. It has been studied in the management of acute pain following surgeries such as abdominal, dental, or orthopedic. The early studies showed an advantage over placebo in reduction of overall pain scores and postoperative opioid use.[76] The half-life of IN ketorolac is similar to that of IM ketorolac, around 5 to 6 hours. Dosing is 1 spray per nostril per dose. Each spray provides 15.75 mg ketorolac tromethamine. Side effects for IN ketorolac are similar to that of other routes of administration with the addition of potential nasopharyngeal irritation. Surgical site infiltration with ketorolac and local anesthetic has shown favorable results[77] and is widely used clinically in orthopedic surgery.

Diclofenac

Diclofenac is a carboxylic acid functional group with rapid and complete absorption. Substantial concentrations of drug are attained in synovial fluid, which has been hypothesized as one of the sites of action of diclofenac.[78] Concentration–effect relationships have been established for total bound, unbound, and synovial fluid diclofenac concentrations.[79] Diclofenac is eliminated following biotransformation to glucuronidated and sulfated metabolites that are excreted in urine with very little drug eliminated unchanged. Diclofenac may have a significantly higher incidence of hepatotoxicity than other NSAIDs. The excretion of conjugates may be related to renal function. Conjugate accumulation occurs in end-stage renal disease; however, no accumulation is apparent on comparison of young and elderly individuals.[80] Dosage adjustments for the elderly, children, or patients with certain comorbidities (e.g., hepatic disease, rheumatoid arthritis) may not be required. Significant drug interactions occur with aspirin, lithium, digoxin, methotrexate, cyclosporin, cholestyramine, and colestipol.[81]

Parenteral diclofenac has been used in Europe for several years and was recently approved for use in the United States. The pharmacokinetics and precautions are similar to that of oral, immediate-release formulations. IV diclofenac has proven to be useful in treating postsurgical pain after abdominopelvic surgery[82] and third molar extraction.[83] In comparison to ketorolac, IV diclofenac demonstrated a superior effect with regard to not only both reduction in pain scores but also lower opioid requirements following orthopedic surgery.[84] In vitro assessments of hemostasis have shown that diclofenac (IV and oral [PO]) produces less platelet dysfunction than aspirin or IV ketorolac.[85]

Topical diclofenac comes in many forms: liquid, gel, and patch. Liquid diclofenac comes in a 2% formulation and uses dimethyl sulfoxide (DMSO) as a driving agent. One percent diclofenac gel has demonstrated a 17-fold reduction in systemic absorption compared to oral diclofenac with repeated administration.[86] The patch form of topical diclofenac 1.3% has also shown little systemic absorption and slow times to peak effect (10 to 20 hours). Systemic exposure is <1% that of a single oral diclofenac 50-mg dose.[87] They have been shown to be effective in treating acute musculoskeletal pain—such as that from sprains, strains, and overuse injuries.[88] There has also been suggestion of its use in acute postoperative pain.[89] However, the beneficial effects of topical NSAIDs tend to be limited to acute pain as reviews of topical diclofenac in chronic pain states have largely yielded mixed results with the exception of

its use in chronic osteoarthritis.[90] Recommended dosing among the topical formulations of diclofenac varies between products and specific applications of the products.

PROPIONIC ACID DERIVATIVES

This class of NSAIDs includes ibuprofen, fenoprofen, ketoprofen, flurbiprofen, and naproxen. A newer drug in this class is oxaprozin, which permits once-daily dose regime, but it has no other advantage over other NSAIDs.[91]

Ibuprofen

Ibuprofen was the first NSAID to become available without prescription in the United States. It is well absorbed; peak plasma levels of 15 to 20 μg/mL are achieved about 1 to 2 hours after a single dose. The half-life is about 3.5 hours. The drug is primarily hepatic metabolized with less than 10% excreted unchanged in the urine and bile.[92] Ibuprofen at a dose of 1,200 mg per day has a predominately analgesic effect in arthritis patients. Normally, a minimum dose of 1,600 mg a day is needed for clinically useful anti-inflammatory activity. At 2,400 mg per day, it produces GI side effects of which nausea and dyspepsia are predominant. Renal side effects of ibuprofen appear to be dose-dependent and were not reported at the recommended dosage as over-the-counter drug (200 to 800 mg per day). Even at anti-inflammatory doses of more than 1,600 mg per day, renal side effects are almost exclusively encountered in patients with low intravascular volume and low cardiac output, particularly in the elderly.[93] Concomitant administration of ibuprofen and aspirin antagonizes the irreversible platelet inhibition induced by aspirin. Therefore, the treatment with ibuprofen in patients with increased cardiovascular (CV) risk may limit the cardioprotective effects of aspirin.[94]

In 2009, IV ibuprofen was approved for use in the United States. The pharmacokinetics of the IV form has a half-life (2 hours) similar to that of the oral formulation but show a nearly twofold increase in peak plasma concentration that occurs at a more rapid rate. Early studies have shown an ability of IV ibuprofen to reduce pain scores and opioid use following orthopedic surgery and gynecologic surgery.[95] The recommended dose is 400 to 800 mg every 6 hours as needed, not to exceed 3,200 mg in a 24-hour period. The drug must be diluted prior to administration and infused over a minimum of 30 minutes.

Ketoprofen

Oral ketoprofen reaches peak plasma levels in 1.5 to 2 hours. The half-life is 2.4 hours with an analgesic duration of 4 to 6 hours.[96] The maximum recommended dose is 300 mg. An investigational topical patch contains 100 mg of the drug. Pharmacokinetic data indicate that the plasma levels of ketoprofen 100 mg administered orally are higher than when applied by patch. Because the patch facilitates ketoprofen delivery over a full day, the drug remains continually present in the tissue adjacent to the site of application. High-tissue but low-plasma ketoprofen concentrations produce a therapeutic effect, whereas plasma concentrations remain low enough to minimize systemic adverse events.[97]

Fenoprofen

The calcium salt of fenoprofen is more common; it is well absorbed and achieves a peak plasma level of 20 to 30 μg/mL 2 hours after a single oral dose with a plasma half-life of 2 to 3 hours.[98] Steady-state plasma levels are reached within the first 24 hours of therapy. Fenoprofen is well tolerated compared to aspirin and causes minimal occult GI bleeding; nevertheless, dyspepsia remains the most common side effect. Most of the drug is excreted as glucuronide in the urine.

Naproxen

Naproxen sodium is also available without a prescription in the United States. Naproxen is well absorbed from the upper

GI tract. Its long half-life of 13 hours makes it suitable for twice-daily administration,[99] and it takes more than 2 days to reach steady-state serum levels. Excretion is almost entirely renal, primarily as an inactive glucuronide metabolite.

Naproxen has been used for the treatment of arthritis and other inflammatory diseases with superior efficacy to aspirin.[100] It causes less GI irritation than aspirin. Naproxen increases bleeding time by inhibiting platelet aggregation. When given during pregnancy, it can cross the placenta in 20 minutes and cause neonatal jaundice. Naproxen appears to have one of the safest CV profiles of all NSAIDs.

Oxaprozin

Oxaprozin is approved for the management of adult rheumatoid arthritis, osteoarthritis, ankylosing spondylitis, soft tissue disorders, and postoperative dental pain. Oxaprozin has a high oral bioavailability (95%), with peak plasma concentrations at 3 to 5 hours after dosing.[101] It is metabolized in the liver by oxidative and conjugative pathways and readily eliminated by the renal and fecal routes. Oxaprozin inhibits nuclear translocation of NF-κB and metalloproteases and modulates the endogenous cannabinoid system.[102] In a randomized study of patients with refractory shoulder pain, oxaprozin (1,200 mg) once a day was superior to three doses per day of diclofenac (50 mg) in reducing pain and improving quality of life.[103]

Oxaprozin diffuses readily into inflamed synovial tissues after oral administration.[104] Although discovered more than 20 years ago, it is now under intensive investigation because of its unusual pharmacodynamic properties. Other than being a nonselective COX inhibitor, the drug is capable of inhibiting both anandamide hydrolase in neurons, with consequent potent analgesic activity and NF-κB activation in inflammatory cells.[102] Moreover, oxaprozin induces apoptosis of activated monocytes in a dose-dependent manner. As monocyte–macrophages and NF-κB pathways are crucial for synthesis of pro-inflammatory and histotoxic mediators in inflamed joints, oxaprozin appears to have pharmacodynamic properties exceeding those presently assumed as markers of classical NSAIDs.[105]

OXICAM DERIVATIVES

Piroxicam, the first drug in this class, provides peak serum concentration following oral dosing slowly and has a long elimination half-life of 48.5 hours. This allows once-daily dosing, but piroxicam may take up to 1 week to achieve steady-state blood concentrations.[106]

Meloxicam

Meloxicam is approved for the treatment of osteoarthritis in the United States. It has also been evaluated for the treatment of rheumatoid arthritis, ankylosing spondylitis, and acute rheumatic pain.[107] Meloxicam is a nonselective COX inhibitor that has been shown to be somewhat COX-2 preferential at low therapeutic dose. It is unclear that this is clinically meaningful at normal therapeutic doses. Therefore, meloxicam should be considered a nonselective NSAID.

In clinical trials at a low dose, meloxicam was as effective as piroxicam, diclofenac, and naproxen with less GI toxicity,[108] but this may not hold true at the commonly required higher dose. Meloxicam's half-life of approximately 20 hours makes it appropriate for once-daily dosing.[108] Meloxicam has not been reported to cause deterioration in renal function in patients with moderate renal failure, and there is no evidence of drug accumulation with continued use. However, the FDA-approved labeling recommends that only the 7.5-mg dose be used in patients with renal insufficiency. Dose adjustment is not required in the elderly. Meloxicam interacts with some medications, including cholestyramine, lithium, and some inhibitors of cytochrome P450: 2C9 and 3A4. Consequently, increased clinical vigilance

is indicated when using it concurrently with other medications metabolized by those enzymes. Concentration-dependent therapeutic and toxicologic effects have yet to be extensively elucidated for meloxicam.[109] Its pharmacokinetic profile is characterized by a prolonged, almost complete absorption, and the drug is more than 99.5% bound to plasma proteins. Meloxicam is metabolized primarily to four biologically inactive metabolites, which are excreted in both urine and feces. Steady-state plasma concentrations are achieved within 3 to 5 days. The pharmacokinetic parameters of meloxicam are linear over the dose range 7.5 to 30 mg, and bioequivalence has been shown for a number of different formulations.

Studies are underway investigating an IV formulation of meloxicam for acute pain following major surgery. Given the efficacy of oral meloxicam and its COX-2 specificity, the results of the trial are an exciting area of interest for the further application of NSAIDs in the acute care setting.

COX-2 SELECTIVE NSAIDs

COX-2 selective NSAIDs were developed to reduce the incidence of serious GI adverse effects associated with the administration of traditional NSAIDs on the assumption that these side effects were COX-1–mediated. Marketing efforts to differentiate these drugs from nonselective NSAIDs led to the term COX-2 specific inhibitors. That is misleading because these drugs are selective, not specific, in their COX-2 affinity. The initial COX-2 selective NSAIDs approved by FDA were celecoxib and rofecoxib.

Celecoxib

Celecoxib, the first COX-2 selective NSAID, was approved by the FDA on the last day of December 1998. It now has approval for the relief of pain from osteoarthritis, rheumatoid arthritis, acute pain, dysmenorrhea, and for familial adenomatous polyposis. It has good selectivity for the COX-2 enzyme. Peak plasma levels occur 3 hours after oral administration, and the drug crosses into the CSF.[27] Celecoxib is 97% serum protein bound with an apparent volume of distribution of 400 L. It is metabolized via cytochrome P450 2C9 and eliminated predominantly by the liver. It is not indicated for pediatric use and is a category C drug for pregnancy. The drug has a half-life of about 11 hours.[110] Adverse events noted in the various clinical trials include headache, edema, dyspepsia, diarrhea, nausea, and sinusitis. It is contraindicated in patients who have a sulfonamide allergy or a known hypersensitivity to aspirin or other NSAIDs.

Because celecoxib does not interfere with platelet function[111] (there is no COX-2 in human platelets), it can be administered perioperatively as a multimodal analgesic without increased risk of bleeding.

The efficacy and upper GI safety of celecoxib compared with nonselective NSAIDs was evaluated in 13,274 patients with osteoarthritis (SUCCESS-I study).[112] Patients were randomly assigned to receive either celecoxib 100 or 200 mg twice daily or nonselective NSAID therapy (diclofenac 50 mg twice daily or naproxen 500 mg twice daily) for 12 weeks. Both celecoxib doses were as effective as the nonselective NSAIDs in treating osteoarthritis and significantly more gastric ulcer–related complications occurred in the nonselective NSAID patients (0.8/100 patient-years) compared with the celecoxib group (0.1/100 patient-years) (odds ratio = 7.02; $P = .008$). The number of CV thromboembolic events was low and not different between the groups. The results of the SUCCESS-I study are different from the "CLASS" trial,[113] which did not demonstrate an advantage of celecoxib in reducing the incidence of upper GI ulcer complications, which is attributed by the SUCCESS-I study authors to the low dropout rate and design of the newer study.

Etoricoxib

Used in more than 80 countries worldwide, etoricoxib is yet to be approved by the FDA for use in the United States. A selective COX-2 inhibitor, etoricoxib, has a near 100% bioavailability. It is primarily metabolized by cytochrome P450 system to water-soluble metabolites. Etoricoxib is excreted in the urine (70%) and feces (20%). Half-life of etoricoxib is 22 hours, and peak plasma concentrations are obtained at 1 hour in a fasting state or 2 hours in a fed state.[114] Etoricoxib is produced in 30-, 60-, 90-, and 120-mg tablets. The efficacy of single daily dosages of 60 or 120 mg have been shown to substantially reduce acute pain following dental surgery and total joint arthroplasty and limit opioid use without any increased incidence of adverse events compared to placebo.[115] Despite worldwide experience with this drug, there are currently no clinical trials underway in the United States to further investigate safety and efficacy of etoricoxib.

Valdecoxib and Parecoxib

Valdecoxib is a derivative of isoxazole and binds noncovalently to COX-2, forming a tight and relatively stable enzyme–inhibitor complex. It is a potent inhibitor of PGE_2 production in humans.[116] Valdecoxib has good oral bioavailability (83%) and a minimal first-pass effect. It achieves maximal plasma concentration in 3 hours with an elimination half-life of about 8 to 11 hours.[117] Valdecoxib was approved for use in osteoarthritis (10 mg), rheumatoid arthritis (10 mg),[118] and acute pain (up to 40 mg). Clinical studies in high-risk cardiac patients demonstrated a significantly increased incidence of major CV adverse events, and the identification of increased risk for serious skin reactions (toxic epidermal necrolysis, Stevens-Johnson syndrome, erythema multiforme) led the FDA to recommend the withdrawal of this COX-2 inhibitor from the US market in 2003. Parecoxib is a parenteral derivative of valdecoxib that has not been approved for marketing in the United States due largely to CV toxicity concerns.

ACETAMINOPHEN

Acetaminophen is a para-aminophenol derivative with analgesic and antipyretic properties similar to aspirin. Antipyresis is likely from direct action on the hypothalamic heat-regulating centers via inhibiting action of endogenous pyrogen.[119] Its exact mechanism of action is unknown, but it is hypothesized to act centrally through pathways that involve serotonin, nitric oxide, eicosanoids, or opioids.[120] Although equipotent to aspirin in inhibiting central PG synthesis, acetaminophen has no significant peripheral PG synthetase inhibition. Therefore, it lacks clinically useful peripheral anti-inflammatory activity, which makes it less desirable than NSAIDs for painful, inflammatory disorders. Doses of 600 to 650 mg are more effective than doses of 300 to 325 mg, but little additional benefit is seen at doses above 1,000 mg, indicating a possible ceiling effect.[121]

Acetaminophen has few side effects in the usual dosage range; no significant GI toxicity or platelet functional changes occur. However, recent studies demonstrate that acetaminophen can cause blood pressure elevations. It is not clear if this presents risk of CV side effects similar to NSAIDs in light of the finding that NSAID-induced blood pressure elevation over time is associated with CV thrombotic effects.[122]

Nephrotoxicity also can occur with acetaminophen but less frequently than it occurs with NSAIDs. Acetaminophen is almost entirely metabolized in the liver, and the minor metabolites are responsible for the hepatotoxicity seen in overdose.[123] Inducers of the cytochrome P450 enzyme system in the liver (such as alcohol) increase the formation of metabolites and therefore increase hepatotoxicity. In certain patients (chronic ethanol users, malnutrition, and fasting patients), repeating therapeutic or slightly excessive doses may precipitate hepatotoxicity. More recently, the maximum allowable content of acetaminophen in a pill form was limited to 325 mg by the FDA with further recommendations to limit the daily dose of acetaminophen to 3 g per day.[124] Toxic doses appear to be a function of baseline glutathione levels and other dose-related factors. Genetically determined glutathione is an important factor in overdose toxicity. Patients with high glutathione stores may tolerate much higher doses, but the daily limit is important for safety because many patients lack sufficient glutathione stores to safely tolerate higher daily doses. Clinicians should carefully inquire and educate patients about other over-the-counter symptom-control products that patients may be taking and which also contain acetaminophen as many over-the-counter and prescription analgesics contain acetaminophen as a component.

Acetaminophen is completely and rapidly absorbed following oral administration, with bioavailability around 85% to 95% after first-pass metabolism. Peak serum concentrations are achieved within 2 hours and therapeutic serum concentrations are 10 to 20 µg/mL.[125] About 90% of acetaminophen is hepatically metabolized to sulfate and glucuronide conjugates for renal excretion with a small amount secreted unchanged in the urine.[126]

IV paracetamol (acetaminophen) has achieved widespread use following its introduction in Europe and eventual use in the United States. Compared to oral dosing, IV paracetamol has a 70% higher maximum concentration. The half-life is approximately 2.5 hours and increases with lower age groups. Metabolism is identical to oral dosing. IV paracetamol offers a unique opportunity for patients who are nothing by mouth (NPO) or anesthetized. It is without surprise that many perioperative multimodal pain protocols have been developed that incorporate this drug. In fact, it has been considered the foundation for perioperative, multimodal analgesia protocols. Injectable paracetamol has been shown to reduce opioid consumption by about 35% to 45%[127] in postoperative pain studies[127,128] including after cardiac surgery.[129] Other beneficial effects have been seen with reductions in postoperative nausea and vomiting.[130] However, it should be noted that these results have not been consistently reproduced. Propacetamol, an injectable prodrug of paracetamol, is hydrolyzed within 6 minutes of administration and 1 g of propacetamol yields 0.5 g of paracetamol.

The bioavailability of rectal acetaminophen is variable and is approximately 80% of that following oral administration. The rectal rate of absorption is slower, with maximum plasma concentration occurring 2 to 3 hours after administration.[131] Doses of 40 to 60 mg/kg of rectal acetaminophen have been shown to have opioid-sparing effect in postoperative pain models.[132] Widespread use of rectal acetaminophen has not gain popularity in the United States largely due to cultural preferences (Fig. 78.2).

NSAID Combination Medications

Combination NSAIDs have been developed with the intent to reduce GI-related side effects. As such, combinations including a histamine receptor antagonist, proton pump inhibitor, and PG analogs have been developed.

Naproxen plus esomeprazole, a proton pump inhibitor, is one of such combinations and was approved by the FDA in 2010. It is available in 375/20 mg and 500/20 mg combinations. Dosing is suggested as one tablet twice daily for pain symptoms stemming from osteoarthritis, rheumatoid arthritis, and ankylosing spondylitis. Small studies have shown an analgesic effect superior to placebo, but similar to celecoxib, in the treatment of these conditions. The addition of esomeprazole has resulted lower upper GI-related adverse events, such as gastric or duodenal ulcers, at 1, 3, and 6 months.[133] However, there is no significant difference in reducing gastroduodenal

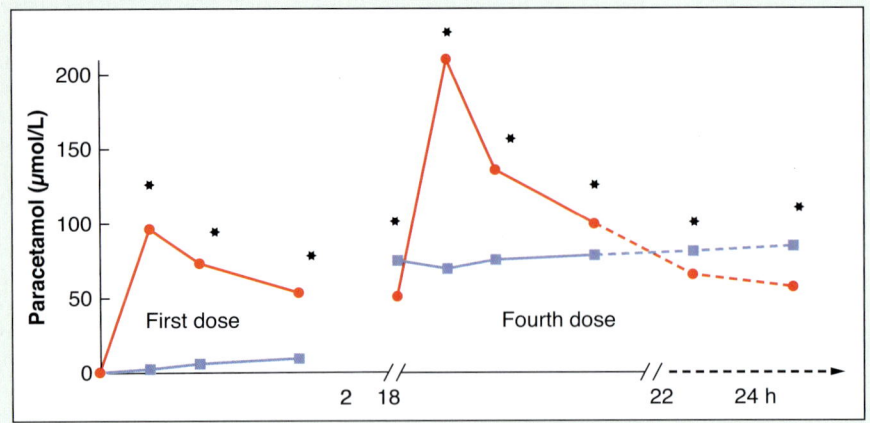

FIGURE 78.2 Paracetamol after heart surgery. Mean maximal plasma paracetamol concentration at times 0, 20, 40, and 80 minutes after 1 g of rectally and intravenously (IV) administered paracetamol (N = 12 + 12 patients) and 6 hours after the third dose, corresponding to before the fourth dose and at 20, 40, and 80 minutes and at 4 and 6 hours after the fourth dose in (N = 12 + 12 patients). ●, IV administered paracetamol; ■, rectally administered paracetamol; ✳, significant difference between groups. *(From Holmér Pettersson P, Jakobsson J, Owall A. Plasma concentrations following repeated rectal or intravenous administration of paracetamol after heart surgery. Acta Anaesthesiol Scand 2006;50[6]:673–677. Copyright © 2006 The Acta Anaesthesiologica Scandinavica Foundation. Reprinted by permission of John Wiley & Sons, Inc.)*

ulcers when compared to COX-2 selective NSAIDs, such as celecoxib and etoricoxib.[134] The addition of a proton pump inhibitor can actually compound GI toxicity of NSAIDs; there is an increase of small intestine mucosal damage when combining the two medications.[135] Furthermore, there appears to be no advantage in mitigating CV toxicity.

An ibuprofen/famotidine combination has also been available in the United States since 2011. This combination is available in an 800/26.6-mg tablet. It is also approved for use in osteoarthritis and rheumatoid arthritis, with three-times-daily dosing. Ibuprofen maintains its pharmacokinetics when administered with famotidine, a histamine-2 receptor antagonist. Early studies show that combining famotidine with ibuprofen reduces gastric ulcers and ulcers within the upper GI tract when compared to ibuprofen alone.[136]

Lastly, the addition of a PG to diclofenac has been developed to accomplish more gastroprotective effects when coadministered. Diclofenac/misoprostol is formulated in 50 mg/200 μg and 75 mg/200 μg tablets. It is also approved for osteoarthritis and rheumatoid arthritis. Dosing is two to four times daily (Fig. 78.3).

SIDE EFFECTS, WARNINGS, AND CONTROVERSIES
Cardiovascular Effects
The risk of major CV events from NSAIDs has garnered much attention since valdecoxib and rofecoxib were removed from the market following evidence of increased rates of stroke and myocardial infarction (MI). On April 7, 2005, the FDA announced a series of labeling changes for all NSAIDs, including over-the-counter forms. This included an FDA boxed warning

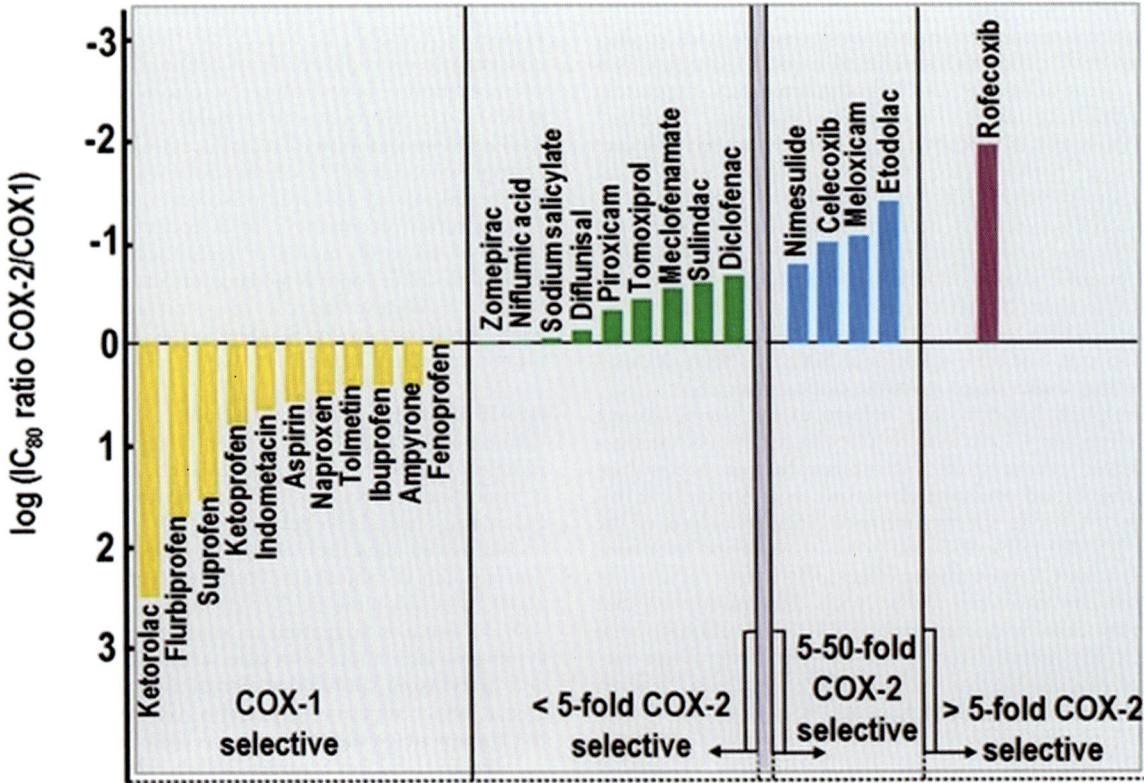

FIGURE 78.3 A comparison of cyclooxygenase (COX) isozyme selectivity of nonsteroidal anti-inflammatory drugs. *(Reprinted from Rang HP, Dale MM. Rang & Dale's Pharmacology. 6th ed. Philadelphia, PA: Churchill Livingstone; 2007. Copyright © 2007 Elsevier. With permission.)*

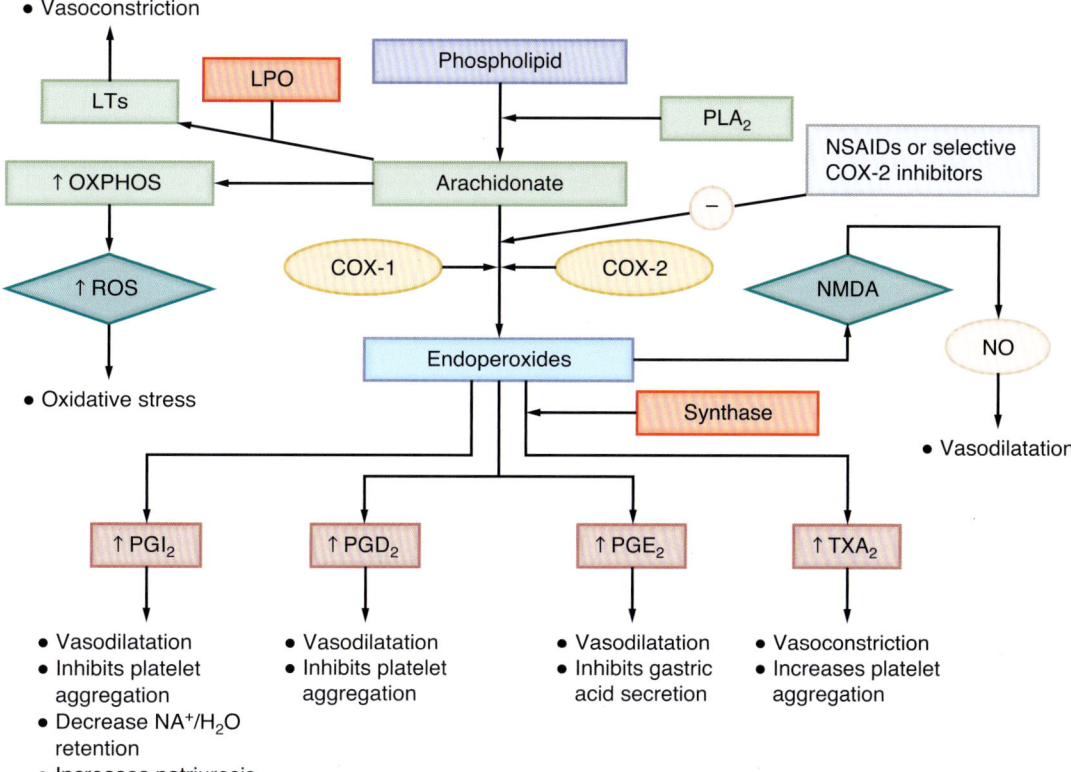

FIGURE 78.4 Assessment of nonsteroidal anti-inflammatory drug (NSAID)-induced cardiotoxicity. Schematic representation of the pharmacologic effects related to cyclooxygenase inhibition. COX-1, cyclooxygenase 1; COX-2, cyclooxygenase 2; LPO, lipoxygenase; LTs, leukotrienes; NMDA, N-methyl-D-aspartic acid; NO, nitric oxide; OXPHOS, oxidative phosphorylation; PGD$_2$, prostaglandin D$_2$; PGE$_2$, prostaglandin E$_2$; PGI$_2$, prostacyclin; PLA$_2$, phospholipase A$_2$; ROS, reactive oxygen species; TXA$_2$, thromboxane A$_2$. *(From Singh BK, Haque SE, Pillai KK. Assessment of nonsteroidal anti-inflammatory drug-induced cardiotoxicity. Expert Opin Drug Metab Toxicol 2014;10[2]:143–156. Reprinted by permission of Taylor & Francis Ltd. http://www.tandfonline.com.)*

for the potential increased risk of CV events and GI bleeding associated with all prescription NSAIDs, including celecoxib. Manufacturers were asked to revise their labeling to include a medication guide for patients to help make them aware of the potential for CV and GI adverse events. In addition, the FDA asked manufacturers of all over-the-counter NSAIDs to revise their labels to include more specific information about potential CV and GI risks and information to assist consumers in the safe use of these drugs. CV toxicity is not completely understood, but it has been postulated that COX inhibition may disrupt the balance between antithrombotic substances like PGI$_2$ and prothrombotic thromboxane A$_2$ (TXA$_2$) in platelets (Fig. 78.4).[137]

On July 7, 2015, the FDA strengthened its NSAID warning, and labeling was updated to state, "non-aspirin NSAIDs increase the chance of a heart attack or stroke." Additional information includes the risk of MI or stroke can occur as early as the first weeks of using an NSAID and may increase with extended use. In fact, the risks of CV mortality and morbidity peak soon after MI and gradually decline to match the risk of the general population after 5 to 10 years.[138] The risk appears to be dose-related, and no difference between individual drugs was noted at the time of the safety announcement (Fig. 78.5).[139]

These labeling updates are challenging to providers, as NSAIDs remain such an integral part to managing both acute and chronic pain conditions. Research has failed to determine an NSAID that stands alone as being safer than others in reducing major CV events. Celecoxib, naproxen, and ibuprofen all have been shown to have similar rates of CV events.[140] The drug dosage may indeed play a role as low doses of diclofenac (50 to 75 mg per day) have shown negligible effects on CV effects.[141]

The interaction between NSAIDs and antihypertensive medication has also been highlighted as cause for concern. There appears variability between individual medications as celecoxib seems to have little effect in patients already taking angiotensin-converting enzyme (ACE) inhibitors,[142] whereas others like diclofenac appear to have an effect on both blood pressure and glomerular filtration rate (GFR).[143] The negative effect of NSAIDs on blood pressure may be limited to those patients taking ACE inhibitor and β-blockers but not calcium channel blockers or diuretics.[144] There is even suggestion that acetaminophen can do the same.[145,146]

The risk of congestive heart failure is ill defined with use of NSAIDs; however, there are correlations between use of these drugs and clinical decompensation[147] and preceding hospital

2015 U.S. Food and Drug Administration NSAID Warning

- Risk of heart attack/stroke can occur as early as first week after starting NSAID and may increase with prolonged use.
- Risk appears to increase with higher doses.
- There is insufficient evidence to determine the risk of individual NSAIDs.
- NSAIDs increase the risk of heart attack/stroke regardless of existing heart disease or risk factors for heart disease.
- NSAID use in patients with risk factors for heart disease increases the likelihood of heart attack or stroke.
- Patients prescribed NSAIDs following a first heart attack were more likely to die within that first year compared to patients who did not receive NSAIDs.
- NSAID use increases risk of heart failure.

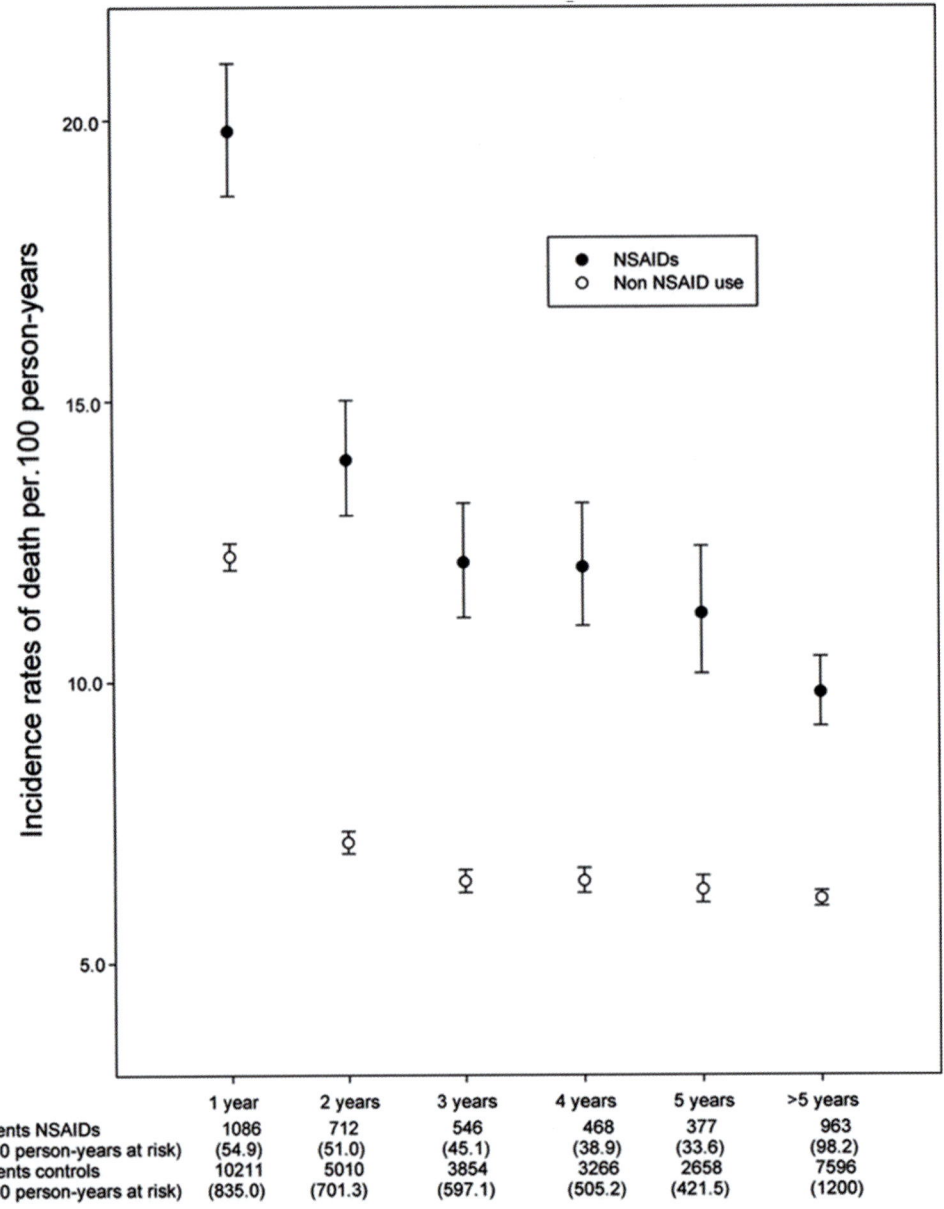

	1 year	2 years	3 years	4 years	5 years	>5 years
Events NSAIDs	1086	712	546	468	377	963
(100 person-years at risk)	(54.9)	(51.0)	(45.1)	(38.9)	(33.6)	(98.2)
Events controls	10211	5010	3854	3266	2658	7596
(100 person-years at risk)	(835.0)	(701.3)	(597.1)	(505.2)	(421.5)	(1200)

Time after discharge from MI
(Vertical bars indicate indicate 95% CI)

FIGURE 78.5 Incidence of death during nonsteroidal anti-inflammatory drug (NSAID) treatment. *(Reprinted with permission from Olsen AMS, Fosbøl EL, Lindhardsen J, et al. Long-term cardiovascular risk of nonsteroidal anti-inflammatory drug use according to time passed after first-time myocardial infarction: a nationwide cohort study. Circulation 2012;126[16]:1955–1963. Copyright © 2012 American Heart Association, Inc.)*

admissions due to heart failure decompensations.[148] The true mechanism is still elusive but is thought to revolve around sodium and fluid retention.

NSAID-induced CV toxicity should be taken seriously. Patients who have experienced an acute CV event in the past year or at risk for heart failure or hypertension should be prescribed with caution or avoided altogether. Reevaluation for efficacy, appropriate dosing, and need for continual administration should be considered on a regular basis by prescribers. With appropriate monitoring, use of the lowest effective dose, and for the shortest duration necessary, patient safety will be optimized.

Allergy and Hypersensitivity

All NSAIDs hypersensitivity (NHS) reactions occur in two general forms. One syndrome is characterized by asthmatic at-

tacks in patients with vasomotor rhinitis, nasal polyposis, and bronchial asthma. It is estimated to occur in 4.3% to 11% of asthmatics.[149] The second includes a syndrome of urticaria and angioedema, occurring in 27% to 35% of patients with chronic urticaria.[150] PGE_2 is a bronchodilator that stabilizes histamine stores in mastocytes and thus helps to inhibit the inflammatory response.[151] In a susceptible person, the result of the inhibition of PG biosynthesis may be spontaneous degranulation of mastocytes with release of histamine in the respiratory tract and skin, leading to bronchoconstriction and asthma as well as urticaria called syndrome called Samter's triad which is COX-1 mediated. Therefore, COX-2 selective NSAIDs may be safely administered to these patients. Other mechanisms have been postulated which include T cell activation, oxidative stress, and platelet activation as causes for the phenotypic response seen in NHS.[152]

As mentioned previously, our general recommendation is to use any NSAID for the shortest time and at the lowest dose that is clinically appropriate. For many patients with chronic, painful, inflammatory disorders, long-term NSAID therapy continues to present a favorable risk-to-benefit ratio.

Gastrointestinal Toxicity

The first evidence that aspirin could damage the stomach was reported in 1938 based on endoscopic observations.[153] In the 1950s and 1960s, case-control studies demonstrated NSAID-associated melena. NSAIDs cause hemorrhagic gastric erosions in the corpus and antrum. The mortality rate attributed to NSAID-related GI toxicity is 0.22% per year with an annual relative risk of 4.21. An estimated that 16,500 NSAID-related deaths occur due to gastric complications, which is similar to the number from acquired immunodeficiency syndrome (16,685) and exceeds the number deaths due to multiple myeloma and asthma. Risk factors identified for the development of NSAID-induced ulcers include advanced age, history of ulcer, concomitant use of corticosteroids, higher doses of NSAIDs including the use of more than one NSAID, concomitant administration of anticoagulation, serious systemic disorder, cigarette smoking, consumption of alcohol, and concomitant infection with *Helicobacter pylori*.

The mechanisms by which NSAIDs cause ulceration in the stomach are contact irritation of the epithelium and suppression of PG synthesis.[154] NSAID-induced gastropathy correlates with the time and dose for gastric PG suppression.[155] Inhibition of PG synthesis reduces the gastric mucosa ability to defend itself against luminal irritants because bicarbonate secretions, blood flow, and epithelial cell turnover are influenced by PG. Gastric bleeding from preexisting ulcers can also occur due to NSAID suppression of platelet aggregation.[156] Mediators in the pathway by which decreased PG levels cause gastric irritation and damage have been extensively studied. These include leukotrienes,[157] tumor necrosis factor (TNF)-∝,[158] and neutrophil adherence substances.[158]

NSAID-induced enteropathy has been documented in the small intestine and colon, although the exact mechanism is not fully understood. Various strategies can reduce NSAID gastroenteropathy.[159] Agents used to prevent NSAID-induced ulcers include sucralfate (efficacy controversial), histamine-2 receptor antagonists (famotidine), proton pump inhibitors (omeprazole), and PGs (misoprostol). Enteric-coated and slow-release NSAID dosage forms have not reduced ulcer risk.

NSAID-induced gastric complications prompted development of COX-2 selective agents. Preferential use of those selective agents to minimize gastropathy resulted in increased CV toxicity as mentioned previously, but the COX-2 NSAIDs have lower risk of GI complications. Nonselective NSAIDs increase the risk of GI complications by a factor of 3.7, whereas COX-2 inhibitors increase the risk by a factor of 2.6.[160] This confirms prior studies that suggest use of COX-2 NSAIDs results in an improved and a better GI side effect profile compared to nonselective NSAIDs.[161] The American Gastroenterological Association has strongly recommended concomitant use of histamine-2 receptor antagonists, proton pump inhibitors, or misoprostol in patients chronically receiving NSAIDs.[162] Other authors have provided additional recommendations to consider probiotics in addition to a gastroprotective agent.[135] According to a recent systematic review, the ideal combination to reduce upper GI complications may be a COX-2 inhibitor plus proton pump inhibitor.[163]

Hematologic Effects

NSAIDs inhibit PG formation, and individual PGs have different, sometimes opposing, functions. TXA_2 is a platelet activator and vasoconstrictor, whereas PGI_2 is a platelet inhibitor and vasodilator. Furthermore, activated platelets divert some of their endoperoxides to vascular cells to further provide substrate for PGI_2 formation.[164] Platelet activity results from a balance between PGI_2 effects on endothelium and TX_{A2} effects on platelets. Platelets are especially vulnerable to NSAIDs because, unlike most other cells, platelets cannot regenerate the COX enzyme. Aspirin irreversibly acetylates the COX enzyme and that inhibits platelet aggregation for the 10 to 14 day lifespan of the platelet.[164] Other nonselective NSAIDs reversibly inhibit COX causing only a transient reduction in TX_{A2} formation. As a result, platelet activation inhibition resolves after most of the drug is eliminated.[164] A single 300- to 900-mg dose of ibuprofen can inhibit platelet aggregation for 2 hours after administration, and the effect is largely dissipated by 24 hours.[165] Similarly, both sulindac and diclofenac also inhibit platelet aggregation for less than 24 hours. The antiplatelet effects of long-acting NSAIDs such as piroxicam can last for several days after the drug is discontinued.[166] Overall, non-aspirin NSAIDs cause "transient, dose-dependent, and modest bleeding time abnormalities," which often do not exceed normal limits.[164]

Although in vitro studies examining the effect of NSAIDs on platelet function provide useful information, the clinical effect in patients is more important. The test primarily used to assess platelet function is bleeding time, but this test is largely operator-dependent and subject to technical artifact. In addition, its clinical utility as a preoperative tool for predicting intraoperative bleeding remains controversial. Studies show variable effects of NSAIDs on bleeding. In one total hip arthroplasty study, 140 patients taking NSAIDs had more intraoperative and postoperative blood loss than those who did not.[167] Unbalanced biosynthesis of PGI_2 and TXA_2 may also play a role in atherogenesis and thrombosis. By inhibiting PGI_2, blood pressure increases which initiates early development of atherosclerosis and the architectural and functional response of blood vessels to stress. These effects predispose individuals to an exaggerated thrombotic response upon rupture of an atherosclerotic plaque.[168] Aspirin and nonselective NSAIDs suppress both COX-1 and COX-2 and therefore reduce both TXA_2 and PGI_2. In contrast, COX-2 selective NSAIDs suppress PGI_2 production without affecting TXA_2 synthesis.[169] Some authors posit that this may increase acute MI risk that has been observed with prolonged use of some of the COX-2 selective agents.

There are differences between individual NSAIDs and their ability to promote GI complications, largely due to COX-1 and COX-2 selectivity. NSAIDs with greater COX-1 activity have higher relative risks of GI complications; an exact dosage where risk increases remains ill defined. Using lower doses appears to result in fewer GI side effects; however, the efficacy of using the drugs may be lost.[170] The duration of therapy is another consideration; what we know is that gastroduodenal bleeding can occur very soon after initiation of NSAID therapy in patients with a history of upper GI ulcers.[171] Additionally, patients with a history of *H. pylori* infection may be at increased risk for developing peptic ulcers.[172] At present, we lack an ideal NSAID; however, there are thoughts that NSAIDs that target microsomal PGE_2 synthase 1 or those that contain nitric oxide donor groups may provide analgesia while sparing GI side effects (Fig. 78.6).[173]

Renal Toxicity

Aspirin and all other NSAIDs can transiently decrease renal function. This effect may occur more often in patients with chronic kidney disease (CKD).[169] The postulated mechanism is the inhibition of the renal PG synthesis, which may be important in the autoregulation of renal blood flow. Aspirin may also block the diuretic effect of spironolactone by inhibiting its binding to the tubular-cell receptor.

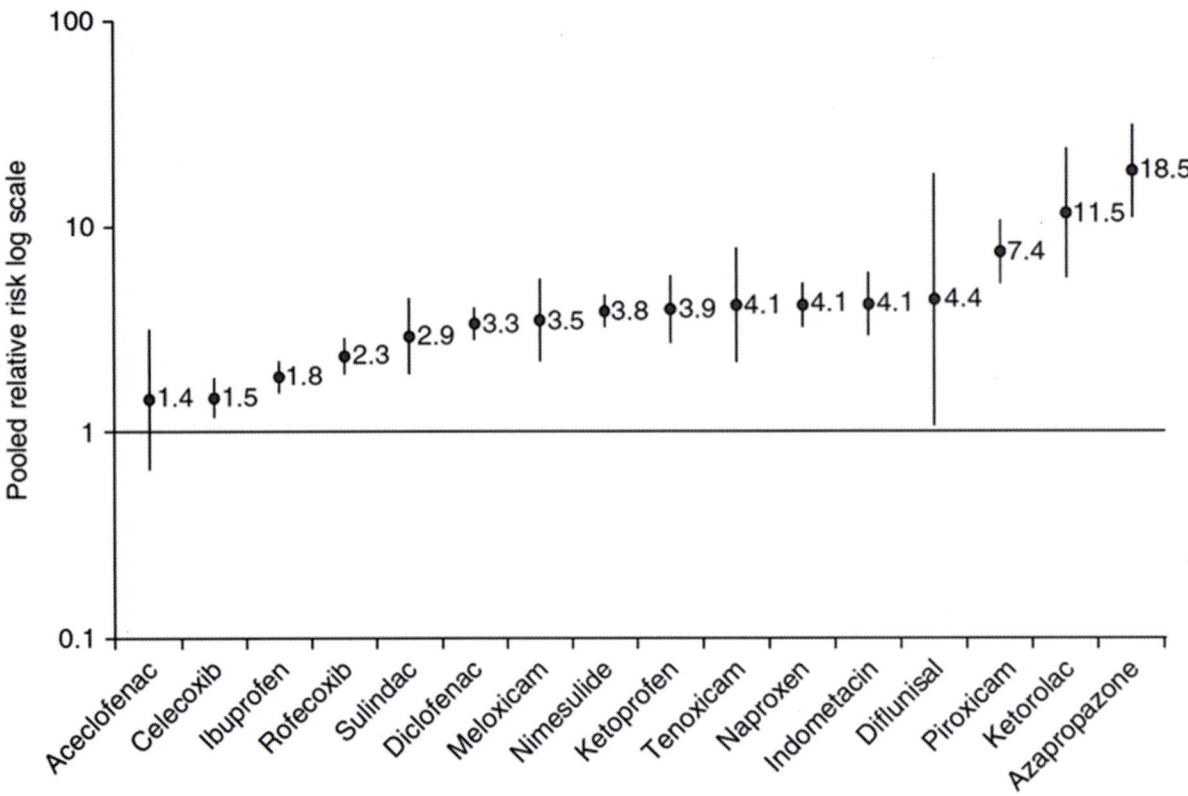

FIGURE 78.6 Nonsteroidal anti-inflammatory drugs. *(Reprinted by permission from Springer: Castellsague J, Riera-Guardia N, Calingaert B, et al. Individual NSAIDs and upper gastrointestinal complications: a systematic review and meta-analysis of observational studies [the SOS project]. Drug Saf 2012;35[12]:1127–1146. Copyright © 2012 Springer International Publishing AG.)*

The renal profile of NSAIDs appears related to sodium retention which is COX-2 inhibition–mediated, and GFR changes due to inhibition of COX-1/COX-2. All NSAIDs are associated with hypertension and edema. Most of these events are of minor clinical significance with discontinuation rates due to hypertension and edema when used for short term.[174] The majority of cases resolve with discontinuation of therapy, generally seen between 1 and 8 weeks. The risk factors for NSAID-induced renal toxicity include the following: chronic NSAID use, multiple NSAID use, dehydration, volume depletion, congestive heart failure, vascular disease, hyperreninemia, shock, sepsis, systemic lupus erythematosus, hepatic disease, sodium depletion, nephrotic syndrome, diuresis, concomitant drug therapy (diuretics, ACE inhibitors, β-blockers, potassium supplements), and age 60 years or older.[169] It should be noted that long-term, regular use of NSAIDs in the absence of risk factors has not been associated with the development of chronic renal impairment.[175]

Some authors have advocated that short-term use of NSAIDs is advisable in patients with stage 1 or 2 CKD. More caution should be exercised in patients with stage 3. In stage 4 or 5 CKD, they should avoided altogether.[176] In those with end-stage renal disease, it is recommended to avoid NSAIDs as the uremic effect on platelets combined with NSAID-induced platelet dysfunction promotes hemorrhage from the GI tract.[177]

Hepatic Toxicity

It has long been known that the cytochrome pathway of metabolism of acetaminophen in the liver can lead to development of N-acetyl-P-benzoquinoneimine (NAPQI) when glutathione stores are low. Patients with liver disease demonstrate prolonged acetaminophen half-life and reduced plasma clearance. However, cytochrome activity is not increased, and glutathione stores remain adequate negating the development of NAPQI.[178] As a result, some authors have made the recommendation that acetaminophen is safe in patients with liver cirrhosis at reduced doses.[179] Given that the FDA recommendations for maximum daily dose is 3 g per day, 2 g per day has been suggested.

NSAIDs are metabolized by the cytochrome system in the liver and are highly protein-bound, >95% to albumin. Cirrhotic patients are sensitive to PG inhibition, which leads to decrease in GFR and increased sodium retention. The constellation of downstream effects reduces kidney perfusion and potentially hepatorenal syndrome, which is often fatal.[179] Advanced liver disease is also associated with thrombocytopenia and coagulopathy leading to spontaneous hemorrhage. NSAIDs compound the problem by inducing platelet dysfunction as mentioned previously. Cirrhotic patients should not receive NSAIDs.

Central Nervous System Effects

Direct toxic reactions are of several types. Tinnitus or deafness are often early warning signs of toxicity. Toxic manifestations are directly related to free drug levels, and those vary inversely with albumin levels. The adverse event is typically reversed when the dose is reduced or discontinued. NSAIDs are the most frequently implicated drugs in hypersensitivity-induced aseptic meningitis. Ibuprofen, sulindac, tolmetin, and naproxen have been implicated in causing drug-induced aseptic meningitis. Patients typically complain of fever, headache, and stiff neck that generally commences within weeks of beginning therapy.[180]

Stages Of Chronic Kidney Disease	
Stage	Glomerular Filtration Rate
1	≥90
2	60–90
3	30–59
4	15–29
5	<15 or receiving dialysis

Surgical Complications

Adverse effects of NSAIDs go beyond the package inserts as complications from surgical procedures can be increased by these medications. One such complication is anastomotic leakage following colon surgery. Three observational studies have shown an increased incidence of anastomotic failure following colonic and/or rectal anastomosis.[181] The exact mechanism is unclear; however, a reduction in leukocyte migration resulting in infection at the site of the anastomosis has been postulated.

Impaired bone healing is another potential drawback to NSAID use. Bone healing can occur in two ways. Natural fracture healing begins with a cartilage callus around the fracture site, ultimately being replaced with bone. This process is called endochondral ossification. The second method is called intramembranous ossification (or primary bone healing), such as that in total joint arthroplasties does not appear to be related to NSAID use. COX-2 appears to be involved, as animal models without COX-1 activity do not have this problem.[182] Proposed mechanisms of this phenomenon that leads to delayed or incomplete bone union may be due to multiple downstream effects of NSAIDs. PGs stimulate osteoblast activity, lure mesenchymal cells to sites of bone injury, and stimulate angiogenesis, which is necessary for endochondral ossification.[183] Additionally, inhibition of COX-2 also prevents terminal differentiation of chondrocytes in fracture callus.[184] Current opinions suggest that in the setting of primary bone healing, a short course of NSAIDs is probably safe in the absence of other risk factors for delayed union.[185]

Delay of tendon-to-bone healing has also been suggested, but currently, clinical evidence is lacking. Lastly, soft tissue healing appears to be unaffected by NSAIDs.[186]

Conclusion

NSAIDs are important drugs that provide excellent analgesic, antipyretic, and anti-inflammatory effects and can be especially useful as part of a multimodal regimens for acute and chronic pain. Acetaminophen does much of the same but lacks clinically useful anti-inflammatory activity. For patients without recent MI, a history of NSAID-exacerbated respiratory disease or asthma, renal insufficiency, cirrhosis of the liver, or iatrogenic or inherited coagulopathy, a short-course of NSAIDs appears to be safe. Long-term prescribing requires critical evaluation of the patient's risk factors for developing adverse events and routine monitoring. Equally important, patients must be apprised of the risks, benefits, and alternatives of NSAID therapy.

DEDICATION

Art was a dear friend and colleague. His patience, guidance, and contributions to this field will be long remembered. It is with heavy hearts and fond memories that we dedicate this piece of work to his memory.

—Adam and Kumar

References

1. EvaluatePharma. *World Preview 2015, Outlook to 2020*. Available at: http://www.evaluategroup.com. Accessed September 9, 2016.
2. Park JY, Pillinger MH, Abramson SB. Prostaglandin E2 synthesis and secretion: the role of PGE2 synthases. *Clin Immunol* 2006;119:229–240.
3. Samad TA, Sapirstein A, Woolf CJ. Prostanoids and pain: unraveling mechanisms and revealing therapeutic targets. *Trends Mol Med* 2002;8:390–396.
4. Cashman J, McAnulty G. Nonsteroidal anti-inflammatory drugs in perisurgical pain management: mechanisms of action and rationale for optimum use. *Drugs* 1995;49:51–70.
5. Ferreira SH, Vane JR. New aspects of the mode of action of non-steroidal anti-inflammatory drugs. *Annu Rev Pharmacol* 1974;14:57–73.
6. Ferreira SH. Prostaglandins, aspirin-like drugs and analgesia. *Nat New Biol* 1972;240:200–203.
7. Gerritsen ME, Cheli CD. Arachidonic acid and prostaglandin endoperoxide metabolism in isolated rabbit and coronary microvessels and isolated and cultivated coronary microvessel endothelial cells. *J Clin Invest* 1983;72:1658–1671.
8. Giuliano F, Warner TD. Origins of prostaglandins E2: involvement of cyclooxygenase (COX)-1 and COX-2 in human and rat systems. *J Pharmacol Ther* 2002;303:1001–1006.
9. Higgs GA. Arachidonic acid metabolism, pain and hyperalgesia: the mode of action of non-steroid mild analgesics. *Br J Pharmacol* 1980;10:233S–235S.
10. Dray A, Bevan S. Inflammation and hyperalgesia: the team effort. *Trends Pharm Sci* 1993;14:287–290.
11. Mancini JA, Blood K, Guay J, et al. Cloning, expression, and up-regulation of inducible rat prostaglandin E synthase during lipopolysaccharide-induced pyresis and adjuvant-induced arthritis. *J Biol Chem* 2001;276:4469–4475.
12. Jakobsson PJ, Morgenstern R, Mancini J, et al. Common structural features of MAPEG—a widespread superfamily of membrane associated proteins with highly divergent functions in eicosanoid and glutathione metabolism. *Protein Sci* 1999;8:689–692.
13. O'Banion MK, Sadowski HB, Winn V, et al. A serum and glucocorticoid-regulated 4-kilobase mRNA encodes a cyclooxygenase-related protein. *J Biol Chem* 1991;266:23261–23267.
14. Smith WL, DeWitt DL, Garavito RM, et al. Cyclooxygenases: structural, cellular biology. *Annu Rev Biochem* 2000;69:145–182.
15. Kraemer SA, Meade EA, DeWitte DL. Prostaglandin endoperoxide synthase gene structure: identification of the transcriptional start site and 5' flanking regulatory sequences. *Arch Biochem Biophys* 1992;293:391–400.
16. O'Banion MK. Cyclooxygenase-2: molecular biology, pharmacology and neurobiology. *Crit Rev Neurobiol* 1999;13:45–82.
17. Yaksh TL, Dirig DM, Conway CM, et al. The acute antihyperalgesic action of nonsteroidal, ant-inflammatory drugs and release of spinal prostaglandin E2 is mediated by the inhibition of constitutive spinal cyclooxygenase-2 (COX-2) but not COX-1. *J Neurosci* 2001;21:5847–5853.
18. Chandrasekharan NV, Dai H, Roos KL, et al. COX-3, a cyclooxygenase-1 variant inhibited by acetaminophen and other analgesic/antipyretic drugs: cloning, structure and expression. *Proc Natl Acad Sci U S A* 2002;99:13926–13931.
19. Qin N, Zhang SP, Reitz TL, et al. Cloning, expression and functional characterization of human cyclooxygenase-1 splicing variants: evidence for intron 1 retention. *J Pharmacol Exp Ther* 2005;315:1298–1305.
20. Vane JR. The mode of action of aspirin and similar compounds. *J Allergy Clin Immunol* 1976;58:691–712.
21. Kroin JS, Buvanendran A, McCarthy RJ, et al. Cyclooxygenase-2 (COX-2) inhibitor potentiates morphine antinociception at the spinal level in a post-operative pain model. *Reg Anesth Pain Med* 2002;27:451–455.
22. Dai YQ, Jin DZ, Zhu XZ, et al. Triptolide inhibits COX-2 expression via NF-kappa B pathway in astrocytes. *Neurosci* 2006;55:154–160.
23. Samad TA, Moore KA, Sapirstein A, et al. Interleukin-1beta mediated induction of COX-2 in the CNS contributes inflammatory pain hypersensitivity. *Nature* 2001;410:471–475.
24. Laflamme N, Lacroix S, Rivest S. An essential role of interleukin-1beta in mediating NF-kappaB activity and COX-2 transcription in cells of the blood-brain barrier in response to a systemic and localized inflammation but not during endotoxemia. *J Neurosci* 1999;9:10923–10930.
25. Buvanendran A, Kroin JS, Berger RA, et al. Up-regulation of prostaglandin E$_2$ and interleukins in the central nervous system and peripheral tissue during and after surgery in humans. *Anesthesiology* 2006;104:403–410.
26. Kroin JS, Ling ZD, Buvanendran A, et al. Upregulation of spinal cyclooxygenase-2 in rats after surgical incision. *Anesthesiology* 2004;100:364–369.
27. Dembo G, Park SB, Kharasch ED. Central nervous system concentration of cyclooxygenase-2 inhibitors in humans. *Anesthesiology* 2005;102:409–415.
28. Buvanendran A, Kroin JS, Tuman KJ, et al. Cerebrospinal fluid and plasma pharmacokinetics of the cyclooxygenase 2 inhibitor rofecoxib in humans: single and multiple oral drug administration. *Anesth Analg* 2005;100:1320–1324.
29. Bartfai T. Immunology telling the brain about pain. *Nature* 2001;410:425–427.
30. Bonati M, Kanto J, Tognoni G. Clinical pharmacokinetics of cerebrospinal fluid. *Clin Pharmacokinet* 1982;7:312.
31. Gaucher A, Netter P, Faure G, et al. Diffusion of oxyphenbutazone into synovial fluid, synovial tissue, joint cartilage and cerebrospinal fluid. *J Clin Pharmacol* 1982;25:107–112.
32. Bannwarth B, Netter P, Pourel J, et al. Clinical pharmacokinetics of nonsteroidal anti-inflammatory drugs in the cerebrospinal fluid. *Biomed Pharmacother* 1989;43:121–126.
33. Netter P, Lapicque F, Bannwarth B, et al. Diffusion of intramuscular ketoprofen into the cerebrospinal fluid. *Eur J Clin Pharmacol* 1985;29:319–321.
34. Cooke AR, Hunt JN. Relationship between pH and absorption of acetylsalicylic acid from the stomach. *Gut* 1969;10:77–78.
35. Eller MG, Wright C III, Della-Coletta AA. Absorption kinetics of rectally and orally administered ibuprofen. *Biopharm Drug Dispos* 1989;10:269–278.
36. Tramèr M, Williams J, Carroll D, et al. Comparing analgesic efficacy of non-steroidal anti-inflammatory drugs given by different routes for acute and chronic pain. *Acta Anaesth Scand* 1998;42:71–79.
37. Moore RA. Topical nonsteroidal anti-inflammatory drugs are effective in osteoarthritis of the knee. *J Rheumatol* 2004;31:1893–1895.
38. Lin J, Zhang W, Jones A, et al. Efficacy of topical nonsteroidal anti-inflammatory drugs in the treatment of osteoarthritis: meta-analysis of randomized controlled trials. *BMJ* 2004;329:324.
39. Galer BS. Topical NSAIDs not created equal—understanding topical analgesic drug formulations. *Pain* 2008;139:237–238.

40. Drover DR, Hammer GB, Anderson BJ. The pharmacokinetics of ketorolac after single postoperative intranasal administration in adolescent patients. *Anesth Analg* 2012;114:1270–1276.

41. Bullingham R, Juan A. Comparison of intranasal ketorolac tromethamine pharmacokinetics in younger and older adults. *Drugs Aging* 2012;29:899–904.

42. Evans AM, Hussein Z, Rowland M. Influence of albumin on the distribution and elimination kinetics of diclofenac in the isolated perfused rat liver: analysis by the impulse-response technique and the dispersion model. *J Pharm Sci* 1993;82:421–428.

43. Soren A. Kinetics of salicylates in blood and joint fluid. *J Clin Pharmacol* 1957;15:173–177.

44. Mäkelä AL, Lempiäinen M, Ylijoki H. Ibuprofen levels in serum and synovial fluid. *Scand J Rheumatol Suppl* 1981;39:15–17.

45. Fowler PD, Shadforth MF, Crook PR, et al. Plasma and synovial fluid concentrations of diclofenac sodium and its major hydroxylated metabolites during long-term treatment of rheumatoid arthritis. *Eur J Clin Pharmacol* 1983;25:389–394.

46. Davies NM, Skjodt NM. Choosing the right nonsteroidal anti-inflammatory drug for the right patient: a pharmacokinetic approach. *Clin Pharmacokinet* 2000;38:377–392.

47. Gibaldi M. Drug distribution in renal failure. *Am J Med* 1977;62:471–474.

48. Verbeeck RK. Pathophysiologic factors affecting the pharmacokinetics of nonsteroidal anti-inflammatory drugs. *J Rheumatol Suppl* 1988;17:44–57.

49. Cook ME, Wallin JD, Thakur VD. Comparative effects of nabumetone, sulindac, and ibuprofen on renal function. *J Rheumatol* 1997;24:1137–1144.

50. Menkes CJ. Renal and hepatic effects of NSAIDs in the elderly. *Scand J Rheumatol Suppl* 1989;83:11–13.

51. Levy G. Clinical pharmacokinetics of aspirin. *Pediatrics* 1978;62:867–872.

52. Flower RJ. Drugs which inhibit prostaglandin biosynthesis. *Pharmacol Rev* 1974;26:33–67.

53. Farrell G, ed. Liver disease produced by nonsteroidal anti-inflammatory drugs. In: *Drug-Induced Liver Disease*. Edinburgh: Churchill Livingstone; 1994:371.

54. Huskisson EC, Williams TN, Shaw LD, et al. Diflunisal in general practice. *Curr Med Res Opin* 1978;5:589–592.

55. Duggan DE, Hogans AF, Kwan KC, et al. The metabolism of indomethacin in man. *J Pharmacol Exp Ther* 1972;181:563–575.

56. Wood LJ, Mundo F, Searle J, et al. Sulindac hepatotoxicity: effects of acute and chronic exposure. *Aust N Z J Med* 1985;15:397–401.

57. Huskisson EC, Franchimont P, eds. Clinoril in the treatment of rheumatic disorders. In: *Proceedings of a symposium held at the 8th European Rheumatology Congress, Helsinki, Finland, 1–7 June 1975*. New York: Raven Press; 1976.

58. Quintero E, Ginés P, Arroyo V, et al. Sulindac reduces the urinary excretion of prostaglandins and impairs renal function in cirrhosis with ascites. *Nephron* 1986;42:298–303.

59. Grindel JM, Migdalof BH, Plostnieks J. Absorption and excretion of tolmetin in arthritic patient. *Clin Pharmacol Ther* 1979;26:122–128.

60. Pena M. Etodolac analgesic effects in musculoskeletal and postoperative pain. *Rheumatol Int* 1990;10:9–16.

61. Schattenkirchner M. An updated safety profile of etodolac in several thousand patients. *Eur J Rheumatol Inflamm* 1990;10:56–65.

62. Forbes JA, Kehm CJ, Grodin CD, et al. Evaluation of ketorolac, ibuprofen, acetaminophen, and an acetaminophen-codeine combination in postoperative oral surgery pain. *Pharmacotherapy* 1990;10:94S–105S.

63. Gills JC, Brogden RN. Ketorolac. A reappraisal of its pharmacodynamics and pharmacokinetic properties and therapeutic use in pain management. *Drugs* 1997;53:139–188.

64. Toradol IV/IM [Package insert]. Nutley, NJ: Roche Laboratories; 1994.

65. Gordon SM, Brahim JS, Rowan J, et al. Peripheral prostanoid levels and nonsteroidal anti-inflammatory drug analgesia: replicate clinical trials in a tissue injury model. *Clin Pharmacol Ther* 2002;72:175–183.

66. Rice ASC, Lloyd J, Bullingham RE, et al. Ketorolac penetration into the cerebrospinal fluid of humans. *J Clin Anesth* 1993;5:459–462.

67. Stouten E, Armbruster S, Houmes RJ, et al. Comparison of ketorolac and morphine for postoperative pain after major surgery. *Acta Anaesthesiol Scand* 1992;36:716–721.

68. Greer I. Effects of ketorolac tromethamine on hemostasis. *Pharmacotherapy* 1990;10:71S–76S.

69. Stephens DM. Is ketorolac safe to use in plastic surgery? A critical review. *Aesthet Surg J* 2015;35:462–466.

70. Strom BL, Berlin JA, Kinman JL, et al. Parenteral ketorolac and risk of gastrointestinal and operating site bleeding. A postmarketing surveillance study. *JAMA* 1996;275:376–382.

71. Choo V, Lewis S. Ketorolac doses reduced. *Lancet* 1993;342:109.

72. Severino FB, Sinatra RS, Paige D, et al. The efficacy of intramuscular ketorolac in combination with intravenous PCA morphine for postoperative pain relief. *J Clin Anesth* 1992;4:285–288.

73. Reuben SS, Connelly NR, Lurie S, et al. Dose-response of ketorolac as an adjunct to patient-controlled analgesia morphine in patients after spinal fusion surgery. *Anesth Analg* 1998;93:98–102.

74. Quadir M, Zia H, Needham TE. Development and evaluation of nasal formulation of ketorolac. *Drug Deliv* 2000;7:223–229.

75. Vyas TK, Shahiwala A, Marathe S, et al. Intranasal drug delivery for brain targeting. *Curr Drug Deliv* 2005;2:165–175.

76. Garnock-Jones KP. Intranasal ketorolac: for short-term pain management. *Clin Drug Investig* 2012;32:361–371.

77. Kroin JS, Li J, Moric M, et al. Local infiltration of analgesics at surgical wound to reduce postoperative pain after laparotomy in rats. *Reg Anesth Pain Med* 2016;41:691–695.

78. Elmquist WF, Chan KK, Sawchuk RJ. Transsynovial drug distribution: synovial mean transit time of diclofenac and other nonsteroidal antiinflammatory drugs. *Pharm Res* 1994;11:1689–1697.

79. Chan KK, Vyas KH, Brandt KD. In vitro protein binding of diclofenac sodium in plasma and synovial fluid. *J Pharm Sci* 1987;76:105–108.

80. Morgan GJ, Poland M, DeLapp RE. Efficacy and safety of nabumetone versus diclofenac, naproxen, ibuprofen, and piroxicam in the elderly. *Am J Med* 1993;9:19S–27S.

81. Davies NM, Anderson KE. Clinical pharmacokinetics of diclofenac. Therapeutic insights and pitfalls. *Clin Pharmacokinet* 1997;33:184–213.

82. Gan TJ, Daniels SE, Singla N, et al. A novel injectable formulation of diclofenac compared with intravenous ketorolac or placebo for acute moderate-to-severe pain after abdominal or pelvic surgery: a multicenter, double-blind, randomized, multiple-dose study. *Anesth Analg* 2012;115:1212–1220.

83. Christensen K, Daniels S, Bandy D, et al. A double-blind placebo-controlled comparison of a novel formulation of intravenous diclofenac and ketorolac for postoperative third molar extraction pain. *Anesth Prog* 2011;58:73–81.

84. Daniels S, Melson T, Hamilton DA, et al. Analgesic efficacy and safety of a novel injectable formulation of diclofenac compared with intravenous ketorolac and placebo after orthopedic surgery: a multicenter, randomized, double-blinded, multiple-dose trial. *Clin J Pain* 2013;29:655–663.

85. Bauer KA, Gerson W, Wright C IV, et al. Platelet function following administration of a novel formulation of intravenous diclofenac sodium versus active comparators: a randomized, single dose, crossover study in healthy male volunteers. *J Clin Anesth* 2010;22:510–518.

86. Voltaren Gel [Package insert]. Parsippany, NJ: Novartis AG; 2009.

87. Flector [Package insert]. Mission, KS: Pfizer; 2016.

88. Derry S, Moore RA, Gaskell H, et al. Topical NSAIDs for acute musculoskeletal pain in adults. *Cochrane Database Syst Rev* 2015;(6):CD007402.

89. Alessandri F, Lijoi D, Mistrangelo E, et al. Topical diclofenac patch for postoperative would pain in laparoscopic gynecologic surgery: a randomized study. *J Min Invav Surg* 2006;13:195–200.

90. Derry S, Conaghan P, Da Silva JA, et al. Topical NSAIDs for chronic musculoskeletal pain in adults. *Cochrane Database Syst Rev* 2016;(4):CD007400.

91. Miller L. Oxaprozin: a once-daily nonsteroidal anti-inflammatory drug. *Clin Pharm* 1992;11:591–603.

92. Brooks CD, Schlagel CA, Sekhar NC, et al. Tolerance and pharmacology of ibuprofen. *Curr Ther Res* 1973;15:180–181.

93. Mann JF, Goerig M, Brune K, et al. Ibuprofen as an over-the-counter drug: is there a risk for renal injury? *Clin Nephrol* 1993;39:1–6.

94. Catella-Lawson F, Reilly MP, Kapoor SC, et al. Cyclooxygenase inhibitors and the antiplatelet effect of aspirin. *N Engl J Med* 2001;345:1809–1817.

95. Atkinson TJ, Fudin J, Jahn HL, et al. What's new in NSAID pharmacotherapy: oral agents to injectables. *Pain Med* 2013;14(suppl 1):S11–S17.

96. Geisslinger G, Menzel S, Wissel K, et al. Pharmacokinetics of ketoprofen enantiomers after different doses of the racemate. *Br J Clin Pharmacol* 1995;40:73–75.

97. Mazieres B. Topical ketoprofen patch. *Drugs* 2005;6:337–344.

98. Gruber CM Jr. Clinical pharmacology of fenoprofen: a review. *J Rheumatol* 1976;2:8–17.

99. Ryley NJ, Lingam G. A pharmacokinetic comparison of controlled-release and standard naproxen tablets. *Curr Med Res Opin* 1988;11:10–15.

100. Sevelius H, Segre E, Bursick K. Comparative analgesic effects of naproxen sodium, aspirin, and placebo. *J Clin Pharmacol* 1980;20:480–485.

101. Davies NM. Clinical pharmacokinetics of oxaprozin. *Clin Pharmacokinet* 1998;35:425–436.

102. Kean WF. Oxaprozin: kinetic and dynamic profile in the treatment of pain. *Curr Med Res Opin* 2004;20:1275–1277.

103. Heller B, Tarricone R. Oxaprozin versus diclofenac in NSAID-refractory periarthritis of the shoulder. *Curr Med Res Opin* 2004;20:1279–1290.

104. Kurowski M, Thabe H. The transsynovial distribution of oxaprozin. *Agents Actions* 1989;27:458–460.

105. Dallegri F, Bertolotto M, Ottonello L, et al. A review of the emerging profile of the anti-inflammatory drug oxaprozin. *Expert Opin Pharmacother* 2005;6:777–785.

106. Caldwell JR. Comparison of the efficacy, safety, and pharmacokinetic profiles of extended-release ketoprofen and piroxicam in patients with rheumatoid arthritis. *Clin Ther* 1994;16:222–235.

107. Fleischmann R, Iqbal I, Slobodin G. Meloxicam. *Expert Opin Pharmacother* 2003;3:1501–1512.

108. Vidal L, Kneer W, Baturone M, et al. Meloxicam in acute episodes of soft tissue rheumatism of the shoulder. *Inflamm Res* 2001;50:S24–S29.

109. Gates BJ, Nguyen TT, Setter SM, et al. Meloxicam: a reappraisal of pharmacokinetics, efficacy and safety. *Expert Opin Pharmacother* 2005;6:2117–2140.

110. Kessenich C. Cyclooxygenase 2 inhibitors: an important new drug classification. *Pain Manag Nurs* 2001;2:13–18.

111. Leese PT, Hubbard RC, Karim A, et al. Effects of celecoxib, a novel cyclooxygenase-2 inhibitor, on platelet function in healthy adults: a randomized, controlled trial. *J Clin Pharmacol* 2000;40:124–132.

112. Singh G, Fort JG, Goldstein JL, et al. Celecoxib versus naproxen and diclofenac in osteoarthritis patients: SUCCESS-I study. *Amer J Med* 2006;119:255–266.

113. Silverstein FE, Faich G, Goldstein JL, et al. Gastrointestinal toxicity with celecoxib vs nonsteroidal anti-inflammatory drugs for osteoarthritis and rheumatoid arthritis: the CLASS study: a randomized controlled trial. Celecoxib Long-term Arthritis Safety Study. *JAMA* 2000;284:1247–1255.

114. Etoricoxib [Package insert]. Whitehouse Station, NJ: Merck & Co; 2014.

115. Clark R, Derry S, Moore RA. Single dose oral etoricoxib for acute postoperative pain in adults. *Cochrane Database Syst Rev* 2012;(4):CD004309.

116. Alsalameh S, Burian M, Mahr G, et al. The pharmacological properties and clinical use of valdecoxib, a new cyclo-oxygenase-2 selective inhibitor. *Aliment Pharmacol Ther* 2003;17:489–501.

117. Jain KK. Evaluation of intravenous parecoxib for the relief of acute postsurgical pain. *Expert Opin Invest Drugs* 2000;9:2717–2723.

118. Fenton C, Keating GM, Wagstaff AJ, et al. Valdecoxib: a review of its use in the management of osteoarthritis, rheumatoid arthritis, dysmenorrhoea and acute pain. *Drugs* 2004;64:1231–1261.

119. Lipton JM, Rosenstein J. Thermoregulatory disorders after removal of a craniopharyngioma from the third cerebral ventricle. *Brain Res Bull* 1981;7:369–373.

120. Smith HS. Potential analgesic mechanisms of acetaminophen. *Pain Physician* 2009;12:269–280.

121. Skoglund LA, Skjelbred P, Fyllingen G. Analgesic efficacy of acetaminophen 1000 mg, acetaminophen 2000 mg, and the combination of acetaminophen 1000 mg and codeine phosphate 60 mg versus placebo in acute postoperative pain. *Pharmacotherapy* 1991;11:364–369.

122. Gaziano JM. Nonnarcotic analgesics and hypertension. *Am J Cardiol* 2006;97(9A):10–16.

123. Stewart DM, Dillman RO, Kim HS, et al. Acetaminophen overdose: a growing health care hazard. *Clin Toxicol* 1979;14:507–513.

124. U.S. Food and Drug Administration. FDA Drug Safety Communication: prescription acetaminophen products to be limited to 325 mg per dosage unit; boxed warning will highlight potential for severe liver failure. Available at: https://www.fda.gov/Drugs/DrugSafety/ucm239821.htm. Published January 13, 2011.

125. Douglas DR, Sholar JB, Smilkstein MJ. A pharmacokinetic comparison of acetaminophen products (Tylenol Extended Relief vs regular Tylenol). *Acad Emerg Med* 1996;3:740–744.

126. Steventon GB, Mitchell SC, Waring RH. Human metabolism of paracetamol (acetaminophen) at different dose levels. *Drug Metabol Drug Interact* 1996;13:111–117.

127. Delbos A, Boccard E. The morphine-sparing effect of propacetamol in orthopedic postoperative pain. *J Pain Symptom Manage* 1995;10:279–286.

128. Sinatra RS, Jahr JS, Reynolds LW, et al. Efficacy and safety of single and repeated administration of 1 gram intravenous acetaminophen injection (paracetamol) for pain management after major orthopedic surgery. *Anesthesiology* 2005;102:822–831.

129. Cattabriga L, Pacini D, Lamazza G, et al. Intravenous paracetamol as adjuvant treatment for postoperative pain after cardiac surgery: a double blind randomized controlled trial. *Eur J Cardiothorac Surg* 2007;32:527–531.

130. Apfel CC, Turan A, Souza K, et al. Intravenous acetaminophen reduces postoperative nausea and vomiting: a systematic review and meta-analysis. *Pain* 2013;154:677–689.

131. Blume H, Ali SL, Elze M, et al. Relative bioavailability of paracetamol in suppositories preparations in comparison to tablets [in German]. *Arzneimittelforschung* 1994;44:1333–1338.

132. Peduto VA, Ballabio M, Stefanini S. Efficacy of propacetamol in the treatment of postoperative pain. Morphine-sparing effect in orthopedic surgery. *Acta Anaesthesiol Scand* 1998;42:293–298.

133. Dhillon S. Naproxen/esomeprazole fixed-dose combination: for the treatment of arthritic symptoms and to reduce the risk of gastric ulcers. *Drugs Aging* 2011;28:237–248.

134. Datto C, Hellmund R, Siddiqui MK. Efficacy and tolerability of naproxen/esomeprazole magnesium tablets compared with non-specific NSAIDs and COX-2 inhibitors: a systematic review and network analyses. *Open Access Rheumatol* 2013;26:1–19.

135. Marlicz W, Loniewski I, Grimes DS, et al. Nonsteroidal anti-inflammatory drugs, proton pump inhibitors, and gastrointestinal injury: contrasting interactions in the stomach and small intestine. *Mayo Clinic Proc* 2014;89:1699–1709.

136. Bello AE. DUEXIS® (ibuprofen 800 mg, famotidine 26.6 mg): a new approach to gastroprotection for patients with chronic pain and inflammation who require treatment with a nonsteroidal anti-inflammatory drug. *Ther Adv Musculoskelet Dis* 2012;4:327–339.

137. Singh BK, Haque SE, Pillai KK. Assessment of nonsteroidal anti-inflammatory drug-induced cardiotoxicity. *Expert Opin Drug Metab Toxicol* 2014;10:143–156.

138. Olsen AM, Fosbøl EL, Lindhardsen J, et al. Long-term cardiovascular risk of nonsteroidal anti-inflammatory drug use according to time passed after first-time myocardial infarction: a nationwide cohort study. *Circulation* 2012;126:1955–1963.

139. U.S. Food and Drug Administration. FDA Drug Safety Communication: FDA strengthens warning that non-aspirin nonsteroidal anti-inflammatory

drugs (NSAIDs) can cause heart attacks or strokes. Available at: https://www.fda.gov/Drugs/DrugSafety/ucm451800.htm. Published July 9, 2015.

140. Nissen SE, Yeomans ND, Solomon DH, et al. Cardiovascular safety of celecoxib, naproxen, or ibuprofen for arthritis. *N Engl J Med* 2016;375:2519–2529.

141. Brune K. Diclofenac: increase of myocardial infarctions at low doses? *Pharmacoepidemiol Drug Saf* 2014;23:326–328.

142. White WB, Kent J, Taylor A, et al. Effects of celecoxib on ambulatory blood pressure in hypertensive patients on ACE inhibitors. *Hypertension* 2002;39:929–934.

143. Izhar M, Alausa T, Folker A, et al. Effects of COX inhibition on blood pressure and kidney function in ACE inhibitor-treated blacks and Hispanics. *Hypertension* 2004;43:573–577.

144. Whelton A, White WB, Bello AE, et al. Effects of celecoxib and rofecoxib on blood pressure and edema in patients ≥65 years of age with systemic hypertension and osteoarthritis. *Am J Cardiol* 2002;90:959–963.

145. Forman JP, Stampfer MJ, Curhan GC. Non-narcotic analgesic dose and risk of incident hypertension in US women. *Hypertension* 2005;46:500–507.

146. Forman JP, Rimm EB, Curhan GC. Frequency of analgesic use and risk of hypertension among men. *Arch Intern Med* 2007;167:394–399.

147. Feenstra J, Heerdink ER, Grobbee DE, et al. Association of nonsteroidal anti-inflammatory drugs with first occurrence of heart failure and with relapsing heart failure: the Rotterdam Study. *Arch Intern Med* 2002;162:265–270.

148. Page J, Henry D. Consumption of NSAIDs and the development of congestive heart failure in elderly patients: an underrecognized public health problem. *Arch Intern Med* 2000;160:777–784.

149. Kasper L, Sladek K. Prevalence of asthma with aspirin hypersensitivity in the adult population of Poland. *Allergy* 2003;58:1064–1066.

150. Erbagci Z. Multiple NSAID intolerance in chronic idiopathic urticaria is correlated with delayed, pronounced and prolonged autoreactivity. *J Dermatol* 2004;31:376–382.

151. Szczklik A, Gryglewski RJ, Czerniawska-Mysik G. Clinical patterns of hypersensitivity to nonsteroidal anti-inflammatory drugs and their pathogenesis. *J Allergy Clin Immunol* 1977;60:276–284.

152. Le Pham D, Kim JH, Trinh TH, et al. What we know about nonsteroidal anti-inflammatory drug hypersensitivity. *Korean J Intern Med* 2016;31:417–432.

153. Douthwaite AH, Lintott GAM. Gastroscopic observation of the effect of aspirin and certain other substances on the stomach. *Lancet* 1938;2:1222–1225.

154. Wallace JL, McCafferty DM, Carter L, et al. Tissue-selective inhibition of prostaglandin synthesis in rat by tepoxalin: anti-inflammatory without gastropathy. *Gastrenterology* 1993;105:1630–1636.

155. Lanza FL. A review of gastric ulcer and gastroduodenal injury in normal volunteers receiving aspirin and other nonsteroidal anti-inflammatory drugs. *Scand J Gastroenterol* 1989;24:24–31.

156. Hawkey CJ, Hawthrone AB, Hudson N, et al. Separation of the impairment of haemostasis by aspirin from mucosal injury in the human stomach. *Clin Sci* 1991;81:565–573.

157. Vaananen PM, Keenan CM, Grisham MB, et al. A pharmacological investigation of the role leukotrienes in the pathogenesis of experimental NSAID-gastropathy. *Inflammation* 1992;16:227–240.

158. Santucci L, Fiorucci S, Giansanti M, et al. Pentoxifylline prevents indomethacin induced acute gastric mucosal damage in rats: role of tumour necrosis factor alpha. *Gut* 1994;35:909–915.

159. Wallace JL. Nonsteroidal anti-inflammatory drugs and gastroenteropathy: the second hundred years. *Gastroenterology* 1997;112:1000–1016.

160. García Rodríguez LA, Barreales Tolosa L. Risk of upper gastrointestinal complications among users of traditional NSAIDs and COXIBs in the general population. *Gastroenterology* 2007;132:498–506.

161. Conaghan PG. A turbulent decade for NSAIDs: update on current concepts of classification, epidemiology, comparative efficacy, and toxicity. *Rheumatol Int* 2012;32:1491–502.

162. Lanza PL, Chan FK, Quigley EM. Guidelines for prevention of NSAID-related ulcer complications. *Am J Gastroenterol* 2009;104:728–738.

163. Yuan JQ, Tsoi KK, Yang M, et al. Systematic review with network meta-analysis: comparative effectiveness and safety of strategies for preventing NSAID-associated gastrointestinal toxicity. *Aliment Pharmacol Ther* 2016;43:1262–1275.

164. Schafer A. Effects of nonsteroidal anti-inflammatory drugs on platelet function and systemic hemostasis. *J Clin Pharmacol* 1995;35:209–219.

165. Lind S. The bleeding time does not predict surgical bleeding. *Blood* 1991;77:2547–2552.

166. Weintraub M, Case K, Kroening B. Effects of piroxicam on platelet aggregation. *Clin Pharmacol Ther* 1978;23:134–135.

167. An H, Mikhail W, Jackson W, et al. Effects of hypotensive anesthesia, nonsteroidal anti-inflammatory drugs, and polymethylmethacrylate on bleeding in total hip arthroplasty patients. *J Arthroplasty* 1991;6:245–250.

168. Egan KM, Wang M, Fries S, et al. Cyclooxygenases, thromboxane, and atherosclerosis: plaque destabilization by cyclooxygenase-2 inhibition combined with thromboxane receptor antagonism. *Circulation* 2005;111:334–342.

169. Taber SS, Mueller BA. Drug-associated renal dysfunction. *Crit Care Clin* 2006;22:357–374.

170. McCarberg B, Gibofsky A. Need to develop new nonsteroidal anti-inflammatory drug formulations. *Clin Ther* 2012;34:1954–1963.

171. Takeuchi K, Smale S, Premchand P, et al. Prevalence and mechanism of nonsteroidal anti-inflammatory drug-induced clinical relapse in patients with inflammatory bowel disease. *Clin Gastroenterol Hepatol* 2006;4:196–202.

172. Patricio JP, Barbosa JP, Ramos RM, et al. Relative cardiovascular and gastrointestinal safety of non-selective non-steroidal anti-inflammatory drugs versus cyclo-oxygenase-2 inhibitors: implications for clinical practice. *Clin Drug Investig* 2013;33:167–183.

173. Narsinghani T, Sharma R. Lead optimization on conventional nonsteroidal anti-inflammatory drugs: an approach to reduce gastrointestinal toxicity. *Chem Biol Drug Des* 2014;84:1–23.

174. Barkin RL, Buvanendran A. Focus on the COX-1 and COX-2 agents: renal events of nonsteroidal and anti-inflammatory drugs-NSAIDs. *Am J Ther* 2004;11:124–129.

175. Yaxley J, Liftin T. Non-steroidal anti-inflammatories and the development of analgesic nephropathy: a systematic review. *Ren Fail* 2016;38:1328–1334.

176. Curiel RV, Guzman NJ. Challenges associated with the management of gouty arthritis in patients with chronic kidney disease: a systematic review. *Semin Arthritis Rheum* 2012;42:166–178.

177. O'Connor NR, Corcoran AM. End-stage renal disease: symptom management and advance care planning. *Am Fam Physician* 2012;85:705–710.

178. Imani F, Motavaf M, Safari S, et al. The therapeutic use of analgesics in patients with liver cirrhosis: a literature review and evidence-based recommendations. *Hepat Mon* 2014;14:e23539.

179. Chandok N, Watt K. Pain management in the cirrhotic patient: the clinical challenge. *Mayo Clin Proc* 2010;85:451–458.

180. Marinac J. Drug and chemical-induced aseptic meningitis: a review of the literature. *Ann Pharmacolother* 1992;26:813–822.

181. Rushfeldt CF, Sveinbjørnsson B, Søreide K, et al. Risk of anastomotic leakage with use of NSAIDs after gastrointestinal surgery. *Int J Colorectal Dis* 2011;26:1501–1509.

182. Simon AM, Manigrasso MB, O'Connor JP. Cyclo-oxygenase 2 function is essential for bone fracture healing. *J Bone Miner Res* 2002;17:963–976.

183. Pountos I, Georgouli T, Calori GM, et al. Do nonsteroidal anti-inflammatory drugs affect bone healing? A critical analysis. *ScientificWorldJournal* 2012;2012:606404.

184. Su B, O'Connor JP. NSAID therapy effects on healing of bone, tendon, and the enthesis. *Appl Physiol* 2013;115:892–899.

185. Giannoudis PV, Hak D, Sanders D, et al. Inflammation, bone healing, and anti-inflammatory drugs: an update. *J Orthop Trauma* 2015;29(suppl 12):S6–S9.

186. Chen MR, Dragoo JL. The effect of nonsteroidal anti-inflammatory drugs on tissue healing. *Knee Surg Sports Traumatol Arthrosc* 2013;21:540–549.

CHAPTER 79

Opioid Analgesics

CHARLES E. INTURRISI, DAVID S. CRAIG, and **ARTHUR G. LIPMAN**

Opioid analgesics remain an important component of the multimodality management of moderate to severe acute pain and cancer pain. The use of opioids for chronic noncancer pain has become controversial due to the lack long-term clinical trials designed to provide evidence of the long-term effectiveness and limited reliable data on the safety of long-term opioid use.[1,2] Not every pain patient will benefit from opioid therapy, and more patients benefit from these strong analgesics when the drugs are used as one component of multimodal therapy that includes nonopioid analgesics and nonpharmacologic treatments.[3] The decision to initiate opioid therapy requires a comprehensive evaluation.[4,5] In this chapter, we address the principles that should guide the appropriate use of opioids.[6] During the past 20 years, there has been a dramatic increase in our knowledge of the sites and mechanisms of action of opioids.[7] The development of analytical methods has also been of great importance by facilitating pharmacokinetic studies of the disposition and fate of opioids in patients. These pharmacokinetic studies and recent discoveries about pain and opioid receptor–related genetic polymorphisms have begun to provide a better understanding of some of the sources of interindividual variation in the response to opioids and suggest ways to minimize some of their adverse effects.[6,8] Pain management with or without opioids requires individualization of treatment and one of the next steps in improving opioid therapy depends on identifying phenotypic and genotypic patient characteristics that are associated with better or worse treatment outcomes.[9,10]

The term *analgesic* (from the Greek *an-*, without + *algesis*, sense of pain) refers to a drug that relieves pain without a significant loss of other sensations. *Opioid* (the preferred term) is any compound that binds to an opioid receptor. Opioids include the exogenous opioid receptor agonists, for example, morphine, and antagonists as well as the endogenous opioid peptides (EOPs), for example, endorphins. The term *opiate* originally referred to any drug derived from opium but now includes the natural opium products (e.g., morphine), the semisynthetic derivatives (e.g., hydromorphone), or completely synthetic congeners (e.g., methadone). The term *narcotic* was originally associated with the opioids. It is now used in a legal context to refer to any drug considered to possess abuse or addictive potential. Because it is a value-laden word, avoidance of the term *narcotic* when discussing opioids with patients is often advisable.

Classification Based on Interactions with an Opioid Receptor

Opioid analgesics can be classified based on their interactions with opioid receptors, namely, mu (μ), delta (δ), and kappa (κ). A fourth member of the opioid receptor family is the nociception (NOPr) receptor.[11] μ-Opioid receptor (MOR) agonists (agents that occupy and activate the receptor) are the major source of clinically used opioid agonist partial agonist and antagonist drugs (Table 79.1). Numerous κ-opioid receptor ligands have been developed and studied; three have been commercially available in the United States. The clinical pharmacology of κ agonists is complicated by concurrent MOR antagonist activity (see the following text and Table 79.1). δ-Opioid receptor

(DOR) ligands have been identified in preclinical studies, but currently, none is available for clinical use.

Each of the opioid receptors is a G protein-coupled receptor (GPCR) and signals via a second messenger, cyclic adenosine monophosphate (cAMP), or an ion channel.[7] Alterations in the levels of cAMP and the transcription factor, cAMP response element binding protein (CREB) during chronic morphine treatment, are associated with numerous cellular changes, some of which can lead to the development of tolerance and physical dependence.[12] Molecular genetic approaches have used gene-targeting (knockout) technology to disrupt the gene that codes for each of the three opioid receptors[13] as well as all three receptors simultaneously.[14] Mice that lack the MOR (MOR-deficient mice) do not respond to morphine with analgesia, respiratory depression, constipation, physical dependence, reward behaviors, or immunosuppression.[13] These results confirm and extend previous pharmacologic and receptor binding studies and demonstrate that the μ receptor mediates the analgesic and adverse effects of morphine. Recent advances in techniques for studying these receptors in vivo and in vitro, including splice variant characterization, high-resolution crystallography, Designer Receptors Exclusively Activated by Designer Drugs (DREADD) receptors, and optogenetic approaches, are expanding and transforming our understanding of opioid receptor function.[7,15]

Pharmacologic evaluation of the effects of the microinjection of morphine and other opioids has been combined with anatomic characterization of the distribution of opioid receptors to provide insight into the sites of action of morphine and other clinically used μ-opioids. Thus, MORs are found in the periphery (following inflammation), at pre- and postsynaptic sites in the spinal cord dorsal horn, and in the brain stem, thalamus, and cortex, in what constitutes the ascending pain transmission system (Fig. 79.1A).[16] In addition, MORs are found in the midbrain periaqueductal grey, the nucleus raphe magnus and the rostral ventral medulla where they comprise a descending inhibitory system that modulates spinal cord pain transmission (Fig. 79.1B).[16]

Opioids inhibit GABAergic neurons and remove the tonic inhibition of the pain inhibitory neurons (PIN) that project from the rostral ventral medulla to the spinal cord dorsal horn. Thus, opioids produce a disinhibition of the PIN, which results in the activation of descending inhibition and the descending modulation of pain transmission (Fig. 79.1C).

Using molecular genetic approaches, Bardoni and colleagues[17] have identified circuitry in the spinal cord dorsal horn wherein DOR activation at the central terminals of myelinated mechanoreceptors depresses synaptic input to the spinal cord dorsal horn, via the inhibition of voltage-gated (VG) calcium (CA++) channels. This circuitry may provide a basis for a more rational use of MOR agonists and the design of analgesic strategies that involve targeting the DOR for touch-evoked neuropathic pain and movement or pressure-evoked pain, two major clinical problems.

MORs are also located peripherally, and the development of peripheral μ-opioid antagonists has provided a new class of drugs to manage opioid bowel dysfunction. For example, activation of the high density of MORs in the human colon appears to be a major mechanism of opioid-induced constipation.[18] This has led to the approval and use of methylnaltrexone and naloxegol for managing opioid-induced constipation and alvimopan for postoperative ileus. More recently, lubiprostone, a drug

TABLE 79.1   Opioid Analgesics Commonly Used for Severe Pain

Name	Equianalgesic Parenteral Dose (mg)[a]	Equianalgesic Oral Dose (mg)[b]	Starting Oral Dose Range (mg)[a]	Comments	Precautions
μ (Morphine-like) Agonist Opioids					
Morphine	10	30	15–30	Standard of comparison for opioid analgesics; IR and ER dosage (MS Contin and Kadian)	Those with impaired ventilation, bronchial asthma, increased intracranial pressure, and liver failure; lower doses for elderly
Hydromorphone (Dilaudid)	1.5	7.5	2–4	Slightly shorter acting than morphine (IR formulations); ER dosage (Exalgo)	Like morphine
Methadone (Dolophine)	10	20	2.5–5	Good oral potency; long and variable plasma half-life; NMDA receptor antagonist activity. Rotation dose depends on prior opioid dosage. See text.	Like morphine; LA; may accumulate over 5–7 d with repetitive dosing causing excessive sedation; can prolong QT interval
Levorphanol	—	2	2–4	Like methadone; long plasma half-life; NMDA receptor antagonist activity	Like methadone; LA; may accumulate over 2–3 d)
Oxymorphone (Opana)	1	10	5–10	IR (Opana) and ER (Opana ER) oral dosage	Like morphine. Do not take with food or alcohol
Oxycodone	—	20	5–20	IR (Roxicodone and OxyIR); for ER dosage, see abuse-deterrent formulations in text and table; also in lower doses in fixed combination with nonopioids for less severe or acute pain	Like morphine; concomitant use with CYP 450 3A4 inducers could decrease while CYP 450 3A4 inhibitors can increase effects.
Fentanyl	0.1[c]	—	—	TD (Duragesic); also as oral trans-mucosal dosage forms (Abstral, Actiq, Fentora, Onsolis, and Sub-sys) and a nasal spray (Lazanda) for breakthrough cancer pain	TD creates a tissue reservoir of drug that results in at least a 12-h delay in onset and offset. Fever and other external heat sources increases absorption.
Meperidine, pethidine (Demerol)	75	300	Not recommended	Slightly shorter acting than morphine. Used orally for less severe pain	Normeperidine, a metabolite, accumulates with repetitive dosing causing CNS excitation; not for patients with impaired renal function or receiving monoamine oxidase inhibitors
Codeine	130	300	30–60	Used orally in combination with nonopioids (e.g., acetaminophen) for less severe or acute pain	Like morphine; subject to CYP 450 2D6 polymorphism variability; see text.
Hydrocodone	—	20	2.5–10	Used orally in combination with nonopioids for less severe or acute pain (Vicodin, Lorcet, Lortab, and many others)	Like morphine and codeine
Centrally Acting μ Agonists					
Tramadol (Ultram)	100	150	50–100	Weak μ agonism, significant serotonin reuptake inhibition; a prodrug; IR and ER dosage, also in combination with acetaminophen	Risk of seizures in patients with seizure disorders; serotonin syndrome, avoid TCAs and SSRIs; subject to CYP 450 2D6 polymorphism variability; see text.
Tapentadol (Nucynta)	—	100	50–100	Analgesia appears to be due to modest μ agonism, significant norepinephrine reuptake inhibition, and weaker serotonin reuptake inhibition; IR and ER dosage	Risk of seizures in patients with seizure disorders
Mixed κ Agonist-μ Antagonist Opioids					
Pentazocine (generics only)	—	100	50 (oral dosing) 30–60 (IM dosing)	Used orally for less severe pain; a mixed agonist-antagonist; see precautions; only available orally as naloxone + pentazocine	May cause psychotomimetic effects; may precipitate withdrawal in μ-opioid–dependent patients; not for myocardial infarction pain
Nalbuphine (generics only)	10	- See comments -	10 (IM, SC, or IV dosing)	Not available orally	Incidence of psychotomimetic effects lower than with pentazocine; may precipitate withdrawal in μ-opioid-dependent patients
Butorphanol (generics only)	2	- See comments -	2–4 (IM dosing) 1 (IV or intranasal)	Not available orally (available generically as a nasal spray)	Like nalbuphine

TABLE 79.1	(Continued)				
Name	Equianalgesic Parenteral Dose (mg)[a]	Equianalgesic Oral Dose (mg)[b]	Starting Oral Dose Range (mg)[a]	Comments	Precautions
Partial μ Agonist Opioid					
Buprenorphine	0.13	0.400	0.075–0.300 (buccal film) 0.200–0.400 (sublingual tablet) 0.005 mg/h (TD)	Belbuca (buccal film) 12-h dosing and Temgesic (sublingual tablet) 6- to 8-h dosing (Temgesic not available in the United States) Butrans (TD) 7-d dosing Also used for the treatment of opioid dependence (Suboxone) (naloxone + buprenorphine combination)	May precipitate withdrawal in opioid-dependent patients; not readily reversed by naloxone Long T$_{1/2}$

NOTE: Some of these equianalgesic parenteral doses may be based on studies that used the intramuscular (IM) route, so that in contrast to intravenous (IV) dosing, the time of peak analgesia in nontolerant patients will range from one-half to 1 hour and the duration from 4 to 6 hours. Compared to the IV or IM routes of administration, the peak analgesic effect is delayed and the duration prolonged after oral administration.

[a]These doses are recommended starting parenteral or oral doses from which the optimal dose for each patient is determined by titration and the maximal dose limited by adverse effects.

[b]The equianalgesic oral dose is provided for comparative purposes (see Starting Oral Dose Range column).

[c]See package insert for dosing information.

CNS, central nervous system; ER, extended-release; IR, immediate-release; LA, long-acting; NMDA, N-methyl-D-aspartate; SC, subcutaneous; SSRI, selective serotonin reuptake inhibitor; TCA, tricyclic antidepressant; TD, transdermal.

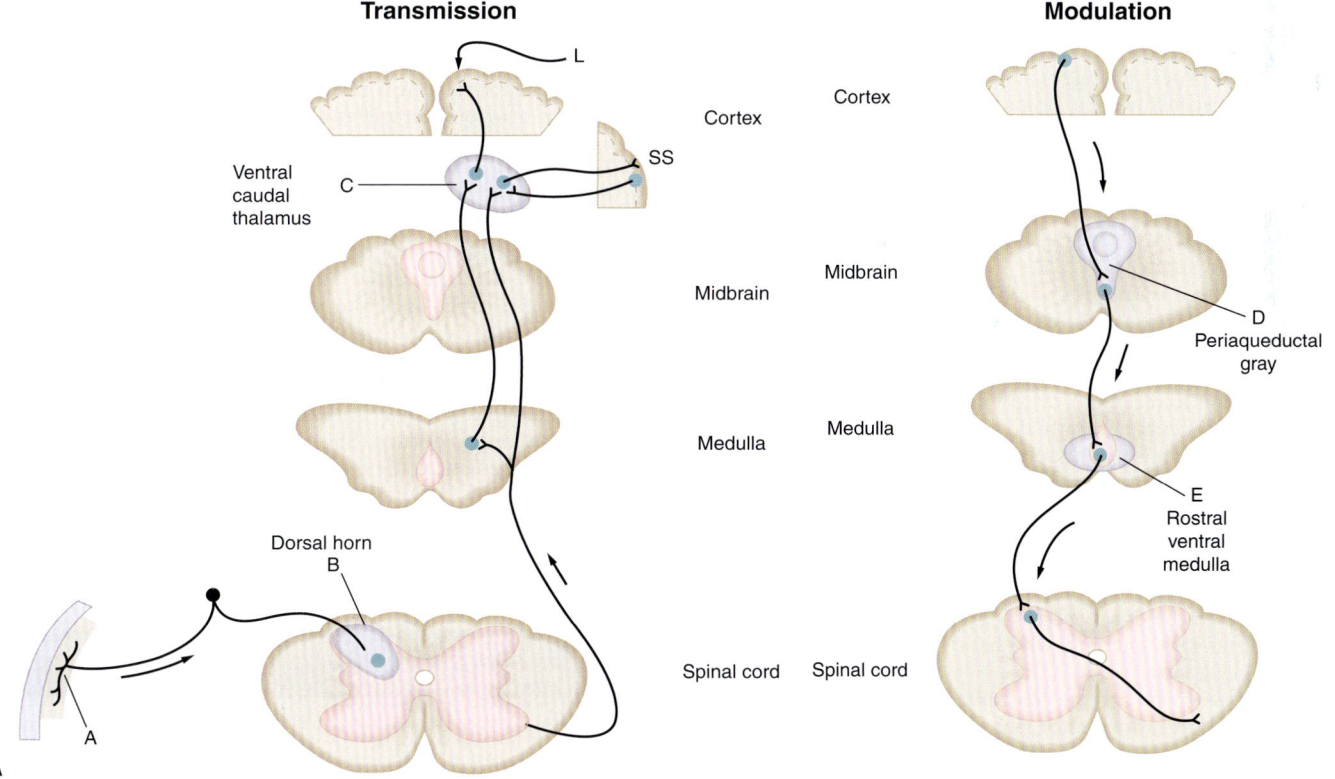

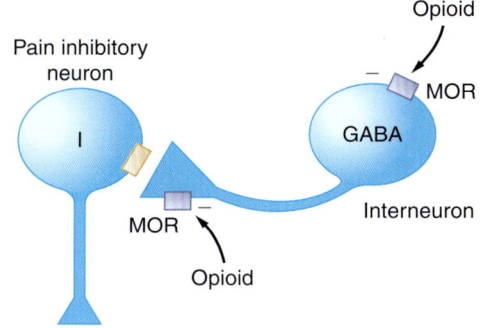

FIGURE 79.1 **A:** Sites of action common to all μ opioids. The location of μ-opioid receptors (MORs). Modulation of ascending pain transmission pathways. MORs are found (A) in the periphery following inflammation, (B) at pre- and postsynaptic sites in spinal cord dorsal horn, and (C) in the thalamus and in the limbic (L) and somatosensory (SS) cortex. **B:** Descending modulation of pain transmission. The location of MORs. MORs are found in (D) the midbrain periaqueductal grey, the nucleus raphe magnus, and (E) the rostral ventral medulla. μ-Opioids activate a descending inhibitory system that modulates spinal cord dorsal horn pain transmission. **C:** Descending modulation of pain transmission. GABAergic neurons and descending inhibition. A brainstem pain inhibitory neuron (I) is tonically inhibited by a GABAergic neuron. Opioids inhibit GABAergic neurons and remove the inhibition of the pain inhibitory neurons (PIN) that project from the rostral ventral medulla to the spinal cord dorsal horn. Thus, opioids produce a disinhibition of the PIN which results in the activation for descending inhibition.

that activates chloride (ClC-2) channels in the intestines suggests a second mechanism of opioid-induced constipation.[19] See also "Peripheral Effects of Opioids" section.

The opioid receptors are part of an endogenous system that includes a large number of EOP ligands. Based on cloning, three distinct families of classical opioid peptides, the enkephalins, endorphins, and dynorphins, have been identified.[7] The physiologic roles of the EOPs are not completely understood. They appear to function as neurotransmitters, neuromodulators, and, in some cases, as neurohormones.[13] When EOP mutant mice are compared to wild-type mice, phenotypes indicative of EOP tone have been observed in major opioid functions including locomotion, nociception, and emotional responses. For example, no change in baseline sensitivity to thermal pain was found in mice devoid of β-endorphin, whereas Penk and Pdyn mutant mice showed increased pain response in the hot plate and tail flick tests, respectively.[13] They also play a role in some forms of stress-induced analgesia and in the analgesia produced by electrical stimulation of discrete brain areas such as the periaqueductal grey.

Classification Based on Opioid Agonist or Antagonist Activity

The expression of agonist or antagonist activity is an important pharmacodynamic property used to classify opioids. The morphine-like agonist drugs represent one end of the pharmacodynamic spectrum. They bind predominately or exclusively to MORs and produce analgesia and the other MOR-mediated effects described below. The opioid antagonists, such as naloxone, represent the other end of the spectrum since their binding to an opioid receptor does not trigger the signaling cascade that leads to the pharmacodynamic effects seen with opioid agonists. Rather, receptor occupancy by a sufficient concentration of an opioid antagonist prevents or reverses opioid receptor–mediated agonist effects.

Between these two types of pharmacodynamic actions fall the effects of the partial agonists, the mixed agonist-antagonists and the centrally acting μ agonist drugs. The mixed agonist-antagonist opioid drugs (see Table 79.1) can demonstrate agonist (at the κ receptor) or antagonist (at the μ receptor) activity. What occurs clinically depends on whether the patient is opioid-naive or has prior exposure to a μ-opioid agonist. Buprenorphine is a partial agonist opioid. This classification derives principally from its pharmacodynamic activity observed in preclinical test systems wherein the difference in efficacy between a full agonist and a partial agonist can be more readily measured. Clinically, the consequences of buprenorphine's partial agonism can be observed as its ability to precipitate opioid withdrawal in some patients who have been receiving repeated doses of a μ agonist.

The newest group are the centrally acting μ agonist analgesics, tramadol and tapentadol (see Table 79.1). The analgesic effects of these drugs appear to result from dual actions: weak opioid receptor activity and blockade of neurotransmitter reuptake, predominately serotonin for tramadol and norepinephrine for tapentadol.[20] Neither mechanism alone appears to be sufficient; rather, the synergistic effects of the dual actions is necessary for analgesia.

Opioid Pharmacodynamics

CELLULAR, SYNAPTIC, AND CIRCUIT LEVEL EVENTS THAT INHIBIT PAIN TRANSMISSION

At the cellular level, activation of an opioid receptor (μ, κ, or δ) by an opioid inhibits of VG Ca++ channels and the opening of certain potassium (K+) channels. The presynaptic block of

VG Ca++ channels reduces transmitter release, whereas the increase in outward K+ currents hyperpolarizes postsynaptic neurons (increasing an inhibitory postsynaptic potential). These effects on transmitter release are believed to decrease synaptic transmission of pain signals in the spinal cord dorsal horn.

At the neuronal circuit level, opioids can disinhibit an inhibitory interneuron. This is the basis of descending modulation of pain transmission as discussed earlier.

The Pharmacodynamic Effects of Opioids

The pharmacodynamic effects of opioids are discussed using the prototype morphine and the morphine-like opioids. In some cases, the term *opioids* refers to properties common to both morphine-like and mixed agonist-antagonist opioids. Later, individual opioids are discussed in the context of how they compare to and differ from morphine and other morphine-like opioids.

The desirable and undesirable effects of morphine can be divided into those that may occur with a single dose and those that occur with repeated administration including tolerance, physical dependence, and addiction (Table 79.2).

Central Nervous System Opioid Effects

ANALGESIA

The relief of pain by opioids such as morphine is relatively selective in that other sensory modalities are not affected. Although continuous dull pain has been relieved more effectively than sharp intermittent pain, morphine-like opioids can relieve severe, acute pain associated with renal or biliary colic. Some patients report that they still perceive pain but that it is no longer as distressing as it was prior to their receiving morphine. Recent reports as well as long-standing clinical observations support the concept that pain includes both sensory-discriminative aspects (e.g., perception of the location, type, intensity) and reactive or affective meaning of the pain experience (e.g., its unpleasantness). Under experimental conditions, positron emission tomography (PET) imaging studies localized and separated these two dimensions of pain. The sensory-discriminative aspects are processed in the somatosensory cortex (SSC), whereas the affective component is processed in the anterior cingulate cortex (ACC).[21] The presence of MORs in both of these brain areas is consistent with the ability of morphine-like opioids to alter both dimensions of pain. Pain relief activates mesolimbic

TABLE 79.2	The Desirable and Undesirable Properties of Morphine as an Analgesic	
Desirable	**Undesirable**
Analgesic	Sedation
Mood effects	Mental clouding
Sedation	Dizziness
	Mood effects
	Dysphoria
	Nausea and vomiting
	Respiratory depression
	Suppression of the cough reflex
Tolerance (to respiratory depression)	Tolerance (to analgesia)
	Physical dependence
	Substance dependence or addiction
	Spasmogenic
	Constipation

reward/motivation circuitry. In animal models of pain, behavioral measures that capture affective and motivational aspects of pain appear to accurately reflect the effectiveness of treatments that are useful clinically (bedside to bench translation). Navratilova and colleagues[22] found that the relief of ongoing pain requires opioid signaling in the ACC and subsequent downstream activation of dopamine neurotransmission in the nucleus accumbens (NAc) that mediates the reward of pain relief. These studies provide a neural explanation for the preferential effects of systemic and endogenous opioids on pain affect and demonstrate that engagement of NAc dopaminergic transmission by nonopioid pain-relieving treatments depends on upstream ACC opioid circuits. Endogenous opioid signaling in the ACC appears to be both necessary and sufficient for relief of pain averseness.[22]

In contrast to nonopioid analgesics, there is no easily measurable ceiling to the dose-dependent analgesic effects of morphine-like opioids. Nevertheless, there is often a practical ceiling imposed by dose-dependent adverse effects including sedation, mental clouding, nausea, vomiting, and respiratory depression (see Table 79.2). The actual dose required for analgesia can vary greatly depending on the type or source of pain and a variety of patient factors. The most important principle that derives from these properties of the morphine-like opioids is the need to titrate the dose for each patient to an acceptable level of analgesia that balances the degree of pain relief with the limits that are imposed by concomitant adverse effects. In the United States, both state (e.g., Washington State Agency Medical Directors' Group[23]) and national guidelines[5] for primary care providers who are prescribing opioids for chronic pain recommend caution in increasing opioid dosage above specified dosages.

MOOD EFFECTS

The morphine-like opioids can produce mood alterations including the relief of anxiety, euphoria (pleasant feelings), as well as dysphoria (unpleasant feelings). Chronic pain patients receiving opioids often report initial relief of depression (a common concomitant of chronic pain), but this usually proceeds to exacerbation of depression after a few days to weeks. Thus, the mood effects appear as both desirable and undesirable effects in Table 79.2. Reports of euphoria or dysphoria usually depend on the individual and the circumstances of the morphine experience. Most "normals" not in pain as well as many patients in pain report some dysphoria after receiving morphine. That is associated with difficulty in mental activities, dizziness, and decrease in physical activity.

The reinforcing and rewarding properties of these drugs that are associated with opioid abuse involve the mesolimbic dopamine system and appear to be distinct from those systems involved in analgesia and the production of physical dependence.[24]

SEDATION

Morphine-like opioids produce drowsiness and sedation, which may be useful in certain clinical situations (e.g., preanesthesia) but usually are not desirable concomitants of analgesia, particularly in ambulatory patients. The central nervous system (CNS) depressant actions of these drugs are at least additive to the sedative and respiratory depressant effects of sedative-hypnotics such as alcohol, barbiturates, and benzodiazepines. Dasgupta et al.[25] using data from the North Carolina Prescription Drug Monitoring Program (PDMP) estimated that the rate of overdose deaths among those codispensed benzodiazepines and opioids were 10 times higher compared to opioids alone.

Reducing the dose and interval, that is, giving a lower dose more frequently, produces a lower peak opioid serum concentration, which may counteract excessive sedation. In addition,

other CNS depressants including sedative hypnotics and antianxiety agents that add to or potentiate the sedative effects of opioids should be discontinued if possible. Concurrent administration of a central stimulant (e.g., dextroamphetamine, methylphenidate) twice daily helps counteract the sedative effects of opioids. Tolerance usually develops to the sedative effects of opioid analgesics within the first several days of repeated administration.

NAUSEA AND VOMITING

The morphine-like analgesics produce nausea and vomiting by stimulating the chemoreceptor trigger zone (CTZ) in the area postrema of the medulla. The incidence of nausea and vomiting is markedly greater in ambulatory patients suggesting that these drugs also alter vestibular sensitivity. The ability of opioid analgesics to produce nausea and vomiting appears to vary with drug and among patients; some advantage may result from opioid rotation. Alternately, a centrally acting antiemetic such as a phenothiazine (e.g., prochlorperazine), a gastric prokinetic agent (e.g., metoclopramide), or a serotonin (5-HT3) receptor antagonist (e.g., ondansetron) may be used in combination with the opioid. For some patients, initiating treatment by the parenteral route and then switching to the oral route may reduce emetic symptoms.[26]

Use of a dual mechanism opioid analgesic (e.g., tapentadol) allows less μ agonist activity due to the synergistic effect of the second mechanism—in this case, norepinephrine reuptake inhibition—while maintaining the full analgesic effect. For patients highly sensitive to gastrointestinal (GI) adverse effects of opioids who cannot tolerate therapeutic doses of morphine or other μ agonists, a dual mechanism opioid can be useful.[27]

RESPIRATORY DEPRESSION

Respiratory depression is potentially the most serious adverse opioid effect. The morphine-like agonists act on brainstem respiratory centers to produce dose-related respiratory depression to the point of apnea. In humans, death due to overdose of a morphine-like agonist is nearly always due to respiratory arrest. Therapeutic doses of morphine may depress all phases of respiratory activity (rate, minute volume, and tidal exchange). However, as carbon dioxide (CO_2) accumulates, it stimulates central chemoreceptors, resulting in a compensatory increase in respiratory rate, which masks the degree of respiratory depression. At equianalgesic doses, the morphine-like agonists produce an equivalent degree of respiratory depression. Therefore, individuals with impaired respiratory function or bronchial asthma are at greater risk of experiencing clinically significant respiratory depression in response to usual doses of these drugs. Respiratory depression and CO_2 retention produces cerebral vasodilation and increased cerebrospinal fluid pressure unless the partial pressure of carbon dioxide (P_{CO_2}) is normalized by artificial ventilation. Respiratory depression occurs most commonly in opioid-naive patients following acute opioid administration, and it is associated with other signs of CNS depression including sedation and mental clouding. It bears repeating that opioids in combination with CNS depressants such as the benzodiazepines can exacerbate opioid-induced respiratory depression and increase risk for overdose.[5] Patients 65 years and older and those with anxiety disorders and other mental health conditions are more likely to be receiving benzodiazepines and therefore at greatest risk of an interaction when opioids are initiated or the dosage is increased. With repeated drug administration, some tolerance often develops to the respiratory depressant effects. Whether this tolerance actually reduces the risk of opioid-CNS depressant combinations has not been established and appears unlikely.[25] Opioids can both exacerbate obstructive sleep apnea and cause central sleep apnea.[28] Obstructive sleep apnea is common in overweight chronic pain patients, and it presents risk for opioid-induced respiratory depression, especially when the patients are sleeping. Recent reports suggest that opioids, and perhaps more so methadone, may induce potentially life-threatening central sleep apnea.[29,30] Respiratory depression can be reversed by timely administration of the opioid antagonist naloxone.[31] In patients chronically receiving opioids who develop respiratory depression, naloxone should be diluted 1:10 (i.e., 400 μg in 10 mL of 0.9% sodium chloride = 40 μg/mL) with each 40-μg dose (1 mL) given in 1- to 2-minute intervals to prevent the precipitation of severe withdrawal symptoms while reversing the respiratory depression. An endotracheal tube should be placed in the comatose patient before administering naloxone to prevent aspiration associated respiratory compromise with excessive salivation and bronchial spasm. In patients receiving meperidine chronically, naloxone may precipitate seizures by blocking the depressant action of meperidine and allowing the convulsant activity of the active metabolite, normeperidine, to be manifest.

The mixed agonist-antagonists, pentazocine, nalbuphine, butorphanol, and the partial agonist buprenorphine have different dose–response characteristics for their respiratory depression curves from the morphine-like opioids. Although therapeutic doses of pentazocine produce respiratory depression equivalent to that of morphine, increasing the dose does not ordinarily produce a proportional increase in respiratory depression. Whether this apparent ceiling to respiratory depression offers any significant clinical advantage has not been determined. Also, naloxone reversal of the respiratory depression produced by buprenorphine requires relatively large doses (5 to 10 mg), is delayed in onset,[32] and is not always effective. In addition, the respiratory depression from buprenorphine or methadone may outlast the effects of a single dose of naloxone, continuous infusions of naloxone may be required to maintain reversal of respiratory depression.[33,34]

CONSTRICTION OF THE PUPIL

Opioids stimulate the Edinger-Wesphal (parasympathetic) nucleus of the oculomotor nerve to produce miosis. Pinpoint pupils (along with respiratory depression and loss of consciousness) are the three pathognomonic signs of opioid overdose. These effects are antagonized by the opioid antagonist, naloxone. However, severe anoxia results in mydriasis.

ANTITUSSIVE EFFECT

Opioids depress the cough centers in the medulla and, in turn, depress the cough reflex. However, the receptor mechanisms involved with cough differ from those involved with other opioid effects such as analgesia. Therefore, the dextrorotatory isomers of opioids (e.g., dextromethorphan), which do not bind to opioid receptors are nevertheless effective antitussives.

HYPOTHALAMIC EFFECTS

Morphine affects both body temperature and circulating neuroendocrine hormone levels by actions on the hypothalamus. Morphine alters hypothalamic heat regulation resulting in a slightly lower body temperature. The release of corticotrophin-releasing hormone (CRH) and gonadotropin-releasing hormone (GnRH) are inhibited, causing a decrease in luteinizing hormone (LH), follicle-stimulating hormone (FSH), and adrenocorticotropic hormone (ACTH). Prolactin and antidiuretic hormone (ADH) release are increased. Based on observations in methadone maintenance patients, tolerance develops to the effects of morphine on these hypothalamic releasing factors.

The term *opioid-induced androgen deficiency* (OPIAD) describes clinically meaningful decrease in testosterone levels that occurs primarily in men receiving ongoing morphine or other potent μ agonist opioid pharmacotherapy for chronic nonmalignant pain[35] or those receiving methadone or buprenorphine

maintenance therapy.[36] Worsening of pain, depressed mood, sexual dysfunction, and refractoriness to treatment are common in such patients. Trials of testosterone replacement therapy have been helpful at improving sexual dysfunction, pain, and quality of life[37,38]; however, the effects of testosterone replacement on improving spermatogenesis or sperm motility are unclear. Inhibition of ovarian sex hormone and adrenal androgen production has been reported among women chronically consuming sustained-action opioids.[39]

CENTRAL NERVOUS SYSTEM EXCITATION

In contrast to the obvious opioid CNS depressant effects, there are excitatory effects. Dose-dependent convulsions occur in rodents but are rare in humans. However, normeperidine, a principal metabolite of meperidine, causes anxiety, tremors, myoclonus, and generalized seizures when it accumulates with repetitive dosing.[40] Naloxone does not reverse, and may even exacerbate, this hyperexcitability. Likewise, the metabolites morphine-3-glucuronide (M3G) and hydromorphone-3-glucuronide can cause movement disorders ranging from myoclonus to grand mal seizures when the metabolite accumulates, typically following relatively high-dose intravenous (IV) administration.[41]

OPIOID TOLERANCE, DEPENDENCE, AND ADDICTION

The properties of the opioid analgesics that are most likely to lead to their being misused, or the patient mistreated, are effects mediated in the CNS that are seen following chronic administration. These include tolerance, physical dependence, and opioid use disorders addiction (see Table 79.2).[42,43] It must be emphasized that although the development of tolerance and physical dependence are predictable pharmacologic effects seen in humans and laboratory animals in response to repeated administration of an opioid, these effects are distinct from the behavioral pattern seen in some individuals and described by the terms *opioid use disorder* and *addiction*. See Chapters 59 and 60 for more on addiction and dependence.

THE OPIOID-TOLERANT PATIENT AND OPIOID-INDUCED HYPERALGESIA
Clinically Observable Tolerance

Tolerance to opioid effects occurs, but it is widely misunderstood. It is useful to subdivide tolerance into three dimensions: (1) tolerance to analgesia, (2) tolerance to other CNS-depressing effects and nausea, and (3) tolerance to opioid-induced constipation. Effective ongoing opioid therapy for chronic pain often requires increasing the dose numerous times in the first days to weeks of therapy until a consistently effective dose is found. This may be initial tolerance or simply reflect a dose-finding period. Once an effective dose is found which keeps the patient reasonably comfortable for a few days, it is relatively uncommon to have to increase the dose further unless the painful pathology increases or a new painful disorder occurs, the patient skips doses, the dosage form is changed, a drug interaction occurs, or some other nonpharmacologic event such as diversion occurs. These types of events probably account for the majority of patient requests for increasing opioid doses. Clinically meaningful tolerance to analgesia occurs unpredictably in a minority of patients receiving opioids chronically for management of pain with a physiologic basis. Many chronic cancer and noncancer pain patients remain comfortable without increasing pain complaints for months or even years without an increase in opioid dose. A minority require escalating opioid doses for reasons that remain unclear. When a patient no longer responds to increasing doses of a particular opioid that was previously effective, consider rotation to another opioid. The management of acute postoperative pain in an opioid-tolerant patient is addressed in recent guidelines.[44]

Conversely, nearly everyone develops some meaningful degree of tolerance to opioid-induced sedation, respiratory depression, nausea, and inhibition of coordination after 5 to 7 days of ongoing (around the clock) opioid pharmacotherapy. At the initiation of opioid therapy, an antiemetic may be needed, but commonly, it is not needed after a few days of therapy. Many patients cannot safely drive a motor vehicle or operate machinery in the first days of opioid treatment. However, after a week of regularly scheduled opioid, most people can drive safely.[45] When the dose is increased or if patient abstains from the medication for a few days, another week may be required to reacquire tolerance to impaired eye-foot-hand coordination.

Tolerance to opioid-induced constipation does not appear to occur. Management of this common and sometimes debilitating side effect is discussed in the following text.

Proposed Mechanisms of Tolerance

Opioid tolerance may be classified as associative or pharmacologic. Associative or contextual tolerance refers to changes in response that result when an opioid is administered in the presence of specific environmental cues that can induce tolerance specific to that setting.[46] Pharmacologic (nonassociative) tolerance is divided into pharmacodynamic tolerance, which is the result of neuronal adaptations that reduce the sensitivity of the system to the drug, and pharmacokinetic tolerance wherein the disposition of the drug is increased so that the effective concentration is reduced. Generally, pharmacodynamic mechanisms are thought to be most responsible for in vivo opioid tolerance. However, a contribution by associative tolerance cannot be excluded.

In the clinical setting, pharmacodynamic tolerance (hereafter, simply tolerance) develops when a given dose of an opioid produces a decreasing effect or when a larger dose is required to maintain the original effect. Some reports suggest that a degree of tolerance to analgesia appears to develop in most patients receiving opioid analgesics chronically.[47] Although tolerance to opioid analgesia appears to develop rapidly in animal models, it does so much more slowly in humans.[48] Other reports, however, document that many patients do not experience tolerance to analgesia, that is, the same dose of opioid continues to provide effective analgesia over days to years unless there is increase in the pathology associated with the pain.[49]

An early sign of the development of tolerance is the patient's complaint of a decrease in the duration of effective analgesia. The rate of tolerance development varies greatly among cancer patients; some demonstrate tolerance within days of initiating opioid therapy, whereas others will remain well controlled for many months on the same dose.[50] Unfortunately, pharmacodynamic tolerance cannot be adequately evaluated in the clinical situation. Factors described earlier as causing "apparent tolerance" should be considered and addressed before concluding that pharmacodynamic tolerance has occurred. Both an increase in pain and the development of tolerance often respond to an increase in the opioid dose. Because the analgesic effect is a logarithmic function of the dose of opioid, a doubling of the dose may be required to restore full analgesia. Although controversial, the experience with cancer patients suggests that there appears to be no limit to the development of tolerance, and with appropriate adjustment of dose, many, but not all, patients can continue to obtain pain relief without intolerable adverse effects. Titration to effect remains the hallmark of effective opioid therapy.

The mechanisms believed to underlie opioid tolerance may be classified into two categories: within-systems and between-systems.[51] These mechanisms of tolerance are not necessarily mutually exclusive, as there is abundant evidence in support of anatomical and functional overlap of both processes. These adaptations can include modifications of the receptor, its

coupling to G proteins and additional signal transduction events including μ-opioid agonist–induced phosphorylation of the MOR, followed by desensitization, receptor internalization, endocytosis, and downregulation.[51] Bohn et al.[52] found that β-arrestin-2 knockout mice fail to develop antinociceptive tolerance to morphine and desensitization of the MOR does not occur after chronic morphine treatment. Interestingly, deletion of the β-arrestin-2 gene does not prevent the chronic morphine-induced upregulation of adenylyl cyclase activity, a cellular marker of dependence, and the mutant mice still become physically dependent to morphine.[52] These observations have led to the design and evaluation of new opioids that activate the μ receptor signaling pathways relevant to analgesia but not β-arrestin signaling (see "Biased Ligands" section).[53] In vitro studies indicate that μ-opioid–mediated stimulation leads to translocation of protein kinase C to the plasma membrane and phosphorylation of the N-methyl-D-aspartate (NMDA) receptor.[51] Between-systems processes of tolerance, on the other hand, are characterized by interactions that antagonize or compensate for the effects of an opioid, usually via some direct antiopioid mechanism. These antiopioid factors may include nonopioid receptors, neurotransmitters, ion channels, and second messengers (see Inturrisi and Gregus[51]) for additional details and references.

Preclinical studies suggest that apparent opioid tolerance may result from excitatory CNS changes that facilitate transmission of and increase sensitivity to pain.[54] This condition is termed *opioid-induced hyperalgesia* (OIH). The basic phenomenon appears to result from the upregulation of antiopioid, pronociceptive systems. The neuroanatomical substrates and signaling pathways involved in OIH are emerging.[54] However, the magnitude of the contribution of OIH to clinical opioid tolerance and its consequences for continued opioid therapy remain controversial. Case reports of OIH describe severe allodynia in patients on high-dose (IV) opioids that resolve with dose reduction. Eisenberg et al.[55] has described a set of clinical criteria for diagnosing OIH. There is general agreement that during opioid withdrawal, OIH may occur and contribute to an exacerbation of pain.[56] Therefore, avoid acute withdrawal. Switching from a morphine-like opioid to a mixed agonist-antagonist (pentazocine, nalbuphine, and butorphanol) or the partial agonist buprenorphine must be avoided or preceded by tapering of the μ-opioid because of the ability of these antagonist drugs to induce abrupt opioid withdrawal and cause concomitant hyperalgesia in opioid-dependent individuals.[6]

A number of opioid-sparing strategies can be used to reduce the rate of the development of tolerance and to restore analgesia in high-dose opioid-tolerant patients. The combination of an opioid with a nonopioid analgesic can enhance analgesia and reduce the rate of development of tolerance because tolerance does not develop to the nonopioid component of the combination. For example, coanalgesics are a diverse group of nonopioid analgesics that can enhance the effects of opioids and have independent analgesic activity in certain painful conditions by nonopioid mechanisms. The coanalgesics include the anticonvulsants (e.g., gabapentin and pregabalin), the tricyclic antidepressants (e.g., amitriptyline, nortriptyline), the selective serotonin reuptake inhibitors (SSRIs) (e.g., paroxetine, citalopram), the selective norepinephrine reuptake inhibitors (SNRIs) (e.g., duloxetine, venlafaxine), the corticosteroids (e.g., dexamethasone, methylprednisolone), the topical local anesthetics and others (e.g., lidocaine patches, capsaicin cream), and the antispasmodics (baclofen) (see American Pain Society[3]). Rotation to an alternative μ-opioid agonist usually results in a relative reduction of opioid dosage due to incomplete cross-tolerance (see the following text) among these opioids.[57] The use of bolus or continuous epidural local anesthetics or peripheral local anesthetic blocks in patients with localized pain, for example, perineal pain, can sometimes dramatically reduce the need for systemic opioids and thus diminish opioid tolerance. However, a recent review concluded that the efficacy of therapeutic nerve blocks for many chronic pain conditions, other than headache, has not been adequately studied.[58] Ketamine is an NMDA receptor antagonist, and NMDA receptors are involved in the facilitation of pain transmission—a phenomenon known as central sensitization which leads to an increased sensitivity to pain following injury. Therefore, NMDA antagonists have antihyperalgesic effects in neuropathic pain states and reduce morphine tolerance in rodents.[59] Ketamine is associated with limiting psychotomimetic effects so that dose titration must be carefully controlled. These approaches may, in some high-dose opioid-tolerant patients, allow a reduction of the opioid dose with a reduction of dose-related adverse effects without a loss of analgesia that may open the therapeutic window. However, a Cochrane systematic review[60] concluded that current evidence is insufficient to assess the benefits and harms of ketamine as an adjuvant to opioids for the relief of cancer pain.

Animal study data on tolerance often do not translate well to humans. The rates of development and loss of tolerance are not well defined in patients. The rate and extent of tolerance can vary greatly among different opioids and among patients receiving the same doses of a single opioid.

Cross-tolerance refers to the effects of one drug that confers tolerance to another drug, usually of the same class. Although some cross-tolerance appears to occur among μ-opioid agonists, the more relevant observation is that this cross-tolerance is incomplete. Therefore, when rotating from one opioid to another, this phenomenon must be taken into account in dosage calculations by initiating dosage, depending on the opioid, with 50% to 90% dose reduction of the calculated equianalgesic dose and titrating as required for pain relief.[57] Patients may have unique pharmacokinetic, pharmacodynamic, or pharmacogenetic differences that make opioid dose conversions less predictable.[57] Therefore, clinical judgment is paramount when converting one opioid to another.

THE OPIOID-DEPENDENT PATIENT

Physical dependence is the term used to describe an altered physiologic state produced by repeated administration of an opioid which requires the continued administration of an opioid to prevent the emergence of a stereotypical withdrawal or abstinence syndrome that is characteristic for the particular opioid. The signs and symptoms of opioid withdrawal are described elsewhere. The administration of an opioid antagonist to a physically dependent individual produces an immediate withdrawal syndrome. Patients who have received repeated doses of a morphine-like agonist, to the point at which they are physically dependent, may experience an opioid withdrawal reaction when given a mixed agonist-antagonist. Prior exposure to a morphine-like drug can greatly increase a patient's sensitivity to the antagonist component of a mixed agonist-antagonist. The severity of withdrawal is a function of the dose and duration of administration of the opioid just discontinued, that is, the patient's prior opioid exposure. The time course of the withdrawal syndrome is a function of the elimination half-life of the opioid to which the patient has become dependent (Table 79.3). Abstinence symptoms will appear within 6 to 12 hours and reach a peak at 24 to 72 hours, following cessation of a short half-life drug such as morphine, whereas onset may be delayed for 36 to 48 hours with methadone, a long half-life drug. Therefore, even for a patient in whom pain has been relieved by a procedure or treatment, it is necessary to slowly decrease the opioid dose to prevent withdrawal.

TABLE 79.3 Plasma Half-life (T$_{1/2}$) Values for Selected Opioids and Their Active Metabolites

Shorter T$_{1/2}$ Opioids	T$_{1/2}$ (h)
Morphine	2–3.5
Morphine-6-glucuronide	2
Hydromorphone	2–3
Oxycodone	2–4
Fentanyl	3.7
Codeine	3
Meperidine	3–4
Pentazocine	2–3
Butorphanol	2.5–3.5
Nalbuphine	5
Hydrocodone	3–4
Tramadol	5
Tapentadol	4
Longer T$_{1/2}$ Opioids	
Oxymorphone	7.5–9.5
Levorphanol	12–16
Normeperidine	14–21
Buprenorphine	22–28
Methadone	13–50

There is not one best method to taper opioids. Several different approaches have worked well. For patients who are anxious about tapering an opioid and those who may be especially sensitive to mild withdrawal effects, a slower taper may be indicated. A decrease of 10% of the original dose per week is a reasonable starting point. Some patients who have taken opioids for a long time might find even slower tapers (e.g., 10% per month) easier.[18]

Experience indicates that the usual daily dose required to prevent withdrawal is approximately one-fourth of the previous daily dose.[61] This dose called, for want of a better term, the detoxification dose is typically given in four divided parts. Commonly, the initial detoxification dose is given for 2 days and then decreased by one-half (administered in four divided doses) for 2 days until a total daily dose of 10 to 15 mg per day (in morphine equivalents) is reached. After 2 days on this dose, the opioid can be discontinued. Thus, a patient who had been receiving 240 mg per day of morphine equivalent for pain would require an initial detoxification dose of 60 mg given as 15 mg every 6 hours. This dose is decreased by 50% per day over the next 3 to 5 days. Buprenorphine is also being used to taper patients from prescription opioids.[62]

Cross-dependence refers to the ability of one opioid to substitute for another in preventing the withdrawal syndrome. Cross-dependence among the opioids allows rotation as described earlier and allows detoxification with an alternate opioid. For example, methadone can be substituted for morphine earlier example by switching the patient to oral methadone at one-fourth to one-eighth of the patient's morphine dose and decreasing the dosage as described earlier.

THE OPIOID-ADDICTED PATIENT WITH PAIN

The term *opioid use disorder* or *addiction* describes a pattern of drug use characterized by a continued craving for an opioid that is manifested as compulsive drug-seeking behavior leading to an overwhelming involvement with the use and procurement of the drug.[43] Within these definitions most, but not all, individuals who are addicted to opioids will have acquired some degree of physical dependence. However, the converse is not true, so that an individual can be physically dependent on an opioid analgesic without being addicted. Fear of addiction is a major concern limiting the use of appropriate doses of opioids.

Recent national surveys indicate a significant increase in nonmedical use of prescription opioids.[63] Increased reports of this problem coincided with attempts to make opioids more widely available to patients in pain. It is important to recognize the responsibility of clinicians to assess and monitor patients who are receiving long-term opioid treatment for pain to limit the abuse of these drugs. We now have the concurrence of two "perfect storms," that is, a continuing epidemic of undertreated pain[64] and, in some countries, such as the United States, a more recent epidemic of prescription drug abuse and overdose deaths.[65] It is also important to recognize that although opioids are sometimes overprescribed, especially for noncancer pain, opioids are sometimes inappropriately withheld when they should be used to manage severe opioid-responsive pain, especially in patients with advanced disease.[66]

PERIPHERAL EFFECTS OF OPIOIDS

In addition to the central effects, opioids have several important peripheral effects. The colon contains a dense population of MORs, and opioid-induced constipation can be a difficult clinical problem. Occupation and activation of those receptors by μ-opioid agonists inhibits peristalsis. Stimulating laxatives are the most appropriate type of laxative to manage this, and they often, but not always, are effective. Stool softeners alone usually are not.

Peripherally acting MOR antagonists are indicated for the treatment of opioid-induced constipation in patients who have failed conventional laxative therapy.

Methylnaltrexone (Relistor) is a quaternary ammonium cation derivative of naltrexone that is charged and therefore confined to peripheral sites. It is available for subcutaneous administration (dosage 8 or 12 mg) and has a rapid onset of action. In July 2016, the U.S. Food and Drug Administration (FDA) approved an oral formulation (450 mg once daily). Methylnaltrexone is approved for opioid-induced constipation in adults with advanced illness who are receiving palliative care and adults with chronic noncancer pain.

Naloxegol (Movantik) is a PEGylated derivative of naloxone and is a substrate for the P-glycoprotein transporter. Due to the reduced GI permeability (i.e., oral absorption) and increased efflux of naloxegol out of the CNS, the CNS penetration of naloxegol appears to be negligible. It is available for oral administration (25 mg once daily). Naloxegol is biotransformed by CYP3A4 so that caution with CYP3A4 poor metabolizers or inhibitors of CYP3A4. Naloxegol is approved for opioid-induced constipation in adults with chronic noncancer pain. Entereg (Alvimopan) owes its selectivity to its slow dissociation kinetics from for peripheral μ receptors. It is indicated for the inpatient management of postoperative ileus. Contraindicated in patients that have taken an opioid regularly for the past 7 days. The most common adverse reactions with these agents are abdominal pain, diarrhea, nausea, flatulence, vomiting, and headache.

A second class of drugs approved by the FDA for the management of opioid-induced constipation is believed to act on chloride 2 channels in the intestines. The one such drug available for clinical use is lubiprostone which is also approved for the management of irritable bowel syndrome with constipation (IBS-C) and idiopathic constipation.[67]

EFFECTS ON SMOOTH MUSCLE AND THE CARDIOVASCULAR SYSTEM

Other peripheral opioid effects include contraction of biliary tract smooth muscle, spasm of the sphincter of Oddi, increased ureteral and bladder sphincter tone, and a reduction in uterine tone. Except for bradycardia, most opioids have no significant effects on the heart or on cardiac rhythm. Methadone dose dependently can prolong the electrocardiographic QTc interval.[68] The 2014 American College of Cardiology/American Heart Association clinical practice guide concludes that morphine sulfate has potent analgesic and anxiolytic effects, as well as hemodynamic actions, that are potentially beneficial in myocardial infarction and unstable angina.[69] Patients with decreased blood volume are at risk of opioid-induced hypotension.

PRURITUS

Itching can result from opioid use and the probability is increased when opioids are given by epidural or intraspinal injection. Although previously thought to be due to the release of histamine from mast cells, more recently, a centrally mediated neurogenic contribution to opioid-induced pruritus has been described.[70] Data from primate studies indicate that κ-opioid agonists and μ-opioid antagonists can block the centrally mediated opioid-induced itch.[71] Antihistamines are used to manage this symptom, but they may also be sedating, thus limiting analgesic administration or placing the patient at greater risk of opioid-related respiratory depression. Dilute infusions of opioid antagonists reverse or decrease opioid-induced pruritus especially that due intraspinal opioids.[70] 5-HT3 receptor antagonists reduced the incidence of pruritus after neuraxial morphine injection but not after neuraxial lipid-soluble opioids injection. Parenteral nalbuphine has also been used for opioid-induced pruritus and may be more effective than antihistamines for this indication.[72] However, avoid mixed agonist-antagonists in μ-opioid–dependent patients. Most opioid-induced itching resolves within a few days. However, opioid rotation, dose reduction, or nondrug treatments such as cool compresses or moisturizers may be necessary for certain patients.

OPIOID EFFECTS IN PREGNANCY AND ON THE NEONATE

Using a private health insurance database representative of the United States beneficiaries from 2005 to 2011, Bateman et al.[73] found that opioids were dispensed to 14% of women during the antepartum period with approximately 6% of women receiving opioids during each of the three trimesters. Although most opioid exposure represented short courses of treatment, 2.2% of women received three or more opioids during pregnancy. Pregnant opioid treated pain patients on low-dose opioid regimes can and usually are taken off the opioid. Pregnant opioid treated pain patients on high-dose opioid regimes are sometimes kept on their opioid because rapid taper can induce miscarriage. The prevalence of opioid use (prescription and nonprescription) among pregnant women has been estimated to range from 1% to 2% to as high as 21%.[74] Pregnant women taking opioids at term may deliver an opioid-dependent infant, and those taking illicit opioids often require treatment to limit the impact of their opioid abuse on the newborn. A systematic review[74] did not find sufficient significant differences between methadone and buprenorphine or slow-release morphine to allow a conclusion that one treatment is superior to another for all relevant outcomes. Whereas methadone seems superior in terms of retaining patients in treatment, buprenorphine seems to lead to less severe neonatal abstinence syndrome.

ROUTES FOR OPIOID ADMINISTRATION

The oral route is generally the preferred route for opioid administration in ambulatory care due to convenience and relatively low cost. Immediate-release oral opioid dosage forms include solutions, compressed tablets, and gelatin capsules. Although solutions are absorbed more promptly, it is not clear that this offers a clinically important advantage for most patients. The risk of patients incorrectly measuring the volume producing inconsistent and sometimes excessive doses is real.

Opioids can be administered by oral, parenteral, rectal, sublingual, transdermal, and transmucosal routes. The μ agonists can be categorized as short-acting, long-acting, and ultra-short acting. Short half-life morphine-type opioids require frequent administration to maintain analgesia. Immediate-release morphine products provide about 4 hours of pain relief and need to be dosed accordingly. Pharmaceutically formulated long-acting, extended-release, or controlled-release formulations (see Table 79.1) provide alternatives to frequent opioid administration of inherently short-acting drugs. Pharmacologically long-acting opioids (i.e., methadone and levorphanol) that have longer half-lives (see Table 79.3) can provide analgesia in some patients for 6 to 12 hours when steady-state dosing is reached. Although methadone protects against opioid withdrawal for 24 or more hours, an oral dose only provides effective analgesia for a much shorter time, typically only about 8 hours. The pharmacologically long-acting opioids, methadone and levorphanol, require an understanding of safe dosing (see the following text).

Clinicians should be cautious about using extemporaneously compounded sustained-release opioids. Although there are franchised compounding pharmacies that prepare these—and some market them aggressively—most release the active ingredient inconsistently and unreliably over time. Uneven pain control, exacerbation of pain, withdrawal, and even overdose may result. The rapid onset of action of fentanyl series μ agonists favors their use as a perioperative adjuncts and their high lipophilicity facilitates transdermal, transmucosal, and subcutaneous administration. When these highly lipophilic opioids are absorbed through or injected under the skin, they create a depot in subcutaneous fat from which the drug is slowly released. This depot effect also makes them very difficult to titrate to response.[75] However, when these medications are administered transmucosally or sublingually, they are rapidly absorbed due to the lack of the buccal and sublingual fat. This prompt onset makes those routes useful in managing breakthrough pain. Buprenorphine also has been formulated as a long-acting transdermal patch and buccal film (Belbuca) (see Table 79.1). The IV route of administration is generally preferred in immediate postoperative and intensive care settings and for a pain crisis. Intramuscular (IM) injection is painful and may produce uneven absorption; it should generally be avoided. The subcutaneous (SC) route is preferred for injection when the IV route is impractical. The pharmacokinetics of SC administered opioids result in levels comparable to the IM route with the advantages that the SC route is far simpler to use and more comfortable for the patient. There is little or no rationale for IM opioid injections.

Table 79.1 lists relative equianalgesic doses and the starting doses recommended for commonly used opioids.

ALTERNATIVE NONINVASIVE ROUTES

When oral administration is not possible, consider alternative noninvasive routes before resorting to injections, infusions, or the placement of epidural or intrathecal catheters.

SUBLINGUAL ADMINISTRATION

Transmucosal absorption occurs following sublingual administration of a reasonably lipophilic opioid. Oral transmucosal dosing may provide less consistent absorption than oral administration due to anatomical and physiologic variability in the mucosa (e.g., thickening due to pathology, pH). This route generally should not be considered when patients can take medications orally because oral administration is simpler and oral solid dosage forms provide more exact doses than liquid doses that must be measured before administration.

Sublingual administration entails placing of a small volume of concentrated liquid or a readily dissolvable solid dosage form or film under the tongue. Other locations in the mouth that can be used are the cheek pouch (buccal administration) and the anterior lip pouch (transmucosal administration). Clinical experience supports these routes, but they have not been systematically studied. Patients should not eat or drink anything for about 15 minutes after taking an oral transmucosal dose. Doing so may increase the amount of drug that is swallowed, causing inconsistent interdose absorption.

Because opioids often cause dry mouth, it is important to counsel patients about this restriction. Some oral transmucosal dose tends to trickle down the throat or be actively swallowed, in which case that portion will undergo normal GI absorption. Factors that influence the percentage of the dose that is swallowed include the volume of liquid and the condition of the oral mucosa. In general, no more than 1 mL of liquid should be placed under the tongue or in a mucosal pouch. Larger volumes tend to increase the amount of drug that is swallowed. Additional doses can be administered in a few minutes if necessary. It is necessary to moisten the mouth before dosing if it is dry idiopathically or due to disease or therapy. Stomatitis and excessive keratinization of the oral mucosa may make absorption inconsistent. The oral pH can influence absorption across the oral mucosa. Whereas normal mouth pH is 6.5, for many cancer patients receiving therapy, it is above 7. The percentage of sublingual opioid absorbed increases with higher pH.[76] Because recently ingested foods and liquids can influence oral cavity pH, it is advisable to rinse the mouth with water before taking or administering an oral transmucosal dose and to not eat or drink anything for the next 15 to 20 minutes.

The rectal route of administration is an alternative for patients unable to take drugs orally. Although used commonly in the early days of modern hospice care (i.e., the 1970s to 1980s), it is less commonly used today due to alternative, nonoral dosage forms becoming available. The rectal route is simple to use and inexpensive. Some patients, however, find it esthetically unpleasant. Table 79.4 lists rectal opioid times to peak and duration of action. This route of administration

TABLE 79.4 Rectal Opioid Times to Peak and Duration of Action

Morphine immediate release oral tablets	
Peak	1.1 h
Duration	<6 h
Morphine controlled release oral tablets	
Peak	5.4 h
Duration	8–12 h
Morphine oral solution	
Peak	0.5 h
Duration	4–6 h
Morphine rectal suppositories	
Peak	1.1 h
Duration	<6 h
Hydromorphone rectal suppositories	
Peak	1 h
Duration	4–6 h
Methadone oral tablets	
Peak	2 h
Duration	6–8 h
Oxycodone oral tablets and solution	
Peak	3.1 h
Duration	8–12 h

Table adapted from Warren D. Practical use of rectal medications in palliative care. *Pain Symptom Manage* 1996;11:378–387.

is generally acceptable for short-term use and in care of terminal patients. Advantages of the rectal route include ease of use, lack of equipment that patients and families often perceive as reinforcing the sick role, and low cost. Rectal administration is contraindicated for patients with painful anal lesions.[77]

Extemporaneously compounded rectal dosage forms can be made by compounding pharmacies for those unable to tolerate orally administered opioids. For such extemporaneously prepared forms, the rate and consistency of release of active ingredient from the dosage form and the risk of dose dumping resulting in toxicity are concerns.[78]

Rectally and orally administered morphine provides similar analgesic effect and serum levels. Although there is far less absorption following a rectal dose, a significant portion of an orally administered dose undergoes first-pass metabolism which is avoided with rectal administration. This effect may be unique to morphine and may not apply to other opioids. Immediate-release oral tablets, liquids, and suppositories of morphine have been used rectally with good effect.[79] Do not assume dose equivalency for other oral opioid dosage forms given rectally because of differences in physicochemical and pharmacokinetic properties. Controlled-release dosage forms do not necessarily have the same effects and duration of action when administered orally and rectally. Lower peak serum levels and more interpatient variability occur with all controlled-release dosage forms when they are given rectally rather than orally. MS Contin administered rectally produces clinical effects similar to those obtained with the same dose taken orally and may produce less rectal irritation than the previously available rectal morphine suppositories.[80] Some palliative care nurses administer tablets rectally in a small mass of butter or an empty gelatin capsule. This is unnecessary and may delay absorption of the opioid. Simply ensure that the rectum is empty before inserting the tablets.

Oxycodone produces similar areas under the curve (AUCs) when administered rectally and orally.[81] Although rectal oxycodone suppositories are available in some countries, only oral solid and liquid forms are marketed in the United States. The commercially available oral liquid could be used rectally, but administration would be required every 3 to 4 hours for continual analgesia.

Informal, anecdotal reports of both immediate-release and controlled-release oral solid dosage forms administered via the vagina and through colostomy and ileostomy stomas also have been mentioned, but no data to support such use have been published. A comparative study of morphine administered rectally and through a colostomy led the investigators to conclude that the opioid should not be given through a colostomy due to poor and inconsistent absorption.[82] Animal studies of methadone administered vaginally indicate possible usefulness of that route.[83] But clinical data to support that hypothesis were not identified in a comprehensive literature search.

Nebulized opioids have been used and may provide good pain relief. However, that is not a cost-effective administration method for analgesia. Nebulized opioids are sometimes used as an alternative to sublingual administration to treat dyspnea (air hunger) in advanced disease[84]; however, there appears to be no benefit of using nebulized versus oral morphine for dyspnea.[85]

Very small particles are needed to deliver drug to the alveoli. Use of an administration method other than a high-quality small particle nebulizer can result in drug deposition on the palate with little or very inconsistent clinical effect. Handheld, squeeze bulb devices are not useful. Nebulized opioid administration requires sterile solutions, which increase expense as compared to oral and sublingual routes.

EPIDURAL, INTRATHECAL, AND INTRAVENTRICULAR ADMINISTRATION

Neuraxial or spinal administration refers to the use of epidural or intrathecal routes of administration. Both of these spinal routes are widely used, the former commonly for postoperative pain control and the latter more for chronic administration. In obstetrical analgesia, a single intrathecal opioid dose followed by continuous or intermittent epidural administration often is used. Epidural patient-controlled analgesia also is used in some settings.[86] In addition to opioids, spinal administration for pain may include local anesthetics, ziconotide, baclofen, clonidine, or ketamine (see American Pain Society[3] for details).

The epidural space is a fat-filled potential space that contains blood vessels (Fig. 79.2). Therefore, epidural opioid administration can cause systemic effects, albeit much more slowly and less than with IV and other systemic routes. The intrathecal route avoids some of the supraspinally mediated toxicity associated with the systemic delivery of these medications. The epidural and intrathecal routes each have advantages and disadvantages. Epidural administration allows opioid placement at any dermatomal level and does not require puncturing of the dura. However, larger doses are required and systemic effects may occur with epidural administration, increasing the risk of adverse effects. For morphine, intrathecal doses are typically one-tenth of those needed for an equianalgesic epidural dose. Intrathecal administration requires puncturing the dura, which delivers drug closer to the spinal cord receptors. Disadvantages of intrathecal use include increased potential for meningitis and risk of postdural puncture headaches. Dose-related problems associated with spinal analgesia include pruritus, urinary retention, and delayed respiratory depression.

Intraventricular administration has been used in cancer patients unresponsive to opioids administered by other routes.[87] The Ommaya reservoir has been used for this method of drug delivery.

With any direct central administration method, the pharmacokinetics of the opioids can vary greatly from systemic administration. Physicochemical drug characteristics, especially lipophilicity, become very important with these routes.

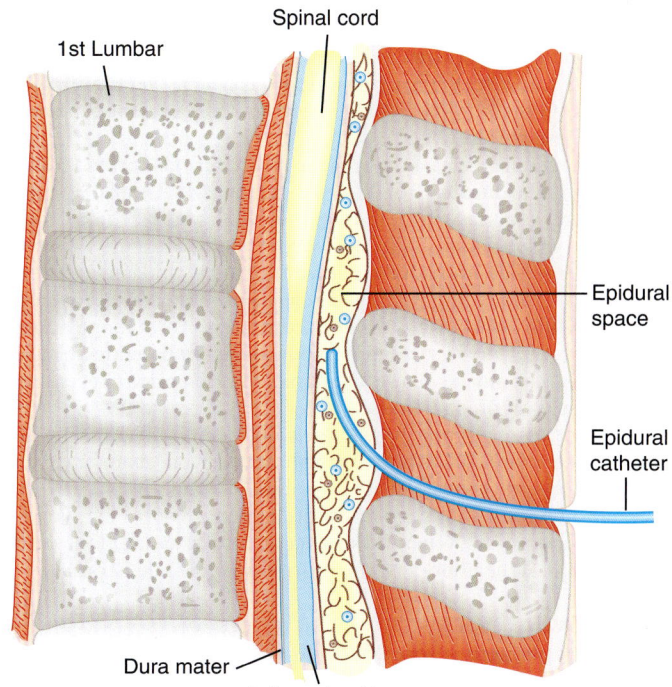

FIGURE 79.2 Drug delivery catheter in the epidural space.

Characteristics of Specific Opioids

MORPHINE

The oral bioavailability of morphine varies from 35% to 75%, which helps to explain some of the interpatient variability in response. Its average plasma half-life of 3 hours is somewhat shorter than its 4- to 6-hour duration of analgesia; this limits accumulation. With repetitive administration, its pharmacokinetics remains linear, and there does not appear to be auto-induction of biotransformation even following large chronic doses.[88] These pharmacokinetic properties contribute to the safe use of morphine over time. The two major morphine metabolites are M3G and morphine-6-glucuronide (M6G). M6G appears to contribute to the analgesic activity of morphine.[89,90] M6G appears to exert its analgesic action through a different splice variant of the MOR than morphine.[7] M6G is eliminated by the kidney and, because it has a somewhat longer half-life than the parent compound, will accumulate relative to morphine in patients with renal insufficiency. A survey of steady-state morphine and M6G levels and adverse effects in 109 cancer patients indicated that myoclonus or cognitive impairment was not associated with M6G accumulation.[91] For a subset of the 20 patients with the highest M6G levels (>2,000 μg/mL), the M6G level and concurrent organ failure was associated with the most severe toxicity (respiratory depression and/or obtundation).[91] It is appropriate to consider an alternate opioid for a patient receiving morphine who experiences a decrease in renal function and a concomitant increase in undesirable effects.

M3G is the predominate metabolite of morphine in humans. It lacks opioid analgesic activity but has excitatory effects in animals after direct injection into the CNS. This has led to the suggestion that M3G may be responsible for the neuroexcitatory effects sometimes seen with large chronic morphine dosing.[41] M3G has an elimination half-life even longer than M6G, and accumulated M3G has been associated with myoclonus and hyperalgesia, although that association is not clear.[92]

Based on single-dose studies in patients with either acute or chronic pain the relative potency of intramuscular to oral morphine is 1:6. However, with repeated administration, when patients are dosed on a regular schedule (around the clock), the parenteral to oral dose ratio is reduced to 1:2 or 1:3 (see Table 79.1). This presumably is due to accumulation of the M6G metabolite, which is active and has a longer half-life than the parent drug.

The extended-release morphine preparations provide analgesia with a duration of 8 to 12 hours (MS Contin) or 12 to 24 hours (Kadian) and allow patients greater freedom from repetitive dosing, especially during the night. Patients may be titrated using the immediate-release morphine and, once stabilized, converted to the sustained-release preparation according to a schedule appropriate for the form used. To manage acute "breakthrough" pain "rescue" medication (immediate-release morphine) should be made available to the patient receiving delayed-release preparations.

Allergy to morphine has historically been associated more with trace plant protein in morphine derived from natural sources (opium). Today, most morphine formulations are very pure and contain so little plant protein that this problem is relatively uncommon. When it does occur, a fully synthetic opioid is indicated. True allergy to the morphine molecule is rare.

HYDROMORPHONE

Hydromorphone is a short half-life opioid used as an alternative to morphine by the oral and parenteral routes. It is available as both immediate-release and extended-release dosage forms. It is more soluble than morphine and is available in a concentrated parenteral dosage form at 10 mg/mL which can be advantageous for opioid-tolerant patients and cachectic patients in whom the volume of the opioid solution must be limited. Although hydromorphone is converted to a 3-glucuronide metabolite, it has not consistently been associated with neurotoxic effects in vivo, although this toxicity has occurred. The dose should be decreased by 25% to 50% in patients with renal impairment.

METHADONE

Methadone use in pain management has dramatically increased in recent years with mixed effects. The original interest in methadone was based on its high (1:2) oral to parenteral potency ratio, which is a reflection of its high oral bioavailability that averages 85%. It was found to be useful in opioid rotation because its incomplete cross-tolerance with opioids like morphine allow a reduction in dose to approximately 10% to 25% of the estimated equianalgesic dose when switching from morphine to methadone (see American Pain Society[3(p49)]). Methadone is relatively inexpensive, and its metabolites do not have opioid activity or apparent toxicity. As with other opioids, it may provide a larger therapeutic window in a particular patient, although this cannot be determined prior to a therapeutic trial. Preclinical studies demonstrate NMDA receptor antagonist activity of both isomers of methadone. In animals, this NMDA receptor antagonist activity included antihyperalgesic activity and the ability to prevent the development of morphine tolerance.[6,93] However, it remains to be determined whether these effects occur in humans at the doses of methadone used clinically. The weak NMDA antagonist effect of methadone has been anecdotally reported to be advantageous in managing neuropathic pain; however, studies have failed to demonstrate its superiority to other opioids.

A major limitation on the use of methadone as a first-line opioid for pain management relates to its safety. Its population pharmacokinetics is variable with a plasma half-life averaging 24 hours, but that may range from 13 to 50 hours. Because initially, the duration of analgesia is often only 4 to 8 hours, repetitive analgesic dosing of methadone can lead to drug accumulation because of this discrepancy between its plasma half-life and the duration of analgesia during initial dosing. Sedation, confusion, and even death can occur when patients are not carefully monitored and dosage adjusted during the accumulation period that can last from 5 to 10 days.

Opioid-naive patients should be started on a low oral dose (e.g., 2.5 mg) every 8 hours. Opioid-tolerant patients should be switched to an oral morphine equivalent dose based on guidelines described on American Pain Society.[3(p49)]

A second safety issue relates to concerns about the potential for methadone to prolong the QTc interval and predispose patients to torsade de pointes (TdP), a life-threatening arrhythmia. This requires consideration of the baseline risk of QTc prolongation, monitoring of the electrocardiogram during dosing with methadone, and appropriate adjustments as described in a clinical practice guideline.[68] This effect is more common at higher doses (e.g., 90 to 120 mg a day), sometimes used for pain due to advanced disease. It is very uncommon with the typical doses used for chronic, nonmalignant pain management (e.g., 7.5 to 60 mg a day).

Finally, there persists a stigma among pain patients and the public attached to the use of methadone for the treatment of opioid addiction due to its association with managing opioid use disorder (addiction).

LEVORPHANOL

Levorphanol is a relatively longer half-life opioid (see Table 79.3) that sometimes can be a useful alternative to morphine, but, like methadone, it must be used cautiously to prevent accumulation.

Like methadone, levorphanol appears to have NMDA receptor blocking activity.

OXYMORPHONE

Oxymorphone, a congener of morphine that is parenterally approximately 10 times more potent than morphine. Opana is available as immediate- and extended-release oral formulations and for parenteral administration (see Table 79.1). The extended-release dosage form (Opana ER) is indicated for every 12-hour dosing. Food enhances the oral bioavailability, so Opana ER should be taken 1 hour prior to a meal or 2 hours after a meal. Coingestion of alcohol with Opana ER may also increase plasma levels of oxymorphone. It is contraindicated in patients with severe hepatic impairment.

OXYCODONE

Oxycodone is available for oral dosing as immediate and extended (controlled)-release (ER) dosage forms for the treatment of severe pain. The abuse of the ER formulation by extracting the active ingredient from crushed tablets and injection of large and sometimes fatal doses by abusers led the manufacturer, Purdue Pharma, in 2010 to reformulate the ER tablets (OxyContin OP) using an abuse-resistant polymer designed to decrease abuse by crushing and extraction of the drug. Oxycodone is also available in lower doses in combination with acetaminophen for mild to moderate pain. Inhibition of CYP3A4 activity by its inhibitors, such as macrolide antibiotics (e.g., erythromycin), azole-antifungal agents (e.g., ketoconazole), and protease inhibitors (e.g., ritonavir), may increase concentrations of oxycodone and prolong opioid effects. CYP450 inducers, such as rifampin, carbamazepine, and phenytoin, may induce the metabolism of oxycodone and, therefore, may cause increased clearance of the drug which could lead to a decrease in oxycodone plasma concentrations, lack of efficacy or, possibly, development of an abstinence syndrome in a patient who had developed physical dependence to oxycodone.

FENTANYL

Fentanyl is a member of the phenylpiperidine family of synthetic opioids. It is approximately 100 times more potent that morphine when given parenterally (see Table 79.1). In addition to parenteral formulations, available dosage forms include a transdermal patch (Duragesic), a sublingual tablet (Abstral), a lozenge or "lollipop" (Actiq), a buccal film (Onsolis), a buccal tablet (Fentora), sublingual spray (Subsys), and a nasal spray (Lazanda). The oral transmucosal and nasal spray dosage forms are approved to treat breakthrough cancer pain (see Table 79.1). Substantial differences exist in the pharmacokinetic profiles of transmucosal dosage forms; patients should not be converted from one fentanyl form to another on a microgram-per-microgram basis. Rather, the manufacturers dosing recommendation for each product should be followed.

Fentanyl is a lipophilic opioid than can be absorbed through the skin. The rate of absorption is controlled, and 12 to 16 hours are required to achieve a therapeutic effect and 48 hours to achieve steady-state serum levels.[94] This lag in onset means that when switching from other routes of opioid administration to a transdermal (TD) dosage form, pain relief should be monitored to be sure analgesia is maintained. Conversely when TD fentanyl is discontinued, plasma levels will slowly decline over the subsequent 24 hours.[94] TD fentanyl can reduce fluctuations of plasma drug levels and avoids the need for repeated injections or use of the oral route. The FDA-approved labeling (package insert) provides information on equianalgesic conversions, but these are all approximate. Like the ER opioids, the TD fentanyl should be avoided in opioid-naive patients. It is "used to manage pain severe enough to require daily around-the-clock, long-term treatment with an opioid, in people who are already regularly using opioid pain medicine, when other pain treatments such as non-opioid pain medicines or immediate-release opioid medicines do not treat your pain well enough or you cannot tolerate them" (Duragesic package insert).

MEPERIDINE

The primary metabolite of meperidine (pethidine), normeperidine, has a unique neurotoxicity, which can lead to symptoms ranging from irritability to grand mal seizures.[40] Because the half-life of normeperidine is approximately four times longer than the parent compound, normeperidine accumulates rapidly following oral administration and in patients with compromised renal function.[95] Therefore, meperidine should not be used for longer than 24 to 48 hours. In patients receiving meperidine chronically, naloxone may precipitate seizures by blocking the depressant action of meperidine and allowing the convulsant activity of the active metabolite, normeperidine, to be manifest. Meperidine administration to patients receiving monoamine oxidase inhibitors has resulted in a fatal hyperthermia and other symptoms of serotonin syndrome.[96] For all of these reasons, many hospitals and health centers have restricted the use of meperidine or removed it from their formularies.

Meperidine has been reported to be the drug of choice to treat both postoperative rigors (shivering and shaking chills associated with antigenic drugs or blood products). More recently, clonidine and physostigmine were also found effective shivering suppressants, suggesting that opioid, α_2 adrenergic, and anticholinergic systems were possibly involved in this adverse effect.[97]

CODEINE

Codeine is widely available and inexpensive. Its use is controversial, in part because codeine is prodrug that is often not effective in patients who cannot convert it to its active metabolite (morphine) by CYP2D6 and because of potential drug interactions resulting from this genetic polymorphism. Although a discussion of the complex polymorphisms of CYP2D6 is beyond the scope of this review (see Zahari and Ismail[98]), it is important to recognize that the poor metabolizer phenotype (seen in 5% to 10% of Caucasians) inhibits conversion of codeine to morphine and resulting in codeine not producing an analgesic response. Whereas the ultrarapid metabolizer phenotype (seen in 1% to 2% of Caucasians) may overdose as a result of the excessive conversion of codeine to morphine,[99] these estimates of CYP2D6 phenotype distributions may differ substantially for other ethnicities.[99] In addition, the induction of CYP2D6 by other drugs will increase the effectiveness of codeine, whereas drugs that inhibit CYP2D6 will decrease codeine's effects inhibition. Codeine should not be taken by nursing mothers; levels that occur in breast milk can be toxic to nursing babies. For a list of drugs that interact with CYP2D6 and other relevant CYP450s, see the Flockhart Table at http://medicine.iupui.edu/clinpharm/ddis/main-table/. Consortium Guidelines for Cytochrome P450 2D6 Genotype and Codeine Therapy[99] recommends using alternative analgesics to codeine in patients who are CYP2D6 poor or ultrarapid metabolizers. Unfortunately genotyping of pain patients is still uncommon and codeine combinations with nonopioids are commonly prescribed.

HYDROCODONE

Hydrocodone is a pure μ agonist much like morphine or oxycodone. It is commonly available as a combination dosage form (e.g., hydrocodone plus acetaminophen); in addition, there are several newly approved long-acting abuse-deterrent pure hydrocodone oral formulations. When combination hydrocodone/acetaminophen products are used, the daily dose limit is primarily due to the acetaminophen, not the opioid.

PROPOXYPHENE

Propoxyphene has been removed from many leading hospital formularies—no longer available in the European Union, New Zealand, and the United Switzerland.

TRAMADOL

Tramadol is a weak μ agonist and weak norepinephrine serotonin reuptake inhibitor. Neither mechanism alone explains its analgesic efficacy. The probable mechanism is synergism between these two weak effects. In some patients, tramadol at a dose of 100 mg four times daily may produce analgesia similar to that of oral morphine 5 to 10 mg four times daily. Higher doses of tramadol offer no advantage and produce greater toxicity. Due to its mechanism, tramadol is more useful in neuropathic than nociceptive pain, and it appears more appropriate as a chronic than acute use analgesic because the dose must be titrated up slowly to minimize risk of lowering seizure threshold.[100] A combination of tramadol 75% with acetaminophen 25% appears to be as effective as the single-ingredient analgesic. Tramadol has recently become a controlled substance in the United States and can be highly toxic when misused.[101]

TAPENTADOL

Like tramadol, tapentadol is a centrally acting dual mechanism μ-opioid agonist and norepinephrine reuptake inhibitor. This dual mechanism likely explains its analgesia beyond its MOR activity. It has several advantages over other opioids; it is not a prodrug which requires biotransformation, has no known active metabolites, and is not metabolized by CYP450 enzyme system; which makes the possibility of CYP450 drug–drug interactions unlikely. It is available in immediate- and extended-release oral formulations. Tapentadol has comparable efficacy to morphine despite having 50-fold lower affinity to the MOR[102] and has better GI tolerability (nausea, vomiting, and constipation) versus oxycodone.[103] Tapentadol IR 50 mg and 75 mg were noninferior to oxycodone 10 mg for the treatment of acute pain with significantly less nausea and vomiting.[104]

PENTAZOCINE, NALBUPHINE, AND BUTORPHANOL

The mixed agonist-antagonist analgesics (see Table 79.1) include pentazocine, butorphanol, and nalbuphine. They produce analgesia as a result of their κ-opioid receptor agonist activity and show μ antagonist activity in the presence of a μ-opioid agonist. This receptor dualism is manifest in the opioid-naive patient as opioid analgesia and as opioid withdrawal in patients who are dependent on a μ-opioid. Therefore, they are not appropriate choices for patients who have been receiving a μ-opioid agonist for pain management or for the maintenance treatment of opioid substance use disorder. There is a ceiling effect on the ability of the mixed agonist-antagonists to produce respiratory depression, and they have a significantly lower abuse liability than the μ-opioid agonists. In therapeutic doses, they may produce certain self-limiting psychotomimetic effects, including confusion and hallucinations. Pentazocine is the mixed agonist-antagonist associated most commonly associated with these psychotomimetic effects. These drugs play a very limited role in the management of persistent pain because the incidence and severity of the psychotomimetic effects increase with dose escalation and because except for pentazocine, they are not currently available in oral dosage forms. Butorphanol is available for both parenteral and intranasal use. Nalbuphine is available only for parenteral use (see Table 79.1). A systematic review concluded that in patients with opioid-induced pruritus as a result of receiving neuraxial opioids for acute pain related to surgery or childbirth, nalbuphine is superior when compared with placebo, control, diphenhydramine, naloxone, or propofol.[72]

BUPRENORPHINE

Buprenorphine is a semisynthetic opioid with relative high affinity for and slow disassociation from the MOR. It appears to fit the pharmacologic profile of a partial MOR agonist in that it has an analgesic ceiling, particularly in acute pain management, and can precipitate opioid withdrawal in patients dependent on μ-opioids. It is available for pain management as Belbuca, a buccal film; Temgesic, a sublingual tablet; and Butrans, a 7-day TD patch (see Table 79.1). Because of the concerns with opioid withdrawal in patients taking more than 80 mg morphine equivalents per day, the dosage and conversion schedules for each formulation should be carefully observed. The buprenorphine T/1/2 is very long[105] (see Table 79.3) and will accumulate with repetitive dosing. Buprenorphine does not require dose reduction in renal failure patients.[106] The slow disassociation kinetics of buprenorphine from the MOR is reflected in the need to use a naloxone infusion to reverse buprenorphine—induced respiratory depression.[33] Buprenorphine is also used for the treatment of opioid dependence (see Table 79.1). Table 79.5 lists metabolites of commonly used opioids.

Abuse-Deterrent Opioid Formulations

Nonmedical use of prescription opioid analgesics worldwide has continued to rise over the past decade. In the United States, approximately 15 million people aged 12 years or older used prescription drugs nonmedically in the past year, and 6.5 million did so in the past month.[107] Prescription drugs are now misused and abused more often than any other drug, except marijuana and alcohol.[107] These trends have driven interest in the development of abuse-deterrent formulations (ADFs) of opioids, in an attempt, to reduce opioid-related abuse, overdose, and death. The currently available products (Table 79.6) reduce the ability to extract the opioid from the formulation, prevent administration through alternative routes like crushing or injecting, and/or make abuse of the manipulated product less attractive and more difficult. However, all of the currently available products can be abused without manipulation (e.g., ingesting large quantities orally) and do not prevent abuse, but rather reduce the likelihood of abuse. In addition, there is no currently available evidence that these formulations reduce the risk of opioid overdose. Table 79.7 lists various technologies currently used to deter abuse with their unique advantages and limitations.

Selecting among the Opioids for Clinical Use

Tables 79.1 and 79.4 list other morphine-like agonists that may be substituted for morphine. An alternative opioid to morphine may be selected based on the need with a particular patient to overcome an adverse effect of morphine (e.g., vomiting or sedation). Other reasons include the cost, a patient's favorable prior experience with another opioid, or even local availability of other morphine-like opioids. There is no evidence to suggest that any other opioid has greater analgesic efficacy than morphine in the population as a whole, but interpatient variability does exist. Only clinical trial can adequately determine the opioid that is the best choice for a specific patient.

Conclusions and Insights into the Future of Opioids for Pain

Opioids are essential analgesics for the management of severe pain. The risk-to-benefit ratio can be favorable when they are used properly. Respiratory depression is a risk particularly in

TABLE 79.5 Opioid Metabolites

Parent Drug (% Eliminated Unchanged)	Duration of Analgesia (h)	Metabolites (% if Known)	Metabolite Half-lives (h)	Primary Metabolite Elimination	Comments
Morphine (~7.2% IV), (~3.7% PO)	4–6				In renal failure, Vd may be smaller producing increased plasma levels; enterohepatic circulation of parent drug and glucuronide metabolites
		Morphine-3-glucuronide (57–74)	2.8–4	Renal	$T_{1/2}$—41–141 h in renal failure
		Morphine-6-glucuronide (4.7–12)	Duration 2 × longer than parent drug	Renal	$T_{1/2}$—89–136 h in renal failure; may cause narcosis in renal failure; intrathecally—100 times more potent than morphine; accumulates with chronic dosing
		Morphine-3-ethereal sulfate (5–10)			
		Normorphine (3.5)			May cause myoclonus and allodynia
		Morphine-N-oxide			
Codeine 11.1%	4–6	Codeine-6-glucuronide		Renal	Primary elimination form; profound narcosis has occurred in chronic renal failure
		Norcodeine			Equipotent to codeine in analgesic activity
		Morphine (10)			Formation dependent on CYP 450 2D6; genetic polymorphism impacts effectiveness and toxicity
Fentanyl (<10%)	1–2	Norfentanyl		Renal, hepatic	May be extensively liver metabolized
					Metabolized to despropionyl fentanyl
		4-N-anilinopiperidine			May cause neurotoxic side effects
					Structurally similar to normeperidine
Hydromorphone (5.6%)		Hydromorphone-3-glucuronide		Renal	Clearance dependent on hepatic blood flow
		Hydromorphone-6-glucuronide			Shown to accumulate in renal failure in one patient
		Normetabolites			Formed from intermediate metabolites, dihydroisomorphine and dihydromorphine
Levorphanol 5%	6–8	Levorphanol glucuronide		Renal	Liver metabolized by glucuronide conjugation
Meperidine 5% (uncontrolled urine pH)	2.5–3.5	Normeperidine (5–30)	15–30	Renal, hepatic	Bioavailability increases from 50% to 80% in cirrhosis; $T_{1/2}$ of meperidine and normeperidine prolonged in cirrhosis; urinary pH effects elimination of unchanged meperidine in urine; 25% in acidic urine vs. 1%–2% in alkaline urine
		Meperidine acid			$T_{1/2}$ prolonged in renal failure (>30 h); double the CNS excitatory effects and half the analgesic effect of meperidine; urinary elimination is pH dependent: uncontrolled pH f_e = 0.05–0.06, acidic urine f_e = 0.30, alkaline urine f_e <0.031
					Inactive metabolite
Methadone 21% (acidic urine increases the fraction of elimination [f_e])	4–6 initially; 6–12 after steady state (1–2 d)	1,5-demethyl-2-ethyl-3,3-iphenyl-1-pyrroline		Renal, biliary	In an anephric patient, 98% of methadone was found in feces as metabolite, suggesting a shift in metabolism from renal to fecal urinary excretion of methadone and metabolites is dose-dependent and is the major route of elimination in doses >55 mg/d; 10%–45% of methadone is eliminated in feces as metabolites
		2-ethyl-5-methyl-3,3-diphenyl-1-pyrroline		Renal, biliary	Unpredictable $T_{1/2}$ with chronic dosing long-term analgesia is 10 times morphine; major metabolite f_e = 0.30
		methadone-N-oxide			Minor metabolite
Oxycodone	3–6	Noroxymorphone		Hepatic, renal	Minor metabolite
		Oxymorphone			Renally excreted, primarily as metabolites
					Active metabolite; renally excreted as oxymorphone-glucuronide

(continued)

TABLE 79.5   (Continued)

Parent Drug (% Eliminated Unchanged)	Duration of Analgesia (h)	Metabolites (% if Known)	Metabolite Half-lives (h)	Primary Metabolite Elimination	Comments
		Noroxycodone			
		Norpropoxyphene (25)	22.9–36.6	Renal	Local anesthetic properties; cardiac conduction abnormalities can result with accumulation (not reversed by naloxone); not hemodialyzable
Buprenorphine	6–8				One source says it is almost completely metabolized in the liver, but another source says the majority is excreted unchanged in feces and undergoes enterohepatic circulation with metabolites.
		Glucuronidation products		Renal	May have weak analgesic properties
		Norbuprenorphine		Renal	Primary route of elimination is renal; hepatic, biliary, and fecal routes also involved
Butorphanol 5%	3–4	Norbutorphanol		Biliary	Extensively liver metabolized; Cl_{Cr} <30 mL/min half-life increased from 5.75 to 10.5 h in single-dose, intranasal administration
		Hydroxybutorphanol		renal	No analgesic activity
Nalbuphine 7%	3–6				Analgesic activity; major metabolite; 60%–80% renally excreted
					Hepatic metabolism; metabolites and parent compound excreted in urine and feces
					Major route of elimination is biliary secretion
Pentazocine 4.9%	3–6	Alcoholic and carboxylic acid metabolites		Renal	(l) Isomer responsible for analgesic activity; large interpatient variability in metabolism and oral bioavailability
					Bioavailability in cirrhotic patients increased to 60%–70%
					Inactive metabolites
		Pentazocine glucuronide		Renal	Inactive metabolite

Cl_{Cr}, creatinine clearance; IV, intravenous; Vd, volume of distribution.

Table adapted from the following references: McEvoy G, ed. *AHFS Drug Information 2008.* Bethesda, MD: American Society of Health-System Pharmacists; 2008; Babul N, Darke A. Putative role of hydromorphone metabolites in myoclonus. *Pain* 1993;52:123; Chan G, Matzke G. Effects of renal insufficiency on the pharmacokinetics and pharmacodynamics of opioid analgesics. *Drug Intell Clin Pharm* 1987;21:773–783; Lötsch J, Stockmann A, Brune K, et al. Pharmacokinetics of morphine and its glucuronides after intravenous infusion of morphine and morphine-6-glucuronide in healthy volunteers. *Clin Pharmacol Therap* 1996;60:316–325; Mulvana D, Duncan G, Shyu W, et al. Quantitative determination of butorphanol and its metabolites in human plasma by gas chromatography-electron capture negative-ion chemical ionization mass spectrometry. *J Chromatogr* 1996;682:289–300; Gutstein HB, Akil H. Opioid analgesics. In: Brunton LL, Lazo JS, Parker KL, eds. *Goodman and Gilman's The Pharmacological Basis of Therapeutic.* 11th ed. New York: McGraw-Hill; 2006:547–589; Shyu W, Morgenthien E, Barbhaiya R. Pharmacokinetics of butorphanol nasal spray in patients with renal impairment. *Br J Clin Pharmacol* 1996;41:397–402; Steinberg R, Gilman D, Johnson F. Acute toxic delirium in a patient using transdermal fentanyl. *Anesth Analg* 1992;75:1014–1016.

TABLE 79.6 Currently Available Abuse-Deterrent Opioid Formulations (as of December 2016)

Trade Name	ADF Technology	Abuse-Deterrent Properties	Comments
OxyContin (oxycodone HCl)	Physical and chemical barriers	Difficult to crush or break; resistant to ethanol dose dumping and other chemical extraction techniques; forms a viscous gel when dissolved	
Targiniq ER (oxycodone HCl + naloxone HCl)	Agonist/antagonist combination	Naloxone exhibits extremely low oral bioavailability due to significant first-pass hepatic metabolism and therefore has very little effect if the product is taken orally as prescribed. Naloxone is absorbed if administered intranasally or intravenously, blocking the euphoric effects of oxycodone.	Approved but not currently marketed
Embeda (morphine sulfate + naltrexone HCl)	Agonist/antagonist combination	Naltrexone, an opioid antagonist, is sequestered in the pellets core which is released with manipulation by crushing. Absorption of crushed naltrexone may precipitate withdrawal, thus deterring abuse.	
Hysingla ER (hydrocodone bitartrate)	Physical and chemical barriers	Difficult to crush or break; resistant to ethanol dose dumping and other chemical extraction techniques; forms a viscous gel when dissolved	
Morphabond (morphine sulfate)	Physical and chemical barriers	Designed to present multiple barriers to abuse through widely used methods of physical and chemical manipulation as well as various routes of administration; does not contain an opioid antagonist	
Xtampza ER (oxycodone)	Physical and chemical barriers	Designed to protect against common methods of manipulation, such as chewing, rushing, insufflation, and extraction for intravenous injection	
Troxyca ER (oxycodone HCl + naltrexone HCl)	Agonist/antagonist combination	Upon manipulation, naltrexone is released blocking the euphoric effects of oxycodone.	

ADF, abuse-deterrent formulation.
Reference: Hale ME, Moe D, Bond M, et al. Abuse-deterrent formulations of prescription opioid analgesics in the management of chronic noncancer pain. *Pain Manag* 2016;6(5):497–508.

the opioid-naive, whereas the chronic toxicity may be related to endocrinopathy, especially androgen deficiency.

Pain management with or without opioids requires individualization of treatment. So that titration to response remains the only effective way to determine the optimal opioid and dose for a specific patient. The initial opioid should be based on past patient experience, dosing schedule compatibility with the patient's life style and probable adherence to the regimen, and cost. Regular observation for adverse effects is essential. When adverse events occur, consider whether changing to a different opioid may be preferable to additional drugs to treat the adverse effect. If opioid efficacy wanes, consider whether nonopioid therapy might then suffice and if androgen deficiency

is a contributor. Opioid rotation also should be considered. Because of the comorbidities that occur with chronic pain, opioid monotherapy is seldom indicated; rather, additional pharmacotherapies, concurrent physical therapy, and psychotherapy are often required for appropriate pain management.

Opioid pharmacokinetics and pharmacodynamics are well characterized at all stages of life. Caution is indicated in very young, the elderly, and renally impaired patients due to the potential for opioid accumulation. Additive and synergistic effects with other CNS depressant medications are common. All opioid regimens should be reevaluated at regular intervals, and the medication should be tapered off if it is no longer needed or is no longer providing more benefits than adverse effects.

TABLE 79.7 Advantages and Limitations of Current Abuse-Deterrent Formulations (ADFs)

ADF Technology	Advantages	Limitations
Physical and chemical barriers	May prevent chewing, crushing, grating, or grinding. May prevent accidental crushing or chewing in compliant patients. May resist extraction by solvents. No adverse effects in compliant patients.	Does not deter abuse of intact tablets
Agonist/antagonist combinations	Antagonist may be formulated to be clinically active only when manipulated. May curb euphoria when formulation is compromised.	Inadvertent chewing or crushing may reduce analgesic effects and/or precipitate side effects or opioid withdrawal symptoms.
Aversion	Aversive agents may be combined with the opioid to create unpleasant side effects when manipulated or taken at higher doses. May prevent abuse by chewing or crushing.	Potential for unpleasant adverse effects in compliant patients who take product as intended. Adverse effects with intact tablets may prevent legitimate dose increases. Adverse effects may not be sufficient to deter a motivated abuser.
Delivery system	The method of drug delivery can offer resistance to abuse (e.g., depot formulations or subcutaneous implants).	It may still be possible to extract the opioid from the formulation.
Prodrug	A prodrug that lacks opioid activity until transformed in the GI tract may be unattractive for intravenous or intranasal routes of abuse.	
Combination	A combination of two or more of the above approaches	

GI, gastrointestinal.
Reference: U.S. Food and Drug Administration. Abuse-deterrent opioids—evaluation and labeling guidance for industry. Available at: https://www.fda.gov/downloads/Drugs /Guidances/UCM334743.pdf. Accessed April 11, 2018.

BIASED LIGANDS

We have always maintained that the ideal opioid would relieve moderate to severe pain with the efficacy of morphine without producing the undesirable effects of morphine and other μ-opioids. These adverse effects include respiratory depression, tolerance, and addiction (see Table 79.2). Today more than ever, the focus is on improving the adverse effect profile of newer opioids, and the abuse-deterrent formulations are a step in the right direction. However, the very recent recognition that opioids can be designed that act on MORs to activate signaling pathways that produce analgesia (the Gi/o signaling proteins) without simultaneous activating those pathways (the β-arrestin signaling proteins) that transduce the major limiting adverse effects of opioids.[53,108,109] With the advent of these biased ligands, we appear to be on the threshold of a new era in opioid pharmacology, clinical drug development, and pain therapy.

Pain remains a major public health problem, and opioids are an important part of the analgesic armamentarium. Used wisely, opioids have great value.

DEDICATION

We dedicate this chapter to our friend and colleague, Dr. Arthur Lipman. Art was a tireless advocate for evidence-based pain management.

References

1. Chapman CR, Lipschitz DL, Angst MS, et al. Opioid pharmacotherapy for chronic non-cancer pain in the United States: a research guideline for developing an evidence-base. *J Pain* 2010;11:807–829.
2. Chou R, Turner JA, Devine EB, et al. The effectiveness and risks of long-term opioid therapy for chronic pain: a systematic review for a National Institutes of Health Pathways to Prevention Workshop. *Ann Intern Med* 2015;162:276–286.
3. American Pain Society. *Principles of Analgesic Use*. Chicago, IL: American Pain Society; 2016.
4. Chou R, Fanciullo GJ, Fine PG, et al. Opioids for chronic noncancer pain: prediction and identification of aberrant drug-related behaviors: a review of the evidence for an American Pain Society and American Academy of Pain Medicine clinical practice guideline. *J Pain* 2009;10:131–146.
5. Frieden TR, Houry D. Reducing the risks of relief—the CDC opioid-prescribing guideline. *N Engl J Med* 2016;376:1501–1504.
6. Inturrisi CE. Clinical pharmacology of opioids for pain. *Clin J Pain* 2002;18:S3–S13.
7. Pasternak GW, Pan YX. Mu opioids and their receptors: evolution of a concept. *Pharmacol Rev* 2013;65:1257–1317.
8. Lotsch J, Geisslinger G. Current evidence for a genetic modulation of the response to analgesics. *Pain* 2006;121:1–5.
9. Bruehl S, Apkarian AV, Ballantyne JC, et al. Personalized medicine and opioid analgesic prescribing for chronic pain: opportunities and challenges. *J Pain* 2013;14:103–113.
10. Witkin LR, Zylberger D, Mehta N, et al. Patient-reported outcomes and opioid use in outpatients with chronic pain. *J Pain* 2017;18:583–596.
11. Lutfy K, Zaveri NT. The nociceptin receptor as an emerging molecular target for cocaine addiction. *Prog Mol Biol Transl Sci* 2016;137:149–181.
12. Nestler EJ. Reflections on: "A general role for adaptations in G-proteins and the cyclic AMP system in mediating the chronic actions of morphine and cocaine on neuronal function." *Brain Res* 2016;1645:71–74.
13. Kieffer BL, Gaveriaux-Ruff C. Exploring the opioid system by gene knock-out. *Prog Neurobiol* 2002;66:285–306.
14. Clarke S, Czyzyk T, Ansonoff M, et al. Autoradiography of opioid and ORL1 ligands in opioid receptor triple knockout mice. *Eur J Neurosci* 2002;16:1705–1712.
15. Bruchas MR, Roth BL. New technologies for elucidating opioid receptor function. *Trends Pharmacol Sci* 2016;37:279–289.
16. Basbaum AI, Bautista DM, Scherrer G, et al. Cellular and molecular mechanisms of pain. *Cell* 2009;139:267–284.
17. Bardoni R, Tawfik VL, Wang D, et al. Delta opioid receptors presynaptically regulate cutaneous mechanosensory neuron input to the spinal cord dorsal horn. *Neuron* 2014;81:1312–1327.
18. Fakata KL, Lipman AG. Gastrointestinal opioid physiology and pharmacology. In: Yuan SH, ed. *Opioid Bowel Dysfunction*. Binghamton, NY: Haworth Medical Press; 2005:7–28.
19. Sarosiek I, Bashashati M, Alvarez A, et al. Lubiprostone accelerates intestinal transit and alleviates small intestinal bacterial overgrowth in patients with chronic constipation. *Am J Med Sci* 2016;352:231–238.
20. Sanchez Del Aguila MJ, Schenk M, Kern KU, et al. Practical considerations for the use of tapentadol prolonged release for the management of severe chronic pain. *Clin Ther* 2015;37:94–113.
21. Rainville P, Duncan GH, Price DD, et al. Pain affect encoded in human anterior cingulate but not somatosensory cortex. *Science* 1997;277:968–971.
22. Navratilova E, Xie JY, Meske D, et al. Endogenous opioid activity in the anterior cingulate cortex is required for relief of pain. *J Neurosci* 2015;35:7264–7271.
23. Washington State Agency Medical Directors' Group. Interagency guideline on prescribing opioids for pain. Available at: www.agencymeddirectors.wa.gov. Accessed April 11, 2018.
24. O'Brien CP, Gardner EL. Critical assessment of how to study addiction and its treatment: human and non-human animal models. *Pharmacol Ther* 2005;108:18–58.
25. Dasgupta N, Funk MJ, Proescholdbell S, et al. Cohort study of the impact of high-dose opioid analgesics on overdose mortality. *Pain Med* 2016;17:85–98.
26. Foley KM. Problems of overarching importance which transcend organ systems. In: Bennett JC, Plum F, eds. *Cecil's Textbook of Medicine*. Philadelphia: Saunders; 1996:100–107.
27. Knezevic NN, Tverdohleb T, Knezevic I, et al. Unique pharmacology of tapentadol for treating acute and chronic pain. *Expert Opin Drug Metab Toxicol* 2015;11:1475–1492.
28. Van Ryswyk E, Antic NA. Opioids and sleep-disordered breathing. *Chest* 2016;150:934–944.
29. Webster LR, Choi Y, Desai H, et al. Sleep-disordered breathing and chronic opioid therapy. *Pain Med* 2008;9:425–432.
30. Yue HJ, Guilleminault C. Opioid medication and sleep-disordered breathing. *Med Clin North Am* 2010;94:435–446.
31. Boyer EW. Management of opioid analgesic overdose. *New Engl J Med* 2012;367:146–155.
32. Gal TJ. Naloxone reversal of buprenorphine-induced respiratory depression. *Clin Pharmacol Ther* 1989;45:66–71.
33. van Dorp E, Yassen A, Sarton E, et al. Naloxone reversal of buprenorphine-induced respiratory depression. *Anesthesiology* 2006;105:51–57.
34. Goldfrank L, Weisman RS, Errick JK, et al. A dosing nomogram for continuous infusion intravenous naloxone. *Ann Emerg Med* 1986;15:566–570.
35. O'Rourke TK Jr, Wosnitzer MS. Opioid-induced androgen deficiency (OPIAD): diagnosis, management, and literature review. *Curr Urol Rep* 2016;17:76.
36. Bliesener N, Albrecht S, Schwager A, et al. Plasma testosterone and sexual function in men receiving buprenorphine maintenance for opioid dependence. *J Clin Endocrinol Metab* 2005;90:203–206.
37. Blick G, Khera M, Bhattacharya RK, et al. Testosterone replacement therapy outcomes among opioid users: the Testim Registry in the United States (TRiUS). *Pain Med* 2012;13:688–698.
38. Daniell HW. DHEAS deficiency during consumption of sustained-action prescribed opioids: evidence for opioid-induced inhibition of adrenal androgen production. *J Pain* 2006;7:901–907.
39. Daniell HW. Opioid endocrinopathy in women consuming prescribed sustained-action opioids for control of nonmalignant pain. *J Pain* 2008;9:28–36.
40. Kaiko RF, Foley KM, Grabinski PY, et al. Central nervous system excitatory effects of meperidine in cancer patients. *Ann Neurol* 1983;13:180–185.
41. Smith MT. Neuroexcitatory effects of morphine and hydromorphone: evidence implicating the 3-glucuronide metabolites. *Clin Exp Pharmacol Physiol* 2000;27:524–528.
42. Schuckit MA. Treatment of opioid-use disorders. *N Engl J Med* 2016;375:357–368.
43. Kampman K, Jarvis M. American Society of Addiction Medicine (ASAM) National Practice Guideline for the use of medications in the treatment of addiction involving opioid use. *J Addict Med* 2015;9:358–367.
44. Chou R, Gordon DB, de Leon-Casasola OA, et al. Management of postoperative pain: a clinical practice guideline from the American Pain Society, the American Society of Regional Anesthesia and Pain Medicine, and the American Society of Anesthesiologists' Committee on Regional Anesthesia, Executive Committee, and Administrative Council. *J Pain* 2016;17:131–157.
45. Fishbain DA, Cutler RB, Rosomoff HL, et al. Are opioid-dependent/tolerant patients impaired in driving-related skills? A structured evidence-based review. *J Pain Symptom Manage* 2003;25:559–577.
46. Mitchell JM, Basbaum AI, Fields HL. A locus and mechanism of action for associative morphine tolerance. *Nat Neurosci* 2000;3:47–53.
47. McQuay H. Opioids in pain management. *Lancet* 1999;353:2229–2232.
48. Petersen KL, Meadoff T, Press S, et al. Changes in morphine analgesia and side effects during daily subcutaneous administration in healthy volunteers. *Pain* 2008;137:395–404.
49. Lipman AG, Jackson KC. Opioid pharmacotherapy. In: Warfield C, Bajwa Z, eds. *Principles and Practice of Pain Management*. New York: McGraw Hill; 2004:583–600.
50. Kanner RM, Foley KM. Patterns of narcotic drug use in a cancer pain clinic. *Ann N Y Acad Sci* 1981;362:161–172.
51. Inturrisi CE, Gregus AM. Mechanisms of opioid tolerance. In: Bell R, Paice JD, Soyannwo O, eds. *The Eighth IASP Research Symposium: A Global Problem: Cancer Pain from the Laboratory to the Bedside*. Seattle, WA: IASP Press; 2010:123–139.
52. Bohn LM, Gainetdinov RR, Lin FT, et al. Mu-opioid receptor desensitization by beta-arrestin-2 determines morphine tolerance but not dependence. *Nature* 2000;408:720–723.

53. Rominger DH, Cowan CL, Gowen-MacDonald W, et al. Biased ligands: pathway validation for novel GPCR therapeutics. *Curr Opin Pharmacol* 2014;16:108–115.

54. Angst MS, Clark JD. Opioid-induced hyperalgesia: a qualitative systematic review. *Anesthesiology* 2006;104:570–587.

55. Eisenberg E, Suzan E, Pud D. Opioid-induced hyperalgesia (OIH): a real clinical problem or just an experimental phenomenon? *J Pain Symptom Manage* 2015;49:632–636.

56. Carroll IR, Angst MS, Clark JD. Management of perioperative pain in patients chronically consuming opioids. *Reg Anesth Pain Med* 2004;29: 576–591.

57. Inturrisi CE. Opioid rotation. In: Gebhart GF, Schmidt RF, eds. *Encyclopedia of Pain*. New York: Springer; 2013;2459–2463.

58. Curatolo M. Regional anesthesia in pain management. *Curr Opin Anaesthesiol* 2016;29:614–619.

59. Shimoyama N, Shimoyama M, Inturrisi C, et al. Ketamine attenuates and reverses morphine tolerance in rodents. *Anesthesiology* 2016;85:1357–1366.

60. Bell RF, Eccleston C, Kalso EA. Ketamine as an adjuvant to opioids for cancer pain. *Cochrane Database Syst Rev* 2012;(11):CD003351.

61. Berna C, Kulich RJ, Rathmell JP. Tapering long-term opioid therapy in chronic noncancer pain: evidence and recommendations for everyday practice. *Mayo Clin Proc* 2015;90:828–842.

62. Fiellin DA, Schottenfeld RS, Cutter CJ, et al. Primary care-based buprenorphine taper vs maintenance therapy for prescription opioid dependence: a randomized clinical trial. *JAMA Intern Med* 2014;174:1947–1954.

63. Volkow ND, McLellan AT. Mitigation strategies for opioid abuse. *N Engl J Med* 2016;375:96.

64. Institute of Medicine. *Relieving Pain in America: A Blueprint for Transforming Prevention, Care, Education, and Research*. Washington, DC: National Academies Press; 2011.

65. Rich BA. The war on drugs versus the war on pain: surviving two perfect storms. *Pain Manage* 2012;2:523–526.

66. Lipman AG. The opioid abuse blame game. *J Pain Palliat Care Pharmacother* 2016;30:2–3.

67. Jamal MM, Adams AB, Jansen JP, et al. A randomized, placebo-controlled trial of lubiprostone for opioid-induced constipation in chronic noncancer pain. *Am J Gastroenterol* 2015;110:725–732.

68. Chou R, Cruciani RA, Fiellin DA, et al. Methadone safety: a clinical practice guideline from the American Pain Society and College on Problems of Drug Dependence, in collaboration with the Heart Rhythm Society. *J Pain* 2014;15:321–337.

69. Amsterdam EA, Wenger NK, Brindis RG, et al. 2014 AHA/ACC guideline for the management of patients with non-ST-elevation acute coronary syndromes: a report of the American College of Cardiology/American Heart Association Task Force on Practice Guidelines. *J Am Coll Cardiol* 2014;64:e139–e228.

70. Kumar K, Singh SI. Neuraxial opioid-induced pruritus: an update. *J Anaesthesiol and Clin Pharmacol* 2013;29:303–307.

71. Ko MC. Neuraxial opioid-induced itch and its pharmacological antagonism. *Handb Exp Pharmacol* 2015;226:315–335.

72. Jannuzzi RG. Nalbuphine for treatment of opioid-induced pruritus: a systematic review of literature. *Clin J Pain* 2016;32:87–93.

73. Bateman BT, Hernandez-Diaz S, Rathmell JP, et al. Patterns of opioid utilization in pregnancy in a large cohort of commercial insurance beneficiaries in the United States. *Anesthesiology* 2014;120:1216–1224.

74. Minozzi S, Amato L, Bellisario C, et al. Maintenance agonist treatments for opiate-dependent pregnant women. *Cochrane Database Syst Rev* 2013;(12):CD006318.

75. Ashburn MA, Lipman AG. Management of pain in the cancer patient. *Anesth Analg* 1993;76(2):402–416.

76. Weinberg DS, Inturrisi CE, Reidenberg B, et al. Sublingual absorption of selected opioid analgesics. *Clin Pharmacol Ther* 1988;44:335–342.

77. Jacox A CD, Carr DB, Payne R, et al. *Management of Cancer Pain. Clinical Practice Guideline No. 9*. Rockville, MD: Agency for Health Care Policy and Research; 1994. AHCPR publication no. 94-0592.

78. Allen LV Jr. Rectal and stomal administration of analgesic suppositories. *Int J Pharm Compd* 1997;1:12.

79. Maloney CM, Kesner RK, Klein G, et al. The rectal administration of MS Contin: clinical implications of use in end stage cancer. *Am J Hosp Care* 1989;6:34–35.

80. Kaiko RF, Fitzmartin RD, Thomas GB, et al. The bioavailability of morphine in controlled-release 30-mg tablets per rectum compared with immediate-release 30-mg rectal suppositories and controlled-release 30-mg oral tablets. *Pharmacotherapy* 1922;12:107–113.

81. Leow KP, Smith MT, Watt JA, et al. Comparative oxycodone pharmacokinetics in humans after intravenous, oral, and rectal administration. *Ther Drug Monit* 1992;14:479–484.

82. Hojsted J, Rubeck-Petersen K, Rask H, et al. Comparative bioavailability of a morphine suppository given rectally and in a colostomy. *Eur J Clin Pharmacol* 1990;39:49–50.

83. Swanson BN, Gordon WP, Lynn RK, et al. Seminal excretion, vaginal absorption, distribution and whole blood kinetics of d-methadone in the rabbit. *J Pharmacol Exp Ther* 1978;206:507–514.

84. Viola R, Kiteley C, Lloyd NS, et al. The management of dyspnea in cancer patients: a systematic review. *Support Care Cancer* 2008;16:329–337.

85. Barnes H, McDonald J, Smallwood N, et al. Opioids for the palliation of refractory breathlessness in adults with advanced disease and terminal illness. *Cochrane Database Syst Rev* 2016;(3):CD011008.

86. Cata JP, Noguera EM, Parke E, et al. Patient-controlled epidural analgesia (PCEA) for postoperative pain control after lumbar spine surgery. *J Neurosurg Anesth* 2008;20:256–260.

87. Karavelis A, Foroglou G, Selviaridis P, et al. Intraventricular administration of morphine for control of intractable cancer pain in 90 patients. *Neurosurgery* 1996;39:57–62.

88. Inturrisi CE, Hanks GW. Opioid analgesic therapy. In: Doyle D, Hanks GWC, MacDonald N, eds. *Oxford Textbook of Palliative Medicine*. Oxford, United Kingdom: Oxford University Press; 1993:166–182.

89. Lotsch J. Opioid metabolites. *J Pain Symptom Manage* 2005;29:S10–S24.

90. Portenoy RK, Thaler HT, Inturrisi CE, et al. The metabolite morphine-6-glucuronide contributes to the analgesia produced by morphine infusion in patients with pain and normal renal function. *Clin Pharmacol Ther* 1992;51:422–431.

91. Tiseo PJ, Thaler HT, Lapin J, et al. Morphine-6-glucuronide concentrations and opioid-related side effects: a survey in cancer patients. *Pain* 1995;61:47–54.

92. McNicol E, Horowicz-Mehler N, Fisk RA, et al. Management of opioid side effects in cancer-related and chronic noncancer pain: a systematic review. *J Pain* 2003;4:231–256.

93. Davis AM, Inturrisi CE. d-Methadone blocks morphine tolerance and N-methyl-D-aspartate-induced hyperalgesia. *J Pharmacol Exp Ther* 1999; 289:1048–1053.

94. Portenoy RK, Southam MA, Gupta SK, et al. Transdermal fentanyl for cancer pain. Repeated dose pharmacokinetics. *Anesthesiology* 1993;78:36–43.

95. Szeto HH, Inturrisi CE, Houde R, et al. Accumulation of normeperidine, an active metabolite of meperidine, in patients with renal failure of cancer. *Ann Intern Med* 1977;86:738–741.

96. Gillman PK. Monoamine oxidase inhibitors, opioid analgesics and serotonin toxicity. *Br J Anaesth* 2005;95:434–441.

97. Holtzclaw BJ. Shivering in acutely ill vulnerable populations. *AACN Clin Issues* 2004;15:267–279.

98. Zahari Z, Ismail R. Influence of cytochrome P450, family 2, subfamily D, polypeptide 6 (CYP2D6) polymorphisms on pain sensitivity and clinical response to weak opioid analgesics. *Drug Metab Pharmacokinet* 2014;29:29–43.

99. Crews KR, Gaedigk A, Dunnenberger HM, et al. Clinical Pharmacogenetics Implementation Consortium guidelines for cytochrome P450 2D6 genotype and codeine therapy: 2014 update. *Clin Pharmacol Ther* 2014;95:376–382.

100. Christoph T, Kogel B, Strassburger W, et al. Tramadol has a better potency ratio relative to morphine in neuropathic than in nociceptive pain models. *Drugs R D* 2007;8:51–57.

101. Shadnia S, Soltaninejad K, Heydari K, et al. Tramadol intoxication: a review of 114 cases. *Hum Exp Toxicol* 2008;27:201–205.

102. Tzschentke TM, Jahnel U, Kogel B, et al. Tapentadol hydrochloride: a next-generation, centrally acting analgesic with two mechanisms of action in a single molecule. *Drugs Today (Barc)* 2009;45:483–496.

103. Etropolski M, Kelly K, Okamoto A, et al. Comparable efficacy and superior gastrointestinal tolerability (nausea, vomiting, constipation) of tapentadol compared with oxycodone hydrochloride. *Adv Ther* 2011;28:401–417.

104. Daniels S, Casson E, Stegmann JU, et al. A randomized, double-blind, placebo-controlled phase 3 study of the relative efficacy and tolerability of tapentadol IR and oxycodone IR for acute pain. *Curr Med Res Opin* 2009;25:1551–1561.

105. Huestis MA, Cone EJ, Pirnay SO, et al. Intravenous buprenorphine and norbuprenorphine pharmacokinetics in humans. *Drug Alcohol Depend* 2013;131:258–262.

106. Davison SN, Koncicki H, Brennan F. Pain in chronic kidney disease: a scoping review. *Semin Dial* 2014;27:188–204.

107. Substance Abuse and Mental Health Services Administration. *Behavioral Health Trends in the United States: Results from the 2014 National Survey on Drug Use and Health*. Rockville, MD: U.S. Department of Health and Human Services. HHS publication no. SMA 15-4927. NSDUH Series H-50.

108. Kieffer BL. Drug discovery: designing the ideal opioid. *Nature* 2016;537: 170–171.

109. Manglik A, Lin H, Aryal DK, et al. Structure-based discovery of opioid analgesics with reduced side effects. *Nature* 2016;537:185–190.

CHAPTER 80

Skeletal Muscle Relaxants and Analgesic Balms

AUSIM CHAGHTAI and **CHARLES E. ARGOFF**

Skeletal Muscle Relaxants

The class of medications termed *skeletal muscle relaxants* is ill defined leading to much confusion for both clinicians and scientists. This confusion results from the assumption that these medications all act in a similar fashion and produce reliable skeletal muscle relaxation. Neither is true. These medications produce a range of effects that remain poorly defined (Table 80.1).[1-4] The class includes carisoprodol, chlorzoxazone, cyclobenzaprine, metaxalone, methocarbamol, and orphenadrine.[5] These medications are approved by the U.S. Food and Drug Administration (FDA) for indications including spasticity, spasms, and/or musculoskeletal conditions (Table 80.2). Medications are often utilized for off-label uses and skeletal muscle relaxants are no exception. Benzodiazepines, principally diazepam, also are commonly used for adjunctive relief of skeletal muscle spasm. Chief among the challenges to clinicians using these drugs is discerning the role of the agents across the continuum of painful disorders. It should be noted that the order of medications within the subsections do not indicate management priority or expert preference.

Historically, skeletal muscle relaxants have been prescribed for acute and chronic conditions associated with muscle related pain. The majority of these agents are indicated for use during the initial presentation of acute low back pain, which often results from soft tissue mechanical injury and normally occurs in the muscles, ligaments, and/or tendons, structures around the lumbar spine. Acute pain may include local pain and tenderness, muscle spasm, and limited range of motion, but what actually constitutes painful muscle spasm remains controversial.[6] Muscle spasm may be a variant of the myofascial pain presentation, and as such not really a spasm.[7]

To better understand the potential pharmacologic benefit of these agents, consider the regulation of muscle activity in both the peripheral tissues and central nervous system (CNS). At the level of the peripheral muscle, tissues are composed of intrafusal fibers that signal changes in muscle length. These lie

TABLE 80.1	Pharmacotherapies Commonly Used for Muscle Spasm				
Drug	**Onset**	**Duration**	**Common Dosing**	**Side Effects**	**Important Drug Interactions**
Sedative					
Carisoprodol (Soma)	30 min	4–6 h	350 PO QID	Ataxia, dizziness, drowsiness, N/V, withdrawal potential	Additive effects with alcohol and other CNS depressants
Chlorzoxazone (Parafon Forte)	~1 h	3–4 h	250–750 mg PO TID–QID	Dizziness, drowsiness, headache, N/V	
Metaxalone (Skelaxin)	1 h	4–6 h	400–800 mg PO TID	Dizziness, drowsiness, headache, N/V, rash	
Methocarbamol (Robaxin)	30 min (PO)	N/A	750–1,000 mg PO QID	Blurred vision, dizziness, drowsiness	
TCA-like					
Cyclobenzaprine (Flexeril)	~1 h	12–24 h	5–10 mg PO TID	Drowsiness, dizziness, dry mouth	Additive effects with alcohol and other CNS depressants; seizures with tramadol and MAOIs; additive effects with TCAs
Antihistamine					
Orphenadrine (Norflex)	1 h (PO)	4–6 h	100 mg PO BID	Tachycardia, light-headedness, N/V, dry mouth	Additive effects with alcohol and other CNS depressants; coadministration with propoxyphene can lead to confusion, anxiety, and/or tremors
GABA Type					
Diazepam (Valium)	30 min (PO)	Variable, depending on elimination	2–10 mg PO TID	Sedation, fatigue, hypotension, ataxia, respiratory depression	Potentiation of effects when taken with phenothiazines, opioids, barbiturates, MAOIs
Baclofen (Lioresal)	3–4 d (PO) 30 min (IT)	Variable (PO) 4–6 h (IT)	5 mg PO TID titrated up to 40–80 mg/d	Drowsiness, slurred speech, hypotension, constipation, urinary retention	Antidepressants (short-term memory loss); additive effects with imipramine
Central α_2 Agonists					
Tizanidine (Tizanidine)	2 wk	Variable	2–8 mg PO TID–QID	Drowsiness, dry mouth, dizziness, hypotension, increased spasm/tone	Additive effects with alcohol and other CNS depressants; reduced clearance with oral contraceptives

CNS, central nervous system; GABA, γ-aminobutyric acid; IT, intrathecal; MAOIs, monoamine oxidase inhibitors; N/A, not applicable; N/V, nausea/vomiting; PO, orally; QID, four times a day; TCA, tricyclic antidepressant; TID, three times a day.

TABLE 80.2 U.S. Food and Drug Administration-Approved Therapies and Indications

Medication	Indication
Baclofen	Spasticity
Dantrolene	Chronic spasticity
	Malignant hyperthermia
Tizanidine	Muscle spasticity
Carisoprodol	Musculoskeletal conditions
Metaxalone	Musculoskeletal conditions
Chlorzoxazone	Musculoskeletal conditions
Cyclobenzaprine	Muscle spasm
Methocarbamol	Muscle spasm
	Tetanus
Orphenadrine	Muscle spasms

in parallel with extrafusal muscle fibers that normally serve to contract or stabilize joints. When muscle tissue is stretched, the intrafusal fibers stretch resulting in an increase in neural discharges carried by afferent nerve fibers. This signal is transmitted to the dorsal horn and synapses with α-motoneurons in the ventral horn, producing excitatory postsynaptic potentials. The result is a type of negative feedback, with muscle contraction of the intrafusal muscle fibers where the original stretch signal originated. These muscle fibers also maintain an efferent component, facilitated by small γ-motoneurons that originate in the ventral horn of the spinal cord and travel together with the α-motoneurons that innervate extrafusal muscle fibers. The γ-motoneurons adjust the sensitivity of the muscle fibers and regulate muscle tension over a wide range of muscle lengths. This complex system of afferent and efferent signaling through

the motoneurons when at homeostasis leads to stabilization of muscle structures (Fig. 80.1).

In the dorsal horn, a complex network of excitatory and inhibitory interneurons mediates motor reflexes in response to deep and cutaneous stimulation. Such reflexes mediate ipsilateral flexion and contralateral extension in response to noxious stimuli to coordinate a protective or escape response. Impulses from cutaneous afferents travel through the dorsal horn of the spinal cord and terminate on excitatory interneurons, which in turn terminate on presynaptic terminals of the intrafusal fibers further promoting excitation at the ventral horn α-motoneuron. Inhibitory centers in the bulbar reticular formation and facilitatory centers from several brain regions further regulate both corticospinal and reflex muscle activity.[8,9]

Excitatory neurotransmitters in the CNS play a major role in the modulation of movement in the spinal cord and include substances like glutamate, aspartate, and substance P. These neurotransmitters are released from the terminals of primary afferent fibers to mediate reflexes that enhance motor tone at the spinal level.[10] γ-Aminobutyric acid (GABA) is a major inhibitory CNS neurotransmitter that emanates from supraspinal and interneuronal inputs. GABA is believed to play a major role in presynaptic inhibition of motor neurons in the dorsal horn.[10]

Any change in the homeostasis of the peripheral or CNS components related to maintaining proper muscle tone can lead to production of an acute reflex muscle spasm. When this occurs, there are two main potential issues. Either a reflex increase in muscle tone activates polysynaptic reflexes and produces hyperexcitability of α- and/or γ-motoneurons, or there is supraspinal activation of descending facilitatory systems.[11] In settings of chronic muscle spasticity, the processes appear to be

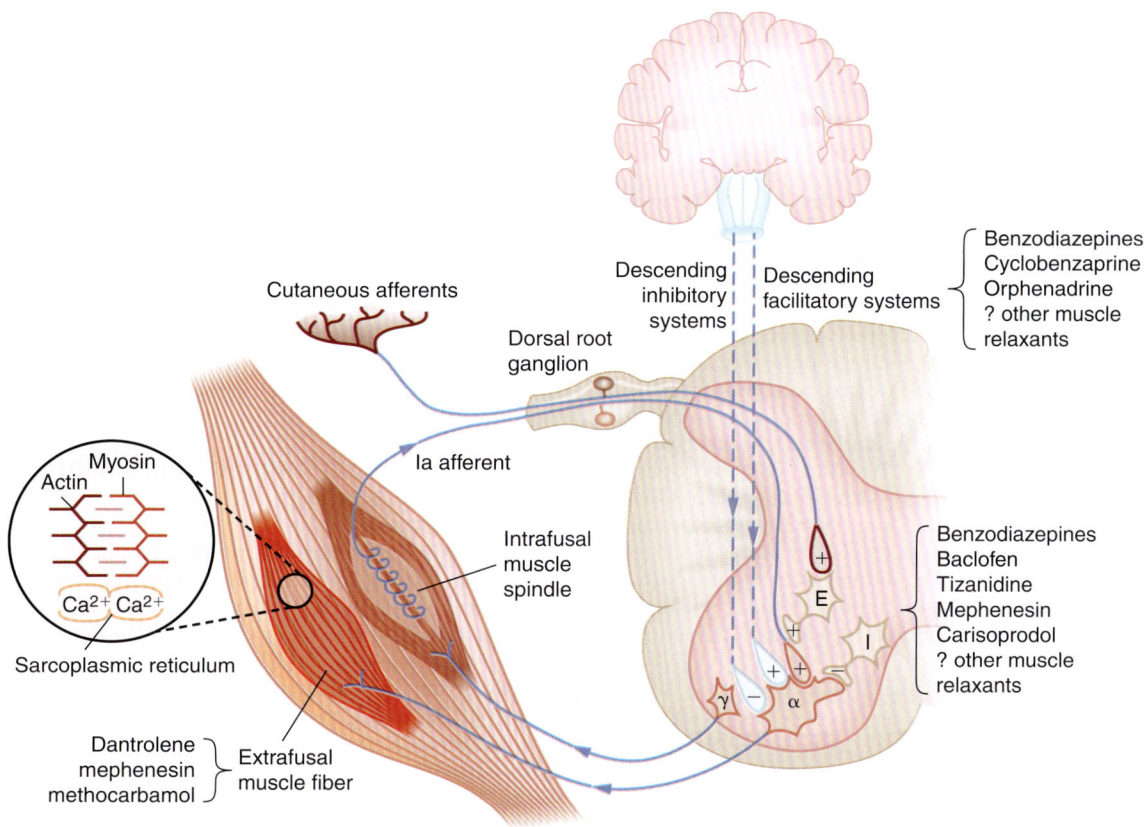

FIGURE 80.1 Neural regulation of muscle tone: possible sites of action of skeletal muscle relaxants. See text for details. +, excitatory effect; −, inhibitory effect; α, α-motoneuron; Ca²⁺, calcium ion; E, excitatory interneuron; γ, γ-motoneuron; I, inhibitory interneuron.

TABLE 80.3   Agents by Proposed Mechanism of Action

CNS Depressants

- Antihistamine
  Orphenadrine
- Sedatives
  Carisoprodol, chlorzoxazone, metaxalone, methocarbamol
- TCA-like
  Cyclobenzaprine

Central α₂ Agonists

Tizanidine

GABA Agonists

Baclofen
Benzodiazepines

CNS, central nervous system; GABA, γ-aminobutyric acid; TCA, tricyclic antidepressant.

more involved, with pathology from supraspinal CNS descending pathways that produce excessive excitation or diminished inhibition of α-motoneurons in the dorsal horn.[12]

MECHANISM OF ACTION

In animal studies, skeletal muscle relaxants act at various CNS sites that are important in muscle activity regulation. The exact mechanism of action for these various agents is not clear. A variety of mechanisms appear to be associated with the activity of this diverse group of agents (Table 80.3). Animal models have historically shown that muscle relaxants exert their activity by blocking polysynaptic neurons in the spinal cord and inhibiting interneuronal activity within the descending reticular formation.[1] Mephenesin, an early predecessor to today's muscle relaxants, in animal models affected monosynaptic and polysynaptic reflexes.[13,14] Subsequent animal data showed that mephenesin and methocarbamol prolonged the refractory period of skeletal muscle by a direct action on skeletal muscle fibers.[15] Very little has been described about the effects of skeletal muscle relaxants such as cyclobenzaprine, methocarbamol, carisoprodol, and chlorzoxazone on neurotransmission. These medications are also known to have a significant sedative profile. This in fact was a quality that was exploited when older treatment paradigms included significant bed rest. Interestingly, other medications with sedative properties are also known to depress polysynaptic reflexes. This situation certainly sheds some degree of confusion as to the specific utility of skeletal muscle relaxants, especially in relation to the purported effects versus nonspecific sedation.

The pharmacologic capacity of other commonly used drugs is less well characterized in specific relation to muscle spasm. Diazepam, a benzodiazepine, suppressed polysynaptic reflexes in cats but required doses higher than would be used clinically.[16] Benzodiazepines act by potentiating the postsynaptic effects of GABA within the CNS.[12] Baclofen (parachlorophenol GABA) is a lipophilic derivative of GABA that binds to GABA_B but not to GABA_A receptors and may exert its effect, in part, by inhibiting the evoked release of excitatory amino acids (e.g., glutamate) and substance P.[10] Tizanidine, a newer antispasticity agent, is an α₂-adrenergic receptor agonist that may also act by decreasing spinal excitatory amino acid release.[16]

Types of Skeletal Muscle Relaxants

CENTRALLY ACTING SEDATIVE-HYPNOTIC MUSCLE RELAXANTS
Chlorzoxazone

Chlorzoxazone may be less effective than the other skeletal muscle relaxants.[17] Chlorzoxazone does not have any significant drug interactions but does have a significant adverse effect profile

that includes a rare idiosyncratic hepatocellular reaction.[18] The use of this agent may be questionable considering the potential lack of efficacy and significant toxicity profile.[19]

Metaxalone

Metaxalone does not have any significant drug interactions and appears to have a fairly benign side effect profile. Hemolytic anemia and impaired liver function may occur but are uncommon. Fatalities attributed to the use of metaxalone have been reported.[20,21] Metaxalone is contraindicated in patients with severe renal or hepatic impairment. Because this drug was FDA-approved over 30 years ago, there are few published placebo-controlled studies of metaxalone for musculoskeletal pain.[22]

Methocarbamol

Methocarbamol is available in an oral form and a parenteral form for intravenous (IV) or intramuscular (IM) use. Complications with the injectable form include pain, skin sloughing, and thrombophlebitis. This drug also was FDA-approved over 30 years ago, and as a result, there are few published studies comparing it to placebo for the treatment of musculoskeletal pain.[23]

Carisoprodol

Carisoprodol is a schedule IV controlled substance in the United States. It is hepatically metabolized to meprobamate. Meprobamate produces physical and psychological dependence.[24–29] Substance abuse appears to be problematic with carisoprodol, probably due to meprobamate formation. In recent years, several states have begun treating carisoprodol as a controlled substance within their state formularies. Due to the dependence potential, carisoprodol should be cautiously tapered as opposed to immediately discontinued following long-term use. At the end of November 2007, the European Medicines Agency recommended the suspension of marketing authorization for carisoprodol-containing products for its 12 member states. Its Committee for Medicinal Products for Human Use concluded that the risk of their use is greater than the benefits.[30] Given the unfavorable risk–benefit balance, which includes a high dependence potential, carisoprodol should generally be avoided.

ANTIHISTAMINE MUSCLE RELAXANT
Orphenadrine Citrate

Orphenadrine is a derivative diphenhydramine and accordingly exhibits antihistaminic and anticholinergic properties. There have been reports of severe adverse reactions with parenteral use (e.g., anaphylactoid reaction). Orphenadrine use with propoxyphene may cause confusion, anxiety, and tremors, perhaps because of additive effects. Orphenadrine's anticholinergic actions have been noted to produce significant adverse effects at high dosages, for example, tachycardia, palpitations, urinary retention, blurred vision.[31]

TRICYCLIC ANTIDEPRESSANT-LIKE MUSCLE RELAXANT
Cyclobenzaprine

Cyclobenzaprine is more structurally and pharmacologically similar to the tricyclic antidepressants than it is to the centrally acting sedative-hypnotic skeletal muscle relaxants. As with the other skeletal muscle relaxants, cyclobenzaprine does not act directly on muscle tissue. Animal data suggest cyclobenzaprine acts primarily at the level of brain stem reducing tonic somatic motor activity.[32] Although no evidence exists in humans to support this mechanism, it is interesting to note that the newer 5-mg dose has yielded similar clinical efficacy with less sedation than the more sedating 10-mg dose.[33] This may prove to be an important distinction from the centrally acting sedative-hypnotic muscle relaxants.

The value of muscle relaxant monotherapy remains the subject of some skepticism; these agents may be used as adjuncts to other therapies. This appears to apply to cyclobenzaprine as well. In an open-label study of patients with acute neck or low back pain associated with muscle spasm who were randomized to be treated for seven days with either cyclobenzaprine 5 mg orally three times daily alone or with cyclobenzaprine 5 mg orally three times daily in combination with ibuprofen at doses of 400 mg orally three times daily or 800 mg three times daily, no significant treatment differences were found among these groups.[34]

Cyclobenzaprine has a similar adverse event profile as the tricyclic antidepressants. Thus, one might want to avoid using cyclobenzaprine and a tricyclic antidepressant concurrently unless the combination is truly clinically indicated. Anticholinergic side effects including dry mouth, urinary retention, and constipation occur with cyclobenzaprine. Use of cyclobenzaprine is contraindicated in the setting of arrhythmias, congestive heart failure, hyperthyroidism, or during the acute recovery phase of a myocardial infarction. Concurrent use with proserotonergic agents such as selective serotonin reuptake inhibitors (SSRIs) may predispose patients to life-threatening serotonin syndrome.[35]

Cyclobenzaprine labeling suggests that concomitant use with tramadol may place patients at higher risk for developing seizures.[32] Concomitant use of cyclobenzaprine with monoamine oxidase inhibitors or use within 14 days after their discontinuation is contraindicated. Cyclobenzaprine can enhance the effects of agents with CNS depressant activity. Older patients appear to have a higher risk for CNS-related adverse reactions, for example, hallucinations and confusion, when using cyclobenzaprine. Withdrawal symptoms have been noted with the discontinuation of chronic cyclobenzaprine use. Use of a medication taper may be warranted for patients with chronic use.

γ-AMINOBUTYRIC ACID AGONIST MUSCLE RELAXANTS

Diazepam

Diazepam is the most commonly prescribed and referenced benzodiazepine in the treatment of muscle spasms.[36] It has hypnotic, anxiolytic, antiepileptic, and antispasmodic properties. Sedation and abuse potential are the main concerns with this agent and class. It is important to slowly taper this agent after long-term use, as opposed to abrupt removal to avoid any withdrawal symptoms. Recent studies have suggested that the addition of diazepam to nonsteroidal anti-inflammatory drugs (NSAIDs) for acute lower back pain have little to no benefit compared to placebo. Use in lower back pain should be cautioned.

Baclofen

Studies have shown baclofen to have superior efficacy than diazepam.[2] Baclofen is unique in that it can be administered intrathecally in cases of severe spasticity and for patients who do not tolerate or have failed oral therapy. Baclofen should be tapered slowly after long-term use to avoid a withdrawal reaction and rebound phenomena. It should be used with caution in the elderly and for patients with renal impairment.

CENTRAL α₂ AGONIST MUSCLE RELAXANTS

Tizanidine

Tizanidine is related chemically to clonidine but has significantly less antihypertensive effect.[37] The main adverse effect for most patients with this agent is sedation.[38] Currently, tizanidine is FDA-approved for the management of increased muscle tone associated with spasticity resulting from CNS disorders, such as multiple sclerosis or spinal cord injury. Two studies report use of tizanidine in of back pain or muscle spasm, either alone or in combination with ibuprofen, and another study reports effectiveness in myofascial pain.[39–42] A multicenter,

placebo-controlled study evaluated the efficacy and safety of tizanidine in the treatment of low back pain; tizanidine was found to provide more pain relief and less restriction of movement than placebo. Drowsiness was the most common side effect, but for acute low back pain patients, this effect may actually be desired, especially at night.[39] A study of 105 patients with acute low back pain who received tizanidine 4 mg orally three times daily with ibuprofen 400 mg orally three times daily or ibuprofen 400 mg orally three times daily compared to placebo. The results suggested that the tizanidine/ibuprofen combination was more effective for moderate or severe acute low back pain than ibuprofen only.[40] Use tizanidine with caution in renal impairment; clearance is decreased by 50% in patients with creatinine clearance <25 mL per minute. Coadministration with alcohol can increase the area under the curve (AUC) of tizanidine by approximately 20% and increase C_{max} by approximately 15%. Use with oral contraceptives can decrease the clearance of tizanidine and place patients at higher risk for sedating adverse effects.

Recent trials of a novel delivery system for tizanidine have been promising. A trial of an intranasal delivery system has shown quicker onset of action and higher serum contractions when compared to oral administration with a similar side effect profile. This may ultimately have efficacy in the management of acute painful muscle spasm syndromes.[41]

Acute Low Back Pain

Available data indicate that skeletal muscle relaxants are more effective than placebo to relieve acute low back pain.[17] Unfortunately, most of the data are dated and are derived form studies for which the designs and analyses that would not be acceptable today. No data clearly show that any one agent as more efficacious than another. Some data suggest that chlorzoxazone may be less effective than other drugs and, as such, puts into question the use of this agent.[17,43]

Most clinical guidelines list skeletal muscle relaxants as optional agents for use individually or in combination with an NSAID. The federal clinical practice guideline published in 1995 specifically noted that skeletal muscle relaxants alone or in combination with an NSAID were no more effective than using an NSAID alone.[44] This conclusion has been supported in systematic reviews by van Tulder and colleagues.[17,43] In the past, skeletal muscle relaxants have been shown to more effective than placebo for patients with acute low back pain with respect to outcomes such as short-term pain relief, global efficacy, and improvement of physical outcomes.[39,45–47] No quality evidence allows a direct comparison of skeletal muscle relaxants to NSAIDs. Most clinicians and researchers agreed that skeletal muscle relaxants may benefit patients with acute low back pain by reducing the duration of their discomfort and accelerating recovery. A meta-analysis of cyclobenzaprine studies for acute low back pain concluded that despite limitations in the available evidence, the combination of an NSAID with cyclobenzaprine appears to be warranted.[48] More recently, NSAIDs prescribed alone or in combination with cyclobenzaprine or oxycodone/acetaminophen for lumbar back pain in the emergency department setting. The addition of cyclobenzaprine or oxycodone/acetaminophen to NSAIDs for lumbar back pain has not shown improvement of functional outcome in short-term follow-up. However, more recently, the use of extended-release cyclobenzaprine alone has suggested benefit for muscle spasm and muscle spasm associated back and neck pain. Further investigation is warranted. It is probably best to consider the use of skeletal muscle relaxants as an adjunct or alternative to NSAIDs, especially in cases where NSAID toxicity is a concern or when NSAID monotherapy proves suboptimal.

Various systematic reviews have been published reviewing the randomized controlled trials of muscle relaxants in the treatment of acute low back pain.[17,43,49] These analyses concur that there is strong evidence that muscle relaxants are more effective than placebo for acute low back pain but do not indicate superiority of a specific type of muscle relaxant. Muscle relaxants also appear to be useful in acute cervical pain presentations.[50–52]

Baclofen and tizanidine are well established for the treatment of spasticity secondary to upper motor neuron or spinal disorders.[10,12,53] Limited clinical evidence exists for the treatment of acute muscle spasm with baclofen. As noted previously, tizanidine has some evidence but can be extremely sedating especially at doses that prove analgesic for acute back pain.

Chronic Low Back Pain

Despite the common use of skeletal muscle relaxants, relatively few data clarify their appropriateness in the treatment of chronic back pain.[17,49] No skeletal muscle relaxant has an indication for use in chronic back pain. Despite this lack of evidence, muscle relaxants are often prescribed on a long-term basis.[54] Only baclofen and tizanidine have FDA-approved indications for spasticity. As a group, these agents may provide some global palliative quality but probably do not effect the course of the underlying morbidity.

Skeletal muscle relaxants have CNS depressant effects and should be used with caution, particularly, for patients with concomitant use of alcohol, anxiolytics, opioid analgesics, or other sedating medications. There is strong evidence that skeletal muscle relaxants are associated with increased risk for total adverse effects, especially those related to the CNS.[17,43,49] Many chronic pain patients appear to benefit from less pharmacotherapy, especially substances that may cloud cognitive and functional capacities.[55] Pill tapers can be used where patients who are appropriate candidates for streamlining can have their muscle relaxant therapy slowly discontinued over a relatively short time, for example, 2 weeks. In some situations, patients may require more interventions, for example, behavioral medicine support. These patients are probably best managed by interdisciplinary pain programs or by a psychiatrist.

Topical Analgesic Balms

Applying medicines topically is an ancient practice that, although often perceived as pragmatic, can become quite problematic. Many ancient cultures utilized a variety of natural substances (e.g., herbs and plants) for a variety of medicinal uses, including analgesia. Today, a variety of topical remedies is available to patients with painful conditions, primarily as over-the-counter (OTC) analgesic balm, many of which have been available for decades. The majority of these preparations contain counterirritants such as camphor, menthol, and salicylates, either alone or in combination with each other or a variety of other medicinal ingredients. Capsaicin, a counterirritant, and nonsalicylate NSAIDs are also available in prescription and OTC topical formulations. Lidocaine and a variety of other substances used topically are discussed elsewhere in this book (see Chapter 82).

Topical drug administration would appear to maintain many potential benefits, especially in pain presentations that have a defined local and peripheral component.[56] The most obvious benefit is avoiding negative systemic effects, for example, adverse drug effects, drug interactions, and need for an effective serum concentration. At the same time, topical administration can be prone to a variety of limitations, often inversely related to the benefits of topical application. Benefits and limitations are summarized in Table 80.4. Direct topical drug

application appears to avoid numerous problems that occur with systemic administration of medications. This is especially true for NSAIDs, where toxicity with systemic administration can be problematic. As described in the following text, topical NSAIDs appear to be useful for some acute pain presentations (e.g., soft tissue injuries and postsurgical pain).

NSAIDs have the strongest evidence base among the topical analgesics. Moore and colleagues[57] conducted a meta-analysis reviewing analgesic efficacy for acute pain related to soft tissue trauma, sprains, and strains. They also analyzed pain relief for chronic pain conditions, such as osteoarthritis and tendonitis. The number needed to treat (NNT) was 3.9 for the acute pain conditions and 3.1 for the chronic pain conditions. The authors noted that local skin reactions were uncommon (3.6% of patients) in the studies. As could be expected, systemic adverse effects were extremely uncommon at less than 0.5% of patients exposed to this drug class. However, the chronic use of topical NSAIDs in osteoarthritis is not entirely clear. A meta-analysis showed benefit in the first 2 weeks but did not sustain in weeks 3 to 4 when compared to placebo.[58] Although topical administration does not appear to afford the same therapeutic profile, this route of administration is also better tolerated and may be of benefit in patients who would not otherwise be able to use an NSAID orally.

TOPICAL COUNTERIRRITANTS

Topical counterirritants comprise a group of substances primarily for use by patients in a variety of OTC analgesic compounds. These include capsaicin, camphor, menthol, and salicylates, which appear to provide analgesic benefit by desensitizing peripheral nociceptive receptors. Galeotti and colleagues[59] suggested that menthol's analgesic properties may be mediated through selective activation of κ-opioid receptors.

Capsaicin appears to have the best evidence for use among the topical analgesics, primarily in osteoarthritis. Analgesic activity for capsaicin is attributed to depletion of substance P from peripheral nerve terminals. This requires both time and consistent dosing. A recent systematic review of topical capsaicin for musculoskeletal pain found an NNT of 8.1 for pain relief.[60] A variety of guidelines list capsaicin as a useful adjunct for use in patients with osteoarthritis. The European League Against Rheumatism (EULAR) and the American College of Rheumatology both recommend capsaicin for the treatment of pain in osteoarthritis.[61,62] The main issue related to capsaicin use is the adverse effect profile, which occurs to some extent with all patients, and is an expected consequence of the mechanism of action. In the aforementioned systematic review, side effects were problematic in approximately one-third of the patients.[60] Typical experiences include local adverse reactions

TABLE 80.4 Benefits and Limitations of Topical Analgesics	
Benefits	**Limitations**
• Avoid need for oral absorption.	• Absorption pharmacokinetic issues due to molecular size, lipophilicity, and skin permeability
• Avoid metabolic complications and systemic adverse effects.	
• Ease of dose termination in the event of untoward side effects	• Topical enzymatic activity may occur and reduce efficacy
• Direct access to the target site	
• Convenient administration	• Localized skin irritation, such as erythema can occur.
• Improved patient acceptance and adherence	
• Alternative route when oral not viable (e.g., patient with emesis)	

Adapted from Hare BD, Lipman AG. Uses and misuses of medication in the treatment of chronic pain. In: Hare BD, Fine P, eds. *Chronic Pain, Problems in Anesthesia.* Philadelphia: J.B. Lippincott Co; 1990.

such as pain upon application, burning, stinging, and redness at the site of application. This adverse effect profile is probably the biggest disadvantage for this medication, causing either early discontinuation or reduced patient compliance leading to absence of efficacy.[63,64]

The other counterirritants can be classified as rubefacients, including salicylates. There are few good efficacy data for these medications, probably in part because these substances have been used for so long. The benefit of these agents may also be due to the actual administration process, that is, rubbing, causing increased stimulation in the area.

Although salicylates may also have activity similar to other NSAIDs, their topical mechanism remains poorly elucidated. Mason and colleagues[65] reviewed the use of topical salicylates for acute musculoskeletal pain. These authors noted that topical salicylates produced a significant reduction in pain compared to placebo, with an NNT of 2.1. The benefit of this medication class for chronic use is limited by both lack of efficacy data and the potential for adverse effects with continued administration.

Conclusion

Skeletal muscle relaxants and topical analgesic balms comprise a cadre of substances that are commonly used for a variety of pain conditions. Skeletal muscle relaxants have value for acute back pain, mainly as adjunctive agents with other forms of analgesia and physical therapy. The use of these agents in chronic pain conditions remains controversial. This is in part due to the lack of efficacy data available for the use of these substances in chronic back pain conditions. Moreover, these agents maintain a substantial adverse effect profile that often is counterproductive for patients with chronic pain. Topical analgesic balms are commonly used for self-care in acute painful conditions.

References

1. Elenbaas JK. Centrally acting oral skeletal muscle relaxants. *Am J Hosp Pharm* 1980;37(10):1313–23.
2. Waldman HJ. Centrally acting skeletal muscle relaxants and associated drugs. *J Pain Symptom Manage* 1994;9(7):434–441.
3. Balano KB. Anti-inflammatory drugs and myorelaxants. Pharmacology and clinical use in musculoskeletal disease. *Prim Care* 1996;23(2):329–334.
4. Patel AT, Ogle AA. Diagnosis and management of acute low back pain. *Am Fam Physician* 2000;61:1779–1786, 1789–1790.
5. Jackson KC. Evaluation of skeletal muscle relaxant use for acute musculoskeletal pain and injury in ambulatory care. *J Pain* 2003;4(2 suppl 1):84.
6. Johnson EW. The myth of skeletal muscle spasm. *Am J Phys Med Rehabil* 1989;68:1.
7. Rivner MH. The neurophysiology of myofascial pain syndrome. *Curr Pain Headache Rep* 2001;5(5):432–440.
8. Magoun HW, Rhines R. An inhibitory mechanism in the bulbar reticular formation. *J Neurophysiol* 1946;9:165–171.
9. Schreiner LH, Lindsley DB, Magoun HW. Role of brain stem facilitatory systems in maintenance of spasticity. *J Neurophysiol* 1949;12:207–216.
10. Davidoff RA. Antispasticity drugs: mechanisms of action. *Ann Neurol* 1985;17:107–116.
11. Stanko JR. A review of oral skeletal muscle relaxants for the craniomandibular disorder (CMD) practitioner. *J Craniomandib Pract* 1990;8:234–243.
12. Young RR, Delwaide PJ. Drug therapy. Spasticity. *N Engl J Med* 1981;304:28–33.
13. Henneman E, Kaplan A, Una K. A neuropharmacological study on the effect of myanesin (Tolserol) on motor systems. *J Pharmacol Exp Ther* 1949;97:331–341.
14. Latimer CN. Action of mephenesin upon three monosynaptic pathways of cat. *J Pharmacol Exp Ther* 1956;118:309–317.
15. Crankshaw DP, Raper C. Some studies on peripheral actions of mephenesin, methocarbamol and diazepam. *Br J Pharmacol* 1968;34:579–590.
16. Ngai SH, Tseng DTC, Wang SC. Effect of diazepam and other central nervous system depressants on spinal reflexes in cats: a study of site of action. *J Pharmacol Exp Ther* 1966;153:344–351.
17. van Tulder MW, Touray T, Furlan AD, et al. Muscle relaxants for non-specific low back pain. *Cochrane Database Syst Rev* 2003;(2):CD004252.
18. Powers BJ, Cattau EL Jr, Zimmerman HJ. Chlorzoxazone hepatotoxic reactions. An analysis of 21 identified or presumed cases. *Arch Intern Med* 1986;146(6):1183–1186.
19. Jackson KC. Low back pain pharmacotherapy. *Drugs Today (Barc)* 2004;40(9):765–772.
20. Moore KA, Levine B, Fowler D. A fatality involving metaxalone. *Forensic Sci Int* 2005;149(2–3):49–51.
21. Poklis JL, Ropero-Miller JD, Garside D, et al. Metaxalone (Skelaxin)-related death. *J Anal Toxicol* 2004;28(6):537–541.
22. Dent RW, Ervin DK. A study of metaxalone (Skelaxin) vs. placebo in acute musculoskeletal disorders: a cooperative study. *Curr Ther Res Clin Exp* 1975;18(3):433–440.
23. Tisdale SA, Ervin DK. A controlled study of methocarbamol (Robaxin) in acute painful musculoskeletal conditions. *Curr Ther Res Clin Exp* 1975;17(6):525–530.
24. Littrell RA, Hayes LR, Stillner V. Carisoprodol (Soma): a new and cautious perspective on an old agent. *South Med J* 1993;86(7):753–756.
25. Bailey DN, Briggs JR. Carisoprodol: an unrecognized drug of abuse. *Am J Clin Pathol* 2002;117(3):396–400.
26. Reeves RR, Carter OS, Pinkofsky HB, et al. Carisoprodol (Soma): abuse potential and physician unawareness. *J Addict Dis* 1999;18(2):51–56.
27. Reeves RR, Carter OS, Pinkofsky HB. Use of carisoprodol by substance abusers to modify the effects of illicit drugs. *South Med J* 1999;92(4):441.
28. Rust GS, Hatch R, Gums JG. Carisoprodol as a drug of abuse. *Arch Fam Med* 1993;2(4):429–432.
29. Elder NC. Abuse of skeletal muscle relaxants. *Am Fam Physician* 1991;44(4):1223–1226.
30. European Medicines Agency. European Medicines Agency recommends suspension of marketing authorizations for carisoprodol-containing medicinal products. Document reference EMEA/520463/2007. Available at: http://www.emea.europa.eu. Accessed March 9, 2017.
31. Gareri P, De Fazio P, Cotroneo A, et al. Anticholinergic drug-induced delirium in an elderly Alzheimer's dementia patient. *Arch Gerontol Geriatr* 2007;44(suppl 1):199–206.
32. Flexeril [package insert]. Fort Washington, PA: McNeil Consumer & Specialty Pharmaceuticals; 2003.
33. Borenstein DG, Korn S. Efficacy of a low-dose regimen of cyclobenzaprine hydrochloride in acute skeletal muscle spasm: results of two placebo-controlled trials. *Clin Ther* 2003;25(4):1056–1073.
34. Childers MK, Borenstein D, Brown RL, et al. Low-dose cyclobenzaprine versus combination therapy with ibuprofen for acute neck or back pain with muscle spasm: a randomized trial. *Curr Med Res Opin* 2005;21(9):1485–1493.
35. Keegan MT, Brown DR, Rabinstein AA. Serotonin syndrome from the interaction of cyclobenzaprine with other serotoninergic drugs. *Anesth Analg* 2006;103(6):1466–1468.
36. Cherkin DC, Wheeler KJ, Barlow W, et al. Medication use for low back pain in primary care. *Spine* 1998;23:607–614.
37. Coward DM. Tizanidine: neuropharmacology and mechanism of action. *Neurology* 1994;44(11 suppl 9):S6–S10.
38. Smith HS, Barton AE. Tizanidine in the management of spasticity and musculoskeletal complaints in the palliative care population. *Am J Hosp Palliat Care* 2000;17(1):50–58.
39. Berry H, Hutchinson DR. A randomized placebo-controlled study in general practice to evaluate the efficacy and safety of tizanidine in acute low-back pain. *J Int Med Res* 1988;16(2):75–82.
40. Berry H, Hutchinson DR. Tizanidine and ibuprofen in acute low back pain: results of a double-blind randomized study in general practice. *J Int Med Res* 1988;16(2):83–91.
41. Vitale DC, Piazza C, Sinagra T, et al. Pharmacokinetic characterization of tizanidine nasal spray, a novel intranasal delivery method for the treatment of skeletal muscle spasm. *Clin Drug Investig* 2013;33(12):885–891.
42. Malanga GA, Gwynn MW, Smith R, et al. Tizanidine is effective in the treatment of myofascial pain syndrome. *Pain Phys* 2002;5(4):422–432.
43. van Tulder MW, Koes BW, Bouter LM. Conservative treatment of acute and chronic nonspecific low back pain. A systematic review of randomized controlled trials of the most common interventions. *Spine* 1997;22:2128–2156.
44. Bigos SJ, Bowyer OR, Braen GR, et al. *Clinical Practice Guideline Number 14: Acute Low Back Problems in Adults.* Rockville, MD: U.S. Department of Health and Human Services, Agency for Health Care Policy and Research; 1994. Publication 95-0642.
45. Barrata R. A double-blind study of cyclobenzaprine and placebo in the treatment of acute musculoskeletal conditions of the low back. *Curr Ther Res* 1982;32(5):646–652.
46. Lepisto P. A comparative trial of dS 103-282 and placebo in the treatment of acute skeletal muscle spasms due to disorders of the back. *Ther Res* 1979;26(4):454–459.
47. Gold R. Orphenadrine citrate: sedative or muscle relaxant? *Clin Ther* 1978;1(6):451–453.
48. Browning R, Jackson JL, O'Malley PG. Cyclobenzaprine and back pain. A meta-analysis. *Arch Intern Med* 2001;161:1613–1620.
49. Chou R, Peterson K, Helfand M. Comparative efficacy and safety of skeletal muscle relaxants for spasticity and musculoskeletal conditions: a systematic review. *J Pain Symptom Manage* 2004;28(2):140–175.
50. Dillin W, Uppal GS. Analysis of medications used in the treatment of cervical disk degeneration. *Orthop Clin North Am* 1992;23(3):421–433.
51. Basmajian JV. Cyclobenzaprine hydrochloride effect on skeletal muscle spasm in the lumbar region and neck: two double-blind controlled clinical and laboratory studies. *Arch Phys Med Rehabil* 1978;59:58–63.

52. Basmajian JV. Reflex cervical muscle spasm: treatment by diazepam, phenobarbital or placebo. *Arch Phys Med Rehabil* 1983;64:121–124.

53. Wagstaff AJ, Bryson HM. Tizanidine: a review of its pharmacology, clinical efficacy and tolerability in the management of spasticity associated with cerebral and spinal disorders. *Drugs* 1997;53:435–452.

54. Dillon C, Paulose-Ram R, Hirsch R, et al. Skeletal muscle relaxant use in the United States; data from the Third National Health and Nutrition Examination Survey (NHANES III). *Spine* 2004;15:29:892–896.

55. Hare BD, Lipman AG. Uses and misuses of medication in the treatment of chronic pain. In: Hare BD, Fine P, eds. *Chronic Pain, Problems in Anesthesia*. Philadelphia: J.B. Lippincott Co; 1990.

56. Stanos SP. Topical agents for the management of musculoskeletal pain. *J Pain Symptom Manage* 2007;33(3):342–355.

57. Moore RA, Tramer D, Carroll PJ, et al. Quantitative systematic review of topically applied non-steroidal anti-inflammatory drugs. *Br Med J* 1998;316(7128):333–338.

58. Lin J, Zhang LW, Jones A, et al. Efficacy of topical non-steroidal anti-inflammatory drugs in the treatment of osteoarthritis: meta-analysis of randomized controlled trials. *Br Med J* 329:324–326.

59. Galeotti N, DiCesare Mannelli L, Mazzanti G, et al. Menthol: a natural analgesic compound. *Neuruosci Lett* 2002;322(3):145–148.

60. Mason L, Moore RA, Derry S, et al. Systematic review of topical capsaicin for the treatment of chronic pain. *Br Med J* 2004;328:991–994.

61. Jordan KM, Arden NK, Doherty M, et al. EULAR recommendations 2003: an evidence based approach to the management of knee osteoarthritis. Report of a Task Force of the Standing Committee for International Clinical Studies Including Therapeutic Trials (ESCISIT). *Ann Rheum Dis* 2003;6(12):1145–1155.

62. American College of Rheumatology Subcommittee on Osteoarthritis Guidelines. Recommendations for the medical management of osteoarthritis of the hip and knee: 2000 update. *Arthritis Rheum* 2000;43(9):1905–1915.

63. Bley KR. Recent developments in transient receptor potential vanilloid receptor 1 agonist-based therapies. *Expert Opin Investig Drugs* 2004;13(11):1445–1456.

64. Szallasi A. Vanilloid (capsaicin) receptors in health and disease. *Am J Clin Pathol* 2002;118(1):110–121.

65. Mason L, Moore RA, Edwards JE, et al. Systematic review of efficacy of topical rubefacients containing salicylates for the treatment of acute and chronic pain. *Br Med J* 2004;328(2004):995–997.

CHAPTER 81

Neuropathic Pain Pharmacotherapy

ELON EISENBERG, SIMON VULFSONS, and **DAVID M. PETERSON**

Neuropathic pain is pain caused by a lesion or disease affecting the somatosensory nervous system.[1,2] According to a recent systematic review of epidemiologic studies on neuropathic pain, the estimated prevalence of neuropathic pain is between 6.9% and 10% of the general population.[3] Neuropathic pain may result from a large variety of insults, examples of which are listed in Table 81.1. Common examples of peripheral neuropathic pain include lumbar radiculopathy, painful diabetic neuropathy (PDN), postherpetic neuralgia (PHN), and posttraumatic/surgical neuropathy. Neuropathic pain of central origin includes central poststroke pain, pain due to multiple sclerosis, and post-spinal cord injury pain.

Neuropathic pain may be continuous or intermittent and is often described as burning or hot, electric shocks or shooting, pricking or pins, and needles. Pain evoked by nonpainful stimuli such as light touching or cold (allodynia) and accompanying nonpainful sensations such as numbness and tingling are all suggestive of neuropathic pain. The combination of several descriptors is a strong indicator of neuropathic pain. The neurologic examination is aimed primarily at detecting reproducible negative sensory signs, such as partial or complete loss to one or several sensory modalities (e.g., light touch, cold sensation) with distinct neuroanatomical borders. Positive sensory signs, especially when accompanying negative signs, are also supportive of neuropathic pain.[1]

Neuropathic pain has negative effects on multiple domains of life resulting in poor quality of life, comparable to that experienced by patients suffering from cancer or chronic heart failure. This is explained, at least in part, by misdiagnosis, undertreatment, and lack of substantial analgesic efficacy of most existing treatments.[4,5]

Neuropathic pain pharmacotherapy is a key therapeutic element, which involves different drug classes including, but not limited to, antidepressants, anticonvulsants, opioids, and topical agents. However, even with the newest of these drugs, effective pain relief occurs in less than half of patients with chronic neuropathic pain.[1] Meta-analyses of trials in neuropathic pain commonly report outcomes in terms of the number needed to treat (NNT) to provide 50% pain relief for one patient. Even highly recommended first-line agents result in NNTs ranging from 3.6 to 7.7, meaning that only 1 out 3.6 to 7.7 patients will experience a 50% reduction in pain.[6] Most clinical trials related to neuropathic pain pharmacotherapy were conducted with a specific agent in patients who had a specific cause of the underlying disorder, with PDN or PHN being the most frequently tested disorder. At the same time, meta-analyses show that the efficacy of any given drug is generally not dependent on the cause of the underlying disorder.[1] In patients with refractory neuropathic pain, combination therapy with two or more agents possessing different mechanisms has been suggested.[7]

A different approach of selecting patients to clinical trials, not based on the specific causes of the underlying disorder, has recently been introduced. According to this approach, standardized quantitative sensory testing (QST) is used for subgrouping patients with peripheral neuropathic pain of different etiologies into different clusters. For example, patients with sensory loss, patients with thermal hyperalgesia and those with mechanical hyperalgesia, regardless of the underlying cause. It is proposed that these profiles may be related to different pathophysiologic mechanisms and may be useful in future clinical trial design.[8]

This chapter reviews pharmacotherapy for neuropathic pain and emphasizes the strengths and the limitations of different treatments. It also addresses unresolved issues related to pharmacologic treatment of neuropathic pain.

Antidepressants

Four classes of antidepressant medications have been studied in neuropathic pain treatment: tricyclic antidepressants (TCAs), selective serotonin and norepinephrine reuptake inhibitors (SNRIs), selective serotonin reuptake inhibitors (SSRIs), and monoamine oxidase inhibitors (MAOIs). Certain drugs in the first two classes are commonly considered first-line recommended treatments for neuropathic pain.[6,9,10] Table 81.2 lists major properties of common antidepressants.

TRICYCLIC ANTIDEPRESSANTS

Table 81.3 summarizes the placebo-controlled trials of various drugs for neuropathic pain and shows efficacy for amitriptyline, imipramine, nortriptyline, desipramine, clomipramine, and maprotiline at daily doses ranging from 30 to 200 mg for PHN, PDN, postmastectomy pain, central poststroke pain, and mixed type neuropathies. These results are commonly extrapolated to all types of neuropathic pain, and clinical experience suggests some broad utility for the drugs. A recent systematic review and meta-analysis found TCAs the most efficacious antidepressants for neuropathic pain with an overall NNT of 3.6 (95% confidence interval [CI], 3.0 to 4.4) and the number needed to harm (NNH) was 13.4 (95% CI, 9.3 to 24.4). The level of evidence was considered moderate.[6] A Cochrane collaboration review of the efficacy of amitriptyline for neuropathic pain found evidence for a statistically significant benefit with an NNT of 4.6 (95% CI, 1.8 to 3.1) and NNH of 4.1 (95% CI, 3.2 to 5.7),[29] and finally, another Cochrane collaboration review found the NNT of TCAs for neuropathic pain to be 3.6 (95% CI, 3.0 to 4.5).[30] However, a few trials failed to demonstrate TCA efficacy for spinal cord injury pain,[13] cisplatin-induced neuropathy,[31] HIV neuropathy,[16,17] phantom limb pain,[15] lumbar radiculopathy,[20] and neuropathic cancer pain.[32]

TABLE 81.1 Causes of Neuropathic Pain (Examples)

- Trauma (surgery, frostbite, amputation)
- Inflammation (Guillain-Barré syndrome)
- Infection (AIDS neuropathy, acute zoster, postherpetic neuralgia)
- Degenerative spine disease
- Ischemic disorders
- Metabolic disorders (diabetes mellitus)
- Neoplastic disorders (tumor invasion, paraneoplastic)
- Congenital disorders (Fabry's disease)
- Toxicity (chemotherapy)
- Immunologic disorders

TABLE 81.2 Comparison of Antidepressants in Neuropathic Pain[11,12,233–238]

Agent	Normal Adult Daily Dose in Psychiatric Disorders[a]	Usual Number of Doses per Day	Elimination Half-life ($t_{1/2}$)	Dosing Adjustments	Serotonin: Norepinephrine Selectivity Ratio[b]
Selective Serotonin Receptor Inhibitors					
Citalopram	20–40 mg	1	35 h	20 mg/d in hepatic impairment or elderly	3,500–3,900
Escitalopram	10–20 mg	1	27–32 h	10 mg/d in hepatic impairment or elderly	7,100
Fluoxetine	20–80 mg	1	24–72 h (acute), 96–144 h (chronic), norfluoxetine 96–384 h	Decrease dose in hepatic impairment.	300–545
Fluvoxamine	100–300 mg	1–2	16 h	Decrease dose in hepatic impairment and elderly.	580–620
Paroxetine HCL	20–60 mg	IR: 1 XR: 1	21 h	Maximum dose = 40 mg/d in hepatic impairment or elderly	300–450
Paroxetine mesylate	20–60 mg	1	33 h	Maximum dose = 40 mg/d in renal or hepatic impairment or elderly	300–450
Sertraline	50–200 mg	1	62–104 h	Decrease dose in hepatic impairment and elderly.	1,400–2,750
Serotonin and Norepinephrine Reuptake Inhibitors					
Desvenlafaxine	50–100 mg	1	11 h	Decrease dose in moderate or severe renal disease.	85
Duloxetine	40–120 mg	1–2	8–17 h	Do not give to patients with hepatic impairment. Decrease dose in severe renal disease.	9
Venlafaxine	75–375 mg	IR: 2–3 XR: 1	3–7 h, ODV 9–13 h	Decrease dose in hepatic or renal impairment.	115–120
Tricyclic Antidepressants[c]					
Amitriptyline	100–300 mg	1–4	9–27 h	Lower doses in elderly and hepatic impairment	8
Clomipramine	100–300 mg	1–3	15–60 h	Lower doses in elderly and hepatic impairment	130
Desipramine	75–300 mg	1–3	10–30 h	Lower doses in elderly and hepatic impairment	0.05
Imipramine	100–300 mg	1–4	5–30 h	Lower doses in elderly and hepatic impairment	27
Maprotiline	100–225 mg	1–3	25–50 h	Lower doses in elderly and hepatic impairment	0.002
Nortriptyline	50–150 mg	1–4	20–55 h	Lower doses in elderly and hepatic impairment	0.24

[a]Dosing is per product U.S. approved dosing; dosing in pain syndromes may vary from that listed.
[b]These are estimates of selectivity ratio; actual selectivity ratios are concentration-dependent; numbers <1 indicate greater affinity for norepinephrine than serotonin.
[c]Tricyclic antidepressants may be safely administered once daily; some practitioners prefer to dose them more frequently.
IR, immediate release; ODV, O-desmethylvenlafaxine; XR, extended release.

Inability to demonstrate effectiveness of the TCAs in these neuropathic pain types may represent a true lack of therapeutic benefit, or it may be due to study design weaknesses or other factors. More studies are needed to clarify the value of specific TCAs in different types of neuropathic pain.

In many countries, TCAs may be overlooked as first-line neuropathic pain drugs because they are generic and are not actively marketed. Newer, more expensive drugs for neuropathic pain may be selected despite comparatively lower effectiveness (higher NNTs). The analgesic efficacy of the TCAs is likely to be independent of their antidepressant effect.[14] In a large survey, over one-fifth (21%) of the patients with chronic pain have been diagnosed with depression associated with their pain.[33] Concomitant chronic pain and depression favor the use of an antidepressant (TCA or another) over other medication classes.

TCAs are associated with dose-dependent adverse events, the most common being sedation, constipation, dry mouth, urinary retention, and orthostatic hypotension. TCAs can be administered once daily, usually at bedtime, exploiting their sedating properties. The dose used for neuropathic pain, typically 75 mg a day or less, is below the antidepressant dose for most patients, lowering the risk of side effects. Secondary amine TCAs (e.g., desipramine, nortriptyline) are better tolerated than tertiary amine TCAs (e.g., amitriptyline, imipramine) but are equally effective.[24,28] Nonetheless, TCAs may not be tolerated by many patients. The anticholinergic effects of TCAs are a relative contraindication in patients with benign prostatic hyperplasia, cardiac conduction defects, and other morbidities sensitive to parasympatholytic action. Desipramine has only one-quarter of the anticholinergic and sedative activity of amitriptyline at comparable doses, making desipramine a TCA of choice.[34] Use of a low initial dose and slow dose titration of all TCAs is important to minimize premature discontinuation due to side effects. Dry mouth is the most common adverse event, and it is often best managed with sugarless candies or chewing gum, especially sugarless lemon

TABLE 81.3 Summary of Randomized Controlled Trials of Antidepressants in Treatment of Neuropathic Pain Published as Peer-Reviewed Articles

Study	Drug	Diagnosis	Design	Number of Patients Treated with Active Drug	Maximal Dosage (mg) per Day	Treatment Duration (wk)	Results
Leijon and Boivie[239]	Amitriptyline	CPSP	Crossover	15	75	4	A > P
Cardenas et al.[13]	Amitriptyline	SCI	Parallel	44	125	6	A = P
Max et al.[14]	Amitriptyline	PDN	Crossover	29	150	6	A > P
Vrethem et al.[240] .	Amitriptyline	PDN and other polyneuropathies	Crossover	33	75	4	A > P
Watson et al.[241]	Amitriptyline	PHN	Crossover	24	137.5	3	A > P
Max et al.[242]	Amitriptyline	PDN	Crossover	34	150	6	A > P
Robinson et al.[15]	Amitriptyline	Phantom limb	Parallel	39	125	6	A = P
Kalso et al.[243]	Amitriptyline	Postmastectomy	Crossover	15	100	4	A > P
Kieburtz et al.[16]	Amitriptyline	HIV neuropathy	Parallel	46	100	10	A = P
Shlay et al.[17]	Amitriptyline	HIV neuropathy	Parallel	58	75	14	A = P
Kvinesdal et al.[244]	Imipramine	PDN	Crossover	12	100	5	A > P
Sindrup et al.[245]	Imipramine	PDN	Crossover	18	150	2	A > P
Sindrup et al.[18]	Imipramine	PDN	Crossover	29	150	4	A > P
Gomez-Perez et al.[19]	Nortriptyline	PDN	Crossover	18	60	4	A > P
Raja et al.[246]	Nortriptyline	PHN	Crossover	46	140	8	A > P
Panerai et al.[247]	Nortriptyline	Mixed neuropathies	Crossover	24	100	3	A > P
Khoromi et al.[20]	Nortriptyline	Radiculopathy	Crossover	34	100	9	A = P
Sindrup et al.[248]	Clomipramine	PDN	Crossover	19	75	2	A > P
Panerai et al.[247]	Clomipramine	Mixed neuropathies	Crossover	24	100	3	A > P
Sindrup et al.[248]	Desipramine	PDN	Crossover	19	200	2	A > P
Max et al.[249]	Desipramine	PDN	Crossover	20	250	6	A > P
Kishore-Kumar et al.[250]	Desipramine	PHN	Crossover	19	250	6	A > P
Raja et al.[246]	Desipramine	PHN	Crossover	13	160	8	A > P
Vrethem et al.[240]	Maprotiline	PDN and other polyneuropathies	Crossover	33	75	4	A > P
Goldstein et al.[21]	Duloxetine	PDN	Parallel	342	120	12	A > P
Raskin et al.[22]	Duloxetine	PDN	Parallel	232	120	12	A > P
Wernicke et al.[23]	Duloxetine	PDN	Parallel	226	120	12	A > P
Sindrup et al.[18]	Venlafaxine	Mixed neuropathies	Crossover	30	225	4	A > P
Rowbotham et al.[24]	Venlafaxine	PDN	Crossover	163	225	6	A > P
Tasmuth et al.[25]	Venlafaxine	Postmastectomy	Crossover	13	75	4	A = P
Yucel et al.[251]	Venlafaxine	Mixed neuropathies	Parallel	8	150	8	A = P[a]
Sindrup et al.[26]	Paroxetine	PDN	Crossover	20	40	2	A = P
Sindrup et al.[27]	Citalopram	PDN	Crossover	20	40	3	A > P
Max et al.[28]	Fluoxetine	PDN	Crossover	46	40	6	A > P

[a]The study showed significant effect of venlafaxine in the manifestations of hyperalgesia and temporal summation but not on the ongoing pain intensity.
CPSP, central poststroke pain; PDN, painful diabetic neuropathy; PHN, postherpetic neuralgia; SCI, spinal cord injury; A, active drug; P, placebo; > indicates that active drug was superior to the comparator in terms of pain reduction; < indicates that active drug was not superior to the comparator in terms of pain reduction; = indicates that active drug was equal to the comparator in terms of pain reduction.

candy to stimulate serous saliva flow. Sips of water provide only transient relief. The most common starting dose for TCAs is 25 mg, but frail elderly and other highly sensitive patients may tolerate an initial dose of 5 to 10 mg better. Increase the dose by the same number of milligram as the starting dose every 3 to 5 days until some diminution of pain complaints occurs or the daily dose totals 100 mg. The maximal effect often occurs within 3 weeks at that dose, generally before antidepressant effects peak.

The anticholinergic effects of TCAs can cause cardiac toxicity including ventricular ectopic activity, prolonged QT interval, myocardial infarction, and sudden death.[35] A screening electrocardiogram (ECG) might be considered in patients over 40 years of age or who have other risk factors prior to initiating a TCA. Use TCAs with caution in patients with a history of ischemic heart disease or increased risk of sudden cardiac death; if TCA treatment is selected in these patients, consider limiting the maximum dose to 100 mg per day or less.[6,11,36]

SELECTIVE SEROTONIN AND NOREPINEPHRINE REUPTAKE INHIBITORS

The SNRIs duloxetine and venlafaxine are newer antidepressants with effectiveness for neuropathic pain. Results with venlafaxine for neuropathic pain have been inconsistent. Venlafaxine was effective for PDN and for various forms of polyneuropathy at daily doses of 150 to 225 mg.[18,24] In one placebo-controlled trial, perioperative venlafaxine at a daily dose of 75 mg prevented the development of postmastectomy pain syndrome,[37] but in other trials on patients with postmastectomy pain[25] syndrome and mixed type neuropathies, efficacy at a dose range of 75 to 150 mg could not be demonstrated.

Three large randomized controlled trials[21–23] and one open-label 52-week extension trial[38] showed that duloxetine was effective for PDN at daily doses of 60 to 120 mg. Duloxetine 60 mg per day has similar efficacy to duloxetine 120 mg per day, but the lower dose is far more tolerable. It can be administered once daily. At that dose, the drug significantly improved sleep and quality of life. The most common adverse effects reported in these clinical trials were nausea, somnolence, dizziness, and constipation, all of which tended to decrease over time. Initiating treatment at a daily dose of 30 mg for 1 week followed by an increase to 60 mg per day during the second week is likely to improve tolerability.[39] Duloxetine has not been associated with cardiac toxicity. It should not be used concomitantly with MAOIs or in patients with markedly impaired liver function.

A meta-analysis of trials for the SNRIs (i.e., duloxetine, venlafaxine, desvenlafaxine) across neuropathic pain types resulted in an NNT of 6.4 (95% CI, 5.2 to 8.4), indicating that they are less effective than the far less expensive TCAs.[6] In the systematic review and meta-analysis cited earlier, the final quality of evidence for SNRI efficacy in the treatment of neuropathic pain was deemed high. Combined NNT was 6.4 (95% CI, 5.2 to 8.4), and NNH was 11.8 (95% CI, 9.5 to 15.2).[6]

SELECTIVE SEROTONIN REUPTAKE INHIBITORS

Reports of the effectiveness of SSRIs in neuropathic pain management are generally not favorable. Some reports may not have separated analgesic effect from the effects of mood elevation on pain perception. One well-controlled trial documented that fluoxetine was no more effective than placebo, whereas both amitriptyline and desipramine were efficacious.[28] Two other trials support efficacy of citalopram[27] and paroxetine[26] (both at 40 mg per day) in PDN. Although SSRIs show a favorable safety profile compared to TCAs and are generally well tolerated, a meta-analysis of available trials in neuropathic pain did not detect significant overall pain reduction with the SSRIs, and therefore, they should not be regarded as first-line agents.[6]

Antiepileptics

Interest in the antiepileptics for pain management dates back to the 1940s.[40] Dozens of randomized controlled trials have attempted to describe the role of different antiepileptic drugs in neuropathic pain treatment. The majority of antiepileptic trials are in PHN or PDN, with less data available for other neuropathic pain types. Recent meta-analyses strongly support the use of the calcium channel $\alpha_2\delta$ ligands pregabalin and gabapentin (including gabapentin ER and gabapentin enacarbil) as first-line therapy for PHN and PDN.[6,41] Data also support the use of pregabalin for treating central neuropathic pain.[41] Carbamazepine is likely effective for trigeminal neuralgia and possibly for PDN and central poststroke pain, but studies of carbamazepine were generally of short duration (i.e., less than 4 weeks) and poor methodologic quality.[42] Although other antiepileptics may be beneficial in individual patients or specific types of neuropathic pain, pooled data either suggested minimal effectiveness or were inconclusive.[6,41] Table 81.4 summarizes trials of the antiepileptics in neuropathic pain.

PREGABALIN

Pregabalin is the most extensively studied drug of any type for treating neuropathic pain.[6] Pregabalin is believed to exert its analgesic effect by binding to the $\alpha_2\delta$ subunit of voltage-gated calcium channels on primary afferent neurons, reducing the release of neurotransmitters from their central terminals.[132] A recent meta-analysis of 25 placebo-controlled trials of pregabalin in various types of neuropathic pain reported an NNT of 7.7 (95% CI, 6.5 to 9.4).[6] Pregabalin was effective for treating PHN and PDN in numerous multicenter, randomized, controlled trials.[74,97,101–112,116,133,134] Pregabalin was also effective for treating spinal cord injury pain,[114,115] posttraumatic peripheral neuropathy,[113] neuropathic cancer pain,[61,100] and mixed types of neuropathic pain.[116,117,119–122] Pregabalin did not significantly improve acute herpetic neuralgia or prevent progression to PHN in one clinical trial,[96] but it did significantly reduce acute herpetic neuralgia and subacute herpetic neuralgia in another

trial.[118] Pregabalin did not significantly improve neuropathic pain associated with HIV[98,99] or central poststroke pain.[97] The effective daily dose of 300 to 600 mg reduces pain and improves sleep, functioning, and quality of life. Response rates are higher when a maintenance dose of 600 mg per day is used.[6] Pregabalin has several advantages compared to other anticonvulsants: It is usually administered twice daily, can be rapidly titrated, has early onset of analgesic effect, and has linear pharmacokinetics. No common drug interactions occur with pregabalin. The most commonly reported adverse events were dose-dependent and included dizziness, somnolence, dry mouth, abnormal vision, confusion, weight gain, and edema.[11]

GABAPENTIN

There is also strong evidence of gabapentin's effectiveness for PHN and PDN at doses of 900 to 3600 mg per day.[7,54–56,62–64,70–75] Gabapentin is available as immediate-release (IR), extended-release (ER), and gabapentin enacarbil formulations, and available data suggest similar effectiveness for the different formulations.[6] Gabapentin IR is normally dosed thrice daily and is commonly the least expensive dosage form. Gabapentin enacarbil is dosed twice daily, and gabapentin ER may be dosed once daily. Across 14 studies, for all gabapentin dosage forms, the overall NNT to reduce pain intensity by 50% was 7.2 (95% CI, 5.9 to 9.1). For gabapentin IR, the NNT was 6.3 (95% CI, 5.0 to 8.3). The NNT for gabapentin enacarbil and gabapentin ER was 8.3 (95% CI, 6.2 to 13.0).[6] In addition to PHN and PDN, gabapentin has demonstrated efficacy in HIV-associated painful neuropathy, pain in Guillain-Barré syndrome, and phantom limb pain.[57–59,65] Gabapentin was not effective for peripheral nerve injury pain in one trial.[66] An 8-day trial of gabapentin was effective for treating neuropathic cancer pain in one trial,[60] but in a smaller 4-week trial, gabapentin was no more effective than placebo.[61] Results for gabapentin in spinal cord injury were mixed in three small trials.[67–69] Gabapentin is believed to have similar mechanism of action to pregabalin. However, unlike pregabalin, it has nonlinear pharmacokinetics and may take days or weeks to reach an effective dose. Gabapentin is relatively safe, with few clinically relevant drug interactions. The main adverse effects are somnolence, dizziness, and peripheral edema.[11] Some clinicians report that some patients who fail to respond to gabapentin may respond to pregabalin and vice versa.

CARBAMAZEPINE

Carbamazepine is commonly used to treat trigeminal neuralgia. Most carbamazepine studies in trigeminal neuralgia were conducted in the 1960s and 1970s using small samples sizes. In these studies, pain relief was superior with carbamazepine compared to placebo.[45–47,135] In a more recent trial, carbamazepine was more effective than lamotrigine for treating pain associated with trigeminal neuralgia.[48] Carbamazepine was also one of the first anticonvulsants used in PDN and was superior to placebo in two small trials.[43,44] Pain reduction was similar between carbamazepine and the TCA nortriptyline in a more recent trial.[19] Carbamazepine was more effective than placebo in patients with mixed types of neuropathic pain in one controlled trial.[49] Effective doses of carbamazepine ranged from 800 to 2,400 mg per day in trigeminal neuralgia, but lower doses of 200 to 600 mg per day were effective for treating other neuropathic pain types. NNT to achieve 50% pain relief with carbamazepine in a meta-analysis of trials in trigeminal neuralgia, PDN, and central poststroke pain was 1.9 (95% CI, 1.6 to 2.5).[42] However, this figure is based primarily on old trials, most of which were conducted in small patient groups for relatively short treatment periods. All of the carbamazepine trials were classified as third tier trials, and heterogeneity associated with pooling the trials was moderately high ($I^2 = 50\%$).[42] The analgesic mechanism of carbamazepine is related to voltage-dependent sodium

TABLE 81.4 Summary of the Randomized Controlled Trials of Antiepileptic Drugs in Treatment of Neuropathic Pain Published as Peer-Reviewed Articles

Study	Drug	Diagnosis	Design	Number of Patients Treated with Active Drug	Maximal Dosage (mg) per Day	Treatment Duration (wk)	Results
Rull et al.[43]	Carbamazepine	PDN	Crossover	30	400	2	A > P
Wilton[44]	Carbamazepine	PDN	Crossover	40	400	2	A > P
Gomez-Perez et al.[19]	Carbamazepine	PDN	Crossover	16	200	4	A = nortriptyline
Nicol[45]	Carbamazepine	TN	Crossover	20	2,400	2	A > P
Campbell et al.[46]	Carbamazepine	TN	Crossover	77	800	2	A > P
Killian and Fromm[47]	Carbamazepine	TN	Crossover	27	1,000	5 d	A > P
Vilming[252]	Carbamazepine	TN	Parallel	6	900	3	A > tizanidine
Lechin et al.[253]	Carbamazepine	TN	Crossover	48	1,200	8	A < pimozide
Lindstrom[254]	Carbamazepine	TN	Crossover	12	Maximal tolerated	2	A = tocainide
Shaikh et al.[48]	Carbamazepine	TN	Crossover	21	1,200	6	A > lamotrigine[a]
Harke et al.[49]	Carbamazepine	Mixed types	Parallel	43	600	8 d	A > P
Dogra et al.[50]	Oxcarbazepine	PDN	Parallel	69	1,800	16	A > P
Grosskopf et al.[51]	Oxcarbazepine	PDN	Parallel	71	1,200	16	A = P
Beydoun et al.[52]	Oxcarbazepine	PDN	Parallel	258	1,800	16	A = P
Demant et al.[53]	Oxcarbazepine	Mixed types	Crossover	83	2,400	6	A > P
Backonja et al.[54]	Gabapentin	PDN	Parallel	84	3,600	8	A > P
Morello et al.[255]	Gabapentin	PDN	Crossover	26	1,800	6	A = amitriptyline
Dallocchio et al.[55]	Gabapentin	PDN	Parallel	13	2,400	12	A > amitriptyline
Simpson et al.[56]	Gabapentin	PDN	Parallel	30	3,600	8	A > P
Pandey et al.[57]	Gabapentin	GBS	Crossover	18	15 mg/kg	1	A > P
Pandey et al.[58]	Gabapentin	GBS	Parallel	12	900	1	A > P
Hahn et al.[59]	Gabapentin	HIV-N	Parallel	15	2,400	4	A > P
Caraceni et al.[60]	Gabapentin	NCP	Parallel	79	1,800	8 d	A > P
Mishra et al.[61]	Gabapentin	NCP	Parallel	30	1,800	4	A = P A = amitriptyline A < pregabalin[a]
Rice and Maton[62]	Gabapentin	PHN	Parallel	223	2,400	7	A > P
Rowbotham et al.[63]	Gabapentin	PHN	Parallel	113	3,600	8	A > P
Chandra et al.[64]	Gabapentin	PHN	Parallel	34	2,700	8	A = nortriptyline
Bone et al.[65]	Gabapentin	PLP	Crossover	19	2,400	6	A > P
Gordh et al.[66]	Gabapentin	PNI	Crossover	98	2,400	7	A = P
Levendoglu et al.[67]	Gabapentin	SCI	Crossover	20	3,600	8	A > P
Tai et al.[68]	Gabapentin	SCI	Crossover	7	1,800	4	A > P[b]
Rintala et al.[69]	Gabapentin	SCI	Crossover	32	3,600	8	A < amitriptyline A = diphenhydramine (active control)
Gilron et al.[7]	Gabapentin	PDN + PHN	Crossover	57	3,200	5	A > P; A = morphine A < A + morphine
Gilron et al.[70]	Gabapentin	PDN + PHN	Crossover	46	3,600	6	A < A + nortriptyline A = nortriptyline
Smith et al.[256]	Gabapentin	PLP + RLP	Crossover	24	3,600	6	A = P
Serpell[257]	Gabapentin	Mixed types	Parallel	153	2,400	8	A > P
Sandercock et al.[258]	Gabapentin ER	PDN	Parallel	96	3,000	4	A > P
Wallace et al.[71]	Gabapentin ER	PHN	Parallel	269	1,800	10	A = P
Sang et al.[72]	Gabapentin ER	PHN	Parallel	221	1,800	10	A > P
Irving et al.[73]	Gabapentin ER	PHN	Parallel	107	1,800	4	A > P
Jensen et al.[259]	Gabapentin ER	PHN	Parallel	102	1,800	4	A = P[c]
Rauck et al.[74]	Gabapentin Enacarbil	PDN	Parallel	235	3,600	13	A = P A = pregabalin[a]
Backonja et al.[260]	Gabapentin Enacarbil	PHN	Parallel	47	1,200	2	A > P
Zhang et al.[75]	Gabapentin Enacarbil	PHN	Parallel	263	3,600	14	A > P
Rauck et al.[76]	Lacosamide	CPSP	Parallel	60	400	6	A > P
Shaibani et al.[77]	Lacosamide	PDN	Parallel	403	600	18	A = P
Wymer et al.[78]	Lacosamide	PDN	Parallel	277	600	18	A = P
Ziegler et al.[79]	Lacosamide	PDN	Parallel	281	600	18	A = P
Breuer et al.[80]	Lamotrigine	CPMS	Crossover	17	400	11	A = P
Vestergaard et al.[81]	Lamotrigine	CPSP	Crossover	30	200	8	A > P
Vinik et al.[82]	Lamotrigine	PDN	Parallel	360	400	10	A = P
Vinik et al.[82]	Lamotrigine	PDN	Parallel	360	400	10	A = P

(continued)

TABLE 81.4 (Continued)

Study	Drug	Diagnosis	Design	Number of Patients Treated with Active Drug	Maximal Dosage (mg) per Day	Treatment Duration (wk)	Results
Eisenberg et al.[83]	Lamotrigine	PDN	Parallel	29	400	8	A > P
Simpson et al.[84]	Lamotrigine	HIV-N	Parallel	20	300	14	A > P
Simpson et al.[85]	Lamotrigine	HIV-N	Parallel	150	600	11	A = P; A > P[d]
Finnerup et al.[86]	Lamotrigine	SCI	Crossover	22	400	8	A = P; A > P[e]
Zakrzewska et al.[87]	Lamotrigine	TN	Crossover	14	400	2	A > P
Shaikh et al.[48]	Lamotrigine	TN	Crossover	21	400	6	A < carbamazepine[a]
McCleane[88]	Lamotrigine	Mixed types	Parallel	50	200	8	A = P
McCleane[89]	Lamotrigine	Mixed types	Parallel	36	200	8	A = P
Silver et al.[90]	Lamotrigine	Mixed types	Parallel	111	400	14	A = P
Jungehulsing et al.[261]	Levetiracetam	CPSP	Crossover	42	3,000	8	A = P
Rossi et al.[91]	Levetiracetam	CPMS	Parallel	12	3,000	12	A > P
Falah et al.[92]	Levetiracetam	CPMS	Crossover	30	3,000	6	A = P
Vilholm et al.[93]	Levetiracetam	Postmastectomy	Crossover	26	3,000	4	A = P
Finnerup et al.[94]	Levetiracetam	SCI	Crossover	34	3,000	5	A = P
Holbech et al.[95]	Levetiracetam	Mixed types	Crossover	35	3,000	6	A = P
Krcevski and Kamenik[96]	Pregabalin	AHN	Parallel	14	300	3	A = P[f]
Kim et al.[97]	Pregabalin	CPSP	Parallel	110	600	13	A = P, A > P[g]
Simpson et al.[98]	Pregabalin	HIV-N	Parallel	151	600	14	A = P
Simpson et al.[99]	Pregabalin	HIV-N	Parallel	183	600	17	A = P
Mishra et al.[61]	Pregabalin	NCP	Parallel	30	600	4	A > P A > gabapentin[a] A > amitriptyline
Raptis et al.[100]	Pregabalin	NCP	Parallel	60	600	4	A > fentanyl transdermal
Richter et al.[101]	Pregabalin	PDN	Parallel	161	600	6	A > P
Lesser et al.[102]	Pregabalin	PDN	Parallel	240	600	5	A > P
Rosenstock et al.[103]	Pregabalin	PDN	Parallel	76	300	8	A > P
Tolle et al.[104]	Pregabalin	PDN	Parallel	299	600	12	A > P
Arezzo et al.[105]	Pregabalin	PDN	Parallel	82	600	12	A > P
Satoh et al.[106]	Pregabalin	PDN	Parallel	179	600	13	A > P
Rauck et al.[74]	Pregabalin	PDN	Parallel	56	300	13	A = P A = gabapentin enacarbil[a]
Irving et al.[262] and Tanenberg et al.[263]	Pregabalin	PDN	Parallel	134	300	12	A = duloxetine A = duloxetine + gabapentin
Smith et al.[107]	Pregabalin	PDN	Parallel	99	300	15	A = P A = carisbamate
Raskin et al.[108]	Pregabalin	PDN	Crossover	301	300	6	A = P
Sabatowski et al.[109]	Pregabalin	PHN	Parallel	157	300	8	A > P
Dworkin et al.[110]	Pregabalin	PHN	Parallel	89	600	8	A > P
van Seventer et al.[111]	Pregabalin	PHN	Parallel	273	600	13	A > P
Stacey et al.[112]	Pregabalin	PHN	Parallel	179	600	4	A > P
Achar et al.[264]	Pregabalin	PHN	Parallel	25	150	8	A > amitriptyline
van Seventer et al.[113]	Pregabalin	PNI	Parallel	127	600	8	A > P
Siddall et al.[114]	Pregabalin	SCI	Parallel	70	600	12	A > P
Cardenas et al.[115]	Pregabalin	SCI	Parallel	108	600	16	A > P
Freynhagen et al.[116]	Pregabalin	PDN + PHN	Parallel	273	600	12	A > P
Vranken et al.[117]	Pregabalin	CPSP + SCI	Parallel	20	600	4	A > P
Liang et al.[118]	Pregabalin	AHN + SHN	Parallel	150	600	4	A > P
Guan et al.[119]	Pregabalin	PDN + PHN	Parallel	206	600	8	A > P
Moon et al.[120]	Pregabalin	Mixed types	Parallel	162	600	9	A > P
Holbech et al.[265]	Pregabalin	Mixed types	Crossover	61	300	5	A > P A < imipramine A < imipramine + pregabalin
Haanpaa et al.[121]	Pregabalin	Mixed types	Parallel	277	600	8	A = capsaicin 8% patch
Gatti et al.[266]	Pregabalin	Mixed types	Parallel	134	290[h]	13	A < oxycodone CR A < A + oxycodone CR
Gilron et al.[122]	Pregabalin	Mixed types	Parallel	80	600	4–9	A > P
Kochar et al.[123]	Sodium valproate	PDN	Parallel	29	1,200	4	A > P

TABLE 81.4 (Continued)

Study	Drug	Diagnosis	Design	Number of Patients Treated with Active Drug	Maximal Dosage (mg) per Day	Treatment Duration (wk)	Results
Kochar et al.[124]	Sodium valproate	PDN	Parallel	21	500	12	A > P
Kochar et al.[125]	Valproic acid + sodium valproate	PHN	Parallel	22	1,000	8	A > P
Drewes et al.[126]	Sodium valproate	SCI	Parallel	20	2,400	3	A = P
Otto et al.[127]	Valproic acid	Mixed types	Crossover	31	1,500	4	A = P
Thienel et al.[128]	Topiramate	PDN	Parallel	878	400	22	A = P[i]
Raskin et al.[129]	Topiramate	PDN	Parallel	214	400	12	A > P
Khoromi et al.[130]	Topiramate	LR	Crossover	42	400	8	A = P; A > P[j]
Atli and Dogra[131]	Zonisamide	PDN	Parallel	13	600	12	A = P

[a]Trial compared two antiepileptics to each other, and the same trial is displayed twice in this table (once for each antiepileptic).
[b]A significant decrease of "unpleasant feeling" and a trend toward a decrease in both the "pain intensity" and "burning sensation."
[c]Significant difference in "itchy pain sensations" but no difference in global pain intensity or other measures of pain.
[d]Lamotrigine was superior to placebo in patients who received antiviral neurotoxic therapy but not in patients who did not receive this therapy.
[e]Lamotrigine was superior to placebo in patients with incomplete spinal cord injury and evoked pain but equal to placebo in patients with complete injury and without evoked pain.
[f]Pregabalin was not effective for preventing subacute herpetic neuralgia or postherpetic neuralgia.
[g]No significant difference between pregabalin and placebo in pain score (primary outcome measure) but significant difference in sleep, anxiety, and clinical global impression scores.
[h]Mean dose reported rather than maximum.
[i]Findings from three double-blind, placebo-controlled trials.
[j]No significant difference between topiramate and placebo in pain score (primary outcome measure) but significant difference in global pain relief score.
AHN, acute herpetic neuralgia; CPMS, central pain due to multiple sclerosis; CPSP, central poststroke pain; ER, extended release; GBS, Guillain-Barré syndrome; HIV-N, HIV neuropathy; LR, lumbar radiculopathy; NCP, neuropathic cancer pain; PDN, painful diabetic neuropathy; PHN, postherpetic neuralgia; PLP, phantom limb pain; PNI, peripheral nerve injury; RLP, residual limb pain; SCI, spinal cord injury; SHN, subacute herpetic neuralgia; TN, trigeminal neuralgia; A, active drug; P, placebo; > indicates that active drug was superior to the comparator in terms of pain reduction; < indicates that active drug was not superior to the comparator in terms of pain reduction; = indicates that active drug was equal to the comparator in terms of pain reduction.

channel blocking, which results in decreased ectopic nerve discharges and neural membrane stabilization.[136] Adverse events are common and include dizziness, nausea, drowsiness, blurred vision, and ataxia.[44] Carbamazepine can cause Stevens-Johnson syndrome (SJS), toxic epidermal necrolysis (TEN), and drug reaction with eosinophilia and systemic symptoms (DRESS). Rare, but serious, side effects include blood dyscrasias, impairment of liver function, and reduction of sodium plasma levels and require routine blood tests to monitor them. Serum carbamazepine concentration monitoring is recommended to maximize efficacy, monitor compliance, and reduce toxicity.[11]

OXCARBAZEPINE
Oxcarbazepine is a carbamazepine analog that is likely to have a similar analgesic mechanism.[137] Oxcarbazepine has primarily been studied in PDN.[50-52] In one PDN trial, oxcarbazepine at a maximal daily dose of 1,800 mg produced greater pain relief than placebo, with an NNT to achieve 50% pain relief of 6.0 (95% CI, 3.3 to 41.0).[50,138] Two other PDN trials, including one much larger trial, found no significant difference in pain relief between oxcarbazepine and placebo.[51,52] Oxcarbazepine 1,800 to 2,400 mg per day was more effective than placebo for treating mixed types of peripheral neuropathy in one trial.[53] Adverse events are generally of mild or moderate severity, but serious adverse events and adverse events leading to treatment withdrawal were more common with oxcarbazepine than placebo in patients with PDN.[138] The most common adverse events with oxcarbazepine are dizziness, drowsiness, headache, ataxia, altered vision, and nausea and vomiting. Hyponatremia can occur with oxcarbazepine, making sodium concentration monitoring important.[11] In summary, results are mixed for oxcarbazepine in PDN, and data are limited for other types of neuropathic pain.

LAMOTRIGINE
Lamotrigine has been studied in several types of neuropathic pain. In a few small trials, lamotrigine 200 to 400 mg per day

was effective for treating central poststroke pain, PDN, HIV neuropathy, or trigeminal neuralgia.[81,83,84,87] However, lamotrigine 200 to 600 mg per day was not effective for treating central or peripheral neuropathic pain in several other trials, some of which included much larger sample sizes.[48,80,82,85,86,88-90] A meta-analysis calculated an NNT of 17.8 (95% CI, 9.3 to 210) for 50% pain reduction across several types of neuropathic pain for lamotrigine.[6] The overall safety profile is dose-related. Common side effects include nausea, vomiting, sedation, drowsiness, dizziness, headaches, malaise, visual disturbances, and ataxia. Skin rash that may deteriorate to dangerous or life-threatening SJS or TEN is the most serious adverse event of lamotrigine. Slow titration may reduce the risk of developing these syndromes. Skin rash development requires discontinuation of lamotrigine.[11]

VALPROATE
Five small trials examined the effects of valproic acid or sodium valproate in neuropathic pain.[123-127] Valproic acid and sodium valproate at a daily dose of 1,000 mg were superior to placebo in reducing PHN in one study.[125] Sodium valproate 500 mg or 1,200 mg significantly improved pain associated with PDN in two trials.[123,124] In contrast, 1,500 mg of valproic acid failed to show superiority to placebo for mixed types of neuropathic pain in one randomized controlled trial,[127] and 2,400 mg of sodium valproate was ineffective for treating central pain associated with spinal cord injury in another trial.[126] The NNT for 50% reduction in pain intensity across all neuropathic pain types was 4.3 (95% CI, 2.7 to 9.9), but this figure was based on a limited number of trials with small sample sizes and therefore may not reflect its actual efficacy.[6]

OTHER ANTICONVULSANTS
Topiramate was effective for PDN in one controlled trial[129] but not in another, much larger trial.[128] Topiramate also yielded equivocal results in one randomized controlled trial in patients

with painful lumbar radiculopathy.[130] Topiramate was titrated up to a daily dose of 400 mg in all three trials. Clinicians were hopeful that levetiracetam would be a useful agent for treating neuropathic pain, but available evidence are not supportive of this use. One very small trial described significant pain relief in patients with central pain associated with multiple sclerosis,[91] but another trial in central pain of multiple sclerosis[92] as well as trials in central poststroke pain, postmastectomy pain, spinal cord injury pain, and other neuropathic pain types found no significant differences between levetiracetam and placebo.[93-95] Lacosamide was effective for reducing pain compared to placebo in one trial in central poststroke pain,[76] but results were similar between lacosamide and placebo in three much larger PDN trials.[77-79] Zonisamide and tiagabine have been used in open-label studies or small-scale randomized controlled trials,[131] but currently available data are too limited to confidently assess the efficacy of these drugs.

Opioids

Sixteen randomized controlled trials tested the efficacy of oral opioids for PDN, PHN, phantom pain, nerve root pain, and neuropathic pain of diverse etiologies (Table 81.5). Six different opioids including morphine, oxycodone, methadone, levorphanol, hydromorphone, and dihydrocodeine were tested in these trials. Most trials found the tested opioid to be superior to placebo in reducing spontaneous neuropathic pain. In one trial, dihydrocodeine was found advantageous to a synthetic cannabinoid nabilone in patients with mixed neuropathies[139] and to mexiletine in another trial on patients with phantom and residual leg pain.[143] Dose-dependent analgesic responses to methadone and levorphanol were demonstrated in patients with mixed neuropathies in two independent trials.[141,142] Two negative studies have been published: In one, morphine, up to 90 mg per day, administered for 8 days, was not more efficacious

TABLE 81.5 Summary of Randomized Controlled Trials of Opioids, Tramadol, and Tapentadol in Treatment of Neuropathic Pain Published as Peer-Reviewed Articles

Study	Drug	Diagnosis	Design	Number of Patients Treated with Active Drug	Maximal Dosage (mg) per Day	Treatment Duration (wk)	Results
Frank et al.[139]	DHC vs. nabilone	Mixed neuropathies	Crossover	96	DHC 240 Nabilone 2	6	DHC > nabilone
Nalamachu et al.[140]	Hydromorphone	Neuropathic LBP	Parallel	43	64	12	A > P
Rowbotham et al.[141]	Levorphanol low-dose vs. levorphanol high-dose	Mixed neuropathies	Parallel	38 43	Low dose 3.15 High dose 15.75	8	A high-dose > A low-dose
Raja et al.[246]	Methadone	PHN	Crossover	26	80	8	A > P
Morley et al.[142]	Methadone low-dose Methadone high-dose	Mixed neuropathic	Crossover	19 17	Low dose 10 High dose 20	20 d	A low dose = P A high dose > P
Huse et al.[267]	Morphine	Phantom limb	Crossover	12	300	4	A > P
Harke et al.[49]	Morphine	Mixed peripheral	Parallel	21	90	8 d	A = P
Raja et al.[246]	Morphine	PHN	Crossover	38	225	8	A > P
Gilron et al.[7]	Morphine vs. gabapentin vs. placebo	PDN + PHN	Crossover	57	Morphine 120 Gabapentin 3,200	5	A > P Morphine = gabapentin
Khoromi et al.[20]	Morphine	Radiculopathy	Crossover	41	90	9	A = P
Wu et al.[143]	Morphine vs. mexiletine	Phantom + residual leg pain	Crossover	60	Morphine 240 Mexiletine 1,200	8	Morphine > mexiletine
Gilron et al.[144]	Morphine vs. nortriptyline	PDN + PHN	Crossover	Morphine 47 Nortriptyline 45	Morphine 100 Nortriptyline 100	6	Morphine = nortriptyline
Watson and Babul[268]	Oxycodone	PHN	Crossover	50	60	4	A > P
Gimbel et al.[269]	Oxycodone	PDN	Parallel	82	120	6	A > P
Watson et al.[270]	Oxycodone	PDN	Crossover	45	80	4	A > P
Jensen et al.[271]	Oxycodone	PDN	Parallel	82	120	6	A > P
Boureau et al.[145]	Tramadol	PHN	Parallel	63	400	6	A > P
Harati et al.[146]	Tramadol	PDN	Parallel	65	400	6	A > P
Sindrup et al.[147]	Tramadol	Mixed neuropathic	Crossover	43	400	4	A > P
Wilder-Smith et al.[148]	Tramadol	Postamputation	Parallel	33	594	1 mo	A > P
Norrbrink and Lundeberg[149]	Tramadol	Spinal cord injury	Parallel	23	400	4	A > P
Sindrup et al.[150]	Tramadol	Mixed	Crossover	64	400	4	A > P
Schwartz et al.[151]	Tapentadol	PDN	Parallel	196	500	12	A > P
Vinik et al.[152]	Tapentadol	PDN	Parallel	166	500	12	A > P
Niesters et al.[153]	Tapentadol	PDN	Parallel	12	500	4	A > P

DHC, dihydrocodeine; LBP, low back pain; PHN, postherpetic neuralgia; PDN, painful diabetic neuropathy; A, active drug; P, placebo; > indicates that active drug was superior to the comparator in terms of pain reduction; < indicates that active drug was not superior to the comparator in terms of pain reduction; = indicates that active drug was equal to the comparator in terms of pain reduction.

than placebo in reducing peripheral neuropathic pain of mixed origin.[49] In a more recent trial, morphine at the same maximal daily dose showed no superiority over placebo in patients with chronic lumbar radicular pain.[20] Notably, a more recent contradictory study showed efficacy of hydromorphone in patient with "neuropathic back pain."[140] Ten trials were recently pooled together in a meta-analysis yielding a combined NNT of 4.3 (95% CI, 3.4 to 5.8).[6] A systematic review of seven short-term (less than 24 hours) and two intermediate-term (4 weeks) randomized controlled trials concluded that opioids can reduce the intensity of dynamic mechanical allodynia and perhaps of cold allodynia in patients with peripheral neuropathic pain. These findings are clinically relevant because dynamic mechanical allodynia and cold allodynia are the most prevalent types of evoked neuropathic pain.[154]

Although opioids clearly reduce neuropathic pain, several questions related to chronic opioid use in neuropathic pain remain unanswered. First, opioids did not demonstrate improvement in many aspects of emotional or physical functioning, as measured by various validated questionnaires.[155] Second, studies were limited to 12 weeks or less. Therefore, no high-quality data on long-term safety and efficacy of opioids in the treatment of neuropathic pain are available. This is particularly important because of emerging reports, coming mainly from North America, on hazards associated with long-term opioid use such as addiction and death.[156]

Tramadol

Tramadol is a synthetic, "weak opioid" analogue with a dual mechanism of analgesia: It has a weak affinity for μ-opioid receptors, and it weakly inhibits serotonin and norepinephrine reuptake.[12,137] Randomized controlled trials show that tramadol can reduce pain in patients with PHN,[145] PDN,[146] mixed forms of painful polyneuropathy,[147,150] spinal cord injury pain,[149] and postamputation pain[148] (see Table 81.5). Its overall efficacy in PHN seems somewhat lower than that of other opioids with an NNT of 4.7 (95% CI, 3.6 to 6.7).[6] Due to dose-dependent adverse effects, a gradual titration from 50 mg two to three times daily to a maximal daily dose of 400 mg is generally required. Common adverse events include drowsiness, nausea, constipation, dizziness, and potential for abuse. Concomitant use of serotonin reuptake inhibitors may increase the risk for serotonergic syndrome. Tramadol is metabolized in the liver by CYP3A4 and CYP2D6 and will likely interact with any drug able to inhibit or induce these enzymes.[12,137]

Tapentadol

Tapentadol is a new synthetic centrally acting, "strong opioid" analgesic with both μ-opioid receptor agonist and norepinephrine reuptake inhibition mechanisms of action.[157] Tapentadol at a maximal daily dose of 500 mg was superior to placebo in three randomized controlled trials in patients with PDN.[151-153] Tapentadol is available as an extended-release formulation. Reported side effects were similar to those of other "strong opioids," including nausea, vomiting, anxiety, diarrhea, dizziness, and abuse potential. Yet, it may have a superior gastrointestinal tolerability profile compared to that of strong opioids.[158]

NMDA Receptor Antagonists

In spite of numerous animal studies in which N-methyl-D-aspartic acid (NMDA) receptor antagonists yielded promising results, clinical trials with oral drugs were generally negative (Table 81.6). Three small trials showed efficacy of the NMDA receptor antagonist dextromethorphan for PDN but not for PHN or neuropathies of mixed etiologies.[159-161] Memantine, which also has NMDA receptor blocking properties, was not effective in PDN, PHN, or chronic phantom limb pain.[163,164] A small trial (n = 19) found that a 4-week course of memantine during the immediate postamputation period reduced phantom limb pain for up to 6 months postamputation but did not attenuate phantom limb pain in the long term (12 months).[162] In contrast, intravenous administration of subanesthetic doses of ketamine produced short-term analgesia (lasting for hours) in multiple forms of neuropathic pain.[165] In one trial, thrice-daily ketamine infusions for 1 week significantly reduced pain scores during treatment and for 2 weeks after the last infusion in patients with neuropathic pain attributed to spinal cord injury who were receiving oral gabapentin.[166] Regardless of the difference in outcomes between short- and long-term studies, one trial showed that short-term intravenous administration of ketamine may be useful in predicting long-term response to oral dextromethorphan.[167] Among other physiologic actions, magnesium sulfate is a natural NMDA receptor antagonist. In one study, a similar number of patients with PHN responded to a single dose of intravenous magnesium sulfate (7/15) compared with a single dose of intravenous ketamine (10/15).[164] A recent meta-analysis determined that results for NMDA antagonists in neuropathic pain treatment were inconclusive.[6] There is interest in developing less-invasive systemic ketamine dosage forms (e.g., oral, sublingual, intranasal), but long-term efficacy data are not yet available for these dosage forms.[168,169]

Systemic Sodium Channel Blockers

Carbamazepine, oxcarbazepine, mexiletine, intravenous lidocaine, and topical lidocaine are all sodium channel blockers. Carbamazepine and oxcarbazepine have already been reviewed earlier in this chapter, and topical lidocaine will be discussed with other topical agents.

Mexiletine, an orally available analog of lidocaine with antiarrhythmic properties,[12] was evaluated in several randomized controlled trials for the treatment of PDN. These trials are summarized in Table 81.7. With the exception of one trial in which a relatively high dose of the drug produced modest effect, no significant pain relief was demonstrated.[170-172] High doses of mexiletine are commonly associated with adverse effects such as chest pain, dizziness, gastrointestinal disturbances, palpitations, tremor, and potential for worsening of existing arrhythmia.[27]

A meta-analysis of randomized controlled trials demonstrated the effectiveness of intravenous lidocaine for various types of peripheral neuropathic pain syndromes. Pain was reduced by about 10 mm more (on a 100-mm scale) with lidocaine than with placebo.[173] Major drawbacks of this therapy are the lack of data on long-term efficacy and the apparent necessity for repeated infusions for sustained pain relief. This may therefore be an impractical approach for many patients. Interestingly, a positive correlation between the response to a single lidocaine infusion and long-term response to oral mexiletine has been reported.[174]

Simple Analgesics

Acetaminophen (paracetamol) is a popular analgesic due to availability and low cost. At or below the recommended dose, adverse effects are limited. However, acetaminophen has not been studied as a treatment option for neuropathic pain in any randomized controlled trials.[6] Based on clinical experience, acetaminophen is unlikely to provide a clinically meaningful benefit in the treatment of neuropathic pain.

TABLE 81.6 Summary of Randomized Controlled Trials of NMDA Receptor Antagonists in Treatment of Neuropathic Pain Published as Peer-Reviewed Articles

Study	Drug	Diagnosis	Design	Number of Patients Treated with Active Drug	Maximal Dosage (mg) per Day	Treatment Duration (wk)	Results
Nelson et al.[159]	Dextromethorphan	PDN	Crossover	13	960	6	A > P
Sang et al.[160]	Dextromethorphan	PDN	Crossover	19	400[a]	9	A = lorazepam (active control) A = memantine[b]
Nelson et al.[159]	Dextromethorphan	PHN	Crossover	13	960	6	A = P
Sang et al.[160]	Dextromethorphan	PHN	Crossover	17	400[a]	9	A = lorazepam (active control) A = memantine[b]
McQuay et al.[161]	Dextromethorphan	Mixed neuropathies	Crossover	17	81	20 d	A = P
Kim et al.[272]	Ketamine IV	PHN	Parallel	15	1 mg/kg	2[c]	A = magnesium sulfate IV[b]
Kim et al.[272]	Magnesium sulfate IV	PHN	Parallel	15	30 mg/kg	2[c]	A = ketamine IV[b]
Sang et al.[160]	Memantine	PDN	Crossover	19	55[a]	9	A = lorazepam (active control) A = dextromethorphan[b]
Sang et al.[160]	Memantine	PHN	Crossover	17	35[a]	9	A = lorazepam (active control) A = dextromethorphan[b]
Eisenberg et al.[273]	Memantine	PHN	Parallel	12	20	5	A = P
Nikolajsen et al.[274]	Memantine	PLP	Crossover	15	20	5	A = P
Maier et al.[275]	Memantine	PLP	Parallel	18	30	4	A = P
Schley et al.[162]	Memantine	PLP	Parallel	10	30	4	A > P[d]
Wiech et al.[276]	Memantine	PLP	Crossover	8	30	4	A = P
Schwenkreis et al.[277]	Memantine	PLP	Parallel	8	30	3	A = P
Galer et al.[278]	Riluzole	Mixed neuropathies	Crossover	22	100	2	A = P
Galer et al.[278]	Riluzole	Mixed neuropathies	Crossover	21	200	2	A = P

[a]Median dose reported rather than maximum dose.
[b]Trial compared two NMDA receptor antagonists to each other, and the same trial is displayed twice in the table (once for each NMDA antagonist).
[c]Patients received a single dose of ketamine or magnesium sulfate and outcomes were tracked for 2 weeks.
[d]Memantine superior to placebo at 1 and 6 months postamputation but not at 1 year.
NMDA, N-methyl-D-aspartic acid; PDN, painful diabetic neuropathy; PHN, postherpetic neuralgia; PLP, phantom limb pain; A, active drug; P, placebo; > indicates that active drug was superior to the comparator in terms of pain reduction; < indicates that active drug was not superior to the comparator in terms of pain reduction; = indicates that active drug was equal to the comparator in terms of pain reduction.

TABLE 81.7 Summary of Randomized Controlled Trials of Systemic Sodium Channel Blockers in Treatment of Neuropathic Pain Published as Peer-Reviewed Articles

Study	Drug	Diagnosis	Design	Number of Patients Treated with Active Drug	Maximal Dosage (mg) per Day	Treatment Duration (wk)	Results
Kieburtz et al.[16]	Mexiletine	HIV-N	Parallel	48	600	10	A = P
Kemper et al.[279]	Mexiletine	HIV-N	Crossover	16	600	6	A = P
Dejgard et al.[280]	Mexiletine	PDN	Crossover	16	10 mg/kg	26	A > P
Stracke et al.[170]	Mexiletine	PDN	Parallel	47	675	5	A = P
Oskarsson et al.[171]	Mexiletine	PDN	Parallel	95	675	3	A = P
Wright et al.[172]	Mexiletine	PDN	Parallel	14	600	3	A = P
Chabal et al.[281]	Mexiletine	PNI	Crossover	11	750	9	A > P
Chiou-Tan et al.[282]	Mexiletine	SCI	Crossover	11	450	4	A = P
Wallace et al.[283]	Mexiletine	Mixed neuropathies	Crossover	20	900	10 d	A = P

HIV-N, HIV neuropathy; PDN, painful diabetic neuropathy; PNI, peripheral nerve injury; SCI, spinal cord injury; A, active drug; P, placebo; > indicates that active drug was superior to the comparator in terms of pain reduction; < indicates that active drug was not superior to the comparator in terms of pain reduction; = indicates that active drug was equal to the comparator in terms of pain reduction.

Nonsteroidal Anti-inflammatory Agents

There is a major discrepancy between the perceived lack of efficacy of nonsteroidal anti-inflammatory drugs (NSAIDs) for neuropathic pain and the widespread use of these drugs for this diagnosis.[175] Although evidence for the role of inflammation in neuropathic pain is emerging and it is estimated that half of all clinical cases of neuropathic pain are associated with inflammation of the peripheral nerves,[176] no controlled clinical trials that tested the effectiveness of NSAIDs for neuropathic pain exist. Animal models of nerve injury display inflammatory responses that are attenuated by the use of NSAIDs.[177,178] In humans, a pilot, randomized, open-label clinical trial which showed comparable effectiveness of lidocaine patch 5% to that of naproxen 500 mg twice daily for the treatment of neuropathic pain associated with carpal tunnel syndrome is available.[179] An open-label study comparing ibuprofen (2,400 mg daily), sulindac (400 mg daily), and placebo in patients suffering from PDN found efficacy for the NSAIDs compared to placebo.[180] Some conditions with a clear inflammatory basis such as acute herpes zoster have been targeted for NSAID treatment.[181] In contrast, a recent Cochrane collaboration report found no evidence for the treatment of acute radicular pain (sciatica) with NSAIDs,[182] although this treatment is quite prevalent.[183]

Topical Agents

CAPSAICIN

Capsaicin is a natural vanilloid that derives from the capsicum plant. It selectively binds to the transient potential vanilloid receptor 1 (TRPV1) and causes initial nociceptor depolarization with acute exposure, followed by substance P depletion and reduced nociceptor functionality with chronic use.[184] Topical low-concentration capsaicin cream (0.075%) applied three to four times daily was effective in three of five published randomized controlled trials in PDN, in two PHN trials, one trial in postsurgical pain and one in patients with mixed neuropathies. Topical capsaicin was not superior to placebo in randomized controlled trials for postmastectomy pain syndrome and for HIV neuropathy. Capsaicin application is associated with burning sensation, particularly during the first weeks of treatment, an adverse event that may often limit its required long-term use.

More recently, single application of 8% capsaicin patch for 30 to 60 minutes was introduced to the market. It has been tested in seven clinical trials in patients with PHN or HIV-related distal sensory polyneuropathy (see Table 81.8). Positive results showing sustained efficacy for up to 12 weeks following a single application were reported in most of these trials. Topical application of the 8% capsaicin patch is frequently associated local side effects including transient burning sensation and pain, pruritus, erythema, and swelling as well as transient alterations in blood pressure. Preapplication of local anesthetics and systemic analgesic administration reduce pain and burning sensations in the treated site.

TOPICAL LIDOCAINE PATCHES

Application of lidocaine gel/cream yielded inconsistent results in neuropathic pain (Table 81.8). The topical lidocaine 5% patch is an attractive option: It is applied for 12 hours and protects the skin from incidental touch, which might be important for patients who experience tactile allodynia. The lidocaine patch was effective for PHN in four short-term randomized controlled trials[185–188] and also in patients with other focal peripheral neuropathies.[179,188] The maximal recommended daily dose is three patches applied simultaneously every 12 hours. With the exception of mild skin reactions, lidocaine patches are not associated with adverse reactions, although caution is required in patients receiving oral Class I antiarrhythmic medications (e.g., mexiletine) and in patients with severe hepatic dysfunction.[192]

TOPICAL KETAMINE

In a small study, ketamine 1% was compared to placebo in patients with PHN, but no difference in pain reduction was found between treatments.[191] Several other studies tested the effect of topically applied ketamine either alone or in combination with other agents against placebo for postchemotherapy neuropathies or mixed neuropathies under randomized controlled conditions. All studies, but one,[193] failed to demonstrate superior efficacy of ketamine over the placebo,[189–190,194–195] thus putting into question the efficacy of topical ketamine for neuropathic pain.

Cannabinoids

The past decade has seen a real surge of interest in the treatment of pain with cannabinoids. This interest has been fueled by two separate phenomena: the increased mortality rate in patients taking prescription opioid drugs[196–198] and the increasing acceptance and legalization of recreational and "medical" cannabis.[199] Although boundaries between medical and recreational cannabis use have become blurred,[200] with increasing recreational use fueling medical acceptance of cannabis and vice versa, it has become apparent that conventional wisdom concerning cannabis use is being challenged by decreased opioid mortality in states with legalized access to medical cannabis.[201]

Another issue of importance is the mode of drug delivery. Cannabis for therapeutic purposes (CTP) can be administered via smoking or ingesting the raw plant, vaporizing the raw plant, or in cannabis-based medicines with known quantities of active agents: delta (9) tetrahydrocannabinol (THC) with or without cannabidiol (CBD).[202] A recent international survey of forms of administration of CTP across countries found that pulmonary delivery of cannabis is the preferred route of administration used by 86.6% (62.9% for smoking and 23.7% for vaporizing) of the participants. The oral mode of delivery of cannabis in edibles was used by 10.3% of the participants, whereas only 2.3% participants used either cannabis extracts delivered by oromucosal route (Sativex) or synthetic cannabinoids (Marinol and Nabilone) delivered orally in tablet forms.[203] This is clearly a strange state of affairs: Pharmacologic administration of cannabis in reproducible doses is very uncommon, whereas the use of raw plant, with no pharmacologic standardization, is the leading mode of administration. Over the last two decades, there has been a regular increase in the potency of illicit cannabis.[204,205] Use of high-potency breeds is common in Europe, Canada, and Australia for both recreational and medicinal purposes.[206] Users of CTP often seek different concentrations of active ingredients in the cannabis that is smoked, and although this might be a very positive trend, it makes comparison of cannabis across studies very complicated.[207]

Although cannabinoids are not formally approved for the treatment of neuropathic pain by drug regulatory agencies, many patients use cannabis for pain relief. In a meta-analysis of cannabis-based treatments for neuropathic and multiple sclerosis–related pain, 7 randomized, double-blind, placebo-controlled trials were included (n = 298).[208] The overall quality of the studies was very good. In general, the overall reductions in pain were in excess of 1.5 on an 11-point scale, and all were statistically significant. The difference in effect size in comparison to placebo was 0.8.

In a systematic review of cannabinoids for the treatment of noncancer pain, 18 trials published between the years of 2003 and 2010 involving 766 participants were included.[209] The quality of the trials was good, and in 15 of the 18 trials, there was a significant analgesic effect for the cannabinoid being

TABLE 81.8 Summary of Randomized Controlled Trials of Topical Agents in Treatment of Neuropathic Pain Published as Peer-Reviewed Articles

Study	Drug	Diagnosis	Design	Number of Patients Treated with Active Drug	Maximal Dosage (mg) per Day	Treatment Duration (wk)	Results
Chad et al.[284]	Capsaicin cream	PDN	Parallel	28	0.075% × 4 a day	4	A = P
Scheffler et al.[285]	Capsaicin cream	PDN	Parallel	19	0.075% × 4 a day	8	A > P
Capsaicin study group[286]	Capsaicin cream	PDN	Parallel	138	0.075% × 4 a day	8	A > P
Tandan et al.[287]	Capsaicin cream	PDN	Parallel	11	0.075% × 4 a day	8	A > P
Low et al.[288]	Capsaicin cream	PDN	Parallel	40	0.075% × 4 a day	12	A = P
Bernstein et al.[289]	Capsaicin cream	PHN	Parallel	16	0.075% × 3–4 a day	6	A > P
Watson et al.[290]	Capsaicin cream	PHN	Parallel	74	0.075% × 4 a day	6	A > P
Watson and Evans[291]	Capsaicin cream	Postmastectomy	Parallel	14	0.075% × 4 a day	6	A = P
Ellison et al.[292]	Capsaicin cream	Postsurgical	Parallel	49	0.075% × 4 a day	8	A > P
Paice et al.[293]	Capsaicin cream	HIV neuropathy	Parallel	15	0.075% × 4 a day	4	A = P
McCleane[88]	Capsaicin cream	Mixed neuropathic	Parallel	33	0.025% × 4 a day	4	A > P
Simpson et al.[294]	Capsaicin patch	HIV polyneuropathy	Parallel	225	8% vs. 0.04% (active placebo)	12	A > P
Backonja et al.[295]	Capsaicin patch	PHN	Parallel	206	8% vs. 0.04% (active placebo)	12	A > P
Backonja et al.[296]	Capsaicin patch	PHN	Parallel	38	8% vs. 0.04% (active placebo)	4	A > P
Webster et al.[297]	Capsaicin patch	PHN	Parallel	222	8% vs. 0.04% (active placebo)	12	A > P
Webster et al.[298]	Capsaicin patch	PHN	Parallel	102	8% vs. 0.04% (active placebo)	12	A = P
Irving et al.[299]	Capsaicin patch	PHN	Parallel	212	8% vs. 0.04% (active placebo)	12	A > P
Clifford et al.[300]	Capsaicin patch	HIV polyneuropathy	Parallel	322	8% vs. 0.04% (active placebo)	12	A = P
Rowbotham et al.[185]	Lidocaine gel	PHN	Crossover	39	5%	9	A > P
Rowbotham et al.[301]	Lidocaine patch	PHN	Crossover	35	5%	24 h	A > P
Galer et al.[186]	Lidocaine patch	PHN	Crossover	32	5%	2–14	A > P
Galer et al.[302]	Lidocaine patch	Focal neuropathies	Crossover	96	5%	3	A > P
Estanislao et al.[303]	Lidocaine gel	HIV neuropathy	Crossover	61	5%	2	A = P
Binder et al.[187]	Lidocaine patch	PHN	Parallel	36	5%	2	A > P
Meier et al.[188]	Lidocaine patch	Focal neuropathies	Crossover	39	5%	1	A > P
Lynch et al.[189,190]	Ketamine cream	Mixed neuropathies	Parallel	22	1%	3	A = P
Barros et al.[191]	Ketamine ointment	PHN	Crossover	12	1%	2	A = P

PDN, painful diabetic neuropathy; PHN, postherpetic neuralgia; A, active drug; P, placebo; > indicates that active drug was superior to the comparator in terms of pain reduction; < indicates that active drug was not superior to the comparator in terms of pain reduction; = indicates that active drug was equal to the comparator in terms of pain reduction.

tested. Four of the trials examined the effect of smoked cannabis on neuropathic pain, all reporting positive effects with minimal or no serious adverse effects. The mean treatment duration was only 8.5 days. Seven trials examined the effects of oromucosal extracts of cannabis-based medicine. Five trials examined the effect on participants with neuropathic pain, and four of these reported positive analgesic effects. Nabilone 2 mg has been found to be as effective as dihydrocodeine 240 mg for patients with neuropathic pain.[139] Dronabinol 10 mg has been found to be effective for central pain in multiple sclerosis (Table 81.9).[210]

Reported adverse events for CTP have included the following: central nervous system–related events such as alterations in perception (blurred vision, visual hallucinations, tinnitus, disorientation, confusion, dissociation, and acute psychosis), alterations in motor function (speech disorders, ataxia, muscle twitching, numbness), and altered cognitive function (impaired memory, disturbance in attention, disconnected thought).[211]

In summary, it appears the cannabis-based medications including smoked cannabis have a positive effect on pain reduction in patients suffering from chronic neuropathic pain. Effect sizes are small, and adverse effects are not uncommon. More study will clearly be done in the future to clarify the most efficient mode and methods of administration, minimizing the recreational effects and enhancing meaningful clinical outcomes.

Drug Combinations

Not uncommonly, administration of a single drug does not produce adequate analgesia. Pharmacologically, it seems reasonable to coadminister drugs with different mechanisms of action. Although combination therapy is commonly used in clinical practice, available data regarding the efficacy and safety of this practice is relatively limited (Table 81.10).

Five trials compared combinations of oral opioids with an agent from another class, typically an antidepressant[7,212,214]

TABLE 81.9 **Summary of Randomized Controlled Trials of Cannabinoids in Treatment of Neuropathic Pain Published as Peer-Reviewed Articles**

Study	Drug/Formulation	Diagnosis	Design	Number of Patients Treated with Active Agent	Maximal Dosage (mg) per Day	Treatment Duration	Results
Karst et al.[304]	1′,1′dimethylheptyl-delta8-tetrahydrocannabinol-11-oic acid (CT3)	Mixed neuropathies	Crossover	19	80	7 d	A > P
Wade et al.[305]	Oromucosal Sativex (THC:CBD) placebo	Neurogenic symptoms MS, spinal cord injury, brachial plexus injuries, limb amputation	Crossover	24	Spray: 2.7 mg of THC and 2.5 mg of CBD up to 120 mg THC a day	2 wk	A > P
Zajicek et al.[306]	Marinol, Cannador, placebo	Symptoms related to MS pain)	Parallel	403	2.5 mg THC 1.25 CBD	14 wk	A > P
Wade et al.[307]	Oromucosal Sativex (THC:CBD)	Pain in MS	Parallel	80	Spray: 2.7 mg of THC and 2.5 mg of CBD up to 120 mg THC a day	6 wk	A = P
Abrams et al.[308]	Cannabis	HIV neuropathy	Parallel	27	3.65 mg smoked three times a day	5 d	A > P
Berman et al.[309]	THC ± CBD	Brachial plexus avulsion	Parallel	93	129.6 ± 120	14 d	A > P
Svendsen et al.[210]	Dronabinol	Central pain (MS)	Crossover	24	10	3 wk	A > P
Rog et al.[310]	THC + CBD	Central pain (MS)	Parallel	34	67.5 + 62.5	4 wk	A > P
Wissel et al.[311]	Nabilone	Spasticity-related pain	Crossover	11	Nabilone 1 mg/d placebo	4 wk	A > P
Nurmikko et al.[312]	Oromucosal Sativex (THC:CBD)	Neuropathic pain of peripheral origin	Parallel	63	Spray: 2.7 mg of THC and 2.5 mg of CBD	5 wk	A > P
Wilsey et al.[313]	Cigarette	Central and peripheral neuropathic pain	Crossover	38	High-dose (7%), low-dose (3.5%), or placebo cannabis	1 d	A > P
Frank et al.[139]	Nabilone vs. dihydrocodeine	Chronic neuropathic pain	Crossover	96	Nabilone 2 mg (dihydrocodeine 240 mg)	6 wk	N < D
Narang et al.[314]	Dronabinol	Chronic pain including neuropathic mixed neuropathic nociceptive	Crossover	30	Dronabinol 10 mg, 20 mg (placebo)	1 d each treatment	A > P
Skrabek et al.[315]	Nabilone	Fibromyalgia	Parallel	40	Nabilone 0.5–1 mg twice daily (placebo)	4 wk	A > P
Ellis et al.[316]	Cigarette	HIV-associated distal sensory predominant polyneuropathy	Crossover	34	1% and 8% delta-9-tetrahydrocannabinol	10 d	A > P
Ware et al.[317]	Cigarette	Neuropathic pain	Crossover	23	0%, 2.5%, 6%, 9.4% (placebo)	14 d	A > P
Pini et al.[318]	Nabilone, ibuprofen	Medication overuse headache	Crossover	26	Nabilone 0.5 mg/d; ibuprofen 400 mg	8 wk	A > P
Corey-Bloom et al.[319]	Cigarette	MS pain	Crossover	30	4% THC, placebo	Single dose	A > P
Toth et al.[320]	Nabilone	Diabetic peripheral neuropathic pain	Parallel	13	Nabilone 1–4 mg	9 wk	A > P
Zajicek et al.[321]	Oral cannabis extract (Cannador), placebo	MS pain	Parallel	224	2.5–25 mg THC	12 wk	A > P
Langford et al.[322]	Oromucosal Sativex (THC:CBD)	MS neuropathic pain	Parallel	167	Spray: 2.7 mg of THC and 2.5 mg of CBD	14 wk	A > P
Wilsey et al.[323]	Vaporized cannabis	Neuropathic pain	Crossover	39	Medium dose (3.53% THC), low dose (1.29% THC), and placebo cannabis	Single exposure	A > P
Lynch et al.[324]	Oromucosal Sativex (THC:CBD)	Chemotherapy-induced neuropathic pain	Crossover	16	2.5–25 mg THC	4 wk	A = P
Serpell et al.[325]	Oromucosal Sativex (THC:CBD)	Peripheral neuropathic pain	Parallel	128	Spray: 2.7 mg of THC and 2.5 mg of CBD	14 wk	A > P
Turcotte et al.[326]	Nabilone adjunct to gabapentin, placebo	MS pain	Parallel	14	Gabapentin ≥1,800 mg + nabilone 0.5–2 mg or placebo	9 wk	A > P

CBD, cannabidiol; MS, multiple sclerosis; N, nabilone; THC, tetrahydrocannabinol; A, active drug; P, placebo; > indicates that active drug was superior to the comparator in terms of pain reduction; < indicates that active drug was not superior to the comparator in terms of pain reduction; = indicates that active drug was equal to the comparator in terms of pain reduction.

TABLE 81.10 Summary of Randomized Controlled Trials of Drug Combinations in Treatment of Neuropathic Pain Published as Peer-Reviewed Articles

Study	Drugs	Diagnosis	Design	Number of Patients Treated with Active Agent	Maximal Dosage (mg) per Day	Treatment Duration (wk)	Results
Opioid Plus Another Agent							
McCleane[327]	Cholecystokinin-2 antagonist + morphine Morphine	NP	Crossover	47	30 or 120 + 40 40	2	C = morphine
Gilron et al.[7]	Gabapentin + morphine vs. gabapentin vs. morphine	Mixed neuropathies	Crossover	49 48 49	60 + 2,400 3,600 120	5	C > morphine = gabapentin > P[a]
Khoromi et al.[20]	Morphine + nortriptyline vs. morphine vs. nortriptyline	Radiculopathy	Crossover	34 41 34	90 + 100 90 100	9	C = morphine = nortriptyline = P[b]
Hanna et al.[212]	Gabapentin + oxycodone vs. gabapentin + placebo	PDN	Parallel	163 165	3,600 + 80 4,800	12	Gabapentin + oxycodone > gabapentin + P[c]
Freeman et al.[213]	Tramadol + acetaminophen vs. placebo	PDN	Parallel	160 153	37.5/325	66 d	C > P
Zin et al.[214]	Oxycodone + pregabalin vs. placebo + pregabalin	PHN + PDN	Parallel	26 29	10 + 600 600	5	C = pregabalin + placebo
Harrison et al.[215]	Duloxetine + methadone vs. duloxetine vs. methadone vs. placebo	HIV neuropathy	Crossover	15	60 + 30 60 30	4	Study terminated prematurely
Gilron et al.[144]	Morphine + nortriptyline vs. morphine vs. nortriptyline	PHN + PDN	Crossover	44 47 45	100 + 100 100 100	6	C > morphine C > nortriptyline
Baron et al.[216]	Tapentadol + pregabalin Tapentadol	LBP + neuropathic component	Parallel[d]	159 154	300 + 300 300	8	C = tapentadol
Other Combinations							
Tonet et al.[217]	Amitriptyline + carbamazepine + ketamine vs. amitriptyline + carbamazepine + placebo	Mixed neuropathies	Parallel	15 15	25 + 600 + 30 25 + 600	4	C = amitriptyline + carbamazepine + P
Gilron et al.[70]	Gabapentin + nortriptyline vs. gabapentin vs. nortriptyline	PHN + PDN	Crossover	50 50 46	3,600 + 100 3,600 100	6	C > gabapentin C > nortriptyline
Tesfaye et al.[218]	Pregabalin + duloxetine vs. pregabalin vs. duloxetine	PDN	Parallel	170 97 73	300 + 60 600 120	8	C = pregabalin = duloxetine[e]

Topical Formulations

Study	Drug	Condition	Design	N	Dose	Duration	Result
McCleane[88]	Doxepin + capsaicin (topical)	NP	Parallel	36	3.3% + 0.025%	4	C = doxepin = capsaicin > P
	vs. doxepin			41	3.3%		
	vs. capsaicin			33	0.25%		
	vs. placebo			41			
Lynch et al.[189,190]	Ketamine + amitriptyline (topical)	Mixed neuropathies	Parallel	23	2% + 1% cream	3	C = ketamine = amitriptyline = P[d]
	vs. ketamine			22	1% cream		
	vs. amitriptyline			22	2% cream		
Lynch et al.[194]	Amitriptyline + ketamine (topical)	NP	Crossover	18	1% + 0.5%	2	C = amitriptyline = ketamine = P
	vs. topical amitriptyline			18			
	vs. topical ketamine			18			
Gewandter et al.[195]	Ketamine + amitriptyline vs. placebo (topical)	Postchemotherapy neuropathy	Parallel	229	2% + 4%	6	C = P
	vs. topical placebo			18			
Agrawal et al.[219]	Glyceryl trinitrate (topical) + valproate	PDN	Parallel	22	0.4 mg + 20 mg/kg/d	12	C = glyceryl trinitrate = valproate > P
	vs. glyceryl trinitrate (topical)			20			
	vs. valproate			20			
	vs. placebo			21			
Barton et al.[193]	Ketamine + baclofen + amitriptyline (topical)	Chemotherapy-induced neuropathy	Parallel[d]	101	20 mg + 10 mg + 40 mg	4	C > P
	vs. placebo			102			
Lynch et al.[194]	Amitriptyline + ketamine (topical)	NP	Crossover	18	1% + 0.5%	2	C = amitriptyline = ketamine = P

Drugs Administered as Infusions

Study	Drug	Condition	Design	N	Dose	Duration	Result
Eichenberger et al.[220]	Ketamine + calcitonin (infusions)	Phantom limb pain	Crossover	20	0.4 mg/kg + 200 IE	48 h	C = ketamine; C > calcitonin; C > P
	vs. ketamine infusion			20	0.4 mg/kg		
	vs. calcitonin infusion			20	200 IE		
	vs. placebo infusion			20			
Amr[166]	Ketamine (infusion) + oral gabapentin	Spinal cord injury pain	Parallel	20	80 IV + 900 (oral)	5	C > P + gabapentin
	vs. placebo (infusion) + gabapentin			20			

[a]Combination therapy superior to each drug alone: all are superior to placebo.
[b]Combination, each drug alone, and placebo showed similar efficacy.
[c]Combination of gabapentin + oxycodone was superior to the combination of gabapentin + placebo.
[d]Combination of ketamine + amitriptyline cream, each drug alone and their combination showed similar efficacy.
[e]Combination showed superiority over each drug in secondary outcomes only.
NP, neuropathic pain; PDN, painful diabetic neuropathy; PHN, postherpetic neuralgia; LBP, low back pain; C, combination of drugs; A, active drug; P, placebo; > indicates that active drug(s) was superior to the comparator in terms of pain reduction; = indicates that active drug(s) was equal to the comparator in terms of pain reduction; < indicates that active drug(s) was not superior to the comparator in terms of pain reduction.

or an anticonvulsant[20,144] against each drug alone. Three trials showed superiority of the combinations over each treatment alone,[7,144,212] whereas the two others[20,214] failed to demonstrate similar results. One of the two negative studies[214] compared 600 mg of pregabalin plus 10 mg of oxycodone against 600-mg pregabalin plus a placebo. The 10-mg oxycodone dose might have been too small to demonstrate an analgesic effect especially because less than 30 patients were included in each treatment arm. In the other negative study, Khoromi et al.[20] could not demonstrate superiority of morphine, nortriptyline, or their combination over placebo in patients with chronic lumbar root pain, thus questioning the efficacy of any of these drugs in this type of neuropathic (radicular) pain. Baron et al.[216] compared the effectiveness of tapentadol prolonged release (PR) 500 mg per day or tapentadol PR 300 mg per day plus pregabalin 300 mg per day during a concurrent 8-week, double-blind comparative period in patients with low back pain with a neuropathic component. The analgesic effectiveness provided by tapentadol monotherapy was noninferior to that provided by the combination therapy. Using a different study design, Freeman et al.[213] found the combination of tramadol and acetaminophen advantageous relative to placebo in patients with PDN, but monotherapy arms of the active drugs were not included in this trial.

Two other trials compared combinations of an antidepressant with an anticonvulsant against monotherapies. One[70] showed superiority of gabapentin and nortriptyline over each drug alone in a mixed group of patients with PHN or PDN. In contrast, another large study showed no difference in efficacy between pregabalin combined with duloxetine at moderate dosages compared with high dosages (600-mg pregabalin, 120-mg duloxetine daily) of each drug alone in patients not responsive to monotherapy at moderate dosages.[218] Notably, secondary outcome measures in this study showed superiority of the combination treatment.

Three trials assessed the efficacy of combining the NMDA receptor antagonist ketamine with other drug classes. A small trial found equal efficacy of the combination of oral amitriptyline, carbamazepine, and ketamine compared to amitriptyline, carbamazepine, and placebo in patients with mixed neuropathies.[217] Eichenberg et al.[220] combined ketamine and calcitonin infusions in 20 patients with phantom limb pain and found the combination to be equally effective to ketamine alone but more efficacious than calcitonin or placebo infusions alone. Adding ketamine infusion to oral gabapentin provided better pain relief than placebo infusion in a small study on patients with central neuropathic pain.[166]

Five trials compared the effect of different combinations of topical agents (ketamine, capsaicin, amitriptyline, doxepin, valproate, topiramate, glycerol) to their single components and to placebo.[88,190,194,195,219] Studies failed to show superiority of the combinations over monotherapies. Three of these studies also failed to show superiority of both the combinations and/or monotherapies over placebo,[190,194,195] whereas the two others and an additional study[193] reported opposing results.

Another reason for considering combining drugs from different classes rather than increasing the dose of a single drug is reducing side effects. This consideration was not tested in many of the drug combination studies, as the maximal allowed dose in the monotherapy arm was equivalent to that of the combination arm.[20,70,214,215] Not surprisingly, the incidence of adverse effects in the combination arms in these trials often exceeded that of the monotherapies. When high doses of monotherapy were compared to lower doses of combination treatments, the combinations did not reduce[7,218] or even increased[212,216] the incidence of side effects.

In summary, although some studies demonstrated superiority of drug combinations over monotherapy, others have not. Hence, the concept according to which combining different classes of drugs is clearly more efficacious or a safer alternative to monotherapy for patients with neuropathic pain has not been proven.

Future Drugs

Several new medications are being evaluated for treating neuropathic pain. Mirogabalin is an $\alpha_2\delta$ ligand being studied in PDN. Unlike the other $\alpha_2\delta$ ligands (i.e., gabapentin, pregabalin), mirogabalin is selective for the $\alpha_2\delta$-1 subunit, which investigators are hopeful will improve analgesic effects and limit central nervous system side effects (e.g., dizziness).[221,222] Cebranopadol is a combined central opioid and nociception/orphanin FQ peptide agonist. Preclinical trials suggest potent effects for cebranopadol in neuropathic pain. In addition to increased activity in neuropathic pain, cebranopadol may produce less respiratory depression and drug tolerance than other opioids.[223] The Nav1.7 sodium channel plays a potentially important role in pain sensing. Early trials of TV-45070, a potent Nav1.7 sodium channel inhibitor, demonstrated analgesic effects in PHN and erythromelalgia.[224,225] Gene therapy and placental cell therapy are areas of interest that may prove valuable in PDN.[226,227]

Evidence-Based Recommendations for Drug Therapy in Neuropathic Pain

Adequate response to drug therapy remains a substantial unmet need in patients with neuropathic pain. Although a considerable number of randomized controlled trials on neuropathic pain pharmacotherapy have been published, the quality of evidence is frequently not very high due to modest efficacy of many drugs, large placebo responses, heterogeneous inclusion criteria, and high level of bias in many trials. Notably, analysis of publication bias suggested a 10% overstatement of treatment effects. Studies published in peer-reviewed journals reported greater effects than did unpublished studies (r^2 9.3%, $P = .009$).[6] For these reasons, there is a clear need for evidence-based recommendations on pharmacologic treatment of neuropathic pain, which are based on systematic reviews and meta-analyses of randomized controlled trials. Indeed, such recommendations have been released over the years by various societies and organizations. Most recommendations are determined by drug treatments rather than by the cause of pain. The recommendations are generally consistent between guidelines, but some differences between them exist.

Perhaps the most recent set of recommendations is that of the International Association for the Study of Pain (IASP's) Neuropathic Pain Special Interest Group (NeuPSIG), which was published in 2015.[6] They recommend TCAs, pregabalin, gabapentin (including extended-release), and duloxetine as first-line for neuropathic pain. Lidocaine patch and high-concentration capsaicin patch are second-line treatments for peripheral neuropathic pain. Strong opioids are recommended as third line, mainly due to safety concerns. A weak recommendation against the use of cannabinoids in neuropathic pain is provided mainly because of negative results, potential misuse, diversion, and long-term mental health risks of cannabis.

The European Federation of Neurological Societies (EFNS) most recent guidelines were published in 2010.[9] They confirm TCAs, gabapentin, and pregabalin as first-line for various neuropathic pain conditions (except for trigeminal neuralgia), lidocaine plasters first-line in PHN particularly in the elderly, and SNRIs first-line in painful diabetic polyneuropathies. Second-line treatments include tramadol and capsaicin cream in PHN. Strong opioids are recommended as second line/third line despite established efficacy in neuropathic noncancer pain because of potential risk for abuse on long-term use.

Capsaicin patches are promising for painful HIV neuropathies or PHN whereas cannabinoids are proposed for refractory cases. Lastly, combination therapy is recommended for patients who show partial response to drugs administered alone.

In 2014, the Canadian Pain Society revised its consensus statement on pharmacologic management of chronic neuropathic pain.[10] They recommend gabapentinoids (gabapentin and pregabalin), TCAs, and SNRIs for first-line treatments. Tramadol and controlled-release opioid analgesics are classified as second-line treatments for moderate to severe pain. Cannabinoids are recommended as third-line treatments. Recommended fourth-line treatments include methadone, anticonvulsants with lesser evidence of efficacy (e.g., lamotrigine, lacosamide), tapentadol, and botulinum toxin. They support some analgesic combinations in selected neuropathic pain conditions. If all fail, more invasive treatments should be considered.

Intrathecal Drugs for Neuropathic Pain

Intrathecal (IT) therapy for patients suffering from chronic refractory pain is well established, and two major drugs, morphine and ziconotide, are U.S. Food and Drug Administration (FDA)-approved for nociceptive, neuropathic, or mixed nociceptive–neuropathic pain states. Other drugs are also used in IT therapy including clonidine, hydromorphone, fentanyl, and bupivacaine. Baclofen, indicated for spasticity, has neuropathic pain–relieving activity but is not indicated as therapy for neuropathic pain without spasticity. The place of IT therapy appears late in the algorithm of pain therapy due not only to the invasive nature of this treatment but also to other important issues such as patient selection, realistic patient expectations, patient compliance, insurance coverage for implantation, and a fully equipped staff able to deal with all aspects of implantation, follow-up, and the handling of complications.[228,229]

Although there is no high-level evidence of randomized controlled trials for the long-term (over 12 months) treatment of patients with IT therapy, the evidence from observational trials indicates efficacy for chronic noncancer pain, both nociceptive and neuropathic.[230] Lack of high-level evidence has spurred on the development of expert consensus through the Polyanalgesic Consensus Conference recommendations for both noncancer and cancer patients.[231,232] For noncancer pain, first-line IT therapy includes morphine, hydromorphone, or ziconotide. Second-line IT therapy includes fentanyl, morphine/hydromorphone plus ziconotide, or morphine/hydromorphone plus baclofen/clonidine.

In summary, IT therapy is a well-accepted treatment option for patients suffering from chronic pain in whom more conservative measures have failed. Patient selection and well-trained staff are essential prerequisites for IT therapy. The paucity of the literature for randomized controlled trials with long-term results necessitates further study.

Neuropathic Pain—Not Only Pharmacotherapy

Although this chapter focuses on neuropathic pain pharmacotherapy, providers should bear in mind that neuropathic pain treatment is not limited to drug therapy and a multidisciplinary treatment approach can often yield better outcomes. Often, the burden on patients with chronic neuropathic pain is huge, and their quality of life is significantly impaired. Above all, pharmacotherapy alone frequently provides insufficient analgesic efficacy and common side effects leading to regular clinic visits for medication titration and changes. The use of additional nonpharmacologic strategies is therefore warranted, preferably with an emphasis on a multidisciplinary approach whenever possible.

References

1. Finnerup NB, Haroutounian S, Kamerman P, et al. Neuropathic pain: an updated grading system for research and clinical practice. *Pain* 2016;157(8):1599–1606.
2. Treede RD, Jensen TS, Campbell JN, et al. Neuropathic pain: redefinition and a grading system for clinical and research purposes. *Neurology* 2008;70(18):1630–1635.
3. van Hecke O, Austin SK, Khan RA, et al. Neuropathic pain in the general population: a systematic review of epidemiological studies. *Pain* 2014;155(4):654–662.
4. Dworkin RH, Panarites CJ, Armstrong EP, et al. Is treatment of postherpetic neuralgia in the community consistent with evidence-based recommendations? *Pain* 2012;153(4):869–875.
5. Torrance N, Ferguson JA, Afolabi E, et al. Neuropathic pain in the community: more under-treated than refractory? *Pain* 2013;154(5):690–699.
6. Finnerup NB, Attal N, Haroutounian S, et al. Pharmacotherapy for neuropathic pain in adults: a systematic review and meta-analysis. *Lancet Neurol* 2015;14(2):162–173.
7. Gilron I, Bailey JM, Tu D, et al. Morphine, gabapentin, or their combination for neuropathic pain. *N Engl J Med* 2005;352(13):1324–1334.
8. Baron R, Maier C, Attal N, et al. Peripheral neuropathic pain: a mechanism-related organizing principle based on sensory profiles. *Pain* 2017;158:261–272.
9. Attal N, Cruccu G, Baron R, et al. EFNS guidelines on the pharmacological treatment of neuropathic pain: 2010 revision. *Eur J Neurol* 2010;17(9):1113–1123.
10. Moulin D, Boulanger A, Clark AJ, et al. Pharmacological management of chronic neuropathic pain: revised consensus statement from the Canadian Pain Society. *Pain Res Manag* 2014;19(6):328–335.
11. Lexi-Drugs Online. Hudson, OH: Lexi-Comp, Inc; 2016.
12. McEvoy GK, Snow EK, Kester L, et al, eds. *AHFS DI (Lexi-Comp Online)*. Bethesda, MD: American Society of Health-System Pharmacists; 2016.
13. Cardenas DD, Warms CA, Turner JA, et al. Efficacy of amitriptyline for relief of pain in spinal cord injury: results of a randomized controlled trial. *Pain* 2002;96(3):365–373.
14. Max MB, Culnane M, Schafer SC, et al. Amitriptyline relieves diabetic neuropathy pain in patients with normal or depressed mood. *Neurology* 1987;37(4):589–596.
15. Robinson LR, Czerniecki JM, Ehde DM, et al. Trial of amitriptyline for relief of pain in amputees: results of a randomized controlled study. *Arch Phys Med Rehabil* 2004;85(1):1–6.
16. Kieburtz K, Simpson D, Yiannoutsos C, et al. A randomized trial of amitriptyline and mexiletine for painful neuropathy in HIV infection. AIDS Clinical Trial Group 242 Protocol Team. *Neurology* 1998;51(6):1682–1688.
17. Shlay JC, Chaloner K, Max MB, et al. Acupuncture and amitriptyline for pain due to HIV-related peripheral neuropathy: a randomized controlled trial. Terry Beirn Community Programs for Clinical Research on AIDS. *JAMA* 1998;280(18):1590–1595.
18. Sindrup SH, Bach FW, Madsen C, et al. Venlafaxine versus imipramine in painful polyneuropathy: a randomized, controlled trial. *Neurology* 2003;60(8):1284–1289.
19. Gomez-Perez FJ, Choza R, Rios JM, et al. Nortriptyline-fluphenazine vs. carbamazepine in the symptomatic treatment of diabetic neuropathy. *Arch Med Res* 1996;27(4):525–529.
20. Khoromi S, Cui L, Nackers L, et al. Morphine, nortriptyline and their combination vs. placebo in patients with chronic lumbar root pain. *Pain* 2007;130(1–2):66–75.
21. Goldstein DJ, Lu Y, Detke MJ, et al. Duloxetine vs. placebo in patients with painful diabetic neuropathy. *Pain* 2005;116(1–2):109–118.
22. Raskin J, Pritchett YL, Wang F, et al. A double-blind, randomized multicenter trial comparing duloxetine with placebo in the management of diabetic peripheral neuropathic pain. *Pain Med* 2005;6(5):346–356.
23. Wernicke JF, Pritchett YL, D'Souza DN, et al. A randomized controlled trial of duloxetine in diabetic peripheral neuropathic pain. *Neurology* 2006;67(8):1411–1420.
24. Rowbotham MC, Goli V, Kunz NR, et al. Venlafaxine extended release in the treatment of painful diabetic neuropathy: a double-blind, placebo-controlled study. *Pain* 2004;110(3):697–706.
25. Tasmuth T, Hartel B, Kalso E. Venlafaxine in neuropathic pain following treatment of breast cancer. *Eur J Pain* 2002;6(1):17–24.
26. Sindrup SH, Gram LF, Brosen K, et al. The selective serotonin reuptake inhibitor paroxetine is effective in the treatment of diabetic neuropathy symptoms. *Pain* 1990;42(2):135–144.
27. Sindrup SH, Bjerre U, Dejgaard A, et al. The selective serotonin reuptake inhibitor citalopram relieves the symptoms of diabetic neuropathy. *Clin Pharmacol Ther* 1992;52(5):547–552.
28. Max MB, Lynch SA, Muir J, et al. Effects of desipramine, amitriptyline, and fluoxetine on pain in diabetic neuropathy. *N Engl J Med* 1992;326(19):1250–1256.
29. Moore RA, Derry S, Aldington D, et al. Amitriptyline for neuropathic pain and fibromyalgia in adults. *Cochrane Database Syst Rev* 2012;(12):CD008242.
30. Saarto T, Wiffen PJ. Antidepressants for neuropathic pain: a Cochrane review. *J Neurol Neurosurg Psychiatry* 2010;81(12):1372–1373.

31. Hammack JE, Michalak JC, Loprinzi CL, et al. Phase III evaluation of nortriptyline for alleviation of symptoms of cis-platinum-induced peripheral neuropathy. *Pain* 2002;98(1–2):195–203.

32. Mercadante S, Arcuri E, Tirelli W, et al. Amitriptyline in neuropathic cancer pain in patients on morphine therapy: a randomized placebo-controlled, double-blind crossover study. *Tumori* 2002;88(3):239–242.

33. Breivik H, Collett B, Ventafridda V, et al. Survey of chronic pain in Europe: prevalence, impact on daily life, and treatment. *Eur J Pain* 2006;10(4):287–333.

34. Lipman AG. Analgesic drugs for neuropathic and sympathetically maintained pain. *Clin Geriatr Med* 1996;12(3):501–515.

35. Zemrak WR, Kenna GA. Association of antipsychotic and antidepressant drugs with Q-T interval prolongation. *Am J Health Syst Pharm* 2008;65(11):1029–1038.

36. Dworkin RH, O'Connor AB, Audette J, et al. Recommendations for the pharmacological management of neuropathic pain: an overview and literature update. *Mayo Clin Proc* 2010;85(3 suppl):S3–S14.

37. Reuben SS, Makari-Judson G, Lurie SD. Evaluation of efficacy of the perioperative administration of venlafaxine XR in the prevention of postmastectomy pain syndrome. *J Pain Symptom Manage* 2004;27(2):133–139.

38. Raskin J, Smith TR, Wong K, et al. Duloxetine versus routine care in the long-term management of diabetic peripheral neuropathic pain. *J Palliat Med* 2006;9(1):29–40.

39. Dunner DL, Wohlreich MM, Mallinckrodt CH, et al. Clinical consequences of initial duloxetine dosing strategies: comparison of 30 and 60 mg QD starting doses. *Curr Ther Res* 2005;66(6):522–540.

40. Blom S. Trigeminal neuralgia: its treatment with a new anticonvulsant drug (G-32883). *Lancet* 1962;1(7234):839–840.

41. Wiffen PJ, Derry S, Moore RA, et al. Antiepileptic drugs for neuropathic pain and fibromyalgia—an overview of Cochrane reviews. *Cochrane Database Syst Rev* 2013;(11):CD010567.

42. Wiffen PJ, Derry S, Moore RA, et al. Carbamazepine for chronic neuropathic pain and fibromyalgia in adults. *Cochrane Database Syst Rev* 2014;(4):CD005451.

43. Rull JA, Quibrera R, Gonzalez-Millan H, et al. Symptomatic treatment of peripheral diabetic neuropathy with carbamazepine (Tegretol): double blind crossover trial. *Diabetologia* 1969;5(4):215–218.

44. Wilton TD. Tegretol in the treatment of diabetic neuropathy. *S Afr Med J* 1974;48(20):869–872.

45. Nicol CF. A four year double-blind study of Tegretol in facial pain. *Headache* 1969;9(1):54–57.

46. Campbell FG, Graham JG, Zilkha KJ. Clinical trial of carbazepine (Tegretol) in trigeminal neuralgia. *J Neurol Neurosurg Psychiatry* 1966;29(3):265–267.

47. Killian JM, Fromm GH. Carbamazepine in the treatment of neuralgia. Use of side effects. *Arch Neurol* 1968;19(2):129–136.

48. Shaikh S, Yaacob HB, Abd Rahman RB. Lamotrigine for trigeminal neuralgia: efficacy and safety in comparison with carbamazepine. *J Chin Med Assoc* 2011;74(6):243–249.

49. Harke H, Gretenkort P, Ladleif HU, et al. The response of neuropathic pain and pain in complex regional pain syndrome I to carbamazepine and sustained-release morphine in patients pretreated with spinal cord stimulation: a double-blinded randomized study. *Anesth Analg* 2001;92(2):488–495.

50. Dogra S, Beydoun S, Mazzola J, et al. Oxcarbazepine in painful diabetic neuropathy: a randomized, placebo-controlled study. *Eur J Pain* 2005;9(5):543–554.

51. Grosskopf J, Mazzola J, Wan Y, et al. A randomized, placebo-controlled study of oxcarbazepine in painful diabetic neuropathy. *Acta Neurol Scand* 2006;114(3):177–180.

52. Beydoun A, Shaibani A, Hopwood M, et al. Oxcarbazepine in painful diabetic neuropathy: results of a dose-ranging study. *Acta Neurol Scand* 2006;113(6):395–404.

53. Demant DT, Lund K, Vollert J, et al. The effect of oxcarbazepine in peripheral neuropathic pain depends on pain phenotype: a randomised, double-blind, placebo-controlled phenotype-stratified study. *Pain* 2014;155(11):2263–2273.

54. Backonja M, Beydoun A, Edwards KR, et al. Gabapentin for the symptomatic treatment of painful neuropathy in patients with diabetes mellitus: a randomized controlled trial. *JAMA* 1998;280(21):1831–1836.

55. Dallocchio C, Buffa C, Mazzarello P, et al. Gabapentin vs. amitriptyline in painful diabetic neuropathy: an open-label pilot study. *J Pain Symptom Manage* 2000;20(4):280–285.

56. Simpson DA. Gabapentin and venlafaxine for the treatment of painful diabetic neuropathy. *J Clin Neuromuscul Dis* 2001;3(2):53–62.

57. Pandey CK, Bose N, Garg G, et al. Gabapentin for the treatment of pain in Guillain-Barré syndrome: a double-blinded, placebo-controlled, crossover study. *Anesth Analg* 2002;95(6):1719–1723, table of contents.

58. Pandey CK, Raza M, Tripathi M, et al. The comparative evaluation of gabapentin and carbamazepine for pain management in Guillain-Barré syndrome patients in the intensive care unit. *Anesth Analg* 2005;101(1):220–225, table of contents.

59. Hahn K, Arendt G, Braun JS, et al. A placebo-controlled trial of gabapentin for painful HIV-associated sensory neuropathies. *J Neurol* 2004;251(10):1260–1266.

60. Caraceni A, Zecca E, Bonezzi C, et al. Gabapentin for neuropathic cancer pain: a randomized controlled trial from the Gabapentin Cancer Pain Study Group. *J Clin Oncol* 2004;22(14):2909–2917.

61. Mishra S, Bhatnagar S, Goyal GN, et al. A comparative efficacy of amitriptyline, gabapentin, and pregabalin in neuropathic cancer pain: a prospective randomized double-blind placebo-controlled study. *Am J Hosp Palliat Care* 2012;29(3):177–182.

62. Rice AS, Maton S. Gabapentin in postherpetic neuralgia: a randomised, double blind, placebo controlled study. *Pain* 2001;94(2):215–224.

63. Rowbotham M, Harden N, Stacey B, et al. Gabapentin for the treatment of postherpetic neuralgia: a randomized controlled trial. *JAMA* 1998;280(21):1837–1842.

64. Chandra K, Shafiq N, Pandhi P, et al. Gabapentin versus nortriptyline in post-herpetic neuralgia patients: a randomized, double-blind clinical trial—the GONIP Trial. *Int J Clin Pharmacol Ther* 2006;44(8):358–363.

65. Bone M, Critchley P, Buggy DJ. Gabapentin in postamputation phantom limb pain: a randomized, double-blind, placebo-controlled, cross-over study. *Reg Anesth Pain Med* 2002;27(5):481–486.

66. Gordh TE, Stubhaug A, Jensen TS, et al. Gabapentin in traumatic nerve injury pain: a randomized, double-blind, placebo-controlled, cross-over, multi-center study. *Pain* 2008;138(2):255–266.

67. Levendoglu F, Ogun CO, Ozerbil O, et al. Gabapentin is a first line drug for the treatment of neuropathic pain in spinal cord injury. *Spine* 2004;29(7):743–751.

68. Tai Q, Kirshblum S, Chen B, et al. Gabapentin in the treatment of neuropathic pain after spinal cord injury: a prospective, randomized, double-blind, crossover trial. *J Spinal Cord Med* 2002;25(2):100–105.

69. Rintala DH, Holmes SA, Courtade D, et al. Comparison of the effectiveness of amitriptyline and gabapentin on chronic neuropathic pain in persons with spinal cord injury. *Arch Phys Med Rehabil* 2007;88(12):1547–1560.

70. Gilron I, Bailey JM, Tu D, et al. Nortriptyline and gabapentin, alone and in combination for neuropathic pain: a double-blind, randomised controlled crossover trial. *Lancet* 2009;374(9697):1252–1261.

71. Wallace MS, Irving G, Cowles VE. Gabapentin extended-release tablets for the treatment of patients with postherpetic neuralgia: a randomized, double-blind, placebo-controlled, multicentre study. *Clin Drug Investig* 2010;30(11):765–776.

72. Sang CN, Sathyanarayana R, Sweeney M. Gastroretentive gabapentin (G-GR) formulation reduces intensity of pain associated with postherpetic neuralgia (PHN). *Clin J Pain* 2013;29(4):281–288.

73. Irving G, Jensen M, Cramer M, et al. Efficacy and tolerability of gastric-retentive gabapentin for the treatment of postherpetic neuralgia: results of a double-blind, randomized, placebo-controlled clinical trial. *Clin J Pain* 2009;25(3):185–192.

74. Rauck R, Makumi CW, Schwartz S, et al. A randomized, controlled trial of gabapentin enacarbil in subjects with neuropathic pain associated with diabetic peripheral neuropathy. *Pain Pract* 2013;13(6):485–496.

75. Zhang L, Rainka M, Freeman R, et al. A randomized, double-blind, placebo-controlled trial to assess the efficacy and safety of gabapentin enacarbil in subjects with neuropathic pain associated with postherpetic neuralgia (PXN110748). *J Pain* 2013;14(6):590–603.

76. Rauck RL, Shaibani A, Biton V, et al. Lacosamide in painful diabetic peripheral neuropathy: a phase 2 double-blind placebo-controlled study. *Clin J Pain* 2007;23(2):150–158.

77. Shaibani A, Fares S, Selam JL, et al. Lacosamide in painful diabetic neuropathy: an 18-week double-blind placebo-controlled trial. *J Pain* 2009;10(8):818–828.

78. Wymer JP, Simpson J, Sen D, et al. Efficacy and safety of lacosamide in diabetic neuropathic pain: an 18-week double-blind placebo-controlled trial of fixed-dose regimens. *Clin J Pain* 2009;25(5):376–385.

79. Ziegler D, Hidvegi T, Gurieva I, et al. Efficacy and safety of lacosamide in painful diabetic neuropathy. *Diabetes Care* 2010;33(4):839–841.

80. Breuer B, Pappagallo M, Knotkova H, et al. A randomized, double-blind, placebo-controlled, two-period, crossover, pilot trial of lamotrigine in patients with central pain due to multiple sclerosis. *Clin Ther* 2007;29(9):2022–2030.

81. Vestergaard K, Andersen G, Gottrup H, et al. Lamotrigine for central post-stroke pain: a randomized controlled trial. *Neurology* 2001;56(2):184–190.

82. Vinik AI, Tuchman M, Safirstein B, et al. Lamotrigine for treatment of pain associated with diabetic neuropathy: results of two randomized, double-blind, placebo-controlled studies. *Pain* 2007;128(1–2):169–179.

83. Eisenberg E, Lurie Y, Braker C, et al. Lamotrigine reduces painful diabetic neuropathy: a randomized, controlled study. *Neurology* 2001;57(3):505–509.

84. Simpson DM, Olney R, McArthur JC, et al. A placebo-controlled trial of lamotrigine for painful HIV-associated neuropathy. *Neurology* 2000;54(11):2115–2119.

85. Simpson DM, McArthur JC, Olney R, et al. Lamotrigine for HIV-associated painful sensory neuropathies: a placebo-controlled trial. *Neurology* 2003;60(9):1508–1514.

86. Finnerup NB, Sindrup SH, Bach FW, et al. Lamotrigine in spinal cord injury pain: a randomized controlled trial. *Pain* 2002;96(3):375–383.

87. Zakrzewska JM, Chaudhry Z, Nurmikko TJ, et al. Lamotrigine (Lamictal) in refractory trigeminal neuralgia: results from a double-blind placebo controlled crossover trial. *Pain* 1997;73(2):223–230.

88. McCleane G. Topical application of doxepin hydrochloride, capsaicin and a combination of both produces analgesia in chronic human neuropathic pain: a randomized, double-blind, placebo-controlled study. *Br J Clin Pharmacol* 2000;49(6):574–579.

89. McCleane G. 200 mg daily of lamotrigine has no analgesic effect in neuropathic pain: a randomised, double-blind, placebo controlled trial. *Pain* 1999;83(1):105–107.

90. Silver M, Blum D, Grainger J, et al. Double-blind, placebo-controlled trial of lamotrigine in combination with other medications for neuropathic pain. *J Pain Symptom Manage* 2007;34(4):446–454.

91. Rossi S, Mataluni G, Codeca C, et al. Effects of levetiracetam on chronic pain in multiple sclerosis: results of a pilot, randomized, placebo-controlled study. *Eur J Neurol* 2009;16(3):360–366.

92. Falah M, Madsen C, Holbech JV, et al. A randomized, placebo-controlled trial of levetiracetam in central pain in multiple sclerosis. *Eur J Pain* 2012;16(6):860–869.

93. Vilholm OJ, Cold S, Rasmussen L, et al. Effect of levetiracetam on the postmastectomy pain syndrome. *Eur J Neurol* 2008;15(8):851–857.

94. Finnerup NB, Grydehoj J, Bing J, et al. Levetiracetam in spinal cord injury pain: a randomized controlled trial. *Spinal Cord* 2009;47(12):861–867.

95. Holbech JV, Otto M, Bach FW, et al. The anticonvulsant levetiracetam for the treatment of pain in polyneuropathy: a randomized, placebo-controlled, cross-over trial. *Eur J Pain* 2011;15(6):608–614.

96. Krcevski Skvarc N, Kamenik M. Effects of pregabalin on acute herpetic pain and postherpetic neuralgia incidence. *Wien Klin Wochenschr* 2010;122(suppl 2):49–53.

97. Kim JS, Bashford G, Murphy TK, et al. Safety and efficacy of pregabalin in patients with central post-stroke pain. *Pain* 2011;152(5):1018–1023.

98. Simpson DM, Schifitto G, Clifford DB, et al. Pregabalin for painful HIV neuropathy: a randomized, double-blind, placebo-controlled trial. *Neurology* 2010;74(5):413–420.

99. Simpson DM, Rice AS, Emir B, et al. A randomized, double-blind, placebo-controlled trial and open-label extension study to evaluate the efficacy and safety of pregabalin in the treatment of neuropathic pain associated with human immunodeficiency virus neuropathy. *Pain* 2014;155(10):1943–1954.

100. Raptis E, Vadalouca A, Stavropoulou E, et al. Pregabalin vs. opioids for the treatment of neuropathic cancer pain: a prospective, head-to-head, randomized, open-label study. *Pain Pract* 2014;14(1):32–42.

101. Richter RW, Portenoy R, Sharma U, et al. Relief of painful diabetic peripheral neuropathy with pregabalin: a randomized, placebo-controlled trial. *J Pain* 2005;6(4):253–260.

102. Lesser H, Sharma U, LaMoreaux L, et al. Pregabalin relieves symptoms of painful diabetic neuropathy: a randomized controlled trial. *Neurology* 2004;63(11):2104–2110.

103. Rosenstock J, Tuchman M, LaMoreaux L, et al. Pregabalin for the treatment of painful diabetic peripheral neuropathy: a double-blind, placebo-controlled trial. *Pain* 2004;110(3):628–638.

104. Tolle T, Freynhagen R, Versavel M, et al. Pregabalin for relief of neuropathic pain associated with diabetic neuropathy: a randomized, double-blind study. *Eur J Pain* 2008;12(2):203–213.

105. Arezzo JC, Rosenstock J, Lamoreaux L, et al. Efficacy and safety of pregabalin 600 mg/d for treating painful diabetic peripheral neuropathy: a double-blind placebo-controlled trial. *BMC Neurol* 2008;8:33.

106. Satoh J, Yagihashi S, Baba M, et al. Efficacy and safety of pregabalin for treating neuropathic pain associated with diabetic peripheral neuropathy: a 14 week, randomized, double-blind, placebo-controlled trial. *Diabet Med* 2011;28(1):109–116.

107. Smith T, DiBernardo A, Shi Y, et al. Efficacy and safety of carisbamate in patients with diabetic neuropathy or postherpetic neuralgia: results from 3 randomized, double-blind placebo-controlled trials. *Pain Pract* 2014;14(4):332–342.

108. Raskin P, Huffman C, Yurkewicz L, et al. Pregabalin in patients with painful diabetic peripheral neuropathy using an NSAID for other pain conditions: a double-blind crossover study. *Clin J Pain* 2016;32(3):203–210.

109. Sabatowski R, Galvez R, Cherry DA, et al. Pregabalin reduces pain and improves sleep and mood disturbances in patients with post-herpetic neuralgia: results of a randomised, placebo-controlled clinical trial. *Pain* 2004;109 (1–2):26–35.

110. Dworkin RH, Corbin AE, Young JP Jr, et al. Pregabalin for the treatment of postherpetic neuralgia: a randomized, placebo-controlled trial. *Neurology* 2003;60(8):1274–1283.

111. van Seventer R, Feister HA, Young JP Jr, et al. Efficacy and tolerability of twice-daily pregabalin for treating pain and related sleep interference in postherpetic neuralgia: a 13-week, randomized trial. *Curr Med Res Opin* 2006;22(2):375–384.

112. Stacey BR, Barrett JA, Whalen E, et al. Pregabalin for postherpetic neuralgia: placebo-controlled trial of fixed and flexible dosing regimens on allodynia and time to onset of pain relief. *J Pain* 2008;9(11):1006–1017.

113. van Seventer R, Bach FW, Toth CC, et al. Pregabalin in the treatment of post-traumatic peripheral neuropathic pain: a randomized double blind trial. *Eur J Neurol* 2010;17(8):1082–1089.

114. Siddall PJ, Cousins MJ, Otte A, et al. Pregabalin in central neuropathic pain associated with spinal cord injury: a placebo-controlled trial. *Neurology* 2006;67(10):1792–1800.

115. Cardenas DD, Nieshoff EC, Suda K, et al. A randomized trial of pregabalin in patients with neuropathic pain due to spinal cord injury. *Neurology* 2013;80(6):533–539.

116. Freynhagen R, Strojek K, Griesing T, et al. Efficacy of pregabalin in neuropathic pain evaluated in a 12-week, randomised, double-blind, multicentre, placebo-controlled trial of flexible- and fixed-dose regimens. *Pain* 2005;115(3):254–263.

117. Vranken JH, Dijkgraaf MG, Kruis MR, et al. Pregabalin in patients with central neuropathic pain: a randomized, double-blind, placebo-controlled trial of a flexible-dose regimen. *Pain* 2008;136(1–2):150–157.

118. Liang L, Li X, Zhang G, et al. Pregabalin in the treatment of herpetic neuralgia: results of a multicenter Chinese study. *Pain Med* 2015;16(1):160–167.

119. Guan Y, Ding X, Cheng Y, et al. Efficacy of pregabalin for peripheral neuropathic pain: results of an 8-week, flexible-dose, double-blind, placebo-controlled study conducted in China. *Clin Ther* 2011;33(2):159–166.

120. Moon DE, Lee DI, Lee SC, et al. Efficacy and tolerability of pregabalin using a flexible, optimized dose schedule in Korean patients with peripheral neuropathic pain: a 10-week, randomized, double-blind, placebo-controlled, multicenter study. *Clin Ther* 2010;32(14):2370–2385.

121. Haanpaa M, Cruccu G, Nurmikko TJ, et al. Capsaicin 8% patch versus oral pregabalin in patients with peripheral neuropathic pain. *Eur J Pain* 2016;20(2):316–328.

122. Gilron I, Wajsbrot D, Therrien F, et al. Pregabalin for peripheral neuropathic pain: a multicenter, enriched enrollment randomized withdrawal placebo-controlled trial. *Clin J Pain* 2011;27(3):185–193.

123. Kochar DK, Jain N, Agarwal RP, et al. Sodium valproate in the management of painful neuropathy in type 2 diabetes—a randomized placebo controlled study. *Acta Neurol Scand* 2002;106(5):248–252.

124. Kochar DK, Rawat N, Agrawal RP, et al. Sodium valproate for painful diabetic neuropathy: a randomized double-blind placebo-controlled study. *QJM* 2004;97(1):33–38.

125. Kochar DK, Garg P, Bumb RA, et al. Divalproex sodium in the management of post-herpetic neuralgia: a randomized double-blind placebo-controlled study. *QJM* 2005;98(1):29–34.

126. Drewes AM, Andreasen A, Poulsen LH. Valproate for treatment of chronic central pain after spinal cord injury. A double-blind cross-over study. *Paraplegia* 1994;32(8):565–569.

127. Otto M, Bach FW, Jensen TS, et al. Valproic acid has no effect on pain in polyneuropathy: a randomized, controlled trial. *Neurology* 2004;62(2):285–288.

128. Thienel U, Neto W, Schwabe SK, et al. Topiramate in painful diabetic polyneuropathy: findings from three double-blind placebo-controlled trials. *Acta Neurol Scand* 2004;110(4):221–231.

129. Raskin P, Donofrio PD, Rosenthal NR, et al. Topiramate vs placebo in painful diabetic neuropathy: analgesic and metabolic effects. *Neurology* 2004;63(5):865–873.

130. Khoromi S, Patsalides A, Parada S, et al. Topiramate in chronic lumbar radicular pain. *J Pain* 2005;6(12):829–836.

131. Atli A, Dogra S. Zonisamide in the treatment of painful diabetic neuropathy: a randomized, double-blind, placebo-controlled pilot study. *Pain Med* 2005;6(3):225–234.

132. Dooley DJ, Donovan CM, Meder WP, et al. Preferential action of gabapentin and pregabalin at P/Q-type voltage-sensitive calcium channels: inhibition of K+-evoked [3H]-norepinephrine release from rat neocortical slices. *Synapse* 2002;45(3):171–190.

133. Strojek K, Floter T, Balkenohl M, et al. Pregabalin in the management of chronic neuropathic pain (NeP): a novel evaluation of flexible and fixed dosing [abstract 804]. *Diabetes* 2004;53(suppl 2):59.

134. Sharma U, Allen R, Glessner C, et al. Pregabalin effectively relieves pain in patients with diabetic polyneuropathy: study 1008-914 [abstract 686-p]. *Diabetes* 2000;40(suppl 1):167.

135. Rockliff BW, Davis EH. Controlled sequential trials of carbamazepine in trigeminal neuralgia. *Arch Neurol* 1966;15(2):129–136.

136. Burchiel KJ. Carbamazepine inhibits spontaneous activity in experimental neuromas. *Exp Neurol* 1988;102(2):249–253.

137. Brunton LL, Chabner BA, Knollmann BC, eds. *Goodman and Gilman's The Pharmacological Basis of Therapeutics.* 12th ed. New York: McGraw-Hill Medical; 2011.

138. Zhou M, Chen N, He L, et al. Oxcarbazepine for neuropathic pain. *Cochrane Database Syst Rev* 2013;(3):CD007963.

139. Frank B, Serpell MG, Hughes J, et al. Comparison of analgesic effects and patient tolerability of nabilone and dihydrocodeine for chronic neuropathic pain: randomised, crossover, double blind study. *BMJ* 2008;336(7637):199–201.

140. Nalamachu S, Hale M, Khan A. Hydromorphone extended release for neuropathic and non-neuropathic/nociceptive chronic low back pain: a post hoc analysis of data from a randomized, multicenter, double-blind, placebo-controlled clinical trial. *J Opioid Manag* 2014;10(5):311–322.

141. Rowbotham MC, Twilling L, Davies PS, et al. Oral opioid therapy for chronic peripheral and central neuropathic pain. *N Engl J Med* 2003;348(13):1223–1232.

142. Morley JS, Bridson J, Nash TP, et al. Low-dose methadone has an analgesic effect in neuropathic pain: a double-blind randomized controlled crossover trial. *Palliat Med* 2003;17(7):576–587.

143. Wu CL, Agarwal S, Tella PK, et al. Morphine versus mexiletine for treatment of postamputation pain: a randomized, placebo-controlled, crossover trial. *Anesthesiology* 2008;109(2):289–296.

144. Gilron I, Tu D, Holden RR, et al. Combination of morphine with nortriptyline for neuropathic pain. *Pain* 2015;156(8):1440–1448.

145. Boureau F, Legallicier P, Kabir-Ahmadi M. Tramadol in post-herpetic neuralgia: a randomized, double-blind, placebo-controlled trial. *Pain* 2003;104 (1–2):323–331.

146. Harati Y, Gooch C, Swenson M, et al. Double-blind randomized trial of tramadol for the treatment of the pain of diabetic neuropathy. *Neurology* 1998;50(6):1842–1846.

147. Sindrup SH, Andersen G, Madsen C, et al. Tramadol relieves pain and allodynia in polyneuropathy: a randomised, double-blind, controlled trial. *Pain* 1999;83(1):85–90.

148. Wilder-Smith CH, Hill LT, Laurent S. Postamputation pain and sensory changes in treatment-naive patients: characteristics and responses to treatment with tramadol, amitriptyline, and placebo. *Anesthesiology* 2005;103(3):619–628.

149. Norrbrink C, Lundeberg T. Tramadol in neuropathic pain after spinal cord injury: a randomized, double-blind, placebo-controlled trial. *Clin J Pain* 2009;25(3):177–184.

150. Sindrup SH, Konder R, Lehmann R, et al. Randomized controlled trial of the combined monoaminergic and opioid investigational compound GRT9906 in painful polyneuropathy. *Eur J Pain* 2012;16(6):849–859.

151. Schwartz S, Etropolski M, Shapiro DY, et al. Safety and efficacy of tapentadol ER in patients with painful diabetic peripheral neuropathy: results of a randomized-withdrawal, placebo-controlled trial. *Curr Med Res Opin* 2011;27(1):151–162.

152. Vinik AI, Shapiro DY, Rauschkolb C, et al. A randomized withdrawal, placebo-controlled study evaluating the efficacy and tolerability of tapentadol extended release in patients with chronic painful diabetic peripheral neuropathy. *Diabetes Care* 2014;37(8):2302–2309.

153. Niesters M, Proto PL, Aarts L, et al. Tapentadol potentiates descending pain inhibition in chronic pain patients with diabetic polyneuropathy. *Br J Anaesth* 2014;113(1):148–156.

154. Eisenberg E, McNicol ED, Carr DB. Efficacy of mu-opioid agonists in the treatment of evoked neuropathic pain: systematic review of randomized controlled trials. *Eur J Pain* 2006;10(8):667–676.

155. McNicol ED, Midbari A, Eisenberg E. Opioids for neuropathic pain. *Cochrane Database Syst Rev* 2013;(8):CD006146.

156. Dowell D, Haegerich TM, Chou R. CDC guideline for prescribing opioids for chronic pain—United States, 2016. *JAMA* 2016;315(15):1624–1645.

157. Raffa RB, Buschmann H, Christoph T, et al. Mechanistic and functional differentiation of tapentadol and tramadol. *Expert Opin Pharmacother* 2012;13(10):1437–1449.

158. Vadivelu N, Kai A, Maslin B, et al. Tapentadol extended release in the management of peripheral diabetic neuropathic pain. *Ther Clin Risk Manag* 2015;11:95–105.

159. Nelson KA, Park KM, Robinovitz E, et al. High-dose oral dextromethorphan versus placebo in painful diabetic neuropathy and postherpetic neuralgia. *Neurology* 1997;48(5):1212–1218.

160. Sang CN, Booher S, Gilron I, et al. Dextromethorphan and memantine in painful diabetic neuropathy and postherpetic neuralgia: efficacy and dose-response trials. *Anesthesiology* 2002;96(5):1053–1061.

161. McQuay HJ, Carroll D, Jadad AR, et al. Dextromethorphan for the treatment of neuropathic pain: a double-blind randomised controlled crossover trial with integral n-of-1 design. *Pain* 1994;59(1):127–133.

162. Schley M, Topfner S, Wiech K, et al. Continuous brachial plexus blockade in combination with the NMDA receptor antagonist memantine prevents phantom pain in acute traumatic upper limb amputees. *Eur J Pain* 2007;11(3):299–308.

163. Finnerup NB, Otto M, McQuay HJ, et al. Algorithm for neuropathic pain treatment: an evidence based proposal. *Pain* 2005;118(3):289–305.

164. Loy BM, Britt RB, Brown JN. Memantine for the treatment of phantom limb pain: a systematic review. *J Pain Palliat Care Pharmacother* 2016;30:276–283.

165. Hocking G, Visser EJ, Schug SA, et al. Ketamine: does life begin at 40? *Pain: Clinical Updates* 2007;XV(3).

166. Amr YM. Multi-day low dose ketamine infusion as adjuvant to oral gabapentin in spinal cord injury related chronic pain: a prospective, randomized, double blind trial. *Pain Physician* 2010;13(3):245–249.

167. Cohen SP, Chang AS, Larkin T, et al. The intravenous ketamine test: a predictive response tool for oral dextromethorphan treatment in neuropathic pain. *Anesth Analg* 2004;99(6):1753–1759, table of contents.

168. Chong C, Schug SA, Page-Sharp M, et al. Development of a sublingual/oral formulation of ketamine for use in neuropathic pain: preliminary findings from a three-way randomized, crossover study. *Clin Drug Investig* 2009;29(5):317–324.

169. Huge V, Lauchart M, Magerl W, et al. Effects of low-dose intranasal (S)-ketamine in patients with neuropathic pain. *Eur J Pain* 2010;14(4):387–394.

170. Stracke H, Meyer UE, Schumacher HE, et al. Mexiletine in the treatment of diabetic neuropathy. *Diabetes Care* 1992;15(11):1550–1555.

171. Oskarsson P, Ljunggren JG, Lins PE. Efficacy and safety of mexiletine in the treatment of painful diabetic neuropathy. The Mexiletine Study Group. *Diabetes Care* 1997;20(10):1594–1597.

172. Wright JM, Oki JC, Graves L III. Mexiletine in the symptomatic treatment of diabetic peripheral neuropathy. *Ann Pharmacother* 1997;31(1):29–34.

173. Tremont-Lukats IW, Challapalli V, McNicol ED, et al. Systemic administration of local anesthetics to relieve neuropathic pain: a systematic review and meta-analysis. *Anesth Analg* 2005;101(6):1738–1749.

174. Galer BS, Harle J, Rowbotham MC. Response to intravenous lidocaine infusion predicts subsequent response to oral mexiletine: a prospective study. *J Pain Symptom Manage* 1996;12(3):161–167.

175. Vo T, Rice AS, Dworkin RH. Non-steroidal anti-inflammatory drugs for neuropathic pain: how do we explain continued widespread use? *Pain* 2009;143(3):169–171.

176. Watkins LR, Maier SF. Neuropathic pain: the immune connection. *Pain: Clinical Updates* 2004;XII(1).

177. Syriatowicz JP, Hu D, Walker JS, et al. Hyperalgesia due to nerve injury: role of prostaglandins. *Neuroscience* 1999;94(2):587–594.

178. Kawakami M, Matsumoto T, Hashizume H, et al. Epidural injection of cyclooxygenase-2 inhibitor attenuates pain-related behavior following application of nucleus pulposus to the nerve root in the rat. *J Orthop Res* 2002;20(2):376–381.

179. Nalamachu S, Crockett RS, Gammaitoni AR, et al. A comparison of the lidocaine patch 5% vs naproxen 500 mg twice daily for the relief of pain associated with carpal tunnel syndrome: a 6-week, randomized, parallel-group study. *MedGenMed* 2006;8(3):33.

180. Cohen KL, Harris S. Efficacy and safety of nonsteroidal anti-inflammatory drugs in the therapy of diabetic neuropathy. *Arch Intern Med* 1987; 147(8):1442–1444.

181. Werner RN, Nikkels AF, Marinovic B, et al. European consensus-based (S2k) guideline on the management of herpes zoster—guided by the European Dermatology Forum (EDF) in cooperation with the European Academy of Dermatology and Venereology (EADV), part 2: treatment. *J Eur Acad Dermatol Venereol* 2017;31(1):20–29.

182. Rasmussen-Barr E, Held U, Grooten WJ, et al. Non-steroidal anti-inflammatory drugs for sciatica. *Cochrane Database Syst Rev* 2016;(10):CD012382.

183. Valat JP, Genevay S, Marty M, et al. Sciatica. *Best Pract Res Clin Rheumatol* 2010;24(2):241–252.

184. Nagy I, Friston D, Valente JS, et al. Pharmacology of the capsaicin receptor, transient receptor potential vanilloid type-1 ion channel. *Prog Drug Res* 2014;68:39–76.

185. Rowbotham MC, Davies PS, Fields HL. Topical lidocaine gel relieves postherpetic neuralgia. *Ann Neurol* 1995;37(2):246–253.

186. Galer BS, Rowbotham MC, Perander J, et al. Topical lidocaine patch relieves postherpetic neuralgia more effectively than a vehicle topical patch: results of an enriched enrollment study. *Pain* 1999;80(3):533–538.

187. Binder A, Bruxelle J, Rogers P, et al. Topical 5% lidocaine (lignocaine) medicated plaster treatment for post-herpetic neuralgia: results of a double-blind, placebo-controlled, multinational efficacy and safety trial. *Clin Drug Investig* 2009;29(6):393–408.

188. Meier T, Wasner G, Faust M, et al. Efficacy of lidocaine patch 5% in the treatment of focal peripheral neuropathic pain syndromes: a randomized, double-blind, placebo-controlled study. *Pain* 2003;106(1–2):151–158.

189. Lynch ME, Clark AJ, Sawynok J, et al. Topical 2% amitriptyline and 1% ketamine in neuropathic pain syndromes: a randomized, double-blind, placebo-controlled trial. *Anesthesiology* 2005;103(1):140–146.

190. Lynch ME, Clark AJ, Sawynok J, et al. Topical amitriptyline and ketamine in neuropathic pain syndromes: an open-label study. *J Pain* 2005;6(10):644–649.

191. Barros GA, Miot HA, Braz AM, et al. Topical (S)-ketamine for pain management of postherpetic neuralgia. *An Bras Dermatol* 2012;87(3):504–505.

192. Dworkin RH, O'Connor AB, Backonja M, et al. Pharmacologic management of neuropathic pain: evidence-based recommendations. *Pain* 2007;132(3):237–251.

193. Barton DL, Wos EJ, Qin R, et al. A double-blind, placebo-controlled trial of a topical treatment for chemotherapy-induced peripheral neuropathy: NCCTG trial N06CA. *Support Care Cancer* 2011;19(6):833–841.

194. Lynch ME, Clark AJ, Sawynok J. A pilot study examining topical amitriptyline, ketamine, and a combination of both in the treatment of neuropathic pain. *Clin J Pain* 2003;19(5):323–328.

195. Gewandter JS, Mohile SG, Heckler CE, et al. A phase III randomized, placebo-controlled study of topical amitriptyline and ketamine for chemotherapy-induced peripheral neuropathy (CIPN): a University of Rochester CCOP study of 462 cancer survivors. *Support Care Cancer* 2014;22(7):1807–1814.

196. Jones CM, Mack KA, Paulozzi LJ. Pharmaceutical overdose deaths, United States, 2010. *JAMA* 2013;309(7):657–659.

197. Dart RC, Surratt HL, Cicero TJ, et al. Trends in opioid analgesic abuse and mortality in the United States. *N Engl J Med* 2015;372(3):241–248.

198. Centers for Disease Control and Prevention. Vital signs: overdoses of prescription opioid pain relievers-United States, 1999-2008. *MMWR* 2011;60:1487–1492.

199. Bachhuber MA, Saloner B, Cunningham CO, et al. Medical cannabis laws and opioid analgesic overdose mortality in the United States, 1999-2010. *JAMA Intern Med* 2014;174(10):1668–1673.

200. Bostwick JM. Blurred boundaries: the therapeutics and politics of medical marijuana. *Mayo Clin Proc* 2012;87(2):172–186.

201. Hayes MJ, Brown MS. Legalization of medical marijuana and incidence of opioid mortality. *JAMA Intern Med* 2014;174(10):1673–1674.

202. Shiplo S, Asbridge M, Leatherdale ST, et al. Medical cannabis use in Canada: vapourization and modes of delivery. *Harm Reduct J* 2016;13(1):30.

203. Hazekamp A, Ware MA, Muller-Vahl KR, et al. The medicinal use of cannabis and cannabinoids—an international cross-sectional survey on administration forms. *J Psychoactive Drugs* 2013;45(3):199–210.

204. Cascini F, Aiello C, Di Tanna G. Increasing delta-9-tetrahydrocannabinol (Delta-9-THC) content in herbal cannabis over time: systematic review and meta-analysis. *Curr Drug Abuse Rev* 2012;5(1):32–40.

205. ElSohly MA, Mehmedic Z, Foster S, et al. Changes in cannabis potency over the last 2 decades (1995-2014): analysis of current data in the United States. *Biol Psychiatry* 2016;79(7):613–619.

206. Ramaekers JG, Kauert G, van Ruitenbeek P, et al. High-potency marijuana impairs executive function and inhibitory motor control. *Neuropsychopharmacology* 2006;31(10):2296–2303.

207. Gruber SA, Sagar KA, Dahlgren MK, et al. Splendor in the grass? A pilot study assessing the impact of medical marijuana on executive function. *Front Pharmacol* 2016;7:355.

208. Iskedjian M, Bereza B, Gordon A, et al. Meta-analysis of cannabis based treatments for neuropathic and multiple sclerosis-related pain. *Curr Med Res Opin* 2007;23(1):17–24.

209. Lynch ME, Campbell F. Cannabinoids for treatment of chronic non-cancer pain; a systematic review of randomized trials. *Br J Clin Pharmacol* 2011;72(5):735–744.

210. Svendsen KB, Jensen TS, Bach FW. Does the cannabinoid dronabinol reduce central pain in multiple sclerosis? Randomised double blind placebo controlled crossover trial. *BMJ* 2004;329(7460):253.

211. Martin-Sanchez E, Furukawa TA, Taylor J, et al. Systematic review and meta-analysis of cannabis treatment for chronic pain. *Pain Med* 2009;10(8):1353–1368.

212. Hanna M, Wilson MC, O'Brien C. Neuropathic pain: optimising patient outcome with combination therapy. Abstract from 5th Congress of the European Federation of IASP Chapters (EFIC). *Eur J Pain* 2006;10(suppl 1):s120.

213. Freeman R, Raskin P, Hewitt DJ, et al. Randomized study of tramadol/acetaminophen versus placebo in painful diabetic peripheral neuropathy. *Curr Med Res Opin* 2007;23(1):147–161.

214. Zin CS, Nissen LM, O'Callaghan JP, et al. A randomized, controlled trial of oxycodone versus placebo in patients with postherpetic neuralgia and painful diabetic neuropathy treated with pregabalin. *J Pain* 2010;11(5):462–471.

215. Harrison T, Miyahara S, Lee A, et al. Experience and challenges presented by a multicenter crossover study of combination analgesic therapy for the treatment of painful HIV-associated polyneuropathies. *Pain Med* 2013;14(7):1039–1047.

216. Baron R, Martin-Mola E, Muller M, et al. Effectiveness and safety of tapentadol prolonged release (PR) versus a combination of tapentadol PR and pregabalin for the management of severe, chronic low back pain with a neuropathic component: a randomized, double-blind, phase 3b study. *Pain Pract* 2015;15(5):455–470.

217. Tonet C, Sakata RK, Issy AM, et al. Evaluation of oral ketamine for neuropathic pain [Avaliacao da cetamina oral para dor neuropatica]. *Revista Brasileira de Medicina* 2008;65(7):214–218.

218. Tesfaye S, Wilhelm S, Lledo A, et al. Duloxetine and pregabalin: high-dose monotherapy or their combination? The "COMBO-DN study"—a multinational, double-blind, parallel-group study in patients with diabetic peripheral neuropathic pain. *Pain* 2013;154(12):2616–2625.

219. Agrawal RP, Goswami J, Jain S, et al. Management of diabetic neuropathy by sodium valproate and glyceryl trinitrate spray: a prospective double-blind randomized placebo-controlled study. *Diabetes Res Clin Pract* 2009;83(3):371–378.

220. Eichenberger U, Neff F, Sveticic G, et al. Chronic phantom limb pain: the effects of calcitonin, ketamine, and their combination on pain and sensory thresholds. *Anesth Analg* 2008;106(4):1265–1273, table of contents.

221. Vinik A, Rosenstock J, Sharma U, et al. Efficacy and safety of mirogabalin (DS-5565) for the treatment of diabetic peripheral neuropathic pain: a randomized, double-blind, placebo- and active comparator-controlled, adaptive proof-of-concept phase 2 study. *Diabetes Care* 2014;37(12):3253–3261.

222. Hutmacher MM, Frame B, Miller R, et al. Exposure-response modeling of average daily pain score, and dizziness and somnolence, for mirogabalin (DS-5565) in patients with diabetic peripheral neuropathic pain. *J Clin Pharmacol* 2016;56(1):67–77.

223. Raffa RB, Burdge G, Gambrah J, et al. Cebranopadol: novel dual opioid/NOP receptor agonist analgesic. *J Clin Pharm Ther* 2017;42:8–17.

224. Price N, Namdari R, Neville J, et al. Safety and efficacy of a topical sodium channel inhibitor (TV-45070) in patients with post herpetic neuralgia (PHN): a randomized, controlled, proof-of-concept, crossover study, with a subgroup analysis of the Nav1.7 R1150W genotype. *Clin J Pain* 2017;33(4):310–318.

225. Goldberg YP, Price N, Namdari R, et al. Treatment of Na(v)1.7-mediated pain in inherited erythromelalgia using a novel sodium channel blocker. *Pain* 2012;153(1):80–85.

226. Kessler JA, Smith AG, Cha BS, et al. Double-blind, placebo-controlled study of HGF gene therapy in diabetic neuropathy. *Ann Clin Transl Neurol* 2015;2(5):465–478.

227. He S, Khan J, Gleason J, et al. Placenta-derived adherent cells attenuate hyperalgesia and neuroinflammatory response associated with perineural inflammation in rats. *Brain Behav Immun* 2013;27(1):185–192.

228. Saulino M, Kim PS, Shaw E. Practical considerations and patient selection for intrathecal drug delivery in the management of chronic pain. *J Pain Res* 2014;7:627–638.

229. Pope JE, Deer TR, Bruel BM, et al. Clinical uses of intrathecal therapy and its placement in the pain care algorithm [published online ahead of print February 23, 2016]. *Pain Pract*. doi:10.1111/papr.12438.

230. Falco FJ, Patel VB, Hayek SM, et al. Intrathecal infusion systems for long-term management of chronic non-cancer pain: an update of assessment of evidence. *Pain Physician* 2013;16(2 suppl):SE185–SE216.

231. Deer TR, Smith HS, Cousins M, et al. Consensus guidelines for the selection and implantation of patients with noncancer pain for intrathecal drug delivery. *Pain Physician* 2010;13(3):E175–E213.

232. Deer TR, Smith HS, Burton AW, et al. Comprehensive consensus based guidelines on intrathecal drug delivery systems in the treatment of pain caused by cancer pain. *Pain Physician* 2011;14(3):E283–E312.

233. Tatsumi M, Groshan K, Blakely RD, et al. Pharmacological profile of antidepressants and related compounds at human monoamine transporters. *Eur J Pharmacol* 1997;340(2–3):249–258.

234. Owens MJ. Selectivity of antidepressants: from the monoamine hypothesis of depression to the SSRI revolution and beyond. *J Clin Psychiatry* 2004;65(suppl 4):5–10.

235. Hardman JG, Limbird LE, eds. *Goodman and Gilman's The Pharmacological Basis of Therapeutics*. 10th ed. New York: McGraw-Hill; 2001.

236. Brungon LL, Lazo JS, Parker KL, eds. *Goodman and Gilman's The Pharmacological Basis of Therapeutics*. 11th ed. New York: McGraw-Hill; 2006.

237. Bymaster FP, Dreshfield-Ahmad LJ, Threlkeld PG, et al. Comparative affinity of duloxetine and venlafaxine for serotonin and norepinephrine transporters in vitro and in vivo, human serotonin receptor subtypes, and other neuronal receptors. *Neuropsychopharmacology* 2001;25(6):871–880.

238. Deecher DC, Beyer CE, Johnston G, et al. Desvenlafaxine succinate: a new serotonin and norepinephrine reuptake inhibitor. *J Pharmacol Exp Ther* 2006;318(2):657–665.

239. Leijon G, Boivie J. Central post-stroke pain—a controlled trial of amitriptyline and carbamazepine. *Pain* 1989;36(1):27–36.

240. Vrethem M, Boivie J, Arnqvist H, et al. A comparison a amitriptyline and maprotiline in the treatment of painful polyneuropathy in diabetics and nondiabetics. *Clin J Pain* 1997;13(4):313–323.

241. Watson CP, Evans RJ, Reed K, et al. Amitriptyline versus placebo in postherpetic neuralgia. *Neurology* 1982;32(6):671–673.

242. Max MB, Schafer SC, Culnane M, et al. Amitriptyline, but not lorazepam, relieves postherpetic neuralgia. *Neurology* 1988;38(9):1427–1432.

243. Kalso E, Tasmuth T, Neuvonen PJ. Amitriptyline effectively relieves neuropathic pain following treatment of breast cancer. *Pain* 1996;64(2):293–302.

244. Kvinesdal B, Molin J, Froland A, et al. Imipramine treatment of painful diabetic neuropathy. *JAMA* 1984;251(13):1727–1730.

245. Sindrup SH, Bach FW, Gram LF. Plasma beta-endorphin is not affected by treatment with imipramine or paroxetine in patients with diabetic neuropathy symptoms. *Clin J Pain* 1992;8(2):145–148.

246. Raja SN, Haythornthwaite JA, Pappagallo M, et al. Opioids versus antidepressants in postherpetic neuralgia: a randomized, placebo-controlled trial. *Neurology* 2002;59(7):1015–1021.

247. Panerai AE, Monza G, Movilia P, et al. A randomized, within-patient, cross-over, placebo-controlled trial on the efficacy and tolerability of the tricyclic antidepressants chlorimipramine and nortriptyline in central pain. *Acta Neurol Scand* 1990;82(1):34–38.

248. Sindrup SH, Gram LF, Skjold T, et al. Clomipramine vs desipramine vs placebo in the treatment of diabetic neuropathy symptoms. A double-blind cross-over study. *Br J Clin Pharmacol* 1990;30(5):683–691.

249. Max MB, Kishore-Kumar R, Schafer SC, et al. Efficacy of desipramine in painful diabetic neuropathy: a placebo-controlled trial. *Pain* 1991;45(1):3–9; discussion 1–2.

250. Kishore-Kumar R, Max MB, Schafer SC, et al. Desipramine relieves postherpetic neuralgia. *Clin Pharmacol Ther* 1990;47(3):305–312.

251. Yucel A, Ozyalcin S, Koknel Talu G, et al. The effect of venlafaxine on ongoing and experimentally induced pain in neuropathic pain patients: a double blind, placebo controlled study. *Eur J Pain* 2005;9(4):407–416.

252. Vilming ST, Lyberg T, Lataste X. Tizanidine in the management of trigeminal neuralgia. *Cephalalgia* 1986;6(3):181–182.

253. Lechin F, van der Dijs B, Lechin ME, et al. Pimozide therapy for trigeminal neuralgia. *Arch Neurol* 1989;46(9):960–963.

254. Lindstrom P. The analgesic effect of carbamazepine in patients with new onset trigeminal neuralgia. *Pain* 1987;4:s85.

255. Morello CM, Leckband SG, Stoner CP, et al. Randomized double-blind study comparing the efficacy of gabapentin with amitriptyline on diabetic peripheral neuropathy pain. *Arch Intern Med* 1999;159(16):1931–1937.

256. Smith DG, Ehde DM, Hanley MA, et al. Efficacy of gabapentin in treating chronic phantom limb and residual limb pain. *J Rehabil Res Dev* 2005;42(5):645–654.

257. Serpell MG. Gabapentin in neuropathic pain syndromes: a randomised, double-blind, placebo-controlled trial. *Pain* 2002;99(3):557–566.

258. Sandercock D, Cramer M, Biton V, et al. A gastroretentive gabapentin formulation for the treatment of painful diabetic peripheral neuropathy: efficacy and tolerability in a double-blind, randomized, controlled clinical trial. *Diabetes Res Clin Pract* 2012;97(3):438–445.

259. Jensen MP, Chiang YK, Wu J. Assessment of pain quality in a clinical trial of gabapentin extended release for postherpetic neuralgia. *Clin J Pain* 2009;25(4):286–292.

260. Backonja MM, Canafax DM, Cundy KC. Efficacy of gabapentin enacarbil vs placebo in patients with postherpetic neuralgia and a pharmacokinetic comparison with oral gabapentin. *Pain Med* 2011;12(7):1098–1108.

261. Jungehulsing GJ, Israel H, Safar N, et al. Levetiracetam in patients with central neuropathic post-stroke pain—a randomized, double-blind, placebo-controlled trial. *Eur J Neurol* 2013;20(2):331–337.

262. Irving G, Tanenberg RJ, Raskin J, et al. Comparative safety and tolerability of duloxetine vs. pregabalin vs. duloxetine plus gabapentin in patients with diabetic peripheral neuropathic pain. *Int J Clin Pract* 2014;68(9):1130–1140.

263. Tanenberg RJ, Irving GA, Risser RC, et al. Duloxetine, pregabalin, and duloxetine plus gabapentin for diabetic peripheral neuropathic pain management in patients with inadequate pain response to gabapentin: an open-label, randomized, noninferiority comparison. *Mayo Clin Proc* 2011;86(7):615–626.

264. Achar A, Chakraborty PP, Bisai S, et al. Comparative study of clinical efficacy of amitriptyline and pregabalin in postherpetic neuralgia. *Acta Dermatovenerol Croat* 2012;20(2):89–94.

265. Holbech JV, Bach FW, Finnerup NB, et al. Imipramine and pregabalin combination for painful polyneuropathy: a randomized controlled trial. *Pain* 2015;156(5):958–966.

266. Gatti A, Sabato AF, Occhioni R, et al. Controlled-release oxycodone and pregabalin in the treatment of neuropathic pain: results of a multicenter Italian study. *Eur Neurol* 2009;61(3):129–137.

267. Huse E, Larbig W, Flor H, et al. The effect of opioids on phantom limb pain and cortical reorganization. *Pain* 2001;90(1–2):47–55.

268. Watson CP, Babul N. Efficacy of oxycodone in neuropathic pain: a randomized trial in postherpetic neuralgia. *Neurology* 1998;50(6):1837–1841.

269. Gimbel JS, Richards P, Portenoy RK. Controlled-release oxycodone for pain in diabetic neuropathy: a randomized controlled trial. *Neurology* 2003;60(6):927–934.

270. Watson CP, Moulin D, Watt-Watson J, et al. Controlled-release oxycodone relieves neuropathic pain: a randomized controlled trial in painful diabetic neuropathy. *Pain* 2003;105(1–2):71–78.

271. Jensen MP, Friedman M, Bonzo D, et al. The validity of the neuropathic pain scale for assessing diabetic neuropathic pain in a clinical trial. *Clin J Pain* 2006;22(1):97–103.

272. Kim YH, Lee PB, Oh TK. Is magnesium sulfate effective for pain in chronic postherpetic neuralgia patients comparing with ketamine infusion therapy? *J Clin Anesth* 2015;27(4):296–300.

273. Eisenberg E, Kleiser A, Dortort A, et al. The NMDA (N-methyl-D-aspartate) receptor antagonist memantine in the treatment of postherpetic neuralgia: a double-blind, placebo-controlled study. *Eur J Pain* 1998;2(4):321–327.

274. Nikolajsen L, Gottrup H, Kristensen AG, et al. Memantine (a N-methyl-D-aspartate receptor antagonist) in the treatment of neuropathic pain after amputation or surgery: a randomized, double-blinded, cross-over study. *Anesth Analg* 2000;91(4):960–966.

275. Maier C, Dertwinkel R, Mansourian N, et al. Efficacy of the NMDA-receptor antagonist memantine in patients with chronic phantom limb pain—results of a randomized double-blinded, placebo-controlled trial. *Pain* 2003;103(3):277–283.

276. Wiech K, Kiefer RT, Topfner S, et al. A placebo-controlled randomized crossover trial of the N-methyl-D-aspartic acid receptor antagonist, memantine, in patients with chronic phantom limb pain. *Anesth Analg* 2004;98(2):408–413, table of contents.

277. Schwenkreis P, Maier C, Pleger B, et al. NMDA-mediated mechanisms in cortical excitability changes after limb amputation. *Acta Neurol Scand* 2003;108(3):179–184.

278. Galer BS, Twilling LL, Harle J, et al. Lack of efficacy of riluzole in the treatment of peripheral neuropathic pain conditions. *Neurology* 2000;55(7):971–975.

279. Kemper CA, Kent G, Burton S, et al. Mexiletine for HIV-infected patients with painful peripheral neuropathy: a double-blind, placebo-controlled, crossover treatment trial. *J Acquir Immune Defic Syndr Hum Retrovirol* 1998;19(4):367–372.

280. Dejgard A, Petersen P, Kastrup J. Mexiletine for treatment of chronic painful diabetic neuropathy. *Lancet* 1988;1(8575–6):9–11.

281. Chabal C, Jacobson L, Mariano A, et al. The use of oral mexiletine for the treatment of pain after peripheral nerve injury. *Anesthesiology* 1992;76(4):513–517.

282. Chiou-Tan FY, Tuel SM, Johnson JC, et al. Effect of mexiletine on spinal cord injury dysesthetic pain. *Am J Phys Med Rehabil* 1996;75(2):84–87.

283. Wallace MS, Magnuson S, Ridgeway B. Efficacy of oral mexiletine for neuropathic pain with allodynia: a double-blind, placebo-controlled, crossover study. *Reg Anesth Pain Med* 2000;25(5):459–467.

284. Chad DA, Aronin N, Lundstrom R, et al. Does capsaicin relieve the pain of diabetic neuropathy? *Pain* 1990;42(3):387–388.

285. Scheffler NM, Sheitel PL, Lipton MN. Treatment of painful diabetic neuropathy with capsaicin 0.075%. *J Am Podiatr Med Assoc* 1991;81(6):288–293.

286. Treatment of painful diabetic neuropathy with topical capsaicin. A multicenter, double-blind, vehicle-controlled study. The Capsaicin Study Group. *Arch Intern Med* 1991;151(11):2225–2229.

287. Tandan R, Lewis GA, Krusinski PB, et al. Topical capsaicin in painful diabetic neuropathy. Controlled study with long-term follow-up. *Diabetes Care* 1992;15(1):8–14.

288. Low PA, Opfer-Gehrking TL, Dyck PJ, et al. Double-blind, placebo-controlled study of the application of capsaicin cream in chronic distal painful polyneuropathy. *Pain* 1995;62(2):163–168.

289. Bernstein JE, Korman NJ, Bickers DR, et al. Topical capsaicin treatment of chronic postherpetic neuralgia. *J Am Acad Dermatol* 1989;21(2 pt 1):265–270.

290. Watson CP, Tyler KL, Bickers DR, et al. A randomized vehicle-controlled trial of topical capsaicin in the treatment of postherpetic neuralgia. *Clin Ther* 1993;15(3):510–526.

291. Watson CP, Evans RJ. The postmastectomy pain syndrome and topical capsaicin: a randomized trial. *Pain* 1992;51(3):375–379.

292. Ellison N, Loprinzi CL, Kugler J, et al. Phase III placebo-controlled trial of capsaicin cream in the management of surgical neuropathic pain in cancer patients. *J Clin Oncol* 1997;15(8):2974–2980.

293. Paice JA, Ferrans CE, Lashley FR, et al. Topical capsaicin in the management of HIV-associated peripheral neuropathy. *J Pain Symptom Manage* 2000;19(1):45–52.

294. Simpson DM, Brown S, Tobias J. Controlled trial of high-concentration capsaicin patch for treatment of painful HIV neuropathy. *Neurology* 2008;70(24):2305–2313.

295. Backonja M, Wallace MS, Blonsky ER, et al. NGX-4010, a high-concentration capsaicin patch, for the treatment of postherpetic neuralgia: a randomised, double-blind study. *Lancet Neurol* 2008;7(12):1106–1112.

296. Backonja MM, Malan TP, Vanhove GF, et al. NGX-4010, a high-concentration capsaicin patch, for the treatment of postherpetic neuralgia: a randomized, double-blind, controlled study with an open-label extension. *Pain Med* 2010;11(4):600–608.

297. Webster LR, Malan TP, Tuchman MM, et al. A multicenter, randomized, double-blind, controlled dose finding study of NGX-4010, a high-concentration capsaicin patch, for the treatment of postherpetic neuralgia. *J Pain* 2010;11(10):972–982.

298. Webster LR, Tark M, Rauck R, et al. Effect of duration of postherpetic neuralgia on efficacy analyses in a multicenter, randomized, controlled study of NGX-4010, an 8% capsaicin patch evaluated for the treatment of postherpetic neuralgia. *BMC Neurol* 2010;10:92.

299. Irving GA, Backonja MM, Dunteman E, et al. A multicenter, randomized, controlled study of NGX-4010, a high-concentration capsaicin patch, for the treatment of postherpetic neuralgia. *Pain Med* 2011;12(1):99–109.

300. Clifford DB, Simpson DM, Brown S, et al. A randomized, double-blind, controlled study of NGX-4010, a capsaicin 8% dermal patch, for the treatment of painful HIV-associated distal sensory polyneuropathy. *J Acquir Immune Defic Syndr* 2012;59(2):126–133.

301. Rowbotham MC, Davies PS, Verkempinck C, et al. Lidocaine patch: double-blind controlled study of a new treatment method for post-herpetic neuralgia. *Pain* 1996;65(1):39–44.

302. Galer BS, Jensen MP, Ma T, et al. The lidocaine patch 5% effectively treats all neuropathic pain qualities: results of a randomized, double-blind, vehicle-controlled, 3-week efficacy study with use of the neuropathic pain scale. *Clin J Pain* 2002;18(5):297–301.

303. Estanislao L, Carter K, McArthur J, et al. A randomized controlled trial of 5% lidocaine gel for HIV-associated distal symmetric polyneuropathy. *J Acquir Immune Defic Syndr* 2004;37(5):1584–1586.

304. Karst M, Salim K, Burstein S, et al. Analgesic effect of the synthetic cannabinoid CT-3 on chronic neuropathic pain: a randomized controlled trial. *JAMA* 2003;290(13):1757–1762.

305. Wade DT, Robson P, House H, et al. A preliminary controlled study to determine whether whole-plant cannabis extracts can improve intractable neurogenic symptoms. *Clin Rehabil* 2003;17(1):21–29.

306. Zajicek J, Fox P, Sanders H, et al. Cannabinoids for treatment of spasticity and other symptoms related to multiple sclerosis (CAMS study): multicentre randomised placebo-controlled trial. *Lancet* 2003;362(9395):1517–1526.

307. Wade DT, Makela P, Robson P, et al. Do cannabis-based medicinal extracts have general or specific effects on symptoms in multiple sclerosis? A double-blind, randomized, placebo-controlled study on 160 patients. *Mult Scler* 2004;10(4):434–441.

308. Abrams DI, Jay CA, Shade SB, et al. Cannabis in painful HIV-associated sensory neuropathy: a randomized placebo-controlled trial. *Neurology* 2007;68(7):515–521.

309. Berman JS, Symonds C, Birch R. Efficacy of two cannabis based medicinal extracts for relief of central neuropathic pain from brachial plexus avulsion: results of a randomised controlled trial. *Pain* 2004;112(3):299–306.

310. Rog DJ, Nurmikko TJ, Friede T, et al. Randomized, controlled trial of cannabis-based medicine in central pain in multiple sclerosis. *Neurology* 2005;65(6):812–819.

311. Wissel J, Haydn T, Muller J, et al. Low dose treatment with the synthetic cannabinoid Nabilone significantly reduces spasticity-related pain: a double-blind placebo-controlled cross-over trial. *J Neurol* 2006;253(10):1337–1341.

312. Nurmikko TJ, Serpell MG, Hoggart B, et al. Sativex successfully treats neuropathic pain characterised by allodynia: a randomised, double-blind, placebo-controlled clinical trial. *Pain* 2007;133(1–3):210–220.

313. Wilsey B, Marcotte T, Tsodikov A, et al. A randomized, placebo-controlled, crossover trial of cannabis cigarettes in neuropathic pain. *J Pain* 2008;9(6):506–521.

314. Narang S, Gibson D, Wasan AD, et al. Efficacy of dronabinol as an adjuvant treatment for chronic pain patients on opioid therapy. *J Pain* 2008;9(3):254–264.

315. Skrabek RQ, Galimova L, Ethans K, et al. Nabilone for the treatment of pain in fibromyalgia. *J Pain* 2008;9(2):164–173.

316. Ellis RJ, Toperoff W, Vaida F, et al. Smoked medicinal cannabis for neuropathic pain in HIV: a randomized, crossover clinical trial. *Neuropsychopharmacology* 2009;34(3):672–680.

317. Ware MA, Wang T, Shapiro S, et al. Smoked cannabis for chronic neuropathic pain: a randomized controlled trial. *CMAJ* 2010;182(14):E694–E701.

318. Pini LA, Guerzoni S, Cainazzo MM, et al. Nabilone for the treatment of medication overuse headache: results of a preliminary double-blind, active-controlled, randomized trial. *J Headache Pain* 2012;13(8):677–684.

319. Corey-Bloom J, Wolfson T, Gamst A, et al. Smoked cannabis for spasticity in multiple sclerosis: a randomized, placebo-controlled trial. *CMAJ* 2012;184(10):1143–1150.

320. Toth C, Mawani S, Brady S, et al. An enriched-enrolment, randomized withdrawal, flexible-dose, double-blind, placebo-controlled, parallel assignment efficacy study of nabilone as adjuvant in the treatment of diabetic peripheral neuropathic pain. *Pain* 2012;153(10):2073–2082.

321. Zajicek JP, Hobart JC, Slade A, et al. Multiple sclerosis and extract of cannabis: results of the MUSEC trial. *J Neurol Neurosurg Psychiatry* 2012;83(11):1125–1132.

322. Langford RM, Mares J, Novotna A, et al. A double-blind, randomized, placebo-controlled, parallel-group study of THC/CBD oromucosal spray in combination with the existing treatment regimen, in the relief of central neuropathic pain in patients with multiple sclerosis. *J Neurol* 2013;260(4):984–997.

323. Wilsey B, Marcotte T, Deutsch R, et al. Low-dose vaporized cannabis significantly improves neuropathic pain. *J Pain* 2013;14(2):136–148.

324. Lynch ME, Cesar-Rittenberg P, Hohmann AG. A double-blind, placebo-controlled, crossover pilot trial with extension using an oral mucosal cannabinoid extract for treatment of chemotherapy-induced neuropathic pain. *J Pain Symptom Manage* 2014;47(1):166–173.

325. Serpell M, Ratcliffe S, Hovorka J, et al. A double-blind, randomized, placebo-controlled, parallel group study of THC/CBD spray in peripheral neuropathic pain treatment. *Eur J Pain* 2014;18(7):999–1012.

326. Turcotte D, Doupe M, Torabi M, et al. Nabilone as an adjunctive to gabapentin for multiple sclerosis-induced neuropathic pain: a randomized controlled trial. *Pain Med* 2015;16(1):149–159.

327. McCleane GJ. A randomised, double blind, placebo controlled crossover study of the cholecystokinin 2 antagonist L-365,260 as an adjunct to strong opioids in chronic human neuropathic pain. *Neurosci Lett* 2003;338(2):151–154.

CHAPTER 82

Local Anesthetics

MICHAEL M. BOTTROS, LARA WILEY CROCK, and **SIMON HAROUTOUNIAN**

Physicochemical Properties of Local Anesthetics

"Cocaine and its salts have a marked anesthetizing effect when brought in contact with the skin and mucous membrane in concentrated solution; this property suggests its occasional use as a local anesthetic, especially in connection with afflictions of the mucous membrane." Cocaine and its potential clinical use as a local anesthetic were described by Sigmund Freud in his 1884 paper "Uber Coca." Almost as an afterthought, he describes cocaine's potential use as a local anesthetic in the very last paragraph[1]: "Indeed, the anesthetizing properties of cocaine should make it suitable for a good many further applications." A friend of Freud, Carl Koller, utilized this property of cocaine for ophthalmologic procedures. Thus, Koller is credited with demonstrating the first local anesthetic in modern clinical practice.[1] Although still somewhat controversial as to when cocaine was first used as a spinal anesthetic, Corning[2] described what he believed was an extradural block using cocaine in 1885, and Bier[3] described a spinal anesthetic effect with cocaine in 1898. Clinically useful due to its properties as both a local anesthetic and vasoconstrictor, cocaine has undesirable side effects that limit its routine use.[4] Other local anesthetics were developed based on the chemical structure of cocaine, and the clinical application of local anesthetics became widespread in modern medicine. The use of local anesthetics has continued to increase in clinical practice, as there is increased interest in the use of regional techniques for surgery as well as in the treatment of chronic pain.

MOLECULAR STRUCTURE

The chemical structure of cocaine was determined by Richard Willstätter in 1898, allowing for the development of the synthetic analogs of cocaine.[5] All currently available local anesthetics have an amine group (usually a tertiary amine) and an aromatic ring. With the exception of benzocaine, these two groups are separated by an intermediate ester or amide linkage (Fig. 82.1). They are classified by their chemical bond as either amino esters (e.g., include cocaine, procaine, chloroprocaine, tetracaine) or amino amides (e.g., lidocaine, prilocaine, bupivacaine, mepivacaine). Esters and amides have distinct properties as a result of their molecular structure. The amino amide bond is more resistant to enzymatic cleavage; therefore, amide local anesthetics are more stable when compared to ester local anesthetics. Amides and esters are metabolized in distinct ways—amides by the liver microsomes and esters by plasma esterases. Chirality, acid–base balance, lipid solubility, and protein binding can all affect the activity of local anesthetics.

CHIRALITY

Stereoisomers have identical sets of atoms that are configured in the same positions with different spatial arrangements. Furthermore, enantiomers are pairs of stereoisomers that appear as nonsuperimposable mirror images, commonly referred to as chiral. More than one-third of synthetic drugs are structurally defined as chiral.[6] Commonly used local anesthetics with the exception of lidocaine are chiral. The body responds to chiral molecules differently because stereoisomers may have different receptor binding properties.

An example of a chiral local anesthetic is bupivacaine, a potent and long-acting local anesthetic with the unfortunate potential for cardiovascular and central nervous system (CNS) toxicity. Bupivacaine is manufactured as a racemic mixture of 50% R-bupivacaine and 50% S-bupivacaine. S- and R-enantiomers have been shown to have unique pharmacodynamic properties (e.g., potency and potential for systemic toxicity). R-enantiomers, like R-bupivacaine, have greater potency for blockade of both neuronal and cardiac sodium (Na^+) channels. R-bupivacaine is 1.5 times more potent when compared to S-bupivacaine (also known as *levobupivacaine*) when the Na^+ channel is in an inactive state.[6] Because of the potential systemic toxicity and higher potency, R-enantiomers are more powerful local anesthetics with

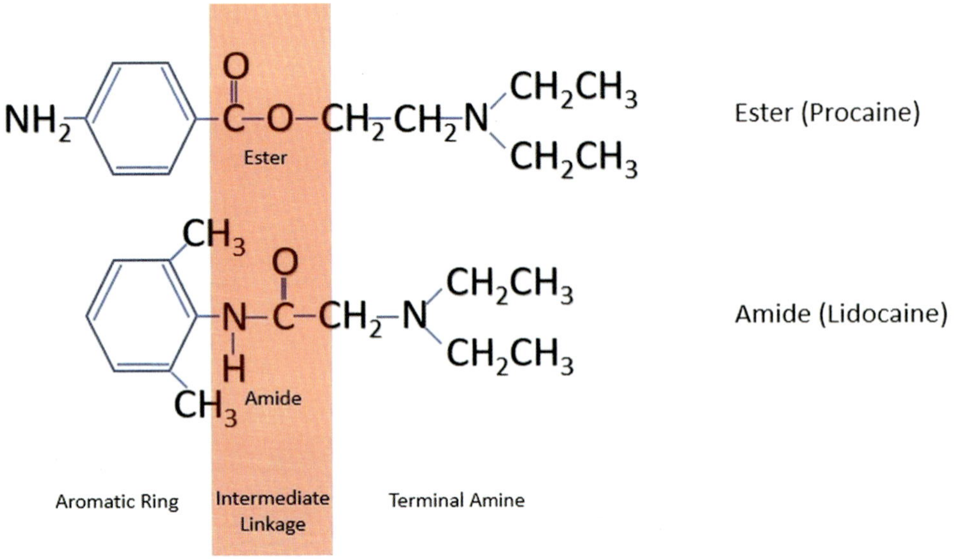

FIGURE 82.1 Local anesthetic structure. Similarities and differences between ester and amide local anesthetics.

a narrower therapeutic index. S-enantiomers on the other hand, have a lower binding potential for cardiac Na$^+$ channels and may be safer.[7] Ropivacaine (a pure S-enantiomer propyl homolog of S-bupivacaine) was developed in response to the need for a long-acting amino amide local anesthetic such as bupivacaine, with a greater margin of safety.[8] It has been shown in both animal and human studies to have similar clinical efficacy compared to bupivacaine but with 30% to 40% less cardiotoxicity.[9–12]

ACID–BASE BALANCE

The pH and acid dissociation constant (pK$_a$) of local anesthetics have a large effect on their onset of action. The pK$_a$ of a specific drug is the pH at which the lipid-soluble neutral form and the charged hydrophilic form are in equilibrium. Most local anesthetics have a pK$_a$ value close to but higher than physiologic pH, making them weak bases. At physiologic pH, local anesthetics exist in a positively charged conjugated acid and an unprotonated neutral form. When unprotonated, the local anesthetic can more easily cross into the cell through the lipid bilayer to reach its receptor binding site. At physiologic pH of 7.4, a drug with a lower pK$_a$ will more readily cross the cell lipid membrane (higher percentage will be in the uncharged, lipophilic form). Thus, the pK$_a$ of a local anesthetic generally correlates with its onset. The pH inside the cell is lower, which shifts the equilibrium toward a higher ratio of positively charged local anesthetic molecules. It is the charged form that binds to the pore of the voltage-gated Na$^+$ channel, causing the anesthetic effects.

Tissue that has been damaged or is infected often produces an acidic extracellular microenvironment, thus increasing the percentage of charged local anesthetic outside the cells. The positively charged local anesthetic cannot easily cross the lipid bilayer and reach the intracellular binding site. For this reason, local anesthetics are not as effective in providing adequate analgesia to infected or damaged tissue.

Just as an acidic extracellular environment can prevent adequate analgesia from reaching the intended target, an acidic intracellular environment can prolong the effect of a local anesthetic. For example, the administration of an accidental overdose of local anesthetic can result in CNS toxicity. At lower toxic doses, central inhibitory neuronal pathways are blocked. This neuronal disinhibition can result in a tonic-clonic seizure, leading to a lactic acidosis in the CNS. As the CNS becomes more acidic, the local anesthetic is essentially trapped inside the cell due to its ionization, exacerbating its CNS toxicity.

LIPOPHILIC–HYDROPHILIC BALANCE

The lipid solubility, or lipophilic nature of a local anesthetic, influences its ability to pass through a lipid bilayer and thus its potency and duration of action. More lipophilic local anesthetics can not only permeate neurons more readily but also result in sequestration of the local anesthetic in lipid-soluble perineural compartments such as the myelin sheath where they are sequestered. The accumulation of local anesthetics in lipid-soluble neuronal components creates a depot of local anesthetics, resulting in a slow release from these lipophilic compartments. Consequently, although the lipophilic local anesthetics may cross membranes more readily, these drugs often have a lower onset of action and prolonged duration of action.[13,14] Increased lipophilicity often translates to greater potency due to drug ability to cross lipid membranes and a greater affinity to bind Na$^+$ channels.[14,15]

Local Anesthetic Pharmacology

PHARMACODYNAMICS

Hodgkin and Huxley used a giant squid axon to determine that electrical signals in the nerves are initiated by voltage-dependent activation of inward sodium currents.[16,17] In 1970, Fraizer used squid giant axons and quaternary compounds to demonstrate

that local anesthetics need to penetrate into the cell to inhibit depolarization and action potentials.[18] It was later discovered that local anesthetics work by binding to and blocking voltage-gated sodium channels (Fig. 82.2). Voltage-gated sodium channels exist in three conformational states: open, closed, and inactivated. Without a stimulus, the channel is in its closed state. In response to a change in membrane potential, the voltage-gated sodium channel will open. After a few milliseconds, an intracellular loop (P) (see Fig. 82.2) will fold inward and occlude the channel pore. This renders the sodium channel inactive, and the channel will temporarily not respond to further changes in membrane potential. Local anesthetics can gain access and bind to the intracellular binding site preferably when the channel is in an open state.[19]

Local anesthetics work by preventing action potential propagation in axons through their inhibitory action on sodium channels.[20] These voltage-gated sodium channels contain a main α-subunit, where the local anesthetics bind and one or more β-subunits.[16,19] Local anesthetics reversibly bind to the α-subunit from inside the cell and inactivate voltage-gated sodium channels, thus preventing channel activation and inhibiting sodium influx, preventing depolarization of the nerve cell membrane (Fig. 82.2). When a local anesthetic binds to the open state of a sodium channel, it stabilizes the inactive state of the channel and prevents further activation. Local anesthetics increase the threshold for electrical excitation in nerves, slow propagation of the impulse, reduce the rate of rise of the action potential, and eventually block conduction.[21]

PHARMACOKINETICS

The pharmacokinetic properties of local anesthetics (i.e., absorption, distribution, metabolism/biotransformation, and excretion), patient factors (i.e., age, overall health, and the functional state of eliminating organs), and clinical circumstances must be combined in order to predict the pharmacokinetic profile of a local anesthetic in a particular patient.

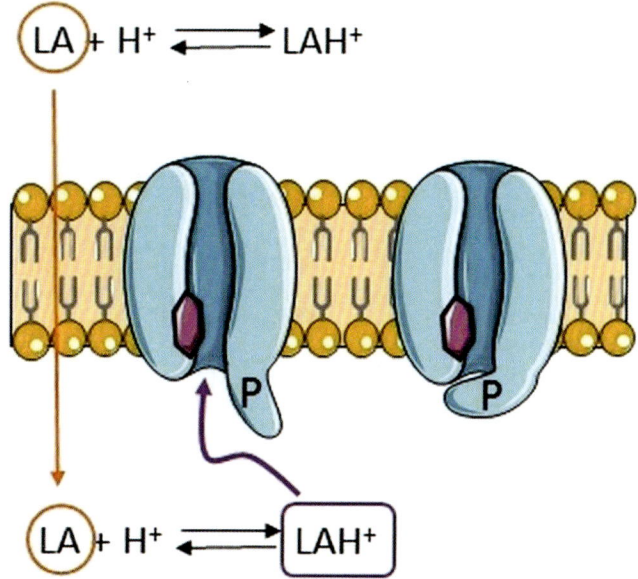

FIGURE 82.2 Diagram of a voltage-gated sodium channel structure and the site of action of local anesthetics. Local anesthetics exist in an equilibrium as a neutral base (LA) and as a charged form (LAH+). The uncharged form (LA) more easily passes through the lipid bilayer to the interior of the cell. Inside the cell, it can be protonated again (LAH+), thus allowing it to bind to, and inhibit (close), the voltage-gated sodium channel. *(Adapted from Drasner K. Local anesthetics. In: Katzung B, Masters SB, Trevor AJ, eds. Basic & Clinical Pharmacology. 12th ed. New York: McGraw-Hill; 2012:452.)*

Absorption

The plasma concentration following systemic absorption of a local anesthetic is highly dependent on the site of administration, the dose, and the physicochemical properties of the drug. The more vascular an injection site, the higher the systemic absorption of the local anesthetic. The highest systemic absorption occurs with intravenous administration. The systemic absorption of local anesthetics after regional anesthesia occurs at decreasing rate after tracheal, intercostal, caudal, paracervical, thoracic/lumbar epidural, brachial plexus, and sciatic nerve blocks and is the lowest with subcutaneous infiltration (Fig. 82.3).[22,23] For example, similar plasma concentrations of lidocaine are achieved after 300 mg delivered as an intercostal nerve block, 500 mg via an epidural block, and 1,000 mg subcutaneously.[24] All local anesthetics produce some level of vasoactivity, with most producing vasodilatation. However, the vasoactivity of local anesthetics is dependent on the drug, the dose, as well as the organ targeted.[24] Vasodilatation increases absorption of the local anesthetic into the systemic circulation. Enhanced absorption reduces the local anesthetic duration and increases the concentration of the drug in the blood. Cocaine is the only local anesthetic that consistently produces vasoconstriction (following initial vasodilatation). The addition of epinephrine to some local anesthetic nerve blocks can reduce absorption by causing vasoconstriction, thus prolonging the nerve block. The extent of this prolongation appears to vary with the site of the nerve block and the vasoconstrictor agent used. For example, 5 μg/mL of epinephrine, added to lidocaine, reduced the peak plasma concentration of subcutaneously infiltrated lidocaine by 50% but only by 20% to 30% when added to intercostal, epidural, and brachial plexus lidocaine blocks.[24] See "Vasoconstrictor Effect" section for further information.

Distribution

Once local anesthetics are absorbed in the blood, they readily cross into all tissues. Organs and tissues and organs with high levels of perfusion (such as the heart and brain) will have higher levels of local anesthetics. Local anesthetics (in their unionized form) are lipophilic and therefore readily cross the blood brain barrier. Depression of the CNS by local anesthetics causes initial sedation. Local anesthetics raise the seizure threshold by decreasing the excitability of cortical neurons in epileptic patients. However, at toxic plasma (and brain) levels, local anesthetics cause seizures.[25]

Biotransformation and Excretion

The primary site of amino amide local anesthetic metabolism is in the liver through hepatic carboxylesterases and cytochrome P450 enzyme. An exception is prilocaine, which is metabolized in both the liver and lungs. Ester local anesthetics, with the exception of cocaine, are hydrolyzed by plasma cholinesterases and tissue esterases.[25,26] The metabolites of both amino ester and amino amide local anesthetics are primarily excreted by the kidneys. Urine concentrations of ester local anesthetics are small due to their metabolism in plasma. Only 2% of procaine is found in urine, whereas 90% is found as its para-aminobenzoate metabolite, para-aminobenzoic acid (PABA).[27]

The rates of hydrolysis of local anesthetics inversely determine their degree of toxicity. A slowly hydrolyzed ester local anesthetic such as tetracaine is more toxic than chloroprocaine, which is hydrolyzed much faster.

Effects of Disease States on Local Anesthetic Pharmacokinetics

Because amide local anesthetics are metabolized primarily in the liver, hepatic perfusion and liver function can affect the rate of amide local anesthetic metabolism. Reduced hepatic function results in a reduced plasma clearance of and prolongation of the elimination half-life of intravenous lidocaine. This does not significantly affect the duration of action but predisposes a patient to the toxic effects.[28] Renal disease has little effect on the pharmacokinetic parameters such as volume of distribution at steady state and total body clearance of intravenous lidocaine.[28] In contrast, patients with cardiac failure had reduced volume of distribution and plasma clearance of intravenous lidocaine.[28] Metabolism byproducts of amide local anesthetics can have clinical effects if allowed to accumulate in the blood. Sedation due to high doses of lidocaine is due to the formation of the metabolites glycine xylidide and monoethylglycinexylidide. Despite ester local anesthetics, biotransformation by plasma cholinesterases, and tissue esterase, at normal doses, there appears to be little effect in patients with pseudocholinesterase deficiency.

Regional Administration of Local Anesthetics for Pain Relief

DIFFERENTIAL BLOCKADE

As sodium channels are expresses in both sensory and motor nerve fibers, the regional administration of local anesthetics can result in blocking conduction along both types of fibers. Therefore, along the desired analgesic effect on sensory fibers, other, less desired effects are often observed. Differential blockade is the gradual and sequential inactivation of differing nerve fiber types when exposed to local anesthetics. A number of factors contribute to this phenomenon:

1. Local anesthetic concentration: Higher concentrations can produce both motor and sensory block, whereas low concentrations produce only sensory block.
2. Nerve fiber size: Small diameter axons are more susceptible to block than large diameter fibers. Sensory nerve fibers are classified as A, B, and C. Type A fibers include afferent fibers responsible for proprioception (Aα), thermal sensation (Aδ), and mechanosensation (Aβ). Type B fibers are mainly visceral sensory fibers and preganglionic

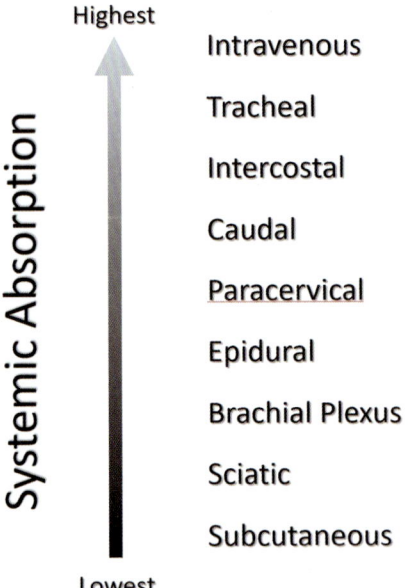

FIGURE 82.3 Degree of systemic absorption based on local anesthetic injection site. The highest systemic absorption occurs with intravenous administration, decreasing after tracheal, intercostal, caudal, paracervical, thoracic/lumbar epidural, brachial plexus, and sciatic nerve blocks and is the lowest with subcutaneous infiltration. (*Based on Drasner K. Local anesthetics. In: Katzung B, Masters SB, Trevor AJ, eds. Basic & Clinical Pharmacology. 12th ed. New York: McGraw-Hill; 2012:452–453.*)

autonomic fibers. Type C fibers are postganglionic autonomic efferents as well as sensory afferents responsible for the transmission of pain and heat signals. Type A fibers are thickest, and type C fibers are thinnest.

3. Degree of nerve fiber myelination: Because local anesthetics exert their effect at the node of Ranvier, myelinated fibers are more sensitive to local anesthetic effects than nonmyelinated ones.

4. Circumferential location of fibers: In nerve bundles, fibers that are located circumferentially are affected first by local anesthetics. In large nerve trunks, motor nerves are usually located circumferentially and may be affected before the sensory fibers. In the extremities, proximal sensory fibers are located more circumferentially than distal sensory fibers. Thus, loss of sensation may spread from the proximal to distal part of the limb.

Gokin et al.[29] studied the preferential block of sensory and motor fibers using lidocaine in a rat sciatic nerve model. They found that the order of fiber susceptibility, ranked by concentrations that gave peak tonic fiber blockade of 50% (IC50s), was $A\gamma > A\delta = A\alpha > A\alpha\beta > C$. Faster conducting C fibers (conduction velocity >1 m/s) were more susceptible than slower ones. Therefore, this does not strictly follow the "size principle" that smaller axons are always blocked first.

SITE OF INJECTION

Local anesthetics are used in a wide variety of anatomical sites. These can generally be grouped into five categories: neuraxial anesthesia, peripheral nerve blockade, intravenous regional anesthesia, infiltration anesthesia, and topical anesthesia.

Neuraxial Anesthesia

Neuraxial anesthesia was first reported for clinical use in the late 19th century by Augustus Karl Gustav Bier, who used intrathecal cocaine on six patients undergoing lower extremity surgery.[30] Since then, neuraxial anesthesia has progressed considerably and has become widely used for surgical anesthesia and pain management in a number of different clinical situations. The term *neuraxial* anesthesia may be further categorized into spinal, epidural, caudal, or combined spinal-epidural (CSE) anesthesia.

Spinal anesthesia involves the administration of local anesthetics into the intrathecal (or subarachnoid) space. As the conus medullaris typically terminates near lumbar nerves L1 or L2, this technique is performed below the L2 level to avoid damage to the spinal cord. As such, this technique may be indicated when the surgical site involves the lower extremities, perineum, or lower trunk. Examples include total hip/knee arthroplasty or cesarean section surgeries.

Epidural anesthesia is categorized by the deposition of local anesthetics via catheter or needle placed into the epidural space, located between the ligamentum flavum and the dura mater (Fig. 82.4). Key differences between epidural and spinal anesthesia include location of drug deposition (epidural vs. intrathecal), onset of action (spinal is generally quicker than epidural), and local anesthetic dose (because of uptake into extraneural fat, blood, and lymphatics, epidural doses are higher than spinal). Epidural catheter analgesia (using low-dose local anesthetics, sometimes with the addition of an opioid) is typically used for truncal or lower extremity postoperative pain relief, such as postthoracotomy or abdominal resection cases.

Caudal epidural anesthesia involves the insertion of a needle through the sacral hiatus in order to gain entrance into the sacral epidural space. Caudal anesthesia is commonly used as a regional technique in neonates and infants for abdominal and pelvic surgeries as it decreases the amount of general anesthetic and intravenous opioids required intraoperatively.[31,32]

A CSE technique may be used in clinical scenarios during surgery at or below the umbilicus requiring prolonged and effective analgesia. This typically entails performing an intrathecal block for the surgical procedure itself while an epidural catheter is placed (subsequent to the intrathecal block) and used during surgery when the intrathecal block is deficient or an extended duration of relief is needed for unanticipated longer surgical procedures. Postoperatively, the epidural catheter may be used for pain control.[33]

Peripheral Nerve Blockade

Peripheral nerve blockade is the deposition of local anesthetic near a nerve or group of nerves associated with the control of sensation and/or movement of a specific part of the body. This may be performed in lieu of or in addition to general anesthesia for surgery. This may be performed as a single-shot technique to facilitate intraoperative and immediate postoperative anesthesia and analgesia. Alternatively, for a longer duration of postoperative analgesia, one can insert a catheter near the nerve/nerves and provide continuous analgesia by supplying an infusion of local anesthetic. Peripheral nerve blockade may be achieved via blind technique, but most are currently performed with concomitant use of either nerve stimulation or ultrasound to guide needle placement.

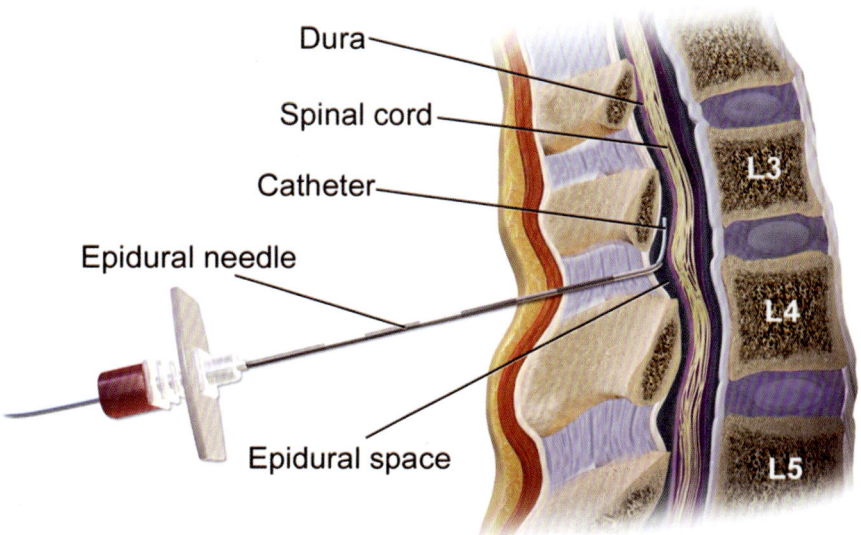

FIGURE 82.4 Epidural anesthesia. A catheter exits the epidural needle in the epidural space where local anesthetics may be deposited. *(From BruceBlaus /Wikimedia Commons/CC-BY-SA-4.0.)*

Intravenous Regional Anesthesia

Intravenous regional anesthesia (IVRA) was first described in 1908 by Augustus Bier, known for his prior work on spinal anesthetics, and is commonly referred to a Bier block.[34] The technique involves exsanguinating the extremity to be anesthetized using passive venous drainage by raising the extremity, followed with active drainage by wrapping an Esmarch bandage around the extremity and subsequently inflating a pneumatic cuff/tourniquet. After this, local anesthetic can be injected through an intravenous catheter placed prior to the initiation of exsanguination on the ipsilateral extremity. The volume of administration can vary based on the potency of the local anesthetic, although 30 to 50 mL of 0.5% lidocaine without epinephrine is typically used.[35] This technique is a useful anesthetic option for short-duration (typically less than 1 hour) upper or lower extremity surgeries, such as carpal tunnel release, Dupuytren contracture release, or neuroma excision.

Infiltration Anesthesia

Infiltration anesthesia is the injection of local anesthetics directly into the area of terminal nerve endings. Its uses include subcutaneous infiltration prior to intravenous catheter placement or suturing, submucosal infiltration prior to laceration repairs or dental procedures, or wound infiltration to facilitate analgesia during a procedure. A "field" block refers to the common technique of infiltrative anesthesia in a circular or diamond pattern around the desired site. Pain reduction on injection can be achieved by warming the local anesthetic solution or "buffering" the solution.[36] Buffering is performed by adding sodium bicarbonate in a local anesthetic-to-bicarbonate ratio of 9:1. This is typically performed with lidocaine as other local anesthetics such as bupivacaine have a tendency to precipitate when increasing the solution pH[37] and is discussed in further detail in "pH Adjustment of Local Anesthetics" section. There appears to be a synergistic effect in pain reduction when warming is coupled with buffering the solution.[38]

Topical Anesthesia

Topical anesthesia is direct application of local anesthetic solutions, ointments, gels, or sprays causing the superficial loss of sensation on skin, mucous membranes, or conjunctiva.[39] These drugs reversibly block nerve conduction at the free nerve endings in the dermis or mucosa, producing anesthesia in a limited area. The main barrier for drug delivery is the stratum corneum. Topical anesthetics cross this layer via the intracellular spaces of cornified keratinocytes, openings of hair follicles and sweat glands, and/or a para- or transcellular route. Clinical applications include local analgesia on intact skin; minimizing discomfort prior to an injection; symptomatic relief of chronic pain; or numbing the outermost layers of the cornea, conjunctiva, or oral tissues. As local anesthetics are poorly absorbed across intact skin, mixtures of local anesthetic agents (called eutectic mixture of local anesthetics, or EMLA) have been used to increase potency, as well as have lower melting points (so that local anesthetic molecules exist in their oil, rather than crystal structure at room temperature), which can promote easier absorption into tissues.[40]

POTENCY, ONSET, AND DURATION

Local anesthetics must cross the lipid membrane to bind to the intracellular portion of the sodium channel, and their anesthetic potency is related to their lipid solubility. In general, more potent local anesthetics are more lipid-soluble.

The onset of action is related to pK_a, dose, and concentration of the drug. As the drug pK_a nears physiologic pH, there is a higher concentration of the drug as a non-ionized base, shortening the onset of action. The administration of a more concentrated local anesthetic typically shortens the onset of the effect and provides a larger degree of nerve blockade.

Degree of protein binding greatly influences duration of action. As local anesthetics target protein receptors, the greater the affinity of the drug to the protein, the longer it will remain bound to its receptor, thereby extending its duration of action (Table 82.1).

pH ADJUSTMENT OF LOCAL ANESTHETICS

The addition of carbon dioxide to a local anesthetic solution accelerates onset of action. There are several reported mechanisms for this: direct effect of CO_2 on the nerve, decrease in the pH of the surrounding environment, and an increase in the base form of the local anesthetic. Commercial local anesthetic solutions are manufactured in acidic pH to maximize their chemical stability and water solubility, thereby increasing their shelf life. Several studies have indicated that adding sodium bicarbonate to local anesthetic solutions enhances onset, increases intensity, and prolongs local anesthetic block duration.[41,42] This is termed *buffering* or *alkalinization*. This increases the proportion of non-ionized drug allowing a theoretical faster rate of diffusion across the cell membrane. Although these buffered solutions

TABLE 82.1	Local Anesthetic Structure and Duration of Action					
Agent	pK_a	Techniques	Concentrations Available	Maximum Dose (mg/kg)	Typical Duration of Nerve Blocks
Esters					
Benzocaine	2.5	Topical	20%	NA	NA
Chloroprocaine	8.7	Epidural, infiltration, peripheral nerve block, spinal	1%, 2%, 3%	12	Short
Cocaine		Topical	4%, 10%	3	NA
Procaine	8.9	Spinal, local infiltration	1%, 2%, 10%	12	Short
Tetracaine	8.5	Spinal, topical (eye)	0.2%, 0.3%, 0.5%, 1%, 2%	3	Long
Amides					
Bupivacaine	8.1	Epidural, spinal, infiltration, peripheral nerve block	0.25%, 0.5%, 0.75%	3	Long
Lidocaine	7.9	Epidural, spinal, infiltration, peripheral nerve block, intravenous regional, topical	0.5%, 1%, 1.5%, 2%, 4%, 5%	4.5 7 (with epinephrine)	Medium
Mepivacaine	7.6	Epidural, infiltration, peripheral nerve block, spinal	1%, 1.5%, 2%, 3%	4.5 7 (with epinephrine)	Medium
Prilocaine	7.9	EMLA (topical), epidural, intravenous regional (outside North America)	0.5%, 2%, 3%, 4%	8	Medium
Ropivacaine	8.1	Epidural, spinal, infiltration, peripheral nerve block	0.2%, 0.5%, 0.75%, 1%	3	Long

EMLA, eutectic mixture of local anesthetics; NA, not applicable.
Data from Liu SS. Local anesthetics and analgesia. In: Ashburn MA, Rice LJ, eds. *The Management of Pain.* New York: Churchill Livingstone; 1997:141.

are typically less painful when injected,[43] there is controversy regarding the clinical utility of this practice as clinical studies have produced inconsistent results.[44] Care must be taken in increasing the pH of bupivacaine and etidocaine, as this may cause precipitation, leading to the injection of particulate along with the solution.[45]

VASOCONSTRICTOR EFFECT

As discussed earlier, the addition of vasoconstrictors to local anesthetic solutions reduces vascular uptake, thereby indirectly increasing the concentration of the drug and increasing the duration of contact with the target nerve. This in turn increases the duration and quality (depth) of anesthetic block. It may also reduce the minimum concentration of anesthetic needed as well as reduce the peak plasma concentration of the drug.[46] Epinephrine is the most commonly used vasoconstrictor, and its addition to neuraxial block also activates endogenous analgesic mechanisms via -adrenergic receptors.[47] Caution should be used with respect to injection site and local anesthetics containing epinephrine, as end organs (e.g., fingers, toes, penis, nose) may have such blood flow compromise that eventual tissue necrosis could occur. The addition of epinephrine has been shown to increase axonal degeneration following intrafascicular bupivacaine injection.[48] However, there is debate about the role of epinephrine and direct peripheral nerve tissue injury, as this has not been proven and clinical observations suggest that this aspect of toxicity generally plays a minor role.[49]

MIXTURES OF LOCAL ANESTHETICS

Local anesthetics are sometimes combined with the goal to achieve longer duration and/or quicker onset than with just one local anesthetic alone. However, there appears to be no clear advantage to mixing different anesthetic compounds as clinical trials have shown inconsistent results. Smith[50] evaluated the combination of chloroprocaine with bupivacaine for brachial plexus block which yielded the desired faster onset and longer duration of action. However, a 1:1 mixture of 1% lidocaine with 0.25% bupivacaine for foot block showed no significant difference in mean onset times compared with either pure anesthetic alone.[51] In the same study, the duration of action was longer with pure bupivacaine, but there was no difference between the pure lidocaine solution and the mixture. Interestingly, nerve blockade characteristics by local anesthetic mixtures appear to be affected by the pH value of the mixture.[52] Using rat sciatic nerve preparation, Galindo and Witcher[52] found that a 1:1 mixture of chloroprocaine 2% and bupivacaine 0.5% resulted in a nerve block with characteristics of a chloroprocaine block. However, changing the pH value of this mixture from 3.60 to 5.56 changed the characteristics to a block resembling bupivacaine.

SPECIAL STATES: PREGNANCY

Local anesthetics have enhanced potency in spinal and epidural anesthesia during pregnancy.[53,54] In addition, the onset of blockade tends to be faster for spinal, epidural, and peripheral nerve blocks. The true mechanism is unknown but is likely due to anatomical changes from pregnancy as well as the effect of progesterone on the sensitivity of the nerve fibers themselves.[55,56] As progesterone levels increase, there is an inverse correlation between the amount of local anesthetic needed and the clinical effect. For example, the dose of local anesthetic should be reduced by 30% regardless of the trimester of pregnancy. A biochemical explanation has been proposed involving pregnancy-induced hyperventilation with a resulting metabolic alkalosis causing local anesthetics to remain in ionized form for a longer time, therefore remaining longer in the area of injection and increasing the time to complete analgesia.[55] In addition, anatomical changes may facilitate spread due to epidural venous distension secondary to increased blood volume during pregnancy, resulting in a decrease of epidural and/or intrathecal volume.[57]

At term, increased intra-abdominal pressure, compression of the inferior vena cava and pelvic veins by a space-occupying effect, and increased epidural pressures have all been implicated in facilitated spread of local anesthetics in the epidural space.

Systemic Administration of Local Anesthetics for Pain Relief

So far, this chapter has discussed the primary mechanism of action of local anesthetics, that is, their action at neuronal voltage-gated sodium channels by local or topical application, infiltration, or regional anesthesia. Considerably less is known about the exact analgesic mechanism of action of local anesthetics such as lidocaine, when administered systemically.

Lidocaine is an U.S. Food and Drug Administration (FDA)-approved Class Ib antiarrhythmic, the intravenous administration of which has been used since the 1950s for the acute management of ventricular arrhythmias.[58] Lidocaine exerts an antiarrhythmic effect by increasing the electrical stimulation threshold of the ventricle during diastole. However, irrespective of its antiarrhythmic effects, intravenously administered lidocaine can exert analgesic activity. This section summarizes the potential use of intravenous lidocaine in the acute and chronic pain settings and discusses the proposed analgesic mechanisms of action.

INTRAVENOUS LIDOCAINE FOR ACUTE POSTOPERATIVE PAIN

Intravenous infusion of lidocaine has been tested as a part of multimodal postoperative analgesic approach in several studies. A recent Cochrane systematic review and meta-analysis has identified 45 randomized controlled trials that have used lidocaine in the perioperative setting,[59] mostly in abdominal surgeries. At early (1 to 4 hours after surgery), and intermediate (24 hours after surgery) time points, lidocaine treatment provided better pain relief and resulted in reduced time to first bowel movement, perhaps related to the reduction in postoperative opioid requirements. In general, the effects on early outcomes 4 hours after surgery (~50% of studies positive) were more substantial than at the 24-hour postoperative time point (~20% of studies positive). About 48 hours after surgery, the outcomes of intravenous lidocaine and placebo were generally not different.

For example, patients undergoing laparoscopic bariatric surgeries were randomized to intraoperative lidocaine (1.5 mg/kg bolus followed by a 2 mg/kg/hour infusion until the end of the surgical procedure) or corresponding placebo. The intervention resulted in less postoperative pain and nausea and reduced opioid consumption.[60] In patients undergoing complex spine surgery, intravenous lidocaine (2 mg/kg/hour, maximum 200 mg per hour, starting at induction of anesthesia and continuing until discharge from the postanesthesia care unit) not only resulted in lower pain scores but also improved quality of life parameters.[61] Other studies, for example, administering intravenous lidocaine in laparoscopic renal surgery,[62] did not demonstrate any difference in lidocaine versus placebo on outcomes such as length of stay, readiness for discharge, opioid consumption, nausea, or return of bowel function. The study used a 1.5 mg/kg bolus dose at anesthesia induction, followed by 2 mg/kg/hour intraoperative infusion, and a 1.3 mg/kg/hour 24-hour infusion.

INTRAVENOUS LIDOCAINE FOR CHRONIC NEUROPATHIC PAIN

Several studies have been published supporting the effectiveness of intravenous lidocaine for the treatment of neuropathic pain. A systematic review and meta-analysis concluded that overall lidocaine was not only more effective than placebo in alleviating neuropathic pain but also resulted in more adverse effects.[63]

The adverse effects seen with intravenous lidocaine usually include dizziness, perioral numbness, drowsiness, blurred vision, and more rarely cardiac rhythm abnormalities and are generally dependent on lidocaine plasma concentration.

Various dosing regimens have been implemented, most of them in the range of 2 to 5 mg/kg, infused over 30 to 60 minutes.

The duration of the analgesic effects is uncertain, with some studies assessing pain relief anywhere between 35 minutes and 6 hours,[64–66] whereas other studies reporting pain reduction in individual patients for up to 1 to 2 weeks.[67,68] However, it is unclear which patients are more likely to have long-term effects with this approach, as daily or weekly treatments with intravenous infusions are not a particularly feasible approach for treating chronic pain.

Mexiletine, which is an orally bioavailable analog of lidocaine, has also been used for the management of chronic neuropathic pain. In a 2005 meta-analysis, the average reduction in pain intensity was demonstrated to be comparable to that of intravenous lidocaine.[63] On the other hand, a recent meta-analysis of high-quality studies found that most (7 of 8) clinical trials with mexiletine in neuropathic pain have been negative, and considering the relatively high incidence of adverse effects, the guidelines currently recommend against the use of mexiletine for managing neuropathic pain.[69]

The exact analgesic mechanism of action of systemic lidocaine is not completely understood. The primary discussed mechanism is the sodium channel–mediated activity affecting signal transduction and transmission in nociceptors, as discussed previously. However, it is unclear whether the main effect in neuropathic pain is peripheral (at the primary afferent fibers), or more centrally (spinal cord or brain). Data from Devor and colleagues suggest that the activity of lidocaine on silencing signal generation in the dorsal root ganglion (DRG) is the primary mechanism by which the drug alleviates pain in peripheral neuropathies.[70,71] This has been demonstrated in a clinical study, where local intraforaminal application of low-concentration lidocaine (0.3%) at the DRG[72] resulted in substantial alleviation of pain and phantom sensations in lower limb amputees.

In addition to sodium channel–mediated mechanisms, several additional mechanisms of lidocaine have been recently been proposed. Microglial hyperactivation at the spinal cord dorsal horn has been shown to contribute to sensitization of somatosensory neurons and accompany the development of thermal and mechanical hypersensitivity after peripheral nerve injury.[73] It was shown both in vitro[74] and in vivo[75] that lidocaine may prevent microglial activation and injury, a mechanism that can possibly contribute to its systemic analgesic effect.

Glycine has been demonstrated as an important neurotransmitter involved in inhibition of sensitization in the spinal cord dorsal horn.[76] GluT1 glycine transporter, expressed on glial cells and a subset of sensory neurons, removes glycine from the synaptic cleft, resulting in disinhibition of sensory neurons.[77] Lidocaine metabolites have been also shown to inhibit the GlyT1 transporter,[78] thus potentially contributing to analgesia by a different mechanism.

Adverse Effects

SYSTEMIC TOXICITY

Local anesthetic systemic toxicity (LAST) is usually a result of an inadvertent intravascular injection of a local anesthetic solution during a regional anesthesia procedure.[79] As stated earlier, the site of injection affects the risk of toxicity as different anatomic locations vary in systemic uptake of each drug. As discussed previously in this chapter, the route of administration of local anesthetics has a direct impact on systemic absorption. Intravenous injection is the highest, whereas subcutaneous is the lowest. However, one must be careful when injecting local anesthetic in multiple places as local anesthetic toxicity is essentially additive.[80]

Local anesthetic toxicity can manifest as CNS excitation (agitation, confusion, seizure), CNS depression (drowsiness, apnea, coma), or nonspecific CNS signs (metallic taste, circumoral numbness, diplopia, tinnitus, and dizziness).[81] In addition to CNS signs, cardiovascular manifestations can include hypertension (that may progress to hypotension), conduction block, bradycardia, ventricular arrhythmias, or asystole.

The key approach to managing LAST is to provide airway management, circulatory support, and diminution of systemic effects of the local anesthetic. If seizures occur, they should be rapidly controlled (preferably with benzodiazepines) to prevent injury to the patient and acidosis.

It is usually recommended to initiate lipid emulsion (20%) therapy as soon as possible, which reduces the concentration of free local anesthetic in the systemic circulation. Studies have shown that this approach is effective in acting as a "lipid sink" to remove lipophilic local anesthetic molecules from the cardiac tissue into the lipid particles.[82,83] Specific dosing guidelines are available via the American Society of Regional Anesthesia and Pain Management (ASRA).[81] A recent study comparing the effectiveness of removing bupivacaine from the systemic circulation by long-chain triglyceride (LCT, e.g., Intralipid) emulsion (Fig. 82.5) versus an emulsion of combined long- and medium-chain triglycerides (LCT/MCT) confirmed that LCT was more effective in clearing bupivacaine from the systemic circulation.[84]

ALLERGIES

Rare individuals are hypersensitive to local anesthetics. The hypersensitivity reactions may appear as allergic dermatitis or as an asthmatic attack.[85] Hypersensitivity seems to occur

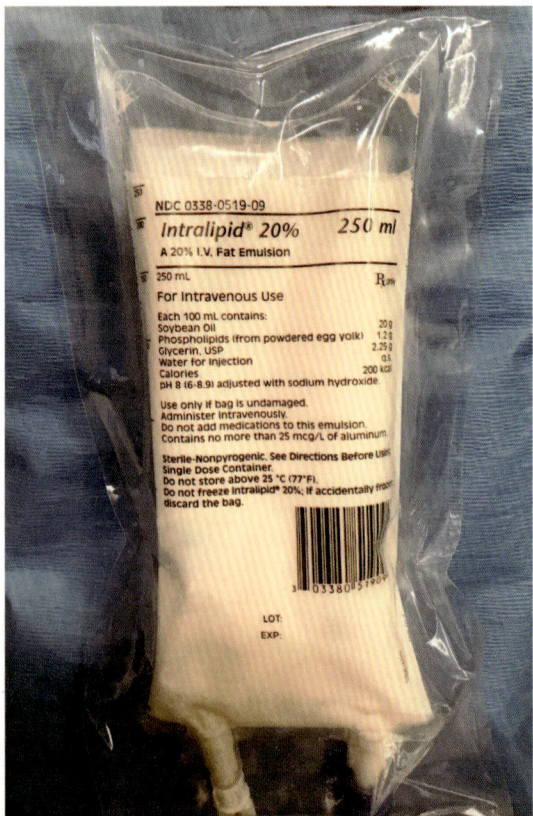

FIGURE 82.5 Intralipid. A long-chain triglyceride emulsion used to clear local anesthetic from systemic circulation during local anesthetic systemic toxicity (LAST) syndrome.

more frequently with ester-type, rather than amide-type, local anesthetics because they are derivatives of PABA, a known allergen. There can also be cross-reactivity, primarily within the same chemical group. For example, a patient hypersensitive to procaine is more likely to develop hypersensitivity to tetracaine than to ropivacaine. Local anesthetic preparations may contain a preservative such as methylparaben (which has a chemical structure similar to PABA), or local anesthetic–vasoconstrictor combinations may contain sulfites added for preventing vasoconstrictor oxidation. Sometimes, these additional compounds may be the cause of hypersensitivity rather the local anesthetic itself.

METHEMOGLOBINEMIA

Local anesthetics such as prilocaine may cause methemoglobinemia. A popular topical local anesthetic—EMLA—contains prilocaine. The metabolism of prilocaine includes derivatives of o-toluidine, which can result in the conversion of hemoglobin (Hb) to methemoglobinemia when seen in doses greater than 10 mg/kg.

Typically, methemoglobin (metHb) concentration is lower than 1% of total Hb concentration. When 3% to 15% of Hb consist of metHb, a slight gray or pale discoloration of the skin may occur. As it increases to 15% to 20%, cyanosis occurs; concentrations >20% substantially increase the risk of headache, dyspnea, respiratory depression, unconsciousness, shock, and seizures. The treatment for methemoglobinemia includes hemodynamic support as well as methylene blue administration (1 to 2 mg/kg over 5 minutes) which reduces metHb to Hb.

Prolonged-Duration Local Anesthetics

Local anesthetics have been extremely effective in providing regional anesthesia and analgesia. One of the main limitations is their temporary effect, which is typically lost within a few hours. Techniques utilizing continuous infiltration of local anesthetics have been developed and are effectively used primarily for managing acute postoperative pain.[86–88] One of the disadvantages of these techniques is the costs associated with catheter placement, maintenance, and the increased risks of infection associated with regional catheter use.

To address these limitations, various pharmaceutical formulations of long-acting local anesthetics have been developed. The formulations are primarily based on liposomes, which release the local anesthetic, for example, bupivacaine, over a prolonged period of time after injection.[89–91] One such formulation of bupivacaine (Exparel) is currently approved by the FDA for local infiltration in the perioperative setting.

The advantages of long-acting local anesthetics include primarily prolonged duration of action, reported to be up to 4 days following a single injection.[92] Some of the disadvantages include stability issues with liposomal formulations[93] and high costs associated with liposome manufacturing.[94] The outcome results have been mixed, and a recent Cochrane review cites lack of evidence to support or refute the use of liposomal bupivacaine in peripheral nerve blocks for the management of postoperative pain.[95] Furthermore, a Cochrane review evaluating surgical site infiltration of liposomal bupivacaine demonstrated superiority over placebo but not to bupivacaine hydrochloride in a comparison of postoperative pain scores.[96] However, more work is currently being done to compare single-shot liposomal bupivacaine to continuous catheters.[97] Recently, novel approaches of simplifying the production process by developing proliposomal formulations have been introduced,[98,99] and they appear to provide a similar long-acting anesthetic and analgesic effect. Future developments will hopefully enable the goal of prolonged analgesic effect with single-dose, low-cost local anesthetic solutions.

References

1. Markel H. Uber coca: Sigmund Freud, Carl Koller, and cocaine. *JAMA* 2011;305(13):1360–1361.
2. Corning JL. Spinal anaesthesia and local medication of the cord. *N Y Med J* 1885;42:483–485.
3. Bier A. Experiments in cocainization of the spinal cord. *Dtsch Z Chir* 1899;51:363–369.
4. Catterall WA, Mackie K. Local anesthetics. In: Brunton LL, Chabner BA, Knollmann BD, eds. *Goodman and Gilman's The Pharmacological Basis of Therapeutics*. 12th ed. New York: McGraw-Hill; 2011:565–582.
5. Calatayud J, González A. History of the development and evolution of local anesthesia since the coca leaf. *Anesthesiology* 2003;98(6):1503–1508.
6. Nau C, Strichartz GR. Drug chirality in anesthesia. *Anesthesiology* 2002;97(2):497–502.
7. Casati A, Putzu M. Bupivacaine, levobupivacaine and ropivacaine: are they clinically different? *Best Pract Res Clin Anaesthesiol* 2005;19(2):247–268.
8. Simpson D, Curran MP, Oldfield V, et al. Ropivacaine: a review of its use in regional anaesthesia and acute pain management. *Drugs* 2005;65(18):2675–2717.
9. Dony P, Dewinde V, Vanderick B, et al. The comparative toxicity of ropivacaine and bupivacaine at equipotent doses in rats. *Anesth Analg* 2000;91(6):1489–1492.
10. Knudsen K, Beckman Suurküla M, Blomberg S, et al. Central nervous and cardiovascular effects of i.v. infusions of ropivacaine, bupivacaine and placebo in volunteers. *Br J Anaesth* 1997;78(5):507–514.
11. Morrison SG, Dominguez JJ, Frascarolo P, et al. A comparison of the electrocardiographic cardiotoxic effects of racemic bupivacaine, levobupivacaine, and ropivacaine in anesthetized swine. *Anesth Analg* 2000;90(6):1308–1314.
12. Stewart J, Kellett N, Castro D. The central nervous system and cardiovascular effects of levobupivacaine and ropivacaine in healthy volunteers. *Anesth Analg* 2003;97(2):412–416.
13. Gissen AJ, Covino BG, Gregus J. Differential sensitivity of fast and slow fibers in mammalian nerve. II. Margin of safety for nerve transmission. *Anesth Analg* 1982;61(7):561–569.
14. Strichartz GR, Sanchez V, Arthur GR, et al. Fundamental properties of local anesthetics. II. Measured octanol:buffer partition coefficients and pKa values of clinically used drugs. *Anesth Analg* 1990;71(2):158–170.
15. Yun I, Cho ES, Jang HO, et al. Amphiphilic effects of local anesthetics on rotational mobility in neuronal and model membranes. *Biochim Biophys Acta* 2002;1564(1):123–132.
16. Catterall WA. Voltage-gated sodium channels at 60: structure, function and pathophysiology. *J Physiol* 2012;590(11):2577–2589. doi:10.1113/jphysiol.2011.224204.
17. Hodgkin AL, Huxley AF. A quantitative description of membrane current and its application to conduction and excitation in nerve. *J Physiol* 1952;117(4):500–544.
18. Frazier DT, Narahashi T, Yamada M. The site of action and active form of local anesthetics. II. Experiments with quaternary compounds. *J Pharmacol Exp Ther* 1970;171(1):45–51.
19. Catterall WA. From ionic currents to molecular mechanisms: the structure and function of voltage-gated sodium channels. *Neuron* 2000;26(1):13–25.
20. Butterworth JF, Strichartz GR. Molecular mechanisms of local anesthesia: a review. *Anesthesiology* 1990;72(4):711–734.
21. Shanes AM, Freygang WH, Grundfest H, et al. Anesthetic and calcium action in the voltage-clamped squid giant axon. *J Gen Physiol* 1959;42(4):793–802.
22. Drasner K. Local anesthetics. In: Katzung B, Masters SB, Trevor AJ, eds. *Basic & Clinical Pharmacology*. 12th ed. New York: McGraw-Hill; 2012:452–453.
23. Liu SS, Lim Y. Local anesthetics. In: Barash PG, Cullen BF, Stoelting RK, eds. *Clinical Anesthesia*. 6th ed. Philadelphia: Lippincott Williams & Wilkins; 2009:531–548.
24. Rosenberg PH, Veering BT, Urmey WF. Maximum recommended doses of local anesthetics: a multifactorial concept. *Reg Anesth Pain Med* 2004;29(6):524, 564–575.
25. Schulman JM, Strichartz GR. Local anesthetic pharmacology. In: Golan DE, Tashjian AH, Armstrong EJ, et al, eds. *Principals of Pharmacology*. 3rd ed. Philadelphia: Lippincott Williams & Wilkins; 2012:147–162.
26. Salinas FV, Liu SL, Scholz AM. Analgesics: ion channel ligands. In: Evers AS, Maze M, eds. *Anesthetic Pharmacology: Physiologic Principles and Clinical Practice*. Philadelphia: Churchill Livingstone; 2004:507–537.
27. Mather LE. Stereochemistry in anaesthetic and analgetic drugs. *Minerva Anestesiol* 2005;71:507–516.
28. Thomson PD, Melmon KL, Richardson JA, et al. Lidocaine pharmacokinetics in advanced heart failure, liver disease, and renal failure in humans. *Ann Intern Med* 1973;78:499–508.
29. Gokin AP, Philip B, Strichartz GR. Preferential block of small myelinated sensory and motor fibers by lidocaine: in vivo electrophysiology in the rat sciatic nerve. *Anesthesiology* 2001;95(6):1441–1454.
30. Marx GF. The first spinal anesthesia. Who deserves the laurels? *Reg Anesth* 1994;19(6):429–430.
31. Dalens B, Hasnaoui A. Caudal anesthesia in pediatric surgery: success rate and adverse effects in 750 consecutive patients. *Anesth Analg* 1989;68(2):83–89.

32. Pullerits J, Holzman RS. Pediatric neuraxial blockade. *J Clin Anesth* 1993;342–354.

33. Rawal N, Holmstrom B. The combined spinal-epidural technique. *Best Pract Res Clin Anaesthesiol* 2003;17(3):347–364.

34. Bier A. Ueber einen neuen weg localanasthesie in den gliedmaassen zu erzeugen [On a new technique to induce local anesthesia in extremities]. *Langenbecks Archiv Klinischirur* 1908;86:1007–1016.

35. Kraus GP, Fitzgerald BM. *Bier Block*. Treasure Island, FL: StatPearls Publishing.

36. Hogan ME, vanderVaart S, Perampaladas K, et al. Systematic review and meta-analysis of the effect of warming local anesthetics on injection pain. *Ann Emerg Med* 2011;58(1):86.e1–98.e1.

37. Cheney PR, Molzen G, Tandberg D. The effect of pH buffering on reducing the pain associated with subcutaneous infiltration of bupivacaine. *Am J Emerg Med* 1991;9(2):147–148.

38. Latham JL, Martin SN. Infiltrative anesthesia in office practice. *Am Fam Physician* 2014;89(12):956–962.

39. Kumar M, Chawla R, Goyal M. Topical anesthesia. *J Anaesthesiol Clin Pharmacol* 2015;31(4):450–456.

40. Lee HS. Recent advances in topical anesthesia. *J Dent Anesth Pain Med* 2016;16(4):237–244. doi:10.17245/jdapm.2016.16.4.237.

41. Fukuda T, Naito H. The effect of pH adjustment of 1% lidocaine on the onset of sensory and motor blockade of epidural anesthesia in nonpregnant gynecological patients. *J Anesth* 1994;8(3):293–296.

42. McMorland GH, Douglas MJ, Axelson JE, et al. The effect of pH adjustment of bupivacaine on onset and duration of epidural anaesthesia for caesarean section. *Can J Anaesth* 1988;35(5):457–461.

43. Hanna MN, Elhassan A, Veloso PM, et al. Efficacy of bicarbonate in decreasing pain on intradermal injection of local anesthetics: a meta-analysis. *Reg Anesth Pain Med* 2009;34(2):122–125.

44. Chassard D, Berrada K, Bouletreau P. Alkalinization of local anesthetics: theoretically justified but clinically useless. *Can J Anaesth* 1996;43(4):384–393.

45. Ikuta PT, Raza SM, Durrani Z, et al. pH adjustment schedule for the amide local anesthetics. *Reg Anesth* 1989;14(5):229–235.

46. Sisk AL. Vasoconstrictors in local anesthesia for dentistry. *Anesth Prog* 1992;39(6):187–193.

47. Bromage PR, Camporesi EM, Durant PA, et al. Influence of epinephrine as an adjuvant to epidural morphine. *Anesthesiology* 1983;58(3):257–262.

48. Selander D, Brattsand R, Lundborg G, et al. Local anesthetics: importance of mode of application, concentration and adrenaline for the appearance of nerve lesions. An experimental study of axonal degeneration and barrier damage after intrafascicular injection or topical application of bupivacaine (Marcain). *Acta Anaesthesiol Scand* 1979;23(2):127–136.

49. Hogan QH. Pathophysiology of peripheral nerve injury during regional anesthesia. *Reg Anesth Pain Med* 2008;33(5):435–441.

50. Smith DL. The evaluation of chloroprocaine in combination with bupivacaine for brachial plexus anesthesia and application of nerve blockade monitor placement. *J Am Osteopath Assoc* 1976;75(8):729–731.

51. Ribotsky BM, Berkowitz KD, Montague JR. Local anesthetics. Is there an advantage to mixing solutions? *J Am Podiatr Med Assoc* 1996;86(10):487–491.

52. Galindo A, Witcher T. Mixtures of local anesthetics: bupivacaine-chloroprocaine. *Anesth Analg* 1980;59(9):683–685.

53. Bromage PR. Continuous lumbar epidural analgesia for obstetrics. *Can Med Assoc J* 1961;85:1136–1140.

54. Datta S, Lambert DH, Gregus J, et al. Differential sensitivities of mammalian nerve fibers during pregnancy. *Anesth Analg* 1983;62(12)1070–1072.

55. Fagraeus L, Urban BJ, Bromage PR. Spread of epidural analgesia in early pregnancy. *Anesthesiology* 1983;58(2):184–187.

56. Flanagan HL, Datta S, Lambert DH, et al. Effect of pregnancy on bupivacaine-induced conduction blockade in the isolated rabbit vagus nerve. *Anesth Analg* 1987;66(2):123–126.

57. Marx GF, Bassell GM. Physiologic considerations of the mother. In: Marx GF, Bassel GM, eds. *Obstetric Analgesia and Anesthesia*. Amsterdam, The Netherlands: Elsevier/North-Holland; 1980:21–54.

58. Weiss WA. Intravenous use of lidocaine for ventricular arrhythmias. *Anesth Analg* 1960;39:369–381.

59. Kranke P, Jokinen J, Pace NL, et al. Continuous intravenous perioperative lidocaine infusion for postoperative pain and recovery. *Cochrane Database Syst Rev* 2015;(7):CD009642.

60. De Oliveira GS Jr, Duncan K, Fitzgerald P, et al. Systemic lidocaine to improve quality of recovery after laparoscopic bariatric surgery: a randomized double-blinded placebo-controlled trial. *Obes Surg* 2014;24(2):212–218.

61. Farag E, Ghobrial M, Sessler DI, et al. Effect of perioperative intravenous lidocaine administration on pain, opioid consumption, and quality of life after complex spine surgery. *Anesthesiology* 2013;119(4):932–940.

62. Wuethrich PY, Romero J, Burkhard FC, et al. No benefit from perioperative intravenous lidocaine in laparoscopic renal surgery: a randomised, placebo-controlled study. *Eur J Anaesthesiol* 2012;29(11):537–543.

63. Challapalli V, Tremont-Lukats IW, McNicol ED, et al. Systemic administration of local anesthetic agents to relieve neuropathic pain. *Cochrane Database Syst Rev* 2005;(4):CD003345.

64. Finnerup NB, Biering-Sørensen F, Johannesen IL, et al. Intravenous lidocaine relieves spinal cord injury pain: a randomized controlled trial. *Anesthesiology* 2005;102(5):1023–1030.

65. Rowbotham MC, Reisner-Keller LA, Fields HL. Both intravenous lidocaine and morphine reduce the pain of postherpetic neuralgia. *Neurology* 1991;41(7):1024–1028.

66. Wallace MS, Dyck JB, Rossi SS, et al. Computer-controlled lidocaine infusion for the evaluation of neuropathic pain after peripheral nerve injury. *Pain* 1996;66(1):69–77.

67. Attal N, Rouaud J, Brasseur L, et al. Systemic lidocaine in pain due to peripheral nerve injury and predictors of response. *Neurology* 2004;62(2):218–225.

68. Kastrup J, Angelo H, Petersen P, et al. Treatment of chronic painful diabetic neuropathy with intravenous lidocaine infusion. *Br Med J (Clin Res Ed)* 1986;292(6514):173.

69. Finnerup NB, Attal N, Haroutounian S, et al. Pharmacotherapy for neuropathic pain in adults: a systematic review and meta-analysis. *Lancet Neurol* 2015;14(2):162–173.

70. Devor M, Wall PD, Catalan N. Systemic lidocaine silences ectopic neuroma and DRG discharge without blocking nerve conduction. *Pain* 1992;48(2):261–268.

71. Sukhotinsky I, Ben-Dor E, Raber P, et al. Key role of the dorsal root ganglion in neuropathic tactile hypersensibility. *Eur J Pain* 2004;8(2):135–143.

72. Vaso A, Adahan HM, Gjika A, et al. Peripheral nervous system origin of phantom limb pain. *Pain* 2014;155(7):1384–1391.

73. Beggs S, Trang T, Salter MW. P2X4R+ microglia drive neuropathic pain. *Nat Neurosci* 2012;15(8):1068–1073.

74. Jeong HJ, Lin D, Li L, et al. Delayed treatment with lidocaine reduces mouse microglial cell injury and cytokine production after stimulation with lipopolysaccharide and interferon gamma. *Anesth Analg* 2012;114(4):856–861.

75. Suzuki N, Hasegawa-Moriyama M, Takahashi Y, et al. Lidocaine attenuates the development of diabetic-induced tactile allodynia by inhibiting microglial activation. *Anesth Analg* 2011;113(4):941–946.

76. Zeilhofer HU. Loss of glycinergic and GABAergic inhibition in chronic pain—contributions of inflammation and microglia. *Int Immunopharmacol* 2008;8(2):182–187.

77. Zeilhofer HU. The glycinergic control of spinal pain processing. *Cell Mol Life Sci* 2005;62(18):2027–2035.

78. Werdehausen R, Kremer D, Brandenburger T, et al. Lidocaine metabolites inhibit glycine transporter 1: a novel mechanism for the analgesic action of systemic lidocaine? *Anesthesiology* 2012;116(1):147–158.

79. Neal JM, Bernards CM, Butterworth JF IV, et al. ASRA practice advisory on local anesthetic systemic toxicity. *Reg Anesth Pain Med* 2010;35(2):152–161.

80. de Jong RH, Bonin JD. Mixtures of local anesthetics are no more toxic than the parent drugs. *Anesthesiology* 1981;54(3):177–181.

81. Neal JM, Mulroy MF, Weinberg GL, et al. American Society of Regional Anesthesia and Pain Medicine checklist for managing local anesthetic systemic toxicity: 2012 version. *Reg Anesth Pain Med* 2012;37(1):16–18.

82. Weinberg GL. Treatment of local anesthetic systemic toxicity (LAST). *Reg Anesth Pain Med* 2010;35(2):188–193.

83. Weinberg GL, Ripper R, Murphy P, et al. Lipid infusion accelerates removal of bupivacaine and recovery from bupivacaine toxicity in the isolated rat heart. *Reg Anesth Pain Med* 2006;31(4):296–303.

84. Tang W, Wang Q, Shi K, et al. The effect of lipid emulsion on pharmacokinetics of bupivacaine in rats: long-chain triglyceride versus long- and medium-chain triglyceride. *Anesth Analg* 2016;123(5):1116–1122.

85. Dewachter P, Mouton-Faivre C, Emala CW. Anaphylaxis and anesthesia: controversies and new insights. *Anesthesiology* 2009;111(5):1141–1150.

86. Chan EY, Fransen M, Parker DA, et al. Femoral nerve blocks for acute postoperative pain after knee replacement surgery. *Cochrane Database Syst Rev* 2014;(5):CD009941.

87. Fredrickson MJ, Leightley P, Wong A, et al. An analysis of 1505 consecutive patients receiving continuous interscalene analgesia at home: a multicentre prospective safety study. *Anaesthesia* 2016;71(4):373–379.

88. Guay J, Nishimori M, Kopp S. Epidural local anaesthetics versus opioid-based analgesic regimens for postoperative gastrointestinal paralysis, vomiting and pain after abdominal surgery. *Cochrane Database Syst Rev* 2016;(7):CD001893.

89. Bulbake U, Doppalapudi S, Kommineni N, et al. Liposomal formulations in clinical use: an updated review. *Pharmaceutics* 2017;9(2):E12.

90. Davidson EM, Barenholz Y, Cohen R, et al. High-dose bupivacaine remotely loaded into multivesicular liposomes demonstrates slow drug release without systemic toxic plasma concentrations after subcutaneous administration in humans. *Anesth Analg* 2010;110(4):1018–1023.

91. Ye Q, Asherman J, Stevenson M, et al. DepoFoam technology: a vehicle for controlled delivery of protein and peptide drugs. *J Control Release* 2000;64(1–3):155–166.

92. Bramlett K, Onel E, Viscusi ER, et al. A randomized, double-blind, dose-ranging study comparing wound infiltration of DepoFoam bupivacaine, an extended-release liposomal bupivacaine, to bupivacaine HCl for postsurgical analgesia in total knee arthroplasty. *Knee* 2012;19(5):530–536.

93. Cohen R, Kanaan H, Grant GJ, et al. Prolonged analgesia from Bupisome and Bupigel formulations: from design and fabrication to improved stability. *J Control Release* 2012;160(2):346–352.

94. Pedoto A, Amar D. Liposomal bupivacaine for intercostal nerve block: pricey or priceless? [published online ahead of print August 30, 2017]. *Semin Thorac Cardiovasc Surg*. doi:10.1053/j.semtcvs.2017.08.016.

95. Hamilton TW, Athanassoglou V, Trivella M, et al. Liposomal bupivacaine peripheral nerve block for the management of postoperative pain. *Cochrane Database Syst Rev* 2016;(8):CD011476.

96. Hamilton TW, Athanassoglou V, Mellon S, et al. Liposomal bupivacaine infiltration at the surgical site for the management of postoperative pain. *Cochrane Database Syst Rev* 2017;(2):CD011419.

97. Sabesan VJ, Shahriar R, Petersen-Fitts GR, et al. A prospective randomized controlled trial to identify the optimal postoperative pain management in shoulder arthroplasty: liposomal bupivacaine versus continuous interscalene catheter. *J Shoulder Elbow Surg* 2017;26(10):1810–1817.

98. Davidson EM, Haroutounian S, Kagan L, et al. A novel proliposomal ropivacaine oil: pharmacokinetic-pharmacodynamic studies after subcutaneous administration in pigs. *Anesth Analg* 2016;122(5):1663–1672.

99. Ginosar Y, Haroutounian S, Kagan L, et al. Proliposomal ropivacaine oil: pharmacokinetic and pharmacodynamic data after subcutaneous administration in volunteers. *Anesth Analg* 2016;122(5):1673–1680.

CHAPTER **83**

Anger and Pain

R. JOSHUA WOOTTON

Cultural Background

Aristotle,[1] referencing Homer's *Iliad*, suggested that "anger may be defined as an impulse, accompanied by pain, to a conspicuous revenge for a conspicuous slight," emphasizing that "the angry man feels pain." There was no suggestion of the separation of emotional distress from its physical consequences. Unlike many of his contemporaries, Aristotle undertook a reasoned approach to the understanding of anger but nevertheless placed it clearly in the context of emotional and physical pain. In his essay *On Anger*, Seneca[2] urged his elder brother Novatus to eschew anger and agreed that he was "right to have a particular dread of this most hideous and frenzied of all emotions," even likening the emotional experience to "a brief insanity." It was a common thematic thread to philosophers and physicians in ancient Greece and Rome that anger tended to reveal itself as a form of madness and that attempts to control it reflected strength of character and spirit.[3] Attempts to control anger in antiquity, however, were usually concerned with altering its often dramatic appearance, not with regulating its impact on the body. The possible harmful effects of managing the expression of anger were paid little consideration.

Scripture, too, characterizes anger as being at the heart of sin or separation from God and admonishes against the dangers of its excesses. In Hebrew, Christian, and Islamic religious writings, God is often portrayed as angry toward those who oppose his will,[2] but the faithful are taught to suppress their angry impulses "for the anger of man does not work the righteousness of God" (James 1:20). The Qur'an teaches that "Allah loves those who restrain anger" ('Al-'Imran 3:134), whereas the Psalms caution us to "be angry, but sin not" (Psalms 4:4). In other passages, we are encouraged not only to avoid expressions of anger but also to resist even the emotion itself. In the Gospel of Matthew, we find that "everyone who is angry with his brother shall be liable to judgment" (Matthew 5:22), whereas elsewhere in the Psalms, we are exhorted to "refrain from anger; and forsake wrath!" (Psalms 37:8), and in the Sunnah of Islam, the Prophet advises, again and again, "Do not become angry and furious" (Hadith-Sahih Al-Bukhari 8.137).

This deeply ingrained cultural awareness—that not only are angry actions dangerous, but the emotion of anger itself can be harmful—led to the inclusion of anger as one of the "seven deadly sins" in the religious West,[4] a theme popularized and later woven into the fabric of Western cultures through literature, drama, and art, including in European cultures the enduring and influential classics of Dante's *Divine Comedy* and Chaucer's *Canterbury Tales*.

Psychoanalytic Background

One important difference between historical and more contemporary discussions of anger is that the former, although often concerned with the negative consequences of expressing anger, were seldom concerned with the possible harmful effects of its inhibition.[3] Anger in psychoanalytic theory does not carry the metaphysical weight of sin, but its expression through hostility and aggressive impulses often lies at the core of conflict, competing drives, and the formation of pathologic symptoms, including pain. Although Freud was an atheist, his frequent excursions into the fields of religion, religious experience, and anthropology are testimony to his respect for the conscious and unconscious impact of culture on the individual; he was the first to emphasize the idea that the individual and culture are linked dynamically and that disturbances may occur in the developmental interaction between the two, leaving behind a disposition to future neuroses.[5] He was also an astute observer of the phenomenon of pain from organic origins being maintained for intrapsychic reasons, long past the point of expectable physical healing and recovery.[6,7]

Early in his work, Freud arrived at the idea that pain is a common symptom of *conversion* and that, although there is usually an organic basis for the onset of pain, it can later be influenced and extended in duration and scope by a process through which mental conflict is displaced onto the body, resulting in the somatic expression of symptoms. Conversion, in this context, is closer to the contemporary term *somatization*, referring both to conversion and psychophysiologic disorders. The repression of negative affects, such as anger, resentment, and guilt, is transmuted into the expression of physical symptoms. The defensive process of somatization continues until relief from the intrapsychic burden of intolerable affect is no longer necessary or desomatization takes place through support—often psychotherapeutic—of the individual's more mature defenses and coping strategies.

Freud's later work was focused more on patients whose pain was less directly associated with an original organic insult and more configured with mood disturbance. In "Mourning and Melancholia," he delineated the intrapsychic origins of depression as a process through which aggression, originally directed toward the lost object, is turned against the self[8]—somewhat oversimplified in the popular formula "anger turned inward." According to this template, pain and mourning may be seen as affective responses to separation and as unconscious defenses against aggression.[8-10] Freud's successors related pain to aggression and hostility more directly, and the idea that the symptom of physical pain can be an unconscious defense against anger and aggression became a widely shared interpretation in psychoanalytic theory; however, as Merskey[7] points out, the evidence has been largely anecdotal, with the relationship between anger and pain often being made more plausible by retrospective analysis.

Like Freud, Engel[11] acknowledged that pain may originate with actual physical injury, but his study of the "pain-prone patient" gave the most enduring and widely influential psychoanalytic expression of chronic pain as a symbolic displacement of anger and aggression. He also suggested that patients are frequently unwilling or unable to acknowledge the hostility and aggressive impulses behind their pain, leaving them with the difficult task of attempting to adjust to symptoms that are borne of conflicts that they can neither recognize nor accept. The presence of chronic pain, then, may reflect underlying conflicts—in turn, giving rise to intolerable affects, which, when repressed, are given dynamic expression through the body. Szasz,[12] as well, held that repression of emotional distress is often the principal mechanism underlying chronic pain and suggested that, by focusing their attention on their pain, many patients are coping with their distress symbolically and through a more socially acceptable expression of their conflicts.

Burns[13,14] summarizes the evidence supporting this view that repression of affect is the mechanism at the heart of chronic pain. First, he cites the phenomenon of the "conversion-V" profile on the Minnesota Multiphasic Personality Inventory (MMPI and MMPI-2), depicted by clinical elevations on scales 1 and 3, Hypochondriasis and Hysteria, with a comparatively lower score on scale 2, Depression. The resulting V configuration suggests the presence of somatic preoccupation and a hysterical constellation of defenses, deployed in the service of relieving depressed affect. Second, he further reports evidence of the link between the tendency to suppress anger and aggression and the symptomatic expression of chronic pain and disability. Finally, he points to the persistent observation that inhibition of emotion, particularly emotions arising in the context of traumatic events, has physiologic consequences.

Where the first of these three lines of evidence is concerned, the conversion-V configuration of scores on the MMPI and MMPI-2 has been studied extensively, and applied to chronic pain, for more than 40 years.[15,16] The first scale of this "neurotic triad" of scores is Hypochondriasis. High scores on Hypochondriasis tend to reflect patterns of neurotic concern over physical health.[17,18] The third scale, Hysteria, was developed specifically as an aid to measuring the predisposition to develop symptoms of conversion or somatization and reflects a high degree of reliance on hysterical defenses.[17,18] When these two scales are clinically elevated and the second scale, Depression, which reflects both mood and neurovegetative aspects of depression, is comparatively lower, the indication of the resulting V configuration is that intolerable affect is being displaced onto somatic concerns, principally through the mechanism of repression.[14–20] Much of this research occurred prior to 2008 and the publication of the revised and restructured form of the MMPI-2. In the MMPI-2-Restructured Form (MMPI-2-RF), the traditional clinical scales are no longer available and have been replaced with restructured scales in an effort to address the shortcomings of the original instrument.[21–25] However, the restructured scales function quite similarly to the original scales in their ability to identify somatization and malingering, albeit without the traditional conversion-V format.[26]

Where the second line of evidence is concerned, Burns's[14] observations of trends in the scientific literature suggesting the link between chronic pain and the inhibition of anger have been replicated and amplified by numerous subsequent studies, although not always with psychoanalytic theory in the foreground.[27–37] The suggestion is that patients with chronic pain are more likely to experience anger than those without pain and more likely also to inhibit their anger.[31–34,36] Burns's[13] third source of evidence concerns the physiologic response, both conscious and unconscious, to efforts at inhibition. Suppression reflects the more obvious example of physiologic cost; however, repression also has a dynamic element that must be balanced in the psychosomatic economy of mind and body interrelationship.[27–29,31–34,36] Within the framework of psychoanalytic theory, the physiologic exertion demanded by inhibition was often seen as related to the persistence of conversion as well as the intensity and duration of somatization.[8,10,38–41]

The following case of a young woman referred for evaluation of her chronic abdominal pain will serve to illustrate the psychoanalytic perspective on inhibition and its relation to anger and pain.

Case 1: Ms. Ostrakova was a 20-year-old single library aide and part-time student at a nearby community college, who presented with a 2-year history of chronic abdominal pain. She had undergone two separate, complete gastroenterologic workups at two different medical centers, without any positive findings. She associated the beginning of her difficulties with a chicken sandwich, prepared by her elder sister, in which the meat was apparently undercooked. She explained that she had become quite ill within a short time, with fever, nausea, and vomiting. These symptoms resolved after a few days, but her abdominal pain persisted and became progressively more debilitating until, by the time she arrived in clinic, she had taken a leave of absence from both college and her job and was attempting to manage her pain with a medication regimen that included short-acting opioids. Ms. Ostrakova was fit and slender and her demeanor, although somewhat subdued, was affable and cooperative. She had no psychiatric history or history of substance abuse, and her medical history was notable only for robust health prior to the onset of her abdominal pain. Her psychosocial history, however, was remarkable for early childhood trauma and abuse and a childhood household of domestic turmoil and violence. She described a history of fighting in school and finally being remanded at age 17 years by the juvenile court system to a residential treatment facility for "anger management" in another state. When asked about the therapeutic aspect of her 1-year treatment program, she replied, "They just taught us how to keep our anger inside, not to let it out, so we wouldn't always get into fights. We had to avoid fighting to prove we had learned how to manage our anger."

As the interview progressed, it became clear that the patient had learned much about recognizing anger when she experienced it, and suppressing it in the moment, but little about the potential cost to herself and her body. A psychometric assessment reflected little endorsement of depressive symptoms on the Beck Depression Inventory or the MMPI-2 but clinically elevated scores on Hypochondriasis and Hysteria, and her history reflected many of the psychosocial factors depicted by Engel as disposing toward "pain proneness." The latter included parents who were abusive toward each other and toward their children, a father who was alcoholic and emotionally and physically domineering, and a mother who was often debilitated by pain of uncertain etiology.[11,40,42]

In her treatment program, the patient appeared to have gotten the message, right or wrong, that, if she showed no outward signs of anger, she would be considered successfully rehabilitated. The experience of anger, therefore, became an obstacle between her court-mandated residential treatment and her successful return home. Over time, the experience of anger was transformed by a developing awareness of intolerable affect—displaced onto her body in the more acceptable symptomatic expression of physical pain. When Ms. Ostrakova's elder sister provided the organic insult of an undercooked chicken sandwich, resulting in gastroenterologic distress, the patient, who might previously have responded with anger leading to physical confrontation, began instead to experience the pain associated with simple repression of her affect—unconsciously "keeping her anger inside." This is the classic picture of somatization, depicted in psychoanalytic theory, which continues to be influential in our assessment of patients with chronic pain.

Current Research in Anger and Its Relation to Pain

The role of anger in exacerbating pain and in disposing toward the development of chronic pain is, in some respects, similar to that of other negative emotions or distressed affective states, such as anxiety and depression.[35,37,43] According to the prevailing gate control and neuromatrix theories of pain, negative emotions can increase the intensity and duration of pain by altering or dysregulating the descending and central pain modulation systems.[44–51] Precisely how this takes place remains an open question for further research, but an integrated neurobiologic model is emerging with implications for treatment of both chronic pain and disorders of anger.

PHYSIOLOGIC MECHANISMS IN ANGER AND PAIN RESEARCH

Merskey[7] noted that pain can make individuals aggressive for purely biologic reasons, associated with the activation of the fight-or-flight mechanisms and high autonomic arousal. He added that we may not need to look much further in our attempts to explain why patients with chronic pain become angry. Whereas angry responses can be adaptive, especially when they prompt the search for constructive solutions to problems within the medical setting, chronically angry reactions of the sort observed in some patients with chronic pain are often seen as maladaptive and disruptive—indicative not of discrete situations of fight or flight but of sustained and simmering autonomic arousal.[33,34,36,37,47,52] Parsing the relationship here has proven challenging because of two related questions: Does chronic pain induce sustained sympathetic arousal and therefore lead to continual expressions of anger? Does the situation of chronic pain arise more easily among individuals who are disposed to express anger and aggression?

Robinson and Riley[43] outlined four models or mechanisms through which the relationship between pain and negative emotion has been usefully described, both from a clinical perspective and as a template for empirical design:

- Negative emotion increases sensitivity.
- Pain is caused by negative emotion.
- Negative affect occurs as a result of chronic pain.
- Pain and negative emotion are concomitant.

The first of these is simply the observation that negative emotion increases somatic sensitivity. In other words, negative emotions increase awareness and recognition of pain. Evidence in support of this mechanism comes from studies in which induced changes in mood have been correlated with increased reports of pain and decreased tolerance for experimentally induced pain, as well as in the clinical observation that depressed patients tend to interpret sensations negatively, experiencing them more often as painful.[43]

The second mechanism—that pain is caused by negative emotion—is most closely allied with the psychoanalytic view of pain as a symptom of underlying or repressed conflict, but inhibition of negative emotion and affect can also result in elevations of autonomic and central nervous system activity, raising serum cortisol levels and leading to neurovegetative dysfunction and increased pain. Cacioppo et al.'s[53] meta-analytic study of the physiologic correlates of negative emotions concluded that the experience of anger, whether expressed or suppressed, tends to be accompanied by increased diastolic blood pressure, skin conductance, stroke volume, cardiac output, peripheral resistance, finger pulse, and heart rate, all suggesting a high sympathetic response. Considering the impact of sustained autonomic arousal, negative emotions, not surprisingly, may also be seen as causal in the expression of stress-related illness and pain in which somatic reactivity can lead to musculoskeletal disorder.[34,36,43,54–57] Robinson and Riley's third mechanism echoes Merskey's suggestion that negative affect may be seen simply as a reaction to the situation of chronic pain, arising within a stress-diathesis framework,[7,43,58] whereas their fourth proposed mechanism posits that pain and negative emotion arise concomitantly from shared neurobiologic pathways.[34,36,43,56]

Taken together, these four mechanisms are broadly consistent with the gate control and neuromatrix theories of pain; however, the last—that anger, anxiety, depression, and pain share neurobiologic pathways—suggests a physiologic context in which negative emotions can alter the descending and central pain modulation processes.[48–50,59] Serotonin, norepinephrine, and dopamine all play roles in the modulation of pain as well as in the development of negative emotions. That pain and depression both respond to certain antidepressant medications has long been cited as evidence of common neurobiologic pathways.[43,60–63] Relative cortisol levels and dopaminergic transfer and regulation have also been implicated in the relationship between anger and pain,[43,64–67] but the key neurotransmitter implicated in the modulation of anger is dopamine, with the focus of activity in the nucleus accumbens.[63,67–71]

From an evolutionary perspective, the emotion of anger is clearly primitive and derived from ancient limbic regions of the brain, as opposed to the cortex and prefrontal cortex, which assume a more modulatory role in its experience and expression.[68] The regions of primary activity for anger—along with its conceptual counterparts, appetitive impulsivity, drive, motivation, pleasure, and psychoticism—appear to be associated with the core regions of temperament: the amygdala and nucleus accumbens or ventral striatum as well as the cingulate cortex.[68,69] Lara and Akiskal[68] suggest that anger is influenced by dopaminergic transfer and regulation in these regions, with high anger being associated with either enhanced postsynaptic response to dopamine or increased synaptic dopamine concentration or both. Wood[67] outlines evidence to suggest that the inhibition of tonic pain is mediated by activation of mesolimbic dopamine neurons, arising from the ventral tegmental area and projecting to the nucleus accumbens.

Ironically, anger may be associated both with an increase or a decrease in the experience of pain.[27,59,72,73] Acute stress may activate mechanisms of pain suppression through the release of endogenous opioids and substance P within the ventral tegmental area, but prolonged exposure to stress—as in the case of sustained anger or proneness to anger—tends to result in a reduction of dopaminergic output in the nucleus accumbens, potentiating the subsequent development of hyperalgesia.[67] The outcome appears to be that inhibition of pain may occur initially when a painful stimulus is first perceived but that, on further exposure and evaluation, sensitization may occur.[59] The experience of anger appears to undergo change over time, leading to associations with both traits and temperament—factors related to the thematic and serial evaluation of stimuli—an observation that has led to the study of anger-related features of both mood and personality disorders.[68,74–80] The influence of anger on the changes involved in mood states suggests a dynamic relationship associated with the tonic and phasic balance of dopaminergic activity.[67,68] In this case, the inhibition of pain may be principally related to physiologic changes occurring in the initial or situational experience of anger, such as changes in cardiovascular reactivity and autonomic arousal that have been shown to modulate the experience of pain.[27] Pain sensitization, on the other hand, appears more associated with the ability to regulate anger and the emotional evaluation of the experience—individual differences that influence dopaminergic output.[59,68] This, in turn, suggests that the experience of anger, relative to personality and temperament, as well as how we manage anger, are important variables in the modulation of pain.[56,59,63,68,70,76]

Other physiologic mechanisms under study include the effects of anger on muscle reactivity, the immune system, and endogenous opioid dysfunction.[47–52] Consideration of the last of these will be deferred to discussion of the related work on anger management, later in this chapter. Where the first is concerned, studies on muscle reactivity have suggested that anger may increase musculoskeletal tension in specific sites that contribute to pain.[33,34,36,37,81,82] The experience of anger, whether inhibited or expressed, and the trait of hostility have been associated with increased likelihood of reporting high levels of tension near the site of pain and injury.[83] A further mechanism through which anger may influence pain is distress-related immune dysregulation.[84] Although brief, situational stressors involving activation of the fight-or-flight mechanisms have been shown to result in potentially beneficial changes to the immune system, exposure to prolonged stress and negative emotion, such as sustained anger and hostility, have been associated with deleterious effects in a broad range of health concerns, immunologic suppression, and generalized inflammatory processes associated with chronic pain.[85–91] Because immunologic changes must be observed longitudinally, this work has tended to emphasize the impact of sustained anger and hostility associated with enduring personality traits and temperament.[87,88]

PSYCHOLOGICAL CONSTRUCTS IN ANGER AND PAIN RESEARCH

The etymology of "anger" is not the same for every modern language, but it appears to have come into modern English usage via Old Norse, *angra*, "to grieve, vex," later *angr*, "distress, grief," Old English, *enge*, "narrow, painful," influenced by the Proto-Indo-European root, *angh-*, "painfully constricted," and finally into Middle English, where its associations with pain endured.[92] The relative importance of the term in ordinary discourse can be illustrated through the frequency of its use: Of the roughly 700,000 words in common English usage, "anger" is ranked 2,382nd in frequency of appearance in spoken and written communication.[93] Focusing on the logic underpinning the ordinary language use of the word *anger*, Smedslund offered a contemporary definition of anger that depicts the psycholinguistic core of the construct rather than emphasizing the characteristic features of its expression: "a feeling involving a *belief* that a person one cares for has, intentionally or through neglect, been treated without respect, and a *want* to have that respect reestablished."[54,55,94] In Smedslund's conceptual framework, the "person one cares for," particularly in the context of pain, is ordinarily the self.

Fernandez emphasizes the dimensions of *action tendency* and *cognitive appraisal* in the study of the relationship between anger and pain.[54,55,95] The former concerns the behavioral tendencies associated with anger, including aggression and impulses directed toward the restoration of control, the removal of obstacles, and the seeking of redress. This becomes an important consideration in the context of whether action is expressed or suppressed and, if expressed, how adaptively. The latter suggests a framework within which the individual seeks to explain otherwise ambiguous interior experiences or changes in arousal. Both of these dimensions are anticipated by and subsumed under Smedslund's ordinary language definition

of anger, and both have proven critical to the study of the relationship between anger and pain.

The cognitive appraisal theory of emotion—perhaps most elegantly and economically portrayed in Lazarus's[96] cognitive-motivational-relational theory—suggests that the experience of an emotion, like anger, is the joint effect of (1) the event of physiologic arousal in response to incoming stimuli and (2) the cognitive appraisal of its meaning with respect to the particular setting in which the event occurs (Table 83.1). Cognitive appraisal, then, is the process through which physiologic states, such as arousal, are interpreted in light of the perceived situation. This becomes critical in the management of anger and, by extension, to the psychotherapeutic treatment of patients with chronic pain, because how events are appraised tends to influence selection and deployment of coping strategies.[97–100] Lazarus[96] further distinguished between primary and secondary appraisals, with the former referring to the interpretation of how a particular situation affects considerations of well-being and the latter, referring to considerations of how to cope with the situation.[96] Secondary appraisals, he suggests, can actually shape the experience of an emotion through the selection of a particular coping strategy.[96,101,102]

ANGER MANAGEMENT STYLE

Much of the research on anger and its relationship to pain has highlighted the related constructs of hostility, aggression, and anger management style.[47,52,103,104] *Anger* is the term denoting the emotion, characterized by physiologic arousal and accompanying conscious and unconscious impulses toward aggression. *Aggression* typically refers to the behavioral expression of the emotion, ordinarily through acts of vindication, punishment, and destruction, directed toward others or objects.[105–107] Freud's focus was ultimately less on anger than on aggression, as one of the two primary instinctual drives.[6,108] In psychoanalytic theory, aggression in its stimulation of defensive functions and coping strategies plays an important role in the development of personality. This distinction between anger and aggression suggests that whereas anger is usually conceived as a transient state, aggression is a more durable and endogenously derived motivational force. The word *anger* can be used in this manner—to denote a more dispositional quality—but, frequently, the term *hostility* is used in reference to the tendency to make consistently negative cognitive appraisals regarding the motivations of others.[55]

Conceptual links with aggression and hostility further raise the distinction between state anger and trait anger, a critical consideration in researching the influence of anger on chronic pain. A good starting point for the distinction is offered by Spielberger,[105] who characterizes state anger as a transitory emotional episode, whereas trait anger is described as a more

TABLE 83.1	Lazarus's Cognitive-Motivational-Relational Theory of Emotion				
Event (Stimulus)	Physiologic Response	Setting/Circumstances	Cognitive Appraisal	Emotion	Secondary Appraisal
Feeling oneself being pushed or shoved	Autonomic arousal, pain	A cashier's line in a busy store where customers are jostling for position	"A stranger has pushed me aside! *This is unfair!*"	Anger (increased pain associated with the unfair slight to one's identity or ego)	The setting may suggest that an angry outburst will prove less effective than a sympathetic, reasoned appeal to civility.
Feeling oneself being pushed or shoved	Autonomic arousal, pain	A pedestrian crosswalk at a busy urban traffic intersection	"A stranger has pushed me out of harm's way! I was nearly struck by that automobile!"	Relief, gratitude (reduced pain); if anger is experienced, it is likely directed toward the impatient motorist or toward oneself for being careless.	The setting may suggest that a personal expression of gratitude toward one's protector is more appropriate than an angry outburst directed toward the fleeing motorist.

NOTE: The same or similar events and physiologic responses may be interpreted or appraised differently, depending on the setting or circumstances, resulting in different emotional responses.

stable pattern of personality attributes, similar to hostility. One way of representing this is that trait anger reflects a relatively stable dimension of proneness to anger in which individual differences are reflected in the frequency, intensity, and duration with which state anger is experienced over time.[33,52,109] This, in turn, suggests that characteristic defensive patterns and reliance on particular coping strategies tend to result in what may be described as more enduring styles of anger management.

Anger management style is a term denoting the relative tendencies of individuals either (1) to suppress or internalize their anger or (2) to express or externalize their anger. The construct of anger management style is often represented in research as anger-in, anger-out, and anger-control.[33,47,103,104] *Anger-in* characterizes the tendency to inhibit the expression of angry thoughts and feelings, whereas *anger-out* describes the tendency to express angry thoughts and feelings directly, whether verbally, physically, or both. High trait anger, according to Deffenbacher,[109] is more associated with the tendency to express anger negatively, less constructively, and with less control than with the tendency to suppress anger; he further notes that there is a stronger connection between the suppressed anger and anxiety than between suppressed anger and forms of expressed anger. *Anger-control* refers to an individual's perceived control over the experience and expression of anger and is usually interpreted as positive, unless too much control approaches no expression at all.[47]

Although the International Association for the Study of Pain (IASP) appears to separate the sensory and emotional dimensions of the experience of pain, when it defines pain as an "unpleasant sensory and emotional experience associated with actual or potential tissue damage,"[110] several studies point to the simultaneous processing of pain in the somatosensory cortex and emotion-related cerebral systems.[59,111–113] Mollet and Harrison[59] summarize the case for the application of emotional theories to the study of pain and propose that emotion may influence the processing of pain in several ways:

- Negative emotion increases pain intensity and decreases threshold and tolerance.
- Positive emotion decreases pain intensity and increases threshold and tolerance.
- Pain may produce negative emotion or increase the memory for negative emotion.

This template emphasizes the relationship between anger and pain and strongly implicates anger in the development and maintenance of chronic pain. It further highlights the role of anger management style as a critical influence in how pain is experienced.

Anger-In

In his study of emotion regulation, Gross[114] utilized a process model to illustrate two features of trait anger-in: First that, while the mechanism of suppression tends to decrease negative emotional expression, it also decreases positive emotional expression and second that although suppression has little impact on the experience of negative emotion, it tends to decrease the experience of positive emotion. In his analysis of emotion regulation, he concluded that, as a means of regulating negative emotion, cognitive appraisal is more adaptive than suppression and tends to decrease both the experience and expression of negative emotion while increasing the experience and expression of positive emotion. He added that there may be times when cognitive appraisal cannot adequately be mobilized, and suppression may be, in the moment, the best available means of regulating negative emotion, but such instances are more likely to involve evaluation in the moment of state anger. The overarching conclusion is that suppression as a trait mechanism for modulating intolerable affect is problematic.

Engel noted that inhibition of anger, whether through repression or suppression, is a common attribute among pain-prone patients, but psychoanalytic theory offered little insight into the causal relationship or cognitive, emotional, and physiologic mechanisms through which inhibited anger can affect pain.[11,31,32] More recent studies of anger-in as a form of emotional regulation confirm that suppression is a prevalent style of management among patients with chronic pain but also point to applications of Wegner's ironic process theory as a means of delineating the mechanisms involved.[31,32,115–117] According to this template, suppression of negative emotion requires the coordination of two distinct cognitive processes: The first represents a resource-dependent operating process that serves to eliminate awareness of unwanted thoughts and feelings, whereas the second represents a monitoring process that remains vigilant to the awareness of unwanted thoughts and feelings to be suppressed (Table 83.2). Under ordinary conditions, the monitor works to identify material to be suppressed, whereas the operating process performs the suppression; however, when under stress or high demand, the operating process may not have sufficient resources to perform its task. Stress, in this context, may be reflected in both cognitive and somatic symptomatology, with cognitive dissonance thwarting both suppression and cognitive appraisal and the corresponding demands on the body being expressed through cardiovascular and musculoskeletal symptoms. Burns et al.[83] reported that patients with chronic low back pain who reflect an anger-in style of management are more likely than other groups to experience high levels of muscle tension at the site of pain and injury when experiencing anger and to show relatively high systolic and diastolic blood pressure.

The irony implicit in Wegner's theory of mental processing is that, under such conditions, the monitor may be serving to bring unwanted thoughts and feelings into conscious awareness without sufficient resources for suppression to take place. The result is that unsuccessful efforts to suppress anger can paradoxically lead to heightened awareness of the cognitive and

TABLE 83.2	**Wegner's Ironic Processes Theory of Mental Control**		
Monitoring Cognitive Processes	**Setting/Circumstances**	**Operating Cognitive Processes**	**Mental Control Outcome**
Vigilance toward unwanted thoughts or reminders of previous events leading to overwhelming anger	*Stress-free* or low-stress circumstances evoking occasional or random thoughts or reminders of previous events leading to anger	Effortful, conscious attempts at suppression of or distraction from unwanted thoughts and reminders	*Successful* suppression of or distraction from monitored thoughts and reminders
	Stress-laden or high-stress circumstances evoking frequent thoughts or reminders of previous events associated with harm or an unfair slight to one's ego or identity leading to anger		*Failed* suppression of or distraction from monitored thoughts and reminders leading to preoccupation and rumination

NOTE: When the operating processes are under high stress, the monitoring processes, which ordinarily serve to identify thoughts to be suppressed, can become the source of continual unwanted reminders of events leading to overwhelming anger.

emotional experience of anger, thereby increasing sensitivity to pain and influencing subsequent perceptions and interpretations of pain according to the unsuccessfully suppressed, unwanted cognitions and intolerable affect.[31,32,116,117] Carson et al. conducted studies on constructs related to anger-in, including the construct of ambivalence of emotional expression (AEE) and the construct of forgiveness.[52,118–120] Theirs and related findings suggest that those who are ambivalent about expressing their emotions and those who cannot forgive others for perceived wrongs and insults may experience higher levels of low back pain and psychological distress, mediated by higher levels of anger. Where treatment is concerned, it is possible that psychotherapeutic interventions designed to resolve patients' ambivalence toward expressing their emotions and to encourage the development of cognitive reappraisals supportive of conciliation and forgiveness may facilitate the management of pain.

Anger-Out

Like anger-in, the emotional regulatory strategy of anger-out— managing anger directly with physical or verbal expression— has been shown repeatedly to be associated with increased responsiveness to pain and higher levels of chronic pain intensity and disability.[47,121,122] It must be noted, here, that anger-out, in this context, usually refers to the trait of immediately responding to the emotional experience of anger with expression of anger—not the same as the considered, constructive expression of anger signifying the mobilization of more mature defensive processes. Hostility and tendencies toward aggression are hallmarks of trait anger-out. Bruehl et al. have done the most complete review of anger-out studies to date and conclude that elevated trait anger-out is associated with heightened chronic pain intensity and low levels of improvement in individuals suffering from a broad range of medical conditions associated with chronic pain.[33,34,36,121] They examine a number of proposed mechanisms underlying the effects of trait anger-out on acute experimental, acute clinical, and chronic pain, but the emphasis here will be on chronic pain.

The authors submit that there is little evidence for the influence of either neuroticism or the psychoanalytic construct of repression.[121] The former—a willingness to overendorse a broad spectrum of symptoms—has sometimes led to spurious correlations between elevated pain and indicators of an anger-out style of management, but the available evidence tends to suggest that the relationship of anger-out to pain is independent of the broader palette of negative affect, including depression and anxiety. Where the latter is concerned, one might expect that trait anger-out would be negatively associated with the classic psychoanalytic constructs of conversion and somatization and therefore consistently lead to an amelioration of pain. As previously noted, however, the hostility and aggression embodied in trait anger-out do not promote the mature and adaptive expressions of anger reflecting successful management that might lead to reduced pain intensity and sensitivity. Other behavioral mechanisms have been considered, including the observation that individuals whose scores are elevated on measures of anger-out show decreased cardiovascular reactivity when encouraged to express their anger versus suppress it, and among a high anger-out group of women, verbal expression of anger during provocation was associated with improved blood pressure recovery, following the stressful event. Although there are some indications that these findings are related to improvement in situations involving acute pain, Bruehl et al.[121] point out that implications for the effect of behavioral anger expression on chronic pain have yet to be fully delineated.

Although not specifically applied to the variable of management style, Greenwood et al.[47] suggest several behavioral mechanisms that may influence the relationship between anger and pain. First, anger may foster the development of pain behaviors

associated with the negative consequences of expressing anger. The high correlation between hostility and absenteeism from work, for example, suggests that anger may contribute to the maintenance of pain-related illness. Second, the effects of anger on marital functioning may lead to spousal responses that exacerbate and maintain pain and pain behaviors. Finally, anger can impact pain by contributing to conflicts and mistrust in relationships between patients and their medical providers. Studies by Burns et al. concluded that high scorers on anger-out and hostility were correlated with patients' reports of weaker alliances with their physicians and with interference in their abilities to improve with pain management.[36,123,124]

Proposed mechanisms underlying the relationship of anger-out and pain have also included a number of physiologically based models.[121] Anger-out has been associated with greater visceral adipose tissue in some studies, a potential source of impact on lower spine mechanics. Like anger-in, anger-out has also been found to be correlated with increases in stress-induced muscle tension among patients with low back pain. Neither of these models, however, can account for the effects of anger-out on acute pain responsiveness and sensitivity. Genetic mechanisms have been suggested as well, but Bruehl et al.[121] assert that none has been adequately investigated, to date, despite promising connections with genetic factors related to personality traits, emotional reactivity, and endogenous opioid system functioning. A related mechanism, referred to as "trait X," suggests that high anger-out individuals express their anger because they believe it is beneficial and it feels better to discharge it than the alternative. The idea is that behaviorally expressing anger for high anger-out individuals actually reduces arousal and restores emotional and physiologic homeostasis more efficiently. The authors comment that trait X state interactions may well reflect some degree of functional regulatory benefit, especially in the immediate aftermath of expressing anger, but the more enduring trait anger dimension has yet to be sufficiently investigated.

Opioid Deficit Hypothesis and the Role of Endogenous Opioid Functioning

Bruehl, in collaboration with others, has also called attention to the role of endogenous opioid dysfunction in the relationship between anger-out and pain.[28,30,121,122,125–131] The essential premise is that mechanisms associated with anger-out may impose an excessive burden or strain on the body's ability to produce endogenous opioids, inhibiting the natural management of chronic pain. Bruehl et al. conducted studies in which subjects with low scores in anger-out reported increased acute pain intensity following opioid blockade with naloxone versus following placebo blockade, whereas subjects high in anger-out reported smaller naloxone blockade effects.[28,30] The implication is that there is less effective endogenous opioid response among those who score high in anger-out, with opioid dysfunction partially mediating the positive correlation between anger-out and chronic pain intensity.[122]

Burns and Bruehl[126] further established that the use of exogenous opioid analgesics remediates opioid deficits such that anger-out is related to chronic pain severity only among patients not taking opioid medications. The results suggest that regular use of opioid medications among those who are high in anger expression may compensate for overtaxed endogenous opioid mechanisms. In another, related study, Bruehl et al.[122] investigated whether impaired central opioid inhibitory functioning, assessed via changes in plasma β-endorphin release, could explain exaggerated pain responsiveness and anger expression in high anger-out subjects. As with the opioid blockade studies and the study of the mediating effects of exogenous opioids, the results of this pain-induced endogenous opioid release study support the opioid deficit hypothesis and demonstrate that greater trait anger-out is associated with higher perceived pain intensity and less endogenous opioid release.

Taken together, these studies provide strong evidence for the idea that patients whose anger management style involves physical and verbal expression show comparative deficits in opioid analgesia because of endogenous opioid dysfunction. Bruehl et al. have taken this one step further with the opioid triggering hypothesis, suggesting that, for individuals high in anger-out, the dramatic expression of anger serves to activate endogenous opioid response that would otherwise remain quiescent when anger associated with pain and stress is either not expressed or only moderately expressed.[121,128–130] Those who are low in anger-out appear to elicit a sufficient endogenous opioid response without expressing their anger, but the expression of anger among high anger-out individuals may actually represent an adaptive mechanism designed to trigger the release of endogenous opioids. Patients high in anger-out may therefore have a higher threshold for the activation of endogenous opioid response, with the increased arousal of dramatic anger expression serving as a triggering mechanism.

Measurement of Anger

Anger, both state and trait, as well as the related constructs of aggression, hostility, and anger management style have been assessed for research purposes with a broad spectrum of tools, ranging from projective tests, like the Rorschach and thematic apperception test (TAT), to physiologic measures principally associated with autonomic arousal.[55,132] Self-report questionnaires and inventories tend to predominate in anger-related research, however, both for their ease of administration and for their more readily documented validity and reliability.

Several of the self-report instruments measuring anger that are more widely utilized or particularly suited to pain research are reviewed in the following discussion. Extensive commentary on each, as well as critical reviews of many instruments designed to measure some aspect of anger, are available in *Tests in Print VII*[133] and the *The Seventeenth Mental Measurements Yearbook, 17th ed.*[134] The instruments discussed in the following text are summarized in Table 83.3.

STATE-TRAIT ANGER EXPRESSION INVENTORY-2

The State-Trait Anger Expression Inventory-2 (STAXI-2) was developed by Spielberger and is widely regarded as the most psychometrically sound and comprehensive tool in the assessment of anger and hostility.[55,105,135] It represents the integration and culmination of several precursors developed by Spielberger, including the State-Trait Anger Scale (STAS), the Anger Expression Scale (AES), and the first version of the STAXI-2. The instrument consists of six scales: Trait Anger, Anger Expression-Out, Anger Expression-In, Anger Control-Out, Anger Control-In, and State Anger as well as five subscales and an Anger Expression Index. It can be administered in 5 to 10 minutes and is scored by hand, making it practical for clinical applications as well as research. The STAXI-2 purports to measure tendencies toward angry action, as well as more dispositional or trait-based hostility, along with tendencies to suppress or express the experience of anger. This makes the inventory well suited for research in anger management styles and clinically well adapted to assess the needs of patients for psychotherapeutic applications of anger management. Normative data are published for adolescents, adults, and psychiatric patients, and evidence for high reliability and validity are detailed in the testing manual.

TABLE 83.3	Instruments Designed to Assess Anger		
Instrument	**Format**	**Administration**	**Availability**
State-Trait Anger Expression Inventory (STAXI-2)	57 items distributed across 6 scales, 5 subscales, and an anger expression index; ages 16 years and up	5–10 min; scored by hand	PAR: Psychological Assessment Resources Inc (www4.parinc.com)
Targets and Reasons for Anger in Pain Sufferers (TRAPS)	10-point Likert scale assessing degree or intensity of anger toward a variety of common objects of anger (e.g., self, significant others, employer, physician) and 10 common reasons for anger	10–20 min for an interactive administration; has been adapted for briefer self-administration; scored by hand	Fernandez E, Salinas N, Swift P, et al. Psychosocial factors that predict anger in chronic pain sufferers. *Ann Behav Med* 1995;17:S164. Fernandez E, Salinas N, Swift P, et al. Psychosocial factors that predict anger in chronic pain sufferers. Paper presented at: Sixteenth Annual Scientific Meeting of the Society of Behavioral Medicine; 1995; San Diego. (Used with permission of primary author.)
Multidimensional Anger Inventory (MAI)	30-item instrument, with multiple variations, assessing the duration, frequency, and magnitude of anger, including differentiation between anger-in and anger-out expression and common situations leading to anger	10–20 min; scored by hand	Siegel JM. The multidimensional anger inventory. *J Pers Soc Psychol* 1986;51:191–200. (Used with permission of author.)
Novaco Anger Scale and Provocation Inventory (NAS-PI)	60 items distributed across 3 subscales (cognitive, arousal, behavioral) plus a 25-item inventory eliciting responses to specific situations	25 min; scored by hand	WPS: Western Psychological Services (www.wpspublish.com/app/)
Anger Disorders Scale (ADS)	70 items distributed over 5 categories (provocations, cognitions, arousal, motives, behaviors)	Short form, 5–10 min; long form, 10–20 min; scored by hand or software	MHS: Multi-Health Systems Inc (http://www.mhs.com)
Minnesota Multiphasic Personality Inventory-2-Restructured Form (MMPI-2-RF)	338 true–false items distributed across multiple validity and clinical scales, with multiple scales assessing some aspect of anger, hostility, or aggression	35–50 min; scored by hand or software	Pearson Inc (http://www.pearson clinical.com)

THE TARGETS AND REASONS FOR ANGER IN PAIN SUFFERERS

Although the STAXI-2 is applied to the study of pain more frequently than other inventories of anger, it was not designed for use with chronic pain patients and does not assess specifically pain-related dimensions of anger. Fernandez[55] developed a structured inventory, the Targets and Reasons for Anger in Pain Sufferers (TRAPS), later adapted for self-administration by Okifuji et al.,[136] that allows chronic pain patients to rate their levels of anger on a Likert-type scale toward a variety of common objects or targets of their anger: whole world, self, God/destiny, significant other, employer, insurance company, attorney or legal system, health care providers, and person who caused the accident. Patients may also be instructed to identify and rank their reasons for being angry toward these targets. The results, especially when the TRAPS is administered in a structured interview, allow clinicians and patients to explore together the relative importance of specific targets of and reasons for anger, suggesting interventions and strategies for reducing the impact of anger on pain. Normative data and information on reliability and validity are not yet available.

MULTIDIMENSIONAL ANGER INVENTORY

Siegel developed the Multidimensional Anger Inventory (MAI) as a brief instrument designed to assess responses to anger-eliciting situations in an attempt to increase sensitivity to the multidimensional nature of the construct.[55] Factor analytic solutions arrived at the following dimensions or factors: anger arousal, hostile outlook, range of anger-eliciting situations, and anger expression, the last being divided into anger-in and anger-out. Although it was developed specifically to assess anger in cardiovascular patients, factor analytic replications in more heterogeneous populations suggest its utility on a broader scope, especially with other health-related groups. Reliability and scale validity information are available through the author's report.[137]

NOVACO ANGER SCALE AND PROVOCATION INVENTORY

This inventory, developed by Novaco,[138] consists of two principal sections: The Novaco Anger Scale (NAS) purports to measure the general inclination toward reacting with anger, whereas the Provocation Inventory (PI) asks patients to respond to descriptions of specific situations that tend to elicit anger. The NAS contains 60 items divided equally over three subscales: (1) a cognitive subscale, measuring anger justification, rumination, hostile attitude, and suspicion; (2) an arousal subscale, measuring anger intensity, duration, somatic tension, and irritability; and (3) a behavior subscale, measuring impulsive reaction, verbal aggression, physical confrontation, and direct expression. The PI contains 25 items, each describing a situation that tends to elicit anger, with subjects being instructed to rate their degree of anger or annoyance on a 5-point Likert-type scale. The situations include scenarios such as "getting your car stuck in the mud or sand" and "being joked about or teased." The items are grouped into five subscales summarizing the theme of the provocation: disrespectful treatment, unfairness, frustration, annoying traits of others, and irritations. The Novaco Anger Scale and Provocation Inventory (NAS-PI) attempts to characterize how an individual experiences anger and what sorts of situations provoke it. The instrument has been widely used to evaluate the role of anger in diverse environments, from community based to correctional settings, and may prove useful in evaluating the role of anger in health care settings. Normative data, reliability, and validity are well documented in the testing manual.[138]

ANGER DISORDERS SCALE

The Anger Disorders Scale (ADS) is a self-report instrument consisting of 70 items distributed over five categories characterizing human emotion: provocations, cognitions, arousal, motives, and behaviors.[139] A short form consisting of only 18 items may be used as a screening tool to obtain scores on three factors: reactivity/expression, anger-in, and vengeance.[140] The ADS is designed to assess and identify dimensions of anger that are associated with dysfunction and impairment in clinical populations. It yields information concerning the duration that an individual stays angry, the breadth of stimuli that may serve as triggers for an individual's anger, and the frequency of angry episodes. Information on reliability and concurrent and discriminative validity are available in the testing manual.

MINNESOTA MULTIPHASIC PERSONALITY INVENTORY-2-RESTRUCTURED FORM

The MMPI-2-RF is a 338-item, true–false, self-report instrument designed to assess a broad range of psychopathology and personality traits and characteristics.[24,25] It is arguably the best known and most widely used psychometric assessment tool available, and it and its predecessors, the MMPI and MMPI-2, have been applied to the investigation of pain in hundreds of empirical studies.[15] Several MMPI-2-RF scales are relevant to the study of anger and its relationship to pain, with all scales relating to anger being well validated and designed to reflect some aspect of trait anger (e.g., anger proneness [ANP] and aggressiveness, revised [AGGR-r] scales).

Psychotherapeutic Management

When anger and problems with the management of anger are aspects of a patient's presentation with chronic pain, ignoring the indication for psychotherapeutic intervention may well jeopardize any chance of successfully treating or managing his or her pain.[141] As we have seen, trait anger and certain styles of anger management are fertile ground for the development of chronic pain, but anger may emerge as a critical factor in response to chronic pain as well. The following case of a middle-aged patient with chronic headaches will serve to illustrate the mutually influential roles of anger and pain in the context of treatment.

Case 2: Mr. Alvarez was a 45-year-old single man, referred to the Pain Center by his new primary care physician and his new neurologist for the treatment of long-standing chronic daily headaches with tension-type and migrainous features. He arrived for his initial evaluation more than an hour late but loudly insisted upon being seen, saying that the traffic was not his fault and that he had a severe headache requiring immediate attention. He was irritable in his exchanges with support staff and paced back and forth in the waiting area, to the discomfiture and consternation of other patients. When he was finally escorted to an examination room, he informed the nurse that he hoped he did not have to wait long to see the physician. Once his pain physician joined him for the evaluation, he seemed deferential and cooperative, as he related his medical history and the history of his headaches. His physician noted, however, that he expressed considerable anger toward previous providers, toward his wife and children, and toward his employer, none of whom, according to the patient, responded with adequate sympathy to his distress or provided any respite from his pain. As his physician rose to conclude the interview, the patient looked at the prescriptions he had been given as a first line of intervention and, tossing them onto the desk, said, "I didn't come here for more pills. I told you, I came for Botox injections, and I'm not leaving here without them." When it was explained that authorization from his insurance carrier had to be obtained and that he might well respond favorably to a less invasive procedure, the patient's anger became increasingly confrontational. When it became clear that he was not going to get what he wished, he vociferously decried "the incompetence of doctors" and stormed from the examining room, upsetting a chair and waste bin in the process.

In the succeeding days, as the patient's stricken pain physician consulted with Mr. Alvarez's referring providers and assembled his medical records, several points became clear. This was not the patient's only reported angry exchange in health care settings and, indeed, it appeared that Mr. Alvarez frequently changed primary care physicians and specialists, whether by his own decision or mutual agreement.

It was a surprise when Mr. Alvarez made and kept a follow-up appointment but less surprising when the outcome was much the same, with the patient discharging his anger and frustration toward staff and his pain physician. It was at the conclusion of his second appointment that he was referred to the pain psychologist to do biofeedback and learn relaxation techniques. This puzzled but did not threaten him because the physiologic benefit of treatment was emphasized, and he was affable enough during the initial visit and anamnesis, which revealed much about the relationship between his anger and his pain. He exhibited many of the behavioral mechanisms, previously mentioned, through which anger can exercise influence over pain.[47] His anger toward his employer led to frequent arguments and resulting exacerbations of his headaches, in turn resulting in high absenteeism, which led to further conflicts at work. His anger toward his wife frequently led to retaliation in various forms on her part, which, again, resulted in exacerbations of his pain and the development of pain behaviors designed both to justify his disability and to elicit sympathy. Finally, his anger in the medical setting led to inconsistent and poorly planned care that, in turn, thwarted his attempts to gain relief, allowing his headache and associated behavioral patterns to become firmly entrenched.

It was nevertheless an unexpected development to Mr. Alvarez when the pain psychologist suggested that his anger may be exerting a dramatic impact on his headaches. The patient characterized himself as "quick to anger but quick to get over it" and cited trends within his family of origin, especially his own parents, to be dramatically expressive of anger. He added with irony, "I thought that's what you psychologists were always saying—'to get it off my chest and not hold it in.'" He portrayed himself honestly and clearly as a high anger-out individual, a style of anger management shown repeatedly to be associated with increased responsiveness to pain and higher levels of pain intensity and disability.[34,36,47,52,103,121,122] In addition to doing biofeedback training and learning relaxation techniques, the goal of psychotherapy in this second case was to encourage the patient to adopt and practice more adaptive strategies for anger management. Neither Mr. Alvarez's anger-out style nor Ms. Ostrakova's anger-in style, depicted in the first case, was conducive to the successful management of their chronic pain.

CONSIDERATIONS IN THE SELECTION OF PSYCHOTHERAPY

Where the special practice of pain psychology is concerned, supportive and psychoanalytically informed psychotherapies have been viewed as useful in the management of pain, primarily when behavioral and cognitive-behavioral treatments have failed to bring relief.[142,143] The psychodynamic approach may nevertheless be a logical starting point for patients whose anger, pain, and disability are sustained by intrapsychic conflicts or unconscious motives associated with childhood trauma or primary or secondary gain.[141,144] The drawbacks associated with pursuing such a course of treatment can be manifold, but there may be times when patients are unable to move forward until they are satisfied that their conflicts and motives are revealed and understood. A problem for the successful management of pain, however, is that psychotherapies focusing on the primacy of the experience of emotion are typically long term and may require many months, if not years, to result in meaningful insight and progress. Such treatments, at least near their outset, can also lead patients to an uncritical acceptance

of their feelings, further validating the experience of negative emotions such as anger; therefore, the selection of appropriate psychotherapy and the skill of the psychotherapist are perhaps most critical in cases where a psychodynamic or supportive approach is indicated.

If the principal obstacles to successful adjustment to chronic pain are factors, such as anger management style and negative cognitions underlying anger and hostility, then a more direct approach to treatment would be to challenge the behaviors reflecting and maintaining anger as well as the negative cognitions driving it. Challenging established behaviors with new, more adaptive ones is the goal of behavioral therapy, whereas identifying, examining, and restructuring the negative cognitions behind negative emotions is the work of cognitive therapy. Both are well established as offering greater efficacy in the implementation of change and the modulation of the effects of anger on chronic pain, but both depend on the patient's willingness to collaborate with treatment and his or her readiness for and motivation to change.[141,145,146]

The influence of any psychosocial risk factor, such as trait anger and hostility, may signal reluctance on the part of the patient to give up his or her pain and suffering or relinquish the refuge of disability.[141] In the first case study, Ms. Ostrakova complained of pain, but her symptoms were driven by powerful and enduring unconscious conflicts associated with her history of childhood trauma and abuse. The high correlations between histories of abuse and the subsequent development of difficulties with both anger and chronic pain are well documented in the psychoanalytic and scientific literatures.[11,42,147-156] For patients who have suffered abuse as children or who have been exposed as adults to situations involving catastrophic loss or harm, chronic pain may come to represent a means of psychologically symbolizing and organizing unbearable memories and intolerable affects.[141] In Ms. Ostrakova's case, coming to an understanding of the relationship between her history and the development of her symptoms may well represent an essential step toward taking an active role in her treatment, and the selection of treatment to facilitate this step is likely to involve a form of supportive and psychodynamic psychotherapy. Ironically, a year of inpatient treatment with behavioral and cognitive-behavioral interventions appears only to have altered the patient's style of anger management from anger-out to anger-in.

Investigators have found that patients vary widely regarding how prepared they are to collaborate in their own treatment and make the changes necessary to manage their anger and their pain more effectively. Assessing a patient's *readiness to change* is frequently a critical prelude to effective psychotherapeutic intervention and may shed insight into why some patients never seem to improve. Cognitive therapy often begins with the patient's response to two questions: What do you want (to change)? What are you willing to do to get it?[141,151] The first question is easy for most patients with chronic pain, but the second implies work and sacrifice and is not so easy when patients are prone to anger and preoccupied with their own suffering and deprivation. Assessing a patient's readiness for change is one way of answering the second question.

Kerns et al. applied Prochaska's transtheoretical model of the stages of change to the situation of chronic pain and arrived at four successive levels in patients' willingness to collaborate with treatment and undertake the behavioral changes necessary to manage their pain more effectively[157-160]:

- *Precontemplation*: patients who have no intention of changing their current patterns of behavior—"You're the doctor. Fix my pain!"
- *Contemplation*: patients who have begun to recognize the necessity of making changes in their behavior but have not yet committed to doing so—"I know it's up to me. I just don't know how to do it."

- *Action*: patients who have committed to a plan of action and are engaged in making changes—"I'm doing something about my pain."
- *Maintenance*: patients who are attempting to sustain the changes they have undertaken—"I'm using what I've learned in treatment to manage my pain better."

Angry and hostile patients, in particular, may be stuck in the precontemplative stage of readiness for change, and their often unrealistic expectations of their physicians may lead them to feel that effective treatment is being withheld. This was the case with Mr. Alvarez, whose anger was driven by his disappointment in providers who never seemed willing to do enough to help him manage his pain. Unlike Ms. Ostrakova, however, his style of managing anger did not reflect defensive inhibition of affect, and his chronic pain was not associated with unconscious conflicts. His anger, although more volatile, also proved more tractable to the psychoeducational component of cognitive therapy, and he was ultimately able to make the transition more easily from the precontemplative to the contemplative stage of readiness for change.

BEHAVIORAL AND COGNITIVE-BEHAVIORAL THERAPIES

Templates for behavioral and cognitive-behavioral intervention in cases of chronic pain are offered in succeeding chapters, but it is instructive to note that their number and applications have burgeoned in recent years, largely through the proliferation of acceptance and commitment therapy (ACT), contextual cognitive-behavioral therapy (CCBT), mindfulness-based stress reduction (MBSR), and mindfulness-based cognitive therapies (MBCT) as well as mindfulness-based behavioral techniques, such as meditation.[161-165]

Behavioral approaches to the treatment of anger have tended to revolve around relaxation training and applications of relaxation techniques to reducing autonomic arousal and uncomfortable musculoskeletal tension. Suinn's template for anxiety/anger management training (AMT) represents one of the more enduring expressions of this form of treatment.[166,167] He proposes a brief, structured therapy involving six to eight sessions in which guided imagery directed toward arousing anger is subsequently and serially paired with relaxation techniques designed to deactivate arousal. Patients are first instructed in the elicitation of the body's natural relaxation response—which can be accomplished using meditation, progressive muscle relaxation, body scans or other forms of autogenic training, or diaphragmatic breathing techniques—and, once they have mastered this, the psychotherapist offers structured practice in the use of the technique to contain or defuse sympathetic nervous system reactivity cued by suggestions and visualizations of stressful images. The use of biofeedback technology in the assessment of progress can frequently hasten mastery of this strategy by presenting the patient with tangible evidence of progress.

Fernandez proposes that if the injury or perceived injustice resulting in chronic pain—whether physical or psychological in origin—cannot be altered or undone, then switching the focus to what can be changed becomes the logical object of therapy. What can be changed is the way the patient with chronic pain construes what has transpired.[168,169] Recall that in Lazarus's[96] cognitive appraisal theory of emotion, the experience of anger is the joint effect of (1) the event of physiologic arousal and (2) the cognitive appraisal of its meaning. Whereas much of behavioral therapy directed toward the management of anger is concerned with the former, cognitive therapy is directed toward the latter. As we have seen, anger, by Smedslund's definition, involves the appraisal by the subject that he or she—or a person for whom he or she cares—has been treated without respect.[94] This, of course, may actually be the case in a given situation and therein lies the foundation of the biologic basis for anger,[67,68,114] but anger, as our Greco-Roman and Judeo-Christian roots attest, does not necessarily conform to logic. The experience of anger can quickly and easily become associated with irrational, automatic thoughts and beliefs concerning the motives of others and the sources of threat to our well-being.

The approach of cognitive therapy is to offer a corrective process to the development and maintenance of errors in our thinking and beliefs.[55,141,161,164,170-173] Through the process of cognitive restructuring or reappraisal, patients are led to examine whether, in the process of trying to make sense of their anger and pain, they may be making fundamental errors in their thinking and relying on mistaken beliefs. Patients are encouraged to challenge their automatic thoughts and uncritically held beliefs regarding their experiences of anger through the template of cognitive appraisal theory—that is, that situations are ordinarily neutral until we assign meaning to them. We are often unaware of this step of assigning meaning because we do not usually stop to examine the thoughts and beliefs that influence our emotional responses to certain situations, and even when we do, we may not consider the accuracy of these thoughts and beliefs. The essence of the cognitive model of treatment suggests that much of our emotional distress and self-defeating behavior is based simply on inaccurate and irrational thinking and that once our attention is drawn to these upsetting cognitions, we can test their veracity and value to see whether they form an appropriate basis for our emotions and behavior.

As they learn to identify negative cognitions, patients begin to monitor their cognitive appraisals more rigorously and critically, cognitively restructuring their primary and secondary appraisals of situations resulting in anger. Common reappraisals of the experience of anger might include reexamining the intention of the one toward whom our anger is directed, reconsidering the harm done by the perceived slight or insult, or reinterpreting the outcome of a situation to determine whether a perceived breach of respect actually resulted in harm or injury.[55] Fernandez's proposed cognitive-behavioral affective therapy (CBAT) serves as a model of integrative treatment for anger in the context of chronic pain because it combines behavioral and affective interventions for self-soothing while the patient undertakes the cognitively challenging work of restructuring his or her appraisals of what has transpired.[168,169] These behavioral and affective techniques target the feelings of distress inherent in the experience of anger, providing both support and respite as the often difficult and taxing work of the cognitive therapy progresses.

In the case of Mr. Alvarez, he was taught meditation as a means of assuaging his sometimes high, reactive affect, although several negative cognitions were identified as being based on dysfunctional family-of-origin models and overrehearsed expression. His primary negative cognition—"Everyone is out to take advantage of me"—may have reflected some degree of utility in the gang-controlled streets of his childhood barrio, but it was dysfunctional and even harmful in the medical setting, where his physicians and other providers were genuinely concerned to help him. Their response to his anger was to defend themselves by disengaging and retreating, often to the detriment of his care. A corollary negative cognition—"No one will help you voluntarily; you have to demand what you need from people"—was equally destructive of the medical alliance. Through cognitive reappraisal and the opportunity to test different interpretations, the patient ultimately proved to himself that people, especially people whose job is to take care of him, really are often willing to help and that consistently making demands of others tends to result in less return than welcoming their responses to reasonable requests. Mr. Alvarez's anger-out style, once a barrier to his receiving the best from his medical care, receded and was replaced by a more genuinely collaborative attitude toward his physicians.

Summary

The cultural background of anger lays the groundwork for understanding its role both as an emotion and as a trait, as well as its relationship to pain. Psychoanalytic theory emphasized the harmful effects of inhibiting the experience and expression of anger, placing it at the core of conflicts between competing drives and the formation of pathologic symptoms. More recent research has brought additional clarity to the relationship between anger and pain, suggesting a number of possible mechanisms through which state and trait anger can influence sensitivity to pain and the development and maintenance of chronic pain. This trend, in turn, has led to improved objective psychological measures of anger and the observation that style of anger management may be a principal modulating factor in the relationship between anger and pain. Anger management style has become a critical consideration in the development of effective psychotherapeutic treatments for anger-related psychopathology, with behavioral and cognitive therapies for anger often resulting in improved management of chronic pain.

References

1. Aristotle. *Rhetoric*. Roberts WR, trans. Whitefish, MT: Kessinger Press; 2004:54–63.
2. Seneca. *Moral and Political Essays*. Procope JF, ed. Cooper JM, trans. Cambridge, United Kingdom: Cambridge University Press; 1995:17.
3. Kemp S, Strongman KT. Anger theory and management: a historical analysis. *Am J Psychol* 1995;108:397–417.
4. Thurman RAF. *Anger*. New York: Oxford University Press; 2005.
5. Freud S. On psycho-analysis. In: Strachey J, trans-ed. *Complete Psychological Works*. Vol 12. Standard ed. London: Hogarth Press; 1958:209. (Original work published 1913.)
6. Breuer J, Freud S. Studies on hysteria. In: Strachey J, ed, trans. *Complete Psychological Works*. Vol 2. standard ed. London: Hogarth Press; 1955. (Original work published 1893–1895.)
7. Merskey H. History of psychoanalytic ideas concerning pain. In: Gatchel RJ, Weisberg JN, eds. *Personality Characteristics of Patients with Pain*. Washington, DC: American Psychological Association; 2000:25–35.
8. Freud S. Mourning and melancholia. In: Strachey J, ed, trans. *Complete Psychological Works*. Vol 14. standard ed. London: Hogarth Press; 1957. (Original work published 1917.)
9. Freud S. Beyond the pleasure principle. In: Strachey J, trans-ed. *Complete Psychological Works*. Vol 18. Standard ed. London: Hogarth Press; 1955. (Original work published 1920.)
10. Freud S. Inhibitions, symptoms, and anxiety. In: Strachey J, trans-ed. *Complete Psychological Works*. Vol 20. Standard ed. London: Hogarth Press; 1959. (Original work published 1926.)
11. Engel GL. "Psychogenic" pain and the pain-prone patient. *Am J Med* 1959;26:899–918.
12. Szasz TS. *Pain and Pleasure: A Study of Bodily Feelings*. London: Tavistock; 1957.
13. Burns JW. Repression predicts outcome following multidisciplinary treatment of chronic pain. *Health Psychol* 2000;19:75–84.
14. Burns JW. Repression in chronic pain: an idea worth recovering. *Appl Prev Psychol* 2000;9:173–190.
15. Keller LS, Butcher JN. *Assessment of Chronic Pain Patients with the MMPI-2*. Minneapolis, MN: University of Minnesota Press; 1991.
16. Tarescavage AM, Scheman J, Ben-Porath YS. Reliability and validity of the Minnesota Multiphasic Personality Inventory-2-Restructured Form (MMPI-2-RF) in evaluations of chronic low back pain patients. *Psychol Assess* 2015;27:433–446.
17. Butcher JN. *MMPI-2: A Practitioner's Guide*. Washington, DC: American Psychological Association; 2005.
18. Graham JR. *MMPI-2: Assessing Personality and Psychopathology*. New York: Oxford University Press; 2005.
19. Vendrig AA. The Minnesota Multiphasic Personality Inventory and chronic pain: a conceptual analysis of a longstanding but complicated relationship. *Clin Psychol Rev* 2000;20:533–559.
20. Schlessinger D. MMPI-2 characteristics in a chronic pain population. *Assessment* 2002;9:406–414.
21. Block AR, Ben-Porath YS, Marek RJ. Psychological risk factors for poor outcome of spine surgery and spinal cord stimulator implant: a review of the literature and their assessment with the MMPI-2-RF. *Clin Neuropsychol* 2013;27:81–107.
22. Block AR, Marek RJ, Ben-Porath YS, et al. Associations between pre-implant psychosocial factors and spinal cord stimulation outcome: evaluation using the MMPI-2-RF. *Assessment* 2017;24:60–70.
23. Kato F, Abe T, Kanbara K, et al. Pain threshold reflects psychological traits in patients with chronic pain: a cross-sectional study. *Biopsychosoc Med* 2017;11:13.
24. Ben-Porath YS. *Interpreting the MMPI-2-RF*. Minneapolis, MN: University of Minnesota Press; 2012.
25. Friedman AF, Bolinskey PK. *Psychological Assessment with the MMPI-2/MMPI-2-RF*. 3rd ed. New York: Routledge; 2015.
26. Thomas ML, Youngjohn JR. Let's not get hysterical: comparing the MMPI-2 validity, clinical, and RC scales in TBI litigants tested for effort. *Clin Neuropsychol* 2009;23:1067–1084.
27. Janssen SA, Spinhoven P, Brosschot JF. Experimentally induced anger, cardiovascular reactivity, and pain sensitivity. *J Psychosom Res* 2001;51:479–485.
28. Bruehl S, Burns JW, Chung OY, et al. Anger and pain-sensitivity in chronic low back pain patients and pain-free controls: the role of endogenous opioids. *Pain* 2002;99:223–233.
29. Bruehl S, Chung OY, Burns JW. Differential effects of expressive anger regulation on chronic pain intensity in CRPS and non-CRPS limb pain patients. *Pain* 2003;104:647–654.
30. Bruehl S, Chung OY, Burns JW, et al. The association between anger expression and chronic pain intensity: evidence for partial mediation by endogenous opioid dysfunction. *Pain* 2003;106:317–324.
31. Quartana PJ, Burns JW. Painful consequences of anger suppression. *Emotion* 2007;7:400–414.
32. Quartana PJ, Yoon KL, Burns JW. Anger suppression, ironic processes, and pain. *J Behav Med* 2007;30:455–469.
33. Bruehl S, Liu X, Burns JW, et al. Associations between daily chronic pain intensity, daily anger expression, and trait anger expressiveness: an ecological momentary assessment study. *Pain* 2012;153:2352–2358.
34. Burns JW, Gerhart JI, Bruehl S, et al. Anger arousal and behavioral anger regulation in everyday life among patients with chronic low back pain: relationships to patient pain and function. *Health Psychol* 2015;34:547–555.
35. Sturgeon JA, Dixon EA, Darnall BD, et al. Contributions of physical function and satisfaction with social roles to emotional distress in chronic pain: a Collaborative Health Outcomes Information Registry (CHOIR) study. *Pain* 2015;156:2627–2633.
36. Burns JW, Gerhart JI, Bruehl S, et al. Anger arousal and behavioral anger regulation in everyday life among people with chronic low back pain: relationships with spouse responses and negative affect. *Health Psychol* 2016;35:29–40.
37. Ricci A, Bonini S, Continanza M, et al. Worry and anger rumination in fibromyalgia syndrome. *Reumatismo* 2016;68:195–198.
38. Engel GL. The psychoanalytic approach to psychosomatic medicine. In: Marmor J, ed. *Modern Psychoanalysis: New Directions and Perspectives*. Piscataway, NJ: Transaction Publishers; 1995:251–273. (Original work published 1968.)
39. Taylor GJ. Somatization and conversion: distinct or overlapping constructs? *J Am Acad Psychoanal Dyn Psychiatry* 2003;31:487–508.
40. Silber TJ. Somatization disorders: diagnosis, treatment, and prognosis. *Pediatr Rev* 2011;32:56–63.
41. Wong WS, Fielding R. Suppression of emotion expression mediates the effects of negative affect on pain catastrophizing: a cross-sectional analysis. *Clin J Pain* 2013;29:865–872.
42. Adler RH, Zlot S, Hürny C, et al. Engel's "psychogenic pain and the pain-prone patient": a retrospective, controlled clinical study. *Psychosom Med* 1989;51:87–101.
43. Robinson ME, Riley JL. The role of emotion in pain. In: Gatchel RJ, Turk DC, eds. *Psychosocial Factors in Pain: Critical Perspectives*. New York: Guilford Press; 1999:74–88.
44. Melzack R. From the gate to the neuromatrix. *Pain* 1999;82(suppl 6):S121–S126.
45. Melzack R. Pain and the neuromatrix in the brain. *J Dent Educ* 2001;65:1378–1382.
46. Melzack R. Evolution of the neuromatrix theory of pain. *Pain Pract* 2005;5:85–94.
47. Greenwood KA, Thurston R, Rumble M, et al. Anger and persistent pain: current status and future directions. *Pain* 2003;103:1–5.
48. Melzack R, Katz J. Pain. *Wiley Interdisc Rev Cogn Sci* 2013;4:1–15.
49. Moayedi M, Davis KD. Theories of pain: from specificity to gate control. *J Neurophysiol* 2013;109:5–12.
50. Mendell LM. Constructing and deconstructing the gate theory of pain. *Pain* 2014;155:210–216.
51. Cárdenas FR. The neuromatrix and its importance in pain neurobiology [article in Spanish]. *Invest Clin* 2015;56:109–110.
52. McDermott KA, Smith HL, Matheny NL, et al. Pain and multiple facets of anger and hostility in a sample seeking treatment for problematic anger. *Psychiatry Res* 2017;253:311–317.
53. Cacioppo JT, Bernston GG, Klein DJ, et al. The psychophysiology of emotion across the lifespan. *Annu Rev Gerontol Geriatr* 1997;17:27–74.
54. Fernandez E, Turk DC. The scope and significance of anger in the experience of chronic pain. *Pain* 1995;61:165–175.
55. Fernandez E. *Anxiety, Depression, and Anger in Pain: Research Findings and Clinical Options*. Dallas, TX: Advanced Psychological Resources; 2002.
56. Nusslock R, Miller GE. Early-life adversity and physical and emotional health across the lifespan: a neuroimmune network hypothesis. *Biol Psychiatry* 2016;80:23–32.

57. Hostinar CE, Nusslock R, Miller GE. Future directions in the study of early-life stress and physical and emotional health: implications of the neuroimmune network hypothesis. *J Clin Child Adolesc Psychol* 2018;47:142–156.

58. Banks SM, Kerns RD. Explaining high rates of depression in chronic pain: a diathesis-stress framework. *Psychol Bull* 1996;119:95–110.

59. Mollet GA, Harrison DW. Emotion and pain: a functional cerebral systems integration. *Neuropsychol Rev* 2006;16:99–121.

60. Mico JA, Ardid D, Berrocoso E, et al. Antidepressants and pain. *Trends Pharmacol Sci* 2006;27:348–354.

61. Maizels M, McCarberg B. Antidepressants and antiepileptic drugs for chronic pain. *Am Fam Physician* 2005;71:483–490.

62. Gebhardt S, Heinzel-Gutenbrunner M, König U. Pain relief in depressive disorders: a meta-analysis of the effects of antidepressants. *J Clin Psychopharmacol* 2016;36:658–668.

63. Sheng J, Liu S, Wang Y, et al. The link between depression and chronic pain: neural mechanisms in the brain. *Neural Plast* 2017;2017:9724371.

64. Hagelberg N, Forssell H, Aalto S, et al. Altered dopamine D2 receptor binding in atypical facial pain. *Pain* 2003;106:43–48.

65. Hagelberg N, Jääskeläinen SK, Martikainen IK, et al. Striatal dopamine D2 receptors in modulation of pain in humans: a review. *Eur J Pharmacol* 2004;500:187–192.

66. Field T, Hernandez-Reif M, Diego M, et al. Cortisol decreases and serotonin and dopamine increase following massage therapy. *Int J Neurosci* 2005;115:1397–1413.

67. Wood PB. Stress and dopamine: implications for the pathophysiology of chronic widespread pain. *Med Hypotheses* 2004;62:420–424.

68. Lara DR, Akiskal HS. Toward an integrative model of the spectrum of mood, behavioral and personality disorders based on fear and anger traits: II. Implications for neurobiology, genetics and psychopharmacological treatment. *J Affect Disord* 2006;94:89–103.

69. Salamone JD, Correa M, Mingote SM, et al. Beyond the reward hypothesis: alternative functions of nucleus accumbens dopamine. *Curr Opin Pharmacol* 2005;5:34–41.

70. Svrakic DM, Cloninger R. Classification of personality disorders: implications for treatment and research. In: Soares JC, Gershon S. eds. *Handbook of Medical Psychiatry*. New York: Marcel Dekker Inc; 2003:117–148.

71. Joyce PR, McHugh PC, Light KJ, et al. Relationships between angry-impulsive personality traits and genetic polymorphisms of the dopamine transporter. *Biol Psychiatry* 2009;66:717–721.

72. Janssen SA. Negative affect and sensitization to pain. *Scand J Psychol* 2002;43:131–137.

73. Burns JW, Bruehl S, Caceres C. Anger management style, blood pressure reactivity, and acute pain sensitivity: evidence for "trait x situation" models. *Ann Behav Med* 2004;27:195–204.

74. Cloninger CR. Antisocial personality disorder: a review. In: Maj M, Akiskal HS, Messich JE, eds. *Personality Disorders*. New York: Wiley; 2005: 125–169.

75. Serretti A, Mandelli L, Lorenzi C, et al. Temperament and character in mood disorders: influence of DRD4, SERTPR, TPH, and MAO-A polymorphisms. *Neuropsychobiology* 2006;53:9–16.

76. Dersh J, Polatin PB, Gatchel RJ. Chronic pain and psychopathology: research findings and theoretical considerations. *Psychosom Med* 2002;64:773–786.

77. Baer RA, Sauer SE. Relationships between depressive rumination, anger rumination, and borderline personality features. *Personal Disord* 2011;2:142–150.

78. DiGiuseppe R, McDermut W, Unger F, et al. The comorbidity of anger symptoms with personality disorders in psychiatric outpatients. *J Clin Psychol* 2012;68:67–77.

79. Tomko RL, Brown WC, Tragesser SL, et al. Social context of anger in borderline personality disorder and depressive disorders: findings from a naturalistic observation study. *J Pers Disord* 2014;28:434–448.

80. Lubke GH, Ouwens KG, de Moor MH, et al. Population heterogeneity of trait anger and differential associations of trait anger facets with borderline personality features, neuroticism, depression, attention deficit hyperactivity disorder (ADHD), and alcohol problems. *Psychiatry Res* 2015;230:553–560.

81. Turk DC, Monarch ES. Biopsychosocial perspective on chronic pain. In: Turk DC, Gatchel RJ, eds. *Psychological Approaches to Pain Management: A Practitioner's Handbook*. New York: Guilford Press; 2002:3–29.

82. Burns JW. Arousal of negative emotion and symptom-specific reactivity in chronic low back pain patients. *Emotion* 2006;6:309–319.

83. Burns JW, Bruehl S, Quartana PJ. Anger management style and hostility among patients with chronic pain: effects upon symptom-specific physiological reactivity during anger- and sadness-recall interviews. *Psychosom Med* 2006;68:786–793.

84. Kiecolt-Glaser JK, McGuire L, Robles TF, et al. Emotions, morbidity, and mortality. *Annu Rev Psychol* 2002;53:83–107.

85. Segerstrom SC, Miller GE. Psychological stress and the human immune system: a meta-analytic study of 30 years of inquiry. *Psychol Bull* 2004; 130:601–630.

86. Kop WJ. The integration of cardiovascular behavioral medicine and psychoneuroimmunology. *Brain Behav Immun* 2003;17:233–237.

87. Graham JE, Robles TF, Kiecolt-Glaser JK, et al. Hostility and pain are related to inflammation in older adults. *Brain Behav Immun* 2006;20:389–400.

88. Boyle SH, Jackson WG, Suarez EC. Hostility, anger, and depression predict increases in C3 over a 10-year period. *Brain Behav Immun* 2007;21:816–823.

89. Grace PM, Hutchinson MR, Maier SF, et al. Pathological pain and the neuroimmune interface. *Nat Rev Immunol* 2014;14:217–231.

90. Generaal E, Vogelzangs N, Macfarlane GJ, et al. Basal inflammation and innate immune response in chronic multisite musculoskeletal pain. *Pain* 2014;155:1605–1612.

91. Ji RR, Xu ZZ, Gao YJ. Emerging targets in neuroinflammation-driven chronic pain. *Nat Rev Drug Discov* 2014;13:533–548.

92. Harper D, ed. Anger. In: *Online Etymology Dictionary*. Available at: http://www.etymonline.com/index.php?allowed_in_frame=0&search=anger. Accessed August 6, 2017.

93. Corpus of Contemporary American English. Word frequency data. Available at: http://www.wordfrequency.info/free.asp?s=y. Accessed August 6, 2017.

94. Smedslund J. How shall the concept of anger be defined? *Theory Psychol* 1993;3:5–33.

95. Fernandez E, Johnson SL. Anger in psychological disorders: prevalence, presentation, etiology and prognostic implications. *Clin Psychol Rev* 2016;46:124–135.

96. Lazarus RS. Cognitive-motivational-relational theory of emotion. In: Hanin YL, ed. *Emotions in Sport*. Champaign, IL: Human Kinetics; 2000:39–64.

97. Anshel MH, Jamison J, Raviv S. Cognitive appraisals and coping strategies following acute stress among skilled competitive male and female athletes. *J Sport Behav* 2001;24:128–143.

98. Grant LD, Long BC, Willms JD. Women's adaptation to chronic back pain: daily appraisals and coping strategies, personal characteristics, and perceived spousal responses. *J Health Psychol* 2002;7:545–563.

99. Uphill MA, Jones MV. Antecedents of emotions in elite athletes: a cognitive motivational relational theory perspective. *Res Q Exerc Sport* 2007;78:79–89.

100. Caselli G, Offredi A, Martino F, et al. Metacognitive beliefs and rumination as predictors of anger: a prospective study. *Aggress Behav* 2017;43:421–429.

101. Cheng C, Cheung MW. Cognitive processes underlying coping flexibility: differentiation and integration. *J Pers* 2005;73:859–886.

102. Ysseldyk R, Matheson K, Anisman H. Forgiveness and the appraisal-coping process in response to relationship conflicts: implications for depressive symptoms. *Stress* 2009;12:152–166.

103. Fishbain DA, Lewis JE, Bruns D, et al. Exploration of anger constructs in acute and chronic pain patients vs. community patients. *Pain Pract* 2011;11:240–251.

104. Jasinski MJ, Lumley MA, Latsch DV, et al. Assessing anger expression: construct validity of three emotion expression-related measures. *J Pers Assess* 2016;98:640–648.

105. Spielberger CD. *The State-Trait Anger Expression Inventory-2*. Odessa, FL: Psychological Assessment Resource; 1999.

106. Ramírez JM, Andreu JM. Aggression, and some related psychological constructs (anger, hostility, and impulsivity); some comments from a research project. *Neurosci Biobehav Rev* 2006;30:276–291.

107. Ahmed AG, Kingston DA, DiGiuseppe R, et al. Developing a clinical typology of dysfunctional anger. *J Affect Disord* 2012;136:139–148.

108. Freud S. New introductory lectures on psychoanalysis. In: *Complete Psychological Works*. Vol 22. standard ed. London: Hogarth Press; 1964. (Original work published 1913.)

109. Deffenbacher JL. Trait anger: theory, findings, and implications. In: Spielberger CD, Butcher JN, eds. *Advances in Personality Assessment*. Vol 9. Hillsdale, NJ: Lawrence Erlbaum; 1990:177–202.

110. International Association for the Study of Pain. IASP Task Force on Taxonomy. In: Merskey H, Bogduk N, eds. *Classification of Chronic Pain: Description of Chronic Pain Syndromes and Definition of Pain Terms*. Seattle, WA: IASP Press; 1994.

111. Chapman CR, Nakamura Y, Donaldson G, et al. Sensory and affective dimensions of phasic pain are indistinguishable in the self-report and psychophysiology of normal laboratory subjects. *J Pain* 2001;2:279–294.

112. Yoshino A, Okamoto Y, Onoda K, et al. Sadness enhances the experience of pain and affects pain-evoked cortical activities: an MEG study. *J Pain* 2012;13:628–635.

113. Yang L, Symonds LL. Neural substrate for facilitation of pain processing during sadness. *Neuroreport* 2012;23:911–915.

114. Gross JJ. Emotion regulation: affective, cognitive, and social consequences. *Psychophysiology* 2002;39:281–291.

115. Wegner DM. Ironic processes of mental control. *Psychol Rev* 1994;101: 34–52.

116. Burns JW, Quartana P, Gilliam W, et al. Effects of anger suppression on pain severity and pain behaviors among chronic pain patients: evaluation of an ironic process model. *Health Psychol* 2008;27:645–652.

117. Burns JW, Quartana PJ, Gilliam W, et al. Suppression of anger and subsequent pain intensity and behavior among chronic low back pain patients: the role of symptom-specific physiological reactivity. *J Behav Med* 2012;35:103–114.

118. Carson JW, Keefe FJ, Goli V, et al. Forgiveness and chronic low back pain: a preliminary study examining the relationship of forgiveness to pain, anger, and psychological distress. *J Pain* 2005;6:84–91.

119. Carson JW, Keefe FJ, Lowry KP, et al. Conflict about expressing emotions and chronic low back pain. *J Pain* 2007;8:405–411.

120. Offenbaecher M, Dezutter J, Kohls N, et al. Struggling with adversities of life: the role of forgiveness in patients suffering from fibromyalgia. *Clin J Pain* 2017;33:528–534.

121. Bruehl S, Chung OY, Burns JW. Anger expression and pain: an overview of findings and possible mechanisms. *J Behav Med* 2006;29:593–606.

122. Bruehl S, Chung OY, Burns JW, et al. Trait anger expressiveness and pain-induced beta-endorphin release: support for the opioid dysfunction hypothesis. *Pain* 2007;130:208–215.

123. Burns J, Higdon L, Mullen J, et al. Relationships among patient hostility, anger expression, depression, and the working alliance in a work hardening program. *Ann Behav Med* 1999;21:77–82.

124. Burns JW, Johnson BJ, Devine J, et al. Anger management style and the prediction of treatment outcome among male and female chronic pain patients. *Behav Res Ther* 1998;36:1051–1062.

125. Bruehl S, McCubbin J, Hardin R. Theoretical review: altered pain regulatory systems in chronic pain. *Neurosci Biobehav Rev* 1999;23:877–890.

126. Burns JW, Bruehl S. Anger management style, opioid analgesic use, and chronic pain severity: a test of the opioid-deficit hypothesis. *J Behav Med* 2005;28:555–563.

127. Bruehl S, Burns JW, Chung OY, et al. Pain-related effects of trait anger expression: neural substrates and the role of endogenous opioid mechanisms. *Neurosci Biobehav Rev* 2009;33:475–491.

128. Burns JW, Bruehl S, Chung OY, et al. Endogenous opioids may buffer effects of anger arousal on sensitivity to subsequent pain. *Pain* 2009;146:276–282.

129. Bruehl S, Burns JW, Chung OY, et al. Interacting effects of trait anger and acute anger arousal on pain: the role of endogenous opioids. *Psychosom Med* 2011;73:612–619.

130. Burns JW, Bruehl S, Chont M. Anger regulation style, anger arousal and acute pain sensitivity: evidence for an endogenous opioid "triggering" model. *J Behav Med* 2014;37:642–653.

131. Burns JW, Bruehl S, France CR, et al. Endogenous opioid function and responses to morphine: the moderating effects of anger expressiveness. *J Pain* 2017;923–932.

132. Fernandez E, Day A, Boyle GJ. Measures of anger and hostility in adults. In: Boyle GJ, Saklofsky DH, Matthews G, eds. *Measures of Personality and Social Psychological Constructs*. London: Elsevier; 2015:74–100.

133. Murphy LL, Plake BS, Spies RA, eds. *Tests in Print VII: An Index to Tests, Test Reviews, and the Literature on Specific Tests*. Vol 7. Lincoln, NE: Buros Institute of Mental Measurements; 2006.

134. Spies RA, Plake BS, Geisinger KF, et al, eds. *The Seventeenth Mental Measurements Yearbook*. 17th ed. Lincoln, NE: Buros Institute of Mental Measurements; 2007.

135. Lievaart M, Franken IH, Hovens JE. Anger assessment in clinical and non-clinical populations: further validation of the State-Trait Anger Expression Inventory-2. *J Clin Psychol* 2016;72:263–278.

136. Okifuji A, Turk DC, Curran SL. Anger in chronic pain: investigations of anger targets and intensity. *J Psychosom Res* 1999;47:1–12.

137. Siegel JM. The multidimensional anger inventory. *J Pers Soc Psychol* 1986; 51:191–200.

138. Novaco RW. *Novaco Anger Scale and Provocation Inventory (NAS-PI)*. Los Angeles, CA: Western Psychological Services; 2003.

139. DiGiuseppe R, Tafrate R. *Understanding Anger and Anger Disorders*. New York: Oxford University Press; 2004.

140. DiGiuseppe R, Tafrate RC. *Anger Disorders Scale: Short (ADS:S)*. North Tonawanda, NY: Multi-Health Systems Inc; 2004.

141. Wootton RJ, Caudill-Slosberg MA, Frank JB. When psychotherapy is indicated in the management of pain. In: Bajwa ZH, Wootton RJ, Warfield CA, eds. *Principles and Practice of Pain Medicine*. 3rd ed. New York: McGraw-Hill; 2017:179–191.

142. Grzesiak RC, Ury GM, Dworkin RH. Psychodynamic psychotherapy with chronic pain patients. In: Gatchel RJ, Turk DC, eds. *Psychological Approaches to Pain Management: A Practitioner's Handbook*. New York: Guilford Press; 1996;148–178.

143. Postone N. Psychotherapy with cancer patients. *Am J Psychother* 1998; 52:412–424.

144. Wootton RJ. Supportive dynamic and existential therapy. *J Cancer Pain Symptom Palliation* 2005;1:73–78.

145. Howells K, Day A. Readiness for anger management: clinical and theoretical issues. *Clin Psychol Rev* 2003;23:319–337.

146. Norcross JC, Wampold BE. What works for whom: tailoring psychotherapy to the person. *J Clin Psychol* 2011;67:127–132.

147. Linton SJ, Lardén M, Gillow AM. Sexual abuse and chronic musculoskeletal pain: prevalence and psychological factors. *Clin J Pain* 1996;12:215–221.

148. Goldberg RT. Childhood abuse, depression, and chronic pain. *Clin J Pain* 1994;10:277–281.

149. Whitehead WE, Crowell MD, Davidoff AL, et al. Pain from rectal distention in women with irritable bowel syndrome: relationship to sexual abuse. *Dig Dis Sci* 1997;42:796–804.

150. Nickel R, Egle UT, Hardt J. Are childhood adversities relevant in patients with low back pain? *Eur J Pain* 2002;6:221–228.

151. Wessler R, Hankin S, Stern J. *Succeeding with Difficult Clients: Applications of Cognitive Appraisal Therapy*. San Diego, CA: Academic Press; 2001.

152. McBeth J, Tomenson B, Chew-Graham CA, et al. Common and unique associated factors for medically unexplained chronic widespread pain and chronic fatigue. *J Psychosom Res* 2015;79:484–491.

153. Kamiya Y, Timonen V, Kenny RA. The impact of childhood sexual abuse on the mental and physical health, and healthcare utilization of older adults. *Int Psychogeriatr* 2016;28:415–422.

154. Ortiz R, Ballard ED, Machado-Vieira R, et al. Quantifying the influence of child abuse history on the cardinal symptoms of fibromyalgia. *Clin Exp Rheumatol* 2016;34(2 suppl 96):S59–S66.

155. Mehta S, Rice D, Chan A, et al. Impact of abuse on adjustment and chronic pain disability: a structural equation model. *Clin J Pain* 2017;33:687–693.

156. Sachs-Ericsson NJ, Sheffler JL, Stanley IH, et al. When emotional pain becomes physical: adverse childhood experiences, pain, and the role of mood and anxiety disorders. *J Clin Psychol* 2017;73;1403–1428.

157. Prochaska JO, DiClemente CC. The transtheoretical approach. In: Norcross JC, Goldfried MR, eds. *Handbook of Psychotherapy Integration*. New York: Basic Books; 1992:300–334.

158. Prochaska JO, Velicer WF. The transtheoretical model of health behavior change. *Am J Health Promotion* 1997;12:38–48.

159. Kerns RD, Rosenberg R, Jamison RN, et al. Readiness to adopt a self-management approach to chronic pain: the pain stages of change questionnaire (PSOCQ). *Pain* 1997;72:227–234.

160. Norcross JC, Krebs PM, Prochaska JO. Stages of change. *J Clin Psychol* 2011;67:143–154.

161. McCracken LM, Vowles KE. Acceptance and commitment therapy and mindfulness for chronic pain: model, process, and progress. *Am Psychol* 2014;69:178–187.

162. Barrett K, Chang Y. Behavioral interventions targeting chronic pain, depression, and substance use disorder in primary care. *J Nurs Scholarsh* 2016; 48:345–353.

163. Castelnuovo G, Giusti EM, Manzoni GM, et al. Psychological treatments and psychotherapies in the neurorehabilitation of pain: evidences and recommendations from the Italian Consensus Conference on pain in neurorehabilitation. *Front Psychol* 2016;7:115.

164. Veehof MM, Trompetter HR, Bohlmeijer ET, et al. Acceptance- and mindfulness-based interventions for the treatment of chronic pain: a meta-analytic review. *Cogn Behav Ther* 2016;45:5–31.

165. Gilpin HR, Keyes A, Stahl DR, et al. Predictors of treatment outcome in contextual cognitive and behavioral therapies for chronic pain: a systematic review. *J Pain* 2017;18;1153–1164.

166. Suinn R. *Anxiety Management Training: A Behavior Therapy*. New York: Plenum Press; 1990.

167. Suinn RM. Anxiety/anger management training. In: Koocher GP, Norcross JC, eds. *Psychologists' Desk Reference*. New York: Oxford University Press; 2005:271–273.

168. Fernandez E. Toward an integrative psychotherapy for maladaptive anger. In: Potegal M, Stemmler G, Spielberger C, eds. *The International Handbook of Anger: Constituent and Concomitant Biological, Psychological, and Social Processes*. New York: Springer; 2010:499–514.

169. Fernandez E, Kerns RD. New prospects for alleviation of anger in the context of chronic pain. In: Bajwa ZH, Wootton RJ, Warfield CA, eds. *Principles and Practice of Pain Medicine*. 3rd ed. New York: McGraw-Hill; 2017:210–215.

170. Turk DS. Cognitive behavioral approach to the treatment of chronic pain patients. *Reg Anesth Pain Med* 2003;28:573–579.

171. Winterowd C, Beck AT, Gruener D. *Cognitive Therapy with Chronic Pain Patients*. New York: Springer; 2003.

172. Thorn BE. *Cognitive Therapy for Chronic Pain: A Step-by-Step Guide*. 2nd ed. New York: Guilford Press; 2017.

173. Vlaeyen JW, Morley S. Cognitive-behavioral treatments for chronic pain: what works for whom? *Clin J Pain* 2005;21:1–8.

CHAPTER 84

Cognitive-Behavioral Therapy for Chronic Pain

LAYNE A. GOBLE, CHRISTOPHER D. SLETTEN, TAYLOR CROUCH, and **KELLY BARTH**

Introduction

Cognitive-behavioral therapy (CBT) is an evidence-based treatment approach that has been effectively applied to the management of chronic pain. This approach is influenced by behavioral techniques (i.e., relaxation therapies, time-based pacing, and behavioral activation) combined with cognitive therapies (i.e., cognitive restructuring) with a goal of better integrating pain management within a biopsychosocial model of care. Additional components that address common comorbidities such as sleep and relationship difficulties are often included in treatment protocols. The main outcome of CBT for chronic pain (CBT-CP) is development of healthy coping techniques to improve functioning in the face of ongoing pain complaints.

For the past three decades, the vast majority of research on psychological approaches to chronic pain has focused on traditional CBT. However, there has been a growing interest in recent years on interventions that include mindfulness and acceptance-based components, which have been called the "third wave" of behavioral and cognitive psychotherapies. As a brief (and certainly incomplete) background review, "first wave" treatments employed classic behavioral therapy, including methods such as contingency management and operant conditioning, to change behavior (e.g., Zinbarg and Griffith[1]). "Second wave" treatments integrated cognitive methods (i.e., identifying and modifying maladaptive cognitions) into behavioral treatment in order to change problematic behaviors and emotions (e.g., Beck[2]). "Third wave" treatments can also be considered cognitive-behavioral interventions, but they collectively emphasize *mindfulness* and *acceptance-based* processes while deemphasizing cognitive change or control. Each of these is reviewed within this chapter.

HISTORY AND DEVELOPMENT OF COGNITIVE-BEHAVIORAL THERAPY FOR PAIN

CBT-CP developed out of a need for an approach outside of the traditional biomedical model. Clinicians and researchers recognized that psychosocial factors had an influence on pain-related behaviors that significantly impacted treatment outcomes. Henry Beecher[3] was a pioneer in pain management who first recognized the impact of psychosocial factors on chronic pain while serving in the Army Medical Corps during World War II. During this time, he first observed that the individuals in his care responded very differently to their traumatic injuries. Namely, he observed that soldiers with serious wounds reported less pain than did his postoperative patients at Massachusetts General Hospital. In interviews with his patients, he found that their pain experiences were mediated by the meaning that they had attributed to their injuries. He concluded, "There is no simple relationship between the wound per se and the pain experienced. The pain is in very large part determined by other factors, and of great importance here is the significance of the wound." He found that only one in four injured soldiers requested analgesic medications despite experiencing severe wounds. Many of these soldiers were grateful to have survived their injuries and directed their thoughts to the positive aspects of their situation—namely, gratitude for having survived their injuries and thoughts of going home. He also found that similar attributions to injury also impacted individuals with injuries outside of combat settings. Beecher was one of the first researchers to acknowledge the complex interplay of the physical, psychological, and sociocultural factors that impact the chronic pain experience. This interplay of factors affected not only the experience of pain but also the behaviors and disability that accompanied chronic pain. This theory would later become the biopsychosocial model of chronic pain.

By the 1960s and 1970s, the health care community began to adopt a new view of chronic pain; first, by distinguishing acute and chronic pain as separate entities and then by developing behavioral and rehabilitation approaches to chronic pain. During this time, Wilbert Fordyce worked with John Bonica to develop groundbreaking behavioral therapies for chronic pain based on operant conditioning approaches. Essentially, he encouraged (i.e., reinforced) individuals with chronic pain to reengage in exercise and other physical activities while reducing (i.e., extinguishing) their maladaptive pain behaviors.[4,5] His approach encouraged individuals to take a more active role in their recovery, thereby helping them to experience a greater sense of control over their chronic pain complaints. This approach was considered revolutionary at the time because these basic changes in behavior led to a reduction in their use of analgesic medications and improved function during their time in treatment.

The growth of cognitive therapy[6] likewise expanded our understanding of psychosocial factors that impact chronic pain. This model addresses the influence that thoughts can have on our emotions, behaviors, and even physiologic processes. Albert Ellis[7] and Aaron Beck[6] first addressed *catastrophizing* as a factor that impacts the development and maintenance of depressive and anxiety disorders. Catastrophizing thoughts are irrational beliefs that one's current or anticipated situation is exaggerated to be far worse than it actually is. Michael Sullivan[8] later developed the Pain Catastrophizing Scale to assess for catastrophizing beliefs in chronic pain patients. His measure is widely used in both clinical and research settings to assess for catastrophizing beliefs in chronic pain patients. Beverly Thorn[9] has also been instrumental in developing cognitive interventions for chronic pain patients.

EVIDENCE FOR COGNITIVE-BEHAVIORAL THERAPY FOR CHRONIC PAIN

There is significant evidence that CBT-CP is effective for a number of chronic pain conditions, including headache, rheumatic diseases, chronic pain syndrome, chronic low back pain, and irritable bowel syndrome.[10–12]

In 2016, Centers for Disease Control and Prevention (CDC) published an update to their "Guidelines for Prescribing Opioids for Chronic Pain."[13] Their first recommendation that the authors emphasized as being of primary importance was "nonpharmacologic and nonopioid pharmacologic therapy are preferred for chronic pain . . . ." This recommendation was based on a contextual review of nonpharmacologic and nonopioid therapies,[14] which cites 13 guidelines and 18 systematic reviews of randomized or quasi-randomized trials of nonpharmacologic and nonopioid therapies, including studies with follow-up periods from 2 weeks to 6 months (with some CBT studies "assessing outcomes at 6 months or longer"). The overall quality of the evidence as informally rated by study authors was felt to be "moderate."

The contextual review found that CBT had significant positive effects on disability and catastrophizing with effects lasting up to 6 months in back pain and osteoarthritis, and biopsychosocial rehabilitation was effective for both pain and disability.[14] The authors concluded that these approaches should be considered first-line treatments for chronic pain.

Components of Cognitive-Behavioral Therapy for Chronic Pain

Several widely used CBT treatment protocols have been developed to bring together the various psychosocial interventions into a coherent approach for treating chronic pain.[15,16] Treatment involves a comprehensive psychosocial assessment that is used to guide treatment planning. The assessment focuses on an individual's pain history, along with psychosocial factors that may be impacting their pain experience. Providers use this assessment as an opportunity to tailor their treatment approach to the needs of the patient. The main components of CBT-CP typically include the following:

- *Chronic pain psychoeducation* to inform patients about the biopsychosocial model of chronic pain, to introduce the components of treatment, to address common barriers to treatment, and to increase self-efficacy for engaging in new pain self-management behaviors
- *Relaxation techniques* for stress management and to decrease muscle tension
- *Behavioral activation coupled with time-based pacing* to encourage increased engagement in pleasant, physical, social, and otherwise meaningful activities while reducing the likelihood of experiencing a painful flare-up and excessive fatigue
- *Sleep hygiene* to improve sleep quality and to improve daytime alertness and activity
- *Cognitive restructuring* to identify and address maladaptive thought patterns and develop strategies to promote adaptive cognitions
- *Communication skills* to help improve and increase positive social interactions and reduce solicitous pain behaviors from family and friends
- *Maintenance and relapse prevention* to increase self-efficacy for using the pain self-management techniques developed in treatment, to address potential barriers and specific difficulties to using these techniques over time

Treatment protocols for CBT-CP are most often tailored for individual therapy, although it has also been adapted into a group therapy approach, as is employed in some pain rehabilitation programs (PRPs). Family members and close friends may also be engaged in treatment to address communication skills and reinforce behavioral activation. Adaptations have also been developed to increase access to CBT for pain, such as delivery via telehealth.

CHRONIC PAIN PSYCHOEDUCATION

The dilemma of chronic pain and its often intractable nature is that it is poorly understood, frustrating, isolating, and confusing for patients, families, and medical providers. A paramount structural element of CBT-CP is psychoeducation. Like many educational approaches, this can be efficiently and effectively accomplished in a group setting. The interaction with other group members, realizing one is "not alone" in their chronic pain, hearing similar questions and concerns, and the repetition of complex material are invaluable elements in the psychoeducational model. The isolation of chronic pain and the feeling that no one else has similar struggles is directly eliminated with this group-based approach. In addition to normalizing the patient's symptoms and experience, the major benefit of the psychoeducational approach is that it can foster motivation and sustained change.[17–20]

Education about the Neurobiology of Chronic Pain

Successful psychoeducational approaches incorporate information about the neurobiology of pain. This includes description of the differences between acute pain and chronic pain and an explanation of central sensitization. Central sensitization is the process by which many chronic symptom conditions are thought to be (1) precipitated and (2) maintained in the central nervous system.[21] The primary goal is to convey to the patients, in an understandable format, how their pain transitioned from acute to chronic, a rationale for how to manage the problem and direction for improving future functioning. Beginning with the physical origins of their problem can remove the stigma that chronic pain is purely psychological or "made up." For example, starting with education about central sensitization followed by an explanation of how treatment can be delivered in the following simplified format: "The main precipitating factor to the development of central sensitization is a pain signal that lasts longer than it should or greater than 3 months (definition of chronic pain)." This causes an upregulated pain signal from the body and a sensitized pain receiver in the brain. As a result of these changes, four responses to chronic pain logically follow: (1) physical deconditioning, (2) emotional distress, (3) behavioral dysregulation, and (4) chemical use. Pivoting from the causative focus and instead looking at these four factors begins to shape the emphasis of the CBT model. All patients benefit from physical reconditioning to improve endurance, strength, and ability to do daily activities. Treating the emotional distress of chronic pain incorporates CBT strategies for stress, anxiety, depression, and anger management. Reducing emotional distress has obvious psychological and social benefits but is also associated with reduced symptom burden.[22] Two major behavioral issues are also introduced during the psychoeducational sessions: overactivity followed by prolonged recovery ("pushing and crashing") and pain behaviors. Patients are educated that addressing both of these behavior patterns yields less distress and fewer symptoms.

Resetting Expectations about the Outcomes of Chronic Pain—the A-B-C Model

It is not uncommon that a patient with chronic pain will lament, "I wish I could go back to the way I was before having chronic pain." In fact, the current medical approach to chronic pain (i.e., offering repeated trials of medications, interventions, and surgeries to "cure" chronic pain) actually fosters this belief that somehow, with enough trials, a cure for one's pain is waiting to be found. For many patients with chronic pain, this will not be the case. The Mayo Clinic's Pain Rehabilitation Center, Florida (MCPRC-F) uses the A-B-C model of the chronic pain experience (Table 84.1). This model illustrates and validates the patient experience and serves as a foundational explanation of the way people change as they experience the suffering of chronic pain. The "A" version is the person's functional status before his or her pain symptoms became chronic. This version is generally characterized by independence, productivity, fitness, and social engagement. The "B" version is the patient's functional status with chronic pain. This version is characterized by "pushing and crashing," reliance on medication or interventions, decreased independence and productivity, deconditioning, and more emotional distress. The goal of CBT for pain is to help the patient move toward the "C" version of functioning. The "C" version is characterized by increasing fitness, independence, productivity, and mood, with additional emphasis on acceptance, moderation, flexibility, and stability.[23]

TABLE 84.1 A-B-C Versions of a Patient with Chronic Pain		
A—Pre-Pain	**B—Pain**	**C—Post–CBT-P**
Active	Depressed	More active
Productive	Deconditioned	More productive
Social	Discouraged	Stable
Motivated	Drugged	Moderation
Independent	Dependent	More independent

CBT-P, cognitive-behavioral therapy for pain.

This model has been an effective clinical tool to educate patients, providers, and family members about the trajectory of treatment. When teaching this model, specific emphasis is placed on the linearity and intentional movement from the "B" version to the "C" version. This concept allows for the discussion that returning to the "A" version is no longer possible, and continued emphasis and expectations in that direction are counterproductive.

Changing Behaviors—SMART Method

One final element from a behavior therapy perspective is the implementation of goal setting. Using the A-B-C model outlined previously, patients can be shown how their goal setting behaviors were likely altered by their chronic pain. Persons who could previously set and achieve goals easily often find themselves at a loss for how to effectively do so in their "B" version. With the unpredictability of symptoms and decreased functional capacity, goal setting can become frustrating and futile. One common method to reinstitute effective goal setting is to use the SMART method.[24] The SMART acronym stands for Specific, Measurable, Attainable, Relevant, and Time bound. Adapted from business management, this model is easy to explain and translates well to the needs of a chronic pain patients. This model can be implemented during treatment and then modified as needed after treatment has ended. The element patients seem to struggle with the most is M—Measurable. Often, a brief explanation about behavioral coding and having the patient determine if the goal is a discrete activity or an ongoing one (i.e., posture, attitude). If it is an ongoing activity, then instructing them in the use of time sampling can be helpful.

Although comprehensive, psychoeducation is a critical foundation for CBT-CP. In our current health care model, patients with chronic pain are often fearful and skeptical about trying an intervention that does not involve medications or interventions and concerned that engaging in CBT-CP will mean that their pain is "in their head." Spending the time to provide education to the patient about chronic pain and how CBT-CP can address the neurobiology of pain is essential for getting patients engaged in this evidence-based treatment.

RELAXATION TECHNIQUES

Relaxation training was one of the earliest techniques to be integrated into CBT-CP treatment protocols. Clinicians use relaxation training to help individuals become more aware of sympathetic arousal that likely increases their pain severity and then induce a relaxation response to counter the effect of this arousal. Although these techniques may be used with biofeedback, it is important for individuals to recognize that they can be used independent of costly equipment or the assistance of a biofeedback specialist. Relaxation techniques should be presented as an active pain management strategy that individuals should practice regularly and utilize when needed. It is important for the clinician to explain relaxation training as a specific technique that actively induces a relaxation response because some people may interpret relaxation as just passively resting.

It is often very easy for individuals with chronic pain to recognize life stressors that relate to their chronic pain experience,

although it may be more challenging for them to recognize the mind–body connections that impact physical sensations through sympathetic arousal (i.e., muscle contraction, dilation of the pupils, constricted blood flow to many parts of the body, and increased heart and breathing rates). Individuals will often see how prolonged stress can lead to fatigue, poor sleep, and tension in their muscles. Having individuals experience a relaxation response is often a helpful step in helping them recognize that they can take an active role in managing their chronic pain complaints. Although there are many relaxation techniques used in clinical settings, we focus on some of the most commonly used techniques in this section.

Herbert Benson[25] is often credited with popularizing relaxation techniques with his book *The Relaxation Response* in 1975. He systematically looked at ways to counter the sympathetic arousal through meditation. His work has promoted relaxation techniques such as diaphragmatic breathing, progressive muscle relaxation, guided imagery, autogenic training, and other meditation techniques. There are several useful guidelines for individuals engaging in these techniques to follow. It is often recommended that individuals beginning this practice should find a quiet location that is free from distractions. Individuals new to these techniques often benefit from being guided through the induction by someone else. Although this was traditionally done by a clinician, there is a wide array of audio and video recordings that are also helpful. It is often helpful to instruct individuals to begin using these techniques at a quiet time when they are more likely to experience the relaxation response. Later, they might try to use the relaxation techniques in more challenging situations.

Diaphragmatic breathing is a simple technique that most individuals can master with regular practice. Individuals practicing this technique learn to recognize the sensation of contracting their diaphragm by engaging in slow, deep breaths paired with stomach and chest expansion. The parasympathetic drive is thought to override the sympathetic as the individual becomes more relaxed.

In 1938, Edmund Jacobson[26] published *Progressive Relaxation* to introduce his work with progressive muscle relaxation. This is a technique developed to increase neuromuscular awareness based on the idea that muscles respond to stressors with tension. Many chronic pain patients recognize muscle tension, stiffness, or chronic guarding of their muscles. This may lead to tension headaches, low back pain, temporomandibular joint disorder, and misaligned posture. Progressive muscle relaxation consists of a series of isometric muscle contractions followed by efforts to completely relax the muscles by focusing on one muscle group at a time. It is also common for individuals to combine diaphragmatic breathing techniques while doing progressive muscle relaxation. This process is thought to intercept the stress response through a direct and conscious inhibition of the excitatory neural drive to muscle fibers.

Guided imagery is another commonly used relaxation technique. Individuals are instructed to close their eyes and use their cognitive skills to imagine a peaceful and relaxing place. Individuals are instructed to use each of their senses when creating this setting to include the sensory perceptions of sight, sound, touch, smell, and even tastes if possible. Individuals often benefit from a discussion of the place they intend to use prior to using this technique for the first time.

Mindfulness meditation is another technique that has been effectively applied to chronic pain. Jon Kabat-Zinn[27] first popularized the use of this technique for health conditions with his book *Full Catastrophe Living*. The purpose of this technique is to assist the individual to bring their attention to the present moment without having a specific judgment about the experience. This can be particularly challenging when an individual perceives his or her experience in that moment to be negative, such as focusing on the pain sensation. The body scan meditation is often a useful technique for chronic pain patients as it allows the individual to practice focusing attention on different areas of the body, including painful areas, without judgment. Mindfulness meditation is also a component of acceptance and commitment therapy (ACT), reviewed at the end of this chapter.

BEHAVIORAL ACTIVATION AND TIME-BASED PACING

Many individuals with chronic pain come to treatment having developed a pervasive pattern of behavioral avoidance. Perhaps, the most important aim of CBT-CP is reducing this behavioral avoidance by enhancing individuals' level of daily functioning and activity. To accomplish this goal, the *behavioral activation* component of treatment involves gradual exposure to previously avoided physical, recreational, and social activities. Behavioral activation has been most frequently used as a treatment approach for depression and generally involves increasing contact with valued and pleasurable environments and activities in order to provide more opportunities for reward and enjoyment.[28] In chronic pain treatment, increasing activity engagement can help disconfirm negative expectations about pain and harm and disrupt the harmful cycle involving fear, avoidance, pain, and low mood.[29]

In order to help patients understand why increasing their activity level is important, they are first introduced to the concept of *hurt versus harm*. Many chronic pain patients believe that activities will lead to increased physical damage and increased pain. Although this belief is typically true for acute pain, it is almost always inaccurate when it comes to chronic pain. Patients are taught about *kinesiophobia*, or the fear of movement, and the negative impacts of avoiding activity on maintenance of pain and distress. The chronic pain cycle is reviewed in detail.

Patients are encouraged to begin an exercise program (once they have been cleared by their primary care physician or other treating medical provider) in order to begin to reduce the unhelpful cycle of pain and avoidance. They are taught about the benefits of exercise in improving flexibility and strength, decreasing pain, and enhancing mood. Walking is the most commonly chosen physical activity because it is low impact and accessible to almost everyone. Swimming, biking, yoga, and other forms of exercise are also encouraged if preferred by the patient. Patients are asked to set a specific goal for walking (or other exercise program) and monitor their progress.

For the patient suffering with chronic pain, it is important to couple behavioral activation with time-based pacing. Time-based pacing is a practical behavioral technique to help individuals to engage in physical activity while reducing the possibility of a painful flare-up or excessive fatigue. This technique is often introduced when a patient is first engaging in a rehabilitation program such as physical or occupational therapy, although it can be applied to any physical activity where a painful flare-up may occur. Individuals are encouraged to identify specific physical activities that are likely to lead to a painful flare-up and then develop time-based pacing schedules to use with these activities. The total time for the activity is interrupted by episodes of rest so that muscle groups can recover before resuming the activity again. It is also important to note that some patients who experience flare-up while sitting or lying down for extended periods of time can also apply time-based pacing.

Individuals with chronic pain often decrease physical activity due to the negative consequences of a painful flare-up. The perception that future activity will then lead to a flare-up will often result in avoidance of physical activity. Time-based pacing can be used in a useful way to expose patients to reengaging in a physical activity. Individuals can build on the SMART goals that they set earlier in treatment to choose an activity and then develop a schedule that is achievable so that the activity is likely to be repeated (i.e., positive reinforcement). Time-based pacing builds on William Fordyce's[30] original behavioral modification techniques for physical activity

where physical activity is rewarded, whereas prolonged inactivity is disregarded.

In addition to physical activity, a later component of treatment involves increasing engagement in *pleasurable activities*. Due to pain and associated distress, many individuals begin avoiding social and recreational activities that they used to enjoy, which can further contribute to the cycle of decreased mood, reduced activity level, and increased pain. Patients are asked to consider pleasurable activities they would be willing to begin engaging in more frequently. To explore options, they are given a list of pleasant activities to choose from, or they can choose their own. They then create a specific plan for implementing these activities while utilizing their pacing skill to maintain a balanced approach to activity. For most individuals, getting back to valued and enjoyable activities that were previously avoided due to pain contributes to mood improvement and increased energy and motivation to stay active.

SLEEP HYGIENE

Patients with chronic pain often report poor sleep due to their pain or associated anxiety. Chronic poor sleep contributes to low energy and reinforces the reduction in functioning often seen in the chronic pain cycle. The sleep hygiene component of treatment involves reviewing current sleep habits and providing basic education about sleep hygiene principles. Patients are encouraged to create a sleep-conducive environment, including minimal noise, a comfortable temperature, and appropriate light. They are guided to use the bed only for sleep (and sex), establish a calming bedtime routine, and set a regular sleep/wake schedule. Sleep-interfering behaviors are introduced and discouraged, including daytime napping, drinking caffeine after midday, consuming alcohol or a large meal prior to bedtime, and watching television or utilizing a laptop (or tablet/cell phone) in bed. Patients are taught to avoid clock watching and get out of the bed if unable to sleep. The use of relaxation techniques (introduced earlier in treatment) prior to sleep is encouraged, with a goal of reducing tension and inducing sleepiness. Additionally, the benefits of exercise are further reinforced by discussing the positive impact of daytime exercise on sleep quality. Finally, the connection between stress and sleep problems is reviewed. For many individuals, worries surface in the context of a quiet bed, which can interfere with sleep onset, so patients are encouraged to set aside time earlier in the day to engage in problem-solving and planning. After reviewing healthy sleep habits, patients select a few sleep behaviors to change and are instructed to monitor these behaviors and their impact on sleep over the next week.

COGNITIVE RESTRUCTURING

Cognitive therapy approaches are grounded in the theoretical and clinical work of Albert Ellis[7] and Aaron Beck[6] and were initially developed to treat anxiety and depressive disorders. These approaches are based on the premise that thoughts, emotions, and behaviors are interrelated. When individuals experience dysfunctional thoughts, they are very likely to then experience related negative emotions and maladaptive behaviors that lead to a mood disorder. Applications were later developed to address dysfunctional thoughts specific to the experience of living with chronic pain. Beverly Thorn's[9] work has been central in forwarding cognitive therapy as a treatment for individuals with chronic pain through her book *Cognitive Therapy for Chronic Pain: A Step-by-Step Guide*, second edition. Individuals with chronic pain may experience dysfunctional thoughts and beliefs related to their experience with chronic pain that impact their engagement in treatment. They may experience avoidance behaviors, catastrophizing, or become excessively focused on a cure.

Cognitive therapy for chronic pain often begins by working with individuals to develop techniques to better identify dysfunctional or inaccurate thoughts related to their chronic pain experience. These thoughts are referred to as automatic

TABLE 84.2 Common Pain-Related Thoughts		
Types of Unhelpful Thoughts	**Examples of Unhelpful Thoughts**	**Examples of Helpful Thoughts**
Catastrophizing: Believing something is the worst it could possibly be	When my pain is bad, I cannot do anything.	Even when my pain is bad, there are still some things I can do.
Should statements: Thinking in terms of how things should, must, or ought to be	My doctor should be able to cure my pain.	There is no cure for chronic pain, but I can use skills to cope with my pain.
All or none thinking: Seeing things as "either or" or "right or wrong" instead of in terms of degrees	I can only be happy if I am pain free.	Even if I am in pain, I can still be happy. There is always something that I can do to have a better quality of life.
Overgeneralization: Viewing one or two bad events as an endless pattern of defeat	I tried doing exercises for my back pain before, and it did not help. So, it is not going to help now.	Although physical therapy did not help much before, maybe this time, it will help. I might as well try.
Jumping to conclusions: Making negative conclusions of events that are not based on fact	When I move, my back hurts, so it must be bad for me to move.	Hurt does not equal harm.
Emotional reasoning: Believing how you feel reflects how things really are	I feel useless, so I am useless.	Even though I cannot do all the things I used to do, it does not mean I cannot do anything.
Disqualifying the positive: Focusing on only the bad and discounting the good	So what if I am doing more, I am still in pain.	Doing more is important for me to live the life I want to live.

Used with permission from KM Phillips, PhD.

because they happen so quickly that individuals are often not fully aware of their presence. In fact, it is more likely that individuals are aware of the shifts toward negative emotions that accompany these automatic thoughts, so they are asked to identify their thoughts that accompany strong negative emotions such as sadness, despair, guilt, fear, or anxiety. Thought records are a valuable tool for identifying automatic negative thoughts, and they are designed to be used outside of the therapy session where individuals are engaged in their daily routines. Individuals are first taught to begin by writing down their stressful events. They will then want to identify the subsequent physical and emotional changes that happen in connection to these events. Finally, they will record the automatic negative thoughts. It is important for individuals to have a reference to common dysfunctional thoughts to provide a reference for them to record their own experiences. A list of common dysfunctional thoughts and associated adaptive thoughts are listed in Table 84.2.

Cognitive restructuring is the next phase in this approach, and this is usually done in the subsequent visit. Once patients have better identified dysfunctional thoughts and beliefs related to their pain experience, they can begin to develop techniques to better test the reality of these thoughts and beliefs. Developing more adaptive thoughts will then lead to shifts in negative emotions and maladaptive behaviors. Individuals are asked to evaluate their thoughts to better determine the extent that their thoughts are correct or inaccurate. It is often important to note that there will likely be some degree of truth in their thoughts, although the thought becomes dysfunctional once the negative beliefs are overexaggerated. The individual can then come to a more balanced conclusion. Individuals are often encouraged to develop coping statements based on their adaptive thoughts that might help them remember this exercise when they experience stressful situations in the future.

COMMUNICATION SKILLS

Communication style and content are important in CBT-CP, in the general management of chronic pain, and in the interactions between patients with chronic pain and their families. Much of the literature in this area focuses on physician–patient communication, but the themes conveyed in this literature apply to the management of the patient in general, including themes that may arise in CBT-CP regarding communication with and between family members and support system.

It is known that words used to communicate with people suffering with chronic pain about their pain affect their outcomes.

For example, words that carry strong, negative connotations have been hypothesized to increase probability that acute pain will progress to chronic pain.[31] It has also been shown that expressed or perceived spouse criticism or hostility can worsen chronic pain symptoms, especially among women and patients with depression.[32] Conversely, positive communication can also be a vital component of effective pain management and relief. For example, it has been shown that improvement in communication between a patient and his or her partner can improve pain severity and relationship discord.[33]

Approaches to improving family communication and support around chronic pain can be done formally not only through family therapy with specific feedback about communication styles and language[33] but also through modeling provided from in-office patient–provider interactions and communication with the family member present. Modeling motivational interviewing strategies including the use of open-ended questions, questions that incite reflection, empathic statements, affirming change talk, and asking permission to share information is suggested and can be successfully adopted by family members.[33]

It is therefore important that the provider treating the patient with chronic pain utilizes and models effective communication during treatment. It has been shown that providing clinicians with communication training in the area of chronic pain increases patient satisfaction and that improved communication predicts improved patient satisfaction more than an actual decrease in pain score.[31]

When evaluating effective components of provider communication with patients with chronic pain, it has been shown that it is vital for a provider to listen to the patient's pain history and show empathy in order to communicate that the patient's pain is "real" and important. It is also helpful to couple validation of the patient's pain experience with the acknowledgment that the provider may not have all the answers for how to manage chronic pain and working with the patient to gently accept that chronic pain may be an ongoing part of his or her life (e.g., there might not be a "cure").[34]

MAINTENANCE AND RELAPSE PREVENTION
Maintaining Treatment Gains

An integral part of any CBT intervention is helping the individual maintain the therapeutic changes. This includes a strong emphasis on self-monitoring and self-management as well as planning for future difficulties and setbacks. This is especially important for individuals with chronic pain. Their struggle with a diverse and complex set of issues makes maintenance planning essential.

Whether done individually or in a group setting, there needs to be sufficient time and effort dedicated to maintaining treatment gains. For the sake of illustration, a group-based PRP is discussed. As mentioned elsewhere, a comprehensive pain rehabilitation approach includes physical therapy, occupational therapy, medication reduction, and CBT. The strength of this interdisciplinary approach is that the patient is exposed in an organized program to the elements that need to change for there to be an improvement in functioning.

One of the core elements of successful maintenance is to help the individual be as independent as possible. This can be achieved by linking the active elements of treatment with how they translate to the home environment. The schedule and intensity of a PRP cannot and should not have to be replicated when the patient is discharged. However, incorporating elements of the program in the home is essential. What follows are examples from a CBT perspective of maintenance tools.

There are three tools that are extensions of treatment goals that are addressed during the PRP: time management, exercise, and managing symptom flares. Before dismissal, the patient is asked to establish a 2-week plan. This plan is designed to ensure continued engagement in moderation, exercise, daily activities, and self-care. They are also given a home-based physical therapy program that is a continuation of the exercises and behavioral activation done during treatment. The patient is asked to maintain this program for 3 months before advancing exercise. Finally, the patient is asked to make a plan for how to handle future symptom flares. This is done for several reasons: to normalize the possibility of flares after treatment, to have a preexisting plan and schedule to maintain functioning, and so the patient's friends and family know what to do during the flare.

The second set of maintenance strategies are more universal CBT principles that are applied to this population: stimulus control, social support, and reinforcement strategies. The use of stimulus control is a behavioral strategy to help an individual not return to previous behavior patterns by limiting exposure to "tempting" stimuli. An example would be having an ex-smoker "pay at the pump" for gas rather than go into the clerk where there are ample smoking-related cues. For pain patients, stimulus control could include avoiding retail pharmacies, limiting internet use (no more symptom/cure searches), and not returning to practitioners who were solely focused on symptom relief.

Social support as a maintenance strategy is extremely important. Patients need several types of support to ensure ongoing treatment success. The primary support group, friends, and family are coached and encouraged to support the behavioral changes, stop symptom-focused talk, and remain neutral to any remaining maladaptive behaviors. In addition, patients are encouraged to increase community involvement, volunteering, school, work for distraction, other focus, and opportunities for new relationships. Finally, it is recommended that patients establish someone to be accountable to regarding adherence to the exercise and activity management.

Lastly, incorporating some form of reinforcement for treatment adherence is strongly recommended. Having the patient set up a reward system (e.g., weekly cash deposits to a vacation/gift account for every week that exercise was done) can add some incentive to the maintenance process.

THIRD-WAVE THERAPIES—ACCEPTANCE AND COMMITMENT THERAPY

Third-wave interventions include such treatments as ACT, mindfulness-based cognitive therapy (MBCT), and dialectical behavior therapy (DBT), among others. As applied to chronic pain, third-wave interventions focus less on controlling pain or changing maladaptive pain-related thoughts and emotions and more on mindful awareness of internal processes and living well despite pain.

ACT,[35] which can be considered a treatment within the family of CBT, is one of the more commonly employed and well-studied third-wave intervention for chronic pain.[36] In general, ACT focuses on behavior change and *psychological flexibility* rather than symptom (i.e., pain) reduction. Psychological flexibility is broadly defined as the ability to remain in contact with present moment experiences (both internal and external) in a way that allows behavior to continue or change consistent with one's goals and values.[37] When applied to chronic pain, ACT aims to help individuals respond more flexibly to pain and distress, reduce unhelpful attempts to control pain, and increase engagement in behaviors that are consistent with one's goals and values.[38] Thus, individuals are guided to alter their expectations from pain elimination to living a "values-based" life despite pain. Important components of treatment typically include exploration of personal values, examination of the ways in which struggling with pain prevents engagement in values-based behaviors, and choosing specific behavioral goals in line with one's values. Mindfulness practices are employed with an aim of enhancing present moment awareness of thoughts, sensations, emotions, and behaviors in order to enhance psychological flexibility. With regard to the cognitive component of treatment rather than teaching patients to *challenge and change* irrational thoughts about their pain or abilities, which is often difficult, patients are guided to mindfully notice and "defuse from" these thoughts in a way that allows them to engage in values-based activities anyway. In other words, the focus is less on trying to control thoughts and more on disallowing thoughts from controlling them, whether that process involves a natural restructuring of the thought or not. Additionally, ACT typically involves less of a didactic approach and more *experiential*, or practice-based, components within sessions.[36]

A recent systemic review and meta-analysis of 11 clinical trials found that ACT for chronic pain is effective in increasing pain acceptance, improving functioning, and reducing depression and anxiety.[39] Research comparing CBT and ACT is limited but has generally found few differences, suggesting that either approach is appropriate. One randomized clinical trial comparing ACT to CBT found that both treatments decreased depression, anxiety, and pain interference (i.e., improved functioning), and those assigned to the ACT condition reported higher levels of satisfaction.[40]

TREATING COMORBID CONDITIONS

Chronic pain and mental health disorders frequently co-occur,[41] and it is important to manage both conditions in order to optimize recovery for patients with chronic pain.

Depression and Anxiety

The link between chronic pain and depression has been well established in the literature.[42] In fact, chronic pain and depression are the most commonly occurring physical and psychological conditions, respectively, with co-occurrence rates of 30% to 50%.[43] Their link is sometimes referred to as the depression–pain dyad, or depression–pain syndrome,[44] given their frequent co-occurrence, tendency to respond similarly to medical and behavioral treatments, and overlap in neurobiologic underpinnings.[42] The link seems to be particularly strong for pain conditions without a specific origin; for example, individuals with fibromyalgia are 3 times as likely to have a major depression diagnosis than individuals without fibromyalgia.[45] Research has also demonstrated a link between pain and anxiety, with 35% of chronic pain patients having an anxiety disorder diagnosis compared to 18% of the general population.[46]

Unfortunately, depression and anxiety have historically been associated with poorer pain treatment outcomes.[47–49]

As discussed earlier in this chapter, CBT was originally developed and evaluated as a treatment for emotional disorders.[6] Thus, the treatment is well suited for chronic pain patients with depression and/or anxiety, as the intervention directly targets cognitions and behaviors that influence affect. The link between physical and emotional factors is explained to patients from the onset of treatment through education about the pain cycle and is repeatedly reinforced throughout treatment. Accordingly, meta-analyses have demonstrated that CBT-CP has a significant impact on both pain outcomes as well as depression and anxiety symptoms.[10] Aggressive treatment of both depression and anxiety to remission is important, as coping with chronic pain can be particularly challenging among patients with active mood disturbance.

Posttraumatic Stress Disorder

Chronic pain also frequently co-occurs with posttraumatic stress disorder (PTSD). Studies have shown that 34% to 50% of patients seeking pain treatment also have PTSD,[50] and 45% to 80% of patients seeking PTSD treatment also have chronic pain.[51,52] The conceptual relationship between PTSD and pain has been explained via the "shared vulnerability" model, which proposes that the fear of physical symptoms predisposes patients to both pain and PTSD as well as the "mutual maintenance" hypothesis, which suggests that pain triggers traumatic memories, and traumatic hyperarousal worsen pains.[53] The link between pain and PTSD has been widely studied in the military veteran population in particular, given the physical and emotional trauma that is often endured in battle.[54] Thus, many veterans, including those from the most recent Operation Enduring Freedom/Operation Iraqi Freedom/Operation New Dawn (OEF/OIF/OND) era, return from deployment with both physical pain and posttraumatic stress symptoms.[55]

Given the frequent co-occurrence and shared fear-avoidance-based vulnerabilities of PTSD and chronic pain, CBT-CP can be appropriately utilized with patients who also have PTSD.[56] Although the specific trauma is not specifically processed or targeted in traditional CBT-CP, the cognitive restructuring, emotional processing, and behavioral skills patients learn in the treatment can be generalized to aid in recovery from PTSD along with chronic pain.[56] Recently, integrated cognitive-behavioral treatments have been developed to concurrently address both PTSD and chronic pain among veterans,[54] and preliminary data shows therapies incorporating behavioral activation can benefit both pain and PTSD.

COGNITIVE-BEHAVIORAL THERAPY WITHIN INTERPROFESSIONAL PAIN PROGRAMS AND PAIN REHABILITATION PROGRAMS

The broad and diverse impact of chronic pain on physical impairment, emotional distress, and social dysfunction can make chronic pain management overwhelming for individual health care providers. This phenomenon has been recognized from the earliest days of pain medicine and has led to the development of the interprofessional team-based approach as the standard of care for chronic pain management. PRPs, which employ an interprofessional approach (psychology, physical therapy, occupational therapy, medical treatment) in an intensive outpatient setting, are reviewed separately,[17] but it is worth noting the recent renewed interest in PRPs in the midst of this nation's opioid crisis. Historically, the number of interprofessional pain programs dramatically decreased from over 1,000 programs in the United States in 1999, when they were at their highest number, to approximately 90 programs in 2015 (this number does not include military and the veterans' administration centers).[57] Much of this decrease can be attributed to the rise in the use of opioid analgesics and economic forces favoring interventional

pain management.[58] The culture of diagnostic and interventional pain management at the time had as its premise, "help the patient to feel better so they can function better." This message has inadvertently led to frustration, patient blaming, and assumptions of psychosomatics and has directly fed the opioid epidemic we are currently battling. As prescriptions for opioid analgesics are now being curbed across the nation, there is now a renewed national interest in PRPs. In fact, the CDC guidelines for pain in 2016[13,14] cited PRPs as an evidence-based alternative to using opioids for chronic pain.

Effectiveness of Interprofessional Pain Management Programs and Pain Rehabilitation Programs

The treatment outcomes of the interprofessional pain programs and PRPs have been well documented and studied and have been shown to improve pain,[59–64] mood,[59] physical functioning,[60] and return to work[18,59,65] and have been shown to decrease medication use[59] and health care utilization and costs.[20,59,66,67] There have been multiple meta-analytic and systematic review types of studies summarizing the effects of interdisciplinary programs and PRPs and their effects on different chronic pain conditions,[61,68,69] and showing effects were durable on pain, mood, employment, and general health, evident even after 13-year follow-up.[19]

COGNITIVE-BEHAVIORAL THERAPY TO PREVENT THE TRANSITION FROM ACUTE TO CHRONIC PAIN

Close to one-third of acute low back pain patients report continued moderate to severe pain 1 year later.[70] Given the high morbidity and health care costs associated with chronic pain, identifying interventions helpful in reducing the progression of acute to chronic pain could greatly reduce burden of disease, disability, and associated health care costs. There has been appreciable literature identifying psychosocial risk factors for developing chronic pain, such as pain catastrophizing,[71,72] fear-avoidance beliefs,[72–75] and depression.[76,77] Additionally, the complex interaction between pain and disability can be associated with additional risk factors, such as self-reported pain and disability, personality traits, and worker's compensation or personal injury status.[78]

The definition of acute and subacute pain varies in the literature from <6 weeks to <3 months, and the studies that have evaluated psychosocial interventions to prevent progression from acute to chronic pain focus on nonspecific back pain and vary in rigor. Physiotherapy or exercise therapy are recommended for acute and subacute back pain that is not improving with conservative treatments (heat, massage, nonsteroidal anti-inflammatory drugs [NSAIDs]) or for patients with risk factors for developing chronic low back pain (e.g., poor functional or health status, psychiatric comorbidities)[79] and has been shown to reduce recurrence of back pain.[80] Therefore, many of the studies evaluate the effects of adding CBT to physiotherapy in improving outcomes for acute/subacute back pain. Earlier studies showed that patient who received CBT reported significantly lower levels of pain and disability compared to those who received electromyography (EMG) biofeedback[81] and a ninefold reduction in sickness time at 1 year when compared to information only.[82]

In a series of studies aimed at identifying and intervening on patients with acute low back pain at high risk for development of chronic pain and disability, Gatchel and colleagues found that high-risk patients who received an early biopsychosocial intervention combining six to nine sessions of physical therapy and six to nine sessions of CBT delivered by a behavioral medicine psychologist demonstrated significantly less pain and disability (including work, health care utilization, and medication use) and improved psychosocial functioning and coping ability when compared to standard care patients at 1 year.[70,83] However, when evaluating general patients (not necessarily high risk for chronic pain and disability), a trial examining exercise + CBT versus exercise alone found that despite significantly more reported exercise and self-efficacy in the combination group, there were no between-group differences in pain intensity between the exercise-only group and the exercise + CBT group.[84] When evaluating health care utilization and work absenteeism, another study showed that CBT, alone or in combination with physiotherapy, resulted in less health care utilization and fewer missed work days for nonspecific back pain than minimal treatment (reassurance and activity advice) with a fivefold lower risk for developing long-term disability.[85]

Because access to mental health providers to perform CBT can be limited, and physical therapists are a common provider for acute and subacute pain, there have been studies evaluating the delivery of specific cognitive-behavioral interventions (pacing, goal setting, relaxation, challenging unhelpful thoughts) by trained physical therapists. Results show that physical therapist–delivered cognitive-behavioral interventions can significantly improve both pain and disability, with the conclusion that physiotherapy interventions targeting both physical and psychological factors should be routinely employed.[86]

Summary

As the pendulum swings away from opioid management for chronic pain in the United States, there continues to be limited access to nonprocedural, nonopioid pain management, including guideline-recommended nonpharmacologic treatments for chronic pain such as CBT and biopsychosocial rehabilitation. There is an acute need for more research on safe and effective treatments for chronic pain as well as an increased multilevel focus on improving access to these evidence-based nonpharmacologic and noninterventional treatments, so that these treatments that tend to be more time intensive and less well reimbursed can become mainstream, first-line interventions for chronic pain. CBT-CP is a first-line treatment for chronic pain and, especially when offered within an interprofessional PRP, offers a cost-effective approach to stopping the ineffective cycle of seeking an interventional "cure" for chronic pain while patients improve long-term biopsychosocial functioning by addressing cognitive distortions and pain behaviors that lead to "crashing and burning." Essential to addressing the nation's opioid crisis comprehensively will be improving access to these nonpharmacologic treatments and fostering their incorporation as early in the pain process as possible.

References

1. Zinbarg RE, Griffith JW. Behavior therapy. In: Lebow JL, ed. *Twenty-first Century Psychotherapies: Contemporary Approaches to Theory and Practice.* Hoboken, NJ: John Wiley & Sons; 2008:8–42.
2. Beck S. *Cognitive Therapy: Basics and Beyond.* New York: Guilford Press; 1995.
3. Beecher HK. Relationship of significance of wound to pain experienced. *J Am Med Assoc* 1956;161(17):1609–1613.
4. Main CJ, Keefe FJ, Jensen MP, et al. *Fordyce's Behavioral Methods for Chronic Pain and Illness: Republished with Invited Commentaries.* Philadelphia: Lippincott Williams & Wilkins; 2015.
5. Patterson DR. Behavioral methods for chronic pain and illness: a reconsideration and appreciation. *Rehabil Psychol* 2005;50(3):312.
6. Beck AT, Rush AJ, Shaw BF, et al. *Cognitive Therapy of Depression.* New York: Guilford Press Google Scholar; 1979.
7. Ellis A. *Reason and Emotion in Psychotherapy.* Secaucus, NJ: Lyle Stuart; 1962.
8. Sullivan MJ, Martel MO, Tripp D, et al. The relation between catastrophizing and the communication of pain experience. *Pain* 2006;122(3):282–288.
9. Thorn BE. *Cognitive Therapy for Chronic Pain: A Step-by-Step Guide.* 2nd ed. New York: Guilford Publications; 2017.
10. Hoffman BM, Papas RK, Chatkoff DK, et al. Meta-analysis of psychological interventions for chronic low back pain. *Health Psychol* 2007;26(1):1.
11. Otis JD, Sanderson K, Hardway C, et al. A randomized controlled pilot study of a cognitive-behavioral therapy approach for painful diabetic peripheral neuropathy. *J Pain* 2013;14(5):475–482.
12. Buhrman M, Syk M, Burvall O, et al. Individualized guided internet-delivered cognitive-behavior therapy for chronic pain patients with co-morbid depression and anxiety: a randomized controlled trial. *Clin J Pain* 2015;31(6):504–516.
13. Dowell D, Haegerich TM, Chou R. CDC guideline for prescribing opioids for chronic pain—United States, 2016. *JAMA* 2016;315(15):1624–1645.
14. Dowell D, Haegerich TM, Chou R. CDC guideline for prescribing opioids for chronic pain—United States, 2016. *MMWR Recomm Rep* 2016;65(1):1–49.
15. Otis J. *Managing Chronic Pain: A Cognitive-Behavioral Therapy Approach.* Oxford, United Kingdom: Oxford University Press; 2007.
16. Murphy JL, McKellar JD, Raffa SD, et al. *Cognitive Behavioral Therapy for Chronic Pain Among Veterans: Therapist Manual.* Washington, DC: US Department of Veterans Affairs; 2014.
17. Stanos S. Focused review of interdisciplinary pain rehabilitation programs for chronic pain management. *Curr Pain Headache Rep* 2012;16(2):147–152.
18. Ektor-Andersen J, Ingvarsson E, Kullendorff M, et al. High cost-benefit of early team-based biomedical and cognitive-behaviour intervention for long-term pain-related sickness absence. *J Rehabil Med* 2008;40(1):1–8.
19. Patrick LE, Altmaier EM, Found EM. Long-term outcomes in multidisciplinary treatment of chronic low back pain: results of a 13-year follow-up. *Spine (Phila Pa 1976)* 2004;29(8):850–855.
20. Lambeek LC, Anema JR, van Royen BJ, et al. Multidisciplinary outpatient care program for patients with chronic low back pain: design of a randomized controlled trial and cost-effectiveness study [ISRCTN28478651]. *BMC Public Health* 2007;7(1):254.
21. Yunus MB. Role of central sensitization in symptoms beyond muscle pain, and the evaluation of a patient with widespread pain. *Best Pract Res Clin Rheumatol* 2007;21(3):481–497.
22. Rome JD, Townsend CO, Bruce BK, et al. Chronic noncancer pain rehabilitation with opioid withdrawal: comparison of treatment outcomes based on opioid use status at admission. *Mayo Clin Proc* 2004;79(6):759–768.
23. Bailey JC, Kurklinsky S, Sletten CD, et al. The effectiveness of an intensive interdisciplinary pain rehabilitation program in the treatment of post-laminectomy syndrome in patients who have failed spinal cord stimulation. *Pain Med* 2018;19(2):385–392.
24. Doran GT. There's a SMART way to write management's goals and objectives. *Management Review* 1981;70(11):35–36.
25. Benson H, Klipper MZ. *The Relaxation Response.* New York: Harper Collins; 1975.
26. Jacobson E. *Progressive Relaxation.* Chicago, IL: University of Chicago Press; 1938.
27. Kabat-Zinn J. *Full Catastrophe Living: Using the Wisdom of Your Body and Mind to Face Stress, Pain, and Illness.* New York: Bantam Dell; 2013.
28. Dimidjian S, Barrera M Jr, Martell C, et al. The origins and current status of behavioral activation treatments for depression. *Annu Rev Clin Psychol* 2011;7:1–38.
29. Philips HC. Avoidance behaviour and its role in sustaining chronic pain. *Behav Res Ther* 1987;25:273–279.
30. Fordyce WE, Fowler RS Jr, Lehmann JF, et al. Some implications of learning in problems of chronic pain. *J Chronic Dis* 1968;21(3):179–190.
31. Frantsve LM, Kerns RD. Patient-provider interactions in the management of chronic pain: current findings within the context of shared medical decision making. *Pain Med* 2007;8(1):25–35.
32. Burns JW, Post KM, Smith DA, et al. Spouse criticism and hostility during marital interaction: effects on pain intensity and behaviors among individuals with chronic low back pain. *Pain* 2018;159(1):25–32.
33. Miller-Matero LR, Cano A. Encouraging couples to change: a motivational assessment to promote well-being in people with chronic pain and their partners. *Pain Med* 2015;16(2):348–355.
34. Evers S, Hsu C, Sherman KJ, et al. Patient perspectives on communication with primary care physicians about chronic low back pain. *Perm J* 2017;21. doi:10.7812/TPP/16-177.
35. Hayes SC. Acceptance and commitment therapy, relational frame theory, and the third wave of behavior therapy. *Behav Ther* 2004;35:639–665.
36. McCracken LM, Vowles KE. Acceptance and commitment therapy and mindfulness for chronic pain. *Am Psychol* 2014;69(2):178–187.
37. Hayes SC, Luoma JB, Bond FW, et al. Acceptance and commitment therapy: model, processes and outcomes. *Behav Res Ther* 2006;44(1):1–25.
38. Vowles KE, Thompson M. Acceptance and commitment therapy for chronic pain. In: McCracken L, ed. *Mindfulness and Acceptance in Behavioral Medicine: Current Theory and Practice.* Oakland, CA: New Harbinger; 2011:31–60.
39. Hughes LS, Clark J, Colclough JA, et al. Acceptance and commitment therapy (ACT) for chronic pain: a systematic review and meta-analyses. *Clin J Pain* 2017;33(6):552–568.
40. Wetherell JL, Afari N, Rutledge T, et al. A randomized, controlled trial of acceptance and commitment therapy and cognitive-behavioral therapy for chronic pain. *Pain* 2011;152(9):2098–2107.
41. Gatchel RJ. Comorbidity of chronic pain and mental health disorders: the biopsychosocial perspective. *Am Psychol* 2004;59(8):795–805.
42. Bair MJ, Robinson RL, Katon W, et al. Depression and pain comorbidity: a literature review. *Arch Intern Med.* 2003;163(20):2433–2445.

43. Miller LR, Cano A. Comorbid chronic pain and depression: who is at risk? *J Pain* 2009;10(6):619–627.
44. Lindsay PG, Wyckoff M. The depression-pain syndrome and its response to antidepressants. *Psychosomatics* 1981;22(7):571–577.
45. Haviland MG, Banta JE, Przekop P. Fibromyalgia: prevalence, course, and co-morbidities in hospitalized patients in the United States, 1999–2007. *Clin Exp Rheumatol* 2011;29(6 suppl 69):S79–S87.
46. McWilliams LA, Cox BJ, Enns MW. Mood and anxiety disorders associated with chronic pain: an examination in a nationally representative sample. *Pain* 2003;106(1–2):127–133.
47. Gatchel RJ, Gardea MA. Psychosocial issues: their importance in predicting disability, response to treatment, and search for compensation. *Neurol Clin* 1999;17(1):149–166.
48. Bair MJ, Wu J, Damush TM, et al. Association of depression and anxiety alone and in combination with chronic musculoskeletal pain in primary care patients. *Psychosom Med* 2008;70(8):890–897.
49. Hansen JS, Bendtsen L, Jensen R. Predictors of treatment outcome in headache patients with the Millon Clinical Multiaxial Inventory III (MCMI-III). *J Headache Pain* 2007;8(1):28–34.
50. Asmundson GJ, Norton GR, Allerdings MD, et al. Posttraumatic stress disorder and work-related injury. *J Anxiety Disord* 1998;12(1):57–69.
51. McFarlane AC, Atchison M, Rafalowicz E, et al. Physical symptoms in post-traumatic stress disorder. *J Psychosom Res* 1994;38(7):715–726.
52. Beckham JC, Crawford AL, Feldman ME, et al. Chronic posttraumatic stress disorder and chronic pain in Vietnam combat veterans. *J Psychosom Res* 1997;43(4):379–389.
53. Gauntlett-Gilbert J, Wilson S. Veterans and chronic pain. *Br J Pain* 2013; 7(2):79–84.
54. Otis JD, Keane TM, Kerns RD, et al. The development of an integrated treatment for veterans with comorbid chronic pain and posttraumatic stress disorder. *Pain Med* 2009;10(7):1300–1311.
55. Lew HL, Otis JD, Tun C, et al. Prevalence of chronic pain, posttraumatic stress disorder, and persistent postconcussive symptoms in OIF/OEF veterans: polytrauma clinical triad. *J Rehabil Res Dev* 2009;46(6):697–702.
56. Bosco MA, Gallinati JL, Clark ME. Conceptualizing and treating comorbid chronic pain and PTSD. *Pain Res Treat* 2013;2013:174728.
57. Schatman ME. The American chronic pain crisis and the media: about time to get it right? *J Pain Res* 2015;8:885–887.
58. Jeffery MM, Butler M, Stark A, et al. *Multidisciplinary Pain Programs for Chronic Noncancer Pain*. Rockville, MD: Agency for Healthcare Research and Quality; 2011.
59. Flor H, Fydrich T, Turk DC. Efficacy of multidisciplinary pain treatment centers: a meta-analytic review. *Pain* 1992;49(2):221–230.
60. Häuser W, Bernardy K, Arnold B, et al. Efficacy of multicomponent treatment in fibromyalgia syndrome: a meta-analysis of randomized controlled clinical trials. *Arthritis Rheum* 2009;61(2):216–224.
61. Scascighini L, Toma V, Dober-Spielmann S, et al. Multidisciplinary treatment for chronic pain: a systematic review of interventions and outcomes. *Rheumatology (Oxford)* 2008;47(5):670–678.
62. Gaul C, Liesering-Latta E, Schäfer B, et al. Integrated multidisciplinary care of headache disorders: a narrative review. *Cephalalgia* 2016;36(12):1181–1191.
63. Momsen AM, Rasmussen JO, Nielsen CV, et al. Multidisciplinary team care in rehabilitation: an overview of reviews. *J Rehabil Med* 2012;44(11):901–912.
64. Norrbrink Budh C, Kowalski J, Lundeberg T. A comprehensive pain management programme comprising educational, cognitive and behavioural interventions for neuropathic pain following spinal cord injury. *J Rehabil Med* 2006;38(3):172–180.
65. Norlund A, Ropponen A, Alexanderson K. Multidisciplinary interventions: review of studies of return to work after rehabilitation for low back pain. *J Rehabil Med* 2009;41(3):115–121.
66. Gatchel RJ, Okifuji A. Evidence-based scientific data documenting the treatment and cost-effectiveness of comprehensive pain programs for chronic nonmalignant pain. *J Pain* 2006;7(11):779–793.
67. Sletten CD, Kurklinsky S, Chinburapa V, et al. Economic analysis of a comprehensive pain rehabilitation program: a collaboration between Florida Blue and Mayo Clinic Florida. *Pain Med* 2015;16(5):898–904.
68. Guzmán J, Esmail R, Karjalainen K, et al. Multidisciplinary rehabilitation for chronic low back pain: systematic review. *BMJ* 2001;322(7301): 1511–1516.
69. Kamper SJ, Apeldoorn AT, Chiarotto A, et al. Multidisciplinary biopsychosocial rehabilitation for chronic low back pain. *Cochrane Database Syst Rev* 2014;(9):CD000963.
70. Whitfill T, Haggard R, Bierner SM, et al. Early intervention options for acute low back pain patients: a randomized clinical trial with one-year follow-up outcomes. *J Occup Rehabil* 2010;20:256–263.
71. Picavet HS, Vlaeyen JW, Schouten JS. Pain catastrophizing and kinesiophobia: predictors of chronic low back pain. *Am J Epidemiol* 2002;156(11):1028–1034.
72. Boersma K, Linton SJ. Psychological processes underlying the development of a chronic pain problem: a prospective study of the relationship between profiles of psychological variables in the fear-avoidance model and disability. *Clin J Pain* 2006;22(2):160–166.
73. Grotle M, Vøllestad NK, Brox JI. Screening for yellow flags in first-time acute low back pain: reliability and validity of a Norwegian version of the Acute Low Back Pain Screening Questionnaire. *Clin J Pain* 2006;22(5): 458–467.
74. Iles RA, Davidson M, Taylor NF. Psychosocial predictors of failure to return to work in non-chronic non-specific low back pain: a systematic review. *Occup Environ Med* 2008;65(8):507–517.
75. Dawson AP, Schluter PJ, Hodges PW, et al. Fear of movement, passive coping, manual handling, and severe or radiating pain increase the likelihood of sick leave due to low back pain. *Pain* 2011;152(7):1517–1524.
76. Neubauer E, Junge A, Pirron P, et al. HKF-R 10–screening for predicting chronicity in acute low back pain (LBP): a prospective clinical trial. *Eur J Pain* 2006;10(6):559–566.
77. Henschke N, Maher CG, Refshauge KM, et al. Prognosis in patients with recent onset low back pain in Australian primary care: inception cohort study. *BMJ* 2008;337:a171.
78. Gatchel RJ, Polatin PB, Mayer TG. The dominant role of psychosocial risk factors in the development of chronic low back pain disability. *Spine (Phila Pa 1976)* 1995;20(24):2702–2709.
79. Hill JC, Whitehurst DG, Lewis M, et al. Comparison of stratified primary care management for low back pain with current best practice (STarT Back): a randomised controlled trial. *Lancet* 2011;378(9802):1560–1571.
80. Choi BK, Verbeek JH, Tam WW, et al. Exercises for prevention of recurrences of low-back pain. *Cochrane Database Syst Rev* 2010;(1):CD006555.
81. Hasenbring M, Ulrich HW, Hartmann M, et al. The efficacy of a risk factor-based cognitive behavioral intervention and electromyographic biofeedback in patients with acute sciatic pain. An attempt to prevent chronicity. *Spine (Phila Pa 1976)* 1999;24(23):2525–2535.
82. Linton SJ, Andersson T. Can chronic disability be prevented? A randomized trial of a cognitive-behavior intervention and two forms of information for patients with spinal pain. *Spine (Phila Pa 1976)* 2000;25(21):2825–2831.
83. Gatchel RJ, Polatin PB, Noe C, et al. Treatment- and cost-effectiveness of early intervention for acute low-back pain patients: a one-year prospective study. *J Occup Rehabil* 2003;13(1):1–9.
84. Göhner W, Schlicht W. Preventing chronic back pain: evaluation of a theory-based cognitive-behavioural training programme for patients with subacute back pain. *Patient Educ Couns* 2006;64(1–3):87–95.
85. Linton SJ, Gross D, Schultz IZ, et al. Prognosis and the identification of workers risking disability: research issues and directions for future research. *J Occup Rehabil* 2005;15(4):459–474.
86. Hall A, Richmond H, Copsey B, et al. Physiotherapist-delivered cognitive-behavioural interventions are effective for low back pain, but can they be replicated in clinical practice? A systematic review. *Disabil Rehabil* 2018; 40(1):1–9.

CHAPTER 85

Pain and Anxiety and Depression

LIN YU and **LANCE M. McCRACKEN**

The experience of chronic pain is upsetting, frightening, discouraging, and demoralizing and creates significant suffering for those who experience it. Chronic pain sufferers struggle with proving the legitimacy of their conditions, constructing an explanation for their suffering, and negotiating health care system. They also perceive an uncertain future and even a loss of sense of self.[1] As chronic pain persists, these experiences can lead to the experience of significant anxiety and depression, among other conditions. The purpose of this chapter is to examine anxiety and depression in the context of chronic pain. It briefly describes the extent of these problems, their impact on individuals who experience them, and the processes in the interaction of these emotional experiences and pain. It also briefly reviews treatments applied to anxiety and depression, with a focus on forms of cognitive-behavioral therapy (CBT). This particularly includes the recent developments in CBT.

Prevalence of Anxiety and Depressive Disorders in Chronic Pain

Estimations of the extent and significance of anxiety and depressive disorders in chronic pain sufferers are not always consistent. Differences in the definition of chronic pain, regarding pain intensity, pain duration, and pain sites as well as differences in sampling methods, including setting and geographical location, can all contribute to variance in prevalence estimates and other measures. Nevertheless, conventionally defined anxiety and depressive disorders appear significantly more frequent among people with chronic pain than those without.

A national survey in the United States showed that among chronic pain sufferers, 35.1% experienced anxiety disorders and 20.2% experienced depressive disorders in the past year, whereas the respective numbers in the general population are 18.1% and 9.3%.[2] Another national survey[3] found similar rates for anxiety, 26.5%, and depression, 17.5%. Again, these estimates are roughly 1.5 to 2 times as high as those in the general community, which are 18.1% and 9.5% for anxiety and depression, respectively, in the United States.[4]

A large household survey in Canada[5] also showed that the rate of depression present in people with chronic pain, 19.8%, is more than 3 times as great as in those without pain (5.9%).

Demyttenaere et al.[6] carried out 18 surveys in 17 countries representing all five continents (N = 85,088). It was reported that "mental disorders" are more common in people with chronic pain than those without, with a pooled odds ratio (OR) of 2.7 for anxiety disorder, 2.1 for agoraphobia or panic disorder, 1.9 for social phobia, 2.6 for posttraumatic stress disorder (PTSD), 2.3 for major depression, and 2.8 for dysthymia. With further analyses of the same data, the researchers found that mood and anxiety disorders are more prevalent in people with multiple pain sites than those without one pain site and those without.[7] Relative to people without pain, the pooled estimates of odd ratios were 1.8 and 1.9 for mood disorder and anxiety, respectively, among people with single pain site and 3.6 and 3.7 among people with multiple pain sites.[7]

Ohayon and Schatzberg[8] conducted a survey in five European countries, including the United Kingdom, Germany, Italy, Portugal, and Spain. It was found that 43.4% of the subjects with major depressive disorder suffer from chronic pain, which is 4 times more often than in subjects without major depressive disorder.

Another large survey representing 15 European countries suggested that the prevalence of self-report diagnosis of depression associated with chronic pain is 21%.[9]

The results reported earlier are from population-based studies. It is perhaps not surprising that the estimates of the prevalence of anxiety and depression are higher in pain sufferers identified in clinical settings than those in the general population. A survey of patients (N = 5,808) visiting a primary care clinic showed that chronic pain is more commonly reported in people with major depressive disorder, 66%, than those without, 43%. In particular, disabling chronic pain is substantially more common in people with major depressive disorder, 41%, than those without, 10%.[10] In a study of 1,204 consecutive adults attending a specialty pain service in London, 60.8% met screening criteria for probable depression, and 33.8% met criteria for severe depression on a commonly used, validated, screening questionnaire.[11] In a literature review of depression and pain comorbidity,[12] the rates for concurrent major depression in pain sufferers were identified as 18% (4.7% to 22%) in population-based settings and an average of 13% to 85% in various clinical settings. Among the 42 studies reviewed, 33 explicitly focused on chronic pain.

Impact of Anxiety and Depressive Disorders on Functioning

The high rates of anxiety and depression in chronic pain are worrying, particularly given that the consequences of these disorders with respect to overall health. In the most updated World Health Organization (WHO)[13] report of global health, depression is ranked as the single largest contributor to global disability, and anxiety disorders the sixth. Depression was also reported to be the major contributor to suicide deaths, with number close to 800,000 per year. It was estimated that 4.4% of the global population are suffering from depression and 3.6% from anxiety.[13] However, in contrast to the high prevalence and significant consequent health loss of these mental disorders, results from WHO surveys also showed that the proportion of people with access to treatment for mental disorders are far lower than that for physical disorders in developed countries, even more so in developing countries, and even for those people assessed as having a severely disabling condition.[14]

The association between the concurrence of depression and pain and the impairment in functioning has been well documented. In a large-scale survey representing five European countries (N = 21,425), it was reported that people with pain and depression experience decreased work productivity on more than twice as many days per month as those with either condition alone, and more than 5 times as many days per month as those without either condition.[6] It has also been reported that patients with pain and depression have higher unemployment rates.[11,12,15,16] In a review of 22 studies on comorbidity between depression and pain, it was identified that patients with depression and pain experience impaired social functioning; functional limitations, such as limited mobility and limitation in activities; more days of illness; and more hospitalizations compared to those with pain alone.[12]

In people seeking specialty treatment for chronic pain, those screening positive for probable depression incur 60% higher total health care costs compared to those who do not screen positive.[11] In this study, the significantly greater costs remained for those with severe depression even after adjustment for the role of age, gender, occupational status, the presence of generalized pain, pain interference, and pain acceptance.

Although it is based on fewer smaller studies, there is also evidence showing the impact of anxiety disorders in combination with pain. In a recent survey of 80 patients with chronic neck pain, it was observed that anxiety is associated with greater functional disability.[17] In a study of 250 chronic musculoskeletal pain patients in a primary care in the United States,[18] 45% of the patients screened positive for at least one anxiety disorder and, as compared to those without any anxiety disorder, showed significant worse health status on a range of pain, psychological, and other quality of life–related outcomes. These patients with anxiety conditions also showed substantial functional impairment, the extent of which was strongly associated with the extent of anxiety disorders, in that higher numbers of anxiety conditions were associated with more severe pain-related interference, worse mental health, and more days of disability.

An expanding body of literature has also shown associations between chronic pain conditions, comorbidity with mental health problems, and suicide.[19–24] A survey suggested that 50% of chronic pain patients had serious thoughts of committing suicide due to their pain disorder.[19] Specific pain-related risk factors, such as pain severity and comorbidity with depression, have been suggested as accounting for the increased rates of suicidal behavior in chronic pain patients.[20] Data from a large-scale survey of Canadian population[23] showed that after controlling for demographics, Axis I mental disorders, and comorbidity (three or more mental disorders), the presence of one or more chronic pain conditions was associated with both suicidal ideation and suicidal attempt. Among those with a mental disorder, comorbidity with one or more chronic pain conditions was also associated with suicidal ideation and suicidal attempt.[23] Braden and Sullivan[21] investigated the independent association between noncancer chronic pain conditions and the risk for suicidal behavior, using data from a national survey (n = 5,692). The results suggested that after controlling for medical, mental health, and demographic variables, the presence of any pain condition was associated with lifetime suicidal ideation, OR 1.4 (95% confidence interval [CI], 1.1 to 1.8). Data from the same survey similarly identified head pain and a summary pain score as potentially independent risk factors for suicidal ideation and suicide attempt.[22]

The comorbidity of chronic pain with depression and anxiety has also shown association with problematic substance use (e.g., Feingold et al.[25]). In a study including 888 individuals receiving treatment for chronic pain,[25] depression was found present in 88% of the participants with problematic use of opioids and 46.5% of those with problematic use of cannabis, and the prevalence of anxiety was 74.5% and 41.9%, respectively. The results also revealed that any diagnosis of depression, particularly moderate to severe and severe depression, and also generalized anxiety disorder (GAD), again more so with greater severity, were significantly associated with problematic use of opioids and cannabis.

A general finding is that chronic pain sufferers with anxiety and/or depression demonstrate significantly worse quality of life compared to those without.[26] Together with the aftermath of suicide, or problems in the wake of substance abuse, they reflect what is arguably the worst possible quality of life.

Once again, there is significant variability in the evidence surrounding rates and impacts of anxiety and depressive disorders in chronic pain sufferers. For instance, in patients suffering from pain and co-occurring depression, depression may be misdiagnosed due to shared symptoms between pain and depression (e.g., sleep disturbance and weight and appetite changes). Caution is warranted in any attempts at higher precision interpretations of these findings. Nevertheless, numerous studies generally demonstrate a high rate of concurrence of anxiety and depressive disorders with pain as well as the additional important burden of anxiety and depression disorders on chronic pain suffers, as observed in a wide range of outcomes.

The Interaction of Anxiety, Depression, and Chronic Pain

There has been a long running debate about the relationship between chronic pain and psychopathology associated with anxiety and depression in terms of which comes first or whether one ought to be appropriately regarded as the cause of the other. Available evidence allows for contrasting interpretations. For instance, patients with preexisting depression were found to be more likely to develop chest pain and headache.[27] On the other hand, in a related review of available evidence at the time, it was suggested that depression is most often a consequence and follows the development of pain.[28] More than 20 years ago, a model called the "diathesis-stress model" was proposed,[29,30] consistent with this view. In this model, the diatheses are conceptualized as preexisting semidormant characteristics of the individuals before the onset of chronic pain that are then activated by the stress of chronic pain condition. Bank and Kerns[29] identified the experience of chronic pain itself as the stress component of the model. The researchers also suggested that chronic pain is more likely to result in depression than other chronic medical conditions due to the uniquely challenging nature of stressor associated with chronic pain.[29] Dohrenwend et al.[31] investigated this hypothesis with a family study for people with myofascial face pain, using psychiatric interviews. The conclusions were consistent with this hypothesis, suggesting that living with myofascial face pain contributes to the elevated rate of depression. On the other hand, a more recent study investigating the comorbidity of fibromyalgia (FM) and PTSD produced an alternative interpretation for the interaction between chronic pain and anxiety.[32] In this study, surveys were conducted among community-dwelling women before and after the 9/11 attack in New York City. The odds of probable PTSD were more than 3 times greater in women with FM-like symptoms than those without, assessed after 9/11. The OR was not reduced after controlling for FM-like symptoms before 9/11 or for the potentially confounded symptoms of PTSD specifically related to arousal. As mentioned, most of this research is now 10 to 20 years old, and some of these conceptualizations are certainly due for an update.

In some ways, it may not be important to know which came first, pain or depression or anxiety, in the early history of the events observed. Instead, an understanding of how this pattern of suffering is maintained and worsened, on a day-to-day basis, may be more practical. This effort should perhaps include identifying the circumstances that give rise to these behavioral patterns, and the most manipulable elements in the patients' experiences, where impacts on these are most likely to lead to significant and durable improvement in functioning and well-being.

THE FEAR-AVOIDANCE MODEL

Anxiety, or its related more particular form, fear, has been integrated into what is by now a very well-known model of chronic pain and disability, referred to as the *fear-avoidance model*.[33–35] The basic assumption of the fear-avoidance model is that the way in which pain is interpreted may lead to one of two different pathways. When acute pain is perceived as nonthreatening, patients are likely to remain engaged in daily activities, which can essentially prevent significant disability or facilitate functional recovery when some disruption is functioning has occurred. On the other hand, when acute pain is perceived as threatening, as a kind of catastrophe, this interpretation may give rise to pain-related fear, which may lead to avoidance behaviors and hypervigilance to bodily sensations, followed by disruption of functioning, including disuse, disability, and depression.[35] In this model, processes including respondent and operant-based learning, in combination with processes of physical deconditioning (loss of physical capacity), possibly muscular reactivity, as well as cognitive processes such as, again, hypervigilance and pain catastrophizing, are proposed as entailing a cycle of mutual influence between behavioral, cognitive, emotional, and muscular processes and reduced functioning.

Numerous studies have investigated the relationships between components of the fear-avoidance model (see review[36]). Associations were reported for pain with disability (e.g., Boersma and Linton,[37] Leeuw et al.[38]), pain catastrophizing with pain disability (e.g., Peters et al.,[39] Sullivan et al.[40]), and excessive attention with pain and pain-related fear (e.g., Goubert et al.,[41] Goubert et al.[42]). Pain-related fear is positively associated with disability (e.g., Goubert et al.,[42] Boersma et al.[43]) and pain intensity (e.g., Buer and Linton,[44] Turner et al.[45]) as well escape/avoidance behavior (e.g., Goubert et al.,[42] Al-Obaidi et al.[46]). A systematic review showed moderate evidence for the moderating role of fear-avoidance beliefs in treatment efficacy in people with low back pain.[47] Overall data appear to suggest the relationships between the components of the fear-avoidance models. In addition to the evidence from chronic pain, there has also been evidence for the role of pain-related fear in various stages of pain. For instance, Picavet et al.[48] showed that both heightened pain-related fear and pain catastrophizing during the acute phase increased the risk of future chronic low back pain and disability. Heightened initial levels of pain-related fear were also shown to be related to decreased probability of returning to work and greater probability of being on sick leave[43,49,50] and to the recurrence of low back pain and care seeking 4 years later.[51]

A Contextual Behavioral Approach to Anxiety and Depressive Disorders

From a contextual behavioral perspective, to improve health and functioning in people who demonstrate the complex and highly varying pathologic behavior patterns in what we call depression and anxiety disorders, requires identifying functionally important factors, or processes, that contribute to the maintenance and exacerbation of these patterns. One such process proposed is experiential avoidance.[52] Experiential avoidance refers to the behavior pattern reflected when a person is unwilling to remain in contact with particular private events, such as bodily sensations, emotions, thoughts, and memories, and takes action to alter the form or frequency of these events or the contexts that occasion them.[52] Experiential avoidance has been proposed as a functional dimension underlying a wide range of behavioral disorders,[52] including anxiety disorders[53] and depression.[54,55] It is suggested that experiential avoidance, regardless of its form (e.g., elaborate rituals observed in people with obsessive-compulsive disorder [OCD], or work absence observed in people with chronic pain), generally reflects the same function, avoiding or escaping from unacceptable private events, such as anxiety. This type of response, in turn, can be additionally negatively reinforced by the avoidance of related undesirable thoughts and other private events that occasion or follow these.[53,55]

In depression, experiential avoidance appears to be a particularly active ingredient related to the perpetuation and exacerbation of the depressive condition, even though this is less typical to consider depression as an avoidance-related disorder. Certainly, the "social withdrawal" aspect of depression is avoidant in quality, and the irritable mood that is often present can function to drive others away, resulting in reduced contact with others. Withdrawing in one's activities after some types of losses can be acquired from a history of avoiding further losses, such as when being withdrawn allows some prevailing threats to pass. Kanter et al.[54] suggested that the core experiences of depression, the elicited emotional or affective experiences, are normal and adaptive. For instance, the capacity to experience low mood or sadness in appropriate situations can have short-term benefits such as initiating social support. So-called "clinical" or pathologic variants of depression then are simply cases of maladaptive dysregulation or overextensions of this adaptive pattern. Here, experiential avoidance is proposed to be one process by which initial emotional responses can lead to chronic and maladaptive depression in the absence of chronically maladaptive environments.[54,55] In this view, the emotional experiences, once elicited and then maintained may play a role in maintaining, exacerbating and creating additional "symptoms" of depression. To say this more succinctly, when the initially elicited private responses to loss are functionally aversive, they can evoke behaviors that function to avoid or escape the private responses. The avoidance of these experiences, even when it works to keep feelings muted in the short term, can in turn produce additional long-term problems.

Indeed, a contextual behavioral analysis of anxiety and depressive disorders does not yet constitute a complete account. Even so, a complete review of this effort is beyond the scope of this chapter. One point that should be clear in this effort is that it is somewhat unconventional, less devoted to diagnoses and disorder, and more devoted to functionally meaningful factors or dimensions that give rise to, maintain, and exacerbate the pathologic behavioral patterns. This approach is inherently transdiagnostic, applicable equally to all the people who experience these "disorders" discussed earlier, regardless of the surface symptoms. In this effort, experiential avoidance has been identified as a potential functional dimension underlying these disorders. There are others, particularly facets of what is called psychological flexibility, to be discussed in a subsequent section of this chapter.

Treatment of Anxiety and Depressive Disorders

EVIDENCE FROM PHARMACOLOGIC APPROACHES
Pharmacologic treatments are commonly used in depressive disorders. However, there have been ongoing debates about their relatively small effects as compared to placebos observed in clinical trials and whether these are clinically meaningful.[56] A recent systematic review including 66 studies (n = 15,161) investigated the efficacy and acceptability of pharmacologic treatments for depressive disorders in primary care.[57] Most of these studies were of short duration (up to 12 weeks). Meta-analyses suggested that more patients responded (showing at least 50% reduction in scores from depression measures) to some forms of pharmacologic treatment, including tricyclic antidepressants (TCAs), selective serotonin reuptake inhibitors (SSRIs), a serotonin norepinephrine reuptake inhibitor (SNRI), a low-dose serotonin antagonist and reuptake inhibitor (SARI), and hypericum extracts, as compared to placebo, but effects were relatively small, with estimated ORs between 1.69 (corresponding to a number needed to treat [NNT] of 7 to 8) and 2.03. Meta-analyses of acceptability of treatments suggested

that some drugs including TCAs, SSRIs, SNRI, norepinephrine reuptake inhibitor (NRI), and noradrenergic and specific serotonergic antidepressant agents (NaSSAs) were associated with significantly more study discontinuations, resulting from adverse effects, than placebo. Overall, these results are comparable with findings from a previous review,[58] suggesting a statistically significant but small short-term effect of antidepressants for depression, and higher risk of harm for patients in pharmacologic treatments as compared to placebo. Pharmacologic treatments may help in preventing subsequent relapse and recurrence[59] but only for so long as one stays on them.

Medications do not appear superior to nonpharmacologic treatments for depression. For instance, a recent review including 44 trials compared second-generation antidepressants (SGAs) with various forms of nonpharmacologic treatments for adults with major depressive disorder.[60] It was reported that SGAs and CBT lead to similar rates of response to treatment (relative risk = 0.91, 0.77 to 1.07). However, patients treated with SGAs have a higher risk of experiencing adverse events or discontinuing treatment because of adverse events, as compared to CBT, acupuncture, or St. John's wort.

The evidence from pharmacologic treatment for anxiety disorders appears to demonstrate a similar pattern. For example, a Cochrane review of antidepressants for GAD[61] suggested the efficacy of antidepressants in reducing anxiety symptoms, with an NNT of 5.7, indicating six patients need to be treated to lead to an additional one achieving clinical improvement. However, antidepressants were found associated with significantly more side effects such as nausea, dry mouth, constipation, drowsiness, insomnia, anorexia, sexual dysfunction, and flatulence. A more recent Cochrane review of second-generation antipsychotics for anxiety disorders suggested comparable results.[62] Participants with GAD responded significantly better to quetiapine than to placebo (OR = 2.21; 95% CI, 1.10 to 4.45). However, they were more likely to drop out due to adverse events, to gain weight, to suffer from sedation or to suffer from extrapyramidal side effects. Again, as in depression, most of these studies were of short duration.

It is worth mentioning that antidepressant medications, typically used to treat depression and anxiety disorders, are also used as first-line analgesics, in such pain conditions as neuropathic pain.[63] The best performance from these medications achieve a modest NNT for 50% pain relief of 6.4 (95% CI, 5.2 to 8.4) for SNRIs in these conditions.[64] In clinical practice, there is often a presumption that these medications might help the patient to achieve multiple improvements, in pain, depression, anxiety, and sleep, where needed. This seems certain to provide some efficiency in treatment and to be practically useful, particularly where alternative mental health services are difficult to access. We only add that the rates of response from these medications, both for pain and for depression, for example, leave many patients remaining in need of relief and support.

EVIDENCE FROM PSYCHOLOGICAL APPROACHES

In addition to pharmacologic treatments, psychological treatments, as well as treatment combining pharmacologic and psychological treatments, are also commonly used for anxiety and depressive disorders.

A group of researchers comprehensively reviewed the meta-analyses for the efficacy of CBT applied to a variety of problems,[65] and CBT for anxiety disorders was identified as among those with the strongest supportive evidence, with medium to large effect sizes reported for a variety of anxiety disorders.

In a systematic review of CBT for anxiety disorders,[66] CBT was identified to be superior to placebo with a medium effect size (Hedges' g = .73) for anxiety disorder severity and a pooled OR of 4.06 (95% CI, 2.78 to 5.92; z = 7.26; P < .001) for treatment response. In addition, no significant difference in attrition rates

between CBT and placebo was observed. When analyzed using intention to treat samples, the effect size became smaller, yet still significant. CBT was also identified as superior to active controls, such as applied relaxation[67] and counseling.[68] Evidence for some secondary symptoms, such as sleep dysfunction and anxiety sensitivity, also supports the efficacy of CBT.[69] In addition, there is evidence from meta-analyses supporting the short-to-medium term effect of CBT for anxiety disorders, such as social phobia.[70,71] CBT has been found similarly effective compared to medications for depression[72] as well as for anxiety disorders.[73]

When psychological and pharmacologic treatments are combined, meta-analysis suggest the combined treatments are superior to either treatment alone at the acute treatment stage, but not more effective than psychological treatment alone in long term, particularly considering the harm due to medication side effects.[74] These results led experts to speculate that having active medication in the system during treatment may undermine the enduring effect of CBT.[75] Naturally, more studies are needed to test this hypothesis. Nevertheless, some patients did appear to respond to pharmacologic treatments, and pharmacologic treatments also showed enduring effect of preventing patients from relapse, as long as the medications are continued. Although caution against the harm to patients due to the side effect of medications should be taken, evidence for psychological treatment, CBT in particular, supports its enduring effectiveness with little risk of harm to participants.

In a relatively new set of developments, Internet-delivered therapist-guided forms of CBT, which are regarded more accessible and cost-effective compared to face-to-face treatment modality, show promise in the treatment of anxiety. A recent Cochrane review of Internet-delivered therapist-guided CBT for anxiety disorders, suggested the superiority of Internet-delivered therapist-guided CBT, in reducing anxiety symptoms at posttreatment, in comparison with a waiting list, attention, information, or online discussion group control.[76] Low-quality evidence also suggests no significant difference between face-to-face CBT and Internet-delivered therapist-guided CBT.[76] However, an overall low quality of evidence and short-duration investigations represent important caveats.

The evidence of CBT for depression appears less consistent. CBT for depression was reported more effective than inactive controls, such as waiting list or no treatment, with a medium effect size.[77,78] However, when compared to other active treatments, such as psychodynamic treatment, problem-solving therapy, and interpersonal psychotherapy, CBT produced mixed results. Some evidence from meta-analyses suggested that CBT is equally effective as other psychological treatments.[78,79] However, evidence in favor of CBT also exists.[80,81] For instance, CBT was found superior to relaxation techniques at posttreatment.[80] CBT was also reported to be superior to psychodynamic therapy at both posttreatment and at 6-month follow-up, although depression and anxiety symptoms were examined together here.[81]

COGNITIVE-BEHAVIORAL THERAPY FOR CHRONIC PAIN: EFFECTS ON DEPRESSION AND ANXIETY

The application of CBT to chronic pain also produces some evidence for the effectiveness of CBT in improving depression and anxiety, albeit with limited effect sizes. In a Cochrane review of psychological treatments for chronic pain,[82] 35 studies were included in the analyses. When compared with active controls, the overall effect of CBT was significant on disability, standard mean difference (SMD) = −.19, and catastrophizing, SMD = −.18, with small effect sizes, but not on pain or mood (depression and anxiety) at posttreatment. The effect of CBT was only significant on disability at follow-up with a small effect size, SMD = −.15. When compared with treatment as usual, the overall effect of CBT was significant on all outcomes examined, including pain, SMD = −.21; disability, SMD = −.26; mood,

SMD = −.38; and catastrophizing, SMD = −.53, at posttreatment. However, the effect disappeared at follow-up, except for a small effect on mood, SMD = −.26.

Developments in Cognitive Behavioral Therapy

There are current developments within CBT. One of these is called contextual cognitive-behavioral therapy (CCBT), including acceptance and commitment therapy (ACT),[55] and often referred to as the "third wave" CBT. CCBT stems from the philosophy and worldview of functional contextualism.[55,83] In this view, behavioral events are ongoing acts, having meaning only with reference to its historical and situational context. Therefore, thoughts and feelings may be related to particular behaviors, but only in historical and situational contexts that give rise to these experiences and their relation to the subsequent actions. In other words, the contents of thoughts and feelings are not problematic unless the context lends the thoughts influences on actions that undermine one's goals and values.[84] Therefore, CCBT as a treatment approach does not focus on creating changes in the content or frequency of one's thoughts and feelings, rather one's "relations" to these thoughts and feelings. CCBT specifically aims at reducing experiential avoidance[85] and related pathologic processes in behavior. All of this means CCBT includes a very different way of looking at depression and anxiety compared to what is usually done.

A reliable and valid measure of experiential avoidance, the Acceptance and Action Questionnaire (AAQ),[85] was developed to assess various aspects of experiential avoidance and shows moderate to high correlations with measures of general psychopathology, such as measures of general health and quality of life, as well as standardized measures of anxiety and depression. In the domain of pain, pain-related avoidance also has been widely explored, in the form of its polar opposite, pain acceptance.[86–88] For example, Vowles and McCracken[88] found that the improvement in acceptance of pain was significantly correlated with the reduction in pain intensity, depression, pain-related anxiety, physical and psychological disability, and physical functioning, with a small to medium effect size during the treatment. The correlations remained significant at 3-month follow-up for pain intensity, depression, pain-related anxiety, and physical and psychological disability. In addition, McCracken and Gutiérrez-Martínez[89] reported the significant associations between general psychological acceptance and pain acceptance, and depression, pain-related anxiety, physical disability, and psychosocial disability, independent from pain. Overall, these empirical findings support the association between experiential avoidance and anxiety, depression, and other aspects of functioning and well-being in pain sufferers. Again, it is beyond the scope of the chapter to provide a complete contextual behavioral account of anxiety or depression, or the pattern of concurrence of these problems and pain. Nevertheless, as outlined earlier, and shown here in evidence, experiential avoidance appears to be a relevant functional dimension related to these complex behavior patterns.

Although the specific application of CCBT to anxiety and depressive disorders is still, as we say, incomplete at this stage, evidence from a meta-analyses show that the "third wave" CBT, regardless of treatment modality, appears to be superior to treatment as usual,[90] and as effective as other psychological treatments[91] for depression.

Accumulating studies of the application of CCBT to chronic pain have produced supportive evidence for effects on depression, anxiety, and other aspects of functioning in chronic pain sufferers. In a systematic review of contextual, "acceptance-based," treatment for chronic pain, 19 studies (9 RCTs, 5 clinically controlled studies with randomization, and 5 noncontrolled studies) were identified and included.[92] When all studies were included in the analysis, significant moderate pooled effect sizes were found for pain, physical functioning and disability, depression, anxiety, and quality of life, SMD = .47 to .69. Pooled effect sizes from all controlled studies suggested a significant and small effect on these outcomes, SMD = .24 to .41. Pooled effect sizes from RCTs suggested a small and significant effect on pain and depression, SMD = .26. Overall, these findings suggested that CCBT is good alternative to CBT.

In an update of the previous review,[93] 25 RCTs were identified and included in the main analyses. Significant and small effects were found for pain intensity, SMD = .24; disability, SMD = .40; and depression, SMD = .43, and significant and moderate effects for pain-related interference, SMD = .62, and anxiety, SMD = .51, at posttreatment. A small effect was found for quality of life, SMD = .44, but not to a statistically significant extent. Improvements in all outcomes maintained or increased at follow-up with small to large effect sizes for pain intensity, SMD = .41; for pain-related interference, SMD = 1.05; for disability, SMD = .39; for depression, SMD = .53; for anxiety, SMD = .59; and for quality of life, SMD = .66.

A recent systematic review identified 11 RCTs of ACT for chronic pain.[94] When compared to controls, ACT was favored at posttreatment with an overall large effect size for the key processes of ACT, including pain acceptance, SMD = .84, and psychological flexibility, SMD = −.87, as well as a small effect size observed for functioning, SMD = −.45; a medium effect size for anxiety, SMD = −.57; and a large effect size for depression, SMD = −.84, but not quality of life or pain intensity. The effect sizes are generally smaller at follow-ups. When ACT was compared to active treatments, ACT was favored over applied relaxation at posttreatment on pain acceptance, SMD = .84; quality of life, SMD = .40; and functioning, SMD = .70, and the effect sizes at follow-up were generally similar or smaller.

Again, overall findings from reviews show CCBT is a good alternative to conventional CBT. Perhaps more importantly, these promising findings suggest the potential of CCBT to address the complex, multiproblem, behavior patterns observed in chronic pain sufferers, including the problems included with categories of depression and anxiety.

Summary

The suffering of anxiety and depressive disorders, as these are conventionally conceived, is evident in people with chronic pain in the community and even more so in the clinic. These conditions impose limits on the physical functioning of people who experience them, interfere with their work and social functioning, reduce quality of life, and lead to significant disability and suffering. Despite the high prevalence of these problems and the significant burden they impose on individuals, communities, and national resources, these problems are not yet adequately addressed.

In general, pharmacologic treatments and psychological treatments, including CBT, focused on reducing anxiety and depression, most consistently produce at least small benefits, mostly in the short term. Medication for depression does not appear to be superior to CBT, even though it appears more frequently applied, and in fact, CBT has fewer adverse side effects. CBT for anxiety disorders in particular produces larger benefits, medium effect sizes, or better. Psychological treatments for chronic pain, again typically CBT, can also produce benefits for depression and anxiety, again on average small in magnitude.

Over time, depression and anxiety are increasingly looked at not only as disorders or syndromes reflected as sets of symptoms but also as complex patterns of behavior that result from multiple psychological processes. Talking about depression and anxiety problems as separate categories of symptoms, separate from other domains of functioning, has clinical utility to a certain extent but may be inadequate to address the complex pathologic patterns of emotions and overt behavior observed in people with these problems. Calling a problem "depression," for example, can create the sense of a "real entity" around the elements and a sense of a unifying cause for the whole set. On the other hand, a functional analysis of how these elements interrelate with each in other, with and in a context that is both situational and historical, can provide a different perspective. This could include a contextual analysis of how the pattern of responses is maintained and worsened, including identifying underlying functional dimensions, and related manipulable events that can create the basis for intervention. Such an analysis could serve practical clinical purposes better. Included in this effort currently is the exploration of a process or functional dimension called experiential avoidance, for example.

The investigation of experiential avoidance is still at early stage. However, as a potentially shared functional process among these emotional experiences, chronic pain, and other related problems in human functioning and well-being, this process appears potentially important and useful for addressing suffering in people with chronic pain. It is, as implied, a fully transdiagnostic process, the kind often called for to improve approaches to treatment development.

A recent development in CBT, a functional contextual approach to human functioning and well-being, called CCBT, is producing promising results. CCBT does not focus on creating changes to one's thoughts and feelings, or one's moods, but rather in one's "relations" to one's thoughts and feelings and the contexts that support those relations. Hence, rather unconventionally, it is not focused on reducing symptoms of anxiety and depression as such and even reflects little interest in disorders named according to, and defined by, the experience of emotions. This is a defining feature of CCBT. It is focused on processes of pathology and well-being and not on diagnoses and syndromes. Perhaps most radically, in this approach, experiences of anxiety and depression are regarded as normal within the realms of being human, and it is just the impacts on behavior from these experiences that are targeted for change.

In chronic pain, CCBT has been applied and has produced promising results in a wide range of outcomes including physical and emotional functioning, work and social functioning, and quality of life, among others (e.g., Hughes et al.,[94] McCracken and Morley[95]). The accumulating evidence appears to suggest significant potential for CCBT in addressing various problems that come with the experience of chronic pain, including the different varieties of how people suffer emotionally with it.

References

1. Toye F, Seers K, Allcock N, et al. Patients' experiences of chronic nonmalignant musculoskeletal pain: a qualitative systematic review. *Br J Gen Pract* 2013;63(617):e829–e841.
2. McWilliams LA, Cox BJ, Enns MW. Mood and anxiety disorders associated with chronic pain: an examination in a nationally representative sample. *Pain* 2003;106(1):127–133.
3. Von Korff M, Crane P, Lane M. Chronic spinal pain and physical–mental comorbidity in the United States: results from the national comorbidity survey replication. *Pain* 2005;113(3):331–339.
4. Kessler RC, Chiu WT, Demler O, et al. Prevalence, severity, and comorbidity of 12-month DSM-IV disorders in the National Comorbidity Survey Replication. *Arch Gen Psychiatry* 2005;62(6):617–627.
5. Currie SR, Wang J. Chronic back pain and major depression in the general Canadian population. *Pain* 2004;107(1):54–60.
6. Demyttenaere K, Bonnewyn A, Bruffaerts R, et al. Comorbid painful physical symptoms and depression: prevalence, work loss, and help seeking. *J Affect Disord* 2006;92(2):185–193.
7. Gureje O, Von Korff M, Kola L, et al. The relation between multiple pains and mental disorders: results from the World Mental Health Surveys. *Pain* 2008;135(1):82–91.
8. Ohayon MM, Schatzberg AF. Using chronic pain to predict depressive morbidity in the general population. *Arch Gen Psychiatry* 2003;60(1):39–47.
9. Breivik H, Collett B, Ventafridda V, et al. Survey of chronic pain in Europe: prevalence, impact on daily life, and treatment. *Eur J Pain* 2006;10(4):287.
10. Arnow BA, Hunkeler EM, Blasey CM, et al. Comorbid depression, chronic pain, and disability in primary care. *Psychosom Med* 2006;68(2):262–268.
11. Rayner L, Hotopf M, Petkova H, et al. Depression in patients with chronic pain attending a specialized pain treatment centre: prevalence and impact on health care costs. *Pain* 2016;147:1472–1479.
12. Bair MJ, Robinson RL, Katon W, et al. Depression and pain comorbidity: a literature review. *Arch Intern Med* 2003;163(20):2433–2445.
13. World Health Organization. Depression and other common mental disorders: global health estimates. Available at: http://www.who.int/mental_health/management/depression/prevalence_global_health_estimates/en/. Accessed August 20, 2017.
14. Ormel J, Petukhova M, Chatterji S, et al. Disability and treatment of specific mental and physical disorders across the world. *Br J Psychiatry* 2008;192(5):368–375.
15. Dolce JJ, Crocker MF, Doleys DM. Prediction of outcome among chronic pain patients. *Behav Res Ther* 1986;24(3):313–319.
16. Sullivan MJ, Reesor K, Mikail S, et al. The treatment of depression in chronic low back pain: review and recommendations. *Pain* 1992;50(1):5–13.
17. Elbinoune I, Amine B, Shyen S, et al. Chronic neck pain and anxiety-depression: prevalence and associated risk factors. *Pan Afr Med J* 2016;24(1):89.
18. Kroenke K, Outcalt S, Krebs E, et al. Association between anxiety, health-related quality of life and functional impairment in primary care patients with chronic pain. *Gen Hosp Psychiatry* 2013;35(4):359–365.
19. Hitchcock LS, Ferrell BR, McCaffery M. The experience of chronic nonmalignant pain. *J Pain Symptom Manage* 1994;9(5):312–318.
20. Fishbain DA. The association of chronic pain and suicide. *Sem Clin Neuropsychiatry* 1999;(3):221–227.
21. Braden JB, Sullivan MD. Suicidal thoughts and behavior among adults with self-reported pain conditions in the National Comorbidity Survey replication. *J Pain* 2008;9(12):1106–1115.
22. Ilgen MA, Zivin K, McCammon RJ, et al. Pain and suicidal thoughts, plans and attempts in the United States. *Gen Hosp Psychiatry* 2008;30(6):521–527.
23. Ratcliffe GE, Enns MW, Belik SL, et al. Chronic pain conditions and suicidal ideation and suicide attempts: an epidemiologic perspective. *Clin J Pain* 2008;24(3):204–210.
24. Cheatle MD, Wasser T, Foster C, et al. Prevalence of suicidal ideation in patients with chronic non-cancer pain referred to a behaviorally based pain program. *Pain Phys* 2014;17(3):E359–E367.
25. Feingold D, Goor-Aryeh I, Bril S, et al. Problematic use of prescription opioids and medicinal cannabis among patients suffering from chronic pain. *Pain Med* 2017;18(2):294–306.
26. Castro M, Quarantini LC, Daltro C, et al. Comorbid depression and anxiety symptoms in chronic pain patients and their impact on health-related quality of life. *Arch Clin Psychiatry* 2011;38(4):126–129.
27. Von Korff M, Le Resche L, Dworkin SF. First onset of common pain symptoms: a prospective study of depression as a risk factor. *Pain* 1993;55(2):251–258.
28. Fishbain D, Cutler R, Rosomoff H, et al. Chronic pain associated depression: antecedent or consequence of chronic pain? A review. *Clin J Pain* 1993;13(2):116–137.
29. Banks SM, Kerns RD. Explaining high rates of depression in chronic pain: a diathesis-stress framework. *Psychol Bull* 1996;119:95–110.
30. Dersh J, Polatin PB, Gatchel RJ. Chronic pain and psychopathology: research findings and theoretical considerations. *Psychosom Med* 2002;64(5):773–786.
31. Dohrenwend BP, Raphael KG, Marbach JJ, et al. Why is depression comorbid with chronic myofascial face pain? A family study test of alternative hypotheses. *Pain* 1999;83(2):183–192.
32. Raphael KG, Janal MN, Nayak S. Comorbidity of fibromyalgia and posttraumatic stress disorder symptoms in a community sample of women. *Pain Med* 2004;5(1):33–41.
33. Lethem J, Slade PD, Troup JDG, et al. Outline of a fear-avoidance model of exaggerated pain perception—I. *Behav Res Ther* 1983;21(4):401–408.
34. Philips HC. Avoidance behaviour and its role in sustaining chronic pain. *Behav Res Therap* 1987;25(4):273–279.
35. Vlaeyen JW, Linton SJ. Fear-avoidance and its consequences in chronic musculoskeletal pain: a state of the art. *Pain* 2000;85 (3):317–332.
36. Leeuw M, Goossens ME, Linton SJ, et al. The fear-avoidance model of musculoskeletal pain: current state of scientific evidence. *J Behav Med* 2007;30(1):77–94.
37. Boersma K, Linton SJ. How does persistent pain develop? An analysis of the relationship between psychological variables, pain and function across stages of chronicity. *Behav Res Ther* 2005;43(11):1495–1507.
38. Leeuw M, Houben RM, Severeijns R, et al. Pain-related fear in low back pain: a prospective study in the general population. *Eur J Pain* 2007;11(3):256–266.
39. Peters ML, Vlaeyen JW, Weber WE. The joint contribution of physical pathology, pain-related fear and catastrophizing to chronic back pain disability. *Pain* 2005;113(1):45–50.
40. Sullivan MJ, Lynch ME, Clark AJ. Dimensions of catastrophic thinking associated with pain experience and disability in patients with neuropathic pain conditions. *Pain* 2005;113(3):310–315.
41. Goubert L, Crombez G, Van Damme S. The role of neuroticism, pain catastrophizing and pain-related fear in vigilance to pain: a structural equations approach. *Pain* 2004;107(3):234–241.

42. Goubert L, Crombez G, Lysens R. Effects of varied-stimulus exposure on overpredictions of pain and behavioural performance in low back pain patients. *Behav Res Therapy* 2005;43(10):1347–1361.

43. Boersma K, Linton SJ. Screening to identify patients at risk: profiles of psychological risk factors for early intervention. *Clin J Pain* 2005;21(1):38–43.

44. Buer N, Linton SJ. Fear-avoidance beliefs and catastrophizing: occurrence and risk factor in back pain and ADL in the general population. *Pain* 2002;99(3):485–491.

45. Turner JA, Mancl L, Aaron LA. Pain-related catastrophizing: a daily process study. *Pain* 2004;110(1):103–111.

46. Al-Obaidi SM, Al-Zoabi B, Al-Shuwaie N, et al. The influence of pain and pain-related fear and disability beliefs on walking velocity in chronic low back pain. *Int J Rehab Res* 2003;26(2):101–108.

47. Wertli MM, Rasmussen-Barr E, Held U, et al. Fear-avoidance beliefs—a moderator of treatment efficacy in patients with low back pain: a systematic review. *Spine J* 2014;14(11):2658–2678.

48. Picavet HS, Vlaeyen JW, Schouten JS. Pain catastrophizing and kinesiophobia: predictors of chronic low back pain. *Am J Epidemiol* 2002;156:1028–1034.

49. Fritz JM, George SZ, Delitto A. The role of fear avoidance beliefs in acute low back pain: relationships with current and future disability and work status. *Pain* 2001;94:7–15.

50. Storheim K, Brox JI, Holm I, et al. Predictors of return to work in patients sick listed for sub-acute low back pain: a 12-month follow-up study. *J Rehabil Med* 2005;37:365–371.

51. Burton AK, McClune TD, Clarke RD, et al. Long-term follow-up of patients with low back pain attending for manipulative care: outcomes and predictors. *Manual Ther* 2004;9:30–35.

52. Hayes SC, Wilson KG, Gifford EV, et al. Experiential avoidance and behavioral disorders: A functional dimensional approach to diagnosis and treatment. *J Consult Clin Psychol* 1996;64(6):1152.

53. Friman PC, Hayes SC, Wilson KG. Why behavior analysts should study emotion: the example of anxiety. *J Appl Behav Anal* 1998;31(1):137–156.

54. Kanter JW, Busch AM, Weeks CE, et al. The nature of clinical depression: symptoms, syndromes, and behavior analysis. *Behav Anal* 2008;31(1):1–21.

55. Hayes SC, Strosahl KD, Wilson KG. *Acceptance and Commitment Therapy: The Process and Practice of Mindful Change.* New York: Guilford Press; 2001.

56. Adli M, Hegerl U. Do we underestimate the benefits of antidepressants? *Lancet* 2014;383(9926):1361.

57. Linde K, Kriston L, Rücker G, et al. Efficacy and acceptability of pharmacological treatments for depressive disorders in primary care: systematic review and network meta-analysis. *Ann Fam Med* 2015;13(1):69–79.

58. Arroll B, Elley CR, Fishman T, et al. Antidepressants versus placebo for depression in primary care. *Cochrane Database Syst Rev* 2009;(3):CD007954.

59. Hansen R, Gaynes B, Thieda P, et al. Meta-analysis of major depressive disorder relapse and recurrence with second-generation antidepressants. *Psychiatr Serv* 2008;59(10):1121–1130.

60. Gartlehner G, Gaynes BN, Amick HR, et al. *Nonpharmacological Versus Pharmacological Treatments for Adult Patients with Major Depressive Disorder.* Rockville, MD: Agency for Healthcare Research and Quality; 2015.

61. Kapczinski F, Lima MS, Souza JS, et al. Antidepressants for generalised anxiety disorder (GAD). *Cochrane Database Syst Rev* 2003;(2):CD003592.

62. Depping AM, Komossa K, Kissling W, et al. Second-generation antipsychotics for anxiety disorders. *Cochrane Database Syst Rev* 2010;(12):CD008120.

63. Finnerup NB, Sindrup SH, Jensen TS. The evidence for pharmacological treatment of neuropathic pain. *Pain* 2010;150:573–581.

64. Finnerup NB, Attal N, Haroutounain S, et al. Pharmacotherapy for neuropathic pain in adults: a systematic review and meta-analysis. *Lancet Neurol* 2015;14:162–173.

65. Hofmann SG, Asnaani A, Vonk IJ, et al. The efficacy of cognitive behavioral therapy: A review of meta-analyses. *Cognit Ther Res* 2012;36(5):427–440.

66. Hofmann SG, Smits JA. Cognitive-behavioral therapy for adult anxiety disorders: a meta-analysis of randomized placebo-controlled trials. *J Clin Psychiatr* 2008;69(4):621.

67. Haby MM, Donnelly M, Corry J, et al. Cognitive behavioural therapy for depression, panic disorder and generalized anxiety disorder: a meta-regression of factors that may predict outcome. *Aust N Z J Psychiatry* 2006;40:9–19.

68. Bisson J, Andrew M. Psychological treatment of post-traumatic stress disorder (PTSD). *Cochrane Database Syst Rev* 2007;(3):CD003388.

69. Ghahramanlou M. *Cognitive behavioral treatment efficacy for anxiety disorders: A meta-analytic review [dissertation].* Teaneck, NJ: Fairleigh Dickinson University; 2003.

70. Gil PJM, Carrillo FXM, Meca JS. Effectiveness of cognitive-behavioural treatment in social phobia: a meta-analytic review. *Psychol Spain* 2001;5:17–25.

71. Fedoroff I, Taylor S. Psychological and pharmacological treatments of social phobia: a meta-analysis. *J Clin Psychopharm* 2001;21:311–324.

72. Vos T, Haby MM, Barendregt JJ, et al. The burden of major depression avoidable by longer-term treatment strategies. *Arch Gen Psychiatr* 2004;61(11):1097–1103.

73. Eddy KT, Dutra L, Bradley R, et al. A multidimensional meta-analysis of psychotherapy and pharmacotherapy for obsessive-compulsive disorder. *Clin Psychol Rev* 2004;24:1011–1030.

74. Furukawa TA, Watanabe N, Churchill R. Combined psychotherapy plus antidepressants for panic disorder with or without agoraphobia: systematic review. *Cochrane Database Syst Rev* 2007;(1):CD004364.

75. Hollon S. Psychological interventions and medications. *Clin Sci* 2016;19(2):2–4.

76. Olthuis JV, Watt MC, Bailey K, et al. Therapist-supported Internet cognitive behavioural therapy for anxiety disorders in adults. *Cochrane Database Syst Rev* 2016;(3):CD01565.

77. Van Straten A, Geraedts A, Verdonck-de Leeuw I, et al. Psychological treatment of depressive symptoms in patients with medical disorders: a meta-analysis. *J Psychom Res* 2010;69:23–32.

78. Beltman MW, Voshaar RC, Speckens AE. Cognitive-behavioural therapy for depression in people with a somatic disease: meta-analysis of randomised controlled trials. *Br J Psychiatry* 2010;197:11–19.

79. Cuijpers P, Smit F, Bohlmeijer E, et al. Efficacy of cognitive-behavioural therapy and other psychological treatments for adult depression: meta-analytic study of publication bias. *Br J Psychiatry* 2010;196:173–178.

80. Jorm AF, Morgan AJ, Hetrick SE. Relaxation for depression. *Cochrane Database Syst Rev* 2008;(4):CD007142.

81. Tolin DF. Is cognitive-behavioral therapy more effective than other therapies? A meta-analytic review. *Clin Psychol Rev* 2010;30:710–720.

82. Williams AC, Eccleston C, Morley S. Psychological therapies for the management of chronic pain (excluding headache) in adults. *Cochrane Database Syst Rev* 2012;(11):CD007407. doi:10.1002/14651858.CD007407.pub3.

83. Pepper SC. *World Hypotheses: A Study in Evidence.* California: University of California Press; 1942.

84. Hayes SC, Luoma JB, Bond FW, et al. Acceptance and commitment therapy: model, processes and outcomes. *Behav Res Ther* 2006;44(1):1–25.

85. Hayes SC, Strosahl K, Wilson KG, et al. Measuring experiential avoidance: a preliminary test of a working model. *Psychol Rec* 2004;54(4):553–578.

86. McCracken LM. Learning to live with the pain: acceptance of pain predicts adjustment in persons with chronic pain. *Pain* 1988;74(1):21–27.

87. McCracken LM, Vowles KE, Eccleston C. Acceptance of chronic pain: component analysis and a revised assessment method. *Pain* 2004;107(1):159–166.

88. Vowles KE, McCracken LM. Acceptance and values-based action in chronic pain: a study of treatment effectiveness and process. *J Consult Clin Psychol* 20088;76(3):397.

89. McCracken LM, Gutiérrez-Martínez O. Processes of change in psychological flexibility in an interdisciplinary group-based treatment for chronic pain based on acceptance and commitment therapy. *Behav Res Ther* 2011;49(4):267–274.

90. Churchill R, Moore TH, Furukawa TA., et al. 'Third wave' cognitive and behavioural therapies versus treatment as usual for depression. *Cochrane Database Syst Rev* 2013;(10):CD008705.

91. Hunot V, Shinohara K, Honyashiki M, et al. Behavioural therapies versus other psychological therapies for depression. *Cochrane Database Syst Rev* 2013;(10);CD008696.

92. Veehof MM, Oskam MJ, Schreurs KM, et al. Acceptance-based interventions for the treatment of chronic pain: a systematic review and meta-analysis. *Pain* 2011;152(3):533–542.

93. Veehof MM, Trompetter HR, Bohlmeijer ET, et al. Acceptance-and mindfulness-based interventions for the treatment of chronic pain: a meta-analytic review. *Cogn Behav Ther* 2016;45(1):5–31.

94. Hughes LS, Clark J, Colclough JA, et al. Acceptance and commitment therapy (ACT) for chronic pain. *Clin J Pain* 2017;33(6):552–568.

95. McCracken LM, Morley S. The psychological flexibility model: a basis for integration and progress in psychological approaches to chronic pain management. *J Pain* 2014;15:221–234.

CHAPTER 86

Hypnosis

History of Hypnosis in Pain and Symptom Control

Hypnosis is a word derived from the Greek word meaning "sleep." The fairly ancient practice was used by the Druids, the Celts, and by the Egyptians who frequented "sleeping temples" for relaxation and healing. In the 1770s, the Austrian physician Franz Friedrich Anton Mesmer (1734–1815) was interested in the effect of physical energy and magnetism on the body and spirit. He placed his patients in a tub of iron filings and with wide sweeps of his arm made "passes" up and down the patients' bodies. The success of the practice, termed *mesmerism*, was attributed to animal magnetism, whereas the benefits were probably due to the hypnotic effect of his arm-waving ritual. In the 1830s, practical uses of mesmerism were discussed by Oliver in the United States and by the French Academy of Medicine. James Braid (1795–1860) in Scotland termed the word *hypnosis* in 1843, thinking it to be a stage of sleep that influenced the nervous system and distinguishing it from the state of mental concentration. Braid concluded that the relaxing suggestions diverted the patients away from critical thinking and led them into trance. Pavlov in the early 1900s also viewed hypnosis as an incomplete sleep state that allowed patients to mentally separate off from what was going on around them.

John Esdaile (1808–1859)[1] began using trance inductions with surgery patients in 1845 in India, where there were not anesthetics available; he found the hypnotized patients to have increased resistance to infection, greater comfort, and quicker recovery times. In Europe, the School of Hypnotic Study was being formed in Nancy, France, where the view was that suggestion led to hypnotic trance states that were quite normal phenomena. Neurologist Jean-Martin Charcot (1825–1893) also noted that hysteria was effectively treated with hypnotism; although he brought hypnotism into favorable light, he viewed it as a part of the hysteria process and not a normal healthy phenomena. However, there does appear to be a high proportion of patients with hysteria-related psychopathology who are highly hypnotizable.[2]

Pierre Janet (1849–1947) saw hypnosis as dissociation or a split away from cognitive consciousness, which was sometimes normal and healthy and other times related to dissociative states or multiple personalities. Freud in the late 1800s became interested in accessing repressed memories through hypnosis, recognizing it as a pathway to the unconscious mind. However, he was not a good hypnotist and therefore abandoned it; in doing so, he led others away as well. However, he did continue his interest in the hypnotic properties of dreams and free associations.

In the mid-1840s, the introduction of chloroform and ether into surgical practice was another reason for the apparent hiatus in the use and study of hypnosis in medicine. In the 1950s, its use in understanding the workings of the mind and its application to psychotherapy began to pick back up. In the United States, psychologist Clark Hull[3] documented its use for anesthesia, posthypnotic amnesia, and pain relief. Milton Erickson conducted many of these experiments and went on to study the mechanisms of trance practices brought to him by Jay Haley and Margaret Meade. Erickson had an exquisite understanding of the mechanisms of the unconscious mind, and his personal understanding of its effectiveness for reducing physical pain, through his personal use of self-hypnosis, left him well-poised to research, practice, and teach hypnosis for symptom control and pain management. The American Society of Clinical Hypnosis (ASCH) was founded in 1957 as a spinoff from the Society for Clinical and Experimental Hypnosis (SCEH), founded in 1949. Hypnosis was endorsed by both the American Psychological Association (APA) and the American Medical Association (AMA) in the late 1950s. The British Medical Association in 1958 endorsed its use as an anesthetic in certain surgical situations.

In a way, there is a great difference between the linear and precise thinking of modern medicine and the spiritual and imagination-rich mosaic thinking of the hypnotherapist; yet, in this chapter, they come together in the discussion of pain as a psychological event and of the role of expectancy and hope in pain management and general wellness. The early researchers and practitioners identified that the spiritual and magical element of hypnosis were somehow related to positive expectation as noted in the early practices of Mesmer with his magnets, Freud with his dream work, and Erickson with his positive mind-set of hope and respect for the patients. These men all identified the role of the unconscious mind in psychosomatic symptom formation and, in doing so, let down the Cartesian wall between the mind and the body. They also recognized that the highly hypnotizable person may be more likely to develop psychosomatic symptoms but also may be more likely to benefit from hypnotic treatment. Upcoming sections in this chapter discuss pain as a psychological event that is moderately plastic and open to suggestion. Research shows that the triggered memory of pain and the expectation of future pain can be as painful as injury-induced pain. In 1970s, there began to be an interest and upsurge in multidisciplinary pain management. Fordyce,[4] Bonica, and many others were at the forefront of the physicians, scholars, and researchers who moved the field forward in the 1980s. Although the ideal was for patients to be holistically treated by all disciplines together, psychological management is still usually done separate from medical treatment. Turk[5] reviewed outcome data for patients receiving care from interdisciplinary chronic pain and rehabilitation programs (ICPRPs) compared with other care. He found that pain reduction and activity level of patients in ICPRPs was as good as or better than patients receiving standard medical treatment, and that iatrogenic complications, medication use, and health care utilization was less, with more patients returning to work. Other studies demonstrate that the outcomes of psychological treatment for chronic pain compare favorably to more invasive measures and to narcotic use. A systematic Cochrane review concluded that cognitive interventions combined with exercise are recommended for chronic low back pain,[6] and this is discussed in detail in Chapter 73. There is also strong evidence that intensive multidisciplinary biopsychosocial rehabilitation improves function when compared with inpatient or outpatient nonmultidisciplinary treatments as summarized in Chapter 90.[7] A study reconfirms the cost-effectiveness of perioperative hypnosis when used for patients in their hospitals.[8] Given the evidence, we may expect that less invasive and less costly treatments may become the preferred options of patients, their providers, and insurance companies. An extensive review of the research[9] found hypnosis to meet the APA's criteria as an effective pain treatment for pain and superior to medication.

In the remainder of this chapter, I will explain hypnotic trance as a state of mind and describe its use in behavioral medicine in general. I will then discuss current understanding of how hypnosis works at the unconscious level in general and for pain relief, citing literature on brain mechanisms of pain. I will outline research suggesting hypnosis application to specific types and locations of pain and some commonly used hypnotic techniques to treat them. Even though some studies discuss symptom relief (tension, twitches, allergies, anxiety, rashes) as separate from pain itself, usually symptom relief leads to pain relief down the road. This chapter describes both traditional and newer practices of pain hypnosis and provides information on certification and training. I conclude with a discussion on chronic pain, where the emotional suffering related to pain, is a notable dynamic.

Hypnosis by Definition

Hypnosis is a process of bypassing the critical thinking cognitive mind to access unconscious processes. Without the critical thinking filters, the hypnotized person may be more suggestible and more easily influenced by the hypnotist. During hypnotic trance, a person can focus intently on just one aspect of an experience or dissociate from the experience to the point of losing track of his body and his whereabouts. Succinctly, hypnosis is simply a programmed entrance into "trance," which is itself a perfectly normal state that we engage in whenever we are totally absorbed in a task or experience and are not reviewing the characteristics of our experience. Formally, hypnosis is "a social interaction in which one person, designated the subject, responds to suggestions offered by another person, designated the hypnotist, for experiences involving alterations in perception, memory, and voluntary action,"[10] hopefully for the sake of some change the patient desires. Professionals should be thoroughly trained in hypnosis before practicing it and should work only in the areas of their professional expertise. ASCH and SCEH train and certify professionals in medical hypnosis; certification requires a professional degree in health or mental health and specific training that includes the ethical uses of hypnosis.

CONSCIOUS, UNCONSCIOUS, AND CONTENT OF CONSCIOUSNESS

A brief review of the conscious and unconscious minds will serve as the groundwork for discussing the mechanisms of hypnosis itself as well as the psychosomatic process of interpreting and feeling an emotional experience as physical pain.

A. Consciousness: what you are oriented toward in the present
   1. Content of consciousness (i.e., perceptions and specific thoughts): what is on your mind and in your thoughts, including what is "on the back burner"
   2. Selective consciousness: what you choose to have in the front rather than in the back or periphery of your mind
B. Unconscious
   1. Long-term memory: which you may or may not access when necessary
   2. Short-term memory: which has happened recently
   3. Automatic functioning that usually but not always bypasses your conscious mind. This is sometimes called the *primary process* or body language that demonstrates when you are angry, happy, or frightened. It also includes behavior such as scratching an itch or catching yourself before you fall.
   4. Programmed physiology that you have little or no access to in normal thinking state, such as your heart beating, breathing, allergic responses, healing rate, etc.
   5. Deeper processes such as the essential self, (the "essence" of you or your sense of who you are at the core). Other parts of the self are the immune system and the neurologic map or the body.

We might say that the conscious mind includes awareness and cognition, and the unconscious mind includes everything else, including your physical self. Cognition is a tool to help with survival and with the expression of your sense of yourself; it is a small part of the whole self-constellation in a somewhat figure–ground relationship. The unconscious mind is adaptive and capable of profound change, potentially with both positive and negative outcomes.

When you are "associated" to a situation, you see it through your own eyes, and you are fully present to it; an example of this is the child who is involved in a task but is not monitoring himself and who needs an adult to oversee his behavior. In reflective thinking, you are in both the conscious and unconscious minds and processes at once, contemplating an idea or situation by looking into your unconscious mind to find new perspectives for viewing or approaching it. The conscious and unconscious processes can operate autonomous of one another, in the condition of dissociation (dis-"associated"), occurring when ideas are split off from the normal (associated) experience and when, to some extent, you are not paying attention. When dissociated, you may take a global experience of the situation and break it down into parts, amplifying one part while diminishing concentration on the other part—when, for instance, you notice one aspect of the situation and no longer notice others. You may see the situation and also see yourself in the situation, or you may see the situation differently. This can occur during trauma or during hypnosis; for instance, during surgery, you can dissociate from pain by imagining yourself at the beach and seeing the beach at the same time or dissociate from a body part during surgery and believe it to be having surgery or recuperating across the room. In an internally directed trance state, the patient may shut off pain and influence healing, immune functions, heart rate, blood flow, and autoimmune responses not commonly accessed in normal consciousness. Again, hypnosis is merely the programmed entrance into trance or dissociation at some level, and hypnotherapy is the programmed entrance into trance for therapeutic purposes.

Actually, the hypnotist or hypnotherapist is merely guiding the patient to self-hypnosis. Unless the state is induced with hypnotic medications or other psychoactive substances, the patient is the one to suspend vigilance, and his ability to do so is likely to depend on (1) the relationship that he has with the hypnotist, (2) the skill of the hypnotist inducing the trance, (3) the safety of the situation and environment, (4) the patient's level of hypnotizability, (5) the patient's expectancy that he will receive benefit and relief, (6) the patient's need for the trance—pain itself can be a trance state to tap into, and (7) the patient's past experience with trance states —ranging from dissociative disorders leading from experienced trauma to meditation and past hypnosis training.

Complementarity, the quantum physics concept of relativity, helps explain the use of hypnosis for pain control. Basically, it is impossible to be wholly in one state (fully present and focused in one perspective, such as the dissociative state) and keep another state (e.g., being in pain) fully in mind at the same time; the difference is being *in* the moment versus *thinking about* the moment. When you are fully locked into pain, you cannot get perspective to solve the pain problem; you need to dissociate from the pain somewhat to get a better perspective on it. Once you dissociate from it, you can no longer feel it. The hypnotherapist facilitates the process. Other examples of split consciousness or going back and forth between the conscious and the unconscious minds are the rewriting the endings of dreams (lucid dreaming), remembering that the stove is on while watching television (split concentration), and accessing memories—all of which are normal functioning but also, in a way, related to hypnosis. These principles of trance and hypnotic states are important to understanding hypnotic pain management. The more access to the unconscious mind one can gain by self or guided hypnosis, to imagine or create another way of being or feeling, the more control of pain and physiologic symptoms one may have.

Central Mechanisms

CENTRAL MECHANISMS OF HYPNOSIS

Hypnosis has been viewed as magical, energy related, sleep related (Braid and Pavlov), psychosomatic, pathologic (Charcot), dissociative,[11-13] and the consequence of normal suggestibility[14]—all of which are partly true. Recent brain research using functional magnetic resonance imaging (fMRI) and positron emission tomography (PET) scans shed more light on the process. In general, the studies show that there are many brain areas involved in the hypnotic process, including simultaneous increased activities in some areas and selective shutting down of others. We can conclude that high- and low-hypnotizable people show different brain response patterns to hypnotic analgesic suggestions. However, there is no specific area of the brain that controls pain.[15] Some studies look at performance on certain tasks (learning, verbal, auditory) and in certain situations (pain, for example) before and during hypnosis, whereas others compare high- and low-hypnotizable patients or subjects.

Clinicians as far back as Freud have known that some people are more suggestible or susceptible to hypnosis than others. About 15% of people are highly suggestible, 65% are moderately, and 20% are not very suggestible.[12] Although hypnotizability is a fairly stable trait and not related to intelligence, people can learn or improve on their ability to develop or maintain trances, use self-hypnosis, and relax vigilance. Furthermore, hypnotizability is somewhat variable within individuals depending on factors such as the situation, the hypnotist's skill, the patient's motivation level and expectancies, the relevance of the induction and trance to the patient, and patient's physical and psychological state. Experienced hypnotists help patients lower their vigilance by addressing all of the aforementioned factors and, even more important, by sensing and identifying the way their patients unconsciously process information in order to help them be maximally at ease (see Haley[16] and Bandler and Grinder[17] or an introductory manual on hypnosis for examples of hypnotic inductions).

HIGH AND LOW HYPNOTIZABILITY

Over the last two decades, Gruzelier[18] has been involved in numerous experiments studying high- and low-hypnotizable patient's brain responses to experimental tasks during pain episodes and other situations. His studies seemed to show that in a hypnotic state, subjects can selectively ignore what is in their perceptual field while still knowing what is there. This is important regarding pain, in that often the patient's focus is as much on misery and helplessness as it is on his physiology; the clinician may not be able to change the physical condition, but he may help the patient selectively disregard the pain and the suffering. Gruzelier[18] found that in general, highly hypnotizable subjects exhibit more neurophysiologic and cognitive flexibility (see also Evans[19]), which include "superior abilities in absorption, creativity, dissociation, attention, and vividness of imagery; these are all well-known correlates of hypnotizability." Regarding hemisphere involvement, highly hypnotizable persons (highs) under hypnosis demonstrate more right hemispheric frontolimbic influence. Furthermore, there is more neuronal flexibility going from the right to left and from the left to right hemispheres, and, according to Gruzelier,[18] "in stimulus repetitions, highs showed a shift from an initial right-sided preference, in line with the right hemisphere's role in global orienting, to a left hemisphere preference, in line with the left-sided involvement in the local orienting process," indicating absorption. One study found greater informational exchange in the prefrontal areas of highs during hypnosis.[20] Highs were better able to inhibit pain from their conscious awareness. fMRIs showed them to have a significantly larger rostrum area, the corpus callosum area involved in transferring problem-solving information between the left and the right hemispheres. Gruzelier emphasized another difference between "highs" and persons with low hypnotizability (lows) during an auditory attention task: Prehypnosis, highs increased event-related potential (ERP) N100 activity (engaging frontal attentional circuits), whereas lows had little activity, indicating distraction; under hypnosis, highs had little activity, indicating disengagement of the frontal process or distraction, whereas lows' activity progressively increased.[21]

Other studies involving mental tasks showed increased activity in the anterior cingulate under hypnosis in highs more than in lows (indicating that they were monitoring the task) and a decrease in the inferior frontal gyrus activity (indicating that they were disengaging from executive functioning).[18] In other words, highs under hypnosis are relatively better at actively not paying attention to what they still know is in the field; they seem to let go of attending it. This seems to represent frontolimbic inhibition on the left side and a shift to the right brain, engaging the patients' ability to feel or imagine things different than they were before. Hypnosis involves activation of the hippocampus and inhibition of the amygdala activity at the same time.[22] A fractal analysis of electroencephalography (EEG) in patients under hypnosis showed dissociation of centralized activity and a loss of the normal patterns of integrated physiologic responses, which results in a trance state.[23]

CENTRAL MECHANISMS OF HYPNOTIC ANALGESIA

Price et al.[24] provided a statistical path analysis to show four necessary elements of hypnotic analgesia—relaxation; absorption; disorientation from time, space, or sense of self; and automaticity—and their relationship order. Automaticity is the condition in which the suggestion bypasses cognition and leads directly to the sensation or experience, such that the suggestion of sinking into a warm bathtub will allow you to relax your back muscles and smile, without having to think about it or consciously relax or lower your shoulders. Studies show that imagining heat actually increases blood flow that relaxes muscles, thereby validating automaticity. The principle is similar to direct suggestion and to suggestion through expectancy and placebo. As well, those who exhibit more θ brain waves, which would lead to easier visualization and creativity and relaxation, *prior* to introduction of hypnotic analgesia, get better pain relief.[25]

Some suggest that hypnotic analgesia works by activating endogenous pain inhibitory systems that descend to the spinal cord, where it prevents transmission to the brain of pain coming from nociception. One study evoked experimental pain in subjects by stimulating the sural nerve, causing the nociceptive flexion reflex (NFR).[26] Hypnotic suggestion could both increase and decrease the NFR, leading the researchers to conclude that their hypnotic suggestion actually controlled the response at the spinal level by activating descending antinociceptive mechanisms. However, this does not appear to stem from the opioid system alone,[27,28] in that the administration of naloxone, an opioid antagonist, does not reverse hypnotic analgesia. It would seem, then, that there are nonopiate cortical fugal or brain-to-spinal-cord descending control mechanisms.

The relationship between pain and hypnotic or dissociative faculties of the brain is made clearer in recent studies of complex regional pain syndrome (CRPS), which begins with excruciating pain and can progress to include dramatic physiologic changes and neglect or dissociation from the painful limb. According to studies, within moments of an injury or absence of sensory input, there is a reorganization of the somatosensory cortex representation of the injured limb that leads the patient to behaviorally isolate or "favor" the limb. fMRI studies show that the degree of change in the somatosensory cortex is directly related to the degree of perceived pain.[29,30] Even when there is painless stimulation in the CRPS patient's uninjured counterpart limb, there is pain-related activation all through the brain, including cerebral, motor, parietal, bilateral S2, and frontal lobe and the anterior and posterior bilion of the cingulate cortex (aACC and pACC).[31] When the CRPS pain lessens, however, both the cortical reorganization and impaired tactile sensation return to normal.[32,33] Wobst[34] summarizes the PET, fMRI, and evoked potential studies on pain, concluding that the ACC, insular, frontal cortices, amygdala, S1 and S2, and the lateral thalamus are all involved in pain and how the body processes the pain in regard to location and duration. The studies show that the affective (cognitive and evaluative) components of pain are processed in the medial thalamus and progress back to the ACC (also see Derbyshire et al.,[35] Vogt et al.,[36] Vogt et al.,[37] and Peyron et al.[38]).

At the same time, other areas of the brain work to calm and heal. Following awareness of physical or emotional pain, the right ventral prefrontal cortex is involved with soothing responses that are triggered by hypnotic therapeutic suggestions and messages of comfort or healing, which proceed to help the right parietal lobe to reorganize and to perceive the body intact and comfortable (see section on CRPS and phantom limb pain).

In a hypnosis study of experimentally induced pain, high- and low-hypnotizable patients responded differently.[39] Under hypnosis, with the low-hypnotizable patients, as the pain ratings increased, so did frontal γ oscillations; however, with high-hypnotizable patients, as the pain ratings increased, the γ oscillations did not increase. The γ frequencies were noted primarily in the bilateral anterior cingulum (within the limbic system), which supports the understanding of pain being tied in with a complex of emotional responses. The midcingulate cortex may modulate and influence sensory, affective, cognitive, and behavioral aspects of nociception at least in the hypnotic state.[40] Raij et al.[41] used fMRI to compare brain mechanistic responses to noxious stimulation perceptions versus hypnotically hallucinated pain; they found that both real and imagined pain produced similar brain responses, although perception of hallucinated pain was less than the actual induced pain. In both cases, there was activity in the rostral and perigenual ACC and in the pericingulate regions of the medial prefrontal cortex. They conclude that the medial prefrontal cortex is involved in monitoring real and hallucinated pain, which then influences how noxious stimuli are experienced and processed. A study exposed subjects to pain (1) in the waking state, (2) with hypnotic relaxation, or (3) with hypnosis suggesting depersonalization (out of body experiences).[42] All the subjects showed somatosensory, insular, and cerebral activation with pain; however, the depersonalization group showed less activation in the contralateral somatosensory, parietal, and prefrontal cortex; putamen; and ipsilateral amygdala. De Pascalis et al.[43] have shown somatosensory event-related increase during pain, followed by a reduction when subjects were administered hypnotic analgesia. De Pascalis[44] found that highs experiencing hypnotic analgesia showed smaller total, δ and β amplitudes in the right hemisphere; they experienced more θ activity in the left hemisphere during pain and more in the right hemisphere with hypnotic analgesia, decreasing both the sympathetic activity and the overall experience of pain. Meier et al.[45] showed that hypnotic hypalgesia decreased subjects' experimental pain; when suggestions about increasing pain were made, somatosensory evoked potentials, auditory evoked potentials, and EEGs remained unchanged from the hypalgesic state, indicating that the physical response to pain and its affective component can indeed be separated. Thus, hypnotizability level certainly appears to impact on the ultimate outcome of hypnosis in general as well as for pain management.

Pain as a Plastic Experience

Why is hypnosis particularly appropriate for acute and chronic pain management? How can it be that Jensen and Barber[46] showed hypnotic analgesia to be more effective than other analgesics, including morphine, for reducing pain? We can begin to answer this by viewing pain as a perception or conclusion derived from a complex interweaving of a real physiologic signal and psychological responses based on expectations and memories of similar past experiences; the perception itself generates feedback to the body. Physical injury and disease cannot fully predict the amount of perceived pain a patient experiences; other determining factors are anxiety and trauma, context of the injury, depression, expectation, social support, and numerous other personality factors and cognitive styles. Interestingly, as is discussed elsewhere in this chapter, those who are highly hypnotizable are often the most likely to experience psychosomatic symptoms of the overlap of psychological interpretation with nociception, but they are also most likely to benefit by hypnosis and other well-applied psychological treatment.

Chapman[47] describes nociception as an unconscious messaging about tissue damage through the nervous system, not to be equated with pain, which is the conscious awareness of that nociception. He defines pain as "a complex, compelling unpleasant bodily awareness normally associated with tissue trauma." One purpose of pain is to engage the cognitive problem solving part of the brain in a plan to resolve the tissue damage. Biologically, pain is a cascade of neurotransmitter and biochemical responses to nociception, involving the hypothalamo-pituitary-adrenocortical (HPA) axis and the limbic system, and causing changes in blood pressure and blood sugar, serotonin and nor-epinephrine levels, effecting concentration, mood, behavior, healing, and sleep. Pain can interfere with psychological and physical well-being. When the nociception is not medically treated and stopped, the body's unconscious responses to it can continue to cause permanent change and damage in other physiologic and psychological systems. At the same time, psychological stress and suffering can lead to the same cascade of physiologic stress responses and even lead to the construction of the sense of pain where no damage exists, which helps to explain why some events, physical or otherwise, cause pain to some people more than others.[47]

Hypnotherapy for pain aims to disengage pain from suffering and soothe both the physical and emotional stress. In the case of acute pain during surgery or procedures and after injury, the patient's focus can be directed away from the experience, or the experience can be reframed as a beneficial and healing, and one not to be feared. Directing the patient's focus away from the pain and back into himself is also a way to alleviate suffering, in that the pain would then be differentiated from the patient's sense of self. Whereas pain is stressful, hypnotherapy is a relaxing and comforting experience that induces brain waves and levels of autonomic functioning that soothe the sympathetic nervous system and enhance healing and resistance to disease (see Gruzelier as mentioned in Liossi[48]) by changing the cognitive mind's and body's responses to nociception. Patients may simultaneously alleviate pain, promote healing, and learn to manage future pain better, all within the same cost-effective applications. For a detailed review of techniques according to medical problem, see Brown and Fromm[49] and Hammond.[50]

Testing Hypnotizability

Hypnotizability level does appear to influence hypnotic pain management and the outcome of hypnosis in general, although there are ways for the experienced hypnotist to work with it successfully. Researchers may be more likely than clinicians to use hypnotizability scales before engaging in subject or patient interactions. Some say that testing for hypnotizability may actually interfere with the research because testing itself is hypnotic training and subjects become more hypnotizable with practice.[51] Nonetheless, when hypnotizability is very important, such as before attempting intraoperative hypnotic analgesia, it may be wise to use the Stanford Hypnotic Susceptibility Scale (SHSS), Form C,[52] which is a fairly long (over an hour) and stringent test with a broad sampling of hypnotic suggestions. The Stanford Hypnotic Clinical Scale (SHCS)[53] is a shorter version that gives scores for adults in 25 minutes; there are also versions for children. The Hypnotic Induction Profile (HIP)[54] gives scores for adults and children in 5 to 15 minutes; it is based on a simple procedure (the eye roll) that goes beyond suggestibility to autonomic function. The Harvard Group Scale of Hypnotic Susceptibility[55] may be read or administered by tape recording and should be used when there is a need to maintain a pool of subjects of varying suggestibility. The Waterloo-Stanford Group C (WSGC) scale of hypnotic susceptibility[56] is a group version of the SHSS, Form C that may be best used for measuring suggestibility. The Hypnotic State Assessment Questionnaire (HSAQ)[57] assesses patients' hypnotic state at one point in time and may be used during clinical or experimental sessions. The Elkins Hypnotizability Scale[58] takes 25.8 minutes, identifies four factors, and has good clinical and research correlation with the Stanford Hypnotic Susceptibility scale. Weitzenhoffer[59] points out that suggestibility and hypnotizability are different and that some research has failed because subjects were not really hypnotized but rather merely followed suggestions. To be sure of hypnotizability, he recommends administering the Stanford Profile Scales of Hypnotic Susceptibility, Forms I and II,[52] or at least one of them, and the next best assurance that the patient is in a hypnotic state would be to use a score of 10 as a cutoff on SHSS, Form C.

Lynn et al.[60] outline various hypnotherapists' views on assessing hypnotizability levels. Many (see Yapko[51]) object to the use of such tests, stating that they are obtrusive, undermine the therapeutic relationship, and do not adequately measure hypnotic capacity or take into consideration change in hypnotizability over time. Other options to using tests are to assess the patient's success with the first induction[61] or to use a conversational assessment of hypnotizability.[62] A series of questions can give the clinician a good idea of how easy it will be to get a patient into a hypnotic state (i.e., questions about past hypnotic states or trauma, dissociative tendencies in various realms of life, and right/left brain characteristics).

A scale that may be informative to a psychologist treating pain patients is the Tellegen Absorption Scale,[63] a 34-item true–false test that correlates well with hypnotic susceptibility. Wickramasekera[64] found that patients scoring high on absorption scales or tests of hypnotic susceptibility and also scoring high on neuroticism as measure by the Marlowe-Crowne Social Desirability Scale[65] were more likely to develop psychosomatic pain or symptoms, by dissociating traumatic or undesirable experiences and converting them into somatic symptoms or pain, creating what Damasio termed "psychological markers." Wickramasekera developed a 25-item scale to be used to identify patients who were more likely to somatize. He points to the neural flexibility and "ideational fluency" that Gruzeleir[18] suggested was related to a propensity to dissociate that can leave one vulnerable to schizotypy, affective distress, mood disorders, and somatic markers or memories that stay beyond conscious awareness. In simpler terms, highly hypnotizable patients are more likely to create a somatic marker for a psychological event and are more likely to trigger a memory of previous pain when they experience a new pain (see Chapman[47]). A meta-analysis[66] shows classic, modern, and mixed forms of hypnosis to be effective for treating psychosomatic disorders (those which

meet the criteria for somatoform disorder), which would include both hypersensitivity to pain, hyperawareness of symptoms and to body processes in general, and the transduction or conversion of emotions and memories into somatic markers. This is remarkable given the range of disorders and symptoms included: tinnitus, duodenal ulcers, asthma, irritable bowel syndrome (IBS), osteoarthritis, chronic pain, and dyspepsia. Also, DuHamel et al.[67] found that their high-hypnotizable burned patients had significantly more intrusive avoidance and arousal symptoms with their injury-related trauma. Roelofs et al.[68] showed that they could use hypnosis to induce catalepsy and altered perception of the cataleptic limb in high-hypnotizable subjects, suggesting the formation of conversion disorders or psychosomatic illness. Younger et al.[69] show a linear correlation between hypnotizability and somatic complaints commonly assumed to be of a psychosomatic nature.

Current Research and Applications of Medical Hypnosis for Pain

The applications of hypnosis to medicine are numerous and go beyond the scope of this chapter because not all involve pain; Table 86.1 outlines common applications of hypnosis in medicine in general. Information on the effect of hypnosis on emotional pain and on physical pain, related or not to medical conditions, is undoubtedly not best found in the medical research but rather in books, articles, and trainings offered by the clinicians who regularly use it but who are not researchers. This is in part because every effective hypnotherapy session is, in research terms, an N of 1. However, research in hypnosis and its clinical use in medicine are increasing due to the recent surge in brain research and the increased understanding of what pain is and due to increased attention to the number of the people in chronic pain and in health care utilization and costs. Hypnosis research is important, for without published results, it is difficult for hospitals and insurance companies to justify reimbursing and endorsing its use in medicine.

Earlier research on psychological treatment of medical conditions often compares such treatment to standard care practices with and without the addition of cognitive-behavioral therapy (CBT). CBT often consists of a standardized program that is more applicable to research than hypnosis. CBT differs from hypnosis in that the therapist intends to speak directly to the patient's cognitive conscious mind, without deliberately sending any direct or indirect messages to his or her unconscious mind. A hypnosis session may likely include behavioral

TABLE 86.1 Common Applications of Hypnosis in Medicine	
Headaches	Smoking cessation
Muscles cramps	Eating disorders
Pain disorders such as CRPS	Perioperative preparation
Chronic diseases	Postoperative pain and
Burns	recuperation
Minor procedures—analgesic	Allergies
or anesthetic	Wound care
Colonoscopies	Hypertension
Blood drawing	Chronic disease management
Dentistry	Cancer-related anxiety and
Surgery—anesthetic	depression
Cancer	Nausea and emesis
Labor and delivery	Dental and needle phobia
Bone growth and healing	Skin rashes and warts
	Immune and autoimmune
	disorders

CRPS, complex regional pain syndrome.

suggestions in and out of trance and messages to the conscious and the unconscious mind at the same time. Both may include homework. Kirsch et al.[61] looked at 18 studies of CBT with and without additional hypnosis. The addition of hypnosis to CBT substantially enhanced treatment outcome, such that the patients who received additional hypnosis did better than 70% of those with just CBT treatment. In most cases, the authors mean CBT administered in the medium of hypnosis.

As we go on to discuss the research on medical hypnosis, there are some points to bear in mind. First, we expect there to be quite a difference between the methods and benefits of hypnosis in clinical practice and the process of studying it in research. We must assume that a clinician in his or her office would not exactly follow a research protocol and that he or she would modify even a hypnotic script to fit his or her patient's situation. Also, pain hypnosis is used primarily for chronic pain, less often for procedural and least for surgical pain, where hypnosis is usually used as an adjunct to medicine. Under strict standards, for hypnosis to be considered the dependent variable in research, it must deliver suggestions that could not be just as well delivered to the patient cognitive behaviorally (as in telling the patient what to do). However, some highly hypnotizable or well-trained patients have ready access to the unconscious mind and absorb even a CBT message quite deeply or literally; a good example of this is the patient who testifies that he always gets all the side effects mentioned on the inserts of his medications. Finally, most patients in severe pain or in traumatic conditions are already in a trance and in a manner of speaking hypnotized, so that the comparison between CBT and hypnosis is muddy at best. A recent study found that multiple sclerosis (MS) patients who tried hypnosis for pain relief had more success than did those who tried opioids, benzodiazepines, or nerve blocks.[70] But in general and in effect, the strict standards of the research may dilute the power of hypnosis. Fortunately, clinical success with hypnosis does not depend wholly on the results of research studies.

EFFICACY AND EFFECTIVENESS

To move the practice of hypnosis in medicine along, research on effectiveness—how hypnosis works in the real world, in quasi-experimental design—should be as methodical as the research on efficacy—how a technique works within the controlled research situation (see Wild and Espie,[71] Nash,[72] Chaves and Dworkin,[73] and Gay et al.[74]). A 1982 article[75] reported skepticism about the effect of hypnosis on pain due to the lack of controlled studies comparing hypnosis with credible placebos or other treatment methods. Hawkins[76] updated that article with a review of research articles up to the year 2000 and was able to conclude that hypnosis is effective for pain related to cancer, burns, gastrointestinal problems, and for invasive medical procedures. He also noted that poor-quality reviews were not more likely to produce positive conclusions about efficacy and that there was a paucity of good studies in the areas of obstetrics, headache, and chronic pain. Montgomery et al.[9] did a meta-analysis of pain analgesia studies using healthy subjects and patient samples and taking into consideration hypnotizability levels; they concluded hypnosis to be effective in both areas for 75% of their population. Hypnotic analgesia compared favorably in effect to standard care and to attention.[77] Hypnosis has compared favorably to empathic attention[78] and to autogenic training (AT) for psychosomatic and medical disorders.[79] Yapko,[51] however, suggests that AT is in itself a hypnotic induction and that the comparison of the two treatments presents a problem.

The research process itself raises some concerns. One is that research studies focus on the precise content of the intervention, not how it can be flexibly adapted to the real-life patient situation. Another concern is the outcome measure itself: We intend

for patients to be noticing pain less, but then we ask them to tune into it and rate it at the end of the study. Also, many studies do not account for hypnotizability, which would color research results and which in clinical practice that therapist could address. Another issue is expectancy—the patient's expectation that hypnosis will resolve his pain, which seems to predict pain relief. Jensen and Patterson[80] suggest that most of hypnosis studies lack adequate controls for expectancy and placebo effects, even though the studies find that hypnotic analgesia is effective in treating chronic pain. Clearly, raising the patient's expectancy is a good thing, as are raising his levels of self-efficacy and curiosity about finding new ways to cope and encouraging the placebo effect. A study looking at changes in various psychological responses to pain postoperatively and after 3 months found hypnosis to be effective. The positive effect was not significantly related to hypnotic ability, concentration of treatment (e.g., daily vs. up to weekly), or initial response pattern to treatment, but it was moderately related to the participants' expectancy ratings of treatment after the first session.[81]

All of this being said, Amundson et al.[82] point out that research probably underestimates the effectiveness of clinical hypnosis. Many are concerned about the randomized controlled trial (RCT) approach to hypnosis research that is so distinct from the patient-centered and cooperative relationship–based nature of clinical hypnotherapy.[83,84] Clinical one-on-one hypnotic sessions take patient's unique issues and personal variables into consideration, and scripted or standardized protocols cannot address the psychological and emotional issues intertwined with the pain. Spiegel and Kahn[85] discuss the difficulties inherent in using an outside hypnotherapist as the interventionist in research or therapy, which lacks the all-important therapeutic relationship; they also point out that the relationship between the hypnotherapist and the treating physician is important. It would seem that hypnotic protocols would be most effective when designed for each patient by a therapist who is interactively responsive to the patient, for according to one extensive study, 30% of therapy outcome is based on the therapeutic relationship, even when the treatment is medication; another 15% is due to expectancy.[86] Nonetheless, research showing the effectiveness of hypnosis must be stringent if it is to be widely available in medicine and adequately reimbursed by insurance companies. In fact, when comparing the delivery of hypnotic analgesia by sessions with the hypnotist present, manualized protocols, standardized audiotapes, or individualized audiotapes (as would be prepared for patients in clinical practice), a meta-analysis indicates that any delivery is better than none[87]; however, since clinicians understand the importance of being fully present and flexible in a hypnotic session, more research in this area is needed. Interesting delivery formats are now on the horizon. Patterson et al.[88] have attempted to improve absorption that may be missing with audiotapes by creating virtual reality (VR) computer-based presentations that immerse patients in a three dimensional computer-generated environment to absorb the patients' attention and divert it away from the pain experience. VR induces and sustains a hypnotic state without a therapist. Questions arise as to whether this intervention satisfies the research definitions for hypnosis and whether the same effect could be accomplished by naturalistic absorption or with audiotapes alone.

Here is an example of a clinical application of hypnosis that is distinct from research protocol. A female patient in her 30s had been extensively evaluated for her deep, sharp right-side pelvic pain that came on for 15 to 20 minutes as often as every hour, even during the night. She rarely has pain when she was on birth control pills, other than after sexual intercourse. There was a small area of endometriosis, successfully removed, and one cyst that ruptured, but otherwise, no diagnoses explained the pain. She and her husband were anxious to be off birth control pills in order to conceive. She also exhibited generalized high vigilance. She asked a hypnotherapist to help find any unconscious motivations for the pain. She was highly hypnotic and motivated, with high expectancy. The therapist worked interactively with her on a wide range of techniques to find what worked uniquely for her in managing and accepting the nerve pain, which she practiced self-hypnotically at home. Hypnosis helped with vigilance, and therapy helped other issues about trust. The therapeutic relationship supported the work with hypervigilance and trust, and specific fears that related to pregnancy.

Clinically and in research, even when patients do not receive pain relief with hypnotic analgesia, they seem to receive satisfaction from the sessions. Jensen et al.[89] reported that out of the benefits listed by subjects in their pain hypnosis study, 23% reported pain-related benefits as the reason for satisfaction, 58% reported other than pain benefits, 13% were neutral, and 8% reported a negative experience. Subjects cited increased sense of control and positive shifts in perspective, with no subjects reporting dissatisfaction. Dawson et al.[90] have said that pain treatment satisfaction in general has more to do with the provider–patient relationship than pain-related outcome.

We will briefly mention two other variables. Direct versus indirect hypnotic suggestions for pain or symptom relief (e.g., to progressively relax muscles vs. imagining lying on a beach at a peaceful island, which would warm and relax muscles) both seem to be effective. In regard to whether hypnosis is more effective when labeled as hypnosis or introduced using other terms, Jensen and Patterson[80] concluded that in the short term, there is probably no difference, but over time, there may be a benefit for the patient in attributing improvement to hypnosis or self-hypnosis.

REVIEW OF RESEARCH STUDIES ACCORDING TO PAIN PROBLEMS OR SITUATIONS

Research on hypnosis has waxed and waned over the years and varied in focus. Many of the new studies are physician driven and are looking for nonmedicinal, noninvasive self-management treatments that improve medical outcome. Even though pain is common to most medical disorders and procedures, each carries a unique cluster of symptoms that might indicate a different psychological or hypnotic approach for healing and management, differing lengths of treatment time and varying depths of trance. Research and clinical reports show the importance of matching the appropriate protocol to the type of pain experienced.[91] The following sections will outline recent research on hypnosis when used as one of the treatment modes, grouped according to medical condition. Under each heading, research findings, primarily since the year 2000, will be followed by some suggestions and techniques for use in clinical practice. Most of the articles address acute and procedural pain. Hopefully, the sections will serve as a background and a resource for hypnotherapists and clinicians and for those planning to embark on such medical research.

Perioperative and Procedural Uses

As described earlier, hypnotic analgesia was first reported as successful in surgery before there were any chemical anesthetic alternatives. In this century, although there are sporadic reports of its successful use as the only anesthetic,[92] it is now most often as an adjunct to chemical anesthetics or to analgesics. Studies have looked at improved well-being or enhanced healing and recovery time after surgery or procedures and reduction in hospital costs. Hypnosis successfully targets a number of surgical and postsurgical variables, such as anxiety, blood pressure, and patients' sense of control over their feelings[93]; pain, nausea, vomiting, blood loss, and wound healing[94]; pain, knee

strength, edema, inflammation, and postsurgical anxiety after anterior cruciate ligament (ACL) surgery[95]; both objectively and subjectively rated healing, when level of hypnotizability was controlled[96]; postoperative anxiety and pain level, even after a single session of hypnosis before surgery[97]; pain and distress, where the effects were mediated by patient expectancy[98]; and shorter hospital stays and less parenteral narcotic use.[99] A study showed hypnosis to lessen procedural pain and result in a speedier medical procedure; positive results did not correlate with hypnotizability, possibly because the hypnotist facilitated self-hypnosis before and during the procedure, such that subjects received individualized treatment.[100]

Three studies used hypnosis because it might be used clinically. Enqvist and Fischer[101] aimed to reduce preoperative stress that might influence healing and recovery from a surgery, specifically to reduce medication use, inflammation, infection, postoperative pain, and edema. Using one surgeon, who was blind to the grouping, patients were given a 20-minute tape containing an induction and suggestions of finding a safe place, having control of bodily responses to surgery, dissociating, and alleviating pain. Subjects were also asked to use their chosen way of relaxing for 2 minutes and to let soft music bring them back to awareness. In a controlled study, Dyas[102] used a conversational induction containing positive language patterns and suggestions that included counting down (into trance), relaxing breathing, finding a safe place, and dissociating from the surgical procedure; reinforcing words were used during surgery, and posthypnotic suggestions addressed continued relaxation and comfort. Another controlled study used music with or without the audio taped voice of a hypnotherapist during surgery under general anesthesia[103]; the addition of hypnosis was beneficial, and the author suggests the results would be even more significant using individualized tapes and in situations where less anesthesia is used.

Obviously, both physical and emotional pain during surgery can present a problem because pain is both traumatic and stressful and relief from it can improve healing, save money, and make for happier patients and surgeons. The most important patient variable to consider for use in surgery as the sole or primary anesthesia seems to be hypnotizability. To be sure the patient is highly hypnotizable and can go into a deep state, stringent testing should be done (see Weitzenhoffer and Hilgard[52] and Lynn et al.[60]). The sole use of hypnosis should be reserved for the patient who is highly hypnotizable, experienced with hypnosis, and for whom the payoff is likely to be great. Preoperative preparation for surgery described by Kessler and Dane[104] is also effective and satisfying to many patients. Kessler also found that the most significant variable related to the anxiety in surgery that can affect the surgical outcome variables related earlier was the expectation of negative surgical outcomes, coming either from patients' previous experiences or to those close to him or her. He designed a short screening questionnaire to identify patients who are in most need of hypnotic preparation (Kessler, personal communication, 1996). Subsequent perioperative hypnotic treatment can be done with any level of trance, even conversational,[62] to assure that the anxiety level regarding the procedure is optimally low and that the mind-set is positive; this can speed up healing and recovery and allay concerns about procedure and recovery processes. During such perioperative preparations, I have twice discovered male patients who fully expected to die because they were grieving the death of fathers who died during the same procedure or at their like chronologic age; we took the time to work through those issues before surgery took place.

Perioperative hypnosis to lower anxiety and its related biologic components should address positive expectancy of the surgical outcome and the positive interpretation of the surgical events and sounds the patient may unconsciously notice.

The optimal protocol will include some critical details of the surgery that the patient can interpret positively, such as

> *When you feel the surgeon touch your stomach with a knife, that will be an indication that he is finding the best place on your belly for the smallest opening to allow him to remove the part of your intestine that needs to come out so that he can reattach the healthy tissue and allow your intestines to work normally again,* or

> *When you feel a little tugging, that will be an indication that he is closing the opening with a nice line of little stitches,* or

> *Since you will be hungry after not eating before surgery, you can begin to look forward to your favorite food soon after surgery,* and

> *You can let your thoughts be on that beach you love so much, and you can listen only to sentences from your own doctor and that begin with your first name.*

In that way, the surgeon can request the patient to lower his blood pressure and divert blood away from the surgical site, and he can prepare the patient for any changes in the surgical plan and even imbed suggestions to lose interest in unhealthy food or cigarettes. For a review of other "patient-friendly" terms, see Bennett and Disbrow.[105]

Complex Regional Pain Syndrome

CRPS is one of two pain syndromes responsive to hypnosis that are particularly interesting because they demonstrate the brain mechanisms of pain. CRPS is a complicated condition wherein pain persists after injury and is disproportionate to the injury or level of stimulus following healing of the injury; the continuing severe pain has no confirmed mechanism.[106] Even when there is neuropathology, which can lead to muscle atrophy and bone demineralization, the symptoms can be sympathetically driven. Treatment usually includes some psychotherapy to manage anxiety and often to disclose a series of emotional events that trigger a flight-or-flight or psychophysiologically defensive response. The psychological meanings attached to a nociception or to perceived pain may trigger the brain to temporarily rewrite the neurosensory map of the pain area. This in turn leads to a relative neglect syndrome of that limb, which can establish, in lay terms, a "cry for help" in the form of pain and distress symptoms.[29,107,108]

Psychosomatic treatment should include psychologically working through the incidents in the patient's life that led to the need for the defensiveness,[109,110] addressing anxiety and stress management, and counteracting the neglect of the injured limb in order to reintegrate it back into the body. This can be done using mental imagery,[111] desensitization training,[112] or hypnosis, which can accomplish all of the aforementioned at the same time. The process of neglect is a dissociative process beginning at a deep level. Given work on hypnotizability and psychosomatic disorders, we can hypothesize that highly hypnotizable people may be more likely to develop CRPS under the right conditions and also assume that hypnosis would more readily help them resolve the complex syndrome. Using hypnosis while undergoing physical therapy for CRPS showed improvement in pain, stiffness, and strength, as well as patient satisfaction.[113]

Phantom Limb Pain

The other pain disorder responding to psychologically addressing brain mechanisms is phantom limb pain. Pain in an amputated limb can come from damaged nerve endings that are at the stump or that connect with the neurons in the spinal cord. It can also come from a change in the somatosensory cortex map of the body that results either from lack of sensory input from the missing or paralyzed limb or from a peripheral nerve injury that leads to lack of sensation.[114] This may lead to a neurologic need or a cry out to find the missing limb that takes the form of pain sensation.[115]

Long before there were fMRI studies, Erickson said, "If you can have phantom limb pain you can have phantom limb pleasure," implying the power of the unconscious mind to change the interpretation of information from the periphery or the somatosensory cortex, from negative to positive. The patient can do this with self-hypnosis or with deep trance hypnotherapy to resolve pain by creating a more positive mind/body messaging system (to counteract pain) and a better transfer of information between the cognitive and the unconscious areas of the brain (this may counteract neglect due to changes in the somatosensory mapping). Giraux and Sirigu[116] have patients imagine that they are still using the missing or paralyzed limb to relieve pain. This is similar to the positive rehabilitative effects found when asking patients to imagine doing the physical therapy if they are not yet ready to actually do it. Flor et al.[117] had patients touch the stump for sensory stimulation; both studies[16,17] demonstrated pain relief. This works along the same lines as having CRPS patients gently stroke and soothe (desensitize) their limbs that were previously too painful to touch in order to restore the somatosensory map that was altered due to excruciating pain (J. Hernandez, unpublished data, 2008). Evidence for the relationship between the somatosensory cortex and pain comes from research where the somatosensory map was reorganized back to the original somatosensory map by using an electrical prosthetic limb[118] or by use of a mirror image of the remaining limb to "trick" the mind to thinking there were two functioning limbs.[119] Hypnosis may also be used to accomplish the end goal of resolving the need to find the missing limb. Older and more traditional hypnotic trances for phantom pain may be found in Hammond.[50] However, a recent systematic review of the literature including RCTs showed limited research and hence limited evidence supporting the effectiveness of hypnosis.[120]

> *Case Study: This author used hypnosis to assist a young college student patient who had lost his leg in an automobile accident. He felt positional pain leading him to believe that his leg was bent in a painful position under his body. First, we discussed the actual cause of the pain as a somatosensory reorganization that was his mind's first attempt to help him survive that he could now revise; this mini-lecture was partly informational and partly a hypnotic confusion technique and an induction into trance. He was guided to imagine moving the leg to a more comfortable position and then soothing it so that it would recover from the bent position. This reduced some but not all the pain. In the next session, we used a technique of connecting spiritually with the limb as a valuable part of himself (J. Hernandez, unpublished data, 2008) for further description of this technique). He was hypnotically guided to bring his attention into his leg ("go down your leg to the injury") and gently nurse and soothe the injury. He was guided to recognize that his leg was a valuable part of himself that he could always have relationship with (as he did with elders who had passed on) and he was guided to watch his leg go to a spiritual place to rest outside of his body where he knew it would be safe in the universe and would wait for the rest of his body in the future at the end of his life. He was then guided to visualize the perimeter (the map) of his body at present (without the leg), and to see and feel the body moving without the leg, and to practice this in his mind, free from pain. His guided imagery had him sensing himself going to class and doing in the future the things he had done in the past. This lengthy set of sessions helped with the majority of his pain; his keen focus on getting back to his life, and on to his active career certainly helped him to take positive suggestions. The treatment is in line with the research on the brain mechanisms discussed earlier and in line with trends toward success reported by Oakley et al.[121]*

Burns

There is relatively long history of using hypnosis for burn pain, which can be very intense for an extended period of time. Wound care procedures necessary for recovery from burns is painful as well, and pain medication usually does not cover all of the pain. Burn pain is often severe enough to evoke a negative trauma-related trance state in itself, if not shock, at the very same time that a positive mind-set is important for recovery. As mentioned earlier, distraction is a useful pain management technique for certain situations, but hypnosis appears to afford more pain relief than distraction alone during dressing changes. Frenay et al.[122] also found it more effective for pain reduction than stress reducing strategies for decreasing pain and anxiety during wound care; in that study, the wording was individualized according to the hypnotherapist's observations and her judgment of the patient's clinical needs. One case study has experimented with immersive VR (mentioned earlier in this chapter).[88] In that study, patients engaged in the VR during wound care; those who remained with the program enjoyed the experience and had no medication side effects, and their pain and anxiety significantly dropped with the VR.

Clinicians will appreciate the work of Ewin,[123-125] a teaching surgeon and psychiatrist who, in addition to using hypnosis during procedures and surgery, also used hypnotic imagery to prevent the symptom formation after skin is burned. He would immediately give suggestions to counteract the body's response to a burn (reddening and blistering), such as swimming in a cold stream in the evening, and he took advantage of the trauma-induced trance state after a burn incident.

Case Study: I used the technique for a hand burn resulting from picking up a frying pan that had been on the stove. I imagined moving my hand in a cool mountain stream visited during childhood, and when that cold was fully reexperienced, I imagined a sequence of events to include swimming pool that day, on through time to the very near future (watching TV in the next room), skipping the episode of the burn completely; I rehearsed the sequence a few times, letting the unconscious mind do the work of deleting the burn experience. Also, to regain my body's trust and prevent avoidance or resistance in the future, I immediately telepathically sent my hand an apology and an assurance about taking better care of the hand from then on.

For débridement and healing of burns, good techniques might include imagining anesthesia or numbness in the area and displacing the limb or area of the body that is in pain to another side of the room or to a special imaginary healing place, so that the body can rest easy and be ready for its return after trance; trance can be extended by posthypnotic suggestion to last as long as is necessary. There may be a place as well for amnesia for the more painful and traumatic events of the accident, which would have to be addressed in trance individually. Trance phenomenon will allow for the conscious and unconscious minds to work together to know that an accident occurred while conveniently forgetting about parts of it, both at the same time; it is also possible for a patient to know he is being treated for a pain injury and to forget the pain, both at the same time.

Dentistry

Hypnosis has been successfully resolving pain and anxiety surrounding dental work for over 80 years and was arguably used as much for dental work as for other purposes through World War II. Kay Thompson, a dentist who was also an Ericksonian hypnotherapist, pointed out potential psychosomatic element of pain in the oral cavity, as the mouth is the first infant connection to the mother, the first source of gratification, and the

first experience of getting attention to one's needs (through crying).[126,127] For whatever reasons, pain in or near the head may be more likely to result in anxiety and a loss of self-control and efficacy, and patients are relatively quick to appreciate caring support and attention.

A study comparing Ericksonian hypnosis to progressive muscle relaxation tapes, education about procedures, and a control group showed the Ericksonian hypnosis group to have less anxiety about dental procedures; in the protocol, negative thoughts were restructured (the sound of the dentist drill as a suggestion to go deeper into trance) and patients were to visualize success over pain and to use age regression to a painless time in the past.[128] A study comparing patient's pain before and after dental work offered five hypnosis sessions which included relaxation imagery, catalepsy, analgesia, and anesthesia, with posthypnotic suggestions to patients; they were also given self-hypnosis tapes.[129] The patients showed less pain frequency and duration and an increase in daily functioning compared to baseline, even at 6-month follow-up. A study comparing educational sessions or occlusal appliances to hypnorelaxation for temporomandibular joint (TMJ) pain showed that the hypnosis group reduced current and worst pain significantly more than the control groups did.[130] Hypnosis has been shown to be an effective adjunct in dental surgery to reduce pain, pain medication use, and anxiety,[87,131] and pre- and intraoperative hypnosis audiotapes used for third molar extraction with anesthesia reduced anxiety and pain medication use.[101]

For surgery and procedures, a depth of hypnosis is often used wherein the patient is responsive to the dentist's requests (to open wider, close, etc.) but does not feel the procedure itself. Hypnotic suggestions may be for relaxation, for creating numbing, for going by trance to another place while safely leaving the tooth with the dentist, and for feeling pressure rather than pain. In addition to dental procedural pain and anxiety, many dentists learn hypnosis for needle phobia, gagging, bruxism, saliva control, and TMJ, all of which will necessitate specific suggestions.

Pediatric Pain

Children are, in general, more hypnotizable than adults for a number of reasons. They have much richer fantasy lives, are relatively more curious, and are encouraged to use imagination in play; there are fewer parameters and fixed interpretations of the world in general, as they are still learning and are relatively trusting of adults and authority. Critical thinking develops as the brain matures, and it is only in adolescence where society demands more realistic and responsible thinking. In general, peak hypnotizability may be as late as latency (8 to 12 years of age), when children are the most open-minded, curious, imaginative, and willing to suspend judgment and when they are reasonably knowledgeable. Learning pain management and self-control early can help children tolerate medical procedures (shots, fracture settings, etc.) and eliminate negative associations to pain that may remain with them as adults. Children are not reflective thinkers, and so they are more likely to be psychosomatic in presentation of emotional or situational problems; the bank of literature on childhood stomach aches tells us that for them, stomach aches may be a benchmark for distress that may otherwise go unexpressed.

Training in self-hypnosis improved children's functional abdominal pain by 80%,[132] and self-hypnosis tapes improved the respiratory functioning of anxious children in a pulmonary center by 95%.[133] A prospective controlled trial explored the efficacy of adding self-hypnosis training to the use of analgesic cream for lumbar puncture-induced pain and anxiety in 6- to 16-year-old cancer patients[134]; the additional hypnosis led to a decrease in anticipatory and procedure-related pain and anxiety. A retrospective study found a significant decrease in self-reported pain intensity, duration, and frequency of headaches, with no adverse effects, after adolescents were taught self-hypnosis.[135] An hour of self-hypnosis training given to children, along with instructions to practice several times a day, led to less stressful and speedier urologic procedures, by both parental and staff report.[136] Manual-based clinical hypnosis has been found more effective than distraction,[137] cognitive-behavioral treatments,[138] and play and distraction.[139] Hypnosis can also help children undergo acupuncture.[140] However, reviews of the research still found hypnosis to be not robust enough to fall within best practice guidelines for managing procedure-related pain in pediatric oncology[71]; several researchers call for more RCT for the clear-cut benefits of hypnosis and other psychological interventions to be shown, although no studies refute the likelihood that it is beneficial and shows a better side effect profile.[141-143]

Designing trances or trance experiences for children will of course involve taking their developmental age into consideration as well as the degree of trauma and fear involved in what they will be experiencing. First, it is important to remember that children are highly suggestible and are still vulnerable to trauma long before they can understand its context or verbalize their problem. On the other hand, even babies can be lulled or stroked into a soothing situation and be spoken to in reassuring words, songs, and sounds. Olness and Gardner[144] suggest framing therapeutic suggestions and stories in the context of what they know, such as bubbles, pop-up books, dolls, and stories, and utilizing storybook figures as the characters of the stories. Nature, favorite pleasant places, cars, magical travel, music, and repetitive action such as ball bouncing or yoyo tossing can be used in inductions. For adolescents and older children who are more interested in relationships, stories and images could include peer groups. All aged children may be quite intrigued with some of the classic induction techniques such as the pendulum, arm levitation, and the coin drop. It is particularly important to speak to the child in language he or she can understand, to consider play as a way to make the experience more pleasant, to speak with a tone of voice that allows the child to feel supported and respected, and to add suggestions about self-control and self-efficacy and safety. For detailed discussion of hypnosis with children, see Olness and Kohen.[145]

Case Study: A case example is a 13-year-old patient who broke his nose while playing baseball; his mother brought him to a facial trauma doctor I was working with at the time. Concern for his anxiety was relatively great since the same surgeon in the same hospital had previously done surgery on the youngster's throat after a near-fatal small airplane crash. Before trance, any fears or discomfort was discussed so that he would be safe in the procedure room. As the room was being set up for him, we discussed any of his concerns and his baseball game. I hypnotically coached him to go back in his mind to complete the game as he wanted it to end, and along the way, I suggested to him that he could forget about whatever parts of the whole afternoon that would make him more comfortable and that he did not need to remember. I gave him permission to suggest to me how to make the experience safer and more comfortable for him. He proceeded to ask one resident to leave because she was talking about trivial personal issues and not paying attention to his procedure. To our surprise, when the patient woke up the next morning, he removed all the bandages and packing and went down to breakfast without mentioning or questioning the bandages or the hospital experience, but he did remember some pretty girls he saw on the way there. Since that incident, the author includes suggestions to follow his doctor's instructions, so that any necessary aftercare does not also go by the wayside!

Irritable Bowel Syndrome

Most IBS patients have low thresholds of pain in their bowels, along with abnormal autonomic nervous system functioning and considerable symptom discomfort.[146] Hypnotherapy has been shown to improve pain, autonomic symptom dysfunction, and well-being,[147] even at follow-ups beyond 5 years.[148] A recent study shows hypnosis to reduce short-term and long-term IBS symptoms themselves in 50% of patients even a year after treatment.[149] The Manchester Model[150] hypnosis protocol has been consistently effective for treatment of bowel and other physical symptoms, depression, and anxiety[151,152]; improvement in symptom scores is associated with improvement in IBS-related thoughts.[153] When Palsson's North Carolina hypnotic protocol[146] is administered to IBS patients, their daily diary reports show an approximate 50% reduction in pain.[154] In a study comparing the North Carolina protocol[146,154] administered with the manual presentation versus with individually tailored presentation, the manualized induction group had less emotional stress after the treatment, but the individualized induction group continued to improve and did better at 10 months than the group who received the scripted trance and showed less emotional distress.[155] Recently, a study showed that home-based gut-directed hypnotherapy with an audio recording for treatment of pediatric abdominal pain and IBS was as effective as therapist-administered hypnotherapy.[156]

Hypnotic suggestions to improve gut symptoms and IBS pain can include those to warm hands, progressively relax, move attention away from gut symptoms, and to calm and comfort the gut, in addition to suggestions for enhanced over-all well-being, self-efficacy, self-management, and control. The North Carolina protocol is lengthy; it includes all the aforementioned and also suggests dissociation away from the pain and to a carefree place. This appears to break the cycle of pain, and patients reset their perceptions of pain. The protocol is seven scripted, therapist-guided sessions and an audiotape for home use. The Manchester Model[150] now has 12 scripted sessions and an audiotape for home use; the scripts include suggestions to warm the hands and transfer the warmth mechanically to the gut, for control and normalization of gut functions, as well as suggestions for ego strengthening and self-control in handling IBS symptoms.

Headaches

In general, migraine, tension, and mixed headaches respond to hypnosis.[157] Migraine headache frequency, duration, and severity decreased in one study when patients were given one group hypnosis session and 12 weeks of follow-up with hypnosis audiotapes.[158] Tension headache pain, vitality, and mental health improved when patients were offered guided imagery audiotapes.[159] There have been many comparisons of AT to hypnosis for headache control. AT focuses specifically on relaxing muscles, which is in part what hypnosis would address, so that similar effectiveness is expected. Studies show AT to be more effective,[160] less effective,[161] or equally effective for headache pain.[162] Both treatments seem to help patients perceive more self-control of pain[163]; improvement in pain scores seems to be related to hypnotizability, and formal hypnosis with a formal induction seems to improve the chances of success.[161]

To treat a headache, it is usually important to know whether the patient has tension, migraine, or cluster headaches. For tension headaches, direct suggestions could be to breath in and out through the skin in the head and neck, to loosen the scalp, to let the hair fall naturally directly from the scalp, or to cool or warm the inside of the head (depending on the type of headache). Indirect suggestions might be to imagine being in a relaxing place or in a cold place, with cool wet rag at the neck. For migraines, Gibbons[164] suggests diving into water, because this lowers blood pressure and heartbeat and may alleviate circulatory congestion in the head. Suggestions for cold (skiing, hiking in the snow) may also be helpful. Patients may also constrict blood vessels by imagining them to become tight, cool, and narrower. Tension headaches may respond to suggestions that help to open the blood vessels, such as warm climates, relaxation, or warm water. Hammond[157] finds self-hypnosis effective for tension headache management; he suggests that patients who report daily morning headaches may respond well to the use of self-hypnosis tapes at bedtime, which aim to allay tension while they are sleeping.

Cancer

Cancer pain may be distinct from other long-term or chronic pain, in that changes or increases in pain may trigger end-of-life concerns, grief, depression, and anxiety. In addition, there are very often painful and bothersome side effects to cancer treatment, such as nausea, vomiting, tissue or nerve damage, weakness, and fatigue, many of which respond to hypnosis quite well. The feedback loop between diseases such as cancer, negative cognitions, and suffering are discussed elsewhere, as is the effect of stress and distress on immunosuppression, which can compromise patients' recovery times and resistance to secondary illnesses.

Hypnosis is particularly effective in reducing stress through direct and indirect suggestions to relax and through enhancing patients' sense of self-efficacy and self-control. Spiegel and Bloom[165] showed positive effects with hypnosis in terminal cancer patients, possibly including giving patients a slightly longer life span; the latter benefit was not replicated in the recent study, possibly due to the improved medical treatments that extend the lives of all patients who were subjects.[166] This does point out the importance of alternative medicine therapists ensuring that patients are not discounting or ignoring medical care.

A number of studies compared hypnosis to CBT for control of cancer pain. One showed bone marrow transplant patients to benefit more from hypnosis than from CBT or attentional control because they had less pain at worst times and for shorter durations.[167] Other studies show the benefits of hypnosis over CBT for pain, anxiety, and overall distress.[98,137,168] A prospective randomized study with advanced-stage cancer patients showed that a manualized presentation of four weekly hypnosis sessions with addition of audiotapes for home use significantly decreased pain; suggestions were comprehensive, including relaxation, comfort, dissociation, and more specific pain control techniques.[169]

Quality of life is particularly important with cancer because for end-of-life patients; there may be grieving to do as well as personal, relationship, and spiritual business to tend. To address this, one study randomly assigned patients to 10-minute self-hypnosis audiotapes teaching either progressive relaxation (a passive coping strategy) or breathing exercises (an active coping strategy) to be used three times a week.[170] Positive attitudes increased and negative attitudes and anxiety decreased in both groups, with more improvement shown with the active coping strategy; this may have had to do, again, with perceived self-control. Quality of life, particularly vitality, improved for metastatic breast cancer patients who were given 4 weeks of self-hypnosis training, in comparison to those offered 4 weeks of training in a Japanese healing method called *Johrei* and to wait-list controls[171]; both treatment groups improved in mood and anxiety scores. Other studies have shown quality of life improvement for cancer patients using hypnosis.[172,173] The latter study's protocol looks similar to what might occur in a clinical setting; it offered four 30-minute sessions of hypnosis weekly, using traditional inductions and individualized suggestions for symptom management and ego strengthening. Hypnotic suggestions that foster or support existential,

religious or other beliefs about life after death for patients, and for those who socially support them, might be given early in treatment (see Spira[174]).

Osteoarthritis

The research literature on the use of hypnosis with arthritic pain is sparse. One study found Erickson hypnosis to compare favorably to Jacobson relaxation and control conditions for treatment of osteoarthritis pain.[74] Pain relief was directly related to imagery and hypnotic susceptibility but not to expectancy. Hypnotic suggestions addressed relaxation, positive imagery, and age regression to a more comfortable time; the authors used the words of *mental imagery* rather than *hypnosis*, and the words *pain* and *analgesia* were not used.

Clinically, suggestions to alleviate arthritis pain may include warm water, warm blankets, warm sun, and stroking the area with arm hands. Also, suggestions to initiate moving arthritic parts or walking while exhaling and to keep the breath flowing can alleviate unnecessary tensing. The patient may self-hypnotically rehearse moving the arthritic area, thereby limbering the body before actually moving, to help the mind and body work together. Patients might move around while keeping in mind the image of themselves at a much younger age and at pain-free times. They might also focus more intently on the *goal* for moving (specifically what they will do on the other side of the room once they get there) rather than on the sensation of moving. Time distortion to a pain-free time in the past or future, and getting involved with increased focus on what they are doing, may also distract them from physical feelings. Other suggestions might be to let go of the sensation of gravity in the body and to lighten their steps.

There are references to anger as a psychosomatic link to some arthritis pain. As with other emotional links to pain, hypnotic treatment is likely to be even more successful when such psychological or emotional components are addressed. Often, defensiveness or fear underlie the anger and can lead to body tension; the extent of this would be relatively easy to discover during the very important pretreatment assessment.

Medical Hypnosis Techniques

PRINCIPLES OF PREPARATION, INDUCTION, AND SUGGESTIONS

The traditional hypnotherapy session may be divided into four phases: induction, a period of deepening involvement of the unconscious mind while lessening involvement of the conscious mind, the therapy itself, and then a gradual transition back to conscious awareness. Beforehand, a pretreatment assessment should include learning the patient's analogies or metaphors about the pain (stabbing, slicing, cold, daggers, or tingling) and learning what the pain means to the patient in terms of suffering; insult; guilt; religious beliefs; associations to past traumas; future expectations and fears; and social, cultural, or familial losses. That information will help the therapist know the extent of the patient's fears and concerns and the nature of his suffering and determine the appropriate therapy and support that is needed. It will also tell the therapist what specific words or metaphors to use in his messages and suggestions to the patient and what overall approach to use. The better the therapist understands the mechanisms of the unconscious mind, particularly where pain, stress, and memories are concerned, the easier it may be to do effective pain management work.

Ethics for using hypnosis are even more stringent than when using other psychological techniques, in that trances allowing access to unconscious processes can potentially leave the patient more vulnerable. ASCH guidelines also include preparing the patient for hypnosis by dispelling myths about what hypnosis is and is not, advising them of what they might experience, and ensuring that hypnosis is not against their religious beliefs or that it will not violate safety boundaries; this protects both the patient and the clinician. They should know that the therapist will not shield them from any pain they should keep in order to protect themselves; it is sometimes best to allow patients to keep a certain small percentage of their pain and to recognize any pain that they might need to address. Patients should be advised and comforted to know that the therapist is guiding them into a condition of self-hypnosis and is not *doing* hypnosis *to* them. They should also be advised that everyone has his own level of susceptibility that is independent of intelligence and emotional or moral fortitude and that can vary according to day or time. They should also be given permission to stop the session and to talk to the therapist whenever they need to do so.

One variable to consider is the level of involvement in treatment the patient desires. Some patients are proactive in their treatment and cope best by knowing everything there is to know about the process and prognosis, whereas others avoid knowing the clinical details. Giving the patient the amount of detail he wants to keep him comfortable will help in keeping good rapport. In one study, researchers found that over time, patients who attributed the pain control to themselves did better with pain.[163] For the benefit of positive expectancy, using the word *hypnosis* may benefit the patient outcome because some patients prefer handing over the pain management to the clinician, as in the often heard phrases "Just hypnotize me and make me stop (smoking) or (eating) so much." That mind-set signifies an external locus of control, which is not a good indicator of pain management in general or for therapeutic success; however, it may indicate success with hypnosis in that the patient may be willing to suspend vigilance with little resistance.

It is best to provide a quiet, pleasant, and emotionally safe space for the hypnosis sessions, which, of course, may be compromised in many clinical, surgical, and emergency settings. Again, the most important element is the patient–clinician relationship, and there are techniques health care providers can use to gain rapport and help anxious and traumatized patients relax in emergency rooms (ERs), operating rooms (ORs), and busy clinics (see http://www.anodyne.net). In the clinical setting, proper posture helps patients truly "let go" and relax; they may do best when sitting with both feet on the floor and with hands resting on the knees, so that they are not likely to fall asleep but they do not have to work at balancing. An emotionally safe one-on-one session would facilitate the patient's recovery of memories and hidden associations to the pain. Setting up positive expectancy, including the clinician's and the rest of the treatment staff's positive belief in success, also improves the success of hypnosis; this is the variable that confounds many research studies, according to Jensen and Patterson.[80]

Styles of hypnosis vary depending on the preferred approach of the therapist, the context, and the needs of the patient. Research indicates that all therapy techniques work more or less equally well, and that the most effective is the one the therapist feels most comfortable using, as he directs his attention toward the patient's chosen outcome and remains flexible about changing approaches as the patient's needs change.[175] In hypnosis, the patient is suspending vigilance and giving over access in his unconscious mind, so that the onus is on the therapist to choose words carefully and to maintain the safe therapeutic space. That being said, the inductions, certainly the messages, and the length of the sessions will necessarily differ according to the circumstance of pain—chronic, acute, surgical, or trauma-induced pain. Emergency situations are often best handled with a very direct authoritarian approach. In emergencies and where pain is suddenly acute, the patient may be anxious and may want someone to take charge, and he may need suggestions for quick

relief; indeed, the pain and trauma involved may already have induced a trance state. Depth of trance is not necessarily related to outcome; the purpose of the trance is to get suggestions to the unconscious mind efficiently, and hypnosis aims to facilitate that at whatever level. Hypnotic anesthesia for surgery demands a deep trance and a longer induction. For other medical procedures where the patient is to be conversant (such as with epidural injections or spinal cord stimulator placements or brain surgery), a lighter trance may be in order. Light trances may allow patients to observe and learn self-hypnosis, whereas the therapist can gain information on how the work is going and even explore sensations in the pain area to gain more diagnostic information. Conversational trances can occur when the therapist establishes very good rapport with the patient, when the patient is already in an altered state of mind, and when the therapist talks directly to the unconscious mind using hypnotic language and techniques (e.g., the Ericksonian techniques described in the following discussion). Hypnosis may bring up unexpected memories or associations that should be addressed and resolved when they occur or when they are recognized; this might necessitate varying levels of trance during the session.

COMMON INDUCTION PROCEDURES

Inductions can be done conversationally, naturalistically, using rituals or chanting, by directing the patient inward, or by using objects such as a coin or crystal on a chain. In general, the induction involves fixating or narrowing the patient's attention and deepening his involvement while at the same time suggesting dissociation from conscious awareness of the field. Good rapport-building skill and the use of hypnotic phrasing and words allow a seamless transition from induction into therapy. Therapy can begin during induction or after the patient is at the necessary level of trance.

A number of classic induction procedures are often taught in hypnosis training:

- Chiasson induction: The patient is asked to hold his hand out in front of him and to notice his arm or hand move slowly toward his face. The therapist suggests that the patient's eyes feel so heavy that he wants to close. When the hand comes closer to the face and as the fingers open, trance will also occur.
- Reversed arm levitation induction: The patient starts with his arm out in front of him, and as it slowly drops to the table (lap, chair arm) and rests there, he will go deeper into trance.
- Catalepsy induction: The patient holds the arm out in front of him and is given the suggestion that he will lose the feeling of it being there and that he will not be able to move it.
- Chevreul pendulum technique[176]: The patient holds a shiny object in front of him at eye level and has his eyes follow the swinging movement; the therapist suggests that the arm is getting tired and will slowly sink to the table. The moment the pendulum hits the table, the patient will go deeper into trance and may close his eyes for comfort.
- Coin technique: The patient holds a coin in his fist out at arm's length. The therapist may suggest that the coin is a balloon that expands, so that the hand opens; eventually the coin drops, which the patient knows is the signal to enter into trance.
- Magnetic hands: The patient holds his two hands out in front of him, with the suggestion to watch how they slowly come together like magnets, eventually touching one another, which is the invitation into trance.
- Imagery induction: The patient is asked to go in his mind to a personally ideal, specific place or location, and to hear, sense, smell, and totally be *in* the setting.

- Going down a staircase: The patient is guided to walk slowly down a flight of stairs (often 20); as the therapist talks, inducing trance, he imbeds a countdown of the number of stairs until the patient gets to the bottom, when he will drop into trance. The lead out of trance will be to reverse the numbers (from 0 to 20) as the patient walk back up into the conscious mind.
- Progressive relaxation: The patient is guided to relax muscle groups progressively, starting at his feet and working upward or starting at his head and working down. The advantage of this technique is that it is easily used self-hypnotically.
- Eye fixation: The patient is asked to watch something intently until he cannot anymore, and when the eyes decide to close, he may go into trance.
- Rapid eye roll[177]: The technique is also an indicator of hypnotizability. The patient is asked to take a deep breath and hold it, then to roll the eyes upward to look into the top of the eye sockets, then to close the eyes, and as he slowly breathes out, he will relax into a trance.

When there is a sufficient level of trance, therapy can continue to help the patient feel better and give him tools to forget pain, change the perception, put it into perspective, or view the sensations constructively.

SUGGESTIONS AND IMAGERY

The link between thoughts, feelings, behaviors, physiologic state, and pain can allow any of them to change when any of the others does. Curiosity and imagination can be essential keys to change, and change can happen for the patient when he imagines that he is in the state of mind or body that will allow the change to occur. For instance, when I want to be relaxed, I can imagine being at the beach, to put me in the right frame of mind, or I can go to the beach. If I want someone to like me, I can imagine that they already do to show them how to treat me. If I want to dance gracefully, I can imagine myself gracefully gliding across a dance floor to access body memories. Body states, behaviors, and feelings are modified more easily in trance than out of trance. When patients use their his or her own images, they are more likely to be relevant to them and more likely to be successfully used in future self-hypnosis sessions. To encourage dissociation away from the body, the suggestion may be a very detailed trip up in the air in a balloon, off into the clouds, on a rowboat in a magical lake, on a magic carpet over a peaceful place, up on a mountain top, or down on a beach. Any of these can help move the focus out of here and now and out of the body. Turning inward, but still dissociating away from pain, suggestions might be to take a journey from the top of the spine all the way down the back to the sit bones,[178] to go inside the organ or area of the body that has pain, and do something soothing (expand the space, add a healing potion, stroke the inside walls of the area) according to the patient's image of the pain problem[179] or to go into (working with) the inner workings of the brain to change the interpretation or sensation of pain.[180] All these use the complementarity principle, to be discussed in the following text.

For hypnosis to be effective, the message or suggestion needs to go (1) from the conscious to the unconscious mind, reflectively or by self-hypnosis; (2) directly to the unconscious mind while the conscious mind is in deep trance; or (3) indirectly to the unconscious mind by confusing the conscious mind or by some otherwise subliminal technique. Techniques to do the latter include (1) imbedded commands ("If *you* are like me, you *will feel* that the couch is *better* than the chair for going *into trance*.")—here, the italic words are said a bit louder and will be heard by the listener, at an unconscious level, as the dominant or "take home" message; (2) suggestions of dissociation ("While you are aware of the pain at a conscious level, your unconscious mind is already

beginning the healing process all by itself without you having to do anything."); (3) the "yes" set, wherein the therapist says a series of truisms the patient will endorse and then presents the therapeutic message that the patient may have otherwise doubted ("You did well last week, and you did well yesterday, and you are doing well now, and you will continue to do well tonight as well."); (4) implied causatives, which assume that when the patient does A, B will follow ("Whenever you begin the healing, you will probably notice the pain that leads to the automatic healing responses in your unconscious mind that know how to resolve pain all on their own."); and (5) confusion, which forces one to suspend the conscious mind so as to think through and resolve the cognitive conflict the confusion created (see section on Erickson). Direct versus indirect style of suggestion is exemplified by whether the patient is told, for instance, to "Lower your shoulders" or "Take the creases out of your forehead" as opposed to "You may remember the pleasure of a very warm shower on your back and shoulders at the end of a winter day" or "If you have ever had a soothing massage, would your shoulders remember that now?" and "Does your forehead remember how it was so smooth when you were a baby, sleeping peacefully in your cradle?" or "As your eyes slowly begin to close, it is as though you can feel the day's tension roll right down your face, from your hair and all down over your chest and onto the floor in front of you."

The unconscious mind operates more in machine language than the sophisticated conscious mind, so keeping language extremely simple, using metaphors and sparing words, is usually more effective, unless you are accessing the patient's unconscious mind by using a confusion technique, imbedding two conversations and hidden messages at the same time, or creating a state of boredom so that the patient will go deeper into unconsciousness. Whatever the purpose for the trance, it is usually a good idea to add in suggestions to enhance self-esteem and self-efficacy. *Convincers* can assist the effect of therapy by raising the patient's level of positive expectancy that hypnosis works. Traditional ways to do this might include glove anesthesia, wherein the therapist guides the patient to create numbness in one hand, catalepsy or the arm raise as discussed earlier, or simply calling attention to the lost sense of time that occurs during trance. Finally, *fractionation* involves changing the patients' depth of trance, coming out and back into trance, which effectively deepens the trance, may make the trance more effective and may show the patient that he is an interactive partner in the process.

For surgical and procedural anesthesia or analgesia and for trauma situations, acute pain relief is the primary concern. However, the suggestions made for trust and emotional comfort during and after surgery, speedy recovery, ease with the hospital and healing processes, reduction in anesthetic and pain medications, self-confidence, amnesia for presurgical pain, and future well-being can be posthypnotic and address postsurgical issues. With chronic pain, posthypnotic suggestions can help the patient process and reframe nociception that continues to occur after the hypnotic session. The suggestions can be general or specific, suggesting that whenever the patient feels x, he can automatically do y ("In the future, whenever you feel tension in your head, you can automatically say your special releasing words to yourself, release, and relax," or "Whenever you want relief from daily tension, you can say the word "ease" to yourself, and you will automatically feel the wave of release throughout your neck area.").

Finally, the patient can be guided out of trance with suggestions that encourage more cognitive thought and less unconscious processing. References to recognizing time, temperature of the room, the therapist's voice ("as distinct from your own"), or feeling the heartbeat, as the therapist picks up the pace and volume of his speech, can all guide the patient back to conscious awareness. There may be side effects to trance which are not convenient, such as foggy thinking, lethargy, disorientation, slow heartbeat, lack of vibrancy, and a temporary amnesia for what was going on before the trance. They may be erased with another brief series of suggestions so that the patient feels refreshed and in control at the end of trance.

Chronic Pain Management

Jensen and Patterson[80] reviewed 19 studies on the efficacy of hypnosis for chronic pain and outlined the control conditions used for comparison. Eight studies involved headache pain alone and others included cancer; sickle cell; low back, temporomandibular, and mixed chronic pain problems. There were six types of control conditions: measuring change from baseline; hypnosis versus standard care; hypnosis added to another treatment, including physical therapy, medication, education or advice, or an occlusal appliance; hypnosis versus biofeedback; an attentional control condition; and minimal effect control conditions (this allows for passage of time and patient expectancy that a change could occur). They also addressed conditions (or independent variables) that effect success with hypnosis, namely, suggestibility, frequency of treatment sessions, frequency of self-hypnosis practices, patient-rated outcome expectations, initial treatment response, and diagnostic group. The overall conclusion was that hypnotic analgesia was significantly more effective than no treatment and other standard care conditions, although other hypnotic-like treatments, such as progressive relaxation and AT, produced similarly effective pain control.

We have mentioned chronic pain as distinct from acute and procedural pain throughout this chapter, although almost all the techniques mentioned also may apply to chronic pain. Chronic pain carries the expectation that it may never go away and the extra burden of itself as a prolonged physiologic stressor. In addition, its emotional suffering component may magnify with time.[180-182] To that aim, Hilgard et al.[181] asked their patients to rate their suffering and pain separately so that they might learn to differentiate them. Chronic pain is of the type that the patient can well afford to disregard, forget, or modify; there are hypnotic techniques for all those possibilities. Treatment may include dissociation from the nociception and from the awareness of pain; time distortion, which allows the patient to mentally "be" in the future or in the past when he does not feel good; selective amnesia for the original injury that cause the pain; displacement of the pain to a place outside the body; imaginary numbing of the pain; and altered perception of the pain that recognizes nociception as just a signal and nothing more.

Brown and Fromm[49] outline group pain therapy sessions, which may be done in 8- to 12-week formats. The techniques are taught to the patient through personal experience during sessions and then the patients practice them for home use. Brown classifies pain management techniques in four categories—alleviation, alteration, avoidance, and awareness.

1. *Alleviation* of the sensations or symptoms involves making direct or indirect suggestions to make the pain go away, to substitute pain sensations for other sensations or for different ones, to create numbness, or to imagine analgesia.
2. *Alteration* involves changing the overall experience of pain by temporary forgetting it or losing sensation of it, by altering the meaning of it, such as aching after winning a sports event, or changing the sensation (from pain to pressure or tingling), or by dissociating from the pain, or by depersonalizing from the body.
3. *Avoidance* involves taking pain away using distraction, engaging in fantasy, distorting time, age regression or progression, by getting absorbed in a mental task, or by imagining the pain somewhere else in the body.

4. *Awareness* techniques include focusing the conscious mind on the component parts of the pain, and studying the component parts of one's pain awareness, or the component parts of the mind and body's nociception process itself. Brown's awareness techniques also highlight complementarity, in that when a patient thinks about his thinking, he tends to go into trance and cannot pay attention to pain.

Brown suggests having patients pinch the skin between the thumb and the forefinger[54] to induce just enough pain to test out each of the aforementioned techniques and to find out which ones work best; in subsequent practice sessions, each patient will hone the techniques that worked best for him personally. Brown suggests beginning with secondary pain areas (for instance, the leg pain that accompanies back pain or compensatory pain) before working with the primary one.

Finally, pain management training should include relapse prevention, to help patients come back from handling occasional relapses in pain or in personal pain management as well as the more challenging times when patients' pain feels more intense due to stress. Patients do best when they are prepared to manage the psychological and behavioral triggers in their lives that exacerbate pain and when they have a variety of techniques to use for different situations, types, and levels of pain.

Spira and Spiegel[183] discuss practical ways hypnotherapists can work with patients' varying levels of hypnotizability, presenting a tabular outline of techniques to use according to the patients' hypnotizability (low, moderate, and high) and pain levels (mild, moderate, or severe). The table shows strategies that help low hypnotizable patients, who will do best learning to release tension for mild pain, differentiate pain from their responses to moderate pain and distract themselves during severe pain bouts. Moderately hypnotic patients may best attend to their own positive coping resources to managing pain and other problems; as pain increases, they may imagine themselves to be in a positively resourceful state. Patients who are highly hypnotizable can alter mild pain directly by triggering memories of past successful alterations to go directly to that state; as pain progresses, they may dissociate from the experience.

ERICKSONIAN NATURALISTIC APPROACHES TO PAIN AND SYMPTOM MANAGEMENT

Erickson was an expert at pain management from personal and professional experience; his techniques and philosophies are taught worldwide and through The Milton H. Erickson Foundation. Neurolinguistic programming (NLP) developed as an attempt to understand how and what Erickson knew about the unconscious minds of his patients; a good part of NLP's focus is on getting into rapport with the patient's unconscious processes to help him make changes that other parts of his mind are resisting (see http://www.NLPU.com for more information on medical and pain-related applications). Erickson believed that hypnotic trance should be cooperative and interactive and that induction should guide the patient inside himself or herself. He believed patients were unique and resourceful in resolving their own pain and suffering, if they could become "unstuck" and open up to doing so. He oriented patients toward positive change, and his rapport with patients was a study in and of itself. He spoke directly to the patient's unconscious mind (or body processes) and bypassed conscious *and* unconscious resistance by utilizing the patient's language, posture, mood, words, and thinking patterns; this requires the attentive listening and observation skills. To treat pain and symptoms, particularly psychosomatic pain, he stressed the importance of seeing the symptom as a valid part of the patient's experience with some positive purpose that the therapist must welcome in order to work with it.

Erickson managed his own pain by absorbing himself deeply into the awareness of his pain and verbalizing his perceptions of it; this advanced technique diverted his attention away from the sensation itself. His other pain management techniques included altering or reinterpreting the signal, reframing it as a positive thing, eliciting positive early memories to replace the present feelings, or disregarding conscious awareness of pain signal. He was also a master at introducing confusion at the cognitive level, to send the patient into trance, and then confusing perception of pain signals. He disengaged the conscious mind with techniques the conscious mind could not follow. Examples of confusion techniques include the following:

- Including syntactical errors into conversation ("wondering how *you will* it will happen for you . . . to *go into trance*")
- Putting two opposing ideas in the same sentence ("You can use self-hypnosis or I will lead you there") or offering like alternatives ("You can go into trance all by yourself or you can go into self-hypnotic trance".)
- Distracting with strange wording ("Isn't it always the way it is when you think you have control.")
- Making blatant suggestions and negating them ("Maybe you were kind of hysterical, or that really doesn't make sense at all.")
- Using double meanings (such as in a story about shattering window panes or taking them out to let air through the frame)
- Interspersing an important suggestion into a sentence ("It's apparent [*as a parent*] that *you do a good job* at work anywhere.")
- Leading the patient away from his or her train of thought with surprise or humor ("Wow, I just remembered . . . sorry to interrupt . . . and you were saying . . . or is there another way you wanted to feel?)
- Suggesting the obvious ("Sooner or later you will feel relaxed and drop into trance," or "You may not yet know how you will get relief, but as your pain waxes and wanes . . .")
- Reframing the experience ("You know you are still alive when you are lucky enough to still feel your pain.")
- Paradoxical states of being to make feeling pain inconsistent with some other state of mind the patient can remember experiencing.
- Describing the pain in a sentence and saying it backward
- Reversing the perceived direction or pathway of the pain

Lankton and others[184-186] use a number of Erickson's tools for treatment of pain that include metaphors, stories and anecdotes, or jokes to pull attention away and disconnect from cognitive control. Lankton and Lankton[184,185] devised the triple imbedded metaphor technique that begins with a naturalistic trance induction and then progresses deeper with the use of three concurrent stories. The technique relies on excellent rapport and the design of stories and language specific to the patient and imbeds suggestions for cognitive, behavioral, emotional, and physiologic changes at deep levels. The use of metaphors fosters a shift to the right side (more hypnotic and feeling) of the brain. Lankton's hypnotic trances for treatment of physical pain highlight confusion of the pain perception, time distortion, humor for distraction and rapport, and posthypnotic suggestion.[186]

Kay Thompson,[187] an Ericksonian who was also a dentist, used distraction techniques with children and played many word games, such as "panes" of glass that could shatter and be disposed of, seeing through a pain of glass, "untying the knots to not feel" pain, and her famous phrase to start the process of pain management, "When everything that can and should be done about the pain has already been done, you can forget about the pain now."

Obviously, there is overlap in the pain management tools that practitioners use; what differs is the style of presentation, the particular suggestions for physiologic healing according to the specific type and site of pain. Above all, the patient needs to know that his or her pain and suffering are acknowledged by the therapist; trust, rapport, safety, confidence, and expectancy are all beneficial to the outcome.

Conclusions

Trance is a natural phenomenon, and health care providers have been using hypnosis to guide the patients into pain relieving trances for over 200 years. Recent research on the central mechanisms of pain and of hypnosis has highlighted a role for hypnosis in many medical disciplines, concluding that patients prepared hypnotically for surgery do better than 89% of other patients, and that 75% of both healthy subjects and patients respond positively to hypnotic analgesia, even when hypnotizability is not controlled. Ongoing efficacy and effectiveness studies on hypnosis have improved techniques such that even in the wake of the improved medicines and procedures that modern pain clinics have to offer, hypnosis is still poised to take a respectable role in interdisciplinary pain medicine.

References

1. Esdaile J. *Mesmerism in India and its Practical Application in Surgery and Medicine*. London: Longman, Brown, Green & Longmans; 1846.
2. Dell PF. Is high hypnotizability a necessary diathesis for pathological dissociation? *J Trauma Dissociation* 2017;18(1):58–87. doi:10.1080/15299732.2016.1191579.
3. Hull CH. *Hypnosis and Suggestibility: An Experimental Approach*. 2nd ed. Carmarthen, Wales: Crown House Publishing; 2002.
4. Fordyce WE. *Behavioral Methods for Chronic Pain and Illness*. St. Louis, MO: Mosby; 1976.
5. Turk D. Cost effectiveness. From: Past and current state of multidisciplinary treatment programs. Presented at: 26th Annual Scientific Meeting of the American Pain Society; May 2–5 2007; Washington DC.
6. Van Tulder M, Becker A, Bekkering T, et al. Chapter 3. European guidelines for the management of acute nonspecific low back pain in primary care. *Eur Spine J* 2006;15(suppl 2):S169–S191.
7. Guzmán J, Esmail R, Karjalainen K, et al. Multidisciplinary rehabilitation for chronic low back pain: systematic review. *BMJ* 2001;322(7301):1511–1516.
8. Montgomery GH, Bovbjerg DH, Schnur JB, et al. A randomized clinical trial of a brief hypnosis intervention to control side effects in breast surgery patients. *J Natl Cancer Inst* 2007;99(17):1304–1312.
9. Montgomery GH, DuHamel KN, Redd WH. A meta-analysis of hypnotically induced analgesia: how effective is hypnosis? *Int J Clin Exp Hypn* 2000;48:138–153.
10. Kihlstrom JF. Hypnosis. *Annu Rev Psychol* 1985;36:385–418.
11. Janet P. The subconscious. In: Badger RG, ed. *Subconscious Phenomena*. Boston, MA: Gorham Press; 1910.
12. Hilgard ER. *Hypnotic Susceptibility*. New York: Harcourt, Brace & World; 1965.
13. Bowers K. Imagination and dissociation in hypnotic responding. *Int J Clin Exp Hypn* 1992;40:253–275.
14. Bernheim H. *Hypnosis and Suggestion in Psychotherapy*. 1884. New edition translated, New York: University Books; 1963.
15. Jensen MP, Adachi T, Tomé-Pires C, et al. Mechanisms of hypnosis: toward the development of a biopsychosocial model. *Int J Clin Exp Hypn* 2015;63(1):34–75.
16. Haley J. *Uncommon Therapy: The Psychiatric Techniques of Milton H. Erickson, MD*. New York: W.W. Norton & Co; 1986.
17. Bandler R, Grinder J. *Patterns of the Hypnotic Techniques of Milton H. Erickson, M.D*. Lewisville, WA: Grinder & Associates; 1996.
18. Gruzelier JH. Frontal function, connectivity and neural efficiency underpinning hypnosis and hypnotic susceptibility. *Contemp Hypn* 2006;23(1):1513–1532.
19. Evans FJ. Hypnotisability: individual differences in dissociation and the flexible control of psychological processes. In: Lynn SJ, Rhue JW, eds. *Theories of Hypnosis*. London: Guilford Press; 1991:144–168.
20. Horton JE, Crawford HJ, Harrington G, et al. Increased anterior corpus callosum size associated positively with hypnotizability and the ability to control pain. *Brain* 2004;127(8):1741–1747.
21. Gruzelier JH, Gray M, Horn P. The involvement of frontally modulated attention in hypnosis and hypnotic susceptibility: cortical evoked potential evidence. *Contemp Hypn* 2002;19:179–189.
22. DeBenedittis G, Sironi VA. Arousal effects of electrical deep brain stimulation in hypnosis. *Int J Clin Exp Hypn* 1988;36:96–106.
23. Lee J, Spiegel D, Kim S, et al. Fractal analysis of EEG in hypnosis and its relationship with hypnotizability. *Int J Clin Exp Hypn* 2007;55(1):14–31.

24. Price DD, Barber J, Harkins S. Path analysis of the hypnotic experience, 1988. Unpublished manuscript described in Barber J. *Hypnosis and Suggestion in the Treatment of Pain.* New York: W.W. Norton & Co; 1996.

25. Jensen MP, Patterson DR. Hypnotic approaches for chronic pain management: clinical implications of recent research findings. *Am Psychol* 2014;69(2):167–177.

26. Danziger N, Fournier E, Bouhassira D, et al. Different strategies of modulation can be operative during hypnotic analgesia: a neurophysiological study. *Pain* 1998;75:85–92.

27. Barber J, Mayer D. Evaluation of the efficacy and neural mechanism of a hypnotic analgesia procedure in experimental and clinical dental pain. *Pain* 1977;4:41–48.

28. Goldstein A, Hilgard ER. Failure of the opiate antagonist naloxone to modify hypnotic analgesia. *Proc Natl Acad Sci U S A* 1975;72:2041–2043.

29. Maihöfner C, Handwerker HO, Neundörfer B, et al. Patterns of cortical reorganization in complex regional pain syndrome. *Neurology* 2003; 61(12):1707–1715.

30. Pleger B, Ragert P, Schwenkreis P, et al. Patterns of cortical reorganization parallel impaired tactile discrimination and pain intensity in complex regional pain syndrome. *Neuroimage* 2006;32(2):503–510.

31. Kupers R. Functional imaging of allodynia in complex regional pain syndrome. *Neurology* 2006;67(8):1526.

32. Maihöfner C, Handwerker HO, Neundörfer B, et al. Cortical reorganization during recovery from complex regional pain syndrome. *Neurology* 2004;63(4):693–701.

33. Pleger B, Tegenthoff M, Ragert P, et al. Sensorimotor retuning [corrected] in complex regional pain syndrome parallels pain reduction. *Ann Neurol* 2005;57:425–429.

34. Wobst AH. Hypnosis and surgery: past, present, and future. *Anesth Analg* 2007;104(5):1199–1208.

35. Derbyshire SW, Whalley MG, Stenger VA, et al. Cerebral activation during hypnotically induced and imagined pain. *Neuroimage* 2004;23(1):392–401.

36. Vogt BA, Berger GR, Derbyshire SW. Structural and functional dichotomy of human midcingulate cortex. *Eur J Neurosci* 2003;18:3134–3144.

37. Vogt BA, Derbyshire S, Jones AK. Pain processing in four regions of human cingulate cortex localized with co-registered PET and MR imaging. *Eur J Neurosci* 1996;8:1461–1473.

38. Peyron R, Laurent B, García-Larrea L. Functional imaging of brain responses to pain. A review and meta-analysis (2000). *Neurophysiol Clin* 2000;30:263–288.

39. Croft RJ, Williams JD, Haenschel C, et al. Pain perception, hypnosis and 40 Hz oscillations. *Int J Psychophysiol* 2002;46:101–108.

40. Faymonville M, Roediger L, Del Fiore G, et al. Increased cerebral functional connectivity underlying the antinociceptive effects of hypnosis. *Brain Res Cogn Brain Res* 2003;17(2):255–262.

41. Raij T, Numminen J, Närvänen S, et al. Brain correlates of subjective reality of physically and psychologically induced pain. *Proc Natl Acad Sci U S A* 2005;102(6):2147–2151.

42. Röder CH, Michal M, Overbeck G, et al. Pain response in depersonalization: a functional imaging study using hypnosis in healthy subjects. *Psychother Psychosom* 2007;76(2):115–121.

43. De Pascalis V, Magurano MR, Bellusci A. Pain perception, somatosensory event-related potentials and skin conductance responses to painful stimuli in high, mid, and low hypnotizable subjects: effects of differential pain reduction strategies. *Pain* 1999;83:499–508.

44. De Pascalis V. Psychophysiological correlates of hypnosis and hypnotic susceptibility. *Int J Clin Exp Hypn* 1999;47(2):117–143.

45. Meier W, Klucken M, Soyka D, et al. Hypnotic hypo- and hyperalgesia: divergent effects on pain ratings and pain-related cerebral potentials. *Pain* 1993;53:175–181.

46. Jensen MP, Barber J. Hypnotic analgesia of spinal cord injury pain. *Austral J Clin Exp Hypn* 2000;28:150–168.

47. Chapman CR. Psychological aspects of pain: a consciousness studies perspective. In: Pappagallo M, ed. *The Neurological Basis of Pain.* New York: McGraw-Hill; 2005:157–167.

48. Liossi C. Hypnosis in cancer care. *Contemp Hypn* 2006;23(1):47–57.

49. Brown DP, Fromm E. *Hypnosis and Behavioral Medicine.* Hillside, NJ: Lawrence Erlbaum Associates; 1987.

50. Hammond DC. *Handbook of Hypnotic Suggestions and Metaphors.* New York: W.W. Norton & Co; 1990.

51. Yapko MD. *Trancework: An Introduction to the Practice of Clinical Hypnosis.* 3rd ed. New York: Brunner-Routledg; 2003.

52. Weitzenhoffer AM, Hilgard ER. *Stanford Hypnotic Susceptibility Scale, Form C to be Use in Conjunction with Forms A and B in Research Investigations.* Palo Alto, CA: Consulting Psychologists Press; 1959.

53. Morgan AH, Hilgard ER. Stanford Hypnotic Clinical Scale (for children, and for adults). *Am J Clin Hypn* 1978–1979;21:134–147,148–169.

54. Spiegel H, Spiegel H, Spiegel D. *Trance and Treatment: Clinical Uses of Hypnosis.* New York: Basic Books; 1978.

55. Shor RE, Orne MT. *Harvard Group Scale of Hypnotic Susceptibility.* Palo Alto, CA: Consulting Psychologists Press; 1962.

56. Bowers K. The Waterloo-Stanford Group C (WSGC) scale of hypnotic susceptibility: normative and comparative data. *Int J Clin Exp Hypn* 1993;41(1):35–46.

57. Kronenberger WG, LaClave L, Morrow C. Assessment of response to clinical hypnosis: development of the Hypnotic State Assessment Questionnaire. *Am J Clin Hypn* 2002;44(3–4):257–272.

58. Elkins GR, Johnson AK, Johnson AJ, et al. Factor analysis of the Elkins Hypnotizability Scale. *Int J Clin Exp Hypn* 2015;63(3):335–345.

59. Weitzenhoffer AM. Scales, scales and more scales. *Am J Clin Hypn* 2002;44:209–219.

60. Lynn SJ, Council JR, Green JP. Assessing hypnotic responsiveness in clinical and research settings. *Am J Clin Hypn* 2002;44:181–183.

61. Kirsch I, Montgomery G, Sapirstein G. Hypnosis as an adjunct to cognitive-behavioral psychotherapy: a meta-analysis. *J Consult Clin Psychol* 1995; 63(2):214–220.

62. Kessler RS, Dane JR, Galper DI. Conversational assessment of hypnotic ability to promote hypnotic responsiveness. *Am J Clin Hypn* 2002; 44(3&4):273–282.

63. Tellegen A, Atkinson G. Openness to absorbing and self-altering experiences ("absorption"), a trait related to hypnotic susceptibility. *J Abnorm Psychol* 1974; 83:268–277.

64. Wickramasekera I. Secrets kept from the mind but not from the body or behavior: the unsolved problems identifying and treating somatization and psychophysiological disease. *Adv Mind-Body Med* 1998;14:81–132.

65. Crowne DP, Marlowe D. A new scale of social desirability independent of psychopathology. *J Consult Psychol* 1960;24:349–354.

66. Flammer E, Alladin A. The efficacy of hypnotherapy in the treatment of psychosomatic disorders: meta-analytical evidence. *Int J Clin Exp Hypn* 2007;55(3):251–274.

67. DuHamel KN, Difede J, Foley F, et al. Hypnotizability and trauma symptoms after burn injury. *Int J Clin Exp Hypn* 2002;50(1):33–50.

68. Roelofs K, Hoogduin KA, Keijsers GP. Motor imagery during hypnotic arm paralysis in high and low hypnotizable subjects. *Int J Clin Exp Hypn* 2002;50(1):51–66.

69. Younger JW, Rossetti GC, Borckardt JJ, et al. Hypnotizability and somatic complaints: a gender-specific phenomenon. *Int J Clin Exp Hypn* 2007; 55(1):1–13.

70. Ehde DM, Alschuler KN, Osborne TL, et al. Utilization and patients' perceptions of the effectiveness of pain treatments in multiple sclerosis: a cross-sectional survey. *Disabil Health J* 2015;8(3):452–456.

71. Wild MR, Espie CA. The efficacy of hypnosis in the reduction of procedural pain and distress in pediatric oncology: a systematic review. *J Dev Behav Pediatr* 2004;25(3):207–213.

72. Nash M. Salient findings: pivotal reviews and research on hypnosis, soma, and cognition. *Int J Clin Exp Hypn* 2004;52:82–88.

73. Chaves JF, Dworkin SF. Hypnotic control of pain: historical perspectives and future prospects. *Int J Clin Exp Hypn* 1997;45:356–376.

74. Gay MC, Philippot P, Luminet O. Differential effectiveness of psychological interventions for reducing osteoarthritis pain: a comparison of Erickson hypnosis and Jacobson relaxation. *Eur J Pain* 2002;6:1–16.

75. Turner JA, Chapman CR. Psychological interventions for chronic pain: a critical review. II. Operant conditioning, hypnosis, and cognitive-behavioral therapy. *Pain* 1982;12(1):23–46.

76. Hawkins RMF. A systemic meta-review of hypnosis as an empirically supported treatment for pain. *Pain Rev* 2001;8:47–73.

77. Patterson DR, Jensen MP. Hypnosis and clinical pain. *Psychol Bull* 2003; 129:495–521.

78. Lang EV, Berbaum KS, Faintuch S, et al. Adjunctive self-hypnotic relaxation for outpatient medical procedures: a prospective randomized trial with women undergoing large core breast biopsy. *Pain* 2006;126(1–3):155–164.

79. Stetter F, Kupper S. Autogenic training: a meta-analysis of clinical outcome studies. *Appl Psychophysiol Biofeedback* 2002;27(1):45–98.

80. Jensen M, Patterson D. Control conditions in hypnotic-analgesia clinical trials: challenges and recommendations. *Int J Clin Exp Hypn* 2005;53(2):170–197.

81. Jensen M, Hanley M, Engel J, et al. Hypnotic analgesia for chronic pain in persons with disabilities: a case series. *Int J Clin Exp Hypn* 2005;53(2): 198–228.

82. Amundson JK, Alladin A, Eamon G. Efficacy vs. effectiveness research in psychotherapy: implications for clinical hypnosis. *Am J Clin Hypn* 2003;46:11–29.

83. Iphofen R, Corrin A, Ringwood-Walker C. Design issues in hypnotherapeutic research. *Eur J Clin Hypn* 2005;6(2):30–36.

84. Roberts LM. Trial design in hypnotherapy: does the RCT have a place? *Eur J Clin Hypn* 2005;6(2):16–19.

85. Spiegel SB, Kahn S. Being "the other therapist": the varieties of adjunctive experience with hypnosis. *Int J Clin Exp Hypn* 2001;49(4):339–351.

86. Hubbe M, Duncan B, Miller S. *Heart and Soul of Change.* Washington, DC: American Psychological Association; 1999.

87. Montgomery GH, David D, Winkel G, et al. The effectiveness of adjunctive hypnosis with surgical patients: a meta-analysis. *Anesth Analg* 2002;94(6):1639–1645.

88. Patterson DR, Wiechman SA, Jensen M, et al. Hypnosis delivered through immersive virtual reality for burn pain: a clinical case series. *Int J Clin Exp Hypn* 2006;54(20):130–142.

89. Jensen MP, McArthur KD, Barber J, et al. Satisfaction with, and the beneficial side effects of hypnotic analgesia. *Int J Clin Exp Hypn* 2006;54(4): 432–447.

90. Dawson R, Spross JA, Jablonski ES, et al. Probing the paradox of patients' satisfaction with inadequate pain management. *J Pain Symptom Manage* 2002;23:211–220.

91. Patterson DR. Treating pain with hypnosis. *Curr Dir Psychol Sci* 2004; 13:252–255.

92. Wain HJ. Reflections on hypnotizability and its impact on successful surgical hypnosis: a sole anesthetic for septoplasty. *Am J Clin Hypn* 2004;46(4): 313–321.

93. Hart RR. The influence of a taped hypnotic induction treatment procedure on the recovery of surgery patients. *Int J Clin Exp Hypn* 1980;28(4): 234–332.

94. Gurgevich S. Clinical hypnosis and surgery. *Alternative Med Alert* 2003; 6(10):109–120.

95. Cupal DD, Brewer BW. Effects of relaxation and guided imagery on knee strength, reinjury, anxiety, and pain following anterior cruciate ligament reconstruction. *Rehab Psychol* 2001;46(1):28–43.

96. Ginandes C, Brooks P, Sando W, et al. Can medical hypnosis accelerate post-surgical wound healing? Results of a clinical trial. *Am J Clin Hypn* 2003;45:91–102.

97. Massarini M, Rovetto F, Tagliaferri C. A controlled study to assess the effects on anxiety and pain in the postoperative period. *Eur J Clin Hypn* 2005;6(1):8–15.

98. Montgomery GH, Weltz CR, Seltz M, et al. Brief presurgery hypnosis reduces distress and pain in excisional breast biopsy patients. *Int J Clin Exp Hypn* 2002;50(1):17–32.

99. Lobe TE. Perioperative hypnosis reduces hospitalization in patients undergoing the Nuss procedure for pectus excavatum. *J Laparoendosc Adv Surg Tech A* 2006;16(6):639–642.

100. Lang EV, Joyce JS, Spiegel D, et al. Self-hypnotic relaxation during interventional radiological procedures: effects on pain perception and intravenous drug use. *Int J Clin Exp Hypn* 1996;44(2):106–119.

101. Enqvist B, Fischer K. Preoperative hypnotic techniques reduce consumption of analgesics after surgical removal of third mandibular molars: a brief communication. *Int J Clin Exp Hypn* 1997;45(2):102–108.

102. Dyas R. Augmenting intravenous sedation with hypnosis, a controlled retrospective study. *Contemp Hypn* 2001;18(3):128–134.

103. Nilsson U, Rawal N, Unestähl LE, et al. Improved recovery after music and therapeutic suggestions during general anaesthesia: a double-blind randomised controlled trial. *Acta Anaesthesiol Scand* 2001;45:812–817.

104. Kessler R, Dane JR. Psychological and hypnotic preparation for anesthesia and surgery: an individual differences perspective. *Int J Clin Exp Hypn* 1996;44(3):189–207.

105. Bennett H, Disbrow EA. Preparing for surgery and medical procedures. In: Goleman D, Gurin J, eds. *Mind–Body Medicine: How to Use your Mind for Better Health.* Yonkers, NY: Consumer Reports Books; 1993:401–427.

106. Harden RN, Bruehl S, Stanton-Hicks M, et al. Proposed new diagnostic criteria for complex regional pain syndrome. *Pain Med* 2007;8(4): 326–331.

107. Moseley GL. Why do people with complex regional pain syndrome take longer to recognize their affected hand? *Neurology* 2004;62:2182–2186.

108. Galer BS, Butler S, Jensen MP. Case reports and hypothesis: a neglect-like syndrome may be responsible for the motor disturbance in reflex sympathetic dystrophy (complex regional pain syndrome-1). *J Pain Symptom Manage* 1995;10:385–391.

109. Gainer MJ. Somatization of dissociated traumatic memories in a case of reflex sympathetic dystrophy. *Am J Clin Hypn* 1993;36(2):124–131.

110. King JH, Nuss S. Reflex sympathetic dystrophy treated by electroconvulsive therapy: intractable pain, depression, and bilateral electrode ECT. *Pain* 1993;55:393–396.

111. Birklein F, Maihöfner C. Use your imagination: training the brain and not the body to improve chronic pain and restore function. *Neurology* 2006;67(12):2115–2116.

112. Burton AW, Hassenbusch SJ III, Warneke C, et al. Complex regional pain syndrome (CRPS): survey of current practices. *Pain Pract* 2004;4(2):74–83.

113. Lebon J, Rongières M, Apredoaei C, et al. Physical therapy under hypnosis for the treatment of patients with type 1 complex regional pain syndrome of the hand and wrist: retrospective study of 20 cases. *Hand Surg Rehabil* 2017;36(3):215–221.

114. Melzack R. Phantom limbs. *Sci Am* 1992;266:120–126.

115. Wall PD. *Pain: The Science of Suffering.* London: Weidenfeld & Nicolson; 1999.

116. Giraux P, Sirigu A. Illusory movements of the paralyzed limb restore motor cortex activity. *Neuroimage* 2003;20:S107–S111.

117. Flor H, Denke C, Schaefer M, et al. Effect of sensory discrimination training on cortical reorganisation and phantom limb pain. *Lancet* 2001;357: 1763–1764.

118. Lotze M, Flor H, Grodd W, et al. Phantom movements and pain. An fMRI study in upper limb amputees. *Brain* 2001;124:2268–2277.

119. Ramachandran VS, Rogers-Ramachandran D. Synaesthesia in phantom limbs induced with mirrors. *Proc Biol Sci* 1996;263:377–386.

120. Batsford S, Ryan CG, Martin DJ. Non-pharmacological conservative therapy for phantom limb pain: a systematic review of randomized controlled trials. *Physiother Theory Pract* 2017;33(3)173–183.

121. Oakley DA, Whitman LG, Halligan PW. Hypnotic imagery as a treatment for phantom limb pain: two case reports and a review. *Clin Rehabil* 2002;16(4):368–377.

122. Frenay MC, Faymonville ME, Devlieger S, et al. Psychological approaches during dressing changes of burned patients: a prospective randomised study comparing hypnosis against stress reducing strategy. *Burns* 2001; 27(8):793–799.

123. Ewin D. The effect of hypnosis and mental set on major surgery and burns. *Am J Clin Hypn* 1986;26:5–8.

124. Ewin D. Emergency room hypnosis for the burned patient. *Am J Clin Hypn* 1986;29:7–12.

125. Ewin D. The use of hypnosis in the treatment of burn patients. *Psychiatr Med* 1992;10(4):79–87.

126. Thompson K. *The Use of Hypnosis for Pain.* Phoenix, AZ: Milton H. Erickson Congress; 1992.

127. Kane S, Olness K, eds. *The Art of Therapeutic Communication: The Collected Works of Kay F. Thompson.* Bethel, CT: Crown House Publishers; 2004.

128. Moore R, Brødsgaard I, Abrahamsen R. A 3-year comparison of dental anxiety treatment outcomes: hypnosis, group therapy and individual desensitization vs. no specialist treatment. *Eur J Oral Sci* 2002;110:287–295.

129. Simon EP, Lewis DM. Medical hypnosis for temporomandibular disorders: treatment efficacy and medical utilization outcome. *Oral Surg Oral Med Oral Pathol Oral Radiol Endod* 2000;90:54–63.

130. Winocur E, Gavish A, Emodi-Perlman A, et al. Hypnorelaxation as treatment for myofascial pain disorder: a comparative study. *Oral Surg Oral Med Oral Pathol Oral Radiol Endod* 2002;93:429–434.

131. Montenegro G, Alves L, Zaninotto AL, et al. Hypnosis as a valuable tool for surgical procedures in the oral and maxillofacial area. *Am J Clin Hypn* 2017;59(4):414–421.

132. Anbar RD. Self-hypnosis for the treatment of functional abdominal pain in childhood. *Clin Pediatr (Phila)* 2001;40:447–451.

133. Anbar R, Geisler S. Identification of children who may benefit from self-hypnosis at a pediatric pulmonary center. *BMC Pediatr* 2005;5(1):6.

134. Liossi C, White P, Hatira P. Randomized clinical trial of local anesthetic versus a combination of local anesthetic with self-hypnosis in the management of pediatric procedure-related pain. *Health Psychol* 2006;25(3):307–315.

135. Kohen DP, Zajac R. Self-hypnosis training for headaches in children and adolescents. *J Pediatr* 2007;150(6):635–639.

136. Butler LD, Symons BK, Henderson SL, et al. Hypnosis reduces distress and duration of an invasive medical procedure for children. *Pediatrics* 2005;115:e77–e85.

137. Liossi C, Hatira P. Clinical hypnosis versus cognitive behavioral training for pain management with pediatric cancer patients undergoing bone marrow aspirations. *Int J Clin Exp Hypn* 1999;47:104–116.

138. Zeltzer L, Lebaron S. Hypnosis and nonhypnotic techniques for reduction of pain and anxiety during painful procedures in children and adolescents with cancer. *J Pediatr* 1982;101(6):1032–1035.

139. Wall VJ, Womack W. Hypnotic versus active cognitive strategies for alleviation of procedural distress in pediatric oncology patients. *Am J Clin Hypn* 1989;31(3):181–191.

140. Zeltzer LK, Tsao JC, Stelling C, et al. A phase I study on the feasibility and acceptability of an acupuncture/hypnosis intervention for chronic pediatric pain. *J Pain Symptom Manage* 2002;24(4):437–446.

141. Ladas EJ, Post-White J, Hawks R, et al. Evidence for symptom management in the child with cancer. *J Pediatr Hematol Oncol* 2006;28(9): 601–615.

142. Lassetter JH. The effectiveness of complementary therapies on the pain experience of hospitalized children. *J Holist Nurs* 2006;24(3):196–208.

143. Uman LS, Chambers CT, McGrath PJ, et al. Psychological interventions for needle-related procedural pain and distress in children and adolescents. *Cochrane Database Syst Rev* 2006;(4):CD005179.

144. Olness K, Gardner GG. *Hypnosis and Hypnotherapy with Children.* 2nd ed. New York: Grune and Stratton; 1988.

145. Olness K, Kohen DP. *Hypnosis and Hypnotherapy with Children.* 3rd ed. New York: Guilford Press; 1996.

146. Palsson OS. Standardized hypnosis treatment for irritable bowel syndrome: the North Carolina protocol. *Int J Clin Exp Hypn* 2006;54(1):51–64.

147. Simrén M, Ringström G, Björnsson ES, et al. Treatment with hypnotherapy reduces the sensory and motor component of the gastrocolonic response in irritable bowel syndrome. *Psychosom Med* 2004;66(2):233–238.

148. Gonsalkorale WM, Miller V, Afzal A, et al. Long term benefits of hypnotherapy for irritable bowel syndrome. *Gut* 2003;52:1623–1629.

149. Surdea-Blaga T, Baban A, Nedelcu L, et al. Psychological interventions for irritable bowel syndrome. *J Gastrointestin Liver Dis* 2016;25:359–366.

150. Whorwell PJ, Prior A, Faragher EB. Controlled trial of hypnotherapy in the treatment of severe refractory irritable-bowel syndrome. *Lancet* 1984;2:1232–1234.

151. Gonsalkorale WM, Houghton LA, Whorwell PJ. Hypnotherapy in irritable bowel syndrome: a large-scale audit of a clinical service with examination of factors influencing responsiveness. *Am J Gastroenterol* 2002;97: 954–961.

152. Lea R, Houghton LA, Calvert EL, et al. Gut-focused hypnotherapy normalizes disordered rectal sensitivity in patients with irritable bowel syndrome. *Aliment Pharmacol Thera* 2003;17:635–642.

153. Gonsalkorale WM, Toner BB, Whorwell PJ. Cognitive change in patients undergoing hypnotherapy for irritable bowel syndrome. *J Psychosom Res* 2004;56(3):271–278.

154. Palsson OS, Turner MJ, Johnson DA, et al. Hypnosis treatment for severe irritable bowel syndrome: investigation of mechanism and effects on symptoms. *Dig Dis Sci* 2002;47(11):2605–2614.

155. Barabasz A, Barabasz M. Effects of tailored and manualized hypnotic inductions for complicated irritable bowel syndrome patients. *Int J Clin Exp Hypn* 2006;54(1):100–102.

156. Rutten JMTM, Vlieger AM, Frankenhuis C, et al. Home-based hypnotherapy self-exercises vs individual hypnotherapy with a therapist for treatment of pediatric irritable bowel syndrome, functional abdominal pain, or functional abdominal pain syndrome: a randomized clinical trial. *JAMA Pediatr* 2017;171(5):470–477.

157. Hammond DC. Review of the efficacy of clinical hypnosis with headaches and migraines. *Int J Clin Exp Hypn* 2007;55(2):207–219.

158. Emmerson GH, Trexler G. A hypnotic intervention for migraine control. *Aust J Clin Exp Hypn* 1999;27:54–61.

159. Mannix LK, Chandurkar RS, Rybicki LA, et al. Effect of guided imagery on quality of life for patients with chronic tension-type headache. *Headache* 1999;39:326–334.

160. Ter Kuile. High hypnotizables showed more improvement than lows. AT was slightly more effective for headache pain. *Headache* 1995;35:630–636.

161. Zitman FG, Van Dyck, Spinhoven P, et al. Hypnosis and autogenic training in the treatment of tension headaches: a two-phase constructive design study with follow-up. *J Psychosom Res* 1992;36(3):219–228.

162. VanDyck R, Zitman FG, Linssen AC, et al. Autogenic training and future oriented hypnotic imagery in the treatment of tension headache: outcome and process. *Int J Clin Exp Hypn* 1991;39:6–23.

163. Spinhoven P, Linssen AC, Van Dyck R, et al. Autogenic training and self-hypnosis in the control of tension headache. *Gen Hosp Psychiatry* 1992;14:408–415.

164. Gibbons DE. Suggestions for pain control. In: DC Hammond, ed. *Handbook of Hypnotic Suggestions and Metaphors*. New York: W.W. Norton & Co; 1990.

165. Spiegel D, Bloom JR. Group therapy and hypnosis reduce metastatic breast carcinoma pain. *Psychosom Med* 1983;45:333–339.

166. Spiegel D, Butler LD, Giese-Davis J, et al. Effects of supportive-expressive group therapy on survival of patients with metastatic breast cancer: a randomized prospective trial. *Cancer* 2007;110:1130–1138.

167. Syrjala KL, Cummings C, Donaldson GW. Hypnosis or cognitive behavioral training for the reduction of pain and nausea during cancer treatment: a controlled clinical trial. *Pain* 1992;48(2):137–146.

168. Mundy EA, DuHamel KN, Montgomery GH. The efficacy of behavioral interventions for cancer treatment–related side effects. *Semin Clin Neuropsychiatry* 2003;8(4):253–275.

169. Elkins GR, Cheung A, Marcus J, et al. Hypnosis to reduce pain in cancer survivors with advanced disease: a prospective study. *J Cancer Integ Med* 2004;2:167–172.

170. Laidlaw TM, Willett MJ. Self-hypnosis tapes for anxious cancer patients: an evaluation using personalized emotional index (PEI) diary data. *Contemp Hypn* 2002;19(1):25–33.

171. Laidlaw T, Bennett BM, Dwivedi P, et al. Quality of life and mood changes in metastatic breast cancer after training in self hypnosis or Johrei: a short report. *Contemp Hypn* 2005;22(2):84–93.

172. Classon C, Butler LD, Koopman C, et al. Supportive-expressive group therapy and distress in patients with metastatic breast cancer: a randomized clinical intervention trial. *Arch Gen Psychiatry* 2001;58:494–501.

173. Liossi C, White P. Efficacy of clinical hypnosis in the enhancement of quality of life of terminally ill cancer patients. *Contemp Hypn* 2001;18(3):145–160.

174. Spira JL. *Group Therapy for Medically Ill Patients*. New York: Guilford Press; 1997.

175. Duncan BL, Miller SD, Sparks JA. *The Heroic Client: Revolutionary Way to Improve Effectiveness Through Client-Directed Outcome-Informed Therapy*. San Francisco, CA: Jossey-Bass; 2004.

176. Easton RD, Shor RE. Information processing analysis of the Chevreul pendulum illusion. *J Exp Psychol: Human Percept Perform* 1975;1(3):231–236.

177. Ewin DM. Rapid eye roll induction. In: Hammond DC, ed. *Hypnotic Induction and Suggestion: An Introductory Manual*. Des Moines: American Society of Clinical Hypnosis; 1998:49–50

178. Lankton S. *Ericksonian Approach to Hypnotherapy*. Pensacola, FL; Advanced Training Workshops; 1994.

179. Hernandez J. The use of self-relations therapy in pain management. In: Gilligan S, Simon D, eds. *Walking in Two Worlds: the Relational Self in Theory, Practice, and Community*. Phoenix, AZ: Zeig Tucker & Theisen Inc; 2002.

180. Hernandez J. *Dialogues with Pain: Internal Body Conversations That Resolve Suffering*. Carmarthen, United Kingdom: Crown House Publishing; 2008.

181. Hilgard ER, Hilgard J, Barber J. *Hypnosis in the Relief of Pain*. Rev ed. New York: Brunner–Mazel; 1994.

182. Chapman CR, Gavrin J. Suffering: the contribution of persistent pain. *Lancet* 1999;353(9171):2233–2237.

183. Spira JL, Spiegel D. Hypnosis and related techniques in pain management. *Hosp J* 1992;8:89–119.

184. Lankton S, Lankton C. *The Answer Within: A Clinical Framework of Ericksonian Hypnotherapy*. New York: Brunner–Mazel Publishers; 1983.

185. Lankton C, Lankton S. *Tales of Enchantment: Goal Oriented Metaphors for Adults and Children*. New York: Brunner–Mazel Publishers; 1989.

186. Lankton S. *Pain Management*. Phoenix, AZ: Milton H. Erickson Congress; 2007.

187. Thompson K. The curiosity of Milton H. Erickson, M.D. In: Zeig JK, ed. *Ericksonian Approaches to Hypnosis and Psychotherapy*. New York: Brunner–Mazel; 1982:413–421.

CHAPTER 87

Group Therapy for Chronic Pain

MELISSA A. DAY and **BEVERLY E. THORN**

Group therapy continues to be an appealing and common method of chronic pain treatment delivery both in clinical and research settings.[1] First appearing over three decades ago in the pain management literature, case reports[2] and open clinical trials[3,4] began reporting on adapted individual treatments applied in small-group settings that explored the patient acceptability of a group format. Since that time, controlled trials have demonstrated the utility, efficacy, and cost-effectiveness of this mode of delivery, and the group format is commonly used in interdisciplinary pain management clinics for helping patients manage heterogeneous chronic painful conditions.

Although there are multiple levels of evidence, and each has advantages and disadvantages, in an evidence-based practice, randomized controlled trials (RCTs) provide stronger support.[5] Therefore, the primary findings presented in this chapter are based on evidence emerging from searches of the scientific literature that were performed as recommended within the practice of evidence-based medicine.[6] Specifically, the search implemented in the prior edition of this chapter that searched the literature dating back to 1980 until 2007 was extended to identify literature published between 2007 and August 2017. As per the prior edition, combinations of controlled vocabulary terms, keywords, and methodologic filters were used in an effort to identify the highest level of evidence currently available on group treatment of chronic pain. Details of these searches may be found in Appendix 87.1.

These literature searches revealed that RCTs have primarily evaluated five different types of groups: (1) cognitive-behavioral therapy (CBT) groups that focus on teaching pain self-management skills; (2) mindfulness-based interventions (MBIs) including mindfulness-based stress reduction (MBSR) and mindfulness-based cognitive therapy (MBCT); (3) acceptance-based approaches, primarily acceptance and commitment therapy (ACT); (4) education groups; and (5) supportive/expressive groups. Although the evidence has rapidly evolved to add further support to mindfulness and acceptance-based approaches since the last edition of this chapter, the vast majority of well-controlled trials of group-delivered treatments for chronic pain continue to be dominated by CBT, which has been shown to be an efficacious treatment of chronic pain; as a result, the focus of this chapter is on group CBT for the management of chronic pain conditions.

Rationale and Basic Considerations of Group Treatment for Pain

EVIDENCE FOR EFFICACY OF GROUP TREATMENT FOR CHRONIC PAIN MANAGEMENT

The highest level of evidence from an evidence-based practice viewpoint is meta-analyses and systematic reviews that quantitatively synthesize the evidence. To our knowledge, no meta-analyses or systematic reviews specifically of group CBT for chronic pain management have been published to date, although reviews of both individual- and group-delivered CBT (combined) have been published.[7,8] Our literature search revealed numerous controlled studies (both RCTs and non-RCTs) of cognitive and behavioral approaches that have compared (1) group treatment to individual treatment; (2) group treatment to wait-list controls, to treatment as usual, and to other

kinds of group treatment (e.g., relaxation or education/support groups); and (3) behavioral group treatments to group exercise and physical therapy treatments. These are reviewed in the following text, followed by a description of the current evidence for group mindfulness- and acceptance-based approaches.

GROUP VERSUS INDIVIDUAL TREATMENT

Table 87.1 summarizes the controlled studies that have directly compared the efficacy of group-administered treatment to individually administered treatment for chronic pain.[9–16] Relatively few studies have compared group to individual treatment, and we found only one further RCT specifically addressing this question since the prior edition,[10] and one further RCT that compared group in-person delivered CBT to individually delivered CBT via the Internet.[9] These studies have consistently demonstrated few meaningful differences in outcome between the two treatment modalities, and no differences were observed in the one study comparing in-person group therapy and online individual therapy.

One of the earliest RCTs comparing group to individual treatment[14] found no differences in outcome between the two modes of treatment for headache patients with the exception that at the 6-month follow-up, participants in the group condition showed less of a tendency to drift back toward baseline levels of pain ratings. Because participants knew prior to treatment that they would be randomly assigned to group or individual treatment formats, posttreatment interviews queried their perceptions regarding the treatment modality to which they were ultimately assigned. Patients in group treatment highlighted the benefit of being able to share openly with other headache sufferers and to discuss their progress with others in the group. Patients in individual treatment valued the personalized attention given via the dyadic therapeutic relationship and expressed concern that group treatment would not have offered sufficient therapist time for each individual. Thus, patients who participated in each treatment modality seemed to highlight the positive aspects of the treatment modality to which they were assigned as the reasons why this would be the preferred mode of treatment.

Another early RCT focusing on patients with pain in the upper extremities also demonstrated minimal overall differences between individual and group treatment.[15] At 6-month and 2-year follow-up, those who received the group treatment reported less pain-related interference than those who were treated individually, and treatment outcome was otherwise equally efficacious.[15,16] It is interesting to note that posttreatment satisfaction ratings were higher for individually treated patients, and individual treatment was more effective than group treatment on the outcome measure of self-reported coping strategies. One limitation of these early RCTs, however, was the relatively low number of participants in each condition, which limited the statistical power. A benefit of the studies was the collection of patient satisfaction data.

Several later trials confirmed these general findings. In patients with chronic low back pain, Rose et al.[13] reported few differences in an RCT comparing patients treated individually and those treated in groups. Another RCT by Kääpä et al.[10] examined group-delivered multidisciplinary treatment compared to individual physiotherapy for chronic low back pain and found few differences in outcome immediately following treatment

TABLE 87.1 Individual Versus Group Therapy

Authors	Study	Treatment Type	Treatment Components	Duration	Outcome Measures	Results	Limitations	Follow up (f/u)
de Boer et al.[9]	RCT	Group in-person CBT vs. individual Internet-delivered CBT	Same treatment components across conditions, included psychoeducation on CBT model and pain, graded activity, pain-stress connection, relaxation, pain cognitions, cognitive restructuring, disengaging attention from pain. Online treatment group received personal feedback from psychologist via e-mail with the option for additional e-mail/phone contact in the case of technical problems, aggravated symptoms or additional questions.	Group CBT: seven 2-h weekly sessions and a booster session at 2 mo	Pain Catastrophizing Scale, VAS pain intensity, fatigue and interference, Pain Coping and Cognition List (PCCL), RAND-36	In ITT analyses, group = Internet on PCS pain catastrophizing, pain intensity, PCCL catastrophizing, pain coping, internal and external pain management, and aspects of global health-related QOL, with both significance improved at posttreatment and 2-mo f/u; in completer analyses, Internet > group on PCS, pain intensity, pain coping, and select QOL dimensions. No significant change in interference or fatigue. Internet course was considered cost-effective relative to group delivery.	Brief f/u; time spent with psychologist in the online condition was not recorded.	2 mo
Kääpä et al.[10]	RCT	Group multidisciplinary rehabilitation (n = 59) vs. individual physiotherapy (n = 61)	Group treatment included physical training, workplace interventions, back school, relaxation training, and cognitive-behavioral stress management; individual treatment included physical exercise, massage, spine traction, manual spine mobilization, ultrasound	Group program was 70 h over 8 wk; individual program was ten 1-h sessions over 6–8 wk.	NRS for pain intensity, sciatic pain intensity, subjective working capacity; Oswestry disability; sick leave due to pain; health care consumption due to back pain; depression symptoms, belief in future working ability, and well-being	Group = individual at posttreatment and f/u, except for general well-being, which was better in the group condition at posttreatment. Both groups showed significant improvements in disability and health care consumption. Within group, the individual condition showed significantly improved pain intensity, whereas group-delivered showed improved subjective working ability, belief in future working ability.	Treatment dose and intervals differed according to group or individual assignment; some measures lacked adequate psychometric properties.	6, 12, and 24 mo
Turner-Stokes et al.[11]	RCT	Group CBT (N = 66) vs. individual CBT (N = 47)	Group and individual: relaxation, cognitive coping strategies, activity pacing, encouraged to exercise by building up with achievable goals	Group: 1 full afternoon per week for 8 wk Individual: 1-h sessions every other week for 8 wk	West-Haven Yale Multidimensional Pain Inventory (WHYMPI), State-Trait Anxiety Inventory (STAI), Beck Depression Inventory (BDI), general activities, analgesic medication consumption, and pain severity	Both groups: significant improvements in pain interference, control over pain, and depression. Group = individual at f/u. Rapid improvements in group, slower improvements in individual. Differences leveled off at f/u. Group = individual overall	Treatment intervals differ according to group or individual assignment.	6–12 mo

Study	Design	Population	Intervention	Components	Duration	Outcome Measures	Results	Limitations	Follow-up
Frettlöh and Kröner-Herwig[12]	Non-RCT[a]	102 with mixed chronic pain	Group CBT (N = 34) vs. individual CBT (N = 34) vs. control (TAU) (N = 34)	Education, relaxation, imagery, cognitive restructuring	12 wk	Subjective disability, catastrophizing, depression, coping, pain diary	Group and individual > control for majority of outcomes. Group = individual for depression and most other measures. Larger effect sizes for group compared to individual at f/u.	Session duration not specified	6 mo
Rose et al.[13]	RCT	84 with chronic low back pain	Part 1: group CBT (N = 26) vs. individual CBT (N = 24) Part 2: compared 15-h (N = 22), 30-h (N = 22), or 60-h duration treatments	Education, cognitive therapy, graded aerobic exercise, relaxation	15, 30, or 60 h duration	VAS pain severity scale (0 to 100), Roland-Morris Disability Questionnaire, Modified Somatic Perception Questionnaire (MSPQ), Modified Zung Depression Inventory, Pain Locus of Control Scale, Pain Self-Efficacy Questionnaire	Individual = group treatments on outcome measures. Individual treatment more strongly associated with changes in disability and on MSPQ. No differences in program duration on outcome.	No control for baseline differences on some variables	6 mo
Johnson and Thorn[14]	RCT	22 with headache	Group CBT (GCBT) (N = 7) vs. individual CBT (ICBT) (N = 7) vs. wait-list control (WLC) (N = 8)	Psychoeducation, cognitive coping strategies, relaxation	5 weekly 90-min sessions	McGill Pain Questionnaire (MPQ), Brief Symptom Inventory (BSI), self-monitoring cards (for pain intensity, number of prescribed medications, number of OTC medications, number of prescribed pills consumed, number of OTC pills consumed)	Improvement in pain ratings and decrease in anxiety across groups from Times 1 to 2. Decreases in number of times individuals took medication and in number of different medications taken. GCBT = ICBT overall	Small sample size, limited power	1, 3, and 6 mo
Spence[15,16] (2-y f/u)	RCT	45 chronic work-related pain of the upper extremity (19 followed at 2 y)	GCBT (N = 13) vs. ICBT (N = 14) vs. WLC (N = 15)	Goal setting, cognitive restructuring, relaxation, cognitive skills training, dealing with sleep problems, assertiveness training	9 weekly sessions at 1.5 h	BDI, STAI, Coping Strategies Questionnaire (CSQ), McGill Pain Rating Index (PRI), Sickness Impact Profile (self-report and other-report) Daily Self-Monitoring	GCBT and ICBT > WLC for reductions on all outcome measures. Improvements maintained at f/u. GCBT = ICBT 2-y f/u: less relapse for GCBT for pain ratings and interference, GCBT = ICBT for other outcomes	Small sample size, limited power	6 mo, 2 y

[a]Information obtained from English abstract only.
CBT, cognitive-behavioral therapy; ITT, intention-to-treat; NRS, Numerical Rating Scale; OTC, over-the-counter; PCS, Pain Catastrophizing Scale; QOL, quality of life; RCT, randomized controlled trial; TAU, treatment as usual; VAS, visual analog scale.

and at 6-, 12-, and 24-month follow-up; however, this study was limited by design features with the two conditions receiving different treatment doses and intervals. In a sample of patients with mixed chronic pain, Frettlöh and Kröner-Herwig[12] also found few statistically significant differences in treatment outcome between individual and group modalities, although the effect sizes in improvement at follow-up suggested that group treatment may have been superior to individual treatment.[12]

In another RCT of individuals with mixed chronic pain, Turner-Stokes et al.[11] compared outpatient group and individual therapies and found that both treatments resulted in improvements on measures of depression, anxiety, medication consumption, general activity, and pain severity. Those treated in a group showed greater initial gains than those treated individually, but these treatment differences were not sustained over time. Patients treated individually showed slower initial gains but evidenced the same benefits as those who had been treated in a group at the end of treatment. These authors also reported less of a tendency for the treatment gains made by individually treated patients to drift back toward baseline over time. In this study, however, group treatment was delivered for more hours at a time and over a shorter duration (8 weeks) than individual treatment (spread over 16 weeks), and this difference could explain the slower treatment gains witnessed with the individually treated patients.

Finally, one recent RCT compared group-delivered, in-person CBT to individual, Internet-delivered CBT.[9] The results showed that both formats resulted in significant improvements across a number of important pain-related outcomes, with the Internet-delivered condition outperforming group therapy on some domains in the completer analyses, although the longevity of these effects was not fully examined. Other research now in progress is examining the utility and efficacy of group-delivered telepain management programs that implement videoconferencing interfaces; these innovative delivery platforms have the potential to improve access to CBT in the future.[17] Overall, the research comparing group to individually delivered treatment has generally concluded that there are very few meaningful differences between outcomes resulting from group and individually administered treatments for chronic pain.

GROUP COGNITIVE-BEHAVIORAL THERAPY VERSUS WAIT-LIST, TREATMENT AS USUAL, OR OTHER GROUP TREATMENTS

Table 87.2 summarizes the controlled studies that have compared the effects of group-administered CBT to wait-list control conditions, treatment as usual conditions, or other group treatments such as relaxation, education, or supportive/expressive group therapy.[18-64] Trials comparing CBT to MBIs and ACT are reported in Tables 87.3 and 87.4, respectively. There are an impressive number of controlled trials that have been carried out by different research groups focusing on different populations of individuals with pain that together establish the efficacy of CBT for chronic pain. Systematic reviews of these trials have been conducted that include both individual and group-delivered CBT formats across pain types and in children and adult populations; due to space limitations, not all of the studies reported in these reviews are included here.[7,8,65,66] In most cases, RCTs that compared group CBT to other types of group treatments also included a wait-list condition to control for the natural progression of the chronic pain disorder. In the following text, we highlight findings from select studies reported in Table 87.2 comparing group CBT to other types of group treatment because they have played an important role in identifying the effects of CBT; later in this chapter, we also describe a selection of studies that have examined the mechanisms underlying CBT treatment efficacy.

CBT is a generic term used to describe a complex and multifaceted treatment, and the included treatment components

within group CBT protocols vary across studies and research groups. However, the general principles associated with CBT are typically consistent across studies (i.e., that one's thoughts and feelings influence one's ability to cope with pain and teaching pain self-management strategies). An overarching component of CBT includes strategies to educate patients about how the brain processes pain and psychological factors affecting pain perception. Furthermore, training in specific pain management skills almost always includes one or more modules on recognizing and modifying maladaptive or distorted pain-related automatic cognitions and beliefs, enhancing cognitive coping, learning relaxation strategies (including one or more types of relaxation techniques such as biofeedback, autogenic relaxation, progressive or passive muscle relaxation, meditation, and/or self-hypnosis), and completing regular homework assignments such as thought records or guided relaxation for skills acquisition. Frequently, but less consistently, CBT includes modules focusing on stress management (sometimes referred to as stress inoculation), paced physical activity, assertive communication, pleasant activity scheduling, and coping self-statements.

Because of the varied approaches that have all been subsumed under the label of CBT in the literature, it has historically been difficult to identify the specific treatment components that account for treatment efficacy, and this continues to be the case. There are a limited number of dismantling studies that have evaluated specific CBT components for pain management. However, controlling for nonspecific treatment effects (e.g., attention from therapist, expectations of health care provider and patient) is an important step toward determining the specific components of treatment efficacy as well as for elucidating specific and shared treatment mechanisms. Comparing patients receiving group treatment for chronic pain to those on a wait-list does not allow for this type of analysis, although wait-lists do control for the natural progression of the disorder over time and potential reactivity associated with self-monitoring or keeping pain diaries (if included as part of the study). The social context in which the treatment is administered is of particular relevance for the study of the active components of group treatment approaches. Therefore, studies comparing one type of group treatment to another type of group "attention control" treatment (e.g., support group) provide better evidence for disentangling the specific versus nonspecific treatment effects of CBT. Furthermore, comparing CBT to other active treatments demonstrates the relative effects and also allows for examination of whether the treatments exert benefit for the reasons proposed by the respective theory.

Although there is strong evidence for CBT delivered in nongroup formats in nonadult populations, most of the group CBT research to date has been conducted within adult populations with chronic back pain, headache, orofacial pain, or arthritis-related pain and to a lesser degree across an array of other pain conditions.[67] Systematic reviews of the CBT literature typically collapse across most pain types (indicative that the treatment approach and effects are sufficiently similar across these conditions to do so); however, headache and migraine are usually reviewed separately due to differences in the overall approach as well as history.[8] More recently, the treatment of neuropathic pain was isolated within a systematic review and results showed that compared to nociceptive pain, neuropathic pain is particularly recalcitrant to treatment.[7] The primary focus here is on adult populations; the specific type of pain investigated in each study is reported in the corresponding Table 87.2.

There continues to be a limited number of studies in which one group treatment for pain has been compared to another. One study in patients with fibromyalgia, for example, compared group education plus CBT versus group education plus group discussion (which controlled for the effects of attention).[44]

TABLE 87.2   Group Cognitive and Behavioral Therapy Studies

Authors	Study	N	Treatment Type	Treatment Components	Duration	Outcome Measures	Results	Limitations	Follow up (f/u)
Thorn et al.[18]	RCT	290 with mixed chronic pain	Literacy-adapted CBT (n = 95) vs EDU (education) (n = 97) vs. treatment as usual (TAU) (n = 98)	CBT: psychoeducation, cognitive restructuring, activity pacing, relaxation, motivational reinforcement EDU: pain-related information provided, no specific skills-building exercises	Ten 1.5-h weekly sessions	Brief Pain Inventory intensity and interference, Patient Health Questionnaire-9	CBT = EDU at posttreatment, both > TAU on pain intensity and physical function; gains in intensity maintained at f/u for EDU but not CBT, gains in physical function maintained for both CBT and EDU. No significant changes in depression.	Participants were recruited from a single health care system, so a self-selection bias was possible.	6 mo
Helminen et al.[19]	RCT	111 with knee osteoarthritis, aged 35–75 y	CBT (n = 55) vs. medical TAU (n = 56)	CBT: psychoeducation on pain, problem-solving skills, relaxation, scheduling activities, cognitive appraisals and beliefs, assertiveness training	Six 2-h weekly sessions	Western Ontario and McMaster Universities Osteoarthritis Index Pain Scale, Pain Self-Efficacy Questionnaire, RAND-36 emotional well-being, Pain Catastrophizing Scale, Tampa Scale for Kinesiophobia (TSK), Beck Depression Inventory (BDI)	CBT = TAU on pain and function; CBT > TAU on well-being, TAU > CBT on self-efficacy. No significant differences at f/u.	Lack of fidelity monitoring, low recruitment to enrollment rate; baseline self-efficacy was high at baseline for both groups.	3 mo 12 mo
Linden et al.[20]	RCT	103 with chronic low back pain	CBT (n = 53) vs. unspecified occupational therapy (OT; n = 50)	All participants treated for 21 d in an inpatient interdisciplinary rehabilitation unit. In addition: CBT group: gate control theory, stress reduction, problem solving, self-monitoring, cognitive restructuring, reducing avoidance, increasing activities, relaxation OT: additional OT sessions, playing games, motivated to engage in activities	Six 90-min sessions (3/wk)	Symptom Checklist-90, Rating of Health Locus of Control Attributions, Fear Avoidance Belief Questionnaire, VAS pain	All outcomes significantly improved in both groups; CBT > OT on pain and fear avoidance beliefs.	Lack of fidelity monitoring; effect of CBT in isolation from other interdisciplinary treatments not established; no f/u	—

(continued)

TABLE 87.2 (Continued)

Authors	N	Study	Treatment Type	Treatment Components	Duration	Outcome Measures	Results	Limitations	Follow up (f/u)
Seminowicz et al.[21]	13 with mixed chronic pain vs. 13 healthy and age-matched controls (baseline only)	Nonrandomized trial	CBT (n = 13)	Self-regulatory skills such as relaxation, cognitive coping strategies such as cognitive restructuring, attention diversion methods, activity pacing, scheduling pleasant events, exercise, methods for enhancing social support	Eleven 1.5-h weekly sessions	Structural neuroplasticity (i.e., gray matter, GM), McGill Pain Questionnaire-Short-Form, Treatment Outcomes in Pain Survey, Short-Form Health Survey (SF-36), BDI, Coping Strategies Questionnaire	Increased GM post-CBT in the bilateral dorsolateral prefrontal, posterior parietal, subgenual anterior cingulate/orbitofrontal, and sensorimotor cortices as well as hippocampus; reduced GM in supplementary motor area. Most increases in GM became significantly greater than GM in controls. CBT-related reductions in pain catastrophizing and increases in pain control were correlated with several of these regional GM changes.	Small sample size; no comparison or randomization; lack of f/u	—
Slavin-Spenny et al.[22]	147 with mixed headaches	RCT	Anger awareness and expression training (AAET; n = 50) vs. relaxation (n = 48) vs. WL (n = 49)	AAET: psychoeducation on stress-headache connection, experiential exercises for emotional awareness, assertive communication Relaxation: psychoeducation on stress-headache connection, progressive muscle relaxation, deep breathing, brief relaxation	Three 1-h weekly sessions	Self-Assessment Manikin, Headache Management Self-Efficacy Scale, Toronto Alexithymia Scale, Rathus Assertiveness Schedule, Emotional Approach Coping Scales, Migraine Disability Assessment Scale, headache frequency, severity and duration, Brief Symptom Inventory	AAET = relaxation on self-efficacy and headache outcomes, both > control. AAET significantly improved alexithymia, emotional processing, and assertiveness, compared to the other two conditions.	Lack of f/u; lack of fidelity monitoring; use of a college sample limits generalizability; no headache diagnostic information obtained; no daily diaries of headache outcomes	—
Heutink et al.[23]	61 with neuropathic pain after SCI	RCT	CBT (n = 31) vs. WL (n = 30)	CBT: psychoeducation, ABC model, stress, movement and pain, assertiveness, relaxation, goals, social aspects; significant other attended first 2 sessions	Ten 3-h sessions over 10 wk and booster session 3 wk post-treatment	Chronic Pain Grade Questionnaire, Hospital Anxiety and Depression Scale, Utrecht Activities List, Life Satisfaction Questionnaire	CBT = WL on intensity and disability; CBT > WL on anxiety and participation in activities	Small sample size	3 and 6 mo

Study	Design	Population	Intervention	Intervention content	Sessions	Measures	Results	Notes	Time
Thorn et al.[24]	RCT	83 with mixed chronic pain	Literacy-adapted CBT (n = 49) vs. EDU (n = 34)	CBT: stress-pain connection, automatic thoughts, challenging automatic thoughts and beliefs, relaxation, coping statements, expressive writing, assertive communication. EDU: psychoeducation on chronic pain, gate control theory, costs of pain, acute vs. chronic pain, sleep, mood changes, pain behaviors, communication, working with health providers	Ten 1.5-h sessions over 10 wk	Brief Pain Inventory, Roland-Morris Disability Questionnaire (RMDQ), Pain Catastrophizing Scale, Center for Epidemiologic Studies Depression Scale, Quality of Life Scale	CBT = EDU; completer analysis showed CBT > EDU on catastrophizing and depression. Gains maintained at 6-mo f/u	Higher dropout rate in CBT; underpowered to detect effects of CBT compared to active treatment	6 mo
Lamb et al.[25]	RCT + cost-effectiveness	701 with subacute or chronic low back pain	Active management consultation + CBT (n = 468) vs. active management consultation only	Active management: active advice on remaining active, avoiding bed rest, medication/symptom management, also provided with The Back Book. CBT: challenging negative thoughts and beliefs, pacing, graded activity, relaxation, activity, and avoidance	Active management: 15 min CBT: an individual 1.5-h assessment, six 1.5-h CBT sessions	Change in RMDQ and modified Von Korff scores at 12 mo	Consultation + CBT > consultation only on both primary outcomes; inclusion of CBT > cost-effectiveness	CBT delivered by a range of professionals with a 2-d training (physiotherapists, nurses, occupational therapists, psychologists)	12 mo
Van Koulil et al.[26]	RCT	158 with fibromyalgia (FM)	Tailored CBT + exercise training vs. wait-list control	Pain avoidance or pain persistence treatment based on baseline cognitive-behavioral pattern. Patient's significant other attended 3rd, 9th, and 15th sessions	16 sessions of CBT (2 h) + exercise training (2 h) over 10 wk and 1 booster session at 3 mo	Pain, fatigue, functional disability, negative mood, and anxiety scales of the Impact of Rheumatic Diseases on General Health and Lifestyle (IRGL), Pain Coping Inventory	CBT + exercise > WL on all primary outcomes, with large effect sizes	Did not compare "tailored" to nontailored treatment; inert comparison	6 mo
Falcão et al.[27]	RCT	60 females aged 18–65 y with FM	CBT (n = 30) vs. TAU (n = 30)	CBT: relaxation training, cognitive restructuring, stress management	CBT: 10 weekly 3-h sessions	VAS for pain, SF-36, State-Trait Anxiety Inventory, BDI, Fibromyalgia Impact Questionnaire, paracetamol	CBT > TAU on improved depression, mental health, and paracetamol. Both groups showed significant improvements on all indicators over time.	Dropouts were excluded from the analyses; limited f/u; participants had not received any prior treatment.	3 mo

(continued)

TABLE 87.2 (Continued)

Authors	N	Study	Treatment Type	Treatment Components	Duration	Outcome Measures	Results	Limitations	Follow up (f/u)
Ersek et al.[28]	256 with non-cancer pain, ≥65 y	RCT	Pain self-management (n = 133) vs. EDU (n = 123)	Self-management: education about persistent pain, problem solving, exercise for pain, relaxation training, pacing and activity scheduling, challenging negative thoughts, medication management, hot/cold packs EDU: read an assigned book, *The Chronic Pain Workbook* or *Managing Your Pain Before It Manages You*	Self-management, 7 weekly 90-min group sessions	Primary: RMDQ. Secondary: Geriatric Depression Scale, Brief Pain Inventory (intensity and interference)	Pain self-management = EDU at posttreatment and 6- and 12-mo f/u. Use of relaxation and exercise/stretching significantly increased in self-management	The number of strategies covered in self-management may have limited effectiveness.	6, 12 mo
Thorn et al.[29]	34 with headache	RCT compared order of treatment modules.	CBT (N = 22) vs. WLC (N = 11)	Cognitive restructuring, cognitive coping, relaxation, assertiveness, behavioral pacing, homework	Ten 90-min group sessions	Pain Catastrophizing Scale (PCS), Pain Anxiety Symptoms Scale (PASS), Beck Depression Inventory–II (BDI-II), Headache Management Self-Efficacy Scale (HMSE), pain and medication via pain diaries; no difference in outcome based on order of treatment	CBT > WLC for improvements in catastrophizing, anxiety, headache management self-efficacy. 50% treated patients showed clinically significant reductions in headache frequency, medication use.	Small sample size rendered limited power to detect potential differences in order of treatment modules.	6, 12 mo
Li et al.[30]	64 with work-related injuries	RCT	Training on work readiness (T) (N = 34) vs. control (C) (N = 30)	T: individual vocational counseling (3 sessions), CBT, pain and stress management, relaxation, stages of change assessment, job acquisition, pre-employment training	T: 3 weekly group sessions at 2–3 h, three 1-h individual sessions	Spinal Function Sort (SFS), Loma Linda University Medical Centre Activity Sort (LLUMC), Chinese Lam Assessment of Stages of Employment Readiness (C-LASER), Chinese State Trait and Anxiety Inventory (C-STAI), SF-36	T > C for improvements in anxiety, work readiness, readiness to change, and perceived health status T: within-group improvements from baseline for most SF-36 subscales and physical capacity	Lack of f/u, stages of change may require longer time period for assessment	None specified
Linton et al.[31]	185 workers with back/neck pain	RCT	CBT (N = 69) vs. CBT and physical therapy (CBT 1 PT) (N = 69) vs. minimal treatment (N = 47)	CBT: problem solving, homework, skills training, stress management, relaxation CBT + PT: CBT plus personalized exercise program Minimal: medical visit and advice, educational booklet	6 weekly 2-h sessions	Sick absenteeism, health care visits, Outcome Evaluation Questionnaire, VAS pain ratings, HAD, PCS, TSK, activities of daily living (ADLs), RMDQ	CBT + PT = CBT for most measures. CBT + PT > Minimal for reductions in health care visits. At f/u: CBT + PT fewest sick days, followed by CBT and Minimal. Both treatment groups 5 times less likely to be on long-term sick leave than Minimal.	Different intervention lengths	1 y

Study	Population	Design	Intervention	Session	Outcomes	Results	Limitations	f/u
Gold et al.[32]	185 with vertebral fracture	RCT	Part 1: Intervention (I) (N = 94) vs. education control (EC) (N = 91) Part 2: Crossover: EC becomes I group after 6 mo. Initial I group self-maintenance	I: exercise, coping skills (relaxation), stress reduction; EC: education of health issues for women	Part 1: I: 5 weekly exercise and coping sessions (225 min) EC: 1 weekly session at 45 min Part 2: I: self-maintain EC = I group	Trunk extension strength, Functional Status Index (FSI), Global Severity Index of Hopkins Symptom Checklist-Revised	Part 1: I > EC for improvement in trunk extension and psychological symptoms. EC: worse for all three outcomes. Part 2: EC showed within-group improvements in trunk extension and psychological symptoms after intervention. I: decrease in back strength from post-treatment, improvement in psychological state maintained	Different session lengths for I and EC, no control group at f/u. I group did not receive education in cross-over design.	6 mo
van Lankveld et al.[33]	59 with rheumatoid arthritis (RA)	RCT compared couples to patient-only group	Couples (C) (N = 31) vs. patient-only (P) (N = 28)	Education, cognitive restructuring, encouragement to use active coping skills	C: 2 weekly 1.5-h sessions for 4 wk	Disease Activity Score (DAS); swollen joint count IRGL, Coping with Rheumatoid Stressors Questionnaire (CORS), Maudsley Marital Questionnaire (MMQ)	Sample improvements in disease activity, cognitions, coping, physical and psychological function (C = P). At f/u: C > P for improvements in disease-related communication with spouse.	Possible selection bias of highly invested couples because of study design	6 mo
Ersek et al.[34]	45 elderly with chronic pain	RCT	Self-management (SM) (N = 17) vs. educational booklet (control) (EB) (N = 23)	SM: education, self-monitoring, communication, relaxation, individualized goals, homework EB: booklet with information about pain, medications, instructions for self-management, and pain resources	SM: 7 group sessions at 90 min	SF-36, Graded Chronic Pain Scale, Geriatric Depression Scale, Survey of Pain Attitudes (SOPA), survey assessing use of pain management strategies, treatment usefulness scales	SM > EB for improvements in pain intensity and physical role function (pre- to post-change); clinically significant improvement in 43% SM and 13% EB; SM = EB at f/u.	Brief f/u	3 mo
Tkachuk et al.[35]	28 with irritable bowel syndrome (IBS)	RCT	CBT (n = 14) vs. home-based symptom monitoring with weekly telephone contact (SMTC) (n = 14)	CBT: education, relaxation, cognitive restructuring, assertiveness training SMTC: daily symptom monitoring, discussion of symptom patterns	Ten 90-min sessions for 9 wk	Daily monitoring IBS scores, BDI-II, cognitive emotional distress (CSFBD), trait anxiety (STAI-T), discomfort with assertion (AQ), quality of life (SF-36)	CBT > SMTC for pain relief ratings, improvement in GI symptoms, quality of life. Maintained at f/u. One-third treated patients experienced clinically significant improvement.	Brief f/u	3 mo

(continued)

TABLE 87.2 (Continued)

Authors	N	Study	Treatment Type	Treatment Components	Duration	Outcome Measures	Results	Limitations	Follow up (f/u)
Mishra et al.[36]	94 with chronic TMD	Urn method of assignment	CBT (n = 22), biofeedback (n = 23), CBT + biofeedback (n = 24), no treatment (n = 25)	CBT: self-change plain; relaxation training; distraction; pleasant activity scheduling; cognitive restructuring; social skills and assertive communication. Biofeedback: 15 min of temperature feedback and 15 min of electromyography (EMG) biofeedback Combined: include components of both of the above	12 sessions of 1.5 h, except for combined treatment which was 2 h; 2/wk for first 4 wk, 1/wk for other 4-wk	Characteristic Pain Intensity (CPI), Graded Chronic Pain Score (GCPS), Profile of Mood States (POMS)	CBT = biofeedback = combined and all 3 greater than no treatment on CPI and POMS. No significant pre- to posttreatment change was observed for GCPS across any group. Biofeedback improved the most compared to the no treatment control on CPI.	Combined treatment was a higher dose. Lack of f/u	—
Leibing et al.[37]	55 with RA	RCT	CBT (N = 19) vs. TAU (N = 36), change in medication-matched control group (CN) (N = 20)	CBT: education, relaxation, cognitive restructuring, pain management, pleasant activity scheduling	CBT: 12 weekly sessions at 90 min	C-reactive protein (CRP), blood sedimentation rate (Westergren), swollen joint count, Hannover Functional Ability Questionnaire (HFAQ), medication types, VAS pain intensity, affective pain score, pain diary, STAI, Depression Scale (DS), Arthritis Helplessness Scale (AHI), Bernese Coping Modes	Overall increase in disease activity across sample CBT less progressive inflammation than TAU. CBT > CN for pain reduction, improvements in depression, anxiety, helplessness; CBT: improved depression, helplessness, positive coping from baseline	Potential type I error from multiple significance tests; lack of f/u	None specified
Potts et al.[38]	60 with noncardiac chest pain	RCT	CBT (N = 34) vs. WLC (N = 26)	CBT: education, relaxation, biofeedback, graded exercise, challenging automatic thoughts, homework WLC: delayed treatment	6 sessions at 2 h	HADS, Nijmegen hyperventilation scale, Sickness Impact Profile (SIP), Nottingham Health Profile (NHP), chest pain diaries, hyperventilation: portable carbon dioxide monitor, exercise electrocardiography (ECG)	CBT > C for improvements in chest pain frequency, pain-free days, anxiety, and depression, disability, and exercise tolerance. Similar results for delayed treatment group once treated. Overall, 76% had improvements in chest pain. Maintained at f/u.	Lack of control group at f/u	6 mo
Cole[39]	113 with mixed chronic pain	Non-RCT	CBT (N = 88) vs. TAU (N = 25)	Coping skills, pain self-management, stress management, relaxation, self-esteem, positive thinking	75 min, 1 per week for 16 wk	Multidimensional Pain Inventory (MPI), Minnesota Multiphasic Personality Inventory-2 (MMPI-2), BDI Reported narcotic medication usage, health care visits, work status	CBT: decreases in BDI and MPI scores, and health care visits from baseline, increase in return to work f/u: medication decreased from 75% at baseline to 44%, health care visits decreased from 5/mo to 1/mo. Work status increased from 10% to 31%.	Patients not randomly assigned. No direct comparison between CBT and control groups.	1 y

Study	Design	Sample	Intervention	Treatment duration	Measures	Results	Follow-up	Comments
Keel et al.[40]	RCT	27 with FM	CBT (N = 14) vs. autogenic (N = 13)	CBT: stress inoculation, cognitive restructuring, activities for pain diversion, information, relaxation, group discussion, stretching, aerobic exercise. Autogenic: practice relaxation	15 weekly sessions lasting 1–2 h	Freiburg Personality Inventory, Locus of Control Scale, Rosenzweig Picture-Frustration Diary (of active hours, resting hours, sleep index, pain intensity, and medication consumption), General Symptom Checklist	2 CBT clients vs. 1 autogenic had clinically-significant improvement in medication consumption, physical therapies, sleep, pain scores, general symptoms. At f/u, CBT > autogenic for improvement in pain ratings. 4 CBT vs. 0 autogenic had clinically significant improvements at f/u.	3 mo	Small sample size; statistical analyses not described
Keel et al.[41]	Non-RCT	411 with low back pain	Experimental (E) (N = 243) vs. standard physiotherapy (S) (N = 168). E: coping strategies, stress management, relaxation, simulated work situations fitness training, education and group activity, individual physiotherapy or psychotherapy for acute pain. S: mostly individual physiotherapy	E: 4-wk (27 d) inpatient program. S: 3-wk (20 d) inpatient program	Work situation, physical activities, pain history, VAS pain rating, pain drawing, RMDQ, Psychological General Well-Being Index (PGWB), health costs, quality of life, impairment	E = S for improvements in functional ability, limitations in daily life, health care visits. E: higher proportion of individuals in work rehabilitation (23% work incapacity decrease), E > S daily hours worked, decrease in professional handicaps; at f/u, larger proportion of S worsened	3 mo, 1 y	Preexisting differences between groups on demographic variables; different predominant treatment modalities in each condition (E = group, S = individual)
Basler et al.[42]	RCT	94 with low back pain	CBT (N = 36) vs. TAU (N = 40)	Education, relaxation, modifying thoughts and feelings, pleasant activity scheduling, postural training	12 weekly sessions at 150 min	Pain diary (pain intensity, control over pain, medication consumption), Heidelberg Coping Scale (HCS), Dusseldorf Disability Scale (DDS)	CBT: decreases in pain intensity, improvements in coping with pain, mental performance, and disability. Gains maintained at 6-mo f/u. TAU: little or no change	6 mo	High attrition rate at f/u
van Dulmen et al.[43]	Non-RCT	45 with IBS	CBT (N = 25) vs. WLC (N = 20)	Patient education (e.g., roles of cognitions, behaviors, in IBS), homework, discussion, progressive muscle relaxation	8 weekly sessions lasting for 2 h	Diary (duration of pain, daily avoidance behavior, GI complaints), Abdominal Complaint Inventory, Symptom Checklist 90 (SCL-90)	CBT > WLC for improvement in Daily Abdominal Complaint Score (DAC), duration, avoidance, and number of successful coping strategies delayed treatment group: decreases in DAC; improvements maintained at f/u	Mean = 2.25 y	No WLC at f/u, wide range of f/u assessment times (6 mo–4 y)

(continued)

TABLE 87.2 (Continued)

Authors	N	Study	Treatment Type	Treatment Components	Duration	Outcome Measures	Results	Limitations	Follow up (f/u)
Vlaeyen et al.[44]	131 with FM	RCT	Cognitive educational intervention (ECO; N = 47) vs. attention control condition of education and discussion (EDI; N = 39) vs. WLC (N = 40)	ECO: imaginative transformation of pain, relaxation and biofeedback, homework. EDI: education, sharing thoughts with group members, listening to music, homework	ECO and EDI = 12 90-min sessions conducted in 6 wk	Pain cognition list, Coping Strategies Questionnaire (CSQ), Behavioral Approach Test, Pain Behavior Scale, McGill Pain Questionnaire (MPQ), Multidimensional Pain Locus of Control Scale, Checklist for Interpersonal Pain Behavior, Fear Survey Schedule, BDI	ECO = EDI for improvements in pain coping and knowledge. EDI > WLC on knowledge and pain control. At 12-mo f/u, ECO = EDI, although ECO had an increase in pain intensity.	Potential confounding of treatment (EDI group shared thoughts, completed homework). Low education level of participants may have made ECO difficult.	12 mo
Newton-John et al.[45]	44 with chronic back pain	RCT	CBT (N = 16) vs. electromyographic biofeedback (EMGBF; N = 16) vs. WLC (N = 12)	CBT: education, goal setting, relaxation, cognitive restructuring, homework. EMGBF: education, diaphragmatic breathing, adaptation, homework	8 sessions at 1 h (2 sessions per week)	BDI, STAI, CSQ, Pain Disability Index, Pain Beliefs Questionnaire (PBQ)	CBT and EMGBF > WLC for improvements in intensity, disability, adaptive beliefs, and depression. Improvements maintained at f/u, along with improvements in anxiety and active coping	Small sample size per group	6 mo
James et al.[46]	33 with headache	RCT	CBT with goals (goal group) (N = 13) vs. CBT with no goals (open group) (N = 13) vs. WLC (N = 7)	Both CBT groups: education, coping, developing appropriate self-talk, generalization of skills, relaxation. Goal: specific time goals for coping with pain/stress. Open: instructions to cope as long as possible	6 weekly sessions at 90 min	Goal specificity: coping with daily stressors and pain, daily self-monitoring, pain index, medication intake, downtime, Pain Behavior Questionnaire, SCL-90, SIP, BDI, STAI, Cognitive Coping Index	Goal and open groups > WLC for improvements in pain coping skills, goal group > open and WLC group for reduction of headache and nonnarcotic medication use	Lack of f/u period	None specified
Turner and Jensen[47]	102 with low back pain	RCT	Relaxation (R) (N = 17) vs. cognitive therapy (C) (N = 21) vs. cognitive therapy and relaxation (CR) (N = 16) vs. WLC (N = 18)	R: imagery, progressive muscle relaxation (PMR). C: identify negative thoughts, counter negative automatic thoughts. CR: combined treatment	6 weekly sessions at 2 h	VAS pain ratings, SIP, BDI, Observed Pain Behaviors, Cognitive Errors Questionnaire, BDI	R, C, and CR > WLC for improvements in pain ratings and disability. At f/u: all three patient groups improved. At both f/u, patients in all groups improved R = C = CR.	No comparison to control group at f/u, attrition rates for control condition	6, 12 mo

Study	Design	Sample	Intervention	Sessions	Measures	Results	Comments	Follow-up
Kneebone and Martin[48]	Non-RCT Compared couples to standard noncouple and control groups	35 with headache	Partners involved (PI) (N = 12) vs. no partners (NPI) (N = 10) vs. no treatment control (NTC) (N = 13)	PI and NPI: self-monitoring, relaxation, cognitive restructuring, assertiveness, group process (e.g., support), homework. PI: partners educated in reinforcement principles	10 weekly sessions at 1.5–2 h	Headache activity, intensity, medication usage, relaxation practice, Partner Involvement Questionnaire, Dyadic Adjustment Scale (DAS), self-monitoring forms	PI = NPI for relaxation time, PI > NPI for partner involvement: spouse assisted with relaxation. PI: decrease headache activity from baseline. NPI: decreased medication usage from baseline. NTC increased medication usage. At f/u: NPI > NTC for reductions in medication. Other measures: PI = NPI at f/u.	Potential for type 1 inflation; low motivation across treatment groups to practice relaxation	2, 12 mo
Nicholas et al.[49]	RCT	58 with low back pain	Cognitive therapy (CT) + relaxation (N = 8) or CT (N = 10) vs. behavior therapy + relaxation (N = 9) or BT (N = 10) vs. attention (ATC; N = 10) and no attention control (N = 11)	All groups: physiotherapy, education, exercise. CT: cognitive restructuring, distraction, imagery, self-monitoring. BT: activity pacing, medication reduction, reinforcement. Relaxation: PMR. ATC: group discussion about back pain	Five 1.5- to 2-h sessions twice per week	Pain Rating Chart, STAI, PBQ, CSQ, SIP, SIP-Others (SIP-O), medication intake, report of alternative treatments, visits to health care facilities	Sample improved on affective distress, functional impairment, medication use, and active coping. Both CBT groups and both BT groups > ATC and control for improvements in pain intensity, self-reported disability, pain beliefs, and active coping. BT > CBT for improvements in impairment. Improvements somewhat maintained at f/u.	Physiotherapy included as part of all treatments Small sample size	6, 12 mo
Subramanian[50,51]	RCT	39 with mixed chronic pain Long-term f/u = 22	Structured group therapy (N = 19) vs. WLC (N = 20)	Therapy: stress management, relaxation cognitive restructuring (coping thoughts, self-defeating, self-enhancing thoughts), assertiveness training	8 weekly 2-h sessions	SIP, Pain level (0–10 scale) used a control variable Profile of Mood States (POMS), Social Support Questionnaire	Therapy > WLC for improvements in physical and psychosocial dysfunction, negative mood states. With-ingroup improvements also apparent. Long-term f/u: improvements maintained, improvement in pain severity observed, 77% improved from post-treatment to f/u, 36% reduction in prescription medication usage	No comparison group at long-term f/u	6 mo Long-term: 18–22 mo

(continued)

TABLE 87.2 (Continued)

Authors	N	Study	Treatment Type	Treatment Components	Duration	Outcome Measures	Results	Limitations	Follow up (f/u)
Peters and Large[52]	68 with chronic pain	RCT	Group inpatient program (IPMP) (N = 29) vs. Group outpatient program (OPMP) (N = 23) vs. control (C) (N = 16)	IPMP: education, pain management, relaxation, cognitive restructuring, exercise, vocational counseling, reinforcement, OPMP: education, activity goal setting, exercise, medication and stress management, relaxation	Inpatient: 4 wk Outpatient: 9 weekly sessions at 2 h	BDI, MPQ, General Health Questionnaire (GHQ), SIP, Pain Behaviour Checklist, pain drawings, VAS ratings, VAS stair climbing test, physiologic measures, physical endurance	Sample improvements in disability, GHQ scores, BDI, and MPQ scores IPMP and OPMP > control for improvements in disability, VAS pain ratings, and pain behavior	Results may have been influenced by timing of the assessments; lack of f/u	None specified
Turner et al.[53]	96 chronic low back pain patients	RCT	Group behavioral and aerobic exercise (BE) (N = 18) vs. behavioral therapy only (B) (N = 18) Aerobic exercise only (E) (N = 21) vs. WLC (N = 23)	BE: behavioral intervention followed by exercise in each session B: reinforcement role-playing, discussion, homework, communication E: Exercises 5 times per week	BE and B: 8 weekly 2-h sessions E: 5 weekly sessions	MPQ, SIP, Pain Behavior Checklist (PBC), PBC-spouse ratings, Physical Work Capacity (PWC), Center for Epidemiologic Studies—Depression Scale (CES-D), recorded pain behaviors	All three groups improved more than the WLC from pre- to posttreatment, BE > WLC from pre- to posttreatment on self-report and observer rated pain behavior measures, BE > E on PBC Spouse ratings F/u: all treatment groups improved over time	Interaction with therapists varied by condition	6, 12 mo
Linton et al.[54]	66 nurses with back pain	RCT	Physical and behavioral preventive intervention (PBI) (N = 36) vs. WLC (N = 30)	PBI: physical therapy, "low back school," relaxation, pain control instruction, goal setting, problem solving, coping, identifying high-risk situations	PBI: 8 h/d for 5 wk	Daily pain diaries, VAS intensity, fatigue, anxiety, sleep, pain behavior, ADLs, BDI, AHI, marital satisfaction, absenteeism, medication intake	PBI > WLC for improvements in pain intensity, fatigue, pain behavior, sleep, ADLs, helplessness Most differences maintained at f/u	Use of non-standardized measures of sleep quality, ADLs, marital satisfaction	6 mo
Puder[55]	69 with mixed chronic pain	RCT	Stress inoculation training (SIT) (N = 31) vs. WLC (N = 38)	SIT: explaining treatment, reviewing progress, problem solving	10 weekly 2-h group sessions	Daily pain diary, non-treatment technique usage: psychological support, exercise, heat/cold, massage, TENS, injections	SIT > WLC for improvements in pain interference, coping, decreased analgesic intake, discontinuation of heat/cold, and home traction technique. No difference according to age. Improvements maintained at f/u.	Use of non-standardized measures	1, 6 mo

Study	Design	Population	Intervention	Treatment content	Measures	Results	Limitations	Follow-up
Bradley et al.[56]	RCT	53 with RA	Biofeedback-assisted CBT (N = 17) vs. structured group social support therapy (SGT) (N = 18), no adjunct treatment (NAT) (N = 18)	CBT: thermal biofeedback, education, relaxation, behavioral goal setting, self-rewards. SGT: education, discussion of coping strategies, encouragement to develop improved strategies. CBT: 5 thermal sessions, 10 family/friend meetings. SGT: 15 sessions family/friends	STAI, Depression Adjective Checklist (DACL), Health Locus of Control Scale (HLCS), AHI, pain behaviors, rheumatologist ratings of disease activity level, rheumatoid factor titers, sedimentation rate (Westergren)	CBT > SGT and NAT for decreases in pain behavior, pain ratings, rheumatoid activity (RAI), NAT: lower RAI scores than SGT. SGT and NAT increased in depression and rheumatoid factor titer across assessments. CBT and SGT > NAT for improvement in anxiety. CBT maintained improvement at f/u	Session duration not specified	6 mo
Larsson et al.[57]	RCT	36 high school students with tension/migraine headaches	Self Help Relaxation (SHR) (N = 12) vs. Problem Discussion Condition (PDC) (N = 10) vs. Untreated Self-Monitoring Condition (SM) (N = 12)	SHR: relaxation programs, rapid cue-controlled strategy, homework, help solving problems during relaxation. PDC: discussion of conflicts in everyday life, role-play, identifying stressors, assertiveness. 5 weekly sessions SHR = 3 h PDC = 7 h	Headache diary: frequency, duration headache free days, peak intensity, modified Depression Scale for Female adolescents, Children's Manifest Anxiety Scale, Social Relationship-Competence Questionnaire (SRCQ)	Headache activity: Greatest reductions for SHR group, SHR > SM and PDC. Headache sum and peak intensity: SHR > PDC during pre-f/u interval. Headache duration and headache-free days: SHR > SM and PDC	Small sample size, different therapist interaction for two interventions	5 mo
Bradley et al.[58]	RCT	33 with RA	Thermal biofeedback and group cognitive behavioral (CB = 11) vs. social support (SS = 10) vs. NAT (N = 12)	CB: thermal biofeedback, education, skills acquisition, self-instructional training, application. SS: education, support, encouragement to develop own coping strategies. NAT = control. CB: 5 individual thermal sessions, 10 family meetings. SS: 15 family meetings	STAI, DACL, VAS ratings of pain intensity, unpleasantness, severity of morning stiffness, pain behaviors, HLCS, rheumatoid factor titers, Westergren, rheumatologist ratings of disease activity	CB > NAT group for significant decreases in pain intensity, pre- to posttreatment: CB less pain behavior from pre- to posttreatment, less rheumatoid activity, and rheumatoid factor titer. CB and SS less anxiety and depression. SS increase in sedimentation rate NAT: significant reduction in morning stiffness.	Small sample size, lack of f/u	None specified
Linton et al.[59] and Melin and Linton[60]	RCT Long-term f/u	28 with heterogeneous chronic pain 26 with heterogeneous chronic pain	Regular treatment (RT) vs. applied relaxation and operant activities (RT + BT) vs. WLC	RT: prescribed treatment plan. RT + BT: plan and relaxation training, operant training, reinforcement of well behaviors, decrease in medication. 12 sessions	BDI, Activities of Daily Living questionnaire, self-monitoring of pain, medication consumption, sleep f/u measures also included pain, health, activity, level, sleep, occupation	RT + BT > RT and WLC for improvements in pain level and leisure activity Improvements maintained at f/u	Small sample size Long-term f/u: WLC group received individual treatment prior to assessment	14–16 mo

(continued)

TABLE 87.2 (Continued)

Authors	N	Study	Treatment Type	Treatment Components	Duration	Outcome Measures	Results	Limitations	Follow up (f/u)
Moore and Chaney[61]	43 with mixed chronic pain	RCT	Couples group therapy (CBT) (N = 17) vs. patient-only group therapy (N = 14) vs. WLC (N = 12)	Couples and patient only: education, goal setting, problem solving, relaxation and controlled breathing, direct pain reduction method, coping strategies, homework	16-h program, couples: 8 biweekly 2-h sessions	VAS pain severity (patient and spouse) MMPI Hs, D, and Hy scales only, SIP, PARS IV Community Adjustment Scale (spouses), Locke-Wallace Marital Adjustment Test (LMAT), utilization of medical resources medication usage	Couples and patient-only groups > WLC for improvements in VAS ratings, pain severity and pain behavior ratings, somatization, and PARS (spouse rating) Patient-only groups > controls on LMAT and SIP scores Treatment gains maintained at f/u Couples = patient-only therapy	Small sample sizes for each condition	3, 7 mo
Cohen et al.[62]	25 with chronic low back pain	RCT	Behavioral intervention (BT) (N = 13) vs. physical therapy (PT) (N = 12)	PT: pain control strategies, relaxation, exercise, pool therapy, use of body mechanics BT: goal setting, activity pacing, problem solving, assertiveness	10 weekly 2-h sessions	Physical Abilities and Walking Abilities testing, Knowledge and Functional Measure of Body Mechanics, CES-D, Psychological Adjustment to Role Scale (PARS-V)	PT: greater low back control and decreases in CES-D score. BT and PT: lower anxiety and depression per patients and significant others on PARS-V, others. Decreases in physical and activity limitations for both groups	Small sample size, validity data for some instruments not provided	None specified
Figueroa[63]	15 tension headache patients	RCT	Behavior therapy (BT) (N = 5) vs. psychotherapy (P) (N = 5) vs. self-monitoring (SM; N = 5)	BT: problem solving, relaxation, anxiety management training, stress inoculation P: discussion, conflict resolution, discussion of stressful events	BT: seven 90-min sessions P: seven 90-min sessions (twice weekly)	Headache questionnaire, headache checklist (e.g., level of relaxation, number of headaches, duration, severity, medication usage, disability), self-monitoring forms	Pre to f/u: B > P and SM for improvements in perceived disability BT > SM for reductions in headache frequency and duration, medication usage, level of relaxation, and pain severity	Small sample size, use of nonstandardized measures	Time not specified
Turner[64]	36 chronic low back pain patients	RCT	CBT (N = 13), vs. relaxation training (N = 14), WLC/attention conditions (N = 9)	CBT: stress inoculation, behavioral goals, cognitive and affective responses to pain, coping self-statements, relaxation Wait-list/attention: gave daily pain ratings to therapist in weekly phone calls	5 weekly 90-min sessions	SIP, SIP Significant Other (SIP-O), VAS ratings, self-ratings of improvement, BDI, work hours, health care usage	CBT and relaxation groups > WLC for improvements in pain, depression, disability, and spousal ratings of physical and psychosocial function At f/u: CBT improved on SIP, SIP-O, pain severity, relaxation: worse pain severity 1.5- to 2-y f/u: both groups retain improvements, CBT > in hours worked per week	Small sample size	1 mo, 1.5–2 y

AQ, Assertiveness Questionnaire; CBT, cognitive-behavioral therapy; CSFBD, Cognitive Scale for Functional Bowel Disorders; GI, gastrointestinal; HADS, Hospital Anxiety and Depression Scale; IPMP, inpatient pain management program; OPMP, outpatient pain management program; RAI, Rheumatoid Activity Index; RCT, randomized controlled trial; SCI, spinal cord injury; STAI-T, State-Trait Anxiety Inventory–Trait Scale; TMD, temporomandibular disorder; VAS, Visual Analog Scale; WL, wait-list; WLC, wait-list control.

These authors found that both groups showed equal improvements in pain coping and knowledge, and both were superior to a wait-list control condition. An economic evaluation of the treatments resulted in the authors' suggestion that the extra health care costs associated with the addition of the CBT modules were not warranted based on the outcomes.[44,68] It is important to note that the education modules that were offered to all participants included structured physical fitness training after each of 12 sessions, and this behavioral component may have served to increase the overall outcome efficacy of both groups. Furthermore, the discussion modules (attention control) included weekly homework assignments, which is typical of CBT groups but atypical of control conditions. The authors suggest that the homework assignments may have served as a form of graded exposure for the fearful participants, thereby resulting in treatment gains in the control group. It is also important to mention that both treatment groups in the mentioned study used limited therapist time in an effort to reduce treatment costs. It may be that the principles associated with cognitive-behavioral change require some threshold amount of therapeutic intervention in order to be successfully implemented. These findings and others led Vlaeyen and colleagues[44] raise the important point that the active components of group treatment need further careful study.

Another study assessed the efficacy of group CBT for pain using education booklets as the control condition[34] and found significant pre- to posttreatment differences in favor of the CBT self-management groups. Although the use of education booklets does not control for the nonspecific treatment effects of group interaction or support, this study suggests that merely offering facts about pain and pain management outside a therapeutic context does not appear to be efficacious. However, another study that compared cognitive-behavioral pain self-management to a condition that was assigned a book to read on managing chronic pain found that both conditions similarly showed clinically significant changes over time.[28] A limitation of such an approach is that to read a book requires a certain level of literacy, as does participating in a traditional CBT program.

Thorn and colleagues addressed the literacy treatment barrier via developing literacy-adapted CBT and education programs and tested their relative efficacy in a series of two RCTs within low-literacy, low-socioeconomic status (SES), predominantly minority populations.[18,24] Results of the initial RCT[24] showed that delivering education *within* a therapeutic context (i.e., that included factors such as therapeutic rapport and group support, as opposed to bibliotherapy) was particularly beneficial and both groups improved significantly across a number of outcomes; no significant differences between the literacy-adapted CBT and pain education treatment were observed in the intent to treat sample. In Thorn and colleagues' most recent trial[18] that included a larger sample size and several methodologic enhancements, again, both the literacy-adapted CBT and education interventions performed similarly on the primary outcome of pain intensity and the secondary outcome of pain interference, with both significantly outperforming the treatment as usual control. Maintenance of gains in pain interference was observed in both groups; although benefits in pain intensity were maintained in education at follow-up, this was not the case for CBT. However, participants in CBT were less likely to be depressed at follow-up. Comparison of effect sizes and clinically meaningful improvement (>30% reductions in pain intensity, pain interference, and depression) suggested a slight advantage of CBT over education, but overall, these findings suggest that both literacy-adapted CBT *and* pain education are suitable for implementation in highly disadvantaged populations. Patient workbooks and therapist supplements for these literacy-adapted treatments are freely available at pmt.ua.edu/publications.html.

Several other studies have compared group CBT to relaxation training or another group condition. In one study of patients with low back pain, patients receiving group CBT and those receiving relaxation training improved compared to wait-list controls, although at follow-up, those who received CBT showed greater treatment gains than those receiving relaxation training.[64] In a similar study with individuals with fibromyalgia, those who received group CBT showed greater improvement in pain ratings than those who received autogenic relaxation training.[40] Focusing on high school students with migraine and tension-type headaches, Larsson et al.[57] compared self-help relaxation groups to problem discussion groups and untreated self-monitoring groups and found self-help relaxation to be superior to the other two conditions. Contrary findings were reported by Mishra and colleagues[36] who compared CBT versus biofeedback versus CBT + biofeedback versus no treatment in a temporomandibular disorder population and found that although all three active treatments significantly outperformed the no treatment arm, there were no significant differences in outcomes across the active treatments. Together, these studies suggest tentative evidence supporting CBT groups as conferring greater benefit than relaxation-only groups and that relaxation groups alone may be superior to groups offering only education or discussion in some settings.

A specialized subset of studies comparing one type of group treatment to another are those that have compared group CBT offered only to the patient, to group CBT offered to both the patient and his or her partner. Moore and Chaney[61] found that among patients with mixed chronic pain syndromes, couples group therapy and patient-only group therapy were both superior to a wait-list control group, but the patient-only groups showed significant improvement on more outcome variables than did the couples groups. Another study found similar improvements in physical and psychological functioning, cognitions, and coping among both couples groups and patient-only groups, although at 6-month follow-up, patients in the couples groups reported greater improvement in communication with their spouse than did patients in the patient-only groups.[33] Patients with chronic headache differ in some ways from those with other chronic pain syndromes, and therefore, it is interesting to note that one study found that partner involvement in chronic headache management groups actually reduced efficacy compared to nonpartner involvement.[48] Further research is necessary to determine whether this finding is unique to individuals with chronic headache pain or if other variables are associated with this outcome.

Another line of research has examined potential algorithms for tailoring CBT to the specific baseline symptom profiles of individuals entering treatment. van Koulil and colleagues[26] conducted an RCT within a fibromyalgia sample and compared tailored CBT + exercise to a wait-list control. Specifically, patients were classified at baseline into two groups, (1) pain avoidance (i.e., individuals who avoid activities due to fear of pain) or (2) pain persistence (i.e., individuals who persist in activities despite pain), and were then randomized. Those in the intervention condition received treatment that was tailored to their cognitive-behavioral pattern. Specifically, individuals with a pain-avoidance profile received group-delivered treatment theorized to explicitly target increasing daily activities, reducing pain and avoidance behaviors, and increasing physical condition. Whereas those individuals with a pain persistence profile received group treatment targeted toward regulating daily activity, increasing activity pacing, restructuring pain-persistence cognitions, and increasing physical condition. Results showed that the tailored treatment resulted in large effect sizes and significantly greater improvements across all primary outcomes as compared to the wait-list control. Unfortunately, this study did not include a "mismatched" arm; hence, the utility of matching patients to these tailored treatments is not fully known. However, in a recent study by Kerns et al.[69] that examined individually delivered tailored CBT to standard CBT, no significant outcomes were observed; to the best of our knowledge, no research has examined similar research questions in a group setting. Future research identifying the optimal approach to tailoring group-delivered CBT to specific profiles is needed as this has the capacity to more efficiently and effectively engender positive changes.

Finally, one promising study by Seminowicz and colleagues[21] showed that group-delivered CBT resulted in increased gray matter in several areas of the brain related to pain processing following an 11-week treatment. Many of these increases were correlated with treatment-related reductions in pain catastrophizing, suggesting that successfully targeting this cognitive mechanism may be a powerful way to harness neuroplasticity and potentially reverse a selection of brain-related changes associated with central sensitization and worse pain outcomes. Although the sample size was small and the design lacked randomization and follow-up, these promising results provide preliminary evidence to support CBT as an intervention that effectively retrains the brain to enhance top–down control of pain and cognitive reappraisal of pain as well as alters the perception of noxious signals. Although reduced pain catastrophizing was found to be a critical correlate of these changes, it is not clear if cognitive change in catastrophizing is a mechanism specific to CBT.

BEHAVIORAL VERSUS EXERCISE AND PHYSICAL THERAPY GROUP TREATMENTS

Physical therapy has long been considered an essential component of chronic pain management, and as a result, it is important to consider its role in treatment groups for chronic pain. Although most studies have focused on the efficacy of physical therapy and exercise in an individual context, we located two RCTs specifically comparing group behavioral approaches to group physical therapy. In one study, individuals with chronic low back pain who received group behavioral treatment and those who received group physical therapy both showed significant decreases in activity limitations, anxiety, and depression.[62] In another study, Turner et al.[53] examined the differential efficacy of group behavioral therapy alone, group aerobic exercise training alone, group behavioral therapy plus group aerobic exercise, and a wait-list control group. The three treatment groups showed greater improvement than the wait-list control group, and all groups showed increasing improvement over the 6- and 12-month follow-ups. It is important to note that in this study, the combined behavioral plus exercise group treatment showed the greatest improvement overall, suggesting that physical activity may be an important component to incorporate into group treatment for chronic pain.

However, in another study by van der Roer et al.[70] that compared a combined exercise therapy, back school and operant-conditioning behavioral principles condition to physiotherapy, no significant differences in outcome were observed on any outcome measure during the complete follow-up period. Similarly, in an RCT by Smeets and colleagues,[71] the advantage of combining cognitive and behavioral interventions (primarily graded activity) with active physical therapy was also not observed; this study found no significant differences in outcomes between the combined treatment and the individual components, but all three significantly outperformed the wait-list control.[71] The van der Roer et al.[70] study and research by Smeets et al.[71] was not included in Table 87.2, however, as the treatments compared in these studies entailed both individual and group delivery components.

To summarize, converging lines of evidence described earlier and in Table 87.2 provide strong evidence that individuals with chronic pain benefit significantly more from group CBT than from being on a waiting list or receiving medical treatment as usual. The specific mechanisms of treatment efficacy have yet

to be clearly identified, but studies to date have shed some light on these mechanisms, which are described in more detail later in this chapter. As efficacy research moves from open trials to RCTs designed specifically to compare group CBT to other active group treatments, future studies are likely to emerge that will help identify the active components of CBT treatment.

MINDFULNESS-BASED APPROACHES TO PAIN MANAGEMENT

The past decade has witnessed an exponential growth in the amount of research directed toward understanding the effects of MBIs for chronic pain management.[72] Although this body of research continues to be limited due to common methodologic issues such as small sample sizes, and lack of randomization and comparison conditions, the number of quality RCTs on mindfulness-based pain and stress reduction or other meditative therapies for chronic pain is steadily increasing. A recent meta-analytic review by Veehof and colleagues[73] examined the evidence of mindfulness- and acceptance-based interventions for pain. Nearly all of the studies reporting on the effects of MBIs for various chronic pain conditions that were included in this review involved group-delivered treatment, except for a small selection that examined modes of online delivery in an individual format. Regarding group meditation treatments specific to chronic pain, we were able to locate 17 RCTs[74–90] and 3 non-RCTs[91–93] (see Table 87.3 for a summary). Most of these studies compared group meditation (usually in integrated packages such as MBSR and more recently, MBCT) to standard care and found meditation to be more beneficial with respect to pain interference, pain perception, pain coping, and measures of affect immediately posttreatment and also at follow-up. However, most follow-up periods were relatively short (i.e., 3 to 6 months), and although pain interference is the recommended primary outcome for MBIs, a number of studies did not include a measure of this outcome.[96] Furthermore, there is a large range in the size of the groups examined in the MBI for chronic pain literature, ranging from as small as 4 all the way up to 25 group members; although yet to be empirically examined, this variability in group size is likely an important factor influencing potential differences in outcomes observed across studies.

Given the promising preliminary evidence of group-delivered MBIs for chronic pain as compared to inert comparison conditions, a more recent focus has been on comparing MBIs to attention control conditions (such as social support), psychoeducation, and to other active treatments—primarily to CBT, given this is the "gold standard" treatment in the field.[67] In one of the largest RCTs conducted to date, Cherkin and colleagues[94] compared MBSR versus CBT versus usual care in a population with chronic low back pain. The results found that MBSR was as effective as CBT (both of which were significantly better than the control) for improving back pain and associated functional limitations, and the benefit in both active treatment conditions was maintained at the 52-week long-term follow-up. In a 2-year follow-up, participants in CBT compared with usual care showed greater improvement in function, whereas MBSR did not differ from usual care at 2 years.[95] Clearly, further well-controlled trials comparing MBIs to other active treatments with adequately powered samples and long-term follow-up assessment time points are needed. However, the literature to date suggests that group-delivered MBIs are efficacious approaches for chronic pain management and, although not typically superior to CBT, do provide a viable alternative.

ACCEPTANCE-BASED APPROACHES TO PAIN MANAGEMENT

As with MBIs, the body of research devoted to acceptance-based interventions such as ACT[97] and contextual cognitive-behavioral therapy (CCBT)[98] has rapidly increased since the prior edition

TABLE 87.3 Mindfulness Based Group Interventions

Authors	N	Study	Treatment Type	Treatment Components	Duration	Outcome Measures	Results	Limitations	Follow up (f/u)
Cherkin et al.[94,95]	342 with chronic low back pain	RCT	MBSR (n = 116) vs. CBT (n = 113) vs. usual care (n = 113)	MBSR: training in mindfulness meditation (MM) and yoga CBT: training to change maladaptive pain-related thoughts and behaviors Usual care: continuation of what is typically received	8 weekly 2-h sessions	Percentage of participants with ≥30% improvement on Roland-Morris Disability Questionnaire (RMDQ), and 0–10 back pain bothersome scale	MBSR = CBT; both MBSR and CBT > usual care; however, at the 2-y f/u, CBT > usual care in function, whereas MBSR = usual care at 2-y f/u.	Participants were recruited from single health care system and were highly educated—limits generalizability; 20% in MBSR and CBT lost to f/u	26 wk, 52 wk; then a 2-y f/u
Davis et al.[77]	143 with rheumatoid arthritis (RA)	RCT	CBT (n = 52) vs. MBI (n = 48) vs. EDU (n = 44)	CBT: training in cognitive reappraisal, relaxation, pacing MBI: training in mindfulness skills and skills to boost affective engagement such as savoring positive events EDU: information on etiology, pathophysiology and treatment of RA, healthy lifestyles and patient–physician communication	8 weekly 2-h sessions	Daily diary of pain and fatigue NRS, morning disability, interpersonal distress, pain catastrophizing and pain control, serene and anxious affect (PANAS items)	MBI > CBT and EDU in daily pain-related catastrophizing, morning disability, and fatigue and greater reductions in daily stress-related anxious affect. On days of high pain, CBT showed less pronounced declines in daily pain-related perceived control than MBI or EDU.	Sample was mostly white and female, so generalizability may be limited; lack of fidelity monitoring; differences between conditions were small in magnitude; lack of f/u	—
Cash et al.[78]	91 women with fibromyalgia (FM)	RCT	MBSR (n = 51) vs. WL (n = 40)	MBSR: formal and information mindfulness practice, and yoga	8 weekly 2.5-h sessions and a half-day meditation retreat after session 6	BDI, Perceived Stress Scale, VAS Pain, Stanford Sleep Questionnaire, Fatigue Symptom Inventory, Fibromyalgia Impact Questionnaire, neuroendocrine function (salivary cortisol)	MBSR > WL on perceived stress, sleep disturbance, symptom severity with gains maintained at f/u; no significant differences in pain, physical functioning, or cortisol profiles	Sample was all female and predominantly well-educated, so generalizability is limited; lack of fidelity monitoring; attrition rate; brief f/u	2 mo
Cathcart et al.[79]	58 with chronic tension-type headache	RCT	MBI (n = 29) vs. WL (n = 29)	MBI: MM	Six 2-h sessions over 3 wk	Five facet mindfulness questionnaire, headache diary (intensity, frequency, duration), Depression Anxiety Stress Scales	MBI > WL on reduction in headache frequency and increase in mindfulness observe facet	Lack of f/u	—
Garland et al.[80]	115 with chronic pain	RCT	MBI (n = 57) vs. support/EDU (n = 58)	MBI: mindfulness training, positive psychology Support: discussion/information on topics of chronic pain, long-term opiate use, dimensions of pain, coping with pain and emotions, stress, acceptance	Eight 2-h weekly sessions	Brief Pain Inventory Intensity and Interference, Current Opioid Misuse Measure, Five Facet Mindfulness Questionnaire nonreactivity scale	MBI > support on pain intensity and interference at posttreatment and f/u; stress arousal and desire for opioids reduced at posttreatment but not maintained	Lack of quantitative fidelity monitoring; attrition rate	3 mo

(continued)

TABLE 87.3 (Continued)

Authors	N	Study	Treatment Type	Treatment Components	Duration	Outcome Measures	Results	Limitations	Follow up (f/u)
Day et al.[81]	36 with primary headache	RCT	MBCT (n = 19) vs. delayed treatment (DT) (n = 17)	MBCT: MM, mindful walking and movement, cognitive therapy–oriented exercises, pleasant and stressful event monitoring	Eight 2-h weekly sessions	Daily headache diary, Brief Pain Inventory, Pain Catastrophizing Scale, Mindful Attention Awareness Scale, Chronic Pain Acceptance Questionnaire, Headache Management Self-Efficacy Scale	MBCT > DT in self-efficacy, pain acceptance; in completers, MBCT > DT also on pain interference and pain catastrophizing	Lack of f/u, small sample size	—
Parra-Delgado and Latorre-Postigo[82]	31 females with FM	RCT	MBCT (n = 17) vs. TAU (n = 16)	MBCT: MM, yoga, psychoeducational activities on anxiety and depression, cognitive therapy–oriented content on automatic thoughts	8 weekly 2.5-h sessions	Beck Depression Inventory (BDI), Fibromyalgia Impact Questionnaire, VAS Pain Intensity	MBCT > TAU on Fibromyalgia Impact Questionnaire and BDI, maintained at f/u; no significant changes in pain intensity	Limited measures of pain-related outcomes; small sample size; brief f/u	3 mo
Brown and Jones[83]	28 with musculoskeletal pain	RCT	MBI (n = 15) vs. TAU (n = 13)	MBI: MM and mindful movement, pacing, kindness meditation	8 weekly 2.5-h sessions	SF-36, Pain Stages of Change Questionnaire, Survey of Pain Attitudes, Short-Form McGill Pain Questionnaire, Mindful Attention and Awareness Scale; EEG and experimental pain manipulation	MBI > TAU on mental health, perceived control of pain, anticipatory and pain evoked event-related potentials to experimental pain	Lack of f/u	—
Wong et al.[84]	99 with chronic pain	RCT	MBSR (n = 51) vs. multidisciplinary pain intervention (MPI; n = 48)	MBSR: training in MM and yoga MPI: educational instructions on management of chronic pain	8 weekly 2.5-h sessions and a 7-h retreat	NRS Pain Intensity and Pain-Related Distress, Profile of Mood States, Center for Epidemiologic Studies Depression Scale, State-Trait Anxiety Inventory, Short-Form Health Survey 12 (SF-12)	MBSR = MPI on pain intensity and pain-related distress; both improved significantly	Fidelity was not monitored in the study.	3, 6 mo
Schmidt et al.[85]	177 females with FM	RCT	MBSR vs. control of nonspecific effects versus WL	MBSR: training in MM and yoga Control: progressive muscle relaxation and FM-specific gentle stretching exercises	8 weekly 2.5-h sessions and all-day retreat for MBSR	Quality of Life Profile for the Chronically Ill, Fibromyalgia Impact Questionnaire, Center for Epidemiologic Studies depression inventory, State-Trait Anxiety Inventory, Pittsburgh Sleep Quality Index, Pain Perception Scale, Freiburg Mindfulness Inventory, Giessen Complaint Questionnaire	MBSR = control = WL on primary outcome, all improved significantly. On secondary outcomes, MBSR significantly improved 6 of 8 outcomes vs. the control condition improved 3 and WL 2 out of 8.	Fidelity was not monitored in the study; brief f/u	2 mo

Study	Design	Sample	Groups	Intervention	Format	Measures	Results	Limitations	Follow-up
Morone et al.[86]	RCT	40 with low back pain, ≥65 y	MBI (n = 20) vs. EDU (n = 20)	MBI: MM and walking practice EDU: session topics on pain medications, complementary treatments, types of back pain, role of physical therapist, nutrition, Alzheimer	8 weekly 90-min sessions	McGill Pain Questionnaire Short-Form, Chronic Pain Self-Efficacy Scale, SF-36, Roland-Morris Disability Questionnaire, Mindfulness Attention Awareness Scale, global impressions of change	MBI = EDU for disability, pain, psychological function at posttreatment and f/u—both conditions significantly improved	High functioning at baseline leading to possibility of ceiling effects; sample was predominantly high functioning, white and well-educated, limiting generalizability	4 mo
Zautra et al.[87]	RCT	144 with RA	CBT (n = 52) vs. MBI (n = 48) vs. EDU (n = 44)	EDU: information on ways to manage RA CBT: psychoeducation, relaxation training; activity pacing; cognitive coping; problem solving MBI: mindfulness and model of emotion; awareness; emotional well-being; acceptance and reframing; pleasant event scheduling; social relations; intimacy; stress	8 weekly 2-h sessions	NRS daily pain; Positive and Negative Affect Schedule; depressive symptoms; coping efficacy; pain catastrophizing; perceived pain control; laboratory outcomes.	CBT > MBI and EDU on self-reported pain control and IL-6; CBT and MBI > EDU on coping efficacy. Participants with recurrent depression benefited most from MBI for negative and positive affect and physicians' ratings of joint tenderness.	Low to moderate baseline levels of pain—not clear if results generalize to more impaired populations; multiple analyses raises issue of potential α inflation.	6 mo
Morone et al.[88]	RCT	37 with low back pain, ≥65 y	MBI (n = 19) vs. WL (n = 18)	MBI: MM and walking practice	8 weekly 90-min sessions	McGill Pain Questionnaire Short-Form, Chronic Pain Acceptance Questionnaire, SF-36, Roland-Morris Disability Questionnaire	MBI > WL on Chronic Pain Acceptance Questionnaire total score and Activity Engagement subscale, SF-36 Physical Function	No f/u data on WL as immediately crossed over to treatment	3 mo
Pradhan et al.[89]	RCT	63 with RA	MBSR (n = 31) vs. WL (n = 32)	MBSR: MM and yoga, mindful walking	8 weekly 2.5-h sessions with 3 booster sessions over following 4 mo	Symptom Checklist-90-Revised, Disease Activity Score 28, Psychological Well-Being Scales, Mindful Attention Awareness Scale	MBSR = WL at posttreatment; MBSR > WL at f/u on psychological distress and well-being; no change on RA disease activity	Possible floor effect as sample had low distress and RA activity at baseline	6 mo
Grossman et al.[91]	Non-RCT	58 females with FM	MBSR (n = 39) vs. Active Social Support (n = 13)	MBSR: mindfulness practice, awareness during yoga, stressful situations, social interactions, homework Support: social support, relaxation training, stretching exercises, discussion, homework	8 weekly 2.5-h sessions plus 1 all-day session	Quality of Life Profile for the Chronically Ill (QoL), Hospital Anxiety and Depression Scale (HADS), Pain Perception Scale (PPS), Inventory of Pain Regulation (IPR), visual analog ratings (VAS)	MBSR > support for improvements in VAS pain, QoL subscales, pain coping, depression, and somatic complaints Improvements maintained at f/u	Unequal n limits statistical power	3 y

(continued)

TABLE 87.3 (Continued)

Authors	N	Study	Treatment Type	Treatment Components	Duration	Outcome Measures	Results	Limitations	Follow up (f/u)
Carson et al.[74]	43 with low back pain	RCT	Loving-kindness meditation (Medi) (N = 18) vs. standard care (TAU) (N = 25)	Medi: silent mental phrases to direct positive feelings toward others attend to feelings of love instead of anger/resentment, discussion, practice	8 weekly 90-min sessions	McGill Pain Questionnaire (MPQ), Brief Pain Inventory (BPI), State-Trait Anger Expression Inventory (STAXI), Anger Expression and Control, Brief Symptom Inventory (BSI), diary, VAS ratings of pain and anger, affect, pain, and fatigue	Medi: improvement in pain intensity, usual pain, psychological distress, and anxiety from baseline. TAU: little change. Pre to f/u: Medi improved in usual pain, anxiety, psychological distress, and the phobia scale of the BSI	No direct comparison between intervention and TAU group	3 mo
Plews-Ogan et al.[75]	30 with musculoskeletal pain	RCT	MBSR (N = 10) vs. massage (N = 10) vs. standard care (TAU) (N = 10)	MBSR: meditation and yoga, nonjudgmental awareness, practice. Massage: Swedish, deep tissue, neuromuscular, pressure point	MBSR: 8 weekly 2.5-h sessions. Massage: 8 weekly 1-h sessions	Pain intensity, pain unpleasantness, SF-12	Posttreatment: Massage > TAU for improvements in unpleasantness and mental status. MBSR = TAU. At f/u: MBSR > TAU for improvement in mental health score	Small sample size limits statistical power	4 wk
Sagula and Rice[93]	57 with mixed chronic pain	Non-RCT	MM (N = 39) vs. Control (C) (N = 18)	MM: 20-min daily meditation (body scan, mindfulness on breath, Hatha yoga), meditation log, development of resources for self-healing	8 weekly 90-min sessions	Response to Loss Scale (RTL) (e.g., Growth, Cope/Awareness), BDI, STAI	MM > C for reductions in depression, state anxiety, and intensity of grief from loss associated with pain. Growth: MM = C	Unequal sample sizes limits statistical power lack of f/u	None specified
Astin et al.[90]	65 with FM	RCT	MBSR + Qigong (n = 32) vs. EDU/support (n = 33)	MBSR + Qigong: MM training and Qigong practices. EDU: information on stress, exercise, pain/emotions	8 weekly 2.5-h sessions	Pain via SF-36, BDI; Fibromyalgia Impact Questionnaire; 6-min walk test; tender point count	MBSR + Qigong = EDU at both posttreatment and f/u	High attrition	6 mo
Kabat-Zinn et al.[92]	90 with mixed chronic pain	Non-RCT	Stress reduction and relaxation (SR and RP) (N = 69) vs. Pain Clinic control group (PC) (N = 21)	SR and RP: meditation training, Hatha yoga, homework, 45-min daily meditation	10 weekly 2-h sessions	McGill-Melzack Pain Rating Index (PRI), Body Parts Problem Assessment (BPPA) scale, medically oriented symptom checklist (MSCL), Profile of Mood States (POMS), revised Hopkins Symptom Checklist (SCL-90R)	Sample improvements in pain indices, mood, and psychological symptoms. SR and PR > PC for improvements in anxiety, hostility, and somatization. SR and PR: larger proportion of individuals with clinically significant improvements. Maintenance at f/u	Wide range in f/u assessments	2.5-15 mo

CBT, cognitive-behavioral therapy; EDU, education; EEG, electroencephalogram; IL-6, interleukin 6; MBCT, mindfulness-based cognitive therapy; MBI, mindfulness-based intervention; MBSR, mindfulness-based stress reduction; NRS, Numerical Rating Scale; RA, rheumatoid arthritis; RCT, randomized controlled trial; SF-36, Short-Form Health Survey; STAI, State-Trait Anger Inventory; TAU, treatment as usual; VAS, visual analog scale; WL, wait-list.

of this book. In the aforementioned review by Veehof and colleagues,[73] several of the included ACT studies entailed group treatment delivery; in total, we identified six RCTs[99–104] that examined group-delivered acceptance-based approaches for heterogeneous chronic pain conditions (see Table 87.4 for a summary). Across these studies, the most consistently reported benefits of group-based ACT applied to chronic pain include improved physical and emotional functioning and increased pain acceptance, and although follow-up periods were short, the benefits observed were maintained.

Several other nonrandomized trials of interdisciplinary treatment outcomes where the orientation was ACT-based have also found support for this approach; these studies were not included in Table 87.4 as it was not possible to determine the effect of group-based ACT as a standalone (i.e., ACT in the absence of combined physiotherapy, activity/exercise, nursing and anesthesiology, etc.).[98,105–109] However, these studies do provide further preliminary evidence for the potential efficacy of group-delivered ACT across a range of chronic pain conditions. To summarize these findings, results generally found interdisciplinary ACT resulted in significantly improved physical performance and quality of life; fewer sick days; and reduced pain intensity, disability, medical utilization, daytime rest, distress, depression, and pain-related anxiety, with these benefits typically maintained at follow-up.

Similar to the mindfulness literature, the research examining group-delivered ACT approaches for chronic pain has more recently transitioned to comparing ACT to other active treatments. Within a fibromyalgia sample, Luciano and colleagues[100] reported that ACT resulted in significantly greater improvements across a number of pain-related outcomes in comparison to both the recommended pharmacologic treatment for fibromyalgia, as well as a wait-list control; these effects were maintained at 6-month follow-up. One RCT by Loebach-Wetherell et al.[104] compared ACT to CBT in a mixed chronic pain sample and reported similar significant benefits for both treatments across physical and emotional functioning outcomes immediately following treatment and at 6-month follow-up; however, ACT outperformed CBT in terms of client satisfaction, whereas treatment credibility ratings were significantly higher for CBT than ACT. Moreover, in a secondary analysis, it was found that although older adults were more likely to respond to ACT, younger adults were more likely to respond to CBT, both immediately following treatment and at follow-up.[110] Across the group-delivered acceptance-based literature as a whole (including open trials), there is a large amount of variability in the number of sessions delivered, and the frequency and length of sessions per week, and much of the research has examined ACT-oriented interdisciplinary programs as opposed to ACT as a stand-alone psychosocial approach. However, the evidence to date is particularly promising and suggests that group-delivered ACT (especially as delivered within an interdisciplinary context) may perform as well as CBT for chronic pain management.

Factors Affecting Psychotherapeutic Outcome

Although evidence for the efficacy of a number of group-delivered psychosocial treatments is accumulating, the approach with the most well developed body of research to support its use continues to be CBT. Thus, here, we focus on examining the literature that has investigated the mechanisms underlying the well-documented effects of CBT for chronic pain. Although there are many potential factors affecting group CBT treatment outcome for pain management, we have chosen to highlight four: the importance of changing cognitions, the importance of practicing skills to maintain treatment gains, the need for sufficient therapist contact to promote change, and the role of the group process itself.

THE IMPORTANCE OF COGNITIVE CHANGE

The CBT approach is based on the underlying theoretical assumption that emotions and behavior are largely determined by cognitive perceptions of the world. Based on this premise, although there is no "standard" CBT protocol, a critical component of CBT for chronic pain is promoting more adaptive and realistic appraisals of pain and stress. Specifically, the basis of cognitively focused CBT for pain is on helping patients become aware of, examine, and gain control over the thoughts that influence their feelings, coping behavior, and physiology.[111] Given the plethora of research that has consistently found that pain catastrophizing is a robust predictor of a range of negative outcomes (above and beyond other factors such as disease severity, pain intensity, anxiety, and neuroticism), this construct represents a key cognitive mechanism targeted in many CBT programs.[112–119] Research has found that treatment-related reductions in pain catastrophizing during CBT-oriented interdisciplinary treatment correlate with improvement in pain-related outcomes.[120,121] In another study by Thorn and colleagues,[29] it was found that tailoring CBT specifically toward the reduction of catastrophizing is particularly effective for headache pain, with treatment-related reductions in pain catastrophizing correlating with improvement in several treatment outcome variables. Furthermore, Burns and colleagues[122,123] used lagged and cross-lagged analyses and found that early treatment reductions in pain catastrophizing predicted late-treatment improvements in pain-related outcomes, but not vice versa during CBT-oriented interdisciplinary treatment programs. Additional cognitive variables that have been found to correlate with improved outcomes during CBT include self-efficacy,[29,124] perceived pain control,[120,125] pain helplessness,[126] and other pain-related beliefs.[120] Other research has also shown CBT to shift implicit pain self-associations, and this shift was correlated with improved self-esteem.[127]

More recent research has identified that changes in cognitions, such as pain catastrophizing is likely not a mechanism *specific* to group CBT for pain, however. For example, Thorn and colleagues conducted secondary analyses of the RCT described earlier[128] (within the low-income population with low health literacy skills[24]) and found that the observed similar efficacy between group CBT and education might have been accomplished through similar mechanisms, with pain catastrophizing found to account for pre- to posttreatment differences in outcomes across both conditions. Smeets et al.[129] found that treatment-related changes in pain catastrophizing similarly mediated outcome across both CBT as well as physical treatments for chronic low back pain. Turner et al.[130] also found that pain catastrophizing similarly improved across both group-delivered CBT and MBSR.[130] Moreover, this same study by Turner's group identified similar effects on mindfulness, acceptance, and pain management self-efficacy for both CBT and MBSR. Consistent with this, other research examining group CBT-based multidisciplinary pain programs has found that pain acceptance (which is a treatment target theoretically specific to acceptance-based treatments) was correlated with improvement in pain outcomes,[131,132] and another study showed CBT-related changes in mindfulness was associated with improved pain outcomes.[133] Taken together, this research suggests that beneficial outcomes during group-delivered CBT (as well as other psychosocial treatments) might be due to widespread changes across a range of both theory-specific and theory-nonspecific, as well as adaptive and maladaptive, pain-related cognitions of which pain catastrophizing is just one (albeit potent) factor.[134] These findings have led some researchers to posit that global changes in cognitions associated with CBT

TABLE 87.4   Group Acceptance and Commitment Therapy

Authors	Study	N	Treatment Type	Treatment Components	Duration	Outcome Measures	Results	Limitations	Follow up (f/u)
Clarke et al.[99]	RCT	31 with knee or hip osteoarthritis	Acceptance and commitment therapy (ACT) (n = 16) vs. TAU (n = 15)	ACT: psychoeducation on pain, acceptance, values, goals and committed action, mindfulness	Six 90-min sessions	Intermittent and Constant Osteoarthritis Pain Scale, General Health Questionnaire, Pain Anxiety Symptoms Scale, NRS Pain Intensity, Chronic Pain Acceptance Questionnaire	ACT > TAU on NRS, constant and intermittent pain, pain-related anxiety, sleep and well-being at 4 mo; ACT > TAU on activity engagement at 2 mo but not 4 mo	Small sample size, brief f/u, lack of fidelity monitoring, low recruitment: enrollment ratio	2 and 4 mo
Luciano et al.[100]	RCT	104 with fibromyalgia	ACT (n = 51) vs. Pharmacologic treatment (n = 52) vs. wait-list (n = 53)	ACT: problem of control, acceptance vs. resignation, values, avoidance, mindfulness, committed action Pharm: pregabalin + duloxetine for those also with major depression	Eight 2.5-h weekly sessions	VAS Pain Intensity, Hospital Anxiety and Depression Scale, Fibromyalgia Impact Questionnaire, Pain Catastrophizing Scale, Chronic Pain Acceptance Questionnaire, EuroQol	ACT > pharm and WL at both posttreatment and f/u for functional impairment, catastrophizing, anxiety, depression, subjective pain, pain acceptance, and quality of life	Lack of formal fidelity monitoring and therapist allegiance	6 mo
Wicksell et al.[101]	RCT	40 females with fibromyalgia	ACT (n = 23) vs. WL (n = 17)	ACT: avoidance, valued living, clarification of values, acceptance, values-based committed action and behavioral goals, acceptance, cognitive defusion	12 weekly 90-min sessions	Pain Disability Index, Fibromyalgia Impact Questionnaire, SF-36, Self-Efficacy Scale, BDI, Spielberger State-Trait Anxiety Inventory, NRS Pain, Psychological Inflexibility in Pain Scale	ACT > WL on pain disability, fibromyalgia impact, mental health-related QOL, self-efficacy, depression, anxiety, psychological flexibility at posttreatment and f/u	Brief f/u; inclusion of only females limits generalizability	3 mo
McCracken et al.[102]	RCT	73 with fibromyalgia or depression or chronic pain	ACT (n = 37) vs. TAU (n = 36)	ACT: acceptance, cognitive defusion, values-based committed action with experiential exercises and metaphors	Four 4-h sessions, 3 sessions in week 1 and 1 session a week later	Roland-Morris Disability Questionnaire, Patient Health Questionnaire-9, SF-36 Physical Function, NRS Pain Intensity, Chronic Pain Acceptance Questionnaire, Acceptance and Action Questionnaire-II	ACT > WL on depression at posttreatment; ACT > WL on depression, pain acceptance, and disability at f/u	Fidelity not reported; brief f/u; large number of analyses for small sample	3 mo
Mo'tamedi et al.[103]	RCT	30 females with primary chronic headache	ACT (n = 15) vs. TAU (n = 15)	ACT: problem of control, engagement in meaningful activities, avoidance, values, mindfulness	8 weekly 90-min sessions	Short-Form McGill Pain Questionnaire, Migraine Disability Assessment Scale, State-Trait Anxiety Inventory	ACT > TAU on disability and affective distress; no change in pain	Lack of f/u, small sample	—
Loebach-Wetherell et al.[104]	RCT	114 with mixed chronic pain	Cognitive-behavioral therapy (CBT) (N = 57) vs. ACT N = 57	In CBT: monitoring of thoughts, feelings, behaviors and pain; challenging negative thoughts; relaxation training; pain-fatigue cycle; pacing; problem-solving skills; assertive communication; and pleasant event scheduling. In ACT: limits of control, focus on experience; values; cognitive defusion; mindfulness of raisin exercise; committed action	Eight 90-min, weekly group sessions	Brief Pain Inventory (BPI); Short-Form Interference Scale, Short-Form Health Survey (SF-12); Multidimensional Pain Inventory; Beck Depression Inventory-II (BDI-II); Pain Anxiety Symptoms Scale Short-Form (PASS-20); Client Satisfaction Questionnaire, Chronic Pain Acceptance Questionnaire, Survey of Pain Attitudes	CBT = ACT at both posttreatment and f/u; both led to significant improvements on interference, depression, and pain-related anxiety that were maintained at f/u. ACT > CBT on client satisfaction; CBT > ACT on treatment credibility	Lack of long-term f/u; generalizability may be limited as sample was predominantly veterans with higher levels of medical and psychiatric co-morbidity, on a high number of medications	6 mo

BDI, Beck Depression Inventory; NRS, numerical rating scale; QOL, quality of life; RCT, randomized controlled trial; SF-36, Short-Form Health Survey; TAU, treatment as usual; WL, wait-list.

(e.g., the way one relates to and conceptualizes chronic pain, appraisal processes, confidence in one's ability to cope, altered pain self-associations) may be more important to positive outcome than increases in the performance of specific skills taught in CBT per se.[135,136] However, this view is yet to be empirically tested, and as discussed in more depth in the next section, it is more commonly theorized that skills practice is a necessary but perhaps not sufficient factor (i.e., cognitive change is also needed) for improving outcomes.

COMPLIANCE WITH HOMEWORK AND SKILLS PRACTICE TO MAINTAIN TREATMENT GAINS

The CBT approach is designed to be an empowering intervention that teaches patients skills that they themselves can continue to use to self-manage pain, long after completion of treatment delivery. Thus, when considering whether a valid clinical trial of CBT has been conducted, there must be some demonstration that patients are independently practicing these coping skills at an adequate level as this is theorized to be a key precipitating factor in engendering the earlier described cognitive changes. Treatment enactment refers to the extent that clients actually apply what they have learned out of the treatment session. Homework or practice of skills learned in treatment is one way to measure treatment enactment. Scharff and Marcus[137] found that individuals with headache pain who practiced the skills taught in treatment (which included physical therapy, headache-free diets, and relaxation) were more likely to maintain their treatment gains when measured at follow-up. Likewise, completion of homework assignments were significantly related to treatment outcome in patients with irritable bowel syndrome (IBS) participating in group CBT.[35] Vlaeyen et al.[44] compared group education plus CBT to group education plus attention control (group discussion) and noted that in the CBT group, compliance with completion of homework assignments was quite low, which might increase risk for relapse long-term.

Indeed, research underscores the problem of relapse following CBT and other psychosocial pain interventions.[138] Although it has been assumed that posttreatment variability in maintenance trajectories depends at least in part on the maintenance of coping skills practice, few studies have empirically examined if this is the case. One important study comparing individually delivered CBT to treatment as usual that examined a 2-week posttreatment epoch identified that on average, continued use of active cognitive and behavioral coping, positive affect, self-efficacy, and perceived control over pain was associated with maintenance of gains, and pain catastrophizing and negative affect were associated with loss of gains.[139] Although innovative approaches to enhancing skills practice have been applied, the beneficial effects of these maintenance model approaches has been somewhat limited.[140,141] The less than optimal efficacy of these relapse prevention interventions may stem from a lack of understanding of the mechanisms of posttreatment improvement, maintenance, and relapse, and future research in this area is critically needed.

IMPORTANCE OF THERAPIST SKILL AND ADEQUATE TIME WITH THERAPIST

Given the lack of compelling evidence to date in regard to change in cognitions being *specific* to CBT, it has been postulated that beneficial effects may be wrought via change in nonspecific factors.[134,142] From the inception of CBT, Beck and colleagues[143] ascribed importance to the presentation of a convincing treatment rationale in the first CBT session. In this context, it has been argued that more experienced/skillful therapists will deliver a more credible and persuasive rationale and will more likely be perceived as "experts." Importantly, this treatment rationale also functions to foster a collaborative therapeutic alliance and generate positive expectations—factors which have

repeatedly been demonstrated to influence outcome across a range of studies and population types.[69,144,145] Furthermore, although trials specifically designed to evaluate the contribution of therapist expertise/skill in group CBT for chronic pain in relation to outcomes are lacking, in the CBT for depression literature, it has been found that compared to those treated by less experienced clinicians, patients of experienced clinicians tend to show more improvements.[146]

Within the group CBT for chronic pain literature included in Table 87.2, there was a large amount of variability across studies regarding the professional discipline of the delivering interventionist (i.e., psychologist, nurse, physiotherapist, etc.), the length and form of therapist training procedures specific to the study protocol, the degree of therapist expertise/experience (i.e., graduate student, postdoctoral student, licensed clinical psychologist), and the amount of time therapists spend with patients (i.e., treatment dose) as well as in the number of therapists in the room leading any one group. Moreover, treatment fidelity (also known as treatment integrity) was not routinely reported, and when fidelity ratings *were* reported, there was also variability in what precisely was coded and described (i.e., adherence, appropriateness and quality, or any combination of the three). Thus, the specific role of therapist factors along with the "dose" of time a patient spends with the therapist is not well quantified in group CBT for pain research.[67] However, available evidence across other population types suggests such therapist factors play a critical role in outcomes, and it will be important for future research to establish the size of these effects in the context of group CBT for chronic pain.

IMPORTANCE OF GROUP PROCESS

Research across various populations (i.e., not specific to pain) has shown that group processes developed during treatment, such as cohesion and social learning, have the capacity to become agents of change in and of themselves.[147] In our review of the group pain management literature, we located one open clinical trial and one RCT that offered interesting qualitative information regarding the importance of group process. Moore et al.[148] identified that failure to improve during a multidisciplinary treatment depended in part on whether other members of the same treatment group also failed to respond (or left the program prematurely due to dissatisfaction). In another study by Day et al.,[149] qualitative data from recorded semistructured interviews with participants who completed either group CBT or pain education (as a component of Thorn et al.'s[24] earlier described RCT among low-income patients who generally had low health literacy) were thematically analyzed. Group cohesion emerged as one of the most robust themes identified across both CBT and education, and within this overarching theme, subtheme processes of "learning together/sharing" and a "feeling of not being alone" were identified as exceptionally valued aspects of both treatments. A sense of "feeling like a family" was a further subtheme reported by participants who completed CBT but not education. More research is needed to clarify the role of such nonspecific treatment factors in treatment outcome. However, the earlier studies highlight the importance of social factors in chronic pain and underscore the caveat that group treatment should be designed to capitalize on these social influences.

Advantages of Group Treatment

EFFICIENCY AND COST-EFFECTIVENESS

Given the general lack of difference in treatment outcomes between group and individual CBT, it could reasonably be argued that group treatment is a more efficient modality of therapy for chronic pain disorders. Certainly, group treatment is cheaper in terms of practitioner time and patient expense. Indeed, in a study by Bruns and colleagues[150] that used Medicare reimbursements rates to compare the cost of a typical lumbar spinal fusion to the cost of a 10-session group-delivered CBT program, it was found that the surgical costs alone were 168 times greater than the costs of delivering the CBT program. However, *cost-effectiveness* depends not only on cost but also on relative effects.

Reviews of the literature have identified that psychosocial approaches such as CBT are at least as efficacious as surgery and medication management for pain.[151,152] Other research[153] has examined the cost-effectiveness of adding CBT to an inpatient rehabilitation program compared to standard rehabilitation without CBT; there were no significant differences between direct medical or nonmedical costs, and CBT showed lower indirect costs. Furthermore, 6 months following treatment, those who additionally received CBT were absent from work an average of 5.4 days less than those who received standard care.[153] Similar results were reported in an outpatient setting by Lamb and colleagues[25] who examined the cost-effectiveness of adding six sessions of group CBT to a standard active management advisor consultation versus the consultation alone; over 1 year, the group who had additionally received CBT had a sustained benefit in pain-related disability at low-cost to the health care provider. However, "more is not always better," as described by Smeets and colleagues[154] who compared the cost-effectiveness of active physical treatment versus graded activity and problem solving versus a combination of these treatments; the combination treatment did not result in significantly greater improvements in quality adjusted life years or disability as compared to the single treatment modalities, and it was not deemed cost-effective.

SOCIAL PROXIMITY AND SUPPORT

There are several other advantages to using a group modality with patients who have chronic pain-related conditions: A group approach provides social interaction and support from others who share common distressing experiences including the pain itself as well as secondary stressors associated with the pain such as frustrating interactions with the health care system, economic hardship, and deteriorating family relationships. Individuals struggling with chronic pain often feel isolated and misunderstood. Disclosing thoughts and feelings to others who share similar concerns offers patients a greater sense of legitimacy than might be experienced by sharing thoughts and feelings with a therapist or significant other who does not experience pain. More times than not, other patients in the group will have had similar experiences that they also share, which is validating to the person who originally disclosed their concerns, leading to a sense of "not being alone." Qualitative studies of people who have previously completed group-delivered CBT have found that sharing experiences and learning together, as well as being listened to, understood, accepted, tolerated, and affirmed, were highly valued perceived benefits of the group approach for pain management.[149,155]

Beyond the social support provided by others who share similar concerns (which is considered a nonspecific treatment factor), group CBT seems to offer additional benefits. Studies have shown group CBT to be superior to group relaxation sessions[64] and to group discussion sessions,[57] both of which offer the type of social support received in group CBT. Maunder and Esplen[156] reported that a supportive-expressive group for patients with inflammatory bowel disease did not improve symptoms of gastrointestinal (GI) distress/pain, patient quality of life, anxiety, or depression, and they concluded that, at least for this population, supportive-expressive group therapy alone is not efficacious.

VICARIOUS LEARNING AND MODELING OF COLLABORATIVE APPROACH

Group treatment provides clinicians with multiple scenarios to choose from and build on during group discussions, which is helpful when illustrating a particular teaching point.

Taking advantage of a salient example and using it for the benefit of the entire group maximizes the likelihood that patients will understand the intervention through vicarious learning (i.e., other group members observing a therapeutic interaction between an individual patient and the therapist).

Moreover, group treatment provides a fertile venue for modeling a collaborative approach to treatment between the patient and the practitioner. Early in the group process, the leader establishes the expectation that patients will actively participate in group discussions, self-monitor their activities, and complete homework assignments. Through selective reinforcement of patients who actively engage in their treatment by participating in the group and completing the homework assignments, the leader can strive to increase active coping in all of its members. A qualitative study of group CBT treatment with women suffering from chronic pelvic pain revealed that this collaborative approach facilitates a therapeutic progression beginning with developing self-knowledge, followed by assuming responsibility for self-management, and ending with increasing self-control and personal mastery of emotions.[157] Similar results were found by Day and colleagues[149] in their qualitative analysis of literacy-adapted CBT versus pain education in a rural, minority population. Participants reported valuing the collaborative rapport and group learning environment, and many found that working through thought record homework activities in session on a flip chart with the therapist was particularly important for acquiring the cognitive restructuring skill set.[149]

INTERPERSONAL GROUP PROCESS

A final potential advantage of group treatment is the use of group process to facilitate treatment gains (i.e., utilizing the interpersonal exchange between group members in addition to the exchange between therapist and the patient). A group of patients provides an opportunity to capitalize on the moment-by-moment interchanges among group members as well as the interpersonal relationships that develop over time. It is noteworthy that group members will often accept positive feedback, negative feedback, and confrontation from other group members better than from the group leader. This may not only be due in part to feeling more understood by a fellow patient (someone who has "walked in my shoes") but may also be due to the power of the interpersonal process that occurs in group settings.

Practical Issues

OPEN VERSUS CLOSED GROUPS

Most controlled studies in the literature have focused on time-limited, closed groups. In research, this is a necessity to control for a number of confounding variables that ongoing, open groups would introduce into a research design. There are also clinical advantages to running a closed group where all members start and end group treatment at the same time. From a practical perspective, however, running closed groups can prove difficult in some clinical settings because new patients would be required to wait until a new group starts to begin treatment. In response to this concern, Thorn[111] adapted her 10-session CBT manual so that the modules were less dependent on each other, with an introductory session provided to any patient just starting out (i.e., before he or she joins an ongoing group). The feasibility and effectiveness of such an approach has not been tested but may hold particular importance for patients such as injured workers, who are under pressure to return to work. Furthermore, such practical adaptations, if found to be effective, would also increase the probability of implementation in real-world settings.

LENGTH OF GROUP

The length of the groups varied in the RCTs reviewed for this chapter, ranging from 5 to 12 sessions, with a modal number of 10 sessions. Most RCTs reported meeting weekly for 90-minute sessions. Time-limited groups are the accepted standard in research trials because treatment manuals are usually highly structured, and demonstrating fidelity of treatment through therapist adherence to the protocol is an important component of treatment implementation.[158] Furthermore, treatment groups of varying lengths would introduce variance that would reduce the statistical power required to detect real differences between treatment and control groups. On the other hand, clinical realities often necessitate varying the length of a particular treatment component based on whether or not the intervention has been understood by the group members. In clinical settings, there may indeed be some situations in which it would be well advised to repeat a particular unit, continue coverage of a particular topic, or adapt the treatment protocol in some other way. An example of this is Thorn's research described earlier, where the CBT and pain education materials were adapted for patients attending low-income clinics, many of whom also had low health literacy.[18,24]

NUMBER OF PARTICIPANTS

A group composed of approximately five to six members is of sufficient size to facilitate interaction among group members, accommodate the absence of a member without jeopardizing group cohesiveness, and provide enough time to attend to each patient during the individual sessions. Most CBT groups will have more women than men because women have more chronic pain problems, present more frequently for pain treatment than men,[159] and may be more receptive to group interventions based on their tendency to cope via a communal support process.[160] Indeed, one study found that women improved more than men on a number of pain-related outcomes during a multimodal pain management program that included both individual as well as group therapy components.[161] Differences in age, ethnicity, and cultural background do not appear to jeopardize the group process perhaps because chronic pain serves as a unifying factor, making other potentially divisive issues less important. We were unable to identify any studies addressing the issue of whether it is important to racially match group leaders with participants. In an unpublished follow-up qualitative study using posttreatment key informant interviews with African American members of a CBT headache management group 2 years after the RCT had been completed,[29] those interviewed thought that including therapists of different racial and ethnic backgrounds as group leaders would enhance the comfort level of participants and thus increase both their willingness to participate and their chances of treatment completion. In mixed race groups, it is probably preferable to have at least one of the cotherapists be a person of different racial and/or ethnic background.

INDIVIDUALS WHO MAY BE INAPPROPRIATE FOR GROUPS

Almost anyone deemed appropriate for individual CBT for pain management is appropriate for group treatment, but there are a few exceptions. Patients with moderate to severe dementia or other cognitive impairment, psychosis, or chronic interpersonal relationship problems have typically been considered inappropriate for group treatment. However, a published protocol by Kennedy et al.[162] described a mixed methods controlled trial that they were conducting to investigate an adapted group CBT program for women with mild to moderate intellectual disabilities and menstrual pain; to the best of our knowledge, although the trial is listed as completed on the trial registry, the results have not been published. Further research to examine modified

CBT programs to reduce the cognitive load and needed literacy level for effective participation is needed.

In addition, it is not unusual for individuals with chronic pain to have problems managing anger, and in some cases, the degree of anger and hostility may be a contraindication for group treatment. In these cases, however, it is often possible to help the patient learn to regulate his or her anger and hostility in individual treatment and then invite him or her to participate in a group at a later date. Keefe et al.[1] noted that they sometimes use a "time-out" strategy for group members whose anger is disruptive or in other ways countertherapeutic, in which patients meet individually with group leaders while continuing to attend the group but remaining silent for two to three sessions. Clearly, if a patient expresses a strong preference for individual treatment or if his or her schedule prohibits involvement at the prescribed group time, an individual approach will need to be employed.

Summary and Conclusions

Group treatment approaches for pain management have been clearly established as efficacious. Although the evidence for MBIs and ACT has grown exponentially over the past decade, the vast majority of controlled research studies continue to be focused on CBT group approaches. The available research suggests that there are few differences in treatment outcome between group and individual CBT for chronic pain. Thus, because group treatment is more efficient in terms of therapist time and more economical for patients, we suggest that group treatment is generally the favored modality. Certainly, not all patients are appropriate for group pain management, and logistical difficulties in organizing and running a group prevent the universal adoption of group treatment as the only method of appropriate treatment. Relatedly, some patients may need more intensive psychotherapy than what the typical group approach has to offer. It is therefore quite appropriate to refer certain patients for individual treatment after the completion of group treatment.

Future Directions

It is important to note that although the extant research literature has established the efficacy of group CBT for pain management, the external validity of research-based efficacy trials has yet to be studied (i.e., effectiveness studies). Because the efficacy studies cover a wide range of pain problems and come from a variety of research laboratories both inside and outside the United States, we may feel more confident in the generalizability of the results. Methodologically, an important next step would be to move toward pragmatic randomized controlled trials (pRCT), which would help provide information necessary for implementation in routine clinical practice. Furthermore, future research such as that initiated by Thorn and colleagues exploring appropriate adaptations for local populations with special needs will help establish the effectiveness of group approaches for real-world settings.[18,24] Other important issues include enhancing access, durability of treatment effects, and identifying and facilitating reliable mechanisms for reimbursement.

Recently published national clinical practice guidelines stress nonpharmacologic evidence-based alternatives to pain medications and specifically list CBT as one of those options.[163–166] Notably, the 2017 MD Chronic Pain Guidelines reviewed all available high-quality research on 364 treatment × condition pairs. Of these, CBT and only seven other treatments are listed as having consistent evidence of efficacy, no risk of mortality, limited or no side effects, and low cost.[166] Although other formats for treatment delivery of CBT have been developed to increase accessibility (e.g., online resources), the power of group participation in patients who are socially isolated cannot be underestimated.

Two other areas in need of more research are cost-effectiveness studies and research examining the specific mechanisms associated with treatment efficacy. Regarding cost-effectiveness, such research is particularly difficult to carry out in health care settings without readily available (electronic and universal) health care utilization information. Regarding the identification of specific treatment factors responsible as the agent of change, the research conducted up to this point offers a promising start that efficacious group CBT is more than simply therapeutic and social support. However, the mechanisms that may be specific to CBT versus shared across all active treatments for chronic pain need further investigation. Also lacking is well-formulated algorithms for tailoring CBT to the specific baseline cognitive and behavioral profiles of patients in order to most effectively and efficiently target change mechanisms to optimize outcomes. Although yet to be empirically tested a priori, the limit, activate and enhance model recently proposed by Day et al.,[167] provides a theory-driven moderation model for guiding the matching of patients to the evidence-based treatment mostly likely to be of benefit on the basis of key baseline characteristics. The determination of the need for preparatory-oriented interventions (i.e., such as motivational interviewing to prepare readiness to change) is also integrated into this framework. This model provides the first theory-driven framework for algorithm-based interventions within the pain management context; further research testing this model is needed to further refine and optimize its tenets.

Finally, there is a clear need for improvements in the reporting of group-delivered treatments across the chronic pain literature. Current reports often omit details regarding theory, design, and delivery features that have been shown to be of importance in the group setting. Indeed, a recent review identified that only 12% of studies investigating group-based behavioral change programs for chronic musculoskeletal pain reported a theoretical basis for the intervention(s) delivered.[168] The insufficient reporting of critical design, implementation, and evaluation processes impedes efforts to compare group-delivered psychological treatments across studies, reduces the capacity to replicate effective treatments, and limits the capacity to synthesize the evidence of effects.[169] Although systematic reviews and meta-analysis of group treatments for chronic pain are lacking, to assist in the future conduct of such studies, it is recommended that future RCTs of group-delivered treatments follow the reporting guidelines for group-delivered interventions proposed by Borek et al.[169] As health care practitioners of all disciplines become more and more reliant on systematic reviews to support evidence-based practice, comprehensive reporting of design and delivery features and a thorough systematic review and meta-analysis of group treatments for chronic pain would represent certain contributions to the literature.

Appendix 87.1: Search Strategies

The search strategy implemented in the prior edition of this chapter was extended to search the updated literature published since the end point of the prior review (March 2007, dating back to 1950) until August 2017. Specifically, the Cochrane Database was searched along with MEDLINE, PsycINFO, PsycARTICLES, CINAHL Complete, and Academic Search Complete using EBSCOhost as an interface to search for group treatments for (1) gastrointestinal disorders; (2) back, facial, neck, neuralgia, and intractable pain; (3) pelvic pain, dysmenorrheal, and vulvar diseases; and (4) headache disorders. The search was limited to "human" studies published in "English."

1. Search strategy
   1. exp psychotherapy, group (15,111)
   2. exp colonic diseases (208)
   3. 1 and 2 (7)
2. Search strategy
   1. exp psychotherapy, group/ (4,397)
   2. back pain/ or facial pain/ or neck pain/ or neuralgia/ or pain, intractable/(36,108)
   3. 1 and 2 (186)
3. Search strategy
   1. exp psychotherapy, group/ (4,689)
   2. exp pelvic pain/ or exp dysmenorrhea/ or vulvar diseases (3890)
   3. 1 and 2 (5)
4. Search strategy
   1. exp group psychotherapy/ (4860)
   2. exp Headache/ (15,574)
   3. 1 and 2 (5)

References

1. Keefe FJ, Beupre PM, Gil KM. Group therapy for patients with chronic pain In: Turk DC, Gatchel RJ, eds. *Psychological Approaches to Pain Management: A Practitioner's Handbook.* 2nd ed. New York: Guilford Press; 2002:234–256.
2. Gamsa A, Braha RE, Catchlove RF. The use of structured group therapy sessions in the treatment of chronic pain patients. *Pain* 1985;22(1):91–96.
3. Blanchard EB, Schwarz SP. Adaptation of a multicomponent treatment for irritable bowel syndrome to a small-group format. *Biofeedback Self Regul* 1987;12(1):63–69.
4. Herman E, Baptiste S. Pain control: mastery through group experience. *Pain* 1981;10(1):79–86.
5. Straus SE, Richardson WS, Glasziou P. *Evidence-Based Medicine: How to Practice and Teach EBM.* 3rd ed. London: Elsevier/Churchill Livingstone; 2005.
6. McKibbon A. *PDQ: Evidence-Based Principles and Practice.* Hamilton, Canada: B.C. Decker; 1999.
7. Eccleston C, Hearn L, Williams AC. Psychological therapies for the management of chronic neuropathic pain in adults. *Cochrane Database Syst Rev* 2015;(10):CD011259.
8. Williams AC, Eccleston C, Morley S. Psychological therapies for the management of chronic pain (excluding headache) in adults. *Cochrane Database Syst Rev* 2012;(11):CD007407.
9. de Boer MJ, Versteegen GJ, Vermeulen KM, et al. A randomized controlled trial of an Internet-based cognitive-behavioural intervention for non-specific chronic pain: an effectiveness and cost-effectiveness study. *Eur J Pain* 2014; 18:1440–1451.
10. Kääpä EH, Frantsi K, Sarna S, et al. Multidisciplinary group versus individual physiotherapy for chronic nonspecific low back pain. *Spine* 2006;31(4):371–376.
11. Turner-Stokes L, Erkeller-Yuksel F, Miles A, et al. Outpatient cognitive behavioral pain management programs: a randomized comparison of a group-based multidisciplinary versus an individual therapy model. *Arch Phys Med Rehabil* 2003;84(6):781–788.
12. Frettlöh J, Kröner-Herwig B. Individual versus group training in the treatment of chronic pain: which is more efficacious? *J Clin Psychol* 1999;28: 256–266.
13. Rose MJ, Reilly JP, Pennie B, et al. Chronic low back pain rehabilitation programs: a study of the optimum duration of treatment and a comparison of group and individual therapy. *Spine* 1997;22(19):2246–2251.
14. Johnson PR, Thorn BE. Cognitive behavioral treatment of chronic headache: group versus individual treatment format. *Headache* 1989;29(6):358–365.
15. Spence SH. Cognitive-behavior therapy in the management of chronic, occupational pain of the upper limbs. *Behav Res Ther* 1989;27(4):435–446.
16. Spence SH. Cognitive-behaviour therapy in the treatment of chronic, occupational pain of the upper limbs: a 2 year follow-up. *Behav Res Ther* 1991;29(5):503–509.
17. Palyo SA, Schopmeyer KA, McQuaid JR. Tele-pain management: use of video-conferencing technology in the delivery of an integrated cognitive-behavioral and physical therapy intervention. *Psychol Serv* 2012;9(2):200–202.
18. Thorn BE, Eyer JC, Van Dyke BP, et al. Literacy-adapted cognitive-behavioral therapy vs education for chronic pain at low-income clinics: a randomized controlled trial [published online ahead of print February 27, 2018]. *Ann Intern Med.* doi:10.7326/M17-0972.
19. Helminen E, Sinikallio SH, Valjakka AL, et al. Effectiveness of a cognitive-behavioural group intervention for knee osteoarthritis pain: a randomized controlled trial. *Clin Rehabil* 2015;29(9):868–881.
20. Linden M, Scherbe S, Cicholas B. Randomized controlled trial on the effectiveness of cognitive behavior group therapy in chronic back pain patients. *J Back Musculoskelet Rehabil* 2014;27:563–568.
21. Seminowicz D, Shpaner M, Keaser ML, et al. Cognitive-behavioral therapy increases prefrontal cortex gray matter in patients with chronic pain. *J Pain* 2013;14(12):1573–1584.
22. Slavin-Spenny O, Lumley MA, Thakur ER, et al. Effects of anger awareness and expression training versus relaxation training on headaches: a randomized trial. *Ann Behav Med* 2013;46:181–192.

23. Heutink M, Post MW, Bongers-Janssen HM, et al. The CONECSI trial: results of a randomized controlled trial of a multidisciplinary cognitive behavioral program for coping with chronic neuropathic pain after spinal cord injury. *Pain* 2012;153(1):120–128.

24. Thorn BE, Day MA, Burns J, et al. Randomized trial of group cognitive behavioral therapy compared with a pain education control for low-literacy rural people with chronic pain. *Pain* 2011;152(12):2710–2720.

25. Lamb SE, Hansen Z, Lall R, et al. Group cognitive behavioral treatment for low-back pain in primary care: a randomised controlled trial and cost-effectiveness analysis. *Lancet* 2010;375:916–923.

26. Van Koulil S, van Lankveld W, Kraaimaat FW, et al. Tailored cognitive-behavioral therapy and exercise training for high-risk patients with fibromyalgia. *Arthritis Care Res* 2010;62:1377–1385.

27. Falcão DM, Sales L, Leite JR, et al. Cognitive behavioral therapy for the treatment of fibromyalgia syndrome: a randomized controlled trial. *J Musulosket Pain* 2008;16(3):133–140.

28. Ersek M, Turner JA, Cain KC, et al. Results of a randomized controlled trial to examine the efficacy of a chronic pain self-management group for older adults. *Pain* 2008;138:29–40.

29. Thorn BE, Pence LB, Ward LC, et al. A randomized clinical trial of targeted cognitive behavioral treatments to reduce catastrophizing in chronic headache sufferers. *J Pain* 2007;8(12):938–949.

30. Li EJ, Li-Tsang CW, Lam CS, et al. The effect of a "training on work readiness" program for workers with musculoskeletal pain: a randomized control trial (RCT) study. *J Occup Rehabil* 2006;16(4):529–541.

31. Linton SJ, Boersma K, Jansson M, et al. The effects of cognitive-behavioral and physical therapy preventive interventions on pain-related sick leave: a randomized controlled trial. *Clin J Pain* 2005;21(2):109–119.

32. Gold DT, Shipp KM, Pieper CF, et al. Group treatment improves trunk strength and psychological status in older women with vertebral fractures: results of a randomized, clinical trial. *J Am Geriatr Soc* 2004;52(9):1471–1478.

33. van Lankveld W, van Helmond T, Näring G, et al. Partner participation in cognitive-behavioral self management group treatment for patients with rheumatoid arthritis. *J Rheumatol* 2004;31(9):1738–1745.

34. Ersek M, Turner JA, McCurry SM, et al. Efficacy of a self-management group intervention for elderly persons with chronic pain. *Clin J Pain* 2003;19(3):156–167.

35. Tkachuk G, Graff L, Martin GL, et al. Randomized controlled trial of cognitive-behavioral group therapy for irritable bowel syndrome in a medical setting. *J Clin Psychol Med Settings* 2003;10(1):57–69.

36. Mishra KD, Gatchel RJ, Gardea MA. The relative efficacy of three cognitive-behavioral treatment approaches to temporomandibular disorders. *J Behav Med* 2000;23(3):293–309.

37. Leibing E, Pfingsten M, Bartmann U, et al. Cognitive-behavioral treatment in unselected rheumatoid arthritis outpatients. *Clin J Pain* 1999;15(1):58–66.

38. Potts SG, Lewin R, Fox KA, et al. Group psychological treatment for chest pain with normal coronary arteries. *QJM* 1999;92(2):81–86.

39. Cole JD. Psychotherapy with the chronic pain patient using coping skills development: outcome study. *J Occup Health Psychol* 1998;3(3):217–226.

40. Keel PJ, Bodoky C, Gerhard U, et al. Comparison of integrated group therapy and group relaxation training for fibromyalgia. *Clin J Pain* 1998;14(3):232–328.

41. Keel PJ, Wittig R, Deutschmann R, et al. Effectiveness of in-patient rehabilitation for sub-chronic and chronic low back pain by an integrative group treatment program (Swiss Multicentre Study). *Scand J Rehabil Med* 1998;30(4):211–219.

42. Basler HD, Jäkle C, Kröner-Herwig B. Incorporation of cognitive-behavioral treatment into the medical care of chronic low back patients: a controlled randomized study in German pain treatment centers. *Patient Educ Couns* 1997;31(2):113–124.

43. van Dulmen AM, Fennis JF, Bleijenberg G. Cognitive-behavioral group therapy for irritable bowel syndrome: effects and long-term follow-up. *Psychosom Med* 1996;58(5):508–514.

44. Vlaeyen JW, Teeken-Gruben NJ, Goossens ME, et al. Cognitive-educational treatment of fibromyalgia: a randomized clinical trial. I. Clinical effects. *J Rheumatol* 1996;23(7):237–245.

45. Newton-John TR, Spence SH, Schotte D. Cognitive-behavioural therapy versus EMG biofeedback in the treatment of chronic low back pain. *Behav Res Ther* 1995;33(6):691–697.

46. James LD, Thorn BE, Williams DA. Goal specification in cognitive-behavioral therapy for chronic headache pain. *Behav Ther* 1993;24:305–320.

47. Turner JA, Jensen M. Efficacy of cognitive therapy for chronic low back pain. *Pain* 1993;53:169–177.

48. Kneebone II, Martin PR. Partner involvement in the treatment of chronic headaches. *Behav Change* 1992;94:201–215.

49. Nicholas MK, Wilson PH, Goyen J. Operant-behavioural and cognitive-behavioural treatment for chronic low back pain. *Behav Res Ther* 1991;29(3):225–238.

50. Subramanian K. Structured group work for the management of chronic pain: an experimental investigation. *Res Soc Work Pract* 1991;1:32–45.

51. Subramanian K. Long-term follow up of a structured treatment for the management of chronic pain. *Res Soc Work Pract* 1994;4(2):32–45.

52. Peters JL, Large RG. A randomised control trial evaluating in- and out-patient pain management programmes. *Pain* 1990;41(3):283–293.

53. Turner JA, Clancy S, McQuade KJ, et al. Effectiveness of behavioral therapy for chronic low back pain: a component analysis. *J Consult Clin Psychol* 1990;58(5):573–579.

54. Linton SJ, Bradley LA, Jensen I, et al. The secondary prevention of low back pain: a controlled study with follow-up. *Pain* 1989;36(2):197–207.

55. Puder RS. Age analysis of cognitive-behavioral group therapy for chronic pain outpatients. *Psychol Aging* 1988;6(2):204–207.

56. Bradley LA, Young LD, Anderson KO, et al. Effects of psychological therapy on pain behavior of rheumatoid arthritis patients. Treatment outcome and six-month followup. *Arthritis Rheum* 1987;30(10):1105–1114.

57. Larsson B, Melin L, Lamminen M, et al. A school-based treatment of chronic headaches in adolescents. *J Pediatr Psychol* 1987;12(4):553–566.

58. Bradley LA, Turner RA, Young LD, et al. Effects of cognitive-behavioral therapy on pain behavior of rheumatoid arthritis (RA) patients: preliminary outcomes. *Scand J Behav Ther* 1985;14:51–64.

59. Linton SJ, Melin L, Stjernlöf K. The effects of applied relaxation and operant activity training on chronic pain. *Behav Psychother* 1985;13:87–100.

60. Melin L, Linton SJ. A follow-up study of a comprehensive behavioural treatment programme. *Behav Psychother* 1988;16(4):313–321.

61. Moore JE, Chaney EF. Outpatient group treatment of chronic pain: effects of spouse involvement. *J Consult Clin Psychol* 1985;53(3):326–334.

62. Cohen MJ, Heinrich RL, Naliboff BD, et al. Group outpatient physical and behavioral therapy for chronic low back pain. *J Clin Psychol* 1983;39(3):326–333.

63. Figueroa J. Group treatment of chronic tension headaches: a comparative treatment study. *Behav Modif* 1982;6:229–239.

64. Turner JA. Comparison of group progressive-relaxation training and cognitive-behavioral group therapy for chronic low back pain. *J Consult Clin Psychol* 1982;50(5):757–765.

65. Lami MJ, Martinez MP, Sanchez AI. Systematic review of psychological treatment in fibromyalgia. *Curr Pain Headache Rep* 2013;17:345.

66. Fisher E, Heathcote L, Palermo TM, et al. Systematic review and meta-analysis of psychological therapies for children with chronic pain. *J Pediatr Psychol* 2014;39(8):763–782.

67. Ehde DM, Dillworth TM, Turner JA. Cognitive behavioural therapy for individuals with chronic pain: efficacy, innovations and directions for research. *Am Psychol* 2014;69(2):153–166.

68. Goossens ME, Rutten-van Mölken MP, Leidl RM, et al. Cognitive-educational treatment of fibromyalgia: a randomized clinical trial. II. Economic evaluation. *J Rheumatol* 1996;23(7):1246–1254.

69. Kerns RD, Burns JW, Shulman M, et al. Can we improve cognitive-behavioral therapy for chronic back pain treatment engagement and adherence? A controlled trial of tailored versus standard therapy. *Health Psychol* 2014;33(9):938–947.

70. van der Roer N, van Tulder M, Barendse J, et al. Intensive group training protocol versus guideline physiotherapy for patients with chronic low back pain: a randomised controlled trial. *Eur Spine J* 2008;17:1193–1200.

71. Smeets RJ, Vlaeyen JW, Hidding A, et al. Active rehabilitation for chronic low back pain: cognitive-behavioral, physical, or both? First direct post-treatment results from a randomized controlled trial. *BMC Musculoskelet Disord* 2006;20:7.

72. Day MA, Jensen MP, Ehde DM, et al. Toward a theoretical model for mindfulness-based pain management. *J Pain* 2014;15(7):691–703.

73. Veehof MM, Trompetter HR, Bohlmeijer ET, et al. Acceptance- and mindfulness-based interventions for the treatment of chronic pain: a meta-analytic review. *Cogn Behav Ther* 2016;45(1):5–31.

74. Carson JW, Keefe FJ, Lynch TR, et al. Loving-kindness meditation for chronic low back pain: results from a pilot trial. *J Holist Nurs* 2005;23(3):287–304.

75. Plews-Ogan M, Owens JE, Goodman M, et al. A pilot study evaluating mindfulness-based stress reduction and massage for the management of chronic pain. *J Gen Intern Med* 2005;20(12):1136–1138.

76. Cherkin DC, Eisenberg D, Sherman KJ, et al. Randomized trial comparing traditional Chinese medical acupuncture, therapeutic massage, and self-care education for chronic low back pain. *Arch Intern Med* 2001;161(8):1081–1088.

77. Davis MC, Zautra AJ, Wolf LD, et al. Mindfulness and cognitive-behavioral interventions for chronic pain: differential effects on daily pain reactivity and stress reactivity. *J Consult Clin Psychol* 2015;83(1):24–35.

78. Cash E, Salmon P, Weissbecker I, et al. Mindfulness meditation alleviates fibromyalgia symptoms in women: results of a randomized clinical trial. *Ann Behav Med* 2015;49:319–330.

79. Cathcart S, Galatis N, Immink M, et al. Brief mindfulness-based therapy for chronic tension-type headache: a randomized controlled pilot study. *Behav Cogn Psychother* 2014;42:1–15.

80. Garland EL, Manusov EG, Froeliger B, et al. Mindfulness-oriented recovery enhancement for chronic pain and prescription opioid misuse: results from an early-stage randomized controlled trial. *J Consult Clin Psychol* 2014;82(3):448–459.

81. Day MA, Thorn BE, Ward LC, et al. Mindfulness-based cognitive therapy for the treatment of headache pain: a pilot study. *Clin J Pain* 2014;30(2):152–161.

82. Parra-Delgado PM, Latorre-Postigo JM. Effectiveness of mindfulness-based cognitive therapy in the treatment of fibromyalgia: a randomised trial. *Cogn Ther Res* 2013;37:1015–1026.

83. Brown CA, Jones AK. Psychobiological correlates of improved mental health in patients with musculoskeletal pain after a mindfulness-based pain management program. *Clin J Pain* 2013;29(3):233–244.

84. Wong SY, Chan FW, Wong RL, et al. Comparing the effectiveness of mindfulness-based stress reduction and multidisciplinary intervention programs for chronic pain: a randomized comparative trial. *Clin J Pain* 2011; 27(8):724–734.

85. Schmidt S, Grossman P, Schwarzer B, et al. Treating fibromyalgia with mindfulness-based stress reduction: results from a 3-armed randomized controlled trial. *Pain* 2011;152(2):361–369.

86. Morone NE, Rollman BL, Moore CG, et al. A mind-body program for older adults with chronic low back pain: results of a pilot study. *Pain Med* 2009;10(8):1395–1407.

87. Zautra AJ, Davis MC, Reich JW, et al. Comparison of cognitive behavioral and mindfulness meditation interventions on adaptation to rheumatoid arthritis for patients with and without history of recurrent depression. *J Consult Clin Psychol* 2008;76:408–421.

88. Morone NE, Greco CM, Weiner DK. Mindfulness meditation for the treatment of chronic low back pain in older adults: a randomized controlled pilot study. *Pain* 2008;134(3):310–319.

89. Pradhan EK, Baumgarten M, Langenberg P, et al. Effect of mindfulness-based stress reduction in rheumatoid arthritis patients. *Arthritis Rheum* 2007;57(7):1134–1142.

90. Astin JA, Berman BM, Bausell B, et al. The efficacy of mindfulness meditation plus Qigong movement therapy in the treatment of fibromyalgia: a randomized controlled trial. *J Rheumatol* 2003;30(10):2257–2262.

91. Grossman P, Tiefenthaler-Gilmer U, Raysz A, et al. Mindfulness training as an intervention for fibromyalgia: evidence of postintervention and 3-year follow-up benefits in well-being. *Psychother Psychosom* 2007;76:226–233.

92. Kabat-Zinn J. The clinical use of mindfulness meditation for the self regulation of chronic pain. *J Behav Med* 1985;8(2):163–190.

93. Sagula D, Rice KG. The effectiveness of mindfulness training on the grieving process and emotional well-being of chronic pain patients. *J Clin Psychol Med Sett* 2004;11:333–342.

94. Cherkin DC, Sherman KJ, Balderson BH, et al. Effect of mindfulness-based stress reduction vs cognitive behavioral therapy or usual care on back pain and functional limitations in adults with chronic low back pain: a randomized controlled trial. *JAMA* 2016;315(12):1240–1249.

95. Cherkin DC, Anderson ML, Sherman KJ, et al. Two-year follow-up of a randomized clinical trial of mindfulness-based stress reduction vs cognitive behavioral therapy or usual care for chronic low back pain. *JAMA* 2017;317(6):642–644.

96. Veehof MM, Oskam MJ, Schreurs KM, et al. Acceptance-based interventions for the treatment of chronic pain: a systematic review and meta-analysis. *Pain* 2011;152(3):533–542.

97. Hayes SC. Acceptance and commitment therapy, relational frame theory, and the third wave of behavioral and cognitive therapies. *Behav Ther* 2004;35:639–664.

98. McCracken LM, MacKichan F, Eccleston C. Contextual cognitive-behavioral therapy for severely disabled chronic pain sufferers: effectiveness and clinically significant change. *Eur J Pain* 2007;11(3):314–322.

99. Clarke SP, Poulis N, Moreton BJ, et al. Evaluation of a group acceptance and commitment therapy intervention for people with knee or hip osteoarthritis: a pilot randomized controlled trial. *Disabil Rehabil* 2017;39(7):663–670.

100. Luciano JV, Guallar JA, Aguado J, et al. Effectiveness of group acceptance and commitment therapy for fibromyalgia: a 6-month randomized controlled trial (EFFIGACT study). *Pain* 2014;155:693–702.

101. Wicksell RK, Kemani M, Jensen K, et al. Acceptance and commitment therapy for fibromyalgia: a randomized controlled trial. *Eur J Pain* 2013;17:599–611.

102. McCracken LM, Sato A, Taylor GJ. A trial of a brief group-based form of acceptance and commitment therapy (ACT) for chronic pain in general practice: pilot outcome and process results. *J Pain* 2013;14(11):1398–1406.

103. Mo'tamedi H, Rezaiemaram P, Tavallaie A. The effectiveness of a group-based acceptance and commitment additive therapy on rehabilitation of female outpatients with chronic headache: preliminary findings reducing 3 dimensions of headache impact. *Headache* 2012;52:1106–1119.

104. Loebach-Wetherell JL, Afari N, Rutledge T, et al. A randomized, controlled trial of acceptance and commitment therapy and cognitive-behavioral therapy for chronic pain. *Pain* 2011;152(9):2098–2107.

105. Vowles KE, Kink B, Cohen L. Acceptance and commitment therapy for chronic pain: a diary study of treatment process in relation to reliable change in disability. *J Context Behav Sci* 2014;3:74–80.

106. Vowles KE, Witkiewitz K, Sowden G, et al. Acceptance and commitment therapy for chronic pain: evidence of mediation and clinically significant change following an abbreviated interdisciplinary program of rehabilitation. *J Pain* 2014;15(1):101–113.

107. Vowles KE, McCracken LM, O'Brien LZ. Acceptance and values-based action in chronic pain: a three-year follow-up analysis of treatment effectiveness and process. *Behav Res Ther* 2011;49(11):748–755.

108. McCracken LM, Vowles KE. A prospective analysis of acceptance of pain and values-based action in patients with chronic pain. *Health Psychol* 2008;27(2):215–220.

109. Vowles KE, McCracken LM. Acceptance and values-based action in chronic pain: a study of treatment effectiveness and process. *J Consult Clin Psychol* 2008;76(3):397–407.

110. Loebach-Wetherell JL, Petkus AJ, Alonso-Fernandez M, et al. Age moderates response to acceptance and commitment therapy vs. cognitive behavioral therapy for chronic pain. *Int J Geriatr Psychiatry* 2016;31:302–308.

111. Thorn BE. *Cognitive Therapy for Chronic Pain: A Step-By-Step Guide.* 2nd ed. New York: Guilford Press; 2017.

112. Geisser ME, Robinson ME, Keefe FJ, et al. Catastrophizing, depression and the sensory, affective and evaluative aspects of chronic pain. *Pain* 1994;59(1):79–83.

113. Sullivan MJ, Rodgers WM, Kirsch I. Catastrophizing, depression and expectancies for pain and emotional distress. *Pain* 2001;91(1–2):147–154.

114. Day MA, Thorn BE. The relationship of demographic and psychosocial variables to pain-related outcomes in a rural chronic pain population. *Pain* 2010;151(2):467–474.

115. Flor H, Behle DJ, Birbaumer N. Assessment of pain-related cognitions in chronic pain patients. *Behav Res Ther* 1993;31(1):63–73.

116. Keefe FJ, Rumble ME, Scipio CD, et al. Psychological aspects of persistent pain: current state of the science. *J Pain* 2004;5(4):195–211.

117. Sullivan MJ, Thorn B, Haythornthwaite JA, et al. Theoretical perspectives on the relation between catastrophizing and pain. *Clin J Pain* 2001;17(1):52–64.

118. Edwards RR, Cahalan C, Mensing G, et al. Pain, catastrophizing, and depression in the rheumatic diseases. *Nat Rev Rheumatol* 2011;7(4):216–224.

119. Drahovzal D, Stewart S, Sullivan M. Tendency to catastrophize somatic sensations: pain catastrophizing and anxiety sensitivity in predicting headache. *Cogn Behav Ther* 2006;35(4):226–235.

120. Jensen M, Turner JA, Romano JM. Changes in beliefs, catastrophizing and coping are associated with improvement in multidisciplinary pain treatment. *J Consult Clin Psychol* 2001;69:655–662.

121. Craner JR, Sperry JA, Evans MM. The relationship between pain catastrophizing and outcomes of a 3-week comprehensive pain rehabilitation program. *Pain Med* 2016;17:2026–2035.

122. Burns JW, Glenn B, Bruehl S, et al. Cognitive factors influence outcome following multidisciplinary chronic pain treatment: a replication and extension of a cross-lagged panel analysis. *Behav Res Ther* 2003;41(10):1163–1182.

123. Burns JW, Kubilus A, Bruehl S, et al. Do changes in cognitive factors influence outcome following multidisciplinary treatment for chronic pain? A cross-lagged panel analysis. *J Consult Clin Psychol* 2003;71(1):81–91.

124. Holroyd KA, Labus JS, Carlson B. Moderation and mediation in the psychological and drug treatment of chronic tension-type headache: the role of disorder severity and psychiatric comorbidity. *Pain* 2009;143:213–222.

125. Spinhoven P, Ter Kuile M, Kole-Snijders AM, et al. Catastrophizing and internal pain control as mediators of outcome in the multidisciplinary treatment of chronic low back pain. *Eur J Pain* 2004;8:211–219.

126. Burns JW, Johnson BJ, Mahoney N, et al. Cognitive and physical capacity process variables predict long-term outcome after treatment of chronic pain. *J Consult Clin Psychol* 1998;66:434–439.

127. Grumm M, Erbe K, von Collani G, et al. Automatic processing of pain: the change of implicit pain associations after psychotherapy. *Behav Res Ther* 2008;47:701–714.

128. Burns JW, Day MA, Thorn BE. Is reduction in pain catastrophizing a therapeutic mechanism specific to cognitive-behavioral therapy for chronic pain? *Trans Behac Med Pract Pol Res* 2012;2:22–29.

129. Smeets RJ, Vlaeyen JW, Kester AD, et al. Reduction of pain catastrophizing mediates the outcome of both physical and cognitive-behavioral treatment in chronic low back pain. *J Pain* 2006;7(4):261–271.

130. Turner JA, Anderson ML, Balderson BH, et al. Mindfulness-based stress reduction and cognitive-behavioral therapy for chronic low back pain: similar effects on mindfulness, catastrophizing, self-efficacy, and acceptance in a randomized controlled trial. *Pain* 2016;157:2434–2444.

131. Akerblom S, Perrin S, Fischer MR, et al. The mediating role of acceptance in multidisciplinary cognitive-behavioral therapy for chronic pain. *J Pain* 2015;16:606–615.

132. Baranoff J, Hanrahan S, Kapur D, et al. Acceptance as a process variable in relation to catastrophizing in multidisciplinary pain treatment. *Eur J Pain* 2013;17:101–110.

133. Cassidy EL, Atherton RJ, Robertson N, et al. Mindfulness, functioning and catastrophizing after multidisciplinary pain management for chronic low back pain. *Pain* 2012;152(3):644–650.

134. Burns J, Nielson WR, Jensen MP, et al. Does change occur for the reasons we think it does? A test of specific therapeutic operations during cognitive-behavioral treatment of chronic pain. *Clin J Pain* 2015;31:603–611.

135. Sil S, Kashikar-Zuck S. Understanding why cognitive-behavioral therapy is an effective treatment for adolescents with juvenile fibromyalgia. *Int J Clin Rheumatol* 2013;8(2).

136. Hofmann SG, Asmundson GJ. Acceptance and mindfulness-based therapy: new wave or old hat? *Clin Psychol Rev* 2008;28(1):1–16.

137. Scharff L, Marcus DA. Interdisciplinary outpatient group treatment of intractable headache. *Headache* 1994;34(2):73–78.

138. Turk DC, Rudy TE. Neglected topics in the treatment of chronic pain patients - relapse, noncompliance, and adherence enhancement. *Pain* 1991;44:5–28.

139. Litt MD, Shafer DM, Ibanez CR, et al. Momentary pain and coping in temporomandibular disorder pain: exploring mechanisms of cognitive behavioral treatment for chronic pain. *Pain* 2009;145:160–168.

140. Naylor MR, Keefe FJ, Brigidi B, et al. Therapeutic interactive voice response for chronic pain reduction and relapse prevention. *Pain* 2008;134(3):335–345.

141. Keefe F, Van Horn Y. Cognitive-behavioral treatment of rheumatoid arthritis pain. *Arthritis Care Res* 1993;6(4):213–222.

142. Day MA, Thorn BE, Burns J. The continuing evolution of biopsychosocial interventions for chronic pain. *J Cogn Psychother* 2012;26(2):114–129.

143. Beck AT, Rush AJ, Shaw B, et al. *Cognitive Therapy of Depression*. New York: Guilford Press; 1979.

144. Jensen M, Nielson WR, Kerns RD. Toward the development of a motivational model of pain self-management. *J Pain* 2003;4:477–492.

145. Day MA, Halpin J, Thorn BE. An empirical examination of the role of common factors of therapy during a mindfulness-based cognitive therapy intervention for headache pain. *Clin J Pain* 2016;32(5):420–427.

146. Ilardi SS, Craighead WE. The role of nonspecific factors in cognitive-behavioral therapy for depression. *Clin Psychol Sci Pract* 1994;1(2):138–155.

147. Yalom ID, Leszcz M. *The Theory and Practice of Group Psychotherapy*. 5th ed. New York: Basic Books; 2005.

148. Moore ME, Berk SN, Nypaver A. Chronic pain: inpatient treatment with small group effects. *Arch Phys Med Rehabil* 1984;65(7):356–361.

149. Day MA, Thorn BE, Kapoor S. A qualitative analysis of a randomized controlled trial comparing a cognitive-behavioral treatment with education. *J Pain* 2011;12(9):941–952.

150. Bruns D, Mueller K, Warren PA. Biopsychosocial law, health care reform, and the control of medical inflation in Colorado. *Rehabil Psychol* 2012;57(2):81–97.

151. Eccleston C, Palermo TM, Williams AC, et al. Psychological therapies for the management of chronic and recurrent pain in children and adolescents. *Cochrane Database Syst Rev* 2009;(2):CD003968.

152. Morley S, Williams A. New developments in the psychological management of chronic pain. *Can J Psychiatry* 2015;60(4):168–175.

153. Schweikert B, Jacobi E, Seitz R, et al. Effectiveness and cost-effectiveness of adding a cognitive behavioral treatment to the rehabilitation of chronic low back pain. *J Rheumatol* 2006;33(12):2519–2526.

154. Smeets RJ, Severens JL, Beelen S, et al. More is not always better: cost-effectiveness analysis of combined, single behavioral and single physical rehabilitation programs for chronic low back pain. *Eur J Pain* 2009;13(1):71–81.

155. Steihaug S, Ahlsen B, Malterud K. "I am allowed to be myself": women with chronic muscular pain being recognized. *Scand J Public Health* 2002; 30(4):281–287.

156. Maunder RG, Esplen MJ. Supportive-expressive group psychotherapy for persons with inflammatory bowel disease. *Can J Psychiatry* 2001;46(7):622–626.

157. Albert H. Psychosomatic group treatment helps women with chronic pelvic pain. *J Psychosom Obstet Gynaecol* 1999;20(4):216–225.

158. Lichstein KL, Riedel BW, Grieve R. Fair tests of clinical trials: a treatment implementation model. *Adv Behav Res Ther* 1994;16:1–29.

159. Unruh AM. Gender variations in clinical pain experience. *Pain* 1996;65: 123–167.

160. Lyons RF, Mickelson KD, Sullivan MJ, et al. Coping as a communal process. *J Soc Pers Relat* 1998;15(5):579–605.

161. Pieh C, Altmeppen J, Neumeier S, et al. Gender differences in outcomes of a multimodal pain management program. *Pain* 2012;153:197–202.

162. Kennedy S, O'Higgins S, Sarma K, et al. Evaluation of a group based cognitive behavioural programme for menstrual pain management in young women with intellectual disabilities: protocol for a mixed methods controlled clinical trial. *BMC Womens Health* 2014;14:107.

163. Institute of Medicine. *Relieving Pain in America: A Blueprint for Transforming Prevention, Care, Education, and Research*. Washington, DC: National Academies Press; 2011.

164. Dowell D, Haegerich TM, Chou R. CDC guideline for prescribing opioids for chronic pain—United States, 2016. *JAMA* 2016;315(15):1624–1645.

165. The Opioid Therapy for Chronic Pain Word Group. *VA/DoD Clinical Practice Guideline for Opioid Therapy for Chronic Pain*. Washington, DC: U.S. Department of Veterans Affairs, Office of Quality and Performance, Office of Evidence Based Practice; 2017.

166. Qaseem A, Wilt TJ, McLean RM, et al. Noninvasive treatments for acute, subacute, and chronic low back pain: a clinical practice guideline from the American College of Physicians. *Ann Intern Med* 2017;166(7): 514–530.

167. Day MA, Ehde DM, Jensen MP. Psychosocial pain management moderation: the limit, activate and enhance model. *J Pain* 2015;16(10):947–960.

168. Keogh A, Tully MA, Matthews J, et al. A review of behaviour change theories and techniques used in group based self-management programmes for chronic pain and arthritis. *Manual Ther* 2015;20:727–735.

169. Borek A, Abraham C, Smith JR, et al. A checklist to improve reporting of group-based behaviour-change interventions. *BMC Public Health* 2015;15:963.

CHAPTER 88

Motivating Chronic Pain Patients for Behavioral Change

AKIKO OKIFUJI, EMILY HAGN, CHRISTINA ELISE BOKAT, and **DENNIS C. TURK**

Motivation is a primary determinant of human behavior, influencing its initiation, direction, intensity, and persistence.[1] Historically, motivation has not been a central issue in health care as the modal approach to treat illness was believed to require very little active participation from patients beyond complying with advice. However, as our appreciation of the growing number of chronic diseases for which there are no cures, the importance of helping patients become active in a treatment has been increasingly noted. Patients have described the importance of motivation and accountability, particularly when they become discouraged or have difficulty with treatment adherence.[2,3] This realization has led to motivation and motivation enhancement being given greater attention. Self-management approaches for managing health have gained in importance as potential methods to increase motivation for self-management and to facilitate long-term health-relevant behaviors. There is a large volume of literature indicating that even relatively simple behaviors, such as taking medication in the prescribed manner, can be problematic. Studies have reported that depending on how it is defined and measured, the rates of nonadherence to medication in adults range anywhere from 8% to 62%.[4,5] In general, one-third of patients can be expected to be nonadherent.[6] Treatment nonadherence is also a significant behavioral health problem and public health concern in pediatric populations. Approximately 50% of children[7] and 65% to 90% of adolescents[8,9] are nonadherent across pediatric conditions.

For patients with chronic pain, rehabilitation rather than complete cure is most realistic. One of the critical requirements for successful rehabilitation is that patients adopt an active, participatory role in their treatments, coping with symptoms and life changes, and adjustment to their circumstances. Literature consistently acknowledges that multidisciplinary pain care, which includes an activating therapy, is helpful for restoring functioning and improving quality of life, without complete elimination of pain.[10] However, such a treatment requires patients to make significant lifestyle changes including the incorporation of various functional activities in their daily routines. Maintaining these changes over long periods of time is often difficult even for healthy individuals. For example, two-thirds of those who sign up with gyms never use the facility,[11] and 50% drop out of physical activity programs within the first 6 months.[12] Thus, it is hardly surprising that patients with chronic pain find it difficult to adhere to regular physical activity regimens, use of coping skills, engaging in problem solving, and modifying communication patterns with family, friends, and coworkers as well as health care providers. In the one study that directly examined the issue of adherence to pain rehabilitation recommendations, Lutz et al.[13] followed patients 8 months after they had been successfully treated at pain rehabilitation and found that, based on self-report, the rates of adherence with each of the specifically recommended behaviors (e.g., progressive ambulation and stretching exercises, regular application of ice and heat, relaxation) averaged about 42% and with all of the recommendations proscribed by the treatment program was only 12.2%.

Another dilemma for successful implementation of activating therapy is that it can be contrary to the very nature of pain where the motivational drive is to avoid or escape from any activities that might increase pain. Furthermore, most people including many health care providers have learned "if something hurts, don't do it." This approach may be appropriate for acute pain care where may pain serve a protective role. However, for chronic pain, equating hurt with harm often becomes a barrier for successful rehabilitation and even increases disability following loss of mobility, strength, and endurance from inactivity. Thus, clinicians are frequently faced with the challenge of how to motivate patients to actively engage in the treatment recommendations that may seem counter to patients' acquired beliefs. Long-term treatment success, in particular, depends on regular adherence to recommended self-care regimens,[6,14,15] although how close to the recommendations is an open question.[16,17] Historically, clinicians have invested less energy in patients who show little commitment to follow through with recommended therapies. "You can lead a horse to water, but you can't make it drink" was a typical way of conceptualizing the issue.[18] However, as noted earlier, motivation to commit to the treatment plan and adherence with regimen are essential in successful pain rehabilitation (pharmacologic as well as rehabilitative).[17] Thus, motivating patients for behavioral change is essential and a critical clinical issue in successful pain management. In this chapter, we review the two approaches to optimize motivation and engagement of patients: motivation enhancement therapy (MET) and implementation intentions (IIs).

Neural Mechanisms of Motivation

Neural mechanisms of motivation are complex, involving multiple brain systems.[19] Although motivation is a critical component of recovery from chronic pain, how specific neural factors underlie the motivational factors relevant to people with chronic pain is not well understood. However, we may consider how chronic pain itself as well as comorbid dysfunctions could contribute to the motivational state of chronic pain patients to adhere to specific recommendations.

Chronic pain commonly outlives peripheral tissue injury or actual neural damage; yet, long-lasting changes in the modulations of pain due to neural plasticity and central sensitization have been well documented in various chronic pain conditions.[20,21] Neuroimaging studies in humans have demonstrated alterations in the reward, motivational, emotional, and cognitive brain centers that may play a role in establishing and/or maintaining chronic pain.[22–24] In addition, it has been hypothesized that some chronic pain syndromes may be maintained by dysregulation of homeostatic reward processes similar to those described in addiction neurobiology.[25] Addiction and chronic pain disorders may share central reward deficiency and motivational maladaptation patterns secondary to hypodopaminergic states in the nucleus accumbens core (NAc) and medial prefrontal cortex (mPFC) and alterations in endogenous pain transmission pathways.[26–28] Furthermore, a study in mice by Schwartz et al.[29] suggests that chronic pain induces synaptic changes within the NAc, which plays a central role in the neural circuitry that modulates motivation.[29,30] Such pain-induced synaptic changes can have a negative impact on patients' motivation,[29,31,32] which in turn could lead to difficulty in adhering to a treatment plan for their chronic pain.

In addition to the painful symptoms, individuals who have chronic pain often experience a multitude of quality of life–altering symptoms such as anxiety, depression, fatigue, sleep disturbance, elevated stress levels, activity reduction, and cognitive deficits.[31–34] Such comorbidities can further decrease motivation to initiate and complete goal-directed and higher order mental and physical tasks.[29] Thus, individuals can experience a twofold impairment of motivation secondary to both chronic pain itself and its comorbidities.

Concept of Readiness to Change: Transtheoretical Model of Behavior Change

The transtheoretical model of behavior change was developed in an attempt to understand motivation to adhere to health care regimens. The model offers an integrative framework describing the process of behavior change.[35] It was originally developed to understand how people change their addictive behaviors. The model, however, has been extended to many medical problems including chronic pain.[36] The basic assumptions underlying the model are the notions that people differ in their readiness and willingness to take on behavioral change and that there are certain processes of changes that facilitate the advancement of one's readiness. The model is organized around a major construct: stages of change.

According to the model, patients attempting to change health-related behavior move from one stage to another, often in a cyclic fashion (Fig. 88.1; description of each stage is in Table 88.1), although the movement through these stages is not necessarily linear or unidirectional. Some behaviors are easier to change than others; it is reasonable to assume that several attempts may be necessary to achieve significant behavioral change. A good example of the nonlinear change of stages may occur in smoking cessation where average smokers take seven to eight attempts to quit before succeeding.[37] The description of each stage as well as typical patient behavior seen at each stage point is listed in Table 88.1.

The model has been adapted to chronic pain. Kerns and colleagues[36] developed a self-report inventory "Pain Stages of Change Questionnaire" to assess the level of readiness to adopt self-management approach in chronic pain patients. Research has found the significant association between the stages of change and coping as well as disability of chronic pain patients.[38] Furthermore, improvement of the stages corresponds with better outcomes of pain rehabilitation.[39]

TABLE 88.1	Stages of Change	
Stages	**Descriptions**	**Patients' Behaviors**
Precontemplation	Patient does not perceive a need to change and actively resists change.	• Unwilling to discuss • "Who? Me?"
Contemplation	Patient begins to see a need for change and may consider making a change in the future.	• Somewhat ambivalent or fearful of change • "Yes, but . . . "
Preparation	Patient feels ready to change and takes a first concrete (behavioral) change.	• Sees more pros for change than cons • "I'll start this on Sunday!"
Action	Patient actively engages in behaviors consistent with regimen.	• Feels more confident
Maintenance	Patient executes plans to sustain the changes made.	• Feels comfortable with the change • Identifies self as the changed entity
Relapse	Some patients fail to sustain the effort.	Variable

There are three critical parameters of the model that determines the likelihood of advancing one's readiness.

1. **Processes of change** are one of the dimensions of the transtheoretical model that enables understanding of *how* shifts in behavior may be achieved. Change processes involve both covert and overt activities and experiences that patients engage in when they attempt to change their behavioral patterns. Each process is a broad category, and an eclectic collection of techniques, methods, and interventions can be recommended to facilitate the change process. Ten processes are cluster into two groups: the cognitive-experiential cluster of processes and the behavioral processes (Table 88.2). As can be seen (right-hand column of Table 88.2), there are various strategies that come from the disparate theoretical orientations to target each process.

2. **Self-efficacy** is defined as personal confidence in one's ability to change problematic situations.[40] If people think that there is no way that they can perform the prescribed activities, it is highly unlikely that they will initiate or persist in the desired behaviors and that the treatment will be successful.

3. **Decisional balance** is defined as a personal "balance sheet" of gains (benefits) and losses (costs) for changing and not changing their behaviors.[41] People are likely to advance their change stages when they (1) perceive themselves to have adequate skills to cope, (2) feel confident

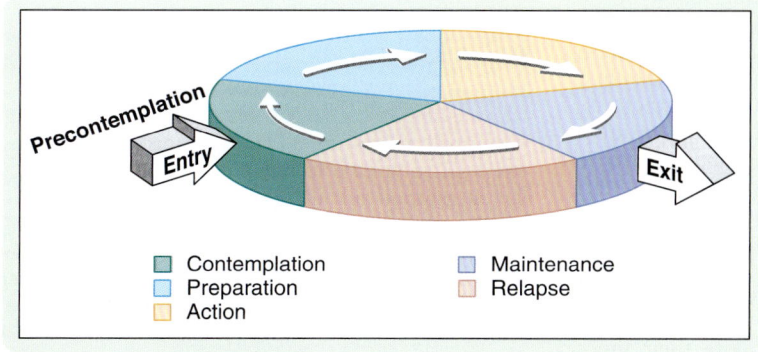

FIGURE 88.1 Stages of changes.

Contemplation
Preparation
Action
Maintenance
Relapse

TABLE 88.2	Processes of Change	
Processes	**Definition**	**Therapeutic Strategies That May Help Targeting the Process**
Experiential Processes		
Consciousness raising	Increasing information about self and problem	Observations, confrontations, interpretations, bibliotherapy
Self-reevaluation	Assessing how one feels and thinks about oneself with respect to a problem	Value clarification, imagery, corrective emotional experience
Dramatic relief	Experiencing and expressing feelings about one's problem and solutions	Role playing, psychodrama, grieving losses
Environmental reevaluation	Assessing how one's problems affect the physical environment	Empathy training, documentaries
Social liberation	Increasing alternatives for nonproblem behaviors available in society	Advocating for rights of repressed, empowering, policy interventions
Behavioral Processes		
Counterconditioning	Substituting alternatives for problem and anxiety related behaviors	Relaxation, desensitization, assertion, positive self-statements
Helping relationships	Being open and trusting about problems with someone who cares	Therapeutic alliance, social support, self-help groups
Reinforcement management	Rewarding oneself or being rewarded by others for making changes	Contingency contracts, overt and covert reinforcement, self-reward
Stimulus control	Avoiding stimuli that elicit problem behaviors	Adding stimuli that encourage alternative behaviors, restructuring one's environment, avoiding high-risk cues, fading techniques
Self-liberation	Choosing and committing to act or believe in ability to change	Decision-making therapy, resolution

in executing those skills (i.e., high efficacy belief), *and* (3) perceive more gains of changing and losses of not changing than more losses of changing and gains of not changing (decisional balance). We discuss the decisional balance process later in this chapter as a part of reviewing some motivational enhancement techniques.

Some of the behavioral strategies such as counterconditioning and stimulus control are generally a major part of the rehabilitation for chronic pain. The cognitive-behavioral self-management skill training that is typically a part of the pain rehabilitation also improves self-efficacy[42]; however, baseline levels of self-efficacy vary across patients, and there is a linear relationship between the baseline level of self-efficacy and posttreatment level of self-efficacy and subsequent treatment benefit self-management skill training.[43] Strategies targeting experiential processes are recommended as the primary approach to help people with low level of treatment readiness and self-efficacy.[44] Thus, using the concept of the change process seems a promising way to optimize the clinical outcomes of pain rehabilitation.

MOTIVATION ENHANCEMENT THERAPY

MET, developed by Miller,[45] is one of the therapeutic methods to target motivation and patient engagement with therapy. This approach is based on the transtheoretical model that people vary in their readiness to adhere to treatment regimen and provides a problem-focused, patient-centered, clinician-directed approach with the aim of helping patients move through the stages-of-change readiness. Although some of the techniques and approaches overlap with those of cognitive-behavioral therapy (CBT), one of the most prevalent behavioral medicine approaches in treating chronic pain patients, the two therapy approaches have some distinct characteristics. The nature of the therapy course is no doubt variable depending on the personal styles of the clinicians, and there is a danger of oversimplification of complex therapy modalities; however, for the sake of comparison and contrast, we summarize the characteristics of MET as compared to CBT in Table 88.3.

MET is nonconfrontational and patient-centered, exploring and reaching resolution of ambivalence toward behavior change. A MET clinician helps patients explore their inner phenomenology that is explored without judgment or criticism. In order to facilitate this process, MET encourages a clinician to exercise empathetic listening and to ask open-ended questions.

Asking open-ended questions helps the clinician to better understand the individualized phenomenology of the patient regarding the problem that is the target of behavior change in a nonthreatening manner. It also aids the patient to achieve a clearer view on the issue. Asking open-ended questions, however, is not time-efficient; asking questions that can be responded with a short "yes" or "no" answer can save time. As you can see in the following sections describing the MET techniques, however, asking open-ended questions is vital in successful implementation of MET. Some examples of open-ended and close-ended questions are listed in Table 88.4.

The MET offers a collection of therapeutic techniques to help patients (1) clearly recognize their problems, (2) perform decisional balance work, and (3) produce self-motivational statements and internalize those motivational statements by means of improved self-efficacy. MET also provides the guidance for how to handle resistance and setbacks. In the following section, we describe the basic MET methods, including how to deal with resistance and what not to do while engaging in MET. Although MET might be a treatment within itself, it may also serve as a complement to CBT and set the stage for patients to benefit from the skills included in CBT.

TABLE 88.3	Motivation Enhancement Therapy (MET) Versus Cognitive-Behavioral Therapy (CBT) Approaches	
	MET	**CBT**
Orientation	Patient-centered	Goal-oriented
Therapist–patient relationship	Collaborative	Top-down
Focus	Stage change	Action
Therapist's task	More listening	More talking
Dealing with ambivalence	Explore ambivalence	Direct persuasion
Approaches to reasons for change	Elicit reasons for change	Give reasons for change

TABLE 88.4 Close-ended Questions Versus Open-ended Questions: Examples

Close-ended Questions	Open-ended Questions
Are you having a problem exercising?	Tell me about the problem you are having about exercising.
Do you overuse your pain medications when your pain is really bad?	What do you do when your pain is really bad?
Would you be able to come to the clinic every week for trigger point injections?	How would you feel about coming to the clinic for trigger point injections?

Help Patients Recognize the Problems and Goals

Patients come to clinics with various expectations and goals. Some patients expect to be pain-free, whereas some patients focus on improving the quality of life even if pain is not totally resolved. However, many patients are often unaware of what should happen to achieve their goals and what their role should be for meeting the expectation. The next step to help patients become more aware of what needs to happen is to delineate the gap between where they are now and where they want to be when they get better. For example, the discussion may start with questions such as:

- How is your life different from your life before pain began?
- How has your pain stopped you from doing what you want to do?
- What are you now doing to cope with your pain problem? How is that working for you?
- How do you think your pain and disability impact your relationship with your spouse/family?
- What do you miss most about your life before the pain began?

Then, the discussion should be turned into what patients want to see happen through treatment. For example:

- What would your life look like with better pain management?
- What change would you like to see most?
- What are you doing now that is helping you to make these things happen?
- What other things could you do, or do more of, to help achieve your goal?

This line of discussion can also help identify specific discrepancy between what a patient wants from therapy (e.g., "I want to get well") and what he or she is doing (e.g., "I can't do my exercise because I am not well"). The process facilitates the realization of the possibility that patients' own behaviors contribute to the maintenance of pain and prevent them from obtaining their goal of "getting better." Such realization in turn can form a background on which motivation for behavioral change can be built.

Not only can clarification of the gap between a present state and a goal state help drive the motivation to change but it also serves to create the opportunity to move to specific plans. A clinician and patient can start "brainstorming" as to what possible ways there are to make the change probable. Plans can be prioritized by patients' preference and practical concerns as well as perceived effectiveness of the actions. Possible problems and obstacles should also be thoroughly explored to better prepare the patient.

It is common to find that the patient, after years of functional impairment and other related problems, feels very helpless and convinced that there is nothing they can do to manage their plight. Such resistance can seriously arrest the process of behavioral change. We discuss some ways to deal with resistance later in this chapter.

DECISIONAL BALANCE

Motivation for behavioral changes is rarely linear. Often, we may understand the need for behavioral change but remain reluctant to commit ourselves to do the things needed for the change. People experiencing persistent pain are no exception. Nearly all pain patients would want to improve, and many of them may intuitively understand how behavioral changes can help their pain. Despite this, many patients may remain feeling ambivalent or conflicted about committing themselves for behavioral change. One often hears comments like "I know I need to be more active, *but* . . . ."

To a large extent, activating rehabilitation and self-management pain care requires daily practice of the learned skills and modification of lifestyle, aiming at the long-term, gradual improvement. Thus, activities required for these approaches typically do occur immediately despite substantial effort involved. This tends to lead patients to focus more on immediate "cost" of self-management activities, such as postexercise soreness and time commitment. Decisional balance helps people explore all sides of the story on the consequences of not only "doing" but also "not doing" activities that they think need to be done.

The decisional balance procedure involves creating a personal "balance sheet" of both advantages and disadvantages of committing to change compared to not committing. For example, suppose that a clinician would like to facilitate a more active lifestyle for a patient who has dealt with pain by remaining sedentary and resting for years. The patient will be asked to list what they think are good things and not so good things about maintaining the status quo, in other words, not changing and keeping doing what they have been doing. The patient will also be asked to list good and not so good things about changing their way to be more active and keep functioning despite pain. An example of a "balance sheet" is shown in Table 88.5. The clinician can help patients explore the impact of the change and no change on various life domains and the emotional and cognitive consequences of their action (or nonaction). The sheet will help facilitate the resolution of the potential "I want to, but . . . " conflict. The section of "not so good" things about change can also help the clinician see what areas of coping and other supportive care can be implemented to increase the sense of self-efficacy for the change.

TABLE 88.5 Decisional Balance Sheet

Staying in Bed or Resting Every Time I Feel Pain (Status Quo)		Trying to Stay Active (Change)	
Good Things	**Not so Good Things**	**Good Things**	**Not so Good Things**
• Helps me rest • I will not get tired or sore.	• Life has to come to a halt. • I do not feel that good anyway. • I may get even more deconditioned. • I have to ask for help from others. • Cannot participate in social things • More depression • May gain weight • Will never be able to go back to work	• Things can get done • Keep in touch with friends • Feel better about the day • Feel more independent • May gain physical strength • Less burden on family	• I may feel worse. • I may feel stressed out.

SELF-MOTIVATIONAL STATEMENTS

Self-motivational statements or "change talks" by patients represent an important step toward better readiness for behavioral change. In MET, it is critical that thoughts reflecting their intention to change are discussed and help them internalize such thoughts. There are three steps in this phase. First, such thoughts should be elicited and verbalized. Then the thoughts need to be elaborated, as such thoughts, if remaining abstract, may result in perpetual wishful thinking with no actual behavioral change. And finally, elicitation and elaboration of such thoughts need to be reinforced. Going through this process helps patients identify problems and goals, and they then explore what it would mean to change versus not change. At this point, the patients may spontaneously come up with statements reflecting their willingness and intention to commit themselves for behavioral changes. If so, the therapy can start with the second step. However, for many chronic pain patients whose maladaptive habitual patterns are so ingrained in their lifestyles, some time may be devoted to help patients feel comfortable with change talks.

In order to guide a patient through this process, the clinician may ask questions such as:

- What encourages you that you can change if you want to?
- What do you think would work for you, if you decided to change?
- What will make (engaging in exercise program, etc.) it easier for you?

One of the supportive yet effective methods for the elicitation of self-motivational statements is to review past success. By recognizing that they were able to commit to change and were successful in doing so, it breeds the ground for optimism and improves the sense of self-efficacy. For example, in the earlier phase in treatment, the clinician may ask patient to list what and how they were able to change something in their lives, and guide the patient by asking

- What do you remember when you were able to . . . ?
- What was it like when you changed . . . ?
- When else in your life have you made a significant change? How did you do it?

Some patients may have a tendency to disregard past success and instead focus exclusively on past failures. It is also common to encounter the extremely negative cognitive style in which patients generalize past failure to all or many future actions. In a case like this, it is helpful to explore their previous failures and help them reframe the experience. Provision of education regarding outcome literature and how certain behaviors increase their probability of recovery may also be beneficial as serve as a means of encouragement and facilitate persistence even when initial positive effects may be modest.

It is extremely important for a clinician to recognize and acknowledge self-motivational statements. Typically, initial self-motivational statements are rather only vaguely directed toward the perceived needs (e.g., "I know I really need to take the home exercise program more seriously," "I am wondering if I should start thinking of how I can manage my anxiety better," "It may not be a bad idea for me to go back to work"). How such statements are responded to by the clinician can determine whether they can be transformed to more concrete motivation and actual behavioral actions. Basic responses by the clinicians should clarify the issue at hand in terms of how the change can be made based on what concerns. The statements can further be elaborated with responses like:

- Tell me in what ways *you* think you can do that.
- Sounds like *you* have some thoughts about it. What other concerns have *you* noticed about this problem?
- What are some reasons why *you* want to do this?
- How do you think *you* can enjoy this change?

Note that these statements focus on the patient's thoughts and not the clinicians. They are designed to engage the patient in the process of exploration.

The clinician must remain cautious during the process of elaboration. It is common to see that premature or presumptuous encouragement by the clinician can result in undue pressure for the patient. A discouraged patient is likely to become resistant to change. It is important to remember that MET is clinician-directed but patient-centered.

The attempts at self-motivational statements and subsequent elaborations should be positively reinforced. The clinician's encouraging responses can significantly impact the patient's frame of mind about the change. Simple comments such as "I think it's a wonderful idea," "I see how important this is to you," "You have a point there," and "You seem to have some useful insights" can help the process of eliciting self-motivational statements conclude in a positive and productive manner.

What Not to Do in Motivation Enhancement Therapy

One of the important aspects in MET is to avoid placing a patient in a passive role in the clinician–patient interaction. This is a very easy trap for the clinician to get in. For example:

Clinician: How long have you had this pain?
Patient: Seven years.
Clinician: Where does it hurt?
Patient: My back.
Clinician: Are you working now?
Patient: No.
Clinician: Are you receiving disability?
Patient: Yes.

The process like this is counterproductive for activating rehabilitation because it sets a tone of the treatment where the clinician is the expert who can tell what to do, whereas the patient is the passive recipient of the treatment.

We are not saying that a clinician should never provide advice. As an expert, a clinician can provide options and choices. What is important here is to emphasize that there are options and to help the patient achieve their own conclusion of what would work for him or her. Ultimate responsibility of behavioral change lies with the patient, and it should be communicated clearly through the MET process.

Value judgment by the clinician can also be detrimental in helping the patient increase motivation for behavioral change. Consider the following interaction:

Clinician: It seems that you are only interested in getting medications from us. You have not done anything we asked you to do such as exercise, habit change, and mood monitoring; no wonder you are not doing so well.
Patient: Well, I need my medicine because it takes some edge off my pain. I am not doing that badly. I am doing fine.

Value judgments by clinicians can elicit defensiveness, often leading patients to discount the very problem that needs to be addressed. "Oh, it's no big deal," and the change stage could return all the way back to the precontemplative stage (see Table 88.1 for the description of the stage). When the patients consider the problem "no problem," it is very hard, if not impossible, to motivate them for behavioral changes.

Dealing with Setbacks and Resistance

Changes are hard to make. As noted earlier, patients are likely to hold some ambivalence about committing to change, particularly when the change involves the fundamental part of their lifestyle. Resistance should be anticipated and is expected. It can occur at any phase of MET and may take various forms such as arguing, interrupting, denying, ignoring, challenging, minimizing, and sidetracking. Some example behaviors of these

TABLE 88.6   Examples of Resistance

Resistance	Behaviors
Arguing	Contests the accuracy of information or the clinician's expertise
Interrupting	Interrupts the clinician in a defensive manner
Denying	Shows unwillingness to admit/recognize problems
Ignoring	Does not follow the discussion or conversational direction
Challenging	Challenges the accuracy, effectiveness, or applicability of what the clinician says
Minimizing	Minimizes the risk of problem behaviors (or not doing something) or minimizing the benefit of change
Sidetracking	Changes the direction of the conversation away from the direction that the clinician was pursuing
Blaming	Blames others for the problem and does not acknowledge any responsibility for him or herself
Nonanswering	Gives a response that is no answer to the question asked
Disagreeing	"Yes, but . . . "—disagrees with a suggestion without offering any constructive alternative

resistance forms are listed in Table 88.6. One of the hallmarks of MET is that a clinician does not fight resistance but works with it. Too often, an eager clinician gets overdriven to argue for the change, only to find that the patient backs off from the previous self-motivational stance and becomes reluctant to commit. MET requires a clinician to direct a patient to move toward the behavioral change without imposing, ordering, or arguing for it. How do we do this? The approach here is to stay on the same side with patients yet help them to argue for change themselves. There are several specific techniques that a clinician can employ to work with resistance.

SIMPLE REFLECTION

In simple reflection, clinicians express their acknowledgment of the patients' comments that reflects resistance in a nonconfrontational manner. For example, patients may argue that they are too exhausted and sore to do the home exercise program after taking care of the household chores; the clinician may respond:

- I see that you are frustrated for not being able to make the change you want.
- It is hard for you to work out after a long day.

The simple reflection method is to provide the sense that the patient is heard and understood. Notice that the reflection does not have any hint of value judgment (e.g., "It is really too bad that you cannot save any energy to exercise because we are not asking you to do that much, you know"), which would defeat the purpose of the simple reflection technique that is to be used to signal that the patient's concern was heard and taken seriously.

AMPLIFIED REFLECTION

Amplified reflection is an applied variation of simple reflection in which the clinician reflects back the patient's comment in an overexaggerated manner. With the example of not being able to do the home exercise earlier, the clinician may respond, "You feel/believe that it is absolutely impossible for you to do the exercise."

The amplified reflection adds the core meaning or intensity of the emotion associated with the patient's statement. By doing so, it helps patient better see the balance of their ambivalence. Facing the exaggerated form of their own statement

often helps them focus more on the other side of their original comment. Consider a case where a patient complains of postexercise soreness.

Patient: I am so sore after doing those exercises that I cannot do anything but lay in bed for the rest of the day. The house is a mess and I do not feel better.
Clinician: There is absolutely no way that the exercise can help you get better.

The amplification must be done in an empathetic manner. There can be a fine line between empathetic amplification and sarcasm. The same statement earlier, with a slightly different tone, can be delivered as a sarcastic criticism. If the patient feels that the clinician is being sarcastic or inpatient, the reflection will likely encourage further resistance and retard the process of change.

DOUBLE-SIDED REFLECTION

Double-sided reflection is used to highlight the ambivalent feeling that the patient has expressed. With the example earlier, the clinician may respond, "On the one hand, you find it very difficult to incorporate exercise in your life, and at the same time, it is frustrating because you really want to do it."

Miller and Rollnick[46] recommend the use of "and" rather than "but" to bridge the two sides of the ambivalence. It also seems advisable that one ends the reflection with the motivational side, perhaps reflecting the motivational statement the patient has previously used.

AGREEMENT WITH TWIST

This is another variation of the reflection in which the clinician initially reflects and then reframes the patient's statement. Initial reflection is typically presented as an empathetic agreement, affirming that the patient was well heard. Then, the clinician offers a reframed perspective on the same subject in a nonthreatening manner. For example:

Patient: I know I do not do all the stuff the physical therapist wants me to do. But it is so hard, and I don't think she [the physical therapist] understands how hard it is for me to do the program every day.
Clinician: You have a point there. It is so frustrating for you not to be able to do the exercise, even though you are so anxious to find a way to do it and move forward with your program.

This subtle change in the direction can help the patient move further toward change while maintaining the therapeutic relationship.

PERSONAL CHOICE AND CONTROL

The psychotherapy literature suggests that one of the conditions in which resistance tends to arise is when a patient perceives a loss of, or a threat of losing, personal choice and control.[47] Typically, resistance is stronger when the importance of the threatened freedom is greater, often resulting in people asserting their option by doing something counteractive to the required behavior. In MET, it is essential that the affirmation of personal choice and control be reminded throughout the course of treatment that it is ultimately their choice to follow through the treatment recommendation. For example:

Patient: All of you keep telling me to do the home program, even though I keep telling you I do not want to do it.
Clinician: It is your choice, of course. It is your health after all. We can only make the recommendations and the rest is up to you.

Such an interaction can help the patients understand that the choice is theirs; at the same time, it fosters a sense of responsibility for the patients to commit to the treatment regimen.

SHIFTING FOCUS

Some patients, particularly those with tendency to "catastrophize" (i.e., a cognitive and emotional process that involves magnification of pain-related stimuli, feelings of helplessness, and a negative orientation toward pain) and use the black–white cognitive styles, tend to get trapped into the mode of "cannot do because . . . "; there is always a reason why they cannot do what they need or want to do. For them, obstacles and barriers to advance behavioral changes can become so great that such barriers could be the only thing on which they focus. This may become even more pronounced in the time of flare-up. Once they feel very discouraged by the flare-up episode, motivation to apply coping skills may dwindle. A clinician can defuse such intense focus and help the patient move out of the trap and onto the step necessary to make the desired change. For example:

Patient: I can't believe this! I thought I was doing so well with this program, but it must have been just all illusion! There is absolutely no way I am getting better. Pain always wins! I just should give up.
Clinician: I see your frustration. Having a bad day feels like such a setback. It sounds like pain really influences your life. Tell me more about the kind of things you would like to do in your life.

Shifting focus can help defuse the resistance and instead shift attention onto something that can be workable and supportive for behavioral change.

Research Outcomes

A growing body of research supports the conclusion that MET is effective in promoting healthful behaviors. Past research has shown that MET has been effective for facilitating change to reduce problem behaviors, such as smoking,[48,49] alcohol abuse,[50,51] problem gambling,[52] behaviors related to eating disorders,[53] and high-risk sexual behaviors.[54,55] MET has also been shown to increase wellness behaviors such as promoting exercise in myocardial infarction patients[56] and cancer survivors,[57] adherence with self-management regimen in diabetics,[58] and attendance for mammography screening.[59] MET has become a popular method to address obesity and research shows its efficacy for children[60] as well as adult diabetic patients.[61] MET has been shown to help normalize the lipid profiles of hyperlipidemic individuals via increased fitness.[56]

MET can easily be integrated in various clinical settings and with pain-oriented treatments such as CBT and physical therapy. Brief MET counseling in a primary care setting may reduce substance use among high-risk adolescents.[62] In a busy clinical setting, clinicians may regard a full course of MET difficult to implement. There is some evidence, however, that implementing even a small part of MET can be efficacious in promoting behavioral change. A recent study has reported that a brief MET provided at the emergency room setting significantly decreased aggressive behaviors in high-risk adolescents.[63] MET can also be implemented through phone counseling. Phone-based MET has been shown to help medication adherence[64] and promote healthy lifestyle in diabetics.[64]

Unfortunately, MET has not been extensively tested for pain patients, although there are some excellent chapters describing MET,[65–67] reflecting the growing awareness of the importance of motivation in pain treatment. Available evidence strongly suggests that the state of motivation for change is critical in better treatment outcomes for pain patients.[68] Furthermore, a recent study suggests that implementing MET prior to the initiation of the CBT-based self-management skill training for pain patients may enhance the treatment attendance.[47] A single-group study shows significant symptom reduction in fibromyalgia patients undergoing a brief exercise program with phone-based MET.[69]

A recent case series[70] for back pain patients also showed significant pain and medication reduction following MET combined with CBT.

Volitional Approach: Implementation Intentions

The idea of IIs aims to address the imperfect relationship between intentions to perform a certain behavior and actual behavioral engagement.[71] IIs involve practical action plans to deal with a range of contingencies; they require construction of "if-then" plans for foreseeable barriers and problems that may interfere with attaining the behavioral goal. Thus, IIs encompass a process of identifying potential barriers and situations and planning potential responses by means of resource findings and problem solving.[72] IIs typically involve two types of planning: action and coping.[73] Action planning involves determining when, where, and how to execute the target behavior, whereas coping planning offers a series of problem-solving exercises to handle potential barriers.

Suppose that one of the therapy goals is to help a patient become more physically active. The patient is well aware of the importance of activation and would very much like to be able to tolerate a greater level of activities so she could enjoy her life with her family. In this case, her intention to be active is strong. What IIs can do for her is to fill a gap between her strong intention and actual implementation of the behavior.

As suggested previously, IIs approaches have two phases: action planning and coping planning. For the action planning, all parameters of behaviors will be determined, including when, where, and how the target behaviors are executed. Action plans should be detailed, feasible, and practical. It should not be overly ambitious; starting out at the level that the patient can easily experience initial success may help foster a sense of self-efficacy.

Coping planning involves identification of potential barriers and preparation to address them. A portion of the session should be spent on identifying specific barriers that may keep the actualization of the behavior from happening. Barriers in various areas need to be considered, such as pain-related issues (e.g., actual or anticipated postactivity flare-ups), lack of time or resources, or interpersonal issues (e.g., family/friends support).

In order for effective coping planning, patients may benefit from acquiring basic problem solving skills. Typical problem-solving skill training[74] begins with the identification of specific problems; for each problem, the patient is asked to generate as many potential solutions as they can, no matter how implausible impossible they may seem. Then, the patient in collaboration with the therapist can systematically evaluate the feasibility and potential consequence of each approach. Based on the evaluation, the patient rank-orders the options and is encouraged to start trying one at the time from the highest ranked solution.

Similarly, acquisition of specific behavioral or cognitive skills that are typically included in a multimodal self-management rehabilitation for chronic pain may also be helpful. For example, self-management skill training for pain flare-ups, effective communication and social skills training, relaxation, and time management can be incorporated in the IIs coping planning to help address specific barriers. Applications of these skills should be well integrated in the coping planning by developing if (barrier)–then (coping) scenarios. For some barriers, behavioral rehearsal may be applied to help patient gain confidence for carrying out the planned behavior.

Each person likely has unique barriers to his or her situation. Those unique barriers also need to be identified and addressed in advance, anticipating the most likely difficulties they will encounter in trying to implement planned behavior. Clinicians should work collaboratively with patients to explore emotional, cognitive, and physical cues that are associated with barriers. Examples of IIs outlines are described in Table 88.7.

IMPLEMENTATION INTENTIONS: OUTCOMES

The IIs approach has been used to promote the patients' active involvement in modifying their own health behaviors including better eating habits,[75] addictive behaviors,[76] smoking,[77] weight loss,[78] medication adherence,[79] cancer screening,[80] vaccination,[81] and dental flossing.[82] A meta-analysis of 94 studies[72] found that II formation had a medium-to-large effect on goal attainment ($d = .65$). IIs have also been incorporated in a number of trials aiming to activate people with or without health concerns. A recent meta-analysis review also showed a large effect of IIs ($d = .99$) for achieving the goal behaviors among those with psychiatric conditions.[83] IIs may be particularly useful adjunct for activation therapy; IIs have been shown to be effective for improving physical activity levels in healthy young adults,[84] sedentary women,[85] obese elderly people,[86] cardiac patients,[87] and diabetic patients.[88] The meta-analytic review of the IIs on physical activity from 24 studies shows encouraging results with a pooled effect of .31 at posttreatment and .24 for follow-up visit with a higher effects shown with a program involving specific barrier management.[73] Interestingly, the coping pattern acquired through the IIs approach appears to generalize over and beyond the target behaviors,[89] likely helping patients become proficient to handle a range of challenges on their own. Although there is no study yet to show the effectiveness of the IIs approach for patients with chronic pain, the available evidence strongly suggests that the approach should be beneficial for improving

their ability to actively engage in the treatment and maintain their effort to perform self-management skills and is worth systematic investigation.

Conclusion

In this chapter, we have described and reviewed the approaches to address patients' motivation and engagement for treatments. Effective pain management often requires active engagement and adherence to prescribed regimens over long periods of time. We reviewed the theoretical basis of behavioral change and the basics of the therapeutic approaches to enhance motivation for change, MET and IIs. There are multiple areas of treatments that require significant behavioral, cognitive, and emotional changes for pain patients. Pain clinicians, across disciplines, often face behavioral issues, such as maladaptive behaviors related to medication use and resistance and nonadherence to exercise and other self-management behaviors, all of which become a significant hindrance for optimal treatment implementation. MET and IIs are two approaches that are designed help patients achieve behavioral goals and optimize treatment benefit. Although there is limited empirical evidence for MET and IIs in pain medicine, there are a growing number of studies in other areas demonstrating the efficacy of MET and IIs in reducing maladaptive behaviors and increasing wellness behaviors, suggesting that these approaches can be a powerful tool for pain clinicians as well. Although we present MET and IIs as stand-alone treatments, the concepts and strategies can be used to complement more traditional rehabilitation treatments.

References

1. Geen R. *Human Motivation: A Social Psychological Approach*. Pacific Grove, CA: Brooks/Cole; 1995.
2. Matthias MS, Bair MJ, Nyland KA, et al. Self-management support and communication from nurse care managers compared with primary care physicians: a focus group study of patients with chronic musculoskeletal pain. *Pain Manag Nurs* 2010;11:26–34.
3. Matthias MS, Miech EJ, Myers LJ, et al. An expanded view of self-management: patients' perceptions of education and support in an intervention for chronic musculoskeletal pain. *Pain Med* 2012;13:1018–1028.
4. Masek BJ. Compliance and medication. In: Doleys DN, Meredith RL, Ciminero AR, eds. *Behavioral Medicine: Assessment and Treatment Strategies*. New York: Plenum Press; 1982:527–545.
5. Timmerman L, Stronks DL, Groeneweg JG, et al. Prevalence and determinants of medication non-adherence in chronic pain patients: a systematic review. *Acta Anaesthesiol Scand* 2016;60:416–431.
6. Turk DC, Rudy TE. Neglected topics in the treatment of chronic pain patients—relapse, noncompliance, and adherence enhancement. *Pain* 1991;44:5–28.
7. Rapoff MA. *Adherence to Pediatric Medical Regimens*. 2nd ed. New York: Springer; 2010.
8. Logan D, Zelikovsky N, Labay L, et al. The Illness Management Survey: identifying adolescents' perceptions of barriers to adherence. *J Pediatr Psychol* 2003;28:383–392.
9. Hommel KA, Davis CM, Baldassano RN. Objective versus subjective assessment of oral medication adherence in pediatric inflammatory bowel disease. *Inflamm Bowel Dis* 2009;15:589–593.
10. Gatchel RJ, Okifuji A. Evidence-based scientific data documenting the treatment and cost-effectiveness of comprehensive pain programs for chronic nonmalignant pain. *J Pain* 2006;7:779–793.
11. Statistic Brain. Gym membership statistics. Available at: https://www.statisticbrain.com/gym-membership-statistics/. Accessed June 20, 2017.
12. U.S. Department of Health and Human Services. *Physical Activity and Health: A Report of the Surgeon General*. Atlanta, GA: Centers for Disease Control and Prevention, National Center for Chronic Disease Prevention; 1996.
13. Lutz RW, Silbret M, Olshan N. Treatment outcome and compliance with therapeutic regimens: long-term follow-up of a multidisciplinary pain program. *Pain* 1983;17:301–308.
14. Hayden JA, van Tulder MW, Malmivaara A, et al. Exercise therapy for treatment of non-specific low back pain. *Cochrane Database Syst Rev* 2005;(3):CD000335.
15. Oliver K, Cronan T. Predictors of exercise behaviors among fibromyalgia patients. *Prev Med* 2002;35:383–389.
16. Curran C, Williams AC, Potts HW. Cognitive-behavioral therapy for persistent pain: does adherence after treatment affect outcome? *Eur J Pain* 2009;13:178–188.

TABLE 88.7 Examples of Implementation Intentions Outlines for Specific Barriers to Activation Therapy

Barriers	Outline

Time management	• Clarifying values of exercise
	• If–then problem solving and action plans
	  • If there is not enough time to exercise because . . .
	    • Apply problem solving
	    • Develop action plans
	• Combating procrastination
	  • How procrastination happen
	  • Apply problem solving
	  • Develop action plans

Flare-ups	• Flare-up management
	  • What can we do
	  • Skill training for flare-up management
	  • If–then exercise
	  • Develop action plans

Support from others	• Interpersonal effectiveness
	  • Effective communication training
	  • Interpersonal effectiveness to improve relation with others
	  • If–then exercise
	  • Develop action plans

Resource management	• Available resources
	  • What are available within 10 min from home
	    • Parks, recreation centers, shopping area, trails
	• Things that make difficult to stick with regimen
	  • Weather, pain, stress, time, low motivation
	  • If–then exercise
	• Develop action plans using available resources

Adapted by permission from Springer: O'Donohue W, James L, Snipes C. *Practical Strategies and Tools to Promote Treatment Engagement*. 1st ed. Cham, Switzerland : Springer International Publishing; 2017:229–251. Table 14-2. Copyright © 2017 Springer International Publishing AG.

17. Nicholas MK, Asghari A, Corbett M, et al. Is adherence to pain self-management strategies associated with improved pain, depression and disability in those with disabling chronic pain? *Eur J Pain* 2012;16:93–104.

18. Meichenbaum DH, Turk DC. *Facilitating Treatment Adherence: A Practitioner's Guidebook*. New York: Plenum Press; 1987.

19. Schmidt L, Lebreton M, Clery-Melin ML, et al. Neural mechanisms underlying motivation of mental versus physical effort. *PLoS Biol* 2012;10:e1001266.

20. Kim W, Kim SK, Nabekura J. Functional and structural plasticity in the primary somatosensory cortex associated with chronic pain. *J Neurochem* 2017;141:499–506.

21. Tajerian M, Clark JD. Nonpharmacological interventions in targeting pain-related brain plasticity. *Neural Plast* 2017;2017:2038573.

22. Apkarian AV, Baliki MN, Farmer MA. Predicting transition to chronic pain. *Curr Opin Neurol* 2013;26:360–367.

23. Apkarian AV, Baliki MN, Geha PY. Towards a theory of chronic pain. *Prog Neurobiol* 2009;87:81–97.

24. Ng SK, Urquhart DM, Fitzgerald PB, et al. The relationship between structural and functional brain changes and altered emotion and cognition in chronic low back pain: a systematic review of MRI and fMRI studies. *Clin J Pain* 2018;34(3):237–261.

25. Elman I, Borsook D. Common brain mechanisms of chronic pain and addiction. *Neuron* 2016;89:11–36.

26. Maarrawi J, Peyron R, Mertens P, et al. Differential brain opioid receptor availability in central and peripheral neuropathic pain. *Pain* 2007;127:183–194.

27. Harris RE, Clauw DJ, Scott DJ, et al. Decreased central mu-opioid receptor availability in fibromyalgia. *J Neurosci* 2007;27:10000–10006.

28. Marbach JJ, Richlin DM, Lipton JA. Illness behavior, depression and anhedonia in myofascial face and back pain patients. *Psychother Psychosom* 1983;39:47–54.

29. Schwartz N, Temkin P, Jurado S, et al. Chronic pain. Decreased motivation during chronic pain requires long-term depression in the nucleus accumbens. *Science* 2014;345:535–542.

30. Mogenson GJ, Jones DL, Yim CY. From motivation to action: functional interface between the limbic system and the motor system. *Prog Neurobiol* 1980;14:69–97.

31. Nicholson B, Verma S. Comorbidities in chronic neuropathic pain. *Pain Med* 2004;5(suppl 1):S9–S27.

32. Turk DC, Audette J, Levy RM, et al. Assessment and treatment of psychosocial comorbidities in patients with neuropathic pain. *Mayo Clin Proc* 2010;85:S42–S50.

33. Bushnell MC, Ceko M, Low LA. Cognitive and emotional control of pain and its disruption in chronic pain. *Nat Rev Neurosci* 2013;14:502–511.

34. Jonsson T, Christrup LL, Hojsted J, et al. Symptoms and side effects in chronic non-cancer pain: patient report vs. systematic assessment. *Acta Anaesthesiol Scand* 2011;55:69–74.

35. Prochaska J, DiClemente C. *The Transtheoretical Approach: Towards a Systematic Eclectic Framework*. Homewood, IL: Dow Jones Irwin; 1984.

36. Kerns RD, Rosenberg R, Jamison RN, et al. Readiness to adopt a self-management approach to chronic pain: the Pain Stages of Change Questionnaire (PSOCQ). *Pain* 1997;72:227–234.

37. Crane R. The most addictive drug, the most deadly substance: smoking cessation tactics for the busy clinician. *Prim Care* 2007;34:117–135.

38. Jensen MP, Nielson WR, Turner JA, et al. Readiness to self-manage pain is associated with coping and with psychological and physical functioning among patients with chronic pain. *Pain* 2003;104:529–537.

39. Kerns RD, Rosenberg R. Predicting responses to self-management treatments for chronic pain: application of the pain stages of change model. *Pain* 2000;84:49–55.

40. Bandura A. Self-efficacy: toward a unifying theory of behavioral change. *Psychol Rev* 1977;84:191–215.

41. Mann L. Use of a "balance sheet" procedure to improve quality of personal decision making: a field experiment with college applicants. *J Vocat Behav* 1972;2:291–300.

42. Gowans SE, deHueck A, Voss S, et al. A randomized, controlled trial of exercise and education for individuals with fibromyalgia. *Arthritis Care Res* 1999;12:120–128.

43. Buckelew SP, Huyser B, Hewett JE, et al. Self-efficacy predicting outcome among fibromyalgia subjects. *Arthritis Care Res* 1996;9:97–104.

44. Prochaska J, Velicer W, DiClemente C, et al. Pattens of change: dynamic typology applied to smoking cessation. *Multivariate Behav Res* 1991;26:83–107.

45. Miller W. Motivational interviewing with problem drinkers. *Behav Psychother* 1983;11:147–172.

46. Miller W, Rollnick S. *Motivational Interviewing: Preparing People for Change*. 2nd ed. New York: Guilford Press; 2002.

47. Brehm SS, Brehm JW. *Psychological Reactance: A Theory of Freedom and Control*. New York: Wiley; 1981.

48. Auer R, Gencer B, Tango R, et al. Uptake and efficacy of a systematic intensive smoking cessation intervention using motivational interviewing for smokers hospitalised for an acute coronary syndrome: a multicentre before-after study with parallel group comparisons. *BMJ Open* 2016;6:e011520.

49. Lindson-Hawley N, Thompson TP, Begh R. Motivational interviewing for smoking cessation. *Cochrane Database Syst Rev* 2015;(3):CD006936.

50. Walker DD, Walton TO, Neighbors C, et al. Randomized trial of motivational interviewing plus feedback for soldiers with untreated alcohol abuse. *J Consult Clin Psychol* 2017;85:99–110.

51. Brown TG, Dongier M, Ouimet MC, et al. Brief motivational interviewing for DWI recidivists who abuse alcohol and are not participating in DWI intervention: a randomized controlled trial. *Alcohol Clin Exp Res* 2010;34:292–301.

52. Yakovenko I, Quigley L, Hemmelgarn BR, et al. The efficacy of motivational interviewing for disordered gambling: systematic review and meta-analysis. *Addict Behav* 2015;43:72–82.

53. Macdonald P, Hibbs R, Corfield F, et al. The use of motivational interviewing in eating disorders: a systematic review. *Psychiatry Res* 2012;200:1–11.

54. Tucker JS, D'Amico EJ, Ewing BA, et al. A group-based motivational interviewing brief intervention to reduce substance use and sexual risk behavior among homeless young adults. *J Subst Abuse Treat* 2017;76:20–27.

55. Rongkavilit C, Wang B, Naar-King S, et al. Motivational interviewing targeting risky sex in HIV-positive young Thai men who have sex with men. *Arch Sex Behav* 2015;44:329–340.

56. Hardcastle SJ, Taylor AH, Bailey MP, et al. Effectiveness of a motivational interviewing intervention on weight loss, physical activity and cardiovascular disease risk factors: a randomised controlled trial with a 12-month post-intervention follow-up. *Int J Behav Nutr Phys Act* 2013;10:40.

57. Spector D, Deal AM, Amos KD, et al. A pilot study of a home-based motivational exercise program for African American breast cancer survivors: clinical and quality-of-life outcomes. *Integr Cancer Ther* 2014;13:121–132.

58. Chen SM, Creedy D, Lin HS, et al. Effects of motivational interviewing intervention on self-management, psychological and glycemic outcomes in type 2 diabetes: a randomized controlled trial. *Int J Nurs Stud* 2012;49:637–644.

59. Bernstein J, Mutschler P, Bernstein E. Keeping mammography referral appointments: motivation, health beliefs, and access barriers experienced by older minority women. *J Midwifery Womens Health* 2000;45:308–313.

60. Resnicow K, Harris D, Wasserman R, et al. Advances in motivational interviewing for pediatric obesity: results of the Brief Motivational Interviewing to reduce body mass index trial and future directions. *Pediatr Clin North Am* 2016;63:539–562.

61. West DS, DiLillo V, Bursac Z, et al. Motivational interviewing improves weight loss in women with type 2 diabetes. *Diabetes Care* 2007;30:1081–1087.

62. Mason M, Pate P, Drapkin M, et al. Motivational interviewing integrated with social network counseling for female adolescents: a randomized pilot study in urban primary care. *J Subst Abuse Treat* 2011;41:148–155.

63. Carter PM, Walton MA, Zimmerman MA, et al. Efficacy of a universal brief intervention for violence among urban emergency department youth. *Acad Emerg Med* 2016;23:1061–1070.

64. Palacio AM, Uribe C, Hazel-Fernandez L, et al. Can phone-based motivational interviewing improve medication adherence to antiplatelet medications after a coronary stent among racial minorities? A randomized trial. *J Gen Intern Med* 2015;30:469–475.

65. Jensen M. Enhancing motivation to change in pain treatment. In: Gatchel R, Turk D, eds. *Psychological Approaches to Pain Management*. New York: Guilford Press; 1996:78–111.

66. Jones KD, Burckhardt CS, Bennett JA. Motivational interviewing may encourage exercise in persons with fibromyalgia by enhancing self efficacy. *Arthritis Rheum* 2004;51:864–867.

67. Turk D, Okifuji A, Sherman J. Psychologic aspects of back pain: implications for physical therapists. In: Twomey L, Taylor J, eds. *Physical Therapy of the Low Back*. New York: Churchill Livingstone; 2000:351–384.

68. Heapy A, Otis J, Marcus KS, et al. Intersession coping skill practice mediates the relationship between readiness for self-management treatment and goal accomplishment. *Pain* 2005;118:360–368.

69. Ang D, Kesavalu R, Lydon JR, et al. Exercise-based motivational interviewing for female patients with fibromyalgia: a case series. *Clin Rheumatol* 2007;26:1843–1849.

70. Jerome J, Topham R, Dematatis A, et al. Treatment outcomes after combination interventional and cognitive motivational counseling on analgesic medication use in patients with chronic spine pain. *Pain Physician* 2015;18:287–297.

71. Gollwitzer PM. Goal achievement: the role of intentions. *Eur Rev Soc Psychol* 1993;4:141–185.

72. Gollwitzer PM, Sheeran P. Implementation intentions and goal achievement: a meta-analysis of effects and processes. *Adv Exp Soc Psychol* 2006;38:69–119.

73. Belanger-Gravel A, Godin G, Amireault S. A meta-analytic review of the effect of implementation intentions on physical activity. *Health Psychol Rev* 2013;7:23–54.

74. Nezu AM, Perri MG. Social problem-solving therapy for unipolar depression: an initial dismantling investigation. *J Consult Clin Psychol* 1989;57:408–413.

75. Adriaanse MA, Vinkers CD, De Ridder DT, et al. Do implementation intentions help to eat a healthy diet? A systematic review and meta-analysis of the empirical evidence. *Appetite* 2011;56:183–193.

76. Webb TL, Sniehotta FF, Michie S. Using theories of behaviour change to inform interventions for addictive behaviours. *Addiction* 2010;105:1879–1892.

77. Armitage CJ. A volitional help sheet to encourage smoking cessation: a randomized exploratory trial. *Health Psychol* 2008;27:557–566.

78. Armitage CJ, Alganem S, Norman P. Randomized controlled trial of a volitional help sheet to encourage weight loss in the Middle East. *Prev Sci* 2017;18:976–983.

79. Meslot C, Gauchet A, Hagger MS, et al. A randomised controlled trial to test the effectiveness of planning strategies to improve medication adherence in patients with cardiovascular disease. *Appl Psychol Health Well Being* 2017;9:106–129.

80. Browne JL, Chan AY. Using the theory of planned behaviour and implementation intentions to predict and facilitate upward family communication about mammography. *Psychol Health* 2012;27:655–673.

81. Milkman KL, Beshears J, Choi JJ, et al. Using implementation intentions prompts to enhance influenza vaccination rates. *Proc Natl Acad Sci U S A* 2011;108:10415–10420.

82. Schuz B, Wiedemann AU, Mallach N, et al. Effects of a short behavioural intervention for dental flossing: randomized-controlled trial on planning when, where and how. *J Clin Periodontol* 2009;36:498–505.

83. Toli A, Webb TL, Hardy GE. Does forming implementation intentions help people with mental health problems to achieve goals? A meta-analysis of experimental studies with clinical and analogue samples. *Br J Clin Psychol* 2016;55:69–90.

84. Prestwich A, Perugini M, Hurling R. Can implementation intentions and text messages promote brisk walking? A randomized trial. *Health Psychol* 2010;29:40–49.

85. Arbour KP, Martin Ginis KA. A randomised controlled trial of the effects of implementation intentions on women's walking behaviour. *Psychol Health* 2009;24:49–65.

86. Belanger-Gravel A, Godin G, Bilodeau A, et al. The effect of implementation intentions on physical activity among obese older adults: a randomised control study. *Psychol Health* 2013;28:217–233.

87. Sniehotta FF, Scholz U, Schwarzer R. Action plans and coping plans for physical exercise: a longitudinal intervention study in cardiac rehabilitation. *Br J Health Psychol* 2006;11:23–37.

88. Thoolen BJ, de Ridder D, Bensing J, et al. Beyond good intentions: the role of proactive coping in achieving sustained behavioural change in the context of diabetes management. *Psychol Health* 2009;24:237–254.

89. Bieleke M, Legrand E, Mignon A, et al. More than planned: implementation intention effects in non-planned situations. *Acta Psychol (Amst)* 2017;184:64–74.

CHAPTER **89**

Basic Concepts in Biomechanics and Musculoskeletal Rehabilitation

MAUREEN YOUNG SHIN NOH, BENJAMIN C. SOYDAN, and **ANAND B. JOSHI**

Clinical pain training has historically focused on the following categories: type, location (usually tied to a specific offending joint), and psychological components of pain. Musculoskeletal pain generators do not neatly fit into these categories. These pain generators are often regional, a consequence of the body's biomechanical function against Earth's gravitational pull, and subject to the will and desire of the individual person. For example, the pain generator in medial compartment knee osteoarthritis can be viewed as the knee joint complex in which targeted treatments such as medications, injections, or surgery can be considered. Alternately (or perhaps ideally, simultaneously), the pain generator could be viewed as all the biomechanical considerations of strength, flexibility, and gait which lead the patient to place increased mechanical stress on the medial knee compartment, therefore worsening pain and joint pathology. In that light, a combination of exercise, weight loss, and specific gait training can decrease medial knee joint loads and therefore treat the painful area.[1]

By emphasizing biomechanical principles, the contents of this chapter represent a fundamental change from the customary emphasis on the use of passive physical therapy and physical modalities in treating musculoskeletal pain. Patients are often treated for musculoskeletal disorders with passive modalities such as hot packs, cold packs, massage, electrical stimulation, and deep heat. Unfortunately, these passive therapies are overused. Although they certainly can play an important role in providing symptomatic relief of musculoskeletal pain, passive modalities should be used only as methods to facilitate active rehabilitation. The patient most needs to become actively involved in a therapeutic exercise program specifically designed to improve musculoskeletal functioning.

Musculoskeletal rehabilitation is a process whereby poor posture, muscle imbalances, and other biomechanical deficits are corrected using specific exercises to gain better static and dynamic control of the musculoskeletal system. The physical restoration process may involve passive therapeutic modalities to facilitate the exercise program. Clinicians treating musculoskeletal pain and dysfunction must identify and work to correct deficits in the patient's biomechanics.

The goal of this chapter is to provide an overview of a biomechanical approach to assessing and managing patients with musculoskeletal pain. This chapter reviews basic concepts in biomechanical assessment, followed by examples of common painful syndromes and their biomechanical considerations. Clinical applications of physical modalities are outside the intention of this chapter and are discussed elsewhere in this book.

Basic Considerations

Key considerations in musculoskeletal rehabilitation include but are not limited to the following concepts: kinetic chain theory, adverse neural tension, and neuromuscular control. In addition, biomechanical considerations in the setting of common physical examination techniques can aid the clinician in evaluating ineffective movement patterns which can precipitate or reinforce pain. As the patient is an active participant in the examination, he or she too is made aware of his or her alternate movement patterns which may positively reinforce the process for correction.

KINETIC CHAIN THEORY

The underpinning of modern kinetic chain theory was pioneered by Franz Reuleaux, a German mechanical engineer as well as author. Reuleaux's works in the late 1800s, inclusive of *The Kinematics of Machinery*, emphasized the relationship among mechanical links or "kinematic pairings." He theorized that any mechanistic movement could be broken down into these fundamental pairings and that the sequences of movement within and between these pairs produced a resultant "kinematic chain" directly related to constraints placed on them.[2] Therefore, movements at one location directly affected movements at another location in the mechanical link.[3] Although kinematics relate more strictly to description of movement, it can be assumed that kinetics (forces that cause motion) can be used to explain kinematic relationships.

Arthur Steindler, an orthopedic surgeon and professor at the University of Iowa, adapted these theories into the analysis of human movement.[4] Steindler was very involved in analysis of movement and pain associated with a variety of orthopedic diagnoses, including scoliosis, foot deformities, and back pain as well as upper and lower extremity reconstruction.[5] Steindler proposed that the segments in the human body be thought of as rigid, overlapping units in series, where successively arranged joints create an overlying kinetic chain and ultimately a collection of multisegmental movement patterns. He divided these movements into two categories: open kinetic (where the terminal segment moves freely) and closed kinetic (the terminal segment is restrained from free motion). It is acknowledged, however, that, unlike machines, no motion of the human body is "true" closed chain, as there always exist some component or segment that is unrestricted during movement (whether it be upper or lower body).[4]

Regardless of whether or not a kinetic chain is open or closed, in order to achieve a desired human movement pattern two kinetic chain variables of interest are considered: adequate range of motion (ROM) (kinematic element) and adequate force production (kinetic element). In the assessment of musculoskeletal pain, it should not and cannot be assumed that each joint has adequate freedom and/or strength to achieve the desired movement pattern (neuromuscular control plays a significant role but is to be discussed in a later section in more detail). One may present with inadequate strength and/or inadequate ROM at a particular joint, thereby lending to a compensatory faulty movement pattern (and likely undue tissue stress) at any given joint involved in the movement.

A prime example of a faulty closed chain movement pattern is that of a flexible foot deformity leading to excessive subtalar joint (STJ) pronation and/or delayed return to supination during gait propulsion. In a weight-bearing position, STJ pronation is correlated with a position of knee flexion, valgus, and medial tibial rotation.[6] If one is unable to adequately control STJ pronation during the initial loading phase or propulsion phase of gait, the knee will be placed in a position of excessive medial tibial rotation, valgus, and flexion. This may lend to excessive stress on supporting structures such as the medial collateral ligament and patellofemoral joint. However, if tissue structures at the knee fail to control motion adequately, the femur may then incur excessive internal rotational forces, and in such cases, the hip or even the sacroiliac (SI) joint may be affected.[6]

In this example, the variable of concern is not a restricted ROM but rather inadequate strength or control to adequately maintain proper positions within a closed kinetic chain movement. This is one isolated example but lends insight into concerns of any multijoint movement (running, walking, bending, throwing, etc.). Although a patient may present with a localized tissue or joint insult, it is paramount that any clinician receiving a patient reporting localized pain acknowledge the role of faulty movement mechanics in the assessment of pain etiology and appropriate management.

ADVERSE NEURAL TENSION

When observing an athletic contest or a performance art, one can appreciate movement of the human body. Although the primary function of the nervous system is to conduct impulses, the nervous system must also be able to move along with the rest of the body. However, in addition to movement alone, nervous system function is also dependent on normal physiology. *Neurodynamics* refers to the interactions between nervous system mechanics and physiology.[7] *Adverse neural tension* is a subset of neurodynamic theory that specifically deals with abnormal mechanical responses of the nervous system as its tissues are taken through a ROM.[8] Due to commonality of use, we use the term *adverse neural tension* (ANT) in this chapter.

Literature on "nerve stretching" can be found as far back as the 1880s.[9,10] Although a full review of the underpinnings of ANT theory is beyond the scope of this book, a bedrock principle for the pain clinician is that abnormalities in nervous system movement or physiology can provoke symptoms.[7] Failure to engage in the protective adaptions mentioned earlier renders the nervous system vulnerable to edema, ischemia, fibrosis, and hypoxia.[11,12]

Testing for ANT can be made a part of the clinical evaluation based on the patient's presentation. The best known test is the straight-leg raise (SLR). However, evaluations for many other peripheral nerves are possible and should be considered when a patient presents with limb pain or paresthesia with movement, or restricted ROM. The nervous system's sensitivity to movement can be considered as a proxy of its physiology, including blood flow, ion channel activity, and inflammation.[13] Therefore, the aim of a neural tension evaluation is to test the mechanics and physiology of the nervous system.[13] Findings of ANT may suggest the need for *neural mobilization*, which aims

to facilitate nerve gliding, reduce nerve adherence, disperse noxious fluids, increase nerve vascularity, and improve axoplasmic flow.[11]

Shacklock[7] has elegantly summarized the connection between the musculoskeletal and nervous systems: Very simply, the musculoskeletal system is felt to be the mechanical interface to the nervous system. This interface occurs at both central and peripheral levels. Centrally, the mechanical interface consists of the cranial and spinal canals, which contain the central nervous system, cranial nerves, and spinal nerve roots. Peripherally, the nervous system interfaces with bone, muscle, joints, and other tissues. The critical concept for the clinician to recollect when evaluating pain is that as the body moves, the mechanical interface between the musculoskeletal and nervous systems changes dimensions, placing force and deformation on nerve structures, which may potentially generate pain or other symptoms.[7]

The nervous system must be able to adapt to mechanical loads and may undergo a variety of adaptations in order to do so, such as nerve elongation, sliding, cross-sectional change, angulation, and compression.[11] As an example, the SLR is a commonly used provocation test that has been shown to displace not only the lumbar nerve roots[14,15] but more proximal structures such as the conus medullaris as well.[16–18] During elbow flexion, the ulnar nerve will lengthen while the median and radial nerves will shorten.[12] Additionally, sliding movements are also possible. The median nerve has a mean displacement of 2.09 mm with fist motion of healthy volunteers.[19] Median nerve displacement is reduced in patients with carpal tunnel syndrome (CTS) when compared to normal volunteers, with smaller amounts of median nerve motion seen when comparing mild to severe CTS.[20]

Several physical examination maneuvers are available to assist the clinician in determining whether ANT is present and related to the patient's presenting complaints. Commonly used neural tension tests are detailed in the following text (images courtesy of Michael Schmidt, PT, DPT, and Preston Roundy, PT, DPT).

Lower Limb

Straight-leg raise: The SLR is among the most commonly performed evaluations of patients with neuropathic leg pain. Performance is straightforward: The patient is positioned supine. The knee of the symptomatic leg is kept extended, and the leg is flexed at the hip (Fig. 89.1).

A positive response will provoke the patient's typical leg pain, frequently cited as being between 30 and 70 degrees.[13]

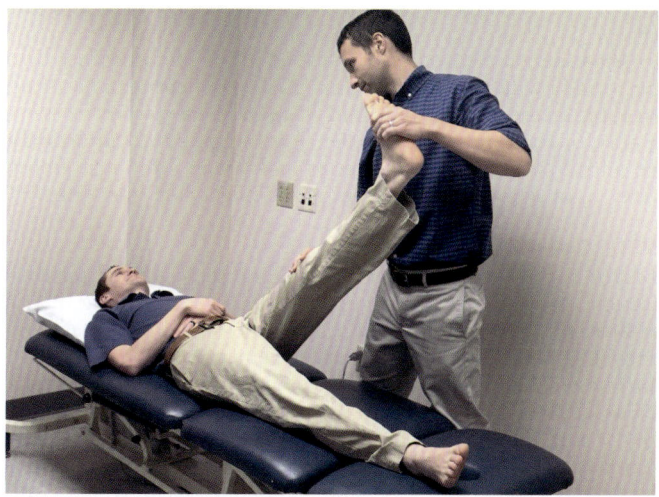

FIGURE 89.1 Straight-leg raise.

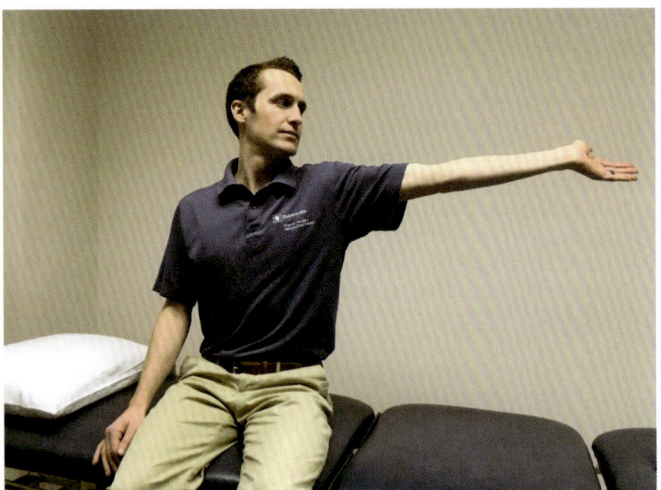

FIGURE 89.2 Median nerve A.

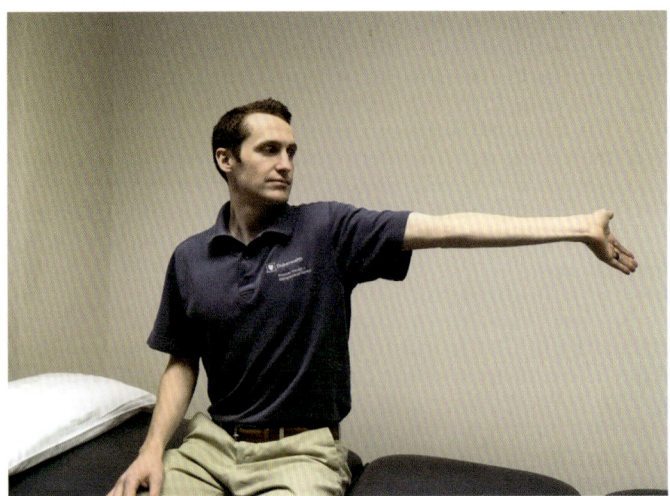

FIGURE 89.3 Median nerve B.

Upper Limb

Neurodynamic testing of the upper limb can be likened to straight-leg raising of the arm. The median, ulnar, and radial nerves can all be evaluated. Although passive positioning of the patient is possible, patients actively positioning themselves is most straightforward. If provocation of symptoms is not achieved with limb positioning alone, additional stress may be incorporated through neck or shoulder positioning.

Median nerve: Neurodynamic testing of the median nerve may be considered when upper limb pain is speculated to be neuropathic and possibly localized to the median nerve pathways, provoked with forearm pronation or supination, or nerve conduction testing suggests median nerve injury.[13] The patient can be asked to look at the palm, extend the elbow, and then extend the arm until it comes level to the head. A positive test would provoke the patient's typical arm symptoms at any step of this test (Figs. 89.2 and 89.3).

Radial nerve: Neurodynamic evaluation of the radial nerve may be considered when the patient presents with lateral elbow pain or a diagnosis of lateral epicondylitis. A very straightforward way to perform this test is for the patient to actively perform it. The patient can be instructed to hold the arm to the side, flex the wrist, internally rotate the arm, and look at the palm over the shoulder. Subsequently, the patient should be asked to depress the shoulder girdle (by "pushing the wrist to the floor") and to laterally flex the neck (by "looking away"). A positive test would provoke typical lateral arm symptoms (Fig. 89.4).[13]

Ulnar nerve: Neurodynamic testing of the ulnar nerve is best performed with the elbow in flexion. The patients can be asked to look at their hand and hold it up as if they were carrying a tray of food at their shoulder. Additional provocation may be added by asking the patient to look away, add more elbow flexion, or depress the shoulder girdle (Figs. 89.5 and 89.6).[13]

NEUROMUSCULAR CONTROL

Motor control is often overlooked in musculoskeletal rehabilitation. A muscle or muscle group may be quite strong, but if it does not fire at the appropriate time (within a synergistic movement pattern), the proper movement pattern is already forfeited. The muscle might as well not fire at all. Neuromuscular control is a combination of sensory feedback from the body part, premotor planning, and motor execution.[21,22] Impairments in any of these pathways can lead to altered mechanics of movement with a resultant musculoskeletal dysfunction and pain.

This is commonly seen in persistent pain after ankle inversion injuries as well as patellofemoral pain. Normal neuromuscular control can be lost through injury or disuse and but can be regained through appropriate retraining.[23] In addition, the effects of neuromuscular training can be seen in those without pain, in the setting of sports performance enhancement independent of strength gains.[24]

Proprioceptive neuromuscular facilitation uses predictable patterns to facilitate efficient muscle movement. These exercises are often prescribed as balance or proprioceptive in nature. Proper movement patterns require properly timed muscle activation. For example, when lifting an object, a person must first fire the foot and ankle muscles to stabilize the feet on the ground. Then, one must fire the thigh muscles to stabilize the

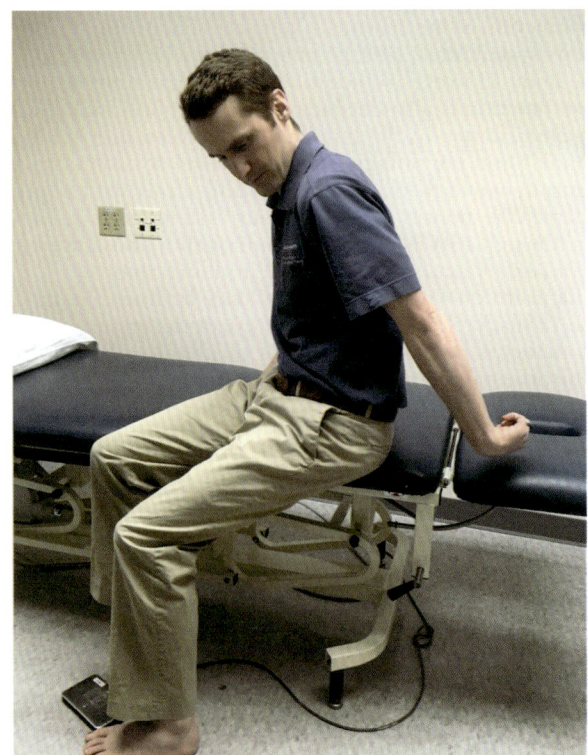

FIGURE 89.4 Radial nerve.

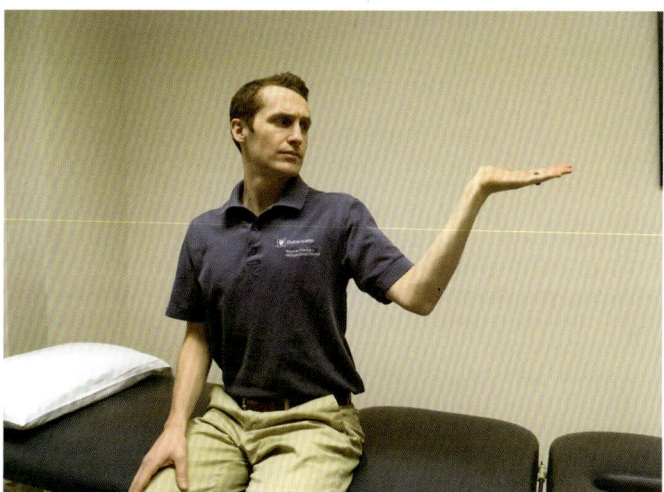

FIGURE 89.5   Ulnar nerve A.

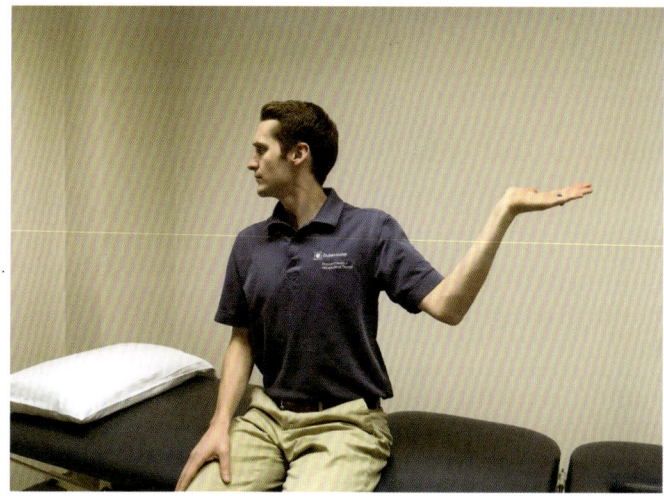

FIGURE 89.6   Ulnar nerve B.

knee. Next, the hip girdle muscles must stabilize the pelvis before the spine extensors can elevate the torso. If the gluteus maximus fails to fire before the erector spinae fires, the pelvis will remain anteriorly tilted and abnormal motion will occur in the lumbar spine.

Corrective technique focuses on the pattern of movement rather than the overall strength gains, which can explain why traditional gym exercises do not necessarily correlate to improvement in pain. This is a key concept in explaining why use of physical and occupational therapy for pain syndromes can be helpful even in the active population.

BIOMECHANICAL CONSIDERATIONS IN THE SETTING OF COMMON PHYSICAL EXAMINATION TECHNIQUES

In the setting of pain, the goal of any proper patient examination is to not only elucidate the painful complaint but also hypothesize causation of pain. In doing so, one must consider the biomechanical nature of musculoskeletal pain syndromes. Basic tenets such as inspection, palpation, and ROM may be highly informative and help achieve a more comprehensive interventional plan.

Inspection: Evaluation of the patient begins with visual inspection. Pattern of shoe wear, assistive device usage, brace needs, general posture, and habitus as well as gross movement patterns during standing, walking, and transfers are significant considerations. These observations provide an overall view of how the patient moves about his or her environment and help the clinician to discern what may be gross mechanical abnormalities.

Palpation: Palpation provides the clinician with information about generalized tenderness, potential targets for injection, tissue texture, and also pain patterns. Kinetic chain abnormalities will often present with palpable pain patterns. For example, patellofemoral pain has been associated with iliotibial band, hamstring, and gastrocsoleus restrictions as well as leg length discrepancies, hip muscle dysfunction, overpronation, patellar malalignment, and patellar hypermobility.[25] Given these biomechanical correlations, a patient with patellofemoral pain has the potential to demonstrate tenderness about the ipsilateral SI joint, greater trochanter, iliotibial band, pes anserine, or medial tibial structures as well. The clinician is thus cued to treat distant areas of dysfunction in order to affect pain at the site of concern.

Range of motion: Lack of adequate ROM may be the most common biomechanical deficit seen and one of the easiest to address. Deficits in ROM can cause pain directly or may lead to pain elsewhere. The musculoskeletal clinician must have knowledge of normative values, employ adequate examination skills to identify major ROM limitations, decide which of these contribute most significantly to the patient's symptoms, and implement appropriate therapies to correct the deficits. For example, during gait, an ankle plantar flexion contracture can cause excessive knee extension and resultant increased hip flexion and forward trunk lean. According to kinetic chain theory, one must address ankle mechanics to normalize the dysfunction at the knee, hip, and spine. This may be required to facilitate adequate pain intervention.[26] ROM restrictions can be due to shortening of muscle-tendon units, restrictions in joint capsule distensibility, ANT, or bone-on-bone contact at joint interfaces. The first three conditions are almost always amenable to specific stretching techniques. ROM deficits due to bone-on-bone contact are generally not improved with therapeutic exercise or physical modalities but at times can be addressed by compensatory strategies.

In addition, quality of ROM can be assessed in the setting of functional movements. For example, functional forward bending is a combination of hip, pelvis, and a spinal movement. This is often clinically evaluated by having a patient bend forward and measuring the distance between the patient's fingertips and the floor. A subject with restricted hamstrings and gluteal muscles will present with increased lumbar and thoracic flexion to reach as low as a subject with highly flexible hamstrings and gluteal muscles. This second subject may exhibit minimal motion through the spine as he or she is able to achieve the required amount of "bend" using predominantly hip flexion.

Strength: Strength assessment is another part of comprehensive patient examination. Whether it is through manual muscle testing (MMT), or a more formal dynamometric assessment, the goal of strength testing is threefold: (1) determining etiology of strength deficits (i.e., deconditioning, pain inhibition, poor neuromuscular control; these often improve with repeated cueing) or neural deficit, (2) painting a clinical picture of overall strength, and (3) demonstration/determination of kinesiophobia (an important factor in chronic pain). As a general rule, the patient should be examined with regard to muscles surrounding the region that is painful and in the regions immediately proximal and distal to the painful region. For example, in a patient with elbow pain, the clinician should evaluate strength in the shoulder, elbow, and wrist. Given that strength deficits are relative, contralateral strength values should be used as an internal control.

Additionally, because many pain complaints are concerning for an underlying spine etiology (e.g., a radiculopathy), it is often useful to examine the key myotomes in the affected region. Using the same example of elbow pain, the clinician would evaluate muscle strength of the C5–T1 myotomes bilaterally to assess for focal weakness. These have been covered earlier in this book.

Admittedly, MMT is a faster method than more formal strength measurement such as dynamometry or manual sphygmomanometry. However, one must acknowledge that the MMT grading scale of 0 to 5 consists only of ordinal values. These values represent directional relationship only and should not be used as replacement for interval or ratio measures, such as torque, force, or percentage of muscle activity. In fact, Beasley[27] noted that a knee extensor strength loss of 50% is needed before clinicians reported a grade change within MMT.

With regard to kinetic chain theory and altered neuromuscular control, the testing of muscles distant to the presenting complaint becomes important during the development of a rehabilitation plan. Just as patients with patellofemoral pain present with distant palpable tender sites, they will often demonstrate weakness as well, typically about the hip abductors, hip extensors, and hip external rotators.[28] This evaluation process is a joint experience, one undertaken by both the clinician and the patient, which may ultimately improve patient compliance in a physiotherapy program.

Two primary factors contribute to relative strength deficits in ambulatory patients without major nerve or muscle injury. The first might be considered a relative disuse weakness. In relative disuse, the body part is not immobilized but is infrequently used in a manner that develops strength. Triceps weakness in sedentary office workers is a good example of this. Although these individuals may be "pushing papers" all day long, they may go for decades without ever performing elbow extensions against enough resistance to prevent gradual weakness from developing.

The second primary factor that contributes to relative strength deficits in ambulatory patients without major nerve or muscle injury is a process sometimes referred to as muscle de-education.[29] This is a process in which the individual fails to activate or abnormally activates a given muscle because of pain, fatigue, maladaptive biomechanics, or psychological basis. Over time, the normal neuromuscular engram for the intended movement becomes more difficult to retrieve, and in time, the neuromuscular control system essentially "forgets" the normal motor control pattern for that requested movement. Most often, muscle de-education involves the patient losing the ability to fire a muscle with the correct timing or with enough synchronous motor units for the intended movement. The patient adopts a maladaptive neuromuscular firing pattern and substitutes other muscles to perform the task. Proper motor synergy and contraction/relaxation timing is lost. Ultimately, it is the clinician's responsibility to identify all strength deficits, determine rationale (neuromuscular or musculoskeletal etiology), decide which are clinically relevant to the patient's symptoms, and implement an appropriate rehabilitation plan.

ENDURANCE

Endurance refers to the capacity to continue to functionally exert oneself. Although patients with pain complaints may occasionally be limited by cardiovascular endurance, the more common context for assessing endurance in a pain patient is local muscular endurance.

As an individual bears weight during a functional activity, the forces of his or her activity (e.g., the ground reaction force while walking) have to be borne by the different structures throughout the kinetic chain. These include bone, joints, articular cartilage, ligaments, and muscles. Ideally, muscles bear a substantial amount of these reactive forces, which reduces the forces transmitted across other structures. However, with repetitive iterations, local anaerobic energy systems are stressed and loading muscles will fatigue. Although these muscles may be able to bear reactive forces initially, with each repetition, these same muscles may lose their ability to attenuate force and, hence, allow transmission to other structures.

The phenomenon of muscle fatigue has important implications both diagnostically and therapeutically. Oftentimes, patients will complain of pain presentations that are initially mild but worsen with increased activity. This is seen especially in the case of postural muscles, which must have sustained exertion against gravity and may present with pain by the end of the day or with any prolonged positioning. Strength measurements may initially appear "normal" on physical examination; however, recall that MMT inherently does not test muscle endurance. Therefore, it may be necessary during examination to exercise a patient to fatigue to simulate those circumstances when the patient is having pain. For example, if a patient complains of knee pain that worsens with walking long distances or climbing stairs, a component of the pain complaint may be poor muscular endurance in the quadriceps and hip abductors. When testing knee extension and hip abduction by MMT, the "strength" may appear normal because the patient's limitation is muscular endurance rather than peak torque production (as tested via MMT). Therefore, the patient may be better assessed by performing repetitive single-leg squats. This can fatigue the quadriceps and hip abductors relatively quickly within the time frame of the examination and allow the clinician to assess whether poor muscular endurance is contributing to the patient's pain complaint. If the clinician assesses that poor muscular endurance is contributing to a patient's pain complaint, improving muscular endurance should be a focus in the patient's physical therapy protocol.

Biomechanical Considerations in Common Musculoskeletal Pain Syndromes

The first part of this chapter highlights key concepts underlying the biomechanical evaluation of pain. Following are selected common axial musculoskeletal pain syndromes that are often ameliorated by the patient engaging in a focused, active rehabilitation program. This list is not exhaustive but serves as a basis for the application of the concepts discussed earlier. The goal of this section is to enlighten the reader on the clinical utility of a biomechanical evaluation of patients presenting with musculoskeletal pain. It will be noted that these anatomic regions overlap in their presentation and redundancy is a product of the very nature of the interrelatedness of biomechanical evaluation.

CERVICALGIA

Patients presenting with chronic atraumatic neck pain often have a history of constant posterior neck, suboccipital, and/or upper trapezius area pain with qualities of pressure, tightness, and spasm. Often, the symptoms are present upon waking and decrease somewhat with movement and a warm shower but worsen as the day progresses. This may be exacerbated by various sedentary positions such as driving, sitting in class or meetings, computer work, reading, or knitting. The pain is usually temporarily improved with lying down or reclining with the head supported as in a lounge chair but may return or worsen with prolonged inactivity, prompting the subject to get up and move about to reduce the pain. In addition, they may have had a prior diagnosis of cervicogenic headaches. To further evaluate, one must understand the functional role of the neck and common pitfalls in daily living.

The obvious functional role of the neck is to hold the head. On second pass, however, that role becomes more nuanced, as the head's role is to house a large and heavy brain, position eyes for binocular vision, position ears for hearing in stereo, and place the nose and mouth for their respective roles. In addition, it positions the head to maximize facial expression due to social human nature. As seen earlier, positioning of the lower spine affects head posture; postural muscles that are suboptimally positioned will have to work harder but maintain the same endurance than those kept in more agreeable alignment with gravity. Slouched sitting will cause excessive thoracic flexion; in this posture, the arms and scapulae slide off the body and the shoulders round forward. This positions the head more forward than intended. Compensatory strategies for this forward head posture include excessive proximal neck extension to raise eye gaze off the floor and facilitation of the upper trapezius and levator scapulae. Muscle balance theory states that a strong, tight muscle group will reflexively inhibit the antagonist group.[29] Thus, as the cervical and thoracic paraspinals along with the upper trapezius and levator scapulae become chronically hyperactive, hypertrophied, and facilitated, reflex inhibition of the middle and lower trapezius, rhomboids, and deep cervical flexors are seen. This pattern was coined by Dr. Vladimir Janda as "upper crossed syndrome."[30] Of note, this neuromusculoskeletal pattern can present clinically as pain in multiple regions, including cervical, thoracic, and periscapular regions, as well as in the presentation of rotator cuff impingement.

There are several clinical patterns in addition to myofascial cervical and upper trapezius pain common to this posture that can be amenable to an *active* physical therapy and biomechanical restoration program which are highlighted in the following text.

Occipital neuralgia: The greater and lesser occipital nerves can become entrapped as they pierce through suboccipitals that have become hypertrophied and shortened. Occipital nerve blocks have been used in this setting; however, providers may find that patients receive temporary relief. From a positioning standpoint, a forward head posture with hypertrophied/facilitated posterior cervical musculature will continue to produce entrapment of the nerves unless the tension is removed from the suboccipital region. Restoration of the head over the neck (as opposed to in front of it) will reduce tension in this region. Due to kinetic chain theory, optimization of this cervical posture requires improvement of the positioning of the lumbopelvic, thoracic, and periscapular region. This positional effort is largely patient-driven following adequate instruction and can help free the patient from cyclical pain relief by external forces (i.e., injections).

Cervical facet pain: In the sagittal plane, the typical cervical vertebrae (C3–C7) are limited in extension by the zygapophysial (facet) joints.[31] The forward head posture produces increased lower cervical flexion and upper cervical extension than a neutral to retracted head posture, and efforts at neck extension in the forward head posture lead to decreased extension at the lower cervical segments compared to the neutral head posture.[32] (It is of note that segmentally, the atlantoaxial joint has paradoxical motion in flexion and extension when compared with the typical vertebral segments.)[31] Increased efforts at neck extension in the forward head posture will presumably increase the segmental extension seen at all, but the lower cervical segments due to this inhibition and are more likely to affect facet loading. Restoration of the neutral head posture can alleviate some of this excessive upper cervical extension.

Cervical radiculopathy: Similarly, the classic neural tension and distraction signs for cervical radiculopathy are Spurling's test, which is described by placing the neck in extension and rotation with an axial load.[33] In patients with poor cervical posture, the typical upper cervical vertebrae are already in a relatively extended position, and addition of rotation in this position essentially reproduces the Spurling's maneuver. Cervical extension has been shown to decrease the cross sectional area of the neuroforamen in particularly C3–C4 and C4–C5.[34] Additional rotation in this position can further compromise the exiting nerve, and clinically, a patient with poor neck posture may complain of radicular symptoms with daily functional tasks such as turning his or her head with driving as he or she is already in a relatively extended position.

PERISCAPULAR AND THORACIC PAIN

In pain management involving the thoracic region (inclusive of the shoulder complex and upper extremity related referral), the attending clinician may have the tendency to direct intervention at a specific location or tissue of concern. Just as with other body regions (discussed within this chapter), this approach is not unwarranted. Musculoskeletal trigger points are an obvious concern, incurring a local pain response associated with the area of hypertonicity. A variety of interventions (not covered in this chapter) exist to manage these trigger points, inclusive of injection, dry needling, manual therapy, and thermomodalities. However, in discussing these abnormal musculoskeletal soft tissue states, one must explore the etiology from multiple perspectives.

Although the exact mechanism of soft tissue trigger point development is not fully understood, there is general consensus that these myofascially derived trigger points (or "taut bands") are related to localized muscle overuse syndrome, such as that following a novel, repetitive, or excessive cyclical loading task.[35–37] This is not surprising, given that a general "training effect" is based on principles, outlined by Hans Selye in the "general adaptation syndrome."[38] The patient may report performing large amounts of repetitive or intense loading, such as typing, repeated lifting, pulling, or pushing, which would serve to create an "overtraining" condition and negative tissue response. However, if the stimulus activity does not appear to fully justify the patient's current presentation, the question must be posed: "Is there some force or some movement pattern lending to an inappropriate amount of stress being placed on the problematic structure(s)?" This is where the clinician must consider biomechanics associated with the movement at hand.

Periscapular pain: The attending clinician's consideration of faulty movement pattern is paramount in assessing etiology of the patient's current localized complaints. This is especially true with regard to the shoulder and thoracic region complex. Although the labrum serves to deepen the glenoid fossa to an extent, the humeral head is roughly 3 to 4 times as large as the admittedly shallow glenoid fossa, lending to the glenohumeral (GH) joint's significant amount of mobility.[39] The tremendous amount of movement available to the GH joint lends itself to risk of injury. If structures that are designed to stabilize this joint are not performing properly, the region is at risk. One must consider the stability of the GH joint, neuromuscular control, and scapulohumeral rhythm as well as patient posture.

As an example, let us consider a patient with subacromial region pain and upper trapezius region pain. One may be concerned about impingement (primary or secondary) as well as upper trapezius trigger point presentation. First, the anterior-posterior force coupling created by the infraspinatus, teres minor, and subscapularis, when operating symmetrically, serve to compress the humeral head into the glenoid fossa during dynamic activity. This limits aberrant arthrokinematic translation that may be associated with impingement. However, research has noted that overdevelopment of the internal rotators and subscapularis musculature (especially within a throwing population) typically lend to an imbalance in this coupling.[40] It would behoove the clinician to consider this proper strength and activation coupling with regard to pain.

A second consideration is that of proper scapular dynamic stability. A generally accepted ratio of humeral to scapular movement is 2 to 1 (in that for every 2 degrees of humeral movement, the scapula moves 1). This needs to be maintained and appropriately timed to ensure proper GH joint position. Researchers has shown that in those with shoulder impingement, the serratus anterior has decreased levels of activity, the lower and middle trapezius have delayed activation, and there exists an overtly dominant activation of the upper trapezius.[41,42] This thereby lends to faulty scapular mechanics, altered scapulohumeral rhythm, and hence a potentially excessive stress to subacromial structures.

Additionally, static and postural concern warrants attention. If a patient, such as that mentioned earlier, is continuously performing an overhead reaching task in an excessively kyphotic position, he or she may be "asking" the shoulder complex to perform a significantly larger amount of relative overhead flexion than capable of (an amount potentially not available passively) regardless of proper scapula-humeral rhythm. The patient may present with a dysfunctional scapular position, such as medial border dysfunction, where in the scapula is excessively internally rotated such that the medial border is raised from the rib cage. This posture has been associated with GH instability.[43] Such a posture may imply weakened, inhibited, excessively stretched supportive structures (serratus anterior musculature, middle and lower trapezius musculature, rhomboid musculature) or even restricted pectoralis minor musculature, such as that noted in the commonly termed *upper crossed syndrome*. Such concern would then warrant tests to rule in/out neuromuscular concerns in activation or pure musculoskeletal concerns in length, strength, or restriction. Patients may complain of thoracic region pain; however, the treatment requires correction of dysfunctions of the GH and scapulothoracic regions for long-term improvement: Simply injecting trigger points will not resolve the offending process.

Furthermore, if an excessively kyphotic resting position were evident, he or she would be required to achieve correlating and likely excessive amount of cervical lordosis in order to maintain gaze forward on the horizon. Such a pathologic resting state may lend toward the muscle overuse scenario as etiology of trigger points (i.e., prolonged levator scapulae, scalene, and/or deep posterior cervical musculature activation) and may even lend to excessive cervical facet joint closure stresses (as discussed in further detail within other sections of this chapter).

Thoracic pain: Interestingly, pure thoracic region spinal pain is reported much more rarely than other spinal region complaints regardless of the previously mentioned postural and dynamic concerns. One report noted that out of all spinal pain reports, only 15% of those resided within the thoracic region (vs. 44% in the neck and 56% in the low back).[44] Although not common, and typically experienced unilaterally and localized,[45] pain related to thoracic spine dysfunction must be mentioned, given that the contractile structures making up the scapulothoracic complex utilize both the ribs and vertebral segments as points of attachment (serratus anterior, trapezius musculature, pectoralis major, and anterior scalenes to name a few), thereby lending to relative scapular or relative rib movement. Clinicians should be versed in, aware of, and able to assess concern for abnormal rib positions and consider postural abnormalities and muscle activation patterns within the kinetic chain when ruling out thoracic positional concerns.

Proper shoulder and thoracic biomechanics *must* be considered in lieu of localized management of irritable structures. However, this is not to say that local tissue management is to be overlooked or minimized. In fact, literature has shown a correlation between local musculature trigger points and correlating muscle inhibition as well-altered motor activation patterns.[35] The cause-and-effect relationship becomes muddied to

some extent as one considers this correlation. Local injection is not by any means contraindicated as it is a valuable intervention for pain management with a soft tissue, myofascial component. Rather, it is recognized as valuable only within a comprehensive approach, acknowledging that there may be a complex interplay among causality and perpetuation of complaints involving mechanics of movement.

LUMBAR PAIN

Low back pain is the leading cause of disability in the world and is the sixth leading contributor to global disease burden.[46,47] The cause of chronic low back pain can be frustratingly difficult to elucidate. Although various studies have documented the primacy of the intervertebral disk,[48,49] followed by the zygapophysial[48,50,51] and SI[48,52] joints, these diagnoses can require invasive techniques, such as provocation discography or image-guided diagnostic injections. Axial low back can occur with or without leg pain. When leg symptoms are present, they may signify radiculopathy, radicular pain, or somatically referred pain. These entities have been defined by the International Association for the Study of Pain[53] and have been more recently articulated by Bogduk.[54] Briefly, radiculopathy implies a conduction block along a spinal nerve or its roots and may or may not be painful.[53] Radicular pain is evoked by ectopic discharges from a dorsal root or its ganglion and does not suggest the presence of an objective neurologic deficit.[53] Somatically referred pain is not dermatomal and signifies the convergence of nociceptive afferents on second-order neurons in the spinal cord.[53] The variability of these clinical presentations may lead treating providers to obtain cross-sectional imaging to help localize the source of pain. Yet, the situation is hardly helped by magnetic resonance imaging (MRI), which can commonly show abnormalities, even in asymptomatic individuals.[55] The confluence of these factors illustrates a common clinical reality: Identifying the pathoanatomic source of low back pain is often difficult, resource-intensive, and may be impossible. In these scenarios, the treating provider may wish to use a biomechanical and active rehabilitation approach for both diagnostic and therapeutic purposes.

Core stability: Perhaps, no single intervention for chronic, axial low back pain has received as much as attention as core stability. The "core" has been defined as a box with the abdominals in the front, paraspinals and gluteals in the back, diaphragm as the roof, and the pelvic floor/hip girdle as the floor.[56] Clinical instability is defined as a significant decrease in the capacity of the stabilizing system of the spine to maintain the intervertebral neutral zones within the physiologic limits.[57] Objective changes of core musculature have been demonstrated in patients with chronic low back pain. The lumbar multifidus muscles are important extensors of the lumbar spine. The lumbar multifidi have been noted to atrophy and become replaced with fatty tissue in patients with chronic low back pain.[58–60] When noted, a stabilizing program directed at activating the lumbar multifidi is an important part of the rehabilitation of a patient with chronic low back pain. In addition to muscular dysfunction, impaired neural feedback control may also lead to instability. A basic framework may be conceptualized as follows. The central nervous system, upon sensing a lack of intervertebral stiffness, may compensate by increasing trunk muscle activation to maintain stability, and static contractions prolonged over a period of time may lead to pain.[61] The goal of core stabilization is to achieve muscular contraction to achieve stability.[62] Although a variety of core stabilizing programs are possible, many seem to incorporate elements from the Saal and Saal's protocol on conservative treatment of patients with lumbar disk herniations.[62,63] Per their description, stabilization exercises may be divided into basic and advanced levels. Basic levels of core stabilization involve supine and prone positioning. Patients may be advanced through transitional, kneeling, and standing positions. The goal of this program was to develop isolate and cocontraction muscle patterns to stabilize the lumbar spine in neutral position. Although core stabilization exercise has strong construct validity, further research will be needed to determine its efficacy.[64]

Mechanical diagnosis and therapy: A patient may present with leg pain, which may be radicular or somatically referred. The history and examination, which may include an evaluation for ANT, can assist with this distinction. The mechanical diagnosis and therapy (MDT) is a paradigm that was developed by Robin McKenzie in the 1950s.[65] The MDT provides a means for treating the patient's symptoms without necessarily establishing a pathoanatomic source. A key portion of establishing a mechanical diagnosis hinges on patients performing repeated end-range lumbar movements to establish whether leg pain may "centralize." McKenzie[66] himself has defined centralization as the phenomenon "whereby the intensity of pain reduces or disappears distally but remains or moves (and in some cases increases) proximally." The "directional preference" is that direction of testing that elicits a centralization response. Once the directional preference that achieves centralization is identified, the patients are then empowered to self-manage their problem through the use of directional exercises that match their directional preference.[67] The value of this approach is that it allows the patients to transition to self-care and affords them the ability to control their symptoms. The prevalence of centralization and directional preference has been reported to be 70% to 87% for acute low back pain and 32% to 52% for chronic or radicular low back pain.[67] If a directional preference exists, patients will benefit the most from exercise that matches their directional preference. One protocol had matched patients to exercise that was opposite of their directional preference.[68] One-third of this group had to withdraw from the study within 2 weeks due to nonimproving or worsening symptoms. Additionally, the presence of centralization and directional preference is a predictor of outcome. In a study of 243 subjects, those who centralized had significantly greater pain reductions and return-to-work rates than those who did not centralize.[69] In addition to being therapeutic, the presence of centralization and directional preference may be diagnostic as well. The only conclusive test for discogenic pain remains provocation discography which is invasive and of debatable clinical value. However, one study has found the presence of centralization to correlate with positive discography. In this study of 63 patients, 47 expressed a directional preference and 16 did not.[70] Of the 16 who did not show a directional preference, only 2 had positive discography. Of the 47 who did show a directional preference, 34 showed had positive discography. This study demonstrates the strong correlation between the presence of a directional preference and discogenic pain.

In summary, the cause or treatment of chronic low back pain is often not illuminated through history, exam, or advanced imaging. However, the need to establish a pathoanatomic diagnosis may be eliminated through active biomechanical techniques, which may serve both a diagnostic and therapeutic value.

SACROILIAC AND HIP GIRDLE PAIN

If there is one theme that has emerged through this discussion of pain and biomechanics, it is that one cannot completely isolate a specific joint or region with regard to etiology of musculoskeletal pain when repetitive movement is involved. The human body, as a functional closed chain system of joints, works synergistically, with the proper amount of joint excursion, proper amount of muscle activation, and in the correct temporal sequence in order to successfully carry out the task at hand. These functional tasks could be as simple as everyday ambulation or as unique as repeated single-leg squatting in an

attic, hopping down a step or rapidly sidestepping to in sport. One could argue that during daily activity, the loading of the lower extremity and lumbopelvic complex is more relevant to pain management than any other region. Although it is beyond the scope of this chapter to fully delve into the biomechanics of the lower extremity and lumbopelvic complex, the correlation between faulty loading mechanics, dysfunctional muscle activation, and pain must be acknowledged and discussed.

There is a body of literature drawing kinetic/kinematic connections between the foot, ankle, knee, femoroacetabular joint, and pelvic complex. As cited previously in this chapter, the pronated STJ is associated with a position of medial tibial rotation, knee valgus, femoral medial rotation, and a hip adduction.[6] Loading of the foot is associated with a pronation moment, serving to increase the impulse time and reduce the amount of force placed through the lower extremity during loading. Accordingly, the body is required to oppose all associated moments (at the knee, hip, and pelvis) throughout the loading chain. This entails producing subtalar supination, ankle plantarflexion, lateral tibial rotation, lateral femoral rotation, femoral abduction, and femoral extension (for our purposes, innominate and SI movement are not discussed here). More recent bodies of literature have confirmed these multijoint correlations, noting that lateral tibial rotation assists in raising the medial longitudinal arch of the foot[71] and that proximal (hip) musculature is highly involved in controlling both femoral and tibial rotation.[72] The musculature within the lower extremity must work synergistically and with proper synchronicity to maintain alignment. Just as in the shoulder complex, if one region is restricted, weakened, or activated with an improper timing sequence, the other regions are required to overcompensate or suffer faulty mechanics, either of which may lend to stress of musculoskeletal structures and potential pain.

Patellofemoral joint pain is a prime example. In the setting of patellofemoral joint pain, literature emphasizes deficiency in quad activation/strength[73] and poor hip stability (with emphasis on gluteus maximus deficiency)[74] as well as poor foot control and excessive pronation[75] as contributing factors to continued complaints. It would behoove the clinician managing such a patient to attend to these biomechanical concerns. If, in fact, the hip cannot compensate for a weakened gluteus musculature, one may note development of Trendelenburg gait, potential bursal irritation, and/or glut medius overuse pathology. Scenarios such as this must be pursued and considered for proper long-term remediation. However, select populations of patients may have faulty mechanics, poor musculature activation, and/or altered motor control/timing in the lower extremity but *without* painful presentation in the lower extremity. One must be concerned about manifestation more proximally (i.e., lumbopelvic region). There is a biomechanical correlation between the lower extremity and the lumbopelvic region. As an example, deficits at the hip may manifest proximally rather than distally depending on that patient's abilities to compensate, and this must be acknowledged, thereby drawing attention to the pelvic ring.

As discussed in earlier sections, the lumbosacral region is a common site of pain management. However, one cannot discount the importance of loading forces placed on the entire pelvic complex during weight bearing. The relationship between the lumbar spine, SI joints, and femoroacetabular joints are inseparable when it comes to movement and determination of pain etiology. Current thinking acknowledges the pelvic girdle as a load-transfer system[76] and, as such, able to both attenuate and generate forces. The proper function of this system depends on the stability of both hip joints and SI joints. The hip joints have a multitude of muscular support and an obvious congruency associated with the ball and socket–type joint. However, the SI joints, being planar, rely heavily on a system of dense ligamentous structure as well as less direct muscular elements connected via fascia tensioning. These elements are in a delicate balance, serving to tension across the SI joints and create stability.

Literature has reported a multitude of structures highly involved in SI joint and general pelvic ring stability. It is beyond the scope of this chapter to discuss these in full detail. However, emphasis has been placed on myofascial attachments of the latissimus dorsi and the multifidus as well as the "guy wire system" of dynamic stabilization created by the deep erector spinae, the psoas major, and the quadratus lumborum.[77] Given a general understanding of anatomy, one can understand how integrated the lumbar and pelvic region become given such information. To complicate matters further, the gluteus maximize has been recognized as a dynamic link between the thoracolumbar fascia and the tensor fascia lata, thereby emphasizing the connection to the lower extremity loading during tensioning of the pelvic girdle.[78]

As noted earlier, the SI joint's planar shape dictates that adequate pelvic girdle function relies very heavily on the concept of dynamic stability. Adequate muscle force generation is required each loading bout, local muscular endurance is needed for repetitive activation, and effective neuromuscular control is required and must ensure proper timing of each muscle activation. If any one attribute is in deficit (i.e., a relevant structure is inflexible, overly flexible, weak, or activated improperly), the system begins to fail, and the patient may become symptomatic due to overstress of any single structure.

Although it is not the purpose of this chapter to explore in detail true medical diagnoses, pain at the SI region cannot be assumed to stem from the SI joint. Referral patterns as mentioned previously (with regard to the lumbar spine) must be considered. Furthermore, pain at the SI joint is not synonymous with true sacroiliitis (as potentially ruled in/out with intra-articular injection). Both the dorsal SI and interosseous ligament have been implicated as an overlooked source of pain in the setting of lumbopelvic dysfunction.[79]

Ultimately, poor dynamic stability, passive restrictions, or altered neuromuscular control within the entire lower closed chain system have the potential to affect the pelvic ring structures and vice versa. It may be thought of as "uncommon" for overpronation to lend to pelvic stress and resultant dysfunction or for weakened gluts to lend to SI region pain. However, such biomechanical-based concerns should be entertained and ruled out. With regard to pain, mechanics, and effective long-term management, the mindful clinician must acknowledge, assess, and implement intervention to address these concerns.

Conclusion

Thorough evaluation of neuromusculoskeletal pain requires the use of biomechanical evaluation and principles to guide pain treatment and patient expectations. The principles of kinetic chain theory, ANT, and neuromuscular control form the groundwork whereupon pain syndromes can be addressed. The clinician should have raised suspicion for kinetic chain dysfunction in patients with neuromusculoskeletal pain whose symptoms are recalcitrant to focal treatment modalities, that are only temporarily improved with passive treatments, or that are poorly defined by anatomic structures. Treatment begins with educating the patient on the global nature of the body dysfunction and includes the patient actively engaging in improving found deficits. Improvement is sustained through the patient continuing with active management techniques over time, often with a physical or occupational therapist–prescribed home exercise program, and adherence begins with the patient recognizing the clinician's understanding of the biomechanical interface of the body with its environment.

References

1. Khalaj N, Abu Osman NA, Mokhtar AH. Effect of exercise and gait retraining on knee adduction moment in people with knee osteoarthritis. *Proc Inst Mech Eng H* 2014;228(2):190–199.
2. Reuleaux F. *The Kinematics of Machinery.* New York: Macmillan and Company; 1876.
3. Ellenbecker TS, Davies GJ. *Closed Kinetic Chain Exercise: A Comprehensive Guide to Multiple Joint Exercise.* Champaign, IL: Human Kinetics; 2001.
4. Steindler A, ed. *Kinesiology of the Human Body Under Normal and Pathological Condition.* 3rd ed. Springfield, IL: Charles C Thomas Books; 1955.
5. Buckwalter J. Arthur Steindler: founder of Iowa Orthopedics. *Iowa Orthop J* 1981;1:5–12.
6. Tibero D. Pathomechanics of structural foot deformities. *Phys Ther* 1988;68:1840–1849.
7. Shacklock M. Neurodynamics. *Physiotherapy* 1995;81:9–16.
8. Butler D, Gifford L. The concept of adverse mechanical tension in the nervous system part 1: testing for "dural tension." *Physiotherapy* 1989;71(11):622–629.
9. Cavafy J. A case of sciatic nerve-stretching in locomotor ataxy: with remarks on the operation. *Br Med J* 1881;2(1094):973–974.
10. Marshall J. Bradshaw lecture on nerve-stretching for the relief or cure of pain. *Br Med J* 1883;2(1198):1173–1179.
11. Ellis R, Hing W. Neural mobilization: a systematic review of randomized controlled trials with and analysis of therapeutic efficacy. *J Man Manip Ther* 2008;16(1):8–22.
12. Pitt-Brooke J. *Rehabilitation of Movement: Theoretical Basis of Clinical Practice.* Philadelphia: Saunders; 1998.
13. Butler D. *The Sensitive Nervous System.* Adelaide, Australia: Neuro Orthopaedic Institute; 2000.
14. Gilbert K, Brismee J, Collins D, et al. 2006 Young Investigator Award Winner: lumbosacral nerve root displacement and strain: part 1. A novel measurement technique during straight leg raise in unembalmed cadavers. *Spine (Phila Pa 1976)* 2007;32(14):1513–1520.
15. Gilbert K, Brismee J, Collins D, et al. 2006 Young Investigator Award Winner: lumbosacral nerve root displacement and strain: part 2. A comparison of 2 straight leg raise conditions in unembalmed cadavers. *Spine (Phila Pa 1976)* 2007;32(14):1521–1525.
16. Rade M, Kononen M, Vanninen R, et al. 2014 Young Investigator Award Winner: in vivo magnetic resonance imaging measurement of spinal cord displacement in the thoracolumbar region of asymptomatic subjects: part 1: straight leg raise test. *Spine (Phila Pa 1976)* 2014;39:1288–1293.
17. Rade M, Kononen M, Vanninen R, et al. 2014 Young Investigator Award Winner: in vivo magnetic resonance imaging measurement of spinal cord displacement in the thoracolumbar region of asymptomatic subjects: part 2: comparison between unilateral and bilateral straight leg raise tests. *Spine (Phila Pa 1976)* 2014;39(16):1294–1300.
18. Rade M, Kononen M, Vanninen R, et al. In vivo MRI measurement of spinal cord displacement in the thoracolumbar region of asymptomatic subjects: part 3: developing methods of in vivo MRI measurement of spinal cord displacement in asymptomatic subjects with unilateral and bilateral SLR tests. *Spine (Phila Pa 1976)* 2015;40(12):935–941.
19. Yoshii Y, Villarraga H, Henderson J, et al. Ultrasound assessment of the displacement and deformation of the median nerve in the human carpal tunnel with active finger motion. *J Bone Joint Surg Am* 2009;91(12):2922–2930.
20. Kuo T, Lee M, Liao Y, et al. Assessment of median nerve mobility by ultrasound dynamic imaging for diagnosing carpal tunnel syndrome. *PLoS One* 2016;11(1):e0147051.
21. Rutherford O, Jones D. The role of learning and coordination in strength training. *Eur J Appl Physiol Occup Physiol* 1986;55(1):100–105.
22. Schaible H, Grubb B. Afferent and spinal mechanisms of joint pain. *Pain* 1993;55(1):5–54.
23. O'Sullivan P, Twomey L, Allison G. Dysfunction of the neuromuscular system in the presence of low back pain—implications for physical therapy management. *J Man Manip Ther* 1997;5:20–26.
24. Kototolis N, Vrabas I, Vamvakoudis E, et al. Proprioceptive neuromuscular facilitation training induced alterations in muscle fibre type and cross sectional area. *Br J Sports Med* 2005;39(3):e11.
25. Halabchi F, Mazaheri R, Seif-Barghi T. Patellofemoral pain syndrome and modifiable intrinsic risk factors: how to assess and address? *Asian J Sports Med* 2013;4(2):85–100.
26. Perry J, Burnfield JM. *Gait Analysis: Normal and Pathological Function.* 2nd ed. Thorofare, NJ: Slack; 2010.
27. Beasley W. Quantitative muscle testing: principle and applications to research and clinical services. *Arch Phys Med Rehabil* 1961;42:398–425.
28. Robinson R, Nee R. Analysis of hip strength in females seeking treatment for unilateral patellofemoral pain syndrome. *J Orthop Sports Phys Ther* 2007;37(5):232–238.
29. Janda V. Muscle weakness and inhibition (pseudoparesis). In: Grieve G, ed. *Back Pain Syndrome in Modern Manual Therapy of the Vertebral Column.* New York: Churchill Livingstone; 1986:197–201.
30. Janda V. Muscles and cervicogenic pain syndromes. In: Grand R, ed. *Physical Therapy of the Cervical and Thoracic Spine.* New York: Churchill Livingstone; 1988:153–166.

31. Bogduk N, Mercer S. Biomechanics of the cervical spine. I: normal kinematics. *Clin Biomech* 2000;15:633–648.
32. Takasaki H, Hall T, Kaneko S, et al. A radiographic analysis of the influence of initial neck posture on cervical segmental movement at end-range extension in asymptomatic subjects. *Man Ther* 2011;16(1):74–79.
33. Landes P, Malanga G, Nadler S, et al. Physical examination of the cervical spine. In: Malanga G, Nadler S, eds. *Musculoskeletal Physical Examination: An Evidence-Based Approach*. Philadelphia: Elsevier; 2006:33–57.
34. Mao H, Driscoll S, Li JS, et al. Dimensional changes of the neuroforamina in subaxial cervical spine during in vivo dynamic flexion-extension. *Spine J* 2016;16(4):540–546.
35. Dommerholt J, Fernández de-las-Peñas C, eds. *Trigger Point Dry Needling: An Evidence and Clinical-Based Approach*. Edinburgh: Churchill Livingstone; 2013.
36. Gerwin R, Dommerholt J, Shah JP. An expansion of Simons' integrated hypothesis of trigger point formation. *Curr Pain Headache Rep* 2004;8:468–475.
37. Gerwin R. The taut band and other mysteries of the trigger point: an examination of the mechanisms relevant to the development and maintenance of the trigger point. *J Musculoskelet Pain* 2008;16:115–121.
38. Selye H. Stress and the general adaptation syndrome. *Br Med J* 1950;1:1383–1392.
39. Hadler A, Iteo E, An K. Anatomy and biomechanics of the shoulder. *Orthop Clin N Am* 2000;39:151–176.
40. Ellenbecker T, Cools A. Rehabilitation of shoulder impingement syndrome and rotator cuff injuries: an evidence-based review. *Br J Sports Med* 2010;44:319–327.
41. Lidewig P, Cook T. Alterations in shoulder kinematics and associated muscle activity in people with symptoms of shoulder impingement. *Phys Ther* 2000;80:276–291.
42. Cools A, Witvrouw E, Declercq G, et al. Scapular muscle recruitment patterns: trapezius muscle latency with and without impingement syndrome. *Am J Sports Med* 2003;31:542–549.
43. Kibler B. Role of the scapula in the overhead throwing motion. *Contemp Orthop* 1991;22:525.
44. Linton S, Hellsing A, Halden K. A population-based study of spinal pain among 35-45-year-old individuals. *Spine* 1998;23:1457–1463.
45. Fukui A, Ohseto K, Shiotani M. Patterns of pain induced by distending the thoracic zygapophyseal joints. *Reg Anesth* 1997;22:332–336.
46. Buchbinder R, Blyth F, March L, et al. Placing the global burden of low back pain in context. *Best Pract Red Clin Rheumatology* 2013;27(5):575–589.
47. Vos T, Flaxman A, Naghavi M, et al. Years lived with disability (YLDs) for 1160 sequelae of 289 diseases and injuries 1990-2010: a systematic analysis for the Global Burden of Disease Study 2010. *Lancet* 2012;380(9859):2163–2196.
48. DePalma M, Ketchum J, Saullo T. What is the source of chronic low back pain and does age play a role? *Pain Med* 2011;12(2):224–233.
49. Schwarzer A, Aprill C, Derby R, et al. The presence and clinical features of internal disc disruption in patients with chronic low back pain. *Spine (Phila Pa 1976)* 1995;20(17):1878–1993.
50. Schwarzer A, Aprill C, Derby R, et al. Clinical features of patients with pain stemming from the lumbar zygapophysial joints. Is the lumbar facet syndrome a clinical entity? *Spine (Phila Pa 1976)* 1994;19(10):1132–1137.
51. Schwarzer A, Rang S, Bogduk N, et al. Prevalence and clinical features of lumbar zygapophysial joint pain: a study in an Australian population with chronic low back pain. *Ann Rheum Dis* 1995;54(2):100–106.
52. Maigne J, Aivaliklis A, Pfefer F. Results of sacroiliac joint double block and value of sacroiliac pain provocation tests in 54 patients with low back pain. *Spine (Phila Pa 1976)* 1996;21(16):1889–1892.
53. Merskey H, Bogduk N, eds. *Classification of Chronic Pain: Descriptions of Chronic Pain Syndromes and Definitions of Pain Terms*. 2nd ed. Seattle, WA: IASP Press; 1994.
54. Bogduk N. On the definitions and physiology of back pain, referred pain, and radicular pain. *Pain* 2009;147(1–3):17–19.
55. Jensen M, Brant-Zawadzki M, Obuchowski N, et al. Magnetic resonance imaging of the lumbar spine in people without back pain. *New Engl J Med* 1994;331(2):69–73.
56. Richardson C. *Therapeutic Exercise for Spinal Segmental Stabilization in Low Back Pain: Scientific Basis and Clinical Approach*. Edinburgh: Churchill Livingstone; 1999.
57. Panjabi M. The stabilizing system of the spine. Part II. Neutral zone and instability hypothesis. *J Spinal Disord* 1992;5(4):390–397.
58. Kjaer P, Bendix T, Sorensen J, et al. Are MRI-defined fat infiltrations in the multifidus associated with low back pain? *BMC Med* 2007;5:2.
59. Kader D, Wardlaw D, Smith F. Correlation between the MRI changes in the lumbar multifidus muscles and leg pain. *Clin Radiol* 2000;55(2):145–149.
60. Barker K, Shamley D, Jackson D. Changes in the cross-sectional area of multifidus and psoas in patients with unilateral back pain: the relationship to pain and disability. *Spine (Phila Pa 1976)* 1994;29(22):E515–E519.
61. Reeves B, Narendra K, Cholewicki J. Spine stability: the six blind men and the elephant. *Clin Biomech* 2007;22(3):266–274.
62. Akuthota V, Nadler S. Core strengthening. *Arch Phys Med Rehabil* 2004; 85(suppl 1):86–92.
63. Saal JA, Saal JS. Nonoperative treatment of herniated lumbar intervertebral disc with radiculopathy: an outcome study. *Spine (Phila Pa 1976)* 1989;14(4):431–437.
64. Akuthota V, Standaert C, Chimes G. The role of core strengthening for chronic low back pain. *PM R* 2011;3(7):664–670.
65. MeKenzie R, May S. *The Lumbar Spine Mechanical Diagnosis & Therapy*. 2nd ed, Vol 1. Waikanae, New Zealand: Spinal Publications; 2003.
66. McKenzie R. Understanding centralization. *J Orthop Sports Phys Ther* 1999;29(8):487–489.
67. Donelson R. Mechanical diagnosis and therapy for radiculopathy. *Phys Med Rehabil Clin North Am* 2011;22(1):75–89.
68. Long A, Donelson R, Fung T. Does it matter which exercise? A randomized control trial of exercise for low back pain. *Spine (Phila Pa 1976)* 2004;29(23):2593–2602.
69. Long A. The centralization phenomenon. Its usefulness as a predictor of outcome in conservative treatment of chronic low back pain (a pilot study). *Spine (Phila Pa 1976)* 1995;20(23):2513–2521.
70. Donelson R, Aprill C, Medcalf R, et al. A prospective study of centralization of lumbar and referred pain. A predictor of symptomatic discs and anular competence. *Spine (Phila Pa 1976)* 1997;22(10):1115–1122.
71. Gross M. Lower quarter screening for skeletal malalignment—suggestions for orthotics and footwear. *J Orthop Sports Phys Ther* 1995;21(6):289–405.
72. Snyder K, Earl J, O'Connor K, et al. Resistance training is accompanied by hip strength and changes in lower extremity biomechanics during running. *Clin Biomech* 2009;24(1):26–34.
73. Fulkerson J. Diagnosis and treatment of patients with patellofemoral pain. *Am J Sports Med* 2002;447–456.
74. Natri A, Kannus P, Jarvinen M. Which factors predict the long-term outcome in chronic patellofemoral pain syndrome? A 7-year prospective follow up. *Med Sci Sports Exerc* 1998;30:1572–1577.
75. Ireland M, Willson J, Ballantyne B, et al. Hip strength in females with and without patellofemoral pain. *J Orthop Sports Phys Ther* 2003;33:671–676.
76. Snijders C, Vleeming A, Stoeckart R. Transfer of lumbosacral load to iliac bones and legs. Part 1: biomechanics of self-bracing of the sacroiliac joints and its significance for treatment and exercise. *Clin Biomech* 1993;8(6): 285–294.
77. Jackson R, Porter K. The pelvis and sacroiliac joint: physical therapy patient management utilizing current evidence. In: Hughes C, ed. *Current Concepts of Orthopaedic Physical Therapy*. 3rd ed. Alexandria, VA: American Physical Therapy Association; 2011:12–14.
78. DeRosa C. Anatomical linkages and muscle slings of the lumbopelvic region. In: Vleeming A, Mooney V, Stoeckart R, eds. *Movement, Stability, and Lumbopelvic Pain: Integration of Research and Therapy*. 2nd ed. New York: Churchill Livingstone; 2007:47–62.
79. Borowsky C, Fagen G. Sources of sacroiliac pain: insights gained from a study comparing standard intra-articular injection with a technique combining intra- and peri-articular injection. *Arch Phys Med Rehabil* 2008;89(11):2048–2056.

CHAPTER 90

Pain Rehabilitation

STEVEN P. STANOS and **WILSON J. CHANG**

"Rehabilitation is a continuous process."[1]
Rehabilitation may be described as a "return to ability . . . the return to the fullest physical, mental, social, vocational, and economic usefulness that is possible for the individual."[2]
The focus is placed more on one's abilities rather than their disabilities.[2]

Historical Overview: Pain Rehabilitation and Functional Restoration

In 2016, in response to the Institute of Medicine's (IOM)[3,4] recommendations to improve the scope and breath of pain management, the National Pain Strategy (NPS), a call to develop a comprehensive population health level strategy to address pain prevention, care, education, and research, was released. Included in the plan is a need to focus on biopsychosocial-based self-management and more formal multidisciplinary team-based models of care. NPS defined "high-impact pain" as pain associated with "substantial restriction of participation in work, social, and self-care activities." This chapter is a foundation to apply a "rehabilitation model" to address the critical needs facing those patients suffering with the debilitating effects of chronic pain, including high-impact chronic pain. In this approach, "function" and "restoration" of previous activity remains the focus of providers in the rehabilitation team.

HISTORY OF PAIN REHABILITATION

Early evidence of a rehabilitation approach to the injured person or worker dates back to the Egyptians under Ramses II in 1500 BC where organized treatments of injured workers, fees for treatment, and compensation for injury were established.[5] The development of more expertise and a more rational treatment and management approach of pain was delayed until the birth of the field of anesthesia in the 1840s and the isolation and synthesis of morphine by Serturner in 1806 and salicylates from willow bark in the late 1800s.[6] The modern development of a rehabilitation model evolved only after World War I and World War II with the birth of the fields of physical and occupational therapy as a means to "rehabilitate" injured returning soldiers.[7] Pain rehabilitation developed in the context of evolution of the medical specialties of physical medicine and rehabilitation, anesthesia, psychiatry, and occupational medicine during the 20th century. John Bonica championed

a more comprehensive "multidisciplinary" approach in the United States in 1947 and later at the University of Washington in 1960.[8] Wilbert Fordyce, a psychologist and collaborator of Bonica, incorporated operant conditioning and other behavioral approaches with more specialized 8-week inpatient programs in the late 1960s. In 1982, John Loeser formalized a more "structured program" at the University of Washington, a 3-week daily program, which has become a model for "interdisciplinary" treatment. A more biopsychosocial approach to pain rehabilitation has also been facilitated by the merging of behavioral and cognitive fields and the subsequent cognitive-behavioral approach to the assessment and treatment of pain in the 1980s and 1990s.[9–11] A proliferation of pain treatment facilities was seen between 1980 and 1995 and included the advancement of interventional procedures.[12] A more recent conceptualization of pain focuses on behaviors within the pain system, a biopsychomotor model of pain, which incorporates three interdependent behavioral subsystems: (1) communicative, (2) protective, and (3) social response behaviors.[13] This model assumes that a pain system can only be adaptive if the sensory component of the pain system is accompanied by behaviors designed to act on the source or cause of injury or illness. This may help to explain the wide variability observed in pain behaviors seen across different patients despite relatively similar levels of reported pain intensity and objective tissue pathology. The biopsychomotor model of pain can be extended to include behavioral factors such as communicative behavior (grimacing), protective behaviors (i.e., withdrawing a limb from the fire), and behaviors designed to elicit social responses (i.e., empathy and solicitous behavior from others). This model, like the biopsychosocial one, emphasizes that dysfunction may develop in behavioral systems separate from pain sensation, and subsequent treatments targeting pain behavior would more likely lead to greater clinical outcomes and provide a more pragmatic and inclusive model for the spectrum of pain rehabilitation (Fig. 90.1).

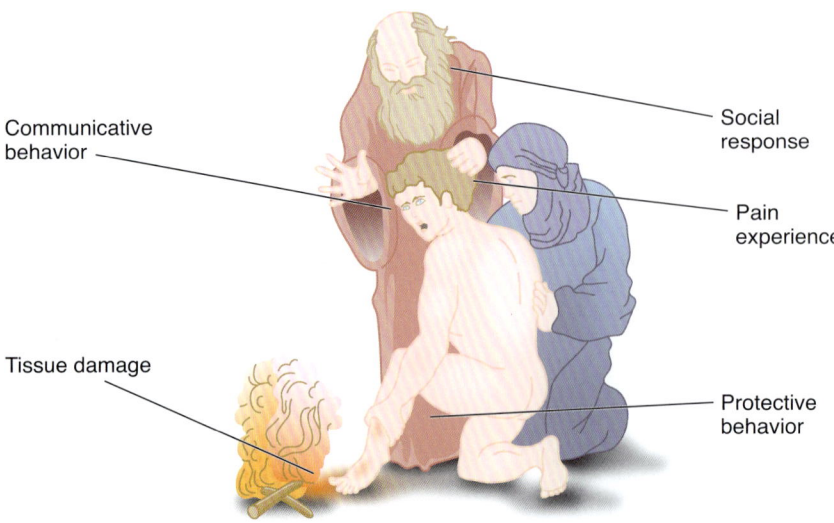

Communicative behavior

Tissue damage

Social response

Pain experience

Protective behavior

FIGURE 90.1 Biopsychomotor response to pain. *(Redrawn from Sullivan MJ. Toward a biopsychomotor conceptualization of pain.* Clin J Pain *2008;24[4]: 281–290, with permission.)*

HISTORY OF FUNCTIONAL RESTORATION AND WORK REHABILITATION

Functional restoration (FR) programs, based on a return-to-work model, evolved along with advancements in occupational medicine beginning in the 1970s. Prior to this, programs of "habit training" focused on restoring workers affected by disease or injury in the 1920s and later by the incorporation of vocational rehabilitation mandated at the federal level in 1923 and the Vocational Rehabilitation Act. In the 1950s, more objective measures were used to track progress and measure outcomes and served as the starting point for more formal work conditioning and work hardening programs championed by Lillian Wegg and Florence Cromwell.[14,15] In the 1970s, work hardening emerged as a formal industrial management service[16] and adopted a similar multidisciplinary approach used in the management of chronic pain and disability. Standardized work stimulation equipment, assessment, and treatment protocols were incorporated into standard practice in the 1980s and led to formal accreditation by the Commission on Accreditation of Rehabilitation Facilities (CARF) in the late 1980s and early 1990s.[17–19]

Gatchel et al.[20] described eight classic critical elements of an FR approach which serves as the foundation for most multi- and interdisciplinary rehabilitation-based programs. Elements include quantification of physical deficits on an ongoing basis, psychosocial and socioeconomic assessment used to individualize and monitor progress, and an emphasis on reconditioning of the injured area or body part. The team-centered FR approach also includes generic simulation of work or activity, disability management with cognitive-behavioral approaches, psychopharmacologic management focusing on improving analgesia, sleep, and affective distress, many times detoxifying patients from medications (i.e., opioids or benzodiazepines).[20]

WHAT IS PAIN REHABILITATION?

A pain rehabilitation model can be applied to the entire spectrum of pain conditions, from acute musculoskeletal injuries, to subacute and recurrent injuries aggravated by poor ergonomics and/or physical impairments, to more complex chronic pain conditions where interplay of biologic, psychologic, and social influences is more apparent. Pain rehabilitation is based on a structured, individualized approach. The formal assessment identifies specific problems and needs most relevant to the patient and relates the problem to impairments and psychosocial factors, selecting appropriate measures to monitor progress and treatment. The rehabilitation program includes planning and coordinating various interventions with a focus on treating the specific impairments by restoring function and identifying compensatory strategies. Additionally, addressing activity limitations by addressing environmental and personal factors may help in restoring patients to previous levels of functioning and preventing or limiting disability.[1]

A traditional definition of rehabilitation, based on a biomedical model, places the concept of rehabilitation as a secondary intervention, used to restore patients to their previous level of (residual) physical, psychologic, and social functioning, and, if possible, return them to (modified) work.[21] Waddell and Burton[22] question this assumption in that the biomedical definition assumes that disability is a "matter of permanent impairment," that sickness and disability imply an incapacity to work, that rehabilitation focuses on "irremediable permanent impairment," and that rehabilitation is a second-stage process following acute medical management and only is carried out after treatment ceases. Waddell and Burton[22] have implied this may be inappropriate in that in many chronic pain conditions (i.e., low back pain), objective factors (pathology and impairment) accounts for a small part of the incapacity. These chronic conditions are characterized more by "symptoms and distress"

than tissue abnormality.[22] A number of biopsychosocial risk factors (i.e., lower level of education, higher preoperative pain, low work satisfaction, longer duration of sick leave, somatic complaints, and passive avoidance coping) have been identified as predictors of poor outcomes after surgical interventions contributing to loss of function, increased disability, and persistent elevated levels of subjective reports of pain.[23,24] These biopsychosocial risk factors may serve as important potential targets for pain rehabilitation.

STAKEHOLDERS IN REHABILITATION

Pain rehabilitation also involves the coordination of a number of important stakeholders involved in the care of the individual patient or worker. Stakeholders may include various health care providers, managed care organizations and insurers, the workers' compensation carrier, society, the individual patient, and family members. This complex health care process and related list of stakeholders involved may sometimes add, as described by Shultz et al.[25] and Gatchel et al.,[20] a political dimension to the individual patient's assessment and treatment process. Success in treatment may vary depending on stakeholder and may indirectly lead to antagonistic, confrontational, and misinterpreted feelings by the patient suffering with pain. Criteria of success may vary significantly depending on whether it is assessed by the patient or by society in general (Fig. 90.2). Many times, contrary to what is seen in other areas of clinical medicine, the pain rehabilitation clinician may find himself or herself in a potentially conflicting role in the treatment of patients with chronic pain (Table 90.1). The focus of care should remain on providing appropriate clinical services, serving as a patient advocate or adjudicator, without crossing ethical boundaries resulting in harm to the client.[26]

This chapter focuses on an overview of assessment and treatment strategies included in a pain rehabilitation–based approach to acute and chronic pain conditions. As part of the clinical continuum, the more comprehensive and integrated treatment approaches commonly referred to as multidisciplinary, interdisciplinary, and/or FR[27] will be examined. Important psychological factors related to chronic pain and disability, the continuum of treatment models from more acute to integrative approaches, specific responsibilities of members of a pain rehabilitation team (i.e., physical and occupational

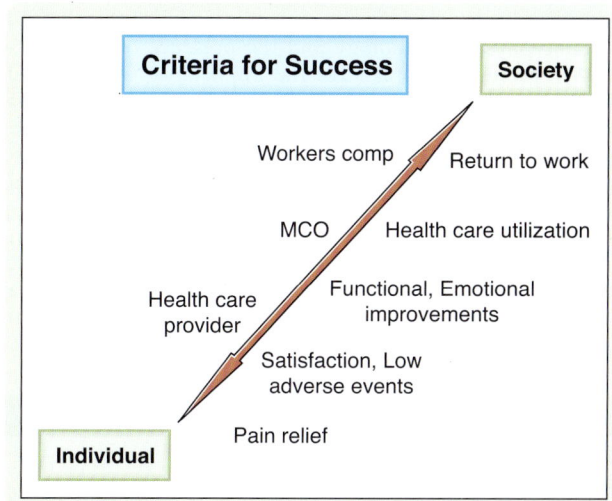

FIGURE 90.2 Criteria for success in comprehensive pain programs. (Redrawn from Gatchel RJ, Okifuji A. Evidence-based scientific data documenting the treatment and cost-effectiveness of comprehensive pain programs for chronic nonmalignant pain. J Pain 2006;7[11]:779–793. Copyright © 2006 American Pain Society. With permission.)

TABLE 90.1 Conflicting Roles of Rehabilitation Specialist

1. Clinical service provider working to reduce the client's suffering
2. Client's advocate working to protect the client in conflicts with an insurer
3. An adjudicator working to help the insurer detect evidence of client's fraudulent behavior

From Sullivan MJL, Main C. Service, advocacy and adjudication: balancing the ethical challenges of multiple stakeholder agendas in the rehabilitation of chronic pain. *Disabil Rehabil* 2007;29(20–21):1596–1603. Reprinted by permission of Taylor & Francis Ltd. http://www.tandfonline.com.

therapist, psychologist, relaxation therapist, and vocational specialist), and an overview of more specific work rehabilitation approaches including work conditioning, work hardening, and functional capacity testing will be reviewed.

Models of Rehabilitation

Conceptual models of pain rehabilitation are based on historical advances that initially described pain as a purely sensory phenomenon evolving to include a more mind–body approach to understanding disability and function (Table 90.2). Hippocrates and Galen (c. 150 AD) described an imbalance of bodily "humors" as a means of developing chronic pain and distress as a model for understanding suffering.[28] In the 1600s, a dualistic mechanistic model emerged. René Descartes (1596–1650) theorized damage to the body would stimulate specific neural pathways, giving rise to the sensation of pain.[28] Through the mid-19th century, medicine focused on the individual's unique manifestations of the disease process. In the mid-1800s, the expanding understanding of pathologic anatomy shifted the focus to a more biomedical model. In 1965, Melzack and Wall[29] proposed the gate control theory of pain which proposed that pain experience was determined by physical, motivational, cognitive, and emotional factors, and transmission of nerve impulses could be modulated by spinal gating mechanisms at the level of the dorsal horn. Melzack[30] elaborated on this more dynamic role of pain networks further with the "neuromatrix" model, arguing that the brain and central nervous system play a dominant role in the pain experience.

BIOPSYCHOSOCIAL APPROACH VERSUS BIOMEDICAL MODEL FOR PAIN MANAGEMENT

The biomedical model assumes a causal relationship between a specific physical pathology and the presence or intensity of pain symptoms. It emphasizes the importance of eliminating pain by restoring normal function in the organ or body part from which pain is thought to emanate. Although the more disease-based biomedical model enabled the medical sciences to flourish and improved our ability to treat infection and other disease processes, its fundamentally limited scope led to less profound success and relative treatment resistance in the treatment of many chronic pain states. A biomedical model may be more advantageous in treating more acute pain states, where interventional procedures, pharmacotherapy, and

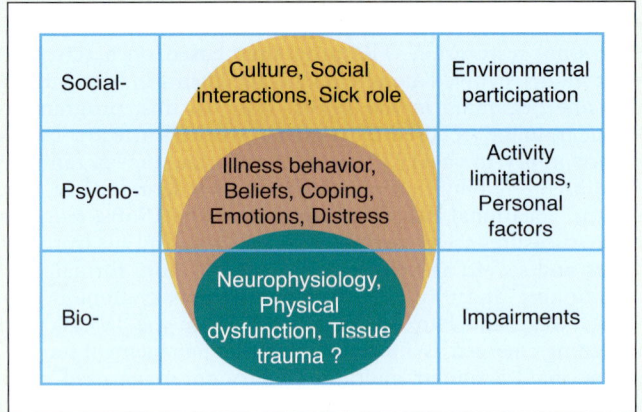

FIGURE 90.3 Domains of the biopsychosocial approach to pain rehabilitation. (*Redrawn from Waddell G, Burton AK. Concepts of rehabilitation for the management of low back pain.* Best Pract Res Clin Rheum *2005;19[4]:655–670. Copyright © 2005 Elsevier. With permission.*)

surgical interventions may lead to recovery of pain or hasten time to recovery. But the biomedical model poorly addresses related mental health issues and frequently relies on dualistic decision pattern, whereby if the patient does not respond to an intervention, then the pain may be not be "real" or just "in their heads."[31] Many more complex pain conditions remain resistant to a purely biomedical approach (i.e., chronic low back pain, neuropathic pain, and fibromyalgia).[32] George Engel[33] helped to shift the thinking from a purely biomedical model of disease management to a more comprehensive biopsychosocial model of illness. Recently, the World Health Organization[34] has embraced a biopsychosocial model of disability (Fig. 90.3), which incorporates a dynamic interaction between the individual health condition and contextual factors.

The pain rehabilitation approach is based on a fundamental understanding of the individual's unique condition as it relates to (1) impairment, (2) disability, and (3) functional limitation. Impairment is the loss of normality psychologically, physically, or functionally at the level of the organs and body systems.[35] Examples of physiologic impairments include muscle weakness, loss of range of motion, and pain. Disability is a restriction or lack of ability to perform activities due to related impairments such as inability to function in a specific vocation, as a spouse, student, or parent. *Functioning* has been described as an umbrella term for body functions, body structures, activities, and participation, denoting a positive interaction between the individual or patient and contextual factors (i.e., background of the individual's life and current situation). Functional limitation is a deviation from the normal behavior of performing activities of daily living (ADLs) and may include problems with transfers, standing, ambulation, running, and stair climbing.[35] A formal model proposed by the International Classification of Functioning, Disability and Health integrates the individual components into a biopsychosocial-based model where a "health condition" is substituted by "chronic pain" (Fig. 90.4). Chronic pain is affected by body function, activities, and participation as well as influences from the environment and personal factors.

A patient-centered approach is necessary if one is to effectively address these important individual concepts. A team-centered approach focuses on helping patients to achieve individual goals, which enable them to improve physical and psychosocial function, decrease pain, and improve quality of life. By working together, the rehabilitation team is able to help patients achieve better outcomes than could be achieved

TABLE 90.2 Historical Overview: Models of Pain

Hippocrates and Galen[28]	Bodily humors
Descartes[28]	Dualistic theory
Melzack and Wall[29]	Gate control theory
Engel[30]	Biopsychosocial approach in medicine
Melzack and Wall[30]	Neuromatrix model
Turk and Gatchel[9]	Biopsychosocial approach
Sullivan[13]	Biopsychomotor approach

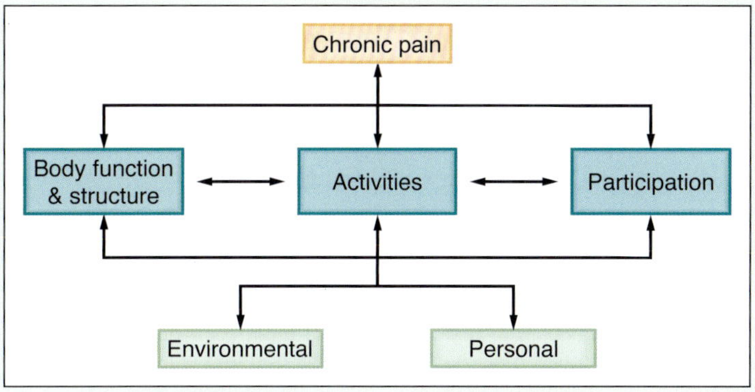

FIGURE 90.4 A formal model demonstrating the relationship among individual components that affect an individual's function was proposed by the International Classification of Functioning, Disability and Health. This model was proposed for any "health condition," and here, we have substituted "chronic pain" for the more generic term. *(Redrawn from Weigl M, Cieza A, Cantista P, et al. Physical disability due to musculoskeletal conditions. Best Pract Res Clin Rheum 2007;21[1]:167–190. Copyright © 2006 Elsevier. With permission.)*

by an individual practitioner or intervention (i.e., surgical procedure, injection, pharmacotherapy). Basic treatment goals of both acute and chronic pain rehabilitation programs focus on functional improvement; improved abilities to perform ADLs, return to leisure, sport, or vocational activities; and improved pharmacologic management of pain and related affective distress (Table 90.3).

TREATMENT APPROACHES: PAIN REHABILITATION

A pain rehabilitation approach encompasses a wide range of treatment options including more directed therapies for acute pain conditions to more comprehensive and collaborative multi- and interdisciplinary approaches (Table 90.4).

Acute Rehabilitation

An approach to managing acute pain conditions relies on a more focused understanding of causative and aggravating factors, changes to affected tissues and related overload stresses, and includes three important phases: (1) acute, (2) recovery, and (3) functional. Within each phase, specific treatment focuses are applied by the therapist or clinician, and tools or skills are taught by the treating therapist with a goal of ongoing self-management and practice. Acute management may involve relative rest, passive modalities (ice, heat, ultrasound), interventional procedures (i.e., trigger point injections, epidural, and facet injections), and oral and topical analgesics. Recovery phases focus on more advanced stretching and strengthening, increasing endurance, and assessing and treating postural changes that may be contributing to chronic pain.[36]

More Comprehensive Team Models: A Pain Continuum

Rehabilitation treatment models include a continuum of care based on patient severity and needs with increasing complexity of treatment philosophies, a need for greater communication, and decreasing individual team member autonomy.[37] Each of these models occupies a position along a continuum of care based on increasing levels of coordination, diversity of philosophies, and decreased hierarchical structure and practitioner autonomy. The left side of the treatment continuum (Fig. 90.5) shows the least collaborative model, parallel practice, where health care providers function quite independently.

As one moves to the right, services become more coordinated with decreasing level of autonomy and increasing diversity of philosophies. From a structure standpoint, moving left to right increases the complexity of care, whereas reliance on hierarchy and clearly defined roles decreases. Complexity and diversity of outcomes increases while, from a process perspective, communication, participants, synergy, and importance of consensus building increases. Multi- and interdisciplinary treatment is even more structured, usually involving a number of specialties with less evidence of practitioner autonomy.

With parallel practice, independent health care practitioners are working within their defined scope of practice such as in an emergency room setting or an acute cardiac unit (i.e., nurse, phlebotomist, physician, radiology technician) where the goal is rapid assessment and treatment in the most efficient manner. Consultation may include a pain physician referring a patient to an addiction specialist or surgeon for recommendations and shared treatment responsibilities. Collaborative practice may include the use of a case manager to help coordinate treatment between the patient and physical therapist. In a collaborative approach, information is shared on an ad hoc basis; practitioners normally practice independently sharing information regarding a particular patient. In coordinated treatment, patient records are shared among clinicians providing treatment for a specific therapy where the case coordinator or case manager is responsible for ensuring information is transferred to all team members. Differentiating between multi- and interdisciplinary treatment will be reviewed in greater detail in the following text. Although commonly used interchangeably, the terms *interdisciplinary* and *multidisciplinary* have important distinguishing features.

Multidisciplinary Treatment

Focused treatment programs for acute conditions may involve individual physical therapy directed by the pain physician, followed by a coordinated program including ongoing communication with the patient's case manager and therapist. With chronic pain conditions, more diverse assessment and treatment teams include multi- and interdisciplinary programs. In the

TABLE 90.3   Pain Rehabilitation Goals
1. Functional improvement
2. Improvement in activities of daily living
3. Relevant psychosocial improvement
4. Rational pharmacologic management (analgesia, mood, and sleep)
5. Return to leisure, sport, work, or other productive activity

TABLE 90.4   Pain Rehabilitation Levels of Care
Unimodal (acute)
Collaborative
Coordinated
Multidisciplinary
• Work conditioning
• Work hardening
Interdisciplinary
Integrative

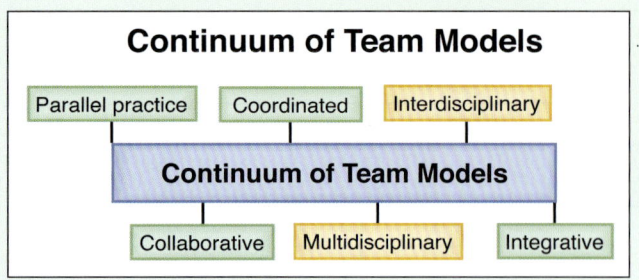

FIGURE 90.5 Continuum of team models. The most common practice model is parallel practice in which each practitioner oversees only the problems within their isolated discipline with little or no interaction with other practitioners caring for the same patient. The most effective models for caring for those with chronic pain involve programs designed to allow for frequent, direct, and repeated interactions among the providers caring for each patient in the form of multidisciplinary and interdisciplinary treatment programs. *(Redrawn from Boon H, Verhoef M, O'Hara D, et al. From parallel practice to integrative health care: a conceptual framework.* BMC Health Serv Res *2004;4[1]:15. © Boon et al; licensee BioMed Central Ltd. 2004. https://doi.org/10.1186/1472-6963-4-15.)*

multidisciplinary model, patient care is planned and managed by a team leader, usually a pain specialist (anesthesiologist, physiatrist, neurologist, psychiatrist, or primary care provider) or a psychologist and is often hierarchical with one or two individuals directing the services of a range of team members, many with individual goals. Treatment may be delivered at different facilities or centers where individual patient progress is not regularly shared between distinct disciplines. The growth of multidisciplinary pain treatment centers in the 1980s led to the need for development of standards and formal accreditation processes. A committee on standards for Pain Treatment Facilities was established by the American Pain Society in the early 1980s, and a process was subsequently developed to accredit multidisciplinary pain centers (MPCs) by the CARF. Non–CARF-accredited programs also exist. Furthermore, the International Association for the Study of Pain delineated four levels of pain programs[38]: MPCs, multidisciplinary pain clinics, pain clinics, and modality-oriented clinics. Multidisciplinary pain clinics and centers, many of which include an even more integrated comprehensive interdisciplinary approach, include similar basic treatment disciplines; however, the MPCs are usually associated with major health science institutions with an additional focus on pain-related research and outcomes.

Interdisciplinary Treatment

Even more collaborative, the interdisciplinary model involves team members working together toward a common goal. Team members are able to communicate and consult with other team members on an ongoing basis, facilitated by regular face-to-face meetings. Incorporation of the cognitive and behavioral psychological approaches along with the development and emergence of the field of health psychology led to the development of more interdisciplinary models under the more general "multidisciplinary" umbrella. Interdisciplinary pain programs may also be referred to as FN programs, which provide outcome-focused, coordinated, goal-oriented services. FR as an approach implies an emphasis on quantification and graded increases in function versus pain reduction, cognitive-behavioral therapy (CBT), occupational therapy, and work conditioning. FR programs were developed in the mid-1980s by Mayer et al.[27] in the United States and have been incorporated with the basic program structure of interdisciplinary programs. The basic treatment model is based on Fordyce's classic contingency management techniques and graded activity related to operant learning processes. FR aims at decreasing or eliminating learned pain behaviors.[39]

The interdisciplinary model provides practical strategies for assessing and treating pain-related deconditioning, psychosocial distress, and socioeconomic factors related to disability. An interdisciplinary team model is characterized by team members working together for a common goal, making collective therapeutic decisions, and having face-to-face meetings and patient team conferences to facilitate communication and consultation. Importantly, in this model, team members possess a combination of skills that no single individual demonstrates alone. Interdisciplinary teams may be led by a physician (medical director), psychologist, or nurse and include comprehensive assessment including pain medicine, pain psychology, and vocational rehabilitation. In some institutions, physical and occupational therapy assessments are also included in the formal assessment. Interdisciplinary programs are usually housed in one facility with periodic interdisciplinary team meetings to assess and adjust treatment progress, program coordination, and discharge planning. Programs primarily focus on restoring joint mobility, muscle strength, endurance, and conditioning and cardiovascular fitness. Coordinated vocational and therapeutic recreation services are also important aspects of care and focus on aiding patients in returning to work, improving behavioral factors (i.e., coping, catastrophizing, and problem solving) in the workplace, clarifying return-to-work level of functioning, and many times, individual occupational therapy.

In general, formal interdisciplinary programs vary in intensity and may include 3 to 8 weeks of 4- to 8-hours-per-day programs with tailored group and individual therapies usually provided in an outpatient or, less often, in an inpatient hospital setting. Long-term follow-up studies of interdisciplinary treatment programs have demonstrated improved return-to-work rates, pain reduction, and quality of life.[40,41] The reader is referred to the chapter on interdisciplinary pain treatment (see Chapter 106).

Outcomes of Multi- and Interdisciplinary Treatment Programs

An early prospective trial documented high rates of return-to-work versus control subjects with improved physical capacities, self-reported disability, depression, and pain scores.[42] Maintained posttreatment improvements in pain, perceived health, and psychological and physical function have been demonstrated in long-term studies (6 months and 5 years).[43,44] The interdisciplinary treatment approach is supported by evidence suggesting these programs are more cost-effective and provide at least equal or greater efficacy than other pain treatments (i.e., spinal cord stimulation and implantable devices, conservative care, and surgery).[45] Additional evidence-based studies have demonstrated outcomes and treatment cost-effectiveness data supporting FR treatment which included multidisciplinary and interdisciplinary treatment programs.[46–48] A recent analysis examined the cost utility of interdisciplinary treatment of chronic spinal pain.[49] Cost utility involved the calculation of cost of the specific treatment relative to desired treatment goal (increased functioning and decreased pain) relative to pharmacologic treatment with or without anesthetic interventions. Interdisciplinary treatment was associated with better cost utility supporting interdisciplinary treatment as both less costly and more effective.[49] Patients undergoing complex lumbar spine surgeries have also demonstrated improvements in pain and function.[50] Although early intervention and referral for pain rehabilitation treatment should intuitively favor greater outcomes as compared to referrals late in the treatment process, studies have demonstrated that patients with long-term disability, many of whom have a greater incidence of pretreatment surgery, may still benefit from comprehensive treatment with similar improved return-to-work rates and decreased lost time rates.[51] Rehabilitation-based multidisciplinary treatment has demonstrated high cost-benefit with regard to decreasing treatment costs and increasing workplace return to work.[52,53] Sustained improvement in pain, mood, function, and opioid reduction or discontinuation was demonstrated in a large cohort of patients enrolled in a structured FR program. Patients entering treatment on opioids retained similar benefits regardless of opioid dose (i.e., high or low daily morphine equivalent doses).[54]

Team Building and Stakeholder Coordination

CASE MANAGEMENT

Case management involvement is an important resource in the management of work-related injuries. Case management has been conceptualized as a system-based approach based on Bronfenbrenner's[55] systems theory, which incorporates an interaction of microsystems (worker factors), mesosystems (workplace, health care utilization, insurance system factors), and macrosystems (economic, social, and legislative factors). Case managers are primarily assigned to injured workers' cases to help facilitate communication between stakeholders and medical providers and coordinate and clarify issues related to return to work and job description, respectively. A practical problem-based approach in rehabilitation management process is the rehabilitation cycle and includes four important interdependent steps: assessment, assignment, intervention, and evaluation (Fig. 90.6).[56] Case management assessment includes identification of patient problems and modification and adjustment of goals. The assignment step involves the assignment to specific health care professionals who understand intervention principles and goals. Intervention more specifically refers to treatment disciplines and interventions with specific goals and milestones. Finally, evaluation refers to the evaluation of goals and level of achievement.[57]

Tate et al.[58] suggested success of any collaborative workplace rehabilitation relationship is contingent on (1) company policy endorsing a commitment to rehabilitation, (2) educational opportunities offered or available for the injured worker by the employer, and (3) identification of key decision-making points involved in the ongoing relationship. Training the nurse case managers in basic fundamentals led to improved work placement as compared to untrained case managers who were more likely to place the injured worker in a sedentary or light duty job position.

Applying a continuum of care model, many times facilitated by strong case management presence, includes a coordination of disciplines, services, providers, and care levels. A continuum of care model developed in Canada for the treatment of musculoskeletal conditions included medical management, active physical therapy, chiropractic management, and multidisciplinary assessment and rehabilitation. Implementation of the program resulted in more rapid and sustained recovery, greater patient satisfaction, and dramatic cost savings as compared to usual care.[59]

APPLYING TEAM VALUES

Decision making in pain rehabilitation has been found to incorporate common decision values shared by the team members, worker, and stakeholders. Shared "general values," as described by Loisel et al.,[60] are those that stress work is therapeutic, pain is multidimensional, and interventions should be graded. These values should in turn be shared by the team members, the worker, and stakeholders facilitated by reassurance and the delivering of a single message as a way of more successfully returning a patient to work or previous level of function.[60] These same values can be applied to the many barriers presented to the individual patient and stakeholder (Table 90.5).

Assessment, Goal Setting, and Progression through Treatment

PAIN REHABILITATION PRINCIPLES

Assessment of patients prior to entering a rehabilitation program is based on a comprehensive examination of physical, psychological, and social or relevant vocational factors. Also, the evaluating clinician must work to develop trust and rapport with the patient in order to understand barriers to recovery (i.e., contentious relationships involving family, employer, case manager, and/or the legal system) that may potentially lead to a delay or reduction of clinical improvement. Many times, the success of developing that relationship starts at the initial evaluation. Understandably, patients undergoing a rehabilitation program are often asked to make significant changes in the ways they cope with pain and function. Readiness to make such important changes has been found to be associated with treatment success,[61,62] and readiness to self-manage pain increases from pre- to post-MPC treatment.[63] Based on the transtheoretical model of behavior change, individuals are seen to progress through a number of stages involving decisions about change and include precontemplation, contemplation, action, maintenance, and acceptance phases.[64] These basic concepts are important for the physician to explore during the evaluation and often become a focus of discussion between other potential treatment disciplines (i.e., pain psychologist, physician, and vocational counselor) when deciding whether the patient is an appropriate candidate for treatment. The pain rehabilitation clinician must be consistent and clear in promoting exercise and activity as essential, safe, and effective for the correction of functional impairments. The clinician must also be aware of various fears, negative attitudes, financial, and vocational stressors many chronic pain working and nonworking patients

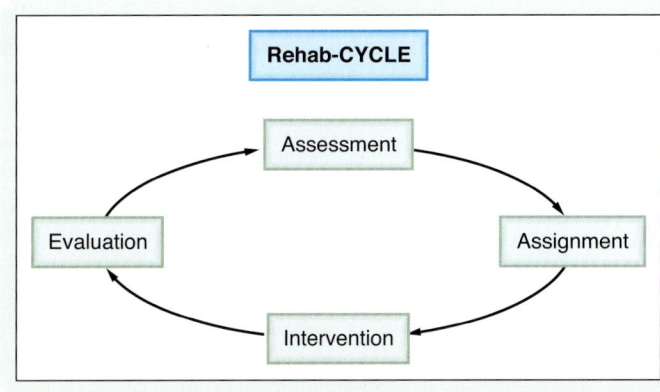

FIGURE 90.6 The rehabilitation cycle. *(Redrawn from Stucki G. International Classification of Functioning, Disability, and Health (ICF): a promising framework and classification for rehabilitation medicine. Am J Phys Med Rehab 2005;84[10]:733–740, with permission.)*

TABLE 90.5   Strategies Applied by the Rehabilitation to Overcome Barriers to Collaboration

Stakeholders	Strategies Applied
Worker	Pain management Relaxation Education Confrontation Rational polypharmacy: analgesia, sleep, mood
Employer	Education Asking for employer's opinion on the TRW setting Sensitizing the employer to its support role in relation to the worker Asking the insurer to use its authority to exert influence on the employer
Insurer	Education Sensitize to the issues involved in the intervention Clarification of the roles and objectives Meeting with the insurer's case worker before meeting the worker or the employer to ensure consistency in information delivered Acting without interfering Choosing convincing information Asking for the case worker's support for the intervention
Physician	Inform the physician about the rehabilitation process Convincing him or her to take action to facilitate return to work Recommendation that worker find another physician if too great a hindrance to the TRW process

TRW, therapeutic return to work.
Adapted by permission from Springer: Loisel P, Durand M, Baril J, et al. Interorganizational collaboration in occupational rehabilitation: perceptions of an interdisciplinary rehabilitation team. *J Occup Rehab* 2005;15(4):581–590. Copyright © 2005 Springer Science + Business Media, Inc.

are sometimes struggling with and be able to confront the patients on these issues in an open and understanding manner (Table 90.6).[65]

Rehabilitation Specialists: Activities and Conceptual Models

A pain rehabilitation team may include a pain physician (i.e., anesthesiologist, physiatrist, psychiatrist, neurologist, and/or primary care physician), physical and/or occupational therapist, a pain psychologist, relaxation (biofeedback) therapist, vocational and therapeutic recreational therapists, social workers, and nurses. Ongoing communication between treating disciplines, including monitoring of progress and adjustment of patient goals, is coordinated by the pain physician. A rehabilitation model is based on a clear, concise, and consistent therapeutic message, which focuses on the patient assuming a more active role in self-management, flare-up management,

and exercise progression. Goals of treatment remain somewhat consistent across all disciplines and focus on improving function and decreasing pain. More specialized roles of individual therapists (i.e., physical and occupational therapy, pain psychology, and vocational rehabilitation) and treatment goals are reviewed in the following text based on an FR approach.

THE THERAPIST'S ROLE: BUILDING AN EFFECTIVE THERAPEUTIC RELATIONSHIP

Besides obvious clinical skills and application of therapies by specific disciplines, the relationship between treating therapist (i.e., physical therapist, occupational therapist, psychologist, etc.) and patient is based on an ability to establish a mutually effective relationship based on ongoing respect, collaboration, and exchange of ideas. A successfully established working alliance will only help to improve outcomes. A process model for patient–practitioner collaboration includes a four-component model based on initially developing a therapeutic relationship, followed by mutual inquiry, problem solving, and negotiation.[66] The therapist must also be cognizant of the patient's beliefs, skills, emotional state, and expectations in effectively developing and adjusting a specific treatment plan and subsequent interventions.[67] A therapeutic relationship involves the establishment of clear and attainable short- and long-term goals, the therapy intervention and training, and discharge planning (i.e., home exercise program). Therapists involved in pain rehabilitation treatment must be adept in their ability to assess initial levels of functional ability and then monitor and progressively increase the individual patient's level and complexity of therapeutic exercises. Therapists assess secondary impairments in addition to their primary pain-related diagnoses (i.e., general inflexibility, deconditioning, regional myofascial pain and dysfunction, and other related postural abnormalities), which expands the area of treatment. Physical and occupational therapists apply a more functional cognitive and behaviorally mediated therapeutic approach and help the patient slowly integrate other aspects of the program into his or her home program.

The basic principles of CBT are also introduced and facilitated by the physical and occupational therapy team members and may include goal setting, education, monitoring and documenting exercise and conditioning progress, and ongoing challenging and redirecting of maladaptive thoughts and behaviors.[68–70] The integration of these approaches may help foster patient optimism, may decrease the fear of reinjury, and may maximize patient compliance. Common cognitive-behavioral objectives may be applied across disciplines as well as by pain psychology professionals in helping the pain rehabilitation patient change maladaptive thoughts and behaviors and include helping patients to combat demoralization, view pain as more manageable, alter or unlearn maladaptive thoughts or behaviors, bolster confidence, and improve problem solving (Table 90.7).

TABLE 90.6   Patient Perceptions

Pathways to Becoming Injured	Seeking Treatment	Seeking Return to Adequate Work	Living as an Injured Worker
Work, workplace, and degree of unsafe practices lead to injury	Desperate for a diagnosis; difficulty accessing appropriate and timely treatment	Returned to modified work yet disillusioned to find accommodations short-lived or nonexistent	Financial hardships; loss of marriages; change in family structure
Fear of unemployment; continued hazardous job	Negative attitudes by doctors and other health practitioners toward the injured worker	Lack of choice and control over vocational issues	Legal action with compensation system drained of financial resources, adding to distress
Lack of knowledge about reporting injuries	Medical uncertainty led to different diagnoses from different specialists; uncertainty led to more doctor shopping and inconsistent message regarding level of activity and restrictions.	Workers believed employer-based actions on the need of company rather than the workers	Psychological deterioration; limitation in self-care activities led to feelings of dependency and social isolation

Reprinted with permission from Beardwood BA, Kirsh B, Clark NJ. Victims twice over: perceptions and experiences of injured workers. *Qual Health Res* 2005;15(1):30–48. Copyright © 2005 SAGE Publications.

TABLE 90.7 Pain Team Shared Primary Objectives of a Cognitive-Behavioral Approach for Pain Patients

1. To combat demoralization by assisting patients to change their view of their pain from overwhelming to manageable
2. To teach patients the coping strategies and techniques to help them to adapt and respond to pain and the resultant problems
3. To assist patients to reconceptualize themselves as active, resourceful, and competent
4. To learn the associations between thoughts, feelings, and behavior and subsequently to identify and alter automatic, maladaptive patterns
5. To utilize more adaptive ways of thinking, feeling, and behaving
6. To bolster self-confidence and patients' attribution of successful outcomes to their own efforts
7. To help patients anticipate problems proactively and generate solutions, thereby facilitating maintenance and generalization

Adapted from Main CJ, Sullivan JM, Watson PJ. *Pain Management: Practical Application of the Biopsychosocial Perspective in Clinical and Occupational Settings.* 2nd ed. Edinburgh: Churchill Livingstone; 2007 and Turk DC, Okifuji A. A cognitive-behavioral approach to pain management. In: Melzack R, Wall PD, eds. *Handbook of Pain Management: A Clinical Companion to Wall and Melzack's Textbook of Pain.* Edinburgh: Churchill Livingstone; 2003:533–541.

INCORPORATING BEHAVIORAL APPROACHES IN PAIN REHABILITATION

Pain rehabilitation approaches rely heavily on incorporating behavioral principles and approaches (i.e., operant, cognitive, and respondent) into active therapies. The cornerstone of operant therapy is graded activity. The basic premise of a graded activity program is based on Fordyce's combined use of graded activity progression and contingency management techniques. This treatment targets helping patients to increase healthy behaviors with positive reinforcement while, at the same time, decreasing maladaptive pain behaviors and beliefs and increasing tolerance for activity.[39,71] Often, graded activity programs are also incorporated with exercise therapy and problem-solving training.[72]

PHYSICAL THERAPY

Physical therapists specialize in gait training, locomotion, core strengthening and stability, joint deficiencies, and proper biomechanics. Active treatments include instruction in strengthening, postural reeducation, and related therapeutic exercise (see Chapter 93). Passive treatment modalities (i.e., local application of heat, cold modalities) may be more efficacious for acute injuries; they are used more judiciously with chronic pain conditions. The use of modalities with chronic pain rehabilitation should shift to an emphasis on facilitating increased activity before or after formal treatment sessions or exercise and as a means of managing pain flare-ups more independently.

Manual therapy, the manipulation of soft tissues, continues to occupy a large part of the modern physical therapist's scope of practice. Not necessarily new to medicine, manual techniques were described by Hippocrates (460 BC) with traction and immobilization as a means of reducing fractures.[73] Galen later recommended techniques to treat "outwardly dislocated" vertebrae.[74] Modern physical therapy's use of manual techniques is based on principles of osteopathic medicine introduced by Andrew T. Still in 1871 and chiropractic treatment pioneered by Daniel Palmer in the late 1800s. Today, many therapists receive special training and certification from a number of "schools" of manual therapy including Maitland, Paris, Kaltenborn, and McKenzie (Table 90.8).[75–77]

Cortical reorganization is coming in to focus for chronic pain management through physical therapy. Evidence of neuroplasticity in amputees with restructured primary sensory cortex receptive fields has been well established.[78] Techniques include graded motor imagery and mirror therapy. These efforts target a rehabilitation program designed for synaptic exercises through the use of tactile and visual stimuli (i.e., computer, flashcards, mirror) and behavioral relevance (i.e., imagined movements, education) controlling for attention.[79]

THERAPEUTIC EXERCISE

Therapeutic exercises targets muscle and joint deficiencies (i.e., weakness, decreased conditioning, and contracture) and serves as the basis for rehabilitation of patients with acute or chronic musculoskeletal, postoperative, and posttraumatic rehabilitation protocols (Table 90.9). The pain clinician must be cognizant of basic principles of physiology and guiding a patient through an individualized active strengthening program. This section reviews important definitions and concepts related to therapeutic exercise. With rehabilitation of any injury, strength and endurance are important targets for assessment and treatment. Muscular strength is the ability of a muscle to generate force against resistance. Maintenance of strength of one's muscle, or, more importantly, muscle groups, will help to improve function and prevent new or reinjury. Strength training also incorporates balance and coordination of movement. Muscular endurance is the ability to perform repetitive muscular contractions against some resistance over time. Endurance will tend to increase with strength. Improvements in muscular endurance may be more advantageous with regard to improving daily function.

In general, skeletal muscular contraction can be divided into three types of contractions: isometric, concentric, and eccentric.[80] Isometric contraction occurs when the muscle contracts without changing length. Isometric or static strength is necessary for performing many ADLs and in functional tasks or sports activities where a stable base of support is necessary

TABLE 90.8 Manual Therapy

Manual Therapy Theories	Basic Principles	Key Terminology
Maitland (Australian)	Graded oscillatory movements to evaluate and treat joint stiffness and restore lost mobility	"S.I.N.S." algorithm *S*everity, *I*rritability, *N*ature of the complaint, *S*tage of the pathology
Paris, Stanley B. (New Zealand)	Focus on examination of spine, facet joint primary source for dysfunction in spine	Incorporates Maitland and Kaltenborn principles
Kaltenborn (Norwegian)	Arthrokinematics principles (e.g., concave-convex, closed-loosely packed positions), treat hypomobility even if asymptomatic	
McKenzie, R (Australia)	Directional preference • "Centralization" vs. "peripheralization" of symptoms • Overpressure	
Cyriax, James (United Kingdom)	Identify "lesion" Heat and friction massage for contractile structures and forceful manipulation with manual distraction to treat intra-articular displacement	

TABLE 90.9	Common Therapeutic Exercises	
Exercise Type	**Description**	**Therapeutic Uses**
Closed kinetic chain	Proximal segment of the extremity moves on a fixed distal segment (e.g., leg press, squats, elliptical walker)	Shoulder and knee rehabilitation, dynamic stability
Concentric	Muscle contracts as it shortens (e.g., flexion phase of a biceps or hamstring curl)	Increase muscle mass and strength
Core stability	Targets low back, trunk, and abdominal muscles (e.g., sit up, back extension, abdominal crunch, Pilates)	Relief of low back pain or pregnancy-related pelvic pain
Eccentric	Muscle contracts as it lengthens (e.g., extension phase of biceps or hamstring curl)	Sport-specific strengthening to prevent injury
Isometric	Muscle contracts, but its length stays the same (e.g., holding a weight in a stationary position for a few seconds)	Muscle toning and strengthening when joint mobility is not advised; quadriceps exercises to treat patellofemoral pain syndrome
Isotonic	Constant resistance applied to a muscle through a joint range of motion (e.g., free-weight lifting)	General muscle conditioning
Open kinetic chain	Distal segment of the extremity moves about the proximal segments (e.g., long arc quadriceps extension, most weight-lifting exercises using the arms)	Functional improvement in activities of daily living

From Rand SE, Goerlich C, Marchand K, et al. The physical therapy prescription. *Am Fam Physician* 2007;76(11):1661–1666. Copyright © 2007 American Academy of Family Physicians. All rights reserved.

for effective and efficient movement of joints. In pain rehabilitation, isometrics may be useful when joint motion is painful, a joint or joints are immobilized, or muscle or muscle groups are weak. In concentric contraction, the muscle shortens in length while tension increases to overcome or move some resistance. With eccentric contraction, resistance is greater than the muscular force being produced, lengthening the muscle while producing tension. This type of muscle activation may be associated with a higher incidence of delayed-onset muscle soreness after exercise.[81] Thus, concentric exercises may be the focus of the program prior to progressing to more eccentric, unloaded ones.

Strength and muscular endurance are dependent on size of muscle or muscle groups, number of muscle fibers, neuromuscular function and efficiency, and biomechanical factors. Neuromuscular training (NT) is a growing area of practice with most work in rehabilitation of musculoskeletal injuries including anterior cruciate ligament reconstruction. NT can include balance exercises, plyometrics, agility training, and joint mobility exercises. Plyometric exercise, initially used to enhance sports performance, may also be used in later stages of an active therapy program as a means of returning the patient to previous levels of sport or work. Plyometric exercise causes a lengthening of the muscle-tendon unit followed immediately by shortening, hence called the stretch-shortening cycle. Plyometrics are used with various demands placed on the musculoskeletal system, usually initiated at lower intensity and progressed to more difficult and physically challenging higher intensity levels. The higher intensity levels may serve to resolve postinjury neuromuscular impairment and prepare the body to respond more effectively and safely to rapid changes in position and movement as well as greater levels of force seen in higher intensity exercise and physically demanding work tasks.[82]

EXERCISE PRESCRIPTION

The goal of an exercise prescription is to maximize the benefit for the patient with pain. Four basic goals include[36,83]:
1. Changing sedentary behaviors to more active ones
2. Modifying risk factors for disability (e.g., obesity, hypertension, deconditioning)
3. Maintaining or improving exercise capacity as it relates to strength, aerobic capacity, balance, and flexibility
4. Enhance psychosocial function

Exercise prescription and focus may vary depending on the patient's age, medical comorbidities, and individual pain-related impairments (i.e., muscle strength, joint pain, joint contracture). Clinicians should be able to optimize therapeutic treatment by balancing the focus of therapy while being mindful of potentially harmful activities. Stretching has been known to increase range of motion of joints, enhance muscle coordination, reduce muscle tension, and increase circulation/energy levels.[84] Strengthening enhances the integrity of muscle, tendons, and other connective tissues, which in turn, improve motor performance and decrease injury risk. Endurance exercise may help to reverse the cycle of deconditioning and weakness commonly seen with chronic pain patients and is an important part of the pain rehabilitation program. Circuit exercise programs, popular with the elderly population, have been shown to provide significant improvements in cardiorespiratory fitness, muscular strength, body composition, and serum cholesterol levels.[85] Aquatic-based therapies offer a partial reduction of stress throughout weight-bearing joints by lowering gravitational burden.[86] This can be considered for patients who have limited range of motion, generalized weakness, poor motor coordination, and/or at a fall risk due to impaired postural deficits (i.e., balance issues, spatial/proprioceptive deficits, sensory disorders). Temperature-controlled facilities can be recommended for additional physiologic effects of exercise have been shown to have analgesic effects, enhance mood, and improve self-efficacy.

OCCUPATIONAL THERAPY
Activities of Daily Living

Occupational therapy focuses primarily on functional mobility and ADLs as well as activity tolerance and ergonomic retraining. Occupational therapists typically concentrate on educating patients regarding proper posture and ergonomics related to upper limb functional activities such as lifting and computer usage as well as proper standing, sitting, carrying, and lifting postures (Table 90.10).

In general, occupational therapists address upper extremity–related ADLs including feeding, hygiene, grooming, bathing, and dressing. Occupational therapists spend considerable time with the patient, educating them on the potential for increases in pain with reinitiation of movement early in the treatment process. Focus may later change to lifting training and tolerance building. Coaching on proper body mechanics could include a basic assessment of maladaptive movement patterns, restriction in joint and soft tissue structures, as well as abnormal postures and bending or lifting techniques, which may exacerbate and/or be the cause of ongoing pain and dysfunction. Occupational therapists are also responsible for managing and directing more individualized work conditioning and work hardening programs as well as administering functional capacity evaluations (FCEs), often in coordination with the vocational rehabilitation team and employer.

TABLE 90.10	Desktop Ergonomics	
	Environment Set up	**Reasoning**
Keyboard	• Position keyboard align to forearms to be parallel to thighs at 90- to 110-degree elbow angle • Elbows held close to trunk • Wrists should be neutral. • Keyboard "legs" collapsed	• Decreases shoulder/neck tension and strain • Prevents nerve compression (i.e., carpal tunnel) and tendonitis of wrists and fingers
Chair	• Sitting as far back in the chair as possible keeping in contact with backrest at all times • Knees at 90-degree angle with feet flat on floor • Backrest at 10- to 15-degree recline • Hips at 100- to 105-degree angle • Use of footrest if chair is elevated. • Avoid leaning forward.	• Decreases stress on mid/low back muscles • Hip and knee angles keep the low back posture in neutral position • Aligns head and neck over spine • Reduces forward head posture/neck tension and headaches
Monitor	• Centered directly in front, not to the side • Eyes should align with a point 1–2 in below the top of screen. • Arm length distance with middle finger just touching the screen • Bifocals: place monitor slightly lower without bending neck or tilting the chin to view screen • Invest in full-lens computer glasses.	• Avoids forward head posture/neck tension and shoulder impingement • Spine in neutral posture without rotational forces
Mouse	• Place mouse on dominant side or more comfortable side. • Elbows tucked and wrist in neutral • Maneuver with full arm/shoulder motion; not isolated wrist motion	• Decreases shoulder/neck tension and strain • Prevents nerve compression and tendonitis at the wrist
Phone	• Placed in arm's length while in chair. • Avoid cradling headset between neck and shoulder. • Consider hands-free headset.	• Decreases shoulder/neck tension and strain • Avoids cervical nerve impingement
Lighting	• Avoid glare by placing screen parallel to light source such as windows. • Tilt 5–15 degrees downward to avoid glare from overhead lights. • Turn off backlighting behind the computer screen.	• Reduces eye strain and fatigue • Reduces migraine/headache triggers
Writing surface	• Separate writing surface from computer station • Keep chest upright and arms resting comfortably with elbow at 90- to 100-degree angle. • Avoid forward posture of head or neck.	• Decreases shoulder/neck tension and strain • Reduces forward head posture and back strain

Pacing

Another important concept occupational therapists are primarily responsible for is directing and instructing patients on activity, work, and leisure pacing. Pacing may be either an appropriate or a maladaptive behavior. Good pacing may include activity scheduling, taking breaks to complete a pain-inducing activity as compared to overdoing activities, and the "crashing and burning" approach with prolonged periods of rest and "down time" in order to recover from activity related flare-ups (Table 90.11).

The therapist is then able to work with the patients in improving their daily routines, incorporating pacing, taking appropriate breaks, and prioritizing activities while incorporating self-management skills learned in other disciplines such as relaxation techniques and stretching into the patient's daily routine at work, at home, and in leisure activities.

TABLE 90.11	Pacing: Useful versus Maladaptive Responses	
Useful	**Maladaptive**
1. Gradual increase in activity	• Overdo activities
2. Increase on a quota system	• Increase activity until "intolerable" pain
3. Varies mixed activities and rest	• "Crash and burn": take extended periods of rest or prolonged down time after an activity or pain flare-up
4. Realistic and manageable	• Too busy to incorporate

Adapted from Harding VR, Williams AC. Extending physiotherapy skills using a psychological approach: cognitive-behavioral management of chronic pain. *Physiotherapy* 1995;81(11):681–688. Copyright © 1995 Chartered Society of Physiotherapy. With permission.

Occupational therapists may also provide job site interventions, which include assessing ergonomics and monitoring for job site safety issues. Services may also include job site training where a trained occupational or physical therapist accompanies the injured worker.

PAIN PSYCHOLOGY

Psychological interventions as part of a pain rehabilitation program have been shown to enhance recovery, decrease disability, and enhance psychosocial functioning.[87–90] Psychological interventions focus on addressing maladaptive cognitions, passive avoidance, depression, anger, and pain-related anxiety. Initial focus of psychological treatment includes challenging patients to change maladaptive thoughts and behaviors. As stated earlier, an individual's readiness to make important changes has been hypothesized to be an important factor in treatment success and serves as an important initial clinical question posed by the treating psychologist.[61,63,91] Over time, patients are also challenged to consider taking a more active role in management and incorporating nonpharmacologic and pharmacologic therapies into their individualized program. Problem-solving training may help to teach patients to choose more effective responses to pain and improve function.[72] Incorporating group pain psychology interventions with an active physical therapy program has been shown to enhance posttreatment outcomes as compared to physical therapy alone on measures of functional impairment, employment of active coping strategies, medication use, and self-efficacy beliefs.[92]

One of the more critical elements of pain psychology involves CBT. As regarded as first-line psychosocial treatment for individuals with chronic pain,[93] CBT techniques include relaxation training, setting and working toward behavioral goals/activation, problem solving, and cognitive restructuring.[94,95] Symptom associations of pain-related beliefs

Respiration

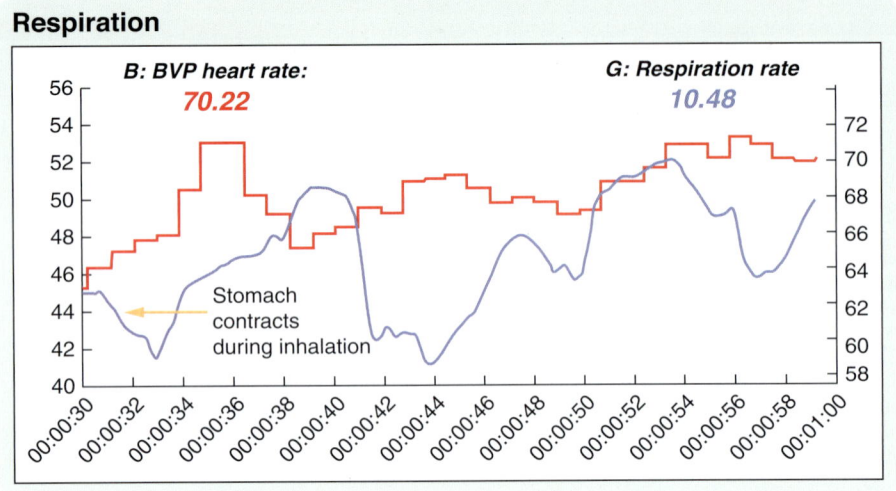

Representation of reverse breathing. X-axis is time. Y-axis is blood volume pulse heart rate. Notice the discordant inhalation/exhalation and respiratory rate (*blue line*) patterns in relation to heart rate. (*Source: Adapted from Chapter 16 Respiration Assessment. Shaffer F. HRV Biofeedback Tutor 2018. biosourcesoftware.com.*)

and appraisals regarding pain intensity, depression, physical disability, and activities/social role limitations are indicated for CBT.[96] In particular, catastrophizing—magnification and rumination about the source of pain and perceived inability to cope with pain—has consistently been found to be associated with physical and psychosocial dysfunction.[97]

Combining group CBT and relaxation therapy with an individually based multidisciplinary treatment (CBT, physical and occupational therapy, and social work) program demonstrated an additive effect with greater improvement on measures of pain, sleep, activity levels, and medication use.[98,99]

Chronic pain frequently accompanied by underlying psychiatric/psychological disorders often benefit from mindfulness meditation.[100] It is characterized by paying attention to the present moment with openness, curiosity, and acceptance.[101] The premise behind mindfulness meditation to target the high prevalence and refractory nature of chronic pain in conjunction with negative consequences of maladaptive behavior, which improved self-referential processing, leads to increased interest in treatment plan including adjunct to therapy and alternative interventions.[100,102] The goal is to refocus the mind on the present, thereby increasing awareness of one's external surroundings and inner sensations, allowing the individual to step back and reframe experiences. Clinical applications of mindfulness meditation include substance use, stress reduction, tobacco, fixation, and chronic pain.

RELAXATION TRAINING

Furthermore, incorporating relaxation techniques (i.e., deep breathing, progressive muscle relaxation) with therapeutic stretching can help the patient progress in the exercise program and improve activity tolerance. Biofeedback is a treatment that has been shown to be quite effective in the management of pain.[103] The treatment serves to help a patient become more aware of their physiologic responses to pain or other stressors. In general, relaxation training focuses on helping the patient to acquire self-management tools for reducing tension and decreasing pain. Initial treatment involves basic education explaining how biofeedback-assisted therapies work and helping the patient to understand they are able to control or modulate physiologic functioning of their own bodies by "seeing" or "hearing" their own physiologic function (i.e., breathing, limb temperature, and sweat).

Respiration assessment should always precede heart rate variability (HRV)-related biofeedback due to potential for dysfunctional breathing. Stimulation of the parasympathetic system through biofeedback produces autonomic relaxation, which in turn, directly counteracts stress effects.[104] Clinical application of breathing assessment includes postural or biomechanical deficits such as clavicular or reverse breathing, thoracic versus inappropriate abdominal usage, hyperventilation, or transient apnea.

Skills training include training with basic biofeedback technologies such as respiratory biofeedback, surface electromyography, and/or thermal biofeedback. Techniques include

Respiration

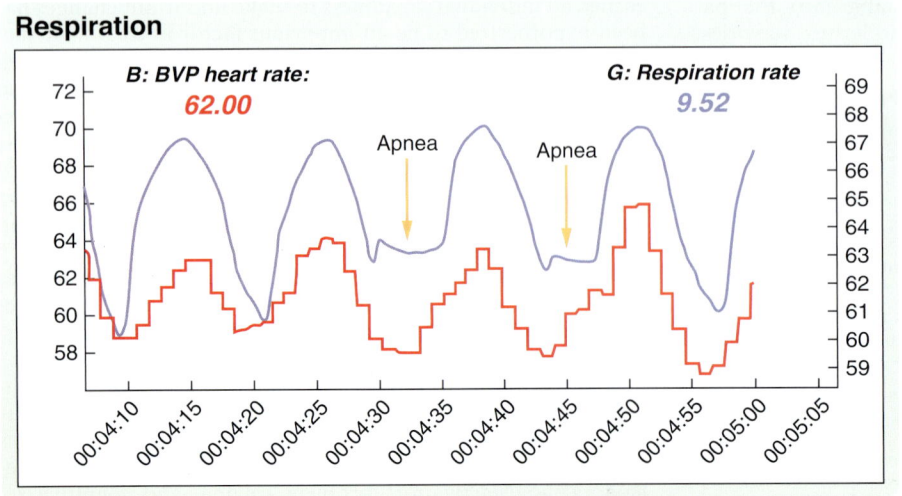

Representation of transient apnea. X-axis is time. Y-axis is blood volume pulse heart rate. Notice two successive periods of transient apnea indicated by *yellow arrows*. (*Source: Adapted from Chapter 16 Respiration Assessment. Shaffer F. HRV Biofeedback Tutor 2018. biosourcesoftware.com.*)

diaphragmatic breathing, progressive muscle relaxation, and autogenic techniques. Patients are encouraged to log their practice sessions in their relaxation practice log. Relaxation training is provided in one-on-one and in group settings usually provided by a health psychologist, biofeedback specialist, or physical or occupational therapist. At the conclusion of formal treatment, patients should be independent with relaxation self-management techniques and be able to incorporate practice and technique integration with normal daily activities and during times of symptom flare-up or elevated levels of distress.

Work Rehabilitation: Work Conditioning and Work Hardening

Work conditioning and work hardening are an important core component of work therapy in the field of industrial and pain rehabilitation. This field of modern occupational therapy developed after World War II with a focus of FR in wounded veterans as a means of securing employment in the civilian world after returning from duty. Work therapy also includes acute treatment, job analysis and placement, and FCE. Multidisciplinary principles were applied to occupational therapy–based work rehabilitation in the 1950s with the development of improved assessment tools and systems and the addition of vocational counseling, medical management, and industrial engineering. In the 1970s, work hardening and conditioning programs were combined with behavioral medicine approaches that focused on reducing abnormal illness behaviors in a more comprehensive treatment of injured workers primarily with low back pain. Eventually, standards were established and subsequently updated by CARF in the late 1989s and early 1990s, respectively. Work rehabilitation usually begins once a patient has reached a treatment plateau in active physical therapy and is unable to return to work due to pain-related impairments (Table 90.12).

Work conditioning is usually concentrated on the physical components of flexibility, strength, coordination, and endurance and involves one discipline of treatment (i.e., physical or occupational therapy). A more multidisciplinary approach is seen with work hardening, which incorporates behavioral and vocational components with a formal focus on return to job-specific tasks or positions. Work conditioning is routinely coordinated with acute medical management as compared to work hardening, which is usually provided later in therapy within the rehabilitation phase of treatment.

Work hardening programs were initially described by Matheson[19] at Rancho Los Amigos Hospital as a work-oriented program focused on improvement in the client's productivity versus symptom reduction or increased physical capacity.

A "client" can be described as an injured worker with impairments that do not match their job position, a worker with disease-based impairments with diminishing physical capacity, a job applicant who may not have the physical abilities to perform the intended job, or a currently employed worker in transition to a job requiring higher physical function.[105]

Work hardening is an individualized, work-specific, multi- and interdisciplinary program centered primarily on returning patients (i.e., the injured worker) to their previous level of work or work demands. Work hardening uses real or simulated work tasks and progressively increasing conditioning, flexibility, neuromuscular control, and tolerances (Tables 90.13 and 90.14). Goals of work hardening include (1) attaining optimal physical tolerances and abilities, (2) maximizing cognitive and psychosocial functioning, (3) developing appropriate worker behaviors, (4) reducing fear and increasing confidence for the resumption of productive work, and (5) identifying problems that may necessitate placement in an alternative job.[106,107]

An individualized work hardening program incorporates a three-step process which includes an initial formal job analysis to determine specific duties, completion of a baseline work tolerance evaluation, and establishment of the individual work hardening plan. Work hardening standards have been established by a number of groups and may vary depending on the state or the federal governing body.[108]

Occupational therapy manages most work conditioning and work hardening treatments as part of the pain rehabilitation program. Assessment of the injured worker is more comprehensive than the assessment done during standard occupational therapist evaluations. Patients are placed in programs of a set number of days, usually 4 to 5 days per week over a 4- to 8-week period. Both programs are highly based on objective measures obtained during the program evaluation which includes tolerances and capacities for lifting, pulling, standing, sitting, reaching, climbing, kneeling, and/or crawling. The treatment program is based on the individual patient's own job demands and work level (sedentary, light, medium, heavy) and developing improved conditioning and tolerances for activities (Table 90.15). Although formal psychological counseling is not a core discipline, these programs are based on helping patients work through and unlearn fear-avoidance beliefs and movement patterns, pain-related fear, catastrophizing, and pain-related anxiety.

OUTCOMES OF WORK CONDITIONING AND WORK HARDENING PROGRAMS
Reviews of work conditioning and work hardening programs have found evidence of improved return-to-work rates and fewer work days off in treated patients versus controls.[109–111]

Measuring Physical Capacity

Functional capacity testing provides a means of measuring function by obtaining objective and subjective data with performance-based testing. Testing can be divided into two groups of tests including examining isolated parts of the body or "functional units" (i.e., lumbar spine, shoulder) and the ability of the functional unit to interact with other bodily functional units or activities such as lifting capacity. Lifting capacity many times involves the interplay of the biomechanical chain of a number of systems. A common example of the biomechanical chain includes transferring forces from a simple lifting task from the ground. Here, forces of the biomechanical chain include transferring forces from the hands through the elbow and shoulder (upper extremity functional unit) to the lumbar spine and hips (lower extremity functional unit) to placing the object and transmitting forces to the floor.

TABLE 90.12	Work Rehabilitation
Musculoskeletal exercise	Stability–mobility
	Strength–endurance
	Balance–coordination
Aerobic training	Equipment based
	Aerobic classes
	Functional activities
Education	Principles
	Technique training
	Problem solving
Work activity	Simulated activity
	Actual equipment
	Actual work

From Isernhagen SJ. Work hardening. In: Demeter SL, Andersson GB, eds. *Disability Evaluation.* 2nd ed. St. Louis: Mosby; 2003:769–780. Reprinted with permission of Dr. Gunnar Andersson.

TABLE 90.13   Components in a Typical Work Hardening Program

Step I Job Analysis	Step II Establishing Work Tolerance Baseline	Step III Individual Work Hardening Plan/Goals
• Understand worker's specific job requirements • Critical job tasks • Physical job demands • Psychosocial demands • High-risk job factors • If job analysis available: review and validate primary job functions • If job analysis not available: on-site job task analysis	• Medical history • Worker interview • Job description with critical job demands • Pain assessment • Physical assessment • Work posture and mobility • Strength, sensation, coordination, lifting, reaching, carrying, pushing and pulling, stooping, bending, kneeling, sitting and standing, work task stimulation	1. Increase duration of daily participation 2. Increase physical tolerances to the level of critical job demands 3. Improve body mechanics and postures 4. Develop pain management strategies 5. Develop problem-solving skills for self-management at the work site 6. Facilitate appropriate worker behaviors

FUNCTIONAL CAPACITY TESTING

FCE is a process where the individual's ability to perform a specific task or physical demands of a job is assessed, bridging the gap between observed physical impairment and work capacity. Matheson[112] describes the FCE as "a systematic method of measuring an individual's ability to perform meaningful tasks in a safe and dependable basis." FCEs have three specific purposes: (1) to improve the likelihood that the patient will be safe in a job task, (2) to assist in improving role performance through assessing and identifying functional decrements as a means of providing appropriate treatment or therapy, and (3) to determine presence of disability for bureaucratic or legal entities that may assign a quantifiable level of impairment or apportionment or deny monetary or medical disability benefits.[113]

The FCE is a valuable tool for the physician, vocational counselor, therapist, or employer to establish a specific attainable work goal based on objective data. In theory, by comparing performance demonstrated on the FCE to the required physical job demands of the individual worker, meeting or exceeding all job requirements simulated during testing will help

to determine if the patient is safe to return to work.[114] Better performance on an FCE, many times defined by lower number of failed tasks during testing, may be associated with lower risk of recurrence after return to work.[115,116]

Various types of FCEs can be performed as a means of obtaining specific vocational goals including establishing functional goal setting, disability rating, job and occupation matching, and work capacity evaluation.[117] In general, the FCE can be done before treatment and usually once a patient has reached a treatment plateau or has completed a formal acute or subacute therapy program. As a means of determining impairment of disability, an FCE may compare measured functional capacity either to the patient's preinjury baseline abilities or population norms. Accurate measurements of a worker's preinjury capacities rarely exist, and health care providers are many times inaccurate in estimating the worker's preinjury functional level or physical capabilities.[118]

The FCE is used to establish a final level of functioning and includes a statement regarding validity, effort, and pain behaviors. A number of validated FCE tests and programs are available from a number of vendors and are individually designed for specific disorders such as low back pain or upper extremity conditions. These tests can be incorporated into a larger battery of tests used in the formal FCE.

Strength testing may include assessing lifting, carrying, pushing and pulling, work stimulation, and circuit testing (Table 90.16).

Common assessment and job simulation devices include the Purdue Pegboard Test, the Crawford Small Parts Dexterity Test, and the Jebsen Hand Dexterity Test. Testing usually lasts between 2 and 6 hours and may also be performed over a number of days to observe for fluctuations in performance depending on change in pain or to make sure the patient meets the demands of more continuous work-related physical activity.

Performance reliability is used to determine performance credibility based on the assumption an individual will produce similar outcomes in a series of trials.[119] Additional objective measures may also be assessed including increase in heart rate during and immediately following performance of a strenuous task. Performance credibility can be subjectively determined by assessing for consistency and incongruity between specific tasks and tests. Reports of pain and pain behavior should be specific to the body part and correlate with the level or area of injury.[120] Performances that do not follow normal or expected patterns may also be indicative of less than sincere effort.

Subjective credibility measures may include the individual's perceived physical strain or effort and may be rated on a number of Ratings of Perceived Exertion scales. In one example, scores range from 6 to 19 (e.g., 6 ["no exertion"], 7 ["very, very light"], 15 ["hard"], to 19 ["very, very hard"]) and increase linearly with exercise intensity. Values of the scale correlate to heart rate (0.8 to 0.9), ranging from 60 to 200 beats per minute.[121]

TABLE 90.14   Work Hardening Program Standards

1. Improve strength and endurance in relation to return to work goal
2. Simulation of critical work demands, tasks, and environment of the job worker will return to
3. Education: body mechanics, pacing, safety, and injury prevention, promoting worker responsibility and self-management
4. Assess for need for job modifications (i.e., equipment changes or additions, ergonomic modification); availability for on-site job modification assessments
5. Individualized written plan which includes observable and measurable goals
6. Safe work or therapy environment that is appropriate for reaching vocational goals
7. Quality assurance system; outcomes based on program and worker goals
8. Documentation or reporting system that includes initial plan, regularly scheduled team conference notes with monitoring of progress, record of attendance, and compliance
9. Evaluation and modification of work behaviors (i.e., timeliness, attendance, interpersonal relationships)
10. Criteria for admission includes physical recovery sufficient to allow for progressive reactivation and participation for a minimum of 4 h/d for 3 to 5 d/wk along with a defined work goal
11. Criteria for discharge clearly stated (i.e., patient met goal stated in plan, patient did not participate according to program plan, goals not feasible to attain)

Adapted from State of Washington Department of Labor and Industries. Work hardening program standards. Available at: http://www.lni.wa.gov/ClaimsIns/Files/ReturnToWork/WhStds.pdf. Accessed October 12, 2008.

TABLE 90.15 Physical Demand and Level of Job Duty

Physical Demand	Occasionally	Frequently	Constantly
Sedentary duty	Lift or carry up to 10 lb Sit 6–8 h Stand or walk 0–2 h	Negligible — —	Negligible — —
Light duty	Lift or carry up to 20 lb Stand 4–8 h Walk 0–4 h	Up to 10 lb — —	Negligible — —
Medium duty	Lift or carry up to 50 lb Stand or walk 8 h	Up to 20 lb —	Up to 10 lb —
Heavy duty	Lift or carry up to 100 lb Stand or walk 8 h	Up to 50 lb —	Up to 20 lb —
Very heavy duty	Lift or carry over 100 lb	Over 50 lb —	Over 20 lb

From U.S. Department of Labor. *Dictionary of Occupational Titles.* Washington, DC: U.S. Government Printing Office; 1986.

Grip strength assessment in the FCE serves two important purposes: to assess handgrip strength and to document performance of maximum voluntary efforts. A common test used in many clinics and mentioned in FCE reports is the Jamar hand dynamometer (Sammons Preston Rolyan, Bolingbrook, IL), a calibrated hydraulic hand dynamometer, which measures static grip strength at five grip spans. The therapist is able to produce a graphical representation of the forces produced at five grip positions, revealing a classic "biomechanical curve," with the lowest force values occurring in positions 1 and 5 and the highest at positions 2, 3, or 4. Inability to produce this bell-shaped curve could cast doubt on the individual's sincerity of full maximal effort. Force variability of multiple trials can be applied to normative data and can also be used to indicate noncredible performance.[122]

FUNCTIONAL CAPACITY TESTING UTILITY

An important and controversial area of FCE results lies in its ability to demonstrate validity, reliability, and accuracy.[123,124] Lemstra et al.[125] examined the tester's ability to judge maximal effort in a standard lifting protocol. They found high specificity but low sensitivity (62%), with only a small number of commonly used maximal lifting tests (5 of 17) able to differentiate between maximal and submaximal effort.[125] Results of a functional capacity test can be used in conjunction with a more detailed understanding of the individual's job description as a means of establishing return-to-work restrictions and formal levels of work (see Table 90.15).[125,126]

What Does an "Invalid" Test Mean?

In clinical practice, "invalid" test results may be related to the patient demonstrating less than full effort in performance. Although not always consistent with malingering, a number of other causes (i.e., physical ability, disability, pain intensity, and fear of reinjury) have been identified and should be considered when interpreting and making clinical decisions based on an invalid test or test with evidence of less than "full" or "maximal" effort" (Table 90.17).[127–131]

The result of an FCE can have far-reaching consequences including injured workers having compensation terminated or losing their job or seeing a reduced medicolegal settlement in patients believed to be exhibiting submaximal effort.[132] In order to establish one's functional capacity, the injured worker must perform at his or her maximal ability or effort. A number of tests have been used as a means of validating effort. Methods used to assess sincerity of effort include Waddell nonorganic signs, pain behavior description, symptom magnification, coefficients of variation, correlations between physical evaluation and function, grip measurements, and temporal relationship between heart rate and increased levels of pain with activity.[132]

Role of Opioid Management in Pain Rehabilitation

The role of chronic opioid management in pain rehabilitation remains a controversial topic. Pain rehabilitation programs as early as the 1960s focused primarily in reducing and/or eliminating opioids secondary to fears of tolerance and development of iatrogenic addiction. This approach still characterizes many interdisciplinary programs today. However, the shift to more liberal use of opioids for chronic noncancer pain in the 1990s and the assumption that risk for addiction was minimal led to increased use of opioids in the treatment of chronic pain.[133–136] The more recent reappraisal of the benefits and potential harms of chronic opioid use has also led to more questions regarding the accuracy of predicting aberrant behavior, and quantifying rates of addiction[137–140] use has been complicated by an appreciation for not only the potential risk for developing aberrant behaviors, misuse, abuse, and opioid use disorders, including

TABLE 90.16 Functional Capacity Evaluation Lifting Protocols

Test	Test of	Specific tests	Progression	End Point/Outcome
Isoinertial lifting evaluation	Occasional lifting tolerance	4 lifts: floor to knuckle, 12 in to knuckle, waist to shoulder, shoulder to overhead carry	Weight increased in 10-lb increments, if too much pain, decrease by 5 lb	
Dynamic carrying, pushing and pulling tests		1. Carrying 2. Pushing (sled) 3. Pulling (sled)	Resistance increased in 10-lb increments	
Progressive isoinertial lifting evaluation (PILE)	Frequent lifting capacity	Lumbar PILE: (floor to 30-in-high shelf) Cervical PILE: (30-in shelf to 54-in shelf)	Starting weight 13 lb (male), 8 lb (female)	End points: 85% of max predicted age adjusted heart rate, 55% to 60% body weight

TABLE 90.17 Causes of Invalid Functional Capacity Evaluation Tests/Less Than Full Effort

1. Malingering syndrome
2. Factitious disorder
3. Learned illness behavior
4. Conversion disorder, pain disorder, or other somatoform disorders
5. Depressive disorders
6. Test anxiety
7. Fear of symptom exacerbation or injury
8. Fatigue
9. Medication and psychoactive substance effects
10. Lowered self-efficacy expectations
11. Need to gain recognition of symptoms

Reprinted with permission from Gaudino E, Mael F, Matheson L. *Synthesis of Research and Development of Prototypes for a New Disability Determination Methodology: Measurement Concepts and Issues Relevant to the Social Security Administration's Disability Determination Process.* Washington, DC: American Institutes for Research; 1999. Table 90.17: Causes of Invalid Functional Capacity Evaluation Tests/LessThan Full Effort.

TABLE 90.19 Behavioral Treatment Techniques for the Chemically Dependent Patient

- Psychotherapeutic strategies
  - Supportive-expressive psychotherapy
  - Multidimensional family therapy
  - Motivational enhancement therapy
- Mind–body therapies
  - Cognitive-behavioral therapy
  - Relaxation techniques
    - Meditation, guided, or self-guided imagery, progressive muscle relaxation, deep breathing

Adapted from Wooten J. Behavioral medicine treatment in the management of the chemically dependent patient. In: Smith HS, Passik SD, eds. *Pain and Chemical Dependency.* New York: Oxford University Press; 2008:253–258.

overdose-related deaths. Common adverse effects include cognitive impairment, endocrine dysfunction (sexual dysfunction and opioid induced hypogonadism), mood disorders,[141–145] and hyperalgesia. In 2016, the Centers for Disease Control and Prevention (CDC) published guideline for opioid management in primary care and recommending nonpharmacologic therapy, including biopsychosocial-based rehabilitation approaches, as preferred first-line treatment to opioid therapy, and if opioid therapy is necessary, their use should be in conjunction with nonpharmacologic interventions.[146] Unfortunately, patients referred for pain rehabilitation treatment include many opioid treatment "failures" and/or patients additionally managed with other controlled substances (i.e., benzodiazepines and hypnotics). A number of reasons for "failing" should be considered during the evaluation and subsequent treatment planning and include ruling out improper or maladaptive opioid or controlled substance use, poorly designed opioid and/or pharmacologic regimen, poor or limited analgesic response with adverse effects, opioid-induced pain sensitivity, or a combination of these factors (Table 90.18).

A pain rehabilitation approach may also offer a patient self-management treatment tools with potentially similar or even greater clinical outcomes than those achieved by his or her opioids. Concurrent pharmacologic management may include a structured taper off the currently used opioid, conversion to methadone, or conversion to buprenorphine products. Use of U.S. Food and Drug Administration-approved buprenorphine products for opioid dependence (i.e., buprenorphine and buprenorphine and naloxone) requires specialized licensure by clinicians. Treatment of withdrawal signs and symptoms

TABLE 90.18 Potential Scope and Spectrum of Use of Opioids in Pain Rehabilitation

1. Rule out improper or maladaptive use of opioids for their nonanalgesic reasons (i.e., depression, psychological tolerance, anxiety)
2. Adjust regimen, limit short-acting, limit total daily dose while patient learns additional nonpharmacologic skills to manage pain and pain-related disability
3. Detoxification secondary to failed analgesia, poor functional outcomes related to use
4. Slow taper down in total daily dose while monitoring for changes in mood and cognition
5. Detoxification secondary to development of possible opioid-induced hyperalgesia
6. Detoxification secondary to pain condition not fully or partially responsive to opioid analgesics

primarily includes the use of oral or transdermal clonidine, an α_2-adrenergic agonist,[147] and adjuvants for withdrawal-related myalgias, insomnia, anxiety, and gastrointestinal distress.[148]

The advantage of a structured and relatively controlled environment of most multi- and interdisciplinary treatment programs is that it offers an opportunity for patients with limited or maximized improvement on chronic opioids to reduce or eliminate opioids while at the same time learning to apply new nonpharmacologic approaches to management of their pain. This structured environment is ideal for more successfully integrating a more rational polypharmacy approach.

Behavioral medicine treatments can be effectively incorporated into a structured multi- or interdisciplinary rehabilitation-based program. Treatment of the chemically dependent patient can include two types of therapies: (1) psychotherapeutic strategies and (2) mind–body therapies.[149] Psychotherapeutic strategies include supportive-expressive psychotherapy, drug counseling, family therapy, and motivational enhancement therapy. Mind–body therapies, in general, include CBT, group support and education therapy, and relaxation therapy (i.e., deep breathing, imagery, hypnosis, and biofeedback) (Table 90.19).

Patients can be successfully weaned or have their opioid dose decreased during an FR rehabilitation-based approach. Active opioid withdrawal did not adversely impact short-term outcomes following a 3-week outpatient pain program,[150] and physical and emotional functioning were favorable in a fibromyalgia cohort that completed an interdisciplinary pain rehabilitation program which included withdrawal of opioids, nonsteroidal anti-inflammatory drugs, benzodiazepines, and muscle relaxants.[151]

Conclusion

Rehabilitation is a continuous process, relying on a comprehensive, pragmatic approach that focuses on an individual's physical impairments and function-related disability. The field of modern pain rehabilitation developed along with the growth of a number of medical specialties (i.e., anesthesia, rehabilitation medicine, psychiatry, neurology, and occupational medicine), physical and occupational therapy, and health psychology. Pain rehabilitation assessment and treatment is based on a biopsychosocial model. A narrower dualistic biomedical model may fail to adequately assess and help patients to manage the complexities of ongoing pain, affective distress, and environmental and social issues. Treatment goals in pain rehabilitation programs include improving psychosocial functioning; decreasing pain; improving aerobic conditioning; and facilitating safe and successful return-to-work status, return to leisure pursuits, and activities at home and in the community.

A pain rehabilitation approach includes planning and coordinating various medical interventions (i.e., pharmacologic and nonpharmacologic), educational activities, and coordinating a patient's participation with specific rehabilitation-based disciplines (i.e., physical and occupational therapy, pain psychology, relaxation, and other mind–body therapies). Vocational rehabilitation can serve as an additional treatment option and may be coordinated in patient-specific work-based therapies such as work conditioning and work hardening programs. Work conditioning and work hardening may be more specific levels of treatment for the injured worker as a bridge to progress patients after completing acute rehabilitation and more closely simulating work activities, respectively, prior to returning to previous levels of sport, function, or work. Functional capacity testing may be used as a more objective means of establishing a baseline level of function, establish treatment and work goals, or finalize return-to-work level of functioning. Validity measures may also help to identify physical and psychosocial factors that are contributing to the injured worker's level of functioning and clarify discrepancies in tolerances and effort.

The pain rehabilitation clinician must work with the patient in conjunction with various stakeholders (i.e., case managers, insurance providers and adjustors, legal personnel, and family members). The clinician's role may include additional responsibilities beyond not only working to help patients decrease pain and increase function but also as an advocate for the patient with insurers, employers, and rare circumstances as adjudicator, helping the insurer or employer to decrease or identify inconsistent or fraudulent patient behavior. Optimal patient outcomes are facilitated by the clinician and team members establishing a therapeutic environment with the patient characterized by ongoing coordination of care, communication between treatment team members and the patient, providing consistency of message, and collaboration between team members.

References

1. Weigl M, Cieza C, Cantista P, et al. Physical disability due to musculoskeletal conditions. *Best Pract Res Clin Rheumatol* 2007;21:167–190.
2. Hopkins HL, Smith HD, Tiffany EG. Rehabilitation. In: Hopkins HL, Smith HD, eds. *Willard and Spackman's Occupational Therapy*. 6th ed. Philadelphia: JB Lippincott; 1983:267–333.
3. Institute of Medicine. *Relieving Pain in America: A Blueprint for Transforming Prevention, Care, Education, and Research*. Washington, DC: National Academies Press; 2011.
4. Interagency Pain Research Coordinating Committee. *National Pain Strategy: A Comprehensive Population Health-Level Strategy for Pain*. Bethesda, MD: Interagency Pain Research Coordinating Committee; 2011.
5. Foley BS, Buschbacher RM. Occupational rehabilitation. In: Braddom RL, ed. *Physical Medicine and Rehabilitation*. 3rd ed. Philadelphia: Saunders Elsevier; 2007:1047–1054.
6. Zimmermann M. The history of pain concepts and treatment before IASP. In: Merskey H, Loeser J, Dubner R, eds. *The Paths of Pain, 1975–2005*. Seattle, WA: IASP Press; 2005:1–21.
7. Murphy W. *Healing the Generations: A History of Physical Therapy and the American Physical Therapy Association*. Alexandria, VA: American Physical Therapy Association; 1995.
8. Bonica JJ. Organization and function of a pain clinic. *Northwest Med* 1950;49:593–596.
9. Turk DC. Biopsychosocial perspective on chronic pain. In: Gatchel RJ, Turk DC, eds. *Psychological Approaches to Pain Management: A Practitioner's Handbook*. New York: Guilford Press; 1996:33–52.
10. Keefe FJ, Dunsmore J, Burnett R. Behavioral and cognitive-behavioral approaches to chronic pain: recent advances and future directions. *J Consult Clin Psychol* 1992;60:528–536.
11. Weiner BK. The biopsychosocial model and spine care. *Spine* 2008;33:219–223.
12. Brena SF. Pain control facilities: patterns of operation and problems of organization in the USA. *Clin Anesth* 1985;3:183–195.
13. Sullivan MJ. Toward a biopsychomotor conceptualization of pain. *Clin J Pain* 2008;24:281–290.
14. Curry R. Understanding patients with chronic pain in work hardening programs. *Work Program Spec Interest Section Newsl* 1989;3:3.
15. Wegg L. Role of occupational therapist in vocational rehabilitation. *Am J Occup Ther* 1957;11:4.
16. Wegg L. Essentials of work evaluation. *Am J Occup Ther* 1960;14:65.
17. Commission on Accreditation of Rehabilitation Facilities. *Standards Manual for Organizations Serving People with Disabilities*. Tucson, AZ: Author; 1989.
18. Commission on Practice. *Occupational Therapy Services in Work Practice: Official Statement*. Bethesda, MD: American Occupational Therapy Association; 1992.
19. Matheson LN. Work hardening for patients with back pain. *J Musculoskelet Med* 1993;10:53–63.
20. Gatchel RG, Mayer TG, Hazard RG, et al. Editorial: functional restoration. Pitfalls in evaluating efficacy. *Spine* 1992;17:988–994.
21. Nocon A, Baldwin S. *Trends in Rehabilitation Policy. A Review of the Literature*. London: Kings Fund; 1998.
22. Waddell G, Burton AK. Concepts of rehabilitation for the management of low back pain. *Best Pract Research Clin Rheum* 2005;19:655–670.
23. den Boer JJ, Oostendorp RA, Beems T, et al. Reduced work capacity after lumbar disc surgery: role of cognitive-behavioral related risk factors. *Pain* 2006;126(1–3):72–78.
24. Donceel P, DuBois M. Predictors of work incapacity continuing after disc surgery. *Scand J Work Environ Health* 1999;25:264–271.
25. Schultz IZ, Stowell AW, Feurstein M, et al. Models of return to work for musculoskeletal disorders. *J Occup Rehabil* 2007;17:327–352.
26. Sullivan JM, Main C. Service, advocacy and adjudication: balancing the ethical challenges of multiple stakeholder agendas in the rehabilitation of chronic pain. *Disabil Rehabil* 2007;29:1596–1603.
27. Mayer T, Gatchel R, Kishino N, et al. Objective assessment of spine function following industrial injury. A prospective study with comparison group and one year follow-up. *Spine* 1985;10:482–493.
28. Descartes R. *De Homine*. Leyden, The Netherlands: Moyardus & Leffen; 1662.
29. Melzack R, Wall P. Pain mechanisms: a new theory. *Science* 1965;150:971–979.
30. Melzack R. From the gate to the neuromatrix. *Pain* 1999;6:S121–S126.
31. Pransky G, Shaw WS, Franche R, et al. Disability prevention and communication among workers, physicians, employers, and insurers: current models and opportunities for improvement. *Disabil Rehabil* 2004;26:625–634.
32. Carragee EJ. Persistent low back pain. *N Engl J Med* 2005;352:1891–1898.
33. Engel GL. The need for a new medical model: a challenge for biomedicine. *Science* 1977;196:129–136.
34. World Health Organization. *International Classification of Functioning, Disability and Health*. Geneva, Switzerland: World Health Organization; 2001. Available at: http://www3.who.int/icf/icftemplate/cfm. Accessed August 28, 2009.
35. American Physical Therapy Association. The guide to physical therapist practice, 2nd ed. *Phys Ther* 2001;81(1):9–738.
36. Fiatarone MA. Exercise to prevent and treat functional disability. *Clin Geriatr Med* 2002;18:431–462.
37. Boon H, Verhoef M, O'Hara D, et al. From parallel practice to integrative health care: a conceptual framework. *BMC Health Serv Res* 2004;4:15.
38. Loeser JD. Desirable characteristics for pain management facilities. In: Bond MJ, ed. *Pain Research and Management*. Amsterdam, The Netherlands: Elsevier; 1991;411–416.
39. Fordyce WE. *Behavioral Methods for Chronic Pain and Illness*. St. Louis, MO: Mosby; 1976.
40. Norrefalk JR, Linder J, Ekholm J, et al. A 6-year follow-up study of 122 patients attending a multiprofessional rehabilitation programme for persistent musculoskeletal-related pain. *Int J Rehabil Res* 2007;30(1):9–18.
41. Angst F, Brioschi R, Main CJ, et al. Interdisciplinary rehabilitation in fibromyalgia and chronic back pain: a prospective outcome study. *J Pain* 2006;7:807–815.
42. Mayer TG, Gatchel RJ, Mayer H, et al. A prospective two-year study of functional restoration in industrial low back injury. An objective assessment procedure. *JAMA* 1987;258:1763–1767.
43. Westman A, Linton S, Theorell T, et al. Quality of life and maintenance of improvements after early multimodal rehabilitation: a 5-year follow-up. *Disabil Rehabil* 2006;28:437–446.
44. Grahn B, Ekdahl C, Borgquist L. Effects of a multidisciplinary rehabilitation programme on health-related quality of life in patients with prolonged musculoskeletal disorders: a 6-month follow-up of a prospective controlled study. *Disabil Rehabil* 1998;20:285–297.
45. Turk DC. Clinical effectiveness and cost effectiveness of treatment for patients with chronic pain. *Clin J Pain* 2002;18:355–365.
46. Chou R, Qaseem A, Snow V, et al. Diagnosis and treatment of low back pain: a joint clinical practice guideline from the American College of Physicians and the American Pain Society. *Ann Intern Med* 2007;147(7):478–491.
47. Gatchel RJ, Okifuji A. Evidence-based scientific data documenting the treatment and cost-effectiveness of comprehensive pain programs for chronic nonmalignant pain. *J Pain* 2006;7(11):779–793.
48. Guzman J, Esmail R, Karjalaninen K. Multidisciplinary rehabilitation for chronic low back pain: systematic review. *BMJ* 2001;322:1511–1516.
49. Hatten A, Gatchel R, Polatin P, et al. A cost-utility analysis of chronic spinal pain treatment outcomes: converting SF-36 data into quality-adjusted life years. *Clin J Pain* 2006;22:700–711.
50. Mayer T, Gatchel R, Brede E, et al. Lumbar surgery in work-related chronic low back pain: can a continuum of care enhance outcomes? *Spine J* 2014;14:263–274.

51. Jordan K, Mayer TG, Gatchel RJ. Should extended disability be an exclusion criterion for tertiary rehabilitation? Socioeconomic outcomes of early versus late functional restoration in compensation spinal disorders. *Spine* 1998;23:2110–2116.

52. Ekto-Andersen J, Ingvarsson E, Kullendorff M, et al. High cost-benefit of early team-based biomedical and cognitive-behavior intervention for long-term pain-related sickness absence. *J Rehabil Med* 2008;40:1–9.

53. Norrefalk JR, Ekholm K, Linder J, et al. Evaluation of a multiprofessional rehabilitation programme for persistent musculoskeletal-related pain: economic benefits of return to work. *J Rehabil Med* 2008;40:15–22.

54. Huffman K, Rush T, Fan Y, et al. Sustained improvements in pain, mood, function and opioid use post interdisciplinary pain rehabilitation in patients weaned from high and low dose chronic opioid therapy. *Pain* 2017;158;1380–1394.

55. Bronfenbrenner U. *The Ecology of Human Development: Experiments by Nature and Design*. Cambridge, MA: Harvard University Press; 1979.

56. Stucki G. International Classification of Functioning, Disability, and Health (ICF): a promising framework and classification for rehabilitation medicine. *Am J Phys Med Rehab* 2005;84(10):733–740.

57. Steiner WQ, Ryser L, Huber E, et al. Use of the ICF model as a clinical problem-solving tool in physical therapy and rehabilitation medicine. *Phys Ther* 2002;82:(11):1098–1107.

58. Tate DG, Habeck RV, Schwartz G. Disability management: a comprehensive framework for prevention and rehabilitation in the workplace. *Rehabil Lit* 1986;47:230–235.

59. Stephens B, Gross DP. The influence of a continuum of care model on the rehabilitation of compensation claimants with soft tissue disorders. *Spine* 2007;32:2898–2904.

60. Loisel P, Falardeau M, Baril R, et al. The values underlying team decision-making in work rehabilitation for musculoskeletal disorders. *Disabil Rehabil* 2005;27:561–569.

61. Jensen MP. Enhancing motivation to change in pain treatment. In: Turk DC, Gatchel RJ, eds. *Psychological Approaches to Pain Management: A Practitioner's Handbook*. New York: Guilford Press; 1996:78–111.

62. Kearns RD, Rosenberg R, Jamison RN, et al. Readiness to adopt a self-management approach to chronic pain: the Pain Stages of Change Questionnaire (PSCOQ). *Pain* 1997;72:227–234.

63. Jensen MP, Nielson WR, Turner J, et al. Changes in readiness to self-manage pain are associated with improvement in multidisciplinary pain treatment and pain coping. *Pain* 2004;111:84–95.

64. Prochaska J, DiClemente C. *The Transtheoretical Approach: Crossing Traditional Boundaries of Therapy*. Homewood, IL: Dow Jones Irwin; 1984.

65. Beardwood BA, Kirsh B, Clark NJ. Victims twice over: perceptions and experiences of injured workers. *Qual Health Res* 2005;15:30–48.

66. Jensen GM, Lorish CD. Promoting patient cooperation with exercise programs: linking research, theory, and practice. *Arthritis Care Res* 1994;4: 181–189.

67. Meichenbaum D, Turk DC. *Facilitation Treatment Adherence: A Practitioner's Guidebook*. New York: Plenum; 1987.

68. Harding V, Williams AC. Extending physiotherapy skills using a psychological approach: cognitive-behavioral management of chronic pain. *Physiotherapy* 1995;81:681–688.

69. Main CJ, Sullivan JM, Watson PJ. *Pain Management: Practical Application of the Biopsychosocial Perspective in Clinical and Occupational Settings*. 2nd ed. Edinburgh: Churchill Livingstone; 2007.

70. Turk DC, Okifuji A. A cognitive-behavioral approach to pain management. In: Melzack R, Wall PD, eds. *Handbook of Pain Management: A Clinical Companion to Wall and Melzack's Textbook of Pain*. Edinburgh: Churchill Livingstone; 2003:533–541.

71. Fordyce WE, Fowler RS, Lehmann JF, et al. Operant conditioning in the treatment of chronic pain. *Arch Phys Med Rehabil* 1973;5:399–408.

72. van den Hout JH, Vlaeyen JW, Heuts PH, et al. Secondary prevention of work-related disability in nonspecific low back pain: does problem-solving therapy help? A randomized clinical trial. *Clin J Pain* 2003;29:87–96.

73. Ackerknecht EH. *A Short History of Medicine*. New York: Ronald Press; 1975.

74. Schiotz EH, Cyriax J. *Manipulation: Past and Present*. London: William Heinemann; 1978.

75. Hall RC, Nitz AJ. Basic concepts of orthopedic manual therapy. In: Malone T, McPoil T, Nitz A, eds. *Orthopedic and Sports Physical Therapy*. 3rd ed. St. Louis, MO: Mosby; 1997:191–209.

76. Maitland GD. *Vertebral Manipulation*. 4th ed. Boston, MA: Butterworth; 1984.

77. McKenzie R. *The Lumbar Spine: Mechanical Diagnosis and Therapy*. Waikane, New Zealand: Spinal Publications; 1981:95–106.

78. Florence SL, Jain N, Kaas JH. Plasticity of somatosensory cortex in primates. *Semin Neurosci* 1997;9:3–12.

79. Bowering KJ, O'Connell NE, Tabor A, et al. The effects of graded motor imagery and its components on chronic pain: a systematic review and meta-analysis. *J Pain* 2013;14:3–13.

80. Prentice WE. Impaired muscle performance: regaining muscular strength and endurance. In: Voight M, Hoogenboom B, Prentice WE, eds. *Musculoskeletal Interventions. Techniques for Therapeutic Exercise*. New York: McGraw-Hill Medical; 2007:135–152.

81. Gabriel D, Kamen G, Frost G. Neural adaptations to resistive exercise: mechanisms and recommendations from training practices. *Sports Med* 2006;36:133–149.

82. Chmielewski TL, Myer GD, Kauffman D, et al. Plyometric exercise in the rehabilitation of athletes: physiological responses and clinical application. *J Orthop Sports Phys Ther* 2006;36(5):308–319.

83. Rand SE, Goerlich C, Marchand K, et al. The physical therapy prescription. *Am Fam Physician* 2007;76:1661–1666.

84. Shellock FG, Prentice WE. Warming-up and stretching for improved physical performance and prevention of sports-related injuries. *Sports Med* 1985;2:267–278.

85. Takeshima N, Rogers ME, Islam MM, et al. Effect of concurrent aerobic and resistance circuit exercise training on fitness in older adults. *Eur J Appl Physiol* 2004;93:173–182.

86. Konlian C. Aquatic therapy: making a wave in the treatment of low back injuries. *Orthop Nurs* 1999;18:11–18.

87. Evers QW, Kraaimaat FW, van Riel PL, et al. Tailored cognitive-behavioral therapy in early rheumatoid arthritis for patients at risk: a randomized controlled trial. *Pain* 2002;100:141–153.

88. Morley S, Williams A. A systematic review and meta-analysis of randomized clinical trials of cognitive behavior therapy and behavior therapy for chronic pain in adults, excluding headache. *Pain* 1990;80:1–13.

89. Tulder can MW, Ostelo RW, Vlayen JW, et al. Behavioral treatment for chronic low back pain: a systematic review within the framework of the Cochrane back review group. *Spine* 2001;26:270–281.

90. Ostelo RW, Tulder M, Vlaeyen J, et al. Behavioral treatment for chronic low-back pain. *Cochrane Database Syst Rev* 2005;(1):CD002014.

91. Kerns RD, Rosenberg R, Jamison RN, et al. Readiness to adopt a self-management approach to chronic pain: the Pain Stages of Change Questionnaire (PSOCQ). *Pain* 1997;72:227–234.

92. Nichoal MK, Wilson PH, Goyen J. Comparison of cognitive-behavioral group treatment and an alternative non-psychological treatment for chronic low back pain. *Pain* 1992;48:339–347.

93. Ehde DM, Dillworth TM, Turner JA. Cognitive-behavioral therapy for individuals with chronic pain. *Am Psychol* 2014;69:153–166.

94. Thorn BE. *Cognitive Therapy for Chronic Pain: A Step-by-step Guide*. New York: Guilford Press; 2004.

95. Turner JA, Romano JM. Cognitive behavioral therapy for chronic pain. *Bonica's Management of Pain*. 3rd ed. Philadelphia: Lippincott Williams & Wilkins; 2001:1751–1758.

96. Gatchel RJ, Peng YB, Peters ML, et al. The biopsychosocial approach to chronic pain: find the figure advances in future directions. *Psychol Bull* 2007;133:581–624.

97. Edwards RR, Cahalan C, Mensing G, et al. Pain, catastrophizing, and depression in the rheumatic diseases. *Nat Rev Rheumatol* 2011;7:216–224.

98. Linton SJ, Melin L, Stjernlof K. The effects of applied relaxation and operant activity training on chronic pain. *Behav Psychother* 1985;13:87–100.

99. Nicholas MK, Wilson PH, Goyen J. Comparison of cognitive-behavioral group treatment and an alternative non-psychological treatment for chronic low back pain. *Pain* 1992;48:339–347.

100. Chiesa A, Serretti A. Mindfulness-based interventions for chronic pain: systematic review of evidence. *J Altern Complement Med* 2011;17:83–93.

101. Kabat-Zinn J, Lipworth L, Burney R. The clinical use of mindfulness meditation for the self-regulation of chronic pain. *J Behav Med* 1985;8: 163–190.

102. Hilton L, Hempel S, Ewing BE, et al. Mindfulness meditation for chronic pain: systemic review and meta-analysis. *Ann Behav Med* 2017;51:199–213.

103. Astin JA. Mind-body therapies for the management of pain. *Clin J Pain* 2004;20:27–32.

104. Shaffer F. *HRV Biofeedback Tutor: Fulfill BCIA's Heart Rate Variability Biofeedback Didactic Requirement*. Kirksville, MO: Biosource Software; 2018.

105. Isernhagen SJ. Work hardening. In: Demeter SL, Andersson GB, eds. *Disability Evaluation*. 2nd ed. St. Louis, MO: Mosby; 2003:769–780.

106. Maultsy Burt C. Work evaluation and work hardening. In: Pedretti LC, Early MB, eds. *Occupational Therapy: Practice Skills for Physical Dysfunction*. 5th ed. St. Louis, MO: Mosby; 2001:337–381.

107. Lindstrom I, Ohlund C, Eek C, et al. The effect of graded activity on patients with subacute low back pain: a randomized prospective clinical study with an operant-conditioning behavioral approach. *Phys Ther* 1002;72:279–290.

108. State of Washington Department of Labor and Industries. Work hardening program standards. Available at: http://www.lni.wa.gov/ClaimsIns/Files /ReturnToWork/WhStds.pdf. Accessed October 12, 2008.

109. Bendix AF, Bendix T, Baegter K, et al. Comparison of three intensive programs for chronic low back pain patients: a prospective, randomized, observer-blinded study with one year follow-up. *Scand J Rehab Med* 1997;29:81–89.

110. Schonstein E, Kenny D, Keating J, et al. Physical conditioning programs for workers with back and neck pain: a Cochrane systematic review. *Spine* 2003;28:E391–E395.

111. Schonstein E, Kenny DT, Keating J, et al. Work conditioning, work hardening and functional restoration for workers with back and neck pain. *Cochrane Database Syst Rev* 2003;(1):CD001822.

112. Matheson L. Functional capacity evaluation. In: Andersson G, Demeter S, Smith G, eds. *Disability Evaluation*. Chicago: Mosby Yearbook; 1996: 168–177.

113. Matheson LN, Mooney V, Grant JE, et al. Standardized evaluation of work capacity. *J Back Musculoskelet Rehabil* 1996;6:249–264.

114. Innes E, Straker L. A clinician's guide to work-related assessments: 1—purposes and problems. *Work* 1998;11:183–189.

115. Isernhagen SJ. *The Comprehensive Guide to Work Injury Management.* Gaithersburg, MD: Aspen Publishers; 1995:821.

116. Gross DP, Battié MC. The prognostic value of functional capacity evaluation in patients with chronic low back pain: part 2. *Spine* 2004;29:920–924.

117. Matheson LN. The functional capacity evaluation. In: Demeter SL, Andersson GB, eds. *Disability Evaluation.* 2nd ed. St. Louis, MO: Mosby; 2003:311–325.

118. Fishbain D, Khalil T, Abdel-Moty E, et al. Physician limitations when assessing work capacity: a review. *J Back Musculoskelet Rehabil* 1995;5: 107–113.

119. Matheson LN. How do you know that he tried his best? The reliability crisis in industrial rehabilitation. *Industrial Rehab Quart* 1988;1:10–12.

120. Owens KA, Buchholz RL. Functional capacity assessment, worker evaluation strategies, and the disability management process. In: Shrey DE, Lacerte M, eds. *Principles and Practices of Disability Management in Industry.* Boca Raton, FL: CRC Press; 1995:269–299.

121. Borg GA. Psychophysical bases of perceived exertion. *Med Sci Sports Exerc* 1982;14:377–381.

122. Matheson L, Carlton R, Niemeyer L. Grip strength in the disabled sample: reliability and normative standards. *Industrial Rehab Quart* 1988;1(3):9.

123. Vasudevan SV. Role of functional capacity assessment in disability evaluation. *J Back Musculoskelet Rehabil* 1996;6:265–276.

124. Vlozo CA. Work evaluations: critique of the state of the art of functional assessment of work. *Am J Occup Ther* 1993;47:203–209.

125. Lemstra M, Olszynski WP, Enright W. The sensitivity and specificity of functional capacity evaluations in determining maximum effort. *Spine* 2004;29:953–959.

126. U.S. Department of Labor. *Dictionary of Occupational Titles.* Washington, DC: U.S. Government Printing Office; 1986.

127. Gross DP, Battié MC. Factors influencing results of functional capacity evaluations in workers' compensation claimants with low back pain. *Phys Ther* 2005;85:315–322.

128. Gross DP, Battié MC. The construct validity of a functional capacity evaluation administered within a workers' compensation environment. *J Occup Rehab* 2003;13:287–295.

129. Cutler RB, Fishbain DA, Steele-Rosomoff R, et al. Relationships between functional capacity measures and baseline psychological measures in chronic pain patients. *J Occup Rehab* 2003;13:249–258.

130. Lackner JM, Carosella AM. The relative influence of perceived pain control, anxiety, and functional self efficacy on spinal function among patients with chronic low back pain. *Spine* 1999;24:2254–2260.

131. Geisser ME, Robinson ME, Miller QL, et al. Psychosocial factors and functional capacity evaluation among persons with chronic pain. *J Occup Rehab* 2003;13:259–276.

132. Lechner DE, Bradbury SF, Bradley LA. Detecting sincerity of effort: a summary of methods and approaches. *Phys Ther* 1998;78:867–888.

133. Moulin DE, Iezzi A, Amireh R, et al. Randomised trial of oral morphine for chronic non-cancer pain. *Lancet* 1996;347:143–147.

134. Tennant FS, Uelmen GF. Narcotic maintenance for chronic pain. Medical and legal guidelines. *Postgrad Med* 1983;73:81–94.

135. Portenoy RK. Chronic opioid therapy in nonmalignant pain. *J Pain Symptom Manage* 1990;5:46–62.

136. Porter J, Jick HN. Addiction rare in patients treated with narcotics. *N Engl J Med* 1980;302:123.

137. Kalso E, Edwards JE, Moore RA, et al. Opioids in chronic non-cancer pain: systematic review of efficacy and safety. *Pain* 2004;112:372–380.

138. Eisenberg E, McNicol ED, Carr DB. Efficacy and safety of opioid agonists in the treatment of neuropathic pain of nonmalignant origin: systematic review and meta-analysis of randomized controlled trials. *JAMA* 2005;293:3043–3052.

139. Fishbain DA, Bole B, Lewis J, et al. What percentage of chronic nonmalignant pain patients exposed to chronic opioid analgesic therapy develop abuse/addiction and/or aberrant drug-related behavior? A structured evidence-based review. *Pain Med* 2008;9:444–459.

140. Furlan A, Sandoval J, Mailis-Gagnon A, et al. Opioids for chronic noncancer pain: a meta-analysis of effectiveness and side effects. *CMAJ* 2006;174:1589–1594.

141. Ballantyne JC, Mao J. Opioid therapy for chronic pain. *N Engl J Med* 2003; 349:1943–1953.

142. Mao J. Opioid-induced abnormal pain sensitivity: implications in clinical opioid therapy. *Pain* 2002;100:213–217.

143. Angst MS, Clark JD. Opioid-induced hyperalgesia: a qualitative systematic review. *Anesthesiology* 2006;104(3):570–587.

144. Daniell HW. Hypogonadism in men consuming sustained-action oral opioids. *J Pain* 2002;3:377–384.

145. Michna E, Ross EL, Hynes WL, et al. Predicting aberrant drug behavior in patients treated for chronic pain: importance of abuse history. *J Pain Symptom Manage* 2004;28:250–258.

146. Dowell D, Hagerich TM, Chou R. CDC guideline for prescribing opioids for chronic pain—United States, 2016. *MMWR Recomm Rep* 2016;65 (RR-1):1–49.

147. Charney DS, Heninger GR, Kleber HD. The combined use of clonidine and naltrexone as a rapid, safe, and effective treatment of abrupt withdrawal from methadone. *Am J Psychiatry* 1986;143:831–837.

148. Collins ED. Pharmacologic approaches to opioid dependence and withdrawal. In: Smith HS, Passik SD, eds. *Pain and Chemical Dependency.* New York: Oxford University Press; 2008:247–251.

149. Wooten J. Behavioral medicine treatment in the management of the chemically dependent patient. In: Smith HS, Passik SD, eds. *Pain and Chemical Dependency.* New York: Oxford University Press; 2008:253–258.

150. Rome JD, Townsend CO, Bruce BK, et al. Chronic noncancer pain rehabilitation with opioid withdrawal: comparison of treatment outcomes based on opioid use status at admission. *Mayo Clin Proc* 2004;79:759–768.

151. Hooten WM, Townsend CO, Sletten CD, et al. Treatment outcomes after multidisciplinary pain rehabilitation with analgesic medication withdrawal for patients with fibromyalgia. *Pain Med* 2007;8:8–16.

CHAPTER 91

Assessment and Treatment of Substance Use Disorders

ANDREW J. SAXON, JAMES P. ROBINSON, and **MARK D. SULLIVAN**

This chapter on assessment and treatment of substance use disorders provides guidance, particularly for practitioners interested in pain medicine, on how various forms of substance use disorders are diagnosed and managed clinically. Because detection and management of opioid use disorder poses a major concern for physicians using opioids to treat patients, and because diagnosis of opioid use disorder in this context is often confounded by pain issues, the chapter focuses special attention on this complex clinical conundrum. More specifically, the chapter focuses on patients with chronic nonmalignant pain (CNMP) because issues related to opioid use disorder are more vexing in these patients than in patients with cancer or other life-threatening illnesses.

Various surveys indicate that individuals with chronic pain disorders are more likely to have substance use disorders than are individuals in the general population,[1,2] and individuals with substance use disorders also have high rates of pain disorders.[3] Therefore, practitioners treating pain disorders are likely to encounter patients with substance use disorders and will need to know how to screen for and recognize these disorders, diagnose these disorders, make appropriate referrals for and/or treat these disorders, monitor for these disorders during ongoing pain treatment, and manage therapy for chronic pain in the context of these disorders.

The first section of the chapter presents the assessment and treatment of all major forms of substance use disorders from the perspective of addiction medicine. The second section focuses on assessment and treatment of opioid use disorder from the perspective of the pain specialist.

Assessment and Treatment of Substance Use Disorders—Addiction Medicine Perspective

The panoply of substance-related disorders includes intoxication, withdrawal, substance use disorder (otherwise known as addiction), and substance induced psychiatric disorders (e.g., psychosis, mood disturbance, or anxiety caused directly by the use of the substance). Substance use disorders occur with a variety of commonly used substances such as alcohol, cannabis, cocaine, opioids, sedative/hypnotics, stimulants like amphetamines and methylphenidate, inhalants, psychedelic agents, and tobacco. A standardized set of criteria characterizing these disorders is provided in the *Diagnostic and Statistical Manual of Mental Disorders* (5th ed., *DSM-5*).[4] Intoxication and withdrawal obviously differ by substance and can generally be diagnosed through history and physical examination. The criteria for substance use disorder which will be covered in greater detail in the following text are identical across substances.

What is currently termed a *substance use disorder* in *DSM-5* was known as either substance *abuse* or *dependence* in prior versions of the *DSM*, with abuse being considered a milder form of the disorder. The use of the term *dependence* generated some confusion and controversy. In contrast to a commonly held conception of "dependence" as notating purely physiologic changes that occur in response to repeated exposure to a substance, in prior versions of the *DSM*, "dependence" referred to a syndrome of physiologic signs and symptoms combined with an array of behavioral disturbances. Prior to the advent of *DSM-5*, some suggested that the phrase "substance dependence" referring to the *Diagnostic and Statistical Manual of Mental Disorders* (4th ed., text rev., *DSM-IV-TR*) syndrome be replaced with the term *addiction* to avoid confusion between purely physiologic dependence and the syndrome of substance dependence.[5] Others felt that the term *addiction* has negative connotations leading to stigmatization. A compromise was settled on with *DSM-5* using the term *substance use disorder*. It is commonly understood that the terms *addiction* and *substance use disorder* are essentially synonymous and interchangeable.

SCREENING AND RECOGNITION

Clearly, some initial evidence must arise through screening to suggest that a patient has a substance use disorder to trigger a thorough diagnostic assessment. In many cases, screening and diagnostic evaluation may overlap. The idea of "universal precautions" in pain medicine has been advanced as one way to detect potential substance use problems in all pain patients, so there may be some value in routine use of some or all of these screening procedures.[6] However, it is often too time-consuming and cumbersome to perform them in primary care, and there is no strong evidence that universal precautions or routine screening leads to better outcomes.

History

Generally, a thorough history of substance use obtained through a matter-of-fact, nonjudgmental interviewing style will provide a great deal of information or even a formal diagnosis. Most patients are not aware of guidelines for safe quantities of alcohol consumption and will readily divulge the amount of their drinking. Many patients are more reluctant to discuss use of illicit substances, but some will freely admit to such use if they do not fear sanctions or punishment. Oftentimes, this openness is more likely to occur during initial intake. Patients may be less forthright during the course of treatment if they believe they have something to lose by admitting to use. If time allows, it is worth asking explicitly about frequency and quantity of use for each class of substance along with route of administration. It is also quite important to ask about any history of current and past problematic substance use, as such problematic use is known to increase the risk of recurrence in the context of pain management. It is useful to know what types of substance use disorders treatment, if any, have been helpful for the patient in the past.

Recommended safe quantities of alcohol use consist of no more than four standard drinks per day (or more than 14 total per week) for men and three standard drinks (or more than 7 total per week) for women.[7] The recommended quantities are less for women because women tend to have less total body water and thus a lower volume of distribution for alcohol.[8] Quantities of different forms of alcohol that define a standard drink are listed in Table 91.1. If patients acknowledge regularly consuming more than the recommended amounts or describe heavy drinking such as five or more drinks on one occasion for men or four or more for women, a more thorough diagnostic evaluation for alcohol use disorder should be pursued.

TABLE 91.1   Quantities of Alcohol that Define a Standard Drink (14 g Pure Alcohol)

Beverage	Percent Alcohol	Quantity in Standard Drink (in Fluid Ounces)
Beer	5%	12
Malt liquor	7%	8.5
Table wine	12%	5
Fortified wine	17%	3.5
Liqueur	24%	2.5
Brandy	40%	1.5
Spirits (gin, vodka, whiskey)	40%	1.5

For illicit substances, any suggestion of more than occasional recreational use of marijuana should prompt a more thorough diagnostic evaluation. It is also important to look for tobacco use disorder, as this disorder has been associated with increased risk of opioid misuse in a number of studies.[1,9]

Physical Examination

Signs of possible substance use problems evident on physical exam include hypertension (common with excessive alcohol use), track marks indicative of recent or past injection drug use, pupillary constriction or dilation, inflamed nasal turbinates from intranasal substance insufflation, wheezes or rhonchi on lung exam from substance smoking, enlarged, tender liver from excessive alcohol use, other substance toxicity or hepatitis, or any stigmata of excessive alcohol use such as flushed facies, spider angiomas, palmar erythema, etc. Any of these findings should trigger further screening and possible thorough diagnostic evaluation.

Laboratory

Routine blood work can provide an indication of excessive alcohol use. Suggestive findings include elevations in liver transaminases or macrocytic, hyperchromic red blood cells related to alcohol's interference with folate absorption, and subsequent folate deficiency. Positive serologies for past or current hepatitis B or C infection or HIV infection would raise concerns about a substance use–related mode of transmission.

In addition, specific laboratory testing to detect presence of substances in body fluids offers a convenient component of screening. Typically, urine is tested,[10] although tests can also be readily performed in oral fluid or blood.[11,12] Substances that have been used are likely to remain present in urine for a longer period than they will in other body fluids (Table 91.2). For urine testing, a screening test is typically performed via immunoassay. When needed, confirmatory tests using high-performance liquid chromatography/mass spectrometry or gas chromatography/mass spectrometry can be ordered. It is important to note that the routine urine assay for opioids does not detect oxycodone, methadone, buprenorphine, or fentanyl which each requires a specific screening test. Heroin can only be detected shortly after use if its intermediate metabolite, 6-monoacetylmorphine, is present. Subsequently, 6-monoacetylmorphine is rapidly metabolized to morphine. If morphine appears in a urine toxicology specimen, it could represent either pharmaceutical morphine use or heroin use. It is difficult to detect alcohol in urine, blood, oral fluid, or breath unless the use has been quite recent. However, the alcohol metabolites, ethyl glucuronide or ethyl sulfate, indicating recent alcohol use can be detected in urine, blood, or hair.[13]

Self-report Questionnaires

A number of self-report questionnaires have been designed to help in screening for substance use disorders, and these can be

TABLE 91.2   Drug Detection Times in Urine and Drug Plasma Half-lives

Drug	Detection Time in Urine (Based on Standard Cutoff Values)	Plasma Half-life
Amphetamine	2–3 d	12 h
Cocaine metabolite (Benzoylecgonine)	2–3 d	7.5 h
Opioids		
Morphine glucuronide	2 d	7.5 h
Codeine glucuronide	3 d	12 h
Heroin metabolite (6-monoacetylmorphine)	2–4 h	20 min
Methadone	3 d single use 7–9 d maintenance dosing	24 h
Oxycodone	2 d	5 h
Hydromorphone	1–2 d	2.5 h
Hydrocodone	1–2 d	4 h
Barbiturates		
Short acting	1 d	25 h
Intermediate acting	2–3 d	38 h
Long acting	≥16 d	100 h
Benzodiazepines		
Short acting	1 d	1.5 h
Intermediate acting	2–4 d	10 h
Long acting	≥7 d	48 h
Cannabis single use	3 d	20 h
Cannabis chronic use	≥30 d	20 h

utilized prior to, concurrent with, or subsequent to the history, physical, and laboratory evaluation to help determine whether a patient warrants more thorough diagnostic evaluation. Although the instruments described in the following text have definite utility in primary care and general populations as well as selected samples such as psychiatric patients, they have not been tested in pain patients.

In screening for alcohol use disorders, the currently most frequently used instruments are the Alcohol Use Disorders Identification Test (AUDIT)[14] and the Michigan Alcoholism Screening Test (MAST).[15] The AUDIT has 10 items related to quantity and frequency of alcohol consumption and to maladaptive behaviors associated with alcohol use and can be completed in about 5 minutes. Each item is scored 0 to 4. A score of 8 or more for men under age 60 years or 4 or more for women or men over age 60 years are considered positive screens indicative of need for further assessment. A shorter version of the AUDIT, the AUDIT-C, which asks only 3 questions related to consumption has also been validated as a screening instrument in primary care settings.[16] The MAST contains 25 questions and focuses more on problem behaviors associated with alcohol use. Each item counts for 1 point, and a score of 6 or more indicates a positive screen with need for further assessment. There are shorter versions of the MAST which also appear to function as adequate screening instruments.

In the context of managing pain patients where urine toxicology should be readily available, self-report instruments to screen for drug use problems are probably less useful than a positive urine toxicology. However, if use of a self-report screening instrument is desired, a commonly used instrument is the Drug Abuse Screening Test (DAST).[17] The DAST is based on the MAST and has 28 items concerning both intensity and frequency of drug use and problematic behaviors associated with drug use. As with the MAST, each item counts for 1 point, and a score of 6 or more points to the needs for further assessment. Shorter versions of the DAST also exist.

A much briefer option to screen for a possible drug use disorder is the single item question, "How many times in the past year have you used an illegal drug or used a prescription medication for nonmedical reasons?" This single item performed as well as the DAST-10 at detecting a substance use disorder.[18]

One recently validated instrument that screens for all major substances is the Tobacco, Alcohol, Prescription Medication, and Other Substance Use (TAPS) tool, which is reasonably brief and can be self-administered.[19]

PRESCRIPTION DRUG MONITORING PROGRAM

Most states in the United States provide prescription drug monitoring programs (PDMPs). How they function and what the requirements are to access them vary widely from state to state. They do provide information on most controlled substance prescriptions that individual patients have obtained. Checking the PDMP can be very helpful in verifying the prescription medications that the patient is reporting via history.[20]

DIAGNOSTIC ASSESSMENT

As noted earlier, criteria provided in *DSM-5* represent the most standard way to make a diagnosis of a substance use disorder. At times, it proves fruitful to interview family members if the patient is not forthcoming.

Table 91.3 contains *DSM-5* criteria for opioid use disorder as an example. The criteria for a substance use disorder are identical across all substances. To determine the presence or absence of the diagnosis, the interviewer should focus one by one in turn on each substance of potential relevance and systematically go over each of the criteria with the patient for each substance.

TABLE 91.3   *Diagnostic and Statistical Manual of Mental Disorders*, 5th Edition, Diagnostic Criteria for Opioid Use Disorder

A problematic pattern of opioid use leading to clinically significant impairment or distress, as manifested by at least two of the following occurring within a 12-mo period:

1. Opioids are often taken in larger amounts or over a longer period than was intended.
2. There is a persistent desire or unsuccessful efforts to cut down or control opioid use.
3. A great deal of time is spent in activities necessary to obtain the opioid, use the opioid, or recover from its effects.
4. Craving, or a strong desire or urge to use opioids
5. Recurrent opioid use resulting in a failure to fulfill major role obligations at work, school, or home
6. Continued opioid use despite having persistent or recurrent social or interpersonal problems caused or exacerbated by the effects of opioids
7. Important social, occupational, or recreational activities are given up or reduced because of opioid use.
8. Recurrent use of opioids in situations in which it is physically hazardous
9. Continued opioid use despite knowledge of having a persistent or recurrent physical or psychological problem that is likely to have been caused or exacerbated by the substance
10. Tolerance,[a] as defined by either of the following:
    a. A need for markedly increased amounts of opioids to achieve intoxication or desired effect
    b. A markedly diminished effect with continued use of the same amount of opioid
11. Withdrawal[a] as manifested by either of the following:
    a. The characteristic opioid withdrawal syndrome
    b. Opioids (or a closely related substance) are taken to relieve or avoid withdrawal symptoms

[a]This criterion is not considered to be met for those taking the substance solely under appropriate medical supervision.
Mild = 2–3 symptoms.
Moderate = 4–5 symptoms.
Severe = 6 or more symptoms.

There are 2 physiologic criteria, tolerance and withdrawal, and 9 behavioral criteria. Two or more of the 11 criteria must be present at any one time over a 12-month period to make the diagnosis. If 2 to 3 criteria are present, the disorder is classified as mild; if 4 to 5 are present, as moderate; and if 6 or more, as severe. The physiologic criteria are not considered to be met for individuals taking the substance under medical supervision. For example, a pain patient treated chronically with opioids who is taking them precisely as prescribed might display tolerance to the effects of opioids and withdrawal signs and symptoms if the medication is stopped, but in this situation, these two criteria would not be applied to the diagnosis of opioid use disorder. Similarly, this scenario could occur with an attention-deficit/hyperactivity disorder patient treated chronically with stimulants, or with an anxiety disorder patient treated chronically with benzodiazepines. Conversely, an individual might not have either tolerance or withdrawal but could have the *DSM-5* defined substance use if he or she meets at least two of the behavioral criteria, although this scenario occurs rarely in clinical practice. Inspection of the criteria reveals that questions about each criterion are unlikely to be interpreted by patients as critical or threatening and unlikely to engender resistance or deception, particularly if posed in a matter-of-fact, nonjudgmental fashion. Although this procedure sounds time-consuming, it frequently can be accomplished in a matter of minutes for each substance of concern. As mentioned at the outset, the diagnosis of opioid use disorder in a patient with CNMP being treated with opioids may not be as straightforward as simple application of the *DSM-5* criteria and is discussed in detail in the following text.

Diagnosis of a substance use disorder certainly should not preclude appropriate interventions for a pain problem and in rare instances, with appropriate monitoring and safeguards, may not categorically preclude opioid treatment of chronic pain.

Co-occurring Psychiatric Disorders

Mental health disorders frequently co-occur with substance use disorders.[21,22] It is likely that chronic pain patients who have substance use disorders will have another non–substance-related co-occurring mental health disorder.[23] Oftentimes, co-occurring mental health and substance use disorders interact with negative synergy so that exacerbation of one disorder in turn exacerbates the other.[24] Thus, if a pain patient does have a substance use disorder, it is imperative to evaluate that patient for other co-occurring mental health disorders and provide appropriate clinical intervention (including pharmacotherapy and/or psychotherapy) for any that are diagnosed.

MONITORING DURING ONGOING PAIN TREATMENT

Even if a patient does not manifest a substance use disorder at the onset of chronic pain treatment, a disorder can certainly arise during the course of treatment. Maintaining vigilance for the development of a disorder involves both observation of the patient for behavioral evidence and routine monitoring techniques.[6] Behaviors that may increase the index of suspicion include missing appointments, having medication shortages, failure to pay bills, or a markedly changed affect during appointments.

Depending on the setting and resources available, it may prove worthwhile to establish routine, monitoring procedures for all pain patients even in the absence of concern. This approach normalizes these procedures, allows patients to expect them, and creates structure that may actually help the patient to feel supported while removing any sense of stigma or accusation that may supervene if the procedures are applied only for cause. The procedures that will be utilized should be specified at the outset of treatment in a written treatment agreement.

One obvious routine monitoring procedure to consider is urine toxicology testing as described earlier.[25]

Another potential procedure is unscheduled medication call backs. For this procedure, patients are telephoned and asked to return to the office within 24 hours with all their outstanding medication. When the patients come in, pill counts are performed to ensure that all expected outstanding medication is accounted for. It is also possible to obtain a urine toxicology specimen at that time.

TREATMENT AND/OR REFERRAL

Some general comments about treatment and referral will be made, and then specific interventions for use disorders involving each particular class of substances will be outlined. Most physicians get virtually no training or experience in treatment of substance use disorders and, therefore, often feel helpless or hopeless in the face of these disorders. Although many patients with these disorders who do get treatment get it in specialized settings that operate in parallel to and oftentimes outside of mainstream medicine, many patients will refuse a referral to such settings, and a growing body of literature supports the efficacy of physician intervention as a reasonable first attempt at treating these disorders.

Brief Interventions

Brief office interventions conducted by physicians have demonstrated efficacy in reducing alcohol consumption for patients with problematic alcohol use that does not rise to the level of an alcohol use disorder but very limited if any benefit for alcohol use disorder.[26,27] Motivational interventions (see following text) which can be incorporated into brief office interventions have demonstrated modest efficacy in nonalcohol substance use disorders.[28]

Brief interventions should be delivered in a manner that is matter-of-fact, nonjudgmental, supportive, and empathic and definitely not in a manner that is confrontational. The first step consists of stating concern about the patient's level of alcohol use (or any level of illicit drug use). It is helpful to give the patient direct examples from his or her medical record including bothersome symptoms, physical findings, specific diseases, or lab abnormalities. The next step involves giving direct advice to cut down (or quit) the substance use along with an offer to help. If the patient is not receptive to this advice, and the situation is not emergent, the physician can encourage him or her to consider it carefully and reflect on why he or she considers ongoing use to be a reasonable course of action. A follow-up can be arranged for further discussion.

If the patient appears receptive to advice to cut down or quit, the physician helps the patient to establish a specific goal to cut down or abstain (for a use disorder). Also, the physician provides explicit behavioral suggestions such as avoiding acquaintances who use, avoiding places where use has previously occurred, or seeking social support for quitting, including attending mutual-help groups such as Alcoholics Anonymous or Narcotics Anonymous. A follow-up appointment should be scheduled to monitor progress.

If the patient has alcohol use disorder and is willing to try for abstinence, the brief intervention could be combined with prescription of an appropriate alcohol treatment medication as described in the following text. If the patient has developed opioid use disorder, the brief intervention could be combined with a recommendation to try buprenorphine also described in the following text. If the pain physician treating the patient has a federal waiver to prescribe buprenorphine, arrangements could be made to stop any opioid analgesic the patient may currently be taking and make a switch to buprenorphine.

Specialty Substance Use Disorders Treatment

If a referral to a specialized substance use disorders treatment provider is needed, the referral could be made to an individual practitioner, another physician, psychologist, social worker, or chemical dependency counselor who specializes in substance use disorders treatment and could work with the patient in a private office setting using one or more of the psychotherapeutic or behavioral interventions detailed in the following text. Frequently, the referral will be made to an addiction treatment or substance use disorders program or agency. The American Society of Addiction Medicine publishes Patient Placement Criteria that can aid in determining what level of addiction treatment is appropriate for a given patient. These criteria have not, however, been fully scientifically validated and are based largely on expert opinion.[29,30]

Medically Supervised Withdrawal

Some patients, who manifest withdrawal when stopping their substance use, may need medically supervised withdrawal (also known as *detoxification*) to stop the substance safely and engage in treatment. The most common substances which require supervised withdrawal are alcohol, sedative-hypnotics, and opioids, although patients may have very unpleasant withdrawal symptoms from marijuana, cocaine, or amphetamines and need some support and monitoring. Medically supervised withdrawal can be accomplished on an outpatient or inpatient basis depending on the severity of the withdrawal. Clearly, alcohol or sedative-hypnotic withdrawal can be life-threatening. Usually, benzodiazepines are prescribed over several days in tapering doses.[31] Supervised opioid withdrawal for physiologic dependence on opioids can be accomplished using methadone in a licensed treatment program[32] (see the following text) or with buprenorphine[33] by appropriately qualified physicians. Alternatively, the α_2-adrenergic agonist, clonidine, can be prescribed to attenuate opioid withdrawal signs and symptoms and tapered over several days.[34] Some paradigms, known as *ultrarapid opioid withdrawal*, have been developed whereby opioid withdrawal is precipitated with an opioid antagonist such as naloxone or naltrexone under sedation or general anesthesia to complete the withdrawal in a brief period of time. These rapid procedures have no better outcomes than more gradual withdrawal but do have more adverse events such as pulmonary problems and psychiatric instability so they are not recommended.[35] It is very important to understand that medically supervised withdrawal (detoxification) alone does not constitute treatment. If medically supervised withdrawal is not immediately followed by more definitive substance use disorders treatment, relapse is almost universal.

Opioid Maintenance Treatment

Many patients with primary opioid use disorder do not want to undergo withdrawal or have tried it previously with subsequent relapse. These patients might be referred to a federally licensed opioid treatment program.[36] These programs provide opioid maintenance therapy with either methadone or buprenorphine. Because these medications have long half-lives, they can prevent the emergence of opioid withdrawal when taken on a once a day basis. (More detail on the clinical use of these medications for the treatment of opioid use disorder is provided in the following text.) The structure of the program is largely dictated by federal and state regulations. Patients must have a minimum of a 1-year history of opioid use disorder. In the early stages of treatment, patients must come to the clinic daily for observed doses of medication with take home doses of medication for weekend days when the clinic is closed. The maximum allowed first dose of methadone is 30 mg with subsequent gradual dose escalation to an optimally therapeutic dosage. A physical examination and basic laboratory tests are required as is periodic urine toxicology testing. Regular counseling visits are delivered as needed. As patients stabilize in treatment, as evidenced by regular attendance at dosing visits and other appointments, remaining on a stable dose of medication, and ceasing illicit substance use as demonstrated by drug-free toxicology specimens, take home doses of medication become available so that patients do not have to attend clinic every day. After 2 years of continuous treatment, stable patients on methadone may receive up to a maximum of 1 month's take home doses. Patients treated with buprenorphine in these settings can gain access to take home doses whenever they meet criteria for stability without regard to time in treatment. Opioid maintenance treatment has exceptionally good outcomes not only in terms of reducing illicit opioid use but also in terms of reducing other substance use, reducing mortality and morbidity, reducing criminal justice involvement, and improving employment.[37,38] It is considered to be as cost-effective as other potential life saving treatments such as coronary bypass surgery or renal dialysis.[39] All physicians are permitted to prescribe methadone for pain management, but only specially licensed facilities can order and dispense methadone specifically for opioid use disorder. Prescription of methadone for pain in patients with signs of opioid use disorder has obvious inherent risks and should be undertaken with careful monitoring precautions in place.

Intensive Outpatient Treatment

For patients who do not have opioid use disorder or who have opioid use disorder but decline maintenance therapy and have completed withdrawal, intensive outpatient treatment is often employed. This type of treatment is generally abstinence-based in that it emphasizes the goal of total abstinence from alcohol and all illicit substances. Some programs would accept pain patients on prescribed opioid therapy if the patient has a goal of abstinence from other substance use. Intensive outpatient treatment involves behavioral interventions usually via a group format with several meetings per week over a 4- to 12-week period so that patients receive up to 72 or more hours of total treatment.[40] Frequent urine toxicology testing is also typically performed. The therapeutic content of the group sessions varies but often includes one or more of the types of behavioral interventions described in the following text. Attendance at mutual help groups such as Alcoholics Anonymous is strongly encouraged. Not surprisingly, patients who complete these programs have better outcomes than those who drop out. Depending on the setting and patient characteristics, the dropout rate can be substantial.

Inpatient Treatment

For patients who fail outpatient treatment and who can obtain funding for it, inpatient treatment is an option. Inpatient treatment could be as brief as a few days[41] but frequently lasts 28 days and can be extended for many months in a model known as a therapeutic community[42] for patients who have severe, intractable substance use disorders that do not respond to any other interventions. Ongoing outpatient treatment subsequent to completion of inpatient treatment is recommended. Inpatient treatment, like intensive outpatient treatment, is almost always abstinence-based. Many short-term inpatient programs would accept pain patients on opioid therapy if the patients committed to abstinence from other substances. Most therapeutic communities would not accept patients receiving opioid therapy even for pain. The content of the care in inpatient treatment does not differ substantially from the content delivered in intensive outpatient treatment, but the inpatient setting provides a controlled environment that minimizes the risk of relapse and can compress more hours of actual treatment into a shorter overall time frame.[43] In the aggregate, it appears that the quantity or "dose" of behavioral treatment

received rather than the setting in which it occurs serves as the key mediator of outcome.

Specific Behavioral Treatments

Numerous types of behavioral interventions are used to treat substance use disorders, and many have been empirically validated. Mastery of specific techniques often requires considerable training and practice. Most studies comparing various behavioral intervention techniques find, as with setting, that the specific technique is less important than the total amount of behavioral intervention received. Many practitioners do not deliver the specific interventions in their pure form. In addition to the amount of intervention received, other important mediators of success are the skill of the specific therapist and the therapeutic alliance achieved between the therapist and patient regardless of what technique is used.[44] To impart at least passing knowledge of the names and basic philosophies of the more common techniques, brief descriptions are provided.

Motivational Interviewing

Motivational interviewing is a directive, patient-centered counseling style for eliciting behavior change by helping patients explore and resolve ambivalence. Compared with nondirective counseling, it is more focused and goal-directed. The examination and resolution of ambivalence is its central purpose, and the counselor is intentionally directive in pursuing this goal using the following techniques.[45]

- Seeking to understand the person's frame of reference, particularly via reflective listening
- Expressing acceptance and affirmation
- Eliciting and selectively reinforcing the client's own self motivational statements expressions of problem recognition, concern, desire and intention to change, and ability to change
- Monitoring the client's degree of readiness to change and ensuring that resistance is not generated by jumping ahead of the client
- Affirming the client's freedom of choice and self-direction

Relapse Prevention Therapy

Relapse prevention is a cognitive-behavioral intervention based on the notion that learning processes play an important role in the development of maladaptive behavior patterns. As applied to substance use disorders, relapse prevention explores the positive and negative consequences of continued substance use, encourages self-monitoring to recognize substance cravings early on, identifies high-risk situations for use, and develops strategies for coping with and avoiding high-risk situations and the desire to use.[46] A central element of this treatment is anticipating the problems that patients are likely to meet and helping them develop effective coping strategies. The skills that patients learn through relapse prevention therapy remain after the completion of treatment, and many maintain the gains they made in treatment throughout the year following treatment.

Drug Counseling

Drug counseling focuses directly on reducing or stopping the patient's substance use. It also addresses related areas of impaired functioning such as employment status, illegal activity, and family/social relationships as well as the content and structure of the patient's recovery program. Through its emphasis on short-term behavioral goals, drug counseling helps the patient develop coping strategies and tools for abstaining from substance use and then maintaining abstinence. The addiction counselor encourages 12-step participation and makes referrals for needed supplemental medical, psychiatric, employment, and other services. Individuals are encouraged to attend sessions one or two times per week.[47]

12-Step Facilitation Therapy

Twelve-step facilitation consists of a structured and manual-driven approach to facilitating early recovery from substance use disorders. It is intended to be implemented on an individual basis in 12 to 15 sessions and is based in behavioral, spiritual, and cognitive principles that form the core of 12-step fellowships such as Alcoholics Anonymous and Narcotics Anonymous. Twelve-step facilitation seeks to achieve two general goals in patients with substance use disorders: acceptance of the need for abstinence from substances and surrender, or the willingness to participate actively in 12-step fellowships as a means of sustaining sobriety. These goals are in turn broken down into a series of cognitive, emotional, relationship, behavioral, social, and spiritual objectives.[48] Twelve-step facilitation has shown excellent results for patients with alcohol use disorder but shows less promise for patients with drug use disorders.[49]

Contingency Management

Contingency management treatments are based on operant conditioning principles as elucidated by B.F. Skinner: If a behavior is reinforced or rewarded, it is more likely to occur in the future.[50] In many contingency management treatments, patients leave urine specimens multiple times each week and receive explicit rewards for each specimen that tests negative for drugs. These rewards often consist of vouchers that have a monetary value and can be exchanged for retail goods. However, contingencies that lack monetary value can also be used. For example, in opioid treatment programs or office-based buprenorphine treatment, the frequency of attendance can be contingent on drug-free urine specimens. Patients who provide drug-negative urine specimens get more take home medication or larger prescriptions, and those who provide drug-positive specimens have their take home privileges reduced or have to pick up a prescription more frequently. Contingency management has been demonstrated to reduce substance use significantly in numerous studies, but its implementation in clinical practice has lagged,[51] although it has now been implemented widely and successfully throughout the Veterans Affairs health care system.

Pharmacotherapies

Currently, there are three U.S. Food and Drug Administration (FDA)-approved medications for the treatment of alcohol use disorder (disulfiram, acamprosate, and naltrexone) and three available FDA-approved medications for the treatment of opioid use disorder (methadone, buprenorphine, and naltrexone). All of the alcohol treatment medications can be used by all physicians, including pain specialists if desired, within the scope of their own practice. Although methadone can be ordered and dispensed for the treatment of opioid use disorder only within licensed clinics, buprenorphine can be prescribed by appropriately qualified physicians (as described in the following text) outside of licensed clinics. Naltrexone for either alcohol or opioid use disorders is not likely to have much utility in pain patients because of its antagonism of μ-opioid receptors and its tendency either to precipitate opioid withdrawal in patients on opioids or to block the effects of opioid analgesics. Nevertheless, it may rarely have potential benefit in selected pain patients not currently on opioids. There are currently no FDA-approved pharmacotherapies for use disorders involving other substances such as cocaine, methamphetamine, sedative-hypnotics, or cannabis, so these disorders must be treated with behavioral interventions alone.

Disulfiram

By inhibiting aldehyde dehydrogenase, a key enzyme in the major metabolic pathway for ethanol, disulfiram causes accumulation of acetaldehyde after alcohol ingestion. The buildup of acetaldehyde usually causes an "alcohol–disulfiram reaction" that typically ensues within minutes of alcohol ingestion.[52]

Different individuals exhibit varying degrees of the reaction which may last for several hours. Signs and symptoms of the alcohol–disulfiram reaction include diaphoresis, flushing, tachycardia, hypotension, nausea, vomiting, and headache. The concept behind the idea of disulfiram is that patients taking disulfiram will fear getting an uncomfortable reaction and thus will be deterred from drinking alcohol. To some extent, change occurs during the informed consent discussion between physician and patient at the time the patient agrees to take disulfiram. During that discussion, the patient may, by agreeing to try disulfiram, be arriving at a decisive interest in achieving abstinence from alcohol.

Obviously, patients must have achieved some time of abstinence before starting disulfiram to avoid provoking the alcohol–disulfiram reaction. Typically, 48 hours of abstinence proves sufficient. The usual starting dose of disulfiram is 250 mg per day. Genetic variability may determine sensitivity to the medication, and patients with high levels of aldehyde dehydrogenase may be less sensitive to the effects of disulfiram and require higher doses of medication, up to 500 mg per day. Some patients may not tolerate 250 mg per day and should have the dose reduced to 125 mg per day.

Disulfiram is associated with a number of mild side effects such headache, metallic aftertaste, erectile dysfunction, mild fatigue or sedation, and rash. Such side effects frequently dissipate spontaneously or with a dosage decrease. Much more serious adverse events such as optic neuritis, peripheral neuropathy, hepatic injury, or psychotic symptoms or delirium, although rare, necessitate immediate disulfiram discontinuation. Disulfiram-induced hepatic injury can occur idiosyncratically at an estimated rate of 1/25,000 to 1/30,000 patient treatment years.[53] Disulfiram-induced hepatic injury can rapidly proceed to total liver failure. It most usually occurs within the first 6 months of treatment. Symptoms include extreme fatigue, malaise, anorexia, fever, jaundice, scleral icterus, nausea, vomiting, and bilirubinuria. Baseline liver function tests should be obtained prior to initiation of disulfiram treatment and then at 1- to 2-month intervals during the first 6 months of treatment. With the decreased risk of disulfiram-induced hepatic injury after the first 6 months of treatment, liver monitoring can subsequently be done every 3 to 6 months if treatment continues. Many patients who might be considered for disulfiram therapy present with moderately elevated transaminases related to alcohol use (particularly in the context of hepatitis C). These modest transaminase elevations do not represent a total contraindication to disulfiram therapy. Very rapid rises in bilirubin and transaminases occur in disulfiram-induced hepatic injury and indicate the need to stop disulfiram at once. If the medication is discontinued promptly, the signs and symptoms of liver injury typically fully resolve. If the medication is not stopped, total hepatic failure and death can supervene unless a liver transplant is performed.

Patients with preexisting cirrhosis or other serious liver disease generally are not good candidates for disulfiram. Other contraindications include pregnancy or lactation, history of prior hypersensitivity to disulfiram, or significant coronary artery disease. The latter group could experience myocardial ischemia during a severe alcohol–disulfiram reaction.

Disulfiram has greater benefit with monitoring of medication administration. Although the largest study to date demonstrated that disulfiram dosed at 250 mg per day over 1-year did not lead to increased abstinence rates or longer time to first drink compared to placebo, it did lead to significantly fewer drinking days over the study year.[54]

Acamprosate

Acamprosate, which has seen widespread use in Europe for many years, received FDA approval for the treatment of alcohol use disorder in 2004. Acamprosate is believed to modulate both the major excitatory system in the brain, the glutamate system, as well as the major inhibitory system, the γ-aminobutyric acid (GABA) system. Alcohol interacts with these systems as well, but when alcohol is stopped after chronic exposure, glutamatergic hyperactivity and GABA hypoactivity contribute substantially to the alcohol withdrawal syndrome. Acamprosate theoretically acts to counteract these imbalances and so may attenuate symptoms associated with subsyndromal, prolonged alcohol withdrawal such as insomnia, anxiety, and restlessness which could provoke alcohol cravings and relapse.[55,56] Acamprosate also may diminish reinforcement derived from alcohol ingestion[55] and the amount of alcohol consumed by patients in treatment who do experience relapse.[57] Numerous controlled studies of acamprosate demonstrated higher total abstinence rates and longer time to relapse for acamprosate compared to placebo.[58] For reasons that remain incompletely understood, acamprosate failed to show efficacy in two large clinical trials conducted in the United States.[59,60] It has been proposed that subjects in the US studies may not have experienced sufficient prolonged subsyndromal withdrawal to benefit from acamprosate.[61]

Acamprosate has very limited oral bioavailability. It achieves steady state after 5 days and is not metabolized by the liver but excreted unchanged in the urine. The usual dose is 666 mg (two 333-mg tablets) three times daily. The labeling indicates that acamprosate should be started after a modicum of abstinence has been achieved, but there are no safety issues if acamprosate is taken concomitantly with alcohol and abstinence is not essential. In fact, acamprosate should be continued in the patient who relapses to alcohol use.

It is recommended that a serum creatinine level to evaluate kidney function be obtained prior to initiation of therapy because the dose should be lowered in patients with impaired kidney function. Acamprosate is FDA category C, so women of childbearing age must use an effective method of birth control when on acamprosate. All patients should be monitored for suicidal thoughts because such thoughts occurred more frequently among acamprosate treated patients than among placebo-treated patients in clinical trials. Diarrhea is the only common side effect noted with acamprosate.

It is recommended that acamprosate treatment be continued for 12 months, and follow-up studies show increased abstinence rates that persist 1 year after cessation of treatment.[62] Advantages of acamprosate include its lack of drug–drug interactions and the fact that it is not contraindicated in patients with serious liver disease.

Naltrexone

The μ-opioid antagonist, naltrexone, originally developed to treat opioid use disorder (see the following text) was subsequently approved to treat alcohol use disorder in 1994 and is now available in an oral generic formulation. An involvement of the endogenous opioid systems in the reinforcing effects of alcohol seems likely based on the fact that opioid antagonists block the alcohol-induced release of dopamine into the nucleus accumbens.[63] The ability of alcohol to promote the release of endogenous opioids[64,65] or to affect opioid receptor binding[66] may account for dopamine release engendered by alcohol and for the blockade of this event by opioid antagonists. Naltrexone changes the subjective experience of alcohol consumption in humans rendering it less reinforcing and more sedating.[67] Naltrexone has demonstrated efficacy in delaying and preventing relapse to heavy drinking and reducing the percentage of drinking days but not in promoting total abstinence in numerous (but not all) clinical trials.[68]

Naltrexone is rapidly and almost fully absorbed after oral administration, achieves its peak effect after 1 hour, and has a half-life of approximately 4 hours (metabolite half-life = 12 hours). The usual dose is 50 mg per day which is sufficient to occupy the majority of μ-opioid receptors.[69] Many clinicians begin naltrexone at 25 mg per day for a few days to minimize side effects and then titrate up to 50 mg per day. Although data are sparse, some clinicians will also increase naltrexone to 100 mg per day if a suboptimal response occurs at 50 mg per day, and the 100 mg per day dose demonstrated modest efficacy in the COMBINE Study.[59]

Common side effects of naltrexone include nausea, headache, dizziness, fatigue, sedation, and anxiety and typically resolve with continued treatment. Oral naltrexone does have a boxed warning for acute hepatitis, although most of these events occurred at doses of 300 mg per day in clinical trials for obesity, and there is little evidence of hepatotoxicity at currently recommended doses for alcohol use disorder. Nevertheless, given the boxed warning, it is judicious to obtain liver function tests prior to initiation and then at months 1, 3, 6, and 12 during therapy.

Because naltrexone blocks μ-opioid receptors, opioid medications will be much less effective in the situation in which an injury or serious medical condition calls for acute pain control. If given in adequate doses (usually higher than would otherwise be required), opioids can generally overcome the blockade, but close monitoring of the patient in an inpatient setting to observe for and manage respiratory depression is advised. Also, naltrexone is quite obviously contraindicated in patients taking opioids for chronic pain.

Long-Acting Injectable Naltrexone

Although oral naltrexone generally appears efficacious compared to placebo in reducing relapse to heavy drinking, it has not performed well in some studies. However, when patients found to be nonadherent for oral naltrexone are factored out in several other studies, naltrexone demonstrates efficacy for treatment of alcohol use disorder compared to placebo.[70,71] Consequently, long-acting intramuscular naltrexone, FDA-approved in 2006 for treatment of alcohol use disorder, may eliminate concerns about adherence and has been shown to be effective compared to placebo in reducing heavy drinking.[72] Additional advantages of long-acting intramuscular naltrexone include lower rates of first-pass hepatic metabolism, exposing the liver to significantly lower peak dosages than daily oral dosing. The injectable formulation does not have a boxed warning for hepatic injury. The reduced first-pass metabolism of intramuscular naltrexone leads to lower levels of the active metabolite 6β-naltrexone, which has been correlated with side effects such as nausea. Lower levels of this metabolite may lead to better tolerability of naltrexone's intramuscular form. Long-acting injectable naltrexone is indicated for patients who have achieved some period of abstinence which could be as brief as several hours. The dosage is one 380-mg gluteal injection every 4 weeks. Patients can be started directly on the injection without a trial on oral medication. In addition to typical side effects seen with oral naltrexone, injection site reactions can occur with the injectable formulation.

Naltrexone for Opioid Use Disorder

For patients with opioid use disorder who have withdrawn from opioids and who do not wish to continue opioid therapy, naltrexone offers, from a theoretical standpoint, an ideal pharmacotherapy. Once a state of full withdrawal is achieved as verified by a naloxone challenge test, naltrexone can be started. With naltrexone on board, the effect of exogenously administered opioids will be blocked so that no euphoria is experienced and physiologic dependence cannot be reestablished. Unfortunately, very few patients with opioid use disorder remain on oral naltrexone for an extended period so that it performs only slightly better than placebo.[73] Some populations such as individuals with legal mandates or impaired professionals may do better on oral naltrexone. Obviously, as noted in the preceding text, naltrexone represents a poor choice of pharmacotherapy for some pain patients because it prevents the use of opioid analgesics. If the oral formulation is prescribed, the typical dose is 50 mg per day.

The injectable formulation was approved for opioid use disorder in 2010. A double-blind randomized, controlled trial conducted in Russia showed that active naltrexone injection compared to placebo produced significantly fewer days of using illicit opioids and better retention in treatment.[74] The only sizable randomized trial conducted in the United States was open label among criminal justice involved patients with opioid use disorder and did show benefit of the injectable formulation compared to treatment as usual, which typically did not include medication.[75]

Methadone

As noted earlier, methadone can only be ordered and dispensed for the treatment of opioid use disorder through federally licensed and regulated clinics. Thus, in most cases, patients with chronic pain who need methadone treatment must be referred to one of these clinics. Such clinics are not available in many geographic regions and at times also have waiting lists.

Methadone is ordered and dispensed quite differently when used to treat opioid use disorder than when prescribed for pain. Typically, for treatment of opioid use disorder, a single daily dose is provided in liquid form. The maximum initial dose is 30 mg. The lowest effective dose of methadone for treatment of opioid use disorder is approximately 50 mg per day, with an optimum average dose for most patients of approximately 80 mg per day (±20 mg), although some patients require a dose higher than this range. The daily dose should be sufficient to prevent emergence of withdrawal symptoms at least through the 24-hour dosing period. The dose should be sufficient to greatly diminish or eliminate opioid cravings and opioid use (as determined by both self-report and urine toxicology testing). The dose should create sufficient tolerance such that illicit opioid use does not cause euphoria. The dose should not be so high that side effects such as sedation, constipation, or loss of libido occur.[36]

Patients who do not stabilize within a few weeks should be evaluated both at the end of the 24-hour dosing cycle just prior to the next scheduled dose to assess the presence of withdrawal signs and symptoms and at 4 hours postdose to observe the patient for any evidence of intoxication or excessive opioid effect at the time of peak plasma levels.[36] If the patient does have withdrawal signs prior to the dose and no intoxication postdose, an upward adjustment in dose is probably warranted. When patients fail to stabilize after successive dose increases, consideration could be given to obtaining a trough (predose) serum methadone level. Levels below 100 ng/mL are associated with withdrawal symptoms and inadequate dosage.[76] There are rare ultrarapid metabolizers of methadone who will not become stable on a single daily dose and will exhibit low trough serum levels of methadone. For this small group of patients, splitting the dose by giving them half of the dose observed and the other half as a take-home for the evening generally promotes stabilization.

For patients on methadone maintenance, their daily dose of methadone will rarely be fully, if at all, efficacious in managing acute or chronic pain. These patients may often benefit from additional analgesics, either methadone tablets or another opioid of choice, given throughout the day in appropriately divided doses given in addition to the daily dose of methadone. For acute pain, these additional opioids can be discontinued when the pain subsides. For chronic pain, the additional opioids will need to be ongoing in most cases. Alternatively, or additionally, nonopioid pharmacotherapies and/or behavioral interventions for pain can be applied.

Buprenorphine

Although buprenorphine can be ordered and dispensed through licensed clinics, its pharmacologic characteristics make it a very attractive medication for office-based therapy. Its partial agonist action means that it has a ceiling effect for central nervous system and respiratory depressive effects, making it is far safer in overdose than methadone and other full μ-opioid agonists.[77] This partial agonist property also makes it easier to withdraw from this medication than from methadone. Withdrawing from methadone can take months or years and be difficult for patients.

In addition, buprenorphine has slow onset when administered sublingually (1.5 to 3 hours to peak plasma levels), a long half-life, and high affinity plus slow dissociation from the receptor.[78,79] Thus, it prevents the emergence of withdrawal symptoms for 24 hours or longer, and by occupying the majority of receptors, it makes very few receptors available for binding of full agonists. Buprenorphine's long half-life allows for once-daily or even thrice-weekly dosing. Buprenorphine is poorly absorbed by the oral route and undergoes extensive first-pass hepatic metabolism, so for treatment of opioid dependence, it is administered sublingually, buccally, or via a subdermal implant.

Buprenorphine prescription in the office setting was made possible in the United States by the Drug Addiction Treatment Act of 2000 (DATA). DATA allows for office-based opioid maintenance therapy for opioid use disorder using Schedule III, IV, or V medications approved for this use by the FDA. In 2002, the FDA approved buprenorphine and buprenorphine/naloxone for this purpose, and they are the only medications at this time with this indication. In order to prescribe buprenorphine, physicians must obtain a waiver from the DEA, which requires specialty training in addictions or completion of approximately 8 hours of training in management of opioid use disorder, and physicians must be able to refer patients to appropriate counseling and ancillary services. The waiver allows physicians to prescribe buprenorphine to up to 100 patients at a given time with the potential to increase the patient limit to 275 as of 2016.

Buprenorphine is available for sublingual or buccal administration as a single agent or as a combination buprenorphine–naloxone preparation with a ratio of 4 mg buprenorphine to 1 mg of naloxone. (There are also buccal and transdermal formulations available with a pain indication, but the doses are approximately an order of magnitude lower than the doses used to treat opioid use disorder.) The advantage of the combination buprenorphine–naloxone preparation is the prevention of misuse. Buprenorphine has adequate bioavailability sublingually, whereas naloxone is minimally bioavailable sublingually, so the naloxone has no effect on patients when administered as intended. If the combination medication is dissolved in an attempt to inject buprenorphine, however, naloxone, which also has a high affinity for the μ receptor, will exert its antagonist properties resulting in withdrawal instead of euphoria. The single agent should be reserved for use only in situations where there is no concern for potential misuse, such as in an inpatient setting or for pregnant women to avoid any potential exposure of the developing fetus to even trace amounts of naloxone. Due to the partial agonist properties of buprenorphine, patients need to be clearly educated that they should not take this medication soon after taking other opioid drugs because buprenorphine in that situation may precipitate withdrawal.

An important component of the clinical skill in using buprenorphine involves the induction procedures. Patients who have been taking full agonist opioids must abstain from their full agonist opioids long enough to evidence signs of mild opioid withdrawal. If patients take the first dose of buprenorphine when not in active opioid withdrawal, there is a risk that buprenorphine as a partial agonist will precipitate more severe opioid withdrawal. Patients often require a fair amount of empathic emotional support to assure them that they can handle a period of several hours without opioids and can tolerate a brief episode of mild withdrawal prior to starting buprenorphine. Usually, it is not the mild withdrawal symptoms themselves that are troublesome, so much as the anxiety about more severe withdrawal. If patients are in mild to moderate withdrawal at the time of starting buprenorphine, the first dose usually alleviates much of the withdrawal within 30 to 60 minutes.

Induction of buprenorphine should thus begin approximately 12 to 24 hours after last use of a short-acting opioid drug or 24 to 48 hours after last use of a long-acting opioid drug, and patients should be showing objective signs of withdrawal at the time of initiation of therapy. On the first day of induction, the maximum dose should usually not exceed 8 to 12 mg. Because the transition from methadone to buprenorphine is more difficult than the transition from short-acting opioids, patients who are receiving methadone for pain and wish to transition can be first switched from methadone to a short-acting opioid and then inducted onto buprenorphine. For patients receiving methadone in a licensed clinic for the treatment of opioid use, this switch to a short-acting opioid is not legally permissible, and such patients must be inducted directly from methadone to buprenorphine.

If, after beginning buprenorphine, patients still have withdrawal symptoms after receiving the maximum first day dose, they should be treated symptomatically with adjunctive agents such as clonidine, antiemetics, antidiarrheals, and benzodiazepines for specific withdrawal symptoms. Over the course of the next 2 to 6 days, patients should be assessed for signs and symptoms of withdrawal with increases in buprenorphine given for persistent symptoms up to a total of 16 mg on the second day and a maximum of 32 mg per day by the end of the first week. Withdrawal symptoms beyond this time typically indicate persisting illicit opioid use.

Following induction, patients will stabilize on a dose over the following weeks, and the dose should be adjusted to the lowest effective dose to prevent withdrawal symptoms, prevent craving of opioids, and suppress illicit opioid abuse. Once this dose is established, patients can be maintained on this medication indefinitely or may choose to taper off.[80]

Numerous studies have found buprenorphine to be effective in retaining patients in treatment and reducing illicit opioid abuse. A systematic review of studies, which compared 31 studies involving 5,430 subjects in trials of buprenorphine versus either placebo or methadone, found buprenorphine to be effective as a maintenance therapy for opioid use disorder when compared to placebo.[81] Compared with methadone, however, especially at higher doses of methadone, buprenorphine may not be quite as effective at maintaining patients in treatment, although this difference is less pronounced at higher buprenorphine doses. Nevertheless, because buprenorphine is a safer medication than methadone, it often makes clinical sense to use buprenorphine as a first-line agent. If a patient fails buprenorphine treatment, the patient can be transitioned to methadone maintenance in a licensed clinic.[82] Transition from methadone to buprenorphine is clinically more difficult than transition from buprenorphine to methadone.

As a partial agonist, buprenorphine has analgesic properties, but its analgesic effects may not always be as powerful as those of a full agonist. However, recent evidence suggests that buprenorphine produces less hyperalgesia than full agonist opioids[83] and so may have some benefit for pain control in patients not responding well to full agonists. Also, although buprenorphine has a ceiling on its respiratory depressant action, it does not appear to have a ceiling on its analgesic activity so higher doses should continue to elicit greater analgesia.[84] Thus, buprenorphine has tremendous potential for management of patients who have combined chronic pain and opioid use disorder. It allows the physician treating such a patient to continue to manage the patient in his or her own office for

both disorders along with referral for ancillary counseling if needed rather than terminating such a patient or sending the patient to an addiction treatment provider or facility with the risk of a failure to follow through. As noted, some clinical skill is required to support the patient in abstaining from full agonist opioids long enough to evidence signs of opioid withdrawal such that buprenorphine induction can take place. Patients being treated with buprenorphine for combined pain and opioid use disorder may get better analgesia by taking the buprenorphine in divided doses throughout the day rather than as a single daily dose. Although more data on the treatment of combined pain and opioid use disorder are needed, preliminary reports indicate a positive response for many patients.[85]

Conceptions of Opioid Use Disorder—The Pain Medicine Perspective

The pain management perspective on opioid use disorder provides observations on the historical changes in the attitudes toward and practice of using opioids for chronic pain and on integration of perceptions from pain medicine with those from addiction medicine.

HISTORY OF OPIOID USE FOR CHRONIC PAIN AS IT RELATES TO IDENTIFYING OPIOID USE DISORDER

Ambiguities related to the definition of opioid addiction in CNMP patients and the practical problems associated with identifying this disorder as of 2006 were detailed in the chapter on addiction in the fourth edition of *Bonica's Management of Pain*. In the present chapter, we focus on changes that have occurred during the past decade in our understanding of addiction in these patients and in attitudes toward the use of opioids in the treatment of CNMP.

There is no simple way to gauge the attitudes and beliefs of the various stakeholders with an interest in opioid therapy (e.g., physicians, regulators, law enforcement officers, patients with CNMP), but initiatives undertaken by legislative bodies and regulators can be viewed as indicators of prevailing attitudes. Because these differ from one community to another, the present discussion focuses on initiatives undertaken in the State of Washington in the United States.[86] The practical reason for this is that we are familiar with these initiatives. There is also evidence that the State of Washington has been a leader in opioid policy. For example, the Centers for Disease Control and Prevention (CDC) opioid guidelines are largely based on the earlier Washington State guidelines.

In the years since 2007, there has been a sea change in these attitudes, and it appears that opioid prescribing by clinicians peaked in 2011 or 2012 and is now declining.[86,87] With the benefit of hindsight, we can now identify three periods regarding these attitudes.

1. Early history (prior to the 1990s): Before the mid-1990s, Washington State Department of Health regulations prohibited physicians from providing long-term opioid therapy for CNMP patients. This regulation existed in many other states as well and reflected the prevailing view that the risks of such therapy outweighed the benefits.

2. The period of enthusiasm (1990 to 2007): As discussed in *Bonica's Management of Pain*, 4th edition, some pain specialists made the case during the late 1980s and early 1990s that opioids were safe and effective in the treatment of CNMP. In 1995, a committee was formed to change the Washington State Department of Health's regulations regarding opioid therapy. The result, published in 1996, was a regulation that stated, "Under generally accepted standards of medical practice, opioids may be prescribed for the treatment of acute or chronic pain including chronic pain associated with cancer and

other non-cancer pain conditions. . . . It is the position of the Department of Health that opioids may be prescribed, dispensed, or administered when there is an indicated medical need without fear of injudicious discipline." This regulation reflected an emerging viewpoint that opioid therapy was safe and effective in the treatment of chronic pain. In 1996, the American Pain Society and the American Academy of Pain Medicine issued a joint statement endorsing the use of opioids in care of patients with CNMP. This time frame is also the when long-acting opioids were aggressively marketed by pharmaceutical companies as less prone to abuse and addiction. Marketing of OxyContin was especially conspicuous,[88] but other opioids were also aggressively marketed. As a result of the mentioned influences, there was a dramatic increase in opioid prescribing, both nationally[89] and in Washington State.[90]

3. The period of retrenchment (2007 to present): As indicated in the discussion in *Bonica's Management of Pain*, 4th edition, by 2006, some pain specialists had become skeptical that the benefits of opioid therapy for CNMP outweighed the risks. The medical director of the Washington State workers' compensation system noticed an increase in deaths among injured workers that were concentrated among those receiving high-dose, long-term opioid therapy. He convened a group of academic and community pain specialists who wrote the first Washington State opioid guideline, which was released in 2007. Since then, skepticism about the benefits of long-term opioid therapy has grown enormously. The CDC has declared that we are in the midst of an opioid epidemic that is killing Americans at a higher rate than HIV ever did. In 2014, the National Institutes of Health held a consensus conference that declared that there was no good evidence of the effectiveness of long-term opioid therapy.

As the aforementioned dates suggest, the chapter section on addiction from the perspective of pain medicine in the fourth edition of *Bonica's Management of Pain* was written as physicians and regulators were becoming skeptical of opioid therapy for CNMP and were moving into the period of retrenchment. Thus, the discussion reflected ambivalence about opioid therapy for CNMP but did not provide any definite conclusions about the pros and cons of the therapy.

Since that chapter was written, several discoveries have occurred and initiatives have been undertaken that have changed the social environment surrounding opioid therapy for CNMP. The most significant are as follows:

1. Changes in the criteria for the diagnosis of "addiction" (formally called substance use disorder) in the *DSM-5*[4]: These changes were discussed previously. They have dealt to some extent with concerns that we voiced in *Bonica's Management of Pain*, 4th edition, about the *DSM-IV* criteria. However, they do not fully resolve the ambiguities and inconsistencies of usage among investigators for a variety of terms that describe problematic use of prescription opioids—including misuse, abuse, aberrancy, dependence, and addiction.[91] Also, as discussed later in text, the *DSM-5* definition does not fully resolve problems that clinicians face in the identification of opioid use disorder in patients with chronic pain.

2. Research on addiction and aberrant behaviors associated with prescription opioids: During the period of enthusiasm for opioid therapy, many pain specialists argued that addiction is uncommon when patients take opioids for their pain. A brief report on an inpatient sample by Porter and Jick[92] was frequently cited to buttress this argument. Recent research has emphatically challenged this assertion. It has been demonstrated that a high

proportion of CNMP patients on opioid therapy have abnormal urine drug screens,[93] strongly suggesting aberrant behaviors (Table 91.4). Our best conservative estimate is now that 25% of patients on long-term opioid therapy will misuse their opioids, and 10% will develop opioid use disorder.[94] Also, there is now evidence that a substantial proportion of people using heroin report that they got started on the path to heroin use via consumption of prescription opioids.[95]

3. Research demonstrating adverse effects of opioids: Research has now documented a litany of adverse effects of opioid therapy that were either unknown or not fully appreciated during the period of enthusiasm. These include overdoses requiring emergency room care, myocardial infarctions, low testosterone levels, and injuries in motor vehicle accidents.[96] Worst of all, there is now convincing evidence of substantial mortality from overdoses of prescription opioids.[97,98] Thus, although practitioners and researchers have been aware for decades that opioids can cause harm, recent evidence has highlighted the frequency with which adverse effects occur. This emerging evidence has led the CDC and other agencies to use the term *opioid epidemic* to describe the current situation with respect to prescription opioids for CNMP.[99]

4. Questionable efficacy: Many RCTs, often sponsored by drug companies, have been performed over the past 25 years. They have generally supported the efficacy of various opioids in the treatment of chronic pain conditions.[100,101] However, these studies almost uniformly examined the effects of an opioid for a limited period of time—usually 8 to 12 weeks. In fact, one recent review concluded that no well-controlled studies have been done addressing the efficacy of opioid therapy over a time interval of greater than 1 year.[96] Moreover, research employing large insurance databases to assess longer term outcomes of opioid therapy has presented a bleak picture. For example, multiple investigators have examined the effects of opioid therapy on injured workers by looking at return to work rates (or termination of disability benefits) among workers with common injuries

TABLE 91.4 **Examples of Aberrant Behaviors Related to Opioid Use**
1. Used additional opioids than those prescribed
2. Used additional opioids than those prescribed more than once
3. Forged prescription
4. Sold prescription
5. Admitted to seeking euphoria from opioids
6. Admitted to wanting opioids for anxiety
7. Overdose and death
8. Injected drug
9. Abnormal urine/blood screen
10. Abnormal urine/blood screen positive for two or more substances
11. Solicited opioids from other providers
12. Unauthorized ER visits
13. Concurrent abuse of alcohol
14. Unauthorized dose escalation
15. Resisted therapy changes/alternative therapy
16. Reported lost or stolen prescriptions
17. Canceled clinic visit
18. Requested early refills
19. Requested refills instead of clinic visit
20. Abused prescribed drug
21. Was discharged from practice (because of aberrant behavior)
22. No-show or no follow-up
23. Third party required to manage patient's medications

ER, emergency room.

such as back injuries who are prescribed opioids versus who are not prescribed them. These studies have consistently found that workers receiving opioids are less likely to return to work than those not receiving them.[102,103]

5. Monitoring: Clinicians have been able to monitor patients taking opioids via urine drug screens for many years. However, it is very likely that clinicians are ordering urine drug screens more frequently now than at the time of *Bonica's Management of Pain*, 4th edition, because during the past few years, several expert panels have recommended their use.[98,104] In contrast, PDMPs were virtually nonexistent at the time when the fourth edition of *Bonica's Management of Pain* was written. As noted earlier, PDMPs are now available in 49 states.[87] Recent studies have shown that PDMPs reduce opioid use among Medicare beneficiaries[105] and in the general patient population.[20] Another study showed that Florida's PDMP and pill mill laws were associated with modest decreases in opioid prescribing and use. The decreases were greatest among prescribers and patients with the highest initial opioid prescribing and use.[106]

6. Policy initiatives: As noted earlier, several initiatives have been undertaken in Washington State to rein in opioid prescribing for CNMP. The first of these was a guideline published by the Agency Medical Directors' Group (AMDG). The AMDG consists of medical directors of the four Washington State–run medical insurance programs—Medicaid, the Department of Labor and Industries (the main Washington State workers' compensation carrier), the Department of Corrections, and Uniform Medical (the health insurance plan for state employees). In 2006, the AMDG formed a committee to address opioid use for beneficiaries of the mentioned insurance programs who suffered from CNMP. The resulting guideline, published in 2007, recommended that primary care physicians obtain consultations from pain specialists regarding opioid use for CNMP and expressed the view that opioid doses for CNMP patients should rarely exceed a morphine equivalent dose (MED) of 120 mg per day.[107] This guideline was the first in a series of initiatives to curb the excesses of the period of enthusiasm. Updated AMDG guidelines were published in 2010[108] and again in 2015.[109] These reiterated many of the recommendations given in the 2007 guideline and buttressed them with data about adverse effects of opioid therapy. Other initiatives included legislation that incorporated principles in the AMDG guideline[110] and the development of a state PDMP. At a national level, the most visible policy initiative was the publication of a guideline by the CDC in 2016.[104] It incorporated many of the principles articulated in the AMDG guidelines.

7. Changes in opioid prescribing practices: Data from Washington State document that in recent years, clinicians have curtailed opioid prescribing, and there has been a corresponding drop in accidental deaths attributable to opioid use.[86] We are not aware of recent data on opioid prescribing in other states. We anticipate that reductions comparable to those in Washington State will occur, but there may well be a time lag because the CDC guideline was not published until 2016.

IMPLICATIONS FOR THE IDENTIFICATION OF OPIOID USE DISORDER

Given the changes that have occurred during the past 11 years in our understanding of the risks and benefits of opioid therapy for CNMP, it is less likely that patients will be intentionally started on long-term opioids for treatment of CNMP in the future. However, many patients are started on opioids for acute pain and then provided refills indefinitely, which leads to de facto long-term opioid therapy.[111] Also, there are millions of CNMP patients who are already taking opioids on a long-term basis. Opioid use disorder occurs frequently enough among these patients that clinicians who prescribe opioids need to be vigilant for its presence. For example, in a large Australian sample of patients prescribed opioids for CNMP, 8.9% met lifetime criteria for opioid dependence using *DSM-IV* criteria, 8.5% fulfilled International Statistical Classification of Diseases and Related Health Problems, 10th revision (ICD10) criteria, and 9.9% met International Statistical Classification of Diseases and Related Health Problems, 11th revision (ICD11) criteria. Using *DSM-5*, 8.9% met criteria for moderate or severe opioid use disorder. Another 11.8% met criteria for mild opioid use disorder.[112]

During the period of widespread use of long-term opioid therapy for CNMP, it is almost certain that many patients who actually had opioid use disorder were not identified. At least two factors contributed to this misidentification. First, if a patient has opioid use disorder but is getting opioids on a regular basis from a physician, drug craving, extreme efforts to get opioids, and other indicators of opioid use disorder are likely not to be present. Second, because there was widespread social support for opioid therapy during the period of enthusiasm, a patient's demands for opioids could be construed not as an indicator of opioid use disorder but, rather, as reasonable demands for therapy that was widely available. This is the essence of the now discredited "pseudoaddiction" concept that has been popular in the pain management community.[113,114] Thus, it is reasonable to anticipate that as opioid therapy is discontinued for patients who previously received opioids, it will become apparent that many of them have opioid use disorder. This expectation is supported by data suggesting that heroin usage has surged in response to the reduced availability of prescription opioids.[115]

But even if it is true that many patients have hidden opioid use disorder that is being unmasked as their clinicians taper and discontinue opioid therapy, this does not resolve the challenges that the clinicians face when they decide whether or not to diagnose opioid use disorder in individual patients receiving opioids for pain. Clinical experience strongly suggests that when patients who have been receiving opioids plead for continuation of the treatment, they will emphasize the tremendous burden that pain places on them and the respite that they get from continued or increased doses of their opioids. In fact, as described in *Bonica's Management of Pain*, 4th edition, they are likely to say that their pain affects them so powerfully that they are "forced" to take opioids.

CLINICAL PREVENTION AND MANAGEMENT OF OPIOID USE DISORDER IN PATIENTS RECEIVING OPIOIDS FOR CHRONIC PAIN

As noted earlier, medication treatment with opioid agonists like buprenorphine or methadone is the best treatment for patients with moderate to severe opioid use disorder. It is not clear how patients with mild opioid use disorder should be treated. Some patients might be tapered gradually to safer low-dose opioid use aligned with the CDC guidelines. Other patients might be tapered off opioids completely. There is evidence that when patients on long-term opioid therapy express motivation to reduce or discontinue their opioids, an opioid taper, combined with motivational interviewing, cognitive-behavioral, and psychopharmacologic support (largely consisting of initiating or adjusting antidepressant medication), can be successful and can be carried out without exacerbation of pain or increase in functional impairment.[116] However, there is a caveat. Of the patients referred to the Sullivan et al.[116] study, 76% were either found to be ineligible to participate or refused to do so. At this point, there is no evidence to guide clinicians as they consider opioid tapers for these patients.

In managing prescription for opioid recipients having problem opioid use, clinicians must first decide if the management should take place in their clinics or the patients should be referred to addiction medicine programs such as the ones described earlier in this chapter. There are no clear-cut criteria for making this decision. Among patients whom pain clinicians continue to treat, the boundary between those who should be tapered off their opioids versus those who should be maintained on methadone or buprenorphine is also not well defined. Experienced clinicians often make an attempt at opioid taper and transition those patients who cannot complete a taper onto buprenorphine-naloxone for long-term maintenance.

Conclusions: Bridging the Gap between Addiction and Pain Medicine

There remain significant barriers to overcome in addressing addiction to prescribed opioids. Since the passage of the Harrison Act in 1914, addiction treatment has been separate from the rest of medical treatment. Treatment facilities are separate, funding is different, and the role of private insurance and public payers is different. Patients with pain typically must accept the label of addiction or opioid use disorder to get treatment in addiction facilities or to get insurance coverage for buprenorphine/naloxone. Many are not willing to do this, and clinicians are often hesitant to force the label on them because of uncertainty about how to construe the patients' requests for continued opioid therapy. Thus, although patients prescribed opioids for pain might benefit in multiple ways (safety, toxicity, emotional stabilization) from transition to buprenorphine/naloxone or methadone, they are often prevented from making the transition by financial considerations.

Just as addiction facilities are reluctant to treat patients who do not accept the opioid use disorder label, pain facilities are reluctant to welcome addiction services under their roof. Health administrators, clinical staff, and patients in pain facilities are resistant to welcoming those with addiction into their clinics. This results in a great chasm between pain and addiction health services into which many patients with problem or high-risk opioid use fall. These patients are poorly served by the present diagnostic and health services system. We will not be able to reverse the opioid epidemic until this chasm between pain and addiction services has been bridged.

References

1. Michna E, Ross EL, Hynes WL, et al. Predicting aberrant drug behavior in patients treated for chronic pain: importance of abuse history. *J Pain Symptom Manage* 2004;28(3):250–258.
2. Manchikanti L, Cash KA, Damron KS, et al. Controlled substance abuse and illicit drug use in chronic pain patients: an evaluation of multiple variables. *Pain Physician* 2006;9(3):215–225.
3. Rosenblum A, Joseph H, Fong C, et al. Prevalence and characteristics of chronic pain among chemically dependent patients in methadone maintenance and residential treatment facilities. *JAMA* 2003;289(18):2370–2378.
4. American Psychiatric Association. *Diagnostic and Statistical Manual of Mental Disorders.* 5th ed. Arlington, VA: American Psychiatric Association; 2013.
5. O'Brien CP, Volkow N, Li TK. What's in a word? Addiction versus dependence in DSM-V. *Am J Psychiatry* 2006;163(5):764–765.
6. Gourlay DL, Heit HA, Almahrezi A. Universal precautions in pain medicine: a rational approach to the treatment of chronic pain. *Pain Med* 2005;6(2):107–112.
7. Dawson DA, Grant BF, Li TK. Quantifying the risks associated with exceeding recommended drinking limits. *Alcohol Clin Exp Res* 2005;29(5):902–908.
8. Swift R. Direct measurement of alcohol and its metabolites. *Addiction* 2003;98(suppl 2):73–80.
9. Butler SF, Budman SH, Fernandez K, et al. Validation of a screener and opioid assessment measure for patients with chronic pain. *Pain* 2004;112 (1–2):65–75.
10. Heit HA, Gourlay DL. Urine drug testing in pain medicine. *J Pain Symptom Manage* 2004;27(3):260–267.
11. Dolan K, Rouen D, Kimber J. An overview of the use of urine, hair, sweat and saliva to detect drug use. *Drug Alcohol Rev* 2004;23(2):213–217.
12. Wolff K, Farrell M, Marsden J, et al. A review of biological indicators of illicit drug use, practical considerations and clinical usefulness. *Addiction* 1999;94(9):1279–1298.
13. Jatlow PI, Agro A, Wu R, et al. Ethyl glucuronide and ethyl sulfate assays in clinical trials, interpretation, and limitations: results of a dose ranging alcohol challenge study and 2 clinical trials. *Alcohol Clin Exp Res* 2014; 38(7):2056–2065.
14. Berner MM, Kriston L, Bentele M, et al. The Alcohol Use Disorders Identification Test for detecting at-risk drinking: a systematic review and metaanalysis. *J Stud Alcohol Drugs* 2007;68(3):461–473.
15. Selzer ML. The Michigan Alcoholism Screening Test: the quest for a new diagnostic instrument. *Am J Psychiatry* 1971;127(12):1653–1658.
16. Bradley KA, DeBenedetti AF, Volk RJ, et al. AUDIT-C as a brief screen for alcohol misuse in primary care. *Alcohol Clin Exp Res* 2007;31(7):1208–1217.
17. Gavin DR, Ross HE, Skinner HA. Diagnostic validity of the drug abuse screening test in the assessment of DSM-III drug disorders. *Br J Addict* 1989; 84(3):301–307.
18. Smith PC, Schmidt SM, Allensworth-Davies D, et al. A single-question screening test for drug use in primary care. *Arch Intern Med* 2010;170(13):1155–1160.
19. McNeely J, Wu LT, Subramaniam G. et al. Performance of the Tobacco, Alcohol, Prescription Medication, and Other Substance Use (TAPS) tool for substance use screening in primary care patients. *Ann Intern Med* 2016; 165(10):690–699.
20. Bao Y, Pan Y, Taylor A, et al. Prescription drug monitoring programs are associated with sustained reductions in opioid prescribing by physicians. *Health Aff (Millwood)* 2016;35(6):1045–1051.
21. Tiet QQ, Mausbach B. Treatments for patients with dual diagnosis: a review. *Alcohol Clin Exp Res* 2007;31(4):513–536.
22. Brooner RK, King VL, Kidorf M, et al. Psychiatric and substance use comorbidity among treatment-seeking opioid abusers. *Arch Gen Psychiatry* 1997;54(1):71–80.
23. Manchikanti L, Giordano J, Boswell MV, et al. Psychological factors as predictors of opioid abuse and illicit drug use in chronic pain patients. *J Opioid Manage* 2007;3(2):89–100.
24. Brady KT, Sinha R. Co-occurring mental and substance use disorders: the neurobiological effects of chronic stress. *Am J Psychiatr* 2005;162(8):1483–1493.
25. Manchikanti L, Manchukonda R, Pampati V, et al. Does random urine drug testing reduce illicit drug use in chronic pain patients receiving opioids? *Pain Physician* 2006;9(2):123–129.
26. Moyer A, Finney JW, Swearingen CE, et al. Brief interventions for alcohol problems: a meta-analytic review of controlled investigations in treatment-seeking and non-treatment-seeking populations. *Addiction* 2002;97(3): 279–292.
27. Kaner EF, Beyer F, Dickinson HO, et al. Effectiveness of brief alcohol interventions in primary care populations. *Cochrane Database Syst Rev* 2007;(2):CD004148.
28. Carroll KM, Ball SA, Nich C, et al. Motivational interviewing to improve treatment engagement and outcome in individuals seeking treatment for substance abuse: a multisite effectiveness study. *Drug Alcohol Depend* 2006;81(3):301–312.
29. Staines G, Kosanke N, Magura S, et al. Convergent validity of the ASAM Patient Placement Criteria using a standardized computer algorithm. *J Addict Dis* 2003;22(suppl 1):61–77.
30. Magura S, Staines G, Kosanke N, et al. Predictive validity of the ASAM Patient Placement Criteria for naturalistically matched vs. mismatched alcoholism patients. *Am J Addict* 2003;12(5):386–397.
31. Mayo-Smith MF. Pharmacological management of alcohol withdrawal. A meta-analysis and evidence-based practice guideline. American Society of Addiction Medicine Working Group on Pharmacological Management of Alcohol Withdrawal. *JAMA* 1997;278(2):144–151.
32. Sees KL, Delucchi KL, Masson C, et al. Methadone maintenance vs 180-day psychosocially enriched detoxification for treatment of opioid dependence: a randomized controlled trial. *JAMA* 2000;283(10):1303–1310.
33. Oreskovich MR, Saxon AJ, Ellis ML, et al. A double-blind, double-dummy, randomized, prospective pilot study of the partial mu opiate agonist, buprenorphine, for acute detoxification from heroin. *Drug Alcohol Depend* 2005;77(1):71–79.
34. Gold MS, Redmond DE Jr, Kleber HD. Clonidine blocks acute opiate-withdrawal symptoms. *Lancet* 1978;2(8090):599–602.
35. Collins ED, Kleber HD, Whittington RA, et al. Anesthesia-assisted vs buprenorphine- or clonidine-assisted heroin detoxification and naltrexone induction: a randomized trial. *JAMA* 2005;294(8):903–913.
36. Center for Substance Abuse Treatment. *Medication-Assisted Treatment for Opioid Addiction in Opioid Treatment Programs. Treatment Improvement Protocol (TIP) Series 43.* Rockville, MD: Substance Abuse and Mental Health Services Administration; 2005. DHHS publication no. (SMA) 12-4214.
37. Gunne LM, Gronbladh L. The Swedish methadone maintenance program: a controlled study. *Drug Alcohol Depend* 1981;7(3):249–256.
38. Kakko J, Svanborg KD, Kreek MJ, et al. 1-year retention and social function after buprenorphine-assisted relapse prevention treatment for heroin dependence in Sweden: a randomised, placebo-controlled trial. *Lancet* 2003;361(9358):662–668.

39. Barnett PG. The cost-effectiveness of methadone maintenance as a health care intervention. *Addiction* 1999;94(4):479–488.

40. McLellan AT, Hagan TA, Meyers K, et al. "Intensive" outpatient substance abuse treatment: comparisons with "traditional" outpatient treatment. *J Addict Dis* 1997;16(2):57–84.

41. Broome KM, Simpson DD, Joe GW. The role of social support following short-term inpatient treatment. *Am J Addiction* 2002;11(1):57–65.

42. Smith LA, Gates S, Foxcroft D. Therapeutic communities for substance related disorder. *Cochrane Database Syst Rev* 2006;(1):CD005338.

43. McKay JR, Donovan DM, McLellan T, et al. Evaluation of full vs. partial continuum of care in the treatment of publicly funded substance abusers in Washington State. *Am J Drug Alcohol Abuse* 2002;28(2):307–338.

44. Meier PS, Barrowclough C, Donmall MC. The role of the therapeutic alliance in the treatment of substance misuse: a critical review of the literature. *Addiction* 2005;100(3):304–316.

45. Miller WR, Rollnick S. *Motivational Interviewing: Preparing People for Change.* 2nd ed. New York: Guilford Press; 2002.

46. Marlatt GA, Dennis DM, eds. *Relapse Prevention: Maintenance Strategies in the Treatment of Addictive Behaviors.* 2nd ed. New York: Guilford Press; 2005.

47. Mercer DE, Woody GE. *An Individual Drug Counseling Approach to Treat Cocaine Addiction: The Collaborative Cocaine Treatment Study Model.* Washington, DC: U.S. Government Printing Office; 1999.

48. Nowinski J, Baker S, Carroll K. *Twelve Step Facilitation Therapy Manual: A Clinical Research Guide for Therapists Treating Individuals with Alcohol Abuse and Dependence.* Rockville, MD: U.S. Department of Health and Human Services, Public Health Service, National Institutes of Health, National Institute on Alcohol Abuse and Alcoholism; 1995.

49. Donovan DM, Daley DC, Brigham GS, et al. Stimulant abuser groups to engage in 12-step: a multisite trial in the National Institute on Drug Abuse Clinical Trials Network. *J Subst Abuse Treat* 2013;44(1):103–114.

50. Skinner BF. *The Behavior of Organisms: An Experimental Analysis.* New York: D. Appleton-Century Company; 1938.

51. Petry NM. Contingency management treatments. *Br J Psychiatry* 2006;189:97–98.

52. Wright C, Moore RD. Disulfiram treatment of alcoholism. *Am J Med* 1990;88(6):647–655.

53. Bjornsson E, Nordlinder H, Olsson R. Clinical characteristics and prognostic markers in disulfiram-induced liver injury. *J Hepatol* 2006;44(4):791–797.

54. Fuller RK, Branchey L, Brightwell DR, et al. Disulfiram treatment of alcoholism. A Veterans Administration cooperative study. *JAMA* 1986;256(11):1449–1455.

55. Myrick H, Anton R. Recent advances in the pharmacotherapy of alcoholism. *Curr Psychiatry Rep* 2004;6(5):332–338.

56. Litten RZ, Fertig J, Mattson M, et al. Development of medications for alcohol use disorders: recent advances and ongoing challenges. *Expert Opin Emerg Drugs* 2005;10(2):323–343.

57. Chick J, Lehert P, Landron F. Does acamprosate improve reduction of drinking as well as aiding abstinence? *J Psychopharmacol* 2003;17(4):397–402.

58. Mann K, Lehert P, Morgan MY. The efficacy of acamprosate in the maintenance of abstinence in alcohol-dependent individuals: results of a meta-analysis. *Alcohol Clin Exp Res* 2004;28(1):51–63.

59. Anton RF, O'Malley SS, Ciraulo DA, et al. Combined pharmacotherapies and behavioral interventions for alcohol dependence: the COMBINE study: a randomized controlled trial. *JAMA* 2006;295(17):2003–2017.

60. Mason BJ, Goodman AM, Chabac S, et al. Effect of oral acamprosate on abstinence in patients with alcohol dependence in a double-blind, placebo-controlled trial: the role of patient motivation. *J Psychiatr Res* 2006;40(5):383–393.

61. Kiefer F, Mann K. Pharmacotherapy and behavioral intervention for alcohol dependence. *JAMA* 2006;296(14):1727–1729.

62. Sass H, Soyka M, Mann K, et al. Relapse prevention by acamprosate. Results from a placebo-controlled study on alcohol dependence. *Arch Gen Psychiatry* 1996;53(8):673–680.

63. Benjamin D, Grant ER, Pohorecky LA. Naltrexone reverses ethanol-induced dopamine release in the nucleus accumbens in awake, freely moving rats. *Brain Res* 1993;621(1):137–140.

64. De Waele JP, Gianoulakis C. Enhanced activity of the brain beta-endorphin system by free-choice ethanol drinking in C57BL/6 but not DBA/2 mice. *Eur J Pharmacol* 1994;258(1–2):119–129.

65. Mitchell JM, O'Neil JP, Janabi M, et al. Alcohol consumption induces endogenous opioid release in the human orbitofrontal cortex and nucleus accumbens. *Sci Transl Med* 2012;4(116):116ra6.

66. Tabakoff B, Hoffman PL. Alcohol interactions with brain opiate receptors. *Life Sci* 1983;32(3):197–204.

67. McCaul ME, Wand GS, Eissenberg T, et al. Naltrexone alters subjective and psychomotor responses to alcohol in heavy drinking subjects. *Neuropsychopharmacology* 2000;22(5):480–492.

68. Jonas DE, Amick HR, Feltner C, et al. Pharmacotherapy for adults with alcohol use disorders in outpatient settings: a systematic review and meta-analysis. *JAMA* 2014;311(18):1889–900.

69. Lee MC, Wagner HN Jr, Tanada S, et al. Duration of occupancy of opiate receptors by naltrexone. *J Nucl Med* 1988;29(7):1207–1211.

70. Volpicelli JR, Rhines KC, Rhines JS, et al. Naltrexone and alcohol dependence. Role of subject compliance. *Arch Gen Psychiatry* 1997;54(8):737–742.

71. Chick J, Anton R, Checinski K, et al. A multicentre, randomized, double-blind, placebo-controlled trial of naltrexone in the treatment of alcohol dependence or abuse. *Alcohol Alcohol* 2000;35(6):587–593.

72. Garbutt JC, Kranzler HR, O'Malley SS, et al. Efficacy and tolerability of long-acting injectable naltrexone for alcohol dependence: a randomized controlled trial. *JAMA* 2005;93(13):1617–1625.

73. Minozzi S, Amato L, Vecchi S, et al. Oral naltrexone maintenance treatment for opioid dependence. *Cochrane Database Syst Rev* 2011;(4):CD001333.

74. Krupitsky E, Nune EV, Ling W, et al. Injectable extended-release naltrexone for opioid dependence: a double-blind, placebo-controlled, multicentre randomised trial. *Lancet* 2011;377(9776):1506–1513.

75. Lee JD, Friedmann PD, Kinlock TW, et al. Extended-release naltrexone to prevent opioid relapse in criminal justice offenders. *N Engl J Med* 2016;374(13):1232–1242.

76. Bell J, Seres V, Bowron P, et al. The use of serum methadone levels in patients receiving methadone maintenance. *Clin Pharmacol Ther* 1988;43(6):623–629.

77. Walsh SL, Preston KL, Stitzer ML, et al. Clinical pharmacology of buprenorphine: ceiling effects at high doses. *Clin Pharmacol Ther* 1994;55(5):569–580.

78. Greenwald MK, Johanson CE, Moody DE, et al. Effects of buprenorphine maintenance dose on mu-opioid receptor availability, plasma concentrations, and antagonist blockade in heroin-dependent volunteers. *Neuropsychopharmacology* 2003;28(11):2000–2009.

79. Johnson RE, McCagh JC. Buprenorphine and naloxone for heroin dependence. *Curr Psychiatry Rep* 2000;2(6):519–526.

80. Center for Substance Abuse Treatment. *Clinical Guidelines for the Use of Buprenorphine in the Treatment of Opioid Addiction. Treatment Improvement Protocol (TIP) Series 40.* Rockville, MD: Substance Abuse and Mental Health Services Administration; 2004.

81. Mattick RP, Breen C, Kimber J, et al. Buprenorphine maintenance versus placebo or methadone maintenance for opioid dependence. *Cochrane Database Syst Rev* 2014;(2):CD002207. doi:10.1002/14651858.CD002207.pub4.

82. Kakko J, Gronbladh L, Svanborg KD, et al. A stepped care strategy using buprenorphine and methadone versus conventional methadone maintenance in heroin dependence: a randomized controlled trial. *Am J Psychiatry* 2007;164(5):797–803.

83. Koppert W, Ihmsen H, Korber N, et al. Different profiles of buprenorphine-induced analgesia and antihyperalgesia in a human pain model. *Pain* 2005;118(1–2):15–22.

84. Cowan A. Buprenorphine: new pharmacological aspects. *Int J Clin Pract Suppl* 2003;133:3–8, 23–24.

85. Malinoff HL, Barkin RL, Wilson G. Sublingual buprenorphine is effective in the treatment of chronic pain syndrome. *Am J Ther* 2005;12(5):379–384.

86. Franklin G, Sabel J, Jones CM, et al. A comprehensive approach to address the prescription opioid epidemic in Washington State: milestones and lessons learned. *Am J Public Health* 2015;105(3):463–469.

87. Gellad WF. Commentary on Daubresse et al. (2017): an epidemic of outdated data. *Addiction* 2017;112(6):1054–1055.

88. Van Zee A. The promotion and marketing of OxyContin: commercial triumph, public health tragedy. *Am J Public Health* 2009;99(2):221–227.

89. Warner M, Hedegaard H, Chen LH. *Trends in Drug-Poisoning Deaths Involving Opioid Analgesics and Heroin: United States, 1999–2012.* Hyattsville, MD: National Centers for Health Statistics; 2014. Available at: www.cdc.gov/nchs/data/hestat/drug_poisoning/drug_poisoning_deaths_1999-2012.pdf. Accessed June 14, 2007.

90. Washington State Department of Health. Drug poisoning and overdose, 2013. Available at: http://www.doh.wa.gov/portals/1/Documents/2900/DOH530090Poison.pdf. Accessed June 14, 2017.

91. Smith SM, Dart RC, Katz NP, et al. Classification and definition of misuse, abuse, and related events in clinical trials: ACTTION systematic review and recommendations. *Pain* 2013;154(11):2287–2296.

92. Porter J, Jick H. Addiction rare in patients treated with narcotics. *N Engl J Med* 1980;302(2):123.

93. Setnik B, Roland CL, Pixton GC, et al. Prescription opioid abuse and misuse: gap between primary-care investigator assessment and actual extent of these behaviors among patients with chronic pain. *Postgrad Med* 2017;129(1):5–11.

94. Vowles KE, McEntee ML, Julnes PS, et al. Rates of opioid misuse, abuse, and addiction in chronic pain: a systematic review and data synthesis. *Pain* 2015;156(4):569–576.

95. Peavy KM, Banta-Green CJ, Kingston S, et al. "Hooked on" prescription-type opiates prior to using heroin: results from a survey of syringe exchange clients. *J Psychoactive Drugs* 2012;44(3):259–265.

96. Chou R, Turner JA, Devine EB, et al. The effectiveness and risks of long-term opioid therapy for chronic pain: a systematic review for a National Institutes of Health Pathways to Prevention Workshop. *Ann Intern Med* 2015;162(4):276–286.

97. Calcaterra S, Glanz J, Binswanger IA. National trends in pharmaceutical opioid related overdose deaths compared to other substance related overdose deaths: 1999–2009. *Drug Alcohol Depend* 2013;131(3):263–270.

98. Agarin T, Trescot AM, Agarin A, et al. Reducing opioid analgesic deaths in America: what health providers can do. *Pain Physician* 2015;18(3): E307–E322.

99. Paulozzi LJ, Budnitz DS, Xi Y. Increasing deaths from opioid analgesics in the United States. *Pharmacoepidemiol Drug Saf* 2006;15(9):618–627.

100. Santos J, Alarcão J, Fareleira F, et al. Tapentadol for chronic musculoskeletal pain in adults. *Cochrane Database Syst Rev* 2015;(5):CD009923.

101. Deyo RA, Von Korff M, Duhrkoop D. Opioids for low back pain. *BMJ* 2015;5:350:g6380. doi:10.1136/bmj.g6380.

102. Volinn E, Fargo JD, Fine PG. Opioid therapy for nonspecific low back pain and the outcome of chronic work loss. *Pain* 2009;142(3):194–201.

103. Franklin GM, Stover BD, Turner JA, et al; for Disability Risk Identification Study Cohort. Early opioid prescription and subsequent disability among workers with back injuries: the Disability Risk Identification Study Cohort. *Spine* 2008;33(2):199–204.

104. Dowell D, Haegerich TM, Chou R. CDC guideline for prescribing opioids for chronic pain—United States, 2016. *MMWR Recomm Rep* 2016;65(1): 1–49.

105. Moyo P, Simoni-Wastila L, Griffin BA, et al. Impact of prescription drug monitoring programs (PDMPs) on opioid utilization among Medicare beneficiaries in 10 U.S. states. *Addiction* 2017;112:1784–1796. doi:10.1111/add.13860.

106. Rutkow L, Chang HY, Daubresse M, et al. Effect of Florida's prescription drug monitoring program and pill mill laws on opioid prescribing and use. *JAMA Intern Med* 2015;175(10):1642–1649.

107. Washington State Agency Medical Directors' Group. *Interagency Guideline on Opioid Dosing for Chronic Non-Cancer Pain.* Olympia, WA: Washington State Department of Labor and Industries; 2007. Available at: www.agencymeddirectors.wa.gov. Accessed June 16, 2017.

108. Washington State Agency Medical Directors' Group. *Interagency Guideline on Opioid Dosing for Chronic Non-Cancer Pain.* Olympia, WA: Washington State Department of Labor and Industries; 2010. Available at: www.agencymeddirectors.wa.gov. Accessed June 16, 2017.

109. Washington State Agency Medical Directors' Group. *Interagency Guideline on Prescribing Opioids for Pain.* Olympia, WA: Washington State Department of Labor and Industries; 2015. Available at: www.agencymeddirectors .wa.gov. Accessed June 16, 2017.

110. Washington State Legislature. Engrossed Substitute House Bill 2876— an act relating to pain management. Available at: http://apps.leg.wa.gov /documents/billdocs/2009-10/Pdf/Bills/Session%20Laws/House/2876-S .SL.pdf. Accessed June 16, 2017.

111. Shah A, Hayes CJ, Martin BC. Characteristics of initial prescription episodes and likelihood of long-term opioid use—United States, 2006-2015. *MMWR Morb Mortal Wkly Rep* 2017;66(10):265–269.

112. Degenhardt L, Bruno R, Lintzeris N, et al. Agreement between definitions of pharmaceutical opioid use disorders and dependence in people taking opioids for chronic non-cancer pain (POINT): a cohort study. *Lancet Psychiatry* 2015;2(4):314–322.

113. Weissman DE, Haddox JD. Opioid pseudoaddiction—an iatrogenic syndrome. *Pain* 1989;36(3):363–366.

114. Greene MS, Chambers RA. Pseudoaddiction: fact or fiction? An investigation of the medical literature. *Curr Addict Rep* 2015;2(4):310–317.

115. Smith DE. Medicalizing the opioid epidemic in the U.S. in the era of health care reform. *J Psychoactive Drugs* 2017;49(2):95–101.

116. Sullivan MD, Turner JA, DiLodovico C, et al. Prescription opioid taper support for outpatients with chronic pain: a randomized controlled trial. *J Pain* 2017;18(3):308–318. 166(19):2087–2093.

CHAPTER 92

Biophysical Agents for Pain Management in Physical Therapy

ROGER J. ALLEN

The primary focus of physical therapy is functional restoration via physical reactivation.[1] Therapeutic exercise, movement, and physical reactivation have been demonstrated not only to be central components in restoration of function following injury and disease but are also efficacious elements of managing both acute pain and chronic pain syndromes.[1-4] In concert with the functional physical restoration activities, physical therapists may also utilize therapeutic biophysical agents (previously referred to as physical *agents* or *modalities*) to complement other treatment elements as part of a comprehensive patient care plan.[5,6] Philosophies and approaches to pain management vary across practitioners and clinical facilities; yet, the use of biophysical agents is widespread.[2,5] The Centers for Medicare & Medicaid Services reported in 2014 that electrical stimulation and ultrasound therapy ranked among the top 10 procedures receiving Medicare payments to rehabilitation providers.[5] All physical therapists and physical therapist assistants receive clinical training in the biophysics and safe therapeutic application of biophysical agents as required for licensure and by the Commission on Accreditation in Physical Therapy Education (CAPTE).[6-8]

Biophysical agents traditionally involve application of some form of heat, cold, light, electromagnetic, or acoustic energy to the body tissue involved in generating pain.[6,9] In the context of pain management, delivery of energy to tissue may modify the underlying pathophysiologic process generating pain or alter the transmission, central processing, or perception of the pain message.[6] They may assist in causing temporary analgesia,[4] resolving inflammation and facilitating tissue repair,[6,9] modifying axonal conduction,[6] generating a counterirritant,[6] altering muscle activation, or increasing extensibility.[6] Biophysical agents may also curb the development of maladaptive central neuropathic changes that could precipitate secondary chronic pain generators[10-13] or provide other means of palliative relief via modified pain perception.[11]

Selection of specific biophysical agents for pain management should be done on a case-by-case basis predicated on clinical impressions regarding the loci and underlying pathophysiologic processes of pain generation.[5,14] For a particular agent to be therapeutically useful, its effects must either address the pathophysiologic changes occurring at the tissue level or alter neural pain transmission or central processing.[14] If the origin of nociceptive pain is due to damaged and/or inflamed tissue, then locally operating agents are indicated. However, if pain is being generated by peripheral neuropathic factors or a central neuroplastic remodeling component, then potentially effective agents should be chosen from those capable of influencing neural transmission or central processing.[15]

Although distal pathophysiology is the primary consideration in the selection of biophysical agents for acute or subacute pain, additional factors must be addressed when considering biophysical agents for use in treating patients with chronic pain. As distal subacute lesions evolve into chronic pain syndromes, the loci of pain generation may migrate.[14,16-18] Restrictions in activity and mobility in response to initial pain from the inciting lesion may lead to connective tissue changes and alterations in vascular physiology that develop into secondary pain generation sites.[16,18] Central pain generators may further develop from neuroplastic remodeling of the dorsal horn, thalamus, or cerebral cortex.[13,17] The application of biophysical agents to the original lesion site may prove ineffective if the sources of the chronic pain are secondary generation sites or neural remodeling that are rostral to the location of perceived pain.[15]

The use of a passive modality as a sole treatment approach is unlikely to lead to long-term improvement in a patient's functional status. In treatment planning for pain management, thoughtful use of biophysical agents coordinates their application with physical restoration activities. In 2014, the American Physical Therapy Association established the position that biophysical agents do not effectively represent stand-alone treatments, stating that clinicians should not "employ passive physical agents except when necessary to facilitate participation in an active treatment program," reinforcing their earlier position that "exclusive use of physical agents in the absence of other skilled therapeutic, or educational intervention, should not be considered."[5]

Thoughtful case-by-case consideration should be given to providing patients experiencing chronic pain an external source of passive palliative relief.[3,5,14,19] Temporary pain relief via the use of biophysical agents may create a therapeutic window for the therapist to mobilize tissue or address movement impairments.[3] For some patients, however, a maladaptive cycle of pain behavior may develop from psychologic dependence on passive external palliative agents. Ultimately, this may reduce progress toward functional restoration by hindering the motivation to actively engage in therapeutic physical activity.[3,14] Passive agents may not only provide disincentives for the patient to approach pain management from an active or functional perspective but may also reinforce an external locus of control, whereby the patient attributes pain relief to procedures unrelated to his or her own actions or pacing.[3] This underscores the importance of utilizing palliative agents as components of comprehensive treatment planning rather than as stand-alone interventions for short-lived pain relief.

Biophysical agents currently in use by physical therapists for the management of pain include superficial heat and cold, light (such as low-level laser or monochromatic infrared energy [MIRE]), therapeutic ultrasound, electrical currents (such as transcutaneous electrical nerve stimulation [TENS] and interferential current [IFC]), materials used to facilitate multimodal somatosensory desensitization, and new techniques for influencing central neuroplastic remodeling of pain perception.

Superficial Thermal Agents

THERMOTHERAPY

Superficial heat, or "thermotherapy," is used to facilitate soft tissue extensibility, increase circulation, enhance healing, induce relaxation, reduce muscle spasms, prepare stiff muscles and tight joints for exercise, and/or control pain.[20] Heat is delivered to superficial tissues via conduction with clinical applications such as moist hot packs and paraffin wax dips, or for home therapy with electric heating pads, air-activated wearable heat wraps, microwavable gel packs, or rice-filled cloth bags. Superficial heat can also be applied via convection using agents such as dry heat fluidotherapy or warm whirlpool hydrotherapy.[20] Thermotherapy is quite commonly utilized by physical therapists across the world, with studies reporting daily use of therapeutic heating agents ranging between 36.5% and 95% across diverse practice settings.[20,21]

As an adjunct to pain management, therapeutic benefits of superficial heat are due to its effects on metabolic, neuromuscular, and hemodynamic processes. Although the physiologic effects of superficial heat primarily influence tissue healing and acute nociceptive pain generation, thoughtfully applied thermotherapy may have utility in the comprehensive management of chronic pain.[14] The oxygen–hemoglobin dissociation curve shifts to the right with mild increases in tissue temperature, making more oxygen available for tissue repair. Increases in enzymatic activity increase oxygen uptake by the cell, thus enhancing healing.[6,20] Increased skeletal muscle temperature (to 42° C) has been reported to decrease firing rates of gamma and type II muscle spindle efferents while increasing Golgi tendon organ type Ib fiber firing rates.[22] This may reflexively lower skeletal muscle tone and spasms. Reduced skeletal muscle activity may assist in breaking the pain–spasm–pain exacerbation cycle.[6,23] Analgesic benefits of superficial heating of the skin may be centrally mediated, as evidenced by functional magnetic resonance imaging (fMRI) findings that warming of distal tissue increases activity of the thalamus and posterior insula, thus initiating a potentially beneficial psychosomatic effect.[24,25]

Elevations in nociceptive threshold have been reported due to superficial heat.[20,26] By increasing activity of afferent thermoreceptive fibers, superficial heat may produce inhibitory modulation of dorsal horn pain gates.[6] Indirectly, pain may be influenced via local vasomotor effects and increased blood flow. Dorsal horn synapses from first-order thermal receptor afferents inhibit sympathetic vasomotor efferents in the spinal intermediolateral grey area, thus decreasing vasoconstriction neurogenically.[6] When sympathetic vasomotor outflow is decreased, local vasodilation and increased vascular perfusion may influence pain further by decreasing tissue ischemia,[27] returning nociceptors to normal firing thresholds by helping to resolve hyperalgesia, and clearing exacerbating metabolites such as prostaglandins from the region. Blood flow increases of as much as 30 mL per 100 g of tissue have been reported.[22] However, these effects influence primarily superficial blood vessels and the tissues they supply. Less evident is vasodilation in deep muscle vasculature because of the limited ability of superficial agents to increase temperature in deeper structures.[6]

Superficial heat, applied in forms such as hot packs, paraffin, hydrotherapy, and fluidotherapy, has been broadly evaluated for effectiveness in the treatment of both rheumatoid and osteoarthritis. Seven controlled studies have found it a beneficial adjunct[28–34] whereas two found it ineffective[35,36] and possibly harmful by increasing collagenase activity which may have damaged compromised articular cartilage.[36] Comparative studies report beneficial effects of superficial heat for trigger point pain in the neck and back,[37] neck and shoulder pain,[37] and chronic low back pain.[38,39]

Local tissue temperatures required to achieve therapeutic outcomes are in the range of 40° to 45° C (104° to 113° F).[20,22,40] Exceeding this range places tissue at risk for damage because at local temperatures >45° C (113° F) metabolic activity required for repair cannot keep pace with protein denaturation.[20] At therapeutic temperatures, applying heat is contraindicated over hemorrhagic areas; regions of acute injury, acute inflammation, peripheral vascular disease, malignancy, impaired sensation, or thrombophlebitis; the abdomens of pregnant women; tissues that have been devitalized by x-ray therapy: or with patients with existing fever, confusion, sedation, coma, or relevant cognitive impairments.[6,9,41,42] Caution should be used when applying heat over areas of impaired circulation, edema, superficial metal implants, where topical counterirritants have been applied, or over open wounds.[41] Also, exercise proper caution during use with children under 4 years old or older adult patients; patients manifesting poor thermal regulation, cardiac insufficiency, or acute inflammatory disorders; or with hypotensive patients, those manifesting orthostatic hypotension, or anyone prone to syncope when heating large body surface areas.[6,9,14,36,42]

CRYOTHERAPY

Application of cold, whether via water immersion, ice, gel, or vapor-coolant sprays, is one of the most effective and cost efficient modalities for managing pain and acute injury.[43] Its therapeutic use has been traced as far back as in Egypt around 2500 BCE.[44] Termed *cryotherapy*, the therapeutic use of cold can be used to control pain, minimize edema, reduce inflammation, enhance movement, and attenuate spasticity.[6]

A primary indication for cryotherapy is to minimize secondary hypoxic injury to adjacent tissue areas immediately following acute trauma.[9] By lowering metabolism of damaged and surrounding cells, they become more resistant to hypoxia resulting from disrupted blood supply to the region, making this the primary reason that cold is the agent of choice for the first 24 to 48 hours after injury.[45] This mechanism of minimizing the extent of tissue damage is dependent on immediate application of cold following trauma and is not a mechanism likely to contribute to the management of chronic pain states. It may also elevate pain thresholds and decrease muscle spasms and tension secondary to myofascial trigger points.[43,46]

Cryotherapy can be administered using conductive agents such as ice bags, superficial ice massage, bags of frozen corn or peas, cold compression units, cold whirlpool immersion, or via contrast baths, in which alternating heat and cold are used. It can also be administered with convective agents such as vapor-coolant sprays.[46] Different cryotherapeutic modalities can produce a varied range of tissue cooling ability.[43] Following 20-minute exposure over the gastrocnemius muscle, skin surface temperature was reportedly lowered by 19.6° C (35.0° F) using crushed ice, 17.0° C (30.6° F) following ice water immersion, 14.6° C (26.0° F) from contact with a bag of frozen peas, and 13.0° C (23.5° F) using a cold gel pack.[47] Following 15-minute exposure, superficial ice massage decreased intramuscular temperature by 4.3° C (7.7° F) compared to contact with ice bag that lowered temperature by 2.3° C (4.1° F).[48] Depth of intervening adipose tissue layers has a significant influence on the rate of intramuscular cooling and subsequent rewarming.[43] It has been found that 10 minutes are required to produce a decrease in intramuscular temperature of 7.0° C (12.5° F) with a 1-cm layer of intervening adipose tissue, whereas given adipose thickness of 3 to 4 cm, 60 minutes are required to achieve the same temperature reduction.[49]

The therapeutic effects of cold result from its actions on metabolic, neuromuscular, and hemodynamic processes.[6] Decreases in nociceptive input and pain perception via application of cold may occur because of influences in both local and central nervous system mechanisms.[14] Vasoconstrictive response to cold decreases local release of vasodilating substances and chemical mediators, which in turn decreases nociceptor sensitization.[6,23] For every 1° C drop in interstitial temperature, nerve conduction velocity of somatosensory afferent fibers drops approximately 2 m/s due to metabolic changes in the axon.[50] It has been reported that at a skin surface temperature of 10° C (50° F) there is a 33% reduction in nerve conduction velocity[50] and that local analgesia may be produced by lowering skin surface temperature to 13.6° C (56.5° F).[51] Aδ nociceptive fibers display the most sensitivity to cold mediated velocity attenuation, whereas blocking conduction of C fibers requires considerably colder temperatures.[22,43] The effects of application of a cryotherapy agent for 10 to 15 minutes may transcend immediate changes and produce pain reductions for more than an hour.[6] Prolonged analgesia may be the result of Aδ conduction block and the maintenance of subnormal deep tissue temperature for 1 to 2 hours following cold exposure.[6,52] Extended cold application has been shown to produce reversible neurapraxia.[53] Theoretically, by interrupting the pain–spasm–pain cycle, cold application may reduce muscle spasm, thus continuing pain relief after tissue temperature has recovered to precryotherapy levels.[6] Finally, by applying vapor-coolant sprays over skeletal muscle and combining it with stretch, evaporative cooling may reduce muscle spasm and allow muscle with excess neurogenic tone to be stretched for increased range of motion.[6,46,54] The vapor-coolant spray has been hypothesized to be effective in this capacity by providing a counterirritation to cutaneous afferents, which in turn leads to a reflex decrease in motor neuron activity and resistance to stretch.[6]

Existing literature is clear in support of the efficacy of cryotherapy in acute trauma management. It may also play a role in treating some manifestations of chronic pain; however, at the current time, there is little well-controlled literature supporting its efficacy.[43] Uncontrolled comparative studies and case studies have reported that in the treatment of muscle spasms and myofascial pain, cryotherapy may be a beneficial adjunct.[46,55,56] Additional comparative studies have reported it to be a useful clinical tool in managing chronic headache,[57] trigeminal neuralgia,[58] chronic osteoarthritis,[59] and low back pain.[39]

Cryotherapy is contraindicated for patients with Raynaud's disease or phenomenon; cryoglobulinemia or paroxysmal cold hemoglobinuria; angina pectoris; those prone to cold urticaria, cold intolerance, or hypersensitivity; or over skin areas of impaired somatosensory discrimination, deep open wounds, areas of circulatory compromise or peripheral vascular disease, and regenerating peripheral nerves.[6,9,42,43] Cryotherapy should be used with caution over the main branch of a superficial nerve, on individuals with unstable hypertension, those with significant loss of superficial sensation, poor thermoregulation, aversion or intolerance to cold, poor cognition, or in the very young or very old.[6,9,42,43] Note that with applications to the lower extremity, proprioception and joint stability will be temporarily compromised following treatment, so caution should be exercised with ambulation or return to sports participation quickly after cryotherapy.[41]

Light Therapy

LASER

Laser light is in current use for a variety of medical conditions. The U.S. Food and Drug Administration (FDA) has three classifications for medical lasers:

- Class 4 (IV)—surgical lasers (>500 mW)
- Class 3B (IIIb)—nonsurgical lasers (5 to 500 mW)
- Class 3R (IIIr)—nonsurgical lasers (<5 mW)

The Class 3 lasers are not of sufficient intensity to damage cells (with the exception of the retina) and are used to help heal superficial wounds (3A), or provide sufficient penetration to address deeper tissue and joint problems (3B). The first FDA approval for the use of Class 3 lasers for pain management was granted in February 2002 for the treatment of carpal tunnel syndrome.[60] Specific low-level laser devices have FDA approval[60] for treatment of the following pain conditions:

- Muscle and joint pain
- Pain associated with muscle spasm
- Hand and wrist pain associated with carpal tunnel syndrome
- Neck pain
- Lower back pain

Since FDA clearance, physical therapists have utilized laser to treat a range of painful and inflammatory conditions.[61] Low-level Class 3 laser therapy (LLLT), or "cold laser," is used in rehabilitation settings to promote healing and manage pain utilizes lasers with power outputs ≤500 mW at a power density of ≤50 mW/cm².[9]

Laser therapy utilizes light energy that has the unique properties of monochromaticity, coherence, and collimation.[6,61] These properties allow laser light to deliver electromagnetic energy to tissue depths slightly below the dermis.[62] Indirect physiologic effects occur at deeper levels due to the promotion of chemical reactions that mediate processes at greater tissue depths.[6,61,62]

Lasers most frequently utilized for LLLT are of the semiconductor diode configuration that produces light in the red and near-infrared portions of the electromagnetic spectrum, utilizing wavelengths ranging from 632.8 to 904 nm.[9] Diode lasers are usually hand held probes that allow for treatment of small, localized areas. Superluminous diodes (SLDs) also produce light in the red and near-infrared portions of the electromagnetic spectrum. They are brighter but less powerful than diode lasers. The advantage of SLDs is to allow hands-free operation and the ability to treat larger surface areas.[62] Single-laser diodes may be mounted in a wand for treatment of small areas, or in a cluster arrangement, which may contain a mix of diodes, for treating larger areas.[9] Depth of penetration for therapeutic laser light is determined by both absorption and scattering of the specific light frequency by body tissue. Visible red laser light (wavelength of 632.8 nm) has a depth of tissue penetration <1 cm, whereas infrared (wavelengths of 780 to 860 nm and 904 nm) can reach depths <5 cm.[9] Infrared lasers typically combine with a red laser light source to both let the therapist and patient know the laser is on and to help visually guide the invisible infrared beam.

Although the mechanisms by which low-level lasers may modulate pain are not definitively established, there is consensus in the literature that LLLT can induce photomodulation effects of chromophores within affected tissue.[6,9,62,63] Cellular chromophores (light absorbing molecules) absorb photons from laser light as it penetrates the skin. Via influence over respiratory chain enzymes, chromophores may then undergo photobiomodulation in the form of either photobiostimulation or photobioinhibition.[9,64] A dose–response interaction effect occurs based on the Arndt-Schultz law of photobiologic activation.[9,64] Low doses of laser light activate photobiostimulation responses that are potentially efficacious for wound healing, whereas higher doses of laser light initiate a photobioinhibition response that may be beneficial for pain management.[9,64]

With possible application to temporary pain relief, LLLT has been hypothesized to influence nerve conduction velocity. There are reports in the literature indicating both slight increases and decreases in peripheral nerve conduction velocity due to low-level laser application with resulting changes in distal latencies.[65,66] Other studies report no effect on nerve conduction velocity following LLLT.[67,68] The influence of LLLT on clinically significant changes in nerve conduction velocity appears uncertain. Other mechanisms by which LLLT may influence perceived pain remain to be explored.

Numerous studies have addressed the effects of LLLT with respect to treating a wide array of pain-generating conditions. For most disorders, the literature is somewhat divided between studies showing some clinically significant beneficial effects over controls and those that do not. Based on a critical review and preponderance of quality evidence from 157 studies, Belanger[9] concluded that the therapeutic effectiveness of LLLT may be considered substantiated with strong evidence for the following conditions: rheumatoid arthritis,[69,70] osteoarthritis,[71–73] herpes/postherpetic neuralgia,[74,75] myofascial/trigger point pain,[76–78] and neck and low back pain.[79,80] Controlled human studies reporting benefits from LLLT have been published that address pain conditions originating from various specific loci. Examples include carpal tunnel syndrome,[81,82] temporomandibular disorders,[83] postsurgical abdominal pain,[84] trigeminal neuralgia,[85,86] plantar fasciitis,[87] chondromalacia,[88] orofacial pain,[89] ankle sprains,[90] and tendinopathies.[91,92] However, at the present time, there appears to be insufficient evidence supporting the use of LLLT for treating acute muscle soreness.[9]

Contraindications to LLLT include exposing any of the following to laser light: photosensitive skin areas; hemorrhagic areas; any area within 4 to 6 months after radiation therapy; neoplastic lesions; unclosed fontanelles or epiphyseal growth plates in children; the abdomens of pregnant women; over the heart, vagus nerve, or sympathetic innervation routes to the heart of cardiac patients; or locally to endocrine glands.[6,9,42,61] Eye exposure is also contraindicated, so both patient and therapist must utilize protective eye wear that must be precisely matched with the frequency of light emitted by the therapeutic laser to afford protection. LLLT should be used with caution over areas with compromised sensation, reproductive organs, infected areas, and with patients displaying fever, epilepsy, or mental confusion.[6,9,42]

MONOCHROMATIC INFRARED ENERGY

Infrared radiation, once widely used as a superficial heating agent, has recently emerged as form of light therapy that may have effects on processes leading to pain relief, tissue repair, and restoration of protective sensation.[93] Current infrared devices produce MIRE from the near-infrared portion of the electromagnetic spectrum at a wavelength of 890 nm through a series of gallium aluminum arsenide diodes in a flexible pad.[61] Infrared light may also be presented as pulsed infrared light therapy (PILT).[93]

The physiologic effects of MIRE on biologic tissues are thought to be due to photochemical reactions in the skin similar to LLLT rather than thermal reactions. Light energy from MIRE devices causes an increase in plasma nitric oxide (NO) from red blood cells, leading to vasodilation and increased circulation. NO is thought to facilitate vascular perfusion, resulting in improved tissue oxygenation, delivery of nutrients, and removal of waste products of metabolism.[94-96] The vascular effects and increased oxygenation to the tissues may facilitate wound healing and potentially explain the promotion of nerve growth and resultant improvement in sensation that has been observed in some individuals with mild peripheral neuropathy.[61,94,97]

The small volume of literature available on MIRE suggests that it has potential for the treatment of pain and spasm associated with temporomandibular joint dysfunction and healing of chronic wounds.[61] It has also been widely promoted as a treatment for the pain and sensory loss associated with diabetic peripheral neuropathy (DPN).[93,98] In a systematic review of randomized controlled trials assessing the effectiveness of MIRE or PILT on diabetic neuropathy, four studies assessed self-reported pain symptoms, with three finding no significant improvement.[93] One study reported improved peripheral sensation and as well as decreased foot pain in an experimental group with less severe peripheral neuropathy but not in a group with more severe peripheral neuropathy.[95] Infrared therapy was found to improve sensation in three studies[97,99,100] and three reported no improvement.[101-103] Infrared therapy was not found to improve nerve conduction, blood flow, tissue temperature, and transcutaneous oxygen pressure[94,99,102] and was not found to improve most measures of quality of life or self-reported disease severity.[102] There appears to be a lack of consistent evidence at this time supporting the use of infrared light therapy as a treatment for DPN in a physical therapy setting.[93]

The precautions and contraindications to MIRE include avoiding placement over the low back or pelvic regions of pregnant women, cancerous lesions, anesthetic skin fields, areas of active hemorrhage, epiphyseal growth plates in children, and anterior neck region over the thyroid.[61] Goggles are not required during treatment because the diode arrays block the infrared radiation from the eyes. However, the pads should not be placed over the eyes.[61]

Therapeutic Ultrasound

Ultrasound is one of the most commonly employed thermal agents in rehabilitation medicine. It is widely used, and sometimes misused, as an adjunct to the management of pain and inflammation by physical therapists.[4,104] Recent studies have found that 82.4% of physical therapists report using it in clinical practice with 40% of their patients and 36.4% of therapists employ it on a daily basis.[104,105] However, this level of implementation represents a decline in the nearly ubiquitous level of usage two decades ago.[104]

Ultrasound is the generation of high-frequency mechanical waves via acoustic energy.[104] As acoustic waves pass through body tissue, their kinetic energy may be converted to thermal energy as the waves encounter tissues of varying sonic impedance. Clinically, ultrasound is capable of producing elevations in temperature at tissue depths of up to 5 cm through the conversion of acoustic energy into heat.[6] Therapeutic ultrasound can be used as a thermal agent to increase deep tissue temperature or increase pain threshold, or as a nonthermal agent to address inflammation and facilitate tissue repair.[6] Ultrasound is also utilized to deliver medication, such as steroid or analgesic preparations, into the tissues.[6]

Therapeutic ultrasound utilizes a reverse piezoelectric effect. Acoustic waves are generated by a crystal sound head at frequencies of either 1 MHz or 3 (or 3.3) MHz.[14,104] Amplitude densities are typically between 0.1 and 3 W/cm^2.[14] Frequency and depth of penetration of the therapeutic ultrasound beam are inversely related. That is, 3 MHz ultrasound is capable of producing heat in tissues up to 2.5 cm from the skin surface, whereas ultrasound delivered at 1 MHz can reach depths of up to 6 cm.[104,106] These parameters are in contrast to the ultrasound sources used for diagnostic imaging whose purpose is not to generate heat. Diagnostic ultrasound beams carry higher frequencies and lower wattage.[14]

Molecules within soft tissue vibrate due to rarefaction and compression as ultrasonic acoustic waves pass through them. Heat is generated, and thus increased tissue temperature, from microfriction caused by this increased vibratory movement of molecules.[9,104] Sonic impedance variations within body tissue facilitate heat generation in the presence of acoustic waves. In general, tissues with high absorption coefficients (i.e., those with low water content or collagen-rich structures such as tendon, cartilage, and bone) will attenuate more ultrasound energy than tissues with low absorption coefficients such as fat or muscle.[6,107] The thermal effects of ultrasound, which include acceleration of metabolic rate, increased circulation, reduction of pain and muscle spasm, changes in nerve conduction velocity, and increases in collagen tissue extensibility, are essentially the same as those of superficial thermal agents except that the structures heated are different.[104]

Nonthermal effects of ultrasound are theoretically thought to be caused by the processes of cavitation, microstreaming, and acoustic streaming.[6,104,107] As oscillating acoustic waves pass through soft tissue, microscopic bubbles, or cavities, are formed from the effect of cyclic drops in pressure on normally present minute gas pockets. Ultrasound produces a state of stable cavitation such that the microscopic bubbles formed pulsate without imploding. A flow of fluid is then established around the pulsating microbubbles, which is referred to as microstreaming, along with acoustic streaming which is the circular flow of cellular fluids.[6,9] These processes have been reported to alter vascular wall permeability and cell membrane activity and facilitate soft tissue healing.[9,107] In order to produce the beneficial nonthermal effects of ultrasound without causing an appreciable rise in tissue temperature, a pulsed mode with a duty cycle of 20% or less is used.[6]

The primary clinical indications for continuous (thermal) ultrasound are soft tissue shortening due to decreased collagen tissue extensibility in structures within 6 cm of the skin surface or pain attenuation. Via alterations in tertiary molecular bonding, heating collagen increases its extensibility. This property allows therapists to utilize ultrasound in treating structural contributors to chronic pain,[16] such as maladaptive shortening of connective tissue, joint contractures, scar tissue, and tissue adhesions.[6,9]

Pain is commonly treated with ultrasound due to its potential to influence inflammatory conditions, edema, or lack of connective tissue extensibility.[104] Increased nociceptive thresholds may occur with exposure to continuous thermal ultrasound, thus giving the agent the potential to reduce perceived pain by influencing peripheral nociceptive activation and transmission.[6,9,14,22] Hypothesized mechanisms for increased nociceptive threshold include heat activation of large diameter afferent fibers, alteration of nociceptor receptor sensitivity, and counterirritation.[14]

Nonthermal (pulsed) ultrasound has been demonstrated in vitro and in animal models to influence many cellular parameters of tissue healing, including increases in blood flow, intracellular calcium levels, skin and cell membrane permeability, rate of protein synthesis by fibroblasts, NO synthesis in endothelial cells, proteoglycan synthesis by chondrocytes, mast cell degranulation, and release of chemotactic factor and histamine.[6] The majority of human trials exploring these effects have been limited to individuals with a variety of chronic wounds that may not, however, respond to the ultrasonic energy in the same way.[104,107] Due to promising in vitro findings,[108,109] low-intensity pulsed ultrasound, or "LIPUS" (frequency between 1 and 1.5 MHz, duty cycle ≤20% and intensity ranging from 0.03 to 0.8 W/cm²),[109] has been investigated as a potential means to promote tissue healing in humans for conditions ranging from skeletal fractures to tendinopathies.[110] However, in vivo studies[111,112] and systematic review[110] have found insufficient evidence that LIPUS is effective in managing inflammation or facilitating soft tissue healing. Its use for these purposes in clinical practice cannot be recommended at this time.[110] There is, however, a preponderance of evidence substantiating the use of LIPUS for facilitating fracture healing.[9,112–114]

Noncontact low-frequency ultrasound (NCLFUS) employs low-frequency ultrasound energy to deliver a saline mist to dermal wounds.[115] It is used to débride and cleanse tissue covering a wound; remove fibrin, exudates, and bacteria; and increase cell membrane permeability to accelerate chronic wound healing.[9] Reviews of efficacy studies indicate that the use of NCLFUS for promoting dermal wound healing may be considered substantiated based on current "moderate" evidence, with a notable absence of studies reporting no benefit.[9,115,116]

Another application of nonthermal ultrasound is for treating pain and inflammation via phonophoresis to enhance topical agent absorption through the skin.[104] Ultrasound is hypothesized to alter the permeability of the stratum corneum which may facilitate the passage of the medication transdermally into the tissues.[6,117] Steroid preparations such as dexamethasone and hydrocortisone or analgesics such as salicylates and lidocaine are used between the sound head and the skin surface within a coupling medium.[6] Although the purpose of this mode of medication delivery is to facilitate local tissue effects, drugs administered via phonophoresis do enter general circulation and systemic contraindications must be taken into account.[6] Current evidence is quite divided, however, regarding whether delivery of corticosteroids or analgesics via phonophoresis promotes either a decrease in perceived pain or increases skin analgesia,[104] with some studies reporting improvement in pain conditions[118,119] and others showing little or no effect.[120,121]

In controlled human studies, ultrasound has been reported to be an effective clinical tool with substantiated benefits in the management of pain associated with arthritic disorders,[122,123] shoulder pain,[124] adhesive capsulitis,[125] soft tissue lesions,[126] prolapsed intervertebral discs,[127] and back pain.[128] Mixed results have been reported in controlled studies for its effectiveness in the management of carpal tunnel syndrome,[124,129] elbow epicondylitis,[130,131] and shoulder calcific tendonitis.[124,132] Limited evidence suggests positive benefits from ultrasound in treating phantom limb pain,[133] postherpetic neuralgia,[134] and myofascial pain.[135] No significant benefit over controls has been reported in studies reviewed assessing the effectiveness of ultrasound for treating subacromial bursitis,[136] shoulder peritendonitis,[137] postextraction dental pain,[138] and perineal postlabor pain.[139] There is a strong consensus of evidence that ultrasound is not effective in the treatment of postexercise muscle soreness, delayed onset muscle soreness, or ankle sprains.[9,140,141]

The potential influences that therapeutic ultrasound may have on pain mechanisms primarily occur at the tissue level. It is therefore of little potential value for treating central pain states or chronic pain conditions perpetuated by neuroplastic remodeling.[14] Consideration of utilizing this biophysical agent with patients experiencing long-standing pain should be based on individual evidence that the patient's pain generation has a nociceptive component due to an active peripheral lesion or inflammation.[14]

Contraindications include the direction of ultrasonic acoustic energy over reproductive organs; pregnant abdomens; eyes; epiphyseal growth plates in skeletally immature patients; fractures; malignant lesions; hemorrhagic, ischemic, thrombotic, insensate, or infected regions; tuberculosis infection; plastic implants or cemented areas of prosthetic joints; areas exposed to radiotherapy within 6 months; central nervous system tissue; spinal cord region postlaminectomy; and electronic implants and neurostimulators.[6,104,142] Caution should be exercised to use only pulsed low doses over areas of acute inflammatory pathology to avoid increased inflammatory response.[41]

Electrical Current

Electroanalgesia is the use of electrical stimulation for pain modulation.[143] The majority of analgesic biophysical agents have their therapeutic effects at the tissue level or site of the lesion, whereas electroanalgesia is thought to primarily operate by interrupting the neural propagation of pain.[144] The most frequently utilized forms of electroanalgesia in clinical settings are TENS,[144] IFC,[41] and the delivery of analgesic medication to subcutaneous tissue via iontophoresis.[145]

TRANSCUTANEOUS ELECTRICAL NERVE STIMULATION

TENS is an attractive therapeutic option for pain management. It is nonpharmacologic, noninvasive, easy to use, low cost, and presents no side effects.[9,146] It can be delivered in different ways to modulate various types of pain. For example, sensory– or motor-level stimulation is used to modulate peripheral nociceptive or neurogenic pain, whereas noxious-level stimulation may be used if pain is centrally mediated.[6,144]

There are four different modes of TENS currently in clinical use that may produce electroanalgesia: sensory-level stimulation, motor-level stimulation, brief-intense stimulation, and noxious-level stimulation.[6,146] Sensory-level stimulation is used for immediate temporary relief of acute, chronic, or postoperative pain. This type of stimulation, which is also known as high-frequency or "conventional" TENS, delivers high-frequency (80 to 110 Hz), short-duration (50 to 100 microseconds) pulses at an amplitude just below the motor threshold that causes comfortable paresthesia in the area of the electrodes.[146] Conventional TENS affects primarily large diameter Aβ afferent fibers and is thought to work via the "gate control" theory proposed by Melzack and Wall.[9,147,148] As Aβ fibers are stimulated, the patient experiences a reasonably comfortable paresthesia. Constant modulation of the parameters of the electrical stimulus by the TENS unit is essential to minimize habituation to the analgesic effects.[9] This type of TENS is appropriate for use during exercise, work, or functional activities. It should be noted that for a given patient, determination of an optimally effective TENS electrode placement site requires some time and exploration by an experienced therapist.[14]

Motor-level stimulation is used for the management of chronic pain or in instances where longer duration pain relief is desired. This type of TENS, also known as "acupuncture-like," delivers a current intensity sufficient to generate visible muscle contractions using low pulse frequencies (typically 1 to 4 pulses per second) and long pulse durations (~200 microseconds).[146] It is proposed to control pain by stimulating the production and release of endogenous opiates such as enkephalins and endorphins as well as activating μ-opioid receptors.[146,148] Acupuncture-like TENS is usually applied over a trigger point, motor point, or acupuncture point related to the painful region. Another type of stimulus presentation for motor-level TENS is called "burst train." This approach is something of a hybrid combining conventional and acupuncture-like TENS. It delivers a long-duration (~200 microseconds) series of high-frequency (~100 Hz) pulses, at a low pulse rate (1 to 4 pulses per second), using an amplitude sufficient to cause muscle twitches.[146] Due to its reported ability to produce more comfortable muscle contractions, this presentation is preferred by some patients.[146] Motor-level TENS is not recommended for use during activities of daily living or exercise because of interference from muscle twitching.[148]

Brief-intense TENS combines the stimulus parameters that cause both sensory- and motor-level stimulation, which is then delivered at the highest tolerable intensity. It is most often used during painful procedures such as wound débridement, wound dressing changes, joint mobilization, suture removal, or venipuncture.[146,148] Brief-intense TENS is high-frequency (100 to 150 Hz), long-duration (150 to 250 microseconds) pulses at an amplitude that will cause strong paresthesia and a motor response under or between the electrodes, applied over a brief period of time (typically <15 minutes).[146]

Noxious-level stimulation, which is sometimes called "hyperstimulation," is thought to lead to analgesia via activation of the descending pain suppression system mediated by the release of endogenous opiates.[148] This mode of TENS is usually only attempted if other types of stimulation have not been effective. Noxious-level stimulation requires low– or high-frequency, long-duration (250 microseconds to 1 second) pulses at an amplitude that causes a painful sensation that is maintained for 30 to 60 seconds. It is reported to produce a concurrent depolarization of sensory (Aβ), motor (Aα), and nociceptive (Aδ and C) peripheral nerve fibers.[9] This mode is typically applied over acupuncture, motor, or trigger points. It is generally quite uncomfortable, producing both muscle contractions and brief pain just below level of intolerance. It should only be used with patients who are fully aware of, and agreeable to, the expected discomfort.[148]

The primary indication for TENS is attenuation of acute and subacute pain; yet, it has theoretical utility for chronic pain conditions where peripheral nociception is not the primary mechanism of pain generation. TENS has been suggested as a treatment option used to reduce painful input to the spine as early as possible in order to fight central pain generation via dorsal horn remodeling of N-methyl-D-aspartate receptors. It has also been hypothesized to use early sensory-level TENS over long stretches of time to body regions other than the painful locus, thus providing a competing attentional stimulus to decrease the probability of long-term cortical remodeling.[14] As yet, there is no efficacy data available to assess the viability of these hypothesized approaches.

Prolonged usage of either high- or low-frequency TENS has been demonstrated in both animal[149] and human[150] studies to produce tolerance, thereby decreasing analgesic effectiveness. Cross-tolerance may also occur between TENS and opioid use due to adaptive changes at μ-opioid receptors in the spinal cord.[146] There is evidence that low-frequency TENS operates centrally by triggering descending inhibitory pathways from the ventral lateral periaqueductal gray area which then projects to the ventral horn of the spine and activates μ-opioid receptors in the rostral ventral medial medulla,[151] spine,[152] and periphery.[153] Because opioid drugs that activate μ-opioid receptors are commonly used, the tolerance developed by many people taking opioids may render low-frequency TENS ineffective for them.[146] One early study demonstrated that people who had developed presurgical tolerance to opioid use experienced no postsurgical analgesic benefit from TENS.[154]

Significant clinical effectiveness has been reported in controlled human studies for TENS in the management of postoperative abdominal pain,[155] postoperative thoracic pain,[156] osteoarthritis,[157,158] postoperative orthopedic pain,[159] neck pain,[160] trigeminal neuralgia,[161] migraine headache,[162] postamputation and phantom limb pain,[163] dysmenorrheal pain,[164] peripheral neurogenic pain,[165,166] and shoulder pain secondary to stroke.[167] There is less consistency in the clinical efficacy literature for the use of TENS to help manage low back pain,[168–170] labor and postlabor pain,[171,172] myofascial pain,[173,174] and pain associated with rheumatoid arthritis.[175,176]

Over-the-counter FDA-approved TENS units are now available and have become widely popular for independent home use. Costs range from around $25 for self-contained patch units for specific regional analgesia (e.g., shoulder or low back pain) to over $200 for higher quality, feature-loaded devices (e.g., multichannel, electromassage). Although TENS units are generally quite safe, it should be emphasized that proper usage and electrode placement are essential elements of effectiveness. It is highly recommended that potential users of these home electrotherapy devices schedule a session with experienced physical therapist to go over proper use, discuss tolerance issues, and determine hands-on the optimal electrode placement for the individual.

INTERFERENTIAL CURRENT

IFC was developed in the 1950s by Hans Nemec[177] and first appeared in American clinics in the 1980s.[41,143] It is one of the most commonly used electroanalgesic modalities in rehabilitation clinics.[146] Its potential clinical advantages over other forms of electroanalgesia is theorized to be its ability to deliver therapeutic electrical stimulation to deeper tissue areas and with greater comfort for patients. To accomplish this, IFC utilizes two intersecting kilohertz-frequency AC carrier currents (~2,000 to 5,000 Hz) typically delivered via a cross-quadripolar placement of four electrodes.[144] Skin resistance to these middle-frequency currents is much lower than for the range of frequencies utilized in conventional TENS units. Skin impedance to a 4,000-Hz current has been measured at ~40 Ω, compared to ~3,200 Ω for a 50-Hz current.[178] This decreased skin resistance allows a middle-frequency current to be delivered deeper into the tissue while using significantly reduced required current amplitude at the skin surface and, therefore, keeping the current amplitude at a very comfortable level for the patient.[6,41]

Fundamental to IFC is that the two intersecting carrier currents differ in frequency by up to 250 Hz. As the currents intersect within the body tissue, there are moments when they are out of phase and cancel each other out (destructive interference) and other moments when they are in phase (constructive interference).[41] This results in a deep wave whose frequency is the difference between frequencies of the two carrier currents, termed the *beat frequency* (typically 20 to 250 Hz). Given the heterogeneity of body tissue conductance, the precise location of the beat current varies yet is usually strongest beneath the electrodes.[41] Most instrument configurations fix the carrier frequency of one channel and allow a frequency "sweep" of the second channel to both limit habituation effects and allow the beat current to migrate to different locations between the electrodes, thus expanding the field of analgesia.[179]

The precise mechanisms for electroanalgesic effects of IFC are speculative at this time and have not been experimentally confirmed.[180] The most often cited mechanism is large-fiber pain inhibition via the gate theory of pain.[146,147] Other hypotheses include increased blood flow, physiologic blockade of neural conduction, activation of descending analgesic pathways, and placebo effects.[146,180] It appears unlikely that IFC produces any physiologic effects that are different from TENS units.[180] However, due to its potential ability to cover larger and deeper fields, IFC may be indicated for deep diffuse pain, whereas TENS may be more appropriate for more superficial, focal areas of pain.[178] It is frequently reported that analgesic effects of IFC are of short duration and are usually limited to when IFC is actually being applied (typically in 10- to 20-minute sessions).[178]

IFC is one of the most commonly used electroanalgesic modalities used in rehabilitation clinics[143] and is utilized clinically for a wide range of disorders.[144] Earlier literature has been inconclusive regarding IFC efficacy for pain modulation, with studies reporting conflicting findings.[14] However, over the past decade, a number of randomized controlled investigations are beginning to show some consistent effects for a limited number of conditions. Controlled studies assessing the ability of IFC to modulate induced pain in healthy subjects have reported decreased pain sensitivity to muscle pressure[181] and increased pain thresholds to mechanical pressure in skeletal muscles following induction of delayed onset muscle soreness.[182] In randomized, placebo-controlled trials investigating the treatment of pain associated with knee osteoarthritis, IFC was found to be effective over controls[183] and as effective as TENS and short-wave diathermy[184] in studies involving 203 and 30 participants, respectively. IFC was also reported to be effective for knee osteoarthritis over sham IFC for improving stationary pain, pain with movement, perceived disability measures, and walking velocity.[185] Investigating responses from a combined total of 300 participants, similar randomized, controlled findings are in evidence for treating chronic low back pain, with IFC providing a significant level of measured pain relief, over placebo, roughly equal to that of TENS[186] and decreased pain medication utilization.[187] In a controlled study of 63 patients with carpal tunnel syndrome, both IFC and TENS improved visual analog pain ratings, electrodiagnostically assessed median nerve distal latencies and sensory nerve conduction velocities compared to splinting therapy, and compared to TENS, IFC showed increases in functional capacity and decreased perceived symptom severity.[188] IFC has been demonstrated in a study of 30 hemiplegic patients to provide decreased pain intensity during movement of the hemiplegic shoulder and increased pain-free range of motion compared to placebo.[189] It should be noted that due to the temporary nature of IFC effects, studies are typically assessing and reporting episodic or short-term attenuation of pain,

with one low back pain study finding IFC pain reduction effectiveness occurring only during the first treatment session.[187] Beyond temporary palliative relieve, IFC's long-term efficacy or ongoing utility for chronic pain syndromes appears to be an open question.

IONTOPHORESIS

Electrical currents can also be utilized to resolve inflammation, enhance healing, and facilitate delivery of topical medication transdermally.[6,145] As early as 1741, Pivati hypothesized that an electromotive force could be used to deliver medications through the skin.[190] The validity of this idea was first demonstrated with animals by Leduc in 1900.[190,191] Iontophoresis is the utilization of direct current to facilitate transdermal delivery to target tissues of local ionizable anesthetics and anti-inflammatories.[143,145] It allows local medication delivery without the use of a needle. Ionic medications carrying a positive electrical charge are drawn to cathode electrodes and repelled by anode electrodes, whereas negatively charged medication compounds display the reverse behavior.[148] Iontophoresis was originally thought to drive the ions through the skin and into deeper tissues via electromigration.[143] Recent work suggests that iontophoresis may promote transdermal penetration through electroporation, by increasing the permeability of the stratum corneum, similar to phonophoresis.[6,143] Although iontophoresis has been demonstrated to effectively deliver select medications to target tissues,[192,193] the actual depth of penetration of drug delivery is uncertain. Several studies have found diffusion of various drugs at tissue depths ranging from 3 to 20 mm.[6]

For managing pain conditions via iontophoresis, several ionic compounds are in use. Negatively charged medications include dexamethasone (4 mg/mL in aqueous solution) for inflammation and salicylates (2% to 3% sodium salicylate solution or 10% trolamine salicylate ointment) for analgesia, inflammation, and chronic muscle and joint pain.[143,145] Positively charged medications include hydrocortisone (1% ointment or solution) for inflammation, lidocaine (4% to 5% ointment or solution) for soft tissue pain and inflammation, and magnesium sulfate (2% ointment or solution) for skeletal muscle spasms.[145] Physical therapy clinics are typically equipped to administer medication via iontophoresis. However, the patient must bring the ionic medication preparation prescribed by the referring physician to the clinic.[14]

The most salient precaution regarding the use of iontophoresis is based on the fact that it utilizes direct current.[143] Sustained application of DC iontophoresis will result in a hydrogen ion concentration beneath the anode and hydroxyl ions beneath the cathode.[145] When used to excess, the accumulated pH changes may result in electrochemical acid or base burns to the skin.[143] These subdermal pH changes also have the potential to affect drug ionization and stability.[14] There exist iontophoresis delivery units that utilize alternating current with a "DC offset" to potentially ameliorate this concern; however, efficacy evidence for this approach is lacking.[143]

A relatively recent advance is the availability of small, wireless battery-operated iontophoresis devices, or "iontophoresors."[9] These may be worn at home by the patient and reduce the need to be present in the clinic in order to utilize this transdermal form of medication delivery. These compact single-adhesive patch devices deliver DC from a button size 0.1 to 4 mA battery via a microcircuit integrated to anode and cathode electrodes with imbedded ionized medication in a saline suspension. The very low amplitude current can deliver medication for periods up to 24 hours.[143]

Although there are few controlled studies in the literature addressing the use of iontophoresis for managing chronic pain, there are reports of significant clinical effectiveness in treating arthritic disorders with dexamethasone[194] and salicylate.[195]

There are individual clinical studies reporting success with dexamethasone delivered using this method in treating post-herpetic neuralgia,[192] epicondylitis,[196] plantar fasciitis,[193] carpal tunnel syndrome,[197] and Achilles tendonitis.[198]

Contraindications to the use of electroanalgesia include its use in individuals with a known cardiac arrhythmia; over the anterior cervical region or carotid sinuses; over a gravid uterus; over infected areas or sites of active bleeding; in the presence of an implanted defibrillator, demand-inhibited cardiac pacemaker, or any other implanted electrical device; and for individuals with venous or arterial thrombosis or thrombophlebitis.[6,41] The use of iontophoresis is contraindicated for patients with sensitivity to ionic medications and over open skin lesions.[9,145]

Precautions should be exercised when using electrical stimulation in the presence of skin irritation or open wounds, malignancies, osteoporosis (with motor-level TENS), or cardiomyopathies; with transthoracic electrode placement (potential for inducing cardiac arrhythmias); over areas of heavy scarring; over tissues susceptible to hemorrhage or hematoma; on patients with movement control disorders or impaired cognition; on areas of anesthetic skin; over superficial metal implants; on craniofacial regions for patients with a history of stroke or seizures; and on patients who are driving or operating heavy machinery.[6,41,42] Limited duration drops in arterial blood pressure have been reported during stimulation to the pelvic floor.[41] With the use of adhesive electrodes, precautions should be taken to prevent skin damage due to adhesive irritants and pH changes under electrodes when using direct current for iontophoresis or for prolonged applications such as TENS.[6,14]

Somatosensory Desensitization

Somatosensory desensitization, utilized extensively by physical therapists and occupational therapists, is considered a requisite component of standard care in the treatment of complex regional pain syndrome (CRPS) and phantom limb pain.[199–201] Desensitization therapy involves exposing a patient's painful skin region to direct physical contact with a progression of materials that have the potential to trigger somatosensory irritation.[14,202] This intervention belongs to a family of treatment approaches for chronic neuropathic pain that paradoxically involve patient exposure to increases in pain that may be linked to physical restoration and functional activity.[203] Other approaches in this category include "pain exposure physical therapy" (PEPT) and "graded exposure" (GEXP), which are showing promise in pain reduction via functional restoration involving carefully dosed exposure to progressive-loading exercise programs coupled with management of pain-avoidance behavior.[203] These strategies are based on the idea that behavioral avoidance of mobility, tactile contact, and functional activity may in some cases maintain the pain condition.[203,204] Therapeutically managed graded pain exposure may help "reduce peripheral and central sensitization and may restore the local autonomic regulation and cortical representation."[203]

The indication for this therapeutic tool is treatment of allodynia associated with chronic pain conditions such as CRPS.[3,200,202] Allodynia is a painful response to nonnoxious somatosensory stimulation.[204,205] One of the hallmarks of CRPS, allodynia is not the same phenomenon as the normal hyperalgesia that follows tissue damage.[204,205] Patients experiencing allodynia may avoid the most seemingly innocuous tactile contact, sometimes refraining from wearing even delicate clothing over the affected area.[10] Allodynia treatment via desensitization aims to attenuate this abnormal somatosensory response and help the patient return the affected area (typically a limb) to normal somatosensory exposure and functional usage.[3,200,202,206] Somatosensory desensitization is also used in the treatment and prevention of postamputation phantom limb pain.[202,206,207]

Traditional somatosensory desensitization protocols involve having the patient lightly rub the painful skin field with a progressive series of coarse or irritating materials.[200,202,208] Early desensitization therapy for CRPS used the chemical irritant capsaicin as the desensitizing agent.[209] In current practice, materials may progress from soft fabrics to items such as small pebbles or dry pasta.[10] Twice daily, the patient rubs the material over the affected area for approximately 3 minutes, then rests for 2 to 3 minutes, and finally rubs again for 3 more minutes.[10,14] Each week, the patient advances to a coarser or potentially more irritating material. Treatment course may span 2 to 4 months and includes home application and in-clinic checks at least weekly.[14,208] Somatosensory desensitization is contraindicated over an active lesion that may be harmed by contact with physically irritating materials or mechanical pressure.[14]

Attenuation of allodynia via desensitization may be due to multifaceted mechanisms. These have been hypothesized to involve somatosensory habituation,[210] reintroduction of large fiber diameter afferent pain inhibition,[14] altered central processing of somatosensory input either at the dorsal horn or parietal lobe,[211] prevention of the development of new permanent neuroplastic pain pathways in the neuromatrix,[206,212] normalization of exposure to the distal environment,[201,206] and management of pain avoidance behavior.[3] During the course of desensitization, the patient is encouraged to begin reintroduction of the limb or body area into normalized functional usage. With direction from the therapist, this reintroduced usage may facilitate a positive spiral of ascending exogenous analgesia and activity. Normal activities of daily living then become a continuation of the desensitization therapy and its ongoing effectiveness.[10,14]

Many patients who have undergone successful desensitization to light touch or who never manifested light touch allodynia may still find nonnoxious levels of pressure, vibration, or thermal variation to be painfully intolerable.[10,208,213] Desensitization therapy may therefore be specific to a given somatosensory modality.[214] Therapeutic desensitizing agents must be matched to the type of somatosensory stimulation triggering the allodynia.[208,213]

Studies have reported success in managing tactile,[10,215–217] thermal,[213] vibratory,[218] and pressure-related allodynia.[208] A 2016 systematic review investigated the current state of evidence on somatosensory desensitization, representing 10 studies and a combined total of 68 patients.[200] This review reported that conclusive efficacy evaluation is limited due to small sample sizes, frequent lack of controls, and inconsistency in desensitization protocols across investigations and that many studies combined desensitization therapy with multimodal treatments.[200] Although currently available research is limited, the consistency of positive results supports the utilization of desensitization in the treatment of people with CRPS while stronger efficacy evidence is sought.[200]

In addition to attenuating allodynia, case study findings report the total body area of reported pain distribution decreasing. or retreating, as a function of desensitization,[219] as quantified using a pain distribution scale.[220] It is also meaningful to note that a study on the effects of pressure desensitization found that increased usage of analgesic medication during the desensitization trial did not appear to diminish the effectiveness of treatment.[208] Significant reductions in subsequent pain medication usage and pain intensity, combined with improved functional usage, suggested that use of analgesics to tolerate the desensitization therapy may not interfere with the treatment's effectiveness.[208]

Desensitization of painful regions may additionally impact somatosensation in proximal limb areas unaffected by pain.[219] There is emerging evidence that as a result of chronic pain in distal limb segments, proximal limb regions may develop diminished somatosensory thresholds and acuity.[10,219]

This is plausible if remodeling of the somatosensory cortex has resulted in increased representation of painful regions at the expense of diminished cortical representation of proximal non-painful areas of the limb.[212,221] A 2017 study of somatosensation in nonpainful limb regions of CRPS patients found notable improvements (toward normalization) in both somatosensory acuity and perceptual thresholds in proximal limb areas that paralleled distal pain reduction over the course of desensitization treatment.[219] These findings suggest expanding the scope of what may be considered affected body regions in patients with chronic pain to include not only painful sites but also adjacent nonpainful areas that are manifesting decreased somatosensation as a result of the ongoing focus on the painful areas and likely cortical remodeling. Potential impact may include previously unrecognized proprioceptive attenuation, limb placement impairments, and reduced functional limb usage.

Emerging Interventions

MANUAL LYMPHATIC DRAINAGE

There is growing clinical interest in the application of lymphedema reduction techniques for the management of both sub-acute and chronic pain conditions.[222] Referred to as *complete decongestive therapy* (CDT), these techniques have been utilized to manage edema and related pain resulting from primary lymphedema conditions such as Milroy disease, Park-Weber syndrome, and Klippel-Trenaunay syndrome, or secondary lymphedema resulting from causes such as surgery, trauma, radiation, obesity, or infection.[223,224] CDT involves a systematic approach utilizing manual lymphatic drainage (MLD), short stretch compression bandaging, decongestive exercise prescription, compression garments, and patient education.[223,224]

Early resolution of edema and prevention of fibrosis development can be an important factor in recovery and pain management for subacute conditions.[16] It may also be a useful element for addressing pathophysiologic deactivation mechanisms integral to the development of chronic pain states such as CRPS.[16,18] A key feature of this sequela is that disuse of distal skeletal musculature leads to venous stasis, followed by edema, decreased arterial perfusion, the establishment of an anaerobic environment, local acidosis, and finally fibrotic tissue changes.[16] It has been hypothesized that introduction of CDT early in this process, to break the cycle of chronic lymphostasis, may be beneficial in treating CRPS, or in some cases perhaps interrupting its development.[225]

Studies assessing the efficacy of CDT for treating CRPS are limited at this time. An initial prospective, randomized investigation compared 35 outpatients experiencing CRPS type I of less than 6 months standing who received either physical therapy with MLD or physical therapy exercises alone.[225] The symptoms of patients with high pain levels in the lymphatic drainage group were reported to show improvement.[225] A randomized trial involving 34 patients with CRPS demonstrated statistically significant short-term reductions in edema after MLD treatment.[226] The long-term efficacy of this treatment approach for CRPS has not yet been established.

Protocols described in efficacy studies and structured interviews conducted with certified lymphedema therapists experienced with the utilization of CDT for patients with CRPS have yielded implementation recommendations. As a general rule, decongestive therapies for CRPS may be most beneficial in the early stages before fibrosis has developed (<12 months following acute injury). In the presence of allodynia, a course of somatosensory desensitization should precede usage of CDT elements. Compression bandaging and/or garments should be the last treatment element introduced.[225,226]

General contraindications for lymphedema therapy include history of peripheral vascular disease, chronic venous insufficiency, thrombosis or other venous blockage, ongoing thrombophlebitis, hemorrhage, acute enuresis, malignant tumors, renal insufficiency/failure, and congestive heart failure.[223,224]

CUPPING

Cupping is an ancient technique whose therapeutic application has been traced as far back as the Egyptian "Ebers Papyrus" (circa 1500 BC) and has a history of reported usage in Chinese medicine extending at least 2,000 years.[227,228] Traditionally, it involved heating small cups of glass, earthenware, or bamboo that were then placed on the skin where the cooling of air within the "cups" created a partial vacuum, thus drawing the skin deeply into the cups while rupturing small blood vessels and creating a local area of ecchymosis.[227,228] Current techniques involve either traditional heat or a vacuum apparatus using unheated glass or compressible silicone cups to create the partial vacuum.[228] Western applications frequently refer to cupping as "myofascial decompression."[229]

Cupping is widely performed by current practitioners of traditional Chinese medicine and across the world, particularly in eastern Asia and the Middle East.[230,231] Interest in the technique is growing in Western countries[230] and physical therapy clinics, in part highlighted by the number of athletes appearing at the 2016 Summer Olympics in Rio de Janeiro conspicuously displaying numerous circular skin welts derived from the use of cupping purported to aid in muscle recovery following intense training. It has been applied as a treatment modality for a broad spectrum of conditions such as facial paralysis, respiratory disorders, postexercise muscular soreness, herpes zoster, and cervical spondylosis and diverse pain conditions ranging from carpal tunnel syndrome and nonspecific low back pain to fibromyalgia syndrome.[227] One factor in its growing popularity as a potential therapeutic adjunct to pain management may be due to the fact that patient surveys have consistently cited pain as the most common reason for people seeking therapeutic alternatives to conventional medicine.[232]

Fundamentally, cupping is performed using one of two methods, either "dry" or "wet." Dry cupping simply draws a small skin field into the cup via the partial vacuum. In traditional Chinese medicine, cups are applied over acupuncture points.[228] Cups are left in place for varying amounts of time anywhere from less than 3 to as long as 15 minutes.[233] Other procedural variations may be used depending on the desired therapeutic effect, such as pulsating (or "pneumatic pulsation therapy"),[234] "quick," "shaking," and "balanced" cupping.[233] A dry form of "moving cupping" involves sliding the cups along a skin surface that has been lubricated with massage oil.[228] This method has been explored for use in mobilizing subcutaneous connective tissue to break down adhesions or scar tissue and possibly facilitate myofascial release. Theoretically, cupping may be advantageous in this regard because other methods of mobilizing or releasing underlying connective tissue (e.g., deep tissue massage or Graston Technique) involve compressing tissue, whereas cupping acts to pull and separate tissue. Although there is a recent proliferation of instructional resources on how to use cupping for "myofascial decompression," to date, there is not adequate published research demonstrating whether cupping can mechanically generate specific force necessary to address adhered tissue below the skin surface or clinical evidence establishing its effectiveness for this purpose.

Wet cupping, which is widely used in eastern Asia and the Middle East,[230,235] involves first making skin incisions beneath where the cups will be placed so that the technique may withdraw blood and, in theory, extract "harmful substances."[228] There does not appear to be a research foundation at this time establishing specifically what harmful substances are extracted and whether the quantities withdrawn are sufficient to produce therapeutic benefit. Due to its invasive nature, wet cupping is not within the licensure parameters or practice domain of most physical therapists, unless they have additional training and certification.

The mechanisms of action for therapeutic benefits associated with cupping are unclear,[228,229] with those currently offered in the literature being primarily untested speculative hypotheses or vague generalizations.[236] It is often stated that the basis of cupping is to "regulate and promote movement of qi and blood."[228,235] The assertion is that, "by doing so, cupping is able to alleviate pain, caused by blood stasis and qi blockage. Cupping may also accelerate microcirculation and relieve muscular spasm."[228] No physiologic evidence has been cited for these mechanisms.[228,231] Physiologically, cupping is creating a skin region of negative pressure resulting in rupture of superficial capillaries and a defined area of ecchymosis. Without supporting evidence, this effect has been cited as increasing blood circulation,[228,235] modulating lymph flow,[236] and reducing blood stasis.[235] It is also thought to provide stretch to nerve and muscle,[237] thought to remove waste products (e.g., lactate) from the body via wet cupping,[235] and theorized to release "a chemical transmitter that can block pain, such as serotonin, endorphin, and cortisol."[237] Alteration of local metabolism as a result of cupping was assessed in a study of six healthy individuals and six with chronic neck pain, which found slight increases in pain threshold immediately postcupping and creation of a local anaerobic state evidenced by increased lactate and lactate/pyruvate ratio occurring between 160 and 280 minutes following the procedure, with no signs of a change in pain thresholds during this anaerobic period.[229] Suggested perceptual mechanisms for potential analgesic effects from cupping have included a counterirritant effect to increase pain thresholds and stimulate inhibitory nociceptive pathways,[236] triggering of "diffuse noxious inhibitory control" (DNIC),[235] tactile stimulation from the procedure producing an analgesic effect via the gate theory,[235] and the influence of a powerful placebo effect.[236–238]

Because of expanding interest in cupping as a therapeutic option for pain management, a thoughtful assessment of research into its potential efficacy and knowledge of verified plausible mechanisms of action are warranted prior to clinical implementation. To date, there have been a notable number of randomized controlled studies (RCTs) and at least six systematic reviews published related to the efficacy of cupping for treating a very wide variety of disorders, including both acute and chronic pain conditions. The majority of research has addressed wet cupping. However, due to generally low methodologic quality of studies, there exists broad consensus among both investigators and reviewers that evidence for cupping is inconclusive at this time.[227,228,230,231,233,236,238,239]

Cao et al.[227] published a 2012 review of 135 RCTs addressing cupping efficacy (132 appearing in Chinese). "Meta-analysis showed cupping therapy combined with other traditional Chinese medicine treatments was significantly superior to other treatments alone in increasing the number of 'cured' patients with herpes zoster, facial paralysis, acne, and cervical spondylosis."[227] The reviewers discussed a "lack of well-designed investigations." This was due in part to the finding that according to application of the Cochrane risk of bias tool,[240] none of the 135 trials reviewed were "low risk of bias" and "nearly all" determined to be "high risk of bias."[227] This review was updated in 2014 with 16 additional studies involving 921 total participants.[228] All trials were assessed via Cochrane criteria[240] as "low risk of bias," and addressed nonspecific low back pain, chronic neck pain herpes zoster, osteoarthritis, shoulder pain, shoulder–hand syndrome, scapulohumeral periarthritis, carpal tunnel syndrome, acute ankle sprain, and headache. The review concluded that cupping therapy may reduce pain intensity in chronic or acute pain.[228] Based on systematic review of 14 RCTs, Al Bedah et al.[230] reported in 2016 that there

exists "promising evidence in favor of the use of wet cupping for musculoskeletal pain, specifically neck pain, carpal tunnel syndrome, nonspecific low back pain, and brachialgia." In an overview of five earlier systematic reviews, Lee et al.[239] concluded that "cupping is only effective as a treatment for pain, and even for this indication doubts remain." In addition to those cited in systematic reviews, trials suggesting positive responses to cupping therapy impacting measures such as decreased subjective pain intensity ratings, pain-related function, pain medication usage, and improved quality of life have been reported for chronic tension and migraine headaches,[241] carpal tunnel syndrome,[236] osteoarthritis of the knee,[242] chronic neck pain,[234,243] and nonspecific low back pain.[233,235]

Available studies have yielded "suggestive evidence for the effectiveness of cupping in the management of pain conditions."[231] However, the consistent view in current literature is that the limited quality of studies does not yet provide convincing evidence that the effects of cupping on pain is sufficient to draw firm conclusions.[233,235] Due to methodologic quality, most cupping studies have been published in low-impact journals.[230] The quality of available studies is primarily limited by inadequate placebo controls and resultant lack of blinding.[228,231] For this type of treatment, it is difficult to implement an effective placebo in that participants can readily tell the difference between actual cupping and sham procedures.[236] One of the few attempts to provide a placebo control was in a recent study of patients with fibromyalgia syndrome, where patients were told they would receive either "traditional cupping" or "modern gentle cupping."[238] The "modern gentle cupping" control utilized silicone cups with small holes that would very quickly release the negative pressure inside the cup. The authors reported "effects of cupping therapy were small and comparable to those of a sham treatment, and as such cupping cannot be recommended for fibromyalgia at the current time."[238]

The vast majority of published trials, including all of the 135 studies cited in Cao et al.'s[227] 2012 systematic review, report patients experiencing no serious adverse effects from cupping.[227,234–236] Resulting ecchymosis is considered a natural response to the procedure and is reported to typically resolve in 2 to 5 days or may persist up to 2 weeks.[228] Potential adverse effects may include burns (with heated cups), mildly increased pain,[238] skin infections (with wet cupping), or fainting (three cases reported).[231]

Cupping is contraindicated for patients with congestive heart failure, renal failure, systemic inflammatory conditions (e.g., rheumatoid arthritis), hemophilia or other blood coagulation disorders, or those taking anticoagulant medication; over the eyes; over skin areas with burns, open wounds, active inflammation, infections; or with underlying severe edema, neural tissue sensitivity, large or varicose veins, hernia, or severe edema.

MIRROR THERAPY AND GRADED MOTOR IMAGERY

Treatment modalities utilized by physical therapists to address chronic pain conditions have broadened in scope to include interventions that target cortical reorganization.[5,9,15] It is recognized that in the development of chronic pain, there is a progression from nociception of distal tissue damage to a dominance of maladaptive neuroplastic remodeling[17,244] of the spine's dorsal horn and the body representation of both somatosensory[245] and motor[246,247] cortical areas. Physical agents that influence pain mechanisms associated with distal tissue damage may be of limited effectiveness, or inappropriate, for treating chronic pain states where the central nervous system is playing the primary role in the generation and/or perpetuation of pain.[14,15] An emerging treatment approach for cortical remodeling is "mirror therapy," sometimes used in conjunction with graded motor imagery.[11,12]

Mirror therapy was first introduced in 1996 by Ramachandran and Rogers-Ramachandran,[248] who hypothesized that individuals with phantom limb pain had a visual–proprioceptive dissociation in the brain. They found that patients experienced a reduction in symptoms by simply viewing a mirrored reflection of their intact limb.[248] This approach has since been utilized for patients with cancer, stroke, focal dystonia, and chronic neuropathic pain conditions such as CRPS types I and II.[12]

The technique of mirror therapy involves positioning a mirror on a midsagittal line in front of a patient so that the painful, or amputated, limb is blocked from view. In place of the distal painful limb, what the patient sees is a reflection of the intact nonpainful limb.[11] The simple technique creates a vivid visual illusion for the patient, such that somatosensory stimulation or movements and functional activities of the nonpainful limb appear as though they are being conducted with the affected limb.[249] This perceptual slight-of-hand provides a visual and somatosensory message to the neuromatrix that the involved limb can be perceived, is performing movement, and engaged in activity without triggering pain, thereby theoretically contributing to cortical reorganization in opposition to the maladaptive remodeling that is perpetuating the pain experience.[249,250] Detailed guidelines for the clinical implementation of mirror therapy with phantom limb pain, based on extensive evidence review, have recently been published by Rothgangel et al.[11]

Mirror therapy is frequently implemented by first taking the patient through preparatory laterality recognition training and then graded motor imagery practice prior to utilization of mirrors.[12,251] It has been suggested that until patients experiencing chronic pain can establish "an accurate cortical representation of their body," they should not proceed with graded motor imagery or mirror therapy.[251] This is theoretically due to a common "neglect-like" response,[3] whereby the patient cognitively walls off the involved limb to help affectively cope with the pain, resulting in a distorted body image evidenced by an impaired ability to distinguish left from right.[251] Clinical studies report enhanced efficacy findings when mirror exercises are prefaced by laterality training and graded motor imagery practice.[252–254]

Case reports and small uncontrolled studies have reported reductions in the intensity, or resolution, of phantom limb pain, sometimes after as little as 3 weeks of therapy.[255,256] Randomized controlled trials investigating the impact of mirror therapy on phantom limb pain have reported significant reductions in phantom pain,[250,257] attenuation of phantom pain that was not significantly different from the use of TENS,[258] and no significant reduction in phantom pain or phantom sensations, yet increased conscious awareness of the phantom limb.[249] Three single-blind randomized controlled trials using mirror therapy combined with laterality training and graded motor imagery found that at 6 weeks, patients with upper limb CRPS type I reported significant decreases in pain,[252–254] swelling,[252] and disability.[253] One of these studies reported significantly decreased pain associated with increased function at 6 weeks and at 6-month follow-up.[254]

Perceiving the illusion of two intact limbs has been reported to trigger emotional reactions in some patients.[259,260] In at least one study, patients experienced significantly increased cognitive focus on the painful limb.[249] Additional reported reactions that reported when viewing the mirror-image limb have included nausea, dizziness, and sweating.[11] Those reactions may be addressed via graded exposure to the treatment.[11]

Either with or without laterality training and graded motor imagery, mirror therapy is a simple, safe, noninvasive, and cost-effective intervention whose efficacy in the long-term management of chronic neuropathic pain has yet to be fully explored.[11]

Conclusion

There is a broad spectrum of therapeutic biophysical agents available to aid in the management of both acute and chronic pain conditions. Determination of the suitability of biophysical agents and selection of the appropriate modality should be made with careful consideration of the mechanism of pain generation for the individual patient and pursued with careful treatment response monitoring.[14] It should be reemphasized that although the use of biophysical agents for treating pain is common in physical therapy settings, their use should be viewed as adjunctive.[5,19] Effective pain management involves not only the attenuation of pain perception but also restoration of compromised or lost function. Appropriate, comprehensive treatment integrates the application of biophysical agents with other indicated therapeutic activities and patient education to address the mechanisms of pain generation and perception while facilitating functional restoration.

References

1. Powers A, Brown LM, Allen RJ. Effectiveness of therapies emphasizing movement in the treatment of complex regional pain syndrome type I: a systematic review. *J Ortho Sport Phys Ther* 2014;44(1):A155.
2. Loeser JD. Multidisciplinary pain programs. In: Loeser JD, ed. *Bonica's Management of Pain*. 3rd ed. Baltimore, MD: Lippincott Williams & Wilkins; 2001:255–264.
3. Galer BS, Schwartz L, Allen RJ. The complex regional pain syndromes: type I: reflex sympathetic dystrophy and type II: causalgia. In: Loeser JD, ed. *Bonica's Management of Pain*. 3rd ed. Baltimore, MD: Lippincott Williams & Wilkins; 2001:388–411.
4. Strong J, Unrugh AM, Wright A, et al, eds. *Pain: A Textbook for Therapists*. Edinburgh: Churchill Livingstone; 2002.
5. Bellew JW. Therapeutic modalities past, present, and future: their role in the patient care management model. In: Bellew JW, Michlovitz SL, Nolan TP, eds. *Michlovitz's Modalities for Therapeutic Intervention*. 6th ed. Philadelphia: FA Davis; 2016:3–18.
6. Cameron MH. *Physical Agents in Rehabilitation: From Research to Practice*. 4th ed. Philadelphia: WB Saunders; 2013.
7. Commission on Accreditation in Physical Therapy Education. Evaluative criteria: PT programs accreditation handbook. Available at: http://www.capteonline.org/AccreditationHandbook/. Accessed April 6, 2017.
8. American Physical Therapy Association. Minimum required skills of physical therapist graduates at entry-level. Available at: http://www.apta.org/uploadedFiles/APTAorg/About_Us/Policies/Education/MinimumRequiredSkillsPTGrads. Accessed April 6, 2017.
9. Belanger AY. *Therapeutic Electrophysical Agents*. 3rd ed. Baltimore, MD: Lippincott Williams & Wilkins; 2015.
10. Allen RJ, Hulten JM. Effects of tactile desensitization on allodynia and somatosensation in a patient with quadrilateral complex regional pain syndrome. *Neuro Rep* 2001;25(4):132–133.
11. Rothgangel A, Braun S, de Witte L, et al. Development of a clinical framework for mirror therapy in patients with phantom limb pain: an evidence-based practice approach. *Pain Pract* 2016;16:422–434.
12. Pelton RD, Williams EE, Allen RJ. Effectiveness of mirror therapy to alleviate symptoms of unilateral neuropathic pain: a systematic review. *J Ortho Sport Phys Ther* 2014;44:A157–A158.
13. Flor H, Nikolajsen L, Jensen T. Phantom limb pain: a case of maladaptive CNS plasticity? *Nat Rev Neurosci* 2006;7:873–881.
14. Allen RJ. Physical agents used in the management of chronic pain by physical therapists. *Phys Med Rehabil Clin N Am* 2006;17:315–345.
15. Pollard C. Physiotherapy management of complex regional pain syndrome. *N Zealand J Physiother* 2013;41:65–72.
16. Allen RJ, Koshi LR. Post-traumatic development of chronic limb pain secondary to excessively restricted activity: a deactivation pain model. *Eur J Pain* 2009;13:S124.
17. Chandler EH, Bonica JJ. Supraspinal mechanisms of pain & nociception. In: Loeser JD, ed. *Bonica's Management of Pain*. 3rd ed. Baltimore, MD: Lippincott Williams & Wilkins; 2001:153–179.
18. Butler SH, Nyman M, Gordh T. Immobility in volunteers transiently produces signs and symptoms of complex regional pain syndrome. In: Devor M, Rowbotham MC, Wiesenfeld-Hallin Z, eds. *Proceedings of the 9th World Congress on Pain. Progress in Pain Research and Management*. Vol 16. Seattle, WA: IASP Press; 2000:657–660.
19. American Physical Therapy Association. *Guide to Physical Therapy Practice*. Fairfax, VA: American Physical Therapy Association; 2001.
20. Rennie S, Michlovitz SL. Therapeutic heat. In: Bellew JW, Michlovitz SL, Nolan TP, eds. *Michlovitz's Modalities for Therapeutic Intervention*. 6th ed. Philadelphia: FA Davis; 2016:61–88.

21. Chipchase LS, Williams MT, Roberson VJ. A national study of the availability and use of electrophysical agents by Australian physiotherapists. *Physiother Theory Pract* 2009;25:279–296.

22. Lehmann JF, DeLateur BJ. Therapeutic heat. In: Lehmann JF, ed. *Therapeutic Heat and Cold*. Baltimore, MD: Williams & Wilkins; 1990:429–432.

23. Newton RA. Contemporary views on pain and the role played by thermal agents in managing pain symptoms. In: Michlovitz SL, ed. *Thermal Agents in Rehabilitation*. Philadelphia: FA Davis; 1990:18–42.

24. Nadler SF, Weingand K, Druse RJ. The physiologic basis and clinical application of cryotherapy and thermotherapy for the pain practitioner. *Pain Physician* 2004;7:395–399.

25. Davis KD, Kwan CL, Crawley AP, et al. Functional MRI study of thalamic and cortical activations evoked by cutaneous heat, cold, and tactile stimuli. *J Neurophysiol* 1998;80:1533–1546.

26. Benson TB, Copp EP. The effects of therapeutic forms of heat and ice on the pain threshold of the normal shoulder. *Rheumatol Rehabil* 1974;13:101–104.

27. Kramer JF. Ultrasound: evaluation of its mechanical and thermal effects. *Arch Phys Med Rehabil* 1984;65:223–227.

28. Ayling J, Marks R. Efficacy of paraffin wax baths for rheumatoid arthritic hands. *Physiotherapy* 2000;86:190–201.

29. Mainardi CL, Walter JM, Spiegel PK, et al. Rheumatoid arthritis: failure of daily heat therapy to affect its progression. *Arch Phys Med Rehab* 1979;60:390–393.

30. Sukenik S, Buskila D, Neumann L, et al. Mud pack therapy in rheumatoid arthritis. *Clin Rheumatol* 1992;11:243–247.

31. Sukenik S, Buskila D, Neumann L, et al. Sulfur bath and mud pack treatment for rheumatoid arthritis in the Dead Sea area. *Ann Rheum Dis* 1990;49:99–102.

32. Sukenik S, Newmann L, Flusser D, et al. Balneotherapy for rheumatoid arthritis at the Dead Sea. *Isr J Med Sci* 1995;31:210–214.

33. Cetin N, Aytar A, Atalay A, et al. Comparing hot pack short-wave diathermy, ultrasound, and TENS on isokinetic strength, pain, and functional status of women with osteoarthritic knees: a single-blind, randomized, controlled trial. *Am J Phys Med Rehabil* 2008;87:443–351.

34. Myrer JW, Johnson AW, Mitchell UH, et al. Topical analgesic added to paraffin enhances paraffin bath treatment of individual with hand osteoarthritis. *Dis Rehabil* 2011;33:467–474.

35. Dellhag B, Wollersjö I, Bjelle A. Effect of hand exercise and wax bath treatment in rheumatoid arthritis patients. *Arthritis Care Res* 1992;5:87–92.

36. Harris ED Jr, McCroskery PA. The influence of temperature and fibril stability on degradation of cartilage collagen by rheumatoid synovial collagenase. *N Engl J Med* 1974;290:1–6.

37. Cordray YM, Krusen EM Jr. Use of hydrocollator packs in the treatment of neck and shoulder pains. *Arch Phys Med Rehab* 1959;40:105–108.

38. Constant F, Collin JF, Guillemin F, et al. Effectiveness of spa therapy in chronic low back pain: a randomized clinical trial. *J Rheumatol* 1995;22:1315–1320.

39. Landen BR. Hear or cold for the relief of low back pain? *Phys Ther* 1967;47:1126–1128.

40. Robertson VJ, Ward AR, Jung P. The effect of heat on tissue extensibility: a comparison of deep and superficial heating. *Arch Phys Med Rehabil* 2005;86:819–825.

41. Hayes KW, Hall KD. *Manual for Physical Agents*. 6th ed. Boston, MA: Pearson; 2012.

42. Batavia M. *Contraindications in Physical Rehabilitation: Doing No Harm*. St. Louis, MO: Saunders; 2006.

43. Fruth SJ, Michlovitz SL. Cold therapy modalities. In: Bellew JW, Michlovitz SL, Nolan TP, eds. *Michlovitz's Modalities for Therapeutic Intervention*. 6th ed. Philadelphia: FA Davis; 2016;21–60.

44. Licht S. *History of Therapeutic Heat and Cold*. 3rd ed. Baltimore, MD: Williams & Wilkins; 1982.

45. Knight KL. *Cryotherapy in Sports Injury Management*. Champaign, IL: Human Kinetics; 1995.

46. Travell J. Ethyl chloride for painful muscle spasm. *Arch Phys Med Rehabil* 1952;33:291–298.

47. Kennet J, Hardaker N, Hobbs S, et al. Cooling efficiency of 4 common cryotherapeutic agents. *J Athl Train* 2007;42:343–348.

48. Zemke JE, Anderson JC, Guion WK, et al. Intramuscular temperature responses in the human leg to two forms of cryotherapy: ice massage and ice bag. *J Ortho Sports Phys Ther* 1998;27:301–307.

49. Otte J, Merrick M, Ingersoll C, et al. Subcutaneous adipose tissue thickness alters cooling time during cryotherapy. *Arch Phys Med Rehabil* 2002;83:1501–1505.

50. Algafly A, George K. The effect of cryotherapy on nerve conduction velocity, pain threshhold, and pain tolerance. *Br J Sports Med* 2007;41:365–369.

51. Jutte L, Merrick M, Ingersoll C, et al. The relationship between intramuscular temperature, skin temperature, and adipose thickness during cryotherapy and rewarming. *Arch Phys Med Rehabil* 2001;82:845–850.

52. Douglas WW, Malcolm JL. The effect of localized cooling on cat nerves. *J Physiol* 1955;130:53–54.

53. Bassett FH III, Kirkpatrick JS, Engelhardt DL. Cryotherapy-induced nerve injury. *Am J Sport Med* 1992;22:516–518.

54. Prentice WE. An electromyographic analysis of the effectiveness of heat or cold and stretching for inducing relaxation in injured muscle. *J Ortho Sports Phys Ther* 1982;3:133–140.

55. Mennel J. Spray-stretch for the relief of pain from muscle spasm and myofascial trigger points. *J Am Podiatr Assoc* 1976;66:873–876.

56. Nielson AJ. Case study: myofascial pain of the posterior shoulder relieved by spray and stretch. *J Ortho Sports Phys Ther* 1981;3:21–26.

57. Robbins LD. Cryotherapy for headache. *Headache* 1989;29:598–600.

58. De Coster D, Bossuyt M, Fossion E. The value of cryotherapy in the management of trigeminal neuralgia. *Acta Stomatol Belg* 1993;90:87–93.

59. Halliday SM, Littler TR, Littler EN. A trial of ice therapy and exercise in chronic arthritis. *Physiotherapy* 1969;55:51–56.

60. U.S. Food and Drug Administration. Device approvals, denials and clearances. Available at: www.fda.gov/medicaldevices/productsandmedical procedures/deviceapprovalsandclearances. Accessed March 18, 2017.

61. Post R, Nolan TP. Electromagnetic waves—laser, diathermy, and pulsed electromagnetic fields. In: Bellew JW, Michlovitz SL, Nolan TP, eds. *Michlovitz's Modalities for Therapeutic Intervention*. 6th ed. Philadelphia: FA Davis; 2016:167–238.

62. Enwemeka CS. Therapeutic light. *Rehab Manag* 2004;17(1):20–25.

63. Schindl A, Schindl M, Pernerstorfer-Schön H, et al. Low intensity laser therapy: a review. *J Investig Med* 2000;48:312–326.

64. Baxter GD. *Therapeutic Lasers: Theory and Practice*. New York: Churchill Livingstone; 1994.

65. Baxter GD, Walsh DM, Allen JM, et al. Effects of low-intensity infrared laser irradiation upon conduction in the human median nerve in vivo. *Exp Physiol* 1994;79:227–234.

66. Snyder-Mackler L, Bork CE. Effect of helium-neon laser irradiation on peripheral sensory nerve latency. *Phys Ther* 1988;68:223–225.

67. Greathouse DG, Currier DP, Gilmore RL. Effects of clinical infrared laser on superficial radial nerve conduction. *Phys Ther* 1985;65:1184–1187.

68. Basford JR, Daube JR, Hallman HO, et al. Does low-intensity helium-neon laser irradiation alter sensory nerve action potentials or distal latencies? *Lasers Surg Med* 1990;10:35–39.

69. Palmgren N, Jensen GF, Kaa K, et al. Low-power laser therapy in rheumatoid arthritis. *Laser Med Sci* 1989;4:193–196.

70. Goats GC, Flett E, Hunter JA, et al. Low-intensity laser and phototherapy for rheumatoid arthritis. *Physiotherapy* 1996;82:311–320.

71. Gur A, Sarac AJ, Cevik R, et al. Efficacy of different therapy regimes of low-power laser in painful osteoarthritis of the knee: a double-blind and randomized-controlled trial. *Lasers Surg Med* 2003;33:330–338.

72. Ozdemir F, Birtane M, Kokino S. The clinical efficacy of low-power laser therapy on pain and function in cervical osteoarthritis. *Clin Rheumatol* 2001;20:181–184.

73. Stelian J, Gil I, Habot B. Improvement of pain and disability in elderly patients with degenerative osteoarthritis of the knee treated with narrow-band light therapy. *J Am Geriatr Soc* 1992;S40:23–26.

74. Schindl A, Neumann R. Low-intensity laser therapy is an effective treatment for recurrent herpes simplex infection. Results from a randomized, double-blind, placebo-controlled trial. *J Invest Dermatol* 1999;113:221–223.

75. Moore KC, Hira N, Kumar PS, et al. A double-blind crossover trial of low-level laser therapy in the treatment of post herpetic neuralgia. *Laser Ther* 1988;1:7–9.

76. Ilbuldu E, Cakmak A, Disci R, et al. Comparison of laser, dry needling, and placebo laser treatments in myofascial pain syndrome. *Photomed Laser Surg* 2004;22:306–311.

77. Ceylan Y, Hizmetli S, Silig Y. The effect of infrared laser therapy and medical treatments on pain and serotonin degradation products in patients with myofascial pain syndrome: a controlled trial. *Rheumatol Int* 2004;24:201–210.

78. Gur A, Consut A, Sarac AJ, et al. Efficacy of 904 nm gallium arsenide low level laser therapy in the management of chronic myofascial pain in the neck: a double-blind and randomized-controlled trial. *Lasers Surg Med* 2004;35:229–235.

79. Basford JB, Sheffield CG, Harmsen WS. Laser therapy: a randomized, controlled trial of the effects of low-intensity Nd:YAG laser irradiation on musculoskeletal back pain. *Arch Phys Med Rehabil* 1999;80:647–652.

80. Chow RT, Barnsley LB, Heller GZ. The effect of 300 mW, 830 nm laser on chronic neck pan: a double-blind, randomized, placebo-controlled study. *Pain* 2006;124:201–210.

81. Naeser MA, Han KA, Lieberman BE, et al. Carpal tunnel syndrome pain treated with low-level laser and microamperes transcutaneous electric nerve stimulation: a controlled study. *Arch Phys Med Rehabil* 2002;83:978–988.

82. Evcik D, Kavuncu V, Cakir T, et al. Laser therapy in the treatment of carpal tunnel syndrome: a randomized controlled trial. *Photomed Laser Surg* 2007;25:34–39.

83. Mazzetto MO, Carasco TG, Bidinelo EF, et al. Low intensity laser application in temporomandibular disorders: a phase I double-blind study. *Cranio* 2007;25:186–192.

84. Moore KC, Hira N, Broome IJ, et al. The effect of infrared diode laser irradiation on the duration and severity of postoperative pain. A double-blind trial. *Laser Ther* 1992;4:145–150.

85. Eckerdal A, Bastian HL. Can low reactive-level laser therapy be used in the treatment of neurogenic facial pain? A double-blind, placebo-controlled investigation of patients with trigeminal neuralgia. *Laser Ther* 1996;8: 247–252.

86. Walker JB, Akhanjee LK, Cooney MM. Laser therapy for pain of trigeminal neuralgia. *Clin J Pain* 1987;3:183–187.

87. Basford JR, Melanga GA, Krause DA, et al. A randomized controlled evaluation of low-intensity laser therapy: plantar fasciitis. *Arch Phys Med Rehab* 1998;79:249–254.

88. Rogvi-Hansen B, Ellitsgaard N, Funch M, et al. Low-level laser treatment of chondromalacia patellae. *Int Orthop* 1991;15:359–361.

89. Hansen HJ, Thorøe U. Low-power laser biostimulation of chronic oro-facial pain. A double-blind, placebo controlled cross-over study in 40 patients. *Pain* 1990;43:169–179.

90. de Bie RA, de Vet HC, Lenssen TF, et al. Low-level laser therapy in ankle sprains: a randomized clinical trial. *Arch Phys Med Rehab* 1998;79:1415–1420.

91. Lam KL, Cheing GL. Effects of 904-nm lo-level laser therapy in the management of lateral epicondylitis: a randomized controlled trial. *Photomed Laser Surg* 2007;25:65–71.

92. Stergioulas A, Stergioulas M, Aarskog R, et al. Effects of low-level laser and eccentric exercises in the treatment of recreational athletes with chronic Achilles tendinopathy. *Am J Sports Med* 2008;36:881–887.

93. Wimett K, Souvall S, Whitfeield J, et al. Effectiveness of infrared light therapy in the treatment of diabetic peripheral neuropathy: a systematic review. Paper presented at: American Physical Therapy Association NEXT Conference & Exposition; June 2015; National Harbor, MD.

94. Franzen-Korzendorfer H, Blackinton M, Rone-Adams S, et al. The effect of monochromatic infrared energy on transcutaneous oxygen measurements and protective sensation: results of a controlled, double-blind, randomized clinical study. *Ostomy Wound Manage* 2008;54(6):16–31.

95. Leonard DR, Farooqi MH, Myers S. Restoration of sensation, reduced pain, and improved balance in subjects with diabetic peripheral neuropathy: a double-blind, randomized, placebo-controlled study with monochromatic near-infrared treatment. *Diabetes Care* 2004;27:168–172.

96. Mak M, Cheing G. Immediate effects of monochromatic infrared energy on microcirculation in healthy subjects. *Photomed Laser Surg* 2012;30(4):193–199.

97. Kochman AB, Carnegie DH, Burke TJ. Symptomatic reversal of peripheral neuropathy in patients with diabetes. *J Am Podiatr Assoc* 2002;92:125–130.

98. Harkless LB, DeLellis S, Carnegie DH, et al. Improved foot sensitivity and pain reduction in patients with peripheral neuropathy after treatment with monochromatic infrared photo energy-MIRE. *J Diabetes Complications* 2006;20(1):81–87.

99. Arnall DA, Nelson AG, Lopez L, et al. The restorative effects of pulsed infrared light therapy on significant loss of peripheral protective sensation in patients with long-term type 1 and type 2 diabetes mellitus. *Acta Diabetologica* 2006;43(1):26–33.

100. Swislocki A, Orth M, Bales M, et al. A randomized clinical trial of the effectiveness of photon simulation on pain, sensation, and quality of life in patients with diabetic peripheral neuropathy. *J Pain Symptom Manage* 2010;39(1):88–99.

101. Clifft JK, Newton TS, Kasser RJ, et al. The effect of monochromatic infrared energy on sensation in patients with diabetic peripheral neuropathy. *Diabetes Care* 2005;28(12):2896–2900.

102. Lavery LA, Williams J, Murdoch D, et al. Does anodyne light therapy improve peripheral neuropathy in diabetes: a double blind, sham-controlled, randomized trial to evaluate monochromatic infrared photoenergy. *Diabetes Care* 2008;31(2):316–321.

103. Nawfar SA, Yacob NBM. Effects of monochromatic infrared energy therapy on diabetic feet with peripheral sensory neuropathy: a randomized controlled trial. *Singapore Med J* 2011;52(9):669–672.

104. Lake D. Therapeutic ultrasound. In: Bellew JW, Michlovitz SL, Nolan TP, eds. *Michlovitz's Modalities for Therapeutic Intervention*. 6th ed. Philadelphia: FA Davis; 2016:89–134.

105. Amijo-Olivo S, Fuentes J, Muir I, et al. Usage patterns and beliefs about therapeutic ultrasound by Canadian physical therapists: an exploratory population-based cross-sectional survey. *Physiother Can* 2013;65:289–299.

106. Hayes BT, Merrick MA, Sandrey MA, et al. Three-MHz ultrasound heats deeper into the tissues than originally theorized. *J Athl Train* 2004;39:230–234.

107. Sparrow KJ. Therapeutic ultrasound. In: Michlovitz SL, Nolan TP, eds. *Modalities for Therapeutic Intervention*. 4th ed. Philadelphia: FA Davis; 2006:79–96.

108. Bashardoust Tajali S, Hought P, MacDermic JC, et al. Effects of low-intensity pulsed ultrasound therapy on fracture healing: a systematic review and meta-analysis. *Am J Phys Med Rehabil* 2012;91(4):349–367.

109. Martin E. The cellular bioeffects of low intensity ultrasound. *Ultrasound* 2009;17:214–19.

110. Khanna A, Nelmes RT, Gougoulias N, et al. The effects of LIPUS on soft-tissue healing: a review of literature. *Br Med Bull* 2009;89:169–182.

111. Watson JM, Kang'ombe AR, Soares MO, et al. Use of weekly, low dose, high frequency ultrasound for hard to heal venous leg ulcers: the VenUS III randomised controlled trial. *BMJ* 2011;342:d1092.

112. Warden SJ, Metcalf BR, Kiss ZS, et al. Low-intensity pulsed ultrasound for chronic patellar tendinopathy: a randomized, double-blind, placebo-controlled trial. *Rheumatol* 2008;47(4):467–471.

113. Dudda M, Hauser J, Huhr G, et al. Low-intensity pulsed ultrasound as a useful adjuvant during distraction osteogenesis: a prospective, randomized controlled trial. *J Trauma* 2011;71:1276–1380.

114. Ricardo M. The effect of ultrasound on the healing of muscle-pediculated bone graft in scaphoid non-union. *Int Orthop* 2006;30:123–127.

115. Smith EK, Craven A, Wilson AM. Effect of noncontact low-frequency ultrasound on wound healing: a systematic review. *J Acute Care Phys Ther* 2014;5:36–44.

116. Escandon J, Vival AC, Perez R, et al. A prospective pilot study of ultrasound therapy effectiveness in refractory venous leg ulcers. *Int Wound J* 2012;9:570–578.

117. Bommannan D, Okuyama H, Stauffer P, et al. The use of high frequency ultrasound to enhance transdermal drug delivery. *Pharm Res* 1992;9:559–564.

118. Bakhtiary AH, Fatemi E, Emami M, et al. Phonophoresis of dexamethasone sodium phosphate may manage pain and symptoms of patients with carpal tunnel syndrome. *Clin J Pain* 2013;29:348–353.

119. Ustun N, Arslan F, Mansuroglu A, et al. Efficacy of EMLA cream phonophoresis comparison with ultrasound therapy on myofascial pain syndrome of the trapezius: a single-blind, randomized clinical study. *Rheumatol Int* 2014;34:453–457.

120. Donovan L, Selkow NM, Rupp K, et al. The anesthetic effect of lidocaine after varying times of phonophoresis. *Am J Phys Med Rehabil* 2011;90:1056–1063.

121. Onuwe HA, Amadi K, Odeh SO. Comparison of the therapeutic efficacy of double-modality therapy. Phonophoresis and cryotherapy in the management of musculoskeletal injuries in adult Nigerian subjects. *Niger J Physiol Soc* 2013;28:153–158.

122. Huang MH, Lin YS, Lee CL, et al. Use of ultrasound to increase effectiveness of isokinetic exercise for knee osteoarthritis. *Arch Phys Med Rehabil* 2005;86:1545–1551.

123. Ozgonenel L, Aytekin E, Durum OL, et al. A double-blind trial of clinical effects of therapeutic ultrasound in knee osteoarthritis. *Ultrasound Med Biol* 2009;35:44–49.

124. Ebenbichler GR, Erdogmus CB, Resh KL, et al. Ultrasound therapy for calcific tendinitis of the shoulder. *N Engl J Med* 1999;340:1533–1538.

125. Roden D. Ultrasonic waves in the treatment of chronic adhesive subacromial bursitis. *J Irish Med Assoc* 1952;30:85–88.

126. Van der Heijden GJ, Leffers P, Wolters PJ, et al. No effect of bipolar interferential electrotherapy and pulsed ultrasound for soft tissue shoulder disorders: a randomised controlled trial. *Ann Rheum Dis* 1999;58:530–540.

127. Nwunga VC. Ultrasound in treatment of back pain resulting from prolapsed intervertebral disc. *Arch Phys Med Rehab* 1983;64:88–89.

128. Ansari NN, Ebadi S, Talebian S, et al. A randomized single blind placebo controlled clinical trial on the effect of continuous ultrasound on low back pain. *Electomyogr Clin Neurophysiol* 2006;46:329–336.

129. Yildiz N, Atalay NS, Gungen GO, et al. Comparison of ultrasound and ketoprofen phonophoresis in the treatment of carpal tunnel syndrome. *J Back Musculoskelet Rehabil* 2011;24:39–47.

130. Binder A, Hodge G, Greenwood AM, et al. Is therapeutic ultrasound effective in treating soft tissue lesions. *BMJ* 1985;290:512–514.

131. Haker E, Lundeberg T. Pulsed ultrasound treatment in lateral epicondylalgia. *Scand J Rehab Med* 1991;23:115–118.

132. Perron M, Malouin F. Acetic acid iontophoresis and ultrasound for the treatment of calcifying tendonitis of the shoulder: a randomized control trial. *Arch Phys Med Rehab* 1997;78:379–384.

133. Tepperberg I, Marjey EJ. Ultrasound therapy of painful postoperative neurofibromas. *Am J Phys Med* 1953;32:27–30.

134. Garrett AS, Garrett M. Ultrasound therapy for herpes zoster pain. *J R Coll Gen Pract* 1982;32:709, 711.

135. Talaat AM, El-Dibany MM, El-Garf A. Physical therapy in the management of myofascial pain dysfunction syndrome. *Ann Otol Rhinol Laryngol* 1995;95:225–228.

136. Downing DS, Weinstein A. Ultrasound therapy of subacromial bursitis. A double blind trial. *Phys Ther* 1986;66:194–199.

137. Flax HJ. Ultrasound treatment of peritendinitis calcarea of the shoulder. *Am J Phys Med* 1964;43:117–124.

138. Hasish I, Hai HK, Harvey W, et al. Reduction of postoperative pain and swelling by ultrasound treatment: a placebo effect. *Pain* 1988;33:303–311.

139. Everett T, McIntosh J, Grant A. Ultrasound therapy for persistent post-natal perineal pain and dyspareunia: a randomized placebo-controlled trial. *Physiotherapy* 1992;78:263–267.

140. Brock Symons T, Clasey JL, Gater DR, et al. Effects of deep heat as a preventive mechanism on delayed onset muscle soreness. *J Strength Cond Res* 2004;18:155–161.

141. Zammit E, Herrington I. Ultrasound therapy in the management of acute lateral ligament sprains of the ankle joint. *Phys Ther Sports* 2005;6:116–121.

142. Houghton PE, Nussbaum IL, Hoens AM. Electrophysical agents: contraindications and precautions. 3. Continuous and pulsed ultrasound. *Physiother Can* 2010;62:13–25.

143. Bellew JW. Clinical electrical stimulation. In: Bellew JW, Michlovitz SL, Nolan TP, eds. *Michlovitz's Modalities for Therapeutic Intervention*. 6th ed. Philadelphia: FA Davis; 2016:287–327.

144. Manal TJ, Snyder-Mackler L. Electrical stimulation for pain modulation. In: Robinson AJ, Snyder-Mackler L, eds. *Clinical Electrophysiology: Electrotherapy and Electrophysiologic Testing*. 3rd ed. Baltimore, MD: Williams & Wilkins; 2008:151–197.

145. Ciccone CD. *Pharmacology in Rehabilitation*. 5th ed. Philadelphia: FA Davis; 2016.
146. Liebano RE. Mechanisms of pain and use of therapeutic modalities. In: Bellew JW, Michlovitz SL, Nolan TP, eds. *Michlovitz's Modalities for Therapeutic Intervention*. 6th ed. Philadelphia: FA Davis; 2016:331–356.
147. Melzack R, Wall PD. Pain mechanisms: a new theory. *Science* 1965;150:971.
148. Nolan TP. Electrotherapeutic modalities: electrotherapy and iontophoresis. In: Michlovitz SL, Nolan TP, eds. *Modalities for Therapeutic Intervention*. 4th ed. Philadelphia: FA Davis; 2006:97–121.
149. Chandran P, Sluka KA. Development of opioid tolerance with repeated transcutaneous electrical nerve stimulation administration. *Pain* 2003;102: 195–201.
150. Liebano RE, Rakel B, Vance CG, et al. An investigation of the development of analgesic tolerance to TENS in humans. *Pain* 2011;152:335–342.
151. Kalra A, Urban MO, Sluka KA. Blockade of opioid receptors in rostral ventral medulla prevents antihyperalgesia produced by transcutaneous electric nerve stimulation. *J Pharmacol Exp Ther* 2001;298:257–263.
152. Sluka KA, Deacon M, Stibal A, et al. Spinal blockade of opioid receptors prevents the analgesia produced by TENS in arthritic rats. *J Pharmacol Exp Ther* 1999;289:840–846.
153. Sabino GS, Santos CM, Francischi JN, et al. Release of endogenous opioids following transcutaneous electric nerve stimulation in an experimental model of acute inflammatory pain. *J Pain* 2008;9:157–163.
154. Solomon RA, Viernstein MC, Long DM. Reduction of postoperative pain and narcotic use by transcutaneous electric nerve stimulation. *Surgery* 1980;87:142–146.
155. Desantana JM, Santana-Filho VJ, Guerra DR, et al. Hypoalgesic effect of transcutaneous electrical nerve stimulation following inguinal herniorrhaphy: a randomized, controlled trial. *J Pain* 2008;9:623–629.
156. Emmiler M, Solak O, Kogogullari C, et al. Control of acute postoperative pain by transcutaneous electrical nerve stimulation after open cardiac operations: a randomized placebo-controlled prospective study. *Heart Surg Forum* 2008;11:E3000–E3003.
157. Ng MM, Jeung M, Poon DM. The effects of electro-acupuncture and transcutaneous electrical nerve stimulation on patients with painful osteoarthritic knees: a randomized controlled trial with follow-up evaluation. *J Altern Complement Med* 2003;9:641–649.
158. Grimmer K. A controlled double-blind study comparing the effects of strong burst mode TENS and high rate TENS on painful osteoarthritic knees. *Austr J Physiother* 1992;38:49–56.
159. Lang T, Barker R, Steinlechner B, et al. TENS relieves acute posttraumatic hip pain during emergency transport. *J Trauma* 2007;62:184–188.
160. Nordemar R, Thörner C. Treatment of acute cervical pain–a comparative group study. *Pain* 1981;10:93–101.
161. Taylor DN, Katims JJ, Ng LK. Sine-wave auricular TENS produces frequency-dependent hypoesthesia in the trigeminal nerve. *Clin J Pain* 1993;9:216–219.
162. Solomon S, Guglielmo KM. Treatment of headache by transcutaneous electrical stimulation. *Headache* 1985;25:12–15.
163. Katz J, Melzack R. Auricular transcutaneous electrical nerve stimulation (TENS) reduces phantom limb pain. *J Pain Symptom Manage* 1991;6:73–83.
164. Dawood MY, Ramos J. Transcutaneous electrical nerve stimulation (TENS) for the treatment of primary dysmenorrhea: a randomized crossover comparison with placebo TENS and ibuprofen. *Obstet Gynecol* 1990;75:656–660.
165. Cheing GL, Luk ML. Transcutaneous electrical nerve stimulation for neuropathic pain. *J Hand Surg Br* 2005;30:50–55.
166. Kumar D, Marshall HJ. Diabetic peripheral neuropathy: amelioration of pain with transcutaneous electrical nerve stimulation. *Diabetes Care* 1997;20:1702–1705.
167. Leandri M, Parodi CI, Corrieri N, et al. Comparison of TENS treatments in hemiplegic shoulder pain. *Scand J Rehab Med* 1990;22:69–72.
168. Bertanlanffy A, Kober A, Bertalanffy P, et al. Transcutaneous electrical nerve stimulation reduces acute low back pain during emergency transport. *Acad Emerg Med* 2005;12:607–611.
169. Deyo RA, Walsh NE, Martin DC, et al. A controlled trial of transcutaneous electrical nerve stimulation (TENS) and exercise for chronic low back pain. *N Engl J Med* 1990;322:1627–1634.
170. Marchand S, Charest J, Li J, et al. Is TENS purely a placebo effect? A controlled study on chronic low back pain. *Pain* 1993;54:99–106.
171. Chao AS, Chao A, Wang TH, et al. Pain relief by applying transcutaneous electrical nerve stimulation (TENS) on acupuncture points during the first stage of labor: a randomized double-blind placebo-controlled trial. *Pain* 2007;127:214–220.
172. Olsen MF, Elden H, Janson ED, et al. A comparison of high- versus low-intensity, high-frequency transcutaneous electric nerve stimulation for painful postpartum uterine contractions. *Acta Obstet Gynecol Scand* 2007;86:310–314.
173. Graff-Radford SB, Reeves JL, Baker RL, et al. Effects of transcutaneous electrical nerve stimulation on myofascial pain and trigger point sensitivity. *Pain* 1989;37:1–5.
174. Kruger LR, van der Linden WJ, Cleaton-Jones PE. Transcutaneous electrical nerve stimulation in the treatment of myofascial pain dysfunction. *S Afr J Surg* 1998;36:35–38.
175. Abelson K, Langley GB, Sheppeard H, et al. Transcutaneous electrical nerve stimulation in rheumatoid arthritis. *N Z Med J* 1983;96:156–158.
176. Møystad A, Krogstard BS, Larheim TA. Transcutaneous electrical nerve stimulation in a group of patients with rheumatic disease involving the temporomandibular joint. *J Prosthet Dent* 1990;64:596–600.
177. Cazejust J, DeVille R, Paleirac R. Preliminary therapeutic results from the application of interferential medium frequency currents (Nemec current). *J Radiol Electrol Arch Electr Medicale* 1956;37:606–607.
178. Knight KL, Draper DO. *Therapeutic Modalities: The Art and Science*. Baltimore, MD: Lippincott Williams & Wilkins; 2008.
179. Johnson MI, Tabasam G. A single-blind investigation into the hypoanalgesic effects of different swing patterns of interferential current on cold-induced pain in healthy volunteers. *Arch Phys Med Rehabil* 2003;84:350–357.
180. Palmer S, Martin D. Interferential current. In: Watson T, ed. *Electrotherapy: Evidence-Based Practice*. 12th ed. Philadelphia: Churchill Livingstone; 2008:297–315.
181. Fuentes JP, Armijo-Olivo S, Magee DJ, et al. A preliminary investigation into the effects of active interferential current therapy and placebo on pressure pain sensitivity: a random crossover placebo controlled study. *Physiother* 2011;97:291–301.
182. Rocha CS, Lanferdini FJ, Kolberg C, et al. Interferential therapy effect on mechanical pain threshold and isometric torque after delayed onset muscle soreness induction in human hamstrings. *J Sport Sci* 2012;30:733–742.
183. Adedoyin RA, Olaogun MOB, Fagbeja OO. Effect of interferential current stimulation in management of osteoarthritic knee pain. *Physiother* 2002;88:493–499.
184. Atamaz FC, Durmaz B, Baydar M, et al. Comparison of the efficacy of transcutaneous electrical nerve stimulation interferential currents, and shortwave diathermy in knee osteoarthritis: a double-blind, randomized, controlled, multicenter study. *Arch Phys Med Rehabil* 2012;93:748–756.
185. Gundog M, Atamaz F, Kanyilmaz S, et al. Interferential current therapy in patients with knee osteoarthritis. *Am J Phys Med Rehabil* 2012;91: 107–113.
186. Facci LM, Nowotny JP, Tormen F, et al. Effects of transcutaneous electrical nerve stimulation (TENS) and interferential currents (IFC) in patients with nonspecific chronic low back pain: randomized clinical trial. *Sao Paulo Med J* 2011;129:206–216.
187. Correa JB, Costa LO, Oliveira NTB, et al. Effects of the carrier frequency of interferential current on pain modulation and central hypersensitivity in people with chronic nonspecific low back pain: a randomized placebo-controlled trial. *Eur J Pain* 2016;20:1653–1666.
188. Koca I, Boyaci A, Tutoglu A, et al. Assessment of the effectiveness of interferential current therapy and TENS in the management of carpal tunnel syndrome: a randomized controlled study. *Rheumatol Int* 2014;34:1639–1645.
189. Suriya-amarit D, Gaogasigam C, Siriphorn A, et al. Effect of interferential current stimulation in management of hemiplegic shoulder pain. *Arch Phys Med Rehabil* 2014;95:1441–1446.
190. Licht S. History of electrotherapy. In: Stillwell GK. *Therapeutic Electrotherapy and Ultraviolet Radiation*. 3rd ed. Baltimore, MD: Williams & Wilkins; 1993:1–64.
191. Leduc S. Introduction of medicinal substances into depth of tissues by electrical current. *Ann Electrobiol* 1900;3:545–560.
192. Ozawa A, Haruki Y, Iwashita K, et al. Follow-up of clinical efficacy of iontophoresis therapy for postherpetic neuralgia (PHN). *J Dermatol* 1999;26:1–10.
193. Gudeman SD, Eisele SA, Heidt RS, et al. Treatment of plantar fasciitis by iontophoresis of 0.4% dexamethasone. A randomized, double-blind, placebo-controlled study. *Am J Sports Med* 1997;25:312–316.
194. Akinbo SR, Aiyejunusie CB, Akinyemi OA, et al. Comparison of the therapeutic efficacy of phonophoresis and iontophoresis using dexamethasone sodium phosphate in the management of patients with knee osteoarthritis. *Nig Postgrad Med J* 2007;14:190–194.
195. Aiyejusunie CB, Kola-Korolo TA, Ajiboye OA. Comparison of the effects of TENS and sodium salicylate iontophoresis in the management of osteoarthritis of the knee. *Nig Q J Hosp Med* 2007;17:30–34.
196. Nirsch RP, Rodin DM, Ochiai DH, et al. Iontophoretic administration of dexamethasone sodium phosphate for acute epicondylitis. *Am J Sports Med* 2003;31:189–195.
197. Gurcay E, Unlu E, Gurcay AG, et al. Assessment of phonophoresis and iontophoresis in the treatment of carpal tunnel syndrome: a randomized controlled trial. *Rheumatol Int* 2012;42:717–722.
198. Neeter C, Thomee R, Sillbernagel KG, et al. Iontophoresis with and without dexamethasone in the treatment of acute Achilles tendon pain. *Scand J Med Sci Sports* 2003;13:376–382.
199. Franklin GM, Glass L, Javaher SP, et al. *Work-Related Complex Regional Pain Syndrome: Diagnosis and Treatment*. Tumwater, WA: Washington State Department of Labor and Industries. Available at: http://www.lni.wa.gov/ClaimsIns/Files/OMD/CRPSdraft061711.pdf. Accessed March 12, 2017.
200. Verberne O, Donnelly K, Helmers L, et al. Effectiveness of desensitization therapy for individuals with complex regional pain syndrome: a systematic review. *J Ortho Sport Phys Ther* 2016;46:A147.
201. Barnhoorn KJ, Oostendorp RA, van Dongen RT, et al. The effectiveness and cost evaluation of pain exposure physical therapy and conventional therapy in patients with complex regional pain syndrome type 1. Rationale and design of a randomized controlled trial. *BMC Musculoskelet Disord* 2012;13:58.

202. Waylett-Rendall J. Desensitization of the hand. In: Hunter JM, Macklin EJ, Callahan AD, eds. *Rehabilitation of the Hand*. 4th ed. St. Louis, MO: Mosby; 1995:693–700.

203. van de Meent H, Oerlemans M, Bruggeman A, et al. Safety of "pain exposure" in patients with complex regional pain syndrome type 1. *Pain* 2011;152:1431–1438.

204. Harden R, Bruehl S, Perez R, et al. Validation of proposed diagnostic criteria (the "Budapest Criteria") for complex regional pain syndrome. *Pain* 2010;150:268–274.

205. Mailis-Gagnon A, Lakha S, Allen M, et al. Characteristics of complex regional pain syndrome in patients referred to a tertiary pain clinic by community physicians, assessed by the Budapest Clinical Diagnostic Criteria. *Pain Med* 2014;15:1965–1974.

206. Melzack R. From the gate to the neuromatrix. *Pain* 1999;6(suppl): S121–S126.

207. Loeser JD. Pain after amputation: phantom limb and stump pain. In: Loeser JD, ed. *Bonica's Management of Pain*. 3rd ed. Baltimore, MD: Lippincott Williams & Wilkins; 2001:412–423.

208. Allen RJ, Wu C, Horiuchi G, et al. Somatosensory specific desensitization in the treatment of patients with complex regional pain syndrome: effects of pressure desensitization. *J Ortho Sports Phys Ther* 2005;35(1):A27.

209. Ribbers GM, Stam HJ. Complex regional pain syndrome type I treated with topical capsaicin: a case report. *Arch Phys Med Rehabil* 2001;82:851–852.

210. Harden RN. Complex regional pain syndrome. *Br J Anaes* 2001;87(1): 99–106.

211. Taub E, Uswatte G, Mark VW, et al. The learned nonuse phenomenon: implications for rehabilitation. *Eura Medicophys* 2006;42:241–256.

212. Moseley GL. A pain neuromatrix approach to patients with chronic pain. *Man Ther* 2003;8:130–140.

213. Allen RJ, Stephenson KM, Sundahl BT, et al. Thermal desensitization for treatment of severe thermal sensitivity and associated functional deficits secondary to complex regional pain syndrome of the upper limb. *Phys Ther Case Reports* 2001;4(2):59–66.

214. Allen RJ. Multimodal allodynia treated with somatosensory-specific desensitization in patients with complex regional pain syndrome. *Eur J Pain* 2009;13:S144–S145.

215. Cuchiarro G, Craig K, Marks K, et al. Diffuse complex regional pain syndrome in an adolescent: a novel treatment approach. *Clin J Pain* 2013; 29:42–45.

216. Pandita M, Arfath U. Complex regional pain syndrome of the knee: a case report. *BMC Sports Sci Med Rehabil* 2013;5:1–5.

217. Lewis JS, Coales K, Hall J, et al. 'Now you see it, now you do not': sensory-motor re-education in complex regional pain syndrome. *Hand Ther* 2011; 16:29–38.

218. Lundeberg T, Nordemar R, Ottoson D. Pain alleviation by vibratory stimulation. *Pain* 1984;20(1):25–44.

219. Allen RJ, Vento M, Hoffman J, et al. Effects of desensitization on pain distribution and normalization of somatosensation in a patient with quadrilateral complex regional pain syndrome. *J Ortho Sport Phys Ther* 2017;47:A58.

220. Allen RJ, Soterakopoulos C, Fugere KJ, et al. Pain distribution quantification using enhanced 'rule-of-nines': reliability and correlations with intensity, sensory, affective, and functional pain measures. *Physiotherapy* 2011;97(suppl 1):309.

221. Weiss T. Plasticity and cortical reorganization associated with pain. *Z Psychol* 2016;224:71–79.

222. Smart KM, Wand BM, O'Connell NE. Physiotherapy for pain and disability in adults with complex regional pain syndrome (CRPS) types I and II. *Cochrane Database Syst Rev* 2016;(2):CD010853.

223. Földi E, Földi M, Strößenreuther C, et al. *Földi's Textbook of Lymphology: For Physicians and Lymphedema Therapists*. 3rd ed. München, Germany: Urban & Fischer; 2012.

224. Zuther JE, Norton S. *Lymphedema Management: The Comprehensive Guide for Practitioners*. 3rd ed. Stuttgart, Germany: Georg Theime; 2013.

225. Uher EM, Vacariu G, Schneider B, et al. Comparison of manual lymph drainage with physical therapy in complex regional pain syndrome, type I. A comparative randomized controlled therapy study. *Wien Klin Wochenschr* 2000;112:133–137.

226. Duman I, Ozdemir A, Tan AK, et al. The efficacy of manual lymphatic drainage therapy in the management of limb edema secondary to reflex sympathetic dystrophy. *Rheumatol Int* 2009;29:759–763.

227. Cao H, Li X, Liu J. An updated review of the efficacy of cupping therapy. *PLoS One* 2012;7:e31793.

228. Cao H, Li X, Yan X, et al. Cupping therapy for acute and chronic pain management a systematic review of randomized clinical trials. *J Trad Chin Med Sci* 2014;1:49–61.

229. Emerich M, Braeunig M, Clement HW, et al. Mode of action of cupping—local metabolism and pain thresholds in neck pain patients and healthy subjects. *Complement Ther Med* 2014;22:148–158.

230. Al Bedah AM, Khalil MK, Posadzki P, et al. Evaluation of wet cupping therapy: systematic review of randomized clinical trials. *J Altern Complement Med* 2016;22:768–777.

231. Kim JI, Lee MS, Lee DH, et al. Cupping for treating pain: a systematic review. *Evid Based Complement Altern Med* 2011;2011:e467014.

232. Astin JA. Why patients use alternative medicine: results of a national study. *JAMA* 1998;279:1548–1543.

233. Huang CY, Choong MY, Li TS. Effectiveness of cupping therapy for low back pain: a systematic review. *Acupuncture Med* 2013;31:336–337.

234. Cramer H, Lauche R, Hohmann C, et al. Randomized controlled trial of pulsating cupping (pneumatic pulsation therapy) for chronic neck pain. *Comp Med Res* 2011;18:327–334.

235. Kim JI, Kim TH, Lee MS, et al. Evaluation of wet-cupping therapy for persistent non-specific low back pain: a randomized, waiting-list controlled, open-label, parallel-group pilot trial. *Trials* 2011;12:146.

236. Michalsen A, Bock S, Ludtke R, et al. Effects of traditional cupping therapy in patients with carpal tunnel syndrome: a randomized controlled trial. *J Pain* 2009;10:1–8.

237. Yi J, Park J, Kim H, et al. Comparison of the effects of muscle stretching exercises and cupping therapy on pain thresholds, cervical range of motion and angle: a cross-over study. *Phys Ther Rehab Sci* 2017;6:83–89.

238. Lauche R, Spitzer J, Schwahn B, et al. Efficacy of cupping therapy in patients with the fibromyalgia syndrome: a randomized placebo controlled trial. *Sci Rep* 2016;6:e37316.

239. Lee MS, Kim JI, Ernst E. Is cupping an effective treatment? An overview of systematic reviews. *J Acupunct Meridian Stud* 2011;4:1–4.

240. Higgins JPT, Green S. *Cochrane Handbook for Systematic Reviews of Interventions*. West Sussex, United Kingdom: Wiley; 2008.

241. Ahmadi A, Schwebel DC, Rezaei M. The efficacy of wet-cupping in the treatment of tension and migraine headaches. *Am J Chin Med* 2008;36:37.

242. Teut M, Kaiser S, Ortiz M, et al. Pulsatile dry cupping in patients with osteoarthritis of the knee—a randomized, controlled, exploratory trial. *BMC Complement Altern Med* 2012;12:184.

243. Chi LM, Lin LM, Chen CL, et al. The effectiveness of cupping therapy on relieving chronic neck and shoulder pain: a randomized controlled trial. *Evid Based Complement Altern Med* 2016;2016:e7358918.

244. Pergolizzi J, Ahlbeck K, Aldington D, et al. The development of chronic pain: physiological change necessitates a multidisciplinary approach to treatment. *Curr Med Res Opin* 2013;29:1127–1135.

245. Flor H, Elbert T, Knecht S, et al. Phantom-limb pain as a perceptual correlate of cortical reorganization following arm amputation. *Nature* 1995;375:482–484.

246. Karl A, Birbaumer N, Lutzenberger W, et al. Reorganization of motor and somatosensory cortex in upper extremity amputees with phantom limb pain. *J Neurosci* 2001;21:3609–3618.

247. Koppelstaetter F, Siedentopf CM, Rhomberg P, et al. Functional magnetic resonance imaging before motor cortex stimulation for phantom limb pain. *Nervenarzt* 2007;78:1435–1439.

248. Ramachandran VS, Rogers-Ramachandran D. Synaesthesia in phantom limbs induced with mirrors. *Proc Biol Sci* 1996;263:377–386.

249. Brodie E, Whyte A, Niven A. Analgesia through the looking-glass? A randomized controlled trial investigating the effect of viewing a 'virtual' limb upon phantom limb pain, sensation and movement. *Eur J Pain* 2007;11: 428–436.

250. Chan B, Witt R, Charrow A, et al. Mirror therapy for phantom limb pain. *N Engl J Med* 2007;357:2206–2207.

251. Priganc V, Stralka SW. Graded motor imagery. *J Hand Ther* 2011;24: 164–169.

252. Moseley GL. Graded motor imagery is effective for long-standing complex regional pain syndrome: a randomized controlled trial. *Pain* 2004;108: 192–198.

253. Moseley GL. Is successful rehabilitation of complex regional pain syndrome due to sustained attention to the affected limb? A randomized clinical trial. *Pain* 2005;114:54–61.

254. Moseley GL. Graded motor imagery for pathologic pain: a randomized controlled trial. *Neurology* 2006;67:2129–2134.

255. Seidel S, Kasprian G, Furtner J, et al. Mirror therapy in lower limb amputees—a look beyond primary motor cortex reorganization. *Fortschr Rontgenstr* 2011;183:1051–1057.

256. Darnall B, Li H. Home-based self-delivered mirror therapy for phantom pain: a pilot study. *J Rehabil Med* 2012;44:254–260.

257. Foell J, Bekrater-Bodmann R, Diers M, et al. Mirror therapy for phantom limb pain: brain changes and the role of body representation. *Euro J Pain* 2014;18:729–739.

258. Tilak M, Isaac SA, Fletcher J, et al. Mirror therapy and transcutaneous electrical nerve stimulation for management of phantom limb pain in amputees - a single blinded randomized controlled trial. *Physiother Res Int* 2016;21:109–115.

259. Casale R, Damiani C, Rosati V. Mirror therapy in the rehabilitation of lower-limb amputation: are there any contraindications? *Am J Phys Med Rehabil* 2009;88:837–42.

260. Hagenberg A, Carpenter C. Mirror visual feedback for phantom pain: international experience on modalities and adverse effects discussed by an expert panel: a Delphi Study. *PMR* 2014;6:708–715.

CHAPTER 93

Exercise Therapy for Low Back Pain

ELLEN McGOUGH and **JOYCE M. ENGEL**

Exercise is a frequently prescribed nonpharmacologic intervention for low back pain (LBP).[1,2] Exercise for therapeutic purposes is defined as the systematic, planned performance of bodily movements, postures, or physical activities.[3] Regular exercise improves general fitness, results in a sense of well-being, and is associated with lower incidence and severity of comorbid conditions such as depression, fatigue, and insomnia, which are often associated with persistent pain.[4] The purpose of this chapter is (1) to describe clinical evaluation and decision making for the development of exercise interventions for individuals with LBP, (2) to discuss physical and psychosocial elements of exercise interventions that ultimately impact outcomes, and (3) to present available evidence for exercise therapy approaches across stages of LBP.

LBP of musculoskeletal origin is a common problem and a major cause of disability. More than 56% of American adults (125 million) had a musculoskeletal pain complaint in 2012.[5] Eighty percent of the population report LBP at some time during their lives,[6] and LBP is the most common cause of work-related disability in people under 45 years of age.[7] Annual financial costs (direct medical expenses, lost income, lost productivity) of all persistent pain syndromes exceed $500 billion annually.[8] Over and above the financial cost of LBP, the human cost, in terms of suffering and impact upon quality of life, cannot be estimated.

According to the American Chronic Pain Association, "persistent" pain is a more accurate description than "chronic" pain, as the former includes information on how pain can interrupt functioning, well-being, and quality of life.[9] The term *persistent pain* therefore is used throughout this chapter. LBP is considered a condition, rather than a disease,[6] with multiple physical and psychosocial factors that impact the prognosis for recovery across the continuum of acute to persistent LBP conditions.[10] LBP not originating from serious spinal pathology or nerve root pain is often classified as "nonspecific LBP" due to our current inability to identify pathologic changes.[11] However, several classification systems have been developed to provide a framework for selecting rehabilitation interventions for the treatment of musculoskeletal LBP, including approaches to exercise.[12–15] Despite the fact that the majority of patients with isolated LBP cannot be given a precise pathoanatomic diagnosis, exercise interventions hold promise for reduction of pain and disability.[1,16,17]

Exercise for musculoskeletal LBP is just one component of a multimodal treatment program which often includes education of anatomy and pathomechanics, postural modification, body mechanics training, manual therapy, functional training, and physical modalities (e.g., thermotherapy, cryotherapy, electrical stimulation). Due to the complex nature of persistent pain, multidisciplinary interventions are often indicated which typically include exercise, relaxation training, cognitive restructuring, vocational counseling, and medication management.[18–20]

Designing an individualized exercise program is a dynamic process initially based on the patient's impairments and exercise tolerance and then adapted to address functional goals. Specific exercises are used for the purpose of addressing LBP symptoms and physical impairments. A specific exercise approach is often selected based on a movement-based diagnosis or theory of contributing pathophysiology, for example, disk pathology,[21] lack of segmental motor control,[22–25] or dysfunction in joint mechanics.[26,27] Exercise interventions designed to address body region impairments are often based on theories of movement dysfunction and muscle imbalance that contribute to mechanically induced LBP and focuses on the correction of postural alignment, modifications of faulty movement patterns, and improvement of neuromuscular control.[15,28]

As acute symptoms subside, patients should transition from specific exercises to global exercise that emphasizes fitness and prevention of relapse. Global exercise programs include components of aerobic, flexibility, strengthening, coordination, and agility exercises. A progressive exercise prescription should be incorporated as soon as the patient demonstrates adequate tolerance and regional movement control, with the ultimate goal of integrating regular exercise into the patient's daily routine.

The overall goal of rehabilitation programs for individuals with LBP is to restore function, assist patients in returning to activity and social participation, and prevent recurrence. Functional restoration involves not only improving physical performance but also the integration of skills into the individual's social and physical environments. In addition to physical factors, psychosocial, environmental, and personal factors should be taken into consideration when prescribing exercise.[29–31]

There is broad agreement that LBP and disability should be managed according to a biopsychosocial model which includes health-related, personal, psychological, and social dimensions and the interactions between them.[10,19,31] Although the origin of LBP and disability may be caused by a biologic condition, the development of persistent LBP and incapacity are subject to dominant psychosocial influences.[10] The International Classification of Functioning Disability and Health model is a biopsychosocial model designed to measure health and disability at the individual and population levels.[32]

Disability is an umbrella term for impairments, activity limitations, and participation restrictions.[33] Three dimensions related to functioning and disability include (1) body functions and structures, (2) activities at the individual level, and (3) participation in society. Impairments of body functions and structures are defined as problems with physiologic functions and/or anatomic parts, such as loss of joint range of motion or reduced muscle strength. Activity restrictions are problems with executing a task or action and reduced participation includes lessened involvement in lived situations such as work, recreation, or social activities. Contextual factors include aspects of the human-built, social, and attitudinal environments that create the lived experience of functioning and disability as well as personal factors such as sex, age, coping styles, social background, education, and overall behavior patterns that may influence how disablement is experienced by the individual.[30] Environmental factors may include physical or social barriers or facilitators to activity and participation.[32]

Changes in attitudes and beliefs may have as much impact as physiologic changes, resulting from exercise, on the activity and participation of individuals.[10,34–36] This indicates that physical, psychosocial, environmental, and personal factors should all be considered when designing individualized exercise programs (Fig. 93.1).

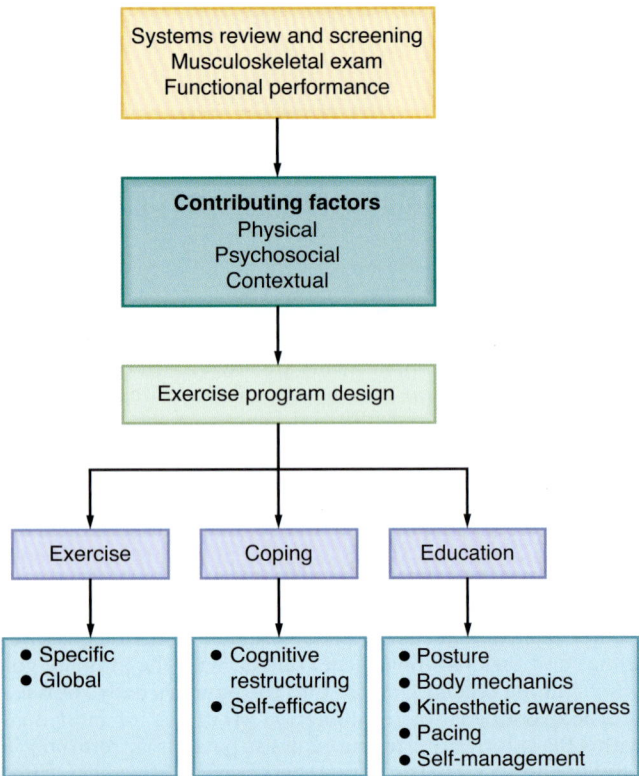

FIGURE 93.1   Patient evaluation.

Individualized Exercise Programs

MUSCULOSKELETAL EXAMINATION FOR LOW BACK PAIN

A systematic musculoskeletal examination involves the patient's history, a systems review, special tests, and measurements.[37] The goals of the clinical examination include (1) to identify contributing impairments; (2) to screen for serious medical problems and precautions related to physical activity; (3) to implement validated outcome measures; (4) to establish baseline status and assess their response to intervention; (5) to establish baseline exercise tolerance; (6) to identify barriers to activity and participation; and (7) to understand the patient's

goals, preferences, and resources to successfully follow through with in exercise program.[38]

In addition to questions regarding pain patterns and the nature of the back problems, the examination should include inquiry related to medical history (including previous musculoskeletal problems and interventions used), psychosocial issues, and environmental barriers to activities and participation. A systems review is also conducted to screen for red flags and to identify potential problem areas. Screening of the neurologic system through testing of key muscles, sensation, and reflexes is an essential component of an LBP evaluation. Current guidelines also emphasize attention to psychosocial factors, at acute through chronic stages of nonspecific LBP, that may impact rehabilitation prognosis and intervention planning.[11,39] Learning about the patient's understanding and beliefs related to their back problem is important. For example, screening for yellow flags, psychosocial factors including fear, unhelpful beliefs in severity of health conditions, catastrophizing, and poor problem solving is helpful in identifying patients at risk for persistent pain and disability.[40,41]

Anatomical structures that may contribute to pain should be tested with a systematic approach including tests of active and passive movement, tissue palpation, end range testing, repeated movements, and sustained postures.[21,37,42] Examination of a patient's postural alignment, willingness to move, body mechanics, and movement patterns should also be incorporated to gain an understanding of problems related to posture and general mobility.[37] Functional performance tests and task analysis provide information related to the ability to perform activities needed to return to activity and participation, including employment.[37,42]

The results of a comprehensive musculoskeletal examination are used to identify physical impairments and psychosocial factors for which purposeful exercise interventions can be aimed. Key elements of an individualized prescription, including exercise interventions, coping strategies, and education, are based on evaluation (Table 93.1). The patient's ability to perform specific exercises serves as an additional source of feedback for both the patient and clinician. During the acute stage of management, specific exercises are selected and modified based on the patient's responses to body position, direction of movement, and dose (intensity, duration, and frequency).

Individualizing the exercise program by mutual goal setting, to meet both physical and psychosocial needs, is essential in maximizing adherence and achieving patient satisfaction.[43] Supervision and adequate compliance are common aspects of randomized clinical trials that have demonstrated positive outcomes for exercise interventions for persistent LBP.[2]

TABLE 93.1 **Elements of Exercise Programs**		
Exercises	**Coping**	**Education**
Specific exercise modes	Cognitive restructuring	Anatomy
Neuromuscular control	Reduce fear of moving	Pathomechanics
Spinal stabilization	Clarify misconceptions	Body mechanics
Movement directional preference	Self-management	Postural alignment
Submaximal strengthening	Self-efficacy	Exercise technique
Regional mobility/flexibility		Kinesthetic awareness
Symptom reduction		Exercise progression
Global exercise modes		Activity modification
Aerobic conditioning		Pacing
Progressive resistance		
Endurance training		
General stretching		
Coordination and agility training		
Aquatic therapy		
Balance training		
Pilates		
Yoga		

DESIGNING INDIVIDUALIZED EXERCISE PROGRAMS

The purpose of exercise interventions refers to the patient's and clinician's goals: (1) specific exercises designed for symptom reduction or addressing physical impairment, for example, impaired muscle performance, joint mobility, flexibility, or kinesthetic awareness and (2) global exercises for improving overall strength, flexibility, and endurance. It is important to adapt an individualized program for the stage of management and exercise capacity.[38,44]

Depending on the stage of management, an exercise program for LBP may comprise specific exercises alone, specific and global exercises, or primarily global exercises. At any stage of management, matching the patient's baseline exercise and pain tolerance is essential to facilitate program adherence.[43]

EXERCISE RECOMMENDATIONS BASED ON THE CLINICAL COURSE

Acute Lower Back Pain

Acute pain is often defined on the basis of the duration of an episode of LBP as well as the suspicion of inflammation because signs and symptoms including pain, muscle guarding, and tissue irritability are typically present.[11,45] The acute episode is generally considered to be within 4 to 6 weeks; however, relapse or recurrence is common. During acute episodes of LBP, advice to stay active is recommended over bed rest because inactivity does not promote recovery and may even be detrimental to recovery.[10,11] Moderate-quality evidence exists for small improvements in pain relief and functional status in favor of advice to stay active in patients with acute LBP, but minimal effect has been reported in patients with sciatica.[46] In general, advice to continue typical activities and participation including work, when reasonable, is also recommended for the management of acute LBP[11]; however, modification to reduce compressive and tensile forces on injured tissues is often needed.

During the acute stage, low-intensity and specific exercises are recommended including direction-specific and submaximal isometric muscle contractions performed in a neutral spine position or within the pain-free ROM.[11,24,38,45,47] Moderate- to strong-intensity muscle contractions are poorly tolerated due to pain and inflammation.[11,45] Gentle active and/or passive exercises specific for symptom reduction are recommended during the acute stage of LBP.[38,48,49] Additional treatments such as manual therapy, electrical stimulation, and cryotherapy may be used for symptom management during the acute stage of management.[38,45]

Subacute Lower Back Pain

Subacute pain is defined as LBP persisting 4 to 12 weeks and/or reduced tissue irritability and increased tolerance for movement.[11,45] As acute pain and muscle guarding subside, impairment may persist in muscle function, motor control, postural awareness, and functional activities.[50] The patient is encouraged to gradually increase activity, performing exercises in the pain-free range to avoid further tissue irritation. Submaximal strengthening and gentle stretching can be incorporated. Progression to postural and kinesthetic awareness and education in body mechanics, ergonomics, and relaxation can also be progressed at this stage of management.[38] In addition, education on relapse prevention and self-management of acute pain episodes is important.[38] Manual therapy, electrical stimulation, and cryotherapy may be used for symptoms management during the subacute stage of management.[38,45]

RECURRENT LOWER BACK PAIN STAGE OF MANAGEMENT

Relapse of LBP after an acute episode is frequently reported.[38,51,52] In an acute exacerbation or recurring LBP exercise interventions of neuromuscular reeducation to promote dynamic (muscular) stability to maintain the involved lumbosacral structures in less symptomatic, midrange position is indicated.[38] Specific exercises to reduce symptoms and promote trunk mobility and coordination, are indicated along with promotion of activity and education to reduce the frequency and intensity of symptoms.[38]

PERSISTENT LOWER BACK PAIN STAGE OF MANAGEMENT

Persistent pain and disability are associated with physical deactivation and deconditioning, influenced by both physical and psychosocial factors.[53] Guidelines for persistent LBP emphasize promotion of activity and participation rather than a focus on protection of structures and pain relief. Supervised exercise, cognitive-behavioral therapy, body mechanics education, and progressive general fitness programs are recommended.[38,39] Current evidence suggests that exercise is an intervention with few adverse events that may improve physical function in individuals with persisting pain of musculoskeletal origin.[54] Progressive moderate- to high-intensity exercise is recommended for patients without generalized pain (due to neural sensitivity), and low- to moderate-intensity exercise for patients with conditions associated with generalized pain.[38] Behavioral interventions aimed at improving coping strategies and assisting patients in changing beliefs and attitudes about their pain in conjunction with exercise prescription are highly recommended.[38,39] In general, individualized exercise programs with regular clinician follow-up and a higher exercise dosage are associated with clinically significant improvement in function in patients with persistent LBP.[1]

During chronic (persistent) stages of LBP, some experts have recommended that exercise programs be guided not by the patient's pain complaints but instead by a predetermined stepwise system for exercise and activity progression. Fordyce[55] outlined such an approach when he applied operant conditioning principles to a graded exercise program for persons with persistent pain. An individual's tolerance to activity is achieved through the use of a quota system.

Quota Programs for Exercise Dosage

Persons with persistent pain often disengage from routine activities. A quota system is a practical approach to making baseline exercise recommendations and progressively increasing the patient's tolerance for activity. Intervention should begin with a series of baseline trials in which the patient is asked to perform a demonstrated exercise to his or her tolerance. Tolerance is defined as the point at which a patient stops exercising due to pain or fatigue. The physical therapist then establishes a quota for each prescribed exercise or activity to be performed daily. Typically, initial quotas are slightly lower than baseline trials (e.g., approximately 75% of baseline mean) and are increased by predetermined small increments (e.g., about 10% every few days). The patient is praised for meeting his or her goal. Unlike traditional exercise programs in which the patient exercises to his or her perceived tolerance, the patient instead achieves a quota. The quota system eliminates the linking of pain with function that might result in overdoing on "good days" and avoiding exercise or activity on "bad days." Rest breaks are scheduled instead of according to the patient's perceived need. Resting at the time of the individual's reported pain onset or exacerbation is avoided as it reinforces pain behaviors.[55,56] A gradual increase in activity also lessens the likelihood of an exacerbation of pain. Quota programs have been effective in increasing functional performance in persons with LBP.[57-59] Modalities (heat or cold) may be applied to prepare the patient for therapeutic exercise or to initiate activities.[4]

RELAPSE MANAGEMENT

Frequently, patients with persistent pain experience an acute pain episode or a significant exacerbation of their pain resulting from increased activity. Until the patient has recovered from the acute incident, the intensity of strength, flexibility, and aerobic conditioning exercises should be reduced, but the patient should be encouraged to maintain a tolerable level of exercise to avoid deconditioning from inactivity. The patient may return to specific exercises to manage symptoms and regain mobility. An incremental, gradual increase in conditioning exercises can then be implemented.[60] The individual should be encouraged to increase his or her use of coping and self-management strategies throughout the flare-up.[61]

THE APPLICATION OF COMMON EXERCISE APPROACHES FOR LOWER BACK PAIN

Specific Exercise

Through one-on-one evaluation and specific exercise instruction, the patient will ideally develop an understanding of principles for movement control and activity progression that will lay the foundation for progressing to a global exercise program and facilitate return to activity and participation. Specific exercise such as spinal stabilization or direction-specific exercise may play a mediating role in reactivation through mechanisms involving early symptom management, improved kinesthetic awareness, and spinal region motor control.[25,62]

Spinal Stabilization Exercise Application

Submaximal training of deep lumbar musculature for the purpose of segmental muscular stabilization and movement control has also been referred to as motor control exercise for the lumbar region.[22,25,62,63] Research suggests that local impairments in the muscle system may be a problem of motor control and coordination rather than simply a strength deficit.[38,62] Spinal stabilization is a specific exercise approach designed to enhance the control of spinal orientation and intervertebral movement via training of deep trunk muscles, specifically the lumbar multifidus and transversus abdominis[23] and sometimes also the rectus abdominis, quadratus lumborum, internal oblique abdominals, and erector spinae.[64] The ultimate goal of spinal stabilization exercises is to integrate local motor control into global functional movements, especially to prevent potential mechanical stress or pain.[64]

Spinal stabilization (or motor control) exercises should be administered with direct one-on-one supervision, sometimes using ultrasound imaging, surface electromyography, or pressure monitoring devices to provide feedback to the clinician and patient about desired muscle recruitment.[25,65] The exercises are low intensity and designed to be completed frequently throughout the day and integrated into daily activities.[23] Usually starting in the supine position with the hips and knees flexed, the therapist assists the patient in finding a neutral lumbopelvic position defined by anatomic landmarks and patient comfort. The patient is then asked to perform submaximal muscle contractions of the deep abdominal or multifidi muscles. Exercise progression proceeds from static (isometric) exercise in a supported position (supine or prone) to static exercise in less supported positions (e.g., 4-point, kneeling, or standing). The application of spinal stabilization during functional activities is emphasized across all stages of management, such as transitions from supine to sitting, sitting to standing, and ultimately to activities addressing the patient's participation goals (e.g., home, work, leisure). To facilitate improved functional mobility, the patient is instructed to perform submaximal muscle contractions during functional activities, especially when anticipating positions of potential mechanical stress.[64]

Directional Preference Exercise

Another form of specific exercise is the McKenzie approach to LBP. Exercises based on directional preference (DP) are at the foundation of the McKenzie approach.[14] DP is identified as a posture or repeated end-range movement in a single direction (flexion, extension, or side-glide/rotation) that immediately decreases lumbar midline pain or reduces the extent of referred symptoms to the extremities.[14] Exercises effective for symptom reduction are selected following a systematic examination in which the patient performs a series of repeated and sustained movements.[21] Patients are instructed to perform specific exercises that reduce peripheralization of symptoms and minimize LBP.[21] Peripheralization of symptoms occurs when movements or positions cause symptoms to radiate away from the midline of the back, into the buttock, or into the lower extremity. This applies to axial LBP as well as symptoms associated with sciatica. Centralization of symptoms occurs when symptoms move toward the midline of the spine, away from the periphery.[21,66] The patient is instructed that if centralization occurs during exercise, they are performing the exercise correctly. Conversely, exercises that cause symptoms to radiate away from the midline of the back, and perhaps into the buttock or low extremity, involve the wrong movement direction and/or incorrect position.[66]

In conjunction with DP exercises, postural correction and body mechanics instruction are a major component of an intervention using the McKenzie approach. For example, a common condition of mechanical LBP presents when pain increases during flexed postures and movements.[21,66] In this case, the patient would be assisted in an exercise progression that facilitates lumbar extension. Education to maintain posture with a bias toward lumbar extension with the use of lumbar rolls or back supports would be emphasized. Instruction would also be provided to maintain lumbar lordosis during all functional movements.

In summary, specific exercises such as DP and spinal stabilization are typically used for symptom relief, early mobility, and local motor control. Specific exercises are beneficial not only during the acute phase of management but also in addressing specific impairments at any stage of recovery. For example, a patient with persistent pain may benefit from spinal stabilization exercises along with a general strengthening and conditioning for impaired spinal region motor control.[25,67] Similarly, a patient with persistent pain may address a local impairment, through symptom reduction and improving mobility, with the use of DP exercise.[48,49] While maintaining a focus on increasing activity and participation, an individual with persistent LBP may be able to manage local impairments through the use of specific exercises.

Global Exercise

With the resolution of acute symptoms, a gradual progression to global exercise is indicated to improve strength and endurance of large muscle groups, optimize general flexibility, and increase aerobic capacity. Emphasis on neutral spine mechanics and motor control is recommended during movement and exercise activities to avoid a relapse of acute symptoms.[44] During therapy sessions, the clinician is able to provide feedback to assist patients to integrate principles of motor control and body mechanics into the performance of daily functional activities.[44] The overall goal of a global exercise program is to develop a regular exercise routine that is integrated into one's daily life and promotes well-being, prevention of injury, and enhanced activity and social participation. Matching the patient's goals and personal preferences for exercise is essential for maximizing exercise program adherence. In addition, considering physical and psychosocial barriers and facilitators to exercise is critical.[29]

A minimum of 150 minutes of aerobic exercise at moderate intensity (30 minutes per day, 5 days per week) or 60 minutes of vigorous-intensity exercise (20 minutes per day, 3 days per week) is recommended by the American College of Sports Medicine (ACSM) and the American Heart Association (AHA) to prevent chronic health conditions. Moderate intensity is defined as physical activity that involves exercising with enough intensity to raise one's heart rate and break a sweat but still be able to carry on a conversation.[68] Types of aerobic training may include brisk walking, running, cycling, or aquatic exercise. Exercise that allows partial unloading of joints such as aquatic exercises, use of an elliptical trainer, or low-resistance cycling are recommended for patients with difficulty with high-impact weight-bearing exercise (e.g., spinal stenosis, lower extremity osteoarthritis). Postural alignment as well as impact forces should be considered for all patients with LBP including education about shock-absorbing footwear and exercise surfaces. Walking and other low-impact activity (e.g., aquatic exercise) are feasible for most people, but exercise often needs to be adapted to the individual's needs.[69] Walking typically results in extension movements of the spine[15]; therefore, patients who have no change in symptoms or reduced symptoms with extension may benefit from walking, if impact force is controlled (footwear, angle of the treadmill platform, quality of the platform used). In contrast, patients demonstrating increased pain with extension movements of the spine may do better with aerobic exercises in which the spine is neutral or slightly flexed (e.g., stationary bike).

A minimal strength training intensity of 8 to 12 repetitions, 2 days per week is recommended by the ACSM and AHA for all adults.[68] Muscle-strengthening activities may include resistance exercises to strengthen major muscle groups; progressive open kinetic chain weight-training exercises (e.g., free weights, pulleys, weight machines); progressive closed kinetic chain exercises (e.g., squats, lunges, push-ups); or methods of controlled movement that target strength, flexibility, and body alignment, including Pilates and yoga.[70–72]

Recommendations regarding exercise dosage are similar for adults of all age groups, but older adults will need more attention to balance and safety issues for exercise.[68] As patients become more active, their general health improves, but the risk of musculoskeletal injury increases.[68] Therefore, guidance in pacing of activity, self-management of symptoms, and safe body mechanics are critical in facilitating ongoing activity and participation. It is essential that guidelines for exercise performance and progression be provided to each patient (Table 93.2).

TABLE 93.2 Exercise Guidelines

Exercise Guidelines for Patients

- Starting and ending position
- Exercise dosage
  - Intensity
  - Frequency
  - Duration
- Quality of movement
  - Speed
  - Accuracy
  - Movement control
- System for progression
  - Guide by symptoms and/or impairments (acute and subacute LBP)
  - Quota (persistent LBP)
  - Physiologic (e.g., heart rate)
  - Formula for progression
- Strategies to overcome barriers
  - Physical environment
  - Psychosocial environment
  - Integration into daily routine

LBP, low back pain.

Psychological and Educational Approaches

Traditional medical and rehabilitation interventions have failed to reduce persistent pain, primarily because of their focus on impairments and body structures rather than addressing the complexity of the problem.[73] Psychological and educational treatments may be used in conjunction with exercise to alleviate severe pain and associated distress, pain interference with activities, and disability.[74]

Behavioral strategies, a common intervention, assume pain and disability are influenced by psychological and social factors. Treatment emphasizes removing the underlying organic pathology, reducing disability through environmental modifications, and cognitive processes. Three behavioral interventions are used: respondent, operant, and cognitive.[57]

According to Fordyce,[55] pain behavior is classified as respondent if its onset and frequency of occurrence were due to tissue damage. Respondent treatment modifies the physiologic response directly (e.g., reduction of muscle tension). As illustrated, the patient is taught relaxation training and electromyographic biofeedback. Therapeutic exercise, physical agent modalities, splinting, adaptive equipment, and consumer education in proper posture, body mechanics, and energy conservation principles for routine activities of daily living are other respondent interventions.[61]

Operant interventions use positive reinforcement of well (healthy) behaviors (e.g., praise for exercising) and withdrawal of attention toward pain behaviors (e.g., limping), time-contingent versus pain-contingent pain management, and significant other involvement. Outcome measures for operant treatment programs have emphasized return to work, increased activity levels and participation, decreased pain-related health care utilization, reduction of pain behaviors, and increased well behaviors.[61] The previously described quota program is based on operant treatment principles.

Cognitive-behavioral strategies strive to identify and modify patient's cognitions (thoughts) regarding the pain and associated disability. Imagery, attention diversion, and modification of maladaptive thoughts (e.g., fear of pain), feelings, and beliefs can be used to restructure the negative thoughts.[75] A 2012 Cochrane review concluded that cognitive-behavioral therapy, compared with treatment as usual or wait-list control conditions, had small yet statistically significant effects on pain and disability and moderate effects on mood and catastrophizing posttreatment. By 6- to 12-month follow-up, however, the only significant effect was for mood.[73] In addition, brief educational interventions using an educational booklet have positive effects on patients' beliefs about LBP and have shown improved physical outcomes.[76]

Evidence to Support Exercise Therapy for Lower Back Pain

There is support for the efficacy of exercise interventions for LBP; however, there is not yet a clear understanding concerning which components of exercise account for its benefits. Several possible reasons exist for the lack of clarity around the efficacy of various exercise interventions, including (1) research study design and methodology problems[1,54,77]; (2) unclear definitions for acute, subacute, recurrent, and persistent (or chronic) LBP[1,50]; (3) the inclusion of heterogeneous study populations in many studies[38,54]; (4) multimodal treatment interventions in addition to exercise[1,17]; and (5) the main effect of exercise programs may be a result of factors other than physiologic changes (i.e., psychosocial factors).[34]

EVIDENCE FOR SPECIFIC EXERCISE APPROACHES
Efficacy of Spinal Stabilization Exercises

In a study by Hides et al.,[24] fewer recurrences of LBP occurred following spinal stabilization exercises for first-episode LBP patients when compared to no exercise intervention. In patients with persistent LBP, supervised trunk strengthening or stabilization exercise programs incorporating flexibility and body mechanics instruction have been shown to be more effective than a waiting list, transcutaneous electrical nerve stimulation (TENS), advice to take regular walks, or to independently complete a home program.[2] The greatest benefits of spinal stabilization occur during the initial phases of the rehabilitation process,[67] whether the stage of management is considered acute, subacute, recurrent, or persistent.[19]

Immediate or short-term benefits of incorporating spinal stabilization exercises have been shown, but there are limited long-term benefits beyond those of a general (global) exercise program. In a randomized controlled trial (RCT) involving patients with LBP, patients who participated in a spinal stabilization exercise program or manipulation treatment reported higher function and global perceived effects at 8 weeks versus patients participating in programs that included aerobic, strengthening, and stretching exercises. In addition, the immediate effect of stabilization did not differ from the effect of manipulation, and there were no between-group differences at 6- and 12 months follow-up.[25] A meta-analysis of exercise studies in patients with LBP reported that stabilization exercises were as efficient as manual therapy for reducing pain and disability.[78]

The groups performing spinal stabilization exercises in addition to global exercises had similar long-term outcomes to those performing group exercises or participating in a conventional physical therapy (PT) program (i.e., exercise, manual therapy, education, modalities).[79,80] In addition, general (or global) exercises reduced disability in the short term to a greater extent than a stabilization-enhanced exercise approach in patients with recurrent LBP.[79] Another RCT demonstrated no additional benefit, in terms of pain, function, or disability, of adding specific stabilization exercises to conventional PT treatment.[81]

Proprioceptive neuromuscular facilitation (PNF) exercises applied to the lumbar region could be considered a form of specific exercise for local neuromuscular retraining. Improved trunk range of motion, muscle endurance, and decreased pain were reported in women with persistent LBP after completing a 4-week program of PNF exercises.[82] Improvement was reported after 4 weeks of training with dynamic resistance exercises, demonstrating better outcomes than static muscle recruitment (isometric).[82]

Efficacy of Directional Preference Exercises

The application of specific exercises based on DP shows potential benefit for patients early in the rehabilitation process during the acute, subacute, and persistent stages of management.[48,49] Pooled results of four trials comparing passive therapy with McKenzie exercises for acute LBP showed a statistically significant decrease in pain and disability favoring the McKenzie approach at 1-week follow-up. At 4 weeks, however, no difference in disability levels was noted between treatments.[47] At the 12-week follow-up, patients advised to stay active produced superior results over the McKenzie exercises. A study in patients with persistent LBP to evaluate the effect of 8 weeks of the McKenzie exercise approach versus intensive dynamic strengthening showed a greater reduction in pain at 2 weeks in the McKenzie exercise group. At the 8-week and 8-month follow-up, however, there were no significant differences between groups in self-reported disability, global change of back-related quality of life, over-the-counter pain medications, or the number of visits to a general practitioner.[49] A more recent RCT in patients with persistent LBP that compared the McKenzie method to a placebo-controlled group and reported that the McKenzie group had a small but significant reduction in pain intensity (immediately after a 5-week intervention) but no difference in disability or function.[83]

EVIDENCE FOR USING CLASSIFICATION SYSTEMS FOR EXERCISE SELECTION
Matching the Exercise Program to the Patient

Treatment-based classification systems for LBP that match exercise approaches to patient baseline characteristics and impairments have been studied.[12,27,84] Patients with acute and subacute LBP who received specific exercise interventions matched to their baseline impairments (manipulation, spinal stabilization exercises, or DP exercises) showed a significantly greater improvement on a disability scale after 4 weeks of treatment than those randomly assigned to a treatment group.[67] Long et al.[48] reported significantly greater short-term (2 weeks) improvement in pain and function when patients were matched to a specific exercise direction based on symptom relief compared to those matched with the opposite direction or multidirectional exercises. Because 46% of patients were considered to have chronic complaints, it appears that exercises based on DP have the potential to produce at least short-term improvement during all stages of LBP (acute, subacute, recurrent, or persistent stages of management).[19,48] Fritz et al.[26] reported lower disability scores among patients receiving stabilization exercises who were classified with segmental hypermobility compared to those classified with segmental hypomobility.

Selecting specific exercises, based on subgroups of baseline characteristics, appears to improve outcomes for acute and subacute stages of management, but these subgroups do not hold up for persistent LBP.[67] Instead, persistent pain is more closely associated with psychosocial factors.[67] Elevated baseline scores on the Fear-Avoidance Beliefs Questionnaire[85] (indicating fear of movement) during the acute stage of LBP have been associated with altered movement patterns, activity limitations, and reduced participation at later stages of management.[36,86] A psychosocial approach to fear-avoidance beliefs involves a reduced emphasis on anatomic findings, encourages the patient to take an active role in his or her rehabilitation, and educates the patient to view back pain as a condition, rather than a serious disease, and that pain does not equal harm.[87] George et al.[87] randomly assigned patients (<8 weeks of symptoms) to receive fear-avoidance–based PT (psychosocial approach + standard care PT) or standard care PT for a 4-week intervention period. Scores on the Oswestry Disability Questionnaire[88] at 4 weeks and 6 months were found to be dependent on an interaction between the type of PT (PT + fear-avoidance approach vs. standard PT) and the initial level on the Fear-Avoidance Beliefs Questionnaire.[85] Therefore, baseline fear-avoidance beliefs remained a significant predictor of disability at 4-week and 6-month follow-up. Fear-avoidance beliefs have been found to be a significant predictor of patients' disability, even after adjusting for age, sex, and pain intensity.[36] It follows that patients with elevated levels of fear-avoidance beliefs related to their back pain may be more successful when cognitive restructuring interventions are incorporated into the delivery of exercise programs.

EVIDENCE FOR GLOBAL EXERCISE APPROACHES

Aerobic training, muscle strengthening, stretching, and skill training (e.g., work tasks, sport-specific activities) are associated with decreased pain, improved function, and reduced disability

TABLE 93.3 The Benefits of Exercise for Lower Back Pain
• Reduce risk for musculoskeletal injury
• Reduce risk of comorbidity
• Improve mood
• Increase sense of well-being
• Improve activity and participation
• Reduce the risk of reoccurrence or relapse of low back pain

TABLE 93.4	The Purpose of Specific versus Global Exercises

- Specific exercises are used for the purpose of reducing symptoms, improving mobility, and enhancing motor control. This creates the foundation for the performance of global exercises and functional activities.
- Global exercise programs encompass exercises for general fitness including aerobic, flexibility, strengthening, and endurance exercises for the purpose of promoting well-being, preventing injury, and enhancing activity and social participation. The ultimate goal is to integrate a global exercise program into one's daily routine.

in patients with LBP.[16,17] Twelve weeks, 3 times per week of moderate- to high-intensity aerobic exercise, individualized by activity type (treadmill, walking, stair climbing, cycling) and baseline fitness was more effective in reducing pain, disability, and psychological strain in individuals with chronic LBP compared to those randomized to a 12-week passive modality program (electrophysiologic agents and thermotherapy).[89] A review of exercise benefits in overweight and obese individuals with persistent LBP reported that resistance, aquatic, and Pilates exercise programs demonstrated the greatest benefits and resistance, aquatic, and walking exercises had relatively high adherence rates and minimal adverse events, suggesting that these modes of exercise may lead to better outcomes.[90]

Although the quality of evidence examining exercise for persistent LBP is low, there is consistent evidence that global exercise programs have a small to moderate effect on improving pain, physical function, and disability levels, and minimal adverse affects.[54] Yoga and Pilates programs, designed specifically for individuals with back pain, are more effective than nonexercise interventions but no more effective than other exercise interventions.[71,91,92] Taken together, this suggests that the selection of an exercise approach is best determined by considering individual preferences and capacity to exercise.

Global exercise programs are generally accepted as an effective intervention for subacute and persistent LBP, particularly when patients have been advised in program progression, self-management of symptoms, and safe body mechanics. Exercise intensity, mode, and individualization of exercise prescription have been identified as elements that positively impact outcomes in adults with persistent LBP.[1]

Conclusion

The four core topics of the chapter are summarized in Tables 93.3 through 93.6.

TABLE 93.5	Individualized Exercise Programs

- Individually designed exercise programs with a higher dose (intensity, frequency, duration) and regular follow-up are associated with improved pain, function, and disability in patients with persistent pain.
- Individualizing the exercise program by mutual goal setting to meet both physical and psychosocial needs is essential in maximizing exercise adherence and achieving patient satisfaction.
- Exercise program delivery should be adjusted to meet the patient's psychosocial needs and goals.
- Adherence and satisfaction are likely to be enhanced by considering the patient's goals, environmental barriers, interests, and preferences.
- Cognitive-behavioral strategies integrated into an exercise program may improve mood, enhance participation, and reduce disability.

TABLE 93.6	Efficacy of Exercise Interventions for Low Back Pain (LBP)

Classification Systems

- Developing subgroups or classification systems may aid in specific exercise selection.
- Physical impairments may be most important when designing exercise programs for patients during the acute and subacute stages of management.
- Psychosocial factors become more important in the management of chronic or persistent pain, although it should still be considered during acute episodes of LBP. For example, catastrophizing and fear-avoidance beliefs need to be addressed.

Specific Exercises

- Specific exercises demonstrate efficacy for short-term improvement in pain and function during the acute, subacute, recurrent, and persistent stages of management.
- Spinal stabilization exercises have not demonstrated long-term efficacy beyond that of global or general exercise programs. However, there may be clinical value at all stages of management that is not easily measured.
- Spinal stabilization exercises have demonstrated short-term benefits in all stages of management and in preventing recurrence of LBP.
- Exercises based on directional preference (e.g., McKenzie approach) show potential benefit for symptom reduction during the first few weeks of the acute, subacute, recurrent, or persistent stages of management.

Global Exercises

- Consistent small to moderate effects of global exercise programs have been reported for improvements in pain, physical function, and disability in patients with LBP, especially persistent LBP.
- Aerobic conditioning, muscle strengthening, stretching, and skill-training exercises are associated with decreased pain, improved function, and reduced disability.
- Attention to program progression, self-management of symptoms, postural alignment, and body mechanics are important for enhancing long-term activity and participation in global exercise programs.

References

1. Hayden JA, van Tulder MW, Tomlinson G. Systematic review: strategies for using exercise therapy to improve outcomes in chronic low back pain. *Ann Intern Med* 2005;142:776–785.
2. Liddle SD, Baxter GD, Gracey JH. Exercise and chronic low back pain: what works? *Pain* 2004;107:176–190.
3. Kisner C, Colby L. *Therapeutic Exercise Foundations and Techniques.* 6th ed. Philadelphia: F. A. Davis; 2013.
4. Engel JM. Relaxation and related techniques. In: Hertling D, Kessler RM, eds. *Management of Common Musculoskeletal Disorders: Physical Therapy Principles and Methods.* 4th ed. Philadelphia: Lippincott Williams & Wilkins; 2006;261–266.
5. Clarke TC, Nahin RL, Barnes PM, et al. *Use of Complementary Health Approaches for Musculoskeletal Pain Disorders among Adults: United States, 2012.* Hyattsville, MD: National Center for Health Statistics; 2016.
6. Cieza A, Stucki G. New approaches to understanding the impact of musculoskeletal conditions. *Best Pract Res Clin Rheumatol* 2004;18:141–154.
7. Deyo RA, Weinstein JN. Low back pain. *N Engl J Med* 2001;344:363–370.
8. Institute of Medicine. *Relieving Pain in America: A Blueprint for Transforming Prevention, Care, Education, and Research.* Washington, DC: National Academies Press; 2011.
9. American Chronic Pain Association. Welcome to the American Chronic Pain Association. Available at: https://theacpa.org. Accessed April 30, 2018.
10. Waddell G, Burton AK. Concepts of rehabilitation for the management of low back pain. *Best Pract Res Clin Rheumatol* 2005;19:655–670.
11. van Tulder M, Becker A, Bekkering T, et al. Chapter 3. European guidelines for the management of acute nonspecific low back pain in primary care. *Eur Spine J* 2006;15(suppl 2):S169–S191.
12. Fritz JM, Cleland JA, Childs JD. Subgrouping patients with low back pain: evolution of a classification approach to physical therapy. *J Orthop Sports Phys Ther* 2007;37:290–302.
13. Fritz JM, Delitto A, Erhard RE. Comparison of classification-based physical therapy with therapy based on clinical practice guidelines for patients with acute low back pain: a randomized clinical trial. *Spine (Phila Pa 1976)* 2003;28:1363–1372.

14. McKenzie R, Stephen M. *The Lumbar Spine Mechanical Diagnosis & Therapy.* Wellington, New Zealand: Spinal Publications New Zealand; 2003.

15. Sahrmann SA. *Diagnosis and Treatment of Movement Impairment Syndromes.* St. Louis, MO: Mosby; 2002.

16. Taylor NF, Dodd KJ, Shields N, et al. Therapeutic exercise in physiotherapy practice is beneficial: a summary of systematic reviews 2002-2005. *Aust J Physiother* 2007;53:7–16.

17. Hayden JA, van Tulder MW, Malmivaara A, et al. Exercise therapy for treatment of non-specific low back pain. *Cochrane Database Syst Rev* 2005;(3):CD000335.

18. Jousset N, Fanello S, Bontoux L, et al. Effects of functional restoration versus 3 hours per week physical therapy: a randomized controlled study. *Spine (Phila Pa 1976)* 2004;29:487–494.

19. Moffett JK, Mannion AF. What is the value of physical therapies for back pain? *Best Pract Res Clin Rheumatol* 2005;19:623–638.

20. Molton IR, Graham C, Stoelb BL, et al. Current psychological approaches to the management of chronic pain. *Curr Opin Anaesthesiol* 2007;20:485–489.

21. Donelson RG, McKenzie RA. Mechanical assessment and treatment of spinal pain. In: Frymoyer JW, ed. *The Adult Spine: Principles and Practice.* Vol 2. New York: Raven Press; 1997:1627–1639.

22. Jull GA, Richardson CA. Motor control problems in patients with spinal pain: a new direction for therapeutic exercise. *J Manipulative Physiol Ther* 2000;23:115–117.

23. Richardson CA, Jull GA. Muscle control-pain control. What exercises would you prescribe? *Man Ther* 1995;1:2–10.

24. Hides JA, Jull GA, Richardson CA. Long-term effects of specific stabilizing exercises for first-episode low back pain. *Spine (Phila Pa 1976)* 2001;26:E243–E248.

25. Ferreira ML, Ferreira PH, Latimer J, et al. Comparison of general exercise, motor control exercise and spinal manipulative therapy for chronic low back pain: a randomized trial. *Pain* 2007;131:31–37.

26. Fritz JM, Whitman JM, Childs JD. Lumbar spine segmental mobility assessment: an examination of validity for determining intervention strategies in patients with low back pain. *Arch Phys Med Rehabil* 2005;86:1745–1752.

27. Hicks GE, Fritz JM, Delitto A, et al. Preliminary development of a clinical prediction rule for determining which patients with low back pain will respond to a stabilization exercise program. *Arch Phys Med Rehabil* 2005;86:1753–1762.

28. Maluf KS, Sahrmann SA, Van Dillen LR. Use of a classification system to guide nonsurgical management of a patient with chronic low back pain. *Phys Ther* 2000;80:1097–1111.

29. Rimmer JH. Use of the ICF in identifying factors that impact participation in physical activity/rehabilitation among people with disabilities. *Disabil Rehabil* 2006;28:1087–1095.

30. Jette AM. Toward a common language for function, disability, and health. *Phys Ther* 2006;86:726–734.

31. World Health Organization. *International Classification of Functioning, Disability and Health.* Geneva, Switzerland: World Health Organization; 2001.

32. Ustun TB, Chatterji S, Bickenbach J, et al. The International Classification of Functioning, Disability and Health: a new tool for understanding disability and health. *Disabil Rehabil* 2003;25:565–571.

33. Cieza A, Stucki G, Weigl M, et al. ICF core sets for low back pain. *J Rehabil Med* 2004;44:69–74.

34. Mannion AF, Muntener M, Taimela S, et al. A randomized clinical trial of three active therapies for chronic low back pain. *Spine (Phila Pa 1976)* 1999;24:2435–2448.

35. Woby SR, Watson PJ, Roach NK, et al. Are changes in fear-avoidance beliefs, catastrophizing, and appraisals of control, predictive of changes in chronic low back pain and disability? *Eur J Pain* 2004;8:201–210.

36. Woby SR, Watson PJ, Roach NK, et al. Adjustment to chronic low back pain—the relative influence of fear-avoidance beliefs, catastrophizing, and appraisals of control. *Behav Res Ther* 2004;42:761–774.

37. Magee DE. *Orthopedic Physical Assessment.* Philadelphia: Saunders; 2002.

38. Delitto A, George SZ, Van Dillen LR, et al. Low back pain. *J Orthop Sports Phys Ther* 2012;42:A1–A57.

39. Airaksinen O, Brox JI, Cedraschi C, et al. Chapter 4. European guidelines for the management of chronic nonspecific low back pain. *Eur Spine J* 2006;15(suppl 2):S192–S300.

40. Waddell G, Somerville D, Henderson I, et al. Objective clinical evaluation of physical impairment in chronic low back pain. *Spine (Phila Pa 1976)* 1992;17:617–628.

41. Nicholas MK, Linton SJ, Watson PJ, et al; for "Decade of the Flags" Working Group. Early identification and management of psychological risk factors ("yellow flags") in patients with low back pain: a reappraisal. *Phys Ther* 2011;91:737–753.

42. Hertling D. Lumbar spine. In: Hertling D, Kessler RM, eds. *Management of Common Musculoskeletal Disorders: Physical Therapy Principles and Methods.* 4th ed. Philadelphia: Lippincott Williams & Wilkins; 2006:843–934.

43. Bergman S. Management of musculoskeletal pain. *Best Pract Res Clin Rheumatol* 2007;21:153–166.

44. Hall CM. Patient management. In: Hall CM, Thein Brody L, eds. *Therapeutic Exercise: Moving Toward Function.* 2nd ed. Philadelphia: Lippincott Williams & Wilkins; 2005:10–34.

45. Albright J, Allman R, Bonfiglio RP, et al. Philadelphia Panel evidence-based clinical practice guidelines on selected rehabilitation interventions for low back pain. *Phys Ther* 2001;81:1641–1674.

46. Dahm KT, Brurberg KG, Jamtvedt G, et al. Advice to rest in bed versus advice to stay active for acute low-back pain and sciatica. *Cochrane Database Syst Rev* 2010;(6):CD007612.

47. Machado LA, de Souza M, Ferreira PH, et al. The McKenzie method for low back pain: a systematic review of the literature with a meta-analysis approach. *Spine (Phila Pa 1976)* 2006;31:E254–E262.

48. Long A, Donelson R, Fung T. Does it matter which exercise? A randomized control trial of exercise for low back pain. *Spine (Phila Pa 1976)* 2004;29:2593–2602.

49. Petersen T, Kryger P, Ekdahl C, et al. The effect of McKenzie therapy as compared with that of intensive strengthening training for the treatment of patients with subacute or chronic low back pain: a randomized controlled trial. *Spine (Phila Pa 1976)* 2002;27:1702–1709.

50. Pengel HM, Maher CG, Refshauge KM. Systematic review of conservative interventions for subacute low back pain. *Clin Rehabil* 2002;16:811–820.

51. Bergquist-Ullman M, Larsson U. Acute low back pain in industry. A controlled prospective study with special reference to therapy and confounding factors. *Acta Orthop Scand* 1977;170:1–117.

52. Carey TS, Garrett JM, Jackman A, et al. Recurrence and care seeking after acute back pain: results of a long-term follow-up study. North Carolina Back Pain Project. *Med Care* 1999;37:157–164.

53. Verbunt JA, Seelen HA, Vlaeyen JW, et al. Disuse and deconditioning in chronic low back pain: concepts and hypotheses on contributing mechanisms. *Eur J Pain* 2003;7:9–21.

54. Geneen LJ, Moore RA, Clarke C, et al. Physical activity and exercise for chronic pain in adults: an overview of Cochrane Reviews. *Cochrane Database Syst Rev* 2017;(4):CD011279.

55. Fordyce WE. *Behavioral Methods for Chronic Pain and Illness.* St. Louis, MO: Mosby; 1976.

56. Turner J, Romano J. Psychological and psychosocial evaluation. In: Loeser J, Butler SH, Chapman CR, et al, eds. *Bonica's Management of Pain.* 3rd ed. Baltimore, MD: Lippincott Williams & Wilkins; 2001:329–341.

57. Henschke N, Ostelo RW, van Tulder MW, et al. Behavioural treatment for chronic low-back pain. *Cochrane Database Syst Rev* 2010;(7):CD002014.

58. Schwartz L, Engel JM, Jensen MP. Pain in persons with cerebral palsy. *Arch Phys Med Rehabil* 1999;80:1243–1246.

59. Keefe FJ, Williams DA, Smith SJ. Assessment of pain behaviors. In: Turk DC, Melzack R, eds. *Handbook of Pain Assessment.* 2nd ed. New York: Guilford; 2001:170–187.

60. Engel JM. Chronic pain management in the adult. In: Hertling D, Kessler RM, eds. *Management of Common Musculoskeletal Disorders: Physical Therapy Principles and Methods.* Philadelphia: Lippincott Williams & Williams; 2006:53–59.

61. Engel JM. Pain management. In: Pendleton HM, Schultz-Krohn W, eds. *Pendretti's Occupational Therapy: Practice Skills for Physical Dysfunction.* 8th ed. St. Louis, MO: Mosby; 2017:701–709.

62. Hodges PW, Richardson CA. Inefficient muscular stabilization of the lumbar spine associated with low back pain. A motor control evaluation of transversus abdominis. *Spine (Phila Pa 1976)* 1996;21:2640–2650.

63. Macedo LG, Saragiotto BT, Yamato TP, et al. Motor control exercise for acute non-specific low back pain. *Cochrane Database Syst Rev* 2016;(2):CD012085.

64. McGill SM. *Rehabilitation of the Spine: A Practitioner's Manual.* Baltimore, MD: Lippincott Williams & Williams; 2007.

65. Hides J, Richardson C, Jull G, et al. Ultrasound imaging in rehabilitation. *Aust J Physiother* 1995;41:187–193.

66. McKenzie R. *Treat Your Own Back.* Waikanae, New Zealand: Spinal Publications; 1985.

67. Brennan GP, Fritz JM, Hunter SJ, et al. Identifying subgroups of patients with acute/subacute "nonspecific" low back pain: results of a randomized clinical trial. *Spine (Phila Pa 1976)* 2006;31:623–631.

68. Garber CE, Blissmer B, Deschenes MR, et al. American College of Sports Medicine position stand. Quantity and quality of exercise for developing and maintaining cardiorespiratory, musculoskeletal, and neuromotor fitness in apparently healthy adults: guidance for prescribing exercise. *Med Sci Sports Exerc* 2011;43:1334–1359.

69. Sluka KA. *Mechanisms and Management of Pain for the Physical Therapist.* Philadelphia: Lippincott Williams & Wilkins; 2016.

70. Cramer H, Lauche R, Haller H, et al. A systematic review and meta-analysis of yoga for low back pain. *Clin J Pain* 2013;29:450–460.

71. Miyamoto GC, Costa LO, Cabral CM. Efficacy of the Pilates method for pain and disability in patients with chronic nonspecific low back pain: a systematic review with meta-analysis. *Braz J Phys Ther* 2013;17:517–532.

72. Miyamoto GC, Costa LO, Galvanin T, et al. Efficacy of the addition of modified Pilates exercises to a minimal intervention in patients with chronic low back pain: a randomized controlled trial. *Phys Ther* 2013;93:310–320.

73. Ehde DM, Dillworth TM, Turner JA. Cognitive-behavioral therapy for individuals with chronic pain: efficacy, innovations, and directions for research. *Am Psychol* 2014;69:153–166.

74. Williams AC, Eccleston C, Morley S. Psychological therapies for the management of chronic pain (excluding headache) in adults. *Cochrane Database Syst Rev* 2012;(11):CD007407.

75. Turner JA, Jensen MP. Efficacy of cognitive therapy for chronic low back pain. *Pain* 1993;52:169–177.

76. Burton AK, Waddell G, Tillotson KM, et al. Information and advice to patients with back pain can have a positive effect. A randomized controlled trial of a novel educational booklet in primary care. *Spine (Phila Pa 1976)* 1999;24:2484–2491.

77. van Tulder M, Malmivaara A, Hayden J, et al. Statistical significance versus clinical importance: trials on exercise therapy for chronic low back pain as example. *Spine (Phila Pa 1976)* 2007;32:1785–1790.

78. Gomes-Neto M, Lopes JM, Conceicao CS, et al. Stabilization exercise compared to general exercises or manual therapy for the management of low back pain: a systematic review and meta-analysis. *Phys Ther Sport* 2017;23:136–142.

79. Koumantakis GA, Watson PJ, Oldham JA. Trunk muscle stabilization training plus general exercise versus general exercise only: randomized controlled trial of patients with recurrent low back pain. *Phys Ther* 2005;85:209–225.

80. Critchley DJ, Ratcliffe J, Noonan S, et al. Effectiveness and cost-effectiveness of three types of physiotherapy used to reduce chronic low back pain disability: a pragmatic randomized trial with economic evaluation. *Spine (Phila Pa 1976)* 2007;32:1474–1481.

81. Cairns MC, Foster NE, Wright C. Randomized controlled trial of specific spinal stabilization exercises and conventional physiotherapy for recurrent low back pain. *Spine (Phila Pa 1976)* 2006;31:E670–E681.

82. Kofotolis N, Kellis E. Effects of two 4-week proprioceptive neuromuscular facilitation programs on muscle endurance, flexibility, and functional performance in women with chronic low back pain. *Phys Ther* 2006;86:1001–1012.

83. Garcia AN, Costa L, Hancock MJ, et al. McKenzie method of mechanical diagnosis and therapy was slightly more effective than placebo for pain, but not for disability, in patients with chronic non-specific low back pain: a randomised placebo controlled trial with short and longer term follow-up. *Br J Sports Med* 2018;52(9):594–600.

84. Fritz JM, Lindsay W, Matheson JW, et al. Is there a subgroup of patients with low back pain likely to benefit from mechanical traction? Results of a randomized clinical trial and subgrouping analysis. *Spine (Phila Pa 1976)* 2007;32:E793–E800.

85. Waddell G, Newton M, Henderson I, et al. A Fear-Avoidance Beliefs Questionnaire (FABQ) and the role of fear-avoidance beliefs in chronic low back pain and disability. *Pain* 1993;52:157–168.

86. Thomas JS, France CR. Pain-related fear is associated with avoidance of spinal motion during recovery from low back pain. *Spine (Phila Pa 1976)* 2007;32:E460–E466.

87. George SZ, Fritz JM, Bialosky JE, et al. The effect of a fear-avoidance-based physical therapy intervention for patients with acute low back pain: results of a randomized clinical trial. *Spine (Phila Pa 1976)* 2003;28:2551–2560.

88. Fairbank JC, Pynsent PB. The Oswestry Disability Index. *Spine (Phila Pa 1976)* 2000;25:2940–2952.

89. Murtezani A, Hundozi H, Orovcanec N, et al. A comparison of high intensity aerobic exercise and passive modalities for the treatment of workers with chronic low back pain: a randomized, controlled trial. *Eur J Phys Rehabil Med* 2011;47:359–366.

90. Wasser JG, Vasilopoulos T, Zdziarski LA, et al. Exercise benefits for chronic low back pain in overweight and obese individuals. *PMR* 2017;9:181–192.

91. Wieland LS, Skoetz N, Pilkington K, et al. Yoga treatment for chronic non-specific low back pain. *Cochrane Database Syst Rev* 2017;(1):CD010671.

92. Yamato TP, Maher CG, Saragiotto BT, et al. Pilates for low back pain. *Cochrane Database Syst Rev* 2015;(7):CD010265.

CHAPTER 94

Complementary and Integrative Health

CHARLES A. SIMPSON

This chapter looks at therapies that historically have been classified as being "unorthodox," "complementary," or "alternative" to conventional medical interventions for pain. A contemporary definition of "complementary and integrative health" (IH) will be considered in the context of the complex and clinically challenging field of evidence-based pain medicine. A rationale for studying these unorthodox treatments of pain is presented. The challenges of an evidence-based approach to incorporating these "integrative" therapies into pain management are explored. And finally, a brief survey of several commonly available complementary and IH therapies and the evidence regarding their utility in pain treatment are provided.

What Is Complementary and Integrative Health?

Identifying and defining nonmainstream approaches to health and healing have been problematic for decades. How these various professions, therapies, and approaches to healing have been characterized by the dominant, conventional medical mainstream is emblematic of the history of antagonisms and misunderstandings between the two. How the IH disciplines have come to define themselves is also instructive of both their differences and similarities. Drawing meaningful distinctions between conventional biomedicine and the array of alternative methods may be useful to illuminate how each can contribute to better care for patients in pain.

Integrative medicine practitioners tend to consider their approaches as holistic and in contrast to a reductionistic approach that is ascribed to modern, specialty-driven biomedicine. Holistic practitioners use

> Rather than focusing on illness or specific parts of the body, this ancient approach to health considers the whole person and how he or she interacts with his or her environment. It emphasizes the connection of mind, body, and spirit. The goal is to achieve maximum well-being, where everything is functioning the very best that is possible. With Holistic Health people accept responsibility for their own level of well-being, and everyday choices are used to take charge of one's own health.[1]

In contrast, the reductionist approach of conventional medicine (CM) adheres to the theory that every complex phenomenon in medicine can be explained by reducing the complexity of health and disease into simple, basic, physical mechanisms and applying a treatment intended to correct the abnormalities, primarily through the use of drugs and surgery.

The Divide

The emergence of organized medicine early in the last century marginalized a large number of existing healing disciplines at that time. Some of these had enjoyed long and successful traditions treating the public. As Cohen[2] points out,

> Although American colonies began with pluralistic notions of health care, the poor state of science, paltry qualifications of many would-be physicians, general lack of medical

standards, and a cornucopia of charlatans eventually led to state regulation of healers—largely through the mechanism of licensure—and thereby to the triumph of biomedicine over competing communities of healers such as naturopathic and homeopathic physicians. Legally, state statutes made unlawful practice of medicine a crime and defined medicine in broad terms, encompassing any activity that potentially could be construed as diagnosis and treatment.

As a result, Western, scientific, reductionist biomedicine became the "real" medicine in legal terms. The resulting cultural authority of CM discounted traditional healers. The hegemony of this dominant paradigm was not seriously challenged until the last few decades of the 20th century.

FRINGE MEDICINE AND QUACKERY

In the early 1960s, British author Brian Inglis developed a model in his book entitled *Fringe Medicine*.[3] This title consigned nonstandard approaches to healing to the periphery of science and the health care system. Inglis[3] considered such professions as homeopathy, bone setting, herbalists, and psychotherapy as fringe medicine. Being on the fringe implied that healers of this stripe were so far removed from the mainstream as to pose no threat to the public or to the dominance of biomedicine.

In the succeeding 30 years, many of these fringe approaches to healing persisted and grew despite persistent opposition from the dominant medical establishment. For example, in the 1950s, the American Medical Association (AMA) developed ethics policies that forbade physicians from interacting with "unscientific, cult practitioners" such as chiropractors. The AMA Committee on Quackery was formed in 1963 targeting vitamins, homeopathy, chiropractic, naturopathy, all alternative cancer treatments, and other practices which compete with the drug sales of pharmaceutical companies.[4] The chiropractic profession fought back in the courts. In the case of *Wilk v. American Medical Association*, the AMA was found to have engaged in an unlawful restraint of trade under the Sherman Antitrust Act. And although the AMA's Committee on Quackery was disbanded, other groups have taken up the charge to criticize and marginalize these therapies (see http://www.quackwatch.com).

"UNORTHODOX" MEDICINE

This unhappy stand-off persisted until Eisenberg et al.'s[5] seminal study in 1993 revealed the depth and breadth to which these fringe practices had penetrated health care delivery. This paper reported a survey of respondents' use of a variety of what Eisenberg termed "*unorthodox medical practice*." These were defined by Eisenberg in exclusionary terms, that is, in terms of what these therapies are *not*. Unorthodox medicine in Eisenberg's view is *not* taught in medical schools, *not* available in hospitals, and *not* generally considered real medicine.

Today, neither of these perspectives, fringe or unorthodox, provide meaningful distinctions between mainstream conventional biomedicine and those forms of healing that are different. Neither perspective bears up to careful scrutiny of the current state of complementary and alternative medicine. Eisenberg et al.[5] amply demonstrated that the volume of visits for health

TABLE 94.1 Terminology	
Conventional medicine	A system in which medical doctors and other health care professionals (such as nurses, pharmacists, and therapists) treat symptoms and diseases using drugs, radiation, or surgery. Also called allopathic medicine, biomedicine, mainstream medicine, orthodox medicine, and Western medicine.
Alternative medicine	"Alternative" connotes that these alternative treatments are used in place of conventional medicine.
Complementary medicine	A group of diagnostic and therapeutic disciplines that are used together with conventional *medicine* in the management of disease.
CAM	*Complementary and alternative medicine* (CAM) is the popular term for health and wellness therapies that have typically not been part of conventional Western medicine.
Integrative medicine	There are many definitions of "integrative" health care, but all involve bringing conventional and complementary approaches together in a coordinated way.
Complementary and integrative health	An integrative approach aims to enhance overall health, prevent disease, and alleviate debilitating symptoms such as pain and stress and anxiety management that often affects patients coping with complex and chronic disease.
Integrative health	A collaborative approach to health care delivery that is characterized by a high level of communication between patients and their health care providers as well as between their conventional and integrative health providers.

care delivered outside of the orthodox mainstream exceeds that of conventional care provided in physician offices—hardly an image of a fringe factor in the overall picture of the health care delivery system.

The popularity of complementary medicine with the public has not gone unnoticed by conventional medical institutions either. Health insurance plans, hospitals, and academic medical centers have integrated, to one extent or another, nontraditional health care providers and therapies into their programs. A 2001 survey of regional health plans in the northeast United States found nearly universal coverage for chiropractic, with just under half of insurers covering acupuncture (usually for chronic pain) and massage therapy (MT).[6] A 2005 American Hospital Association survey revealed that 370 of 1,394 respondent institutions (26.5%) offer some form of complementary health care.[7] A similar survey in 2010 found 42% of responding hospitals offered at least one integrative medicine service.[8]

Integrative medicine topics are being introduced into the curricula of up to 64% of US medical schools.[9] The American Medical Student Association has developed the Educational Development for Complementary and Alternative Medicine program to promote medical school education on alternative medicine topics. The Academic Consortium for Integrative Medicine and Health is composed of 69 academic medical centers and health plans including Harvard, Duke, Stanford, Thomas Jefferson, and Yale medical schools as well as health plans including Cleveland Clinic, Mayo Clinic, Memorial Sloan Kettering, and Veterans Health Administration. The stated mission of the consortium is to "advance integrative medicine and health through academic institutions and health systems." With a vision of "a transformed healthcare system promoting integrative medicine and health for all."[10]

These developments indicate the trend of increasing integration of conventional and integrative medicine. Contemporary integrative medicine has moved well beyond the "unorthodox" label offered by Eisenberg.

COMPLEMENTARY AND ALTERNATIVE MEDICINE

The fringe and unorthodox labels are a carryover from more contentious times. Over time, other labels have included "nontraditional" medicine in supposed contrast to traditional conventional medical care. However, considering that some of these nontraditional therapies predate conventional interventions, for example in the case of acupuncture by 3,000 years, traditional versus nontraditional seems irrational. "Integrative" and "integrated" medicines have had some currency as well. The term *alternative medicine* suggests that the therapies are used in place of CM. *Integrative medicine* often refers to alternative medicine therapies delivered by CM practitioners

or at least in conventional medical settings. *Integrated medicine* implies the thoughtful collaboration of conventional and alternative medicine providers in the treatment of patients. The notion of *complementary medicine* is supported by evidence showing that most patients use both conventional and complementary interventions, seeking to integrate their own care. The favored terminology until 2015 by the National Institutes of Health (NIH) has been *complementary and alternative medicine* (CAM) with the National Center for Complementary and Alternative Medicine (NCCAM) (Table 94.1).

COMPLEMENTARY AND INTEGRATIVE HEALTH

Recognition of the growing volume of integrative medicine use, the accumulating research evidence, and how patients actually use the medicine ultimately led to a name change for NCCAM. The December 2014 Congressional omnibus budget measure renamed the Center the National Center for Complementary and Integrative Health (NCCIH). As the Center's Web site notes,

> The change was made to more accurately reflect the Center's research commitment to studying promising health approaches that are already in use by the American public. Since the Center's inception, complementary approaches have grown in use to the point that Americans no longer consider them an alternative to medical care. For example, more than half of Americans report using a dietary supplement, and Americans spend nearly four billion dollars annually on spinal manipulation therapy. The name change is in keeping with the Center's existing Congressional mandate and is aligned with the strategic plan currently guiding the Center's research priorities and public education activities.[11]

BRIDGING THE DIVIDE: ONE KIND OF MEDICINE

The work of NCCIH is reflective of increasing the quality of research-focused complementary and IH interventions. The current trend toward evidence-based medicine (EBM) may eventually point the way to a reconception and resolution of the distinction between CM and IH. IH is frequently dismissed by critics as being unscientific and without evidence of its safety, efficacy, and effectiveness. However, over the last decade, the emergence of complementary medicine on the national research agenda through the NCCIH and other institutions has furthered the development of academic and intellectual infrastructure of IH that can explore the scientific evidence which demonstrates the utility of complementary therapies.

Originally formed as the Office of Complementary Medicine, the federal budget for NCCIH grew from $2 million in fiscal year 1992 to $121.4 million in fiscal year 2007. The body of research is growing. There are currently thousands of clinical trials of IH interventions. A 2000 survey of over 5,000 controlled trials found "The overall quality of evidence for IH RCTs is poor but improving slowly over time, *about the same as that of biomedicine* [emphasis added]."[12] Systematic reviews of the IH literature are prevalent. There are hundreds of Cochrane Collaboration reviews of alternative therapies (see http://www.cochranelibrary.com/topic/Complementary%20%26%20alternative%20medicine/).

Angell and Kassirer[13] noted several years ago in *The New England Journal of Medicine* editorial that in the future, medicine will be divided into those approaches to health and healing that are backed by scientific evidence and those that are not. They conclude that "there cannot be two kinds of medicine—conventional and alternative. There is only medicine that has been adequately tested and medicine that has not, medicine that works and medicine that may or may not work. Once a treatment has been tested rigorously, it no longer matters whether it was considered alternative at the outset."

A 2005 Institute of Medicine report on complementary medicine emphasizes, "The committee recommends that the same principles and standards of evidence of treatment effectiveness apply to all treatments, whether currently labeled as conventional medicine or CAM."[14] This evidence-based perspective will continue to erode the barriers between health care that is provided in the tradition of Western scientific medicine and the healing disciplines that, in some instances, predate modern medicine by millennia. This perspective may well put to rest the arbitrary and, at times, antagonistic differentiation between IH and CM.

WHAT IS DIFFERENT ABOUT COMPLEMENTARY AND ALTERNATIVE MEDICINE?

There clearly are differences between health care available in conventional medical physician offices, clinics, and hospitals and that provided by IH practitioners. There are three features of IH that tend to distinguish it from CM. In general, IH therapies are individualized to each patient rather than using a standardized clinical protocol. IH almost universally incorporates a philosophy of health that emphasizes and leverages the innate capacity for healing in every individual. And finally, IH tends to acknowledge the existence of properties of living systems that are resistant to understanding by contemporary reductionist scientific methods of inquiry.

These distinguishing features present significant challenges to research methods and thus to assembling meaningful evidence. They also create opportunities to develop more effective, efficient, and humanizing care for a very difficult population of patients—especially those with pain. Some have recognized the limitation of CM. For example, an editorial observation by Cicerone[15] on evidence-based practice and the limits of rational rehabilitation points out that "we need to acknowledge the subjective meanings of illness and disability to the patients we serve. Any efforts to build our practice based on the best available systematic evidence are unlikely to succeed unless we include patients' values and beliefs and incorporate this perspective into our rehabilitation research. This aspect of evidence-based rehabilitation raises important questions about our fundamental roles and how we will choose to practice and define our field in the future."

Individualized treatment is a hallmark of most IH therapies. For example, an acupuncture practitioner may evaluate two patients, both with the same CM diagnosis, but develop two radically different treatment plans based on the oriental medicine (OM) examination findings and assessment. This approach seems to work well for patients as revealed by observational studies. Studies of patients who obtain care from IH practitioners reveal high levels of satisfaction with the practitioners and the outcome of the therapies. IH providers spend time with their patients, and they are successful in explaining to patients the nature of their health problems. Treatment planning tends to be collaboration between therapist and patient. Interventions are developed that are consistent with each patient's own needs and preferences.

Philosophy of care is not something that most CM practitioners ponder extensively. However, philosophical discourse underlies many IH therapies. Chiropractic, for example, contains an extensive literature that can only be described as philosophy. Beginning with the founder, D. D. Palmer, chiropractic thinkers have historically focused on not so much the rational scientific underpinnings of this healing art but on the art itself. Innate intelligence is posited by Palmer and his successors as a fundamental life force that when fully expressed without interference, maximized expression of health occurs, naturally and without need of intrusion from outside agents like drugs and surgery. In this chiropractic philosophical worldview, the aim of the chiropractor is to locate and correct interferences with this natural expression of the life force. Other IH disciplines have identified this life force known as "qi" in acupuncture and oriental medicine (AOM), "prana" in yoga, "doshas" in Ayurvedic medicine, and "vix medica naturae" in naturopathic medicine, each discipline has elaborated some measure of a conceptual life force that guides and propels healing and health.

CM, with its intellectual traditions anchored in Western scientific thought, is understandably skeptical of notions of innate intelligence, qi, or other conceptualization of a putative life force. Finding no testable hypotheses to investigate a possible life force, CM has largely dismissed such philosophical musing. Oschman[16] provides a comprehensive review of this seeming impenetrable intellectual barrier between the IH and CM worldviews.

WHO USES COMPLEMENTARY AND INTEGRATIVE HEALTH?

The research on IH utilization is often confusing and contradictory. Research is complicated by a number of factors, including a lack of consensus on what therapies, interventions, and practitioner types constitute IH. Varying methodologies for collecting data, the variety of populations, and settings in which data are gathered provide sometimes contradictory conclusions. Further challenges to IH research is when it is studied in different countries where the availability of IH may vary considerably due to tradition, licensure, and cultural acceptance.

However, despite the inconsistent nature of research efforts, it is certain that IH use is widespread across populations, clinical conditions, settings, and sociodemographic groups. In 1993, Eisenberg and colleagues'[5] paper alerted the CM community to the magnitude of IH utilization. This discovery revealed an ongoing phenomenon in the general population that has been verified and replicated in many subpopulations. A search of PubMed for "IH utilization" returned over 1,500 citations.[17] These include abstracts referring to various clinical populations (cancer, inflammatory bowel disease, autoimmune deficiency syndrome, diabetes, hypertension, allergies, rheumatic conditions, chronic fatigue, fibromyalgia, emergency department patients) and sociodemographic groups (veterans, racial and ethnic groups, geriatrics, women, children, athletes). In short, no matter what population is examined, IH use is prevalent.

IH use is particularly widespread among patients with chronic pain conditions. Nayak et al.[18] reported on a small sample of spinal cord injury patients with chronic pain. About 40% of respondents had used some form of IH during the preceding year. Forty-four percent of chronic pain patients being treated with opioids reported concomitant IH use.[19] Twenty-seven percent of veterans with cancer or chronic pain reported IH use.[20] More veterans would have used IH had it been covered by insurance.

Tsao et al.[21] found that, given a choice of several IH interventions, over 60% of pediatric patients (and their parents) opted to try at least one IH approach in addition to CM treatments. A survey of 43 pediatric anesthesia fellowship training programs showed 38 (86%) offered one or more IH therapies.[22]

CATEGORIZING COMPLEMENTARY AND INTEGRATIVE HEALTH THERAPIES

There is considerable diversity in IH practices and deciding which discipline to include under the rubric IH and which to exclude can be problematic and markedly affects the study results of IH utilization. In 1993, Eisenberg et al.[5] limited his survey inquiries to 16 commonly used interventions but included "relaxation therapy . . . lifestyle diets, spiritual or religious healing by others." Eisenberg et al.[5] do note a categorical difference, however, between IH therapies that are delivered by a professional, such as massage and acupuncture, and those that are largely self-administered without the involvement of a trained and licensed provider, such as lifestyle diets and intercessory prayer. Hospitals reporting the integration of IH most frequently identify massage, body movement therapies (qigong, yoga, tai chi), relaxation, acupuncture, guided imagery, and therapeutic touch (TT) as the IH modalities of choice.[7] Conspicuous by their absence from the hospitals are some of the most frequently encountered IH modalities, such as chiropractic, nutraceutical, and herbal therapies.

NCCIH has categorized IH in two domains: natural products such as nutritional supplements, probiotics, and herbs and mind–body interventions such as massage, yoga, manipulation, acupuncture, and movement therapies.[23] The array of CAM therapies can be further categorized by their intellectual and philosophical nature as being either essentially biologically based or energy-based. Biologically based therapies are explained and practiced fundamentally in ways that are familiar to practitioners trained in the CM model of Western scientific inquiry. Clinical conditions are mostly described in terms of disturbed anatomy and physiology. Treatment interventions are categorized by their physiologic effects. Outcomes are measured in objective clinical terms. These disciplines, such as chiropractic and natural medicine, often view themselves as being within the context of orthodox scientific thought. Many chiropractors, for example, have rejected the theories of Palmer. Some of these therapies have been rigorously scrutinized through the lens of conventional medical scientific investigation. Many of these disciplines are developing intellectual, administrative, and physical infrastructure to conduct research in the mold of CM as part of a commitment to evidence-based practices.

In contrast, energy-based therapies are most often founded on putative notions of natural systems of "invisible energetic relations and connections that govern living form and function."[16] Although some of these energy-based therapies have undergone scientific inquiry, most notably acupuncture, the fundamental worldview of energy-based healers has not been altered to conform to the understandings offered by rational reductionist methods. For example, science has attempted to understand the physiologic basis of acupuncture in terms of its neuroendocrine effects. However, few acupuncture practitioners endorse or, more importantly, practice within this intellectual context. Most acupuncture practitioners prefer instead to explain what they do in the language of AOM, such as the flow of chi throughout the meridians of the body.

For purposes of the discussion in this chapter, consideration of IH therapies is limited to those commonly accessible in the community to chronic pain patients and, for the most part, administered under the guidance of licensed health care professionals. Although this approach may exclude some valuable and frequently used therapies, it does encompass IH therapies that are in regular use by chronic pain patients, have been evaluated by research, are at least somewhat institutionalized, have been used or referred to by CM providers, and are capable of being integrated clinically and administratively into the CM care of chronic pain patients.

Why Consider Complementary and Integrative Health Therapies in Pain Management?

There is a compelling case for why CM physicians, especially in the challenging field of pain medicine, should better understand IH therapies. Based on the study results of IH utilization, it is quite likely that any given pain patient is using at least one IH therapy concurrently with CM treatments. Clinical inquiry into IH use is important because patients often fail to reveal their use of IH therapies to their CM providers. There are potential complications that arise with the combination of IH and CM therapies, and awareness of these enhances safety and quality of care. Understanding the rationale for and evidence that supports IH use in pain conditions places the clinician in a helpful role of providing objective information to pain patients. And, perhaps most significantly, integration of IH therapies can be effective and improve the quality of care for chronic pain patients.

Some 50 million Americans suffer from chronic or severe pain.[24] It is estimated that 40% of them fail to achieve adequate relief.[25] Surveys of IH users note a high prevalence of chronic conditions, including chronic pain. Observers of IH note that "consumers will continue to use IH, particularly in chronic conditions, in which patients struggle to find any treatment that may cure their condition or improve their quality of life."[26]

Most IH interventions are "low-tech, high-touch" in nature. They are often perceived as inherently safe and natural by patients and practitioners. However, there is a growing body of evidence that illuminates adverse reactions to commonly used IH therapies either by themselves or when combined with CM. Drug–herb interactions, for example, present potential challenges to patient safety and compromises of therapeutic intent. In 1993, Eisenberg noted that patients use IH and CM concurrently for the same condition upward of 83% of the time however IH users failed to disclose IH use to CM physicians. Subsequent investigation by Eisenberg et al.[27] indicates that this failure to disclose has not improved over time. Better understanding by both CM and IH practitioners of risks can modify the potential for adverse outcomes.

Avoiding adverse CM–IH interactions can obviously improve patient care. Asking patients about their use of IH, especially from an objective and evidence-based perspective, can enhance patient communication. The cultural competency of being able to provide nonjudgmental acknowledgment of IH use, particularly when it can be supported by objective evidence of safety and effectiveness, can reinforce a productive therapeutic relationship between patients and their CM physician.

It is well recognized that effective physician–patient communication is a critical element in predicting better patient satisfaction and compliance with chronic pain treatment.[28] Moreover, as reliable evidence of IH effectiveness emerges, CM physicians may be in a position to better integrate evidence-based IH approaches in an active manner rather than passively accepting what chronic pain patients may already be attempting to integrate on their own.

CHALLENGES OF EVIDENCE-BASED COMPLEMENTARY AND ALTERNATIVE MEDICINE THERAPIES

Developing the evidence about IH therapies for chronic pain is problematic from a number of perspectives. IH therapies are often inherently resistant to analysis by commonly used clinical research methods. For example, in the hierarchy of evidence, the randomized controlled trial (RCT) is considered to be the criterion standard. Yet, many argue that this methodology, although well suited to the study of drugs, may not be the best research design to study complex, individualized treatments routinely offered by CAM practitioners.[29,30]

For instance, trials of manipulative therapy have been plagued by the difficulty in developing a "sham" manipulation and concurrently controlling for the nonspecific effects of the hands-on practitioner–patient interaction with the theoretically inert sham treatment. Similarly, acupuncture research using sham acupuncture points irritates acupuncture practitioners who note that any needling at any point on the body affects the flow of chi and therefore cannot be considered an inert intervention in the same way that a placebo pill is used in a clinical trial of drug therapy. Functional magnetic resonance imaging and positron emission tomography imaging studies have demonstrated brain changes with sham acupuncture procedures compared to "true" acupuncture.[31]

Furthermore, evidence about treatment interventions for chronic pain is confounded by the complex nature of the condition itself. Patient selection is often a significant challenge to study validity. For example, aggregating patients with mechanical low back pain (LBP) into a conceptually uniform study group may satisfy a study methodology, but it ignores the wide variety of disorders that produce this pain population. Given this clinical heterogeneity, it is no wonder that trials with this fundamental design flaw frequently come up with equivocal results and fail to reveal significant differences in effectiveness between treatments. A conventional medical analog would be treating undifferentiated chest pain as gastroesophageal reflux disease (GERD).

The challenges of applying evidence of this nature to the practical realities of treating patients have been increasingly recognized.[32] Fortunately, researchers in the IH fields are actively developing research methodologies that are more appropriate both for the individualized nature of CAM interventions and the complex, multifactorial nature of chronic pain. Pragmatic controlled trials, for example, evaluate interventions in real-world settings that involve the specific effects of the intervention as well as the nonspecific effects of the therapeutic relationship, expectations, values, and beliefs that combine to affect the clinical outcomes of interest.

Publication and indexing biases also are obstacles to assembling high-quality evidence about IH therapies.[32] As is the case with CM, studies with positive results are more likely to be submitted for publication. Many studies of IH are in foreign language journals, thus limiting their exposure to English-speaking audiences. A subtler bias also is observed in CM-published research on IH. As one IH researcher put it, "A negative study of acupuncture concludes that 'acupuncture doesn't work.' The analogue would be a negative drug trial that concluded 'pharmaceuticals do not work'" (R. Hammerschlag, personal communication, February 20, 2005).

Despite these challenges in developing an evidence-based approach to the use of IH therapies in chronic pain conditions, clinical evidence is accumulating. Many formerly unproven and unscientific therapies have, in fact, been shown to be safe and effective. Achieving the goal of Angell and Kassirer's[13] "one kind of medicine" is becoming a reality in health care and in the treatment of chronic pain.

The Complementary and Integrative Health Therapies: The Evidence

The following is a brief overview of commonly available IH therapies and the evidence that supports them. Evidence from systematic reviews, especially from the Cochrane Collaboration (http://www.cochrane.org), and from clinical practice guidelines is noted. These therapies are categorized as biologically based and energy-based.

BIOLOGICALLY BASED THERAPIES

These therapies are based mainly on concepts of biology and physiology commonly accepted in conventional biomedicine. These therapies rely on clinical theories, therapeutic approaches, and rationales that are couched in terms consistent with current scientific understanding of biology and physiology familiar to CM.

Manipulation

Manipulation is the most frequently used IH therapy.[33] It is widely practiced by a variety of specialties including doctors of chiropractic (DC), osteopathic physicians (DO), medical doctors (MD), physical therapists, and some lay practitioners. It is estimated that DCs deliver over 90% of all manipulative therapy.[34] According to the 2007 National Health Interview Survey (NHIS), patients spent an estimated $3.9 billion on visits to practitioners for chiropractic or osteopathic manipulation.[35] Chiropractic training in manipulative techniques is arguably the most extensive among manipulation practitioners.

Manipulation is thought to improve pain by locating and treating disturbed joint and muscle function described as dysfunction, subluxation, fixation, and other terminology that may vary by discipline, training, and technique. Manipulation practitioners primarily treat spine pain and dysfunction, but these techniques are also applied to the rest of the musculoskeletal system.

Historically, manipulation has also been applied to nonmusculoskeletal disorders. It is hypothesized that somatoautonomic reflexes activated by manipulation can modulate visceral function. This linkage has not been elucidated nor confirmed in the paucity of current research. Despite the lack of a comprehensive neurobiologic rationale, there have been some studies that suggest weak but favorable evidence for positive effects of manipulation for a number of conditions including asthma, hypertension, infantile colic, otitis media, cervicogenic vertigo, and others.[36]

Of the CAM therapies, manipulation has been studied the most extensively. NCCIH has identified over 500 clinical trials of manipulative and other body work therapies such as massage. Although the results are often and predictably inconclusive, there is clear evidence that manipulation is superior to sham treatment and equivalent to other conservative interventions for acute spinal pain.[34] Systematic reviews of acute and chronic LBP conclude that the evidence supporting manipulation is on par with other interventions typically employed in conventional medical practice.[37,38] Other systematic reviews show long-term benefit for neck pain,[39] headaches,[40] and chronic mechanical spine pain.[41]

A 2007 clinical practice guideline from the American Pain Society (APS) and the American College of Physicians (ACP) recommends manipulation, among other IH treatments, for both acute and chronic LBP.[42] An updated 2017 ACP systematic review and clinical practice guideline reinforced the recommendations for nonpharmacologic interventions for acute and chronic LBP including manipulation as well as yoga, tai chi, acupuncture, and MT. The ACP systematic review concluded, ". . . several non-pharmacologic therapies for low back pain were associated with small to moderate, primarily short-term effects on pain."[43] In contrast, the ACP review of drug therapy concluded, "Several systemic medications for low back pain are associated with small to moderate, primarily short-term effects on pain."[44] Of interest as well is a 2016 Cochrane review[45] that ". . . found high quality evidence that paracetamol [acetaminophen] is no better than placebo for relieving acute low back pain . . ." and despite practice guidelines and recommendations that include acetaminophen as a first-line treatment.

Therapeutic Massage

MT encompasses more than 150 named body work systems and perhaps thousands of variations and individual techniques. Therapeutic, clinical, or medical massage is engaged to treat specific clinical conditions. The physiologic effects of massage are well documented, including muscular relaxation, improved blood and lymph circulation, and neuro-hormonal-immunologic effects.

There are numerous clinical trials of massage for pain. However, clinical trials of MT are difficult methodologically because of the impossibility of blinding subjects or therapists, a lack of an effective placebo and often small numbers of subjects in the trials. Physical Medicine and Rehabilitation Clinics of North America reviewed therapeutic massage in 1999. A 2007 review concluded that there is robust evidence in favor of MT for chronic LBP and more modest support for massage in the treatment of chronic headache, shoulder pain, mixed pain conditions, fibromyalgia, and carpal tunnel syndrome.[46]

A recent Cochrane Review of massage for LBP concluded that although the evidence was of generally low quality, MT did provide short-term improvement in pain for acute, subacute, and chronic LBP. Short-term improvement in function was also observed.[47] An "evidence map" developed by the Veterans Affairs identified some high-quality systematic reviews that noted "potential benefits" for pain related to labor, shoulder, neck, back, cancer, fibromyalgia, and temporomandibular joint.[48] Reported methods often do not qualify the type of MT provided. A recent review of complementary health approaches to pain management in the September 2016 Mayo Clinic Proceedings concluded that the preponderance of positive versus negative trials of MT showed at least short-term benefit for neck pain. Lower quality trials showed benefit for LBP as well.[49]

Natural Medicine Therapies

A number of IH interventions use nutritional supplements and herbs (known collectively as nutraceuticals) in the treatment of chronic pain. Although these natural medicine approaches are most commonly identified with naturopathic physicians (ND), herbs and supplements are frequently used by acupuncture/OM and chiropractic providers as well. Many nutraceutical interventions are thought to modify disturbed metabolism that underlie chronic pain conditions such as fibromyalgia. Although much nutraceutical information on the Internet is proprietary and commercial in nature, there are evidence-based sources of information for a number of painful conditions.[50]

Natural medicine can be used directly for analgesia (white willow bark, for example), anti-inflammatories (omega-3 fatty acids), and antispasmodics (valerian and passiflora are examples). Nutritional and herbal interventions are most commonly applied to modify perceived underlying physiologic disturbances such as fibromyalgia, depression, osteoarthritis, and rheumatoid arthritis.[50] Of commonly used nutritional approaches, glucosamine and chondroitin sulfate have been most extensively studied. Glucosamine has been shown to slow cartilage deterioration and relieve pain in knee osteoarthritis.[51,52] A 2014 Cochrane review concluded that some herbal preparations (cayenne, devils claw, white willow bark) reduced LBP more than placebo and in one (white willow bark) about the same as rofecoxib.

Body Awareness Therapy

A number of approaches to chronic pain treatment involve the idea of improving postural coordination by using conscious processes to alter automatic postural coordination and ongoing muscular activity. These body awareness therapies (BAT) may be practiced by physical and occupational therapists, massage therapists, as well as nonlicensed body work professionals. Two common BAT have been described: Alexander technique (AT) and Feldenkrais method (FM).

AT is described as "a method that works to change (movement) habits in our everyday activities. It is a simple and practical method for improving ease and freedom of movement, balance, support, and coordination. The technique teaches the use of the appropriate amount of effort for a particular activity, giving you more energy for all your activities. It is not a series of treatments or exercises, but rather a reeducation of the mind and body."

A 2003 systematic review of AT revealed few high-quality RCTs but noted promising results with Parkinson disease and back pain.[53] A 2008 RCT published in *BMJ* conducted a cost-effectiveness analysis of a number of body work interventions and concluded that AT followed by exercise was the most clinically effective and cost-effective intervention.[54] A more recent systematic review found "strong evidence" supporting the effectiveness of AT for chronic LBP.[55]

FM is a technique said to improve function by "expanding the self-image through movement sequences that bring attention to the parts of the self that are out of awareness and uninvolved in functional actions. Better function is evoked by establishing an improved dynamic relationship between the individual, gravity, and society."[56] In 2004, Jain and colleagues[57] provided a "critical overview" of the method, its use and the relevant research, and research gaps concerning this BAT. A 2014 systematic review found "further promising evidence" for the effectiveness of FM in improving balance in the elderly as well as in reducing pain.[58]

Breath Pattern Retraining

In 1975, Lum[59] introduced the concept of disordered breathing patterns as the underlying cause of "a collection of bizarre and unrelated symptoms" including cardiovascular, neurologic, respiratory, gastrointestinal, musculoskeletal, psychologic, and other syndromes. More recently, Chaitow[60] has emphasized disturbed breathing patterns as the cause of chronic pain. Proposed mechanisms are summarized as "respiratory alkalosis, leading to reduced oxygenation of tissues (including the brain), smooth muscle constriction, heightened pain perception, speeding up of spinal reflexes, increased excitability of the corticospinal system, hyperirritability of motor and sensory axons, changes in serum calcium and magnesium levels, and encouragement of myofascial trigger points." Breath pattern retraining therapists note that the respiratory mechanism is the only physiologic function that is under both autonomic and voluntary control.

A 2005 RCT involving chronic LBP patients revealed equivalent improvement from 12 sessions of breath therapy as measured on a visual analogue scale (VAS), Roland-Morris Scale, and 36-Item Short Form Survey (SF-36) when compared to high-quality, extended physical therapy. Breath therapy was found to be safe.[61]

Prolotherapy

The use of proliferation therapy (prolotherapy) has waxed and waned in popularity for nearly a century. Often provided by CM practitioners, prolotherapy is also frequently in the therapeutic armamentarium of naturopathic medicine (ND). The underlying theory is that following an injury, failure of adequate tendon or ligament healing results in instability, connective tissue insufficiency, or lack of tensile strength. Normal use of these compromised structures causes pain. Prolotherapy consists of injections of an array of substances intended to trigger growth factors in local connective tissue and restart the repair sequence that results in more normal and functional tissue.

A 2005 critical review of prolotherapy retrieved over 30 studies of prolotherapy for spinal pain.[62] These reflected wide variation in treatment protocols and concluded that "clinical studies published to date indicate that it may be effective at reducing spinal pain." Case reports, case series, and non-randomized trials suggest that prolotherapy is helpful for a variety of musculoskeletal disorders. RCT evidence, however, is conflicting.[63,64] A Cochrane review concluded that "if used alone, prolotherapy injections do not have a role in the treatment of chronic low-back pain. When combined with other treatments, they may give prolonged partial relief of pain and disability."[65]

The Tensegrity Model

Tensegrity (or biotensegrity) is not a therapy in itself but rather a concept of how biologic systems function from the ultra-structure of the cell to the organism. The concept is attributed to sculptor Kenneth Snelson, and the term was coined by Buckminster Fuller to represent "tensional integrity." Snelson[66] noted, "Tensegrity describes a closed structural system composed of a set of three or more elongate compression struts within a network of tension tendons, the combined parts mutually supportive in such a way that the struts do not touch one another, but press outwardly against nodal points in the tension network to form a firm, triangulated, pre-stressed, tension and compression unit." Donald E. Ingber of Harvard Medical School and Stephen M. Levin, an orthopedic surgeon, have applied tensegrity concepts to biology and medicine. Ingber has postulated that cell function is regulated mechanically via tensegrity. Levin[67] contends that the integrity of the musculoskeletal system "is a function of continuous tension, discontinuous compression, so that the skeleton, rather than being a frame of support to which the muscles and ligaments and tendons attach, has to be considered as compression components suspended within a continuous tension network." Many body work practitioners including physical therapists, chiropractors, massage therapists, martial artists, and others have incorporated the tensegrity model into evaluation and treatment approaches.

The Fascia Model

The tensegrity "model" in some respects is similar to other concepts founded perhaps initially by Andrew Taylor Still, the founder of osteopathy. Other generations of "body workers" have proposed similar models of the human locomotor system including D. D. Palmer's formulation of chiropractic being founded on "tone." More contemporary practitioners have elaborated further models such as Ida Rolf's concepts of "structural integration." Ultimately, these various fields of clinical study and practice came to suggest fascia as an underlying anatomical and physiologic structures and processes that help explain the often-remarkable success of various manual techniques from massage, soft tissue and joint manipulations, to acupuncture and physical therapy.

Fascia is something of a stepchild in anatomy. Students of human dissection are well aware of the prevalence of the layers of fascia that invest the organs and tissues. However, fascia has historically been disregarded and considered merely an impediment to dissection. Research over the past few decades has begun to illuminate the role of the fascia as a continuous connective tissue system throughout the body. It is postulated that far from being passive, inert structures, the continuum of fascia allows it to serve as a body-wide mechanosensitive signaling system.[68] Stecco and colleagues[69] provide a summary of contemporary research on the characteristics of the human fascial system. Knowledge of this body-wide connective tissue system "may contribute to clinicians' understanding of the myofascial system and the role which the deep fasciae may play in musculoskeletal dysfunctions."[69] Beginning in 2007, the Fascia Research Society has sponsored a series of Fascia Research Congress meetings dedicated to the emerging field of fascia studies.[70]

Trigger Point Manipulation

Travell and Simons[71] offered an early treatise on myofascial trigger points (TrPs) which were defined originally as "a hyperirritable spot in skeletal muscle that is associated with a hypersensitive palpable nodule in a taut band. The spot is tender when pressed and can give rise to characteristic referred pain, motor dysfunction, and autonomic phenomena."[71]

Although the existence of this clinical finding is well recognized, the understanding of the etiology of TrPs is evolving. McPartland[72] offered "molecular and osteopathic perspectives" on the TrP phenomenon in 2004. They postulated that "TrPs are evoked by the abnormal depolarization of motor end plates . . . presynaptic, synaptic, and postsynaptic mechanisms of abnormal depolarization (i.e., excessive release of acetylcholine [ACh], defects of acetylcholinesterase, and upregulation of nicotinic ACh-receptor activity, respectively)." More recent work by Shah and colleagues[73] at the NIH Rehabilitation Medicine Department have developed microdialysis techniques that have confirmed "that biochemicals associated with pain, inflammation, and intercellular signaling are elevated in the vicinity of active MTrPs."

In sharp contrast,[74] in a "critical evaluation of the trigger point phenomenon," the authors claim to have debunked these perspectives as well as other putative explanations of TrPs. They concluded that the TrP phenomenon "has no scientific basis. . . ."[74] More recent work has begun to suggest the relationship of central sensitization to the creation and maintenance of TrPs.[75]

No objective diagnostic tests for TrPs are available. TrPs are diagnosed by manual palpation to identify a tender nodule, often at characteristic locations in muscle that, when stimulated, produce characteristic radiating pain as reported by the patient. Despite this low-tech diagnostic method, TrP detection has good test–retest reliability.[76] Various approaches to treating TrPs have been elaborated including manual compression, "spray and stretch," injection, dry needling, and modalities (ultrasound, electric stimulation, low-level laser). TrP treatment is often rendered by certain CM physical medicine practitioners, but most frequently by chiropractors, acupuncturists, massage practitioners, and other IH providers.

ENERGY-BASED THERAPIES

In contrast to the biologically based therapies, a number of "energy-based" interventions are common among IH practitioners as well as some CM clinicians. Energy medicine is a domain in health care that deals with putative energy fields of two types: veritable, which can be measured, and putative, which have yet to be measured.

The veritable energies include mechanical vibrations (such as sound) and electromagnetic forces, including visible light, magnetism, monochromatic radiation (such as laser beams), and rays from other parts of the electromagnetic spectrum. These veritable energy-based therapies involve the use of specific, measurable wavelengths and frequencies to treat patients.

In contrast, putative energy fields are based on the concept that human beings are infused with a subtle form of energy. This vital energy or life force is known under different names in different cultures and traditions, such as "qi" in traditional Chinese medicine (TCM), "ki" in the Japanese Kampo system, "doshas" in Ayurvedic medicine, and elsewhere as "prana," "etheric energy," "fohat," "orgone," "odic force," "mana," and "homeopathic resonance." Vital energy is believed to flow throughout the material human body, but it has not been unequivocally measured by means of conventional instrumentation. Nonetheless, therapists claim that they can work with this subtle energy, see it with their own eyes, feel it, and otherwise sense its presence and quality and then use it to effect changes in another's physical body to influence health.

Veritable Energy Therapies
Magnetic Therapy

Magnetic therapy has a long and controversial history in medicine. It has recently regained popularity in the marketplace. Application is by way of various devices such as electromagnetic coil and static magnets worn in garments or jewelry or held in place with adhesive patches. Magnetic therapy is typically applied to the skin overlying the affected area. The popular press indicates the use of magnets for treating a wide variety of chronic pain problems such as migraine, osteoarthritis, and injury to muscles, ligaments, and tendons. Contraindications are few but do include pregnancy, pediatric age, and presence of implantable electronic devices.

Contemporary clinical trials of magnet therapy have produced conflicting results. A study of carpal tunnel syndrome in 2002 found no statistically significant difference between magnets and placebo. But the authors did note, "Although this study did not show magnets to be more effective than the placebo, the reduction in pain with this simple intervention was remarkable."[77] In a double blind, placebo-controlled trial, static magnets produced statistically significant ($P < .05$) short-term pain relief in osteoarthritis of the knee.[78] Systematic reviews of magnet therapy are scarce, and EBM reviews for magnet therapy for pain are lacking.

Transcranial magnetic stimulation is a recent development in CM for the therapeutic use of magnetic energy. Cochrane reviews of this intervention have looked at applications for tinnitus, schizophrenia, depression, poststroke, epilepsy, and others.[79] These reviews have been unable to either support or refute magnetic energy therapies.

Microcurrent Stimulation

Microcurrent stimulation generally involves apparatus that can supply electrical current usually below 1 mA in various frequency ranges. Microcurrent has been used in CM for the treatment of nonunion fracture and delayed bone healing. The exact mechanism of action is unknown but may involve intracellular regulation of calcium. A narrative review of microcurrent in physical therapy found good support for its use in bone and skin lesion healing. Other applications have only scant evidence.

Microcurrent has found application in the treatment of soft tissue disorders as well. McMakin has published three studies of this modality, which is termed *frequency-specific microcurrent* (FSM), in chronic pain patients. The studies are case series reports involving head, neck, and facial pain[80]; chronic LBP[80,81]; and fibromyalgia associated with cervical spine trauma.[82] In this study, McMakin and colleagues also began to explore the mechanisms of FSM. Their subjects revealed reductions in inflammatory cytokines, increase in β-endorphins, as well as subjective reports of pain relief in fibromyalgia with FSM.

Low-Level Laser Therapy

Low-level laser therapy (LLLT) is a form of phototherapy that involves the application of low-power laser light to areas of the body in order to stimulate healing and relieve pain. It is also known as cold laser, soft laser, or low-intensity laser. It is hypothesized that photons are absorbed in the mitochondria. The light energy is converted to chemical energy within the cell affecting the permeability of the cell membrane, which in turn produces various physiologic effects. These physiologic changes affect a variety of cell types including macrophages, fibroblasts, endothelial cells, and mast cells.

Although the underlying physiologic mechanisms are incompletely understood, LLLT is widely used in physical therapy, chiropractic, and other physical medicine disciplines. Although reportedly safe, the modality is relatively new and is still controversial with respect to its effectiveness. A 2005 Cochrane review of LLLT used in rheumatoid arthritis suggested that LLLT "could be considered for relief of pain and morning stiffness for RA patients, particularly since it has few side-effects."[83] A 2009 systematic review and meta-analysis of 16 RCTs in *The Lancet* showed "that LLLT reduces pain immediately after treatment in acute neck pain and up to 22 weeks after completion of treatment in patients with chronic neck pain."[84] A 2017 systematic review of LLLT for musculoskeletal pain concluded that despite heterogeneous study methodology, LLLT "appears to be an effective treatment modality to achieve pain relief in adult patients with musculoskeletal disorders."[85]

Putative Energy Therapies
Acupuncture and Oriental Medicine

Among the putative energy therapies, none has received more notice and scrutiny than acupuncture. Acupuncture, the use of fine wire needles inserted into various points along meridians, is but one therapy within broader field of OM. The practice of OM includes a range of systems, interventions, schools of thought, and techniques. One such system, TCM, is widely taught and practiced in the United States. TCM encompasses herbs, massage, qigong, and acupuncture.

In the TCM view, the body is a delicate balance of two opposing and inseparable forces: yin and yang. Yin represents the cold, slow, or passive principle, whereas yang represents the hot, excited, or active principle. Among the major assumptions in TCM are that health is achieved by maintaining the body in a "balanced state" and that disease is due to an internal imbalance of yin and yang. This imbalance leads to blockage in the flow of qi (or vital energy) and of blood along pathways known as meridians. TCM practitioners typically use herbs, acupuncture, and massage to help unblock qi and blood in patients in an attempt to bring the body back into harmony and wellness.[86] These therapies are intended to balance the flow of qi rather than to produce a specific physiologic effect.

Although not synonymous with TCM, needle acupuncture has received the most attention in the research and clinical communities. It is the most common OM therapy received by patients. Acupuncture describes a family of procedures involving stimulation of anatomic locations on the skin by a variety of techniques. There are a number of approaches to diagnosis and treatment in American acupuncture that incorporate medical traditions from China, Japan, Korea, and other countries. The most studied mechanism of stimulation of acupuncture points employs penetration of the skin by thin, solid, metallic needles, which are manipulated manually or by electrical stimulation.[87]

The body of research literature on acupuncture is robust. A search on PubMed for "acupuncture" returned more than 25,000 citations. Limiting the search terms to "acupuncture and chronic pain" returned more than 1,500 citations. The Cochrane Collaboration lists over 200 reviews for "acupuncture" and 18 EBM reviews specifically for "acupuncture and chronic pain." A comprehensive review of this literature base is well beyond the scope of this chapter, but it is apparent that there is conclusive evidence of the effectiveness and safety of this therapy for pain and other clinical conditions.

It is clear that acupuncture is widely used by chronic pain patients. A telephone survey from a decade ago by Breivik et al.[88] found 13% of chronic pain patients in Europe were using acupuncture. Research methodology challenges in the investigation of acupuncture stubbornly persist. Meta-analyses frequently conclude that although acupuncture can be shown to be effective for pain relief, the therapy itself has not been shown to be superior to other therapies.

Craniosacral Therapy

Craniosacral therapy (CST) developed from the work of an American osteopath, William Sutherland, in the early 1900s. It is founded on the notion of the primary respiratory mechanism that involves intrinsic motions of the cranial bones, the dura, and the flow of cerebrospinal fluid. Rhythmic motions are said to be measurable with instruments, but in clinical practice, it is by palpation that a CST practitioner identifies disturbed cranial rhythms and applies corrective gentle manipulations. Restricted motion of the cranial bones at the sutures is thought to impede cerebrospinal fluid flow and lead to disordered function and disease.

CST is known in the osteopathic profession preferentially as cranial osteopathy. The chiropractic profession has a technique that encompasses much of CST and others as well, known as sacro-occipital technique. CST is also practiced by a variety of other hands-on practitioners including physical therapists, massage therapists, dentists, and lay practitioners.

CST is included under the putative energy category in that the motions of the primary respiratory mechanism have not been irrefutably demonstrated. Skeptics and critics have challenged the existence of these subtle rhythms.[89] Reliability studies of the manual diagnosis of disturbed cranial rhythms have been disappointing.[90] CST has been studied in clinical trials addressing fibromyalgia,[91] asthma,[92] urinary tract signs in multiple sclerosis,[93] and others. The Cochrane Collaboration contains no EBM reviews of CST. A 2012 systematic review of CST identified only three RCTs and four observational studies that met criteria of the Downs and Black checklist. The review concluded that CST "has the potential of providing valuable outcomes. . . . However, due to the current moderate methodological quality of the included studies, further research is needed."[94]

Homeopathy

Homeopathy is a system of diagnosis and treatment founded by Samuel C. Hahnemann in Germany in the late 18th century. Homeopathy is currently practiced widely in Europe and Great Britain and by many practitioner types in the United States including MD, DO, DC, ND, and lay providers. Clinical evaluations include detailed history interviews that lead to individualized treatment regimens depending on a host of physical, emotional, and psychological factors. The therapies include the use of homeopathic remedies which are derived from plant, mineral, and other extracts that have been serially diluted, often to the point where, statistically at least, no physical molecules of the original substance remain.

This fact challenges fundamentally the notions of science and the physical universe that underlie CM. Most CM practitioners simply cannot accept the idea that a substance that has nothing physically "there" can have any real effect beyond that attributable to placebo. Nonetheless, a number of studies in reliable scientific journals report the apparent effectiveness of the medicine.

There is an extensive literature on homeopathy. A search of the National Library of Medicine for "homeopathy" returned over 6,000 citations. A strictly nonscientific sampling of these abstracts indicates that pain and chronic pain conditions have not typically been studied. A search of the *Homeopathy: The Journal of the Faculty of Homeopathy* for "pain management" retrieved only 197 results.[95] The challenge of submitting homeopathy to rigorous research designs revolves around the highly individualized treatments encountered in practice. As with other natural medicine approaches to pain treatment, a homeopathic practitioner is more likely to be evaluating and treating underlying causes of pain rather than treating pain itself.

Ayurvedic Medicine

Ayurveda, which literally means "the science of life," is a natural healing system developed in India. Ayurvedic texts claim that the sages who developed India's original systems of meditation and yoga developed the foundations of this medical system. It is a comprehensive system of medicine that places equal emphasis on the body, mind, and spirit and strives to restore the innate harmony of the individual. Some of the primary Ayurvedic treatments include diet, exercise, meditation, herbs, massage, exposure to sunlight, and controlled breathing. In India, Ayurvedic treatments have been developed for various diseases (e.g., diabetes, cardiovascular conditions, and neurologic disorders). However, a survey of the Indian medical literature indicates that the quality of the published clinical trials generally falls short of contemporary methodologic standards with regard to criteria for randomization, sample size, and adequate controls.[96]

In the prebiblical Ayurvedic origins, every creation, inclusive of a human being, is a model of the universe. In this model, the basic matter and the dynamic forces (dosha) of nature determine health and disease, and the medicinal value of any substance (plant and mineral). The Ayurvedic practices (chiefly that of diet, life style, and the Panchakarma) aim to maintain the dosha equilibrium. Despite a holistic approach aimed to cure disease, therapy is customized to the individual's constitution (Prakruti). Numerous Ayurvedic medicines (plant-derived in particular) have been tested for their biologic (especially immunomodulation) and clinical potential using modern ethno-validation, and thereby setting an interface with modern medicine.[96]

A PubMed search for "Ayurvedic medicine" returned over 2,800 results. A 2005 systematic review of Ayurvedic medicine for treatment of rheumatoid arthritis concluded that "there is a paucity of RCTs of Ayurvedic medicines for rheumatoid arthritis. The existing RCTs fail to show convincingly that such treatments are effective therapeutic options for rheumatoid arthritis."[97] In contrast, a 2011 pilot RCT comparing Ayurvedic medicine with CM (methotrexate) or their combination found "all 3 treatments were approximately equivalent in efficacy."[98]

However, as with many other CAM therapies, especially the energy-based modalities, the issues raised by double-blind methodologies and placebo effects have not been thoroughly accounted for. For example, the spiritual strength of the Ayurvedic healer and the utility of the placebo effect are both acknowledged and considered significant in many non-Western healing traditions.[99]

Biofield Therapies

Biofield therapies encompass modalities such as TT, Reiki, and healing touch (HT). They are based on the idea that humans exhibit nonphysical energy that can be sensed and modulated by a practitioner to affect health. These vital energy concepts are expressed as prana in yoga, chi in OM, qi in Japanese acupuncture, and as spirit in Western traditions. Survey research estimates about 3.7 U.S. adults have used biofield therapies at some point in their life.[100]

The significant challenges to valid clinical research on biofield therapies are similar to found in many other IH fields of study. Primary among them is a lack of biologic plausibility for the existence of biofields in terms that conventional Western medical thought can grasp. Further challenges emerge when considering the issues of patient and therapist blinding, identifying a suitable placebo, differentiating placebo from therapeutic effects, and lack of standardized treatment protocols.

Therapeutic Touch

Touch is a fundamental human sense. The skin is arguably the largest sensory organ of the body. The power of human touch has been recognized throughout the history of medicine. TT and its derivatives are energy-based therapies that have become common in some hospitals and other clinical settings.

From the TT Web site:

Therapeutic Touch is based on the idea that human beings are energy in the form of a field. When you are healthy, that energy is freely flowing and balanced. In contrast, disease is a condition of energy imbalance or disorder. The human energy field extends beyond the level of the skin, and the Therapeutic Touch practitioner attunes him or herself to that energy using the hands as sensors.

Exact methods vary between practitioners, but generally, they will pass their hands over your body from head to toe, front and back, holding them between 2-6 inches from the skin. This is done to assess the condition of the human energy field. They may use rhythmical, sweeping motions with the hands, as if they are smoothing out wrinkles in your energy field. The practitioner may or may not touch you physically.[101]

The evidence supporting TT is inconclusive. Two Cochrane reviews found insufficient evidence that TT is effective in the management of anxiety disorder or dementia.[102,103] However, a pilot trial of TT in a cognitive-behavioral therapy (CBT) program found chronic pain patients who received TT in addition to relaxation and CBT fared better in terms of enhanced self-efficacy and unitary power, as well as having lower attrition rates than patients who only received relaxation training and CBT.[104]

A study at the University of Wisconsin-Eau Claire studied another touch therapy (Tellington touch) in patients about to undergo venipuncture.[105] The intervention is described as "gentle physical touch and consisting of four components: a mental attitude of openness, use of the hands and fingers, breath awareness, and moderate finger/hand pressure." Analysis of qualitative descriptions by patients and the phlebotomist-nurse demonstrated that this massage-like, caring touch promoted relaxation and produced a helpful distraction in patients about to undergo a potentially painful procedure. Although further study is warranted, the implications for physicians and others who have hands-on contact with patients of any sort, and chronic pain patients in particular seem obvious. Human-to-human contact can have powerful effects in relieving anxiety and pain. The development of these skills by physicians and other caregivers may be of significant benefit to patients.

Reiki and Energy Healing Therapies

Reiki (pronounced RAY-kee) is Japanese for universal life energy. It is derived from *rei*, meaning "free passage" or "transcendental spirit," and *ki*, meaning "vital life force energy" or "universal life energy." Reiki is based on the belief that when spiritual energy is channeled through a Reiki practitioner, the patient's spirit is healed, which in turn heals the physical body.[106] Reiki practice usually involves no direct physical contact between practitioner and recipient. By the practitioner holding his or her hands over the patient's body, the recipient is said to draw energy from the universal life force through the practitioner.

In the late 1800s, Mikao Usui developed modern Reiki from ancient Asian healing traditions said to be thousands of years old. Introduced to the West in the 1970s, Reiki has become a popular IH therapy in the United States.[107] Reiki and other energy healing (EH) therapies have also attracted the attention of CM practitioners and researchers.

Reiki is practiced by a variety of licensed health care practitioners including CM and CAM physicians, allied health care providers, psychotherapists, massage practitioners, as well as nonlicensed Reiki masters. Although Reiki and other EH therapies are not without their critics,[108] these high-touch, low-tech interventions are being adopted by hospitals, clinics, and physician offices as useful adjuncts to patient care.[109] Higher patient satisfaction, improved clinical outcomes, and lower costs are ascribed to implementing Reiki and other EH therapies.[110]

Healing Touch

HT was developed by Janet Mentgen, an "energetically sensitive" nurse. A certificate program through the Healing Touch Program sponsored by the American Holistic Nurses Association. Mentgen advocated for an evidence-based approach to HT. A 2009 best evidence synthesis concluded that although biofield therapies (Reiki, TT, and HT) are widely used, review of 66 clinical studies showed strong evidence for reducing pain and less convincing evidence for improvement in anxiety, fatigue and quality of life.[111]

Conclusion

Far from being on the fringes of modern health care, many IH therapies have been in regular and frequent use especially by many chronic pain patients. Patients may seek out these therapies on their own from IH practitioners, but they are increasingly provided in conventional health care settings as well.

Many of these unconventional therapies are being subjected to the same rigorous investigation that is expected of all contemporary evidence-based medical practices. Arguably, many IH therapies hold up very well to this scrutiny and do so certainly as well as many commonly prescribed CM treatments (Table 94.2).

The fact that IH therapies are in common use by chronic pain patients suggests the need to better understand them. The emerging evidence that they are safe, clinically effective, and cost-effective when appropriately rendered further recommends them. That IH therapies explicitly incorporate the power of intention, awareness, and healing in the human interaction of the therapeutic encounter may well be the key to achieving a more individualized, sensitive, and humanized approach to the treatment of a most difficult and challenging patient population—those with chronic pain.

TABLE 94.2 Evidence in Cochrane Reviews	
Clinical Intervention for Spine Pain	**Cochrane Collaboration Review Conclusions**
Paracetamol (acetaminophen), for example, Tylenol	Paracetamol does not produce better outcomes than placebo for people with acute LBP, and it is uncertain if it has any effect on chronic LBP.
Opioids	There are no placebo RCTs supporting the effectiveness and safety of long-term opioid therapy for treatment of CLBP.
Radiofrequency (RF) denervation	There is no high-quality evidence that RF denervation provides pain relief for patients with chronic low back pain.
Acupuncture	Acupuncture is more effective for pain relief than no treatment or sham treatment. When added to other conventional therapies, it relieves pain and improves function better than the conventional therapies alone.
Chiropractic	Combined chiropractic interventions slightly improved pain and disability in the short-term and pain in the medium-term for acute and subacute LBP.

CLBP, chronic low back pain; LBP, low back pain.

References

1. Walter S. *The Illustrated Encyclopedia of Body–Mind Disciplines.* New York: Rosen; 1999.
2. Cohen M. *Healing at the Borderland of Medicine and Religion.* Chapel Hill, NC: University of North Carolina Press; 2006.
3. Inglis B. *Fringe Medicine.* London: Faber and Faber; 1964.
4. Kent M. False cry of quackery. Available at: http://askwaltstollmd.com/body_quackery.html. Accessed May 15, 2007.
5. Eisenberg D, Kessler RD, Foster C, et al. Unconventional medicine in the United States—prevalence, cost, and patterns of use. *N Engl J Med* 1993;328(4):426–525.
6. Cleary-Guida M, Okvat HA, Oz MC, et al. A regional survey of health insurance coverage for complementary and alternative medicine: current status and future ramifications. *J Altern Complement Med* 2001;7(3):269–273.
7. Ananth S, Martin W. *Health Forum 2005 Complementary and Alternative Medicine Survey.* Chicago, IL: American Hospital Association; 2006.
8. Anath S. 2010 Complementary and alternative medicine survey of hospitals: summary of results. Available at: http://www.samueliinstitute.org/File%20Library/Our%20Research/OHE/CAM_Survey_2010_oct6.pdf. Accessed February 27, 2017.
9. Consortium of Academic Health Centers for Integrative Medicine. March 16, 2008. Consortium of Academic Health Centers for Integrative Medicine. June 12, 2007. Available at: http://www.imconsortium.org/cahcim/home.html. Accessed August 27, 2009.
10. Academic Consortium for Integrative Medicine and Health. Available at: http://www.imconsortium.org/about/mission.cfm. Accessed February 28, 2017.
11. National Center for Complementary and Integrative Health. Frequently asked questions: name change. Available at: https://nccih.nih.gov/news/name-change-faq. Accessed February 28, 2017.
12. Bloom BS, Retbi A, Dahan S, et al. Evaluation of randomized controlled trials on complementary and alternative medicine. *Int J Technol Assess Health Care* 2000;16(1):13–21.
13. Angell M, Kassirer JP. Alternative medicine—the risks of untested and unregulated remedies. *N Engl J Med* 1998;339(12):839–841.
14. Committee on the Use of Complementary and Alternative Medicine by the American Public. *Complementary and Alternative Medicine in the United States.* Washington, DC: National Academies Press; 2005.
15. Cicerone KD. Evidence-based practice and the limits of rational rehabilitation. *Arch Phys Med Rehabil* 2005;86(6):1073–1074.
16. Oschman J. *Energy Medicine in Therapeutics and Human Performance.* Edinburgh: Butterworth-Heinemann; 2003.
17. PubMed. IH utilization. Available at: https://www.ncbi.nlm.nih.gov/pubmed/?term=IH+utilization. Accessed February 18, 2017.
18. Nayak S, Matheis RJ, Agostinelli S, et al. The use of complementary and alternative therapies for chronic pain following spinal cord injury: a pilot survey. *J Spinal Cord Med* 2001;24(1):54–62.
19. Fleming S, Rabago DP, Mundt MP, et al. CAM therapies among primary care patients using opioid therapy. *BMC Complement Altern Med* 2007;7:15.
20. McEachrane-Gross F, Liebschutz JM, Berlowitz D. Use of selected complementary and alternative medicine (CAM) treatments in veterans with cancer or chronic pain: a cross-sectional survey. *BMC Complement Altern Med* 2006;6:34.
21. Tsao J, Meldrum M, Kim S, et al. Treatment preferences for CAM in children with chronic pain. *Evid Based Complement Alternat Med* 2007;4(3):367–374.
22. Lin YC, Lee AC, Kemper KJ, et al. Use of complementary and alternative medicine in pediatric pain management service: a survey. *Pain Med* 2005;6:452–458. doi:10.1111/j.1526-4637.2005.00071.x.
23. National Center for Complementary and Integrative Health. Complementary, alternative, or integrative health: what's in a name? Available at: https://nccih.nih.gov/health/integrative-health#types. Accessed February 28, 2017.
24. Nahin R. Estimates of pain prevalence and severity in adults: United States, 2012. *J Pain* 2015;16(8):769–780.
25. Whitten CE, Evans CM, Cristobal K. Pain management doesn't have to be a pain: working and communicating effectively with patients who have chronic pain. *Perm J* 2005;9(2):41–48.
26. Lundgren J, Ugalde V. The demographics and economics of complementary alternative medicine. *Phys Med Rehabil Clin N Am* 2004;15(4):955–961.
27. Eisenberg DM, Davis RB, Ettner SL, et al. Unconventional medicine in the U.S.: prevalence, costs, and patterns of use. *JAMA* 1998;290:1569–1575.
28. Hirsh AT, Atchison JW, Berger JJ, et al. Patient satisfaction with treatment for chronic pain: predictors and relationship to compliance. *Clin J Pain* 2005;21(4):302–310.
29. Sullivan MD. Placebo controls and epistemic control in orthodox medicine. *J Med Philos* 1993;18(2):213–231.
30. Paterson C, Dieppe P. Characteristic and incidental (placebo) effects in complex interventions such as acupuncture. *BMJ* 2005;330(7501):1202–1205.
31. Langevin H, Hammerschlag R, Lao L, et al. Controversies in acupuncture research: selection of controls and outcome measures in acupuncture clinical trials. *J Altern Complement Med* 2006;12(10):943–953.
32. Shekell P, Morton SC, Suttorp MJ, et al. Challenges in systematic reviews of complementary and alternative medicine topics. *Ann Intern Med* 2005;142(12 pt 2):1042–1047.
33. Barnes P, Powell-Griner E, McFann K, et al. Complementary and alternative medicine use among adults: United States, 2002. *Adv Data* 2004;343:1–19.
34. Koes B, van Tulder M. Low back pain (acute). *Clin Evid* 2006;15:1619–1633.
35. National Center for Complementary and Integrative Health. Chiropractic: in depth. Available at: https://nccih.nih.gov/health/chiropractic/introduction.htm. Accessed February 28, 2017.
36. Clar C, Tsertsvadze A, Court R, et al. Clinical effectiveness of manual therapy for the management of musculoskeletal and non-musculoskeletal conditions: systematic review and update of UK evidence report. *Chiropr Man Therap* 2014;22:12. doi:10.1186/2045-709X-22-12.
37. Rubinstein SM, Terwee CB, Assendelft WJJ, et al. Spinal manipulative therapy for acute low-back pain. *Cochrane Database Syst Rev* 2012;(9): CD008880. doi:10.1002/14651858.CD008880.pub2.
38. Rubinstein SM, van Middelkoop M, Assendelft WJJ, et al. Spinal manipulative therapy for chronic low-back pain. *Cochrane Database Syst Rev* 2011(2):CD008112. doi:10.1002/14651858.CD008112.pub2.
39. Bronfort G. The effectiveness of cervical adjustment for acute and chronic neck pain: excerpts from a systematic review and best evidence synthesis. *J Am Chiropr Assoc* 2003;40:42.
40. McCrory DC, Penzien DB, Hasselblad V, et al. *Evidence Report: Behavioral and Physical Treatments for Tension-Type and Cervicogenic Headache.* Des Moines, IA: Foundation for Chiropractic Education and Research; 2001.
41. Muller R, Giles LG. Long-term follow-up of a randomized clinical trial assessing the efficacy of medication, acupuncture, and spinal manipulation for chronic mechanical spinal pain syndromes. *J Manipulative Physiol Ther* 2005;28(1):3–11.
42. Chou R, Huffman LH; for American Pain Society, American College of Physicians. Nonpharmacologic therapies for acute and chronic low back pain: a review of the evidence for an American Pain Society/American College of Physicians clinical practice guideline. *Ann Intern Med* 2007;147(7):492–504.
43. Chou R, Deyo R, Friedly J, et al. Nonpharmacologic therapies for low back pain: a systematic review for an American College of Physicians clinical practice guideline. *Ann Intern Med* 2017;166:493–505. doi:10.7326/M16-2459.
44. Chou R, Deyo R, Friedly J, et al. Systemic pharmacologic therapies for low back pain: a systematic review for an American College of Physicians clinical practice guideline. *Ann Intern Med* 2017;166(7):480–492. doi:10.7326/M16-2458.
45. Saragiotto BT, Machado GC, Ferreira ML, et al. Paracetamol for low back pain. *Cochrane Database Syst Rev* 2016;(6):CD012230. doi:10.1002/14651858.CD012230.
46. Tsao J. Effectiveness of massage therapy for chronic, non-malignant pain: a review. *Evid Based Complement Alternat Med* 2007;4(2):165–179.
47. Furlan AD, Giraldo M, Baskwill A, et al. Massage for low-back pain. *Cochrane Database Syst Rev* 2015;(9):CD001929. doi:10.1002/14651858.CD001929.pub3.
48. Department of Veterans Affairs Health Services Research & Development Service. Evidence-based Synthesis Program. Massage for pain: an evidence map. Available at: https://www.hsrd.research.va.gov/publications/esp/massage.pdf. Accessed April 16, 2018.
49. Nahin RL, Boineau R, Khalsa PS, et al. Evidence-based evaluation of complementary health approaches for pain management in the United States. *Mayo Clin Proc* 2016;91(6):1292–1306.
50. Holdcraft LC, Assefi N, Buchwald D. Complementary and alternative medicine in fibromyalgia and related syndromes. *Best Pract Res Clin Rheumatol* 2003;17:667–683.
51. Clegg DO, Reda DJ, Harris CL, et al. Glucosamine, chondroitin sulfate, and the two in combination for painful knee osteoarthritis. *N Engl J Med* 2006;354(8):795–808.
52. Hochberg MC, Zhan M, Langenberg P. The rate of decline of joint space width in patients with osteoarthritis of the knee: a systematic review and meta-analysis of randomized placebo-controlled trials of chondroitin sulfate. *Curr Med Res Opin* 2008;24(1):3029–3035.
53. Erntst E, Canter PH. The Alexander technique: a systematic review of controlled clinical trials. *Forsch Komplementarmed Klass Naturheilkd* 2003; 10(6):325–329.
54. Hollinghurst S, Sharp D, Ballard K, et al. Randomised controlled trial of Alexander technique lessons, exercise, and massage (ATEAM) for chronic and recurrent back pain: economic evaluation. *BMJ* 2008;337:a2656.
55. Woodman JP, Moore NR. Evidence for the effectiveness of Alexander Technique lessons in medical and health-related conditions: a systematic review. *Int J Clin Pract* 2012;66:98–112. doi:10.1111/j.1742-1241.2011.02817.x.
56. The Feldenkrais Educational Foundation of North America and the Feldenkrais Guild of North America. The Feldenkrais method of somatic education. Available at: http://www.feldenkrais.com/method/standards/index.html#what. Accessed March 24, 2017.
57. Jain S, Janssen K, DeCelle S. Alexander technique and Feldenkrais method: a critical overview. *Phys Med Rehabil Clin N Am* 2004;15(4):811–825, vi.
58. Hillier S, Worley A. The effectiveness of the Feldenkrais method: a systematic review of the evidence. *Evid Based Complement Alternat Med* 2015; 2015:752160. doi:10.1155/2015/752160.
59. Lum LC. Hyperventilation: the tip of the iceberg. *J Psychosom Res* 1975; 19(5–6):375–383.
60. Chaitow L. Breathing pattern disorders, motor control, and low back pain. *J Osteopath Med* 2004;7(1):34–41.

61. Mehling WE, Hamel KA, Acree M, et al. Randomized, controlled trial of breath therapy for patients with chronic low back pain. *Altern Ther Health Med* 2005;11(4):44–52.

62. Dagenais S, Haldeman S, Wooley JR. Intraligamentous injection of sclerosing solutions (prolotherapy) for spinal pain: a critical review of the literature. *Spine J* 2005;5(3):310–328.

63. Rabago D, Best T, Beamsley M, et al. A systematic review of prolotherapy for chronic musculoskeletal pain. *Clin J Sports Med* 2005;15(5):376–380.

64. Hauser R, Hauser M, Baird N, et al. Evidence-based use of dextrose prolotherapy for musculoskeletal pain: a scientific literature review. *J Prolother* 2011;3(4):765–789.

65. Dagenais S, Yelland MJ, Del Mar C, et al. Prolotherapy injections for chronic low-back pain. *Cochrane Database of Syst Rev* 2007;(2):CD004059.

66. Snelson K. Weaving, mother of tensegrity. Available at: http://www.kenneth snelson.net/icons/struc.htm. Accessed March 27, 2017.

67. Levin S. Continuous tension, discontinuous compression: a model for biomechanical support of the body. A presentation to the North American Academy of Manipulative Medicine in 1980. Available at: http://www .biotensegrity.com/index.php?option=com_content&task=view&id=14&It emid=29. Accessed March 27, 2017.

68. Langevin H. Connective tissue: a body-wide signaling network? *Med Hypotheses* 2006;66(6):1074–1077.

69. Stecco C, Macchi V, Porzionato A, et al. The fascia: the forgotten structure. *Ital J Anat Embryol* 2011;116(3):127–138.

70. Fascia Research Society. Available at: https://fasciaresearchsociety.org/. Accessed March 27, 2018.

71. Travell JG, Simons DG. *Myofascial Pain and Dysfunction: The Trigger Point Manual: The Upper Extremities.* Vol 1. Baltimore, MD: Williams & Wilkins; 1983.

72. McPartland J. Travell trigger points—molecular and osteopathic perspectives. *J Am Osteopath Assoc* 2004;104(6):244–249.

73. Shah JP, Thaker N, Heimur J, et al. Myofascial trigger points then and now: a historical and scientific perspective. *PM R* 2015;7(7):746–761. doi:10.1016 /j.pmrj.2015.01.024.

74. Quinter J, Bove J, Cohen M. A critical evaluation of the trigger point phenomenon. *Rheumatology* 2015;54(3):392–399. Available at: https://academic .oup.com/rheumatology/article/54/3/392/1796114/A-critical-evaluation -of-the-trigger-point. Accessed April 16, 2018.

75. Fernández-de-las-Peñas C, Dommerholt J. Myofascial trigger points: peripheral or central phenomenon? *Curr Rheumatol Rep* 2014;16:395. doi:10.1007/s11926-013-0395-2.

76. Al-Shenqiti AM, Oldham JA. Test-retest reliability of myofascial trigger point detection in patients with rotator cuff tendonitis. *Clin Rehabil* 2005;19(5):482–487.

77. Carter R, Hall T, Aspy CB, et al. The effectiveness of magnet therapy for treatment of wrist pain attributed to carpal tunnel syndrome. *J Fam Pract* 2002;51(1):38–40.

78. Wolsko PM, Eisenberg DM, Simon LS, et al. Double-blind placebo-controlled trial of static magnets for the treatment of osteoarthritis of the knee: results of a pilot study. *Altern Ther Health Med* 2004;10(2):36–43.

79. The Cochrane Collaboration. Transcranial magnetic stimulation. Available at: http://www.cochrane.org/search/site/magnetic%20therapy. Accessed April 16, 2018.

80. McMakin C. Microcurrent treatment of myofascial pain in the head, neck, and face. *Top Clin Chiropr* 1998;5:29–35.

81. McMakin C. Microcurrent therapy: a novel treatment method for chronic low back myofascial pain. *J Bodyw Mov Ther* 2004;8(2):143–153.

82. McMakin C, Gregory WM, Phillips TM. Cytokine changes with microcurrent treatment of fibromyalgia associated with cervical spine trauma. *J Bodyw Mov Ther* 2005;9(3):169–176.

83. Brosseau L, Welch V, Wells GA, et al. Low level laser therapy (Classes I, II and III) for treating rheumatoid arthritis. *Cochrane Database Syst Rev* 2005;(4):CD002049.

84. Chow R, Johnson MI, Lopes-Martins RA, et al. Efficacy of low-level laser therapy in the management of neck pain: a systematic review and meta-analysis of randomised placebo or active-treatment controlled trials. *Lancet* 2009;374(9705):1897–1908.

85. Clijsen R, Brunner A, Barbero M, et al. Effects of low-level laser therapy on pain in patients with musculoskeletal disorders: a systematic review and meta-analysis. *Eur J Phys Rehabil Med* 2017;53:603–610.

86. National Center for Complementary and Integrative Health. Traditional Chinese medicine: in depth. Available at: https://nccih.nih.gov/health/whatiscam /chinesemed.htm#intro. Accessed March 29, 2017.

87. NIH Consensus Development Program. Acupuncture. Available at: https:// consensus.nih.gov/1997/1997acupuncture107html.htm. Accessed March 29, 2017.

88. Breivik H, Collett B, Ventafridda V, et al. Survey of chronic pain in Europe: prevalence, impact on daily life, and treatment. *Eur J Pain* 2006;10(4):287–333.

89. Bledsoe BE, Licciardone JC. The elephant in the room: does OMT have proved benefit? *J Am Osteopath Assoc* 2004;104(10):405–406.

90. Moran RW, Gibbons P. Intraexaminer and interexaminer reliability for palpation of the cranial rhythmic impulse at the head and sacrum. *J Manipulative Physiol Ther* 2001;24(3):183–190.

91. Castro-Sánchez A, Matarán-Peñarrocha GA, Sanchez-Labrace G, et al. A randomized controlled trial investigating the effects of craniosacral therapy on pain and heart rate variability in fibromyalgia patients. *Clin Rehabil* 2011;25:25–35.

92. Mehl-Madrona L, Kligler B, Silverman S, et al. The impact of acupuncture and craniosacral therapy interventions on clinical outcomes in adults with asthma. *Explore* 2007;3(1):28–36.

93. Raviv G, Shefi S, Nizani D, et al. Effect of craniosacral therapy on lower urinary tract signs and symptoms in multiple sclerosis. *Complement Ther Clin Pract* 2009;15:72–75.

94. Jäkel A, von Hauenschild P. A systematic review to evaluate the clinical benefits of craniosacral therapy. *Complement Ther Med* 2012;20:456–465.

95. Homeopathy. Available at: http://www.homeopathyjournal.net/. Accessed April 16, 2018.

96. Chopra A, Doiphode VV. Ayurvedic medicine. Core concept, therapeutic principles, and current relevance. *Med Clin North Am* 2002;86(1):75–89, vii.

97. Park J, Ernst E. Ayurvedic medicine for rheumatoid arthritis: a systematic review. *Semin Arthritis Rheum* 2005;34(5):705–713.

98. Furst DE, Venkatraman MM, McGann M, et al. Double-blind, randomized, controlled, pilot study comparing classic ayurvedic medicine, methotrexate, and their combination in rheumatoid arthritis. *J Clin Rheumatol* 2011;17(4):185–92. doi:10.1097/RHU.0b013e31821c0310.

99. Jonas WB, Levin JS. *Essentials of Complementary and Alternative Medicine.* Baltimore, MD: Lippincott Williams & Wilkins; 1999:210.

100. Centers for Disease Control and Prevention. National Health Interview Survey: 2012 data release. Available at: http://www.cdc.gov/nchs/nhis/nhis _2012_data_release.htm. Accessed March 2, 2017.

101. Therapeutic Touch International Organization. The process of therapeutic touch. Available at: http://therapeutictouch.org/what-is-tt/history-of-tt/. Accessed April 1, 2017.

102. Robinson J, Biley FC, Dolk H. Therapeutic touch for anxiety disorders. *Cochrane Database Syst Rev* 2007;(3):CD006240.

103. Hansen NV, Jørgensen T, Ørtenblad L. Massage and touch for dementia. *Cochrane Database Syst Rev* 2006;(4):CD004989.

104. Smith D, Arbstein P, Rosa K, et al. Effects of integrating therapeutic touch into a cognitive behavioral pain treatment program. *J Holist Nurs* 2002;20(4):367–387.

105. Wendler MC. Effects of Tellington touch in healthy adults awaiting venipuncture. *Res Nurs Health* 2003;26:40–52.

106. Holisticonline.com. Reiki infocenter. Available at: http://www.holistic-online .com/Reiki/hol_reiki_introduction.htm. Accessed April 1, 2017.

107. Chu DA. Tai Chi, Qi gong and Reiki. *Phys Med Rehabil Clin N Am* 2004;15(4):773–781.

108. Science-Based Medicine. Reiki. Available at: https://sciencebasedmedicine .org/?s=reiki&category_name=&submit=Search. Accessed April 1, 2017.

109. Notte B, Fazzini C, Mooney, et al. Reiki's effect on patients with total knee arthroplasty: a pilot study. *Nursing* 2016;46(2):17–23.

110. Birocco N, Guillame C, Storto S, et al. The effects of Reiki therapy on pain and anxiety in patients attending a day oncology and infusion services unit. *Am J Hosp Palliat Care* 2012;29(4):290–294.

111. Shamini J, Mills P. Biofield therapies: helpful or full of hype? A best evidence synthesis. *Int J Behav Med* 2010;17:1–16. doi:10.1007/s12529-009-9062-4.

IMPLANTED ELECTRICAL STIMULATORS

CHAPTER 95

Stimulation of the Peripheral Nervous System for Pain Relief

MATTHEW S. WILLSEY, SRINIVAS CHIRAVURI, LYNDA J. YANG, and **PARAG G. PATIL**

Electrical stimulation of the peripheral nervous system for medically intractable pain dates from ancient times. Scribonius Largus reported that pain could be relieved by standing on an electric fish. In the 16th through the 18th century, many scientists, including Benjamin Franklin, advocated using various electrostatic devices for headache and other pains. Development of modern stimulation began with transcutaneous electrical nerve stimulation (TENS), which is generally credited to C. Norman Shealy.[1] This battery-powered, pain-relieving device delivers a small electrical current via electrical leads that can be attached to the skin overlying the painful area. In 1965, Melzack and Wall[2] introduced the concept of "gate-control theory," which hypothesized that stimulating peripheral nerves would block the transmission of pain in the dorsal horn of the spinal cord. Based on this theory, the first peripheral nerve stimulation (PNS) for pain relief in humans was reported by Wall and Sweet,[3] and the first implantable leads were placed by Sweet and Wepsic in 1968.[4] In the 1970s, the applications for PNS expanded with the work of Long, Nashold, Picaza, and others and included mononeuropathy, often posttraumatic or postsurgical, sciatica, reflex sympathetic dystrophy, causalgia, and amputation stump pain.[5–10] Weiner and Reed[11] were the first to report transcutaneous implantation techniques for treatment of occipital neuralgia in 1999. Recently, several groups have combined percutaneous approaches with real-time image guidance to achieve accurate lead placement from a minimally invasive approach.[12] (For a detailed history, see Slavin.[13])

Whereas PNS directs stimulation of a peripheral nerve, peripheral field stimulation (PFS) targets terminal nerve branches and pain receptors in the subcutaneous tissue. Goroszeniuk et al.[14] introduced this concept in a case series in 2006, although the success of peripheral stimulation reported by others was likely mediated through subcutaneous stimulation.[15] This method has proven to relieve pain effectively and is especially useful in cases where the painful area lies outside clearly demarcated dermatomes or peripheral nerve distributions. Patients undergoing PFS are estimated to have a 50% average reduction of pain.[16]

The final modality of peripheral stimulation is dorsal root ganglion stimulation (DRGS) that has been used since the mid-2000s.[17,18] The dorsal root ganglion had previously been a target of resection and ablative techniques to control pain,[19] but neuromodulation of the dorsal root ganglion became possible and easy to access with percutaneous leads. In 2016, the U.S. Food and Drug Administration (FDA) approved the use of DRGS for complex regional pain syndrome (CRPS) of the groin and lower extremities, which can be difficult to treat with other forms of neuromodulation such as spinal cord stimulation (SCS).

Figure 95.1 graphically depicts all the modalities of neuromodulation of the peripheral nervous system.

Pathophysiology and Mechanisms of Analgesia

Afferent pain pathways begin in the peripheral nervous system and are carried by myelinated Aδ and unmyelinated C fibers into the spinal cord, where they synapse in the posterior horn of the spinal cord. Second-order neurons cross to the contralateral spinal cord and ascend to synapse primarily in the ventroposterior lateral (VPL) nucleus of the thalamus via the lateral spinothalamic tract. From the VPL nucleus, third-order neurons project to the somatosensory cortex, cingulate gyrus, and insula. In addition to this pathway, sharp pain can also be carried by Aδ fibers to the spinal cord to ascend up the dorsal column–medial lemniscus pathway, where synapses are made in the cuneate and gracile nucleus of the medulla and VPL nucleus of the thalamus on way to the somatosensory cortex.

The mechanism of TENS is thought to be primarily mediated through neurotransmitters and not by modulating electrical activity. Both high- and low-frequency TENS likely mediate their effects through opioid and muscarinic receptors.[20,21] High-frequency stimulation has been shown to involve γ-aminobutyric acid (GABA),[22] and low-frequency stimulation involves serotonin.[23]

The mechanism of PNS is very different from that of analgesic pain medications and TENS units. The gate-control theory proposes that neuromodulation occurs in the dorsal horn of the

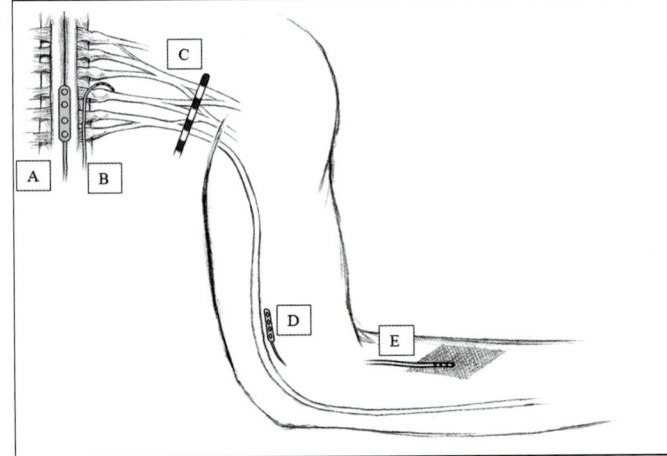

FIGURE 95.1 Peripheral stimulation modalities. The graphic illustrates the nervous system from the spinal cord to peripheral nerve. A, spinal cord stimulation is not a form of peripheral stimulation but shown in the graphic for completeness; B, dorsal root ganglion stimulation; C, brachial plexus stimulation; D, peripheral nerve stimulation; E, peripheral field stimulation.

spinal cord.[2] Electrical activation of Aβ fibers has been shown to block transmission of pain via Aδ and C fibers at the substantia gelatinosa in the dorsal horn of the spinal cord—closing the "gate."[24,25] Furthermore, in contrast to SCS, which modulates only the dorsal column pathway, peripheral stimulation may modulate both the spinothalamic tract and the dorsal column pathway because peripheral stimulation blocks both Aδ and C fibers that travel to the spinothalamic pathway.[26]

There is evidence for both short- and long-term modulation of dorsal horn activity. Short-term effects may be mediated by modulating electrical activity and further support the gate-control theory.[25] Long-term depression of dorsal horn activity may be mediated through gene expression,[27] and it has been demonstrated by both low- and high-frequency (1 to 100 Hz) stimulation.[27,28]

In addition to the dorsal horn, nerve fibers might also be affected by stimulation. Stimulation of Aδ and C fibers has been shown to reduce excitability.[29] This may potentially be mediated by decreased conduction velocities, decreased amplitude (especially Aδ fibers), and increased the threshold needed to trigger an action potential.[30,31] Peripheral stimulation has also been shown to reduce nociceptive and neuropathic pain.[32] Nociceptive inhibition may result from blocking Aδ afferents consistent with gate-control theory or from decreased excitability of Aδ fibers.[30,32]

The mechanism of PFS is largely unknown. Some believe the mechanism to follow that of the gate-control theory.[33] However, others suggest the subcutaneous stimulation blocks depolarization of sensory afferents, inhibits axonal conduction, or modulates the effect of endogenous endorphins.[34] In their study of visceral abdominal pain, Paicius et al.[34] suggest that subcutaneous stimulation affects the response of visceral fibers that merge with the subcutaneous fibers in the same dermatome. Like in PNS, PFS is presumed to affect both neuropathic and nociceptive pain pathways.[35]

As with other methods of peripheral stimulation, the exact mechanism for how DRGS alleviates pain is not well understood. Stimulation of dorsal roots has been shown to affect multiple spinal levels.[36] Many believe that the dorsal root ganglion neurons are hyperexcitable in pain syndromes and lead to excess activity in the dorsal horn of the spinal cord and, in turn, to increased pain.[17,37,38] The hyperexcitability is thought to be at least partially mediated by alterations in ion channels.[39] Some preliminary work has shown that direct stimulation of the dorsal root ganglion stabilizes the excitable neurons.[40] Detailed mechanistic reviews are available.[38]

Stimulation Technologies

The initial lead implantation techniques for PNS skeletonized the nerve and placed a lead in contact with the nerve. Many of these techniques also included direct stimulation of the nerve to determine the sensory fascicles supplying the painful area.[8] A variety of electrodes have been used, including "plate" electrodes,[41] "button" electrodes,[8] and electrodes that can be wrapped around the nerve.[5] In addition to their various shapes, the electrodes can be monopolar, bipolar, quadripolar, or octapolar. The nerves can be anchored in proximity by directly suturing the electrode to the nerve,[8] wrapping the nerve in mesh and then fastening to the electrode,[42] or suturing to the surrounding subcutaneous tissue often with a fascial flap between the electrode and nerve.[41]

Traditionally, the leads are connected to an implantable pulse generator (IPG) that is placed in a subcutaneous pocket. The leads are tunneled to the implantation site, typically located in the infraclavicular area, abdominal wall, or superior gluteal region, among other locations.[43,44] New wireless systems have been recently introduced to eliminate challenges and complications related to tunneled leads.[45,46]

Less invasive techniques of percutaneous implantation methods were first introduced by Weiner and Reed.[11] Since then, percutaneous techniques have been reported for a variety of peripheral nerves and can include insertion of electrodes through a cannulated needle or insertion of a thin electrode toward the nerve after blunt surgical dissection.[11,47-60]

Placing the electrode in proximity to the nerve is a challenge with percutaneous techniques where the nerve is not visualized. Often, electrodes are placed perpendicular to the trajectory of the nerve, making it more likely that at least some electrodes will be in proximity to the nerve,[43] and many percutaneous techniques rely heavily on anatomic landmarks and fluoroscopic guidance.[11,55] Nerve stimulation inducing appropriate distribution of paresthesia verifies percutaneous placement. Even with these techniques, the separation between electrode and nerve is difficult to control, particularly with high rates of lead migration.[61]

Real-time imaging with ultrasound has improved the accuracy of subcutaneous electrode placement, and many groups now rely on this imaging modality.[12] Several studies have shown that ultrasound-guided percutaneous placement can successfully place leads in proximity to target nerves.[56,62-64] Rauck et al.[56] have shown that leads can be placed within 2 mm of the target nerve and also suggest that leads at least 5 mm away from the target nerve may increase selectivity to desired fibers. Others have successfully utilized ultrasound guidance to place electrodes next to deep targets such as the brachial plexus.[56,65] Combining ultrasound guidance with percutaneous placement allows accuracy close to that achieved with open procedures without the tissue damage and risk required in skeletonizing the nerve.

As previously mentioned, PFS allows treatment of painful areas not well covered with PNS and targets subcutaneous afferents and receptors rather than the nerve itself.[14,15] A major procedural difference in PFS is that the painful region is mapped out and subcutaneous electrodes are placed to maximally cover this area. As in PNS, a trial is performed where the area is stimulated with temporary probes or electrodes. Temporary electrodes are then placed for the outpatient portion of the trial. If pain is improved with stimulation, permanent electrodes are typically implanted. A cannulated needle, such as a Tuohy needle, is used to place cylindrical-type leads that are connected to the IPG.

Placement of the subcutaneous leads at the correct depth is of fundamental importance in PFS. Too superficial can lead to burning or lack of efficacy, and too deep can lead to muscle contractions.[66] Abejón et al.[66] uses a radiofrequency probe to determine the appropriate depth and passes the electrode to the tip of the probe. Ultrasound-guided placement of leads is another option to place leads at a prespecified depth—especially useful in patients with high body mass index.[67]

Largely due to the lack of efficacy of SCS and PNS for some indications (e.g., CRPS) and ease of lead implantation, DRGS was introduced. The implantation of leads in DRGS is typically performed percutaneously and under fluoroscopic guidance, and cylindrical leads as shown in Figure 95.2 are typically used. Some groups insert the leads and pulse generator through a single incision.[68]

Early approaches to implanted percutaneous leads used both anterograde (inserting leads from caudally and advancing cranially) and retrograde (advancing from cranial to caudal). Anterograde insertion aimed to place cylindrical leads in the lateral recess to span multiple spinal levels, whereas retrograde techniques aim for the lead to exit the foramen of a single targeted spinal root.[18] Current techniques and at our institution usually advance leads in an anterograde fashion toward a target dorsal root ganglion as will be explained in detail in the following discussion.[69]

FDA approval of PNS devices is primarily limited to radio frequency coupled devices where pulse generator and battery

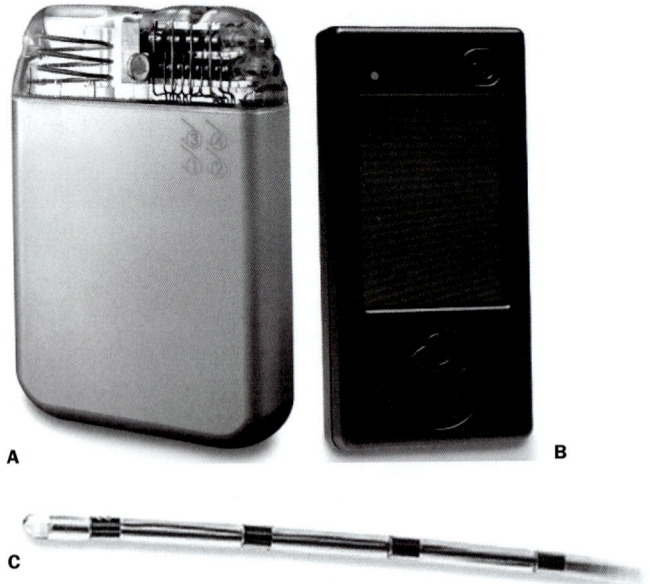

FIGURE 95.2 Hardware photos. The pictures illustrate the types of implantable devices. **A:** Implantable pulse generator associated with a dorsal root ganglion lead. **B:** Patient programmer. **C:** Dorsal root ganglion lead.

pack communicate to the stimulating leads through the skin. However, no fully implantable PNS or PFS devices are FDA-approved for the United States, although these full-implantable devices have been approved for use in Europe in the early 2010s.[70] As previously mentioned, the FDA approved DRGS for treatment of CRPS of the lower extremities in 2016.[17]

Implantation Techniques

There are numerous target nerves and techniques for placing stimulating electrodes, and techniques vary from institution to institution. In this chapter, we provide our experience with electrode implantation for a few sample procedures in the following discussion. For additional information on techniques, comprehensive surgical references are available.[43,44]

OPEN SURGICAL PLACEMENT

In the first stage of the procedure, and as shown in Figure 95.3A, the target nerve is exposed and skeletonized, with the length of exposure depending on the size of the electrode. After exposure, the electrode can be placed underneath the traversing nerve, and often, an interleaving plane of fascia is placed between the nerve and electrode.[43,44] To reduce the likelihood of lead migration, the electrode is secured to the surrounding tissue, and a tension relieving loop is created.

In the second stage of the procedure, the electrode leads are connected to an IPG in a subcutaneous pocket. The lead is tunneled to the IPG implantation location, which depends on surgeon preference and the target nerve. Typical locations include, but are not limited to, the infraclavicular area, abdominal wall, and superior gluteal region.[43,44]

PERCUTANEOUS PLACEMENT WITH FLUOROSCOPIC GUIDANCE

For occipital nerve stimulation, the patient is placed with the head turned laterally in Mayfield pins under general anesthesia. A lateral incision immediately inferior to the mastoid notch and in line with the atlas is planned with the assistance of fluoroscopy. A Tuohy needle or peel-away sheath introducer is passed through the subcutaneous tissue superior to the underlying fascia perpendicular to the trajectory of the occipital nerves toward

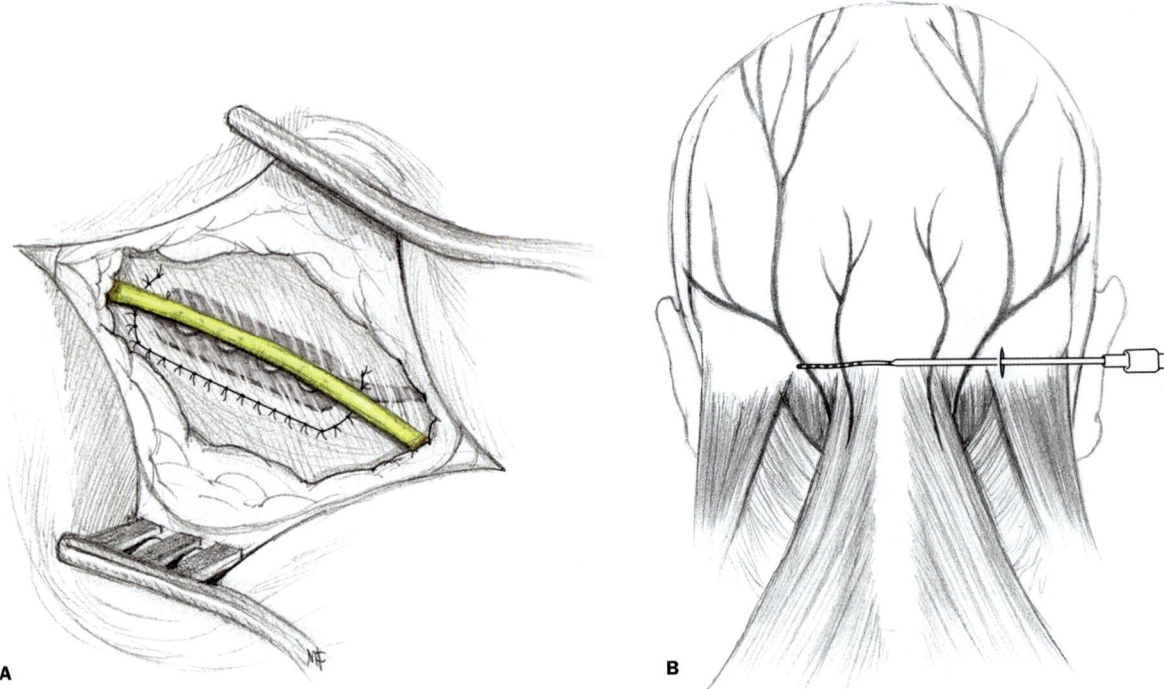

FIGURE 95.3 Illustrations of procedures. **A:** Traditional paddle electrodes applied to peripheral nerves. The dissection is carried down to the peripheral nerve (*in yellow*) to be stimulated. A paddle electrode is placed underneath the nerve. Often, fascial tissue is laid between the nerve and electrode to help secure the electrode. **B:** Percutaneous placement of cylindrical leads for occipital nerve stimulation. As seen in the depiction, the occipital nerve exits the trapezius and travels above the muscular fascia that becomes the galea/aponeurosis. The occipital leads are placed in the subcutaneous tissue superficial to the exiting greater and lesser occipital nerve. Although the lead in this cartoon entered laterally, others choose to insert the leads in the midline and point the leads laterally toward the painful side.

(continued)

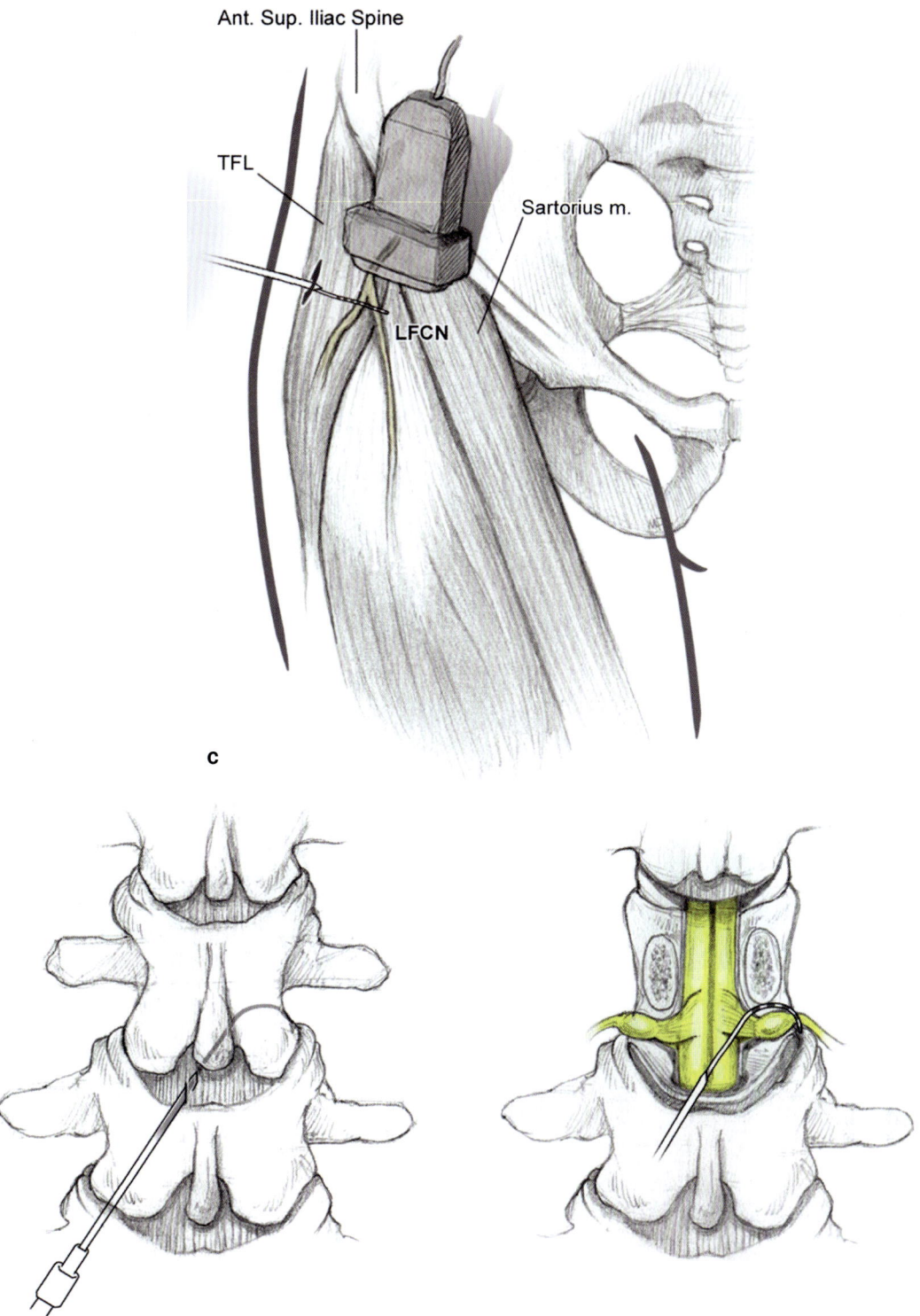

FIGURE 95.3 *(continued)* **C:** Use of ultrasound to visualize the sartorius and tensor fasciae latae (TFL). The lateral femoral cutaneous nerve (LFCN), *in yellow*, travels between these two muscles and can be targeted with a percutaneous lead as seen here. **D:** Insertion of dorsal root ganglion leads. First, a hollow bore needle is passed through the interlaminar space **(left)**. Once the ligamentum flavum is entered and before entering the dura, the needle is stopped, and an electrode is passed laterally toward the neural foramen to be in proximity to the dorsal root ganglion **(right)**. The dorsal root, dorsal root ganglion, and spinal cord (all enclosed in dura) are *in yellow*.

the contralateral side, as shown in Figures 95.3B and 95.4C. Given the reliability of the anatomic landmarks, we forgo intraoperative stimulation of the occipital nerves. A small subcutaneous pocket on top of the fascia is created, and a tension-relieving loop is secured to the fascia. The leads are then tunneled to an infraclavicular pocket where the IPG is implanted.

PERCUTANEOUS PLACEMENT WITH ULTRASOUND GUIDANCE

At our institution, patients undergoing PNS typically undergo an ultrasound-guided trial of stimulation to evaluate efficacy. The most successful location for stimulation is captured with ultrasound imaging.

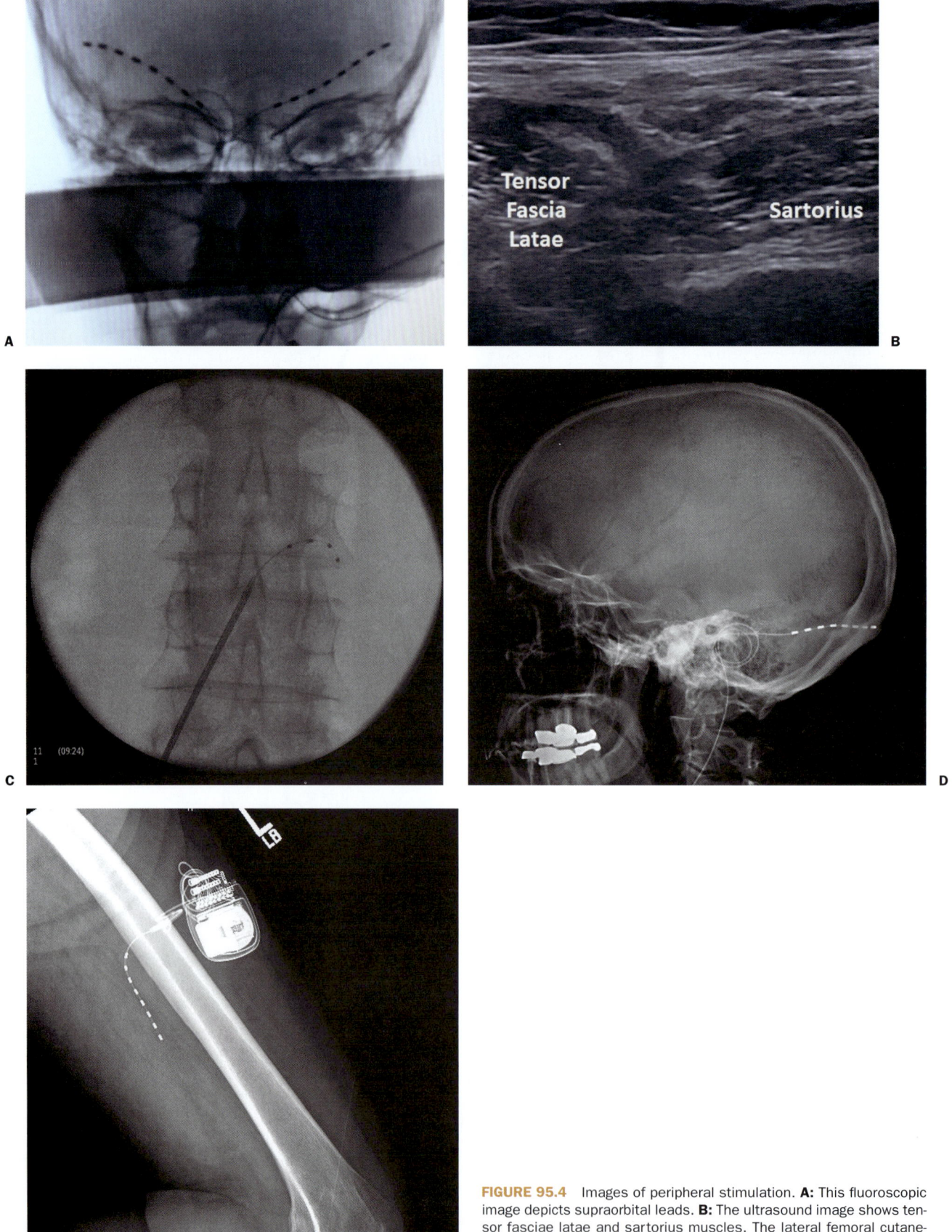

FIGURE 95.4 Images of peripheral stimulation. **A:** This fluoroscopic image depicts supraorbital leads. **B:** The ultrasound image shows tensor fasciae latae and sartorius muscles. The lateral femoral cutaneous nerve (LFCN) traverses between these two muscles which serve as a landmark to target the LFCN. **C:** The fluoroscopic image shows a cylindrical lead being advanced into the neural foramen. **D:** This image shows a percutaneously implanted occipital nerve stimulator (note the tension-relieving loops near the entry site). **E:** This shows implanted saphenous nerve stimulator.

Permanent implantation begins with visualization of the lateral femoral cutaneous nerve (LFCN) between sartorius and tensor fasciae latae, as shown in Figure 95.4B. A small incision only big enough to allow the entry of a needle is made in the skin. A hollow bore needle with stylet is passed toward the nerve, as shown in Figure 95.3C. The stylet is removed, and a cylindrical lead is advanced through the needle toward the LFCN. The cylindrical lead is shown in Figure 95.2. The distal portion of the lead is ideally placed in close proximity to the nerve (within a few millimeters), and the proximal portion is several millimeters deep to the incision. The hollow bore needle is removed, and the skin is closed with dressing. The external stimulator is applied with one end overlying the distal electrodes and one end overlying the proximal leads.

PLACEMENT AT THE NERVE ROOT/DORSAL ROOT GANGLION

For a patient to undergo L1 DRGS, the needle with stylet is placed in the skin at the level below (L2 to L3) on the opposite side of pain; this means that if a patient needs stimulation of left-sided L1 DRG, the needle is inserted from the right side at L2/3. The needle targets the L1 to L2 interlaminar space under fluoroscopic guidance. As the needle is passed through the ligamentum flavum, less resistance is encountered, which indirectly identifies the epidural space. A J-catheter is passed through the needle and is positioned to pass the tip outside the neural foramen. The foramen is entered and requires an interval increase force to "pop" through the foramen. The electrode is then passed through the J-catheter with the radiopaque leads positioned immediately inferior to the pedicle (see Figs. 95.3D and 95.4C). On lateral fluoroscopy, the lead should be in the foramen; it should not cross the disk/vertebral body because this is more likely to induce motor spasms due to stimulation of ventral root. An "S"-shaped tension-relieving loop is then created in the epidural space by twisting the J-catheter. The catheter and the needle are then removed, leaving only the lead. The leads are then tunneled to the IPG, and the incision is closed.

Patient Selection and Preoperative Workup

A typical workup should include detailed history, psychological evaluation, and thorough physical exam. Routine lab work is helpful to screen for systemic disorders or clotting diatheses. As is the case for many pain conditions, a psychological evaluation is necessary to evaluate whether psychiatric condition may be clouding the clinical picture, and if psychiatric condition is found, successful treatment may also reduce the pain experienced.

Radiographs and computed tomography (CT) scans may demonstrate compressive osseous structures or bony entrapments. Magnetic resonance (MR) neurography may show mass lesions or intrinsic lesions that result in pain. Ultrasound is also useful for diagnosing entrapments, compressive mass lesions, and traumatic injuries. Electromyography (EMG) can aid in localizing the nerve, especially to avoid missing a case of entrapment. However, this test can be painful especially for those experiencing neuropathic pain in the area being studied.

PNS is almost never a first-line treatment for pain conditions but follows exhaustive conservative measures, including physical therapy, analgesic/antiepileptic medications, and anesthetic blocks/injections. Injections provide not only a therapeutic effect but also can aid diagnosis (diagnostic blocks) by providing evidence for the target lesion causing pain. Surgical intervention is usually offered prior to neuromodulation to correct the underlying condition if possible.

Many factors influence the efficacy of peripheral stimulation. Prior to permanent implantation of peripheral nerve stimulators, trial stimulators are used to evaluate whether the painful areas are responsive to electrical stimulation. Only if the area is responsive to temporary stimulation does one consider permanent implantation. Poor response to nerve block is also widely considered a poor prognostic sign.[71] Other negative prognostic factors include sensory loss, allodynia, and pain exacerbation with TENS; positive prognostic factors include successful diagnostic nerve block.[16]

Generally speaking, insertions of peripheral stimulators are relatively straightforward procedures that do not require general anesthesia. Thus, clinical judgment should be employed to determine whether the patient is an acceptable surgical candidate. Specific to implantation of peripheral stimulators, the need for frequent MR imaging scans and a remote infection would be relative contraindications.

Clinical Indications and Outcomes

Commonly reported indications for peripheral stimulation are discussed in the following text and include neuropathy (nerve entrapment, postoperative/posttraumatic injuries, or amputation), head/face pain (occipital neuralgia, chronic migraines, cluster headaches, trigeminal neuropathy), back pain, pelvic pain, CRPS, and brachial plexus injury. Peripheral stimulation, however, has also been reported in a number of other pain conditions such as fibromyalgia,[72] phantom limb pain,[56] poststroke pain,[73] postherpetic pain,[74,75] cardiac/visceral pain,[76,77] hemicrania continua,[57] and posttraumatic headaches.[57] Major clinical indications are outlined in Table 95.1.

EXTREMITY PAIN

Extremity pain can be treated with a wide variety of stimulation modalities that are detailed below.

Peripheral Nerve Stimulation

Large peripheral nerves provide excellent targets for peripheral stimulation. Sensory nerves in particular are especially suitable targets because they avoid unwanted motor recruitment, although mixed motor and sensory nerves can be stimulated at the

TABLE 95.1 Major Clinical Indications for Each Modality of Peripheral Stimulation	
Stimulation Technology	**Indication**
Peripheral Nerve Stimulation	**Extremity Pain**
	Neuropathy: entrapment, postoperative, posttraumatic
	Electrical burns
	Amputation pain
	Complex regional pain syndrome
	Headache/Facial Pain
	Occipital neuralgia
	Chronic migraine
	Cluster headache
	Trigeminal neuropathy
	Postherpetic trigeminal neuropathic pain
	Frontal headaches
Brachial/Lumbar Plexus Stimulation	**Extremity Pain**
	Complex regional pain syndrome
	Neuropathy: post posttraumatic (including traction), postamputation
Peripheral Field Stimulation	**Truncal Pain**
	Axial back pain
	Groin neuralgia
Dorsal Root Ganglion Stimulation	**Extremity Pain**
	Complex regional pain syndrome
	Truncal Pain
	Axial back pain with or without radiculopathy
	Groin neuralgia

risk of motor recruitment at stimulation amplitudes. Indications include nerve injuries causing neuropathic pain (entrapment, posttraumatic, iatrogenic),[71] electrical burns,[10] amputational pain,[56] and CRPS.[78] Target nerves include axillary, median, ulnar, and radial nerves in the upper extremities and sciatic, femoral, posterior tibial, peroneal, and LFCNs in the lower extremities.

Many case reports and case series describe promising results for PNS in medically refractory extremity pain. However, no long-term, prospective, randomized studies have been completed. In general, it could be challenging to evaluate stimulation in large, randomized studies because patients typically can sense therapeutic stimulation. In most studies, a majority of patients report 50% to 80% improvement in pain, although there are reports of full pain relief with follow-up ranging from weeks to two decades.[8,10,42,52,56,65,71,78–80] In a 1998 meta-analysis, Long[6] found that 82.5% reported a "good" response.

Some studies have suggested that stimulation of nerves of the lower extremity, specifically the sciatic and posterior tibial nerves, are more likely to fail.[8,42] Nashold et al.[8] suggested stimulation might be more difficult for the sciatic nerve because sensory fascicles are deep in the sciatic trunk, and that failures could also be due to nerve length, tethering of the nerve, or compression in the tarsal tunnel. Regardless, other studies have achieved acceptable results for lower extremity PNS, and Eisenberg et al.[71] reported that 8 of 10 patients had ≥50% improvement in pain.

Brachial and Lumbar Plexus Stimulation

Stimulation of the brachial plexus has been attempted for posttraumatic injury (including traction)[26,81] and CRPS,[65] and stimulation of the lumbar plexus has been reported for traumatic/amputation neuropathy.[82] Traditional treatments for posttraumatic injury include medical management, anesthetic blocks, and implantation of pain catheters.[26] Implantation at the brachial plexus offers several advantages over stimulation of distal nerves such as broad area of coverage, possibility for a single incision for lead and pulse generator, and protection from migration provided by deep location.[81] Compared to SCS, implantation of the PNS lead is less invasive. Both posterior and supraclavicular approaches are reported.[26,83]

In posttraumatic neuropathy, Law et al.[81] published a series of 22 patients implanted with brachial plexus stimulators at the cords and trunks. Thirteen patients achieved pain control at 25 months. Goroszeniuk et al.[26] reported percutaneous cylindrical leads at the brachial plexus for a patient with traction injury. The patient stopped all pain medications and at 21-month follow-up noticed improvement in sensory and motor loss from the original accident.

Bouche et al.[65] reported that 10 of 17 patients implanted for CRPS type 2 had ≥50% reduction of pain at 1 to 2 years. The study noted no cases of lead migration. Only one patient required surgical correction for an adverse event, a surgical site infection; the stimulator was removed and then reimplanted after the infection cleared.

Dorsal Root Ganglion Stimulation

DRGS is especially helpful for neuropathic pain of the trunk and extremities. It is FDA-approved for CRPS of the lower extremities and groin.[17] Other reported indications include amputational pain,[84,85] neuropathy of the lower extremities,[68,86] postherpetic pain,[87] and postthoracotomy syndrome.[17]

CRPS is a pain condition commonly treated with neuromodulation—traditionally SCS. However, pain in the lower extremities is difficult to cover with SCS, and DRGS is often successful in cases refractory to SCS.[88] In one of the few prospective studies, 152 patients with CRPS of the lower extremities were randomized to either DRGS or SCS, and efficacy was defined as a 50% drop in visual analog scale (VAS) pain scores

at 3 months. The DRG group had a statistically significant superior result, with an 81.2% response rate compared to a 55.7% response rate for SCS. The efficacy of DRGS was also found to be less dependent on lead position than SCS.[89] Successful DRGS has been demonstrated in several case reports and case series.[90,91]

Similar to CRPS, many physicians have turned to DRGS for amputation stump pain when other forms of neuromodulation, like SCS, are unsuccessful. Several small series have shown early success.[84,85] As mentioned previously, PNS can also be used for amputation stump pain.[56,79]

Our institution uses DRGS for several pain conditions previously treated with other forms of neuromodulation. We favor L5 DRGS over SCS for CRPS of the foot because we have found it more efficacious and less invasive. For improved efficacy, we use L3 DRGS for neuropathic pain in the distribution of the LFCN and L2 to L4 DRGS for femoral neuralgia.

TRUNCAL PAIN
Axial Back Pain

Historically, low back pain from failed back surgery is an excellent indication for SCS. Typically, the radicular component of the pain is more responsive than the axial component, and stimulating the dorsal columns does not easily provide coverage in the low back, chest wall, or abdominal wall.[92,93] Obviously, direct stimulation of peripheral nerves is not effective, given that axial back pain is not isolated to the distribution of one nerve or spinal root. However, PFS and DRGS effectively cover the painful area of the back.

Several case reports and case series describe successful control of back pain with PFS. Paicius et al.[94] reported improvement of intractable, axial low back pain in six patients, and in one patient, Krutsch et al.[92] reported improvement of pain severity to 1 on a 10-point VAS without oral pain medications. Two large series[95,96] and one small series of patients with variable painful conditions that included low back pain found significant improvement in pain with PFS with up to 1-year follow-up.

In the only prospective, blinded, randomized study, McRoberts et al.[33] placed trial stimulators in 32 patients with chronic, intractable low back pain and divided patients into groups with minimal stimulation, subtherapeutic stimulation, low-frequency stimulation, and standard stimulation. At short-term follow-up, there was a statistically significant decrease in VAS between groups with effective stimulation and those without stimulation. Subsequently, the 23 responders underwent permanent implantation, with 69.5% of patients reporting "excellent" to "good" pain control at 1 year.

Recently, DRGS has been applied to intractable back pain, radiculopathy, or failed back syndrome.[69,97] Deer et al.[69] implanted trial DRG stimulators in five patients with primarily back pain who experienced, on average, an 84% improvement in VAS pain scores at 3 to 7 days. The average decrease in pain was 80% in the leg and 70% in the foot. Liem et al.[97] permanently implanted 32 patients with DRG stimulators for back and lower extremity pain attributable to CRPS, failed back surgery syndrome, chronic postsurgical pain, disk pain, radicular pain, and lumbar stenosis. The patients were followed prospectively, and at 12 months, VAS scores for the back, leg, and foot had decreased by 42%, 62%, and 80%, respectively. Our current practice is to use PFS for axial low back pain without radicular pain and multicolumn SCS or high-frequency SCS for back pain with radicular pain.

Pelvic and Groin Pain

Pelvic pain is another common pain syndrome, as roughly 10% of gynecology visits are related to chronic pelvic pain.[98] Previously, SCS was employed mainly to control the visceral component of pelvic pain. Tamimi et al.[99] demonstrated the successful use of PFS in two patients with chronic pelvic pain and one with laparoscopically diagnosed endometriosis. The subcutaneous leads were placed in the distribution of the L1 root and ilioinguinal nerve.

Stinson et al.[15] reported the implantation of subcutaneous leads in three patients, not with deep visceral pain but chronic groin pain associated with open herniorrhaphy. The incidence of intractable, postherniorrhaphy inguinal pain was estimated in 2001 to be 6,800 to 13,600 new cases annually in the United States. Although not referred to as PFS, the method of implantation is similar to PFS because the leads are implanted into the subcutaneous tissue of the painful area and not directly to the nerve proximal to the area of pain. All three patients had 75% to 100% pain relief at 3, 10, and 12 months.[15] Rauchwerger et al.[24] reported successful pain relief in three patients with medically refractory postsurgical ilioinguinal neuralgia who were implanted with subcutaneous leads at 6 to 12 months.

Recently, many have used DRGS to treat groin neuralgia. Although there are no randomized comparisons between DRGS and other modalities of neuromodulation, several series and reviews report success.[100–103] Regarding postoperative etiologies, Zuidema et al.[101] reported 90% to 100% improvement in postherniorrhaphy at 2 to 3 months and also reported 80% pain reduction in intractable groin pain after resection of Bartholin's cyst.[102] Rowland et al.[100] successfully used a DRG stimulator at L1 and L2 for chronic and intractable pelvic girdle pain after pregnancy.

We favor DRGS over PFS for most groin neuralgias. We feel the implantation is easier, and efficacy is the same or better. Specifically, L1 DRG is used for ilioinguinal neuralgia and L1 and L2 DRG for genitofemoral neuralgia. However, for neuropathic pain in the pudendal distribution, we use epidural stimulation within the sacral spinal canal of the sacral roots for ease of implementation.

Other Truncal Pain Syndromes

In addition to back and pelvic pain, case reports and small series have successfully demonstrated PFS in chronic neck pain,[35] postthoracotomy pain,[104] and chronic abdominal pain.[34] Given the high incidence of postthoracotomy pain (up to 50%),[105] neuromodulation techniques such as SCS[106] and PFS[104] have become useful techniques for these difficult-to-control pain syndromes. Finally, in our experience, DRGS has been helpful for postherpetic pain at the level above the painful dermatome.

HEADACHE AND FACIAL PAIN

A major application for PNS is relief of headache, facial pain, and head pain. The target nerves in this region are the occipital nerve and branches of the trigeminal nerves, including the supraorbital, infraorbital, and supratrochlear nerves.

Occipital nerve stimulation is a major target of PNS and one of the first targets of percutaneous nerve stimulation.[9,11,12,49,51,53,59,61,107] Since its original use, the occipital nerve has been the target for not only occipital neuralgia but also triggered migraine headaches,[48,54,57,108–113] cluster headaches,[47,54,55,114,115] hemicrania continua,[57] and posttraumatic headaches.[57]

It is not well understood why stimulating the occipital nerve relieves pain outside of its sensory distribution such as migraine headaches. As explained by Goroszeniuk and Pang,[116] convergence of common pathways (cervico-trigeminal relay) in the brainstem may allow the occipital nerve to act as an access point to modulate various brainstem afferents. This theory is further evidenced by preliminary studies such as Busch et al.,[117] which shows that the trigeminal-mediated blink reflex is impeded by occipital block. In response to occipital nerve stimulation, preliminary positron emission tomography (PET) studies suggest central changes, including regional blood flow variations to the anterior cingulate, cuneus, rostral-dorsal midbrain, and pulvinar nucleus.[109] Magis et al.[115] showed on 18-fluorodeoxyglucose-PET that occipital nerve stimulation normalized elevated metabolism

of the midbrain and lower pons but did not decrease elevations of hypothalamus. Additionally, elevations in the metabolism of the anterior cingulate cortex correlated with better response to stimulation. Finally, further proof of a shared occipital nerve and central pathway lies in a study by Aló and Holsheimer[118] that showed that cervicogenic headaches in the C1 to C3 distribution can transform into chronic migraines.

Other major targets of PNS in the face are the branches of the trigeminal nerve. The supraorbital nerve is a branch of the ophthalmic nerve (V1). The nerve has been stimulated for pain syndromes, including neuropathic facial pain in the trigeminal distribution that is postherpetic or secondary to surgical/traumatic injury,[60,74,119–121] chronic cluster headache,[122] and frontal headaches.[123]

Occipital Neuralgia

Much of the early work on occipital nerve stimulation for pain was reported for large series in which the occipital nerve was just one of several nerves stimulated, and the approach was an open procedure that identified the nerve and placed an electrode in proximity to the nerve.[9,107] In 1999, Weiner and Reed[11] placed leads at the occipital nerve via a percutaneous approach for patients with occipital neuralgia. Recent studies have demonstrated success in the majority of patients, with follow-up times between 3 months and 6 years. These studies primarily include series from a single institution and usually report success as ≥50% decrease in VAS scores.[49,51,59,61,107,124] A detailed review of occipital nerve stimulation for occipital neuralgia can be found in Liu et al.[53] The occipital nerve is not the only target for occipital neuralgia, as Chivukula et al.[125] stimulated the spinal roots and spinal cord for relief of occipital neuralgia.

Migraine Headache

Stimulation of the occipital nerve for patients with migraine headaches is an option for patients with migraines refractory to conservative medical treatments. Silberstein et al.[112] performed one of the first prospective, multicenter, blinded studies, which involved 157 patients. At 12 weeks, stimulated patients had decreased headache severity and decreased number of headache days compared to controls, although the primary outcome, defined as a 50% decrease in VAS scores, shows no significant difference between treated patients and controls. At 12 months, all patients were moved to the stimulation group, and roughly half had either decreased headache severity, decreased frequency of headache, or both. A downside of the study was the large number of adverse events—41% required surgical management of an adverse event.[48]

In the occipital nerve stimulation for the treatment of intractable chronic migraine headache (ONSTIM) trial, the multicenter, randomized study of 66 patients by Saper et al.,[111] patients with occipital nerve stimulation had a 39% response rate compared to medically treated controls with a 0% response rate. Response rate was defined as either a >50% reduction in headache days or a 3-point drop in headache intensity (VAS). Patients who responded to occipital nerve block were randomly assigned to stimulation and control groups. The stimulation group consisted of patients with an occipital nerve stimulator who adjusted the intensity of the stimulation to minimize pain. The control groups included both medically managed patients and those with occipital nerve stimulation that was turned on for only 1 minute per day and were told that stimulation intensity was at a preset level. Although the number of patients responding to stimulation was significant, the stimulation and control groups did not differ significantly when the number of headache days and overall intensity were averaged over the respective groups.[111]

In another randomized study, Slotty et al.[113] showed that a small group of eight patients treated for chronic migraines had a statistically significant drop in VAS score when compared to controls. The stimulation group was divided into a suprathreshold group and subthreshold group; threshold was set at the level of the patient's perception of stimulation. VAS score decreased from 8.2 ± 1.22 preoperatively to 1.98 ± 1.56 in suprathreshold stimulation and 5.65 ± 2.11 in subthreshold stimulation. Only patients with a stable response to occipital nerve stimulation were selected for this study,[113] in which intensity of stimulation correlated with reduction in pain.

The aforementioned results contrast with those of Lipton et al.[108] in the PRecision Implantable Stimulator for Migraine (PRISM) study of 132 patients with medication refractory chronic migraines. Compared to patients with sham stimulation, those with occipital nerve stimulation (active arm) had no statistically significant decrease in number of headache days. In the active arm, 5 to 10 days of percutaneous trial stimulation prior to implantation was moderately predictive of stimulation success at 12 weeks.[108] Unlike Silberstein et al.,[112] Lipton et al.[108] did not use trial stimulation to screen patients for permanent implantation, which is a major difference in study design.

In addition to these larger studies, several case series demonstrate relief of pain from chronic migraines. Popeney and Alo[110] implanted 25 patients with occipital nerve stimulators, with an average improvement in Migraine Disability Assessment score of 89% at mean follow-up of 18 months. Oh et al.[124] implanted 10 patients with chronic migraines, with near complete resolution of pain at 6 months.

Cluster Headache

Neuromodulation for cluster headaches has been previously reported by Franzini et al.,[126] who used deep brain stimulation of the posterior hypothalamus. However, occipital nerve stimulation for cluster headaches has also demonstrated success and is less invasive. Several series show promising results.[47,54,114] In these studies, the majority of 41 patients responded well to stimulation at varying follow-up times (3 to 47 months). Additional prospective, randomized trials are needed to further validate this application of neurostimulation technology.

Other targets of neuromodulation to relieve pain from cluster headaches have been studied. Narouze and Kapural[127] employed supraorbital stimulation for both early abortion of cluster headaches and prevention of recurrent attacks up to 14 months later. Schoenen et al.[128] targeted the sphenopalatine ganglion for transorally placed electrical stimulators.

Trigeminal Neuralgia and Facial Pain

Facial pain syndromes have long been a source of chronic suffering for patients, and recently, neuromodulation has been applied toward their relief. Johnson and Burchiel[74] found $\geq 50\%$ pain relief in 7 of 10 patients with primarily posttraumatic or postherpetic neuropathic pain in the V1 and V2 branches. Eight of these patients had implantation of leads at the supraorbital foramen and two at the infraorbital foramen. Slavin et al.[59] implanted 22 patients with peripheral nerve stimulators for postsurgical, posttraumatic, or unknown nerve injury, targeting the occipital, supraorbital, or infraorbital nerve. Fifteen of the 22 had $\geq 50\%$ reduction in pain. The results are not subcategorized by nerve, but 4 patients had supraorbital stimulators, and 1 had a combination of occipital and supraorbital nerve stimulators.[119] In a separate report, Slavin et al.[59] implanted supraorbital/infraorbital stimulators in 8 patients with facial pain, and 7 of the 8 experienced $\geq 50\%$ improvement in pain. Amin et al.[123] was the first study of supraorbital stimulation for frontal headaches. Ten patients underwent implantation, and VAS scores decreased from 7.5 ± 1.2 to 3.5 ± 1.2 at 30 weeks. Additional small case reports and series include studies of supraorbital neuralgia[120] and postherpetic neuralgia.[121]

Other targets for facial pain include the trigeminal ganglion itself. Studies have demonstrated stimulation of the ganglion for

facial pain from peripheral neuropathy, stroke, or postherpetic neuralgia.[129,130] A thorough review of this topic was presented by Holsheimer,[131] who found $\geq 50\%$ improvement in VAS scores in 48% of patients with atypical trigeminal neuralgia; the response rate for those with postherpetic neuropathy was $<10\%$.

Complications

The anticipated complications for any implantable stimulator include infection, lead migration, hardware failure, and lead/wire fracture. Specific complications are reviewed in the following text for each modality of stimulation.

PERIPHERAL NERVE STIMULATION

Complication rates vary widely for large studies that implanted electrodes via open techniques. Nashold et al.[8] implanted sutured button electrodes directly to the fascicles to be stimulated in 35 patients and reported an 8.6% complication rate, but no patients required surgical revision. Eisenberg et al.[71] also directly sutured leads to the nerve, with 5 of 46 patients (11%) having a complication leading to additional surgery. Mobbs et al.,[42] who wrapped the nerve in mesh in PNS for chronic pain, had an 18% rate of complication requiring surgery. In Hassenbusch et al.,[78] the electrode "with a layer of free fascia covering its surface was placed in apposition" to the nerve, and the rate of complication was 27%.

Historically, open procedures use paddle electrodes placed in proximity to the nerve. These paddle electrodes can be complicated by compression neuropathy[44] and perineural fibrosis. However, this outcome is much less likely with newer cylindrical electrodes and percutaneous placement.[43]

Some have suggested that percutaneous placement of cylindrical leads may be more prone to migration than open techniques with paddle electrodes, although no studies directly compare open versus percutaneous techniques.[61,124] The migration of cylindrical leads can be reduced by looping the electrode in the subcutaneous pocket.[44] In the ONSTIM trial using percutaneous leads in 51 patients, the migration rate was 26%.[111] Dodick et al.[48] reported that 71% of 157 patients experienced an adverse event, including 29 lead migration events, in their study of occipital nerve stimulation for chronic migraines. Eighty-five (41%) of the adverse events required additional procedures. On the other hand, in Mueller et al.'s[54] study of occipital nerve stimulation, only 1 of 27 patients had lead migration. More data and better strategies are needed to reduce the number of adverse events from lead migration.

PERIPHERAL FIELD STIMULATION

Complications of PFS are similar to those of PNS and include infection, lead migration or fracture, lead erosion, hardware failure, and postoperative pain. Several large series have noted adverse events, including lead migration rates of 4%,[96] 13%,[95] and 22%.[33] Reoperation rates are not widely reported, but McRoberts et al.[33] reported a high rate of 13 of 23 patients (56%). Seventy-four percent of 111 patients in the retrospective study of Sator-Katzenschlager et al.[95] had no complications, but the rate of reoperation was not given. Further studies will help to better understand the side-effect profile of PFS.

DORSAL ROOT GANGLION STIMULATION

Although generic risks for DRGS include those previously mentioned (infection, lead migration/fracture, device failure, and postoperative pain), cerebrospinal fluid (CSF) leak is a unique risk for this procedure given the proximity of the dorsal root ganglion to the thecal sac. Although the rate of serious adverse events (life-threatening risks, disability, or need for invasive procedure) have been shown to be comparable to SCS,[89] the total number of adverse events is likely higher. Deer et al.[89] reported a 10.5% rate of serious adverse events in 76 patients without any deaths, although the rate of total adverse events was higher in DRGS (46%) than SCS (26%). Postoperative incisional pain was the most common procedure-related event, and pain at the IPG was the most common device-related event. Likewise, Liem et al.[97] recorded 86 events in 29 of 51 patients, with 14.6% experiencing temporary motor recruitment, 8.5% CSF leak, and 8.5% infection. Clearly, more studies are needed as this technique improves and evolves.

Conclusion and Future Directions

Painful conditions are a source of tremendous patient suffering and high health care costs. Patients in pain often turn to addictive narcotic medications that do not relieve pain long term due to medication tolerance and that also have unwanted side effects. Electrical stimulation has been used for many years and provides effective pain relief for those with refractory pain conditions, without the side effects of narcotic medications. PNS has been used for many decades, and in recent years, implantation has become less invasive. PFS has been proposed to treat conditions such as axial back pain that are not effectively covered by a single peripheral nerve. Likewise, DRGS has shown tremendous efficacy in conditions with pain distributed across multiple peripheral nerve roots.

Finally, just as the field has experienced exponential growth recently, new technologies and strategies using peripheral stimulation continue to emerge. Recently, some have combined the use of peripheral stimulation with other forms of electrical stimulation, such as SCS. Furthermore, implantation techniques are becoming less invasive, and many investigators have proposed either small or wireless IPG devices that are easier to implant.

References

1. Shealy CN. Transcutaneous electrical nerve stimulation: the treatment of choice for pain and depression. *J Altern Complement Med* 2003;9(5):619–623.
2. Melzack R, Wall PD. Pain mechanisms: a new theory. *Science* 1965;150(3699): 971–979.
3. Wall PD, Sweet WH. Temporary abolition of pain in man. *Science* 1967;155(3758):108–109.
4. Sweet WH, Wepsic JG. Treatment of chronic pain by stimulation of fibers of primary afferent neuron. *Trans Am Neurol Assoc* 1968;93:103–107.
5. Campbell JN, Long DM. Peripheral nerve stimulation in the treatment of intractable pain. *J Neurosurg* 1976;45(6):692–699.
6. Long D. The current status of electrical stimulation of the nervous system for the relief of chronic pain. *Surg Neurol* 1998;49(2):142–144.
7. Long DM. Electrical stimulation for relief of pain from chronic nerve injury. *J Neurosurg* 1973;39(6):718–722.
8. Nashold BS Jr, Goldner JL, Mullen JB, et al. Long-term pain control by direct peripheral-nerve stimulation. *J Bone Joint Surg Am* 1982;64(1):1–10.
9. Picaza JA, Cannon BW, Hunter SE, et al. Pain suppression by peripheral nerve stimulation. Part II. Observations with implanted devices. *Surg Neurol* 1975;4(1):115–126.
10. Racz GB, Browne T, Lewis R Jr. Peripheral stimulator implant for treatment of causalgia caused by electrical burns. *Tex Med* 1988;84(11):45–50.
11. Weiner RL, Reed KL. Peripheral neurostimulation for control of intractable occipital neuralgia. *Neuromodulation* 1999;2(3):217–221.
12. Skaribas I, Aló K. Ultrasound imaging and occipital nerve stimulation. *Neuromodulation* 2010;13(2):126–130.
13. Slavin KV. History of peripheral nerve stimulation. In: *Peripheral Nerve Stimulation*. Switzerland: Karger; 2011:1–15.
14. Goroszeniuk T, Kothari S, Hamann W. Subcutaneous neuromodulating implant targeted at the site of pain. *Reg Anesth Pain Med* 2006;31(2):168–171.
15. Stinson LW Jr, Roderer GT, Cross NE, et al. Peripheral subcutaneous electrostimulation for control of intractable post-operative inguinal pain: a case report series. *Neuromodulation* 2001;4(3):99–104.
16. Deogaonkar M, Slavin KV. Peripheral nerve/field stimulation for neuropathic pain. *Neurosurg Clin Am* 2014;25(1):1–10.
17. Deer TR, Pope JE. Dorsal root ganglion stimulation approval by the Food and Drug Administration: advice on evolving the process. *Expert Rev Neurother* 2016;16(10):1123–1125.
18. Haque R, Winfree CJ. Spinal nerve root stimulation. *Neurosurg Focus* 2006;21(6):E4.
19. Pope JE, Deer TR, Kramer J. A systematic review: current and future directions of dorsal root ganglion therapeutics to treat chronic pain. *Pain Med* 2013;14(10):1477–1496.
20. Sluka KA, Deacon M, Stibal A, et al. Spinal blockade of opioid receptors prevents the analgesia produced by TENS in arthritic rats. *J Pharmacol Exp Ther* 1999;289(2):840–846.

21. Radhakrishnan R, Sluka K. Spinal muscarinic receptors are activated during low or high frequency TENS-induced antihyperalgesia in rats. *Neuropharmacology* 2003;45(8):1111–1119.
22. Maeda Y, Lisi T, Vance C, et al. Release of GABA and activation of GABA(A) in the spinal cord mediates the effects of TENS in rats. *Brain Res* 2007;1136:43–50.
23. Sluka KA, Lisi TL, Westlund KN. Increased release of serotonin in the spinal cord during low, but not high, frequency transcutaneous electric nerve stimulation in rats with joint inflammation. *Arch Phys Rehabil* 2006;87(8): 1137–1140.
24. Rauchwerger JJ, Giordano J, Rozen D, et al. On the therapeutic viability of peripheral nerve stimulation for ilioinguinal neuralgia: putative mechanisms and possible utility. *Pain Pract* 2008;8(2):138–143.
25. Hanai F. Effect of electrical stimulation of peripheral nerves on neuropathic pain. *Spine (Phila PA 1976)* 2000;25(15):1886–1892.
26. Goroszeniuk T, Kothari SC, Hamann WC. Percutaneous implantation of a brachial plexus electrode for management of pain syndrome caused by a traction injury. *Neuromodulation* 2007;10(2):148–155.
27. Randić M, Jiang M, Cerne R. Long-term potentiation and long-term depression of primary afferent neurotransmission in the rat spinal cord. *J Neurosci* 1993;13(12):5228–5241.
28. Sandkühler J, Chen J, Cheng G, et al. Low-frequency stimulation of afferent Adelta-fibers induces long-term depression at primary afferent synapses with substantia gelatinosa neurons in the rat. *J Neurosci* 1997;17(16): 6483–6491.
29. Torebjörk HE, Hallin RG. Responses in human A and C fibres to repeated electrical intradermal stimulation. *J Neurol Neurosurg Psychiatry* 1974;37(6):653–664.
30. Ignelzi RJ, Nyquist JK. Direct effect of electrical stimulation on peripheral nerve evoked activity: implications in pain relief. *J Neurosurg* 1976;45(2):159–165.
31. Ignelzi RJ, Nyquist JK. Excitability changes in peripheral nerve fibers after repetitive electrical stimulation. Implications in pain modulation. *J Neurosurg* 1979;51(6):824–833.
32. Ellrich J, Lamp S. Peripheral nerve stimulation inhibits nociceptive processing: an electrophysiological study in healthy volunteers. *Neuromodulation* 2005;8(4):225–232.
33. McRoberts WP, Wolkowitz R, Meyer DJ, et al. Peripheral nerve field stimulation for the management of localized chronic intractable back pain: results from a randomized controlled study. *Neuromodulation* 2013;16(6): 565–575.
34. Paicius RM, Bernstein CA, Lempert-Cohen C. Peripheral nerve field stimulation in chronic abdominal pain. *Pain Physician* 2006;9(3):261–266.
35. Lipov EG, Joshi JR, Sanders S, et al. Use of peripheral subcutaneous field stimulation for the treatment of axial neck pain: a case report. *Neuromodulation* 2009;12(4):292–295.
36. Pinto V, Szucs P, Lima D, et al. Multisegmental Aδ-and C-fiber input to neurons in lamina I and the lateral spinal nucleus. *J Neurosci* 2010;30(6): 2384–2395.
37. Liem AL, Krabbenbos IP, Kramer J. Dorsal root ganglion stimulation: a target for neuromodulation therapies. In: Knotkova H, Rasche D, eds. *Textbook of Neuromodulation: Principles, Methods and Clinical Applications*. New York: Springer; 2015:53–59.
38. Krames ES. The dorsal root ganglion in chronic pain and as a target for neuromodulation: a review. *Neuromodulation* 2015;18(1):24–32.
39. Wang W, Gu J, Li YQ, et al. Are voltage-gated sodium channels on the dorsal root ganglion involved in the development of neuropathic pain? *Mol Pain* 2011;7:16.
40. Koopmeiners AS, Mueller S, Kramer J, et al. Effect of electrical field stimulation on dorsal root ganglion neuronal function. *Neuromodulation* 2013; 16(4):304–311.
41. Slavin KV, Burchiel KJ. Peripheral nerve stimulation for painful nerve injuries. *Contemp Neurosurg* 1999;21(19):1–6.
42. Mobbs RJ, Nair S, Blum P. Peripheral nerve stimulation for the treatment of chronic pain. *J Clin Neurosci* 2007;14(3):216–223.
43. Slavin KV. Peripheral nerve stimulation for neuropathic pain. *Neurotherapeutics* 2008;5(1):100–106.
44. Weiner RL. Peripheral nerve neurostimulation. *Neurosurg Clin N Am* 2003; 14(3):401–408.
45. Deer TR, Levy RM, Rosenfeld EL. Prospective clinical study of a new implantable peripheral nerve stimulation device to treat chronic pain. *Clin J Pain* 2010;26(5):359–372.
46. Deer T, Pope J, Benyamin R, et al. Prospective, multicenter, randomized, double-blinded, partial crossover study to assess the safety and efficacy of the novel neuromodulation system in the treatment of patients with chronic pain of peripheral nerve origin. *Neuromodulation* 2016;19(1):91–100.
47. Burns B, Watkins L, Goadsby PJ. Treatment of medically intractable cluster headache by occipital nerve stimulation: long-term follow-up of eight patients. *Lancet* 2007;369(9567):1099–1106.
48. Dodick DW, Silberstein SD, Reed KL, et al. Safety and efficacy of peripheral nerve stimulation of the occipital nerves for the management of chronic migraine: long-term results from a randomized, multicenter, double-blinded, controlled study. *Cephalalgia* 2015;35(4):344–358.
49. Johnstone CS, Sundaraj R. Occipital nerve stimulation for the treatment of occipital neuralgia-eight case studies. *Neuromodulation* 2006;9(1):41–47.

50. Jones RL. Occipital nerve stimulation using a Medtronic Resume II electrode array. *Pain Physician* 2003;6(4):507–508.

51. Kapural L, Mekhail N, Hayek SM, et al. Occipital nerve electrical stimulation via the midline approach and subcutaneous surgical leads for treatment of severe occipital neuralgia: a pilot study. *Anesth Analg* 2005;101(1):171–174.

52. Kothari S, Goroszeniuk T. Percutaneous permanent electrode implantation to ulnar nerves for upper extremity chronic pain: 6 years follow up: 201. *Reg Anesth Pain Med* 2006;31(5):16.

53. Liu A, Jiao Y, Ji H, et al. Unilateral occipital nerve stimulation for bilateral occipital neuralgia: a case report and literature review. *J Pain Res* 2017;10:229–232.

54. Mueller O, Diener HC, Dammann P, et al. Occipital nerve stimulation for intractable chronic cluster headache or migraine: a critical analysis of direct treatment costs and complications. *Cephalalgia* 2013;33(16):1283–1291.

55. Mueller O, Hagel V, Wrede K, et al. Stimulation of the greater occipital nerve: anatomical considerations and clinical implications. *Pain Physician* 2013;16(3):E181–E189.

56. Rauck RL, Cohen SP, Gilmore CA, et al. Treatment of post-amputation pain with peripheral nerve stimulation. *Neuromodulation* 2014;17(2):188–197.

57. Schwedt TJ, Dodick DW, Hentz J, et al. Occipital nerve stimulation for chronic headache—long-term safety and efficacy. *Cephalalgia* 2007;27(2):153–157.

58. Shetty A, Pang D, Mendis V, et al. Median nerve stimulation in forearm for treatment of neuropathic pain post reimplantation of fingers: a case report. *Pain Pract* 2012;12:92.

59. Slavin KV, Nersesyan H, Wess C. Peripheral neurostimulation for treatment of intractable occipital neuralgia. *Neurosurgery* 2006;58(1):112–119.

60. Slavin KV, Wess C. Trigeminal branch stimulation for intractable neuropathic pain: technical note. *Neuromodulation* 2005;8(1):7–13.

61. Magown P, Garcia R, Beauprie I, et al. Occipital nerve stimulation for intractable occipital neuralgia: an open surgical technique. *Clin Neurosurg* 2009;56:119–124.

62. Huntoon MA, Huntoon EA, Obray JB, et al. Feasibility of ultrasound-guided percutaneous placement of peripheral nerve stimulation electrodes in a cadaver model: part one, lower extremity. *Reg Anesth Pain Med* 2008;33(6):551–557.

63. Huntoon MA, Burgher AH. Ultrasound-guided permanent implantation of peripheral nerve stimulation (PNS) system for neuropathic pain of the extremities: original cases and outcomes. *Pain Med* 2009;10(8):1369–1377.

64. Kent M, Upp J, Spevak C, et al. Ultrasound-guided peripheral nerve stimulator placement in two soldiers with acute battlefield neuropathic pain. *Anesth and Analg* 2012;114(4):875–878.

65. Bouche B, Manfiotto M, Rigoard P, et al. Peripheral nerve stimulation of brachial plexus nerve roots and supra-scapular nerve for chronic refractory neuropathic pain of the upper limb. *Neuromodulation* 2017;20(7):684–689.

66. Abejón D, Deer T, Verrills P. Subcutaneous stimulation: how to assess optimal implantation depth. *Neuromodulation* 2011;14(4):343–348.

67. Burgher AH, Huntoon MA, Turley TW, et al. Subcutaneous peripheral nerve stimulation with inter-lead stimulation for axial neck and low back pain: case series and review of the literature. *Neuromodulation* 2012;15(2):100–107.

68. van Velsen V, van Helmond N, Levine ME, et al. Single-incision approach to implantation of the pulse generator and leads for dorsal root ganglion stimulation: a case report. *A A Pract* 2017;10(1):23–27.

69. Deer TR, Grigsby E, Weiner RL, et al. A prospective study of dorsal root ganglion stimulation for the relief of chronic pain. *Neuromodulation* 2013;16(1):67–72.

70. Birk DM, Yin D, Slavin KV. Regulation of peripheral nerve stimulation technology. *Prog Neurol Surg* 2015;29:225–237.

71. Eisenberg E, Waisbrod H, Gerbershagen HU. Long-term peripheral nerve stimulation for painful nerve injuries. *Clin J Pain* 2004;20(3):143–146.

72. Thimineur M, De Ridder D. C2 area neurostimulation: a surgical treatment for fibromyalgia. *Pain Med* 2007;8(8):639–646.

73. Wilson RD, Gunzler DD, Bennett ME, et al. Peripheral nerve stimulation compared with usual care for pain relief of hemiplegic shoulder pain: a randomized controlled trial. *Am J Phys Med Rehabil* 2014;93(1):17–28.

74. Johnson MD, Burchiel KJ. Peripheral stimulation for treatment of trigeminal postherpetic neuralgia and trigeminal posttraumatic neuropathic pain: a pilot study. *Neurosurgery* 2004;55(1):135–142.

75. Yakovlev AE, Peterson AT. Peripheral nerve stimulation in treatment of intractable postherpetic neuralgia. *Neuromodulation* 2007;10(4):373–375.

76. Buiten MS, DeJongste MJ, Beese U, et al. Subcutaneous electrical nerve stimulation: a feasible and new method for the treatment of patients with refractory angina. *Neuromodulation* 2011;14(3):258–265.

77. Goroszeniuk T, Khan R. Permanent percutaneous splanchnic nerve neuromodulation for management of pain due to chronic pancreatitis: a case report. *Neuromodulation* 2011;14(3):253–257.

78. Hassenbusch SJ, Stanton-Hicks M, Schoppa D, et al. Long-term results of peripheral nerve stimulation for reflex sympathetic dystrophy. *J Neurosurg* 1996;84(3):415–423.

79. Miles J, Lipton S. Phantom limb pain treated by electrical stimulation. *Pain* 1978;5(4):373–382.

80. Novak CB, Mackinnon SE. Outcome following implantation of a peripheral nerve stimulator in patients with chronic nerve pain. *Plast Reconstr Surg* 2000;105(6):1967–1972.

81. Law JD, Swett J, Kirsch WM. Retrospective analysis of 22 patients with chronic pain treated by peripheral nerve stimulation. *J Neurosurg* 1980;52(4):482–485.

82. Petrovic Z, Goroszeniuk T, Kothari S, et al. Percutaneous lumbar plexus stimulation in the treatment of intractable pain. *Reg Anesth Pain Med* 2007;32(5):11.

83. Goroszeniuk T, Pang D, Krol A, et al. T701 a novel technique of percutaneous brachial plexus stimulation for chronic neuropathic pain. *Eur J Pain Suppl* 2011;5(suppl 1):95.

84. Eldabe S, Burger K, Moser H, et al. Dorsal root ganglion (DRG) stimulation in the treatment of phantom limb pain (PLP). *Neuromodulation* 2015;18(7):610–617.

85. Hunter CW, Yang A, Davis T. Selective radiofrequency stimulation of the dorsal root ganglion (DRG) as a method for predicting targets for neuromodulation in patients with post amputation pain: a case series. *Neuromodulation* 2017;20(7):708–718.

86. Maino P, Koetsier E, Kaelin-Lang A, et al. Efficacious dorsal root ganglion stimulation for painful small fiber neuropathy: a case report. *Pain Physician* 2017;20(3):E459–E463.

87. Lynch PJ, McJunkin T, Eross E, et al. Case report: successful epiradicular peripheral nerve stimulation of the C2 dorsal root ganglion for postherpetic neuralgia. *Neuromodulation* 2011;14(1):58–61.

88. Yang A, Hunter CW. Dorsal root ganglion stimulation as a salvage treatment for complex regional pain syndrome refractory to dorsal column spinal cord stimulation: a case series. *Neuromodulation* 2017;20(7):703–707.

89. Deer TR, Levy RM, Kramer J, et al. Dorsal root ganglion stimulation yielded higher treatment success rate for complex regional pain syndrome and causalgia at 3 and 12 months: a randomized comparative trial. *Pain* 2017;158(4):669–681.

90. Van Buyten JP, Smet I, Liem L, et al. Stimulation of dorsal root ganglia for the management of complex regional pain syndrome: a prospective case series. *Pain Pract* 2015;15(3):208–216.

91. van Bussel CM, Stronks DL, Huygen FJ. Successful treatment of intractable complex regional pain syndrome type I of the knee with dorsal root ganglion stimulation: a case report. *Neuromodulation* 2015;18(1):58–60.

92. Krutsch JP, McCeney MH, Barolat G, et al. A case report of subcutaneous peripheral nerve stimulation for the treatment of axial back pain associated with postlaminectomy syndrome. *Neuromodulation* 2008;11(2):112–115.

93. Barolat G. A prospective multicenter study to assess the efficacy of spinal cord stimulation utilizing a multi-channel radio-frequency system for the treatment of intractable low back and lower extremity pain. Initial considerations and methodology. *Neuromodulation* 1999;2(3):179–183.

94. Paicius RM, Bernstein CA, Lempert-Cohen C. Peripheral nerve field stimulation for the treatment of chronic low back pain: preliminary results of long-term follow-up: a case series. *Neuromodulation* 2007;10(3):279–290.

95. Sator-Katzenschlager S, Fiala K, Kress HG, et al. Subcutaneous target stimulation (STS) in chronic noncancer pain: a nationwide retrospective study. *Pain Pract* 2010;10(4):279–286.

96. Verrills P, Vivian D, Mitchell B, et al. Peripheral nerve field stimulation for chronic pain: 100 cases and review of the literature. *Pain Med* 2011;12(9):1395–1405.

97. Liem L, Russo M, Huygen FJ, et al. One-year outcomes of spinal cord stimulation of the dorsal root ganglion in the treatment of chronic neuropathic pain. *Neuromodulation* 2015;18(1):41–49.

98. Reiter RC, Gambone JC. Demographic and historic variables in women with idiopathic chronic pelvic pain. *Obstet Gynecol* 1990;75(3):428–432.

99. Tamimi MA, Davids HR, Langston MM, et al. Successful treatment of chronic neuropathic pain with subcutaneous peripheral nerve stimulation: four case reports. *Neuromodulation* 2009;12(3):210–214.

100. Rowland DC, Wright D, Moir L, et al. Successful treatment of pelvic girdle pain with dorsal root ganglion stimulation. *Br J Neurosurg* 2016;30(6):685–686.

101. Zuidema X, Breel J, Wille F. Paresthesia mapping: a practical workup for successful implantation of the dorsal root ganglion stimulator in refractory groin pain. *Neuromodulation* 2014;17(7):665–669.

102. Zuidema X, Breel J, Wille F. S3 dorsal root ganglion/nerve root stimulation for refractory postsurgical perineal pain: technical aspects of anchorless sacral transforaminal lead placement. *Case Rep Neurol Med* 2016;2016:8926578.

103. Schu S, Gulve A, ElDabe S, et al. Spinal cord stimulation of the dorsal root ganglion for groin pain-a retrospective review. *Pain Pract* 2015;15(4):293–299.

104. Al Tamimi M, Davids HR, Barolat G, et al. Subcutaneous peripheral nerve stimulation treatment for chronic pelvic pain. *Neuromodulation* 2008;11(4):277–281.

105. Pluijms W, Steegers M, Verhagen A, et al. Chronic post-thoracotomy pain: a retrospective study. *Acta Anaesthesiol Scand* 2006;50(7):804–808.

106. Segal R, Stacey B, Rudy T, et al. Spinal cord stimulation revisited. *Neurol Res* 1998;20(5):391–396.

107. Waisbrod H, Panhans C, Hansen D, et al. Direct nerve stimulation for painful peripheral neuropathies. *J Bone Joint Surg Br* 1985;67(3):470–472.

108. Lipton R, Goadsby P, Cady R, et al. PRISM study: occipital nerve stimulation for treatment-refractory migraine. *Cephalalgia* 2009;29:30.

109. Matharu MS, Bartsch T, Ward N, et al. Central neuromodulation in chronic migraine patients with suboccipital stimulators: a PET study. *Brain* 2004;127(pt 1):220–230.

110. Popeney CA, Alo KM. Peripheral neurostimulation for the treatment of chronic, disabling transformed migraine. *Headache* 2003;43(4):369–375.

111. Saper JR, Dodick DW, Silberstein SD, et al. Occipital nerve stimulation for the treatment of intractable chronic migraine headache: ONSTIM feasibility study. *Cephalalgia* 2011;31(3):271–285.

112. Silberstein SD, Dodick DW, Saper J, et al. Safety and efficacy of peripheral nerve stimulation of the occipital nerves for the management of chronic migraine: results from a randomized, multicenter, double-blinded, controlled study. *Cephalalgia* 2012;32(16):1165–1179.

113. Slotty PJ, Bara G, Kowatz L, et al. Occipital nerve stimulation for chronic migraine: a randomized trial on subthreshold stimulation. *Cephalalgia* 2015;35(1):73–78.

114. Magis D, Allena M, Bolla M, et al. Occipital nerve stimulation for drug-resistant chronic cluster headache: a prospective pilot study. *Lancet Neurol* 2007;6(4):314–321.

115. Magis D, Bruno MA, Fumal A, et al. Central modulation in cluster headache patients treated with occipital nerve stimulation: an FDG-PET study. *BMC Neurol* 2011;11:25.

116. Goroszeniuk T, Pang D. Peripheral neuromodulation: a review. *Curr Pain Headache Rep* 2014;18(5):412.

117. Busch V, Jakob W, Juergens T, et al. Functional connectivity between trigeminal and occipital nerves revealed by occipital nerve blockade and nociceptive blink reflexes. *Cephalalgia* 2006;26(1):50–55.

118. Alò KM, Holsheimer J. New trends in neuromodulation for the management of neuropathic pain. *Neurosurgery* 2002;50(4):690–704.

119. Slavin KV, Colpan ME, Munawar N, et al. Trigeminal and occipital peripheral nerve stimulation for craniofacial pain: a single-institution experience and review of the literature. *Neurosurg Focus* 2006;21(6):E5.

120. Asensio-Samper JM, Villanueva VL, Pérez AV, et al. Peripheral neurostimulation in supraorbital neuralgia refractory to conventional therapy. *Pain Pract* 2008;8(2):120–124.

121. Dunteman E. Peripheral nerve stimulation for unremitting ophthalmic postherpetic neuralgia. *Neuromodulation* 2002;5(1):32–37.

122. Narouze SN, Zakari A, Vydyanathan A. Ultrasound-guided placement of a permanent percutaneous femoral nerve stimulator leads for the treatment of intractable femoral neuropathy. *Pain Physician* 2009;12(4):E305–E308.

123. Amin S, Buvanendran A, Park K, et al. Peripheral nerve stimulator for the treatment of supraorbital neuralgia: a retrospective case series. *Cephalalgia* 2008;28(4):355–359.

124. Oh MY, Ortega J, Bellotte JB, et al. Peripheral nerve stimulation for the treatment of occipital neuralgia and transformed migraine using a c1-2-3 subcutaneous paddle style electrode: a technical report. *Neuromodulation* 2004;7(2):103–112.

125. Chivukula S, Tempel ZJ, Weiner GM, et al. Cervical and cervicomedullary spinal cord stimulation for chronic pain: efficacy and outcomes. *Clin Neurol Neurosurg* 2014;127:33–41.

126. Franzini A, Ferroli P, Leone M, et al. Stimulation of the posterior hypothalamus for treatment of chronic intractable cluster headaches: first reported series. *Neurosurgery* 2003;52(5):1095–1101.

127. Narouze SN, Kapural L. Supraorbital nerve electric stimulation for the treatment of intractable chronic cluster headache: a case report. *Headache* 2007;47(7):1100–1102.

128. Schoenen J, Jensen RH, Lantéri-Minet M, et al. Stimulation of the sphenopalatine ganglion (SPG) for cluster headache treatment. Pathway CH-1: a randomized, sham-controlled study. *Cephalalgia* 2013;33(10):816–830.

129. Taub E, Munz M, Tasker RR. Chronic electrical stimulation of the gasserian ganglion for the relief of pain in a series of 34 patients. *J Neurosurg* 1997;86(2):197–202.

130. Young RF. Electrical stimulation of the trigeminal nerve root for the treatment of chronic facial pain. *J Neurosurg* 1995;83(1):72–78.

131. Holsheimer J. Electrical stimulation of the trigeminal tract in chronic, intractable facial neuralgia. *Arch Physiol Biochem* 2001;109(4):304–308.

CHAPTER 96

Spinal Cord Stimulation

RICHARD B. NORTH and **BENGT LINDEROTH**

History

In antiquity, some healers successfully treated pain by placing electrogenic fish on or near the painful area of the patient's body.[1] This crude form of electrotherapy enjoyed a measure of success but was limited in scope by the geographic and ecologic constraints associated with keeping the fish alive and available. Thus, electrotherapy was not widespread until creation of the Leyden jar in 1745 made it possible for physicians not only to deliver electrotherapy at will but also to exert a modicum of control over how much electrical current the patient received. This was an exciting medical advance, and by the 19th century, physicians were considered well equipped only if they had a portable generator and could provide electrotherapy for a wide range of indications. The advent of empirical medicine in the 20th century, however, caused most physicians to abandon the application of electrical shocks to treat pain. In the mid-1960s, however, neurosurgeon C. Norman Shealy et al.[2] recognized that Melzack and Wall's newly published *Gate Control Theory of Pain*[3] provided a theoretical basis for a new form of electrotherapy that could be delivered with implanted electrodes. Shealy et al.[2] called the innovation "dorsal column stimulation"; today, we know it as spinal cord stimulation (SCS).

Melzack and Wall's[3] Gate Control Theory proposed that the balance of activity between large and small nerve fibers in the peripheral nervous system determines whether or not pain signals are transmitted centrally. According to the theory, when small fiber input is dominant, a pain "gate" opens in the dorsal horn (DH) of the entrance segment of the spinal cord; this gate closes when large fiber activity is dominant. Because electrical stimulation depolarizes large fibers before it affects small fibers, the theory suggests that it should be possible for stimulation to close the pain gate. This hypothesis inspired Shealy et al.[2] to deliver current directly to a terminal cancer patient's spinal cord with an implanted electrode and external pulse generator in a successful bid to relieve the patient's otherwise intractable pain.

Although the electrical stimulation therapies inspired by the Gate Control Theory have succeeded, the theory itself remains controversial. It predicts that all types of pain will be inhibited, but clinical experience has shown that SCS is more effective for neuropathic pain than for acute or nociceptive pain.[4,5] Furthermore, large fiber activity can itself signal pain (e.g., the pain of sunburn).[6]

Despite the fact that the Gate Control Theory does not adequately explain all aspects of the therapies it inspired, it provides a useful description of the general concept of the transmission of pain signals and has stood the test of time to a remarkable degree.[7]

Within a few years of the introduction of SCS, it was reported that coverage of each patient's areas of pain by stimulation-evoked paresthesia was necessary for pain relief.[8,9] For many years thereafter, technical advances in SCS were directed at optimizing this, scaling amplitude to the range from perception of paresthesia to discomfort from the paresthesia.[10] More recently, automated methods have been developed to maintain amplitude below discomfort threshold based on either postural sensing or evoked potentials.[11,12]

As shown in Figure 96.1, since 2010, frequencies as high as 10 kHz as well as "burst" (to be distinguished from conventional monotonic) waveforms have been introduced. The therapeutic range for these new waveforms can begin below perceptual threshold, and this is fortuitous, as some patients prefer paresthesia-free stimulation, and as perceptual threshold can coincide with discomfort threshold for frequencies >800 Hz.[13] It also is now appreciated that even with conventional (monotonic, <1,500 per second) waveforms relief can be achieved at amplitudes below perceptual threshold.[14] Relevant basic science and clinical experiences will be detailed in the following discussion.

Today, SCS is a minimally invasive, reversible therapy implemented with sophisticated techniques and implanted equipment, including a variety of electrodes and multiple-output pulse generators. Unlike most surgical procedures undertaken to relieve pain, SCS does not ablate pain pathways or result in anatomic change. SCS also offers its candidates the advantage of undergoing a screening trial with a temporary SCS system before proceeding (or not) to implantation.

Pain and its relief by SCS vary by condition and from patient to patient. When SCS is delivered to the right patient by the right (experienced) clinician in the right setting using the right equipment, pain relief is optimized and can be sustained for decades. It is important to remember, however, that SCS is expected to reduce, not eliminate, pain, particularly pathologic (neuropathic) pain which itself is a disease. SCS is not expected or intended to relieve nociceptive or biologically useful pain.

Investigators are continually improving SCS patient care by refining techniques and equipment, and as we learn more about the mechanisms of action of SCS, we will be able to optimize its application.

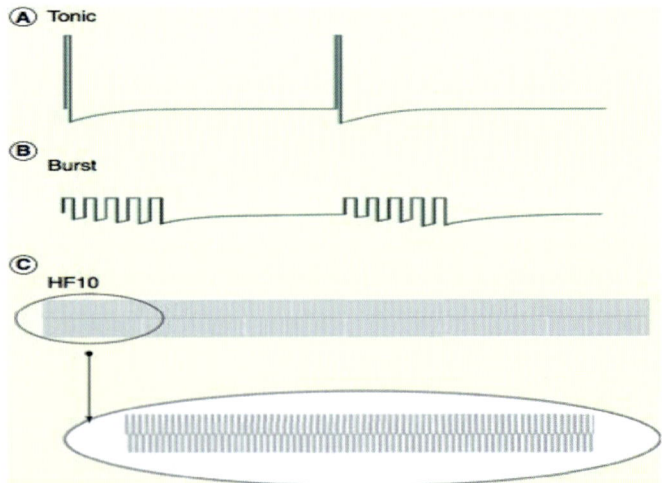

FIGURE 96.1 The presently used spinal cord stimulation (SCS) waveforms. **A:** Traditional SCS frequency of about 30 to 80 Hz. **B:** Burst SCS with internal pulse frequency of 500 Hz and burst repetition rate of 40 Hz. **C:** High-frequency stimulation—usually 10 kHz. (*From Pope JE, Falowski S, Deer TR. Advanced waveforms and frequency with spinal cord stimulation: burst and high-frequency energy delivery. Expert Rev Med Devices 2015;12[4]:431–437. Adapted by permission of Taylor & Francis Ltd. http://www.tandfonline.com.*)

Basic Science of Conventional Spinal Cord Stimulation

INTRODUCTION

The work of several investigative teams in the five decades since Shealy et al.[2] implanted the first "dorsal column stimulation" electrode has helped us identify promising avenues of research, refine experimental techniques, and develop evidence in support of hypotheses that explain aspects of the mechanisms of action of SCS. The challenge in experimental studies is to mimic the human painful condition and deliver stimulation, for example in rats, with parameters that would be clinically relevant in humans. Even in a homogeneous population of laboratory animals, however, the yield of neuropathic pain models is uncertain, and clinical studies must grapple with even greater variability among human subjects and painful pathologies. Furthermore, as already mentioned earlier, the clinical application of SCS elicits a discernible tingling, known as paresthesia, which confounds experimental blinding. An additional challenge is the fact that the universally agreed on measurement of the effectiveness of SCS (reduction in pain) is subjective and depends to an uncomfortable degree on a patient's ability to remember the intensity of past pain in order to make a valid comparison with current pain. Pain assessment also relies on rather crude measurements, such as verbal rating scales and the Visual Analogue Scale. Thus, patient assessment has to be assisted by measures of medication use, physical activity, well-being, general perception of change, etc.

Despite these obstacles, researchers have learned enough to propose distinct mechanisms of action for the therapeutic effects of SCS in the treatment of neuropathic, ischemic, and visceral pain.

NEUROPHYSIOLOGY AND NEUROCHEMISTRY

SCS affects both spinal and supraspinal circuits[15–21] and thus does not rely solely on antidromic activation of the dorsal columns.[17,22] Some SCS effects actually survive disruption of supraspinal circuits by transection of the dorsal columns, the dorsolateral funiculi, and even the entire spinal cord rostral to a lumbar electrode.[23–25]

SCS modulates DH and/or supraspinal neurotransmitters; thus, the beneficial effects of SCS often outlast the period of active stimulation (see following discussion).

Most studies indicate that endogenous opioids are not involved in the pain-relieving effects of conventional SCS; for example, the effects of SCS are not reversed by the opioid antagonist naloxone,[26] and the neuropathic pain of SCS patients is usually resistant to opioid therapy.

SCS might[27] or might not[28] cause release of spinal opioids. There is some experimental evidence that only stimulation with very low frequencies (e.g., 4 Hz) might involve the release of endogenous opioids.[29]

Additionally, in patients with angina, SCS during atrial pacing and at rest has been demonstrated to release the opioid peptide β-endorphin into cardiac circulation, indicating that SCS affects "local myocardial turnover of the opioid peptides leu-enkephalin, β-endorphin, and calcitonin gene-related peptide (CGRP), a powerful vasodilator."[30]

Nerve or nervous system injury can lead to neuropathic pain, which is often radiating, generally described as "burning," and in some cases involves hyperalgesia (an extreme sensitivity to pain) and allodynia (pain from normally nonpainful stimuli). In contrast, dull, aching nociceptive pain, which is mediated by receptors in skin, muscle, bone, viscera, etc., is responsive to opioids. Because SCS, in most cases, is not thought to cause the release of endogenous opioids,[28] the clinical expectation is that SCS will be more effective as a treatment of neuropathic, ischemic, and visceral pain than of nociceptive pain. The fact that SCS is effective in treating ischemic pain, which is considered a form of nociceptive pain, does not necessarily mean that SCS directly affects this type of pain. Instead, SCS seems to exert a beneficial effect on the underlying ischemic condition and pain relief in considered as secondary to that (see following discussion).

Among the things rats and humans have in common are that nerve injury alone sometimes causes allodynia (in neuropathic pain cases merely around 20% report allodynia[31]) and that SCS is not universally therapeutic. Only in single clinical studies have the SCS effects on allodynia been monitored, but in selected material presented by Harke et al.,[32] the therapeutic effect on allodynia was similar to that on continuous pain.

Investigators also used models of painful neuropathy to explore the impact of SCS on the pain threshold in rats and found that during and after SCS, the threshold of withdrawal from innocuous mechanical stimuli increases and that SCS affects only the component of the flexor reflex mediated by A fibers (not the late component mediated by C fibers).[33] Thus, current thinking holds that, to a large extent, SCS acts at a segmental spinal level,[34] although additional inhibitory influences might be transmitted by descending serotonergic and noradrenergic pathways. A related study used the partial sciatic nerve ligation model to examine how SCS affects the response to innocuous stimuli in postligation rats with and without allodynia and in controls. Only in the allodynic rats did SCS significantly depress abnormal responses and spontaneous discharge of wide dynamic range (WDR) neurons.[35] The same research group introduced acetylcholine (ACH) into the list of transmitters possibly involved in the beneficial effects of SCS after a microdialysis study demonstrated that ACH is released in the DHs of rats whose pain-related symptoms after nerve injury decreased in response to stimulation.[36] These effects seem to be caused by activation of muscarinic M4 and M2 receptors in the DH.[36,37] This finding might lead to new ways to enhance an otherwise inadequate effect of SCS in certain patients. Allodynia occurs when the activation of nerve fibers in the periphery causes hyperactivity of WDR neurons in the superficial laminae of corresponding DHs.[38] SCS relieves allodynia by suppressing this hyperactivity.[35] Treatment with γ-aminobutyric acid (GABA) agonists also has this effect, and SCS induces GABA release in the DH of rats[18] and activates the GABA-B receptor.[39,40] SCS also decreases DH release of the excitatory amino acids glutamate and aspartate in rats.[40] One probable mechanism would be that release of GABA binding to presynaptic GABA-B receptors could inhibit the release of excitatory amino acids (e.g., glutamate).

Investigators have also proposed that SCS might relieve pain by blocking conduction of primary afferents at the branch points of dorsal column fibers and collaterals.[6] This explanation is insufficient, however, because the effect of SCS extends beyond the dorsal columns and electrical stimulation does not inhibit every type of pain.[21] Dorsal column activation, however, is more successful than ventral stimulation,[41] which might exert effects on the spinothalamic tract fibers that transmit nociception.

SCS inhibition of the pathologic response (increased firing frequency of WDR neurons, afterdischarge in response to pressure, etc.) of DH neurons in rats exhibiting symptoms of allodynia after peripheral nerve injury continues for more than 10 minutes,[35] consistent with SCS-induced release of DH and cerebral neurotransmitters, and changes the concentration of neurotransmitters and their metabolites in cerebrospinal fluid.[41–44]

Through the use of microdialysis and immunohistochemical techniques, investigators have examined the effects of SCS on the cerebral neurotransmitter serotonin. In decerebrate cats, SCS applied with clinical parameters evokes a DH release of serotonin.[42]

It was recently demonstrated in neurophysiologic studies with microelectrode recordings from different brainstem regions that both the "serotonergic cells" and the OFF-cells in the rostroventromedial medulla (RVM) are selectively activated by lumbar SCS in neuropathic rats, and this happens only in animals responding to the stimulation in previous behavioral studies.[45] In SCS-responding animals, the tissue concentration of 5 hydroxytryptamine (5-HT) is increased in lumbar DHs following stimulation.[46] The behavioral effects of the 5-HT release in the DHs seem to be mediated by 5-HT2A, 5-HT3, and the 5-HT4 receptors.[47,48]

Similarly, a massive activation of neurons induced by SCS occurs in the locus coeruleus, another brainstem center, where many noradrenergic cell bodies are gathered. In contrast to the RVM where 5-HT release could be observed at the spinal level, there was no sign of direct projection of noradrenergic neurons activated by SCS to the DHs (as demonstrated by several methods[49]).

Based on the finding that spinal extracellular GABA levels are lower in allodynic rats than in controls but increase in allodynic rats that respond to SCS,[50] investigators have attempted to potentiate the therapeutic effect of SCS in nonresponding rats with concurrent intrathecal administration of normally subtherapeutic levels of GABA or the GABA-B agonist baclofen.[39] This strategy caused a marked increase in the rats' threshold for paw withdrawal from innocuous mechanical stimulation. Intrathecal administration of the selective α_1-adenosine receptor agonist R-phenyl isopropyl adenosine produced similar results.[40] Administration of subtherapeutic doses of these agents as adjunct therapy with SCS causes nonresponding rats to respond to SCS.[51]

In the first clinical study based on this response, however, the addition of intrathecal baclofen and/or adenosine in small doses was effective, but the latter potentiated SCS in only 2 of 5 patients.[52]

This result caused investigators to try instead other drugs administered orally in man for neuropathic pain. In rodents, the drugs were given intrathecally and intravenously instead: gabapentin and pregabalin in per se ineffective doses in non-SCS-responding rats with partial sciatic nerve lesion. In these rats, the drugs together with SCS reduced tactile allodynia in a dose-dependent manner and enhanced suppression of hyperexcitability of WDR neurons.[53]

Accordingly, investigators conducted a pilot study that offered intrathecal baclofen (and, in a few cases, intrathecal adenosine) to 48 patients who did not successfully respond to technically adequate SCS.[54] Although 20 patients achieved satisfactory pain relief with baclofen plus SCS or baclofen alone, only 11 continued treatment: 7 with a combination SCS system and intrathecal baclofen pump and 4 with only a baclofen pump. At mean 67 months postimplant, 2 SCS/intrathecal patients had their pumps removed and the remaining 9 in the group (5 SCS/intrathecal, 4 intrathecal) reported continued pain relief. The baclofen dose was increased 160% from baseline, but 5 patients reduced their use of other analgesics.

A similar dose-dependent effect occurred in rodents with intrathecal administration of an otherwise subtherapeutic dose of clonidine, which partially exerts its effects via release of ACH in the DH.[36,55] A small randomized, double-blind prospective clinical study reportedly indicated that clonidine could be equally useful as low-dose baclofen to enhance the effect of SCS.[56]

We have yet to identify all of the neurotransmitters and neuromodulators affected by SCS, let alone to decipher their doubtless complicated interactions.[40,42,57] The mechanisms and neurotransmitters known or hypothesized (so far) to be involved in the effects of conventional SCS in neuropathic pain are illustrated in Figure 96.2.

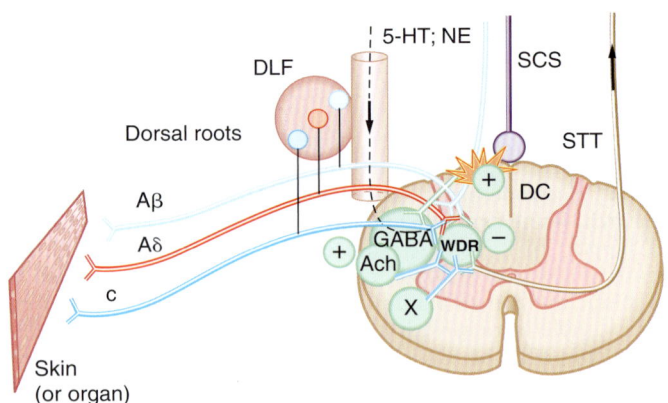

FIGURE 96.2   Schematic illustration of mechanisms and neurotransmitters possibly involved in the effects of spinal cord stimulation (SCS) in neuropathic pain. SCS activation of dorsal column collaterals secondarily induces release of γ-aminobutyric acid (GABA) from dorsal horn (DH) interneurons, activating mainly GABA-B receptors and decreasing the release of excitatory amino acids from hyperexcited second-order DH wide dynamic range (WDR) neurons. SCS also causes cholinergic neurons to activate M4 and M2 muscarinic type receptors (Ach). Several other transmitters, adenosine, and hitherto unknown substances are also likely involved. Furthermore, the orthodromic SCS-induced activity in the dorsal columns might—via neuronal circuitry in the brainstem (or even more rostrally)—induce descending inhibition via serotonergic (5-HT) and noradrenergic (NE) pathways in the dorsolateral funiculus (DLF), which might contribute to inhibitory influences in the DHs. c, c fibers accompanying Aδ and Aβ fibers; DC, dorsal columns; STT, spinothalamic tract; X, unknown transmitters probably modulated by spinal stimulation.

Basic Science of New Spinal Cord Stimulation Waveforms

HIGH-FREQUENCY SPINAL CORD STIMULATION

In principle, high-frequency (HF) sinusoidal stimulation applied to a nerve or an axon provides a local conduction block (e.g., Kilgore and Bhadra[58,59]). In contrast to HF current application to a peripheral nerve, HF SCS applied to the dorsal spinal cord of lightly anesthetized rats with the pulse width (PW) and the low amplitudes used clinically induced no block of transmission in the dorsal columns (DCs) nor any activation.[60]

Clinical HF SCS is applied via bipolar stimulation at a pulse repetition rate of 10 kHz and a short PW of about 30 microseconds at an amplitude that is below perceptual threshold (see Fig. 96.1).

The "working hypotheses" for HF SCS so far have been (1) a transmission block or (2) activation of some pathways in the spinal cord. However, a recent computer simulation study[61] has demonstrated that both these hypotheses require high stimulation amplitudes that are at the upper end or outside of the ranges used clinically in HF SCS.

A third hypothesis was based on observations from studies of the auditory system in cats and on some few patients with cochlear implants. HF stimulation seemed to be able to induce a desynchronization of neural signals from groups of neurons firing in synchrony. This interesting hypothesis has, to the best of our knowledge, never been studied in nociception (review Linderoth and Foreman[62]).

Furthermore, a study by Song et al,[60] has shown that transmission in the DCs is not affected because there is neither fiber recruitment nor block with HF SCS. Another recent study[63] where recordings from rats with nerve injury were performed with tungsten electrodes on single DC fibers provided data supporting the view that no blockade of the DCs is obtained with HF SCS at clinically relevant amplitudes.

It seems that there is a therapeutic effect of HF SCS, but so far, it has not been found superior to that of traditional SCS in our own animal model using monophasic pulses.[60] Because the DCs are neither activated nor blocked by the HF SCS, the mechanisms hypothesized may be segmental. In a rat study with biphasic stimulation, Shechter et al.[64] compared 20%, 40%, and 80% of motor threshold (MT) as stimulation amplitudes. They used 50 Hz, 1 kHz, and 10 kHz applied for 30 minutes on 3 consecutive days. The only amplitude producing relevant data was 40% of the MT. For this amplitude, some effects of SCS emerged over the 3 days, and actually, the frequency 1 kHz proved slightly better—or at least equally effective as the 10 kHz SCS.

It must be remembered that clinical experiences demonstrate that HF SCS (>800 Hz) might result in uncomfortable sensory experiences as soon as the amplitude is beyond the sensory (paresthetic) threshold.[13]

Very recent preclinical studies (unpublished data[65,66]) using HF SCS (2 to10 kHz) where DC activation was also studied have yielded interesting results. Application of 10-kHz SCS in the rat through conductive agar from needle electrodes directly over the L5 segment demonstrated no evidence of a DC fiber conduction block nor activation. Stimulation for several hours did not induce asynchronous firing in myelinated primary sensory neurons. In an inflammatory pain model producing more long-lasting pain, SCS using 20% MT for up to 135 minutes, which was verified to be subthreshold for activation of Aβ projection neurons, occurred after 45 to 90 minutes when compared to control.

The present view of HF SCS mechanisms may be summarized as follows: HF SCS must be applied with low amplitude—below paresthesia threshold; otherwise, it can be very uncomfortable. There seems to be neither activation nor block of the dorsal columns with HF SCS. Although PW is short and amplitude low, HF delivers more energy, and thus, rechargeable or wireless devices have to be used.

The dorsal columns do not seem to be involved in the effect,[63,67] thus clearly distinguishing HF SCS from conventional SCS. As yet unpublished data indicate that HF SCS might induce a slowly building up, inhibitory effect directly onto superficial neurons in the DH.[65,66]

BURST SPINAL CORD STIMULATION

The use of irregular stimulation patterns including "burst stimulation" originates from De Ridder's work with cortical stimulation, but "modulated stimulation" has been used earlier in the clinic. In the 1970s, burst transcutaneous electrical stimulation (TENS) was launched as a variant to steady frequency TENS with very low "electro-acupuncture-like" frequency (1 to 5 Hz) as compared to normal TENS at about 100 Hz.[68] At this time, hypotheses about different mechanisms for burst and HF TENS were discussed, and the burst TENS was applied more for nociceptive pain types, and some data pointed to a possible mediation by release of endogenous opioids. As already mentioned, recent animal studies further indicate that the antinociceptive effect of low-frequency SCS may depend on opioid mechanisms.[29] One manufacturer marketed for a period during the 1980s an external stimulator that could give variable stimulation patterns ("modulated SCS"), but it never became popular, and the apparatus disappeared from the market.

Burst SCS was presented as a stimulation mode, which would also be effective for the midline or axial low back pain component of failed back surgery syndrome (FBSS).[69,70] De Ridder argues that bursts or irregular firing are similar to normal nerve activity and exert more prominent effects on supraspinal relays (e.g., the thalamus, as "a wake-up call to the brain" to activate neurons).[71] De Ridder et al.[70] have, on the basis of "source localized electroencephalogram (EEG)" investigations of patients with burst SCS, advanced the idea that burst SCS could activate cortical areas involved in the modulation of pain perception (Fig. 96.3). In a very recent study, De Ridder and Vanneste[72] presented data from five patients undergoing tonic, burst, and sham stimulation. In a source-localized EEG subtraction and conjunction analysis, they showed that burst and tonic stimulation share activation of some cortical areas

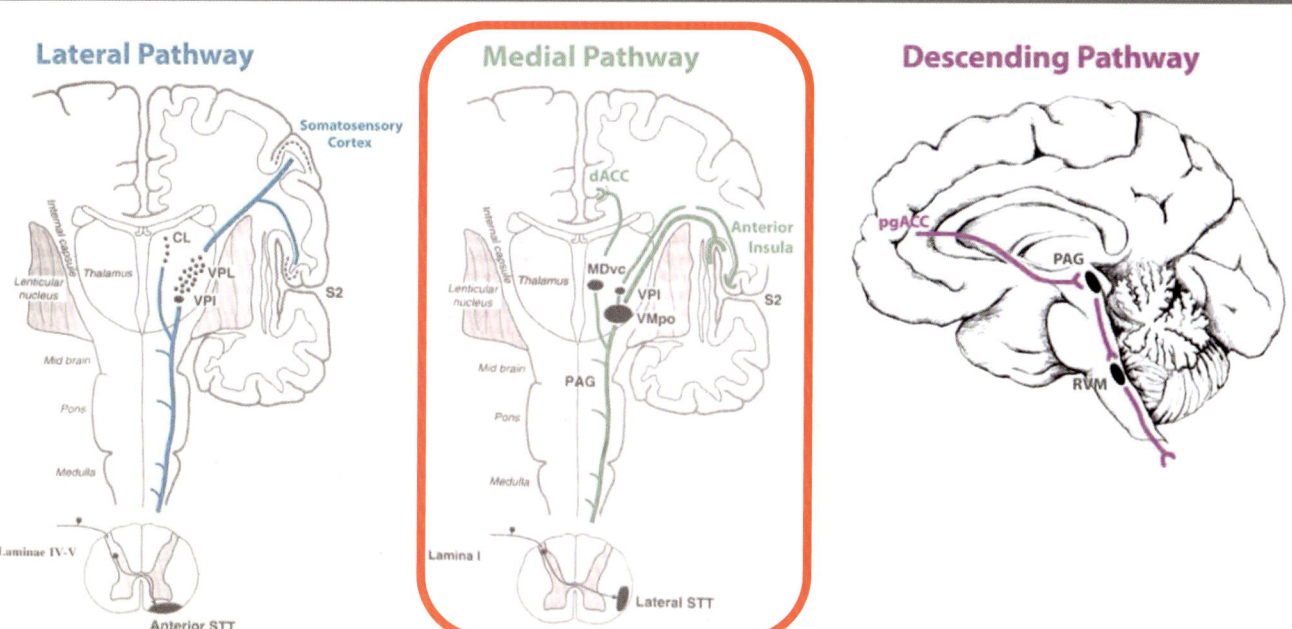

FIGURE 96.3 Present hypotheses for mechanisms behind effects of burst stimulation of the spinal cord. Burst spinal cord stimulation (SCS) is hypothesized to especially modulate the activation of the medial (affective/attentional) pathway **(right)**. Conventional SCS more acts on the lateral spinothalamic tract which conveys information of nociception (strength; site). *(Adapted from De Ridder D, Vanneste S. Burst and tonic spinal cord stimulation: different and common brain mechanisms. Neuromodulation 2016;19[1]:47–59. Copyright © 2015 International Neuromodulation Society. Reprinted by permission of John Wiley & Sons, Inc.)*

such as the pregenual anterior cingulate cortex, whereas only burst SCS reduced the connectivity between the dorsal anterior cingulate and the parahippocampal cortices.

The originators of the burst paradigm[72] claim that the burst type of SCS preferentially modulates the medial spinothalamic pathway leading to activity changes in subcortical centers involved in emotions, whereas conventional SCS acts more on the lateral tract leading to the lateral thalamic nuclei and eventually to the sensory cortex. They hypothesize that burst stimulation modulates the medial pain pathway by actions of C fibers synapsing onto lamina I neurons with projections to the dorsomedial nucleus of the thalamus and from there to the dorsal anterior cingulum. An earlier functional magnetic resonance imaging (fMRI) study[73] demonstrated that conventional SCS predominantly modulated the lateral pain pathways as judged by changes in blood oxygen levels in the somatosensory cortices.

Burst SCS, at least in rat models, does not seem to involve the DC system[74]—another difference to conventional paresthetic SCS. More recent data indicate that the effects of burst SCS do not rely on activation of GABA-B receptors[75] as has been claimed for conventional SCS (e.g., Cui et al.,[39] Cui et al.,[40] Meyerson et al.,[44] Cui et al.,[76] Ultenius et al.[77]).

Burst SCS is commonly administered at amplitudes that do not produce paresthesia. In spite of this, as the average frequency is higher, the energy consumption is larger than that of conventional SCS. A recent finding is that the efficacy of burst SCS seems to relate to the electric charge per burst, at least as found in a rat model of neuropathic pain.[78]

In conclusion, burst SCS as now most often used clinically (5 pulses at 500 Hz repeated with 40-Hz rate at subparesthetic amplitude) cannot be completely explained on the basis of physiologic mechanisms activated or inhibited by stimulation of the dorsal aspect of the spinal cord. Preclinical and clinical studies are underway to shed more light on mechanisms of these novel algorithms.

MODERATE CHANGES OF CONVENTIONAL SPINAL CORD STIMULATION PARAMETERS

At present, almost all manufacturers produce stimulators that can generate stimulation frequencies up to and above 1 kHz and PWs up to 1 μsec. Higher frequencies than those typically used for SCS have been available for many years[79] but have been used and reported for pain only anecdotally. A few centers during the 80s applied high cervical SCS (around 1,000 Hz) for torticollis.[80]

Because the higher frequencies and longer PWs were available already in the existing stimulators, many centers tried to adapt the stimulation parameters especially in cases with therapy failure after some time with conventional SCS but eventually also in new cases during trials.

It must be kept in mind that frequencies above 800 Hz with stimulation-induced paresthesias can be perceived as very unpleasant,[13] and so these parameters usually were used at subparesthetic amplitude. In this way, higher amounts of electric charge could be transmitted from the electrode poles to the neural tissue without discomfort or damage to the nervous system.[81]

Recent experiments in the rat have demonstrated that subsensory SCS can exert clear effects on symptoms of neuropathic pain.[60,64,67] These studies also show that moderately increased frequencies of 1,000 Hz can be as effective at the subsensory level as 10-kHz SCS. Such changes in SCS parameters to increase transfer of electric charge have been tried clinically in recent years referring to the fact that pulse density (i.e., the percentage active stimulation during a pulse cycle) can be increased from just 1% to 2% up to 20% to 25% for the maximal available settings at a subsensory mode.

The few clinical reports on this type of stimulation now available[14,82–84] will be discussed below. Furthermore, some recent studies also illustrate that for each patient, the SCS therapy could be optimized by the use of "individualized" settings and that some patients actually like to keep their paresthetic SCS as part of their stimulation program.[14,84] In conclusion to this section, it must be admitted that we are just at the beginning of exploration of the efficacy of slightly changed SCS parameters, and only short-term results are available so far. The mechanisms behind an increased effect has not been studied (besides using higher frequencies; e.g., 500 and 1,000 Hz), and the neurophysiologic/neurochemical correlates are not known.

COMPUTER MODELING STUDIES

Finite element computer models of SCS electrical fields in the spinal cord[85–87] have confirmed the current and voltage distribution measurements previously obtained in cadavers and primates.[88] Application of these models has also led to the prediction that (1) an electrode's longitudinal position governs its segmental effect; (2) bipolar stimulation with contacts separated by 6 to 8 mm optimizes selection of midline, longitudinally oriented fibers (a longer distance reduces therapeutic effect by favoring dorsal root stimulation); and (3) the electrical field between two cathodes placed on either side of the physiologic midline does not sum constructively in the midline. Clinical experience confirms that the correct position and spacing of SCS electrodes is essential for therapeutic success and that, instead of expanding the area of paresthesia, positioning electrodes cephalad to the involved spinal levels commonly elicits unwanted, excessive, local segmental effects.[10]

The first computerized models developed to study the spinal canal represented the meninges, cerebrospinal fluid, fiber tracts, and gray matter with geometric shapes.[89,90] The equally simplistic, two-dimensional initial computer models of dorsal epidural stimulation[91–93] were soon replaced by a three-dimensional model that took into account fiber tracts, their branch points, and dorsal roots.[85,94]

In 1991, Holsheimer and Struijk[95] developed a new model that merged this three-dimensional construct with a McNeal-type[96] cable model of the electrical behavior of myelinated nerve fibers and data derived from mammalian myelinated fibers.[97] The resulting "University of Twente SCS Computer Model" allowed investigators to determine the impact of the location and configuration (anode/cathode, on/off) of SCS electrodes (e.g., to maximize recruitment of deep, midline, longitudinal axons rather than of the lateral, or dorsal root, fibers that can cause discomfort and motor responses) and to suggest ways to optimize SCS equipment design.

The University of Twente model was further refined when the investigators were able to apply data from human sensory fibers.[98] This improved the accuracy of predictions about the impact of various SCS threshold voltages.[99] An additional improvement streamlined the mathematical techniques used to predict stimulation effects when computing the three-dimensional action potential field.[100] Model predictions for "transverse tripole" electrode performance have been validated in part by clinical studies.[101]

Lempka et al.[61] recently applied a similar model to kilohertz frequency SCS and reported that at intensities used clinically, stimulation probably does not cause the direct activation or conduction block of dorsal column or dorsal root fibers.[61] Arle et al.[102] on the other hand, inferred from a similar model that because of an interaction between ion gate dynamics and the anodal current distribution over axons, larger fibers that cause paresthesia in low-frequency simulation are blocked at higher frequencies, whereas medium and smaller fibers are recruited, leading to pain relief by inhibiting centrally projecting WDR cells in the DH.

CONVENTIONAL SPINAL CORD STIMULATION MECHANISMS IN ISCHEMIC PAIN

SCS is thought to induce vasodilatation and improve microperfusion in patients with ischemic pain, which is sharp, aching, heavy, and tiring[103] and a signal of local ischemia. Thus, SCS has a beneficial effect on the cause, not merely the symptoms, of ischemic pain. This might explain why ischemic pain is one of the few types of nociceptive pain known to respond to SCS and why the mechanisms seem to be fundamentally distinct from those that provide relief of neuropathic pain.[28,42,104]

PERIPHERAL VASCULAR DISEASE

To investigate the mechanism of SCS in the treatment of peripheral vascular disease (PVD), better renamed "peripheral arterial occlusive disease" (PAOD) (especially because if the vascular problem affects the venous side, standard SCS produces little or no effect), investigators developed a new animal model that involves applying mechanical pressure to an artery in the groin of rats.[105] Using this model, SCS delivered with clinically relevant stimulation parameters recovered normal microcirculation in 100% of treated rats versus 28% of controls. In addition, administering SCS preemptively reduced the amplitude of the invoked spasm and significantly shortened the time to recovery of microcirculation. In skin flaps with severely compromised arterial blood supply, application of SCS could significantly increase the flap survival as judged 1 week after the provocation. If a CGRP receptor antagonist was given before the SCS treatment, the survival rate decreased considerably, implicating this vasodilatory compound in the effect.[106]

SCS also suppresses efferent sympathetic activity (maintained by nicotinic ganglionic receptors and α_1-adrenoreceptors)[104] and might activate antidromic mechanisms at intensities far below the MT,[107–111] thus causing peripheral vasodilation by stimulating release of CGRP[106–108] from the terminals of sensory fibers that contain transient receptor potential vanilloid-1 (TRPV1) receptors[112,113] and the release of nitric oxide from endothelial cells.[113]

The balance between these two mechanisms seems to depend on the activity level of the sympathetic nervous system, the intensity of SCS, and individual patient factors (genetic differences, diet, etc.).[111]

In fact, antidromic activation dominated at low autonomic baseline activity, whereas the sympatholytic effects of SCS were clear with high baseline activity.[111,114] Later studies have indicated that even small-diameter fibers are involved at SCS intensities much below the MT[112,113] and have pointed toward additional mechanisms.

The observation that SCS has a powerfully beneficial effect on vasospastic conditions, such as Raynaud's syndrome, is consistent with theories that the cause of this syndrome is a combination of heightened sensitivity or increased density of α-adrenergic receptors[115] and CGRP-system dysfunction.[116] A stimulation-induced "normalization" of function in each system could underlie the efficacy of SCS in treating this condition.

Up to the present, most animal studies have utilized SCS frequencies that are routinely applied in the clinic (i.e., 40 to 80 Hz), but in a more recent study, higher SCS frequencies up to 500 Hz were tried at intensities 30% to 90% of MT.[89] This study showed that although the MTs for SCS at all frequencies were similar, SCS at 500 Hz induced a significantly larger blood flow elevation in the hind paw than did SCS at 50 Hz. The effects of these frequencies and intensities seem to depend on activation of TRPV1-containing fibers and the release of CGRP. Thus, further trials with new stimulation parameters should be undertaken to increase benefits of SCS.

A review of the mechanisms involved in SCS-induced vasodilation is included in a report by Wu et al.[117] and by Foreman and Lindertoh.[118]

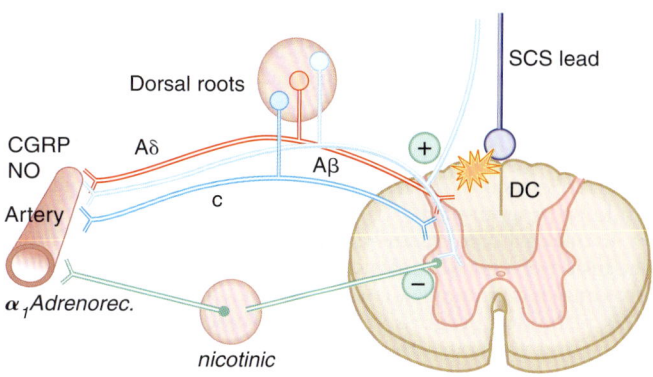

Sympathetic Efferent Fibers

FIGURE 96.4 Schematic illustration of mechanisms and neurotransmitters possibly involved in effects of spinal cord stimulation (SCS) in ischemic pain. SCS probably indirectly exerts inhibition onto medullary neurons, thus perpetuating sympathetic efferent vasoconstriction via nicotinic ganglionic receptors, mainly α_1 (α_1Adrenorec. = adrenoreceptors) peripheral receptors. In parallel, SCS activates an antidromic loop inducing peripheral release of calcitonin gene-related peptide (CGRP), probably also involving small-diameter fibers. An inhibition of nociceptive transmission has also been indicated in experimental studies but is clinically unlikely. c, small diameter unmyelinated "c-fibers"; DC, dorsal columns; NO, nitric oxide.

The mechanisms and neurotransmitters known or hypothesized to be involved in the effects of SCS in ischemic pain are depicted in Figure 96.4.

SPINAL CORD STIMULATION FOR ANGINA PECTORIS AND CARDIAC DISEASE

Investigators studying the mechanism of action of SCS in patients with otherwise refractory angina agree that SCS reduces ischemia[119] but disagree about how this occurs. Positron emission tomography has indicated that SCS causes a redistribution of coronary blood flow in patients with refractory angina[120,121] (even though other experimental studies have failed to demonstrate this effect).[122] On the other hand, the decrease in the depression extending from the end of the S wave to the beginning of the T wave (ST-segment depression) that appears on electrocardiograms (ECGs) during SCS treatment and the observed SCS-induced reversal of lactate production to extraction might indicate an accompanying decrease in cardiac myocyte oxygen demand.[123]

The SCS-induced protective changes that increase myocardial resistance to critical ischemia[124] are manifest by the improved tolerance of patients to a deliberately paced increase in heart rate[119] and by increased time-to-angina in exercise tests.[119,123] This effect might signal an SCS-induced inhibition of the excitatory effect of ischemia on the intrinsic cardiac nervous system (such an excitatory effect might lead to dysrhythmia and increased ischemia).[124–126] The possibility that SCS modulates cardiac neurons is supported by the finding that transcutaneous electrical nerve stimulation increases blood flow in intact human hearts but not in transplanted, denervated hearts.[127]

There is no proper animal model of angina pectoris mimicking the syndrome in humans. The animal studies discussed in the following text are instead focused onto various deleterious effects of experimentally induced chronic and/or acute coronary ischemia.

Because SCS reduces total body, but not cardiac-specific, norepinephrine spillover during pacing to moderate angina,[128] part of the anti-ischemic effect of SCS might owe its potency to an overall reduction in sympathetic activity. An experimental study using induced cardiac infarcts in a rabbit model, however, indicates that the decrease in infarct size with SCS therapy shares some mechanisms with "ischemic preconditioning" but, notably, does not cause cardiac ischemia.[129]

In order to mimic the development of chronic ischemic heart disease in an animal model of myocardial ischemia, progressive occlusion of the arterial blood supply by a device or creation of cardiac infarction of moderate size could be used, after which a period of acute ischemia provocation with or without SCS could be programmed.

In one early canine study, a slowly expanding material lining the inside of a metal constrictor ring was implanted around the proximal left circumflex coronary artery of a group of dogs.[124] This technique progressively reduces blood flow through the artery and facilitates the development of collaterals creating a collateral-dependent myocardial ischemia substrate. In subsequent acute experiments, the exposed heart was paced at a basal rate of 150 beats per minute. An ECG plaque was used to record from multiple sites on the left ventricle supplied by the left coronary artery occluded by the constrictor. In order to stress the heart, either angiotensin II, administered via the local arterial supply to the right atrial ganglionated plexus, was used, or rapid ventricular pacing applied via a standard pacemaker. Both these maneuvers produced an elevation of the ST segments that was markedly attenuated during SCS. In a similar way, ST-segment responses were largely unchanged when rapid ventricular pacing (240 beats per minute during 60 seconds) was induced during SCS. These experiments indicate that SCS may attenuate the deleterious effects that stressors, especially chemical activation of the intrinsic cardiac nervous system, exert on a myocardium with reduced reserve capacity. This observation led to the conclusion that SCS produces anti-ischemic effects that contribute to improved cardiac function.

Further evidence to support the anti-ischemic effects of SCS on the heart is the observation that preemptive SCS appears to have a protective effect on the myocardium, which makes it more resistant to critical ischemia as demonstrated by rabbit experiments with left anterior descending (LAD) artery occlusion lasting 30 minutes. In these studies, the infarct size was markedly reduced by preemptive SCS. However, the protective effects of SCS therapy were lost if SCS was begun after ischemia induction.[129] Patients with SCS therapy for chronic therapy-resistant angina are recommended to use their stimulators at low amplitude most of the day or at least for 6 to 8 hours and to increase the amplitude when needed during an angina attack or when physical stress is expected to produce angina. Thus, the validity of this clinical recommendation is substantiated by experimental data.

In experimental cardiology, there is a well-known phenomenon that a short ischemic episode preceding a longer occlusion of a coronary vessel induces complicated protective processes in the myocardium that diminishes the resulting infarct size. This phenomenon is called ischemic preconditioning, and the details are still not completely known (e.g., Foreman[130]). Recent studies indicate that SCS-induced local release of catecholamines in the myocardium may trigger protective changes related to mechanisms behind such ischemic preconditioning but without producing any signs of ischemic changes in the heart. There are also other signs indicating that SCS may induce a state similar to that following a short ischemic period, for example, by activating protein kinase C, a substance which is pivotal in ischemic preconditioning.[129]

An important part of the "general common pathways" in the communication between the CNS and the heart is the intrinsic cardiac nervous system (ICNS). The ICNS is located in the cardiac ganglionated plexuses covered by epicardial fat pads situated on the myocardium.[131] The ICNS plexuses are composed of mixed somatosensory, sympathetic, and parasympathetic fibers. The ICNS plays a critical role in coordinating regional cardiac function and providing rapid reflex coordination of autonomic

neuronal inflow to the heart. In critical ischemia, the ICNS is vigorously activated.[126] The ICNS responds to ischemic stress by marked activity increase even if the ischemic region is situated far away from the neuron population.[125] If the increased activity persists, it may result in spreading dysrhythmias that may lead to more generalized ischemia and/or to ventricular fibrillation. Several experimental studies have clearly shown that SCS may potently inhibit and stabilize the activity of the ICNS especially during a critical ischemic challenge.

In patients with angina, SCS can relieve the symptoms and signs of ischemia for long periods after the stimulation is terminated which may relate to prolonged effects of SCS on ICNS activity observed at least up to 45 to 60 minutes after SCS stimulation off in dogs.[131]

Modulation of the ICNS may be one mechanism that protects the heart from more severe ischemic threats due to generalized arrhythmias. Others have confirmed the observation that experimental animals display less arrhythmia during ischemic provocation when being subjected to SCS. Experiments by Lopshire et al.[132] demonstrated that SCS might improve cardiac function in canine heart failure following an experimental myocardial infarction and continued stress by HF pacing over 8 weeks. In addition, acute experiments with experimental occlusion of the LAD carried out with or without SCS on landrace pigs showed that the stimulation provided positive effects as displayed in the vectorized ECG.[133]

In several of the studies mentioned earlier, the ischemic challenge induced arrhythmias, but in virtually all studies, these were less severe during SCS treatment. This observation was recently supported by a new study.[134]

The use of SCS for angina reached a peak in the 1990s and early 2000s (when it was the best indication for SCS with outcomes >80% of patients clearly helped by the therapy), but thereafter, the use of this technique has diminished considerably also in Europe due largely to increased use of stenting.

It also should be noted that angina pectoris is presently not a U.S. Food and Drug Administration (FDA)-approved indication for SCS in the United States.

Some of the pathways and mechanisms behind beneficial effects of SCS on cardiac function discussed earlier are schematically summarized in Figure 96.5, which illustrates the mechanisms and neurotransmitters known or hypothesized to be involved in the effects of SCS in angina.

MECHANISMS OF SPINAL CORD STIMULATION IN VISCERAL ABDOMINAL PAIN

The treatment of visceral pain is a relatively new application for SCS, and investigators have proposed that SCS might exert its positive effect on visceral pain (and dysfunction) by moderating the so-called "brain–gut" axis (the neural circuitry thought to control the interface among visceral afferent sensation, intestinal motor function, and the brain).[130,135–137]

In fact, moving an active SCS electrode along the neuraxis demonstrates that electric activation occurs at various levels; thus, in addition to its beneficial effects on pain and ischemia, SCS inhibits the viscerosomatic reflexes involved with the particular spinal segmental level being stimulated (Fig. 96.6).

Some rodent studies in experimental colonic pain[137,138] demonstrated that SCS applied with conventional clinical stimulation parameters significantly decreased the painful symptoms (measured by monitoring of abdominal contractions as response to balloon inflation in the distal colon). Based on these observations, first a case of irritable bowel symptom was successfully treated by SCS,[139] and thereafter, a prospective randomized clinical study in a small series confirmed the beneficial findings in a pilot study.[140]

In fact, as shown in Figure 96.6, SCS might have many as yet unexplored positive effects on visceral problems.

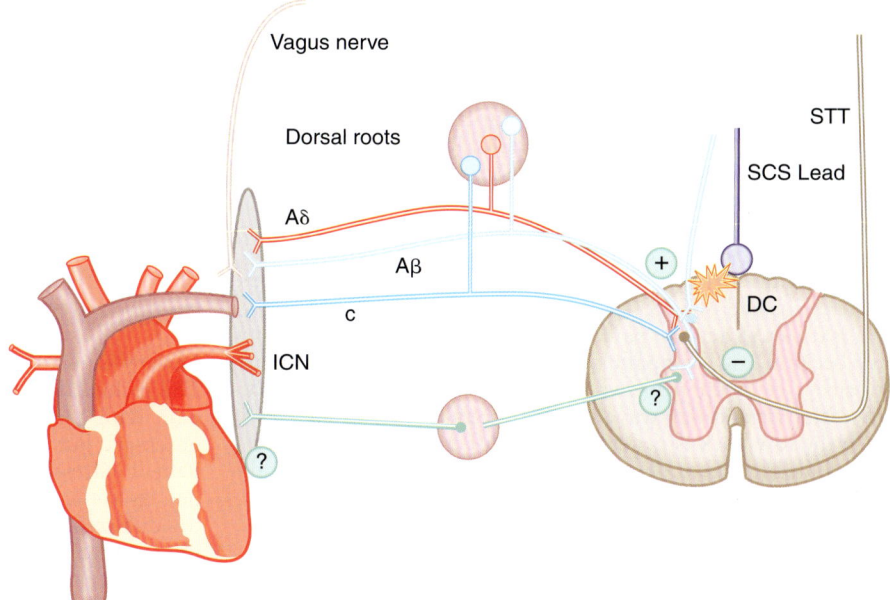

FIGURE 96.5 Schematic illustration of some mechanisms possibly involved in the effects of spinal cord stimulation (SCS) on coronary ischemic pain. SCS might exert indirect inhibitory effects on nociceptive transmission to higher centers and on the level of sympathetic activity; SCS might also have antidromically transmitted effects. Intrinsic cardiac nervous system (ICNS) are deeply involved in monitoring ischemic events in the heart, and this function is drastically influenced by SCS. The interplay between somatosensory and autonomic influences and the effects of SCS is presently largely unknown but is the subject of intense investigation. DC, dorsal columns; STT, spinothalamic tract.

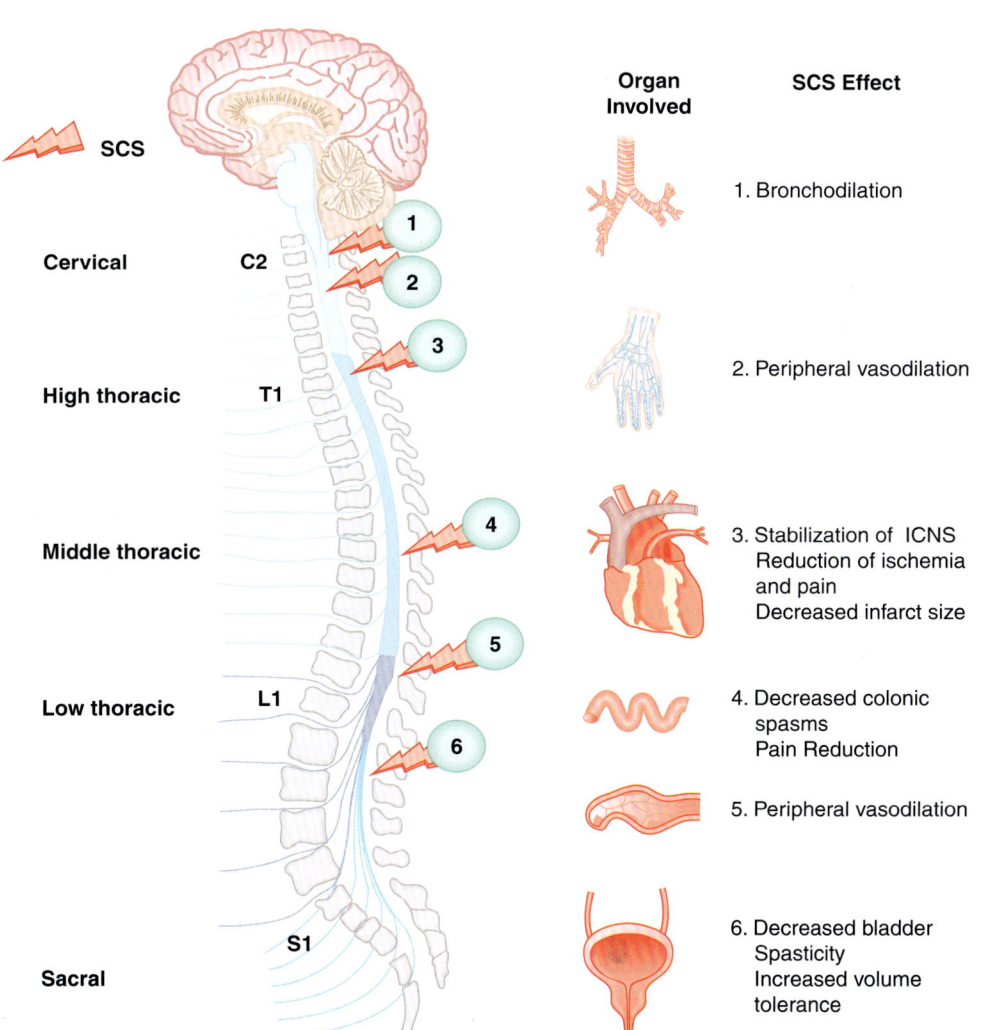

FIGURE 96.6 Spinal cord stimulation (SCS) applied at different levels of the neuraxis might, in addition to affecting pain and peripheral blood flow, induce changes in different target organs mediated via stimulation induced changes in local autonomic activity, dorsal root reflexes, or viscerosomatic eflexes. Some of these changes in target organ function might be beneficial. ICNS, intrinsic cardiac nervous system. *(Redrawn after Linderoth B, Foreman RD. Mechanisms of spinal cord stimulation in painful syndromes: role of animal models. Pain Med 2006;7[suppl 1]:S14–S26. Reproduced by permission of American Academy of Pain Medicine.)*

Indications

NEUROPATHIC PAIN

In the United States, the major indication for SCS is the treatment of FBSS, particularly with a component of neuropathic pain. Two randomized controlled trials (RCTs) have demonstrated the superiority of treating FBSS with SCS versus reoperation[141] or optimized conventional medical management.[142] Of course, an FBSS patient with gross instability or a neurologic deficit caused by neural compression that is evident on an imaging study would undergo a corrective surgical procedure before or instead of SCS.

It is easier to achieve pain relief in the limbs than in the low back because low back pain is more likely than leg pain to have a nociceptive component, which is not expected to respond to SCS with conventional waveforms; also, pain/paresthesia overlap in the low back is generally more difficult to achieve, even with complex electrode arrays and detailed psychophysical tests. At one time, achieving low back pain relief with SCS was considered rare; however, Law's[143] research on techniques to guide paresthesia coverage kept the low back available as an SCS therapeutic target, and clinicians have built on his work to define the best electrodes[144] and contact combinations[86] for achieving pain relief in the low back.

Over the past 5 years, 10-kHz stimulation has been reported to be highly effective for FBSS and in one head-to-head RCT comparison to be superior to conventional SCS.[145–148] The most recent such comparisons, however, have shown conventional and high frequencies to be equally effective.[146,149] "Burst" SCS also has been reported to be highly effective for FBSS,[69,70,150] and most recently, an RCT comparing burst with conventional waveforms showed burst to be superior, but in crossover comparisons, a substantial fraction (20%) of patients preferred the conventional waveform, showing the clinical importance of a device which delivers multiple waveforms.[151]

The use of SCS to treat pain in the limbs arising from complex regional pain syndrome type I (CRPS I) (reflex sympathetic dystrophy) is also supported by data from an RCT.[152,153] In that study, 5 years posttreatment, the 20 patients remaining in the group that actually received SCS reported better pain relief and superior global perceived effect than did those patients remaining in the alternate group who did not receive SCS.[154] More recently, HF and burst SCS also have been reported to be effective for CRPS, with individual patients showing preferences for one or the other, or for conventional waveforms.[84]

Other neuropathic pain indications for SCS include phantom limb/postamputation syndrome, postherpetic neuralgia, root injury pain, and pain/spasm arising from spinal cord injury or lesion.

ISCHEMIC PAIN

In Europe, clinicians have gathered evidence on the efficacy of SCS in the treatment of ischemic pain caused by refractory angina (including syndrome X),[155–158] PVD,[159,160] Raynaud's syndrome, and diabetic neuropathy. As noted earlier, in patients with ischemia, SCS not only treats the pain but also has a positive effect on the underlying ischemia. Thus, the outcome criteria used to document the impact of SCS on critical limb ischemia arising from PVD include survival, limb salvage, and measures of microcirculation[161] as well as pain relief.

In Raynaud's syndrome, the few published studies (all of which involve small numbers of patients) demonstrate the positive effect of SCS therapy.[162–166] This is not surprising because, compared with PVD patients, patients with vasospastic conditions are relatively young, present with relatively few obliterative vessel wall processes, and have symptoms that are often temporarily relieved by destroying or blocking the corresponding sympathetic ganglia.

Some clinicians are using cervical SCS in exploratory trials to improve cerebral blood flow in patients recovering from stroke,[167] coma,[168] or brain tumors.[169]

VISCERAL PAIN AND DYSFUNCTION

SCS and other forms of neurostimulation are also being used to treat visceral dysfunction and pain associated with such diseases as interstitial cystitis,[170] pancreatitis,[171] motility disorders, urinary urgency and frequency,[172] pelvic pain,[173] vulvodynia,[174] and pelvic floor dysfunction.[175]

Potential Beneficial Outcomes

TECHNICAL GOAL

The technical goal of conventional SCS is to cover a patient's pain with a comfortable level of paresthesia; this has been a necessary but not sufficient condition for therapeutic success. Recent paresthesia free waveforms and settings have continued to use paresthesia mapping data, whether historical or individualized, to optimize electrode placement. If an electrode migrates or if pain changes location, appropriate paresthesia coverage can be lost. Thus, contemporary SCS systems are designed to allow adjustment of stimulation parameters postimplant to steer paresthesia to a new location or to recapture coverage. Only occasionally does readjustment for these purposes require a surgical intervention.

It is possible for paresthesia to cover the painful area without providing an analgesic effect. Such clinical failure can become evident during the screening trial or can arise after a period of success. On rare occasions, a patient who experiences technical success and pain relief dislikes the sensation of paresthesia and decides not to continue the therapy. New waveforms offer additional options for these patients.

CLINICAL GOALS

A commonly used definition of "success" in treatment for pain is a minimum of 50% pain relief, but this and other measures all have limitations.[176] Additional reported benefits of SCS include (1) reduced consumption of medication and other health care resources; (2) improved ability to engage in the activities of daily living, quality of life, neurologic function, and symptoms of emotional depression; and (3) return to work when uncontrolled chronic pain was the only impediment (and generally when the patient has been out of work for less than 2 years).[177,178]

In patients suffering from ischemic pain, SCS can improve microcirculation and tissue oxygenation. This, in turn, can promote the healing of ischemic ulcers and increase the possibility of limb salvage.

Prognostic Factors

Demographics are of little help in choosing the ideal SCS candidate. Age is only a factor in children, where the safety and effectiveness of SCS is not established, and in the elderly, who might have difficulty dealing with the patient interface (or recharging a battery), but, as for example with driving cars, the effect of advanced age must be assessed on an individual basis.

Researchers have reported some outcome differences between men and women, but these have been minor and of little if any practical value. Thus, the only sex-related caveat is that the safety of SCS during pregnancy is not established (although pregnant women have continued to use SCS rather than suffer known and suspected adverse effects of alternative pain treatments). Even a very short life expectancy does not rule out SCS, which can be cost-effective for short-term use if an external stimulator is used.

Also, we cannot reliably predict SCS outcome based on worker's compensation or litigation status, but some clinicians consider the unresolved possibility of secondary gain a relative contraindication to allowing a patient to undergo a screening trial in clinical practice and an exclusionary factor for clinical trials.

For FBSS patients, it seems that the chance of success with SCS decreases as the number of prior surgical procedures and the time since the last surgical procedure increases. The type of surgical procedure the patient has experienced is also important; some ablative procedures, such as rhizotomy, dorsal root gangli-onectomy, or dorsal root entry zone lesioning, might obliterate the neural substrate on which SCS is thought to depend.[179]

For patients with PVD, investigators have reported that 1-year limb salvage is more likely to occur if the baseline supine transcutaneously measured oxygen tension ($TcPO_2$) is >10 mm Hg, the baseline sitting-supine score is >17 mm Hg, and the treatment difference is >4 mm Hg.[180] Some investigators believe that a 50% improved $TcPO_2$ score during a 2-week screening period predicts limb salvage[181] regardless of baseline score or disease stage.[182] In the case of diabetic neuropathy, however, these investigators found the stage of neuropathy to be inversely related to SCS treatment success,[183] independent of the stage of the disease.[184]

Patient Selection

One of the first things we learned about SCS was that achieving a successful outcome required the right patient. In any diagnostic group, the presence of seemingly identical pain syndromes was not enough to predict identical (or even any) SCS success in each individual. A major advantage of SCS, however, is that it is possible to perform a screening trial, which involves temporary (typically 7 to 10 days) placement of an electrode to determine the extent of pain/paresthesia overlap and the resulting therapeutic effect. In some European countries, a trial period of several weeks is required for reimbursement.

The screening trial offers the most meaningful prognostic sign of the outcome of SCS, but, of course, not all potential SCS patients proceed to a screening trial. Information to determine a patient's suitability for a screening trial is gathered from the patient's history and from the results of a physical examination and imaging studies.

Among the important aspects of the patient's history are the location, intensity, duration, and characteristics of the pain and the patient's psychological status. Radiating pain that has an objective basis, is distributed in a manner consistent with information gleaned from a physical examination and imaging studies, and can be labeled with a specific diagnosis is the most straightforward to treat. Imaging studies that are useful for diagnostic purposes can also provide anatomic information, namely, as to spinal canal diameter, that can be helpful or even vital during SCS implantation.

In the United States, Medicare and many health insurance companies require SCS candidates to undergo a routine psychological evaluation. Although no psychological test reliably predicts the result of SCS treatment (and physicians routinely expect new patients to meet reasonable psychological/behavioral standards), patients who have been living with chronic pain often benefit from psychological screening with the attendant possibility of therapy. Any major psychiatric comorbidity should be addressed before a patient undergoes an SCS screening trial.

Relative contraindications include the following:
Unresolved major psychiatric comorbidity
Unresolved possibility of secondary gain
Inappropriate dependency on pharmaceuticals
Inconsistency among the history, pain ratings and description, physical examination, and diagnostic studies
Abnormal pain ratings
A predominance of nonorganic signs (e.g., Waddell's signs)
Alternative therapies with a risk–benefit ratio comparable to that of SCS remain to be tried
Pregnancy
Occupational risk (e.g., of falling)
Local or systemic infection
Presence of a demand pacemaker or cardioverter defibrillator
Foreseeable need for MRI particularly if high field strength will be required and/or the implant will be in or near the area to be imaged. Some contemporary implants allow MRI on a limited basis.
Presence of a major comorbid chronic pain syndrome
Anticoagulant or antiplatelet therapy
Absolute contraindications include the following:
　Inability to control the device
　Gross spinal instability at risk for progression, or nerve compression causing a potentially disabling neurologic deficit, amenable to corrective surgery
　Coagulopathy, immunosuppression, or other condition associated with an unacceptable surgical risk
　Need for therapeutic diathermy

Technique

A discussion of techniques used for the various types of SCS screening trials and for SCS implantations is beyond the scope of this chapter. Instead, we refer the reader to previous publications.[185–187]

Screening Trial

Before the introduction of percutaneous catheter electrodes in the 1970s, physicians used a variety of methods to screen potential SCS candidates, including TENS, which were found to lack prognostic value. The percutaneous electrodes developed to facilitate a screening trial were immediately adopted for chronic use as well. Today, SCS systems in the United States are generally only implanted in patients who pass a screening trial. In Europe, the screening trial is commonly bypassed in patients with typical angina pectoris, a shortcut that reflects the fact that more than 80% of these patients enjoy significant pain relief with SCS.

Beyond indicating that SCS therapy might be successful, the benefits of a screening trial include allowing a patient to experience the sensation of paresthesia before undergoing implantation of the expensive pulse generator. The trial also provides important information that will dictate the choice of a permanent electrode and pulse generator and the optimum stimulating configuration. A successful screening trial commonly is defined by at least 50% patient-reported pain relief despite appropriate (provocative) physical activity and stable or reduced analgesic consumption. Patient satisfaction is another vital outcome. Medicare and many third-party payers require a successful screening trial before implantation.

SCREENING ELECTRODE CHOICE

A percutaneous catheter electrode placed under fluoroscopy provides easy access to multiple target spinal levels and facilitates mapping of pain/paresthesia overlap to determine the optimal longitudinal level for the electrode.

An insulated surgical plate/paddle electrode inserted by laminectomy limits access to spinal levels and mapping but is required if a percutaneous catheter electrode does not access the epidural space satisfactorily. Screening with a surgical plate/paddle electrode is also necessary in some patients to eliminate uncomfortable extraneous stimulation or provide sufficient pain/paresthesia overlap.

ELECTRODE POSITIONING

Ideally, patients remain conscious during trial electrode placement under local anesthesia in order to describe paresthesia coverage and have the opportunity to react to changes in stimulation parameters or unanticipated intraoperative events. Evoked potential techniques may be used when general anesthesia is required, as for example in some cases of paddle electrode implantation.[188]

PARAMETER ADJUSTMENT

Trained professionals work with patients to adjust simulation parameters during the screening trial and after implantation to find the settings that maximize comfortable pain/paresthesia overlap, reduce or eliminate extraneous stimulation, and minimize power requirements. Even when paresthesia-free stimulation settings will ultimately be used, this may be presumed to be the best method for selection of the electrode contacts. Patients are instructed at each stage so as to operate the device appropriately.

PROCEDURAL RISK REDUCTION

Implanting an electrode for a screening trial or chronic stimulation is associated with certain risks, including spinal cord or nerve injury, dural puncture, epidural hematoma, and infection. Risk can be reduced by ordering a preimplant MRI of the target spinal levels, performing the procedure under fluoroscopy with the patient conscious, maintaining a meticulously sterile environment, administering prophylactic antibiotics, and observing the patient for a reasonable length of time postprocedure (e.g., overnight). Discharge instructions must indicate when and how patients should contact their physicians, the device manufacturer, and emergency care providers.

TRIAL DURATION

A typical screening trial with a temporary percutaneous electrode lasts a week. In some circumstances, a shorter trial will be adequate, whereas in others, a longer trial might be beneficial. The role of a screening trial is subject to change with recent technical developments: As more and more waveforms become available, and as some patients need to try multiple settings to achieve a satisfactory result, trial duration can increase to an extent causing undue risk of infection. Externally powered implants which can be inserted in their entirety through a needle might mitigate this problem.[189]

REMOVAL OF TRIAL ELECTRODE

Using the same percutaneous catheter electrode for screening and permanent stimulation would reduce the cost of the hardware, but this savings would be offset by the increased cost of anchoring the electrode, which must take place in an operating room. Anchoring a trial electrode for potential permanent stimulation also increases incisional pain, which might confound interpretation of the trial; anchoring also requires use of a percutaneous extension cable, which increases the risk of infection. On the other hand, a percutaneous catheter electrode designed solely for screening is relatively inexpensive, can be inserted under sterile conditions with fluoroscopy, and can be removed easily.

Using the same electrode for the screening trial and permanent stimulation might eliminate the possibility that the replacement electrode will not reproduce the pain/paresthesia overlap, but this strategy also eliminates the opportunity to improve on the results of the screening trial—which can inform the patient as well as the physician.

Device Options

In alphabetical order, the major manufacturers of SCS equipment are Abbott (previously St. Jude's Medical, previously Advanced Neuromodulation Systems, Plano, TX), Boston Scientific (previously Advanced Bionics Inc, Natick, MA), Medtronic Inc (Minneapolis, MN), Nevro Corp (Redwood City, CA), Nuvectra Corp (Plano, TX), and Stimwave (Pompano Beach, FL).

CHOICE OF ELECTRODE

Percutaneous catheter electrodes are available with up to 16 contacts and can be implanted singly, creating a one-dimensional array or multiply, creating a two-dimensional array. Multiple percutaneous electrodes can be introduced one by one through a Tuohy needle to rest side by side. Use of three or more such electrodes in parallel permits programming of lateral anodes "guarding" a central cathode, which might mitigate dorsal root recruitment causing uncomfortable side effects; however, it can be difficult to achieve and maintain appropriate spacing between electrodes. Figure 96.7 illustrates a selection of available electrodes.

An important role remains for plate/paddle electrodes, which cannot be introduced through a needle and thus require surgical exposure via laminectomy. These electrodes have as many as 32 contacts in multi-column configurations and are insulated to prevent excess stimulation of dorsal structures.[189] The spacing of the columns is fixed, precluding adjustment as well as postoperative migration of one column with respect to another.

Factors that dictate choice of electrode include the location of the pain, the amount of extraneous stimulation that must be managed, and the physician's qualifications and experience (anesthesiologists, e.g., might be expected to use only percutaneous electrodes).

CHOICE OF PULSE GENERATOR

Pulse generators are distinguished by their power sources and output configurations. The earliest systems incorporated a small radiofrequency receiver with no implanted battery,

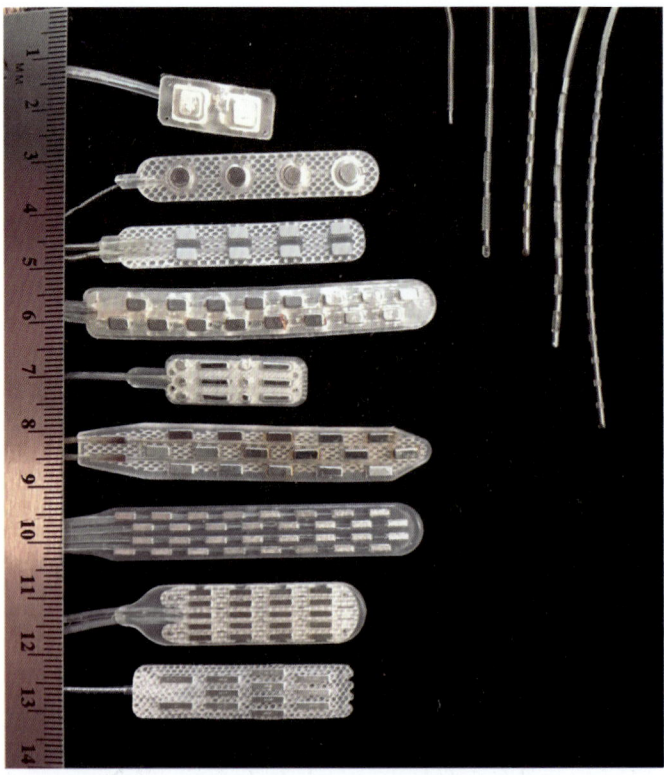

FIGURE 96.7 Percutaneous catheter electrodes **(top left)** have as many as 16 cylindrical contacts designed for introduction through a needle. Laminectomy electrodes **(bottom)** have evolved **(left to right)** from a single column of contacts to as many as seven columns or centerlines, with as many as 32 contacts.

powered by an external transmitter and antenna worn by the patient. The development of lithium primary cells made the internally powered generator (IPG) feasible in the 1980s; it was marketed as "totally implanted," although it still required an external remote control device. Early IPGs required surgical replacement when the battery was exhausted, but newer generators, introduced in 2004, have rechargeable batteries. Most recently, advances in microwave power and microcircuit technology have led to development of a wireless implant which can be inserted through a needle and which, as it is passive, need not be modified to accommodate new waveforms delivered by the external transmitter.

Since the 1980s, all generators have allowed noninvasive postoperative reassignment of each electrode contact (to anode, cathode, or off), and generators now support up to 32 independent contacts. The newest "multichannel" generators are capable of simultaneously or sequentially delivering pulses with different amplitudes and widths to different combinations of contacts, which of course consumes more energy compared with the simpler generators and thus motivates use of the rechargeable devices.

Factors that dictate the choice of stimulator/power generator include the patient's ability to control the device, the amount of power required, and patient convenience.

PROGRAMMING A SPINAL CORD STIMULATION SYSTEM

The number of contact combinations possible with either a surgical plate/paddle or percutaneous catheter electrode has grown markedly as the number of contacts has increased. In fact, more programming options exist than can be tested (e.g., whereas a four-contact electrode offers 50 functional bipolar combinations of anodes and cathodes, an eight-contact electrode increases the choices to 6050). Thus, all three SCS manufacturers employ computerized equipment to find the best options for an individual patient and save these settings for subsequent use. Not only is initial programming important, skillful reprogramming can compensate for changes in impedance (e.g., due to postural changes or fibrosis), electrode migration, and changes in pain location or intensity.

Although each manufacturer's adjustment system is unique, each asks the patient to describe the area of pain and paresthesia and (for conventional SCS) to rate pain overlap and intensity at various settings. Figure 96.8 shows a prototype developed in the 1990s to automate this process and interact directly with patients.

Patient Management

The patient should have a postoperative surgical check and SCS adjustment and on postoperative day 7 to 14 return for suture or staple removal and any needed additional adjustment.

From that point on, monthly visits should gradually taper to yearly visits.

Patients should understand that SCS is expected to reduce, not eliminate, pain. It is, therefore, important for clinicians to remember that other pain treatments remain available, especially those designed to treat nociceptive pain, for which SCS might not be so effective.

On/off time has a direct effect on battery longevity, but there are no studies of the impact of an imposed duty cycle on pain relief. In some patients, pain relief persists for a week or more after the device is turned off; others must operate the stimulator continuously. It is possible but rare for an SCS patient to achieve complete resolution of pain and request removal of the system.

Stimulation can induce subtle loss of normal sensation in SCS patients, but this loss is not sufficient to cause undesirable side effects, such as Charcot joints.[4,190] A change in paresthesia intensity corresponding to a change in posture is a normal, generally benign, side effect of SCS related to normal movement of the spinal cord with respect to the electrode(s).[191] Automated methods have been developed to mitigate this.[11,12]

These side effects might, however, make certain activities hazardous; thus, we instruct patients to turn off SCS before driving a car or climbing a ladder, etc. The incidence of SCS side effects increases as stimulation amplitude and recruitment increase.[192]

As is standard practice, except in emergency cases that require immediate attention, a physician has the discretion to accept or reject any new patient who was implanted elsewhere. The device manufacturers provide all SCS patients with identification cards with the necessary contact information to facilitate appropriate emergency treatment.

SPINAL CORD STIMULATION PATIENT PRECAUTIONS

SCS systems might affect or be affected by electromagnetic fields, and this necessitates certain precautions. When MRI was first introduced, it was generally contraindicated in SCS patients; some systems are now "MRI contingent." Manufacturers generally recommend that implants be disabled before a patient enters an electromagnetic field produced by antitheft devices, a metal detector, or any other security scanning device. A patient with an IPG must also refrain from scuba diving more than (typically) 10 m deep or entering hyperbaric chambers with an absolute pressure above (typically) 2.0 atmospheres. Everyday precautions include avoiding placing excessive mechanical stress on the system.

Special steps must be taken before an SCS patient undergoes certain routine medical tests (such as cardiac monitoring) or radiation therapy with the pulse generator in the active field. Radiofrequency ablation, electrocautery, and lithotripsy also require caution. Ultrasound over the device and diathermy in any location are contraindicated in SCS patients.

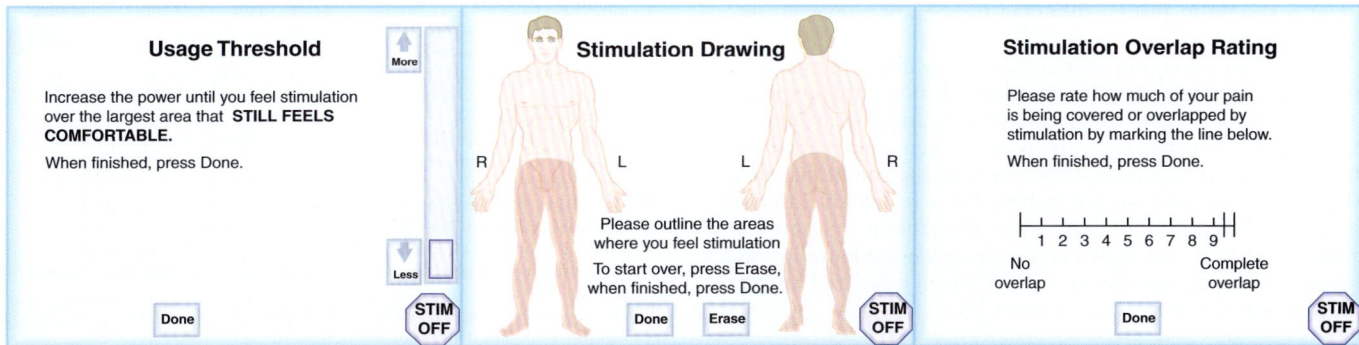

FIGURE 96.8 This computerized patient-interactive system allows the patient to (1) adjust amplitude to a specified level, (2) draw the area of paresthesia to be compared with a pain drawing, and (3) rate pain/paresthesia overlap.

Spinal Cord Stimulation Treatment Challenges

CLINICAL FAILURE

The loss of pain relief despite pain/paresthesia overlap in a functioning system occurs in a minority of patients. This clinical failure might have a neurochemical basis, and it might respond to adjuvant medical therapy with baclofen or gabapentin. Clinical failure can also occur if the patient develops (1) pain in a new location that cannot be covered by paresthesia unless the equipment is revised surgically, (2) troublesome postural changes in paresthesia coverage, or (3) excessive pain/irritation at the implant site that is not caused by infection and cannot be treated locally.

BIOLOGIC FAILURE

Infection, the most common biologic failure, is almost always treated successfully (treatment, however, is expensive because it generally requires removal and replacement of the SCS system). The risk of infection is small, however, and is reduced by maintaining sterility and administering prophylactic intravenous antibiotics. Should an infection occur, specimen culture will guide antibiotic therapy. Unless the infection is limited to the skin over the implant, the entire SCS system should be removed until the infection resolves, when a new system can be implanted. Clinicians have reported patients with an "allergic reaction" to the implant, but this is rare and might be undiagnosed infection. A second biologic failure, the development of fibrosis around implanted electrodes, can impede treatment, but this problem generally can be overcome through reprogramming.

PSYCHOLOGICAL FAILURE

Psychological problems, such as conversion disorder,[193] can require system removal.

TECHNICAL FAILURE

Technical failure, the inability to achieve or loss of clinically useful pain/paresthesia overlap, can result from suboptimal electrode choice or placement, from electrode migration, or from equipment malfunction. Technical failure can be mitigated by increasing clinician skill and experience, which includes adoption of the best implantation techniques; for example, the risk of percutaneous electrode migration can be nearly eliminated by applying an adhesive to the anchor/strain relief during implantation,[187,194] and the risk of fatigue fracture can be lessened by implanting the pulse generator in the lateral abdomen instead of the buttock and by creating strain relief coils in appropriate places.

In patients with suspected spinal stenosis or another anatomic anomaly that increases the risk of spinal cord or nerve injury, it is prudent to obtain an MRI of the target spinal areas before implantation of a surgical plate/paddle electrode. With the SCS system in place, computed tomography myelography is an alternative.

The risk of dural puncture is reduced by using an anesthetic technique that permits patient feedback during implantation of an electrode and avoiding placement in scarred areas, and the risk of epidural hematoma is reduced by preoperative review of the patient's coagulation history, medications, and blood chemistry and by monitoring the patient for a reasonable amount of time. Uncomfortable extraneous paresthesia or motor responses can be avoided by careful electrode implantation and postoperative adjustment or by use of an insulated surgical plate/paddle electrode.

EQUIPMENT FAILURE

Every part of an SCS system can fail. The electrode/lead/extension conductors can develop an open circuit through fatigue, fracture, or corrosion; insulation might fail; the generator battery can be depleted prematurely; or the generator itself can fail (e.g., by supplying excessive or unacceptable stimulation).[195,196]

Cost-effectiveness

Although the initial expense of implanted SCS equipment creates a potential barrier to patient access, investigators have established that SCS is cost-effective in the treatment of FBSS,[197–200] CRPS,[201] PVD, and angina.[156,202] Cost recovery occurs in approximately 3 years in patients with FBSS or CRPS, after 1 year in patients with angina who are not candidates for coronary artery bypass surgery, and immediately in patients with angina who would otherwise receive coronary artery bypass surgery only for symptom relief.

The cost-effectiveness of SCS will be improved by the development of new equipment and techniques and can be enhanced by minimizing the incidence of complications (especially those, such as infection, that require surgical intervention and system replacement) and by careful patient selection.

The incidence of complications can be reduced if the specialist is meticulous, technically proficient, and knowledgeable (e.g., a simple technique nearly eliminates percutaneous electrode migration).[187] One improvement that has had a direct impact on cost-effectiveness is the development of equipment designed to facilitate noninvasive reprogramming to optimize pain/paresthesia overlap. Another improvement, the introduction of rechargeable batteries, is intended to extend the life of expensive implanted pulse generators.[203]

Spinal Cord Stimulation Challenges

In common with most medical therapies, we can improve patient outcomes with SCS by improving patient selection criteria, equipment design, implantation techniques, and clinician training. Continued investigation of the mechanisms of action of SCS will allow us to potentiate the benefits of the therapy, and developing refined outcome measures and appropriate research techniques will help us to optimize clinical application.

The increasing presence of magnetic fields in our environment and in the use of higher field strengths in MRI investigations motivates the development of electrodes and pulse generators that will tolerate the magnetic fields.

SCS remains an underused therapy that should be considered early in the treatment continuum for a large group of patients.

References

1. Largus S. *Compositiones*. Helmreich G, ed. Leipzig: Tuebner; 1887.
2. Shealy CN, Mortimer JT, Reswick JB. Electrical inhibition of pain by stimulation of the dorsal columns: preliminary clinical report. *Anesth Analg* 1967;46(4):489–491.
3. Melzack P, Wall PD. Pain mechanisms: a new theory. *Science* 1965;150(3699):971–978.
4. Lindblom U, Meyerson BA. Influence on touch, vibration and cutaneous pain of dorsal column stimulation in man. *Pain* 1975;1:257–270.
5. Linderoth B, Meyerson BA. Dorsal column stimulation: modulation of somatosensory and autonomic function. In: McMahon SB, Wall PD, eds. *The Neurobiology of Pain. Seminars in the Neurosciences.* London: Academic Press; 1995:263–277.
6. Campbell JN, Davis KD, Meyer RA, et al. The mechanism by which spinal cord stimulation affects pain: evidence for a new hypothesis. *Pain* 1990;5:S228.
7. Dickenson AH. Gate control theory of pain stands the test of time. *Br J Anaesth* 2002;88(6):755–757.
8. Nashold B, Somjen G, Friedman H. Paresthesias and EEG potentials evoked by stimulation of the dorsal funiculi in man. *Exp Neurol* 1972;36(2):273–287.
9. Hosobuchi Y, Adams JE, Weinstein PR. Preliminary percutaneous dorsal column stimulation prior to permanent implantation. *J Neurosurg* 1972;37(2):242–245.
10. Law JD. Spinal stimulation: statistical superiority of monophasic stimulation of narrowly separated bipoles having rostral cathodes. *Appl Neurophysiol* 1983;46:129–137.

11. Schultz DM, Webster L, Kosek P, et al. Sensor-driven position-adaptive spinal cord stimulation for chronic pain. *Pain Physician* 2012;15(1):1–12.

12. Parker JL, Karantonis DM, Single PS, et al. Compound action potentials recorded in the human spinal cord during neurostimulation for pain relief. *Pain* 2012;153(3):593–601.

13. Abejon D, Rueda P, Vallejo R. Threshold evolution as an analysis of the different pulse frequencies in rechargeable systems for spinal cord stimulation. *Neuromodulation* 2016;19:276–282.

14. North JM, Hong KJ, Cho PY. Clinical outcomes of 1 kHz subperception spinal cord stimulation in implanted patients with failed paresthesia-based stimulation: results of a prospective randomized controlled trial. *Neuromodulation* 2016;19(7):731–737. doi:10.1111/ner.12441.

15. Saadé NE, Tabet MS, Atweh SF, et al. Modulation of segmental mechanisms by activation of a dorsal column brainstem spinal loop. *Brain Res* 1984;310:180–184.

16. Saadé NE, Jabbur SJ. Nociceptive behavior in animal models for peripheral neuropathy: spinal and supraspinal mechanisms. *Prog Neurobiol* 2008; 86:22–47.

17. El-Khoury C, Hawwa N, Baliki M, et al. Attenuation of neuropathic pain by segmental and supraspinal activation of the dorsal column system in awake rats. *Neuroscience* 2002;112(3):541–553.

18. Stiller CO, Linderoth R, O'Connor WT, et al. Repeated spinal cord stimulation decreases the extracellular level of gamma-aminobutyric acid in the periaqueductal gray matter of freely moving rats. *Brain Res* 1995;699(2):231–241.

19. Hautvast RW, Ter Horst GJ, DeJong BM, et al. Relative changes in regional cerebral blood flow during spinal cord stimulation in patients with refractory angina pectoris. *Eur J Neurosci* 1997;9(6):1178–1183.

20. De Jongste MJ, Hautvast RW, Ruiters MH, et al. Spinal cord stimulation and the induction of c-fos and heat shock protein 72 in the central nervous system of rats. *Neuromodulation* 1998;2:73–85.

21. Linderoth B, Foreman RD. Physiology of spinal cord stimulation: review and update. *Neuromodulation* 1999;2(3):150–164.

22. Saadé NE, Atweh SF, Jabbur SJ, et al. Effects of lesions in the anterolateral columns and dorsolateral funiculi on self-mutilation behavior in rats. *Pain* 1990;42(3):313–321.

23. Yakhnitsa V, Linderoth B, Meyerson BA. Modulation of dorsal horn neuronal activity by spinal cord stimulation in a rat model of neuropathy: the role of the dorsal funicles. *Neurophysiology* 1998;30:424–427.

24. Barchini J, Tchagchagian S, Shmaa F, et al. Spinal segmental and supraspinal mechanisms underlying the pain-relieving effects of spinal cord stimulation: an experimental study in a rat model of neuropathy. *Neuroscience* 2012;215:196–208.

25. Saadé NE, Barchini J, Tchachaghian S, et al. The role of the dorsolateral funiculi in the pain relieving effect of spinal cord stimulation: a study in a rat model of neuropathic pain. *Exp Brain Res* 2015;233:1041–1052.

26. Freeman TB, Campbell JN, Long DM. Naloxone does not affect pain relief induced by electrical stimulation in man. *Pain* 1983;17:189–195.

27. Tonelli L, Setti T, Falasca A, et al. Investigation on cerebrospinal fluid opioids and neurotransmitters related to spinal cord stimulation. *Appl Neurophysiol* 1988;51(6):324–332.

28. Meyerson BA, Linderoth B. Spinal cord stimulation: mechanisms of action in neuropathic and ischemic pain. In: Simpson BA, ed. *Electrical Stimulation and the Relief of Pain.* New York: Elsevier; 2003:161–182.

29. Sato KL, King EW, Johanek LM, et al. Spinal cord stimulation reduces hypersensitivity through activation of opioid receptors in a frequency-dependent manner. *Eur J Pain* 2013;17:551–561.

30. Eliasson T, Mannheimer C, Waagstein F, et al. Myocardial turnover of endogenous opioids and calcitonin-gene-related peptide in the human heart and the effects of spinal cord stimulation on pacing-induced angina pectoris. *Cardiology* 1998;89(3):170–177.

31. Hansson P. Difficulties in stratifying neuropathic pain by mechanisms. *Eur J Pain* 2003;7:353–357.

32. Harke H, Gretenkort P, Ladleif HU, et al. Spinal cord stimulation in sympathetically maintained complex regional pain syndrome type I with severe disability. A prospective clinical study. *Eur J Pain* 2005;9:363–373.

33. Meyerson BA, Ren B, Herregodts P, et al. Spinal cord stimulation in animal models of mononeuropathy: effects on the withdrawal response and the flexor reflex. *Pain* 1995;61(2):229–243.

34. Ren B, Linderoth B, Meyerson BA. Effects of spinal cord stimulation on the flexor reflex and involvement of supraspinal mechanisms: an experimental study in mononeuropathic rats. *J Neurosurg* 1996;84(2):244–249.

35. Yakhnitsa V, Linderoth B, Meyerson BA. Spinal cord stimulation attenuates dorsal horn neuronal hyperexcitability in a rat model of mononeuropathy. *Pain* 1999;79(2–3):223–233.

36. Schechtmann G, Song Z, Ultenius C, et al. Cholinergic mechanisms in the pain relieving effect of spinal cord stimulation in a model of neuropathy. *Pain* 2008;139(1):136–145.

37. Song Z, Meyerson BA, Linderoth B. Muscarinic receptor activation potentiates the effect of spinal cord stimulation on pain related behaviour in rats with mononeuropathy. *Neurosci Lett* 2008;436:7–12.

38. Hanai F. C fiber responses of wide dynamic range neurons in the spinal dorsal horn. *Clin Orthop Relat Res* 1998;349:256–267.

39. Cui JG, Linderoth B, Meyerson BA. Effects of spinal cord stimulation on touch-evoked allodynia involve GABAergic mechanisms: an experimental study in the mononeuropathic rat. *Pain* 1996;66:287–295.

40. Cui JG, O'Connor WT, Ungerstedt U, et al. Spinal cord stimulation attenuates augmented dorsal horn release of excitatory amino acids in mononeuropathy via a GABAergic mechanism. *Pain* 1997;73:87–95.

41. Linderoth B. *Dorsal Column Stimulation and Pain: Experimental Studies of Putative Neurochemical and Neurophysiological Mechanisms* [doctoral thesis]. Stockholm, Sweden: Karolinska Institute; 1992.

42. Linderoth B, Gazelius B, Franck J, et al. Dorsal column stimulation induces release of serotonin and substance P in the cat dorsal horn. *Neurosurgery* 1992;31:289–297.

43. Cui JG, Sollevi A, Linderoth B, et al. Adenosine receptor activation suppresses tactile hypersensitivity and potentiates spinal cord stimulation in mononeuropathic rats. *Neurosci Lett* 1997;223:173–176.

44. Meyerson BA, Brodin E, Linderoth B. Possible neurohumoral mechanisms in CNS stimulation for pain suppression. *Appl Neurophysiol* 1985;48:175–180.

45. Song Z, Ansah OB, Meyerson BA, et al. Exploration of supraspinal mechanisms in effects of spinal cord stimulation: role of the locus coeruleus. *Neuroscience* 2013;253:426–434.

46. Song Z, Ultenius C, Meyerson BA, et al. Pain relief by spinal cord stimulation involves serotonergic mechanisms: an experimental study in a rat model of mononeuropathy. *Pain* 2009;147(1–3):241–248.

47. Song Z, Meyerson BA, Linderoth B. Spinal 5-HT receptors that contribute to the pain-relieving effects of spinal cord stimulation in a rat model of neuropathy. *Pain* 2011;152:1666–1673.

48. Song Z, Meyerson BA, Linderoth B. Interaction between antidepressant drugs and the pain relieving effect of spinal cord stimulation in a rat model of neuropathy. *Anesth Analg* 2011;113(5):1260–1265.

49. Song Z, Ansah OB, Meyerson BA, et al. The rostroventromedial medulla is engaged in the effects of spinal cord stimulation: a study in a rodent model of neuropathic pain. *Neuroscience* 2013;247C:134–144.

50. Stiller CO, Cui JG, O'Connor WT, et al. Release of gamma-aminobutyric acid in the dorsal horn and suppression of tactile allodynia by spinal cord stimulation in mononeuropathic rats. *Neurosurgery* 1996;39(2):367–374.

51. Cui JG, Meyerson BA, Sollevi A, et al. Effect of spinal cord stimulation on tactile hypersensitivity in mononeuropathic rats is potentiated by simultaneous GABA(B) and adenosine receptor activation. *Neurosci Lett* 1998;247:183–186.

52. Meyerson BA, Cui JG, Yakhnitsa V, et al. Modulation of spinal pain mechanisms by spinal cord stimulation and the potential role of adjuvant pharmacotherapy. *Stereotact Funct Neurosurg* 1997;68(1–4 pt 1):129–140.

53. Wallin J, Cui JG, Yakhnitsa V, et al. Gabapentin and pregabalin suppress tactile allodynia and potentiate spinal cord stimulation in a model of neuropathy. *Eur J Pain* 2002;6:261–272.

54. Lind G, Schechtmann G, Winter J, et al. Baclofen-enhanced spinal cord stimulation and intrathecal baclofen alone for neuropathic pain: long-term outcome of a pilot study. *Eur J Pain* 2008;12:132–136.

55. Schechtmann G, Wallin J, Meyerson BA, et al. Intrathecal clonidine potentiates suppression of tactile hypersensitivity by spinal cord stimulation in a model of neuropathy. *Anesth Analg* 2004;99:135–139.

56. Schechtmann G, Lind G, Winter J, et al. Intrathecal clonidine and baclofen enhance the pain relieving effect of spinal cord stimulation: a placebo-controlled randomized trial. *Neurosurgery* 2010;67:173–181.

57. Linderoth B, Stiller CO, O'Connor WT, et al. An animal model for the study of brain transmittor release in response to spinal cord stimulation in the awake, freely moving rat: preliminary results from the periaqueductal grey matter. *Acta Neurochir Suppl (Wien)* 1993;58:156–160.

58. Kilgore KL, Bhadra N. Nerve conduction block utilising high-frequency alternating current. *Med Biol Eng Comput* 2004;42:394–406.

59. Kilgore KL, Bhadra N. Reversible nerve conduction block using kilohertz frequency alternating current. *Neuromodulation* 2014;17:242–254.

60. Song Z, Viisanen H, Meyerson BA, et al. Efficacy of kilohertz-frequency and conventional spinal cord stimulation in rat models of different pain conditions. *Neuromodulation* 2014;17(3):226–234.

61. Lempka SF, McIntyre CC, Kilgore KL, et al. Computational analysis of kilohertz frequency spinal cord stimulation for chronic pain management. *Anesthesiology* 2015;122:1362–1376.

62. Linderoth B, Foreman RD. Conventional and novel spinal stimulation algorithms: hypothetical mechanisms of action and comments on outcomes. *Neuromodulation* 2017;20(6):525–533.

63. Crosby ND, Janik JJ, Grill WM. Modulation of activity and conduction in single dorsal column axons by kilohertz-frequency spinal cord stimulation. *J Neurophysiology* 2017;117:136–147.

64. Shechter R, Yang F, Xu Q, et al. Conventional and kilohertz-frequency spinal cord stimulation produces intensity- and frequency-dependent inhibition of mechanical hypersensitivity in a rat model of neuropathic pain. *Anesthesiology* 2013;119:422–432.

65. McMahon S. Effect of different frequency spinal cord stimulation on pain-model rodent superficial dorsal horn neuronal excitability. Paper presented at: North American Neuromodulation Society's 21st Annual Meeting; 2018; Las Vegas, NV.

66. McMahon S, Jones M, Lee D, et al. Effects of 10kHz spinal cord stimulation on pain-model rodent deep dorsal horn neuronal excitability. Paper presented at: North American Neuromodulation Society's 21st Annual Meeting; 2018; Las Vegas, NV.

67. Song Z, Meyerson BA, Linderoth B. High-frequency (1 kHz) spinal cord stimulation—is pulse shape crucial for the efficacy? A pilot study. *Neuromodulation* 2015;18(8):714–720.

68. Eriksson MB, Sjölund BH, Nielzén S. Long term results of peripheral conditioning stimulation as an analgesic measure in chronic pain. *Pain* 1979;6:335–347.

69. De Ridder D, Vanneste S, Plazier M, et al. Burst spinal cord stimulation: toward paresthesia-free pain suppression. *Neurosurgery* 2010;66:986–990.

70. De Ridder D, Plazier M, Kamerling N, et al. Burst spinal cord stimulation for limb and back pain. *World Neurosurg* 2013;80:642–649.

71. De Ridder D, van der Loo E, Van der Kelen K, et al. Do tonic and burst TMS modulate the lemniscal and extralemniscal system differentially? *Int J Med Sci* 2007;9:242–246.

72. De Ridder D, Vanneste S. Burst and tonic spinal cord stimulation: different and common brain mechanisms. *Neuromodulation* 2016;19(1):47–59.

73. Stancák A, Kozák J, Vrba I, et al. Functional magnetic resonance imaging of cerebral activation during spinal cord stimulation in failed back surgery syndrome patients. *Eur J Pain* 2008;12:137–148.

74. Tang R, Martinez M, Goodman-Keiser M, et al. Comparison of burst and tonic spinal cord stimulation on spinal neural processing in an animal model. *Neuromodulation* 2014;17:143–151.

75. Crosby N, Weisshaar C, Smith J, et al. Burst and tonic spinal cord stimulation differentially activate GABAergic mechanisms to attenuate pain in a rat model of cervical radiculopathy. *IEEE Trans Biomed Eng* 2015;62(6):1604–1613.

76. Cui JG, Linderoth B, Meyerson BA. Incidence of mononeuropathy in rats is influenced by pre-emptive alteration of spinal excitability. *Eur J Pain* 1997;1:53–59.

77. Ultenius C, Song Z, Meyerson BA, et al. Spinal GABAergic mechanisms in the effects of spinal cord stimulation in a rodent model of neuropathic pain: is GABA synthesis involved? *Neuromodulation* 2013;16(2):114–120.

78. Crosby ND, Goodman Keiser MD, Smith JR, et al. Stimulation parameters define the effectiveness of burst spinal cord stimulation in a rat model of neuropathic pain. *Neuromodulation* 2015;18:1–8.

79. Shealy CN. Dorsal column electrohypalgesia. *Headache* 1969;9(2):99–102.

80. Waltz JM. Spinal cord stimulation. A quarter century of development and investigation. A review of its development and effectiveness in 1,336 cases. *Stereotact Funct Neurosurgery* 1997;69(1–4 pt 2):288–299.

81. Miller J, Eldabe S, Buchser E, et al. Parameters of spinal cord stimulation and their role in electrical charge delivery: a review. *Neuromodulation* 2016;19(4):373–384.

82. Sweet J, Badjatiya A, Tan D, et al. Paresthesia-free high density spinal cord stimulation for postlaminectomy syndrome in a prescreened population: a prospective case series. *Neuromodulation* 2016;19:260–267.

83. Wille F, Breel JS, Bakker EW, et al. Altering conventional to high density spinal cord stimulation: an energy dose-response relationship in neuropathic pain therapy. *Neuromodulation* 2017;20:71–80.

84. Kriek N, Groeneweg JG, Stronks DL, et al. Preferred frequencies and waveforms for spinal cord stimulation in patients with complex regional pain syndrome: a multicentre, double-blind, randomized and placebo-controlled crossover trial. *Eur J Pain* 2017;21(3):507–519.

85. Coburn B, Sin W. A theoretical study of epidural electrical stimulation of the spinal cord—part I. Finite element analysis of stimulus fields. *IEEE Trans Biomed Eng* 1985;32:971–977.

86. Holsheimer J, Struijk JJ, Rijkhoff NJ. Contact combinations in epidural spinal cord stimulation: a comparison by computer modeling. *Stereotact Funct Neurosurg* 1991;56:220–233.

87. Holsheimer J, Wesselink WA. Effect of anode-cathode configuration on paresthesia coverage in spinal cord stimulation. *Neurosurgery* 1997;41:654–660.

88. Sances A, Swinotek TJ, Larson SJ, et al. Innovations in neurologic implant systems. *Med Instrum* 1975;9:213–216.

89. Ranck JB, BeMent SL. The specific impedance of the dorsal columns of the cat: an anisotropic medium. *Exp Neurol* 1965;11:451–463.

90. Geddes LA, Baker LE. The specific resistance of biological material—a compendium of data for the biomedical engineer and physiologist. *Med Biol Eng* 1967;5:271–293.

91. Coburn B. Electrical stimulation of the spinal cord: two-dimensional finite element analysis with particular reference to epidural electrodes. *Med Biol Eng Comput* 1980;18:573–584.

92. Rusinko JB, Walker CF, Sepulvedo NG. Finite element modeling of potentials within the human thoracic spinal cord due to applied electrical stimulation. In: *Frontiers of Engineering in Health Care.* Vol. 3. Houston, TX: Proceedings of the IEEE Transactions on Biomedical Engineering Conference; 1981:76–81.

93. Sin WK, Coburn B. Electrical stimulation of the spinal cord: a further analysis relating to anatomic factors and tissue properties. *Med Biol Eng Comput* 1983;21:264–269.

94. Coburn B. A theoretical study of epidural electrical stimulation of the spinal cord—part II. Effects on long myelinated fibers. *IEEE Trans Biomed Eng* 1985;32:978–986.

95. Holsheimer J, Struijk JJ. How do geometric factors influence epidural spinal cord stimulation? A quantitative analysis by computer modeling. *Stereotact Funct Neurosurg* 1991;56:234–249.

96. McNeal DR. Analysis of a model for excitation of myelinated nerve. *IEEE Trans Biomed Eng* 1976;23:329–337.

97. Chiu SY, Ritchie JM, Rogart RB, et al. A quantitative description of membrane currents in rabbit myelinated nerve. *J Physiol* 1979;292:149–166.

98. Wesselink WA, Holsheimer J, Boom HB. A model of the electrical behaviour of myelinated sensory nerve fibres based on human data. *Med Biol Eng Comput* 1999;37(2):228–235.

99. Struijk JJ, Holsheimer J, Barolat G, et al. Paresthesia thresholds in spinal cord stimulation: a comparison of theoretical results with clinical data. *IEEE Trans Rehab Eng* 1993;1:101–108.

100. Hoekema R, Venner K, Struijk JJ, et al. Multigrid solution of the potential field in modeling electrical nerve stimulation. *Comput Biomed Res* 1998;31:348–362.

101. Oakley JC, Espinosa E, Bothe H, et al. Transverse tripolar spinal cord stimulation: results of an international multicenter study. *Neuromodulation* 2006;9(3):183–191.

102. Arle JE, Mei L, Carlson KW, et al. High-frequency stimulation of dorsal column axons: potential underlying mechanism of paresthesia-free neuropathic pain relief. *Neuromodulation* 2016;19(4):385–397.

103. Kimble LP, McGuire DB, Dunbar SB, et al. Gender differences in pain characteristics of chronic stable angina and perceived physical limitation in patients with coronary artery disease. *Pain* 2003;101:45–53.

104. Linderoth B. Spinal cord stimulation in ischemia and ischemic pain. In: Horsch S, Claeys L, eds. *Spinal Cord Stimulation III: An Innovative Method in the Treatment of PVD and Angina.* Darmstadt, Germany: Steinkopff Verlag; 1995:19–35.

105. Linderoth B, Gherardini G, Ren B, et al. Preemptive spinal cord stimulation reduces ischemia in an animal model of vasospasm. *Neurosurgery* 1995;37(2):266–271.

106. Gherardini G, Lundeberg T, Cui JG, et al. Spinal cord stimulation improves survival in ischemic skin flaps: an experimental study of the possible mediation via the calcitonin gene-related peptide. *Plast Reconstr Surg* 1999;103(4):1221–1228.

107. Croom JE, Foreman RD, Chandler MJ, et al. Cutaneous vasodilation during dorsal column stimulation is mediated by dorsal roots and CGRP. *Am J Physiol* 1997;272:H950–H957.

108. Croom JE, Foreman RD, Chandler MJ, et al. Reevaluation of the role of the sympathetic nervous system in cutaneous vasodilatation during dorsal spinal cord stimulation: are multiple mechanisms active? *Neuromodulation* 1998;1:91–101.

109. Tanaka S, Barron KW, Chandler MJ, et al. Low intensity spinal cord stimulation may induce cutaneous vasodilatation via CGRP release. *Brain Res* 2001;896:183–187.

110. Tanaka S, Barron KW, Chandler MJ, et al. Role of primary afferent in spinal cord stimulation-induced vasodilatation: characterization of fiber types. *Brain Res* 2003;959(2):191–198.

111. Tanaka S, Barron KW, Chandler MJ, et al. Local cooling alters neural mechanisms producing changes in peripheral blood flow by spinal cord stimulation. *Auton Neurosci* 2003;104(2):117–127.

112. Wu M, Komori N, Qin C, et al. Sensory fibers containing vanilloid receptor-1 (VR-1) mediate spinal cord stimulation-induced vasodilation. *Brain Res* 2006;1107:177–184.

113. Wu M, Komori N, Qin C, et al. Roles of peripheral terminals of transient receptor potential vanilloid-1 containing sensory fibers in spinal cord stimulation-induced peripheral vasodilation. *Brain Res* 2007;1156:80–92.

114. Tanaka S, Komori N, Barron KW. Mechanisms of sustained cutaneous vasodilatation induced by spinal cord stimulation. *Auton Neurosci* 2004;114(1–2):55–60.

115. Freedman RR, Sabharwal SC, Desai N, et al. Increased α-adrenergic responsiveness in idiopathic Raynaud's disease. *Arthritis Rheum* 1989;32:61–65.

116. Bunker CB, Terenghi G, Springall DR, et al. Deficiency of calcitonin gene-related peptide in Raynaud's phenomenon. *Lancet* 1990;336:1530–1533.

117. Wu M, Linderoth B, Foreman RD. Putative mechanisms behind effects of spinal cord stimulation on vascular diseases: a review of experimental studies. *Auton Neurosci* 2008;1381(1–20):9–23.

118. Foreman RD, Linderoth B. Neural mechanisms of spinal cord stimulation. In: Hamani C, Moro E, eds. *Emerging Horizons in Neuromodulation.* London: Elsevier; 2012:87–113. *International Review of Neurobiology*; vol 107.

119. Mannheimer C, Eliasson T, Andersson B, et al. Effects of spinal cord stimulation in angina pectoris induced by pacing and possible mechanisms of action. *BMJ* 1993;307:477–480.

120. Mobilia G, Zuin G, Zanco P, et al. Effects of spinal cord stimulation on regional myocardial blood flow in patients with refractory angina. A positron emission tomography study [in Italian]. *G Ital Cardiol* 1998;28(10):1113–1119.

121. Hautvast RW, Blanksma PK, DeJongste MJ, et al. Effect of spinal cord stimulation on myocardial blood flow assessed by positron emission tomography in patients with refractory angina pectoris. *Am H Cardiol* 1996;77:462–467.

122. Kingma JG Jr, Linderoth B, Ardell JL, et al. Neuromodulation therapy does not influence blood flow distribution or left-ventricular dynamics during acute myocardial ischemia. *Auton Neurosci* 2001;91(1–2):47–54.

123. Eliasson T, Augustinsson LE, Manneheimer C. Spinal cord stimulation in severe angina pectoris: presentation of current studies, indications and practical experience. *Pain* 1996;65:169–179.

124. Cardinal R, Ardell J, Linderoth B, et al. Spinal cord activation differentially modulates ischemic electrical responses to different stressors in canine ventricles. *Autonom Neurosci* 2004;111(1):34–47.

125. Foreman RD, Linderoth B, Ardell JL, et al. Modulation of intrinsic cardiac neuronal activity by spinal cord stimulation (SCS) in the dog: implications for the use of SCS in angina pectoris. *Cardiovasc Res* 2000;47(2):367–375.

126. Foreman RD, DeJongste MJL, Linderoth B. Integrative control of cardiac function by cervical and thoracic spinal neurons. In: Armour JA, Ardell JL, eds. *Basic and Clinical Neurocardiology*. London: Oxford University Press; 2004:153–186.

127. Chauhan A, Mullins PA, Thuraisingham SI, et al. Effect of transcutaneous electrical nerve stimulation on coronary blood flow. *Circulation* 1994;89(2):694–702.

128. Norrsell H, Eliasson T, Mannheimer C, et al. Effects of pacing-induced myocardial stress and spinal cord stimulation on whole body and cardiac norepinephrine spillover. *Eur Heart J* 1997;18(12):1890–1896.

129. Southerland EM, Milhorn D, Foreman RD, et al. Preemptive, but not reactive, spinal cord stimulation mitigates transient ischemia-induced myocardial infarction via cardiac adrenergic neurons. *Am J Physiology Heart Circ Physiol* 2007;292(1):H311–H317.

130. Foreman RD. Mechanisms of visceral pain: from nociception to targets. *Drug Dis Today: Dis Mech* 2004;1:457–463.

131. Armour JA, Linderoth B, Arora RC, et al. Long-term modulation of the intrinsic cardiac nervous system by spinal cord stimulation in normal and ischemic hearts. *Auton Neurosci* 2004;95(1–2):71–79.

132. Lopshire JC, Zhou X, Dusa C, et al. Spinal cord stimulation improves ventricular function and reduces ventricular arrhythmias in a canine postinfarction heart failure model. *Circulation* 2009;120:286–294.

133. Odenstedt J, Linderoth B, Bergfeldt L, et al. Spinal cord stimulation on myocardial ischemia, infarct size, ventricular arrhythmias, and noninvasive electrophysiology in a porcine ischemia-reperfusion model. *Heart Rhythm* 2011;8(6):892–898.

134. Howard-Quijano K, Takamiya T, Dale EA, et al. Spinal cord stimulation reduces ventricular arrhythmias during acute ischemia by attenuation of regional myocardial excitability. *Am J Physiol Heart Circ Physiol* 2017;313(2): H421–H431.

135. Qin C, Farber JP, Linderoth B, et al. Neuromodulation of thoracic intraspinal visceroreceptive transmission by electrical stimulation of spinal dorsal column and somatic afferents in rats. *J Pain* 2008;9(1):71–78.

136. Guru K, Mailis A, Ashby P, et al. Postsynaptic potentials in motoneurons caused by spinal cord stimulation in humans. *Electroencephalogr Clin Neurophysiol* 1987;66(3):275–280.

137. Greenwood-Van Meerveld B, Johnson AC, Foreman RD, et al. Attenuation by spinal cord stimulation of a nociceptive reflex generated by colorectal distention in a rat model. *Auton Neurosci* 2003;104(1):17–24.

138. Greenwood-Van Meerveld B, Johnson AC, Foreman RD, et al. Spinal cord stimulation attenuates viscero-motor reflexes in a rat model of post-inflammatory colonic hypersensitivity. *Auton Neurosci* 2005;122(102):69–76.

139. Krames E, Mousad DG. Spinal cord stimulation reverses pain and diarrheal episodes of irritable bowel syndrome: a case report. *Neuromodulation* 2004;7:82–88.

140. Lind G, Winter J, Linderoth B, et al. Therapeutic value of spinal cord stimulation in irritable bowel syndrome: a randomized cross-over pilot study. *Am J Physiol Regul Integr Comp Physiol* 2015;308(10):R887–R894.

141. North RB, Kidd DH, Farrokhi F, et al. Spinal cord stimulation versus repeated lumbosacral spine surgery for chronic pain: a randomized, controlled trial. *Neurosurgery* 2005;56(1):98–106.

142. Kumar K, Taylor RS, Jacques L, et al. Spinal cord stimulation versus conventional medical management for neuropathic pain: a multicentre randomised controlled trial in patients with failed back surgery syndrome. *Pain* 2007;132(1–2):179–188.

143. Law JD. Spinal stimulation in the "failed back surgery syndrome": comparison of technical criteria for palliating pain in the leg vs. in the low back. *Acta Neurochir* 1992;117:95.

144. North RB, Kidd DH, Olin J, et al. Spinal cord stimulation for axial low back pain: a prospective, controlled trial comparing dual with single percutaneous electrodes. *Spine* 2005;30(12):1412–1418.

145. Van Buyten JP, Al-Kaisy A, Smet I, et al. High-frequency spinal cord stimulation for the treatment of chronic back pain patients: results of a prospective multicenter European clinical study. *Neuromodulation* 2013;16:59–65.

146. Al-Kaisy A, Van Buyten JP, Smet I, et al. Sustained effectiveness of 10 kHz high-frequency spinal cord stimulation for patients with chronic, low back pain: 24-month results of a prospective multicenter study. *Pain Med* 2014;15:347–354.

147. Kapural L, Yu C, Doust MW, et al. Novel 10-kHz high-frequency therapy (HF10 therapy) is superior to traditional low-frequency spinal cord stimulation for the treatment of chronic back and leg pain: the SENZA-RCT randomized controlled trial. *Anesthesiology* 2015;123(4):851–860.

148. Kapural L, Yu C, Doust MW, et al. Comparison of 10-kHz high-frequency and traditional low-frequency spinal cord stimulation for the treatment of chronic back and leg pain: 24-month results from a multicenter, randomized, controlled pivotal trial. *Neurosurgery* 2016;79(5):667–677.

149. Thomson S, Zadeh MT, Love-Jones S, et al. The PROCO randomised controlled trial: effects of pulse rate on clinical outcomes in kilohertz frequency spinal cord stimulation: a multicentre, double-blind, crossover study. Paper presented at: International Neuromodulation Society; May 2017; Edinburgh, United Kingdom.

150. Schu S, Slotty PJ, Bara G, et al. A prospective, randomised, double-blind, placebo-controlled study to examine the effectiveness of burst spinal cord stimulation patterns for the treatment of failed back surgery syndrome. *Neuromodulation* 2014;17(5):443–450.

151. Deer T, Slavin KV, Amirdelfan K, et al. Success using neuromodulation with burst (SUNBURST) study: results from a prospective, randomized controlled trial using a novel burst waveform. *Neuromodulation* 2018;21(1):56–66. doi:10.1111/ner.1.2698.

152. Kemler MA, Barendse GA, van Kleef M, et al. Spinal cord stimulation in patients with chronic reflex sympathetic dystrophy. *N Engl J Med* 2000;343(9):618–624.

153. Kemler MA, De Vet HC, Barendse GA, et al. The effect of spinal cord stimulation in patients with chronic reflex sympathetic dystrophy: two years' follow-up of the randomized controlled trial. *Ann Neurol* 2004; 55(1):13–18.

154. Kemler MA, de Vet HC, Barendse GA, et al. Effect of spinal cord stimulation for chronic complex regional pain syndrome Type I: five-year final follow-up of patients in a randomized controlled trial. *J Neurosurg* 2008;108(2):292–298.

155. Mannheimer C, Eliasson T, Augustinsson LE, et al. Electrical stimulation versus coronary artery bypass surgery in severe angina pectoris: the ESBY study. *Circulation* 1998;97(12):1157–1163.

156. Andréll P, Ekre O, Eliasson T, et al. Cost-effectiveness of spinal cord stimulation versus coronary artery bypass grafting in patients with severe angina pectoris—long-term results from the ESBY study. *Cardiology* 2003;99(1):20–24.

157. Ekre O, Eliasson T, Norrsell H, et al. Long-term effects of spinal cord stimulation and coronary artery bypass grafting on quality of life and survival in the ESBY study. *Eur Heart J* 2002;23(24):1938–1945.

158. Norrsell H, Pilhall M, Eliasson T, et al. Effects of spinal cord stimulation and coronary artery bypass grafting on myocardial ischemia and heart rate variability: further results from the ESBY study. *Cardiology* 2000;94(1): 12–18.

159. Ubbink DT, Vermeulen H. Spinal cord stimulation for non-reconstructable chronic critical leg ischaemia. *Cochrane Database Syst Rev* 2005;(3): CD004001.

160. Ubbink DT, Vermeulen H. Spinal cord stimulation for critical leg ischemia: a review of effectiveness and optimal patient selection. *J Pain Symptom Manage* 2006;31(4 suppl):S30–S35.

161. Ubbink DT, Spincemaille GH, Prins MH, et al. Microcirculatory investigations to determine the effect of spinal cord stimulation for critical leg ischemia: the Dutch multicenter randomized controlled trial. *J Vasc Surg* 1999;30(2):236–244.

162. Barolat G, Myklebust JR, Wenninger W. Effects of spinal cord stimulation on spasticity and spasms secondary to myelopathy. *Appl Neurophys* 1988;51:29–44.

163. Augustinsson LE, Linderoth B, Mannheirmer C. Spinal cord stimulation in various ischaemic conditions. In: Illis L, ed. *Spinal Cord Dysfunction. III: Functional Stimulation*. Oxford, United Kingdom: Oxford Medical Publications; 1992:272–295.

164. Robaina FJ, Dominguez M, Diaz M, et al. Spinal cord stimulation for relief of chronic pain in vasospastic disorders of the upper limbs. *Neurosurgery* 1989;24:63–67.

165. Ktenidis K, Claeys L, Bartels C, et al. Spinal cord stimulation in the treatment of Buerger's disease. In: Horsch S, Claeys L, eds. *Spinal Cord Stimulation: An Innovative Method in the Treatment of PVD and Angina*. Darmstadt, Germany: Springer-Verlag Telos; 1995:207–214.

166. Francaviglia N, Silvestro C, Maiello M, et al. Spinal cord stimulation for the treatment of progressive systemic sclerosis and Raynaud's syndrome. *Br J Neurosurg* 1994;8:567–571.

167. Robaina F, Clavo B. Spinal cord stimulation in the treatment of post-stroke patients: current state and future directions. *Acta Neurochir Suppl* 2007;97(pt 1):277–282.

168. Kuwata T. Effects of the cervical spinal cord stimulation on persistent vegetative syndrome: experimental and clinical study [in Japanese]. *No Shinkei Geka* 1993;21(4):325–331.

169. Robaina F, Clavo B. The role of spinal cord stimulation in the management of patients with brain tumors. *Acta Neurochir Suppl* 2007;97(pt 1): 445–453.

170. Peters KM. Neuromodulation for the treatment of refractory interstitial cystitis. *Rev Urol* 2006;4:S121–S125.

171. Khan YN, Raza SS, Khan EA. Spinal cord stimulation in visceral pathologies. *Pain Med* 2006;7:S121–S125.

172. Elabbady AA, Hassouna MM, Elhilali MM. Neural stimulation for chronic voiding dysfunctions. *J Urol* 1994;152:2076–2080.

173. Kapural L, Narouze SN, Janicki TI, et al. Spinal cord stimulation is an effective treatment for the chronic intractable visceral pelvic pain. *Pain Med* 2006;7(5):440–443.

174. Whiteside JL, Walters MD, Mekhail N. Spinal cord stimulation for intractable vulvar pain. A case report. *J Reprod Med* 2003;48(10):821–823.

175. Kenefick NJ. Sacral nerve neuromodulation for the treatment of lower bowel motility disorders. *Ann R Coll Surg Engl* 2006;88(7):617–623.

176. North RB. The glass is half full [commentary on the fallacy of 50% pain relief]. *Pain Forum* 1999;8:195–197.

177. Waddell G. The clinical course of low back pain. In: *The Back Pain Revolution*. Edinburgh: Churchill Livingstone; 1998:103–107.

178. Waddell G, Burton AK. Occupational health guidelines for the management of low back pain at work: evidence review. *Occup Med (Lond)* 2001;51(2):124–135.

179. North RB, Ewend MG, Lawton MT, et al. Failed back surgery syndrome: 5-year follow-up after spinal cord stimulator implantation. *Neurosurgery* 1991;28(5):692–699.

180. Ubbink DT, Gersbach PA, Berg P, et al. The best TcPO2 parameters to predict the efficacy of spinal cord stimulation to improve limb salvage in patients with inoperable critical leg ischemia. *Int Angiol* 2003;22(4):356–363.

181. Petrakis IE, Sciacca V. Transcutaneous oxygen tension (TcPO₂) in the testing period of spinal cord stimulation (SCS) in critical limb ischemia of the lower extremities. *Int Surg* 1999;84(2):122–128.

182. Petrakis IE, Sciacca V. Spinal cord stimulation in critical limb ischemia of the lower extremities: our experience. *J Neurosurg Sci* 1999;43(4):285–293.

183. Petrakis IE, Sciacca V. Spinal cord stimulation in diabetic lower limb critical ischaemia: transcutaneous oxygen measurement as predictor for treatment success. *Eur J Vasc Endovasc Surg* 2000;19(6):587–592.

184. Petrakis IE, Sciacca V. Does autonomic neuropathy influence spinal cord stimulation therapy success in diabetic patients with critical lower limb ischemia? *Surg Neurol* 2000;53(2):182–188.

185. North RB. Spinal cord stimulation. In: Connolly ES, McKhann GM, Huang J, et al, eds. *Fundamentals of Operative Techniques in Neurosurgery*. 2nd ed. New York: Thieme; 2011:622–625.

186. North RB, Linderoth B. Spinal cord stimulation for chronic pain. In: Schmidek HH, Roberts D, eds. *Schmidek & Sweet: Operative Neurosurgical Techniques: Indications, Methods, and Results*. 5th ed. Vol. 2. Philadelphia: Elsevier; 2005:2165–2186.

187. Renard VM, North RB. Prevention of percutaneous electrode migration in spinal cord stimulation by a modification of the standard implantation technique. *J Neurosurg Spine* 2006;4(4):300–303.

188. Falowski SM, Celii A, Sestokas AK, et al. Awake vs. asleep placement of spinal cord stimulators: a cohort analysis of complications associated with placement. *Neuromodulation* 2011;14(2):130–134.

189. North RB, Kidd DH, Zahurak M, et al. Spinal cord stimulation for chronic, intractable pain: two decades' experience. *Neurosurgery* 1993;34:384–395.

190. Marchand S, Bushnell MC, Molina-Negro P, et al. The effects of dorsal column stimulation on measures of clinical and experimental pain in man. *Pain* 1991;45:249–257.

191. Olin JN, Kidd DH, North RB. Postural changes in spinal cord stimulation thresholds. *Neuromodulation* 1998;1(4):171–175.

192. Law JD, Kirkpatrick AF. Pain management update: spinal cord stimulation. *Am J Pain Manage* 1991;2:34–42.

193. Parisod E, Murray RF, Cousins MJ. Conversion disorder after implant of a spinal cord stimulator in a patient with a complex regional pain syndrome. *Anesth Analg* 2003;96(1):201–206.

194. North RB, Recinos VR, Attenello FJ, et al. Prevention of percutaneous spinal cord stimulation electrode migration: a 15-year experience. *Neuromodulation* 2014;17(7):670–676.

195. Cameron T. Safety and efficacy of spinal cord stimulation for the treatment of chronic pain: a 20-year literature review. *J Neurosurg* 2004;100(3 suppl):254–267.

196. Kumar K, Bucher E, Linderoth B, et al. Spinal cord stimulation: avoiding complications from spinal cord stimulation: practical recommendations from an international panel of experts. *Neuromodulation* 2007;10(1):24–33.

197. Bell GK, Kidd D, North RB. Cost-effectiveness analysis of spinal cord stimulation in treatment of failed back surgery syndrome. *J Pain Symptom Manage* 1997;13:286–295.

198. North RB, Kidd D, Shipley J, et al. Spinal cord stimulation versus reoperation for failed back surgery syndrome: a cost effectiveness and cost utility analysis based on a randomized, controlled trial. *Neurosurgery* 2007;61(2):361–369.

199. Blond S, Buisset N, Dam Hieu P, et al. Cost-benefit evaluation of spinal cord stimulation treatment for failed-back surgery syndrome patients [in French]. *Neurochirurgie* 2004;50(4):443–453.

200. Kumar K, Malik S, Demeria D. Treatment of chronic pain with spinal cord stimulation versus alternative therapies: cost-effectiveness analysis. *Neurosurgery* 2002;51(1):106–116.

201. Kemler MA, Furnée CA. Economic evaluation of spinal cord stimulation for chronic reflex sympathetic dystrophy. *Neurology* 2002;59:1203–1209.

202. Yu W, Maru F, Edner M, et al. Spinal cord stimulation for refractory angina pectoris: a retrospective analysis of efficacy and cost-benefit. *Corno Artery Dis* 2004;15(1):31–37.

203. Hornberger J, Kumar K, Verhulst E, et al. Rechargeable spinal cord stimulation versus nonrechargeable system for patients with failed back surgery syndrome: a cost-consequences analysis. *Clin J Pain* 2008;24(3):244–252.

CHAPTER 97

Deep Brain and Motor Cortex Stimulation

JIMMY CHEN YANG, ATHAR N. MALIK, and **EMAD N. ESKANDAR**

Deep brain stimulation (DBS) and motor cortex stimulation (MCS) have both been used as invasive neuromodulatory therapies in the treatment of medication-refractory pain. Although each has its own specific mechanism of action, both types of therapy have been employed in the treatment of a wide variety of neuropathic pain diagnoses. In addition, DBS has demonstrated additional effects in the pain "neuromatrix" and has also been used to treat nociceptive pain and to modulate the affective components of pain. Despite being used for similar diagnoses, MCS targets primary motor cortex, whereas DBS may involve different targets singly or in combination, including the sensory or ventral posterior (VP) thalamus, the periaqueductal or periventricular gray matter (PAG/PVG), and the anterior cingulate cortex (ACC). Although many published studies have demonstrated the effectiveness of both DBS and MCS, many of these have been in the form of case series rather than randomized, well-controlled, blinded trials.

Both MCS and DBS have been used worldwide as neurosurgical techniques in the management of pain, although studies utilizing DBS tend to be seen from European or Canadian centers. The reason for fewer published studies from the United States is likely secondary to DBS for pain having an "off-label" status due to initial trials that suggested its lack of efficacy. However, recent studies and ongoing research have demonstrated that both MCS and DBS may be effective in the treatment of pain, although further work in the form of large, randomized, blinded, and well-controlled trials are still needed. Ultimately, the demonstration of efficacy will hopefully lead to guidelines that will provide patients with additional options in the treatment of medication-refractory pain. At the same time, concomitant research in noninvasive therapies such as repetitive transcranial magnetic stimulation (rTMS) may offer another option for therapy and act as a screening tool for surgical candidates.

Deep Brain Stimulation

BASIC CONSIDERATIONS

DBS has been used in a number of targets for pain, although recent literature suggests a focus on the sensory thalamus or VP thalamus, the PAG/PVG, and the ACC. DBS has been used to treat a number of pain diagnoses, including phantom limb pain, brachial plexus injury, stroke, cephalalgias, multiple sclerosis, spine injury, failed low back surgery syndrome, and chronic cluster headaches, as reviewed in several studies.[1-6]

The use of PAG/PVG targets began from animal research that demonstrated analgesia from stimulation of these areas, with subsequent translation to patients.[7-11] Initial studies suggested that DBS in this region acted via opioidergic mechanisms, supported by a reported effect reversal with naloxone, but later studies challenged these conclusions.[1,12] Current models suggest that the ventral PAG works via influencing coping behavior, whereas the dorsal PAG has sympathomimetic effects, which may also have opioidergic effects.[12,13] Overall, the PAG target has been primarily used for nociceptive pain.[2,14]

DBS for sensory thalamic targets, the ventral posterior lateral and medial (VPL/VPM) nuclei, arose from initial work that

demonstrated symptomatic relief from ablative procedures.[12,15-17] In these patients, pain is thought to result in increased thalamic firing,[17] and DBS to this region likely affects thalamo-corticofugal descending pathways.[5] Recordings at these sites have demonstrated increased spike density as well as possible neural hyperactivity when these regions are stimulated.[18] Overall, this target has been favored for neuropathic pain.[2,14]

DBS to both VP and PAG/PVG targets is also thought to exert effects by either disrupting synchronous pathologic high frequencies or by enhancing low frequencies.[1,12] Studies have demonstrated that at both VP and PAG targets, reduction in pain results from lower frequencies ≤50 Hz, whereas increased sensitivity to pain results from higher frequencies >70 Hz.[4,12] One group, which has published extensively on DBS for pain, suggests that only demonstrable efficacy should guide the decision for implanting an electrode at the PAG, VP, or both sites,[1,17] although their own practice is to target the PAG site initially, except in cases of head and facial pain.[19] Importantly, some patients may have components of both neuropathic and nociceptive pain and may therefore derive benefit from DBS therapy to both PAG and VP sites.[2]

The ACC has also been reported as a successful DBS target for pain based on the effectiveness of cingulotomy.[20-24] The ACC is thought to modulate pain processing and is involved in the affective component of pain. As a result, DBS therapy to this target likely affects emotional components to pain rather than nociceptive perception, thereby reducing the "unpleasantness" of pain rather than the pain itself.[1,4,6,25]

Other targets that have additionally been reported in the literature include the internal capsule,[26,27] ventral striatum and internal capsule,[28,29] centromedian parafascicular complex and the intra-laminar zone,[30] and posterior hypothalamus.[31,32]

EFFICACY OF DEEP BRAIN STIMULATION

Initial studies of DBS for pain in the United States were based on two multicenter trials from 1989 to 1995, which were not randomized or case controlled.[1,33] Neither trial met criteria for efficacy, with the first trial defining effective therapy as ≥50% of patients with ≥50% pain relief at 1-year follow-up and the second trial defining efficacy as ≥50% of patients with ≥30% pain relief and decrease in the usage of analgesia medication.[33] Multiple reviews have subsequently commented on the limitations of these trials, which include patient heterogeneity, lack of blinded assessment, and lack of standardization among centers.[1,17] Nevertheless, as a result of these studies, DBS for pain in the United States has been used with an off-label status.[33]

Subsequent studies, reviews, and meta-analyses have provided a mixed picture regarding the efficacy of DBS for pain. Many published studies have limited numbers of patients, with few centers reporting larger numbers. Ultimately, long-term efficacy has been reported in ~83% of patients,[1] with one large case series by a well-published center suggesting an overall long-term efficacy of 67% at their center, with no significant differences in efficacy based on stimulation site.[19]

Several meta-analyses have suggested efficacy of DBS for pain. A 2010 meta-analysis examined 13 studies and estimated that 50% of patients had long-term relief with DBS, with a 61% success rate for nociceptive pain diagnoses and 42% success rate with neuropathic pain diagnoses.[2] A 2005 meta-analysis of 6 older studies (from 1977 to 1997) had also demonstrated 55% to 70% pain relief at >1-year follow-up.[13] This meta-analysis suggested good to excellent results with PAG stimulation, with further increases in success when combined with thalamic or internal capsule stimulation, a strategy that has been seen in other studies.[34]

However, there have been limitations to in-depth analysis of both individual studies and meta-analyses due to factors such as heterogeneity in patient diagnoses and selection criteria, DBS sites, stimulation parameters, and use of unblinded assessments. These limitations have been reflected in recent recommendations from the European Academy of Neurology (EAN) in 2016 and the European Federation of Neurological Societies (EFNS) in 2007.[5,35] The EAN's meta-analysis of studies from 2006 to 2014 that used DBS for a variety of pain diagnoses determined that there was very low quality of evidence.[35] Overall, the EAN gave a recommendation of "inconclusive," highlighting the further need for additional prospective, randomized, controlled trials. Nevertheless, they noted that the overall pain intensity reduction was close to 50% in their included studies.[35] This was an update to the EFNS 2007 study, which had calculated an overall 46% long-term success rate of DBS for pain.[5] Further investigations will be required to determine whether specific DBS targets are best suited for particular diagnoses, as there has been lack of consensus.[5,35,36]

Few studies have also utilized randomized or placebo-controlled experimental designs. Marchand et al.[37] studied thalamic stimulation and examined the effects of placebo stimulation, ultimately demonstrating a significant placebo effect from thalamic DBS. Rasche et al.[34] included placebo testing during the trial stimulation phase; ultimately, 57% of patients passed this phase with demonstrated analgesic effects and were implanted with a pulse generator. Fontaine et al.[38] reported a randomized, placebo-controlled, double-blind trial to study the effects of hypothalamic DBS in cluster headache and found that although there was lack of efficacy during the randomized phase of the trial, patients derived a reduction in their attacks during the open phase. Finally, Lempka et al.[28] targeted the ventral striatum/anterior limb of the internal capsule in a prospective, double-blind, randomized, placebo-controlled, crossover study and did not meet its primary endpoint of ≥50% improvement in ≥50% of patients with active DBS compared to placebo. However, there were improvements in other measures such as depression, anxiety, and quality of life. These studies have suggested legitimate effects from DBS, although its effects may not be adequately measured purely by pain intensity ratings.

Overall, there have been persistent limitations to comparing published studies, which have included diverse patient selection criteria and diagnoses, heterogeneous methodology, and diversity of intracranial targets. In addition, certain effects may not have been fully studied or reported. For example, DBS for pain may result in substantial insertional effects.[39] As increasingly examined by recent published studies, future investigations may also benefit from assessing patient improvements in areas other than pain, such as mood, anxiety, and quality of life, which may improve to a significant degree.[40] Although a number of studies have suggested that DBS may be more effective for particular diagnoses, or identified particular targets as being more effective for specific diagnoses, there does not yet appear to be general consensus.[13,17,36]

Some studies have demonstrated loss of efficacy over time, with some series noting that up to a half of patients who have success during the trial stimulation period do not have sustained benefit at ≥1 year follow-up, which may be attributed to factors such as scarring around electrode targets, brain plasticity, and inconsistent patient reporting.[17,25] To mitigate these effects, groups have resorted to intensive reprogramming, with authors noting that stimulation parameters may increase with time.[1,41] Strategies for reprogramming include changing pulse width or frequency or allowing for cycled stimulation or "off" periods.[17]

SURGICAL TECHNIQUE

Optimal patient selection has been important in ensuring that those who undergo DBS benefit from therapy. A multidisciplinary approach is used to screen potential patients who may benefit from DBS, and neuropsychological testing is a key component, with patients who have psychological etiologies excluded. Patients are also typically medication refractory ≥2 years, but there are no restrictions on whether patients have undergone other surgical procedures.[1,17] Some groups examine patients' responses to analgesics prior to DBS.[18] Quantitative and qualitative assessment of pain is required, as well as quality of life assessments, which may allow clinicians and patients to best see changes that occur after DBS. Contraindications include medical conditions that would make surgery unsafe or anatomic factors such as ventriculomegaly that would prevent placement of an electrode into the surgical target.

DBS electrodes are implanted stereotactically, using either a frame or frameless approach (Fig. 97.1).[2] As a result, high-resolution magnetic resonance imaging (MRI) is required to allow for accurate targeting. Surgery is performed with

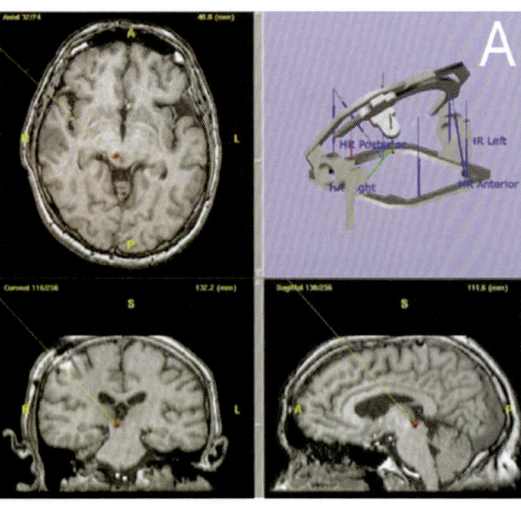
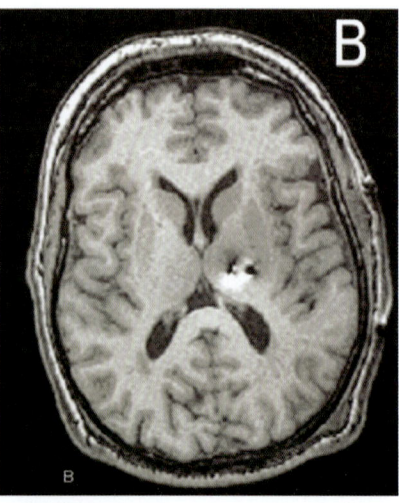

FIGURE 97.1 A: T1-weighted magnetic resonance imaging (MRI) showing planned trajectory ad target for placement of a periaqueductal or periventricular gray matter (PAG/PVG) in the axial, frontal, and sagittal planes. **B:** Postoperative MRI showing ventral posterior lateral (VPL) electrode (lateral) and the wire to the PVG electrode (medial and inferior). *(Reprinted with permission from Owen SL, Green AL, Stein JF, et al. Deep brain stimulation for the alleviation of post-stroke neuropathic pain. Pain 2006;120[1–2]:202–206.)*

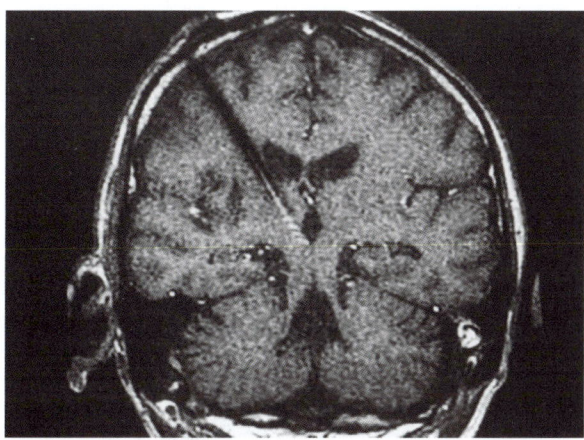

FIGURE 97.2 T1 coronal image with implanted periventricular gray matter electrode. *(Reprinted with permission from Owen SL, Green AL, Stein JF, et al. Deep brain stimulation for the alleviation of post-stroke neuropathic pain. Pain 2006;120[1–2]:202–206.)*

sedation and local anesthesia; however, some targets, such as the ACC, can be performed under general anesthesia. Targets in the thalamus and midbrain are contralateral to the symptomatic side, whereas the ACC target requires bilateral electrode implantation.[1]

For targeting coordinates, the PAG is typically found 2 to 3 mm lateral to the third ventricle at the level of the posterior commissure and 10 mm posterior to the midcommissural point and 0 mm vertical; the VP target is typically found 10 to 13 mm posterior to the midcommissural point, 14 to 18 mm lateral, and from 5 mm below to 2 mm above the midcommissural line (Fig. 97.2).[1,4] To isolate a particular limb, studies have suggested that the arm representation of the VPL is 2 to 3 mm medial to the internal capsule, whereas the leg representation is 1 to 2 mm medial to the internal capsule.[4] The ACC target is typically 20 to 25 mm posterior to the anterior horns of the lateral ventricles, with the electrode tip near the corpus callosum and the electrode in the cingulum bundle.[4,25]

Intraoperative physiologic stimulation is used to refine the final target, with microelectrode recording, microstimulation, and macrostimulation. This step is considered critical in order to obtain adequate coverage of the symptomatic region. For instance, patients undergoing VP stimulation should experience paresthesias in previously painful areas, whereas those undergoing PAG stimulation should note a sensation of warmth or analgesia.[4,13] Once targets are identified, the electrodes are introduced, and the leads are externalized for trial stimulation. Patients undergo postoperative imaging, typically via computed tomography (CT), to look for possible complications.

A trial assessment period typically lasts from 5 to 9 days, during which physicians may test different combinations of stimulation parameters to optimize patient effects.[2] Different approaches have been taken for assessing effectiveness, with some authors using an "N-of-1 trial" approach, in which a patient undergoes randomized pairs of treatments to elucidate the effects of DBS and placebo.[17] Overall, a large percentage of patients typically pass the trial stimulation period.[36,39,42] Some authors have noted that DBS to the ACC may take an extended period to demonstrate effectiveness.[4] Stimulation parameters have varied across the literature, with some groups reporting bipolar stimulation parameters in the range of 5 to 50 Hz with pulse widths from 100 to 450 μs and amplitudes from 0.1 to 3 V, although ACC stimulation may require higher settings.[1,17] Afterward, the most effective electrodes are internalized and connected to either an infraclavicular or abdominal pulse generator.

Overall, DBS is considered to be a generally safe procedure, with adverse events occurring in 8% to 9% of cases.[35] One of the more serious complications is hemorrhage, which has been reported in 1.9% to 4.1% of cases.[2,43] Device malfunction may also occur. There is a risk of infection, which has been reported in 1.9% to 13.3% of cases.[14,43] Other minor risks include diplopia and visual gaze effects, headache, and nausea.[14,17] The risk of permanent neurologic deficit has ranged from 2% to 3.4%, and mortality is rare, ranging from 0% to 1.6%.[2]

Motor Cortex Stimulation

BASIC CONSIDERATIONS

The use of MCS was initiated after a study by Tsubokawa et al.[44] in 1991, with the demonstration that chronic stimulation of the motor cortex with epidural electrodes inhibited thalamic hyperactivity and ultimately led to symptom control. Following this study, neuromodulation of the motor cortex was examined as an option for the treatment of medically intractable central and peripheral neuropathic pain.[45,46] Based on these initial studies, MCS has been subsequently made an option for patients who have failed pharmacologic therapy or other stimulation techniques like spinal cord stimulation.[47]

Interestingly, MCS is able to achieve pain reduction at voltages below the threshold for muscle contraction, and, at these voltages, it can induce paresthesias.[47] Numerous studies have sought to determine the mechanism of action of MCS, with several proposed explanations. Its effects have been attributed to modulation of connections among somatosensory cortex, thalamus, spinothalamic tract, and motor cortex.[48–51] MCS results in both direct and indirect waves, with anodal stimulation resulting in direct stimulation and cathodal stimulation resulting in depolarization of horizontal interneurons that trigger indirect waves of stimulation.[45,48,52] Ultimately, the indirect waves are thought to result in analgesia via top–down inhibition.[52,53] Thalamic hypersensitivity is reduced by antidromic modulation, endogenous opioids in the periaqueductal gray and cingulate are released,[54] and regions that modulate pain, such as the orbitofrontal cortex, are activated.[48,55–58]

A common inclusion criterion for MCS includes a diagnosis of neuropathic pain with the identification of a lesion within the central nervous system.[48] A consensus meeting suggested that central and peripheral causes are both treatable and can be of a variety of etiologies including trauma or injury from procedures as well as vascular, inflammatory, degenerative, and oncologic causes.[48] Notably, candidates for MCS should have psychological or psychiatric diagnoses and morbidities evaluated, and patients generally have a pain Visual Analog Scale (VAS) of at least 5.[48]

Specifically, centers have used MCS for indications including poststroke pain (including facial, upper and lower extremity, and dystonias),[47,59–63] plexus avulsion pain, atypical facial pain, post-irradiation pain for treatment of arteriovenous malformations, phantom limb pain,[47,60,61,64] lumbar plexus pain, chronic regional pain syndrome,[64] root lesions of the upper extremity,[47,64] multiple sclerosis,[47] syringomyelia,[47,63] postherpetic pain,[64,65] trigeminal neuropathic pain and anesthesia dolorosa,[46,47,60,61,66] sciatic pain, and spinal cord injury,[62,63] as reviewed in a recent study.[48] Atypical facial pain is felt to be heterogeneous and therefore may have limited treatment success.[48]

Despite heterogeneity, most published studies have demonstrated positive responses to MCS, although this may be due to publication bias.[61] In addition, centers have also varied in terms of their definition of a "good" result, which may or may not depend on the VAS and therefore make comparisons across studies challenging.[48]

Predictive factors have been inconsistently identified. One study found that the only predictive factor was the patient's response in the first month after the procedure.[67] Other studies have suggested that motor weakness in the region of pain may be tied to reduction in efficacy,[47,48,68] although this did not play a significant role in other studies.[67,69,70]

There is increasing evidence that rTMS may be used as a tool to determine which patients may benefit from MCS, although consensus groups have felt that it was less useful for excluding patients from MCS.[48,55,71] rTMS provides high positive predictive value for response to MCS but has a high rate of false negatives and lower negative predictive value,[72] although the predictive value of rTMS may be better at examining long-term effects.[73]

EFFICACY OF MOTOR CORTEX STIMULATION

Success rates of MCS for pain have been analyzed through case reviews and meta-analyses. Examination of case series that used MCS for chronic neuropathic pain published from 1991 to 2006 demonstrated that ≥40% improvement in pain relief from MCS was seen in 56.7% of patients, with long-term benefit in 45% of patients at ≥1 year.[74] Another meta-analysis of 22 studies from 1960 to 2007 found that 64% of patients undergoing MCS responded to therapy.[51] Finally, a review that specifically examined MCS for facial chronic neuropathic pain indications found that 84% of patients who had implantation of the system had good pain control at the end of the study with long-term follow-up of 30.7 months.[56]

The effects of MCS have also been examined in specific diagnoses, in case it may be applied more effectively for specific indications, although the results have been inconsistent.[47,60,62] For instance, some authors believe that MCS for poststroke pain leads to good relief in approximately two-thirds of patients, whereas therapy for trigeminal neuropathic pain leads to good relief in >75% of patients.[2,75] Some studies have suggested that the use of MCS for diagnoses related to spinal cord injury or brachial plexus pain may be more challenging.[47,62]

Study of long-term outcomes has been necessary, as many investigations have shown that MCS can lose efficacy at extended time points as patients develop "tolerance."[47,48,51,74] Reasons for this gradual loss of efficacy have included brain remodeling and plasticity or scar build up at the surgical site.[76] Further intensive stimulator reprogramming may lead to return of analgesic effects.[48,76] However, even with longer follow-up periods, one study found that on the order of 1 to 6 years of follow-up, >50% of patients still had benefit from MCS, with patients with thalamic central pain felt to have the best result.[47]

Several trials have been conducted with MCS, although there have been inconsistent results. One crossover trial that examined MCS for refractory peripheral pain in 16 patients demonstrated a mean rate of pain relief, as assessed by VAS scores, of 48%, with 60% having a satisfactory or good result with MCS therapy (>40% VAS score reduction) after prolonged stimulation after a crossover phase.[70] However, during the crossover period which allowed comparison between "on" versus "off" conditions, there were no significant differences, which were attributed to carry-over effects.[70] A second crossover trial that tested "on" versus "off" stimulation in patients found that patients had significant benefit from MCS only in the "on" setting, with 60% of patients ultimately experiencing >40% pain reduction at follow-up.[77] A third crossover trial that also studied "on" versus "off" stimulation settings found that patients had pain reduction only in the "on" setting, with return of pain in the "off" setting.[78] Improvement at 1 year was >40% for all tested patients.[78] However, in contrast to these studies, a recent randomized study that examined conditions of low stimulation (subtherapeutic levels) versus high stimulation (therapeutic levels) was stopped due to lack of efficacy.[64] No differences were seen between the two groups, and a possible nocebo effect was also discovered; however, the

diagnoses of the patients involved in the study were limited.[64] Some authors have noted the importance of a double-blind testing phase during MCS trial stimulation. For example, one study of MCS for trigeminal neuropathic pain in 36 patients included a double-blind testing phase.[79] Seventeen percent of patients were found to be false-positive responders and did not have permanent implantation of the device, and ultimately, 57.6% of patients had >30% pain reduction.[79]

Reasons for poor response to MCS have included the need for more intensive programming or the need for an extended testing period prior to permanent implantation.[47,61] One study that did not use a trial period in all patients noted that this may be required in order to increase the rate of successful therapy in patients with permanent implantations[61]; one author noted that typically only about 50% of patients who undergo trial stimulation go on to have the device permanently implanted.[75] In addition, many authors have noted that MCS can have significant placebo effects, with up to 35% of patients experiencing a placebo effect. Nevertheless, one study queried patients as to whether they would proceed with surgery again, and 70% stated that they would.[67]

SURGICAL TECHNIQUE

Preoperative evaluation includes assessment of pain intensity as well as psychological evaluation in order to assess for risk factors that may affect surgical outcome.[47,60] TMS, as discussed previously, is used at some centers to help predict which patients may have better response to MCS.[48,72,73]

Preoperative studies aim to improve target selection and include high-resolution MRI for identification of anatomic landmarks and functional MRI to ensure optimal placement of electrodes over motor cortex.[48,55,60,65,80] For instance, cases of phantom limb pain and thalamic pain may result in plasticity-related changes that may complicate optimal electrode placement over the motor strip.[47,55] Neuronavigation is typically employed to accurately determine the surgical site and to allow for anatomic localization.

The procedure can be performed under either local or general anesthesia. A craniotomy or burr hole allows access to the epidural space. From here, mapping is performed to identify the N20-P20 phase reversal that characterizes the location of the central sulcus, which is considered the gold standard for identifying the motor cortex.[48,55] Additional intraoperative electrophysiology with somatosensory evoked potentials (SSEPs) or motor evoked potentials can further verify the optimal location of the electrode (Figs. 97.3 and 97.4).[47,48,61]

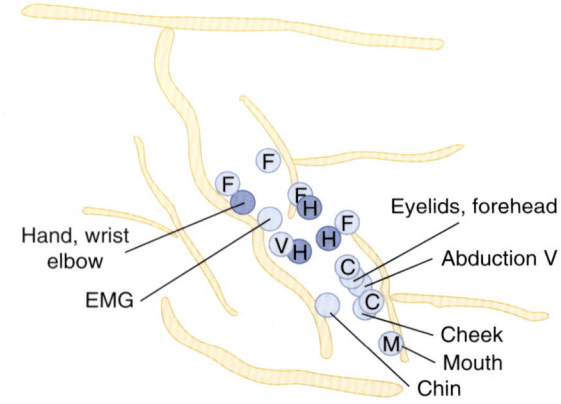

FIGURE 97.3 Blue circles correspond to position of motor cortex stimulation. Dark blue, hand; light blue, face; F, fingers; H, hand; V, abduction of fifth finger; C, cheek; M, mouth; EMG, electromyography responses. *(Reprinted from Nguyen JP, Lefaucher JP, Le Guerinel C, et al. Motor cortex stimulation in the treatment of central and neuropathic pain. Arch Med Res 2000;31[3]:263–265. Copyright © 2000 IMSS. With permission.)*

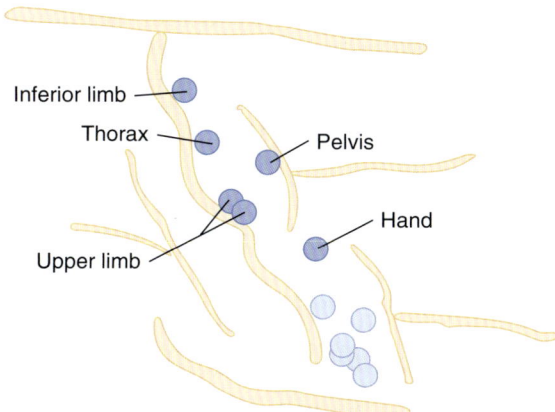

FIGURE 97.4 Circles correspond to the position of motor cortex stimulation that resulted in good or excellent pain reduction. Dark blue, hand; light blue, face. *(Reprinted from Nguyen JP, Lefaucher JP, Le Guerinel C, et al. Motor cortex stimulation in the treatment of central and neuropathic pain.* Arch Med Res *2000;31[3]:263–265. Copyright © 2000 IMSS. With permission.)*

At some centers, the dura is opened under certain circumstances. For instance, the dura may need to be opened to access the interhemispheric fissure for providing therapy to the lower extremities or if there is a significant distance between the dura and cortex.[47,60] Many different types of electrodes have been used, including 4 and 8 contact electrodes, as well as grids, and both parallel and perpendicular orientations have been used.[47,48,60,61,64] Electrode location can be subsequently confirmed by stimulating through the contacts, and motor threshold testing can be carried out in the operating room.[55,75] Some centers choose to coagulate the dura underneath the electrode in order to avoid possible headache that can arise from dural nerve stimulation.[48]

Once the leads are secured in place, they can be either passed to an infraclavicular chest or abdominal pocket to a pulse generator or they can be tunneled out from the skin for postoperative testing (Fig. 97.5). Trial periods for MCS vary, with some centers not performing any trial period, and others typically trialing stimulation for 3 to 7 days, with longer periods having a possible increased infection risk.[2,48,56,60,61,63,64] Patients who have a response have the electrodes permanently implanted, although improvement thresholds that would allow for permanent implantation can range at different centers. As mentioned earlier, patients may develop tolerance to the MCS and require ongoing adjustments or stimulation holiday periods.

Stimulation regimens vary widely, as reviewed recently.[48,55] Voltage can range from 2 V to ≥8 V, and typically a cyclic mode is used. Generally, the best orientation arises from cathodal stimulation of the precentral gyrus and anodal stimulation of the anterior border of the central sulcus.[48] Frequencies vary, from 20 to 80 Hz, with pulse duration from 90 to 450 μs.[48,55] Subsequent programming after pulse generator implantation can take an extended period of time, lasting >3 months at some centers.

Complications of MCS include seizures, wound infection, hardware malfunction, hematomas, and paresthesias.[47,55,60,61,63,64] Seizures have typically occurred in the setting of increased voltages.[60,61,64] A large number of studies have reported no adverse events,[75] and the complication rate overall is considered to be about 5%, with the most common complications being seizure and wound infection.[55,56] One large examination of case series published from 1991 to 2006 found that infection occurred in about 5.7% of cases and hardware-related issues were found in 5.1%, with seizures occurring in 12% of patients in the early postoperative period.[74] There may be higher risk of complications with subdural placement of electrodes.[55]

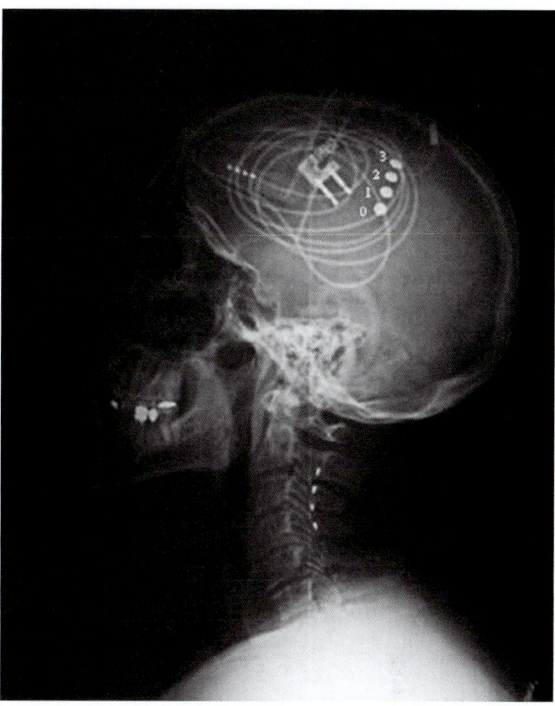

FIGURE 97.5 Skull radiograph of a patient with an epidural electrode over the right motor cortex for motor cortex stimulation. *(Reprinted from Di Lazzaro V, Oliviero A, Pilato F, et al. Comparison of descending volleys evoked by transcranial and epidural motor cortex stimulation in a conscious patient with bulbar pain.* Clin Neurophysiol *2004;115[4]:834–838. Copyright © 2004 International Federation of Clinical Neurophysiology. With permission.)*

Transcranial Magnetic Stimulation

BASIC CONSIDERATIONS

rTMS has been applied to a variety of diagnoses and has been identified as a possible therapy for neuropathic chronic pain. The procedure involves placing a stimulating coil adjacent to the scalp, with the changing magnetic fields subsequently inducing electric currents in local neurons and resulting in depolarization (Fig 97.6).[81,82]

The rationale for rTMS has been derived from MCS, in which stimulation of the motor cortex corresponding to the region of pain results in pain relief, and the two therapies may share basic mechanisms, although their different stimulation

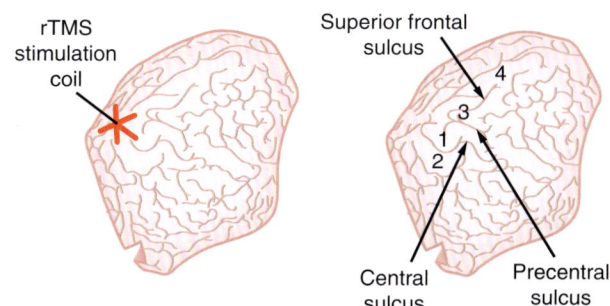

FIGURE 97.6 The use of a navigation system for repetitive transcranial magnetic stimulation (rTMS). The stimulation coil **(left)** is centered over the motor cortex; the *numbers* on the right show motor cortex (1), relative to the sensory cortex (2), the premotor area (3), and the supplementary motor area (4). *(Reprinted with permission from Hirayama A, Saitoh Y, Kishima H, et al. Reduction of intractable deafferentation pain by navigation-guided repetitive transcranial magnetic stimulation of the primary motor cortex.* Pain *2006;122[1–2]:22–27.)*

parameters may recruit different substrates.[53,83,84] Specific rTMS settings can trigger varying effects; for instance, rTMS at ≥5 Hz can increase excitability and potentiate transmission, but rTMS at ≤1 Hz can decrease it, thereby leading to either long-term potentiation or depression.[81,84,85] Other factors such as pulse waveform and coil orientation can also lead to differing effects.[84,86]

rTMS has been investigated as a therapy for several etiologies, including central pain,[71,87,88] facial neuropathic pain,[88] postherpetic neuralgia,[81] fibromyalgia,[89,90] brachial plexus and peripheral nerve related pain,[71,88] spinal cord lesions,[88] and phantom limb pain.[91] A majority of rTMS studies have targeted primary motor cortex.[82] For pain, ≥5 Hz frequency has been the most common.[81,82] Intensity of the pulses is typically tailored to individual motor thresholds; the number of pulses can vary, as can the orientation of the coil. Notably, the effects of rTMS may be temporary, and maintenance protocols will need to be developed.[84,86,92]

EFFICACY OF REPETITIVE TRANSCRANIAL MAGNETIC STIMULATION FOR PAIN

Recent large-scale reviews of rTMS have demonstrated heterogeneous results.[82,86] A notable 2014 Cochrane review suggested that although high-frequency stimulation of the motor cortex can result in short-term effects in single doses, multiple dose studies have not shown a significant effect. In addition, the review failed to demonstrate meaningful clinical effect of rTMS, although it was limited by significant variation among studies and conflicting results.[82]

Another large review similarly found that low-frequency rTMS was ineffective, but high-frequency rTMS likely results in significant analgesic effects.[86] This review also suggested that comparison among studies may be affected by variation in therapy time course and posttherapy evaluation, as the effects from rTMS may be most significant after a few days. In addition, there is some debate over whether rTMS is best for particular diagnoses. An earlier meta-analysis had suggested that rTMS for pain that originates from central, rather than peripheral, sources may be more effective.[93] Notably, however, it has been difficult to perform double-blind studies of rTMS because there are auditory, visual, and sensation changes that occur during the course of therapy which may be difficult to replicate.[81]

There are typically few complications from rTMS.[94] The most important adverse events can arise from damage to or heating of implants that are nearby; otherwise, the only significant risk is seizure, which has a very small risk, <1%.[81] In order to avoid this, high-frequency therapy is typically used in trains of pulses.[81] Other adverse events may include headache, pain at the stimulation site, muscle pain, dizziness, nausea, and tiredness, although these may be experienced in both therapeutic and sham settings.[95]

Conclusion

Challenges with treating chronic neuropathic pain have prompted a call for the development of additional therapies that go beyond medical management. Although definitive evidence supporting the use of neuromodulation for pain will require ongoing research, data collection, and additional trials, DBS and MCS offer nonablative options that have demonstrated a degree of efficacy in existing literature. However, it has been difficult to optimize these invasive neuromodulatory procedures due to limitations in reported studies, as described earlier. In addition, similar to the limitations of the majority of studies that have been published regarding DBS and MCS, comparisons among neuromodulatory techniques (such as comparisons among DBS, MCS, and spinal cord stimulation)

have been affected by aspects such as heterogeneous patient populations and diagnoses, which have made it challenging to effectively compare these different procedures. Ultimately, ongoing research and well-designed trials are needed to provide more definitive recommendations and guidelines for both practitioners and patients.

References

1. Pereira EA, Aziz TZ. Neuropathic pain and deep brain stimulation. *Neurotherapeutics* 2014;11(3):496–507.
2. Levy R, Deer TR, Henderson J. Intracranial neurostimulation for pain control: a review. *Pain Phys* 2010;13(2):157–165.
3. Deer TR, Mekhail N, Petersen E, et al. The appropriate use of neurostimulation: stimulation of the intracranial and extracranial space and head for chronic pain. Neuromodulation Appropriateness Consensus Committee. *Neuromodulation* 2014:551–570.
4. Boccard SG, Pereira EA, Aziz TZ. Deep brain stimulation for chronic pain. *J Clin Neurosci* 2015;22(10):1537–1543.
5. Cruccu G, Aziz TZ, Garcia-Larrea L, et al. EFNS guidelines on neurostimulation therapy for neuropathic pain. *Eur J Neurol* 2007;14(9):952–970.
6. Russo JF, Sheth SA. Deep brain stimulation of the dorsal anterior cingulate cortex for the treatment of chronic neuropathic pain. *Neurosurg Focus* 2015;38(6):E11.
7. Mayer DJ, Wolfle TL, Akil H, et al. Analgesia from electrical stimulation in the brainstem of the rat. *Science* 1971;174(4016):1351–1354.
8. Reynolds DV. Surgery in the rat during electrical analgesia induced by focal brain stimulation. *Science* 1969;164(3878):444–445.
9. Richardson DE, Akil H. Pain reduction by electrical brain stimulation in man. Part 1: acute administration in periaqueductal and periventricular sites. *J Neurosurg* 1977;47(2):178–183.
10. Richardson DE, Akil H. Pain reduction by electrical brain stimulation in man. Part 2: chronic self-administration in the periventricular gray matter. *J Neurosurg* 1977;47(2):184–194.
11. Hosobuchi Y, Adams JE, Linchitz R. Pain relief by electrical stimulation of the central gray matter in humans and its reversal by naloxone. *Science* 1977;197(4299):183–186.
12. Pereira EA, Boccard SG, Aziz TZ. Deep brain stimulation for pain: distinguishing dorsolateral somesthetic and ventromedial affective targets. *Neurosurgery* 2014;61(suppl 1):175–181.
13. Bittar RG, Kar-Purkayastha I, Owen SL, et al. Deep brain stimulation for pain relief: a meta-analysis. *J Clin Neurosci* 2005;12(5):515–519.
14. Falowski SM. Deep brain stimulation for chronic pain. *Curr Pain Headache Rep* 2015;19(7):27.
15. Mark VH, Ervin FR, Hackett TP. Clinical aspects of stereotactic thalamotomy in the human. Part I. The treatment of chronic severe pain. *Arch Neurol* 1960;3:351–367.
16. Hosobuchi Y, Adams JE, Rutkin B. Chronic thalamic stimulation for the control of facial anesthesia dolorosa. *Arch Neurol* 1973;29(3):158–161.
17. Pereira EA, Green AL, Aziz TZ. Deep brain stimulation for pain. *Handb Clin Neurol* 2013;116:277–294.
18. Yamamoto T, Katayama Y, Obuchi T, et al. Thalamic sensory relay nucleus stimulation for the treatment of peripheral deafferentation pain. *Stereotact Funct Neurosurg* 2006;84(4):180–183.
19. Boccard SG, Pereira EA, Moir L, et al. Long-term outcomes of deep brain stimulation for neuropathic pain. *Neurosurgery* 2013;72(2):221–231.
20. Foltz EL, White LE. Pain "relief" by frontal cingulumotomy. *J Neurosurg* 1962;19:89–100.
21. Hassenbusch SJ, Pillay PK, Barnett GH. Radiofrequency cingulotomy for intractable cancer pain using stereotaxis guided by magnetic resonance imaging. *Neurosurgery* 1990;27(2):220–223.
22. Pillay PK, Hassenbusch SJ. Bilateral MRI-guided stereotactic cingulotomy for intractable pain. *Stereotact Funct Neurosurg* 1992;59(1–4):33–38.
23. Viswanathan A, Harsh V, Pereira EA, et al. Cingulotomy for medically refractory cancer pain. *Neurosurg Focus* 2013;35(3):E1.
24. Spooner J, Yu H, Kao C, et al. Neuromodulation of the cingulum for neuropathic pain after spinal cord injury. Case report. *J Neurosurg* 2007;107(1):169–172.
25. Boccard SG, Prangnell SJ, Pycroft L, et al. Long-term results of deep brain stimulation of the anterior cingulate cortex for neuropathic pain. *World Neurosurg* 2017;106:625–637.
26. Adams JE, Hosobuchi Y, Fields HL. Stimulation of internal capsule for relief of chronic pain. *J Neurosurg* 1974;41(6):740–744.
27. Fields HL, Adams JE. Pain after cortical injury relieved by electrical stimulation of the internal capsule. *Brain* 1974;97(1):169–178.
28. Lempka SF, Malone DA, Hu B, et al. Randomized clinical trial of deep brain stimulation for poststroke pain. *Ann Neurol* 2017;81(5):653–663.
29. Moore NZ, Lempka SF, Machado A. Central neuromodulation for refractory pain. *Neurosurg Clin N Am* 2014;25(1):77–83.
30. Hollingworth M, Sims-Williams HP, Pickering AE, et al. Single electrode deep brain stimulation with dual targeting at dual frequency for the treatment of chronic pain: a case series and review of the literature. *Brain Sci* 2017;7(1):9.

31. Franzini A, Ferroli P, Leone M, et al. Hypothalamic deep brain stimulation for the treatment of chronic cluster headaches: a series report. *Neuromodulation* 2004;7(1):1–8.

32. Schoenen J, Di Clemente L, Vandenheede M, et al. Hypothalamic stimulation in chronic cluster headache: a pilot study of efficacy and mode of action. *Brain* 2005;128(pt 4):940–947.

33. Coffey RJ. Deep brain stimulation for chronic pain: results of two multicenter trials and a structured review. *Pain Med* 2001;2(3):183–192.

34. Rasche D, Rinaldi PC, Young RF, et al. Deep brain stimulation for the treatment of various chronic pain syndromes. *Neurosurg Focus* 2006;21(6):E8.

35. Cruccu G, Garcia-Larrea L, Hansson P, et al. EAN guidelines on central neurostimulation therapy in chronic pain conditions. *Eur J Neurol* 2016;23(10):1489–1499.

36. Owen SL, Green AL, Nandi DD, et al. Deep brain stimulation for neuropathic pain. *Acta Neurochir Suppl* 2007;97(pt 2):111–116.

37. Marchand S, Kupers RC, Bushnell MC, et al. Analgesic and placebo effects of thalamic stimulation. *Pain* 2003;105(3):481–488.

38. Fontaine D, Lazorthes Y, Mertens P, et al. Safety and efficacy of deep brain stimulation in refractory cluster headache: a randomized placebo-controlled double-blind trial followed by a 1-year open extension. *J Headache Pain* 2010;11(1):23–31.

39. Hamani C, Schwalb JM, Rezai AR, et al. Deep brain stimulation for chronic neuropathic pain: long-term outcome and the incidence of insertional effect. *Pain* 2006;125(1–2):188–196.

40. Gray AM, Pounds-Cornish E, Eccles FJ, et al. Deep brain stimulation as a treatment for neuropathic pain: a longitudinal study addressing neuropsychological outcomes. *J Pain* 2014;15(3):283–292.

41. Abreu V, Vaz R, Rebelo V, et al. Thalamic deep brain stimulation for neuropathic pain: efficacy at three years' follow-up. *Neuromodulation* 2017;20(5):504–513.

42. Pereira EAC, Boccard SG, Linhares P, et al. Thalamic deep brain stimulation for neuropathic pain after amputation or brachial plexus avulsion. *Neurosurg Focus* 2013;35(3):E7.

43. Falowski S, Ooi YC, Smith A, et al. An evaluation of hardware and surgical complications with deep brain stimulation based on diagnosis and lead location. *Stereotact Funct Neurosurg* 2012;90(3):173–180.

44. Tsubokawa T, Katayama Y, Yamamoto T, et al. Treatment of thalamic pain by chronic motor cortex stimulation. *Pacing Clin Electrophysiol* 1991;14(1):131–134.

45. DosSantos MF, Ferreira N, Toback RL, et al. Potential mechanisms supporting the value of motor cortex stimulation to treat chronic pain syndromes. *Front Neurosci* 2016;10:18.

46. Meyerson BA, Lindblom U, Linderoth B, et al. Motor cortex stimulation as treatment of trigeminal neuropathic pain. *Acta Neurochir Suppl (Wien)* 1993;58:150–153.

47. Sokal P, Harat M, Zieliński P, et al. Motor cortex stimulation in patients with chronic central pain. *Adv Clin Exp Med* 2015;24(2):289–296.

48. Kurt E, Henssen DJHA, Steegers M, et al. Motor cortex stimulation in patients suffering from chronic neuropathic pain: summary of an expert meeting and pre-meeting questionnaire, combined with a literature review. *World Neurosurg* 2017;108:254–263.

49. Garcia-Larrea LG, Peyron R, Mertens P, et al. Positron emission tomography during motor cortex stimulation for pain control. *Stereotact Funct Neurosurg* 1997;68(1–4):141–148.

50. Garcia-Larrea L, Peyron R, Mertens P, et al. Electrical stimulation of motor cortex for pain control: a combined PET-scan and electrophysiological study. *Pain* 1999;83(2):259–273.

51. Lima MC, Fregni F. Motor cortex stimulation for chronic pain: systematic review and meta-analysis of the literature. *Neurology* 2008;70(24):2329–2337.

52. Lefaucheur J-P, Holsheimer J, Goujon C, et al. Descending volleys generated by efficacious epidural motor cortex stimulation in patients with chronic neuropathic pain. *Exp Neurol* 2010;223(2):609–614.

53. Nguyen J-P, Nizard J, Keravel Y, et al. Invasive brain stimulation for the treatment of neuropathic pain. *Nat Rev Neurol* 2011;7(12):699–709.

54. Maarrawi J, Peyron R, Mertens P, et al. Motor cortex stimulation for pain control induces changes in the endogenous opioid system. *Neurology* 2007;69(9):827–834.

55. Ostergard T, Munyon C, Miller JP. Motor cortex stimulation for chronic pain. *Neurosurg Clin N Am* 2014;25(4):693–698.

56. Monsalve GA. Motor cortex stimulation for facial chronic neuropathic pain: a review of the literature. *Surg Neurol Int* 2012;3(suppl 4):S290–S311.

57. Fonoff ET, Hamani C, Ciampi de Andrade D, et al. Pain relief and functional recovery in patients with complex regional pain syndrome after motor cortex stimulation. *Stereotact Funct Neurosurg* 2011;89(3):167–172.

58. Peyron R, Faillenot I, Mertens P, et al. Motor cortex stimulation in neuropathic pain. Correlations between analgesic effect and hemodynamic changes in the brain. A PET study. *Neuroimage* 2007;34(1):310–321.

59. Tsubokawa T, Katayama Y, Yamamoto T, et al. Chronic motor cortex stimulation for the treatment of central pain. *Acta Neurochir Suppl (Wien)* 1991;52:137–139.

60. Buchanan RJ, Darrow D, Monsivais D, et al. Motor cortex stimulation for neuropathic pain syndromes: a case series experience. *Neuroreport* 2014;25(9):715–717.

61. Sachs AJ, Babu H, Su Y-F, et al. Lack of efficacy of motor cortex stimulation for the treatment of neuropathic pain in 14 patients. *Neuromodulation* 2014;17(4):303–311.

62. Im S-H, Ha S-W, Kim D-R, et al. Long-term results of motor cortex stimulation in the treatment of chronic, intractable neuropathic pain. *Stereotact Funct Neurosurg* 2015;93(3):212–218.

63. Son B-C, Kim D-R, Kim H-S, et al. Simultaneous trial of deep brain and motor cortex stimulation in chronic intractable neuropathic pain. *Stereotact Funct Neurosurg* 2014;92(4):218–226.

64. Radic JA, Beauprie I, Chiasson P, et al. Motor cortex stimulation for neuropathic pain: a randomized cross-over trial. *Can J Neurol Sci* 2015;42(6):401–409.

65. Esfahani DR, Pisansky MT, Dafer RM, et al. Motor cortex stimulation: functional magnetic resonance imaging-localized treatment for three sources of intractable facial pain. *J Neurosurg* 2011;114(1):189–195.

66. Raslan AM, Nasseri M, Bahgat D, et al. Motor cortex stimulation for trigeminal neuropathic or deafferentation pain: an institutional case series experience. *Stereotact Funct Neurosurg* 2011;89(2):83–88.

67. Nuti C, Peyron R, Garcia-Larrea L, et al. Motor cortex stimulation for refractory neuropathic pain: four year outcome and predictors of efficacy. *Pain* 2005;118(1–2):43–52.

68. Katayama Y, Fukaya C, Yamamoto T. Poststroke pain control by chronic motor cortex stimulation: neurological characteristics predicting a favorable response. *J Neurosurg* 1998;89(4):585–591.

69. Fagundes-Pereyra WJ, Teixeira MJ, Reyns N, et al. Motor cortex electric stimulation for the treatment of neuropathic pain. *Arq Neuropsiquiatr* 2010;68(6):923–929.

70. Lefaucheur J-P, Drouot X, Cunin P, et al. Motor cortex stimulation for the treatment of refractory peripheral neuropathic pain. *Brain* 2009;132(pt 6):1463–1471.

71. André-Obadia N, Peyron R, Mertens P, et al. Transcranial magnetic stimulation for pain control. Double-blind study of different frequencies against placebo, and correlation with motor cortex stimulation efficacy. *Clin Neurophysiol* 2006;117(7):1536–1544.

72. Lefaucheur J-P, Ménard-Lefaucheur I, Goujon C, et al. Predictive value of rTMS in the identification of responders to epidural motor cortex stimulation therapy for pain. *J Pain* 2011;12(10):1102–1111.

73. André-Obadia N, Mertens P, Lelekov-Boissard T, et al. Is life better after motor cortex stimulation for pain control? Results at long-term and their prediction by preoperative rTMS. *Pain Phys* 2014;17(1):53–62.

74. Fontaine D, Hamani C, Lozano A. Efficacy and safety of motor cortex stimulation for chronic neuropathic pain: critical review of the literature. *J Neurosurg* 2009;110(2):251–256.

75. Levy RM. Motor cortex stimulation for chronic pain: panacea or placebo? *Neuromodulation* 2014;17(4):295–299.

76. Stadler JA, Ellens DJ, Rosenow JM. Deep brain stimulation and motor cortical stimulation for neuropathic pain. *Curr Pain Headache Rep* 2011;15(1):8–13.

77. Nguyen J-P, Velasco F, Brugières P, et al. Treatment of chronic neuropathic pain by motor cortex stimulation: results of a bicentric controlled crossover trial. *Brain Stimul* 2008;1(2):89–96.

78. Velasco F, Argüelles C, Carrillo-Ruiz JD, et al. Efficacy of motor cortex stimulation in the treatment of neuropathic pain: a randomized double-blind trial. *J Neurosurg* 2008;108(4):698–706.

79. Rasche D, Tronnier VM. Clinical significance of invasive motor cortex stimulation for trigeminal facial neuropathic pain syndromes. *Neurosurgery* 2016;79(5):655–666.

80. Pirotte B, Voordecker P, Neugroschl C, et al. Combination of functional magnetic resonance imaging-guided neuronavigation and intraoperative cortical brain mapping improves targeting of motor cortex stimulation in neuropathic pain. *Neurosurgery* 2005;56(2 suppl):344–359.

81. Klein MM, Treister R, Raij T, et al. Transcranial magnetic stimulation of the brain: guidelines for pain treatment research. *Pain* 2015;156(9):1601–1614.

82. O'Connell NE, Wand BM, Marston L, et al. *Non-Invasive Brain Stimulation Techniques for Chronic Pain*. Hoboken, NJ: Wiley; 2014.

83. Lefaucheur J-P. Principles of therapeutic use of transcranial and epidural cortical stimulation. *Clin Neurophysiol* 2008;119(10):2179–2184.

84. Lefaucheur J-P, Antal A, Ahdab R, et al. The use of repetitive transcranial magnetic stimulation (rTMS) and transcranial direct current stimulation (tDCS) to relieve pain. *Brain Stimul* 2008;1(4):337–344.

85. Di Lazzaro V, Dileone M, Pilato F, et al. Modulation of motor cortex neuronal networks by rTMS: comparison of local and remote effects of six different protocols of stimulation. *J Neurophysiol* 2011;105(5):2150–2156.

86. Lefaucheur J-P, André-Obadia N, Antal A, et al. Evidence-based guidelines on the therapeutic use of repetitive transcranial magnetic stimulation (rTMS). *Clin Neurophysiol* 2014;125(11):2150–2206.

87. Hasan M, Whiteley J, Bresnahan R, et al. Somatosensory change and pain relief induced by repetitive transcranial magnetic stimulation in patients with central poststroke pain. *Neuromodulation* 2014;17(8):731–736.

88. Lefaucheur J-P, Drouot X, Menard-Lefaucheur I, et al. Neurogenic pain relief by repetitive transcranial magnetic cortical stimulation depends on the origin and the site of pain. *J Neurol Neurosurg Psychiatry* 2004;75(4):612–616.

89. Boyer L, Dousset A, Roussel P, et al. rTMS in fibromyalgia: a randomized trial evaluating QoL and its brain metabolic substrate. *Neurology* 2014;82(14):1231–1238.

90. Marlow NM, Bonilha HS, Short EB. Efficacy of transcranial direct current stimulation and repetitive transcranial magnetic stimulation for treating fibromyalgia syndrome: a systematic review. *Pain Pract* 2013;13(2):131–145.

91. Malavera A, Silva FA, Fregni F, et al. Repetitive transcranial magnetic stimulation for phantom limb pain in land mine victims: a double-blinded, randomized, sham-controlled trial. *J Pain* 2016;17(8):911–918.

92. Hodaj H, Alibeu J-P, Payen J-F, et al. Treatment of chronic facial pain including cluster headache by repetitive transcranial magnetic stimulation of the motor cortex with maintenance sessions: a naturalistic study. *Brain Stimul* 2015;8(4):801–807.

93. Leung A, Donohue M, Xu R, et al. rTMS for suppressing neuropathic pain: a meta-analysis. *J Pain* 2009;10(12):1205–1216.

94. Rossi S, Hallett M, Rossini PM, et al. Safety, ethical considerations, and application guidelines for the use of transcranial magnetic stimulation in clinical practice and research. *Clin Neurophysiol* 2009;120:2008–2039.

95. Maizey L, Allen CPG, Dervinis M, et al. Comparative incidence rates of mild adverse effects to transcranial magnetic stimulation. *Clin Neurophysiol* 2013;124(3):536–544.

CHAPTER 98

Diagnostic and Therapeutic Nerve Blocks

MICHELE CURATOLO and **NIKOLAI BOGDUK**

Local anesthetic blocks are procedures in which a local anesthetic agent is deliberately injected onto a peripheral nerve in order to temporarily stop conduction of action potentials. Local anesthetic agents block conduction of action potentials by acting on the sodium channels of the nerve cell membranes. Their effect is temporary because their pharmacologic action is reversible.

Nerve blocks are an attractive tool in pain medicine because they are the only means by which to stop pain completely. Analgesics may reduce pain, but only local anesthetics stop it.

Virtually any nerve in the body can be blocked in order to relieve pain. All that is required is an access to the nerve and the agent with which to anesthetize it. Many textbooks and manuals have been published that describe the techniques used to do so, and it is not the intention or purpose of this chapter to duplicate these publications. Many of the available procedures have an application in anesthesia for surgical procedures, but they are not germane to the practice of pain medicine. Some procedures have a role in securing relief of pain postoperatively of after a trauma; for those, the distinction between the discipline of pain medicine and the practice of anesthesia is uncertain. These procedures will not be the focus of this chapter.

The short duration of action of local anesthetic agents limits the utility of local anesthetic blocks in pain medicine. For acute pain, their premier utility lies in providing protection from incident pain. For chronic pain, their most straightforward use is as a diagnostic test. Otherwise, they have putative roles as prognostic tests and as therapeutic interventions.

This chapter focuses on the principles of local anesthetic blocks used in pain medicine. It illustrates the more commonly used and useful procedures and reviews the evidence concerning their validity and utility.

Common Principles

Irrespective of the purpose for which local anesthetic blocks are used, certain principles apply. These pertain to the physician, the patient, the preparation for the procedure, its contraindication, the procedure itself, and its complications.

PHYSICIAN

Any physician who performs nerve blocks should be suitably trained and experienced. He or she needs to understand the pain problem being addressed and how the proposed procedure relates to the patient's management. He or she needs to be familiar with the patient, the patient's complaints, and how the patient expresses him- or herself. The physician should be able to explain to the patient the nature and significance of the procedure to be undertaken and, together with the patient, be able to assess and interpret the response. These requirements require training in more than the execution of the procedure.

The physician needs a detailed knowledge of the anatomic basis of the procedure not only to execute it accurately but also to avoid complications. Similarly, he or she needs to be able to deal with the possible side effects and complications of local anesthetic agents. For procedures performed under image guidance, the physician needs to be able to obtain the correct views and to interpret them accurately.

More difficult to define and to achieve is technical excellence to perform the procedure expeditiously yet accurately with the minimum of stress to the patient. This includes avoiding painful structures during the insertion of the needle and keeping the number of adjustments during its course to a minimum. Acquisition of these skills requires good mentoring and forethought on the part of the practitioner and takes years of training.

PATIENT

The patient should understand the purpose of the procedure to be undertaken. This requires distinguishing between diagnostic and therapeutic procedures. Unless they are properly informed, patients may mistake a diagnostic block as a treatment and be disappointed when it appears not to have worked when the effect wears off. They should understand the limitations of prognostic and therapeutic blocks as outlined in the corresponding sections of this chapter. In this regard, there is a difference between a patient consenting to a procedure and being fully informed about it.

The patient should be aware of the potential side effects and complications of the procedures, what actions are to be taken to avoid them, and what will be done in the event that they occur.

Both for diagnostic blocks and therapeutic blocks, the patient will be required to assess and report their response. Therefore, before the procedure, the patient should be instructed in how to use instruments such as pain-rating scales and measurements of function. Patients who have pain in multiple sites but who undergo blocks for only one site need to understand which pain is being tested and must be able to report the effects of the block on that particular site of pain. Relief of pain will need to be corroborated by testing activities that usually are limited by pain. For this purpose, the patient must be able to specify a set of suitable activities before the block and be able to test for their restoration after the block.

PREPARATION

The preparation of the patient differs according to the nature of procedure to be undertaken and the region in which the target nerve lies. Orders for "nil by mouth" are indicated only for procedures in which loss of consciousness and aspiration of gastric contents are possible complications. Examples include cervical transforaminal blocks and procedures that involve high doses of local anesthetic. In the opinion and experience of the authors, the majority of nerve blocks can be performed safely with the patient having had a light meal even before the procedure. Indeed, fasting may compromise the procedure if the patient is uncomfortable or distressed for not having eaten.

For most local anesthetic blocks, establishing an intravenous line is not indicated, nor is continuous monitoring of respiratory and cardiovascular function required. The doses of local anesthetic typically administered do not pose hazards that require these preparations. However, appropriate precautions are indicated for procedures that are performed close to vital structures, such as the spinal cord or the vertebral artery, or when large doses of a local anesthetic agent are to be administered. In such cases, an intravenous line should be placed before the procedure in order to ensure access for the rapid administration of fluids and resuscitation drugs, should these be necessary. Vital functions should be monitored (i.e., electrocardiogram, pulse oximetry, and blood pressure). A means of ventilating the patient with 100% oxygen with a bag and mask or via endotracheal tube and suction should be available, along with drugs and equipment to manage a cardiac arrest.

Local anesthetic blocks do not require routine sedation. Proper explanation, continuous communication, and good technique will provide patient comfort without the need for systemic medication. In the case of diagnostic and prognostic blocks, using sedation may confound the validity of response by increasing the rate of false-positive blocks,[1] for which reason it is best avoided.

Only occasional patients will require sedation: those who are markedly apprehensive or who have a manifest anxiety over needles or invasive procedures. In such cases, sedation can be secured by oral agents (benzodiazepines) or intravenous administration of modest doses of sedatives (midazolam, propofol). If needed, analgesia can be provided by short-acting opioids (fentanyl, alfentanil, remifentanil), provided that the procedure is not diagnostic or prognostic. The dose should be titrated to provide sufficient sedation only for the duration of the procedure; the patient should be fully awake or be readily awakened during the procedure in order to be able to report its effects. If intravenous sedation or analgesia is used, it should be complemented with monitoring of respiratory and cardiovascular function. Supplemental oxygen may be required.

CONTRAINDICATIONS

Blocks are contraindicated in patients who are unwilling to undergo the procedure or who have attributes that compromise the safe execution of the procedure. The latter include inability to lie still despite sedation, allergy to the drugs to be used, infection at the site of injection, and anatomic abnormalities, among others.

A coagulation disorder or anticoagulation therapy is a relative contraindication. Blocks of superficial nerves in easily accessible parts of the body may be safely undertaken. Reservations apply for blocks of deep nerves in sites where hemorrhage could compromise vital structures. Guidelines on the management of patients under antithrombotic therapy have been published.[2] Patients with compromised cardiovascular function are more susceptible to either the toxic effects of local anesthetic or the effects of blockade of sympathetic nerves. Appropriate precautions should be taken with such patients if large volumes of a local anesthetic agent are to be used.

COMPLICATIONS

The potential complications of local anesthetic blocks can be categorized as systemic effects of the drugs injected, physiologic effects of the procedure, inadvertent damage to structures other than nerves, and damage to nerves.

Systemic Effects

Allergy to local anesthetic agents is rare. The physiologic consequences and treatment are as for any anaphylactic reaction.

Local anesthetics have direct toxic effects on the central nervous system (CNS) and cardiovascular system (CVS). These effects become increasingly pronounced as blood levels of the offending agent rise. High or rapidly rising blood levels can occur because of inadvertent intravascular injection of the local anesthetic, unusually rapid absorption from a highly vascular region, or the administration of an excessive dose of agent.

Several precautions can be taken to reduce the risk of intravascular injection. For procedures performed under fluoroscopic guidance, a test dose of contrast medium can be administered before injecting the local anesthetic agent. This will likely show vascular uptake. For procedures where the uptake may be to a small but vital vessel, such as a radicular artery, digital subtraction angiography serves to demonstrate the vessel more clearly. For procedures performed under ultrasound guidance, lack of fluid visualization may be a sign of intravascular injection. In this case, injection should be stopped immediately and the needle should be repositioned.

The needle should be aspirated before injection and after each 2 to 5 mL of injectate, if such volumes are used, in order to ensure no bloody return. For blocks using large volumes, 3 to 4 mL of a mixture of local anesthetic plus 1:200,000 epinephrine may be injected as an initial test dose. If injected intravascularly, such a mixture will cause, with a high degree of probability, a brief and transient (2 to 3 minutes) rise in the heart rate of 20 to 25 beats per minute and a rise in systolic blood pressure of 20 to 30 points because of the β and α effects of the epinephrine.[3] This precaution was originally developed to detect inadvertent intravascular injection during epidural anesthesia, but it applies equally well for other regional techniques.

A rising, or high, blood level of local anesthetic is typically manifest by the onset of CNS features such as anxiety, agitation, tinnitus, muscle twitching, perioral numbness or tingling, and dizziness. As plasma levels rise, tonic-clonic seizures can occur. At even higher plasma levels, neuronal inhibition occurs, leading to respiratory arrest, coma, and cardiovascular collapse. Although most anesthetics produce signs of CNS toxicity prior to either seizure or CVS toxicity, this is not always the case. With highly lipophilic, highly protein bound agents (e.g., bupivacaine), CVS collapse may even precede CNS symptoms.[4]

If a patient manifests features of toxicity during the course of an injection, the injection should be stopped immediately and assistance should be enlisted or summoned. Oxygen (100%), via a bag and mask, should be commenced immediately. If the patient's oxygen saturation, as judged from pulse oximetry, falls below 90%, positive pressure ventilation should be instituted. A small, anticonvulsant dose of propofol (50 to 100 mg) should be administered. Cardiovascular parameters should be monitored and adverse effects treated: hypotension with fluids and vasopressors (ephedrine 5 to 10 mg), hypertension with vasodilators (labetalol 5 to 10 mg), and tachycardia with β-blockers (esmolol 5 mg, metoprolol 2.5 to 5 mg).

These measures will often abort progressive local anesthetic toxicity. However, if the toxicity appears to be proceeding toward convulsions (agitation, limb jerking, loss of consciousness), further measures are necessary. Positive pressure ventilation with oxygen should be commenced in order to ensure oxygen saturation greater than 90%. If ventilation is difficult, or if the patient convulses, muscle paralysis with 50 to 100 mg succinylcholine should be administered to ensure adequate ventilation. Cardiovascular monitoring and treatment of adverse CVS effects should continue. Intravenous lipid emulsion therapy should be used if these measures fail.[5]

Physiologic Effects

Although undertaken to relieve pain, nerve blocks will, or may, block other sensory functions, motor function, balance, and sympathetic function. When these are to be expected but pose no immediate hazard, the patient should be warned to expect them and to not be alarmed by their onset. Appropriate precautions should be taken to compensate against loss of function and to avoid injury. Examples of side effects pertinent to blocks used in pain medicine are numbness or weakness in the limb following spinal nerve blocks, ataxia following third occipital nerve blocks, and hypotension or Horner syndrome following sympathetic nerve blocks.

Blocks targeting particular nerves may spill over to adjacent nerves and produce unwanted effects (e.g., paravertebral nerve blocks may produce inadvertent epidural blockade). Patients undergoing such blocks should be closely monitored for adverse effects and treated early and vigorously in the event that they do occur.

Damage to Nonneural Structures
The needles used for local anesthetic blocks have the potential to pierce and damage structures along the course of the insertion or near the target point. Examples include pneumothorax following intercostal nerve block or thoracic spinal nerve block, piercing the esophagus during stellate ganglion blocks, piercing pelvic viscera during sacral spinal nerve blocks, and penetrating the aorta or inferior vena cava during celiac plexus blocks.

Piercing a blood vessel has the potential to produce bleeding or hematoma. In patients with normal clotting mechanisms, it is rare for such bleeding or hematoma to produce significant sequelae. In patients with abnormal coagulation, bleeding may produce hypovolemia, and hematoma may exert pressure effects on adjacent structures. For these reasons, coagulopathy is a relative contraindication for local anesthetic blocks.

Damage to Nerves
Targeting a nerve with an injection carries the risk of nerve damage. The resultant symptoms range from minor paresthesia to severe pain. The damage may be caused by piercing the nerve with the needle or by what is injected. Components of the injectate, such as preservative, may be neurotoxic, epinephrine may cause spasm of the vasa nervorum and result in ischemic damage, or the pressure of injection may damage the nerve physically. The incidence of long-term injury remains extremely low, ranging 2 to 4 per 10,000 blocks.[6]

PROCEDURE
In order to be valid or effective, nerve blocks need to be accurate. This involves placing the injection as close as possible to the target nerve. Several techniques are available to secure accurate placement. They differ for unaided (i.e., "blind") techniques and for image-guided techniques.

Blind Techniques
For blind techniques, the oldest method of correct needle placement is to probe the nerve gently with the tip of the needle. This maneuver produces a paresthesia in the area of distribution of the nerve. Once paresthesia is elicited, the needle is held steady and the local anesthetic is injected. This technique, however, has now become obsolete. Probing some nerves (e.g., autonomic nerves) does not elicit paresthesia and, more importantly, probing nerves risks damaging them.

Mixed nerves, containing sensory and motor fibers, can be located by using an insulated needle connected to a peripheral nerve stimulator. By passing an electric current through the needle, the motor fibers in the nerve are stimulated, producing a twitch in the muscles supplied by the nerve. This stimulation is usually not painful because motor fibers are activated at lower current intensity than sensory fibers. A typical setting is a frequency of 1 to 2 Hz and a current strength of 1 mA. At this setting, a twitch will be produced as the needle approaches

the nerve but still lies some distance from it. Reducing the current to 0.4 to 0.5 mA allows the needle to be advanced further. A well-defined twitch at this intensity of current implies that the needle is close to the nerve.

Data from clinical anesthesia practice show a high success rate of blocks facilitated by a nerve stimulator.[7] However, large volumes of local anesthetic are typically administered for operative anesthesia, and it is unclear if these data can be extrapolated to blocks in pain medicine, in which small volumes of local anesthetic are used in order to maximize the selectivity of the block. Although rare, neurologic complications may occur even when nerve stimulators are used.[8]

For some blocks, palpable landmarks can be used to secure the accuracy of the block. A classic example is the intercostal block, for which the rib is an adequate landmark for the target site.

Fluoroscopy-Guided Techniques
When nerves and landmarks are not palpable and precision is required, unaided techniques do not ensure accuracy and selectivity of the block. In such circumstances, image guidance should be used to secure safety, accuracy, and selectivity.

Fluoroscopy is the most commonly used form of image guidance in pain medicine. Its main limitation is that fluoroscopy shows only bones. Therefore, it is suitable only for target nerves that bear a dependable relationship to a bony landmark. The accuracy of the block is achieved by directing the needle to the landmark. Safety is achieved both by choosing a course that does not incur intervening structures that should not be damaged and by having the needle not stray from the intended target. Selectivity is achieved by administering a test dose of contrast medium to establish that the injectate will flow into the region of the target nerve and will not flow onto other structures where anesthetization might compromise the selectivity of the block (Fig. 98.1). The advantages of fluoroscopy are that it demonstrates a wide field of view around the target region; with C-arm fluoroscopy, views of any orientation can be obtained in order to define the location of the needle during its course or at its target point; intermittent images are rapidly applied and continuous imaging is possible, if required; and the apparatus is not excessively expensive. A particular advantage of fluoroscopy is that in the event of intravascular injection, it will reveal rostral or caudal flow of contrast medium away from the target point. This facility is not available from devices that produce planar images.

Computed Tomography–Guided Techniques
Some operators use computed tomography (CT) guidance instead of fluoroscopy. They are attracted by the definition that CT provides of viscera and vessels that should be avoided by the needle. Ostensibly, this allows for a safer placement of the needle. For injections into narrow joint cavities or irregularly oriented joints such as the sacroiliac joint, CT offers the virtue of depicting the cavity and its orientation directly. Consequently, a path for the needle can be planned to coincide directly with the joint. The disadvantages of CT guidance are numerous. Each time the needle position is checked, the patient must be rescanned. This interrupts the procedure, prolongs it, and involves considerable radiation exposure. More critically, planar image does not reveal flow of contrast medium in vessels that run out of the plane of view. Serial reconstruction does not compensate for this because by the time the images are acquired, the contrast medium will have left the field of view. Safety with respect to inadvertent intravascular injection has not been demonstrated for CT guidance. CT is far more expensive than fluoroscopy. For these reasons, fluoroscopic guidance remains preferable. Only in selected cases would CT guidance be justified.

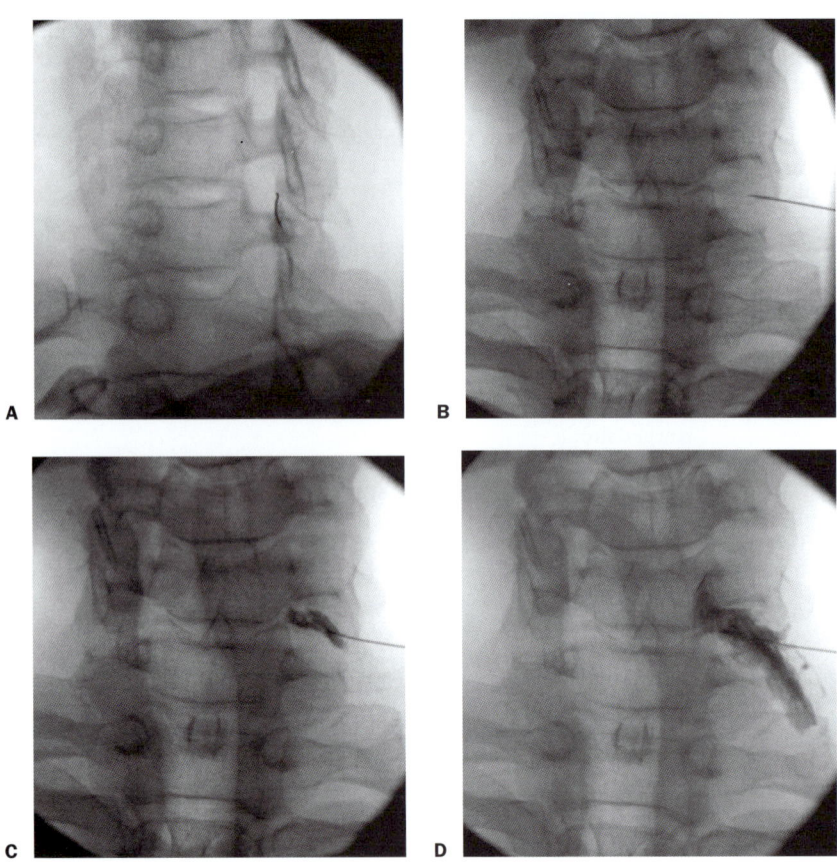

FIGURE 98.1 Steps in the execution of a C7 spinal nerve block. **A:** Oblique view showing a needle in position tangential to the superior articular process of C7. **B:** Anteroposterior view of the needle, showing its tip midway across the width of the articular pillars. **C:** Anteroposterior view of a test dose of contrast medium injected into the intervertebral foramen. **D:** Anteroposterior view after injection of sufficient contrast medium to reach the dural sac. *(Radiographs provided by Dr. Paul Dreyfuss, Seattle, WA, and reproduced with permission from Bogduk N, ed.* Guidelines for Spinal Diagnostic and Treatment Procedures. *San Francisco, CA: International Spine Intervention Society; 2004.)*

Ultrasound-Guided Techniques

Ultrasound guidance is being increasingly used and explored in pain medicine. It demonstrates muscles, ligaments, vessels, joints, and bones (Fig. 98.2). Moreover, if high-resolution transducers are used, thin nerves can be directly visualized (Fig. 98.3). Ultrasound does not involve radiation exposure, either to the patient or to the operator, and continuous screening can be used. Fluid injected can be visualized in a real-time fashion. Ultrasound is less expensive than CT, and most ultrasound devices suitable for pain procedures are much less expensive than fluoroscopy. For these reasons, ultrasound guidance is emerging as an attractive alternative to other modalities of image guidance. Its main limitations, at present, are poor resolution of narrow-gauge needles (although, with experience, operators can infer the location of the needle from the movements of the soft tissues); echoes from overlying structures, such as bones, interfere with the image of the target area; decreasing image resolution with increasing depth; and requirement of substantial training and experience to be able to perform the blocks effectively and safely.

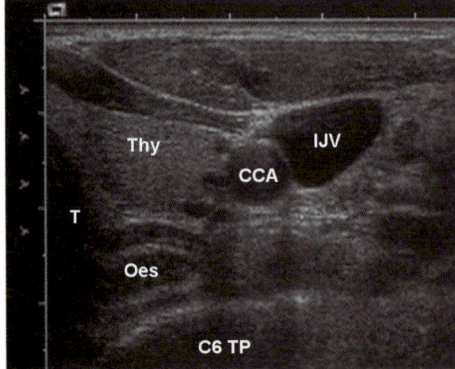

FIGURE 98.2 Ultrasound anatomy of the neck in the plane used for stellate ganglion block. Note how an anteroposterior approach, using either the traditional blind technique or fluoroscopy guidance, carries the risk of incurring the thyroid gland (Thy), common carotid artery (CCA), internal jugular vein (IJV), or esophagus (Oes). Under ultrasound guidance, an oblique approach lateral to the great vessels is possible. T, trachea; TP, transverse process of C6. *(Illustration kindly provided by Dr. Urs Eichenberg, Balgrist University Hospital, Zurich, Switzerland.)*

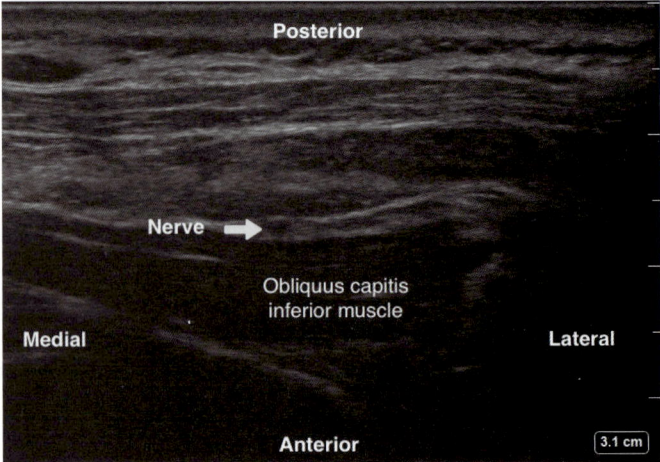

FIGURE 98.3 Ultrasound image of the greater occipital nerve (*arrow*), visible as hypoechoic round structure posterior to the obliquus inferior capitis muscle. The ultrasound anatomy and technique has been described by Greher et al.[114]

From the first reports of ultrasound-guided nerve blocks in pain medicine,[9] the number of published papers has skyrocketed and practice has expanded enormously. Most of the research has focused on techniques, that is, on how to perform blocks of different nerves. More recently, randomized controlled trials have evaluated the value of ultrasound guidance in relation to patient-relevant outcomes. When comparing fluoroscopy-guided with ultrasound-assisted epidural steroid injections, the two techniques were found to be similar in terms of mean procedure time, number of needle insertion attempts or needle passes, mean pain intensity, and degree of disability scores at 1 and 3 months postprocedure.[10] For perioperative thoracic epidural injections, the use of ultrasound to identify the epidural space resulted in a decreased number of needle punctures to achieve loss of resistance and in lower pain scores after surgery compared with the use of palpation.[11] A systematic review on the use of ultrasound in lumbar spinal and epidural anesthesia found significant evidence supporting the role of ultrasound in improving the precision and efficacy of neuraxial anesthetic techniques.[12] With fluoroscopy as reference standard, ultrasound imaging was found to be an accurate technique for performing cervical facet joint nerve blocks, with some improvements regarding time to perform the block.[13–15] Ultrasound-guided piriformis injections provided similar outcomes to fluoroscopically guided injections without differences in imaging, needling, or overall procedural times.[16] Similarly, there was no differences in patient-related outcomes at 7 days to 3 months between fluoroscopy- and ultrasound-guided sacroiliac joint injections.[17] Although ultrasound guidance may decrease the risk of local anesthetic toxicity and of pneumothorax, the incidence of peripheral nerve damage is not decreased.[18]

Taken together, these data indicate that ultrasound guidance has an emergent evidence-based role in pain medicine, representing for several procedures a valuable alternative to fluoroscopy. For procedures in which fluoroscopy has no role, such as nerve blocks of the extremities, ultrasound guidance is likely superior to nerve stimulation.

Test Blocks

Test blocks are ones that are not therapeutic injections, prognostic tests, or diagnostic tests in the strict and correct sense of those terms. They are performed simply to test if a particular nerve is involved in the patient's symptoms. A nerve is anesthetized and the response is either that the patient's pain is relieved or not. The block is not prognostic because it is not used to predict the outcomes of any subsequent treatment. Nor is it diagnostic because the block is not used to distinguish one source of pain from another. It is used only to see if the nerve anesthetized is involved in the patient's symptoms.

Virtually any nerve in the body can be blocked in this way. Examples include supraorbital blocks for headache; blocks of the median, ulnar, or radial nerves for pain in the hand; ilioinguinal and iliohypogastric nerve blocks for pain after herniorrhaphy; and tibial nerve blocks for pain in the foot.

The nature of the information derived by test blocks, and its utility, have been poorly elaborated. In some cases, the blocks are used to "confirm" the diagnosis, but the diagnosis will already be evident from other clinical information. The pivotal question—both clinically and philosophically—is what then.

If the patient's response is used to predicate a subsequent treatment, the test must convert to a prognostic block (see following section). In that event, however, the block and the response to it need to be valid, and the treatment needs to be effective. If those requirements are not satisfied, the utility of the blocks remain unclear.

Prognostic Blocks

A prognostic block is one undertaken to test if a definitive treatment will be successful. The rationale is that if a nerve block with local anesthetic relieves the pain, then a treatment capable of interrupting conduction along the nerve should relieve the pain for a prolonged period, if not permanently.

For prognostic blocks to be valid, evidence is required to complete a table like that depicted in Table 98.1. There needs to be a strong association between a positive response to the block and a successful outcome from treatment and between a negative response to the block and failure of treatment. Such data are hard to produce and, to the authors' knowledge, are not available. They would require a study in which patients undergo treatment irrespective of their response to blocks. They also require a treatment that is dependably effective. Unless that is the case, failures may be due to the failure of treatment rather than an error in the response to blocks. Few such treatments exist.

In the absence of proper evidence, practitioners who use prognostic blocks assume that a positive response to a block should be predictive of a favorable outcome to treatment. This has not always proven to be the case. For instance, prognostic blocks of peripheral somatic nerves may be used to test the outcome of surgical neurectomy. However, there is no evidence for validity of these prognostic blocks to predict the efficacy of neurectomy. Furthermore, neuroma formation and deafferentation pain complicate the treatment, and worsening due to the treatment can occur also in the presence of positive prognostic blocks. Positive responses to sympathetic blocks are unclearly associated with favorable or sustained outcomes from sympathectomy—either surgical or chemical.

SPINAL NERVE BLOCKS

In some patients with radicular pain, medical imaging is not diagnostic. CT or magnetic resonance imaging (MRI) may show more than one spinal nerve affected by a disk herniation or by foraminal stenosis, and the clinical features do not help to determine which nerve is the source of symptoms. Spinal nerve blocks were developed to assist surgeons to determine the symptomatic level in such cases so that surgery could be directed at the correct segmental level.

Spinal nerve blocks involve placing a needle, under fluoroscopic guidance, into the intervertebral foramen that lodges the target nerve. If anesthetizing that nerve relieves the patient's pain, then that nerve is implicated as the source of pain. If anesthetizing the nerve does not relieve the pain, then that nerve is excluded as the source of pain, and investigations can be redirected to another nerve. Steps in the execution of a cervical spinal nerve blocks are shown in Figure 98.1.

Because of the proximity of the medullary arteries and the spinal cord, and of the vertebral artery in the cervical spine, spinal nerve blocks require consummate skill in obtaining the correct view, delivering the needle, and checking its location. Guidelines for the safe conduct of the procedure have been published.[19,20]

Data on the validity of spinal nerve blocks are limited because of two factors. First, nerve blocks should be performed under

TABLE 98.1 Contingency Table Illustrating the Nature of Evidence Required to Establish the Validity of a Prognostic Block			
		Response to Treatment	
		Relief	**No relief**
Response to Prognostic Block	Relief	a	b
	No relief	c	d

controlled conditions in order to guard against false-positive responses, but only one study of spinal nerve blocks has used control blocks.[21] Second, the predictive validity of blocks requires a study in which patients with positive responses to blocks and patients with negative responses both be submitted to treatment. Only such a study would provide proper data on the sensitivity and specificity of the blocks. Such studies are difficult to justify ethically and, to the authors' knowledge, have not been conducted.

Partial data are available from studies that report the proportion of patients with positive responses to blocks in whom pathology is found at surgery. This proportion is not the sensitivity of the test but its positive predictive value in the sample tested. Because that value is dependent on the nature of the sample studied, it is not generalizable to other samples or to practice at large.

For lumbar spinal nerve blocks, various studies have reported positive predictive values that ranged between 80% and 100%.[22,23] These high values imply that the false-positive rate of lumbar spinal nerve blocks is low and, therefore, that their specificity is likely to be high. In one study, a small number of patients with negative responses to blocks nevertheless underwent surgery.[23] Pathology was found in all cases but not at the level tested; in no case did surgery find pathology at the level tested when the block had been negative. These patients proved to have multilevel disease or anomalous nerve roots. This implies that the false-negative rate of lumbar spinal nerve blocks is low and, therefore, that their sensitivity is high.

One study measured sensitivity by performing lumbar spinal nerve blocks in 46 patients with clinical and radiologic evidence of nerve root compression, subsequently confirmed at surgery.[24] The sensitivity was 100%, with 95% confidence intervals of 88% to 100%. That same study measured specificity by performing blocks in 23 patients at levels known by radiology not to be symptomatic. No false-positive responses were encountered, and the specificity of lumbar spinal nerve blocks was estimated at "around 90%.[24]

The one study that used controlled blocks enlisted 18 patients with cervical radiculopathy and 83 with lumbar radiculopathy but did not stratify the results according to region investigated.[21] Using a criterion standard of good outcome from surgery, it found a sensitivity of 93% but a specificity of only 33%. Spinal nerve blocks were no better than MRI in predicting good outcome, but the particular advantage of spinal nerve blocks demonstrated in this study was the ability of negative responses to blocks to predict poor outcome, particularly when MRI was negative or ambiguous.

SYMPATHETIC BLOCKS

Blocks of various elements of the sympathetic nervous system have a status somewhere intermediate between diagnostic and prognostic. They are not diagnostic in the strict sense of that adjective, for the cause of pain is usually evident from clinical assessment or other investigations. Fundamentally, they are used to test if the patient's clinical features are mediated by sympathetic nerves. Knowing this does not affect management unless the response to blocks is used to prognosticate the response to neurolytic treatment of the sympathetic nerves.

Cervical sympathetic blocks have been used largely in the evaluation of patients with complex regional pain syndromes of the upper limb. Other applications have been for patients with pain in the face or head. The procedure requires delivering an aliquot of local anesthetic onto the stellate ganglion. The traditional approach has been a blind technique based on surface markings and palpation. The blind technique classically involved injecting a large volume of local anesthetic in order to ensure saturation of the ganglion. Large volumes compromise the validity of cervical sympathetic blocks because structures other than the target nerve are anesthetized. In a study of eight volunteers, MRI showed that injectate was not delivered to the stellate ganglion but passed anterior to it.[25] Several complications following stellate ganglion blocks have been described, mostly due to inadvertent puncture of sensitive structures.[26–30] For these reasons, image-guided techniques are preferred.

Ultrasound guidance is an alternative to fluoroscopic guidance and offers certain advantages in this region. Ultrasound demonstrates the common carotid artery, internal jugular vein, thyroid gland, and esophagus—all of which need to be avoided during passage of the needle (Fig. 98.2). In a study that compared ultrasound guidance with the blind technique, the volume of local anesthetic required was reduced to 5 mL, the onset of block was sooner, and hematoma was avoided (but occurred in 3 out of 12 cases with the blind technique).[31] A study in healthy volunteers showed that the esophagus, the vertebral artery, and other arteries are located in the needle path of the traditional blind technique and that manual dislocation did not displace these structures from the needle path in the majority of cases.[32] Although comparative studies are lacking, it is reasonable to avoid the blind approach. Ultrasound seems preferable to fluoroscopy due to its ability to visualize structures that must be avoided during the needle passage.

Lumbar sympathetic blocks involve anesthetizing the lumbar sympathetic trunk, typically at the L3 level. They have traditionally been used to test if they relieve pain or other features of complex regional pain syndrome. The standard technique is fluoroscopically guided (Fig. 98.4).

The use of fluoroscopy or ultrasound establishes the face validity of sympathetic blocks (i.e., the sympathetic trunk is accurately and selectively infiltrated). Face validity can be confirmed physiologically by observing a rise in skin temperature in the limb of the target side, which suggests that the sympathetic trunk has indeed been anesthetized.

What has not been shown is that sympathetic blocks have construct validity (i.e., that the physiologic response is due to the effects of the local anesthetic and not to nonspecific factors such as placebo). This requires the execution of controlled blocks. Failing to use controlled blocks in the past may have led to overestimates of so-called sympathetic-mediated pain. Unless and until studies are conducted using controlled blocks, its true prevalence will not be known. To the authors' knowledge, no studies have tested the validity of lumbar sympathetic blocks. Nor has the prognostic validity of sympathetic blocks—cervical or lumbar—in predicting the outcomes of sympathectomy been demonstrated by rigorous research.

Other blocks of the sympathetic nervous system are practiced, ostensibly widely. These include blocks of the celiac plexus, splanchnic nerves, hypogastric plexuses, and blocks of the ganglion impar. However, there is no evidence on their validity as either diagnostic or prognostic procedures.

Diagnostic Blocks

Many conditions associated with chronic pain have no detectable anatomical correlate. The cause of pain is not evident on conventional medical imaging. For some such conditions, although the cause might not be evident, the source of pain can be established using diagnostic blocks.

The rationale for diagnostic, local anesthetic blocks is that if a structure is the source of pain, then anesthetizing it or its nerve supply should relieve the pain. If the suspected structure is not the source of pain, then anesthetizing it should not relieve the pain.

Two types of blocks have been used to pinpoint sources of pain: intra-articular blocks and nerve blocks. Intra-articular blocks involve injecting local anesthetic into a joint suspected of being the source of pain. Diagnostic nerve blocks are restricted to small nerves that have a limited and specific distribution.

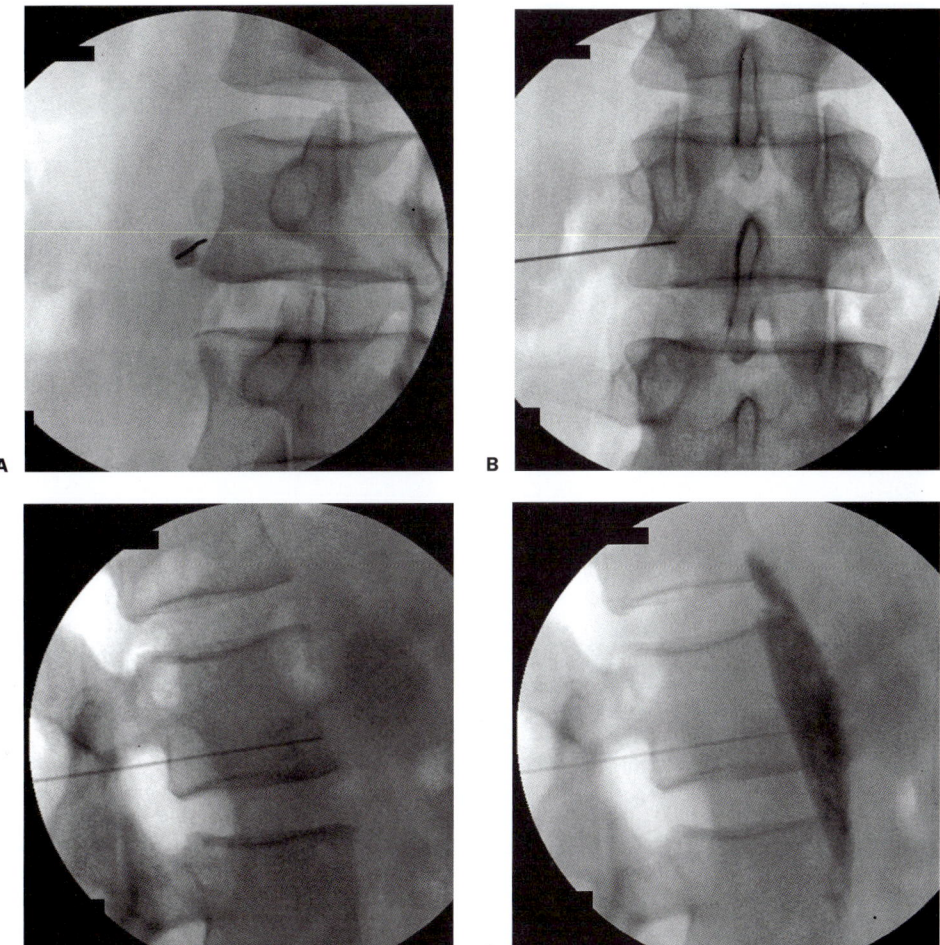

FIGURE 98.4 Stages in the conduct of a lumbar sympathetic block. **A:** An oblique view showing a needle passing tangential to the lower anterolateral surface of the L3 vertebral body. **B:** Anteroposterior view, showing the needle in place over the anterolateral aspect of the L3 vertebral body. **C:** Lateral view showing the needle in place over the anterolateral aspect of the L3 vertebral body. **D:** Lateral view showing contrast medium spreading longitudinal over the anterior surface of the psoas major muscle. *(Illustrations kindly provided by Dr. Milton Landers.)*

Blocks of larger nerves or of nerves that supply multiple tissues are not diagnostic of a particular source because of their widespread distribution; they fall under the category of test blocks.

PRINCIPLES
Controls

There are no objective tests for the presence of pain or for its relief. Investigators rely only on what the patient reports, but patients can report relief of pain for reasons other than the effect of a local anesthetic injected during a diagnostic block. They may have an expectation that the block will relieve their pain, particularly if they have been coached or instructed to expect a positive response. Unprompted, they might want the response to be positive so that they qualify for the resultant treatment that promises to relieve their pain in the long term. Patients with medicolegal claims might choose to report relief in order to vindicate their claim.

Because of these extraneous, confounding factors, a positive response to a block cannot be summarily attributed to the effect of the local anesthetic injected. Some form of control is necessary if the response is to be valid and for the interpretation of the response to be correct. The most rigorous form of control is a placebo control in which an inactive agent is injected to test for spurious responses. However, for two reasons, placebos cannot be administered in an arbitrary manner. In the first instance, administering a placebo on a single-blind basis is considered unethical in some jurisdictions. Patients would need to be informed that they might receive an inactive agent. Furthermore, a positive response to placebo does not necessarily rule out that the tested structure is symptomatic.

Comparative local anesthetic blocks can be used as alternatives to placebo-controlled blocks. These involve administering a particular agent on the occasion of the first block but using a different agent on a second occasion. The agents advocated are lidocaine and bupivacaine. The paradigm maintains that a genuine patient will report short-lasting relief when lidocaine is used and long-lasting relief when bupivacaine is used. However, it is unclear whether a discordant response truly rules out a positive diagnosis. Patients may display prolonged pain relief after lidocaine for different reasons: The block may reduce central sensitization processes that contribute to pain intensity; the pain relief may have positive psychological effects, leading to long-lasting pain relief; the patient may experience prolonged pain relief because he or she will rest after the block, giving the false impression that the block is responsible for the absence of pain; etc.

Despite the limitations associated with placebo-controlled and comparative blocks, data on diagnostic blocks for zygapophysial joint pain presented in the following sections have shown that single blocks are associated with high false-positive rates. Therefore, a form of control is currently an appropriate standard of care.

Criteria for Positive Response

For a response to a diagnostic block to be valid, certain criteria should be satisfied. On each occasion that the nerve is blocked, the patient should obtain substantial relief of pain. That should be validated by recording the intensity of pain before and after the block. Moreover, for the block to be physiologically and pharmacologically meaningful, the pain should return as the

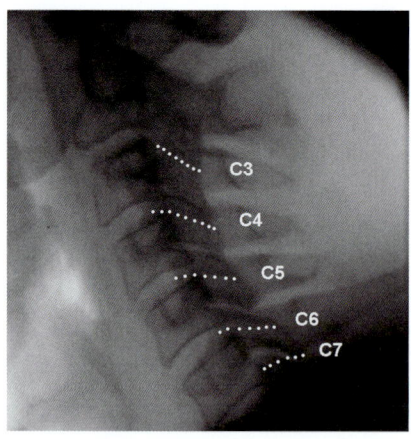

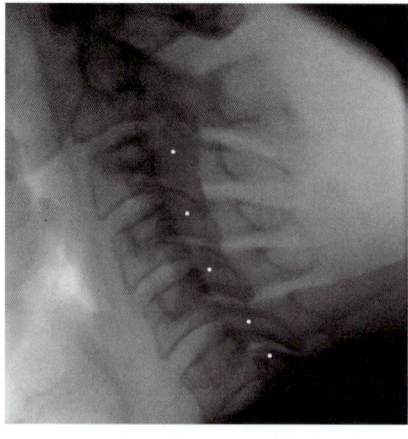

FIGURE 98.5 A lateral radiograph of the cervical spine on which the courses of the cervical medial branches and the target points for medial branch blocks have been depicted. **A:** The courses of the typical cervical medial branches are plotted by *dotted lines.* **B:** The *dots mark* the target points for medial branch blocks.

effect of the local anesthetic wears off. Recording the return of pain, therefore, becomes part of the assessment. A painful structure should resume being painful once the local anesthetic has ceased to operate. Prolonged relief of pain, lasting days, weeks, or months, occasionally occurs but is of difficult interpretation. Prolonged responses suggest either a placebo effect or some sort of modulatory effect on pain perception, the nature of which has not been determined.

A positive response to blocks should be corroborated by narrative and activity. The patients should volunteer that they feel distinctly better, and they should be able to undertake and demonstrate activities that previously were prevented or restricted by their pain. If activities are not restored, the utility of the block is questionable. If activities, ostensibly restricted by the pain, are not restored when pain is relieved, some factor other than the pain must still be responsible for the restriction.

APPLICATIONS

Nerve Blocks for Cervical Zygapophysial Joint Pain

The largest body of evidence on the validity of diagnostic nerve blocks has been produced in the context of zygapophysial (facet) joint pain. The cervical facet joints are supplied by the medial branches of the dorsal rami, with the exception of the C2–C3 joint that is supplied by the third occipital nerve.[33] It has been shown that cervical medial branch blocks are target-specific. Material injected onto the target points floods the location of the target nerve but does not spread to adjacent nerves or the spinal nerves.[34] Nor do cervical medial branch blocks anesthetize the posterior neck muscles in a nonspecific manner. The standard technique for cervical medial branch blocks is fluoroscopy-guided (Figs. 98.5 and 98.6). Ultrasound-guided techniques have been described and validated, but only very experienced practitioners can safely and effectively perform them.[13–15,35,36]

The construct validity of the comparative block paradigm has been tested in the context of diagnostic blocks of the medial branches. Concordant responses (i.e., effect lasting longer with bupivacaine than with lidocaine) have a high specificity (88%) when compared with placebo-controlled blocks.[37] This means that positive responses are very unlikely to be false. However, concordant responses have a low sensitivity (54%).[37] This means that they do not detect all patients with cervical zygapophysial joint pain who do not have placebo responses. Discordant responses (i.e., effect lasting longer with lidocaine than with bupivacaine) have a high sensitivity (100%), implying that they detect all patients who have zygapophysial joint pain.[37] However, their specificity is limited (65%), meaning that positive responses can include some placebo responses.[37]

In studies using concordant comparative blocks as reference standard, single medial branch blocks had false-positive rates

of 27%.[38] However, as mentioned earlier ("Controls" section), it is unclear whether a discordant response truly rules out facet joint pain. The false-positive rate of single blocks may therefore be lower than 27%. Nevertheless, it is safe to say that single medial branch blocks are of questionable validity due to high false-positive rate and that the diagnostic confidence is improved by the practice of controlled blocks.

These different sensitivities and specificities make little difference in clinical practice because the prevalence of cervical zygapophysial joint pain is high, around 60%.[39–41] Given a concordant response, a practitioner can be 88% confident that the positive response is true positive (Table 98.2). In comparison, although a discordant response has a lower specificity, its sensitivity is high, which means that the practitioner can be 81% confident that a positive response is true positive (see Table 98.2).[42]

Cervical medial branch blocks have established utility. They are the only means by which to diagnose the most common cause of chronic neck pain. Moreover, patients correctly diagnosed can be treated successfully with percutaneous radiofrequency neurotomy: Those patients who obtain complete relief from cervical medial branch blocks can expect a 70% chance of achieving complete relief of pain after cervical medial branch neurotomy.[43–48]

The C2–C3 zygapophysial joint is innervated by the third occipital nerve, which is the superficial medial branch of the C3 dorsal ramus. Third occipital nerve blocks, therefore, are a particular subset of cervical medial branch blocks. They are used in patients with upper cervical pain and headache to test if the pain stems from the C2–C3 zygapophysial joint.

The utility of third occipital blocks lies in the investigation of cervicogenic headache. In patients with posttraumatic neck pain, in whom headache is the dominant complaint, the prevalence of pain from the C2–C3 zygapophysial joint is 53%.[49] No other blocks and no other diagnostic tests have established

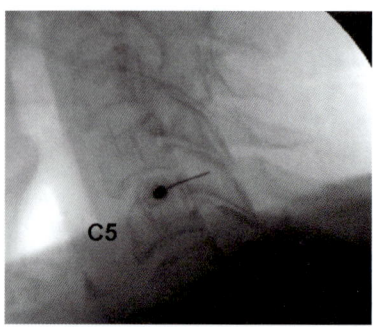

FIGURE 98.6 A lateral fluoroscopic view of the cervical spine showing a needle in place on the articular pillar of C5 for a C5 medial branch block.

TABLE 98.2 Contingency Table Showing the Effect on Diagnostic Confidence of Different Specificities and Sensitivities of a Diagnostic Test in Detecting a Condition with a Prevalence of 60%

Specificity	Sensitivity	Prevalence	Blocks	Condition Present	Condition Absent	Diagnostic Confidence
0.88	0.54	60%	Positive	324	48	88%
			Negative	276	352	
				600	400	
0.65	1.00	60%	Positive	600	140	81%
			Negative		260	
				600	400	

Diagnostic confidence is the measure of how confident the practitioner can be that the condition really is present when a test is positive. It amounts to the positive predictive value that applies for a particular prevalence and is derived from the specificity and sensitivity of the test by the equations[42]:

$$\text{posttest odds} = \text{pretest odds} \times \text{positive likelihood ratio}$$
$$\text{positive likelihood ratio} = \text{sensitivity} / (1 - \text{specificity})$$
$$\text{pretest odds} = \text{prevalence} / (1 - \text{prevalence})$$
$$\text{diagnostic confidence} = [(\text{posttest odds}) / (\text{posttest odds} + 1)] \times 100\%$$

any other source of cervicogenic headache with a prevalence that rivals this figure. A positive response to controlled, third occipital nerve blocks is prognostic of an 88% success rate for completely relieving headache by third occipital radiofrequency neurotomy.[44]

Nerve Blocks for Lumbar Zygapophysial Joint Pain

Lumbar medial branch blocks are the only means available by which either to implicate or to refute the lumbar zygapophysial joints as the source of back pain. The validity of lumbar medial branch blocks has been studied more than any other diagnostic block in pain medicine. The blocks are target-specific. Provided that the correct target points are used and provided that small volumes are used, the injectate remains exclusively on the target nerve.[50] Placements more proximal along the nerve risk having the injectate spread into the intervertebral foramen.[50] Construct validity has been demonstrated. Medial branch blocks protect normal volunteers from experimentally induced zygapophysial joint pain.[51]

As for the cervical region, the standard technique for lumbar medial branch blocks is fluoroscopy-guided (Figs. 98.7 and 98.8). Ultrasound-guided techniques have been described and validated, but they require excellent expertise.[52–54]

In order to be valid in patients, the blocks should also be controlled. Single blocks of the lumbar medial branches have false-positive rates of between 25% and 41%.[55–57] This means that if the prevalence of lumbar zygapophysial joint pain is 15% (see the following text), for every three blocks that appear to be positive, two will be false positive. If the prevalence is 5%, five out of every six blocks will be false positive. A caveat applies to these calculations. As for cervical zygapophysial joint pain, the prevalence and false-positive rates have been computed based

on concordant responses of comparative blocks, implying that only cases in which bupivacaine effects last longer than lidocaine effects are true positives. As mentioned earlier, we cannot rule out zygapophysial joint pain in the presence of discordant responses, that is, in those cases in which lidocaine duration of effect exceeds bupivacaine effect. This consideration suggests that the prevalence of lumbar zygapophysial joint pain may be higher than reported and, accordingly, the false-positive rates of single blocks may be lower than we currently estimate. Nevertheless, they likely remain clinically significant, indicating that a valid diagnosis cannot be made using a single diagnostic block.

Comparative local anesthetic blocks have been advocated and used as controls for lumbar medial branch blocks on the grounds that they have been validated for the cervical spine. In the cervical spine, comparative blocks have a specificity of either 65% or 88%, depending on the stringency of the criteria for a positive response.[37] These values are acceptable for cervical medial branch blocks because cervical zygapophysial joint pain is so common. However, in the lumbar spine, where zygapophysial joint pain is far less common, comparative blocks result in inordinate numbers of false-positive results.

For a specificity of 65%, and a prevalence of 40%, the diagnostic confidence of positive comparative blocks is only 66% (Table 98.3). For a prevalence of 15%, this confidence drops to 32% and is even less for lower prevalence rates. For a specificity of 88% and a prevalence of 15%, the diagnostic confidence is only 60% but rises to 85% if the prevalence is 40% (see Table 98.3). These calculations show that for comparative blocks to be valid in the lumbar spine, the prevalence of zygapophysial joint pain must be substantial, and strict criteria for a positive response must be applied (e.g., the patient must have substantial relief of pain on each occasion that the nerves are

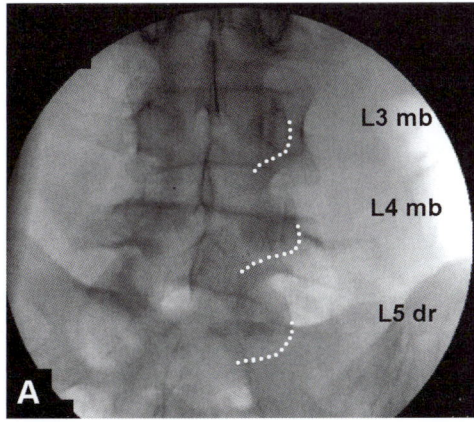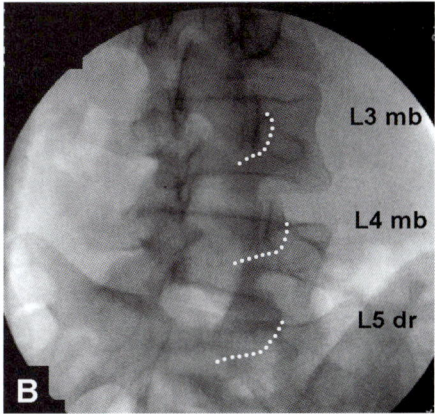

FIGURE 98.7 Radiographs of the lower lumbar spine on which the courses of the medial branches (mb) of the lower lumbar dorsal rami and the L5 dorsal ramus (dr) have been depicted. **A:** Anteroposterior view. **B:** Oblique view.

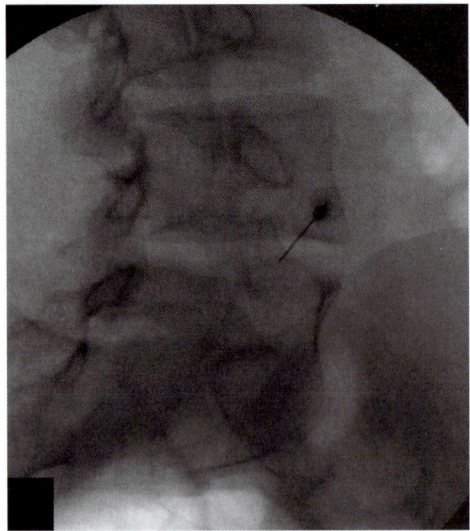 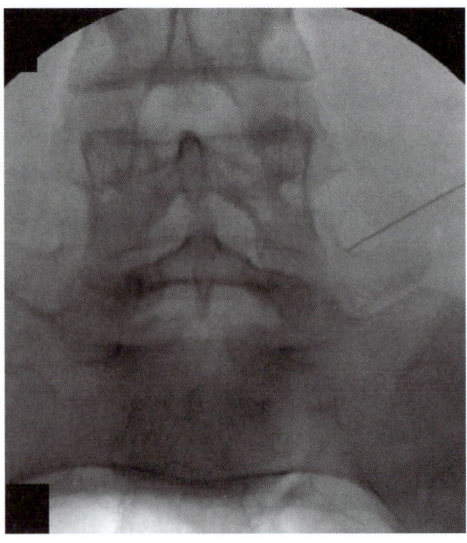

FIGURE 98.8 Radiographs of an L4 medial branch block. **A:** Oblique view showing a needle resting on the neck of the superior articular process of L5. **B:** Declined view showing the needle aiming obliquely onto the neck of the superior articular process at its junction with the transverse process.

blocked and function has to be restored). Unless these conditions apply, the false-positive rates render the diagnostic confidence unacceptably low.

The available data on the prevalence of lumbar zygapophysial joint pain is mixed and contentious and differs according to the sample studied and the criteria used to define a positive response. Using the criterion of 50% relief of pain, the prevalence has been reported as 15% (10% to 20%) among younger, injured workers.[58] Using a criterion of 75% relief of pain, the prevalence was 45% (39% to 54%) in patients attending a pain clinic,[57] and for a criterion of 90% relief, the prevalence was 40% (27% to 53%) in elderly patients with no history of trauma.[59] These data leave the prevalence of lumbar zygapophysial joint pain in doubt. It appears to be low in injured young patients but may approach 40% in elderly patients.

Because of the relatively low prevalence of lumbar zygapophysial joint pain, the pretest likelihood is that the patient will have a negative response to lumbar medial branch blocks. Consequently, it would be inappropriate in most cases to test each joint one at a time. A more efficient use of lumbar medial branch blocks would be initially to perform a screening block, in which the L3 medial branch, L4 medial branch, and L5 dorsal ramus (supplying the L4–L5 and L5–S1 joint) are blocked simultaneously. If these blocks prove negative, zygapophysial joint pain is effectively refuted. Joints are most often symptomatic at L4–L5 and L5–S1,[59] and an investigator would need good cause to test joints at higher segmental levels. If the screening blocks are positive, controlled blocks at single segments may be pursued to determine if the response is valid and to establish which particular joint is the source of pain.

TABLE 98.3 Contingency Table Showing the Effect on Diagnostic Confidence of Different Specificities of a Diagnostic Test and Decreasing Prevalence Rates

| Specificity | Prevalence | Blocks | Condition | | Diagnostic Confidence |
			Present	Absent	
0.88	40%	Positive	400	72	85%
		Negative		528	
			400	600	
	15%	Positive	150	102	60%
		Negative		748	
			150	850	
	5%	Positive	50	114	30%
		Negative		846	
			50	950	
0.65	40%	Positive	400	210	66%
		Negative		528	
			400	600	
	15%	Positive	150	328	32%
		Negative		748	
			150	850	
	5%	Positive	50	333	13%
		Negative		846	
			50	950	

The calculations assume a sensitivity of 100%. Diagnostic confidence is the measure of how confident the practitioner can be that the condition really is present when a test is positive. It amounts to the positive predictive value that applies for a particular prevalence and is derived from the specificity and sensitivity of the test by the equations[42]:

$$\text{posttest odds} = \text{pretest odds} \times \text{positive likelihood ratio}$$
$$\text{positive likelihood ratio} = \text{sensitivity} / (1 - \text{specificity})$$
$$\text{pretest odds} = \text{prevalence} / (1 - \text{prevalence})$$
$$\text{diagnostic confidence} = [(\text{posttest odds}) / (\text{posttest odds} + 1)] \times 100\%$$

Establishing a diagnosis of lumbar zygapophysial joint pain allows treatment to be offered in the form of lumbar radiofrequency medial branch neurotomy. If they are selected on the basis of positive responses to controlled blocks, 60% of patients so treated can expect to obtain at least 80% relief of pain lasting 12 months, and 80% can expect at least 60% relief.[60] If pain recurs, neurotomy can be repeated in order to reinstate relief.[61] A systematic review of randomized controlled trials that compared radiofrequency neurotomy with blockades, infiltrations, or placebo found low to moderate evidence in favor of radiofrequency neurotomy.[62] Unfortunately, patient selection using controlled diagnostic blocks was not considered as criterion to include studies in the analysis, and therefore, several investigations enrolled patients who were unlikely to have zygapophysial joint pain. This has likely reduced the overall effect size of the procedure. A more recent randomized controlled trial found very limited benefit of adding radiofrequency neurotomy to an exercise program.[63] However, the study has severe limitations that are summarized in a following commentary.[64] A single diagnostic block was performed, and the effect of the diagnostic block was based solely on pain relief (50%), with no evaluation of function. This practice likely resulted in high false-positive rates and therefore in the enrollment of patients with no pain stemming from the zygapophysial joints. Furthermore, based on the description of the technique, the radiofrequency electrode was not placed parallel to the nerve, which is essential to maximize the chances of coagulating the nerve.[65] This technical flaw has likely prevented the procedure from being effective in patients with true zygapophysial joint pain. The results of this recent study are nevertheless important, as they confirm that lack of strict selection criteria and expeditious practice are not associated with successful outcomes of radiofrequency neurotomy.

The selection of patients for radiofrequency neurotomy is a crucial process. A multicenter randomized controlled trial compared the outcomes of lumbar radiofrequency medial branch neurotomy in patients selected with three different criteria: clinical findings (without diagnostic block), positive response to a single diagnostic block, and positive response to comparative blocks.[66] Denervation success rates in the three groups were 33%, 39%, and 64%, respectively, indicating that controlled blocks led to better outcomes. However, the most cost-effective paradigm was proceeding to radiofrequency denervation without a diagnostic block. Due to the very low morbidity of radiofrequency denervation, economic considerations may encourage the practice of skipping diagnostic blocks and proceed directly to radiofrequency neurotomy. The authors of this chapter do not support this practice. A success rate of 33% is ethically unacceptable, considering that selection of patients with diagnostic blocks would substantially increase the chance of a positive outcome.

Which type of control an investigator chooses to use and which criteria should be used to assess comparative blocks is a matter of preference depending on the circumstances, that is, whether the blocks are performed for research or clinical purposes, the nature of the planned research, or the clinical circumstances. The choice ranges from placebo-controlled blocks to comparative blocks with more or less strict criteria regarding the relative duration of pain relief with the two different anesthetic agents.

Substantial controversy exists regarding the amount of pain relief that has to be achieved by diagnostic blocks in order to categorize a response as positive. In theory, zygapophysial joint pain is expected to be completely relieved by nerve blocks. However, there is widespread practice of considering 50% pain relief as sufficient to enroll patients for radiofrequency neurotomy. This approach may be associated with increased risk of false-positive responses and, consequently, failure of radiofrequency neurotomy. However, a study that evaluated the

relationship between degree of pain relief after the blocks and denervation outcomes found no significant differences in radiofrequency outcomes based on any pain relief cutoff over 50% with the diagnostic blocks.[67] Based on the results, the authors raised concerns that adopting the very stringent selection criterion of 80% to 100% pain relief as screening for radiofrequency ablation would result in withholding a beneficial procedure from a substantial number of patients.

Other Diagnostic Nerve Blocks

Unfortunately, most of the nerve blocks that can be technically performed have not been tested for their diagnostic utility. Therefore, despite wide use, the validity of most diagnostic nerve blocks remains undetermined. One example is the block of the greater occipital nerve for the diagnosis of occipital neuralgia. The causes of occipital neuralgia are mostly unclear, the most straightforward one being injury to the nerve caused by trauma or surgery. However, patients who fulfill the criteria for the clinical diagnosis of occipital neuralgia[68] do not necessarily have a history of trauma or surgery. In these patients, the rationale for greater occipital nerve blocks as a diagnostic test is unclear. The block cannot establish or rule out the diagnosis of occipital neuralgia. At best, greater occipital nerve blocks can only be used to establish that afferent activity in this nerve, in some way, "modulates" the perception of pain. As mentioned in the section on therapeutic blocks, this modulatory effect can play a role also in forms of headache other than occipital neuralgia, such as migraine or cluster headache, which challenges the validity of occipital nerve blocks for the diagnosis of occipital neuralgia.

Diagnostic Intra-articular Blocks

Intra-articular injections are performed on joints of the appendicular skeleton for a variety of reasons. These include therapeutic injections and diagnostic arthrography. However, diagnostic intra-articular blocks, using local anesthetic agents, are not common practice. The diagnosis of peripheral joint pain is established largely on the basis of physical examination and medical imaging, and there is no requirement for diagnostic blocks in routine practice. Some practitioners might use joint blocks in patients in whom the source of pain is ambiguous, such as hip joint blocks to distinguish hip joint pain from referred pain to the groin or buttock, but such practices are not widely used, and their validity and utility have still to be established.

Diagnostic joint blocks have a greater application in the diagnosis of spinal pain because the joints of the spine are less accessible to physical examination, and medical imaging is typically unhelpful in pinpointing a particular joint as the source of pain. In the past, intra-articular blocks of the zygapophysial joints were used as a means of diagnosing zygapophysial joint pain. The practice still continues in some circles. However, intra-articular blocks of the spine have never been validated and have not been shown to have therapeutic utility. They have been supplanted by medial branch blocks, which have been validated and which do have therapeutic utility.

It is unclear whether joint pain is the result of intra- or periarticular pathology or both. If periarticular lesions are involved, intra-articular blocks would not be sensitive for the diagnosis of joint pain. Periarticular infiltrations are performed in clinical practice, but their validity and therapeutic utility are unknown.

There are two spinal joints for which nerve blocks are not practical and for which intra-articular blocks remain the only means to determine if that joint is the source of pain. They are the lateral atlantoaxial joint and the sacroiliac joint.

Experimental studies in normal volunteers have shown that the lateral atlantoaxial joint (C1–C2) can produce pain in the upper cervical spine and in the head.[69] In principle, therefore, this can be a source of cervicogenic headache and neck pain.

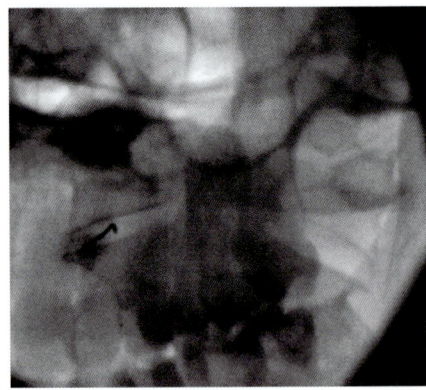
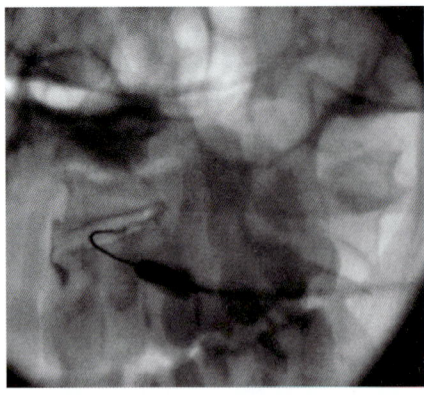

A   **B**

FIGURE 98.9 Anteroposterior fluoroscopy views of a lateral atlantoaxial joint injection. **A:** The needle has been advanced into the cavity of the joint. **B:** Contrast medium outlines the joint cavity and the internal surface of the lateral capsule.

Lateral atlantoaxial joint blocks involve delivering a needle into the cavity of the joint. The technique involves a posterior approach, using fluoroscopic guidance.[70] The proximity of the target area to the dural sac, spinal cord, internal carotid artery, and vertebral artery poses significant risks during lateral atlantoaxial joint injection. Misplaced injections of local anesthetic could result in a high spinal block. Intra-arterial injection of depot corticosteroids could result in embolism and stroke. Therefore, the technique for lateral atlantoaxial joint blocks does not allow for any but minimal deviations of the needle from a straight course from the skin to the target point. These blocks should be performed only by operators who can use bevel control to restrict movements to less than a few millimeters from a straight course. Contrast medium is injected in order to establish that the injectate enters the joint cavity and does not escape from it (Fig. 98.9). This establishes the face validity of the injection. Once correct placement has been confirmed, about 1 mL of local anesthetic can be injected. A positive response is one in which the injection substantially relieves the patient's pain.

The validity of lateral atlantoaxial joints has not been tested. Single diagnostic blocks may have a false-positive rate which has not yet been measured. In principle, controlled blocks are required in order to maximize validity. Controls using comparative local anesthetic blocks might be used, but the validity of comparative blocks inside joints, where blood flow is low, has not been established. Anatomic controls might be an alternative, in which the control is to block an adjacent joint (e.g., C2–C3), but the results of such controls have not yet been reported.

There are few prevalence studies of lateral atlantoaxial joint pain, but the available data indicate a nonzero prevalence. One study, using single diagnostic blocks, found that at least 16% of patients presenting with headache responded to lateral atlantoaxial joint blocks.[70] Another study found a prevalence of at least 13%.[71] Each of these may be underestimates because not all eligible patients underwent diagnostic blocks. Conversely, the figures might be lower because controlled blocks were not used.

Lateral atlantoaxial joint blocks have therapeutic utility because patients can be treated by atlantoaxial arthrodesis. Follow-up studies have reported that arthrodesis succeeds in providing sustained relief of pain.[72–74] Intra-articular injections of corticosteroids are a more conservative alternative but benefit only about 1 in 8 patients over the long term.[71]

Sacroiliac joint blocks are a test for back pain stemming from a sacroiliac joint. They involve introducing a needle under fluoroscopic[75] or ultrasound[76] control into the lower end of the cavity of the joint (Fig. 98.10). With fluoroscopy, a test dose of contrast medium establishes that the injectate lies within the joint cavity and does not escape from it. Ultrasound has emerged as an alternative to fluoroscopy as image guidance,[76] with a randomized controlled trial showing that ultrasound-guided

sacroiliac joint injection has similar accuracy and efficacy to fluoroscopy-guided injection.[17] With either technique, a local anesthetic can be injected in order to anesthetize the joint. A positive response is substantial relief of the patient's pain.

Two types of controls have been used in order to maximize the validity of sacroiliac joint blocks. One study used anatomic controls by previously anesthetizing lumbar zygapophysial joints.[77] Another study used comparative local anesthetic blocks.[78] Respectively, these studies found a prevalence (95% confidence intervals) of 13% (6% to 20%) and 19% (9% to 29%).

The lateral sacral branches contribute to the innervation of the sacroiliac joint[79,80] and are therefore potential targets of diagnostic blocks. However, the intra-articular portion of the sacroiliac joint is innervated also from ventral nerves.[79] Therefore, lateral sacral nerve blocks are unlikely suitable to diagnose sacroiliac joint pain. They should rather be considered a potential tool to predict the effect of lateral branch radiofrequency neurotomy.[81] The block can be performed under either fluoroscopy or ultrasound guidance.[82] A systematic review found some evidence for the face validity of sacral lateral branch blocks to diagnose posterior sacroiliac complex pain, and some evidence of moderate quality for the efficacy of lateral branch radiofrequency neurotomy.[83] Three randomized controlled studies found lateral branch radiofrequency neurotomy to be superior to a placebo treatment.[84–87]

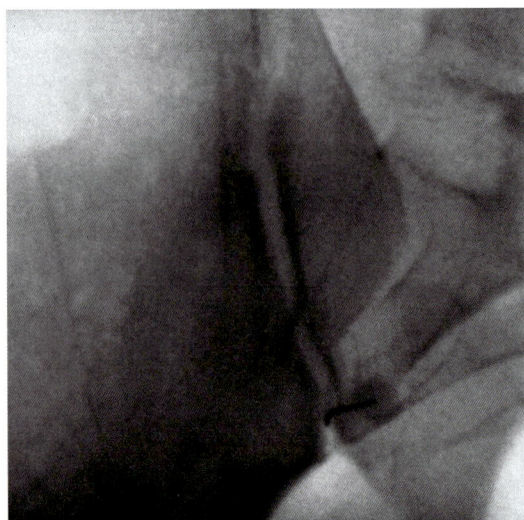

FIGURE 98.10 An anteroposterior fluoroscopy view of a needle placed for an intra-articular block of sacroiliac joint. *(Radiograph provided by Dr. Paul Dreyfuss, Seattle, WA, and reproduced with permission from Bogduk N, ed.* Practice Guidelines for Spinal Diagnostic and Treatment Procedures. *San Francisco, CA: International Spine Intervention Society; 2004.)*

Therapeutic Nerve Blocks

Local anesthetics have a limited duration of action, and their effects are expected to wear off. Therefore, the most straightforward application of therapeutic nerve blocks is acute pain: The pain is treated while spontaneous healing is anticipated. Examples include femoral nerve blocks for a fractured femur,[88] intercostal blocks to permit deeper breathing in patients with painful fractures of the ribs,[89] and various nerve blocks, with or without indwelling catheter, for the management of postoperative pain.[90,91] As mentioned in the introduction, these blocks are not the focus of this chapter.

For chronic pain, nerve blocks can be used to temporarily facilitate function or enhance the efficacy of other treatments. Examples include brachial plexus blocks to facilitate rehabilitation in patients with complex regional pain syndromes of the upper limb[92] and suprascapular nerve blocks to facilitate mobilization of frozen shoulder.[93] In these examples, it is recognized that the period of relief required is temporary and that other interventions will eventually treat the pain. If required, the blocks can be repeated to facilitate rehabilitation, but the blocks are not repeated ad infinitum.

In addition to serving as a complement to other treatments, nerve blocks have a long tradition as therapeutic tools per se in chronic pain conditions. The basis for this practice has been the anecdotal evidence that in some patients, repeating blocks can lead to prolonged periods of relief well beyond the duration of action of the agent used. This is supported by a systematic review that found the effect of local anesthetic injections to consistently exceed the duration of the conduction blockade.[94] However, all the articles included in that review were single case reports or case series, preventing firm conclusions. As a matter of fact, neither the proportion of patients who respond with long-term benefits or the mechanism of this effect is known. It may be a peculiar effect of local anesthetic on open sodium channels in patients with chronic pain. It may be a placebo effect. It may be due to a settling effect on CNS pathways. Notwithstanding this lack of information, therapeutic nerve blocks are an attractive option for some practitioners and for some patients when other options are not available or impractical.

To date, the best evidence for the efficacy of therapeutic nerve blocks is for blocks of the greater occipital nerve in the treatment of headache. Several studies using local anesthetics alone or in combination with a steroid have shown efficacy in reducing pain intensity and/or frequency of pain attacks in different forms of headache. The study design has been heterogenic. Most studies have been conducted as prospective case series or audits, using single injections or a series of procedures at variable intervals.[95-97] An observational study on the effect of repeated greater occipital nerve and supraorbital nerve blocks with bupivacaine (without a steroid) for migraine found that 85% of patients had a positive response during a 6-month observation period.[98] One randomized controlled trial on cervicogenic headache found occipital nerve blocks with a mixture of local anesthetic, opioid, and clonidine to be superior to placebo at 2-week follow-up.[99] A greater occipital nerve injection with steroid (without local anesthetic) was superior to placebo in preventing cluster headache attacks.[100] Another randomized controlled trial in chronic daily headache found a significant reduction in pain up to 4 weeks after the injection, with no difference between local anesthetic alone and its combination with a steroid.[101] Lastly, a more recent placebo-controlled trial on chronic headache showed superiority of a series of greater occipital nerve blocks with a local anesthetic at 4-week follow-up.[102] A caveat applies to placebo-controlled trials on occipital nerve blocks, namely, the limited ability to blind patients to the group allocation due to the cutaneous numbness caused by the nerve block.

The mechanisms underlying long-term effects of occipital nerve blocks in headache are unclear. The nerve does not supply structures that are potential primary triggers of headache syndromes. The functional connections between cervical and trigeminal system[103,104] may be involved in the effect of greater occipital nerve blocks in headache: Reducing the sensory input to the cervical system may lead to reduced nociceptive activity in the trigeminal system. This is supported by studies that explored the nociceptive trigeminal transmission with the nociceptive blink reflex, showing reduction in the reflex responses following nerve block.[105,106] Furthermore, greater occipital nerve block reduces allodynia at both trigeminal and cervical areas not primarily supplied by the nerve,[107] further supporting a modulatory effect of the block on central nociceptive pathways involved in headache.

The sphenopalatine ganglion is another potential target of local anesthetic blocks for the treatment of headache. The rationale is its anatomical connections with the trigeminal and parasympathetic system that are involved in symptoms associated with different forms of headache, in particular trigeminal autonomic cephalalgia. Block of the sphenopalatine ganglion has a long tradition in the treatment of headache.[108] The ganglion can be blocked via either the transnasal route or infrazygomatic percutaneous puncture. Some evidence for efficacy has been produced. According to a recent review, the published data support efficacy of the block for cluster headache and migraine in both the short and long term, although the data are not very robust.[108]

There are data on nerve blocks for the treatment of chronic shoulder pain. A randomized placebo-controlled trial on the treatment of shoulder pain after hemiplegic stroke found a single suprascapular nerve block with bupivacaine and steroid to be superior to placebo in terms of pain relief.[109] The number-needed-to-treat for 50% pain relief at 4 weeks was 4. Another randomized placebo-controlled trial studied the effect of suprascapular nerve block with bupivacaine, performed three times every 7 days, on frozen shoulder.[93] Both the bupivacaine and placebo group underwent a home exercise program. After 1 month, the bupivacaine and placebo group displayed a 64% and 13% pain reduction, respectively, with 15.8% improvement in shoulder function in the bupivacaine group versus 4% in the placebo group. This reproduced the results of a previous randomized placebo-controlled trial on shoulder pain in rheumatoid arthritis and degenerative disease of the shoulder. This study found clinically and statistically significant improvements in pain scores, disability scores, and range of movement in the group receiving suprascapular nerve block, compared with the placebo group, at weeks 1, 4, and 12.[110] A recent meta-analysis came to the conclusion that suprascapular nerve blocks provide better pain relief for 12 weeks compared with physical therapy and placebo injections in patients with chronic shoulder pain but is not superior to intra-articular injections.[111] The same review found evidence for better clinical outcomes when the block is performed under ultrasound guidance, compared to blind techniques and fluoroscopy guidance. In this regard, an ultrasound-guided technique of suprascapular nerve block has been developed that approaches the nerve at the supraclavicular region, resulting in better visualization of the nerve, compared with the traditional suprascapular technique.[112]

Several caveats apply to the mentioned data on therapeutic blocks. Most of the studies have not been performed in a randomized controlled manner. The few randomized controlled trials are characterized by small sample sizes, heterogenic clinical regimens, and the aforementioned difficulty in ensuring blinding to the group allocation. These factors limit our ability to attribute the positive outcomes to a specific effect of the local anesthetic blocks. Factors other than the blocks may account for the positive outcome or contribute to them. They include placebo effects, spontaneous healing, and regression to the mean. Furthermore, the basic science supporting the therapeutic efficacy of nerve blocks is almost inexistent, making explanations of the underlying mechanisms largely speculative.

In these authors' opinion, the earlier limitations should not prohibit the use of therapeutic blocks. The limited data available allow consideration of this practice for selected patients. Careful evaluation of alternative treatments, expected benefits, risks and costs associated with the procedure, and thorough patient information are mandatory. It is reasonable to predict that only a minority of patients have long-term relief of pain. Therefore, the indication for therapeutic nerve blocks should be restrictive. Alternative more evidence-based treatments must be tried or at least discussed with the patient before planning blocks. In the light of the weak literature and the small proportion of patients who benefit in the long term, the procedures should be of very low risk and performed by, or under supervision of, very experienced practitioners. This will minimize the risk–benefit ratio.

Realistic expectations have to be discussed with the patient. Nerve blocks cannot be expected to "fix" a chronic pain problem. Many patients will experience for the first time complete pain relief for few hours after the block. This may generate the unrealistic expectation that pain can be cured in this way. Patients have to be informed that complete pain relief is very rarely achieved in the long term.

There is no purpose in performing repeated nerve blocks for a chronic condition if the effects are short lasting, and blocks should not be offered indefinitely in patients who do not display long-term benefits. Also, restoration of activities is an important goal, for if function does not improve, the risk–benefit or cost–benefit ratio may be considered as unfavorable.

The use of therapeutic nerve blocks is an area of pain medicine that has potential but suffers of very limited scientific background. The availability of more data presented in this chapter, compared with the previous edition of this book, is encouraging but far from providing solid support for an evidence-based practice. Hopefully, future research will provide further support to clinical decision making.

Conclusion

Anesthesiologists were prominent among those who founded the discipline of pain medicine. From their background and training in surgical anesthesia, they brought with them the art of local anesthetic blocks. In a new discipline, these blocks were a powerful tool: They could stop the symptom of which the patient complained. Over the last 40 years, however, the standards of science in medicine have escalated. The art of local anesthetic blocks has not kept pace with the science required of them.

Most of the publicity concerning evidence-based medicine has centered on the standards set and expected for studies of the efficacy of treatments. For such studies, rules apply concerning randomization, blinding, controls, follow-up, outcome measures, and intention-to-treat analysis. These same rules do not apply to diagnostic tests, but others do.

The rules for operative anesthesia are straightforward and easy to apply. In operative anesthesia, the objective is to protect the patient from feeling pain once the surgery commences. Adequacy of anesthesia can be tested by applying a noxious stimulus and asking the patient of any effect. If they are numb, the patient, the anesthetist, and the surgeon are all satisfied. At a philosophical level, it does not matter if the patient had a placebo effect. The block, nevertheless, served its purpose.

A different set of rules applies to pain medicine. The situation differs in that the objective of local anesthetic blocks is to stop ongoing pain, be that for diagnostic, prognostic, or therapeutic purposes. This is a different idiom from that of securing surgical anesthesia.

Paramount is the validity of the local anesthetic block, and placebo effect is a serious, potential, confounding factor. It does matter if the patient has a placebo response when diagnostic and therapeutic decisions are based on that response. Notwithstanding the mysteries of the placebo response and what it means, a placebo response is likely a false-positive response. It means that any decision about diagnosis may not be correct and any decision about treatment may be wrong.

Because false-positive responses can occur, sometimes commonly, practitioners cannot assume that all positive responses to blocks are true positive. A block cannot be held to be valid unless it is subjected to some sort of control.

It is in this regard that the art of local anesthetic blocks has lagged behind the pace of contemporary science. Eminent authorities in the past have described a vast litany of the types of blocks that could be performed; some even implied that they should be done. At a scientific and clinical level, however, those recommendations pertained only to the execution of blocks. They did not address their validity and interpretation.

For prognostic blocks, the assumption has been that uncontrolled blocks will faithfully predict the outcome of treatment. This assumption may be convenient for expeditious practice, but it does not amount to evidence-based practice. Two confounding influences apply. The prediction of the blocks may be incorrect because the response to blocks is not valid, and the treatment may not work because its efficacy has not been established.

It is for these reasons that the present chapter does not resemble corresponding chapters in other books. Local anesthetic blocks have not been described just because they can be done. Instead, the present chapter has focused on why blocks might be done. Some degree of evidence is required to find the answer to that question. As a result, the present chapter does not describe blocks for which there is barely anecdotal evidence. Prominence has been given to those blocks for which there is evidence and in proportion to the volume and quality of evidence available.

The foundations of pain medicine in general and interventional pain medicine in particular depend on the validity of local anesthetic blocks. The evidence, at present, would indicate that whereas diagnostic medial branch blocks are sound, all other diagnostic blocks have uncertain validity. Medial branch blocks have been shown to protect healthy volunteers from experimentally induced pain, they have been shown to have target specificity, their false-positive rates are known and are large but can be reduced by using controls, and positive responses are associated with successful outcomes of treatment. For no other local anesthetic block have these requirements been satisfied.

In comparison with the previous version of this chapter,[113] some more evidence on the efficacy of therapeutic blocks has emerged, but the sparse data are in sobering contrast with the 8 years that have elapsed. The challenge, if not duty, of experts in this discipline is to make up the difference. It is often said that no evidence of efficacy is not evidence of no efficacy, but a retort applies. Assumption is not a substitute for evidence. Hopefully, future editions of this chapter can be enriched by a greater, appropriate body of evidence.

References

1. Cohen SP, Hameed H, Kurihara C, et al. The effect of sedation on the accuracy and treatment outcomes for diagnostic injections: a randomized, controlled, crossover study. *Pain Med* 2014;15(4):588–602.
2. Narouze S, Benzon HT, Provenzano DA, et al. Interventional spine and pain procedures in patients on antiplatelet and anticoagulant medications: guidelines from the American Society of Regional Anesthesia and Pain Medicine, the European Society of Regional Anaesthesia and Pain Therapy, the American Academy of Pain Medicine, the International Neuromodulation Society, the North American Neuromodulation Society, and the World Institute of Pain. *Reg Anesth Pain Med* 2015;40(3):182–212.
3. Moore DC, Batra MS. The components of an effective test dose prior to epidural block. *Anesthesiology* 1981;55(6):693–696.

4. Nancarrow C, Rutten AJ, Runciman WB, et al. Myocardial and cerebral drug concentrations and the mechanisms of death after fatal intravenous doses of lidocaine, bupivacaine, and ropivacaine in the sheep. *Anesth Analg* 1989;69(3):276–283.

5. Hoegberg LCG, Gosselin S. Lipid resuscitation in acute poisoning: after a decade of publications, what have we really learned? *Curr Opin Anaesthesiol* 2017;30:474–479.

6. Neal JM, Barrington MJ, Brull R, et al. The second ASRA practice advisory on neurologic complications associated with regional anesthesia and pain medicine: executive summary 2015. *Reg Anesth Pain Med* 2015;40(5):401–430.

7. Fanelli G, Casati A, Garancini P, et al. Nerve stimulator and multiple injection technique for upper and lower limb blockade: failure rate, patient acceptance, and neurologic complications. Study Group on Regional Anesthesia. *Anesth Analg* 1999;88(4):847–852.

8. Auroy Y, Benhamou D, Bargues L, et al. Major complications of regional anesthesia in France: the SOS Regional Anesthesia Hotline Service. *Anesthesiology* 2002;97(5):1274–1280.

9. Eichenberger U, Greher M, Curatolo M. Ultrasound in interventional pain management. *Tech Reg Anesth Pain Manage* 2004;8:171–178.

10. Evansa I, Logina I, Vanags I, et al. Ultrasound versus fluoroscopic-guided epidural steroid injections in patients with degenerative spinal diseases: a randomised study. *Eur J Anaesthesiol* 2015;32(4):262–268.

11. Auyong DB, Hostetter L, Yuan SC, et al. Evaluation of ultrasound-assisted thoracic epidural placement in patients undergoing upper abdominal and thoracic surgery: a randomized, double-blind study. *Reg Anesth Pain Med* 2017;42(2):204–209.

12. Perlas A, Chaparro LE, Chin KJ. Lumbar neuraxial ultrasound for spinal and epidural anesthesia: a systematic review and meta-analysis. *Reg Anesth Pain Med* 2016;41(2):251–260.

13. Siegenthaler A, Mlekusch S, Trelle S, et al. Accuracy of ultrasound-guided nerve blocks of the cervical zygapophysial joints. *Anesthesiology* 2012;117(2):347–352.

14. Finlayson RJ, Etheridge JPB, Vieira L, et al. A randomized comparison between ultrasound- and fluoroscopy-guided third occipital nerve block. *Reg Anesth Pain Med* 2013;38(3):212–217.

15. Finlayson RJ, Gupta G, Alhujairi M, et al. Cervical medial branch block: a novel technique using ultrasound guidance. *Reg Anesth Pain Med* 2012;37(2):219–223.

16. Fowler IM, Tucker AA, Weimerskirch BP, et al. A randomized comparison of the efficacy of 2 techniques for piriformis muscle injection: ultrasound-guided versus nerve stimulator with fluoroscopic guidance. *Reg Anesth Pain Med* 2014;39(2):126–132.

17. Soneji N, Bhatia A, Seib R, et al. Comparison of fluoroscopy and ultrasound guidance for sacroiliac joint injection in patients with chronic low back pain. *Pain Pract* 2016;16(5):537–544.

18. Neal JM. Ultrasound-guided regional anesthesia and patient safety: update of an evidence-based analysis. *Reg Anesth Pain Med* 2016;41(2):195–204.

19. Benzon HT, Huntoon MA, Rathmell JP. Improving the safety of epidural steroid injections. *JAMA* 2015;313(17):1713–1714.

20. Rathmell JP, Benzon HT, Dreyfuss P, et al. Safeguards to prevent neurologic complications after epidural steroid injections: consensus opinions from a multidisciplinary working group and national organizations. *Anesthesiology* 2015;122(5):974–984.

21. Sasso RC, Macadaeg K, Nordmann D, et al. Selective nerve root injections can predict surgical outcome for lumbar and cervical radiculopathy: comparison to magnetic resonance imaging. *J Spinal Disord Tech* 2005;18(6):471–478.

22. Haueisen DC, Smith BS, Myers SR, et al. The diagnostic accuracy of spinal nerve injection studies. Their role in the evaluation of recurrent sciatica. *Clin Orthop Relat Res* 1985(198):179–183.

23. Dooley JF, McBroom RJ, Taguchi T, et al. Nerve root infiltration in the diagnosis of radicular pain. *Spine* 1988;13(1):79–83.

24. van Akkerveeken PF. The diagnostic value of nerve root sheath infiltration. *Acta Orthop Scand Suppl* 1993;251:61–63.

25. Hogan QH, Erickson SJ, Haddox JD, et al. The spread of solutions during stellate ganglion block. *Reg Anesth* 1992;17(2):78–83.

26. Bruyns T, Devulder J, Vermeulen H, et al. Possible inadvertent subdural block following attempted stellate ganglion blockade. *Anaesthesia* 1991;46:747–749.

27. Higa K, Hirata K, Hirota K, et al. Retropharyngeal hematoma after stellate ganglion block: analysis of 27 patients reported in the literature. *Anesthesiology* 2006;105(6):1238–1245.

28. Rathmell JP, Michna E, Fitzgibbon DR, et al. Injury and liability associated with cervical procedures for chronic pain. *Anesthesiology* 2011;114(4):918–926.

29. Vadodaria B, Bridgens J, Richmond M. Pyogenic cervical epidural abscess and discitis following stellate ganglion block. *Anaesthesia* 2001;56:871–872.

30. Wulf H, Maier C. Complications and side effects of stellate ganglion blockade. Results of a questionnaire survey. *Anaesthesist* 1992;41:146–151.

31. Kapral S, Krafft P, Gosch M, et al. Ultrasound imaging for stellate ganglion block: direct visualization of puncture site and local anesthetic spread. A pilot study. *Reg Anesth* 1995;20:323–328.

32. Siegenthaler A, Mlekusch S, Schliessbach J, et al. Ultrasound imaging to estimate risk of esophageal and vascular puncture after conventional stellate ganglion block. *Reg Anesth Pain Med* 2012;37(2):224–227.

33. Bogduk N. The clinical anatomy of the cervical dorsal rami. *Spine* 1982;7:319–330.

34. Barnsley L, Bogduk N. Medial branch blocks are specific for the diagnosis of cervical zygapophyseal joint pain. *Reg Anesth* 1993;18:343–350.

35. Eichenberger U, Greher M, Kapral S, et al. Sonographic visualization and ultrasound-guided block of the third occipital nerve: prospective for a new method to diagnose C2-C3 zygapophysial joint pain. *Anesthesiology* 2006;104:303–308.

36. Siegenthaler A, Schliessbach J, Curatolo M, et al. Ultrasound anatomy of the nerves supplying the cervical zygapophyseal joints: an exploratory study. *Reg Anesth Pain Med* 2011;36(6):606–610.

37. Lord SM, Barnsley L, Bogduk N. The utility of comparative local anesthetic blocks versus placebo-controlled blocks for the diagnosis of cervical zygapophysial joint pain. *Clin J Pain* 1995;11:208–213.

38. Barnsley L, Lord S, Wallis B, et al. False-positive rates of cervical zygapophysial joint blocks. *Clin J Pain* 1993;9:124–130.

39. Barnsley L, Lord SM, Wallis BJ, et al. The prevalence of chronic cervical zygapophysial joint pain after whiplash. *Spine* 1995;20(1):20–25.

40. Lord SM, Barnsley L, Wallis BJ, et al. Chronic cervical zygapophysial joint pain after whiplash. A placebo-controlled prevalence study. *Spine* 1996;21:1737–1745.

41. Speldewinde GC, Bashford GM, Davidson IR. Diagnostic cervical zygapophyseal joint blocks for chronic cervical pain. *Med J Aust* 2001;174:174–176.

42. Sackett D, Haynes R, Guyatt G, et al. *Clinical Epidemiology: A Basic Science for Clinical Medicine.* Boston, MA: Little Brown; 1991.

43. Barnsley L. Percutaneous radiofrequency neurotomy for chronic neck pain: outcomes in a series of consecutive patients. *Pain Med* 2005;6(4):282–286.

44. Govind J, King W, Bailey B, et al. Radiofrequency neurotomy for the treatment of third occipital headache. *J Neurol Neurosurg Psychiat* 2003;74:88–93.

45. Lord SM, Barnsley L, Wallis BJ, et al. Percutaneous radio-frequency neurotomy for chronic cervical zygapophyseal-joint pain. *N Engl J Med* 1996;335(23):1721–1726.

46. MacVicar J, Borowczyk JM, MacVicar AM, et al. Cervical medial branch radiofrequency neurotomy in New Zealand. *Pain Med* 2012;13(5):647–654.

47. McDonald GJ, Lord SM, Bogduk N. Long-term follow-up of patients treated with cervical radiofrequency neurotomy for chronic neck pain. *Neurosurgery* 1999;45:61–68.

48. Siegenthaler A, Eichenberger U, Curatolo M. A shortened radiofrequency denervation method for cervical zygapophysial joint pain based on ultrasound localization of the nerves. *Pain Med* 2011;12(12):1703–1709.

49. Lord SM, Barnsley L, Wallis BJ, et al. Third occipital nerve headache: a prevalence study. *J Neurol Neurosurg Psychiatry* 1994;57(10):1187–1190.

50. Dreyfuss P, Schwarzer AC, Lau P, et al. Specificity of lumbar medial branch and L5 dorsal ramus blocks. A computed tomography study. *Spine* 1997;22:895–902.

51. Kaplan M, Dreyfuss P, Halbrook B, et al. The ability of lumbar medial branch blocks to anesthetize the zygapophysial joint. A physiologic challenge. *Spine* 1998;23:1847–1852.

52. Greher M, Moriggl B, Peng PW, et al. Ultrasound-guided approach for L5 dorsal ramus block and fluoroscopic evaluation in unpreselected cadavers. *Reg Anesth Pain Med* 2015;40(6):713–717.

53. Greher M, Scharbert G, Kamolz LP, et al. Ultrasound-guided lumbar facet nerve block: a sonoanatomic study of a new methodologic approach. *Anesthesiology* 2004;100:1242–1248.

54. Shim JK, Moon JC, Yoon KB, et al. Ultrasound-guided lumbar medial-branch block: a clinical study with fluoroscopy control. *Reg Anesth Pain Med* 2006;31(5):451–454.

55. Schwarzer AC, Aprill CN, Derby R, et al. The false-positive rate of uncontrolled diagnostic blocks of the lumbar zygapophysial joints. *Pain* 1994;58:195–200.

56. Manchikanti L, Pampati V, Fellows B, et al. Prevalence of lumbar facet joint pain in chronic low back pain. *Pain Physician* 1999;2(3):59–64.

57. Manchikanti L, Pampati V, Fellows B, et al. The diagnostic validity and therapeutic value of lumbar facet joint nerve blocks with or without adjuvant agents. *Curr Rev Pain* 2000;4(5):337–344.

58. Schwarzer AC, Aprill CN, Derby R, et al. Clinical features of patients with pain stemming from the lumbar zygapophysial joints. Is the lumbar facet syndrome a clinical entity? *Spine* 1994;19:1132–1137.

59. Schwarzer AC, Wang SC, Bogduk N, et al. Prevalence and clinical features of lumbar zygapophysial joint pain: a study in an Australian population with chronic low back pain. *Ann Rheum Dis* 1995;54:100–106.

60. Dreyfuss P, Halbrook B, Pauza K, et al. Efficacy and validity of radiofrequency neurotomy for chronic lumbar zygapophysial joint pain. *Spine* 2000;25:1270–1277.

61. Schofferman J, Kine G. Effectiveness of repeated radiofrequency neurotomy for lumbar facet pain. *Spine* 2004;29:2471–2473.

62. Poetscher AW, Gentil AF, Lenza M, et al. Radiofrequency denervation for facet joint low back pain: a systematic review. *Spine* 2014;39(14):E842–E849.

63. Juch JNS, Maas ET, Ostelo R, et al. Effect of radiofrequency denervation on pain intensity among patients with chronic low back pain: the Mint randomized clinical trials. *JAMA* 2017;318(1):68–81.

64. Provenzano DA, Buvanendran A, de Leon-Casasola OA, et al. Interpreting the MINT randomized trials evaluating radiofrequency ablation for lumbar

facet and sacroiliac joint pain: a call from ASRA for better education, study design, and performance. *Reg Anesth Pain Med* 2018;43(1):68–71.

65. Bogduk N, Macintosh J, Marsland A. Technical limitations to the efficacy of radiofrequency neurotomy for spinal pain. *Neurosurgery* 1987;20:529–535.

66. Cohen SP, Williams KA, Kurihara C, et al. Multicenter, randomized, comparative cost-effectiveness study comparing 0, 1, and 2 diagnostic medial branch (facet joint nerve) block treatment paradigms before lumbar facet radiofrequency denervation. *Anesthesiology* 2010;113(2):395–405.

67. Cohen SP, Strassels SA, Kurihara C, et al. Establishing an optimal "cutoff" threshold for diagnostic lumbar facet blocks: a prospective correlational study. *Clin J Pain* 2013;29(5):382–391.

68. Headache Classification Committee of the International Headache Society. The International Classification of Headache Disorders, 3rd edition (beta version). *Cephalalgia* 2013;33(9):629–808.

69. Dreyfuss P, Michaelsen M, Fletcher D. Atlanto-occipital and lateral atlanto-axial joint pain patterns. *Spine* 1993;19:1125–1131.

70. Aprill C, Axinn MJ, Bogduk N. Occipital headaches stemming from the lateral atlanto-axial (C1-2) joint. *Cephalalgia* 2002;22:15–22.

71. Narouze SN, Casanova J, Mekhail N. The longitudinal effectiveness of lateral atlantoaxial intra-articular steroid injection in the treatment of cervicogenic headache. *Pain Med* 2007;8(2):184–188.

72. Joseph B, Kumar B. Gallie's fusion for atlantoaxial arthrosis with occipital neuralgia. *Spine* 1994;19(4):454–455.

73. Ghanayem AJ, Leventhal M, Bohlman HH. Osteoarthrosis of the atlanto-axial joints. Long-term follow-up after treatment with arthrodesis. *J Bone Joint Surg Am* 1996;78(9):1300–1307.

74. Schaeren S, Jeanneret B. Atlantoaxial osteoarthritis: case series and review of the literature. *Eur Spine J* 2005;14(5):501–506.

75. Kennedy DJ, Engel A, Kreiner DS, et al. Fluoroscopically guided diagnostic and therapeutic intra-articular sacroiliac joint injections: a systematic review. *Pain Med* 2015;16:1500–1518.

76. Klauser A, De Zordo T, Feuchtner G, et al. Feasibility of ultrasound-guided sacroiliac joint injection considering sonoanatomic landmarks at two different levels in cadavers and patients. *Arthritis Rheum* 2008;59(11):1618–1624.

77. Maigne JY, Aivaliklis A, Pfefer F. Results of sacroiliac joint double block and value of sacroiliac pain provocation tests in 54 patients with low back pain. *Spine* 1996;21(16):1889–1892.

78. Bogduk N, Bartsch T. Headaches of cervical origin: focus on anatomy and physiology. In: Goadsby P, Silberstein S, Dodick D, eds. *Chronic Daily Headache for Clinicians*. London: BC Decker; 2005:369–381.

79. Grob KR, Neuhuber WL, Kissling RO. Innervation of the sacroiliac joint of the human. *Z Rheumatol* 1995;54:117–122.

80. Roberts SL, Burnham RS, Ravichandiran K, et al. Cadaveric study of sacroiliac joint innervation: implications for diagnostic blocks and radiofrequency ablation. *Reg Anesth Pain Med* 2014;39(6):456–464.

81. Dreyfuss P, Henning T, Malladi N, et al. The ability of multi-site, multi-depth sacral lateral branch blocks to anesthetize the sacroiliac joint complex. *Pain Med* 2009;10(4):679–688.

82. Finlayson RJ, Etheridge JB, Elgueta MF, et al. A randomized comparison between ultrasound- and fluoroscopy-guided sacral lateral branch blocks. *Reg Anesth Pain Med* 2017;42(3):400–406.

83. King W, Ahmed SU, Baisden J, et al. Diagnosis and treatment of posterior sacroiliac complex pain: a systematic review with comprehensive analysis of the published data. *Pain Med* 2015;16(2):257–265.

84. Cohen SP, Hurley RW, Buckenmaier CC III, et al. Randomized placebo-controlled study evaluating lateral branch radiofrequency denervation for sacroiliac joint pain. *Anesthesiology* 2008;109(2):279–288.

85. Patel N. Twelve-month follow-up of a randomized trial assessing cooled radiofrequency denervation as a treatment for sacroiliac region pain. *Pain Pract* 2016;16(2):154–167.

86. Patel N, Gross A, Brown L, et al. A randomized, placebo-controlled study to assess the efficacy of lateral branch neurotomy for chronic sacroiliac joint pain. *Pain Med* 2012;13(3):383–398.

87. van Tilburg CW, Schuurmans FA, Stronks DL, et al. Randomized sham-controlled double-blind multicenter clinical trial to ascertain the effect of percutaneous radiofrequency treatment for sacroiliac joint pain: three-month results. *Clin J Pain* 2016;32(11):921–926.

88. Schiferer A, Gore C, Gorove L, et al. A randomized controlled trial of femoral nerve blockade administered preclinically for pain relief in femoral trauma. *Anesth Analg* 2007;105(6):1852–1854.

89. Osinowo OA, Zahrani M, Softah A. Effect of intercostal nerve block with 0.5% bupivacaine on peak expiratory flow rate and arterial oxygen saturation in rib fractures. *J Trauma* 2004;56(2):345–347.

90. Ilfeld BM. Continuous peripheral nerve blocks: an update of the published evidence and comparison with novel, alternative analgesic modalities. *Anesth Analg* 2017;124(1):308–335.

91. Curatolo M. Regional anesthesia in pain management. *Curr Opin Anaesthesiol* 2016;29(5):614–619.

92. Detaille V, Busnel F, Ravary H, et al. Use of continuous interscalene brachial plexus block and rehabilitation to treat complex regional pain syndrome of the shoulder. *Ann Phys Rehabil Med* 2010;53(6–7):406–416.

93. Dahan TH, Fortin L, Pelletier M, et al. Double blind randomized clinical trial examining the efficacy of bupivacaine suprascapular nerve blocks in frozen shoulder. *J Rheumatol* 2000;27(6):1464–1469.

94. Vlassakov KV, Narang S, Kissin I. Local anesthetic blockade of peripheral nerves for treatment of neuralgias: systematic analysis. *Anesth Analg* 2011;112(6):1487–1493.

95. Afridi SK, Shields KG, Bhola R, et al. Greater occipital nerve injection in primary headache syndromes—prolonged effects from a single injection. *Pain* 2006;122(1–2):126–129.

96. Peres MF, Stiles MA, Siow HC, et al. Greater occipital nerve blockade for cluster headache. *Cephalalgia* 2002;22:520–522.

97. Jurgens TP, Muller P, Seedorf H, et al. Occipital nerve block is effective in craniofacial neuralgias but not in idiopathic persistent facial pain. *J Headache Pain* 2012;13(3):199–213.

98. Caputi CA, Firetto V. Therapeutic blockade of greater occipital and supra-orbital nerves in migraine patients. *Headache* 1997;37:174–179.

99. Naja ZM, El-Rajab M, Al-Tannir MA, et al. Occipital nerve blockade for cervicogenic headache: a double-blind randomized controlled clinical trial. *Pain Pract* 2006;6(2):89–95.

100. Ambrosini A, Vandenheede M, Rossi P, et al. Suboccipital injection with a mixture of rapid- and long-acting steroids in cluster headache: a double-blind placebo-controlled study. *Pain* 2005;118(1–2):92–96.

101. Ashkenazi A, Matro R, Shaw JW, et al. Greater occipital nerve block using local anaesthetics alone or with triamcinolone for transformed migraine: a randomised comparative study. *J Neurol Neurosurg Psychiat* 2008;79(4):415–417.

102. Inan LE, Inan N, Karadas O, et al. Greater occipital nerve blockade for the treatment of chronic migraine: a randomized, multicenter, double-blind, and placebo-controlled study. *Acta Neurol Scand* 2015;132:270–277.

103. Bartsch T, Goadsby PJ. The trigeminocervical complex and migraine: current concepts and synthesis. *Curr Pain Headache Rep* 2003;7(5):371–376.

104. Piovesan EJ, Kowacs PA, Oshinsky ML. Convergence of cervical and trigeminal sensory afferents. *Curr Pain Headache Rep* 2003;7(5):377–383.

105. Busch V, Jakob W, Juergens T, et al. Functional connectivity between trigeminal and occipital nerves revealed by occipital nerve blockade and nociceptive blink reflexes. *Cephalalgia* 2006;26(1):50–55.

106. Busch V, Jakob W, Juergens T, et al. Occipital nerve blockade in chronic cluster headache patients and functional connectivity between trigeminal and occipital nerves. *Cephalalgia* 2007;27(11):1206–1214.

107. Ashkenazi A, Young WB. The effects of greater occipital nerve block and trigger point injection on brush allodynia and pain in migraine. *Headache* 2005;45(4):350–354.

108. Robbins MS, Robertson CE, Kaplan E, et al. The sphenopalatine ganglion: anatomy, pathophysiology, and therapeutic targeting in headache. *Headache* 2016;56(2):240–258.

109. Adey-Wakeling Z, Crotty M, Shanahan EM. Suprascapular nerve block for shoulder pain in the first year after stroke: a randomized controlled trial. *Stroke* 2013;44(11):3136–3141.

110. Shanahan EM, Ahern M, Smith M, et al. Suprascapular nerve block (using bupivacaine and methylprednisolone acetate) in chronic shoulder pain. *Ann Rheum Dis* 2003;62(5):400–406.

111. Chang KV, Hung CY, Wu WT, et al. Comparison of the effectiveness of suprascapular nerve block with physical therapy, placebo, and intra-articular injection in management of chronic shoulder pain: a meta-analysis of randomized controlled trials. *Arch Phys Med Rehabil* 2016;97(8):1366–1380.

112. Siegenthaler A, Moriggl B, Mlekusch S, et al. Ultrasound-guided suprascapular nerve block, description of a novel supraclavicular approach. *Reg Anesth Pain Med* 2012;37(3):325–328.

113. Curatolo M, Bogduk N. Diagnostic and therapeutic nerve blocks. In: Fishman SM, Ballantyne JC, Rathmell JP, eds. *Bonica's Management of Pain*. 4th ed. Philadelphia: Lippincott William & Wilkins; 2010:1401–1423.

114. Greher M, Moriggl B, Curatolo M, et al. Sonographic visualization and ultrasound-guided blockade of the greater occipital nerve: a comparison of two selective techniques confirmed by anatomical dissection. *Br J Anaesth* 2010;104(5):637–642.

CHAPTER 99

Epidural Steroid Injections

TIMOTHY PHILIP MAUS and NIKOLAI BOGDUK

Definition

Lumbar epidural steroid injections (ESIs) are a minimally invasive procedure designed to treat lumbar radicular pain. They involve inserting a needle into a location from which medication can be delivered onto the affected spinal nerve, the dorsal root ganglion, or its roots. The medication delivered includes a corticosteroid preparation but variously may also contain a local anesthetic preparation or normal saline.

Steroid preparations are used in the belief that radicular pain is caused not just by compression but also by inflammation of the target nerve. There is both clinical and experimental evidence that an inflammatory component is necessary for the expression of radicular pain.[1] Clinically, large disk herniations with significant neural compression may be asymptomatic,[2] whereas severe radicular pain may exist without detectable root compression.[3] The size or shape of a disk herniation, or change in size or shape over time, does not correlate with clinical presentation or course.[4] Experimentally, it is well established that the natural history of disk herniation is resolution, mediated by macrophage-produced metalloproteases, abetted by neovascularization also induced by chemical signalling.[5] The disk nucleus pulposus is known to be immunogenic with inflammatory mediators (phospholipase A_2; prostaglandin E_2; interleukins 1α, 1β, 6; tumor necrosis factor, and nitric oxide) all detected in relationship to disk herniations.[1] Available evidence suggests that both mechanical compression and an inflammatory component are necessary for radicular pain.[6,7] This provides a rationale for the use of an anti-inflammatory corticosteroid preparation as a therapeutic agent.

Over the years, various steroid preparations, in various dosages, have been used. The original agent was hydrocortisone.[8] Subsequently, depot preparations were introduced, such as those of methylprednisolone, betamethasone, and triamcinolone. Of late, dexamethasone has enjoyed resurgence.

These preparations have typically been injected along with local anesthetic agents, but the rationale for using local anesthetics has never been expressly articulated. Ostensibly, early practitioners used local anesthetics in order to make the injection less painful, but modern experience shows that epidural injections are largely painless if performed carefully, and in those cases in which injection is painful, the sources of pain are not ones that are simply anesthetized by adding local anesthetic to the injected medication.

In some procedures, local anesthetic is used to provide what some practitioners call a "diagnostic phase." The belief is that steroids do not take effect until days after their injection and that any immediate relief of pain must be due to the local anesthetic and, therefore, that relief serves as a diagnostic block that proves that the correct nerve was targeted. The rationale for this belief is mitigated by the reciprocal facts that steroids can have a local anesthetic effect[9] and that local anesthetics have an anti-inflammatory effect.[10] Consequently, the routine use of local anesthetic may not be well founded. Additionally, simultaneous optimization of diagnostic and therapeutic effects is not possible. Evidence supports greater therapeutic effect with central delivery of corticosteroids to the ventral epidural space.[11] Centrally delivered injectate is not segment specific; true selective blocks must be performed at and peripheral to the neural foramen.[12]

Background

The history of ESIs is characterized by tension. For a long time, the tension was between reported experience and evidence from controlled trials. Most recently, it has been tension between different types of systematic reviews of the evidence. At the heart of these tensions are driving forces and various differences.

A fundamental driving force is that many physicians want epidural steroids to be an accepted treatment because it is an intervention that is simple to perform, is not time consuming, and which they can readily provide. Many observational studies fed this desire with reports of good success rates, so much so that ESI became entrenched as common, if not standard, practice. This established the basis for the first tension. The evidence from controlled trials did not corroborate the great success rates and in many instances questioned if steroids had any appreciable attributable effect.

The contemporary tension lies between reviews of the literature, both systematic and otherwise, that produce conflicting conclusions. Authors of reviews differ in the techniques that they apply, the literature that they retrieve, their interpretations of that literature, and the severity of their critical analysis. Whereas some reviews include all of the literature, others—including ones called Cochrane reviews—restrict their retrieval to randomized controlled trials (RCT), even though Cochrane himself called for reviews to include all studies, not just controlled trials.[13]

A fundamental difference, however, is that many reviews lump the literature; they do not distinguish between procedures on technical grounds. Yet, there are at least seven different ways of delivering epidural steroids. Each differs by route of administration, the accuracy of needle placement, and the dispersal of injectate. Each of these factors can affect the effectiveness of the treatment, either potentially or actually. Furthermore, the available evidence for different procedures differs in quantity and quality.

Techniques

The various techniques for ESIs differ primarily according to target and route of administration. In the caudal route, the needle is inserted through the sacral hiatus, and the target is the epidural space. In the interlaminar route, the needle is inserted between consecutive laminae, and the target is the dorsal epidural space, with the hope for ventral distribution. In the transforaminal (TF) route, the needle is placed just inside an intervertebral foramen, and the target is the spinal nerve, the dorsal root ganglion, and its roots, which traverse that foramen.

A second distinction is whether the needle is inserted under image guidance or without imaging (i.e., "blind"). A third distinction is if that image guidance is fluoroscopy or computed tomography (CT).

As a result of these several technical distinctions, at least seven versions of "epidural steroids" can be recognized (Table 99.1). TF injections are performed only under image guidance; there is no "blind" version of this procedure. Caudal injections are performed blind or under fluoroscopy; although CT or ultrasound guidance might be used, there is no substantial literature on CT or ultrasound-guided caudal injections.

TABLE 99.1   Technical Variants of Epidural Steroid Injections

Guidance	Route		
	Caudal	Interlaminar	Transforaminal
Blind	Yes	Yes	—
Fluoroscopy	Yes	Yes	Yes
CT	—	Yes	Yes

NOTE: Techniques that are commonly practiced and reported in the literature are indicated by YES.
CT, computed tomography.

CAUDAL INJECTIONS: TECHNIQUE

The purported attraction of caudal injections is that they are easy to perform, and because the needle is placed distal to the dural sac, unintended penetration of the dural sac is avoided. Another advantage is that multiple nerves can be targeted with a single injection, if and when that is the desired outcome. The corollary of these advantages, however, is that the steroid preparation has to be propelled by a large volume of injectate in order to disperse it rostrally toward the target nerve or nerves, and hence, it will be of reduced concentration at a given epidural site.

When caudal injections are performed "blind," the sacral hiatus is located by palpation, and the needle is introduced through the overlying skin until it is felt to penetrate the membrane that encloses the hiatus. Once the needle is placed, a steroid preparation mixed with local anesthetic or normal saline, is injected. Typical volumes are 10 to 15 mL, but volumes as large as 64 mL have been reported.[14]

When caudal injections are performed under fluoroscopy, the sacral hiatus is visualized directly, and a needle is introduced

into it. Correct depth of penetration and entry into the sacral canal can be determined using a lateral view (Fig. 99.1). A test dose of contrast medium can then be injected in order to confirm flow into the sacral canal, exclude intravascular injection, and determine the volume of injection required to reach the target level. Thereafter, the therapeutic agent and its vehicle can be injected.

The cardinal liability of the "blind" technique is that the physician has no means of verifying the final location of their needle. Consequently, caudal injections can fail to enter the sacral canal in up to 35% of cases.[15–19] Injections can lie dorsal to the sacrum or coccyx (Fig. 99.2A), or be intravascular (Fig. 99.2B),[20] the latter despite no blood appearing on aspiration before injection. For these reasons, many physicians now prefer to perform caudal injections under image guidance.

CAUDAL INJECTIONS: EVIDENCE

The evidentiary support for epidural steroid administration by the caudal route for radicular pain is limited and contradictory. Very few studies have used image guidance; hence, the unguided and image-guided evidence will be considered here collectively. In four nonimage-guided, randomized controlled explanatory trials with 12 months follow-up from 1971 to 2009, there was no long-term efficacy of caudal epidural injections.[21–24] For example, a double-blind RCT of nonimage-guided caudal administration of steroid and local anesthetic versus saline (N = 23) showed an improvement in the steroid group in pain and function at 4 weeks relative to the control arm; at 1 year, there was no difference in pain and functional outcomes.[22] A short-term, randomized trial of caudal epidural steroid plus local anesthetic versus local anesthetic alone (N = 48, unguided) showed no difference between the

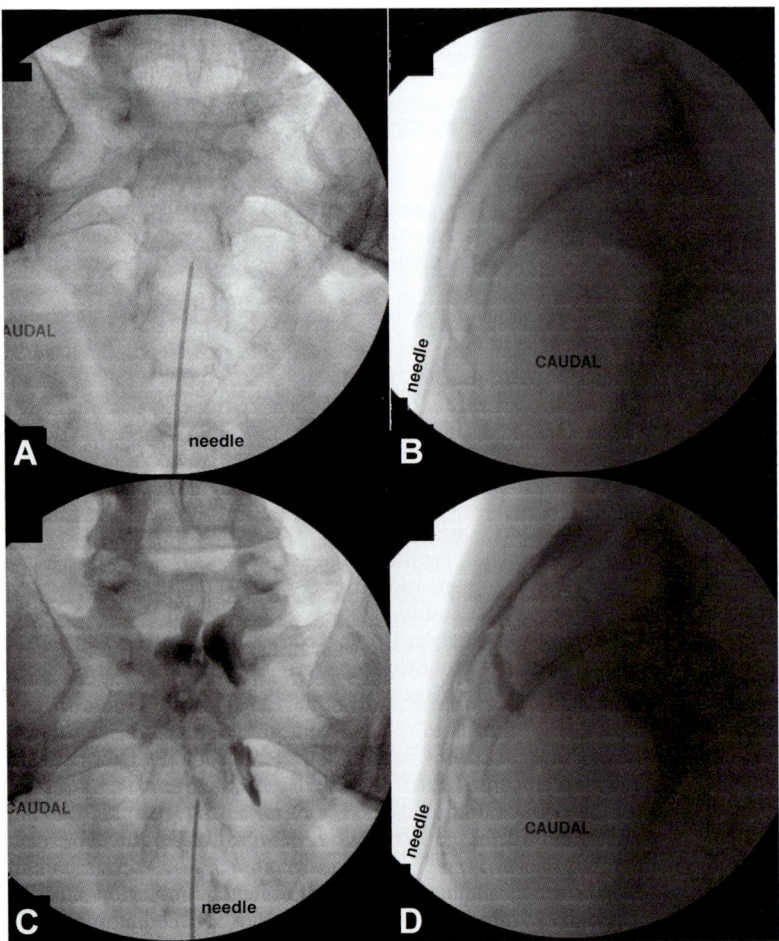

FIGURE 99.1 Fluoroscopy images of a caudal injection of steroids. **A:** Posterior view showing a needle inserted into the sacral hiatus. **B:** Lateral view showing the needle correctly placed in the sacral canal. **C:** Posterior view after injection of contrast medium, showing flow of contrast medium as far as the L5 nerves. **D:** Lateral view after injection of contrast medium, showing flow of contrast medium within the sacral canal and epidural space. *(Images kindly provided by Dr. Milton Landers, of Wichita, KS.)*

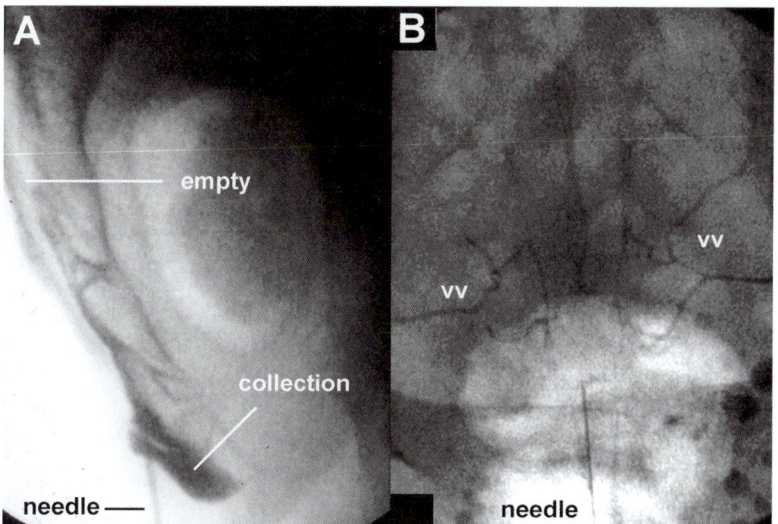

FIGURE 99.2 Fluoroscopy views of needles placed in the wrong location during the conduct of a caudal injection. **A:** Lateral view showing a needle that missed the sacral canal and passed dorsal to the sacrum. When injected, contrast medium forms a collection dorsal to the sacrum caudally, and the sacral canal is empty of contrast medium. **B:** Posterior view showing a needle correctly having entered the sacral canal but entering an epidural vein (vv). Subsequent injection of contrast medium is intravenous. *(Images kindly provided by Dr. Paul Dreyfuss, of Seattle, WA.)*

groups at follow-up of 1 to 3 months.[25] In another randomized trial of steroid plus local anesthetic versus local anesthetic plus saline (N = 183, unguided), the corticosteroid group had greater improvements in functional recovery than the control arm out of 1 year, but the magnitude of the differential improvement was not clinically relevant.[26]

In the current decade, a randomized, double-blind, controlled trial of caudal epidural steroid plus local anesthetic versus local anesthetic alone (N = 120, fluoroscopic guidance) showed both groups improved, and there was a significantly greater but quantitatively modest improvement in pain and functional recovery at 3 months for the steroid group, but no differences at 6 and 12 months, and no difference in opioid use at any time point.[27] The improvement noted in both groups is confounded by multiple repeat injections over the year with no reporting of the temporal relationship between the repeat injections and the pain and functional assessments.[27] A high-quality randomized controlled, blinded (patients, assessors) trial compared epidural corticosteroids versus epidural saline versus subcutaneous saline (N = 116, ultrasound guidance). There were no statistically nor clinically significant differences in pain, function, or quality of life (EuroQol) at 6 weeks, 12 weeks, or 52 weeks follow-up. All groups improved, in that at entry, all patients had a clinically documented radiculopathy; at 52 weeks, 27% of patients persisted with a radiculopathy, without difference between the groups.[28] A short-term (12 weeks, N = 163, unguided) randomized trial compared three different steroid preparations plus local anesthetic versus local anesthetic alone. There were no differences in pain and functional recovery at 4 weeks, whereas measurements at 12 weeks favored the steroid groups.[29]

A systematic review[30] identified only one RCT addressing caudal ESIs in neurogenic claudication patients.[31] This trial (N = 40, fluoroscopic guidance) compared caudal administration of steroid plus local anesthetic versus local anesthetic alone, with 1 year follow-up. Both groups improved, but there was no difference between the groups in pain relief, function recovery, or opioid use.[31] This study is another confounded by multiple injections with uncertain temporal relationship to assessment. A retrospective study of neurogenic claudication patients (N = 95, fluoroscopic guidance, follow-up 5 to 76 months, mean 32 months) receiving caudal epidural injections showed very modest improvements, with only 35% of patients having a 50% improvement in pain and only 36% having a 2-point improvement in the Roland-Morris Disability Questionnaire.[32] A small prospective cohort study (N = 34, follow-up 1 year, mean 2.2 fluoroscopically guided injections) reported 54% of patients had 50% pain relief and 51% had improved waking tolerance at 1 year.[33]

CAUDAL INJECTIONS: ADVERSE EVENTS

Adverse events with caudal ESIs are uncommon but do occur. In a series of 257 fluoroscopically guided injections in 139 patients, no major adverse events were noted.[34] There were 15.6% minor adverse events per injection, primarily consisting of transient central steroid effects (flushing, nonpositional headache, insomnia). There were no dural punctures. An explanatory trial of 441 caudal injections in 120 patients reported no major adverse events; minor adverse events were not recorded.[27] A more detailed reporting of minor adverse events in a series of 100 patients undergoing fluoroscopically guided caudal injections described minor complications in 24% of patients; the most commonly reported was soreness at the injection site (18%).[20]

A recent single-center adverse event study reported 10,151 caudal injections over the span of a decade.[35] There were three major adverse events in this series: one epidural hematoma, one paracoccygeal abscess, and one case of infectious spondylitis with epidural abscess. The most common minor adverse event was symptom aggravation in 11 patients (0.1%). Numerous case reports have described rare events, including transient blindness, retinal necrosis, chemical meningitis, arachnoiditis, epidural hematoma, and epidural abscess.[30]

INTERLAMINAR INJECTIONS: TECHNIQUE

For interlaminar ESI, a needle is passed through an interlaminar space that is closest to the target nerve. The needle is inserted usually along the midline through the interspinous ligament or slightly to the side of this ligament. The procedure requires that the needle penetrates the ligamentum flavum to enter the epidural space but falls short of piercing the dural sac.

When performed "blind," the physician relies on "loss of resistance" to detect entry into the epidural space. A syringe, filled with air or normal saline, or both, is attached to the needle and pressurized as the needle advances. When the tip of the needle is in the ligamentum flavum, the ligament resists injection, but once the tip enters the epidural space, the resistance suddenly drops. Upon loss of resistance, the medication is injected. A steroid preparation can be injected alone or mixed with local anesthetic or normal saline, in total volumes of 2 mL to 43 mL,[14] with volumes of 2 to 5 mL being typical.

When performed under fluoroscopy, interlaminar injection starts with inserting a needle, in a posterior view, onto the lower lamina of the interlaminar space that is the target segmental level.[36] Noting the depth of this insertion serves to determine the depth of the ligamentum flavum. The needle is then readjusted to aim at the interlaminar space and is inserted as far as the previously noted depth plus a touch more,

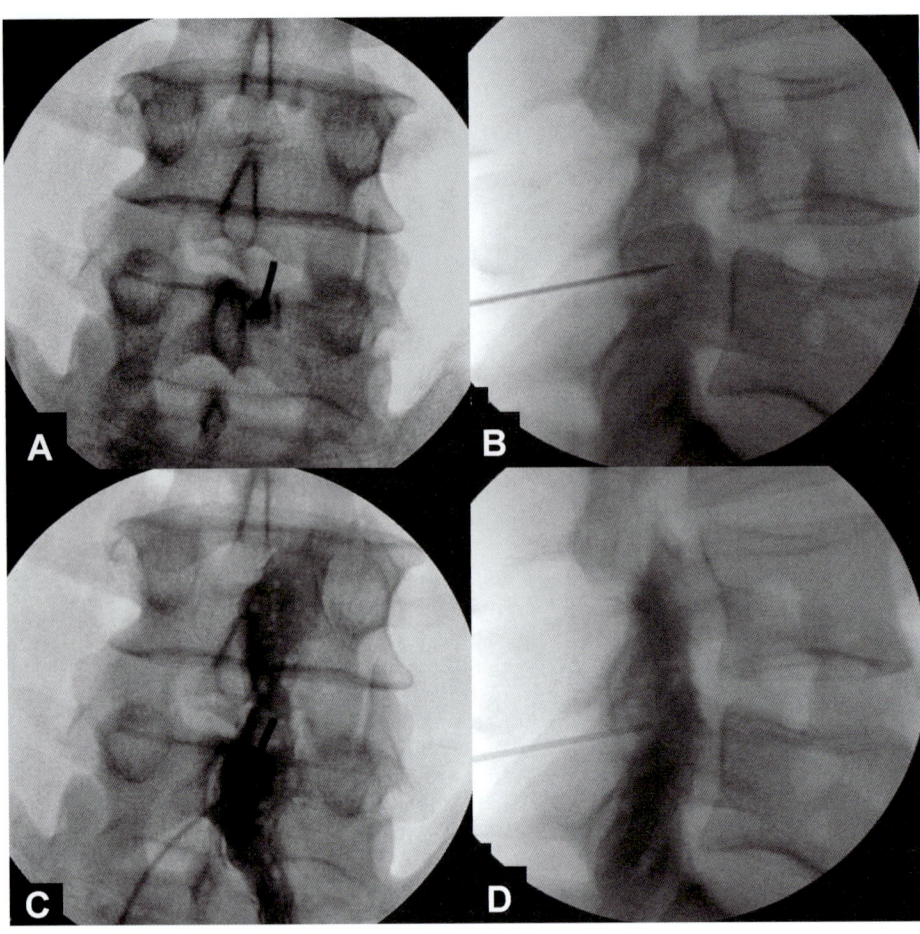

FIGURE 99.3 Stages in the conduct of an interlaminar injection under fluoroscopy. **A:** A posterior view showing a spinal needle inserted through an interlaminar space. **B:** A lateral view showing the tip of the needle just reaching the epidural space. **C:** A posterior view after injection of contrast medium showing correct spread of contrast medium across the epidural space. **D:** A lateral view showing spread of contrast medium across the epidural space. *(Images kindly provided by Dr. Milton Landers, Wichita, KS and reproduced with permission from International Spine Intervention Society. Lumbar interlaminar access. In: Bogduk N, ed. Practice Guidelines for Spinal Diagnostic and Treatment Procedures. 2nd ed. San Francisco, CA: International Spine Intervention Society; 2013:443–456.)*

so that the tip engages the ligament (Fig. 99.3). This step guards against testing loss of resistance at too shallow depth. Final depth of insertion can then be determined by either of two methods.

If loss of resistance is used, a pressurized syringe is used as the needle is advanced through the ligamentum flavum. Once loss of resistance is felt, insertion is stopped, and the depth of insertion is checked on a lateral or contralateral oblique view. The tip of the needle should project just beyond the spinolaminar line or interlaminar line, respectively (see Fig. 99.3).

An alternative technique relies on imaging rather than loss of resistance. The needle is inserted while monitoring its progress on lateral screening. Insertion is stopped once the tip projects just past the spinolaminar line.

Once the tip of the needle is in the epidural space, aspiration is performed to check for cerebrospinal fluid (CSF). Thereafter,

a test dose of contrast medium is injected to confirm that it spreads in the epidural space and is not intravascular (see Fig. 99.3). If correct placement is confirmed, the desired medication can be injected.

Many physicians prefer fluoroscopic guidance because it avoids the liabilities of the blind technique. Without image guidance, injections can be subdural or superficial to the ligamentum flavum in some 17% of cases,[15,37] or they can be intravascular (Fig. 99.4). Errors are more common in patients with large body mass index,[18] when landmarks are difficult to palpate.[17] Furthermore, even if the needle is accurately placed in the epidural space, the injectate can fail to reach the target level[38,39] or can remain in the posterior epidural space and not reach the disk nerve root interface.[38] Image guidance checks for these liabilities before any therapeutic agents are injected.

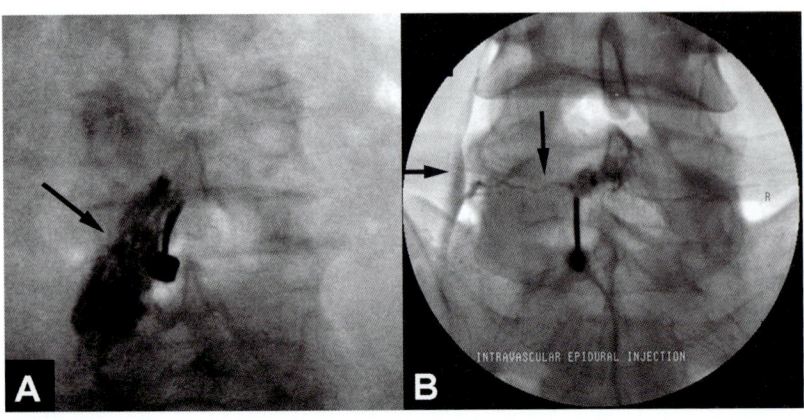

FIGURE 99.4 Fluoroscopy views of misplaced needles in the conduct of a lumbar interlaminar injection. **A:** Posterior view showing injection of contrast medium into the multifidus muscle (*arrow*). **B:** Posterior view showing injection of contrast medium into an epidural vein and drained into an ascending lumbar vein (*arrows*). *(Images kindly provided by Dr. Milton Landers, Wichita, KS and reproduced with permission from International Spine Intervention Society. Lumbar interlaminar access. In: Bogduk N, ed. Practice Guidelines for Spinal Diagnostic and Treatment Procedures. 2nd ed. San Francisco, CA: International Spine Intervention Society; 2013:443–456.)*

NONIMAGE-GUIDED INTERLAMINAR TECHNIQUE: EVIDENCE

A recent systematic review of nonimage-guided interlaminar injections examined 21 observational, 9 pragmatic, and 9 explanatory studies. There was no evidence supporting benefit for unguided injections beyond 3 to 6 weeks in either radicular pain or neurogenic claudication.[40] An RCT (N = 228, radicular pain) series of three unguided steroid injections versus interspinous saline control injections showed an improvement in leg pain and a nonstatistically significant improvement in function, at 3 weeks only. There was no significant benefit in any pain or functional measure, return to work, or need for surgery from 6 to 52 weeks. There was no benefit of three over one injection.[41,42] Another explanatory trial (N = 158, one to three injections, radicular pain) used epidural saline as the control. Mean leg pain scores improved at 6 weeks but not at 12 weeks. There was no difference in categorical outcomes of global improvement at any time point out of 12 weeks. Secondary outcomes were no different between the active and control groups at 12 weeks.[43] A third RCT (N = 85, three injections, radicular pain) compared epidural steroid to epidural saline injections. The primary outcome was a semiquantitative global perceived effect measure, which was not different between the two groups at 35 days (study endpoint). Secondary measures of pain and functional improvement also did not differ between the groups.[44]

The evidence supporting short-term benefit was conflicting and of low quality, culminating in a recommendation that nonimage-guided injections should be restricted to the rare settings where fluoroscopy is not available.[40] This is in concert with the recommendations of the U.S. Food and Drug Administration (FDA) Safe Use Initiative on ESIs, that multiplanar image guidance is recommended for all epidural injections.[45]

IMAGE-GUIDED INTERLAMINAR TECHNIQUE: EVIDENCE

Even image-guided interlaminar injections are challenged by the inability of the operator to control the distribution of delivered medications. This is particularly problematic with midline interlaminar injections, where spread from the insensate dorsal epidural space to the target of epidural injections, the ventral epidural space, lateral recess, and neural foramen may occur only infrequently and unpredictably. Injectate has been documented reaching the ventral epidural space in only 36% to 51% of injections.[46,47] A systematic review of fluoroscopically guided interlaminar injections revealed no explanatory trials and documented only modest short-term improvements in pain.[48]

An RCT (N = 120, radicular pain) compared the interlaminar epidural injection of steroid plus local anesthetic versus local anesthetic alone.[49] This was considered a pragmatic trial given the potential therapeutic effects of the local anesthetic. Both groups demonstrated significant improvement (50% decrement) over baseline in pain and function at 3, 6, and 12 months. There was no difference between the groups at 3 and 12 months; scores at 6 months favored the steroid group. This study allowed multiple injections and is again confounded by no reporting of the temporal relationship of the injections to the assessments.[49] A small observational trial (N = 21, radicular pain) noted that 28% of patients had complete pain relief at 3 months, whereas 38% achieved 50% pain relief.[50] A retrospective trial (N = 40, radicular pain) compared interlaminar versus TF ESIs. There was more short-term improvement in pain in the TF group, and over 12-month follow-up, more interlaminar patients progressed to surgical intervention.[51]

Four pragmatic studies addressed the efficacy of lateral parasagittal interlaminar injections in comparison to midline injections or TF injections.[52–55] The evidence suggests that parasagittal interlaminar injections have improved outcomes when compared to midline injections in radicular pain patients

and approach the outcomes achieved with TF injections. This is likely due to the greater delivery of injectate to the ventral epidural space with parasagittal versus midline injections. This promotes parasagittal interlaminar injections as a useful strategy in the face of foraminal stenosis, which may make effective TF injections more difficult.

INTERLAMINAR TECHNIQUE: ADVERSE EVENTS

Adverse events may be segregated into major (neurologic injury, intraspinal hemorrhage, spinal infections) and minor events (vasovagal syncope, dural puncture, acute systemic steroid effects, contrast reactions). Serious adverse events have been limited to case reports, including intraspinal hematoma, spondylodiscitis with epidural abscess, chemical meningitis following inadvertent intrathecal delivery, paraplegia, and transient blindness.[48] Fortunately, large prospective series reporting adverse event rates have identified few major complications. No major adverse events were seen in a multi-institutional cohort of >1,500 interlaminar injections.[56] Dural punctures were seen in 0.2% of patients, vasovagal reactions in 0.5%, and a central steroid effect (transient flushing, sleeplessness, nonpositional headache) was observed in 2.6%. A recently reported single-center 12-year experience in >9,800 lumbar interlaminar injections identified single cases (0.01%) each of intraspinal hematoma, spondylodiscitis, and septic shock.[35] Dural puncture with CSF leak was seen in six patients (0.06%); vasovagal reactions and systemic steroid effects were not described.

TRANSFORAMINAL INJECTIONS

Caudal and interlaminar injections rely on medication spreading to the target nerve or nerve roots from the point of injection. Because the spread of injectate into the epidural space is uncontrolled and unpredictable, only a fraction of the medication administered may actually reach the target nerve. TF injections differ in that the needle is placed next to the target nerve, virtually or actually touching it. Thereby, all the medication is delivered onto the target nerve.

There is no "blind" version of TF injections. They are performed under image guidance.[57] Image guidance is also critical for safety. The most serious danger of TF injections is injection into a radicular artery that reinforces the blood supply of the conus medullaris. Therefore, steps must be taken to guard against complications from such intra-arterial injections.

When lumbar spinal nerves are the target, the target zone is the intervertebral foramen that lodges that nerve. Along a posterior or posterior oblique view, a spinal needle is delivered into that foramen, at a location where the target spinal nerve does not lie (Fig. 99.5). The classical placement is subpedicular (i.e., tangential to the inferior surface of the pedicle) as deeply as the back of the vertebral body (see Fig. 99.5).

Alternative placements are supraneural, retroneural, and infraneural (Fig. 99.6). These can be used if and when the spinal nerve is displaced onto the pedicle, in patients with foraminal stenosis, or to avoid arteries in the rostral sectors of the foramen.

When sacral nerves are the target, a technique analogous to that for lumbar nerves is used. The needle is inserted through the posterior sacral foramen and placed in a retroneural position (Fig. 99.7).

Once the needle has been placed, one or more safety checks are performed to avoid injection into a radicular artery. Such tests are necessary because infarction of the conus medullaris is the most catastrophic complication of TF injection of steroids, and circumstantial evidence implicates intra-arterial injection of particulate steroids as the cause.

Laboratory studies have shown that agents such as triamcinolone, betamethasone, and methylprednisolone form particles or aggregates that are large enough to block end arteries

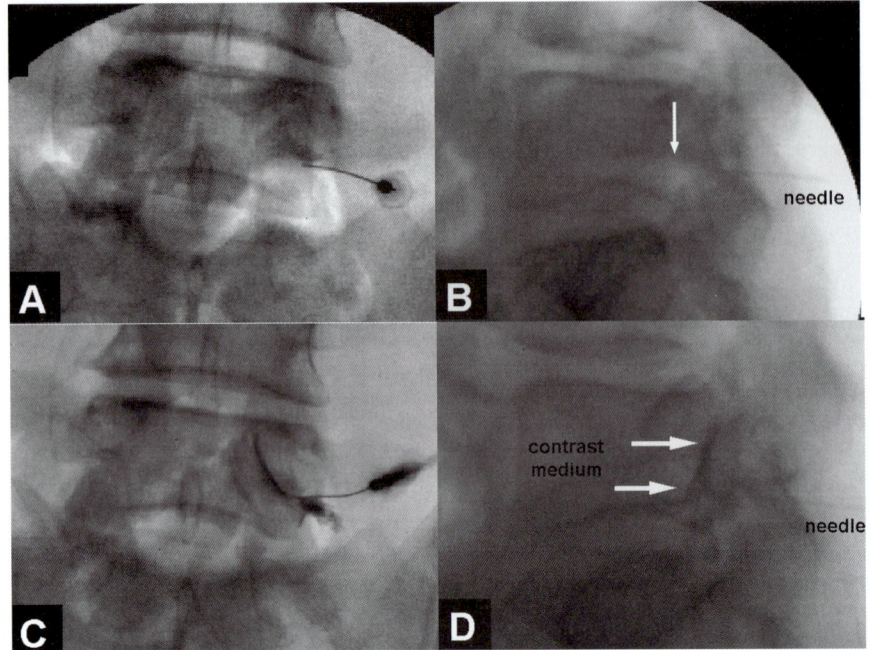

FIGURE 99.5 Fluoroscopy views of stages in the conduct of a lumbar transforaminal injection. **A:** Posterior view showing a needle directed to a subpedicular position in a right L5–S1 intervertebral foramen. **B:** Lateral view showing the needle tangential to the pedicle, with its tip (*arrow*) resting on the back of the vertebral body. **C:** Posterior view after injection of contrast medium which outlines the parapedicular course of the L5 spinal nerve and the dural sleeve covering its roots. **D:** Lateral view after injection of contrast medium. The contrast medium (*arrows*) surrounds the nerve and flows rostrally, around the pedicle and under the lamina. (*Images from International Spine Intervention Society. Lumbar interlaminar access. In: Bogduk N, ed.* Practice Guidelines for Spinal Diagnostic and Treatment Procedures. *2nd ed. San Francisco, CA: International Spine Intervention Society; 2013:443–456.*)

or capillaries.[58] By implication, these particles could act as emboli if injected into an artery that supplies the spinal cord. More recent evidence suggests that particulate steroids may cause stasis in a microvascular bed due to red blood cell agglutination as a consequence of red cell membrane effects.[59] Studies in animals have shown that injection of particulate steroids into cerebral arteries universally causes fatal stroke, whereas the nonparticulate steroid, dexamethasone, does not.[60,61] In virtually all cases of spinal cord infarction after lumbar TF injection of steroids, a particulate steroid was used.[62] Only one case report records this complication after the use of dexamethasone.[63] Dexamethasone, however, is known to precipitate into particles if mixed with ropivacaine.[64,65] Additionally, there is some evidence that steroid preparations can have a direct neurotoxic effect without forming emboli.[60]

The foremost test for intra-arterial injection is the injection of a test dose of contrast medium. In the first instance, contrast medium is injected in order to show that injectate will flow in the appropriate direction, which is centrally, along the course of the target nerves and the dural sleeve that encloses its roots (see Fig. 99.5). It also serves to reveal aberrant flow if the needle has not been placed correctly. Aberrant flow can be into the subarachnoid space or the subdural space if the dural sleeve has been punctured; it may be externally, away from the nerve, if the intervertebral foramen is blocked or stenosed; or it may be into an epidural vein. Guidelines for what to do in the face of aberrant flow are elaborated elsewhere.[57]

Notwithstanding normal flow, if the needle has punctured a radicular artery, the contrast medium will briefly flow within the artery before it is washed away. Intra-arterial injection is an indicated to terminate the procedure in order to avoid the risk of injecting potentially offensive medications into the artery and, therefore, into the circulation of the spinal cord. However, given that these arteries are tiny, it may be difficult to visualize arterial uptake of the contrast medium against a background of contrast medium in the epidural space (Fig. 99.8A). For this

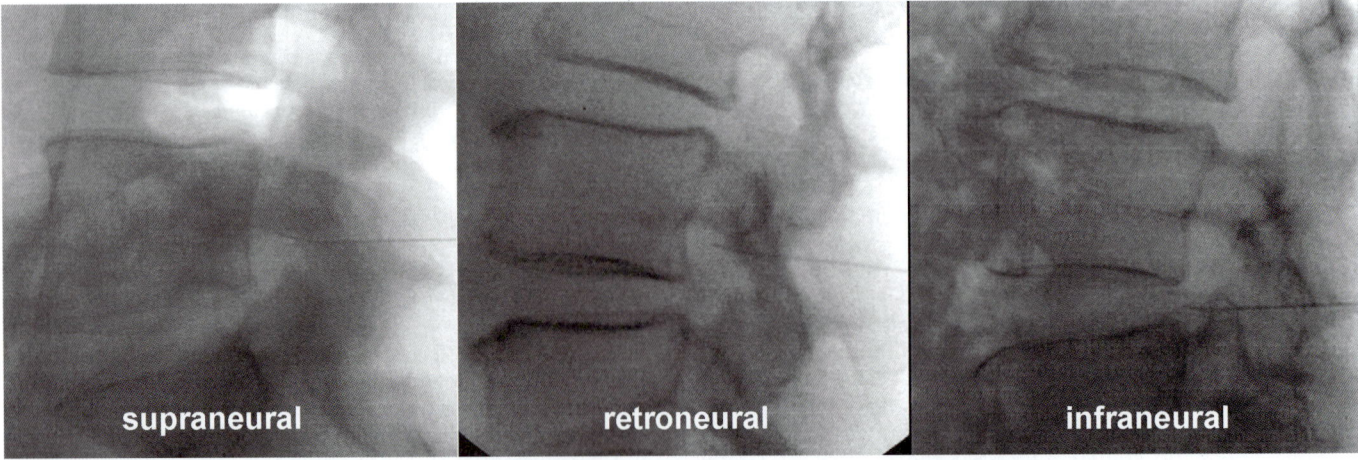

FIGURE 99.6 Alternative placements of a needle in the intervertebral foramen for transforaminal injections. In the supraneural placement, the tip of the needle lies above the nerve. For the retroneural placement, the tip of the needle lies behind the nerve. For infraneural placement, the tip of the needle lies below the nerve, opposite the intervertebral disk. (*Images reproduced with permission from International Spine Intervention Society. Lumbar interlaminar access. In: Bogduk N, ed.* Practice Guidelines for Spinal Diagnostic and Treatment Procedures. *2nd ed. San Francisco, CA: International Spine Intervention Society; 2013:443–456.*)

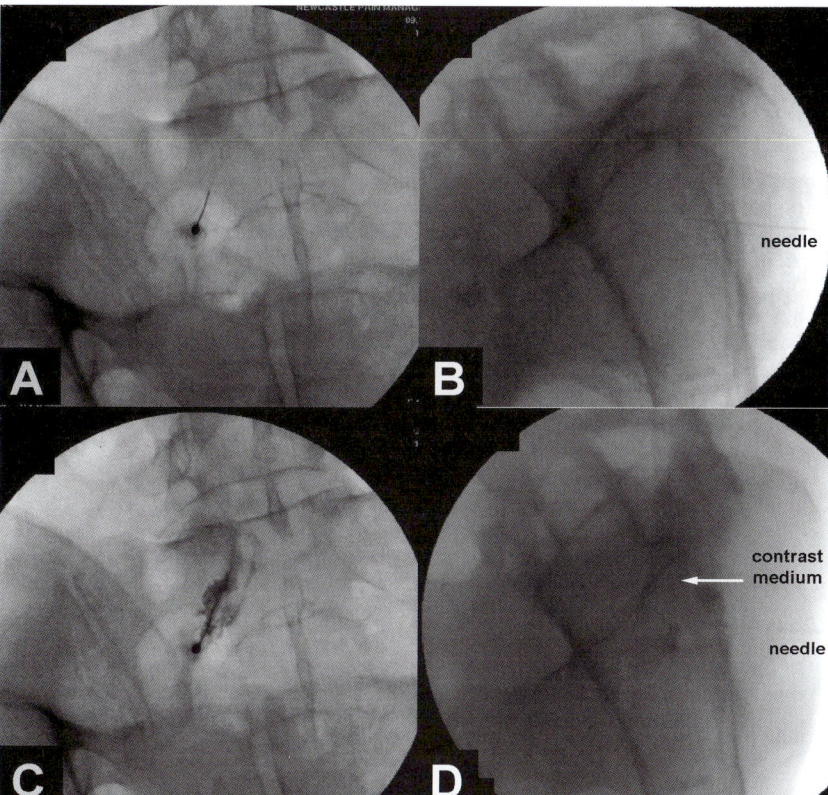

FIGURE 99.7 Fluoroscopy views of stages in the conduct of a sacral transforaminal injection. **A:** Posterior view showing a needle directed to a subpedicular position through a left S1 posterior sacral foramen. **B:** Lateral view showing the needle tangential to the pedicle, with its tip resting on the floor of the sacral canal. **C:** Posterior view after injection of contrast medium which outlines the parapedicular course of the S1 spinal nerve and the dural sleeve covering its roots. **D:** Lateral view after injection of contrast medium showing contrast medium surrounding the nerve and flowing rostrally.

reason, some physicians repeat the injection of contrast medium under digital subtraction imaging (DSI). Under DSI, tiny arteries are brought into stark relief (Fig. 99.8B). Although adding DSI increases the amount of radiation to which the patient is exposed, the amount is small and well within notionally safe limits.[66]

Some physicians perform an additional test, although its validity is contentious. The test is to administer a small dose (1 mL) of lidocaine 2%; wait 2 minutes and examine the patient for sensory of motor loss in the lower limbs. The rationale for this test is that if the needle has punctured a radicular artery but the artery

has not been noticed during the injection of contrast medium, the local anesthetic will be injected into the artery and will cause temporary neurologic deficits on the spinal cord being anesthetized. Incurring a temporary neurologic deficit protects the patient from permanent damage that would occur had hazardous medications been administered. The test is loosely based on a single case report of temporary neurologic deficit after injection of local anesthetic during a cervical TF injection[67] and a retrospective study of cervical TF injections that found that four patients in a series of 532 were positive to the local anesthetic test even though contrast medium had not shown arterial uptake.[68]

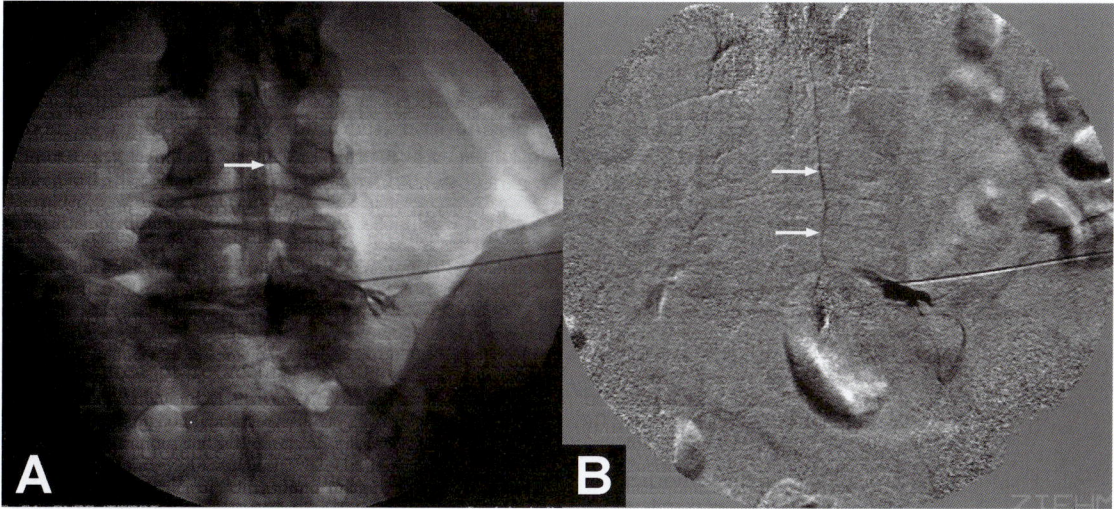

FIGURE 99.8 Injection into a radicular artery during a lumbar transforaminal injection. **A:** Posterior view during injection of contrast medium. The tiny artery (*arrow*) is difficult to see. **B:** Digital subtraction imaging brings the artery into starker relief (*arrows*). (*Images kindly provided by Dr. Way Yin, Bellingham, WA and reproduced with permission from International Spine Intervention Society. Lumbar interlaminar access. In: Bogduk N, ed.* Practice Guidelines for Spinal Diagnostic and Treatment Procedures. *2nd ed. San Francisco, CA: International Spine Intervention Society; 2013:443–456.*)

Once the needle has been correctly placed and safety checks have reduced the likelihood of intra-arterial injection, the chosen medication can be administered. In the past, the agents used had been methylprednisolone (40 or 80 mg), triamcinolone (40, 50, or 80 mg), or betamethasone (5.7, 8.55, or 11.4 mg). Until recently, these particulate steroids were preferred over dexamethasone (6 or 7.5 mg) because they were regarded as being more effective. Indeed, the early literature supported this view because the studies with the best outcome data all used particulate steroids, whereas outcomes were poor in the few studies that used dexamethasone. However, that situation has changed.

Multiple large studies[69-71] and reviews[72,73] have shown that the success rates of TF injection of steroids are not significantly different statistically when dexamethasone is used instead of particulate steroids. This has promoted dexamethasone as a safer alternative for lumbar TF injections.

Concerned about the safety profile of TF injections, the FDA commissioned an expert panel to publish recommendations designed to reduce the risk of spinal cord injury.[45] In the essence, those recommendations are the following:

- All lumbar interlaminar ESIs should be performed using image guidance, with appropriate anteroposterior (AP), lateral, or contralateral oblique views and a test dose of contrast medium.
- Lumbar TF ESIs should be performed by injecting contrast medium under real-time fluoroscopy and/or DSI, using an AP view, before injecting any substance that may be hazardous to the patient.
- A nonparticulate steroid (e.g., dexamethasone) should be used for the initial injection in lumbar TF epidural injections.
- There are situations where particulate steroids could be used in the performance of lumbar TF ESIs.

TRANSFORAMINAL INJECTIONS UNDER FLUOROSCOPIC GUIDANCE: EVIDENCE

TF injections require image guidance, but fluoroscopy facilities are not generally available to pain physicians for relatively minor injections. Therefore, the practice of TF injections has not been as widespread as the practice of blind caudal injections or blind interlaminar injections. Nevertheless, there is an abundant literature on the outcomes of TF injections of steroids for radicular pain.

A systematic review reviewed all of the literature until 2013, covering observational studies as well as pragmatic trials and explanatory trials.[74] It found that the evidence differed in volume and in conclusions for radicular pain due to disk herniation compared with neurogenic claudication associated with spinal stenosis.

For spinal stenosis, the literature and evidence were largely limited to observational studies. There was one pragmatic trial but no explanatory trials. Several observational studies did not provide meaningful evidence because, although they claimed success, they did not define successful relief of pain or because follow-up was only for 2 weeks. Two outcome studies respectively reported 26 of 48 patients[75] and 6 of 10 patients[76] having 50% relief of pain at 6 months. From the single, pragmatic trial data on success rates could not be calculated, but outcomes were not significantly different between patients treated with either TF injections or fluoroscopically guided interlaminar epidural injections of methylprednisolone.[77]

For disk herniation, the review[74] found that the literature is sufficiently abundant to show that lumbar TF injection of steroids is not universally effective but, nevertheless, benefits a substantial proportion of patients and is not a placebo.

The original study of TF steroids reported that 47% of 30 patients obtained complete relief of pain, which was maintained for 2 years, and only 20% of patients required surgery.[78]

The surgery-sparing effect was corroborated by a subsequent study in which 53 (77%) of 69 patients avoided surgery for 12 months after treatment.[79]

Seven other observational studies provided reliable estimates of success rates for achieving at least 50% relief of pain at the times after treatment indicated: 100% of 53 patients at 1 month[80]; 52% of 40 patients[81] and 62% of 41 patients at 90 days; 60% of 20 patients[76] and 62% of 191 patients[75] at 6 months; 75% of 69 patients at 12 months[82]; and 78% of 40 patients at 1 month, reducing to 67% at 6 months and 55% at 12 months.[83]

Although the review[74] found several pragmatic studies, most did not provide data on success rates. Of the two that did, one reported 66% of patients achieved 50% relief of pain at 2 months,[84] and the other reported 33% having this outcome at 6 months.[11] These results are consistent with those of the observational studies.

Of the five explanatory trials, three[85-87] used TF injection of bupivacaine as the comparison treatment, but it is not known if TF bupivacaine is strictly an inactive treatment. Ostensibly, local anesthetic might have only a temporary relieving effect on pain, but long-lasting effects have not been formally excluded.

A fourth study used intramuscular saline as the control treatment,[88] which should be acceptable as a suitably inactive treatment for radicular pain, but this control treatment was administered in a different manner—as an office procedure—from that of fluoroscopically guided TF steroids. As well, patients were randomized according to patient choice. Both of these factors compromise the internal validity of the study and demote it to providing only weak evidence of efficacy of TF steroids.

A fifth study used TF normal saline as the control treatment.[89] With respect to pharmacologic activity, this served as an appropriate, inactive control, but it does not control for possible irrigation effects of TF injections.

The sixth study[90] addressed all of these concerns. It randomized patients to TF steroids or TF bupivacaine, TF normal saline, intramuscular steroids, or intramuscular normal saline, each performed in a fluoroscopy suite with intramuscular injections mimicking TF injections. Under these conditions, TF bupivacaine controlled for the addition of steroids to a TF injection, TF normal saline controlled for the possible effects of simply irrigating the affected nerve, intramuscular steroids controlled for systemic effects of steroids, and intramuscular saline served as a credible sham control.

The first explanatory study[85] did not report on relief of pain or other conventional outcomes. It used avoidance of surgery as the single outcome measure. It showed that TF steroids spared patients from surgery significantly more often than did TF bupivacaine alone. Only 29% (±17%) of 29 patients required surgery during the 13 months after treatment with TF steroids compared with 66% (±18%) of those treated with bupivacaine. Furthermore, the surgery-sparing effect was maintained during a subsequent 5-year follow-up.[91]

The weak explanatory study[88] found that 84% (±14%) of 25 patients treated with TF steroids achieved at least 50% reduction of pain, accompanied by improvements of at least 5 points on the Roland-Morris Disability Questionnaire, persisting for 12 months. In comparison, only 48% (±20%) achieved these outcomes after intramuscular injections of normal saline.

The double-blind trial that compared TF steroids and TF bupivacaine followed patients for 12 weeks[86] and was supplemented by a 1-year follow-up.[87] It found no differences in outcome, based on group scores, but success rates were not reported. However, patients who underwent surgery or a repeat injection before 3 months were excluded from the analysis, as were 16 patients who failed to attend for review at 3 months. It is not evident the extent to which these exclusions may have compromised the comparisons of outcomes.

The study that compared TF steroids with TF normal saline initially found no differences between outcomes based on group data.[89] However, a later analysis revealed several features.[92] First, TF steroids were not universally successful. They were no more effective than sham treatment in patients with extruded or sequestrated disk herniations, but they were effective in those patients with contained disk herniations. TF steroids were significantly more effective than control treatment for reducing leg pain at 2 weeks and 1 month. As well, patients treated with TF steroids tended to have fewer sick days, fewer resorted to surgery, and twice as many had at least 75% reduction in pain (44% ± 20% compared with 21% ± 16%), but for these latter differences, statistical significance did not emerge because of the small sample sizes involved (25 and 24). However, what did emerge is that for those patients with contained herniations, TF steroids were significantly cost-effective at 12 months, achieving a cost reduction of $12,666 per responder.

The sixth randomized, controlled study was designed primarily to test if the effects of TF steroids could be attributed to placebo.[90] For that purpose, it evaluated responses at 1 month after treatment, but it also provided subsequent 12-month data. It found that the various control treatments had success rates for providing at least 50% relief of pain that were statistically indistinguishable. Some 15% (8% to 22%) of patients obtained at least 50% relief after treatment with TF bupivacaine, TF normal saline, intramuscular steroids, or intramuscular saline. The success rate for TF steroids was significantly greater at 54% (36% to 72%). Furthermore, this study showed that successful relief of pain was accompanied by restoration of function and clinically significant reduction—or elimination—of the need for other health care for radicular pain. All patients recruited for the study came from a neurosurgery unit, and all were destined for surgical treatment. Successful relief of pain by transforaminal injection of steroid (TFIS) avoided the need for surgery. During the 12 months after treatment, the success rate from the initial treatment deteriorated, but at 12 months, 11% of patients still had at least 50% relief of pain and a further 14% still had complete relief.

This latter study also revealed a pertinent feature about reporting outcomes. The study clearly showed that TF steroids had a success rate that was significantly greater than those of any of the compared treatments, both statistically and clinically. However, the distribution of outcomes was distinctly bimodal: success or no success. Consequently, the group data did not produce a statistically significant difference because they camouflaged this bimodal distribution. Only if and when success rates were compared did significant differences appear. For these reasons, studies that report only group data may miss detecting statistically and clinically significant data.

Since the publication of this review,[74] a systematic review reinforced the surgery-sparing effects of TF injection of steroids for radicular pain due to disk herniation,[93] and several studies have corroborated the observed success rates. One study found success rates of 70% at 3 months and at 6 months, with success defined as greater than 50% reduction of pain, coupled with 50% reduction in disability.[70] A large study of 2,634 patients had a success rate of 52% at 2 months and 50% reduction in pain, coupled with 40% improvement in disability.[69] A companion study of 1,078 patients had a success rate of 45% for these same outcomes.[94]

An additional study demonstrated that repeat injection could increase the success rate of an initial injection that provided partial relief or could reinstate relief if initial relief waned.[95] Importantly, this study also showed that if TF steroids were used in a disciplined manner, few patients actually required more than three injections per year in order to benefit from repeat injections.

In patients with neurogenic claudication due to spinal stenosis, a large double-blind multisite pragmatic trial (N = 400) compared epidural administration of corticosteroid plus lidocaine versus lidocaine alone by both TF and interlaminar routes.[96] In this patient population, there was no detectable difference between the groups in pain reduction or functional recovery.

TRANSFORAMINAL INJECTIONS: DETERMINANTS OF EFFICACY

It would be clinically useful to identify patient, imaging, or procedural characteristics which are predictive of a positive response to TF ESIs. Spinal cord physiologic changes of central sensitization may amplify intensity and duration of perceived pain; pain chronicity may be a clinical marker of this process. A systematic review[74] pooled data from three studies and noted a significant, although weak, association; patients having pain less than 6 months had better outcomes after TF injections. Another study of >2,000 lumbar TF injections had ~60% responders for pain and functional recovery in patients with pain <3 months. For patients with pain greater than 6 months, there were ~35% responders for both measures.[94]

Two studies on disk herniation patients demonstrated an association between the degree of neural compression and outcomes; patients with lesser degrees of neural compression on magnetic resonance imaging (MRI) had better outcomes.[97,98] This was not, however, confirmed in a subsequent analysis of over 500 injections in a more heterogeneous population that includes fixed bony lesions as well as disk herniations.[99] This study also demonstrated an association between the nature of the compressive lesion and outcomes; there were more responders in the entire cohort for functional recovery in disk herniation patients than in those with a fixed lesion. When data was stratified by steroid preparation, however, patients with fixed lesions who received dexamethasone were indistinguishable from disk herniation patients. Patients with tandem lesions—a proximal zone of significant central canal compromise with a second lateral recess or foraminal lesion—did less well than those with single level lesions.

The targeted delivery of the steroid preparation to the site of neural compression, in the ventral epidural space, lateral recess, or foramen, has also been shown to be associated with better clinical outcomes after TF injections.[11,100,101] The clinical assessment of response to an epidural injection, and hence further decision making, can occur at 2 weeks postinjection, as pain and functional recovery responses at this time are strongly associated with longer term response.[102]

TRANSFORAMINAL INJECTIONS: ADVERSE EVENTS

The safety concerns leading to the adoption of the nonparticulate steroid dexamethasone are discussed earlier; it must be recalled that this was prompted by case reports of spinal cord infarction. All used particulate steroids except a recent report describing a cord infarct with dexamethasone, but this report[63] is incomplete in its description of the injection procedure and the injectate.

More revealing are large prospective studies collecting adverse event data on consecutive patients. A multi-institutional study reported on 15,000 consecutive TF injections performed using Spine Intervention Society procedural guidelines; there were no neurologic events, intraspinal hematomas, or infections.[56] The most common minor adverse events were vasovagal reactions (1.3%), central steroid effects (2.6%), and transient increased pain (2.1%). A single-center study reported on >22,000 lumbar TF injections; there were no major adverse events.[35] Symptom aggravation was described in 0.43%. In another single-center study of 1,300 lumbar TF injections, there were no major adverse events; minor events, primarily vasovagal reactions, were reported in 11.5%.[103] An additional single-center study reported on nearly 4,000 lumbar TF injections.[104] There were no major adverse events; the most common minor adverse event was transient increase in pain in 0.01% of injections. Thus, despite the concerns raised by case reports, TF injections are very safe when performed according to evidence-based procedural guidelines.

TRANSFORAMINAL INJECTIONS UNDER COMPUTED TOMOGRAPHY GUIDANCE: EVIDENCE, ADVERSE EVENTS

A systematic review found that, although there were several publications that promoted the use of TF injections under CT guidance, most did not provide evidence either of efficacy or of effectiveness.[105] Variously, the published studies assessed several interventions but without stratifying outcomes, claimed success but without defining success, and claimed success but did not provide baseline data or numerical outcome data to corroborate that claim.

Of the four accepted studies, the first treated patients with radicular pain due to disk herniation[106] and second treated patients with spinal stenosis.[107] Both reported significant decreases in pain scores but did not provide any data on success rates. The third study treated patients with disk herniation or foraminal stenosis.[108] It reported that 62% ($\pm$16%) had 50% relief at 6 months. The fourth study[109] reported results in a confusing manner. A distillation of those results suggests the following:

- Of 49 patients with disk herniation, 24 obtained lasting relief, with 90% of these having at least 50% relief, which amounts to a success rate of 44% $\pm$ 14%.
- Of 59 patients with foraminal stenosis, 22 had lasting relief, with 90% of these having at least 50% relief, which amounts to a success rate of 34% $\pm$ 12%.
- Of those patients with lasting relief, only 78% also ceased medications. Thus, the success rate for relieving pain and also ceasing medications may be lower than the success rates for relieving pain alone.

Conspicuously, the review[105] found no evidence to support the claims of proponents that CT-guided TF injections were "more accurate" and "safer" than fluoroscopically guided injections. Although CT shows the target nerve, this feature does not make the procedure "more accurate" than placing a needle under fluoroscopy. Meanwhile, the existing literature actually refutes claims of CT guidance being safer.

In the first instance, CT guidance incurs radiation exposure that is some five times greater than that of fluoroscopic guidance.[105] Secondly, CT guidance is not immune to serious vascular complications. At least half of the complications described in case reports have occurred under CT guidance, but all were prior to the recognition of the risks associated with particulate steroids. Critical to the avoidance of vascular complications is the administration of a test dose of contrast medium in order to check for arterial uptake. Conventional CT guidance does not allow for this safety check.[105] The single-plane, axial view of conventional CT guidance does not show arteries running cephalad of the point of injection. However, if multislice CT fluoroscopy is employed, with image acquisition as the injection is performed, and immediately following cessation of the injection, vascular uptake can be evaluated under CT.[110] When performed in this fashion, rates of detection of vascular uptake approached those seen with DSI. In a large prospective series of consecutive patients using this technique, in all spine segments, no major adverse events were noted.[56]

TRANSFORAMINAL EPIDURAL STEROID INJECTIONS: THEIR ROLE IN TREATING THE RADICULAR PAIN PATIENT

ESIs can never be seen as an isolated therapeutic intervention; they must be part of a holistic spine care program. Their role in the disk herniation patient is to diminish the inflammatory response that causes neural irritation and to allow time for the natural history of involution of the herniated disk material to play out. TF ESIs have also been demonstrated to enable more vigorous and effective participation in a rehabilitation program. In a prospective cohort study, patients who had failed conservative therapy and were consented for surgery were offered up to two TF injections followed by a rigorous rehabilitation program.[111] At 1 year, 78% had avoided surgery, and 62% had minimal pain (Visual Analog Scale [VAS] <10/100) and near complete functional recovery (Roland-Morris Disability Questionnaire <3/24).

Epidural corticosteroids may thus be effective in symptom control, but they do not treat the underlying lesion, whether it be disk herniation causing radicular pain/radiculopathy, with a favorable natural history, or fixed stenotic lesions, causing radicular pain or neurogenic intermittent claudication, whose natural history is less favorable, and where outcomes with epidural steroids are accordingly less positive. When positive outcomes for pain and functional recovery are achieved, but prove to be temporary, epidural steroids can be used as part of a longer term management program, being mindful of the endocrine side effects of chronic steroid use.

References

1. Mulleman D, Mammou S, Griffoul I, et al. Pathophysiology of disk-related sciatica. I. Evidence supporting a chemical component. *Joint Bone Spine* 2006;73(2):151–158.
2. Boden SD, Davis DO, Dina TS, et al. Abnormal magnetic-resonance scans of the lumbar spine in asymptomatic subjects. A prospective investigation. *J Bone Joint Surg Am* 1990;72:403–408.
3. Boos N, Rieder R, Schade V, et al. 1995 Volvo Award in clinical sciences. The diagnostic accuracy of magnetic resonance imaging, work perception, and psychosocial factors in identifying symptomatic disc herniations. *Spine (Phila Pa 1976)* 1995;20(24):2613–2625.
4. Modic MT, Obuchowski NA, Ross JS, et al. Acute low back pain and radiculopathy: MR imaging findings and their prognostic role and effect on outcome. *Radiology* 2005;237(2):597–604.
5. Haro H, Crawford HC, Fingleton B, et al. Matrix metalloproteinase-7-dependent release of tumor necrosis factor-alpha in a model of herniated disc resorption. *J Clin Invest* 2000;105:143–150.
6. Kuslich SD, Ulstrom CL, Michael CJ. The tissue origin of low back pain and sciatica: a report of pain response to tissue stimulation during operations on the lumbar spine using local anesthesia. *Orthop Clin North Am* 1991;22:181–187.
7. Olmarker K, Størkson R, Berge OG. Pathogenesis of sciatic pain: a study of spontaneous behavior in rats exposed to experimental disc herniation. *Spine (Phila Pa 1976)* 2002;27:1312–1317.
8. Robecchi A, Capra R. L'idrocortisone (composto F). Prime esperienze cliniche in campo reumatologico. *Minerva Med* 1952;43(98):1259–1263.
9. Johansson A, Hao J, Sjölund B. Local corticosteroid application blocks transmission in normal nociceptive C-fibres. *Acta Anaesthesiol Scand* 1990;34:335–338.
10. Yabuki S, Kawaguchi Y, Nordborg C, et al. Effects of lidocaine on nucleus pulposus-induced nerve root injury. A neurophysiologic and histologic study of the pig cauda equina. *Spine (Phila Pa 1976)* 1998;23:2383–2389.
11. Ackerman WE III, Ahmad M. The efficacy of lumbar epidural steroid injections in patients with lumbar disc herniations. *Anesth Analg* 2007;104(5):1217–1222.
12. Furman MB, Lee TS, Mehta A, et al. Contrast flow selectivity during transforaminal lumbosacral epidural steroid injections. *Pain Physician* 2008;11(6):855–861.
13. Cochrane A. *Effectiveness and Efficiency*. Cambridge, United Kingdom: Cambridge University Press; 1977.
14. Bogduk N, Aprill C, Derby R. Epidural steroid injections. In: White AH, ed. *Spine Care: Diagnosis and Conservative Treatment*. Vol 1. St. Louis, MO: Mosby; 1995:322–343.
15. White AH, Derby R, Wynne G. Epidural injections for the diagnosis and treatment of low-back pain. *Spine (Phila Pa 1976)* 1980;5:78–86.
16. el-Khoury GY, Ehara S, Weinstein JN, et al. Epidural steroid injection: a procedure ideally performed with fluoroscopic control. *Radiology* 1988;168:554–557.
17. Stitz MY, Sommer HM. Accuracy of blind versus fluoroscopically guided caudal epidural injection. *Spine (Phila Pa 1976)* 1999;24:1371–1376.
18. Price CM, Rogers PD, Prosser AS, et al. Comparison of the caudal and lumbar approaches to the epidural space. *Ann Rheum Dis* 2000;59:879–882.
19. Bartynski WS, Grahovac SZ, Rothfus WE. Incorrect needle position during lumbar epidural steroid administration: inaccuracy of loss of air pressure resistance and requirement of fluoroscopy and epidurography during needle insertion. *AJNR Am J Neuroradiol* 2005;26:502–505.

20. Manchikanti L, Cash KA, Pampati V, et al. Evaluation of fluoroscopically guided caudal epidural injections. *Pain Physician* 2004;7:81–92.

21. Breivik H, Hesla P, Molnar I, et al. Treatment of chronic low back pain and sciatica: comparison of caudal epidural injections of bupivacaine and methylprednisolone with bupivacaine followed by saline. *Adv Pain Res Ther* 1976;1:927–932.

22. Bush K, Hillier S. A controlled study of caudal epidural injections of triamcinolone plus procaine for the management of intractable sciatica. *Spine (Phila Pa 1976)* 1991;16(5):572–575.

23. Mathews JA, Mills SB, Jenkins VM, et al. Back pain and sciatica: controlled trials of manipulation, traction, sclerosant and epidural injections. *Br J Rheumatol* 1987;26(6):416–423.

24. Manchikanti L, Singh V, Cash KA, et al. Preliminary results of a randomized, equivalence trial of fluoroscopic caudal epidural injections in managing chronic low back pain: part 2—disc herniation and radiculitis. *Pain Physician* 2008;11(6):801–815.

25. Béliveau P. A comparison between epidural anaesthesia with and without corticosteroid in the treatment of sciatica. *Rheumatol Phys Med* 1971;11(1):40–43.

26. Sayegh FE, Kenanidis EI, Papavasiliou KA, et al. Efficacy of steroid and nonsteroid caudal epidural injections for low back pain and sciatica: a prospective, randomized, double-blind clinical trial. *Spine (Phila Pa 1976)* 2009;34(14):1441–1447.

27. Manchikanti L, Singh V, Cash KA, et al. A randomized, controlled, double-blind trial of fluoroscopic caudal epidural injections in the treatment of lumbar disc herniation and radiculitis. *Spine (Phila Pa 1976)* 2011;36(23):1897–1905.

28. Iversen T, Solberg TK, Romner B, et al. Effect of caudal epidural steroid or saline injection in chronic lumbar radiculopathy: multicentre, blinded, randomised controlled trial. *BMJ* 2011;343:d5278.

29. Datta R, Upadhyay KK. A randomized clinical trial of three different steroid agents for treatment of low backache through the caudal route. *Med J Armed Forces India* 2011;67(1):25–33.

30. Conn A, Buenaventura RM, Datta S, et al. Systematic review of caudal epidural injections in the management of chronic low back pain. *Pain Physician* 2009;12(1):109–135.

31. Manchikanti L, Cash KA, McManus CD, et al. Preliminary results of a randomized, equivalence trial of fluoroscopic caudal epidural injections in managing chronic low back pain: part 4—spinal stenosis. *Pain Physician* 2008;11(6):833–848.

32. Barre L, Lutz GE, Southern D, et al. Fluoroscopically guided caudal epidural steroid injections for lumbar spinal stenosis: a retrospective evaluation of long term efficacy. *Pain Physician* 2004;7(2):187–193.

33. Botwin K, Brown LA, Fishman M, et al. Fluoroscopically guided caudal epidural steroid injections in degenerative lumbar spine stenosis. *Pain Physician* 2007;10(4):547–558.

34. Botwin KP, Gruber RD, Bouchlas CG, et al. Complications of fluoroscopically guided caudal epidural injections. *Am J Phys Med Rehabil* 2001;80(6):416–424.

35. Lee JW, Lee E, Lee GY, et al. Epidural steroid injection-related events requiring hospitalisation or emergency room visits among 52,935 procedures performed at a single centre. *Eur Radiol* 2018;28(1):418–427.

36. International Spine Intervention Society. Lumbar interlaminar access. In: Bogduk N, ed. *Practice Guidelines for Spinal Diagnostic and Treatment Procedures.* 2nd ed. San Francisco, CA: International Spine Intervention Society; 2013:443–456.

37. Mehta M, Salmon N. Extradural block. Confirmation of the injection site by X-ray monitoring. *Anaesthesia* 1985;40:1009–1012.

38. Whitlock EL, Bridwell KH, Gilula LA. Influence of needle tip position on injectate spread in 406 interlaminar lumbar epidural steroid injections. *Radiology* 2007;243:804–811.

39. Fredman B, Nun MB, Zohar E, et al. Epidural steroids for treating "failed back surgery syndrome": is fluoroscopy really necessary? *Anesth Analg* 1999; 88:367–372.

40. Vorobeychik Y, Sharma A, Smith CC, et al. The effectiveness and risks of non-image-guided lumbar interlaminar epidural steroid injections: a systematic review with comprehensive analysis of the published data. *Pain Med* 2016;17(12): 2185–2202.

41. Arden NK, Price C, Reading I, et al. A multicentre randomized controlled trial of epidural corticosteroid injections for sciatica: the WEST study. *Rheumatology (Oxford)* 2005;44(11):1399–1406.

42. Price C, Arden N, Coglan L, et al. Cost-effectiveness and safety of epidural steroids in the management of sciatica. *Health Technol Assess* 2005; 9(33):1–58.

43. Carette S, Leclaire R, Marcoux S, et al. Epidural corticosteroid injections for sciatica due to herniated nucleus pulposus. *N Engl J Med* 1997;336(23):1634–1640.

44. Valat JP, Giraudeau B, Rozenberg S, et al. Epidural corticosteroid injections for sciatica: a randomised, double blind, controlled clinical trial. *Ann Rheum Dis* 2003;62(7):639–643.

45. Rathmell JP, Benzon HT, Dreyfuss P, et al. Safeguards to prevent neurologic complications after epidural steroid injections: consensus opinions from a multidisciplinary working group and national organizations. *Anesthesiology* 2015; 122:974–984.

46. Botwin KP, Natalicchio J, Hanna A. Fluoroscopic guided lumbar interlaminar epidural injections: a prospective evaluation of epidurography contrast patterns and anatomical review of the epidural space. *Pain Physician* 2004;7(1):77–80.

47. Weil L, Frauwirth NH, Amirdelfan K, et al. Fluoroscopic analysis of lumbar epidural contrast spread after lumbar interlaminar injection. *Arch Phys Med Rehabil* 2008;89(3):413–416.

48. Sharma AK, Vorobeychik Y, Wasserman R, et al. The effectiveness and risks of fluoroscopically guided lumbar interlaminar epidural steroid injections: a systematic review with comprehensive analysis of the published data. *Pain Med* 2017;18(2):239–251.

49. Manchikanti L, Singh V, Cash KA, et al. The role of fluoroscopic interlaminar epidural injections in managing chronic pain of lumbar disc herniation or radiculitis: a randomized, double-blind trial. *Pain Pract* 2013;13(7):547–558.

50. Furman MB, Kothari G, Parikh T, et al. Efficacy of fluoroscopically guided, contrast-enhanced lumbosacral interlaminar epidural steroid injections: a pilot study. *Pain Med* 2010;11(9):1328–1334.

51. Schaufele MK, Hatch L, Jones W. Interlaminar versus transforaminal epidural injections for the treatment of symptomatic lumbar intervertebral disc herniations. *Pain Physician* 2006;9(4):361–366.

52. Ghai B, Vadaje KS, Wig J, et al. Lateral parasagittal versus midline interlaminar lumbar epidural steroid injection for management of low back pain with lumbosacral radicular pain: a double-blind, randomized study. *Anesth Analg* 2013;117(1):219–227.

53. Ghai B, Bansal D, Kay JP, et al. Transforaminal versus parasagittal interlaminar epidural steroid injection in low back pain with radicular pain: a randomized, double-blind, active-control trial. *Pain Physician* 2014;17(4):277–290.

54. Ghai B, Kumar K, Bansal D, et al. Effectiveness of parasagittal interlaminar epidural local anesthetic with or without steroid in chronic lumbosacral pain: a randomized, double-blind clinical trial. *Pain Physician* 2015;18(3):237–248.

55. Hashemi SM, Aryani MR, Momenzadeh S, et al. Comparison of transforaminal and parasagittal epidural steroid injections in patients with radicular low back pain. *Anesth Pain Med* 2015;5(5):e26652.

56. El-Yahchouchi CA, Plastaras CT, Maus TP, et al. Adverse event rates associated with transforaminal and interlaminar epidural steroid injections: a multi-institutional study. *Pain Med* 2016;17(2):239–249.

57. International Spine Intervention Society. Lumbar transforaminal access. In: Bogduk N, ed. *Practice Guidelines for Spinal Diagnostic and Treatment Procedures.* 2nd ed. San Francisco, CA: International Spine Intervention Society; 2013:377–442.

58. Derby R, Lee SH, Date ES, et al. Size and aggregation of corticosteroids used for epidural injections. *Pain Med* 2008;9:227–234.

59. Laemmel E, Segal N, Mirshahi M, et al. Deleterious effects of intra-arterial administration of particulate steroids on microvascular perfusion in a mouse model. *Radiology* 2016;279(3):731–740.

60. Dawley JD, Moeller-Bertram T, Wallace MS, et al. Intra-arterial injection in the rat brain: evaluation of steroids used for transforaminal epidurals. *Spine (Phila Pa 1976)* 2009;34:1638–1643.

61. Okubadejo G, Talcott M, Schmidt R, et al. Perils of intravascular methylprednisolone injection into the vertebral artery. An animal study. *J Bone Joint Surg Am* 2008;90:1932–1938.

62. Kennedy DJ, Dreyfuss P, Aprill CN, et al. Paraplegia following image-guided transforaminal lumbar spine epidural steroid injection: two case reports. *Pain Med* 2009;10:1389–1394.

63. Gharibo C, Fakhry M, Diwan S, et al. Conus medullaris infarction after a right l4 transforaminal epidural steroid injection using dexamethasone. *Pain Physician* 2016;19:E1211–E1214.

64. Watkins TW, Dupre S, Coucher JR. Ropivacaine and dexamethasone: a potentially dangerous combination for therapeutic pain injections. *J Med Imaging Radiat Oncol* 2015;59:571–577.

65. Hwang H, Park J, Lee WK, et al. Crystallization of local anesthetics when mixed with corticosteroid solutions. *Ann Rehabil Med* 2016;40:21–27.

66. Maus T, Schueler BA, Leng S, et al. Radiation dose incurred in the exclusion of vascular filling in transforaminal epidural steroid injections: fluoroscopy, digital subtraction angiography, and CT/fluoroscopy. *Pain Med* 2014;15:1328–1333.

67. Karasek M, Bogduk N. Temporary neurologic deficit after cervical transforaminal injection of local anesthetic. *Pain Med* 2004;5:202–205.

68. Smuck M, Maxwell MD, Kennedy D, et al. Utility of the anesthetic test dose to avoid catastrophic injury during cervical transforaminal epidural injections. *Spine J* 2010;10:857–864.

69. El-Yahchouchi C, Geske JR, Carter RE, et al. The noninferiority of the nonparticulate steroid dexamethasone vs the particulate steroids betamethasone and triamcinolone in lumbar transforaminal epidural steroid injections. *Pain Med* 2013;14:1650–1657.

70. Kennedy DJ, Plastaras C, Casey E, et al. Comparative effectiveness of lumbar transforaminal epidural steroid injections with particulate versus nonparticulate corticosteroids for lumbar radicular pain due to intervertebral disc herniation: a prospective, randomized, double-blind trial. *Pain Med* 2014;15:548–555.

71. Denis I, Claveau G, Filiatrault M, et al. Randomized double-blind controlled trial comparing the effectiveness of lumbar transforaminal epidural injections of particulate and nonparticulate corticosteroids for lumbosacral radicular pain. *Pain Med* 2015;16:1697–1708.

72. Diehn FE, Murthy NS, Maus TP. Science to practice: what causes arterial infarction in transforaminal epidural steroid injections, and which steroid is safest? *Radiology* 2016;279:657–659.

73. Feeley IH, Healy EF, Noel J, et al. Particulate and non-particulate steroids in spinal epidurals: a systematic review and meta-analysis. *Eur Spine J* 2017;26:336–344.

74. MacVicar J, King W, Landers MH, et al. The effectiveness of lumbar transforaminal injection of steroids: a comprehensive review with systematic analysis of the published data. *Pain Med* 2013;14:14–28.

75. Jeong HS, Lee JW, Kim SH, et al. Effectiveness of transforaminal epidural steroid injection by using a preganglionic approach: a prospective randomized controlled study. *Radiology* 2007;245:584–590.

76. Narozny M, Zanetti M, Boos N. Therapetuic efficacy of selective nerve root blocks in the treatment of lumbar radicular leg pain. *Swiss Med Wkly* 2001;131:75–80.

77. Smith CC, Booker T, Schaufele MK, et al. Interlaminar versus transforaminal epidural steroid injections for the treatment of symptomatic lumbar spinal stenosis. *Pain Med* 2010;11:1511–1555.

78. Weiner BK, Fraser RD. Foraminal injection for lateral lumbar disc herniation. *J Bone Joint Surg Br* 1997;79:804–807.

79. Wang JC, Lin E, Brodke DS, et al. Epidural injections for the treatment of symptomatic lumbar herniated discs. *J Spinal Disord Tech* 2002;15:269–272.

80. Park CH, Lee SH, Kim BI. Comparison of the effectiveness of lumbar transforaminal epidural injection with particulate and nonparticulate corticosteroids in lumbar radiating pain. *Pain Med* 2010;11:1654–1658.

81. Viton JM, Peretti-Viton P, Rubino T, et al. Short-term assessment of periradicular corticosteroid injections in lumbar radiculopathy associated with disc pathology. *Neuroradiology* 1998;40:59–62.

82. Lutz GE, Vad VB, Wisneski RJ. Fluoroscopic transforaminal lumbar epidural steroids: an outcome study. *Arch Phys Med Rehabil* 1998;79:1362–1366.

83. Kabatas S, Cansever T, Yilmaz C, et al. Transforaminal epidural steroid injection via a preganglionic approach for lumbar spinal stenosis and lumbar discogenic pain with radiculopathy. *Neurol India* 2010;58:248–252.

84. Lee JH, Moon J, Lee SH. Comparison of effectiveness according to different approaches of epidural steroid injection in lumbosacral herniated disk and spinal stenosis. *J Back Musculoskelet Rehabil* 2009;22:83–89.

85. Riew KD, Yin Y, Gilula L, et al. The effect of nerve-root injections on the need for operative treatment of lumbar radicular pain. A prospective, randomized, controlled, double-blind study. *J Bone Joint Surg Am* 2000;82-A:1589–1593.

86. Ng L, Chaudhary N, Sell P. The efficacy of corticosteroids in periradicular infiltration for chronic radicular pain: a randomized, double-blind, controlled trial. *Spine (Phila Pa 1976)* 2005;30:857–862.

87. Tafazal S, Ng L, Chaudhary N, et al. Corticosteroids in peri-radicular infiltration for radicular pain: a randomised double blind controlled trial. One year results and subgroup analysis. *Eur Spine J* 2009;18:1220–1225.

88. Vad VB, Bhat AL, Lutz GE, et al. Transforaminal epidural steroid injections in lumbosacral radiculopathy: a prospective randomized study. *Spine (Phila Pa 1976)* 2002;27:11–16.

89. Karppinen J, Malmivaara A, Kurunlahti M, et al. Periradicular infiltration for sciatica: a randomized controlled trial. *Spine (Phila Pa 1976)* 2001;26:1059–1067.

90. Ghahreman A, Ferch R, Bogduk N. The efficacy of transforaminal injection of steroids for the treatment of lumbar radicular pain. *Pain Med* 2010;11:1149–1168.

91. Riew KD, Park JB, Cho YS, et al. Nerve root blocks in the treatment of lumbar radicular pain. A minimum five-year follow-up. *J Bone Joint Surg Am* 2006;88:1722–1725.

92. Karppinen J, Ohinmaa A, Malmivaara A, et al. Cost effectiveness of periradicular infiltration for sciatica: subgroup analysis of a randomized controlled trial. *Spine (Phila Pa 1976)* 2001;26:2587–2595.

93. Bhatti A, Kim S. Role of epidural injections to prevent surgical intervention in patients with chronic sciatica: a systematic review and meta-analysis. *Cureus* 2016;8(8):e723.

94. Kaufmann TJ, Geske JR, Murthy NS, et al. Clinical effectiveness of single lumbar transforaminal epidural steroid injections. *Pain Med* 2013;14:1126–1133.

95. Murthy NS, Geske JR, Shelerud RA, et al. The effectiveness of repeat lumbar transforaminal epidural steroid injections. *Pain Med* 2014;15:1686–1694.

96. Friedly JL, Comstock BA, Turner JA, et al. A randomized trial of epidural glucocorticoid injections for spinal stenosis. *N Engl J Med* 2014;371(1):11–21.

97. Ghahreman A, Bogduk N. Predictors of a favorable response to transforaminal injection of steroids in patients with lumbar radicular pain due to disc herniation. *Pain Med* 2011;12(6):871–879.

98. Choi SJ, Song JS, Kim C, et al. The use of magnetic resonance imaging to predict the clinical outcome of non-surgical treatment for lumbar intervertebral disc herniation. *Korean J Radiol* 2007;8:156–163.

99. Maus TP, El-Yahchouchi CA, Geske JR, et al. Imaging determinants of clinical effectiveness of lumbar transforaminal epidural steroid injections. *Pain Med* 2016;17(12):2176–2184.

100. Desai MJ, Shah B, Sayal PK. Epidural contrast flow patterns of transforaminal epidural steroid injections stratified by commonly used final needle-tip position. *Pain Med* 2011;12(6):864–870.

101. Lee JW, Kim SH, Lee IS, et al. Therapeutic effect and outcome predictors of sciatica treated using transforaminal epidural steroid injection. *AJR Am J Roentgenol* 2006;187(6):1427–1431.

102. El-Yahchouchi C, Wald J, Brault J, et al. Lumbar transforaminal epidural steroid injections: does immediate post-procedure pain response predict longer term effectiveness? *Pain Med* 2014;15(6):921–928.

103. Karaman H, Kavak GO, Tüfek A, et al. The complications of transforaminal lumbar epidural steroid injections. *Spine (Phila Pa 1976)* 2011;36(13):E819–E824.

104. McGrath JM, Schaefer MP, Malkamaki DM. Incidence and characteristics of complications from epidural steroid injections. *Pain Med* 2011;12(5):726–731.

105. Bui J, Bogduk N. A systematic review of the effectiveness of CT-guided, lumbar transforaminal injection of steroids. *Pain Med* 2013;14:1860–1865.

106. Lee KS, Lin CL, Hwang SL, et al. Transforaminal periradicular infiltration guided by CT for unilateral sciatica—an outcome study. *Clin Imaging* 2005;29:211–214.

107. Karaeminoğullari O, Sahin O, Boyvat F, et al. Transforaminal epidural steroid injection under computed tomography guidance in relieving lumbosacral radicular pain [in Turkish]. *Acta Orthop Traumatol Turc* 2005;39:416–420.

108. Wewalka M, Abdelrahimsai A, Wiesinger G, et al. CT-guided transforaminal epidural injections with local anesthetic, steroid, and tramadol for the treatment of persistent lumbar radicular pain. *Pain Physician* 2012;15:153–159.

109. Berger O, Dousset V, Delmer O, et al. Évaluation de l'efficacité des infiltrations foraminales de croticoïdes guides sous tomodensitoméétrie, dans le traitement des radiculagies par conflit foraminal. *J Radiol* 1999;80:917–925.

110. Kranz PG, Amrhein TJ, Gray L. Incidence of inadvertent intravascular injection during CT fluoroscopy-guided epidural steroid injections. *AJNR Am J Neuroradiol* 2015;36(5):1000–1007.

111. van Helvoirt H, Apeldoorn AT, Ostelo RW, et al. Transforaminal epidural steroid injections followed by mechanical diagnosis and therapy to prevent surgery for lumbar disc herniation. *Pain Med* 2014;15(7):1100–1108.

CHAPTER 100

Intrathecal Drug Delivery in the Management of Pain

EDGAR ROSS and **DAVID ARCELLA**

During the past 25 to 30 years, implantable drug delivery devices designed for long-term continuous infusion of medications have become an increasingly important part of the armamentarium for physicians involved in the treatment of patients with intractable pain. Intrathecal drug delivery systems (IDDSs) are an important and effective tool for use in the management of noncancer pain, spasticity, and cancer-related pain, and potentially for other central nervous system (CNS) disorders. Over the past several years, there has been a shift away from utilizing IDDS for nonmalignant pain, but recent studies suggesting the usefulness of far lower drug doses than previously employed (microdosing) might change the current trend.

History of the Development of Intrathecal Drug Delivery Systems

The development of IDDS devices represents one of the most significant advances of the past several decades in the field of chronic pain management. The advent of intraspinal opioid therapy is directly linked to the discovery and isolation of opioid receptors in the early 1970s and the discovery of their existence in both the brain and spinal cord. Yaksh and Rudy.[1] discovered that direct application of morphine to the spinal cord in experimental animals produced measurable analgesic effects, and several years later, it was shown that the intraspinal injection of morphine, epidurally or intrathecally, produced effective analgesia in humans. In 1981, the first report describing the continuous infusion of intrathecal (IT) morphine in patients with intractable pain due to underlying malignancy was published.[2] Since this initial publication, a sizeable body of literature has amassed detailing the application, safety, and efficacy of intraspinal opiates in the management of both acute and chronic pain.[3]

Basic Pharmacology of Intrathecal Drug Administration

The safe and effective use of IT infusion therapy is predicated on a thorough knowledge of the pharmacology of the individual drugs and an understanding of the pharmacodynamics of IT or epidural drug delivery.

The distribution and absorption of a drug delivered directly to the cerebrospinal fluid (CSF) within the IT space is based on multiple variables. These can be divided into patient characteristics (age, height, weight, gender, spinal anatomy, and CSF volume and circulation), drug characteristics (baricity, volume, dose, concentration, temperature of solution, viscosity, and additives), and injection technique (patient position, level of injection, needle type and alignment, use of an IT catheter, and fluid dynamics) (Fig. 100.1). When reviewing the patient characteristics, one must consider the nature of the patient's pain complaint and the desired drug target. Central receptors within the spinal cord itself are the target for IT drug infusion, whereas brain receptors are the desired target in systemic drug therapy. CSF characteristics are also consequential. The choroid plexus produces CSF at a rate of about 0.3 to 0.4 mL per minute, and the CSF itself circulates through the cerebral ventricles and is ultimately reabsorbed into the venous system through the arachnoid villi.

CSF drug distribution was once thought to be primarily through bulk flow but now is thought to be mixing within the CSF produced by pulsatile blood flow (Fig. 100.2). Because of the relatively small volume of CSF in the spinal canal (about 75 mL) and the relatively slow clearance of hydrophilic drugs from the CSF, infusions of even small doses of hydrophilic compounds can result in relatively high concentrations of that drug at the target site of action within the spinal cord as well as significant concentrations within the brain, potentially leading to side effects. Lipid solubility of drugs plays an important role in determining both the spread of the drug within the IT space and its rate of clearance from the CSF. More water-soluble (hydrophilic) substances like morphine do not readily cross the blood–brain barrier, and infusion into the lumbar IT space produces high lumbar CSF concentrations of the infused agent in a gradient from the caudal to rostral direction. In contrast, compounds that are more lipid soluble (hydrophobic) will be preferentially absorbed into the substance of the spinal cord or diffuse across the subarachnoid-dural barrier to the epidural space. Lipophilic drugs like fentanyl and sufentanil usually do not reach significant concentrations within the CSF and may be useful in producing more segmental analgesia without the supraspinal effects that occasionally occur with more hydrophilic drugs.

A continuous implanted IT drug infusion has significant theoretical and practical advantages over bolus administration. The use of an implanted continuous IT drug delivery system provides a continuously consistent concentration of drug within the CSF. This is advantageous because the concentration gradient is the primary driving force for diffusion of a drug to its target site in the spinal cord. This method also results in more predictable concentration gradient and is generally associated with fewer adverse side effects than intermittent bolus administration of the same drug.

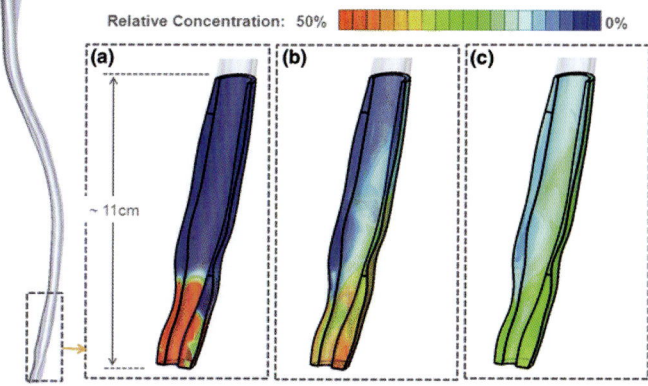

FIGURE 100.1 Three-dimensional drug propagation in the lower thoraco-lumbar regions starting from a concentration distribution simulated in a separate injection analysis. Contour plots (scaled to 50% of the initial concentration) after 0 minutes (A), 20 minutes (B), and 20 minutes (C) show decreased and homogenized drug concentration levels. *(Reprinted by permission from Springer: Kuttler A, Dimke T, Kern S, et al. Understanding pharmacokinetics using realistic computational models of fluid dynamics: biosimulation of drug distribution within the CSF space for intrathecal drugs. J Pharmacokinet Pharmacodyn 2010;37[6]:629–644. Copyright © 2010 The Author[s].)*

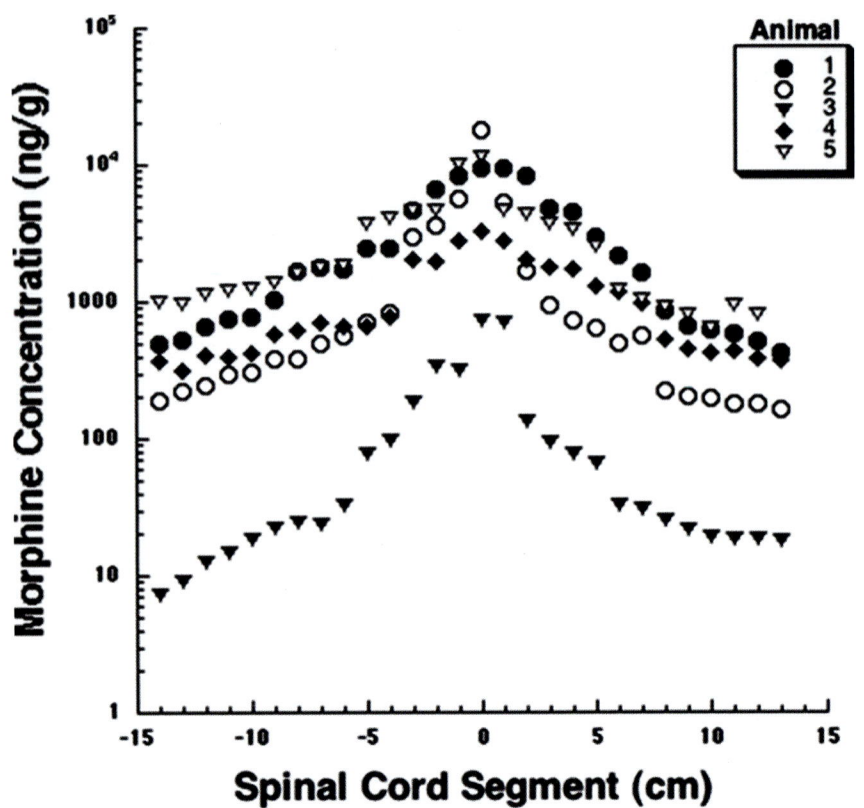

FIGURE 100.2 Morphine concentration (log scale) in each spinal segment from each animal. Animal 3 received one-tenth of the morphine dose in comparison with the other animals. *(Reprinted with permission from Flack SH, Anderson CM, Bernards C. Morphine distribution in the spinal cord after chronic infusion in pigs. Anesth Analg 2011;112[2]:460–464.*

Selection of Agents for Intrathecal Drug Delivery

Many drugs have been developed specifically for continuous IT delivery; however, only three have been approved by the U.S. Food and Drug Administration (FDA) for use with IDDS: morphine, ziconotide, and baclofen. Although there have been many scientific studies examining the use of other drugs published in the scientific literature, their use is considered "off label," as they have not undergone the rigorous testing required for regulatory approval.

The Polyanalgesic Consensus Conference (PACC) is composed of a group of experts in the use of IDDS that convenes every several years to update recommendations about the evidence-based use of IT drugs for the treatment of pain. The most recent PACC recommendations on IT drug infusion systems were revised in May 2016. This group recommends selecting the appropriate agent based on the nature of each patient's pain. Decision making should include an effort to differentiate nociceptive, neuropathic, spastic, or mixed pain syndromes. The PACC recommends that use of FDA-approved agents should precede any off-label drug use, alone or in combination with other agents; off-label use should be reserved for those patients who cannot tolerate or fail to respond to FDA-approved agents. In selecting a drug or drug combination, the PACC used the available scientific evidence and expert input to develop two distinct algorithms: one for neuropathic pain and one for nociceptive pain. The regimens are ranked from first-line recommended therapy (supported by extensive clinical experience and published literature) through fifth-line treatment approaches (anecdotal evidence alone). Neuropathic pain generally responds to ziconotide, opioid plus local anesthetic, local anesthetic alone, clonidine plus opioid, and clonidine alone. Nociceptive pain generally responds to opioid, ziconotide, opioid plus local anesthetic, and local anesthetic alone. Care should be given to selection of medication or compounded medications because granuloma formation has been associated with higher concentrations and total daily doses of all opioids except fentanyl.

The PACC further makes distinct recommendations to allow for variations including localized and diffuse pain, cancer or terminal illness, and noncancer pain. Thus, it is important to consider age, type of pain, and anticipated duration of therapy when selecting an agent. Table 100.1 details these recommendations.

Specific Agents for Intrathecal Drug Delivery

OPIOIDS
Morphine
The discovery of spinal opioid receptors in the 1970s represents the initial event that spawned interest in the IT administration of morphine. Several types of opioid receptors have been identified (μ, δ, κ). μ Receptors are the most important subtype in so far as the major clinical effects of morphine are concerned.[4] Indeed, high concentration of μ receptors have been identified in the dorsal horn of the spinal cord, the presumed spinal site of action of morphine and other opioids used for IT infusion. IT morphine is considered to be about 10 times more potent than the same dose administered epidurally and approximately 100 times as potent as the same dose given IV. The most commonly used conversion values for morphine are 1 mg IT morphine = 10 mg epidural morphine = 100 mg IV morphine = 300 mg oral morphine. It should be clearly understood that these figures represent estimates and that the relative potency of morphine administered by different routes may not be the same in all patients or in patients who have been receiving chronic systemic therapy.

TABLE 100.1	2017 Polyanalgesic Consensus Conference Dosing and Concentration Guidelines				
Drug	Starting Dose Range	Recommended Maximum Concentration	Recommended Maximum Dose per Day	Guidelines: Localized Nociceptive or Neuropathic Pain	Guidelines: Diffuse Nociceptive or Neuropathic Pain
Morphine	0.1–0.5 mg/d	20 mg/mL	15 mg	First line alone Second line + bupivacaine Third line + clonidine Fourth line + clonidine and bupivacaine	First line +/− bupivacaine Second line + clonidine
Hydromorphone	0.01–0.5 mg/d	15 mg/mL	10 mg	First line alone Second line + bupivacaine Third line + clonidine Fourth line + clonidine and bupivacaine	Second line +/− bupivacaine or clonidine
Fentanyl	25–75 µg/d	10 mg/mL	1,000 µg	First line alone Second line + bupivacaine Third line + clonidine Fourth line + clonidine and bupivacaine	Third line +/− bupivacaine or clonidine
Sufentanil	10–20 µg/d	5 mg/mL	500 µg	Third line alone Fourth line + bupivacaine Fifth line + bupivacaine and clonidine	Not recommended
Bupivacaine	1–4 mg/d	30 mg/mL	15–20 mg	Second line + opioid Fourth line + opioid and clonidine Fifth line + sufentanil and clonidine	First line + morphine Second line + hydromorphone Third line + fentanyl Fourth line + clonidine +/− opioid
Clonidine	20–100 µg/d	1,000 mcg/mL	600 µg	Third line + opioid Fourth line + opioid and bupivacaine *or* + sufentanil Fifth line + sufentanil + bupivacaine	Second line + morphine or hydromorphone Third line + fentanyl Fourth line + bupivacaine + opioid
Ziconotide	0.5–1.2 µg/d (to 2.4 µg/d per product labeling)	100 mcg/mL	19.2 µg	First line alone Second line + opioid	First line alone Third line + opioid
Baclofen	50–100 µg/d	5,000 mg/mL	1,000 µg (highest dose studied as an analgesic)	Not recommended	Fifth-line monotherapy

The advantages of IT drug administration include the lack of an absorption phase and essentially 100% bioavailability. Because of the small volume of distribution (spinal CSF volume is approximately 75 mL) of morphine when injected or infused into the CSF, a dose of IT morphine yields significantly higher CSF concentration than that which occurs when given epidurally where significant vascular absorption occurs. In addition, because the rate of elimination of morphine from the CSF and plasma is similar, the duration of action of IT morphine is relatively long. Following IT administration, morphine is not detectable in serum for the first 2 hours.[5] Because morphine is a hydrophilic compound, there is slow rostral spread of the drug through bulk flow of CSF, one factor responsible for clearance of morphine from the CSF. This slow rostral spread is also thought to be responsible for the delayed respiratory depression that can occur following IT administration, particularly in opioid-naive patients. Studies have indicated that following IT infusion of morphine in the upper lumbar region, a steady-state concentration gradient develops over a period of about 72 hours, with a lumbar:cervical concentration ratio of around 7 to 8:1. Elimination of IT morphine occurs through vascular absorption through the blood supply of the spinal cord. CSF elimination of opioids in general is biexponential and dependent on the lipid solubility of the drug. With a single bolus injection of morphine, there is thought to be little metabolism of the drug. However, with chronic infusion, morphine is metabolized to morphine-6-glucuronide (M6G) which has been shown in animal studies to have a potency

10 to 45 times that of morphine itself.[5] Preservative-free morphine is currently the only opioid that is approved for IT use by the FDA.

Hydromorphone
Despite the paucity of clinical studies, the use of IT hydromorphone as an alternate opioid has steadily increased. Hydromorphone was initially utilized for IDDS in patients who manifested intolerable side effects to IT morphine or inadequate analgesia. Indeed, based on the large clinical experience with hydromorphone, this agent has been recommended as a "line 1" agent by the most recent Polyanalgesia Consensus Conference.[6] IT hydromorphone is approximately 5 to 6 times more potent than IT morphine and is somewhat more lipophilic.[4] Perhaps its main attraction is that IT hydromorphone is generally associated with fewer side effects than is IT morphine.

Fentanyl and Sufentanil
There has been considerable human and animal research regarding the IT use of both fentanyl and sufentanil.[4] Both fentanyl and sufentanil are highly potent µ receptor agonists which are highly lipid soluble. Both have a rapid onset (approximately 10 minutes) and relatively long duration of action (1 to 4 hours for fentanyl, 2 to 6 hours for sufentanil) following acute IT administration. Because of the lipid solubility of these agents, it is important that the tip of the delivery catheter be positioned within a few spinal segments of the segmental pain level. Although this is not particularly critical for treatment of axial lumbar and/or lower extremity pain, it is important for treatment of

pain at more rostral levels. In such cases, if the catheter is not located relatively close to the segmental level of pain, the drug will be absorbed into the spinal cord preventing the development of adequate concentration at the intended target site.

Overall, the analgesic response to long-term infusion to either agent was favorable and relatively well tolerated. Effective dosages have been in the microgram range: 10 to 115 µg per day for fentanyl and 12 to 77 µg per day for sufentanil.

Opioid-Induced Hyperalgesia and Intrathecal Opioids

Opioid-induced hyperalgesia is a condition that is manifest by a dramatically augmented sensitivity to stimuli and often appears in those receiving long-term IT therapy with opioids. This is manifest as *hyperalgesia*, an exaggerated pain response to a stimuli that would normally be considered mildly noxious, like a pinprick and *allodynia*, pain that is produced by a normally nonnoxious stimulus, like light touch. This phenomenon has been increasingly recognized in patients who have been treated with long-term opioid therapy and is yet another potential cause loss of analgesia with IT drug infusion. Opioid-induced hyperalgesia is not simply an escalation of the patient's original pain condition. Rather, the "abnormal" pain often originates from an area that is anatomically distinct from the original pain. In some patients, pain seems to increase and become more diffuse over time despite gradual escalation in their opioid doses. It has recently been shown that opioid-induced hyperalgesia may also develop in the context of short-term therapy in the absence of physical dependence or withdrawal.[7]

LOCAL ANESTHETICS

Local anesthetics have played a central role in the treatment of pain for decades, although it was not until the 1990s that continuous infusion of these agents was routinely used.[8] Currently, local anesthetics such as bupivacaine are commonly given by continuous chronic IT infusion, often combined with opiates for the treatment of both cancer and nonmalignant pain. In low concentrations, local anesthetics such as bupivacaine are nontoxic and alter neurotransmission in a predictable and reversible fashion.

Bupivacaine is the most common local anesthetic used for continuous IT infusion. It appears to be most effective in patients with a neuropathic component of pain, although it may also provide some degree of benefit for patients with nociceptive pain. The utilization and dose escalation of bupivacaine is mainly limited by its side effects, which include sensorimotor blockade at higher doses and hemodynamic instability. Usually, clinically relevant side effects do not occur with doses less than 15 mg per day, although administration of doses as high as 118 mg per day has been reported with apparently no adverse effects. Optimal dosing is reached with progressive titration beginning with a daily dose of 3 to 5 mg per day. There has been some interest in liposomal encapsulation for local delivery by the IT route because this tends to reduce the toxicity and cardiovascular effects while increasing the anesthetic duration.

Ropivacaine is a long-acting amide type of local anesthetic that is unique in that it blocks sensory nerve fibers to a greater extent than motor fibers. It is similar to bupivacaine in onset and duration of sensory blockade. The potential advantage of ropivacaine is that it produces less motor block and has less cardiac toxicity than bupivacaine. As of yet, there have been no clinical studies published on the long-term use of IT ropivacaine for the management of chronic pain.[6]

Tetracaine is another local anesthetic that acts through blockade of sodium channels. Unfortunately, tetracaine has been shown to have direct neurotoxicity in animals manifested by damage to both the dorsal and ventral roots, chromatolytic deterioration of motor neurons, and vacuolation of the spinal cord. Because of the potential neurotoxicity, tetracaine should not be used for long-term IT drug delivery.[6,9]

α₂-ADRENERGIC AGONISTS

α_2-Adrenergic receptors play an important role in spinal antinociception. α_2-Receptor agonists in general, and clonidine in particular, are believed to produce their antinociceptive effects through inhibitory interactions with both pre- and postsynaptic primary afferent nociceptive projections onto secondary neurons in the spinal dorsal horn. Clonidine in particular has been felt to act by postsynaptic activation of descending noradrenergic inhibitory systems. It has also been suggested that the analgesic effects of this class of drugs might also be produced through the inhibition of substance P (SP) release.[10] Clonidine-induced spinal analgesia is reversed by α-adrenergic antagonists such as yohimbine but not by naloxone, providing further evidence of its mechanism of action.

Clonidine is one of the best studied of the nonopioid agents that have been adapted for intraspinal delivery. Clonidine has been shown to have analgesic action in both cancer and nonmalignant pain syndromes when administered intraspinally.[4] Clonidine is a highly lipid-soluble drug that is rapidly absorbed and eliminated from CSF. Bolus administration of IT clonidine results in dose-dependent analgesia at doses of 150, 300, and 450 µg, and effective analgesia has also been shown with continuous IT infusion. Intraspinal clonidine appears to be devoid of any local neurotoxicity. The rapid onset of antinociceptive action when given intrathecally provides a strong argument that the major pharmacologic effects occur at the segmental spinal level. However, delayed supraspinal analgesic effects cannot be completely discounted because it has been shown that application of clonidine to the locus coeruleus results in analgesia. Because IT injection does not usually result in high cisternal concentrations of clonidine, these supraspinal effects might be explained by systemic absorption and central redistribution of the drug.

Although clonidine is the most common drug in this class to be used for spinal analgesia, other agents such as epinephrine, tizanidine, and dexmedetomidine continue to be studied for spinal infusion. Because the antinociceptive actions of the α_2-adrenergic agonists (and most of the other alternative agents discussed later) occur through a nonopioid mechanism, they are often effective in individuals who have become tolerant to morphine or other opiates. These agents (clonidine in particular) shift the opioid dose–response curve to the left and appear to be synergistic with opioids; in other words, the analgesia produced by the combination of clonidine with an opiate often results in a magnitude of analgesia greater than that produced by either agent alone. The major side effects of spinal clonidine include hypotension, bradycardia, and sedation. The hypotensive effects most commonly occur with lower and moderate doses and are generally counteracted at higher doses by a direct peripheral vasoconstrictive effect.[11] Unlike the opiates, clonidine does not cause respiratory depression. Clonidine has been studied in various animal models for possible neurotoxicity prior to its clinical use and has been found safe.[12]

Clonidine has become a popular agent for spinal infusion in patients with reflex sympathetic dystrophy (RSD), now known as complex regional pain syndrome (CRPS) type I. Rauck et al.[13] studied the efficacy of epidural clonidine in 26 patients with severe pain from CRPS I using a randomized, double-blind, placebo-controlled design. Cervical or lumbar catheters were placed in patients with upper or lower extremity RSD, respectively. Epidural clonidine (300 or 700 µg) and placebo were randomly administered on 3 consecutive days, and the analgesic response assessed at specified intervals for 6 hours following injection using Visual Analog Scale (VAS) scores and the McGill Pain Questionnaire (MPQ). Patients considered positive responders were offered entry into a trial of continuous epidural clonidine infusion. Within 20 minutes of injection, both doses of clonidine but not placebo-produced significant reductions in both VAS and MPQ scores that persisted for the

6-hour study period. Blood pressure was reduced by a similar amount with both clonidine doses. Nineteen patients were subsequently treated with continuous clonidine infusion (32 ± 6 µg per hour; range 14 to 50 µg per hour) for 43 ± 8 days (range 7 to 225 days). Their VAS scores, which were measured at weekly intervals during infusion, were significantly reduced compared with those recorded prior to clonidine therapy. Clonidine is currently approved by the FDA for continuous epidural infusion. Clonidine is not currently approved for IT infusion.

Although clonidine has been the most widely studied of the α_2-agonists, several other agents have also received attention as potential spinal analgesic agents. Tizanidine is another α_2-agonist that has shown promise as a potential analgesic substance. Leiphart et al.[14] studied the effects of tizanidine in a rat model of mononeuropathic pain that is believed to mimic the hyperalgesia and allodynia typical of many neuropathic pain syndromes in humans. Tizanidine increased the intensity of the mechanical stimulus required to induce paw withdrawal and reduced the duration of limb withdrawal from both normal temperature and cooled surfaces in a dose-dependent fashion. The effects of tizanidine were limited to the hyperalgesic limb and served only to normalize reactive latencies. However, morphine affected both the experimental and unaffected hind limb and increased withdrawal latencies to supernormal values. These findings suggest that IT tizanidine may be more specific for the hyperalgesia and allodynia associated with neuropathic pain states and perhaps may be valuable in managing patients that exhibit these findings.

Dexmedetomidine, another α_2-agonist with a higher α_2-receptor affinity than clonidine, has been studied experimentally for its effects on neuropathic pain.[15] A dose of 1 µg of dexmedetomidine or 10 µg of clonidine administered intrathecally following sciatic nerve section resulted in a significant reduction in autotomy behavior (self-mutilation thought to be a sign of neuropathic pain) compared with both IT morphine and saline controls. Interestingly, morphine (but not α_2-agonists) caused a significant reduction in autotomy behavior when given prophylactically or before sciatic nerve section. This finding suggests that morphine may prevent autotomy if administered prophylactically, whereas α_2-agonists may be useful for treating established pain on a chronic basis. This observation could potentially have practical implications on the prevention or treatment of certain pain states such as pain following peripheral nerve injury or phantom pain. To date, there have been no studies in humans to investigate the efficacy or toxicity of this agent when given intrathecally.

CALCIUM CHANNEL ANTAGONISTS

Calcium is a critical element in the regulation of intracellular processes, including modulation of neuronal excitability, release of neurotransmitters, activation of second messenger systems, and gene transcription. Calcium has been found to play an important role in nociception and pain transmission. Regulation of calcium entry into cells is controlled by voltage-sensitive calcium channels (VSCCs) consisting of at least six neuronal subtypes (L, N, P, Q, R, and T). VSCCs are abundantly expressed on presynaptic nerve terminals where they regulate the calcium-dependent release of neurotransmitters that control synaptic transmission. N-type VSCCs are concentrated in the most superficial laminae of the dorsal horn of the spinal cord, where most primary nociceptive afferent fibers (Aδ and C fibers) terminate. Selective antagonists of N-type calcium channels such as ziconotide (also known as SNX-111), a synthetic agent derived from ω-conopeptide that selectively binds to N-type VSCC, have consistently been antinociceptive in animal models of acute, chronic, and neuropathic pain.[16,17] Based on animal studies, numerous studies of ziconotide have been conducted in humans to determine both safety and efficacy. Based on these studies, ziconotide was ultimately approved by the FDA for IT use in humans.[18,19]

The most common side effects included mental confusion, word-finding difficulties, nystagmus, gait, and balance problems. The frequent side effects associated with IT ziconotide have limited the overall use of this agent.

N-METHYL-D-ASPARTATE RECEPTOR ANTAGONISTS

The involvement of excitatory amino acids (EAAs) and the N-methyl-D-aspartate (NMDA) receptor system in nociceptive transmission, along with a clearer understanding of the development of central sensitization and wind-up phenomena, have generated considerable interest in developing antagonists of this receptor for the treatment of chronic pain, particularly neuropathic pain states. NMDA receptors alter opioid receptor sensitivity in a variety of pain states and have been implicated in the development of both opioid tolerance and opioid-induced hyperalgesia. Ketamine has been the most studied and has been used both epidurally and intrathecally for the treatment of postoperative and chronic pain.

To date, the use of NMDA receptor antagonists has been limited due to side effects. All of the NMDA receptor antagonists to some extent produce phencyclidine-like side effects such as disinhibition, hallucinations, paranoid delusions, and rises in arterial blood pressure.[20] There is also animal data suggesting that some of the NMDA antagonists may be neurotoxic when administered intrathecally. Using a sheep model for IT infusion, Hassenbusch et al.[21] conducted a randomized, double-blind toxicity study of three NMDA antagonists: dextrorphan, dextromethorphan, and memantine. Gross and histologic examination as well as neurologic measures demonstrated that all three agents produced a dose-dependent chronic inflammatory response of the spinal cord that led to necrosis. Although these agents are not currently suited for widespread use in humans, their beneficial effects, especially on wind-up pain and hyperalgesia, suggest that further efforts should be directed toward developing an agent that retains its analgesic properties while eliminating most of the side effects.

γ-AMINOBUTYRIC ACID AGONISTS

γ-Aminobutyric acid (GABA) and glycine are inhibitory neurotransmitters that are widely distributed throughout the nervous system. The beneficial effects of GABA agonists such as baclofen in reducing both spinal- and cerebral-origin spasticity have been well chronicled. Less well known are the potential analgesic effects of these agents. GABA can be readily found within the pain transmission system, particularly in Lissauer's tract, and in laminae I, II, and III of the dorsal horn of the spinal cord. Baclofen is a GABA-B agonist and has been shown to be analgesic when administered intrathecally in animals. The antinociceptive effects of GABA agonists are not reversed by naloxone, suggesting that GABA-aminergic analgesia is not mediated through endogenous opiates. IT baclofen diminished allodynic behavioral responses following IT administration of prostaglandin (PG) F$_{2\alpha}$ and reduced c-*fos* gene expression in an animal model of neurogenic pain.[22]

GABAPENTIN

The use of IT gabapentin has been evaluated in a number of rodent models.[9] Injection of an IT bolus of gabapentin resulted in reduction in mechanical allodynia and thermal hyperalgesia. There was no demonstrable effect on acute nociceptive pain assessed by the formalin or hot plate test. IT gabapentin produced no deleterious hemodynamic effects but did lead to mild neurologic dysfunction when dose in excess of 300 µg were used.

SOMATOSTATIN AND SOMATOSTATIN ANALOGUES

Somatostatin is a tetradecapeptide that is widely distributed throughout the CNS. Somatostatin was initially discovered by virtue of its ability to inhibit the secretion of growth hormone from the pituitary gland. However, its distribution is not limited to the pituitary axis. Indeed, somatostatinergic neurons can be found in the spinal cord, primarily in the substantia gelatinosa where they seem to exert inhibitory effects on nociceptive neurons.[23] Somatostatin is also present in other areas of the CNS concerned with pain transmission and modulation such as the periaqueductal gray (PAG) and both ascending and descending pain-modulating systems in the brainstem. The presence of somatostatin in primary afferent axons that terminate in lamina II of the dorsal horn of the spinal cord, spinal interneurons, descending inhibitory pathways, and PAG presents a strong circumstantial argument for an antinociceptive role of this substance. Single cell recordings have indicated that somatostatin inhibits the responses of dorsal horn neurons to noxious stimulation.[24] Somatostatin has been shown to elevate pain thresholds in experimental animals and has been reported to produce analgesia in humans when administered by either an epidural or IT route.[25–28] The exact mechanism of action is unclear, although it does not appear to be opioid-mediated because the antinociceptive effects of somatostatin are not antagonized by naloxone.

Octreotide, a stable, nonenzymatically degraded, nontoxic analogue of somatostatin, has yielded promising results as a spinal analgesic for cancer pain. Penn et al.[25] reported the efficacy and preclinical neurotoxicity of IT octreotide in six patients with terminal cancer. At a concentration of 500 μg/mL, octreotide was found to be stable within the SynchroMed model 8611 programmable infusion pump (Medtronic Neurological, Minneapolis, Minnesota) over a 4-week period. Insignificant concentration changes were measured at the catheter tip and within the pump drug reservoir. Preclinical toxicity testing in dogs showed no evidence of histopathologic changes. Based on the stability and toxicity studies, six patients were treated with IT octreotide. Dosing was initiated at 2.5 to 5.0 μg per hour and increased by increments of 2.5 to 5.0 μg per hour to a maximum dose of 20 μg per hour or 240 μg per day as necessary to achieve pain control. Treatment was continued for periods of 13 to 91 days (mean duration 45.5 days). Baseline mean VAS scores of 9.7 were significantly reduced to 1.7 after 1 week of treatment. Although VAS scores increased to 3.6 at 1 month, the improvements remained statistically significant. The same authors have reported long-term experience with octreotide in two patients with nonmalignant pain.[26] Although this experience is modest if not anecdotal, it nevertheless provides additional evidence for a sustained analgesic effect of IT octreotide in nonmalignant disease states.

There does appear to be some element of tolerance, necessitating upward titration of the dose over time. Although octreotide does in fact produce analgesia, many factors currently make this agent impractical for widespread clinical use. First, the commercially available preservative-free preparation comes at a concentration of 500 μg/mL, necessitating frequent refills. Additionally, in order to avoid damaging the infusion device, the pH must be adjusted. Perhaps the most important factor is the extreme cost—in excess of $20,000 per year—which makes this agent unsuitable. Notwithstanding the limitations of octreotide, these results should prompt further investigation into the development of other somatostatin analogues that might be equally effective but more practical for clinical development.

TRICYCLIC ANTIDEPRESSANTS

Tricyclic antidepressants (TCAs) have long been known to participate in the modulation of pain transmission. The analgesic effects of TCAs are believed to be mediated through effects on monoaminergic and serotonergic pathways in the CNS, specifically, prevention of reuptake of these transmitters. In vitro testing has also shown that the TCAs bind with the NMDA receptor complex, possibly meaning that the antiallodynic and hyperalgesic effects of the TCAs are mediated via an NMDA

receptor mechanism.[29] The effect of IT TCAs on pain behavior has been studied in several animal models. Presently, IT administration of TCAs in humans is not possible due to the lack of preclinical toxicity data, the observed development of motor impairment at high doses in rat experiments, and the unavailability of preservative-free preparations. However, the profound reduction in hyperalgesia and the synergistic effect with opiates provide ample reason to pursue and develop this class of agents as an effective mode of pain control.

ACETYLCHOLINESTERASE INHIBITORS

Acetylcholine (ACH) is a ubiquitous neurotransmitter in all parts of both the central and peripheral nervous systems. Choline acetyltransferase, the rate-limiting enzyme in the synthesis of ACH, is abundant in nerve terminals within the dorsal horn of the spinal cord. Moreover, the presence of acetylcholinesterase in certain descending raphe-spinal projections implies that ACH may be implicated in the modulation of nociception. ACH diminishes the response of dorsal horn interneurons to EAAs. Some neurons are depolarized by cholinergic substances, whereas others become hyperpolarized. IT administration of both muscarinic and nicotinic agents has indicated that analgesic effects are mediated only through muscarinic receptors. Animal studies have shown that spinal neostigmine produces analgesia (albeit transiently) and also enhances the analgesia provided by IT clonidine but with fewer side effects.

Based on animal data, human applications of the use of IT neostigmine have been performed. Hood et al.[30] studied the effects of IT neostigmine in 28 healthy volunteers. Although IT administration of neostigmine was antinociceptive to a noxious cold stimulus, significant side effects occurred, including nausea, vomiting, reversible lower extremity weakness, and, at larger doses, tachycardia and hypertension. Although neostigmine alone is probably not suitable based on the side-effect profile, further studies may be warranted using this agent in patients who have become tolerant to opiates.

ADENOSINE

Although the results have been conflicting, some studies have demonstrated that adenosine, an endogenous nucleoside, and its analogues may participate in pain modulation. Belfrage et al.[31] performed an open-label trial to determine the safety and efficacy of IT adenosine in 14 patients with neuropathic pain accompanied by tactile hyperalgesia or allodynia.[31] Patients were given IT injections of either 500 or 1,000 μg of adenosine (n = 9), and areas of tactile pain were mapped. Spontaneous and evoked pain were assessed (VAS scale of 0 to 100) before and 1 hour after injection. Median VAS scores for spontaneous and evoked pain were reduced from 65 to 24 ($P < .01$) and 71 to 12 ($P < .01$), respectively. Parallel increases in tactile pain thresholds in areas of allodynia were also observed. The median reduction in the area of tactile hyperalgesia/allodynia was 90% ($P < .001$). Twelve of the 14 patients experienced pain relief for a median of 24 hours. The only noted side effect was transient lumbar pain at the site of injection.

NITRIC OXIDE

Nitric oxide (NO) is synthesized from L-arginine by activation of NO synthase. Because NO easily penetrates cell membranes, it has been identified as a substance that may potentially act like a neurotransmitter. Because synthesis of NO is induced through an NMDA receptor mechanism, and because NMDA receptors have been implicated in the wind-up phenomenon, NO may in fact participate in the development of this pathologic state. There is evidence of increased synthesis of NO in the dorsal root ganglion animal models of neuropathic pain. Malmberg and Yaksh[32] have injected arginine analogues that functionally inhibit NO synthesis intrathecally and found that they induce a dose-dependent reduction in the formation of the hyperalgesic state. Although there are currently no human trials to evaluate the role of NO synthesis inhibitors, this may represent fertile ground for future research.

PROSTAGLANDIN INHIBITORS

PGs are another well-known group of substances that participate as neurotransmitters. PGs are synthesized at the spinal cord level in the identical way to that which occurs systemically. Activation of the NMDA receptor and subsequent calcium influx are thought to lead to activation of phospholipase A_2 and ultimately to the formation of cyclooxygenase products. PGs increase calcium conductance in dorsal root ganglion cells, thereby increasing the release of SP and other peptides. Potentially, inhibition of IT PG formation might result in a reduction in neurotransmitters such as SP, thereby decreasing nociception. The effects of nonsteroidal anti-inflammatory agents are mediated through inhibition of PG synthesis. In fact, recent attention has been directed toward evaluating the analgesic effects of IT nonsteroidal agents. Malmberg and Yaksh[33] have studied the effects of IT ketorolac on nociception. IT ketorolac was found to inhibit the development of hyperalgesia in a rat model of neuropathic pain, but it had minimal effect on the acute phase of pain. When administered concomitantly with morphine, ketorolac produced a synergistic analgesic effect on both the fast and slow components of pain. Further research is obviously needed to define the exact role of the various PG substances as they relate to pain transmission as well as to study the potential for spinal toxicity.

CALCITONIN GENE-RELATED PEPTIDE ANTAGONISTS

Calcitonin gene-related peptide (CGRP) is another neuropeptide found in dorsal root ganglion cells, Aδ and C fibers, Lissauer's tract, and the terminals of primary afferents in laminae I, II, and V of the dorsal horn.[29] There are two types of CGRP and perhaps as many as four receptor subtypes. A noxious thermal stimulus has been shown to result in increased levels of CGRP in lamina II or the substantia gelatinosa. Moreover, some studies have shown that IT administration of CGRP actually increases nociceptive transmission, although the data on this are conflicting. It has been suggested that CGRP may enhance the effects of SP by either inhibition of the enzyme that degrades SP or augmentation of SP release. Yu et al.[34] showed that, although IT administration of CGRP does not produce any apparent effect on pain transmission, IT injection of CGRP 8-37, a known CGRP receptor antagonist, does induce a dose-dependent reduction in nociception. Notwithstanding the work of Yu et al.,[34] the conflicting evidence regarding CGRP indicates that the role of this substance needs to be more clearly defined before human trials of CGRP antagonists can be conducted.

SUBSTANCE P ANTAGONISTS

SP belongs to the family of substances known as the tachykinins. It is believed to be involved in the transmission or modulation of nociceptive information. SP is stored in synaptic vesicles in primary afferents located in laminae I and II of the dorsal horn and preferentially binds to the NK1 receptor. Based on SP's presumed role in pain transmission, studies have focused on whether antagonists of SP may be effective in producing analgesia. Again, data are conflicting regarding the effects of IT SP antagonists. Unfortunately, further studies have been hampered by the fact that these substances are neurotoxic and subject to rapid biodegradation, thus hindering application to human clinical trials.

Patient Selection for Intrathecal Drug Delivery

In selecting appropriate patients to undergo trial and ultimately permanent implantation of an IT drug delivery device and continuous IT infusion therapy, appropriate patient selection is

TABLE 100.2 Common Diagnosis Treated with Intrathecal Therapy

• Axial neck or back pain; not a surgical candidate
  • Multiple compression fractures
  • Discogenic pain
  • Spinal stenosis
  • Diffuse multiple-level spondylosis
• Failed back surgery syndrome
• Abdominal/pelvic pain
  • Visceral
  • Somatic
• Extremity pain
  • Radicular pain
  • Joint pain
• Complex regional pain syndrome (CRPS)
• Trunk pain
  • Postherpetic neuralgia
  • Postthoracotomy syndromes
• Cancer pain, direct invasion, and chemotherapy related
• Analgesic efficacy with systemic opioid delivery complicated by intolerable side effects

critical to success. Proper patient selection includes consideration of disease-specific indications, comorbid disease, previous systemic medication use, sustainability, economics and anticipated duration of IT therapy, patient goals of care, as well as psychological assessment and social support evaluation. When assessing potential candidacy for implantation, one needs to ensure that the patient candidate has already participated in multidisciplinary care and has tried the maximum oral therapeutic medications available. Of these patients, potential implantation candidates are those who have failed optimization of oral therapy or are not able to tolerate the adverse side effects of systemic medications.

Disease-specific indications include patients who have chronic intractable axial neck or back pain and are not candidates for surgical intervention and patients with failed back surgery syndrome, abdominal/pelvic pain, extremity pain, CRPS, trunk pain, or cancer pain either caused by direct invasion of tumor or as a result of therapy directed against malignancy. Patients may also be considered for IT drug delivery if they receive moderate pain relief with use of systemic opioids but are not able to tolerate the adverse effects of systemic therapy. Table 100.2 lists some of these common diagnosis.[35]

Comorbid conditions should be carefully considered in patient selection. Patients who are undergoing radiation or chemotherapy for treatment of malignancy may exhibit poor wound healing or be more susceptible to infection from therapy-induced neutropenia. A patient may be a good candidate for implanted IT drug delivery but may require coordination of implantation timing to coincide with a break in other therapies to allow for optimal conditions to undergo the surgery of implantation itself. Presence of coagulopathy or concomitant use of anticoagulants must be closely considered (e.g., a patient who has an extensive history of thrombotic events with any cessation or decrease in anticoagulation therapy might not be a candidate for implantation), as the risks of stopping anticoagulation might exceed the potential benefit of IT pain therapy. Care must also be given to the review of a candidate's medication list and various comorbidities. Specifically, one must assess any perturbations in the cardiopulmonary system that may be impacted by the introduction of sedating and respiratory depressant IT medications as well as their interactions with the patient's current regimen.

Previous systemic medication use comes into play in assessing the potential efficacy of utilizing implanted IT drug delivery systems. If a patient has shown evidence of analgesia with the use of a systemic opioid medication but is intolerant of the systemic adverse effects of opioid medication, they may be considered a stronger candidate than one who has not shown any relief with the use of systemic opioid medications. The patient's previous systemic medication usage also comes into play when attempting to determine dosing for both the trial phase and after implantation.

Sustainability, economics, and anticipated duration of therapy are important consideration in patient selection. The up-front cost of implantation of IDDS can be quite significant. The combined cost of the implanted device itself, along with operating room time and associated staff costs and the total hospital stay all figures into determining the total financial impact of employing this therapy. Hasselbusch et al.[36] in 2013 determined that when treating cancer pain, implanted IDDS achieved cost equivalence at an average of 7.4 months when compared to high-cost conventional therapies including high-dose opioids, nongeneric drugs, and parenteral drug administration. Kumar et al.[37] determined that the cross-over point where conventional therapy exceeded IDDS in treating nonmalignant pain was at 28 months.

Patient goals of care, psychological assessment, and social support evaluation are important to consider in evaluating a patient for potential implantation. With most patients treating malignant pain, the goals are usually palliative and in line with improving the patient's quality of life in their remaining time. An implanted IT drug delivery device should strongly be considered if a patient's main goal of care is to remain at home in the company of their family, as it can aid in achieving this goal. In patients with intractable pain associated with advanced illness, detailed psychological screening is often omitted. However, in selecting patients with nonmalignant pain, it is important to perform careful psychological screening while discussing and defining clear patient expectations of treatment and making clear the need for ongoing close follow-up for IDDS refill and management (see Chapter 76 for a detailed discussion of psychological screening in selecting patients for IDDS). It should be emphasized that the purpose of the psychological evaluation is not to simply "clear" or, for that matter, exclude the patient for an implant but rather to gain an understanding of the psychological factors that might influence the outcome in a particular patient. It is also important to realize that although a given patient might initially be noted to have an unfavorable psychological profile, this does not necessarily constitute an absolute contraindication to implantation at some time in the future. Patients who are willing to work with a psychologist and/or psychiatrist can progress to the point where they are appropriate candidate for IDDS at some point in the future. Table 76.3 lists referral guidelines for presurgical psychological screening.

Each patient should undergo a detailed pain history that includes a review of all prior pain treatments and the results of such treatments. A history of lack of benefit from all prior treatment is a poor prognostic sign. A relatively recent spinal imaging study should be reviewed to exclude obvious, surgically correctable conditions such as spinal stenosis or spinal instability and to assure that there is no pathology that would otherwise preclude safe placement of an IT catheter.

Contraindications to pump implantation include the presence of systemic infection, local cutaneous infection near the potential surgical sites, uncorrectable coagulopathy, known allergies to components of either the pump or catheter, and active IV drug use. Further challenges include emaciation or patients with a body habitus that may not be conducive to an implant in standard locations (i.e., inadequate subcutaneous tissue to create a pocket for the implanted pump). Careful consideration must be given to patients receiving anticoagulation therapy. Although implantation is not contraindicated in these patients, all anticoagulations must be reversed prior to any type of invasive procedure. Patients with an unfavorable psychological profile should not be considered for IDDS until any psychological concerns have been addressed and resolved. Although recovering drug addiction is not an absolute contraindication, these patients need careful assessment prior to proceeding with this therapy; it is important to understand that placement of an IDDS device does not lead directly or inevitably to cessation of all oral opioids.

Trialing Techniques for Intrathecal Drug Delivery

Prior to implantation of a permanent IDDS device, patients should undergo some type of screening trial to determine the effectiveness and potential drug-related side effects. Even before proceeding with the trial, it is imperative that the patient and physician establish the specific goals for determining success of the trial. Goals are not necessarily uniform across all patients but must be individualized on a case-by-case basis, depending on the particular circumstances. One of the goals, and probably the most important goal from the patient's point of view, is pain reduction. Most of the published literature defines a successful trial as a 50% reduction in the patient's pain. Although 50% pain reduction would seem to be a reasonable achievement in the chronic pain population, this figure should not be used as the sole determining factor of the success or failure of an individual trial. There are patients for whom a lesser reduction in pain is sufficient and results in improvement in activities, reduction in medication use, and other beneficial effects. There are also patients who will be disappointed with the outcome if they experience anything short of complete pain resolution. Some patients have difficulty with the realization that they will have some degree of pain for the duration of their life. These patients often struggle with discontinuing systemic opioids following pump implantation, demand frequent increases in their IT drug dose, and generally do not demonstrate the kind of improvement in function commensurate with their stated degree of pain reduction. Such patients often pose difficult long-term management problems; thus, it is imperative that the implanting physician clearly outlines the *reasonable* benefits and expectations of the therapy *before* proceeding with the trial. By establishing reasonable goals and expectations at the outset, future problems can often be avoided. Clinicians who fail to follow this basic principle will, more often than not, be left to deal with an unhappy and frustrated patient.

Although pain reduction is important, perhaps the more important and revealing outcome measure is improvement in function. The type and degree of functional improvement will vary between patients. Nonetheless, it is important to establish reasonable goals for functional improvement that can be measured and confirmed after institution of IT drug delivery. Physical and occupational therapists can be quite valuable in assisting the clinician in developing achievable goals and monitoring the patient during therapy. These individuals also provide an independent evaluator in evaluating the outcome of treatment. Besides improvement in physical function, other important and useful measures of outcome include improvements in vocational activity(i.e., return to work, increase in social and vocational activities, improvement in sleep patterns, improvement in mood/affect, reduction in adjuvant medication use, and reduction in health care utilization). There exist a number of valuable standardized and validated measurement tools that can be utilized to assess outcomes. These include tools such as Short Form Health Survey (SF-36), the Brief Pain Inventory (BPI), various mood scales, etc. These questionnaires can be administered prior to treatment and at various intervals thereafter to provide objective measurements that can then be correlated with the patient's reported degree of pain reduction. Careful patient

TABLE 100.3 Trial Approaches and Doses for Intrathecal Therapy

Trialing Techniques	Intrathecal		Epidural
	Single Shot/Multiple Shot	Continuous	Continuous
Drug: recommended trialing doses			
Morphine	0.1–0.5 mg	0.1–0.5 mg/d	2.8–14.4/d Need reference
Hydromorphone	0.025–0.1 mg	0.01–0.15 mg/d	2.8–14.4 mg/d
Ziconotide	15 µg	0.5–2.4 µg/d	
Fentanyl	15–75 µg	25–75 µg/d	144–480 µg/d
Bupivacaine	0.5–2.5 mg	0.01–4 mg/d	90–300 mg/d
Clonidine	5–20 µg	20–100 µg/d	72–120 µg/d
Sufentanil	5–20 µg	10–20 µg/d	
Baclofen	25–100 µg (0.5–1.0 µg/kg)		
Note	Starting dose of medication in the opioid-naive patient for outpatient bolus delivery should not exceed 0.15 mg morphine, 0.04 mg hydromorphone, or 25 µg fentanyl.	Starting doses of continuous IT delivery should be half of the trial dose for opioid-based medications.	Infusions of 0.0625%–0.125% bupivacaine mixed with 20–60 µg/mL are often run starting at 6 mL/hr.

selection is the key to success of IDDS. Table 100.3 lists various approaches and doses for IT or epidural trials.

Aside from the criteria that will be used to determine the success or failure of the trial, there are a number of issues to consider in designing an IT trial, including (1) the method that will be used for screening, (2) duration of the trial, (3) which drug to use and what starting dose, (4) the potential use of a placebo, and (5) what to do with systemic opioids during the trial. There are several accepted screening methods available for IT trials including single IT bolus injection, multiple IT boluses, continuous epidural, or IT infusion.

There is currently no clear consensus among clinicians as to the ideal trial technique. Each has its advantages and disadvantages. The single IT bolus represents the simplest, most cost-effective method of screening for IT drug delivery. However, depending on the dose injected, bolus injection may result in subanalgesic drug levels, thus producing a "false-negative trial." Additionally, drug-related adverse side effects are generally more common following bolus injection than continuous infusion, and these side effects may obscure the analgesic response. There is also a higher likelihood of a placebo response when using a single injection technique. Even though a single low-dose bolus of opioid produces a positive response, it is difficult to determine an accurate starting dose for the implanted pump. Finally, although single shot bolus trials are simple to perform, they do not provide the ability to evaluate the effect of the therapy on function as well as some of the other outcome measures that have been discussed. Although multiple IT boluses are more costly and time-consuming, they do provide the ability to titrate the dose and establish a dose–response curve. It is also possible to employ placebo injections for comparison with active drug administration using multiple boluses during the trial. On the other hand, multiple boluses are often associated with an increased incidence of side effects, lack of correlation with the results of continuous infusion, and require multiple dural punctures unless a temporary IT catheter is used.

The continuous or functional trial is probably the one preferred by the majority of implanters. In fact, in a survey of implanters at academic teaching institutions conducted in 1999, 52% indicated they preferred continuous infusion for performing screening trials. Fifty-nine percent of implanters utilized the IT route, 17% used epidural infusion, and 22% employed both routes at various times.[38] Intuitively, it would seem that continuous infusion would have clear advantages over bolus techniques. Continuous infusion can be performed using either the IT or epidural route. Although either is acceptable, it is important to

understand the difference between IT and epidural drug delivery (Table 100.4). Regardless of the route chosen, continuous infusion allows for controlled dose titration and assessment of a reasonable starting dose once the pump is implanted. On balance, there is a lower risk of side effects with continuous infusion. There is also less chance of a placebo response because continuous infusion allows for the placebo response to dissipate over time as the trial is continued. Perhaps, most importantly, a continuous trial, particularly if continued for a sufficient period of time, allows for assessment of functional outcome which is perhaps the most important determining factor of success. Notwithstanding the advantages, there are some relative disadvantages to continuous infusion. It is more complicated and requires greater expertise for placement of a tunneled catheter and is obviously more costly to perform than a bolus trial.

For opioid-naive patients or those on relatively low oral doses, a tunneled externalized IT catheter can be placed in the operating room and a continuous functional outpatient trial conducted for anywhere between 2 and 4 weeks. By providing the patient a drug holiday, it is possible to begin the IT infusion at very low doses (usually around 0.25 to 0.5 mg per day of IT morphine) of medication. For patients with nociceptive pain or mixed nociceptive/neuropathic pain, an opioid is typically used. If the pain is predominantly neuropathic, bupivacaine or clonidine is added to the infusion. The patient is evaluated at least three times per week to determine the analgesic response, degree of functional improvement, and the development of side effects. Incremental dose escalation is performed and if a significant degree of pain reduction

TABLE 100.4 Comparison of Epidural versus Intrathecal Drug Infusion

Criterion	Intrathecal	Epidural
Onset of action	Faster onset	Slower onset
Systemic effects	Minimal systemic effects	Larger systemic effects
Duration of effect	Long-lasting	Short-lasting
dosage	Smaller dose (1/10 epidural dose for morphine)	Larger dose required
Adverse effects	Post-LP headache	More systemic side effects
	Risk of meningitis	Risk of epidural abscess Respiratory depression

LP, lumbar puncture.

or functional improvement is not realized by the time the patient reaches 2 to 4 mg of IT morphine (or its equivalent) per day, the trial is terminated and the catheter is removed. The success or failure of the trial is based on the goals that have been agreed on by the clinician and patient prior to proceeding with the trial. If the trial is deemed a success, the patient is then returned to the operating room for revision of the catheter and implantation of the pump. Patients are provided short-acting opioids during the immediate postoperative period for management of surgical pain and these are weaned and discontinued over a 2-week period. Patients are routinely counseled that they may experience incident pain that will typically be transient depending on their daily activities and are provided with nonpharmacologic coping strategies for managing these situations.

Of note, the 2017 PACC consensus guidelines on IT drug delivery states that no single study has shown that a continuous IT trial is superior to other methods of IT trialing in noncancer pain.[39] There are equal levels of evidence for single shot trialing, bolus trialing, and continuous infusion. Other issues that need to be addressed include the duration of the trial, the specific medication(s) and dosages administered, and the handling of baseline systemic opiates during the trial.

There is currently no standard protocol that defines the optimal trial duration, trialing with specific medications, or how to handle baseline opioids during the trial. According to the 2017 PACC consensus guidelines, there are four possible scenarios for managing oral/systemic opioids during and after the IT drug trial.[39] The first scenario is that the patient remains on oral systemic opioids throughout the trial and implantation of the IT drug delivery device. The second scenario is that systemic opioids are eliminated prior to trialing and implantation. The third scenario is that the systemic opioids are reduced during the trial/implant. The fourth scenario is that the systemic opioids are reduced during the trial and eliminated after the implant. There are advocates for employing each of these strategies, but great caution should be employed when considering concurrent use of IT and systemic opioid medications as there is an increased risk for adverse effects from additive effects. Ideally, patients should be positioned for dose reduction and or elimination of systemic opioids when considered for implanted IT drug delivery. The majority of patients being considered for implanted IT drug devices have been on or are currently taking chronic systemic opioid medication, and many will have opioid tolerance and hyperalgesia. In this set of patients, it may be very difficult to assess the efficacy of therapy during the trial, and consideration should be given to weaning or eliminating systemic opioid medications prior to trial.

Implantable Pump Technology

Fully implantable infusion pumps were first used for the continuous delivery of heparin, insulin, and intraarterial chemotherapy and later applied to intraspinal drug infusion. There are two basic types of fully implantable devices for continuous delivery of IT medications: constant flow pumps and programmable pumps.[40,41]

The first-generation pumps were constant flow devices preprogrammed to deliver medication at a single, fixed, constant rate. The initial prototype of the constant flow pump consists of a hollow titanium two-chambered device which consists of a drug reservoir and a chamber that contains a volatile two-phase fluorinated hydrocarbon (FHC) which functions as a propellant. Installation of medication into the drug reservoir results in compression of the propellant which transforms it to a liquid state. As the propellant is warmed by the patient's body temperature, the FHC is transformed from liquid to vapor which then exerts continuous pressure on a system of bellows which expand and force the drug out of the reservoir and into the IT catheter. The standard pump holds a volume just under 50 mL and is filled

TABLE 100.5 Factors Affecting Drug Delivery with Constant Flow Infusion Pumps
• Body temperature
• Calibrated for 37° C
• 10% to 13% increase in flow per 1° C rise
• Geographical elevation
• Calibrated for elevation of implanting center
• Flow increases at higher altitudes
• Blood pressure (at site of drug discharge)
• Inversely proportional
• 3% change for every 10 mm Hg mean arterial pressure
• Drug viscosity
• Reservoir capacity
• Flow rate calibrated for 50% capacity
• 4% variability at extremes of volume
• Pump "dead space"
• 4 mL "dead volume"
• Correction factor for concentration

by puncturing a special inlet septum with a noncoring Huber needle. Flow rates designed to deliver 1.0 to 6.0 mL per day are preset and calibrated at the factory. Although this pump is relatively simple and inexpensive compared to fully programmable devices, the major disadvantage is that dosage alterations require the pump to be drained and refilled with a different concentration of drug. Also, flow rates can be altered by certain physical and physiologic factors, and these fluctuations in drug delivery rate can result in parallel fluctuations in analgesia (Table 100.5).

The second type of fully implanted drug delivery device is a fully programmable pump such as the SynchroMed infusion system (Medtronic Neurological, Minneapolis, Minnesota) or a Flowonix infusion system (Mt. Olive Township, New Jersey). The current model (SynchroMed II) consists of a collapsible drug reservoir into which the drug is injected through a self-sealing septum. The pump is powered by a lithium–cadmium battery which drives an internal peristaltic pump. The pump contains an electronic module with a computer chip which allows one to program variable infusion rates, bolus injections, etc. A small radiofrequency antenna allows the pump to be noninvasively interrogated by telemetry and programmed with an external handheld programmer. The pump can be programmed for a variety of delivery modes which can be tailored to the individual circumstances. The pump comes with a catheter access port (CAP) side port which is extremely valuable for troubleshooting catheter-related problems.

SURGICAL TECHNIQUE OF PUMP IMPLANTATION

Implantation of an IDDS system is usually a straightforward procedure for the properly trained and experienced implanter. Despite the perceived simplicity of the implant procedure, there are numerous pitfalls that can lead to complications. Many complications can be avoided through attention to meticulous aseptic operative technique, gentle tissue handling, and adherence to certain technical points during catheter insertion and pump implantation.[42]

Implantation of an IDDS can be performed either under local anesthesia with IV sedation or general anesthesia, depending on the clinician's preference and the overall condition of the patient. All patients should receive a single dose of prophylactic antibiotics directed toward the normal skin flora within 30 minutes of incision. Typically cefazolin 1 to 3 g based on the patient's weight (clindamycin 600 mg IV if they have an allergy to β-lactam medication) is sufficient for prophylaxis. The patient is positioned and secured in a lateral decubitus position taking care to pad the patient's pressure points and using an axially roll to alleviate pressure to the dependent brachial plexus. The pump can be placed on either side, either in the subcostal region or lower quadrant of the abdomen. It is important to position the pump such that it does not impinge on or sit directly over any bony prominence (e.g., iliac crest, or rib cage, as this is likely to result in local pain and the need for revision of the pump pocket site). Other factors that occasionally need to be taken into account include the presence of either current or expected ostomies and body habitus. Although implantation of a pump is not absolutely contraindicated in those with ostomies, there is likely a higher risk of infection and every effort should be made to implant the pump as far from these sites as possible.

Prior to pump implantation, all patients should undergo an appropriate imaging study of the spine (computed tomography [CT] with IV contrast, CT myelography, or magnetic resonance imaging [MRI]) to ensure there is no anatomical obstruction that might preclude safe catheter insertion. The first step is to insert and properly position the catheter in the subarachnoid space.[42] This should always be performed with the use of intraoperative C-arm fluoroscopy to verify the correct position of the catheter. A small stab incision is made in the midlower lumbar region based on fluoroscopic imaging. Keeping in mind that the spinal cord terminates at the T12 or L1 vertebral level, needle entry should be caudal to this level, ideally at L2–L3 or L3–L4. The exact insertion site may vary depending on the

spinal anatomy and the presence of spinal instrumentation. A lumbar puncture is performed using a paramedian approach with a shallow insertion angle (the angle between the plane of the skin's surface and the axis of the needle shaft) to facilitate catheter advancement and reduce the chance of kinking and fracture. After obtaining good flow of CSF, the catheter is inserted through the needle and is threaded rostrally. Either a one- or two-piece catheter can be used, depending on the clinical situation and the preference of the implanter. The catheter should pass easily with minimal resistance. Under no circumstances should the catheter be forced passed the point of an apparent obstruction or withdrawn. Advancing the catheter against resistance can lead to inadvertent entry of the catheter into the substance of the spinal cord, resulting in serious neurologic sequelae; withdrawing the catheter through the needle can lead to shearing of the catheter. The tip of the catheter should generally be positioned in the uppermost portion of the lumbar cistern (Fig. 100.3). The guide wire is then removed by straightening the catheter and applying gentle traction to the guide wire. CSF should be flow spontaneously from the end of the catheter; occasionally, it is necessary and to insert a blunt-bevel needle in to the catheter and attach a syringe to, then

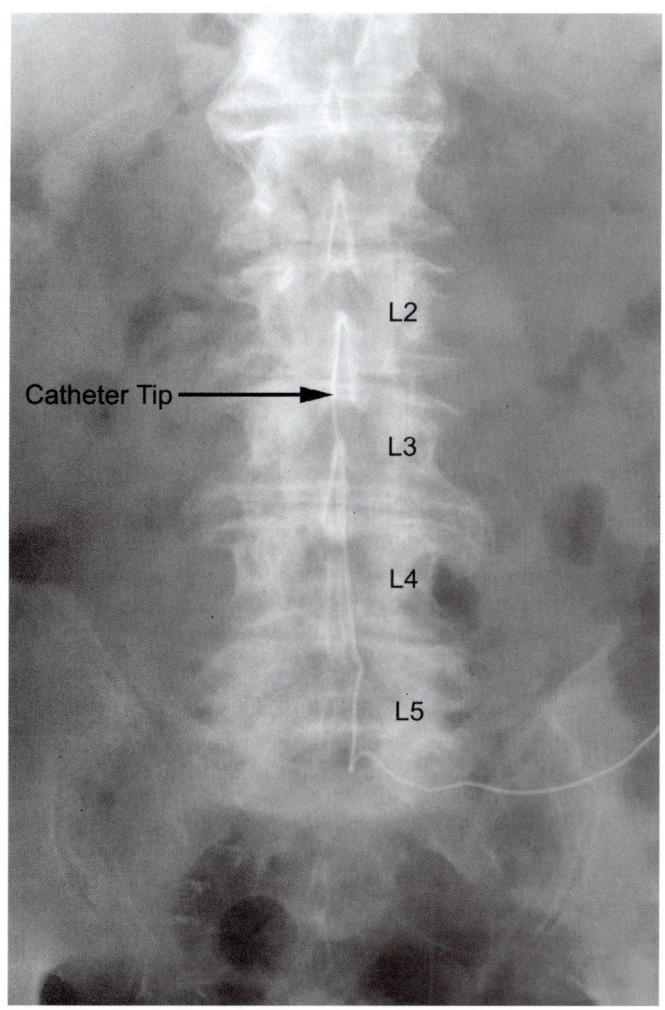

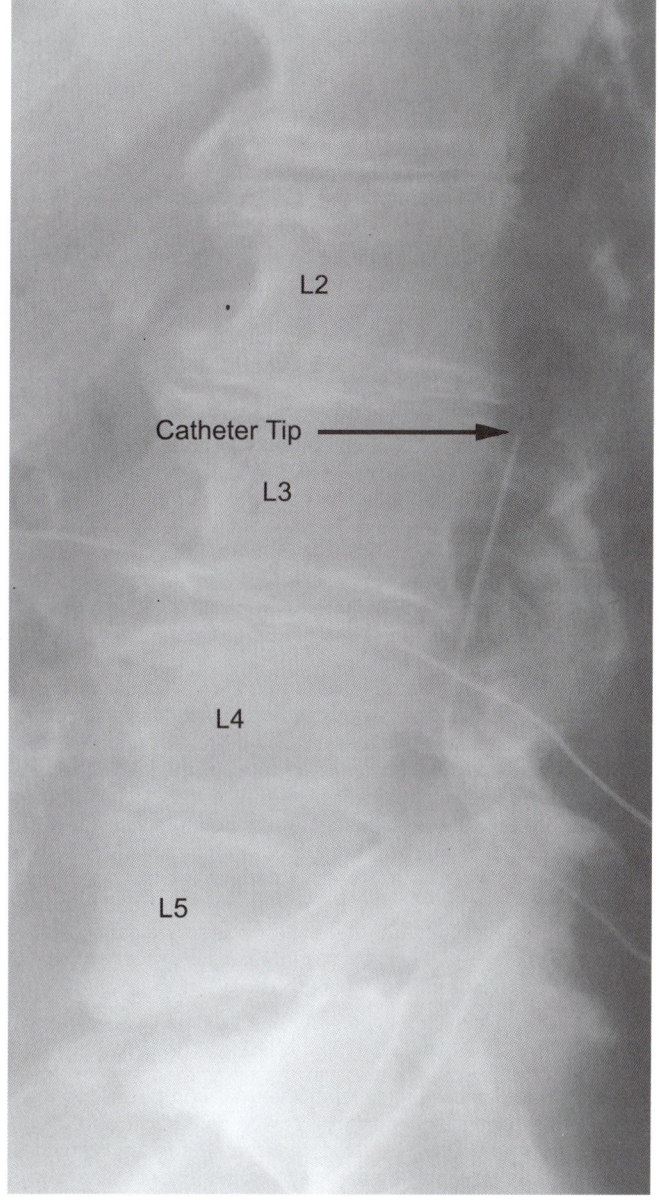

FIGURE 100.3 **A:** Anteroposterior radiograph of the intrathecal catheter tip (*arrow*) in final position with tip adjacent to the L2/L3 intervertebral disc. **B:** Lateral radiograph of the intrathecal catheter tip (*arrow*) in final position with tip adjacent to the L2/L3 intervertebral disc. (*Reprinted with permission from Rathmell JP. Atlas of Image-Guided Intervention in Regional Anesthesia and Pain Medicine. Philadelphia, PA: Lippincott Williams & Wilkins; 2006:164–165, Figures 15.5 and 15.6.*)

gently aspirate to establish CSF flow. Once CSF flow is confirmed, the tubing is temporarily occluded with an atraumatic clamp to prevent CSF loss.

The Tuohy needle is left in place to prevent inadvertent damage to the catheter during dissection. A skin incision is made incorporating the needle, and dissection is carried down to the lumbodorsal fascia. A small pocket is then fashioned to accommodate a loop of catheter in the subcutaneous tissue of the lumbar region. This loop prevents kinking and reduces strain between the distal and proximal portions of the catheter that can occur as the patient flexes and extends the lumbar region after implantation. The needle is then withdrawn leaving the catheter in place. The catheter is anchored using a standard anchoring devices close to where the catheter enters the fascia to prevent migration using nonabsorbable suture.

With the catheter secured in place, the next step is to create a subcutaneous pocket in the abdominal region to accommodate the pump. The pocket should be sufficiently large to easily accommodate the pump and allow closure of the wound without any significant tension. Care should be taken to avoid making the pocket too large as this can lead to the pump inverting within the pocket. Once an adequate pocket has been created, a tunneling device is passed through the subcutaneous tissues from the pocket to the lumbar paraspinous incision. Care must be taken to palpate the tip as the tunneling device is advanced to prevent the device from penetrating in to the abdominal cavity. The catheter is then passed through the hollow tunneling device and the device is removed, leaving the catheter in the subcutaneous tunnel with the tip now exiting from the abdominal pocket. Continued flow of CSF should be confirmed from the end of the catheter. If a two-piece catheter is used, the distal (i.e., IT) catheter is trimmed by an appropriate amount (if so desired) and then connected to the proximal catheter using a pin connector; this connection is then covered with a strain relief sleeve to prevent kinking at the connection site. This pin connector is then used as a second anchoring site, thereby creating a gentle strain relief loop between the fascial anchor and the pin connector. The amount of the distal catheter that is trimmed should be measured and recorded to be able to accurately calculate the catheter volume for subsequent drug delivery programming. Once the pump has been prepared and filled with drug (the technique will vary depending on the type of pump), it is brought onto the surgical field and connected to the catheter. The pump is then placed into the subcutaneous pocket, ensuring that the refill side is toward the skin and secured in place with nonabsorbable sutures, utilizing either the suture loops attached to the pump or by placing the pump into a Dacron pouch and securing the pouch to the fascia. Securing the pump to the fascia significantly reduces the chance of the pump inverting. Any excess proximal catheter should be gently beneath the pump, taking care to avoid kinking the catheter. A generous amount of catheter should be left in the pouch, as this will create an additional strain relief loop in the system. After securing the catheter and anchoring the pump, the CAP (if there is one) should be entered with a 24-gauge noncoring needle and CSF aspirated. A small amount of nonionic preservative-free contrast can be injected to confirm patency of the system. If contrast is used, it should be flushed from the catheter using preservative-free saline. The surgical wounds are then closed in anatomical layers. The pump can then be programmed to infuse a bolus to bring active drug to the tip of the catheter.

Complications of Spinal Drug Delivery

A thorough understanding of the potential complications that might occur during the course of device placement and long-term use of spinal drug infusion is essential for any clinician involved in the implantation and/or management of spinal drug

---

TABLE 100.6	Complications of Intrathecal Drug Delivery

Surgical Complications
- Wound hematoma or seroma
- Intraspinal hematoma
- Wound infection
- Meningitis
- Epidural abscess
- Postdural puncture headache
- Persistent cerebrospinal fluid leak
- Malposition of subcutaneous pump pocket
- Neurologic injury

Device-Related Complications
- Catheter-related problems
  - Migration
  - Fracture
  - Occlusion
- Mechanical pump failure

Pharmacologic Complications
- Drug-related side effects
- Tolerance
- Withdrawal and abstinence syndromes
- Opioid-induced hyperalgesia
- Inflammatory catheter tip mass (granuloma)

Complications Associated with Pump Refill
- Contamination of pump reservoir
- Accidental subcutaneous administration
- Accidental intrathecal bolus during intended refill

---

delivery systems. Although complications can and do occur, early detection can minimize the harm that results. Complications associated with IDDS can be divided into surgical complications related to the implant procedure, device-related complications, and pharmacologic complications (Table 100.6).[43]

SURGICAL COMPLICATIONS
Wound Hematoma/Seroma and Epidural Hematoma
Bleeding is an obvious risk for any surgical procedure and can occur intraoperatively or in the postoperative period. The bleeding can be superficial or deep and related to either surgical or systemic factors. Severe bleeding is rare. Prior to proceeding with insertion of a catheter for screening or implantation of an IDDS, all patients should be screened for risk factors that could cause intraoperative or postoperative bleeding. A careful medical history including family history of bleeding, screening for coagulation disorders should be conducted. Laboratory studies such as prothrombin and partial thromboplastin times, platelet function assays, and specialized bleeding tests should be reserved for those patients where a specific bleeding disorder is suspected. If the patient is being treated with anticoagulant medications, they should be stopped for a sufficient period of time prior to the procedure based on the pharmacology of each drug. It is important to coordinate cessation of anticoagulant therapy with each patient's treating physician to assure that the risks and benefits of discontinuing therapy have been carefully weighed.

Intraoperative bleeding is rare as the degree of tissue dissection necessary to place IDDS is minimal, and the anatomical areas that are involved are not particularly vascular. Most of the bleeding problems associated with IDDSs involve the subcutaneous tissues, particularly the pump pocket. Failure to assure hemostasis in the subcutaneous tissues can lead to complications wound hematoma, seroma, and/or infection. Infiltration of the surgical sites with local anesthetic containing 1:200,000 epinephrine can be helpful to reduce superficial bleeding. Use of electrocautery for the majority of the dissection will also minimize bleeding. Excessive use of electrocautery in any one location can destroy and devitalize tissue making it a potential nidus for infection. Electrocautery should be avoided near skin edges and the IT access. This can lead to poor wound healing and subsequent wound breakdown and/or infection or spinal cord injury.

Clinically significant intraspinal bleeding related to needle or catheter insertion is rare. The risk of intraspinal bleeding can be reduced by minimizing the number of needle passes. Tumors can be vascular and should be avoided. A small amount of epidural bleeding is unlikely to be clinically significant. However, accumulation of sufficient blood in the epidural space as an epidural hematoma can lead to the development of neurologic injury. Epidural hematoma should be suspected in a patient who reports severe, escalating back pain and progressive symptoms of neurologic dysfunction. Any patient who develops neurologic symptoms or signs in the immediate postoperative period should undergo an immediate imaging study (CT or MRI) of the spine, and neurosurgical consultation should be obtained.

Wound hematoma and/or seroma are more common and usually due to inadequate hemostasis. A wound hematoma is usually manifest by local pain, pressure, and swelling over the surgical wound and may or may not be accompanied serous or serosanguineous drainage. Most wound hematomas or seromas can be managed conservatively and will resolve spontaneously. However, in the event of a large collection, either surgical evacuation or percutaneous aspiration may be necessary. In the event of a wound hematoma or seroma, early pump refills should be limited because puncture of the skin may increase the risk of infection. A large hematoma overlying the pump will make accessing the refill port more difficult and increase the chances of subcutaneous injection of the medication.

Infectious Complications
The incidence of infection following implantation of an IDDS is low, and the presence of an active systemic infection or localized soft tissue infection near the site of implantation may increase the risk of a surgical site infection. Most wound infections present early, typically within 1 to 4 weeks after implantation. The usual presentation includes pain, swelling, erythema, and tenderness over the surgical incision, sometimes accompanied by purulent drainage. Although fever may be present, absence of fever should not rule out an infection. In the absence of systemic symptoms and/or signs of infection, a period of conservative management for several weeks, including percutaneous aspiration, IV antibiotics, and, in some cases, instillation of antibiotics directly into the pump pocket should be considered. However, if an infection of the pump pocket occurs involving more than the superficial tissues, explantation of the device (including the catheter) is typically required. If there is no evidence of extension of the infection from the subcutaneous tissues surrounding the pump toward the lumbar catheter insertion site, it is possible to remove just the pump and leave the IT catheter in situ. The catheter is exposed in the lumbar paraspinous region far from the site of the pocket infection, cut and occluded just above the fascial insertion site. In this way, once the infection has resolved, the catheter can be revised without having to replace the IT segment of the original catheter and a new pump implanted in a site remote from the previous infection. However, the safest approach is to remove the entire system and consider reimplantation once the infection has resolved. Once the pump has been explanted, systemic analgesics must be started to prevent withdrawal.

Meningitis is another rare infectious complication that has been reported after IDDS placement. The clinical presentation of bacterial meningitis includes fever, chills, intractable headache, malaise, nausea/vomiting, neck/back pain, and nuchal rigidity.

Most patients who develop meningitis look ill, and progression can be extremely rapid. The key to treatment is early recognition of clinical signs followed by a lumbar puncture and early institution of broad-spectrum antibiotics. Urgent removal of the IT infusion system should be strongly considered.

Epidural abscess is rare following IDDS implantation, although there are numerous case reports of epidural abscess following insertion of epidural catheters. The clinical presentation of epidural abscess is similar to that of an epidural hematoma, although the onset is generally more delayed and the progression of symptoms may be slower. Early diagnosis requires a high degree of suspicion; any patient who develops unexplained neurologic signs or symptoms should undergo an imaging study to exclude this problem. If an epidural abscess is confirmed and the patient demonstrates signs of neurologic dysfunction, neurosurgical consultation should be obtained immediately and consideration given toward surgical decompression. Although epidural abscess has traditionally been considered a neurosurgical emergency, an increasing number of reports of nonoperative management of this condition have appeared in recent years. If the patient has no sign of neurologic dysfunction, it may be possible to manage the patient with an epidural abscess with antibiotics combined with close clinical observation. This approach is probably most applicable to abscesses that occur in the lumbar region since the cauda equina, where expansion of the abscess is less likely to produce immediate neurologic compromise. As is the case with more superficial infections, the most conservative approach regarding the implant is removal. Most postoperative epidural abscesses are due to *Staphylococcus aureus* and should be treated with at least 6 weeks of IV antibiotics.

Cerebrospinal Fluid Leak and Postdural Puncture Headache
Insertion of the IT catheter requires performing a lumbar puncture with large Tuohy needle. CSF leak and postdural puncture headache (PDPH) are risks associated with pump implantation. This problem may occur as a result of multiple dural punctures or as a result of a CSF leak around the catheter where it enters the dura. Some implanters try to minimize this risk by placing a purse-string suture around the catheter below the fascial insertion site. If this technique is employed, one must be careful to avoid occlusion of the IT catheter that can result if the purse-string suture is cinched too tightly, occluding the catheter.

PDPH is classically described as a severe postural headache, but this postural change is not always present. Initial management includes bed rest, fluids including caffeinated beverages, and the use of an abdominal binder. If conservative measures fail to eliminate the problem, an epidural blood patch can be considered. Placing a blood patch in a patient with an IDDS requires fluoroscopic guidance in order to avoid damaging the IT catheter. If the leak persists, surgical exploration to seal the leak may be required.

Occasionally, patients will present with a CSF hygroma beneath the lumbar incision. In most cases, this will resolve spontaneously with time. It is usually not necessary nor recommended that these collections be aspirated as there is risk of infection or damage to the catheter. If the collection is large and/or the patient is symptomatic, then surgical exploration to close the leak around the catheter might be required.

Neurologic Injury
Neurologic injury during and after IDDS placement is most commonly associated with the development of an epidural hematoma or abscess. Although uncommon, direct neurologic injury can also occur from insertion of the needle or IT catheter. Neurologic injury can be minimized by preoperative imaging study of the spine, preferably an MRI, to ensure that the spinal

canal is patent and that the catheter can be inserted safely. This is especially important in patients with cancer and spinal metastases. Imaging will also exclude the presence of problems such as a low-lying or tethered cord. To minimize the risk of neural injury, the needle should be inserted in the lower to midlumbar region in order to avoid direct injury to the conus medullaris (which usually terminates around T12 or L1) or the spinal cord itself. Once the needle has been inserted and free flow of CSF confirmed, the catheter should be inserted and positioned using fluoroscopy. The catheter should be gently advanced; under no circumstance should the catheter be forced if undue resistance is met. If this occurs, the entire catheter and needle assembly should be removed and the process repeated. The position of the catheter tip should be confirmed with fluoroscopy. Ideally, the catheter tip should be positioned in the upper portion of the lumbar cistern. By keeping the catheter caudal to the conus medullaris, the risk of cord compression due to subsequent development of an IT granuloma will be minimized. If the catheter passes retrograde toward the sacrum, it should be removed and repositioned with the introducer needle to avoid shearing of the catheter. If the catheter remains low in the lumbar region, it can potentially "knot" and damage the nerve roots of the cauda equina in the event it needs to be removed. It is not uncommon for the catheter to cause transient nerve root irritation that is usually manifest by radicular symptoms. This is usually self-limited and resolves over several days to weeks. In the event it persists, it may become necessary to remove the catheter.

DEVICE-RELATED COMPLICATIONS
Catheter and Pump Problems
Complications related to the catheter system represent a considerable source of morbidity in patients with IDDS. Catheter-related problems include fracture, migration, kinking, occlusion, and dislodgment. In three separate clinical trials conducted by Medtronic, catheter-related complications were reported in 20% to 25% of patients who received an implant. This included both one- and two-piece catheters. During a 1- to 2-year follow-up period, approximately 80% of the catheters remained complication-free. Correction of a catheter complication not only requires additional surgery but also results in interruption of therapy with the possibility that withdrawal symptoms will develop. The device-manufacturing companies consistently maintain that only the FDA-approved IT pump medications should be used with their devices, which reduces pump failure rates. When a patient presents with a sudden loss of pain relief after an IDDS has been functioning well, a sequential and systematic approach will usually identify the problem. First, proper function of the pump itself can generally be confirmed using telemetry. The pump should be interrogated to ensure that the information is as expected from prior records and accurate. The accuracy of the pump prescription is checked, and the device is refilled with new medication. The residual drug volume is checked against that predicted by the telemetry, and these volumes should agree. Plain radiographs that include the entire catheter and pump system are then obtained to exclude disconnection of the catheter from the pump as well as fracture, migration, or kinking of the catheter. Although most catheter fractures can be seen with plain radiographs, some leaks are small and cannot be seen with plain x-rays. MRI imaging can be ordered to exclude the presence of a catheter granuloma, especially where new neurologic signs or symptoms are noted or large pump volume discrepancies are evident. If this evaluation fails to reveal the source of the problem, then a contrast study can be done to further evaluate the catheter. The CAP (Fig. 100.4) is accessed using either a 24- or 25-gauge needle provided in the CAP kit. Prior to anything being injected, the catheter should be aspirated to confirm CSF flow and several

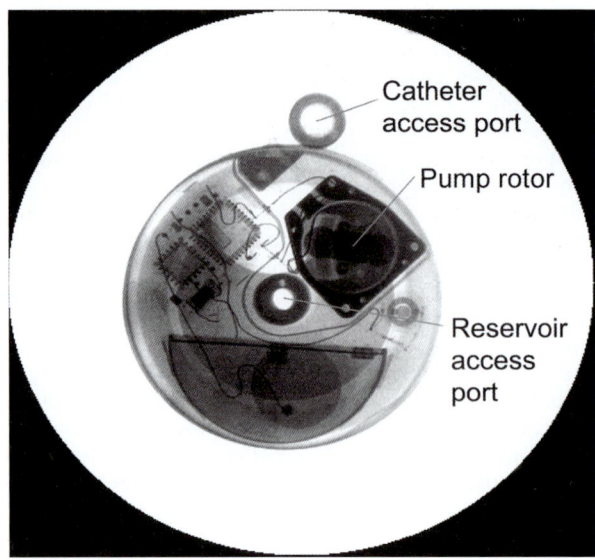

FIGURE 100.4   Plain radiograph of the Medtronic SynchroMed programmable intrathecal drug delivery pump. *(Used with permission from the manufacturer. The pump shown is the most common pump in use worldwide in 2009, the SynchroMed pump manufactured by Medtronic Neurological, Minneapolis, MN.) (Reprinted with permission from Ferrante FM, Rathmell JP. Complications associated with intrathecal drug delivery systems. In: Neal JM, Rathmell JP, eds.* Complications in Regional Anesthesia and Pain Medicine. *2nd ed. Philadelphia, PA: Lippincott Williams & Wilkins; 2013:278. Figure 25-6.)*

milliliters of CSF should be removed. Remember, the length of the catheter extending from the CAP on the pump to the distal tip within the CSF is filled with highly concentrated drug. When CSF cannot be aspirated, injection is likely to push drug within the catheter directly into the CSF, resulting in a drug overdose. Assuming one can easily aspirate CSF, a small amount of nonionic, radiographic contrast can then be slowly injected and the spread observed under fluoroscopy. If the catheter is patent and there is no obstruction at the tip, contrast should be seen to flow from the catheter and then dissipate quickly in the subarachnoid space. It is also possible to study the catheter by placing a radioisotope such as indium-111 in the drug reservoir and imaging the system over a sufficient period of time to allow for tracer movement into the CSF based on the flow rate of the pump.

Complications Associated with Refill of the Pump Reservoir
Complications related to refilling a drug delivery device include inadvertent subcutaneous administration, accidental IT injection, and pump programming errors. All of these complications are avoidable by adhering to a strict protocol for pump refills. The danger during initiation of IDDS and refilling of the reservoir is apparent from a recent postmarketing study carried out by Medtronic. This report revealed that mortality after initiation of IDDS or device interventions (reprogramming, refilling of the drug reservoir) typically occurred as a result of multiple factors, including excessive IT morphine dosing during initiation of IDDS, lack of close supervision of concomitant opioid or respiratory depressant drug intake, and early hospital discharge preventing monitoring for respiratory depression early after initiation of IDDS.[44] Before refilling any drug delivery device, one should check to ensure that the drug prescription matches that currently in the pump. Refills should be performed sterilely to avoid contamination of the drug reservoir. Refills should only be performed with the appropriate needles provided in the manufacturer's pump refill kit. The drug reservoir is accessed with 22-gauge Huber needle and the CAP with a 24- or 25-gauge needle, depending on the model of the pump.

The needle intended for entering the CAP should *never* be utilized for accessing the drug reservoir. If the smaller needle is used and accidentally inserted into the CAP, the entire volume of medication can be directly injected into the IT space. The CAP bypasses the drug reservoir and pump and cannot be accessed with the larger 22-gauge needle. If there is any question that the needle is in the appropriate port, it is prudent to confirm this with fluoroscopy. The provider performing the refill should confirm that the residual volume of the reservoir matches that predicted by telemetry. Once the refill has been completed and the pump reprogrammed, the pump prescription should again be rechecked for accuracy.

Inadvertent injection into the subcutaneous tissues around the pump as well as injection through the CAP directly into the IT space have both been reported. This can lead to significant respiratory depression, which is likely to be delayed in onset and occur after the patient has left the office. If subcutaneous injection occurs in patients already receiving chronic opioid therapy, treatment with an opioid antagonist should be instituted, with careful observation with incremental doses to avoid excessive reversal; overly aggressive reversal could precipitate acute withdrawal leading to hypertension, cardiac arrhythmias, and pulmonary edema. In the event that direct injection into the CSF does occur and it is recognized, the drug infusion should be stopped and the patient admitted to the hospital for observation and close monitoring for signs of respiratory or hemodynamic compromise. Judicious use of opioid antagonists as described is warranted. If the patient develops signs of respiratory compromise, there should be no hesitation in proceeding with endotracheal intubation of the patient and providing mechanical ventilatory support until the drug effects have dissipated. If subcutaneous injection occurs in patients receiving baclofen, the patient may exhibit signs of overdose including CNS depression, somnolence, hallucinations, agitation, mydriasis, nausea and vomiting and may progress to severe bradycardia, hypotension, and respiratory failure. If baclofen overdose is suspected, immediate admission to the hospital is warranted. These patients should be closely monitored and can require supportive care to maintain hemodynamic and respiratory function. A nonspecific reversal agent for baclofen overdose is physostigmine which should be administered in incremental doses.

PHARMACOLOGIC COMPLICATIONS AND DRUG-RELATED SIDE EFFECTS
Side Effects of Intrathecal Opioids

It is commonly held misconception that switching from systemic to IT delivery of opioids alleviates all of the clinically significant side effects. However, IT opioid infusion is commonly associated with side effects. Often, these side effects are mild and well tolerated and do not interfere with therapy. As patients develop tolerance to the analgesic effects of the drug, they also tend to develop tolerance to the side effects. Nonetheless, some patients develop side effects that may be so bothersome as to have a significant impact on the treatment. The most common side effects experienced by patients receiving IDDS include respiratory depression, gastrointestinal symptoms, urinary dysfunction, hormonal alterations, and itching.

Aside from true anaphylaxis, which is rare with the use of opioids, respiratory depression is the most clinically concerning drug-related side effect. Respiratory depression results from the supraspinal interaction of the drug with μ-opioid receptors in the brainstem. It can occur from rostral spread of the drug and is probably more common when using hydrophilic agents which can attain significant concentrations in the CSF. Respiratory depression can also occur with systemic absorption from the CSF into the blood and redistribution to the CNS. It is most likely to occur in patients who are opioid naive. There are relatively few reports of clinically significant respiratory depression in patients who have been exposed to opioids before instituting IDDS. Additional risk factors for development of respiratory depression include advanced age, absence of severe pain, debilitated physical condition, preexisting pulmonary disease, sleep apnea, and use of additional opioids delivered by alternative routes. Respiratory depression can occur as early as 4 hours following IT dosing, although it is often delayed in onset up to 24 hours. Treatment consists of support of respiration and the judicious use of a μ-receptor antagonist such as naloxone and employing appropriate precautions as outlined previously in this chapter.[45]

Urinary retention is another common side effect of IT opioids, reported in 20% to 40% of patients. It is a direct spinal side effect caused by reduction in detrusor muscle tone and detrusor-urethral sphincter dyssynergia. It does occur with the intraventricular administration of morphine. It is believed to be mediated primarily through μ- and δ-receptors. It is more common in males and rare in women and individuals who are opioid tolerant. It is often self-limited and usually resolves within 24 to 48 hours. Treatment entails intermittent bladder catheterization until the problem resolves. One can also consider adjunct pharmacologic treatment with opioid antagonists and/or phenoxybenzamine. If the problem persists, an alternative strategy involves switching to another opioid.[45]

Gastrointestinal side effects such as nausea, vomiting, and constipation are less common than with systemic delivery. However, they still occur in up to 25% to 30% of patients, especially those who are opioid naive. Nausea and vomiting are mediated by the interaction of opioids with the chemoreceptor trigger zone. Treatment is usually symptomatic with antiemetic agents.

Pruritus occurs in about 25% of patients exposed to IT opioids and may be more common in opioid-naive individuals. It is more common with morphine than other opioids and is believed to result from degranulation of mast cells. The problem is usually self-limited and can be managed with antihistamines albeit with mixed results. In the case of severe persistent itching, the best approach is to switch to an alternative opioid such as hydromorphone or fentanyl. It is important to differentiate opioid-induced pruritus from true allergy. Most patients and many clinicians not familiar with the actions of IT opioids will misconstrue itching as an allergic reaction. In fact, true allergic reactions to morphine or its congeners is unusual.[45]

Finally, there is compelling evidence that opioids can have a negative effect on neuroendocrine function.[46] Morphine has been shown to inhibit the release of gonadotropin- and corticotrophin-releasing hormones from the hypothalamus, resulting in reduced circulating levels of luteinizing hormone (LH), follicle-stimulating hormone (FSH), adrenocorticotropic hormone (ACTH), and β-endorphin. The end result is reduction in serum levels of cortisol and testosterone. Clinically, the end effect is reduction in libido and/or impotency. In men, reductions in testosterone can also result in decreased muscle mass and increased fat mass. In addition to these effects, IT morphine administration can also produce significant fluid retention, likely due to alterations in antidiuretic hormone function.

Opioid Tolerance

Tolerance can be defined as the requirement for progressively escalating doses of medication in order to achieve the same degree of clinical effect. In pharmacologic terms, tolerance represents a pharmacodynamic effect manifested by a rightward shift in the dose–response curve. Two mechanisms for opioid tolerance have been proposed: desensitization (i.e., decreased activation) of opioid receptors following prolonged exposure to opioids and opioid receptor downregulation.[7] Desensitization involves changes in opioid receptor physiology that are believed to result from alterations in G-protein coupled receptor (GPCR) function. The end result is a decrease in analgesia.

Like many other GCPRs, downregulation, the second mechanism believed to produce opioid tolerance occurs when opioid receptors are internalized from the cell membrane by endocytosis, is mediated through the β-arrestin pathway.

Although tolerance is discussed mostly in terms of loss of analgesia, it should be noted that tolerance also occurs to other effects of a given drug. Tolerance is believed to be an important causal factor in the loss or complete failure of analgesia in patients with implanted drug delivery systems, particularly those patients primarily receiving opioid medications. Tolerance usually develops over the course of time, and the rate at which tolerance develops may vary between individuals. Moreover, tolerance does not usually develop equally to all effects of a given drug at the same rate. Before concluding that loss of analgesia is indeed related to tolerance, it is important for the clinician to exclude other reasons such as problems with the delivery system or progression of disease.

Management of tolerance depends to large degree on the baseline treatment protocol for a given patient.[45] In some cases, simple dose titration by 10% to 30% per day will overcome the problem. If indeed the problem is simply a tolerance issue, then increasing the dose should result in demonstrably improved pain control, at least for some period of time. Depending on the delivery system, dose escalation will be limited by the volume that can be safely infused. The maximum infusion rate generally recommended for an epidural infusion is around 10 to 15 mL per hour; for IT infusion, the rate should not exceed more than 10% of the patient's calculated CSF volume (typically 75 mL total, limiting the daily infusion to 7.5 mL per day). These limitations can make restoration of analgesia impossible by dose titration alone unless the infusion prescription can be prepared in a higher concentration, although there are also limits to this (Table 100.7).

It has been suggested that continuous drug delivery is less likely or will less rapidly lead to the development of tolerance, although there are no studies that clearly demonstrate this to be the case. Switching to a more potent opioid may result in a slower development of tolerance by reducing the rate of receptor downregulation. One can also consider switching to a different opioid assuming there is incomplete cross tolerance between the two drugs. Another strategy is to add other agents such as clonidine that act through alternative spinal modulating systems and therefore might have some opiate-sparing effects. Finally, some experts have suggested that a local anesthetic be substituted for the opioid to provide for an opioid-free interval.

Intrathecal Inflammatory Masses (Intrathecal Granuloma)

Inflammatory masses associated with the tip of an IT catheter is a potentially serious complication that, if not promptly recognized and managed, can result in neurologic injury. IT granuloma was first reported in 1991 and, over the course of time, additional case reports and small case series appeared in the literature. By 2000, 41 cases had been reported. Due to growing concern about this problem, a consensus panel met and subsequently published recommendations on the management of catheter-tip inflammatory masses. A similar consensus panel was reconvened in 2007 and the recommendations and guidelines of this panel were recently published.[47] The panel reviewed the pertinent literature including preclinical data, information on pathophysiology of inflammatory mass formation, and clinical data, and ultimately developed an algorithm for prevention, early detection, and treatment.

An inflammatory catheter tip mass typically is composed of both acute and chronic reactive inflammatory cells derived from the arachnoid and/or fibrosis that does not directly involve the spinal cord parenchyma. Although these masses represent a buildup of granulation tissue and have been termed "granulomas," they do not fit the classical histopathologic description of a true granuloma. An infectious agent has never been associated with these inflammatory masses. There are a number of preclinical studies in both dogs and sheep that demonstrate that catheter-tip inflammatory masses occur predictably in animals receiving IT morphine infusions. Based on preclinical studies, the panel concluded that these masses likely occurred as a result of infusion of high concentrations and/or high daily doses of IT morphine.

Although most of the preclinical evidence implicated the use of morphine, more recent data indicate that other opioid infusions may be associated with inflammatory catheter tip masses. There has also been a more recent report implicating IT baclofen as a potential causative agent.

Although the occurrence of inflammatory masses in humans is less predictable than in animal models, it is believed that the incidence in humans increases with the duration of IT therapy, ranging between 0.4% after 2 years of treatment up to 1.16% after 6 years of treatment. Moreover, animal data fails to clarify whether there is dose in humans below which granuloma formation will not occur. Available data do support the concept that both concentration and total dose of all opioids, with the exception of fentanyl, are important in the development of inflammatory masses. Based on the available data, the 2007 consensus panel has published recommendations for maximum doses and concentrations of the currently used IT agents (see Table 100.7).

The first clinical clue of the development of an inflammatory catheter tip mass in a patient who has otherwise been doing well is often an increase in the patient's pain and the requirement for repeated and rapid dose escalations. In such cases, absent an obvious progression of disease, one should begin to consider that diagnosis of an inflammatory mass. Any patient who develops new neurologic symptoms should be evaluated with spinal imaging, preferably MRI. A catheter-tip inflammatory mass can usually be detected with MRI (Fig. 100.5).

Management of the patient with an inflammatory catheter tip mass depends on the clinical situation but is primarily related to the presence or absence of neurologic signs and/or symptoms. If a mass is detected and the patient does not have neurologic symptoms, it is possible to retract the catheter caudally a few centimeters out of the granuloma and reduce the drug dose and/or concentration. One additional suggestion has been to switch to a "safer" medication such as fentanyl or ziconotide. If symptoms persist despite these changes, the patient should be rapidly weaned off all IT opioids, the medication should be removed from the pump, and the pump filled with saline. One needs to pay close attention to signs of withdrawal, not only from opioids but also from adjuvant medications that may also be in the pump such as clonidine and/or baclofen. If the symptoms resolve after removing the catheter from the

TABLE 100.7	**Current Suggested Dose and Concentration Limitations for It Drug Delivery**	
Drug	**Maximum Concentration**	**Maximum Daily Dose**
Morphine	20 mg/mL	15 mg/d
Hydromorphone	10 mg/mL	4 mg/d
Fentanyl	2 mg (2,000 μg)/mL	Unknown
Sufentanil[a]	50 μg/mL	Unknown
Bupivacaine	40 mg/mL	30 mg/d
Clonidine	2 mg (2,000 μg)/mL	1.0 mg (1,000 μg)/d
Ziconotide[b]	100 μg/mL	19.2 μg/d

[a]Sufentanil is not available for compounding.
[b]Maximum daily dose based on recommendations of Jazz Pharmaceuticals.
From Deer T, Krames EJ, Hassenbusch SJ, et al. Polyanalgesic consensus conference 2007: recommendations for the management of pain by intrathecal (intraspinal) drug delivery: report of an interdisciplinary expert panel. *Neuromodulation* 2007;10(4):300–328. Adapted by permission of John Wiley & Sons, Inc.

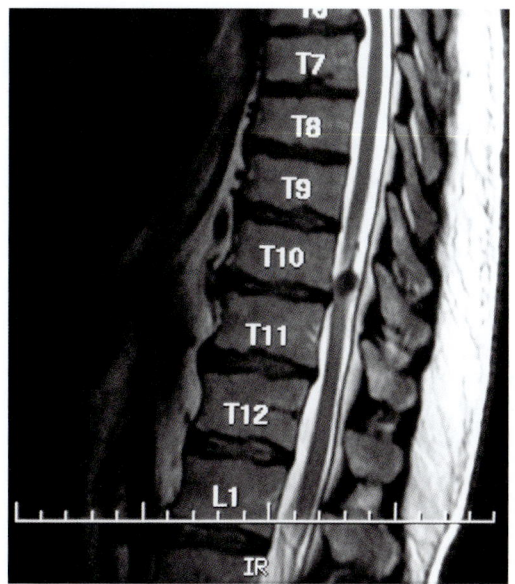
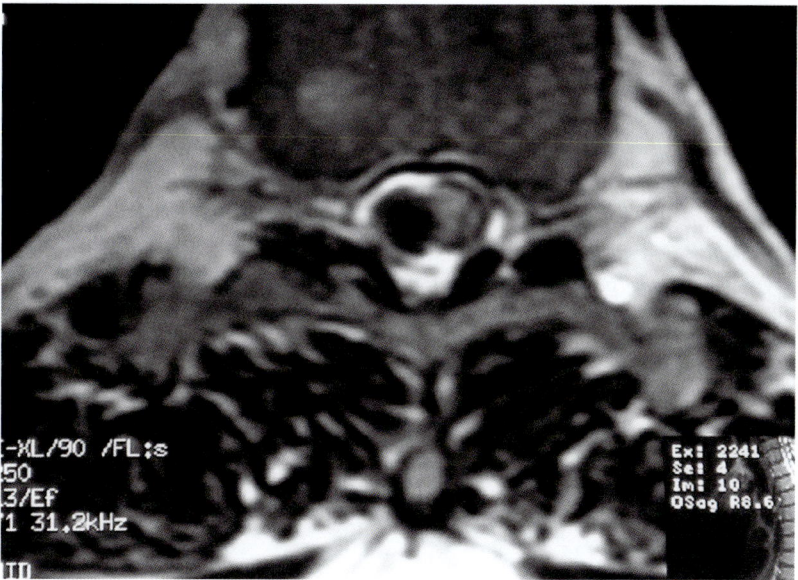

FIGURE 100.5 Magnetic resonance imaging (MRI) study of a patient with an inflammatory mass surrounding the tip of an implanted intrathecal drug delivery catheter. **A:** Midline, sagittal, T2-weighted image. The inflammatory mass involves the dorsal aspect of the spinal cord at the level of the inferior end plate of T10. **B:** Axial, T2-weighted image through the inflammatory mass. The mass displaces the spinal cord toward the left. *(Reprinted with permission from Ferrante FM, Rathmell JP. Complications associated with intrathecal drug delivery systems. In: Neal JM, Rathmell JP, eds.* Complications in Regional Anesthesia and Pain Medicine. *Philadelphia, PA: Lippincott Williams & Wilkins; 2013:279. Figure 25-7.)*

mass, the patient should be reimaged in 6 months to confirm resolution of the granuloma before reinstituting the therapy. If a small granuloma is still evident, one must decide between further retraction or removal of the catheter. If neurologic signs and symptoms persist or in the event that a granuloma is detected that is producing significant neural compression, then the system should be removed. In patients with a large granuloma compressing the spinal cord and producing neurologic dysfunction, consultation with a neurosurgeon should be obtained to determine whether removal of the granuloma itself is warranted.

Drug Withdrawal

Disruption of the IT catheter, pump battery failure, and human error during refill and reprogramming can all lead to sudden cessation of drug delivery and result in drug withdrawal. Of the medications that are currently used for IT delivery, distinct abstinence syndromes are most commonly associated with opioids, baclofen, and clonidine. There are currently no reports of withdrawal associated with the use of IT ziconotide.

The clinical symptoms and signs associated with opioid withdrawal include any or all of the following: increased lacrimation and rhinorrhea, diaphoresis, mydriasis, pilomotor erection, restlessness, irritability or agitation, gastrointestinal symptoms (nausea, vomiting, diarrhea), tremor, abdominal cramping, and, of course, increased pain levels.[45] In severe cases, acute opioid withdrawal can lead to pulmonary edema or cardiovascular collapse resulting in death. The most common causes of opioid withdrawal are catheter disruption and pump refill/programming errors. Because of the risk of opioid withdrawal, antagonist medication must be used with caution in patients undergoing chronic opioid therapy. Treatment should be aimed at respiratory and hemodynamic support with restoration of the drug infusion as soon as possible.

Baclofen withdrawal is a serious complication that, if unrecognized, can be life-threatening. It is usually heralded by increase in spasticity, sometimes to the point of rigidity, pruritus, hyperthermia, drowsiness progressing to obtundation, respiratory depression, rhabdomyolysis, acute renal failure, acute multiorgan failure, and even death.[45] Early recognition is the key to treatment. The treatment of baclofen withdrawal

requires urgent attention, the goal being restoration of the IT baclofen infusion as soon as possible. For patients with signs of severe baclofen withdrawal, it is not sufficient to merely provide oral medication until the problem can be fixed. In such cases, it may be prudent to place a temporary lumbar drain and restart the infusion until such time as the problem can be correctly diagnosed and treated. Abrupt cessation of clonidine can also be associated with adverse effects such as rebound hypertension, particularly in patients receiving higher doses. All patients receiving clonidine should be provided a prescription for either oral or transdermal clonidine and advised to contact the implanting physician should they develop any symptoms or signs of clonidine withdrawal.

Patient Outcomes and Intrathecal Drug Infusion

CANCER PAIN

Continuous IT infusion of opioids was first used for the management of cancer pain in the early 1980s and, over the next decade, remained the single most common indication for IDDS. During the past several years, it seems the use of IT opioids for cancer pain has declined due in large measure to the development of more effective long-acting oral opioids as well as the development of less expensive drug infusion reservoirs. Nevertheless, continuous IT opiate infusion remains one of the most effective methods of controlling cancer pain and affording patients, maximal independence.

IT opioids are indicated for the management of cancer pain in two circumstances: (1) in patients whose pain is refractory to reasonable doses of oral opioids and (2) in patients who are unable to tolerate sufficient doses of oral medications needed to adequately treat their pain due to undesirable systemic side effects, mainly sedation. Although appropriate management of the patient is the paramount goal, the current climate of health care in the United States has dictated an ever increasing recognition of the cost of care. In order to justify the cost of an implanted system, potential candidates for pump implantation should have a life expectancy of at least 3 to 6 months. Cost analysis studies comparing implanted programmable pumps to external infusion systems have shown that for patients requiring treatment more than 3 months, an IDDS is the more cost-effective device.[48,49]

Continuous infusion of IT opiates has proven to be an effective and safe method for controlling cancer pain.[2,50–52] Adequate pain control that results in significant reduction in oral narcotic intake and increase in activity can be achieved in the majority of patients. A retrospective multicenter survey regarding intraspinal opiate therapy revealed the average reduction in pain to be just over 60% (n = 382) regardless of etiology.[52] Increase in activity was noted in nearly 82% of patients (n = 399) with 59% realizing moderate to significant increases in activities of daily living (ADL). Just over 95% of patients reported either good (42.9%) or excellent (52.4%) pain relief. There were no significant differences in the level of pain relief reported between patients with cancer and those with nonmalignant pain syndromes. Complications related to the delivery system occurred in 21.6% of patients (n = 380) and were most often related to the catheter. Adverse drug effects were reported in approximately one quarter of the patients. The most common adverse effects were nausea and vomiting (25.2%) and pruritus (13.3%).

Perhaps the best evidence for the use of IDDS in patients with cancer pain comes from the study of Smith et al.[48] The authors performed a randomized controlled trial of IDDS versus conventional medical management (CMM) in a cohort of 202 patients. Entry criteria include inadequately controlled pain of 5 or greater (0 to 10 VAS scale). Clinical success was defined as either a 20% reduction in baseline VAS score or equivalent VAS score accompanied by at least a 20% reduction in toxicity following 4 full weeks of treatment. Nearly 85% (60 of 71) of patients randomized to IDDS achieved clinical success compared to 70% (51 of 72) of patients who received CMM (P = .05). Mean pain scores fell from 7.8 to 3.7 (52%) for the IDDS group compared to 7.8 to 4.8 in the CMM group (P = .055). Toxicity scores fell 50% for the IDDS group compared with only 17% for the CMM group (P = .004). Interestingly, the IDDS also showed improved survival, with 54% alive at 6 months compared with 37% in the CMM group.

INTRATHECAL DRUG DELIVERY FOR CHRONIC NONCANCER PAIN

During the past two decades, there has been an increasing trend toward the use of chronic IT opiates in the management of refractory noncancer pain syndromes.[6,8,52–60] Noncancer pain related to failed back surgery syndrome is now the most common indication for the use of IDDS. However, in spite of encouraging results in carefully selected patients with noncancer-related pain, the use of intraspinal opiates for these chronic pain conditions has remained a controversial issue among clinicians, lay persons, and government regulators. Indeed, much of the fear regarding this issue has been born of the belief that the use of opioids in noncancer pain invariably leads to tolerance and drug abuse. However, numerous retrospective and prospective studies suggest that these previously held beliefs may have been overly critical. Noncancer pain syndromes for which IT opiates have been and might be used are outlined in Table 100.8. The treatment strategy in patients with noncancer pain syndromes should obey the principle that the least invasive and least costly interventions should be attempted first, reserving more invasive and expensive therapies for patients who fail the former. Unfortunately, patient selection for IT administered opiates is not as straightforward as in patients with cancer. Although there are ample reports of significant pain reduction using IDDS, translation of pain reduction into functional improvement has been more difficult to achieve.

Winkelmüller and Winkelmüller[56] reported on 120 patients with noncancer pain syndromes managed with long-term

TABLE 100.8 Chronic Pain States Currently Treated with Chronic Spinal Drug Infusion
• Cancer pain
• Postlaminectomy syndrome
• Nerve root injury
• Adhesive spinal arachnoiditis
• Brachial or lumbosacral plexitis
• Complex regional pain syndrome
• Type I (reflex sympathetic dystrophy)
• Type II (causalgia)
• Spinal cord injury pain
• Phantom pain
• Postherpetic neuralgia
• Painful peripheral neuropathy
• Poststroke pain
• Intractable angina
• HIV-related pain

IT opiates with an average follow-up of more than 3 years. Nearly three-quarters (74.2%) of the patients derived benefit from the therapy, with a mean pain reduction of 58%. Overall, 92% of patients were satisfied with the treatment and 81% reported an improvement in their quality of life. The incidence of tolerance was low, only 5.8% (seven patients) and was successfully managed in four patients by means of "drug holidays." Anderson and Burchiel[57] investigated the long-term efficacy and safety of IT morphine in 33 patients with noncancer pain. These investigators noted a significant reduction in pain which persisted up to 2 years. Although the daily IT of morphine appeared to increase for the initial months of treatment, this tended to stabilize and remain constant after 1 year.

Roberts et al.[58] reported their results of IDDS for noncancer pain in 84 patients who were followed on average for 3 years. Nearly two-thirds of their patients suffered from low back and/or radicular pain. Mean pain reduction was around 60%, and 74% of patients self-reported increased activity levels as well as significant reduction in oral medication. These gains were not accompanied by change in work status. Technical complications requiring an additional surgical procedure occurred in 40% of patients. These patients were initially receiving relatively high doses of morphine (9.95 mg per day) and by the end of 6 months, the mean daily dose had escalated to 15.3 mg per day.

Finally, Deer et al.[59] reported the results of IDDS for the treatment of low back pain from the National Outcomes Registry for Low Back Pain. Out of 166 patients enrolled to be trialed for an IDDS system, 136 (82%) received a permanent implant. Scores for back and leg pain fell by an average of 47% and 31% respectively at 12 months follow-up for those who received an implant. In addition, more than 65% of patients demonstrated reduction in Oswestry scores by at least one level compared with baseline. At 1-year follow-up, 80% of patients indicated they were "satisfied" with the therapy, and 87% said they would undergo the procedure again for the same outcome.

Conclusion

IT drug delivery has evolved since its inception more than 30 years ago. This technique represents a viable option for patients with intractable pain conditions. Although once viewed solely as a salvage treatment, this is no longer the case. The surgical procedure for IDDS placement is relatively simple, yet the management of patients with IDDS is has many associated challenges. IDDS, particularly for patients with noncancer pain, represents a long-term commitment on the part of both the patient and clinician. Multiple problems will inevitably develop over the course of treatment, including drug-related side effects and system complications that must be addressed. Consequently, this therapy should be reserved for those who do not respond to less invasive treatments. In spite of the potential problems associated with this therapy, IDDS can be useful and beneficial to patients who fail to respond to simpler pain treatments, so long as one adheres to the principles of judicious patient selection, meticulous surgical technique, and diligent patient management.

ACKNOWLEDGMENT

The authors would like to thank Richard K. Osenbach for his contributions to the previous edition of this chapter.

References

1. Yaksh T, Rudy TA. Analgesia mediated by a direct spinal action of narcotics. *Science* 1976;192:1357–1358.
2. Onofrio BM, Yaksh TL, Arnold PG. Continuous low-dose intrathecal morphine administration in the treatment of chronic pain of malignant origin. *Mayo Clin Proc* 1981;56:516–520.
3. Cousins MJ, Mather LE. Intrathecal and epidural administration of opioids. *Anesthesiology* 1984;61:276–310.
4. Bennett G, Serafini M, Burchiel K, et al. Evidence-based review of the literature on intrathecal delivery of pain medications. *J Pain Symptom Manage* 2000;20:S12–S36.
5. Nordberg G, Hedner T, Mellstrand T, et al. Pharmacokinetic aspects of intrathecal morphine analgesia. *Anesthesiology* 1984;60:448–454.
6. Deer T, Krames EJ, Hassenbusch SJ, et al. Polyanalgesic Consensus Conference 2007: recommendations for the management of pain by intrathecal (intraspinal) drug delivery: report of an interdisciplinary expert panel. *Neuromodulation* 2007;10:300–328.
7. DuPen A, Shen D, Ersek M. Mechanisms of opioid-induced tolerance and hyperalgesia. *Pain Manag Nurs* 2007;8:113–121.
8. Krames ES, Lanning RM. Intrathecal infusion analgesia for nonmalignant pain: analgesic efficacy of intrathecal opioid with or without bupivacaine. *J Pain Symptom Manage* 1993;8:539–548.
9. Hassenbusch SJ, Portnoy RK, Cousins M, et al. Polyanalgesic Consensus Conference 2003: an update on the management of pain by intraspinal drug delivery-report of an expert panel. *J Pain Symptom Manage* 2004;27: 540–563.
10. Eisenach JC. Three novel spinal analgesics: clonidine, neostigmine, amitriptyline. *Reg Anesth* 1996;21:81–83.
11. Eisenach J, Detweiler D, Hood D. Hemodynamic and analgesic actions of epidurally administered clonidine. *Anesthesiology* 1993;78:277–287.
12. Gordh T, Post C, Olsson Y. Evaluation of the toxicity of subarachnoid clonidine, guanfacine, and a substance P-antagonist on rat spinal cord and nerve roots: light and electron microscopic observations after chronic intrathecal administration. *Anesth Analg* 1986;65:1303–1311.
13. Rauck RL, Eisenach JC, Jackson K, et al. Epidural clonidine treatment for refractory reflex sympathetic dystrophy. *Anesthesiology* 1993;179: 1163–1169.
14. Leiphart JW, Dills CV, Zikel OM, et al. A comparison of intrathecally administered narcotic and nonnarcotic analgesics for experimental chronic neuropathic pain. *J Neurosurg* 1995;92:595–599.
15. Puke MJ, Zsuzanna W. The differential effects of morphine and the alpha-2 adrenoreceptor agonists clonidine and dexmedetomidine on the prevention and treatment of experimental neuropathic pain. *Anesth Analg* 1993;77:104–109.
16. Bowersox S, Gadbois T, Singh T, et al. Selective N-type neuronal voltage-sensitive calcium channel blocker, SNX-111, produces spinal antinociception in rat models of acute, persistent, and neuropathic pain. *J Pharmacol Exper Ther* 1996;279:1243–1249.
17. Malmberg A, Yaksh TL. Voltage-sensitive calcium channels in spinal nociceptive processing: blockade of N- and P-type channels inhibits formalin-induced nociception. *J Neurosci* 1994;14:4882–4890.
18. Brose WG, Gutlove DP, Luther RR, et al. Use of intrathecal SNX-111, a novel, N-type, voltage-sensitive, calcium channel blocker, in the management of intractable brachial plexus avulsion. *Clin J Pain* 1997;13:256–259.
19. McGuire D, Bowersox S, Fellman JD, et al. Sympatholysis after neuron-specific, N-type, voltage-sensitive calcium channel blockade: first demonstration of N-channel function in humans. *J Cardiovasc Pharmacol* 1997;30: 400–403.
20. Muir K, Lees K. Clinical experience with excitatory amino acid antagonist drugs. *Stroke* 1995;26:503–513.
21. Hassenbusch S, Satterfield WC, Gradert TL, et al. Preclinical toxicity study of intrathecal administration of the pain-relievers dextrorphan, dextromethorphan, and memantine in the sheep model. *Neuromodulation* 1999;2:230–239.
22. Taira T, Kawamura H, Tanikawa T, et al. A new approach to control central deafferentation pain: spinal intrathecal baclofen. *Stereotact Funct Neurosurg* 1995;65:101–105.
23. Terenius L. Somatostatin and ACTH are peptides with partial antagonist-like selectivity for opiate receptors. *Eur J Pharmacol* 1976;38:211–213.
24. Sandkühler J, Fu QG, Helmchen C. Spinal somatostatin superfusion in vivo affects activity of cat nociceptive dorsal horn neurons: comparison with spinal morphine. *Neuroscience* 1990;34:565–576.
25. Penn RD, Paice JA, Kroin JS. Octreotide: a potent new non-opiate analgesic for intrathecal infusion. *Pain* 1992;49(1):13–19.
26. Paice J, Penn RD, Kroin JS. Intrathecal octreotide for relief of intractable nonmalignant pain: 5-year experience with two cases. *Neurosurgey* 1996;38: 203–207.
27. Meynadier J, Chrubasik J, Dubar M, et al. Intrathecal somatostatin in terminally ill patients. A report of two cases. *Pain* 1985;23:9–12.
28. Mollenholt P, Rawal N, Gordh T, et al. Intrathecal and epidural somatostatin for patients with cancer. Analgesic effects and postmortem neuropathological investigations of spinal cord and nerve roots. *Anesthesiology* 1994;81:534–542.
29. Staats P, Mitchell VD. Future directions for intrathecal therapies. *Prog Anesthesiol* 1997;11:367–382.
30. Hood DD, Eisenach JC, Tuttle R. Phase I safety assessment of intrathecal neostigmine methylsulfate in humans. *Anesthesiology* 1995;82:331–343.
31. Belfrage M, Segerdahl M, Arnér S, et al. The safety and efficacy of intrathecal adenosine in patients with chronic neuropathic pain. *Anesth Analg* 1999;89:136–142.
32. Malmberg AB, Yaksh TL. Spinal nitric oxide synthesis inhibition blocks NMDA-induced thermal hyperalgesia and produces antinociception in the formalin test in rats. *Pain* 1993;54(3):291–300.
33. Malmberg AB, Yaksh TL. Pharmacology of the spinal action of ketorolac, morphine, ST-91, U50488H, and L-PIA on the formalin test and an isobiologic analysis of the NSAID interaction. *Anesthesiology* 1993;79: 270–281.
34. Yu LC, Hansson P, Lundeberg T. The calcitonin gene-related peptide antagonist CGRP8-37 increases the latency to withdrawal responses in rats. *Brain Res* 1994;653:223–230.
35. Saulino M, Kim PS, Shaw E, et al. Practical considerations and patient selection for intrathecal drug delivery in the management of chronic pain. *J Pain Res* 2014;7:627–638.
36. Hassenbusch SJ, Paice JA, Patt RB, et al. Clinical realities and economic considerations: economics of intrathecal therapy. *J Pain Symptom Manage* 1997;14(3 suppl):S36–S48.
37. Kumar A, Maitra S, Khanna P, et al. Clonidine for management of chronic pain: a brief review of the current evidences. *Saudi J Anaesth* 2014;8(1): 92–96.
38. Fanciullo GJ, Rose RJ, Lunt PG, et al. The state of implantable pain therapies in the United States: a nationwide survey of academic teaching programs. *Anesth Analg* 1999;88(6):1311–1316.
39. Deer TR, Pope JE, Hayek SM, et al. The Polyanalgesic Consensus Conference (PACC): Recommendations for intrathecal drug delivery: guidance for improving safety and mitigating risks. *Neuromodulation* 2017;20:155–176. doi:10.1111/ner.12579.
40. Johnston J, Reich S, Baily A, et al. Shiley INFUSAID pump technology. *Ann N Y Acad Sci* 1988;531:57–65.
41. Synchromed Infusion System. *Clinical Reference Guide for Pain Therapy*. Minneapolis, MN: Medtronic Neurological; 1998.
42. Follett KA, Burchiel KJ, Deer T, et al. Prevention of intrathecal drug delivery catheter-related complications. *Neuromodulation* 2003;6:32–41.
43. Narang S, Srinivasan SK, Zinboonyahgoon N, et al. Upper antero-medial thigh as an alternative site for implantation of intrathecal pumps: a case series. *Neuromodulation* 2016;19(6):655–663.
44. Coffey RJ, Divisions of Neuromodulation Clinical Research, Regulatory Vigilance, and Biostatistics, Medtronic Inc, Minneapolis, MN. Mortality associated with implantation and management of intrathecal opioid drug infusion systems to treat non-cancer pain: identification, analysis and mitigation of risk factors. Oral presentation during the American Society of Regional Anesthesia and Pain Medicine Annual Pain Meeting, Huntington Beach, California, November 20, 2008.
45. Patt RB, Hassenbusch SJ. Implantable technology for pain control: identification and management of problems and complications. In: Waldman SW, ed. *Interventional Pain Management*. 2nd ed. Philadelphia, PA: WB Saunders; 2001:654–670.
46. Cole BE. Neuroendocrine implications of opioids therapy. *Curr Pain Headache Rep* 2007;11:89–92.
47. Deer T, Krames ES, Hassenbusch SJ, et al. Management of intrathecal catheter-tip inflammatory masses: an updated 2007 consensus statement from an expert panel. *Neuromodulation* 2008;11:77–91.
48. Smith TJ, Staats PS, Deer T, et al. Randomized clinical trial of an implantable drug delivery system compared with comprehensive medical management for refractory cancer pain: impact on pain, drug-related toxicity, and survival. *J Clin Oncol* 2002;20(19):4040–4049.
49. Bedder MD, Burchiel KJ, Larson A. Cost analysis of two implantable narcotic delivery systems. *J Pain Symptom Management* 1991;6:368–373.

50. Krames ES, Gershow J, Glassberg A, et al. Continuous infusion of spinally administered narcotics for the relief of pain due to malignant disorders. *Cancer* 1985;56:696–702.

51. Onofrio BM, Yaksh TL. Long-term pain relief produced by intrathecal morphine infusion in 53 patients. *J Neurosurg* 1990;72:200–209.

52. Paice JA, Penn RD, Shott S. Intraspinal morphine for chronic pain: a retrospective, multicenter study. *J Pain Symptom Manage* 1996;11(2):71–80.

53. Krames ES. Intrathecal infusional therapies for intractable pain: patient management guidelines. *J Pain Symptom Manage* 1993;8:36–46.

54. Krames ES. Intraspinal opioid therapy for chronic nonmalignant pain: current practice and clinical guidelines. *J Pain Symptom Manage* 1996;11:333–352.

55. Tutak U, Doleys DM. Intrathecal infusion systems for treatment of chronic low back and leg pain of noncancer origin. *South Med J* 1996;89: 295–300.

56. Winkelmüller M, Winkelmüller W. Long-term effects of continuous intrathecal opioid treatment in chronic pain of nonmalignant etiology. *J Neurosurg* 1996;85:458–467.

57. Anderson A, Burchiel KJ. A prospective study of long-term intrathecal morphine in the treatment of nonmalignant pain. *Neurosurgery* 1999;44: 289–301.

58. Roberts LJ, Finch PM, Goucke CR, et al. Outcome of intrathecal opioids in chronic non-cancer pain. *Eur J Pain* 2001;5:353–361.

59. Deer T, Chapple I, Classen A, et al. Intrathecal drug delivery for treatment of chronic low back pain: report from the National Outcomes Registry for Low Back Pain. *Pain Med* 2004;5:6–13.

60. Turner JA, Sears JM, Loeser J. Programmable intrathecal opioid delivery systems for chronic non-cancer pain: a systematic review of effectiveness and complications. *Clin J Pain* 2007;23:180–195.

CHAPTER 101

Intradiscal Therapies for Low Back Pain

YAKOV VOROBEYCHIK and **NIKOLAI BOGDUK**

Intradiscal therapies are interventions in which agents—physical or chemical—are delivered into an intervertebral disk, either to stop pain or to reverse or remove processes responsible for the pain. Fundamental to the use of such interventions is the belief that the lumbar intervertebral disks are a common source of chronic low back pain. This belief has a long history and is based on a variety of circumstantial and direct evidence.

Discogenic Pain

The proposition that lumbar disks could be a source of back pain has been espoused at least since as long ago as 1940.[1] Over the ensuing years, opponents have raised various arguments against the concept. However, each of these arguments has been systematically refuted.[1]

Originally, the argument was that disks could not hurt because they lacked a nerve supply. This argument was maintained as recently as 1980[2,3] despite the fact that studies published in 1940[4] and 1959[5] had shown that the lumbar disks were, indeed, innervated. Studies in 1980[6] and 1981[7] confirmed that innervation and established its source. Later studies, using modern techniques, confirmed the presence of nociceptive nerves in the outer third of the anulus fibrosus of normal disks.[8–11] Other studies showed that, in addition to their normal innervation, damaged or degenerated disks can attract an ingrowth of new nerves, which follow blood vessels and granulation tissue.[12–14]

The second argument was that, although disks might be innervated, they did not hurt (the innervation being vasomotor or serving some function other than nociception). This was refuted by observations that back pain could be provoked by noxious stimulation of disks. When discography was developed as a diagnostic test for disk herniation, investigators noted that injections of contrast medium into affected disks reproduced the patients' low back pain.[15–18] Others, when operating on patients under local anesthesia, observed that probing the disk evoked back pain.[19,20] A modern study found that, of all the structures in the lumbar spine submitted to mechanical provocation, the disks were the most potent source of back pain.[21]

The third argument was that, although disks might hurt, there are no means of diagnosing the condition. This argument is correct if the diagnostic test relies on detecting degenerative changes on imaging of the disk. So-called degenerative changes are almost as prevalent in patients with back pain as in asymptomatic subjects and have no clinically significant, statistical association with pain.[22] For this reason, those who pursue discogenic pain rely on disk stimulation as the diagnostic test.

Disk stimulation is an adaptation of discography.[23] Discography was originally developed in order to demonstrate the internal morphology of the disk, but this is largely irrelevant to diagnosis. Disk stimulation differs in that its emphasis is on the patient's response to stimulation of the disk with injections of contrast medium or normal saline. Morphologic changes are of secondary importance.

The operational guidelines for disk stimulation[23] are that for a disk to be deemed to be the source of pain:

- Stimulating the disk must reproduce the patient's pain (known as a concordant response).
- Stimulation of adjacent disks does not reproduce pain.
- Pain is evoked at low thresholds of stimulation: less than 20 psi (0.14 kPa).
- The evoked pain is clinically significant, that is, rated as greater than 7 out of 10 on a numerical pain rating scale or its equivalent.

These guidelines were developed on the basis of various studies that were performed in order to ensure consistency of practice and interpretation and to minimize false-positive rates caused by excessive stimulation or by hyperalgesia.[1]

The validity of disk stimulation was challenged by studies that reported purportedly high false-positive rates.[24] However, when the data of those studies were analyzed according to operational guidelines, the false-positive rates all but disappeared.[1] A systematic review showed that the false-positive rate of disk stimulation was less than 10% and probably closer to 6%,[25] which is a tolerably low rate.

The final argument against lumbar discogenic pain has been that there is no pathology that renders the disk painful. This has now been comprehensively refuted,[1] as shown in the following section.

Pathology

It is now evident that the lumbar disk responds to a variety of nutritional, metabolic, and mechanical insults in a similar manner.[26,27] Those responses are expressed as what, to date, have been called degenerative changes.

The disk matrix is produced by chondrocytes in the nucleus pulposus, and synthesis is promoted by factors such as transforming growth factor (TGF) and insulin-like growth factor (IGF), which reside in the matrix (Fig. 101.1). Under normal conditions, the matrix is continually renewed. For this to occur, old matrix has to be degraded. The chondrocyte produces enzymes—known as matrix metalloproteinases (MMPs), which degrade the matrix. These enzymes are controlled by tissue inhibitors of matrix metalloproteinases (TIMMPs).[26,27]

Injury disturbs the normal balance between synthesis and degradation toward degradation[26,27] (see Fig. 101.1). Injury results in the liberation of phospholipases (PLAs), which in turn act on arachidonic acid to produce prostaglandins (PGs) and leukotrienes (LTs). LTs are chemotactic and attract macrophages. Macrophages release superoxide and cytokines such as tumor necrosis factor alpha (TNFα), interleukins (IL), and interferon (IFN). These cytokines stimulate the chondrocyte to produce more MMPs and, thereby, promote matrix degradation. The cytokines also stimulate nitric oxide synthetase to produce nitric oxide (NO). NO not only inhibits the chondrocyte but also combines with superoxide to produce peroxynitrite, which inhibits the tissue inhibitors of MMPs, thereby promoting matrix degradation. Superoxide itself inhibits the chondrocyte and directly degrades the matrix.

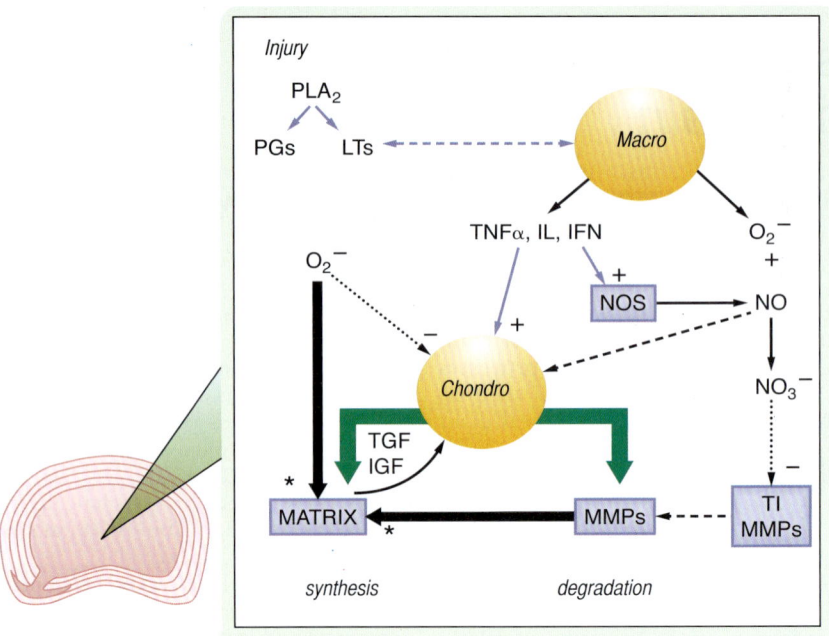

FIGURE 101.1 The molecular biology of disk degeneration and internal disk disruption. *Bold arrows* and *plus signs* (+) indicate production, promotion, or stimulation. *Dashed arrows* indicate attraction. *Dotted arrows* and *minus signs* (−) indicate inhibitory influences. *Open arrows* and *asterisks* (*) indicate degradative effects. Chondro, chondrocyte; IFN, interferon; IGF, insulin-like growth factor; IL, interleukins; LTs, leukotrienes; NOS, nitric oxide synthetase; NO_3, peroxynitrite; NO, nitric oxide; O_2^-, hyperoxide; PGs, prostaglandins; PLA_2, phospholipase A_2; Macro, macrophage; MMPs, matrix metalloproteinases; TFG, transforming growth factor; TIMMPs, tissue inhibitors of MMPs; TNFα, tumor necrosis factor alpha.

As the nucleus degrades, it is no longer able to retain water and loses its hydrostatic properties. Pressures within the nucleus become irregular and reduced[28,29] (Fig. 101.2), and the nucleus is less able to sustain compression loads. Meanwhile, compression loads are increasingly borne by the posterior anulus, which is subjected to loads substantially above normal[28,29] (see Fig. 101.2). Irregular pressures in the nucleus and increased stresses in the posterior anulus are each independently associated with the disk being painful.[30]

The depressurized nucleus is unable to brace the anulus internally. As a result, the inner anulus buckles and delaminates.

Progressive disruption of the anulus leads to the development of radial fissures, which are characteristic of the condition known as internal disk disruption.[31–33] The severity of disruption can be graded according to the extent to which fissures penetrate the anulus (Fig. 101.3). Grade III fissures reach the outer third of the anulus and become grade IV fissures if they extend circumferentially around the outer anulus. These fissures are the hallmark of internal disk disruption. They do not represent age changes[34] and are most likely features of previous injury. Grade III or grade IV fissures are imperfectly but nonetheless significantly associated with the disk being painful on disk stimulation.[1,34–39]

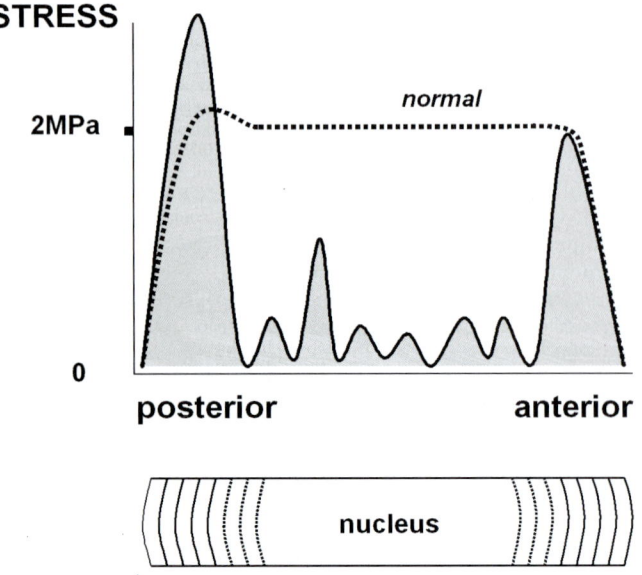

FIGURE 101.2 The internal stress profile across a diameter of an injured intervertebral disk. Stresses are normal in the anterior anulus, decreased and irregular across the nucleus, and raised in the posterior anulus.

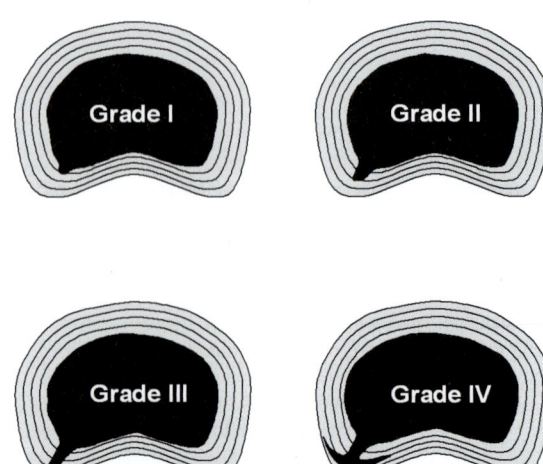

FIGURE 101.3 The grading of radial fissures in internal disk disruption.

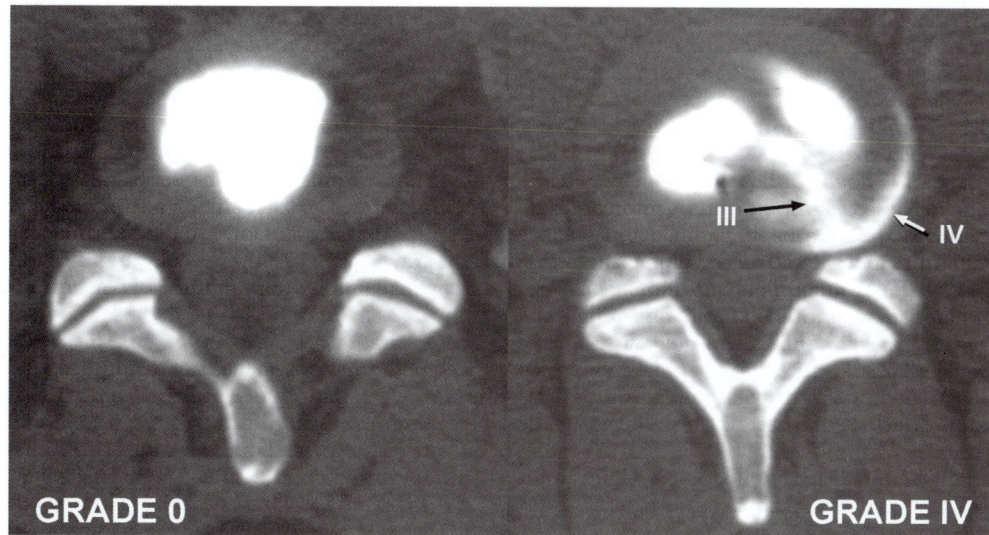

FIGURE 101.4 Postdiscography computed tomography scans showing Grade 0 and a Grade IV internal disk disruption. In the Grade 0 disk, the contrast medium is contained in the nucleus pulposus, with a regular, smooth perimeter. In the Grade IV disk, a Grade III radial fissure has penetrated the anulus fibrosus and has spread circumferentially to become a Grade IV fissure. *(Images kindly provided by Dr. Milton Landers, Wichita, Kansas.)*

Experimental studies have now produced internal disk disruption in laboratory animals.[40,41] The initiating injury was fracture of the vertebral endplate. This injury precipitates the biochemical and morphologic changes of internal disk disruption. Biomechanics studies in cadavers have shown that endplate fractures can be precipitated by fatigue failure.[28] Immediately after fracture of the endplate, the disk expresses the biophysical features of internal disk disruption.[28] Endplate fractures are caused by repeated compression loading and can occur after as few as 100 cycles of compression at 50% to 80% of ultimate tensile strength of the endplate.[42,43] This level of stress is well within the range experienced during normal occupational heavy lifting.

Internal disk disruption can be diagnosed in patients. Radial and circumferential fissures can be demonstrated by computed tomography (CT) discography, in which a CT scan is obtained after contrast medium has been injected into the disk (Fig. 101.4). Demonstrating such fissures converts the diagnosis from discogenic pain to painful internal disk disruption. Otherwise, certain features evident on magnetic resonance imaging (MRI) are consistent with features of internal disk disruption.

High-intensity zones (HIZ) in the posterior anulus (Fig. 101.5) represent the cross-sectional appearance of a circumferential fissure. They occur in 20% to 30% of patients with chronic low back pain and correlate with the affected disk being painful. Although figures differ between studies (Table 101.1), the pooled data show that an HIZ has a positive likelihood ratio greater than 3 for the affected disk being the source of pain.

Modic lesions occur in the spongiosa of the vertebral body above an abnormal disk (Fig. 101.6). Type 1 lesions appear dark on T1-weighted images but bright on T2-weighted images and represent bone marrow edema. Type 2 lesions appear bright both on T1-weighted images and T2-weighted images and represent fat deposition (implicitly postinflammatory). They occur in about 33% of patients with chronic back pain and correlate significantly with the affected disk being painful, the pooled data indicating a positive likelihood ratio of about 3 (Table 101.2).

In patients with chronic low back pain, the prevalence of internal disk disruption is about least 40%.[56,57] The diagnostic features are reproduction of the patient's pain by disk stimulation and demonstration of a radial fissure on postdiscography CT scan.[1]

The mechanism of pain in internal disk disruption appears to be a combination of mechanical and chemical factors. The increased pressures in the posterior anulus provide a basis for mechanical pain. The inordinate pressures in the posterior anulus would stimulate the nociceptive nerve endings in the outer anulus. Inflammatory mediators from the degraded nucleus provide a basis for chemical pain. Mediators that track through the radial fissure would reach the nerve endings in the outer anulus. They could stimulate the nerve endings to produce chemical nociception or they could sensitize the endings and lower their threshold to mechanical stimulation. Both mechanisms could be amplified if new nerve fibers are attracted into the disk by the radial fissure.[12–14]

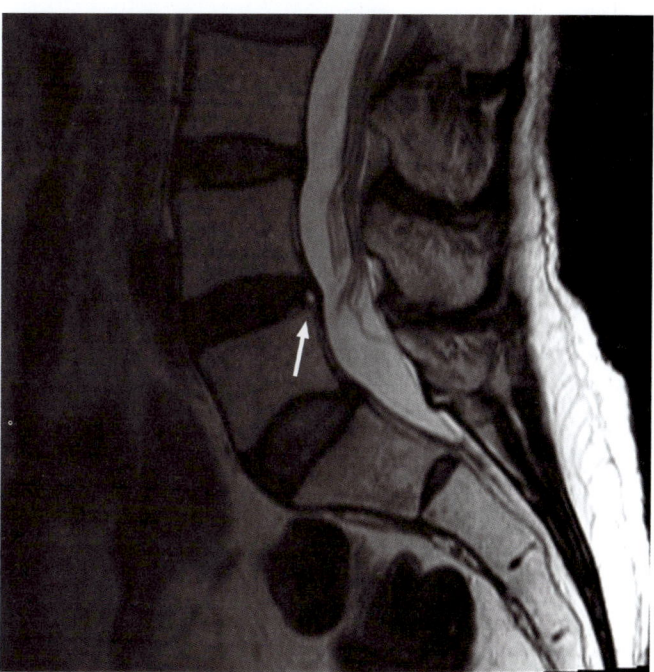

FIGURE 101.5 A T2-weighted, midline, sagittal magnetic resonance scan showing a high-intensity zone (*arrow*) in the anulus fibrosus of the L4–L5 disk. *(Image kindly provided by Dr. Milton Landers, Wichita, Kansas.)*

TABLE 101.1 The Sensitivity, Specificity, and Likelihood Ratio of the High-intensity Zone as a Predictor of the Affected Disc being Painful, as Reported by 12 Studies

Sample Size	Sensitivity	Specificity	Likelihood Ratio	95% CI	Source
142	0.37	1.00	∞	—	Peng et al.[44]
120	0.82	0.89	7.5	4.0–14.1	Aprill et al.[36]
256	0.45	0.94	7.5	3.7–15.1	Chen et al.[45]
152	0.27	0.95	5.4	1.7–17.1	Saifuddin et al.[46]
101	0.52	0.90	5.2	2.4–11.2	Ito et al.[47]
155	0.81	0.79	3.9	2.5–6.0	Lam et al.[48]
178	0.57	0.84	3.6	2.2–5.7	Kang et al.[49]
109	0.45	0.84	2.8	1.4–5.5	Carragee et al.[50]
152	0.26	0.90	2.6	1.2–5.8	Kokkonen et al.[39]
97	0.56	0.70	1.9	1.2–3.0	Lim et al.[38]
116	0.27	0.85	1.8	0.9–3.8	Weishaupt et al.[51]
80	0.09	0.93	1.3	0.3–5.4	Ricketson et al.[52]
1,658	0.45	0.88	3.8	3.1–4.5	ALL

95% CI, 95% confidence interval, the prevalence represents the number of disks studied that showed the sign.

Therapies

The recognition of lumbar discogenic pain and internal disk disruption has attracted the exploration of a number of therapies that specifically target this condition. Variously they involve ablating the nerves that mediate the pain, injecting drugs or chemicals to suppress chemical nociception, or injecting agents intended to reverse the degradative processes within the disk.

ABLATION

Attempts have been made to denervate painful disks at a variety of sites, using a variety of means. Most have proved unsuccessful.

Ramus Communicans Lesions

A prospective, controlled study compared the effects of thermal radiofrequency lesioning in the region of the ramus communicans with those of injections of lidocaine over the same site.[58] Statistically, significant differences arose in favor of radiofrequency treatment, at 4 months following intervention. However, the degree of relief afforded by radiofrequency therapy was modest, amounting to only a 46% mean decrease in pain, and the authors did not report the number of patients experiencing high-grade relief (75% to 100%). Moreover, the study was confounded because patients who received radiofrequency therapy also received an injection of triamcinolone (40 mg) at the site treated, which the control group did not receive. It is,

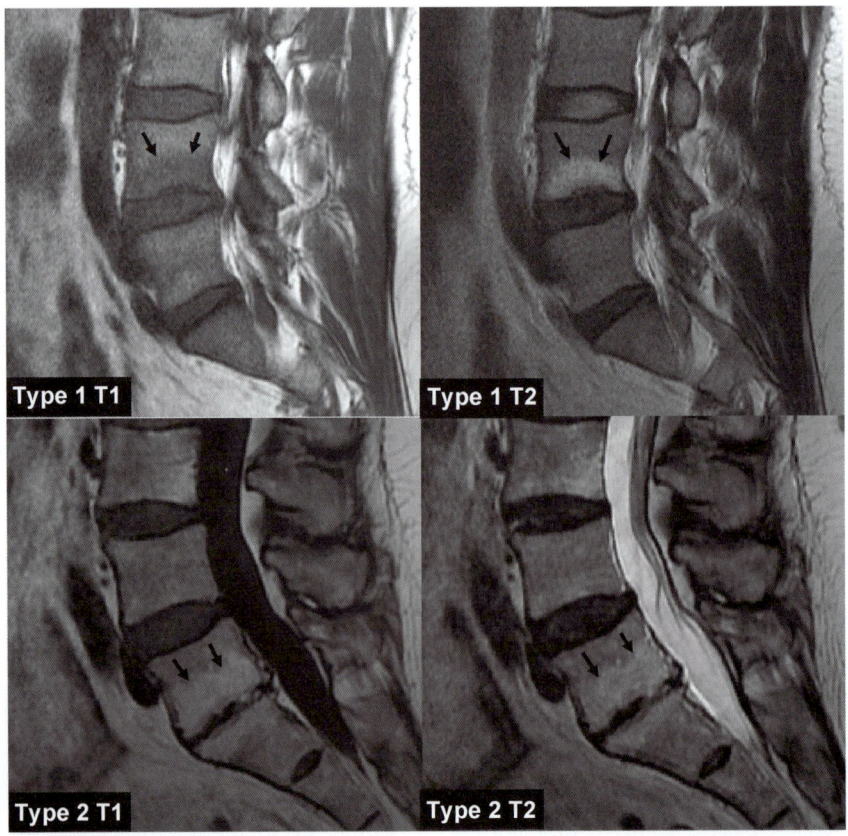

FIGURE 101.6 Sagittal magnetic resonance scans showing the appearance of type 1 and type 2 Modic lesions on T1-weighted and T2-weighted scans. *(Images kindly provided by Dr. Tim Maus, Mayo Clinic, Rochester, Minnesota.)*

TABLE 101.2 The Sensitivity, Specificity, and Likelihood Ratio of Modic Changes as Predictors of the Affected Disc being Painful, as Reported by 12 Studies

Sample	Sensitivity	Specificity	Likelihood Ratio	95% CI	Source
2,457	0.25	0.94	4.2	3.3–5.2	Thompson et al.[53]
152	0.23	0.97	7.7	1.9–31.6	Braithwaite et al.[54]
101	0.22	0.95	4.4	1.3–15.0	Ito et al.[47]
255	0.18	0.90	1.8	0.9–3.5	Sandhu et al.[55]
178	0.14	0.87	1.1	0.5–2.6	Kang et al.[49]
97	0.09	0.83	0.52	0.2–1.8	Lim et al.[38]
3,240	0.24	0.83	3.4	2.8–4.1	ALL

95% CI, 95% confidence interval of likelihood ratio, the prevalence represents the number of disks studied that showed the sign.

therefore, not evident if the modest improvements seen in the study group arose from the radiofrequency lesion created, or the injection of corticosteroids.

Intranuclear Radiofrequency

The nucleus pulposus is normally devoid of nerve endings. Therefore, placing radiofrequency lesions in the nucleus has no prospect of coagulating nerves in the immediate vicinity of the electrode. However, proponents of intranuclear radiofrequency argued that the electric field produced around the electrode would be sufficient to heat and destroy nerve fibers in the outer anulus fibrosus, and thereby provide relief of pain[59]; but cadaver studies have dispelled this notion.[60,61] Significant heating does not occur in the outer anulus. A controlled trial demonstrated that intranuclear radiofrequency achieved no greater relief of pain than sham therapy.[62] What were promoted as successful outcomes in earlier observational studies amounted to no more than placebo responses.

PERCUTANEOUS INTRADISCAL RADIOFREQUENCY THERMOCOAGULATION

Percutaneous intradiscal radiofrequency thermocoagulation (PIRFT) involves inserting a flexible radiofrequency electrode into the posterior anulus fibrosus in order to coagulate fissures and nociceptors with a heat lesion.[63] Good results were reported in a pilot study, with some 40% of patients achieving at least 50% relief of pain, coupled with improvement in disability.[63] However, a controlled trial later found minimal improvements in pain and no differences in outcome between active and sham treatment.[64]

Intradiscal Electrothermal Therapy

Intradiscal electrothermal therapy (IDET) was a treatment developed in the mid-1990s that involved threading a flexible heating element into the posterior anulus fibrosus or along the nucleus–anulus boundary in order to ablate nociceptors in the posterior anulus and to seal fissures.[65–69] The procedure attracted attention in the form of observational and controlled studies.[69–74]

In observational studies, the proportion of patients who achieved greater than 50% relief ranged from 50%[75–77] to 70%,[78,79] and up to 20% of patients achieved complete relief.[75,76] In some studies, outcomes were maintained for 2 years.[76,80,81]

Two randomized, placebo-controlled trials had different results.[82,83] In one trial, a clear difference was demonstrated between placebo and experimental groups, although success rates were modest.[82] Greater than 50% relief was achieved in 40% of patients, among whom 22% experienced 75% to 100% relief of pain. These outcomes were consonant with those reported from observational studies. The other controlled study[83] found no effect, either from active treatment or from sham treatment. This lack of any response is dissonant with the outcomes of observational studies, and the lack of any placebo effect is curious and unexplained. However, because no placebo effects

were demonstrated, this study does not provide evidence that the responses in other studies were due to placebo effects.

Despite these data, the popularity of IDET has all but evaporated. To some extent, that could be because successful outcomes occurred in only a modest proportion of patients or because many patients suffer exacerbation of the pain rather than relief. The principal factor, however, seems to be the failure of the procedure to attract reimbursement in the US health system.

L'DISQ

L'DISQ is the proprietary name for a flexible and navigable electrode that can be used to deliver thermal lesions into an anulus fibrosus. It differs from its predecessors in that the tip of the electrode can be bent by an internal mechanical device in order to change its course as it is pushed across the anulus. A single case series reported that 11 of 20 patients treated with this device achieved 50% relief of pain at 24 weeks and 48 weeks after treatment.[84] From the data published, it is not clear the extent to which these same patients reduced their disability or improved their function.

Coblation

Coblation is a procedure that uses an electrode bathed in saline that produces a so-called "plasma field" around the tip of the electrode consisting of ionized particles. The electrode can be used to dissolve and remove ("coblate") tissues. When used for discogenic pain, the electrode is inserted into the outer anulus fibrosus ostensibly to remove material in radial fissures. One study reported that 10 of 17 patients so treated achieved at least 50% reduction in pain,[85] but no outcome data were reported on restoration of function or continuing health care.

Biacuplasty

Intradiscal biacuplasty is a procedure in which cooled, radiofrequency electrodes are inserted into opposite, posterolateral corners of the anulus fibrosus of the target disk (Fig. 101.7). The rationale for the procedure is that arcing a heat lesion between the electrodes will ablate nociceptors in the posterior anulus or around fissures traversing the anulus. This procedure has received sustained attention from one particular group.

A pilot study of 15 patients reported that 6 had greater than 50% relief of pain at 6 months, coupled with improvement in physical function.[86] A subsequent letter reported that 7 patients had this same response at 12 months.[87] In a randomized study, biacuplasty was shown to be more effective than sham therapy,[88] but success rates were modest. With success being defined as a reduction of pain by 2 points out of 10 and improvement in physical function by 15 points out of 100, 8 of 27 patients (30%) achieved a successful outcome after biacuplasty compared with only 1 of 30 after sham treatment. At 12 months follow-up of 22 patients, group scores for pain and physical function continued to improve, but only 4 patients (18% of those followed, or 15% of those originally treated) satisfied the criteria for successful outcome.[89]

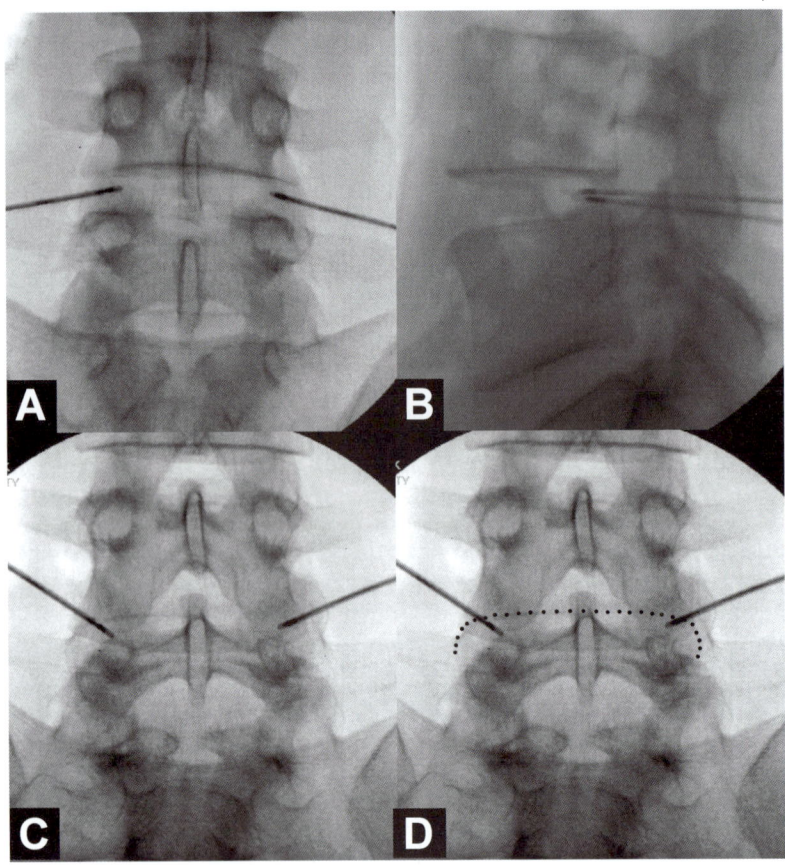

FIGURE 101.7 Fluoroscopy images of electrodes placed for intradiscal biacuplasty. **A:** Anteroposterior view. **B:** Lateral view. **C:** Declined view, with the x-ray beam passing to view the L4–L5 disk from behind and below. **D:** Declined view on which the posterior margin of the disk has been drawn as a *dotted line,* in order to show how the electrodes are inserted radially across the posterolateral corners of the anulus fibrosus. *(Reproduced with permission from International Spinal Intervention Society. Lumbar disc access: Appendix 2: Transdiscal Biacuplasty. In: Bogduk N, ed. Practice Guidelines for Spinal Diagnostic and Treatment Procedures. 2nd ed. San Francisco, CA: International Spine Intervention Society; 2013:417–419.)*

Similar, modest outcomes have been reported by others. In one study, 8 of 15 patients had 50% relief of pain or better.[90] In another study, 4 of 14 patients had greater than 60% relief at 6 months, sustained for 12 months, with 1 having complete relief over this period.[91]

Although the outcomes of biacuplasty appear to be modest, they can be viewed in the context of alternatives for patients with discogenic pain. A randomized controlled study showed that, despite modest success rates, biacuplasty coupled with conventional medical management was clearly superior to conventional medical management alone, in terms of group scores for pain and function.[92,93] Some 42% of patients treated with biacuplasty had at least 50% relief of pain at 6 months, compared with only 7% treated by conventional medical management.[92] This outcome was largely sustained at 12 months.[93] Furthermore, the group scores for relief of pain and improvement in function were not appreciably different from those for surgery for the same condition.[93]

Taken in context, the outcomes of biacuplasty make it an entertainable option for patients with discogenic pain. It is a remarkably safe procedure that is easy to perform and tolerated by patients. No alternatives have proven to offer better prospects of relief. A technical issue limits the efficacy of biacuplasty. The iliac crests can prevent optimal placement of electrodes into L5–S1 disks, such that not all of the posterior anulus can be adequately encompassed by the thermal lesion delivered. If this can be overcome, success rates might be improved.

CHEMICAL THERAPIES

Various chemicals have been used for discogenic pain. For some, there is a reasonable rationale because the drug administered targets one or other of the agents involved in disk degradation. For others, a solid rationale is lacking.

Intradiscal Steroids

Because phospholipase A_2 (PLA_2) has been implicated in disk degeneration and disk injury, intradiscal injection of corticosteroids has a rationale. By inhibiting PLA_2, steroids prevent the arachidonic acid cascade and the production of PGs and LTs (see Fig. 101.1).

In early studies, investigators claimed good results when they used intradiscal steroids to treat patients with a variety of complaints described as back pain and/or sciatic but without a diagnosis of discogenic pain having been made objectively.[94–97] In later studies, a diagnosis of discogenic pain was established by discography, and therapeutic injections were performed at the time of discography.[98–100]

Two controlled trials have refuted any attributable effect from intradiscal steroids for discogenic pain diagnosed solely by disk stimulation. The first compared the therapeutic effects of intradiscal methylprednisolone (80 mg) with those of 1.5 mL intradiscal bupivacaine (0.5%).[98] At 10 to 14 days after treatment, improvements in pain and disability occurred in similar, small proportions of patients in both groups. In the second trial, responses to intradiscal injections of either 40-mg methylprednisolone or 1-mL normal saline were compared. At 1-year follow-up, there were no discernible improvements in disability or pain scores in either group.[99]

A different picture has emerged for the treatment of painful disks that exhibit Modic changes. In one study at 1 month after intradiscal injection of 25 mg prednisolone, 1 of 11 patients with type 2 lesions reported greater than 50% relief of pain, whereas 18 of 33 patients with type 1 lesions and 13 of 25 patients with combined lesions reported that degree of relief.[101] Another study found significant improvements in pain 1 day after intradiscal injection of steroids in patients with type 1 lesions,[102] but improvements attenuated over 12 months or longer follow-up. However, a controlled trial has provided support for intradiscal steroids in such patients.

Patients with Modic type 1 or Modic type 2 lesions were randomized to receive intradiscal injections of saline, betamethasone, or betamethasone mixed with a Chinese medicine extract.[103] No significant improvements occurred in patients treated with normal saline, but at 3 and 6 months, significant improvements in pain scores and in disability occurred in all groups treated with betamethasone, with or without extract, and regardless of lesions being type 1 or type 2. In those groups, no significant differences arose according to type of treatment or type of Modic lesion. At 6 months, mean pain scores dropped from 7 to 2, and disability scores dropped from 35 to 15. However, the authors did not report the success rates for any given definition of success.

Had there been no placebo-controlled trial, the observational studies of intradiscal steroids for Modic lesions could be dismissed as showing no more than placebo responses. However, there being a positive, placebo-controlled trial, the treatment cannot be summarily dismissed as a placebo. What is still required, however, is evidence that this treatment obviates need for other health care and evidence either that it has long-term effects or can be repeated safely in order to reinstate relief if it wanes.

Etanercept

Because TNFα is involved in the degradation of lumbar disks (see Fig. 101.1), there is a rationale for using TNF-blocking agents to treat discogenic pain. One such agent is etanercept, which binds TNF receptors.

A placebo-controlled study assessed the efficacy of intradiscal injection of etanercept in doses increasing from 0.1 to 1.5 mg.[104] No differences were found at 1 month, either within or between patients treated with etanercept or normal saline, with respect to relief of pain or disability. A second controlled trial compared the effects of 10 mg etanercept plus bupivacaine with those of bupivacaine alone.[105] At 4 weeks after treatment, improvements in pain scores and disability were significantly greater in the etanercept group. Moreover, 56% of patients treated with etanercept achieved at least 50% relief of pain, compared with only 23% of those treated with bupivacaine alone. However, at 8 weeks, the therapeutic benefits had extinguished.

Thus, there is evidence that a high dose of etanercept has therapeutic effects beyond those of placebo, but those effects occur only in some patients and are not lasting. By inference, it seems that etanercept can block the inflammatory processes of internal disk disruption, but a single dose is not enough to overcome continued production of TNFα.

Methylene Blue

Methylene blue has weak neurolytic effects and inhibits guanylate cyclase and nitric oxide synthesis. The latter property affords it a role in the treatment of discogenic pain by blocking the degradative effects of NO (see Fig. 101.1).

In a pilot study, a team of investigators in China reported astounding results from the use of intradiscal methylene blue for discogenic back pain.[106] They subsequently published a sham-controlled trial that corroborated these results. At 24 months, 19% of the patients treated with methylene blue had complete relief of pain and no restriction in activities; a further 72% had only slight pain and mild restriction of activities.[107] Of the sham control group, only 15% had slight pain; the remainder had continuing pain. Later, another study from China echoed these results but published only group data that showed improvements in pain scores and disability.[108]

These results have not been reproduced in open-label studies by others. One study had only 1 patient out of 8 who obtained complete relief of pain, which continued for 12 months; the other 7 patients had no relief or various grades of relief that lasted no longer than 6 months.[109] A second study reported success rates based on 2 points reduction of pain but did not report

the proportions of patients achieving 50% relief or complete relief.[110] A third study provided 50% relief to 5 of 15 patients.[111] A fourth study had 3 of 16 patients achieve 50% relief or greater at 2 months, dwindling to 1 of 16 patients at 6 months.[112]

Observational studies are considered a low level of evidence when results are positive, but when results are negative, such studies constitute strong evidence. In the process of scientific enquiry, reproduction of results is essential for credibility. The failure to match the results of the original studies from China is enigmatic, if not curious.

Antibiotics

A group of investigators explored the conjecture that back pain in patients with Modic lesions was due to infection of the disk by anaerobic organisms. On this assumption, they conducted a pilot study, followed by a placebo-controlled trial of antibiotic therapy for back pain in patients with disk herniations and Modic lesions affecting the same level.[113] Their group data showed significantly greater improvements in pain and disability in those patients treated with antibiotics. Despite these results, however, some 67% of their patients still had pain at 1 year. Although heralded as a major breakthrough in the treatment of back pain, this study has attracted criticism on several counts.[114,115] A later study, using ribosomal assays of herniated disk material, found no evidence of bacterial infection.[116]

Proliferants

Some investigators have sought to ameliorate disk pain through the injection of substances purported to enhance healing of diseased disk tissue. Typically, solutions have been used that contain chondroitin sulfate, glucosamine hydrochloride, dimethyl sulfoxide (DMSO), bupivacaine, and hypertonic dextrose[117,118] or hypertonic dextrose alone.[119]

The literature on using these agents is limited to isolated publications that claimed good outcomes but which provided little objective data. Although they reported various degrees of relief of pain, for various durations, none provided data on function or subsequent use of other health care. So, it is not evident from the literature if these interventions make any impact on the burden of illness.

Although authors have referred to injection of these agents as "regenerative" or "proliferative" therapies, chondroitin and glucosamine have not been shown to have any specific anabolic effect on the disk, and DMSO is neurolytic rather than restorative. The term *regenerative* seems more appropriate for emerging intradiscal therapies that have a known positive effect on connective tissue metabolism.

BIOLOGICS

The term *biologics* is used to refer to elements, naturally found in blood or bone marrow as cells or proteins, that are known from studies *in vitro* and in laboratory animals to promote healing of connective tissues or to inhibit cytokines or degradative enzymes. Jointly or severally, such elements have been used extensively to treat musculoskeletal disorders such as tendon injuries and osteoarthritis. Based on their reputed success in these conditions, they have been explored for the treatment of discogenic pain.

Sealant

A proprietary preparation of fibrinogen, referred to as a sealant, has been used to control bleeding in neurosurgery, but it also inhibits cytokines and MMPs. These properties made it an attractive agent ostensibly to seal radial fissures and inhibit the degradative processes of internal disk disruption. A pilot study of intradiscal injection of sealant in 15 patients provided 7 patients with greater than 50% relief of pain, accompanied with improvements in disability, at 1 year after treatment, with 6 maintaining this response to 2 years.[120]

Platelet-Rich Plasma

Platelet-rich plasma (PRP) contains high concentrations of TGF, IGF, basic fibroblast growth factor, and platelet-derived growth factor, which promote matrix synthesis (see Fig. 101.1) and connective tissue healing.[121] It has, therefore, been used in attempts to produce these responses in internal disk disruption.

The first study compared the effects of intradiscal PRP with those of a control injection of contrast medium.[122] Statistically significant differences in favor of PRP were found in some outcome measures, although not for "current pain" or physical function. Success rates of treatment were not reported. An open-label study provided 9 out of 22 patients with greater than 50% relief of pain, coupled with greater than 30% improvement in disability, at 6 months after treatment.[123]

α_2 Macroglobulin

Fibronectin-aggrecan complex (FAC) is a marker of cartilage degradation. Its formation is inhibited by α_2 macroglobulin (A2M). A study explored the effects of intradiscal injection of plasma rich in A2M in 24 patients in whom disk lavage detected FAC or not.[124] At 6 months after treatment, significantly greater improvements in pain and in disability were found in those patients who were FAC positive.

Stem Cells

Of all the biologics, intradiscal stem cell therapy has attracted the greatest amount of attention. There is an abundant literature on the effects of stem cells on disk tissue in vitro and in laboratory animals.[125-127] In these models, stem cells suppress genes for synthesis of degradative enzymes, increase proteoglycan content and extracellular matrix, improve the histologic appearance of the disk, increase disk height, and improve MRI appearance.[125-127] Several small studies have established the feasibility and safety of intradiscal injection of stem cells in humans.[125]

With respect to effectiveness, an observational study found that 16 of 26 patients achieved greater than 50% relief of pain at 12 months after intradiscal stem cells, with 2 of these patients being completely pain free. Relief was accompanied by improvements in disability.[128] These outcomes were largely sustained at 2 years.[129]

An earlier study compared the outcomes from intradiscal stem cells with those of sham therapy.[130] It claimed that stem cell therapy was effective on the grounds that patients had greater and more sustained relief of pain after treatment with intradiscal stem cells. However, pain scores and disability scores were not compared statistically between groups. Inspection of the published data suggests that stem cell therapy reduced the mean values of pain scores to levels slightly lower than those achieved by sham therapy at 6 months after treatment but not at 3 or 12 months. Furthermore, although 5 of 12 treated patients had good relief of pain, so did 4 of 12 control patients. The authors were concerned that active treatment appeared to work in only 40% of patients and were not able to explain this phenomenon.

A leading possibility stems from the fact that all of the preliminary and subsequent studies of intradiscal injection of stem cells selected patients on the basis of MRI features of disk degeneration, but disk degeneration occurs commonly in asymptomatic subjects and has no clinically significant association with the affected disk being painful.[22] Therefore, the disks that were treated may not have been the source of pain in many of the patients treated. The prospect arises that the success rates of intradiscal stem cell therapy might be substantially improved if the treatment was applied to disks shown to be painful by disk stimulation or likely to be painful on the basis of Modic changes or HIZs on MRI.

Discussion

A common theme in most of the studies of treatments for discogenic pain is that many investigators seem intent on discovering a cure for discogenic pain. Some have affiliations with or proprietary interests in the device, technique, or agent that they have investigated or promoted.

Another theme is "50% relief in 50% of patients." This seems to be offered as sufficient evidence that the treatment is successful. However, what is missing from the literature is any evidence that such outcomes actually reduce the burden of illness: that patients return to normal function or near normal but satisfying function and require no continuing health care for their back pain.

These themes create points of resistance among consumers of research data. Tutored consumers would be wary of reporting bias and generous definitions of success. Developments in this field would be more compelling if and once independent, third parties conducted replication studies to determine how well a new treatment works, for how long, and in which types of patients.

A parallel theme is the hope that ablating parts of a disk, or injecting something into it, will be enough to produce a cure. This overlooks the fact that disrupted disks continue to be subject to offending compression loads during normal activities of daily living. Biomechanics continues to drive degradative processes and threatens to overwhelm the effects of single-shot interventions. Thus, although thermal interventions might temporarily ablate fissures and degrade cytokines, continued compression threatens to create new fissures and cytokines. Thermal interventions might destroy nociceptors, but they will likely regenerate. Chemicals might inhibit agents currently active in the disk, but the dose will not be enough to antagonize newly secreted agents. Biologics might promote synthesis of new matrix, but will they be strong enough to overcome continued degradation? In that regard, what is seen in a Petri dish is not what happens in vivo. Cells that benefit from biologics in a Petri dish are not constantly subjected to offensive compression loads. These considerations warn that the current battery of interventions for discogenic pain might have partial or temporary effects, but none are designed to stop permanently the biochemical and morphologic responses to biomechanical injury.

References

1. Bogduk N, Aprill C, Derby R. Lumbar discogenic pain: state-of-the-art review. *Pain Med* 2013;14:813–836.
2. Lamb DW. The neurology of spinal pain. *Phys Ther* 1979;59:971–973.
3. Wyke B. The neurology of low back pain. In: Jayson MIV, ed. *The Lumbar Spine and Back Pain*. 2nd ed. Tunbridge Wells, United Kingdom: Pitman; 1980:265–339.
4. Roofe PG. Innervation of anulus fibrosus and posterior longitudinal ligament. *Arch Neurol* 1940;44:100–103.
5. Malinsky J. The ontogenetic development of nerve terminations in the intervertebral discs of man. *Acta Anat* 1959;38:96–113.
6. Yoshizawa H, O'Brien JP, Thomas-Smith W, et al. The neuropathology of intervertebral discs removed for low-back pain. *J Pathol* 1980;132:95–104.
7. Bogduk N, Tynan W, Wilson AS. The nerve supply to the human lumbar intervertebral discs. *J Anat* 1981;132:39–56.
8. Korkala O, Grönblad M, Liesi P, et al. Immunohistochemical demonstration of nociceptors in the ligamentous structures of the lumbar spine. *Spine* 1985;10:156–157.
9. Konttinen YT, Grönblad M, Antti-Poika I, et al. Neuroimmunohistochemical analysis of peridiscal nociceptive neural elements. *Spine* 1990;15:383–386.
10. Ashton IK, Walsh DA, Polak JM, et al. Substance P in intervertebral discs: binding sites on vascular endothelium of the human annulus fibrosus. *Acta Orthop Scand* 1994;65:635–639.
11. Roberts S, Eisenstein SM, Menage J, et al. Mechanoreceptors in intervertebral discs. Morphology, distribution, and neuropeptides. *Spine* 1995;20:2645–2651.
12. Freemont AJ, Peacock TE, Goupille P, et al. Nerve ingrowth into diseased intervertebral disc in chronic back pain. *Lancet* 1997;350:178–181.
13. Coppes MH, Marani E, Thomeer RT, et al. Innervation of "painful" lumbar discs. *Spine* 1997;22:2342–2350.

14. Freemont AJ, Watkins A, Le Maitre C, et al. Nerve growth factor expression and innervation of the painful intervertebral disc. *J Pathol* 2002;197:286–292.

15. Lindblom K. Diagnostic disc puncture of intervertebral disks in sciatica. *Acta Orthop Scand* 1948;17:231–239.

16. Lindblom K. Technique and results in myelography and disc puncture. *Acta Radiol* 1950;34:321–330.

17. Hirsch C. An attempt to diagnose the level of a disc lesion clinically by disc puncture. *Acta Orthop Scand* 1949;18:132–140.

18. Gardner WJ, Wise RE, Hughes CR, et al. X-ray visualization of the intervertebral disk with a consideration of the morbidity of disk puncture. *Arch Surg* 1952;64:355–364.

19. Wiberg G. Back pain in relation to the nerve supply of the intervertebral disc. *Acta Orthop Scand* 1949;19:211–221.

20. Falconer MA, McGeorge M, Begg AC. Observations on the cause and mechanism of symptom-production in sciatica and low-back pain. *J Neurol Neurosurg Psychiatry* 1948;11:13–26.

21. Kuslich SD, Ulstrom CL, Michael CJ. The tissue origin of low back pain and sciatica: a report of pain response to tissue stimulation during operations on the lumbar spine using local anesthesia. *Orthop Clin North Am* 1991;22:181–187.

22. Bogduk N. Degenerative joint disease of the spine. *Radiol Clin North Am* 2012;50:613–628.

23. International Spine Intervention Society. Lumbar disc access. In: Bogduk N, ed. *Practice Guidelines for Spinal Diagnostic and Treatment Procedures.* 2nd ed. San Francisco, CA: International Spine Intervention Society; 2013:317–375.

24. Carragee EJ, Tanner CM, Khurana S, et al. The rates of false-positive lumbar discography in select patients without low back symptoms. *Spine* 2000;25:1373–1381.

25. Wolfer LR, Derby R, Lee JE, et al. Systematic review of lumbar provocation discography in asymptomatic subjects with a meta-analysis of false-positive rates. *Pain Physician* 2008;11:513–538.

26. Peng B, Wu W, Hou S, et al. The pathogenesis of discogenic low back pain. *J Bone Joint Surg Br* 2005;87:62–67.

27. Hadjipavlou AG, Tzermiadianos MN, Bogduk N, et al. Pathophysiology of disc degeneration: a unified theory. *J Bone Joint Surg* 2008;90:1261–1270.

28. Adams MA, McNally DS, Wagstaff J, et al. Abnormal stress concentrations in lumbar intervertebral discs following damage to the vertebral bodies: cause of disc failure? *Eur Spine J* 1993;1:214–221.

29. McNally DS, Adams MA. Intervertebral disc mechanics as revealed by stress profilometry. *Spine* 1992;17:66–73.

30. McNally DS, Shackleford IM, Goodship AE, et al. In vivo stress measurement can predict pain on discography. *Spine* 1996;21:2580–2587.

31. Crock HV. A reappraisal of intervertebral disc lesions. *Med J Aust* 1970;1:983–989.

32. Crock HV. Internal disc disruption: a challenge to disc prolapse fifty years on. *Spine* 1986;11:650–653.

33. Bogduk N. The lumbar disc and low back pain. *Neurosurg Clin North Am* 1991;2:791–806.

34. Moneta GB, Videman T, Kaivanto K, et al. Reported pain during lumbar discography as a function of anular ruptures and disc degeneration. A re-analysis of 833 discograms. *Spine* 1994;17:1968–1974.

35. Vanharanta H, Sachs BL, Spivey MA, et al. The relationship of pain provocation to lumbar disc deterioration as seen by CT/discography. *Spine* 1987;12:295–298.

36. Aprill C, Bogduk N. High-intensity zone: a diagnostic sign of painful lumbar disc on magnetic resonance imaging. *Br J Radiol* 1992;65:361–369.

37. Smith BMT, Hurwitz EL, Solsberg D, et al. Interobserver reliability of detecting lumbar intervertebral disc high-intensity zone on magnetic resonance imaging and association of high-intensity zone with pain and anular disruption. *Spine* 1998;23:2074–2080.

38. Lim CH, Jee WH, Son BC, et al. Discogenic lumbar pain: association with MR imaging and CT discography. *Eur J Radiol* 2005;54:431–437.

39. Kokkonen SM, Kurunlahti M, Tervonen O, et al. Endplate degeneration observed on magnetic resonance imaging of the lumbar spine: correlation with pain provocation and disc changes observed on computed tomography discography. *Spine* 2002;27:2274–2278.

40. Holm S, Kaigle-Holm A, Ekstrom L, et al. Experimental disc degeneration due to endplate injury. *J Spinal Disord Tech* 2004;17:64–71.

41. Cinotti G, Della Rocca C, Romeo S, et al. Degenerative changes of porcine intervertebral disc induced by vertebral endplate injury. *Spine* 2005;30:174–180.

42. Hansson TH, Keller TS, Spengler DM. Mechanical behaviour of the human lumbar spine. II. Fatigue strength during dynamic compressive loading. *J Orthop Res* 1987;5:479–487.

43. Liu YK, Njus G, Buckwalter J, et al. Fatigue response of lumbar intervertebral joints under axial cyclic loading. *Spine* 1983;8:857–865.

44. Peng B, Hou S, We W, et al. The pathogenesis and clinical significance of a high-intensity zone (HIZ) of lumbar intervertebral disc on MR imaging in the patient with discogenic low back pain. *Eur Spine J* 2006;15:583–587.

45. Chen J, Ding Y, Lv R, et al. Correlation between MR imaging and discography with provocative concordant pain in patients with low back pain. *Clin J Pain* 2011;27:125–130.

46. Saifuddin A, Braithwaite I, White J, et al. The value of lumbar spine magnetic resonance imaging in the demonstration of anular tears. *Spine* 1998;23:453–457.

47. Ito M, Incorvaia KM, Yu SF, et al. Predictive signs of discogenic lumbar pain on magnetic resonance imaging with discography correlation. *Spine* 1998;23:1252–1260.

48. Lam KS, Carlin D, Mulhollad RC. Lumbar disc high-intensity zone: the value and significance of provocative discography in the determination of the discogenic pain source. *Eur Spine J* 2000;9:36–41.

49. Kang CH, Kim YH, Lee SH, et al. Can magnetic resonance imaging accurately predict concordant pain provocation during provocative disc injection? *Skeletal Radiol* 2009;38:877–885.

50. Carragee EJ, Paragoudakis SJ, Khurana S. Lumbar high-intensity zone and discography in subjects without low back problems. *Spine* 2000;25:2987–2992.

51. Weishaupt D, Zanetti M, Hodler J, et al. Painful lumbar disk derangement: relevance of endplate abnormalities at MR imaging. *Radiology* 2001;218:420–427.

52. Ricketson R, Simmons JW, Hauser BO. The prolapsed intervertebral disc. The high-intensity zone with discography correlation. *Spine* 1996;21:2758–2762.

53. Thompson KJ, Dagher M, Eckel TS, et al. Modic changes on MR images as studied with provocative diskography: clinical relevance—a retrospective study of 2457 disks. *Radiology* 2009;250:849–855.

54. Braithwaite I, White J, Saifuddin A, et al. Vertebral end-plate (Modic) changes on lumbar spine MRI: correlation with pain reproduction at lumbar discography. *Eur Spine J* 1998;7:363–368.

55. Sandhu HS, Sanchez-Caso LP, Parvataneni HK, et al. Association between findings of provocative discography and vertebral endplate changes as seen on MRI. *J Spinal Disord* 2000;13:438–443.

56. Schwarzer AC, Aprill CN, Derby R, et al. The prevalence and clinical features of internal disc disruption in patients with chronic low back pain. *Spine* 1995;20:1878–1883.

57. DePalma M, Ketchum J, Saullo R. Multivariable analyses of the relationships between age, gender, and body mass index and the source of chronic low back pain. *Pain Med* 2012;13:498–506.

58. Oh WS, Shim JC. A randomized controlled trial of radiofrequency denervation of the ramus communicans nerve for chronic discogenic low back pain. *Clin J Pain* 2004;20:55–60.

59. Van Kleef, Barendse GAM, Wilmink JT. Percutaneous intradiscal radiofrequency thermocoagulation in chronic non-specific low back pain. *Pain Clin* 1996;9:259–268.

60. Troussier B, Lebas JF, Chirossel JP, et al. Percutaneous intradiscal radiofrequency thermocoagulation. A cadaveric study. *Spine* 1995;20:1713–1718.

61. Houpt JC, Conner ES, McFarland EW. Experimental study of temperature distributions and thermal transport during radiofrequency current therapy of the intervertebral disc. *Spine* 1996;21:1808–1813.

62. Barendse GA, van den Berg SG, Kessels AH, et al. Randomized controlled trial of percutaneous intradiscal radiofrequency thermocoagulation for chronic discogenic back pain: lack of effect from a 90-second 70° C lesion. *Spine* 2001;26:287–292.

63. Finch PM, Price LM, Drummond PD. Radiofrequency heating of painful annular disruptions: one-year outcomes. *J Spinal Disord Tech* 2005;18:6–13.

64. Kvarstein G, Måwe L, Indahl A, et al. A randomized double-blind controlled trial of intra-annular radiofrequency thermal disc therapy—a 12-month follow-up. *Pain* 2009;145:279–286.

65. Kleinstueck FS, Diederich CJ, Nau WH, et al. Acute biomechanical and histological effects of intradiscal electrothermal therapy on human lumbar discs. *Spine* 2001;26:2198–2207.

66. Kleinstueck FS, Diederich CJ, Nau WH, et al. Temperature and thermal dose distributions during intradiscal electrothermal therapy in the cadaveric lumbar spine. *Spine* 2003;28:1700–1709.

67. Freeman BJ, Walters RM, Moore RJ, et al. Does intradiscal electrothermal therapy denervate and repair experimentally induced posterolateral annular tears in an animal model? *Spine* 2003;28:2602–2608.

68. Karasek M, Bogduk N. Intradiscal electrothermal annuloplasty: percutaneous treatment of chronic discogenic low back pain. *Tech Reg Anesth Pain Manag* 2001;5:130–135.

69. Bogduk N, Lau P, Govind J, et al. Intradiscal electrothermal therapy. *Tech Reg Anesth Pain Manag* 2005;9:25–34.

70. Freeman BJ. IDET: a critical appraisal of the evidence. *Eur Spine J* 2006;15(suppl 3):S448–S457.

71. Andersson GB, Mekhail NA, Block JE. Treatment of intractable discogenic low back pain. A systematic review of spinal fusion and intradiscal electrothermal therapy (IDET). *Pain Physician* 2006;9:237–248.

72. Andersson GB, Mekhail NA, Block JE. Intradiscal electrothermal therapy (IDET). *Spine* 2006;31:1402–1403.

73. Appleby D, Anderson G, Totta M. Meta-analysis of the efficacy and safety of intradiscal electrothermal therapy (IDET). *Pain Med* 2006;7:308–316.

74. Assietti R, Morosi M, Block JE. Intradiscal electrothermal therapy for symptomatic internal disc disruption: 24-month results and predictors of clinical success. *J Neurosurg Spine* 2010;12:320–326.

75. Karasek M, Bogduk N. Twelve-month follow-up of a controlled trial of intradiscal thermal anuloplasty for back pain due to internal disc disruption. *Spine* 2000;25:2601–2607.

76. Bogduk N, Karasek M. Two-year follow-up of a controlled trial of intradiscal electrothermal anuloplasty for chronic low back pain resulting from internal disc disruption. *Spine J* 2002;2:343–350.

77. Cohen SP, Larkin T, Abdi S, et al. Risk factors for failure and complications of intradiscal electrothermal therapy: a pilot study. *Spine* 2003;28: 1142–1147.

78. Kapural L, Mekhail N, Korunda Z, et al. Intradiscal thermal annuloplasty for the treatment of lumbar discogenic pain in patients with multilevel degenerative disc disease. *Anesth Analg* 2004;99:472–476.

79. Kapural L, Hayek S, Malak O, et al. Intradiscal thermal annuloplasty versus intradiscal radiofrequency ablation for the treatment of discogenic pain: a prospective matched control trial. *Pain Med* 2005;6:425–431.

80. Lee MS, Cooper G, Lutz GE, et al. Intradiscal electrothermal therapy (IDET) for treatment of chronic lumbar discogenic pain: a minimum 2-year clinical outcome study. *Pain Physician* 2003;6:443–448.

81. Saal JA, Saal JS. Intradiscal electrothermal treatment for chronic discogenic low back pain: prospective outcome study with a minimum 2-year follow-up. *Spine* 2002;27:966–974.

82. Pauza KJ, Howell S, Dreyfuss P, et al. A randomized, placebo-controlled trial of intradiscal electrothermal therapy for the treatment of discogenic low back pain. *Spine J* 2004;4:27–35.

83. Freeman BJ, Fraser RD, Cain CM, et al. A randomized, double-blind, controlled trial: intradiscal electrothermal therapy versus placebo for the treatment of chronic discogenic low back pain. *Spine* 2005;30:2369–2378.

84. Lee SH, Derby R, Sul D, et al. Effectiveness of a new navigable percutaneous disc decompression device (L'DISQ) in patients with lumbar discogenic pain. *Pain Med* 2015;16:266–273.

85. He L, Hu X, Tang Y, et al. Efficacy of coblation annuloplasty in discogenic low back pain: a prospective observational study. *Medicine* 2015;94:e846.

86. Kapural L, Ng A, Dalton J, et al. Intervertebral disc biacuplasty for the treatment of lumbar discogenic pain: results of a six-month follow-up. *Pain Med* 2008;9:60–67.

87. Kapural L. Intervertebral disk cooled bipolar radiofrequency (intradiskal biacuplasty) for the treatment of lumbar diskogenic pain: a 12-month follow-up of the pilot study. *Pain Med* 2008;9:407–408.

88. Kapural L, Vrooman B, Sarwar S, et al. A randomized, placebo-controlled trial of transdiscal radiofrequency, biacuplasty for treatment of discogenic lower back pain. *Pain Med* 2013;14:362–373.

89. Kapural L, Vrooman, B, Sarwar S, et al. Radiofrequency intradiscal biacuplasty for treatment of discogenic lower back pain: a 12-month follow-up. *Pain Med* 2015;16:425–431.

90. Karaman H, Tüfek A, Kavak GÖ, et al. 6-month results of transdiscal biacuplasty on patients with discogenic low back pain: preliminary findings. *Int J Med Sci* 2011;8:1–8.

91. Bogduk N, Lau P, Gowaily K. An audit of radiofrequency biacuplasty for back pain due to internal disc disruption. *Pain Med* 2009;10:947.

92. Desai MJ, Kapural L, Petersohn JD, et al. A prospective, randomized, multicenter, open-label clinical trial comparing intradiscal biacuplasty to conventional medical management for discogenic lumbar back pain. *Spine* 2016;41:1065–1074.

93. Desai MJ, Kapural L, Petersohn JD, et al. Twelve-month follow-up of a randomized clinical trial comparing intradiscal biacuplasty to conventional medical management for discogenic lumbar back pain. *Pain Med* 2017;18:751–763.

94. Feffer HL. Treatment of low-back and sciatic pain by the injection of hydrocortisone into degenerated intervertebral discs. *J Bone Joint Surg Am* 1956;38-A:585–590.

95. Feffer HL. Therapeutic intradiscal hydrocortisone. A long-term study. *Clin Orthop Relat Res* 1969;67:100–104.

96. Graham CE. Chemonucleolysis: a double blind study comparing chemonucleolysis with intra discal hydrocortisone: in the treatment of backache and sciatica. *Clin Orthop Relat Res* 1976;117:179–192.

97. Wilkinson HA, Schuman N. Intradiscal corticosteroids in the treatment of lumbar and cervical disc problems. *Spine* 1980;5:385–389.

98. Simmons JW, McMillin JN, Emery SF, et al. Intradiscal steroids. A prospective double-blind clinical trial. *Spine* 1992;17:S172–S175.

99. Khot A, Bowditch M, Powell J, et al. The use of intradiscal steroid therapy for lumbar spinal discogenic pain: a randomized controlled trial. *Spine* 2004;29:833–836.

100. Yavuz F, Taşkaynatan MA, Aydemir K, et al. The efficacy of intradiscal steroid injections in degenerative lumbar disc disease. *Turk J Phys Med Rehab* 2012;58:88–92.

101. Fayad F, Lefevre-Colau MM, Rannou F, et al. Relation of inflammatory Modic changes to intradiscal steroid injection outcome in chronic low back pain. *Eur Spine J* 2007;16:925–931.

102. Beaudreuil J, Dieude P, Poiraudeau S, et al. Disabling chronic low back pain with Modic type 1 MRI signal: acute reduction in pain with intradiscal corticotherapy. *Ann Phys Rehabil Med* 2012;55:139–147.

103. Cao P, Jiang L, Zhuang C, et al. Intradiscal injection therapy for degenerative chronic discogenic low back pain with end plate Modic changes. *Spine J* 2011;11:100–106.

104. Cohen SP, Wenzell D, Hurley RW, et al. A double-blind, placebo-controlled, dose-response pilot study evaluating intradiscal etanercept in patients with chronic discogenic low back pain or lumbosacral radiculopathy. *Anesthesiology* 2007;107:99–105.

105. Sainoh T, Orita S, Miyagi M, et al. Single intradiscal administration of the tumor necrosis factor-alpha inhibitor, etanercept, for patients with discogenic low back pain. *Pain Med* 2016;17:40–45.

106. Peng B, Zhang Y, Hou S, et al. Intradiscal methylene blue injection for the treatment of chronic discogenic low back pain. *Eur Spine J* 2007; 16:33–38.

107. Peng B, Pang X, Wu Y, et al. A randomized placebo-controlled trial of intradiscal methylene blue injection for the treatment of chronic discogenic low back pain. *Pain* 2010;149:124–129.

108. Zhang X, Hao J, Hu ZM, et al. Clinical evaluation and magnetic resonance imaging assessment of intradiscal methylene blue injection for the treatment of discogenic low back pain. *Pain Physician* 2016;19: E1189–E1195.

109. Gupta G, Radhakrishna M, Chankowsky J, et al. Methylene blue in the treatment of discogenic low back pain. *Pain Physician* 2012;15:333–338.

110. Kim SH, Ahn SH, Cho YW, et al. Effect of intradiscal methylene blue injection for the chronic discogenic low back pain: one year prospective follow-up study. *Ann Rehabil Med* 2012;36:657–664.

111. Kallewaard JW, Geurts JW, Kessels A, et al. Efficacy, safety, and predictors of intradiscal methylene blue injection for discogenic low back pain: results of a multicenter prospective clinical series. *Pain Pract* 2016;16:405–412.

112. Levi DS, Horn S, Walko E. Intradiskal methylene blue treatment for diskogenic low back pain. *PM R* 2014;6:1030–1037.

113. Albert HB, Sorensen JS, Christensen BS, et al. Antibiotic treatment in patients with chronic low back pain and vertebral bone edema (Modic type 1 changes): a double-blind randomized clinical controlled trial of efficacy. *Eur Spine J* 2013;22:697–707.

114. O'Dowd J, Casey A. Antibiotics a cure for back pain, a false dawn or a new era? *Eur Spine J* 2013;22:1694–1697.

115. Lings S. Antibiotics for low back pain? *Eur Spine J* 2014;23:469–472.

116. Alamin TF, Munoz M, Zagel A, et al. Ribosomal PCR assay of excised intervertebral discs from patients undergoing single-level primary lumbar microdiscectomy. *Eur Spine J* 2017;26:2038–2044.

117. Klein RG, Eek BC, O'Neill CW, et al. Biochemical injection treatment for discogenic low back pain: a pilot study. *Spine J* 2003;3:220–226.

118. Derby R, Eek B, Lee SH, et al. Comparison of intradiscal restorative injections and intradiscal electrothermal treatment (IDET) in the treatment of low back pain. *Pain Physician* 2004;7:63–66.

119. Miller MR, Mathews RS, Reeves KD. Treatment of painful advanced internal lumbar disc derangement with intradiscal injection of hypertonic dextrose. *Pain Physician* 2006;9:115–121.

120. Yin W, Pauza K, Olan WJ, et al. Intradiscal injection of fibrin sealant for the treatment of symptomatic lumbar internal disc disruption: results of a prospective multicenter pilot study with 24-month follow-up. *Pain Med* 2014;15:16–31.

121. Monfett M, Harrison J, Boachie-Adjei K, et al. Intradiscal platelet-rich plasma (PRP) injections for discogenic low back pain: an update. *Int Orthop* 2016;40:1321–1328.

122. Tuakli-Wosornu YA, Terry A, Boachie-Adjei K, et al. Lumbar intradiskal platelet-rich plasma (PRP) injections: a prospective, double-blind, randomized controlled study. *PM R* 2016;8:1–10.

123. Levi D, Horn S, Tyszko S, et al. Intradiscal platelet-rich plasma injection for chronic discogenic low back pain: preliminary results from a prospective trial. *Pain Med* 2016;17:1010–1022.

124. Montesano PX, Cuellar JM, Scuderi GJ. Intradiscal injection of an autologous alpha-2-macroglobulin (A2M) concentrate alleviates back pain in FAC-positive patients. *Ortho & Rheum Open Access* 2017;4:555634.

125. Oehme D, Goldschlager T, Ghosh P, et al. Cell-based therapies used to treat lumbar degenerative disc disease: a systematic review of animal studies and human clinical trials. *Stem Cells Int* 2015;946031.

126. Priyadarshani P, Li Y, Yao L. Advances in biological therapy for nucleus pulposus regeneration. *Osteoarthritis Cartilage* 2016;24:206–212.

127. Zeckser J, Wolff M, Tucker J, et al. Multipotent mesenchymal stem cell treatment for discogenic low back pain and disc degeneration. *Stem Cells Int* 2016;3908389.

128. Pettine KA, Murphy MB, Suzuki RK, et al. Percutaneous injection of autologous bone marrow concentrate cells significantly reduces lumbar discogenic pain through 12 months. *Stem Cells* 2015;33:146–156.

129. Pettine K, Suzuki R, Sand T, et al. Treatment of discogenic back pain with autologous bone marrow concentrate injection with minimum two year follow-up. *Int Orthop* 2016;40:135–140.

130. Noriega DC, Ardura F, Hernández-Ramajo R, et al. Intervertebral disc repair by allogeneic mesenchymal bone marrow cells: a randomized controlled trial. *Transplantation* 2017;101:1945–1951.

CHAPTER 102

Neurolytic Blockade for Noncancer Pain

JOHN MACVICAR and **NIKOLAI BOGDUK**

Introduction

DEFINITION

Stedman's Medical Dictionary defines *neurolysis* as either the selective, iatrogenic destruction of neural tissue to secure the relief of pain, or a procedure in which the nerve is electively freed surgically from inflammatory tissue.[1] This chapter deals with the former half of this definition. It covers using chemical or physical means to damage peripheral nerves focally in order to prevent the transmission of nociceptive information along the target nerve in order to provide relief of pain. Surgical interventions are described in Chapters 103–105.

Etymologically, the term *neurolysis* actually means teasing apart or dissolving a nerve, and *neurotomy* means opening a nerve, but no superior term has been advanced and accepted to refer to producing focal damage to a nerve while leaving it intact. In this chapter, the term *neurolytic blockade* has been adopted, as a general term, to refer to all procedures whose intent is to prevent the conduction of nociceptive traffic along it. Reflecting convention, rather than good etymologic practice, "neurolysis" has been retained in the context of chemical procedures and "neurotomy" in the context of physical procedures.

PRINCIPLES

Neurolytic blockade is a therapeutic option when the actual source of pain cannot be treated. The objective is to relieve the pain by blocking the nerves that transmit nociception from its source.

The primary indication for neurolytic blockade is complete relief of pain when the target nerve is anesthetized temporarily with controlled, local anesthetics (see Chapter 98). Longer lasting relief can then putatively be achieved by neurolysis or neurotomy.

Of the chemical agents, phenol and alcohol are the most commonly used, and there are no comparative outcome data by which to choose between the two. Glycerol has a special application in the management of trigeminal neuralgia.

Of the physical modalities, heat and cold have both been used to interrupt conduction along peripheral nerves. In both instances, a probe or an electrode is placed on the nerve and is used to produce a small lesion that incorporates a segment of the nerve. Cold lesions (cryoneurotomy) are produced by passing carbon dioxide through a probe. Thermal lesion (thermal neurotomy) are produced by passing a radiofrequency (RF) current through an electrode. Variants of RF neurotomy have been developed in which the emphasis lies in the frequency and modulation of the current applied rather than the heat that it generates.

HISTORY AND TRENDS

The earliest form of neurolytic blockade was surgical neurectomy, in which the nerves from a source of pain were simply transected. This approach has largely been abandoned for several reasons. Neurectomy did not achieve long-term results, and when pain returned, the procedure could not be repeated, painful neuromas could develop on the proximal stump of transected nerve, and transecting large nerves could result in deafferentation pain.

Chemical and physical neurolytic blockades were developed to overcome or circumvent these problems. Neuroma formation could be avoided by not transecting the nerve. If the nerve recovered, and pain recurred, the neurolytic procedure could be repeated. Small nerves, not readily accessed surgically, could be targeted with electrodes or injections in order to avoid having to target their larger, parent nerves.

LIMITATIONS

Classical pathology teaching describes how nerves recover after they have been transected. Wallerian degeneration occurs in the distal stump and is completed within 24 hours in small nerve fibers and in 48 hours in larger nerve fibers. In the proximal stump, regeneration of axon tubules occurs within hours of the transection. The process is driven by neurotrophic agents, such as tumor necrosis factor α (TNF-α), T cells, macrophages, leukocyte inhibitory factor (LIF), and cell adhesion molecules, which are expressed in a highly coordinated fashion.[2-4] A growth cone, containing mitochondria, vesicular elements, neurofilaments, and endoplasmic reticulum, emerges from the proximal stump and proceeds into the distal stump, if it is accessible; Schwann cells undergo mitotic activity and form a framework for developing fibers.[2] Regeneration occurs at a rate of approximately 1 mm per day so that reinnervation of a structure 5 cm away would take approximately 50 days. This process requires an intact dorsal root ganglion to synthesize the regenerative proteins and other nutrients.

Neurolytic blockade involves a different pathology, much of which has not been explored and explained. The differences arise according to where in the nerve the lesion is made, the nature of the lesion, and its size.

If the dorsal root ganglion is destroyed, regeneration will not occur because the cell nucleus is not available to drive the process. Consequently, not only permanent relief of pain but also permanent side effects and complications can be expected from neurolytic procedures that target a dorsal root ganglion.

If a peripheral nerve is targeted, chemical neurolysis does not destroy it. Instead, the chemical applied denatures the components of the axons, in one way or another, and only focally. Chemicals can bind to membrane proteins or other elements, or they can exert an osmotic effect which focally desiccates the nerve. From such processes, the nerve can recover. All that is required is that the damaged elements be replaced in the normal course of endocellular maintenance of the cell membrane or other constituents. The rate at which this happens, however, has not been established.

Cryoneurotomy works by freezing intracellular water; the ice expands and essentially fractures the nerve membrane, thereby preventing conduction along it. From this effect, the nerve can recover by reconstituting the damaged segment of membrane. Based on the duration of relief of pain following cryoneurotomy, this recovery process appears to be relatively fast: measurable in weeks.

Thermal RF neurotomy denatures all the proteins in the segment of nerve incorporated in the lesion made. Nevertheless, the nerve remains macroscopically intact. Regeneration does not occur by classical processes because the nerve is sealed by the coagulated proteins, not transected, and left open. Therefore, growth cones cannot emerge. Before the nerve can regenerate, the coagulated material has to be removed by endocellular repair mechanisms. The rate of this process has not been determined but appears to be measurable in months based on the duration of effect of thermal RF neurotomy. Critical in this regard is the length of nerve affected. It is axiomatic that, if a short segment (1 to 2 mm) is coagulated, recovery will be faster than if a longer segment (10 to 15 mm) is coagulated. An appropriate simile is that endocellular repair is like tunneling a mineshaft that has caved in; it takes longer to tunnel a longer length of caved-in shaft.

Chemical Neurolytic Blockade

PRINCIPLES

Phenol, alcohol, and glycerol are locally neurotoxic in a dose-dependent manner. These dehydrating agents cause a nonselective destruction of neuronal tissues followed by necrosis, nonsegmental demyelination, wallerian degeneration, and complete conduction block occurs within 10 minutes of application.[5-12]

PHENOL

First introduced by Lister in 1867 as an antiseptic, phenol (carbolic acid) is a neurolytic agent with local anesthetic properties. Concentrations of less than 1% produce local anesthesia without toxicity or neurolysis and may be used as a topical anesthetic. Phenol can be injected directly onto peripheral nerves or into the subarachnoid space in order to target dorsal root ganglia. Nonselective neuronal destruction leading to wallerian degeneration is its principle mode of action.

ALCOHOL

Alcohol (absolute alcohol, ethanol, ethyl alcohol) is a clear volatile hygroscopic liquid that exerts its analgesic effect by nonselective neuronal destruction.[8-10] Because of its irritant effect, alcohol may exacerbate local pain on injection and may produce dose-dependent burning and dysesthesia. Prior injection of local anesthetic may minimize this effect. Alcohol has produced variable results, and some consider that the risk of complications outweighs its benefits.[8]

APPLICATIONS

Alcohol or phenol has been widely used to perform neurolytic blockades of various parts of the sympathetic nervous system of the abdomen. Targets have included the lumbar sympathetic trunks and the splanchnic nerves but most commonly the celiac plexus and ganglia.

In patients with visceral disorders, neurolytic blocks of the celiac ganglion or plexus are most commonly used to treat the pain of carcinoma of the pancreas. Various techniques are available by which to block the celiac plexus, ranging between anterior or posterior approaches, using fluoroscopy, computed tomography (CT), or endoscopic ultrasound, for guidance.[13] For carcinoma of the pancreas, neurolytic blocks are often helpful to reduce pain[14-17] but are not necessarily more effective than treatment with analgesics and opioids.[17-20]

For the pain of chronic pancreatitis, the evidence is less robust and less heartening. Response rates are low,[13,15] and unequivocal data on efficacy, and long-term outcomes are lacking.[21]

Descriptive studies promoted neurolytic lumbar sympathetic blocks as a worthwhile treatment for rest pain in patients with peripheral vascular disease, particularly those in whom surgery could not be performed.[22-24] A controlled trial showed that neurolytic blocks were far more effective than local anesthetic blocks,[25] but higher levels of evidence have not appeared.

Phenol or alcohol can be injected intrathecally in order to target particular nerve roots. Mixing the neurolytic agent with glycerine produces a hyperbaric solution, which can be guided under gravity to the target nerve or nerves. Adding contrast medium to the solution allows the movement of the solution to be monitored. With skillful technique, the solution can even be guided into a single nerve root pouch by appropriately tilting the patient. In case reports and book chapters, such injections have been promoted as a treatment for cancer pain, but there have been no controlled trials.[26] The treatment provides complete relief of pain in up to half of the patients treated.[27] The duration of effect is measurable in weeks or months, which may be sufficient for patients with short life expectancy. Intrathecal injections of phenol have not been promoted for the treatment of noncancer pain.

Neurolytic blocks of the lumbar or cervical sympathetic chains have been used, at times, for the treatment of complex regional pain syndromes, albeit on the basis of very little published evidence. A systematic review concluded that there is no good evidence for the effectiveness of sympathectomy—particularly with regard to long-term effectiveness outcomes—and it should be used with great caution if at all outside a research context, in carefully selected patients after thorough assessment and probably only after failure of other treatment options.[28] A narrative review concluded that no high-level evidence exists to support the widespread use of neurolytic blocks for complex regional pain syndromes, particularly because there is evidence to support other forms of treatment.[29]

Although injections of phenol have been used to treat lumbar zygapophysial joint pain,[30] this treatment has not been widely adopted by others and has neither been corroborated nor validated by controlled trials.

GLYCEROL

Propane-1,2,3 triol, or glycerol, is a colorless hygroscopic, syrupy liquid that has a unique application in the management of trigeminal neuralgia. Percutaneous retrogasserian glycerol rhizolysis is achieved by the instilling, under fluoroscopic guidance, no more than 0.3 mL of glycerol into the gasserian cistern. Glycerol nonselectively damages both the axons and the myelin sheath,[11] and 30% to 76% of patients suffer sensory loss.[12] Some achieve good pain relief without detectable facial numbness.[31] Onset of analgesia takes about 1 to 10 days to occur but can be delayed for up to 6 weeks.[31] It provides excellent pain relief while largely sparing trigeminal nerve function in most patients.[32] As many as 72% of patients can be totally free of pain for 3 years, and in one series, 60% remained pain-free for more than 10 years after a single injection.[31] Within the first year, 10% to 53% recur,[32] whereas 25% to 83% recur between 2 and 5 years.[33] These long durations of effect are concordant with the trigeminal ganglion being the target of the treatment. Damaging ganglion cells prevents or impedes regeneration of the peripheral nerve fibers that they subtend.

Glycerol is preferred when pain is localized to the first division as it rarely produces corneal anesthesia, but the overall effectiveness is less than for RF neurotomy.[34] In the elderly or where microvascular decompression is contraindicated, glycerol ganglion lysis is safer, more effective than stereotactic surgery and is more cost-effective.[35] Head-to-head comparisons of effectiveness indicate that glycerol is at least as effective as RF neurotomy,[36] but balloon compression may be slightly more effective than either of these procedures.[37]

Cryoneurotomy

Cryoneurotomy relieves pain by causing a variable degree of nerve injury. Freezing is achieved by a simultaneous reduction in pressure and temperature as expanding carbon dioxide is forced through a specialized probe. An ice ball averaging 3.5 to 5.5 mm in diameter rapidly forms at temperatures as low as

−50° to −70° C. Subzero temperatures cause nonselective but reversible conduction block, and the effect is prolonged when the intracellular contents are crystallized. There is little clinical difference provided that the temperature is maintained below −20° C for 1 minute.[38,39]

Nerve injury is dose dependent and ranges from a mild "neurapraxia" to changes of wallerian degeneration, associated with very minimal inflammatory reaction. Within a few days of freezing, the lesion is seen as a dense cellular matrix of macrophages.[40] In contrast to chemical neurolysis, painful neuromas, neuritis or dysesthesia is avoided as exact regeneration is facilitated by an intact epineurium and perineurium.[38,39] The duration of the block depends on the rate of nerve regeneration at the proximal stump, which averages 1 to 3 mm per day.[38,39] Cryolesioning is a safe, simple, and repeatable procedure: It produces a temporary block, and its therapeutic effect may last for many weeks. The main disadvantage is that the relief of pain is often of short duration and unpredictable.[41]

Cryotherapy has been used by some as an effective adjunct to the pharmacologic management of trigeminal neuralgia when other more invasive treatments are contraindicated. In most patients, the relief of pain is immediate, and in one series, at least 58% remained pain free for 12 months with a mean time to recurrence of 20 months.[42]

For chronic lumbar zygapophysial joint pain, modest outcomes have been noted in two studies. One study claimed a 72% success rate 6 weeks after cryotherapy.[43] The other found that 62% of patients reported at least 50% relief of pain for 12 months, with parallel improvements in activities of daily living.[44]

Cryoneurotomy has been reported as useful for the management of postthoracotomy pain and intercostal neuralgia.[45] In these conditions, the short duration of relief obtained may be enough to render patients comfortable while natural healing occurs or other measures are implemented.

Thermal Radiofrequency

INTRODUCTION

Thermal (continuous) percutaneous RF procedures have now evolved as one of the better and more practical neurosurgical procedures for the management of chronic disabling pain. With modern imaging and the development of sophisticated equipment, precise ablation of neural pathways is possible. When meticulously executed in correctly selected patients, RF neurotomy with temperature monitoring has proven itself to be safer and more effective than any other procedure. The technique required principally depends on the source of nociception and the accessibility of the nerves that innervate it. Critical to its correct application is an understanding and appreciation of its limitations, the pathophysiology of the primary condition, and a valid diagnosis.

PHYSICS

Thermal RF should not be confused with electrocautery. Tissues are not burned or oxidized. Rather, they are coagulated in situ by the application of a high-frequency, alternating electric field.[46] The objective of RF lesioning is to deliver sufficient heating power into biologic tissue such that the tissue temperature is raised above the "lethal temperature" range of 45° to 50° C. Neural cells exposed to these temperatures for 20 seconds or more will be destroyed by heat.[47,48] This requires an RF generator, an insulated electrode with an exposed ("active") tip of 2 to 10 mm, and a ground or dispersive ("passive") plate with a large surface area.[49] The electrode is placed either into (central nervous system) or onto (peripheral nerve) the target structure. The larger dispersive plate is placed at a convenient location of the body remote from the electrode. The patient completes

the electrical circuit, and the generator delivers the alternating current between exposed tip of the insulated electrode and the large dispersive plate.

The passage of low-energy, high-frequency alternating current (100,000 to 500,000 Hz) causes intense oscillation of ions. This oscillation heats charged molecules, notably proteins.[50] The exposed, active tip of the electrode acts as an antenna, around which the current concentrates into a greater density. Consequently, greater heating occurs in the tissues around the electrode, and it is the tissue about the electrode tip, rather than the electrode itself, that becomes the source of heat. The tissues heat the electrode, and a thermocouple, built into the electrode, monitors the temperature generated. Once a certain temperature is reached, lesion formation ("coagulation") occurs.

Tissue temperature (T) is related directly to current density (I) but inversely to the fourth power of the radius (R) from the electrode, that is, $T = IR^{-4}$. Current density is less at the distal tip of the electrode than at its sides. Therefore, the lesion extends little, if at all, in a longitudinal direction from the tip. Rather, it extends radially around the circumference of the exposed shaft and generally assumes the shape of a prolate spheroid (football).[50] However, because the tissue temperature drops rapidly with distance from the electrode, the lesion is limited in size, to 2 mm or less beyond the surface of the electrode (Fig. 102.1).

The physical variables that govern lesion size include current density, its rate of application, lesioning temperature, electrode size, the duration of heating, and impedance.[48,50–52] Temperature is the fundamental lesioning parameter, and temperature monitoring remains central to the safety of the procedure and quantification of lesion size.[53,54] Because there is no consistent relation between temperature and voltage, temperature-controlled RF lesioning is preferred to voltage-controlled lesioning in order to create reproducible and well-defined lesion sizes.[55] The use of lower temperatures may not be acceptable in the clinical setting because it may not produce a permanent or long-term or sufficiently extensive lesion. Above 60° C,[56,57] soft tissues generally will coagulate, and if the surface temperature of the electrode is elevated to 80° to 85° C, then tissues within a short distance from

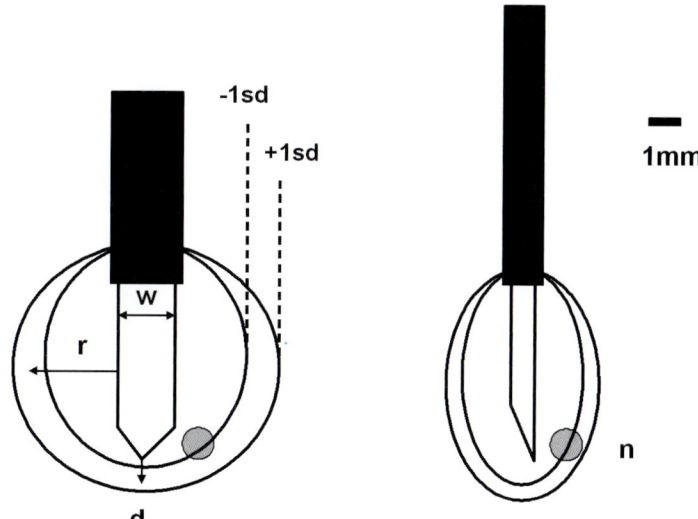

FIGURE 102.1 Longitudinal sections through thermal radiofrequency electrodes, showing the geometry of the lesions that they produce. The lesion has a transverse radius (r) that is proportional to the width (w) of the electrode. Less lesion is produced distally (d). For the same electrode on different occasions, the size of the lesion varies around a mean value in a normal distribution. Smaller electrodes generate smaller lesions. Smaller lesion may fail to incorporate a target nerve (n) completely, even if the electrode is placed close to the nerve.

the surface will be heated to 60° to 65° C or more. Once the electrode surface temperature reaches 80° C, lesion size increases with time as the temperature is maintained. Most of the increase in size occurs within 60 seconds, but an appreciable growth continues between 60 and 90 seconds.[57] After 90 seconds, further growth is prevented because the coagulated tissues present an increasing impedance (resistance) to flow of current and, therefore, the generation of any further lesion.

The lesion should be generated by increasing the temperature by about 1° C per second. This avoids cavitation, steam formation, microexplosions, and charring,[48,50,51] but more critically in the event that the patient experiences adverse sensations, heating can be aborted promptly, before the temperature rises too high and any damage is done.[49]

The size of the lesion is directly proportional to the diameter (width) of the electrode. Because lesions develop from the surface of the electrode, those formed by a larger electrode will reach further away from its center. Lesions made by small-diameter electrodes will extend only a short distance from their surface (see Fig. 102.1). In practice, the radius of a lesion is equal in length to between 1 and 2 times the width of the electrode used. Beyond this range, tissues may escape coagulation.[49,57]

Because electrodes generate lesions radially, they must be placed close and parallel to the target nerve in order for the lesion to be optimally effective.[49,56] If the electrode is placed perpendicular to the nerve, the lesion made may fail to incorporate the target nerve (Fig. 102.2). Throughout the lesioning process, the electrode must be held in place lest it dislodges, and its proper placement should be checked by periodic fluoroscopic monitoring.

PATHOLOGY

Heating by RF causes many cells to die rapidly at temperatures greater than 45° C. Similar effects are produced irrespective of whether the electrode is placed either inside the dorsal root ganglion or onto a peripheral nerve. Above 55° C, there is an indiscriminate destruction of both small and large myelinated fibers, focal necrosis, hemorrhages, extensive edema, and features of wallerian degeneration.[58–63] Even with a low voltage of 0.1 V, an electrode placed inside a dorsal root ganglion and heated to 67° C causes a total loss of myelinated fibers, with hemorrhages.[63]

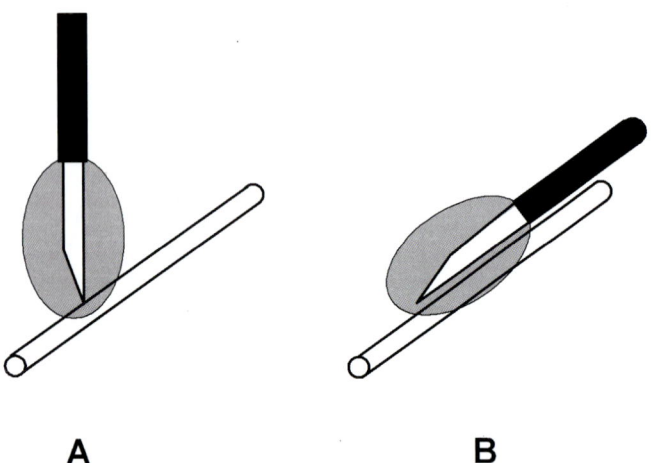

A   **B**

FIGURE 102.2 The influence of orientation on the effects of thermal radiofrequency neurotomy. **A:** If an electrode is placed perpendicular to the target nerve, it may coagulate the nerve only partially and for a short length because of the limited range over which the electrode generates a lesion distally. **B:** If an electrode is placed parallel to a nerve, it incorporates a large volume of the nerve along a greater length.

PHYSIOLOGY

The study by Letcher and Goldring[64] is often misrepresented as showing that RF neurotomy selectively destroys small-diameter fibers while preserving large-diameter fibers. Rather, what the study showed was that depression of C-fiber and Aδ-fiber action potentials preceded depression of the potentials of Aβ fibers, but, within in a short time, all fibers were ultimately and equally affected, and the disappearance of action potentials was independent of fiber size. No class of fiber was exempt from the effects of heat.[64] These findings were confirmed in two independent clinical studies which showed that RF neurotomy of the medial branches of the lumbar dorsal rami resulted in electromyographic abnormalities in over 80% of patients.[65,66] These abnormalities indicated that large-diameter α motor neurons were not spared by RF neurotomy.

APPLICATIONS

In general medicine, thermal RF is widely used for the treatment of supraventricular tachyarrhythmias.[67] Water-cooled electrodes permit the generation of larger lesions to ablate thick ventricular muscle effectively.[68] In pain medicine, thermal RF has been used to treat trigeminal neuralgia, to interrupt pain pathways in the spinal cord or brainstem, and to treat various types of spinal pain and miscellaneous other types of pain.

Trigeminal Neuralgia

For the symptomatic treatment of trigeminal neuralgia, various descriptors, such as RF trigeminal neurolysis, RF thermocoagulation of the gasserian ganglion, or retrogasserian thermorhizotomy, each refer to the generation of thermal lesions in an area between the trigeminal ganglion and its sensory root. Under fluoroscopic guidance, the electrode is introduced via the foramen ovale until the active tip sits at the posterior end of Meckel's cave, the average depth of insertion being 5 to 6 cm. Once the electrode appears to be adequately placed, a test electric stimulus is delivered to the nerve. If the electrode has been accurately placed, test stimulation will evoke pain in the area in which the patient normally experiences pain. Lesioning temperature may range between 55° and 90° C,[33,69,70] and the current may be applied either continuously for up to 300 seconds[69] or in 45- to 90-second cycles.[70]

The evidence of effectiveness for trigeminal RF neurotomy consists of several, large, observational studies, some encompassing over 1,000 patients.[71] In one series, 41% of patients sustained relief for 20 years.[70] However, because of methodologic inconsistencies, a systematic review[72] found only four studies on which sound conclusions could be based.[69,70,73,74] Nevertheless, collectively, these studies reaffirmed the general, favorable impression conveyed by the literature at large. Compared with other, commonly used, ablative techniques, RF neurotomy provided the highest rate of complete pain relief: Some 75% of patients were free of all pain for at least 6 months. At 12 months, RF provided a higher rate of complete pain relief than stereotactic radiosurgery.[72] In a later, unrelated study,[75] 90% of patients reported complete pain relief from their first RF, and a significant proportion continued to enjoy excellent relief some 15 years later. Presumably due to neuronal regeneration, the success rate diminishes and pain returns such that just over 50% remain completely relieved at 5 years[72] with a 14-year recurrence rate of 25% in one series.[75]

Common side effects are sensory loss, sufficient to affect quality of life, in more than 30% of patients; keratitis in some 10%; and dysesthesia in 4% to 10%. Although rare, reported complications include cranial nerve palsies, brainstem injury, meningitis, and vascular fistula formations.[76–79]

Central Ablative Procedures

In conditions where pain is intractable and refractory to most forms of nonsurgical and minimally invasive interventions, relief may be secured by interrupting pathways in the spinal cord.[80] The most common target sites are the dorsal root entry zones, the spinothalamic tract, and trigeminal pathways.

Dorsal Root Entry Zone Lesions

Dorsal root entry zone (DREZ) lesioning is performed for the relief of central (deafferentation) and peripheral (neuropathic) pain caused by disease of peripheral nerves or injuries to them.[80,81] In these conditions, deafferentation results in spontaneous activity in the apical neurons of the dorsal gray column of the segments to which the affected nerves relay.[82] DREZ lesioning involves inserting a small electrode into this region in order to ablate the spontaneously active cells.[81] Multiple lesions are usually required in order to capture all the active neurons. Better outcomes are obtained when the dorsal root and the dorsal horn are primarily affected by the injury and both the pain and the pathology are topographically well defined. Conversely, DREZ lesioning is contraindicated where pain is poorly localized because identifying the level at which the operation should be performed is difficult.[80] The ablative process includes the central portion of the dorsal root, the tract of Lissauer, and layers I to V of the dorsal horn. In this manner, the lateral portion of the dorsal horn, where C fibers predominate, is destroyed. By sparing the medial portion of the dorsal horn, tactile and proprioception senses are preserved.

Better outcomes are obtained if test electrical stimulation is used. Stimulation not only confirms the relevant segments but also identifies additional zones of dorsal horn electrical hyperactivity which would have been missed if topographical landmarks alone are used.[83,84]

Controlled trials have not been performed, but this may be understandable given the nature of the disorder and the nature of the intervention. Advocacy is based on multiple observational studies in which significant proportions of recipients report remarkable relief. DREZ lesioning has been particularly effective for the pain of brachial plexus avulsion with 66% and 87% patients affirming more than 70% relief,[85–94] and an appreciable proportion not requiring supplementary medication.[86] For traumatic spinal cord injuries, percentage relief of pain can range from at least 50% to complete relief with no limitation of activity or the need for opioids,[94–96] but a recent review found the published evidence to be limited.[97] With respect to postamputation pain, the outcomes are better for phantom pain than for stump pain alone.[86] DREZ lesioning has not been particularly effective for postherpetic neuralgia. Some 18% to 47% report complete pain relief, but such relief is not consistently maintained.[85] The close neuroanatomical relationship between the site of DREZ lesioning, the lateral corticospinal tract, and the dorsal column can lead to severe neurologic complications such as motor weakness, bladder or sexual dysfunction, and dysesthesia (see Chapter 107).[98]

Brainstem Procedures

Pain subtended by the nucleus caudalis of the trigeminal nerve can be treated by ablating various sites within the brainstem, such as the descending trigeminal tract (trigeminal tractotomy), the nucleus caudalis (trigeminal nucleotomy), or all of the substantia gelatinosa of the nucleus caudalis (nucleus caudalis dorsal root entry zone, NCDrez). Nociceptive type pain is most sensitive to NCDrez ablation.[85] Indications have included severe glossopharyngeal neuralgia, craniofacial dysesthesia, posttraumatic neuropathy, atypical facial pain, complex craniofacial pain, and anesthesia dolorosa.[94,99–101] For intractable facial pain, such as "end-stage" trigeminal neuralgia that has failed all other means of treatment including microvascular decompression, DREZ lesioning of the nucleus caudalis has been successful in 60% to 70% of cases.[102,103]

Cordotomy

Percutaneous cordotomy can be used to treat unilateral intractable pain transmitted by the lateral spinothalamic tract.[99] A lesion made in the anterolateral segment of the spinal cord totally abolishes pain and temperature in one-half of the body below the lesion.[99] The procedure is typically performed percutaneously at the C1–C2 level, using a lateral approach to insert the electrode. Indications for these procedures have included severe neuropathic pain arising from brachial plexus root avulsion imitating phantom pain, electric burns, postherpetic neuralgia, and cancer pain.[104] In patients with cancer pain, some 70%[105] or more[106,107] initially obtain worthwhile relief. This relief wanes with time but persists in most for the duration of remaining life.

Medial Branch Neurotomy

Medial branch neurotomy is a procedure in which an RF electrode is used to coagulate one or more medial branches of the dorsal rami of the spinal nerves.[108,109] The strictest, taxonomically purest definition of the indication for the procedure is that it is used to treat pain mediated by one or more medial branches. A corollary of this definition is that the indication requires complete relief of pain when the target nerve or nerves is anesthetized using controlled diagnostic blocks (see Chapter 98).

However, the medial branches of the dorsal rami have a restricted distribution. They supply the zygapophysial joints and certain of the posterior spinal muscles. These muscles, however, are innervated in a myotomal fashion such that only those fascicles stemming from a particular spinous process are innervated by the nerve of the same segmental number. There are no known disorders that affect selectively only particular myotomes of the back muscles.[110,111] Therefore, the most likely sources of pain mediated by medial branches are the zygapophysial joints. Consequently, medial branch neurotomy has come to be regarded as a treatment for zygapophysial joint pain. However, stipulating the actual source of pain is immaterial, for the indication for treatment is relief of pain after blocking the nerve or nerves that mediate the pain.

Lumbar Medial Branch Neurotomy

Background. The history of lumbar medial branch neurotomy is replete with misconceptions, errors, and misrepresentations. These apply both to surgical technique and to patient selection.

The original version of the procedure—known as "facet denervation"[112–115]—was based on the concept that coagulating articular nerves would relieve pain from the zygapophysial ("facet") joints. An abundant literature followed, with many studies claiming remarkable success for relieving back pain.[108] However, it was subsequently shown that there were no nerves in the location where electrodes were placed.[116,117] This converted the procedure to a sham.

At the same time, it was shown that the only suitable targets for denervating a zygapophysial joint were the medial branches that supplied the joint.[116,117] Consequently, the procedure was renamed medial branch neurotomy.[117] Furthermore, the practice became to place the electrode perpendicular to the nerve.[118] However, some 7 years later, it was shown that perpendicular placements risked missing the nerve, or capturing it only partially (see Fig. 102.2).[56] The resultant revision was to place the electrode parallel to the nerve in order to capture a maximal thickness of the nerve and a maximal length of it in the lesion created by the electrode.[56]

Studies showed[56,57,119] that large-gauge (16 gauge) electrodes made larger lesions and were more likely to capture the target nerve than would small-gauge (20- to 22-gauge) electrodes. If smaller electrodes were used, they had to be in direct contact with the nerve in order to capture it. Displacements as little as 1 mm could result in failure to capture the nerve.

Furthermore, it became apparent that the exact location of the nerve could vary, by up to a few millimeters.[119] Therefore, a single target point could not be used. Instead, in order to capture the nerve, multiple lesions need to be made across the target zone in which the nerve could lie. The smaller the gauge of the electrode used, the greater the number of lesions that needed to be made in order to fully coagulate the target zone.[108]

Despite the research over 20 years that established these principles, not all surgeons have heeded them. They have developed, used, and continue to use flawed techniques, despite warnings publicizing these flaws.[120,121] Electrodes have been placed in locations where nerves are not located, which renders the procedure a sham. Electrodes have continued to be placed perpendicular to the nerve, which risks coagulating the nerve inadequately and, therefore, lowering the success rate, the degree of relief, and its duration.

A different set of confounding influences pertains to patient selection. They relate to the validity of diagnosis and its subsequent effects on the success of treatment.

The paradigm of medial branch neurotomy is that the patient's pain must be relieved by prior diagnostic blocks.[108] If the pain is not relieved, there is no logic using medial branch neurotomy to treat the pain, for the patient does not have the condition for which the treatment is designed.

The strictest operational criteria for diagnostic medial branch blocks are that the patient's pain must be completely relieved by double-blind controlled blocks and that relief is accompanied by restoration of activities of daily living previously impeded by the pain.[122] Any deviation from these criteria threatens the validity of the blocks.

Single diagnostic blocks are not valid. Not only do single blocks fail to identify the 34% or so of patients who fail to get any relief when a block is repeated,[123] they also have false-positive rates that range between 25% and 45%.[124–129] Depending on the prevalence of the condition, such false-positive rates mean that even if the patient reports complete relief of pain, up to 60% or more of patients will not actually have the condition being tested. In turn, that means that up to 60% of patients will not respond to treatment, except perhaps through a placebo effect.

For diagnosis to be valid, diagnostic blocks must be controlled. Vexatious, however, is the type of control that should be used. That, too, depends on the prevalence of the condition. For common conditions, such as cervical zygapophysial joint pain, lesser controls are adequate. For less common conditions, such as lumbar zygapophysial joint pain, tighter controls are required in order to ensure validity.

For common conditions, comparative local anesthetic blocks are practical.[130,131] They provide a credibility of 75% if agents are fully randomized or 50% if agents are only routinely alternated.[131] For less common conditions, diagnostic confidence plummets such that when the prevalence is only 30% or less, as many as two-thirds of positive responses to comparative blocks will be false.[122,131] For those conditions, placebo-controlled blocks are required for consummate diagnostic accuracy.[130,131]

The degree of relief from a diagnostic block is also critical. Optimally, the relief should be complete. In that regard, nuances apply. In a patient with pain stemming from consecutive zygapophysial joints, a physician might have initiated investigations by anesthetizing the upper of the two levels. In that event, the patient may report complete relief but only in the upper part of his or her region of pain.[122,132] Reciprocally, if the physician anesthetizes the lower of the two joints, the patient may report complete relief but only in the lower region of his or her pain. However, once both sources of pain have been correctly identified, complete relief can be achieved by performing diagnostic blocks simultaneously of both sources of pain. Detailed protocols for these situations are available elsewhere.[122,132]

That situation is different from a patient reporting only, say, 50% relief of all of his or her pain. Without further information, such a response is uninterpretable. A physician cannot tell if the patient is reporting some sort of placebo response; is uncertain of the effect of the block; does not understand the purpose and significance of the block; or has some other, unknown, concurrent source of pain. Although it might be convenient to assume that the patient has a concurrent source of pain, that assumption cannot be held to be true unless and until that other source of pain is identified in a valid manner. However, regardless of the reason, 50% relief pain from a diagnostic block means that, at best, the patient could not expect better than 50% relief following treatment.

Witnessing restoration of activities of daily living is a critical requirement of diagnostic blocks. Relief of pain is a subjective phenomenon, but restoration of activities previously limited by pain renders the response to a block objective[122] For example, seeing a patient being able to move freely without pain serves to confirm the positive response to the block. Not being able to move is incongruous with a positive response to the block.

If these various requirements are not satisfied, the validity of a block is compromised, and poorer outcomes from medial branch neurotomy can be expected. If blocks are not repeated in order to confirm the response, or if controlled blocks are not used, the resultant false-positive responses mean that large proportions of patients will not respond to medial branch neurotomy because they do not have the condition that the treatment is designed to treat or they will have only placebo responses to treatment. If the patient does not get complete relief from a block, they cannot expect complete relief from the treatment. If a block does not restore the patient's activities of daily living, they cannot expect the treatment to do so. These various features have confounded much of the literature concerning the evidence for the effectiveness of medial branch neurotomy.

Technique. The one technique for lumbar medial branch neurotomy that is based on the research literature concerning the anatomical basis for this procedure, and for which there is evidence of effectiveness, is that described by the Practice Guidelines of the International Spine Intervention Society.[108] Details for the conduct of that procedure are provided in those guidelines. Figure 102.3 illustrates the critical features.

The electrode must be inserted so that its tip lies parallel to the target nerve. This requires an insertion from below, along a ventrorostral trajectory (Fig. 102.3A). The electrode must also avoid the mamilloaccessory ligament. Therefore, the trajectory must also be slightly abducted (Fig. 102.3C). The electrode is inserted until its tip enters the target zone for the medial branch, which lies opposite the middle two-quarters of the neck of the superior articular process.[108,119]

Because of idiosyncrasies in anatomy, for the L1–L4 nerves, the target is the medial branch. At L5, the target is actually the L5 dorsal ramus itself. It is the L5 dorsal ramus, rather than the L5 medial branch, that crosses the target zone opposite the middle two-quarters of the neck of the S1 superior articular process.[108,110,119]

Once the electrode has been placed, the tissues surrounding its tip are coagulated by raising the temperature of the electrode to 80° to 85° C for 90 seconds. However, for optimal outcomes, adjustments have to be made to cater for the gauge of the electrode and the length of its exposed tip. A single lesion may not be adequate to ensure capturing the entire nerve. Because the nerve may lie slightly higher or slightly lower on the neck of the superior articular process, lesions may need to be placed high and low in the target zone. This is less of an issue if large-gauge electrodes are used, for such electrodes form large lesions that can encompass the entire height of the target zone, but if smaller electrodes are used, two or three placements may be required

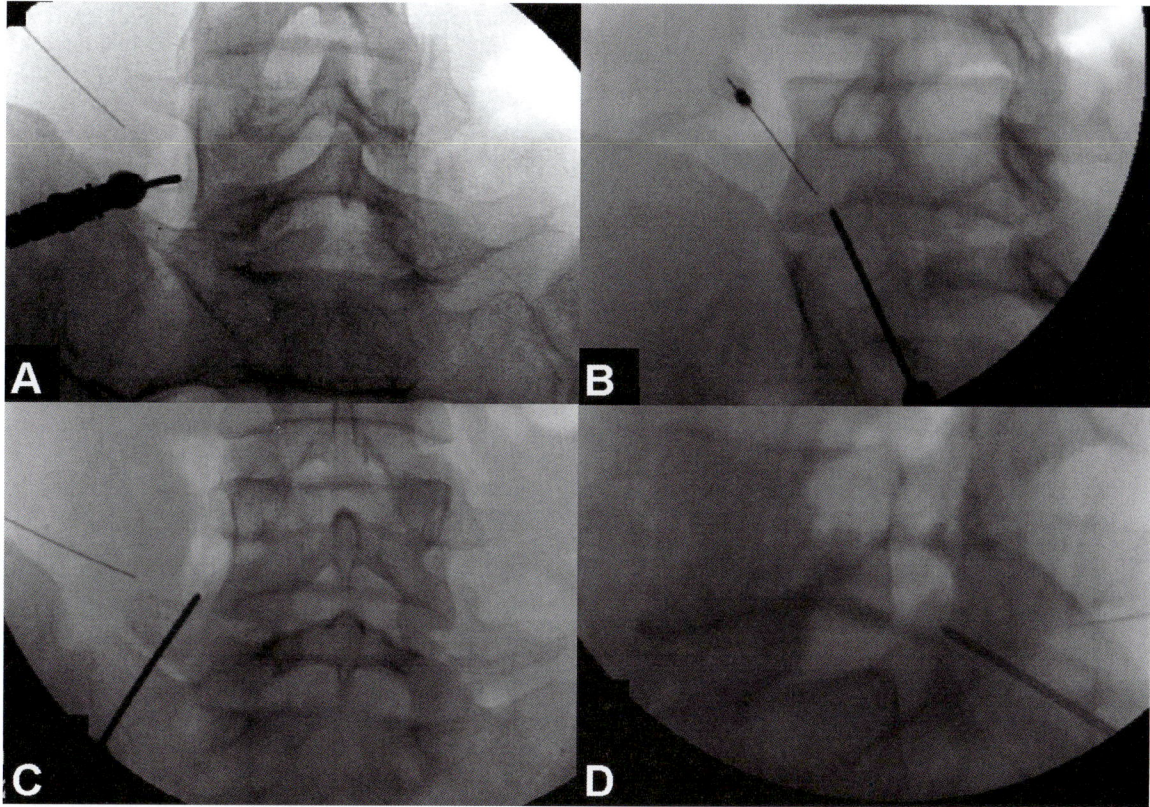

FIGURE 102.3 Fluoroscopy views of an electrode in place for an L4 medial branch radiofrequency neurotomy. **A:** Declined (pillar) view showing the tip of the electrode lodged in the notch between the superior articular process and transverse process of L5. **B:** Oblique view showing the tip of the electrode crossing the junction of the superior articular process and transverse process. **C:** Posteroanterior view showing the electrode orientated obliquely, cephalad and medially, against the lateral surface of the superior articular process. **D:** Lateral view showing the active tip of the electrode lying opposite the middle two-fourths of the neck of the superior articular process.

in order to encompass the entire target zone.[108] If the exposed tip of the electrode is only 5 mm, lesions may need to be made both distally and proximally along any given insertion, in order to capture a maximal length of the nerve.[108] If these precautions are not taken, either the nerve may escape coagulation or be only partially coagulated, either of which consequence compromises the outcome of the treatment.

Effectiveness. The effectiveness of this technique of lumbar medial branch neurotomy was benchmarked by two studies. Both studies selected patients for treatment on the basis of responses to comparative local anesthetic blocks. Both placed large-gauge electrodes parallel to the target nerves, across the target zone for each nerve.

The earlier study selected patients on the basis of greater than 80% relief from pain following each of two diagnostic blocks.[66] Anatomical success in coagulating the target nerves was confirmed by postoperative electromyography of the myotomes of the nerves coagulated. At 12 months after treatment, 80% of patients continued to have at least 60% relief of pain, and 80% had at least 60% relief.

The later study was conducted in two neighboring practices.[133] The data from each practice differed only in that one practice performed treatments over a longer period of survey and performed more repeat treatments when pain recurred. Patients were selected on the basis of complete relief of pain following comparative local anesthetic blocks. Successful outcome was defined as complete relief of pain for at least 6 months, accompanied by restoration of activities of daily living and no need for continuing care for back pain. In the two practices, the initial success rates were 58% (44% to 72%) and

53% (40% to 66%). In the first practice, the median duration of relief from the first treatment was 15 months, with an interquartile range of 10 to 28 months. In the second practice, the corresponding figures were 15 (10 to 29) months. Repeat treatments were performed to reinstate relief if pain recurred after the first treatment. A total of 35 treatments in 29 patients were performed in the first practice, and 66 treatments in 30 patients in the second practice, resulting in a median duration of relief, per treatment, of 13 months, over a 5-year period.

These data established that good outcomes could be achieved if patients were correctly selected using controlled diagnostic blocks and if meticulous surgical technique was used. Moreover, a success rate of over 50% for achieving complete relief of pain, with restoration of activities of daily living and no need for continuing care is unprecedented in the treatment of back pain.

Other studies, including controlled trials, have not matched these outcomes, but nor have they applied the same discipline and rigor, either for selection of patients, for surgical technique, or both. Consequently, none of the other literature constitutes legitimate evidence concerning the effectiveness or efficacy of lumbar medial branch neurotomy as prescribed by the International Spine Intervention Society. Any evidence that other studies provide pertain to other variants of this procedure.

This distinction has been overlooked or ignored by authors of systematic reviews. Any objective appraisal of the evidence requires stratifying the data according patient selection and surgical technique, for variations in those domains seriously compromises the outcomes achieved. Not making the distinctions creates a false impression of the effectiveness of lumbar medial branch neurotomy.

Relying on single blocks to select patients and not using controlled blocks does not provide a valid diagnosis. The high false-positive rates of single blocks means that the study sample will be contaminated by patients who are unlikely to have the condition that lumbar medial branch neurotomy is designed to treat. Indeed, it has been shown that success rates are significantly lower in patients selected by single blocks, than in those selected by controlled blocks.[134] This flaw does not compromise the outcomes on those patients who do have the condition, but it reduces the power of the study, particularly if it is a controlled trial. Genuine responses to treatment will be swamped and obscured by patients with no response or placebo responses.

Using less-than-complete relief of pain as a selection criterion compromises the validity of diagnosis and the outcomes achieved by treatment. A criterion of 50% relief means that no patient can be expected to achieve the benchmark standard of complete relief of pain. Nor can they be expected to restore activities of daily living or cease health care, which are also the benchmark standards for lumbar medial branch neurotomy. For statistical purposes, this may or may not be a fatal problem in controlled trials. The trial could still show that a greater proportion of patients achieved 50% relief after active treatment, but such an outcome would be of questionable value if it does not reduce the burden of illness, that is, the patients still have a complaint that requires continuing treatment.

Placing the electrode perpendicular to the target nerve incurs the risk of not coagulating the nerve adequately. In turn, this risks reducing the success rate for achieving complete relief of pain or reducing the duration of relief. Likewise, creating a single lesion at a single target site, rather than coagulating an entire target zone, risks inadequate coagulation of the target nerve. The same applies to using small-gauge electrodes. In both instances, both the success rate and the duration of relief can be compromised.

A fatal flaw applies to techniques in which the electrode is placed at locations remote from any known nerve or insufficiently close to the target nerve to capture it. Such techniques, by definition, constitute a sham procedure. Neurotomy cannot be a genuine procedure if no nerve is coagulated.

Throughout the literature, outcomes inferior to those of the benchmark studies can be traced to one or more of these flaws. In some instances, the flaws disqualify the study from providing any evidence. In others, certain conclusions can be drawn but not others.

In two explanatory controlled trials, electrodes for active treatment were placed remote from any target nerve.[135,136] These studies constitute comparing one sham with another. The authors of one of these studies later acknowledge this flaw.[137]

Perpendicular placement of electrodes is characteristic of studies emanating from The Netherlands or influenced by them. The earliest of these studies described but did not illustrate the technique used,[138] so it is not exactly clear where the electrode was placed. Nevertheless, sham treatment was rigorously compared with active treatment. The success rate of active treatment was low, ostensibly because single blocks were used to select patients or because a single lesion was made perpendicular to the target nerve, using a small electrode. Consequently, it was difficult to show statistically significant difference by a simple comparison of success rates. However, survival analysis clearly showed that success over time was significantly greater after active treatment.[138]

Another explanatory study from The Netherlands found no significant difference in favor of active treatment.[139] However, small-gauge electrodes were used; single lesions were made, perpendicular to the target nerve; and the illustration of the technique showed that electrodes were not placed sufficiently near to the target nerve.[121] The authors acknowledged these limitations but explained that they tested how RF neurotomy was performed in their community, that is, The Netherlands.[140] Therefore, the conclusions from this study cannot be generalized to other techniques of lumbar medial branch neurotomy; they expressly apply only to how it is practiced in The Netherlands.

A second explanatory study from The Netherlands found no attributable effect from active RF neurotomy compared with sham.[141] However, patients were selected on the basis of a decrease in pain of only 2/10 following a single diagnostic block, small-gauge electrodes were placed perpendicular to the target nerve, and only a single lesion was made at each site.

A more recent study from The Netherlands reported that adding neurotomy to conservative treatment did not improve outcomes.[142] However, patients were selected by single blocks, and although the surgical technique used was not illustrated, the authors—when challenged[143-145]—responded that they studied how neurotomy was practiced in The Netherlands.[146] Therefore, although their conclusion might apply to practice in The Netherlands, they do not apply to other techniques of lumbar medial branch neurotomy.

One controlled study used correct surgical technique but selected patients by single blocks only.[147] Consequently, the data do not lack validity but are compromised by less than optimal success rates. Even so, the study showed that lumbar medial branch neurotomy was significantly more often effective than a credible sham comparator.

Two studies selected patients by comparative local anesthetic blocks, and each used correct surgical technique. The first was an observational study.[148] Patients were selected if they reported at least 70% relief of pain following comparative medial branch blocks. Of 174 patients reviewed over a 10-year period, 35% (29% to 41%) of patients had at least 50% relief of pain, and a further 22% (16% to 28%) had 80% relief of pain, at 6 months after treatment. The proportions of patients with enduring relief decreased between 6 months and 2 years after treatment, but the median duration of relief was 12 months. A later, placebo-controlled trial[149] showed that patients reported significantly greater relief of back pain after active treatment, but this study was compromised because patients had other complaints of pain, such as radicular pain. Consequently, a success rate for complete elimination of pain could not be determined.

No controlled trial has shown that the results of lumbar medial branch neurotomy—when performed correctly—are attributable to placebo. Yet, a small number of controlled trials, with limitations, have shown that the outcomes of lumbar medial branch neurotomy cannot be attributed to placebo. Those controlled trials that claim no benefit beyond that of placebo are all compromised by suboptimal selection of patients and discredited surgical technique.

Cervical Medial Branch Neurotomy

Background. The principles of surgical precision that beset lumbar medial branch neurotomy were established before cervical medial branch neurotomy was extensively used. Therefore, its literature is less affected by errors and misrepresentations. Nonetheless, some problems still apply.

In strictest terms, cervical medial branch neurotomy is used to treat pain mediated by one or more of the medial branches of the cervical dorsal rami.[109] In practical terms, it is used to treat cervical zygapophysial joint pain. At typical cervical levels, each zygapophysial joint is supplied by the two medial branches with the same segmental numbers as the joint.[111] The C2–C3 joint is supplied by one nerve: the third occipital nerve, which is the superficial medial branch of the C3 dorsal ramus.[111]

The singular indication for cervical medial branch neurotomy is complete relief of pain when one or more medial branches is anesthetized by controlled diagnostic blocks.[109,132]

Typically, this means both of the nerves that innervate a particular zygapophysial joint or the third occipital nerve when the C2–C3 joint is the source of pain.

Technique. A particular idiosyncrasy that affects cervical medial branch neurotomy is that cervical medial branches follow a curved path around the waist of the cervical articular pillars. Therefore, in order to capture fully a long length of the target nerve, electrodes have to be placed along each of two paths: a sagittal path to capture the nerve on the lateral aspect of the articular pillar and an oblique path to capture it on the anterolateral aspect.[111,132,150]

The one technique that has been based on original anatomical and laboratory research is that promoted in the Practice Guidelines of the International Spine Intervention Society.[109] It is also the only technique that has been validated in clinical studies and trials. The Practice Guidelines describe in detail how cervical medial branch neurotomy should be performed.[109] Figure 102.4 illustrates the key features.

In order to reach the proximal end of the target nerve, the electrode is inserted along a 30-degree oblique path so that its tip lies against the anterolateral aspect of the articular pillar (see Figs. 102.3A and 102.3B). That portion of the nerve is coagulated by raising the temperature around the tip of the electrode to 80°C for 90s. In order to reach the next section of the nerve, the electrode is inserted along a sagittal path so that its tip lies tangential to the lateral aspect of the articular pillar (see Figs. 102.3C and 102.3D).

For nerves at different segmental levels the target zone differs.[57,109] At the C4 and C5 levels, the target zone lies opposite the central half of the articular pillar. At higher and lower segmental levels, the target zones lie progressively higher on the pillar.

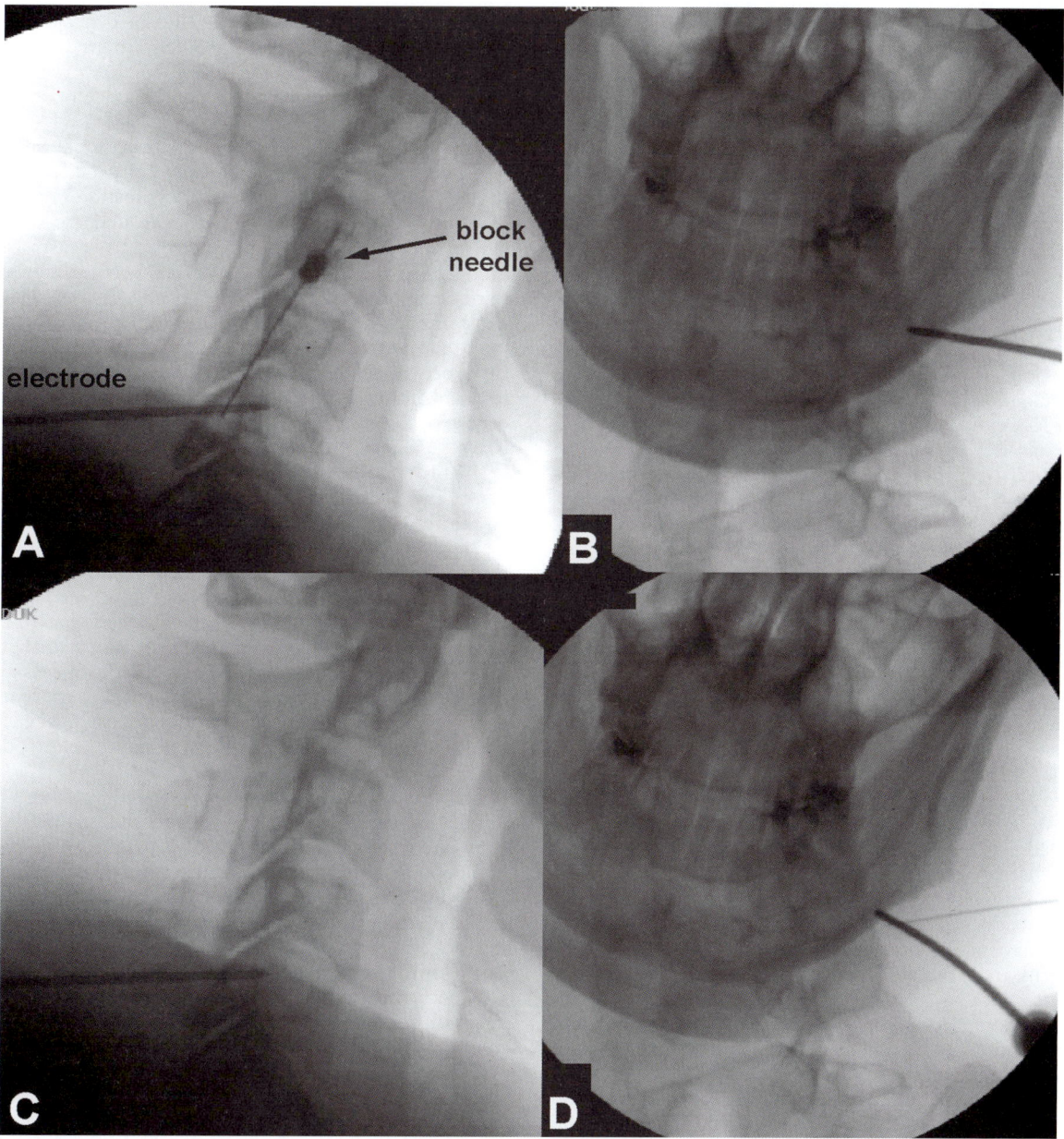

FIGURE 102.4 Fluoroscopy view of electrode placements in the execution of a C5 medial branch radiofrequency (RF) neurotomy. **A:** Lateral view of an oblique insertion. The tip of the electrode lies over the anterolateral surface of the C5 articular pillar. (A block needle remains in place over the target area, in case supplementary local anesthesia is required.) **B:** Posteroanterior view of an oblique insertion. The tip of the electrode lies just medial to lateral margin of the silhouette of the C5 articular pillar. **C:** Lateral view of a sagittal insertion. The tip of the electrode lies over the lateral surface of the C5 articular pillar. **D:** Posteroanterior view of a sagittal insertion. The tip of the electrode lies tangential to the lateral surface of the C5 articular pillar.

Efficacy. This technique was developed initially on the basis of anatomical studies[111] but subsequently refined in the light of pilot clinical studies.[150] Once perfected, it was rapidly subjected to a placebo-controlled trial.[151] That trial showed that active treatment was significantly more effective than sham treatment both in terms of success rate and duration of relief. In that study, and in those that followed, the definition of success was complete relief of pain, accompanied by restoration of activities of daily living and no need for other health care.

Subsequent studies performed long-term follow-up of the patients treated in the placebo-controlled trial and patients treated after the trial.[152] Other studies corroborated the outcomes and provided additional details.[153,154]

Complete relief of pain is achieved in some 70% of patients treated.[150-154] Errors in diagnosis account for the failures. Some patients have false-positive responses to diagnostic blocks, even when these are controlled. In other patients, neurotomy unmasks latent or previously undiagnosed sources of pain, for example, at adjacent segmental levels.

The pooled data indicate that about 60% of patients maintain complete relief of pain at 6 months, and between 30% and 50% do so at 12 months.[155] Success rates are not demonstrably different between patients with legal claims and those without.[151-154] Recurrence of pain is to be expected because the treated nerves regenerate, but repeat neurotomy reinstates relief. Repetition has been reported to reinstate relief up to seven times, with the average duration of relief ranging between 8 and 18 months per repetition.[57,152-154]

Complete relief of pain is accompanied by restoration of activities of daily living and no need for other health care.[57,154,155] These outcomes occur only if the technique recommended by the International Spine Intervention Society[109] is used and only if the selection criteria are complete relief of pain following controlled diagnostic blocks of the medial branches to be targeted.[155] If lesser diagnostic criteria are used, success rates and the degree of relief are substantially lower.[156,157]

Conspicuously, RF medial branch neurotomy is the only treatment that has been shown to provide complete relief of chronic neck pain, with restoration of activities of daily living and no other need for health care.[57,151,155] Moreover, it also resolves psychological distress immediately upon relieving pain[158,159] and reduces central sensitization and hyperalgesia.[160] No other treatment for chronic neck pain has been shown to have these properties. A Cochrane review found that the evidence for cervical RF neurotomy was limited, but only in the sense that there have not been more controlled trials; there was no dispute concerning the quality of the published studies.[161] An independent review reported that RF neurotomy sets a benchmark for the treatment of chronic neck pain.[162]

The rare side effects of cervical medial branch neurotomy include vasovagal syncope, dermoid cyst, Koebner phenomenon, and so-called neuritis: ostensibly, irritation of one of the target nerves.[57,163] More common side effects are numbness or dysesthesia in the cutaneous territory of one of the target nerves.[57,163] These have been self-limiting and not requiring treatment. None is permanent because the target nerve regenerates.

Skin burns are avoided by using a firmly applied dispersive/ground plate with a large surface area rather than a spinal needle to dissipate electrical energy. Meticulous technique and strict asepsis should guard against infection and hematoma formation. Neurologic complications are avoided by ensuring that electrodes always remain external to the vertebral column and do not reach either the vertebral artery or the intervertebral foramen.[109]

Concerns that denervating a zygapophysial joint could cause Charcot joints[164,165] are unfounded. There are no published reports of Charcot arthropathy directly attributable to RF neurotomy. Modern pathophysiology implicates a neurovascular mechanism, and diabetes has replaced tertiary syphilis as the most common cause of Charcot arthropathy,[166] and arthropathy can occur in advance of abnormal neurology.[167,168] Charcot joints classically occur in weight-bearing joints of the lower limb in which all the surrounding muscles are insensate, resulting in instability.[169] This does not occur with spinal RF neurotomy. The medial branches innervate only the deep paramedian muscles. The superficial and lateral muscles are spared. Thus, the spinal motion segment is not rendered insensate. Meanwhile, the disk and articular processes maintain stability passively.

Catastrophic, spinal cord injuries have occurred only when electrodes have been egregiously misplaced.[170] They are avoided by careful placement of electrodes into the correct target zone and monitoring their location during the generation of lesions.

Third Occipital Neurotomy

RF third occipital neurotomy is a companion procedure to conventional cervical medial branch neurotomy. Its distinction is that the target nerve is the third occipital nerve (see Fig. 102.4), and the pain problem treated is cervicogenic headache. The singular indication for the procedure is complete relief of headache after controlled blocks of the third occipital nerve.[171]

The Practice Guidelines of the International Spine Intervention Society describe in detail how third occipital neurotomy should be performed.[109] Figure 102.5 illustrates the key features.

The third occipital nerve wraps around the waist or lower half of the C2–C3 zygapophysial joint.[111] It furnishes articular branches to the joint from its deep aspect. The location of the third occipital nerve is quite variable but in a predictable area.[57] Most often, it lies along the equator of the C2–C3 zygapophysial joint, but it can also lie low on the joint, toward the waist of the C3 articular pillar. Consequently, there is no single target point for neurotomy. Rather, a target zone has to be coagulated, in order to accommodate variations in the exact location of the nerve.[109]

In order to reach the proximal end of the third occipital nerve, the electrode is inserted along a 30-degree oblique path so that its tip tucks across the ventrolateral aspect of the joint (see Fig. 102.5). To reach the more distal segment of the nerve, the electrode is inserted along a sagittal path so that its tip rests tangential to the lateral aspect of the joint (see Fig. 102.5).

Along each path, the tip of the electrode has to be adjusted into two or more, higher or lower locations so that the entire target zone is coagulated. Fewer such adjustments are required if large-gauge (16G) electrodes are used, but more lesions need to be made if small-gauge electrodes are used. At each location, the target zone is coagulated by holding the electrode temperature at 80 to 85°C for 90 seconds.[109]

This intervention has not been subjected to a placebo-controlled trial because it is not possible to mask the procedure. Active treatment produces a patch of anesthesia in the cutaneous territory of the third occipital nerve. However, the procedure has been benchmarked by an observational study.

That study showed that when patients were selected on the basis of complete relief of headache following controlled blocks of the third occipital nerve and when third occipital neurotomy was performed according to prescribed standards,[109] complete relief of headache was achieved in 88% of patients, for a median duration of some 297 days.[172] That relief was associated with restoration of activities of daily living and no need for other health care. Such results have been corroborated by other studies,[152-154] which included patients with cervicogenic headache but did not focus explicitly on them. For patients in whom headaches recur, relief can be reinstated by repeating the neurotomy. By repeating neurotomy as required, some patients have been able to maintain relief of their headache for longer than 2 years,[172] for up to 5 years,[154] and beyond.[152]

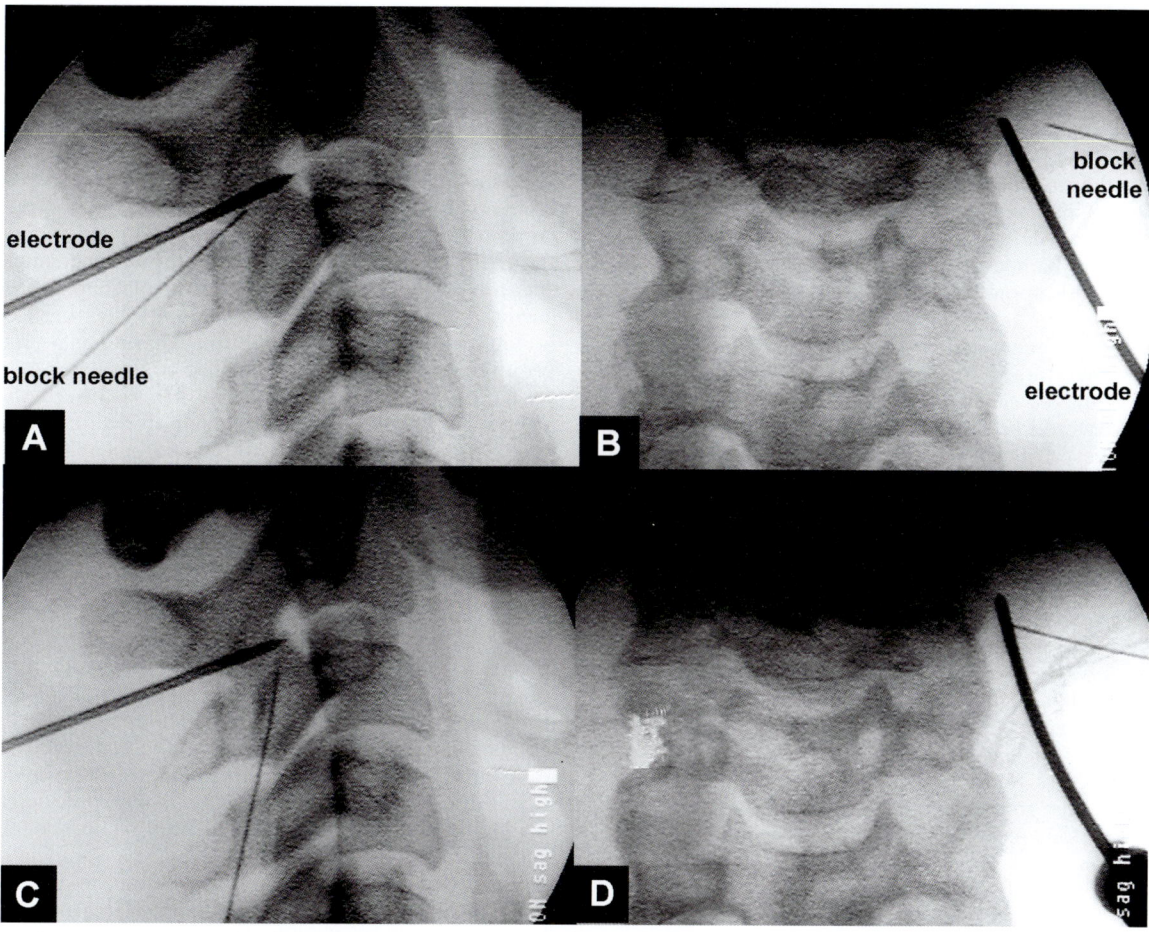

FIGURE 102.5 Fluoroscopy views of electrode placement for third occipital radiofrequency neurotomy. **A:** Lateral view of oblique insertion of electrode. The electrode tip lies over the anterolateral aspect of the C2–C3 zygapophysial joint. The electrode lies in the higher of two positions required to encompass the third occipital nerve thoroughly. (A block needle overlies the target zone in case supplementary anesthesia is required.) **B:** Posteroanterior view of an oblique insertion. The tip of the electrode lies medial to the lateral margin of the silhouette of the C2–C3 zygapophysial joint. **C:** Lateral view of a sagittal insertion. The tip of the electrode lies over the lateral aspect of the C2–C3 zygapophysial joint. The electrode lies in the highest of three positions required to encompass the third occipital nerve thoroughly. **D:** Posteroanterior view of a sagittal insertion. The electrode lies tangential to the C2–C3 zygapophysial joint.

Others who have purported to study cervicogenic headache in controlled trials have not matched these benchmarks,[173–175] but in those studies,

- Patients were selected simply on the basis of clinical criteria.
- Nerves were indiscriminately targeted, without having been subjected previously to controlled blocks.
- None of the surgical techniques has ever been validated anatomically or clinically.

So, there was no evidence in these controlled trials that any of the patients had third occipital headache and no evidence that the technique used could successfully and thoroughly coagulate the third occipital nerve. Consequently, these controlled trials do not contribute any evidence concerning the efficacy or effectiveness of third occipital neurotomy when performed correctly.

Third occipital neurotomy is associated with distinctive side effects: notably numbness, ataxia, and dysesthesia.[172] Numbness is to be expected because the third occipital nerve has a cutaneous distribution that is larger and more constant than that of typical cervical medial branches. Touch-evoked hypersensitivity and dysesthesia typically resolve spontaneously, usually within a fortnight, but may last up to 6 weeks. The third occipital nerve also innervates the semispinalis capitis and contributes substantially to cervical proprioception and tonic neck reflexes. Therefore, neurotomy is commonly associated with a mild ataxia. Generally, this ataxia is not disabling, for

patients can rely on visual cues to locate horizontal objects and thereby stabilize the orientation of their head. No long-term effects have been reported.

Because of possible problems with ataxia, presumptive bilateral neurotomy is not recommended in patients with bilateral third occipital headache. If bilateral neurotomy is indicated, it is recommended that one side be treated first and the other side be tested with a prognostic block to test that subsequent neurotomy on this side does not produce disabling ataxia.[171]

Sacral Lateral Branch Neurotomy

Sacral lateral branch neurotomy is a procedure devised for the treatment of sacroiliac pain. It involves coagulating the lateral branches of the S1–S3 dorsal rami where they emerge from their dorsal sacral foramina.

A variety of methods have been used to coagulate these nerves, ranging from conventional, monopolar electrodes to bipolar electrodes, cooled electrodes, and special multipronged electrodes. None has emerged as the preferred method, and outcomes have been less than impressive. Moreover, the indications for the procedure have not been rigorous.

The most unambiguous indication for lateral branch neurotomy would be complete relief of pain from controlled, diagnostic blocks of the sacral lateral branches, but no one has followed this paradigm. Instead, a variety of other indications have been used.

One indication has been a positive response to intra-articular blocks of the sacroiliac joint, in the belief that lateral branch neurotomy should be a treatment for sacroiliac joint pain. Indeed, a recent Appropriate Use Criteria listed relief from intra-articular blocks as a prime indication for lateral branch neurotomy.[176] However, this belief is inconsistent with the available evidence.[177] Anesthetizing the lateral branches does not protect normal volunteers from experimental pain from the sacroiliac joint.[178] Consequently, lateral branch neurotomy cannot be a logical treatment for sacroiliac joint pain, and positive sacroiliac joint blocks cannot be a logical indication for lateral branch neurotomy.

Anesthetizing the lateral branches protects normal volunteers from experimental pain from the posterior sacroiliac ligaments.[178] Therefore, a logical indication for lateral branch neurotomy would be sacroiliac ligament pain, for which the diagnostic test would be controlled blocks of the sacral lateral branches. However, in that regard, several problems arise.

No one has systematically determined the prevalence of sacroiliac ligament pain. So, we do not know if this is a common or a rare condition. No one has determined if the condition occurs in isolation or concurrently with sacroiliac joint pain. The previously conventional technique, using single-site blocks, has been shown to be flawed, in that it often fails to capture the target nerves.[179] More accurate is a multisite, multidepth technique,[178] but no one has applied this technique to determine the prevalence of sacroiliac ligament pain. In principle, single blocks—by any technique—would be liable to false-positive responses, but no one has reported using controlled diagnostic blocks of the sacral lateral branches, and the false-positive rate is not known, either for single blocks or controlled blocks.

For these various reasons, sacral lateral branch neurotomy lacks a firm foundation. Although a rationale for lateral branch neurotomy can be formulated, data consistent with this rationale are few.

Most studies selected patients on the ill-founded basis of positive responses to one or two intra-articular blocks.[180–188] For achieving at least 50% relief of pain, they variously reported success rates of 50% to 80% at 2 or 3 months, reducing to 30% to 60% at 6 and 9 months.

One study selected patients on the basis of an initial intra-articular block, supplemented by a single lateral branch block.[189] It reported 50% of patients having at least 50% relief at 9 months.

The only study that used lateral branch blocks alone, selected patients who had at least 75% relief from each of two blocks that were not in any way controlled.[190] At 6 months after lateral branch neurotomy, 27% of patients had greater than 50% relief of pain, and 18% reported being totally free of pain. At 9 months, these figures were 52% and 15%. The proportion of patients who achieved good outcomes at 1 month was nearly six times greater than that of patients who underwent sham therapy, but the small sample size prevented demonstrating an absolute statistically significant difference.

Although the development of sacral lateral branch neurotomy was inspired by the success of cervical and lumbar medial branch neurotomy, the outcomes of lateral branch neurotomy have not mirrored those achieved by medial branch neurotomy. Most studies have reported only the achievement of 50% relief of pain. No evidence has appeared that such an outcome is sufficient to reduce the burden of illness.

The one study that most closely adhered to the rationale for lateral branch neurotomy[191] achieved complete relief of pain in only 18% of patients. The reason for this low yield is not known. There may be limitations to surgical technique, or it may be that 75% relief from diagnostic blocks is not a sufficiently rigorous selection criterion. For medial branch neurotomy, the best outcomes have been achieved after complete relief of pain following controlled diagnostic blocks.

Discussion

The published evidence shows that of all the neurolytic procedures, thermal RF neurotomy is the most widely successful in terms of the diversity of pain problems for which it can be used, its success rate for achieving complete or near-complete relief of pain, and the duration of effect than can be achieved, either from a single application or by repeating the treatment in order to reinstate relief.

The effectiveness of RF neurotomy for trigeminal neuralgia has not been questioned despite no placebo-controlled trials having been conducted. Its success rate has been consistently so high, and its effects so enduring, that it has been exempt the requirement for placebo-controlled trials.

RF medial branch neurotomy has also been shown to be successful. Of all treatments for any form of spinal pain, it is the only one that has been shown to be capable of achieving complete relief of pain accompanied by restoration of function and eliminating the need for other health care. In that regard, it is the only treatment for spinal pain that has been shown to reduce the burden of illness.

However, RF medial branch neurotomy is not a treatment for nonspecific spinal pain. It is applicable only for pain mediated by one or more medial branches of the dorsal rami. For the treatment of that condition, the diagnosis must be rigorously established using controlled diagnostic blocks, and the treatment must be performed meticulously. Only under those conditions can optimal outcomes be achieved.

Unfortunately, both in the published literature and in practice, these conditions are not always met. Taking shortcuts in diagnosis, and imprecision of surgical technique, decrease the success rate and effectiveness of medial branch neurotomy, which gives the procedure a poor reputation. These problems, however, are an indictment of how the treatment is practiced but not an indictment of its effectiveness.

References

1. Stedman TL. *Stedman's Medical Dictionary*. 27th ed. Philadelphia: Lippincott Williams & Wilkins; 2000.
2. Stoll G, Jander S, Myers RR. Degeneration and regeneration of the peripheral nervous system: from Augustus Waller's observations to neuroinflammation. *J Peripheral Nervous System* 2002;7:13–27.
3. Ramer MS, Priestley JV, McMahon SB. Functional regeneration of sensory axon into the adult spinal cord. *Nature* 2000;403:312–316.
4. Chen ZL, Yu WM, Strickland S. Peripheral regeneration. *Annu Rev Neurosci* 2007;30:209–233.
5. Iggo A, Walsh EG. Selective block of small fibers in the spinal roots by phenol. *Brain* 1960;83:701–708.
6. Wood KM. The use of phenol as a neurolytic agent: a review. *Pain* 1978;5:205–229.
7. Nathan PW, Sears TA, Smith MC. Effect of phenol solution on the nerve roots of the cat: an electrophysiological and histological study. *J Neuro Science* 1965;2:7–29.
8. Gregg RV, Costantini MD, Douglas JF, et al. Electrophysiologic investigation of alcohol as a neurolytic agent. *Anesthesiology* 1985;63:A250.
9. Taylor JJ, Woolsey RM. Dilute ethyl alcohol: effect on the sciatic nerve of the mouse. *Arch Phy Med Rehabil* 1976;57:233–237.
10. Woolsey RM, Taylor JJ, Nagel JH. Acute effects of topical ethyl alcohol on the sciatic nerve of the mouse. *Arch Phy Med Rehabil* 1972;53:410–414.
11. Burchiel KJ, Russell LC. Glycerol neurolysis: neurophysiologic effects of topical glycerol application in a rat saphenous nerve. *J Neurosurg* 1985;63:784–788.
12. Lunsford LD. Percutaneous retrogasserian glycerol rhizotomy. In Rovit RL, Muralie R, Jannetta PJ, eds. *Trigeminal Neuralgia*. Baltimore, MD: Williams & Wilkins; 1990:145–164.
13. Noble M, Gress FG. Techniques and results of neurolysis for chronic pancreatitis and pancreatic cancer pain. *Curr Gastroenterol Rep* 2006;8:99–103.
14. Eisenberg E, Carr DB, Chalmers TC. Neurolytic celiac plexus block for treatment of cancer pain: a meta-analysis. *Anesth Analg* 1995;80:290–295.
15. Kaufman M, Singh G, Das S, et al. Efficacy of endoscopic ultrasound-guided celiac plexus block and celiac plexus neurolysis for managing abdominal pain associated with chronic pancreatitis and pancreatic cancer. *J Clin Gastroenterol* 2010;44:127–134.
16. Puli SR, Reddy JB, Bechtold ML, et al. EUS-guided celiac plexus neurolysis for pain due to chronic pancreatitis or pancreatic cancer pain: a meta-analysis and systematic review. *Dig Dis Sci* 2009;54:2330–2337.

17. Lo SK. Endoscopic palliation of pancreatic cancer. *Gastroenterol Clin N Am* 2012;41:237–253.

18. Yan BM, Myers RP. Neurolytic celiac plexus block for pain control in unresectable pancreatic cancer. *Am J Gastroenterol* 2007;102:430–438.

19. Johnson CD, Berry DP, Harris S, et al. An open randomized comparison of clinical effectiveness of protocol-driven opioid analgesia, celiac plexus block or thoracoscopic splanchnicectomy for pain management in patients with pancreatic and other abdominal malignancies. *Pancreatology* 2009;9:755–756.

20. Arcidiacono PG, Calori G, Carrara S, et al. Celiac plexus block for pancreatic cancer pain in adults. *Cochrane Database Syst Rev* 2011;(3):CD007519. doi:10.1002/14651858.CD007519.pub2.

21. Bhutani MS, Pasricha PJ. Neurolytic approaches for the treatment of pain in patients with chronic pancreatitis. *Curr Treat Options Gastroenterol* 2003;6:375–379.

22. Löfstrom B, Zetterquist S. Lumbar sympathetic blocks in the treatment of patients with obliterative arterial disease of the lower limb. *Int Anesthesiol Clin* 1969;7:423–438.

23. Cousins MJ, Reeve TS, Glynn CJ, et al. Neurolytic lumbar sympathetic blockade: duration of denervation and relief of rest pain. *Anaesth Intensive Care* 1979;7:121–135.

24. Mashiah A, Soroker D, Pasik S, et al. Phenol lumbar sympathetic block in diabetic lower limb ischemia. *J Cardiovasc Risk* 1995;2:467–469.

25. Cross FW, Cotton LT. Chemical lumbar sympathectomy for ischemic rest pain. A randomized prospective controlled clinical trial. *Am J Surg* 1985;150:341–345.

26. Candido K, Stevens RA. Intrathecal neurolytic blocks for the relief of cancer pain. *Best Pract Res Clin Anaesthesiol* 2003;17:407–428.

27. Ischia S, Luzzani A, Ischia A, et al. Subarachnoid neurolytic block (L5-S1) and unilateral percutaneous cervical cordotomy in the treatment of pain secondary to pelvic malignant disease. *Pain* 1984;20:139–149.

28. Straube S, Derry S, Moore RA, et al. Cervico-thoracic or lumbar sympathectomy for neuropathic pain and complex regional pain syndrome. *Cochrane Database Syst Rev* 2013;(9):CD002918. doi:10.1002/14651858.CD002918.pub3.

29. Harden RN, Oaklander AL, Burton AW, et al. Complex regional pain syndrome: practical diagnostic and treatment guidelines, 4th edition. *Pain Medicine* 2013;14:180–229.

30. Silver HR. Lumbar percutaneous facet rhizotomy. *Spine* 1990;15:36–40.

31. Liu JK, Apfelbaum RI. Treatment of trigeminal neuralgia. *Neurosurg Clin N Am* 2004;15:319–334.

32. Peters G, Nurmikko TJ. Peripheral and gasserian ganglion-level procedures for the treatment of trigeminal neuralgia. *Clin J Pain* 2002;18:28–34.

33. Brown JA. Percutaneous techniques: part IV trigeminal neuralgia. In: Winn HR, ed. *Youmans Neurological Surgery.* 5th ed. New York: Saunders; 2004:2996–3004.

34. Molet J. Neurosurgical treatment of facial neuralgias and neuropathic pain of the face. *Pain Rev* 1999;6:35–51.

35. Pollock B, Ecker R. A prospective cost-effectiveness study of trigeminal neuralgia surgery. *Clin J Pain* 2005;21:317–322.

36. Udupi BP, Chouhan RS, Dash HH, et al. Comparative evaluation of percutaneous retrogasserian glycerol rhizolysis and radiofrequency thermocoagulation techniques in the management of trigeminal neuralgia. *Neurosurgery* 2012;70:407–412.

37. Noorani I, Sparrow O, Vajramani G. Comparing percutaneous treatments of trigeminal neuralgia with long-term outcomes. *Neurosurgery* 2016;63(suppl 1):175–176.

38. Evans P, Lloyd J, Green C. Cryoanalgesia. The response to alterations in the freeze cycle temperature. *Br J Anaesthesia* 1981;53:1121–1127.

39. Lloyd J, Barnard J, Glynn C. Cryoanalgesia: a new approach to pain relief. *Lancet* 1976;2:932–934.

40. Collins GH, West NR, Parmely JD, et al. The histopathology of freezing injury to the rat spinal cord. A light microscope. I. Early degenerative changes. *J Neuropathol Exp Neurol* 1986;45:721–741.

41. Evans PJ. Cryoanalgesia. *Anaesthesia* 1981;36:1003–1013.

42. Zakrzewska JM, Nally FF. The role of cryotherapy (cryoanalgesia) in the management of paroxysmal trigeminal neuralgia: a six-year experience. *Brit J Oral Maxillofacial Surg* 1988;26:18–25.

43. Barlocher CB, Krauss JK, Seiler RW. Kryorhizotomy: an alternative technique for lumbar medial branch rhizotomy in lumbar facet syndrome. *J Neurosurg* 2003;98:14–20.

44. Birkenmaier C, Veihelmann A, Trouillier H, et al. *Int Orthop* 2007;31:525–530.

45. Wang JK. Cryoanalgesia for painful peripheral nerve lesions. *Pain* 1985;22:191–193.

46. Committee on Man and Radiation. Medical aspects of radiofrequency radiation overexposure. *Health Phys* 2002;82:387–391.

47. Foster KR. Thermal and non-thermal mechanisms of interaction of radiofrequency energy with biological systems. *IEEE Trans Plasma Sci* 2000;28:15–23.

48. Cosman ER, Blaine S, Nashold MD, et al. Theoretical aspects of radiofrequency lesions in the dorsal root entry zone. *Neurosurgery* 1984;15:945–950.

49. International Spine Intervention Society. Principles of thermal radiofrequency neurotomy. In: Bogduk N, ed. *Practice Guidelines for Spinal Diagnostic and Treatment Procedures.* 2nd ed. San Francisco, CA: International Spine Intervention Society; 2013:15–25.

50. Organ LW. Electrophysiological principles of radiofrequency lesion making. *App Neurophysiol* 1976;39:69–76.

51. Alberts WW, Wright EW, Feinstein B, et al. Experimental radiofrequency brain lesion size as a function of physical parameters. *J Neurosurgery* 1966;25:421–423.

52. Cosman ER, Ritman WJ, Nashold BS, et al. Radiofrequency generation and its effects on tissue impedance. *App Neurophysiol* 1988;51:230–242.

53. Haines DE, Watson DD. Tissue heating during radiofrequency catheter ablation: a thermodynamic model and observations in isolated perfused and superfused canine right ventricular free wall. *Pacing Clin Electrophysiol* 1989;12:962–976.

54. Jain MK, Wolf PD. Temperature-controlled and constant power radiofrequency ablation: what affects lesion growth? *IEEE Trans Biomed Eng* 1999;46:1405–1412.

55. Buijs EJ, Roelof MA, van Wijk AW, et al. Radiofrequency lumbar facet denervation: a comparative study of the reproducibility of lesion size after 2 current radiofrequency techniques. *Reg Anesth Pain Med* 2004;29:400–407.

56. Bogduk N, Macintosh J, Marsland A. Technical limitations to the efficacy of radiofrequency neurotomy for spinal pain. *Neurosurgery* 1987;20:529–535.

57. Lord SM, McDonald GJ, Bogduk N. Percutaneous radiofrequency neurotomy of the cervical medial branches: a validated treatment for cervical zygapophysial joint pain. *Neurosurgery* 1998;8:288–308.

58. Hamann W, Hall S. Acute effect and recovery of primary afferent nerve fibres after graded radiofrequency lesions in anaesthetized rats. *Br J Anaesthesia* 1992;68:443P.

59. Zervas NT, Kuwayama A. Pathological characteristics of experimental thermal lesions. Comparison of induction heating and radiofrequency electrocoagulation. *J Neurosurg* 1972;37:418–422.

60. Kanpolat Y, Onol B. Experimental percutaneous approach to the trigeminal ganglion in dogs with histopathological evaluation of radiofrequency lesions. *Acta Neurochirurgica Suppl* 1980;30:363–366.

61. Podhajsky RJ, Sckiguchi Y, Kikuchi S, et al. The histologic effects of pulsed and continuous radiofrequency lesions at 42°C to rat dorsal root ganglion and sciatic nerve. *Spine* 2005;30:1008–1013.

62. Smith HP, Whorter JM, Challa VR. Radiofrequency neurolysis in a clinical mode: neuropathological correlation. *J Neurosurg* 1981;55:246–253.

63. de Louw AJ, Vles HS, Freling G, et al. The morphological effects of a radiofrequency lesion adjacent to the dorsal root ganglion (RF-DRG)—an experimental study in the goat. *Eur J Pain* 2001;5(2):169–174.

64. Letcher FS, Goldring S. The effect of radiofrequency current and heat on peripheral nerve action potential in the cat. *J Neurosurg Sci* 1968;29:42–47.

65. Oudenhoven RC. Paraspinal electromyography following facet rhizotomy. *Spine* 1977;2:299–304.

66. Dreyfuss P, Halbrook B, Pauza K, et al. Efficacy and validity of radiofrequency neurotomy for chronic lumbar zygapophysial joint pain. *Spine* 2000;25:1270–1277.

67. Kuck KH, Akhtar M. New horizons for electrical therapy in managing ventricular and supraventricular tachyarrhythmias [editorial]. *Pacing Clin Electrophysiol* 1993;16:505–506.

68. Ruffy R, Imran MA, Sanrel DJ, et al. Radiofrequency delivery through a cooled catheter allows the creation of larger endomyocardial lesions in the ovine heart. *J Cardiovasc Electrophysiol* 1995;6:1089–1096.

69. Zakrzewska JM, Jassim S, Bulman JS. A prospective longitudinal study on patient with trigeminal neuralgia who underwent radiofrequency theromocoagulation of the Gasserian ganglion. *Pain* 1999;79:51–58.

70. Kanpolat Y, Savas A, Bekar A, et al. Percutaneous controlled radiofrequency trigeminal rhizotomy for the treatment of idiopathic trigeminal neuralgia: a 25 year experience with 1600 patients. *Neurosurg* 2001;48:524–534.

71. Wilkins RH. Trigeminal neuralgia: historical overview, with emphasis on surgical treatment. In: Burchiel K, ed. *Surgical Management of Pain.* New York: Thieme Medical; 2002:288–303.

72. Lopez BC, Hamlyn PJ, Zakrzewska JM. Systematic review of ablative neurosurgical techniques for the treatment of trigeminal neuralgia. *Neurosurgery* 2004;54:973–982.

73. Latchaw JP, Hardy RW, Forsythe SB, et al. Trigeminal neuralgia treated by radiofrequency coagulation. *J Neurosurg* 1983;59:479–484.

74. Oturai AB, Jensen K, Eriksen J, et al. Neurosurgery for trigeminal neuralgia: comparison of alcohol block, neurectomy, and radiofrequency coagulation. *Clin J Pain* 1996;12:311–315.

75. Taha JM, Tew J, Buncher CR. A prospective 15-year follow-up of 154 consecutive patients with trigeminal neuralgia treated by percutaneous stereotactic radiofrequency thermal rhizotomy. *Neurosurg Focus* 2005;18:1–5.

76. Harrigan M, Chandler WF. Abducens nerve palsy after radiofrequency rhizolysis for trigeminal neuralgia: case report. *Neurosurgery* 1998;43:623–625.

77. Berk C, Honey CR. Brain stem injury after radiofrequency trigeminal rhizotomy. *Acta Neurochirurgica* 2004;146:635–636.

78. Torroba L, Moreno S, Lorenzana L, et al. Purulent meningitis after percutaneous radiofrequency trigeminal rhizotomy. *J Neurol Neurosurg Psychiatry* 1987;50:1081–1082.

79. Kaplan M, Erol FS, Ozveren MF, et al. Review of complications due to foramen ovale puncture. *J Clin Neurosci* 2007;14:563–568.

80. Romanelli P, Ersposito V, Adler J. Ablative procedures for chronic pain. *Neurosurg Clin N Am* 2004;15:335–342.

81. Nashold JRB, Nashold BS Jr, Pearlstein RD. The DREZ operation for the relief of deafferentation pain. In: Kaye AH, Black PM, eds. *Operative Neurosurgery*. London: Churchill Livingstone; 2000:1521–1537.

82. Guenot M, Bullier J, Sindou M. Clinical and electrophysiological expression of deafferentation pain alleviated by dorsal root entry zone lesion in rats. *J Neurosurg* 2002;97:1402–1409.

83. Falci S, Best L, Bayles R, et al. Dorsal root entry zone micro-coagulation for spinal cord injury-related central pain: operative intramedullary electrophysiological guidance and clinical outcome. *J Neurosurg* 2002;97:193–200.

84. Tomas R, Haninec P. Dorsal root entry zone (DREZ) localization using direct spinal cord stimulation can improve results of the DREZ thermocoagulation procedure for intractable pain relief. *Pain* 2005;116:159–163.

85. Gorecki JP. Dorsal root entry zone and brainstem ablative procedures. In Winn HR, ed. *Youmans Neurological Surgery*. 5th ed. New York: Saunders; 2004:3045–3058.

86. Sindou MP, Mertens P. Surgery in the dorsal root entry zone for pain. *Semin Neurosurg* 2004;15:221–232.

87. Sindou MP, Blondet E, Emery E, et al. Microsurgical lesioning in the dorsal root entry zone for pain due to brachial plexus avulsion: a prospective series of 55 patients. *J Neurosurg* 2005;102:1018–1028.

88. Blumenkopf B. Neuropharmacology of the dorsal root entry zone. *Neurosurgery* 1984;15:900–903.

89. Parry CB. Pain in avulsion of brachial plexus. *Neurosurg* 1984;15:960–965.

90. Ruiz-Juretschke F, García-Salazar F, García-Leal R, et al. Treatment of neuropathic deafferentation pain using DREZ lesions; long-term results. *Neurologia* 2011;26:26–31.

91. Zheng Z, Hu Y, Tao W, et al. Dorsal root entry zone lesions for phantom limb pain with brachial plexus avulsion: a study of pain and phantom limb sensation. *Stereotact Funct Neurosurg* 2009;87:249–255.

92. Takai K, Taniguchi M. Modified dorsal root entry zone lesioning for intractable pain relief in patients with root avulsion injury. *J Neurosurg Spine* 2017;27:178–184.

93. Haninec P, Kaiser R, Mencl L, et al. Usefulness of screening tools in the evaluation of long-term effectiveness of DREZ lesioning in the treatment of neuropathic pain after brachial plexus injury. *BMC Neurol* 2014;14:225.

94. Chivukula S, Tempel ZJ, Chen CJ, et al. Spinal and nucleus caudalis dorsal root entry zone lesioning for chronic pain: efficacy and outcomes. *World Neurosurg* 2015;84:494–504.

95. Sindou MP. Microsurgical DREZotomy. In: Schmidek HH, Sweet WH, eds. *Operative Neurosurgical Techniques*. 3rd ed. Philadelphia: Saunders; 1995:1585–1594.

96. Denkers M, Biagi H, O'Brieb A, et al. Dorsal root entry zone lesioning used to treat central neuropathic pain with traumatic spinals cord injury: a systematic review. *Spine* 2002;27:E177–E184.

97. Mehta S, Orenczuk K, McIntyre A, et al; and SCIRE Research Team. Neuropathic pain post spinal cord injury part 2: systematic review of dorsal root entry zone procedure. *Top Spinal Cord Inj Rehabil* 2013;19:78–86.

98. Sampson JH, Cashman RE, Nashold BS Jr, et al. Dorsal root entry zone lesions for intractable pain after trauma to the conus medullaris and cauda equina. *J Neurosurg* 1995;82:28–34.

99. Kanpolat Y. The surgical treatment of chronic pain: destructive therapies in the spinal cord. *Neurosurg Clin N Am* 2004;15:307–317.

100. Sharma M, Shaw A, Deogaonkar M. Surgical options for complex craniofacial pain. *Neurosurg Clin N Am* 2014;25:763–775.

101. Rahimpour S, Lad SP. Surgical options for atypical facial pain syndromes. *Neurosurg Clin N Am* 2016;27:365–370.

102. Bullard DE, Nashold BS Jr. The caudalis DREZ for facial pain. *Stereotact Funct Neurosurg* 1997;68:168–174.

103. Bernard EJ Jr, Nashold BS Jr, Caputi F, et al. Nucleus caudalis DREZ lesions for facial pain. *Br J Neurosurg* 1987;1:81–91.

104. Kanpolat Y. Cordotomy for pain. In: Winn HR, ed. *Youmans Neurological Surgery*. 5th ed. New York: Saunders; 2004:3059–3071.

105. Sanders M, Zuurmond W. Safety of unilateral and bilateral percutaneous cervical cordotomy in 80 terminally ill cancer patients. *J Clin Oncol* 1995;13:1509–1512.

106. Crul BJ, Blok LM, van Egmond J, et al. The present role of percutaneous cervical cordotomy for the treatment of cancer pain. *J Headache Pain* 2005;6:24–29.

107. Ischia S, Luzzani A, Ischia A, et al. Role of unilateral percutaneous cervical cordotomy in the treatment of neoplastic vertebral pain. *Pain* 1984;19:123–131.

108. International Spine Intervention Society. Lumbar medial branch thermal radiofrequency neurotomy. In: Bogduk N, ed. *Practice Guidelines for Spinal Diagnostic and Treatment Procedures*. 2nd ed. San Francisco, CA: International Spine Intervention Society; 2013:489–522.

109. International Spine Intervention Society. Cervical medial branch thermal radiofrequency neurotomy. In: Bogduk N, ed. *Practice Guidelines for Spinal Diagnostic and Treatment Procedures*. 2nd ed. San Francisco, CA: International Spine Intervention Society; 2013:133–176.

110. Bogduk N, Wilson AS, Tynan W. The human lumbar dorsal rami. *J Anat* 1982;134:383–397.

111. Bogduk N. The clinical anatomy of the cervical dorsal rami. *Spine* 1982;7:319–330.

112. Shealy CN. Facets in back and sciatic pain. *Minn Med* 1974;57:199–203.

113. Shealy CN. The role of the spinal facets in back and sciatic pain. *Headache* 1974;14:101–104.

114. Shealy CN. Percutaneous radiofrequency denervation of spinal facets. *J Neurosurg* 1975;43:448–451.

115. Shealy CN. Facet denervation in the management of back sciatic pain. *Clin Orthop* 1976;115:157–164.

116. Bogduk N, Long DM. The anatomy of the so-called 'articular nerves' and their relationship to facet denervation in the treatment of low back pain. *J Neurosurg* 1979;51:172–177.

117. Bogduk N, Long DM. Percutaneous lumbar medial branch neurotomy. A modification of facet denervation. *Spine* 1980;5:193–200.

118. Bogduk N. Lumbar dorsal ramus syndrome. *Med J Aust* 1980;2:537–541.

119. Lau P, Mercer S, Govind J, et al. The surgical anatomy of lumbar medial branch neurotomy. *Pain Med* 2004;5:289–298.

120. Bogduk N, Dreyfuss P, Govind J. A narrative review of lumbar medial branch neurotomy for the treatment of back pain. *Pain Med* 2009;10:1035–1045.

121. Bogduk N. Lumbar radiofrequency neurotomy. *Clin J Pain* 2006;22:409.

122. International Spine Intervention Society. Lumbar medial branch blocks. In: Bogduk N, ed. *Practice Guidelines for Spinal Diagnostic and Treatment Procedures*. 2nd ed. San Francisco, CA: International Spine Intervention Society; 2013:457–488.

123. Lord SM, Barnsley L, Bogduk N. The utility of comparative local anaesthetic blocks versus placebo-controlled blocks for the diagnosis of cervical zygapophysial joint pain. *Clin J Pain* 1995;11:208–213.

124. Barnsley L, Lord S, Wallis B, et al. False-positive rates of cervical zygapophysial joint blocks. *Clin J Pain* 1993;9:124–130.

125. Schwarzer AC, Aprill CN, Derby R, et al. The false-positive rate of uncontrolled diagnostic blocks of the lumbar zygapophysial joints. *Pain* 1994;58:195–200.

126. Manchikanti L, Pampati V, Fellows B, et al. Prevalence of lumbar facet joint pain in chronic low back pain. *Pain Phys* 1999;2:59–64.

127. Manchikanti L, Pampati V, Fellows B, et al. The diagnostic validity and therapeutic value of lumbar facet joint nerve blocks with or without adjuvant agents. *Curr Rev Pain* 2000;4:337–344.

128. Manchikanti L, Boswell MV, Singh V, et al. Prevalence of facet joint pain in chronic spinal pain of cervical, thoracic, and lumbar regions. *BMC Musculoskelet Disord* 2004;5:15.

129. Manchukonda R, Manchikanti KN, Cash KA, et al. Facet joint pain in chronic spinal pain: an evaluation of prevalence and false-positive rate of diagnostic blocks. *J Spinal Disord Tech* 2007;20:539–545.

130. Bogduk N. On the rational use of diagnostic blocks for spinal pain. *Neurosurgery* 2009;19:88–100.

131. Engel AJ, Bogduk N. Mathematical validation and credibility of diagnostic blocks for spinal pain. *Pain Med* 2016;17:1821–1828.

132. International Spine Intervention Society. Cervical medial branch blocks. In: Bogduk N, ed. *Practice Guidelines for Spinal Diagnostic and Treatment Procedures*. 2nd ed. San Francisco, CA: International Spine Intervention Society; 2013:85–113.

133. MacVicar J, Borowczyk JM, MacVicar AM, et al. Lumbar medial branch radiofrequency neurotomy in New Zealand. *Pain Med* 2013;14:639–645.

134. Cohen SP, Williams KA, Kurihara C, et al. Multicenter, randomized, comparative cost-effectiveness study comparing 0, 1, and 2 diagnostic medial branch (facet joint nerve) block treatment paradigms before lumbar facet radiofrequency denervation. *Anesthesiology* 2010;113:395–405.

135. Gallagher J, Petriccione di Valdo PL, Wedley JR, et al. Radiofrequency facet joint denervation in the treatment of low back pain: a prospective controlled double-blind study to assess its efficacy. *Pain Clin* 1994;7:193–198.

136. Leclaire R, Fortin L, Lambert R, et al. Radiofrequency facet joint denervation in the treatment of low back pain: a placebo-controlled clinical trial to assess efficacy. *Spine* 2001;26:1411–1416.

137. Dreyfuss P, Baker R, Leclaire R, et al. Radiofrequency facet joint denervation in the treatment of low back pain: a placebo-controlled clinical trial to assess efficacy. *Spine* 2002;27:556–557.

138. van Kleef M, Barendse GA, Kessels A, et al. Randomized trial of radiofrequency lumbar facet denervation for chronic low back pain. *Spine* 1999;24:1937–1942.

139. van Wijk RM, Geurts JW, Wynne HJ, et al. Radiofrequency denervation of lumbar facet joints in the treatment of chronic low back pain. A randomized, double-blind sham lesion-controlled trial. *Clin J Pain* 2004;21:335–344.

140. van Wijk RM, Geurts JW, Groen GJ. Comments on efficacy of radiofrequency facet denervation procedures. *Pain Med* 2012;13:843–845.

141. van Tilburg CW, Stronks DL, Groeneweg JG, et al. Randomised sham-controlled double-blind multicentre clinical trial to ascertain the effect of percutaneous radiofrequency treatment for lumbar facet joint pain. *Bone Joint J* 2016;98-B:1526–1533.

142. Juch JNS, Maas ET, Ostelo RWJG, et al. Effect of radiofrequency denervation on pain intensity among patients with chronic lowback pain the Mint randomized clinical trials. *JAMA* 2017;318:68–81.

143. Vorobeychik Y, Stojanovic MP, McCormick ZL. Radiofrequency denervation for chronic low back pain. *JAMA* 2017;318:2254–2255.

144. Rimmalapudi V, Buchalter J, Calodney A. Radiofrequency denervation for chronic low back pain. *JAMA* 2017;318:2255–2256.

145. Ming-Chih Kao MC, Leong MS, Mackey S. Radiofrequency denervation for chronic low back pain. *JAMA* 2017;318:2256.

146. Maas E, Juch J, Huygen F. Radiofrequency denervation for chronic low back pain. *JAMA* 2017;318:2256–2257.

147. Tekin I, Mirzai H, Ok G, et al. A comparison of conventional and pulsed radiofrequency denervation in the treatment of chronic facet joint pain. *Clin J Pain* 2007;23:235–249.

148. Gofeld M, Jitendra J, Faclier G. Radiofrequency denervation of the lumbar zygapophysial joints: 10-year prospective audit. *Pain Phys* 2007;10:291–300.

149. Nath S, Nath CA, Pettersson K. Percutaneous lumbar zygapophysial (facet) joint neurotomy using radiofrequency current, in the management of chronic low back pain: a randomized double-blind trial. *Spine* 2008;33:1291–1297.

150. Lord SM, Barnsley L, Bogduk N. Percutaneous radiofrequency neurotomy in the treatment of cervical zygapophysial joint pain: a caution. *Neurosurgery* 1995;36:732–739.

151. Lord SM, Barnsley L, Wallis B, et al. Percutaneous radiofrequency neurotomy for chronic cervical zygapophysial joint pain. *N Engl J Med* 1996; 335:1721–1726.

152. McDonald G, Lord SM, Bogduk N. Long-term follow-up of patients treated with cervical radiofrequency neurotomy for chronic neck pain. *Neurosurgery* 1999;45:61–68.

153. Barnsley L. Percutaneous radiofrequency neurotomy for chronic neck pain: outcomes in a series of consecutive patients. *Pain Med* 2005;6:282–286.

154. MacVicar J, Borowczyk J, MacVicar AM, et al. Cervical medial branch radiofrequency neurotomy in New Zealand. *Pain Med* 2012;13:647–654.

155. Engel A, Rappard G, King W, et al; for Standards Division of the International Spine Intervention Society. The effectiveness and risks of fluoroscopically-guided cervical medial branch thermal radiofrequency neurotomy: a systematic review with comprehensive analysis of the published data. *Pain Med* 2016;17:658–669.

156. Royal M, Wienecke G, Movva V, et al. Retrospective study of efficacy of radiofrequency neurolysis for facet arthropathy. *Pain Med* 2001;2:249.

157. Shin WR, Kim HI, Shin DG, et al. Radiofrequency neurotomy of cervical medial branches for chronic cervicobrachialgia. *J Korean Med Sci* 2006;21:119–125.

158. Wallis BJ, Lord SM, Bogduk N. Resolution of psychological distress of whiplash patients following treatment by radiofrequency neurotomy: a randomised, double-blind, placebo-controlled trial. *Pain* 1997;73:15–22.

159. Smith AD, Jull G, Schneider G, et al. Cervical radiofrequency neurotomy reduces psychological features in individuals with chronic whiplash symptoms. *Pain Phys* 2014;17:265–274.

160. Smith AD, Jull G, Schneider G, et al. Cervical radiofrequency neurotomy reduces central hyperexcitability and improves neck movement in individuals with chronic whiplash. *Pain Med* 2014;15:128–141.

161. Niemisto L, Kalso EA, Malmivaara A, et al. Radiofrequency denervation for neck and back pain. *Cochrane Database Syst Rev* 2003;(1):CD004058. doi:10.1002/14651858.CD004058.

162. Basset K, Sibley LM, Anton H, et al. Percutaneous radio-frequency neurotomy treatment of chronic cervical pain following whiplash injury: reviewing evidence and needs. Vancouver, Canada: University of British Columbia, British Columbia Office of Health Technology Assessment; 2001.

163. Lord SM, McDonald GJ, Bogduk N. Side effects and complications of cervical percutaneous radiofrequency neurotomy-an audit of 83 procedures [abstract]. *Anaesth Intensive Care* 1998;26:322–328.

164. Merrill DG. Hoffman's glasses: evidence-based medicine and the search for quality in the literature of interventional pain medicine. *Reg Anesth Pain Med* 2003;28:547–560.

165. Drinka PJ, Jaschob K. Treatment of chronic cervical zygapophysial joint pain [letter]. *N Engl J Med* 1997;336:1530.

166. Hutton CW. Osteoarthritis. In: Weatherall DJ, Wedingham JGG, Warrell DA, eds. *Oxford Textbook of Medicine*. 3rd ed. New York: Oxford University Press; 1996:2979.

167. Norman A, Robins H, Milgram JE. The acute neuropathic arthropathy-a rapid severely disorganising form of arthritis. *Radiology* 1968;90:1159–1164.

168. Kate I, Rabinowitz JG, Dziadiw B. Early changes in Charcot's joints. *AJR* 1961;86:965–974.

169. Lord SM, Bogduk N. Treatment of chronic zygapophysial joint pain (letter). *N Engl J Med* 1997;336:1531.

170. Bogduk N, Dreyfuss P, Baker R, et al. Complications of spinal diagnostic and treatment procedures. *Pain Med* 2008;9:S11–S34.

171. International Spine Intervention Society. Third occipital nerve blocks. In: Bogduk N, ed. *Practice Guidelines for Spinal Diagnostic and Treatment Procedures*. 2nd ed. San Francisco, CA: International Spine Intervention Society; 2013:141–163.

172. Govind J, King W, Bailey B, et al. Radiofrequency neurotomy for the treatment of third occipital headache. *J Neurol Neurosurg Psychiat* 2003; 74:88–93.

173. Haspeslagh SR, van Suijlekom HA, Lame IE, et al. Randomised controlled trial of cervical radiofrequency lesions as a treatment for cervicogenic headache. *BMC Anesthesiol* 2006;6:1.

174. Stovner LJ, Kolstad F, Helde G. Radiofrequency denervation of facet joints C2-C6 in cervicogenic headache: a randomised, double-blind, sham-controlled study. *Cephalalgia* 2004;24:821–830.

175. van Suijlekom HA, van Kleef M, Barendse GAM, et al. Radiofrequency cervical zygapophyseal joint neurotomy for cervicogenic headaches: a prospective study of 15 patients. *Funct Neurol* 1998;13:297–303.

176. MacVicar J, Kreiner DS, Duszynski B, et al. Appropriate use criteria for fluoroscopically guided diagnostic and therapeutic sacroiliac interventions: results from the spine intervention society convened multispecialty collaborative. *Pain Med* 2017;18:2081–2095.

177. Bogduk N. A commentary on appropriate use criteria for sacroiliac pain. *Pain Med* 2017;18:2055–2057.

178. Dreyfuss P, Henning T, Malladi N, et al. The ability of multi-site, multi-depth sacral lateral branch blocks to anesthetize the sacroiliac joint complex. *Pain Med* 2009;10:679–688.

179. Dreyfuss P, Snyder BD, Park K, et al. The ability of single site, single depth sacral lateral branch blocks to anesthetize the sacroiliac joint complex. *Pain Med* 2008;9:844–850.

180. Buijs EJ, Kamphuis ET, Groen GJ. Radiofrequency treatment of sacroiliac joint-related pain aimed at the first three sacral dorsal rami: a minimal approach. *Pain Clin* 2004;16:139–147.

181. Jung JH, Kim UI, Shin DA, et al. Usefulness of pain distribution pattern assessment in decision-making for the patients with lumbar zygapophyseal and sacroiliac joint arthropathy. *J Korean Med Sci* 2007;22: 1048–1054.

182. Speldewinde GC. Outcomes of percutaneous zygapophysial and sacroiliac joint neurotomy in a community setting. *Pain Med* 2001;12:209–218.

183. Stelzer W, Aiglesberger M, Stelzer D, et al. Use of cooled radiofrequency lateral branch neurotomy for the treatment of sacroiliac joint-mediated low back pain: a large case series. *Pain Med* 2013;14:29–35.

184. Kapural L, Nageeb F, Kapural M, et al. Cooled radiofrequency (RF) system for the treatment of chronic pain from sacroiliitis: the first case-series. *Pain Pract* 2008;8:348–354.

185. Karaman H, Kavak GO, Tüfek A, et al. Cooled radiofrequency application for treatment of sacroiliac joint pain. *Acta Neurochir* 2011;153: 1461–1468.

186. Cheng J, Pope JE, Dalton JE, et al. Comparative outcomes of cooled versus traditional radiofrequency ablation of the lateral branches for sacroiliac joint pain. *Clin J Pain* 2013;29:132–137.

187. Cohen SP, Hurley RW, Buckenmaier CC, et al. Randomized placebo-controlled study evaluating lateral branch radiofrequency denervation for sacroiliac joint pain. *Anesthesiology* 2008;109:279–288.

188. Burnham RS, Yasui Y. An alternate method of radiofrequency neurotomy of the sacroiliac joint: a pilot study of the effect on pain, function, and satisfaction. *Reg Anesth Pain Med* 2007;32:12–19.

189. Cohen SP, Abdi S. Lateral branch blocks as a treatment for sacroiliac joint pain: a pilot study. *Reg Anesth Pain Med* 2003;28:113–119.

190. Cohen SP, Strassels SA, Kurihara C, et al. Outcome predictors for sacroiliac joint (lateral branch) radiofrequency denervation. *Reg Anesth Pain Med* 2009;34:206–214.

191. Patel N, Gross A, Brown L, et al. A randomized, placebo-controlled study to assess the efficacy of lateral branch neurotomy for chronic sacroiliac joint pain. *Pain Med* 2012;13:383–398.

CHAPTER 103

Surgery of the Peripheral Nervous System as a Treatment for Pain

JAMES MICHAEL MOSSNER and PARAG G. PATIL

In this chapter, we consider ablative and decompressive surgical approaches to pain that target the peripheral nervous system. Ablative procedures interrupt signal flow between pain generators in the periphery and brain. For example, cutting a peripheral nerve may prevent transmission of pain-encoding signals from an injured region to the spinal cord. By contrast, nonablative procedures may relieve pain due to compression of nerves by adjacent connective tissue.

There are five major categories of pain surgery involving the peripheral nervous system: peripheral neurectomy, nerve entrapment release, dorsal rhizotomy and ganglionectomy, sympathectomy, and neurostimulation. The treatment of trigeminal neuralgia, one of the most prevalent pain diseases successfully treated with surgery, is presented in Chapter 104. Ablative procedures aimed at the spinal cord, such as the dorsal root entry zone operation for brachial plexus avulsion or cordotomy for cancer pain, are presented in Chapter 105. Neurostimulation procedures, including dorsal column stimulation, nerve root stimulation, and peripheral nerve/field stimulation, are presented in Chapter 96.

There are two fundamental approaches to control intractable pain: attempts to palliate symptoms and attempts to eliminate pain definitively. Pharmacologic, psychological, physiotherapeutic, neuromodulation, and neurointerventional approaches each attempt to reduce the severity of pain symptoms. Surgical approaches have great appeal for their potential to eliminate pain altogether. In fact, nerve decompressions are among the most common peripheral nerve surgeries. By contrast, ablative procedures such as neurectomy and ganglionectomy are notorious for achieving only short-term benefits, a reputation that undermines their appeal. In support of such skepticism, animal research suggests that axotomy alone may be sufficient to induce pain.[1] However, regardless of the perception that inappropriate patient selection may lead to considerable morbidity, the experience of some clinicians remains that ablative procedures have the capacity to relieve pain enduringly and that ablative procedures are useful therapeutic ventures in properly selected patients.

Peripheral Neurectomy

BASIC CONSIDERATIONS

There are two reasons that a nerve may be cut to eliminate pain. One reason is to denervate a peripheral pain-producing structure to treat nociceptive pain. For example, facet rhizotomy denervates the facet joint as a treatment for axial spine pain. A second reason to cut a nerve is to remove an abnormal focus of nerve injury (e.g., excision of a neuroma). In this case, there is some irony in the use of neurectomy to treat pain, as transection of a somatic nerve may have been the original cause of the pain. To understand how neurectomy may relieve pain, we must consider some aspects of the pathophysiology of neuropathic pain.

Pathophysiology of Neuropathic Pain

When sensory nerve fibers are severed, the proximal axons remain in continuity with cell bodies in the dorsal root ganglion. These axons sprout and seek Schwann-cell guides. Schwann cells are believed to upregulate expression of neurotrophic factors, which induce axonal growth.[2-5] If the perineurium of the injured nerve has remained intact, as in the case of crush or certain thermal injuries, the sprouts may successfully reinnervate the target tissue. Successful regeneration may also occur when the transected ends of the nerve are surgically reapproximated (neurorrhaphy). However, when Schwann-cell guides are not present, the axon sprouts are unable to reach the target tissue and randomly double back on themselves. This disordered process of growth ultimately results in a densely packed cluster of nerve sprouts known as a *neuroma*.

Weir Mitchell[6] brought attention to the problem of painful nerve injury after caring for wounded soldiers during the American Civil War. A century later, Denny-Brown and Kirk[2] presented one of the first studies demonstrating that axotomy can induce behavioral signs of pain in an animal model. More recent studies have suggested that axotomy of a major nerve, by itself, may induce hyperalgesia in animals. Although nontraumatic neuropathies may induce pain in diverse ways, the single nerve lesion offers a useful model through which to understand the mechanisms of neuropathic pain.

At least four pathophysiologic mechanisms appear to play a role in nerve injury pain.

Ectopic generation of action potentials: Although normally silent, nociceptive afferents may become spontaneously active following nerve injury, producing action-potential activity in the absence of a stimulus.[3] This activity may be experienced as spontaneous pain. In addition to abnormal signaling in the nerve itself, the activity may sensitize central neurons, such that inputs from nonnociceptive, tactile afferents produce pain (allodynia).[7]

Ectopic excitability: Uninjured nerve trunks are minimally sensitive to mechanical stimuli. Gentle percussion over a nerve is not painful. Following injury, however, regenerating fibers may abnormally respond to mild, mechanical stimuli. Such ectopic mechanical excitability gives rise to Tinel sign, an electrical sensation in the nerve's original target distribution, elicited by mechanical stimulation at the location of regenerating axons. Furthermore, ectopic excitability to mechanical stimuli may be accompanied by chemical sensitization. For example, injured nociceptive axons may become abnormally sensitive to catecholamines. As a result, the physiologic release of norepinephrine from sympathetic terminals may induce pain (sympathetically maintained pain [SMP]).[4,5]

Nervi nervorum: Nerves themselves appear to be innervated by nociceptive fibers. These nervi nervorum fibers may be sensitized to mechanical stimuli following nerve injury. Such a mechanism may explain, for example, the local tenderness and mechanical hyperalgesia of the ulnar nerve when it is entrapped at the elbow or the local tenderness of nerves entrapped by scar tissue.[8]

Ephaptic conduction: Under normal conditions, signals in adjacent afferent nerve fibers are insulated from each other. Activity in an injured nerve fiber may cross to a nearby fiber, through a direct electrical connection between the two. During such ephaptic transmission, or cross-talk, a nonnoxious sensory stimulus may evoke activity in nociceptive fibers and thereby cause pain.

Some of the mechanisms of ectopic generation of action potentials and ectopic excitability have been described. When an axon is severed, the axonal transport of sodium channels and other ion channels from the neuronal cell body to the sensory terminal is interrupted. As a result, channels may be expressed ectopically in the neuroma formed at the nerve injury site. Nociceptive fibers in the neuroma thereby become sensitive to normally nonpainful stimuli, producing pain when these stimuli are present.[9,10] In addition, nerve injury may lead to profound changes in gene expression, promoting ectopic excitability.[11]

Other mechanisms may also contribute to neuropathic pain. Although inflammatory and neuropathic pain syndromes are traditionally considered separately, immunologic studies have implicated several pathways through which inflammatory responses may alter nociceptive processing, resulting in neuropathic pain.[12] Evidence supports what may be termed the *wallerian degeneration hypothesis*.[13] According to this hypothesis, uninjured nociceptors that are adjacent to nerves undergoing wallerian degeneration may become spontaneously active and develop sensitivity to catecholamines, resulting in spontaneous pain and SMP. To the extent that neuropathic pain results from these mechanisms, peripheral neurectomy may be expected to worsen pain because the nerve undergoes wallerian degeneration distal to the site of neurectomy.

Rationale for Neuroma Relocation Surgery

The concept of surgery to *remove* a neuroma as a treatment of nerve injury pain is a flawed one. Neuromas arise from nerve fibers proximal to a region of transection or severe injury, which remain in continuity with their cell bodies in the dorsal root ganglia. Cutting the nerve at a location that is proximal to the site of nerve injury to remove the neuroma results in the formation of a new neuroma at the proximal location. Surgery in which neuromas are "removed" should therefore be termed *neuroma relocation surgery*.

Not all neuromas are painful. The tissue milieu surrounding the nerve may determine whether a neuroma becomes painful or remains painless. The use of peripheral neurectomy as a treatment for painful neuromas is therefore predicated on the hope that relocation of the neuroma may convert it from a painful one to a painless one. For example, relocating a neuroma to a non–pressure-sensitive area may alleviate pain in some patients. Relocation of neuromas into muscle was first described in 1918. Since that time, the identification of anatomic locations appropriate for nerve relocation has improved outcomes substantially.[14–22]

Thus, an important consideration in peripheral neurectomy is the role of location in the production of pain. If the location of nerve injury contributes to pain, then relocating the neuroma to a mechanically favorable area may be advantageous. However, to the extent that there is location-independent ectopic generation of action potentials in the neuroma, neuroma relocation surgery will fail. Additionally, some investigators have argued that central mechanisms may account for pain in many nerve injuries.[23] In this circumstance, neuroma relocation surgery may also fail. However, our observations as well as those of other experienced clinicians suggest that in patients with nerve injury pain, where anesthetic block of the injured nerve relieves pain, peripheral neurectomy may provide significant pain relief.

CLINICAL CONSIDERATIONS
Preoperative Evaluation

Clinical scenarios favoring peripheral neurectomy may be broadly divided into two circumstances: neuropathic pain resulting from nerve injury and nociceptive pain from a diseased tissue other than nerve. Nerve injury pain is characterized by numbness, burning, and allodynia. Tinel sign may be present at the site of a painful neuroma. Candidates for neuroma relocation surgery should respond to local anesthetic blockade.

Successful anesthetic blockade is an important prerequisite for effective neuroma relocation surgery. If blockade of the putative, pain-generating neuroma fails to relieve pain nearly entirely, the rationale for neuroma relocation surgery is precarious. The decision to operate may be made with more confidence if more than one block is done. Once candidate nerves are identified, local anesthetic blocks indicate the level of benefit that can be obtained following nerve ablation. A successfully applied block should induce anesthesia in the distribution of each target nerve, but not beyond, to indicate the specificity of the blockade. Injection of saline or injections away from the nerve may enhance blockade specificity by identifying nonspecific responses (e.g., placebo responses).

Findings associated with complex regional pain syndrome (CRPS), such as edema, hyperalgesia, and trophic changes, also suggest that neurectomy will not alleviate pain. Notably in such cases, peripheral nerve blockade typically produces little relief. Patients should be additionally assessed for hyperalgesia to cooling stimuli. This finding is suggestive of SMP, discussed in the following text. Finally, local tenderness in combination with Tinel sign suggests nerve entrapment. In this instance, nerve decompression would be indicated rather than neurectomy. It is important to note that even subtle entrapments without significant motor or sensory loss may induce severe pain.

Even after one has identified a specific nerve as the pain generator, and one has determined that there are no contraindications to neuroma relocation surgery, a wait-and-see approach may remain most appropriate. For example, where injury is relatively recent and the nerve relatively minor, one may choose to observe. The pain may resolve spontaneously. Where there is only partial nerve injury with remaining function, neurectomy may sacrifice function without any assurance that the new neuroma will be less painful than the old one. In this circumstance, nerve repair should be considered before performing neuroma relocation surgery.

Nerve repair has the potential to relocate neuromas with the advantage of restoring neurologic function. The clinician sometimes faces the ironic situation that to repair an injured nerve, a normal nerve (e.g., sural nerve) may be sacrificed to provide donor grafts. In effect, nerve repair is, in a sense, still a neuroma relocation operation—the neuroma is relocated to the donor nerve. Repair of an injured nerve, when feasible, is generally preferable to permanent transection. By contrast, if a nerve has already been completely severed, the risk of relocating the neuroma is low. Thus, in a case of a well-defined neuroma, when an anesthetic block relieves pain, surgical neurectomy may be the preferred first line of surgical therapy.

Careful analysis may lead to rewarding outcomes. The following case presents the history, preoperative evaluation, and treatment of a patient with neuropathic pain.

A 44-year-old woman presented with a chief complaint of right vaginal pain. This problem had been present for 3 years and originated with an excisional biopsy of a right-sided vaginal ulcer near the introitus. The pain was always present, but especially disturbing were lightning attacks of pain that occurred unpredictably several times a day. Examination disclosed a subtle sensory loss in the right vulvar area. Medication trials were minimally helpful. An anesthetic block of the right pudendal nerve led to 50% pain relief. A combined ilioinguinal and genitofemoral nerve block also led to 50% pain relief. A local anesthetic block of all three nerves together led to 100% pain relief. As treatment, the right pudendal nerve was severed distal to the sacral spinous ligament through a perivulvar approach, and the patient, predictably, had 50% of her pain relieved. At a separate surgery, the right ilioinguinal and genitofemoral nerves were severed through a retroperitoneal approach. At 3-year follow-up, the patient had complete relief. There were no adverse sequelae.

In this case, both lumbosacral neural segments provided innervation to the painful neuromas. Failure to appreciate this would have led to a less than satisfactory result. This case underscores the need for complete blockade of pain during the application of local anesthetic to ensure that all involved nerves are identified.

Operative Technique

Once peripheral neurectomy has been selected as the treatment of choice, the primary surgical issue is where to relocate the neuroma. Troublesome neuromas typically are in areas near joints, scars, and structures that may tether the nerve. The idea of surgery is to relocate the neuroma to a new location where tethering does not occur.[17] Nerves may be cut back to locations such that the ends can be placed in healthy, well-vascularized muscle. Some have also advocated that neuromas be placed in holes in bone. Placement of a cut nerve into these environments does not change the fact that the cut ends of the nerve will sprout and that a neuroma will form. However, with relocation of the neuroma into muscle or bone, chances are reduced that the new neuroma will be subject to the tension and shearing forces likely to play a role in pain generation.

Alternatives to neuroma relocation exist. The nerves may be cauterized, frozen, burned, or injected with toxic chemicals. These options have been reported to be successful, but their advantages over surgical neurectomy have not been demonstrated. A surgical procedure where the neurectomy is done sharply, with limited damage to the surrounding environment of the nerve, is most appealing from a mechanistic perspective. Damage to the surrounding tissues, such as necrosis due to phenol injection, may create a new focus for pain generation.[24]

INDICATIONS AND OUTCOMES FOR TREATMENT OF NEUROPATHIC PAIN

Ordinarily, neurectomy should be reserved for those situations in which nerve decompression is unlikely to provide a satisfactory result and nerve repair is not possible. Division of major nerves can cause significant motor deficits, sensory deficits, and pain. Ablation of such nerves as a treatment of pain should ordinarily be considered only if the nerve is already divided. Nerve graft repair should be considered as an alternative to repeat transection. Neurectomy of minor nerves has a role in pain treatment, and the risk–reward ratio may be favorable.

Amputation Stump Pain

In cases of stump pain, it is worthwhile to examine the patient for tender neuromas. A prosthetic device, for example, may apply pressure to the neuroma, causing pain. Surgical relocation of neuromas to more proximal or protected locations, often in conjunction with nerve wrapping, may provide significant benefit in these cases.[25,26]

Intercostal and Intercostobrachial Pain

Chest trauma or thoracotomy may damage intercostal nerves. Shoulder trauma and axillary node dissection may damage the intercostobrachial nerve. Motor deficits associated with intercostal

and intercostobrachial neurectomy are clinically insignificant. Hence, neurectomy is usually without significant drawbacks. This procedure can be safely accomplished through video-assisted thoracoscopy as well as through an open procedure.[27]

Perineal and Inguinal Pain

Injuries to the pudendal, ilioinguinal, iliohypogastric, and genitofemoral nerves may result in severe pain. These injuries are often due to abdominal and pelvic surgery, episiotomy, hernia repair, entrapment, or blunt trauma. For example, the Pfannenstiel transverse incision may injure the ilioinguinal/iliohypogastric nerves. Groin pain from inguinal herniorrhaphy is not uncommon. Stulz and Pfeiffer[28] reported relief of pain with neurectomy in 70% (16 of 23) of patients with ilioinguinal and iliohypogastric neuralgia as a complication of prior surgery. Starling and Harms[29] reported similar rates of success: 89% (17 of 19) for ilioinguinal neuralgia and 71% (12 of 17) for genitofemoral neuralgia. In the largest series to date, Amid[30] reported 95% improvement in pain among 225 patients. Our own experience supports the use of neurectomy, but the incidence of long-term favorable outcomes is much more modest.[31] Recently, Chen and colleagues[32] reported that patients who underwent a laparoscopic retroperitoneal triple neurectomy for inguinal pain over open and standard procedures for inguinal herniorrhaphy showed superior outcomes in terms of postoperative pain scores and recovery time.

Meralgia Paresthetica

Entrapment or injury of the lateral femoral cutaneous nerve, meralgia paresthetica, may result in pain and dysesthesia in the anterolateral thigh. In cases where the diagnosis is unclear, local anesthetic blockade may be helpful. Transection should ordinarily be considered as a backup procedure when decompression is not feasible and nonsurgical approaches, such as weight loss, have failed.[33] A study comparing neurolysis to neurectomy for the treatment of meralgia paresthetica found that only 60% of patients who underwent neurolysis reported being pain free compared to 87.5% of patients treated with neurectomy.[34]

Saphenous Neuralgia

Entrapment of the saphenous nerve in the subsartorial canal[35] may occur with or without a history of trauma. Damage to the saphenous nerve may occur when the saphenous vein is harvested during revascularization procedures.[36] Risk factors associated with the development of saphenous neuralgia after saphenous vein harvest include younger age, female sex, diabetes mellitus, higher body mass index, distal-to-proximal dissection of the saphenous vein, and closure of the leg wound in two layers.[37] The condition is associated with pain (with or without numbness) along the anterior and medial leg and the dorsum of the foot. Proximal neurectomy may be used if the nerve has been directly injured. Otherwise, in our experience, the nerve should be decompressed as the first-line treatment.

Morton's Neuroma

This condition involves compression of the digital nerve, typically between the third and fourth tarsal bones. The compression leads to a swelling of the nerve, which is mistakenly called a neuroma. Patients present with pain in this region worsened by wearing shoes and walking. If conservative measures (e.g., orthotics) fail, neurectomy may be offered. Indeed, this operation is a common procedure for this condition. Johnson et al.[38] reported relief of pain in 67% (22 of 33) of patients, with 6 years average follow-up, following excision of the plantar interdigital neuroma. Others have reported surgical success rates of up to 90%.[39,40] A recent consecutive cohort study reported that ultrasound-guided radiofrequency ablation of

Morton's neuroma provided pain relief in 25 out of 30 patients. This procedure can be completed on an outpatient basis and is less invasive than traditional neurectomy.[41]

General Results of Neurectomy for Neuropathic Pain

What are the predicted results of neurectomy for nerve injury pain? The question is difficult to answer because the patients undergoing this treatment are heterogeneous. In addition, measurement of patient outcome varies greatly among studies with regard to methodologic rigor, length of follow-up, and technique. As suggested by the studies cited earlier, success rates vary from modest to high.

Burchiel and colleagues[42] have taken a systematic approach to the treatment of nerve injury pain, moving the field toward a definition of the indications for neuroma surgery. In their study, 42 patients with nerve injury pain were divided into four treatment groups:

- Patients with distal sensory neuromas treated by excision of the neuroma and implantation of the proximal nerve into muscle or bone marrow
- Patients with *suspected* distal sensory neuromas in which the involved nerve was sectioned proximal to the injury site and implanted into muscle or bone
- Patients with proximal neuromas-in-continuity of major sensorimotor nerves treated by neuroplasty, which frees a nerve from adjacent tissue
- Patients with nerve injuries at points of anatomic entrapment treated by neuroplasty and transposition

Surgical success (rated as a greater than 50% subjective improvement in pain levels, subjectively rated pain relief as "good" or "excellent," and no postoperative narcotic usage) varied between the groups. In the 40 patients who received postoperative follow-up care over 2 to 32 months (average of 11 months), 16 (40%) met these criteria. By group, successful pain relief was accomplished in 44% (8 of 18) of group 1, 40% (4 of 10) of group 2, 0% (0 of 5) of group 3, and 57% (4 of 7) of group 4.

After obtaining these results, Burchiel et al.[42] attempted to determine retrospectively the extent to which indicators of nerve injury predicted surgical success. Such indicators included Tinel sign, hyperalgesia, a "discrete nerve syndrome," litigation, and prior procedures. Some predictors showed promise. For example, a *discrete nerve syndrome*, defined as a condition in which a single nerve could account for all the neurologic findings and pain distribution, tended to predict success. However, none of the relationships between preoperative diagnostic variables and treatment success achieved statistical significance at the $P < .05$ level. Another prospective study found that employment status, duration of pain, CRPS, smoking, and improvement with nerve block were all prognostic factors for surgical management of neuroma pain.[43]

One can only speculate why the results of this series differ substantially from those of other series. Perhaps patient selection accounts for differences, yet Burchiel and colleagues[42] appeared to discriminate patients at high risk for failure. Surgical technique could also play a role, but there is no evidence on which to base such a statement. In some cases, neuromas are innervated by more than one nerve. For example, proximal resection of the superficial radial nerve to treat dorsoradial wrist neuromas often relieves pain only temporarily. Further inspection reveals that the lateral antebrachial cutaneous nerve may also innervate these neuromas, and thus, success may require sectioning this nerve as well.[44]

Another reason for failure in neuroma relocation surgery may relate to the discovery that the *distal* side of a severed nerve may also form a neuroma at the site of injury. Plexus formation distal to the neurectomy may allow intact nerve fibers from other nerves to sprout in retrograde fashion to innervate this distal site. This retrograde sprouting may create a potentially painful neuroma on the "wrong" side.[45] Neuroma relocation surgery should perhaps attend to neuroma formation on both sides of a severed nerve.

INDICATIONS AND OUTCOMES FOR TREATMENT OF NOCICEPTIVE PAIN

Neurectomy may be performed to interrupt the flow of pain signals through intact nerves from a diseased, pain-generating tissue to the spinal cord. In these cases, a balance is sought between elimination of input from the pain-generating tissue and the potential formation of a painful neuroma. Following neurectomy, regrowth of the transected nerve and invasion of the diseased tissue by surrounding nerves may result in a return of pain. In addition, intact and otherwise "normal" nerve fibers may be sensitized by the release of growth factors in partially denervated tissues. Progression of the underlying disease process may also enlarge the injured tissue region, producing pain beyond the region of surgery. In spite of these considerations, in the following disease processes, neurectomy may be an effective treatment of nociceptive pain.

Axial Spine Pain

The medial branches of dorsal rami innervate the paraspinal muscles, the interspinous ligament, and the zygapophyseal (facet) joints. Pain associated with movement of the lower back, which is relieved by rest and is not attributable to other spine pathology, may be relieved through bilateral, percutaneous radiofrequency or chemical ablation of these branches in the lumbar spine.[46,47] A success rate of 85% with mean duration of relief of 10.5 months was reported by Schofferman and Kine[48] through this procedure. In addition, neck pain associated with whiplash injury may benefit from a similar procedure in the cervical spine.[49] The mechanism of pain relief is thought to relate to denervation of the facet joint. Because the dorsal ramus innervates several structures, other mechanisms are possible. Evidence is indeterminate for similar pain of thoracic origin.

Many experts suggest diagnostic anesthetic blocks of the facets prior to a facet denervation procedure. Good results are expected only in patients who get excellent benefit from the blocks. Patients who have axial pain in addition to radicular symptoms tend not to benefit from facet denervation procedures alone. Among preexisting symptoms, only paraspinal tenderness has been shown to predict treatment success, whereas increased pain with facet loading maneuvers predicts less favorable outcomes.[50,51]

The procedure is performed percutaneously with radiofrequency heat lesions. The advantages of this procedure are that it can be done on an outpatient basis and morbidity is low. The disadvantage is that the procedure often confers only temporary relief or often no relief at all regardless of the temporary effects of diagnostic facet blocks. In addition to continuous, high-temperature radiofrequency medial branch ablation, pulsed radiofrequency, cryodenervation, and phenol neurolysis have also been used to provide intermediate to long-term pain relief.

In patients with no prior spine surgery, these procedures have been reported to provide initial relief for 60% to 70% of patients.[36,49,50,52] Rates are reported to be considerably lower, 20% to 50%, for patients with prior spine surgery.[36,52,53] However, a history of spine surgery is associated with treatment failure not only for radiofrequency denervation but other interventions as well, including epidural steroid injection and open surgery. Our view is that this is a low-morbidity procedure that can provide effective, albeit impermanent, pain relief for patients with axial spine pain. Recurrence of pain following denervation can be treated with repeated neurotomy with comparable efficacy. See Chapter 102 for a detailed discussion of neurolytic blocks, including radiofrequency neurolysis.

Extremity Joint Pain

Denervation procedures aim to eliminate pain arising from degenerative processes in the joint while preserving functions that may be lost after other forms of joint surgery. Buck-Gramcko[54] reported retention of wrist mobility with substantial reduction of pain in 69% (135 of 195) of patients following wrist denervation surgery. Wilhelm[55] reported success in 90% of patients with tennis elbow treated by denervation. Dellon et al.[56] reported satisfaction in 86% (60 of 70) of patients following partial denervation surgery for persistent, postoperative knee pain. Pulsed radiofrequency denervation has also been used to provide relief although generally with shorter effect when compared to conventional radiofrequency ablation and limited evidence to support the efficacy of this approach.[57]

Pelvic Pain

Neurectomy of the superior hypogastric (presacral) plexus has been advocated as a treatment for medically refractory pelvic pain. In 1948, Ingersoll and Meigs[58] reported complete relief of primary dysmenorrhea in 81% (72 of 89) of women treated with neurectomy. More recently, with the development of more effective analgesics, ablative approaches to pelvic pain have been largely limited to patients with secondary dysmenorrhea associated with endometriosis. Nezhat et al.[59] reported at least 50% relief from pain in 70% to 85% of patients with various stages of endometriosis, with 1-year follow-up, following presacral neurectomy combined with excision and vaporization of endometriotic lesions. Debate over the proper role of presacral neurectomy has been ongoing for well over 50 years. Introduction of the biopsychosocial model of chronic pain has potential to spare many women from surgery.

Cancer Pain

Peripheral neurectomy is infrequently used in the treatment of pain due to cancer. This is due to the availability of alternative strategies with low morbidity and higher success rates, such as spinal opiates or percutaneous radiofrequency cordotomy.[60,61] Transecting a peripheral nerve may fail to relieve pain because of overlapping receptive fields of adjacent nerves or central plasticity. Sectioning major peripheral nerves results not only in numbness but also in unacceptable motor loss. Peripheral neurectomies are rarely indicated in the extremities. However, localized chest or abdominal wall pain can successfully be treated with intercostal neurectomies. Alcohol injection, cryoprobe, or radiofrequency lesions provide similar success to open surgery and lowered morbidity for the treatment of cancer pain.

Nerve Entrapment Release

BASIC CONSIDERATIONS
Pathophysiology of Nerve Entrapment Pain

Nerve entrapment syndromes result from pressure applied directly to a nerve, causing pain, paresthesias, or weakness in the sensory distribution of the nerve.[44,62,63] Entrapment commonly develops where peripheral nerves traverse confined anatomic spaces, rest in superficial locations or in proximity to joints, or become tethered to adjacent tissues. Structural factors such as anomalous nerves, cervical ribs, muscles, or connective tissue bands also may contribute. Repetitive motion, nerve traction due to joint position, chronic vibration, and high force constitute physical stressors that increase the risk of symptomatic entrapment.

Although the degree of compression required to cause nerve injury may vary, axonal degeneration follows pressure in a dose-dependent relationship.[64] Symptoms can arise following a few significant events or after a longer period of repetitive mild insults. The time course and force of injury are just two of the prognostic considerations. The length of the affected nerve

region as well as the presence and severity of nerve ischemia are important factors in the development of symptomatic nerve entrapment. Finally, nerves become more vulnerable to injury in the presence of concurrent systemic metabolic disease, and nerves lose their regenerative capacity with age.

Several pathophysiologic mechanisms have been proposed to explain pain associated with peripheral nerve entrapment at the cellular level. Evidence for these mechanisms arises from studies of animal models.[64–66] Following local nerve compression, internodes along myelinated fibers distort in shape. Demyelination appears earliest in the segment nearest to the point of compression.[67,68] Eventually, segmental demyelination leads to diffuse demyelination and, ultimately, axonal degradation. Compressive injury usually affects larger, more peripherally located myelinated nerves as opposed to smaller or unmyelinated fibers.

Nerve ischemia may also play an important role in nerve entrapment pain syndromes. Focal pressures of 20 to 30 mm Hg may impede venous blood flow, whereas higher pressures may reduce arterial supply.[69,70] Within 4 hours of extraneural compression, increasing permeability of the blood–nerve barrier leads to development of subperineurial edema.[71–74] As there is no lymphatic drainage of the endoneurial space, sustained intraneural pressure elevations persist for at least 24 hours after compressive forces are removed. Following such injury, reactive inflammation, fibrin deposition, and proliferation of endoneurial fibroblasts and capillary endothelial cells lead to intraneural fibrosis of perineurial and epineurial tissues.

Ischemia does not appear to play a role in the initial demyelination associated with acute compressive injury.[75,76] Rather, nodes of Ranvier adjacent to the point of compression are outwardly displaced and disrupt the myelin sheath. Segmental demyelination follows, stemming from these sites of myelin invagination.[77,78] Disruption of anterograde axoplasmic flow of vital nutrient proteins reduces terminal membrane excitability. Long-standing ischemia thereby results in replacement of funicular contents with fibrotic tissue, producing derangements in electrical conductivity.[79]

Nerve Entrapment and Systemic Disease

Several endocrine and rheumatologic diseases show an association with increased risk for nerve entrapment. Approximately 15% of upper extremity nerve entrapment patients have diabetes. This may result from an increased association of peripheral neuropathies with entrapment. Both hypo- and hyperthyroidism have been shown to pose an increased risk for nerve entrapment, which is thought to result from glycogen deposition in Schwann cells.[80] Up to 30% of acromegalics are diagnosed with nerve entrapment syndromes, which often resolve with treatment of the underlying acromegaly.[81,82] Obesity and pregnancy have well-documented associations with entrapment syndromes, with as many as two-thirds of pregnant women experiencing temporary symptoms.[83] Rheumatoid arthritis is also thought to contribute to entrapment in anatomic locations where synovial overgrowth can produce compression of a nerve. There is an estimated 45% incidence of entrapment neuropathy in rheumatoid arthritis patients.[84,85] Amyloidosis, carcinomatosis, gout, mucopolysaccharide storage diseases, and polymyalgia rheumatica are all suspected to pose an increased risk for exacerbation of nerve entrapment.

CLINICAL CONSIDERATIONS
Preoperative Evaluation

Clinical findings: Patients suffering from nerve entrapment syndromes present with pain, paresthesias, or motor weakness along a specific nerve distribution. Nocturnal pain, either sharp or burning, classically develops before the onset of daytime or persistent symptoms. Muscular changes, such as atrophy or fasciculation, as well as sensory alterations, such as altered two-point discrimination or temperature sensation, can occur in advanced cases. Specific symptoms result from the location and severity of compression.

On physical examination, Tinel sign may be present. Tinel sign is an electric radiating sensation in the distribution of the nerve, produced by percussion over the nerve. Tinel sign represents ectopic excitability, a hallmark of nerve entrapment, and may be accompanied by local tenderness. Provocative maneuvers may reproduce or exacerbate symptoms and have significantly positive predictive value in the diagnosis of entrapment syndromes.

In many cases, diagnosis of a specific entrapment syndrome may be difficult to make. Compensation of one muscle group by another may create uncertainty in identifying etiology of the entrapment. Furthermore, entrapment syndromes may be accompanied by concurrent radiculopathy, producing synergistic pain, thereby adding to the diagnostic challenge.[86] In addition, pain associated with entrapment syndromes may not be well localized. For example, radial nerve entrapment may present with global arm pain. Finally, results of electrodiagnostic studies may be normal in some cases, further increasing the diagnostic dilemma.

Electrodiagnostic studies: Physical findings may be supported by electrodiagnostic studies. Nerve conduction studies (NCS) measure action potentials along axons, whereas electromyography studies (EMG) measure muscle fiber activity. In sensory NCS, a stimulus is applied to the nerve and a sensory nerve action potential (SNAP) is measured at various distal points along the nerve. Alterations in axon number, diameter, myelination, or temperature all affect the magnitude and temporal profile of the SNAP. In motor NCS, a stimulus is applied to the nerve and a compound motor action potential (CMAP) is measured from the innervated muscle. Changes in conduction velocity, amplitude of CMAP, and distal motor latency suggest that conduction inhibition exists between the point of initial stimulation and the site of recording. Needle EMG examines the spontaneous electrical activity of individual muscle fibers resulting from denervation, reinnervation, or acute muscle injury.

These studies aid in the differentiation of peripheral nerve entrapments from brachial plexopathy and radiculopathy by defining the nature and extent of neurologic dysfunction. For example, although NCS cannot be performed in structures like the brachial plexus due to an inability to record and stimulate across the region of compression, a plexus lesion would be expected to affect the function of multiple peripheral nerves. In entrapment neuropathy, large myelinated sensory fibers are typically affected before motor fibers. Hence, NCS are most often effective earlier in the disease than motor conduction studies (ulnar compression at the elbow is a notable exception to this rule). Entrapment is represented by abnormal recordings of evoked SNAPs along a short nerve segment. Prolonged latency or reduced motor conduction velocity is also indicative of injury, although they are less sensitive measures. Fibrillation seen on EMG occurs as a result of wallerian degeneration of distal nerve segments and suggests advanced entrapment. In general, a combination of studies and measurement points yields the best information with which to form a diagnosis.

Comparison among the nerves of interest and a nearby unaffected nerve is often more accurate than comparison of a nerve with normal reference values. Cooler temperature, increasing age, and patient size all serve to prolong sensory latencies, confounding reference values. As a result, and to avoid such confounding factors, it is common to perform sensory latency comparisons at as many as three sites (median-ulnar midpalmar, median-ulnar ring finger, and median-radial thumb) in the diagnosis of carpal tunnel syndrome (CTS).[87] Although the greater number of studies increases the likelihood of false-positive results,[88] summation of the latencies of these three studies has proven to be the most sensitive and specific test for CTS.[89]

Following entrapment release, it is notable that clinical improvement may not correlate reliably with electrodiagnostic studies. However, in patients with persistent symptoms following treatment, comparison with pretreatment studies may be helpful. If earlier studies are unavailable, a series of postoperative studies over several months should be obtained.

Imaging studies: Developments in ultrasonography and magnetic resonance imaging (MRI) have resulted in a potentially expanded role for imaging in the diagnosis of entrapment neuropathies. Ultrasonography now offers the highest available resolution for visualizing the location of entrapment (Fig. 103.1). However, ultrasound is unable to show pathologic changes within nerves. In contrast, signal and configuration characteristics seen in chronically compressed or tethered peripheral nerves have been well characterized by MRI (Fig. 103.2). On MRI, indicators for nerve abnormality include focal enlargement, T2 hyperintensity, and an indistinguishable or nonuniform fascicular pattern. In addition, MRI simultaneously visualizes muscular alterations due to atrophy and neurogenic edema.

Specific MRI findings have been correlated with clinical findings, electrodiagnostic findings, and postoperative outcomes for several nerve entrapment syndromes.[90–93] With current technology, MRI may be a useful adjunct in the diagnosis of entrapment. Specific indications for MRI may include ulnar entrapment, entrapment in the presence of superimposed neuropathy, entrapment where other tests are equivocal, and postoperative evaluation of entrapment.[94] The value of MRI imaging in the setting of uncommon entrapments is less clear.

Operative Technique

Substantial experimental evidence supports three treatments of peripheral nerve entrapment: splinting, local corticosteroid injection, and surgical release. Splinting reduces the offending stimulus through postural correction and reduction of repetitive injury, thereby decreasing reactive inflammation. Local corticosteroid injections have been shown to be helpful in mild cases. Surgical release of anatomic compression is the mainstay of treatment in more advanced cases of peripheral nerve entrapment.[95]

In general, operative release of entrapment can be quite rewarding, as the risks of surgery are typically low and pain improvement is often dramatic. Avoidance of additional trauma to the compressed nerve is of great importance to surgical outcome. Occasionally, unexpected sources of entrapment may be found during surgical exposure, such as cysts, soft tissue masses, and bony prominences. Choices of surgical approach and operative technique are based largely on individual surgeon preferences.[96] Rates of success and complications vary with the location of entrapment and the etiology of pain.

INDICATIONS AND OUTCOMES
Entrapments of the Median Nerve

Carpal tunnel syndrome: CTS results from compression of the median nerve between bones of the wrist and the flexor retinaculum. CTS is the most common nerve compression syndrome, with an annual incidence of 150 per 100,000 population and a 2:1 female predominance.[97,98] Patients with CTS present with pain along the radial half of the hand, particularly at night, and weakness of median innervated muscles. Phalen's sign—recreation of pain through complete wrist flexion for 30 to 60 seconds—is a sensitive and specific marker of mild to moderate CTS.[99,100] Electrodiagnostic studies typically demonstrate decreased median-nerve conduction velocity at the wrist. Imaging findings on MRI, when performed, may demonstrate increased

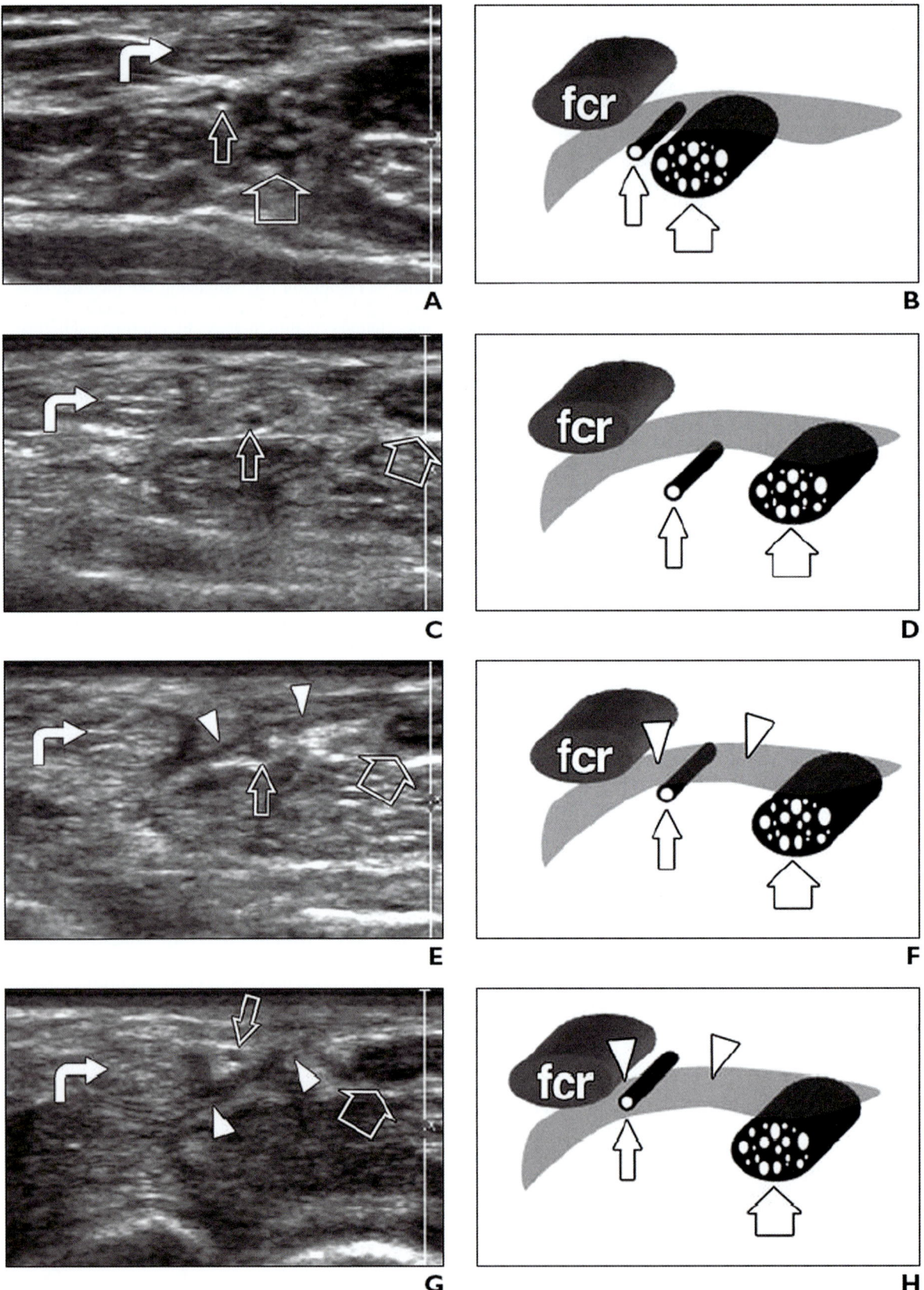

FIGURE 103.1 Series of transverse 17.5 MHz sonography images obtained from proximal to distal over palmar cutaneous branch of median nerve (MN) in 35-year-old healthy man with corresponding diagrams. Relationships of palmar cutaneous branch of MN (*thin arrows*) with MN (*thick arrows*), flexor carpi radialis tendon (*curved arrow* in **A**, **C**, **E**, and **G**; *fcr* in **B**, **D**, **F**, and **H**), and antebrachial fascia (*arrowheads*, **E–H**) are shown. **A,B:** Palmar cutaneous branch of MN detaches from MN as one of its most radial fascicles. **C,D:** Palmar cutaneous branch of MN gradually deflects to approach flexor carpi radialis tendon. **E,F:** Palmar cutaneous branch of MN runs slightly deep in relation to antebrachial fascia. **G,H:** Palmar cutaneous branch of MN lies adjacent to flexor carpi radialis tendon after piercing fascia. (*From Tagliafico A, Pugliese F, Bianchi S, et al. High-resolution sonography of the palmar cutaneous branch of the median nerve. Am J Roentgen 2008;191[1]:107–114. Reprinted with permission from the American Journal of Roentgenology.*)

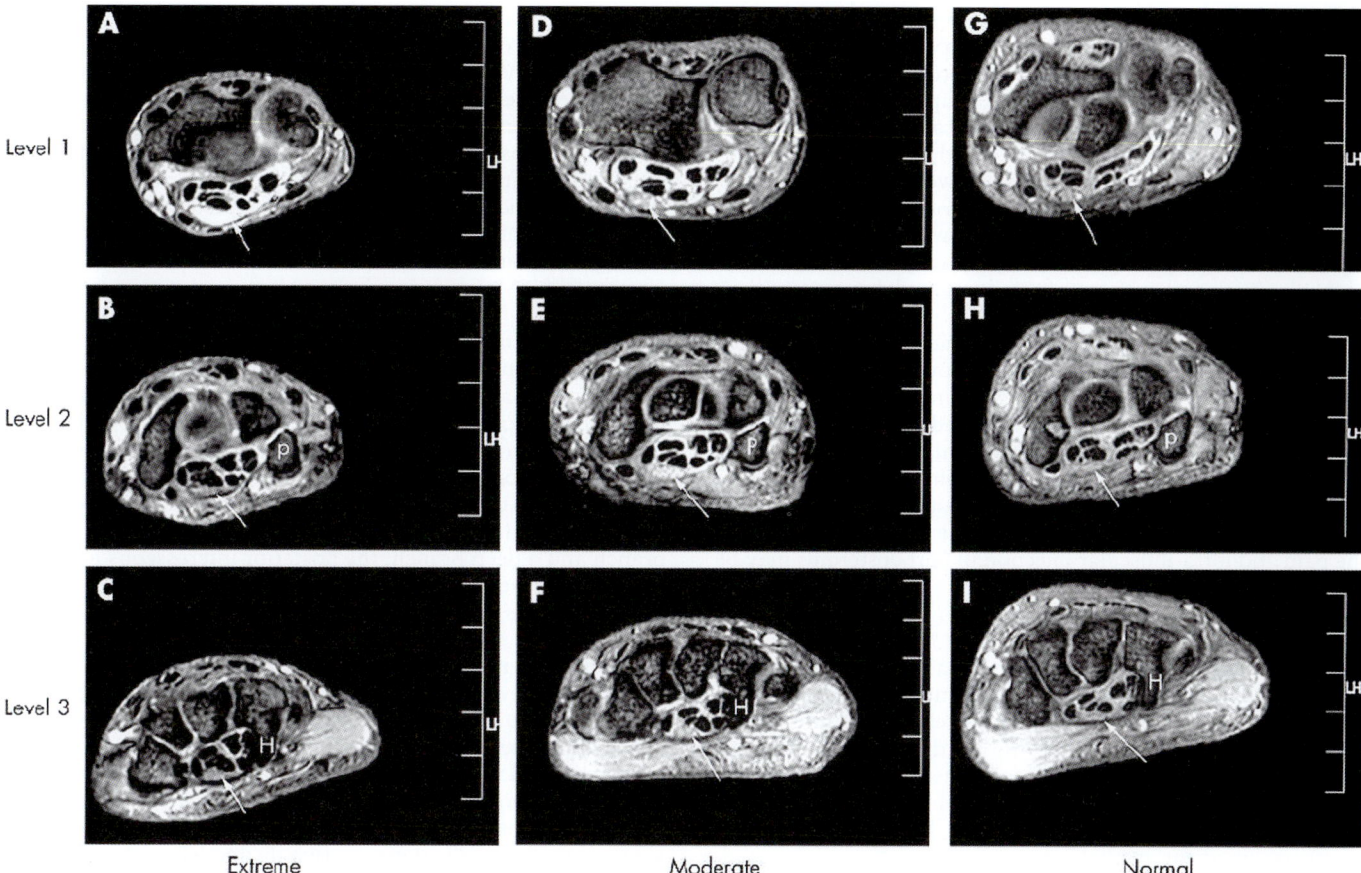

FIGURE 103.2 T2-weighted gradient echo images at the distal part of the distal radioulnar joint level (DRUJ) (level 1), at the level of the pisiform (level 2), and at the level of the hook of the hamate (level 3) in three different stages of idio pathic carpal tunnel syndrome. *Solid arrow* indicates the cross section of the median nerve. **Upper part** represents the dorsal side, and the **right-hand side** represents the ulnar side. H, hook of the hamate; P, pisiform bone. **A–C:** Extreme stage. Enlargement and high signal intensity of the flattened median nerve are seen at level 1, and enlargement of the median nerve at levels 2 and 3. Palmar bowing of the transverse carpal ligament (TCL) is evident. **D–F:** Moderate stage. Enlargement and high signal intensity of the median nerve are seen at level 2. They are slightly appreciated at level 3 and still not seen at level 1. Palmar bowing of the TCL is well appreciated. **G–I:** Normal wrist. Enlargement of the median nerve is not seen at any level. Isointensity of the nerve to the hypothenar muscle is seen throughout the cross sections. Palmar bowing of the TCL is not seen. *(Reprinted from Uchiyama S, Itsubo T, Yasutomi T, et al. Quantitative MRI of the wrist and nerve conduction studies in patients with idiopathic carpal tunnel syndrome. J Neurol Neurosurg Psych 2005;76[8]:1103–1108, with permission from BMJ Publishing Group Ltd.)*

signal intensity in the nerve, volar bowing of the flexor retinaculum, and flattening of the median nerve at the level of the hamate.[101]

Initial therapy includes splinting, activity modification, and nonsteroidal anti-inflammatory medications for mild disease. Corticosteroid injections offer nearly a 70% positive response initially, although eventual recurrence of symptoms is high.[102]

Surgical decompression of the carpal tunnel is indicated in cases that have failed conservative management or in cases with severe or rapid onset of symptoms. Some 80% of patients achieve excellent pain relief with surgery, whereas another 10% achieve partial relief; less than 1% of patients experience worsening of their pain symptoms. For patients with motor weakness, similar results have been reported with 84% of patients returning to baseline function and another 9% experiencing some improvement.[100,103–105] Early surgery in patients with ongoing pain has been associated with improved resolution of symptoms.

Incomplete decompression of the nerve is seen in the majority of cases in which pain relief is incomplete, absent, or transient. Another cause of recurrent pain includes postoperative fibrosis. Failure to appreciate the path of the recurrent motor (thenar) branch of the nerve can result in postoperative weakness following release. Injury to the palmar cutaneous branch can result in postoperative pain in the wrist and proximal

thenar eminence.[106,107] A 2010 review attempted to identify optimal outcome prognostic factors for patients undergoing carpal tunnel release. They discovered that having comorbid conditions such as diabetes, poor health status, thoracic outlet syndrome (TOS), double crush, alcohol, and smoking led to a worse prognosis. However, they were unable to identify any positive prognostic indicators that would predict an optimal outcome in patients with CTS undergoing carpal tunnel release.[108]

Anterior interosseus syndrome: Anterior interosseus syndrome results from isolated injury or entrapment of this largely motor branch of the median nerve.[109] The nerve arises distal to the medial epicondyle and is vulnerable to injury in supracondylar and forearm fractures.[110–112] In severe cases, there may be weakness of flexor pollicis longus, flexor digitorum profundus to the index finger, and pronator quadratus.

Patients with anterior interosseus syndrome may present with a characteristic pinch as compensation for weakness in the long flexors of the index finger and thumb. The condition may also present with pain in the forearm associated with tenderness in the proximal volar forearm. EMG may confirm changes associated with muscular denervation. Surgical exploration with neuroplasty is most commonly performed for patients whose pain does not respond to anti-inflammatory medications or avoidance of repetitive pronation/supination activity.[113–117]

Entrapment by the ligament of Struthers: Struthers' ligament can cause compression of the median nerve, brachial artery, or brachial vein as they pass beneath it, proximal to the medial epicondyle. A variant bony spicule (supracondylar process) arising from the humerus at this level can place the nerve at risk for entrapment.[118] A rare disorder, this pathology can potentially be mistaken for CTS.[119] Motor weakness of the pronator teres, flexor carpi radialis, and flexor digitorum profundus (to the first two digits), although not always present, indicate a point of compression proximal to the carpal tunnel. Release of the ligament and excision of the supracondylar process typically provides pain relief.

Pronator syndrome: Pronator syndrome presents as a vague, aching pain in the volar aspect of the elbow and forearm that is exacerbated by activities involving grasping or pronation of the forearm.[120] On physical examination, tenderness can usually be elicited by deep palpation over the pronator teres. Compression occurs at the lacertus fibrosus, within the muscle between the two heads of pronator teres, or beneath the flexor superficialis tendon at its origin. Avoiding maneuvers that exacerbate the pain and intra-muscular injection of corticosteroids may be attempted prior to surgical release.

Entrapments of the Ulnar Nerve

Ulnar nerve entrapment at the elbow: Ulnar nerve entrapment at the elbow (UNEE) is the second most common peripheral nerve entrapment syndrome after CTS. At the elbow, the ulnar nerve is bounded medially and anteriorly by the medial epicondyle and laterally by the olecranon. A dense fascial layer overlies this space, forming the cubital tunnel. Entrapment may occur at the cubital tunnel, in the epicondylar groove, beneath the arcade of Struthers, or at the medial intermuscular septum.[121] Antecedent trauma, inflammatory change, and mass lesions increase the risk of UNEE. Subluxation of a hypermobile ulnar nerve over the medial epicondyle may lead to traumatic injury. An anomalous and potentially compressive anconeus epitrochlearis muscle may be found in up to 30% of patients.[122-124]

UNEE typically presents insidiously with paresthesias in the ulnar distribution of the forearm, wrist, and hand. Muscle weakness leads to impaired grip and clumsiness in the hand and, in more severe cases, atrophy of intrinsic hand muscles. Tinel sign and the elbow flexion-pressure test, which is done with manual compression of the ulnar nerve just proximal to the cubital tunnel for 30 seconds, offer significant sensitivity and specificity for UNEE.[125,126] Electrodiagnostic studies may demonstrate reduced sensory and motor conduction velocity across the elbow.

The optimal surgical technique for entrapment release in UNEE has not been established. Options include transposition of the nerve and in situ decompression. For transposition, the ulnar nerve is displaced anterolaterally in order to shorten its course around the medial epicondyle. Transposition may be subcutaneous, intramuscular, or submuscular, with respect to the flexor-pronator muscle mass.[127-135] Among the larger case series, successful surgical results of 90% have been reported regardless of technique.[136-140] Many surgeons favor in situ decompression as an initial surgical treatment, particularly when patients have milder symptoms and isolated compression at only one site.[141-145]

Traumatic etiology, chronic symptoms, absence of sensory potentials, and severe muscular weakness are among the indicators of poor prognosis for surgical outcome. Pain symptoms more often resolve, whereas motor symptoms may only partially improve, after surgery. Persistent pain following ulnar nerve decompression at the elbow may be due to injury of the medial antebrachial cutaneous nerve.

Ulnar nerve entrapment at the wrist: The ulnar nerve and artery course through Guyon's canal and may become entrapped there.[146]

This canal is bounded by the volar and transverse carpal ligaments and palmaris brevis muscle, with the pisiform bone proximally and medially and the hook of the hamate laterally and distally. Common causes of entrapment include local masses, such as ganglion formation, lipomas, and uremic tumoral calcinosis, or anatomic variants, such as the presence of abductor digit minimi within the canal.[147] Evaluation is typically based on physical examination and electrodiagnostic studies. MRI, when a dedicated wrist coil is utilized, offers noninvasive visualization of Guyon's canal.[148] Surgical decompression involves unroofing of the canal and removal of any masses.[149,150]

Entrapments of the Radial Nerve

Compression neuropathy of the radial nerve occurs at the radial tunnel, a 5-cm space extending from the capitulum of the humerus to the distal edge of the supinator muscle. It is bounded anteromedially by the brachialis muscle, anterolaterally by brachioradialis and extensor carpi radialis brevis, and posteriorly by the capitulum. Just distal to the lateral epicondyle, the radial nerve divides into a purely sensory superficial branch and a deep branch, the posterior interosseous nerve.

Whereas the superficial branch passes superior to the supinator muscle, the posterior interosseous nerve courses in a plane between the two heads of the supinator muscle as they both continue into the forearm. Potential sources of compression at this level include the fibrous bands that anchor the radial nerve to the elbow, the recurrent radial artery and its associated vessels and branches (collectively known as the leash of Henry), and the arcade of Frohse at the fibrous origin of the supinator and other muscles.[149,151-153]

Radial tunnel syndrome and posterior interosseous nerve syndrome: Classically, there are two distinct clinical syndromes involving this pathology—one primarily involving pain, and the other, motor dysfunction. Radial tunnel syndrome itself is a frequently cited, yet somewhat controversial diagnosis, as some argue against its existence. It consists of pain symptoms including deep aching pain, often worse at night, in the extensor muscle mass at the lateral elbow. On physical examination, several particular maneuvers are suggestive of this diagnosis: (1) reproduction of pain by resisting extension of the third digit, with the elbow and wrist in full extension; (2) tenderness to palpation over the entry of the posterior interosseous nerve into the supinator muscle, approximately 5 cm distal to the radial head; and (3) reproduction of pain with the application of a tourniquet at this level.[154-157]

In contrast to radial tunnel syndrome, posterior interosseous nerve syndrome is defined primarily by motor symptoms, including progressive weakness of the wrist and digit extensor muscle group. Due to the relatively distal point of compression, innervation to the brachioradialis, extensor carpi radialis muscles, and supinator are typically unaffected. Weakness in wrist extension is incomplete, such that there is radial deviation. Pain, when present, is secondary in this constellation of symptoms.

Development of this entrapment syndrome is associated with repetitive forceful movements involving elbow extension and forearm pronation and supination.[158] Mass lesions, elbow dislocation, vascular malformations, and synovial inflammation are other potential etiologies of compression, and MRI or ultrasound may be useful in the identification of compression. Electrodiagnostic studies are of limited utility for most patients. Hence, the diagnosis is typically clinical.

Operative release of entrapment includes an exploration of all the branches of the radial nerve, such that the posterior interosseous branch can be fully liberated.[159] Few large case series have been analyzed, and reported outcomes vary in the region of 70%. In some series, however, improved functional outcomes have been reported in over 90% of treated patients.[160-162]

Superficial sensory branch entrapment: Entrapment of the superficial sensory branch of the radial nerve can occur through externally compressive apparel such as watchbands. Chronic intermittent compression tends to cause numbness and dysesthesias over the dorsal surface of the hand, whereas blunt injury at this location typically causes highly refractory pain. Operative neuroplasty has yielded significant improvement of symptoms in 74% to 86% of patients.[163–165] Of note, superficial sensory branch entrapment may be associated with De Quervain's tenosynovitis, and release of the extensor compartment is sometimes performed in combination with neuroplasty.

Entrapment of the Suprascapular Nerve

Suprascapular nerve entrapment presents with shoulder pain along the border of the trapezius muscle and often denervation of the associated musculature.[166–169] On physical examination, it is exacerbated with abduction and external rotation of the arm. The suprascapular nerve passes through the suprascapular notch and beneath the suprascapular ligament before entering the supraspinatus fossa.[170] Compression at the suprascapular ligament is common, and thus, a palsy involving both supraspinatus and infraspinatus is more frequently seen than an isolated infraspinatus denervation on EMG. History of trauma such as shoulder dislocation or scapular fracture is usually present. When this is absent, suprascapular ligament compression, tumor, ganglion, or Parsonage-Turner neuritis should be considered. Reported pain relief and strength increase after surgery have been excellent, with improvement in over 90% of patients.[168,169,171–174] Early surgical treatment appears to yield better results than a delayed operation.[175] This is thought to primarily to prevent the progression of nerve injury as well as muscle atrophy; however, a true association between nerve injury and muscle atrophy reversibility and latency from symptom onset to treatment has yet to be shown. Additionally, the approach to decompression of the suprascapular nerve is still hotly debated among physicians.[176]

Thoracic Outlet Syndrome

The term "thoracic outlet syndrome" (TOS) was coined by Peet[177] to describe compression at the thoracic inlet of the neurovascular bundle composed of the brachial plexus, subclavian vein, and subclavian artery. TOS is most commonly neurogenic in origin. In TOS, unlike other upper extremity entrapments, NCS across the putative entrapment site are not feasible. The diagnosis is therefore typically based on clinical criteria.

TOS has been subdivided into three syndromic zones, according to likelihood of entrapment of the brachial plexus, subclavian artery, and subclavian veins. Anterior scalene syndrome occurs with brachial plexus or subclavian artery compression in the interscalene triangle. Costoclavicular syndrome occurs with compression of any nearby structures in the space between the clavicle and the first rib. Retropectoralis minor syndrome can involve any adjacent structure as well, and compression occurs at the attachment site of pectoralis minor at the coracoid process (the subcoracoid tunnel).[178–181]

In cases of pure peripheral nerve compression, insidious onset of pain and paresthesias in the neck, shoulder, arm, or hand is typical, whereas motor weakness occurs in just 10% of patients. Nearly 90% of cases involve the ulnar nerve distribution.[182] Symptoms may be reproduced when assuming a spear-throwing position or with downward pressure on the shoulder. Tenderness (with or without Tinel sign) over the anterior scalene muscle in the supraclavicular fossa may also be present.

Diagnosis can be aided by imaging and electrodiagnostic studies. In particular, a radiograph demonstrating anomalous bony findings, such as a cervical rib, in the presence of corresponding symptoms is highly predictive of good surgical outcome. Comparing MRIs of the thoracic outlet in the standard anatomic position and following hyperabduction and external rotation of the arm may reveal significant narrowing of the costoclavicular space in patients with TOS compared to normal healthy subjects.[179]

With careful attention to patient selection and surgical technique, good results have been reported with surgical management. Surgery can involve first rib resection, anterior scalenectomy, resection of the costoclavicular ligament, or neuroplasty, depending on suspected pathology.[183] The majority of surgeons employ a transaxillary or supraclavicular approach.

In general, immediate pain relief with surgery is good, although results often deteriorate over time. Numerous outcome studies for the transaxillary approach report greater than 90% of patients enjoy initial symptomatic relief. However, long-term follow-up has revealed that less than 50% of patients sustain relief at 5 years, and less than 10% of patients have relief persisting at 20 years.[181,182,184] Although reported in fewer numbers and with shorter follow-up, outcomes for the supraclavicular approach appear to be equally good in terms of initial results.[185,186] Complications of surgery for TOS are unfortunately common and include vascular injury, brachial plexus injury, and thoracic wall injury.[187]

Entrapments of the Lower Extremities

Of the entrapment syndromes seen in the lower extremities, meralgia paresthetica (symptoms along the lateral femoral cutaneous nerve) is the most common. Inciting factors are many, including trauma, weight gain, and clothing. Indeed, trauma is the foremost cause of peripheral nerve injury in the lower extremities, particularly around the pelvic, inguinal, and ankle regions, often involving the femoral, obturator, ilioinguinal, iliohypogastric, genitofemoral, and posterior tibial nerves. Described chronic compressive syndromes include entrapment of the lateral femoral cutaneous, sciatic, saphenous, posterior tibial, common peroneal, deep peroneal, and plantar digital nerves. Results from surgical management of meralgia paresthetica and Morton's neuroma (of a plantar digital nerve) are discussed with other pathologies treated by neurectomy and will be omitted here.

Sciatic nerve entrapment: The posterior L4–S3 sacral plexus nerve roots typically give rise to the sciatic nerve, which travels anterior to the piriformis muscle before passing beneath its inferior border to exit the pelvis through the greater sciatic foramen posterior to the piriformis muscle, along with the superior and inferior gluteal vessels and nerves. When the sciatic nerve instead travels above or even through the piriformis muscle, a syndrome of gluteal region pain, weakness in hip abduction resulting in a lurching gait, and tenderness to palpation just lateral to the greater sciatic notch can be induced.[188] Weakness in knee flexion in the absence of paraspinous muscle weakness can be suggestive of this peripheral injury as well, and there is often discrete tenderness between the greater trochanter and ischium.

This entrapment syndrome is six times more common in women than in men and often associated with repetitive trauma such as horseback riding, muscular hypertrophy or ossification, or with iatrogenic injury to the sciatic nerve.[189] It can closely mimic the sciatica caused by lumbar disk herniation or spinal stenosis, and MRI is particularly helpful in determining the likelihood of a peripheral nerve entrapment in relation to the far more common spinal etiologies. Electrodiagnostic tests are very difficult to perform reliably in this region and are generally of little utility. Focal tenderness directly over the piriformis muscle, together with normal MRI of lumbar spine, is suggestive of sciatic nerve entrapment.

Surgical management involves sectioning of the overlying piriformis muscle and has provided excellent relief in a limited number of reported cases.[190,191] A feared complication of this procedure is complete sectioning of one of the associated gluteal vessels, which can retract into the pelvis, necessitating laparotomy for hemostasis.[192] There have been case reports of spontaneous entrapment neuropathies involving the distal portions of the sciatic nerve in the thigh.[193,194] Endoscopic release of the piriformis muscle has also been shown to be an effective approach to improving pain symptoms for patients with sciatic nerve entrapment.[195]

Saphenous nerve entrapment: Iatrogenic saphenous nerve injury is commonly a result of saphenous vein harvesting. A similar syndrome that also presents as dysesthesias and pain involving the medial aspect of the knee and anterior tibial region has been treated successfully with surgical release in the subsartorial (Hunter's) canal.[35,196] A fascial band between the abductor magnus and vastus medialis muscles is the offending factor, and pain can typically be elicited on examination with palpation over the canal.

Tibial nerve entrapment: Tibial nerve entrapment at the popliteal fossa results from compression by the tendinous arch of the origin of the soleus muscle as well as from nerve tumors, Baker's cyst, and trauma. As it crosses medially in the popliteal fossa, the tibial nerve travels superficially to the popliteus muscle while passing under the tendinous arch of the soleus muscle before entering the space between the heads of the gastrocnemius and plantaris muscles.[197,198]

Symptoms of tarsal tunnel syndrome result from compression of the posterior tibial nerve at the medial malleolus. The tarsal tunnel itself refers to the deep posterior compartments of the distal leg as they pass beneath the flexor retinaculum, which is formed from the superficial and deep aponeuroses of the leg.[199] Symptoms typically include pain and dysesthesias involving the plantar surface of the foot and sometimes the heel, depending on whether the posterior tibial nerve trifurcates and gives rise to the medial calcaneus sensory branch proximal to the point of compression. Tinel sign over the flexor retinaculum is quite sensitive and specific in the diagnosis of entrapment, particularly when combined with the dorsiflexion–eversion maneuver.[200] In fact, a recent study in 2012 found that a positive Tinel sign over the tibial nerve at the tarsal tunnel in a diabetic patient with chronic nerve condition at the aforementioned location predicts significant pain relief and improvement in plantar sensibility.[201] Both MRI and electrodiagnostic studies are extremely helpful in confirming and assessing severity of the pathology, particularly in recurrent cases and in those rare instances refractory to conservative management.[202–206] The differential diagnosis is wide and includes such common etiologies as CRPS, plantar fasciitis, and Achilles tendonitis.

Surgical sectioning of the flexor retinaculum and release of the nerve has demonstrated only moderate success, perhaps in part due to the success of conservative management in such a large proportion of cases.[207–209] Pfeiffer and Cracchiolo[210] reported 44% of patients received significant improvement after decompression, and two subsequent studies showed similar overall benefit. Sammarco and Chang[211] later reported significantly better surgical outcomes in patients with duration of symptoms lasting less than 1 year, compared with disease present for greater than 1 year. Still, Turan et al.[212] demonstrated that surgical management is still of benefit in those with long-standing symptoms, providing excellent results in 61% of patients who experienced symptoms for more than 5 years.

Peroneal nerve entrapment: Once the sciatic nerve reaches the popliteal fossa, it gives rise to the common peroneal nerve, which then wraps around the fibular head and passes into the peroneal tunnel alongside the peroneus longus tendon. There, it trifurcates, giving off superficial and deep peroneal nerve branches as well as a sensory branch to the tibiofibular joint and knee.[213] Entrapment syndromes typically arise due to compression in the knee (due to fatty tissue deposition or Baker's cyst)

or at the peroneal tunnel, but the superficial and deep branches can be compressed at the fascial exit of the superficial branch over the anterolateral aspect of the lower shin[214] and at the anterior tarsal tunnel bounded by the fascial layers over the talus and the inferior extensor retinaculum, respectively. Several small series of patients undergoing decompression of the superficial and deep branches have shown the efficacy of surgical treatment, but large reports guiding decision making in surgical decompression are lacking.[215–219]

The common peroneal nerve rests in a particularly superficial position at the fibular neck and thus is susceptible to external compression as well as to traction injury. It is also a common site of intraneural ganglia.[213] Neuropathy is commonly found in women who habitually sit in a cross-legged position. Similarly, prolonged squatting or kneeling can cause compressive symptoms. Repetitive plantarflexion and inversion of the foot is often the mechanism of traction on the nerve, and a constricting band at the level of the fibular head is often found at the time of operation. Symptoms most commonly include foot drop, weakness of ankle, dorsiflexion and eversion, and pain in the peroneal nerve dermatome along the lateral leg. The pain symptoms can be easily confused with such common ailments as shin splints or tibial stress fracture as well as with an L5 radiculopathy or compartment syndrome. Electrodiagnostic studies are helpful in isolating the region of entrapment.[220]

Surgical decompression must not be delayed, although conservative management is successful in approximately one-third of cases.[221] In one analysis, 87% of patients with motor dysfunction obtained good improvement, whereas only 54% of patients with purely sensory deficits experienced long-term relief.[222] However, the average time between onset of symptoms and operation was 14 months in this study. In another series, surgical intervention was shown to yield a 97% immediate success rate when performed within 2 months of onset of injury, whereas in cases lasting 4 to 8 months, only a 38% benefit was found.[223]

Dorsal Rhizotomy and Ganglionectomy

BASIC CONSIDERATIONS

The Bell-Magendie model describes a dorsal root composed solely of primary afferent fibers, whereas the ventral root contains only efferent fibers. Dorsal rhizotomy and ganglionectomy procedures seek to take advantage of this apparent physiologic segregation to halt the inflow of nociceptive signals to the spinal cord at particular levels while sparing motor outputs. Injury to motor fibers in the ventral root is avoided (Fig. 103.3). No neuroma forms at the cut ends of the rootlets, as nerve fibers that enter the spinal cord are deprived of their cell body and hence degenerate.[224]

Theoretically an appealing treatment option for pain, rhizotomy in practice often fails to confer the lasting benefit that one might expect. Early surgeons performed dorsal rhizotomy for a broad range of conditions including stump pain, intercostal neuralgia, angina, visceral pain, and spastic hemiplegia. After comparing operative results for pain with those for spasticity in 1911, Groves[225] remarked, "Strangely enough, the division of the posterior spinal roots has given the least satisfactory results in those very cases where we should have expected it to be the most efficient . . . the relief of pain."

An important problem with rhizotomy is that the sensory afferents that arise from a region of the body may provide contributions to multiple spinal nerves. Conversely, fibers from a single spinal nerve may innervate multiple segments of the spinal cord. As a result, sensory dermatomes overlap considerably, so that ablation of a single dorsal root produces little sensory deficit.[226] The earliest studies[227,228] of the dermatomes appreciated this complexity, and early surgeons performed rhizotomy

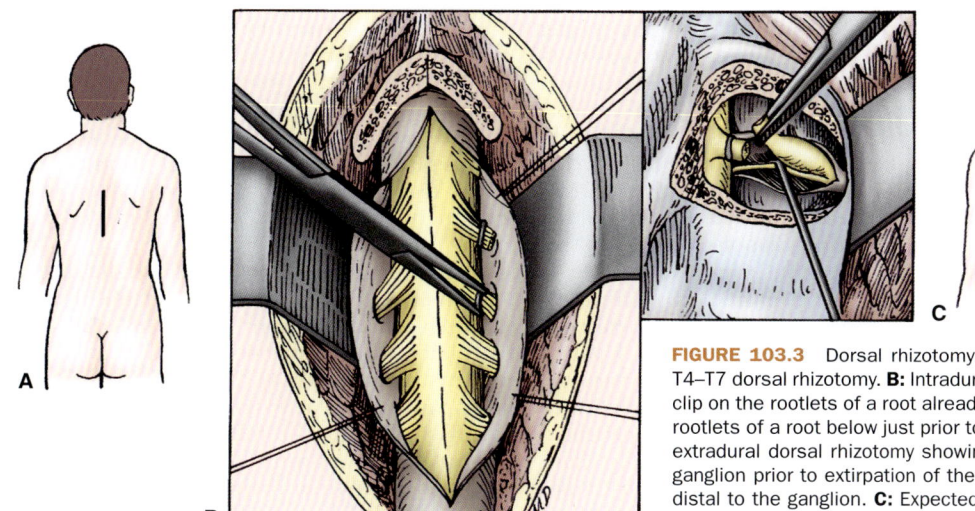

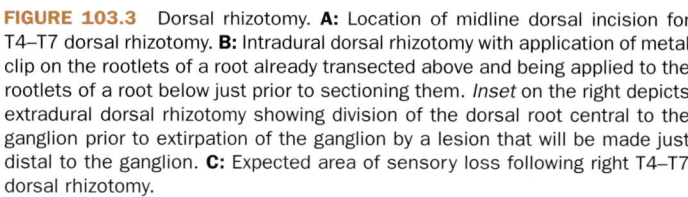

FIGURE 103.3 Dorsal rhizotomy. **A:** Location of midline dorsal incision for T4–T7 dorsal rhizotomy. **B:** Intradural dorsal rhizotomy with application of metal clip on the rootlets of a root already transected above and being applied to the rootlets of a root below just prior to sectioning them. *Inset* on the right depicts extradural dorsal rhizotomy showing division of the dorsal root central to the ganglion prior to extirpation of the ganglion by a lesion that will be made just distal to the ganglion. **C:** Expected area of sensory loss following right T4–T7 dorsal rhizotomy.

at two to three levels or more to achieve pain control.[225] Extensive remodeling of sensory dermatomes, attributed to intraspinal sprouting of dorsal root axons,[229] functional reorganization of existing sensory pathways,[230] and other mechanisms, has since been described.

A second potential explanation of surgical failure involves the presence of unmyelinated sensory fibers in the ventral roots. In 1894, Sherrington noted degeneration of fibers on the cord side of a transected ventral root.[231,232] He suggested that these fibers, which he presumed would double back and reenter the cord through the dorsal root, might provide a physiologic basis for the observation that stimulation of the ventral root results in pain. Microscopy has demonstrated that some fibers do, in fact, enter the cord through ventral roots, cross the ventral horn, and synapse within the dorsal horn or enter the dorsal columns.[233] Thus, dorsal rhizotomy may fail ultimately because of the presence of afferents that reach the spinal cord via the ventral root. However, the actual frequency of ventral root sensory nerves is not known.

To obviate this problem, consideration may be given to performance of a sensory ganglionectomy. The cell body for all primary afferents is believed to reside in the dorsal root ganglion regardless of whether the fibers reach the spinal cord via the dorsal or ventral roots. One report cites a patient with recurrent pain following dorsal rhizotomy that experienced enduring pain relief following removal of the dorsal root ganglia at the same level,[234] providing further evidence that afferents concerned with pain may enter the spinal cord through ventral roots. Ganglionectomy has gained acceptance in the treatment of certain pain disorders.[235] However, including ganglionectomy in a dorsal rhizotomy has not been demonstrated to yield better long-term results, although late recurrence with ganglionectomy is also common.

CLINICAL CONSIDERATIONS
Preoperative Evaluation
Dorsal rhizotomy or sensory ganglionectomy may be attempted for treatment of both nociceptive and neuropathic pain, although in our experience, pain often recurs within a few years. Prediction of the potential effect of an operation can be fairly simple, if only a single level is affected. A number of confounding anatomic situations, such as root-to-root anastomosis or overlap of root innervation, must be considered.[236] Identification of the appropriate spinal level and roots or ganglia for ablation is accomplished through paravertebral local anesthetic

nerve blocks. Spinal epidural or subarachnoid blocks can be used for screening purposes when considering sacral rhizotomy. For greater accuracy in diagnosis, these blocks should be performed at multiple levels, with placebo controls. There is a tendency for the anesthetic to leak into the epidural space, and this may lead to a false-positive result.

Although rhizotomies are now done infrequently for pain, some patients do gain enduring pain relief from rhizotomy or ganglionectomy, with acceptable morbidity. The challenge is to select the patients most likely to benefit. Feasibility dictates the appropriate procedures to some extent. If the clinical problem is limited to one root, ganglionectomy has appeal in order to avoid the problem of ventral root afferents. Unfortunately, surgical ganglionectomy involves destruction of a substantial portion of the facet and therefore may not be practical if two or more roots are involved. Rhizotomy may be preferable in this instance; however, the problem of pain recurrence may be higher. No clinical studies directly compare rhizotomy and ganglionectomy, and differences in outcome between the two procedures are not well understood.

Dorsal rhizotomy and sensory ganglionectomy spare motor efferents and do not lead to the formation of neuromas. However, careful attention must be given to the potential complications of dorsal root surgery. Ablations of the dorsal roots attenuate not only pain but also vibratory, temperature, and proprioceptive inputs. Loss of these sensory functions may be troublesome particularly in the extremities. In addition, with the ablation of the highly vascularized dorsal roots, blood supply to the spinal cord can be jeopardized. Ablation of more than six dorsal roots increases this risk considerably.[226] Finally, dorsal rhizotomy and ganglionectomy, if unsuccessful, preclude the use of dorsal column stimulation as a means of pain treatment because the primary afferents on which the stimulator acts undergo wallerian degeneration.

The following case presents evaluation and treatment of a patient with neuropathic pain, in an ideal setting for performance of a ganglionectomy, although with eventual pain recurrence.

A 42-year-old woman underwent an anterior cervical discectomy and fusion with harvesting of a bone graft from the left iliac crest. An anterior abdominal wall hernia developed at the site of bone harvest. This defect was repaired with mesh, and the patient developed severe pain at the repair site. Eventually, the repair site was explored, and injury to the subcostal nerve (T12) was noted. The neuroma was resected back and relocated to a healthy muscular bed away from scar. Pain was relieved for several weeks and then returned. An additional attempt at neuroma relocation surgery met with the same fate. Opioid treatments as well as other pharmacologic approaches failed to provide satisfactory relief. Nerve root blocks of T12 but not of T11 or L1 led to complete pain relief. A ganglionectomy was performed at T12, and the patient had sustained pain relief for 2 years.

In this case, pain was limited to a single, clearly defined spinal level. The return of pain following neurectomy demonstrated the high likelihood of reformation of a painful neuroma. A single ganglionectomy both eliminated the pain and precluded the reformation of a painful neuroma. However, the pain recurred after 2 years. In our experience, peripheral nerve stimulation, spinal cord stimulation, and intrathecal pain pumps may be preferable and nondestructive first-line therapies for radicular pain prior to performance of sensory rhizotomy or ganglionectomy.

Operative Technique

Dorsal rhizotomy is performed using either an intradural or extradural approach, whereas ganglionectomy is by extradural approach. For intradural rhizotomy, a laminectomy is performed at the levels of interest and the dura is opened, where sensory rootlets are then identified at the intervertebral foramina, followed proximally, and divided. For extradural rhizotomy, the lateral facet is removed and the appropriate nerve roots are exposed laterally. The proximal spinal root is dissected free, and the dorsal rootlet is identified and divided. For ganglionectomy, the dorsal root ganglion is also dissected free and removed. In some cases, separation of the ganglion from the motor root is difficult, and there may be resections of this structure as well, a factor to be borne in mind when selecting the ablative approach. Ganglionectomy can also be performed from a foraminal approach with minor disruption of the facet. Sacral rhizotomy may be accomplished through sacral laminectomy and division of the thecal sac between the S1 and S2 roots.[237]

INDICATIONS AND OUTCOMES

Indications for dorsal rhizotomy or ganglionectomy may be broadly divided into procedures for cancer and noncancer pain[238] and are outlined by the Joint Section on Pain in its 1994 recommendations. In addition, dorsal rhizotomy can be a useful therapy in treatment of certain spasticity disorders, including spastic cerebral palsy. Barrash and Leavens[239] reported success in 70% (50 of 71) of patients with cancer, with 10.5-month average follow-up. By contrast, Onofrio and Campa[240] reported an overall success rate of 41% (46 of 112) in patients with localized idiopathic pain. Wilkinson and Chan[241] reported excellent pain reduction in 74% of patients with dorsal root ganglionectomy alone, with no adverse complications, for pain refractory to other treatments. The differences in success rate between cancer and noncancer pain could potentially result from earlier mortality among patients with cancer-related pain, given the significant incidence of late-recurring pain.

Cranial and Cervical Pain

Rhizotomy of C1–C4 in combination with cranial nerves V, IX, and X may provide effective pain relief from extensive head and neck cancers.[242] In considering such a procedure, one would have to consider the morbidity of such an extensive operation in terms of sensory loss. In some cancer victims, however, sensory loss is already extensive. Dorsal cervical rhizotomy may also be combined with trigeminal tractotomy. Cancers of the lung or breast with brachial plexus involvement, with loss of function in the upper limb, may also benefit from cervical rhizotomy.

Occipital Neuralgia

The greater occipital nerve, formed by the posterior primary ramus of C2, and the lesser occipital nerve, formed by the C2 and C3 roots in the cervical plexus, jointly innervate the occipital region of the scalp. Occipital neuralgia is headache, characterized by severe paroxysmal lancinating or continuous pain, localized to this innervated region.[243] Occipital neuralgia may be due to migraine, compression of the C2 root, entrapment of greater occipital nerve at the superior nuchal line, or nerve injury.[244]

C2 or C3 ganglionectomy, as well as upper intradural cervical rhizotomy, have been used successfully in treatment of occipital neuralgia. Stechison and Mullin[245] reported success in 4 of 4 patients with idiopathic greater occipital neuralgia, with 2-year average follow-up. Lozano et al.[246] reported that patients with occipital neuropathic pain due to trauma are more likely to experience significant pain reduction following C2 ganglionectomy than other patient groups with occipital pain. Onofrio and Campa[240] reported relief from occipital neuralgia in 64% (9 of 14) of patients immediately and 50% (7 of 14) of patients after months to years following ablation of 1 to 3 cervical roots. Dubuisson[247] reported success in 71% (10 of 14) of patients, with 33-month average follow-up, following partial posterior rhizotomy at C1–C3. Cervical nerve block has been shown to be useful for confirmation of occipital neuralgia and possibly as a patient selection tool for rhizotomy.[248] In a recent study, Acar and colleagues reported the return of pain within a year in 65% (13 of 20) of patients undergoing C2 or C3 ganglionectomy.[249] Occipital nerve stimulation may be considered a favorable alternative to C2 or C3 ganglionectomy.[250] However, future work must be completed to further optimize this technology.[251]

All other recent studies recapitulate what is already been said.

Thoracic Pain

Pain associated with chest wall invasion of pleural-based or chest wall malignancies, as well as localized thoracic pain secondary to nerve invasion or compression, can be an indication for dorsal rhizotomy or ganglionectomy. Arbit et al.[252] reported complete pain relief in 64% (9 of 14) and 50% to 100% pain relief in an additional 29% (4 of 14) of patients with cancer pain, with 22-month median follow-up, following thoracic dorsal and ventral rhizotomy. Smith[253] reported success in 10 of 10 patients with intercostal pain due to thoracotomy (7), herpes zoster (2), and cancer (1), following thoracic ganglionectomy.

Postsurgical Truncal Pain

Persistent pain following thoracotomy or laparotomy may be responsive to dorsal rhizotomy. White and Kjellberg[226] reported successful treatment of intercostal neuralgia in 3 of 4 patients, with 8-month median follow-up, following thoracic rhizotomy. Loeser[238] reported success in 33% (1 of 3) of patients at more than 3 months. By contrast, Onofrio and Campa[240] reported on 18 patients with postthoracotomy pain and 5 patients with postlaparotomy pain, none of whom obtained benefit. White and Kjellberg[226] also reported successful treatment of postherniorrhaphy neuralgia in 3 of 4 patients, with 2-year median follow-up, following thoracolumbar rhizotomy. There are no large series of patients on which to base management decisions.

One case report demonstrated complete resolution of pain symptoms from postthoracotomy pain syndrome using spinal cord stimulation at 4-month follow-up. However, the authors cite that this technique must be further researched and refined.[254]

Sacral Pain

Cancers of the colon, rectum, urinary tract, cervix, and prostate may result in pain attributable to sacral roots. Unfortunately, ablation of the second and third sacral roots may affect bladder,

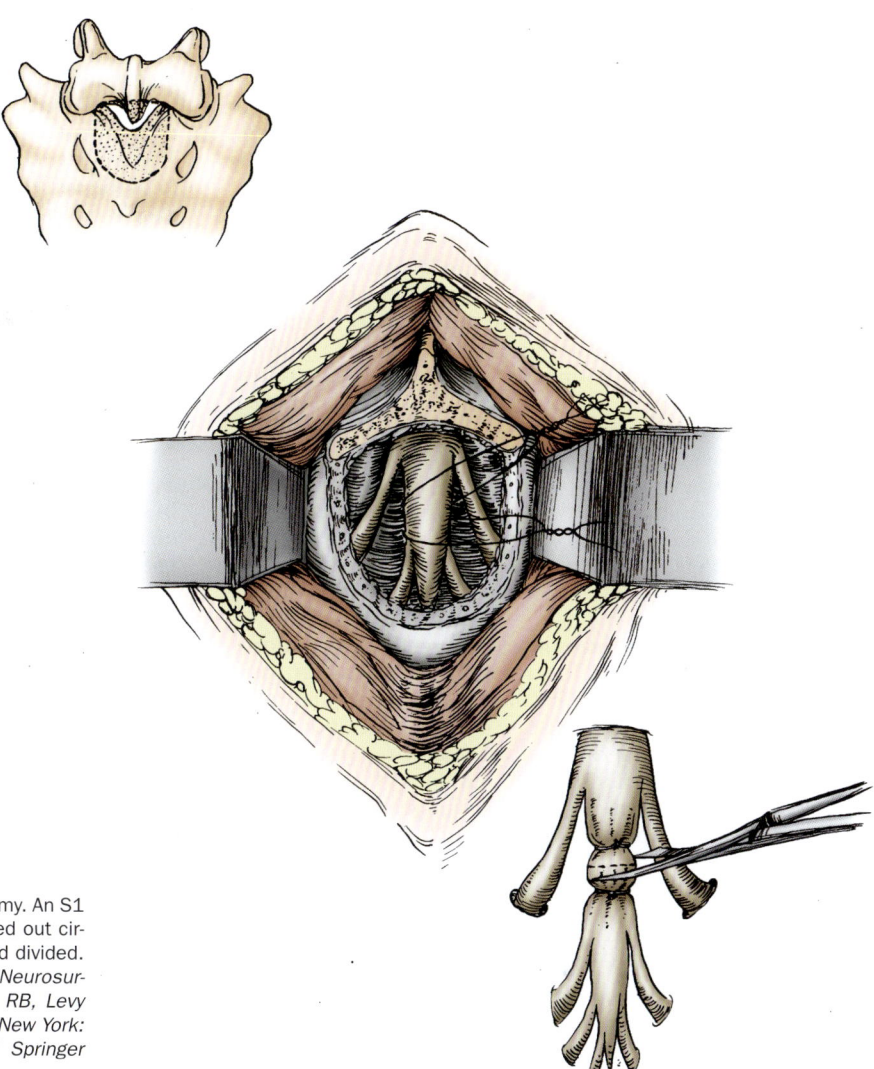

FIGURE 103.4 Technique of extradural sacral rhizotomy. An S1 laminectomy is performed, and thecal sac is dissected out circumferentially between S2 and S3, doubly ligated, and divided. *(Reprinted by permission from Springer: Burchiel KJ. Neurosurgical procedures of the peripheral nerves. In: North RB, Levy RM, eds.* Neurosurgical Management of Pain. *1st ed. New York: Springer-Verlag; 1997:133–161. Copyright © 1997 Springer Science+Business Media New York.)*

sphincter, and sexual function. Thus, sacral root division is indicated in cases of pelvic cancer pain, where patients have already lost bladder and bowel function. It is a simple procedure that may confer striking benefit. Saris et al.[255] reported success in 47% (7 of 15) of patients with colorectal cancer presenting with perianal pain, with 1-year median follow-up, following bilateral S3–S5 rhizotomy. Felsoory and Crue[237] reported satisfactory results in 69% (20 of 28) of patients with colorectal (17), cervical (5), anal (3), and other (3) cancers, with unstated follow-up duration, following transection of the cauda equina at L5/S1. The surgical anatomy is depicted in Figure 103.4.

A 14-year single-center study showed an 87.5%, 84.8%, and 73% improvement in patients with idiopathic urinary retention, urgency urinary incontinence, and painful bladder syndrome with sacral neuromodulation.[256] This technology has, however, been studied and used more in the treatment of fecal incontinence.

Extremity Pain

Rhizotomy or ganglionectomy is indicated for denervation of a functionally useless limb. There are few other indications in the treatment of extremity pain. That multiple roots may be involved, the morbidity of sensory loss, and the problem of frequent pain recurrence, lead to infrequent use of these procedures for extremity pain. Ganglionectomy for monoradicular extremity pain has been proposed but remains unproven.[257]

North et al.[258] reported greater than 50% relief from failed back surgery syndrome in none of the 13 patients they studied, with 5.5-year average follow-up.[258] By contrast, Taub et al.[259] reported success in 59% (36 of 61) of patients with intractable monoradicular sciatica following dorsal root ganglionectomy, with 5- to 9-year median follow-up. This unusually high rate of success likely reflects very careful patient selection.

The choice of rhizotomy or ganglionectomy for treatment of extremity pain requires a balance between compromise of function due to elimination of sensation and the elimination of pain. For the upper extremity, White and Kjellberg[226] reported successful treatment of diffuse upper extremity pain in 50% (7 of 14) of patients, with 3-year median follow-up, following rhizotomy at various levels. Following the procedure, none of the patients complained of unpleasant numbness or clumsiness of the hand, perhaps reflecting the seriousness of the preoperative condition. In the lower extremity, they reported successful treatment of lateral femoral cutaneous neuralgia in 67% (4 of 6) of patients, with 3-year median follow-up, following L2–L3 rhizotomy. Spinal cord stimulation may offer a nondestructive alternative to rhizotomy or ganglionectomy for the treatment of extremity pain. In addition, recent work has shown that stimulation of the dorsal root ganglion at certain spinal levels provides longer lasting relief than does traditional spinal cord stimulation. Yang and Hunter[260] reported successful treatment of traditional spinal cord stimulator failed CRPS in two patients with the use of dorsal root ganglion stimulation. Huygen and colleagues[261] reported 50% improvement in patients with failed back surgery syndrome who had undergone L2–L3 dorsal root ganglion stimulation. Although this technology is continuing to be refined and studied, these nonablative and modifiable methods of improving pain outcomes may indeed show promising outcomes over more traditional ablative procedures.

Visceral Pain

Although rarely used today due to the advent of other techniques, dorsal rhizotomy has been reported to be highly effective in controlling visceral pain. White and Kjellberg[226] reported successful treatment of medically intractable angina in 75% (3 of 4) of patients, with 14-month median follow-up, following T1–T4 rhizotomy. Success was 50% (3 of 6) for treatment of other forms of visceral pain.[226]

Peripheral subcutaneous nerve stimulation has been recently introduced as a new technology to improve the symptoms of abdominal pain from a variety of sources including hernia repair and painful surgical scars. However, no long-term trails have been completed to prove its effectiveness.

Axial Spine Pain

Lumbar median branch rhizotomy via percutaneous radiofrequency ablation is indicated for treatment of facet arthropathy pain and is discussed in detail in Chapter 102. Local and radicular pain due to lumbar spine disease is largely unresponsive, in the longer term, to dorsal rhizotomy. Loeser[238] reported success in 75% (12 of 16) at up to 3 months but only 14% (2 of 14) at more than 3 months for patients with disk disease. Onofrio and Campa[240] reported improvement in 17% (11 of 64) of patients with lumbosacral pain following rhizotomy, with unstated follow-up. Wetzel et al.[262] reported success in 55% (28 of 51) at up to 6 months and 19% (7 of 37) at 2 years for patients with lumbar radiculopathy after lumbar surgery.

Taub and colleagues[259] reported similar findings in that patients with intractable radicular pain who underwent ganglionectomy, 59% achieved reduced or eliminated pain symptoms. However, dysesthesias developed in a significant number (60%) of these patients. Therefore, there may be a role for ganglionectomy in the treatment of axial spine pain, but it must be weighed against the development of other painful symptoms (dorsal root ganglion for intractable monoradicular sciatica).

Postherpetic Neuralgia

Dermatomal pain following herpetic infection responds poorly to dorsal rhizotomy. Loeser[238] reported failure in 2 of 2 patients. Onofrio and Campa[240] reported success in only 20% (1 of 5) of patients, with 5-year follow-up, following unilateral rhizotomy. The treatment of postherpetic neuralgia is discussed in Chapter 27. A 2002 study showed 82% of patients with postherpetic neuralgia treated with spinal cord stimulation showed long-term pain relief and significant improvement in pain-limiting activities of daily living. In fact, 8 patients in the study had their stimulators removed between 3 and 66 months postimplantation because of complete pain relief, possibly suggesting that the stimulation induces some form of plasticity within the central nervous system to achieve complete resolution of pain symptoms.[263]

Sympathectomy

BASIC CONSIDERATIONS
Sympathetic Efferents

Sympathetic efferents reach their target structures in two steps. Preganglionic sympathetic efferents arise in the intermediolateral cell column of the spinal cord at T1–L3. Thinly myelinated fibers emerge in the ventral roots and transit briefly through the

spinal nerve before exiting to form the white rami communicantes, leading to the paravertebral sympathetic ganglia. Some preganglionic fibers form synapses in the sympathetic chain with postganglionic neurons, from which unmyelinated fibers return to the spinal nerves, forming the gray rami communicantes. These postganglionic efferents provide sympathetic innervation to blood vessels, sweat glands, and other structures. Other preganglionic fibers pass through the paravertebral sympathetic chain without forming synapses and continue to the prevertebral ganglia. In the prevertebral ganglia, these efferents synapse with postganglionic effector neurons. From the prevertebral ganglia, unmyelinated fibers innervate the abdominal and pelvic viscera. Sympathectomy has been used in the treatment of pain from the limbs, the heart, and abdominal viscera. Presacral neurectomy and thoracic sympathectomy for cardiac pain are discussed earlier in this chapter and are not further addressed here.

Sympathetically Maintained Pain

In some patients with chronic pain syndromes, the pain depends on the activity of sympathetic efferents in the painful area. This pain, termed *sympathetically maintained pain* (SMP), is defined as that aspect of pain that is relieved by blockade of sympathetic efferents.[264] Pain that is unaffected by the activity of sympathetic efferents is termed *sympathetically independent pain*. The diagnosis of SMP is empiric; that is, it is made based on response to treatment. In any pain syndrome, a portion may be sympathetically maintained, although another part is sympathetically independent. Notably, CRPS and other neuropathic conditions may or may not be associated with SMP.

Traditionally, three distinct mechanisms have been considered as ways through which ablation of sympathetic nerves or ganglia may lead to pain relief:

1. The sympathetic efferents in T1–L3 that pass through paravertebral sympathetic ganglia to abdominal and pelvic viscera do not travel alone. They are accompanied by afferents, with cell bodies in the dorsal root ganglia of T1–L3, which convey sensory information about distension and inflammation of visceral organs to the central nervous system. As a result of this colocalization, ablation of prevertebral ganglia (or the nerves originating from them) interrupts the flow of nociceptive signals from visceral structures to brain, thereby producing pain relief. Hence, as a treatment for visceral pain, sympathectomy is a form of sensory neurectomy.

2. Sympathectomy may improve pain associated with ischemia. Sympathetic efferents maintain arterial tone. In vasospastic and vasoocclusive conditions, the vasodilation consequent to sympathectomy may ameliorate ischemia, thereby decreasing pain.[265]

3. Finally, sympathectomy may eliminate norepinephrine-mediated activation of nociceptors and thereby relieve SMP. In this section, we concentrate on this latter mechanism and extremity pain related to CRPS in which a component of pain has been demonstrated to be sympathetically maintained.

Understanding of the pathophysiologic mechanisms underlying SMP continues to increase. The involvement of both A and polymodal C nociceptors is evident although incompletely elucidated.[266,267] Immunologically mediated mechanisms involving prostaglandin, bradykinin, substance P, neuropeptide Y, and calcitonin gene-related peptide have also been proposed in treatment-resistant patients.[268,269] Increased expression of class I and II human leukocyte antigen in patients diagnosed with reflex sympathetic dystrophy suggests a genetic predisposition to poor treatment response,[270] although a relationship to SMP has not been defined.

By definition, SMP is eliminated by blockade of sympathetic efferent innervation of the painful area. Thus, anesthetic blockade of the relevant sympathetic ganglia relieves pain in patients with SMP. Stimulation of the sympathetic chain evokes pain in patients with SMP but not in those without SMP.[25] Moreover, Walker and Nulson[271] noted that stimulation of the severed distal end of the sympathetic chain evokes pain in those diagnosed with SMP but not in other patients. Thus, the central connections of sympathetic efferent fibers are not required for stimulation of the sympathetic system to evoke pain. These observations establish that efferent sympathetic fibers, rather than afferent sensory fibers that may travel with sympathetic fibers, account for SMP in nonvisceral pain syndromes.

Several independent lines of pharmacologic evidence support the claim that norepinephrine released from sympathetic fibers is critical in SMP. First, regional infusion of guanethidine, which acts to deplete norepinephrine from sympathetic terminals, relieves pain in patients with SMP.[272] Second, in patients whose pain had been relieved by either sympathetic block or sympathectomy, a cutaneous injection of norepinephrine into the previously painful area rekindles the pain and hyperalgesia. However, norepinephrine injected intracutaneously into normal subjects induces less pain and less hyperalgesia.[273,274] Finally, administration of sympathetic β-adrenergic antagonists, such as prazosin, phenoxybenzamine, or phentolamine, relieves SMP.[273,275-277]

Following nerve injury, neuromas that form may acquire sensitivity to norepinephrine. Injection of pH-balanced norepinephrine solution into normal subcutaneous tissues causes little pain. However, injection of norepinephrine onto painful neuromas does induce pain.[278] Thus, nerve injury may be associated with the induction of SMP.

These observations suggest that an abnormal increase in the amount of norepinephrine released from sympathetic terminals is not likely to be the mechanism of SMP. Rather, it is the response to norepinephrine that appears to be critical. Studies continue to support this theory, demonstrating the benefit of perioperative pharmacologic sympathetic block in reducing recurrence.[279,280] Whether this change is due to an upregulation of β-adrenergic receptors or increased receptor sensitivity is unknown.

CLINICAL CONSIDERATIONS
Preoperative Evaluation
SMP cannot be diagnosed purely from history and physical examination of the patient.[281] However, it must be differentiated from similar-appearing chronic pain syndromes, particularly peripheral nerve injury. A number of clinical features are helpful: (1) In general, SMP does not occur in places other than the extremities or face. As a rule, the likelihood of developing SMP parallels the density of sympathetic innervation of the skin. Hence, truncal pain is far less likely to be due to SMP than is extremity pain. (2) Signs that may be inferred to represent increased sympathetic activity in the painful area do not necessarily denote the presence of SMP.[282] For example, limbs associated with SMP may be warmer, cooler, or the same temperature as unaffected limbs. Similarly, differences in sweating, nail growth, and muscle tone do not reliably contribute to the diagnosis of SMP. Nonetheless, sweating abnormalities in particular, as well as temperature alterations in general, may have some diagnostic utility.[283] We have found that among patients with traumatic nerve or soft tissue injury with touch-evoked pain, all patients with SMP and 50% of patients with sympathetically independent pain have striking sensitivity to mild cooling stimuli.[7,284]

Due to adverse effects and lack of definitive supporting evidence, surgical sympathectomy is typically reserved for medically refractory SMP. Careful patient selection is critical to success. Thus, preoperative evaluation is of great importance. Mechanical allodynia with temperature change and cooling hyperalgesia together form an indication for

sympathetic blockade.[282] The effect of sympathetic blockade via regional blockade or systemic infusion, in turn, plays an important role in identifying patients who might benefit from sympathectomy. High rates of recurrence, either due to sympathetic chain regeneration or new-onset CRPS, as well as significant adverse effects of the operation, serve to further highlight the need for discriminating patient selection. Finally, early intervention is important to optimize patient outcomes.

Quantitative sensory testing: Essentially all patients with SMP have cooling hyperalgesia.[281,284] In fact, patients with SMP often spontaneously volunteer that the one stimulus that they most dread is cooling of the painful area. Cooling hyperalgesia occurs less frequently in patients with sympathetically independent pain. This suggests that cooling hyperalgesia is a highly sensitive although not specific, indicator of SMP.

Local anesthetic sympathetic ganglion blocks: The traditional procedure to diagnose SMP is percutaneous injection of local anesthetic onto the sympathetic ganglia serving the painful region. In local anesthetic sympathetic ganglion blocks (LASB), ganglia are localized through anatomic landmarks, ideally under fluoroscopic guidance, and local anesthetic is injected into the region. The presence of local anesthetic at the ganglia prevents norepinephrine from being released into peripheral tissues. Although frequently used to diagnose SMP, LASB results must be interpreted with care: (1) Incomplete block of individual ganglia may falsely underestimate the contribution of SMP to a painful condition. The extent of sympathetic block must be evaluated by assaying for effects of sympathetic block, such as changes in skin temperature. (2) Spread of local anesthetic onto somatic afferents in the nerve roots, or blockade of sensory afferents that accompany sympathetic efferents, may induce pain relief by way of somatic block rather than sympathetic block. Careful sensory examination must be performed to ensure that somatic afferents are not affected by injection of local anesthetic. (3) LASB may evoke a placebo response, causing overestimation of pain relief. In addition to these interpretive issues, LASB has some risk. Complications reported with LASB include pneumothorax, phrenic and laryngeal nerve block, cardiac arrhythmia, kidney injury, hemorrhage, and inadvertent intravascular or epidural injections (see Chapter 98 for a detailed discussion of the role of local anesthetic blocks in the diagnosis of SMP).

Systemic phentolamine infusion: An alternative strategy to assess the potential efficacy of sympathectomy involves intravenous infusion of phentolamine, a short-acting antagonist of α-adrenergic receptors.[273,276] There is good correlation between pain relief with LASB and that with systemic phentolamine infusion (SPI).[281,285] As a systemic infusion, phentolamine does not provide any information about anatomic localization, as is available with LASB. However, SPI has a number of advantages over LASB: (1) The test is painless in that the phentolamine is delivered systemically and does not require fluoroscopy or needles to be placed in the paravertebral space; (2) with SPI, a significant observation period can be used prior to the administration of the drug, and the patient can be blinded to the time of drug administration, allowing a placebo-control period in every trial; and (3) SPI appears to be safer than LASB, with only nasal stuffiness and peripheral vasodilation reported as side effects.[286] Furthermore, because the activity of nearby sensory afferents is preserved, SPI appears to be a more specific diagnostic test for SMP.[281,285]

Intravenous regional block: A third method to detect SMP involves regional intravenous infusion of an agent that impedes peripheral release of norepinephrine,[272] known as a Bier block. Sympatholytic agents studied include bretylium, reserpine, and guanethidine.[284] To avoid systemic circulation of the sympatholytic agent, a tourniquet is applied to the limb during the test. The central advantage of intravenous regional block (IRB) is localization of sympathetic block to the limb of interest.

However, there are shortcomings: (1) Some patients poorly tolerate the required tourniquet application; (2) the dramatic release of sympathetic neurotransmitter accompanying infusion of guanethidine in SMP patients may be severely painful; (3) the blocking agent may leak beyond the tourniquet, in some instances with significant hemodynamic effects; (4) the need for a tourniquet makes IRB difficult to perform either in the trunk or in the lower extremity; and (5) it is difficult to evaluate placebo responses with IRB. Although frequently mentioned as a means to diagnose and to treat SMP, we believe that IRB has few advantages. The same degree of β-receptor blockade can be achieved with systemic phentolamine.

Medical treatment of sympathetically maintained pain: Once the diagnosis of SMP is made, the mainstay of treatment is medical sympatholysis, with surgical intervention reserved for refractory cases. A remarkable feature of SMP is that extended sympathetic blockade may lead to long-term or permanent relief from the disorder. When the goal of blockade is diagnosis, the diagnostic technique should be specific to the sympathetic nervous system. By contrast, when the goal is treatment, there need not be specificity. There are several medical and interventional means by which to achieve sympatholysis. The choice of technique should be based on considerations of safety, comfort, and efficacy.

Multiple sympathetic ganglion blocks with local anesthetics have, in the past, served as the criterion standard for treatment. However, local anesthetic treatment of peripheral nerves may work as well by inducing similar blockade of the distal sympathetic fibers. For example, SMP in the upper extremity could be treated either by LASB of thoracic sympathetic ganglia or by local anesthetic application to the appropriate nerves.

Alternatively, although epidural administration of anesthetic may lack specificity as a means to diagnose SMP, it may provide an effective treatment regimen. Epidural clonidine, although limited by hemodynamic effects, provides extensive analgesia.[287] SPI has been used successfully to treat SMP in a patient with pain in all extremities due to Sjögren's associated polyneuropathy.[288]

When episodic treatments fail to provide adequate relief, chronic treatment with oral sympatholytics may reduce SMP. Both phenoxybenzamine and prazosin have been used in this manner.[275,277] However, the systemic hypotension that frequently accompanies the use of these agents may preclude adequate

sympathetic blockade. Finally, topical clonidine, which is likely to inhibit local norepinephrine release, may be a low-morbidity treatment of SMP in some patients, albeit locally.[273,289] If well tolerated, this and other medical techniques could substantially reduce the need for surgical sympathectomy; indeed the role for surgical sympathectomy remains in question.

Operative Techniques

To achieve sympathectomy of the upper extremity, it is necessary to resect the T2, T3, and T4 sympathetic ganglia. Removal of less than all three ganglia risks inadequate sympathectomy for pain. One of our patients required extension of the sympathectomy to T5. This is best achieved through a thoracoendoscopic technique, although the data on this operation have been acquired through open supraclavicular transaxillary or posterior costotransversectomy approaches. By contrast, the lumbar sympathetic chain, most commonly involving L2 and L3 ganglia, is generally accessed through an anterolateral retroperitoneal surgical approach. Percutaneous approaches have been suggested, but these procedures often do not achieve enduring results. In addition, the scarring produced by these approaches makes later surgical treatment more difficult.

Many clinicians have reported limited success in the treatment of pain by surgical sympathectomy.[290,291] Failure of sympathectomy may reflect inadequacies either of the preoperative evaluation, as discussed earlier, or of the extent of the sympathectomy. For example, sympathetic outflow to the arm derives predominantly from the T2 and T3 ganglia and not from the stellate ganglion. Failure to remove the T2 ganglion, at a minimum, will result in continued sympathetic innervation of the hand. An important feature in the lower extremity is that sympathetic innervation is often bilateral. Bilateral lumbar sympathectomy of L2–L4 is typically necessary (Fig. 103.5). A typical patient history is one of impressive relief of pain lasting several weeks following an ipsilateral lumbar sympathectomy. The pain then returns, and at that time, the pain may be relieved by a contralateral block of the lumbar sympathetic ganglia. Patients will typically have enduring relief of pain following contralateral lumbar sympathectomy.[292,293] As in the upper extremity, complete sympathectomy is required for pain relief; the partial denervation that is successful for vascular diseases is not adequate as a treatment for pain.

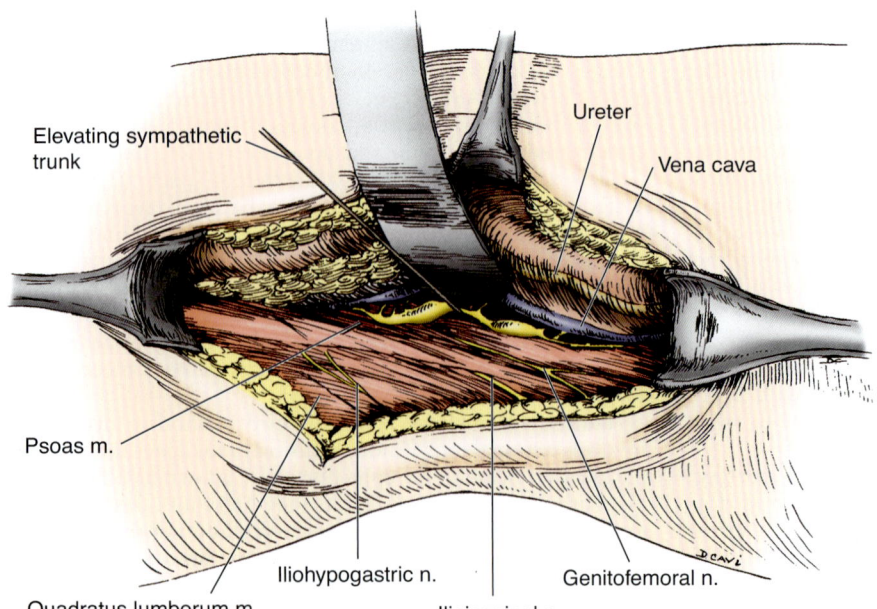

Elevating sympathetic trunk

Ureter

Vena cava

Psoas m.

Quadratus lumborum m.

Iliohypogastric n.

Genitofemoral n.

Ilioinguinal n.

FIGURE 103.5 Open lumbar sympathectomy is done through retroperitoneal exposure of the sympathetic chain. (*Reprinted by permission from Springer: Wilkinson HA. Neurosurgical procedures of the sympathetic nervous system. In: North RB, Levy RM, eds. Neurosurgical Management of Pain. 1st ed. New York: Springer-Verlag; 1997:162–175. Copyright © 1997 Springer Science+Business Media New York.*)

INDICATIONS AND OUTCOMES

Ulmer and Mayfield[294] reported successful treatment of 96% (67 of 70) of soldiers with burning pain due to nerve injury by surgical sympathectomy of appropriate ganglia. In studies of a civilian population, Manart et al.[295] reported a "good" response to thoracic sympathectomy in 59% (13 of 22) of patients with burning posttraumatic pain, even when diagnostic blockades were not typically performed. For patients selected for preoperative diagnostic sympathetic block, Mockus et al.[296] reported improvement in 94% (29 of 31) of patients, with 3.4 years average follow-up. AbuRahma et al.[297] reported 1-year satisfactory improvement of pain in 20 of 21 patients. Overall success rates of 90% or greater with surgical sympathectomy have been reported by several groups.[298] Thompson[299] reported successful surgical treatment in 46% (55 of 120) of patients with SMP following minor trauma, who were unresponsive to medical therapy. Overall, long-term successful outcomes in 70% to 85% of cases of thoracic, and slightly less in lumbar sympathectomy, can be expected.

As noted, results of sympathectomy largely depend on careful patient selection.[277] Our experience has been that patients do extremely well if the pain responds dramatically to sympathetic ganglion block and systemic infusion of phentolamine, and there is provocation of pain with injection of norepinephrine when the patient is under the influence of LASB. Although our conclusions are preliminary, it appears that if one or more of these elements are missing, the patient does not fare as well. The modest response rates to sympathectomy in earlier series may reflect improper patient selection and inadequate sympathectomy (e.g., bilateral sympathectomy required for lower extremity pain) or more extensive unilateral ganglionectomy for total denervation of an extremity.

POSTOPERATIVE COMPLICATIONS

Surgical sympathectomy may be associated with idiosyncratic complications. One frequent complication, affecting up to 20% to 50% of patients, is postsympathectomy pain.[296,300,301] This condition is characterized by the sudden onset, a few weeks after the procedure, of superficial burning pain, deep aching pain, and cutaneous hyperalgesia.[302] The pain arises in the *proximal* regions of limbs and the trunk despite surgical ablation of sympathetic innervation to the *distal* limbs. Fortunately for the majority of patients, postsympathectomy pain resolves spontaneously in several weeks to a few months, and no further surgical intervention is warranted.[300]

Ablation of sympathetic input to a region of skin results in sudomotor paralysis. In the upper extremity, the resultant dryness can be uncomfortable. In the lower extremity, dryness is better tolerated. Postural hypotension also can be a transient problem. However, even in patients with sympathectomy of all four extremities, this problem is usually not enduring. Compensatory hyperhidrosis, as well as pathologic gustatory sweating, may be found in patients following sympathectomy.[303] Two additional complications of sympathectomy include paradoxical vasoconstriction and ileus. Sympathetic fibers arising from the celiac and mesenteric ganglia modulate gastrointestinal motility. Both complications are generally transient.

CRPS is defined as a chronic pain disorder that has a propensity to affect only one limb (arm, leg, etc.) and is disproportionate in terms of how long the pain lasts or how intense the pain is compared to any known trauma or other lesion. It is also a progressive disease that is not confined to a certain nerve territory or dermatome and has a predilection for producing distal sensory and motor symptoms including burning sensations, allodynia, and hyperalgesia.[304]

SCS has been shown to be beneficial in the treatment of CRPS. Although traditional SCS is the primary type of SCS that is used clinically, one study showed that dorsal root ganglion SCS is superior to traditional SCS for the treatment of CRPS.[305] However, traditional SCS has been shown to be superior to other treatments for CRPS. Kemler and Furnee[306] studied a population of patients who were initially unable to work due to severe pain and disability and were refractory to physical therapy (PT) and other medical treatments. These patients were then either randomized to a control group that received only PT or the experimental group that received SCS and PT. The study showed that the patients who were randomized to the SCS-with-PT group had a greater than 50% decrease in their pain at 6 months compared to the PT-only group. Additionally, the study showed that at 1 year, patients in the SCS-with-PT group had a marked improvement in their quality of life compared to the PT-only group. They did not, however, observe any difference in functional status or psychological depression between the two studied groups.[306,307] Another study showed that pain caused by CRPS decreased on average by 45% after treatment with SCS.[308] These studies and others demonstrate that using SCS for medically refractory CRPS is beneficial.

Conclusion

The peripheral nervous system offers a number of attractive strategies for treatment of pain. Peripheral nerves may be transected or released from regions of entrapment. Where regional pain control is required, sensory roots or ganglia may be the targets of therapy. In cases where pain has a significant sympathetically maintained component, sympathectomy may offer significant and long-lasting pain relief.

As for all surgical procedures, careful patient selection and clear establishment of the etiology of the painful condition is critical to ensure successful analgesia. Enthusiasm for these surgical procedures must be tempered by a keen appreciation of potential complications.

Nerve transection may either produce or eliminate pain. This leaves the clinician with the sometimes daunting task of deciding if, when, and how to perform neurectomy. Each patient must be carefully evaluated. In the case of minor nerves previously transected, the clinician should not labor over the decision to relocate the neuroma to a protected, unscarred site. In this instance, there is little to lose.

Pain due to mechanical compression may be relieved through release of nerve root entrapments. Carpal tunnel release and release of UNEE are among the most commonly performed peripheral nerve procedures. However, many less common forms of nerve root entrapment may be overlooked or misdiagnosed. A systematic understanding of peripheral neuroanatomy on the part of the pain clinician is essential to accurate diagnosis and treatment of these pain syndromes.

Dorsal rhizotomy is seldom used in modern practice, but a survey of the existing literature reveals that patients certainly exist in whom rhizotomy conferred long-term benefit. Today's pain clinician does well to keep this option in mind in properly selected cases. Ganglionectomy has certain theoretical advantages over rhizotomy and neurectomy and is still another technique that should be considered in certain cases. However, recurrence of pain several years after surgery may be quite common.

Sympathectomy is helpful in patients with persistent SMP who are refractory to medical management. Recognition of the clinical symptoms of SMP, such as cold allodynia, and appropriate selection of sympathetic blockade modalities are required to make the diagnosis and to provide a successful treatment strategy. Hence, the key to success with this procedure, as with most surgery, is meticulous patient selection and proper execution of the operation.

Peripheral electrical neuromodulation, a nonablative surgical intervention for the treatment of pain, is emerging as a promising therapeutic approach for well-selected patients. This technology is still evolving, and further research will need to be conducted to objectively show improvements in the quality of pain improvement as well as the exact mechanism by which this technique works on a cellular and network basis.

References

1. Kim KJ, Yoon YW, Chung JM. Comparison of three rodent neuropathic pain models. *Exp Brain Res* 1997;113(2):200–206.
2. Denny-Brown D, Kirk E. Hyperesthesia from spinal and root lesions. *Trans Am Neurol Assoc* 1968;93:116–120.
3. Wall PD, Gutnick M. Properties of afferent nerve impulses originating from a neuroma. *Nature* 1974;248(5451):740–743.
4. Wall PD, Gutnick M. Ongoing activity in peripheral nerves: the physiology and pharmacology of impulses originating from a neuroma. *Exp Neurol* 1974;43(3):580–593.
5. Wall PD, Waxman S, Basbaum AI. Ongoing activity in peripheral nerve: injury discharge. *Exp Neurol* 1974;45(3):576–589.
6. Mitchell SW. *Injuries of Nerves and Their Consequences*. Philadelphia: J. B. Lippincott; 1872.
7. Frost SA, Raja SN, Campbell JN. Does hyperalgesia to cooling stimuli characterize patients with sympathetically maintained pain (reflex sympathetic dystrophy)? In: Dubnar R, Gebhart GF, Bond MR, eds. *Proceedings of the Vth World Congress on Pain*. New York: Elsevier; 1988.
8. Lang E, Spitzer A, Pfannmüller D, et al. Function of thick and thin nerve fibers in carpal tunnel syndrome before and after surgical treatment. *Muscle Nerve* 1995;18(2):207–215.
9. Koschorke GM, Meyer RA, Campbell JN. Cellular components necessary for mechanoelectrical transduction are conveyed to primary afferent terminals by fast axonal transport. *Brain Res* 1994;641(1):99–104.
10. Koschorke GM, Meyer RA, Tillman DB, et al. Ectopic excitability of injured nerves in monkey: entrained responses to vibratory stimuli. *J Neurophysiol* 1991;65(3):693–701.
11. Xiao Y, Segal MR, Rabert D, et al. Assessment of differential gene expression in human peripheral nerve injury. *BMC Genomics* 2002;3(1):28.
12. Thacker MA, Clark AK, Marchand F, et al. Pathophysiology of peripheral neuropathic pain: immune cells and molecules. *Anesth Analg* 2007;105(3):838–847.
13. Campbell JN, Meyer RA. Mechanisms of neuropathic pain. *Neuron* 2006;52(1):77–92.
14. Atherton DD, Elliot D. Relocation of neuromas of the lateral antebrachial cutaneous nerve of the forearm into the brachialis muscle. *J Hand Surg Eur Vol* 2007;32(3):311–315.
15. Atherton DD, Leong JC, Anand P, et al. Relocation of painful end neuromas and scarred nerves from the zone II territory of the hand. *J Hand Surg Eur Vol* 2007;32(1):38–44.
16. Dellon AL, Kim J, Ducic I. Painful neuroma of the posterior cutaneous nerve of the forearm after surgery for lateral humeral epicondylitis. *J Hand Surg Am* 2004;29(3):387–390.
17. Dellon AL, Mackinnon SE. Treatment of the painful neuroma by neuroma resection and muscle implantation. *Plast Reconstr Surg* 1986;77(3):427–438.
18. Hazari A, Elliot D. Treatment of end-neuromas, neuromas-in-continuity and scarred nerves of the digits by proximal relocation. *J Hand Surg Br* 2004;29(4):338–350.
19. Novak CB, van Vliet D, Mackinnon SE. Subjective outcome following surgical management of lower-extremity neuromas. *J Reconstr Microsurg* 1995;11(3):175–177.
20. Novak CB, van Vliet D, Mackinnon SE. Subjective outcome following surgical management of upper extremity neuromas. *J Hand Surg Am* 1995;20(2):221–226.
21. Sood MK, Elliot D. Treatment of painful neuromas of the hand and wrist by relocation into the pronator quadratus muscle. *J Hand Surg Br* 1998;23(2):214–219.
22. Stahl S, Rosenberg N. Surgical treatment of painful neuroma in medial antebrachial cutaneous nerve. *Ann Plast Surg* 2002;48(2):154–158.
23. D'Mello R, Dickenson AH. Spinal cord mechanisms of pain. *Br J Anaesth* 2008;101(1):8–16.
24. Kirvelä O, Nieminen S. Treatment of painful neuromas with neurolytic blockade. *Pain* 1990;41(2):161–165.
25. White JC, Sweet WH. *Pain and the Neurosurgeon: A Forty-Year Experience*. Springfield, IL: Charles C. Thomas; 1969.
26. Economides JM, DeFazio MV, Attinger CE, et al. Prevention of painful neuroma and phantom limb pain after transfemoral amputations through concomitant nerve coaptation and collagen nerve wrapping. *Neurosurgery* 2016;79(3):508–513.
27. Lai YY, Chen SC, Chien NC. Video-assisted thoracoscopic neurectomy of intercostal nerves in a patient with intractable cancer pain. *Am J Hosp Palliat Care* 2006;23(6):475–478.
28. Stulz P, Pfeiffer KM. Peripheral nerve injuries resulting from common surgical procedures in the lower portion of the abdomen. *Arch Surg* 1982;117(3):324–327.
29. Starling JR, Harms BA. Diagnosis and treatment of genitofemoral and ilioinguinal neuralgia. *World J Surg* 1989;13(5):586–591.
30. Amid PK. Causes, prevention, and surgical treatment of postherniorrhaphy neuropathic inguinodynia: triple neurectomy with proximal end implantation. *Hernia* 2004;8(4):343–349.
31. Aasvang E, Kehlet H. Surgical management of chronic pain after inguinal hernia repair. *Br J Surg* 2005;92(7):795–801.
32. Chen DC, Hiatt JR, Amid PK. Operative management of refractory neuropathic inguinodynia by a laparoscopic retroperitoneal approach. *JAMA Surg* 2013;148(10):962–967.
33. Williams PH, Trzil KP. Management of meralgia paresthetica. *J Neurosurg* 1991;74(1):76–80.
34. de Ruiter GC, Wurzer JA, Kloet A. Decision making in the surgical treatment of meralgia paresthetica: neurolysis versus neurectomy. *Acta Neurochir (Wien)* 2012;154(10):1765–1772.
35. Luerssen TG, Campbell RL, Defalque RJ, et al. Spontaneous saphenous neuralgia. *Neurosurgery* 1983;13(3):238–241.
36. Lora J, Long DM. So-called facet denervation in the management of intractable back pain. *Spine* 1976;1:121–126.
37. Hakim SM, Narouze SN. Risk factors for chronic saphenous neuralgia following coronary artery bypass graft surgery utilizing saphenous vein grafts. *Pain Pract* 2015;15(8):720–729.
38. Johnson JE, Johnson KA, Unni KK. Persistent pain after excision of an interdigital neuroma. Results of reoperation. *J Bone Joint Surg Am* 1988;70(5):651–657.
39. Dereymaeker G, Schroven I, Steenwerckx A, et al. Results of excision of the interdigital nerve in the treatment of Morton's metatarsalgia. *Acta Orthop Belg* 1996;62(1):22–25.
40. Gauthier G. Thomas Morton's disease: a nerve entrapment syndrome. A new surgical technique. *Clin Orthop Relat Res* 1979;(142):90–92.
41. Chuter GS, Chua YP, Connell DA, et al. Ultrasound-guided radiofrequency ablation in the management of interdigital (Morton's) neuroma. *Skeletal Radiol* 2013;42(1):107–111.
42. Burchiel KJ, Johans TJ, Ochoa J. The surgical treatment of painful traumatic neuromas. *J Neurosurg* 1993;78(5):714–719.
43. Stokvis A, van der Avoort DJ, van Neck JW, et al. Surgical management of neuroma pain: a prospective follow-up study. *Pain* 2010;151(3):862–869.
44. Mackinnon SE, Dellon AL. *Surgery of the Peripheral Nerve*. New York: Thieme Medical Publishers; 1988.
45. Belzberg AJ, Campbell JN. Evidence for end-to-side sensory nerve regeneration in a human. Case report. *J Neurosurg* 1998;89(6):1055–1057.
46. Bogduk N, Long DM. The anatomy of the so-called "articular nerves" and their relationship to facet denervation in the treatment of low-back pain. *J Neurosurg* 1979;51(2):172–177.
47. Shealy CN. Percutaneous radiofrequency denervation of spinal facets. Treatment for chronic back pain and sciatica. *J Neurosurg* 1975;43(4):448–451.
48. Schofferman J, Kine G. Effectiveness of repeated radiofrequency neurotomy for lumbar facet pain. *Spine* 2004;29(21):2471–2473.
49. Lord SM, Barnsley L, Wallis BJ, et al. Percutaneous radio-frequency neurotomy for chronic cervical zygapophyseal-joint pain. *N Engl J Med* 1996;335(23):1721–1726.
50. Cohen SP, Bajwa ZH, Kraemer JJ, et al. Factors predicting success and failure for cervical facet radiofrequency denervation: a multi-center analysis. *Reg Anesth Pain Med* 2007;32(6):495–503.
51. Cohen SP, Hurley RW, Christo PJ, et al. Clinical predictors of success and failure for lumbar facet radiofrequency denervation. *Clin J Pain* 2007;23(1):45–52.
52. Silvers HR. Lumbar percutaneous facet rhizotomy. *Spine* 1990;15(1):36–40.
53. Oudenhoven RC. Paraspinal electromyography following facet rhizotomy. *Spine* 1977;2:299–304.
54. Buck-Gramcko D. Denervation of the wrist joint. *J Hand Surg Am* 1977;2(1):54–61.
55. Wilhelm A. Tennis elbow: treatment of resistant cases by denervation. *J Hand Surg Br* 1996;21(4):523–533.
56. Dellon AL, Mont MA, Mullick T, et al. Partial denervation for persistent neuroma pain around the knee. *Clin Orthop Relat Res* 1996;(329):216–222.
57. Tekin I, Mirzai H, Ok G, et al. A comparison of conventional and pulsed radiofrequency denervation in the treatment of chronic facet joint pain. *Clin J Pain* 2007;23(6):524–529.
58. Ingersoll FM, Meigs JV. Presacral neurectomy for dysmenorrhea. *N Engl J Med* 1948;238:357–360.
59. Nezhat CH, Seidman DS, Nezhat FR, et al. Long-term outcome of laparoscopic presacral neurectomy for the treatment of central pelvic pain attributed to endometriosis. *Obstet Gynecol* 1998;91(5 pt 1):701–704.
60. Hayek SM, Deer TR, Pope JE, et al. Intrathecal therapy for cancer and non-cancer pain. *Pain Physician* 2011;14(3):219–248.
61. Raslan AM, Cetas JS, McCartney S, et al. Destructive procedures for control of cancer pain: the case for cordotomy. *J Neurosurg* 2011;114(1):155–170.
62. Omer GE, Spinner M, Van Beek A. *Management of Peripheral Nerve Problems*. 2nd ed. Philadelphia: Saunders; 1998.
63. Pecina M, Krmpotic-Nemanic J, Markiewitz AD. *Tunnel Syndromes: Peripheral Nerve Compression Syndromes*. 3rd ed. Boca Raton, FL: CRC Press; 2001.

64. Rempel D, Dahlin L, Lundborg G. Pathophysiology of nerve compression syndromes: response of peripheral nerves to loading. *J Bone Joint Surg Am* 1999;81(11):1600–1610.

65. Mackinnon SE, Dellon AL, Hudson AR, et al. A primate model for chronic nerve compression. *J Reconstr Microsurg* 1985;1(3):185–195.

66. Novak CB, Mackinnon SE. Nerve injury in repetitive motion disorders. *Clin Orthop Relat Res* 1998;(351):10–20.

67. Ochoa J, Fowler TJ, Gilliatt RW. Anatomical changes in peripheral nerves compressed by a pneumatic tourniquet. *J Anat* 1972;113(pt 3):433–455.

68. Ochoa J, Marotte L. The nature of the nerve lesion caused by chronic entrapment in the guinea-pig. *J Neurol Sci* 1973;19(4):491–495.

69. Dahlin LB, Lundborg G. The neurone and its response to peripheral nerve compression. *J Hand Surg Br* 1990;15(1):5–10.

70. Rydevik B, Lundborg G, Bagge U. Effects of graded compression on intraneural blood blow. An in vivo study on rabbit tibial nerve. *J Hand Surg Am* 1981;6(1):3–12.

71. Dyck PJ, Lais AC, Giannini C, et al. Structural alterations of nerve during cuff compression. *Proc Natl Acad Sci U S A* 1990;87(24):9828–9832.

72. Lundborg G. Structure and function of the intraneural microvessels as related to trauma, edema formation, and nerve function. *J Bone Joint Surg Am* 1975;57(7):938–948.

73. Lundborg G, Myers R, Powell H. Nerve compression injury and increased endoneurial fluid pressure: a "miniature compartment syndrome." *J Neurol Neurosurg Psychiatry* 1983;46(12):1119–1124.

74. Powell HC, Myers RR. Pathology of experimental nerve compression. *Lab Invest* 1986;55(1):91–100.

75. Abramowitz J, Dion JE, Jensen ME, et al. Angiographic diagnosis and management of head and neck schwannomas. *AJNR Am J Neuroradiol* 1991;12(5):977–984.

76. Rudge P, Ochoa J, Gilliatt RW. Acute peripheral nerve compression in the baboon. *J Neurol Sci* 1974;23(3):403–420.

77. Drake CG. Diagnosis and treatment of lesions of the brachial plexus and adjacent structures. *Clin Neurosurg* 1964;11:110–127.

78. Stull MA, Moser RP Jr, Kransdorf MJ, et al. Magnetic resonance appearance of peripheral nerve sheath tumors. *Skeletal Radiol* 1991;20(1):9–14.

79. Fullerton PM. The effect of ischaemia on nerve conduction in the carpal tunnel syndrome. *J Neurol Neurosurg Psychiatry* 1963;26:385–397.

80. Beard L, Kumar A, Estep HL. Bilateral carpal tunnel syndrome caused by Graves' disease. *Arch Intern Med* 1985;145(2):345–346.

81. O'Duffy JD, Randall RV, MacCarty CS. Median neuropathy (carpal-tunnel syndrome) in acromegaly. A sign of endocrine overactivity. *Ann Intern Med* 1973;78(3):379–383.

82. Schiller F, Kolb FO. Carpal tunnel syndrome in acromegaly. *Neurology* 1954;4(4):271–282.

83. Weimer LH, Yin J, Lovelace RE, et al. Serial studies of carpal tunnel syndrome during and after pregnancy. *Muscle Nerve* 2002;25(6):914–917.

84. Kline DG, Hudson AR. *Nerve Injuries: Operative Results for Major Nerve Injuries, Entrapments, and Tumors*. Philadelphia: W. B. Saunders; 1995.

85. Neary D, Ochoa J, Gilliatt RW. Sub-clinical entrapment neuropathy in man. *J Neurol Sci* 1975;24(3):283–298.

86. Dellon AL, Mackinnon SE. Chronic nerve compression model for the double crush hypothesis. *Ann Plast Surg* 1991;26(3):259–264.

87. Jablecki CK, Andary MT, So YT, et al. Literature review of the usefulness of nerve conduction studies and electromyography for the evaluation of patients with carpal tunnel syndrome. AAEM Quality Assurance Committee. *Muscle Nerve* 1993;16(12):1392–1414.

88. Rivner MH. Statistical errors and their effect on electrodiagnostic medicine. *Muscle Nerve* 1994;17(7):811–814.

89. Robinson LR, Micklesen PJ, Wang L. Strategies for analyzing nerve conduction data: superiority of a summary index over single tests. *Muscle Nerve* 1998;21(9):1166–1171.

90. Britz GW, Haynor DR, Kuntz C, et al. Carpal tunnel syndrome: correlation of magnetic resonance imaging, clinical, electrodiagnostic, and intraoperative findings. *Neurosurgery* 1995;37(6):1097–1103.

91. Hochman MG, Zilberfarb JL. Nerves in a pinch: imaging of nerve compression syndromes. *Radiol Clin North Am* 2004;42(1):221–245.

92. Jarvik JG, Yuen E, Kliot M. Diagnosis of carpal tunnel syndrome: electrodiagnostic and MR imaging evaluation. *Neuroimaging Clin N Am* 2004;14(1):93–102, viii.

93. Maurer J, Bleschkowski A, Tempka A, et al. High-resolution MR imaging of the carpal tunnel and the wrist. Application of a 5-cm surface coil. *Acta Radiol* 2000;41(1):78–83.

94. Grant GA, Britz GW, Goodkin R, et al. The utility of magnetic resonance imaging in evaluating peripheral nerve disorders. *Muscle Nerve* 2002;25(3):314–331.

95. Hughes R. Treatment of peripheral nerve disorders. *Curr Opin Neurol* 2005;18(5):554–556.

96. Lowe JB, Mackinnon SE. Controversies in peripheral nerve surgery. *Neurosurg Clin N Am* 2001;12:267–284.

97. Martin BI, Levenson LM, Hollingworth W, et al. Randomized clinical trial of surgery versus conservative therapy for carpal tunnel syndrome [ISRCTN84286481]. *BMC Musculoskelet Disord* 2005;6:2.

98. Stevens JC, Sun S, Beard CM, et al. Carpal tunnel syndrome in Rochester, Minnesota, 1961 to 1980. *Neurology* 1988;38(1):134–138.

99. Jarvik JG, Yuen E, Haynor DR, et al. MR nerve imaging in a prospective cohort of patients with suspected carpal tunnel syndrome. *Neurology* 2002;58(11):1597–1602.

100. Phalen GS. The carpal-tunnel syndrome. Clinical evaluation of 598 hands. *Clin Orthop Relat Res* 1972;83:29–40.

101. Mackinnon SE, Novak CB, Landau WM. Clinical diagnosis of carpal tunnel syndrome. *JAMA* 2000;284(15):1924–1926.

102. O'Connor D, Marshall S, Massy-Westropp N. Non-surgical treatment (other than steroid injection) for carpal tunnel syndrome. *Cochrane Database Syst Rev* 2003;(1):CD003219.

103. Cseuz KA, Thomas JE, Lambert EH, et al. Long-term results of operation for carpal tunnel syndrome. *Mayo Clin Proc* 1966;41(4):232–241.

104. Gainer JV Jr, Nugent GR. Carpal tunnel syndrome: report of 430 operations. *South Med J* 1977;70(3):325–328.

105. Gerritsen AA, de Vet HC, Scholten RJ, et al. Splinting vs surgery in the treatment of carpal tunnel syndrome: a randomized controlled trial. *JAMA* 2002;288(10):1245–1251.

106. Lanz U. Anatomical variations of the median nerve in the carpal tunnel. *J Hand Surg Am* 1977;2(1):44–53.

107. Werner RA, Andary M. Carpal tunnel syndrome: pathophysiology and clinical neurophysiology. *Clin Neurophysiol* 2002;113(9):1373–1381.

108. Turner A, Kimble F, Gulyas K, et al. Can the outcome of open carpal tunnel release be predicted? A review of the literature. *ANZ J Surg* 2010;80(1–2):50–54.

109. Kiloh LG, Nevin S. Isolated neuritis of the anterior interosseous nerve. *Br Med J* 1952;1(4763):850–851.

110. Collins DN, Weber ER. Anterior interosseous nerve syndrome. *South Med J* 1983;76(12):1533–1537.

111. Spinner M, Schreiber SN. Anterior interosseous-nerve paralysis as a complication of supracondylar fractures of the humerus in children. *J Bone Joint Surg Am* 1969;51(8):1584–1590.

112. Warren JD. Anterior interosseous nerve palsy as a complication of forearm fractures. *J Bone Joint Surg Br* 1963;45:511–512.

113. Lake PA. Anterior interosseous nerve syndrome. *J Neurosurg* 1974;41(3):306–309.

114. Spinner M. The anterior interosseous-nerve syndrome, with special attention to its variations. *J Bone Joint Surg Am* 1970;52(1):84–94.

115. Yasunaga H, Shiroishi T, Ohta K, et al. Fascicular torsion in the median nerve within the distal third of the upper arm: three cases of nontraumatic anterior interosseous nerve palsy. *J Hand Surg Am* 2003;28(2):206–211.

116. Kim DH, Murovic JA, Kim YY, et al. Surgical treatment and outcomes in 15 patients with anterior interosseous nerve entrapments and injuries. *J Neurosurg* 2006;104(5):757–761.

117. Joist A, Joosten U, Wetterkamp D, et al. Anterior interosseous nerve compression after supracondylar fracture of the humerus: a metaanalysis. *J Neurosurg* 1999;90(6):1053–1056.

118. Laha RK, Dujovny M, DeCastro SC. Entrapment of median nerve by supracondylar process of the humerus. Case report. *J Neurosurg* 1977;46(2):252–255.

119. Aydinlioglu A, Cirak B, Akpinar F, et al. Bilateral median nerve compression at the level of Struthers' ligament. Case report. *J Neurosurg* 2000;92(4):693–696.

120. Werner CO, Rosen I, Thorngren KG. Clinical and neurophysiologic characteristics of the pronator syndrome. *Clin Orthop Relat Res* 1985;(197):231–236.

121. Spinner M, Spencer PS. Nerve compression lesions of the upper extremity. A clinical and experimental review. *Clin Orthop Relat Res* 1974;(104):46–67.

122. Clark CB. Cubital tunnel syndrome. *JAMA* 1979;241(8):801–802.

123. Hirasawa Y, Sawamura H, Sakakida K. Entrapment neuropathy due to bilateral epitrochleoanconeus muscles: a case report. *J Hand Surg Am* 1979;4(2):181–184.

124. Matev B. Cubital tunnel syndrome. *Hand Surg* 2003;8(1):127–131.

125. Novak CB, Lee GW, Mackinnon SE, et al. Provocative testing for cubital tunnel syndrome. *J Hand Surg Am* 1994;19(5):817–820.

126. Greenwald D, Blum LC III, Adams D, et al. Effective surgical treatment of cubital tunnel syndrome based on provocative clinical testing without electrodiagnostics. *Plast Reconstr Surg* 2006;117(5):87e–91e.

127. Dellon AL. Operative techniques for submuscular transposition of the ulnar nerve. *Contemp Orthop* 1988;16:17–24.

128. Harrison MJ, Nurick S. Results of anterior transposition of the ulnar nerve for ulnar neuritis. *Br Med J* 1970;1(5687):27–29.

129. Kleinman WB, Bishop AT. Anterior intramuscular transposition of the ulnar nerve. *J Hand Surg Am* 1989;14(6):972–979.

130. Learmonth JR. A technique for transplanting the ulnar nerve. *Surg Gynec Ostet* 1942;75:792–793.

131. Lowe JB III, Novak CB, Mackinnon SE. Current approach to cubital tunnel syndrome. *Neurosurg Clin N Am* 2001;12(2):267–284.

132. Nouhan R, Kleinert JM. Ulnar nerve decompression by transposing the nerve and Z-lengthening the flexor-pronator mass: clinical outcome. *J Hand Surg Am* 1997;22(1):127–131.

133. Pasque CB, Rayan GM. Anterior submuscular transposition of the ulnar nerve for cubital tunnel syndrome. *J Hand Surg Br* 1995;20(4):447–453.

134. Richmond JC, Southmayd WW. Superficial anterior transposition of the ulnar nerve at the elbow for ulnar neuritis. *Clin Orthop Relat Res* 1982;(164):42–44.

135. Siegel DB. Submuscular transposition of the ulnar nerve. *Hand Clin* 1996;12(2):445–448.

136. Bartels RH, Menovsky T, Van Overbeeke JJ, et al. Surgical management of ulnar nerve compression at the elbow: an analysis of the literature. *J Neurosurg* 1998;89(5):722–727.

137. Bartels RH, Verhagen WI, van der Wilt GJ, et al. Prospective randomized controlled study comparing simple decompression versus anterior subcutaneous transposition for idiopathic neuropathy of the ulnar nerve at the elbow: part 1. *Neurosurgery* 2005;56(3):522–530.

138. Dellon AL. Review of treatment results for ulnar nerve entrapment at the elbow. *J Hand Surg Am* 1989;14(4):688–700.

139. Dellon AL. Techniques for successful management of ulnar nerve entrapment at the elbow. *Neurosurg Clin N Am* 1991;2(1):57–73.

140. Kim DH, Han K, Tiel RL, et al. Surgical outcomes of 654 ulnar nerve lesions. *J Neurosurg* 2003;98(5):993–1004.

141. Amadio PC. Anatomical basis for a technique of ulnar nerve transposition. *Surg Radiol Anat* 1986;8(3):155–161.

142. Chan RC, Paine KW, Varughese G. Ulnar neuropathy at the elbow: comparison of simple decompression and anterior transposition. *Neurosurgery* 1980;7(6):545–550.

143. Heithoff SJ. Cubital tunnel syndrome does not require transposition of the ulnar nerve. *J Hand Surg Am* 1999;24(5):898–905.

144. LeRoux PD, Ensign TD, Burchiel KJ. Surgical decompression without transposition for ulnar neuropathy: factors determining outcome. *Neurosurgery* 1990;27(5):709–714.

145. Miller RG. The cubital tunnel syndrome: diagnosis and precise localization. *Ann Neurol* 1979;6(1):56–59.

146. Grantham SA. Ulnar compression in the loge de Guyon. *JAMA* 1966;197(6):509–510.

147. Moneim MS. Ulnar nerve compression at the wrist. Ulnar tunnel syndrome. *Hand Clin* 1992;8(2):337–344.

148. Zeiss J, Jakab E, Khimji T, et al. The ulnar tunnel at the wrist (Guyon's canal): normal MR anatomy and variants. *AJR Am J Roentgenol* 1992;158(5):1081–1085.

149. Kleinert JM, Mehta S. Radial nerve entrapment. *Orthop Clin North Am* 1996;27(2):305–315.

150. Uriburu IJ, Morchio FJ, Marin JC. Compression syndrome of the deep motor branch of the ulnar nerve (Piso-Hamate Hiatus syndrome). *J Bone Joint Surg Am* 1976;58(1):145–147.

151. Chien AJ, Jamadar DA, Jacobson JA, et al. Sonography and MR imaging of posterior interosseous nerve syndrome with surgical correlation. *AJR Am J Roentgenol* 2003;181(1):219–221.

152. Konjengbam M, Elangbam J. Radial nerve in the radial tunnel: anatomic sites of entrapment neuropathy. *Clin Anat* 2004;17(1):21–25.

153. Spinner M. The arcade of Frohse and its relationship to posterior interosseous nerve paralysis. *J Bone Joint Surg Br* 1968;50(4):809–812.

154. Lister GD, Belsole RB, Kleinert HE. The radial tunnel syndrome. *J Hand Surg Am* 1979;4(1):52–59.

155. Moss SH, Switzer HE. Radial tunnel syndrome: a spectrum of clinical presentations. *J Hand Surg Am* 1983;8(4):414–420.

156. Rinker B, Effron CR, Beasley RW. Proximal radial compression neuropathy. *Ann Plast Surg* 2004;52(2):174–180.

157. Verhaar J, Spaans F. Radial tunnel syndrome. An investigation of compression neuropathy as a possible cause. *J Bone Joint Surg Am* 1991;73(4):539–544.

158. Roquelaure Y, Raimbeau G, Dano C, et al. Occupational risk factors for radial tunnel syndrome in industrial workers. *Scand J Work Environ Health* 2000;26(6):507–513.

159. Mayer JH, Mayfield FH. Surgery of the posterior interosseous branch of the radial nerve: analysis of 58 cases. *Surg Gynec Obstet* 1947;84:593–595.

160. Atroshi I, Johnsson R, Ornstein E. Radial tunnel release. Unpredictable outcome in 37 consecutive cases with a 1–5 year follow-up. *Acta Orthop Scand* 1995;66(3):255–257.

161. Hashizume H, Nishida K, Nanba Y, et al. Non-traumatic paralysis of the posterior interosseous nerve. *J Bone Joint Surg Br* 1996;78(5):771–776.

162. Sotereanos DG, Varitimidis SE, Giannakopoulos PN, et al. Results of surgical treatment for radial tunnel syndrome. *J Hand Surg Am* 1999;24(3):566–570.

163. Dellon AL, Mackinnon SE. Radial sensory nerve entrapment in the forearm. *J Hand Surg Am* 1986;11(2):199–205.

164. Kim DH, Kam AC, Chandika P, et al. Surgical management and outcome in patients with radial nerve lesions. *J Neurosurg* 2001;95(4):573–583.

165. Lanzetta M, Foucher G. Entrapment of the superficial branch of the radial nerve (Wartenberg's syndrome). A report of 52 cases. *Int Orthop* 1993;17(6):342–345.

166. Fritz RC, Helms CA, Steinbach LS, et al. Suprascapular nerve entrapment: evaluation with MR imaging. *Radiology* 1992;182(2):437–444.

167. Post M, Grinblat E. Nerve entrapment about the shoulder girdle. *Hand Clin* 1992;8(2):299–306.

168. Rengachary SS, Neff JP, Singer PA, et al. Suprascapular entrapment neuropathy: a clinical, anatomical, and comparative study. Part 1: clinical study. *Neurosurgery* 1979;5(4):441–446.

169. Zehetgruber H, Noske H, Lang T, et al. Suprascapular nerve entrapment. A meta-analysis. *Int Orthop* 2002;26(6):339–343.

170. Rengachary SS, Burr D, Lucas S, et al. Suprascapular entrapment neuropathy: a clinical, anatomical, and comparative study. Part 2: anatomical study. *Neurosurgery* 1979;5(4):447–451.

171. Antoniadis G, Richter HP, Rath S, et al. Suprascapular nerve entrapment: experience with 28 cases. *J Neurosurg* 1996;85(6):1020–1025.

172. Callahan JD, Scully TB, Shapiro SA, et al. Suprascapular nerve entrapment. A series of 27 cases. *J Neurosurg* 1991;74(6):893–896.

173. Fabre T, Piton C, Leclouerec G, et al. Entrapment of the suprascapular nerve. *J Bone Joint Surg Br* 1999;81(3):414–419.

174. Vastamaki M, Goransson H. Suprascapular nerve entrapment. *Clin Orthop Relat Res* 1993;(297):135–143.

175. Post M. Diagnosis and treatment of suprascapular nerve entrapment. *Clin Orthop Relat Res* 1999;(368):92–100.

176. Moen TC, Babatunde OM, Hsu SH, et al. Suprascapular neuropathy: what does the literature show? *J Shoulder Elbow Surg* 2012;21(6):835–846.

177. Peet RM, Hendriksen JD, Anderson TP, et al. Thoracic outlet syndrome: evaluation of the therapeutic exercise program. *Proc Staff Meet Mayo Clin* 1956;31:281–287.

178. Atasoy E. Thoracic outlet syndrome: anatomy. *Hand Clin* 2004;20(1):7–14.

179. Demondion X, Bacqueville E, Paul C, et al. Thoracic outlet: assessment with MR imaging in asymptomatic and symptomatic populations. *Radiology* 2003;227(2):461–468.

180. Urschel HC Jr. Anatomy of the thoracic outlet. *Thorac Surg Clin* 2007;17(4):511–520.

181. Urschel HC, Patel A. Thoracic outlet syndromes. *Curr Treat Options Cardiovasc Med* 2003;5(2):163–168.

182. Urschel HC Jr, Razzuk MA. Neurovascular compression in the thoracic outlet: changing management over 50 years. *Ann Surg* 1998;228(4):609–617.

183. Sheth RN, Campbell JN. Surgical treatment of thoracic outlet syndrome: a randomized trial comparing two operations. *J Neurosurg Spine* 2005;3(5):355–363.

184. Qvarfordt PG, Ehrenfeld WK, Stoney RJ. Supraclavicular radical scalenectomy and transaxillary first rib resection for the thoracic outlet syndrome. A combined approach. *Am J Surg* 1984;148(1):111–116.

185. Dellon AL. The results of supraclavicular brachial plexus neurolysis (without first rib resection) in management of post-traumatic "thoracic outlet syndrome." *J Reconstr Microsurg* 1993;9(1):11–17.

186. Hempel GK, Rusher AH Jr, Wheeler CG, et al. Supraclavicular resection of the first rib for thoracic outlet syndrome. *Am J Surg* 1981;141(2):213–215.

187. Melliere D, Becquemin JP, Etienne G, et al. Severe injuries resulting from operations for thoracic outlet syndrome: can they be avoided? *J Cardiovasc Surg (Torino)* 1991;32(5):599–603.

188. Pecina M. Contribution to the etiological explanation of the piriformis syndrome. *Acta Anat (Basel)* 1979;105(2):181–187.

189. Papadopoulos SM, McGillicuddy JE, Albers JW. Unusual cause of 'piriformis muscle syndrome.' *Arch Neurol* 1990;47(10):1144–1146.

190. Patil PG, Friedman AH. Surgical exposure of the sciatic nerve in the gluteal region: anatomic and historical comparison of two approaches. *Neurosurgery* 2005;56(1 suppl):165–171.

191. Rask MR. Superior gluteal nerve entrapment syndrome. *Muscle Nerve* 1980;3(4):304–307.

192. Russell SM, Kline DG. Complication avoidance in peripheral nerve surgery: injuries, entrapments, and tumors of the extremities—part 2. *Neurosurgery* 2006;59(4 suppl 2):ONS449–ONS456.

193. Banerjee T, Hall CD. Sciatic entrapment neuropathy. Case report. *J Neurosurg* 1976;45(2):216–217.

194. Venna N, Bielawski M, Spatz EM. Sciatic nerve entrapment in a child. Case report. *J Neurosurg* 1991;75(4):652–654.

195. Martin HD, Shears SA, Johnson JC, et al. The endoscopic treatment of sciatic nerve entrapment/deep gluteal syndrome. *Arthroscopy* 2011;27(2):172–181.

196. Mozes M, Ouaknine G, Nathan H. Saphenous nerve entrapment simulating vascular disorder. *Surgery* 1975;77(2):299–303.

197. Mastaglia FL. Tibial nerve entrapment in the popliteal fossa. *Muscle Nerve* 2000;23(12):1883–1886.

198. Sansone V, Sosio C, da Gama Malcher M, et al. Two cases of tibial nerve compression caused by uncommon popliteal cysts. *Arthroscopy* 2002;18(2):E8.

199. Zeiss J, Fenton P, Ebraheim N, et al. Normal magnetic resonance anatomy of the tarsal tunnel. *Foot Ankle* 1990;10(4):214–218.

200. Kinoshita M, Okuda R, Morikawa J, et al. The dorsiflexion-eversion test for diagnosis of tarsal tunnel syndrome. *J Bone Joint Surg Am* 2001;83-A(12):1835–1839.

201. Lee Dellon A, Muse VL, Scott Nickerson D. A positive Tinel sign as predictor of pain relief or sensory recovery after decompression of chronic tibial nerve compression in patients with diabetic neuropathy. *J Reconstr Microsurg* 2012;28(4):235–240.

202. Edwards WG, Lincoln CR, Bassett FH III, et al. The tarsal tunnel syndrome. Diagnosis and treatment. *JAMA* 1969;207(4):716–720.

203. Frey C, Kerr R. Magnetic resonance imaging and the evaluation of tarsal tunnel syndrome. *Foot Ankle* 1993;14(3):159–164.

204. Mondelli M, Morana P, Padua L. An electrophysiological severity scale in tarsal tunnel syndrome. *Acta Neurol Scand* 2004;109(4):284–289.

205. Recht MP, Donley BG. Magnetic resonance imaging of the foot and ankle. *J Am Acad Orthop Surg* 2001;9(3):187–199.

206. Chhabra A, Subhawong TK, Williams EH, et al. High-resolution MR neurography: evaluation before repeat tarsal tunnel surgery. *AJR Am J Roentgenol* 2011;197(1):175–183.

207. Bailie DS, Kelikian AS. Tarsal tunnel syndrome: diagnosis, surgical technique, and functional outcome. *Foot Ankle Int* 1998;19(2):65–72.

208. Day FN III, Naples JJ. Endoscopic tarsal tunnel release: update 96. *J Foot Ankle Surg* 1996;35(3):225–229.

209. Takakura Y, Kitada C, Sugimoto K, et al. Tarsal tunnel syndrome. Causes and results of operative treatment. *J Bone Joint Surg Br* 1991;73(1):125–128.

210. Pfeiffer WH, Cracchiolo A III. Clinical results after tarsal tunnel decompression. *J Bone Joint Surg Am* 1994;76(8):1222–1230.

211. Sammarco GJ, Chang L. Outcome of surgical treatment of tarsal tunnel syndrome. *Foot Ankle Int* 2003;24(2):125–131.

212. Turan I, Rivero-Melian C, Guntner P, et al. Tarsal tunnel syndrome. Outcome of surgery in longstanding cases. *Clin Orthop Relat Res* 1997;(343):151–156.

213. Spinner RJ, Atkinson JL, Scheithauer BW, et al. Peroneal intraneural ganglia: the importance of the articular branch. Clinical series. *J Neurosurg* 2003;99(2):319–329.

214. Yang LJ, Gala VC, McGillicuddy JE. Superficial peroneal nerve syndrome: an unusual nerve entrapment. Case report. *J Neurosurg* 2006;104(5):820–823.

215. Akyuz G, Us O, Turan B, et al. Anterior tarsal tunnel syndrome. *Electromyogr Clin Neurophysiol* 2000;40(2):123–128.

216. Banerjee T, Koons DD. Superficial peroneal nerve entrapment. Report of two cases. *J Neurosurg* 1981;55(6):991–992.

217. Borges LF, Hallett M, Selkoe DJ, et al. The anterior tarsal tunnel syndrome. Report of two cases. *J Neurosurg* 1981;54(1):89–92.

218. Dellon AL. Deep peroneal nerve entrapment on the dorsum of the foot. *Foot Ankle* 1990;11(2):73–80.

219. Kernohan J, Levack B, Wilson JN. Entrapment of the superficial peroneal nerve. Three case reports. *J Bone Joint Surg Br* 1985;67(1):60–61.

220. Singh N, Behse F, Buchthal F. Electrophysical study of peroneal palsy. *J Neurol Neurosurg Psychiatry* 1974;37(11):1202–1213.

221. Kim DH, Kline DG. Management and results of peroneal nerve lesions. *Neurosurgery* 1996;39(2):312–319.

222. Fabre T, Piton C, Andre D, et al. Peroneal nerve entrapment. *J Bone Joint Surg Am* 1998;80(1):47–53.

223. Mont MA, Dellon AL, Chen F, et al. The operative treatment of peroneal nerve palsy. *J Bone Joint Surg Am* 1996;78(6):863–869.

224. Abbott R. Sensory rhizotomy for the treatment of childhood spasticity. *J Child Neurol* 1996;11(suppl 1):S36–S42.

225. Groves EW. On the division of the posterior spinal nerve roots. *Lancet* 1911;2:79–85.

226. White JC, Kjellberg RN. Posterior spinal rhizotomy: a substitute for cordotomy in the relief of localized pain in patients with normal life-expectancy. *Neurochirurgia (Stuttg)* 1973;16(5):141–170.

227. Sherrington CS. Experiments in examination of the peripheral distribution of the fibers of the posterior roots of some spinal nerves. *Proc R Soc (Lond)* 1896;60:403–411.

228. Foerster O. The dermatomes in man. *Brain* 1933;56:1–39.

229. Liu CN, Chambers WW. Intraspinal sprouting of dorsal root axons; development of new collaterals and preterminals following partial denervation of the spinal cord in the cat. *AMA Arch Neurol Psychiatry* 1958;79(1):46–61.

230. Hodge CJ Jr, King RB. Medical modification of sensation. *J Neurosurg* 1976;44(1):21–28.

231. Coggeshall RE. Law of separation of function of the spinal roots. *Physiol Rev* 1980;60(3):716–755.

232. Sherrington CS. On the anatomical constitution of nerves of skeletal muscles; with remarks on recurrent fibers in the ventral spinal nerve-root. *J Physiol (Lond)* 1894;17:211–258.

233. Light AR, Metz CB. The morphology of the spinal cord efferent and afferent neurons contributing to the ventral roots of the cat. *J Comp Neurol* 1978;179(3):501–515.

234. Hosobuchi Y. The majority of unmyelinated afferent axons in human ventral roots probably conduct pain. *Pain* 1980;8(2):167–180.

235. North RB, Levy RM. Consensus conference on the neurosurgical management of pain. *Neurosurgery* 1994;34(4):756–760.

236. Schwartz HG. Anastomoses between cervical nerve roots. *J Neurosurg* 1956;13(2):190–194.

237. Felsoory A, Crue BL. Results of 19 years experience with sacral rhizotomy for perineal and perianal cancer pain. *Pain* 1976;2(4):431–433.

238. Loeser JD. Dorsal rhizotomy for the relief of chronic pain. *J Neurosurg* 1972;36(6):745–750.

239. Barrash JM, Leavens ME. Dorsal rhizotomy for the relief of intractable pain of malignant tumor origin. *J Neurosurg* 1973;38(6):755–757.

240. Onofrio BM, Campa HK. Evaluation of rhizotomy. Review of 12 years' experience. *J Neurosurg* 1972;36(6):751–755.

241. Wilkinson HA, Chan AS. Sensory ganglionectomy: theory, technical aspects, and clinical experience. *J Neurosurg* 2001;95(1):61–66.

242. Dandy WE. Operative relief from pain in lesions of the mouth, tongue, and throat. *Arch Surg* 1929;19:143–148.

243. Hunter CR, Mayfield FH. Role of the upper cervical roots in the production of pain in the head. *Am J Surg* 1949;78(5):743–751.

244. Hammond SR, Danta G. Occipital neuralgia. *Clin Exp Neurol* 1978;15:258–270.

245. Stechison MT, Mullin BB. Surgical treatment of greater occipital neuralgia: an appraisal of strategies. *Acta Neurochir (Wien)* 1994;131(3–4):236–240.

246. Lozano AM, Vanderlinden G, Bachoo R, et al. Microsurgical C-2 ganglionectomy for chronic intractable occipital pain. *J Neurosurg* 1998;89(3):359–365.

247. Dubuisson D. Treatment of occipital neuralgia by partial posterior rhizotomy at C1-3. *J Neurosurg* 1995;82(4):581–586.

248. Kapoor V, Rothfus WE, Grahovac SZ, et al. Refractory occipital neuralgia: preoperative assessment with CT-guided nerve block prior to dorsal cervical rhizotomy. *AJNR Am J Neuroradiol* 2003;24(10):2105–2110.

249. Acar F, Miller J, Golshani KJ, et al. Pain relief after cervical ganglionectomy (C2 and C3) for the treatment of medically intractable occipital neuralgia. *Stereotact Funct Neurosurg* 2008;86(2):106–112.

250. Slavin KV, Nersesyan H, Wess C. Peripheral neurostimulation for treatment of intractable occipital neuralgia. *Neurosurgery* 2006;58(1):112–119.

251. Falowski S, Wang D, Sabesan A, et al. Occipital nerve stimulator systems: review of complications and surgical techniques. *Neuromodulation* 2010;13(2):121–125.

252. Arbit E, Galicich JH, Burt M, et al. Modified open thoracic rhizotomy for treatment of intractable chest wall pain of malignant etiology. *Ann Thorac Surg* 1989;48(6):820–823.

253. Smith FP. Trans-spinal ganglionectomy for relief of intercostal pain. *J Neurosurg* 1970;32(5):574–577.

254. Graybill J, Conermann T, Kabazie AJ, et al. Spinal cord stimulation for treatment of pain in a patient with post thoracotomy pain syndrome. *Pain Physician* 2011;14(5):441–445.

255. Saris SC, Silver JM, Vieira JF, et al. Sacrococcygeal rhizotomy for perineal pain. *Neurosurgery* 1986;19(5):789–793.

256. Al-Zahrani AA, Elzayat EA, Gajewski JB. Long-term outcome and surgical interventions after sacral neuromodulation implant for lower urinary tract symptoms: 14-year experience at 1 center. *J Urol* 2011;185(3):981–986.

257. van Kleef M, Liem L, Lousberg R, et al. Radiofrequency lesion adjacent to the dorsal root ganglion for cervicobrachial pain: a prospective double blind randomized study. *Neurosurgery* 1996;38(6):1127–1131.

258. North RB, Kidd DH, Campbell JN, et al. Dorsal root ganglionectomy for failed back surgery syndrome: a 5-year follow-up study. *J Neurosurg* 1991;74(2):236–242.

259. Taub A, Robinson F, Taub E. Dorsal root ganglionectomy for intractable monoradicular sciatica. A series of 61 patients. *Stereotact Funct Neurosurg* 1995;65(1–4):106–110.

260. Yang A, Hunter CW. Dorsal root ganglion stimulation as a salvage treatment for complex regional pain syndrome refractory to dorsal column spinal cord stimulation: a case series. *Neuromodulation* 2017;20(7):703–707.

261. Huygen F, Liem L, Cusack W, et al. Stimulation of the L2-L3 dorsal root ganglia induces effective pain relief in the low back. *Pain Pract* 2018;18(2):205–213.

262. Wetzel FT, Phillips FM, Aprill CN, et al. Extradural sensory rhizotomy in the management of chronic lumbar radiculopathy: a minimum 2-year follow-up study. *Spine* 1997;22(19):2283–2291.

263. Philip A, Thakur R. Post herpetic neuralgia. *J Palliat Med* 2011;146:765–773.

264. Roberts WJ. A hypothesis on the physiological basis for causalgia and related pains. *Pain* 1986;24(3):297–311.

265. Smithwick RH. The rationale and technic of sympathectomy for the relief of vascular spasm of the extremities. *N Engl J Med* 1940;222:699–703.

266. Cline MA, Ochoa J, Torebjork HE. Chronic hyperalgesia and skin warming caused by sensitized C nociceptors. *Brain* 1989;112(pt 3):621–647.

267. Gracely RH, Lynch SA, Bennett GJ. Painful neuropathy: altered central processing maintained dynamically by peripheral input. *Pain* 1992;51(2):175–194.

268. Schinkel C, Gaertner A, Zaspel J, et al. Inflammatory mediators are altered in the acute phase of posttraumatic complex regional pain syndrome. *Clin J Pain* 2006;22(3):235–239.

269. van der Laan L, ter Laak HJ, Gabreels-Festen A, et al. Complex regional pain syndrome type I (RSD): pathology of skeletal muscle and peripheral nerve. *Neurology* 1998;51(1):20–25.

270. Mailis A, Wade J. Profile of Caucasian women with possible genetic predisposition to reflex sympathetic dystrophy: a pilot study. *Clin J Pain* 1994;10(3):210–217.

271. Walker AE, Nulson F. Electrical stimulation of the upper thoracic portion of the sympathetic chain in man. *Arch Neurol Psych* 1948;59:309–317.

272. Hannington-Kiff JG. Intravenous regional sympathetic block with guanethidine. *Lancet* 1974;1(7865):1019–1020.

273. Davis KD, Treede RD, Raja SN, et al. Topical application of clonidine relieves hyperalgesia in patients with sympathetically maintained pain. *Pain* 1991;47(3):309–317.

274. Torebjork E, Wahren L, Wallin G, et al. Noradrenaline-evoked pain in neuralgia. *Pain* 1995;63(1):11–20.

275. Abram SE, Lightfoot RW. Treatment of long-standing causalgia with prazosin. *Reg Anaesth* 1981;6:79–81.

276. Arner S. Intravenous phentolamine test: diagnostic and prognostic use in reflex sympathetic dystrophy. *Pain* 1991;46(1):17–22.

277. Ghostine SY, Comair YG, Turner DM, et al. Phenoxybenzamine in the treatment of causalgia. Report of 40 cases. *J Neurosurg* 1984;60(6):1263–1268.

278. Chabal C, Jacobson L, Russell LC, et al. Pain response to perineuromal injection of normal saline, epinephrine, and lidocaine in humans. *Pain* 1992; 49(1):9–12.

279. Reuben SS. Preventing the development of complex regional pain syndrome after surgery. *Anesthesiology* 2004;101(5):1215–1224.

280. Reuben SS, Rosenthal EA, Steinberg RB. Surgery on the affected upper extremity of patients with a history of complex regional pain syndrome: a retrospective study of 100 patients. *J Hand Surg Am* 2000;25(6):1147–1151.

281. Dellemijn PL, Fields HL, Allen RR, et al. The interpretation of pain relief and sensory changes following sympathetic blockade. *Brain* 1994; 117(pt 6):1475–1487.

282. Treede RD, Davis KD, Campbell JN, et al. The plasticity of cutaneous hyperalgesia during sympathetic ganglion blockade in patients with neuropathic pain. *Brain* 1992;115(pt 2):607–621.

283. Chelimsky TC, Low PA, Naessens JM, et al. Value of autonomic testing in reflex sympathetic dystrophy. *Mayo Clin Proc* 1995;70(11):1029–1040.

284. Wahren LK, Torebjork E, Nystrom B. Quantitative sensory testing before and after regional guanethidine block in patients with neuralgia in the hand. *Pain* 1991;46(1):23–30.

285. Raja SN, Treede RD, Davis KD, et al. Systemic alpha-adrenergic blockade with phentolamine: a diagnostic test for sympathetically maintained pain. *Anesthesiology* 1991;74(4):691–698.

286. Shir Y, Cameron LB, Raja SN, et al. The safety of intravenous phentolamine administration in patients with neuropathic pain. *Anesth Analg* 1993;76(5):1008–1011.

287. Rauck RL, Eisenach JC, Jackson K, et al. Epidural clonidine treatment for refractory reflex sympathetic dystrophy. *Anesthesiology* 1993;79(6):1163–1169.

288. Galer BS, Rowbotham MC, Von Miller K, et al. Treatment of inflammatory, neuropathic and sympathetically maintained pain in a patient with Sjogren's syndrome. *Pain* 1992;50(2):205–208.

289. Kirkpatrick AF, Derasari M. Transdermal clonidine: treating reflex sympathetic dystrophy. *Reg Anesth* 1993;18(2):140–141.

290. DeSalles AAF, Johnson JP. Sympathectomy for pain. In: Winn HR, Youmans JR, eds. *Youmans Neurological Surgery.* 5th ed. Philadelphia: W. B. Saunders; 2004:3096–3106.

291. Wilkinson HA. Percutaneous radiofrequency upper thoracic sympathectomy. *Neurosurgery* 1996;38(4):715–725.

292. Hoffert MJ, Greenberg RP, Wolskee PJ, et al. Abnormal and collateral innervations of sympathetic and peripheral sensory fields associated with a case of causalgia. *Pain* 1984;20(1):1–12.

293. Howng SL, Loh JK. Long-term follow up of upper dorsal sympathetic ganglionectomy for palmar hyperhidrosis—a scale of evaluation. *Gaoxiong Yi Xue Ke Xue Za Zhi* 1987;3(11):703–707.

294. Ulmer JL, Mayfield FH. Causalgia. *Surg Gynec Obstet* 1946;83:789–796.

295. Manart FD, Sadler TR Jr, Schmitt EA, et al. Upper dorsal sympathectomy. *Am J Surg* 1985;150(6):762–766.

296. Mockus MB, Rutherford RB, Rosales C, et al. Sympathectomy for causalgia. Patient selection and long-term results. *Arch Surg* 1987;122(6):668–672.

297. AbuRahma AF, Robinson PA, Powell M, et al. Sympathectomy for reflex sympathetic dystrophy: factors affecting outcome. *Ann Vasc Surg* 1994;8(4): 372–379.

298. Hassantash SA, Afrakhteh M, Maier RV. Causalgia: a meta-analysis of the literature. *Arch Surg* 2003;138(11):1226–1231.

299. Thompson JE. The diagnosis and management of post-traumatic pain syndromes (causalgia). *Aust N Z J Surg* 1979;49(3):299–304.

300. Litwin MS. Postsympathectomy neuralgia. *Arch Surg* 1962;84:121–125.

301. Raskin NH, Levinson S, Hoffman PM, et al. Postsympathectomy neuralgia. Amelioration with diphenylhydantoin and carbamazepine. *Am J Surg* 1974;128(1):75–78.

302. Kramis RC, Roberts WJ, Gillette RG. Post-sympathectomy neuralgia: hypotheses on peripheral and central neuronal mechanisms. *Pain* 1996; 64(1):1–9.

303. Mailis A, Furlan A. Sympathectomy for neuropathic pain. *Cochrane Database Syst Rev* 2003;(2):CD002918.

304. Turner JA, Loeser JD, Deyo RA, et al. Spinal cord stimulation for patients with failed back surgery syndrome or complex regional pain syndrome: a systematic review of effectiveness and complications. *Pain* 2004;108(1–2): 137–147.

305. Liem L, Russo M, Huygen FJ, et al. One-year outcomes of spinal cord stimulation of the dorsal root ganglion in the treatment of chronic neuropathic pain. *Neuromodulation* 2015;18(1):41–48.

306. Kemler MA, Furnee CA. Economic evaluation of spinal cord stimulation for chronic reflex sympathetic dystrophy. *Neurology* 2002;59(8): 1203–1209.

307. Kemler MA, Barendse GA, van Kleef M, et al. Spinal cord stimulation in patients with chronic reflex sympathetic dystrophy. *N Engl J Med* 2000;343(9):618–624.

308. Calvillo O, Racz G, Didie J, et al. Neuroaugmentation in the treatment of complex regional pain syndrome of the upper extremity. *Acta Orthop Belg* 1998;64(1):57–63.

CHAPTER 104

The Surgical Management of Trigeminal Neuralgia

MATTHEW K. MIAN, SARAH K. BICK, PRATIK A. TALATI, and **EMAD N. ESKANDAR**

Trigeminal neuralgia (TN), formerly known as *tic douloureux*, is a chronic pain disorder affecting the trigeminal nerve. Clinically, TN is characterized by bouts of severe, lancinating pain in a trigeminal distribution, often triggered by light touch or facial movement. A variety of effective medical and surgical therapies exist for TN. Carbamazepine (Tegretol) is considered the first-line treatment; second-line medications include oxcarbazepine and lamotrigine, among others.[1] Opiates are not particularly effective.[2] Surgical therapies include microvascular decompression (MVD), percutaneous rhizotomy, and radiosurgery. In this chapter, we review the surgical management of TN.

Patient Presentation

TN is rare, with an incidence of 2 to 5 per 100,000 per year[3] and a prevalence of 0.03% to 0.3%.[4] Patients typically present in their 60s,[5] although some develop symptoms as early as their late 30s. There is a female preponderance (3:2), and some studies suggest an association with arterial hypertension.[3] Case reports have identified familial forms of TN; these appear to be rare, are sometimes bilateral, and may follow an autosomal dominant inheritance pattern.[6,7]

Patients typically present with one of two clinical syndromes.[8] Type 1 TN ("typical TN") is characterized by a predominance of brief, lancinating, or electrical unilateral pain. Type 1 TN most frequently occurs in the V2 or V3 division, and it does not cross the midline. Triggers may include tactile stimuli or facial movements such as talking or chewing, and there is usually a refractory period during which pain cannot be elicited. The duration of pain is often brief, lasting seconds, but there may be up to several minutes of paroxysms before the pain-free refractory period.[8] The International Headache Society diagnostic criteria for TN are outlined in Table 104.1.[9]

Type 2 TN ("atypical TN") is characterized by a predominance of constant pain, often burning or aching.[10] This pain usually exists in addition to the brief, lancinating pain that occurs in type 1 TN. Although not firmly established, some believe that type 2 TN may emerge from long-standing type 1 TN.[11]

TABLE 104.1 Diagnostic Criteria for Trigeminal Neuralgia from the International Headache Society

A. At least three attacks of unilateral facial pain fulfilling criteria B and C

B. Occurring in one or more divisions of the trigeminal nerve, with no radiation beyond the trigeminal distribution

C. Pain has at least three of the following four characteristics:
- Recurring in paroxysmal attacks lasting from a fraction of a second to 2 minutes
- Severe intensity
- Electric shock-like, shooting, stabbing, or sharp in quality
- Precipitated by innocuous stimuli to the affected side of the face

D. No clinically evident neurologic deficit

E. Not better accounted for by another ICHD-3 diagnosis

ICHD-3, International Classification of Headache Disorders, 3rd edition.

Anatomy

The trigeminal nerve contains motor and sensory fibers that exit the lateral brainstem at the level of the mid-pons. Just distal to the brainstem root entry zone (REZ), the nerve transitions its myelinating cells from central oligodendrocytes to peripheral Schwann cells. This transition zone, which occurs several millimeters from the REZ at about one-third to one-fourth of the distance to Meckel's cave, is believed to be particularly sensitive to mechanical irritation.

The cisternal segment of the nerve traverses the subarachnoid space, traveling anterolaterally to pierce the dura near the petrous apex to enter Meckel's cave, a CSF-filled space between two layers of dura over the petrous portion of the temporal bone.[12] The nerve then splits into three divisions: (1) ophthalmic (V1; sensory only), which travels through the superior orbital fissure to enter the orbit; (2) maxillary (V2; sensory only), which enters the pterygopalatine fossa via the foramen rotundum; and (3) mandibular (V3; motor and sensory), which exits the skull through the foramen ovale (FO).

Pathophysiology

Type 1 TN is classically believed to stem from mechanical irritation of the trigeminal nerve by a blood vessel.[13-15] Under this model, pulsatile vascular compression causes focal irritation and eventually demyelination. The superior cerebellar artery (SCA) is most commonly implicated (75%), with other offenders being the anterior inferior cerebellar artery (10%), posterior fossa veins (12%), vertebral artery (2%), posterior inferior cerebellar artery (1%), and the basilar artery (1%).[16]

Injured trigeminal axons become hyperexcitable, spilling excitatory neurotransmitters that depolarize neighboring cells via ephaptic conduction (the "ignition hypothesis") and incite synchronized afterdischarges.[10,17] Periodic waves of depolarization are experienced as paroxysms of pain in the trigeminal distribution, often corrupting the perception of normal tactile stimuli.

Type 2 TN is posited to result from deafferentation of higher order somatosensory neurons, similar to other types of chronic neuropathic pain.[10] Some have proposed that type 1 and 2 TN sit at opposing ends of a single spectrum.[11] Chronic nerve injury in the setting of type 1 TN may extend proximally to and beyond the REZ, precipitating type 2 TN symptoms.[18]

First-line medical therapy consists of carbamazepine. The mechanism of carbamazepine's efficacy is unknown, although it is speculated that blockade of voltage-sensitive sodium channels may stabilize hyperexcitable cell membranes, reducing aberrant action potential propagation.[19]

MVD, described in the following text, yields immediate cessation of pain in many patients suffering from TN. The mechanism remains a subject of debate, but several hypotheses have been put forward. First, mechanical compression generates ectopic action potentials that may be alleviated by decompression.[20,21] Second, ephaptic conduction may be less effective when a compressive force is removed because there is more relative distance between demyelinated axons. Finally, there may be a pressure-dependent mechanical conduction block on subpopulations of fibers that is dissolved upon decompression.[2]

Evaluation for Surgery

Surgery should be considered for patients with persistent, severe symptoms despite adequate drug therapy or those with intolerable medication side effects. Medication trials at a minimum should include carbamazepine or oxcarbazepine.

An evaluation for surgery should prompt scrutiny of the patient's diagnosis. There exists a cornucopia of facial pain disorders. TN is a clinical diagnosis, and certain red flags should give the clinician pause: pain that does not respect the midline, age <40 years, absence of any *initial* response to carbamazepine, and facial numbness, among others.

Surgical options for TN can be divided into two categories: palliative ablative procedures (e.g., percutaneous rhizotomy, stereotactic radiosurgery) and nondestructive MVD. Neuromodulatory techniques are growing in popularity for a select set of facial pain disorders, but there is insufficient evidence or experience to support their use as a first-line surgical option for type 1 or 2 TN.

Regarding procedure selection, Slavin and colleagues[22] developed a facial pain surgical algorithm that is concordant with our own experience (Fig. 104.1). MVD is best reserved for those patients with type 1 TN, although some data suggest it may alleviate episodic pain in type 2 TN patients as well.[23] Radiofrequency rhizotomy and other percutaneous variants (glycerol, balloon compression) may be used for both type 2 TN patients and those type 1 TN patients in whom medical comorbidities or personal preferences preclude a retrosigmoid craniotomy or those who have already failed an MVD. Radiosurgery is an option for those patients seeking to avoid an invasive procedure.

Imaging is mandatory in the presurgical evaluation, primarily to rule out pathologies that would be symptomatic of TN yet mandate different treatment, namely, posterior fossa tumors or vascular malformations, multiple sclerosis (MS),

and brainstem or thalamic infarctions. The preferred imaging study is a magnetic resonance scan with a thin-cut axial T2-weighted 3D sequence (e.g., constructive interference in steady state [CISS], fast imaging employing steady-state acquisition [FIESTA], or similar) through the brainstem. Such sequences delineate the trigeminal nerve in high resolution. Of particular interest is contact or compression of the cisternal component of the trigeminal nerve by a blood vessel (Fig. 104.2).

Importantly, the presence of a vessel compressing the trigeminal nerve is not an obligate criterion for MVD candidacy, as some TN patients without radiographic neurovascular compression (NVC) are indeed found to have NVC at surgery, and asymptomatic NVC is frequently observed both in healthy controls and on the contralateral (unaffected) side in patients with TN.[24,25] It does appear, however, that imaging features such as nerve displacement and atrophy may be more specific, although less sensitive, for predicting whether radiographic NVC is symptomatic.[26,27]

Microvascular Decompression

MVD remains the preferred surgical treatment for medically suitable patients with type 1 TN. MVD offers a high success rate, the longest duration of pain relief, and is nondestructive, thus avoiding complications associated with deafferentation. The surgical goal is to identify and mechanically isolate an irritating vessel from the cisternal segment of the trigeminal nerve.

After the induction of general anesthesia, the patient is positioned supine with the head turned away from the affected side and secured in pin fixation, with the neck slightly flexed and elevated. The approximate courses of the transverse and sigmoid sinuses are outlined on the scalp (Fig. 104.3). We place electrodes for auditory brainstem responses to monitor for traction on the eighth cranial nerve. We have found facial nerve monitoring unnecessary.

The surgical field is shaved, prepped, and draped. We open a linear incision two fingerbreadths behind the base of the pinna and extending from the top of the pinna, over the digastric notch, and to the level of the mastoid, pointing toward the ipsilateral foot (see Fig. 104.3). A pericranial graft is harvested from above the nuchal line for later use in the dural closure.

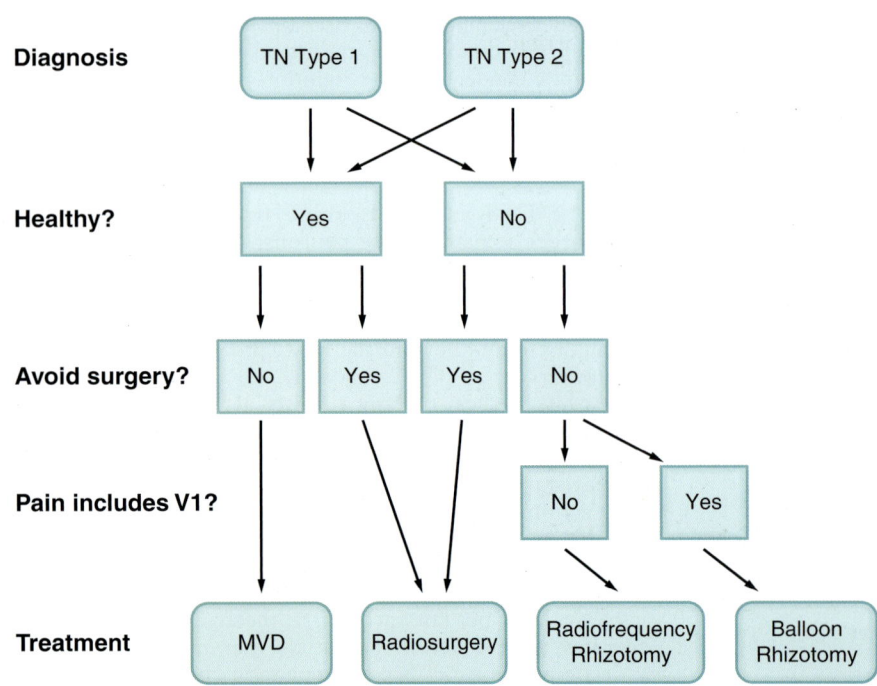

FIGURE 104.1 Surgical treatment algorithm for trigeminal neuralgia (TN) types 1 and 2. *(Adapted from Slavin KV, Nersesyan H, Colpan ME, et al. Current algorithm for the surgical treatment of facial pain.* Head Face Med *2007;3:30).*

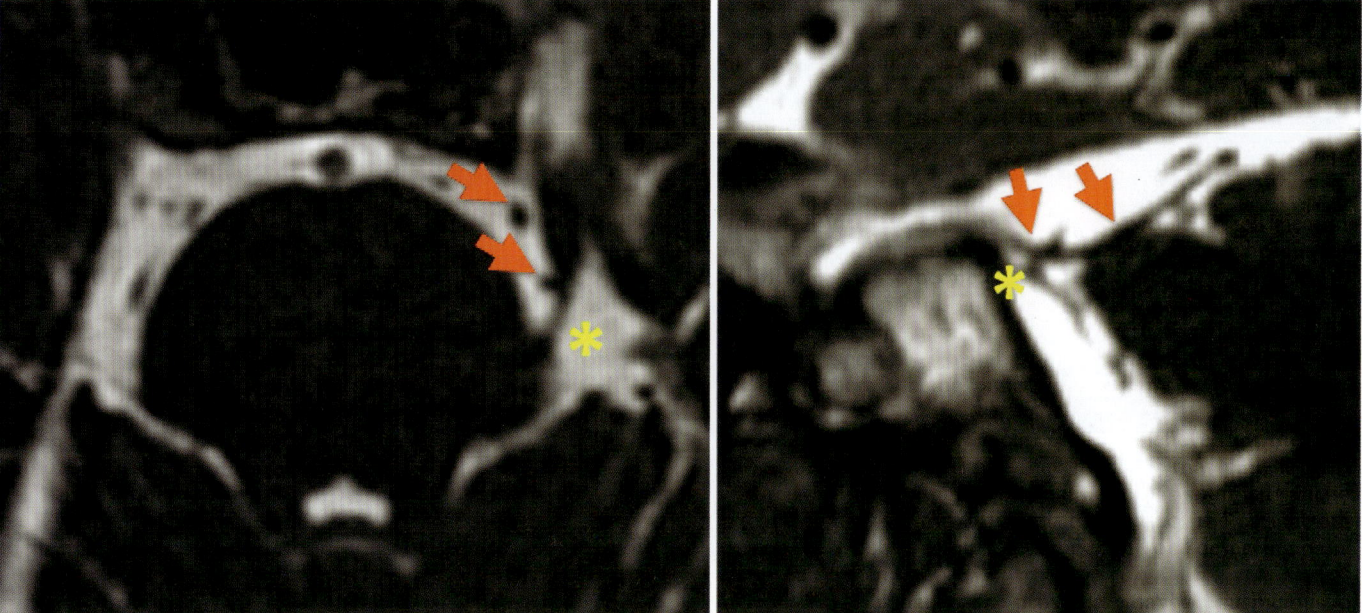

FIGURE 104.2 Axial **(left)** and sagittal **(right)** fast imaging employing steady-state acquisition magnetic resonance imaging sequences demonstrating neurovascular compression of the superior aspect of the left trigeminal nerve (*yellow asterisks*) by a loop of the superior cerebellar artery (SCA; *red arrowheads*). Note the displacement and atrophy of the proximal nerve segment on the axial image. On the sagittal image, only a narrow cross-section of the nerve is captured, but the looping course of the SCA is apparent.

The suboccipital musculature is dissected away, and a burr hole is placed near the junction of the venous sinuses. We use a combination of high-speed drilling and rongeur instruments to create an approximately 3-cm craniotomy, exposing the edges of the transverse and sigmoid sinuses superiorly and laterally, respectively. Mastoid air cells are waxed.

The dura is opened in a stellate manner. A handheld brain retractor is used to depress the cerebellum, and CSF is aspirated from the cisterna magna, slackening the hemisphere. Some surgeons place a lumbar drain at the start of the case or perform a lumbar puncture intraoperatively.

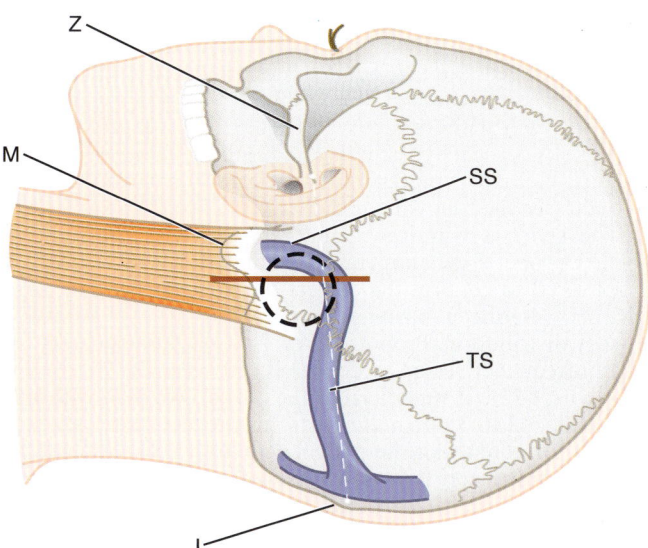

FIGURE 104.3 External landmarks for a left-sided microvascular decompression. The skin incision (*red line*) is vertically oriented, passing from the top of the pinna down and behind the mastoid tip. The transverse sinus can be approximated by a line connecting the zygoma to the inion. A retrosigmoid craniotomy (*black hashed line*) is performed just below the junction of the transverse and sigmoid sinuses.

The operating microscope is brought in, and under constant monitoring of the auditory brainstem responses, a fixed retractor is used to displace the cerebellum from the lateral skull base (Fig. 104.4). We identify the complex of the seventh and eighth nerves coursing out to the internal auditory canal. A petrosal vein or venous complex usually obscures the view of the (deeper) trigeminal nerve; this can be coagulated and divided safely.

Arachnoid adhesions are taken down sharply, and the trigeminal nerve is traced to its entry zone in the lateral pons (see Fig. 104.4). The most common offending vessel is the superior cerebellar artery (>80%), which generally contacts the superomedial surface of the nerve. Other vascular offenders may include the anterior inferior cerebellar artery and posterior fossa veins. The segment of the nerve that is most sensitive to mechanical irritation is the transition zone from central to peripheral myelin, which occurs approximately 1 to 3 mm from the brainstem[27,28]; sometimes an area of demyelination is visually apparent as a discolored patch on the surface of the nerve.

A straight dissector is used to tease any offending vessel away from the nerve. Teflon pledgets are interposed between the vessel and the nerve, with care taken to ensure the vessel is not kinked in the process.

The cerebellar retractor is removed, and the field is irrigated. We close the dura watertight using a pericranial graft. The duraplasty is coated with a layer of fibrin glue, and the bony defect is corrected with bone cement or a titanium mesh. The soft tissue is closed in layers, culminating in an absorbable stitch on the skin. Patients are monitored in the intensive care unit for one night and usually discharge on the second postoperative day. They are initially maintained on their baseline TN medication regimen, which is then weaned later as an outpatient.

OUTCOMES

MVD offers excellent long-term pain control. Eighty percent to 96% of patients experience initial pain relief after MVD.[29–31] At 5 years, pain control is maintained in 72% to 85%.[31–33] One study with extended follow-up reported that 73% of patients were pain free 15 years after surgery.[34]

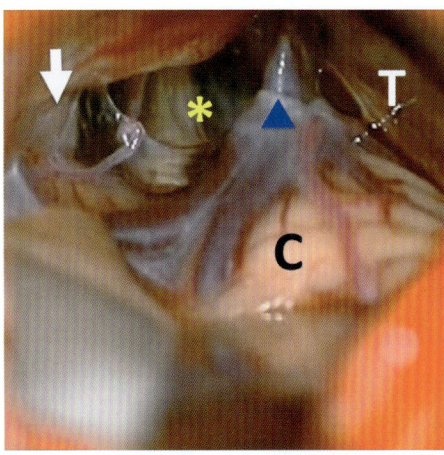 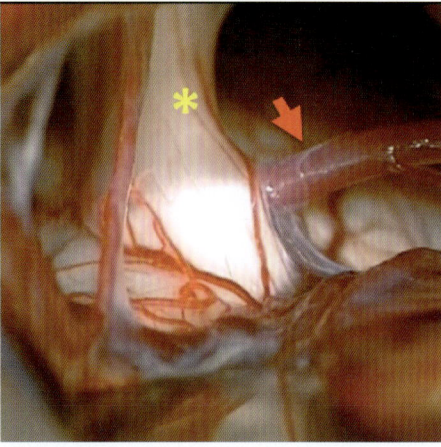 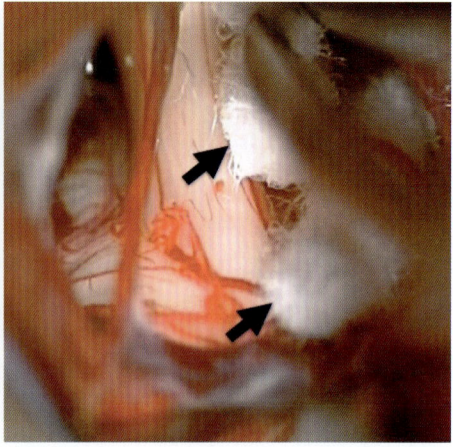

FIGURE 104.4   Intraoperative photographs from a left-sided microvascular decompression. *Left panel*: Relevant anatomic structures visualized after dural opening and placement of a retractor on the lateral cerebellum (*C*). From inferior to superior **(left to right on the image)**: arachnoid membranes overlying the complex of cranial nerves VII and VIII (*white arrowhead*), trigeminal nerve (*yellow asterisk*), petrosal venous complex (*blue triangle*), and tentorium (*T*). *Middle panel*: View of compression of the superior surface of the trigeminal nerve (*yellow asterisk*) by a loop of the superior cerebellar artery (*red arrowhead*). *Right panel*: Teflon pledgets (*black arrowheads*) are interposed between the trigeminal nerve and the artery.

One of the landmark series of MVD for TN reports on the outcomes of 1,185 patients who underwent MVD over a 20-year period with outcomes prospectively evaluated. At 10 years after surgery, 70% of patients were pain free while off of medication.[16] This study found that most recurrences occur during the first 2 years after surgery, with very low recurrence rates later.[16]

MVD has better outcomes in type 1 TN than type 2 TN perhaps because patients with type 2 TN have greater underlying damage to the trigeminal nerve.[35] Presence of arterial compression of the nerve is also associated with better outcomes,[36] with greater degree of compression additionally correlated with positive outcome.[34] Treatment failure is associated with longer symptom duration prior to surgery, presence of venous NVC, and lack of immediate postoperative symptom relief.[16]

Although MVD has a higher complication rate than percutaneous procedures, in experienced hands, the procedure is relatively safe. Mortality is low (0.15% to 0.8%)[37] and related to hospital and surgeon volume.[38] Trigeminal sensory deficit occurs in 1.6% to 22% of cases.[29,33] The incidence of facial weakness is 1.2% to 6.8%.[29,33] Hearing loss occurs in 1.2% to 6.8% but may be decreased by the use of brainstem auditory evoked potential monitoring.[39]

Other serious complications include cerebrospinal fluid leak (1.5% to 4%) and cerebellar infarct or hematoma (<1%).[16,39] Anesthesia dolorosa is very uncommon after MVD, with one large series reporting 0% incidence,[16] although the rate may be higher with internal neurolysis, a procedure involving the longitudinal splitting of trigeminal nerve fibers that is sometimes used when NVC is not identified intraoperatively.[32]

Percutaneous Rhizotomy

Radiofrequency rhizotomy is an excellent surgical option for patients with type 2 TN or for patients with type 1 TN who medically are not candidates for MVD or have already failed MVD. The goal of a rhizotomy is to lesion the retrogasserian trigeminal root, which can be accessed percutaneously through the FO. The procedure is effective, can be performed on an outpatient basis without general anesthesia, and can be repeated. Drawbacks include facial numbness and the risk of deafferentation pain.

The patient is positioned supine on the operative table. Midazolam (1 to 2 mg) is administered for anxiolysis as well as meperidine (25 to 50 mg) to blunt bradycardia that can occur with trigeminal stimulation. The head is turned slightly away from the affected side, and submental vertex fluoroscopy is used to identify the FO near the junction of the pterygoid plate and the petrous ridge.

The face is prepped with alcohol and squared off with sterile towels. Local anesthetic is instilled in the soft tissue along the anticipated needle trajectory. The needle entry point is generally 2.5 cm lateral to and at or just below the labial commissure. A 20G spinal needle is advanced toward the FO, using the midpupil as an approximate external landmark. Fluoroscopy is repeated when the needle contacts the skull base, and the trajectory is adjusted until the FO is entered, which is often signified by a jaw jerk and wince.

The fluoroscope is rotated into a lateral view. Under constant fluoroscopy, the needle is advanced toward the clival line (Fig. 104.5). On the lateral view, V2 fibers are encountered approximately at the clival line, with V1 being deeper and V3 more superficial (see Fig. 104.5). Radiofrequency rhizotomy is best reserved for cases of V2 or V3 TN; V1 fibers can be difficult to reach without a curved needle, and a radiofrequency lesion risks corneal hypesthesia and resulting keratitis; for these reasons, balloon compression is preferred for cases involving V1 pain (see the following text).

The stylet is withdrawn and replaced with the radiofrequency probe. Low-temperature stimulation (40° to 50° C) is delivered to confirm the correct division has been targeted. Patients describe a burning sensation in the corresponding sensory distribution. Propofol (2 to 4 mL) is administered, and a radiofrequency lesion is delivered (60 seconds; 75° C if at the clivus, 85° C if superficial to the clivus). We then withdraw the needle ~2 to 3 mm and repeat this process iteratively, with the goal of abolishing the patient's ability to discriminate between pinprick and light touch (usually two or three lesions per sensory division). When this is achieved, the needle is withdrawn, and the patient is taken to the recovery area.

Balloon compression is a percutaneous rhizotomy variant uniquely indicated for V1 pain; the goal is to compress the trigeminal nerve within the porus trigeminus. Surgical technique is similar to the radiofrequency rhizotomy, except that it is typically done under general anesthesia and requires a larger cannula (14G) to accommodate the balloon. A balloon catheter is

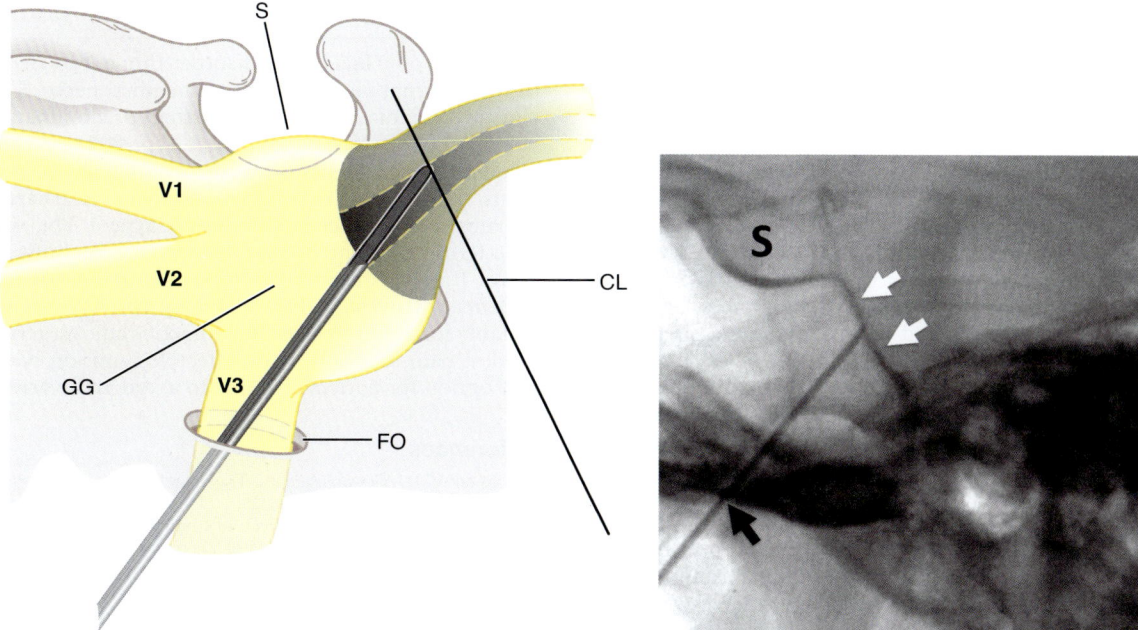

FIGURE 104.5 Percutaneous radiofrequency rhizotomy, lateral view. *Left panel*: The gasserian ganglion (*GG*) is located within Meckel's cave. A spinal needle is used to pierce the foramen ovale, and radiofrequency lesions are created in the retrogasserian fibers. V3 fibers are encountered superficially, with V2 and V1 fibers deeper. *Right panel*: Lateral fluoroscopy demonstrating a spinal needle passing through the foramen ovale (*black arrowhead*). The outline of the sella (*S*) can be seen superiorly. V2 fibers are encountered at the clival line (*white arrowheads*).

introduced after the FO has been cannulated, and it is advanced on the lateral fluoroscopy view until the tip is just past the clival line. The balloon is inflated to 1.5 atmospheres for 60 seconds before being withdrawn.

OUTCOMES

Percutaneous Radiofrequency Rhizotomy

Initial response to percutaneous radiofrequency rhizotomy is excellent, with rates of pain relief up to 97.6%,[40] on par with MVD. However, as with other percutaneous procedures, the response to radiofrequency rhizotomy is less durable, and the procedure may need to be repeated. One of the largest series of radiofrequency rhizotomy followed the results of 1,600 patients with TN who underwent 2,138 radiofrequency rhizotomy procedures over 25 years. This study found that 58% of patients who had undergone a single procedure had complete pain relief at 5-year follow-up, whereas 92% of patients achieved pain relief with multiple procedures at 5 years.[40] At 20 years, 41% of patients who had undergone a single procedure had pain relief, and all of the patients who had undergone multiple procedures and were followed were free from pain.[40]

Type 1 TN may be associated with better outcomes following radiofrequency rhizotomy,[41] as is postoperative facial numbness.[42] One of the relative advantages of radiofrequency rhizotomy is that it allows more selective targeting of specific trigeminal nerve distributions than chemical or balloon rhizotomy.[41]

Radiofrequency rhizotomy has a higher rate of decreased corneal sensation than other percutaneous procedures at 5.7% to 17.3%.[40,43] Anesthesia dolorosa occurs in 0.8%.[40] Higher lesioning temperatures may be associated with higher rates of trigeminal sensory dysfunction.[44] Masseter weakness occurs in 3% to 29% of cases.[42] Some of the adverse effects of radiofrequency rhizotomy are thought to occur via selective damage to small unmyelinated trigeminal pain fibers.[45]

Percutaneous Balloon Compression

Percutaneous balloon compression similarly has a high rate of initial pain control, with up to 94% reporting initial pain relief,[46] with recurrence rates of 20% to 48%.[42] One of the largest published series reported on the outcomes of 901 patients who underwent percutaneous balloon compression at a single institution. This series found a 92.7% rate of significant pain relief at 1 month, with excellent pain relief in 67.1% at 1 year and complete pain relief in 62% at mean 16.5 year follow-up.[47]

The rate of postoperative trigeminal sensory disturbance is high following balloon compression, with initial disturbance in almost all patients, and persistent symptoms in 4.6% to 40% of patients.[37] Trigeminal dysfunction may be related to the rate and duration of balloon compression.[48] Balloon compression has a low rate of decreased corneal sensation, perhaps because it damages medium and large myelinated pain fibers, sparing small fibers important in corneal sensation.[45] As such, it is the percutaneous treatment of choice for V1 distribution TN.

Conversely, the rate of masseter weakness following balloon compression is high at 10% to 50%.[42] Hearing loss is reported in 2.4% to 6.3%.[49] And the rate of intraoperative trigeminal reflex bradycardia and hypotension may be higher in balloon compression than other percutaneous procedures, an important consideration for patients with preexisting cardiac comorbidities.[45]

Radiosurgery

Radiosurgery uses focused radiation to the trigeminal nerve or ganglion to disrupt pain transmission. Several different radiosurgery systems have been used to treat TN. One of the most commonly used is Gamma Knife, which uses 201 cobalt-60 radiation sources arranged in a hemispheric assembly to target energy to a focal point. Linear accelerator–based therapies have also been used in TN and generate high-energy particles that are delivered through a single source that moves relative to the patient around the planned focal point. One such system is CyberKnife, which uses a linear accelerator mounted on a robotic arm, with two orthogonally positioned x-ray detectors that provide movement correction by imaging the patient's bony anatomy.[50] This system has also been used for TN with success.[50] All systems seem to have similar efficacy in TN.

During radiosurgery, the patient's head is fixed using a head frame or facemask, depending on the system being used. The patient's MRI or CT is used in conjunction with planning software to identify the target. Several targeting strategies have been used, including a single isocenter in the REZ,[51] the cisternal portion of the trigeminal nerve,[50,52] a retrogasserian target in the anterior cisternal portion of the trigeminal nerve anterior to the emergence of the nerve,[53,54] or two isocenters in the gasserian ganglion and the REZ.[55] One trial randomized patients to one versus two retrogasserian isocenters and found that two isocenters did not improve pain outcomes but resulted in a higher rate of sensory disturbances.[56] Shorter distance between the target and brainstem may be associated with better pain outcomes.[57] Median doses of 70 to 90 Gy are generally used.[58,59] Higher dose rate may not only be associated with better initial pain relief and lower recurrence rates[59,60] but also be associated with higher rates of trigeminal sensory dysfunction.[60]

One of the disadvantages of radiosurgery is that it has a delayed onset of pain relief, with a median latency of 1 to 2 months,[61] making it less suitable for patients in acute pain crisis. A shorter latency to response may predict longer durability of pain relief.[62] Patients who undergo radiosurgery early in their disease course have decreased latency to response and longer durability of symptom relief.[62]

OUTCOMES

A high proportion of patients have at least some improvement in pain after radiosurgery, with 79% to 92% reporting initial pain improvement.[37] Unfortunately, durability and extent of pain relief are limited. Patients who have not had previous surgery have better pain outcomes.[54,63] Better outcomes are also associated with type 1 TN, previous percutaneous procedures, and older age.[61,64] Interestingly, radiosurgery may also be effective for MS-related TN.[61]

A large study reported on the outcomes of a series of 503 TN patients treated with Gamma Knife. This study found that 89% of patients achieved an initial Barrow Neurological Institute (BNI) pain score of I to IIIb (pain adequately controlled with medication); this rate was 80% at 1 year, 46% at 5 years, and 30% at 10 years.[63] There was a 10.5% rate of new trigeminal sensory disturbance.[63] Another large study reported on 497 patients with type 1 TN not previously treated with radiosurgery and followed for at least 1 year. This study reported that 92% had initial freedom from pain, whereas at 5 and 10 years follow-up, 65% and 45% of patients were pain free off medication, respectively.[54]

The most common side effect after radiosurgery is trigeminal sensory disturbance, with decreasing rates with increasing time after the procedure.[61] Higher radiation dose may be associated with greater rates of sensory disturbance, ranging from 6% to 42%.[37] Importantly, postprocedure facial numbness is a predictor of treatment durability.[61] The rate of anesthesia dolorosa is very low (0.2%).[63] Repeat radiosurgery is associated with a higher rate of sensory dysfunction.[65] Other, rarer complications include masticator weakness and hearing loss.[61]

In patients who have recurrence of symptoms after initial radiosurgery, repeat radiosurgery can provide symptom relief. One study found that 63% of patients were pain free off medication at 1 year after repeat Gamma Knife, whereas at 5 years, the rate had fallen to 37%.[58] Response to initial Gamma Knife and facial numbness after initial Gamma Knife were predictors of response to repeat radiosurgery.[58] Third Gamma Knife procedure has also been reported in a small series, with 47% reporting initial complete pain relief, and 35% maintaining this at mean 22.9 months follow-up.[66] There were no new sensory deficits after third Gamma Knife.[66]

Conclusions

TN is a chronic facial pain disorder thought to stem from NVC of the cisternal segment of the trigeminal nerve. There are two clinical variants: type 1, consisting predominantly of brief, lancinating, or electrical pain, and type 2, chiefly with constant burning or aching pain. Surgery should be considered in patients' refractory to carbamazepine or oxcarbazepine. MVD remains the treatment of choice for type 1 TN, with excellent long-term pain control—even in patients without radiographic NVC. Radiofrequency rhizotomy is suitable for type 2 TN or patients with type 1 TN refractory to MVD or who are not suitable for a craniotomy. Stereotactic radiosurgery offers more modest pain relief rates and effective duration but is an excellent option for patients seeking to avoid an invasive procedure.

References

1. Reddy GD, Viswanathan A. Trigeminal and glossopharyngeal neuralgia. *Neurol Clin* 2014;32:539–552.
2. Fern R, Harrison PJ. The effects of compression upon conduction in myelinated axons of the isolated frog sciatic nerve. *J Physiol* 1991;432:111–122.
3. Manzoni GC, Torelli P. Epidemiology of typical and atypical craniofacial neuralgias. *Neurol Sci* 2005;26(suppl 2):s65–s67.
4. De Toledo IP, Conti Réus J, Fernandes M, et al. Prevalence of trigeminal neuralgia: a systematic review. *J Am Dent Assoc* 2016;147:570.e2–576.e2.
5. Siqueira SR, Teixeira MJ, Siqueira JT. Clinical characteristics of patients with trigeminal neuralgia referred to neurosurgery. *Eur J Dent* 2009;3:207–212.
6. Fleetwood IG, Innes AM, Hansen SR, et al. Familial trigeminal neuralgia. Case report and review of the literature. *J Neurosurg* 2001;95:513–517.
7. Smyth P, Greenough G, Stommel E. Familial trigeminal neuralgia: case reports and review of the literature. *Headache* 2003;43:910–915.
8. Elias WJ, Burchiel KJ. Trigeminal neuralgia and other neuropathic pain syndromes of the head and face. *Curr Pain Headache Rep* 2002;6:115–124.
9. Headache Classification Committee of the International Headache Society. The International Classification of Headache Disorders, 3rd edition (beta version). *Cephalalgia* 2013;33:629–808.
10. Burchiel K. *Surgical Management of Pain.* 2nd ed. New York: Thieme Medical Publishers; 2014.
11. Burchiel KJ, Slavin KV. On the natural history of trigeminal neuralgia. *Neurosurgery* 2000;46:152–154; discussion 154–155.
12. Binder DK, Sonne DC, Fischbein NJ. *Cranial Nerves: Anatomy, Pathology, Imaging.* New York: Thieme Medical Publishers; 2010.
13. Dandy W. Concerning the cause of trigeminal neuralgia. *Am J Surg* 1934;24:447–455.
14. Jannetta PJ. Arterial compression of the trigeminal nerve at the pons in patients with trigeminal neuralgia. *J Neurosurg* 1967;26(suppl):159–162.
15. Jannetta PJ. Neurovascular compression in cranial nerve and systemic disease. *Ann Surg* 1980;192:518–525.
16. Barker FG, Jannetta PJ, Bissonette DJ, et al. The long-term outcome of microvascular decompression for trigeminal neuralgia. *N Engl J Med* 1996;334:1077–1083.
17. Devor M, Amir R, Rappaport ZH. Pathophysiology of trigeminal neuralgia: the ignition hypothesis. *Clin J Pain* 2002;18:4–13.
18. Obermann M, Yoon MS, Ese D, et al. Impaired trigeminal nociceptive processing in patients with trigeminal neuralgia. *Neurology* 2007;69:835–841.
19. Obermann M. Treatment options in trigeminal neuralgia. *Ther Adv Neurol Disord* 2010;3:107–115.
20. Smith KJ, McDonald WI. Spontaneous and mechanically evoked activity due to central demyelinating lesion. *Nature* 1980;286:154–155.
21. Smith KJ, McDonald WI. Spontaneous and evoked electrical discharges from a central demyelinating lesion. *J Neurol Sci* 1982;55:39–47.
22. Slavin KV, Nersesyan H, Colpan ME, et al. Current algorithm for the surgical treatment of facial pain. *Head Face Med* 2007;3:30.
23. Sandell T, Eide PK. Effect of microvascular decompression in trigeminal neuralgia patients with or without constant pain. *Neurosurgery* 2008;63:93–99; discussion 99–100.
24. Chun-Cheng Q, Qing-Shi Z, Ji-Qing Z, et al. A single-blinded pilot study assessing neurovascular contact by using high-resolution MR imaging in patients with trigeminal neuralgia. *Eur J Radiol* 2009;69:459–463.
25. Peker S, Dinçer A, Necmettin Pamir M. Vascular compression of the trigeminal nerve is a frequent finding in asymptomatic individuals: 3-T MR imaging of 200 trigeminal nerves using 3D CISS sequences. *Acta Neurochir (Wien)* 2009;151:1081–1088.
26. Antonini G, Di Pasquale A, Cruccu G, et al. Magnetic resonance imaging contribution for diagnosing symptomatic neurovascular contact in classical trigeminal neuralgia: a blinded case-control study and meta-analysis. *Pain* 2014;155:1464–1471.
27. Donahue JH, Ornan DA, Mukherjee S. Imaging of vascular compression syndromes. *Radiol Clin North Am* 2017;55:123–138.

28. Haller S, Etienne L, Kövari E, et al. Imaging of neurovascular compression syndromes: trigeminal neuralgia, hemifacial spasm, vestibular paroxysmia, and glossopharyngeal neuralgia. *AJNR Am J Neuroradiol* 2016;37:1384–1392.

29. Broggi G, Ferroli P, Franzini A, et al. Microvascular decompression for trigeminal neuralgia: comments on a series of 250 cases, including 10 patients with multiple sclerosis. *J Neurol Neurosurg Psychiatry* 2000;68:59–64.

30. Pamir MN, Peker S. Microvascular decompression for trigeminal neuralgia: a long-term follow-up study. *Minim Invasive Neurosurg* 2006;49:342–346.

31. Tyler-Kabara EC, Kassam AB, Horowitz MH, et al. Predictors of outcome in surgically managed patients with typical and atypical trigeminal neuralgia: comparison of results following microvascular decompression. *J Neurosurg* 2002;96:527–531.

32. Ko AL, Ozpinar A, Lee A, et al. Long-term efficacy and safety of internal neurolysis for trigeminal neuralgia without neurovascular compression. *J Neurosurg* 2015;122:1048–1057.

33. Pollock BE, Stien KJ. Posterior fossa exploration for trigeminal neuralgia patients older than 70 years of age. *Neurosurgery* 2011;69:1255–1260.

34. Sindou M, Leston J, Decullier E, et al. Microvascular decompression for primary trigeminal neuralgia: long-term effectiveness and prognostic factors in a series of 362 consecutive patients with clear-cut neurovascular conflicts who underwent pure decompression. *J Neurosurg* 2007;107:1144–1153.

35. Degn J, Brennum J. Surgical treatment of trigeminal neuralgia. Results from the use of glycerol injection, microvascular decompression, and rhizotomia. *Acta Neurochir (Wien)* 2010;152:2125–2132.

36. Miller JP, Acar F, Burchiel KJ. Classification of trigeminal neuralgia: clinical, therapeutic, and prognostic implications in a series of 144 patients undergoing microvascular decompression. *J Neurosurg* 2009;111:1231–1234.

37. Bick SKB, Eskandar EN. Surgical treatment of trigeminal neuralgia. *Neurosurg Clin N Am* 2017;28:429–438.

38. Kalkanis SN, Eskandar EN, Carter BS, et al. Microvascular decompression surgery in the United States, 1996 to 2000: mortality rates, morbidity rates, and the effects of hospital and surgeon volumes. *Neurosurgery* 2003;52:1251–1262.

39. McLaughlin MR, Jannetta PJ, Clyde BL, et al. Microvascular decompression of cranial nerves: lessons learned after 4400 operations. *J Neurosurg* 1999;90:1–8.

40. Kanpolat Y, Savas A, Bekar A, et al. Percutaneous controlled radiofrequency trigeminal rhizotomy for the treatment of idiopathic trigeminal neuralgia: 25-year experience with 1,600 patients. *Neurosurgery* 2001;48:524–534.

41. Jin HS, Shin JY, Kim YC, et al. Predictive factors associated with success and failure for radiofrequency thermocoagulation in patients with trigeminal neuralgia. *Pain Physician* 2015;18:537–545.

42. Wang JY, Bender MT, Bettegowda C. Percutaneous procedures for the treatment of trigeminal neuralgia. *Neurosurg Clin N Am* 2016;27:277–295.

43. Fraioli B, Esposito V, Guidetti B, et al. Treatment of trigeminal neuralgia by thermocoagulation, glycerolization, and percutaneous compression of the gasserian ganglion and/or retrogasserian rootlets: long-term results and therapeutic protocol. *Neurosurgery* 1989;24:239–245.

44. Tronnier VM, Rasche D, Hamer J, et al. Treatment of idiopathic trigeminal neuralgia: comparison of long-term outcome after radiofrequency rhizotomy and microvascular decompression. *Neurosurgery* 2001;48:1261–1268.

45. Cheng JS, Lim DA, Chang EF, et al. A review of percutaneous treatments for trigeminal neuralgia. *Neurosurgery* 2014;10(suppl 1):25–33.

46. Lobato RD, Rivas JJ, Sarabia R, et al. Percutaneous microcompression of the gasserian ganglion for trigeminal neuralgia. *J Neurosurg* 1990;72:546–553.

47. Abdennebi B, Guenane L. Technical considerations and outcome assessment in retrogasserian balloon compression for treatment of trigeminal neuralgia. Series of 901 patients. *Surg Neurol Int* 2014;5:118.

48. Abdennebi B, Bouatta F, Chitti M, et al. Percutaneous balloon compression of the Gasserian ganglion in trigeminal neuralgia. Long-term results in 150 cases. *Acta Neurochir (Wien)* 1995;136:72–74.

49. de Siqueira SR, da Nobrega JC, de Siqueira JT, et al. Frequency of postoperative complications after balloon compression for idiopathic trigeminal neuralgia: prospective study. *Oral Surg Oral Med Oral Pathol Oral Radiol Endod* 2006;102:e39–e45.

50. Karam SD, Tai A, Snider JW, et al. Refractory trigeminal neuralgia treatment outcomes following CyberKnife radiosurgery. *Radiat Oncol* 2014;9:257.

51. Hitchon PW, Holland M, Noeller J, et al. Options in treating trigeminal neuralgia: experience with 195 patients. *Clin Neurol Neurosurg* 2016;149:166–170.

52. Martinez Moreno NE, Gutierrez-Sarraga J, Rey-Portoles G, et al. Long-term outcomes in the treatment of classical trigeminal neuralgia by Gamma Knife radiosurgery: a retrospective study in patients with minimum 2-year follow-up. *Neurosurgery* 2016;79:879–888.

53. Park SC, Kwon DH, Lee DH, et al. Repeat Gamma-Knife radiosurgery for refractory or recurrent trigeminal neuralgia with consideration about the optimal second dose. *World Neurosurg* 2016;86:371–383.

54. Regis J, Tuleasca C, Resseguier N, et al. Long-term safety and efficacy of Gamma Knife surgery in classical trigeminal neuralgia: a 497-patient historical cohort study. *J Neurosurg* 2016;124:1079–1087.

55. Dai ZF, Huang QL, Liu HP, et al. Efficacy of stereotactic Gamma Knife surgery and microvascular decompression in the treatment of primary trigeminal neuralgia: a retrospective study of 220 cases from a single center. *J Pain Res* 2016;9:535–542.

56. Flickinger JC, Pollock BE, Kondziolka D, et al. Does increased nerve length within the treatment volume improve trigeminal neuralgia radiosurgery? A prospective double-blind, randomized study. *Int J Radiat Oncol Biol Phys* 2001;51:449–454.

57. Massager N, Lorenzoni J, Devriendt D, et al. Gamma Knife surgery for idiopathic trigeminal neuralgia performed using a far-anterior cisternal target and a high dose of radiation. *J Neurosurg* 2004;100:597–605.

58. Helis CA, Lucas JT Jr, Bourland JD, et al. Repeat radiosurgery for trigeminal neuralgia. *Neurosurgery* 2015;77:755–761.

59. Lee JY, Sandhu S, Miller D, et al. Higher dose rate Gamma Knife radiosurgery may provide earlier and longer-lasting pain relief for patients with trigeminal neuralgia. *J Neurosurg* 2015;123:961–968.

60. Pollock BE, Phuong LK, Foote RL, et al. High-dose trigeminal neuralgia radiosurgery associated with increased risk of trigeminal nerve dysfunction. *Neurosurgery* 2001;49:58–64.

61. Wolf A, Kondziolka D. Gamma Knife surgery in trigeminal neuralgia. *Neurosurg Clin N Am* 2016;27:297–304.

62. Mousavi SH, Niranjan A, Huang MJ, et al. Early radiosurgery provides superior pain relief for trigeminal neuralgia patients. *Neurology* 2015;85:2159–2165.

63. Kondziolka D, Zorro O, Lobato-Polo J, et al. Gamma Knife stereotactic radiosurgery for idiopathic trigeminal neuralgia. *J Neurosurg* 2010;112:758–765.

64. Taich ZJ, Goetsch SJ, Monaco E, et al. Stereotactic radiosurgery treatment of trigeminal neuralgia: clinical outcomes and prognostic factors. *World Neurosurg* 2016;90:604.e11–612.e11.

65. Tuleasca C, Carron R, Resseguier N, et al. Decreased probability of initial pain cessation in classic trigeminal neuralgia treated with Gamma Knife surgery in case of previous microvascular decompression: a prospective series of 45 patients with >1 year of follow-up. *Neurosurgery* 2015;77:87–95.

66. Tempel ZJ, Chivukula S, Monaco EA III, et al. The results of a third Gamma Knife procedure for recurrent trigeminal neuralgia. *J Neurosurg* 2015;122:169–179.

CHAPTER 105

Ablative Neurosurgical Procedures for Chronic Pain

BENJAMIN L. GRANNAN, MUHAMED HADZIPASIC, and EMAD N. ESKANDAR

Consideration of an ablative procedure for chronic pain typically follows numerous evaluations for other therapeutic options that have either failed or were deemed not suitable for the patient. The decision tree for deciding a patient's candidacy for surgical ablation hinges on careful consideration of the type of pain present, its mechanism, the anatomic distribution, the desired durability of a cure, and the overall state of health and life expectancy of the patient. This clinical information is then merged with our current framework and understanding of pain signaling pathways to develop a treatment plan with the highest probability of achieving the patient-specific metric for success. The efficacy of ablative procedures depends heavily on our understanding of the physiology of the human pain experience incorporating all elements beginning with the nature of the peripheral stimulus end ending with behavioral and emotional perception of pain. Current theory has evolved from concepts of serial processing defining the "labelled line" theory of pain transmission to more sophisticated, distributed models of a "pain matrix," in which peripheral nociception feeds into multilayered central circuitry that not only localizes painful stimuli but also incorporates emotional and temporal contexts, elicits top–down control, and changes the way future stimuli are perceived.[1] Ablative procedures seek to alter pain processing by removing part of this complex circuitry (Fig. 105.1). In doing so, it is possible to disrupt pain transmission but also to change how it is processed—sometimes leading to initial pain relief followed by recurrence. Because neuroaugmentative procedures incorporating high-frequency stimulation and local analgesic administration have become routine parts of clinical practice, use of neuroablative techniques has decreased.

However, several procedures still provide significant value in certain clinical scenarios. In this chapter, we review the indications, anatomy, techniques, and outcomes in dorsal root entry zone lesioning, cordotomy, stereotactic cingulotomy, thalamotomy, and tractotomies within the brainstem.

Dorsal Root Entry Zone Lesioning

INDICATIONS

Lesioning of the dorsal root entry zone of the spinal cord (DREZ procedure) is performed in patients with refractory neuropathic pain of peripheral origin, most commonly resulting from nerve root avulsion or injury within the brachial plexus. The procedure has also been performed in neuropathic pain resulting from spinal cord injury (SCI), spasticity, and postherpetic neuralgia.[2,3] Although less typical, it has also been performed in patients suffering cancer-related pain. Because the DREZ procedure disrupts afferent pain signaling at a specific level, patients with pain distributions that are focal, only spanning a few dermatomal levels, are considered better candidates for this procedure compared to individuals with more diffuse pain syndromes.[4]

ANATOMY AND PHYSIOLOGY

The DREZ procedure is built on the hypothesis that following injury of primary peripheral neurons and subsequent deafferentation, central second-order neurons in the spinal cord become hypersensitive and produce aberrant afferent pain signals. This occurs in the absence of a real painful stimulus and is therefore neuropathic in nature. The cell bodies of the second-order sensory neurons carrying afferent pain information reside in the

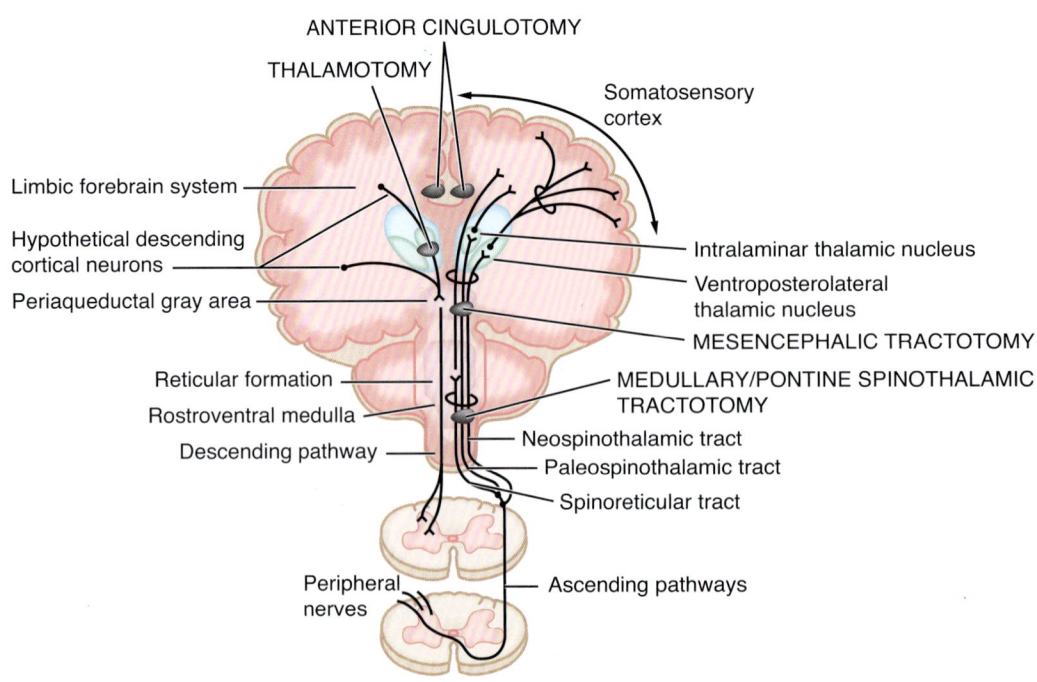

FIGURE 105.1 Specific ablative lesions and their locations relative to the nociceptive pathways.

substantia gelatinosa (Rexed layers 1 and 2) of the dorsal horn throughout the spinal cord.[3] Primary neurons, whose cell bodies reside in the dorsal root ganglion, enter the spinal cord via the DREZ and either immediately synapse in the substantia gelatinosa or travel within Lissauer's tract 1 to 2 levels above or below the level of entry prior to synapsing.[5] The area of synapse lies immediately deep and medial to the entry zone where nerve rootlets enter the spinal cord (Fig. 105.2). Lesioning this area disrupts the abnormal pain signaling of second-order neurons at the associated dermatomal level but does not affect transmission of painful stimuli arising from levels below the lesion that travel within the spinothalamic tract. This is in contrast to cordotomy which specifically targets the ascending spinothalamic tract, thus severing pain transmission of all dermatomal levels whose second-order neurons have already entered and are traveling in the spinothalamic tract. It is important to recognize that the corticospinal tract lies lateral to the dorsal horn and ablations targeted too laterally can result in ipsilateral hemiparesis. Additionally, in cervical levels of the spinal cord, proprioceptive information from the ipsilateral arm runs in the dorsal column just medial to the dorsal horn. Therefore, lesioning aimed too far medially may result in loss of ipsilateral upper extremity proprioception.[5,6]

TECHNIQUE

Under general anesthesia, the patient is placed in the prone position with rigid head fixation. Multiple laminotomies are made to provide adequate access to the spinal cord level of interest and one to two spinal cord levels above and below. A midline durotomy is performed, and the posterolateral sulcus on the affected side is identified. In instances of nerve root or brachial plexus injury, nerve root atrophy can often be observed and used to identify the appropriate level for lesioning. This can be confirmed after placing the radiofrequency ablation (RFA) probe (e.g., Nashold electrode) in the DREZ

and measuring an impedance value between the DREZ of the spinal cord and a peripherally placed grounding electrode. Injured areas have markedly decreased impedance values. This measurement will also serve as a preablation baseline (typically 900 to 1,200 ohms) because the impedance will also decrease after lesioning is performed. To perform the ablation, the Nashold electrode is placed 1 to 2 mm into the area of the entry zone at an angle 20 to 30 degrees medial to lateral relative to the plane perpendicular to the spinal cord surface.[7] Each RFA is then carried out by powering to a temperature of 75° C for 15 to 20 seconds. A total of 40 to 60 lesions centered around the level of interest are performed.[8] Microsurgical technique as well as laser ablation serve as alternatives to RFA.

OUTCOMES

Patients experiencing the most favorable outcomes following the DREZ procedure are those suffering from neuropathic pain related to brachial plexus avulsion injury. A review of the published clinical studies that reported greater than 20 patients identified 62% to 91% patients suffering from brachial plexus avulsion pain to have "good improvement" in symptoms after the surgery,[9–13] where "good improvement" was defined as the need for only minimal ongoing medical management to maintain satisfactory pain relief.[5] The knowledge surrounding the durability of pain control is limited by the length of follow-up in the published studies but has been confirmed to last, in some instances, up to 3 to 5 years. One particular study performed a subgroup analysis to evaluate the effect of intraoperative electrophysiology mapping of the DREZ on outcome and found improved pain control in the group that received intraoperative mapping.[12] Patients undergoing DREZ for SCI-related pain can expect pain relief of localized, end-zone pain occurring just at or above the level of sensory loss. More diffuse and distal pain phenomenon below the level of injury, however, is not as well managed, with efficacy rates falling

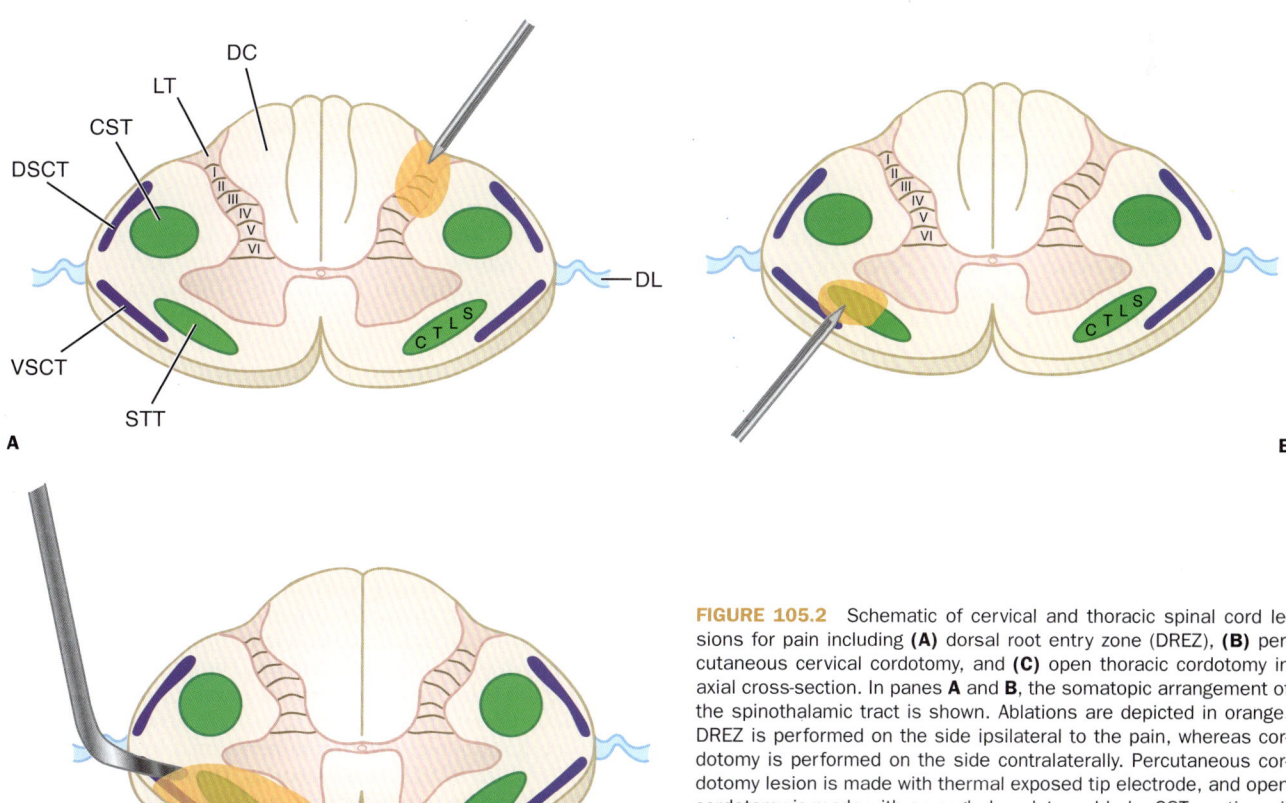

FIGURE 105.2 Schematic of cervical and thoracic spinal cord lesions for pain including **(A)** dorsal root entry zone (DREZ), **(B)** percutaneous cervical cordotomy, and **(C)** open thoracic cordotomy in axial cross-section. In panes **A** and **B**, the somatotopic arrangement of the spinothalamic tract is shown. Ablations are depicted in orange. DREZ is performed on the side ipsilateral to the pain, whereas cordotomy is performed on the side contralaterally. Percutaneous cordotomy lesion is made with thermal exposed tip electrode, and open cordotomy is made with an angled cordotomy blade. CST, corticospinal tract; DC, dorsal columns; DL, dentate ligament; DSCT, dorsal spinocerebellar tract; LT, Lissauer's tract; STT, spinothalamic tract; VSCT, ventral spinocerebellar tract.

to 20% or lower.[5] To improve efficacy of the DREZ procedure in SCI patients, Falci et al.[14] have suggested using intramedullary electrophysiologic guidance to identify regions of spontaneous DREZ hyperactivity to identify optimal lesion placement. In a group of 32 patients who underwent this approach, 84% achieved 100% pain reduction. Pain control following the DREZ procedure in patients suffering from postherpetic neuralgia is felt to be only transient, with only approximately 25% of patients experiencing relief at 1 year.[2] Outcomes are largely comparable for RFA versus laser or microsurgical technique.[15] However, many surgeons utilize the RFA technique because of the reproducible lesions provided by the Nashold electrode.[5]

The most common adverse effect of the DREZ procedure is paresthesia, which is usually transient but can be permanent in a minority of cases. This is estimated to incidence of transient or permanent paresthesias, that is, 15% to 30%.[4] Transient or temporary motor weakness is also a known risk of the procedure which results from an ablation field that extends laterally beyond the DREZ to involve the corticospinal tract. Incidence rates of permanent weakness vary widely, with the majority of studies citing less than 10% risk, with some studies citing up to 40% to 60% according to a review by Konrad.[5]

Cordotomy

INDICATIONS

Destruction of the anterolateral column, or spinothalamic tract, for treatment of chronic pain, was first reported in 1912 by Spiller and Martin.[16] The procedure, referred to as cordotomy, has evolved since that time but exists today in its same conceptual form, with the goal of eliminating the transmission of afferent pain signal by ablating the spinothalamic tract. The most appropriate candidates are those who have localized, unilateral pain that is nociceptive in origin.[17] The most typical, current-day indication would be in the setting of intractable unilateral pelvic, flank, or chest wall pain from metastatic cancer. Cordotomy has become less commonly performed due to the rise of opioid therapies and intrathecal pain pumps for palliation but should continue to be considered in situations in which these initial therapies are ineffective or inappropriate in the setting of the patient's wishes or life expectancy. Additionally, it is important to note that chronic cancer-related pain can develop a neuropathic component due to actual injury to nerve fibers, and it is important to counsel patients regarding the likely persistence of the neuropathic component after cordotomy.[17] The surgery is either performed percutaneously at the C1/2 level with the patient awake to provide sensory feedback or via an open surgical approach at an upper thoracic level with the patient under general anesthesia in the prone position. For percutaneous cervical technique, the patient must be able to tolerate lying flat and still for approximately 45 minutes. For thoracic open cordotomy, the patient must not have other active cardiac, pulmonary, or hematologic medical problems that would contraindicate an open surgery in the prone position.[18]

ANATOMY AND PHYSIOLOGY

The anatomic target of the cordotomy is the spinothalamic tract within the anterolateral quadrant of spinal cord at the high cervical level (C1/2) or mid-to-upper thoracic level (T4) on the side contralateral to the patient's pain.[19,20] Pain-mediating afferent fibers enter the spinal cord through the DREZ on the side of the painful stimulus before synapsing in the substantia gelatinosa of the dorsal horn and decussating via the anterior commissure and joining the ascending fibers of the spinothalamic tract contralateral to the side of pain. The decussation of fibers for a given nerve root entry level can occur over 2 to 5 spinal levels.[17] Therefore, the cordotomy lesion ought to be sufficiently rostral relative to the level of pain in order to fully disrupt nociceptive transmission. As general rule

of thumb, allowing for per-patient variation, a C1/2 cordotomy tends to result in analgesia at C5 and below, whereas a T4 cordotomy will achieve analgesia at T10 and below.[20] The somatotopic arrangement of the spinothalamic tract lends itself to targeted lesioning when percutaneous RFA is performed. The ascending spinothalamic tract accrues fibers decussating from their contralateral entry at its medial-most aspect. This leads to the sacral representation being most dorsal, and lateral and the cervical representation being most ventral and medial, with lumbar and thoracic information arranged accordingly in between. This somatotopy is demonstrated in Figure 105.2.

As a result, in patients with predominant hemipelvis or unilateral lower extremity pain, it is possible to selectively lesion sacral and lumbar fibers while preserving the cervical and thoracic domains of the spinothalamic tract.[17]

The operating surgeon must be keenly aware of critical structures in near proximity to the lesion target. Anterior horn cells controlling level-specific motor function lie deep and medial to the spinothalamic tract throughout the spinal cord and are at risk of being involved in the field of ablation. Therefore, C1/2 and midthoracic levels are preferred because loss of anterior horn cells at these levels is not associated with significant morbidity. However, high cervical lesions near the cervicomedullary junction can involve decussating fibers of the cortical spinal tract and pose the risk of causing contralateral weakness of the lower extremity. Importantly, interneurons involved in respiratory control reside within the upper cervical levels and are located within the ventromedial cord in near proximity to the spinothalamic tract. Because of this, bilateral cervical cordotomies must be judiciously considered in order to avoid the life-threatening sleep-related apnea phenomenon, commonly referred to as Ondine's curse.[17]

TECHNIQUE

Percutaneous cervical cordotomy is performed under either fluoroscopic[21] or computed tomography (CT)-guidance.[17] The patient is placed in the supine position with the head maintained in slight flexion either with a fixation band or rigid frame fixation depending on surgeon preference. A combination of local anesthetic and light sedation is provided for anesthesia. The C1/2 interspace is identified using lateral x-ray or CT imaging. In the case of fluoroscopy or x-ray technique, a 20-gauge spinal needle must first be introduced into the subarachnoid space in order to inject contrast to aid in identification of the dentate ligament, which is the critical landmark in the anterior-posterior dimension for safe localization of the spinothalamic tract. CT myelogram with contrast injection through either lumbar or cervical site provides multiplanar acquisition of imaging to more confidently identify the needle or cannula trajectory with respect to the dentate ligament and spinothalamic tract. Once the dentate ligament is identified, the electrode cannula with stylet is introduced into the spinal cord with a goal target of 1 to 2 mm anterior to the dentate ligament for sacral and lumbar fibers and 2 to 3 mm anterior to the ligament for thoracic and cervical fibers. Repeat CT imaging may be obtained to confirm appropriate cannula positioning. The stylet is then removed, and the noninsulated electrode (2.5 mm in length by 0.25 mm in diameter) is introduced into the spinal cord through the cannula. The electrode impedance is tested to confirm intraparenchymal placement (greater than 800 ohms).[17,21] Stimulation of 0.2 to 1.5 mV can be provided at 100 Hz to obtain neurophysiologic confirmation of electrode placement. The patient will likely experience dysesthesias in the form of inappropriate temperature sensation. Once there is satisfactory confirmation of correct electrode positioning, ablation is performed by heating the tissue to 70° C to 80° C for 60 seconds. Depending on the extent of the patient's pain symptoms, multiple lesions may be performed. Postprocedurally, the patient is monitored closely either in perioperative recovery unit or in the intensive care unit for at least 4 to 6 hours prior to less intensive monitoring or discharge.

Open thoracic cordotomy is performed in the operating room with the patient in the prone position. A bilateral or hemilaminectomy is performed and a durotomy is made to provide access and direct visualization of the spinal cord. The dentate ligament is identified and separated from the dura to facilitate gentle upward rotation of the spinal cord to provide the surgeon access to the anterior spinal cord. An angled cordotomy knife is then inserted anterior to the dentate ligament to a depth of 3 to 4 mm and swept anteriorly to ensure complete disruption of the spinothalamic tract. It is essential that the surgeon respect the dentate ligament as the posterior boundary in order to avoid injury to the corticospinal tract.[5] The dura is then closed in a watertight fashion in order to prevent cerebrospinal fluid (CSF) leak. Figures 105.2b and 105.2c demonstrate the differences in approach and the expected lesion size for percutaneous and open cordotomy. Of note, the ventral spinocerebellar tract is more likely to be involved in the open lesion which may contribute to postoperative ataxia.

OUTCOMES

Compared to other ablative procedures for pain, cordotomy is well studied with over 3,600 patients reported in the literature, including one prospective study.[22] In general, as reviewed by Konrad,[5] immediate pain relief following percutaneous cordotomy occurs in approximately 90% of patients with rates of pain relief falling to 50% to 60%, 1 year after procedure. Similarly, open cordotomy provides high rates of immediate pain relief (up to 93% reported by Cowie and Hitchcock[23]) which fall to 54% to 65% after 1 year follow-up.[23–25] Therefore, cordotomy remains an impactful option for patients with severe pain due to advanced metastatic disease. Its efficacy has also been studied in cases of chronic pain from nonmalignant etiologies. In a study of 122 patients who underwent percutaneous cervical cordotomy, 27 suffered from nonmalignant sources of pain. In this subgroup, only 20% experienced complete pain relief compared to a rate of 66% in cancer patients. Cordotomy, therefore, is felt to be most effective for cancer-related pain but still remains an option for patients suffering from intractable pain due to SCI or other etiologies, in which all other options have been exhausted.

The most common adverse outcomes reported following cordotomy include spinal headache from dural puncture, short duration of "mirror pain" during which time symptoms similar to preoperative pain are experienced on the contralateral side of the body, dysesthesias, ataxia, temporary leg weakness, and temporary bowel and/or bladder dysfunction.[18] Estimated incidences of these side effects are reported to be in the range of 10% to 34%, with ataxia and bladder dysfunction being most commonly reported. Serious adverse events including respiratory impairment and even associated death have been reported even in unilateral procedures. Ischia et al.[26] cites a 0% to 9% risk of mortality rate in unilateral procedures and 11% risk of death in bilateral cervical cordotomy. It is generally felt that the majority of complications arise from poor electrode placement and that the rise of CT guidance has led to decreased rates of severe complication.[17] Open cordotomy comes with the increased risk of CSF leak due to larger durotomy, but the ablation-related neurologic side effects discussed are largely similar in both percutaneous and open approaches.[5]

Cingulotomy

INDICATIONS

Although cingulotomy was first performed for psychiatric disease by Sir Hugh Cairns in 1948, it was not until over a decade later in that the first series on cingulotomy for intractable pain was reported in 1962 by Foltz and White at the University of Washington.[27,28] Motivated by significant reduction of intractable pain in patients who had undergone prefrontal lobotomy in combination with animal studies implicating the frontal cingulum fasciculus as the critical white matter tract involved generating the emotional valence of pain,[29–31] Foltz and White[28] sought to employ stereotactic cingulotomy as a refined ablative approach for pain control. Rather than enrolling patients based on a specific etiology of intractable pain, they worked with psychiatry colleagues to select patients who "showed prominent emotional factors" such that the cingulotomy might "modify the patient's emotional response . . . so that his expressions of fear and anxiety no longer augmented critically whatever pattern of organic pain was present."[28] Following their initial success with their report describing 11 of 16 patients experiencing good pain relief, many other groups explored the role of anterior cingulotomy for chronic medically refractory pain, including applications for both neoplastic and nonneoplastic sources of pain. In recent years, however, the rise of implantable intrathecal pain pumps and neuromodulatory devices, anterior cingulotomy has become less popular.[32] However, anterior cingulotomy continues to offer a widely applicable approach for severe, intractable pain, especially in patients predominantly featuring an affective component to their pain. It may also be most appropriate in patients who are not candidates for implantable devices due to barriers to frequent follow-up care or due to short life expectancy in the setting of end-stage malignancy.

ANATOMY AND PHYSIOLOGY

General pain perception has been described as being divided into two components: a lateral pain system involved in spatial discrimination of pain and a medial pain system involved in the affective and autonomic response to pain.[33] The anterior cingulate is a main component of the medial system. It is located mesial, ventral, rostral, and dorsal relative to the genu of the corpus callosum and has broad connections to many different sites involved in pain processing. These include the medial frontal cortex, thalamic nuclei (anterior, midline, interlaminar, and others), septum, amygdala, basal ganglia, nucleus accumbens, and brain stem sites such as the periaqueductal gray.[34] The anterior cingulate receives nociceptive input and has connections with several sites involved in the affective and attentional component of pain which is supported by a broad range of data. Foltz and White,[28] for example, noted changes in comfort and affect in several patients immediately following lesioning in the operating room. Additionally, functional imaging studies have shown bilateral response within the anterior cingulate in response to pain.[35] Furthermore, intraoperative single neuron recordings in humans undergoing anterior cingulotomy for psychiatric disease have demonstrated modulated activity in response to thermal and mechanical noxious stimuli. Those same neurons did not respond to nonnoxious stimuli.[36] Furthermore, stimulation studies in monkeys and humans have been able to induce responses of fear or happiness in response to anterior cingulate stimulation.[33]

TECHNIQUE

When the procedure was first developed in the 1950s prior to CT and magnetic resonance imaging (MRI) availability, ventriculography was used for anterior cingulate localization relative to the frontal horn of the lateral ventricle. The lesion was frequently performed with the patient awake to allow for continuous assessment of the patient's emotional, affective, and motor function.[28] In current practice, the procedure is performed with either under CT- or MRI-based stereotactic guidance, with MRI becoming progressively more popular. The bilateral anterior cingulate targets are mapped preoperatively with standard coordinates being 20 to 25 mm posterior to tip of frontal horn, 7 mm lateral from midline, and 2 to 3 mm

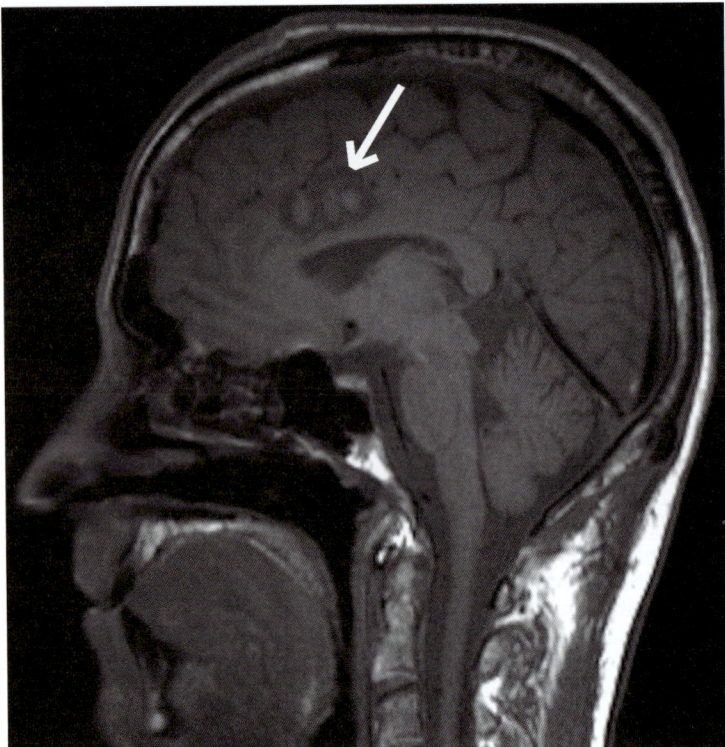
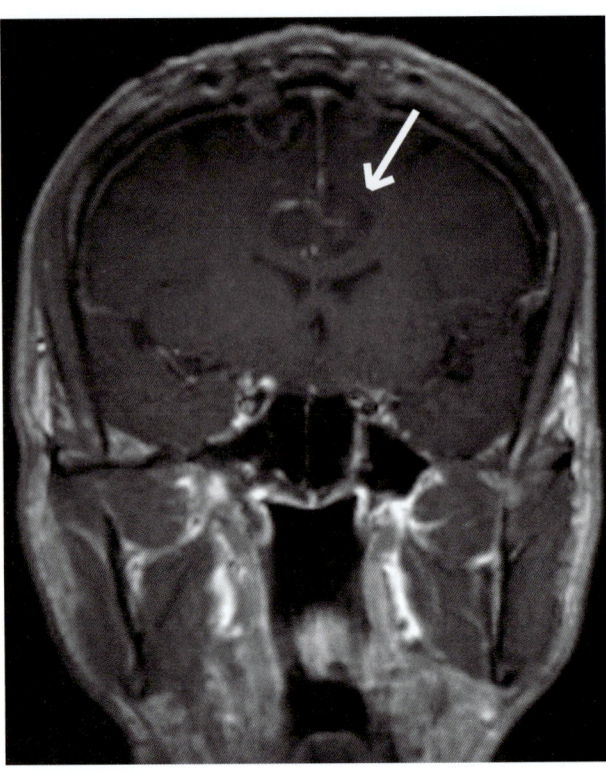

FIGURE 105.3   Postoperative magnetic resonance imaging following stereotactic anterior cingulotomy. **A:** Sagittal T1 sequence reveals three lesions (*white arrow*) within the anterior cingulate gyrus. **B:** Coronal postcontrast T1 sequence shows bilateral lesions within the anterior cingulate gyrus with post-surgical changes along the stereotactic probe trajectories through the bilateral frontal calvarium and frontal lobes.

superior to the corpus callosum.[37] Importantly, two retrospective analyses of patients with lesions ranging from 17.5 mm to 37.5 mm posterior from the tip of the frontal horn showed that patients with more posterior lesions had less effective pain relief.[32,38] In the operating room, the target is accessed through the placement of two burr holes, each approximately 20 to 30 mm from midline just anterior to the coronal suture. Correct stereotactic placement can be confirmed by the use of microelectrode recording. An uninsulated 10-mm radiofrequency thermocoagulation electrode is placed in the target tissue which is then heated to 85° C for 90 seconds. Typically, the electrode is then pulled back 5 mm, and a second lesion is made.[37] Multiple lesions along the cingulate cortex in the anterior-posterior direction can be performed. Figure 105.3 provides postoperative MRI demonstrating ablation of the bilateral anterior cingulate cortex with three lesions on each side. Alternative methods for creating the lesion include radiofrequency thermal ablation and laser interstitial thermal therapy.

OUTCOMES

Anterior cingulotomy has generally been referred to as an option most appropriate for patients suffering from cancer-related nociceptive pain. However, a recent review and meta-analysis by Sharim and Pouratian[32] showed equivalent outcomes in both neoplastic and nonneoplastic populations. In a total of 224 patients (97 with cancer-related pain and 127 with non-cancer pain) across 11 studies, 66.5% reported pain relief after the procedure. This rate was comparable in both cancer patients (65.3%) and noncancer patients (68.0%). Table 105.1, adapted from their review, contains the breakdown of the outcomes on a per study basis. Types of noncancer pain varied widely including neurofibromatosis, thalamic stroke, trauma, failed back syndrome, phantom limb pain, atypical facial pain, and peripheral neuropathy.[32]

Although up to two-thirds of patients will report pain relief at some point postoperatively, the durability of the relief

has been shown to diminish with time. In some instances of persistent pain in the immediate postoperative period, repeat cingulotomy is offered in order to expand the extent of the lesion. The incidence of repeat cingulotomy has been estimated at 7.6% across all published cases[32]; however, the current routine addition of a second ablative site after withdrawing the ablative catheter 5 mm is thought to mitigate this risk.

Temporary postoperative adverse symptoms associated with cingulotomy include urinary incontinence, confusion, and disorientation. More serious reported events include a less than 5% incidence seizure and less than 1% incidence of hemiparesis or personality change.[32] Longer term assessment of effect on

TABLE 105.1   Outcomes of Anterior Cingulotomy Broken Down by Neoplastic versus Nonneoplastic Pain Etiology

Study	Total No. of Patients	Fraction (%) Experiencing Pain Relief	
		Cancer	Noncancer
Foltz and White[28]	16	5/6 (83)	6/10 (60)
Foltz and White[64]	35	9/11 (82)	18/24 (75)
Faillace et al.[65]	9	3/7 (43)	1/2 (50)
Hurt and Ballantine[66]	68	18/32 (56)	16/36 (44)
Voris and Whisler[67]	16	5/5 (100)	8/11 (73)
Pillay and Hassenbusch[68]	10	5/8 (63)	1/2 (50)
Cohen et al.[39]	12	—	8/12 (67)
Wilkinson[69]	23	—	18/23 (78)
Yen et al.[70]	22	12/15 (80)	7/7 (100)
Yen et al.[40]	10	6/10 (60)	—
Patel et al.[71]	3	3/3 (100)	—
TOTAL	224	66/97 (68)	83/127 (65)

Modified from Sharim J, Pouratian N. Anterior cingulotomy for the treatment of chronic intractable pain: a systematic review. *Pain Physician* 2016;19:537–550.

cognition have revealed decrements in executive function that peaks in severity at approximately 3 months postoperatively but tends to resolve by 1 year postprocedure. Persistent impairment in spontaneous word production and speech fluency have also been reported.[39,40]

Thalamotomy

INDICATIONS

The thalamus is a collection of nuclei through which nearly all sensory input passes in order to reach the cortex and conscious perception. As such, the thalamus was recognized early as a logical target for disrupting nociceptive transmission through anatomically precise ablative procedures.[41,42] However, early experience with thalamic lesioning for chronic pain forced a reconsideration of the thalamus as a simple relay station because therapeutic pain relief achieved by thalamotomy frequently waned within 3 to 6 months of the procedure.[43] These observations, combined with other unwanted sensory and psychiatric side effects, and the advent of more sophisticated pharmacologic and deep brain stimulation procedures for chronic pain control have led to a general paucity of rigorous clinical data assessing the efficacy of thalamotomy. It is currently a relatively rare procedure used for chronic, nonmalignant pain and is considered a last-line approach for malignant neuropathic pain.[22] Most typically, it is used in scenarios of limited life expectancy where direct tumor invasion is causing intractable face and/or head pain that is not alleviated by pharmacologic therapy and is not anticipated to be adequately managed by an ablative lesion at the spinal cord or peripheral level. Thalamic targets have evolved from lateral to medial with the observation that ventrocaudal thalamic nucleus lesions tend to produce more unwanted side effects.[44,45] Currently, medial targets including centromedian (CM), parafascicular (PF), and centrolateral (CL) are most common, with the pulvinar nucleus also being targeted.[46] Recently, with the emergence of focused ultrasound (FUS) as a technique for achieving precise ablation, thalamotomy is being revisited as a method for treatment of nonmalignant chronic neuropathic pain.[47] As results using this method become more established and as refinement of FUS technique occurs, reconsideration of thalamic targets for ablation in specific clinical scenarios may be warranted.

ANATOMY AND PHYSIOLOGY

Thalamic nuclei are anatomically organized into medial, lateral, and anterior groups separated internally by the internal medullary lamina (which houses intralaminar nuclei) and contained laterally by the thalamic reticular nucleus.[48] Additional functional characterization of nuclei exists based on the origin of their inputs as well as the specificity of their projections. Medial nuclei receiving peripheral nociceptive inputs include the dorsomedial nucleus (DM), which primarily receives inputs from the amygdala, olfactory cortex, and limbic basal ganglia. The DM also projects to frontal cortex in a diffuse manner. Lateral nuclei receiving nociceptive inputs include the ventral posterolateral nucleus (VPL), the ventral posterior medial nucleus (VPM), and the pulvinar nucleus (PVN). VPL receives inputs from the spinothalamic tract and projects in a precise manner to somatosensory cortex, relaying peripheral nociceptive signals from the body. The VPM analogously receives inputs from the trigeminothalamic tract projecting in an anatomically precise manner to the somatosensory cortex and relaying nociceptive signals originating from the face. The specificity of inputs and projections associated with lateral nuclei may underlie why targeted ablation of these nuclei produce sensory deficits, whereas medial targets with broader inputs and outputs can be ablated without as many obvious side effects. Anterior targets include the anterior nucleus of the thalamus (AT). AT receives

inputs from the hippocampus and amygdala and projects to the cingulate cortex. Intralaminar nuclei receiving peripheral nociceptive inputs include the CL which is part of the rostral intralaminar nuclei as well as the CM and PF which are subsets of the caudal group of intralaminar nuclei.

TECHNIQUES

Stereotactic open approach: The general surgical method for stereotactic ablation of thalamic targets involves awake surgery to simultaneously record from and identify the nucleus of choice and then ablate it using thermal energy. The procedure starts by placing the patient's head in a rigid stereotactic frame. The frame is then fixed to the operating table in final position. A pilot CT scan is obtained via portable or intraoperative CT. This CT image is merged with a previously obtained MRI in order to determine stereotactic coordinates of the target in relation to the line defined by connecting the anterior and posterior commissure (AC-PC coordinates). Coordinates from 6 to 10 mm lateral to the AC-PC line, 7 to 11 mm posterior to the AC-PC midpoint, and from 1 mm below to 2 mm above the AC-PC line have been used to target DM and CM.[49,50] An entry point is typically chosen near the coronal suture 3 cm from midline. A curvilinear incision is made and a burr hole drilled and then dura opened in standard fashion to give access to the brain. Depending on the target and surgeon preference, microelectrode recordings can be used for localization. Although there is not always a clear electrographic correlate to localize the nucleus, in certain cases, neuronal bursting patterns may indicate deafferentation pain.[51] Medial nuclei, in general, provide a large target with no somatotopic projection pattern. Therefore, electrical recording may be of little utility; nonetheless, test stimulation for motor and sensory phenomena can always be conducted as a safety measure prior to lesioning.[46] Using a thermocouple probe, a test lesion is made at a lower temperature (40° C for 25 seconds), and if the patient shows no adverse effects, an ablative lesion is made (70° C for 70 seconds).[46]

Noninvasive radiosurgery and focused ultrasound: Radiosurgery techniques used for thalamotomy include both Gamma Knife and linear accelerator methods. FUS is beginning to emerge as an alternate energy source for creating precise lesions. As imaging technology for lesion localization becomes more accurate, clinical results of noninvasive ablative approaches may near those of stereotactic open approaches.[52] One key difference with respect to radiosurgery approaches is the time needed for lesions to mature following radiation treatment. Young et al.[49] describes a case series in which 24 medial thalamic lesions were created via Gamma Knife using 140 to 180 Gy. The emergence of distinct lesions via MRI occurred 3 to 6 weeks after the initial procedure and did not fully mature until 8 to 12 weeks. Ultimately, 9 out of 15 total patients achieved a greater than 50% pain reduction at 3-month follow-up, which is comparable to the results of stereotactic ablation. However, if shorter term pain relief is needed, such as in the context of severe pain and limited life expectancy, then stereotactic alternatives will need to be considered to provide prompt palliation to the patient. Moreover, recent results of noninvasive thermoablation by FUS suggest that it may represent a tractable alternative. In a case series by Jeanmonod et al.,[47] transcranial MR-guided FUS (tcMRgFUS) was used to perform CL thalamotomies on 12 patients suffering from chronic neuropathic pain. Lesions 3 to 4 mm in size were made using tcMRgFUS to heat the tissue to 51° C to 64° C as monitored by MR thermometry. Six patients experienced some degree of immediate pain relief, whereas a mean pain reduction of 49% was experienced by nine patients at 3-month follow-up. A randomized sham-controlled clinical trial is currently underway to assess the efficacy of ExAblate FUS technology in treatment of refractory chronic trigeminal neuropathic pain of nonmalignant origin (NCT03309813). The key technical barrier to improvement in precision and accuracy

TABLE 105.2 **Core Outcome Results of Studies of Thalamotomy for Cancer Pain from 1966 to 2009**

Authors and Year	No. of Patients	Outcome
Whittle and Jenkinson[46]	2	Adequate pain relief until death
Steiner et al.[72]	52	8 had excellent pain relief, 18 with moderate pain relief.
Hitchcock and Teixeira[73]	16 cancer/53 total	Bilateral center-median superior to basal thalamotomy
Fairman and Llavallol[74]	165	70% had no or satisfactory pain relief.
Richardson[53]	38 total	Favorable outcome
Richardson[54]	24 total	Mixed results but return of chronic pain occurred in all patients
Uematsu et al.[75]	17	3 excellent, 7 good, 3 no benefit
Sugita et al.[55]	44/60	85% had excellent or satisfactory pain relief initially, generally good results in cancer pain patients.
Leksell et al.[76]	25	6 pain free, 4 moderate pain relief, effect noticed after 3 weeks
Shimizu et al.[77]	8/17	6 had complete pain relief until death (3 died <1 month postprocedure); 2 had adequate pain relief, psychological disturbances common
Fairman[78]	15/53	80% had bilateral pain relief.
Ramamurthi and Kalyanaraman[79]	7	All had reasonable pain relief.
Sano et al.[80]	10 total	Lasting effect in 8 cases
Amano et al.[81]	14/47	Good pain relief only in thalamic pain or causalgia
Choi and Umbach[82]	30/37	91% of all cases had excellent or good results.
Voris and Whisler[67]	35/58	Pain relief in most patients, few had long lasting pain relief

Adapted from a systematic review by Raslan AM, Cetas JS, McCartney S, et al. Destructive procedures for control of cancer pain: the case for cordotomy. *J Neurosurg* 2011;114:155–170.

of both radiosurgery and FUS techniques is improvement in MR technology for target localization. Real-time continuous MR imaging and MR thermometry monitoring dictate both lesion accuracy as well as accuracy of thermal effects during FUS ablation. As this technology improves, the noninvasive nature of approach will likely make it a more favorable alternative to stereotactic thermoablation.

OUTCOMES

Although efficacy of medial thalamotomy has been shown in multiple case series and case reports, systematic studies of methods, targets, lesion sizes, and indications have not been conducted. Raslan et al.[22] conducted a systematic review of ablative pain procedure studies including thalamotomy for malignant pain and found only a handful of reports, all case series level evidence. The results of the systematic review for thalamotomy are summarized in Table 105.2, which is adapted from Raslan et al.[22] It is therefore not surprising that there is no consensus as to a specific nucleus to optimally target for ablation. As mentioned, medial targets with less somatotopic mapping seem to produce fewer side effects. In addition, it seems that pain caused by direct tissue damage (nociceptive, for example from malignant invasion) responds more favorably than neuropathic pain, although individual reports vary. Sugita et al.[55] found 85% had excellent or satisfactory pain relief initially, whereas Richardson[53,54] found mixed results with return of chronic pain occurring in all patients. The aforementioned noninvasive techniques seem to produce approximately 50% pain reduction at 3 months postprocedure.[52] As with all ablative procedures, the outcome depends in large part on the circuit pathophysiology prior to intervention and the reaction of the remaining circuit or network after ablation. As our understanding of pain physiology advances; as the technology to interrogate the circuitry prior, during, and after ablation improves; and as our methods of ablation become more precise, it is possible that the seemingly heterogeneous outcomes of thalamotomy will become better understood.

Ablative Procedures of the Brainstem

INDICATIONS

Because the anatomical basis of pain transmission was established throughout the 19th century, surgical procedures for treatment of pain advanced, leading to cordotomy in 1911[16] as well as spinothalamic tractotomy. However, throughout the first half of the 20th century, it became apparent that existing procedures did not provide long-term relief of neck, shoulder, and face pain. This led Spiegel and Wycis to pioneer stereotactic lesioning of the mesencephalon in 1953 and later Hitchcock to use stereotaxis for lesioning of the pons and trigeminothalamic pathways in the brainstem.[56] Here, we discuss mesencephalic tractotomy (lesioning of the spinothalamic tract in the midbrain) and ablation of the trigeminothalamic tract and nucleus caudalis (the caudalmost subdivision of the spinal trigeminal nucleus). These procedures are indicated in cases of facial, head, neck, or shoulder pain which are unresponsive to pharmacologic therapy and more conservative measures. Furthermore, for pain rostral to C5, cordotomy may be limited, in which case mesencephalic tractotomy serves as an alternative. Typically, underlying disorders in which the aforementioned procedures are considered include geniculate or glossopharyngeal neuralgia, failed trigeminal surgery or anesthesia dolorosa, posttraumatic neuropathy, postherpetic dysesthesia, atypical facial pain, and cancer-related pain.[1]

ANATOMY AND PHYSIOLOGY

The trigeminal sensory nuclei not only receive somatic sensory input in large part from the trigeminal nerve but also receive input from the facial nerve (sensation near outer ear), glossopharyngeal nerve (sensation for middle ear, external auditory meatus, pharynx, posterior third of tongue), and vagus nerve (sensation for pharynx, outer ear, infratentorial meninges). The trigeminal nuclear complex extends from the rostral cervical spinal cord to the midbrain and is made up of the mesencephalic, chief sensory, and spinal trigeminal nuclei. These nuclei transmit fine touch, pressure, temperature, and pain sensations from the face to the brain in an analogous manner to posterior columns and anterolateral systems of the spinal cord. Namely, the chief sensory nucleus (located dorsolaterally in the rostral pons) receives synaptic input from large diameter sensory fibers carrying fine touch and pressure transmission. Cell bodies in the nucleus give rise to the trigeminal lemniscus in the rostral aspect of the pons which decussates and travels to the VPM adjacent to the medial lemniscus in the dorsal brainstem. Fibers carrying crude touch, pain, and temperature enter the pons and immediately descend via the spinal trigeminal tract (an analogue of Lissauer's tract) to synapse on the spinal trigeminal nucleus in the dorsolateral brainstem starting at the cervicomedullary junction (the rostral extent of the dorsal horn). The spinal trigeminal nucleus is subdivided from rostral to caudal into the nucleus oralis, nucleus interpolaris, and nucleus caudalis (extending caudally to the C2 segment of spinal cord and substantially overlapping with substantia gelatinosa containing cervical inputs). The spinal trigeminal nucleus gives rise to the trigeminothalamic tract which decussates and ascends to the VPM alongside the spinothalamic tract (in the dorsal pons at the level of the middle cerebral peduncle). Of note, there is somatotopic organization of the trigeminothalamic tract and spinal trigeminal nucleus as described by various authors[1,48,57] with an "onion skin" topology in which the central face is represented rostrally, and the peripheral face is caudal with V1 to V3 organization assuming a ventral to dorsal pattern. The mesencephalic trigeminal nucleus and tract together mediate facial proprioception and are located adjacent to the periaqueductal gray matter in the dorsal pons. The nucleus houses cell bodies of proprioceptive neurons, whereas the tract houses axons of these neurons. Of particular clinical significance is the anatomic relationship of the nucleus caudalis and spinal trigeminal tract to the dorsal spinocerebellar tract which is located just lateral on the dorsal surface of the spinal cord and brainstem as well as the lateral spinothalamic tract, located ventrally. Extensive lesioning at this level can cause an ipsilateral ataxia from damage to the spinocerebellar tract or contralateral anesthesia from spinothalamic tract damage. Similarly, damage to the nucleus cuneatus which receives dorsal column input and is located in a caudal and medial direction would cause ipsilateral proprioceptive and fine touch deficits.[1,57] Finally, extensive lesioning of the spinothalamic tract in the midbrain is known to cause oculomotor deficits as well as ptosis due to proximity to the oculomotor nucleus and Edinger-Westphal nucleus.[58]

TECHNIQUES

Mesencephalic tractotomy is performed using stereotactic lesioning via a radiofrequency probe as previously described.[58] Of note, the procedure is performed under local anesthesia which facilitates intraoperative stimulation prior to lesioning to ensure that the target has been identified. Namely, as described by Frank et al.,[59] prior to lesioning, an evoked feeling of thermal sensation should be obtained to ensure the stimulator is in the spinothalamic tract. Also, while lesioning, sensation and proprioception should be assessed systematically to ensure the medial lemniscus is not inadvertently targeted (which could lead to painful anesthesia following the procedure as observed by Spiegel and Wycis). The spinothalamic tract can be localized using various imaging protocols including CT with ventricular contrast or MRI. Integrated data suggest that most lesions are 5-mm behind the posterior commissure, 5 to 10 mm lateral, and 5 mm below the AC-PC plane.[60] Of note, although the original procedure was designed to target the lateral spinothalamic (and also the trigeminothalamic) tracts, evolution of the procedure has included simultaneous lesioning of the DM of the thalamus in order to disrupt its prefrontal connections thought to carry the affective "suffering" component of pain. Similarly, Spiegel et al.[61] have advocated a more medial target to include spinoreticular pathways, also thought to project an affective component of pain processing to limbic structures.

After satisfactory localization of the spinothalamic tract, a radiofrequency lesion can be created in stepwise manner. It is also crucial to assess eye movements and eyelid function throughout this process because the surrounding oculomotor, abducens, and Edinger-Westphal nuclei can be damaged causing gaze palsies (see in the following discussion). Kanpolat[57] has developed a technique for a CT-guided percutaneous trigeminal tractotomy and nucleotomy. Contrast is injected into the subarachnoid space via lumbar puncture prior to the procedure, and a CT is then obtained with careful measurements taken of the depth from skin to dura. The patient is positioned prone, and local anesthetic is given. The procedure is done percutaneously using the electrode system developed by Kanpolat.[57] Impedance measurements are initially used to guide electrode placement. Stimulation is performed with low and high frequencies, and the patient is monitored for paresthesias of the face indicating the electrode is in projecting trigeminal nerve axons. Once positioning of the electrode is acceptable and confirmed by CT, the patient is given additional anesthesia prior to lesioning, which can be painful. One to three lesions are made in a stepwise manner starting with a temperature of 50° to 60° C and then 60° to 80° C for 60 seconds.

OUTCOMES

In a systematic review of ablative procedures for malignant pain control, Raslan et al.[22] reviewed data for both trigeminal tractotomy and nucleotomy as well as mesencephalotomy (see adapted Table 105.3). Mesencephalotomy and pontine tractotomy (combined) are rarely performed (a total of seven studies were cited up until 2011), but effective pain relief generally achieved in a population of patients with very limited life expectancy. Trigeminal tractotomy for cancer-related pain, similarly, was found to have only a small number of studies qualifying for systematic review with the one noncase series piece of evidence being an open-label prospective study.[62] This study employed standardized outcome measures of pain and reported sustained pain relief in 80% of subjects at 6 months.

More recently, in his case series, Kanoplat[57] described 81 patients who underwent 96 CT-guided trigeminal tractotomy and nucleotomy. Sixty-six (85.7%) patients achieved complete or partial satisfactory pain control, whereas 15 patients (14.3%) responded poorly to the procedure. The largest fraction of patients in this series had glossopharyngeal neuralgia. Of note, at the conclusion of the follow-up period (maximum 216 months), 55 patients (71.4%) achieved sustained pain relief, 13 (16.9%) reported partial pain control, and 9 (11.7%) reported failure of pain control.

Frank et al.[58] describe 14 patients treated with stereotaxic rostral mesencephalotomy (a total of 19 procedures) for unilateral thoracobrachial cancer-related pain with frequent neck and/or face involvement. The mean follow-up time was 4.9 months with 14 procedures leading to good or excellent pain relief, whereas 4 led to only fair or no pain relief. The reported complications include two cases with persistent Parinaud syndrome; one case of bilateral ptosis; and single reports of dysesthesias, painful anesthesia, and mental changes.[58] Kim et al.[60] more recently reported a case of MRI-guided stereotactic mesencephalotomy in which initial pain control was achieved with a subsequent increase in pain at the 2-month mark. From this and preceding evidence, the authors argue that mesencephalotomy is rarely indicated for pain other than cancer pain and thalamic syndrome due to probability of pain recurrence at long-term follow-up.[63]

TABLE 105.3 Results of Studies of Mesencephalotomy for Cancer Pain

Authors and Year	No. of Patients	Outcome
Bosch[83]	40	Effective for nociceptive pain
Frank et al.[59]	202	81% lasting pain relief
Barberá et al.[84]	6	All cases with pain relief in neck and upper extremity
Zapletal[85]	12/16	1 patient with long-term relief
Whisler and Voris[86]	38	92% patients with pain relief until death
Nashold[87]	8	All patients with pain relief and with side effects

Adapted from systematic review by Raslan AM, Cetas JS, McCartney S, et al. Destructive procedures for control of cancer pain: the case for cordotomy. *J Neurosurg* 2011;114:155–170.

Conclusion

With the development of improved pharmacotherapy, intrathecal delivery systems, and high-frequency stimulation, ablative procedures for pain have become less commonly utilized treatment options. Like all functional procedures, their utility is limited by current knowledge of the underlying circuitry. Indeed, with the elucidation of nearly every major element of the pain transmission pathway, there has come a corresponding ablative procedure. Here, we discussed indications, anatomy, techniques, and outcomes regarding the DREZ procedure, cordotomy, cingulotomy, thalamotomy, and tractotomies within the brainstem. Unfortunately, the complexity, inherent feedback, and nonlinearity of the pain transmission circuitry has made durable solutions to chronic pain more difficult than simply ablating component parts of the pain pathway. Systematic study of ablative procedures is still lacking, but the literature, as we discussed here, contains many instances of ablative procedures effectively providing relief to patients with severely intractable pain. As neurosurgical procedures for pain become less invasive, including techniques that allow one to lesion without even entering the skull, the need for a thorough understanding and optimization of ablative approaches is crucial. We anticipate that as technology and understanding of functional anatomy advances, we will have the opportunity to readdress ablative approaches and consider more precise or combination therapies to provide satisfactory pain relief to patients with no reasonable alternative.

References

1. Burchiel KJ. *Surgical Management of Pain*. 2nd ed. New York: Thieme; 2014.
2. Friedman AH, Bullitt E. Dorsal root entry zone lesions in the treatment of pain following brachial plexus avulsion, spinal cord injury and herpes zoster. *Appl Neurophysiol* 1988;51:164–169.
3. Nashold BS Jr, Ostdahl RH. Dorsal root entry zone lesions for pain relief. *J Neurosurg* 1979;51:59–69.
4. Piyawattanametha N, Sitthinamsuwan B, Euasobhon P, et al. Efficacy and factors determining the outcome of dorsal root entry zone lesioning procedure (DREZotomy) in the treatment of intractable pain syndrome. *Acta Neurochir (Wien)* 2017;159:2431–2442.
5. Konrad P. Dorsal root entry zone lesion, midline myelotomy and anterolateral cordotomy. *Neurosurg Clin N Am* 2014;25:699–722.
6. Denkers MR, Biagi HL, Ann O'Brien M, et al. Dorsal root entry zone lesioning used to treat central neuropathic pain in patients with traumatic spinal cord injury: a systematic review. *Spine (Phila Pa 1976)* 2002;27:E177–E184.
7. Schulder M. *Handbook of Stereotactic and Functional Neurosurgery*. Boca Raton: CRC Press; 2003.
8. Eli I, Konrad P, Neimat J. Ablative procedures for neuropathic pain. In: Harbaugh RE, Shaffrey C, Couldwell WT, et al, eds. *Neurosurgery Knowledge Update: A Comprehensive Review*. New York: Thieme; 2015:300–307.
9. Thomas DG, Jones SJ. Dorsal root entry zone lesions (Nashold's procedure) in brachial plexus avulsion. *Neurosurgery* 1984;15:966–968.
10. Samii M, Moringlane JR. Thermocoagulation of the dorsal root entry zone for the treatment of intractable pain. *Neurosurgery* 1984;15:953–955.
11. Samii M, Bear-Henney S, Lüdemann W, et al. Treatment of refractory pain after brachial plexus avulsion with dorsal root entry zone lesions. *Neurosurgery* 2001;48:1269–1277.
12. Tomás R, Haninec P. Dorsal root entry zone (DREZ) localization using direct spinal cord stimulation can improve results of the DREZ thermocoagulation procedure for intractable pain relief. *Pain* 2005;116:159–163.
13. Chen HJ, Tu YK. Long term follow-up results of dorsal root entry zone lesions for intractable pain after brachial plexus avulsion injuries. *Acta Neurochir Suppl* 2006;99:73–75.
14. Falci S, Best L, Bayles R, et al. Dorsal root entry zone microcoagulation for spinal cord injury-related central pain: operative intramedullary electrophysiological guidance and clinical outcome. *J Neurosurg* 2002;97:193–200.
15. Sindou M. Microsurgical DREZotomy (MDT) for pain, spasticity, and hyperactive bladder: a 20-year experience. *Acta Neurochir (Wien)* 1995;137:1–5.
16. Spiller WG, Martin E. The treatment of persistent pain of organic origin in the lower part of the body by division of the anterolateral column of the spinal cord. *JAMA* 1912;58:1489–1490. doi:10.1001/jama.1912.04260050165001.
17. Kanpolat Y, Ugur HC, Ayten M, et al. Computed tomography-guided percutaneous cordotomy for intractable pain in malignancy. *Neurosurgery* 2009;64:187–194.
18. Bain E, Hugel H, Sharma M. Percutaneous cervical cordotomy for the management of pain from cancer: a prospective review of 45 cases. *J Palliat Med* 2013;16:901–907.
19. White JC, Sweet WH. *Pain and the Neurosurgeon: A Forty-Year Experience*. Springfield, IL: C. C. Thomas; 1969.
20. Jones B, Finlay I, Ray A, et al. Is there still a role for open cordotomy in cancer pain management? *J Pain Symptom Manage* 2003;25:179–184.
21. Bellini M, Barbieri M. Percutaneous cervical cordotomy in cancer pain. *Anaesthesiol Intensive Ther* 2016;48:197–200.
22. Raslan AM, Cetas JS, McCartney S, et al. Destructive procedures for control of cancer pain: the case for cordotomy. *J Neurosurg* 2011;114:155–170.
23. Cowie RA, Hitchcock ER. The late results of antero-lateral cordotomy for pain relief. *Acta Neurochir (Wien)* 1982;64:39–50.
24. Piscol K. Open spinal surgery for (intractable) pain. In: Penholz H, Brock M, Hamer J, eds. *Brain Hypoxia*. Vol 3. Berlin Heidelberg: Springer; 1975:157–169.
25. White JC, Sweet WH, Hawkins R, et al. Anterolateral cordotomy: results, complications and causes of failure. *Brain* 1950;73:346–367.
26. Ischia S, Ischia A, Luzzani A, et al. Results up to death in the treatment of persistent cervico-thoracic (Pancoast) and thoracic malignant pain by unilateral percutaneous cervical cordotomy. *Pain* 1985;21:339–355.
27. Ballantine HT Jr, Cassidy WL, Flanagan NB, et al. Stereotaxic anterior cingulotomy for neuropsychiatric illness and intractable pain. *J Neurosurg* 1967;26:488–495.
28. Foltz EL, White LE Jr. Pain "relief" by frontal cingulumotomy. *J Neurosurg* 1962;19:89–100.
29. Scarff JE. Unilateral prefrontal lobotomy for the relief of intractable pain and termination of narcotic addiction. *Surg Gynecol Obstet* 1949;89:385–392.
30. Scarff JE. Unilateral prefrontal lobotomy for the relief of intractable pain. *J Neurosurg* 1950;7:330–336.
31. Meyer A, Beck E, Mclardy T. Prefrontal leucotomy: a neuro-anatomical report. *Brain* 1947;70:18–49.
32. Sharim J, Pouratian N. Anterior cingulotomy for the treatment of chronic intractable pain: a systematic review. *Pain Physician* 2016;19:537–550.
33. Vogt BA, Sikes RW. *The Medial Pain System, Cingulate Cortex, and Parallel Processing of Nociceptive Information*. Vol 122. New York: Elsevier; 2013.
34. Devinsky O, Morrell MJ, Vogt BA. Contributions of anterior cingulate cortex to behaviour. *Brain* 1995;118(pt 1):279–306.
35. Rolls ET, O'Doherty J, Kringelbach ML, et al. Representations of pleasant and painful touch in the human orbitofrontal and cingulate cortices. *Cereb Cortex* 2003;13:308–317.
36. Hutchison WD, Davis KD, Lozano AM, et al. Pain-related neurons in the human cingulate cortex. *Nat Neurosci* 1999;2:403–405.
37. Agarwal N, Choi PA, Shin SS, et al. Anterior cingulotomy for intractable pain. *Interdiscip Neurosurg* 2016;6:80–83.
38. Steele JD, Christmas D, Eljamel MS, et al. Anterior cingulotomy for major depression: clinical outcome and relationship to lesion characteristics. *Biol Psychiatry* 2008;63:670–677.
39. Cohen RA, Kaplan RF, Moser DJ, et al. Impairments of attention after cingulotomy. *Neurology* 1999;53:819–824.2009;16:214–219.
40. Yen CP, Kuan CY, Sheehan J, et al. Impact of bilateral anterior cingulotomy on neurocognitive function in patients with intractable pain. *J Clin Neurosci* 2009;16:214–219.
41. Gorecki JP. Thalamotomy for cancer pain, part I. An overview. In: Gildenberg PL, Tasker RR, eds. *Textbook of Stereotactic and Functional Neurosurgery*. New York: McGraw-Hill; 1998:1439–1442.
42. Amano K. Thalamotomy for cancer pain, part II. Outcome. In: Gildenberg PL, Tasker RR, eds. *Textbook of Stereotactic and Functional Neurosurgery*. New York: McGraw-Hill; 1998:1443–1444.
43. Laitinen LV. Mesencephalotomy and thalamotomy for chronic pain. In: Lunsford LD, ed. *Modern Stereotactic Neurosurgery*. Boston, MA: Springer; 1988:269–277.
44. Mark VH, Ervin FR, Yakovlev PI. Correlation of pain relief, sensory loss, and anatomical lesion sites in pain patients treated with stereotactic thalamotomy. *Trans Am Neurol Assoc* 1961;86:86–90.
45. Mark VH, Ervin FR. Role of thalamotomy in treatment of chronic severe pain. *Postgrad Med* 1965;37:563–571.
46. Whittle IR, Jenkinson JL. CT-guided stereotactic antero-medial pulvinotomy and centromedian-parafascicular thalamotomy for intractable malignant pain. *Br J Neurosurg* 1995;9:195–200.
47. Jeanmonod D, Werner B, Morel A, et al. Transcranial magnetic resonance imaging-guided focused ultrasound: noninvasive central lateral thalamotomy for chronic neuropathic pain. *Neurosurg Focus* 2012;32:E1.
48. Blumenfeld H. *Neuroanatomy Through Clinical Cases*. Sunderland, MA: Sinauer Associates; 2002.
49. Young RF, Jacques DS, Rand RW, et al. Technique of stereotactic medial thalamotomy with the Leksell Gamma Knife for treatment of chronic pain. *Neurol Res* 1995;17:59–65.
50. Niizuma H, Kwak R, Ikeda S, et al. Follow-up results of centromedian thalamotomy for central pain. *Appl Neurophysiol* 1982;45:324–325.
51. Jeanmonod D, Magnin M, Morel A. Thalamus and neurogenic pain: physiological, anatomical and clinical data. *Neuroreport* 1993;4:475–478.
52. Young RF, Jacques DS, Rand RW, et al. Medial thalamotomy with the Leksell Gamma Knife for treatment of chronic pain. *Acta Neurochir Suppl* 1994;62:105–110.

53. Richardson DE. Thalamotomy for intractable pain. *Confin Neurol* 1967; 29:139–145.
54. Richardson DE. Thalamotomy for control of chronic pain. *Acta Neurochir (Wien)* 1974;(suppl 21):77–88.
55. Sugita K, Mutsuga N, Takaoka Y, et al. Results of stereotaxic thalamotomy for pain. *Confin Neurol* 1972;34:265–274.
56. Polin R, Evans R, eds. *Neurosurgical Management of Chronic Pain.* Published November 5, 2005. Available at: http://www.medlink.com/article/neurosurgical_management_of_chronic_pain. Accessed August 31, 2018.
57. Kanoplat Y. Percutaneous stereotactic pain procedures: percutaneous cordotomy, extralemniscal myelotomy, trigeminal tractotomy-nucleotomy. In: Burchiel K, ed. *Surgical Management of Pain.* New York: Thieme; 2002:745–762.
58. Frank F, Tognetti F, Gaist G, et al. Stereotaxic rostral mesencephalotomy in treatment of malignant faciothoracobrachial pain syndromes. A survey of 14 treated patients. *J Neurosurg* 1982;56:807–811.
59. Frank F, Fabrizi AP, Gaist G. Stereotactic mesencephalic tractotomy in the treatment of chronic cancer pain. *Acta Neurochir* 1989;99:38–40.
60. Kim DR, Lee SW, Son BC. Stereotactic mesencephalotomy for cancer-related facial pain. *J Korean Neurosurg Soc* 2014;56:71–74.
61. Spiegel EA, Kletzkin M, Szekely EG. Pain reactions upon stimulation of the tectum mesencephali. *J Neuropathol Exp Neurol* 1954;13:212–220.
62. Watling CJ, Payne R, Allen RR, et al. Commissural myelotomy for intractable cancer pain: report of two cases. *Clin J Pain* 1996;12:151–156.
63. Gildenberg PL. Mesencephalotomy for cancer pain. In: Lozano AM, Gildenberg PL, Tasker RR, eds. *Textbook of Stereotactic and Functional Neurosurgery.* Vol 1. New York: McGraw-Hill; 2009:2533–2540.
64. Foltz EL, White LE. The role of rostral cingulumotomy in "pain" relief. *Int J Neurol* 1968;6:353–373.
65. Faillace LA, Allen RP, McQueen JD, et al. Cognitive deficits from bilateral cingulotomy for intractable pain in man. *Dis Nerv Syst* 1971;32:171–175.
66. Hurt RW, Ballantine HT Jr. Stereotactic anterior cingulate lesions for persistent pain: a report on 68 cases. *Clin Neurosurg* 1974;21:334–351.
67. Voris H, Whisler W. Results of stereotaxic surgery for intractable pain. *Confin Neurol* 1975;37:86–96.
68. Pillay PK, Hassenbusch SJ. Bilateral MRI-guided stereotactic cingulotomy for intractable pain. *Stereotact Funct Neurosurg* 1992;59:33–38.
69. Wilkinson HA. Bilateral anterior cingulotomy for chronic noncancer pain. *Neurosurgery* 2000;46:1535–1536.
70. Yen CP, Kung SS, Su YF, et al. Stereotactic bilateral anterior cingulotomy for intractable pain. *J Clin Neurosci* 2005;12:886–890.
71. Patel NV, Agarwal N, Mammis A, et al. Frameless stereotactic magnetic resonance imaging-guided laser interstitial thermal therapy to perform bilateral anterior cingulotomy for intractable pain: feasibility, technical aspects, and initial experience in 3 patients. *Neurosurgery* 2015;11(suppl 2):17–25.
72. Steiner L, Forster D, Leksell L, et al. Gammathalamotomy in intractable pain. *Acta Neurochir* 1980;52:173–184.
73. Hitchcock ER, Teixeira MJ. A comparison of results from center-median and basal thalamotomies for pain. *Surg Neurol* 1981;15:341–351.
74. Fairman D, Llavallol MA. Thalamic tractotomy for the alleviation of intractable pain in cancer. *Cancer* 1973;31:700–707.
75. Uematsu S, Konigsmark B, Walker AE. Thalamotomy for alleviation of intractable pain. *Confin Neurol* 1974;36:88–96.
76. Leksell L, Meyerson BA, Forster DM. Radiosurgical thalamotomy for intractable pain. *Confin Neurol* 1972;34:264.
77. Shimizu S, Aikawa S, Nishioka S, et al. Stereotaxic thalamotomy for pain relief. *Tohoku J Exp Med* 1968;96:219–234.
78. Fairman D. Unilateral thalamic tractotomy for the relief of bilateral pain in malignant tumors. *Confin Neurol* 1967;29:146–152.
79. Ramamurthi B, Kalyanaraman S. Stereotactic thalamotomy in pain relief. *J R Coll Surg Edinb* 1966;12:46–48.
80. Sano K, Yoshioka M, Ogashiwa M, et al. Thalamolaminotomy. A new operation for relief of intractable pain. *Confin Neurol* 1966;27:63–66.
81. Amano K, Kitamura K, Sano K, et al. Relief of intractable pain from neurosurgical point of view with reference to present limits and clinical indications—a review of 100 consecutive cases. *Neurol Med Chir (Tokyo)* 1976;16(pt 1):141–153.
82. Choi CR, Umbach W. Combined stereotaxic surgery for relief of intractable pain. *Neurochirurgia (Stuttg)* 1977;20:84–87.
83. Bosch DA. Stereotactic rostral mesencephalotomy in cancer pain and deafferentation pain. A series of 40 cases with follow-up results. *J Neurosurg* 1991;75:747–751.
84. Barberá J, Barcia-Salorio JL, Broseta J. Stereotaxic pontine spinothalamic tractotomy. *Surg Neurol* 1979;11:111–114.
85. Zapletal B. Open mesencephalotomy and thalamotomy for intractable pain. *Acta Neurochir (Wien)* 1969;(suppl 18):1.
86. Whisler WW, Voris HC. Mesencephalotomy for intractable pain due to malignant disease. *Appl Neurophysiol* 1978;41:52–56.
87. Nashold BS Jr. Extensive cephalic and oral pain relieved by midbrain tractotomy. *Stereotact Funct Neurosurg* 1972;34:382–388.

PART SIX

Provision of Pain Treatment

C H A P T E R **106**

Interdisciplinary Chronic Pain Management: Overview and Lessons from the Public Sector

JENNIFER L. MURPHY and **MICHAEL E. SCHATMAN**

History of Interdisciplinary Chronic Pain Management

In the 1940s, John J. Bonica became the first physician to publicly recognize the complexity of chronic pain syndromes, understanding that they affect patients not only physically but also across myriad dimensions of their lives. Chronic pain of nonmalignant origin (i.e., noncancer pain) has been noted to be the most unpredictable type when compared to acute and chronic pain due to malignancy, which also makes it the most challenging to address.[1] Bonica found himself frustrated by his inability to effectively treat those with chronic pain and found that consultation with his colleagues seemed to benefit all who were involved.[2] Because of this, Bonica developed the first formal multidisciplinary pain management team at MultiCare Tacoma General Hospital, with members including an anesthesiologist, orthopedist, neurosurgeon, internist, psychiatrist, and radiation therapist. However, the model used was multidisciplinary triage in order to determine which team member would provide treatment and included only physicians with differing specialties versus professionals from entirely different fields.

Concurrently, unbeknownst to Bonica,[3] others were simultaneously developing similar programs in Texas, Oregon, Canada, and Europe. Although some of these programs were successful, Bonica's efforts to change the overall approach to chronic pain management were not so, and he wrote accordingly, "Despite my persistent drum beating, consisting of several hundred lectures and the publication of numerous articles in various parts of the world, the multidisciplinary concept was ignored by the medical profession for two decades."[4] Fortunately, the integration by clinical psychologist Wilbert Fordyce of a strong behavioral medicine into Bonica's team in the late 1960s was instrumental in the development of the first multidisciplinary pain evaluation and triage team, which included disciplines outside of medicine. With the availability of behavioral approaches to assessment and treatment, the focus of pain clinics shifted from the eradication of pain to teaching patients how to *manage* their symptoms and restore a positive quality of life.[5] Behavioral approaches were soon replaced by cognitive-behavioral approaches, which note only were less time-consuming and costly but also emphasized the patient as an *active participant* in his or her rehabilitation who is able to develop the coping skills necessary to restore independence.[2]

Multidisciplinary chronic pain management programs proliferated in the 1970s and 1980s, described as "medicine's new growth industry."[6] Among the most active and prestigious of these facilities was that developed by Bonica at the University of Washington where he was succeeded in directorship by the neurosurgeon, John Loeser. According to Loeser,[7] the great success of the program was due to the interaction between the various disciplines of the team members rather than to any specific intervention that was applied. This encapsulates the magic of interdisciplinary treatment which is often difficult to explain to outsiders but easily understood by those who have worked in the milieu. By the early 1980s, approximately 1,000 multidisciplinary evaluation and treatment centers were in operation in the United States[8] and were becoming more numerous in other parts of the world as well. However, these programs were *multidisciplinary* rather than *interdisciplinary*. Contrary to common belief, the first truly interdisciplinary treatment program was not developed until the early 1980s, when Wilbert Fordyce and John Loeser opened the facility at the University of Washington that resembled the modern concept of the interdisciplinary chronic pain management (ICPM) program (J. Loeser, personal communication, December 2, 2017).

Although third-party payers were initially enthusiastic regarding these programs, they soon became less supportive. It is difficult to specifically determine the point at which the number of interdisciplinary treatment programs and the availability of this type of pain management began to decline; however, Schatman[9,10] has noted that the number of programs in the United States accredited by the Commission on Accreditation of Rehabilitation Facilities (CARF) declined from 210 in 1998 to 84 in 2005; in 2017, the total number of CARF-accredited pain rehabilitation programs has dwindled to 67. The availability of ICPM programs in the United States has flourished only in the Department of Veterans Affairs (VA) with the Department of Defense following step, a phenomenon which will be explored in greater depth later in this chapter.

EMPIRICAL SUPPORT FOR INTERDISCIPLINARY CHRONIC PAIN MANAGEMENT

The evidence to support the clinical efficacy and cost-effectiveness of ICPM is robust, and the studies are numerous; therefore, it is most efficient to focus on meta-analyses and systematic reviews that provide the approach with unequivocal empirical support. These studies will be reviewed briefly, and several prominent and more recent studies will be highlighted. Flor and colleagues[11] performed the earliest meta-analysis of ICPM in 1992. The review of 65 studies identified numerous benefits for participants: reducing medication use, reducing emotional distress, reducing health care utilization, reducing iatrogenic consequences, increasing return to work and physical activity levels, closing disability claims, and an average pain reduction of 20%. Although the figure for pain reduction may not seem impressive, patients in these programs are generally told that pain relief is not the goal of treatment and are taught to focus on functional and emotional benefits. Not surprisingly, ICPM programs were determined to be superior to unimodal treatments as well as to no treatment and waiting list controls. The beneficial effects of the programs appeared to be stable over time. As with most large-scale reviews, it was recommended that results be interpreted with some caution due to inconsistencies in methodologies and quality of research designs and descriptions.

The area of cost-effectiveness for ICPM deserves attention because it is typically regarded as an intensive and concomitantly expensive option for chronic pain management; however, a review of the literature does not support this widely held belief. In 1998, Turk and Okifuji[12] performed a comparative analysis of ICPM programs in order to assess their cost-effectiveness as compared to surgery, chronic opioid therapy, and implantable devices. Most striking was the finding that ICPM programs were up to 21 times more cost-effective than alternative treatments for chronic pain such as surgery.[12] Okifuji and colleagues[13] performed a review of the literature on various treatment approaches to chronic pain, analyzing the cost-effectiveness of ICPM in comparison to surgery or conventional medical treatment. ICPM compared favorably to other treatments in terms of pain reduction, management of opioid analgesics, restoration of function as measured by activity levels and return to work, health care utilization, and closure of disability claims. Additionally, the authors dispelled the myth of ICPM representing an expensive approach to pain management, calculating that its use in lieu of the other typical approaches could result in a cost savings of $5 billion per year in the United States. Turk[14] obtained similar findings in a 2002 review, noting not only that ICPM is comparable to oral medications, surgery, spinal cord stimulation (SCS), and intrathecal drug delivery in terms of pain relief but also that interdisciplinary treatment can provide considerable savings in costs for medications and additional health care utilization. Turk's[14] data on cost-effectiveness are dramatic, as he determined that interdisciplinary care is 6.29 times more cost-effective than surgery, 15 times more so than conventional care, and 25 times more cost-effective than SCS. This opens up the question regarding why insurance would reimburse procedures such as SCS but deny any coverage for ICPM programs when the evidence suggests that this is misguided.

Turk and Swanson[15] performed an "analysis and evidence-based synthesis" of the efficacy and cost-effectiveness of medications, surgery, SCS, intrathecal drug delivery systems, and ICPM in the treatment of chronic pain. The authors found that all of these approaches resulted in roughly the same amount of pain relief, with only ICPM determined to be essentially free of iatrogenic complications and adverse events as well as being numerous times more cost-effective than the other treatments considered in achieving therapeutic goals. Perhaps the most compelling empirical support for ICPM is provided by the 2001 and 2002 systematic[16] and Cochrane[17] reviews by Guzmán and colleagues and the 2003 Cochrane review by Schonstein et al.,[18] as these studies involved careful analyses of trial quality. In each of these reviews, the authors determined that ICPM improves pain and function, which was not determined to be the case for less intensive treatments.

In an ICPM context and beyond, increasing functioning and optimizing quality of life often requires the reevaluation of pharmaceuticals. With a recent emphasis on reducing the use of analgesics that are not always helpful and potentially harmful,

including opioids, it is worthwhile to include several studies demonstrating the role of ICPM programs in this effort. A 2013 study by Murphy et al.[19] examined the outcomes of more than 700 participants who completed the inpatient ICPM program at the VA in Tampa, Florida. Since the program's advent in 1988, veterans who enter the program taking opioids are tapered off during the course of their 3-week participation. The study compared how those who were on opioid medications at program admission fared against those who were not on opioids.[19] There were no significant differences between groups at admission and all participants improved, but those on opioid analgesics at program initiation *benefitted even more* on several domains including catastrophizing and activities of daily living. A study and 6-month follow-up conducted by the ICPM program at Mayo Clinic in Minnesota examined treatment outcomes following opioid analgesic cessation[20,21] and found that although patients on opioid analgesics at admission reported higher levels of pain and depression relative to those not taking opioids, there were no differences in outcomes at discharge or 6-month follow-up. Clearly, further research on the effects of opioid tapering on ICPM outcomes is warranted because the Tampa and Mayo studies suggest a significant and sustained improvement in pain severity and functioning following interdisciplinary treatment regardless of previous opioid status.

Evaluating medications not only is important to patient long-term well-being but also has financial implications. A novel economic analysis was conducted in 2015 by Mayo Clinic's Florida ICPM program in collaboration with Florida Blue, the state branch of Blue Cross Blue Shield.[22] Sletten et al.[22] collaboratively examined the economic impact of participation in an ICPM on health care utilization and expenditures. Results indicated decreases in overall medical costs for up to 18 months including the use of specialty care, tests, and procedures. Of note, unlike many other cost-effectiveness studies that focus on low back pain, this ICPM sample included a broad range of chronic pain conditions with an average pain duration of 8 years. The involvement of a third-party payer in this analysis represents an important model for future studies because this may be the most convincing way to garner the support of insurance companies. This is consistent with Schatman's work on the demise of interdisciplinary pain management in the United States, in which he posited that insurers' exclusive focus on cost-containment and profitability trumps pain patient well-being.[10] In the future, it would be ideal for ICPM programs to partner together and enlist the collaboration of multiple health care plans and payer types to once again demonstrate the economic benefit of interdisciplinary care.

Given these data, the process by which third-party payers determine what is worthy of a cost investment can be puzzling. Procedures such as back surgery, which is costly and risky and yields very mixed empirical outcomes, are typically covered, yet payers are unlikely to reimburse evidence-based and lower risk ICPM programs. This in part speaks to the antiquated yet ongoing biomedical approach that much of the public, providers, and payers apply to chronic pain treatment. Although it is clearly a complex biopsychosocial experience that persists across time, chronic pain continues to be approached in the same manner as acute pain. This error is a significant reason why individuals and systems seek and support medical solutions that "cure" pain rather than understanding that pain can be best minimized and quality of life improved with a whole-person, comprehensive, self-management approach.

THEORETICAL BASIS OF THE INTERDISCIPLINARY APPROACH

Before proceeding, it is important to clarify the distinction between *multidisciplinary* and *interdisciplinary*. Although the terms are often used interchangeably, they are not synonymous.

Multidisciplinary treatment suggests that there are providers from multiple disciplines treating a patient in parallel. Communication may exist, but is not required, and varies widely. Coordination of care and treatment planning is atypical and is unfortunately often fragmented. This is a common approach in primary and secondary care, in which specialists are consulted as needed and work in silos. On the other hand, interdisciplinary care is best reflected in a cohesive team composed of experts from various disciplines who share a philosophy of care and communicate routinely regarding patient treatment. They are ideally colocated, although if not, may use technology for information sharing (e.g., phone calls, e-mails, electronic medical records) as well as holding scheduled and unscheduled in-person meetings. The importance of regular communication among team members cannot be overstated, and consistency in the philosophy of patient care is critical for program success.

All ICPM is based on the biopsychosocial approach that emphasizes the complex and dynamic interaction between physiologic, psychological, and social factors. These variables and how patients respond to them can exacerbate or ameliorate the patient's pain experience. For Bonica, the addition Fordyce contributed to the evolution of the approach by considering the emotional and behavioral sequelae of chronic pain as well as nociceptive experience was invaluable. Chronic pain is a disease of the *person*, and the person is often obscured by using the traditional biomedical approach without the integration of other critically relevant factors.[23] Therefore, to effectively treat chronic pain, the motivational-affective and cognitive-evaluative contributions must be weighed in addition to the nociceptive. ICPM recognizes the bidirectionality of pain and psychosocial factors, considering that emotions and maladaptive behavioral patterns can perpetuate as well as result from persistent physical discomfort. Regardless of the etiology of pain and even its comorbidities, patients who have functional impairments can improve on multiple dimensions if they are provided with appropriate guidance and are motivated by the staff to exert maximal effort. The goal is for participants to achieve management of their pain, with an emphasis on increasing self-efficacy and restoring independence and overall quality of life.

COMPOSITION OF THE INTERDISCIPLINARY TEAM AND ROLES OF MEMBERS

ICPM is based on the premise that no individual or discipline can "cure" the patient of all of the ills associated with his or her pain condition. Although specialization serves to enhance expertise, specialization without diversification results in limitations to what health care can offer patients whose conditions are as complex as chronic pain. This, perhaps, was the greatest wisdom that Bonica contributed to the pain treatment community. Although the specific construction of ICPM programs vary depending on factors such as available resources, the typical treatment provided includes three common elements: (1) medication management, (2) graded physical exercise, and (3) cognitive and behavioral techniques for pain and stress management.[13] The CARF standards[24] identify only two defined disciplines as essential for ICPM rehabilitation programs: the pain team physician and pain team psychologist; additional health care professionals are based on the needs of the persons served. The roles of ICPM team members that are generally identified as constituting the core as well as other members that expand and enrich services provided are reviewed in the following discussion.

Core Team Members
- *Physician/medical director*: The ICPM program medical director provides medical leadership and accepts responsibility for the physical well-being of the patients treated. Although it is important that the physician possesses expertise in the rehabilitation of pain disorders, a survey of programs yields wide variance in the training experience

and practice specialties of their medical directors. These specialties range from physical medicine and rehabilitation to psychiatry, rheumatology to internal medicine. Of note, the CARF standards require that a medical director be a physician who is certified in their recognized board, has met established interdisciplinary training requirements, and is involved in the field of pain and in the ICPM program.[24]

The precise duties of the medical director vary depending on his or her engagement in patient care versus nurse practitioners or physicians' assistants, which is discussed in the following text. If involved in a more hands-on role, the physician may take a medical history, evaluate the patient for purposes of providing or confirming a diagnosis, analyze test results, manage medications, and in some cases provide interventions such as trigger point injections. If nurse practitioners or physicians' assistants provide much of the direct clinical contact, the medical director may be called on to see patients who are most complex or may value from the input of a physician. The medical director also may represent the program to hospital or academic leadership. In general, the physician who is seen as warmer and less directive is likely to foster greater team cohesiveness.[25] Similarly, Spoonhour and Schatman[26] have suggested that selflessness is ideal because the most effective medical directors are those who are willing to allow the team member with certain expertise to function in a manner maximizing the benefit of that expertise.

- *Advanced practice nurses and physicians' assistants*: As mentioned, the day-to-day duties involved in an ICPM may be carried out by a nurse practitioner or physician's assistant. This is done typically to conserve fiscal resources, although nurse practitioners and physicians' assistants often have high levels of pain expertise and need limited input from a physician. They perform duties such as evaluating individuals for program appropriateness, completing histories and physicals, managing medication regimens, evaluating patients during crises, participating in team meetings, and offering input on various impacts of biomedical information regarding the treatment plan. They may communicate with the medical director or other physicians often or seldom, depending on the structure and needs of the specific program.

- *Psychologist*: Pain psychologists on interdisciplinary treatment teams are primarily responsible for the psychosocial aspects and status of patients' care. As patients' pain becomes more chronic, their development of maladaptive emotional and behavioral patterns increases, necessitating expert psychological care if they are to become more functional in their lifestyles. In addition to a medical director, CARF requires a pain psychologist on the team whose qualifications include licensure, completion of established interdisciplinary training requirements, and routine involvement in the ICPM program.[24] Although CARF does not specify the discipline of the pain program director, this is often fulfilled by the psychologist.

The duties of psychologists in ICPM are vast. Initially, they assist in determining whether a patient is appropriate for program participation by evaluating pain-related functional status and psychological stability. Often, they communicate information regarding program benefits and expectations. During the program, the pain psychologist will work with patients on both an individual and group basis, with an emphasis on identifying more adaptive ways to respond to pain, acquiring problem-solving and stress management techniques, decreasing catastrophization, and enhancing self-efficacy. Through these approaches, reductions in depression and anxiety along with more adaptive behavioral responses to pain are typically evidenced.

Although not always the case, psychologists also may serve as the biofeedback therapist on the ICPM team to facilitate reducing patients' psychophysiologic reactivity to stress. Effective use of relaxation techniques (e.g., progressive muscle relaxation, imagery, diaphragmatic breathing) are a cornerstone of pain management and help shift a patient toward internal locus of control[27] as well as reduce tension and pain. In some cases, the biofeedback therapist works in tandem with the physical therapist, using biofeedback technology to help patients improve patterns of muscle activation during physical activities. The ICPM psychologist will also often work with a patient's family during the course of a program because the family may unwittingly be reinforcing the "patient role," thereby enabling the patient. Finally, as psychologists are trained as scientist practitioners, they are likely to coordinate outcomes information and performance improvement projects for the ICPM team.

- *Nurse*: Nurses on ICPM treatment teams often assume diverse responsibilities and are accordingly invaluable. Because of their medical backgrounds, they can potentially serve in a variety of roles. They support other medical staff and often provide education to patients and their families. In a role delineation study, Pellino and colleagues[28] determined that assessing, evaluating, and monitoring pain were nurses' most common activities. Nurses are also the multidisciplinary team members that spend the greatest amount of time with patients.[29] Additionally, as many nurses are trained and experienced in case management, a nurse is often the team member responsible for the day-to-day management of the program.

- *Physical therapist*: Movement-based therapies are an essential element of physical activation that is key for effective pain rehabilitation. The physical therapist on a pain treatment team is responsible for assessing patients' levels of functioning and then designing and monitoring programs of graded therapeutic exercise that will safely increase these levels. Areas of focus may include increasing flexibility and range of motion, restoring appropriate posture and body mechanics, ambulation and gait training, development of core and limb strength and stability, and decreasing pain-related fear of movement. Treatment is typically provided on both an individual and group basis. Modalities such as ultrasound and massage are generally avoided, as the focus of ICPM is on teaching patients *independent* active management of their pain. Stretching and strengthening are emphasized because these exercises have been empirically supported through systematic reviews as being among the most effective treatments for a number of types of chronic pain.[30-35] It is critical that the ICPM physical therapist has received specialized training in chronic pain management emphasizing a behavioral approach, which is not the norm; however, for those who value working on a team and the reward of success with patients with longer standing issues, it can be an excellent fit.

- *Case manager/coordinator*: This is a role versus a discipline and can be performed by those in various areas but is most commonly fulfilled by a nurse. Duties are critical for smooth maintenance of the program and may include triaging referred patients; confirming insurance sponsorship; development of policies and procedures; quality assurance; collection and maintenance of patient data; and correspondence with referral sources, employers, attorneys, health insurance providers, and other health care professionals treating a patient.

Other Team Members

- *Vocational counselor*: The vocational counselor on the treatment team is responsible for evaluating the capacity, goals, and needs of patients in the area of return to work, school, or other meaningful activity. A common aspect of this interaction is helping the patient understand the benefits of returning to the work force because participating in gainful employment is considered a primary goal of many ICPM programs, particularly those that emphasize a *functional restoration* approach.[36] Vocational counselors may serve as case managers who contact employers, obtain and analyze job descriptions, and facilitate return to previous employment. They may also provide testing and counseling in order to prepare patients for vocational retraining. Perhaps even more than other team members, it is important for vocational counselors to understand issues such as primary and secondary gain as well as the role of psychological factors in perpetuating perceived disability.

- *Occupational therapist*: Areas that are considered primarily within the domain of occupational therapists include ergonomic training, upper extremity activities of daily living, work activities, leisure activities, and any other activities that are meaningful and purposeful to the individual patient. Some occupational therapists perform work-site analyses, visiting the work place to which the patient intends to return, observing the specific job-related tasks that he or she will need to perform, and then developing a work simulation component of the ICPM program. If a patient has a specific job to which he or she intends to return, a workplace analysis may be conducted by an occupational therapist and vocational counselor in order to assess the physical and emotional safety of returning to that position.

- *Aquatic therapist*: When available, the use of supervised exercises in a heated therapeutic aquatic environment can be a helpful element of physical rehabilitation and one of those most enjoyed by the patients. It can be conducted by those in various disciplines but is most commonly a physical therapist or kinesiotherapist who is interested and has additional competency in the area. Water-based treatments are complementary to land-based exercises and have various therapeutic benefits that are especially helpful for those with chronic pain, such as buoyancy that reduces the effects of gravity and hydrostatic pressure that offers stability and support.

- *Recreational therapist*: Those programs fortunate enough to have the influence of a recreational therapist reap various patient benefits. Due to the social isolation that many with chronic pain experience, recreational therapy typically offers an opportunity to be around others and practice potentially rusty social skills. Recreational therapists also evaluate pleasurable activities in which patients wish to engage (either through initiation or rekindling) and determine how to help individuals move toward their goals. They often offer options such as crafts and art work as a means to stimulate creativity, improve focus, and distract from pain.

- *Clinical pain pharmacist*: Particularly with the emphasis on analgesics, the presence of a pain pharmacist can be very helpful in providing support to medical and other staff as well as to patients regarding medications. Within the context of ICPM programs, pain pharmacists typically advise on medication choices, provide educational classes, and meet with patients as needed to answer in-depth questions about pharmaceuticals, including addressing issues regarding polypharmacy, adverse events, and side effect profiles.

- *Social worker*: Social workers may play a variety of roles in ICPM programs. They can function in a case manager and coordinator role, tracking patient participation and addressing issues that arise. If participation in the program involves travel, social workers often play an important role in making sure that transportation is arranged and patients are able to access what is needed at the facility. They also provide more traditional guidance on introducing various administrative forms and can teach classes on how to access opportunities in the community. Those who are licensed clinical social workers may have more direct contact to address clinical needs.

In addition to those specialties listed here, many ICPM programs include other professionals, including a dietician who reviews the important role of nutrition and weight in pain management, a chaplain who addresses spiritual needs, a yoga or tai chi instructor who provides guided direction on these active and beneficial treatments, as well as options such as an art therapist, music teacher, and other disciplines that encourage the development of activities that are enjoyable and assist with fostering positive self-esteem and sense of purpose.

The Process of Interdisciplinary Chronic Pain Management

Despite the long history and strong empirical support for ICPM, this form of treatment is often seen as a "last resort" by referral sources, many of whom have a limited understanding of the complexities of and best treatments for chronic pain. This is a reflection of a biomedically based health care system and society that tends to seek passive/receptive interventions for the management of pain rather than approaching it as a chronic condition that requires active self-care by the patient as a foundation for the potential success of other treatment options. ICPM programs are viewed as tertiary, which too often subsumes that all other treatments have "failed"; however, it is a treatment best correlated with complexity and pain-related functional impairment and should be considered as soon as possible when these conditions are met. If individuals had access to ICPM programs earlier in their pain journeys, it is likely that our system could be spared billions of dollars because the chronification and negative impacts for many would be minimized.

Referrals may come from a wide variety of sources, including other physicians and health care providers, attorneys, employers, and insurance carriers. Some ICPM programs are a part of a broader pain management system, in which case triage may be necessary. Due to economic realities, insurance coverage is generally confirmed prior to proceeding. Once this is accomplished, medical records are requested and reviewed to ascertain the patient's appropriateness for evaluation. In systems such as the VA, referrals for evaluation can be made more easily because third-party payer obstacles are removed and shared medical records facilitate screening evaluation processes.

The initial evaluation of a candidate for ICPM may occur in a variety of ways, but the goal is to determine if the individual is appropriate for the treatment, provide education on the treatment approach, and determine collaboratively a plan of care. Typically, providers from more than one discipline are involved in this process so that information regarding all relevant biopsychosocial factors can be assessed. For example, a medical professional gathers information regarding medication use and comorbidities as well as physical fitness and ability, whereas a mental health professional ascertains details regarding pain-related functional impacts and emotional and social factors and shares the program's philosophy, expectations, and potential benefits from participation. Physical therapists or others may also be involved in this evaluation in order to obtain objective measurement of functional capacities. At times, the patient is deemed to be not currently ready for ICPM due to various factors including psychiatric or medical instability (e.g., active suicidal ideation and intention, unmanaged psychosis, cardiac issues). If the ICPM team believes that these factors can be addressed, delaying admission until the patient has received appropriate treatment may be in the best interest of the patient and the program. If the option for reconsideration is not viable, the program should provide treatment recommendations to the patient and the referral source.

ICPM programs tend to be intensive, often requiring patients to participate from 20 to 40 hours per week. Although patients may find the prospect of such a commitment daunting, they will not be asked to perform physical tasks that are beyond their functional capacities. Distinguishing between "hurt" and "harm" and assuring patients that the treatment team considers their physical and emotional safety to be of the greatest importance helps build therapeutic trust, thereby enhancing adherence.[37] The specific "mix of services" that patients receive between and within programs will vary. Typically, patients spend significant time engaging in physical activities that will increase their flexibility, strength, and functional capacities. Patients whose emotional status and behavioral responses to their pain are less unhelpful will likely require less time with the psychologist than will those patients who are struggling psychosocially. Similarly, patients demonstrating limited psychophysiologic reactivity to stress will require less intensive biofeedback training, and those whose vocational issues are more straightforward will require less concentrated vocational counseling services. The frequency with which a patient sees the physician and/or nurse practitioner or physicians' assistant on an individual basis will vary depending on the specific program. Frequent individual physician appointments are generally discouraged because the goal of ICPM is typically reduction of medical services in lieu of enhanced independent self-management of pain.

The patient-centered nature of ICPM requires regular team conferences in which the entire treatment team meets to discuss patient progress, which includes any issues that are potentially limiting gains and therapeutic goals. This may happen with the patient, without the patient, or both. Regardless, feedback to patients should be immediate, consistent, and coherent. In situations in which patients' adherence is considered good and they are making progress, team conference provides a forum in which they are able to receive much-needed positive reinforcement regarding their attitude and effort. Patients with chronic pain are often unjustifiably blamed for the failures of the primary and secondary care systems to help them recover, making appropriate positive reinforcement even more important. Conversely, in cases in which adherence and progress are considered by the team to be inadequate, the conference provides an opportunity for the treatment team to develop an approach for patient feedback and/or to present a united front in addressing the relevant issues and work with patients to remedy any problematic aspects of their programs. Because the literature confirms that individuals with personality disorders are prevalent in ICPM programs,[38,39] it is not unusual to encounter attempts to "split" treatment team members. Because of this, it is particularly important for the program team to develop a coherent plan together and enforce it consistently so that patients receive a unified message throughout their participation. Unfortunately, although ICPM programs work to facilitate success for all patients, some circumstances necessitate early discharge. Stanos[40] has recently suggested that such premature discharge can potentially encourage enhanced compliance or efforts among other patients in the group.

Once a patient has completed an ICPM program, he or she can be neither forgotten nor abandoned. Although programs are typically close-ended, some form of follow-up to determine implementation of what has been learned in the program is important. Additionally, if the program is involved in outcomes research, follow-up provides a source for collection of more data. For the sake of cost-efficiency, selected measures of patients' emotional and behavioral responses to their pain that are administered can be sent to them to determine longer term outcomes and identify any clinical needs. Positive outcomes data should serve as a powerful tool for demonstrating the program's effectiveness to patients and providers which can assist with marketing. Potential referring physicians may be uninformed regarding the wide range of benefits of interdisciplinary treatment for their patients, and well-organized data may help them understand how a program can make their own lives easier as well as helping their more challenging patients. Additionally, although some health insurance programs may argue against the efficacy of ICPM, data that invalidates their arguments will ideally help convince them of the legitimacy of this treatment approach.

Interdisciplinary Chronic Pain Management in Veterans Healthcare Administration: Overview of a Model System

Although ICPM programs have greatly diminished in the United States in the last 20 years, there is one place where they have flourished: the VA health care system.[41] The VA undertook specific efforts to highlight the need for improved pain care in 1998. At that time, leaders in the VA acknowledged that pain was an underrecognized and undertreated issue that impacted veterans across the continuum of care. This led to a series of successful initiatives and collaborations that increased the measurement, tracking, treatment, and overall quality of services available to veterans with pain. One of the most important was a 2003 pain management policy, the first of its kind and an important step toward establishing pain as a high priority for the Veterans Healthcare Administration (VHA).[42] In 2004, pain management was established as a separate organizational entity within VA Central Office under the direction of clinical psychologist, Robert D. Kerns. Among many identified areas of focus was an emphasis on multidisciplinary and interdisciplinary pain care, the least common models previously found in the community.

In 2009, a revised VHA pain directive was established which introduced a stepped care approach to pain management as the standard for the VA.[43] It not only reasserted VHA's commitment to an approach that is informed by a biopsychosocial model of pain and an interdisciplinary, multidimensional, and multimodal approach to pain management but also asserted that improved quality of life, rather than pain relief per se, is the accepted standard outcome measure of effectiveness. In addition to many other recommendations such as establishing facility multidisciplinary pain committees and specific research efforts, the stepped care model delineated the primary level Patient Aligned Care Team (PACT) and reinforced secondary level specialty pain care (e.g., pain medicine, behavioral health). The tertiary level was defined as interdisciplinary care for the most complex, treatment refractory, and at-risk patients. Along with the availability of advanced pain diagnostics, VHA made a commitment to developing at least one interdisciplinary pain rehabilitation program in each Veterans Integrated Service Network (VISN) by the end of September 2014. These programs were to be accredited by CARF, ensuring the highest level of quality for care.

At the time the directive was published,[43] there were only two CARF-accredited programs in the VA system, located in Tampa, Florida, and San Juan, Puerto Rico, both in VISN 8; therefore, developing and implementing programs for the other

20 VISNs was an ambitious mandate. Five years were allotted to accomplish the goal, with no particular pathway defined for how each different region or facility would meet it. Furthermore, no resources were provided by VA Central Office, and the details and timeline of implementation were left to the VISNs. The VA pain team training program was established under the leadership of clinical psychologist, Michael Clark at the James A. Haley Veterans' Hospital in Tampa, Florida, site of the longest standing CARF-accredited pain rehabilitation program in the VA. Over the next 5 years, the program directly assisted facilities with training visits, providing models and advisement in their fulfillment of the directive as well as ongoing consultation as needed. Tampa trained over 30 VA teams in the philosophical and practical foundations of an interdisciplinary pain rehabilitation program, many of whom went on to implement their own versions at local facilities.

In 2017, the VA's 20 programs represent almost a third of the 67 CARF-accredited pain programs that are available in the United States, even though veterans served by the VA represent only a fraction of the nation's population. Although the overall presence of programs has steadily decreased in the United States, the VA has maintained an upward trend and taken steps to coordinate these centers across the country. The first author of this chapter (JLM), the VA's liaison for the development and maintenance of CARF programs, formed a national CARF Pain Programs Leadership Committee in late 2015 which serves as a community of practice and forum for collaboration across CARF sites. Through regularly scheduled calls, members share questions and updates and consult with each other in order to maintain the CARF standards. As an example of collaboration across sites, a group of VA programs established mutually agreeable core outcome measures to foster a means for comparison of program outcomes. Although not required, this effort serves as a model for the level of coordination that may one day become standard across the system as a means for continual program improvement.

The current state of affairs begs the question, "Why is the VA committed to ICPM programs more than the private sector?" There are several explanations which have been reviewed by LaChappelle et al.[42] First, the VHA emphasizes those treatment options such as ICPM, which have the greatest evidence base. This is supported in the mission statement of the VA as well as in the policies for interventions and pharmaceuticals. Undoubtedly, another factor is the cost–benefit analysis of lifelong patient care that takes into account and often prioritizes long-term outcomes over short-term outcomes. Outside the VA, third-party payer health insurance plans will often fund and reimburse care that may be less expensive in the short term but may be more expensive in the long term, since changes in insurance coverage occur routinely. However, a system that treats patients for the span of their lives is more likely to value an initial higher financial cost of multidisciplinary treatment. This investment in the interdisciplinary approach achieves greater health and well-being in the long term rather a than lower cost financial investment in the short term, with poorer health outcomes in the long term.[44,45] Although a number of factors contribute to frequently switching health insurance carriers in the private sector, the behavior results in a disincentive for insurers' coverage of ICPM programs. Despite the literature supporting their cost-efficiency, they are considered a formidable expense in the short term, and accordingly, insurance payers are more likely to cover inferior (and often more dangerous) but less expensive treatment options. Sadly, if insurance companies would recognize that the investment in ICPM care is well worth the cost, these programs would flourish outside of the VA system and all would benefit as demonstrated by the 2015 Mayo Clinic study.[22]

There are numerous lessons to be learned from the growth of ICPM programs in the VA. First, although many in the private sector perceive the VA system to be flushed with endless resources, the limitations of space and personnel are familiar barriers across the system. Because of this, programs have taken a variety of forms, tailored and built to fit the unique picture of each particular facility. For instance, a program that is 2 to 3 days per week may require 25% of a full-time physical therapist who also works in other settings. Others in less routinely incorporated specialties such as a chaplain, dietician, pharmacist, or addictions counselor may be able to provide a group once during the course of a program, something that adds greatly to the richness of program content while not taxing human resources. Although these creative strategies could theoretically be helpful in convincing insurers to reconsider coverage of ICPM programs, "carving out" essential aspects of them has been empirically established as resulting in far less favorable outcomes.[46,47]

In addition, VA's model of setting an administrative mandate for one CARF ICPM program per region was an ambitious goal, yet it has served several purposes. First, it represented formal recognition by leadership of the importance of interdisciplinary care. Second, although the number was insufficient to serve the entire veteran population, the emergence of ICPM programs throughout the country introduced the treatment approach to providers and patients who were previously unfamiliar. This has served to reinforce the need for a biopsychosocial model and increase access to additional pain care options that are not strictly medical or pharmacologic. Because insurance companies appear unlikely to return to coverage of ICPM programs, a legislative mandate supporting ICPM programs is necessary to effect a restoration of reimbursement for this effective mode of chronic pain treatment. As in the VA, it took a national pain directive recognizing a public health need to spur the development of this valued treatment option and a similar call from on high is needed in the private sector.

Future Considerations for Interdisciplinary Chronic Pain Management

Chronic pain is and has been underrecognized and undertreated as a health care need. Although the biopsychosocial model is recognized as the gold standard for pain care, in reality, the biomedical model continues to reign supreme. This means that despite the overall clinical efficacy and cost-effectiveness of ICPM programs, the number in the United States has decreased precipitously since 1999 (A. Whitney, personal communication, July 16, 2007), thereby severely limiting the availability of a treatment approach that has been the most rigorously validated. The demise of these programs is a disturbing phenomenon particularly given the cost of chronic pain and the drastic increase in opioid use disorder and opioid-related overdose deaths. As Chapman states, "Concurrent with the decline of intensive programs is the rise of procedural interventions and medication, which receives a great deal of support from medical technology and pharmaceutical companies."[48] These unfortunate realities only underscore the need for an approach to chronic pain that matches its complexities without defaulting to a unimodal medical attempt to cure something which requires long-term management.

One potentially positive result of America's prescription opioid crisis has been a shift in focus to treatments that are nonpharmacologic. This has significantly increased the interest of some in options such as pain psychology, complementary integrative health (e.g., acupuncture, yoga), and ICPM programs which provide comprehensive care with a decreased focus on medical modalities and an increased emphasis on self-management strategies. It is unfortunate that it took the drastic increase in opioid prescribing and related negative events to propel health

care professionals, systems, and even lawmakers toward considering treatment options that capture the biopsychosocial approach, but the momentum is welcome. Additional funding for treatment options as well as research that considers physiologic as well as other highly relevant factors in the chronic pain experience may lead to improvement in the availability of ICPM options. The growth of interdisciplinary pain rehabilitation programs within the VA demonstrates a cultural transformation within the largest single health care system in the United States, one that should be used as a model for how to walk the walk of whole person pain care across the country.

Conclusion

Seventy years after Bonica introduced the concept of interdisciplinary pain management, those who work in the field sadly continue to encounter similar challenges to those that he faced. The lack of acceptance by the medical community of the interdisciplinary approach that left Bonica ready "to give up" still challenges those that rightly acknowledge the necessity of an interdisciplinary treatment model for optimal patient outcomes. Despite substantial and unequivocal empirical support for its clinical utility and cost-efficiency, in every setting but the VA, the number of programs in the United States has dwindled. Patients have been forced to resort to less effective, more expensive, and often more dangerous treatment options which tend to focus on body parts as opposed to the person in need.

Although third-party payers and some in the field suggest that the ICPM model should be pared down to deintensify the commitment by providers and patients, the evidence suggests the opposite: Providers, payers, and patients should instead embrace the intervention which best matches the treatment needs of those with complex chronic pain. The evidence indicates that the model is not broken—the system is. As one of the most pervasive and costliest health care issues, chronic pain and the ICPM approach deserves the attention and support of legislators, insurance companies, and the health care industry at large. Those who have the privilege of working in a true interdisciplinary framework must be the leaders in this mission: to advocate, to educate, to model, and to celebrate the patients with whom they have the ability to effect change. The noble practitioners of the interdisciplinary approach need to become ICPM "champions" to defend the life of that which science and clinical experience tells us is the closest thing we have to a "cure" for our patients.

References

1. Katz WA. The needs of a patient in pain. *Am J Med* 1998;105:2S–7S.
2. Meldrum ML. A capsule history of pain management. *JAMA* 2003;290:2470–2475.
3. Bonica JJ. Evolution and current status of pain programs. *J Pain Symptom Manage* 1990;5:368–374.
4. Bonica JJ. Oral history interview. *John C. Liebeskind History of Pain Collection*. Los Angeles, CA: Louise M. Darling Biomedical Library, UCLA; 1993.
5. Fordyce WE, Fowler RS, DeLateur B. An application of behavior modification technique to a problem of chronic pain. *Behav Res Ther* 1968;6:105–107.
6. Leff DN. Management of chronic pain: medicine's new growth industry. *Med World News* 1976;54.
7. Loeser JD. Multidisciplinary pain management. In: Merskey H, Loeser JD, Dubner R, eds. *The Paths of Pain, 1975–2005*. Seattle, WA: IASP Press; 2005:503–511.
8. Aronoff GM, Evans WO, Enders PL. A review of follow-up studies of multidisciplinary pain units. *Pain* 1983;16:1–11.
9. Schatman ME. The demise of multidisciplinary pain management clinics? *Practical Pain Manage* 2006;6:30–41.
10. Schatman ME. The demise of the multidisciplinary chronic pain management clinic: bioethical perspectives on providing optimal treatment when ethical principles collide. In: Schatman ME, ed. *Ethical Issues in Chronic Pain Management*. New York: Informa Healthcare; 2007:43–62.

11. Flor H, Fydrich T, Turk DC. Efficacy of multidisciplinary pain treatment centers: a meta-analytic review. *Pain* 1992;49:221–230.

12. Turk DC, Okifuji A. Treatment of chronic pain patients: clinical outcomes, cost-effectiveness, and cost-benefits of multidisciplinary pain centers. *Crit Rev Phy Rehab Med* 1998;10:181–208.

13. Okifuji A, Turk DC, Kalauoklani D. Clinical outcome and economic evaluation of multidisciplinary pain centers. In: Block AR, Kramer EF, Fernandez E, eds. *Handbook of Pain Syndromes: Biopsychosocial Perspectives*. Mahwah, NJ: Lawrence Erlbaum Associates; 1999:77–97.

14. Turk DC. Clinical effectiveness and cost-effectiveness of treatments for patients with chronic pain. *Clin J Pain* 2002;18:355–365.

15. Turk DC, Swanson K. Efficacy and cost-effectiveness treatment for chronic pain: an analysis and evidence-based synthesis. In: Schatman ME, Campbell A, eds. *Chronic Pain Management: Guidelines for Multidisciplinary Program Development*. New York: Informa Healthcare; 2007:15–38.

16. Guzmán J, Esmail R, Karjalainen L, et al. Multidisciplinary rehabilitation for chronic low back pain: a systematic review. *BMJ* 2001;322:1511–1516.

17. Guzmán J, Esmail R, Karjalainen L, et al. Multidisciplinary bio-psycho-social rehabilitation for chronic low back pain. *Cochrane Database Syst Rev* 2002;(1):CD000963.

18. Schonstein E, Kenny DT, Keating J, et al. Work conditioning, work hardening and functional restoration for workers with back and neck pain. *Cochrane Database Syst Rev* 2003;(1):CD001822.

19. Murphy JL, Clark ME, Banou E. Opioid cessation and multidimensional outcomes after interdisciplinary chronic pain treatment. *Clin J Pain* 2013; 29(2):109–117.

20. Rome JD, Townsend CO, Bruce BK, et al. Chronic noncancer pain rehabilitation with opioid withdrawal: comparison of treatment outcomes based on opioid use status at admission. *Mayo Clin Proc* 2004;79:759–768.

21. Townsend CO, Kerkvliet JL, Bruce BK, et al. A longitudinal study of the efficacy of a comprehensive pain rehabilitation program with opioid withdrawal: comparison of treatment outcomes based on opioid use status at admission. *Pain* 2008;140:177–189.

22. Sletten CD, Kurklinsky S, Chinburapa V, et al. Economic analysis of a comprehensive pain rehabilitation program: a collaboration between Florida Blue and Mayo Clinic Florida. *Pain Med* 2015;16(5):898–904.

23. Schatman ME. Psychological assessment of maldynic pain: the need for a phenomenological approach. In: Giordano J, ed. *Maldynia: Inter-disciplinary Perspectives on the Illness of Chronic Pain*. New York: Informa Healthcare; 2009.

24. Committee on Accreditation of Rehabilitation Facilities. *Medical Rehabilitation Standards*. Tucson, AZ: Committee on Accreditation of Rehabilitation Facilities; 2017.

25. Antonuccio DO, Davis C, Lewinsohn PM, et al. Therapist variables related to cohesiveness in a group treatment for depression. *Small Group Behav* 1987;18:557–564.

26. Spoonhour P, Schatman ME. Development of policies and procedures: assurance of consistent chronic pain management practice. In: Schatman ME, Campbell A, eds. *Chronic Pain Management: Guidelines for Multidisciplinary Program Development*. New York: Informa Healthcare; 2007: 189–202.

27. Katz RC, Simkin LR, Beauchamp KL, et al. Specific and nonspecific effects of EMG biofeedback. *Biofeedback Self Regul* 1987;12:241–253.

28. Pellino TA, Willens JS, Polomano RC, et al; and the American Society of Pain Management Nurses. The American Society of Pain Management Nurses role-delineation study. National Association of Orthopaedic Nurses respondents. *Orthop Nurs* 2003;22:289–297.

29. McCaffery M, Ferrell BR, Pasero C. Nurses' personal opinions about patients' pain and their effect on recorded assessments and titration of opioid doses. *Pain Manag Nurs* 2000;1:79–87.

30. Swenson RS. Therapeutic modalities in the management of nonspecific neck pain. *Phys Med Rehabil Clin N Am* 2003;14:605–627.

31. Kay TM, Gross A, Goldsmith C, et al; and the Cervical Overview Group. Exercises for mechanical neck disorders. *Cochrane Database Syst Rev* 2005;(3):CD004250.

32. Arnold LM. Biology and therapy of fibromyalgia. New therapies in fibromyalgia. *Arthritis Res Ther* 2006;8:212.

33. Joines JD. Chronic low back pain: progress in therapy. *Curr Pain Headache Rep* 2006;10:421–425.

34. Gross AR, Goldsmith C, Hoving JL, et al; and the Cervical Overview Group. Conservative management of mechanical neck disorders: a systematic review. *J Rheumatol* 2007;34:1083–1102.

35. Taylor NF, Dodd KJ, Shields N, et al. Therapeutic exercise in physiotherapy practice is beneficial: a summary of systematic reviews 2002–2005. *Aust J Physiother* 2007;53:7–16.

36. Mayer TG, Gatchel RJ. *Functional Restoration for Spinal Disorders: The Sports Medicine Approach*. Philadelphia: Lea & Febiger; 1988.

37. Hatzakis M, Schatman ME. The impact of interventional approaches when used within the context of multidisciplinary chronic pain management. In: Schatman ME, Campbell A, eds. *Chronic Pain Management: Guidelines for Multidisciplinary Program Development*. New York: Informa Healthcare; 2007:101–115.

38. Schatman ME. The challenge of the characterologically disturbed chronic pain patient. *Pain Pract* 2003;13:5–7.

39. Schatman ME. Dramatically disturbed patients in interdisciplinary pain programs. *Pract Pain Manage* 2004;4:24–29.

40. Stanos S. Developing an interdisciplinary multidisciplinary chronic pain management program: nuts and bolts. In: Schatman ME, Campbell A, eds. *Chronic Pain Management: Guidelines for Multidisciplinary Program Development*. New York: Informa Healthcare; 2007:151–172.

41. Schatman ME. Interdisciplinary chronic pain management: international perspectives. *Pain: Clin Updates* 2012;20(7):1–5.

42. LaChappelle K, Boris-Karpel S, Kerns RD. Pain management in the Veterans Health Administration. In: Miller TW, ed. *Veterans' Healthcare: Volume IV. Future Directions for Veterans Healthcare*. New York: Praeger Publishers Inc; 2012.

43. Department of Veterans Affairs Veterans Health Administration. Pain Management. VHA Directive 2009-053. Oct 28, 2009. Available at: https://www.va.gov/painmanagement/docs/vha09paindirective.pdf.

44. Boris-Karpel S. Policy and practice issues in pain management. In: Ebert MH, Kerns RD eds. *Behavioral and Psychopharmacologic Pain Management*. Cambridge, United Kingdom: Cambridge University Press; 2007: 407–433.

45. Martell BA, O'Connor PG, Kerns RD, et al. Systematic review: opioid treatment for chronic back pain: prevalence, efficacy, and association with addiction. *Ann Intern Med* 2007;146:116–127.

46. Gatchel RJ, Noe C, Gajraj N, et al. The negative impact on an interdisciplinary pain management program of insurance "treatment carve out" practices. *J Work Compens* 2001;10:50–63.

47. Robbins H, Gatchel RJ, Noe C, et al. A prospective one-year outcome study of interdisciplinary chronic pain management: compromising its efficacy by managed care policies. *Anesth Analg* 2003;97(1):156–162.

48. Chapman SL. Chronic pain rehabilitation: lost in a sea of drugs and procedures? *Am Pain Soc Bull* 2000;10(suppl 3):8–9.

CHAPTER 107

Spine Clinics

JAMES D. KANG, HAI V. LE, and **KENNETH C. NWOSU**

Back pain is one of the most common chief complaints in the emergency room and primary care clinic. It is composed of a wide range of symptoms with varying characteristics. Patients may present with or without associated neurologic signs or symptoms. Adding to this complexity is the multiple potential pain generators that exist in the spine, which include disks, facets, bones, muscles, ligaments, and nerves. For these reasons, back pain presents a great challenge to health care providers, one where it is difficult to correctly identify an underlying cause and develop an efficacious treatment.

Anatomically, the human spine is a structure of tremendous intricacy. Consider, for example, the primary roles of the spine—support and flexibility. On one hand, it must be strong enough to maintain an upright posture. On the other, its elastic properties should permit broad motion through flexion, extension, lateral bending, and rotation. The spinal column also has a protective function to surround and cushion the delicate structures of the spinal cord and nerve roots. It is capable of accomplishing these tasks through a conglomeration of bones, joints, ligaments, disks, and neural elements. Spinal anatomy is further complicated by the number of mobile segments, the proximity of the spinal cord and nerve roots, the intricate motions of multiple small joints, and the natural changes that occur with aging.

Knowledge of the intricate biochemistry of the intervertebral disk and the role of inflammatory mediators in back pain continues to expand. There is also a significant psychological component that impacts the behaviors of patients with back pain and their recovery from injury. Considering the complexity of the spine, it is understandable that definitively diagnosing the exact source(s) of symptoms is often difficult and sometimes impossible.[1] This task is made even more difficult by the strong impact of personality in reporting and dealing with pain, particularly work-related low back pain.[2]

The spine is continually beset by physical stresses, and once an individual reaches adulthood, it is in a constant state of degeneration. The very complexity of the human spine creates the conditions that make it so difficult to resolve back pain. With so many complex and interacting structures, pain can arise from individual structures, multiple structures, or their dynamic interaction. As noted by Jerome Groopman[3] in his best-selling text, *How Doctors Think*, "given all of these structures, the source of the chronic . . . back pain is often a mystery. Doctors can be hard-pressed to identify why a patient is uncomfortable."

Despite its complexity, back pain is nearly universal in the general population with a lifetime prevalence of 65% to 80% in the United States and an annual economic impact that ranges from $84.1 to $624.8 billion.[4] Using data from the 2002 National Health Interview Survey, Strine and Hootman[5] reported that the 3-month prevalence of back and/or neck pain among adults in the United States was 31%. Understandably, these subjects generally had more comorbid conditions and greater psychological distress than did subjects without back or neck pain. Supportively, some studies have indicated that psychosocial factors have an even more influential contribution than mechanical factors toward back pain.[6] In addition, Fanuele et al.[7] using the Short Form Health Survey (SF-36) general health status questionnaire reported back pain patients were significantly impaired, even when compared to a variety of other health conditions. In order to effectively treat such patients, one must understand the severity of the problems and appreciate that back pain may often be accompanied by a variety of comorbidities.

The patient with chronic back pain is often passed from practitioner to practitioner, at times of widely varying expertise, training, and experience, and each subjecting the patient to his or her own preferred techniques for palliation. As the patient drifts further into disability, pain, and medication use, desperation and the cost of single-modality treatments increase in parallel, whereas the probabilities of overcoming the pain and of improving function diminish. It is, according to Groopman,[3] "as though each approach to diagnosis and treatment is essentially a 'franchise' and that too many franchises are battling for control." Such a state of affairs leads to treatments that are increasingly expensive, unfocused, unsubstantiated, and ineffective.

Thus is the complexity of chronic back pain and the costly, untenable nature of many treatments. All point to the need for a different approach to manage back pain where improvement in value depends on improved performances and accountability among individuals who have a shared goal that unites the interests and activities of all stakeholders. The desired approach is no different now from that developed for general chronic pain by Dr. Bonica, and aptly described by Loeser et al. in the third edition of *Bonica's Management of Pain*.[8] They state that Dr. Bonica

> . . . brought clinical psychologists, pharmacists and other non-physician providers to the conference table with anesthesiologists, neurologists, physiatrists, neurosurgeons, orthopedic surgeons, psychiatrists and others. This blend of perspectives kept each specialist from exercising specialty-specific tunnel vision, and in conferences a group understanding often emerged that greatly exceeded the understanding that the record would yield after a series of serial consultations.

This is an apt description of the multidisciplinary approach to care. Of course, a multidisciplinary approach alone does not guarantee either efficiency or effectiveness. In order to provide maximally effective and efficient treatment, and to limit treatment costs, a spine treatment facility must include practitioners with the highest levels of training and experience, who follow treatment guidelines that are scientifically validated yet flexible enough to address the idiosyncrasies of individual patient problems. The care needs to be carefully coordinated to avoid duplication, unnecessary expense, and use of treatments with limited possibility of success. A number of specific principles should guide the multidisciplinary spine facility:

1. Specific algorithms for evaluation and treatment
2. Ongoing multidisciplinary case management and case discussion
3. Active process of continuous quality improvement including outcome measurement, assessment of patient satisfaction, and use of results to improve treatment algorithms
4. Professional education of treatment team members
5. Participation in active research programs

In this chapter, we discuss the key elements needed to establish and maintain an effective multidisciplinary spine facility.

Treatment Components

The three major components that comprise the clinical aspects of a multidisciplinary spine center are (1) a group of dedicated, highly trained physicians and allied health providers with expertise in spine care, (2) a set of treatment algorithms guiding assessment and intervention, and (3) active and aggressive case management, especially when patients fall outside of established treatment algorithms. One of the keys of a successful center is building a multidisciplinary team that understands and respects the roles and skills of individual team members. In caring for patients with acute or chronic back pain, we emphasize the importance of interprofessional communication and teamwork among all care providers (Fig. 107.1).

Treatment Providers

CONSERVATIVE CARE GATEKEEPERS

Of the many individuals who experience back pain, only about 10% ever undergo spine surgery.[9] It is therefore logical that the initial evaluation of patients presenting to a comprehensive spine center should be conducted by a "conservative care" physician—one who is specially trained in the assessment and treatment of spinal disorders. These physicians should be competent in triaging patients and placing them into appropriate assessment and treatment algorithms. Complicated cases and those requiring urgent or emergent intervention can be promptly identified and referred for appropriate diagnostic workup and intervention. However, the majority of cases will be best handled using standard treatment algorithms in which resolution of the back pain is expected with minimal intervention. Such physicians may include primary care doctors or specialists in anesthesiology, physical medicine and rehabilitation (PM&R), or occupational medicine. All of these providers must be able to recognize the "red flags" of back pain, which warrant further lab or imaging studies and timely intervention.

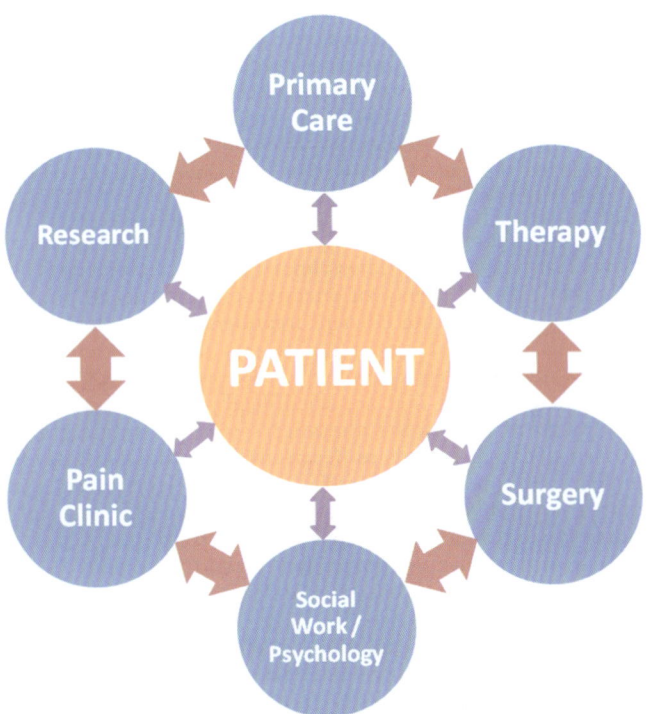

FIGURE 107.1 Illustrative diagram demonstrating the intricate relationships between care providers and the patient at a comprehensive spine center. Close communication among the various providers and the patient is required to provide the highest level of clinical care.

PAIN MANAGEMENT

The most ubiquitous and bothersome indication of spine injury is back pain. Unremitting pain, often fluctuating randomly, can decimate both emotional stability and physical capability. Physicians now have a diverse armamentarium of oral, topical, and injectable medications that may provide immediate, and at times prolonged, relief. The mainstay nonprescription medications for the treatment of back pain are acetaminophen and nonsteroidal anti-inflammatory drugs (NSAIDs). Prescription oral medications include muscle relaxants, opioids, corticosteroids, and certain antidepressants and antiseizure medications. The opioid analgesics, even in recently developed time-release preparations, carry with them both the potential for physical dependence and addiction in up to 40% of chronic pain patients[10] which have been reported to cost upward of $53 billion to treat.[11] Therefore, it is imperative that only one provider in a multidisciplinary team is prescribing and managing the medications. A pain treatment agreement should be implemented early on. Targeted injections are of some value in specific conditions (see Chapters 99 and 100 for a detailed discussion), but their use requires sophisticated equipment and advanced training in order to be used safely and effectively. Physicians with subspecialty training in pain medicine, often specially trained anesthesiologists or PM&R specialists, can effectively use injection therapy, but these treatments must be used in coordination with the other evaluation and treatment efforts, including physical therapy (PT).

PSYCHOLOGY

Patients suffering with spinal injuries and back pain experience dramatic emotional and social changes. Up to 80% of patients with persistent back pain are diagnosable with clinical depression,[12] and many will express anger as the most common emotion they experience.[13] Fear and avoidance of pain often drive patients into unnecessary functional decline. Marriages and relationships can shatter, and spine injuries often leave economic devastation in their wake. For these reasons, specifically trained psychologists often play a pivotal role within the spine center. Numerous studies have shown that psychosocial factors can complicate recovery from spine surgery (see Chapter 76 and Block et al.[14] for a review). Thus, one of the major functions played by psychologists is to perform presurgical psychological screening, providing information to surgeons about the level of psychosocial risk found in patients who are being considered for spine surgery. Such a process allows the surgeon to individualize treatment protocols. In patients who have a high level of identified psychosocial risk, alternatives to spine surgery can be considered. Psychologists often see nonsurgical patients as well, helping them cope with the emotional sequelae of spinal injury and to help them learn new means of coping with pain and its limitations. Social workers can also play a pivotal role in counseling these patients while establishing support network to help them recover.

PHYSICAL THERAPY

Many patients with back pain require little intervention from a physician. Their problems are related to body mechanics and deconditioning. For this reason, a conservative approach to the treatment of back pain incorporates PT as a first-line treatment. Frequently, therapists provide a combination of strengthening, stretching, palliative modalities (such as heat or electrical stimulation), and hands-on muscle activation that offer good pain relief. Fritz et al.[15] found that patients with acute spine pain who have high adherence rates to active PT-based exercise programs achieve excellent reductions in disability and pain. Symptomatic management with structured PT may delay or avoid more invasive interventions altogether.

Another benefit of PT is that patients often continue the activities they learned during therapy well beyond their treatment course. Many rehabilitation centers provide patients a home exercise program as their formal treatment period ends. Additionally, getting into the habit of exercise during PT may encourage patients to continue a more active lifestyle, improving their general health as well as potentially decreasing their back pain.

OCCUPATIONAL THERAPY

One of the most challenging and costly aspects of back pain is effectively managing patients who suffer workplace-related back pain. Patients with pain that is inadequately treated may function poorly at work, which can lead to termination of current employment, unemployment, and disability. Occupational therapists play a central role in conducting structured functional evaluations to determine the patient's current level of performance compared to their job demands. Their primary goal is to help restore patients to their baseline functional status so they can lead a productive lifestyle at home and at work. Of note, in many settings, physical therapists take on part of the role of occupational therapists.

It is important to remember that the response to physical and occupational therapy may vary among patients, as is the duration of therapy required before a response is observed. Therefore, therapy is generally recommended for at least 6 weeks. With regard to conservative management of back pain, if standard treatment modalities are ineffective, patients may be encouraged to explore alternative options such as chiropractic and acupuncture.

SPINE SURGERY

Spine surgery is the topic of much discussion as many surgeons are devoted to developing novel implant designs and operative techniques. As previously noted, only about 10% of patients seeking care for back pain go on to have surgery. The most important, and arguably the most difficult, aspect of spine surgery is choosing the appropriate indications for surgery. Although the outcomes for surgery for radicular leg pain and neurogenic claudication are more predictable and favorable, surgery for back pain without any clear underlying etiology is less so. When patients have exhausted nonoperative treatment options for back pain, the default unfortunately is to resort to surgery. However, operative intervention is generally not recommended for pure mechanical back pain, as surgery can lead to more pain and disability. This dilemma highlights the importance of having an interdisciplinary spine care team that upholds high standards and expectations while holding each member accountable for high-quality patient care. Even when the indications are appropriate to proceed with surgery, the risks involved, as well as the costs, mandate that surgery is used sparingly and only when nonoperative options have failed to provide adequate symptomatic relief.

A spine center of excellence certainly needs a group of well-trained spine surgeons. Although not frequently addressed in the literature, there has been some investigation into the relationship of surgeon experience and complications associated with spine surgery. Wiese et al.[16] found that the complication rate following lumbar microdiscectomy was significantly less among surgeons with a greater level of experience (2.2% vs. 10.7%). In results from a multicenter total disk replacement study, it was reported that among the high-enrolling surgeons and/or centers, the length of hospital stay, operating time, and complication rates were significantly less than among low-enrolling sites.[17] Results of the studies suggest that established spine centers that make use of a team of specialists with varying expertise have an advantage over individual physicians with respect to complication rates.

Although surgery is sometimes viewed as the "end of the road" in treatment, this should not be the case. Although surgery is a dramatic event, it is only one step in a continuum of care.

Treatment does not end with surgery. Most patients who undergo spinal surgery will not have been engaging in typical activities due to pain. Although the surgery may address the structural component of their problem, it cannot address the deconditioning that has occurred. In a spine clinic, there are postoperative rehabilitation protocols for the various types of surgery performed. In this day of escalating surgical options and approaches, physical therapists must gain a clear understanding of each operative intervention and lend their expertise to developing safe and effective rehabilitation protocols that will maximize functional recovery after surgery. For example, a therapist not working closely with spine surgeons may have a difficult time devising the most appropriate and safe program for a patient who has undergone surgery using a nontraditional approach such as the trans-sacral approach to the L5–S1 disk space or extreme lateral interbody fusion for other lumbar disks. Some new procedures require avoidance of specific motions early after surgery with guided progression back to full activity.[18] Without an understanding of the goals and functions of new implants, it is unlikely that a physical therapist working in isolation will be able to design an optimally safe and effective rehabilitation regimen.

Surgeons at a specialty spine center should be slow to adapt new technologies and techniques, and the group's practice should be standardized and evidence-based. One of the advantages of a spine specialty center is the enhanced opportunity for surgeons to participate in clinical trials evaluating new technologies. These centers are often preferred sites due to the expertise of the surgeons and the ability to have a large enough patient population to meet enrollment needs. The benefit to the surgeons is that they can offer patients interventions that would otherwise be unavailable outside of an investigational setting for many years to come. Patients have the benefit of participating in clinical trials if they meet the selection criteria and elect to participate. The multidisciplinary nature of an established spine center offers the optimal atmosphere for testing new and emerging technologies for treating spinal disorders.

CHRONIC PAIN MANAGEMENT PROGRAM

The multifaceted nature of spine injuries points to the importance of approaching spine treatment in a multidisciplinary fashion. After treatment, patients must often resume a life where the very assumptions and boundaries have been greatly distorted, all too often by ongoing pain or marked functional limitations that were not present before illness or injury. With or without surgery for spinal disorders, pain and concomitant limitations often linger and, without proper treatment and planning, these can magnify. The chronic pain management program (CPMP) thus becomes a truly integral component of treatment in most spine centers. Such programs, involving many disciplines (most often pain medicine, PM&R, PT and occupational therapy, and psychology), rely on therapeutic group milieu to assist patients in learning (and helping each other to learn) new ways to deal with pain, minimize its impact on their lives, and overcome psychosocial barriers. Research on the CPMP approach indicates that patients achieve an average pain reduction of approximately 50%, about 75% are able to get off narcotic medications, and the return to work rate from such programs is approximately 67%.[19] Of course, CPMPs vary widely in terms of their composition and effectiveness. The spine center should, at a minimum, be certified by and adhere to the standards set by the Commission on Accreditation of Rehabilitation Facilities (CARF) or a similar international organization.

POTENTIAL BENEFITS OF A SPINE SPECIALTY CLINIC

Many components of treating chronic pain of other origins and back pain are similar. What, then, is the advantage of having a spine specialty clinic? Focusing solely on back pain has several potential advantages.

Although in the past, there may have been more separation between nonsurgical care providers and surgeons, the two can be blended into a comprehensive system. As reported by Rasmussen et al.,[20] the initiation of multidisciplinary "nonsurgical" spine clinics significantly reduced the number of lumbar discectomy surgeries performed. One of the factors that was felt most likely to account for this decline was an improved diagnostic evaluation process.

Considering the wide range of potential pain origins as well as the potential and varying roles of psychosocial factors related to back pain, it is not surprising that patients cover a very broad spectrum of problems and needs. This gives rise to the need for true multidisciplinary care. It is imperative that the care providers have, and maintain, a strong and specific knowledge base regarding spinal disorders. Such skills can only be developed and continually honed by ongoing interaction with patients, continuing professional education, and the cross-training provided by the frequent interaction of professionals from various disciplines caring for similar patients. This is true not only for the physicians involved in the clinic but also for the physical therapists and other members of the treatment team. By building a strong knowledge base in one area, providers can equip patients with a greater level of education in discussing their spinal problems and working together toward effective solutions.

Specialized spine centers require a large patient population to support all the facets required for the multidisciplinary approach to care. Although some painful conditions are relatively rare, back pain is a very common problem. Considering that 80% of people have back pain at some point during their lives and that about 10% go on to develop chronic pain, there are likely to be large enough patient populations in most communities to make a spine center a viable undertaking.

The term *center of excellence* is a determination used in several specialties to provide quality assurance for new procedures or technologies or for those surgeries not widely performed, such as video-assisted thoracic surgery.[21] A number of centers of excellence in spine care have emerged in recent years, but there is no uniform set of criteria used to define a spine center of excellence. Such centers have a multidisciplinary treatment philosophy and are committed to providing the highest quality of care. It is these centers of excellence that should be the lead sites in developing treatment guidelines, participating in registries, performing research, and providing education. Implementation of a structured quality assurance program is a critical element of developing a spine center of excellence. Designing and implementing guidelines, assessing outcomes, and implementing changes for improvement may be more manageable in a spine clinic. This type of program is becoming increasingly needed in this age of increasing demands for ongoing quality assessment and reimbursement initiatives such as pay for performance.

Within the spine clinic, subspecialization will naturally take place. Based on the interests and skills of the professionals involved with patient care, various physicians will gravitate toward treatment of specific spinal disorders. For example, one may take the majority of patients with unusually challenging cervical spine problems, another may be a leader in one or more areas of spine arthroplasty, and there should be at least one surgeon adept at diagnosing the multiply operated failed back patient who eventually arrives at a spine specialty facility. Some physicians may elect to perform injections, whereas others do not. There is a need for advanced interventions such as spinal cord stimulation for pain management. This type of subspecialization within a spine clinic further provides the care provider the opportunity to hone highly specialized skills as well as allowing them to pursue the interventions they are most interested in providing.

The presence of professionals from multiple disciplines in a spine clinic will also increase awareness about alternate pain mechanisms and approaches to treatment. For example, the addition of chiropractic care providers will increase the awareness of all the care providers of problems arising from the sacroiliac joint and the role of manipulative therapy in treating this group of patients with low back pain.

COORDINATION OF CARE

Working one's way through most health care systems can be daunting for patients. A comprehensive spine clinic can reduce confusion and anxiety. Patients can receive a wide variety of services as needed within a single facility. Patients receiving treatment in a single center will become familiar with employees, and they will find less redundant paperwork required for insurance and providing basic history and health data. The best spine centers provide close coordination of care from one provider to another through close communication.

RESEARCH AND EDUCATION

If practicing in a university setting, education and research are built into the framework and environment of patient care. However, the success of programs still depends strongly on the commitment made by the individuals involved. Although this is also true in private practice, the challenges are greater. There is no institutional framework or incentive built into the practice that promotes involvement in either research or education. To create a research environment outside the university setting requires a commitment of time and financial resources. However, a practice cannot hope to become a spine care center of excellence without incorporating research and education. The implementation of a research program is becoming easier with the growing use of electronic medical records and registry systems in spine care facilities. Establishing an infrastructure for data collection complements the current demands for evidence-based medicine and cost-effectiveness information for back pain interventions. Considering the societal costs associated with back pain, these demands may be even greater for spine care specialists than for other disciplines. Although in the past, care providers may have been able to be successful without engaging in organized data collection, this is likely to change. Research also provides a venue to gain recognition in the peer group. This is more easily accomplished in a specialty clinic than in one spread across multiple specialties, unless focused efforts can be made in multiple areas.

The increasing use of electronic medical records and national study registries in spine has greatly facilitated tracking treatment outcomes. Although these mechanisms are far superior to traditional paper data collection, they still require time to harvest the data, address unanticipated scenarios, download, analyze, and prepare reports of the data and write abstracts and manuscripts. One of the greatest advantages of the registries is that some are programmed to contact patients by e-mail up to 24 months after treatment and have patients complete self-assessment forms online without returning to the clinic. Although radiographic follow-up cannot be achieved, the patient's clinical condition can be evaluated.

Another opportunity to become active in spine research is through participation in clinical trials. To do so is a great responsibility for the investigator to ensure that the trials are being conducted in accordance to federal regulations and study protocols. Staff should be hired with experience in conducting clinical trials, regulatory requirements, and experience interacting with institutional review boards or human experimentation ethics committees. Many such trials are financially self-sustaining, as industry sponsors will provide the funding to cover the cost of conducting the trial. Participation in such studies provides the framework for rigorous data collection.

Research is a vital part of quality patient care. Although all care providers want to take the best care of their patients, without measuring and being willing to critically appraise their own outcomes, it is impossible for the individual practitioner to assess and improve the quality of care he or she is delivering. Through the collection of data and ongoing assessment of results, problems, such as spikes in particular complication rates, can be identified and addressed. This is particularly important in a multiple-physician group to assess the complications and clinical outcomes of all the care providers in the practice and to ensure that problems are addressed as soon as they are identified. The emergence of Patient-Reported Outcome Measurement Instrument System (PROMIS) and its associated computer-adaptive test (CAT), which strongly correlates with other "gold standard" spinal outcomes measurement instruments but has a significantly lower completion time, shows immense promise toward making this process more seamless.[22]

Accepting the role of serving as faculty for a residency program or establishing a fellowship program can also enhance the intellectual environment of a spine clinic. Such programs often lead to creating lecture series such as grand rounds and journal clubs, which are relatively inexpensive. Creating forums for discussion among all care providers in the group can strengthen the bonds of the practice, allow more insight into what the other team members' discipline offer to overall care, and enhance care by getting the right patient to the right provider more quickly.

Spine specialty centers have the potential to step to the forefront in shaping the future of spine care on a large-scale basis. Being specialized and focused in one area makes it easier to participate in registry networks and other quality improvement initiatives.

Conclusion

The spine is a complex structure that often presents diagnostic dilemmas and treatment challenges to health care providers. The complexity is compounded by the frequent and profound psychosocial impact of chronic spinal disorders. A spine center of excellence must be designed to address the complexity of these challenges. One of the primary needs is an organized, deliberately planned approach to the evaluation and treatment of the broad spectrum of back pain patients. Members of the multidisciplinary team must be trained and focused on quality spine care. The use of electronic medical records greatly enhances the ability to track patients and events related to their care. The team of providers must understand the role of the other team members and respect what each has to offer in providing quality care to patients. There must be strong leadership to keep the team focused, efficient, and effective.

Part of developing a center of excellence is incorporating research and education. Research efforts can provide patients and practitioners with the opportunity to participate in clinical trials which can enhance the reputation of the center in the community while at the same time providing a means to assess outcomes of various treatments provided in the clinic. Only through incorporating research can providers have access to the latest technology and be involved in continually improving the delivery of patient care. Everyone benefits from education, which can take on many forms including lectures, journal clubs, conferences, fellowship programs, and research.

References

1. Hazard RG. Low-back and neck pain diagnosis and treatment. *Am J Phys Med Rehabil* 2007;86:S59–S68.
2. Pincus T, Burton AK, Vogel S, et al. A systematic review of psychological factors as predictors of chronicity/disability in prospective cohorts of low back pain. *Spine* 2002;27:E109–E120.
3. Groopman J. *How Doctors Think*. New York: Houghton Mifflin Company; 2007.
4. Nwosu KC, Bono CM. Incidence of low back pain in athletes and differential diagnosis and evaluation of the athlete with back and/or leg pain. In: Hecht AC, ed. *Spine Injuries in Athletes*. Philadelphia: Wolters Kluwer; 2017:146–153.
5. Strine TW, Hootman JM. US national prevalence and correlates of low back and neck pain among adults. *Arthritis Rheum* 2007;57:656–665.
6. Frymoyer JW, Pope MH, Costanza MC, et al. Epidemiologic studies of low-back pain. *Spine (Phila Pa 1976)* 1980;5:419–423.
7. Fanuele JC, Birkmeyer NJ, Abdu WA, et al. The impact of spinal problems on the health status of patients: have we underestimated the effect? *Spine* 2000;25:1509–1514.
8. Loeser JD, Butler S, Chapman CR, et al. *Bonica's Management of Pain*. 3rd ed. Philadelphia: Lippincott Williams & Wilkins; 2001.
9. Scientific approach to the assessment and management of activity-related spinal disorders. A monograph for clinicians. Report of the Quebec Task Force on Spinal Disorders. *Spine* 1987;12:S1–S59.
10. Martell BA, O'Connor PG, Kerns RD, et al. Systematic review: opioid treatment for chronic back pain: prevalence, efficacy, and association with addiction. *Ann Intern Med* 2007;146:116–127.
11. Hansen RN, Oster G, Edelsberg J, et al. Economic costs of nonmedical use of prescription opioids. *Clin J Pain* 2011;27:194–202.
12. Lindsay PG, Wyckoff M. The depression-pain syndrome and its response to antidepressants. *Psychosomatics* 1981;22:571–573, 576–577.
13. Fernandez E, Clark TS, Ruddick-Davis D. A framework for conceptualization and assessment of affective disturbance in pain. In: Block AR, Kremer E, Fernandez E, eds. *Handbook of Pain Syndromes: Biopsychosocial Perspectives*. Mahwah, NJ: Lawrence Erlbaum Associates; 1999:123–148.
14. Block AR, Gatchel RJ, Deardorff WW, et al. *The Psychology of Spine Surgery*. Washington, DC: American Psychological Association; 2003.
15. Fritz JM, Cleland JA, Brennan GP. Does adherence to the guideline recommendation for active treatments improve the quality of care for patients with acute low back pain delivered by physical therapists? *Med Care* 2007;45:973–980.
16. Wiese M, Krämer J, Bernsmann K, et al. The related outcome and complication rate in primary lumbar microscopic disc surgery depending on the surgeon's experience: comparative studies. *Spine J* 2004;4:550–556.
17. Regan JJ, McAfee PC, Blumenthal SL, et al. Evaluation of surgical volume and the early experience with lumbar total disc replacement as part of the investigational device exemption study of the Charité Artificial Disc. *Spine* 2006;31:2270–2276.
18. Ozgur BM, Aryan HE, Pimenta L, et al. Extreme Lateral Interbody Fusion (XLIF): a novel surgical technique for anterior lumbar interbody fusion. *Spine J* 2006;6:435–443.
19. Turk DC, Burwinkle TM. Assessment of chronic pain in rehabilitation: outcomes measures in clinical trials and clinical practice. *Rehabil Psychol* 2005;50:56–64.
20. Rasmussen C, Nielsen GL, Hansen VK, et al. Rates of lumbar disc surgery before and after implementation of multidisciplinary nonsurgical spine clinics. *Spine* 2005;30:2469–2473.
21. Chin CS, Swanson SJ. Video-assisted thoracic surgery lobectomy: centers of excellence or excellence of centers? *Thorac Surg Clin* 2008;18:263–268.
22. Hung M, Hon SD, Franklin JD, et al. Psychometric properties of the PROMIS physical function item bank in patients with spinal disorders. *Spine (Phila PA 1976)* 2014;39:158–163.

CHAPTER 108

Pain Management in Primary Care

WILLIAM C. BECKER and **MATTHEW J. BAIR**

Introduction

PREVALENCE OF PAIN IN THE UNITED STATES

Pain is the most common reason cited for patients seeking medical care, and pain accounts for up to 80% of total visits to physicians' offices.[1,2] Although it is difficult to determine the prevalence of pain precisely, recent surveys suggest that 75 to 105 million Americans experience pain daily or intermittently.[3–5] Given this widespread prevalence, the Institute of Medicine (now the National Academy of Medicine)[6] and the U.S. Department of Health and Human Services,[7] among other important stakeholder groups, have called primary care the foundation of pain treatment in the United States, a foundation that should be adequately trained to meet the challenge of delivering high-quality pain care.

ECONOMIC IMPLICATIONS OF CHRONIC PAIN

The National Academy of Medicine estimated the cost of pain to be approximately $565 billion dollars, making it one of the costliest conditions in the United States. Although the precise figure has been debated, there is little argument that the costs associated with pain treatment and the economic impact of missed days of work and unemployment and other societal costs are high and increasing.

Care management plans and disease management programs are abundant for other chronic conditions, such as asthma, hypertension, hyperlipidemia, and diabetes mellitus. Treatment strategies include case management, treatment algorithms, provider education, and patient support groups. In contrast, very little emphasis has been placed on studying and developing such initiatives for chronic pain conditions. Given the large allocation of United States health care dollars for treating patients with these conditions, it is time for the provider, payer, and policymaker communities to take notice; emerging models discussed at the end of this chapter may signal the beginning of a promising trend.

CHRONIC PAIN MANAGEMENT: THE STATUS QUO

With the onset of pain, most patients attempt self-care with over-the-counter products and/or self-help techniques (e.g., distracting activities, rest). When these methods fail to provide adequate relief, the patient generally seeks help from a medical professional. In many cases and particularly in health care systems with limited access to specialty care, the gatekeeping primary care provider is the first medical contact. The primary care provider recommends treatment and refers the patient for appropriate specialty care, such as a physical medicine assessment for low back pain.

When pain becomes chronic and specialty care is ineffective in improving the underlying condition, care management becomes more difficult. In a recent survey, only 34% of internists reported that they felt comfortable with their abilities to manage patients with chronic pain.[2] In a related article, Ballantyne and Mao[8] wrote that the most difficult issue now facing physicians is "whether and how to prescribe opioid therapy for chronic pain that is not associated with terminal disease, including pain experienced by the increasing number of patients with cancer in remission." In part, physicians are hesitant to prescribe opioids because they lack both the understanding of how to comprehensively assess pain and its common comorbidities and the knowledge of available pain therapies.

The varied presentations and manifestations of chronic pain may at times confound primary care providers. Physical exam and radiographic abnormalities are not predictive of pain severity or dysfunction.[9] Many patients experience pain that may be constant and occurs for several years, and yet their life functioning is not changed in major ways. Conversely, there are other patients with similar structural abnormalities who suffer substantially more and cannot maintain their usual levels of activity.[10] Patients whose lives are significantly disrupted by pain engage in behaviors that are maladaptive, anticipate more distress, amplify sensations associated with pain, spend more time resting, and complain of less ability to control pain.[11,12] It may be reassuring to providers to recognize that this same degree of variability is seen in virtually all chronic conditions as a manifestation of the complex interplay of biologic, psychological, and social factors.

At the same time, surveys evaluating the adequacy of pain treatment demonstrate that the current system is dysfunctional.[13] Patients report that they are not asked about pain, that they are afraid to report pain to their primary care providers, and that they are often not offered treatment. In one survey, 22% of patients with pain reported being uncomfortable discussing pain with their personal physicians, 13% said they were denied pain medication or referrals to pain specialists, and 70% reported experiencing continued pain despite treatment.[14] Much of these system problems can be attributed to the treatment of pain at the primary care level.

SEARCHING FOR SOLUTIONS

There have been tremendous advances in the knowledge of pain pathophysiology, the understanding of treatments for pain, and recognition of the value of an interdisciplinary approach to pain management. On the scientific front, there has been an explosion in pain research, and new pharmaceutical agents have become available for treating different types of pain. Complementary and integrative health therapies for pain management have gained recognition and an increasingly robust evidence base. Novel interventional techniques and surgeries have been introduced. Professional pain societies have sprung up, and training is now available to provide physicians and other health care professionals with expertise in pain management. Despite this unprecedented progress, pain care remains inadequate, and undertreatment of pain is still considered pandemic. The reasons for these continuing inadequacies are varied, but it is clear that new solutions must focus on primary care.

A New Approach to Chronic Pain Management

There are many different types of pain that it is difficult for a nonexpert provider to become familiar with and comfortable treating all pain conditions. Current categories for classifying pain include nociceptive versus neuropathic, acute versus persistent, cancer versus noncancer, and area of the body (headache, abdominal pain, chest pain). These categories are simplistic and helpful only in a general way.

We are accustomed to accepted, well-defined, objective measurements to assess the quality of care. For many other chronic conditions, there are standardized outcome measures. In patients with diabetes, we can measure hemoglobin A_1C levels. In patients with asthma, peak flow and the use of inhaled β agonists guide care. Treatment outcomes for pain are often subjective, confusing, and controversial. If a patient's pain severity is better but function is not improved, is this outcome adequate? If the patient is satisfied with treatment but pain intensity levels remain high (e.g., an 8 on the 0 to 10 pain numerical rating scale), is this treatment sufficient? If the patient returns to work but is on high doses of opioids, is this acceptable? All of these questions frequently arise in the primary care and complicate treatment.

WHO TREATS CHRONIC ILLNESS?

When pain becomes chronic, a behavioral syndrome and co-morbidities may emerge including depression, anxiety, helplessness, insomnia, deconditioning, and increased reliance on the health care system, what has been called "high-impact" chronic pain. At this point, chronic pain becomes a disease process that needs chronic disease management.[15] Chronic back pain is not a diagnosis but rather a description of duration and location. In many cases, it is not possible to be more precise in the diagnosis of, for example, low back pain because even experts disagree on the underlying etiology.[16] Neuroscience increasingly points to dysregulated neuroplasticity and central sensitization as common pathways to chronic pain,[17] further underscoring the futility of "imaging" chronic pain in most cases. Providers would do well to learn to message to patients that a lack of imaging findings is important for ruling out sinister causes of pain (e.g., cancer) but does not mean the pain is not real.

Failure to be more precise in the diagnosis should not delay treatment or impede medical management. Treatment in primary care often involves uncertainty, as most of the conditions encountered cannot be diagnosed precisely: Viral illness, rash, or headaches are common, and the etiology unexplained. Chronic pain falls into the group of conditions that often defies definitive diagnosis and is suited to the primary care practice. A patient's suffering can be ameliorated by nonpharmacologic interventions including patient education and self-management skills that may be combined with analgesics such as nonsteroidal anti-inflammatory drugs (NSAIDs).

All primary care physicians must treat patients with a variety of chronic diseases. In fact, most chronic illness is principally managed at the primary care level.[18] Improvements in the medical management of asthma, hypertension, and diabetes have arisen from interventions implemented in primary care. Despite the lack of specialty training and through the use of practice guidelines, following treatment recommendations, conducting chart reviews, discussing shared experience, and providing expert assistance, primary care delivers excellent medical care. Management of persistent pain lends itself to the same paradigm.

WHY PRIMARY CARE IS INVOLVED?

Primary care is based on the elements of trust, therapeutic alliance, advocacy, continuity, care coordination, preventive care, and careful attention to quality of life/lifestyle issues. Motivating patients to strive for better health through exercise, diet, stress management, medication adherence, and disease monitoring is a common role played by the primary care provider—a role that requires the provider to adopt and maintain a nonjudgmental attitude.

Primary care is uniquely positioned to provide care for patients with chronic pain. Of all specialties, primary care providers have the largest geographic distribution. Rather than clustering around medical centers in the largest cities, they are broadly distributed over diverse communities—from urban clinics to suburban medical centers to private practices in small towns and rural areas. Furthermore, primary care providers are trained in patient-centered communication, biopsychosocial assessment, and multimodal treatment planning, all core features of a high-quality approach to chronic pain.

By its very nature, primary care entails continuity by developing a longitudinal experience with patients. Each office visit enables the provider to achieve greater understanding of how individual patients are dealing with their persistent pain. Primary care providers are experienced in providing comfort and disease management for chronic conditions. When clinicians are challenged to broaden their definition of pain as a symptom and begin to view it as a chronic illness,[11] primary care is well equipped to deal with chronic pain.

When a patient's pain becomes persistent and specialty care is either unavailable or ineffective as a treatment option, the providers can continue to play a key role by coordinating care, intervening when symptoms change, and constantly encouraging patients to make lifestyle choices as they do in all other chronic diseases: weight loss, sleep hygiene, anxiety/depression/mood management, physical activity, education, and judicious use of medications.[19]

From a cost and utilization perspective, primary care is the most appropriate setting for chronic pain management. Most types of health insurance, as well as Medicare and Medicaid, cover primary care visits yet may not cover long-term psychosocial treatment or interventional procedures. A classic 1995 study of low back pain examined 1,555 patients cared for by chiropractors, orthopedic surgeons, or primary care providers. Cost, work status, and time to restoration of baseline status were monitored. All groups achieved similar outcomes yet primary care was the least costly.[20] Risks of polypharmacy are better managed within the primary care structure because it is accustomed to dealing with multiple diseases and their treatments in a single patient.

TREATING CHRONIC PAIN IN THE PRIMARY CARE SETTING—WHY A CHALLENGE?
Training in Pain

Much of formal medical training occurs in hospitals where acute symptoms and life-threatening conditions are studied. Historically, very little practice has been offered in the management of chronic pain in the outpatient setting. Training in pain management may be limited to a brief session in a pharmacology or neuroanatomy course during medical school. As a consequence of this limited training, many residency-trained primary care providers are ill equipped and therefore uncomfortable treating patients with persistent pain.[21] This may lead to inadequate assessment, substandard treatment planning, poor follow-up and monitoring, and generally poor quality of care.

However, the opioid crisis has prompted medical schools to re-examine pain management curricula and has spurred widespread calls for medical student and provider education to be cornerstones in addressing the crisis.

Disagreement among Experts—To Treat and Not to Treat

In recognition of the need to improve pain management, the Federation of State Medical Boards issued guidelines on the appropriate workup and treatment of persistent pain.[22] Most states have adopted the Federation's recommendations in the form of Intractable Pain Tratement Acts. The safe and proper use of opioids is the cornerstone of these acts, encouraging providers to assess patients' pain and use medication when necessary. Increasingly, adequate pain relief is being viewed as a patient's right—and a clinician's obligation—sometimes to the point of allowing the patient or family to take legal action against doctors for the undertreatment of pain. On the other hand, the opioid crisis has ushered in a new era of caution in treating pain.

The Centers for Disease Control and Prevention (CDC) released the Guideline for Prescribing Opioids for Chronic Pain in March 2016,[23] a landmark effort that garnered widespread publicity and spurred heated discussions of controversies related to guideline recommendations. For example, the CDC guideline contrasted significantly to the 2009 American Pain Society/American Academy of Pain Management's Clinical Guidelines for the Use of Chronic Opioid Therapy in Chronic Noncancer Pain[24] as decidedly "opioid avoidant." The CDC guideline promoted nonopioid analgesics and nonpharmacologic treatment options as preferred in the treatment of chronic pain, identified recommended limits in opioid doses prescribed, and advocated for heightened vigilance and monitoring for indications to taper down or discontinue opioids especially among patients already on long-term opioid therapy when benefits no longer outweigh harms. The CDC guideline also emphasized the lack of evidence demonstrating long-term efficacy of long-term opioid therapy in contrast to other treatments for chronic pain[25] and the growing evidence of potential harms, especially at higher doses.

It is too early to tell the full impact of the CDC guideline. However, the CDC guideline has already changed many providers' approach to opioid therapy specifically and chronic pain care generally. More providers appreciate that high-quality pain care involves a combination of nonpharmacologic and pharmacologic options. Treatments where patients take an active role (e.g., yoga) are viewed as particularly valuable. Pain self-management skill building is considered low cost and effective and promotes less reliance on the health care system and that it may be in patients' best interests to reduce or avoid taking opioids, especially long term. Avoiding long-term opioid therapy has been informed by consistent observational data and emerging randomized controlled trial (RCT) data that patients may experience accelerated decline in well-being and accrue a variety of bothersome and sometimes serious harms on long-term, and especially high-dose, opioids. That said, for individuals already on long-term opioid therapy for whom benefit *is* outweighing harm, the therapy (and ongoing close monitoring of it) should be continued. Involuntary tapering of patients not experiencing harm is not evidence based, not patient centered, and may have its own set of serious risks and unintended consequences.[26]

Barriers to Treating Pain

Many barriers to the management of pain have been well-documented in this text and others.[27] These obstacles relate to the medical system, providers, patients, and regulatory and governmental agencies, all of which are operant in primary care practices. At the same time, other obstacles are unique to primary care, making pain management more difficult even for the well-trained, conscientious provider.

Time Constraints

Primary care providers often perceive pressure to do more in less time, especially in light of cuts in reimbursement (Medicare, Medicaid, and other types of commercial insurance). Furthermore, the typical 15-minute office visits are crowded by other activities: telephone calls, add-on appointments, emergencies, hospital admissions, serving as preceptor for students or midlevel providers (i.e., interns, residents, nurse practitioners), and reviewing laboratory and x-ray reports.

Patient complexity is also a major contributor to time constraints. Patients may present with multiple medical issues at each visit—ranging from chronic conditions (diabetes, hypertension, and hypercholesterolemia), situational issues (insomnia, stress at work, menopausal symptoms), preventive care needs (immunizations, cancer screening), procedural needs (skin tag removal, knee injections), and other issues (medication refills, disability forms, jury excuses).

Comprehensive assessment and documentation of pain would be difficult in this setting even if the entire 15 minutes were available to address pain during the visit. To address these issues but still harness the wealth of resources that make primary care such a compelling foundational treatment setting, promising new care models described in the following discussion have emerged.

Lack of Guidelines Specific to Primary Care

A variety of well-recognized treatment algorithms and evidence-based guidelines exist for treating other chronic conditions encountered by primary care physicians (e.g., cancer,[28] neuropathy,[29] fibromyalgia syndrome[30]). Although guidelines have been developed for some pain problems, there are relatively few specific recommendations for the treatment of persistent pain and rarely address the practical challenges to managing chronic pain in primary care.

Even when guidelines are available, studies show that often they are not followed by clinicians.[31] This can be explained in part by the nature of chronic pain. When a patient's chronic pain worsens, the cause is frequently undiscoverable, making it difficult to apply a guideline or to decide on a different treatment when so many therapeutic options have been ineffective.

Patient Nonadherence to Treatment

In other diseases, the consequences of nonadherence are not apparent to the patient. Patients with worsening atherosclerosis, hypertension, or diabetes are often asymptomatic. In contrast, nonadherence to medical management has serious implications for patients with persistent pain and their physicians. Detriments to patients' pain intensity, functional status, quality of life, and mental health conditions may occur as a result to nonadherence.

Specialty Referrals

Referrals for patients with persistent pain may differ for other conditions in primary care practice. After referrals to specialists in other conditions, patients may return to the primary care provider after the medical issue has resolved or the chronic illness has an expected treatment course. Some examples include dysfunctional uterine bleeding is diagnosed and treated before referral back to primary care. The fractured bone is set and stabilized, rehabilitation is arranged, and the patient presents back to primary care with restored function. The patient with congestive heart failure has further diagnostic testing, medication adjustments, and returns to primary care when symptoms have improved and the patient is stable.

The workup and treatment of the patient with persistent pain, on the other hand, may be less amenable to these clear benefits and resolution of symptoms. The acupuncturist diagnoses an imbalance of energy or "chi" and treats with needles and herbs. The physiatrist may focus on muscle tightness and nerve injury and offers rehabilitative therapies. The interventionalist uses injections to alleviate radicular pain. The chiropractor focuses on structural imbalance of the skeleton and offers manipulation therapy.

Often, the diagnoses and procedures for chronic pain are less familiar to the primary care provider (e.g., disk disruption, discogram, vertebroplasty, facet arthritis, radiofrequency ablation). Unfamiliar drugs and drug combinations are uncomfortable for physicians to prescribe and monitor. These may include polypharmacy with four or five drugs, such as combinations of multiple anticonvulsants (gabapentinoids), serotonin norepinephrine reuptake inhibitors, multiple opioids, and/or other analgesics; drugs rarely prescribed (e.g., methadone); and doses not used (e.g., high-dose opioids or gabapentin). After referral, patients may return to primary care with unclear parameters on what constitutes treatment "success." Too often, the patient's pain level is as high as when first referred for specialty care, and psychosocial issues such as depression and anxiety may not have been addressed.

Comorbid Conditions

The most commonly occurring comorbid conditions in patients with persistent pain are depression, anxiety, insomnia, and substance misuse or substance use disorders.[32] These comorbidities complicate care. Patients may resist psychiatric care for many reasons including the perceived stigma, the additional cost, or the belief that their pain is unrelated to their mental health comorbidities.

Pain can make depression worse, and depression can make pain worse, both independently.[33] Patients seeking relief from their pain and comorbid conditions may self-medicate with alcohol and other substances such as marijuana, which can further complicate the problem. They may take prescribed pain medications to treat the comorbid condition and temporarily relieve their symptoms but can make them feel worse long term.

Failure to address underlying anxiety, depression, insomnia, and substance use disorders makes pain treatment more difficult. These comorbid conditions are difficult to treat in stable patients. When persistent pain or a chronic illness is also present, the treatment is even more complicated because the pain experience is more severe and less amenable to treatment. It is unlikely that a simple, single-drug regimen or series of epidural steroid injections will be the long-term solution for chronic pain and comorbid conditions.

Adversarial Relationship

Medical practice in primary care is built on trust, respect, and advocacy for the patient. The doctor–patient relationship is fundamental and develops over years of providing preventive care, treating acute conditions, and supporting the patient through life transitions such as the birth of a child, unemployment, and the death of a close family member. This long-term relationship enables the primary care provider to better understand the patient as an individual and allows the provider to more effectively share medical advice and decisions with their patients.

Persistent pain may disrupt this stable pattern and create an unusual relationship that may not emerge in the management of other chronic diseases. The primary care provider may, at times, feel forced into an uncomfortable adversarial position that he or she is not well trained to manage. Patients with chronic pain ask for many things that are not guideline concordant at times the physician must argue against or deny certain diagnostic tests or treatments. For example, the patient wants the doctor to order additional or repeated expensive procedures (e.g., magnetic resonance imaging [MRI]) when his or her pain worsens. The doctor refuses because it is not consistent with guidelines, will not change the treatment plan or lead to a cure for the persistent pain, or is not approved by the patient's health insurance plan.

In this scenario, the provider may find themselves in the difficult role of contradicting the patient's wishes. When the doctor is unable to be supportive, the patient begins to question whether his or her "advocate" still wants to help. The patient–provider relationship may become strained, and the patient may resist potentially beneficial treatment options recommended.

Addressing Barriers to Care

As mentioned earlier in this chapter, primary care providers may lack comfort and confidence in managing chronic pain. In addition to limited training, there are a number of other underlying reasons for this.

MYTHS AND BIASES

Patients—Without conscious intention, people attach meaning to all sensory experiences. The smell of a rose may hold a special meaning to someone who received her first bouquet for the high school prom. The sound of the musical tune "Jingle Bells" may signify happiness, family gatherings, and holiday gifts. Pain, especially when it is persistent, often conveys a sense that the person is being punished for some real or perceived infraction.

Too often, patients with chronic pain believe that they suffer because of some mistake they made or that pain is to be expected as a part of aging. At times, there is so much salience attached to pain that it is difficult to convince the patient otherwise. These beliefs about "needing pain" or "deserving pain" complicate treatment.

Providers—Primary care providers may be suspicious of patients who complain of pain. Physicians understand certain types of pain—cancer pain, end-of-life pain, or acute trauma/illness pain—but are less accepting of the persistent pain that has few objective signs of defined conditions. We ask, "Why do some patients complain while others, with the same pathology or anatomy, do not complain?" "What is the secondary gain?" "Is this pain real?"

Some providers still cling to the outdated notion that most causes of chronic pain should clearly be identifiable on imaging studies. When pain is not easily explained in this paradigm, bias may lead the primary care provider to suspect mental health causes. In addition, mental health comorbidities are common with persistent pain. The primary care provider may believe that the persistence of the pain relates directly to the patient's depression or anxiety, thereby depreciating the pain complaint. Patients perceive this attitude as devaluing their experience.

PATIENT RESISTANCE

The false dichotomy of physical pain versus emotional pain, still often perpetuated by health care providers, affects patients' experiences as well. The patient reasons, "If my doctor cannot find anything wrong with me and if there is no fix for my situation, he or she will assume that I must be crazy." For this reason, feelings such as "you think this is all in my head" are often expressed in patient encounters.

In fact, physical and emotional pain cannot be separated. They coexist and feed on each other. For instance, the most balanced, rational, and accepting patients can still experience high pain levels from fibromyalgia syndrome even when anatomic pathology is lacking on physical exam or diagnostic studies. As noted earlier, advances in neuroscience have elucidated pathways that explain this phenomenon.

Despite wide recognition that mental health comorbidities frequently coexist, patients often resist the suggestion that anxiety and depression may be exacerbating their pain. They equate these diagnoses with hysteria or hypochondria and feel that the physician is depreciating their pain experience. Treating comorbidities is difficult in this setting, especially for providers with inadequate training.

REGULATORY SCRUTINY

Fear of regulatory scrutiny is common in primary care settings, although in reality, very few primary care physician practices are ever investigated by regulatory bodies. Even fewer practices have had their licensure suspended. These few cases and those covered in the media often involve high-profile providers or illegal and unethical activities. Despite this fact, reality sometimes does not mitigate perception, and regulatory scrutiny, as noted in a previous chapter by Gilson in this text, continues to impede more aggressive pain management in many primary care practices.

PATIENT EXPECTATIONS

The paternalistic relationship commonly seen in medical practice is being challenged by consumer activism. Patients have more access to health information than ever before. They have more time and motivation to research their conditions on the Internet and may sometimes know (or believe they know) more about treatment options and a particular disease process than their primary care physician. As is often the case, this is a mixed blessing. On the one hand, an informed patient may be much more amenable to self-management. In some cases, however, an informed patient may have misguided beliefs based on less reputable information sources.

Most patients with persistent pain do best after learning and adopting self-management skills. Acceptance of their chronic condition, developing strategies including conditioning exercises, and making changes in work or hobbies lead to the best results. However, when information-seeking patients are confronted with "miraculous cures" and daily news articles touting advancements in pain treatment, adapting to pain is difficult for the provider to sell. Too often, patients find themselves on a constant search for the next cure or "fix" only to be disappointed when it fails and then moving on to the next "harmless, 100% effective" treatment. As this pattern repeats over and over, the best treatment—acceptance, adaptation, and conditioning—is delayed. The expectations of desperate patients seeking miracle cures create significant barriers to optimal care.

Pain Practitioner: A Primary Care Model

TRAINING

As in other disciplines, training received by primary care providers may become outdated as new knowledge is accumulated and scientific advancements are achieved. Education in all areas of medicine must be lifelong and constantly updated. Medical training provides a knowledge base with courses in neuroanatomy, pathophysiology, and pharmacokinetics. This training serves primarily as a foundation and a method for learning and applying new knowledge.

The process of learning and reapplying new knowledge is well accepted in medicine. Despite all the practice management issues and the multilevel barriers to pain care, primary care providers continue to learn and apply new information in their daily clinical practice.

COLLABORATION WITH PAIN SPECIALISTS

Complex conditions are always better managed when primary care providers and specialists have open lines of communication and clearly delineated systems for coordinating care; pain care is of course no different. For their part, informed and collaborative pain specialists trained in the biopsychosocial approach to pain can be a great asset to primary care by guiding primary care physicians through learning new skills and providing direction regarding when to refer patients back for further specialty care. Such constructive communication can lead to greater self-assurance and competence among primary care physicians as they manage complex pain patients in their practices.

NEW FOCUS

Patients with persistent pain have similarities and differences from patients with other chronic illnesses. They both have chronic conditions where cure is unlikely. Self-management is the key to reaching treatment goals. Denial about the disease and nonadherence to treatment recommendations are common and expected challenges for the provider.

On the other hand, mental health issues are more common in persistent pain and interfere with treatment. Patients may resist psychosocial diagnosis and interventions. Long-term opioid management can be challenging for the patient and the provider. Nonadherence to treatment recommendations increases morbidity and mortality in diabetes, hypertension, and congestive heart failure. In chronic pain, nonadherence increases the clinicians' work stress, by requiring more office visits, documentation, and medication surveillance. Although regulatory scrutiny does not occur often, the perception of legal difficulties increases practice discomfort.

In managing pain, it is important for the physician to understand that pain scores are subjective and that a stronger focus should be placed on function. Although measuring pain is important and mandated in a variety of settings,[34] the physician must not lose sight of the agreed on goals of treatment.

A new pain complaint or worsening symptoms do not necessarily mandate more medication. In treating diabetes, a worsening glycated hemoglobin ($HgBA_1C$) leads the physician to recommend adjustments in diet, exercise, and medication. Similarly, in treating chronic pain, recommendations should take into consideration life stressors, pacing daily activities, depression, anxiety, and worsening of underlying pathology as well as medication. When the primary care provider understands that an increase in pain does not necessarily mean increasing the patient's medications, treatment issues may become easier.

ASSESSMENT AND EVALUATION DURING SHORT VISITS

Given the typically short office visit and the many pressures on the physician's time, chronic illness management is becoming more difficult. In the typical 15-minute appointment, the patient with low back pain must be evaluated, but he or she may have other conditions requiring assessment, such as hypertension, diabetes, a sleep disorder, and fatigue that are also bothersome to the patient and they want addressed. Given an hour for the evaluation and adequate support staff, primary care physicians would all be better pain managers. But given a short time, stressed, and overworked support staff and patients with sometimes myriad complex conditions to be addressed, this is not the case.

Despite the reality of a busy office schedule, primary care is uniquely positioned to take care of the patients with chronic pain. We know our patients through associations developed over years of repeated exposure at routine medical care. We understand our patient's coping strategies, family dynamics, and work stresses. The solution to the dilemma lies in making the typical short office visit more effective for patients needing chronic pain management.

THE 15-MINUTE OFFICE VISIT
Validating the Patient

Validation is straightforward when a patient presents with an ankle sprain or a sore back. The injury is easily identified by the history, and the diagnosis is easily confirmed by physical examination. Diagnostic imaging and/or laboratory reports further support the physician's initial impression, and the patient's chief complaint and the associated pain improve steadily with a short course of uncomplicated therapies—an NSAID, muscle relaxant, application of cold or heat, and rest.

Validation poses problems for primary care when the patient suffers from chronic pain. We are concerned that the patient will request something we cannot deliver, such as total pain relief, additional MRI studies, or unsafe doses of medication. The evidence shows that, in fact, clear, nonjargon-laden, nonjudgmental education makes pain care planning easier. In a study of patients with fibromyalgia syndrome, providing the patient with a diagnosis resulted in the patient making fewer visits to the physician's office and becoming more empowered and proactive.[35]

Once the patient understands that we believe the pain is real, more time can be spent dealing with symptom control, exercise, and other important management issues. At each office visit, make sure that the following steps have been taken:

- Ask about pain intensity but more importantly, pain-related functional interference.
- Determine the functional status of the patient and whether the treatment is improving function.
- Modify the treatment according the patient's response.
- Use a combination of nonpharmacologic and pharmacologic methods for pain control.
- Explain the available options and foster a positive attitude in the patient toward dealing with the pain.
- Normalize the interrelationship between mood and pain and help the patient understand that managing mood disorders and other comorbid conditions will also help the experience of pain and thereby improve quality of life.

Having a set routine with these key goals in mind sets the agenda and can streamline even a difficult, complex visit.

Assessment Tools

Chronic pain usually starts as an acute pain episode. In most cases, the acute episode resolves and the patient returns to normal function. Even fibromyalgia syndrome, defined as widespread pain for months to years, has a beginning. The workup and treatment can take months before the correct diagnosis is discovered, and the physician becomes aware that the problem is long term and likely to present problems in management.

At this point, the physician's attention should focus on chronic disease management (i.e., symptom improvement rather than multiple interventions and cure). How can the physician best do this evaluation in a short office visit? Referral may or may not be an option as specialty referral may not be available, too expensive, and time-consuming for many patients. Evaluation needs to be focused on the desired outcome of pain reduction, functional improvement, and identification and management of comorbidities. Because such an evaluation can easily take up several visits, handouts and questionnaires can be very useful (i.e., The Initial Pain Assessment Tool, Pain Disability Index, Quality of Life Scale, Patient Health Questionnaire-9, Generalized Anxiety Disorder 7 [GAD-7], Zung Self-Rating Depression Scale, and Function and Goal Setting).

Try giving the patient self-assessment forms that measure pain, function, depression, and anxiety and allow the patient to complete the assignment at home. Patients tend to like these questionnaires because they permit patients to describe in detail issues that the physician may not have the time to elicit during the office visit.

A follow-up visit is designed to review the results with the patient. The handouts direct the follow-up visit to the important outcome variables: pain and function. They are helpful in that they let the patient know which outcomes are most important and what each subsequent office visit will address. The patient who demonstrates anxiety or depression on the self-reported questionnaire is more likely to accept treatment, making discussion and treatment of such comorbidities less time-consuming. Assessment is covered in detail elsewhere in this text.

Substance Misuse Screening

Primary care physicians are often hesitant to prescribe opioids. When treating patients with chronic pain, such caution is justified as long-term opioid therapy often offers modest or no benefit, usually involves bothersome side effects, and may lead to serious adverse effects. Substance misuse, particularly involving opioids, is an important comorbidity in chronic pain

management. Fortunately, there are multiple questionnaires available to help assess this risk. Commonly used screening tools practical in primary care include The Screener and Opioid Assessment for Patients with Pain,[36] Opioid Risk Tool,[37] and Drug Abuse Screening Test.[38] Patients who score high on any of these scales are more likely to misuse opioids. If referral to a pain management specialist is an option, the primary care physician might consider this. Such screening is also covered fully elsewhere in this text.

Goal Setting and Plan of Action

Like other chronic illnesses, patient participation and adherence to treatment recommendations predict better outcomes. Chronic pain affects many life activities and, in turn, quality of life. Goal-setting discussions direct the patient to improved activity and a targeted outcome. For example, if the patient wants and agrees to spend more time out of bed, walk 10 minutes a day, or work in the garden, any of these might serve as a goal that can be tracked with each visit. As patients begin to anticipate the questions the physician will ask about their goals, visits become more streamlined and focused on a functional outcome.

After the patient has been evaluated and treatment has been initiated, adequate follow-up of a patient with chronic pain can be difficult to accomplish in a 15-minute visit. Follow-up does not take as much time when the physician stays focused on the desired functional outcome. Consider a routine follow-up for a patient with diabetes. We begin by asking about diet, exercise, foot numbness, vision, and home glucose monitoring. We review the self-monitoring results and then perform a physical exam focused on the blood pressure, eyes, heart, and monofilament exam of the feet. We review the $HgBA_1C$, microalbumin, and low-density lipoprotein. We ensure that the patient is taking recommended medications. We change treatment based on all the information received. All of this is done every day with our patients with diabetes and at each visit; all of this can be accomplished in 15 minutes.

The difference in managing chronic pain, and the reason that visits consume more time, is that often it is unclear what to follow, what to ask, and what outcomes to track at each visit. It is vital that each follow-up session remains focused on symptom management and functional improvement. A patient's pain diary or journal can be helpful in focusing follow-up visits. Pain diaries, available in paper and electronic form, are similar to regular diaries except that the entries focus on pain. Patients record pain-related elements such as the time pain was experienced, pain characteristics (e.g., burning, stabbing, aching), the location of the pain, what he or she did to alleviate the pain, and whether what they did helped. The patient brings the pain diary to each follow-up session, focusing the visit on a particular pain score and whether the recommended treatment was effective.

Activity and sleep questionnaires are also helpful in concentrating the appointment on these quality of life issues. In a mutual goal-setting discussion with the patient, the questions can revolve around previously agreed on and previously documented functional outcomes such as the amount of time spent out of bed, the 10-minute walk, or the time spent working in the garden.

Charts reviewed of primary care visits in patients with pain frequently demonstrate a failure of adequate documentation.[39] Given the time pressures, it is no wonder that documentation often is low on our list of priorities. Handouts and questionnaires filed in the patient's chart enhance this record keeping and save time.

PHARMACOLOGIC TREATMENT

There are many pharmacologic treatment options for persistent pain. Pharmacology in primary care is difficult because of the many treatment choices, the lack of agreement among experts,

TABLE 108.1 The Five As of Treatment Success

A-1 = Analgesia or pain score
A variety of pain scales are available in multiple languages. Pain measurement is the first element in evaluating successful treatment.

A-2 = Activities of daily living or functional outcome that is meaningful to the patient
At the initial and subsequent visits, work activities, household duties, social activities, hobbies, and physical exercise target are recorded and goal setting is discussed. When treating any chronic condition, follow-up visits are necessary to evaluate the effectiveness of the treatment.

A-3 = Adverse events
Anticipating and soliciting feedback from the patient regarding side effects from treatment allows the physician to proactively manage adverse events rather.

A-4 = Aberrant behavior
Patients on long-term opioid therapy may display behaviors that raise concerns, including early refill requests or using analgesic medication with unprescribed controlled substances or illicit substances. When such patient behavior occurs, careful interpretation is needed. Document the behavior in the patient's chart, discuss it with the patient, and come to a mutual understanding of what action will be taken if the behavior occurs again.

A-5 = Adherence to the treatment plan
Providers should engage patients in a shared decision-making process to arrive at a feasible, acceptable multimodal pain care plan that has at its foundation active pain self-management. Providers should follow-up with patients about adherence to that plan to troubleshoot barriers and coach and motivate patients to greater adherence to the agreed on plan.

and the nearly complete absence of data from pragmatic studies where patients have multiple comorbidities and are on multiple medications for other conditions. How and why a particular medication is used in a patient with pain varies based on pain severity, diagnosis, and many other factors. U.S. Food and Drug Administration-approved drugs or randomized trial results could guide prescribing. Primary care often uses past experience even when this experience is inaccurate or inappropriate. An example of this is the common use of ineffective nonsteroidal anti-inflammatory medications in neuropathic pain treatment in the primary care office.[40]

Access to medication is also a major force in pharmacologic options in the primary care setting. Nonformulary drugs or third-tier medications requiring high patient copays are a significant factor in prescribing. If the primary care provider has to obtain a preauthorization or justify a prescription, the medication may not be prescribed because this extra step requires excessive time.

As the Ballantyne and Mao[8] article points out, opioid prescribing is one of the most difficult decisions facing primary care in managing persistent pain. When prescribing opioids for pain management, physicians are often faced with scenarios that mirror those we associate with addiction: early refills, lost or stolen medication, borrowed medication, and urine drug tests that are inconsistent with current therapy. In these cases, documentation is critical. Strategies such as the five As of treatment success enable the primary care physician to concentrate on the outcomes that are essential to the patient's overall quality of life (Table 108.1).[41]

REFERRAL TO AN ADDICTION SPECIALIST
When to refer a patient to specialty care may be a difficult question and is highly variable among different practitioners. Some providers refer whenever long-term opioid management begins. Others refer only when intervention or surgery is needed. When behavior around the use of an opioid becomes problematic, referral is often prudent. At a minimum, documentation of the

behaviors and an understanding between patient and provider is necessary. The five As allow the physician to address the issue and develop a treatment strategy. It is important for the physician to recognize the risk and recommend a corrective action (i.e., an abnormal urine drug test may trigger a referral to an addiction medicine provider). The patient with a substance use disorder may argue and dismiss the risk.

MOTIVATING BEHAVIOR CHANGE IN PATIENTS WITH CHRONIC PAIN
The key message in managing chronic pain is that the way to improve is through changes in lifestyle rather than solely through medication or surgical procedures. This may not always be an easy message for primary care to deliver because patients may expect their physician to give them something to cure their problem. Lifestyle and behavior changes are never easy.

Successful management of chronic pain is much more dependent on what the patient does than on what the physician does to the patient. The issue becomes one of the patient's readiness to accept responsibility and to adopt a self-management approach. This represents a role reversal for the physician whose task is not to treat but to understand and motivate patients for self-management. On occasion, this may include convincing the patient not to look for another doctor or another procedure.

Because of their unique relationships with patients, primary care physicians are well suited in motivating patients to change. We are motivating patients to lose weight, stop smoking, take their medication, and obtain flu shots. A patient-centered approach, emphasizing the importance of considering the patient's perspective when making treatment recommendations, has been shown to be a valuable technique.[42] The goals of a patient-centered approach are to
- Address the patient's concerns
- Enhance a collaborative relationship
- Provide information that the patient is ready to hear
- Refocus the visit from making treatment recommendations to supporting the patient's self-care
- Foster increased patient control of decision making and responsibility for self-care

This technique requires a reorientation of the traditional patient–physician relationship. The physician must learn to view the patient as an autonomous and equal member of the health care team, whose self-knowledge is pivotal to the management of his or her condition (persistent pain).

Reflective listening is a technique that involves making statements that demonstrate the physician's understanding of what the patient has said. There are ways of making reflective statements, including the following:
- Restating what the patient has said
- Paraphrasing what the patient has said
- Anticipating and continuing the patient's thought (i.e., saying what you believe the patient will say next rather than repeating)
- Reflecting the patient's feelings

The patient's readiness to change is the basis of a motivational approach. According to one well-regarded model,[43] patients who strongly believe that their pain only requires a medical or surgical intervention are not ready to accept and adopt self-management. On the other hand, patients who believe that medical and surgical interventions can provide only limited relief from pain are more likely to perceive benefits from self-management techniques. Readiness to self-manage should be assessed on a continuum, and interventions should be tailored to the particular patient's level of readiness to change.

The physician can help the patient to understand the importance of behavior change by guiding him or her through a discussion of the pros and cons, including whether a given change is attainable, how much effort it will take, and how much time it will take given the known obstacles. Motivating the patient involves eliciting the patient's feelings about and reasons for pain self-management and reflecting back statements that support the premise that self-management is possible. Although time-pressed physicians may balk at the prospect of such a dialogue, the consultation time is usually more efficient (e.g., fewer arguments, less resistance) when a patient is encouraged to speak in a focused manner about a specific problem.

Goals for Pain Self-management

In general, primary care physicians are in agreement about health care goals such as encouraging smoking cessation, maintaining blood pressure within normal limits, and controlling blood sugar. Although the goals for pain self-management are not as clear cut, most pain specialists would advise primary care physicians to consider the following as important when motivating a patient:

1. Beginning or maintaining a regular exercise regimen
2. Using medications as prescribed
3. Returning to normal daily activities given the pain condition
4. Practicing appropriate pain and stress-coping strategies (e.g., relaxation techniques, reassuring "self-talk")
5. Returning to or maintaining normal work activities
6. Pacing activities appropriately
7. Monitoring, managing, and/or reporting symptoms of depression as appropriate
8. Practicing good eating habits (e.g., reducing or maintaining an appropriate weight)
9. Engaging in other healthy lifestyle behaviors as necessary (e.g., reducing alcohol consumption, stopping smoking)

Importance and Confidence Scales

Patients will change behavior only when they are convinced that it is important and when they have confidence that the change is possible. Assessing patient perceptions of importance and confidence can be helpful when evaluating motivation. For example, patients who give a low rating to the importance of exercise but a high rating to the belief that exercise could be done would need help to change their views of the importance of exercise before adherence could be expected. On the other hand, brainstorming for solutions may be helpful for those who rate importance high and confidence low.

Strategies for Helping Patients Understand the Importance of Change

Information and advice presented in a lecturing style often leads to patient responses of "Yes, but . . ." and the already too brief visit is taken up with the patient expressing reasons why a recommended change will not work. Social psychology research has shown that, in general, people are more likely to believe what they have said over what others have said to them. It follows that a didactic approach may undermine the physician's attempts to motivate the patient.

Primary care providers are invested in behavior change and motivation. Four strategies have been shown to be effective in helping patients understand the importance of change and increase their confidence to make that change.[44] These uncomplicated strategies are effective because they enable patients to talk themselves into using pain self-management techniques.

1. *Always elicit positive statements from the patient.* Use the "why so high" technique. For example, ask the patient with chronic pain to rate the importance of daily exercise on a scale of 0 (low) to 10 (high). If the patient's answer is 5, ask "Why so high? Why not a 1?" Most patients understand the importance of conditioning and exercise in pain rehabilitation. By asking "why so high," the patient provides the evidence for an exercise program. Once you know the patient's thought process, you can use this to motive a change of behavior.

"You think it is very important for you to make your muscles stronger to make your pain better" (restating what the patient has expressed).

2. *Examine the pros and cons of behavior change.* Patients will feel ambivalent about self-management. This allows the patient to explore feelings and think through self-management in a judgment-free environment. Bear in mind that although this technique is easy to understand, it can be difficult for the physician to do. He or she must listen, encourage, and provide a summary at the end of the visit.

"What do you think will happen if you continue to stay in bed?" The patient may steer the conversation back to you: "Unless you make me better, I cannot get out of bed" or "Unless you give me more pain medication, I will not be able to get out of bed." Be persistent and keep to the same question. The patient has stated earlier that conditioning and exercise are important.

"Your mother was sick all the time. How did that affect you?" Patients may have an environmental background for pain in another family member which impacted them when growing up. Patients may also express concern about the impact of their pain on the other members of the family. The desire to have their pain not have an impact may motivate the patient to different behavior.

3. *Elicit patient concerns about the status quo.* Patients who rate the importance of pain self-management as low may be concerned about their current situation. Ask the patient to talk about the consequences of not making the behavior change. Once the patient has listed as many concerns as he or she can think of, summarize these, using the patient's words if possible. This may help to increase the patient's perception of the importance of the change.

"If things do not change, what will happen?" The patient may try to guide the discussion back to you and the medical profession, disability, or legal issues. Be persistent about "What will happen with your spouse or children; how will you pay the bills?"

4. *Brainstorm for solutions.* Without giving specific advice, remind the patient that there are usually many ways to achieve self-management. Guide the patient in conceptualizing a number of possibilities. Help the patient to decide which possibilities might work best for him or her. Guide the patient to develop plan for achieving his or her goal.

"You spend 16 hours of your day in bed. Any activity makes your pain worse. The last time you tried to exercise, your pain was at a 9/10 and you wanted to go to the hospital. How are you going to get to exercise?" Keep the focus on what the patient can do, or what solutions the patient has. Add suggestions and advice related to the patient's solutions.

Once the patient has adopted a self-management plan with specific goals, the physician can use open-ended questions to encourage the patient to talk about his or her progress. The questions should communicate the physician's interest in the patient's perspective. For instance, "At your last visit, you were thinking about making some changes in pacing your work. I'd be interested in hearing how this is going and whether you've noticed any change in your ability to manage your pain." Such questions enable the physician to conduct an informal assessment of the patient's readiness and also enhance rapport with the patient.

Emerging Models of Care

There is increasing recognition that team-based care, where providers from multiple disciplines collaborate in the care of patients with chronic pain, may be the key to optimizing primary care's foundational role in chronic pain management.[45] Collaborative care models, adopting successful approaches from other conditions like depression and diabetes, have demonstrated promise in integrated health systems for treatment of chronic pain. These successful programs, published as clinical trials, usually feature a care manager, such as a pharmacist, nurse, or advanced practice nurse, who collaborates with a physician to provide referral-based care to a population of patients embedded within group practices. Several recent studies have demonstrated success with these models in terms of pain intensity, pain-related functional interference, use of multimodal pain care, and patient satisfaction.[46–49] Cost-effectiveness studies and implementation trials—to address issues of more widespread dissemination of these models—are underway. Another example of team-based care involved a study where nurses team with primary care providers in an intervention that improved adherence with opioid therapy for chronic pain guidelines.[50] More resource-intensive primary care–based clinics that manage patients with high-risk opioid use and chronic pain have also demonstrated initial promise.[51]

Conclusion

Persistent pain, a highly prevalent condition in the United States, has a significant impact on our health and productivity as a society as well as on our medical and financial resources. Primary care is the most appropriate setting for the management of patients with chronic pain because of the mutual understanding that results from a long-standing physician–patient relationship. The barriers to managing chronic pain are significant but not insurmountable. Persistent pain is similar to other chronic illness but also has many unique differences, making management complicated and difficult in the busy primary care office. A new skill set is required by the provider to help the undertreatment of pain. Available tools (e.g., questionnaires, pain diaries, pain scales) and techniques (e.g., reflective listening, goal setting) make it possible for the primary care physician to provide management for patients with chronic pain in a 15-minute office visit. Diabetes, chronic obstructive pulmonary disease, and other chronic, complicated illnesses require other skills yet have been handled skillfully and competently in the primary care setting.

Some of the most appreciative patients are those who have a sympathetic provider to help them with chronic pain. Yet treating chronic pain patients is rarely met with enthusiasm in primary care. Patients with chronic pain may have complex conditions that are rarely cured. They may have previously made little progress toward normal life functioning and often have complex psychosocial issues that a physician cannot address. There is never sufficient time to adequately follow up patients with pain. The primary care provider is accustomed to dealing with chronic problems through short, focused visits and a longitudinal experience. A treatment plan and mutually agreed on goals allow the physician to conduct a follow-up visit in 15 minutes by focusing discussions on the treatment success that both the physician and patient desire.

References

1. Harstall C. How prevalent is chronic pain? *Pain: Clinical Updates* 2003;X:1–4.
2. O'Rorke JE, Chen I, Genao I, et al. Physicians' comfort in caring for patients with chronic nonmalignant pain. *Am J Med Sci* 2007;333:93–100.
3. Gallup Inc. Pain in America: a research report. Washington, DC: Gallup Inc; 2000.
4. Boström BM, Ramberg T, Davis BD, et al. Survey of post-operative patients' pain management. *J Nurs Manag* 1997;5:341–349.
5. Dworkin R, Backonja M, Rowbotham M, et al. Advances in neuropathic pain: diagnosis, mechanisms, and treatment recommendations. *Arch Neurol* 2003;60:1524–1534.
6. Institute of Medicine Committee on Advancing Pain Research, Care, and Education. *Relieving Pain in America: A Blueprint for Transforming Prevention, Care, Education, and Research*. Washington, DC: National Academies Press; 2011.
7. U.S. Department of Health and Human Services. National pain strategy: a comprehensive population health strategy for pain. Available at: https://iprcc.nih.gov/sites/default/files/HHSNational_Pain_Strategy_508C.pdf. Accessed on July 24, 2018.
8. Ballantyne JC, Mao J. Opioid therapy for chronic pain. *N Engl J Med* 2003;349:1943–1953.
9. Flor H, Turk DC. Chronic back pain and rheumatoid arthritis: predicting pain and disability from cognitive variables. *J Behav Med* 1988;11:251–265.
10. Sanders SH, Brena SF, Spier CJ, et al. Chronic back pain patients around the world: cross-cultural similarities and differences. *Clin J Pain* 1992;8:317–323.
11. Reesor KA, Craig KD. Medically incongruent chronic back pain physical limitations, suffering, and ineffective coping. *Pain* 1988;32:35–45.
12. Pinsky J. Chronic pain syndromes and their treatment. In: Brodwin MG, Tellez F, Brodwin SK, eds. *Medical, Psychosocial and Vocational Aspects of Disability*. Athens, GA: Elliott & Fitzpatrick; 1993:179–194.
13. Dahlman GB, Dykes AK, Elander G. Patients' evaluation of pain and nurses' management of analgesics after surgery. The effect of a study day on the subject of pain for nurses working at the thorax surgery department. *J Adv Nurs* 1999;30:866–874.
14. Drayer R, Henderson J, Reidenberg M. Barriers to better pain control in hospitalized patient. *J Pain Symptom Manage* 1999;17:434–440.
15. Brookoff D. Chronic pain: 1. A new disease? *Hosp Pract (1995)* 2000;35(7):45–59.
16. Deyo R, Rainville J, Kent DL. What can the history and physical examination tell us about low back pain? *JAMA* 1992;268:760–765.
17. Woolf CJ. Central sensitization: implications for the diagnosis and treatment of pain. *Pain* 2011;152(3 suppl):S2–S15.
18. Martin JC, Avant RF, Bowman MA, et al. The future of family medicine: a collaborative project of the family medicine community. *Ann Fam Med* 2004;2(suppl 1):S3–32.
19. Bigos SJ, McKee JE. Reliable care through the activity paradigm for back problems. In: McCarberg B, Passik S, eds. *Expert Guide to Pain Management*. Philadelphia: American College of Physicians; 2005:35–64.
20. Carey TS, Garrett J, Jackman A, et al. The outcomes and costs of care for acute low back pain among patients seen by primary care practitioner, chiropractors, and orthopedic surgeons. The North Carolina Back Pain Project. *New Engl J Med* 1995;333(14):913–917.
21. Cherkin DC, MacCornack FA, Berg AO. Managing low back pain—a comparison of the beliefs and behaviors of family physicians and chiropractors. *West J Med* 1998;149(4):475–480.
22. Federation of State Medical Boards of the United States Inc. Model policy for the use of controlled substances for the treatment of pain. Available at: https://www.ihs.gov/painmanagement/includes/themes/newihstheme/display_objects/documents/modelpolicytreatmentpain.pdf. Accessed July 24, 2018.
23. Dowell DT, Haegerich TM, Chou R. CDC guideline for prescribing opioids for chronic pain—United States, 2016. *MMWR Recomm Rep* 2016;65(1):1–49.
24. Chou R, Fanciullo GJ, Fine PG, et al. Clinical guidelines for the use of chronic opioid therapy in chronic noncancer pain. *J Pain* 2009;10(2):113–130.
25. Tayeb BO, Barreiro AE, Bradshaw YS, et al. Durations of opioid, nonopioid drug, and behavioral clinical trials for chronic pain: adequate or inadequate? *Pain Med* 2016;17(11):2036–2046.
26. Kertesz SG. Turning the tide or riptide? The changing opioid epidemic. *Subst Abus* 2017;38(1):3–8.
27. American Pain Society. *Guideline for the Management of Pain in Osteoarthritis, Rheumatoid Arthritis, and Juvenile Chronic Arthritis*. 2nd ed. Glenview, IL: American Pain Society; 2002.
28. American Pain Society. *Guideline for the Management of Cancer Pain in Adults and Children*. Glenview, IL: American Pain Society; 2005.
29. Argoff C, Bruckenthal P, Charmichael B, et al. *Consensus Recommendations: Neuropathic Pain*. Charlotte, NC: Primary Care Education Consortium; 2004.
30. American Pain Society. *Guideline for the Management of Fibromyalgia Syndrome Pain in Adults and Children*. Glenview, IL: American Pain Society; 2005.
31. McCarberg B. Impact of guidelines on healthcare from the patient and payor perspective: example of the American Pain Society guidelines. *Dis Manage Health Outcomes* 2004;12(1);73–79.
32. Polatin PB, Kinney RK, Gatchel RJ, et al. Psychiatric illness and chronic low-back pain. The mind and the spine—which goes first? *Spine (Phila Pa 1976)* 1993;18(1):66–71.
33. Fishbain DA, Cutler R, Rosomoff HL, et al. Chronic pain-associated depression: antecedent or consequence of chronic pain? A review. *Clin J Pain* 1997;13(2):116–137.
34. Jacox AK, Carr DB, Capman CR, et al. Acute pain management: operative or medical procedures and trauma. *Clinical Practice Guideline No. 1*; 1992. AHCPR publication no. 92-0032.
35. White KP, Nielson WR, Harth M, et al. Does the label "fibromyalgia" after health status, function, and health service utilization? A prospective, within-group comparison in a community cohort of adults with chronic widespread pain. *Arthritis Rheum* 2002;47(3):260–265.

36. Butler SF, Budman SH, Fernandez K, et al. Validation of a screener and opioid assessment measure for patient with chronic pain. *Pain* 2004;112: 65–75.

37. Webster LR, Webster RM. Predicting aberrant behaviors in opioid-treatment patients: preliminary validation of the Opioid Risk Tool. *Pain Med* 2005;6: 432–442.

38. Skinner HA. The drug abuse screening test. *Addict Behav* 1982;7(4): 363–371.

39. Clark JD. Chronic pain prevalence and analgesic prescribing in a general medical population. *J Pain Symptom Manage* 2002;23:131–137.

40. Oster G, Berger A, Dukes E, et al. Use of potentially inappropriate pain-related medications in older adults with painful neuropathic disorders. *Am J Geriatr Pharmacother* 2004;2(3):163–170.

41. Passik SD, Weinreb HJ. Managing chronic nonmalignant pain: overcoming obstacles to the use of opioids. *Adv Ther* 2000;17:70–83.

42. Stewart MA, McWhinney IR, Weston WW, et al. *Patient-Centered Medicine: Transforming the Clinical Method.* Thousand Oaks, CA: Sage Publications; 1995.

43. Prochaska JO, DiClemente CC, Norcoss JC. In search of how people change. Applications to addictive behaviors. *Am Psychol* 1992;47:1102–1114.

44. Rollnick S, Mason P, Butler C. *Health Behavior Change: A Guide for Practitioners.* Edinburgh: Harcourt Publisher; 1999.

45. Seal K, Becker W, Tighe J, et al. Managing chronic pain in primary care: it really does take a village. *J Gen Intern Med* 2017;32(8):931–934.

46. Bair MJ, Ang D, Wu J, et al. Evaluation of stepped care for chronic pain (ESCAPE) in veterans of the Iraq and Afghanistan conflicts: a randomized clinical trial. *JAMA Intern Med* 2015;175(5):682–689.

47. Kroenke K, Krebs EE, Wu J, et al. Telecare collaborative management of chronic pain in primary care: a randomized clinical trial. *JAMA* 2014;312(3):240–248.

48. Kroenke K, Bair MJ, Damush TM, et al. Optimized antidepressant therapy and pain self-management in primary care patients with depression and musculoskeletal pain: a randomized controlled trial. *JAMA* 2009;301(20): 2099–2110.

49. Dobscha SK, Corson K, Perrin NA, et al. Collaborative care for chronic pain in primary care: a cluster randomized trial. *JAMA* 2009;301(12): 1242–1252.

50. Liebschutz JM, Xuan Z, Shanahan CW, et al. Improving adherence to long-term opioid therapy guidelines to reduce opioid misuse in primary care: a cluster-randomized clinical trial. *JAMA Intern Med* 2017;177(9):1265–1272.

51. Becker WC, Edmond SN, Cervone DJ, et al. Evaluation of an integrated, multidisciplinary program to address unsafe use of opioids prescribed for pain [published online ahead of print March 23, 2017]. *Pain Med.* doi:10.1093/pm/pnx041.

CHAPTER 109

Pain Management at the End of Life

JUDITH A. PAICE

Adequate relief of pain at the end of life is an ethical imperative. Studies suggest that although pain may not be the most prevalent symptom during the final days or weeks of life, it is frequently the most distressing.[1-7] In addition to the negative consequences pain has on the patient, inadequate pain control adversely affects the ongoing emotional well-being of family and friends at the bedside. To witness unrelieved pain during the final hours of life leaves long-lasting negative memories of the dying process that can hamper bereavement. The setting of care can dictate whether patients will receive adequate relief during the dying process, and significant change in our systems of care is needed. The majority of end-of-life care is currently provided in institutions, with more than two-thirds of individuals dying in hospitals or nursing homes. In a large survey of surviving family members, more than 25% reported that their loved one received inadequate relief of pain in these settings.[8] The challenge for our health care system is to ensure that regardless of setting, pain management at end of life is provided by skilled professionals who understand the special needs of the dying. These skills include assessment of pain in those who might not be able to verbally describe their pain, awareness of pain syndromes common at end of life, as well as familiarity with the pharmacologic and nonpharmacologic management of pain in the dying. Furthermore, clinicians must be aware of the role of suffering and existential distress as well as management of intractable symptoms.

Introduction

Currently, death in developed countries is more likely to occur after a long chronic illness. This is in contrast to a century ago when people died a more rapid death, often due to infection. Currently, the most common causes of death in high-income countries include ischemic cardiac disease, cerebrovascular disease, and cancer.[9] Globally, more than 70% of deaths are due to chronic, noncommunicable diseases, principally cardiovascular diseases and diabetes, cancers, and chronic respiratory diseases.[9] Thus, people are more likely to die after a long, protracted illness, and pain is a common comorbidity of these illnesses. Several care delivery models exist to address the specialized pain and symptom needs of those with life-threatening illnesses, including palliative care and hospice. Both of these care models focus attention on the patient and family, not unlike the structure of care delivered in truly interdisciplinary pain treatment programs.

PALLIATIVE CARE

Palliative care strives to relieve suffering and improve the quality of life of those individuals with a life-threatening illness.[10] The palliative care movement in the United States originated in academic medical centers but has moved into community hospitals, outpatient clinics, and other centers of care. Palliative care programs are rapidly growing within hospitals, existing in 67% of hospitals in the United States with 50 or more beds and in 90% of hospitals with 300 or more beds.[11] Commitment to early identification, thorough assessment, and effective treatment of pain are key components of palliative care, as is attention to other physical, psychosocial, and spiritual concerns.[12]

The goal is to neither hasten nor prolong death but rather affirm life by offering a support system to patients and families. To that end, palliative care is optimally provided by an interdisciplinary group of professionals, including physicians, nurses, social workers, chaplains, and others.

Confusion persists regarding the timing of appropriate referral to palliative care. Previous models of care incorporated palliative care during the final phases of life, once all curative therapy was completed (Fig. 109.1). It is clear that patients and families benefit greatly when palliative care is integrated into the plan of care early during the course of illness (Fig. 109.2). Effective pain management provided during cancer treatment, for example, can allow patients to complete potentially curative or life-prolonging therapies.[13] Attention to other symptoms associated with the underlying illness, including distressing complications of treatment, can provide improved quality of life during this time. Research supports the feasibility and benefit of integrating palliative and oncology care in ambulatory patients.[14-19]

HOSPICE

The modern concept of hospice care developed from the work of Dame Cicely Saunders and others in the United Kingdom during the 1960s. In this model, freestanding centers of care were developed where patients spent their final days receiving pain and symptom management, along with attention to the emotional and spiritual aspects of the individual's life. A decade later, hospice began in the United States with the same goals of care, but a home-based model quickly took root. In 1982, the Medicare Hospice Benefit was passed to provide reimbursement for these services. A Medicare Part A beneficiary is eligible for this benefit if she or he is determined to have a life expectancy of 6 months or less if the life-limiting disease or combination of comorbid conditions runs its normal course.[20] Studies reveal that patients at end of life and their family members prefer care provided in the home with the support of hospice, reporting improved symptom management and significantly greater satisfaction with the overall quality of care.[8,21] Both of these models, palliative care and hospice, provide support to patients and loved ones. As pain is so prevalent, all health care professionals working with people at this time of life must be exceptionally knowledgeable about common pain syndromes as well as appropriate assessment and management.

Pain Syndromes Common at the End of Life

Pain syndromes specific to cancer have been well characterized; yet, much research is needed to describe pain associated with other life-threatening illnesses. Furthermore, greater attention is needed to identify pain syndromes most common at the very end of life along with appropriate treatment strategies (Table 109.1).

CANCER

Prevalence rates of pain in advanced cancer vary based on the settings of care in which the studies were conducted, the instruments used to measure pain and other symptoms as well as the methods employed in data collection. In general, approximately two-thirds

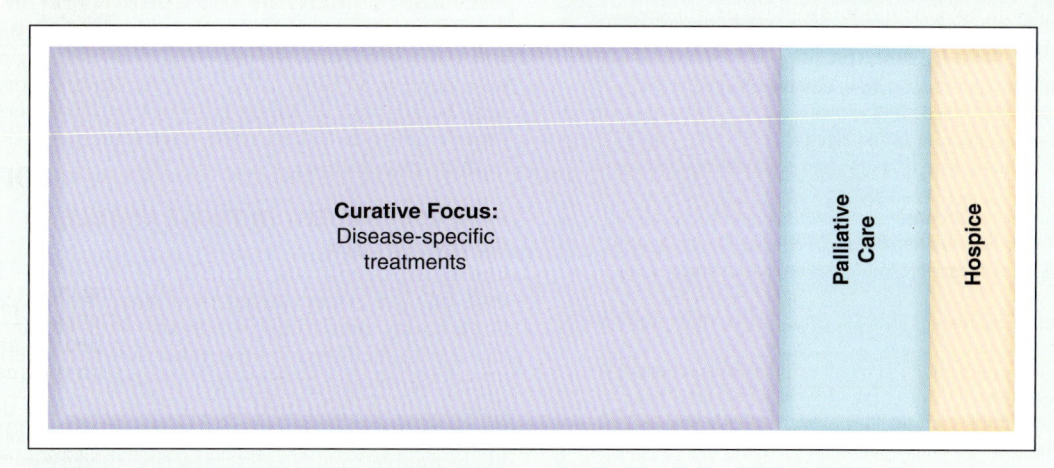

FIGURE 109.1 Previous models of palliative care and hospice.

of patients with advanced malignant disease experience pain.[22–25] Cancer patients referred to palliative care or hospice commonly have a greater prevalence of pain and other symptoms. Regarding the pain trajectory in cancer patients very near the end of life, pain occurred in 54% and 34% at 4 weeks and 1 week prior to death, respectively.[26] Children dying of cancer also are at risk for pain and suffering.[27,28] The result of unrelieved pain and associated interference may include increased desire for hastened death.[29,30]

NONCANCER DIAGNOSES

Many life-threatening illnesses are known to cause pain, including human immunodeficiency virus,[31] multiple sclerosis,[32–35] amyotrophic lateral sclerosis,[36] other neurologic disorders,[37] end-stage renal disease,[38] and heart failure.[39,40] At the end of life, it is apparent that many of the preexisting pain syndromes associated with these disorders can escalate, particularly pain related to progression of disease, immobility, or comorbid complications. Furthermore, many patients with advanced disease are elderly and more likely to have existing chronic pain syndromes, such as osteoarthritis or low back pain.[41] Regrettably, there have been few studies characterizing the prevalence of pain or the types of pain experienced by these individuals with noncancer diagnoses. Greater awareness of the risk and types of pain seen will lead to improved detection, assessment, and treatment.

Pain Assessment at the End of Life

CHALLENGES IN PAIN ASSESSMENT

Comprehensive assessment of pain at the end of life is imperative. As with all pain, assessment must be conducted upon initial presentation, regularly throughout the course of care, and during any changes in the patient's pain state.[42] Documentation of and communication about these findings are crucial. Assessment in patients who are cognitively intact and able to verbalize can incorporate standard intensity tools such as the numeric rating scale (NRS), the verbal descriptor scale (VDS), the visual analogue scale (VAS), or the Brief Pain Inventory (BPI) for more comprehensive evaluation.[43] A panel of international experts in palliative care rated essential components of pain assessment to include intensity, temporal pattern, treatment and exacerbating/relieving factors, location, and interference with health-related quality of life as essential dimensions.[44] In their content evaluation of more than 64 pain assessment tools, none were found to satisfactorily incorporate all of these domains.

Tools exist that measure multiple symptoms seen in life-threatening illness, and the majority include pain. One study demonstrated that using systematic assessment of symptoms in palliative care yielded a 10-fold greater number than when volunteered by the patient. The investigators conclude that

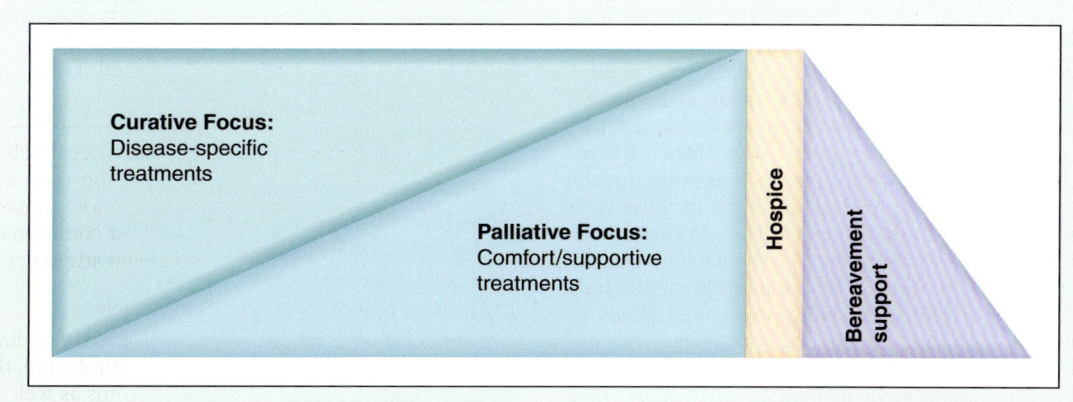

FIGURE 109.2 Proposed model for integration of palliative care.[193]

TABLE 109.1   Pain Syndromes in Palliative Care[194–196]

Pain Related to Underlying Disease

- Tumor-related pain due to pressure or compression
- Chest pain due to end-stage cardiac disease
- Ischemia caused by atherosclerotic disease
- Abdominal pain with referral to thorax and shoulder due to liver failure, cirrhosis
- Abdominal pain due to ascites
- Extremity skin pain due to edema
- Back pain and skin discomfort/pruritus due to end-stage renal disease
- Chest pain due to pulmonary fibrosis, emphysema, other advanced lung disorders
- Central nervous system infection (meningitis, cryptosporidium) leading to headache
- Central pain after stroke, particularly affecting thalamus
- Trigeminal neuralgia in multiple sclerosis
- Vaso-occlusion leading to bone, muscle, and visceral pain in sickle cell disease
- Rapid onset of cachexia leading to peripheral neuropathy
- Spasticity due to neuromuscular disorders

Pain Related to Treatment

- Peripheral neuropathy due to cancer chemotherapy or treatment of HIV/AIDS
- Arthralgias and myalgias due to aromatase inhibitors
- Surgically induced phantom pain, chronic neuropathy
- Immunocompromise leading to postherpetic neuropathy
- Radiation-induced plexopathies, osteoradionecrosis, lymphedema
- Graft-versus-host disease after stem cell transplant leading to skin and mucous membrane lesions
- Aseptic necrosis due to prolonged corticosteroid use

Pain Unrelated to Disease or its Treatment

- Pressure ulcers
- Reduced muscle and fat padding at bony prominences
- Muscle atrophy leading to myalgia
- Immobility leading to joint pain
- Contractures

Adapted from Von Roenn JH, Paice JA, Preodor ME. Pain management in palliative care. In: Von Roenn JH, Paice JA, Preodor ME. *Current Diagnosis & Treatment of Pain.* 1st ed. New York: Lange; 2006.

specific detailed symptom investigation is necessary.[45] Examples of tools include the Edmonton Symptom Assessment Scale,[46] the M.D. Anderson Symptom Inventory,[47] the Memorial Symptom Assessment Scale,[48–50] the Rotterdam Symptom Checklist,[51,52] the Symptom Distress Scale,[53] and others. One constraint of these scales for clinical care at end of life is the length of most of these tools, leading to respondent fatigue. The Brief Hospice Inventory[54] was developed specifically to evaluate symptoms, including pain, and satisfaction with hospice care. Initial testing revealed that patients at end of life could complete the instrument.

A wide range of health-related quality-of-life instruments, such as the European Organisation for Research and Treatment of Cancer QLQ-C30 and the Functional Assessment of Cancer Therapy—General, include symptoms such as pain, but the burden to complete these tools preclude their use in those with advanced disease. Several tools target patients at the end of life: the Hospice Quality of Life Index,[55,56] the McGill Quality of Life Questionnaire, and others.[57] These instruments include symptoms and can be useful in assessing the global needs of dying patients. Although these tools are appropriate for patients who are cognitively intact, many patients at the end of life develop delirium, some have dementia, and others have limited ability to communicate due to intubation or neurologic disorders.

PAIN ASSESSMENT IN THE COGNITIVELY IMPAIRED

Several excellent reviews thoroughly describe tools used to assess pain in cognitively impaired older adults, primarily those with dementia (Table 109.2).[58–60] Although many of these tools may be adapted to assess pain in the dying person with delirium or other disorders, none have undergone extensive testing in these populations.

PAIN ASSESSMENT IN THOSE UNABLE TO COMMUNICATE

One in five people who die in hospitals have used intensive care unit (ICU) services during their final hospitalization.[61,62] In a large multicenter study of patients with serious illness, half of those who died during hospitalization had received ICU care.[63] Thus, significant percentages of people with life-threatening illness will be admitted to the ICU prior to death. Yet, one in five patients in ICU lack decision-making capacity and are likely unable to accurately describe their pain.[64] Furthermore, although a number of these patients may be cognitively intact, the use of mechanical ventilation often complicates pain assessment. Some patients may be able to use an NRS, VDS, or VAS, either by pointing to a chart with numbers or a line representing pain or by nodding "yes" when asked sequentially if pain is "mild," "moderate," or "severe." For those patients who cannot use these techniques, several pain assessment tools have been developed to assess pain in the ICU, including the Behavioral Pain Scale[65] and the Critical-Care Pain Observation Tool.[66,67] For children, several tools exist, including the Faces, Legs, Activity, Cry, Consolability Observational Tool (validated in children 2 months to 7 years and tested in the ICU),[68] Distress Scale for Ventilated Newborn Infants (tested in ventilated newborns), and the COMFORT Behavior Scale (tested in neonates to 3 years of age in ICU).[69]

Although standardized instruments to measure pain at the end of life are needed, several principles can guide clinicians when patients are cognitively impaired and unable to report pain.[58] Behaviors suggestive of pain should be evaluated, including the furrowed brow, guarding, or vocalizing on movement. Consider causes of pain, including the underlying disease and treatments, as well as new complications such as pressure ulcers, constipation, urinary retention, or infection. Ask family members or others who have known the patient if they observe changes in behaviors that might imply discomfort. If any of these indicators suggest that the patient may be in pain, initiate an analgesic trial and reassess. Resolution of the behaviors provides suggestive evidence that pain exists. Regular administration of the analgesic should then be included in the treatment plan.

TABLE 109.2   Pain Assessment Tools in Nonverbal Patients that May Be Useful in End-of-Life Care

Dementia

- Assessment of Discomfort in Dementia Protocol
- Checklist of Nonverbal Pain Indicators
- Nursing Assistant-Administered Instrument to Assess Pain in Demented Individuals
- Pain Assessment Scale for Seniors with Severe Dementia
- Pain Assessment in Advanced Dementia Scale

Intubated or Unconscious Children (Neonates, Infants, Nonverbal Children)

- COMFORT Behavior Scale
- Distress Scale for Ventilated Newborn Infants
- Faces, Legs, Activity, Cry, Consolability Observational Tool

Intubated or Unconscious Adults

- Behavioral Pain Scale
- Critical-Care Pain Observation Tool

PAIN MEASUREMENT IN RESEARCH CONDUCTED AT END OF LIFE

Research in pain at the end of life is hampered by lack of consistency in the use of valid and reliable pain measurement tools. An expert working group convened by the European Association of Palliative Care recommended standardized methods be applied in clinical trials and other pain studies in those with life-threatening illnesses. They recommended unidimensional tools such as the NRS, VAS or verbal rating scales, or, when indicated, multidimensional tools such as the BPI-Short Form or the McGill Pain Questionnaire.[70]

Pain Management Strategies at End of Life

The principles employed in treating other patients in pain should be applied to the dying. These include the use of multimodal therapies based on the underlying pain mechanisms as determined by comprehensive assessment. Of particular challenge at the end of life is the need for alternate routes of administration and a plan of care when pain becomes intractable to standard therapies or adverse effects to the treatment become unmanageable.

ROUTES OF DRUG DELIVERY

Many patients can use the oral route until death. In one study, 43% and 20% of cancer patients were able to take oral opioids at 1 week and 24 hours before death, respectively.[26] When oral delivery is no longer feasible, alternate routes of administration are available. Oral routes, including sublingual, transmucosal, and buccal delivery, as well as enteral, rectal, nasal, parenteral, spinal, topical, and transdermal routes, have all been employed.

Oral, Sublingual, Transmucosal, and Buccal Routes

When patients have difficulty swallowing pills but can take soft food, microsphere formulations of long-acting morphine or oxycodone provide sustained release when the capsule is broken open and the "sprinkles" are placed in applesauce or other soft food. Oral opioid solutions (e.g., morphine, oxycodone, hydromorphone, or methadone) can be swallowed or small volumes (0.5 to 1 mL) of a concentrated solution can be placed sublingually or buccally in patients whose swallowing abilities are limited. Nevertheless, buccal and sublingual uptake of these opioids is slow and not very predictable, particularly with more hydrophilic compounds such as morphine.[71,72] Small studies suggest that most of the analgesic effect of morphine administered in this manner is due to drug dripping down the oropharynx and into the gastrointestinal tract.[73] Conversely, absorption with the use of more lipophilic drugs, such as methadone and fentanyl, is relatively high.[72] Immediate-release fentanyl products will be described in the following text. Topical morphine and methadone mouthwashes have been reported to treat chemotherapy-induced oral mucositis and might be useful for other pain syndromes associated with oral lesions.[74–76]

Transmucosal Immediate-Release Fentanyl Products

Immediate-release fentanyl products are available as lozenges, sublingual tablets and sprays, and buccal tablets and film as well as nasal delivery.[77] The lipid solubility of fentanyl allows more rapid onset when compared with hydrophilic compounds, making these products useful for breakthrough pain. All of these products are approved for patients who are already tolerant to opioids, and in general, the dose of the long-acting opioid does not predict the effective dose of the transmucosal agent. One major obstacle to the use of these products is their cost, limiting use in hospice or other capitated healthcare delivery systems.

In the United States, the U.S. Food and Drug Administration has instituted a Risk Evaluation and Mitigation Strategy (REMS) for transmucosal immediate-release fentanyl (TIRF) products. This program requires prescribers to enroll in the TIRF REMS Access Program after reading educational materials and completing a test knowledge focusing on safe use of these products.[78] This program applies to transmucosal (buccal and sublingual) and nasal fentanyl products.

Oral transmucosal, sublingual, and buccal fentanyl: Oral transmucosal fentanyl citrate (OTFC) is a lipid-soluble (lipophilic) synthetic opioid formulation that consists of a lozenge on a stick. Patients must actively rub the fentanyl-containing lozenge against the oral mucosa to provide rapid absorption of the drug, usually experiencing some relief in 5 to 15 minutes, with a peak effect of 30 minutes.[77,79,80] Too rapid application, usually less than 15 minutes, will result in more of the agent being swallowed rather than being absorbed transmucosally. Some patients develop oral candida due to the high sugar content of the compound, and others complain of the sweet taste and lack of variety in flavor, particularly with prolonged use. Xerostomia can reduce bioavailability of the agent and altered dexterity may complicate use.

Other transmucosal fentanyl products include fentanyl sublingual tablet (FST)[81] and fentanyl sublingual spray (FSS)[82] as well as fentanyl buccal tablet (FBT)[83] and fentanyl buccal soluble film (FBSF).[84]

These products are generally well tolerated and produce more rapid onset of analgesia when compared with immediate-release oral morphine. A randomized study compared FSTs with subcutaneous morphine in people with severe cancer breakthrough pain and found that more than 90% of patients preferred the tablets.[81] Few trials compare these fentanyl products for superiority. In one study, the rate and extent of fentanyl absorption were greater following FBT compared to OTFC, such that approximately 30% less drug was required when administering FBT to achieve similar OTFC systemic drug levels.[80]

Nasal fentanyl: Two nasal fentanyl preparations are accessible globally for breakthrough pain, intranasal fentanyl spray (INFS) and fentanyl pectin nasal spray (FPNS), although in the United States, only FPNS is available. Both of these delivery systems provide significant analgesia within 10 minutes.[85,86]

Enteral and Rectal

Preexisting enteral feeding tubes can be used to deliver medications when patients cannot swallow at the end of life. It is rare that circumstances would require placement of a tube at this time, and doing so may send a contradictory message about the need for enteral nutrition and hydration. The size of the tube and volume of fluid used to mix the "sprinkles" formulation of morphine or oxycodone must be considered when delivering this form of long-acting opioid to avoid obstruction of the tube.[87]

Opioids can be delivered via the rectal route using commercially prepared suppositories, compounded suppositories, or microenemas. Studies suggest a larger area under the curve when morphine suppositories are used when compared with oral sustained-release morphine.[88] Sustained-release morphine tablets have also been used rectally, with resultant delayed time to peak plasma level and approximately 90% of the bioavailability achieved by oral administration.[89] Rectal methadone can be used safely and has bioavailability approximately equal to oral methadone.[90,91] Neutropenia and thrombocytopenia are generally considered contraindications to rectal drug administration, but clinicians must consider the goals of care for delivering these drugs as well as the risks and benefits at this time of life. Painful rectal lesions, such as hemorrhoids or fissures, preclude the use of these routes. Attempting to place agents rectally at home may be difficult for family members when caring for loved ones who cannot move or reposition without significant assistance.

Parenteral

Parenteral administration includes intravenous and subcutaneous delivery of drug. Intramuscular opioid delivery is inappropriate in the palliative care setting due to the pain associated with this route and the variability in systemic uptake of the drug.[42] Intravenous administration of drugs is often used when patients are hospitalized at end of life, as this route provides rapid and predictable drug delivery. For patients being cared for at home, the need for vascular access may be cumbersome. Subcutaneous infusions, including morphine, hydromorphone, and fentanyl, provide an effective and safe alternative.[92] Methadone has been reported to cause local site irritation, although small case reports suggest that lower doses given intermittently are less likely to cause pain.[93] Subcutaneous boluses of morphine have a slower onset and lower peak effect when compared with intravenous boluses, although with continuous infusions they provide similar blood levels and resultant pain relief.[94] Subcutaneous infusions may include up to 10 mL per hour, although most patients absorb 2 to 3 mL per hour with the least difficulty. Volumes greater than 10 mL per hour are often poorly absorbed and can lead to pain or leakage of fluid. Hyaluronidase has been reported to speed absorption of subcutaneously administered fluids, although a randomized trial yielded no difference in pain or edema between treatment and placebo groups.[95] Despite these findings, these investigators and others suggest that hyaluronidase may have utility when subcutaneous absorption is not well tolerated.

Spinal (Epidural/Intrathecal)

Intraspinal routes, including epidural or intrathecal delivery, allow administration of drugs such as opioids, local anesthetics, and/or α-adrenergic agonists more proximate to their respective effector sites.[96,97] A randomized controlled trial demonstrated benefit for ambulatory cancer patients with a life expectancy of at least 3 to 6 months experiencing pain.[98] However, initiating this therapy during the final hours of life requires the availability of experts to place an external catheter as well as caregivers with specialized knowledge to safely and effectively provide care. As with all therapies, the potential risks, including greater caregiver burden, need to be weighed against the benefits. Intraspinal delivery may be considered when patients do not obtain adequate relief from aggressive titration of systemic opioids and other analgesics or they experience intolerable adverse effects. A systematic review of spinal opioids in cancer pain found only weak evidence to recommend this therapy.[99] More information regarding the use of intraspinal drug delivery is available in Chapter 100.

Topical

Topical morphine administration to open areas, such as pressure ulcers, burns, malignant skin lesions, and ulcers associated with venous stasis or sickle cell disease, has been reported to be effective in case reports and open-label trials.[100–102] However, a randomized controlled trial of topical morphine used to treat painful skin ulcers found no benefit when compared with placebo.[103] An analysis of the bioavailability of morphine when delivered to open ulcers found little systemic uptake, a possible explanation for the lack of efficacy.[104] Topical morphine applied to the wrist in a pluronic lecithin organogel (PLO) base for systemic delivery is being used in some settings; yet, evidence of its efficacy is lacking. A bioavailability study of topical morphine in healthy volunteers revealed that morphine was seldom detected in plasma samples after topical administration, and when values were detected, they were below the level of quantification.[105] These results suggest that topical administration of morphine compounded in a PLO base for topical drug delivery is unlikely to provide relief of pain.

Transdermal

Transdermal fentanyl has been used extensively, and a wide range of dosing options (ranging from 12- to 100-μg-per-hour patches) makes this route particularly useful in cancer pain and palliative care.[106] Most individuals experience relief for 3 days, although approximately 25% of patients will consistently report increased pain on the third day, despite adequate use of breakthrough medications. These patients benefit from changing the patch more frequently (every 48 hours). Equianalgesic dosing with other opioids has been unknown; a recent study suggests that a 100-μg patch is approximately equivalent to 240 mg of oral morphine equivalents.[107] Fentanyl is another option when considering opioid rotation, and several reports suggest the resolution of delirium when patients are converted from other opioids to transdermal or intravenous fentanyl.[108,109] Fever, diaphoresis, cachexia, morbid obesity, and ascites may have a significant impact on the absorption, predictability of blood levels, and clinical effects of transdermal fentanyl, although studies are lacking. There is some suggestion in open-label and retrospective studies that transdermal fentanyl may produce less constipation than long-acting morphine.[106,110] A small subset of patients will develop skin irritation due to the adhesive in any patch. Because most topical antihistamines consist of an oil base which would prevent patch adherence, the use of an aqueous based steroid inhaler (intended for the management of asthma) applied prior to patch administration can preclude skin reactions and allows the patch to remain in place.

INTRACTABLE PAIN OR UNMANAGEABLE ADVERSE EFFECTS OF TREATMENT

Although most pain at end of life can be well managed with available therapies, intractable pain or unmanageable adverse effects can occur that can lead to incredible suffering. In some cases, pain escalates due to rapidly increasing disease burden. At other times, pharmacokinetics of the opioids and other analgesics are altered by organ dysfunction associated with the dying process, leading to inadequate relief.

Effect of Organ Dysfunction on Pharmacokinetics

Organ dysfunction at the end of life will alter the absorption, distribution, metabolism, and elimination of analgesic agents, thereby influencing the efficacy of the drug. People with advanced malignancy or other life-threatening illness may undergo changes in any of these phases as a result of extensive disease. Little is known about the alterations in absorption of opioids that occur when people are dying. Factors such as shortened gastrointestinal transit time may delay absorption of oral opioids, particularly long-acting or sustained-release compounds.

Distribution of the drug is in part dependent on plasma proteins within the vasculature, body fat stores, and total body water. These can all be significantly altered in patients who are cachectic and dehydrated at the end of life. Aging patients are known to have decreased volume of distribution of morphine and fentanyl. Additionally, methadone binds avidly to α_1 glycoprotein, which is increased in advanced cancer. This leads to decreasing amounts of unbound methadone and a delayed onset of analgesic effect.

Metabolism of drugs can be changed by advanced age, liver dysfunction, and other factors that are widespread in palliative care.[111] Excretion can be altered as renal failure occurs, particularly because most opioids, with the exception being methadone, are primarily excreted by the kidneys. Patients with renal failure or those receiving dialysis might benefit from the use of agents that are more readily dialyzable, such as fentanyl, as opposed to morphine or codeine.[110,112] Research is needed regarding the effect of advanced disease and the dying process on the pharmacokinetics of analgesics, particularly opioids.

Myoclonus

One consequence of altered pharmacokinetics at the end of life is the development of myoclonus. Myoclonus is a sudden, uncontrollable, nonrhythmic jerking of the extremities. This can be extremely distressing, causing fatigue and sleep disruption and exacerbating the patient's pain. Furthermore, myoclonus can progress to the development of uncontrolled seizures.[113] Myoclonus has been reported to occur after surgery to the brain,[114] in acquired immunodeficiency syndrome,[115] after hypoxia,[116] and after chlorambucil administration.[117] However, myoclonus at end-of-life care is most commonly associated with opioids. Controversy exists regarding whether this is dose dependent and how much of this effect is from parent drug versus metabolites. Most reports of opioid-related myoclonus implicate higher doses, although it has been reported to occur in patients receiving low doses of opioids, particularly hydromorphone.[118,119] Other opioids that have been implicated include methadone[120] and fentanyl.[121] Myoclonus has also been reported during withdrawal from transdermal fentanyl.[122,123]

The underlying mechanism of opioid-induced myoclonus is poorly understood. Myoclonus and seizures have been reported to occur in patients receiving high-dose morphine or hydromorphone administration.[124] However, Fainsinger and colleagues[125] describe a case of myoclonus occurring with stable hydromorphone dosing in the face of acute renal failure. A retrospective chart review found that in terminally ill patients receiving parenteral hydromorphone, the dose and duration of drug were associated with the development of myoclonus, whereas age, gender, and diagnosis were not.[126] These findings point to the role of accumulating neuroexcitatory metabolites that are poorly excreted either due to prolonged dosing, high doses, or concomitant renal failure. The 3-glucuronide metabolites are implicated as contributing to these neuroexcitatory effects.[127] Both morphine-3-glucuronide (M3G) and hydromorphone-3-glucuronide (H3G) are believed to produce excitatory behaviors, including myoclonus, allodynia, and seizures. In a study of cancer patients who developed allodynia and myoclonus during morphine infusions, M3G levels were elevated.[124] Case reports suggest that M3G and H3G plasma levels are greatly increased in the presence of renal failure, with the ratio of metabolite to parent compound four times higher than the ratio seen in patients with normal renal function.[128,129] However, one prospective study found no relationship between myoclonus and renal function.[130] In rodent models, H3G has more potent neuroexcitatory effects when compared with M3G.[131] However, a pilot study of people in hospice receiving morphine and experiencing myoclonus revealed no elevation in M3G levels.[132]

Regardless of the underlying cause, treatment is imperative. The goal is to significantly reduce the dose of the opioid, and this is usually accomplished by rotation to an alternate opioid.[133,134] Methadone has been used as an alternative agent with success, although other opioids may be easier to titrate and methadone also has been found to produce myoclonus.[120] Other strategies include adding adjuvant analgesics and using interventional techniques (e.g., spinal drug administration, nerve blocks) to potentially reduce the amount of total systemic opioid. Ketamine has been suggested as beneficial to rapidly reduce systemic opioid dose.[135] Little research is available regarding agents used to reduce myoclonic jerking. Benzodiazepines, including clonazepam, diazepam, and midazolam, have been recommended.[133,136] The mechanism of action of benzodiazepines is through binding to γ-aminobutyric acid type A (GABA$_A$) receptors within the central nervous system, leading to central nervous system depression. At higher doses, benzodiazepines may also limit repetitive neuronal firing, similar to several anticonvulsant compounds. Clonazepam may be useful in patients who can swallow, with doses starting at 0.5 to 1 mg by mouth every 6 or 8 hours, with upward titration as needed. Lorazepam tablets or solution can be placed sublingually if the patient is unable to swallow. Lorazepam and midazolam can be administered parenterally and are often indicated during the final hours of life.

Intractable Pain at End of Life

When pain is poorly managed despite aggressive titration of available therapies, several other options can be employed.[137] First, thorough assessment is needed to rule out potentially reversible etiologies. Because the pain demands immediate attention, titration of the opioid therapy must be aggressive while carefully preventing and treating adverse effects. Additional therapies should be considered, such as corticosteroids, local anesthetics, ketamine, and other therapies. Bringing in a team approach is crucial, including experts in pain and palliative care, as well as chaplains, social workers, psychologists, and others, to address patient and family suffering. When these interventions are unsuccessful, palliative sedation may be considered.

Intravenous Lidocaine

Systemic administration of local anesthetics, such as lidocaine, has been used to treat chronic pain.[138–140] At subanesthetic doses, lidocaine blocks neuronal function in active or depolarized neurons without interfering with the normal function of other sensory or motor neurons. Although historically used as a monthly infusion in chronic pain clinics, similar protocols have been adapted for use in patients at end of life with intractable pain. The dosage is generally 1 to 3 mg/kg administered intravenously over 20 to 30 minutes.[141] During the bolus infusion, pain intensity scores often decline significantly. If effective, a continuous infusion of 1 to 3 mg/kg/hour will be initiated. Immediate signs of toxicity include numbness around the lips or a sensation of thickness of the tongue. Due to the short half-life of lidocaine, the symptoms of toxicity are transient and easily reversible by lowering the infusion rate. However, toxicity has been reported at very low doses of lidocaine.[142]

In concert with the goals of care at this time of life, cardiac monitoring is not usually performed nor are plasma levels of lidocaine obtained. If subcutaneous administration is indicated due to lack of venous access, the initial loading dose is administered over a longer time period (30 minutes to an hour) and the response may be delayed by a few minutes.[143] If subcutaneous infusion is elected, more concentrated lidocaine solutions allow for lower volumes to be infused. If the bolus dose is ineffective or toxicity is unmanageable, the lidocaine challenge is discontinued and other pain relief modalities must be selected.

The lidocaine infusion technique has been reported to be effective in a child with cancer, using 35 μg/kg/min initially, with an increase to 50 μg/kg/min after several days.[144] Other case reports suggest the efficacy of continuous intravenous lidocaine in pediatric patients with opioid-resistant cancer pain.[145] The only randomized controlled trial of intravenous lidocaine for neuropathic pain from cancer using 5 mg/kg over 30 minutes found no difference in analgesia.[146] Much more research in this particular area is needed.

Ketamine

Ketamine is an N-methyl-D-aspartate antagonist that can be given by a variety of routes: oral, intravenous, subcutaneous, intranasal, sublingual, epidural, intrathecal, and topical. It has been reported to improve pain relief and reduce opioid requirements in a variety of pain syndromes associated with cancer and other life-threatening illnesses.[147–149] Although it can be used earlier in the course of the disease trajectory, ketamine is most commonly trialed in the face of intractable pain at the end of life.

In a small (n = 10) study of cancer patients who reported pain unrelieved with morphine, a slow bolus of ketamine (0.25 mg/kg or 0.50 mg/kg) was evaluated using a randomized, double-blind, crossover, double-dose design. Ketamine, but not saline solution, significantly reduced the pain intensity in almost all the patients at both doses, with the greatest effect being in those treated with higher doses. Adverse effects included hallucinations in 4 patients and an unpleasant cognitive sensation in 2 patients. These adverse effects responded to diazepam 1 mg intravenously. Drowsiness was also significantly more likely to occur, particularly with the higher dose. The investigators concluded that ketamine improved morphine analgesia in a variety of difficult pain syndromes; yet, central adverse effects can limit the use of this therapy.[149]

A study of young children and adolescents who were on high doses of opioids and had uncontrolled cancer pain examined the effect of adding a low-dose ketamine infusion. In 8 of 11 patients, ketamine infusions used as an adjuvant to opioid analgesia provided improvement in pain and was associated with opioid-sparing effects. This allowed reduction in opioid dose that ultimately improved social interaction during this important time.[150]

The usual oral dose of ketamine is 10 to 15 mg every 6 hours. Because oral preparations are not commercially available in the United States, the solution used for injection is administered orally, usually mixed with juice or cola to hide the unpleasant taste. Parenteral dosing is typically 0.04 mg/kg/hour with titration to a maximum of 0.3 mg/kg/hour. When given parenterally or orally, the onset of analgesia is 15 to 30 minutes with a duration of effect ranging between 15 minutes and 2 hours. A general recommendation is to reduce the opioid dose by approximately 25% when starting ketamine to avoid sedation. Severe side effects are generally associated with doses of parenteral ketamine above 0.5 mg/kg and include psychotomimetic phenomena such as dysphoria, nightmares, hallucinations, excessive salivation, and tachycardia.

Although there are many small trials and case series that suggest efficacy from ketamine, a well-designed randomized controlled trial found no benefit.[151] An updated Cochrane review concluded that there was insufficient evidence to conclude that ketamine improves the effectiveness of opioid treatment in cancer pain.[152] Clearly, more research in this area is needed.

Fears of Hastening Death

Pain at the end of life may be poorly managed due to fears of causing respiratory depression. This is particularly true when family members administering opioids at home express fear about causing their loved one's death. It can also occur in institutional settings where clinicians are uncomfortable ordering or administering therapeutic doses of drugs. Clinicians and family members also fear "giving the last dose" of an opioid. Education is desperately needed. Respiratory depression is rare in palliative care as most patients are opioid tolerant. A study of cancer patients undergoing parenteral opioid titration for severe pain revealed no change in end-tidal carbon dioxide, oxygen saturation, or respiratory rate.[153] Sykes and Thorns[154] evaluated 17 studies that examined the use of opioids at end of life. None of the five studies that explored opioid use and survival found any relationship. Their own earlier study also found no relationship between the dose or the timing of the opioid administration and the time of death.[155] These authors conclude that the doctrine of double effect, which suggests it is ethical to employ a treatment intending to obtain its beneficial effect (e.g., analgesia) but at the same time recognizing that it may also have harmful effects (e.g., respiratory depression or death), is not relevant. They also argue that it is potentially harmful to invoke this doctrine as it potentiates a myth: one that can lead to greater fear and

unrelieved pain. A study from the National Hospice Database reported similar result: The dose of opioid had no appreciable impact on the timing of death in patients with far-advanced disease.[156] Several other reviews found a similar lack of association between opioid doses or timing with survival.[157,158]

Suffering and Existential Distress

It may be very difficult to distinguish pain from other causes of suffering in dying patients.[159] Although the trend toward greater attention to pain is positive, there is frequently little attention to the role loss, burden, sadness, fear, isolation, and other existential concerns that can play at this time of life.[160] Several studies support the need for more useful definitions and distinctions and to address the role of suffering in the individual's life. For example, one study asked hospice patients about suffering in an open-ended interview, revealing that in the views of the 100 patients included in this study, relief of pain and relief of suffering are not the same.[161] Another study of health care professionals revealed that suffering was viewed quite differently by chaplains, who defined this in spiritual terms, versus pain professionals, who placed existential issues in the context of pain.[162]

Using semistructured interviews, 381 patients with advanced cancer were asked if they felt they were suffering and were also asked about physical symptoms, social concerns, psychologic problems, and existential issues. Approximately 25% reported they were suffering at a moderate-to-extreme level. This suffering was strongly correlated with general malaise, weakness, pain, and depression. Thus, although many patients with advanced cancer do not consider themselves to be suffering, for those who are suffering, it is a multidimensional experience related most strongly to physical symptoms but with contributions from psychologic distress, existential concerns, and social-relational worries as well.[163] The consequences of unresolved suffering are great, including a wish for hastened death. In a study of 96 terminally ill elders, 15 acknowledged significant suffering that resulted in a wish for a hastened death, and several had even considered strategies to accelerate the dying process. In analyses of the interviews of these individuals, four critical themes emerged: perceived insensitive and uncaring communication of a terminal diagnosis by their health care professional, experiencing unbearable physical pain, unacknowledged feelings regarding undergoing chemotherapy or radiation treatment, and dying in a distressing environment.[164]

Assessment of the whole person should be multidimensional, and an interdisciplinary team is best equipped to address these broad issues. In addition to a thorough pain and symptom assessment, patients should be asked about the meaning of their lives, their sense of hope, the goals they have for this time of their lives, and whether they are suffering. Suffering is a deeply personal experience, accompanied by a wide range of emotions and meanings.[159] Inadequate assessment that only equates pain with suffering can lead to inappropriate increases in opioids, without benefiting their existential concerns, while leading to increased toxicity.[165]

When patients are identified as experiencing suffering, several interventions can be useful. Life review allows the individual to reminisce about life experiences, often leading to self-discovery of meaning in the contributions they have made. Some people benefit by developing letters or videotapes to loved ones to be read at a later date during anticipated landmark events in the loved one's life, such as college graduation, marriage, or the birth of a child. One novel model to address psychosocial and existential distress in the dying is called dignity therapy.[166,167] This brief, individualized approach to end-of-life care allows patients to discuss issues that are most important to them and to describe the things they would most want remembered as death draws near. These discussions are recorded, transcribed, and developed into a document, which can be given to family or loved ones. In one study of people with advanced cancer, 76% reported a heightened sense of dignity, 68% reported an increased sense of purpose, 67% reported a heightened sense of meaning, and 47% reported an increased will to live.[168] Family perceptions were also positive, with the majority stating that the document developed by the dying loved one helped during the grieving process and that the document would continue to be a source of comfort for their families and themselves.[169] Those who are suffering often feel voiceless and having professionals witness and listen to their concerns in an empathic manner can be extraordinarily therapeutic.

NONPHARMACOLOGIC TECHNIQUES

Nonpharmacologic therapies can be particularly useful during the final hours of life. Cognitive-behavioral techniques, physical measures, and education can be used as part of the multimodal treatment plan to reduce pain and suffering, although few have been tested in end-of-life care.[170] The patient's and caregivers' abilities to participate must be considered when selecting any of these therapies, including their fatigue level, interest, cognition, and other factors.[171] Cognitive-behavioral techniques include guided imagery,[172] meditation,[173] hypnosis,[174] music[175-177] and art therapy,[178] and other complementary therapies.[179]

Physical measures, including massage,[180,181] reflexology,[177] heat, and other techniques,[182] can produce relaxation and relieve pain. In a small study of massage in hospice patients, reductions in blood pressure, heart rate, and skin temperature were noted, suggestive of a relaxation effect.[183] A potential benefit of all of these therapies is the ability to include family members who are often seeking methods to provide comfort to their loved one.

Family involvement in all aspects of care is crucial. Family caregivers who rate their self-efficacy, or their ability to care for their loved one, as high report much lower levels of strain as well as decreased negative mood and increased positive mood. Ultimately, the caregiver's self-efficacy in managing the patient's pain related to the patient's physical well-being. In dyads where the family caregiver perceived higher self-efficacy, the patient reported having more energy, feeling less ill, and spending less time in bed.[184] As a result of these findings, Keefe and colleagues[185] developed a partner-guided pain management training intervention that they tested in 78 advanced cancer patients who met criteria for hospice eligibility. Patients and their partners were randomly assigned to the intervention or to usual care as the control condition. The partner-guided pain management training protocol consisted of educational information about cancer pain with systematic training of patients and partners in cognitive and behavioral pain coping skills delivered in the patients' homes over three sessions. The partner-guided pain management protocol significantly increased partners' ratings of their self-efficacy for helping the patient control pain and other symptoms. These family caregivers also showed a trend toward reduced levels of caregiver strain.[185]

Although case reports and open-label trials of cognitive-behavioral, physical measures, and educational interventions are reported to be very effective in relieving symptoms at end of life, more research is needed.[170,186] Furthermore, most existing research has been conducted in patients early in the disease trajectory, so more research is needed to determine the potential value, no less the feasibility, of these interventions in the final days and hours of life.

Palliative Sedation

Although the majority of individuals with pain at the end of life can obtain relief with available therapies, some dying patients experience distressing symptoms that cannot be controlled.

In these cases, palliative sedation may be considered. Several steps are crucial when implementing palliative sedation. First, the team must be confident that all other reasonable options have been explored, the disease is irreversible, and that death would be expected in hours to days.[187] Second, the patient and family should be carefully informed about the risks and benefits of sedation, and they should provide informed consent and agree with these plans. The entire team (physicians, nurses, respiratory therapy, chaplains, social workers, and others involved in the patient's care) must have the opportunity to discuss this option and agree as a team about the justification for the use of palliative sedation and the details of the care to be provided. These are generally complex cases that are emotionally stressful. All involved can benefit from talking about the complex medical, ethical, and emotional issues they raise. Decisions about hydration and nutrition as well as resuscitation status (most centers require that the patient has do not resuscitate orders) should be made prior to initiating sedation. Sedation may be delayed if the patient is awaiting the arrival of a family member from out of town. In some cases, light sedation may be used and reversed once the relative arrives and then restarted and increased once the patient and loved one have had time to say goodbye. The American Academy of Hospice and Palliative Medicine offers a position statement to guide clinicians when opting to initiate palliative sedation.[188]

The agent most commonly employed drug for palliative sedation is midazolam, although other benzodiazepines, propofol, or barbiturates can be administered (Table 109.3).[187] Benzodiazepines have anxiolytic, muscle relaxant, sedative-hypnotic, anticonvulsant, antiemetic, and amnesic effects. Their mechanism of action is through binding to GABA receptors within the central nervous system leading to central nervous system depression. Midazolam is the shortest acting agent within this class, with an onset of action within 3 to 5 minutes after intravenous injection and a half-life of 1 to 4 hours. These attributes, rapid onset and relatively short duration, as well as the ability to administer it either intravenously or subcutaneously makes this a useful drug in instituting palliative sedation.

TABLE 109.3 Doses of Agents Used in Palliative Sedation[189,197]

Drug	Route	Bolus Dose	Continuous Infusion
Midazolam	IV, SQ	5 mg	Starting dose 1 mg/h; usual maintenance dose 20–120 mg/h
Lorazepam	IV, SQ, SL, PO	0.5–2 mg PO, SL every 1–2 h; 2–5 mg SQ or IV	Starting dose 0.5–1.0 mg/h; usual maintenance dose 4–40 mg/h
Chlorpromazine	PO, IV, PR	10–25 mg every 2–4 h	
Haloperidol	PO, IV, SQ	0.5–5 mg PO every 2–4 h; 1–5 mg IV/SQ bolus	Starting dose 0.2 mg/h; maintenance 0.2–0.6 mg/h
Thiopental	IV	5–7 mg/kg/h	20–80 mg/h
Pentobarbital	IV	2–3 mg/kg	Starting dose 1 mg/kg/h; titrate upward as needed
Phenobarbital	IV, SQ	200 mg, can repeat every 10–15 min	25 mg/h; maintenance dose 25–66 mg/h
Propofol	IV	20–50 mg bolus; may repeat	5–10 mg/h; may increase dose by 10 mg/h every 15–20 min

IV, intravenous; PO, oral; PR, rectal; SL, sublingual; SQ, subcutaneous.

Furthermore, it is stable with most other agents but is incompatible with corticosteroids such as dexamethasone, betamethasone, or methylprednisolone.

Propofol is an intravenous nonbarbiturate thought to enhance the activity of GABA. The advantages of propofol include rapid onset and short half-life. Although studies are lacking, the recommended dose of propofol to treat refractory pain/suffering is 1 to 2 mg/kg via intravenous injection over 5 minutes.[189] The bolus may need to be repeated if the first injection is ineffective. Bolus doses are followed by a maintenance intravenous infusion of 2 to 10 mg/kg/hour, using the lowest dose needed to suppress symptoms. Propofol is recommended for intravenous administration; subcutaneous delivery has not been studied. Propofol contains soybean oil and egg yolk phospholipid and therefore is contraindicated for use in patients with egg hypersensitivity or soya lecithin hypersensitivity.[190]

Family members must be provided sufficient information and support during this time. In a multicenter study conducted in Japan, bereaved family members of cancer patients who received sedation in seven palliative care units were surveyed.[191] The families reported that 69% of the patients were considerably or very distressed before sedation. Although the majority of families were satisfied with the treatment, 25% expressed a high level of emotional distress. The factors associated with high levels of family distress were poor symptom control after sedation, feeling the burden of responsibility for the decision, feeling unprepared for changes in the patient's condition, feeling that the physicians and nurses were not sufficiently compassionate, and a shorter time to their loved one's death. Regular monitoring of patient distress with timely modification of the sedation protocol is vital, as is providing sufficient information and sharing the responsibility for the decision. Family members require emotional support to assist with their anticipatory and ongoing grief, although a recent observational study found no negative impact on the well-being of loved ones after witnessing palliative sedation.[192] As the use of palliative sedation increases, guidelines should be developed across settings and disciplines to ensure consistency. These guidelines must articulate that this therapy is not euthanasia but is rather directed toward treatment of symptoms.

Conclusion

The relief of pain during the final phase of life is vital for both the patient who is experiencing this pain and for those at the bedside witnessing this distress. All clinicians have the responsibility to learn how to assess pain in the cognitively impaired and how to employ effective pharmacologic and nonpharmacologic treatments. Empathic listening with attention to suffering and existential distress will help improve the quality of life of the dying. When pain remains severe, despite aggressive use of all appropriate options, the team must carefully consider the use of palliative sedation, along with the patient and their loved ones. All of this care involves the skills of a well-functioning interdisciplinary team, combining the expertise of each individual to provide optimal care to the most vulnerable of all of our patients.

References

1. Kutner JS, Bryant LL, Beaty BL, et al. Time course and characteristics of symptom distress and quality of life at the end of life. *J Pain Symptom Manage* 2007;34(3):227–236.
2. Cooley ME, Short TH, Moriarty HJ. Symptom prevalence, distress, and change over time in adults receiving treatment for lung cancer. *Psychooncology* 2003;12(7):694–708.
3. Chang VT, Hwang SS, Feuerman M, et al. Symptom and quality of life survey of medical oncology patients at a Veterans Affairs medical center: a role for symptom assessment. *Cancer* 2000;88(5):1175–1183.
4. Lo RS, Woo J, Zhoc KC, et al. Quality of life of palliative care patients in the last two weeks of life. *J Pain Symptom Manage* 2002;24(4):388–397.
5. Vainio A, Auvinen A. Prevalence of symptoms among patients with advanced cancer: an international collaborative study. Symptom Prevalence Group. *J Pain Symptom Manage* 1996;12(1):3–10.
6. Hall P, Schroder C, Weaver L. The last 48 hours of life in long-term care: a focused chart audit. *J Am Geriatr Soc* 2002;50(3):501–506.
7. Stromgren AS, Sjogren P, Goldschmidt D, et al. Symptom priority and course of symptomatology in specialized palliative care. *J Pain Symptom Manage* 2006;31(3):199–206.
8. Teno JM, Clarridge BR, Casey V, et al. Family perspectives on end-of-life care at the last place of care. *JAMA* 2004;291(1):88–93.
9. Wang H, Naghavi M, Allen C, et al. Global, regional, and national life expectancy, all-cause mortality, and cause-specific mortality for 249 causes of death, 1980–2015: a systematic analysis for the Global Burden of Disease Study 2015. *Lancet* 2016;388(10053):1459–1544.
10. Center to Advance Palliative Care. About palliative care. Available at: https://www.capc.org/about/palliative-care/. Accessed June 29, 2017.
11. Dumanovsky T, Augustin R, Rogers M, et al. The growth of palliative care in U.S. hospitals: a status report. *J Palliat Med* 2016;19(1):8–15.
12. Morrison RS. Models of palliative care delivery in the United States. *Curr Opin Support Palliat Care* 2013;7(2):201–206.
13. Ferrell BR, Temel JS, Temin S, et al. Integration of palliative care into standard oncology care: American Society of Clinical Oncology clinical practice guideline update. *J Clin Oncol* 2017;35(1):96–112.
14. Smith AK, Thai JN, Bakitas MA, et al. The diverse landscape of palliative care clinics. *J Palliat Med* 2013;16(6):661–668.
15. Bauman JR, Temel JS. The integration of early palliative care with oncology care: the time has come for a new tradition. *J Natl Compr Canc Netw* 2014;12(12):1763–1771.
16. Parikh RB, Temel JS. Early specialty palliative care. *N Engl J Med* 2014;370(11):1075–1076.
17. Davis MP, Temel JS, Balboni T, et al. A review of the trials which examine early integration of outpatient and home palliative care for patients with serious illnesses. *Ann Palliat Med* 2015;4(3):99–121.
18. Nickolich MS, El-Jawahri A, Temel JS, et al. Discussing the evidence for upstream palliative care in improving outcomes in advanced cancer. *Am Soc Clin Oncol Educ Book* 2016;35:e534–e538.
19. Temel JS, Greer JA, El-Jawahri A, et al. Effects of early integrated palliative care in patients with lung and GI cancer: a randomized clinical trial. *J Clin Oncol* 2017;35(8):834–841.
20. National Hospice and Palliative Care Organization. NHPCO's facts and figures: hospice care in America. Available at: https://www.nhpco.org/sites/default/files/public/Statistics_Research/2015_Facts_Figures.pdf. Accessed June 29, 2017.
21. Kumar P, Wright AA, Hatfield LA, et al. Family perspectives on hospice care experiences of patients with cancer. *J Clin Oncol* 2017;35(4):432–439.
22. Wilson KG, Chochinov HM, Allard P, et al. Prevalence and correlates of pain in the Canadian National Palliative Care Survey. *Pain Res Manag* 2009;14(5):365–370.
23. Breivik H, Cherny N, Collett B, et al. Cancer-related pain: a Pan-European survey of prevalence, treatment, and patient attitudes. *Ann Oncol* 2009;20(8):1420–1433.
24. van den Beuken-van Everdingen MH, de Rijke JM, Kessels AG, et al. Prevalence of pain in patients with cancer: a systematic review of the past 40 years. *Ann Oncol* 2007;18(9):1437–1449.
25. van den Beuken-van Everdingen MH, de Rijke JM, Kessels AG, et al. High prevalence of pain in patients with cancer in a large population-based study in The Netherlands. *Pain* 2007;132(3):312–320.
26. Coyle N, Adelhardt J, Foley KM, et al. Character of terminal illness in the advanced cancer patient: pain and other symptoms during the last four weeks of life [comment]. *J Pain Symptom Manage* 1990;5(2):83–93.
27. Wolfe J, Grier HE, Klar N, et al. Symptoms and suffering at the end of life in children with cancer [comment]. *N Engl J Med* 2000;342(5):326–333.
28. Wolfe J, Orellana L, Ullrich C, et al. Symptoms and distress in children with advanced cancer: prospective patient-reported outcomes from the PediQUEST Study. *J Clin Oncol* 2015;33(17):1928–1935.
29. Price A, Lee W, Goodwin L, et al. Prevalence, course and associations of desire for hastened death in a UK palliative population: a cross-sectional study. *BMJ Support Palliat Care* 2011;1(2):140–148.
30. Rosenfeld B, Pessin H, Marziliano A, et al. Does desire for hastened death change in terminally ill cancer patients? *Soc Sci Med* 2014;111:35–40.
31. da Silva JG, da Rocha Morgan DA, Melo FCM, et al. Level of pain and quality of life of people living with HIV/AIDS pain and quality of life in HIV/AIDS. *AIDS Care* 2017;29(8):1041–1048.
32. Drulovic J, Basic-Kes V, Grgic S, et al. The prevalence of pain in adults with multiple sclerosis: a multicenter cross-sectional survey. *Pain Med* 2015;16(8):1597–1602.
33. Heitmann H, Biberacher V, Tiemann L, et al. Prevalence of neuropathic pain in early multiple sclerosis. *Mult Scler* 2016;22(9):1224–1230.
34. Ehde DM, Osborne TL, Hanley MA, et al. The scope and nature of pain in persons with multiple sclerosis. *Mult Scler* 2006;12(5):629–638.
35. Higginson IJ, Hart S, Silber E, et al. Symptom prevalence and severity in people severely affected by multiple sclerosis. *J Palliat Care* 2006;22(3):158–165.

36. Rivera I, Ajroud-Driss S, Casey P, et al. Prevalence and characteristics of pain in early and late stages of ALS. *Amyotroph Lateral Scler Frontotemporal Degener* 2013;14(5–6):369–372.

37. Saleem T, Leigh PN, Higginson IJ. Symptom prevalence among people affected by advanced and progressive neurological conditions—a systematic review. *J Palliat Care* 2007;23(4):291–299.

38. Brkovic T, Burilovic E, Puljak L. Prevalence and severity of pain in adult end-stage renal disease patients on chronic intermittent hemodialysis: a systematic review. *Patient Prefer Adherence* 2016;10:1131–1150.

39. Johnson MJ. Management of end stage cardiac failure. *Postgrad Med J* 2007;83(980):395–401.

40. Swetz KM, Shanafelt TD, Drozdowicz LB, et al. Symptom burden, quality of life, and attitudes toward palliative care in patients with pulmonary arterial hypertension: results from a cross-sectional patient survey. *J Heart Lung Transplant* 2012;31(10):1102–1108.

41. Coelho T, Paul C, Gobbens RJJ, et al. Multidimensional frailty and pain in community dwelling elderly. *Pain Med* 2017;18(4):693–701.

42. American Pain Society. *Principles of Analgesic Use.* 7th ed. Chicago, IL: American Pain Society; 2016.

43. National Comprehensive Cancer Network. Adult cancer pain clinical practice guideline. Available at: https://www.nccn.org/. Accessed January 5, 2017.

44. Holen JC, Hjermstad MJ, Loge JH, et al. Pain assessment tools: is the content appropriate for use in palliative care? [comment]. *J Pain Symptom Manage* 2006;32(6):567–580.

45. Homsi J, Walsh D, Rivera N, et al. Symptom evaluation in palliative medicine: patient report vs systematic assessment. *Support Care Cancer* 2006;14(5):444–453.

46. Hui D, Bruera E. The Edmonton Symptom Assessment System 25 years later: past, present, and future developments. *J Pain Symptom Manage* 2017;53(3):630–643.

47. Cleeland CS, Mendoza TR, Wang XS, et al. Assessing symptom distress in cancer patients: the M.D. Anderson Symptom Inventory. *Cancer* 2000;89(7):1634–1646.

48. Chang VT, Hwang SS, Feuerman M. Validation of the Edmonton Symptom Assessment Scale. *Cancer* 2000;88(9):2164–2171.

49. Portenoy RK, Thaler HT, Kornblith AB, et al. The Memorial Symptom Assessment Scale: an instrument for the evaluation of symptom prevalence, characteristics and distress. *Eur J Cancer* 1994;30A(9):1326–1336.

50. Webber K, Davies AN. Validity of the Memorial Symptom Assessment Scale-Short Form psychological subscales in advanced cancer patients. *J Pain Symptom Manage* 2011;42(5):761–767.

51. Stein KD, Denniston M, Baker F, et al. Validation of a modified Rotterdam Symptom Checklist for use with cancer patients in the United States. *J Pain Symptom Manage* 2003;26(5):975–989.

52. Pelayo-Alvarez M, Perez-Hoyos S, Agra-Varela Y. Reliability and concurrent validity of the Palliative Outcome Scale, the Rotterdam Symptom Checklist, and the Brief Pain Inventory. *J Palliat Med* 2013;16(8):867–874.

53. Stapleton SJ, Holden J, Epstein J, et al. A systematic review of the Symptom Distress Scale in advanced cancer studies. *Cancer Nurs* 2016;39(4):E9–E23.

54. Guo H, Fine PG, Mendoza TR, et al. A preliminary study of the utility of the Brief Hospice Inventory. *J Pain Symptom Manage* 2001;22(2):637–648.

55. McMillan SC, Mahon M. Measuring quality of life in hospice patients using a newly developed Hospice Quality of Life Index. *Quality of Life Research* 1994;3(6):437–447.

56. McMillan SC, Weitzner M. Quality of life in cancer patients: use of a revised Hospice Index. *Cancer Practice* 1998;6(5):282–288.

57. Albers G, Echteld MA, de Vet HC, et al. Evaluation of quality-of-life measures for use in palliative care: a systematic review. *Palliat Med* 2010;24(1):17–37.

58. Herr K, Coyne PJ, McCaffery M, et al. Pain assessment in the patient unable to self-report: position statement with clinical practice recommendations. *Pain Manag Nurs* 2011;12(4):230–250.

59. Booker SQ, Herr KA. Assessment and measurement of pain in adults in later life. *Clin Geriatr Med* 2016;32(4):677–692.

60. Hadjistavropoulos T, Herr K, Prkachin KM, et al. Pain assessment in elderly adults with dementia. *Lancet Neurol* 2014;13(12):1216–1227.

61. Angus DC, Barnato AE, Linde-Zwirble WT, et al. Use of intensive care at the end of life in the United States: an epidemiologic study. *Crit Care Med* 2004;32(3):638–643.

62. Angus DC, Truog RD. Toward better ICU use at the end of life. *JAMA* 2016;315(3):255–256.

63. SUPPORT Principal Investigators. A controlled trial to improve care for seriously ill hospitalized patients. The Study to Understand Prognoses and Preferences for Outcomes and Risks of Treatment (SUPPORT). *JAMA* 1995;274:1591–1598.

64. White DB, Curtis JR, Wolf LE, et al. Life support for patients without a surrogate decision maker: who decides? *Ann Int Med* 2007;147(1):34–40.

65. Payen JF, Bru O, Bosson JL, et al. Assessing pain in critically ill sedated patients by using a Behavioral Pain Scale. *Crit Care Med* 2001;29(12):2258–2263.

66. Gelinas C, Johnston C. Pain assessment in the critically ill ventilated adult: validation of the Critical-Care Pain Observation Tool and physiologic indicators. *Clin J Pain* 2007;23(6):497–505.

67. Rijkenberg S, Stilma W, Endeman H, et al. Pain measurement in mechanically ventilated critically ill patients: Behavioral Pain Scale versus Critical-Care Pain Observation Tool. *J Crit Care* 2015;30(1):167–172.

68. Manworren RC, Hynan LS. Clinical validation of FLACC: preverbal patient pain scale. *Pediatric Nursing* 2003;29(2):140–146.

69. van Dijk M, de Boer JB, Koot HM, et al. The reliability and validity of the COMFORT scale as a postoperative pain instrument in 0 to 3-year-old infants. *Pain* 2000;84(2–3):367–377.

70. Caraceni A, Cherny N, Fainsinger R, et al. Pain measurement tools and methods in clinical research in palliative care: recommendations of an Expert Working Group of the European Association of Palliative Care. *J Pain Symptom Manage* 2002;23(3):239–255.

71. Reisfield GM, Wilson GR. Rational use of sublingual opioids in palliative medicine. *J Palliat Med* 2007;10(2):465–475.

72. Weinberg DS, Inturrisi CE, Reidenberg B, et al. Sublingual absorption of selected opioid analgesics. *Clin Pharmacol Ther* 1988;44(3):335–342.

73. Coluzzi PH. Sublingual morphine: efficacy reviewed. *J Pain Symptom Manage* 1998;16(3):184–192.

74. Sarvizadeh M, Hemati S, Meidani M, et al. Morphine mouthwash for the management of oral mucositis in patients with head and neck cancer. *Adv Biomed Res* 2015;4:44.

75. Vayne-Bossert P, Escher M, de Vautibault CG, et al. Effect of topical morphine (mouthwash) on oral pain due to chemotherapy- and/or radiotherapy-induced mucositis: a randomized double-blinded study. *J Palliat Med* 2010;13(2):125–128.

76. Gallagher R. Methadone mouthwash for the management of oral ulcer pain. *J Pain Symptom Manage* 2004;27(5):390–391.

77. Schug SA, Ting S. Fentanyl formulations in the management of pain: an update. *Drugs* 2017;77(7):747–763.

78. TIRF REMS Access. About the TIRF REMS Access Program. Available at: https://www.tirfremsaccess.com/TirfUI/rems/about.action. Accessed June 29, 2017.

79. Christie JM, Simmonds M, Patt R, et al. Dose-titration, multicenter study of oral transmucosal fentanyl citrate for the treatment of breakthrough pain in cancer patients using transdermal fentanyl for persistent pain. *J Clin Oncol* 1998;16(10):3238–3245.

80. Darwish M, Kirby M, Robertson P Jr, et al. Absolute and relative bioavailability of fentanyl buccal tablet and oral transmucosal fentanyl citrate. *J Clin Pharmacol* 2007;47(3):343–350.

81. Zecca E, Brunelli C, Centurioni F, et al. Fentanyl sublingual tablets versus subcutaneous morphine for the management of severe cancer pain episodes in patients receiving opioid treatment: a double-blind, randomized, noninferiority trial. *J Clin Oncol* 2017;35(7):759–765.

82. Parikh N, Goskonda V, Chavan A, et al. Pharmacokinetics and dose proportionality of fentanyl sublingual spray: a single-dose 5-way crossover study. *Clin Drug Investig* 2013;33(6):391–400.

83. Kleeberg UR, Davies A, Jarosz J, et al. Pan-European, open-label dose titration study of fentanyl buccal tablet in patients with breakthrough cancer pain. *Eur J Pain* 2015;19(4):528–537.

84. Rauck R, North J, Gever LN, et al. Fentanyl buccal soluble film (FBSF) for breakthrough pain in patients with cancer: a randomized, double-blind, placebo-controlled study. *Ann Oncol* 2010;21(6):1308–1314.

85. Fallon M, Reale C, Davies A, et al. Efficacy and safety of fentanyl pectin nasal spray compared with immediate-release morphine sulfate tablets in the treatment of breakthrough cancer pain: a multicenter, randomized, controlled, double-blind, double-dummy multiple-crossover study. *J Support Oncol* 2011;9(6):224–231.

86. Mercadante S, Prestia G, Adile C, et al. Intranasal fentanyl versus fentanyl pectin nasal spray for the management of breakthrough cancer pain in doses proportional to basal opioid regimen. *J Pain* 2014;15(6):602–607.

87. McCarberg BH, Kopecky EA, O'Connor M, et al. An abuse-deterrent, microsphere-in-capsule formulation of extended-release oxycodone: alternative modes of administration to facilitate pain management in patients with dysphagia. *Curr Med Res Opin* 2016;32(12):1975–1982.

88. Du X, Skopp G, Aderjan R. The influence of the route of administration: a comparative study at steady state of oral sustained release morphine and morphine sulfate suppositories. *Ther Drug Monit* 1999;21(2):208–214.

89. Gourlay GK. Sustained relief of chronic pain. Pharmacokinetics of sustained release morphine. *Clin Pharmacokinet* 1998;35(3):173–190.

90. Dale O, Sheffels P, Kharasch ED. Bioavailabilities of rectal and oral methadone in healthy subjects. *Br J Clin Pharmacol* 2004;58(2):156–162.

91. Ripamonti C, Zecca E, Brunelli C, et al. Rectal methadone in cancer patients with pain. A preliminary clinical and pharmacokinetic study. *Ann Oncol* 1995;6(8):841–843.

92. Watanabe S, Pereira J, Hanson J, et al. Fentanyl by continuous subcutaneous infusion for the management of cancer pain: a retrospective study. *J Pain Symptom Manage* 1998;16(5):323–326.

93. Centeno C, Vara F. Intermittent subcutaneous methadone administration in the management of cancer pain. *J Pain Palliat Care Pharmacother* 2005;19(2):7–12.

94. Nelson KA, Glare PA, Walsh D, et al. A prospective, within-patient, crossover study of continuous intravenous and subcutaneous morphine for chronic cancer pain. *J Pain Symptom Manage* 1997;13(5):262–267.

95. Bruera E, Neumann CM, Pituskin E, et al. A randomized controlled trial of local injections of hyaluronidase versus placebo in cancer patients receiving subcutaneous hydration. *Ann Oncol* 1999;10(10):1255–1258.

96. Baker L, Lee M, Regnard C, et al. Evolving spinal analgesia practice in palliative care. *Palliat Med* 2004;18(6):507–515.

97. Burton AW, Rajagopal A, Shah HN, et al. Epidural and intrathecal analgesia is effective in treating refractory cancer pain [comment]. *Pain Med* 2004;5(3):239–247.

98. Smith TJ, Staats PS, Deer T, et al. Randomized clinical trial of an implantable drug delivery system compared with comprehensive medical management for refractory cancer pain: impact on pain, drug-related toxicity, and survival [comment]. *J Clin Oncol* 2002;20(19):4040–4049.

99. Kurita GP, Kaasa S, Sjogren P; for European Palliative Care Research Collaborative. Spinal opioids in adult patients with cancer pain: a systematic review: a European Palliative Care Research Collaborative (EPCRC) opioid guidelines project. *Palliat Med* 2011;25(5):560–577.

100. Zeppetella G, Porzio G, Aielli F. Opioids applied topically to painful cutaneous malignant ulcers in a palliative care setting. *Journal of Opioid Manag* 2007;3(3):161–166.

101. Zeppetella G, Ribeiro MD. Morphine in intrasite gel applied topically to painful ulcers. *J Pain Symptom Manage* 2005;29(2):118–119.

102. Ballas SK. Treatment of painful sickle cell leg ulcers with topical opioids. *Blood* 2002;99(3):1096.

103. Vernassiere C, Cornet C, Trechot P, et al. Study to determine the efficacy of topical morphine on painful chronic skin ulcers. *J Wound Care* 2005;14(6):289–293.

104. Ribeiro MD, Joel SP, Zeppetella G. The bioavailability of morphine applied topically to cutaneous ulcers. *J Pain Symptom Manage* 2004;27(5):434–439.

105. Paice JA, Von Roenn JH, Hudgins JC, et al. Morphine bioavailability from a topical gel formulation in volunteers. *J Pain Symptom Manage* 2008;35(3):314–320.

106. Hadley G, Derry S, Moore RA, et al. Transdermal fentanyl for cancer pain. *Cochrane Database Syst Rev* 2013;(10):CD010270.

107. Reddy A, Yennurajalingam S, Reddy S, et al. The opioid rotation ratio from transdermal fentanyl to "strong" opioids in patients with cancer pain. *J Pain Symptom Manage* 2016;51(6):1040–1045.

108. Morita T, Takigawa C, Onishi H, et al. Opioid rotation from morphine to fentanyl in delirious cancer patients: an open-label trial. *J Pain Symptom Manage* 2005;30(1):96–103.

109. Muijsers RB, Wagstaff AJ. Transdermal fentanyl: an updated review of its pharmacological properties and therapeutic efficacy in chronic cancer pain control. *Drugs* 2001;61(15):2289–2307.

110. Caraceni A, Hanks G, Kaasa S, et al. Use of opioid analgesics in the treatment of cancer pain: evidence-based recommendations from the EAPC. *Lancet Oncol* 2012;13(2):e58–e68.

111. Soleimanpour H, Safari S, Shahsavari Nia K, et al. Opioid drugs in patients with liver disease: a systematic review. *Hepat Mon* 2016;16(4):e32636.

112. Dean M. Opioids in renal failure and dialysis patients. *J Pain Symptom Manage* 2004;28(5):497–504.

113. Golf M, Paice JA, Feulner E, et al. Refractory status epilepticus. *J Palliat Med* 2004;7(1):85–88.

114. Nishigaya K, Kaneko M, Nagaseki Y, et al. Palatal myoclonus induced by extirpation of a cerebellar astrocytoma. Case report. *J Neurosurg* 1998;88(6):1107–1110.

115. Fontoura P, Vale J, Lima C, et al. Progressive myoclonic ataxia and JC virus encephalitis in an AIDS patient. *J Neurol Neurosurg Psychiatry* 2002;72(5):653–656.

116. Frucht SJ. The clinical challenge of posthypoxic myoclonus. *Adv Neurol* 2002;89:85–88.

117. Wyllie AR, Bayliff CD, Kovacs MJ. Myoclonus due to chlorambucil in two adults with lymphoma. *Ann Pharmacother* 1997;31(2):171–174.

118. Patel S, Roshan VR, Lee KC, et al. A myoclonic reaction with low-dose hydromorphone. *Ann Pharmacother* 2006;40(11):2068–2070.

119. Hofmann A, Tangri N, Lafontaine AL, et al. Myoclonus as an acute complication of low-dose hydromorphone in multiple system atrophy. *J Neurol Neurosurg Psychiatry* 2006;77(8):994–995.

120. Sarhill N, Davis MP, Walsh D, et al. Methadone-induced myoclonus in advanced cancer. *Am J Hosp Palliat Care* 2001;18(1):51–53.

121. Bruera E, Pereira J. Acute neuropsychiatric findings in a patient receiving fentanyl for cancer pain. *Pain* 1997;69(1–2):199–201.

122. Andersen G, Jensen NH, Christrup L, et al. Pain, sedation and morphine metabolism in cancer patients during long-term treatment with sustained-release morphine. *Palliat Med* 2002;16(2):107–114.

123. Han PK, Arnold R, Bond G, et al. Myoclonus secondary to withdrawal from transdermal fentanyl: case report and literature review. *J Pain Symptom Manage* 2002;23(1):66–72.

124. Sjøgren P, Thunedborg LP, Christrup L, et al. Is development of hyperalgesia, allodynia and myoclonus related to morphine metabolism during long-term administration? Six case histories. *Acta Anaesthesiol Scand* 1998;42(9):1070–1075.

125. Fainsinger R, Schoeller T, Boiskin M, et al. Palliative care round: cognitive failure and coma after renal failure in a patient receiving captopril and hydromorphone. *J Palliat Care* 1993;9(1):53–55.

126. Thwaites D, McCann S, Broderick P. Hydromorphone neuroexcitation. *J Palliat Med* 2004;7(4):545–550.

127. Smith MT. Neuroexcitatory effects of morphine and hydromorphone: evidence implicating the 3-glucuronide metabolites. *Clin Exp Pharmacol Physiol* 2000;27(7):524–528.

128. Babul N, Darke AC, Hagen N. Hydromorphone metabolite accumulation in renal failure. *J Pain Symptom Manage* 1995;10(3):184–186.

129. Portenoy RK, Foley KM, Stulman J, et al. Plasma morphine and morphine-6-glucuronide during chronic morphine therapy for cancer pain: plasma profiles, steady-state concentrations and the consequences of renal failure. *Pain* 1991;47(1):13–19.

130. Tiseo PJ, Thaler HT, Lapin J, et al. Morphine-6-glucuronide concentrations and opioid-related side effects: a survey in cancer patients. *Pain* 1995;61(1):47–54.

131. Wright AW, Mather LE, Smith MT. Hydromorphone-3-glucuronide: a more potent neuro-excitant than its structural analogue, morphine-3-glucuronide. *Life Sciences* 2001;69(4):409–420.

132. McCann S, Yaksh TL, von Gunten CF. Correlation between myoclonus and the 3-glucuronide metabolites in patients treated with morphine or hydromorphone: a pilot study. *J Opioid Manag* 2010;6(2):87–94.

133. Cherny N, Ripamonti C, Pereira J, et al. Strategies to manage the adverse effects of oral morphine: an evidence-based report. *J Clin Oncol* 2001;19(9):2542–2554.

134. Sjogren P, Jensen NH, Jensen TS. Disappearance of morphine-induced hyperalgesia after discontinuing or substituting morphine with other opioid agonists. *Pain* 1994;59(2):313–316.

135. Winegarden J, Carr DB, Bradshaw YS. Intravenous ketamine for rapid opioid dose reduction, reversal of opioid-induced neurotoxicity, and pain control in terminal care: case report and literature review. *Pain Med* 2016;17(4):644–649.

136. Eisele JH Jr, Grigsby EJ, Dea G. Clonazepam treatment of myoclonic contractions associated with high-dose opioids: case report [comment]. *Pain* 1992;49(2):231–232.

137. Moryl N, Coyle N, Foley KM. Managing an acute pain crisis in a patient with advanced cancer: "this is as much of a crisis as a code." *JAMA* 2008;299(12):1457–1467.

138. Linchitz RM, Raheb JC. Subcutaneous infusion of lidocaine provides effective pain relief for CRPS patients. *Clin J Pain* 1999;15(1):67–72.

139. Wu CL, Tella P, Staats PS, et al. Analgesic effects of intravenous lidocaine and morphine on postamputation pain: a randomized double-blind, active placebo-controlled, crossover trial. *Anesthesiology* 2002;96(4):841–848.

140. Baranowski AP, De Courcey J, Bonello E. A trial of intravenous lidocaine on the pain and allodynia of postherpetic neuralgia. *J Pain Symptom Manage* 1999;17(6):429–433.

141. Ferrini R. Parenteral lidocaine for severe intractable pain in 6 hospice patients continued at home. *J Palliat Med* 1999;3(2):193–201.

142. Tei Y, Morita T, Shishido H, et al. Lidocaine intoxication at very small doses in terminally ill cancer patients. *J Pain Symptom Manage* 2005;30(1):6–7.

143. Seah DSE, Herschtal A, Tran H, et al. Subcutaneous lidocaine infusion for pain in patients with cancer. *J Palliat Med* 2017;20(6):667–671.

144. Massey GV, Pedigo S, Dunn NL, et al. Continuous lidocaine infusion for the relief of refractory malignant pain in a terminally ill pediatric cancer patient. *J Pediatr Hematol Oncol* 2002;24(7):566–568.

145. Gibbons K, DeMonbrun A, Beckman EJ, et al. Continuous lidocaine infusions to manage opioid-refractory pain in a series of cancer patients in a pediatric hospital. *Pediatr Blood Cancer* 2016;63(7):1168–1174.

146. Bruera E, Ripamonti C, Brenneis C, et al. A randomized double-blind crossover trial of intravenous lidocaine in the treatment of neuropathic cancer pain. *J Pain Symptom Manage* 1992;7(3):138–140.

147. Lossignol DA, Obiols-Portis M, Body JJ. Successful use of ketamine for intractable cancer pain. *Support Care Cancer* 2005;13(3):188–193.

148. Kotlinska-Lemieszek A, Luczak J. Subanesthetic ketamine: an essential adjuvant for intractable cancer pain [comment]. *J Pain Symptom Manage* 2004;28(2):100–102.

149. Mercadante S, Arcuri E, Tirelli W, et al. Analgesic effect of intravenous ketamine in cancer patients on morphine therapy: a randomized, controlled, double-blind, crossover, double-dose study. *J Pain Symptom Manage* 2000;20(4):246–252.

150. Finkel JC, Pestieau SR, Quezado ZM. Ketamine as an adjuvant for treatment of cancer pain in children and adolescents. *J Pain* 2007;8(6):515–521.

151. Hardy J, Quinn S, Fazekas B, et al. Randomized, double-blind, placebo-controlled study to assess the efficacy and toxicity of subcutaneous ketamine in the management of cancer pain. *J Clin Oncol* 2012;30(29):3611–3617.

152. Bell RF, Eccleston C, Kalso EA. Ketamine as an adjuvant to opioids for cancer pain. *Cochrane Database Syst Rev* 2017;(6):CD003351.

153. Estfan B, Mahmoud F, Shaheen P, et al. Respiratory function during parenteral opioid titration for cancer pain. *Palliat Med* 2007;21(2):81–86.

154. Sykes N, Thorns A. The use of opioids and sedatives at the end of life. *Lancet Oncol* 2003;4(5):312–318.

155. Thorns A, Sykes N. Opioid use in last week of life and implications for end-of-life decision-making. *Lancet* 2000;356(9227):398–399.

156. Portenoy RK, Sibirceva U, Smout R, et al. Opioid use and survival at the end of life: a survey of a hospice population. *J Pain Symptom Manage* 2006;32(6):532–540.

157. Azoulay D, Jacobs JM, Cialic R, et al. Opioids, survival, and advanced cancer in the hospice setting. *J Am Med Dir Assoc* 2011;12(2):129–134.

158. Lopez-Saca JM, Guzman JL, Centeno C. A systematic review of the influence of opioids on advanced cancer patient survival. *Curr Opin Support Palliat Care* 2013;7(4):424–430.

159. Krikorian A, Limonero JT, Mate J. Suffering and distress at the end-of-life. *Psychooncology* 2012;21(8):799–808.

160. Coyle N. The hard work of living in the face of death. *J Pain Symptom Manage* 2006;32(3):266–274.
161. Terry W, Olson LG. Unobvious wounds: the suffering of hospice patients. *Intern Med J* 2004;34(11):604–607.
162. Strang P, Strang S, Hultborn R, et al. Existential pain—an entity, a provocation, or a challenge? *J Pain Symptom Manage* 2004;27(3):241–250.
163. Wilson KG, Chochinov HM, McPherson CJ, et al. Suffering with advanced cancer. *J Clin Oncol* 2007;25(13):1691–1697.
164. Schroepfer TA. Critical events in the dying process: the potential for physical and psychosocial suffering. *J Palliat Med* 2007;10(1):136–147.
165. Al-Shahri MZ, Molina EH, Oneschuk D. Medication-focused approach to total pain: poor symptom control, polypharmacy, and adverse reactions. *Am J Hosp Palliat Care* 2003;20(4):307–310.
166. Chochinov HM. Dignity and the essence of medicine: the A, B, C, and D of dignity conserving care [comment]. *BMJ* 2007;335(7612):184–187.
167. Chochinov HM, Kristjanson LJ, Breitbart W, et al. Effect of dignity therapy on distress and end-of-life experience in terminally ill patients: a randomised controlled trial. *Lancet Oncol* 2011;12(8):753–762.
168. Chochinov HM, Hack T, Hassard T, et al. Dignity therapy: a novel psychotherapeutic intervention for patients near the end of life [comment]. *J Clin Oncol* 2005;23(24):5520–5525.
169. McClement S, Chochinov HM, Hack T, et al. Dignity therapy: family member perspectives. *J Palliat Med* 2007;10(5):1076–1082.
170. Syrjala KL, Jensen MP, Mendoza ME, et al. Psychological and behavioral approaches to cancer pain management. *J Clin Oncol* 2014;32(16):1703–1711.
171. Kwekkeboom KL, Bumpus M, Wanta B, et al. Oncology nurses' use of nondrug pain interventions in practice. *J Pain Symptom Manage* 2008;35(1):83–94.
172. Kwekkeboom KL, Kneip J, Pearson L. A pilot study to predict success with guided imagery for cancer pain. *Pain Manag Nurs* 2003;4(3):112–123.
173. Lafferty WE, Downey L, McCarty RL, et al. Evaluating CAM treatment at the end of life: a review of clinical trials for massage and meditation. *Complement Ther Med* 2006;14(2):100–112.
174. Spiegel D, Moore R. Imagery and hypnosis in the treatment of cancer patients. *Oncology (Williston Park)* 1997;11(8):1179–1195.
175. Bradt J, Dileo C, Magill L, et al. Music interventions for improving psychological and physical outcomes in cancer patients. *Cochrane Database Syst Rev* 2016;(8):CD006911.
176. Magill L. The meaning of the music: the role of music in palliative care music therapy as perceived by bereaved caregivers of advanced cancer patients. *Am J Hosp Palliat Care* 2009;26(1):33–39.
177. Magill L, Berenson S. The conjoint use of music therapy and reflexology with hospitalized advanced stage cancer patients and their families. *Palliat Support Care* 2008;6(3):289–296.
178. Nainis N, Paice JA, Ratner J, et al. Relieving symptoms in cancer: innovative use of art therapy. *J Pain Symptom Manage* 2006;31(2):162–169.
179. Deng G, Cassileth BR, Yeung KS. Complementary therapies for cancer-related symptoms. *J Support Oncol* 2004;2(5):419–429.
180. Post-White J, Kinney ME, Savik K, et al. Therapeutic massage and healing touch improve symptoms in cancer. *Integr Cancer Ther* 2003;2(4):332–344.
181. Polubinski JP, West L. Implementation of a massage therapy program in the home hospice setting. *J Pain Symptom Manage* 2005;30(1):104–106.
182. Zappa SB, Cassileth BR. Complementary approaches to palliative oncological care. *J Nurs Care Qual* 2003;18(1):22–26.
183. Meek SS. Effects of slow stroke back massage on relaxation in hospice clients. *Image* 1993;25(1):17–21.
184. Keefe FJ, Ahles TA, Porter LS, et al. The self-efficacy of family caregivers for helping cancer patients manage pain at end-of-life. *Pain* 2003;103(1–2):157–162.
185. Keefe FJ, Ahles TA, Sutton L, et al. Partner-guided cancer pain management at the end of life: a preliminary study. *J Pain Symptom Manage* 2005;29(3):263–272.
186. Kwekkeboom KL, Gretarsdottir E. Systematic review of relaxation interventions for pain. *J Nurs Scholarsh* 2006;38(3):269–277.
187. Cherny NI, Group EGW. ESMO Clinical Practice Guidelines for the management of refractory symptoms at the end of life and the use of palliative sedation. *Ann Oncol* 2014;25(Suppl 3):iii143–iii152.
188. American Academy of Hospice and Palliative Medicine. Statement on palliative sedation. Available at: http://aahpm.org/positions/palliative-sedation. Accessed June 29, 2017.
189. Lundstrom S, Zachrisson U, Furst CJ. When nothing helps: propofol as sedative and antiemetic in palliative cancer care. *J Pain Symptom Manage* 2005;30(6):570–577.
190. Baker MT, Naguib M. Propofol: the challenges of formulation. *Anesthesiology* 2005;103(4):860–876.
191. Morita T, Ikenaga M, Adachi I, et al. Family experience with palliative sedation therapy for terminally ill cancer patients. *J Pain Symptom Manage* 2004;28(6):557–565.
192. Bruinsma SM, van der Heide A, van der Lee ML, et al. No negative impact of palliative sedation on relatives' experience of the dying phase and their wellbeing after the patient's death: an observational study. *PLoS One* 2016;11(2):e0149250.
193. World Health Organization. *Cancer Pain Relief.* Geneva, Switzerland: World Health Organization; 1996.
194. Paice JA, Ferrell B. The management of cancer pain. *CA Cancer J Clin* 2011;61(3):157–182.
195. Paice JA, Portenoy R, Lacchetti C, et al. Management of chronic pain in survivors of adult cancers: American Society of Clinical Oncology clinical practice guideline. *J Clin Oncol* 2016;34:3325–3345.
196. Portenoy RK. Treatment of cancer pain. *Lancet* 2011;377(9784):2236–2247.
197. Rousseau P. Palliative sedation in the management of refractory symptoms. *J Support Oncol* 2004;2(2):181–186.

CHAPTER 110

Ethical Principles that Support Decision Making in Pain Management: The Case of Stopping Opioids

FAYE M. WEINSTEIN, CLAUDIA KOHNER, and **STEVEN H. RICHEIMER**

New findings about long-term opioid use, as well as the new Centers for Disease Control and Prevention (CDC) Guidelines for Prescribing Opioids for Chronic Pain,[1] are encouraging physicians to consider tapering or weaning opioid treatment for chronic pain patients.[2,3] This process of weaning opioids can be difficult for both the patient and the physician. The physical difficulties are addressed elsewhere, but the ethical and emotional difficulties are rarely discussed. Although there is information in the literature about ethical considerations and establishing trust with a patient when *starting* a patient on opioids,[4] we also need to understand the issues involved in *stopping* opioid medication in a manner that maintains physician–patient trust and ethical practice. Using a practical framework to address these ethical and emotional issues can help the physician avoid missteps that may result in disruption to the physician–patient relationship and may lead to unwanted results, such as patient lack of receptivity to other treatment options, patient difficulty with the titration regimen, and/or patient dissatisfaction.

Background

Gunderman,[5,6] a physician who writes on the ethics of the business of medicine and leadership in medicine, has used Erik Erikson's ideals as a platform for his formulations. Erikson is credited with contributions to the fields of psychology, religion, and ethics.[7] Erikson's version of the Golden Rule includes a "concern with universal justice and respect for the other, where every person deserves recognition and mutual regard."[8(p153)]

Following Gunderman's[5,6] lead, the authors of this chapter use Erikson's ethical theory to help guide the physician–patient relationship during opioid cessation. Case vignettes of physicians taking patients off opioid medication, along with analyses of the vignettes, are presented in order to guide the reader in ethical analysis grounded in Erikson's ethical theory. Tools for building mutuality in the physician–patient relationship are also covered.

MEDICAL ETHICS AND ERIKSON'S GOLDEN RULE

Medical ethics is typically discussed in terms of autonomy, beneficence, and justice. The authors of this chapter believe that Erik Erikson's approach will provide a more practical framework.

Erikson presented his theory of the Golden Rule at the George W. Gay Lecture Upon Medical Ethics, at Harvard Medical School on May 4, 1962. Erikson's reformulation of the Golden Rule emphasizes mutuality between the physician and patient. For Erikson, medical ethics involves not only rational decision making but also ideals related to a higher good.[9] Ethical acts are grounded in a sense of justice, a universal sense of responsibility toward all human beings, and the need for mutual respect and recognition.[10] Erikson emphasized partnership and mutuality in the physician–patient relationship, which provide the opportunity for growth in both the physician and

patient and bidirectional trust between physician and patient. For Erikson,[10(p233)] the Golden Rule encourages that "it is best to do to another what will strengthen you even as it will strengthen him—that is, what will develop his best potentials even as it develops your own."

Two primary elements of Erikson's Golden Rule are trust and mutuality.[11] Investigating an ethical approach to a medical decision to stop the use of opioids begins with an understanding of these components of ethical practice.

TRUST

According to Erikson, over an individual's life span, an "individual develops the propensity for ethics as he passes through eight (developmental) stages."[12(p171)] Developmental experiences in infancy involving trust with caregivers form the bedrock on which the later seven psychosocial stages will be experienced.[13] To develop a sense of trust, infants must be able to count on their caregivers to feed them, soothe them, arouse or quiet them when needed, and mirror smiles and babbles.[14] In an optimal environment, the infant learns that the world is generally a safe and consistent place and that people are mostly "good." The infant gains the strength of "hope," which is the perception that, even if there is waiting, one's needs will be met and other people can be relied on to be responsive to the one's needs. Over the life span, trust is transformed and provides a guiding principle for daily life and relationships with others.[15]

However, people with less optimal early lives may learn that their needs will not be met and that people are unreliable; these individuals may develop mistrust in their relationships as adults. Chronic pain patients may have a greater likelihood of histories of early challenges in developing trust[16] and, therefore, go through life burdened with vulnerability to mistrust.[17]

Trust is one of the central features of the physician–patient relationship.[18] Sass, a philosopher and ethicist, states that "trust becomes the overriding principle and virtue that establishes and safeguards all expert-lay interactions, particularly in the clinic."[19(p354)]

Patient trust in a physician manifests as the expectation that the physician will behave in a way that makes it safe for the patient to take the risk of sharing personal information. Dimensions of physician behavior on which patients are believed to base their trust in their physician are "competence, compassion, reliability and dependability, and communication."[18(p509)] Pearson and Raeke[18] identify the importance of interpersonal trust, the trust built through repeated interactions with a physician within which the patient learns over time that his or her needs will be met in a predictable and consistent way despite changes in the medical environment that may threaten trust.

O'Neill[20] also describes trust building as a dynamic activity and views physician trust as a partnership. *Physician trust in a patient* is not only determined by the trustworthiness of the patient but can also be influenced by external factors, including media events, current research, racial bias,[21,22] practices of colleagues, and the physicians' own experiences.[23] With each patient, the physician's trust is based on the assumption that the patient's motive is pain reduction and improvement in function and that the patient is truthful in his or her self-report of symptoms and prior treatment. Trust is confirmed via observation of patient adherence to a treatment plan, patient efforts at participation in treatment, and prompt patient communication with the physician if problems arise.[4]

MUTUALITY

According to Erikson,[10(p231)] the relationship between the parent and the infant involves mutuality, which is a bidirectional process by which the "partners depend on each other for the development of their respective strengths." Relevant to the focus of this chapter, Erikson[10(p231)] asserts, "The fact is that the mutuality of adult and baby is the original source of hope, the basic ingredient of all effective as well as ethical human action." The parent tries to understand the variety of needs in the child in regard to soothing, eating, sleeping, and elimination. Parent and infant work to read each other's signals and to learn to regulate the amount of time that passes between the expression of the need and satisfaction of the need. The work of creating mutuality of interaction and communication is characterized as a process of coordination, mismatch, and repair.[24] Mutuality emerges from patterns of physical (e.g., eye gaze, proximity, offering food), verbal (patterns of speaking/vocalizing and responding), and affective (e.g., smiling) expressions. Erikson[10] emphasized that through mutuality, the parent reinforces his or her own sense of trust or revisits issues of mistrust. Thus, mutuality is the focus on the relationship with others that becomes a source of information about one's identity and interactions with others.

Over the life span, mutuality is not exclusive to parent–child relationships but manifests in different types of adult relationships, where mutuality means "personal recognition, joint work, effective communication, and understanding and respect for each other's roles."[25(p741)]

MORALS AND ETHICS

Erikson[10] differentiated between morals and ethics, with ethics emerging developmentally later than morals. In early life, the child not only learns to trust whether needs will be met and comfort will be given. She or he also learns that caregivers are a source of limit setting. The child internalizes these prohibitions, forming the basis of morals, which are identified as behaviors based on fear of consequences, such as "threats of abandonment, punishment and public exposure, or a threatening inner sense of guilt, of shame or of isolation."[10(p222)] In adolescence, an individual starts to transition from moral to ethical behavior, with behaviors and relationships based on rigid ideas and ideologic devotion (e.g., "all my friends do this"). Finally, in adulthood, the individual can become less ruled by rigid ideals and becomes more able to act and relate to others on the basis of individual worth and dignity. According to Erikson,[10] this is the development of the "ethical sense."

Erikson's distinction between morals and ethics resonates with Smith and Newton's[26] three-phase evolution of physician ethics. According to these authors, the Hippocratic Oath was the initial structure for the physician–patient relationship with the "notion of authority,"[26(p47)] or paternalism, toward the patient. Following a cultural shift to individualism, the focus of ethical inquiry turned to patient autonomy, the second phase in Smith and Newton's[26] three-phase evolution of physician ethics. This led to rigid moral rules and formulas for the physician to follow in a heightened climate of the protection of patient rights. Smith and Newton[26] consider this era as the "essential formative period"[26(p44)] for the emergence of the third phase in their three-phase evolution of physicians ethics, one that is

focused less on applying rules and more on valuing "mutuality,"[26(p56)] "reflective experience,"[26(p56)] and "goals of human dignity and dialogue"[26(p56)]—concepts in line with the foci of this chapter.

Erikson's ethical sense has particular relevance when tested during crises in which interactions with others trigger earlier psychosocial tensions about trust. A physician-initiated cessation of a chronic pain patient's opioid prescription is potentially such a crisis. At this medical juncture, issues of trust, mutuality, and the ethical sense are salient for both patient and physician.

With its focus on trust and mutuality, Erikson's Golden Rule can serve as the ethical foundation for the navigation of the medical crossroad of cessation of opioid prescription in chronic pain patients. It provides a way to find resolution to the tension that arises in this situation, to manage the dynamic activity of trust, to build a partnership, and to promote mutual growth.

Case Vignettes and Analysis

Three cases—each involving a type of challenge faced by physicians who deal with cessation of opioid use for chronic pain patients—are presented and evaluated to assess whether Erikson's tenets of trust and mutuality in his concept of the Golden Rule are evident or absent and whether the physician was functioning from a moral sense or an ethical sense.

Table 110.1 lists the criteria—in the form of questions—that will be used in assessing the cases for Erikson's tenets of trust and mutuality in the "Analysis" section for each of the three cases. Criteria numbers in parentheses will be included in the analyses to link the concepts in the analyses to the criteria. The purpose of these criteria is to provide a framework for thinking about the basic concepts of Erikson's ethical theory in relation to the three cases.

CASE 1: OPIOID-INDUCED HYPERALGESIA
Background and First Attempt at Change of Treatment Plan to Opioid Cessation

Ms. R is a 51-year-old married woman with a history of neck and low back pain. She had been treated for about a year by Dr. T for pain related to cervical and lumbar spondylosis, facet arthropathy, myofascial pain, and fibromyalgia. Ms. R travels a long distance to see Dr. T, and she has communicated to her that it is worth spending the time in traffic to see her because Dr. T is the first doctor who really listens to her and takes her needs into account in making medical decisions. Ms. R's pain medications had been oxycodone 30 mg four times a day, gabapentin 600 mg two times a day, and 50 μg fentanyl patch 50 μg per hour every 72 hours. Two visits prior to the visit that is the focus of this discussion, in response to a pain flare, Dr. T increased Ms. R's medication to fentanyl patch 100 μg per hour every 48 hours. In the next visit, Ms. R reported an improved pain score. However, in the following visit, Ms. R was tearful, complained of worse pain, and reported 9 to 10/10 pain on the pain numeric rating scale, and she communicated that she was having trouble getting to the store, socializing, and dealing with her son's move out of the

---

home to college. As Dr. T reviewed prior notes in the computer, she responded that despite the increase in the opioids, Ms. R had not improved in pain level or in function. Dr. T added that the patient may have developed opioid-induced hyperalgesia. Dr. T concluded that the patient needed to titrate completely off the fentanyl patch and go on an opioid holiday before Dr. T could reevaluate Ms. R for the need to be on chronic opioids. Dr. T noted in the computer that Ms. R was very reluctant to follow her advice and told Ms. R that, at this point, she did not think there were other options, saying, "There is nothing more that I can offer you." Dr. T looked up from her computer and recommended an immediate wean of fentanyl from 100 μg per hour to 75 μg per hour patch, decreasing to 50 μg per hour in 1 month, 25 μg per hour in 2 months, and then off. Ms. R said that she could not believe that Dr. T would do this to her at this point, as she is a parent, too, and from their time together, they have talked about the difficulty of a child leaving home. Dr. T and Ms. R had talked in previous visits about the patient's son's impending move from home. Dr. T encouraged Ms. R to find other coping mechanisms to deal with her pain, perhaps regular exercise, such as swimming. Ms. R became tearful, saying that she did not know what went wrong, that before Dr. T was so understanding, and now she is unwilling to help and is acting as if she does not know her anymore. Ms. R challenged the assessment of hyperalgesia and expressed fear that without opioids her pain could not be managed.

Physician Consultation with a Colleague

After the visit, Dr. T felt unsettled by the interaction with Mr. R and consulted with a colleague about the visit. Dr. T said that the visit "just felt wrong" despite her confidence in the treatment plan. She admitted that she felt betrayed by the patient's resistance to her offer of help and that the patient no longer trusted her judgment. Her colleague asked her, "What was different for you in the visit?" Dr. T said that she felt disengaged from the patient and that she was "just doing the mission of medicine." She reflected on what Ms. R's experience of the interaction had been. She pondered whether Ms. R also felt accused of poor judgment or pressured about this sudden treatment change. Dr. T then recalled that she did not engage the patient in their usual discussion about family or how the patient could navigate yet another change.

Dr. T reflected on the themes of trust and betrayal that permeated both her and Ms. R's perspectives. The consultation with her colleague and consequent self-reflection allowed Dr. T to not only attend to her own feelings but also to reevaluate the interaction with Ms. R.

Modification in Engagement with Patient and Treatment Plan following the Consultation and Reflection

During the next visit with Ms. R, Dr. T asked her how her son was doing. Ms. R smiled and responded, and in a few moments, they began to discuss the treatment plan from the last session. Ms. R reported that she felt that she could not yet stop the fentanyl patch, but she proudly reported that, despite sweating from the titration, she had decreased her oxycodone, showing Dr. T the bottle with many pills left over. Dr. T praised Ms. R's success in cutting back on oxycodone. She requested Ms. R's input on what timing for titration of fentanyl would enhance her continued success. Ms. R said that she is going to visit her son so she can see with her own eyes that he has settled in and is doing well. Ms. R expressed that waiting until after she visited her son would be helpful to her. Dr. T praised Ms. R for her self-reflection and insight regarding the postponement of titration until after her visit to her son. Dr. T utilized Ms. R's perspective to reconsider the treatment plan and postponed

weaning off of opioids. Dr. T prescribed a clonidine 0.1 mg patch to help with sweating and communicated to Ms. R the plan to begin the titration after the visit to her son, when she has adjusted better to the stressors currently affecting her life.

Analysis

Within the framework of the ethical principles described earlier, we can see that in the visit in which Dr. T initially changed the treatment plan to stop opioid use, she failed to use trust-building modes of communication with the patient, which disrupted the trust that had been built in this physician–patient relationship (C3). Threats to trust in adulthood may trigger vulnerabilities that formed early in life and lead to frustration in the current situation. Despite this difficulty, Erikson's Golden Rule suggests that challenges to trust, especially in a situation where there is disruption to an expected receipt of care, can be optimized by both the patient and the physician engaging in strategies to facilitate trust, to draw on the history of trust built in the physician–patient relationship (C3). During the disruptive office visit, Dr. T was driven by the pressure and frustration she felt about the appropriate use of opioids (her goal) and failed to consider how her stance would impact Ms. R (C1, C4).

Physicians may adopt various stances when engaging with patients during difficult encounters, especially if the physician feels his or her knowledge is being challenged or if the physician feels that his or her ability to treat the patient is being undermined.[27] Many physicians act in a paternalistic fashion as a first-line response when perceiving urgency to minimize risk and harm.[28] The ethical nature of this type of physician behavior is questionable because it fails to take into account the impact on the patient of the physician's decision making. Time with patients is limited, creating additional pressure to adopt a forceful stance in order to quickly communicate a judgment so that the patient will make a behavior change.[27] And for some physicians, offering up the rules of opioid prescribing is a stance to demonstrate the veracity of their decision.[26] Lorenzetti et al.[27] reinforce the need to adopt principles of empathy and effective communication and thus foster a relationship so that these stances are not needed.

In this case, Dr. T reinforced her decision via an ultimatum that Ms. R must comply or nothing else would be offered in the relationship, which represented a failure to recognize Ms. R's perspective (C4). This ultimatum left no room for Ms. R to consider the rationale behind the decision, and she responded as if she were being punished (C2).

In Dr. T's efforts to provide what she identified as appropriate care, she did not consider that this represented to Ms. R a drastic change in care and in the relationship (C4). Dr. T did not interact with Ms. R as she had in the past, when the context and home life of the patient had been discussed, physician behaviors that promoted Ms. R's trust in Dr. T (C3). Dr. T did not seem to be aware that this shift in style of engagement with Ms. R would be difficult for Ms. R (C4), and Dr. T may have assumed that Ms. R would automatically follow the titration plan. This lack of awareness by Dr. T was interpreted by Ms. R as a violation of the trust in how care was offered. The interaction shifted from being predictable and consistent—an interaction in which Dr. T's empathy was accessible to Ms. R—to Ms. R coming to feel not being known and forced into a care plan not based on her needs (C1, C2, C3, C4). Unfortunately, with this breach of trust, Ms. R expressed reluctance to accept the change in treatment plan that Dr. T recommended (C2). Despite Dr. T's attempt to provide education about the rationale for the change, Ms. R felt as if the "decision had nothing to do with her or her needs" (C4).

As a result of Dr. T's consultation with a colleague, she was able to return to her previous fostering of trust and mutuality in her relationship with Ms. R. This made it more likely for Dr. T to achieve an ethical state with Ms. R (C5). A first step for Dr. T was to identify trust issues for both her and Ms. R (C3). This is a difficult step—it requires the physician to carefully examine the issues. It would be ideal if physicians could do this before a potentially problematic interaction, but at least a distraught patient can be a signal that the doctor should step back and reflect on interpersonal issues with a patient. In fact, Dr. T. took a close look at where she might have missed signals of need and distress from Ms. R. She also identified where there had been disruption in their usual relationship (C4). In the visit after the consultation, which from Dr. T's side included the yield from Dr. T's reflection on what had happened with Ms. R in the previous visit, Dr. T actively engaged with Ms. R, creating a dialogue, asking for Ms. R's perspective, and providing a direct response to Ms. R's feedback (C3, C4). Dr. T validated for Ms. R her attempts to manage her feelings about her son's transition (C4). With renewal of trust and mutuality in the engagement, the effectiveness and ethical quality of the treatment were both enhanced (C5).

CASE 2: CHANGE IN THE CENTERS FOR DISEASE CONTROL AND PREVENTION GUIDELINES

Background

The office manager of a family medicine practice received a call from the Risk Management Department about Mr. B, a patient of Dr. J. Mr. B's complaint stated that his opioid medication had been stopped by Dr. J, a physician in the medical practice, because of the new CDC guidelines. Mr. B has a history of complex regional pain syndrome (CRPS) and had been treated by Dr. J for many years. The office manager recalled their struggle to find a treatment regimen that worked for Mr. B and Mr. B's success at stopping smoking in an effort to control pain symptoms. Mr. B reported to Risk Management that Dr. J told him that Dr. J had become too scared of the CDC and Drug Enforcement Administration (DEA) to prescribe opioids any longer. Mr. B feared not getting adequate pain control without opioids. He started smoking again because he was so upset. Mr. B told Risk Management that Dr. J offered an epidural injection, but Mr. B is still waiting for the insurance company to authorize this treatment.

Analysis

In this case, the physician had difficulty coping with an unexpected change in prescribing guidelines. Dr. J felt angry and trapped. After many years of practice, based on then-current guidelines about the appropriateness of long-term use of opioids, he now had a large cohort of long-term patients who are taking opioids. With the change in CDC guidelines, based on new evidence of the pitfalls of long-term use of opioids, Dr. J felt that he was being blamed by the CDC for getting his patients dependent on a type of medication that is not good for long-term use.

Using the perspective of Erikson's Golden Rule, Dr. J's own sense of trust in the foundations of how to practice ethically in pain management was threatened by shifting CDC guidelines. In this particular case, he may have been revisiting a crisis of trust similar to ones that he had experienced in prior situations where the rules had been changed. His frustration about the unexpected demands from the CDC guidelines impaired his ability to maintain trust in his prescribing of opioid medication. With Mr. B, he made an abrupt decision to stop prescribing opioids based on his perception of the rigid expectation of the CDC authority (meeting Dr. J's goals), instead of engaging in self-reflection and trust-building communication with his patient (C1, C3). Dr. J's conformity to a rigid ideology and his inflexibility in his application of the CDC guidelines left him lost in defensiveness and rejection of his patient, unable to shift into the "unique needs of the present moment" (C5).[12(p172)]

Dr. J functioned with the moral sense of young adulthood rather than with the ethical sense of later adulthood, leaving Mr. B feeling so abandoned by and angry at Dr. J (C2) that Mr. B filed a complaint against Dr. J.

Had Dr. J functioned according to Erikson's Golden Rule, there would have been alternative approaches to dealing with the situation with the potential for more beneficial outcomes for this crisis. Specifically, had Dr. J reflected on his and Mr. B's prior successful experience with smoking cessation, Dr. J could have talked to Mr. B about Mr. B having been able previously to tolerate a painful loss of a substance he had relied on, which would have been an interaction that would have strengthened both patient and physician (C5). This discussion could have laid a foundation for Mr. B facing the prospect of cessation of opioids. Furthermore, Dr. J could have reminded Mr. B that he had been able weather this challenge because of his trust (C3) in Dr. J and that after cessation of smoking, Mr. B had noted some reduction in his pain. By "renewing prior achievements in trust,"[15(p255)] Dr. J could have helped Mr. B counteract his sense of distrust in his ability to manage the situation as well as his sense of distrust in the physician. This alternative approach could have avoided the breakdown in Mr. B's trust in Dr. J and subsequent call to Risk Management (C3).

In terms of the threat of the change in CDC guidelines to Dr. J as a physician, another possibility would have been for Dr. J to reflect on how hard it is for him and for other physicians to cope with the change in CDC guidelines regarding prescribing opioids, especially when what they were taught and practiced is now being identified as wrong. He might have identified that all of these changes make him feel off-kilter and, in addition, that he has to get used to the change in his practice. Although this is difficult, he could have recalled that he had navigated similar challenges in the past. For instance, as a family medicine physician, Dr. J had had to change how he prescribed antibiotics.[29] That transition had been difficult, but Dr. J had felt backed up by science and was able to adapt. If Dr. J could have identified that he has survived prior challenges, he could have drawn on these previous experiences to remind him of his achievements. He could have reapplied the same coping he had used to survive the other situations to the current situation, which would have strengthened both him and his patient (C5).

Applying the concept of mutuality would have been useful. Mr. B may have appreciated hearing Dr. J say that he saw how the change could be upsetting to the patient and that he (Dr. J) is distressed at the changing rules. This bidirectional sharing could have been strengthening for both patient and physician and could have contributed to both the effectiveness and ethicality of the handling of the crisis (C4, C5).

CASE 3: OPIOID PRESCRIPTIONS FROM OTHER PHYSICIANS FOUND IN CHECK OF STATE DRUG MONITORING PROGRAM

Background

Ms. A, a single woman in her 30s, came to Dr. S after extensive treatment by another pain specialist. She had chronic low back pain associated with post-laminectomy, or failed back syndrome. Her insurance no longer covered her prior physician. She was on high doses of opioids—higher than Dr. S usually prescribed. Her prior medical records documented Ms. A's report that she had not responded to various spinal injections or to physical therapy, but she was stable on fentanyl patch, 75 μg every 3 days plus hydrocodone/acetaminophen 10/300 three times a day. Dr. S found himself struggling with issues of prejudging—Ms. A was heavily tattooed and not working, and there was no clear pain source for her chronic pain. Dr. S had to make a conscious effort to not to assume—based on appearances—that the patient was inappropriately seeking opioids. Dr. S explained to Ms. A his concerns for safety given her opioid dose of approximately

180-mg morphine equivalents per day. He specifically addressed the issue of hyperalgesia and his long-term goal of her coming off opioids completely. Ms. A said that the only helpful treatment for her pain is opioids, and she did not want to come off of them completely. They agreed to go down slowly. Dr. S was willing to prescribe her medications if she would agree to lower her fentanyl dose over the next 2 months to 50 μg every 3 days. Ms. A also signed a standardized treatment agreement, which includes informing the signer that all controlled substances must be prescribed by Dr. S. Ms. A also signed that she understood that Dr. S would monitor her for usage of any controlled substances by any other provider.

Dr. S continued to prescribe these medications for the next year, until a check of the state drug monitoring program revealed three extra prescriptions for hydrocodone/acetaminophen 10/300 mg from other physicians. Ms. A's violation of the treatment agreement led Dr. S initially to feel that Ms. A could not be trusted. However, he reminded himself that there is a difference between not being trustworthy at all and not being trustworthy to handle a specific drug. Ms. A might be trusted with other drugs and procedures.

Dr. S anticipated that when he brought the results of the check of the state drug monitoring program to Ms. A's attention, she would angrily deny the problem and then storm out of the office, never to return. Dr. S braced himself for Ms. A's anger at her next office visit. In fact, at first, Ms. A did deny the extra prescriptions, but not angrily, and then she apologized for the "mistake" and promised to not "mess up" again. Dr. S explained to Ms. A that she is not a safe candidate for opioids. He told her that he would be happy to continue to treat her but without opioids. Again, Dr. S braced himself for anger, but to his surprise, Ms. A said, "Okay doc," and she continued to treat with Dr. S.

Over the next few months, Dr. S started Ms. A on physical therapy and pain psychology (which she discontinued after two sessions) and tried facet joint injections. Ms. A reported that none of these treatments was helpful, and after a few months, she started requesting that they resume opioids because the pain is so bad. Dr. S continues to wrestle with himself that perhaps this is one of the relatively few patients who do benefit from long-term opioids, but he reminds himself and Ms. A that opioids are too seductive and dangerous for her. Ms. A is not happy that Dr. S continues to decline to prescribe opioids, but she has continued to treat with Dr. S, and the state drug monitoring program indicates that she is not receiving opioids anywhere else. Dr. S feels good that Ms. A has "stuck with me."

Analysis

In this case, Dr. S's insight and self-reflection, which laid the foundation for sound communications with Ms. A (C3), helped him to effectively and ethically deal with a variety of trust-related issues regarding opioid use and cessation. Some of the trust issues were related to himself, and others stemmed from the patient's presentation and actions. The patient's unclear pain source, use of a high level of opioids, and prejudice-triggering appearance caused concern for Dr. S about whether he could trust Ms. A. In order to clearly see and respond to her needs, Dr. S had to contain his initial reaction that she was an untrustworthy patient. However, Dr. S reflected on his impulse to mistrust and waited for more input before reacting. He saw that the patient spoke reasonably about her use of opioids and that her medical records correlated with her self-report. Dr. S's capacity to wait created (1) a space for more information about the patient to emerge, (2) a physician–patient dialogue about safety, and (3) the patient signing a treatment agreement—three factors that had the potential to enhance mutual trust between patient and physician (C3). This trust

may have helped Ms. A to agree to the initial titration of the fentanyl and have a reasonable reaction when confronted with obtaining opioids from other sources (C2). When Ms. A went against the treatment agreement, Dr. S initially felt a sense that she could not be trusted. However, he tried to understand her perspective of trying many treatments without results (C4). He reminded himself that there is a difference between not being trustworthy at all and being a person who cannot be trusted to handle a specific drug. Dr. S reasoned that Ms. A could be trusted with other drugs and procedures that he offered but not with opioids. His continued relationship with Ms. A enhanced his confidence in his decision not to prescribe opioids for her. Dr. S continues to feel good that the patient has stayed in treatment with him (C5).

Of particular note in this case is Dr. S's success in both avoiding behaviors that could have triggered feelings of abandonment in the patient and in implementing limit setting with the patient—in contrast with Case 1 and Case 2. This resonates deeply with Erikson's Golden Rule. Dr. S's way of engaging with Ms. A is like a parent with an infant who—through fostering trust and communicating mutuality—can instill in the infant the strength of hope.[11] It is hypothesized that Ms. A could sense Dr. S's commitment to working with her and that feeling his commitment helped her in accepting that he would no longer provide opioids as part of the treatment plan (C4).

Case 3, in contrast with Case 1 and Case 2, illustrates Erikson's[10] distinction between moral rules and ethical rules. The physicians in Case 1 and Case 2 were guided by moral rules, "fear of *threats* to be forestalled. These may be outer threats of abandonment, punishment and public exposure, or a threatening inner sense of guilt, or shame or of isolation."[10(p222)] Dr. S's actions were based on a physician–patient relationship, grounded in ideals rather than rigid adherence to rules.[10(p222)] This led to thoughtful action that girded both physician and patient for the vicissitudes of pain management in the face of opioid prescribing and cessation (C5).

Building Trust through Mutuality

Three tools can help physicians build trust through mutuality. These tools are especially helpful for physicians who treat chronic pain patients:

- Dialogue
- Empathy
- Narrative medicine

DIALOGUE

From the analysis of Case 1, we saw the patient's loss of trust in the physician undermining the physician's efforts to help the patient. Smith and Newton[26(p54)] encourage "meaningful dialogue" between patient and physician. They encourage the physician to see the patient as a person, to connect with that person, and to be a person (in addition to a physician) during the interaction.[26]

Reflecting back on Erikson's view of mutuality, what is needed is a willingness on the part of the physician to not only try to read the verbal and nonverbal signals of the patient but also to acknowledge, discuss, and reflect on them. Physicians who can engage in this type of dialogue may also ameliorate their own frustration and promote personal growth in the physician. Thus, both physician and patient may benefit from an ethical interaction. Allowing oneself to participate in dialogue with a patient can be an authentic way of connecting beyond the mask of professionalism. The realization of change is illustrated in Stephen Sondheim's song "It Takes Two" from the musical "Into the Woods," where the baker has become a better and different man by including his wife's input and participation in a critical venture. The baker's wife noted that the baker had become more "daring," confident, "sharing," and "openhearted."[30]

EMPATHY

Physicians who want to have mutuality in their interaction with their patients may need to be refreshed in the skills needed to do this. Empathy is a skill that can promote mutuality.

Hojat et al.[31] uses Mercer and Reynolds's 2002 paper "Empathy and the Quality of Care" to characterize four abilities that a physician uses to engage with a patient with empathy:

- Cognitive. The physician identifies and understands the patient's emotional experience.
- Emotive. The physician imagines and relates the patient's emotional experience to his or her own experience.
- Moral. The physician is motivated to express his or her understanding of the patient's experience to the patient grounded in the physician's humanity.
- Behavioral. The physician communicates to the patient his or her understanding of the patient's experience.

Empathy training offers strategies to bring trust building and mutuality to a difficult physician–patient interaction.[27] Specific communication strategies include (1) techniques to enhance physician–patient dialogue, (2) active listening, (3) validating emotion, and (4) exploring alternative solutions.[27(p423)] For instance, during the visit in which the physician in Case 1 decided to move toward cessation of opioids, the physician was facing her computer, not facing the patient. According to Ambady and Rosental,[32] eye gaze and contact is needed for mutuality and for transmitting empathy.

Researchers believe that it is possible to teach and for physicians to learn and practice empathy, or at the very least act empathetically.[33] A systematic review of published literature on empathy training interventions that were quantitatively evaluated to detect changes in empathy among medical students, residents, fellows, and physicians found that 66% (42 out of 64) of reviewed studies reported a statistically significant increase in empathy.[33]

Practice of empathic techniques may help the physician become genuinely empathic.[34] To further the goal of being able to "treat each patient as a person, not an illness,"[35] the authors of this chapter suggest that pain physicians engage in team meetings that include discussions of the patients' personal histories and the potential difficulties with connection with an individual patient.

NARRATIVE MEDICINE

Charon[36] has written about the use of narrative theory and methods in the practice of bioethics. The goal of these methods, called narrative-based medicine (NBM), per Charon,[36(p1897)] is to "practice medicine with empathy, reflection, professionalism and trustworthiness." It is a pathway toward the "authentic engagement [that] is transformative for all participants,"[36(p1898)] thus invoking the tenet of mutuality that anchors Erikson's Golden Rule. She describes the contributions of NBM to both patient and physician. For the patient, NBM makes the patient feel better understood, more hopeful, and more comfortable asking difficult questions. For physicians who can engage with their patients using NBM, it makes the physicians a reflective practitioner with an enhanced ability to "identify and interpret their own emotional responses to patients, make sense of their own life journeys" and achieve a more accurate understanding of illness and suffering.[36(p1899)] Peterkin[37] offers a list of some of the basic physician behaviors of NBM, which include the following:

1. "Ask open-ended questions."
2. "Do not interrupt."
3. Ask about suffering
4. "Learn your patients' stories."

5. "View noncompliance as a blocked narrative, not as patient stubbornness."
6. Ask the question "What do you think is going on?"
7. Ask yourself, "Where did we leave the thread of our story the last time?"

Charon[36] recommends training in narrative skills as well as reading, reflective writing, and authentic dialogue with patients.

Conclusion

Crises in trust occur during physician–patient encounters involving opioid cessation. By addressing trust issues in these interactions via mutuality, physicians may be able to help with the ethical distress that comes with having to balance their patient's best interests with cultural swings of the pendulum toward and away from opioid prescribing. Erikson's Golden Rule provides a framework for navigating the challenge of cessation of opioids in chronic pain patients.

References

1. Dowell D, Haegerich TM, Chou R. CDC Guideline for Prescribing Opioids for Chronic Pain—United States, 2016. *MMWR Recomm Rep* 2016; 65(1):1–4.
2. Dowell D, Haegerich TM, Chou R. CDC Guideline for Prescribing Opioids for Chronic Pain—United States, 2016. *JAMA* 2016;315(15): 1624–1645.
3. McCarberg B. How opioid prescribing guidelines may affect (help or hinder) a primary care physician's ability to provide pain management. Paper presented at: the American Academy of Pain Medicine 33rd Annual Meeting; March 16–19, 2017; Orlando, FL.
4. Victor L, Richeimer SH. Trustworthiness as a clinical variable: the problem of trust in the management of chronic, nonmalignant pain. *Pain Med* 2005;6:385–391.
5. Gunderman RB. *We Make a Life by What We Give.* Bloomington, IN: Indiana University Press; 2008.
6. Gunderman RB. *Leadership in Healthcare.* London: Springer; 2009.
7. Snarey J, Bell D. Erikson, Erik H. In: Dowling EM, Scarlett WG, eds. *Encyclopedia of Religious and Spiritual Development.* Thousand Oaks, CA: Sage; 2006:146–150.
8. Browning DS. Generativity, ethics, and hermeneutics: revisiting Erik Erikson. In: Browning DS, Witte J, series eds. *Christian Ethics and the Moral Psychologies.* Grand Rapids, MI: Wm. B. Eerdmans; 2006:146–165. *Religion, Marriage, and Family.*
9. Erikson EH. The Golden Rule and the cycle of life. *Harvard Medical Alumni Bulletin.* Winter 1963.
10. Erikson EH. The Golden Rule in the light of new insight. In: *Insight and Responsibility: Lectures on the Ethical Implications of Psychoanalytic Insight.* New York: Norton; 1964:217–243.
11. Conn WE. Erik Erikson: the ethical orientation, conscience and the golden rule. *J Relig Ethics* 1977;5(2):249–266.
12. Piediscalzi N, Erik H. Erikson's contribution to ethics. *J Relig Health* 1973;12(2):169–180.
13. Erikson EH. *Childhood and Society.* 2nd ed. New York: Norton; 1963.
14. Mooney CG. Chapter 3: Erik Erikson. In: *Theories of Childhood: An Introduction to Dewey, Montessori, Erikson, Piaget & Vygotsky.* St. Paul, MN: Redleaf Press; 2000:53–76.
15. Perry TE, Ruggiano N, Shtompel N, et al. Applying Erikson's wisdom to self-management practices of older adults: findings from two field studies. *Res Aging* 2015;37(3):253–274.
16. Van Houdenhove B. Assessing adverse childhood experiences in chronic pain: it does matter. *Clin J Pain* 2006;22:584–585.
17. Vogel-Scibilia SE, McNulty KC, Baxter B, et al. The recovery process utilizing Erikson's stages of human development. *Community Ment Health J* 2009;45(6):405–414.
18. Pearson SD, Raeke LH. Patients' trust in physicians: many theories, few measures, and little data. *J Gen Intern Med* 2000;15:509–513.
19. Sass HM. The clinic as testing ground for moral theory: a European view. *Kennedy Inst Ethics J* 1996;6:351–355.
20. O'Neill O. *Autonomy and Trust in Bioethics.* Cambridge, United Kingdom: Cambridge University Press; 2002.
21. Moskowitz D, Thom DH, Guzman D, et al. Is primary care providers' trust in socially marginalized patients affected by race? *J Gen Intern Med* 2012;26(8):846–851.
22. Thom DH, Wong ST, Guzman D, et al. Physician trust in the patient: development and validation of a new measure. *Ann Fam Med* 2011;9: 148–154.
23. Gooberman-Hill R, Heathcote C, Reid CM, et al. Professional experience guides opioid prescribing for non-cancer pain in primary care. *Fam Pract* 2010;0:1–8.

24. Tronick E, Beeghly M. Infants' meaning-making and the development of mental health problems. *Am Psychol* 2011;66(2):107–119.

25. Watt G. A social institution based on mutuality and trust. *Br J Gen Pract* 2011;61(593):741.

26. Smith DG, Newton L. Physician and patient: respect for mutuality. *Theor Med Bioeth* 1984;5:43–60.

27. Lorenzetti R, Jacques CH, Donovan C, et al. Managing difficult encounters: understanding physician, patient and situational factors. *Am Fam Physician* 2013;87(6):419–425.

28. Genuis SJ. Dismembering the ethical physician. *Postgrad Med J* 2006; 82(966):233–238.

29. Saltzman M, de Melker S. As opioid epidemic worsens, rethinking how doctors are taught to treat pain. *PBS NewsHour*. https://www.pbs.org /newshour/show/as-opioid-epidemic-worsens-rethinking-how-doctors-are -taught-to-treat-pain. Accessed April 29, 2017.

30. Sondheim S. *It Takes Two*. New York: Rilting Music; 1987.

31. Hojat M, Gonnella JS, Mangione S, et al. Empathy in medical students as related to academic performance, clinical competence and gender. *Med Educ* 2002;36:522–527.

32. Ambady N, Rosental R. Nonverbal communication. In: Friedman H, ed. *Encyclopedia of Mental Health*. Vol 2. San Diego, CA: Academic Press; 1998:775–782.

33. Kelm Z, Womer J, Walter JK, et al. Interventions to cultivate physician empathy: a systematic review. *BMC Med Educ* 2014;14:219.

34. Taigman M. Can empathy and compassion be taught? *JEMS* 1996;21(6): 42–48.

35. Hirsch EM. The role of empathy in medicine: a medical student's perspective. *Virtual Mentor* 2007;9(6):423–427.

36. Charon R. The patient-physician relationship. Narrative medicine: a model for empathy, reflection, profession, and trust. *JAMA* 2001;286(15):1897–1902.

37. Peterkin A. Practical strategies for practising narrative-based medicine. *Can Fam Physician* 2012;58(1):63–64.

CHAPTER 111

Training Pain Specialists

JAMES P. RATHMELL and **JAN VAN ZUNDERT**

The Evolution of Pain Medicine as a Subspecialty

It is impossible for any physician to become an expert in every field. As knowledge expands and the need for detailed skills arises, the natural progression is for specialization to ensue. There has long been a discomfort with specialization despite an unflagging progression in that direction. The urge to both specialize and remain unspecialized dates back to the earliest recorded history of medicine. The first specializations were between the barber-surgeons and the internists, and a rivalry of sorts remains to this day. Writing about Ambrose Paré, the 16th century physician who elevated the role of the barber-surgeons to that of other physicians, the present-day surgeon and historian Sherwin Nuland[1] reflects on the ongoing distinction between internist and surgeon:

> Surgery is an exercise in the use of the intellect. Heckling internists, with tongues barely in check, would prefer that surgical specialists be viewed merely as dexterous craftsman who carry out the routing errands assigned to them by their more cerebrally endowed medical overseers. I attribute this teasing raillery to a kind of good-natured fraternal envy, not so much of our celebrity status, but rather of the visibility of the cures we surgeons achieve and the particular personal gratification we have while doing it.

In the United States, anesthesiology has progressed toward further specialization, first with the establishment of critical care; then pain management (now called pain medicine); and more recently, pediatric anesthesiology, cardiothoracic anesthesiology, and obstetric anesthesiology. The addition of pain medicine as a subspecialty of anesthesiology is just one recent example of the growth of medical specialties. With specialization comes a conscious effort to focus practice to become intricately familiar with a more limited realm. The obvious result is a loss of the skills and knowledge needed to practice in the broader parent specialty. In pain medicine, many now view this as a full-time vocation. The scientific meetings and journals that keep pain medicine specialists up-to-date have little overlap with those that are designed to serve anesthesiologists practicing in the operating room. The only common thread between the technical skills needed in the pain clinic and those required for anesthesiology in the operating room is expertise with neural blockade, which is one of several important skill sets needed in pain medicine. The rapid expansion of knowledge in the causes and complications of acute and chronic pain, particularly in the neurobehavioral sciences, has led to a growing recognition that the pain medicine practitioner must acquire a vastly different skill set than those practicing anesthesiology, including expanding their skills as diagnosticians.

Much has been written about the origins of pain medicine as a distinct discipline, and anesthesiologists have played a primary role since the start,[2] as have specialists in neurology, psychiatry, neurosurgery, and physical medicine and rehabilitation.[3] Anesthesiology really started with the introduction of effective general anesthetics in the mid-19th century, when surgical pain could be separated from operation. Almost 100 years later, the late John Bonica, an anesthesiologist and recognized father of the specialty we now call pain medicine, developed his career promoting multidisciplinary pain care and formal training of specialists. From his life's work, we now have extensive ongoing efforts to recognize and treat pain effectively, to train subspecialists, and to conduct basic and clinical research to further our understanding of pain and its treatment. The International Association for the Study of Pain (IASP) founded in 1974; its US chapter, the American Pain Society; and the journal *Pain* are legacies left by Dr. Bonica for our patients. Dr. Bonica began his practice with a focus on regional anesthesia techniques but soon came to realize that these techniques were inadequate to meet the needs of his patients with chronic pain and that he could not incorporate the growing scientific evidence of the importance of neurobehavioral factors. This realization evolved to the belief that developing the field of pain as a separate clinical discipline and treating chronic pain competently required the intellectual input and clinical skills of several other specialties. He published the first edition of this seminal textbook, *The Management of Pain*, toward that end in 1953.[4] It is noteworthy that IASP presidents have backgrounds from anesthesiology, dentistry, neurology, neurophysiology, neurosurgery, psychiatry, and psychology. All share a common intellectual passion and achievement, as well as clinical dedication, to developing pain research, teaching, and clinical care in pain medicine.

Accredited fellowship training in pain medicine is a relatively recent development. Prior to 1992, training was frequently obtained in academic anesthesiology departments, including those of John Bonica, Philip Bridenbaugh, Harold Carron, Daniel Moore, Prithvi Raj, Alon Winnie, and others, and subsequently in programs run by their trainees. These unaccredited programs advanced the specialty, widened interest in pain medicine as a career, and propagated anesthesiology-based pain care in smaller and smaller communities across the country. Other specialists also contributed to the development of the practice model of pain care. Many of the early leaders of pain medicine were from other specialties, and they trained fellows in unaccredited programs as well. Multispecialty entrance into pain medicine training became a tradition in several cities, including Boston, under Daniel Carr (Harvard, Massachusetts General) and Carol Warfield (Harvard, Beth Israel); New York, under Kathy Foley, Russ Portenoy, and Bob Breitbart (Memorial Sloan Kettering Cancer Center); and Seattle, under John Loeser, John Bonica's successor (University of Washington), among others. For example, one of the authors (Rollin M. Gallagher) provided fellowship training in chronic pain rehabilitation at State University of New York at Stony Brook and Drexel University College of Medicine to doctors with residency backgrounds in neurology, psychiatry, physiatry, and family practice before accreditation was possible. Outside of the United States, with the notable exception of Australia, this type of informal training remains the rule for those seeking expertise in pain medicine. In the United States, the American Board of Anesthesiology (ABA) developed interest in certifying pain medicine training. The failure of coalition of the boards of anesthesiology, psychiatry and neurology, physical medicine and rehabilitation, and neurosurgery in 1990 to form a conjoint American Board of Medical Specialties (ABMS) board led the ABA, under the leadership of Bill Owens in his roles on both the ABA and the Residency Review Committee (RRC) for Anesthesiology, and through

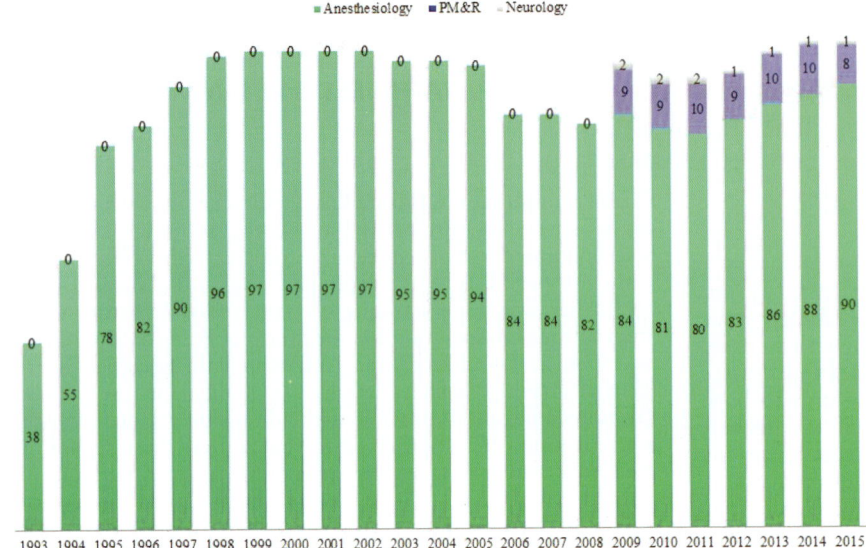

FIGURE 111.1 The Number of Accreditation Council for Graduate Medical Education (ACGME)-accredited pain medicine training programs in the United States by primary sponsoring medical specialty over time through 2015. *(Data provided by the American Council on Graduate Medical Education.)*

his representations of the subspecialty to the ABMS, to begin accrediting formal training programs and certifying physicians in 1992 through the Accreditation Council for Graduate Medical Education (ACGME). Steve Abram and John Rowlingson were both key members of the group that assisted Dr. Owens in moving the new subspecialty forward.

The number of ACGME-accredited programs (Fig. 111.1) and the number of trainees in accredited programs have grown steadily over the past decade, reaching just under 100 training programs by 1999 that train just over 300 new pain specialists each year (Fig. 111.2). The ABA working in parallel with the ACGME developed a subspecialty certification examination in pain medicine, first named the "Certificate of Added Qualifications in Pain Management," now titled "Subspecialty Certification in Pain Medicine." The first exam was given in 1993. The number of candidates sitting for the examination has steadily grown since the first exam was given.

Dr. Bonica's original push to develop multidisciplinary pain care recently evolved into collaboration between four specialties agreeing to a single and unified set of program requirements for all ACGME-accredited pain fellowships regardless of sponsoring specialty. Consequently, in 1999, the ABA invited representatives of the American Board of Psychiatry and Neurology (ABPN) and the American Board of Physical Medicine and Rehabilitation (ABPMR) to join the ABA's Pain Management Examination Committee to broaden the examination beyond its prior focus on regional anesthesia, and, in 2000, the ABPN and ABPMR began issuing certificates of subspecialty certification in pain management to those diplomates who passed the expanded ABA examination. Between 2002 and 2006, the ACGME, working in collaboration with the ABA, ABPN, and ABPMR, developed new program requirements for pain fellowship training programs aimed at improving the quality of education in pain medicine and promoting a multidisciplinary approach to care. The new program requirements were adopted in 2006, and the number of programs achieving ongoing accreditation under these broader and more rigorous requirements initially declined by nearly 20% (see Fig. 111.2) and has rebounded in more recent years, with anesthesiology programs being replaced by those sponsored by physical medicine and rehabilitation. A 2015 snapshot of the distribution of board-certified pain specialties by primary medical specialty is shown in Figure 111.3. Equally important in the evolution of the discipline is the creation of academic physicians within the fellowships who undertake research programs to add new knowledge to this needed field of medical practice.

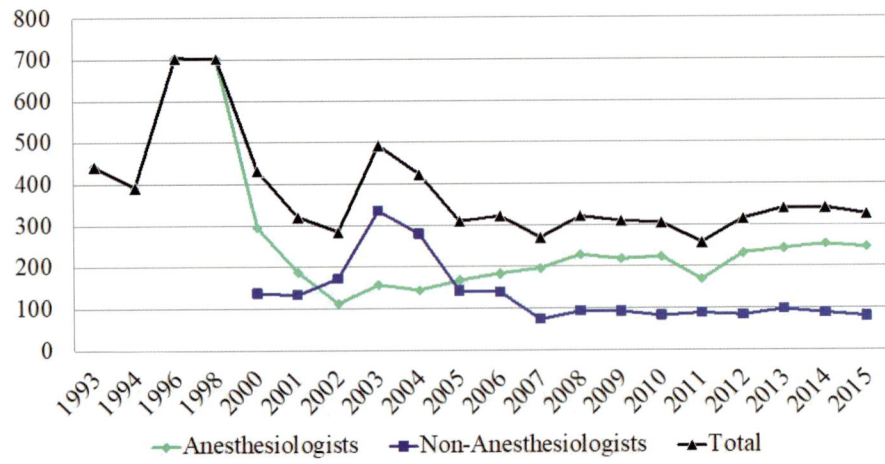

FIGURE 111.2 The number of new board-certified pain medicine specialists in the United States by specialty over time through 2015. ABMS, American Board of Medical Specialties. *(Data provided by the American Board of Anesthesiology.)*

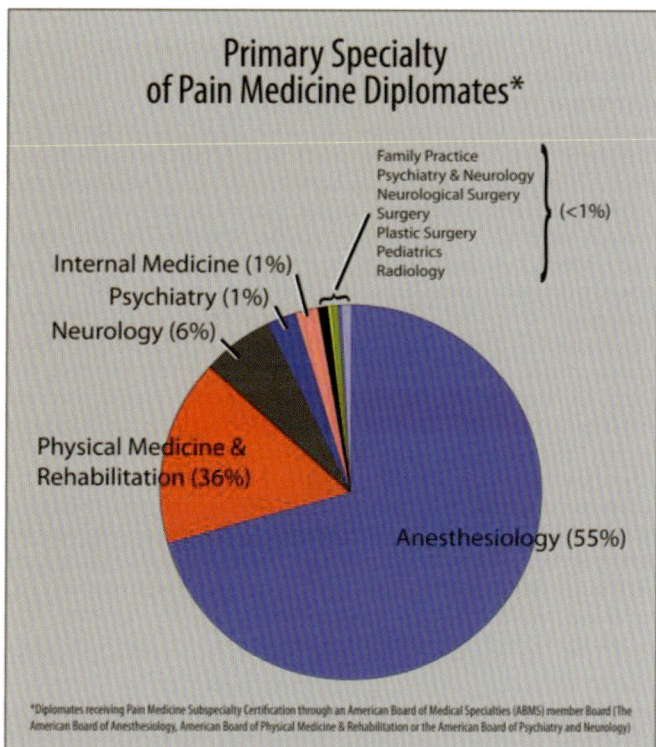

FIGURE 111.3 Distribution of the primary medical specialty of physicians board certified in the subspecialty of pain medicine in the United States in 2015. *(Data provided by the American Board of Anesthesiology.)*

Pain and its consequences draw on resources from all medical disciplines. Dr. Bonica's experiences during World War II suggested that each medical specialist had unique expertise to bring to patients suffering in pain, hence his consistent and effective promotion of a multidisciplinary process for pain care. Also thanks largely to Dr. Bonica, anesthesiology has led the development of formal training programs. Indeed, the majority of currently accredited programs reside within academic anesthesiology departments, and most program directors are anesthesiologists. Specialists from other disciplines have also focused their clinical and research efforts on pain. The most obvious example is neurology where the majority of clinical treatment and research about headache and peripheral neuropathy has arisen. Physical medicine and rehabilitation has also long had a focus and expertise in functional restoration, and physiatrists lead many chronic pain rehabilitation programs. And, of course, psychiatrists have been closely involved where pain, illness behavior, stress, depression, anxiety, and substance abuse overlap. During the last decade, specialists from these other disciplines have been seeking subspecialty training in pain medicine with increasing regularity.

The range of practitioners declaring themselves as pain medicine specialists is extraordinary; from clinics that provide largely or solely cognitive-behavioral approaches to chronic pain through functional restoration programs all the way to the type of clinic that offers nothing more than injections of various sorts. "Interventional pain medicine" is a term that has been coined for those techniques that involve minimally invasive treatments and minor surgery as part of their application, including neural blockade and implantable analgesic devices. Despite the paucity of scientific evidence to guide pain practitioners, particularly, evidence to support the use of many interventional modalities, many techniques appear to have efficacy based on limited observational data and have been adopted into widespread use. As practitioners, we are left to choose among available treatment modalities, often with only anecdote and personal experience to guide us in treating a group of desperate patients with intractable pain who are willing to accept almost any treatment, even those which remain unproven. There is no single practice pattern that any pain specialist can point toward as the correct way to treat patients with chronic pain. Training programs vary widely in the scope of what they train practitioners to do. The best pain medicine practitioners strike a reasonable balance between interventional and noninterventional management. This practice pattern is sustainable, and those adopting a balanced style of practice will be able to adapt to evolving scientific evidence that appears in support of pain treatment regardless of the type of treatment. A balance between treatment modalities also allows practitioners to switch from one mode to another or incorporate multiple treatment approaches simultaneously. Use of these interventional modalities is just a small part of the armamentarium of the skilled pain medicine practitioner.

Pain Medicine as a Primary Medical Specialty

Dr. Bonica developed his multidisciplinary clinic with the understanding that the expertise of several specialties was necessary to successfully manage chronic pain. A detailed history of the intellectual background of pain medicine and particularly Bonica's work in the early development of the field can be found in Baszanger's 1998 book, *Inventing Pain Medicine*.[5]

The rationale for a separate specialty in pain medicine involves the documentation of many factors: public health need,[6–8] a growing consensus of pain treatment as a human right,[9] ethical difficulties that are at the heart of pain medicine practice,[10,11] inadequate education[3] and knowledge[12] and a rapidly growing scientific and practice base,[13] and the need to promote integrated pain medicine with primary care.[14,15] The high costs of inadequately managed pain reverberate in our society's health care crisis and are well documented. Emblematic of the same, it has been our citizens, the victims of inadequate pain management, who have decried this problem and demanded change through legislation at both a state and a national level when organized medicine, itself beset by competition among established specialties, cannot act. The rationale is scientific as well. Since the publication of John Bonica's first edition of *The Management of Pain* in 1953, the problem of pain has challenged some of the best minds in science and medicine. In 1965, Melzack and Wall's[16] seminal paper in *Science* describing the gate theory of pain created a conceptual framework resulting in a relative explosion of science in the physiology, molecular biology, and pharmacology of acute pain and the epidemiology, neurobiology, pathophysiology, genetics, and treatment of chronic pain conditions and diseases at the levels of soma, spinal cord, and brain. Today's pain medicine physician is armed with a tremendous knowledge base as a foundation for the myriad of effective medications, behavioral therapies, physical therapies, neural blockades, neuromodulatory devices, and cross-cultural complementary and alternative treatments such as acupuncture and meditation. A growing number of pain medicine and other specialists in organized medicine believe that longer training, either a 2-year fellowship or a separate 3-year residency, is needed to learn how, when, and in what combinations of these tools can be cost-effectively utilized to competently treat patients with chronic pain, to establish standards for training all physicians, and to lead the development of clinical research and health policy.[17] Although each traditional medical specialty contributes to this knowledge base and skill set, their respective specialists are not trained to manage the entirety of the spectrum of chronic pain contributing to fragmentation not unification of care and failed public health. Table 111.1 outlines the special skills contributed by traditional specialties that converge to define the pain medicine specialist. This specialized knowledge, education, training, and multidisciplinary nature suggest that pain medicine's evolution as a specialty is paralleling that of other disciplines, such as emergency medicine or physical medicine and rehabilitation. Knowledge and skills of the latter disciplines, initially fragmented, later coalesced into primary medical specialties because of the inability of multiple specialties to offer an integrated approach that would best serve patients, medical science, and public health.

The momentum to establish standards for pain medicine as a specialty is now global. For example, in 1998, the government of Australia formally recognized pain medicine as a specialty and endorsed training and credentialing requirements recommended by the newly formed Faculty of Pain Medicine of the Australian and New Zealand College of Anaesthetists.[18] In 2007, the Section and Board of Anaesthesiology of the European Union of Medical Specialists (UEMS) initiated the establishment of the Multidisciplinary Joint Committee on Pain Medicine of the UEMS, which has created a certification examination in pain medicine (see further discussion of training in the European Union later in this chapter). Also in 2007, the Ministry of Health of the People's Republic of China announced the designation of pain medicine as a separate specialty and that there will be a Department of Pain Medicine in all major hospitals in China (R. M. Gallagher and J.-S. Han, December 2007, oral communication). In the United States, the momentum for establishing residency training programs in pain medicine under a new residency review committee has never gained momentum. The simple rationale is that training for 1 year has proven to be inadequate, but the status of pain medicine will remain as a subspecialty with just 1 year of training until leaders in the field find a way to collaboratively improve the depth and breadth of training. Similar to a cardiologist learning the science and clinical practice related to the cardiovascular system, starting with primary prevention of heart disease, by identification and early intervention of risk, and primary and secondary treatment of actual heart disease, the pain medicine specialist who will train in the future could learn about the pain perception and modulation system, from the relatively simple peripheral nociceptor to the system's complex neurobehavioral networks and about the pathophysiologies of this system.[19,20]

TABLE 111.1 Examples of Disease and Treatment Contributions to Pain Medicine from Traditional Specialties

Specialty	Illness/Disease Knowledge Contribution	Medical Skill/Treatment Contribution
Anesthesiology	Acute pain	Regional anesthesia (including neurolytic)
	Chronic pain	Spinal anesthesia
	Cancer pain	Operative anesthesia
Neurology	Peripheral neuropathy	Assessment of neuropathic pain
	Neuropathic pain	Neuropathic pain analgesia
	Central pain	Headache medication
	Headache	
Neurosurgery	Spine disease	Implantable medication pumps
	Central pain	Neurostimulation
		Spine evaluation and surgery
Orthopedic surgery	Low back pain	Spine evaluation and surgery
	Physical disability	Joint surgery
Palliative care	Cancer pain	End-of-life symptom management
		Bioethics
Primary care	Chronic diseases	Chronic disease management
		Biopsychosocial medicine
Psychiatry, behavioral medicine	Psychiatric comorbidity; stress, behavior and emotions	Antidepressant analgesia
	Fibromyalgia	Behavioral rehabilitation
	Personality and coping	Biofeedback and relaxation
		Biopsychosocial formulation
		Psychotherapies (dynamic, cognitive behavioral, group, family, hypnosis)
		Psychiatric diagnosis
		Psychological and psychometric evaluation
		Psychopharmacology
Radiologic medicine		Diagnostic imaging
		Procedure imaging
		Radiotherapy
Rehabilitation medicine, physical therapy	Musculoskeletal medicine	Physical therapy
	Myofascial pain	Physical rehabilitation
	Physical disability	Transcutaneous electrical nerve stimulation
		Trigger point therapy
Rheumatology	Joint diseases	Joint injections
	Fibromyalgia	Peripheral nociceptive analgesia (nonsteroidal anti-inflammatory drugs)
Complementary and alternative medicine		Acupuncture
		Massage
		Meditation
		Tai chi

Training in Pain Medicine in Europe

In Europe, there is no systematic training in pain medicine for medical students. The lack of obligatory training leads to later deficiencies in clinical care. Some countries (e.g., Germany) have made efforts in establishing a core curriculum for medical students. However, the worldwide need for a thorough basic education in pain medicine is underestimated by most health care officials.

The postgraduate training varies widely within Europe. This led to guidelines for anesthesiologist specialist training in pain medicine.[21] In these guidelines, approved by the UEMS, pain medicine is considered to be an area of expertise in anesthesiology. However, simultaneously, it is mentioned that pain medicine is not claimed for anesthesiology alone. It is clearly stated that pain medicine is included in anesthesia specialist training. However, an additional qualification following basic anesthesia training is recommended. The multidisciplinary approach to pain is mentioned, and an initiative to set up a multidisciplinary joint committee on pain medicine within the UEMS has begun.

The proposed duration of pain medicine training is 3 months during the 5 years of basic anesthetic training required in the European Union. In contrast to this relation representing only 5% of the total time of training, it is recommended to occupy a minimum of 10% of the multiple-choice questions on the European Society of Anaesthesiology's European Diploma in Anaesthesiology and Intensive Care.

Some years ago, the Scandinavian Society of Anaesthesiology and Intensive Care Medicine established the Nordic education in advanced pain medicine. The clinical part lasts at least 3 months. The education includes, and this is unique in Europe, a scientific part.[22]

In April 2007, the Royal College of Anaesthetists (United Kingdom) established a faculty of pain medicine and stressed this as a major way point in the last 50 years.[23] However, the question is raised: Should pain medicine strive to be a "stand-alone speciality," or should it be linked to parent specialties like anesthesiology? Additionally, is education also required for the public and the patients? Both the British and the Irish curriculum in pain medicine require similar training and examination. The candidate has to complete a total of 6 months training in pain medicine before ending up with a 2-day written and oral examination with review of actual clinical cases and a practical examination.

As early as 1992, the German Society of Anaesthesiology started a curriculum and specialist training in pain medicine. This included a 2-week theoretical course and a 1-year practical training requirement in a pain clinic. From this first example, a specialty open for all clinical disciplines has been developed. Since 1996, a specialty called "specialized pain therapy" has been established by the German Medical Assembly. A curriculum has been developed by the German Pain Society and approved by the German Medical Assembly. Similar to the Society of Anaesthetists, the specialization demands 1 year of clinical training in a certified institution and an 80-hour theoretical course. Additionally, to maintain specialty certification, physicians must attend multidisciplinary pain conferences regularly, where patients are presented and discussed between several disciplines, including at least one psychological discipline. In 2008, Austria introduced a similar specialty, and the German training is approved by the Austrian Medical Assembly.

The dramatic effect of a thorough education and programmatic work has been demonstrated in Catalonia in Spain within a project sponsored by the World Health Organization. Symptom control and patient satisfaction were both improved, and a striking cost savings of many million Euros per year has been demonstrated as compared to the rest of Spain.[24] Europe has lagged behind the United States in developing formal training for pain medicine specialists.

In 2016, the European Pain Federation EFIC developed a curriculum, predominantly based on the pain curriculum of the Faculty of Pain Medicine of the Australian and New Zealand College of Anaesthetists. The knowledge of the curriculum, pain assessment, and treatment skills are evaluated by a two-part examination: the European Diploma in Pain Medicine (EDPM). The examination is open to all qualified doctors who see and treat patients with pain who have appropriate clinical experience in pain assessment and treatment. The diploma aims to show that the fellow has a firm grounding in the basic skills and knowledge needed to assess and manage the many patients whose pain requires attention in all types of clinical scenario. The EDPM assesses the general knowledge of multidisciplinary pain management. Some countries in Europe have also approved the examination of the World Institute of Pain (WIP) to become Fellow in Interventional Pain Practice (FIPP) as an evaluation of the skills to select and perform interventional pain management techniques.

Training and Credentialing in Interventional Pain Medicine

In our rapidly changing world of modern health care, new technologies are appearing at a dizzying rate. Many of these new treatments require physicians to acquire detailed new knowledge and technical skills. The introduction of new techniques typically extends from centers in the public or private sector, where the ideas are conceived and tested in a limited realm among innovators. From there, anecdote can often take over, and many techniques in pain medicine have blossomed into widespread use with nothing more than word-of-mouth to propagate their use. The use of pulsed radiofrequency treatment for treatment of chronic pain after herniorrhaphy is one such example where clinical application has preceded detailed clinical testing.[25]

In the United States and Europe, industry often leads innovation by testing and leading the introduction of new devices. When the innovation appears to have merit in limited trials, many devices have been introduced to the market with approval through the U.S. Food and Drug Administration's (FDA) 510K "substantially similar device" process with little or no data regarding efficacy. Once on the market, the means by which practitioners decide to adopt new technologies, the speed of progression of these new techniques, and—of great importance—the means by which practitioners gain enough expertise to introduce new techniques into their own practices, are all highly variable and seemingly without any rational or consistent approach.

Interventional pain medicine is evolving as a distinct discipline that requires detailed new knowledge and expertise. Familiarity with radiographic anatomy for the conduct of image-guided injection and the minor surgical skills needed to place implanted devices such as spinal cord stimulators and implanted drug delivery systems are just a few of the techniques that practitioners must master. As we set out to introduce new interventional techniques to our own pain practices, we must assure that we have been properly trained to conduct these techniques to ensure safety and success.

Adequate exposure during the fellowship-training period to these newer treatment alternatives is necessary to assure appropriate application and optimize patient outcomes. Although we do not have scientific data that define the average minimum level of experience that will be necessary to achieve competence, especially for complex procedures that are associated with significant risks, logic dictates that there are a minimum number of these procedures that trainees should be exposed to during a fellowship. The ACGME has established requirements for average minimal numbers of epidural, spinal, and peripheral nerve blocks necessary for accreditation of anesthesiology residency programs. Other medical subspecialties also require a minimum number of specified procedures to achieve and maintain competence: Subspecialty training in gastroenterology has a requirement of performing a minimum of 100 esophagogastroduodenoscopies and 100 colonoscopies with polyp removal[26] during formal training, and subspecialty training in cardiovascular disease requires 100 cardiac catheterizations to demonstrate minimum proficiency.[27] Indeed, in 2017, the ACGME's RRC for Anesthesiology has accepted revised program requirements for pain medicine training programs that specify minimum exposure of trainees for various techniques. For those techniques that are now widely accepted as a core part of pain practice, we must assure that our trainees gain enough experience to conduct these procedures independently. One key element of the ACGME deliberations about unified pain training is to acknowledge that not all pain fellows will have experience in the wide variety of interventional techniques. Rather, it is hoped that these fellows will gain an understanding of all available options for patients with pain and yet demonstrate and have competence documented in only those techniques for which formal training is made available during fellowship training.

It is difficult to define the techniques that are core for a pain practitioner, but it does seem that detailed knowledge of radiographic anatomy of the spine and the minor surgical skills required to implant spinal cord stimulators and place permanent spinal drug delivery systems are among those skills most practicing pain physicians would expect a new graduate from a pain fellowship to emerge with. New techniques are appearing at a staggering rate, and we cannot rely on pain fellowship programs to provide all of the technical training that is needed. Stronger standards for minimal training following fellowship are also urgently needed. Some pain practitioners believe that all too many of their colleagues find it perfectly acceptable to attend a brief weekend course and then introduce a highly technical new treatment into practice without additional study, training, or oversight.[28] The recent proliferation of new approaches to minimally invasive treatment of spinal pain and spinal cord stimulation all require unique knowledge and skills to be used safely and effectively. Practitioners themselves must take the lead in obtaining adequate training *before* proceeding with any new and unfamiliar technique. The weekend workshop is just a start, often a good start—the best will give practitioners a detailed understanding of anatomy; pathophysiology of disease related to the use of the new technique; patient selection; conduct of the procedure; outcomes; and avoidance, management,

and recognition of complications. Here, we would like to suggest a method for practitioners[29] (Table 111.2): (1) *study the new technique*, the published literature, and gain a detailed knowledge of all aspects of the technique; (2) *attend a workshop*, preferably a hands-on cadaver-based workshop that allows introduction to the technique in as realistic a setting that can be assembled; (3) *plan* adequate time for your initial procedures; (4) *get help* at the bedside during initial conduct of new procedures—perhaps another experienced practitioner at your institution, an invited expert to assist, or team up with a colleague in a related discipline; (5) *inform your patients* that you are introducing a new technique and include this discussion as part of the informed consent process; and (6) *examine your outcomes* carefully in the initial stages of using any new technique and compare them with those of your colleagues and the published literature.

Conclusion

The field of evidence-based medicine has emerged as a new paradigm to guide practicing physicians. This field endeavors to educate practitioners about how to frame specific questions based on the clinical problems they are faced with every day. They then venture to the published scientific literature with focused questions about prevention, diagnosis, and treatment of a specific clinical condition. Many evidence-based medicine centers offer concise and periodically updated summaries about specific clinical conditions. The idea is to get the best information available to the practicing clinician. It describes the best available evidence, and if there is no good evidence, it says so. In pain medicine, we are faced with an expanding array of treatment options that strikes us as logical developments that *should* provide pain relief for our patients. However, there is a dearth of clinical evidence to guide rational choice and application of the majority of these emerging treatments. So how are we to decide when to apply them?

Merrill[30] presented a detailed analysis of the current state of evidence guiding the use of interventional treatments in the field of pain medicine. He points out the frequent flaws in existing studies (largely the lack of valid comparators, such as no treatment) and concludes that "the practice of invasive pain medicine teeters at a particularly critical juncture . . . crippled by a lack of vigorous self-evaluation of its role in the treatment of chronic pain." Merrill[30] goes on to detail the means by which we, as scientists and clinicians, can proceed to build a better body of evidence for the treatments we are using. But the field of pain medicine is young and early in development, and it is perhaps unreasonable to expect an accumulation of randomized clinical trials just yet.

New treatments evolve slowly in clinical medicine. Applying the scientific method in clinical medicine begins with an observation. Perhaps a chance observation that a certain drug typically used for another purpose provides analgesia to a given patient. If the drug is readily available, a clinician may choose to try treatment on other patients with similar presentations. If an academic sort, the clinician may choose to report the limited success in a case series. Case series are a valuable beginning: the very beginning of emerging new ideas. If the problem is uniform and prevalent enough, the new treatment may gain the attention of investigators willing to assemble a randomized clinical trial. All too often, sound treatments are never tested for lack of interest or funding. Those that are tested tend to be those under patent where a manufacturer proceeds with these large endeavors understandably in hope of financial return in the event the treatment proves useful. Patients who are suffering from severe and intractable pain are desperate, and they can easily be convinced that desperate measures, however new or unproven, are warranted.

TABLE 111.2 Suggested Training and Experience When Introducing a New Technique in to Clinical Practice

1. *Study the new technique,* the published literature, and gain a detailed knowledge of all aspects of the technique.
2. *Attend a workshop,* preferably a hands-on cadaver-based workshop that allows introduction to the technique in as realistic a setting that can be assembled.
3. *Plan* adequate time for your initial procedures.
4. *Get help* at the bedside during initial conduct of new procedures—perhaps another experienced practitioner at your institution, an invited expert to assist, or team up with a colleague in a related discipline.
5. *Inform your patients* that you are introducing a new technique and include this discussion as part of the informed consent process.
6. *Examine your outcomes* carefully in the initial stages of using any new technique and compare them with those of your colleagues and the published literature.

How, then, are we to proceed? Our patients are begging for us to try anything that offers a glimmer of hope in reducing their pain, and we as scientists embrace the rigor of the scientific method and want desperately to do what is best for our patients. We have treatment after treatment that makes logical sense and shows early promise in case series and observational studies but little data that support an evidence-based approach to practice. The evidence-based medicine movement gives little guidance to practitioners whose tools are still under development. They simply remind us that no evidence regarding many of our techniques exists. Without declaring a moratorium on all of interventional pain, Merrill[30] offers the individual practitioner advice: Monitor your own outcomes using valid measures, be more reflective and systematic in studying your own outcomes and patterns of care, and provide this information to your patients as part of the decision-making process. As pain practitioners, we have an expanding range of treatment options available to us, few with convincing evidence of efficacy superior to alternate treatments. We must evaluate each patient and use the limited evidence available to us today to guide compassionate and rational, if not evidence-based, use of therapy for our desperate patients.

ACKNOWLEDGMENTS

We would like to thank Michael Zenz, Rollin M. Gallagher, and David L. Brown, who contributed to this chapter for *Bonica's Management of Pain*, fourth edition. We have built on the previous edition's chapter to create this updated chapter.

References

1. Nuland SB. The gentle surgeon: Ambrose Paré. In: Nuland SB, ed. *Doctors: The Biography of Medicine*. New York: Knopf; 1988:94.
2. Rathmell JP. American Society of Regional Anesthesia and Pain Medicine 2011 John J. Bonica Award Lecture: the evolution of the field of pain medicine. *Reg Anesth Pain Med* 2012;37(6):652–656.
3. Gallagher RM. Pain education and training: progress or paralysis? *Pain Med* 2002;3(3):196–197.
4. Bonica JJ. *The Management of Pain*. Philadelphia: Lippincott; 1953.
5. Baszanger I. *Inventing Pain Medicine: From the Laboratory to the Clinic*. New Brunswick, NJ: Rutgers University Press; 1998.
6. Latham J, Davis BD. The socioeconomic impact of chronic pain. *Disabil Rehabil* 1994;16:39–44.
7. Burcheil KJ. Social costs of denying access to care. In: Cohen M, Campbell J, eds. *Pain Treatment Centers at Crossroads: A Practical and Conceptual Reappraisal/the Bristol–Myers Squibb Symposium on Pain Research*. Seattle, WA: IASP Press; 1996:125–142.
8. Osterweis M, Kleinman A, Mechanic D. Pain and disability. Clinical, behavioral, and public policy perspectives. In: Institute of Medicine. *Committee on Pain, Disability, and Chronic Illness Behavior*. Washington, DC: National Academies Press; 1987:280–282.
9. Brennan F, Carr DB, Cousins MJ. Pain management: a fundamental human right. *Anesth Analg* 2007;105:205–221.
10. Gallagher RM. Ethics in pain medicine: good for our health, good for the public health. *Pain Med* 2001;2:87–89.
11. Banja J. Empathy in the physician's pain practice: benefits, barriers, and recommendations. *Pain Med* 2006;7:265–275.
12. Green CR, Wheeler JR, LaPorte F, et al. How well is pain managed? Who does it well? *Pain Med* 2002;3:56–65.
13. Fishman S, Gallagher RM, Carr D, et al. The case for pain medicine as a medical specialty. *Pain Med* 2004;5:281–286.
14. Gallagher RM. The pain medicine and primary care community rehabilitation model: monitored care for pain disorders in multiple settings. *Clin J Pain* 1999;15:1–3.
15. Bair MJ. Overcoming fears, frustrations, and competing demands: an effective integration of pain medicine and primary care to treat complex pain patients. *Pain Med* 2007;8:544–545.
16. Melzack R, Wall PD. Pain mechanism: a new theory. *Science* 1965;150:971–979.
17. Follett K, Dubois K. Program requirements for ACGME training in pain medicine released for the first time. *Pain Med* 2008;9:471–472.
18. Cohen M, Goucke R. Pain medicine recognized as a specialty in Australia. *Pain Med* 2006;7:473.
19. Basbaum AI. Distinct neurochemical features of acute and persistent pain. *Proc Natl Acad Sci U S A* 1999;96:7739–7743.
20. Rome HP Jr, Rome JD. Limbically augmented pain syndrome (LAPS): kindling, corticolimbic sensitization, and the convergence of affective and sensory symptoms in chronic pain disorders. *Pain Med* 2000;1:7–23.
21. Cunningham AJ, Knape JT, Adriaensena H, et al. Guidelines for anaesthesiologist specialist training in pain medicine. Section and Board of Anesthesiology, European Union of Medical Specialists. *Eur J Anaesth* 2007;24:568–570.
22. Scandinavian Society of Anaesthesiology and Intensive Care Medicine. SSAI's Nordic education in advanced pain medicine. Available at: http://www.ssai.info/Education/pain.html. Accessed February 1, 2009.
23. Justins DM. The Faculty of Pain Medicine of the Royal College of Anaesthetists. *Br J Anaesth* 2008;101:4–7.
24. Gómez-Batiste X, Porta-Sales J, Pascual A, et al; and the Palliative Care Advisory Committee of the Standing Advisory Committee for Socio-Health Affairs, Department of Health, Government of Catalonia. Catalonia WHO palliative care demonstration project at 15 years (2005). *J Pain Symptom Manage* 2007;33:584–590.
25. Werner MU, Bischoff JM, Rathmell JP, et al. Pulsed radiofrequency in the treatment of persistent pain after inguinal herniotomy: a systematic review. *Reg Anesth Pain Med* 2012;37:340–343.
26. Program requirements for residency education in gastroenterology. Available at: https://www.acgme.org/Portals/0/PFAssets/ProgramRequirements/144_gastroenterology_2017-07-01.pdf?ver=2017-04-27-145620-577. Accessed April 26, 2018.
27. Program requirements for residency education in cardiovascular disease. Available at: https://www.acgme.org/Portals/0/PFAssets/ProgramRequirements/141_cardiovascular_disease_2017-07-01.pdf. Accessed April 26, 2018.
28. Rathmell JP. The injectionists. *Reg Anesth Pain Med* 2004;29:305–306.
29. Lubenow TR, Rathmell JP. Let's take a rational approach to technical training in pain medicine. *Am Soc Anesth News* 2005;69:6–8.
30. Merrill DG. Hoffman's glasses: evidence-based medicine and the search for quality in the literature of interventional pain medicine. *Reg Anesth Pain Med* 2003;28:547–560.

CHAPTER 112

Emergencies in the Pain Clinic

CHRISTOPHER GILLIGAN, MILAN P. STOJANOVIC, RAMSEY SABA, and
JAMES P. RATHMELL

This chapter seeks to provide the pain management specialist with an overview of emergencies and complications that may occur in the course of caring for patients with acute and chronic pain. Throughout this review, we will also emphasize strategies for decreasing risk, specifically, strategies for identifying specific risks and considering alternatives, understanding rare event analysis, and maintaining a comprehensive view of the patient when prescribing specialty specific interventions. A prudent first step for practitioners who will be managing emergencies related to pain therapies is to understand the incidence of each of these emergencies. However, because rates have been relatively low for serious complications, and because minor complications frequently go unreported, measuring the true incidence of most complications is not feasible.

The American Society of Anesthesiologists Closed Claims Project

In the United States, the American Society of Anesthesiologists Closed Claims Project offers a close look at serious adverse events secondary to pain management interventions that lead to malpractice claims, but no incidence can be calculated due to the lack of any knowledge regarding the overall frequency with which the interventions are performed. We can, however, make educated changes to our practice by evaluating trends in these closed claims.

A review of 1,037 total pain medicine malpractice claims of the database between 1980 and 2012 showed that most claims were related to lumbar nonneurolytic injections (n = 273). Other claims included cervical nonneurolytic injections (n = 211); device implantation, management, or removal (n = 146); and medication management (n = 115). Looking just at the claims between the years 2000 and 2012 (n = 505), we find that most claims have trended toward cervical nonneurolytic injections (Table 112.1). Furthermore, the overall percentage of malpractice claims for pain medicine has increased from 3% of all anesthesia malpractice claims between 1980

and 1989 to 18% of all anesthesia malpractice claims between 2000 and 2012 as reviewed from the American Society of Anesthesiologists Closed Claims Project database. Outcomes in pain medicine claims have also grown increasingly more severe in nature over the years. Death and permanent disability increased from 21% of pain medicine claims in the 1980s to 55% of claims in the 2000s.[1]

Nerve damage and pneumothorax were the most common adverse events leading to claims in interventional pain management claims (Fig. 112.1). Serious adverse events leading to brain damage or death occurred at a far lower rate than that seen in surgical and obstetric anesthesia claims. A closer analysis of the subset of claims associated with epidural steroid injections (ESIs) revealed that death and brain damage occurred only when local anesthetic or opioid (or both) were administered in conjunction with the steroid (Fig. 112.2). This likely reflects unintended delivery of local anesthetic or opioid to the subarachnoid space or simply the predictable effects of neuraxial opioids; resultant high spinal anesthesia or neuraxial effects of opioid could both have led to respiratory compromise and underscores the need for close observation following neuraxial administration of local anesthetic or opioid. Not infrequently, claims resulted from the maintenance of spinal drug delivery systems (20/276 claims or 7%); these claims often stemmed from refilling of implanted drug reservoirs with potent opioid by nonphysician personnel in the outpatient or home care settings.

Bleeding Complications

Spinal hematomas have been described in autopsies since 1682 but not as a clinical diagnosis until 1867.[2] Within one decade of August Bier's discovery of spinal anesthesia, the first known epidural hematoma as a complication of spinal anesthesia occurred in a 36-year-old male following unsuccessful neuraxial blockade for excision of a pilonidal cyst.[3] In that case, repeated lumbar puncture revealed blood-tinged cerebrospinal fluid (CSF), and the patient subsequently developed paresthesias and weakness in both lower extremities. The introduction of heparin in 1937 and warfarin in 1941 introduced the possibility of anticoagulation contributing to epidural hematoma formation. Epidural hematoma is a rare but potentially catastrophic complication of spinal or epidural anesthesia or injections. Because the spinal column is an enclosed space, hematoma formation can cause compression and ischemia of neural structures. Bleeding may result from injury to the abundant epidural veins or may be arterial. A retrospective study of central neuraxial blocks in Sweden from 1990 to 1999 identified 33 spinal hematomas, during a period when approximately 1,260,000 spinal blocks and 450,000 epidural blocks were administered. In that study, the incidence of spinal hematoma was 1 in 200,000 after obstetric epidural blockade and 1 in 3,600 among female patients undergoing knee arthroplasty.[4] At a single teaching hospital in Australia, data were collected prospectively over a 16-year period for all epidural catheters placed for postoperative analgesia. During that period, 8,210 epidural catheters were inserted, and 2 spinal hematomas (1:4,105) and 6 epidural abscesses (1:1,368) were diagnosed.[5] In rare instances, spinal epidural hematoma has developed following chiropractic manipulation

TABLE 112.1 Specific Procedures Used for the Treatment of Chronic Pain within the American Society of Anesthesiologists Closed Claims Project that Led to Malpractice Claims (n = 505)

Procedure	Claims 2000–2012	
	n	%
Cervical nonneurolytic injections	134	27
Lumbar nonneurolytic injections	87	17
Medication management	87	17
Devices	83	16
Other nonneurolytic injections	43	9
Neurolytic procedures	33	7
Other procedures	38	8

Reprinted with permission from Pollak KA, Stephens LS, Posner KP, et al. Trends in pain medicine liability. *Anesthesiology* 2015;123(5):1133–1141.

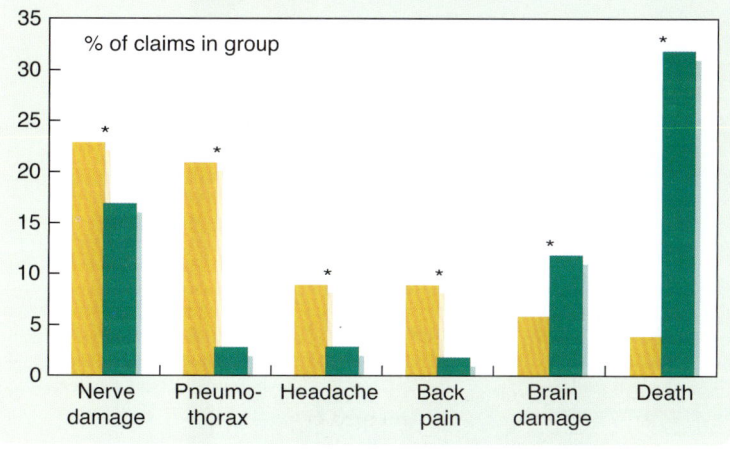

FIGURE 112.1   Primary outcomes within the American Society of Anesthesiologists Closed Claims Project in chronic pain management claims (*yellow bars*) versus surgical/obstetric claims (*green bars*). *$P < 0.05$. (*Reprinted with permission from Fitzgibbon DR, Posner KL, Domino KB, et al; American Society of Anesthesiologists. Chronic pain management: American Society of Anesthesiologists Closed Claims Project. Anesthesiology 2004;100[1]:98–105.*)

and acupuncture therapy.[6,7] Factors that determine whether epidural hematoma results in injury to neural structures include the location in the spinal column (the level of the cauda equina is relatively resistant to injury, whereas the cervical spinal cord is not), and the rate at which the blood accumulates. Tarlov[8] demonstrated in dogs that spinal cord injury due to spinal epidural hematoma depends on both the amount of pressure exerted on the spinal cord and the duration of that pressure elevation. Interestingly, some epidural hematomas cause significant injury despite the fact that their volume is significantly less than that typically used during epidural blood patch placement. Vertebral column neoplasms and vascular malformations are also risk factors. Patients who have an underlying coagulopathy or are being anticoagulated with warfarin, intravenous (IV) heparin, subcutaneous low molecular weight heparin, platelet-inhibiting medications such as clopidogrel or ticlopidine, platelet glycoprotein IIb/IIIa receptor inhibitors, or fibrinolytic agents are at elevated risk of spinal hematoma formation. It should also be noted that with the growing number of patients on novel anticoagulation agents, including but not limited to, apixaban, dabigatran, rivaroxaban, prasugrel, and ticagrelor, a careful consideration of guidelines and practice advisories are necessary prior to any neuraxial procedures. The incidence of spontaneous spinal epidural hematoma estimated by Holtås et al.[9] was 0.1 per 100,000 people, and less than 1% of those with spinal hematomas had their spinal epidural space occupied by lesions. The etiology of these hematomas was unsurprisingly related to coagulopathies, vascular malformations, neoplasms, infections, minor vertebral traumas, and idiopathic causes.[10] In addition, garlic has been shown to inhibit platelet

aggregation and has been linked in one case to the development of a spontaneous epidural hematoma. Ginkgo biloba inhibits platelet-activating factor and has been linked to several cases of spontaneous intracranial bleeding, and ginseng inhibits platelet aggregation and prolongs both thrombin time and activated partial thromboplastin time, although the clinical significance of these findings remain unclear.[11–13]

Timely diagnosis of spinal epidural hematoma is critical but, in many cases, will be challenging. Many patients have few complaints initially, commonly developing progressively worsening back pain as the hematoma expands with or without the immediate or delayed appearance of focal neurologic deficits. A progressive neurologic deficit may develop over a variable interval and with variable severity. Typically, neurologic deficits evolve over the course of several hours, but in some instances, they may develop over several days. In some instances, neurologic deficit rather than pain may be the presenting sign. Physical findings of myelopathy, or the development of the Brown-Sequard syndrome, should be recognized as indicative of spinal cord compression and should prompt emergent diagnostic evaluation and treatment.[14] Intractable leg pain and cauda equina syndrome may develop as well. Urinary retention may precede urinary incontinence. When a spinal epidural hematoma is suspected, a thorough neurologic examination is mandatory. This examination should include evaluation of anal sphincter tone and direct examination in efforts to detect loss of perineal sensation. Furthermore, serial examinations should be performed at short intervals. Findings on physical examination will be variable depending on the level of the lesion. Unilateral or bilateral weakness and/or paresthesias

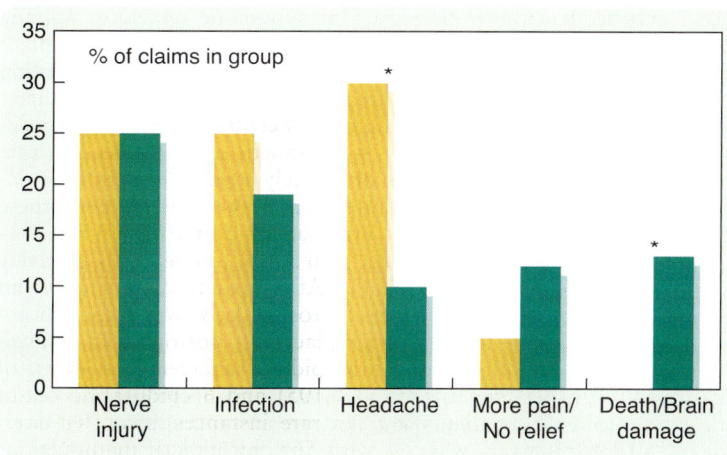

FIGURE 112.2   Most common outcomes within the American Society of Anesthesiologists Closed Claims Project in those claims following epidural steroid injection. *Yellow bars* represent injections with steroids only. *Green bars* indicate injections in which local anesthetic or opioid (or both) were added to the steroid. *$P < 0.05$ between proportion of injection group with that outcome. (*Reprinted with permission from Fitzgibbon DR, Posner KL, Domino KB, et al; American Society of Anesthesiologists. Chronic pain management: American Society of Anesthesiologists Closed Claims Project. Anesthesiology 2004;100[1]:98–105.*)

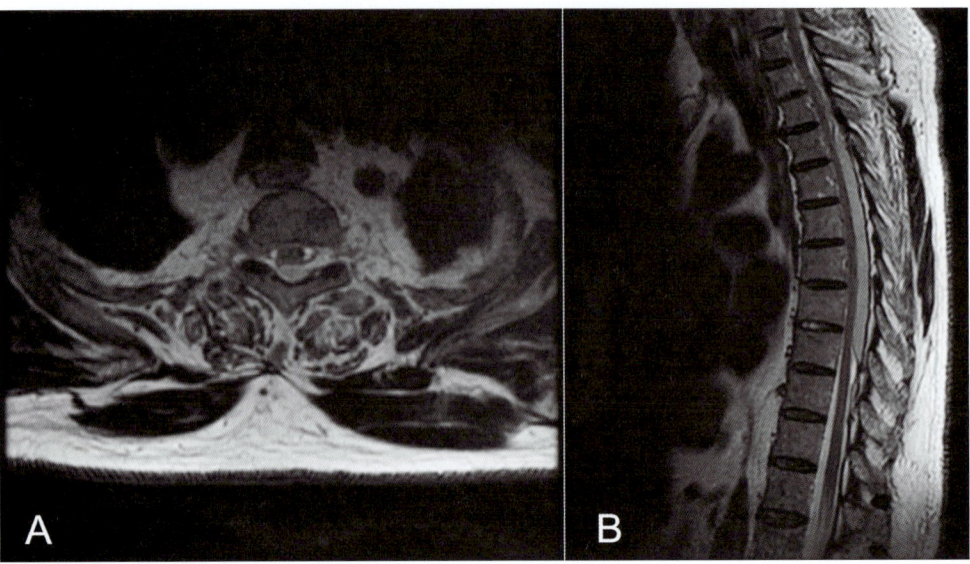

FIGURE 112.3 Magnetic resonance imaging (MRI) of the lumbosacral spine demonstrating a lumbar epidural hematoma. Axial **(A)** and sagittal **(B)** reconstructed T2-weighted MRIs demonstrating a biconvex mass dorsal to the thecal sac extending from the cervicothoracic junction to the low thoracic area, with tapering cephalad and caudad margins, the typical appearance of an epidural hematoma.

may be present. Hyper- or hyporeflexia may also be present. Depending on the clinical context, the differential diagnosis may include spinal epidural abscess. Urgent laboratory studies should include a complete blood count with platelets as well as a prothrombin time and activated partial thromboplastin time. In addition, a blood bank sample should be sent for type and cross-match in preparation for surgery as well as in cases where fresh frozen plasma may be needed to reverse coagulopathies.

Magnetic resonance imaging (MRI) is the preferred radiologic study for diagnosis of spinal epidural hematoma. On sagittal reconstructed computed tomography (CT) or MR images, a spinal epidural hematoma typically appears as a biconvex mass dorsal to the thecal sac, with tapering cephalad and caudal margins (Fig. 112.3). Associated spinal cord edema may also be seen. Acute hemorrhage is characterized by a marked decrease in signal intensity on T2-weighted images. Subacute hematoma is characterized by increased signal intensity on both T1- and T2-weighted images.[15] The dura matter appears as a low-signal curvilinear structure separating the hematoma from the spinal cord on T2-weighted gradient echo sequences. In one retrospective study of 17 patients with acute spinal epidural hematoma, 10 patients' T1-weighted images showed isointensity to the spinal cord, and in 7 patients, the hematomas were slightly hyperintense. T2-weighted images showed hyperintensity with areas of hypointensity. Other MRI findings included hematomas showing direct contiguity with the adjacent osseous spine in 13 patients. Posterolateral location of the hematomas was noted in 13 patients. Additional findings were capping of the epidural fat, compression of the epidural fat and ligamentum flavum, and compression of the thecal sac and/or cord.[16] MRI will also help to identify associated spinal cord tumors or arteriovenous malformations. For patients who cannot undergo MRI scanning or in cases where MRI scanning is not immediately available, CT, with or without myelography, is the study of choice. A spinal epidural hematoma appears as a biconcave dorsal mass typically extending over at least two vertebral levels (see Fig. 112.3).[17] Lumbar puncture does not add to the diagnosis and may worsen the patient's condition in some instances.

When spinal epidural hematoma is entertained as a diagnosis, urgent neurosurgical consultation should be obtained. In a retrospective study of 30 patients who were treated for

spinal epidural hematoma between 1979 and 1993, rapidity of surgical decompression of the spinal cord correlated with neurologic outcome.[16] Patients who were taken to surgery within 12 hours of symptom onset fared significantly better than those whose surgery was delayed beyond 12 hours. In this series, the patients' preoperative neurologic status was also predictive of outcome. Of note, in a series of 30 patients, of 8 patients who had complete loss of neurologic function (Frankel grade A), 6 improved with surgical decompression, and 2 of these regained normal function.[12] Emergent surgical evacuation remains the standard of care and treatment of choice for spinal epidural hematoma. In some instances, spinal epidural hematomas have been successfully conservatively managed, typically in patients whose neurologic examination was spontaneously, steadily improving.[18]

Infectious Complications

Infectious complications may ensue following either peripheral or central neuraxial blockade, although the latter is more likely to lead to catastrophic sequelae such as meningitis or compression of neural structures. Both superficial and deep infections have been reported following epidural injections, facet joint injections, and trigger point injections. In the case of indwelling catheters, the risk of infection increases with increased duration of catheter therapy. One systematic review examining 4,628 cancer patients with indwelling catheters left in place for 7 days or more found that the incidence of deep infection was 1 per 2,391 days of treatment, or 0.4 per 1,000 catheter treatment days. The average catheter duration for these patients was shown to be 74 days with a deep infection rate reaching 2.8%. Four out of 57 of the patients with deep infections related to their indwelling catheters died from these infection complications.[19] When comparing infection rates between cancer and noncancer patients, one study retrospectively examined 131 patients (80% cancer patients) and found no difference in infection rates of spinal cord stimulator and intrathecal drug delivery systems.[20] In the case of implanted spinal cord stimulators and intrathecal drug pumps, a review of four prospective trials found 36 infections in 35 patients out of a total of 700 patients who underwent implantation. The overall infection rate was 5% with 57% to 80% of the infections in the trials involving the pump pocket, 13% to 33% involving the lumbar site, and 0% to 14% leading to meningitis.[21] One study showed that a more skilled/experience operator had a lower infection rate (1.8%) compared to the less skilled/experienced (13%).[22] All patients undergoing interventional therapies for pain treatment should be given explicit written postprocedural guidelines that include a clear description of the signs and symptoms that may herald an infection and a clear process for contacting pain clinic personnel on an urgent basis if such signs and symptoms develop.

The source of the pathogen may be either external, as in the case of contaminated equipment or breaches in sterile technique, or internal, in the case of patients with local or systemic infections such as skin and soft tissue infections or bacteremia. It is not surprising then that occlusive postsurgical dressings and perioperative antibiotics have been shown to decrease the risk of infections.[23] Risk factors for infection include diabetes, alcoholism, smoking, and immunosuppression. Similarly, infections in the epidural space may spread to other areas via hematogenous spread or local extension. Pathogens include skin flora such as *Staphylococcus aureus* and *Staphylococcus epidermidis*. In patients with implanted spinal catheters or devices, the incidence of methicillin-resistant *S. aureus* epidural infection is particularly high. Injury to the neural structures may occur due to direct compression by an abscess or due to ischemia caused by septic thrombophlebitis.

Initially, the patient with an evolving epidural abscess typically presents with back pain at the affected level of the spine. Subsequently, they may develop radicular pain corresponding to the involved level. They may then progress to development of motor and sensory deficits accompanied by bowel and bladder dysfunction and finally to frank paralysis. Back pain will be present in roughly three-quarters of patients, fever in almost half, and neurologic deficits in about one-third. Thus, the classic triad of back pain, fever, and neurologic deficit is seen in only a minority of patients.[24] Both the duration of symptoms prior to presentation and the rate of progression of symptoms can be highly variable. Spinal epidural abscesses typically extend over three to four vertebral levels; however, in rare instances, they may involve the whole spine. Laboratory studies should include a complete blood count with differential as about two-thirds of patients will have leukocytosis. Erythrocyte sedimentation rate and C-reactive protein are almost always elevated, although neither of these tests is specific. Blood cultures should be sent prior to the administration of antibiotics and approximately 60% of patients will be bacteremic. When lumbar puncture is performed, CSF analysis shows elevated protein and pleocytosis in three-quarters of patients. Gram staining and culture of CSF are negative in the majority of patients. Lumbar puncture adds little to the diagnosis and entails risk of causing meningitis if the needle traverses the epidural abscess en route to the thecal space; CSF should be analyzed if myelography is undertaken.

MRI with IV gadolinium is the study of choice to evaluate possible epidural abscess (Fig. 112.4). MRI is highly sensitive for diagnosing epidural abscess and allows evaluation of the dimensions of the abscess which facilitates surgical planning. If MRI is contraindicated or is not readily available, CT myelography is also quite sensitive but is more invasive. Plain x-rays or CT scan of the spine without myelography may demonstrate diminished disk space and/or bony destruction suggestive of discitis and osteomyelitis. These conditions coexist with epidural abscess in up to 80% of cases. Urgent surgical drainage accompanied by administration of systemic antibiotics is the standard of care for epidural abscesses.[25] In rare cases, percutaneous drainage with systemic antibiotics or antibiotic treatment in the absence of surgery may be undertaken.[24]

Superficial infections typically present with local erythema, pain, swelling, and, in some cases, purulent discharge. In some instances, superficial infections associated with catheters can be managed with local drainage and antibiotics without removing the catheter.[26] Some cases of superficial infections and pocket site infections following implantations of spinal cord stimulators and intrathecal drug pumps have been successfully managed using oral and parenteral antibiotics that correspond to antimicrobial sensitivities on the basis of wound cultures, although the implanted device has been left in place.[27,28] However, as other authors have noted, device-related infections are rarely completely eradicated without removal of the device in question.[21] This observation mirrors the extensive experience with infected cardiac pacemakers.[29] In all cases, a high degree of vigilance must be maintained to the possibility that a device-related superficial or pocket infection may spread to the neuraxis with catastrophic results. In the event that signs of infection such as erythema, swelling, fluctuance, or tenderness progress along the course of an implanted lead or catheter, the device with all associated hardware should be surgically removed on an urgent basis. Similarly, urgent device removal should be undertaken if the patient displays signs of systemic infection such as fever or chills, or signs of possible meningitis such as fever, neck pain and stiffness, severe headache, or altered mental status. At the time of surgery, separately labeled wound cultures should be sent from all surgical sites, and all surgical sites should be extensively irrigated. As with spinal epidural hematoma, the patient's preoperative neurologic function is the best predictor of final neurologic outcome.[30] For any patient where there is a significant concern for systemic infection or meningitis, antibiotics should be administered immediately and should not be delayed until cultures can be obtained. Empiric antibiotic coverage should provide coverage of *Staphylococcus* species, preferably with vancomycin to ensure coverage of methicillin-resistant *S. aureus*, Streptococci species, and should also provide coverage of gram-negative microbes with a third- or fourth-generation cephalosporin (such as cefepime or ceftriaxone) or equivalent. When the etiologic agent has been identified, antibiotics should be directed toward the specific pathogen. Five percent of patients with spinal epidural abscesses die secondary to sepsis or other infectious complications signifying the importance of early intervention.[24]

Local Anesthetic Systemic Toxicity

Lidocaine and bupivacaine are amide local anesthetics which are widely used in interventional pain management procedures due to their relative safety. Lidocaine is of relatively lower potency and has a rapid onset of action and an intermediate duration of action. Nonetheless, the potential for lidocaine associated systemic toxicity due to excessive dose, inadvertent intravascular administration, or unanticipated rapid absorption is well recognized. Bupivacaine is of higher potency but has a slower onset and prolonged duration of action. Local anesthetics, including lidocaine and bupivacaine, bind sodium channels and inhibit the sodium permeability that underlies action potentials in both neurons and cardiac myocytes. Local anesthetic inhibition of sodium permeability increases with repeated depolarization. In addition to binding sodium channels, local anesthetics will bind potassium and calcium channels as well as N-methyl-D-aspartate receptors, β-adrenergic receptors, and nicotinic acetylcholine receptors. Indeed, local anesthetic toxicity may be mediated in part through binding to these channels and receptors.[31–33] In general, the anesthetic potency of a local anesthetic correlates with its central nervous system (CNS) toxicity. Local anesthetics appear to cause cardiac toxicity through several different mechanisms including inhibition of calcium and potassium channels and inhibition of β-adrenergic receptors and epinephrine stimulated cAMP formation. Local anesthetics prolong cardiac conduction in a dose-dependent fashion. With increasing serum concentration, bupivacaine provokes QT prolongation, ventricular tachycardia, and ventricular fibrillation. Risk factors for the development of local anesthetic toxicity include the extremes of

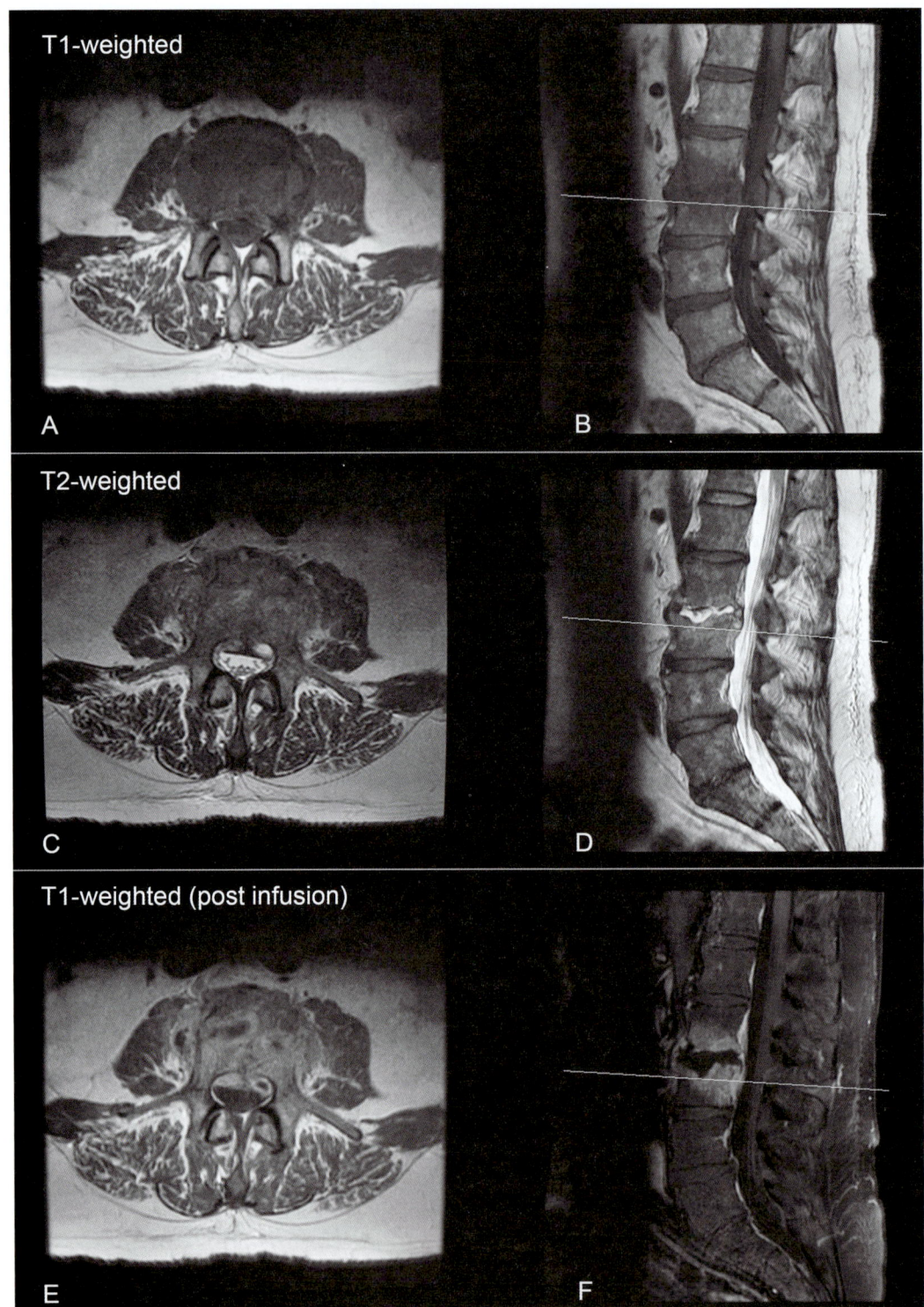

FIGURE 112.4   Magnetic resonance imaging of the lumbosacral spine demonstrating epidural abscess. This is a 64-year-old who presented with worsening axial low back pain 2 weeks following lumbar epidural injection of steroid for treatment of acute radicular pain. Axial **(A)** and sagittal **(B)** T1-weighted images. Axial **(C)** and sagittal **(D)** T2-weighted images. Axial **(E)** and sagittal **(F)** T1-weighted images following intravenous administration of gadolinium. These findings are compatible with diskitis/osteomyelitis at L2–L3, with enhancement of the anterior epidural space and a focus of high T2 and low T1 signal in the left anterior epidural space consistent with epidural abscess.

age, end-organ dysfunction (hepatic, renal, and cardiac), and pregnancy. The threshold dose of local anesthetic required to provoke seizures is affected by the route and rate of injection, the rate of increase of serum drug concentration, the presence of acidosis, and whether the patient is awake or anesthetized. Local anesthetic toxicity may result from systemic absorption of excessive doses following local infiltration; however, toxicity

more commonly occurs due to inadvertent intravascular injection. Intra-arterial injection poses a greater risk of CNS and cardiovascular toxicity than IV injection because, in the latter case, passage through the lung allows for some clearance of the drug. In the case of intra-arterial injection, doses as small as 2.5 mg of bupivacaine or 15 mg of lidocaine have resulted in seizures when injected into the carotid or vertebral arteries, and

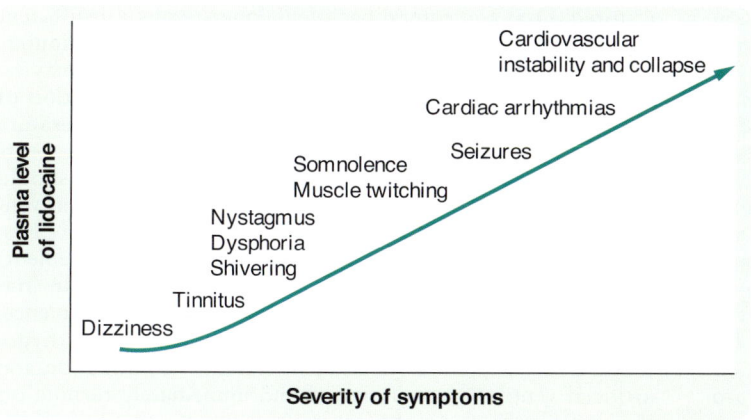

FIGURE 112.5 Relationship between plasma concentration of lidocaine and the development of signs and symptoms of local anesthetic toxicity.

this is felt to result from direct delivery of the local anesthetic to the brain.[34,35]

In the event of lidocaine toxicity, CNS symptoms typically precede cardiovascular symptoms.[36] CNS symptoms are initially characterized by inhibitory neuronal blockade leading to excitatory manifestations such as perioral numbness, a metallic taste, tinnitus, restlessness, confusion, a sense of impending doom, visual disturbances that are most commonly described as oscillations of objects in the visual fields, shivers, tremors, and tonic-clonic seizures (Fig. 112.5). Sympathetic stimulation is also observed during this phase, with resultant tachycardia and hypertension.[37] In patients who are receiving procedural sedation with benzodiazepines or other sedatives, the excitatory phase of local anesthetic toxicity may not be apparent. The excitatory phase is followed in episodes of severe toxicity by a depressed phase characterized by coma and respiratory arrest. Cardiovascular toxicity develops at higher serum levels and may include profound bradycardia, arrhythmias, contractile dysfunction, and asystole.[31] In the case of bupivacaine, doses that are insufficient to provoke seizures will provoke cardiac arrhythmias.[38]

Treatment of local anesthetic–induced seizures focuses on maintaining the airway and oxygenation. The injection or infusion of local anesthetic must be stopped immediately. Lorazepam, midazolam, thiopental, or propofol may be used to terminate the seizure. Cardiovascular depression with resultant hypotension due to local anesthetic toxicity should be treated with IV crystalloids and vasopressors such as norepinephrine, or phenylephrine. In the event of severe contractile dysfunction, epinephrine should be administered. If cardiac arrest occurs, advanced cardiac life support (ACLS) protocol should be pursued, although if epinephrine is used, small initial doses ($\leq$1 μg/kg) are preferred and vasopressin is not recommended. Successful resuscitation following cardiac arrest due to bupivacaine toxicity has included the administration of IV lipid emulsion.[39,40] A 20% lipid emulsion may be administered as a 1.5 mL/kg bolus followed by a 0.25 mL/kg/min infusion for 30 to 60 minutes. A repeat bolus is often administered for persistent cardiovascular collapse. It should be noted that the lipid emulsion infusion should be continued for at least 10 minutes after hemodynamic stability is achieved.[41] Current evidence suggests that lipid emulsion works as a carrier to scavenge local anesthetic away from high blood flow organs that are most sensitive to local anesthetic toxicity (i.e., the heart and brain) and redistribute it to organs that store and eliminate the drug (i.e., muscle and liver, respectively).[42] In the presence of persistent cardiovascular collapse associated with local anesthetic administration, urgent institution of cardiopulmonary bypass can be lifesaving. The American Society of Regional Anesthesia and Pain Medicine recently published their most recent Practice Advisory on Local Anesthetic Systemic Toxicity, and this includes an up-to-date and comprehensive review of this topic.[43]

UNINTENDED DESTINATIONS FOLLOWING LOCAL ANESTHETIC ADMINISTRATION

The direct effects of local anesthetics are critically dependent on where they are applied. Inadvertent intrathecal injection of local anesthetic can result in a high thoracic or cervical level of sensory and motor block or total spinal anesthesia, with transient loss of consciousness and respiratory arrest. This is most likely to occur during cervical injections or when a large volume of local anesthetic is used during lumbar injections. Signs and symptoms of a high spinal progress rapidly and most typically include flaccid paralysis, apnea, hypotension, bradycardia, and dilated pupils. They initially include symptoms of sympathectomy, presenting as light-headedness, dizziness, nausea, and vomiting.[35] In addition, the patient may develop air hunger due to loss of intercostal muscle activity, followed by phrenic nerve paralysis and eventually apnea due to blockade of the respiratory center in the brainstem. Blockade of the cardioaccelerator fibers at T1 to T4 or of the medulla may inhibit sympathetic positive chronotropic effects resulting in bradycardia, hypotension, or arrhythmias.[44] Blockade of the Edinger-Westphal nucleus with subsequent loss of efferent parasympathetic activity produces dilated, nonreactive pupils.[45] In the case of subdural injection, symptoms develop more slowly, typically 15 to 30 minutes after injection, and are commonly asymmetric. When symptoms do occur, they may progress to respiratory and cardiovascular collapse as with intrathecal injection. When a high spinal occurs, ventilation with 100% oxygen with a bag valve mask must be initiated if phrenic nerve blockade or apnea is present. Endotracheal intubation may be required to maintain ventilation or protect the lungs from aspiration. Bradycardia and hypotension should be treated with crystalloids and atropine, ephedrine, phenylephrine, or epinephrine.[44] The patient may remain awake but paralyzed during a high spinal, so reassurance that the condition is temporary is warranted as is consideration of administration of an anxiolytic agent.

VASOVAGAL REACTIONS

Vasovagal reactions, which may include frank syncope, are one of the most common emergencies encountered in a pain center. Fortunately, these episodes typically have a benign natural history. Sir William Gowers first used the term *vasovagal* in 1907, and vasovagal syncope is now accepted as the most common form of syncope, accounting for two thirds of syncopal episodes presenting to the emergency department.[46] The pathogenesis of vasovagal syncope remains uncertain, but the current understanding is that it results from venous pooling and reduced venous return and that vigorous contraction of the heart's chambers when they are inadequately filled provokes the Bezold-Jarisch reflex, resulting in paradoxical hypotension and bradycardia. At the onset of a vasovagal reaction, patients typically appear pale and diaphoretic and complain of light-headedness, sweatiness, nausea, and tunnel vision. Myoclonic jerks may accompany vasovagal syncope and may be clinically indistinguishable from seizure activity. If a patient exhibits signs of a vasovagal reaction during an interventional pain treatment procedure, the procedure should be halted, and the patient should be placed supine if not already in that position. Care should be taken to ensure that the patient will not fall and sustain a secondary injury. Randomized trials have demonstrated that leg crossing, and isometric arm exercises can help prevent progression to vasovagal syncope.[47] Most cases of vasovagal syncope will resolve spontaneously and will require only conservative measures. In the event that blood pressure and heart rate continue to decline, an IV line should be placed, crystalloids and oxygen administered, the patient should be placed on a cardiac monitor and a vasopressor, such as ephedrine (in 5- to 10-mg increments) or an anticholinergic drug such as atropine (0.4 to 1 mg) should be administered.[35]

Complications Associated with Intrathecal Drug Delivery

When drugs are delivered via the intrathecal route, complications may arise either due to withdrawal or due to administration of an excessive dose. In the case of intrathecal baclofen administration, withdrawal may be particularly severe and can even be fatal. Baclofen is an analogue of the inhibitory neurotransmitter γ-aminobutyric acid (GABA). It acts as an agonist of the $GABA_B$ receptors in the brainstem, dorsal horn of the spinal cord, and other CNS regions. Although the mechanism of intrathecal baclofen withdrawal is not established, it may be due to diffuse disinhibition of $GABA_B$-modulated pathways.[48] Although the most common manifestation of under dosage of baclofen is pruritus and return of the patient's spasticity, abrupt baclofen withdrawal may result in a life-threatening syndrome characterized by fever, tachycardia, labile blood pressure or hypotension, malaise, dysphoria, and hallucinations followed by coma, rebound spasticity more severe than the patient's baseline, hyperreflexia or rigidity, paresthesias, priapism in males, and seizures. If not treated adequately and promptly, the patient may develop rhabdomyolysis, brain injury, kidney and liver failure, and disseminated intravascular coagulation.[48,49] In some cases, death ensues.[50] The differential diagnosis of intrathecal baclofen withdrawal includes infection, neuroleptic malignant syndrome, serotonin syndrome, malignant hyperthermia, and autonomic dysreflexia. Paradoxically, the diagnosis may be more difficult to make in more severe cases of withdrawal. Symptoms of intrathecal baclofen withdrawal typically present 1 to 3 days after interruption of baclofen delivery. Interruption of baclofen delivery may be due to an exhausted drug reservoir after missing a scheduled refill, pump malfunction, catheter kinking or disruption, or mistakes in drug formulation or pump programming. Restoration of adequate intrathecal baclofen delivery by addressing pump problems or by lumbar puncture or drain represents the most definitive therapy.[51] If the pump catheter remains intact, intrathecal baclofen may be administered via the side port. Evaluation of the pump should be performed with the manufacturer's interrogation device. If interrogation of the pump does not reveal the underlying problem, a catheter dye study should be undertaken and the pump should be refilled with medication at the correct concentration. To conduct a catheter dye study, radiographic contrast is administered through the side port of the infusion device to assess the integrity and position of the intrathecal catheter. Oral and enteral baclofen administration (up to 120 mg per day of baclofen in six to eight divided doses in adults), accompanied by IV benzodiazepine administration should be undertaken until intrathecal baclofen delivery is

restored. Oral and enteral baclofen alone are often insufficient to treat withdrawal from intrathecal baclofen. Continuous or intermittent infusions of diazepam or midazolam may be rapidly titrated upward until muscle relaxation, cessation of seizure activity, and normal blood pressure and temperature are restored. Propofol infusion and chemical paralytic agents may also be used in the intubated patient.[52] The patient should be treated in a setting where critical care monitoring and ventilator and cardiovascular support is available. In some cases, patients with hyperthermia have been treated with dantrolene. In case reports, cyproheptadine has proven helpful.[48,53] In contrast, baclofen overdose typically presents with somnolence, hypothermia, comas, seizures, respiratory depression, hypotonia, and arrhythmias. Treatment consists of intubation and artificial ventilation as indicated and immediately turning off the pump with the manufacturer's programmer or, if this is not available, emptying the pump reservoir. In cases where the overdose is detected within the first few hours, withdrawal of 30 to 40 mL of CSF via the catheter access port of the pump may reverse the overdose.[54] Physostigmine may reverse drowsiness and respiratory depression (adult dose 0.5 to 2 mg IV over 5 to 10 minutes, may repeat every 10 to 30 minutes as required; pediatric dose 0.02 mg/kg IV, less than 0.5 mg per minute, may repeat every 5 to 10 minutes as required up to 2 mg maximum).

OPIOID WITHDRAWAL

Opioid withdrawal can also occur in patients receiving intrathecal drug delivery or systemic opioids and typically manifests with anxiety, insomnia, yawning, diaphoresis, lacrimation, rhinorrhea, mydriasis, myalgias, piloerection, nausea, vomiting, diarrhea, and abdominal cramping.[55,56] In patients for whom ongoing opioid therapy is indicated, treatment consists of resuming opioid therapy. In some cases, an alternate route of administration may be necessary, such as IV and/or transdermal delivery for a patient who is no longer able to take oral medications. In cases where opioid therapy is not indicated, symptoms of opioid withdrawal may be mitigated with α_2-adrenergic agonists such as clonidine (0.1 to 0.3 mg orally per dose every 6 to 8 hours increasing to a maximum of 1.2 mg per day[57]) or lofexidine (0.4 to 0.8 mg orally per dose increasing to a maximum of 2.4 mg per day). α_2-Adrenergic agonists may cause hypotension, fatigue, lethargy, and dry mouth. Nausea and vomiting may be treated with IV fluids and antiemetics such as metoclopramide or prochlorperazine. Diarrhea and colicky abdominal pain may be treated with loperamide or hyoscine butylbromide.[56] Agitation may be treated with benzodiazepines, although a careful consideration of risks is necessary anytime concurrent benzodiazepines and opioids are prescribed. It should be noted that opioids are not a first-line or routine therapy for chronic, noncancer pain. The Centers for Disease Control and Prevention (CDC) Guidelines for Prescribing Opioids for Chronic Pain include several recommendations for determining when to initiate or continue chronic opioids for chronic pain. Complications from opioid withdrawal are often avoidable simply from a proper assessment prior to clinical prescription. In assessing potential risks, the CDC recommends that clinicians should review their respective state prescription drug monitoring program data periodically during opioid therapy for chronic pain, ranging from every prescription to every 3 months.[58]

Anaphylactic and Anaphylactoid Reactions

At the turn of the 19th century, Charles Richet and Paul Portier coined the term *anaphylaxis* when they observed that several dogs died following repeat challenges with *Physalia* extracts during experiments that they reported while guests on

Prince Albert of Monaco's yacht in the Mediterranean Sea.[59] In an anaphylactic reaction, the inciting allergen binds to previously formed immunoglobulin E (IgE) on the surface of previously sensitized mast cells and basophils. These cells release mediators such as histamine, leukotrienes, prostaglandins, bradykinins, and thromboxanes that cause markedly reduced vascular tone, increased mucous membrane secretions, and increased capillary permeability.[60] Anaphylactoid reactions produce a similar and often indistinguishable clinical picture but are not IgE mediated. Anaphylactoid reactions occur through nonimmune-mediated release of mediators from mast cells and/or basophils or result from direct complement activation.[61] Generalized hypersensitivity reactions may be divided into grade 1 or mild reactions, grade 2 or moderate reactions, and grade 3 or severe reactions.[62] Grades 2 and 3 correspond with anaphylaxis and are clinically similar to anaphylactoid reactions. Grade 1 reactions are defined by generalized erythema, urticaria, periorbital edema, or angioedema. Grade 2 reactions are characterized by dyspnea, stridor, wheezing, nausea and vomiting, dizziness or presyncope, chest or throat tightness, or abdominal pain. Grade 3 reactions are defined by cyanosis or an oxygen saturation less than or equal to 92%, hypotension, confusion, collapse, loss of consciousness, or incontinence. Cutaneous manifestations such as erythema, itch, and urticaria are present in almost all cases, although they may be quite subtle. Therefore, when the diagnosis is unclear, it is crucial to fully undress the patient and carefully examine the skin. In one retrospective study of 1,149 cases of generalized hypersensitivity treated in the emergency department, 250 cases were assessed as being due to medications; 145 cases were believed to be due to antibiotics, with the majority being β-lactam antibiotics. Nonsteroidal anti-inflammatory drugs were implicated in 32 cases, narcotics in 11 cases, radiologic contrast in 7 cases, angiotensin-converting enzyme (ACE) inhibitors in 4 cases, vaccines in 4 cases, and other or unclear medications in 47 cases.[62] The median interval between drug administration and fatal collapse is 5 minutes.[63] The differential diagnosis of anaphylactic and anaphylactoid reactions includes asthma attack, scombroid poisoning, angioedema either secondary to ACE inhibitors or hereditary, panic attack, and vasovagal syncope (these last two conditions do not cause urticaria, angioedema, or bronchospasm).

There are no randomized trials of therapies for these potentially fatal reactions, so most treatment recommendations are on the basis of consensus. The patient undergoing an anaphylactic or anaphylactoid reaction should be administered high flow oxygen. Intramuscular (IM) epinephrine should be given early to all patients with signs of a systemic reaction such as hypotension, airway edema, or dyspnea (0.3 to 0.5 mg, 1:1,000, IM repeated every 15 to 20 minutes if there is no clinical improvement). If the reaction appears to be severe and/or imminently life threatening, IV epinephrine should be given (0.1 mg, 1:10,000, IV over 5 minutes, followed by an IV infusion of 1 to 4 μg per minute as needed). Patients receiving epinephrine should be monitored in an emergency department or intensive care unit. Aggressive fluid resuscitation with isotonic crystalloids such as normal saline should be undertaken.[64] One liter to 2 L should be rapidly infused. Antihistamines such as diphenhydramine should be given (25 to 50 mg per dose IV or IM) as well as H2 blockers (e.g., cimetidine 300 mg IM or IV). Bronchospasm should be treated with inhaled β-adrenergic agents such as albuterol and/or IV/IM epinephrine. High-dose IV corticosteroids should be administered early, although their therapeutic effects are seen 4 to 6 hours after administration. Other therapies which may be considered in anaphylaxis or anaphylactoid reactions include vasopressin, which has been beneficial in case reports for severely hypotensive patients, atropine in the setting of severe bradycardia, and glucagon for patients who are unresponsive epinephrine, particularly if they are taking β-blockers.[60] Pumphrey,[63] who attempted to identify and analyze every fatal anaphylactic reaction in the United Kingdom since 1992, stresses the importance of keeping patients supine with their legs elevated.

CATASTROPHIC NEURAL INJURIES AND THE ADMINISTRATION OF PARTICULATE STEROIDS

In the cervical spine, the carotid and vertebral arteries lie in close proximity to the stellate ganglion, the cervical facet joints, and the cervical intervertebral foramina. The anterior spinal artery provides the principal vascular supply to the spinal cord. The anterior spinal artery arises rostrally from the vertebral arteries and receives input from six to nine radicular arteries. It is located at the anterior central sulcus and supplies the anterior two-thirds of the spinal cord. The posterior spinal arteries supply the posterior one-third of the spinal cord. They are paired and run just medial to the dorsal roots. The arteria radicularis magna (more commonly referred to as the artery of Adamkiewicz) is the largest of the radicular arteries. It is most commonly located at T10 on the left side but may occur anywhere from T8 to L2 and occurs on the right in 17% of subjects.[65] In addition, the ascending cervical artery and the deep cervical artery each furnish spinal branches that enter the intervertebral foramina. These spinal branches not only supply the vertebral column but also give rise to radicular arteries that accompany the dorsal and ventral roots of the spinal nerves (Fig. 112.6). In some individuals, the radicular arteries are substantial in size and reinforce the anterior spinal artery. Such reinforcing arteries can occur at any cervical level and those radicular arteries that supply the spinal cord are termed *spinal medullary arteries*. If reinforcing radicular arteries are compromised by a transforaminal injection, infarction of the cervical spinal cord could ensue. If the vertebral or carotid arteries are entered, infarction of the brainstem and portions of the brain supplied by the posterior circulation may ensue, causing stroke, often resulting in death.

The first report of a complication attributed to cervical transforaminal injection of steroids described a patient who died from a spinal cord infarction.[14] The location of the infarction implied that a radicular artery that reinforced the anterior spinal artery had been compromised, but no evidence was offered about the mechanism by which the artery had been compromised. Images of the placement of the needle were not published.

Reports of spinal cord infarction following cervical[66,67] or lumbar[68,69] transforaminal injection of steroid have appeared, and this topic has been reviewed in detail.[70] Vertebral artery injection with subsequent stroke involving the posterior circulation has also been reported.[71] A similar case of massive infarction involving the posterior cerebral circulation following injection of particulate steroid during attempted intra-articular atlantoaxial joint injection is shown in Figure 112.7.

The exact mechanism of spinal cord injury following transforaminal injections has not been determined. As analyzed using MRI, the pattern of injury strongly implicates a reinforcing radicular artery. Spasm of the artery would seem to be an unlikely mechanism because it is inconsistent with the vasodilatory effect of local anesthetic agents when applied to arterial walls. Embolism of particulate steroids ranks as the leading hypothesis, but direct evidence is still lacking. In cases involving the vertebral artery, a similar uncertainty remains. The injection of contrast medium cannot be an explanation; in the past, direct puncture of the vertebral artery has been used for angiography. Steroid embolism remains the most likely explanation.

The guidelines for the conduct of cervical transforaminal injections[70] are designed to guard against these complications. These guidelines stipulate that the needle must be accurately and correctly placed. Once the needle has been placed, a test dose of contrast medium should be injected and its flow carefully monitored during injection. That injection tests two

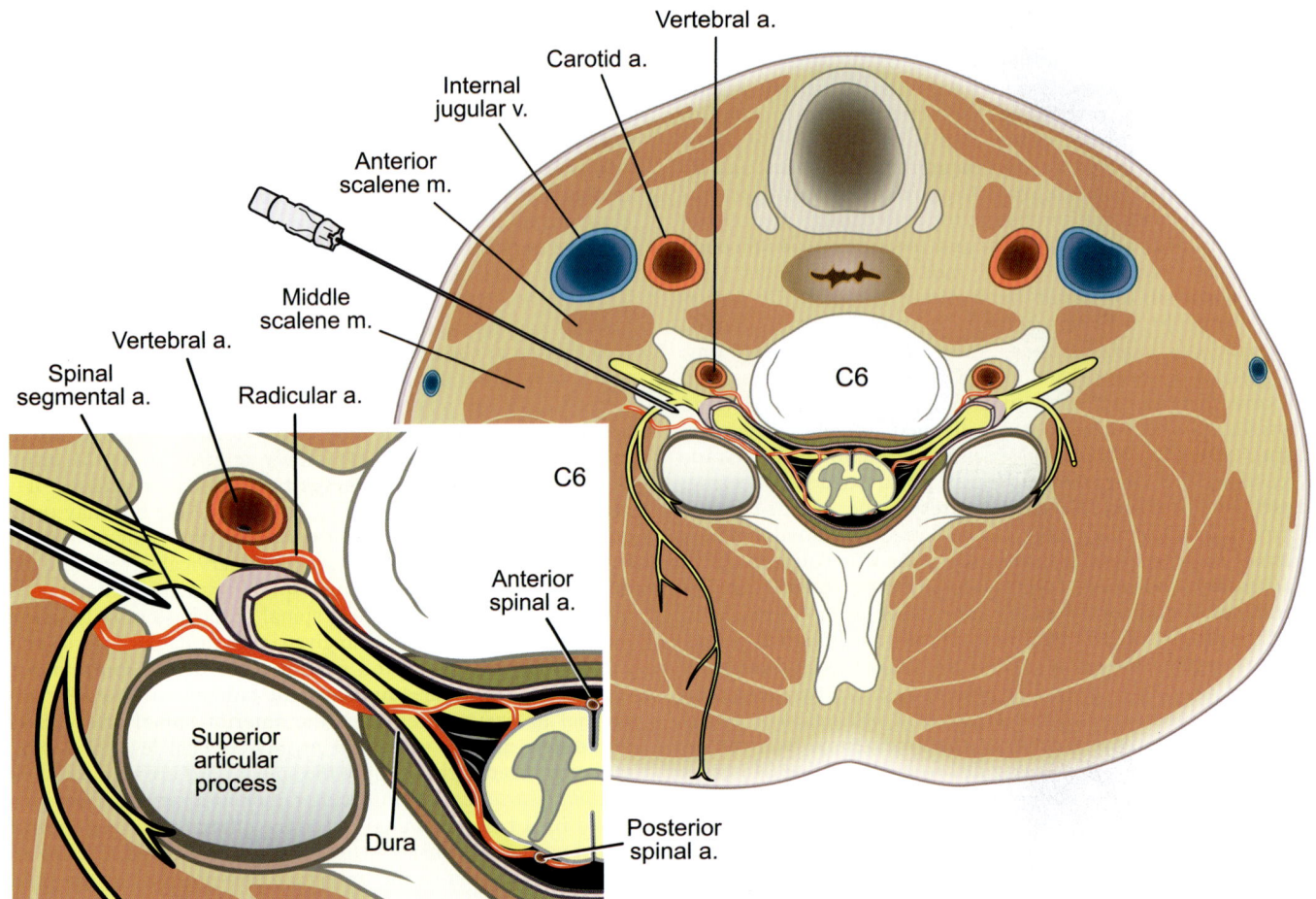

FIGURE 112.6 Axial view of cervical transforaminal injection at the level of C6. The needle has been inserted along the axis of the foramen and is in final position against the posterior aspect of the intervertebral foramen. Insertion along this axis places the needle behind the spinal nerve and behind the vertebral artery, which lies anterior to the foramen. **Inset:** A spinal artery arises from the vertebral artery. It supplies the vertebral column. Another spinal artery enters the intervertebral foramen from the ascending cervical artery or deep cervical artery. It furnishes radicular branches that accompany the nerve roots and ultimately reach the anterior and posterior spinal arteries of the spinal cord. *(Redrawn from Rathmell JP. Atlas of Image-Guided Intervention in Regional Anesthesia and Pain Medicine. 2nd ed. Philadelphia: Lippincott Williams & Wilkins; 2011, with permission. Figure 6-1.)*

things. First, under normal circumstances, it should show that the injectate is correctly flowing around the target nerve and into the lateral epidural space. Simultaneously, but more critically, it shows if an intravascular injection has occurred.

Neurologic complications of transforaminal injections are typically catastrophic. They are clinically obvious on the onset of spinal weakness and numbness. Spinal cord infarction due to embolization of a radicular artery is clinically indistinguishable from the anterior spinal artery syndrome, also known as Beck syndrome. Patients develop abrupt onset of weakness below the level of the infarction, flaccid paralysis, areflexia, loss of pain and temperature perception, and atonic urinary bladder. Position and vibratory sensation will typically be relatively intact. Preserved proprioception at symptom onset has been associated with better outcomes.[72] In contrast to cerebrovascular infarction, spinal cord infarction is frequently painful. Patients may experience a radicular or back pain, and some cases, spinal cord infarction will mimic angina pectoris.[73] Later in the clinical course, the patient may develop spasticity, hyperreflexia, Babinski responses, and clonus.[65] In the setting of possible acute spinal cord infarction, the differential diagnosis may include spinal cord compression by a mass lesion such as a spinal epidural or subdural hematoma or abscess, or a herniated nucleus pulposus. When spinal cord infarction is suspected, emergent MRI of the spinal cord should be undertaken to rule out the presence of any space-occupying lesion that may be

amenable to surgical decompression. If spinal cord infarction is present, sagittal T2-weighted MRI scanning performed at least 4 hours after symptom onset commonly reveals "pencil-like" hyperintensities and cord enlargement. Diffusion weighted imaging is particularly sensitive for detecting ischemic changes in the spinal cord.[74] Common diagnostic pitfalls include failure to image higher levels of the spinal cord when the patient develops a sensory level that is caudal to the infarction.

One collaboration between the U.S. Food and Drug Administration (FDA), an expert multidisciplinary working group, and 13 specialty stakeholder societies reviewed existing evidence and produced a consensus to enhancing the safety of neuraxial injections.[75] A few of these notable endorsed clinical considerations included the following:

A. Cervical and lumbar interlaminar ESIs should be performed using image guidance, with appropriate posteroanterior, lateral, or contralateral oblique views and a test dose of contrast medium.

B. Cervical and lumbar transforaminal ESIs should be performed by injecting contrast medium under real-time fluoroscopy and/or digital subtraction imaging, using an anteroposterior view, before injecting any substance that may be hazardous to the patient.

C. Cervical interlaminar ESIs are recommended to be performed at C7–T1 but preferably not higher than the C6–C7 level.

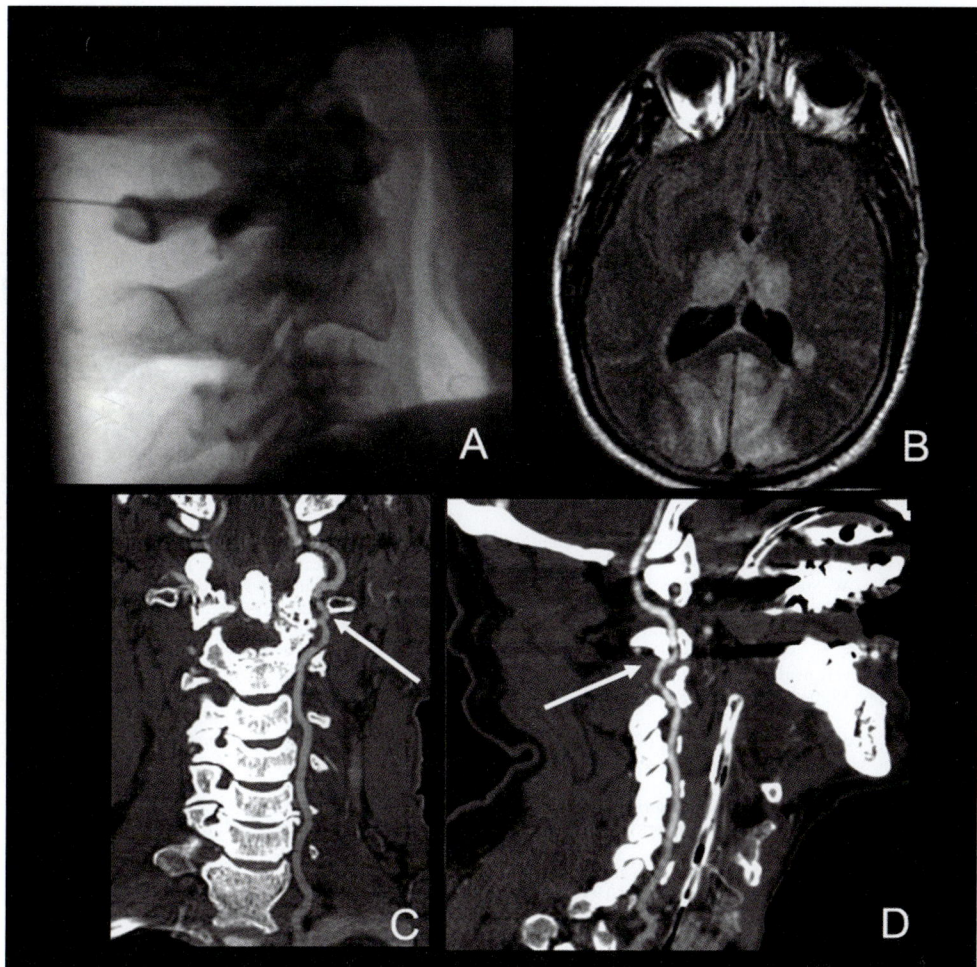

FIGURE 112.7 Cerebrovascular accident following intra-arterial injection of particulate steroid during attempted intra-articular atlantoaxial (C1/C2) joint injection. **A:** Lateral fluoroscopy imaging demonstrating needle position adjacent to the C1/C2 facet joint. **B:** Axial magnetic resonance imaging (T1 FLAIR sequence) of the brain. Frontal **(C)** and axial **(D)** computed tomography angiography of the vertebral arteries; *arrows* point to a small filling defect within the left vertebral artery adjacent to the left C1/C2 facet joint, suggesting the point of needle entry in to the vertebral artery. The proximity of the vertebral artery to the C1/C2 facet joint is immediately apparent from the images.

D. Particulate steroids should not be used in therapeutic cervical transforaminal injections.

E. A face mask and sterile gloves must be worn during the procedure.

F. Moderate-to-heavy sedation is not recommended for ESIs, but if light sedation is used, the patient should remain able to communicate pain or other adverse sensations or events.

There is no emergency management known to reverse spinal cord infarction. Many of the principles guiding treatment of acute spinal cord infarction are derived from experience treating ischemic cerebrovascular accidents. Initially, emphasis should be placed on reducing the likelihood of secondary injury to the spinal cord by preventing hypotension and/or hypoxia. In addition, rapid triage and transport to a definitive care facility with appropriate imaging, critical care, and surgical capabilities should be undertaken. In the case of ischemic cerebrovascular accidents, induced hypertension to achieve a mean arterial pressure of 20% to 30% above baseline or to achieve a predefined target mean arterial pressure has been advocated, although this therapy remains controversial.[76] Although aspirin has been advocated for the treatment of spinal cord infarction related to atherosclerotic disease or dissection, principally on the basis of its use in the treatment of ischemic stroke, there does not appear to be a role for antiplatelet or anticoagulant therapy in the treatment of spinal

cord infarction presumed secondary to embolization of particulate steroids. In a prospective study of 77 patients with acute neurologic deficits secondary to spinal cord injuries, patients treated with 7 days of volume resuscitation with crystalloids, transfusion of blood products to maintain a hematocrit greater than 32, as well as dopamine and norepinephine (Levophed) as needed to maintain a mean arterial blood pressure greater than 85 mm Hg had better neurologic outcomes than historical controls.[77] This therapy has not been studied in prospective randomized controlled trials. One 2014 meta-analysis examining over 13,000 patients found that blood pressure reduction started within 7 days of acute stroke led to an increase in risk of mortality within 30 days,[78] although it had no effect on long-term mortality. Treatment of nonpenetrating acute spinal cord injury with methyl prednisolone remains controversial despite evaluation in three large, prospective randomized double-blind controlled trials.[79–81] At the current time, there is insufficient evidence to advocate routine administration of methylprednisolone to patients with acute spinal cord infarction. Standard measures to prevent complications of acute paraplegia should be implemented, including measures directed at prevention of deep venous thrombosis and pulmonary embolus, as well as bladder catheterization if indicated. Early consultation with physiatrists should be undertaken in order to optimize functional recovery and prevent development of spasticity and decubiti.

Conclusion

Although emergencies in the pain clinic are quite rare, when they do occur they can be catastrophic and even deadly. The pain specialist should be familiar with the most common complications and their mechanisms as well as techniques that can be used to reduce the risk of said complications. Familiarity with common complications, including their clinical presentations and natural histories, will facilitate prompt recognition and treatment, thereby improving the chances of good outcomes. Pain specialists should educate patients about specific signs and symptoms of complications that may ensue from their treatment and provide them with clear instructions for reaching members of the pain clinic staff or emergency health care providers in a timely manner, both during clinic hours and on evenings and weekends, in order to achieve prompt identification and treatment of complications when they arise.

References

1. Pollak KA, Stephens LS, Posner KL, et al. Trends in pain medicine liability. *Anesthesiology* 2015;123(5):1133–1141.
2. Kreppel D, Antoniadis G, Seeling W. Spinal hematoma: a literature survey with meta-analysis of 613 patients. *Neurosurg Rev* 2003;26(1):1–49.
3. Usubiaga JE. Neurological complications following epidural anesthesia. *Int Anesthesiol Clin* 1975;13(2):1–153.
4. Moen V, Dahlgren N, Irestedt L. Severe neurological complications after central neuraxial blockades in Sweden 1990–1999. *Anesthesiology* 2004;101(4):950–959.
5. Cameron CM, Scott DA, McDonald WM, et al. A review of neuraxial epidural morbidity: experience of more than 8,000 cases at a single teaching hospital. *Anesthesiology* 2007;106(5):997–1002.
6. Segal DH, Lidov MW, Camins MB. Cervical epidural hematoma after chiropractic manipulation in a healthy young woman: case report. *Neurosurgery* 1996;39(5):1043–1045.
7. Keane JR, Ahmadi J, Gruen P. Spinal epidural hematoma with subarachnoid hemorrhage caused by acupuncture. *AJNR Am J Neuroradiol* 1993;14(2):365–366.
8. Tarlov IM. Spinal cord compression studies. III. Time limits for recovery after gradual compression in dogs. *AMA Arch Neurol Psychiatry* 1954;71:588–597.
9. Holtås S, Heiling M, Lönntoft M. Spontaneous spinal epidural hematoma: findings at MR imaging and clinical correlation. *Radiology* 1996;199:409–413.
10. Baek BS, Hur JK, Kwon KY, et al. Spontaneous spinal epidural hematoma. *J Korean Neurosurg Soc* 2008;44(1):40–42.
11. Rose KD, Croissant PD, Parliament CF, et al. Spontaneous spinal epidural hematoma with associated platelet dysfunction from excessive garlic ingestion: a case report. *Neurosurgery* 1990;26(5):880–882.
12. Haemorrhage due to Ginkgo biloba? *Prescrire Int* 2008;17(93):19.
13. Friedman JA, Taylor SA, McDermott W, et al. Multifocal and recurrent subarachnoid hemorrhage due to an herbal supplement containing natural coumarins. *Neurocrit Care* 2007;7(1):76–80.
14. Binder DS, Sonne CS, Lawton MD. Spinal epidural hematoma. *Neurosurg Q* 2004;14(1):51–59.
15. Lawton MT, Porter RW, Heiserman JE, et al. Surgical management of spinal epidural hematoma: relationship between surgical timing and neurological outcome. *J Neurosurg* 1995;83(1):1–7.
16. Sklar EM, Post JM, Falcone S. MRI of acute spinal epidural hematomas. *J Comput Assist Tomogr* 1999;23(2):238–243.
17. Boukobza M, Guichard JP, Boissonet M, et al. Spinal epidural haematoma: report of 11 cases and review of the literature. *Neuroradiology* 1994;36(6):456–459.
18. Hentschel SJ, Woolfenden AR, Fairholm DJ. Resolution of spontaneous spinal epidural hematoma without surgery: report of two cases. *Spine* 2001;26(22):E525–E527.
19. Ruppen W, Derry S, McQuay HJ, et al. Infection rates associated with epidural indwelling catheters for seven days or longer: systematic review and meta-analysis. *BMC Palliative Care* 2007;6(1):3.
20. Engle MP, Vinh BP, Harun N, et al. Infectious complications related to intrathecal drug delivery system and spinal cord stimulator system implantations at a comprehensive cancer pain center. *Pain Phys* 2013;16(1533):251–257.
21. Rathmell JP, Lake T, Ramundo MB. Infectious risks of chronic pain treatments: injection therapy, surgical implants, and intradiscal techniques. *Regional Anesth Pain Med* 2006;31(4):346–352.
22. Rudiger J, Thomson S. Infection rate of spinal cord stimulators after a screening trial period. A 53-month third party follow-up. *Neuromodulation* 2011;14(2):136–141.
23. Hoelzer BC, Bendel MA, Deer TR, et al. Spinal cord stimulator implant infection rates and risk factors: a multicenter retrospective study. *Neuromodulation* 2017;20(6):558–562.
24. Darouiche RO. Spinal epidural abscess. *N Engl J Med* 2006;355(19):2012–2020.
25. Curry WT Jr, Hoh BL, Amin-Hanjani S, et al. Spinal epidural abscess: clinical presentation, management, and outcome. *Surg Neurol* 2005;63(4):364–371.
26. Jong PC, Kansen PJ. A comparison of epidural catheters with or without subcutaneous injection ports for treatment of cancer pain. *Anesth Analg* 1994;78(1):94–100.
27. Du Pen S. Complications of neuraxial infusion in cancer patients. *Oncology (Williston Park)* 1999;13(suppl 2):45–51.
28. Du Pen SL, Peterson DG, Williams A, et al. Infection during chronic epidural catheterization: diagnosis and treatment. *Anesthesiology* 1990;73(5):905–909.
29. Wade JS, Cobbs CG. Infections in cardiac pacemakers. *Curr Clin Top Infect Dis* 1988;9:44–61.
30. Lu CH, Chang WN, Lui CC, et al. Adult spinal epidural abscess: clinical features and prognostic factors. *Clin Neurol Neurosurg* 2002;104(4):306–310.
31. Groban L. Central nervous system and cardiac effects from long-acting amide local anesthetic toxicity in the intact animal model. *Reg Anesth Pain Med* 2003;28(1):3–11.
32. Butterworth JF IV, Strichartz GR. Molecular mechanisms of local anesthesia: a review. *Anesthesiology* 1990;72(4):711–734.
33. Hille B. Ionic channels in excitable membranes. Current problems and biophysical approaches. *Biophys J* 1978;22(2):283–294.
34. Kozody R, Ready LB, Barsa JE, et al. Dose requirement of local anaesthetic to produce grand mal seizure during stellate ganglion block. *Can Anaesth Soc J* 1982;29(5):489–491.
35. Mahajan G. Pain clinic emergencies. *Pain Med* 2008;9(suppl 1):S113–S120.
36. Sawyer RJ, von Schroeder H. Temporary bilateral blindness after acute lidocaine toxicity. *Anesth Analg* 2002;95(1):224–226.
37. Brown DL, Ransom DM, Hall JA, et al. Regional anesthesia and local anesthetic-induced systemic toxicity: seizure frequency and accompanying cardiovascular changes. *Anesth Analg* 1995;81(2):321–328.
38. de Jong RH, Ronfeld RA, DeRosa RA. Cardiovascular effects of convulsant and supraconvulsant doses of amide local anesthetics. *Anesth Analg* 1982;61(1):3–9.
39. Rosenblatt MA, Abel M, Fischer GW, et al. Successful use of a 20% lipid emulsion to resuscitate a patient after a presumed bupivacaine-related cardiac arrest. *Anesthesiology* 2006;105(1):217–218.
40. Warren JA, Thoma RB, Georgescu A, et al. Intravenous lipid infusion in the successful resuscitation of local anesthetic-induced cardiovascular collapse after supraclavicular brachial plexus block. *Anesth Analg* 2008;106(5):1578–1580.
41. Hoegberg LC, Bania TC, Lavergne V, et al. Systematic review of the effect of intravenous lipid emulsion therapy for local anesthetic toxicity. *Clin Toxicol* 2016;54(3):167–193.
42. Fettiplace MR, Lis K, Ripper R, et al. Multi-modal contributions to detoxification of acute pharmacotoxicity by a triglyceride micro-emulsion. *J Control Release* 2015;198:62–70.
43. Neal JM, Barrington MJ, Fettiplace MR, et al. The Third American Society of Regional Anesthesia and Pain Medicine Practice Advisory on Local Anesthetic Systemic Toxicity: executive summary 2017. *Reg Anesth Pain Med* 2018;43(2):113–123. doi:10.1097/AAP.0000000000000720.
44. Morgan P. The role of vasopressors in the management of hypotension induced by spinal and epidural anaesthesia. *Can J Anesth* 1994;41(5):404–413.
45. Borgeat A, Blumenthal S. Unintended destinations of local anesthetics. In: Neal JM, Rathmell JP, eds. *Complications in Regional Anesthesia and Pain Medicine*. Philadelphia: Saunders; 2007:157–163.
46. Tan MP, Parry SW. Vasovagal syncope in the older patient. *J Am Coll Cardiol* 2008;51(6):599–606.
47. Krediet CT, van Dijk N, Linzer M, et al. Management of vasovagal syncope: controlling or aborting faints by leg crossing and muscle tensing. *Circulation* 2002;106(13):1684–1689.
48. Meythaler JM, Roper JF, Brunner RC. Cyproheptadine for intrathecal baclofen withdrawal. *Arch Phys Med Rehabil* 2003;84(5):638–642.
49. Coffey RJ, Edgar TS, Francisco GE, et al. Abrupt withdrawal from intrathecal baclofen: recognition and management of a potentially life-threatening syndrome. *Arch Phys Med Rehabil* 2002;83(6):735–741.
50. Green LB, Nelson VS. Death after acute withdrawal of intrathecal baclofen: case report and literature review. *Arch Phys Med Rehabil* 1999;80(12):1600–1604.
51. Duhon BS, Macdonald JD. Infusion of intrathecal baclofen for acute withdrawal. Technical note. *J Neurosurg* 2007;107(4):878–880.
52. Ackland GL, Fox R. Low-dose propofol infusion for controlling acute hyperspasticity after withdrawal of intrathecal baclofen therapy. *Anesthesiology* 2005;103(3):663–665.
53. Zuckerbraun NS, Ferson SS, Albright AL, et al. Intrathecal baclofen withdrawal: emergent recognition and management. *Pediatr Emerg Care* 2004;20(11):759–764.
54. Hsieh JC, Penn RD. Intrathecal baclofen in the treatment of adult spasticity. *Neurosurg Focus* 2006;21(2):e5.
55. Gowing LR, Farrell M, Ali RL, et al. α_2-Adrenergic agonists in opioid withdrawal. *Addiction* 2002;97(1):49–58.

56. Armstrong J, Little M, Murray L. Emergency department presentations of naltrexone-accelerated detoxification. *Acad Emerg Med* 2003;10(8): 860–866.

57. Kampman K, Jarvis M. American Society of Addiction Medicine (ASAM) National Practice Guideline for the Use of Medications in the Treatment of Addiction Involving Opioid Use. *J Addict Med* 2015;9(5):358–367.

58. Centers for Disease Control and Prevention. CDC guideline for prescribing opioids for chronic pain. Available at: http:// www.cdc.gov/drugoverdose /prescribing/guideline.html. Accessed September 1, 2017.

59. Brown AF. Anaphylaxis gets the adrenaline going. *Emerg Med J* 2004;21(2): 128–129.

60. Part 10.6: anaphylaxis. *Circulation* 2005;112(suppl 24):VI-143–VI-145.

61. Lagopoulos V, Gigi E. Anaphylactic and anaphylactoid reactions during the perioperative period. *Hippokratia* 2011;15(2):138–140.

62. Brown SG. Clinical features and severity grading of anaphylaxis. *J Allergy Clin Immunol* 2004;114(2):371–376.

63. Pumphrey R. Anaphylaxis: can we tell who is at risk of a fatal reaction? *Curr Opin Allergy Clin Immunol* 2004;4(4):285–290.

64. Brown SG, Blackman KE, Stenlake V, et al. Insect sting anaphylaxis: prospective evaluation of treatment with intravenous adrenaline and volume resuscitation. *Emerg Med J* 2004;21(2):149–154.

65. Cheshire WP, Santos CC, Massey EW, et al. Spinal cord infarction: etiology and outcome. *Neurology* 1996;47(2):321–330.

66. Baker R, Dreyfuss P, Mercer S, et al. Cervical transforaminal injection of corticosteroids into a radicular artery: a possible mechanism for spinal cord injury. *Pain* 2003;103(1–2):211–215.

67. Brouwers PJ, Kottink EJ, Simon MA, et al. A cervical anterior spinal artery syndrome after diagnostic blockade of the right C6-nerve root. *Pain* 2001;91(3):397–399.

68. Houten JK, Errico TJ. Paraplegia after lumbosacral nerve root block: report of three cases. *Spine J* 2002;2(1):70–75.

69. Somayaji HS, Saifuddin A, Casey AT, et al. Spinal cord infarction following therapeutic computed tomography-guided left L2 nerve root injection. *Spine* 2005;30(4):E106–E108.

70. Rathmell JP, Aprill C, Bogduk N. Cervical transforaminal injection of steroids. *Anesthesiology* 2004;100(6):1595–1600.

71. Rozin L, Rozin R, Koehler SA, et al. Death during transforaminal epidural steroid nerve root block (C7) due to perforation of the left vertebral artery. *Am J Forensic Med Pathol* 2003;24(4):351–355.

72. Masson C, Pruvo JP, Meder JF, et al. Spinal cord infarction: clinical and magnetic resonance imaging findings and short term outcome. *J Neurol Neurosurg Psychiatry* 2004;75(10):1431–1435.

73. Cheshire WP Jr. Spinal cord infarction mimicking angina pectoris. *Mayo Clin Proc* 2000;75(11):1197–1199.

74. Weidauer S, Nichtweiss M, Lanfermann H, et al. Spinal cord infarction: MR imaging and clinical features in 16 cases. *Neuroradiology* 2002;44(10):851–857.

75. Rathmell JP, Benzon HT, Dreyfuss P, et al. Safeguards to prevent neurologic complications after epidural steroid injections. *Anesthesiology* 2015;122(5): 974–984.

76. Adams HP Jr, del Zoppo G, Alberts MJ, et al. Guidelines for the early management of adults with ischemic stroke: a guideline from the American Heart Association/American Stroke Association Stroke Council, Clinical Cardiology Council, Cardiovascular Radiology and Intervention Council, and the Atherosclerotic Peripheral Vascular Disease and Quality of Care Outcomes in Research Interdisciplinary Working Groups: the American Academy of Neurology affirms the value of this guideline as an educational tool for neurologists. *Stroke* 2007;38(5):1655–1711.

77. Vale FL, Burns J, Jackson AB, et al. Combined medical and surgical treatment after acute spinal cord injury: results of a prospective pilot study to assess the merits of aggressive medical resuscitation and blood pressure management. *J Neurosurg* 1997;87(2):239–246.

78. Wang H, Tang Y, Rong X, et al. Effects of early blood pressure lowering on early and long-term outcomes after acute stroke: an updated meta-analysis. *PLoS One* 2014;9(5).

79. Miller SM. Methylprednisolone in acute spinal cord injury: a tarnished standard. *J Neurosurg Anesthesiol* 2008;20(2):140–142.

80. Bracken MB, Shepard MJ, Holford TR, et al. Methylprednisolone or tirilazad mesylate administration after acute spinal cord injury: 1-year follow up. Results of the third National Acute Spinal Cord Injury randomized controlled trial. *J Neurosurg* 1998;89(5):699–706.

81. Rozet I. Methylprednisolone in acute spinal cord injury: is there any other ethical choice? *J Neurosurg Anesthesiol* 2008;20(2):137–139.

CHAPTER 113

Pain Management in the Emergency Department

JAMES R. MINER

The specialties of both emergency medicine and pain medicine are relatively new members of the modern house of medicine. The first academic department of emergency medicine was established in 1971, and the American Board of Medical Specialties recognized emergency medicine as a distinct specialty by conferring primary board status only 30 years ago. The numbers of visits to US emergency departments (EDs) have increased markedly over the past decade. From 2005 to 2015, the annual ED visit volumes increased from 115.3 million to 136.3 million, a 20% increase following a similar increase in the previous decade.[1] There are more than 34,000 active board-certified emergency physicians, 31,000 of whom are represented by the American College of Emergency Physicians (ACEP).

EDs provide care for patients with an extraordinarily broad range of illnesses and injuries associated with both acute and chronic pain. Pain is common in the ED, with up to 42% of ED visits being related to painful conditions.[2] It is commonly believed that injury and trauma are responsible for the majority of ED visits associated with pain; however, this impression is misleading. A landmark multicenter study of adults presenting to EDs in the United States and Canada with moderate to severe pain found that two-thirds of patients presentation with pain from medical, rather than traumatic, conditions.[3] Major categories of discharge diagnoses reported in this study appear in Figure 113.1.

In the United States, the ED serves as a safety net for our fragmented health care system. Pain is but one of many conditions for which emergency physicians not only treat acute clinical presentations but also care for those with chronic or recurrent painful conditions who are unable to access other parts of the health care system. Emergency physicians also frequently manage pain in the course of performing emergent diagnostic and therapeutic procedures.

This chapter discusses the prevalence of acute and chronic pain in the ED, its assessment, barriers to adequate pain treatment, the influence of substance use disorders and aberrant drug-related behaviors on ED pain practices, as well as a variety of commonly employed pain treatment and procedural sedation modalities. Space limits prohibit a discussion of the wide variety of specific painful conditions that present to the ED.

The Prevalence of Pain in the Emergency Department

Pain is the most frequent reason for seeking ED treatment, and as a part of the presenting complaint, pain accounts for over 70% of visits to US EDs.[3-5] A study conducted by Tanabe and Buschmann,[6] found that among adults treated at one Chicago ED, 78% presented with a chief complaint related to pain. Of these patients, only 47% received analgesics. For patients receiving analgesics, an average of 74 minutes elapsed from the time of arrival to the time of treatment.

Cordell et al.[4] reported an analysis of secondary data from an urban, tertiary-care ED using explicit data abstraction rules to determine the prevalence of pain and to assign painful conditions

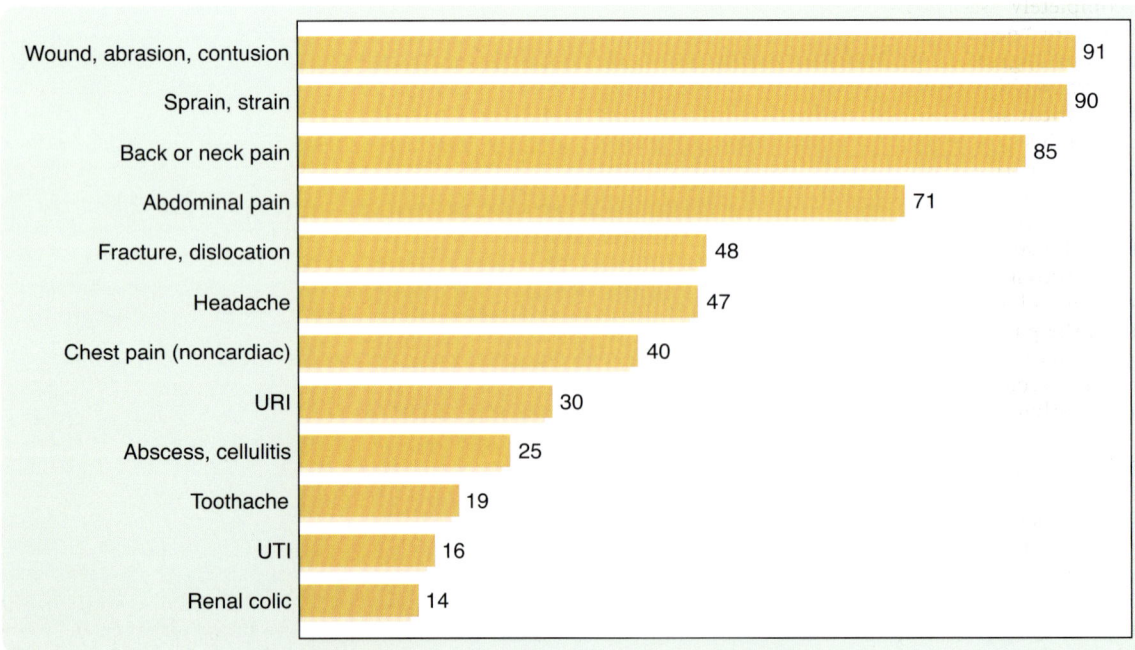

FIGURE 113.1 Major categories of discharge diagnoses among patients presenting to the emergency department (ED) with moderate to severe pain. Note: Other diagnoses present for 243 patients. URI, upper respiratory tract infection; UTI, urinary tract infection. (*Data from Todd KH, Ducharme J, Choiniere M, et al. Pain in the emergency department: results of the Pain and Emergency Medicine Initiative (PEMI) multicenter study. J Pain 2007;8[6]:460–466.*)

into standard categories. With inclusion of all age groups, they found evidence of pain in 61% of patients. Pain was the chief complaint for 52% of patient visits. After excluding patients less than 5 years of age for whom chart reviews are obviously less reliable, almost 70% of patient encounters involved pain complaints.

Although the high prevalence of pain among ED patients is well documented, the underlying conditions responsible for pain in this population are less well characterized. In Cordell et al.'s[4] retrospective study, 11% of patients presenting to the ED were judged to be suffering from pain that was chronic in nature. In a larger prospective multicenter study conducted in the United States and Canada, 44% of ultimately discharged patients presenting to the ED with pain reported underlying chronic pain syndromes. In one-half of these cases, the ED visit was prompted by an exacerbation of this chronic pain condition. Importantly, patients with chronic pain reported three to four times the number of annual physician visits when compared to those without chronic pain. Median and mean durations of symptoms for those reporting chronic pain syndromes were 24 and 52 months, respectively.[3] For physicians who view themselves as experts in the management of acute medical and surgical emergencies, chronic pain may represent a less familiar condition with which to contend.

EDs frequently treat patients with chronic or recurrent pain who are often frustrated by a lack of information about ongoing pain management and poor access to specialty-level care. In a 2007 study, 500 US adults with chronic or recurrent pain and an ED visit within the past 2 years were interviewed.[7] Sixty percent were female, their median age was 54 years, two-thirds were under the care of a physician, and 14% were uninsured. They reported an average of 4.2 ED visits within the past 2 years. Relatively large proportions reported pain relief during the ED visit, and 57% endorsed that "the ED staff understood how to treat my pain" as "definitely true." Although over three-fourths of patients felt receiving that additional information on pain management (82%) or referrals to specialists (74%) was "extremely" or "very" important, only one-half reported receiving such referrals (46%) or information (55%). A significant minority (11%) reported that the "ED staff made me feel like I was just seeking drugs." The majority (55%) were "very" or "completely" satisfied with their medical treatment, whereas 24% were "neutral" to "completely" dissatisfied. In multivariate models, greater age, male gender, higher level of education, shorter waiting time, use of imaging, and pain relief contributed to patient satisfaction with ED care.

Findings from this survey provide a more precise estimate of the prevalence of ED use associated with chronic and recurrent pain in the United States. The final survey incidence rate of adults reporting a recent ED visit for chronic or recurrent pain was 15% of all those reached by phone. Given the US adult population of approximately 225 million, this survey incidence rate suggests that 34 million adults meet our criteria of an ED visit within the past 2 years for chronic or recurrent pain. Within this population, approximately 43%, or 15 million people, experience recurrent pain, whereas 57%, or 19 million people, have underlying chronic pain syndromes.

Pain management in the ED has received increased emphasis over the past two decades, including increased emphasis on patient satisfaction surveys, and The Joint Commission's emphasis on analgesia.[8] There have been a large number of important findings showing that analgesia in the ED is often inadequate, including an Institute of Medicine report,[9] leading to emphasis on improving pain treatment. This emphasis has likely resulted in improvements in pain treatment in the ED but may have had the unintended consequence of increasing the use of opioids in the ED and after ED care.

The high prevalence of acute and chronic pain in the ED, and the increased emphasis on its treatment, has led to the question of the role of EDs in the increasing use of opioids in the United States.[10,11] Among 20- to 29-year-olds, emergency medicine ranks third among specialties in terms of the number of opioid prescriptions, writing 12% of the total number of prescriptions.[12] In one study, 17% of ED patients were discharged with an opioid medication, the majority of which were small pill counts and immediate-release formulations.[13] A recent study found that for opioid-naive patients, the odds ratio for developing recurrent use after a single prescription for opioids versus a nonopioid prescription from the ED was 1.8.[14] This is difficult to interpret because many of the patients who received an opioid may have had more pain or a more severe injury than those who did not, but it highlights the need for attention to the risk of recurrent opioid use when they are used. The risk of opioids from the ED on patients in the ED with chronic or recurrent pain who already use opioids is much likely larger but is difficult to quantify. This complicates pain treatment in the ED and makes it a difficult challenge for emergency physicians.[15]

The increase in deaths associated with opioid abuse has heightened concern[16,17] and has led to the development of some actions to decrease the risk to patients. This includes the U.S. Food and Drug Administration's proposal for the establishment of physician education programs for the prescribing of long-acting and extended-release opioids as part of the national opioid risk evaluation and mitigation strategy (REMS) program.[18] Statewide opioid prescribing guidelines, such as those developed by the Utah Department of Health[19] and the Washington Chapter of the ACEP,[20] and guidelines developed by individual physician groups have shown promise in decreasing opioid prescription overdoses.[21] ACEP has also developed a policy on the use of opioids that clarifies the use of state prescription monitoring programs, the treatment of back pain with opioids, and the use of different opioids.[22] As research advances and policies develop, the role of EDs in opioid abuse will be further explored and the effects mitigated.

The Assessment of Pain in the Emergency Department

Pain is inherently subjective and inevitably complex. Patients experience pain and suffering as individuals; clinicians assess it only indirectly. The emergency provider's task is to use a commonly understood vocabulary and classification system in assessing pain so that our findings can be communicated consistently. Only by quantifying the pain experience in meaningful ways can we move beyond practices that are influenced by myth and opinion toward a scientific approach to our many questions regarding the pain experience. This challenge is at the root of the difficulties in treating pain and not only in the ED; thus, issues surrounding pain assessment should have primacy in our attempts to understand our patients' pain experiences.

EDs employ a number of practical unidimensional pain assessment tools. Viewing pain as the "fifth vital sign," as encouraged by The Joint Commission on Accreditation of Health Care Organizations, has fostered the widespread use of such tools. For those without cognitive impairment, pain intensity is routinely assessed with either an 11-point numerical rating scale (NRS) or a graphical rating scale (GRS). The NRS is sensitive to the short-term changes in pain intensity associated with emergency care and is the most commonly employed pain assessment instrument. GRS or picture scales are particularly useful for populations with limited literacy, including children. The visual analog scale (VAS) is used by some EDs; however, this instrument is more commonly employed in research settings. There is no demonstrated advantage in using a VAS over an NRS in the ED setting; both are reliable and valid measures of pain intensity. A patient's answer to the query "Do you want more pain medication?" however, has been shown to be an unreliable measure of pain or relief, and descriptive pain scales are likely to prove more accurate and reliable.[23]

Among nonverbal patients, including infants or those with cognitive impairment and dementia, a number of observational pain scales are available for use. Both the Face, Legs, Activity, Cry, and Consolability (FLACC) observational scale for use in very young children[24] and the Pain Assessment in Advanced Dementia scale for use in the setting of advanced dementia[25] are used with some frequency in the ED; however, adequate observational pain assessments are less the exception than the rule.

No matter the specific pain scale used, assessments should be repeated after therapeutic interventions and at the time of ED discharge. One multicenter study found that relatively few ED patients are reassessed after an initial pain score, reporting that fewer than one-third of ED patients presenting with moderate to severe pain had repeat pain assessments while in the ED.[3] Despite efforts to promote pain intensity as an outcome measure with which to judge the quality of ED pain practice, the finding that pain intensity is measured only once in most EDs may mirrors medicine's traditional view of pain as a diagnostic indicator rather than an outcome deserving of attention in its own right.

Oligoanalgesia in the Emergency Department

Notwithstanding the clinician's duty to provide compassionate care, pain that is not acknowledged and managed appropriately causes anxiety, depression, sleep disturbances, increased oxygen demands with the potential for end-organ ischemia, and decreased movement with an increased risk of venous thrombosis.[26] Failure to recognize and treat pain may also result in dissatisfaction with medical care, hostility toward the physician, unscheduled returns to the ED, delayed complete return to full function, and, potentially, an increased risk of litigation.[27] Although adequate analgesia in the ED would appear to be an important goal of treatment, the underuse of analgesics, termed "oligoanalgesia" by Wilson and Pendleton[28] in 1989, occurs in a large proportion of ED patients. A variety of factors are felt to give rise to pain under treatment, and these are listed in Table 113.1.

Emergency medicine investigators have identified a number of risk factors for oligoanalgesia, ranging from patient factors to physician variation.[29] As in other settings, the very young or old tend to receive less intensive treatment for pain in ED. Studies have documented oligoanalgesia and delays to analgesic administration among those of minority ethnicity for a variety of painful conditions, even when objective evidence for the presence of pain is obvious (e.g., long-bone fractures).[2,30–33] Although patients' expectations for pain treatment and perceptions of pain intensity don't differ by ethnic groups, when patients are matched for socioeconomic factors, differences have been noted in the manner in which patients of different cultural backgrounds express their pain. Differences in the interactions of physicians and patients of different ethnic groups have been described, and subtle differences within these interactions may affect the physician's pain assessment.[34] When affect, actual patient–physician interaction, and cultural expressions of ethnicity are removed from a case presentation, such as through written clinical vignettes, patients with similar pain tend to be similarly treated by physicians.[35] Cultural discordance between the patient and the physician may hinder the ability of patients to confer an understanding of their pain to the physician.

Of course, any treatment of pain is dependent on the physician's accurate assessment of the patient's pain. In fact, the only predictor of treatment that Bartfield and colleagues[36] found for ED patients with back pain was the physician's assessment, regardless of the patients' ethnicity, age, or insurance status. Disparities in the treatment of pain are more likely to result from variations in physicians' assessment of pain intensity than variations in treatment among patients judged to have similar degrees of pain.

Although emergency physicians may be reluctant to accept a patient's report as the most reliable indicator of pain, and disparities between patient's and physician's pain intensity ratings may lead to inadequately treated pain, even patients themselves may be reluctant to report the presence of pain and its intensity. This may be due to low expectations of obtaining pain relief, fear of analgesic side effects, and perhaps the notion that pain is to be expected as part of an underlying disease or from medical treatments. Some patients exhibit an inappropriate fear of addiction when prescribed opioids or fear the stigma associated with opioid use, even in the short term.

Pain and Opioid Abuse in the Emergency Department

ED personnel commonly identify patients who they feel are attempting to obtain opioids for illegitimate purposes. Although drug addiction occurs in all patient populations, it is likely that the ED sees a higher proportion of such patients than a typical office-based practice. Unfortunately, the true prevalence of addiction and aberrant drug-seeking behaviors in the ED is unknown and difficult to measure.[37] When the prevalence of such problems is overestimated, oligoanalgesia is the predictable result.

Definitions

In discussing issues of chemical dependency and aberrant behaviors related to opioid use, a valid system of nomenclature is necessary for clear communication and measurement. Historically, the meaning of different terms has changed, particularly in light of the increased use of chronic opioid therapy for cancer and noncancer chronic pain conditions. In treating pain in this population of patients with chronic opioids, confusion over the concepts of physical dependence, tolerance, addiction, and pseudoaddiction may constitute a barrier to understanding and to appropriate treatment. These phenomena are discrete, and standard definitions may be helpful in caring for such patients. Currently accepted definitions of these include the following: *Addiction* is a primary, chronic, neurobiologic disease with genetic, psychosocial, and environmental factors influencing its development and manifestations. It is characterized by behaviors that include one or more of the following: impaired control over drug use, compulsive use, continued use despite harm, and craving. *Physical dependence* is a state of adaptation that often includes tolerance and is manifested by a drug class–specific withdrawal syndrome that can be produced by abrupt cessation, rapid dose reduction, decreasing blood level of the drug, and/or administration of an antagonist. *Tolerance* is a state of

TABLE 113.1 Factors Contributing to Emergency Department (ED) Oligoanalgesia
Lack of educational emphasis on pain management
Inadequate ED quality improvement systems
Lack of ED pain research, particularly among geriatric and pediatric populations
Emergency providers' concerns regarding opioid addiction and abuse
Fear of opioid adverse effects
Racial and ethnic bias

adaptation in which exposure to a drug induces changes that result in a diminution of one or more of the drug's effects over time. *Pseudoaddiction* is a term which has been used to describe patient behaviors, including drug-seeking behavior, that may occur when pain is undertreated. Patients with unrelieved pain may become focused on obtaining medications, may "clock watch," and may otherwise seem inappropriately "drug seeking." Even such behaviors as illicit drug use and deception can occur in the patient's efforts to obtain relief. Pseudoaddiction can be distinguished from true addiction in that the behaviors resolve when pain is effectively treated; the use of the term *pseudoaddiction* has fallen out of favor, as it is difficult to discern between the patient who finally achieves adequate pain control and the rare, but worrisome, patient who initially presents with poorly controlled pain and subsequently reports improvement but is actually diverting the opioids prescribed for nonmedical use.

The term *substance abuse* is particularly problematic and resistant to precise definition. The American Psychiatric Association has defined substance abuse as a maladaptive pattern of drug use associated with some manifest harm to the user or others. Other groups using consensus methodology have defined abuse as any use considered to be outside of socially accepted norms. Determining the bounds of "socially accepted norms" within the broad range of social strata treated within any ED is a difficult task. Physicians may believe that they "know abuse when they see it," and its identification may be influenced by subjective judgments that may or may not correspond to socially accepted norms for the index patient's particular social group.[38] Often, the term *substance misuse* is applied to behaviors that are not perceived as particularly extreme (e.g., taking opioid analgesics to relieve symptoms other than pain such as anxiety or boredom).

The difficulty in determining whether a given set of behaviors fall within accepted definitions of substance use, misuse, or abuse has important implications outside the clinical realm. Physicians may prescribe controlled substances for the treatment of pain, whereas patients may use these drugs to treat a broad range of symptoms with varying degrees of relatedness to underlying pain syndromes and may, in fact, use drugs in a manner totally unrelated to the physicians' intent (i.e., to obtain euphoric, rather than analgesic, effects). Given the unclear distinctions between use, misuse, and abuse and a regulatory climate in which practitioners prescribing patterns are increasingly scrutinized, emergency physicians are required to be cautious when the need to prescribe opioids to patients with whom they expect to have only a transitory relationship.

Using any definition, substance abuse is a highly prevalent problem in the ED.[11,39] The National Survey on Drug Use and Health reports that in 2015, an estimated 10.1%, of the population aged 12 years or older used an illicit drug during the month prior to the survey interview.[40] Importantly, the survey documents a 13.6% reported lifetime nonmedical use of pain relievers in 2014. To be considered nonmedical use, the respondent had to take drugs not prescribed for them or take them only for the "experience or feeling" they caused. Specific analgesics included Vicodin, Lortab, or Lorcet (combination analgesics containing hydrocodone); Percocet, Percodan, or Tylox (combination analgesics containing oxycodone); hydrocodone; OxyContin (extended-release oxycodone); methadone; and tramadol.

In contrast to the prominence of ED-based data collection systems in efforts to monitor deleterious outcomes associated with substance abuse, relatively few studies have systematically assessed substance abuse prevalence and treatment needs in the ED population.[41] As an example, the Drug Abuse Warning Network is a federally financed, public health surveillance system that monitors drug-related ED visits and drug-related deaths investigated by medical examiners and coroners. This reporting system involves hundreds of hospital EDs throughout the United States and provides valuable data with which to monitor drug abuse trends. In contrast to this large monitoring research enterprise, relatively little focus has been given to use of the ED as a setting in which to intervene in substance abuse problems.

In a study of trauma patients, Soderstrom et al.[42] assessed the prevalence of psychoactive substance use disorders in a large, unselected group of seriously injured patients treated in one Baltimore ED, using standardized diagnostic interviews and explicit criteria. Psychoactive substance use disorders were diagnosed using the Structured Clinical Interview, an instrument based on the *Diagnostic and Statistical Manual of Mental Disorders*. Of 1,118 patients consenting to the study, 71.8% used alcohol, 45.3% used illegal drugs, 18.8% demonstrated active drug abuse or dependence, and 32.1% demonstrated concurrent alcohol abuse or dependence.[43] The high rate of substance use and abuse among trauma patients, and the fact that trauma usually is associated with pain that requires treatment, complicates the treatment of pain from trauma.

Pain and "Drug-Seeking Behavior" in the Emergency Department

The preceding discussion makes clear the high prevalence of both pain and substance use disorders in the ED. Although acute and chronic pains are far more common than substance use disorders, it is inevitable that emergency physicians will frequently encounter patients presenting with both pain and substance use disorders. Professional discussions of pain treatment in the ED frequently center on concerns of being duped by such patients who fabricate painful symptoms in order to obtain opioids, so-called "drug-seeking behavior."[34,37] Drug-seeking behaviors may represent an entirely appropriate response by those with chronic pain who are routinely undertreated by the medical profession and for who comprehensive pain treatment centers are in short supply. Although the term *drug-seeking behavior* is poorly defined, it is used in the emergency medicine literature and will be used with acknowledgment of its imprecision.

Only a limited amount of emergency medicine research has addressed this problematic issue. In 1996, Zechnich and Hedges[44] attempted to measure community-wide use of ED services by patients at high risk for drug-seeking behavior. In this retrospective, observational study, patients were categorized as exhibiting drug-seeking behavior if they sought care at a university hospital in Portland, Oregon, for a specific pain-related diagnosis (i.e., ureteral colic, toothache, back pain, abdominal pain, or headache) and were either independently identified on at least one other local hospital's "patient alert" list or suffered a drug-related death during the year in question. After identifying 33 such patients, they determined the frequency of their ED visits at each of seven local hospitals and conducted detailed chart reviews of their visits at three of these hospitals. The patients identified as drug seeking were generally young, and one-half of drug seekers were female. This suggests that drug-seeking behaviors are exhibited (or identified) more commonly among female ED patients with substance abuse problems than among males.[39,45] The 33 patients visited EDs, urgent care clinics, or were hospitalized a total of 379 times over the study period, for an average of 12.6 visits per person annually. Interestingly, although chart reviews identified 17 patients who were told that he or she "would receive no further narcotics" at a given facility, these patients subsequently received controlled substances from another hospital in 93% of cases and from even the same facility in 71%. The authors suggested that information sharing between hospitals could help to identify drug-seeking patients and promote more consistent community-wide care and appropriate substance abuse interventions.

The need for information sharing has led to the development of statewide prescription monitoring programs.[46] These programs allow physicians to determine whether a patient has received opioid medications regardless of their individual report, allowing easier identification of patients who are misrepresenting their current opioid use. Such monitoring systems are generally not required and are not universal, but data indicate they are successful, at least more so than the previous attempts at internal lists many EDs had used, and their use should be expanded.[47] It has been shown that the use of such lists alters physicians' prescribing behavior, both by increasing pain medications for patients who do not exhibit frequent use and identifying patients at risk for opioid abuse or dependence related to their treatment.[48,49] Although early versions of these monitoring programs were difficult to access and use, they are becoming increasing usable and are becoming a typically step in the prescribing of opioids in the ED.[50] Prescription drug monitoring programs are generally underused in EDs, and nationwide enrollment is low among emergency physicians. In order to improve this, an expert panel was convened by ACEP and made policy recommendations within these main themes: Enrollment should be mandatory, with an automatic process to mitigate the workload; registration should be open to all prescribers; delegates should have access to prescription drug monitoring program to alleviate workflow burdens; prescription drug monitoring program data should be pushed into hospital electronic health records; prescription drug monitoring program review should be mandatory for patients receiving opioid prescriptions and based on objective criteria; the prescription drug monitoring program content should be standardized and updated in a timely manner; and states should encourage interstate data sharing.[51]

It has been difficult to quantify the overall effect of such systems,[13] and they run the risk of resulting in unfair treatment of the patient if the information is not used properly and it is a context appropriate to the patient.[52] It is likely, however, that improved information will reduce risks to patients and improve care, both in terms of identifying patients who have developed substance abuse problems related to their pain treatment and in terms of avoiding misidentifying patients exhibiting behaviors that appear associated with addiction but are in fact exhibiting pseudoaddiction related to oligoanalgesia.

Pain and Substance Abuse in the Emergency Department: A Balanced Perspective

In managing pain, emergency physicians are responsible for beneficence as well as nonmaleficence. We must treat pain and ameliorate suffering while minimizing the extent to which our treatment strategies enable substance abuse by our patients. For the vast majority of patients presenting with a first episode of acute pain, whether from trauma, acute medical illness, or procedures performed in the ED, there is little danger of enabling substance abuse and a great deal of room for improvement in the quality of analgesic practices. For a small subset of ED patients, particularly for those presenting with chronic or recurrent pain syndromes, the physician may have legitimate concerns regarding underlying substance abuse or related disorder. Our task is to balance the often unclear risk of fostering substance abuse, and even diversion, in this subset of patients with the well-known and well-documented risk of under treating painful conditions.

Certainly, the presence of an obvious painful condition (e.g., appendicitis, fracture) should preempt concerns about illegitimate drug-seeking behaviors. Given the high prevalence of chronic pain and the widespread unavailability of chronic

pain management resources, particularly for populations served by the ED, pseudoaddiction is the most likely cause for a large proportion of drug-related behaviors deemed aberrant. In particular, patient reports of distress associated with unrelieved symptoms, aggressive complaining about the need for higher doses of analgesics, and unilateral dose escalation by the patient are suggestive of pseudoaddiction. Establishing the diagnosis of pseudoaddiction is particularly difficult if the patient has both pain and a comorbid substance use disorder; however, the two can coexist. The signature of pseudoaddiction is that aberrant behaviors disappear when adequate analgesics are given to control pain.

In dealing with complex chronic pain patients, the emergency physician practicing in isolation may exhibit symptoms of despair and direct his or her anger toward the patient with pain, resulting in more alienation of patients who may have already been abandoned by other sectors of the health care system. This is particularly likely to happen in communities without multidisciplinary treatment centers for either substance abuse disorders or chronic pain and for those with inadequate health care insurance. Thus, the patient with chronic pain joins the larger group of those with unmet health care needs that currently crowd our EDs. The hectic nature of emergency medicine practice often does not allow sufficient time for precisely characterizing patients with complex pain complaints, and clinicians may lump legitimate pain behaviors with the ploys of those seeking opioids inappropriately. Both groups of patients may be ultimately mistrusted and treated with disdain.

Aside from considerations of pseudoaddiction, chronic pain is often accompanied by mood disorders and psychiatric comorbidities that complicate the management of these challenging patients.[26] The presence of aberrant drug-related behaviors in patients with borderline personality disorders may represent an expression of fear and anger or an attempt to cope with chronic boredom. Patients may use opioids and alcohol in attempts to lessen symptoms of anxiety, panic disorder, depression, or insomnia. Emergency physicians often receive limited training in dealing with such disorders and the specialty's deficiencies in dealing with such problems have been documented.[53] Psychiatric consultation, if available, may be useful in both suggesting alternative causes for aberrant behaviors and tailoring the physician's therapeutic approach to deal with these complicating factors.

For some patients, aberrant drug-related behaviors represent criminal intent to divert or sell controlled substances. The prevalence of behaviors occasioned by such intent is unknown, and it is likely that in many cases, multiple etiologies of aberrant behaviors coexist.[37,54] Certainly, patients with active or past substance use disorders are at increased risk for injuries and illnesses that can lead to chronic pain (e.g., motor vehicle injury).

Finally, although federal regulators and state medical boards do not perceive emergency medicine as a specialty prone to inappropriate prescribing, and investigations of emergency physicians are rare, if not unheard of, many emergency physicians express fears of such scrutiny or sanctions related to prescribing or administering opioids. Although this concern is often voiced, it seems likely that this fear represents concern about other, less obvious physician uncertainties related to pain management and substance abuse disorders. Emergency physicians may be concerned about being overburdened by the inherent difficulties of managing patients with complicated pain syndromes and the potential of coexisting substance abuse disorders.

The Example of Sickle Cell Disease

The condition that best exemplifies the problem of ED-based pseudoaddiction is sickle cell disease. Vaso-occlusive pain crises are the most common reason for ED visits by patients with sickle cell disease, and the genetics, molecular biology, and pathophysiology of this disease are relatively well understood. Although the management of sickle cell vaso-occlusive pain crises is viewed as challenging by emergency physicians, it has been a relatively neglected area of research investigation by the specialty.[55]

Despite our understanding of the sickle cell disease process, many health professionals are reluctant to prescribe adequate doses of opioids for these patients experiencing pain largely due to addiction concerns, and that care is frequently insufficient and delayed.[56] In one survey study, 53% of emergency physicians were of the belief that more than 20% of patients with sickle cell disease were addicted to opioids, whereas only 23% of hematologists shared this belief. Also, in this survey, 35% of hematologists reported that they followed pain management protocols when treating painful crises as compared to only 17% of emergency physicians.[57,58]

Nurses' attitudes regarding the prevalence of addiction among this patient population are even more extreme, with 63 respondents reporting that addiction was prevalent.[59] Thirty percent of nurses in this survey reported that they were hesitant to administer high-dose opioids for painful vaso-occlusive crises. A hesitant approach to ED opioid administration in the setting of vaso-occlusive pain crises will predictably lead to continued pain, increased anticipation of pain, and increased patient anxiety. This experience may generate pain-avoidance manifestations by patients that are interpreted by physicians as aberrant drug-related behaviors. Eventually, larger doses of opioids may be administered to control pain that is spiraling out of control with resultant excessive sedation. This apparent sedation in the setting of a painful condition may reinforce the physician's disbelief in the reality of his or her patient's initial pain reports.

It has been demonstrated that this cycle of inadequate care can be broken by the institution of pain management protocols that emphasize continuous opioid infusions and sustained courses of orally administered controlled-release opioids. Tanabe et al. demonstrated in several studies that the addition of nurse-initiated protocols, including the use of high-dose opioids, and provider education led to improvements in pain management.[55,56,60,61]

Pain Treatment and Procedural Sedation in the Emergency Department

Effective pain management involves both pharmacologic and nonpharmacologic modalities. Simply asking about pain and validating the pain reports impacts patients' satisfaction with ED pain management. In one study, patient satisfaction with pain management was predicted more strongly by the perception that ED staff asked about pain than by the actual administration of an analgesic.[62] Other nonpharmacologic modalities, such as reassuring the patient that pain will be addressed; immobilizing and elevating injured extremities; and providing quiet, darkened rooms for patients with migraine headaches, are important aspects of quality pain management. Pharmacologic therapies should begin as soon as is practical after presentation to the ED. Analgesic protocols allowing early pain treatment can decrease the time to effective treatment and improve patient outcomes.[63,64]

Analgesics may be administered by a variety of routes; however, the vast majority of medications are administered by the oral or parenteral routes. Oral therapies are most commonly employed as they are convenient and inexpensive for patients who can tolerate oral intake.[64] When pain is severe, analgesics must be given immediately and titrated to effect, generally by parenteral routes. The intravenous, rather than intramuscular, route is indicated in this context. Intramuscular injections are painful, do not allow for rapid titration, exhibit unpredictable absorption,

and result in a slower onset of drug action. Unless intravenous access is elusive, there is little to recommend the intramuscular route. In general, it is inappropriate to delay analgesic use until a diagnosis has been made. In the case of acute abdominal pain, for which surgical dogma historically discouraged adequate analgesia, studies report no deleterious effect of intravenous opioid therapy on our ability to make appropriate diagnoses.[65]

Specific Treatment Modalities

Analgesics are the most commonly administered class of drug in the ED. The National Center for Health Statistics reports that analgesics account for the top three therapeutic classes of drugs used in the ED (Fig. 113.2).[40] The majority of analgesics administered were opioids (59%); morphine being the most commonly used analgesic (20%), followed by ibuprofen (17%) (Table 113.2).

NONOPIOIDS

Commonly used ED analgesics include opioids, acetaminophen, and nonsteroidal anti-inflammatory drugs (NSAIDs). When opioids are required for pain treatment, nonopioids should be included in order to potentiate the opioid analgesic effect and decrease the severity of side effects. Unfortunately, nonopioid agents exhibit an analgesic ceiling effect and cannot be titrated to effect. This limits their usefulness in the setting of severe or fluctuating pain; however, they should be used as an adjunct to opioid therapies unless otherwise contraindicated.

Acetaminophen is indicated for mild to moderate pain and is often combined with opioid agents. Acetaminophen, unlike NSAIDs, has no antiplatelet activity or anti-inflammatory effect. Although a great deal of attention has been paid to acetaminophen hepatotoxicity, especially in the setting of chronic malnutrition, alcoholism, or liver disease, such effects are uncommon, particularly when contrasted to the underappreciated high prevalence of NSAID-related adverse effects

NSAIDs, including salicylates, act to inhibit prostaglandin synthesis by interfering with cyclooxygenase enzymes. They frequently cause gastritis and gastrointestinal (GI) bleeding, cause platelet dysfunction, and can precipitate renal failure in patients with renal insufficiency or volume depletion, a particular concern in the elderly or those presenting to the ED with hemodynamic instability. They have a ceiling effect at relatively low doses.[66] Ketorolac, the only parenteral available in the United States, is commonly used in the ED and is felt to be particularly useful in the setting of renal colic. One study of renal colic in the ED found that a combination or ketorolac and morphine resulted in superior analgesia and reduced adverse effects when compared to the use of either agent alone.[67] A recent study by Motov et al.[66] demonstrated that at dose of 10 mg intravenously has similar analgesic efficacy as 15 or 30 mg, indicating that is likely the safest dose for emergent therapy.

OPIOIDS

Opioid combination analgesics are commonly used for moderate to severe pain. Although the opioid component in these agents does not exhibit ceiling analgesic effects, the nonopioid component dose must be limited; thus, one cannot titrate these analgesics. The convenience of combination therapy must be balanced against this limitation. Hydrocodone and oxycodone combination agents are associated with less nausea and vomiting and are preferable to codeine combinations agents. Also, significant proportions of the population are poor metabolizers of codeine, which must be metabolized to morphine in order to manifest analgesic effects, further limiting its effectiveness.

The tramadol/acetaminophen combination agent is indicated for acute pain; however, experience with this agent in the ED setting is limited. In one recent trial of acute ankle sprains

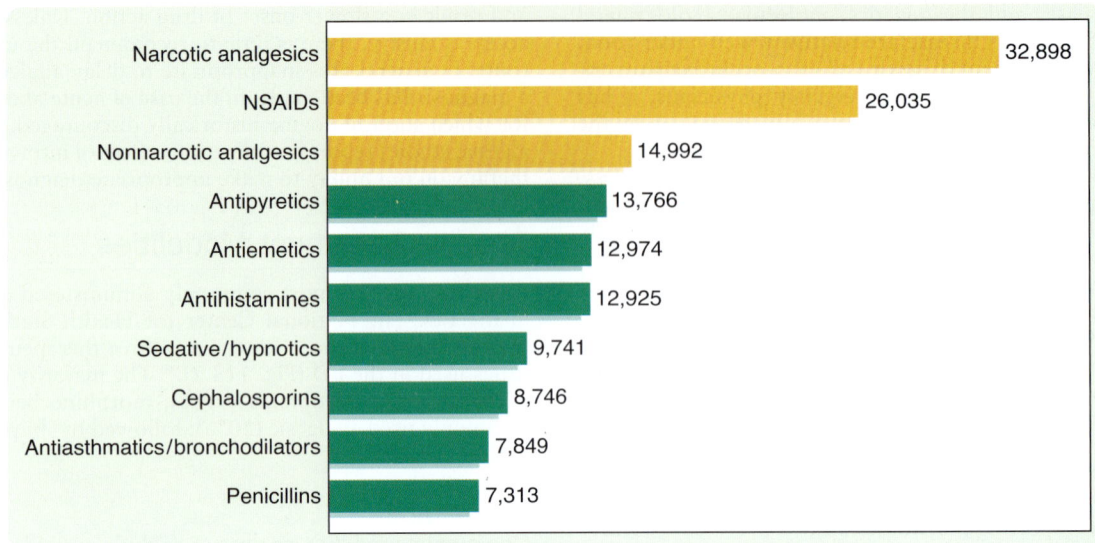

FIGURE 113.2   Top 10 therapeutic drug classes mentioned at emergency department visits. *(Data from National Center for Health Statistics.* National Hospital Ambulatory Medical Care Survey: 2013 Emergency Department Summary Tables. *Atlanta, GA: U.S. Department of Health and Human Services, Centers for Disease Control and Prevention; 2013. Available at: https://www.cdc.gov/nchs/fastats/emergency-department.htm. Accessed September 1, 2017.)*

presenting to the ED, the tramadol/acetaminophen combination agent had comparable clinical utility to that of hydrocodone with acetaminophen.[68] Tramadol's mechanism of action is unclear: It binds only weakly to opioid receptors and inhibits the reuptake of both norepinephrine and serotonin.

Opioids are the mainstay of ED therapy for moderate to severe pain, and morphine is the standard of comparison for all agents of this class. If contraindicated due to allergy or other sensitivity, hydromorphone or fentanyl may be substituted. These opioids can be rapidly titrated intravenously to control severe pain, allowing early institution of an oral regimen. Fentanyl has the advantage of being relatively short acting and is preferred in the setting of multiple trauma, head injury, and potential hemodynamic instability. Intravenous morphine is the standard of treatment for severe pain in the ED. Morphine 0.1 mg/kg bolus has been found to be safe but not usually adequate to effect pain relief.[69] Repeat boluses of 0.05 mg/kg every 5 minutes until pain relief represents a safe incremental strategy. In patients with impaired hepatic function in the elderly, hydromorphone may be superior to morphine because it has less active metabolites. Oral oxycodone has shown to be comparable to intravenous morphine and when compared to the time of ordering has a similar time to analgesia to intravenous morphine due to the time needed to place the intravenous line.[64] It is more difficult to titrate, however, requiring 20 to 30 minutes between doses to observe the full effect rather than 10 to 15 minutes needed for morphine. A common strategy in a patient in severe pain is to start oral oxycodone before the intravenous line is placed and then switch to an intravenous opioid titrated to pain relief.

Agonist-antagonist opioids, such as nalbuphine and butorphanol, have mixed effects on opioid receptor subtypes, exhibiting ceiling effects on both analgesia and respiratory depression. Because clinically important respiratory depression is distinctly rare in the setting of acute pain treatment, it is difficult to justify their routine use. One possible exception is for patients with advanced pulmonary disease. A particular drawback is that one cannot titrate these drugs to maximal effect because of analgesic ceiling effects. Additionally, these drugs are contraindicated and will induce withdrawal symptoms in patients who are physically dependent on opioids, either because of opioid therapy for chronic pain, methadone maintenance therapy, or active opioid addiction.

PATIENT-CONTROLLED ANALGESIA

The use of patient-controlled analgesia (PCA) has been described in emergency medicine for both adults and children.[70] Although no specific advantage has been found over the titration of opioids, PCA is at least as effective in relieving pain. In the setting of high demands on nursing resources, PCA could serve to ensure that patients' pain treatment needs are addressed in a timely fashion. In addition, patients admitted from the ED to inpatient hospital beds often experience a "pain window" between the last dose of an analgesic in the ED and the first dose administered on the hospital ward. Wider use of ED PCA might obviate this common problem.

ALTERNATIVE DELIVERY ROUTES

Multiple alternative delivery routes for the administration of pain medications have been described. The use of nebulized fentanyl has been described and holds promise as a route of opioid delivery that can be initiated before an intravenous line has been placed.[71,72] In addition, intranasal ketamine[73,74]

TABLE 113.2 Analgesics Administered in the Emergency Department[3]	
Analgesic	**N (%)**
Morphine	148 (20.1)
Ibuprofen	127 (17.3)
Hydrocodone; acetaminophen	93 (12.7)
Oxycodone; acetaminophen	83 (11.3)
Ketorolac	60 (8.2)
Acetaminophen	53 (7.2)
Hydromorphone	36 (4.9)
Antacid	26 (3.5)
Meperidine	24 (3.3)
Fentanyl	23 (3.1)
Metoclopramide	13 (1.8)
Codeine; acetaminophen	12 (1.6)
Oxycodone	10 (1.4)
Naproxen	9 (1.2)
Other	18 (2.4)
Total	735 (100)

and intranasal ketorolac have been described and have shown promise.[75] Nebulized pain medications, especially for children who have severe pain but have not had an intravenous line placed, could be of use in the ED.

PROCEDURAL SEDATION AND ANALGESIA

Patients often present to the ED in need of painful or complex procedures that require patient cooperation and must be done emergently. Procedural sedation and analgesia (PSA) practices and policies have evolved rapidly in the ED, and this is a growing area in the practice of emergency medicine.[76] PSA in the ED is complicated by the occurrence of unpredictable concurrent events as well as time and space constraints of the ED. Furthermore, unlike most patients who undergo sedation in other settings, patients in the ED typically have an unpredictable "nothing by mouth" (NPO) status, often have concurrent severe systemic disease, and usually are in severe pain before the procedure begins.[77]

The indications for ED PSA range from pain control for short painful procedures to the need for patient compliance with a complex emergency procedure. The typical target sedation level for ED PSA ranges from minimal through moderate and deep sedation, depending on the demands of specific procedures.[78] Deep sedation can inadvertently result in the patient achieving a level of sedation consistent with general anesthesia, but this is not an intended target level of ED PSA.[79]

Minimal sedation describes a drug-induced state during which patients are sedated but are still able to respond appropriately to verbal commands (according to their developmental age) and whose eyes remain open. Depending on the agent, it is possible to achieve amnesia of the procedure at this level of sedation, but by definition, patients will still respond to their surroundings. It is generally performed for procedures that require patient compliance but are not typically intensely painful when performed with local anesthesia. Minimal sedation is typically used for procedures such as lumbar puncture, evidentiary exams, simple fracture reductions (in combination with local anesthesia), and the incision and drainage of small abscesses.

During minimal sedation, cardiovascular and ventilatory functions are generally maintained, although patients should be monitored for inadvertent oversedation to deeper levels using oxygen saturation monitors and direct observation. Agents typically used for minimal sedation include alfentanil, fentanyl, midazolam, combinations of the two, and low-dose ketamine.

Moderate sedation is performed on patients who would benefit from a deeper level of sedation to augment the procedure. Moderate sedation describes patients sedated to the point at which their eyes are closed but they open in response to verbal commands (appropriately to their developmental age) alone or to light tactile stimulation. Patients at this level usually have an intact airway and maintain ventilatory function without support. As with minimal sedation, inadvertent over sedation to deeper levels can occur with moderate sedation.[80,81] Appropriate monitoring including oxygen saturation, cardiac monitoring, and blood pressure measurements should be done throughout the sedation, and direct observation of the patient's airway should be maintained throughout the procedure. Agents used for moderate sedation in the ED include propofol, etomidate, ketamine, and the combination of fentanyl and midazolam.

Deep sedation is performed on patients who would benefit from a deeper level of sedation, often in order to complete a procedure already begun that requires more patient relaxation than was achieved at a lighter level of sedation. Generally, amnesia of the procedure is similar between moderate and deep sedation, and it is not necessary to sedate patients to a deep level only to obtain amnesia.[82] Deep sedation is achieved in the ED with the same agents as moderate sedation; the difference is

in the intended level of sedation. Monitoring requirements for deep sedation are similar to those for moderate sedation.

End-tidal carbon dioxide monitoring has also been described in ED PSA,[83,84] and it is generally regarded as the monitor most comparable to direct observation of the patients airway for detecting changes in the patients ventilator patterns,[85] especially in patients receiving high-flow oxygen to prevent hypoxia.[85] Deeply sedated patients can develop respiratory depression but generally maintain a patent airway and adequate ventilation.[80,86,87] Patients sedated to this level can progress to a level of sedation consistent with general anesthesia. This can occur after the procedure for which the patient was sedated has been completed. Pain is a powerful stimulant, and after it is removed due to the completion of a procedure or the application of local anesthesia, patients may progress to a deeper level of sedation. There is some evidence that the inadvertent progression to general anesthesia occurs more frequently in patients targeted for deep sedation than in those undergoing moderate sedation.[82] For this reason, and the fact that the occurrence of procedural recall is similar between moderate and deep sedation, it is usually safer to use moderate sedation than deep sedation in the ED unless the procedure requires progressively deeper levels of sedation to complete successfully, such as the reduction of hip dislocations.

Patients who progress to an unintended level of sedation consistent with general anesthesia are not arousable, even to pain. The ability to independently maintain ventilatory function is usually impaired, and patients often require assistance in maintaining a patent airway. Patients can quickly progress to the level of general anesthesia using agents commonly employed for moderate and deep sedation, and physicians performing ED PSA must be prepared to provide ventilatory support until the patient's level of consciousness has improved and they are able to protect their airway and ventilate normally.

In order to decrease the likelihood of aspiration, patients who are undergoing moderate or deep sedation in the ED are often kept NPO. Regardless of the target depth of sedation or the agent administered, there is insufficient evidence to support specific fasting requirements prior to procedural sedation. A guideline for emergency physicians has made recommendations for the proper risk stratification of patients based of their last oral intake.[77] In general, the risk of aspiration from recent oral intake increases with the depth of sedation and must be balanced with the urgency of the procedure when deciding whether or not to delay sedation due to recent oral intake.

Patients who have not had oral intake other than clear liquids for 3 hours prior to their procedure have a low risk of aspiration at any level of sedation. In patients with recent oral intake in need of an emergent procedure, the risk of aspiration is unlikely to outweigh the risk of delaying the procedure. Because the risk of aspiration likely increases with the depth of sedation, it is prudent to target the lightest level of sedation feasible for the necessary procedure. For nonurgent procedures where a time delay is unlikely to have a negative effect on the patient, patients who have eaten more than clear liquids in the prior 3 hours should have the procedure delayed until 3 hours after their last intake. For urgent procedures falling in between emergency and nonurgent procedures, lighter levels and shorter durations of PSA should be used as the size of oral intake taken within 3 hours of the procedure increases.

Patients who are intoxicated, especially with alcohol, can be especially difficult to sedate. They often have food in their stomachs, and the achieved level of sedation can be difficult to predict. In emergent reductions, this increases their risk but does not change the procedure. In patients who can safely have the procedure delayed, intoxicated patients may benefit from a delay in their sedation until the progression of their mental status (getting worse or getting better) can be ascertained through observation.

ED PSA is necessarily used for patients who are medically healthy or have uncomplicated coexisting medical conditions (American Society of Anesthesiologists Physical Classes 1 and 2) and those who have more significant or life-threatening coexisting medical conditions (Classes 3 and 4). PSA for critically ill children has been described using ketamine[88] and in adults using propofol or etomidate.[89] The degree of respiratory depression noted in these patients was similar to patients with physical status scores of 1 or 2, but an increased rate of hypotension was seen in physical status 3 and 4 patients who received propofol. It may be that ketamine and etomidate are better suited for the emergent sedation of critically ill patients, but there is not yet sufficient data to make a definite recommendation.

The ventilatory status of sedated patients must be monitored. This is generally accomplished with pulse oximetry, capnography, and direct observation of the patient's respiratory effort. Pulse oximetry is a sensitive measure of oxygenation. If a patient receives supplemental oxygen prior to starting PSA and during the procedure, this monitor may not be as sensitive to changes in the patient's ventilatory status. End-tidal carbon dioxide has been recommended as an additional modality for the monitoring ventilatory status.[84–86,90] It provides a graphic display of ventilatory status that can be used to detect respiratory depression before it becomes clinically apparent. In the event of hypoventilation, the end-tidal carbon dioxide value increases as the respiratory rate decreases. In the event of increasing airway obstruction, the baseline end-tidal carbon dioxide value decreases along with a blunting of the waveform due to increased mixing of the nasal expiratory sample with ambient air due to the turbulence from the obstruction.

Ketamine use has been described in adults and children undergoing ED PSA.[91,92] Ketamine is a dissociative anesthetic that provides 15 to 20 minutes of sedation when given intramuscularly, with a return to baseline mental status in 30 to 60 minutes. It can be given in doses of 1 to 4 mg/kg intramuscularly and should be combined with atropine 0.01 mg/kg to prevent hypersalivation. The 1 mg/kg dose achieves minimal sedation sufficient for such procedures as lumbar puncture, dressing changes, and simple laceration repair. Doses from 2 to 4 mg/kg result in increasingly deeper levels of moderate to deep sedation. Patients sedated with ketamine usually maintain a patent airway and ventilate normally. Patients receiving ketamine should be monitored for respiratory depression and rare occurrences of laryngospasm.[93] Emergence phenomena, unpleasant perceptual experiences as patients regain consciousness, have been described in both adults and children.[94] The addition of 0.1 mg/kg of midazolam to ketamine has been described to prevent emergence phenomena, but no difference in the occurrence of emergency phenomena has been found with its use.[95] Intravenous ketamine is also used for ED PSA at doses of 1 mg/kg with an onset of 1 to 2 minutes, followed by moderate sedation lasting 8 to 12 minutes. The adverse effects of intravenous ketamine are similar to those of intramuscular use.

The combination of fentanyl and midazolam has been used for minimal, moderate, and deep sedation in the ED.[96–99] This combination results in longer periods of sedation than other agents and carries a higher rate of respiratory depression than other commonly used agents. Although adequate for minimal sedation, the high level of respiratory depression and long duration of action makes this combination less useful for moderate or deep sedation. Dosing for minimal sedation has been described as 0.1 mg/kg intravenous midazolam followed by 0.05 mg/kg intravenous fentanyl, with repeated fentanyl boluses every 1 to 3 minutes until the patient is adequately sedated. The sedation typically lasts 30 to 60 minutes with a return to baseline mental status by 45 to 120 minutes. This method of PSA requires direct ventilatory monitoring.

Pentobarbital is a sedative agent typically used for minimal to moderate sedation for radiologic procedures.[100] This agent has no analgesic properties and patients who appear sedated after its administration can be aroused with less stimuli than is typical for many of the other agents used in ED PSA, which is an excellent characteristic for preventing over sedation for radiologic procedures, but is of limited utility for painful procedures. The medicine is administered at 2.5 mg/kg intravenously, followed by 1.25 mg/kg every 5 minutes until adequate sedation is achieved. Pulse oximetry should be used; however, the rate of respiratory depression is lower than for other agents.

Methohexital has been used for moderate and deep PSA.[101] It is a very short-acting agent with excellent amnestic properties. It is administered at 1 mg/kg intravenously with 0.5 mg/kg repeat boluses every 1 to 2 minutes as needed. It has an onset of 30 seconds, with sedation lasting 2 to 4 minutes and returning to baseline within 5 to 10 minutes. It has been associated with respiratory depression and a quick progression to deeper levels of sedation than intended and can cause over sedation even when carefully titrated. It should therefore be used with close ventilatory monitoring. Compared to propofol, methohexital is similarly effective and safe with single bolus use but is less safe than propofol when multiple doses are required. It should be used principally for very brief procedures expected to last less than 2 to 4 minutes, such as the reduction of simple fractures and dislocations.

Propofol is well described for ED PSA.[79] It is administered as a 1 mg/kg bolus with repeat boluses of 0.5 mg/kg every 2 to 3 minutes until the patient achieves the desired level of sedation. The sedation persists 2 to 5 minutes after a single bolus and longer for patients receiving multiple boluses, with a return to baseline within 10 to 15 minutes. This medication has been associated with rates of clinically apparent respiratory depression from 4.0% to 7.7% in ED PSA. As with similar agents, close ventilatory monitoring is required. Propofol causes hypotension in critically ill patients and should be used with caution in hemodynamically unstable patients.

The combination of propofol and ketamine has also been described. It has been shown to have decreased rates of recovery agitation than ketamine alone, and less hypotension than propofol alone. It is likely that the combination of agents can decrease the associated risk of adverse events and potentiate the benefit of the drugs but that it must be tailored to the needs to the individual patient.[87,96]

Etomidate is also frequently used for ED PSA.[102] It is given as a single bolus of 0.1 to 0.3 mg/kg, with an onset of sedation in 30 to 60 seconds and sedation lasting 7 to 10 minutes. It is not associated with hypotension and is more commonly used when this is an issue; however, its use is associated with myoclonic jerking in up to 25% of patients. This adverse effect can complicate the procedure for which the patient has been sedated, making it inferior to propofol for the sedation of healthy patients. Etomidate, in single boluses of 0.3 mg/kg, has been shown to cause transient adrenal suppression, but no significant changes in cortisol levels occur, and the significance of this finding remains unclear. It has been shown to cause less hypotension in severely ill patients requiring sedation and is likely a better choice in these patients until they are stabilized despite the unclear risk of adrenal suppression.

Evolving Emergency Department Pain Management Practice

Pain management practices in the ED continue to evolve. The ACEP, emergency medicine's principal specialty organization, established its first general policy statement regarding analgesic practices in 2004.[103] Prior to this, data from the National Hospital Ambulatory Medical Care Survey showed that, from 1997 to 2001, there was an impressive 18% increase in analgesic use in US EDs (from 47.2 to 56.2 mentions per 100 visits), with marked increases in both NSAID agents and opioid analgesics.[104]

At the local level, adoptions of pain management guidelines and quality improvement processes have demonstrated dramatic improvements in practices. In one 3-site study, rates of ED analgesic treatment increased from 54% to 84% over 1 year as a result of individual and group feedback.[105] In a study from one Swiss ED, educational programs and guideline implementation led to marked increases in pain intensity documentation, analgesic administration, reduction in pain intensity scores, and improved patient satisfaction over a 4-month period.[106]

We do not know the reasons for the rapid evolution of ED pain management practice. Policy and regulatory initiatives, institutional quality improvement programs, increased attention to the opioid abuse epidemic in the United States, pharmaceutical marketing campaigns, educational efforts, and new knowledge from basic and clinical research are all likely to be influential factors. No matter the cause, emergency medicine pain research is increasing at a rapid pace, and ED pain management practices will continue to evolve.

Conclusion

Relieving pain and reducing suffering are primary responsibilities of emergency medicine and much can be done to improve the care of ED patients in pain. Emergency physicians and nurses continue to refine their approach to the problem of pain, and in time, the current large amount of variability in ED pain practices will no doubt lessen. Clinicians, researchers, and policy makers continue to define specialty-specific standards for emergency medicine pain practice in an effort to both improve the management of pain in emergencies and to decrease the risk to patients from the medications used. Ongoing quality improvement initiatives, education, and research are essential to achieving these goals.

References

1. National Center for Health Statistics. *National Hospital Ambulatory Medical Care Survey: 2013 Emergency Department Summary Tables.* Atlanta, GA: U.S. Department of Health and Human Services, Centers for Disease Control and Prevention; 2013. Available at: https://www.cdc.gov/nchs/fastats/emergency-department.htm. Accessed September 1, 2017.
2. Pletcher MJ, Kertesz SG, Kohn MA, et al. Trends in opioid prescribing by race/ethnicity for patients seeking care in US emergency departments. *JAMA* 2008;299(1):70–78.
3. Todd KH, Ducharme J, Choinere M, et al. Pain in the emergency department: results of the Pain and Emergency Medicine Initiative (PEMI) multicenter study. *J Pain* 2007;8(6):460–466.
4. Cordell WH, Keene KK, Giles BK, et al. The high prevalence of pain in emergency medical care. *Am J Emerg Med* 2002;20(3):165–169.
5. Rupp T, Delaney KA. Inadequate analgesia in emergency medicine. *Ann Emerg Med* 2004;43(4):494–503.
6. Tanabe P, Buschmann M. A prospective study of ED pain management practices and the patient's perspective. *J Emerg Nurs* 1999;25(3):171–177.
7. Todd KH, Cowan P, Homel P, et al. Chronic or recurrent pain in the emergency department: national telephone survey of patient experience. *West J Emerg Med* 2010;11(5):408–415.
8. Phillips DM. JCAHO pain management standards are unveiled. Joint Commission on Accreditation of Healthcare Organizations. *JAMA* 2000;284(4):428–429.
9. Institute of Medicine. *Relieving Pain in America: A Blueprint for Transforming Prevention, Care, Education and Research.* Washington, DC: National Academies Press; 2011.
10. Strayer RJ, Motov SM, Nelson LS. Something for pain: responsible opioid use in emergency medicine. *Am J Emerg Med* 2017;35(2):337–341.
11. Paulozzi LJ, Weisler RH, Patkar AA. A national epidemic of unintentional prescription opioid overdose deaths: how physicians can help control it. *J Clin Psychiatry* 2011;72(5):589–592.
12. Volkow ND, McLellan TA, Cotto JH, et al. Characteristics of opioid prescriptions in 2009. *JAMA* 2011;305(13):1299–1301.
13. Pomerleau AC, Nelson LS, Hoppe JA, et al. The impact of prescription drug monitoring programs and prescribing guidelines on emergency department opioid prescribing: a multi-center survey. *Pain Med* 2017;18(5):889–897.

14. Hoppe JA, Kim H, Heard K. Association of emergency department opioid initiation with recurrent opioid use. *Ann Emerg Med* 2015;65(5):493.e4–499.e4.
15. Perrone J, Mycyk MB. A challenging crossroad for emergency medicine: the epidemics of pain and pain medication deaths. *Acad Emerg Med* 2014;21(3):334–336.
16. Piercefield E, Archer P, Kemp P, et al. Increase in unintentional medication overdose deaths: Oklahoma, 1994-2006. *Am J Prev Med* 2010;39(4):357–363.
17. Porucznik CA, Johnson EM, Sauer B, et al. Studying adverse events related to prescription opioids: the Utah experience. *Pain Med* 2011;12(suppl 2):S16–S25.
18. U.S. Department of Health and Human Services, U.S. Food and Drug Administration. Draft blueprint for prescriber education for long-acting/extended-release opioid class-wide risk evaluation and mitigation strategy. *Fed Regist* 2011;2011(76):68766–68767.
19. Sundwall DN, Rolfs RT, Johnson E. *Utah Clinical Guidelines on Prescribing Opioids for Treatment of Pain.* Salt Lake City, UT: Utah Department of Health; 2009.
20. Washington Chapter of American College of Emergency Physicians, Washington State Emergency Nurse Association, Washington Medical Association, Washington State Hospital Association. *Washington Emergency Department Opioid Prescribing Guidelines.* Available at: http://washingtonacep.org/postings/edopioidabuseguidlinesfinal.pdf. Accessed September 1, 2017.
21. Johnson EM, Porucznik CA, Anderson JW, et al. State-level strategies for reducing prescription drug overdose deaths: Utah's prescription safety program. *Pain Med* 2011;12(suppl 2):S66–S72.
22. Cantrill SV, Brown MD, Carlisle RJ, et al. Clinical policy: critical issues in the prescribing of opioids for adult patients in the emergency department. *Ann Emerg Med* 2012;60(4):499–525.
23. Chauny JM, Marquis M, Paquet J, et al. The simple query "Do you want more pain medication?" is not a reliable way to assess acute pain relief in patients in the emergency department. *CJEM* 2018;20:1–7.
24. Malviya S, Voepel-Lewis T, Burke C, et al. The revised FLACC observational pain tool: improved reliability and validity for pain assessment in children with cognitive impairment. *Paediatr Anaesth* 2006;16(3):258–265.
25. Warden V, Hurley AC, Volicer L. Development and psychometric evaluation of the Pain Assessment in Advanced Dementia (PAINAD) scale. *J Am Med Dir Assoc* 2003;4(1):9–15.
26. Gureje O, Von Korff M, Simon GE, et al. Persistent pain and well-being: a World Health Organization study in primary care. *JAMA* 1998;280(2):147–151.
27. Fosnocht DE, Swanson ER, Barton ED. Changing attitudes about pain and pain control in emergency medicine. *Emerg Med Clin North Am* 2005;23(2):297–306.
28. Wilson JE, Pendleton JM. Oligoanalgesia in the emergency department. *Am J Emerg Med* 1989;(6):620–623.
29. Albrecht E, Taffe P, Yersin B, et al. Undertreatment of acute pain (oligoanalgesia) and medical practice variation in prehospital analgesia of adult trauma patients: a 10 yr retrospective study. *Br J Anaesth* 2013;110(1):96–106.
30. Neighbor ML, Honner S, Kohn MA. Factors affecting emergency department opioid administration to severely injured patients. *Acad Emerg Med* 2004;11(12):1290–1296.
31. Todd KH, Samaroo N, Hoffman JR. Ethnicity as a risk factor for inadequate emergency department analgesia. *JAMA* 1993;269(12):1537–1539.
32. Todd KH, Deaton C, D'Adamo AP, et al. Ethnicity and analgesic practice. *Ann Emerg Med* 2000;35(1):11–16.
33. Bijur PE, Esses D, Chang AK, et al. Dosing and titration of intravenous opioid analgesics administered to ED patients in acute severe pain. *Am J Emerg Med* 2012;30(7):1241–1244.
34. Miner J, Biros MH, Trainor A, et al. Patient and physician perceptions as risk factors for oligoanalgesia: a prospective observational study of the relief of pain in the emergency department. *Acad Emerg Med* 2006;13(2):140–146.
35. Tamayo-Sarver JH, Hinze SW, Cydulla RK, et al. Racial and ethnic disparities in emergency department analgesic prescription. *Am J Public Health* 2003;93(12):2067–2073.
36. Bartfield JM, Salluzo RF, Raccio-Robak N, et al. Physician and patient factors influencing the treatment of low back pain. *Pain* 1997;73(2):209–211.
37. Weiner SG, Griggs CA, Mitchell PM, et al. Clinician impression versus prescription drug monitoring program criteria in the assessment of drug-seeking behavior in the emergency department. *Ann Emerg Med* 2013;62(4):281–289.
38. Cederbaum JA, Guerrero EG, Mitchell KR, et al. Utilization of emergency and hospital services among individuals in substance abuse treatment. *Subst Abuse Treat Prev Policy* 2014;9:16.
39. Beaudoin FL, Baird J, Liu T, et al. Sex differences in substance use among adult emergency department patients: prevalence, severity, and need for intervention. *Acad Emerg Med* 2015;22(11):1307–1315.
40. National Institute of Drug Abuse. National survey of drug use and health. Available at: https://www.drugabuse.gov/national-survey-drug-use-health. Accessed September 1, 2017.
41. Hirabayashi N, Wada K, Kimura T, et al. Prevalence of substance abuse among patients with physical diseases seen in an emergency room in Japan. *Am J Addict* 2004;13(4):398–404.

42. Soderstrom CA, Smith GS, Dischinger PC, et al. Psychoactive substance use disorders among seriously injured trauma center patients. *JAMA* 1997;277(22):1769–1774.

43. Martins SS, Copersino ML, Soderstrom CA, et al. Risk of psychoactive substance dependence among substance users in a trauma inpatient population. *J Addict Dis* 2007;26(1):71–77.

44. Zechnich AD, Hedges JR. Community-wide emergency department visits by patients suspected of drug-seeking behavior. *Acad Emerg Med* 1996;3(4):312–317.

45. Beaudoin FL, Lin C, Guan W, et al. Low-dose ketamine improves pain relief in patients receiving intravenous opioids for acute pain in the emergency department: results of a randomized, double-blind, clinical trial. *Acad Emerg Med* 2014;21(11):1193–1202.

46. Maughan BC, Bachhuber MA, Mitra N, et al. Prescription monitoring programs and emergency department visits involving opioids, 2004-2011. *Drug Alcohol Depend* 2015;156:282–288.

47. Smith RJ, Kilaru AS, Perrone J, et al. How, why, and for whom do emergency medicine providers use prescription drug monitoring programs? *Pain Med* 2015;16(6):1122–1231.

48. Baehren DF, Marco CA, Droz DE, et al. A statewide prescription monitoring program affects emergency department prescribing behaviors. *Ann Emerg Med* 2010;56(1):19.e3–23.e3.

49. Todd KH. Pain and prescription monitoring programs in the emergency department. *Ann Emerg Med* 2010;56(1):24–26.

50. Poon SJ, Greenwood-Ericksen MB, Gish RE, et al. Usability of the Massachusetts Prescription Drug Monitoring Program in the emergency department: a mixed-methods study. *Acad Emerg Med* 2016;23(4):406–414.

51. Greenwood-Ericksen MB, Poon SJ, Nelson LS, et al. Best practices for prescription drug monitoring programs in the emergency department setting: results of an expert panel. *Ann Emerg Med* 2016;67(6):755–764.e4.

52. Marco CA, Venkat A, Baker EE, et al. Prescription drug monitoring programs: ethical issues in the emergency department. *Ann Emerg Med* 2016;68(5):589–598.

53. Simon LJ, Bizamcer AN, Lidz CW, et al. Disparities in opioid prescribing for patients with psychiatric diagnoses presenting with pain to the emergency department. *Emerg Med J* 2012;29(3):201–204.

54. Grover CA, Elder JW, Close RJ, et al. How frequently are "classic" drug-seeking behaviors used by drug-seeking patients in the emergency department? *West J Emerg Med* 2012;13(5):416–421.

55. Tanabe P, Hafner JW, Martinovich Z, et al. Adult emergency department patients with sickle cell pain crisis: results from a quality improvement learning collaborative model to improve analgesic management. *Acad Emerg Med* 2012;19(4):430–438.

56. Tanabe P, Myers R, Zosel A, et al. Emergency department management of acute pain episodes in sickle cell disease. *Acad Emerg Med* 2007;14(5):419–425.

57. Puri Singh A, Haywood C Jr, Beach MC, et al. Improving emergency providers' attitudes toward sickle cell patients in pain. *J Pain Symptom Manage* 2016;51(3):628.e3–632.e3.

58. Shapiro BS, Benjamin LJ, Payne R, et al. Sickle cell-related pain: perceptions of medical practitioners. *J Pain Symptom Manage* 1997;14(3):168–174.

59. Pack-Mabien A, Labbe E, Herbert D, et al. Nurses' attitudes and practices in sickle cell pain management. *Appl Nurs Res* 2001;14(4):187–192.

60. Tanabe P, Martinovich Z, Buckley B, et al. Safety of an ED high-dose opioid protocol for sickle cell disease pain. *J Emerg Nurs* 2015;41(3):227–235.

61. Tanabe P, Artz N, Mark Courtney D, et al. Adult emergency department patients with sickle cell pain crisis: a learning collaborative model to improve analgesic management. *Acad Emerg Med* 2010;17(4):399–407.

62. Todd KH, Sloan EP, Chen C, et al. Survey of pain etiology, management practices and patient satisfaction in two urban emergency departments. *CJEM* 2002;4(4):252–256.

63. Steinberg PL, Nangia AK, Curtis K. A standardized pain management protocol improves timeliness of analgesia among emergency department patients with renal colic. *Qual Manag Health Care* 2011;20(1):30–36.

64. Miner JR, Moore J, Gray RO, et al. Oral versus intravenous opioid dosing for the initial treatment of acute musculoskeletal pain in the emergency department. *Acad Emerg Med* 2008;15(12):1234–1240.

65. Neighbor ML, Baird CH, Kohn MA. Changing opioid use for right lower quadrant abdominal pain in the emergency department. *Acad Emerg Med* 2005;12(12):1216–1220.

66. Motov S, Yasavolian M, Likourezos A, et al. Comparison of intravenous ketorolac at three single-dose regimens for treating acute pain in the emergency department: a randomized controlled trial. *Ann Emerg Med* 2017;70(2):177–184.

67. Safdar B, Degutis LC, Landry K, et al. Intravenous morphine plus ketorolac is superior to either drug alone for treatment of acute renal colic. *Ann Emerg Med* 2006;48(2):173.e1–181.e1.

68. Hewitt DJ, Todd KH, Xiang J, et al. Tramadol/acetaminophen or hydrocodone/acetaminophen for the treatment of ankle sprain: a randomized, placebo-controlled trial. *Ann Emerg Med* 2007;49(4):468.e2–480.e2.

69. Bijur PE, Kenny MK, Gallagher EJ. Intravenous morphine at 0.1 mg/kg is not effective for controlling severe acute pain in the majority of patients. *Ann Emerg Med* 2005;46(4):362–367.

70. Birnbaum A, Schechter C, Tufaro V, et al. Efficacy of patient-controlled analgesia for patients with acute abdominal pain in the emergency department: a randomized trial. *Acad Emerg Med* 2012;19(4):370–377.

71. Miner JR, Kletti C, Herold M, et al. Randomized clinical trial of nebulized fentanyl citrate versus i.v. fentanyl citrate in children presenting to the emergency department with acute pain. *Acad Emerg Med* 2007;14(10):895–898.

72. Borland M, Jacobs I, King B, et al. A randomized controlled trial comparing intranasal fentanyl to intravenous morphine for managing acute pain in children in the emergency department. *Ann Emerg Med* 2007;49(3):335–340.

73. Shimonovich S, Gigi R, Shapira A, et al. Intranasal ketamine for acute traumatic pain in the emergency department: a prospective, randomized clinical trial of efficacy and safety. *BMC Emerg Med* 2016;16(1):43.

74. Yeaman F, Meek R, Egerton-Warburton D, et al. Sub-dissociative-dose intranasal ketamine for moderate to severe pain in adult emergency department patients. *Emerg Med Australas* 2014;26(3):237–242.

75. Arhami Dolatabadi A, Memary E, Kariman H, et al. Intranasal desmopressin compared with intravenous ketorolac for pain management of patients with renal colic referring to the emergency department: a randomized clinical trial. *Anesth Pain Med* 2017;7(2):e43595.

76. Godwin SA, Burton JH, Gerardo CJ, et al. Clinical policy: procedural sedation and analgesia in the emergency department. *Ann Emerg Med* 2014;63(2):247.e18–258.e18.

77. Green SM, Roback MG, Miner JR, et al. Fasting and emergency department procedural sedation and analgesia: a consensus-based clinical practice advisory. *Ann Emerg Med* 2007;49(4):454–461.

78. Miner JR, Huber D, Nichols S, et al. The effect of the assignment of a pre-sedation target level on procedural sedation using propofol. *J Emerg Med* 2007;32(3):249–255.

79. Miner JR, Burton JH. Clinical practice advisory: emergency department procedural sedation with propofol. *Ann Emerg Med* 2007;50(2):182.e1–187.e1.

80. Miner JR, Driver BE, Moore JC, et al. Randomized clinical trial of propofol versus alfentanil for moderate procedural sedation in the emergency department. *Am J Emerg Med* 2017;35:1451–1456.

81. Bellolio MF, Gilani WI, Barrionuevo P, et al. Incidence of adverse events in adults undergoing procedural sedation in the emergency department: a systematic review and meta-analysis. *Acad Emerg Med* 2016;23(2):119–134.

82. Miner JR, Bachman A, Kosman L, et al. Assessment of the onset and persistence of amnesia during procedural sedation with propofol. *Acad Emerg Med* 2005;12(6):491–496.

83. Burton JH, Miner JR, Shipley ER, et al. Propofol for emergency department procedural sedation and analgesia: a tale of three centers. *Acad Emerg Med* 2006;13(1):24–30.

84. Miner JR, Heegaard W, Plummer D. End-tidal carbon dioxide monitoring during procedural sedation. *Acad Emerg Med* 2002;9(4):275–280.

85. Deitch K, Miner J, Chudnofsky CR, et al. Does end tidal CO2 monitoring during emergency department procedural sedation and analgesia with propofol decrease the incidence of hypoxic events? A randomized, controlled trial. *Ann Emerg Med* 2010;55(3):258–264.

86. Miner JR, Moore JC, Plummer D, et al. Randomized clinical trial of the effect of supplemental opioids in procedural sedation with propofol on serum catecholamines. *Acad Emerg Med* 2013;20(4):330–337.

87. Miner JR, Moore JC, Austad EJ, et al. Randomized, double-blinded, clinical trial of propofol, 1:1 propofol/ketamine, and 4:1 propofol/ketamine for deep procedural sedation in the emergency department. *Ann Emerg Med* 2015;65(5):479.e2–488.e2.

88. Green SM, Denmark TK, Cline J, et al. Ketamine sedation for pediatric critical care procedures. *Pediatr Emerg Care* 2001;17(4):244–248.

89. Miner JR, Martel ML, Meyer M, et al. Procedural sedation of critically ill patients in the emergency department. *Acad Emerg Med* 2005;12(1):124–128.

90. Deitch K, Chudnofsky CR, Dominici P, et al. The utility of high-flow oxygen during emergency department procedural sedation and analgesia with propofol: a randomized, controlled trial. *Ann Emerg Med* 2011;58(4):360.e3–364.e3.

91. Green SM, Roback MG, Kennedy RM, et al. Clinical practice guideline for emergency department ketamine dissociative sedation: 2011 update. *Ann Emerg Med* 2011;57(5):449–461.

92. Green SM, Roback MG, Krauss B, et al. Predictors of airway and respiratory adverse events with ketamine sedation in the emergency department: an individual-patient data meta-analysis of 8,282 children. *Ann Emerg Med* 2009;54(2):158.e4–168.e4.

93. Green SM, Roback MG, Krauss B; for Emergency Department Ketamine Meta-Analysis Study Group. Laryngospasm during emergency department ketamine sedation: a case-control study. *Pediatr Emerg Care* 2010;26(11):798–802.

94. Green SM, Sherwin TS. Incidence and severity of recovery agitation after ketamine sedation in young adults. *Am J Emerg Med* 2005;23(2):142–144.

95. Green SM, Roback MG, Krauss B, et al; for Emergency Department Ketamine Meta-Analysis Study Group. Predictors of emesis and recovery agitation with emergency department ketamine sedation: an individual-patient data meta-analysis of 8,282 children. *Ann Emerg Med* 2009;54(2):171.e4–180.e4.

96. Nejati A, Moharari RS, Ashraf H, et al. Ketamine/propofol versus midazolam/fentanyl for procedural sedation and analgesia in the emergency department: a randomized, prospective, double-blind trial. *Acad Emerg Med* 2011;18(8):800–806.

97. McQueen A, Wright RO, Kido MM, et al. Procedural sedation and analgesia outcomes in children after discharge from the emergency department: ketamine versus fentanyl/midazolam. *Ann Emerg Med* 2009;54(2):191.e4–197.e4.

98. Deitch K, Chudnofsky CR, Dominici P. The utility of supplemental oxygen during emergency department procedural sedation and analgesia with midazolam and fentanyl: a randomized, controlled trial. *Ann Emerg Med* 2007;49(1):1–8.

99. Godambe SA, Elliot V, Matheny D, et al. Comparison of propofol/fentanyl versus ketamine/midazolam for brief orthopedic procedural sedation in a pediatric emergency department. *Pediatrics* 2003;112(1 pt 1):116–123.

100. Chun TH, Amanullah S, Karishma-Bahl D, et al. Comparison of methohexital and pentobarbital as sedative agents for pediatric emergency department patients for computed tomography. *Pediatr Emerg Care* 2009;25(10):648–650.

101. Miner JR, Biros M, Krieg S, et al. Randomized clinical trial of propofol versus methohexital for procedural sedation during fracture and dislocation reduction in the emergency department. *Acad Emerg Med* 2003;10(9):931–937.

102. Miner JR, Danahy M, Moch A, et al. Randomized clinical trial of etomidate versus propofol for procedural sedation in the emergency department. *Ann Emerg Med* 2007;49(1):15–22.

103. Pain management in the emergency department. *Ann Emerg Med* 2004;44(2):198.

104. McCaig LF, Burt CW. National Hospital Ambulatory Medical Care Survey: 2002 emergency department summary. *Adv Data* 2004;340:1–34.

105. Sucov A, Nathanson A, McCormick J, et al. Peer review and feedback can modify pain treatment patterns for emergency department patients with fractures. *Am J Med Qual* 2005;20(3):138–143.

106. Decosterd I, Huqli O, Tamchés E, et al. Oligoanalgesia in the emergency department: short-term beneficial effects of an education program on acute pain. *Ann Emerg Med* 2007;50(4):462–471.

CHAPTER 114

Pain Management in the Intensive Care Unit

CURTIS N. SESSLER, KIMBERLY VARNEY GILL, and **KRISTIN MILLER**

Pain, Analgesia, and Critical Illness

Pain is ubiquitous among critically ill patients, yet the nature of critical illness and intensive care unit (ICU) care presents many unique challenges to effective pain management.[1-10] A central responsibility of all ICU clinicians is to provide comfort and mitigate unpleasant sensations including pain as well as anxiety, dyspnea, and other forms of distress.[11-17] Experts have provided guidance regarding managing pain in the ICU, often within the paradigm of sedation and analgesia. In this chapter, we focus on the unique aspects of pain and analgesia in the ICU within the context of a comprehensive textbook on pain.[11-14,17-20]

ICUs are filled with patients who have suffered critical illness or injury and the accompanying discomfort. Many patients have undergone surgery or experienced trauma or burns and are likely to have pain as a direct result of tissue injury and related management such as dressing changes and wound care. Other patients have localized inflammation due to infection or have neuropathies or other specific conditions that produce pain. The majority of ICU patients undergo routine care which can contribute to discomfort or frank pain. Such interventions include the presence of indwelling tubes (i.e., nasogastric, endotracheal, bladder, and rectal tubes) or vascular catheters that can induce pain during their insertion and in some cases continue to produce discomfort by their mere presence.[3-5,21,22] Even simple tasks that are routinely performed many times each day—such as tracheal suctioning or turning of the patient from side to side—are reported as painful by ICU patients.[5,9,22,23]

The nature of critical illness and ICU care can complicate various aspects of pain management. For example, the sensation of pain may be intensified by the concomitant anxiety, sleep deprivation, and delirium.[23-33] It is clear that all of these conditions are commonplace among critically ill patients. Further, immobility and impaired communication can intensify anxiety and perception of pain. Newer integrated approaches to optimize patient comfort and hasten recover comprehensively address analgesia as well as efforts to reduce anxiety yet avoid oversedation, improve sleep quality, prevent delirium, speed liberation from mechanical ventilation, and enhance rehabilitation and mobility.[34-40]

Pain is often poorly recognized and quantified, further challenging effective pain management.[11,12] This can be the result of impaired communication due to a reduced level of consciousness from sedative medications or difficulty with phonation and movement due to oral tubes, physical restraints, or paralysis. Although the presence of pain may be inferred as a result of unexplained autonomic hyperactivity (i.e., tachypnea, tachycardia, or hypertension), these signs have many other causes and thus are nonspecific for pain.[11] Clinicians' evaluation of patients for possible pain include observing behaviors such as grimacing or rigid body positioning, but these are less reliable as sedation deepens.[11,22,41-55] Overt agitated behavior, a not infrequent occurrence among critically ill patients, is typically attributed to delirium, particularly due to alcohol or sedative drug withdrawal, but can also be the result of inadequately managed pain.[56-63]

Pharmacologic management of pain is more complex in the ICU than in many other settings.[11-14,17-20] The majority of ICU patients have organ dysfunction. In particular, the utilization of many opioid and nonopioid analgesics is impacted by the high prevalence of impaired hepatic metabolism or renal clearance, problems with enteral or transdermal drug administration, and concerns for drug interactions with the extensive list of medications required for many ICU patients.[64-67] Recognition and amelioration of adverse effects of analgesics and other medications is often more difficult because of ongoing organ dysfunction and concomitant medical problems as well as the large number of medications utilized. In particular, the high prevalence of impaired gastrointestinal mobility from opioids becomes far more than just the inconvenience and discomfort of constipation and can impact administration of nutrition and enteral medications; can worsen respiratory function; and can lead to additional treatment, tests, and interventions.[68] These many ICU factors elevate the complexity of pain management.

In the ICU setting, opioid administration is often performed for purposes beyond pure pain management, that of providing comfort and tolerance of the ICU interventions along with sedative drugs—called analgosedation. This approach relies on titration of both sedative-hypnotic and opioid analgesic drugs to improve the patient's tolerance of mechanical ventilation and other aspects of the ICU environment and routine ICU care. The target is comfort without oversedation and is often best achieved with a balanced approach that allows selection of medications that are preferred for a specific patient (e.g., organ dysfunction or hemodynamic compromise) and can minimize adverse effects of medications by using lower doses and potentially synergistic effects.[11-20,69-74] Some clinical trials have demonstrated better outcomes when such an approach is used. Although titration of the opioid component to a pain reduction target remains operative, the overall level of consciousness and patient–ventilator interaction often influences the dosing of both sedative and analgesic infusions. Thus, somewhat uniquely to the ICU setting, "pain management" also encompasses management of "analgosedation" and tolerance of mechanical ventilation and other ICU interventions.

Successful management of pain, provision of comfort, and timely recovery from critical illness are highly dependent on the multiprofessional care team implemented in many ICUs. Pain management in particular relies on the effective partnership between the treating physician, the bedside nurse, and the clinical pharmacist. This includes designing a treatment strategy that is patient focused with consideration of the patient's unique analgesic needs and factors like organ dysfunction that influence management. Implementation is enhanced through standardized approaches, order sets, guidelines, and other tools plus ongoing communication and review. The comprehensive ICU team also includes physical therapists, nutritionists, respiratory therapists, and others who contribute to missions of comfort and rapid recovery. Further, utilization of expert consults from palliative care or pain management services can make an important difference in selected patients. Accordingly, effective pain management in the ICU brings the advantages, but also challenges, of a team-based approach.[34-40]

TABLE 114.1 Systemic and Physiologic Consequences of Pain in the Intensive Care Unit

Physiologic System and Effects	Consequences
Immune: cytokines elaboration and leukocyte dysfunction	Decreased ability to fight infection and hemodynamic instability
Cardiovascular: increased adrenergic tone and increased vascular resistance	Increased myocardial oxygen demand, stress, and ischemia; venous stasis
Renal: activation of renin-angiotensin-aldosterone axis	Water and sodium retention, anasarca
Endocrine: hormonal imbalance, especially cortisol and insulin	Hyperglycemia
Respiratory: restrictive physiology, hyperventilation, lowered residual capacity	Patient–ventilator asynchrony, atelectasis, hypoxia, increased pneumonia risk
Psychological and neurologic: altered sleep stage and serotonergic imbalance	Depression, fatigue, psychosis, sleep deprivation, anxiety
Hematologic: hypercoagulability and platelet dysfunction	Bleeding, thromboembolic disease

A final consideration as to the unique aspects of pain management in the ICU is that the physiologic consequences of untreated pain may be particularly detrimental in critically ill patients who already have ongoing shock, tissue injury, and organ failure producing a complex state of physiologic disruption.[75] Pain can cause neurohormonal derangements, catecholamine release, stress response, cytokine production, and other physiologic derangements. These and other pain-induced changes can promote hypercoagulability, altered glucose control, myocardial ischemia, hemodynamic compromise, immune system dysfunction, excessive inflammation, ventilator asynchrony, and disrupted sleep.

There is strong motivation from multiple standpoints to effectively detect and manage pain in a multiprofessional and patient-centered approach. Some of these manifestations are listed in Table 114.1. The core evidence-based recommendations directly related to pain and analgesia from the Society of Critical Care Medicine (SCCM) are displayed in Table 114.2 and form the basis of management.[11]

TABLE 114.2 2013 SCCM Pain, Agitation, and Delirium Guidelines: Statements and Recommendations for Treatment of Pain in the Intensive Care Unit (ICU)

- ICU patients frequently experience pain at rest, with routine ICU care and in association with devices and procedures (B).
- Pain should be routinely monitored in all adult ICU patients (+1B).
- The Behavioral Pain Scale and the Critical-Care Pain Observational Tool are the most valid behavioral pain scales in medical, postoperative, or trauma (with the exception of brain injury) adult ICU patients who are unable to self-report pain (B).
- Vital signs may be used as a cue (+2C) but should not be used alone in the assessment of pain (+2C).
- Preemptive analgesia should be used in adult ICU patients prior to procedures (+2C), including chest tube removal (+1C).
- First-line therapy: intravenous opioids for nonneuropathic pain (+1C).
- Consider nonopioid analgesics as adjunctive therapies to reduce opiates and related side effects (+2C).
- Treat neuropathic pain with gabapentin or carbamazepine (+1A).
- Thoracic epidural anesthesia/analgesia should be considered for abdominal aortic aneurysm postoperative patients (+1B) or patients with traumatic rib fractures (+2B).
- Analgesia-first sedation should be used in mechanically ventilated adult ICU patients (+2B).

NOTE: The quality of evidence for each statement and recommendation was ranked as high (A), moderate (B), or low/very low (C). The strength of recommendations was ranked as strong (1) or weak (2) and either in favor of (+) or against (−) an intervention.

Evaluation and Monitoring of Pain in the Intensive Care Unit

Effective pain management begins with the assumption that pain is common among ICU patients and that caregivers should systematically and repeatedly evaluate each patient for the presence of pain, its intensity, and its characteristics.[11–13,16,41] Unfortunately, research confirms that caregivers tend to underrecognize pain and often fail to preemptively treat pain.[21] Accordingly, clinicians should err on the side of presuming pain is present. Repeated assessment is desirable because conditions change over time and pain management is more effective at an early stage than after pain has become established and more severe.

Ideally, pain should be described in regard to location, duration, type, exacerbating and relieving factors, and intensity. Pain should be also be considered by subtype—including somatic, visceral, and neuropathic—because manifestations and management can be different.[11,41] For example, somatic pain is typically dull and aching, often localized, and responds well to opioids and nonsteroidal anti-inflammatory drugs (NSAIDs). In contrast, visceral pain is often cramping and colicky and may respond to anticholinergic therapy, whereas the burning and shooting neuropathic pain is often best treated with antidepressant and anticonvulsant agents. Repeated and thorough evaluation helps to determine the cause and to appreciate prior responses to therapy.

Because pain is a subjective interpretation by an individual, the ability of that individual to communicate the presence and magnitude of pain is important in guiding evaluation and management when possible.[11,41] Many ICUs employ a strategy of daily interruption of sedation, even in unstable sedated patients, and this brief period of greater awareness by the patient presents an opportunity for communication about pain. Although detailed verbal communication about the presence, intensity, and character of pain is ideal, it is often not possible with ICU patients and the use of simple tools can enhance communications of the presence and intensity of pain. These simple tools, such as numerical rating scales and a series of cartoon faces ranging from smiling to crying like the Wong-Baker FACES scale, can facilitate communication via pointing or nodding by the cognitively intact but nonverbal patient.[42] A simple horizontal 0-to-10 numerical scale with enlarged font was judged to be feasible and valid in one comparison of tools.[43] Other techniques to improve the process of self-reporting of pain include adding descriptive words to the numerical scale, explaining the tool and correcting errors with each encounter, providing needed glasses and hearing aids, and ensuring adequate time for instructions and patient response.[41] Use of a scale that incorporates descriptive pictures, like the FACES scale, can help overcome language barriers as well as mild cognitive dysfunction.

Many ICU patients are cognitively impaired, and self-reporting pain is not feasible. For these patients, utilizing a structured evidence-based approach to infer the presence and severity of pain based on observation can be performed. Tools have been developed based on observed behaviors that have been correlated with self-reported pain and/or with responses to noxious stimuli in prior research.[9,21,44–46] Various combinations of behaviors have been assembled into structured assessment tools—most include facial expressions, body position and movement, and patient–ventilator interaction. Contraction of facial muscles associated with grimacing correlates particularly well with noxious stimuli.[22] The early work in pain assessment for noncommunicative ICU patients was with infants and young children, resulting in the development of the COMFORT Scale, the FLACC Observation tool, and others.[41,76,77] Subsequently, a variety of pain assessment tools for nonverbal critically ill adults have been developed, validated, and critically reviewed.[11,41,47,48] Published pain observation tools for adults in the ICU care include the Critical-Care Pain

TABLE 114.3 The Critical-Care Pain Observation Tool (CPOT)

Indicator	Description	Score	
Facial expression	No muscular tension observed	Relaxed, neutral	0
	Presence of frowning, brow lowering, orbit tightening, and levator contraction	Tense	1
	All of the above facial movements plus eyelid tightly closed	Grimacing	2
Body movements	Does not move at all (does not necessarily mean absence of pain)	Absence of movements	0
	Slow, cautious movements, touching or rubbing the pain site, seeking attention through movements	Protection	1
	Pulling tube, attempting to sit up, moving limb, thrashing, not following commands, striking at staff, trying to climb out of bed	Restlessness	2
Muscle tension	No resistance to passive movements	Relaxed	0
Evaluation by passive flexion and extension of upper extremities	Resistance to passive movements	Tense, rigid	1
	Strong resistance to passive movements, inability to complete them	Very tense or rigid	2
Compliance with the ventilator (intubated patient)	Alarms not activated, easy ventilation	Tolerating ventilator or movement	0
	Alarms stop spontaneously	Coughing but tolerating	1
	Asynchrony: blocking ventilation, alarms frequently activated	Fighting ventilator	2
-OR-			
Vocalization (extubated patient)	Talking in normal tone or no sound	Talking in normal tone or no sound	0
	Sighing, moaning	Sighing, moaning	1
	Crying out, sobbing	Crying out, sobbing	2
Total, range			0–8

NOTE: Subscale scores are summed with a CPOT score ranging from 0 to 8. In one study, CPOT >3 had sensitivity of 67% and specificity of 83% for self-reported pain in conscious ICU patients.[55]

Republished with permission of American Association of Critical-Care Nurses from Gelinas C, Fillion L, Puntillo KA, et al. Validation of the critical-care pain observation tool in adult patients. *Am J Crit Care.* 2006;15(4):420–427; permission conveyed through Copyright Clearance Center, Inc. Copyright © 2006 by the American Association of Critical-Care Nurses.

Observation Tool (CPOT); the Behavioral Pain Scale (BPS); the Behavioral Pain Scale for non-intubated patients (BPS-NI); the Nonverbal Pain Scale (NVPS); the Pain Behavioral Assessment Tool (PBAT); and the Pain Assessment, Intervention, and Notation (PAIN) tool.[49–55] Additionally, the Adaptation to the Intensive Care Environment (ATICE) tool incorporates facial grimacing as one of five components.[78] Following comprehensive testing of psychometric properties and issues of relevance and implementation, the CPOT (Table 114.3) and BPS (Table 114.4) scales were recommended in the 2013 guidelines as the most valid and reliable behavioral pain scales for monitoring pain in adult medical, postoperative, or trauma ICU patients who are unable to self-report and in whom motor function is intact and behaviors are observable.[11] Because these tools all rely on behavioral responses to noxious events, their validity can be influenced by other factors, particularly sedative medications. Specifically, both scores of CPOT and BPS decrease and validity falls with deepening sedation.[50,55] Given the inexact nature of pain evaluation in noncommunicative patients, investigators continue to explore new ways to detect pain including detection of specific muscles during facial movements

like grimacing,[22,79] and various measures of autonomic response to nociceptive stimulation including heart rate variability, pupillary dilatation reflex, and skin conductance.[80,81]

In addition to observable behaviors, pain is often accompanied by readily observed physiologic responses such as tachycardia, hypertension, and tachypnea. However, these changes in vital signs are inconsistently associated with pain, are effected by many confounding factors (such as β-adrenergic antagonists or other medications), and lack specificity for pain with many other common causes including dyspnea, anxiety, and fever.[55] Accordingly, 2013 guidelines recommend against the use of vital signs (or observational pain scales that include vital signs) alone for pain assessment in adult ICU patients.[11] Clinicians should, however, regard unexplained tachycardia, tachypnea, and hypertension as potential clues to the presence of pain, prompting further pain assessment.[11] Other potentially useful approaches include assessing the patient's response to a trial of analgesic medication[41] and use of surrogate (such as family members) report.[2] It should be considered, however, that surrogates may lack reliability and accordingly should not be the sole source for monitoring.[82,83]

Managing Pain and Analgesia in the Intensive Care Unit

The provision of adequate pain control is a core practice for all ICU patients. Ensuring pain relief to patients not only relieves human suffering but additionally mitigates the negative short- and long-term physiologic effects caused by untreated pain. Unfortunately, pain remains inadequately treated in many patients. Some of the barriers to providing adequate pain relief include difficulty with accurate pain assessment, a lack of understanding of dose and dose titration of opioids, presence of adverse effects from opioids, and variations in attitudes toward use of opioids (particularly in patients with an underlying opioid use disorder).[11,12,17,64] Increased education on use of pain assessment tools and a comprehensive understanding of the pharmacokinetic and pharmacodynamic properties of various pain medications may help improve overall outcomes with regard to the treatment of pain in hospitalized patients. Structured approaches and aids such as order sets and guidelines can reduce variability in practice.

TABLE 114.4 The Behavioral Pain Scale (BPS)

Item	Description	Score
Facial expression	Relaxed	1
	Partially tightened (e.g., brow lowering)	2
	Fully tightened (e.g., eyelid closing)	3
	Grimacing	4
Upper limbs	No movement	1
	Partially bent	2
	Fully bent with finger flexion	3
	Permanently retracted	4
Compliance with ventilation	Tolerating movement	1
	Coughing but tolerating ventilation for most of the time	2
	Fighting ventilator	3
	Unable to control ventilation	4

NOTE: Three subscale scores are summed yielding a BPS score ranging from 3 to 12.
Reprinted with permission from Payen JF, Bru O, Bosson JL, et al. Assessing pain in critically ill sedated patients by using a behavioral pain scale. *Crit Care Med.* 2001;29(12):2258–2263.

A considerable challenge during management is balancing adequate pain control against the adverse effects of medications, particularly opioids, in a diverse ICU patient population. Clinicians should consider a multimodal approach to pain control, as some pain may not be responsive to opioid therapy.[84] Proposed opioid-sparing approaches include prioritizing intermittent opioid boluses over continuous infusions when possible, using patient-controlled analgesia when appropriate, and using nonopioid medications when clinically feasible (i.e., low-dose ketamine, α_2 agonists such as clonidine and dexmedetomidine, acetaminophen, NSAIDs, and local treatments such as lidocaine patches).[11,12] Adjuvant nonpharmacologic therapies (i.e., music therapy, relaxation techniques) also play a complementary role and should be considered to help decrease the use of opioids.[11,12,17,85–87] Pharmacologic and other approaches are discussed in detail in the following section, along with approaches to integrate analgesic practices with related care.

PHARMACOLOGIC TREATMENT OF PAIN IN THE INTENSIVE CARE UNIT: PARENTERAL OPIOIDS

The objective of administering opioids in the ICU is to improve patient comfort and outcomes for critically ill patients. The opioid class is considered first-line therapy for ICU patients experiencing nonneuropathic pain.[11,12] This class of medications acts primarily on the μ-opioid receptor to provide analgesia. Opioid receptors are found in the central nervous system within the locus ceruleus, ventral medulla, and substantia gelatinosa of the dorsal horn; they are also found in peripheral tissue of neural and nonneural origin.[66] Most opioids have lipophilic properties and undergo extensive first-pass metabolism, allowing for rapid transference across cell membranes and rapid onset of activity. Important variations in pharmacokinetics and dynamics exist between individual opioids (i.e., drug metabolism, drug interactions, protein binding, lipophilicity, adverse effects) as well as with individual physiologic conditions (i.e., cirrhosis, renal disease, opioid tolerance, older age, genetic polymorphism). These characteristics should be thoughtfully considered when choosing and titrating an opioid medication.[88]

The impact of the adverse effects of opioids on clinical outcomes in the ICU is becoming increasingly recognized.[11,12,17] Examples of adverse effects of opioids include respiratory depression which may delay time to extubation, development of constipation or ileus causing delays to nutrition goals and impairing ventilation and oxygenation, altered mental status including oversedation that can delay progression to liberation from mechanical ventilation, mobility and strength, and the potential for opioid withdrawal or dependence if receiving opioids for a prolonged period of time.

Opioids, like other medications administered for prolonged periods, can manifest protracted durations of effect. Analgesia and sedation can persist for days to weeks after sustained infusions are discontinued, and it is common for patients with hepatic or renal disease to experience oversedation. Evidence-based therapeutic recommendations favor bolus dosing and daily interruption of sedative and analgesic medications except for the dying and those with uncontrolled pain.[11,12]

No specific opioid agent has been demonstrated to be preferable in all ICU patients or across all clinical entities. Selection of initial analgesic therapy should be based on individual patient characteristics and knowledge of prior opiate exposure, experience, and side effects, when available. As is the case for all medications first introduced to the patient in the ICU, it is important to de-escalate opioid doses in a fashion that does not promote withdrawal symptoms but uses the lowest effective dose aiming for transition to nonopioid agents if possible. The devastating impact of the ongoing opioid abuse epidemic certainly provides strong motivation for vigilance in opioid de-escalation.

Fentanyl

Over the last 20 years, fentanyl has supplanted morphine as the most commonly used analgesic in adult ICUs in the United States and is commonly used throughout the world.[89–91] Fentanyl is a potent opioid from the phenylpiperidine class with an onset of action of 1 to 2 minutes and a short duration of action when used in intravenous (IV) bolus form in healthy individuals. It is highly lipophilic and highly protein bound. Fentanyl exhibits a three-compartment distribution model, distributing readily into both muscle and fat tissue. Prolonged IV fentanyl infusions (i.e., >7 days) have led to protracted clearance times and delayed awakening.[92] Fentanyl is devoid of the histamine release seen upon initiation of morphine and therefore is recommended over morphine for patients who are hemodynamically unstable. Clinicians should still use caution in hypotensive patients; however, as studies have demonstrated hypotension associated with fentanyl use, particularly when fentanyl is given in conjunction with other sedatives or when given rapidly in an IV bolus form.[93]

Fentanyl undergoes hepatic metabolism via the cytochrome P450 3A4 isoenzyme, and potential for drug interactions is high causing either inhibition or induction of fentanyl clearance. Fentanyl has a high hepatic extraction ratio; therefore, clearance will be more affected by blood flow through the liver than by intrinsic liver function.[65] Accumulation of the parent drug can occur in patients with cirrhosis, and monitoring for oversedation is recommended.[65] The presence of chest wall rigidity has been described frequently with fentanyl in the pediatric population; it has been reported as a rare but significant adverse effect in adults.[88]

Synthetic opioids from the phenylpiperidine and diphenylheptane classes (i.e., fentanyl, methadone, meperidine, remifentanil, tramadol) exhibit a dose-related increase in norepinephrine release from sympathetic nerve endings and inhibition of neuronal uptake of norepinephrine. These opioids also block reuptake of serotonin and have serotonin receptor agonist activity. This increase in central norepinephrine and serotonin levels can thereby predispose a patient to dangerous reactions if these opioids are administered with serotonergic agents (i.e., antidepressants) or monoamine oxidase inhibitors (i.e., linezolid).[92,94–98] Reactions include serious autonomic and neurologic changes, such as hypertension, tachyarrhythmias, severe hyperpyrexia, spontaneous or inducible clonus, and coma; death has been reported in severe cases. In cases of drug overdose from a serotonergic agent or monoamine oxidase inhibitor, or if there are concerns for serotonin syndrome, certain opioids including fentanyl should be avoided.[99]

These drug interactions need careful consideration if a patient requires an opioid for acute pain control, along with reinitiation of the outpatient antidepressant to avoid withdrawal. Therapeutic options may include starting a lower dose of the serotonergic antidepressant, although this may not prevent withdrawal from the antidepressant, or choosing an alternative to fentanyl (i.e., hydromorphone, morphine, nonopioids). The combination of a monoamine oxidase inhibitor with fentanyl or tramadol should be avoided altogether due to a high risk and severity of adverse events.

Critical care guidelines recommend the choice of opioid be based on specific drug and individual patient characteristics.[11,12] Despite the aforementioned concerns with variable kinetics and drug interactions in a critical care patient, fentanyl has become the most commonly used opioid in adult ICUs, likely due to its quick onset of action, lack of active metabolites, and guideline recommendation over morphine for the hemodynamically unstable patient.[11] Clinicians should familiarize themselves with the pharmacokinetics and dynamics of fentanyl, as it continues to be highly utilized in adult ICUs.

Hydromorphone

Most studies reporting use of IV hydromorphone infusions in the acute adult ICU setting are retrospective or observational in nature. Short- and long-term effects of hydromorphone infusions have not been well described in the adult ICU literature. Although fentanyl is generally the recommended opioid of choice in the acute adult ICU setting, clinicians may opt to use hydromorphone over fentanyl for various clinical scenarios including prior chronic outpatient use of hydromorphone, tachyphylaxis to fentanyl, better pain control with hydromorphone over fentanyl, and the need to administer a serotonergic agent or a monoamine oxidase inhibitor concomitantly.

When administered IV, hydromorphone has an onset of activity of 5 to 10 minutes and a duration of activity of 3 to 4 hours. Hydromorphone is only 10% to 20% protein bound (because it undergoes phase 2 hepatic glucuronidation), has less potential for metabolically based drug interactions, and has more reliable clearance in hepatic failure. Glucuronidation of hydromorphone produces the metabolite hydromorphone-3-glucuronide (H3G). The H3G metabolite is devoid of analgesic activity; however, it maintains neurotoxic effects such as cognitive dysfunction, agitation, confusion, hallucinations, tremors, clonus, and seizures.[100–102] As glomerular filtration rate (GFR) declines, H3G accumulates up to fourfold the initial concentration. Occurrence of neurologic toxicities was seen in approximately 20% of patients with GFR <60 mL per minute in a study of palliative care patients with chronic renal insufficiency.[28] Starting doses of hydromorphone should be adjusted for renal dysfunction, and patients should be closely monitored for signs of neurotoxicity if receiving high doses or continuous infusions of hydromorphone in the presence of renal failure. Hemodialysis clears hydromorphone; however, close monitoring of neurotoxic effects should still be observed for patients on dialysis.

Morphine

Morphine has historically been the opioid of choice for acute pain and is still commonly used in adults ICU patients around the world.[103] Morphine is a low-cost medication with effective analgesic and euphoric effects, making it an attractive alternative in many acute clinical scenarios. Critical care guidelines recommend morphine as an acceptable first-line agent for pain in the ICU but advise that morphine may cause hypotension due to systemic release of histamine.[11] Both animal and human studies have demonstrated significant histamine and nitric oxide release with morphine, with subsequent decreases in systemic vascular resistance, bronchospasm, and urticaria.[104]

Morphine is metabolized in the liver to morphine-3-glucuronide (M3G) and morphine-6-glucuronide (M6G), both of which are subsequently cleared by the kidneys. Similar to the hydromorphone metabolite H3G, M3G does not have analgesic activity but can cause severe neurotoxic symptoms such as cognitive dysfunction, tremors, and seizure activity.[105] However, the M6G metabolite is 2 to 8 times more potent than morphine as an analgesic.[106,107] These metabolites can exhibit prolonged effects in patients with renal dysfunction and in patients receiving dialysis; therefore, scheduled dosing and continuous infusions are not recommended in those settings.[105] In critically ill patients, the altered protein binding resulting from malignancy, renal impairment, and hepatic failure may also alter morphine pharmacokinetics and make dosing titration challenging.[100]

Remifentanil

Remifentanil is a selective μ-opioid receptor agonist approved for use in anesthesia induction and maintenance that may have advantageous properties for ICU care. The novelty in this agent, in contrast to fentanyl, is that remifentanil is metabolized by multiple ubiquitous esterases, and its half-life is not known to be prolonged by critical illness nor organ dysfunction.[108,109] Due to its pharmacokinetic properties, this agent has a terminal half-life of less than 30 minutes and may reduce the incidence of prolonged sedative complications seen with continuous infusions of other opiates. Short-duration studies demonstrate reduced duration of mechanical ventilation when this agent is compared to other opiates.[110–112] Remifentanil can cause bradycardia and hypotension, potentially limiting its use in the ICU. It has been used in traumatic brain injury and neurosurgical settings with favorable effects on neurologic function assessment and a dose-dependent reduction in coughing associated with endotracheal suctioning. Concern remains, however, that the rapid offset of this agent may lead to withdrawal and agitated behavior.[113–115] In one study, remifentanil was associated with a higher rate of moderate or rebound pain upon cessation of a 72-hour infusion compared to fentanyl (33% vs. 9%).[73] There was no difference in mean extubation time in this short-term study.[73] Other published reports suggest remifentanil may be associated with more rapid recovery from respiratory failure. In one randomized controlled trial (RCT), patient who received remifentanil had shorter duration of mechanical ventilation (3.9 vs. 5.1 days).[74] In a 2017 meta-analysis of 23 RCTs of adult mechanically ventilated ICU patients, remifentanil was associated with shorter duration of mechanical ventilation, shorter time to extubation after sedation cessation, and shorter ICU length of stay (LOS).[116]

PHARMACOLOGIC TREATMENT OF PAIN IN THE INTENSIVE CARE UNIT: ADJUVANT THERAPY

Ketamine

Ketamine has been used for decades in bolus IV form for procedural sedation and analgesia, rapid sequence intubation, and brief operating room (OR) cases.[117] It is a well-established anesthetic agent and produces a qualitatively unique state referred to as "dissociative anesthesia." This dissociative anesthesia has been described as having a spectrum of effects, including hypnosis at lower doses, deep sedation and coma with higher doses, potent antinociceptive effects, increased sympathetic tone, and intact respiratory and airway tone. Added benefits include maintenance of normal gastrointestinal motility and less respiratory depression compared to opioids. At the bedside, these clinical effects could prove beneficial for unstable ICU patients and has prompted increased interest in sustained infusion ketamine in the ICU setting.[118]

Ketamine provides these effects via multiple mechanisms including blockade of the N-methyl-D-aspartate (NMDA) channels, neuronal hyperpolarization, δ- and μ-opioid agonism and opioid potentiation, effects on the nitric oxide guanosine monophosphate system, reduction in cholinergic modulation, and central release of dopamine and noradrenaline.[119] Ketamine has a large volume of distribution due to its lipophilic properties but is not highly protein bound. It has a quick onset of action (<5 minutes) and a short duration of activity in bolus form (5 to 15 minutes depending on dose). Hepatic and renal dysfunction can cause accumulation and prolong ketamine's duration of activity.

Emergence from the dissociative effect of ketamine can illicit reactions such as hallucinations, agitation, confusion, and delirium. This emergence reaction may be mitigated by giving a benzodiazepine prior to ketamine boluses or upon discontinuation of continuous ketamine infusions. Because ketamine is a sympathomimetic producing increased levels of circulating dopamine and norepinephrine, ketamine should be avoided in patients with concomitant cardiovascular disease or myocardial infarction. Ketamine may also increase pulmonary vascular pressures and therefore should be used with caution or avoided in this patient population.

Reports of prolonged ketamine use (>24 hours) in the ICU are limited to a few small studies.[117,118] The optimal dose, duration, monitoring parameters, and how ketamine fits into the armamentarium of medications used for analgesia and sedation in the adult ICU remain unclear. Reported ketamine doses described for use in the ICU vary but generally range from 0.05 mg/kg/hour to 0.4 mg/kg/hour, with a maximum of 1.2 mg/kg/hour when used for severe pain.[11,118] Potential benefits of ketamine include additional pain control (opioid sparing), reduced airway resistance, increased lung compliance, minimal effect on respiratory drive at low to moderate doses, and intact gastrointestinal motility.

Methadone

Methadone is a unique analgesic with multiple mechanisms of action which contribute to its antinociceptive effects. These mechanisms are centrally mediated through agonism at the μ-opioid receptor, antagonism at the NMDA receptor, and inhibition of serotonin and norepinephrine reuptake.[120] The primary indications for use of methadone include chronic pain and prevention of opioid withdrawal. Using methadone for acute pain is challenging secondary to the need for slow and gradual uptitration every 2 to 3 days. More frequent titration can lead to higher than expected drug levels with respiratory depression and oversedation as the drug gradually reaches steady state.

Methadone is highly lipophilic leading to its relatively quick onset of action, a "drug-depot" effect throughout the tissues, and an extended half-life. Methadone is highly bound to plasma proteins, in particular to α_1-acid glycoprotein. The dosage forms for methadone include oral tablets, suspension, and an IV formulation. The potency of the IV dose is approximately twice that of the oral dose. There are multiple considerations when using methadone in a complex ICU setting. Methadone undergoes hepatic clearance; therefore, accumulation can occur in acute or chronic liver dysfunction and lower doses should be used. It is a major substrate of enzymes CYP 3A4 and 2B6 and a minor substrate of CYP 2D6, 2C9, and 2C19; thus, medication profiles should be closely scrutinized for multiple drug interactions. Concern for QTc prolongation exists for methadone, which can be problematic in an ICU setting where other risk factors for QTc prolongation are often present (multiple medications which prolong QTc, electrolyte abnormalities, underlying cardiac disease). Common medications which will increase methadone levels, thereby increasing risk for QTc prolongation and serotonin syndrome, include azoles, macrolides, antipsychotics, and antidepressants. The U.S. Food and Drug Administration (FDA) has issued a boxed warning for the use of methadone with benzodiazepines, as this combination has resulted in significant respiratory depression, profound sedation, coma, and death. If using methadone in the ICU, an electrocardiogram should be routinely monitored and electrolytes such as potassium, magnesium, and calcium be maintained within the normal range.[120–122] Patients admitted to ICU from home while receiving chronic methadone treatment and patients in opioid withdrawal may necessitate initiation of methadone in the hospital or ICU—but with significant caution.

Other Analgesics and Adjuvant Agents

Other agents may have a role in the ICU, but many possess properties that limit their utility in critical care settings. Meperidine is associated with neuroexcitation due to a metabolite, normeperidine potentially producing seizures, and thus is rarely used in the ICU setting.[11,12] It has been used in the short term for shivering associated with general anesthesia or to abate drug-induced rigors. Meperidine should not be given for more than 1 day or at a cumulative dose over 600 mg. Codeine is converted to morphine in order to be active, but a proportion of the population lack the necessary enzymatic mechanism.

Oxycodone is pharmacologically similar to morphine but is only available in oral preparations. Oxycodone, along with hydrocodone, have been associated with a high abuse potential in the United States.[123] Consideration for the patient's medical and social history (i.e., history of opioid abuse) should be taken into account upon initiation of these medications.

Ketorolac is an IV nonsteroidal anti-inflammatory medication that may be useful for anti-inflammatory effects but produces gastrointestinal toxicity and increases the risk for gastrointestinal bleeding that limits its use to less than 5 days at a time or not at all in ICU patients already at risk for bleeding. Corticosteroids and adenosine may have opiate-sparing effects as adjuvant therapy but have not been evaluated in the ICU. Lidocaine has also been used as an effective adjuvant for complex or neuropathic syndromes but may be limited in the ICU due to its arrhythmogenic properties.[124] Acetaminophen is a weak analgesic that carries the risk of hepatotoxicity with chronic use that similarly restricts its utility in the ICU.

Clonidine is an α_2-receptor agonist that provides mild sedation and mild analgesia but is an antihypertensive and can cause hypotension. Its cousin, dexmedetomidine, is a selective α_2-receptor agonist with sedative properties similar to benzodiazepines and propofol but, in contrast to other sedatives, has analgesic properties and can be opioid sparing, is sympatholytic potentially producing prominent bradycardia as well as hypotension at higher doses, is associated with a more alert state relative to anxiolytic properties, and has minimal effect on respiratory drive.[125,126] It does not bind γ-aminobutyric acid (GABA) receptors. In a meta-analysis of 24 RCTs comparing dexmedetomidine to alternative sedative drugs, ICU LOS was shorter with dexmedetomidine, whereas duration of mechanical ventilation was not significantly different.[127] Clinical trial results suggest that when compared directly to midazolam, dexmedetomidine may be associated with lower prevalence of delirium.[128]

Anticonvulsants (i.e., gabapentin, carbamazepine) are recommended in guidelines in combination with opioids for confirmed neuropathic pain.[11] However, anticonvulsants have not been studied extensively in the ICU population, and there is a potential for significant adverse effects and drug interactions, requiring close monitoring and follow-up. If the patient is discharged home on an anticonvulsant for neuropathic pain, close follow-up should be performed by the outpatient provider.

NONPHARMACOLOGIC MANAGEMENT OF PAIN IN THE INTENSIVE CARE UNIT

Nonpharmacologic modalities are incompletely studied and infrequently used in the ICU but have the potential to improve pain management.[11,12] Complementary therapies include distraction therapies, behavioral modification, touch therapy, meditation, music therapy, acupuncture or acupressure, and massage, among others. Simply providing information can be beneficial. These approaches are generally safe, easy to provide, and inexpensive; however, evidence of benefit sufficient to justify routine use is weak, and their true impact on pain should not be overestimated.[85–87]

REGIONAL ANESTHETIC APPROACHES TO PAIN IN THE INTENSIVE CARE UNIT

Regional anesthesia and analgesia (RAA) includes continuous epidural analgesia and/or anesthesia (central neuraxial techniques) and continuous peripheral nerve or plexus block. These techniques are reviewed in detail in Chapter 52 and will only be commented on briefly here. RAA techniques provide medication delivery in close proximity to the spinal cord or nerves and thus can result in parenteral opioid sparing, which is associated with less respiratory depression and gastrointestinal hypomotility, and other benefits. These techniques do, however, introduce new issues related to needle and catheter placement and maintenance as well as physiologic derangements related to local anesthetic block and epidural drug administration. Critically ill patients are probably at higher risk for RAA-related complications due to a higher incidence of coagulopathy, thrombocytopenia, sepsis, and hemodynamic instability.

Utilization of RAA techniques in the ICU setting is largely limited to surgical patients who are postoperative or injured. The availability of and success with these techniques is probably closely tied to cumulative experience and expertise of local experts. Peripheral nerve blocks can be useful for anatomically localized pain such as limb injury or operation, but there are few RCTs in ICU patients on which to base recommendations. The largest body of evidence is related to epidural techniques but even that is quite limited. Recommendations regarding RAA published in the 2013 SCCM guidelines were limited by availability of high-level data for ICU patients, but recommendations were provided in several specific scenarios.[11] Thoracic epidural anesthesia and analgesia for postoperative analgesia in patients with abdominal aortic surgery received a strong recommendation as superior to IV opioids.[129] High-level evidence was also available to compare lumbar epidural analgesia to IV opioids in the same population but no benefit was demonstrated, and RAA was not recommended.[130] ICU patients with traumatic rib fractures had superior pain and fewer cases of pneumonia when treated with thoracic epidural analgesia than IV opioids but experienced more hypotension, and this form of RAA was endorsed with a weak recommendation for managing pain from traumatic rib fractures.[131,132] There was insufficient evidence to support RAA in any other ICU clinical setting including after thoracic operations and nonvascular abdominal operations and for medical ICU patients.[11]

Integrated Analgesia Management in the Intensive Care Unit

Pain management and analgesia is a central theme in the comprehensive care of the critically ill patient. The key concepts supported by published evidence and recommended by experts (see Table 114.2) form the framework of integrated analgesia management. First, pain should be routinely monitored in all adult ICU patients, using behavioral pain scales in those who are unable to self-report. Second, preemptive analgesia should be used prior to procedures because it is more effective to prevent pain than to control it once it has developed. Third, analgesia-first sedation (analgosedation) should be used in mechanically ventilated adult ICU patients. Fourth, IV opioids are first-line therapy for nonneuropathic pain, but consider nonopioids analgesics to reduce opioid dosage and side effects, and treat neuropathic pain with gabapentin or carbamazepine.[11]

The following sections will provide additional detail about using combination therapy with opioid analgesics and sedative-hypnotic agents with emphasis on analgesia-first sedation (analgosedation), followed by discussion of the role of analgesia in comprehensive care that integrates management of analgesia, sedation, delirium mitigation, liberation from mechanical ventilation, and mobility and rehabilitation.

ANALGOSEDATION IN THE INTENSIVE CARE UNIT

Analgesic and sedative drug therapy of critically ill, mechanically ventilated patients should focus on careful selection and titration of drugs to achieve optimal patient comfort while avoiding the adverse impact of excessive or unnecessarily prolonged sedation. The use of structured approaches to sedation and analgesia via algorithms and protocols has achieved a prominent place in ICU practice. There are several common themes. One theme is to focus first on analgesia, as discussed earlier.

The 2013 guidelines suggest that analgesia-first sedation be used in mechanically ventilated adult ICU patients.[11] Asking first about pain, before the patient has been sedated and cognitively impaired, is advantageous. Additionally, several RCTs have demonstrated analgesia-based sedation to be associated with shorter duration of mechanical ventilation in comparison to hypnotic-based sedation.[74,109,133] Strom et al.[69] randomized mechanically ventilated adult ICU patients to bolus morphine (analgesia-based, limited sedation) versus morphine plus propofol for the first 48 hours and then midazolam (sedation + analgesia) and found shorter duration of mechanical ventilation and ICU LOS but threefold more agitation when sedative drugs were minimized.

A second major theme is to tailor the sedation to the specific patient, including medication selection based on sedation goals (such as rapid arousal), avoidance of side effects (such as hypotension), and consideration of elimination issues (such as avoiding midazolam in a patient with impaired renal function). In addition to the opioid analgesic medications discussed previously, a variety of sedative drugs have a role in ICU sedation management. However, there is emerging evidence appears to favor using propofol or dexmedetomidine in preference to benzodiazepines in patients for whom continuous infusion sedation is needed.[11] A meta-analysis limited to moderate- or high-quality RCTs demonstrated slightly longer ICU LOS with benzodiazepines in comparison to propofol or dexmedetomidine.[127] Several studies deserve additional comment. A multicenter RCT comparing dexmedetomidine to midazolam demonstrated that dexmedetomidine was associated with shorter time to extubation, lower prevalence of delirium, and fewer infections but no difference in ICU LOS, mortality, or sedation quality.[128] In the two phase-3 multicenter RCTs that compared dexmedetomidine to midazolam, or propofol, patients randomized to dexmedetomidine had shorter duration of mechanical ventilation than with midazolam but not with propofol.[134] Patient interaction (communication, arousability, cooperation) was better with dexmedetomidine than with either other agent, but hypotension and bradycardia were more common. Dexmedetomidine may offer advantages for managing agitation or hyperactive delirium, particularly that related to alcohol withdrawal.[135–138] Propofol, the most widely used sedative agent in the United States,[89] binds GABA and other receptors and produces sedative-hypnotic effects similar to benzodiazepines but no analgesic effects. It has rapid onset and offset of action but has the disadvantages of producing hypotension and depressed respiratory drive.[139] Compared to benzodiazepines, propofol is associated with shorter duration of mechanical ventilation and shorter ICU LOS.[140]

Another theme is to strive for a light level of consciousness and to avoid accumulation of medications and their active metabolites, thus reducing the likelihood of delayed awakening. This approach is strongly recommended in the 2013 guidelines[11] based in part on studies like those of Strom et al.[69] The underlying rationale for this approach arises from the observation that continuous IV sedation and analgesia is associated with delayed recovery from respiratory failure and longer LOS.[141] Although a variety of sedation management strategies have been demonstrated to shorten the duration of mechanical ventilation, the most robust data supports the use of a sedation protocol or the implementation of daily interruption of sedation. Strategies that successfully promote a more alert state have been associated with less medication use and accompanying costs, less delirium, fewer tests for altered mental status, shorter duration of mechanical ventilation, fewer tracheostomies, and shorter time in the ICU and hospital.[11,69,70,142–155] Abrupt withdrawal of sedative (and sometimes analgesic) medications is accompanied by several-fold increases in circulating catecholamines as well as tachycardia and hypertension, but no evidence of triggering cardiac ischemia.[156] Daily interruption of sedation is also not followed by psychological complications like posttraumatic stress disorder.[157] Patients who should probably not undergo daily interruption of sedation includes those with active seizures, alcohol withdrawal, worsening agitation, neuromuscular blockade, acute myocardial ischemia, or elevated intracranial pressure.[158]

ANALGESIA AS A COMPONENT OF COMPREHENSIVE BUNDLED INTENSIVE CARE UNIT CARE

Over the past decade, multiple RCTs have demonstrated the value of linking strategies for managing analgesia and sedation in ICU patients with related components of patient care including weaning and liberation from mechanical ventilation, reducing the prevalence and duration of ICU delirium, and promoting mobility and early rehabilitation. The improved outcomes associated with linking interruption of sedation (or spontaneous awakening trial [SAT]) with testing of the potential for ventilator liberation (spontaneous breathing trial [SBT]),[158] so called "wake up and breathe,"[159] illustrated the value of such an approach. Addition of early mobility and exercise to SAT and SBT has further improved outcomes including less delirium and more rapid recovery.[160] Research and experience has shown that when incorporating these components collectively as a "bundle," the patient has better outcomes, including decreased ventilator days, decreased incidence of delirium, and shortened hospital LOS.[34–40] A crucial aspect of improving patient care revolves around successfully disseminating and implementing the results of compelling research findings through knowledge translation.

The ABCDEF approach (http://www.iculiberation.org) provides an effective framework for patient-centered integrated care, with the components depicted in Table 114.5.[34,35] It is no surprise that a critical part of the ABCDEF bundle is "A," which stands for assessing, preventing, and treating pain. The ABCDEF bundle also incorporate other components that are relevant to the treatment of pain, such as "C" (choice of sedating agent), not only focusing on analgosedation, to ensure pain is controlled, but also recognizing the potential need for short-acting sedatives as adjunctive agents to provide sedation, assisting in minimizing potential adverse side effects of opiate-only sedation. In addition, the importance of daily delirium screening ("D" in the ABCDEF bundles), which may be directly related to sedation choice, is emphasized in the ABCDEF bundles. Furthermore, the many benefits of early mobilization ("E" in the ABCDEF bundles) are also a treatment and pain preventative tool in itself for ICU-related pain, as the pain associated with immobility is a debilitating phenomenon that is often underrecognized. Collectively, one could argue that all the components of the ABCDEF bundle are either directly or indirectly intertwined and interrelated to pain in the ICU, including the direct assessment and anticipation of pain, the pain associated with endotracheal tubes that may be able to be removed sooner with daily awakening and breathing trials, or the pain that accompanies immobility. Therefore, it is imperative that a multimodal, interdisciplinary group become familiar with these guidelines and implementation tools that collectively represent best practice in intensive care medicine.

TABLE 114.5 The ABCDEF Bundle

Each letter of the ABCDEF bundle represents patient-centered, best practice in critical care:
A: assessing, preventing, and managing pain
B: both spontaneous awakening and breathing trials
C: choice of analgesia and sedation
D: assessing, preventing, and managing delirium
E: early mobility and exercise
F: family engagement and empowerment

Pain and Analgesia at the End of Life in the Intensive Care Unit

Unfortunately, critically ill patients die in the ICU, and in some instances, the realization that the end of life is imminent occurs when the patient is receiving life-sustaining interventions such as vasopressors, mechanical ventilation, dialysis, and other life-support devices. The presence of pain, dyspnea, and other unpleasant sensations is not uncommon in the end-of-life setting, particularly with existing invasive ICU interventions, and achieving relief from distress becomes of paramount importance. The principles for pain management at the end of life are discussed in detail in Chapter 109.

In many such cases, the patient has ongoing analgesic and sedative therapy that can be titrated to achieve goals of relieve of pain and suffering without concerns for hemodynamic or respiratory consequences. Providers should administer pain medications and other palliative therapies for the dying patient in the ICU, even if the possibility exists that such treatment could possibly hasten death.[161–163] A doctrine of "double effect" supports adequate and aggressive palliation of pain to be differentiated from active hastening of death and ethically justifiable, as long as the provider's primary intent is mitigating suffering.[164–167]

It is imperative that a patient in the ICU die with dignity and that an individualized treatment plan be used at the end of life.[161–163,166,167] This involves use of preemptive medications aimed at treating pain, dyspnea, anxiety, delirium, and any other symptoms that may be distressing to the patient. It is important that ICU clinicians discuss with family members or other individuals present what to expect during the dying process and continue to provide support to the patient and their family.[166] Some practical recommendations for managing end-of-life issues in the ICU are noted in Table 114.6.

TABLE 114.6 End-of-Life Care and Pain Management in the Dying Intensive Care Unit Patient

- Clarify and document the goals of care.
- Notify interested individuals (surgeon, oncologist, specialty nurse, outpatient physician, or nurse).
- Emphasize to family that care continues but with new goals (i.e., care is not being "withdrawn" but rather is focused on dignity and comfort).
- Discontinue interventions and treatments that do not contribute to comfort (phlebotomy, imaging, remove nonessential devices, silence alarms).
- Provide sufficient analgesia, generally with systemic opioids (assure reliable intravenous access, take into account recent and/or chronic opioid use, avoid arbitrary maximum analgesic dosing, begin with a bolus of drug if planning to remove devices, including the endotracheal tube, that raise the possibility of discomfort).
- Educate and reassure family and staff that the purpose of opioids is to relieve and prevent suffering, not to hasten death.
- Consider removing the endotracheal tube because this can generally be done with no discomfort as long as adequately premedicated.
- Reassess regularly whether the goals of care (comfort) are being met and titrate pharmacologic agents and interventions (clinically examine for signs of discomfort), determine whether vital signs respond to interventions, and solicit family input: Do you feel your loved one is comfortable?
- Invite pastoral care, palliative care, or pain management specialists to participate, when appropriate.
- Consider transfer out of the intensive care unit, particularly to a palliative care unit, for continued comfort care.

Conclusions

Managing pain and providing effective analgesia are critical component of comprehensive care of our ICU patients. Although the core principles of pain management in general certainly apply in the ICU setting, the unique issues related to complex acute and chronic medical illness, organ dysfunction, communication difficulties, and integration with sedative therapy and life support provide sound rationale for utilizing a multiprofessional and patient-centered approach.

ACKNOWLEDGMENTS

The authors are grateful to Richard Mularski, MD, and Gregory Schmidt, MD, who are coauthors of the chapter "Pain Management in the Intensive Care Unit" published in the fourth edition of *Bonica's Management of Pain* in 2009. Their work paved the way for this updated chapter on pain management in the ICU in the fifth edition of *Bonica's Management of Pain*.

References

1. Puntillo KA, Arai S, Cohen NH, et al. Symptoms experienced by intensive care unit patients at high risk of dying. *Crit Care Med* 2010;38: 2155–2160.
2. Desbiens NA, Wu AW, Broste SK, et al. Pain and satisfaction with pain control in seriously ill hospitalized adults: findings from the SUPPORT research investigations. *Criti Care Med* 1996;24(12):1953–1961.
3. Novaes MA, Knobel E, Bork AM, et al. Stressors in ICU: perception of the patient, relatives and health care team. *Intensive Care Med* 1999;25(12): 1421–1426.
4. Turner JS, Briggs SJ, Springhorn HE, et al. Patients' recollection of intensive care unit experience. *Crit Care Med* 1990;18(9):966–968.
5. Puntillo KA. Dimensions of procedural pain and its analgesic management in critically ill surgical patients. *Am J Crit Care* 1994;3(2):116–122.
6. Nelson JE, Meier DE, Oei EJ, et al. Self-reported symptom experience of critically ill cancer patients receiving intensive care. *Crit Care Med* 2001;29(2):277–282.
7. Nelson JE, Meier DE, Litke A, et al. The symptom burden of chronic critical illness. *Crit Care Med* 2004;32(7):1527–1534.
8. Morrison RS, Ahronheim JC, Morrison GR, et al. Pain and discomfort associated with common hospital procedures and experiences. *J Pain Symptom Manage* 1998;15(2):91–101.
9. Puntillo KA, Morris AB, Thompson CL, et al. Pain behaviors observed during six common procedures: results from Thunder Project II. *Crit Care Med* 2004;32(2):421–427.
10. Stanik-Hutt JA, Soeken KL, Belcher AE, et al. Pain experiences of traumatically injured patients in a critical care setting. *Am J Crit Care* 2001;10(4):252–259.
11. Barr J, Fraser GL, Puntillo K, et al. Clinical practice guidelines for the management of pain, agitation, and delirium in adult patients in the intensive care unit. *Crit Care Med* 2013;41(1):263–306.
12. Erstad BL, Puntillo K, Gilbert HC, et al. Pain management principles in the critically ill. *Chest* 2009;135(4):1075–1086.
13. Mularski RA. Pain management in the intensive care unit. *Crit Care Clin* 2004;20(3):381–401.
14. Mularski RA, Sessler CN, Schmidt GA. Pain management in the intensive care unit. In: Rathmell J, Ballantye J, Fishman S, eds. *Bonica's Management of Pain*. 4th ed. Philadelphia: Lippincott Williams & Wilkins; 2009:1587–1602.
15. Sessler CN. Comfort and distress in the ICU: scope of the problem. *Sem Respir Crit Care Med* 2001;22(2):111–113.
16. Sessler CN. Progress toward eliminating inadequately managed pain in the ICU through interdisciplinary care. *Chest* 2009;135(4):894–896.
17. Vincent J, Shhabi Y, Walsh TS, et al. Comfort and patient-centred care without excessive sedation: the eCASH concept. *Intensive Care Med* 2016;42:962–971.
18. Caswell DR, Williams JP, Vallejo M, et al. Improving pain management in critical care. *Jt Comm J Qual Improv* 1996;22(10):702–712.
19. Patel SB, Kress JP. Sedation and analgesia in the mechanically ventilated patient. *Am J Respir Crit Care Med* 2012;185(5):486–497.
20. Reade MC, Finfer S. Sedation and delirium in the intensive care unit. *N Engl J Med* 2014;370:444–454.
21. Puntillo KA, Wild LR, Morris AB, et al. Practices and predictors of analgesic interventions for adults undergoing painful procedures. *Am J Crit Care* 2002;11(5):415–429.
22. Rahu MA, Grap MJ, Cohn JF, et al. Facial expression as an indicator of pain in critically ill intubated adults during endotracheal suctioning. *Am J Crit Care* 2013;22(5):412–422.
23. Darbyshire JL, Young JD. An investigation of sound levels on intensive care units with reference to the WHO guidelines. *Crit Care* 2013;17:R187.
24. Li SY, Wang TJ, Vivienne Wu SF, et al. Efficacy of controlling night-time noise and activities to improve patients' sleep quality in a surgical intensive care unit. *J Clin Nurs* 2011;20(3–4):396–407.
25. Xie H, Kang J, Mills GH. Clinical review: the impact of noise on patients' sleep and the effectiveness of noise reduction strategies in intensive care units. *Crit Care* 2009;13(2):208.
26. van de Leur JP, van der Schans CP, Loef BG, et al. Discomfort and factual recollection in intensive care unit patients. *Crit Care* 2004;8(6):R467–R473.
27. Litton E, Carnegie V, Elliott R, et al. The efficacy of earplugs as a sleep hygiene strategy for reducing delirium in the ICU: a systematic review and meta-analysis. *Crit Care Med* 2016;44:992–999.
28. McAndrew NS, Leske J, Guttormson J, et al. Quiet time for mechanically ventilated patients in the medical intensive care unit. *West J Nurs Res* 2016;38(10):1374–1375.
29. Ely EW, Shintani A, Truman B, et al. Delirium as a predictor of mortality in mechanically ventilated patients in the intensive care unit. *JAMA* 2004;291(14):1753–1762.
30. Girard TD, Jackson JC, Pandharipande PP, et al. Delirium as a predictor of long-term cognitive impairment in survivors of critical illness. *Crit Care Med* 2010;38(7):1513–1520.
31. Gunther ML, Morandi A, Ely EW. Pathophysiology of delirium in the intensive care unit. *Crit Care Clin* 2008;24(1):45–65.
32. Bledowski J, Trutia A. A review of pharmacologic management and prevention strategies for delirium in the intensive care unit. *Psychosomatics* 2012;53(3):203–211.
33. Pandharipande PP, Girard TD, Jackson JC, et al. Long-term cognitive impairment after critical illness. *N Engl J Med* 2013;369(14):1306–1316.
34. Morandi A, Brummel NE, Ely EW. Sedation, delirium and mechanical ventilation: the 'ABCDE' approach. *Curr Opin Crit Care* 2011;17(1):43–49.
35. Ely EW. The ABCDEF bundle: science and philosophy of how ICU liberation serves patients and families. *Crit Care Med* 2017;45:321–330.
36. Louzon P, Jennings H, Ali M, et al. Impact of pharmacist management of pain, agitation, and delirium in the intensive care unit through participation in multidisciplinary bundle rounds. *Am J Health Syst Pharm* 2017;74:253–262.
37. CHECKLIST-ICU Investigators. Effect of a quality improvement intervention with daily round checklists, goal setting, and clinician prompting on mortality of critically ill patients. A randomized clinical trial. *JAMA* 2016;315(14):1480–1490.
38. Dale CR, Bryson CL, Fan VS, et al. A greater analgesia, sedation, delirium order set quality score is associated with a decreased duration of mechanical ventilation in cardiovascular surgery patients. *Crit Care Med* 2013;41:2610–2617.
39. Walsh TS, Kydonaki K, Lee RJ, et al. Development of process control methodology for tracking the quality and safety of pain, agitation, and sedation management in critical care units. *Crit Care Med* 2016;44(3):564–574.
40. Walsh TS, Kydonaki K, Antonelli J, et al. Staff education, regular sedation and analgesia quality feedback, and a sedation monitoring technology for improving sedation and analgesia quality for critically ill, mechanically ventilated patients: a cluster randomized trial. *Lancet Respir Med* 2016;4: 807–817.
41. Puntillo K, Pasero C, Li D, et al. Evaluation of pain in ICU patients. *Chest* 2009;135(4):1069–1074.
42. Jensen MP, Karoly P, Braver S. The measurement of clinical pain intensity: a comparison of six methods. *Pain* 1986;27(1):117–126.
43. Chanques G, Viel E, Constantin JM, et al. The measurement of pain in intensive care unit: comparison of 5 self-report intensity scales. *Pain* 2010;151(3):711–721.
44. Payen JF, Bosson JL, Chanques G, et al. Pain assessment is associated with decreased duration of mechanical ventilation in the intensive care unit: a post hoc analysis of the DOLOREA study. *Anesthesiology* 2009;111(6): 1308–1316.
45. Puntillo KA, Miaskowski C, Kehrle K, et al. Relationship between behavioral and physiological indicators of pain, critical care patients' self-reports of pain, and opioid administration. *Crit Care Med* 1997;25(7):1159–1166.
46. Herr K, Coyne PJ, Key T, et al. Pain assessment in the nonverbal patient: position statement with clinical practice recommendations. *Pain Manag Nurs* 2006;7(2):44–52.
47. Li D, Puntillo K, Miaskowski C. A review of objective pain measures for use with critical care adult patients unable to self-report. *J Pain* 2008;9(1):2–10.
48. Sessler CN, Grap MJ, Ramsay MA. Evaluating and monitoring analgesia and sedation in the intensive care unit. *Crit Care* 2008;12(suppl 3):S2.
49. Gelinas C, Fillion L, Puntillo KA, et al. Validation of the critical-care pain observation tool in adult patients. *Am J Crit Care* 2006;15(4):420–427.
50. Payen JF, Bru O, Bosson JL, et al. Assessing pain in critically ill sedated patients by using a behavioral pain scale. *Crit Care Med* 2001;29(12): 2258–2263.
51. Chanques G, Payen JF, Mercier G, et al. Assessing pain in non-intubated critically ill patients unable to self report: an adaptation of the Behavioral Pain Scale. *Intensive Care Med* 2009;35(12):2060–2067.
52. Odhner M, Wegman D, Freeland N, et al. Assessing pain control in nonverbal critically ill adults. *Dimens Crit Care Nurs* 2003;22(6):260–267.
53. Li D, Miaskowki C, Burkhardt D, et al. Evaluations of physiologic reactivity and reflexive behaviors during noxious procedures in sedated critically ill patients. *J Crit Care* 2009;24(3):472.e9–472.e13.

54. Puntillo KA, Stannard D, Miaskowski C, et al. Use of a pain assessment and intervention notation (P.A.I.N.) tool in critical care nursing practice: nurses' evaluations. *Heart Lung* 2002:31(4):303–314.

55. Gelinas C, Johnston C. Pain assessment in the critically ill ventilated adult: validation of the Critical-Care Pain Observation Tool and physiologic indicators. *Clin J Pain* 2007;23(6):497–505.

56. Woods JC, Mion LC, Connor JT, et al. Severe agitation among ventilated medical intensive care unit patients: frequency, characteristics and outcomes. *Intensive Care Med* 2004;30(6):1066–1072.

57. Fraser GL, Prato BS, Riker RR, et al. Frequency, severity, and treatment of agitation in young versus elderly patients in the ICU. *Pharmacotherapy* 2000;20(1):75–82.

58. Sessler CN, Glass C, Grap MJ. Unplanned extubation: incidence, predisposing factors, and management. *J Crit Illness* 1994;9:609–619.

59. Carrion MI, Ayuso D, Marcos M, et al. Accidental removal of endotracheal and nasogastric tubes and intravascular catheters. *Crit Care Med* 2000;28(1):63–66.

60. Mion LC, Minnick AF, Leipziq R, et al. Patient-initiated device removal in intensive care units: a national prevalence study. *Crit Care Med* 2007;35(12):2714–2720.

61. Fraser GL, Riker RR, Prato BS, et al. The frequency and cost of patient-initiated device removal in the ICU. *Pharmacotherapy* 2001;21(1):1–6.

62. Jaber S, Chanques G, Altairac C, et al. A prospective study of agitation in a medical-surgical ICU: incidence, risk factors, and outcomes. *Chest* 2005;128(4):2749–2757.

63. Chanques G, Jaber S, Barbotte E, et al. Impact of systematic evaluation of pain and agitation in an intensive care unit. *Crit Care Med* 2006;34(6):1691–1699.

64. Murnion BP, Gnijidic D, Hilmer SN. Prescription and administration of opioids to hospital in-patients, and barriers to effective use. *Pain Med* 2010;11(1):58–66.

65. Smith HS. Opioid metabolism. *Mayo Clin Proc* 2009;84(7):613–624.

66. Pathan H, Williams J. Basic opioid pharmacology: an update. *Br J Pain* 2012;6(1):11–16.

67. Devlin JW, Roberts R. Pharmacology of commonly used analgesics and sedatives in the ICU: benzodiazepines, propofol, and opioids. *Crit Care Clin* 2009;25(3):431–449.

68. Mostafa SM, Bhandari S, Ritchie G, et al. Constipation and its implications in the critically ill patient. *Br J Anaesth* 2003;91(6):815–819.

69. Strom T, Martinussen T, Toft P. A protocol of no sedation for critically ill patients receiving mechanical ventilation: a randomised trial. *Lancet* 2010;375(9713):475–480.

70. Sessler CN, Pedram S. Protocolized and target-based sedation and analgesia in the ICU. *Critical Care Clinics* 2009;25(3):489–513.

71. Riker RR, Fraser GL. Altering intensive care sedation paradigms to improve patient outcomes. *Crit Care Clinics* 2009;25(3):527–538.

72. Honiden S, Siegel M. Analytic reviews: managing the agitated patient in the ICU: sedation, analgesia, and neuromuscular blockade. *J Intensive Care Med* 2010;25(4):187–204.

73. Muellejans B, López A, Cross MH, et al. Remifentanil versus fentanyl for analgesia based sedation to provide patient comfort in the intensive care unit: a randomized, double-blind controlled trial. *Crit Care* 2004;8(1):R1–R11.

74. Rozendaal FW, Spronk PE, Snellen FF, et al. Remifentanil-propofol analgo-sedation shortens duration of ventilation and length of ICU stay compared to a conventional regimen: a centre randomised, cross-over, open-label study in the Netherlands. *Intensive Care Med* 2009;35(2):291–299.

75. Epstein J, Breslow MJ. The stress response of critical illness. *Crit Care Clin* 1999;15(1):17–33.

76. Ambuel B, Hamlett KW, Marx CM, et al. Assessing distress in pediatric intensive care environments: the COMFORT scale. *J Pediatr Psychol* 1992;17(1):95–109.

77. Merkel SI, Voepel-Lewis T, Shayevitz JR, et al. The FLACC: a behavioral scale for scoring postoperative pain in young children. *Pediatr Nurs* 1997;23(3):293–297.

78. De Jonghe B, Cook D, Griffith L, et al. Adaptation to the Intensive Care Environment (ATICE): development and validation of a new sedation assessment instrument. *Crit Care Med* 2003;31(9):2344–2354.

79. Heiderich TM, Leslie AT, Guinsburg R. Neonatal procedural pain can be assessed by computer software that has good sensitivity and specificity to detect facial movements. *Acta Paediatr* 2015;104(2):e63–e69.

80. Constant I, Saboudin N. Monitoring depth of anesthesia: from consciousness to nociception. A window on subcortical brain activity. *Paediatr Anaesth* 2015;25(1):73–82.

81. Ledowski T. Analgesia-nociception index. *Br J Anaesth* 2014;112(5):937.

82. McPherson CJ, Addington-Hall JM. Judging the quality of care at the end of life: can proxies provide reliable information? *Soc Sci Med* 2003;56(1):95–109.

83. Seckler AB, Meier DE, Mulvihill M, et al. Substituted judgment: how accurate are proxy predictions? *Ann Intern Med* 1991;115(2):92–98.

84. Wick EC, Grant MC, Wo CL. Postoperative multimodal analgesia pain management with nonopioid analgesics and techniques: a review. *JAMA Surg* 2017;152(7):691–697.

85. Cepeda MS, Carr DB, Lau J, et al. Music for pain relief. *Cochrane Database Syst Rev* 2006;(2):CD004843.

86. Kwekkeboom KL, Gretarsdottir E. Systematic review of relaxation interventions for pain. *J Nurs Scholarsh* 2006;38(3):269–277.

87. Suls J, Wan CK. Effects of sensory and procedural information on coping with stressful medical procedures and pain: a meta-analysis. *J Consult Clin Psychol* 1989;57(3):372–379.

88. Coruh B, Tonelli MR, Park DR. Fentanyl-induced chest wall rigidity. *Chest* 2013;143(4):1145–1146.

89. Wunsch H, Kahn JM, Kramer AA, et al. Use of intravenous infusion sedation among mechanically ventilated patients in the United States. *Crit Care Med* 2009;37(12):3031–3039.

90. Gill KV, Voils SA, Chenault GA, et al. Perceived versus actual sedation practices in adult intensive care unit patients receiving mechanical ventilation. *Ann Pharmacother* 2012;46(10):1331–1339.

91. Mehta S, Burry L, Fischer S, et al. Canadian survey of the use of sedatives, analgesics, and neuromuscular blocking agents in critically ill patients. *Crit Care Med* 2006;34(2):374–380.

92. Insler SR, Kraenzler EJ, Licina MG, et al. Cardiac surgery in a patient taking monoamine oxidase inhibitors: an adverse fentanyl reaction. *Anesth Analg* 1994;78(3):593–597.

93. Kane-Gill SL, LeBlanc JM, Dasta JF, et al. A multicenter study of the point prevalence of drug-induced hypotension in the ICU. *Crit Care Med* 2014;42(10):2197–2203.

94. Pedavally S, Fugate JE, Rabinstein AA. Serotonin syndrome in the intensive care unit: clinical presentations and precipitating medications. *Neurocrit Care* 2014;21(1):108–113.

95. Gillman PK. Monoamine oxidase inhibitors, opioid analgesics and serotonin toxicity. *Br J Anaesth* 2005;95(4):434–441.

96. Ailawadhi S, Sung KW, Carlson LA, et al. Serotonin syndrome caused by interaction between citalopram and fentanyl. *J Clin Pharm Ther* 2007;32(2):199–202.

97. Buckley NA, Dawson AH, Isbister GK. Serotonin syndrome. *BMJ* 2014;348:g1626.

98. Beakley BD, Kaye AM, Kaye AD. Tramadol, pharmacology, side effects, and serotonin syndrome: a review. *Pain Physician* 2015;18(4):395–400.

99. Solhaug V, Molden E. Individual variability in clinical effect and tolerability of opioid analgesics—importance of drug interactions and pharmacogenetics. *Scand J Pain* 2017;17:193–200.

100. Ehieli E, Yalamuri S, Brudney CS, et al. Analgesia in the surgical intensive care unit. *Postgrad Med J* 2017;93(1095):38–45.

101. Dean M. Opioids in renal failure and dialysis patients. *J Pain Symptom Manage* 2004;28(5):497–504.

102. Gagnon DJ, Jwo K. Tremors and agitation following low-dose intravenous hydromorphone administration in a patient with kidney dysfunction. *Ann Pharmacother* 2013;47(7–8):e34.

103. Yassin SM, Terblanche M, Yassin J, et al. A web-based survey of United Kingdom sedation practice in the intensive care unit. *J Crit Care* 2015;30(2):436.e1–436.e6.

104. Baldo BA, Pham NH. Histamine-releasing and allergenic properties of opioid analgesic drugs: resolving the two. *Anaesth Intensive Care* 2012;40(2):216–235.

105. Mazoit JX, Butscher K, Samii K. Morphine in postoperative patients: pharmacokinetics and pharmacodynamics of metabolites. *Anesth Analg* 2007;105(1):70–78.

106. Lotsch J, Geisslinger G. Morphine-6-glucuronide: an analgesic of the future? *Clin Pharmacokinet* 2001;40(7):485–499.

107. Buetler TM, Wilder-Smith OH, Wilder-Smith CH, et al. Analgesic action of IV morphine-6-glucuronide in healthy volunteers. *Br J Anaesth* 2000;84(1):97–99.

108. Scott LJ, Perry CM. Remifentanil: a review of its use during the induction and maintenance of general anaesthesia. *Drugs* 2005;65(13):1793–1823.

109. Breen D, Karabinis A, Malbrain M, et al. Decreased duration of mechanical ventilation when comparing analgesia-based sedation using remifentanil with standard hypnotic-based sedation for up to 10 days in intensive care unit patients: a randomised trial [ISRCTN47583497]. *Crit Care* 2005;9(3):R200–R210.

110. Dahaba AA, Grabner T, Rehak PH, et al. Remifentanil versus morphine analgesia and sedation for mechanically ventilated critically ill patients: a randomized double blind study. *Anesthesiology* 2004;101(3):640–646.

111. Frid I, Haljamäe H, Ohlén J, et al. Brain death: close relatives' use of imagery as a descriptor of experience. *J Adv Nurs* 2007;58(1):63–71.

112. Baillard C, Cohen Y, Le Toumelin P, et al. Remifentanil-midazolam compared to sufentanil-midazolam for ICU long-term sedation [in French]. *Ann Fr Anesth Reanim* 2005;24(5):480–486.

113. Leone M, Albanèse J, Viviand X, et al. The effects of remifentanil on endotracheal suctioning-induced increases in intracranial pressure in head-injured patients. *Anesth Analg* 2004;99(4):1193–1198.

114. Karabinis A, Mandragos K, Stergiopoulos S, et al. Safety and efficacy of analgesia-based sedation with remifentanil versus standard hypnotic-based regimens in intensive care unit patients with brain injuries: a randomised, controlled trial [ISRCTN50308308]. *Crit Care* 2004;8(4):R268–R280.

115. Bauer C, Kreuer S, Ketter R, et al. Remifentanil-propofol versus fentanyl-midazolam combinations for intracranial surgery: influence of anaesthesia technique and intensive sedation on ventilation times and duration of stay in the ICU [in German]. *Anaesthetist* 2007;56(2):128–132.

116. Zhu Y, Wang Y, Du B, et al. Could remifentanil reduce duration of mechanical ventilation in comparison with other opioids for mechanically ventilated patients? A systematic review and meta-analysis. *Crit Care* 2017;21(1):206–217.
117. Patanwala AE, Martin JR, Erstad BL. Ketamine for analgosedation in the intensive care unit: a systematic review. *J Intensive Care Med* 2017;32(6):387–395.
118. Erstad BL, Patanwala AE. Ketamine for analgosedation in critically ill patients. *J Crit Care* 2016;35:145–149.
119. Sleigh J, Harvey M, Voss L, et al. Ketamine: more mechanisms of action than just NMDA blockade. *Trends Anaesth Crit Care* 2014:76–81.
120. Elefritz JL, Murphy CV, Papadimos TJ, et al. Methadone analgesia in the critically ill. *J Crit Care* 2016;34:84–88.
121. Jones GM. Methadone in the critically ill—an unlikely player in intensive care medicine. *J Crit Care* 2016;34:162.
122. Eap CB, Buclin T, Baumann P. Interindividual variability of the clinical pharmacokinetics of methadone: implications for the treatment of opioid dependence. *Clin Pharmacokinet* 2002;41(14):1153–1193.
123. Cicero TJ, Inciardi JA, Munoz A. Trends in abuse of OxyContin and other opioid analgesics in the United States: 2002-2004. *J Pain* 2005;6(10):662–672.
124. Groudine SB, Fisher HA, Kaufman RP Jr, et al. Intravenous lidocaine speeds the return of bowel function, decreases postoperative pain, and shortens hospital stay in patients undergoing radical retropubic prostatectomy. *Anesth Analg* 1998;86(2):235–239.
125. Bhana N, Goa KL, McClellan KJ. Dexmedetomidine. *Drugs* 2000;59(2):263–268.
126. Gerlach AT, Murphy CV, Dasta JF. An updated focused review of dexmedetomidine in adults. *Ann Pharmacotherapy* 2009;43(12):2064–2074.
127. Tan JA, Ho KM. Use of dexmedetomidine as a sedative and analgesic agent in critically ill adult patients: a meta-analysis. *Intensive Care Med* 2010;36:926–939.
128. Riker RR, Shehabi Y, Bokesch PM, et al. Dexmedetomidine vs midazolam for sedation of critically ill patients: a randomized trial. *JAMA* 2009;301(5):489–499.
129. Nishimori M, Ballantyne JC, Low JH. Epidural pain relief versus systemic opioid-based pain relief for abdominal aortic surgery. *Cochrane Database Syst Rev* 2006;(3):CD005059.
130. Block BM, Liu SS, Rowlingson AJ, et al. Efficacy of postoperative epidural analgesia: a meta-analysis. *JAMA* 2003;290:2455–2463.
131. Bulger EM, Edwards T, Klotz P, et al. Epidural analgesia improves outcome after multiple rib fractures. *Surgery* 2004;136(2):426–430.
132. Carrier FM, Turgeon AF, Nicole PC, et al. Effect of epidural analgesia in patients with traumatic rib fractures: a systemic review and meta-analysis of randomized controlled trials. *Can J Anaesth* 2009;56:230–242.
133. Park G, Lane M, Rogers S, et al. A comparison of hypnotic and analgesic based sedation in a general intensive care unit. *Brit J Anaesthesia* 2007;98(1):76–82.
134. Jakob SM, Ruokonen E, Grounds RM, et al. Dexmedetomidine vs midazolam or propofol for sedation during prolonged mechanical ventilation: two randomized controlled trials. *JAMA* 2012;307(11):1151–1160.
135. Mueller SW, Prelaski CR, Kiser TH, et al. A randomized, double-blind, placebo-controlled dose range study of dexmedetomidine as adjunctive therapy for alcohol withdrawal. *Crit Care Med* 2014;42:1131–1139.
136. Bielka K, Kuchyn I, Glumcher F. Addition of dexmedetomidine to benzodiazepines for patients with alcohol withdrawal syndrome in the intensive care unit: a randomized controlled study. *Ann Intensive Care* 2015;5:33.
137. Reade MC, Eastwood GM, Bellomo R, et al. Effect of dexmedetomidine added to standard care on ventilator-free time in patients with agitated delirium: a randomized clinical trial. *JAMA* 2016;315(14):1460–1468.
138. Carrasco G, Baeza N, Cabre L, et al. Dexmedetomidine for the treatment of hyperactive delirium refractory to haloperidol in nonintubated ICU patients: a nonrandomized controlled trial. *Crit Care Med* 2016;44:1295–1306.
139. Marik PE. Propofol: therapeutic indications and side-effects. *Current Pharmaceutical Design* 2004;10(29):3639–3649.
140. Ho KM, Ng JY. The use of propofol for medium and long-term sedation in critically ill adult patients: a meta-analysis. *Intensive Care Med* 2008;34(11):1969–1979.
141. Kollef MH, Levy NT, Ahrens TS, et al. The use of continuous IV sedation is associated with prolongation of mechanical ventilation. *Chest* 1998;114(2):541–548.
142. Brook AD, Ahrens TS, Schaiff R, et al. Effect of a nursing-implemented sedation protocol on the duration of mechanical ventilation. *Crit Care Med* 1999;27(12):2609–2615.
143. Kress JP, Pohlman AS, O'Connor MF, et al. Daily interruption of sedative infusions in critically ill patients undergoing mechanical ventilation. *N Engl J Med* 2000;342(20):1471–1477.
144. de Wit M, Gennings C, Jenvey WI, et al. Randomized trial comparing daily interruption of sedation and nursing-implemented sedation algorithm in medical intensive care unit patients. *Crit Care* 2008;12(3):R70.
145. De Jonghe B, Bastuji-Garin S, Fangio P, et al. Sedation algorithm in critically ill patients without acute brain injury. *Crit Care Med* 2005;33(1):120–127.
146. Mascia MF, Koch M, Medicis JJ. Pharmacoeconomic impact of rational use guidelines on the provision of analgesia, sedation, and neuromuscular blockade in critical care. *Crit Care Med* 2000;28(7):2300–2306.
147. Brattebo G, Hofoss D, Flaatten H, et al. Effect of a scoring system and protocol for sedation on duration of patients' need for ventilator support in a surgical intensive care unit. *Qual Saf Health Care* 2004;13(3):203–205.
148. MacLaren R, Plamondon JM, Ramsay KB, et al. A prospective evaluation of empiric versus protocol-based sedation and analgesia. *Pharmacotherapy* 2000;20(6):662–672.
149. Quenot JP, Ladoire S, Devoucoux F, et al. Effect of a nurse-implemented sedation protocol on the incidence of ventilator-associated pneumonia. *Crit Care Med* 2007;35(9):2031–2036.
150. Skrobik Y, Ahern S, Leblanc M, et al. Protocolized intensive care unit management of analgesia, sedation, and delirium improves analgesia and subsyndromal delirium rates. *Anesth Analg* 2010;111(2):451–463.
151. Bucknall TK, Manias E, Presneill JJ. A randomized trial of protocol-directed sedation management for mechanical ventilation in an Australian intensive care unit. *Crit Care Med* 2008;36(5):1444–1450.
152. Elliott R, McKinley S, Aitken LM, et al. The effect of an algorithm-based sedation guideline on the duration of mechanical ventilation in an Australian intensive care unit. *Intensive Care Med* 2006;32(10):1506–1514.
153. Marshall J, Finn CA, Theodore AC. Impact of a clinical pharmacist-enforced intensive care unit sedation protocol on duration of mechanical ventilation and hospital stay. *Crit Care Med* 2008;36(2):427–433.
154. Mehta S, Burry L, Cook D, et al. Daily sedation interruption in mechanically ventilated critically ill patients cared for with a sedation protocol: a randomized controlled trial. *JAMA* 2012;308(19):1985–1992.
155. Carson SS, Kress JP, Rodgers JE, et al. A randomized trial of intermittent lorazepam versus propofol with daily interruption in mechanically ventilated patients. *Crit Care Med* 2006;34(5):1326–1332.
156. Kress JP, Vinayak AG, Levitt J, et al. Daily sedative interruption in mechanically ventilated patients at risk for coronary artery disease. *Crit Care Med* 2007;35(2):365–371.
157. Kress JP, Gehlbach B, Lacy M, et al. The long-term psychological effects of daily sedative interruption on critically ill patients. *Am J Respir Crit Care Med* 2003;168(12):1457–1461.
158. Girard TD, Kress JP, Fuchs BD, et al. Efficacy and safety of a paired sedation and ventilator weaning protocol for mechanically ventilated patients in intensive care (Awakening and Breathing Controlled trial): a randomised controlled trial. *Lancet* 2008;371(9607):126–134.
159. Sessler CN. Wake up and breathe. *Crit Care Med* 2004;32:1413–1414.
160. Schweickert WD, Pohlman MC, Pohlman AS, et al. Early physical and occupational therapy in mechanically ventilated, critically ill patients: a randomized controlled trial. *Lancet* 2009;373(9678):1874–1882.
161. Downar J, Delaney J, Hawryluck L, et al. Guidelines for the withdrawal of life-sustaining measures. *Intensive Care Med* 2016;42:1003–1017.
162. Cook D, Rocker G. Dying with dignity in the ICU. *N Engl J Med* 2014;370:2506–2514.
163. Connolly C, Miskolei O, Phelan D, et al. End-of-life in the ICU: moving from withdrawal of care to a palliative care, patient-centred approach. *Br J Anaesth* 2016;117(2):143–145.
164. Beauchamp TL, Childress JF. *Principles of Biomedical Ethics*. 5th ed. Oxford, United Kingdom: Oxford University Press; 2001.
165. Paris JJ, Muir JC, Reardon FE. Ethical and legal issues in intensive care. *J Intensive Care Med* 1997;12(6):298–309.
166. Mularski RA, Heine CE, Osborne ML, et al. Quality of dying in the ICU: ratings by family members. *Chest* 2005;128(1):280–287.
167. Mularski RA, Curtis JR, Billings JA, et al. Proposed quality measures for palliative care in the critically ill: a consensus from the Robert Wood Johnson Foundation Critical Care Workgroup. *Crit Care Med* 2006;34(11 suppl):S404–S411.

CHAPTER 115

The Future of Pain Medicine: An Epilogue

SCOTT M. FISHMAN and **JAMES P. RATHMELL**

The creation of this fifth edition of *Bonica's Management of Pain* reflects a major collaboration among many of the world's leading authorities in the basic and clinical sciences. As in prior editions, this text serves as a resource for those who seek to increase their understanding of this aspect of the human condition. However, it also provides an important reference point—an elaboration on how far we have come and how far we have to go in order to prevent, markedly reduce, and perhaps even cure the pervasive problem of pain as a cause of unnecessary suffering, debility, and economic hardship. As in the previous edition, we will again briefly look ahead to where this journey may—and should—lead us before the next edition of this textbook is written and reflect on what has happened since the last edition was published in 2010.

The future is unpredictable; nonetheless, there are many current trends that portend an optimistic course ahead. Foremost is the pivotal recognition that pain is much more than a symptom and that its consequences, in the acute or chronic form, may be devastating at every level of human health. This profound understanding continues to transform the perspective of modern medicine, offering greater possibilities for dealing with the burden of disease than ever before. Soon after publication of the prior edition of this text, the Institute of Medicine (now the National Academy of Medicine) published its landmark report entitled "Relieving Pain in America," reporting that approximately 100 million Americans suffer with chronic pain. It highlighted that clinicians remain substantially undereducated about pain and ill prepared to respond.[1] This education gap has increasingly been seen as a one of the major root causes of the current epidemic of prescription drug abuse, in that US clinicians were advised, if not forced, to recognize pain as a fifth vital sign with woefully inadequate education, science, and clinical resources. Nonetheless, just as pain as the fifth vital sign was a well-intentioned but poorly executed intervention aimed at reversing decades of ignoring pain, the field of pain medicine continues to progress along a notable course. Prior to the first edition of this textbook, there were no pain specialists, pain journals, pain specialty organizations, pain advocacy groups, pain training programs, or laws or regulations specifically addressing the issues involved in delivering pain relief. At the time that the third and most recent edition of this text was written, the number of published reports in the realm of pain within the medical literature was a fraction of those today and there was no pain consortium at the National Institutes of Health (NIH). Clinical training of pain specialists was in its infancy, with minimal guidance from accrediting bodies. Certification of pain specialists through the American Board of Medical Specialties (ABMS) was available only to anesthesiologists, and the immense problem of pain management in primary care had barely been raised.

Ironically, in part due to increased attention related to the opioid crisis in the United States, recent unprecedented events suggest that we are on a trajectory toward improved knowledge about pain and increased commitment to pain relief, particularly care that is not solely focused on opioids. These events include increasing demands for standards for pain-related assessment and safe treatment in all health care facilities as well as mandates for improving education in pain and its management. There is little doubt that the future for pain management is inextricably linked to both science and education. Core competencies for all health professionals have now been established as a tool for educators to guide curriculum and for accreditors to base evaluation of educational institutions. Today, pain has growing representation in the NIH, and professional societies are working diligently to further increase this new commitment. Subspecialty clinical training has become much more integrative and multidisciplinary as a result of groundbreaking revisions to requirements set by the Accreditation Council of Graduate Medical Education (ACGME). Previously, such requirements were predominantly directed by the discipline of anesthesiology but have now been revised through an extraordinary collaboration of multiple disciplines. Subspecialty training for a physician from any primary clinical discipline is now possible in accredited programs that lead to certification as a pain specialist by the ABMS. Similarly, the multidisciplinary field of palliative medicine is designated as a subspecialty that is intertwined within many ABMS primary specialties, a most recent example of medicine's increasing assimilation of symptom management and quality of life interventions. Although pain medicine has also developed as a broad-based, multidisciplinary subspecialty, its place in the overall structure of the field of medicine as a whole is still in evolution. Reform initiatives are well underway to refine the position of this emerging discipline in effort to advance its research, education, and clinical missions. Great debate remains over whether pain medicine should evolve into a more robust subspecialty that integrates parts of many clinical disciplines or whether it should become a primary specialty in its own right, but little progress has been made toward changing the current training paradigm. How pain medicine is ultimately positioned will greatly impact the field of medicine's ability to meet its fundamental obligations to mitigate suffering.

At the time of publication of the prior edition in 2010, the National Pain Care Policy Act of 2008 and 2009 ultimately became part of the US Affordable Care Act in 2010. Since then, we have witnessed unprecedented legislative and regulatory attention to pain and its treatment. Recent developments suggest that states and the federal government remain uncertain how to balance the needs of patients in pain to have appropriate access to controlled substances with safety concerns for the general public. Potential solutions have gained intense scrutiny by the pain and law enforcement communities, respectively. Over time, national policies by the U.S. Drug Enforcement Administration (DEA), U.S. Food and Drug Administration (FDA), and the overarching Departments of Justice and Health and Human Services will hopefully evolve into rational approaches that balance compassion and safety. Evidence suggests that the public health crises of prescription drug abuse and inadequate pain management are receiving unprecedented attention and action. The U.S. Department of Health and Human Services released a National Pain Strategy for addressing the clinical, education, and research needs of current and future Americans in pain.[2] Currently, the US epidemic of prescription opioid abuse and excessive opioid prescribing has led to a high pace of new legislative and regulatory attention. It remains unclear if upcoming legislative and regulatory actions will simply restrict opioid prescribing and access or improve the underlying educational deficiencies that drive most excessive prescribing. The Obama administration appeared to address the prescription drug abuse crisis as a public health issue, whereas the Trump White House seems to see the issue as more of a law enforcement problem. It remains to be seen if this raised awareness and action will translate to improved access to safer and more effective care for patients. Leading clinicians and scientists with expertise in pain recently issued a special publication through the National Academy of Medicine calling for clinicians to rationally counter the opioid epidemic.[3]

The clinical practice of pain management, now more commonly termed *pain medicine*, has changed dramatically since the creation of this textbook in 1953. Under the direction of John Bonica, the establishment of specialized centers that focus on pain management arose from anesthesiology roots. These centers were initially based on an intensive multidisciplinary model of care. Despite several decades of research firmly establishing its effectiveness, such care is expensive and has been largely unsustainable. Centers dedicated to this model have faced drastic reorganization or become extinct.

These same anesthesiology roots of pain medicine also shaped another important aspect of the field. With the influx of anesthesiologists came a rise in the use of specific pain treatments that adopted regional anesthetic or injection based techniques. Although any action taken to manage pain should be considered an "intervention," this new clinical arena based on more invasive procedures, such as analgesic injections in the spine or placement of implantable devices for pain, has been termed *interventional pain medicine*. Currently, some experts contend that general pain medicine and interventional pain medicine should be discrete disciplines with practitioners separated based on interventional and noninterventional pain practice. The heightened role of procedure-based pain practices, and some of the drive to isolate this part of care from the rest of pain medicine, has almost certainly been driven by health care reimbursement systems, such as those in the United States, that reward practitioners with higher payment for procedural care than for almost all other aspects of pain care. Indeed, the reimbursement for pain specialists who perform procedural interventions is often many times that for those who treat the same group of patients and spend the same amount or more time with them but do not provide such interventions regardless of the level of evidence of predictive outcomes that might reasonably justify one type of care over another. With lucrative salaries in the private sector, too few of this new breed of interventional pain physician have stayed in the academic realm and fewer still have gone about conducting meaningful clinical trials to examine the efficacy of their interventions.

Major health reform appeared imminent in the United States back in 2010, and that remains the case in 2018. Pain medicine, particularly interventional pain medicine, stands at a crossroads as many of the treatments that are part of currently accepted pain practice are expensive but have little scientific evidence to support their efficacy. As the forces of health care reform and evidence-based medicine unite to guide clinical practice, many commonly used treatments are facing increased scrutiny by payers. The unbridled growth of interventional pain medicine has already moderated toward a more balanced form, where practitioners provide a broad range of interventional and non-interventional treatment for common pain conditions. Indeed, for economic, medical, social, and ethical reasons, the field has moved toward a more uniform discipline, in which individualized pain care is more similar than dissimilar based on a relatively broad spectrum of mainstream treatment options, with therapeutic choices based on weighing all available evidence and driven by the best interests of each individual patient. Since publication of the fourth edition, new clinical trials have appeared and numerous systematic reviews and clinical practice guidelines have been published highlighting the lack of evidence for sustained benefits from many interventions, such as spinal procedures including epidural steroid injections and radiofrequency ablation. This parallels heightened concerns about the lack of evidence for long-term

safety and efficacy of pharmacologic analgesia. Evidence for opioid use for chronic pain has been shown to be weak or inadequate despite mounting evidence that risks are higher than previously believed, and these risks increase markedly with dose. Taken together, as the field of pain medicine evolves, its evidentiary foundation will be an increasingly important factor in its credibility as a distinct discipline within medicine.

There is widespread agreement that existing systems are inadequate for training clinicians to treat pain. Despite this, today's clinicians are armed with an unprecedented array of effective tools including pharmacologic, behavioral, and physical therapies; invasive procedures; and cross-cultural complementary and alternative treatments such as acupuncture and meditation. Bringing these and new tools to bear on all cases of pain will be a major challenge, requiring education for nonspecialist clinicians at the professional school and postgraduate levels. Mandating substantive pain education for all clinicians has been a missed opportunity that must be corrected. It is to be seen whether or not the US National Pain Strategy will lead to actions that address its pain management goals for improved clinical care, foundational and far-reaching education, and substantially increased research.

Pain will continue to be a pervasive problem for mankind, science will continue its exponential growth in knowledge of pain and its treatment, and society will increasingly recognize that pain management is integral to the humane and economically viable practice of medicine. The current medical, social, and economic crises in health care, if not medicine's covenant to mitigate suffering, demand nothing less than systemic solutions to timely, integrated, and cost-effective pain relief. The current controversies and opportunities in association with better understanding and treatment of pain will likely push us toward a tipping point beyond which the very structure of medicine is likely to have to change.

Currently, medicine possesses greater knowledge and more tools to treat pain than ever before. Despite the inadequate treatment of pain, undereducation of clinicians, and underfunding of research, medicine is much further along today than it was even a decade ago—a trajectory that bodes well for the future. The optimal organizational structure of science and medicine for advancing understanding and treatment of pain is yet to be defined. But it will most certainly require transcending current barriers that serve to fragment care, such as the illogical separation of the mind and body within the whole person or the splintering of core elements of pain management due to obsolete lines that separate one discipline from another. Change will likely be proportionate to the value we place on reducing suffering along with curing disease. Moreover, how general clinicians and pain scientists of the future are supported and trained and how the emerging discipline of pain medicine is positioned for continued development and integration throughout health care will greatly impact medicine's ability to meet its mission to understand and treat pain. Looking to the future, we appear to be headed for sweeping change in health care that may well lead to new heights in medical research, education, and clinical care for pain that is safer and more effective. This, in the light of the remarkable progress that has already been made, is a signal that medicine is rediscovering its fundamental ethos, most assuredly, to cure when possible but to relieve suffering and provide comfort always.

References

1. Institute of Medicine (US) Committee on Advancing Pain Research Care and Education. *Relieving Pain in America: A Blueprint for Transforming Prevention, Care, Education, and Research.* Washington, DC: National Academies Press; 2011.
2. National pain strategy: a comprehensive population health-level strategy for pain. Available at: https://iprcc.nih.gov/sites/default/files/HHSNational_Pain_Strategy_508C.pdf. Accessed May 15, 2018.
3. First, do no harm: marshalling clinician-leadership to counter the opioid-epidemic. Available at: https://nam.edu/first-no-harm-nam-special-publication. Accessed May 15, 2018.

Index

Page numbers followed by *b* indicate boxes; those followed by *f* indicate figures, and those followed by *t* indicate tables.